ALTE Chap 117   RM: 22697
CPV chap 17   RM: 23867

OSKI'S PEDIATRICS

PRINCIPLES & PRACTICE

FOURTH EDITION

OSKI'S PEDIATRICS

PRINCIPLES & PRACTICE

Editor-in-Chief

Julia A. McMillan, MD

Professor of Pediatrics
Vice Chair for Education
Department of Pediatrics
Director, Residency Training Program
Associate Dean for Graduate Medical Education
Johns Hopkins University School of Medicine
Johns Hopkins Hospital
Baltimore, Maryland

Editors

Ralph D. Feigin, MD

Distinguished Service Professor
Baylor College of Medicine
Chairman, Department of Pediatrics
Baylor College of Medicine
Physician-in-Chief
Texas Children's Hospital
Chief, Pediatric Service
Ben Taub General Hospital
Chief, Pediatric Service
The Methodist Hospital
Houston, Texas

Catherine DeAngelis, MD, MPH

Professor of Pediatrics
Johns Hopkins University School of Medicine
Editor-in-Chief
JAMA
Chicago, Illinois

M. Douglas Jones, Jr., MD

Professor
Department of Pediatrics
Section of Neonatology
The University of Colorado School of Medicine
The Children's Hospital
Denver, Colorado

389 Contributors

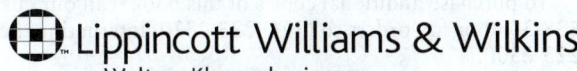

Lippincott Williams & Wilkins
a Wolters Kluwer business

Philadelphia • Baltimore • New York • London
Buenos Aires • Hong Kong • Sydney • Tokyo

Acquisitions Editor: Anne M. Sydor/Sonya Seigafuse
Developmental Editor: Kathleen Scogna
Managing Editor: Nicole T. Dernoski
Editorial Assistant: Sarah Granlund
Project Manager: Nicole Walz
Senior Manufacturing Manager: Benjamin Rivera
Designer Coordinator: Holly Reid McLaughlin
Cover Designer: Christine Jenny
Compositor: TechBooks
Printer: Quebecor World-Taunton

Library of Congress Cataloging-in-Publication Data

Oski's pediatrics : principles & practice / editor-in-chief, Julia A. McMillan ; editors, Ralph
D. Feigin, Catherine D. DeAngelis, M. Douglas Jones, Jr.— 4th ed.
        p. ; cm.
    Includes bibliographical references and index.
    ISBN 0-7817-3894-6 (alk. paper)
    1. Pediatrics.   I. McMillan, Julia A. II. Oski, Frank A. Principles and practice of
pediatrics. III. Title: Pediatrics.
    [DNLM: 1. Pediatrics.   WS 100 O816 2006]
    RJ45.P6754 2006
    618.92—dc22   2006000380

10 9 8 7 6 5 4 3 2 1

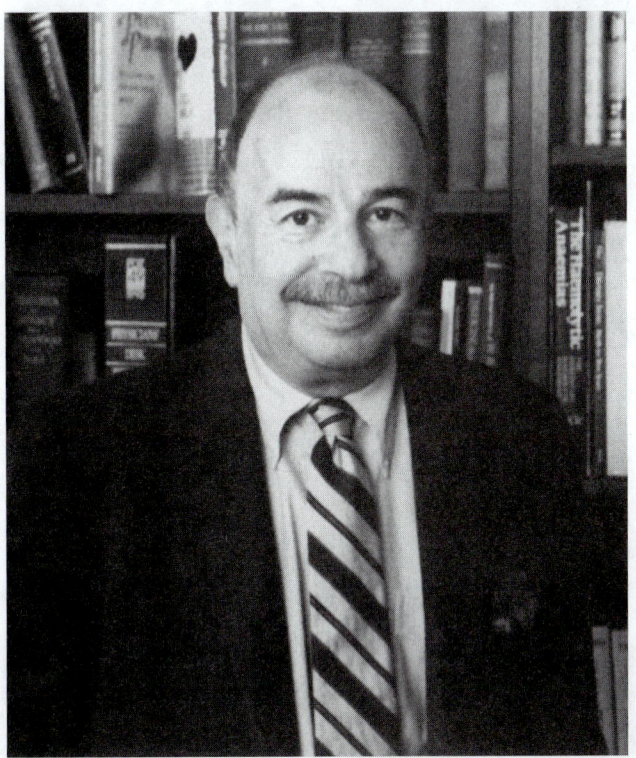

FRANK A. OSKI, MD (1932–1996)

Frank A. Oski was a leader, a mentor, a visionary, a scientist, and a clinician, but most of all he was a teacher. He welcomed students willing to take on the awesome responsibility of providing medical care for children, but he demanded excellence in that endeavor.

Frank was chairman of two departments of pediatrics—at the State University of New York Health Science Center at Syracuse (1972 to 1985) and at Johns Hopkins University School of Medicine (1985 to 1994). He was editor or author of 13 books for pediatricians and hematologists, authored 293 articles, and served on nine editorial boards of pediatric journals and as the editor-in-chief of *The Yearbook of Pediatrics* and *Contemporary Pediatrics*. As the founding editor-in-chief of this textbook, he wrote in the preface of the first edition, "Our goal has been to represent accurately and fully the broad and rich tapestry that is pediatrics today." No thread was more important to that tapestry during the past three decades than Frank.

Pediatricians and children throughout the country and the world have benefited from Frank's teaching, but those fortunate enough to have been his students had their lives changed by him. He reminded his students often that they had an obligation to their patients and to their own students to realize that they could never know as much as they should. Frank's expectations were high, but one of his many particular gifts was that he identified strengths in each of his students and then helped each achieve the potential he knew he or she had. His legacy to the field of pediatrics is that he helped many future pediatricians become stronger, wiser, and more confident than they ever thought they could be. His personal legacy is that, because of him, we know more about what a privilege it is to teach.

Julia A. McMillan, MD
Catherine D. DeAngelis, MD
Ralph D. Feigin, MD
Joseph B. Warshaw, MD

FRANK A. ... MD (1932-1999)

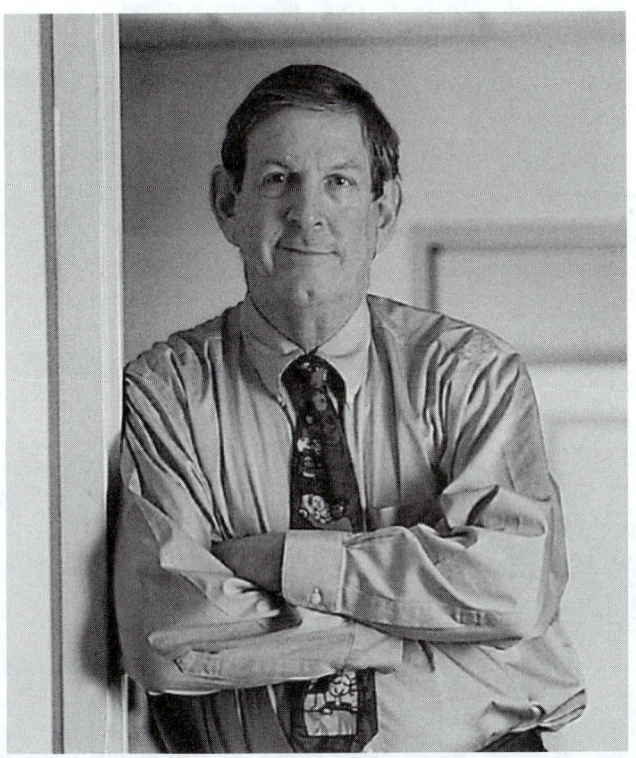

TO JOSEPH B. WARSHAW, MD (1936–2003)

This fourth edition of *Oski's Pediatrics: Principles and Practice* is dedicated to the memory of Joseph B. Warshaw, M.D., one of the editors of the first three editions of this text. Joe died in December, 2003, of multiple myeloma. He was an active participant in the planning and initial revisions for the current edition.

Joe was a pediatrician, a neonatologist, a developmental biologist, and a leader in academic medicine. Most importantly, however, he was an educator with an instinct for creating environments and programs in which young physician scientists could thrive. Joe's research efforts led to improved understanding of fetal growth and development and appreciation for the complexities of neonatal biochemical adaptation. As Chair of the Departments of Pediatrics at the University of Texas Southwestern Medical School at Dallas and at Yale University School of Medicine, he fostered the development of departments of pediatrics whose faculty members forged a consistent link between molecular biology and clinical medicine. Joe helped found the Pediatrician Scientist Development Program, an effort led by the chairs of American departments of pediatrics to encourage pediatricians with particular interest

in and aptitude for scientific exploration to pursue careers that would result in improved health for children throughout the world. At the University of Vermont, where he was Dean of the College of Medicine at the time of his death, he spearheaded the creation of the M.D./Ph.D. program and the school's new medical curriculum.

Joe had enthusiasm and energy that caught everyone around him into its vortex. He loved life and lived it to the fullest. He displayed sincere interest and appreciation for those fortunate enough to work with him or to be part of his family, and he considered everyone part of his family. He was an advocate for students, for trainees, for his faculty, and for children. *Oski's Pediatrics: Principles and Practice* is only a part of the profound legacy Joe leaves to pediatrics, its practitioners, and its scientists.

Julia A. McMillan, MD
Catherine D. DeAngelis, MD
Ralph D. Feigin, MD
M. Douglas Jones, Jr., MD

PREFACE TO THE FIRST EDITION

Principles and Practice of Pediatrics represents a unique departure from current textbooks of pediatrics. Really five books in one, it reflects the way our specialty is learned and practiced today. The book is divided into five parts: "General Pediatrics," "The Fetus and the Newborn," "Ambulatory Pediatrics," "The Sick or Hospitalized Patient," and "The Pediatrician's Companion: Important Things You Forget to Remember."

In Part I, "General Pediatrics," the reader will find the basic topics that are relevant to all aspects of pediatrics, whether the patient is newborn, ambulatory, or acutely ill in the hospital. Examples of these chapters are "The History of Pediatrics," "The Economics of Medicine," "Immunology," "Molecular Genetics," "Ethics," "The Pediatric History and Physical Examination," "The Problem-Oriented Medical Record," "The Diagnostic Process," and even "The Consultation." Such fundamental topics transcend all boundaries and are important to every pediatrics student or practitioner.

Part II, "The Fetus and the Newborn," is a self-contained treatise containing what the physician needs to know once he or she enters a nursery, whether it is a nursery for the normal term infant or a neonatal intensive care unit. The newborn and its problems are discussed from the developmental, physiologic, and pathologic perspective.

Part III, "Ambulatory Pediatrics," provides the necessary information for the conduct of a comprehensive and satisfying office practice that includes infants and adolescents, the well child, and the child with a chronic illness. Chapters in this part discuss topics such as infant feeding, immunizations, developmental assessment, and psychobehavioral disturbances. Part III includes material on the common acute illnesses and sudden emergencies that confront the pediatrician on a daily basis.

Part IV, "The Sick or Hospitalized Patient," is a detailed presentation of the disturbances that may result in the hospitalization of infants and children. This part is a truly encyclopedic work that has been designed to serve as a core reference for every pediatrician treating a sick or hospitalized patient.

The final part of our book, "The Pediatrician's Companion: Important Things You Forget to Remember," provides you with laboratory values and guidelines on how to interpret them, assistance with the identification of 50 of the more common syndromes, and an illustrated manual of pediatric procedures. Part V concludes with a list of common symptoms and signs and their differential diagnoses. We hope that you will turn to this section frequently and find the answers to your problems.

This book is designed to meet the needs of the student of pediatrics, whether he or she is a medical student, a busy pediatric house officer, or a practitioner of our much-valued discipline. We believe the book is both comprehensive and cohesive. Our goal has been to represent accurately and fully the broad and rich tapestry that is pediatrics today.

My colleagues, Catherine D. DeAngelis, Ralph D. Feigin, and Joseph B. Warshaw, join me in wishing you enjoyment and satisfaction in the use of our book.

Frank A. Oski, MD

This fourth edition of *Oski's Pediatrics: Principles and Practice* has been extensively revised, both in content and in format. Chapter authors have worked with the editors to provide basic background information needed by students approaching pediatrics early in their careers, by practitioners seeking answers to questions of management posed by patients they interact with every day, and by pediatric residents and academic pediatricians whose patient care and teaching activities require access to up-to-date biochemical and genetic information. Each chapter has been carefully revised with the needs of all of these readers in mind. New chapters—including Genetics and Pediatric Primary Care, Complementary and Alternative Medicine, and Type 2 Diabetes Mellitus—reflect a society that is increasingly seeking new approaches to medical care and a population whose lifestyle choices uncover underlying genetic vulnerabilities. There is also a new and authoritative chapter on normal infant and child development, and the entire section on mental health in children has been updated. The section on newborn medicine has been extensively revised.

The format of this edition is in response to recognizing the need for ready access to summarized information, whatever the background of the reader. We have provided boxed lists summarizing major points, increased the number of photographs and figures, and highlighted important information using color.

In undertaking this revision, we considered the role of the textbook as a resource for medical information. The accessibility and currency of information available on the Internet has at times been used as an argument against the need for a comprehensive text. We all agreed, however, that there are benefits to the convenience, familiarity, and authenticity of a textbook such as this one. We each continue to reach for books as resources in our everyday work. We hope that students, physicians, and others in need of information about health and illness in children will continue to find this book a valuable resource.

Julia A. McMillan, MD
Catherine D. DeAngelis, MD
Ralph D. Feigin, MD
M. Douglas Jones, Jr., MD

◼ ACKNOWLEDGMENTS

We are all grateful to our families, especially our spouses, Jed Dietz, James Harris, Judith Feigin, and Ann Jones, whose tolerance for the time we spent hunched over computer screens and reading chapter revisions is exceeded only by their pride when seeing the finished product.

We thank the chapter authors, who had the patience and perseverance to stick with us through the longer-than-expected revision process and to add the photos, lists, and other elements that we believe enhance this book. We thank Anne Sydor, Nicole Dernoski, and Kathleen Scogna, who took on this project in mid-course and had the courage to corral four sometimes reluctant editors into making changes that have improved the accessibility of this book for increasingly busy readers. Sarah Granlund was a consistent touch point at Lippincott,

and Mary Campbell and Lee Ligon provided help with correspondence and editorial tasks in Houston.

Finally, Julia McMillan, Cathy DeAngelis, and Ralph Feigin thank Doug Jones for being willing to step into the middle of the revision process and with skill and sensitivity take on the portion of the book overseen in all three previous editions by Joe Warshaw. It was Doug's respect and admiration for Joe that led him to agree immediately when asked, and we are deeply grateful.

Julia A. McMillan, MD
Catherine D. DeAngelis, MD
Ralph D. Feigin, MD
M. Douglas Jones, Jr., MD

■ CONTRIBUTORS

Jennifer A. Accardo
Neurodevelopmental Disabilities Resident
Department of Neurology and
    Developmental Medicine
Kennedy Krieger Institute
Baltimore, Maryland

Pasquale J. Accardo, MD
James H. Franklin Professor of
    Developmental Research in Pediatrics
Department of Pediatrics
Virginia Commonwealth University
Developmental Pediatrician
Children's Hospital
Richmond, Virginia

Stuart P. Adler, MD
Professor and Chair
Department of Pediatrics
Virginia Commonwealth University
Virginia Commonwealth University
    Medical Center
Richmond, Virginia

Gladstone Airewele, MD, MPH
Assistant Professor
Department of Pediatrics
Baylor College of Medicine
Attending Physician
Texas Children's Cancer Center
    and Hematology Service
Texas Children's Hospital
Houston, Texas

Olakunle B. Akintemi, MBBS
Associate Professor
Department of Pediatrics
The University of North Carolina School
    of Medicine
Attending Physician
Department of Pediatrics
Moses Cone Health System
Greensboro, North Carolina

Errol R. Alden, MD
Executive Director
American Academy of Pediatrics
Elk Grove Village, Illinois

Donald C. Anderson, MD
Adjunct Professor of Pediatrics
Baylor College of Medicine
Texas Children's Hospital
Houston, Texas
Chief Medical Officer
ProNAi Therapeutics
Kalamazoo, Michigan

Billy S. Arant, Jr., MD
Professor of Pediatrics
Department of Pediatrics
University of Tennessee College of Medicine
Medical Director
Hypertension Management Center
Erlanger Medical Center
Chattanooga, Tennessee

Robert L. Atmar, MD
Associate Professor
Departments of Medicine, Molecular
    Virology and Microbiology
Baylor College of Medicine
Chairman, Infection Control
Ben Taub General Hospital
Houston, Texas

Yasser M. K. Baghdady, MD
Professor of Cardiology
Cardiology Department
Cairo University
Cairo, Egypt

Carol J. Baker, MD
Professor
Departments of Pediatrics and Molecular
    Virology & Microbiology
Baylor College of Medicine;
Attending Physician
Department of Infectious Diseases
Texas Children's Hospital
Houston, Texas

William F. Balistreri, MD
Dorothy M. Kersten Professor of Pediatrics
Department of Pediatrics
University of Cincinnati College of Medicine
Director of the Pediatric Liver Care Center
Cincinnati Children's Hospital Medical
    Center
Cincinnati, Ohio

Robert S. Baltimore, MD, FAAP
Professor
Departments of Pediatrics and Epidemiology
Yale University School of Medicine
Attending Physician in Pediatrics
Department of Pediatrics
Yale-New Haven Children's Hospital
New Haven, Connecticut

Lawrence M. Barat, MD, MPH
Senior Technical Advisor
Global Health, Population, and Nutrition
    Group
Academy for Educational Development
Washington, District of Columbia

Lewis A. Barness, MD
Department of Pediatrics
University of South Florida College
    of Medicine
Tampa, Florida

Michael A. Barone, MD, MPH
Assistant Professor
Department of Pediatrics
Johns Hopkins University School
    of Medicine
Baltimore, Maryland

Michael Bell, MD
Centers for Disease Control and Prevention
Atlanta, Georgia

Louis I. Bezold, MD
Associate Professor
Department of Pediatrics
University of Kentucky College of Medicine
Associate Chief
Division of Pediatrics Cardiology
Kentucky Children's Hospital
Lexington, Kentucky

Ellen L. Blank, MD
Associate Professor
Department of Pediatrics
Medical College of Wisconsin
Pediatric Gastroenterologist
Department of Pediatrics
Children's Hospital of Wisconsin
Milwaukee, Wisconsin

Margaret J. Blythe, MD
Professor of Pediatrics
Department of Pediatrics/Adolescent
    Medicine
Indiana University Hospital
Professor of Pediatrics
Department of Pediatrics/Adolescent
    Medicine
Riley Hospital of Children
Indianapolis, Indiana

Neil E. Bowles, PhD
Assistant Professor of Pediatrics
Section of Cardiology
Baylor College of Medicine
Texas Children's Hospital
Houston, Texas

Simeon A. Boyadjiev, MD
Assistant Professor
Institute of Genetic Medicine, Pediatrics
Johns Hopkins University
Baltimore, Maryland

Kenneth M. Boyer, MD
Department of Pediatrics
Rush-Presbyterian, St. Lukes Medical
   Center
Chicago, Illinois

Mary L. Brandt, MD
Vice Chairman and Professor
Michael E. DeBakey Department of
   Surgery
Baylor College of Medicine
Texas Children's Hospital
Houston, Texas

Joseph S. Bresee, MD, FAAP
Respiratory and Enteric Virus Branch
Division of Viral and Rickettsial Diseases
National Center for Infectious Diseases
Centers for Disease Control and Prevention
Atlanta, Georgia

Eileen D. Brewer, MD
Professor and Head, Pediatric Renal
   Section
Department of Pediatrics
Baylor College of Medicine
Chief, Renal Service
Texas Children's Hospital
Houston, Texas

J. Timothy Bricker, MD, MBA
Department of Pediatrics
University of Kentucky Medical Center
Lexington, Kentucky

William J. Britt, MD
Charles A. Alford Professor of Pediatrics
Department of Pediatrics
University of Alabama School of Medicine
Attending Physician
Children's Hospital of Alabama
Birmingham, Alabama

Itzhak Brook, MD, MSc
Professor
Department of Pediatrics
Georgetown University School of Medicine
Consultant, Infectious Diseases
Department of Pediatrics
Naval Hospital Bethesda
Bethesda, Maryland

Marilyn R. Brown, MD
Professor of Pediatrics
Department of Pediatrics
Pediatric Gastroenterology Nutrition
University of Rochester School of Medicine
Attending Physician
Pediatrics Strong Memorial Hospital
Golisano Children's Hospital at Strong
Rochester, New York

Iley B. Browning, MD
Director of Respiratory Service
Driscoll Children's Hospital
Corpus Christi, Texas

George R. Buchanan, MD
Professor of Pediatrics
The University of Texas Southwestern
   Medical Center at Dallas
Medical Director
Center for Cancer and Blood Disorders
Children's Medical Center at Dallas
Dallas, Texas

Steven C. Buckingham, MD
Associate Professor
Department of Pediatrics
University of Tennessee Health Science Center
LeBonheur Children's Medical Center
Memphis, Tennessee

Rebecca H. Buckley, MD
J. Buren Sidbury Professor of Pediatrics
Professor of Immunology
Departments of Pediatrics and Immunology
Duke University Medical Center
Department of Pediatrics
Duke University Hospital
Durham, North Carolina

Sergio R. Buzzini, MD, MPH
Assistant Professor of Pediatrics
Division of Adolescent Medicine
Medical University of South Carolina
Attending Physician
Medical University of South Carolina
   Children's Hospital
Charleston, South Carolina

Benjamin B. Cable, MD
Assistant Professor of Surgery
Department of Surgery
Uniformed Services University of the
   Health Sciences
Bethesda, Maryland
Chief, Pediatric Otolaryngology
Department of Surgery
Tripler Army Medical Center
Honolulu, Hawaii

Bryan C. Cannon, MD
Assistant Professor of Pediatrics
Department of Pediatrics, Section
   of Cardiology
Baylor College of Medicine
Texas Children's Hospital
Houston, Texas

Arnold J. Capute, MD, MPH
A.J.C. Professor of Pediatrics
Division of Child Development
Johns Hopkins University School
   of Medicine
Kennedy Krieger Institute
Baltimore, Maryland

John L. Carroll, MD
Professor
Departments of Pediatrics and Physiology
University of Arkansas for Medical Sciences
Section Chief
Division of Pediatric Pulmonary Medicine
Arkansas Children's Hospital
Little Rock, Arkansas

Terrence W. Carver, Jr., MD
Assistant Professor
Department of Pediatrics
University of Missouri-Kansas City
Chief
Pediatric Pulmonology
Children's Mercy Hospital
Kansas City, Missouri

Thomas B. Casale, MD
Assistant Dean, Clinical Research
Professor and Associate Chair
Department of Medicine
Chief, Allergy/Immunology
Creighton University
Creighton University Medical Center
Omaha, Nebraska

James F. Casella, MD
Rainey Professor and Chief of Pediatric
   Hematology
Department of Pediatrics
Johns Hopkins University School
   of Medicine
Johns Hopkins Hospital
Baltimore, Maryland

William J. Cashore, MD
Section of Prenatal Pediatrics
Women and Infants Hospital Rhode Island
Providence, Rhode Island

James T. Cassidy, MD
Department of Child Health
University of Missouri Health Sciences
   Center
Columbia, Misouri

Elizabeth A. Catlin, MD
Associate Professor of Pediatrics
Department of Pediatrics
Harvard Medical School
Neonatologist
Pediatric Service
Massachusetts General Hospital
Boston, Massachusetts

Andreea C. Cazacu, MD
Assistant Professor
Department of Pediatrics
University of Massachusetts
Director, Clinical Affairs
Massachusetts Biologic Laboratory
Jamaica Plain, Massachusetts

Frank Cecchin, MD
Assistant Professor
Department of Pediatrics
Harvard Medical School
Associate in Cardiology
Department of Cardiology
Children's Hospital of Boston
Boston, Massachusetts

Kevin Chapman, MD
Assistant Professor
Department of Pediatrics, Neurology
Baylor College of Medicine
Texas Children's Hospital
Houston, Texas

John P. Cheatham, MD
Professor
Departments of Pediatrics and
   Internal Medicine
The Ohio State University
Director, Cardiac Catheterization
   and Interventions
The Heart Center
Columbus Children's Hospital
Columbus, Ohio

Thomas Cherian, MD
Scientist
Initiative for Vaccine Research, Vaccines
   and Biologicals
World Health Organization
Geneva, Switzerland

James D. Cherry, MD, MSc
Professor
Department of Pediatrics
David Geffen School of Medicine at UCLA
Attending Physician
Mattel Children's Hospital
University of California, Los Angeles
Los Angeles, California

Myra L. Chiang, MD
Associate Professor & Chair
Department of Pediatrics
West Virginia University
Vice Chief
Department of Pediatrics
Charleston Area Medical Center
Charleston, West Virginia

Murali M. Chintagumpala, MD
Associate Professor
Department of Pediatrics
Baylor College of Medicine
Texas Children's Hospital
Houston, Texas

Thomas G. Cleary, MD
Professor, Director of Pediatric Infectious
    Diseases
Department of Pediatrics
The University of Texas-Houston Health
    Science Center
Memorial Hermann Hospital
Houston, Texas

William J. Cochran, MD, FAAP
Vice Chairman
Department of Pediatrics
Geisinger Clinic
Danville, Pennsylvania

Edward V. Colvin, MD
Associate Professor of Pediatrics
University of Alabama School of
    Medicine
Birmingham, Alabama

David W. Cooke, MD
Associate Professor
Department of Pediatrics
Johns Hopkins University School
    of Medicine
Johns Hopkins Hospital
Baltimore, Maryland

Jose C. Cortes, MD
Private Practice
Austin, Texas

Carmen C. Cosio, MD
Assistant Professor
Pediatrics Critical Care
Baylor College of Medicine
Texas Children's Hospital
Houston, Texas

Laurie E. Cutting, PhD
Assistant Professor
Department of Neurology
Johns Hopkins School of Medicine/Johns
    Hopkins University
Research Scientist
Developmental Cognitive Neurology
Kennedy Krieger Institute
Baltimore, Maryland

Mary E. D'Alton, MD
Chair of Department
Obstetrics and Gynecology
Columbia University, College of Physicians
    and Surgeons
New York, New York

Stephen R. Daniels, MD, PhD
Professor and Chairman
Department of Pediatrics
University of Colorado School of Medicine
Pediatrician-in-Chief
The Children's Hospital
Denver, Colorado

Catherine DeAngelis, MD, MPH
Professor of Pediatrics
Johns Hopkins University School
    of Medicine
Editor-in-Chief
JAMA
Chicago, Illinois

Gail J. Demmler, MD
Professor
Department of Pediatrics
Baylor College of Medicine
Attending Physician
Infectious Disease Service
Texas Children's Hospital
Houston, Texas

Martha Bridge Denckla, MD
Professor
Departments of Neurology, Pediatrics,
    and Psychiatry
Johns Hopkins School of Medicine
Developmental Cognitive Neurology
Kennedy Krieger Institute
Baltimore, Maryland

Darryl C. De Vivo, MD
Sidney Carter Professor of Neurology
Professor of Pediatrics
Department of Neurology
Columbia University Medical
    Center-Neurologic Institute
Attending Neurologist and Pediatrician
New York Presbyterian Hospital
New York, New York

William H. Dietz, MD
Director
Division of Nutrition and Physical Activity
Centers for Disease Control and Prevention
Atlanta, Georgia

Harry C. Dietz, III, MD
Professor
Institute of Genetic Medicine
Johns Hopkins University School of
    Medicine
Investigator, Howard Hughes Medical
    Institute
Pediatrics, Medicine, Molecular Biology
    & Genetics, Neurosurgery
Johns Hopkins Hospital
Baltmore, Maryland

Salvatore DiMauro, MD
Lucy G. Moses Professor of Neurology
Columbia University College of
    Physicians and Surgeons
New York, New York

Kenneth L. Dominguez, MD, MPH
Medical Epidemiologist
Surveillance and Epidemiology Branch
Division of HIV/STD/TB Prevention
National Center for HIV/STD/TB Prevention
Centers for Disease Control and Prevention
Atlanta, Georgia

Patricia A. Donohoue, MD
Professor
Department of Pediatrics
University of Iowa, Roy J. and Lucille A.
    Carver College of Medicine
Children's Hospital of Iowa
Iowa City, Iowa

David J. Driscoll, MD
Professor of Pediatrics
Head, Division of Pediatric Cardiology
Department of Pediatrics
Mayo Clinic and Medical School
Rochester, Minnesota

Christopher Duggan, MD
Associate Professor
Department of Nutrition
Harvard Medical School
Department of Nutrition
Children's Hospital
Boston, Massachusetts

Lisa M. Dunkle, MD
Senior Director
Department of Global Clinical Development
Schering-Plough Research Institute
Kenilworth, New Jersey

Morven S. Edwards, MD
Professor
Department of Pediatrics
Baylor College of Medicine
Department of Pediatric Infectious Diseases
Texas Children's Hospital
Houston, Texas

Peyton A. Eggleston, MD
Professor
Department of Pediatrics
Johns Hopkins University
Attending Physician
Johns Hopkins Hospital
Baltimore, Maryland

Richard A. Ehrenkranz, MD
Professor
Department of Pediatrics
Yale University
Clinical Director
Newborn Special Care Unit
Yale-New Haven Children's Hospital
New Haven, Connecticut

Benjamin W. Eidem, MD
Associate Professor
Department of Pediatrics
Section of Pediatric Cardiology and
    Cardiovascular Diseases
Mayo Clinic College of Medicine
Rochester, Minnesota

Ewa Elenberg, MD
Assistant Professor
Department of Pediatrics
Baylor College of Medicine
Attending Physician
Renal Service Department
Texas Children's Hospital
Houston, Texas

Galal M. El-Said, MD
Professor of Cardiology
Cardiology Department
Cairo University
Cairo, Egypt

Howaida G. El-said, MD
Department of Pediatrics
Cairo University
Cairo, Egypt

B. Keith English, MD
Professor
Department of Pediatrics
University of Tennessee Health
    Science Center
Chief, Division of Infectious Diseases
Le Bonheur Children's Medical Center
Memphis, Tennessee

Jose A. Ettedgui, MD
Glenn Chuck Professor of Pediatric
    Cardiology
Department of Pediatrics
University of Florida
Chief of Pediatric Cardiology
Wolfson Children's Hospital
Jacksonville, Florida

Daniel I. Feig, MD, PhD
Assistant Professor
Pediatrics, Renal Section
Baylor College of Medicine
Chief
Pediatrics Hypertension Clinics
Texas Children's Hospital
Houston, Texas

Ralph D. Feigin, MD
Distinguished Service Professor
Chairman
Department of Pediatrics
Baylor College of Medicine
Physician-in-Chief
Texas Children's Hospital
Chief, Pediatric Service
Ben Taub General Hospital
The Methodist Hospital
Houston, Texas

Donna M. Ferriero, MD
Professor
Department of Neurology and
    Pediatrics
University California San Francisco
Director
Department of Child Neurology
University of California San Francisco
    Children's Hospital
San Francisco, California

Laurence Finberg, MD
Clinical Professor
Department of Pediatrics
Univeristy of California, San Francisco
San Francisco, California
Standford University
Palo Alto, California

Laura S. Finn, MD
Assistant Professor
Department of Pathology
University of Washington
Associate Pathologist
Department of Laboratories
Children's Hospital & Regional Medical
    Center
Seattle, Washington

Randall G. Fisher, MD
Associate Professor
Department of Pediatrics
Eastern Virginia Medical School
Medical Director
Department of Pediatric Infectious Diseases
Children's Hospital of the King's
    Daughters
Norfolk, Virginia

Marvin A. Fishman, MD
Professor
Departments of Pediatrics and Neurology
Baylor College of Medicine
Attending Neurologist
Texas Children's Hospital
Houston, Texas

David E. Fixler, MD
Professor
Department of Pediatrics
University of Texas Southwestern
    Medical Center
Attending Cardiologist
Department of Cardiology
Children's Medical Center
Dallas, Texas

Alan R. Fleischman, MD
Senior Advisor
The New York Academy of Medicine
Clinical Professor of Pediatrics,
    Epidemiology and Population Health
Albert Einstein College of Medicine
New York, New York

Craig E. Fleishman, MD
Department of Cardiology
Harvard Medical School
Boston, Massachusetts

Thomas R. Flynn, DMD
Assistant Professor
Department of Oral and Maxillofacial
    Surgery
Harvard School of Dental Medicine
Associate Visiting Surgeon
Massachusetts General Hospital
Boston, Massachusetts

James D. Fortenberry, MD, FAAP, FCCM
Clinical Associate Professor
Department of Pediatrics
Emory University School of Medicine
Medical Director, Pediatric Critical
    Care Medicine
Children's Healthcare of Atlanta
    at Egleston
Atlanta, Georgia

Norman C. Fost, MD, MPH
Professor
Departments of Pediatrics and Bioethics
University of Wisconsin Medical School
University of Wisconsin Hospital
Madison, Wisconsin

Richard A. Friedman, MD
Associate Professor of Pediatrics
Department of Pediatrics
Texas Children's Hospital
Houston, Texas

Junichiro Fukushige, MD
Clinical Professor
Department of Pediatrics
Kyushu University
Chief Executive
Fukuoka Children's Hospital & Medical
    Center for Infectious Disease
Fukuoka, Japan

Glenn T. Furuta, MD
Assistant Professor
Department of Pediatrics
Harvard Medical School
Associate Fellowship Training
    Program Director
Division of Pediatric Gastroenterology
Children's Hospital, Boston
Boston, Massachusetts

Patrick G. Gallagher, MD
Associate Professor
Department of Pediatrics
Yale University
Attending Physician
Yale-New Haven Children's Hospital
New Haven, Connecticut

Joseph M. Gertner, MD, MRCP
Lecturer
Department of Pediatrics
Harvard Medical School
Attending Physician
Department of Medicine
Children's Hospital
Boston, Massachusetts

Mark A. Gilger, MD
Associate Professor of Pediatrics
Section of Gastroenterology, Pediatrics
Baylor College of Medicine
Medical Director, Section of
    Gastroenterology, Hepatology
    and Nutrition
Texas Children's Hospital
Houston, Texas

Daniel G. Glaze, MD
Associate Professor
Departments of Pediatrics and Neurology
Baylor College of Medicine
Medical Director, Children's Sleep Center
Medical Director, The Methodist Hospital
    Sleep Disorders Center
Medical Director, The Blue Bird Circle Rett
    Center
Houston, Texas

W. Paul Glezen, MD
Professor
Molecular Virology and Microbiology
    and Pediatrics
Baylor College of Medicine
Attending Pediatrician
Ben Taub General Hospital
Houston, Texas

Benjamin D. Gold, MD
Associate Professor of Pediatrics and
    Microbiology
Division of Pediatric Gastroenterology,
    Hepatology and Nutrition
Emory University School of Medicine
Chief
Gastroenterology Service
Children's Healthcare of Atlanta
Egleston Children's Hospital
Atlanta, Georgia

Melanie A. Gold, DO
Associate Professor
Department of Pediatrics, Division of
   Adolescent Medicine
University of Pittsburgh School of Medicine
Director of Family Planning Services and
   Adolescent Medicine Research
Children's Hospital of Pittsburgh
Pittsburgh, Pennsylvania

Nira A. Goldstein, MD
Associate Professor
Department of Pediatric Otolaryngology
State University of New York Downstate
   Medical Center
Attending Physician
Department of Otolaryngology
University Hospital of Brooklyn, Long
   Island Hospital, Kings County Hospital
   Center
Brooklyn, New York

Stuart L. Goldstein, MD
Associate Professor
Department of Pediatrics
Baylor College of Medicine
Texas Children's Hospital
Houston, Texas

Edmond T. Gonzales, Jr., MD
Professor
Scott Department of Urology
Baylor College of Medicine
Medical Director, Renal Dialysis Unit
Renal Section
Texas Children's Hospital
Houston, Texas

Robert J. Gorlin, DDS, MS, DSc
Regents Professor, Emeritus
Oral Pathologist
University of Minnesota
Consultant
Fairview University Hospital School
   of Medicine
Minneapolis, Minnesota

Richard J. Grand, MD
Professor of Pediatrics
Harvard Medical School
Director, General Clinical Research Center
Director, Center for Inflammatory Bowel
   Disease
Division of Gastroenterology and Nutrition
The Children's Hospital, Boston
Boston, Massachusetts

Morris Green, MD
Perry W. Lesh Professor of Pediatrics
Department of Pediatrics
Indiana University School of Medicine
Director, Behavioral/Developmental
   Pediatric Section
Department of Pediatrics
James Whitcomb Riley Hospital for
   Children
Indianapolis, Indiana

Adda Grimberg, MD, FAAP
Assistant Professor
Department of Pediatrics
University of Pennsylvania School
   of Medicine
Attending Physician
Division of Pediatric Endocrinology
   and Diabetes
The Children's Hospital of Philadelphia
Philadelphia, Pennsylvania

Charles F. Grose, MD
Professor
Department of Pediatrics
University of Iowa
Director of Infectious Diseases
Department of Pediatrics
Children's Hospital of Iowa
Iowa City, Iowa

Ian Gross, MBBCh
Professor
Department of Pediatrics Division of
   Perinatal Medicine
Yale University School of Medicine
Director, Newborn Special Care Unit
Yale-New Haven Children's Hospital
New Haven, Connecticut

Nicholas G. Guerina, MD, PhD
Director of Perinatal Infectious Diseases
Department of Pediatrics
Turfs University School of Medicine
The Floating Hospital for Children
New England Medical Center
Boston, Massachusetts

Carl H. Gumbiner, MD
Professor
Department of Pediatrics
University of Nebraska Medical Center
Pediatric Cardiologist
University of Nebraska College of Medicine
Creighton University Children's Hospital
Omaha, Nebraska

Howard P. Gutgesell, MD
Professor
Department of Pediatrics
University of Virginia School of Medicine
Attending Physician
University of Virginia Hospital
Charlottesville, Virginia

Steven L. Guthery, MD
Assistant Professor
Department of Pediatrics
University of Utah School of Medicine
Salt Lake City, Utah

Brian E. Hainline, MD, PhD
Clinical Associate Professor of Pediatrics
Assistant Professor of Medical and
   Molecular Genetics
Indiana University School of Medicine
The James Whitcomb Riley Hospital for
   Children
Indianapolis, Indiana

Caroline Breese Hall, MD
Professor
Departments of Pediatrics and Medicine
University of Rochester School of Medicine
   and Dentistry
Professor of Pediatrics and Medicine
Departments of Pediatrics and Medicine
Golisano's Children's Hospital at Strong
Rochester, New York

Neal A. Halsey, MD
Professor
Department of International Health
Johns Hopkins Bloomberg School of Public
   Health
Baltimore, Maryland

Margaret R. Hammerschlag, MD
Professor of Pediatrics and Medicine
Department of Pediatrics
State University of New York Downstate
   Medical Center
Director, Division of Pediatric Infectious
   Diseases
University Hospital of Brooklyn
Kings County Hospital Center
Brooklyn, New York

Ada Hamosh, MD, MPH
Associate Professor of Pediatrics
The McKusick-Nathans Institute of
   Genetic Medicine
Johns Hopkins University School
   of Medicine
Department of Pediatrics
Johns Hopkins Hospital
Baltimore, Maryland

I. Celine Hanson, MD
Professor
Department of Pediatrics
Baylor College of Medicine
Clinic Chief
Allergy and Immunology Section
Texas Children's Hospital
Houston, Texas

James C. Harris, MD
Director, Developmental Neuropsychiatry
Professor of Psychiatry and Behavioral
   Sciences, Pediatrics and Mental Hygiene
Departments of Psychiatry and Behavioral
   Sciences and Pediatrics
Johns Hopkins University School
   of Medicine
Johns Hopkins Hospital
Baltimore, Maryland

John V. Hartline, MD
Clinical Professor, Emeritus
Pediatric and Human Development
Michigan State University College of
   Human Medicine
Kalamazoo Center for Medical Studies
Kalamazoo, Michigan

William W. Hay, Jr., MD
Professor
Department of Pediatrics
University of Colorado School of Medicine
The Children's Hospital
Denver, Colorado

C. Mary Healy, MD, MRCP
Assistant Professor of Pediatrics
Department of Pediatrics
Baylor College of Medicine
Attending Physician
Department of Pediatrics, Section of
   Infectious Diseases
Texas Children's Hospital
Houston, Texas

Andrew J. Healy, MD
Fellow, Division of Maternal Fetal Medicine
Obstetrics and Gynecology
Columbia University, College of Physicians
   and Surgeons
Morgan Stanley Children's Hospital-New
   York Presbyterian Hospital
New York, New York

Mark E. Helm, MD, MBA
Assistant Professor
College of Pharmacy
University of Arkansas
Medical Director
Arkansas Medicaid Evidence-Based
    Prescription Drug Program
Little Rock, Arkansas

Rubina A. Heptulla, MD
Assistant Professor
Department of Pediatrics, Endocrinology
Baylor College of Medicine
Texas Children's Hospital
Houston, Texas

Robert A. Herzlinger, MD
Associate Clinical Professor
Department of Pediatrics
Yale University School of Medicine
New Haven, Connecticut
Director of Neonatology
Department of Pediatrics
Bridgeport Hospital
Bridgeport, Connecticut

Richard B. Heyman, MD
Adjunct Professor of Clinical Pediatrics
Department of Pediatrics, Division of
    Adolescent Medicine
University of Cincinnati College of Medicine
Attending Physician
Department of Pediatrics
Cincinnati Children's Hospital Medical
    Center
Cincinnati, Ohio

Peter W. Hiatt, MD
Associate Professor
Department of Pediatrics
Baylor College of Medicine
Director, Cystic Fibrosis Center
Department of Pulmonary Medicine Service
Texas Children's Hospital
Houston, Texas

M. John Hicks, MD, PhD, DDS, MS, PhD
Professor of Pathology
Department of Pathology
Baylor College of Medicine
Director of Anatomic Pathology
Medical Director of Surgical and Ultra
    Structural Pathology
Department of Pathology
Texas Children's Hospital
Houston, Texas

Leslie M. Higuchi, MD, MPH
Instructor in Pediatrics
Harvard Medical School
Assistant in Medicine
Division of Gastroenterology and Nutrition
Children's Hospital
Boston, Massachusetts

Sharon Hill, ACNP
The Heart Center
Columbus Children's Hospital
Columbus, Ohio

L. Leighton Hill, MD
Professor of Pediatrics, Renal Section
Baylor College of Medicine
Houston, Texas

Anthony M. Hlavacek, MD
Clinical Fellow
Department of Pediatric
Medical University of South Carolina
Department of Cardiology
Medical University of South Carolina
    Children's Hospital
Charleston, South Carolina

Ching Lin Ho, FRCS Ed
Clinical Tutor
Department of Ophthalmology
National University of Singapore
Associate Consultant
Glaucoma Service
Singapore National Eye Center
Singapore

Lewis B. Holmes, MD
Professor of Pediatrics
Harvard Medical School
Chief, Genetics and Teratology Unit
Massachusetts General Hospital for
    Children
Boston, Massachusetts

Todd E. Holmes, MD
Chief Resident
Department of Dermatology
Fletcher Allen Health Care
Burlington, Vermont

Barbara J. Howard, MD
Assistant Professor of Pediatrics
Department of Pediatrics
Johns Hopkins University School
    of Medicine
Baltimore, Maryland

Walter T. Hughes, Jr., MD
Emeritus Chairman
Department of Infectious Diseases
St. Jude Children's Research Hospital
Memphis, Tennessee

James C. Huhta, MD
Professor of Pediatrics and Ob/Gyn
Daicoff-Andrews Chair in Perinatal
    Cardiology-Pediatrics
University of Florida College of Medicine
Noninvasive Lab Medical Director
Department of Cardiology
All Children's Hospital
St. Petersburg, Florida

Sandy T. Hwang, MD
Assistant Professor of Pediatrics
Division of Gastroenterology and Nutrition
Department of Pediatrics
Baylor College of Medicine
Houston, Texas

Ethylin Wang Jabs, MD
Dr. Frank V. Sutland Professor of Pediatric
    Genetics
Institute of Genetic Medicine, and Surgery
Johns Hopkins University
Baltimore, Maryland

W. Daniel Jackson, MD
Associate Professor
Department of Pediatrics
University of Utah School of Medicine
Salt Lake City, Utah

Richard F. Jacobs, MD, FAAP
Horace C. Cabe Professor of Pediatrics
University of Arkansas for Medical Sciences
President
Arkansas Children's Hospital Research
    Institute
Little Rock, Arkansas

Phillip A. Jacobson, MD
Pediatric Intensive Care
Rush University Medical Center
Chicago, Illinois

Tom Jaksic, MD, PhD
The Children's Hospital
Boston, Massachusetts

Joseph Jankovic, MD, PhD
Department of Neurology
Baylor College of Medicine
Houston, Texas

Alain Joffe, MD, MPH
Associate Professor of Pediatrics
Johns Hopkins University School
    of Medicine
Director, Student Health and Wellness
    Center
Johns Hopkins University
Baltimore, Maryland

Sid Johnson, MD
Children's Hospital
Boston, Massachusetts

Anne M. Johnston, MD
Clinical Assistant Professor
Department of Pediatrics/Neonatology
Fletcher Allen Health Care
Burlington, Vermont

M. Douglas Jones, Jr., MD
Professor
Department of Pediatrics
Section of Neonatology
The University of Colorado
The Children's Hospital
Denver, Colorado

Stuart D. Josell, DMD, MDentSC
Associate Professor
Department of Orthodontics
Baltimore College of Dental Surgery, Dental
    School University of Maryland
Associate Professor
Department of Dentistry
University of Maryland Medical System
Baltimore, Maryland

Victoria E. Judd, MD, MBA
Clinical Professor of Pediatrics
Department of Pediatrics
University of Utah School of Medicine
Congenital Cardiologist
Department of Pediatrics
Primary Children's Medical Center
Salt Lake City, Utah

Stephen G. Kahler, MD
Professor
Department of Pediatrics
University of Arkansas for Medical Sciences
Director, Clinical Genetics
Department of Pediatrics
Arkansas Children's Hospital
Little Rock, Arkansas

Arundhati S. Kale, MBBS
Associate Professor
Department of Pediatrics
Baylor College of Medicine
Attending Physician
Texas Children's Hospital
Houston, Texas

Sheldon L. Kaplan, MD
Professor and Vice Chairman for Clinical
    Affairs
Department of Pediatrics
Baylor College of Medicine
Chief, Infectious Disease Service
Texas Children's Hospital
Houston, Texas

Jorge M. Karam, MD
Pediatric Pulmonologist
Allergy and Immunology Service
Hospital Infantil de Mexico
Mexico City, Mexico

Garyfallia Katsavounidou, MS, DMD
Graduate Student
Department of Architecture
Massachusetts Institute of Technology
Cambridge, Massachusetts

Mark L. Kayton, MD
Assistant Member
Department of Surgery
Memorial Sloane-Kettering Cancer Center
Assistant Surgery Service
Memorial Hospital
New York, New York

Haig H. Kazazian, Jr., MD
Chairman, Seymour Gray Professor
    on Molecular Medicine
Department of Genetics
University of Pennsylvania School
    of Medicine
Philadelphia, Pennsylvania

James S. Kemp, MD
Associate Professor
Department of Pediatrics
St. Louis University School of Medicine
Cardinal Glennon Children's Medical Center
St. Louis, Missouri

Kathi J. Kemper, MD, MPH
Caryl J. Guth Chair for Holistic and
    Integrative Medicine
Professor, Public Health Sciences
Professor, Pediatrics
Wake Forest University School of Medicine
Chief, Second Opinion Clinic
Brenner Children's Hospital
Winston-Salem, North Carolina

Kathleen A. Kennedy, MD, MPH
Professor of Pediatrics
Department of Pediatrics
University of Texas Medical School at
    Houston
Houston, Texas

Bradley H. Kessler, MD
Director, Pediatric Gastroenterology
Department of Pediatrics
Good Samaritan Hospital Medical Center
West Islip, New York

Melanie S. Kim, MD
Associate Professor
Department of Pediatrics
Boston University School of Medicine
Associate Residency Program Director
Department of Pediatrics
Boston Medical Center
Boston, Massachusetts

John L. Kirkland, MD
Professor
Department of Pediatrics
Baylor College of Medicine
Endocrine and Metabolism Section
Texas Children's Hospital
Houston, Texas

Rebecca T. Kirkland, MD, MPH
Professor
Chief, Academic General Pediatrics
Department of Pediatrics
Baylor College of Medicine
Medical Director
Department of Ambulatory Services
Texas Children's Hospital
Houston, Texas

Mark W. Kline, MD
Professor
Department of Pediatrics
Baylor College of Medicine
Chief, Retro Virology Clinic
Texas Children's Hospital,
Houston, Texas

William J. Klish, MD
Professor
Department of Pediatrics
Baylor College of Medicine
Department of Gastroenterology
    Hepatology and Nutrition
Texas Children's Hospital
Houston, Texas

Edward C. Kohaut, MD
Professor and Co-Chairman
Department of Pediatrics
Florida State University in Pensacola
Director
Department of Pediatric Nephrology
Nemours Children's Clinic
Pensacola, Florida

Steve Kohl, MD
Clinical Professor
Department of Pediatrics
Oregon Health and Sciences University
Portland, Oregon

Gary S. Kopf, MD
Professor of Surgery
Department of Surgery
Yale University School of Medicine
Chief, Pediatric Cardiac Surgery
Department of Surgery
Yale-New Haven Hospital
New Haven, Connecticut

Andrew J. Kornberg, MBBS, FRACP
Senior Lecturer
Department of Pediatrics
University of Melbourne
Neurologist
Department of Neurology
Royal Children's Hospital
Parkville, Victoria, Australia

John P. Kovalchin, MD
Assistant Professor
Department of Pediatrics
Baylor College of Medicine
Associate Chief of Cardiology Services
Pediatric Cardiology
Texas Children's Hospital
Houston, Texas

Richard E. Kreipe, MD
Professor of Pediatrics
University of Rochester School of Medicine
    & Dentistry
Chief, Division of Adolescent Medicine
Department of Pediatrics
Golisano Children's Hospital at Strong
Rochester, New York

Daniel P. Krowchuk, MD
Professor of Pediatrics and Dermatology
Department of Pediatrics
Chief
Departments of General Pediatrics and
    Adolescent Medicine
Wake Forest University Health Sciences
Winston-Salem, North Carolina

Paul A. Krusinski, MD
Professor and Director
Dermatology Division
University of Vermont
Fletcher Allen Health Care
Burlington, Vermont

Ingrid Kuehnle, MD
Assistant Professor
Department of Pediatrics
Section of Hematology/Oncology
Baylor College of Medicine
Center for Cell and Gene Therapy
Baylor College of Medicine
Texas Children's Hospital
The Methodist Hospital
Houston, Texas

Katherine S. Kula, MS, DMD
Chair
Department of Orthodontics and
    Dentofacial Orthopedics
University of Missouri-Kansas City School
    of Dentistry
Orthodontic Consultant
Mid-America Cleft and Craniofacial
    Program
St. Luke's Hospital
Kansas City, Misouri

Gregory L. Landry, MD
Professor of Pediatrics
University of Wisconsin Medical School
Head, Division General Pediatrics and
    Adolescent Medicine
Department of Pediatrics
University of Wisconsin
Madison, Wisconsin

Claire Langston, MD
Professor
Department of Pathology
Baylor College of Medicine
Pathologist
Department of Pathology
Texas Children's Hospital
Houston, Texas

Marc H. Lebel, MD, FRCPC
Clinical Associate Professor
Division of Infectious Diseases, Department
of Pediatrics
University of Montreal
Sainte Justine Hospital
Montreal, Quebec, Canada

Howard M. Lederman, MD, PhD
Professor
Departments of Pediatrics, Medicine and
Pathology
Johns Hopkins University School of
Medicine
Director, Immunodeficiency Clinic
Division of Pediatric Allergy and
Immunology
Johns Hopkins Hospital
Baltimore, Maryland

Mary M. Lee, MD
Professor of Pediatrics and Cell Biology
Pediatric Endocrine Division
University of Massachusetts Medical School
Director, Pediatric Endocrine Division
Department of Pediatrics
University of Massachusetts Memorial
Health Care
Worcester, Massachusetts

Robert J. Leggiadro, MD
Adjunct Professor
Department of Pediatrics
University of Medicine and Dentistry
of New Jersey
Newark, New Jersey
Chairman
Department of Pediatrics
Lincoln Hospital
Bronx, New York

Rebecca A. Levin-Goodman, MPH
Manager, Injury, Violence, and Poison
Prevention
Division of Safety and Health Promotion
American Academy of Pediatrics
Elk Grove Village, Illinois

Moise L. Levy, MD
Professor
Departments of Dermatology and Pediatrics
Baylor College of Medicine
Chief, Dermatology Service
Texas Children's Hospital
Houston, Texas

Amy Feldman Lewanda, MD
Assistant Professor
Institute of Genetic Medicine, Pediatrics
Johns Hopkins University
Baltimore, Maryland
Clinical Associate Professor
Department of Pediatrics
University of Virginia School of Medicine
Richmond, Virginia
Clinical Assistant Professor Department of
Pediatrics
George Washington University School of
Medicine and Health Sciences
Washington, District of Columbia

Victor A. Lewis, MB, BS
Department of Oncology
Alberta Children's Hospital
Calgary, Alberta, Canada

Carlos H. Lifschitz, MD
Associate Professor
Department of Pediatrics/Nutrition
Baylor College of Medicine
Department of Pediatrics
Texas Children's Hospital
Houston, Texas

Bart L. Loeys, MD, PhD
Associate Professor
Center for Medical Genetics
Ghent University
Gent, Belgium

Sarah S. Long, MD
Professor of Pediatrics
Drexel University College of Medicine
Chief, Section of Infectious Diseases
Department of Pediatrics
St. Christopher Hospital for Children
Philadelphia, Pennsylvania

Martin I. Lorin, MD
Professor
Department of Pediatrics
Baylor College of Medicine
Attending Physician
Department of Pediatrics
Texas Children's Hospital
Houston, Texas

Timothy E. Lotze, MD, BS
Assistant Professor
Department of Pediatrics
Baylor College of Medicine
Division of Child Neurology
Texas Children's Hospital
Houston, Texas

Gerald M. Loughlin, MD
Nancy C. Paduano Professor and Chair
Department of Pediatrics
Weill Medical College of Cornell University
Pediatrician-in-Chief
Phyllis and David Komansky Center for
Children's Health
New York Presbyterian Hospital
New York, New York

Penelope Terhune Louis, MD
Associate Professor
Physical Medicine and Rehabilitation
Baylor College of Medicine
Kelsey-Seybold Clinic
Houston, Texas

Katherine Luzuriaga, MD
Professor
Department of Pediatrics, Program in
Molecular Medicine
University of Massachusetts Medical
School
Chief
Department of Pediatrics
University of Massachusetts Memorial
Hospital
Worcester, Massachusetts

Ruth Lynfield, MD
Medical Director
Infectious Disease Epidemiology, Prevention
and Control Division
Minnesota Department of Health
St. Paul, Minnesota

Donald H. Mahoney, Jr., MD
Professor of Pediatrics
Baylor College of Medicine
Director, Hematology Laboratory
Department of Pediatric
Hematology-Oncology
Texas Children's Hospital
Houston, Texas

Carole L. Marcus, M.B.B.Ch.
Professor of Pediatrics
Department of Pediatrics
University of Pennsylvania School
of Medicine
Director, Sleep Center
Children's Hospital of Philadelphia
Philadelphia, Pennsylvania

M. Michele Mariscalco, MD
Assistant Professor
Department of Pediatrics
Baylor College of Medicine
Staff Physician
Intensive Care Service
Texas Children's Hospital
Houston, Texas

Paul L. Martin, MD, PhD
Associate Clinical Professor
Department of Pediatrics
Duke University Medical Center
Medical Director
Children's Health Center
Durham, North Carolina

Nancy J. Matyunas, PharmD
Clinical Pharmacist
Family Health Center
Louisville, Kentucky

Edward R. B. McCabe, MD, PhD
Executive Chair and Professor
Department of Pediatrics
David Geffen School of Medicine at UCLA
Physician-in-Chief
Department of Pediatrics
Mattel Children's Hospital at UCLA
Los Angeles, California

Kenneth L. McClain, MD, PhD
Professor
Department of Pediatrics
Baylor College of Medicine
Attending Physician
Texas Children's Cancer Center/Hematology
Service
Texas Children's Hospital
Houston, Texas

Colston F. McEvoy, MD
Pediatric Gastroenterologist
Children's Hospital Center for Digestive
Health
Greenville Hospital System University
Medical Center
Greenville, South Carolina

Michael R. McGinnis, PhD
Professor
Department of Pathology
Associate Director, Clinical Microbiology
Department of Pathology
University of Texas Medical Branch
Galveston, Texas

Ross E. McKinney, Jr., MD
Associate Professor of Pediatrics
Duke University Medical Center
Durham, North Carolina

Julia A. McMillan, MD
Professor of Pediatrics, Vice Chair for
    Education
Department of Pediatrics
Johns Hopkins University School of
    Medicine
Baltimore, Maryland

Dennis M. Mello, MD
Assistant Professor
Department of Surgery
University of Connecticut
Farmington, Connecticut
Chief
Department of Cardiothoracic Surgery
Connecticut Children's Hospital
Hartford, Connecticut

Patricia Mena, MD
Assistant Professor
Clinical Nutrition
Instituto Nutricion y Technologia De Los
    Alimentos/University of Chile
Head
Neonatal Unit
Hospital Dr. Sotero Del Rio
Santiago, Chile

Laura R. Ment, MD
Professor
Departments of Pediatrics and Neurology
Yale University School of Medicine
Attending Physician
Department of Pediatrics and Neurology
Yale-New Haven Hospital
New Haven, Connecticut

Denise W. Metry, MD
Associate Professor of Dermatology
    and Pediatrics
Baylor College of Medicine
Chief, Pediatric Dermatology Clinic
Texas Children's Hospital
Houston, Texas

Laurie C. Miller, MD
Associate Professor of Pediatrics
Department of Pediatrics
Tufts University School of Medicine
Director, International Adoption Clinic
New England Medical Center
Boston, Massachusetts

Ryan S. Miller, MD
Clinical Fellow
Department of Pediatrics, Endocrinology
Johns Hopkins University School of
    Medicine
Johns Hopkins Hospital
Baltimore, Maryland

Tara D. Miller, MD
Resident
Department of Dermatology
University of California, San Francisco
San Francisco

Cynthia S. Minkovitz, MD, MPP
Associate Professor
Department of Population and Family
    Health Sciences
Johns Hopkins Bloomberg School
    of Public Health
Department of Pediatrics
Johns Hopkins Hospital
Baltimore, Maryland

John F. Modlin, MD
Professor and Chair
Department of Pediatrics
Medical Director
Dartmouth Medical School
Children's Hospital at Dartmouth
Lebanon, New Hampshire

Mary J. H. Morris, MD
Associate Professor of Clinical Pediatrics
Department of Pediatrics
University of Iowa Hospitals and Clinics
Iowa City, Iowa

Jill H. Morriss, MD
Professor of Clinical Pediatrics
Pediatrics, Division of Pediatric Cardiology
University of Iowa
Department of Pediatrics
Children's Hospital of Iowa
Iowa City, Iowa

W. Robert Morrow, MD
Professor of Pediatrics
Department of Pediatrics
University of Arkansas for Medical Sciences
Chief, Pediatric Cardiology
Arkansas Children's Hospital
Little Rock, Arkansas

Thomas Moshang, Jr., MD
Professor Emeritus
Department of Pediatrics
University of Pennsylvania
Senior Endocrinologist
Department of Endocrinology and Diabetes
Children's Hospital of Philadelphia
Philadelphia, Pennsylvania

Immanuela Ravé Moss, MD, PhD
Professor
Departments of Pediatrics and Physiology
McGill University
Attending Physician
Division of Respiratory Medicine
The Montreal Children's Hospital, McGill
    University Health Centre
Montreal, Quebec, Canada

Stewart H. Mostofsky, MD
Assistant Professor
Departments of Neurology and Psychiatry
Johns Hopkins University School of
    Medicine
Medical Director, Center for Autism and
    Related Disorders
Developmental Cognitive Neurology
Kennedy Krieger Institute
Baltimore, Maryland

Kathleen J. Motil, MD, PhD
Associate Professor
Department of Pediatrics
Baylor College of Medicine
Active Staff
Section of Pediatric Gastroenterology and
    Nutrition
Texas Children's Hospital
Houston, Texas

Edina H. Moylett, MD
Senior Lecturer
Department of Pediatrics
National University of Ireland, Galway
Clinical Science Institute
Consultant Pediatrician
University College Hospital
Galway, Ireland

Charles E. Mullins, MD
Professor
Department of Pediatrics
Baylor College of Medicine
Director Emeritus, Cardiac Catheterization
    Laboratory
Department of Pediatric Cardiology
Texas Children's Hospital
Houston, Texas

Holly J. Mulvey, MA
Director
Division of Graduate Medical Education
American Academy of Pediatrics
Elk Grove Village, Illinois

Prathiba Nanjundiah, MD
Pediatric Gastroenterologist
Department of Pediatrics
Southern California Permanente Medical
    Group
Los Angeles Medical Center
Los Angeles, California

Patricia Mena Nanning, MD
Associate Professor
Department of Human Nutrition
INTA, Universidad de Chile
Chief
Neonatal Sevice
Hospital Dr Sotero del Rio
Santiago, Chile

James P. Nataro, MD, PhD
Professor of Pediatrics and Medicine
Center for Vaccine Development
Associate Chair for Research
Department of Pediatrics
University of Maryland School of
    Medicine
Department of Pediatrics
University of Maryland Hospital for
    Children
Baltimore, Maryland

William H. Neches, MD
Emeritus Professor of Pediatrics
University of Pittsburgh School of
    Medicine
Former Physician Director of Informatics
    and Pediatric Cardiologist
Children's Hospital
Pittsburgh, Pennsylvania

Herbert L. Needleman, MD
Professor
Departments of Psychiatry and Pediatrics
University of Pittsburgh School of
    Medicine
Pittsburgh, Pennsylvania

Umbereen S. Nehal, MD
Harvard Pediatric Health
Boston, Massachusetts

Peter Ngo, MD
Clinical and Research Fellow
Division of Pediatric Gastroenterology
   and Nutrition
Harvard Medical School
Fellow in Pediatric Gastroenterology
Division of Pediatric Gastroenterology
   and Nutrition
Children's Hospital
Boston, Massachusetts

Bruce G. Nickerson, MD
Associate Clinical Professor of Pediatrics
University of California
Director, Pulmonary Medicine
Children's Hospital of Orange County
Orange, California

Donald A. Novak, MD
Professor
Department of Pediatrics
University of Florida
Gainesville, Florida

Edward J. Novotny, Jr., MD
Associate Professor
Department of Pediatrics
Yale University
Director, Pediatric Epilepsy Program
Department of Pediatrics
Yale-New Haven Children's Hospital
New Haven, Connecticut

Jed G. Nuchtern, MD
Associate Professor of Surgery and Pediatrics
Michael DeBakey Department of Surgery
Baylor College of Medicine
Attending Surgeon
Pediatric Surgery
Texas Children's Hospital
Houston, Texas

Theresa J. Ochoa, MD
Assistant Professor
Department of Pediatrics
Univeridad Peruana Cayetano Heredia
Lima Peru

Angela K. Ogden, MD
Texas Children's Hospital
Houston, Texas

Folashade A. Ogunmodede, MD, MPH
Resident in General Internal Medicine
Department of Internal Medicine
Marshfield Clinic and St. Joseph's Hospital
Marshfield, Wisconsin

Donald P. Orr, MD
Professor
Department of Pediatrics, Nursing,
   Nutrition/Dietetics
Indiana University School of Medicine
Director of Adolescent Medicine
Department of Pediatrics
Riley Hospital for Children
Indianapolis, Indiana

Frank A. Oski, MD (Deceased)
Given Professor of Pediatrics
Johns Hopkins University School
   of Medicine
Pediatrician-in-Chief
Johns Hopkins Children's Center
Baltimore, Maryland

Jane A. Oski, MD
Director of Adolescent Health Services
Department of Pediatrics
Tuba City Indian Medical Center
Tuba City, Arizona

James Owens, MD, PhD
Fellow, Clinical Neurophysiology
Department of Neurology
Baylor College of Medicine
Houston, Texas

Charles N. Paidas, MD, MBA
Professor of Surgery
Department of Surgery
University of South Florida
Chief, Division of Pediatric Surgery
Tampa General Hospital
Tampa, Florida

Frederick B. Palmer, MD
Shainberg Professor of Pediatrics
Director, Boling Center for Developmental
   Disabilities
University of Tennessee Health Science
   Center
Memphis, Tennessee

Stephen M. Paridon, MD
Associate Professor
Department of Pediatrics
University of Pennsylvania
Medical Director, Exercise Physiology
   Laboratory
Division of Cardiology
The Children's Hospital of Philadelphia
Philadelphia, Pennsylvania

Sang C. Park, MD
Professor of Pediatrics
University of Pittsburgh School of Medicine
Associate Director, Cardiology Division
Children's Hospital of Pittsburgh
Pittsburgh, Pennsylvania

Julie Thorne Parke, MD
Presbyterian Health Foundation Chair in
   Child Neurology
Professor of Neurology and Pediatrics
Chief, Section of Child Neurology
University of Oklahoma School of Medicine
Oklahoma City, Oklahoma

Yves D. Pastore, MD
Assistant Professor
Department of Pediatrics Hematology/
   Oncology
Baylor College of Medicine
Faculty
Hematology-Oncology
Texas Children's Hospital
Houston, Texas

Christian C. Patrick, MD, PhD
Chief Medical Officer
Senior Vice President for Medical Affairs
Miami Children's Hospital
Miami, Florida

Lori E. R. Patterson, MD
Director, Pediatric Infectious Disease
East Tennessee Children's Hospital
Knoxville, Tennessee

Howard A. Pearson, MD
Professor of Pediatrics Emeritus
Department of Pediatrics
Yale University School of Medicine
Department of Pediatrics
Yale New Haven Children's Hospital
New Haven, Connecticut

Angela J. Peck, MD
Senior Fellow
Department of Pediatrics
Division of Pediatric Infectious Diseases
University of Washington
Seattle, Washington

Walter Pegoli, Jr., MD
Associate Professor
Departments of Surgery and Pediatrics
University of Rochester School of Medicine
Chief, Pediatric Surgery
Golisano Children's Hospital
Rochester, New York

Maria A. Pelidis, MD
Assistant Professor
Tufts University School of Medicine
Assistant Pediatrician
Boston Floating Hospital for Children
New England Medical Center
Boston, Massachusetts

Alan K. Percy, MD
Professor, Departments of Pediatrics,
   Neurology, and Neurobiology
University of Alabama School of Medicine
University of Alabama at Birmingham
Emeritus Director, Child Neurology
Department of Pediatrics
Children's Hospital of Alabama
Birmingham, Alabama

Robert Perelman, MD
Associate Executive Director
Director, Department of Education
American Academy of Pediatrics
Elk Grove Village, Illinois

Jeffrey M. Perlman, MD
Professor
Department of Pediatrics
Weill-Cornell Medical College
Chief, Newborn Medicine
Department of Pediatrics
New York Presbyterian Hospital-Cornell
   Medical Center
New York, New York

Steven M. Peterec, MD
Associate Clinical Professor
Department of Pediatrics (Neonatology)
Yale University School of Medicine
Attending Neonatologist
Department of Pediatrics
Yale-New Haven Children's Hospital
New Haven, Connecticut

Larry K. Pickering, MD, FAAP
Professor
Department of Pediatrics
Emory University of Medicine
Senior Advisor to the Director
National Immunization Program
Centers for Disease Control and Prevention
Atlanta, Georgia

Joseph F. Piecuch, DMD, MD
Clinical Professor
Oral and Maxillofacial Surgery Department
University of Connecticut
Farmington, Connecticut
Director
Oral and Maxillofacial Surgery Section
Hartford Hospital
Hartford, Connecticut

Sharon E. Plon, MD
Department of Pediatric Hematology/
    Oncology
Baylor College of Medicine
Houston, Texas

Leslie P. Plotnick, MD
Professor
Department of Pediatrics
Johns Hopkins University School
    of Medicine
Pediatric Endocrinologist
Johns Hopkins Hospital
Baltimore, Maryland

Barbara R. Pober, MD
Associate Professor
Department of Pediatrics
Harvard School of Medicine
Pediatrician, Pediatric Service
Massachusetts General Hospital for
    Children
Boston, Massachusetts

David R. Powell, MD
Vice President and Director
Endocrinology and Metabolism
Lexicon Genetics incorporated
The Woodlands, Texas

Arthur L. Prensky, MD
Professor Emeritus
Department of Neurology
Washington University School of Medicine
Pediatrician and Neurologist
Department of Pediatric Neurology
St. Louis Children's Hospital
St. Louis, Missouri

Charles T. Quinn, MD
Assistant Professor Pediatrics
Department of Pediatrics
University of Texas Southwest Medical
    Center
Center for Cancer and Blood Disorders
Children's Medical Center, Dallas
Dallas, Texas

Leonard A. Rappaport, MD, MS
Mary Deming Scott Associate Professor
Chief, Division of General Pediatrics
Department of Pediatrics
Harvard Medical School
Director-Developmental Medicine Center
Department of Medicine
Boston Children's Hospital
Boston, Massachusetts

William V. Raszka, Jr., MD
Associate Professor
Department of Pediatrics
University of Vermont College of Medicine
Director, Pediatrics Infectious Disease
    Service
Vermont Children's Hospital
Burlington, Vermont

Robert M. Reece, MD
Clinical Professor of Pediatrics
Tufts University School of Medicine
Department of Pediatrics
Tufts University School of Medicine
Director, Child Protection Program
Department of Pediatrics
Turfs-New England Medical Center
Boston, Massachusetts

Tyler Reimschisel, MD
Post-doctoral Fellow
McKusisk-Nathans Institute
    of Genetic Medicine
Johns Hopkins Hospital
Baltimore, Maryland

Regina M. Reynolds, MD
Fellow, Neonatal-Perinatal Medicine
Department of Pediatrics
University of Colorado Health
    Sciences Center
The Children's Hospital of Denver
Denver, Colorado

Donald A. Riopel, MD
Clinical Professor of Pediatrics
Department of Pediatrics
University of North Carolina at Chapel Hill
    School of Medicine
Chapel Hill, North Carolina
Pediatric Cardiologist
Department of Pediatrics
Carolinas Medical Center
Charlotte, North Carolina

Sharon B. Richter, DO, FAAP
Director, Division of Developmental and
    Behavioral Pediatrics
Department of Pediatrics
The Children's Hospital at Sinai
Baltimore, Maryland

Kenneth B. Roberts, MD
Professor of Pediatrics
Department of Pediatrics
University of North Carolina School
    of Medicine
Chapel Hill, North Carolina
Director, Pediatric Teaching Program
Moses Cone Health System
Greensboro, North Carolina

George C. Rodgers Jr., MD, PhD
Professor of Pediatrics and Pharmacology/
    Toxicology
Departments of Pediatrics and
    Pharmacology/Toxicology
University of Louisville
Louisville, Kentucky

Nathan Rodgers, M.H.A.
Universidad Autonoma de Guadalajara
Guadalajara, Jalisco, Mexico

Carol L. Rosen, MD
Professor
Department of Pediatrics
Case University School of Medicine
Medical Director, Pediatric Sleep Services
Department of Pediatrics
Rainbow Babies and Children's Hospital
Cleveland, Ohio

Adam A. Rosenberg, MD
Professor of Pediatrics
Department of Pediatrics
University of Colorado School of Medicine
Director of Newborn Services
Department of Pediatrics
University of Colorado Hospital
The Children's Hospital
Denver, Colorado

Beryl J. Rosenstein, MD
Professor
Department of Pediatrics
Johns Hopkins University School
    of Medicine
Attending Physician
Cystic Fibrosis Center
Johns Hopkins Hospital
Baltimore, Maryland

N. Paul Rosman, MD
Professor of Pediatrics and Neurology
Departments of Pediatrics and Neurology
Boston University School of Medicine
Pediatric Neurologist
Departments of Pediatrics and Neurology
Boston Medical Center
Boston, Massachusetts

David R. Roth, MD
Professor
Departments of Urology and Pediatrics
Baylor College of Medicine
Texas Children's Hospital
Houston, Texas

Guillermo M. Ruiz-Palacios, MD
Professor and Head
Department of Infectious Diseases
National Institute of Medical Science
    and Nutrition
Infectious Diseases Department
Mexico City, Mexico

Heidi V. Russell, MD
Associate Professor
Department of Pediatrics Hematology/
    Oncology
Baylor College of Medicine
Hematology and Oncology
Texas Children's Hospital/Texas Children's
    Cancer Center
Houston, Texas

Hugh A. Sampson, MD
Professor of Pediatrics & Immunobiology
Department of Pediatrics
Mount Sinai School of Medicine
Staff Physician
Mount Sinai Hospital
New York, New York

Pablo J. Sánchez, MD
Professor of Pediatrics
Department of Pediatrics
Divisions of Neonatal-Perinatal Medicine
    and Pediatric Infectious Diseases
University of Texas Southwestern Medical
    Center
Parkland Memorial Hospital
Children's Medical Center
Dallas, Texas

Nina Sand-Loud, MD
Assistant Professor
Department of Pediatrics
NEOUCOM
Neurodevelopmental Center
Akron Children's Hospital
Akron, Ohio

Mathuram Santosham, MD, MPH
Professor
Department of International Health
Johns Hopkins University
Department of Pediatrics
Johns Hopkins Hospital
Baltimore, Maryland

Bradley L. Schlaggar, MD, PhD
Assistant Professor
Departments of Neurology, Radiology,
    Anatomy and Neurobiology
Washington University School of Medicine
St. Louis Children's Hospital
St. Louis, Misouri

Alison D. Schonwald, MD
Instructor in Pediatrics
Department of General Pediatrics
Harvard Medical School
Assistant in Medicine
Department of Medicine
Boston Children's Hospital
Boston, Massachusetts

Kenneth C. Schuberth, MD
Associate Professor
Department of Pediatrics
Johns Hopkins University School
    of Medicine
Baltimore, Maryland

Heidi Schwarzwald, MD, MPH
Assistant Professor
Department of Pediatrics
Baylor College of Medicine
Section of Retrovirology
Texas Children's Hospital
Houston, Texas

Paula J. Schweich, MD
Clinical Associate Professor
Department of Pediatrics
University of Washington
Attending Physician
Emergency Department
Mary Bridge Children's Hospital
Tacoma, Washington

David T. Scott, PhD
Associate Professor
Department of Psychiatry and Behavioral
    Sciences
University of Washington School of
    Medicine
Chief Psychologist, Clinical Training Unit
Center on Human Development and
    Disability
University of Washington Medical Center
Seattle, Washington

John H. Seashore, MD
Professor of Surgery and Pediatrics
Department of Surgery
Yale University School of Medicine
New Haven, Connecticut

Paul N. Severin, MD, FAAP
Assistant Professor
Department of Pediatrics, Section of
    Pediatric Critical Care Medicine
Rush University Medical Center
Attending Physician
Department of Pediatrics
John H. Stroger, Jr. Hospital of Cook
    County
Chicago, Illinois

Nadeem I. Shafi, MD, BA
Clinical Fellow
Department of Pediatrics, Critical Care
Baylor College of Medicine
Texas Children's Hospital
Houston, Texas

Snehal N. Shah, MD
Epidemic Intelligence Service Officer
Malaria Branch
National Center for Infectious Diseases
Centers for Disease Control and Prevention
Atlanta, Georgia

Bruce K. Shapiro, MD
Associate Professor
Department of Pediatrics
Johns Hopkins University School of Medicine
The Arnold J. Capute Chair in
    Neurodevelopmental Disabilities
Kennedy Krieger Institute
Baltimore, Maryland

William T. Shearer, MD, PhD
Professor
Department of Pediatrics and Immunology
Baylor College of Medicine
Chief, Allergy and Immunology Service
Texas Children's Hospital
Houston, Texas

Ziad M. Shehab, MD
Professor of Clinical Pediatrics
Department of Pediatrics
University of Arizona
Head, Section of Pediatric Infectious Diseases
Department of Pediatrics
University Medical Center
Tucson, Arizona

Rita D. Sheth, MD
Assistant Professor
Department of Pediatrics
Baylor College of Medicine
Attending Physician
Renal Section
Texas Children's Hospital
Houston, Texas

Tracy Shevell
Fellow
Obstetrics and Gynecology
Columbia University, College of Physicians
    & Surgeons
New York Presbyterian Hospital
New York, New York

Robert J. Shulman, MD
Professor
Department of Pediatrics
Baylor College of Medicine
Director, Nutrition Support Team
Texas Children's Hospital
Houston, Texas

Jane D. Siegel, MD
Professor of Pediatrics
University of Texas Southwestern
    Medical Center at Dallas
Attending Physician and Infection Contro
Children's Medical Center of Dallas
Dallas, Texas

Michael J. Silka, MD
Professor of Pediatrics
Keck School of Medicine
The University of Southern California
Chief, Division of Cardiology
Children's Hospital Los Angeles
Los Angeles, California

Richard H. Sills, MD
Professor of Pediatrics
Department of Pediatrics
Albany Medical College
Director, Pediatric Hematology/Oncology
Albany Medical Center
Albany, New York

F. Estelle R. Simons, BSc, MD, FRCPC
Professor
Department of Pediatrics & Child Health
University of Manitoba
Health Sciences Centre—Children's
    Hospital
Winnipeg, Manitoba, Canada

Frank R. Sinatra, MD
Professor of Pediatrics
Keck School of Medicine of the University
    of Southern California
Director, Pediatric Gastroenterology
Women's and Children's Hospital at
    Los Angeles County-USC Medical Center
Los Angeles, California

Timothy C. Slesnick, MD
Pediatric Cardiology Fellow
Department of Pediatrics
Baylor College of Medicine
Department of Pediatric Cardiology
Texas Children's Hospital
Houston, Texas

C. Wayne Smith, MD
Professor
Department of Pediatrics
Baylor College of Medicine
Houston, Texas

Michael B. Smith, MD
Associate Professor
Department of Pathology
University of Texas
Director, Division of Clinical
    Microbiology
Department of Pathology
University of Texas Medical Branch
Galveston, Texas

Richard J. H. Smith, MD
Sterba Hearing Research Professor
Department of Otolaryngology—Head and
    Neck Surgery
University of Iowa College of Medicine
Department of Otolaryngology—Head and
    Neck Surgery
Iowa City, Iowa

Marianna M. Sockrider, MD, DrPH
Associate Professor of Pediatrics
Department of Pediatrics
Baylor College of Medicine
Medical Staff
Pulmonary Medicine Service
Texas Children's Hospital
Houston, Texas

Michael J. G. Somers, MD
Assistant Professor of Pediatrics
Department of Pediatrics
Harvard Medical School
Director of Clinical Services
Division of Nephrology
Children's Hospital
Boston, Massachusetts

Alexandra C. Spadola, MD
Clinical Fellow
Departments of Obstetrics and Gynecology
Columbia University Medical Center
Department of Obstetrics and Gynecology
Morgan Stanley Children's Hospital
New York Presbyterian Hospital
New York, New York

Paul D. Sponseller, MD, MBA
Professor
Department of Orthopedics
Johns Hopkins Medical School
Head, Division of Pediatric Orthopedics
Johns Hopkins Hospital
Baltimore, Maryland

Jeffrey R. Starke, MD
Professor
Department of Pediatrics
Baylor College of Medicine
Chief, Department of Pediatrics
Bed Taub General Hospital
Houston, Texas

Barbara W. Stechenberg, MD
Professor
Department of Pediatrics
Tufts University School of Medicine
Boston, Massachusetts
Director
Pediatric Infectious Diseases
Baystate Medical Center Children's Hospital
Springfield, Massachusetts

Fernando Stein, MD
Associate Professor of Pediatrics
Department of Pediatrics
Baylor College of Medicine
Medical Director
Progressive Care
Texas Children's Hospital
Houston, Texas

C. Philip Steuber, MD
Professor
Department of Pediatrics, Hematology/
  Oncology
Baylor College of Medicine
Director, Leukemia/Lymphoma Team
Hematology-Oncology
Texas Children's Hospital
Houston, Texas

Jeffrey R. Stokes, MD
Assistant Professor
Department of Medicine
Creighton University School of Medicine
Omaha, Nebraska

Stephanie H. Stovall, MD
Fellow, Pediatric Infectious Diseases
Department of Pediatrics
University of Tennessee Health Sciences
  Center
St. Jude Children's Research Hospital
LeBonheur Children's Medical Center
Memphis, Tennessee

Janette F. Strasburger, MD
Professor of Pediatrics
Department of Pediatrics
Medical College of Wisconsin
Director of Cardiology
Children's Hospital of Wisconsin—Fox
  Valley
Milwaukee, Wisconsin

Douglas R. Strother, MD
Associate Professor
Departments of Oncology and Pediatrics
University of Calgary
Alberta Children's Hospital
Calgary, Alberta, Canada

Raymond Sturner, MD
Department of Pediatrics
Johns Hopkins University School
  of Medicine
Johns Hopkins Hospital
Baltimore, Maryland

Jason T. Su, DO
Assistant Professor in Pediatric Cardiology
University of Utah
Primary Children's Medical Center
Salt Lake City, Utah

Gina S. Sucato, MD
Assistant Professor
Department of Pediatrics
University of Pittsburgh
Attending Physician
Department of Pediatrics
Children's Hospital of Pittsburgh
Pittsburgh, Pennsylvania

Frederick J. Suchy, MD
Herbert H. Lehman Professor of Pediatrics
  and Chair
Department of Pediatrics
Mount Siani School of Medicine
New York, New York

John L. Sullivan, MD
Professor of Pediatrics and Molecular
  Medicine
University of Massachusetts Medical School
Department of Pediatrics
University of Massachusetts Memorial
  Health Care
Worcester, Massachusetts

Robert P. Sundel, MD
Associate Professor
Department of Pediatrics
Harvard Medical School
Director of Rheumatology
Department of Pediatrics
Children's Hospital
Boston, Massachusetts

Clifford M. Takemoto, MD
Assistant Professor
Department of Pediatrics
Johns Hopkins University School
  of Medicine
Assistant Professor
Department of Pediatrics
Johns Hopkins Hospital
Baltimore, Maryland

Norman S. Talner, MD
Clinical Professor of Pediatrics
Department of Pediatrics
Duke University School of Medicine
Durham, North Carolina

Herbert B. Tanowitz, MD
Professor
Departments of Pathology and Medicine
Albert Einstein College of Medicine
Attending Physician
Department of Medicine
Weiler Hospital, Montefiore Medical Center
  and Jacobi Medical Center
Bronx, New York

Jonathan E. Teitelbaum, MD
Assistant Professor
Department of Pediatrics
Drexel University School of Medicine
Philadelphia, Pennsylvania
Director
Pediatric Gastroenterology and Nutrition
Monmouth Medical Center
Long Branch, New Jersey

Elizabeth H. Thilo, MD, FAAP
Associate Professor
Department of Pediatrics
University of Colorado School of Medicine
The Children's Hospital
Department of Neonatology
Denver, Colorado

Dan W. Thomas, MD
Associate Professor
Department of Pediatrics
Keck School of Medicine, University of
  Southern California
Head, Division of Gastroenterology
  and Nutrition
Department of Pediatrics
Children's Hospital Los Angeles
Los Angeles, California

Richard G. Topazian, DDS
Professor Emeritus, Oral and Maxillofacial
  Surgery
Professor of Surgery
Department of Oral and Maxillofacial
  Surgery
University of Connecticut, School of Dental
  Medicine
University of Connecticut Health Center
Farmington, Connecticut

Robert J. Touloukian, MD
Professor of Surgery and Pediatrics
Section of Pediatric Surgery
Yale University School of Medicine
Pediatric Surgeon
Department of Surgery
Yale-New Haven Children's Hospital
New Haven, Connecticut

Jeffrey A. Towbin, MD
Professor
Department of Pediatrics
Baylor College of Medicine
Chief of Pediatric Cardiology
Department of Pediatrics
Texas Children's Hospital
Houston, Texas

Elias A. Traboulsi, MD
Professor of Ophthalmology and Pediatrics
Cleveland Clinic, Lerner College of Medicine
Head, Department of Pediatric
  Ophthalmology and Strabismus
Cleveland Clinic Foundation
Cleveland, Ohio

Maria Trent, MD
Assistant Professor of Pediatrics
Department of Pediatrics
Johns Hopkins School of Medicine
Attending Physician
Department of Pediatrics
Johns Hopkins Hospital
Baltimore, Maryland

Theodore F. Tsai, MD, MPH
Senior Director
Global Medical Affairs
Wyeth Research
Collegeville, Pennsylvania

Walter W. Tunnessen, Jr., MD (Deceased)
Children's Hospital of Philadelphia
Philadelphia, Pennsylvania

Jon E. Tyson, MD, MPH
Director, Center for Clinical Research and
    Evidence Based Medicine
Professor of Pediatrics, Obstetrics and
    Internal Medicine
The University of Texas Medical School
Houston, Texas

Ricardo Uauy, MD, PhD
Full Professor
INTA, University of Chile
Santiago, Chile

Anne Marie Valente, MD
Fellow in Cardiology
Departments of Internal Medicine
    and Pediatrics
Duke University School of Medicine
Durham, North Carolina

Jack van Hoff, MD
Associate Professor
Department of Pediatrics
Yale University School of Medicine
Attending Physician
Department of Pediatrics
Yale-New Haven Children's Hospital
New Haven, Connecticut

John A. Vanchiere, MD, PhD
Assistant Professor
Department of Pediatrics, Section of
    Infectious Diseases
Baylor College of Medicine
Houston, Texas

Jon A. Vanderhoof, MD
Professor
Department of Pediatrics
University of Nebraska Medical Center
Omaha, Nebraska

Thomas A. Vargo, MD
Professor
Department of Pediatrics
Baylor College of Medicine
Associate in Cardiology
Department of Cardiology
Texas Children's Hospital
Houston, Texas

Charles P. Venditti, MD, PhD
Staff Clinician
National Human Genome Research Institute
Attending Physician
Mark O. Hatfield Clinical Research Center
National Institutes of Health
Bethesda, Maryland

James Versalovic, MD, PhD, FCAP
Assistant Professor of Pathology
Department of Pathology
Baylor College of Medicine
Director of Microbiology Laboratories
Department of Pathology
Texas Children's Hospital
Houston, Texas

G. Wesley Vick, III, MD, PhD
Associate Professor
Sections of Cardiology and Atherosclerosis
Departments of Pediatrics and Medicine
Baylor College of Medicine
Associate
Department of Pediatric Cardiology
Texas Children's Hospital
Houston, Texas

Ellen R. Wald, MD
Professor and Chair
Department of Pediatrics
University of Wisconsin-Madison
Chief, Department of Pediatrics
University of Wisconsin Children's Hospital
Madison, Wisconsin

W. Allan Walker, MD
Director, Division of Nutrition
Harvard Medical School
Boston, Massachusetts

David S. Walton, MD
Clinical Professor of Ophthalmology
Department of Ophthalmology
Harvard Medical School
Surgeon
Department of Ophthalmology
Massachusetts Eye and Ear Infirmary
Boston, Massachusetts

Rebecca S. Wappner, MD
Professor of Pediatrics
Professor of Medical and Molecular
    Genetics
Director, Pediatric Metabolism and Genetics
Indiana University School of Medicine
The James Whitcomb Riley Hospital
    for Children
Indianapolis, Indiana

Kent E. Ward, MD
Associate Professor of Pediatrics
Department of Pediatrics
University of Oklahoma Health Science
    Center
Attending Physician
Department of Pediatrics
Children's Hospital at Oklahoma University
    Medical Center
Oklahoma City, Oklahoma

Mark A. Ward, MD
Assistant Professor
Department of Pediatrics
Baylor College of Medicine
Houston, Texas

Joseph B. Warshaw, MD (Deceased)
Dean
University of Vermont College
    of Medicine
Burlington, Vermont

David D. Weaver, MD, MS
Professor
Department of Medical and Molecular
    Genetics
Indiana University School of Medicine
Indianapolis, Indiana

Thomas R. Welch, MD
Professor of Medical and
    Molecular Genetics
Division of Nephrology and Hypertension
Children's Hospital Medical Center
Cincinnati, Ohio

Steven L. Werlin, MD
Professor
Department of Pediatric Gastroenterology
Medical College of Wisconsin
Pediatric Gastroenterology
Children's Hospital of Wisconsin
Milwaukee, Wisconsin

David E. Wesson, MD
Professor of Surgery
Department of Surgery
Baylor College of Medicine
Chief, Pediatric Surgery
Department of Surgery
Texas Children's Hospital
Houston, Texas

Patricia G. Wheeler, MD
Assistant Professor
Department of Pediatrics
Tufts University School of Medicine
Attending Geneticist
Department of Pediatrics
Tufts-New England Medical Center,
    Floating Hospital for Children
Boston, Massachusetts

Bernhard L. Wiedermann, MD
Associate Professor and Vice Chair
    for Education
Department of Pediatrics
The George Washington University School
    of Medicine and Health Sciences
Director, Medical Education and Attending
    in Infectious Diseases
Children's National Medical Center
Washington, District of Columbia

James A. Wilde, MD, FAAP
Associate Professor
Departments of Emergency Medicine &
    Pediatrics
Director, Pediatric Emergency Medicine
Medical College of Georgia
Augusta, Georgia

Modena Hoover Wilson, MD, MPH
Director, Department of Committees and
    Sections
American Academy of Pediatrics
Elk Grove Village, Illinois

Jerry A. Winkelstein, MD
Professor of Pediatrics, Medicine and
    Pathology
Department of Pediatrics
Johns Hopkins University School of
    Medicine
Baltimore, Maryland

Scott D. Wissman, MD, MPH
International Pediatrics, P.A.
Private Practice
Rockville, Maryland

Lawrence S. Wissow, MD, MPH
Professor
Department of Health Behavior and Society
Johns Hopkins Bloomberg School of
    Hygiene and Public Health
Associate Staff
Division of Child Psychiatry
Johns Hopkins Hospital
Baltimore, Maryland

Murray Wittner, MD, PhD
Professor of Pathology and
    Parasitology
Department of Pathology
Albert Einstein College of
    Medicine
Director, Parasitology and Tropical
    Medicine Clinic
Attending Physician
Jacobi Medical
Bronx, New York

Patricia Woo, CBE
Professor of Pediatrics
    Rheumatology
Immunology and Molecular
    Pathology
University College of London
Consultant Physician
Department of Rheumatology
Great Ormond Street Hospital
    for Sick Children
    NHS Trust
London, United Kingdom

Charles R. Woods, Jr., MD, MS
Associate Professor of Pediatrics
Department of Pediatrics
Wake Forest University School of
    Medicine
Brenner Children's Hospital
Winston-Salem, North Carolina

Michael J. Wright, MB, ChB, MSc
Professor of Dentistry
Department of Pediatric Dentistry
University of North Carolina at
    Chapel Hill School of
    Dentistry
Chapel Hill, North
    Carolina

Robert H. Yoken, MD
Theodore and Vada Stanley Professor
    of Pediatrics
Johns Hopkins University School
    of Medicine
Director, Stanley Division of
    Develpmental Neurovirology
Johns Hopkins Hospital
Baltimore, Maryland

Richard S. K. Young, MD, MPH
Associate Clinical Professor of Pediatrics
    and Neurology
Departments of Pediatrics and Neurology
Yale University School of Medicine
Neurologist
Department of Pediatrics
Hospital of St. Raphael
New Haven, Connecticut

Joseph H. Zelson, MD
Clinical Professor of Pediatric
Yale University School of Medicine
New Haven, Connecticut

Lori P. Zink, MD, FAAP
Clinical Assistant Professor
Department of Family and Community
    Medicine
University of New Mexico School
    of Medicine
Albuquerque, New Mexico
Active Staff Pediatrician
Department of Pediatrics
Carlsbad Medical Center
Carlsbad, New Mexico

■ CONTENTS

SECTION II ■ DISEASES OF THE RESPIRATORY TRACT

SECTION III ■ DISEASES OF THE CARDIOVASCULAR SYSTEM

SECTION IX ■ INBORN ERRORS OF METABOLISM

SECTION X ■ DISEASES OF THE NERVOUS SYSTEM

APPENDICES ■ PEDIATRICIANS COMPANION: THINGS YOU FORGET TO REMEMBER

CHAPTER 1 ■ THE HISTORY OF PEDIATRICS IN AMERICA

HOWARD A. PEARSON

Pediatrics, or at least the medical care of infants and children, began in America shortly after the founding of the English colonies in the early seventeenth century. In 1677, Rev. Thomas Thacher of Boston, a pastor and part-time physician, wrote the first medical publication of the English colonies, a broadside on smallpox. In 1721, Dr. Zabdiel Boylston, working with Cotton Mather, the great Massachusetts Puritan preacher, introduced variolization (inoculating his own son as well as others) to abort a smallpox epidemic in Boston. John Winthrop, Jr., governor of Connecticut from 1657 to 1675, conducted an extensive medical practice through the colonial mails. The lack of physicians and Winthrop's willingness to prescribe free of charge led to his being consulted frequently. Winthrop's medical letters described a wide range of pediatric problems, such as rashes, jaundice, seizures, and diarrhea, and one of the letters contains a description of child abuse.

Colonial physicians, often uneducated, poorly trained practitioners, wielded a variety of ineffective herbal remedies and anecdotal treatments against the formidable assaults of disease and death. These were perilous times for children. As Dr. Ernest Caulfield, an important American pediatric historian, wrote:

> In addition to diphtheria, dysentery, measles, and scarlet fever, smallpox, influenza, and tuberculosis should certainly be included in the list of common diseases of colonial children. A surprisingly large proportion of them had worms. Deaths from falls, burns, and poisonings were frequent. It seems a little surprising that any of them survived.

Some early American physicians were careful observers and recorders. Dr. Hezikiah Beardsley, writing in the *Cases and Observations by the Medical Society of New Haven County* in 1788, described the clinical course and autopsy findings of a child with a "scirrhus" of the pylorus. In 1903, this early report was rediscovered by Sir William Osler, who said that Beardsley had described the disease of hypertrophic pyloric stenosis

clearly and accurately. Early American universities and colleges emphasized classical and theological curricula; training in secular subjects, such as medicine, came later. The first American medical schools were the University of Pennsylvania in Philadelphia, founded in 1765; King's College of Medicine, established in New York in 1768, which became the College of Physicians and Surgeons in 1814; Harvard, established in Boston in 1783; and Dartmouth, in Hanover, New Hampshire, founded in 1798 by Dr. Nathan Smith, a Harvard graduate who became Dartmouth's one-man faculty.

Teaching about the diseases of children was done sporadically, if at all, and then under the aegis of physic (medicine) or midwifery (obstetrics). At the University of Pennsylvania, Dr. Benjamin Rush, a preeminent American patriot-physician and a signer of the Declaration of Independence, was a professor of medicine between 1789 and 1813. Rush was the most influential American physician of his day. Rush's medical teaching included lectures on "Diseases peculiar to children." He wrote articles describing pediatric diseases, including spasmodic asthma, diseases of the mind, and diphtheria. Rush also coined the term *cholera infantum* for the lethal summer diarrhea that killed thousands of American children well into the middle of the twentieth century.

In 1825, Dr. William Potts Dewees, a professor of midwifery at the University of Pennsylvania, published his *Treatise on the Physical and Medical Treatment of Children*. This text had eight subsequent re-editions and was arguably the first American textbook of pediatrics. The first formal medical school course and the first faculty appointment in the diseases of children in the United States were at Yale College in Connecticut. For nearly 40 years, between 1813 and 1852, Dr. Eli Ives lectured on the diseases of children to an estimated 1,500 Yale medical students. His motivation for teaching this subject was because "diseases and remedies of the infantile state [are] a subject that has received little attention from Enlightened

Physicians. . . . The difficulty of acquiring a knowledge of disease in infants results from their inability to communicate their sensations by language."

Ives' course, recorded by hand in student notebooks, consisted of lectures on subjects ranging from angina to worms. Ives ascribed many medical illnesses to offending substances in the gastrointestinal tract, which had to be removed by inducing vomiting or by purging. Accordingly, Ives' therapeutic anchors were calomel (mercury) and ipecac, plus a variety of herbal remedies. According to Ives, teething either caused or aggravated many diseases of infants, and lancing of the gums was considered essential.

During the latter half of the nineteenth century, American pediatrics began to take on a more defined presence. Children's hospitals were established, some evolving from asylums and foundling homes. The first American children's hospitals were the New York Nursing and Child Hospital, which opened in 1854; the Children's Hospital of Philadelphia, which opened in 1855; and the Boston Children's Hospital, which opened in 1869.

Pediatric progress was most evident in New York City, where Drs. Abraham Jacobi and Job Lewis Smith were contemporaries in the second half of the nineteenth century. Jacobi received his medical training at the University of Bonn, Germany. Imprisoned for 2 years as a suspected revolutionary, he emigrated to New York in 1853. In 1860, he established a children's clinic at the New York Medical College, where he was appointed Professor of Infantile Pathology and Therapeutics. He later became Professor of Pediatrics at Columbia's College of Physicians and Surgeons. Among Jacobi's many contributions were his founding of the Section of Pediatrics of the American Medical Association (AMA) in 1880, and his selection as the first president of the American Pediatric Society (APS) in 1888. He established pediatric services in several New York hospitals and effectively championed causes that promoted the welfare of children. In 1896, he wrote an important textbook, *Therapeutics of Infancy and Childhood*. His drive and enthusiasm were instrumental in establishing pediatrics as a separate discipline in the United States.

Job Lewis Smith, who entered practice in Manhattan at about the same time as Jacobi, also played a major role in early American pediatrics. Smith worked primarily at the Bellevue Medical School, where he was appointed Clinical Professor of Morbid Anatomy in 1861 and Clinical Professor of Diseases of Children in 1876. Smith was a prolific writer, publishing papers on infectious diseases, rickets, and neonatal tetanus.

Between 1869 and 1896, Smith published eight editions of his *A Treatise on the Diseases of Infancy and Childhood*. One of Smith's signal accomplishments was the founding of the APS: In 1887, Smith invited a group of pediatricians to join him in establishing the APS, a goal that was achieved in the following year. Forty-three American physicians were elected as "Founders." For more than 50 years, the APS was the preeminent pediatric organization in the United States. The presentations and discussions that took place at the annual meetings, as recorded in the *Society Transactions,* documented striking progress and advances in the specialty. Smith was very concerned about the dangers of bottle feeding and vigorously promoted milk sterilization. The appalling consequences of the hand (artificial) feeding of foundlings in New York were described poignantly by Smith at the 1889 meeting of the APS: "The steamboat every morning brought foundlings to the (Randall's) Island and every afternoon removed an equal number for burial in Potters' Field."

The availability of safe, pure milk for infant feeding was an overriding concern of pediatricians in the United States. Breastfeeding was advocated strongly, and some foundling hospitals employed wet-nurses. However, the large numbers of abandoned and orphaned infants necessitated cow's milk feeding.

In American cities, much of the milk supply was contaminated and adulterated. Between 1870 and 1920, the need for safe milk for infant feeding became a crusade for the leaders of American pediatrics, and the campaign for safe milk was the first concerted involvement of pediatricians in issues of social welfare and reform.

Nutritional diseases were prevalent among American children in the last decades of the nineteenth century. In 1898, the APS conducted a national survey on the cause of scurvy, the first national study of a pediatric disease. Clinical and dietary information was collected on nearly 400 cases of scurvy. The study concluded that scurvy was probably caused by the extensive use of artificial foods for infants. Although the curative value of orange or lime juice had been described by James Lind in 1757, most American pediatricians did not accept scurvy as a simple dietary deficiency. In 1928, Dr. Albert Szent-Györgyi isolated hexuronic acid which, in 1932, was identified by biochemists Waugh and King as the antiscorbutic factor, vitamin C.

At the turn of the twentieth century, rickets was epidemic in American children, particularly those living in the northeastern cities, where as many as two-thirds of infants were rachitic. An investigative team at Johns Hopkins, Drs. John Howland, Benjamin Kramer, Edwards Park, and Elmer V. McCollum developed those micro-methods for the measurement of phosphate and calcium that defined the biochemical profile of rickets. They developed a rat model of human rickets in which they demonstrated the antirachitic properties of cod liver oil. In 1923, vitamin D was identified as the antirachitic factor in cod liver oil. In 1936, Dr. Philip Jeans persuaded the Committee on Foods of the AMA to recommend the fortification of milk, including evaporated and dried milks, with vitamin D. This was nationally implemented, and rickets was rapidly transformed from a common chronic disease of childhood to a rare one in the United States. Application of the principles of the burgeoning science of bacteriology to infant nutrition in the early twentieth century provided a scientific basis for safe infant feeding. Gastroenteritis was a major contributor to high infant mortality at this time; that the pasteurization of milk could prevent milk-transmitted diseases was appreciated by about 1895. However, some practitioners opposed pasteurization because they believed that heating of milk made it indigestible. It was not until 1908 that Chicago became the first American city to mandate the pasteurization of milk. Soon, pasteurization became nearly universal, and the lives of tens of thousands of children were saved.

In Boston, pediatrics was taught at Harvard Medical School as early as 1871. In 1893, Dr. Thomas Morgan Rotch was appointed Professor of the Diseases of Children. Rotch is remembered best for his textbook *Pediatrics*, published in 1895, and for his "percentage method" of infant feeding. This system was based upon the concept that cow's milk was relatively indigestible and, therefore, had to be diluted. Because dilution reduced fat and carbohydrate content, cream and sugar were added. This logical concept became exquisitely convoluted in Rotch's percentage method, which mandated complex formulations with varying percentages of protein, fat, and carbohydrates, with changes frequently made on a day-to-day basis. (European physicians often wonder why Americans call milk mixtures for infant-feeding *formulas*; the nomenclature derives from the formulas of Dr. Rotch.)

The Rotch system required "almost the equivalence of an advanced degree in higher mathematics employing algebraic equations to compute the food mixture of a baby." This system ultimately collapsed under its own complexity. As Oliver Wendell Holmes quipped, "A pair of substantial mammary glands has the advantage over the two hemispheres of the most learned professor's brain in the art of compounding a nutritious fluid for infants." Jacobi is said to have commented to Rotch at a meeting of the APS, "You can't feed babies with mathematics; you must feed them with brains."

By the end of the first decade of the twentieth century, physicians in the United States developed and employed much more simplified feeding techniques based on the changing caloric needs of growing infants (calorimetric method). The increasing availability of evaporated milk, and later of commercially prepared infant feeding mixtures, reduced the complexities of feeding infants who were not breast-fed. A decreased emphasis on the technicalities of infant feeding resulted in the elimination of the term "baby feeders" to describe pediatricians.

Infectious disease was the other major concern of pediatricians during this era. Diphtheria, scarlet fever, measles, whooping cough, and infant diarrhea were endemic. Diphtheria was particularly lethal because of the laryngeal obstruction caused by the diphtheritic pseudomembrane. Tracheotomy was associated with considerable morbidity and mortality. Dr. Joseph O'Dwyer, a physician at the New York Foundling Hospital, developed a device for laryngeal intubation—the O'Dwyer tube—that reduced the mortality of laryngeal diphtheria from virtually 100% to only 75%. (Intubation became largely unnecessary after the introduction of diphtheria antitoxin.) The discovery of diphtheria antitoxin in 1890 by Dr. Emil von Behring provided the first effective therapy, and von Behring received the first Nobel Prize in Medicine in 1901 for his discovery. Large collaborative studies of the treatment of diphtheria were conducted by the APS in 1896 and 1897, analyzing the records of nearly 6,000 cases of diphtheria. These studies showed that antitoxin treatment decreased the mortality of diphtheria from 27% to 7%. The incidence of diphtheria was subsequently further reduced by active immunization, first with toxin-antitoxin mixtures and, after 1920, with diphtheria toxoid. An intradermal test to determine susceptibility was introduced by Dr. Bela Schick.

Infant diarrhea, or the "summer complaint" (the *cholera infantum* described by Benjamin Rush) was epidemic in American cities well into the twentieth century. It had a distressingly high mortality. Therapy, as summarized by Dr. Grover Powers, was largely symptomatic: "tea, barley water, protein milk, floating hospitals, or country sanatoria."

The Boston Floating Hospital had its origin in 1894, when a rented barge was loaded with hundreds of mothers and infants and towed around Boston harbor for a day. It was believed that sick infants would benefit from a day of clean salt air and cool ocean breezes.

Major advances in the management of fluid and electrolyte disorders of childhood occurred during the first half of the twentieth century. These advances were made possible by the investigations of Drs. L. Emmett Holt Sr., James L. Gamble, Daniel C. Darrow, Allan M. Butler, William McKim Marriot, Alexis Hartman, and Oscar Schloss, among others. The effective treatment of dehydration and electrolyte imbalance greatly reduced the morbidity and mortality of childhood gastroenteritis.

Dr. L. Emmett Holt, Sr. of New York is credited with establishing a scientific basis for pediatrics in the United States. Holt, a 1878 graduate of the College of Physicians and Surgeons, entered private practice in midtown Manhattan and worked in the New York Foundling Hospital. In 1889, he became the medical director of the New York Babies Hospital, which was in danger of closing. Holt's efforts culminated in the opening of a new Babies Hospital in 1910. In addition to outpatient facilities and 70 inpatient beds, the Hospital also had dedicated research laboratories, and Holt appointed experienced chemists to the hospital staff. Holt also played a major role in the founding of the Rockefeller Institute, and he worked with Rockefeller scientists publishing collaborative papers dealing with the chemical analysis of milk and milk proteins, salt and water balance, and the absorption of nutrients and electrolytes

in diarrheal diseases. One of his greatest accomplishments was the authorship of a classic pediatric textbook, *The Diseases of Infancy and Childhood.* First published in 1897, it had 11 subsequent editions during Holt's lifetime (and had its twenty-first re-edition as *Rudolph's Pediatrics* in 2003). It was the standard pediatric textbook of its day, and it was considered the equal of Sir William Osler's monumental *Textbook of Internal Medicine.* Even more widely read than his textbook was Holt's *The Care and Feeding of Children,* a widely distributed and influential manual written for parents.

Dr. John Howland, one of the greatest figures of pediatrics in the United States, graduated from the Cornell Medical School, studied in Europe, and worked with Holt in New York. He assumed the position of professor and full-time head of the pediatric department at Johns Hopkins in 1912. Over the next 14 years, he built and directed the first scientifically based, full-time pediatric department in the United States. The Harriet Lane Home, a Hopkins-affiliated children's hospital, opened in 1912. Because Howland recognized the importance of biochemical investigations of the diseases of children, he ensured that the Harriet Lane Home contained well-equipped biochemistry laboratories and a staff of full-time pediatricians. He and a group of talented clinician-investigators published classic studies on acidosis, fluid and electrolyte balance, rickets, and tetany. Howland's trainees became leaders in U.S. pediatrics for half a century. These notables included Drs. Edwards Park, Kenneth Blackfan, Grover Powers, William McKim Marriott, James Gamble, Ethel C. Dunham, Alfred Shohl, Wilburt C. Davison, Samuel Clausen, Horton Caspairo, Benjamin Kramer, and others. These pediatricians became teachers, investigators, and leaders in medical schools around the country. During the first 50 years of the twentieth century, most medical schools established departments of pediatrics that utilized the clinical resources in affiliated teaching hospitals, and freestanding children's hospitals were opened in many American cities.

Edwards A. Park succeeded John Howland at Johns Hopkins. One of his major achievements was the development of pediatric subspecialty programs. Dr. Helen Taussig became one of the first pediatric cardiologists; Lawson Wilkins was the father of pediatric endocrinology.

One of Howland's proteges, Kenneth D. Blackfan, became professor of pediatrics at Harvard and director of the Boston Children's Hospital. Under Blackfan's leadership, James Gamble continued his important research on fluid and electrolyte physiology, Drs. William E. Ladd and Robert Gross were instrumental in the development of pediatric surgery as a specialty, and Dr. Louis K. Diamond established pediatric hematology as a discipline. Diamond conducted lifelong clinical studies of Rh erythroblastosis; during the course of his own career, he was able to document progress from the initial clinical and laboratory definition of the disease to its effective therapy and, ultimately, to its prevention. Dr. Sidney Farber, a pediatric pathologist, pioneered chemotherapy for acute lymphocytic leukemia and other childhood malignancies.

The psychosocial aspects of pediatrics were increasingly recognized and emphasized during the middle of the twentieth century, as exemplified by Dr. Grover F. Powers. Powers trained under John Howland in Baltimore. In 1921, he accompanied Edwards Park to New Haven, where a new department of pediatrics had been established at Yale. When Park returned to Johns Hopkins in 1926, after Howland's death, Powers was appointed Chairman of Pediatrics at Yale—a position he held for 30 years. Among Powers' unique contributions were his clear definition and articulation of the humanistic and social aspects of pediatrics. He wrote and taught about the many problems associated with mental retardation and emotional disorders. His support of Dr. Edith Jackson resulted in the innovative "Rooming In" program at Yale that humanized the birth experience for new mothers and their infants.

Concerns about children's health received governmental attention during the twentieth century. The first White House Conference on the Care of Dependent Children, convened in 1909 by President Theodore Roosevelt, addressed some of the problems of children. The Conference recommended the formation of a federal agency devoted to children. In 1912, President Taft acted on this recommendation to create the Children's Bureau. The Bureau's charge was to "investigate and report upon all matters pertaining to the welfare of children and child life among all classes of our people and especially to investigate the questions of infant mortality, the birth rate, orphanages, juvenile courts, desertion, dangerous occupations, accidents, and diseases of children."

Congress authorized $25,000 for the Children's Bureau (at the same time approving $650,000 for a study of hog cholera). Although the Bureau was given little administrative or enforcement authority to address the high rates of maternal and infant mortality and the unequal access to medical care by poor families, it had an important influence on many issues relating to child health. Between 1909 and 1991, nine presidents convened White House Conferences on children and their health needs. Each conference issued "strong, sweeping, and perceptive reports which ultimately only gathered dust."

In 1921, Congress enacted the Sheppard-Towner Act authorizing the Children's Bureau to become involved in the health problems of infants and children and to provide grants to states for maternal and child health activities. The intent of the Act was approved unanimously by the Pediatric Section of the AMA in 1922. On the same day, the House of Delegates of the AMA passed a resolution condemning the Sheppard-Towner Act as interfering with the private practice of medicine and as an attempt to introduce socialized medicine. When news of the Pediatric Section's action was received by the AMA House of Delegates, the Pediatric Section was reprimanded and a rule was made that sections could not act independently of AMA policy. The action was viewed by many pediatricians as censorship and became the major impetus for the founding, in 1930, of a new pediatric organization independent of the AMA, the American Academy of Pediatrics (AAP). An indication of the growth of pediatrics in the United States can be seen by comparing the 43 pediatricians who were founders of the APS in 1888, with the 304 pediatricians who were charter members of the Academy of Pediatrics in 1930, and the more than 50,000 pediatricians who are members of the AAP in 2005. Much of this growth reflects the redirection of the role of the pediatrician in the United States from primarily an academic specialist and consultant to a primary care provider.

Dr. Isaac Abt of Chicago was the first president of the AAP. In his inaugural address he noted:

> It is our desire to build an association so that every qualified pediatrician could seek membership. It will be necessary for the Academy to interest itself in undergraduate and postgraduate instruction and to exert a regulatory influence over hospitals. As an organization it should assist and lead in public health measures in society reform and in hospital and educational administration as they affect the welfare of children.

In 1932, the *Journal of Pediatrics*, owned and published by the C.V. Mosby Co., was established as the official journal of the AAP. However, by the early 1940s, conflict between the publisher and the AAP led to the withdrawal of AAP support, and the founding of a new AAP journal called *Pediatrics*. The first American journal devoted entirely to pediatrics was the *Archives of Pediatrics*, initially published in 1884. Today, a plethora of general pediatric journals exists, and many more are devoted to pediatric subspecialties.

One of the first actions of the executive committee of the AAP was to set in motion an initiative that led to the founding of the American Board of Pediatrics (ABP) in 1933. Qualifications for board certification included specific training requirements and an examination. Certification by the ABP, which attested to adequate clinical training and competence, was made a requirement for AAP membership. The ABP examinations consisted of both written and oral examinations until 1989, when the oral examinations were discontinued. In 1988, the certification examinations became time limited, and recertification examinations were required every 7 years. The ABP also assumed responsibility for pediatric subspecialty certification.

As pediatric research increased during the 1920s and 1930s, a need was perceived for a research society to complement the APS. This led, in 1931, to the organization of the Society for Pediatric Research (SPR). Requirements for SPR membership were active involvement in pediatric research and age younger than 45 years. The annual joint meetings of the APS and SPR became important forums for reporting advances in pediatrics during much of the twentieth century. In 1967, the APS/SPR initiated their own journal, *Pediatric Research*. In 1960, the APS and SPR were joined by the Ambulatory Pediatric Society (APA). In 1997, the APS, SPR, and APA became formally affiliated as the Pediatric Academic Societies. The Association of Medical School Pediatric Department Chairmen (AMSPDC) was founded in 1967.

During World War II, concern about the health care of the children of American servicemen motivated the U.S. Congress to enact the Emergency Maternal and Infant Care Act (EMIC) in 1953. Dr. Martha Eliot, director of the Children's Bureau, organized and implemented a national program that subsidized and regulated the pediatric care of these children. At the end of the war, major concerns were voiced among some of the leaders of the AAP that Martha Eliot and the Children's Bureau wanted to have the EMIC extended into peace time. This was viewed by some as an attempt to continue and possibly expand the influence of the government on private pediatric practice. A major confrontation between the AAP and the Children's Bureau was avoided when both agreed to collaborate in a major study of pediatric care in the United States, the *Study of Child Health Services and Pediatric Education*. The study was published in 1958, and provided important information for planning and allocating pediatric health resources over the next decade. It also assured continued communication and cooperation between the AAP, which was the collective voice of practicing pediatricians, and the Children's Bureau, the governmental agency dealing with child-health issues.

Following a slowdown during World War II, a postwar boom in pediatrics occurred. Full-time departments of pediatrics were established and expanded at most American medical schools. The expansion of pediatric research was fueled by federal funds, especially from the National Institutes of Health. The National Institute of Child Health and Human Development (NICHD) was founded in 1960. Under its first director, Dr. Robert Aldrich, the NICHD supported the investigation of a wide range of child-health issues.

The 1954 Nobel Prize–winning discovery by John Enders and his pediatric colleagues, Drs. Frederick C. Robbins and Thomas H. Weller (who at the time were research fellows in Ender's laboratory), that viruses could be grown successfully in tissue culture enabled the development of vaccines against poliomyelitis, first by Dr. Jonas Salk and then by Dr. Albert B. Sabin. The National Foundation for Infantile Paralysis had been established in 1938 by President Franklin D. Roosevelt, himself a victim of paralytic polio, to raise funds to support polio research and treatment. In 1954, the National Foundation financed and conducted a nationwide field trial of the formalin-inactivated Salk vaccine. At the time of the trial, preliminary studies of the Salk vaccine had been undertaken in only a few thousand subjects. Despite the small numbers, these studies were believed to indicate a "high degree of effectiveness and absolute safety." Although the polio field trial was certainly a research study, no truly informed consent was obtained. Because of the public hysteria about paralytic polio prevalent in the mid twentieth century, participation was widely accepted by the American public, and 650,000 American children received either the Salk vaccine or a placebo. The study revealed that the frequency of paralytic polio was reduced in children receiving the Salk vaccine to just over one-quarter of that in the controls. This success was marred because several large batches of vaccine contained live polio virus, and 204 vaccinated children and family contacts developed poliomyelitis. This incident lead to increasing governmental supervision and regulation of vaccine manufacture, ultimately a charge of the Food and Drug Administration. Immunization against polio became common throughout the world, and in 1996, the World Health Organization announced that poliomyelitis had been eradicated from the Western Hemisphere. On a broader scale, because of vaccination, smallpox has been eliminated from the entire world.

Other effective vaccines against infectious disease are being developed continuously. These include vaccines against measles and rubella, and more recently, against varicella and hepatitis B. Effective vaccines against bacterial diseases have made diphtheria, tetanus, pertussis, *Haemophilus influenza* infections, and pneumococcal bacteremia unusual today. Unfortunately, despite the efforts of pediatricians, some American children still are not immunized, and recurrent mini-epidemics of measles and pertussis are cause for continuing concern.

The use of prophylactic antibiotics for the control of beta-hemolytic streptococcal infections was an important factor in the near disappearance of clinical rheumatic fever and carditis in the United States. The neonatal diagnosis of sickle cell anemia, followed by the use of prophylactic penicillin, has markedly reduced the earlier 20% to 30% mortality due to overwhelming pneumococcal sepsis and meningitis in infants with sickle cell anemia.

Pediatric cardiologists, led by the efforts of Drs. Helen Taussig and Maude Abbott, developed the criteria and techniques that permitted the differentiation of various congenital anatomic lesions of the heart during life. This differentiation led to the development of surgical procedures to correct some of these defects, starting with the surgical ligation of the patent ductus arteriosus by Dr. Robert Gross in 1939, and a palliative but effective procedure for tetralogy of Fallot by Drs. Alfred Blalock and Helen Taussig in 1945. Today, the complete correction of even complex congenital heart anomalies often is possible. Ultrasonography has emerged as an important diagnostic tool for pediatric cardiologists. Pediatric surgeons, because of advances in anesthesiology and intra- and postoperative care, are able to treat effectively many congenital anomalies and acquired disorders. Organ transplantation has been successful in saving children with end-stage renal and hepatic diseases.

The treatment of childhood cancer, the major cause of nonaccidental mortality after the neonatal period, has been phenomenal. Beginning with Dr. Sydney Farber's introduction of folic acid antagonists in 1958, to treat acute lymphoblastic leukemia, modern multiagent chemotherapeutic protocols have evolved for the treatment of childhood malignancies. Today, more than 70% of childhood malignancies can be cured.

Some of the most dramatic advances in pediatrics have been in the care of premature infants. In 1943, Dr. Ethel C. Dunham and her colleagues in the Children's Bureau published the landmark *Standards and Recommendations for the Hospital Care of Newborn Infants, Full Term and Premature.* Six revisions of this manual continued to be published by the AAP until 1977. Incubators for newborns were first developed in the late nineteenth century in European hospitals. (These "showcases"

also were centerpieces of commercial "incubator baby" shows at international expositions and World Fairs well into the twentieth century.) Incubators, such as the Isolette, invented by Dr. Charles C. Chapple of Philadelphia, maintained the newborn infant's body temperature and facilitated oxygen administration. Because premature infants within these incubators were often exposed to high oxygen levels, which were shown to be the major cause of retrolental fibroplasia (retinopathy of prematurity) and subsequent blindness, techniques for monitoring oxygen levels and recommendations concerning oxygen usage and concentration were developed to sharply reduce the incidence of this iatrogenic disease after 1955.

Low-birth-weight infants often develop respiratory distress syndrome (hyaline membrane disease) because of lung immaturity. Increasingly improved procedures for respiratory management were developed, including better respirators. The importance of the developmental pattern of lung lipids (pulmonary surfactants) in the pathogenesis of respiratory distress syndrome was suggested by Drs. Mary Ellen Avery and Jere Mead in 1959. Dr. Louis Gluck demonstrated that the levels of phospholipids in the amniotic fluid reflected the degree of maturation of the fetal lung, thus providing a guide for the antenatal treatment of premature infants. These observations led to the development of artificial surfactants that can reduce the severity of respiratory distress and improve survival.

In 1952, Dr. Virginia Apgar of Denver proposed a new method for the assessment of the condition of the newborn 1 and 5 minutes after birth. The Apgar score provides information about the need for active resuscitation and correlates with neonatal morbidity and mortality. Advances in neonatology resulted in increasingly better outcomes of ever smaller premature infants. The survival of very low-birth-weight (VLBW) infants, as small as 500 grams, is being reported with increasing frequency and the definition of fetal viability based on weight has progressively decreased.

Genetic studies flowered during the last half of the twentieth century, and a large catalog of heritable diseases has been developed. Screening for the carrier states of diseases such as Tay-Sach disease and thalassemia combined with genetic counseling and prenatal diagnosis, has markedly reduced the incidence of these serious conditions. The neonatal diagnosis of disorders such as hypothyroidism, congenital adrenal hyperplasia, phenylketonuria, galactosemia, and other rare endocrinologic and metabolic disorders has enabled early therapeutic interventions that prevent severe mental retardation and death.

However, unforeseen challenges still are being presented to pediatricians. Some of these "new" diseases have been defined, understood, and controlled through incisive epidemiologic studies and effective interventions. The recognition that aspirin interaction with a viral infection, such as influenza or varicella, may cause Reye syndrome resulted in the virtual disappearance of this often fatal disease in the United States by restricting aspirin usage in children. The last decades of the twentieth century saw the emergence of human immunodeficiency virus (HIV) infections as a new scourge of children. Although still incurable, life expectancy and improved quality of life in these children has been accomplished with antiretroviral therapy. It is also possible to reduce the incidence of HIV infection through the testing of blood products and by preventing vertical transmission from infected mothers to their newborns with perinatal antiretroviral medications.

By the end of the 20th century, a "new morbidity" emerged, as described by Drs. Morris Green and Robert Haggerty, consisting of those problems resulting from social factors such as child abuse, divorce, violence, substance abuse, and other psychologic issues, and replacing many of the infectious, nutritional deficiency, and organic diseases that, one hundred years ago, made up nearly all of pediatric practice.

TABLE 1.1

SOME IMPORTANT DATES IN THE HISTORY OF PEDIATRICS IN THE UNITED STATES

1721	Introduction of variolization to prevent smallpox	Dr. Zabdiel Boylston; Rev. Cotton Mather, Boston, MA
1788	Publication of description of a child with pyloric stenosis	Dr. Hezikiah Beardsley, New, New Haven, CT
1800	Introduction of Jenner's vaccination for prevention of smallpox	Dr. Benjamin Waterhouse Boston, MA
1813	First medical school course and faculty appointment in The Diseases of Children	Dr. Eli Lves, Yale College New Haven, CT
1825	*Treatise on the Physical and Medical Treatment of Children,* the first American pediatric textbook	Dr. William Potts Dewees Philadelphia, PA
1854–1855	Opening of first children's hospitals in the United States	New York Nursing and Child Hospital; Children's Hospital of Philadelphia
1880	Founding of the Section on Pediatrics of the AMA	Dr. Abraham Jacobi, New York, NY
1888	Founding of the American Pediatric Society	Dr. Job Lewis Smith, New York, NY
1888	Publication of the *Archives of Pediatrics,* the first American pediatric journal	
1890	Discovery of diphtheria toxin and antitoxin	Dr. Emil von Behring, Berlin, Germany
1897	Publication of *The Diseases of Infancy and Childhood* now in its 21st edition as *Rudolph's Pediatrics*	Dr. L. Emmett Holt, Sr. New York, NY
1898	Establishment of the first premature infant incubator station	Dr. Joseph DeLee, Chicago, IL
1908	The city of Chicago mandated pasteurization of milk	
1912	Creation of the Children's Bureau	President William H. Taft
1912	Dr. John Howland appointed as Professor of Pediatrics at the Johns Hopkins School of Medicine and the Harriet Lane Home	Baltimore, MD
1920	U.S. Congress enacted the Sheppard-Towner Act authorizing the Children's Bureau to provide grants to States for meternal and child health activities	
1923	Discovery of vitamin D as the antirichitic factor in cod liver oil	Drs. Edwards Park and Elmer V. McCollum Baltimore, MD
1923	Active immunization with diptheria toxoid implemented widely in the U.S.	
1928	Identification of hexuronic acid (vitamin C) deficiency and the cause of scurvy	Dr. Albert Szent-Gyorgy, Philadelphia, PA
1930	Founding of the American Academy of Pediatrics independent of the American Medical Association	
1931	Founding of the Society for Pediatric Research	
1933	Founding of the American Board of Pediatrics	
1936	Committee on Foods of the AMA recommended fortification of milk with Vitamin D to prevent rickets	Dr. Philip Jeans, Iowa City, IO
1948	Dr. John Enders and associates received the Nobel Prize in Medicine for successful tissue culture of polio virus	Boston, MA
1949	Dr. Sidney Farber induced remissions of acute leukemia with a folic acid antagonist	Boston, MA
1950	Nationwide field trial of formalin-inactivated (Salk) polio vaccine	
1960	Founding of the National Institute of Child Health and Human Development	
1963	First mass testing in neonatal period for a metabolic disease (phenylketonuria)	Dr. Robert Guthrie, Albany, NY
1980	The beginning of the HIV pandemic, soon affecting newborns and hemophiliacs	
1996	World Health Organization announces the elimination of polio from the Western Hemisphere	

Conversely, a true revolution in bioscience, medicine, and pediatrics—the so-called "new biology"—also is occurring. Dazzling new technologies have made it possible to define disease at the cellular, subcellular, and molecular levels. Increasingly sophisticated techniques, such as magnetic resonance imaging (MRI), computed tomography (CT), and ultrasonography have improved diagnosis, and laboratory methods such as radio immunoassay and polymerase chain reaction (PCR) have enhanced the ability to diagnose many pediatric diseases.

The genes responsible for many human diseases are being identified, made increasingly possible by the recent completion of the monumental task of the mapping of the human genome—the DNA of the human chromosomes. Ultimately, this may lead to the prevention and cure of many diseases through genetic engineering, but this bright promise still is unfulfilled.

Pediatric subspecialties and specialists have multiplied, and their special skills have advanced the effective treatment of a wide variety of pediatric disorders. Unfortunately, each subspecialty has developed its own argot that sometimes makes communication between pediatricians difficult. A plethora of subspecialty societies and subspecialty journals has resulted in the fragmentation of general pediatric communication and education. Even more unfortunate is what may be an increasing emphasis on single organ systems or diseases, which may result in the neglect of the whole child, the child's family, and the child's community. One of the greatest challenge of U.S. pediatrics today to preserve the art, empathy, and concern for the whole child that have characterized this discipline over the last century as our technologies become ever more complex and the body of scientific knowledge becomes ever larger. All this in an American society that, despite mouth service, often appears to be unconcerned about the most basic health needs of many of our children.

Table 1.1 presents a timeline of progress in pediatrics in the United States.

Suggested Readings

Abt AF. *Abt-Garrison history of pediatrics*. Philadelphia: W.B. Saunders, 1965.

Baker J. *The machine in the nursery*. Baltimore: Johns Hopkins Press, 1996.

Baker JP, Pearson HA. *Dedicated to the health of all children*. Elk Grove: American Academy of Pediatrics, 2005.

Cone TE Jr. *History of American pediatrics*. Boston: Little Brown, 1979.

Cone TE Jr. *History of the care and feeding of the premature infant*. Boston: Little Brown, 1985.

Faber K, McIntosh R. *History of the American Pediatric Society, 1887-1965*. New York: McGraw-Hill, 1966.

Meckel, R. *Save the babies*. Baltimore: Johns Hopkins Press, 1991.

Parish HJ. *A history of immunization*. Edinburgh: E.S. Livingston, 1965.

Pearson HA. *The centennial history of the American Pediatric Society*. New Haven, Conn.: American Pediatric Society, 1988.

Pearson HA, Annunziato D, Baker JP, et al. AAP committee report: American Pediatrics: Milestones at the Millennium. *Pediatrics* 2001;107:1482–1491.

Pease MC. *A history of the American Academy of Pediatrics*. Chicago: American Academy of Pediatrics, 1951.

Shyrock RH. *Medicine and society in America 1660–1860*. New York: New York University Press, 1960.

Veeder S. *Pediatric profiles*. St. Louis: CV Mosby, 1957.

CHAPTER 2 ■ THE FIELD OF PEDIATRICS

ERROL R. ALDEN, HOLLY J. MULVEY, JOHN V. HARTLINE, AND ROBERT PERELMAN

The field of pediatrics is about the health care of those individuals who will make the future of the world possible. Children are our future, and it is among the highest callings to be involved in their care and nurture.

Pediatrics is concerned with the child's physical, mental, and psychosocial health. In the 1911 edition of his classic textbook, L. Emmett Holt stated that children's health is the product of three factors, "inheritance, surroundings, and food." Of these, the pediatricians can influence environment and nutrition. Holt also stated that observations about growth and development are most important during infancy and early childhood, because through this means, many conditions are detected early. Familiarity with the normal makes perception of the abnormal easier.

What was true in 1911 is true today: The field of pediatrics is about children's health and the factors that affect their health. Growth and development, nutrition, and genetics remain critical components of pediatrics. Although much of the *field* of pediatrics has not changed since the beginning of the century, the *practice* of pediatrics is dramatically different. Universal immunization has reduced the incidence of many diseases (e.g., pertussis, measles, diphtheria, polio) and eliminated others (e.g., smallpox). As a result, pediatrics has become less about the treatment of disease and more about prevention. Today, the highest priorities for pediatricians are to prevent and detect those disorders that cause significant morbidity or death. Preventive services such as immunization, screening, and counseling, now are the cornerstone of pediatric practice, replacing the need to diagnose and treat formerly common childhood diseases.

Despite these dramatic changes, old problems remain, and new challenges have arisen. Poverty—sustained economic hardship—continues to contribute to poor physical, psychological, and cognitive function and has a major effect on the practice of medicine and pediatrics. At the same time, the threat of old diseases has resurfaced (e.g., smallpox) and new diseases (e.g., pediatric human immunodeficiency virus infection) have emerged. As a result, ongoing education remains crucial, and new technologies (e.g., CD-ROM, Internet) have made education more accessible.

In light of these changes and challenges, it can be said that the field of pediatrics is about the health care and well-being of children, about the education of pediatricians, and about research. More precisely, pediatrics addresses what must be known to help each child achieve his or her optimal potential. This chapter discusses childhood populations and the U.S. supply of pediatricians, while also speculating about the future.

THE CHANGING PEDIATRIC POPULATION

Mortality and Morbidity

In the United States, in 2001, life expectancy at birth reached a record high of 77.2 years for all sex and race groups combined. However, the infant mortality rate was slightly higher than in previous years, and mortality for black infants was 2.5 times that for white infants. A large proportion of childhood deaths continue to occur as a result of preventable injuries. [The slightly higher infant mortality is due to an increase in multiple births derived in part from new technologies that help women conceive (Table 2.1).]

Many adult-onset diseases have their origins in childhood. Perhaps no better example exists than obesity, with its many medical complications. Type II diabetes (once a rarity in

TABLE 2.1

INFANT DEATHS AND IMRS FOR THE 10 LEADING CAUSES OF INFANT DEATH IN 2001: UNITED STATES, 2000 AND 2001 AND PERCENTAGE CHANGE, 2000–2001

Cause of Death and International Classification of Diseases, Tenth Revision, Codes	Rank*	2001			2000			% Change 2000–2001
		n	%	Rate[†]	n	%	Rate[†]	
All causes	NA	27 568	100.0	684.8	28 035	100.0	690.7	−0.9
Congenital malformations, deformations, and chromosomal abnormalities	1	5513	20.0	136.9	5743	20.5	141.5	−3.3
Disorders related to short gestation and LBW, not elsewhere classified	2	4410	16.0	109.5	4397	15.7	108.3	1.1
SIDs	3	2234	8.1	55.5	2523	9.0	62.2	−10.8
Newborn affected by maternal complications of pregnancy	4	1499	5.4	37.2	1404	5.0	34.6	7.5
Newborn affected by complications of placenta, cord, and membranes	5	1018	3.7	25.3	1062	3.8	26.2	−3.4
Respiratory distress of newborn	6	1011	3.7	25.1	999	3.6	24.6	2.0
Accidents (unintentional injuries)	7	976	3.5	24.2	881	3.1	21.7	11.5
Bacterial sepsis of newborn [P36]	8	696	2.5	17.3	768	2.7	18.9	−8.5
Diseases of the circulatory system	9	622	2.3	15.4	663	2.4	16.3	−5.5
Intrauterine hypoxia and birth asphyxia	10	534	1.9	13.3	630	2.2	15.5	−14.2
All other causes [residual]	NA	9055	32.8	224.9	8965	32.0	220.9	NA

NA, not applicable; IMR, infant mortality rate; LBW, low birth rate; SIDs, sudden infant death syndrome.
Source: Centers for Disease Control and Prevention/NCHS, 2000–2001 National Vital Statistics System, mortality (unlinked file).
*Rank based on 2001 data. Ranking is shown for 10 leading causes of infant death. For an explanation of ranking procedures, see Technical Appendix in Vital Statistics of the United States, Vol. II, Mortality Part A (published annually).
[†]Rate per 100 000 live births.

children) is directly related to obesity, and it accounts for 8% to 45% of all new cases of diabetes in childhood. It is significant that the time required from recognition of the disease to development of complications is no different in children and adults. Increases in television watching and fast-food consumption, combined with more sedentary endeavors such as computer games, all play major roles in childhood obesity. Early childhood obesity is associated with more severe obesity among adults. Other data suggest that overweight and obese school-aged children are more likely to be the victims and perpetrators of bullying behavior than their normal-weight peers.

Demographics

As pediatrics enters the new millennium, it is appropriate to assess the changes in the demographics of the pediatric population that have taken place. The twentieth century saw a significant growth (approximately 165 million people) in the U.S. population. In 1900, 40.5% of the total U.S. population was under 18 years of age. Over the next several decades, this percentage continued to decline to a low of 30.6% in 1940. Not unexpectedly, the decades following World War II saw an increase in the percent of the population that was under age 18. The increase continued until the 1980 U.S. census, which again demonstrated a decline in the percentage of the total U.S. population under 18 years of age. This decline continued until the close of the century. According to the 2000 census, 25.7% of the U.S. population was under the age of 18. To some extent, this decline in the percentage of the younger population is a result of the increased longevity of the population overall. During these same time periods, an increase occurred in the percent of the population over 65 years of age.

It is important to note, however, that during a century that saw a decline in infants, children, and adolescents under the age of 18 as a *percentage* of the population, the actual *numbers* of individuals in these age groups increased from 30.7 million in 1900 to approximately 72.3 million in 2000. This number is expected to reach 80.3 million in 2020. For the proper allocation of resources and the development of health policy, it is important to make an accurate determination of the percentage of the population under 18 years of age as a part of the total U.S. population. However, the actual number of people in this age group has significant implications for those who provide pediatric health care. Pediatricians of the future will be faced with responsibility for the health care of an increasing absolute number of children at a time when those children represent a smaller fraction of the total population.

Several demographic changes and other related factors have implications for the pediatrician workforce and the pediatric population. The most compelling of these demographic changes are those pertaining to race and ethnicity. The percentage of children who are white and non-Hispanic decreased from 74% in 1980 to 64% in 2000. During the same 20-year period, the percentages of black, Hispanic, and Native American/Alaska Native children have been fairly stable. The percentage of Asian/Pacific Islander children doubled from 2% to 4% of all U.S. children between 1980 and 2000. This percentage is projected to continue to increase to 6% in 2020, although the absolute numbers remain low.

The number of Hispanic children has increased faster than that of any other racial and ethnic group, growing from 9% of the child population in 1980 to 16% in 2000. By 2020, it is projected that more than 1 in 5 children in the United States will be of Hispanic origin. From the 2000 U.S. census, respondents who reported more than one race were more likely to be under age 18 than those who identified only one racial origin. Of the 6.8 million people in the two or more race category, 42% were under age 18. This contrasts with one-race category, in which 25% of these 274.6 million people were under 18 years. In 1979, 1.3 million children spoke their native language at home and had difficulty speaking English. By 1999, it is estimated that this number had doubled. In addition to race and ethnicity, other types of diversity within the pediatric population also will have implications for the allocation of resources as well as access to and utilization of pediatric health care services. These influences include religious diversity, sexual orientation, socioeconomic status, gender, and a host of other attributes.

Social Changes Affecting the Pediatric Population

The lifestyles of children and their families have a large effect on the field of pediatrics. The high rate of divorce, the number of children who live in reconstituted families, and the number of hours children watch television have become critical factors in the health of children and must be taken into account by their health care providers. Approximately 26% of children are living in married, two-parent families, and 8% live in married families where only the father works and the mother stays home. It is estimated that 8 to 10 million children in the United States are living with gay or lesbian parents. The prevention of illness and injury in children, as well as the care of chronically ill children, depends heavily upon caretakers. The practice of pediatrics requires the pediatrician to form a close alliance with the child's primary caretakers. In the past, the latter was almost always the mother, but, in today's world, it may include one or both parents, stepparents, grandparents, or other caretakers.

The high mobility of the family, the fact that fewer married couples have had much experience in rearing children (because of the small size of their own families), and the fact that many families do not live close to parents or other relatives also make the role of the pediatrician or the pediatric caregiver much more challenging and interesting. Simultaneously, the economics of medicine pressures pediatricians to see more patients, to have a larger practice, and to function in more cost-efficient and cost-effective ways.

THE CHANGING PRACTICE OF PEDIATRICS

Technologic Advances

New technologies have had a major effect on pediatric practice. The discovery of new antibiotics and the development of new vaccines continue to reduce the influence of infectious diseases, especially the "common childhood diseases," on modern children and their families. Genetic innovations place pediatricians at the frontier of modern medicine.

Mapping of the human genome has made possible an endless array of advances in the prevention of disease. The diagnosis of propensity for specific cancers and obesity, as well as hypertension, will enable the pediatrician to formulate an individual health prevention plan for each child. Unfortunately, progress and scientific advances have not been matched by concurrent advances in ethical, political, and societal reactions. Thus, the prediction of a potentially debilitating disease such as hypertension may push the cost of insurance to an uncomfortable or unattainable level. To accommodate advances in

medical care and to allow their optimal effects on human health, pediatrics must include advocacy, both for the individual child and for society's public health, so that advancements in science will not be drastically limited due to financial constraints.

Consumer-based interventions also have helped reduce risk for children. For example, aspirin poisoning has virtually disappeared with the advent of safety caps, and car seats have markedly reduced injuries in automobiles. New technologies virtually have eliminated many of those procedures and their complications that used to be commonplace, (e.g., exchange transfusions, pneumoencephalography, and myelography). The development of these new technologies, and the ability to use the Internet to access the literature on a complex topic, has made access to new knowledge at least as important as the simple acquisition of new knowledge itself.

Psychosocial and Developmental Problems

An increase in psychosocial and behavioral problems confront the pediatrician, despite a marked shortage of pediatric psychiatrists. The increase of autism in children, the poor prognosis associated with maternal depression, and the increase of children with attention deficit hyperactivity disorder (ADHD) all must be addressed by pediatricians. ADHD presents interesting challenges to pediatric practice and clinical research. Pediatricians are necessarily concerned with the impact of these conditions on both the child's and the family's psychological health, knowing full well that the families are the single greatest and most enduring influence on children.

Access to Pediatricians

Changes within the health care system also have an effect. One study found that large employers believe that pediatricians are the best primary care givers for the infants and children of their employees. The study also found that parents insist on access to pediatricians, particularly when they consider their child to be ill. On the other hand, a broad perception exists, as indicated by approximately 25% of the employers surveyed, that mid-level practitioners, nurse practitioners, and physician assistants working under the supervision of a physician could substitute for the general pediatrician or family physician with little diminution in quality. The provision of optimal pediatric care depends on a team-based approach, with coordination by a physician leader, preferably a pediatrician. This leadership role is based on the pediatrician's ability to manage, coordinate, and supervise the entire spectrum of pediatric care from diagnosis through all stages of treatment and in all practice settings.

International Issues

Global trends are a cause for change as well. The United States remains a country comprised of immigrants, but the incoming population of newer immigrants tends to be from countries different from those of their predecessors, countries in which diseases uncommon in the United States are prevalent. The frequency of international travel to and from all parts of the world can turn local outbreaks of disease into global concerns; two recent examples being severe acute respiratory syndrome (SARS) and avian influenza. Children seeking care in the United States may have been exposed to diseases elsewhere. To meet their care needs, the field of pediatrics in the United States must be prepared to address worldwide health issues.

If optimal care for children is to be provided, the practice of pediatrics must be culturally effective. This does not necessarily mean that pediatricians need to speak the same language, be of the same race, or hold the same religious beliefs as their patients: It does mean, however, that if optimal care is to be provided, the cultural needs and beliefs of children and their caretakers must be recognized and respected.

THE CHANGING PEDIATRICIAN POPULATION

To completely understand the field of pediatrics, in addition to the projections of future numbers of children and their health care needs discussed earlier, it is important to examine the pediatric workforce. The key factors influencing this workforce include the size of the pediatrician workforce, currently and over time; the influence of gender and lifestyle issues on the pediatric workforce; the age composition of the pediatrician workforce; the role of International Medical Graduates (IMGs) within this workforce; and the racial and ethnic composition of the pediatrician workforce. Two additional considerations also merit review: the role of pediatric subspecialists and the role of nonpediatric clinicians. To provide a contextual framework for the specialty of general pediatrics, it is important to make some comparisons to the overall physician workforce. Data from the American Medical Association (AMA) Masterfile provide the best source for making theses comparisons. They demonstrates that, in most instances, trends in the overall physician population are mirrored in the specialty of pediatrics.

Demographics

Over the past several decades, the total number of physicians has increased dramatically. In 1975, according to the AMA Masterfile, 393,742 physicians practiced in the United States, of which 35,636 were female. By 2002 (December 31), the most recent year for which data exists, the total number of U.S. physicians had increased by 46% to 853,187, of which

215,005 were female, accounting for one-quarter of the total physician population. Three-fifths (60.2%) of all physicians were in 10 specialty fields in 2001, of which the top 5 were internal medicine, family practice, pediatrics, obstetrics/gynecology, and psychiatry. This ranking shifts slightly when only women physicians are considered. For women in medicine, the specialty of pediatrics enjoys the second rank, following internal medicine.

The number of pediatricians has demonstrated strong increases over time. From approximately 22,192 general pediatricians in 1975, the specialty has grown to just over 66,000 in 2002. The specialty of pediatrics also reflects the growing number of women entering medicine. Pediatrics has historically attracted a larger number of female physicians than has other specialties. At the end of 2002, just over 50% of all pediatricians were female. Additionally, the percentage of female pediatric residents currently is over 60%.

What does this say about the field of pediatrics? It speaks to the continuing popularity of this primary care specialty; it also serves as a harbinger of the future of medicine. Pediatrics has the opportunity, now and in the future, to shape medical education, practice, and academic medicine (including research and teaching) to meet the needs of both women and men in the specialty. Recent studies have demonstrated that women pediatricians are more likely to work part-time than their male counterparts, and pediatric residents also have identified a strong interest in working part-time.

American Academy of Pediatricians (AAP) data show virtually no difference between male and female pediatricians in terms of practice location (urban, inner city; urban, not inner city; suburban; and rural). The majority of pediatricians (approximately 39%) are in suburban or urban, not inner city (approximately 28%) locations. No notable gender differences exist in employment settings (solo/two physician; pediatric group/HMO; medical school/hospital; other) for pediatricians, with most (approximately 46%) being in a pediatric group/HMO (Fig. 2.1).

Data for physicians in all specialties reveal that the greatest number belong to the 35 to 44 years of age category, followed closely by the 45 to 54 years of age group. However, looking just at the female physician group, the highest percentage

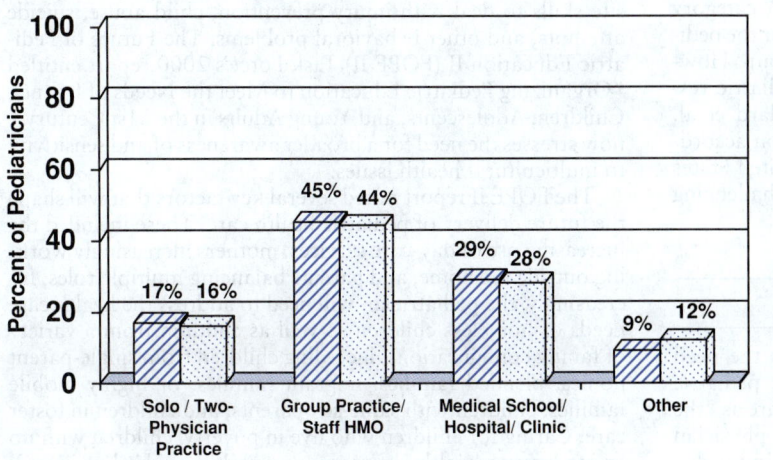

Employment Setting

p<.05 for M v F

FIGURE 2.1. Employment settings in pediatric medicine. (Reproduced with permission from American Academy of Pediatrics, Division of Health Policy Research, Periodic Survey of Fellows #47 thru #50, 2001.)

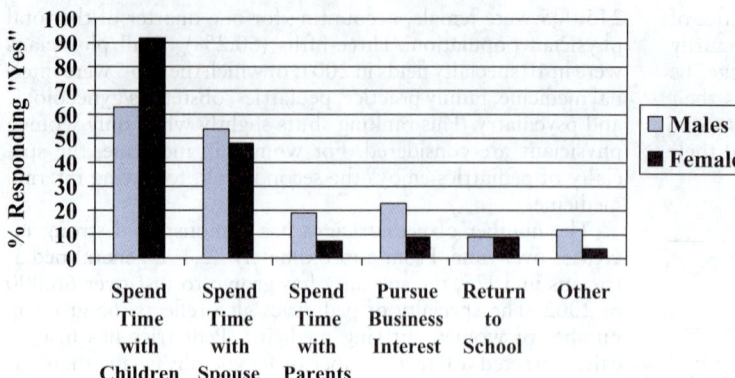

FIGURE 2.2. How would you use your extra time if you were to arrange a part-time or reduced-hours position? (Adapted with permission from Cull WL, Mulvey HJ, O'Connor KG, et al. Pediatricians working part-time: past, present, and future. *Pediatrics* 2002;109(6):1015.)

(41%) is in the under-35 category. This pattern of age distribution also is found in the specialty of pediatrics. It is important to note that 63% of all female pediatricians are age 35 or younger. Tangential to the correlation between gender and part-time employment, it has long been recognized that younger physicians of both genders place a higher premium on balancing their careers and their personal lives, with a strong emphasis placed on the needs of their family, personal health and recreation, and community issues. When the AAP surveyed third-year pediatric residents in 2000, female residents who were interested in part-time employment were significantly more likely than males to identify that they would spend extra time with their children (Fig. 2.2). The Future of Pediatric Education II (FOPE II) Project calls for both practice and academic settings to promote coordinated schedules, fair leave policies, quality day care at or near the workplace, and flexibility in academic promotion and advancement.

Racial and Ethnic Diversity

In addition to gender, age, and practice characteristics, the racial and ethnic diversity of the pediatrician workforce is an important consideration for the specialty of pediatrics. In 2002, an AAP survey found that 76% of post-resident pediatricians were white, non-Hispanic; 12% were Asian-Pacific Islander; 5% were Hispanic/Latino; and 4% were black/African American. Two percent of the pediatricians who responded selected the "other" category, while .4% are Native American/Alaskan. The findings from the pediatric residents who participated in this same survey reveal that fewer (67%) are white, non-Hispanic as compared with the post-resident respondents. Correspondingly, every other racial/ethnic category save one demonstrated a slight percentage increase for the pediatric residents, compared with the post-resident group. However, there were fewer Black/African American pediatric residents than post-residents (3% versus 4%). Stoddard et al. have suggested that "the goal of equal representation according to race/ethnicity among pediatricians in the United States remains elusive and seems to be an increasingly challenging policy goal."

Culturally Effective Practice

Related to any discussion of race and ethnicity is the need for all pediatricians to provide culturally effective pediatric care. The AAP defines culturally effective pediatric care as "the delivery of care within the context of appropriate physician knowledge, understanding, and appreciation of cultural distinctions. Such understanding should take into account the beliefs, values, actions, customs, and unique health care needs of

distinct populations groups. Providers will thus enhance interpersonal and communication skills, thereby strengthening the physician–patient relationship and maximizing the health status of patients." Unlike the more commonly used terms, "cultural sensitivity" and "cultural competence," culturally effective care shifts the emphasis from process to optimal outcomes. To ensure the delivery of optimal pediatric health care, the term "cultural" should be considered in the broadest possible context, and should include a host of attributes, ranging from race/ethnicity to religion to sexual orientation and poverty.

Delivering culturally effective pediatric care becomes all the more important when the cultural attributes of the pediatrician differ from those of the patient and his or her family. Pediatricians will be expected to acquire knowledge, refine their skills, and demonstrate behaviors and attitudes that are appropriate to care for and interact with patients and their families, as well as all members of the health care team. Additionally, pediatricians must be part of the solution as they work not only through the health care delivery system, but also with patients and their families to address situations related to limited English proficiency, the use of medical interpreters, low health literacy, and a host of concerns that will effect health care outcomes.

CHANGING THE EDUCATION OF PEDIATRICIANS

Other characteristics of the pediatric population will require innovative strategies from both current and future pediatricians. The Task Force on the Future of Pediatric Education (1978) correctly identified the need for pediatricians to have requisite skills to deal with injury prevention, child abuse, suicide attempts, and other behavioral problems. The Future of Pediatric Education II (FOPE II) Task Force's 2000 report entitled "Organizing Pediatric Education to Meet the Needs of Infants, Children, Adolescents, and Young Adults in the 21st Century," now stresses the need for a broader awareness of and sensitivity to multicultural health issues.

The FOPE II report noted several key factors that will shape the future delivery of pediatric health care. These included the increasing use of day-care services, mothers increasingly working outside the home, and parents balancing multiple roles. Increasingly, the pediatrician will need to address the health care needs of homeless children as well as children from a variety of family configurations, including children from single-parent homes, blended families, migrant families, or highly mobile families; children with same-sex parents; and children in foster care. Caring for children who live in poverty, children with no or inadequate health insurance, and children who live in geographic areas with limited access to pediatric health care pose challenges to pediatricians.

Pediatricians have a unique opportunity to be part of the solution and provide not only health care, but also guidance and strategies to both individuals and communities, and to serve as advocates for the rights and needs of the pediatric population at every level, from the hospital, to the community, to the national policy arena. Because of the close association of the pediatrician with the needs of the community, advocacy for child and family health priorities extends the influence of the pediatrician from the immediate community into society as a whole.

Integration of care across age and developmental stage epochs via the *medical home* can best mitigate genetic antecedents and influence adult health status. A medical home is not a building, house, or hospital, but rather a concept for providing health care services in a high-quality and cost-effective manner. Children and their families who have a medical home receive the care they need in concert with a pediatrician and other health professionals whom they trust, in a partnership that allows the identification of and access to all the medical and nonmedical services needed to help children and their families achieve their maximum potential.

Residency education is a pivotal step in the lifelong learning continuum of the pediatrician. The field of pediatrics continues to grow ever more challenging. These challenges reflect increases in clinical knowledge, technological advances, and demographic changes. The pediatrician of the future will need to address myriad societal issues as well, ranging from children without access to pediatric health care to children who are exposed to or are the victims of violence. Graduate Medical Education (GME) represents the best opportunity to introduce residents to topics and issues (both clinical and nonclinical) that will serve as a springboard for effective clinical practice, innovative future research, requisite pediatric subspecialization, life-long self-directed learning, and professional development.

CONCLUSIONS

The field of pediatrics has progressed from the treatment of children with disease (e.g., meningitis, whooping cough, measles) to embrace the prevention of disease and injury (e.g., the Back to Sleep Campaign for prevention of sudden infant death syndrome and the use of bicycle helmets). An explosion in biologic science places us in the post-genome era. The new paradigm, as expressed by Sherin U. Devaskar, is for pediatric research to untangle the reams of information gathered for the benefit of children and make practical sense of it. Evidence-based practice parameters, using practical tools such as computer-based quality and evaluation tools (e.g., *e*QIPP), help clinicians assess their practice, compare it to

best practices, and make improvements for the benefit of their patients.

The goals of the field of pediatrics have not changed: Pediatricians working with patients, parents, and caregivers apply the best science and technology to help children maximize their potential and avoid preventable and predictable causes of injury and disease.

Pediatricians believe in the inherent worth of all children. They are our most enduring and vulnerable legacy. The field of pediatric medicine has devoted itself to this most vulnerable and precious segment of the population. Success, for pediatricians, is to ensure a healthy, productive future for the population served. This is a significant yet enticing challenge.

Suggested Readings

American Academy of Pediatrics' Policy Statement. Pediatric Workforce Statement. *Pediatrics* 1998;102(2):418.

American Academy of Pediatrics. Scope of practice issues in the delivery of pediatric health care. *Pediatrics* 2003;111(2):426.

American Academy of Pediatrics. Personal/Practice Characteristics of Pediatricians (U.S. only), 2002. Available at: http//www.aap.org/research/periodicsurvey/practicecharacter2002color.htm. Accessed December 8, 2003.

American Academy of Pediatrics, Committee on Pediatric Workforce. Ensuring culturally effective pediatric care: implications for education and health policy. *Pediatrics* 2004 .

ChildStats.gov. Table POP5. Available at: http://www.childstats.gov/ac2003/tbl.asp?iid=102&id=1&indcode=POP5. Accessed November 25, 2003.

California District IX of the American Academy of Pediatrics study on the managed care initiative, June 1996.

ChildStats.gov. Racial and Ethnic Composition. Available at: http:/www.childstats.gov/ac2003/indicators.asp?IID=100&id=1. Accessed November 25,2003.

Cull WL, Mulvey HJ, O'Connor KG, et al. Pediatricians working part-time: past, present, and future. *Pediatrics* 2002;109(6):1015.

Devaskar SU, Mercier JC. Pediatric research—a look toward the future. *Pediatr Res* 2004;55(2):179. Epub 2004 Jan 08.

Holt EL, Howland J. *The diseases of infancy and childhood. For the use of students and practitioners of medicine.* New York: D. Appleton and Co., 1912.

Pasko T, Smart DR. *Physician characteristics and distribution in the U.S., 2003–2004 ed.* AMA Press.

Stoddard JJ, Back MR, Brotherton SE. The respective racial and ethnic diversity of U.S. pediatricians and American children. *Pediatrics* 2000;105(1):27.

Task Force of the Future of Pediatric Education II (FOPE II) Project. Organizing pediatric education to meet the needs of infants, children, adolescents, and young adults in the 21st century. The changing pediatric practice environment. *Pediatrics* 2000;105(Suppl 2):173.

U.S. Bureau of the Census. Population by age and sex for the United States: 1900 to 2000, Part D. Percent distribution for selected age groups. Available at: http://www.census.gov/prod/2002pubs/censr-4.pdf. Accessed January 8, 2004.

U.S. Bureau of the Census. Population by age and sex for the United States: 1900 to 2000, Part C. Selected age groups. Available at: http://www.census.gov/prod/2002pubs/censr-4.pdf. Accessed January 8, 2004.

U.S. Bureau of the Census. Total population by number of races reported, age, and Hispanic or Latino origin: 2000. Available at: http://www.census.gov/prod/2001pubs/c2kbr01-6.pdf. Accessed January 8, 2004.

CHAPTER 3 ■ ETHICS OF PEDIATRIC MEDICINE

NORMAN C. FOST

Every patient presents ethical problems. How much should be disclosed about the side effects of common drugs? How much authority should parents have in determining the medical management of their children, for trivial or life-threatening conditions? How much autonomy should be given to adolescents regarding their own health care? How should a pediatrician allocate her time, among patients and between practice and personal life?

Many of these problems are generic, in the sense that they arise in any clinical setting. Some are exotic, applying only to small numbers of patients or practitioners. This chapter focuses on problems common in pediatric practice. For discussion of a broader range of ethical problems in health care, the reader is referred to some of the excellent anthologies and introductions to ethical theory that are available (see Selected Readings). A few concepts are so central to pediatric practice that a brief review is necessary here.

AUTONOMY, COMPETENCE, CONSENT, AND PATERNALISM

American health care, and the political and legal milieu in which it exists, is oriented heavily toward autonomy or self-governance. A competent person has a nearly absolute right to decide what shall be done to his or her own body, according to a U.S. Supreme Court decision made 80 years ago. Any touching done without consent, by a doctor or anyone else, is battery. Consent can justify touching, but only if it is meaningful consent, requiring at least that it be informed and uncoerced. The legal requirements for informed consent reflect the widely shared moral belief that individuals should be free to make their own decisions, however foolish they may be.

These principles apply to competent patients. The definition and boundaries of competence are controversial, but clearly exclude many, if not most, children. For such individuals, others must be entrusted with the authority to make decisions on their behalf. This is called *paternalism*, interfering with someone's liberty on the grounds that it is in his interest. To be justified, paternalism requires that the interference be such that the individual plausibly would agree with it if he had a moment of lucidity and could see the issue clearly. Given this condition, imposing health care on people simply on the grounds that it is good for them is not sufficient. If that were the case, consent would be unnecessary.

What are the implications of these principles for pediatrics? For those older adolescents who resemble adults more than they do children (i.e., who would meet standard notions of competence), consent is necessary and sufficient for providing health care for the same reasons that apply to other competent patients. For infants and most young children, who would not meet any common notion of competence, proxy consent, motivated by paternalistic impulses, provides a sufficient basis on which to intervene with standard therapeutic interventions. For children between these extremes, who have an evolving capacity to understand the nature and implications of proposed interventions, a growing claim can be made for involving them in the decision-making process.

SERIOUSLY ILL INFANTS: THE "BABY DOE" PROBLEM

Since the 1970s, no single ethical issue has preoccupied American pediatrics more than the controversy surrounding the withholding of life-sustaining treatment from handicapped or seriously ill newborns. The practice of allowing such infants to die, or even killing them, is thousands of years old, but it became a national debate in the early 1970s with the public disclosure that routine, standard treatment, such as the repair of duodenal atresia, commonly was withheld from infants with birth defects such as Down syndrome. The death of "Baby Doe" in 1982, resulting from untreated esophageal atresia and Down syndrome, triggered a federal statute and regulations requiring that all infants be given medically beneficial treatment, regardless of handicap, unless they are comatose or their death is imminent. The application of these regulations to specific cases, in theory and practice, is controversial.

Whatever the merits or effects of the legal response, the Baby Doe debate appeared to cause a shift in consensus on a fundamental ethical point: that the value to be maximized in considering whether to give or withhold treatment should be the best interest of the infant. This replaced previous notions that parents' wishes should predominate and earlier efforts to rely on distinctions between ordinary and extraordinary means as a basis for making decisions. The "best interest" standard left open questions of how and by whom these interests should be defined and ascertained. In these matters, too, a consensus has been growing. In theory and practice, broad agreement exists that multidisciplinary consultations are more likely to result in ethically sound decisions than would be made by parents and personal physicians making decisions in private. Hospital ethics committees now are used widely to help resolve controversial cases and, in fact, are required (or some similar mechanism) by the Joint Commission on Accreditation of Hospitals. These committees typically do not make decisions, but strive to facilitate consensus among providers and parents. One of their most important functions appears to be improving the factual basis for decisions. Good ethics starts with good facts; many of the most controversial Baby Doe decisions were predicated on inadequate information, which could have been corrected if a more deliberate and collaborative process had been used.

C A S E   1

A 700-g newborn has trisomy 13. He has congestive heart failure and chronic renal failure and is dependent on a ventilator, with severe chronic lung disease, at 5 months of age. His parents ask that the ventilator be discontinued, realizing that he will die.

Comment

The child is unlikely to leave the nursery. He does not appear to be experiencing any of the pleasures of even neonatal life. His parents' request is consistent with his caretakers' view that continued treatment is likely to bring him prolonged suffering with little prospect of relief until death occurs. If disagreement arose among any of his caretakers or family members, consultation with an ethics committee would be advisable. Otherwise, there seems little reason not to discontinue life support. Withholding and withdrawing life support are morally equivalent, although some believe that withdrawal is preferable because it implies a clinical trial to document better the poor prognosis.

CASE 2

A newborn with anencephaly is expected to die. The parents ask that he be used as a heart donor.

Comment

Even more clearly than in case 1, this child has no discernible interests, either in living or dying. He presumably experiences no pain, so continued intensive care or surgery presents no burden to him. If he is breathing, he is not brain dead and, therefore, would not be considered legally dead in any state. Death is not an essential condition for discontinuation of life support, but it is an essential legal condition for removal of vital organs. Removal of the heart before documentation of death would be contrary to traditional attitudes and policies of transplantation. It technically would be homicide. Consultation with an ethics committee, the hospital attorney and, perhaps, a court should occur before the traditional boundary of using only dead donors is crossed.

CASE 3

An infant born at 29 weeks of gestation is breathing rapidly in the delivery room. The parents insist that nothing be done and that the infant be allowed to die.

Comment

Good ethics starts with good facts. Inadequate information is available to support a conclusion that continued treatment is not in the child's interests. A policy should be in place requiring the stabilization of newborns in this situation, with transfer to the NICU, so that an adequate assessment can be made. If withholding or withdrawing treatment is found to be in the child's interests, that decision can be made on a more informed basis.

SCREENING

Screening can be defined as the search for occult disease or the potential for disease to develop in a defined population. The purpose may be treatment [e.g., newborn screening for phenylketonuria (PKU)], counseling (e.g., testing for carrier status for sickle trait or Tay-Sachs disease in a sexually active adolescent), or research. As with all interventions, benefits should be established and shown to be commensurate with risks before application is made to broad populations. The harms of screening usually are indirect and, therefore, under-recognized. These harms can be organic, such as when a positive test result leads to harmful treatment. This occurred in the early days of widespread PKU testing, when the significance of elevated serum phenylalanine was unknown and the toxicity

of a low-phenylalanine diet was not fully understood. Many children were labeled incorrectly as having PKU and were harmed by the diet. Harms more commonly are psychosocial, a result of labeling and stigmatization. This was widespread when sickle cell screening caused parents of carriers to believe falsely that their children had a fatal condition or reduced the children's access to life and health insurance.

Screening has become such a central part of medical care that its risks are underestimated, and its benefits are assumed. Such common tests as the Denver Developmental Screening Test or an annual urine culture may result in undesirable and unwanted consequences. The former may cause the child to be labeled, by parents or others, as retarded. The latter may result in a series of costly and possibly toxic studies and therapies of uncertain benefit. When the benefits are clear, and the risks and costs trivial, little disagreement will arise. But when the benefits have not been established, or when the risks of stigmatization may be serious, the physician should be cautious about routine screening. At the least, parents or patients should be informed of the likelihood and evidence of claimed benefits and of the possibility of risks, and they should be given the opportunity to choose. New screening tests should be thought of as experimental until well-designed trials demonstrate their benefits and assess their risks.

CASE 4

A mother informs her pediatrician that she has been found to carry the BRCA1 gene, which implies a 70% probability of developing breast or ovarian cancer in her lifetime. She asks to have her 6-year-old daughter tested, because a 50% chance exists that the daughter also has the gene.

Comment

The chance of the daughter developing cancer during childhood is very small, and presently no known way to prevent it exists. A positive test result could cause harm to the child, including anxiety and loss of insurability. It also shuts off her opportunity to decide for herself whether to be tested when she becomes mature. Genetic testing of children generally is discouraged unless clear benefits exist.

CASE 5

The hospital laboratory has a new method for screening newborns for 50 biochemical abnormalities, using the same blood taken for PKU screening. The pediatric staff is asked to check and return a form if they want their patients screened.

Comment

The benefits of presymptomatic detection for many of the conditions are unclear. Genetic counseling benefits may exist, depending on the parents' reproductive plans. False-positive test results may have prolonged stigmatizing effects, even if the test done to confirm the diagnosis is negative. The pediatrician should seek expert opinion on the benefits and risks of performing the screening tests. Parents should participate in the decision whether to have their infants screened.

CONFLICTS OF INTEREST

The pediatrician experiences, as do other physicians, those familiar conflicts of interest inherent in charging fees for service or in reducing costs for capitated patients, and in balancing patient needs with personal needs and goals. In addition, because children needing health care typically are represented by their parents, the pediatrician often must distinguish the parents' needs and desires from those of the child. A mother asking for methods to control nocturnal enuresis in a 4-year-old child may be more concerned with her own interests than with her child's. Requests to withhold life-sustaining treatment from a handicapped newborn sometimes are based explicitly on consideration of the welfare of the other family members rather than on the interests of the patient. Contemporary notions of holistic medicine, including advocacy for treating the whole family, compete with traditional ideas of placing the interests of the patient above all others.

The physician who is employed by an institution or by the state has more explicit conflicts. The physician's contract implies that his primary duty is to the employer.

C A S E   6

Dr. Jones is a pediatric sports medicine specialist. He is a paid consultant to the university athletic department, which has asked him to set up a drug-screening program. Athletes with three violations must lose their scholarships and, therefore, for many, their opportunity for an education. Jones does not approve of illegal drug use, but he does not like being a police officer, and he thinks that his duty to his patients, the students, supersedes his duty to the school.

Comment

Having contracted with the school to test for drugs, Dr. Jones is obliged to fulfill his contract. He could try to change the rule requiring expulsion. He could ask the school to hire an outside consultant to administer the drug program. If these approaches fail, and if Jones does not like the heat, he may have to get out of the kitchen—or at least advise his patients of his conflicting interests so that no deception is involved.

The state may impose obligations on the pediatrician that compete with her duty to serve her patients. Requirements for reporting contagious diseases compete with promises of confidentiality and may jeopardize seriously the interests of patients. This has been most dramatic in cases of HIV infection.

Legal requirements that child abuse be reported may expose parents to professionals whose role as double agents prohibits them from respecting the confidentiality of sensitive information. This conflict of interest may work to the detriment of the parent. Physicians often feel, sometimes correctly so, that they cannot serve the interests of patients and simultaneously obey the law.

C A S E   7

Timmy, 3 years old, is in the emergency room with his third fracture in a year, allegedly caused by falling from a tree. The father is president of Mega, Incorporated. The mother seems distracted, defensive, and not nurturing of her son. Dr. Smith, their private pediatrician, suspects abuse, but believes that it would be best to discuss his concerns in the office, when they return for follow-up.

Comment

Smith's explicit duties are to the child and to the state, not to the parents. He clearly is violating the reporting law and is vulnerable to a charge of breaking another law—negligence. He might claim that the law is a bad one, not deserving of respect, but one of the requirements for justified civil disobedience is

openness. As a physician, he has no more claim than any other citizen to decide which laws deserve respect.

CONFIDENTIALITY

Physicians who work for institutions or under the requirements of state laws may have little choice about disclosing confidential information to authorities, without the consent of the patient or parents. Many situations occur, however, in which the decision whether to disclose information is discretionary. The pediatrician who is asked to prescribe contraception or treat sexually transmitted disease in a young adolescent may be legally authorized to do so without disclosure to the parents, but still must decide whether he can promote the child's interests without including the family. Similarly, the physician who discovers that his patient is abusing drugs may feel obliged to inform school or law enforcement officials to recruit their assistance in helping the patient. And the physician who discovers HIV infection in a neonate or school-aged child may feel obliged to inform foster parents, day-care providers, or school officials because of a concern for their health. The general rule is that no information obtained in a doctor–patient relationship should be disclosed without the consent of patient or guardian. Two reasons exist for this ancient rule: First, a public health concern exists that patients will be less likely to seek medical attention if they are not confident that stigmatizing information will be kept confidential. Decreased use of medical resources can impose costs on others, by increasing the spread of contagious diseases or increasing the costs to the community of treating disability. Second, the presumption that personal information will not be disclosed without consent is so widespread, among professionals as well as the public, as to constitute an implied promise. To break that promise for the benefit of others, without warning the patient beforehand, is to deceive the patient into disclosing information when she otherwise would not do so.

As with all principles, exceptions exist. Intervening in suicides and reporting child abuse are the most familiar examples of clinical problems for which nearly everyone supports the disclosure of confidential information. A principled basis exists for such disclosures: When a high probability of serious physical harm, a high likelihood of benefit, and no alternatives exist, and the patient is likely to later appreciate the disclosure, disclosure may be warranted.

ADOLESCENT SEXUALITY

Competent citizens have a nearly absolute right to decide what shall be done with their own bodies, and age is an imperfect measure of competence. Legal notions of majority, therefore, are only guidelines as to whether an adolescent can consent to any medical care. When a minor is emancipated, living independently of his or her parents, a presumption is made that she is competent to consent to medical care. A physician also may make a judgment that a minor is sufficiently mature as to be able to consent to his or her own medical care. In actual practice, the state is extremely deferential to physician judgment in these matters; virtually no legal risks exist for treating anyone older than 15 years.

When reproductive behavior is involved, the state is even more protective of the adolescent's right to health care, regardless of demonstrated competence. The reason for this is twofold. The first concern is that many patients will not seek medical care if parental consent is required and will suffer irreversible harm. Second, broad public concern exists about the epidemic of teenage pregnancy and sexually transmitted disease, with its adverse implications for adolescents and their children. Accordingly, such patients are granted broad access

---

BOX 3.1	Principles in End-of-Life Decisions

- A patient does not have to be brain dead, terminally ill, or comatose to justify discontinuing life support. Many children's interests are not served by prolonged survival. The terminally ill child, by definition, soon will escape the burdens of treatment. The child who faces a long life of continued suffering, with little prospect for the pleasures that make life worth living, may not have his interests served by continued existence.
- Withholding and withdrawing life support are morally equivalent; indeed, withdrawing may be morally preferable, although more difficult psychologically. If treatment is not serving the interest of the patient, it is irrelevant whether or not it is contemplated or in progress. Other things being equal, withdrawing treatment has the advantage of a clinical trial, so the judgment that the patient is not thriving is based on empiric evidence, rather than merely on speculation.
- Retardation or handicap alone is not a sufficient reason for terminating treatment. In the past, Down syndrome and spina bifida, common malformation syndromes with good prospects for long and happy lives, often were considered sufficient reason for allowing a child to die. Whether the

virtual disappearance of such practices is the result of a consensus on ethical issues or a fear of legal repercussions is not clear, but the moral issue does not seem to be in dispute.
- The child's best interest is the strongest argument for discontinuing treatment, not the family's or the community's interest. When treatment is not serving the child's interests, not only is it permissible to discontinue treatment, it is obligatory.
- When the child is incompetent, the parents generally should make decisions, but when such choices appear not to be in the child's interest, the decisions must be reviewed. The trend has been toward collaborative decision making in such matters, particularly when disagreement exists between the medical staff and the family, or within the family or medical staff. Hospital ethics committees are involved increasingly in consensus development in controversial cases. The ethical basis for such committees is the obligation to ensure that decisions are based on the best available facts, that interests other than the patient's are not playing a dominant role, and that the relevant issues are considered in a dispassionate manner.

---

to services for birth control, treatment of sexually transmitted disease, and abortion. An increasing number of states, however, require parental consent, or the approval of a court, before abortion is provided to a minor. Although most professionals advocate including parents in such discussions and decisions whenever possible, there will be an irreducible number of patients for whom parental involvement is not in the child's interest. As stated earlier, legal protection for adolescent access to reproductive services may be based more on public health considerations than on the interests of any specific patient. In some sense, this debate centers on an empiric question; namely, whether access to reproductive services promotes risky sexual behavior and thereby increases the incidence of adverse consequences of early sexuality.

TERMINAL CARE

From the perspective of many patients, there comes a point at which life is no longer worth living, when the burdens outweigh the benefits. Because medical technology is so successful in prolonging life, it usually becomes necessary to decide whether and when to withhold or withdraw treatment, whether it be resuscitation, ventilation, or more specific therapy. For most patients, these questions arise late in life, and the difficult question of defining the patient's best interest can be answered by each patient in his own idiosyncratic way, either at the time decisions must be made or beforehand, through written or spoken advance directives.

Allowing competent patients to participate in such decisions is a recent development in medical practice. Traditionally, physicians treated all patients paternalistically, shielding them from bad news and protecting them from the perceived stress of making hard choices. Similar attitudes persist among some pediatricians, who "protect" parents from active participation

in life-or-death decisions and, more commonly, shield children from facts and from discussion of their terminal care. Empirically, little support exists for the notion that patients are well served by this protection. Ethically, such paternalism precludes them from participating in decisions that affect them more than anyone else.

To include parents and patients in such discussions is not to yield all authority to them. Not all decisions are acceptable, and decision making, therefore, must be collaborative, including the physician, family, and, when appropriate, the pediatric patient. Although controversy abounds over the limits of acceptable decisions, consensus has been increasing over several issues that once were controversial (Box 3.1).

Suggested Readings

American Academy of Pediatrics, Committee on Bioethics. Informed consent, parental permission, and assent in pediatric practice. *Pediatrics* 1995;95:314.

Beauchamp TL, Childress JF. *Principles of biomedical ethics.* New York: Oxford, 1983.

Beauchamp TL, Walters L. *Contemporary issues in bioethics,* 6th edition. Thomson/Wadsworth, Belmont, Calif, 2003.

Buchanan A, Brock D. Minors. In: *Deciding for others: the ethics of surrogate decision making.* Oxford: Cambridge University Press, 1989.

Fost N. Treatment of seriously ill and handicapped newborns. *Crit Care Clin* 1986;2:149.

Gaylin W, Macklin R. *Who speaks for the child.* New York: Plenum, 1982.

Holder AR. *Legal issues in pediatrics and adolescent medicine,* 2nd ed. New Haven: Yale Press, 1985.

Holder AR. Minors' rights to consent to medical care. *JAMA* 1987;257:3400.

Jonsen AR, Siegler M, Winslade WJ. *Clinical ethics: a practical approach to ethical decisions in clinical medicine,* 3rd ed. New York: McGraw-Hill, 1992.

President's Commission for the Study of Ethical Problems in Medicine and Biomedical Research. *Deciding to forego life-sustaining treatment.* Washington, DC: U.S. Government Printing Office, 1983.

Steinbock B, Arras JD, London A, eds. *Ethical issues in modern medicine.* Boston, McGraw Hill, 2003.

Wald M. State intervention on behalf of neglected children. *Stanford Law Rev* 1976;28:623.

CHAPTER 4 ■ READING AND KEEPING UP WITH THE MEDICAL LITERATURE

OLAKUNLE B. AKINTEMI AND KENNETH B. ROBERTS

Many studies have documented a decline in the medical knowledge of physicians after residency and their failure to keep abreast of advances in diagnosis and therapy. Maintaining clinical competence and keeping up with advances in medicine are clearly uphill tasks. Currently, more than 25,000 biochemical journals are in print, with an estimated 6,000 new articles appearing every day and an archive of 6 million articles. To keep up with the medical literature, it is imperative to seek proper balance between browsing, "background" reading, and reading for individualized patient-care decision making (problem solving).

This balanced reading requires clinical information-management and evidence-based medicine (EBM) skills—skills that are important to lifelong, self-directed learning and continuous professional development.

EVIDENCE-BASED MEDICINE

EBM is defined as "the conscientious, explicit and judicious use of the current best evidence in making decisions about the care of individual patients." Essentially, EBM is a method of making clinical decisions by integrating clinical expertise, patient's preferences, circumstances and values, and judicious application of the best available research evidence.

The steps involved in EBM are: (a) formulating a focused and answerable clinical question; (b) identifying the "best evidence" (articles, studies) to answer the question; (c) appraising (reading and analyzing) the studies critically; and (d) integrating the evidence with clinical expertise, patient's (parents') values, preferences, and circumstances.

Background questions (why, what, when, how, who) ask about the general knowledge of a disease and can be answered using textbooks and classical review articles. An example of a background question is "What are the complications of gastroesophageal reflux disease?" *Foreground questions*, however, are answered using EBM skills. The four essential components of foreground questions have been given the acronym PICO: Patient and/or problem (P), the intervention (I), comparison intervention (if relevant) (C), and clinical outcomes (O). The outcomes should be "patient-oriented outcomes that matter" rather than "disease-oriented outcomes." An example of a foreground question is "In a 6-month-old infant with gastroesophageal reflux, do prokinetic agents reduce the frequency of vomiting?"

Clinical foreground questions fall into four categories: therapy (intervention), harm (etiology), diagnosis, and prognosis. A hierarchical classification of evidence according to its strength has been proposed: For example, the hierarchy of evidence regarding therapy questions ranges from unsystematic clinical observations at the bottom (weakest) to systematic reviews at the top (strongest).

The type of question, the topic, and the time available determine the selection of an evidence source. To answer general background clinical questions, a well-referenced and regularly updated textbook is recommended. However, for focused foreground therapy questions, prefiltered, evidence-based resources (e.g., Clinical Evidence, Cochrane Library) are preferred.

Until recently, EBM was a technical, time consuming, and labor intensive endeavor that few physicians had the interest, skills, and will to pursue. But today, with new technologies, many excellent EBM resources are available on the Internet, making EBM more accessible and "doable" in daily medical practice (Box 4.1).

READING CRITICALLY

Because the volume of material is large and time is limited, a method is necessary to identify which articles are worth screening and which among those screened are worth appraising critically. The two major types of studies reported in the medical literature are (a) primary or analytic and (b) secondary or integrative. Primary studies, which can be observational, experimental, or interventional, report original research. Box 4.2 depicts the classification of research designs in primary studies. Secondary (integrative) studies summarize or draw conclusions from the original research (systematic reviews, meta-analyses, clinical guidelines).

A number of formats, guides, questions, checklists, and resources are available for critically appraising the medical literature (Boxes 4.3 through 4.5 and Table 4.1). One of the more user-friendly and popular is the Users' Guides to the Medical Literature, developed by Haynes, Sackett, and Tugwell at McMaster University, Canada. These guides, initially published in *The Journal of the American Medical Association*, have been revised and compiled in a textbook. Other formats include the traditional pre-EBM journal club method and the "How to Read a Paper" series by Greenhalgh, initially published in *The British Medical Journal* and now compiled in a textbook. The Consolidated Standards of Reporting Trials (CONSORT) statement is a checklist for writing, reviewing, and evaluating reports of parallel-group randomized clinical trials. Recently, the Quality of Reports of Meta-analyses (QUOROM) statement was developed and published to improve the quality of the reporting of meta-analyses of randomized controlled trials.

The basic structure of a medical journal article is shown in Box 4.6. Critical appraisal, an essential component of EBM, is a method of assessing the validity, results, and relevance of a medical journal article. The following is offered as one approach to reading the medical literature, based on a series of questions.

Is This Article Worth Reading?

If the title is interesting and relevant, most readers then scan the abstract's introduction and conclusion. The abstract states the purpose of the study, major methods and procedures, findings, and conclusions. Journals increasingly are using structured abstracts to provide information about objectives, study design,

---

BOX 4.1   Selected EBM Resources Available on the Internet

Journals
1. ACP journal club http://www.acpjc.org
2. Evidence-based medicine http://www.ebm.bmjjournals.com
3. Bandolier http://www.jr2.ox.ac.uk/bandolier
4. Evidence-based Practice http://www.ebponline.net

Evidence Summaries
1. Clinical Evidence http://www.clinicalevidence.com
2. The Cochrane Database of Systematic Reviews http://www.cochrane.org/cochrane/revabstr/mainindex.htm
3. DynaMed http://www.dynamicmedical.com
4. FirstConsult http://www.firstconsult.com
5. InfoRetriever http://www.infopoems.com
6. SUMSearch http://sumsearch.uthscsa.edu/
7. TRIP Database (Turning Research Into Practice) http://www.tripdatabase.com
8. The York Database of Abstracts of Reviews of Effects (DARE) http://www.york.ac.uk/inst/crd/darehp.htm
9. EBM Guidelines. Evidence-based Medicine. http://www.ebm-guidelines.com

Clinical Guidelines
1. Institute for Clinical Systems Improvement (ICSI) http://www.icsi.org/knowledge
2. National Guideline Clearinghouse http://www.guidelines.gov
3. US Preventive Services Task Force (USPSTF) Recommendations http://www.ahrq.gov/clinic/uspstfix.htm

Other Useful Sites
1. Netting the Evidence http://www.shef.ac.uk/~scharr/ir/netting
2. Centre for Evidence-Based Medicine http://www.cebm.utoronto.ca
3. Ovid EBM http://www.ovid.com
4. Centre for Evidence-Based Medicine (Oxford) http://www.cebm.net

---

BOX 4.2   Study Designs of Primary Studies

A. Observational
  1. Descriptive
    ■ Case reports
    ■ Case series
    ■ Cross-sectional studies
    ■ Longitudinal studies
  2. Analytic
    ■ Prospective cohort
    ■ Retrospective cohort
    ■ Nested case-control
    ■ Multiple cohort
    ■ Case-control
B. Experimental
  ■ Randomized control trial
  ■ Factorial design
  ■ Randomization of matched pairs
  ■ Group or cluster randomization
  ■ Nonrandomized between groups design
  ■ Within-group designs
  ■ Cross-over designs

BOX 4.3   Resources for Critical Appraisal of Journal Articles

Books
1. Guyatt G, Rennie D. *Users' guides to the medical literature*. Chicago: AMA Press, 2002.
2. Greenhalgh T. *How to read a paper*, London: BMJ Books, 2001.
3. Gehlbach SH. *Interpreting the medical literature*, New York: McGraw-Hill Publishing, 2002.
4. Dawson B, Trapp RG. *Basic and clinical biostatistics*, New York: Lange Medical Books, 2004.
5. Sackett DL, Strauss SE, Richardson WS, et al. *Evidence-based medicine*. Edinburgh: Churchill Livingstone, 2000.
6. Badenoll D, Henegan C. *Evidence-based medicine toolkit*. London: BMJ Books, 2002.

Journals
1. *Journal of the American Medical Association (JAMA)* series, 1993–2000: "User's Guides to the Medical Literature."
2. *British Medical Journal (Br Med J)* series, 1997: "How to Read a Paper."

Web sites
1. Centers for Health Evidence http://www.cche.net
2. Introduction to Evidence-based Medicine http://www.hsl.unc.edu/lm/ebm/index.htm
3. Critical Appraisal and Using the Literature http://www.shef.ac.uk/sharr/ir/units/critapp/index/htm
4. Bandolier–Critical Assessment Skills Program (CASP) http://www.jr2.ox.ac.uk/Bandolier

---

methods, results, and conclusions in separate paragraphs. If the conclusion is intriguing, helpful, applicable, or provocative (e.g., contrary to expectation, experience, or knowledge), pause and think of reasons why the conclusion may be correct and why it may not.

Peer-review is a cursory screen for quality, but not a guarantee. Examples of flawed studies in well-respected journals abound, but the chances are greater that a higher-quality journal will contain higher quality articles.

Review the list of authors. Do they have a proven track record? Do they seem appropriate to do the study? Finally, do the authors or funding source have a vested interest in the outcome of the study? In most journal articles, authors are required to state sources of funding.

What Is the Purpose of This Article?

If the title and abstract suggest a relevant, interesting study worth reading, the next task is to determine the why the study was done; what hypothesis the authors were testing; what is

BOX 4.4   Traditional Pre-EBM Journal Club Framework for Evaluating Journal Articles

Title
1. Is the title succinct and descriptive of the article content?
2. Is it clinically relevant to your practice?

Authors
1. What are the authors' academic background?
2. Are they experts in the subject area?
3. Are they based at well-established academic centers?

Abstract
1. Is the topic of the study important and worth knowing about?
2. What is the aim of the study?
3. What is the main outcome of the study?
4. Is the population of patients relevant to your practice?
5. If results are "statistically significant," are they also clinically meaningful?

Introduction
1. What research has already been done on this topic, and what outcomes were reported?

Methods
1. Is the appropriate study design used?
2. Does the study cover an adequate period of time? Is the follow-up period long enough?
3. Are the criteria for inclusion and exclusion of subjects clear?
4. Were subjects randomly assigned? Was the randomization method described?
5. What were the outcome measures?
6. Are statistical methods outlined? Are they appropriate?
7(a). In a clinical trial:
    How were subjects recruited?
    Are the patients in the study similar to mine?
    Are all the patients who entered the study properly accounted for at its conclusion?
    Were patients analyzed in the group to which they were initially randomized (intention to treat analysis)?
    Is the study "blind"? Was everyone involved in the study (participants and investigators) "blind" to the treatment (double blind)?
    Were treatment and control groups similar at the beginning of the trial?
    Were the groups treated equally (except for the experimental intervention)?
    How is compliance ensured?
    Are the results statistically and clinically significant?

    In a negative study, was power analysis done?
    Were other factors present that might have affected the outcome?
7(b). In a cohort study:
    How were subjects recruited? From a tertiary children's hospital, primary care practice, or the community?
    Were the subjects randomly selected from an eligible pool?
    How rigorously were subject followed?
    How many drop-outs occurred, and who were they?
7(c). In a case-control study:
    Was there a clearly defined comparison group of those at risk for having the outcome of interest?
    Were the exposures and outcomes measured in the same way in the groups being compared?
    Were the observers blinded to the exposure of outcome and to the outcome?
    Was the follow-up sufficiently long and complete?
    Is there a dose-response gradient?
    How strong is the association between exposure and outcome? Is the odds ratio (OR) large?

Results
1. Do the reported findings answer the research questions?
2. Are actual values reported (means, standard deviations, proportions)?
3. Are many P values reported, thus increasing the likelihood that some findings are due to chance?
4. Are groups similar on baseline measures? If not, how did investigators deal with confounding variables?
5. Are the graphs and tables easy to read and understand?
6. If the topic is a diagnostic procedure, or a new test, is information on both sensitivity and specificity, positive and negative likelihood ratios, and positive and negative predictive values given?

Conclusion and Discussion
1. Are the research questions adequately discussed?
2. Are the conclusions of the study justified?
3. Are the conclusions discussed in the context of other relevant research?
4. Are shortcomings of the research addressed?

Adapted from Dawson B, Trapp RG. *Basic and clinical biostatistics,* New York: McGraw-Hill, Inc., 2004; and Misser WF. Critical appraisal of the literature. *J Am Board Fam Pract* 1999;12(4):315–333.

---

already known and what new information the study provides; what type of study (primary or secondary) was conducted; what broad field of research the study covers, and whether the study design and methods were appropriate. The purpose of the article (study) can be found by reading the introduction, methods, and the first paragraph of the discussion. Each of the five major clinical categories of research in primary studies (therapy, diagnosis, screening, prognosis, and causation/etiology) has a particular study design.

Are the Results Valid and Applicable?

The next tasks are to critically assess the article for validity and personal applicability. Although the questions asked

vary depending on the type of article, the Users' Guides recommend asking three core questions: Are the results valid? What are the results? Will the results help me in caring for my patients?

Are the Results Likely to Be Valid?

Validity depends on how the study was designed and conducted to minimize or avoid sources of systematic error or bias. The validity of a study is assessed by reading the methods section. Unfortunately, many lose their will here, intimidated by daunting phrases such as "retrospective cohort," "double-blind," "Wilcoxon signed rank test," "repeated measures ANOVA," and the like. However, for most studies, common sense and a simple line of questioning (Users' Guides) suffice. Threats to a

---

BOX 4.5   EBM Approach

Determine What the Paper Is About

1. Why was the study done? (What clinical question did it address?)
2. What type of study was done (primary or secondary)?
3. Was the research design appropriate to the broad field of research addressed (therapy, diagnosis, screening, prognosis, causation)?
4. Was the study ethical?

Methods Section of the Paper

1. Was the study original?
2. Who is the study about?
   How were subjects recruited?
   Who was included in, and who was excluded from the study?
3. Was the design of the study sensible?
   What intervention or other maneuver was being considered?
   What outcome(s) were measured and how?
4. Was the study adequately controlled?
   If a randomized trial, was randomization truly random?
   If a cohort, case-control, or other nonrandomized comparative study, were the controls appropriate?
   Were the groups comparable in all important aspects except for the variable being studied?
   Was assessment of outcome (or, in a case-control study, allocation of caseness) "blind"?
5. Was the study large enough, and continued long enough, to make the results credible?

Statistical Aspects of a Paper

1. Have the authors set the scene correctly?

Have they determined whether their groups are comparable and, if necessary, adjusted for baseline differences?
What sort of data have they obtained, and have they used appropriate statistical tests?
If the statistical tests in the paper are obscure, why have the authors chosen to use them?
Have the data been analyzed according to the original study protocol?

2. Paired data, tails, and outliers:
   Were paired tests performed on paired data?
   Was a two-tailed test performed whenever the effect on intervention could conceivably be a negative one?
   Were outliers analyzed with both common sense and appropriate statistical adjustments?
3. Correlation, regression, and causation:
   Has correlation been distinguished from regression, and has the correlation coefficient (r value) been calculated and interpreted correctly?
4. Probability and confidence:
   Have P values been calculated and interpreted appropriately?
   Have confidence intervals been calculated and do the authors conclusions reflect them?
5. Have the authors expressed their results in terms of the likely harm or benefit that an individual can expect, such as:
   Relative risk reduction?
   Absolute risk reduction?
   Number needed to treat?
   Odds ratio?

Adapted from Greenhalgh T. *How to read a paper*, London: BMJ Books, 2001.

---

study's validity may be internal (architecture, design) or external (generalization).

Were the Patients Randomized? The randomized double-blind controlled trial (RCT) is the gold standard for quality in studies of therapy. Randomization should allocate patients to treatment groups and avoid bias by ensuring that each patient has an equal chance of being allocated to treatment or control groups. Ideally, it should produce two or more groups that are comparable except for the treatment being studied. For example, if two groups of children with otitis media are similar except for the treatment (i.e., antibiotic and placebo) and the antibiotic group has more rapid improvement, then it is reasonable to associate the antibiotic with the improved outcome. If, however, one group was more likely not to respond to the antibiotic (e.g., because of other coexisting conditions), then a difference in outcome may not be solely attributable to the antibiotic. The methods section should describe the randomization procedure (alternate patients, random number generator). The randomization list or random allocation should be concealed from those individuals responsible for the enrollment of patients into the trial. A table displaying important baseline characteristics (age, sex, risk factors) of the groups provides reassurance that the study groups were comparable.

Were the Participants "Blinded"? The main purpose of blinding (or masking) is to make observations more objective and thus avoid bias. In an ideal trial, physicians, patients, outcome assessors, and biostatisticians should be blinded. Blinding may be single, double, or triple, depending on the research

question. A double-blind trial (in which both patient and physician are unaware of who is receiving treatment or placebo) is the gold standard. Blinding is often impossible or impractical, as in clinical trials in surgery.

Were All Patients Accounted For at the End of the Study? Was an Intention-to-Treat Analysis Performed? Did more patients in one group drop out of the study and, if so, why? Did patients who dropped out feel better or worse than those who remained? Studies have shown that patients who drop out tend to be less compliant with treatment, experience more side effects, and are less motivated. If less than 80% of study patients are accounted for at the conclusion of the study, the study may be invalid.

Was the duration of the study long enough to allow outcomes to manifest? Were patients analyzed in the group to which they were originally randomized? In a RCT, patients should be analyzed as randomized (i.e., by intention-to-treat-analysis or principle) regardless of subsequent events (e.g., withdrawal for adverse effects, failure to take medication).

Were the Comparison Groups Similar? Most articles have an initial table in the results section comparing the groups with reference to a number of variables (age, gender, severity of illness at baseline, and so forth). If the groups do not appear to be comparable in some important way, think about how the results might be affected. Introduced bias may have worked against showing a difference and therefore enhancing the meaningfulness of a demonstrated difference. Stratification and regression analysis are some of the statistical techniques used to address

TABLE 4.1
USERS' GUIDES TO THE MEDICAL LITERATURE

Diagnosis	Therapy	Prognosis	Harm
I. Are the results valid? ■ Was there an independent, blind comparison with a reference standard? ■ Did the patient sample include an appropriate spectrum of patients to whom the diagnostic test will be applied in clinical practice? ■ Did the results of the test being evaluated influence the decision to perform the reference standard? ■ Were the methods for performing the test described insufficient detail to permit replication? II. What are the results? ■ Are the likelihood ratios for the test presented or data necessary for their calculation provided? III. Will the results help me in caring for my patients? ■ Will the reproducibility of the test result and its interpretation be satisfactory in my setting? ■ Will the results change my management? ■ Will patients be better off as a result of the test?	I. Are the results valid? ■ Was the assignment of patients to treatments randomized? ■ Were all patients who entered the trial properly accounted for and attributed at its conclusion? ■ Was follow-up complete? ■ Were patients, health workers, and study personnel "blind" to treatment? ■ Apart from the experimental intervention, were the groups treated equally? II. What were the results? ■ How large was the treatment effect? ■ How precise was the estimate of the treatment effect? III. Will the results help me in caring for my patients? ■ Can the results be applied to my patient care? ■ Were all clinically important outcomes considered? ■ Are the likely treatment benefits worth the potential harms and costs?	I. Are the results valid? ■ Was there a representative and well-defined sample of patients at a similar point in the course of the disease? ■ Was follow-up sufficiently long to complete? ■ Were objective and unbiased outcome criteria used? ■ Was there adjustment for important prognostic factors? II. What were the results? ■ How large is the likelihood of the outcome event(s) in a specified period of time? ■ How precise are the estimates of likelihood? III. Will the results help me in caring for my patients? ■ Were the study patients similar to mine? ■ Will the results lead directly to selecting or avoiding therapy? ■ Are the results useful for reassuring or counseling patients?	I. Are the results valid? ■ Were there clearly defined comparison groups that were similar with respect to important determinants of outcome, other than the one of interest? ■ Were the exposures and outcomes measured in the same way in the groups being compared? ■ Was follow-up sufficiently long and complete? ■ Are the temporal relationships correct? ■ Is there a dose–response gradient? II. What are the results? ■ How strong is the association between the exposure and outcome? ■ How precise is the estimate of the risk? III. Will the results help me in caring for my patients? ■ Are the results applicable to my practice? ■ What is the magnitude of the risk? ■ Should I attempt to stop the exposure?

Reproduced with permission from Guyatt G, Rennie D. *Users' guides to the medical literature*. Chicago: AMA Press, 2002.

BOX 4.6	The Basic Structure of a Journal Article

1. Abstract
2. Introduction
3. Methods
4. Results
5. Discussion
6. References

incomparabilities in the study groups. Did the authors use these methods? Sometimes a big difference between two groups melts away after controlling for another factor (e.g., age, gender).

Are the Statistical Tests Appropriate for the Data? The statistical tests used for hypothesis testing are based on (a) the number of subjects in the groups studied (sample size); (b) the variability of measurement within each group; (c) the type of experiment used to collect the data; and (d) the scale of measurement. Statistical tests commonly used include the Student t test, when data are continuous (such as age or weight); the chi-square test, when data are dichotomous (e.g., obese versus nonobese, or 3-year-old versus 7-year-old subjects); and the Mann-Whitney U test, when data are ordinal (e.g., croup score, wheezing score).

The purpose of statistics is to provide an estimate of how likely it is that the observed findings were (or were not) caused by chance, not to determine whether the findings are clinically important. Statistical tests express chance as P value or significance level. P value is the chance probability of seeing an effect as big as or bigger than that shown in the study. It is a measure of the strength of evidence against the null hypothesis. Historically, the evidence against the null hypothesis has been considered "significant" if $P <0.05$. The use of the word "significant" is unfortunate, because it invites confusion with "meaningful" or "important." The choice of 0.05 (or 5% significance level) remains purely arbitrary. Precise P values are more useful than "significant" or "not-significant." (See the section How Precise Is the Treatment Effect?)

What Are the Results?

How Large Is the Treatment Effect? Several ways exist for expressing the magnitude of association or effect between an exposure (or treatment) and an outcome (or benefit). These include relative risk reduction (RRR), absolute risk reduction (ARR), relative risk (RR), the number needed to treat (NNT), and odds ratio (OR). A "risk" is the probability of an event, and its "odds" is the probability divided by its complement $(1 - \text{probability})$. For example, if a 60% risk of an event is present, the odds of that event is $0.60/(1 - 0.60) = 1.5$.

The RRR is the percentage reduction in risk in the treated group compared with the control group. It is expressed as $1 - \text{RR}$ or $100 - \text{RR}$ depending on whether the RR is presented as a proportion or percentage.

The ARR, or risk difference, is the absolute difference in risk between the control and the treatment group.

The NNT, the reciprocal of ARR, is the number of patients who must be treated to benefit one patient or prevent one patient from developing an adverse target outcome event.

The RR, or risk ratio, is a ratio of the risk in the experimental (treatment) group to the risk in the control group. An RR of less than 1 means that there is less risk of the event occurring in the treatment group (i.e., treatment is beneficial). An RR of 0 means that no harm or benefit derives from the treatment. However, if the RR is greater than 1, the treatment is harmful.

The OR is the odds of an event in the treatment group divided by the odds of the same event in the control or placebo group. In most studies, the OR is approximately the same as the RR when the likelihood of outcomes of interest is small. The more common the outcome, the greater the divergence between OR and RR.

The NNT and the 95% confidence interval (CI) are measures of the impact of a treatment on a patient (i.e., the likelihood that a patient will benefit from a treatment—its effectiveness). Consider, for example, the rate of hospitalization in children with asthma treated with levalbuterol or racemic albuterol. In one study from an emergency department (Fig. 4.1), 36% of children treated with levalbuterol were hospitalized compared with 45% treated with racemic albuterol. The ARR was 9%, RRR was 20%; RR was 0.8, OR was 0.68, and NNT was 12. In this study, then, 12 children with asthma treated with levalbuterol instead of racemic albuterol prevented hospitalization in one.

How Precise Is the Treatment Effect? The results of clinical research (means and differences in means, odds ratios, relative risk, etc.) are presented as P values and/or confidence intervals (CT). Although $P = 0.04$ means that a difference between two groups is unlikely to have occurred by chance, it does not indicate the size or meaningfulness of that difference. The CI—the range within which the true population difference is expected to lie—is a measure of both the magnitude of the difference

| | OUTCOME | | |
	ADMIT	HOME	
Levalbuterol	101	177	278
Racemic Albuterol	122	147	269
	223	324	547

FIGURE 4.1. Levalbuterol versus albuterol in acute asthma. (Reproduced with permission from Carol JC, Myers TR, Kirchner HL, et al. Comparison of racemic albuterol and levalbuterol for treatment of asthma. *J Pediatr* 2003;143:732–736.)

estimate and the precision of that estimate. It can be used to determine both statistical and clinical significance. It also provides clinically useful information even when it includes the null value (0 for differences, 1 for OR and RR).

The 95% CI is the range within which 95% of the true population difference is expected to lie. Traditionally, the 95% CI is used, although the 90% or 99% could be used. The width of the CI depends on the standard error and thus the standard deviation and sample size. The wider the CI, the less precise the results. Studies using large sample size are more precise and have narrower CIs than those using small sample size.

If No Difference Is Found (Negative Study), How Likely Is It That a True Difference (True Positive Effect) Was Missed? A researcher may erroneously conclude that a difference exists in the outcomes between a treatment group and a control group when no difference really exists. This is known as *Type I error*, and the probability of making the error is called the alpha level of the statistical significance. The effect of committing a Type I error is a *false-positive* result or outcome. *Type II* or beta error occurs when the research concludes that no difference exists between a treatment group and a control group when, in fact, a difference does exist. This may result in falsely concluding that an effective treatment is useless (*false-negative* result). The ability to detect that a difference between groups actually exists is called the *power* of a study (e.g., the power to detect a difference if one exists). Power is determined by sample size (a large study has more power than a small study) and beta. By tradition, Type II or beta error is arbitrarily set at 0.20, although values between 0.05 and 0.20 are sometimes used. Power is equal to 1 − beta; a power of 80% usually is considered adequate. Any decrease in Type II error increases power. The goal of hypothesis testing is to make Type I, alpha and Type II, beta as small as possible. As the alpha level is decreased (to decrease the size of a Type I error), the likelihood of making a Type II error is increased.

Will the Results Help Me in Caring for My Patients?

Were the Study Patients Similar to the Patients in My Practice? Even if the study is valid, it must be applicable to be useful. If the subjects of the study were selected from a tertiary-care setting, and the results are applied to children in a community practitioner's office, the outcome may not be the same. Other important population differences include setting (urban, suburban, rural; developed country, developing country), social class (lower, middle, upper) and gender.

Were All Clinically Important Outcomes Considered? The article should identify all outcomes (beneficial and harmful) that were measured during the study, how they were measured, and the objectivity of the measurement. The authors also should state *a priori* the primary and secondary outcome measures. Outcomes that are a proxy for the main or primary outcome of interest (i.e., sinus CT as a proxy for clinical improvement in sinusitis, increase in CD4 counts in AIDS studies) are called *surrogate endpoints* and must be viewed with great skepticism. If a surrogate endpoint is used, assurance is required that it is valid, reproducible, sensitive, specific, a true predictor of disease, and adequately reflects response to therapy.

Are the Likely Treatment Benefits Worth the Potential Harms and Costs? The final step is to decide whether the treatment benefits are worth the potential harms and costs. This involves balancing benefits and adverse effects of treatment with patient and parent values and preferences. Treatments may cause benefits and harms, and the size of the benefit must be weighed against the harms. The threshold NNT is the point at which the risks of treatment equal the benefits, and it is a function of the baseline risk without treatment. Factors that influence the threshold NNT include parent's values and preferences and the severity of the adverse effects of therapy (in other words, Is the harm is too great to treat the patient?). The NNT is low in patients at high baseline risk (without treatment) and high when the baseline risk falls. If a patient's baseline risk is high, and the NNT is below the threshold, treatment should be administered. However, if the baseline risk is low, and the NNT is above the threshold, treatment should not be given. Methods of calculating threshold NNT and the minimum event rate to justify treatment are beyond the scope of this chapter. Interested readers are referred to the Selected Readings section.

KEEPING UP AND CHANGING PRACTICE: THE BOTTOM LINE

Many reasons explain why change in medical practice comes slowly. In general, new findings are reviewed and published in journal articles, confirmed by others in the field, endorsed by acknowledged experts, accepted by influential colleagues, and disseminated locally and through prestigious national and international organizations. Newer systems of rapid communication and electronic access permit the practitioner to keep up with advances more easily than ever, but the sheer volume of material is daunting. What has not changed is the need for physicians to maintain the ability and discipline to read critically, apply a sense of what is relevant and applicable, and utilize a network of trusted colleagues and experts with whom to confer and confirm changes in practice.

Suggested Readings

Altman DG. *Practical statistics for medical research*. London: Chapman and Hall, 1991.

Badenoch D, Heneghan C. *Evidence-based medicine toolkit*. London: BMJ Books, 2002.

Carol JC, Myers TR, Kirchner HL, et al. Comparison of racemic albuterol and levalbuterol for treatment of asthma. *J Pediatr* 2003;143:732–736.

Chatellier G, Zapletal E, Lemaitre D, et al. The number needed to treat: a clinically useful nomogram in its proper context. *Br Med J* 1996;312:426–429.

Christakis D. Evaluating articles about treatment in the medical literature. *Contemp Pediatr* 2003;20(5):79–80, 82, 85–86, 91–92, 95.

Cook RJ, Sackett DL. The number needed to treat: a clinically useful measure of treatment effect. *Br Med J* 1995;310–451.

Dawes M, Davies P, Gray A, et al. *Evidence-based practice*. Edinburgh: Churchill Livingstone, 1999.

Greenhalgh T. *How to read a paper*. London: BMJ Books, 2001.

Guyatt G, Rennie D. *Users' guide to the medical literature*. Chicago: AMA Press, 2002.

Jadad AR. *Randomized controlled trial*. London: BMJ Books, 1998.

Laine C, Weinberg DS. How can physicians keep up-to-date? *Ann Rev Med* 1999; 50:99–110.

McKibbon A, Eady A, Marks S. *PDQ. Evidence-based principles and practice*. Hamilton, Ontario: B.C. Decker, 1999.

Miser WF. Critical appraisal of the literature. *J Am Board Fam Pract* 1999; 12 (4):315–333.

Moher D, Cook DJ, Eastwood S, et al. Improving the quality of reports of meta-analyses of randomized controlled trials: The Quorum Statement. Quality of Reporting of Meta-Analyses. *Lancet* 1999;354:1896–1900.

Moher D, Schultz KF, Alman D. The Consort Statement: revised recommendations for improving the quality of reports of parallel-group randomized trials. *JAMA* 2001;285:1987–1991.

Sackett DL, Straus SE, Richardson WS et al. *Evidence-based medicine. How to practice and teach EBM*. Edinburgh: Churchill Livingstone, 2000.

Silagy C, Haines A. *Evidence-based practice in primary care*. London: BMJ Books, 2001.

Shiffman RN, Shekelle P, Overhage JM, et al. Standardized reporting of clinical practice guidelines: a proposal from the conference on guideline standardization. *Ann Intern Med* 2003;139:493–498.

Sinclair JC. Weighing risks and benefits in treating the individual patient. *Clin Perinatol* 2003;30(2):251–268.

Sinclair JC, Cook RJ, Guyatt GH, et al. When should an effective treatment be used? Derivation of the threshold needed to treat and the minimum event rate for treatment. *J Clin Epidemiol* 2001;54(3):253–262.

GLOSSARY OF EBM TERMINOLOGY

Absolute Risk Reduction (ARR): The difference of the risk of an outcome between treatment and control groups or the absolute difference in experimental event rate and control event rate (EER – CER).

Absolute Risk Increase (ARI): The absolute difference in rates of bad events (i.e., when the experimental treatment harms more patients than the control treatment).

Confidence Interval: A measure of precision; it quantifies the uncertainty in measurement. It is usually reported as 95%. CI is the range of values within which one can be 95% sure that the true value for the whole population lies.

Likelihood Ratio: The probability that a given test would be expected in patients with the target disorder to the probability of that same result in those without the target disorder.

Negative Predictive Value: The proportion of patients with a negative test who are free of a disease.

Null Hypothesis: The statistical hypothesis that one variable has no association with another variable, or that two or more population distributions do not differ from one another. For example, in a comparison of the efficacy of Drug A and Drug B, the null hypothesis is "no difference exists between A and B." In simplest terms, the null hypothesis states that the differences observed between the effects of Drug A and B are no different from what might have occurred as a result of chance alone.

Number Need to Harm (NNH): The number of patients who, if they receive the experimental treatment, would lead to one additional person being harmed, compared with patients who receive the control treatment. It is calculated as $\frac{1}{ARI}$.

Number Needed to Treat (NNT): The number of patients who need to be treated to benefit one patient or prevent one additional bad outcome. It is calculated as $\frac{1}{ARR}$.

Odds Ratio (OR) (cross-product ratio, prevalence odds): The ratio of an event occurring in a treated or exposed group to the odds of the same event occurring in a group that is not treated or exposed. It is a measure of association between an exposure and the outcome of interest. It is a valid measure of the size of an effect in clinical trials, case-control studies, cohort studies, systematic reviews, and meta-analyses. When events or outcomes are rare, the OR approximates the relative risk. However, for common events, it is quite different.

One-Tailed Test: A statistical significance test based on the assumption that the data have only one possible direction of variability. Because of this directionality, it is easier to prove a "one-tailed" hypothesis than a "two-tailed" hypothesis.

Positive Predictive Value: The proportion of people with a positive test who have a disease.

Post-test odds: A patient's likelihood of a disease by taking into account the likelihood ratio of the test used and the patient's pretest probability.

Relative Risk (RR) or Risk Ratio: The ratio of the rate (risk) of disease among those exposed to the rate in those not exposed.

Relative Risk Increase (RRI): The proportional increase in rates of "bad" outcomes between experimental and control patients in a trial.

Relative Risk Reduction (RRR): The proportional reduction in rates of "bad" events or outcomes between experimental and control patients in a trial.

Sensitivity: The proportion of patients with the target disorder who have a positive test.

Specificity: The proportion of patients without the target disease who have a negative test.

Two-Tailed Test: A statistical significance test based on the assumption that the data are distributed in both directions from a central value. For example, if the alternate hypothesis states that "A difference exists between Drug A and B," we have no prior impression as to whether Drug A or B is superior to the other. A "two-tailed" test is therefore used to test this hypothesis.

The Basics of Critically Appraising the Medical Literature

	+ Disease or outcome	– Disease or outcome	
Test + /Treated/ + Exposure	a	b	a + b
Test – /Control/ – Exposure	c	d	c + d
	a + c	b + d	n

$$\text{Sensitivity} = \frac{a}{a+c}$$

$$\text{Specificity} = \frac{d}{b+d}$$

$$\text{Positive Predictive Value (PPV)} = \frac{a}{a+b}$$

$$\text{Negative Predictive Value} = \frac{d}{c+d}$$

$$\text{Positive likelihood ratio (LR}^+) = \frac{\text{sensitivity}}{1 - \text{specificity}} = \frac{a/(a+c)}{b/(b+d)}$$

$$\text{Negative likelihood ratio (LR}^-) = \frac{1 - \text{sensitivity}}{\text{specificity}} = \frac{c/(a+c)}{d/(b+d)}$$

(Rules of Thumb: LR$^+$ >10 and LR$^-$ <0.1 significantly change the post-test odds of a disease.)

$$\text{Experimental event rate (EER)} = \frac{a}{a+b}$$

$$\text{Control event rate (CER)} = \frac{c}{c+d}$$

$$\text{Relative risk (RR) or Risk ratio} = \text{EER/CER}$$
$$= [a/(a+b)] \div [c/(c+d)]$$

$$\text{Relative risk reduction (RRR)} = 1 - \text{RR} \times 100\%$$

Absolute risk reduction (ARR) or Risk difference
$$= \text{EER} - \text{CER} = [a/(a+b)] - [c/(c+d)]$$

$$\text{Number needed to treat (NNT)} = \frac{1}{\text{ARR}}$$

$$\text{Pretest odds} = \frac{\text{prevalence}}{1 - \text{prevalence}}$$

$$\text{Post-test odds} = \text{LR} \times \text{pretest odds}$$

$$\text{Odds ratio} = a/c \div b/d = \frac{ad}{cb}$$

CHAPTER 5 ■ PEDIATRIC HISTORY AND PHYSICAL EXAMINATION

LEWIS A. BARNESS

HISTORY

A complete history on a pediatric patient leads to the correct diagnosis in the majority of children. The history usually is learned from the parent, the older child, or the caretaker of a sick child. After learning the fundamentals of obtaining and recording case history data, the nuances associated with interpreting information must be learned.

For the acutely ill child, a short, rapidly obtained report of the events of the immediate past may suffice temporarily, but as soon as the crisis is stabilized, a more complete history is necessary. A convenient method for obtaining a meaningful history is to ask systematically and directly all the questions outlined in this chapter. After confidence is gained with experience, questions can be directed at specific problems and asked in an order designed to elicit more specific information about a suspected disease state or diagnosis. Some psychosocial implications will be obvious. More subtle details often are obtained by asking open-ended questions. Those patients with organic illness usually have short histories; those with psychosomatic illness generally have a longer list of symptoms and complaints.

During the interview, it is important to convey to the parent interest in the child, as well as the illness. The parent should be allowed to talk freely at first and to express concerns in his or her own words. The interviewer should look directly either at the parent or the child intermittently and not only at the writing instruments or the record generated on the computer. A sympathetic listener who addresses the parent and child by name frequently obtains more accurate information than does a harried, distracted interviewer. Careful observation during the interview may uncover stresses and concerns that otherwise are not apparent.

The written record is not only helpful in determining a diagnosis and making decisions, but also is necessary for observing the growth and development of the child. A well-organized record facilitates the retrieval of information and obviates problems if it is required for legal review.

The following guidelines indicate the information needed. If preferred, a number of printed forms are available that contain similar material, or forms may be modified, as long as consistency is maintained.

General Information

Identifying data include the examination date; the patient's name, age, and birth date, gender, and race; the referral source if pertinent; the relationship of the child and informant, and some indication of the mental state or reliability of the informant. It frequently is helpful to include the ethnic or racial background, address, and telephone numbers of the informants.

Chief Complaint

After the identifying data, the chief complaint should be recorded. Given in the informant's or patient's own words, the chief complaint is a brief statement of the reason why the patient is being seen. The stated complaint often is not the true reason the child was brought for attention. Expanding the question, "Why did you bring the child in?" to "What concerns you?" allows the informant to focus on the complaint more accurately. Carefully phrased questions can elicit information without prying.

History of Present Illness

Next, the details of the present illness are recorded in chronologic order. For the sick child, it is helpful to begin, "The child was well until ___ days before this visit." This is followed by a daily documentation of events leading up to the present time, including signs, symptoms, and treatment, if any. Statements should be recorded in number of days before the visit or specific dates, but not by days of the week, because chronology will be difficult to retrieve even a short time later. If the child is taking medicine, the record should indicate type and brand, the amount being taken, the frequency of administration, how well it has worked, and how long it has been taken.

For the well child, a simple statement such as "No complaints" or "No illness" suffices. A question about school attendance may be pertinent. If the past medical history is significant to the current illness, a brief summary is included. If information is obtained from old records, it should be noted.

Past Medical History

Depending on the age of the patient, some aspects of the past history that follow may not be pertinent. Obtaining the past medical history serves not only to provide a record of data that may be significant to the well-being of the child either now or later, but also to provide evidence of children who are at risk for health or psychosocial problems.

Prenatal History

If a prenatal interview has been held (see following discussion), this information already may be available. Questions to be answered include those regarding the health of the mother during the pregnancy, especially in regard to any infections, other illnesses, vaginal bleeding, toxemia, or exposure to animals (e.g., maternal exposure to cats may raise the possibility of toxoplasmosis), any of which can have permanent effects on the embryo and child. The time and type of fetal movements should be determined. The record should include the number of previous pregnancies and their results, whether radiography was performed, what medications were taken, and whether the mother smoked or abused drugs or alcohol during the pregnancy, results of serology and blood typing of the mother and baby, and results of other tests such as amniocentesis. If the mother's weight gain was excessive or insufficient, this should be noted.

Birth History

The duration of pregnancy, the ease or difficulty of labor, and the duration of labor may be important, especially if there is a question of developmental delay. The type of delivery (spontaneous, forceps-assisted, or cesarean section), type of anesthesia or analgesia used during delivery, attendance by other family members at delivery, and presenting part (if known) are recorded. Note the child's birth order (if there have been multiple births) and birth weight.

Neonatal History

Many informants are aware of Apgar scores at birth and at 5 minutes, any unusual appearance of the child such as cyanosis or respiratory distress, and any resuscitative efforts that took place and their duration. If the mother was delayed in seeing the infant after birth, reasons should be sought. Jaundice, anemia, convulsions, dysmorphic states, and congenital anomalies or infections in the mother or infant are some of the reasons why viewing or handling of the newborn by the mother may be delayed. The time of onset of any of these abnormal states may be significant.

Feeding History

Note whether the baby was breast- or bottle-fed and how well the baby took the first feeding. Poor sucking at the first feeding may be the result of sleepiness, but also is a warning sign of neurologic abnormality, which may not become manifest until much later in life. By the second or third feeding, even brain-damaged children usually nurse well.

If the infant has been bottle-fed, inquire about the type of formula used and the amount taken during a 24-hour period. Ask about the mother's initial reaction to her baby, the nature of bonding and eye-to-eye contact, and the baby's patterns of crying, sleeping, urinating, and defecating. Supplemental feeding, vomiting, regurgitation, colic, diarrhea, or other gastrointestinal or feeding problems should be noted.

Determine the ages at which solid foods were introduced and supplementation with vitamins or fluoride took place, as well as the age at which weaning occurred and the method used to wean. In addition, note the age at which baby foods, toddlers' foods, and table food were introduced, the response to these, and any evidence of food intolerance or vomiting. If feeding difficulties are present, determine the onset of the problem, methods of feeding, reasons for changes, interval between feedings, amount taken at each feeding, vomiting, crying, and weight changes. With any feeding problem, evaluate the effect on the family by asking, "How did you manage the problem?"

For an older child, ask the informant to supply some breakfast, lunch, and dinner menus; likes and dislikes; and response of the family to eating problems.

Developmental History

An estimation of physical growth rate is important. Attempt to ascertain the birth weight and the weights at 6 months, 1 year, 2 years, 5 years, and 10 years. Lengths at similar ages are desirable. These data are plotted on physical growth charts. Any sudden gain or loss in physical growth should be noted, because its onset may correspond to the onset of organic or psychosocial illness. It may be helpful to compare the child's growth with the rate of growth of siblings or parents. Ages at which major developmental milestones were met aid in indicating deviations from normal. Such milestones include following a person with the eyes, holding the head erect, smiling responsively, reaching for objects, transferring objects, sitting alone, walking with support and alone, speaking the first words and sentences, and experiencing tooth eruption. Ages of dressing self, tying own shoes, hopping, skipping, and riding a tricycle and bicycle should be noted, as well as grade in school and school performance.

In addition, note should be made of the age at which bowel and bladder control was achieved. If problems exist, the ages at which toilet teaching began also may indicate reasons for problems.

Behavior History

The amount of sleep and sleep problems and habits such as pica, smoking, and use of alcohol or drugs should be questioned. The informant should state whether the child is happy or difficult to manage and should indicate the child's response to new situations, strangers, and school. Temper tantrums, excessive or unprovoked crying, nail biting, and nightmares and night terrors should be recorded. Question the child regarding masturbation, dating, dealing with the opposite sex, and parents' responses to menstruation and sexual development. Questions should be free of heterosexual assumption, direction of romantic interests, and gender of partners.

Immunization History

The types of immunizations received, with the number, dates, sites given, and reactions should be recorded as part of the history. In addition, it is helpful to record these immunizations with lot numbers on the front of the chart or in a convenient, obvious place.

History of Past Illnesses

A general statement should be made about the child's general health before the present encounter, such as weight change, fever, weakness, or mood alterations. Specific inquiry is helpful regarding the results of any screening tests and any history of infectious or contagious diseases, or any other illness, as well as specific treatment, results, and residua. The history of each past illness should include dates of onset, course, and termination. If hospitalization or surgery was necessary, the diagnoses, dates, and name of the hospital should be included. Questions concerning allergies include the occurrence and type of any drug reactions, food allergies, hay fever, and asthma. Accidents, injuries, and poisonings should be noted.

Review of Systems

The review of systems serves as a checklist for pertinent information that might have been omitted. If information has been obtained previously, simply state, "See history of present illness" or "See history of past illnesses." Questions concerning each system may be introduced with a question such as, "Are there any symptoms related to ... ?"

- Head (e.g., injuries, headache)
- Eyes (e.g., visual changes, crossed or tendency to cross, discharge, redness, puffiness, injuries, glasses)
- Ears (e.g., difficulty with hearing, pain, discharge, ear infections, myringotomy, ventilation tubes)
- Nose (e.g., watery or purulent discharge, difficulty in breathing through nose, epistaxis)
- Mouth and throat (e.g., sore throat or tongue, difficulty in swallowing, dental defects)
- Neck (e.g., swollen glands, masses, stiffness, symmetry)
- Breasts (e.g., lumps, pain, symmetry, nipple discharge, embarrassment)
- Lungs (e.g., shortness of breath, ability to keep up with peers, timing and character of cough, hoarseness, wheezing, hemoptysis, pain in chest)
- Heart (e.g., cyanosis, edema, heart murmurs or "heart trouble," pain over heart)
- Gastrointestinal (e.g., appetite, nausea, vomiting with relation to feeding, amount, color, blood- or bile-stained, or projectile, number and character of bowel movements, abdominal pain or distention, jaundice)
- Genitourinary (e.g., dysuria, hematuria, frequency, oliguria, character of urinary stream, enuresis, urethral or vaginal discharge, menstrual history, attitude toward menses and opposite sex, sores, pain, sexually active, birth control, sexually transmitted disease and protection, abortions)
- Extremities (e.g., weakness, deformities, difficulty in moving extremities or in walking, joint pains and swelling, muscle pains or cramps)
- Neurologic (e.g., headaches, fainting, dizziness, incoordination, seizures, numbness, tremors)
- Skin (e.g., rashes, hives, itching, color change, hair and nail growth, color and distribution, bruises or bleeds easily)
- Psychiatric (e.g., usual mood, nervousness, tension, drug use or abuse)

Family History

The family history provides evidence for considering familial diseases as well as infections or contagious illnesses. A genetic type chart is easy to read and very helpful. It should include parents, siblings, and grandparents, with their ages, health, or cause of death. If problems with genetic implications exist, all known relatives should be inquired about. If a genetic type chart is used, pregnancies should be listed in a series and should include the health of the siblings (Fig. 5.1).

Family diseases include allergy; blood, heart, lung, venereal, or kidney disease; tuberculosis; diabetes; rheumatic fever; convulsions; skin, gastrointestinal, behavioral, or mental disorders; cancer; or other disease the informant mentions. These diseases may have a heritable or contagious effect. Pertinent negative answers should be included.

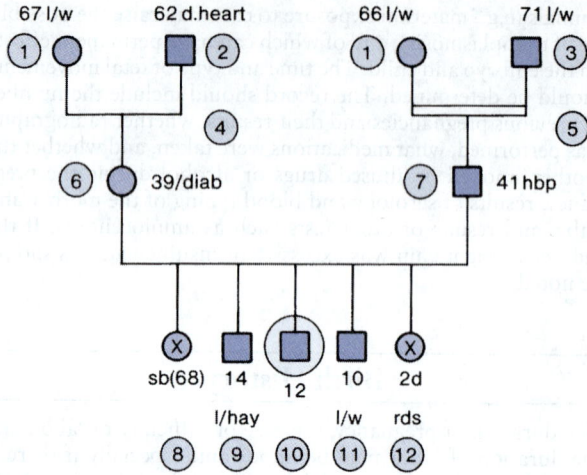

FIGURE 5.1. Genetic type chart. (*Circle*, female; *square*, male.) 1, maternal grandmother, 67 years old, living and well; paternal grandmother, 66, living and well. 2, Maternal grandfather, died at 62 of heart disease. 3, Paternal grandfather, 71, living and well. 4, Single horizontal line, married. 5, Double horizontal line, consanguineous marriage. 6, Mother, 39 years old, living, diabetic. 7, Father, 41 years old, living, hypertensive. 8, Stillbirth, died in 1968. 9, Male sibling, 14 years old, living, hay fever. 10, Patient, 12 years old (note light circle). 11, Brother, 10 years old, living and well. 12, Female, died at 2 days old of respiratory distress (year can be included).

Social History

Details of the family unit include the number of people in the habitat and its size, the presence of grandparents, the marital status of the parents, the significant caretaker, the total family income and its source, and whether the mother and father work outside the home. If it is pertinent to the current problems of the child, inquire about the family's attitude toward the child and toward each other, the type of discipline used, and the major disciplinarian. If the problem is psychosocial and only one parent is the informant, it may be necessary to interview the other parent and to outline a typical day in the life of the child.

Prenatal History

It is desirable, if feasible, to interview the mother and father before the child is born. Not only can some necessary data be obtained, but also the parents can become acquainted with the doctor who will be seeing them shortly after the arrival of their newborn. The health of the mother, whether she will nurse or bottle-feed the baby and whether the husband supports her choice, the preparation for the baby on arrival home, and whether help will be available can be ascertained. Because the father may feel left out of the pregnancy experience, it is important to direct some questions to him (e.g., "Do you want your son circumcised?") and to get the family history of diseases from him first.

History from the Child

Even young children should be asked about their symptoms and their understanding of their problem. This also provides an opportunity to observe the child interact with the parent. For most adolescents, it is important to take part of the history from the adolescent alone after asking for his or her approval. (see Chapter 89 for a more complete discussion of appropriate components of the history in the adolescent patient.) Regardless of your own opinion, obtain the history objectively without any moral implications, starting with open-ended questions related to the initial complaint and then directing the questions.

PHYSICAL EXAMINATION

An examination of the infant and young child begins with observing him or her and establishing rapport. The order of the examination should fit the child and the circumstances. It is wise to make no sudden movements and to complete first those parts of the examination that require the child's cooperation. Painful or disagreeable procedures should be deferred to the end of the examination, and these should be explained to the child before proceeding. For the older child and adolescent, examination can begin with the head and conclude with the extremities. The approach is gentle but expeditious and complete. For the young, apprehensive child, chatter, reassurance, or other communication frequently permits an orderly examination. Some children are best held by the parent during the examination. For others, part of the examination may require restraint by the parent or assistant.

When the complaint includes a report of pain in a certain area, this area should be examined last. If the child has obvious deformities, that area should be examined in a routine fashion without undue emphasis, because extra attention may increase embarrassment or guilt. Because the entire child is to be examined, at some time all of the clothing must be removed. This does not necessarily mean that it must be removed at the same time. Only the part that is being examined needs to be uncovered, and then it can be reclothed. Except during infancy, modesty should be respected, and the child should be kept as comfortable as possible.

With practice, the examination can be completed quickly even in most critical emergency states. Only in those with apnea, shock, absence of pulse, or, occasionally, seizures is the complete examination delayed. Although the method of procedure may vary, the record of examination should be in the same format for all children. This provides easy access to information later. The description that follows is the usual way of recording the examination and not necessarily its required order. When diseases are given with a sign, these are meant as examples and not a complete differential for that sign. The significance of the record of a previous examination cannot be overstressed. A murmur that was not heard a year ago but now is easily audible has far different significance than does a similar murmur heard many years before.

The completion of the history can be accomplished during the physical examination. Talking to the parent frequently reassures the child. Praising the young child, explaining the parts of the examination to the older child, and reassuring the adolescent of normal findings facilitates the examination. Usually, if the examiner enjoys the spontaneity and responsiveness of children, the examination will be easier and more thorough.

Measurements (Vital Signs)

Temperature is taken in the axilla or rectum in the young child and by mouth after 5 or 6 years of age, when the child can understand how to hold the thermometer. Electronic thermometer probes inserted into the mouth or rectum give rapid, accurate determinations. In general, the rectal temperature will be approximately 0.5 degrees higher than the oral temperature. Sometimes body temperature is determined by placing the thermometer under the child's arm, with the upper arm held firmly by the side. Somewhat less accuracy is possible with this method, and in general, the reading that results will be about 1 degree lower than the rectal temperature. There is some controversy about the accuracy of electronic assessment through use of probes in the external ear canal. It is important to correlate the temperature determined by this method with the clinical condition of the child. Elevated temperature occurs with infection, excitement, anxiety, exercise, hyperthyroidism, collagen-vascular disease, or tumor. Decreased temperature occurs with chilling, shock, hypothyroidism, or inactivity. Temperature may be decreased after taking certain drugs, with hypocortisolism, or with overwhelming infection.

The pulse rate can be obtained at any peripheral pulse (femoral, radial, or carotid) or by palpation over the heart. The normal rate varies from 70 to 170 beats per minute at birth to 120 to 140 shortly after birth, and ranges from 80 to 140 at 1 to 2 years, from 80 to 120 at 3 years, and from 70 to 115 after 3 years. The sleeping pulse after the age of 2 years normally is approximately 20 beats per minute less than the awake pulse, but does not decrease with rheumatic fever or thyrotoxicosis. For each centigrade degree of temperature increase, the pulse rate increases approximately 10 beats per minute. The pulse rate is elevated with excitement, exercise, or hypermetabolic states and is decreased with hypometabolic states, hypertension, or increased intracranial pressure. Irregularity may be caused by sinus arrhythmia, but can indicate underlying heart disease. Absence of the femoral pulse is a cardinal sign of postductal coarctation of the aorta.

Respiratory Rate

The respiratory rate should be determined by observing the movement of the chest or abdomen or by auscultating the chest. The normal newborn rate is 30 to 80 breaths per minute; the rate decreases to 20 to 40 in early infancy and childhood, and then to 15 to 25 in late childhood and adolescence. Exercise, anxiety, infection, and hypermetabolic states increase the rate; central nervous system lesions, metabolic abnormalities, alkalosis, depressants, and other poisons decrease the rate.

Blood Pressure

The blood pressure should be measured with a cuff, with the bladder completely encircling the extremity and the width covering one-half to two-thirds of the length of the upper arm or upper leg. The pressure should be recorded and compared with normal readings (Tables 5.1 and 5.2). High systolic pressure occurs with excitement, anxiety, and hypermetabolic states. High systolic and diastolic pressures occur with renal diseases, pheochromocytoma, adrenal disease, arteritis, or coarctation of the aorta. Press and release the child's nail. Normally, color returns in less than 1 second, the capillary refill time. Color returns in 2 to 3 seconds with 50 to 90 mL/kg fluid depletion, and in more than 3 seconds with greater than 90 mL/kg fluid depletion. At more than 90 mL/kg fluid depletion, medical shock ensues.

Height, Weight, and Head Circumference

To obtain height and weight recordings, the infant should be measured supine up to the age of 2 years and standing

TABLE 5.1

BP LEVELS FOR GIRLS BY AGE AND HEIGHT PERCENTILE

Age, y	BP Percentile	SBP, mm Hg Percentile of Height							DBP, mm Hg Percentile of Height						
		5th	10th	25th	50th	75th	90th	95th	5th	10th	25th	50th	75th	90th	95th
1	50th	83	84	85	86	88	89	90	38	39	39	40	41	41	42
	90th	97	97	98	100	101	102	103	52	53	53	54	55	55	56
	95th	100	101	102	104	105	106	107	56	57	57	58	59	59	60
	99th	108	108	109	111	112	113	114	64	64	65	65	66	67	67
2	50th	85	85	87	88	89	91	91	43	44	44	45	46	46	47
	90th	98	99	100	101	103	104	105	57	58	58	59	60	61	61
	95th	102	103	104	105	107	108	109	61	62	62	63	64	65	65
	99th	109	110	111	112	114	115	116	69	69	70	70	71	72	72
3	50th	86	87	88	89	91	92	93	47	48	48	49	50	50	51
	90th	100	100	102	103	104	106	106	61	62	62	63	64	64	65
	95th	104	104	105	107	108	109	110	65	66	66	67	68	68	69
	99th	111	111	113	114	115	116	117	73	73	74	74	75	76	76
4	50th	88	88	90	91	92	94	94	50	50	51	52	52	53	54
	90th	101	102	103	104	106	107	108	64	64	65	66	67	67	68
	95th	105	106	107	108	110	111	112	68	68	69	70	71	71	72
	99th	112	113	114	115	117	118	119	76	76	76	77	78	79	79
5	50th	89	90	91	93	94	95	96	52	53	53	54	55	55	56
	90th	103	103	105	106	107	109	109	66	67	68	69	69	70
	95th	107	107	108	110	111	112	113	70	71	71	72	73	73	74
	99th	114	114	116	117	118	120	120	78	78	79	79	80	81	81
6	50th	91	92	93	94	96	97	98	54	54	55	56	56	57	58
	90th	104	105	106	108	109	110	111	68	68	69	70	70	71	72
	95th	108	109	110	111	113	114	115	72	72	73	74	74	75	76
	99th	115	116	117	119	120	121	122	80	80	80	81	82	83	83
7	50th	93	93	95	96	97	99	99	55	56	56	57	58	58	59
	90th	106	107	108	109	111	112	113	69	70	70	71	72	72	73
	95th	110	111	112	113	115	116	116	73	74	74	75	76	76	77
	99th	117	118	119	120	122	123	124	81	81	82	82	83	84	84
8	50th	95	95	96	98	99	100	101	57	57	57	58	59	60	60
	90th	108	109	110	111	113	114	114	71	71	71	72	73	74	74
	95th	112	112	114	115	116	118	118	75	75	75	76	77	78	78
	99th	119	120	121	122	123	125	125	82	82	83	83	84	85	86
9	50th	96	97	98	100	101	102	103	58	58	58	59	60	61	61
	90th	110	110	112	113	114	116	116	72	72	72	73	74	75	75
	95th	114	114	115	117	118	119	120	76	76	76	77	78	79	79
	99th	121	121	123	124	125	127	127	83	83	84	84	85	86	87
10	50th	98	99	100	102	103	104	105	59	59	59	60	61	62	62
	90th	112	112	114	115	116	118	118	73	73	73	74	75	76	76
	95th	116	116	117	119	120	121	122	77	77	77	78	79	80	80
	99th	123	123	125	126	127	129	129	84	84	85	86	86	87	88
11	50th	100	101	102	103	105	106	107	60	60	60	61	62	63	63
	90th	114	114	116	117	118	119	120	74	74	74	75	76	77	77
	95th	118	118	119	121	122	123	124	78	78	78	79	80	81	81
	99th	125	125	126	128	129	130	131	85	85	86	87	87	88	89
12	50th	102	103	104	105	107	108	109	61	61	61	62	63	64	64
	90th	116	116	117	119	120	121	122	75	75	75	76	77	78	78
	95th	119	120	121	123	124	125	126	79	79	79	80	81	82	82
	99th	127	127	128	130	131	132	133	86	86	87	88	88	89	90
13	50th	104	105	106	107	109	110	110	62	62	62	63	64	65	65
	90th	117	118	119	121	122	123	124	76	76	76	77	78	79	79
	95th	121	122	123	124	126	127	128	80	80	80	81	82	83	83
	99th	128	129	130	132	133	134	135	87	87	88	89	89	90	91
14	50th	106	106	107	109	110	111	112	63	63	63	64	65	66	66
	90th	119	120	121	122	124	125	125	77	77	77	78	79	80	80
	95th	123	123	125	126	127	129	129	81	81	81	82	83	84	84
	99th	130	131	132	133	135	136	136	88	88	89	90	90	91	92

(Continued)

TABLE 5.1
(CONTINUED)

Age, y	BP Percentile	SBP, mm Hg							DBP, mm Hg						
		Percentile of Height							Percentile of Height						
		5th	10th	25th	50th	75th	90th	95th	5th	10th	25th	50th	75th	90th	95th
15	50th	107	108	109	110	111	113	113	64	64	64	65	66	67	67
	90th	120	121	122	123	125	126	127	78	78	78	79	80	81	81
	95th	124	125	126	127	129	130	131	82	82	82	83	84	85	85
	99th	131	132	133	134	136	137	138	89	89	90	91	91	92	93
16	50th	108	108	110	111	112	114	114	64	64	65	66	66	67	68
	90th	121	122	123	124	126	127	128	78	78	79	80	81	81	82
	95th	125	126	127	128	130	131	132	82	82	83	84	85	85	86
	99th	132	133	134	135	137	138	139	90	90	90	91	92	93	93
17	50th	108	109	110	111	113	114	115	64	65	65	66	67	67	68
	90th	122	122	123	125	126	127	128	78	79	79	80	81	81	82
	95th	125	126	127	129	130	131	132	82	83	83	84	85	85	86
	99th	133	133	134	136	137	138	139	90	90	91	91	92	93	93

The 90th percentile is 1.28 SD, the 95th percentile is 1.645 SD, and the 99th percentile is 2.326 SD over the mean.
SBP, systolic blood pressure; DBP, diastolic blood pressure.

TABLE 5.2

BP LEVELS FOR BOYS BY AGE AND HEIGHT PERCENTILE

Age, y	BP Percentile	SBP, mm Hg							DBP, mm Hg						
		Percentile of Height							Percentile of Height						
		5th	10th	25th	50th	75th	90th	95th	5th	10th	25th	50th	75th	90th	95th
1	50th	80	81	83	85	87	88	89	34	35	36	37	38	39	39
	90th	94	95	97	99	100	102	103	49	50	51	52	53	53	54
	95th	98	99	101	103	104	106	106	54	54	55	56	57	58	58
	99th	105	106	108	110	112	113	114	61	62	63	64	65	66	66
2	50th	84	85	87	88	90	92	92	39	40	41	42	43	44	44
	90th	97	99	100	102	104	105	106	54	55	56	57	58	58	59
	95th	101	102	104	106	108	109	110	59	59	60	61	62	63	63
	99th	109	110	111	113	115	117	117	66	67	68	69	70	71	71
3	50th	86	87	89	91	93	94	95	44	44	45	46	47	48	48
	90th	100	101	103	105	107	108	109	59	59	60	61	62	63	63
	95th	104	105	107	109	110	112	113	63	63	64	65	66	67	67
	99th	111	112	114	116	118	119	120	71	71	72	73	74	75	75
4	50th	88	89	91	93	95	96	97	47	48	49	50	51	51	52
	90th	102	103	105	107	109	110	111	62	63	64	65	66	66	67
	95th	106	107	109	111	112	114	115	66	67	68	69	70	71	71
	99th	113	114	116	118	120	121	122	74	75	76	77	78	78	79
5	50th	90	91	93	95	96	98	98	50	51	52	53	54	55	55
	90th	104	105	106	108	110	111	112	65	66	67	68	69	69	70
	95th	108	109	110	112	114	115	116	69	70	71	72	73	74	74
	99th	115	116	118	120	121	123	123	77	78	79	80	81	81	82
6	50th	91	92	94	96	98	99	100	53	53	54	55	56	57	57
	90th	105	106	108	110	111	113	113	68	68	69	70	71	72	72
	95th	109	110	112	114	115	117	117	72	72	73	74	75	76	76
	99th	116	117	119	121	123	124	125	80	80	81	82	83	84	84
7	50th	92	94	95	97	99	100	101	55	55	56	57	58	59	59
	90th	106	107	109	111	113	114	115	70	70	71	72	73	74	74
	95th	110	111	113	115	117	118	119	74	74	75	76	77	78	78
	99th	117	118	120	122	124	125	126	82	82	83	84	85	86	86

(Continued)

TABLE 5.2
(CONTINUED)

Age, y	BP Percentile	SBP, mm Hg							DBP, mm Hg						
		Percentile of Height							Percentile of Height						
		5th	10th	25th	50th	75th	90th	95th	5th	10th	25th	50th	75th	90th	95th
8	50th	94	95	96	99	100	102	102	56	57	58	59	60	60	61
	90th	107	109	110	112	114	115	116	71	72	72	73	74	75	76
	95th	111	112	114	116	118	119	120	75	76	77	78	79	79	80
	99th	119	120	122	123	125	127	127	83	84	85	86	87	87	88
9	50th	95	96	98	100	102	103	104	57	58	59	60	61	61	62
	90th	109	110	112	114	115	117	118	72	73	74	75	76	76	77
	95th	113	114	116	118	119	121	121	76	77	78	79	80	81	81
	99th	120	121	123	125	127	128	129	84	85	86	87	88	88	89
10	50th	97	98	100	102	103	105	106	58	59	60	61	61	62	63
	90th	111	112	114	115	117	119	119	73	73	74	75	76	77	78
	95th	115	116	117	119	121	122	123	77	78	79	80	81	81	82
	99th	122	123	125	127	128	130	130	85	86	86	88	88	89	90
11	50th	99	100	102	104	105	107	107	59	59	60	61	62	63	63
	90th	113	114	115	117	119	120	121	74	74	75	76	77	78	78
	95th	117	118	119	121	123	124	125	78	78	79	80	81	82	82
	99th	124	125	127	129	130	132	132	86	86	87	88	89	90	90
12	50th	101	102	104	106	108	109	110	59	60	61	62	63	63	64
	90th	115	116	118	120	121	123	123	74	75	75	76	77	78	79
	95th	119	120	122	123	125	127	127	78	79	80	81	82	82	83
	99th	126	127	129	131	133	134	135	86	87	88	89	90	90	91
13	50th	104	105	106	108	110	111	112	60	60	61	62	63	64	64
	90th	117	118	120	122	124	125	126	75	75	76	77	78	79	79
	95th	121	122	124	126	128	129	130	79	79	80	81	82	83	83
	99th	128	130	131	133	135	136	137	87	87	88	89	90	91	91
14	50th	106	107	109	111	113	114	115	60	61	62	63	64	65	65
	90th	120	121	123	125	126	128	128	75	76	77	78	79	79	80
	95th	124	125	127	128	130	132	132	80	80	81	82	83	84	84
	99th	131	132	134	136	138	139	140	87	88	89	90	91	92	92
15	50th	109	110	112	113	115	117	117	61	62	63	64	65	66	66
	90th	122	124	125	127	129	130	131	76	77	78	79	80	80	81
	95th	126	127	129	131	133	134	135	81	81	82	83	84	85	85
	99th	134	135	136	138	140	142	142	88	89	90	91	92	93	93
16	50th	111	112	114	116	118	119	120	63	63	64	65	66	67	67
	90th	125	126	128	130	130	133	134	78	78	79	80	81	82	82
	95th	129	130	132	134	135	137	137	82	83	83	84	85	86	87
	99th	136	137	139	141	143	144	145	90	90	91	92	93	94	94
17	50th	114	115	116	118	120	121	122	65	66	66	67	68	69	70
	90th	127	128	130	132	134	135	136	80	80	81	82	83	84	84
	95th	131	132	134	136	138	139	140	84	85	86	87	87	88	89
	99th	139	140	141	143	145	146	147	92	93	93	94	95	96	97

The 90th percentile is 1.28 SD, the 95th percentile is 1.645 SD, and the 99th percentile is 2.326 SD over the mean.
SBP, systolic blood pressure; DBP, diastolic blood pressure.

TABLE 5.3

APGAR SCORE

Rating	0	1	2
Appearance	Pale or blue	Body pink, extremities blue	Pink all over
Pulse	Absent	100	100
Grimace	None	Weak	Strong
Activity (tone)	Limp	Some flexion	Spontaneous movement
Respiratory	Absent Hyproventilation	Weak cry, Hypoventilation	Coordinated effort, vigorous cry

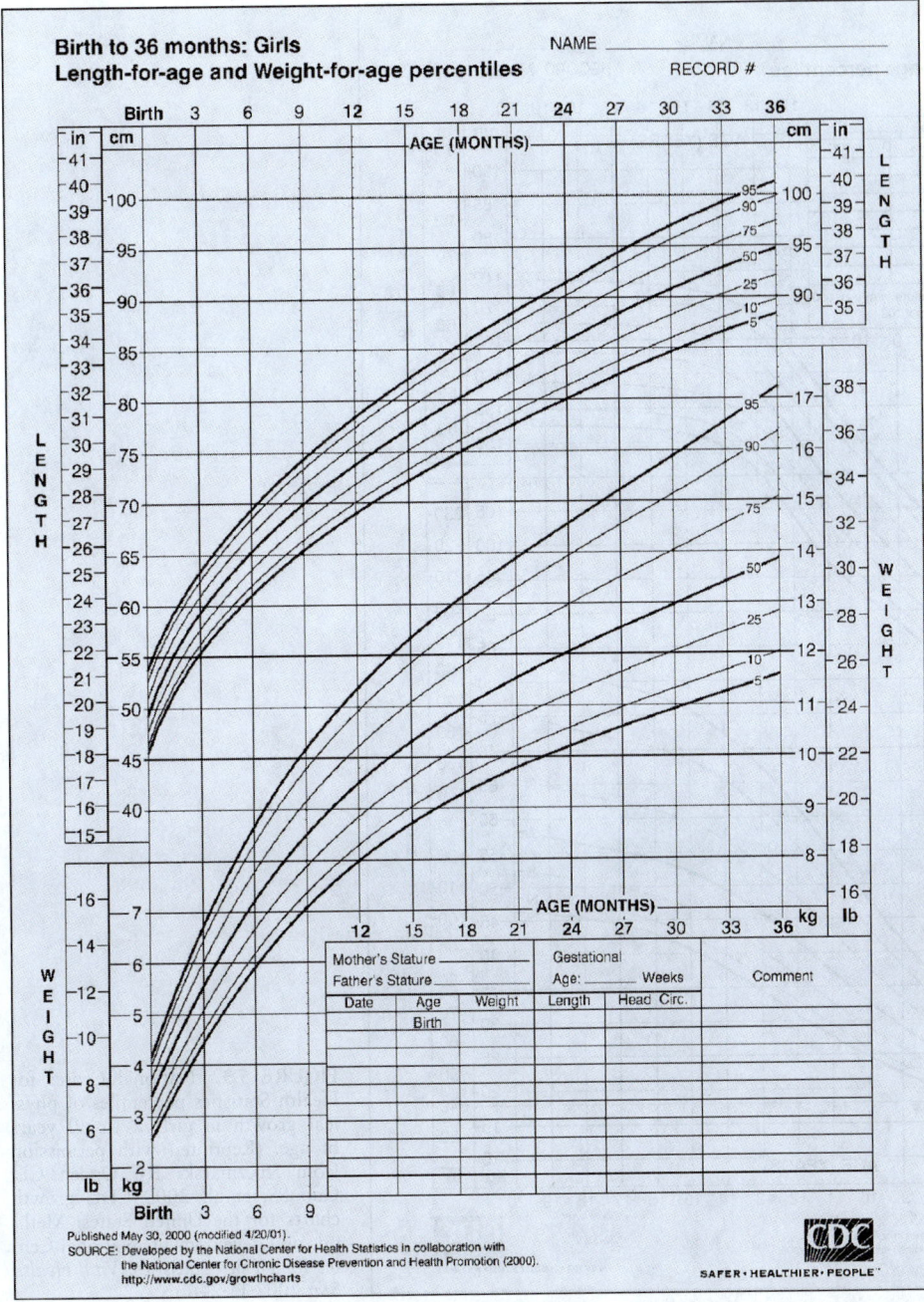

Birth to 36 months: Girls
Length-for-age and Weight-for-age percentiles

NAME _____

RECORD # _____

FIGURE 5.2. National Center for Health Statistics percentiles of physical growth in girls from birth to 36 months of age. (Reprinted with permission from Kuczmarski RJ, Ogden CL, Guo SS, et al. 2000 CDC growth charts for the United States: Methods and development. National Center for Health Statistics. *Vital Health Stat* 2002;11:246).

thereafter. Head circumference should be measured in all infants younger than 2 years and in those with misshapen heads, and measurements should be recorded with percentiles on a chart (Figs. 5.2 through 5.7).

Shortness may be caused by malnutrition, chronic illness, psychosocial deprivation, hormonal disorders, familial patterns, or syndromes with dwarfism. Gigantism may be the result of pituitary abnormalities. Compare sitting height and total height in dwarfs with standard measurements to determine the type of syndrome present.

Decreased weight can be caused by conditions similar to those that cause decreased height. In states of malnutrition, weight percentile is less than height percentile; head circumference remains normal unless the condition is severe and persists. Being overweight usually is exogenous and associated with increased height until epiphyseal closure. Being overweight as a result of endocrine disorders is associated with decreased linear growth.

Skin Fold Measurements

Skin fold measurements are useful in determining obesity and in identifying and following malnutrition. Skin fold calipers are applied over the mid triceps.

General Appearance

A statement should be recorded about the alertness, distress, general development, and nutrition of the child. Mental status, activity, unusual positions, or apprehension or cooperativeness may direct one to consider an acute or chronic illness or no illness at all. The child who lies quietly, staring into space, may be gravely ill. The child who lies quietly but becomes irritable when held by the mother (paradoxic irritability) may have meningitis or pain in motion. Note any unusual odor, which

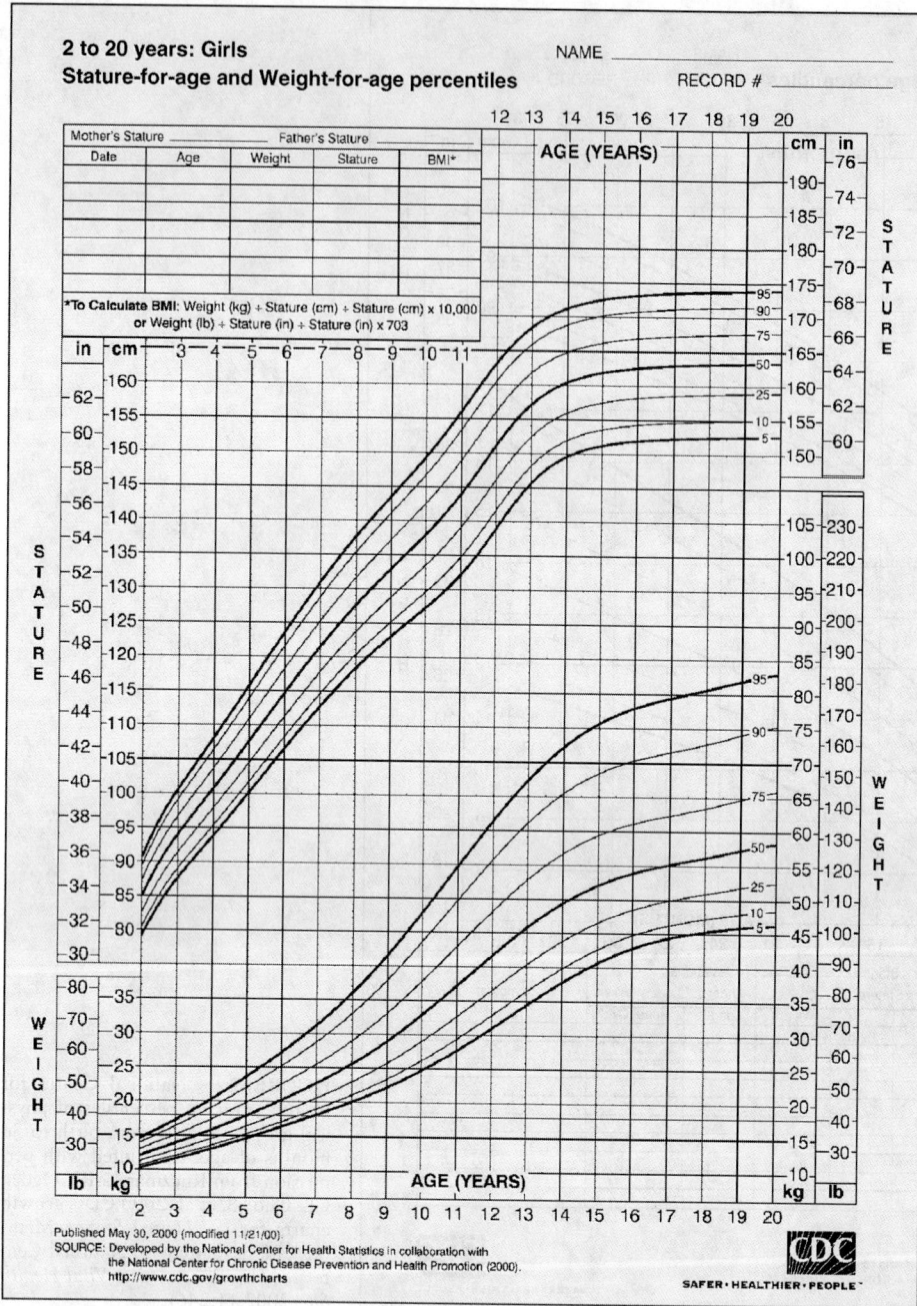

2 to 20 years: Girls
Stature-for-age and Weight-for-age percentiles

NAME _____

RECORD # _____

Mother's Stature _____ Father's Stature _____

Date	Age	Weight	Stature	BMI*

*To Calculate BMI: Weight (kg) ÷ Stature (cm) ÷ Stature (cm) x 10,000
or Weight (lb) ÷ Stature (in) ÷ Stature (in) x 703

AGE (YEARS)

Published May 30, 2000 (modified 11/21/00).
SOURCE: Developed by the National Center for Health Statistics in collaboration with
the National Center for Chronic Disease Prevention and Health Promotion (2000).
http://www.cdc.gov/growthcharts

CDC
SAFER • HEALTHIER • PEOPLE™

FIGURE 5.3. National Center for Health Statistics percentiles of physical growth in girls 2 to 20 years of age. (Reprinted with permission from Kuczmarski RJ, Ogden CL, Guo SS, et al. 2000 CDC growth charts for the United States: Methods and development. National Center for Health Statistics. *Vital Health Stat* 2002:11:246.)

may suggest the presence of a foreign body in one of the orifices or certain metabolic diseases or toxins.

Skin

In examining the skin, record its color and turgor, the type of any lesions, and the condition of body and scalp hair, and nails. The normal color of the skin is the result of the presence of melanin; depigmented areas are vitiligo; absence of pigment occurs in albinism. Cyanosis is caused by desaturation of or abnormal forms of hemoglobin; jaundice is caused by excessive bilirubin deposited in the adipose tissue. Note the size and borders of nevi, which usually are darkly pigmented areas, and café au lait spots, which are brownish areas that may signal neurofibromatosis. White spots shaped like a leaf suggest tuberous sclerosis. Ecchymoses or petechiae and scars may indicate abuse.

Swelling may be caused by edema. Lack of turgor occurs with dehydration or recent weight loss. Describe any rashes, many of which are characteristic of viral or bacterial infection.

Head and Face

Record the shape, symmetry, and any defects of the head; the distribution of hair; and the size and tension of the fontanelles. A large head may be an early sign of hydrocephalus or an intracranial mass. A small head may be the result of early closure of sutures or lack of brain development. For any deviation from normal head size, frequent measurements are necessary. The fontanelles normally are flat. The posterior fontanelle closes by 2 months of age, and the anterior fontanelle closes by 12 to 18 months of age. Unusual hair whorls are associated with severe intracranial abnormalities.

The face may appear distinctive for a number of syndromes. For example, unilateral facial paralysis may be associated with

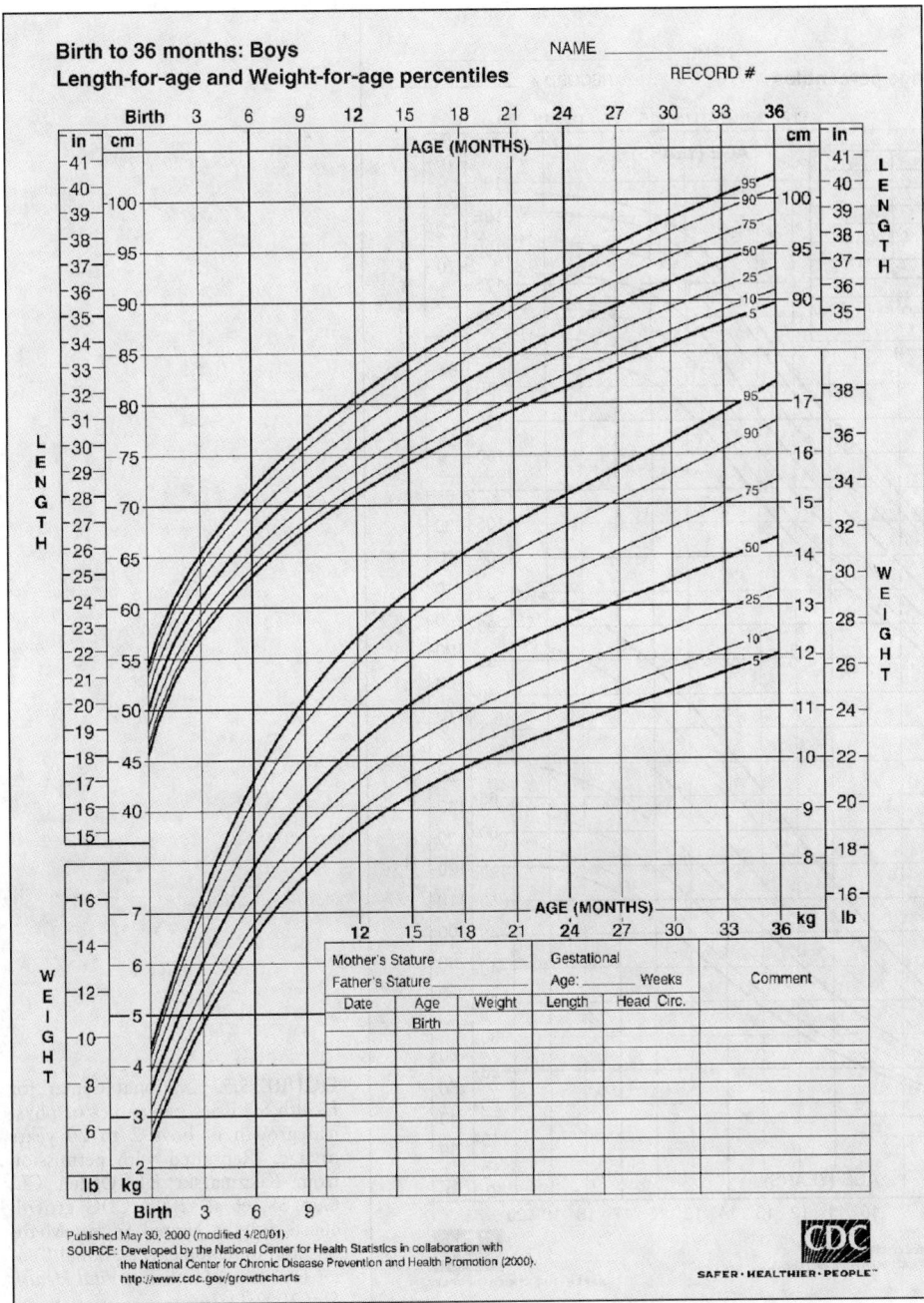

Birth to 36 months: Boys
Length-for-age and Weight-for-age percentiles

NAME _____
RECORD # _____

Published May 30, 2000 (modified 4/20/01).
SOURCE: Developed by the National Center for Health Statistics in collaboration with the National Center for Chronic Disease Prevention and Health Promotion (2000).
http://www.cdc.gov/growthcharts

SAFER · HEALTHIER · PEOPLE™

FIGURE 5.4. National Center for Health Statistics percentiles of physical growth in boys from birth to 36 months of age. (Reprinted with permission from Kuczmarski RJ, Ogden CL, Guo SS, et al. 2000 CDC growth charts for the United States: Methods and development. National Center for Health Statistics. *Vital Health Stat* 2002:11:246.)

congenital heart disease. Coarse facies occur with storage diseases. Epicanthal folds occur in a number of syndromes, including trisomy 21.

Eyes

Test vision grossly in the young child with brightly colored objects. In the older child, test with Snellen's E chart. Evaluate for strabismus by noting the position of the reflection of light on the cornea from a distant source. Evaluate the range of eye movements and the presence of nystagmus. Both eyelids should open equally. Failure to open is ptosis and may be caused by neurologic or systemic diseases. Upward slanting of the palpebral fissures with covering of the inner canthus (epicanthal folds) is a sign of Down syndrome. The conjunctivae should be pink, but not inflamed; the sclerae should be white. Examine the cornea for haziness (a sign of glaucoma) or opac-

ities. Record the size and shape of the pupils, the color of the iris, and the response of the iris to light and accommodation. In the funduscopic examination, use a zero lens and note the presence of a red reflex, or hemorrhages or pigmented areas, and the size of the veins compared to the arteries. Any obstruction, such as a corneal or lenticular cataract, will obliterate part or all of the red reflex. The disc borders should be sharp. They are blurred with increased intracranial pressure. The macula may not be clear, which is a sign of degenerative diseases. Obtain the corneal reflex by lightly touching the cornea with a piece of cotton. Failure to blink indicates trigeminal or facial nerve injury.

Ears

Note the position of the ears and abnormalities of the external ear, the pinna. Low-set ears may suggest the presence of renal agenesis. Tags and deformities frequently are associated with

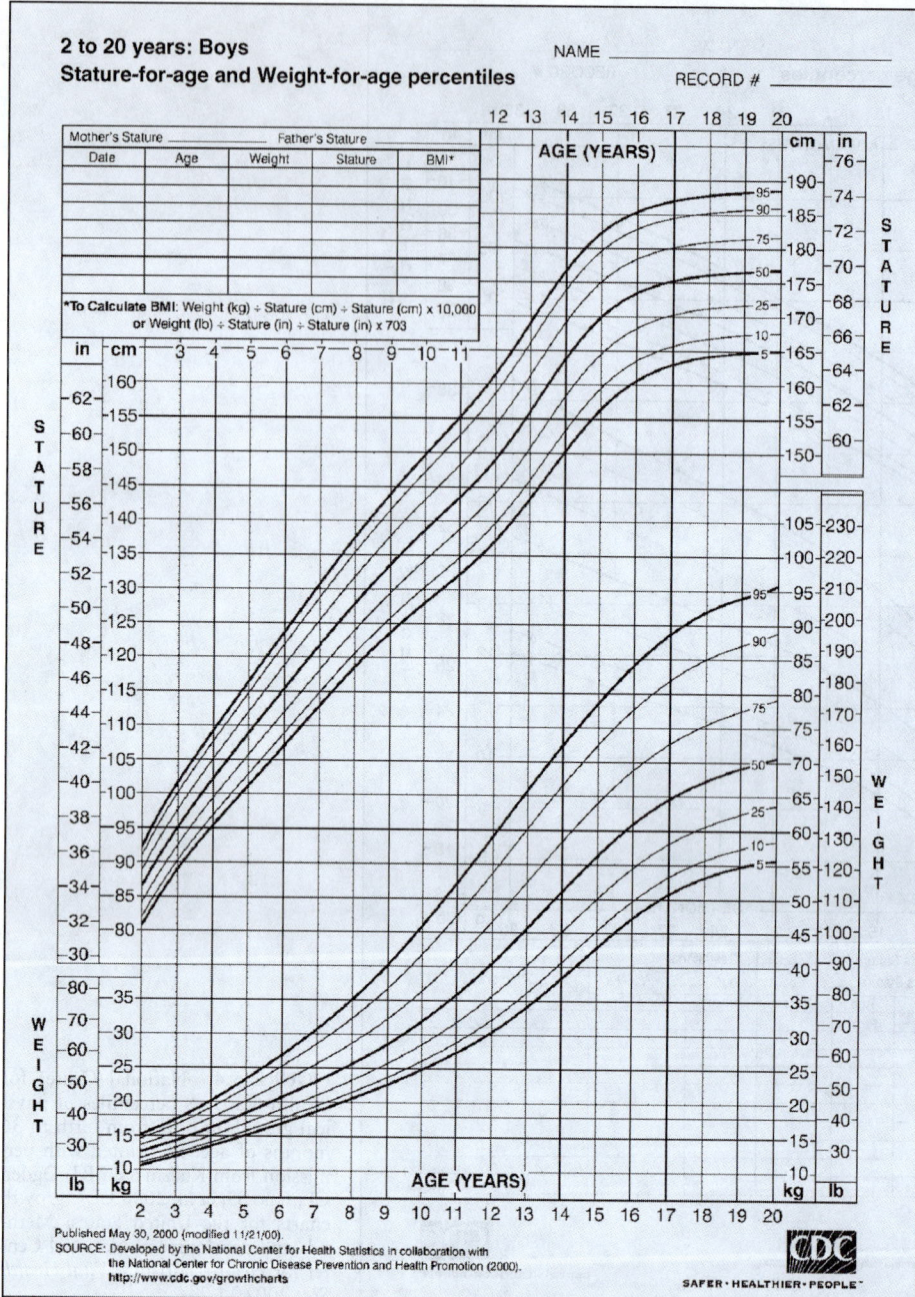

2 to 20 years: Boys
Stature-for-age and Weight-for-age percentiles

NAME _____

RECORD # _____

*To Calculate BMI: Weight (kg) ÷ Stature (cm) ÷ Stature (cm) x 10,000
or Weight (lb) ÷ Stature (in) ÷ Stature (in) x 703

Published May 30, 2000 (modified 11/21/00).
SOURCE: Developed by the National Center for Health Statistics in collaboration with
the National Center for Chronic Disease Prevention and Health Promotion (2000).
http://www.cdc.gov/growthcharts

FIGURE 5.5. National Center for Health Statistics percentiles of physical growth in boys 2 to 20 years of age. (Reprinted with permission from Kuczmarski RJ, Ogden CL, Guo SS, et al. 2000 CDC growth charts for the United States: Methods and development. National Center for Health Statistics. *Vital Health Stat* 2002:11:246.)

other minor or major anomalies. Grossly evaluate hearing, then proceed with examination of the inner ear. Pull the earlobe up and anteriorly. Grasp an otoscope equipped with a bright light so that the hand rests on the child's head and moves with any movement of the head, and use the largest speculum that will fit into the canal. The canal should be clear, and the drum should be pearly gray in color and concave. A cone of light, the malleus, and sometimes the incus can be identified. If the bones are not visualized, the drum is not gray in color or is infected, or the drum is not concave, fluid may be in the ear. Fill the canal firmly with the speculum and give a short burst of air. The tympanic membrane should move. Lack of motion suggests serous or purulent otitis media.

Nose

Raise the tip of the nose and look up the nose with a bright light. Record discharges, bleeding, or deformities of the septum. The normal nasal mucosa is light pink. Tap on the maxillary and frontal sinuses of older children to elicit tenderness. Feel for air egress from both nares.

Mouth and Throat

The young child usually is most resistant during examination of the mouth and throat, so this part of the examination should be performed near the end of the visit. The child should be sitting so that the tongue is less likely to obstruct the pharynx. Deformities or infections around the lips are recorded. Count the number and note the condition of the teeth. Similarly, note the condition and color of the tongue, buccal mucosa, palate, tonsils, and posterior pharynx. Normally, these are pink. Exudate indicates infection by bacteria, viruses, or fungi, but etiology usually cannot be determined by physical examination alone. Note also the presence of the gag reflex

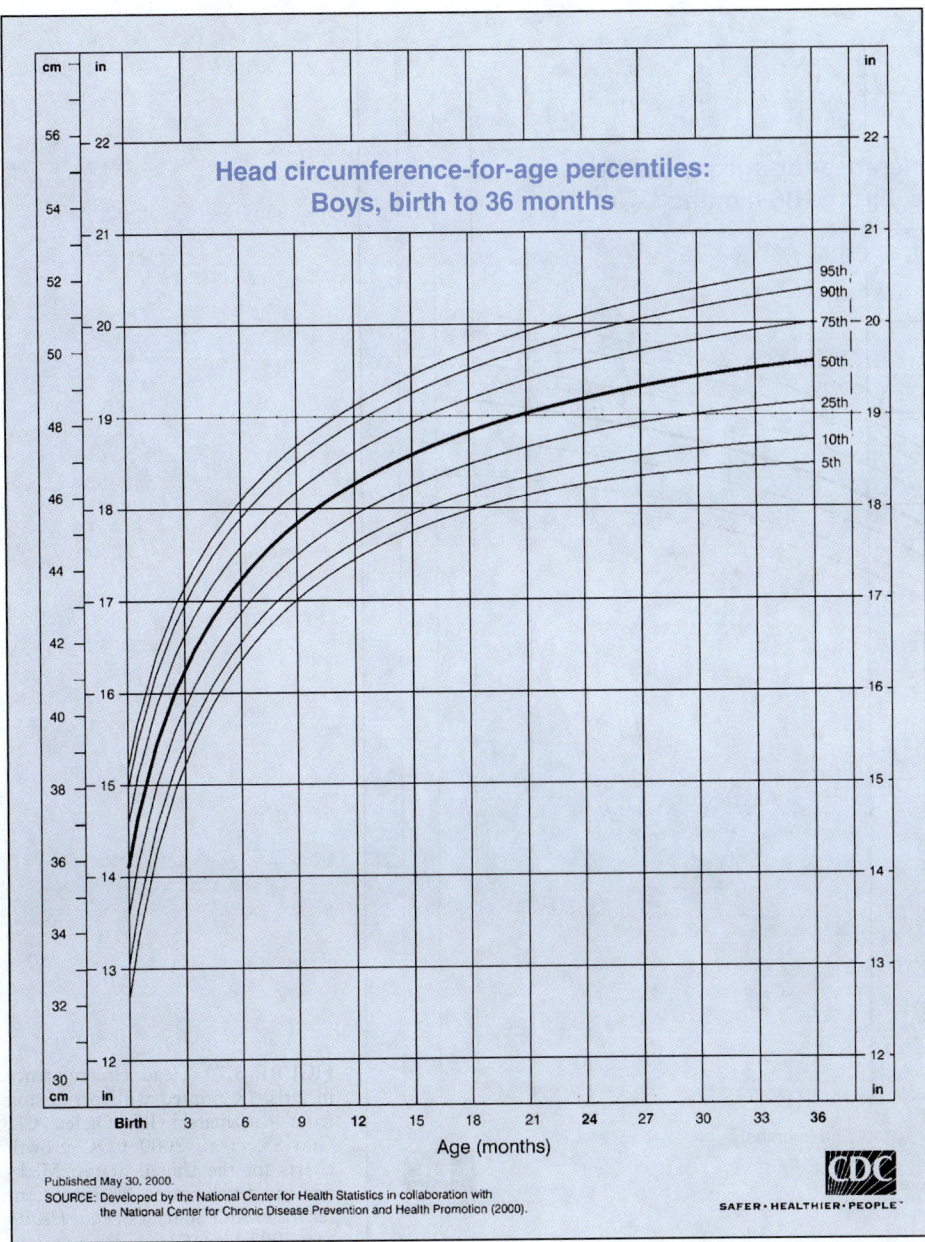

cm in

56 — 22
54 — 21
52 — 20
50
48 — 19
46 — 18
44
42 — 17
40 — 16
38 — 15
36 — 14
34
32 — 13
30 — 12
cm in
Birth 3 6 9 12 15 18 21 24 27 30 33 36

Head circumference-for-age percentiles:
Boys, birth to 36 months

in

22
21
20
19 — 95th
       90th
       75th — 20
       50th
       25th — 19
       10th
       5th
18
17
16
15
14
13
12
in

Age (months)

Published May 30, 2000.
SOURCE: Developed by the National Center for Health Statistics in collaboration with
the National Center for Chronic Disease Prevention and Health Promotion (2000).

CDC
SAFER · HEALTHIER · PEOPLE™

FIGURE 5.6. Head circumference in boys. (Reprinted with permission from Kuczmarski RJ, Ogden CL, Guo SS, et al. 2000 CDC growth charts for the United States: Methods and development. National Center for Health Statistics. *Vital Health Stat* 2002:11:246.)

and the voice or cry. If the child seems hoarse, question the parent concerning the normal voice. Laryngitis can lead to airway obstruction. After the age of 2 years, children should not drool. Chronic drooling may suggest mental deficiency, but acute onset of drooling is a grave sign of epiglottitis or poison ingestion.

Neck

Feel in the neck for lymph nodes, which normally are non-tender and up to 1 cm in diameter in both the anterior and posterior cervical triangles. Larger or tender nodes occur with local or systemic infection or malignancies. Feel the trachea in the midline. Feel for the thyroid. Other masses may be present and are always abnormal. Flex the neck. Resistance to flexion is a cardinal sign of meningitis, but this also occurs with severe infections around the neck or dislocation of the cervical vertebrae.

Lymph Nodes

In addition to the lymph nodes in the neck, palpate inguinal, epitrochlear, supraclavicular, axillary, and posterior occipital nodes. Normally, inguinal nodes may be up to 1 cm in diameter; the others are nonpalpable or less than 5 mm. Larger or tender nodes hold significance similar to that described for abnormal cervical glands.

Chest

Observe the chest for shape and symmetry. The chest wall is almost round in infancy and in children with obstructive lung disease. Respirations are predominantly abdominal until about 6 years of age, when they become thoracic. Note suprasternal, intercostal, and subcostal retractions, which are signs of increased respiratory work. Swelling at the costochondral junctions is an indication of rickets. Edema of the chest wall occurs in children with superior vena cava obstruction. Asymmetry

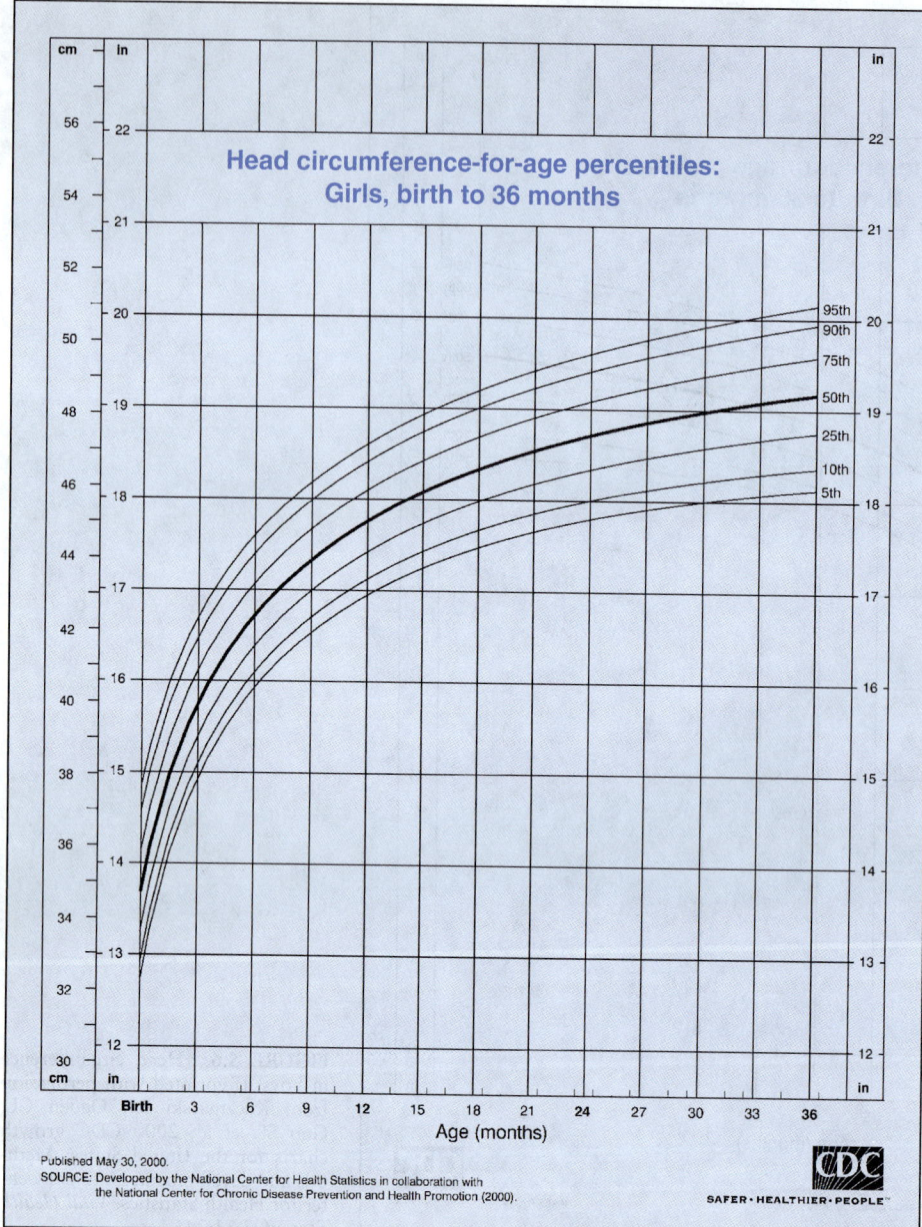

Published May 30, 2000.
SOURCE: Developed by the National Center for Health Statistics in collaboration with
the National Center for Chronic Disease Prevention and Health Promotion (2000).

FIGURE 5.7. Head circumference in girls. (Reprinted with permission from Kuczmarski RJ, Ogden CL, Guo SS, et al. 2000 CDC growth charts for the United States: Methods and development. National Center for Health Statistics. *Vital Health Stat* 2002:11:246.)

of expansion occurs with diaphragmatic paralysis, pneumothorax, or other intrathoracic abnormalities.

Breasts

Breasts normally are hypertrophied at birth; they regress within 6 months and develop with the onset of puberty. Development during adolescence is staged. Breast development in both boys and girls usually begins asymmetrically. Palpate for nodules, which may be cysts or tumors. Redness, heat, and tenderness usually indicate infection.

Lungs

An examination of the lungs includes observation, palpation, percussion, auscultation and, if indicated, transillumination.

Observation

Note the type and rate of the child's breathing. The rate of respiration varies, as described previously. Rapid rates, known as *tachypnea*, are associated with infection, fever, excitement, ex-

ercise, heart failure, or intoxicants. Slower rates are characteristic of intracranial lesions, depression caused by sedative drugs, heart block, or alkalosis. Cheyne-Stokes breathing, which is characterized by periods of deep, rapid respirations followed by slow, shallow respirations, is common in premature and newborn infants, and in those with intracranial or metabolic abnormalities. Dyspnea, or distress during breathing, is associated with flaring of the intercostal spaces and nares. Inspiratory dyspnea is more common with obstruction high in the respiratory system, and expiratory dyspnea is more common with lower respiratory diseases.

Palpation

Feel the entire chest with the palms and fingertips. Note masses or areas of tenderness. Tactile fremitus, a vibratory sensation during crying or speaking, normally is felt over the entire chest. Fremitus is absent if the airway is obstructed.

Percussion

Either direct percussion (tapping the chest wall directly with either the index or middle fingers) or indirect percussion (placing a finger of one hand firmly on the chest wall and tapping that finger with the index or middle finger of the opposite hand) may be used. Percuss the entire chest wall anteriorly, posteriorly, and along the midaxillary line. A resonant sound is obtained over most of the chest except over the scapulae, diaphragm, liver, and heart, where dullness is elicited. Dullness detects consolidation in the lungs, as well as the size and position of the liver and heart. Scratch percussion, which involves tapping the chest wall with a finger while listening with a bell stethoscope over the heart and liver, is especially useful in determining heart and liver size. Increased resonance is found with increased trapped air, emphysema, or air in the pleural space (pneumothorax).

Auscultation

To auscultate the lungs in children, listen with a small bell in small children and with the diaphragm in older children. Normal breath sounds are bronchovesicular and inspiration is twice as long as expiration in young children; breath sounds are vesicular and inspiration is three times as long as expiration in older children. Breath sounds are decreased with consolidation or pleural fluid in the young child and increased with pneumonia in the older child. Fine crackles either in inspiration or expiration (rales) indicate foreign substances, usually fluid, in the alveoli or smaller bronchi, as occurs in bronchitis, pneumonia, or heart failure. Coarse extraneous sounds (rhonchi) are the result of foreign substances in the larger airways, as in crying or upper respiratory infection. Musical extraneous sounds (wheezes) are caused by air flow through compromised larger airways, as in asthma.

Transillumination

If pneumothorax is present, the chest can be transilluminated. This test is especially useful in the newborn.

Heart

In addition to the heart's rate (pulse) and rhythm, and the blood pressure, note the size, shape, sound quality, and presence of murmurs when examining the heart. Precordial bulging is a sign of right-sided enlargement. A cardiac impulse may not be noted in a young child, but in a thin, active child, it may suggest the size and position of the heart. An apex beat outside the midclavicular line in the fifth interspace indicates cardiomegaly, which is a significant sign of heart disease or heart failure. Palpation and percussion were described previously. Auscultate both in the sitting and the supine positions. Determine the heart rate and rhythm if this was not done previously. Auscultate initially over the apex (mitral area), then over the lower right sternal border (tricuspid area), second left intercostal space at the sternal edge (pulmonary area), and second right intercostal space at the sternal edge (aortic area). Next, proceed to the remainder of the precordium, axillae, back, and neck. Note heart sounds and any arrhythmia. A loud first sound at the apex occurs with mitral stenosis, a loud second sound at the pulmonary area occurs with pulmonary hypertension, and a fixed split-second sound in the pulmonary area occurs with an atrial septal defect. Innocent murmurs are systolic, musical, or vibratory and of low intensity, and usually are heard at the third left interspace, just inside the apex, or beneath either clavicle. The latter is a venous hum that may be continuous and that disappears when the patient is supine. Diastolic murmurs almost always are significant. Significant systolic murmurs may be stenotic and are loudest in midsystolic over the aortic or pulmonary areas. Regurgitant murmurs begin immediately after the first sound. Over the mitral or tricuspid area, they indicate valvular insufficiency. A continuous or uneven systolic murmur along the upper left sternal border indicates patent ductus arteriosus.

Abdomen

Observe the shape and tone of the abdomen. A distended abdomen may indicate intestinal obstruction or ascites; a board-like abdominal wall may indicate intraabdominal disease. Auscultate before percussing or palpating. Normally, peristaltic sounds are heard every 10 to 30 seconds. High-pitched frequent sounds occur with obstruction or peritonitis; absent sounds indicate ileus. Next, palpate gently, beginning in the left lower quadrant and proceeding to the left upper, right upper, right lower, and midline areas. Then palpate more deeply in the same areas and follow with palpation in the same areas with the unused hand, pushing toward the front hand from the child's back. Feel especially for the liver in the right upper quadrant and the spleen in the left upper quadrant, and estimate their size. Any other masses are abnormal. Transilluminate other masses to distinguish cystic from solid masses. Determine tenderness and attempt to locate the maximum point of any tenderness, which may indicate intraabdominal infection such as peritonitis, cystitis, or appendicitis, or rapid enlargement of organs, as occurs with enlargement of the liver in heart failure. Percuss to verify findings. Feel in the costovertebral angles to determine kidney size. Tenderness here usually indicates pyelonephritis. Percuss or palpate the bladder for size and tenderness.

Genitalia

A child's stage of pubertal development is estimated from the presence of pubic hair, examination of the genitalia, as well as other features of sexual development (see Chapter 89). Average adolescent development in girls proceeds as follows: breast development after 8 years of age, pubic hair after 12 years of age, increase in height velocity after 12 years of age, and menarche and axillary hair after 13 years of age. Average development in boys proceeds as follows: testicular enlargement at 11.5 years of age, pubic hair at 12.5 years of age, increase in height velocity at 14 years of age, and facial and axillary hair at 14.5 years of age. Variations in order of development suggest hormonal abnormalities. Modesty of the child should be respected during the examination, especially of the breasts and genitalia.

Inspect the genitalia for urethral discharges, which are always pathologic and indicate infection anywhere in the genitourinary system.

In a girl, vaginal bleeding after the newborn period and before puberty may be the result of injury or a foreign body. Fused labia minora usually part with hygiene. Imperforate hymen causes hydrocolpos before puberty and hematocolpos after menarche. Vaginal discharge may be the result of injury or a foreign body in a young girl, usually is normal at the start of puberty, and suggests infection in an older girl. Adolescents with vaginal discharge, dysuria, lower abdominal pain, irregular bleeding, or sexual activity require a complete vaginal examination. The uterus in a younger child is palpated for size, shape, and tenderness with one hand over the lower abdomen and a finger of the other hand in the rectum. For an older child, the cervix is visualized with a vaginoscope or small speculum, and cultures are obtained.

In boys, testes should be in the scrotum after birth, although active cremasteric reflexes may empty the scrotum temporarily. The meatal opening should be slitlike and the urinary stream should be strong. Hydroceles, which do not reduce and do transilluminate, and hernias, which reduce but do not transilluminate, enlarge the scrotum. Testicular tenderness suggests torsion of the testis or epididymitis.

Rectum

Inspect the anus for fissures, inflammation, or lack of tone. The latter may indicate child abuse. The rectum is not examined routinely but is examined in all children with abdominal or gastrointestinal complaints, including diarrhea, constipation, or bleeding from the rectum.

Extremities and Back

Asymmetry, anomalies, unusual size, pain, tenderness, heat, and swelling deformities of the extremities and back must be distinguished from congenital malformations, osteomyelitis, cellulitis, myositis or, rarely, rickets and scurvy. Joint heat, tenderness, swelling, effusion, redness, and limitation or pain on motion may indicate arthritis, arthralgia, synovitis or injury, or septic arthritis (which is a medical emergency). Observe the child walking and look for the presence of a limp. Clubbing of the fingers is a sign of chronic hypoxemia, as in congenital heart or chronic pulmonary diseases.

The spine should be straight, with mild lumbar lordosis. Kyphosis, scoliosis, masses, tenderness, limitation of motion, spina bifida, pilonidal dimples, tufts of hair, or cysts may be caused by injury, malformation, infections, or tumors.

Weakness, tenderness, or paresis of the muscles suggests inflammatory muscle disease, congenital or metabolic neuromuscular diseases, or central nervous system abnormalities.

Neurologic Examination

Mental status and orientation help determine the acuteness of a child's illness, depending on the environmental conditions. Position at rest and abnormal movements such as tremors, twitchings, choreiform movements, and athetosis are characteristic of hyperirritability of the central nervous system. Incoordination of gait usually indicates cerebellar dysfunction. Kernig sign (inability to extend the leg with the hip flexed) and Brudzinski sign (flexing the neck with resultant flexion of the hip or knee) are indications of meningeal irritation.

Cranial nerves can be tested. Dysfunction of olfactory nerve I results in anosmia. Dysfunction of the trigeminal nerve V results in lack of sensation of the face and tongue. Ask the child to smile. With peripheral facial nerve VII paralysis, neither the forehead nor the face moves. With nuclear VII paralysis, the forehead moves. Difficulty in swallowing and loss of pharyngeal reflexes are caused by dysfunction of the glossopharyngeal nerve IX or the vagus nerve X. Patients cannot contract the sternocleidomastoid or trapezius muscles with involvement of the spinal accessory nerve XI. The tongue protrudes to the involved side with hypoglossal nerve XII lesions.

An examination of tendon reflexes (biceps, triceps, patellar, and Achilles) is less important than is observation of general activity. Hyperactive reflexes indicate an upper motor neuron lesion or hypocalcemia. Decreased reflexes are seen in lower motor neuron lesions or the muscular dystrophies.

NEWBORN EXAMINATION

(See Chapter 23 for a more complete discussion of the examination and management of the newborn.)

In the delivery room, a minimal examination is needed. The general appearance is noted and, at 1 and 5 minutes of age, an Apgar score is assigned (Table 5.1). A score of 7 or less indicates that an infant is at risk.

The infant is placed in a warmer. A small catheter is passed through both nares. Secretions are aspirated, and the tube is continued into the stomach and the stomach contents are aspirated. Easy passage of the catheter indicates patency of both nares. Passage into the stomach obviates blind pouch types of tracheoesophageal fistulas. The infant may urinate or defecate, indicating patency of these orifices. The mouth is inspected for cleft palate. Gestational age is assessed based on neurodevelopmental signs. Newborn care then is given and further examination is deferred to the nursery.

Preferably within the first few hours of birth, an admission newborn examination is performed in the presence of the parents. Develop a routine for the newborn examination so that critical areas are never omitted. In the first few hours of life, newborns usually are awake, but after 4 hours, they may be sleepy. The pressing question to be answered in the first examination is, "Is my child normal?" Although the order of the examination may vary, as with the history, initiate an order of recording for easy retrieval of information if it is needed later.

Vital Signs

Vital signs include temperature, heart rate, respiratory rate, blood pressure (using an apparatus for newborns) in an upper and a lower extremity, weight, length, and head, chest, and abdominal circumferences. In addition to recording these, it is essential that they also be plotted on a chart (see Figs. 5.2 and 5.4).

General Appearance

Within a few moments, observe the movement of the four extremities, the appearance of the head and neck, body symmetry, and any gross abnormalities.

Skin

The skin may be covered by a white, greasy, easily removable material, the vernix caseosa. Note skin color, consistency, and hydration. Cyanosis, jaundice, eruptions, edema, bruises, petechiae, and pallor are significant abnormalities. Note also hemangiomas and nevi, their size and location. Mongolian (brown) spots over the back are not suggestive of disease, but café au lait spots, if they are numerous, may be a cardinal sign of neurofibromatosis. Papules and pustules must be identified as either normal eruptions or infections.

Head and Neck

The fontanelle size and head circumference are variable on the first day because of molding. Scalp edema (caput succedaneum) crosses the midline and may be present; this is distinguished from cephalhematoma, which does not cross the midline and is caused by subperiosteal bleeding. Unusual facies suggests dysmorphic syndromes. Peripheral facial nerve palsies are common. Edema of the eyelids is a result of birth processes or reaction to silver nitrate prophylaxis. Subconjunctival and retinal hemorrhages are found frequently. Red reflex from the fundus, if not visible, indicates some obstruction in the preretinal chambers. Malformation of the pinnae of the ears often is accompanied by severe congenital malformations. If the nose was not found to be patent in the first examination, reexamine by passing a catheter through both nares. Reexamine the mouth for cleft palate. Examine the neck for shortening (as in Klippel-Feil syndrome), redundant skin folds (as in gonadal dysgenesis), vertebral anomalies, cysts, sinuses, and limitation of motion (torticollis).

Chest

The chest normally is barrel-shaped and smooth at birth, and expands symmetrically with no retractions. Unequal expansion or asymmetry suggests intrathoracic pathology such as cardiac enlargement, pneumothorax, or diaphragmatic hernia. The respiratory rate normally is less than 60 breaths per minute. Occasional irregularities with apnea up to 10 seconds can be normal. Auscultation may reveal adventitious sounds for the first 4 to 6 hours. Percussion is resonant throughout. Maximal cardiac impulse is felt in the fourth interspace close to the sternum. Thrills, if they are present, usually indicate cardiac abnormalities. Murmurs are present in 60% of normal newborns, but the lack of a murmur does not eliminate a diagnosis of congenital heart disease. Brachial and femoral pulses, if they are not of equal intensity, suggest vascular anomalies such as coarctation of the aorta. If chest expansion is unequal, transilluminate the chest. Transillumination can be detected with pneumothorax and occasionally with diaphragmatic hernia.

Abdomen

Distention of the abdomen occurs with sepsis, intestinal or urinary system obstruction, ascites, tumors, or pneumoperitoneum. Scaphoid abdomen suggests a diaphragmatic hernia. Palpate gently. The liver's edge usually is felt 1 to 2 cm below the costal margin and the spleen tip is barely palpable. The bladder, if it is palpable, should be reexamined after voiding. Palpation of the costovertebral angle with ballottement helps to determine the size of the kidneys. The umbilical cord contains two arteries, which are small and thick walled, and one vein, which is larger and thin walled. A single umbilical artery is associated with an increased incidence of congenital anomalies. Erythema at the base of the cord suggests omphalitis. Note the patency of the urethral meatus by observing voiding and the patency of the anus either by observing the passage of meconium or by inserting a small rubber catheter.

Extremities

Asymmetric posturing requires careful palpation of the clavicles, shoulders, and extremities for fractures or brachial plexus injuries. Anomalies of the hands and feet such as webbing, polydactyly, and clubfoot are noted. Abduct both legs to determine any limitation of movement or instability of the hips, which is characteristic of dysplasia.

Genitalia

Testes normally are in the scrotum of term infants. Determine the position and size of the urethral meatus. The newborn's penis is longer than 2 cm. An enlarged clitoris can be confused with a small penis and requires evaluation for chromosomal sex and other abnormalities of the genitourinary system. The vaginal opening is inspected, and mucosal tags, imperforate hymen, and ambiguous genitalia are sought. A small amount of bleeding from the vagina in infant girls can be normal and is a result of the influence of maternal hormones.

Neurologic Examination

Assess muscle tone and strength. Extremities normally recoil spontaneously when they are extended from a flexed position and thrash about when they are irritated. Moro reflex, which is obtained by loud noise or sudden motion, involves abduction of the upper arms and legs, and extension at the elbows and knees, followed by flexion. Absence of this reflex indicates central nervous system depression. Asymmetry suggests extremity fracture or peripheral nerve injury.

Suggested Readings

Apgar V. A proposal for a new method of evaluation of the newborn infant. *Curr Res Anesth Analg* 1963;32:260.

Zitelli BJ, Davis HW. *Atlas of pediatric physical diagnosis*, 4th ed. Philadelphia: Mosby, 2002.

CHAPTER 6 ■ DIAGNOSTIC PROCESS

FRANK A. OSKI* AND JANE A. OSKI

This chapter on the diagnostic process was written for the first edition of this textbook in 1989. While the content of the essay is essentially timeless, a new edition of a textbook necessitates a re-examination of even the most classical elements. When the first edition appeared, the polymerase chain reaction (PCR) was an evolving laboratory technique, genetic testing was in its infancy, and magnetic resonance imaging (MRI) was just beginning to demonstrate its power to noninvasively study the human body. None of these current realities would have significantly altered Frank Oski's central thesis regarding the physician's role in the diagnostic process. What follows is an attempt to leave the message unchanged while appropriately updating statistical data and diagnostic trends in pediatric medicine.

Diagnosis is one of the most important tasks of the clinician. Problem solving in medicine has been described, somewhat cynically, as "the process of making adequate decisions with inadequate information." If the diagnosis is correct and treatment is available, proper care usually follows. If no specific treatment is available, correct diagnosis is still important, because it provides a basis for prognosis and advice to patients or parents.

The need for a logical approach to medical diagnosis is vitally important to the economy of the United States, where health costs account for more than 10% of the gross national

*Deceased

product. Former U.S. Secretary of Health, Education, and Welfare Joseph A. Califano once observed that "the physician is the central decision maker for more than 70% of health care services." Despite extensive changes in the management of health care resources over the past two decades, the physician remains the principal decision maker. These decisions include that for hospitalization, duration of hospitalization, medications administered, and diagnostic tests used.

BASIC APPROACHES TO DIAGNOSIS

The cognitive processes used in making a diagnosis are not fully understood. Perhaps nowhere else in medicine do the art and science of medicine blend as imperceptibly as they do in the process of making a diagnosis. Physicians use four basic approaches to reach a diagnosis: pattern recognition, sampling the universe, clinical algorithms, and hypothesis generation.

Pattern Recognition

Pattern recognition is the process by which a diagnosis is made based on physical clues or linkage identification. For example, a diagnosis of Down syndrome can be made by recognizing the physical findings that make up this genetic abnormality. Similarly, the diagnosis of Henoch-Schönlein purpura is immediately apparent if the rash has a characteristic pattern and distribution. Diagnosis by pattern identification requires familiarity with diseases through experience or study. The expression "the more you see, the more you know, and the more you know, the more you see" describes how pattern recognition develops.

Linkage identification is a form of pattern recognition. A diagnosis is based on history and physical or laboratory findings. For example, the finding of a micropenis and hypoglycemia in a neonate would result in a prompt diagnosis of congenital hypopituitarism. A history of bloody diarrhea in association with a white blood cell count demonstrating more band forms than mature polymorphonuclear leukocytes would result in an immediate diagnosis of Shigella gastroenteritis. Skill in linkage identification, like pattern recognition, is gained by observation and study. The seemingly intuitive diagnosis, often the hallmark of the older physician, is usually a result of linkage identification.

Sampling the Universe

Sampling the universe refers to the inappropriate ordering of laboratory studies in hopes that an abnormality will appear that can result in a diagnosis. This is a diagnostic process to be decried. In the United States, approximately $30 billion per year are spent on laboratory tests representing approximately 3.5% of total health care spending, and another $2.8 billion per year are spent on chest roentgenography alone. Computed axial tomography (CAT) scans, MRI, and diagnostic ultrasounds are rapidly eclipsing the costs of laboratory studies and, according to many critics of the trend, are replacing the physical exam. An estimated 20% to 60% of these tests are unnecessary. If the estimates are accurate, a minimum of $6 to $18 billion per year are spent on procedures that do not aid in the diagnosis or treatment of illness. As the number of new tests available constantly increases, so will the amount spent on those that are inappropriately ordered. Laboratory tests should be obtained only to support a hypothesis. If the history and physical diagnosis do not suggest an underlying organic disorder, no rationale exists for ordering a battery of laboratory tests in an attempt to uncover an occult disease. As any practitioner who has been guilty of overdoing test order-

ing can vouch, one runs the risk of obtaining a questionable result on any number of laboratory evaluations that can then generate an additional mindless search for an answer to a diagnostically insignificant question. The evaluation of infants and children with failure to thrive is an example of this form of behavior. In a classic 1978 review of 2,607 laboratory studies performed on 185 patients with failure to thrive, Sills found that only 1.4% of the tests were of any positive diagnostic assistance, and all of them were specifically indicated by the history or physical examination. More recent studies on failure to thrive both confirm and uphold the observation that most patients with failure to thrive require very little laboratory evaluation.

Clinical Algorithms

A clinical algorithm is a protocol, presented as a flow chart, that contains branch points requiring decisions. The clinical algorithm enables the user to reach a diagnosis. The clinical algorithm is a byproduct of computer science and is based on the belief that the medical diagnostic process can be automated. A number of clinical situations have been adapted successfully to algorithms, but the majority have not. An example of a clinical algorithm is depicted in Figure 6.1.

Early algorithms were comprehensive and required many laboratory tests and physical findings. Many of these procedures were found to be unnecessary, and algorithms were simplified. An algorithm is not merely a list of symptoms or diagnostic procedures, but a logical flow chart or decision table that helps clinicians make decisions. They often require a precise yes or no answer; not all clinical questions can be answered so crisply. "Maybe" or any other vague answer blocks the progression in the typical algorithm. Algorithms have not been developed for every clinical situation or patient complaint. Algorithms are not yet a substitute for decision analysis or hypothesis generation in the establishment of a diagnosis.

The emergence of clinical practice guidelines and evidence-based medicine holds out the promise of streamlining our approach to the diagnosis of selected diseases. Because the development of these guidelines requires a systematic review of sufficient numbers of studies to generate clinically useful analyses of the accuracy of diagnostic tests, there will inevitably be a considerable lag time between the availability of a new test and a thorough evaluation of its sensitivity, specificity, and predictive value.

Hypothesis Generation

Hypothesis generation—the development of possible explanations for the patient's problem—is the most common and intellectually satisfying technique for arriving at a diagnosis. The development of hypotheses distinguishes the problem-solving process from mere data collection. The stockpiling of facts without a hypothesis has been likened to baseball statisticians with a great number of facts at hand but no way of determining what the facts really mean.

Hypotheses, or potential diagnoses, are generated early in patient encounters. Studies demonstrate that the competent physician begins to generate hypotheses the moment the chief complaint is heard. The generation of hypotheses continues as the remainder of the history unfolds. These hypotheses guide further inquiry. This immediate hypothesis generation directly contradicts the conventional strategy taught to medical students, which is to defer all hypotheses until history taking and physical examination are completed.

Many physicians use a common strategy to analyze presenting complaints. Initially, they interpret complaints anatomically; next, they interpret complaints physiologically; and finally, they interpret major symptoms pathophysiologically.

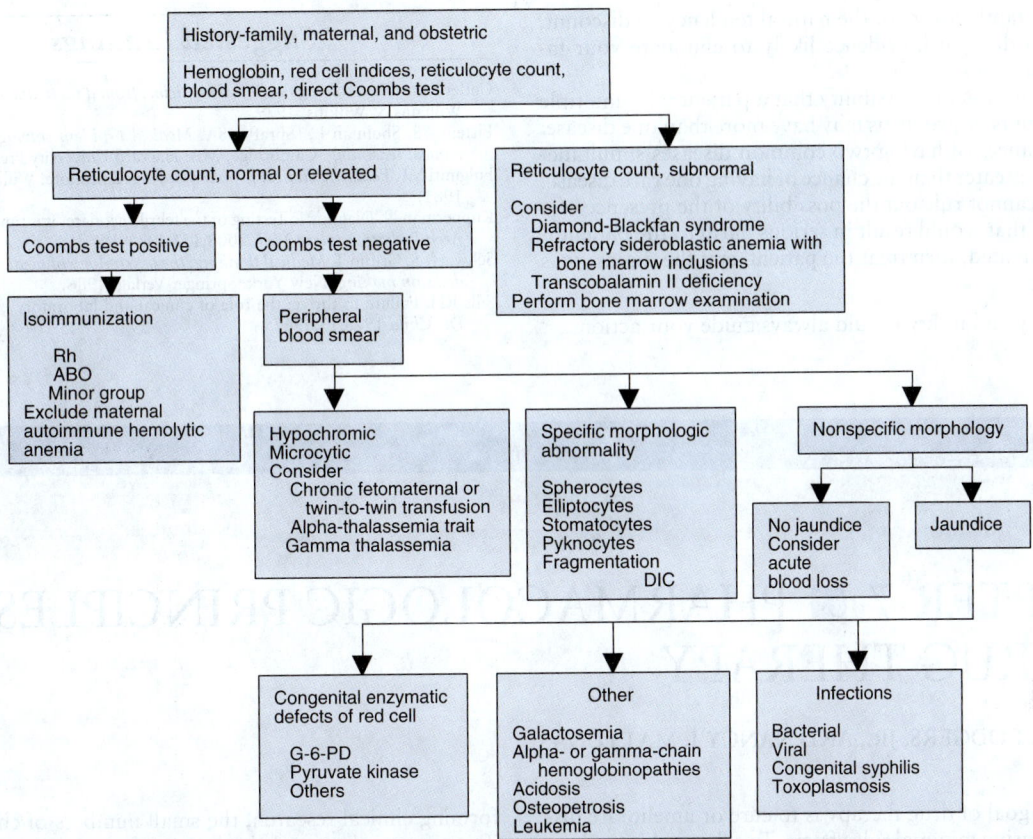

FIGURE 6.1. An approach to the differential diagnosis of anemia in the newborn. DIC, disseminated intravascular coagulation; G6PD, glucose 6-phosphate dehydrogenase. (Reprinted with permission from Oski FA, Naiman JL. *Hematologic problems of the newborn.* Philadelphia: Saunders, 1982:72.)

Fulginiti lists seven principles used to establish a clinical hypothesis:

- Common diseases and conditions occur commonly.
- A single process should be invoked to explain most of the data, if not all of it.
- Simple problems usually have simple explanations.
- Hypotheses should derive from the data and not be imposed on them.
- The hypothesis should be consistent with known pathophysiologic mechanisms.
- Serious consideration of an individual hypothesis should be based on its probability.
- Hypotheses may be formulated, accepted, rejected, or modified at any point in the course of problem solving.

Research reveals that competent physicians tend to generate hypotheses the moment the chief complaint is heard. The same research demonstrates that a limited number of hypotheses are entertained simultaneously. More than five hypotheses usually are not actively retained, and never are more than seven considered. Investigation often is limited to those hypotheses that survive revisions that occur while the history and physical examination are performed. Several things can go wrong: The physician may retain hypotheses that are too general and often not easily tested; facts and findings may be ignored because they are inconsistent with a hypothesis; and physicians may be loath to generate new hypotheses after the initial list is formulated, and equally loath to discard an existing one. The human mind needs to perceive problems as having limited degrees of complexity. We oversimplify by assigning new information to existing hypotheses rather than forming new

hypotheses, even when the information does not fit. The labeling of a condition as atypical or as a form fruste is an example of the parsimony of the human mind and is responsible for the slow recognition of new diseases.

SUGGESTED GUIDELINES FOR ESTABLISHING A DIAGNOSIS

- Always think of a number of diagnostic possibilities that are compatible with the chief complaint or the initial physical findings. Always consider the most common diagnosis first, but always include among your diagnoses those conditions, no matter how rare, for which treatment is available and which, if missed and untreated, would produce irreparable harm or even death to your patient.
- Form a reasoned plan for testing your hypothesis. Sequence laboratory tests to establish, or rule out, the most common diseases first, as well as the diseases requiring urgent treatment.
- Do not rush to make a diagnosis for which no treatment is available.
- Never perform a diagnostic procedure that is not related to any of your diagnostic possibilities (e.g., a urinalysis in a patient being evaluated for inspiratory stridor).
- Do not pursue a differential among diagnoses that will not alter your course of action.
- Always consider the harm that tests might do as well as their costs. Balance the harm and the costs against the information that may be gained.

- Be constantly aware of the natural tendency to discount, or even disregard, evidence likely to eliminate your favored diagnosis.
- Never dismiss the possibility that a patient with multiple complaints or problems may have more than one disease. The chances of having two common diseases simultaneously is greater than the chance of having one rare disease.
- If you cannot rule out the possibility of the presence of a disease that would result in serious harm to the patient if left untreated, then treat the patient as if the disease was present.

Probability and utility should always guide your actions.

Suggested Readings

Cutler P. *Problem solving in clinical medicine: from data to diagnosis.* Baltimore: Williams & Wilkins, 1979.

Elstein AS, Shulman L, Sprafka SA. *Medical problem solving: an analysis of clinical reasoning.* Cambridge, MA: Harvard University Press, 1978.

Fulginiti VA. *Pediatric clinical problem solving.* Baltimore: Williams & Wilkins, 1981.

Kupperman N. Diagnostic Testing of the febrile neonate. It is time to collaborate. *Arch Pediatr Adolesc Med* 2003;157:508.

Schwartz S, Griffin T. *Medical thinking: the psychology of medical judgment and decision making.* New York: Springer-Verlag, 1986.

Sills RH. Failure to thrive: the role of clinical and laboratory evaluation. *Am J Dis Child* 1978;132:967.

CHAPTER 7 ■ PHARMACOLOGIC PRINCIPLES OF DRUG THERAPY

GEORGE C. RODGERS, JR., AND NANCY J. MATYUNAS

The primary goal of drug therapy is to cure or ameliorate disease while causing minimal side effects. To achieve this goal the most appropriate drug is chosen and used in an optimal manner. Often, the result of the improper use of a drug is either therapeutic failure or toxicity. These consequences are preventable if the principles of pharmacodynamics and pharmacokinetics are considered in the selection and monitoring of a treatment regimen. This chapter reviews these principles as they apply to the use of drugs in pediatric patients.

SCIENTIFIC BASIS OF PEDIATRIC CLINICAL PHARMACOLOGY

Decision making in pediatric drug therapy has historically been made on the basis of data gathered in adults, even though it is clear that developmental age directly influences the disposition of drugs and chemicals. Great variability in drug response exists even among preterm and term newborns, infants, toddlers, children and adolescents. These differences have led to such widely publicized problems as the "gray-baby syndrome" due to delayed chloramphenicol metabolism in neonates, severe jaundice from the use of sulfa drugs that displace bilirubin in newborns, and the "gasping syndrome" in newborns treated with drug preparations containing the preservative benzyl alcohol.

The recognized gold standard for evaluating clinical efficacy is the prospective, randomized, controlled trial. A relative lack of good clinical data in children exists because of the difficulties associated with performing such studies. However, the body of clinical drug data in children is growing, in part due to a federal mandate requiring drug manufacturers to provide pediatric drug-use guidelines. Drug manufacturers also must provide data to support the safe and effective use of drugs in children.

Some of the difficulties associated with performing drug studies in children include ethical issues, difficulty obtaining parental or patient consent, lack of pediatrician interest in performing clinical research, the small numbers of children qualifying for studies, and the lack of financial incentive for the pharmaceutical industry because of the limited market potential for most drugs in pediatric patients. Because drug response may be variable across age groups, these differences must be taken into consideration when designing clinical trials, thus adding further complexity to the study design. To gather adequate numbers of patients to ensure statistical power, trials often require the participation of multiple research centers. For similar reasons, few drugs are developed specifically for diseases primarily afflicting children.

In the absence of controlled, randomized clinical trials in children, pediatricians either must extrapolate information from adult studies or from uncontrolled clinical reports in children, both of which sources of data should be used cautiously. Reliance on adult studies may lead to either underdosing or overdosing. Uncontrolled clinical reports in children often can be misleading, because many factors unrelated to the use of the drug may affect outcome. Only a properly designed controlled trial effectively eliminates confounding variables. Pediatricians must bear in mind the uncertainty that the lack of data adds to their drug selection and exercise appropriate caution.

SELECTION OF AN APPROPRIATE DRUG

The selection of the appropriate drug is a four-step process. First, the therapeutic goal must be clearly defined, such as the treatment of infection or maintenance of blood pressure. Second, all of the potentially useful therapeutic agents must be identified. Third, the most appropriate agent must be selected based upon the patient's age, developmental status, history of allergy or previous intolerance, drug resistance (in the case of antibiotics), and the availability and cost-effectiveness of the various agents. Fourth, the optimal dosing regimen and therapeutic monitoring plan must be determined.

For a few diseases, such as Gaucher disease, only one therapeutic option may be available. For most diseases however, several possible options exist. Some drugs should not be used because of age-specific adverse effects. For example, the adverse effect of tetracyclines on tooth development in children younger than 8 years dictates that these drugs generally should not be used in this age range. The lack of a U.S. Food and Drug Administration (FDA)—approved pediatric indication is not a legal prohibition against the use of the drug in children. It is always important to ask patients or family members about possible drug allergy or intolerance. Common, relatively benign effects, such as antibiotic-induced gastrointestinal discomfort, may be an acceptable side effect and should not preclude the use of the drug if absolutely necessary. On the other hand, if a serious reaction, such as an urticarial rash or respiratory difficulty is reported, the offending drug and its chemical analogues should not be used.

The soaring cost of drug therapy, due in part to the introduction of many innovative but expensive agents, has led to increased efforts to control this segment of health care expenditures. An aspect of disease management reviews the value of the drug in the overall management of a particular disease. A drug with a high unit cost may be a better value if it controls the disease more effectively or can be administered in a manner that improves adherence to therapy. Most health care facilities, managed care organizations, and state Medicaid programs use drug formularies that encourage the use of the most cost-effective drug. Formularies can be useful in providing the pediatrician with a reference guide of relative drug costs or cost effectiveness. There will always be patients whose condition requires the use of a drug not included on the formulary, and all programs using formularies provide some mechanism to obtain an alternative agent. Usually, it is to the patient's and pediatrician's advantage to select an agent on the formulary. Because some families may not be able to obtain the prescribed drug because of the high cost, pediatricians should include affordability when considering which drug to use. Increasingly, drug manufacturers provide patient assistance programs that provide maintenance drugs at no cost when the family does not have the resources to purchase them.

PHARMACODYNAMICS

Pharmacodynamics describes how the drug affects the body. It encompasses the mechanism of action, clinical effects measured, and the safety profile of the agent. Most drugs produce their therapeutic (and toxic) effects through interacting with receptors. Children may respond to a drug in a way different from that of an adult because they have increased or decreased numbers of receptors, altered receptor binding affinity for the drug, or the organ may not respond to receptor stimulation in the same fashion as an adult. The result of these alterations may be increased toxicity that precludes use of the drug, decreased clinical response that requires larger doses of the drug, or paradoxical effects. The paradoxical excitability in children caused by phenobarbital is an example of altered receptor response and is independent of the dose administered.

For most drugs, the concentration of unbound or free drug at its site of action is directly proportional to the pharmacologic response. It is assumed that the whole blood, plasma, or serum concentrations measured are proportional to tissue concentrations, and these are used as a surrogate. The manipulation of the dose and dosing interval significantly affects the concentration of the drug at its site of action. In general, a larger dose and more frequent administration produce higher drug concentrations at the site of action. Figure 7.1 shows how varying the dose and/or dosing interval produces very different drug concentrations. Thus, any change in the dose or dosing

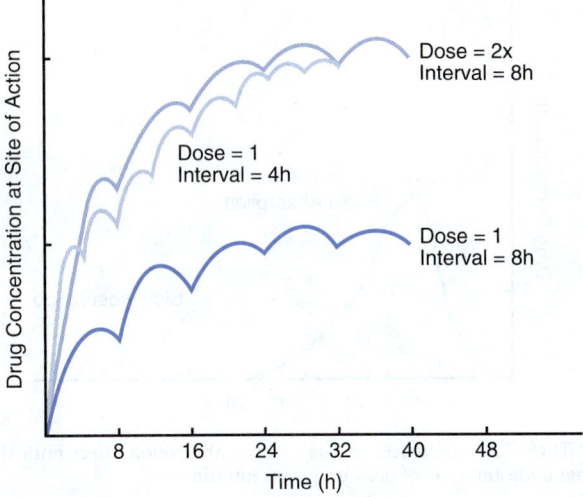

FIGURE 7.1. Influence of drug dose and interval on the concentration of drug at the site of action. Doubling the dose or giving the drug twice as often produces the same result in terms of drug concentration.

interval can result in a change in the drug concentration and potentially alter the efficacy or toxicity of the drug.

The dosage form of the drug also may dictate the choice of dose and dosing interval. To improve adherence to the drug regimen, many sustained-release preparations have been developed. These preparations usually allow for once or twice daily dosing and produce less variation in drug blood levels over the dosing interval. Switching between regular-release and sustained-release formulations usually requires an adjustment in both the dose and dosing interval, although the total daily dose remains the same. Failure to make these adjustments may result in undesirable blood concentrations.

Optimal dosing may be one of the greatest challenges facing pediatricians. Extrapolating a dose from adult studies may result in either underdosing or overdosing, leading to adverse effects. If a dose must be extrapolated from adult data, doses usually are scaled based on weight or body surface area. Generally, the body surface area method better reflects age-dependent physiologic differences and is preferred.

PHARMACOKINETICS

Pharmacokinetics describes the movement of drugs throughout the body. Components include absorption of the drug from its site of administration, distribution to tissues and site of effect, metabolism (biotransformation), and elimination. Pharmacokinetic parameters vary with age and should be taken into consideration in selecting drugs to use, routes of administration, and dosing regimens.

Absorption

The rate of drug absorption depends on the dosage form of the drug, the physical–chemical characteristics of the drug, the route of administration, and the individual patient's physiology. In Figure 7.2, although the total amount of drug absorbed is equivalent based on the area under the curve, the concentration versus time profiles are very different due to differences in the rate of absorption. The time to and magnitude of peak drug concentration and the concentrations achieved at equivalent times differ, which may affect the onset and duration of drug effect. Either profile shown could be desirable, depending on the clinical situation. For example, rapid absorption with higher

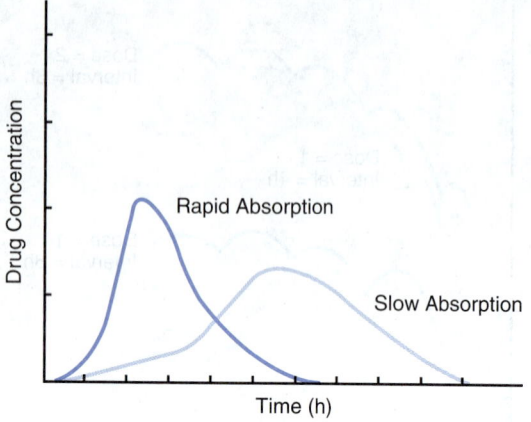

FIGURE 7.2. Differences in rate of drug absorption affect both the magnitude and time of peak drug concentration.

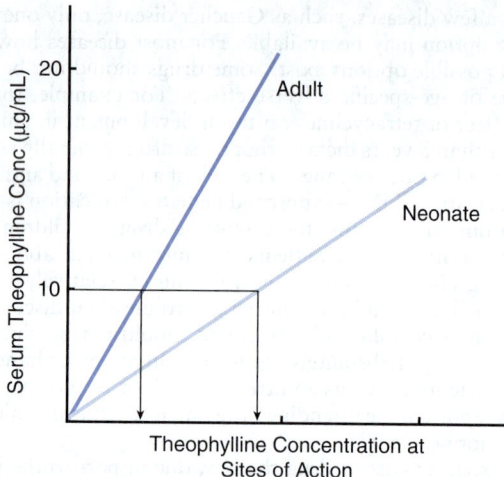

FIGURE 7.3. The effect of differences in plasma protein binding of theophylline on drug action. Because of less serum protein binding of theophylline in neonates, equal serum theophylline concentrations to those in adults actually deliver more drug to sites of action (*arrows*).

peak levels may be desirable for many antimicrobials, anesthetic agents, and analgesics. Slower absorption, with lower peak concentrations but more sustained effects, may be desirable for drugs used to treat chronic conditions such as asthma or hypertension.

Drug concentration versus time profiles may differ for the same drug when given by different routes. Subcutaneous or intramuscular administration of morphine may have an onset of action 15 to 20 times slower than a comparable dose given intravenously. A rapidly administered intravenous dose of morphine may produce such high drug concentration with rapid distribution into the central nervous system that respiratory depression may develop.

Developmental changes in several physiologic parameters important for drug absorption occur as the child grows, including stomach and intestinal pH, gastric emptying time, pancreatic function, intestinal flora, and blood flow to the gut. For several drugs, diminished and erratic absorption has been demonstrated in neonates and infants after oral or intramuscular administration. Comorbidities also can affect drug absorption. For example, hypotension and shock lead to decreased blood flow to both the gut and skeletal muscle, making absorption after oral or intramuscular routes unpredictable.

Some drugs display low oral bioavailability because they undergo high first-pass extraction by the liver. This means that a very high percentage of the drug dose is removed from circulation during the initial passage through the liver. The dosage differences for propranolol document the significance of the first-pass effect: The oral dose is 0.1 mg/Kg versus an intravenous dose of 0.01 mg/Kg.

Distribution

Factors that influence drug distribution to various tissues include the concentration of the drug in the blood; the amount of drug bound to serum proteins such as albumin, alpha-1-acid glycoprotein, bilirubin, and intracellular protein binding sites; blood flow to the particular tissue; the lipophilicity of the drug; and the percentage of fat and water in the body. Many of these factors contribute to age-dependent alterations in the distribution of some drugs.

The degree to which a drug binds to proteins accounts for major differences in the relative distribution of the drug between blood and tissues. A drug that is highly bound to serum proteins tends to remain in the vascular compartment, whereas drugs that bind more avidly to intracellular sites are more highly concentrated outside the vascular compartment. For example, digoxin concentrations within myocardial tissue can be 200 times greater than serum digoxin concentrations.

Neonates and infants generally have lower concentration of several serum proteins, most importantly albumin and alpha-1-acid glycoprotein. Because of reduced serum protein binding of theophylline in neonates and infants, the drug is more likely to distribute into extravascular compartments when compared with adults. Therefore, a serum theophylline concentration of 10 μg/mL in a neonate reflects a greater tissue concentration of the drug when compared with a similar level in an adult. Thus, at any given theophylline serum concentration, a neonate experiences a greater drug response than an adult (Fig. 7.3). Neonates and infants also may have higher concentrations of unconjugated bilirubin and free fatty acids, which can affect the percentage of circulating free drug. Thus, the pediatrician must be cautious when interpreting serum drug concentrations.

Premature infants and neonates have a greater percentage of body water than adults, so water-soluble drugs distribute to a greater degree, necessitating larger doses relative to weight or body surface area. Premature infants also have a lower percentage of body fat when compared with full-term neonates and older children, so lipophilic drugs will not distribute to as great an extent, thus producing higher than expected blood concentrations and possibly a greater therapeutic effect or toxicity. In addition, the blood–brain barrier is not fully developed in neonates (particularly premature infants) and young infants. This may result in the unwanted distribution of some drugs into the central nervous system (CNS), with resulting toxicity.

Metabolism

Drug metabolism (biotransformation) is the conversion of a drug into generally more polar and water-soluble metabolites. Drugs are metabolized primarily by microsomal enzymes in the liver. Other organs (e.g., kidney, blood, lung, and intestine) do have limited drug-metabolizing ability. Drug metabolizing pathways are generally divided into phase I reactions (i.e. oxidation, reduction, and hydrolysis reactions) and phase II reactions (i.e. acetylation, glucuronidation, and other conjugation reactions). Different enzymes are responsible for the various phase I and phase II reactions.

Metabolites may be pharmacologically active, although in general they are either less active than the parent compound or inactive. Drugs differ markedly in the rate and extent to which they are metabolized. Also, large interindividual differences occur in the rate and extent of metabolism and the pattern of metabolites produced. These differences derive from genetics, age-dependent physiologic differences, and the effects of disease states on metabolizing organs. Various liver enzyme systems mature at different rates during the first 2 years of life. In general, the quantity and functionality of microsomal enzymes are decreased in the immature liver, and drug metabolism is reduced. Therefore, lower drug dosages may be required to achieve and maintain therapeutic concentrations in neonates and infants. In older children, metabolism may be increased in comparison with adults, and higher doses of some drugs (e.g., phenytoin), may be required on a per-kilogram body weight basis. Because the metabolism of a given drug may involve several age-dependent enzyme systems, the prediction of metabolic rate is difficult without experimental data from children of various ages.

Some enzymatic reactions are capacity limited. When the metabolizing capacity of liver enzymes is saturated, a proportional relationship between dose and serum concentration no longer exists. In this situation, an increase in drug dosage results in a disproportionate increase in drug concentration, making attempts to optimize therapy difficult.

Certain drugs (e.g., phenobarbital) and xenobiotics (e.g., polycyclic aromatic hydrocarbons) can stimulate hepatic microsomal enzyme activity, whereas others (e.g., cimetidine, erythromycin) may inhibit enzyme activity. A drug that undergoes extensive hepatic metabolism may require a dose or dosing interval adjustment to maintain therapeutic blood concentrations in the presence of either diminished liver function or coadministered drugs.

Pharmacogenetics

A new and important area of pediatric drug research is pharmacogenetics, the study of genetic influences on drug metabolism. The cytochrome P-450 (CYP) system is the major group of enzymes responsible for drug oxidation, the major phase I route of metabolism. Several dozen different CYP enzymes have been described. Genetic polymorphisms are well described for at least two of the important enzymes in this series, CYP2D6 and CYP2C19. These two enzymes are involved in the metabolism of many drugs, including a number of antidepressants and neuroleptics, anticonvulsants, and cardiovascular drugs. Significant polymorphisms also exist for some phase II enzymes, most notably N-acetyltranferase-2. It is clear that for drugs metabolized by these and perhaps other polymorphic enzymes, the development and expression of these polymorphisms may be important in determining how a drug is used in an individual or what drug–drug interactions might be expected. At present, relatively little is known about the age-dependent development and expression of these various enzymes and their isoforms. Phenotyping may become both practical and important for children who are to be treated chronically with drugs whose metabolism is dependent on polymorphic enzymes, and where the therapeutic index is narrow and good markers of therapeutic effect or toxicity do not exist.

Elimination

The primary organ of drug elimination is the kidney. In neonates and infants, kidney function is dependent on the maturity of the organ. The immature kidney is less efficient at drug removal, so drugs may persist in the blood and tissues for longer periods, prolonging the therapeutic effect or producing toxicity. Dose or dosing interval adjustments may be necessary for drugs

TABLE 7.1

GENTAMICIN DOSAGE AND PHARMACOKINETICS IN NEONATES VERSUS ADULTS

	Neonates	Adults
Volume of distribution	400–600 mL/kg	200–300 mL/kg
Peak plasma concentration	6–10 μg/mL	6–10 μg/mL
Elimination half-life	3–4 hours	1.5–3 hours
Dose	7.5 mg/kg/day	3–6 mg/kg/day

that are primarily renally excreted. Gentamicin is an example of a drug with different dosage requirements for neonates and adults because of differences in distribution and elimination (Table 7.1). Although renal elimination of gentamicin is slower in neonates and infants than in adults, the volume of distribution is considerably larger. The net effect is that proportionally larger daily doses are administered in neonates than in adults. All pharmacokinetic parameters should be considered when selecting a dose and dosing interval.

Most drugs exhibit first-order kinetics within their therapeutic range. For such drugs, the concentration of drug in the blood, and therefore at the site of action, is directly proportional to the dose. For instance, doubling the dose doubles the blood concentration. For a few drugs (e.g., phenytoin), zero-order kinetics occur within the therapeutic range. An increase in dose produces a disproportionate increase in blood level. Conversely, a decrease in dose leads to a disproportionate decrease in blood concentration. Drugs such as these must be dosed and monitored very carefully to prevent toxicity or lack of effect.

THERAPEUTIC DRUG MONITORING

Therapeutic drug monitoring can be an effective tool for optimizing drug efficacy and minimizing drug toxicity. Monitoring, however, is useful only if there is a well-established relationship between the serum concentration of the drug and the therapeutic effectiveness or toxicity of the agent. Drug levels should be obtained to document toxicity or investigate lack of therapeutic effect. Obtaining a drug level is rarely justified if standard doses are used, metabolism and elimination can be presumed to be normal, and a short course of therapy is anticipated. For many drugs given chronically, such as phenobarbital, theophylline, and phenytoin, blood levels generally are monitored periodically to adjust doses with growth. A list of drugs commonly used in pediatrics for which therapeutic monitoring is useful and readily available is provided in Table 7.2.

The relationship between serum drug concentration and effect varies depending on the drug. Figure 7.4 illustrates three such relationships. Drug A shows the most common and desirable relationship: first-order kinetics within its therapeutic range. For such drugs, the concentration of drug in the blood, and therefore at the site of action, is directly proportional to the dose. Doubling the dose doubles the blood concentration. Drug C presents a more clinically difficult situation to monitor, because a large change in serum drug concentration produces only small changes in effect. Drug B demonstrates a nonlinear relationship between serum concentration and effect. For a few drugs (e.g., phenytoin), such zero-order kinetics occur within the therapeutic range, and an increase in dose produces a disproportionate increase in blood level. Conversely, a decrease in dose leads to a disproportionate decrease in blood concentration. These drugs must be monitored closely to avoid toxicity and assure efficacy.

TABLE 7.2

GUIDELINES FOR THERAPEUTIC MONITORING OF DRUGS COMMONLY USED IN PEDIATRICS

Drug	Usual Target Ranges		Timing of Samples
	Trough	Peak	
Antibiotics			
Amikacin	<10 μg/mL	20–30 μg/mL	Peak 30 minutes after end of infusion; trough just before dose
Chloramphenicol	5–15 μg/mL	15–25 μg/mL	Peak 90 minutes after end of infusion or 2 hours after oral dose; trough just before dose
Gentamicin	0.5–2.0 μg/mL	4–10 μg/mL	Peak 30 minutes after infusion or 1 hour after IM injection; trough just before dose (peaks not used for once daily doing)
Kanamycin	<5–10 μg/mL	15–30 μg/mL	Peak 30 minutes after infusion or 1 hour after IM injection; trough just before dose
Tobramycin	0.5–2.0 μg/mL	4–10 μg/mL	Peak 30 minutes after infusion or 1 hour after IM injection; trough just before dose
Vancomycin	5–15 μg/mL	25–40 μg/mL	Peak 20–30 minutes after end of infusion; trough just before dose
Anticonvulsants			
Carbamazepine	4–12 μg/mL		Trough just before dose
Ethosuximide	40–100 μg/mL		Trough just before dose
Phenobarbital	15–40 μg/mL		Trough just before dose
Phenytoin	10–20 μg/mL		Trough just before dose
Primidone	8–12 μg/mL		Trough just before dose
Valproic acid	50–100 μg/mL		Trough just before dose
Cardiovascular drugs			
Digoxin	0.8–2.0 ng/mL (age dependent)		Trough just before dose
Lidocaine		1.5–5.0 μg/mL	Level done 3 to 9 hours after initiation of infusion
Procainamide	4–10 μg/mL		Trough just before dose
Quinidine	2–5 μg/mL		Trough just before dose
Miscellaneous			
Caffeine		5–15 μg/mL	Peak levels 1 hour after oral dose
Cyclosporine	100–800 ng/mL (assay and protocol dependent)		Trough just before dose
Lithium	0.4–1.4 mEq/mL (disease dependent)		Trough just before dose
Theophylline		10–20 μg/mL	Peak 30 minutes after end of infusion, 2 hours after standard-release oral dose, or 4 hours after sustained-release oral dose

IM, intramuscular.

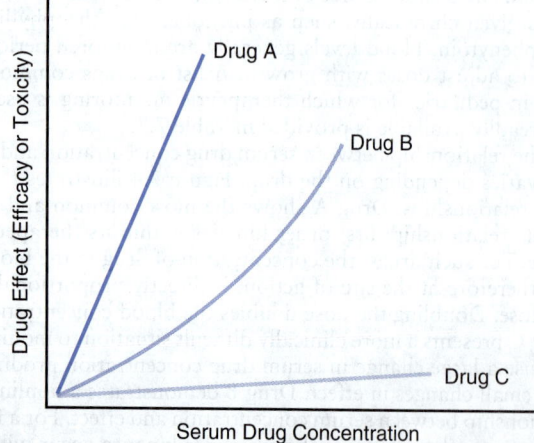

FIGURE 7.4. Potential usefulness of relationship between serum drug concentration and drug effect. Drug A demonstrates a useful relationship and drug B a nonlinear, less predictable situation. Drug C illustrates a difficult circumstance in which major changes in serum drug concentration result in little change in drug effect.

If a predictable relationship between drug concentration and effect or toxicity exists, the target concentrations of drug in the serum can be identified. These concentrations define the therapeutic range (Fig. 7.5) above which toxicity may be expected and below which a loss of efficacy occurs.

The timing of serum sampling is critical, as is the decision on whether to monitor peak or trough levels or both. Peak concentrations of a drug in the serum develop at some time point after drug administration, and trough concentrations occur just before the next dose is given. The time at which peak serum concentrations is reached is not always obvious. The rate and extent of drug absorption influence the time to peak and the magnitude of peak drug concentrations. In practice, peak concentrations are assumed to occur shortly after the completion of an intravenous infusion, although drug residence time in intravenous tubing may make it difficult to tell precisely when an infusion is completed. Peak levels are usually achieved 1 to 2 hours after administration of a regular-release oral preparation, whereas peak levels may be delayed 4 to 12 hours after administration of a sustained-release product. Considerable age and individual variability in the time required to reach peak levels may exist.

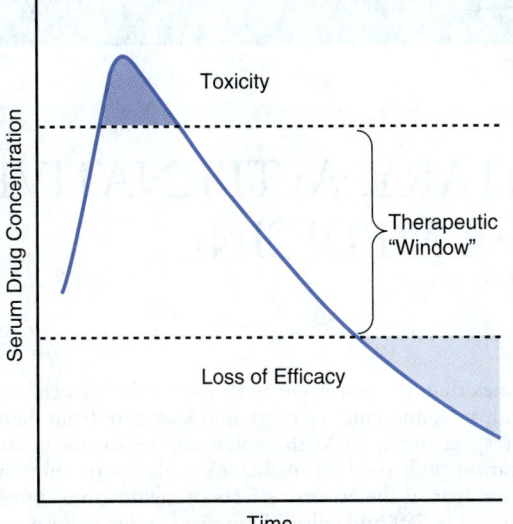

FIGURE 7.5. The concept of therapeutic range: the ideal drug serum concentration above which toxicity is expected and below which efficacy is reduced or lost.

General information on drug-level monitoring is provided in Table 7.2.

The concept of a steady-state concentration (Fig. 7.6) after repeated doses of a drug is important for the appropriate timing of serum sampling in monitoring drug therapy. Blood

levels measured before a steady state is reached do not represent or predict drug concentrations at steady state. Dosage adjustments based on such premature data can result in serious dosage errors. Steady-state blood levels are achieved after approximately five drug half-lives have elapsed since the first dose, if no loading dose is given. A loading dose of drug may be necessary or desirable to rapidly achieve adequate therapeutic drug concentrations. Drugs that commonly require loading dose regimens include digoxin, phenobarbital, theophylline, and chloramphenicol.

CONCLUSIONS

Pediatric drug therapy poses unique problems for the pediatrician. The relative lack of drug data in children, together with the well-recognized age variations in pharmacodynamics and pharmacokinetics, make the selection and appropriate dosing of many drugs difficult. In the absence of good age-dependent data in children, the pediatrician always must bear in mind the basic principles of pediatric clinical pharmacology when selecting which drug and dosing regimen to use.

Suggested Readings

American Academy of Pediatrics Committee on Drugs. Inactive ingredients in pharmaceutical products. *Pediatrics* 1985;76:635.

American Academy of Pediatrics Committee on Drugs. Guidelines for the ethical conduct of studies to evaluate drugs in pediatric populations. *Pediatrics* 1995;95:286.

American Academy of Pediatrics Committee on Drugs. Unapproved uses of approved drugs: the physician, the package insert, and the Food and Drug Administration: subject review. *Pediatrics* 1996;98:143.

Aranda JV, Stern L. Clinical aspects of developmental pharmacology and toxicology. *Pharmacol Ther* 1983;20:1.

Benedetti MS, Baltes EL. Drug metabolism and disposition in children. *Fund Clin Pharmacol* 2003;17:281.

Benitz WE, Tatro DS. *The pediatric drug handbook,* 3rd ed. St. Louis: Mosby–Year Book, 1995.

Gunn V, ed. *The Harriet Lane handbook: a manual for pediatric house officers,* 16th ed. St. Louis: Mosby–Year Book, 2002.

Kearns GL, Reed MD. Clinical pharmacokinetics in infants and children: a reappraisal. *Clin Pharmacokin* 1989;17(Suppl 1):29.

Koren G. Therapeutic drug monitoring principles in the neonate. *Clin Chem* 1997;43:222.

Leeder JS, GL Kearns. Pharmacogenetics in pediatrics. *Pediatr Clinics North Am* 1997;44:55.

Physicians' desk reference, 58th ed. Montvale, NJ: Medical Economics Company, 2004.

Rane A. Phenotyping of drug metabolism in infants and children: potentials and problems. *Pediatrics* 1999;104:640.

Roberts RJ. Drug therapy in infants: pharmacological principles and clinical experience. Philadelphia: Saunders, 1984.

Taketomo CK, Hodding JH, Kraus DM. *Pediatric dosage handbook,* 10th ed. Hudson, OH: Lexi-Comp, 2003.

Warner A. Drug use in the neonate: interrelationships of pharmacokinetics, toxicity and biochemical maturity. *Clin Chem* 1986;32:721.

Yaffe SJ, Aranda JV, eds. *Pediatric pharmacology: therapeutic principles in practice,* 2nd ed. Philadelphia: Saunders, 1992.

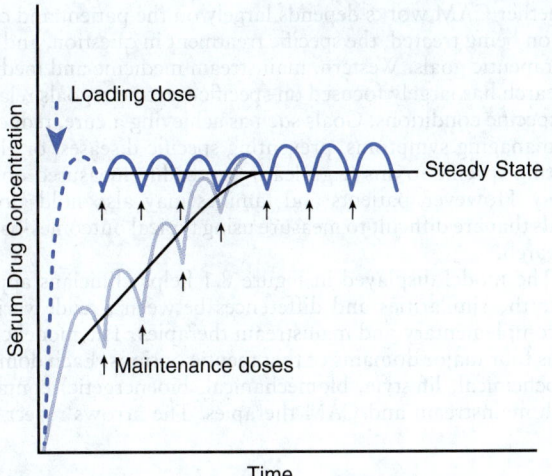

FIGURE 7.6. Steady-state serum concentrations achieved over time with repeated maintenance doses (*solid line*) or more rapidly after a loading dose (*dashed line*).

CHAPTER 8 ■ COMPLEMENTARY, ALTERNATIVE, HOLISTIC, AND INTEGRATIVE MEDICINE

KATHI J. KEMPER

Historically, health care providers considered complementary or unconventional therapies as a nonscientific alternative to mainstream medicine. However, rising patient demand and the recent increase in controlled clinical trials evaluating the efficacy and safety of these therapies have fueled physician interest.

Complementary and alternative medicine (CAM) has been defined as a broad domain of healing practices that encompasses practices other than those intrinsic to the politically dominant health system. These might include specific therapies, such as acupuncture and homeopathy, or entire systems of healing such as Traditional Chinese Medicine, Ayurveda, or Native American healing. *Holistic* medicine refers to care of the whole patient—body, mind, emotions, spirit, and relationships—within the context of the patient's values, beliefs, culture, and community. It is sometimes called patient-centered or humanistic care. *Integrative* medicine refers to comprehensive care that respects patients' choices, integrating CAM into mainstream practice, based on scientific evidence of safety and the uniqueness of patients' cultural and psychosocial context.

EPIDEMIOLOGY

CAM therapies are commonly used across a broad spectrum of pediatric patients. The percentage of American adults in the general population using CAM increased from 34% in 1990 to 42% in 1997; out-of-pocket expenditures increased 45% during this same period. Certain racial and cultural groups, age, gender, and socioeconomic status groups may have even higher use of certain kinds of CAM therapies. For example, in the general public, CAM is most commonly used by middle-aged, white women with above-average income and education. Parental CAM use is one of the strongest predictors of pediatric CAM use. Overall, CAM use in children is least common in healthy community populations, ranging from 2% to 7%; intermediate in clinic patients, ranging from 11% to 20%; and highest in clinics and inpatient settings serving patients with chronic or incurable conditions such as allergies, asthma, attention deficit-hyperactivity disorder (ADHD), autism, cystic fibrosis, cancer, inflammatory bowel disease, rheumatoid arthritis, or complex psychosocial problems, ranging from 25% to more than 70% of children. The use of CAM therapies is more common among patients with worse quality of life and poor prognosis. Fewer than 50% discuss their CAM use with physician.

RATIONALE FOR USING CAM

The most common reasons that parents seek CAM therapies for their children is to relieve symptoms and to be assured that they have tried every reasonable, safe option. Many CAM therapies also are perceived as less expensive and safer than conventional medications and surgical treatments. Patients prefer therapies that are consistent with their values (such as being natural, safe, and empowering), and seek care from therapists who respect them. CAM therapies may be sought because of frustration with modern medicine's inability to cure chronic illnesses, fear of the adverse effects of medications, interest in traditional beliefs and cultural practices, a desire for more natural therapies and more time for discussion with the clinician, a desire to decrease reliance on external, technical solutions, and a desire to enhance one's resilience and natural ability to respond effectively to challenges. Implicitly or explicitly then, the goals many patients seek in CAM are global goals such as connection, respect, support, meaning, harmony, presence, and peace of mind (Box 8.1).

EFFECTIVENESS

Whether CAM works depends largely on the patient and condition being treated, the specific treatment in question, and the therapeutic goals. Western, mainstream medicine and medical research has largely focused on specific treatment goals related to specific conditions. Goals such as achieving a cure, reducing or managing symptoms, preventing specific diseases, or eliminating specific toxins (e.g., lead) are readily measured objectively. However, patients and families may also hold global goals that are difficult to measure using typical outcomes-based research.

The model displayed in Figure 8.1 helps clinicians appreciate the similarities and differences between a wide variety of complementary and mainstream therapies. The model contains four major domains of therapeutic options. Each domain (biochemical, lifestyle, biomechanical, bioenergetic) contains both mainstream and CAM therapies. The arrows reflect the

---

| BOX 8.1 | Therapeutic Goals of CAM |

Specific, Disease-Focused
- Cure
- Relieve or manage symptoms
- Prevent specific disease(s)
- Eliminate specific toxins

Global, Person-Focused
- Trust, connection, support, community
- Peace, harmony, meaning
- Promote health, resilience, vitality
- Empowerment, reduce dependence
- Transcendence

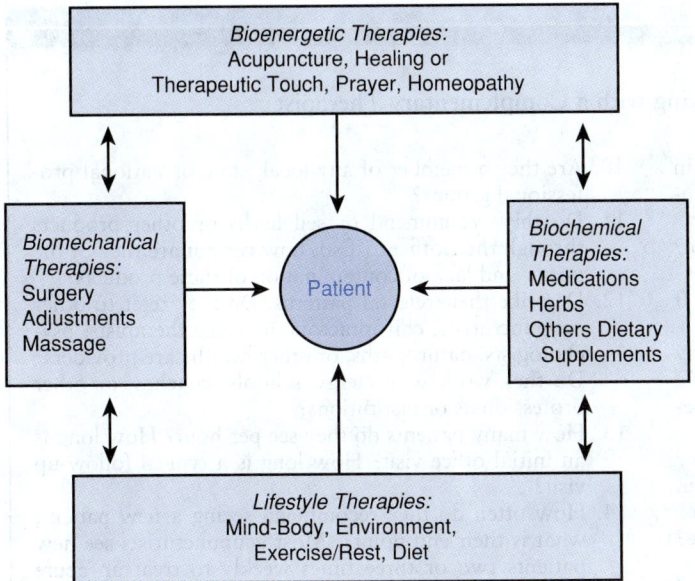

FIGURE 8.1. Integrative model of therapeutic options.

similarities and continuum of adjacent therapies in different domains, such as dietary supplements (Biochemical domain) and diet (Lifestyle domain). CAM therapies are not a cure for cancer, cystic fibrosis, autism, fractured femurs, appendicitis, and congenital or genetic defects. Nor do CAM therapies prevent polio, measles, lead poisoning, substance abuse, child abuse, or anthrax. However, CAM therapies may help with symptoms that trouble many children. Massage has proven helpful in promoting growth in preterm infants, relieving muscle spasm, pain, anxiety, depression, and insomnia, and enhancing lymphatic drainage. Acupuncture has proven effective in treating pain and nausea. Hypnosis, biofeedback, guided imagery, and meditation offer assistance with a variety of behavioral problems, dermatologic disorders, insomnia, and anxiety as well as chronic pain. Certain herbs and dietary supplements may enhance relaxation (chamomile), promote sleep (lavender), reduce gastrointestinal spasms (peppermint), relieve rashes (aloe), and prevent osteoporosis (calcium and vitamin D). Osteopathic manipulation can help prevent recurrent otitis media. Substantial additional research is necessary to define the optimal, cost-effective integration of complementary therapies into conventional practice.

SAFETY

In general, complementary therapies are substantially safer than conventional medications and surgery. Although patients can have minor bleeding or bruising at needle insertion sites, the serious adverse effects of acupuncture are exceedingly rare. Between the years 1981 and 1994, only 193 patients worldwide had reported adverse events from acupuncture. Despite a few well-publicized case reports of serious complications, chiropractic and osteopathic treatments are also very safe, even for young children. Similarly, massage is very safe when common-sense precautions are followed (e.g., no firm pressure in patients with low platelet counts, no massage over indwelling catheter sites or open wounds). Music, guided imagery, Healing Touch, and prayer are practically without side effects. The most serious risk from most professionally provided CAM therapies is that families will forego effective conventional care and rely solely on CAM to treat serious conditions such as cancer or diabetes. Prudent pediatricians ask a series of sensible questions prior to referring patients to CAM providers (Box 8.2).

For several reasons, self-care using herbs and dietary supplements can pose risks to children and adolescents. First, the supplement itself may be harmful; for example ephedra may cause severe cardiac disturbances; comfrey and chaparral can cause hepatotoxicity; pennyroyal can induce miscarriage and cause comas; and aristolochia may lead to renal tumors. Second, because herbal products are not as stringently regulated as medications, their quality may vary, and there is the risk of contamination with heavy metals or pharmaceuticals; this is a particular problem with products imported from developing countries such as China, India, and Mexico. Third, herbs may interact with conventional medications, increasing side effects or interfering with efficacy, requiring adjustments in dose to maintain effective levels while minimizing side effects. For example, St. John's wort enhances metabolic clearance, and thereby reduces the serum levels of many chronically used medications including digoxin, cyclosporine, protease inhibitors, anticonvulsant medications, and oral contraceptives.

RESOURCES

Resources for reliable, evidence-based information about CAM therapies have grown more abundant and available over the last five years (Box 8.3). Human resources may include pharmacists, nurses, physical and occupational therapists, pastoral care counselors, and other physicians as well as CAM providers. Most professional providers of CAM care (e.g., acupuncturists, chiropractors, clinical hypnotists, homeopaths, massage therapists, music therapists, and naturopaths) have professional organizations that maintain active Internet sites describing their membership and/or certification criteria. In addition, the U.S. government has numerous Internet sites sponsored by the National Center for Complementary and Alternative Medicine, the Food and Drug Administration, the Office of Dietary Supplements, and the National Cancer Institute that provide patient-oriented information about CAM. Government and academic sites are far less likely to offer biased information than typical commercial or private Internet sites. However, a few commercial sites, for example ConsumerLab (which offers independent testing of dietary supplements) and Natural Medicines Comprehensive Database (which provides reviews of over 2,000 herbs and supplements) are excellent sources of information. In addition, the National Library of

---

BOX 8.2   Questions to Consider When Working with a Complementary Therapist

1. What are your state's requirements for the practice of in this field? (Individual state requirements vary, particularly for massage and naturopathy.)
2. Has the therapist graduated from an accredited school?
3. Has the therapist passed the national certifying process?
4. Have they had special training in pediatric practice? If yes, describe that training.
5. How long have they been in practice, and how many pediatric patients do they see in a typical week? (We typically recommend a minimum of 12 months of experience, with at least three pediatric visits per week.)
6. Do they practice within a particular style or tradition? (Japanese acupuncture, for example is often gentler, while Chinese acupuncture has a more forceful style.)
7. What are their usual fees? Do they accept insurance? If so, which ones? Do they have a sliding scale? (*Note:* Medicaid pays for CAM services, particularly for chiropractic care in many states, but payments vary geographically and over time.)
8. Do they carry malpractice insurance? Have they ever been sued for malpractice? Have they ever lost privileges or been forced to leave a practice or group?
9. How many continuing education credits have they earned in the past 3 years?
10. Are they a member of any local, state or national professional groups?
11. Do they recommend or sell herbs or other products through their office? (If so, how certain are they of the purity and lack of contamination of these products?)
12. Describe their referral patterns. Do they refer to other acupuncturists, chiropractors, massage therapists, psychologists, naturopaths, or other health care providers? Do they work with clergy, schools, coaches, or other professionals or institutions?
13. How many patients do they see per hour? How long is an initial office visit? How long is a typical follow-up visit?
14. How often do they recommend seeing a new patient; what is their end point? (Most acupuncturists see new patients two or three times weekly to treat an acute problem and expect to see some objective improvement within five treatments.)
15. What are the most common side effects of their treatment, and what do they consider contraindications to treatment? (If they say they've never had a side effect, or if they fail to mention any contraindications, they may not be keen observers or complete reporters.)

Medicine now offers CAM on PUBMED, which offers quick and easy access to thousands of peer-reviewed articles about complementary therapies.

CONCLUSIONS

Complementary therapies are widely used and have been integrated into routine care by many families and holistic physicians. Many of these therapies are aimed at improving patients' global sense of well-being rather than as cures of specific conditions. Their effectiveness varies depending on the patient and condition being treated, treatment goals, and the particular therapy employed. Most are safer on average than conventional therapies as long as effective therapies are not withheld nor treatment delayed for life-threatening conditions. Substantial and growing resources are available to the practicing clinician to answer practical questions in this field.

BOX 8.3   Resources

Internet Sites (Academic or governmental)
Best Health (Wake Forest University School of Medicine): http://www.besthealth.com/

Food and Drug Administration MedWatch (to report adverse effects of herbs and supplements): http://www.fda.gov/medwatch/

Longwood Herbal Task Force (Boston Children's Hospital, Boston Medical Center, Harvard Medical School and Massachusetts College of Pharmacy): http://www.mcp.edu/herbal/

National Cancer Institute, Office of Cancer and Complementary and Alternative Medicine: http://www3.cancer.gov/occam/

National Institutes of Health Office of Dietary Supplements: http://ods.od.nih.gov/

National Institutes of Health, National Center for Complementary and Alternative Medicine: http://altmed.od.nih.gov/health/

U.S. Department of Agriculture, Food and Nutrition Information Center: http://www.nal.usda.gov/fnic/etext/000015.html

Internet Sites (Commercial)
ConsumerLab (independently evaluates dietary supplement products): http://www.consumerlab.com/

Natural Medicine Comprehensive Database (regularly updated, evidence-based source of information on herbs and supplements): http://www.naturaldatabase.com/

TABLE 8.1

COMMON HERBS USED IN PEDIATRICS

Generally Safe

Herb	How Used	Indication	Side Effects/Problems
Aloe vera	Topically	Minor wounds, burns, skin irritation, muscus membrane inflammation	Rare allergies
Chamomile	Topically and as tea	Topically as mild anti-inflammatory; as tea, mild sedative, spasmolytic, anti-inflammatory	Rare allergies; one case of botulism from home grown tea
Cranberry	Juice, dried, capsules	Prevent urinary tract infection	Dislike of taste; substitution of cranberry for antimicrobial therapy
Ginger	Tea	Antiemetic	Heartburn, dislike taste
Lavender	Aromatherapy	Mild sedative, sleep aid	Rare allergies or skin irritation
Peppermint	Topically; as tea or enteric capsules; aromatherapy	Topically on temples for headache; as tea or enteric capsules for intestinal spasms (colonoscopy); as aromatherapy to decrease subjective nasal congestion	Rare allergies; can exacerbate reflux; high amounts directly under nose of newborns may lead to apnea

Products to Avoid

	How Used	Indication	Side Effects/Problems
Any herb imported from developing country	Particularly for oral use	Varied	Risk of misidentification of herb, contamination with heavy metals, adulteration with pharmaceuticals
Very high doses of any herb	Oral use	Varied	E.g., high doses of ephedra lead to cardiac arrhythmias; high doses of ginseng may lead to hypertension and mania; high doses of wintergreen may lead to salicylism
Chronic use of cacscara, senna, medicinal rhubarb	Orally	Constipation	May lead to dependence or pseudo-melanosis coli
Chronic use of coltsfoot or comfrey	Orally	Cough, cuts, bruises	Pyrrolizidine alkaloids may lead to veno-occlusive disease
Chronic use of licorice	Orally	Dyspepsia, anti-inflammatory	May lead to hypokalemia, hypertension, arrhythmias
Aristolochia	Oral use	Cough, asthma, bronchitis, colic	Nephrotoxicity; carcinogenic
Chaparral	Oral use	Anti-inflammatory, antioxidant, pain, cancer	Liver damage
Germander	Oral use	Digestion, stomachache, diarrhea, fever	Liver damage
Pennyroyal oil	Oral use	Antispasmodic, bronchitis, abortifacient, digestive and liver disorders	Hepatic, cardiac and CNS toxicity including coma
St. John's wort	Oral use	Depression	May decrease blood levels of other medications
Wormwood	Oral use	Digestion, tonic	Seizures, hallucinations

Suggested Readings

NIH Consensus Conference. Acupuncture. *JAMA.* 1998;280(17):1518.

Astin JA. Why patients use alternative medicine: results of a national study. *JAMA* 1998;279(19):1548.

Davis MP, Darden PM. Use of complementary and alternative medicine by children in the United States. *Arch Pediatr Adolesc Med* 2003;157(4):393.

Field T. Massage therapy. *Med Clin North Am* 2002;86(1):163.

Gardiner P, Kemper KJ. Herbs in pediatric and adolescent medicine. *Pediatr Rev* 2000;21(2):44.

Kemper K. *The holistic pediatrician,* 2nd ed. New York: Harper Collins, 2002.

Kemper KJ, Wornham WL. Consultations for holistic pediatric services for inpatients and outpatient oncology patients at a children's hospital. *Arch Pediatr Adolesc Med.* 2001;155(4):449.

Pachter LM, Sumner T, Fontan A, et al. Home-based therapies for the common cold among European American and ethnic minority families: the interface between alternative/complementary and folk medicine. *Arch Pediatr Adolesc Med* 1998;152(11):1083.

Sanders H, Davis MF, Duncan B, et al. Use of complementary and alternative medical therapies among children with special health care needs in southern Arizona. *Pediatrics* 2003;111(3):584.

Woolf AD. Herbal remedies and children: do they work? Are they harmful? *Pediatrics* 2003;112(1 Pt 2):240.

CHAPTER 9 ■ FLUID AND ELECTROLYTE PHYSIOLOGY AND THERAPY

MELANIE S. KIM AND MICHAEL J. G. SOMERS

The regulation of body fluids is maintained within a narrow range in healthy children, despite the wide variations that occur in the intake and output of water and solutes. In particular, homeostatic mechanisms control volume and osmolality to provide a stable environment for normal bodily function. Understanding the normal physiology of body fluids is essential so that appropriate therapeutic interventions can be made when disruption occurs due to disease processes.

This chapter reviews our current understanding of normal homeostatic mechanisms that maintain regulation of osmolality, effective circulating volume, and total body water and fluid compartments. The discussion of abnormal electrolyte and fluid states focuses on underlying pathophysiology that should direct clinical evaluation and corrective therapy. In addition, an overview of fluid management in the healthy child and in specific common pathologic clinical conditions is presented.

NORMAL BODY FLUIDS AND HOMEOSTASIS

Total Body Water (TBW)

Water is the largest constituent of the body, and its contribution to body mass or weight varies with age, body size, and body composition. As can be seen in Figure 9.1, the total body water (TBW) of newborn infants is 75% to 80% of body mass, falling to 65% to 70% in toddlers, and to adult levels of 55% to 60% after puberty. Fat has lower water content than muscle; hence TBW as a percent of total weight is lower in prepubertal children and postpubertal young women than in mature adolescent males, who tend to have more muscle mass. Similarly, in individuals who are obese, in poor physical condition, or are elderly, there tends to be less muscle mass with decreased TBW as a percentage of total weight.

Body mass is composed of solid tissues and TBW (Fig. 9.2). TBW is distributed into two main compartments, the intracellular fluid and the extracellular fluid. The relative size of these compartments to overall TBW also varies with age (see Fig. 9.1), with the increased TBW in the neonate reflecting increased extracellular fluid. The intracellular fluid compartment contains the water in all body cells, making up about 60% to 65% of the TBW (see Fig. 9.2). The extracellular fluid compartment, 35% to 40% of the TBW outside the neonatal period, is further subdivided into interstitial fluid (~25% to 30% TBW) that bathes the cells and plasma, or intravascular fluid (~5% TBW). The regulation of intracellular volume and osmolality is important for cellular function and is dependent on *plasma osmolality control*. Extracellular volume is important in maintaining *effective circulating volume* to provide adequate perfusion to all parts of the body.

INTRACELLULAR AND EXTRACELLULAR FLUID COMPARTMENTS

The intracellular and extracellular fluids compartments are separated by the cell membrane, which also maintains different solute compositions within each compartment (see Fig. 9.2). Sodium is the major extracellular cation, with minor contributions from potassium, calcium, and magnesium. Sodium composition is balanced to maintain electroneutrality by the anions chloride (Cl^-) and bicarbonate (HCO_3^{-2}), negatively charged plasma proteins, and organic bases. Sodium also is the major extracellular osmole and, in the healthy individual. Its concentration is the main determinant of extracellular osmolality. Potassium acts in a similar manner as the major intracellular cation and osmole, whereas organic phosphorus is the main intracellular anion.

Each body fluid space is maintained by the separation of solutes, with the distribution of water across the cell membrane as determined by osmotic forces in either direction. The separation of solutes is achieved and maintained by many mechanisms, including electrochemical gradient; selective cell permeability; active transport, such as the sodium-potassium pump (Na^+, K^+-ATPase) transporting potassium into the cell and sodium out; and facilitated solute transport, such as the sodium-inositol and sodium-glucose transporters. Changes in

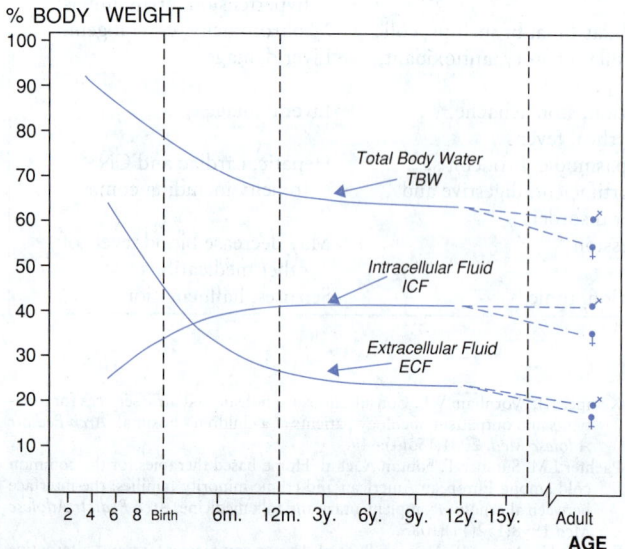

% BODY WEIGHT

FIGURE 9.1. Total body water and its compartments as a percent of total body weight, as it varies with age. (Reprinted with permission from Robert W. Winters, ed. *The body fluids in pediatrics.* Boston: Little Brown and Co., 1973:100.)

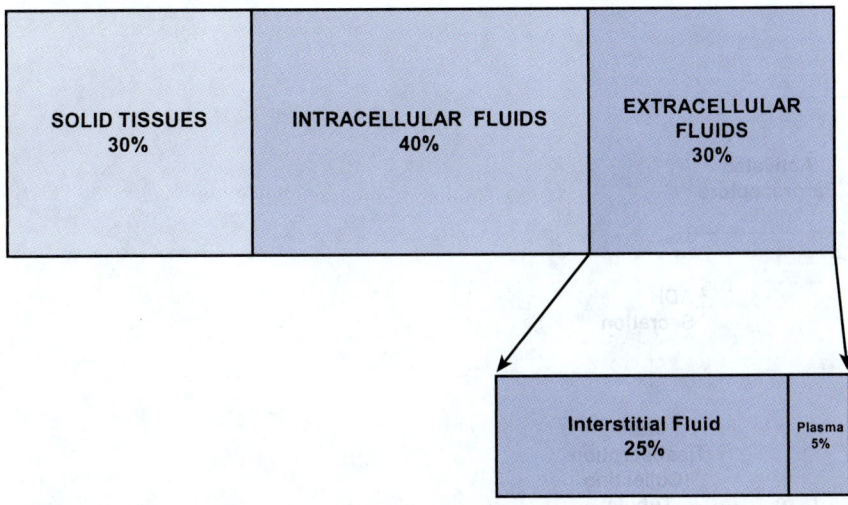

SOLUTE COMPOSITION OF BODY FLUID COMPARTMENTS

SOLUTES	PLASMA mEq/L	INTERSTITIAL FLUID mEq/L	INTRACELLULAR FLUID mEq/L
Na^+	140	145	10
K^+	4	4	150
Ca^{+2}	5	-	3
Mg^{+2}	2	-	26
Cl^-	110	115	3-5
HCO_3^-	24-26	30-31	10
Phosphorus	2	-	95
Organic Acids	6	-	15
Proteins	16	-	5-6

FIGURE 9.2. Body composition as a percent of total mass.

these processes may result in solute flux between compartments. For example, increased insulin availability and activity up-regulates sodium-potassium pump activity, increasing the intracellular uptake of potassium, and decreasing the extracellular potassium concentration.

Although solute composition differs between fluid compartments, total solute concentration is similar due to the free movement of water across the cell membrane. Hence, osmolar changes in one compartment trigger water movement to correct the osmolar gradient, ultimately effecting a change in volume between the fluid compartments. For example, an intravenous infusion of mannitol increases the osmolality of the extracellular fluid compartment, leading to a flow of water from the intracellular fluid to correct the osmotic difference. The net result is a decrease in the intracellular fluid compartment and a commensurate increase in the extracellular fluid compartment.

The intracellular fluid cannot be readily accessed, limiting the ability to determine directly intracellular solute concentration. Moreover, any impact on the intracellular milieu from the external environment must be mediated through the extracellular fluid compartment and, similarly, any excretion of an intracellular product ultimately depends on its transfer and clearance from the extracellular compartment.

As noted, the extracellular fluid is divided into interstitial fluid and plasma water via the vascular capillary bed. Unlike the cell membrane, the capillary is permeable to sodium, potassium, and glucose. As a result, the osmotic pressure difference between the intravascular and interstitial fluids is due to plasma proteins that cannot traverse the capillary wall and are, thus,

able to hold water in the intravascular space. The relative volumes of the interstitial and intravascular spaces are determined by the balance of these osmolar forces generated by plasma proteins and hydrostatic forces, which tend to move fluid out of the intravascular space and into the interstium. Changes in these processes will lead to a redistribution of water within these extracellular compartments. For example, patients with marked hypoalbuminemia, such as children with nephrotic syndrome, have an increased movement of fluid from the intravascular space into the interstitial space due to decreased intravascular oncotic pressure. Clinically, this movement is manifested by ascites and peripheral edema, as a direct result of interstitial space expansion or what is often termed *third-space losses.*

In summary, because perturbations occur in fluids or the electrolyte composition of a body compartment, the clinician must consider these effects in the disease state and how they will continue to change with any corrective action.

EFFECTIVE CIRCULATING VOLUME

Adequate tissue perfusion is critical for normal cell function, providing essential nutrients and oxygen to the cells, and removing metabolites and waste products from the cells. The effective circulating volume (ECV) is that intravascular volume on the arterial side of circulation that actively perfuses tissues. Because tissue perfusion is vital, the body

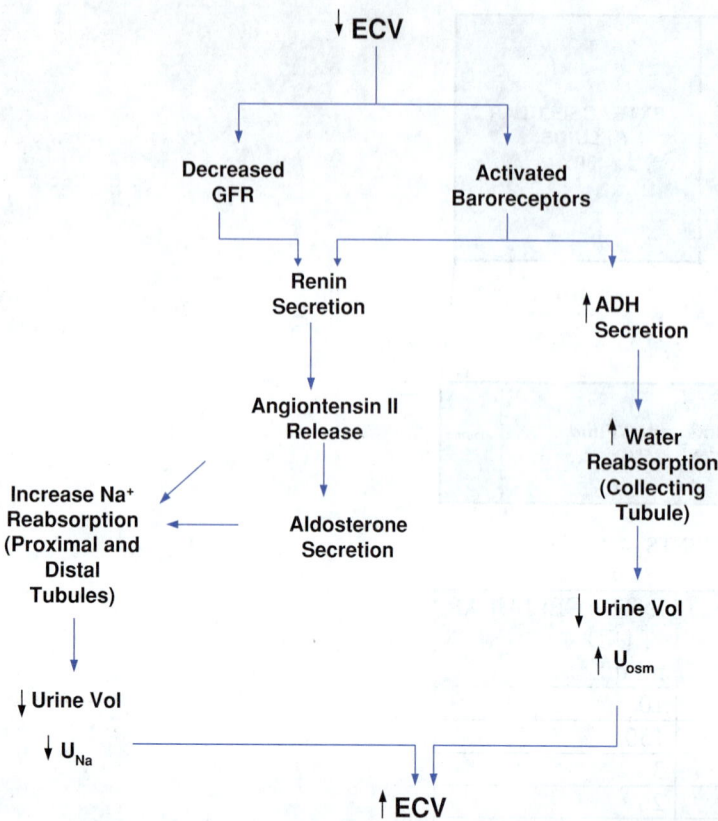

FIGURE 9.3. Regulation of effective circulating volume (ECV). GFR, glomerular filtration rate; U_{Na}, urinary sodium concentration; U_{osm}, urine osmolality.

continuously monitors the ECV through baroreceptors that, when activated, restore ECV by neurohumoral mechanisms that ultimately increase intravascular volume, cardiac output, and blood pressure. Alterations in ECV usually vary directly with similar alterations in the extracellular fluid compartment and with the total body sodium stores, because sodium is the primary extracellular solute that maintains the extracellular fluid. Hence, water and sodium regulation are critical in maintaining ECV.

Baroreceptors, located in the carotid sinuses, atria, and glomerular afferent arterioles, are actually stretch receptors that are sensitive to pressure changes. The activation of these receptors initiates a cascade of homeostatic mechanisms that include the release of antidiuretic hormone (ADH) and increased renal tubular epithelial cell reabsorption of sodium via the renin-angiotensin-aldosterone axis (Fig. 9.3). As these mechanisms increase the retention of sodium and water, the ECV is restored.

Baroreceptors in the carotid sinus mediate the parasympathetic stimulation of the vasomotor center in the medulla, leading to ADH secretion from the paraventricular nuclei. Circulating ADH increases water reabsorption into the distal tubular cells of the kidney by stimulating the insertion of water channels into the luminal membrane of the collecting duct. In the presence of ADH, urine osmolality (U_{osm}) should be high and only small volumes of concentrated urine should be produced.

With decreased ECV, renal hypoperfusion activates glomerular afferent arteriole baroreceptors. Hypoperfusion also results in decreased glomerular filtration, with a decrease in sodium delivery to the macula densa. In response to these stimuli, renin release launches a series of events that results in angiotensin II–mediated vasoconstriction and enhancement of water and sodium reabsorption. Renal sodium reabsorption is modulated directly by angiotensin II–stimulated sodium reabsorption in the proximal tubule and indirectly via aldosterone-stimulated sodium reabsorption distally. The end result is

increased sodium and water retention, low urinary sodium concentration (U_{Na^+}), decreased urine volume, and ultimate correction of the ECV.

An increase in ECV will stretch the atria, releasing atrial natriuretic peptide (ANP). ANP has two major actions. First, it lowers blood pressure by direct vasodilation and second, it increases sodium and water excretion. ANP increases the glomerular filtration rate (GFR) and promotes sodium excretion by inhibiting sodium reabsorption in the medullary collecting tubule and inhibiting renin, aldosterone, and angiotensin II secretion.

CLINICAL SIGNIFICANCE OF CHANGES IN EFFECTIVE CIRCULATING VOLUME

Thus, the tightly controlled regulation of ECV is normally maintained by a number of factors, including the size of the extracellular space, the relative efficacy of perfusion within the intravascular space, and hormonal regulation of sodium and water excretion by the kidney. In certain clinical conditions, these homeostatic mechanisms are altered, resulting in an aberrant fluid and electrolyte balance. For example, children with congestive heart failure have a decrease in their ECV due to decreased cardiac output. Subsequent renal hypoperfusion activates the release of renin and up-regulation of renal sodium and water retention by angiotensin II and aldosterone. Due to cardiac insufficiency, however, the increased vascular volume still does not effectively perfuse the kidney. The end result, then, is total body and extracellular salt and water expansion but no correction of the low ECV. Thus, in these patients, the kidneys respond as though they are volume depleted, with increased sodium avidity (low U_{Na^+}) despite a pathologically expanded TBW.

TABLE 9.1

CAUSES OF LOW EFFECTIVE CIRCULATING VOLUME

Mechanism	Clinical Examples
Loss of sodium and water	Gastroenteritis
	Burns
Loss of vascular tone	Septic shock
Loss of plasma oncotic pressure	Nephrotic syndrome
Loss of intravascular fluid to	Ascites
interstitial space	Pleural effusions
Loss of plasma and blood	Trauma
	Gastrointestinal bleeding

The causes of low ECV are listed in Table 9.1. These include clinical conditions with defects in these homeostatic mechanisms resulting in the ineffective expansion of extracellular volume, such as loss of intravascular osmotic pressure, as seen in nephrotic syndrome, and loss of vascular tone due to decreased systemic resistance, as seen in sepsis. Clearly, in these conditions, an infusion of sodium and water would not correct the ECV and would only exacerbate the volume overload. Rather, detecting and correcting the root cause of the decreased ECV—that may not even be related to extracellular fluid depletion—is the correct clinical approach. For example, in the child with cardiac insufficiency, optimizing inotropy will increase renal perfusion and allow a salt and water diuresis. Similarly, in the child with nephrotic syndrome, restoring intravascular oncotic pressure restores renal perfusion and allows a natriuresis and diuresis.

Without understanding the homeostatic mechanisms regulating ECV and the possible disturbances that can occur, the clinician would not be able to select the most appropriate therapy to restore ECV which, as illustrated, may have nothing to do with the provision of fluid or solute. Decisions based on a careful clinical assessment of ECV and extracellular volume, as well as careful consideration of possible causes of low ECV, will enable the clinician to restore ECV, tissue perfusion, and normal homeostasis.

Osmolality

Plasma osmolality is tightly regulated at 275 to 290 mOsm/L in order to provide the best milieu for cellular function. Plasma or serum osmolality is estimated by the equation:

$$serum\,osms = [(2 \times serum\,sodium) + (serum\,glucose/18)$$
$$+ (serum\,BUN/2.8)]$$

where serum or plasma sodium is measured in mEq/L and serum or plasma glucose and BUN in mg/dL. In the absence of diabetes mellitus or renal insufficiency, the contributions to osmolality of glucose and BUN normally are quite small (for example, a normal serum glucose of 100 mg/dL contributes 5.6 mOsm/L and a normal serum BUN of 10 mg/dL only 3.6 mOsm/L, for a total of 9.2 mOsm/L to total serum osmolality). Sodium is balanced by plasma cations, primarily chloride and bicarbonate, to maintain electroneutrality. Hence, in healthy individuals, the major determinant of plasma osmolality becomes the sodium concentration and its anionic counterparts, as estimated by doubling the sodium concentration. Thus, a normal serum sodium of 140 mEq/L contributes 280 mOsm/L: 140 mOsm from the serum sodium and a further 140 mOsm from the anions electrically balancing the sodium. Sodium concentration is maintained by an intricate balance of water intake and solute excretion (Fig. 9.4) resulting in no more than a 1%

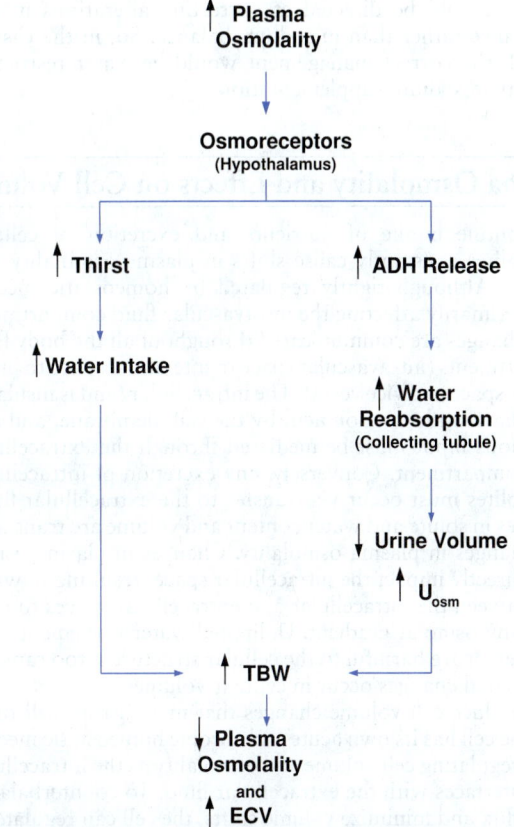

FIGURE 9.4. Regulation of plasma osmolality. ADH, antidiuretic hormone; TBW, total body water; ECV, effective circulating volume; U_{osm}, urine osmolality. (Modified with permission from Rose BD and Post TW. Clinical physiology of acid-base and electrolyte disorders, 5th ed. New York, New York: McGraw-Hill, 2001.)

to 2% normal variation in plasma osmolality, despite wide fluctuations in water and solute intake.

Osmoreceptors in the hypothalamus control thirst and the secretion of antidiuretic hormone (ADH). Normally, the osmotic threshold for ADH release is reached as serum osmolarity exceeds the mid-280 mOsm/L range. Above this level, a progressive and relatively linear rise occurs in ADH secretion from the posterior pituitary. As previously discussed, circulating ADH increases water reabsorption from the collecting tubules with a subsequent increase in U_{osm} and a decrease in urine volume. The increased water retention serves to decrease serum sodium concentration and, as a result, decreases serum osmolality, because sodium is the major determinant of serum osmolality. As previously discussed, hypovolemia also can cause ADH secretion with subsequent increase in ECV. Maximum fluid retention mediated by ADH occurs 90 to 120 minutes after an increase in osmolality. The osmotic threshold for thirst is reported to be 2 to 5 mOsm/L higher than that for ADH release and, thus, usually occurs at a time point after ADH secretion has been stimulated. Thirst will result in water ingestion and, in the presence of ADH, ultimate intravascular volume expansion, resulting in a decrease in plasma osmolality.

Understanding that sodium concentration is mainly regulated by water homeostasis enables the clinician to recognize that hyponatremia (hypo-osmolality) and hypernatremia (hyperosmolality) usually are due to altered water balance rather than a deficit or surfeit of sodium. For example, the syndrome of inappropriate ADH secretion (SIADH) results in hyponatremia because of the inappropriate release of ADH below normal osmotic thresholds. The increased water retention that results causes a low serum sodium concentration. Hence, therapy should be directed at correcting alterations in water balance rather than in sodium balance. So, in the case of SIADH, the correct management would be water restriction rather than sodium supplementation.

Plasma Osmolality and Effects on Cell Volume

The routine intake of nutrients and excretion of cellular metabolites constantly cause shifts in plasma osmolality and volume. Although tightly regulated by homeostatic mechanisms primarily affecting the intravascular fluid compartment, these changes are communicated throughout all the body fluid compartments (intravascular space to interstitial space to intracellular space and vice versa). The intracellular fluid is insulated from the outside environment by the cell membrane, and any exogenous input must be mediated through the extracellular fluid compartment. Conversely, any excretion of intracellular metabolites must occur via transfer to the extracellular fluid. Changes in solute and water content and volume are translated into changes in plasma osmolality. Changes in plasma osmolality directly impact the intracellular space, resulting in water flux between the intracellular and extracellular spaces to minimize any osmolar gradient. Unlimited water movement may, however, prove harmful to the cellular structure if too rapid or unregulated changes occur in cellular volume.

To reduce cell volume changes that may disrupt cell function, the cell has its own acute and chronic homeostatic mechanisms regulating cell volume and osmolality as the intracellular fluid interfaces with the extracellular fluid. To counterbalance water flux and minimize volume shifts, the cell can regulate its osmolality via the transport and production of osmo-effective solutes. When faced with sudden decreases in plasma osmolality, to counteract water flux into the cell and cellular swelling, potassium is acutely transported out of the cell, thus reducing cellular osmolality and limiting net intracellular water gain and swelling. In chronic hypo-osmolar settings, organic osmolytes, such as taurine and inositol, are transported out of the cell. In hyper-osmolar states, to counteract water flux out of the cell and cellular shrinking, electrolytes are transported into the cells acutely, and production of idiogenic osmoles is up-regulated to reduce cellular water loss on a chronic basis.

Despite these regulatory controls, extreme osmotic perturbations or rapid alterations in osmolality can have harmful consequences, especially related to rapid volume shifts within cells of the central nervous system (CNS). Acute osmotic alterations can be corrected more quickly, because electrolyte flow is more rapidly reversible than processes impacting the production and transport of organic osmoles. Such considerations are important when considering the time span over which corrections to abnormalities of fluid and electrolyte should occur.

FLUID AND ELECTROLYTE DERANGEMENTS

Fluid and electrolyte balance is assessed most readily by evaluating volume status and osmolality. Perturbations in the control of either will result in abnormalities in a patient's clinical status. Health care providers should recognize common signs and symptoms in determining whether a change in volume status is present, especially any alteration of ECV and its potential impact on tissue perfusion. In addition, the use of laboratory studies, most notably measurement of sodium concentration, will reveal significant changes in osmolality or tonicity.

Clinically, patients can be categorized into nine states (Fig. 9.5) depending on a patient's volume status and osmolality, all of which potentially can be interconnected by underlying pathology. The goal of fluid and electrolyte therapy is to maintain or return the patient to a state of isovolemia and iso-osmolality, without causing undue harm to the patient in the process of making these corrections. The next section is arranged to discuss changes in osmolality as determined by sodium concentration. Within each section, changes in volume status as they interrelate to changes in osmolality will be addressed, both to focus on possible underlying etiologies and to set a framework for a general approach to therapy. Simple diagnostic tests, such as urine sodium concentration (U_{Na^+}) and urine osmolality (U_{osm}), also are reviewed because they may aid in diagnosing the etiology of alterations of volume and osmolality regulation. Treatment for specific clinical conditions is discussed in the Management section.

Hyponatremia

Hyponatremia is defined as a plasma sodium concentration of less than 130 mEq/L. In the majority of cases, hyponatremia reflects hypo-osmolality and may result in water flux into the cell. Hyponatremia indicates a clinical state in which an excessive amount of free water is present relative to solute (sodium) stores. This may be due to sodium loss in excess of concomitant water loss, with a resultant decrease in TBW, or retention of excess water greater than potential sodium gains, with normal

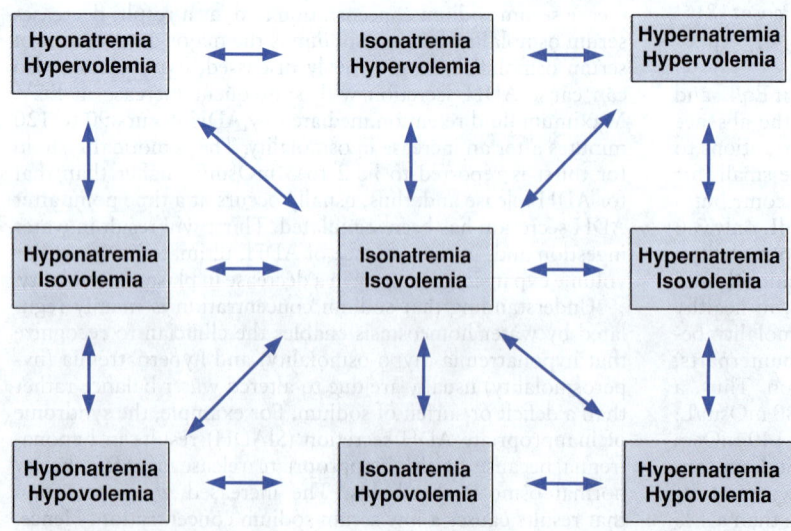

FIGURE 9.5. Fluid and electrolyte clinical states based on volume and electrolyte status. Hyponatremia, serum sodium below 130 mEq/L; isonatremia, serum sodium between 130 to 150 mEq/L; hypernatremia, serum sodium above 150 mEq/L.

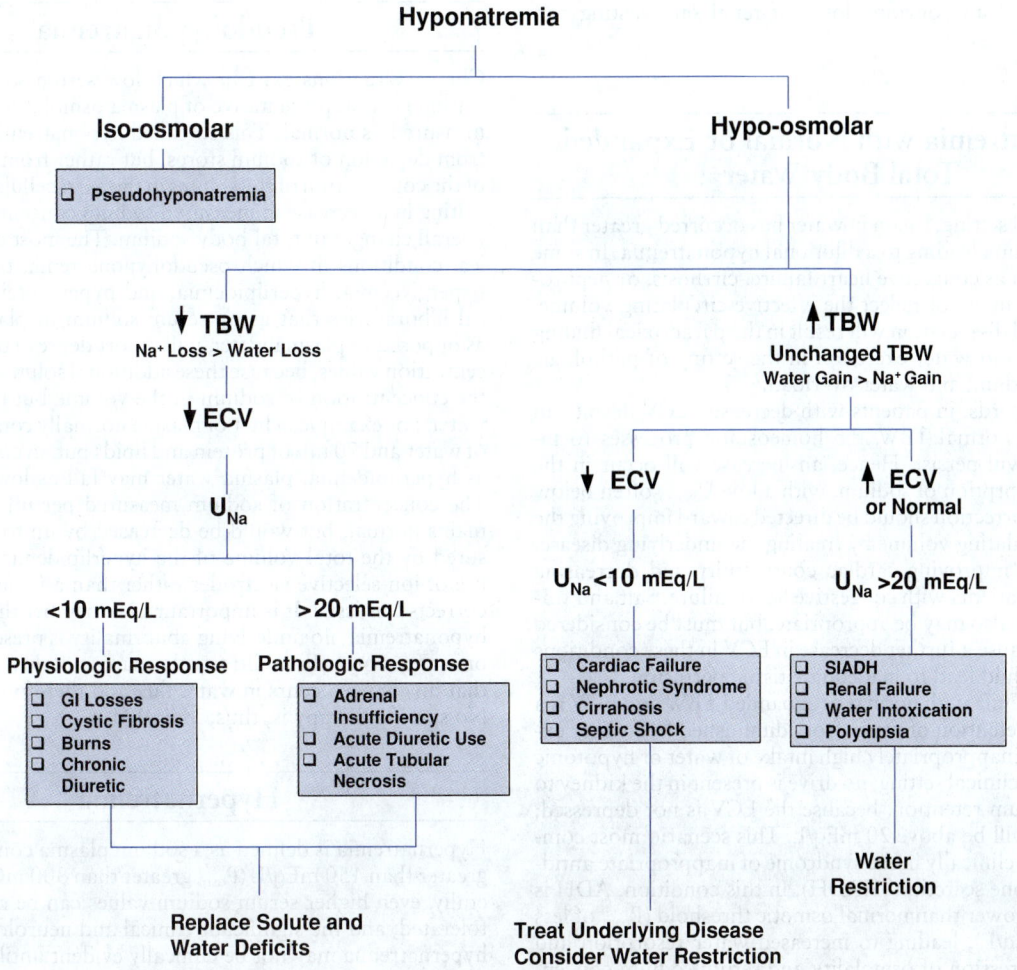

FIGURE 9.6. Hyponatremia: Clinical approach to hyponatremia based on total body water (TBW), effective circulating volume (ECV), and urinary sodium concentration (U_{Na^+}). The boxes list potential diagnoses followed by clinical management.

or expanded TBW. Figure 9.6 is a schematic diagram outlining the clinical approach to and findings associated with hyponatremia, both of which are discussed below.

Hyponatremia with Decrease in Total Body Water

In this setting, a loss of both water and sodium has occurred, but the sodium loss exceeds the water loss and results in a lower than normal serum sodium concentration. With a decrease in both solute and TBW, a decrease in the ECV results. If severe enough, problems with tissue perfusion may occur, and the situation may progress to frank circulatory collapse.

The most common site for nonrenal loss of solute and water is the gastrointestinal tract, usually from diarrhea and vomiting. Another nonrenal site is the skin. Normally, sweat contributes little in the way of effective sodium loss. In pathologic situations, such as cystic fibrosis or burns, however, there may be inappropriately high losses of solute and water. In these clinical conditions, the kidney's homeostatic mechanisms to increase ECV are usually intact, including the capacity to enhance sodium and water renal tubular reabsorption as mediated by the renin-angiotensin-aldosterone system. As a result, urinary sodium reabsorption is avid and can be confirmed by spot U_{Na^+} below 10 mEq/L.

The chronic use of diuretics, particularly the combination of a loop diuretic and a thiazide diuretic, also results in volume depletion and solute loss. Over time, due to the patient's chronic decreased volume status and activation of the renin-angiotensin-aldosterone axis, vigorous proximal tubular reabsorption occurs of any filtered sodium and water. Thus, urinary sodium values are low despite diuretic therapy because so little filtered sodium actually makes its way unabsorbed to those areas of the tubule where diuretics block its reabsorption.

Fluid and electrolyte therapy in a patient with hyponatremia and decreased TBW should be aimed at replenishing both solute and water in the proportion that reflects original losses. This may be accomplished with either appropriate oral or parenteral fluids.

Hyponatremia with decrease in TBW and a U_{Na^+} above 20 mEq/L indicates renal salt wasting. This may be due to intrinsic tubular disease, as seen with acute tubular necrosis (ATN); in children with congenital urologic obstruction; acute diuretic use; or less commonly, in some forms of adrenal insufficiency with decreased mineralocorticoid effect. In all cases, random U_{Na^+} usually exceed 20 mEq/L, regardless of the patient's volume status and the appropriateness of the natriuresis. Therapy should be directed toward hormone replacement in patients with adrenal anomalies. In addition, these patients, as well as those with renal salt wasting from direct injury or diuretics, will require supplementation of sodium to replace past sodium losses and, after this repletion has occurred, replacement of any ongoing losses if renal salt-wasting persists.

Hyponatremia with Normal or Expanded Total Body Water

In this clinical setting, a gain in water has occurred greater than a gain in sodium, leading to a dilutional hyponatremia. In some illnesses, such as congestive heart failure, cirrhosis, or nephrosis, the TBW may not reflect the effective circulating volume. This potential dissociation will result in the paradoxical finding of low U_{Na^+} and water excretion in the setting of pathologic total body sodium and water overload.

In other words, in patients with decreased ECV despite an expanded or normal TBW, the homeostatic processes to increase ECV will persist. Hence, an increase will occur in the tubular reabsorption of sodium, with a low U_{Na^+}, often below 10 mEq/L. Correction should be directed toward improving the effective circulating volume by treating the underlying disease, for example, improving cardiac contractility and decreasing afterload in patients with congestive heart failure. Salt and water restriction also may be appropriate, but must be considered carefully, because a further decrease in ECV in these conditions potentially could lead to inadequate tissue perfusion.

Hyponatremia with normal or expanded TBW and ECV is a result of the retention of water from diminished free-water excretion or an inappropriately high intake of water or hypotonic fluids. In this clinical setting, no drive is present in the kidney to increase sodium retention, because the ECV is not depressed; hence U_{Na^+} will be above 20 mEq/L. This scenario most commonly is seen clinically in the syndrome of inappropriate antidiuretic hormone secretion (SIADH). In this condition, ADH is secreted at a lower than normal osmotic threshold (P_{osm} of less than 285 mEq/L), leading to increased water resorption and a further depression of osmolality and serum sodium concentrations. Patients will have inappropriately low urine volume and high U_{osm} despite the hypo-osmolality and increased TBW, because ADH is present and water is reabsorbed. SIADH can occur in a number of clinical conditions, such as meningitis, encephalitis, following CNS trauma and surgery, with pulmonary diseases including pneumonia and asthma, and in excessive pain. In addition, a number of drugs can potentiate ADH effect, most notably carbamazepine, intravenous cyclophosphamide, or chlorpropamide, and others act as an exogenous source of ADH, such as oxytocin or vasopressin. Therapy includes water restriction and treating the underlying disease that led to SIADH.

Rarer causes of hyponatremia with expanded TBW include chronic renal insufficiency, water intoxication, and polydipsia. As GFR falls and fewer functioning nephrons are present, free-water clearance decreases. This becomes more clinically relevant as the GFR approaches levels nearing the need for dialysis. Polydipsia or water intoxication is rare in children, but may be seen in infants who are given large hypotonic fluid loads by their caretakers. Psychogenic polydipsia is quite rare in children, being nearly nonexistent in the pre-school aged child, and it generally is found in children with other signs and symptoms of emotional disturbance. With water intoxication, water intake is not dependent on the normal thirst mechanism and osmotic threshold and, because of chronic volume expansion, urine output is brisk and dilute with U_{Na^+} of greater than 20 mEq/L.

In all these conditions, because ECV is normal or expanded, therapy includes fluid restriction. Patients should be given a daily fluid limit and educated about sources of water present in many solid foods that are predominantly liquid at room temperature.

Pseudohyponatremia

Clinical situations exist in which low serum sodium concentration is not representative of plasma osmolality which, when measured, is normal. This so-called hyponatremia results, not from depletion of sodium stores, but rather from an alteration of the composition of the solutes in the extracellular volume, resulting in a decrease in measured sodium concentration but no overall changes in total body sodium. The most common clinical conditions in which pseudohyponatremia occurs include hyperglycemia, hyperlipidemia, and hyperproteinemia. Clinical laboratories that assay serum sodium in plasma volume, as opposed to plasma water, will report depressed sodium concentration values, because these additional solutes will decrease the concentration of sodium in the volume but not in plasma water. For example, a liter of plasma normally contains 930 mL of water and 70 mL of protein and lipids but, in conditions such as hyperlipidemia, plasma water may fall as low as 720 mL. The concentration of sodium measured per mL of water remains normal, but would be decreased by up to 25% if measured by the total volume of the hyperlipidemic plasma. The use of ion-selective electrodes rather than a flame photometer corrects this issue. It is important to remember that in pseudohyponatremia, no underlying abnormality is present in sodium or water stores. In addition, plasma osmolality is normal, so that no change occurs in water flux and therefore cell volume. No specific therapy is, thus, indicated.

Hypernatremia

Hypernatremia is defined as a sodium plasma concentration of greater than 150 mEq/L (P_{osm} greater than 300 mOsm/L). Generally, even higher serum sodium values can be relatively well tolerated, and the significant clinical and neurologic effects of hypernatremia may not be clinically evident until sodium concentrations exceed 160 mEq/L. Hypernatremia usually reflects a change in water balance, with water loss in excess of sodium loss; it is rarely a result of a surfeit of sodium. Figure 9.7 is a schematic diagram outlining the clinical approach and findings to hypernatremia, which are discussed below.

Hypernatremia with Increase in Total Body Water

This form of hypernatremia is due to excess sodium intake and is rare in pediatrics. Clinical scenarios include incorrect mixing of infant formula or rehydration solution with excess salt, ingestion of seawater, use of parenteral hypertonic saline solutions, or large repetitive doses of sodium bicarbonate to treat a refractory acidosis. In all these cases, the ECF and TBW are expanded, because water is retained due to the increase in osmolality. Clinical signs and symptoms may include peripheral edema, hypertension, and in severe cases, congestive heart failure and pulmonary edema. Therapy is directed at the elimination of excess sodium and includes the use of diuretics and augmenting free-water intake.

Hypernatremia with Decrease in Total Body Water

In this setting, hypernatremia is due to a loss of free water or a combination of both sodium and water loss, in which the water loss is much greater than sodium loss. TBW is reduced, but ECV will be somewhat preserved initially, at the expense of osmotic water flux from the intracellular fluid. Hence, patients

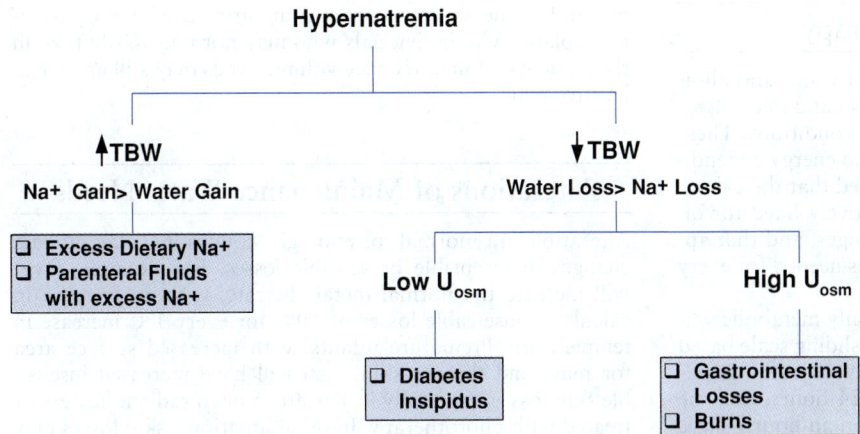

FIGURE 9.7. Hypernatremia: Clinical approach to hypernatremia based on total body water (TBW) and urine osmolality (U_{osm}). The boxes list potential diagnoses.

with hypernatremic dehydration may display fewer and milder symptoms of dehydration than those with either isonatremic or hyponatremic dehydration with similar volumes of overall water loss.

Normally, ADH would be secreted as the osmotic threshold (P_{osm} approaching 285) has been exceeded, resulting in the excretion of concentrated urine in low volumes (see Fig. 9.4). Thus, hypernatremia that presents with inappropriately low U_{osm} is due to impaired ADH function, with an inability to appropriately reabsorb water and lower the sodium concentration and osmolality. This may be due to lack of ADH secretion; central diabetes insipidus, as seen in patients with a CNS disorder; or to the resistance of the collecting tubule to respond to ADH, as seen in nephrogenic diabetes insipidus. Nephrogenic diabetes insipidus either can be congenital, due to genetic defects in either the ADH receptor or the collecting tubule water channels, or acquired, as seen with lithium toxicity. Hormonal replacement is therapeutic in central diabetes insipidus. In nephrogenic diabetes insipidus, ensured access to free water is critical, especially in very young children and infants. In addition, a low-salt diet and thiazide diuretics have been used as adjunctive therapies to try to promote the increased proximal tubular resorption of water by causing chronic volume depletion.

Hypernatremia with high U_{osm} indicates that the ADH-mediated renal concentrating mechanism is intact. Free-water loss has occurred either alone or in combination with sodium loss, in which water loss has significantly exceeded that of sodium. Plasma osmolality exceeds the threshold for ADH release, and the body compensates for the water loss by ADH-mediated water retention and the passage of small volumes of urine with high U_{osm}. In addition, ECV also is decreased, with stimulation of tubular reabsorption of sodium and subsequently a low U_{Na^+} of less than 20 mEq/L. The gastrointestinal tract is the site of the most common loss of hypotonic solution due to diarrheal illnesses. Skin is another site of free-water loss, as in the burn patient or in the very premature infant with thin dermis placed under a radiant heater, which may increase insensible losses without adequate water replacement.

FLUID MANAGEMENT

Fluid therapy, whether parenteral or oral, is intended to maintain the normal volume and composition of body fluids and, as necessary, correct any existing abnormality. Corrective therapy must be given as safely as possible, with the main goal of restoring bodily homeostasis to promote optimal cell and organ function. It has been over two centuries since the use of replacement fluid and electrolyte therapy was first introduced for victims of cholera. During the twentieth century, pediatricians led the way in continued development of fluid therapy, with increasing knowledge of body fluid physiology, including compartmentalization of water and solutes and the ability to identify and measure specific electrolytes. The initial focus on the use of parenteral fluid and electrolyte therapy for children with fluid and electrolyte aberrations has more recently given rise to the development of oral therapy as effective treatment for children with a variety of illnesses in a variety of clinical settings.

Many approaches to fluid therapy have been developed. Many of these are empiric in nature, based on clinical experience and efficacy, and can be used relatively interchangeably. The following broad guidelines should direct clinicians in caring for patients' fluid needs:

- Therapy must be individualized.
- The calculations of necessary fluid volumes or solute loads for either maintenance or replacement therapy are estimates and may not be generalized across clinical scenarios.
- The patient's response is ultimately the gauge of the success of therapy, and the patient must be sequentially re-evaluated during therapy to make any necessary adjustments.
- Simplicity in the design and execution of therapy is essential for accurate and effective treatment.

In the last half of the twentieth century, many of the approaches to fluid and electrolyte therapy in children were based on a tradition of calculating fluid and electrolytes required to cover maintenance needs, alterations in maintenance needs, and corrective therapy for any deficit or replacement needs. Fluid and electrolyte therapy most often was given parenterally. With the advent of oral rehydration therapy, it has been suggested that this approach may be more complicated than needed (Holliday, 1996), and that oral rehydration therapy can be a straightforward and effective therapy for *most* children, particularly those with acute dehydrating diarrheal illnesses.

In the next section, the traditional approach to fluid management, with the more precise calculations for maintenance needs and deficit replacement, is presented. This approach is particularly useful in patients with more complicated fluid and electrolyte issues, in whom such accounting may prevent complications from therapy. The use of oral rehydration solutions will also be reviewed, but should be considered mainly for those patients with diarrheal dehydration, because its effectiveness and safety has been well documented in that clinical setting.

Maintenance Fluid Therapy

Maintenance therapy refers to the volume of water and allotment of electrolytes needed to replace the water and electrolytes that are lost daily under normal physiologic conditions. These requirements are related to metabolic rate and energy expenditure. Holliday and Segar (1957) demonstrated that the caloric expenditure rate/unit weight ratio was relatively fixed for infants and children in three broad weight ranges, and that approximately 100 mL of exogenous water was needed for every 100 kcal of energy expended.

To apply these principles clinically, the daily metabolic water requirements have been translated into a sliding scale based on weight. Two methods of calculation have become popular, one based on a volume calculated for 24 hours, and the other to a volume that would be delivered on an hourly basis (Table 9.2). The total daily volume of fluid prescribed with the hourly format is slightly lower but not of significant clinical relevance. For example, using the 24-hour daily volume calculations, the estimated maintenance fluid requirement for a 13 kg child would be 1,150 mL (1,000 mL for first 10 kg at 100 mL/kg/day and 150 mL for the next 3 kg at 50 mL/kg/day). Using hourly calculations (960 for the first 10 kg at 4 mL/kg/hour and 144 mL for the next 3 kg at 2 mL/kg/hour), a slightly lower volume of 1,104 mL is derived. After 80 kg, the proportion of body weight and water distribution diverges significantly, so that calculations beyond 80 kg will be significantly overestimated by these calculations.

Water needs result from sensible losses from urine and stool, as well as from insensible loss through the skin and respiratory tract. This daily deficit is blunted somewhat by the endogenous water production that occurs with metabolism. Under normal conditions, insensible losses account for one-third of the calculated daily maintenance requirements for fluids, and urinary losses for the other two-thirds. Skin losses are evaporative due to convection and conduction and are increased with high core body temperature. Respiratory water losses occur in the lungs as relatively dry and cool inspired air is humidified and warmed as it reaches the bifurcation of the trachea. Insensible losses are strictly water, with skin accounting for about two-thirds of these losses and the remaining one-third from the respiratory tract. Normally, the water loss from stools is negligible, so that sensible losses are due to daily urine output. In states of increased diarrheal stool loss, however, gastrointestinal (GI) tract losses may be profound. An obligate urine water loss also is needed to excrete the osmotic and solute load generated by the body's metabolism and intake. The minimal obligate urine volume is 25 mL for every 100 kcal of energy expended, and it is dependent on maximal ADH stimulation and urinary concentrating capacity, with U_{osm} of 1,200 to 1,400 mOsm/L. Thus, urine volume comes to be regulated by solute intake and water production, renal function, and the maximally achievable concentration of the urine. The daily maintenance calculation assumes normal solute load with isosthenuric urine (U_{osm} of 300

mOsm/L). The ability to concentrate urine to higher osmolality explains why individuals who may not necessarily take in their calculated maintenance volume needs may still appear to be euvolemic.

Alterations of Maintenance Water Needs

Alterations in normal physiologic conditions may impact changes in insensible or sensible losses. For example, fever will increase the normal metabolic rate, with an increase in calculated insensible losses of 10% for every 1°C increase in temperature. Premature infants, with increased surface area for mass and thinner skin, also will have increased insensible skin losses, especially if they are in open radiant heaters or treated with phototherapy. In these situations, skin losses may double or triple normal losses. On the other hand, patients on ventilators receiving humidified air will have a decrease in their insensible losses. Anuric patients with renal failure will have no urinary fluid losses, whereas those with diabetes insipidus may have more than 5 L of daily urine output. Hence, in ill patients, *maintenance volume* calculations should consider the potential fluctuations from the norm in urinary output and skin and respiratory water losses. These alterations have been referred to as *supplemental therapy*, but it is important to appreciate that these so-called supplemental changes in daily fluid provision may not merely be increased daily fluid provision but may also require subtracting fluid from usual daily needs.

Maintenance Electrolyte/Solute Therapy

Estimates for maintenance electrolyte requirements evolved both from early studies and clinical experience and, like water, are generally calculated based on metabolic or energy needs. Baseline sodium and chloride requirements vary from 2 to 3 mEq/100 mL of water per day for normal homeostasis. The baseline potassium requirement is 1 to 2 mEq/100 mL of water per day. The majority of electrolyte losses are from the urine but, at times, significant losses can occur from the skin or gastrointestinal tract. As is true with water and volume calculation, alterations in maintenance electrolyte needs must be considered based on the clinical context, especially in situations where daily volume needs have changed. Hence, the very low-birth-weight infant who has a doubling of her insensible water losses will not have the same need to double the daily electrolyte requirements relative to water, because the insensible skin losses are essentially all water. In patients who are anuric, a marked decrease in the daily loss of electrolytes needs to be reflected in adjusting replacement therapy. This is especially true with potassium because, without a decrease in intake, these patients may develop hyperkalemia.

Clinically, the standard commercially available parenteral solution of D5 0.25% NaCl with 20 mEq/L of potassium will meet the normal electrolyte maintenance requirements for most children with normal renal function if infused at "maintenance" volume rates. In patients who are only receiving parenteral fluids, dextrose is often added to water as a 5% solution. This provides about 20% of daily caloric needs when full-maintenance daily fluids are infused.

Once the clinician has assessed a patient's fluid needs and chosen the appropriate maintenance fluid regimen, the adequacy of therapy is judged by the patient's response, most notably cardiovascular signs, changes in weight, or changes in serum sodium. For example, in the very low-birth-weight premature infant, decrease in body weight, an increase in serum sodium concentration, and an increased heart rate to maintain

---

TABLE 9.2

CALCULATION OF MAINTENANCE FLUIDS BASED ON BODY WEIGHT

Body Weight (kg)	Maintenance Fluid Requirements mL/day	Maintenance Fluid Requirements mL/hour
1–10	100/kg	4 mL/kg
11–20	1,000 plus 50/kg for weight over 10 kg	40 mL plus 2 mL/kg for weight over 10 kg
21–80	1,500 plus 20/kg for weight over 20 kg	60 mL plus 1 mL/kg for weight over 20 kg

cardiac output will reflect the inadequacy of the fluid therapy to meet unrecognized increased insensible loss.

Replacement Fluid Therapy

In infants and children, the most common fluid disorder is dehydration or hypovolemia. This occurs because children have a higher frequency of illnesses with gastrointestinal tract losses (diarrhea or vomiting); have higher surface area to volume ratios, and thus the potential for increased insensible skin losses with fever; and, especially in the young, may be unable to communicate the need for fluids or have access to fluids, thus limiting their ability to replenish volume losses. In the United States, tens of thousands of admissions are for dehydration; and globally, the problem is even more serious, with deaths due to dehydration numbering in the millions.

In treating a child with dehydration, the following steps should be completed:

- Clinical assessment of the degree of dehydration
- Consideration of the type of dehydration and resulting alterations in osmolality or sodium concentration
- Development of a safe therapeutic plan to correct the fluid and electrolyte deficit and to provide ongoing needs

Clinical Assessment

The degree of dehydration is most objectively measured as a change in weight from baseline. Acute loss of body weight reflects loss of fluids and electrolytes and not lean body mass. In many clinical situations, the clinician will not have a previous weight readily available, and other clinical parameters are used to judge the severity of dehydration (Table 9.3). Similar clinical findings represent different degrees of dehydration in older children compared with infants.

As the ECV is reduced, the signs and symptoms of dehydration become more apparent. Hence, a history of excessive fluid losses may be the sole indication of mild dehydration, because clinical signs may be absent or minimal. Moderate losses will present with more apparent clinical symptoms, such as decreased skin turgor and tears, dry mucous membranes, and irritability and may include findings of decreased ECV, such as orthostatic blood pressure changes and tachycardia. Severe dehydration, a near shock-like state, occurs with further reduction in ECV, with resulting hemodynamic instability, including hypotension, decreased peripheral perfusion, oliguria or anuria, and lethargy. This latter state requires immediate attention using aggressive volume resuscitation to restore ECV

and prevent the development of ischemic and hypoxic tissue damage due to underperfusion of the body's organs and cells.

The degree of dehydration is an important factor in deciding on the type and speed of fluid therapy. Severe dehydration requires the use of rapid parenteral fluid resuscitation until adequate tissue perfusion and some hemodynamic stability is achieved. Oral replacement therapy may be appropriate for mild to moderate dehydration and, in less developed countries, has been given by nasogastric tube to more profoundly dehydrated patients. As the child receives replacement fluid, it is important to assess clinical progress. Initial estimates of the degree of dehydration may need adjustment as the patient responds. Serial weights, urine output and osmolality, patient affect, general appearance, and vital signs are all parameters to assess the adequacy of volume replacement.

In general, laboratory studies have not been useful in assessing the severity of dehydration. Blood urea nitrogen (BUN) rises with an increasing severity of dehydration (prerenal azotemia), but the correlation is not strong enough to be clinically useful for assigning an absolute degree of dehydration based on BUN level.

Type of Dehydration

Serum sodium concentration will define the type of dehydration (see Fig. 9.5): hypotonic (sodium level less than 130 mEq/L), hypertonic (sodium level greater than 150 mEq/L), and isotonic (sodium level between 130 to 150 mEq/L). In most cases of dehydration, especially those with mild to moderate severity, the dehydration will be isotonic. These broad categories are useful in the diagnostic approach to dehydration (see previous sections) and in planning fluid replacement, with special considerations for severe hyponatremia and hypernatremia.

Approach

A number of approaches can be taken to replacement therapy, all based on two phases. The first phase focuses on assessing the perfusion of the patient and, if necessary, *emergently* restoring the ECV to ensure adequate circulation. The second *subsequent* phase replaces fluids and electrolyte losses in those patients whose circulation has been restored or in those patients with mild to moderate dehydration, without impaired circulation, and who did not need initial aggressive fluid resuscitation. The subsequent replacement phase can be either oral or parenteral therapy.

Emergent Therapy. Regardless of the type of dehydration, the first phase is needed in patients with signs and symptoms of ineffective circulating volume, such as orthostasis or frank

TABLE 9.3			
CLINICAL EVALUATION: SEVERITY OF DEHYDRATION			
	Mild	Moderate	Severe
% Wt Loss			
Infant	<5	10	15
Child	<3	6	9
Physical exam			
Behavior	Consolable	Irritable	Lethargic
Blood pressure	Normal	Orthostatic	Hypotensive
Mucous membranes	Normal	Dry	Parched/crack
Tears	Present	Decrease	Absent
Eyes	Normal	Deep set	Sunken
Skin turgor	Normal	Decrease	Tenting
Fontanels	Flat	Slightly depressed	Sunken
Capillary refill	Normal	3–5 seconds	>5 seconds
Urine output	Normal	Decreased	Anuric

TABLE 9.4

ELECTROLYTE COMPOSITION OF COMMON SOLUTIONS

	Sodium mEq/L	Potassium mEq/L	Cl⁻ mEq/L	Buffer mEq/L	Glucose g/L
Parenteral Crystalloids					
NS (0.9%)	154	0	154	0	0
Lactated Ringer's	130	4	109	Lactate/28	0
D5 0.45% NaCl (1/2 Normal saline)	75	0	75	0	50
D5 0.25% NaCl (1/4 Normal saline)	35	0	35	0	50
D5	0	0	0	0	50
Normosol	140	5	98	Acetate/27 Gluconate/23	0
Plasma-Lyte	140	5	98	Acetate/27 Gluconate/23	
Colloids					
5% Albumin	130–160	<1	130–160	0	0
25% Albumin	130–160	<1	130–160	0	0
Fresh frozen plasma	140	4	110	Bicarbonate/25	0
Oral Rehydration Solutions	Citrate				
WHO ORS	75	20	8	30	13.5
Rehydralyte	75	20	65	30	25
Pedialyte	45	20	35	30	25
Ricelyte	30	25	45	34	3*

*Carbohydrate is rice based.

hypotension, tachycardia, and decreased capillary refill. Patients with impaired peripheral circulation or overt shock require emergent treatment to restore their ECV and prevent serious hypoxic tissue injury. This requires rapid parenteral therapy using a bolus infusion of isotonic fluid. NS (0.9% NaCl) at 20 mL/kg is infused over 30 to 60 minutes. Lactated Ringer's solution also can be used but must be used cautiously in patients with lactic acidosis or who are unable to convert lactate to bicarbonate, because this may cause or worsen metabolic acidosis. Because of its potassium content, lactated Ringer's solution also should be avoided in children with known or suspected impaired renal function. Other commercially available crystalloid solutions are rarely used in pediatrics. In addition, colloid therapy may be used. There does not appear, however, to be any increased advantage of colloid versus crystalloid therapy in assessing patient survival after fluid resuscitation, and the increased cost of colloids has further limited their use.

NS, lactated Ringer's, and colloid solutions all have an osmolality near 300 mOsm/L and hence will restore the ECV and remain in the plasma space. Table 9.4 lists commercially available parenteral solutions and their solute composition. The isotonic bolus can be repeated up to two additional times until the patient is hemodynamically stable and adequate perfusion is restored. During the fluid bolus therapy, further clinical assessment and laboratory evaluation to establish both the severity and type of dehydration occurs, allowing planning for the next phase of replacement therapy. Clinicians may also opt to treat initially with a rapid intravenous bolus even in patients without circulatory compromise, as long as the patient has normal cardiac and renal function.

Once the circulation has been stabilized, or as an earlier step in patients with mild to moderate dehydration without impaired circulation, corrective therapy (phase two) to replace the remaining deficit of fluids and electrolytes begins. This therapy can be accomplished in a number of ways, with the type and volume of fluid as well as the route of administration varying according to the patient's specific clinical circumstances.

Oral Rehydration Therapy. Oral rehydration therapy (ORT) has been used successfully throughout the world in children with mild to moderate dehydration and has been extensively studied in children with diarrheal illness. In addition, ORT has been used successfully as corrective therapy after patients receive initial parenteral bolus therapy to restore ECV (phase one). Several commercially prepared ORT solutions are available (see Table 9.4). Each of these solutions contains 2 to 3 g/dL of glucose, the optimal concentration that will facilitate sodium and water uptake from the gut and not produce osmotic diarrhea. The sodium content in the World Health Organization (WHO) Oral Rehydration Solution (ORS) is 75 mEq/L, which was changed from the original formulation of 90 mEq/L. Commercially available solutions contain 45 to 75 mEq/L. The higher sodium concentration has allowed the successful use of WHO ORS in cholera epidemics, in which sodium losses are more profound, as well as in cases of nonsecretory diarrhea. In developed countries, dehydrating diarrheal illness is usually viral in etiology, producing a lower sodium content than the secretory diarrhea seen in underdeveloped country.

The use of ORT has assumed that no severe electrolyte abnormalities are present. Many patients with severe hypernatremia have been treated successfully with ORT; however, there have been reports of seizures secondary to too rapid correction of the serum sodium level when the initial level was greater than 160 mEq/L.

ORT is based on the consistent administration of small volumes of fluids (initial volume of 5 mL) at frequent and regular intervals (every 1 to 2 minutes). If the child tolerates the initial regimen, then the volume can be increased and the frequency decreased with the goal to deliver a prescribed volume over 3 to 4 hours. The plan must be laid out clearly to the care providers, with alternative options available if the plan is not successfully implemented.

Several oral rehydration schemes have been proposed (Table 9.5). The American Academy of Pediatrics (AAP) recommends that children with acute dehydration and extracellular volume contraction be given 40 to 50 mL/kg of a solution containing 2% to 2.5% glucose, 75 to 90 mEq/L of sodium, 20 mEq/L of potassium, and 20 to 30 mEq/L of buffer over 3 to 4 hours. Once the extracellular volume has been restored using this initial intervention, the solution should be changed to decrease the sodium to 40 to 60 mEq/L of sodium at half the rate (20 to

TABLE 9.5

ORAL REHYDRATION REGIMENS

American Academy of Pediatrics	Solution: 75–90 mEq/L sodium, 2% to 2.5% glucose, 20–30 mEq/L potassium, 20 mEq/L of base Rate 40–50 mL/kg over 3 to 4 hours
Murphy	Solution: 60 mEq/L sodium, 2% glucose, 20 mEq/L potassium, 10 mmol/L citrate Rate dependent on type of dehydration over 3 to 4 hours ■ Mild: 30–50 mL/kg ■ Moderate: 50–100 mL/kg ■ Severe: 100–150 mL/kg ■ Shock: First resuscitate with IV normal saline bolus: 20 mL/kg

25 mL/kg over 3 to 4 hours). A more recent proposal based on a review of the literature (Murphy, 1998), treats children in accordance with the degree and type of dehydration, using a solution with 90 mEq/L of sodium, 1.62% glucose, and 10 mmol/L citrate. Fluid volumes of 30 to 150 mL/kg were given over 3 to 12 hours, again depending on the type and severity of dehydration. The WHO also has a treatment regimen that is based on the use of the WHO ORS, with different rates and volumes for moderate and mild dehydration.

A patient with moderate or severe dehydration, with signs indicative of compromised effective circulating volume, should first receive resuscitative therapy restoring circulation. If possible, this should be done using parenteral therapy to restore adequate perfusion in the most rapid and controlled fashion. After hemodynamic stability is re-established, if the patient is able to tolerate oral fluids, they should be transitioned to ORT.

Caregivers should be discouraged against using household beverages such as soft drinks, sports drinks, or tea to treat dehydration. These beverages do not contain adequate sodium and potassium supplementation and often will contain suboptimal carbohydrate concentration or source. The clinician must carefully lay out to care providers an appropriate ORT fluid and a precise schedule of administration, including both timing and volume, to increase the chances of successful oral rehydration. If the care providers are unwilling to follow these directives, or the child is unable to tolerate oral therapy, parenteral therapy must be considered.

Parenteral Therapy. As noted, parenteral therapy is indicated if any sign of impaired circulation is present or if there are impediments to the successful delivery of ORT. In addition, if there is clinical concern that dehydration may be complicated by severe electrolyte abnormalities or underlying medical conditions, parenteral therapy should be considered.

Parenteral therapy is based on initially restoring ECV to maintain adequate perfusion, using rapid boluses of isotonic crystalloid at 20 mL/kg. This may be repeated up to two times. The second next phase of therapy is to continue the replacement of existing deficits and provide maintenance needs (both normal and abnormal needs) of sodium and water. Calculations for sodium and water requirements to replace deficit losses and maintenance needs can be done for the planned time interval of fluid therapy. The type of dehydration also will dictate the length of time over which fluid perturbations will be corrected. For example, severe cases of hypernatremia, with serum sodium levels greater than 160 mEq/L, may take 48 to 72 hours to treat, in comparison to 24 hours in cases of isonatremic dehydration with the same degree of dehydration.

Volume Deficit and Rate

In the setting of acute dehydration, acute weight loss is considered fluid deficit. If weights are not available, the volume deficit is calculated based on the clinical assessment of severity of dehydration (see Table 9.4), minus the volume received emergently. It is important to determine over what time interval replacement losses will be replaced. The total hourly rate of parenteral fluids administrated is the sum of the hourly replacement rate and the hourly maintenance rate. For example: A child with a baseline weight of 10 kg with moderate dehydration (10%) treated emergently with 20 mL/kg NS bolus:

a. Initial Fluid Deficit = 10% of 10 kg = 1,000 mL
b. Emergent Therapy: 20 mL/kg NS boluses = 200 mL
c. Subsequent therapy for next 24 hours:
   i. Remaining Fluid Deficit = 800 mL;
     Rate = 800 mL ÷ 24 hours = 35 mL/hour
   ii. Maintenance Rate (assumes no alterations)
     = 4 cc/kg/hour × 10 kg = 40 mL/hour
   iii. Total Rate 75/mL/hour

Sodium Deficit

In all types of dehydration, the assumption is that acute weight loss represents isotonic fluid loss, reflective of the extracellular fluid. Probably due to homeostatic mechanism with water movement and ion transport, this approach appears to be relatively safe and has been widely adopted in rehydration practices.

In addition, in cases of hypotonic dehydration, additional sodium solute may have been lost. The sodium loss can be determined by calculating the difference in total serum sodium content in the patient's normal or desired condition and the current hyponatremic condition. Total body sodium or solute is the product of the serum sodium concentration (Na^+) and the total body water (TBW).

$$\text{sodium deficit} = [TBW_{desired} \times Na^+_{desired}] - [TBW_{current} \times Na^+_{current}] \quad (1)$$

TBW in most situations is 60% of the total mass ($0.6 \times$ weight in kg), except for babies, in which TBW may be up to 80% in the very low-birth-weight premature infant (see previous section on Total Body Water). Desired sodium is 140 mEq/L, so

$$Na^+ \text{ deficit} = (TBW_{desired} \times 140\,mEq/L) - [TBW_{current} \times Na^+_{current}]$$

In patients with isotonic dehydration, the calculation is simplified, because serum sodium (S_{Na^+}) is 140 mEq/L for both the desired and current states. The difference in TBW is the fluid deficit, hence the serum sodium deficit becomes:

$$Na^+ \text{ deficit} = (TBW_{desired} - TBW_{current}) \times 140\,mEq/L$$
$$= \text{Fluid deficit} \times 140\,mEq/L$$

In hypotonic dehydration, one can also simplify equation 1 by substituting $TBW_{desired}$ with $TBW_{current}$ plus Fluid Deficit. Making this substitution, equation 1 becomes:

$$Na^+ \text{ deficit} = (TBW_{current} + \text{Fluid Deficit}) \times 140 - [TBW_{current} \times Na^+_{current}]$$

$$Na^+ \text{ deficit} = [(TBW_{current}) \times 140 + \text{Fluid Deficit} \times 140] - [TBW_{current} \times Na^+_{current}]$$

$$Na^+ \text{ deficit} = \text{Fluid Deficit} \times 140\,mEq/L + (140\,mEq/L - Na^+_{current}) \times TBW_{current}$$

In both isotonic and hypotonic dehydration, one must consider the solute that already has been replaced with the emergent therapy of rapid infusion of isotonic saline when calculating subsequent replacement. A 10 kg child with moderate dehydration (10%) and a serum sodium level of 130 mEq/L treated with 20 mL/kg NS bolus emergently:

a. Initial Deficit:
  i. Sodium loss in fluid deficit: $1 L \times 140$ mEq/L = 140 mEq
  ii. $TBW_{current} = 0.6$ $TBW_{desired}$ – fluid deficit = 0.6 (10 kg) – 1 L = 5 L; Sodium loss in current TBW: $(140 – 130)$ mEq/L $\times 5 L = 50$ mEq
  iii. Total sodium loss = 190 mEq
b. Emergent therapy: 20 mL/kg bolus NS = 200 mL (150 mEq/L Na) = 30 mEq
c. Subsequent sodium therapy for next 24 hours:
  i. Remaining sodium deficit: 160 mEq
  ii. Maintenance needs (assume no alterations): 3 mEq/kg/day $\times$ 10 kg = 30 mEq
  iii. Total sodium needs: 190 mEq
  iv. Type or salinity of solution: total solute needs/total volume needs = 190 mEq/L

Half of volume can be given as NS (11 mEq/hr $\times$ 12 hrs) and the remaining half with 1/2 NS (5.5 mEq/hr $\times$ 12 hrs) for a total of 193 mEq to restore both the fluid and electrolyte needs of the patient.

Symptomatic Hyponatremia

Symptomatic hyponatremia, most commonly manifested by neurologic dysfunction, relates to both the rate of change of serum sodium from normal, as well as to the absolute level of serum sodium. The more rapid and extensive the degree of change, the less time is available for the regulatory mechanism to minimize cell volume change. As the plasma osmolality (serum sodium) falls, an osmolar gradient develops between the intracellular and extracellular fluids, with a subsequent intracellular water movement and an expansion of cell volume. Due to the limited space in the skull, significant increase in the volume of brain cells will increase intracerebral pressure. As the sodium falls acutely below 125 mEq/L, patients may begin to complain of nausea and malaise. Headache, lethargy, obtundation, and seizures may present as serum sodium levels fall below 120 mEq/L.

Treatment is directed acutely to resolving the neurologic symptoms, especially seizures, by raising the serum sodium acutely by 5 mEq/L. This is one of the few clinical situations in which hypertonic 3% NaCl (sodium 513 mEq/L or 0.5 mEq/mL) is used. The sodium dose needed to increase the serum sodium by 5 mEq/L is calculated, and 3% saline is administered over 3 to 4 hours, raising the serum sodium no more rapidly than 2 mEq/L/hour.

$$Na^+ \text{ dose} = TBW \times (5 \text{ mEq/L})$$

To calculate the volume of 3% NS: 1 mEq of sodium is contained in 2 mL of 3% NS; therefore, the volume of 3% NaCl (in mL) needed to deliver a sodium dose is $(2 \times Na^+ \text{dose})$ mL. For example: A 10 kg child with seizures and a serum sodium of 115 mEq/L. (TBW = 0.6 of Wt.)

a. Sodium dose = TBW $\times$ 5 mEq/L = 0.6 $\times$ 10 kg $\times$ 5 mEq/L = 30 mEq of sodium
b. Volume of 3% NaCl = 2 $\times$ Sodium Dose = 2 $\times$ 30 = 60 mL

Administer 60 ml 3% NaCl over 3 hours = Rate 20 mL/hour.

If symptoms persist, repeat intervention using 3% NaCl can be considered. However, a too rapid correction of hyponatremia can result in central nervous system demyelinization, especially in the pons. Unfortunately, symptoms of pontine demyelinization may not manifest until several days after acute injury. In asymptomatic hyponatremia, or after successful resolution of neurologic symptoms due to severe hyponatremia, the corrective rate of sodium repletion is no more than 12 to 15 mEq/L over 24 hours, using fluid with lower concentrations of sodium. More rapid correction does not improve outcome and may predispose to CNS injury.

Hypernatremia

In hypernatremic dehydration, sodium repletion must be judicious, because a too rapid correction may result in cerebral edema. In cases in which the serum sodium is in excess of 160 mEq/L, sodium should be lowered by 10 to 12 mEq/L each day, or at a rate no greater than 0.5 mEq/L/hour. Because most cases of hypernatremia are due to water loss, correction is based on the replacement of water deficits. Fluid needs can be calculated as isotonic loss or deficit, which includes the sodium loss, and free-water loss. As always, the patient's isotonic losses or deficit is best estimated by weight loss, if known, or otherwise by clinical signs. Free water (CH_2O) calculation is based on the current and desired serum sodium concentration and TBW:

$$CH_2O = [(Na^+_{current}/Na^+_{desired}) \times TBW] - TBW$$
$$\text{Isotonic Fluid Deficit} = \text{Total Fluid Deficit} - CH_2O$$

Determination of fluid needs is based on Calculated Fluid Loss. For example: A 10 kg child who is 10% dehydrated with a serum sodium level of 165 mEq/L. Patient initially receives emergent therapy to stabilize ECV with a 20 mL/kg NS bolus. Plan to correct sodium to 145 mEq/L over next 48 hours at an hourly rate of 0.4 mEq/L. TBW = 0.6 of Wt.

a. Fluid Deficit: 10% of Wt. = 1,000 mL
b. $CH_2O = [(Na^+_{current})/Na^+_{desired}) \times TBW] - TBW$
  $CH_2O = (165/145 \times 6 L) - 6 L = 830$mL
c. Isotonic Loss: Total Fluid Deficit – CH_2O = 1,000 mL – 830 mL = 170 mL
d. Emergent Care: Received 20 mL/kg bolus of NS, 200 mL of isotonic fluid. Hence all of the isotonic sodium loss was restored during emergent therapy.
e. Subsequent Therapy for next 2 days to replace CH_2O and maintenance needs:
  i. Remaining CH_2O: 800 mL
  ii. Maintenance needs: 2,000 mL/2 days
  iii. Total Fluids: 2,800 mL/2 days IV sodium needs: No remaining isotonic losses, replaced during emergent therapy
    Maintenance needs: 3 mEq /kg/day = 60 mEq/ 2 days
  v. Rate: 2,800 mL/48 hours = 60 mL/hr
  vi. Concentration of sodium needed: 60 mEq/2.8 L, 22 mEq/L
  vii. Solution Selected: 0.2% NaCl (1/4 NS)

The serum sodium level should be monitored to ensure that the actual decrease is consistent with the therapeutic plan. If the corrective rate is too rapid, additional adjustments can be made by a decrease in the rate of infusion or by increasing the salinity of the infused fluids.

POTASSIUM

Potassium plays an important role in neuromuscular transmission and cellular function and metabolism, including protein and glycogen synthesis. Potassium is the main intracellular cation; 98% of the total body potassium is intracellular. As a result, the measurement of serum potassium levels is only an indirect assessment of total body potassium and, in some cases, may be misleading.

The gradient of potassium across the cell membrane is the major determinant of the resting membrane potential, the basis for the action potential that is essential for neuronal and muscular function. The gradient is actively maintained by the sodium-potassium (Na^+, K^+-ATPase) pump. Perturbations in potassium levels affect the potassium gradient and the resting membrane potential, conditions that clinically are manifested by muscle weakness or cardiac arrhythmias. Hence, the regulation of potassium is tightly controlled, because as small fluxes of intracellular potassium (as little as 2%) can result in potentially fatal increases of extracellular plasma potassium of 8 mEq/L or above. After exogenous potassium intake, the initial homeostatic response is to rapidly move extracellular potassium into the cell, with eventual renal excretion of any excess extracellular potassium that has been derived from dietary intake or cellular breakdown.

The distribution of potassium between the intracellular and extracellular fluid spaces is influenced by many factors that may have major clinical ramifications (Box 9.1). Insulin and beta-adrenergic catecholamines increase cellular potassium uptake in skeletal muscle and liver, thereby decreasing extracellular or plasma potassium. Similarly, acid–base perturbations cause potassium flux through electrochemical gradients. Alkalosis, either metabolic or respiratory, will promote potassium entry into the cell, whereas acidosis causes intracellular potassium to leave the cell.

The fine-tuning of renal excretion of potassium occurs in the cortical collecting tubule and is dependent on the electrical and concentration gradients across the luminal membrane. Aldosterone enhances sodium resorption from filtrate in the lumen, resulting in the evolution of a negative electrical gradient in the lumen that promotes the flow of cationic potassium down its concentration gradient from the potassium-rich intracellular space. Potassium secretion is diminished if decreased sodium flow to the distal tubule is present, because there is limited sodium presented to reabsorb and establish an electrical gradient between the intracellular space and the lumen. Similarly, potassium secretion is diminished if limited or absent aldosterone secretion is present or there is end-organ resistance to aldosterone, because there will be a reduction in the number of open potassium channels to allow ion exchange.

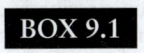

BOX 9.1   Conditions Enhancing Intracellular Potassium Movement

Metabolic alkalosis
Increased insulin activity
Beta-adrenergic stimulation
Periodic paralysis

Hypokalemia

Potassium homeostasis is impacted by exogenous potassium intake, either orally or through intravenous infusion; by potassium storage within the cells; and by potassium excretion in the urine and, to a lesser degree, in the stool. Any abnormality in one of these processes can lead to hypokalemia (Fig. 9.8), generally defined in most clinical laboratories by a serum potassium level of below 3.5 mEq/L.

In the normal diet, it is difficult to decrease potassium intake enough to cause total body potassium depletion resulting in hypokalemia. Potassium is present in meat and most other protein sources, fruits, and many vegetables. As a result, severe and lengthy dietary restrictions would be necessary for diet-associated hypokalemia to ensue. Often, other factors, such as increased renal losses due to diuretics, may exacerbate decreased intake of potassium and contribute to hypokalemia. In an intriguing form of pica that can be seen in rural areas, clay ingestion may limit the dietary intake of potassium and iron by binding these two elements and diminishing their absorption, contributing to a hypokalemic state.

Sudden intracellular movement of extracellular potassium can result in a transiently low serum potassium. Catecholamines activate the beta-adrenergic stimulation of potassium uptake. Potassium levels may fall by 0.5 to 1 mEq/L after the administration of nebulized beta-adrenergic agonists, such as albuterol, or even further in the setting of continuous intravenous beta-agonist therapy using agents such as terbutaline.

Insulin also promotes potassium intake into hepatic and skeletal muscle cells, probably by up-regulating the activity of the sodium-potassium pump. This hypokalemia may be seen with insulin therapy in patients with severe hyperglycemia due to diabetes mellitus, especially if the patient's initial acidosis is corrected more rapidly than the hyperglycemia.

Alkalosis can enhance intracellular potassium movement, compensating electrochemically for the loss of intracellular hydrogen ions that are consumed as a buffer in alkalosis. Plasma potassium levels fall 0.2 to 0.4 mEq/L for each 0.1 increase in plasma pH.

Periodic paralysis is a rare disorder, with recurrent episodes of muscle weakness due to the sudden movement of potassium into the cells, resulting in an acute decrease of potassium to levels as low as 1.5 to 2.5 mEq/L. Concomitant decreases also occur in phosphate and magnesium levels. Hypothermia can also lower potassium levels to below 3.0 mEq/L, due to intracellular movements that may be somewhat enhanced by the catecholamine release accompanying this state.

An increased loss of potassium either in the stool or the urine also can cause hypokalemia. In the setting of a low blood potassium level, if the urine excretion of potassium is low (less than 10 to 20 mEq/L), extrarenal potassium loss is most likely. In addition to the potassium losses that can accompany normal stools, significantly enhanced intestinal potassium excretion can be seen with persistent chronic diarrhea, as the intestines preferentially secrete potassium bicarbonate into the lumen and reabsorb sodium chloride.

In the setting of hypokalemia, if the urine excretion of potassium is high (greater than 20 mEq/L), inappropriate renal potassium wasting occurs. If this is seen in the setting of concomitant increased ECV and hypertension, it suggests an inappropriate activation of the renin-aldosterone axis, with stimulation of sodium and water absorption (volume expansion) and potassium excretion in the distal tubule. The diagnostic evaluation for these patients includes checking plasma renin and aldosterone levels, which should be low in the setting of volume expansion and hypokalemia. If renin is elevated, the diagnostic differential includes renal artery

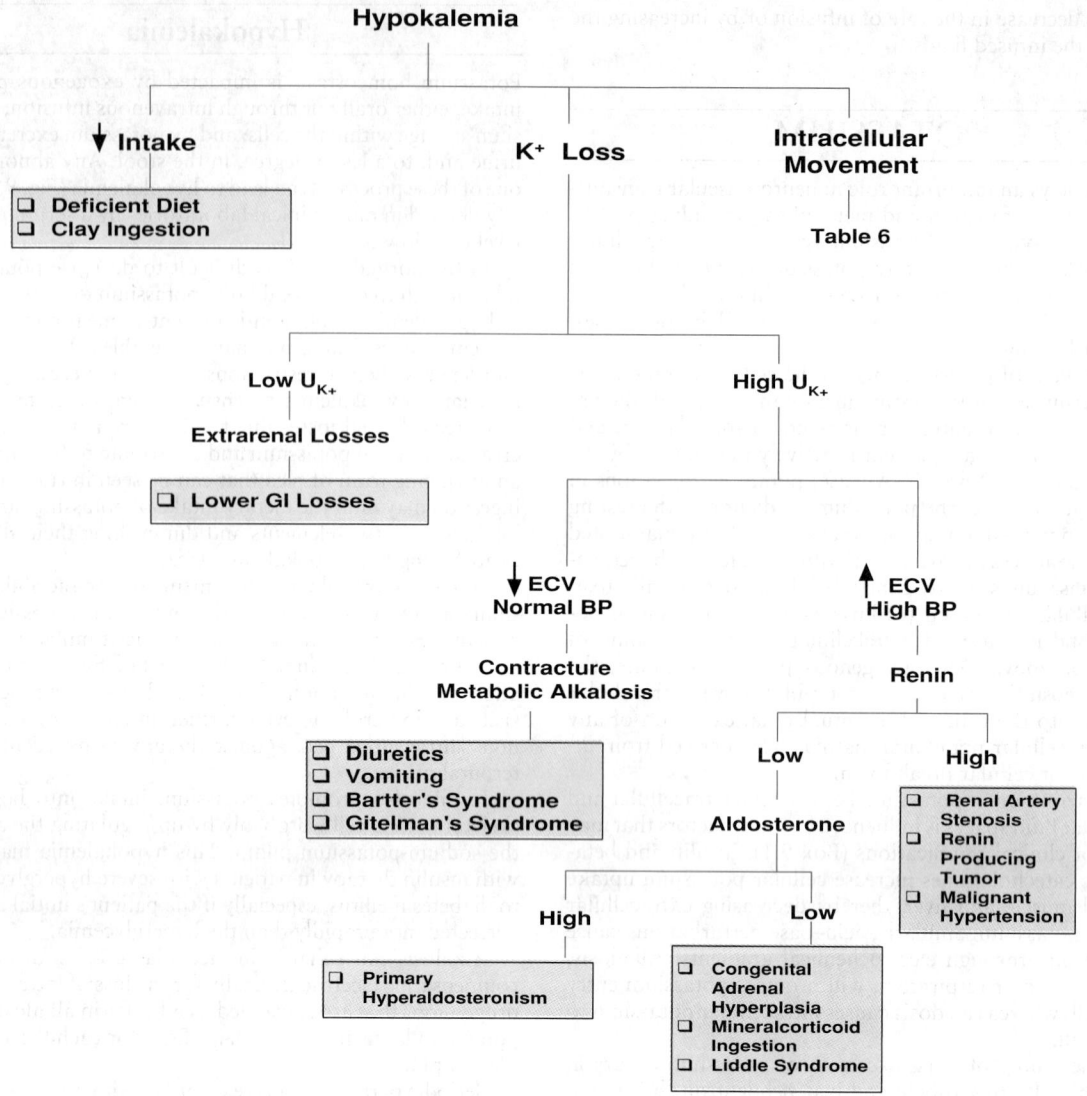

FIGURE 9.8. Hypokalemia: Clinical approach to hypokalemia based on urinary potassium concentration (U_{K+}) and effective circulating volume (ECV). The boxes list potential diagnoses.

stenosis or a renin-producing tumor. If the renin level is appropriately low, but the aldosterone level is high, a diagnosis of hyperaldosteronism is made. If both the renin and aldosterone level are low, the differential diagnosis includes exogenous mineralocorticoid ingestion, congenital adrenal hyperplasia with mineralocorticoid activity, and Liddle syndrome. Liddle syndrome is a rare genetic defect of the collecting tubule sodium channels that enhances sodium absorption, with the subsequent development of hypertension, hypokalemia, and alkalosis.

Hypokalemia, without an increase in ECV or hypertension, and especially in the setting of metabolic contracture alkalosis and normal blood pressure, usually is seen in patients on diuretic therapy or who have had prolonged vomiting. In addition, rare congenital abnormalities may mimic the clinical presentation seen with diuretic use. In Bartter syndrome, defects are found in the furosemide-sensitive sodium transport in the loop of Henle, resulting in possible profound alterations in sodium, potassium, and acid–base balance. In patients with Gitelman syndrome, a defect is present in the thiazide-sensitive sodium transport in the distal tubule, and these patients also may present with laboratory findings similar to chronic thiazide diuretic therapy.

The initial management of hypokalemia depends on an assessment of any functional physiologic defects, such as alterations in muscle strength or electrocardiogram activity. Hypokalemia delays myocyte repolarization after contraction and prolongs the duration of the relative refractory period. In the heart, this predisposes to reentrant arrhythmias. Changes seen in the electrocardiogram with severe hypokalemia (potassium levels of less than 3 mEq/L) include depressed ST segments, decreased T wave amplitude, and increased U wave amplitude. With further depression of serum potassium levels, an increase occurs in the width and amplitude of the P wave, prolongation of the PR interval, and widening of the QRS complex. Muscle weakness, tetany, cramping, and ileus also are other signs of hypokalemia.

The route and amount of potassium administration is difficult to determine, because the clinician is unable to directly determine the potassium deficit and must guard against overshooting desired potassium levels with a too rapid administration of potassium. In patients symptomatic with EKG changes or significant muscle findings, acute management includes the use of intravenous potassium therapy with ongoing cardiac monitoring. Potassium chloride, especially in those patients with contracture alkalosis, is most effective and can be given at doses of 0.5 to 1 mEq/kg up to 20 mEq intravenously over 1 hour. It is essential to monitor potassium serum levels and ascertain that ongoing urine output is occurring in these patients. Asymptomatic patients, or those less profoundly depleted, can be managed with oral potassium supplements at a dose of 1 to 4 mEq/kg/day divided into two times a day or four times a day doses, or potassium can be added to peripheral intravenous fluid infusions at a concentration of 20 to 40 mEq/L.

Hyperkalemia

Hyperkalemia, defined as a serum potassium level greater than 6.5 mEq/L, potentially can be life-threatening. Hence, the body has evolved tight regulation of potassium to avoid elevations of serum potassium to these dangerous levels. After the ingestion of dietary potassium and absorption into the extracellular space, potassium is moved rapidly into the cells and, subsequently, extra potassium either from dietary intake or cell breakdown is excreted by the kidneys. Abnormalities in any of these processes will result in hyperkalemia (Fig. 9.9).

Increased potassium intake alone as the etiology of hyperkalemia is relatively uncommon, given the mechanisms in place to prevent excessive rises in potassium levels. In adults, acute oral potassium intake of 135 to 160 mEq will transiently raise the serum potassium by 2.5 to 3.5 mEq/L. Other than the oral ingestion of concentrated potassium supplements, it is unlikely that this level of oral potassium loading could be achieved within the context of a normal diet. More concerning is the possible rapid intravenous infusion of solutions containing potassium. This is a particular risk in newborns who still have limited GFR and small absolute extracellular volumes that may be substantially affected by the infusion of even modest fluid volumes.

Hyperkalemia can occur from the transcellular movement of potassium. This may be due to intracellular potassium release from cell membrane disruption, as seen in tumor lysis syndrome, hemolysis, or with rhabdomyolysis. In addition, pseudohyperkalemia may result from potassium movement out of cells during or after the drawing of a blood specimen, with mechanical lysis of red blood cells. Transient hyperkalemia can be seen with movement of intracellular potassium from intact cells with insulin deficiency, metabolic acidosis, and the inherited autosomal disease of hyperkalemic periodic paralysis.

As previously discussed, basal potassium excretion is so efficient that even a substantial intake of potassium will not produce hyperkalemia in patients with normal potassium renal excretion. For hyperkalemia to persist, usually a compromise is present in renal potassium excretion. Impaired renal excretion usually is due to one of three causes: hypoaldosteronism, including end-organ unresponsiveness to aldosterone; renal failure with decrease in GFR and potassium clearance; and decreased ECV, leading to avid proximal tubular solute reabsorption and inadequate distal sodium delivery to allow potassium secretion.

Patients with renal failure, indicated by a decrease in GFR, have a decrease in the overall filtration of potassium and also may suffer from decreased sodium delivery to the distal tubule. In other patients, direct injury to the distal tubule may impair potassium secretion. This occurs in sickle cell nephropathy, type 4 renal tubular acidosis (RTA) associated with obstructive uropathy, and cystic dysplastic kidneys. Distal tubular injury may be due to direct structural damage or end-organ unresponsiveness to aldosterone as seen in type 4 RTA. Drugs such as amiloride act to decrease sodium absorption by blocking distal tubular sodium channels, hence indirectly

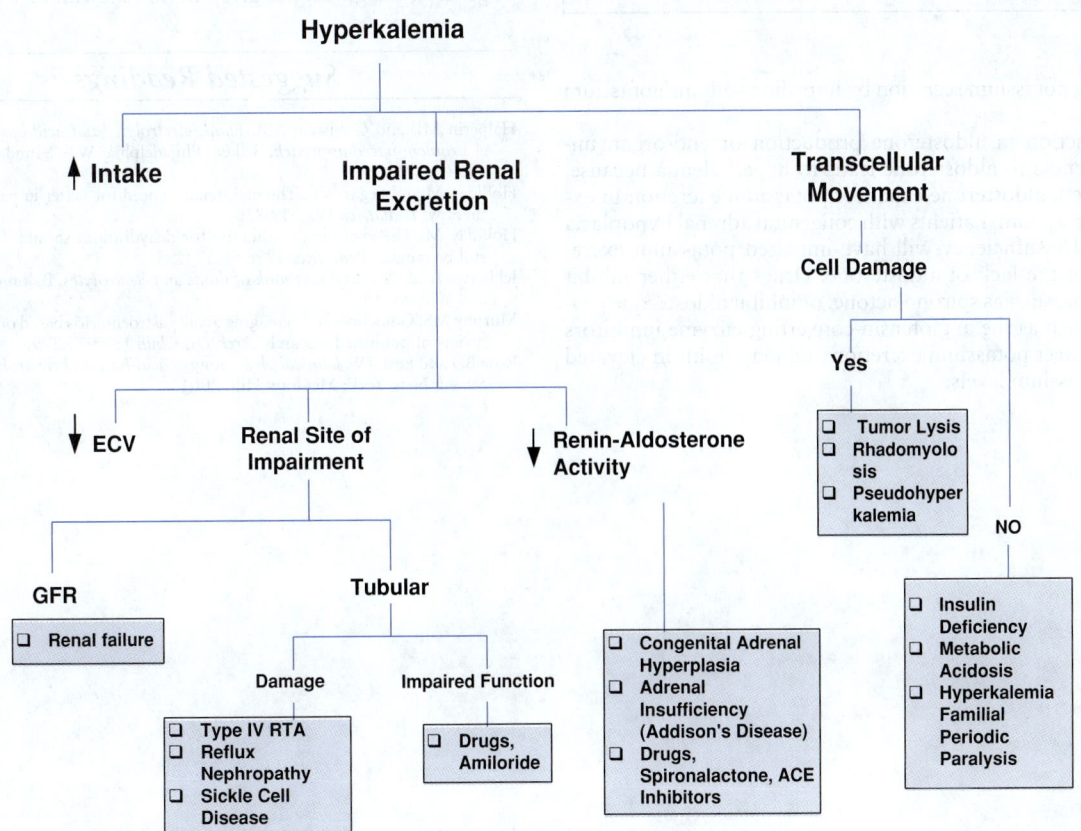

FIGURE 9.9. Hyperkalemia: Clinical approach to hyperkalemia. The boxes list potential diagnoses.

BOX 9.2	Treatment for Hyperkalemia

■ Potassium levels of 6 to 7 mEq/L: No EKG changes or peaked T waves alone;
  Stop potassium intake.
  Enteral cation-exchanger, sodium polystyrene sulfonate (Kayexalate): 1 g/kg up to 40 g q 4 hours, p.o., p.g. or p.r.
  Consider furosemide (Lasix) therapy, 1 mg/kg q 6 hours IV
■ Potassium levels of greater than 7 mEq/L: with significant EKG changes
  Insulin: 0.1 to 0.3 U/kg *and*
  Glucose: D25: 2 to 4 mL/kg IV to promote intracellular potassium movement
  Calcium gluconate (10%): 10 mg/kg IV stabilizes cardiac membrane excitability
  Bicarbonate only after calcium administration: 1 mEq/kg (alkali therapy) will promote intracellular potassium movement but use prior to calcium administration will increase binding of calcium to albumin, decreasing ionized calcium and resulting in increased cardiac membrane excitability.
  Start additional sodium polystyrene sulfonate and furosemide therapy after above therapy is administered.
  Hemodialysis if the patient is in renal failure or above is ineffective.

After the patient's potassium level has been lowered to a safe range, diagnostic evaluation and corrective therapy is needed to prevent further increases in potassium.

Patients with severe volume depletion, with chronic salt depletion, or with an ineffective ECV for other reasons, all will have diminished renal perfusion. In these patients, again due to avid proximal tubular reabsorption of filtered sodium, the distal delivery of sodium is decreased, thus leading to an impairment of potassium exchange for sodium and a decrease in net potassium excretion.

As with hypokalemia, hyperkalemia clinically may affect muscle strength and cardiac conduction and can lead to fatal arrhythmias. Muscle weakness typically does not develop until the plasma potassium concentration is above 8 mEq/L. Of greater concern is the effect of hyperkalemia on cardiac conduction that leads to ventricular fibrillation and asystole. As delineated in the following list, as the serum potassium concentration rises, characteristic changes are seen in the electrocardiogram due to effects on atrial and ventricular depolarization (seen as changes in P waves and QRS complex) and repolarization (changes in T waves).

■ Potassium levels of 6 to 7 mEq/L: No EKG changes or peaked T waves
■ Potassium levels of 7 to 8 mEq/L: Decreased amplitude and widening of P waves (eventually loss of P waves), PR prolongation, and widened QRS complex
■ Potassium levels greater than 8 mEq/L: Sine wave pattern as QRS complex merges with T wave; followed by ventricular fibrillation

The degree of hyperkalemia dictates the therapeutic course, especially in those ranges where significant cardiac arrhythmias may occur. In addition, wide patient variability occurs, so that a clinical assessment for each patient is necessary, including understanding the underlying cause for hyperkalemia. Hence, if the cause is due to an increase in intake, diuretic therapy may be useful in promoting renal excretion but would not be helpful in an anuric patient with renal failure who ingested potassium. In general, the guidelines given in Box 9.2 can be used.

---

decreasing potassium secretion by impeding sodium/potassium exchange.

A reduction in aldosterone production or end-organ unresponsiveness to aldosterone leads to hyperkalemia because, as discussed, aldosterone enhances potassium excretion in exchange for sodium. Patients with congenital adrenal hypoplasia or adrenal insufficiency will have impaired potassium excretion due to the lack of aldosterone. Drugs that either inhibit aldosterone, such as spironolactone, or inhibit aldosterone production, such as the angiotensin-converting enzyme inhibitors will also effect potassium excretion and may result in elevated serum potassium levels.

Suggested Readings

Halperin ML and Goldstein MB. *Fluid, electrolyte, and acid-base physiology. A problem-based approach,* 3rd ed. Philadelphia: W.B. Saunders Company, 1998.

Holliday M and Segar WE. The maintenance need for water in parenteral fluid therapy. *Pediatrics* 1957;19:823.

Holliday M. The evolution of therapy for dehydration: should deficit therapy still be taught? *Pediatrics* 1996;98:171.

Ichikawa I, ed. *Pediatric textbook of fluids and electrolytes.* Baltimore: Williams and Wilkins, 1990.

Murphy MS. Guidelines for managing acute gastroenteritis based on a systematic review of published research. *Arch Dis Child* 1998;79:279.

Rose BD and Post TW. *Clinical physiology of acid-base and electrolyte disorders,* 5th ed. New York: McGraw-Hill, 2001.

CHAPTER 10 ■ MOLECULAR GENETICS

CHARLES P. VENDITTI AND HAIG H. KAZAZIAN, JR.

The golden age of biology and medical science began around 1945, and can be traced to the work, both basic and applied, of many investigators. These investigators forged the foundation of knowledge that is rapidly revolutionizing modern medicine. The primary event that catalyzed the revolution was the discovery of restriction endonucleases, the bacterial enzymes that cut DNA at precise recognition sites specific for each enzyme. This discovery, along with that of another bacterial enzyme that ligates two pieces of DNA together, led to the ability to produce *recombinant DNA*—DNA fragments made up of segments from different species. This ability rapidly led to the cloning of human DNA in vectors known to replicate in bacteria, to the production of libraries of DNA fragments, and to the era of recombinant DNA medicine.

In this chapter, the basic principles of gene structure and the basis of recombinant DNA technology are discussed briefly as a prelude to genomics and the Human Genome Project. An outline of what is known about normal variations in DNA follows. The chapter ends with a discussion of mutations and how the knowledge of specific sites of mutation has helped us learn which nucleotide sequences are important in gene expression and how to diagnose the genetic diseases they produce. Also included in this section is a discussion of nonclassical forms of mutation and some unusual modes of inheritance.

GENE STRUCTURE

Genetic material consists of double-helical DNA, with each strand composed of the deoxyribonucleotides, A, G, T, C (adenylic acid, guanylic acid, thymidylic acid, and cytidylic acid, respectively) and a sugar phosphate backbone (Fig. 10.1). This backbone runs along the outside of the helix; the base components of the nucleotides face into the interior of the helix. In that central portion, the critical hydrogen bonds between A of one strand and its complement T of the other, or G of one strand and its complement C of the other, are formed. The human genome contains about 3 billion of these base pairs. The base-pairing rules (A with T and G with C) are critical in information transfer, both during DNA replication and in the transcription of the DNA code into RNA. Each nucleotide is linked to its neighbor via a sugar–phosphate linkage involving the 3′ carbon of one sugar attached to a phosphate group. That phosphate is linked in turn to the 5′ carbon of the next nucleotide. Thus, the nucleotide linkages are referred to as 3′ to 5′. This linkage gives a DNA (or RNA) strand its polarity or directionality. This polarity determines the direction in which the DNA is synthesized during replication and read during the transcription of DNA into RNA. Thus, a DNA sequence 3′ to 5′ is decoded during transcription in a 5′ to 3′ direction in RNA.

The great majority of mammalian genes coding for a protein product have split coding regions; that is, the coding regions are discontinuous. The beta-globin gene of adult hemoglobin has three coding regions, termed *exons*, and two intervening sequences (IVS), called *introns*. The coding regions are divided

between the codons for amino acids 30 and 31 of the 146 amino-acid chain and the codons for amino acids 104 and 105. Although only about 450 nucleotides are necessary to encode the protein (3 nucleotides/amino acid), because of the introns, the gene contains roughly 1,500 nucleotides. Yet, this is a very simple gene. Many genes now have been described with 10 or more introns (the gene for the pro-alpha 1 collagen chain has more than 50 introns), and some genes have a total size of more than 200 kilobases (kb) or 200 thousand base pairs. In fact, dystrophin, the gene affected in Duchenne muscular dystrophy, has over 2 million base pairs. Some large introns contain entire genes within their boundaries. On the other hand, certain genes, such as those encoding histones and interferons, are small and do not contain introns. These genes are unexplained exceptions to the split gene rule.

EXPRESSION OF GENETIC MATERIAL

The mechanisms of expression for protein-coding genes are exemplified by the globins (Fig. 10.2). The entire gene, including the two introns, is transcribed into a precursor RNA. This RNA is immediately modified at both its ends (called 5′ and 3′ ends). The modification at the 5′ end is an addition of a methylated G in an unusual triphosphate linkage. This modification, which is specific for messenger RNA, is called

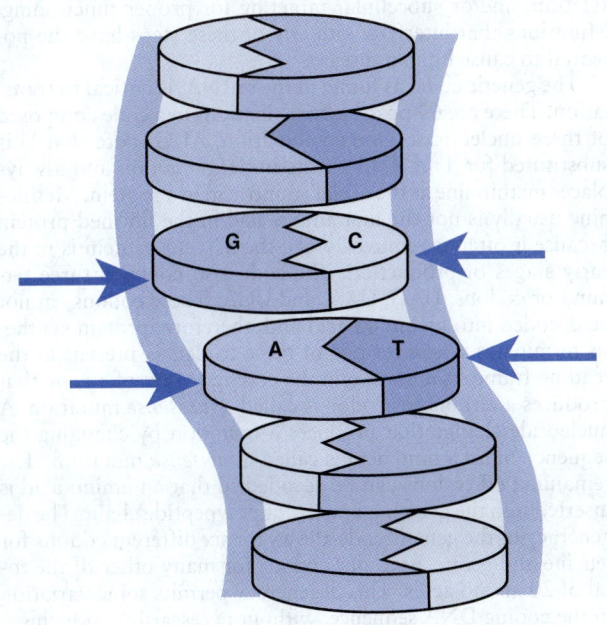

FIGURE 10.1. Base pairing in DNA. As shown, G of one strand pairs by hydrogen bonding with C of the other strand. Likewise, A pairs with T.

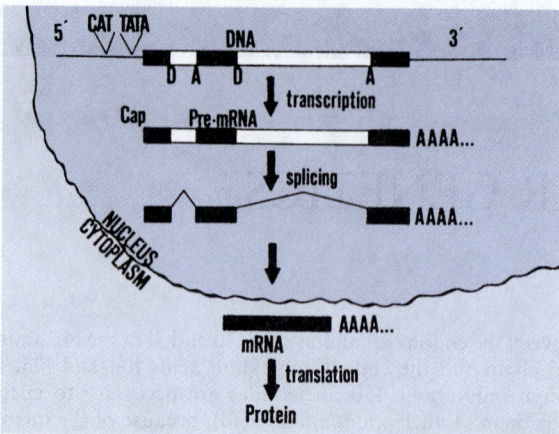

FIGURE 10.2. Gene expression. The dark black bars correspond to exons, the unshaded regions between the D and A represent introns. Steps include (a) transcription of precursor RNA, (b) cap and poly A addition to the ends of the RNA, (c) splicing out of intron sequences, and (d) translation of the mature messenger RNA into protein. CAT and TATA in front of the gene refer to sequences important in transcription, whereas D and A refer to donor and acceptor splice junctions important in RNA splicing.

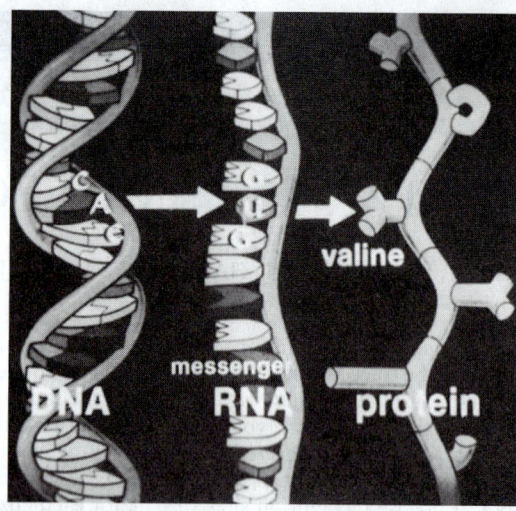

FIGURE 10.3. Relationship between the triplet code in the strand of DNA that is transcribed, the codon in messenger RNA, and the specific amino acid inserted in the polypeptide chain. For example, CAC in the DNA is transcribed into GUG in RNA and the amino acid inserted is valine. Shown here is the mutant sequence in the beta-globin gene for the beta^s or sickle hemoglobin chain. The sequence of normal beta^A-globin DNA for the strand shown is CTC.

5' capping. The modification at the 3' end is the addition of about 150 A residues (the poly A tail). The 5' cap is thought to be important in the translation of the RNA into protein, whereas the 3' poly A tail may have a role in RNA stability. Next, the introns are precisely spliced out of the RNA, thereby approximating the coding region sequences. The precise mechanism, and the enzymes involved in RNA splicing, is now well understood.

RNA splicing also is important in transporting the RNA from the nucleus to the cytoplasm, where it will be translated into protein; nucleotide sequences near the exon–intron junctions are important in normal splicing. Translation then occurs on the fully processed messenger RNA (mRNA) in the cytoplasm to produce the peptide chain, which may need post-translational modification, such as glycosylation or farnysylation, and/or subcellular targeting for proper functioning. Mutations that interfere with any of these steps have the potential to cause human disease.

The genetic code, as found in the mRNA, is critical to translation. There are 64 possible combinations in a code composed of three nucleotides. One combination, AUG (note that U is substituted for T in RNA) is the initiation codon and always places methionine as the initial amino acid in a protein. Methionine usually is not the first amino acid in the finished protein because it often is removed when the nascent protein is in the early stages of production. The code also contains three terminator codons, UAG, UAA, and UGA. These codons cannot be decoded into an amino acid and, therefore, protein synthesis terminates whenever one of these triplets is present in the reading frame. A mutation in the coding region of a gene that produces a terminator codon is called a *nonsense* mutation. A nucleotide change that produces a mutation by changing the sequence of an amino acid is called a *missense* mutation. The remaining 60 codons can be decoded so that an amino acid is inserted into the growing or nascent polypeptide chain. The degeneracy of the genetic code allows for six different codons for leucine and serine, and four codons for many of the total of 20 amino acids. This degeneracy permits some variation in the coding DNA sequence, without necessarily producing a change in the amino acid encoded. The relationship between the nucleotide triplet in DNA, its complement in mRNA, and the amino acid designated by that triplet is demonstrated for

the sixth codon of the beta-globin chain (Fig. 10.3). CTC in DNA is decoded as GAG in mRNA and as glutamate in the protein. A single nucleotide substitution (T to A) causes a missense mutation that leads to sickle cell anemia, as discussed later.

NORMAL VARIATION IN DNA

Any discussion of mutations and their consequences requires a brief introduction to normal variation. Much has been learned about normal variation at the protein or enzyme level. Scientists are learning that variations in the DNA are even more extensive than we imagined from protein data. A number of different types of variation have been found. Originally, common normal variation in DNA was termed *DNA polymorphism*, and it could be detected in the laboratory as a *restriction fragment length polymorphism* (RFLP). This variation usually is the result of single nucleotide substitutions and is detected if the variation affects a restriction endonuclease site. The insertion or deletion of a large number of nucleotides also can be detected as an RFLP. One RFLP that affects a site that is cleaved by the restriction enzyme *HincII* near the beta-globin gene is shown (Fig. 10.4). When genomic DNA is digested with *HincII*, electrophoresed, and hybridized with a radioactive probe containing the beta-globin gene, chromosomes that contain this site yield a 3.7-kb fragment, and those that lack the site demonstrate an 8-kb fragment. Because this polymorphism is very frequent, nearly 50% of individuals in the population are heterozygous and demonstrate both fragments by this analysis.

Southern blotting (Box 10.1) is a technique used to find a number of DNA polymorphisms in a gene cluster and in and around a large number of other genes. Thus, normal variation in DNA is extensive. The 50,000 nucleotides of the paternal beta-globin gene cluster contain 100 or more nucleotide differences from the 50,000 maternal nucleotides of this cluster. In total, the haploid DNA derived from one parent contains 3 to 10 million differences (single nucleotide substitutions) from the genetic material derived from one's other parent.

A
Hinc II map at ε - globin gene

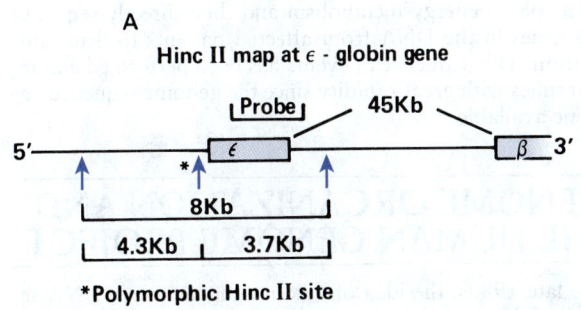

*Polymorphic Hinc II site

B
Hinc II autoradiogram

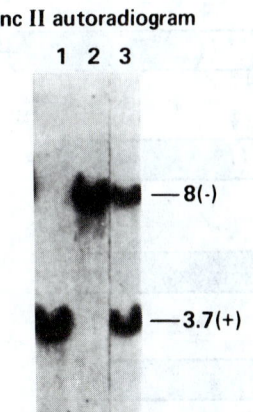

— 8(-)

— 3.7(+)

FIGURE 10.4. A polymorphism of a restriction endonuclease site near the epsilon-globin gene. A: Near many normal epsilon-globin genes is a *Hinc*II site, but this site is often missing in normal individuals. When the site is present, the 8-kb fragment is cut into 3.7- and 4.3-kb fragments. B: The 3.7-kb fragment is readily detected by use of a DNA probe containing the epsilon gene. When the site is absent, the 8-kb fragment is not cleaved. The presence or absence of this *Hinc*II site can be discovered by Southern blotting (see Fig. 10.5).

BOX 10.1	Molecular Techniques: Southern Blotting

Single gene fragments are detected by a technique called Southern blotting. Southern blotting is named for E. M. Southern, inventor of the method, and it can be used to detect single copy genes in as little as 3.5 micrograms of DNA. [See section, General Methods of DNA Analysis, for a discussion of the polymerase chain reaction (PCR), which can detect single genes in 100 nanograms of DNA routinely, and in 10 picograms of DNA in research labs. Ten picograms is the amount of DNA in a single human sperm.] Most Southern blot analyses are carried out on DNA isolated from the leukocytes of peripheral blood, from which one can isolate about 50 to 100 μg/mL of blood (Fig. 1). Usually 5 μg of genomic DNA of an individual is digested with a specific restriction enzyme, and the digested DNA is subjected to electrophoresis in an agarose gel that separates DNA on the basis of size. The DNA is transferred to a nitrocellulose paper and hybridized to a radioactive cloned DNA fragment of interest (the probe). After hybridization with the probe, the filter is washed to remove nonspecific radioactivity, and the washed filter is placed in contact with an x-ray film. After a day or two, the film is removed and developed to demonstrate the bands of interest.

DNA Isolation

DNA

Restriction Endonuclease Digestion

Double-Stranded DNA Fragments

Gel Electrophoresis

Denaturing to Single-Stranded Fragments and Transfer

Filter Paper

Specific mRNA

Reverse Transcriptase

Specific Single-Stranded Complementary DNA

DNA Polymerase

Specific Double-Stranded DNA

Recombinant Plasmid

Amplification in Bacteria

Isolation of Specific DNA Fragments from Plasmids

Radiolabeling and Denaturing

Single-Stranded Probe

Study Pattern

Reference Pattern

BOX 10.1. FIGURE 1. Southern Blotting, or Restriction Endonuclease Analysis. The steps in this procedure are shown, beginning with isolation of DNA from leukocytes to discovery of hybridizing fragments (bands) in that DNA with a specific radioactive probe.

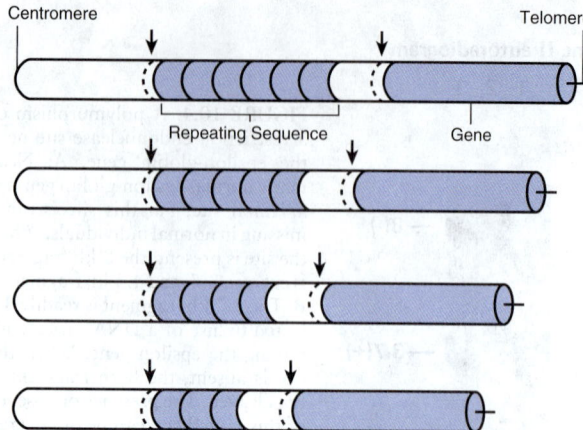

FIGURE 10.5. A VNTR (variable number of tandem repeats) polymorphism adjacent to a gene. A 30-nucleotide sequence has three repeats, four repeats, five repeats, or six repeats in tandem in different chromosomal homologues. The length variation in this region of the genome can be easily detected by Southern blot analysis or the polymerase chain reaction. In an SSR (simple sequence repeat) polymorphism, the polymorphic repeat sequence would contain two to four nucleotides (e.g., the dinucleotide CA), repeated ten to 30 times.

Even more important forms of DNA polymorphisms are variable number of tandem repeats (VNTRs) and simple sequence repeats (SSRs). VNTRs are repeats of 15 to 50 nucleotides, and the repeat number at a locus may vary widely (Fig. 10.5). SSRs are variations in the number of repeats of very short sequences, usually two to four nucleotides. Often, a VNTR locus may contain many possible alleles, perhaps 100 or more, if a population group is studied. SSR loci may contain 5 to 10 alleles. The variation in VNTRs and SSRs contrasts with that of most common RFLPs, which are dimorphisms. Because of the large number of alleles at many VNTR loci, a particular genotype at four or five such loci may be present in only one person in several million individuals in the population. This normal DNA variation has had substantial practical value in the forensic investigation of criminal cases. DNA analysis has played a major role in the conviction or exclusion of many individuals accused of rape or other crimes.

DNA polymorphisms also have been used as markers to trace the inheritance of particular regions of the genome in families. When a large number of such markers are studied in families affected with single-gene diseases, such as Huntington disease, it has been possible to find a single marker that is co-inherited with the disease gene in the affected families. After this marker is mapped to some particular chromosome segment, the disease gene is *ipso facto* mapped to the same location. In this way, the Huntington disease (HD) locus was mapped to the short arm of chromosome 4, the neurofibromatosis locus (NF-1) to the centromeric region of chromosome 17, and the cystic fibrosis locus (CF) to the long arm of chromosome 7, to name a few successful examples of this approach.

The genes responsible for these diseases have been isolated by this method of finding the gene's location in the genome before knowing the function of the encoded product. One of the great promises of the Human Genome Project is that this type of reverse genetic analysis, called *positional cloning,* will be very easy to execute. Once a gene is mapped to a region of the chromosome, and the DNA sequence of that region is known, finding genes in that region can be done quickly using a combination of computational and experimental methods. For example, if a metabolic disorder known to be associated with an electron transport chain defect is localized to a specific chromosomal region, a researcher might examine the DNA sequence in that region carefully for gene products that are predicted to have a role in energy metabolism and then directly sequence those genes in the DNA from affected patients to determine causation. This sequence of events has been performed a number of times with great rapidity since the genome sequence has become available.

GENOME ORGANIZATION AND THE HUMAN GENOME PROJECT

In the late 1980s, the idea of determining the exact DNA sequence of the entire human genome was discussed. By the late 1990s, the project was well underway. Two remarkable reports appeared in February 2001, describing the sequencing and analysis of most of the human genome, completed several years earlier than anticipated. The availability of this sequence or blueprint for life is certain to revolutionize the impact of genetics in pediatrics and in medicine in general. For that reason, we review selected aspects of the human genome sequencing project. The strategies for mapping and sequencing the human genome are described in Box 10.2, Figure 1.

Human Genome Project: Selected Findings

The analysis of the DNA sequence of the human genome has provided fundamental insights into evolution, chromosome structure and recombination, the origin and organization of genes, and DNA and protein polymorphisms. It also has identified the set of protein coding genes.

The human genome is largely composed of interspersed repeat elements of various classes. Long interspersed nuclear elements (LINEs); short interspersed nuclear repeats (SINEs), including the *Alu* elements; long terminal repeats (LTRs); and retrotransposons and DNA transposon copies comprise 21%, 13%, 8%, and 3%, respectively, of the genome sequence and total over 3 million copies—three orders of magnitude greater than the largest multigene family. Retrotransposons are copied into RNA, reverse transcribed into complementary DNA (cDNA), and then inserted into the genome at a new location. Transposons are DNA sequences that are directly "cut and pasted" into another genomic site. *Alu* sequences are the most prevalent constituent of the genome. *Alu* sequences contain an *Alu*I restriction endonuclease site, are about 300 nucleotides in length and, when compared with one another, are roughly 95% homologous.

Transposable elements, once considered "junk" DNA, are thought be a driving force in genome evolution, because they can be associated with recombination, pseudogene formation, and exon shuffling. It is now known that some copies of LINE elements are capable of retrotransposition and have been shown to produce human disease when they are mobilized to a new genomic location (see section, Insertion of Transposable Elements). The occurrence of repeated sequences located in the flanking DNA between functional gene sequences and within introns of genes is a general characteristic of the human genome. It is likely that repetitive DNA is not "junk," but part of an evolutionary engine that has shaped the human genome.

Single Nucleotide Polymorphisms

As discussed, the individual base sequence at any position in the DNA can be either A, T, G, or C. In certain positions, scattered throughout the genome, are variations at only one such nucleotide in a stretch. These changes are called single nucleotide polymorphisms (SNPs). When the draft sequence of the human genome was analyzed, 1.42 million such changes were detected.

BOX 10.2   Molecular Technique: The Human Genome Project

The strategy to map and sequence the human genome relied on an integration of a variety of technologies. A general overview is presented in Figure 1. Genetic and cytogenetic markers were used to define a set of large-insert DNA clones called BACs (bacterial artificial chromosomes) isolated from a library of human DNA. These BACs contained large pieces of human DNA, 100 to 250 kilobase pairs, that could be tracked to the origin and exact location of the specific human chromosome from which they were derived. The BAC clones were then mapped using restriction enzyme digestion and gel electrophoresis to generate "fingerprints" for each clone. Overlapping clones then could be identified with certainty, because they shared a similar fingerprint pattern, thus allowing groups of such clones to be ordered into larger units called *contigs*. These contigs in turn could be assigned to a specific portion of a chromosome and the map position or location also could be verified using other parallel methods, such as fluorescent *in situ* hybridization (FISH) and radiation hybrid (RH) mapping. Thus, the starting material in this approach was a physically mapped collection of overlapping large-insert BAC clones.

To generate the raw sequence for the genome analysis, the mapped BAC clones were then uniformly fragmented by shearing or restriction enzyme digestion and re-cloned as small fragments for random sequencing. Robotic technology and computational advances allowed this process, called *shotgun sequencing*, to be performed on a large scale. One factory-style robotic instrument used in the project was able to process 100,000 sequencing reactions in 12 hours. Considering that, a decade ago, it took one person an entire day to process 10 to 20 similar specimens, the technologic advances required to execute this project can be more fully appreciated. The small overlapping shotgun clone sequences were then assembled by looking for overlap in the DNA sequence output, followed by alignment to generate the entire sequence of the parent BAC clone. A reiteration of this process using DNA sequences from different BACs allowed larger regions to be similarly aligned, eventually connecting all the contiguous large insert clones together.

The genomic sequences generated in this fashion then can be further analyzed using computer programs, as well as other resources, in an attempt to annotate the sequence. One important approach has been to try to correlate the sequence of expressed genes with their location and their intron–exon boundaries by analyzing complementary DNA. Complementary DNA (cDNA) is derived from purified messenger RNA that has been isolated from a tissue, such as white blood cells or muscle, and has been copied into DNA using a retroviral enzyme called *reverse transcriptase*. The resulting cDNA can be transferred into a vector that replicates in bacteria, allowing individual cDNA clones to be isolated and sequenced. Comparisons between the genomic DNA and the sequence of cDNAs from a variety of tissue sources helps define the structure of each gene. Multiple techniques—both computational and experimental—then can be used to define individual genes in the genome. It is important to realize that not all genes can be identified by any one method; therefore, a combination of techniques is required to make robust predictions. Other methods that utilize large-scale analysis of proteins (proteomics) will ultimately be needed to confirm the predictions made from sequence analysis.

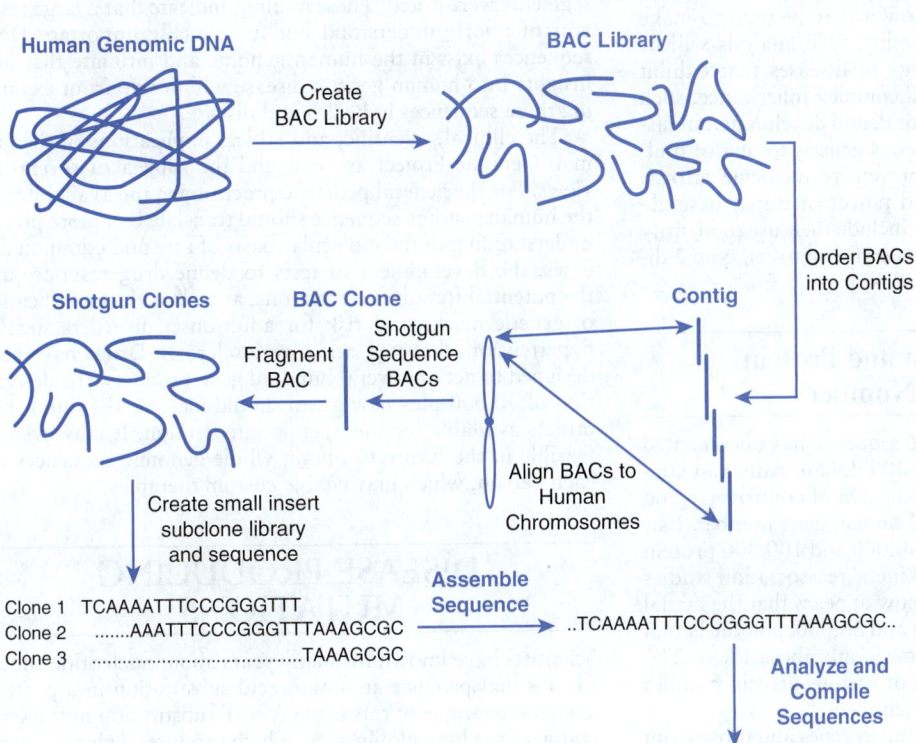

Clone 1 TCAAAATTTCCCGGGTTT
Clone 2 .......AAATTTCCCGGGTTTAAAGCGC
Clone 3 ....TAAAGCGC

..TCAAAATTTCCCGGGTTTAAAGCGC..

GENOMIC DNA SEQUENCE

BOX 10.2. FIGURE 1. An overview of the Human Genome Sequencing Strategy. A large insert DNA library was prepared by size fractionating human genomic DNA. The fragments were cloned as bacterial artificial chromosome (BACs) clones, assembled by a variety of methods, including fingerprinting, into contigs. The ordered BACs were then fragmented and recloned as random small fragments which were then sequenced and assembled to produce the DNA sequence of the genome.

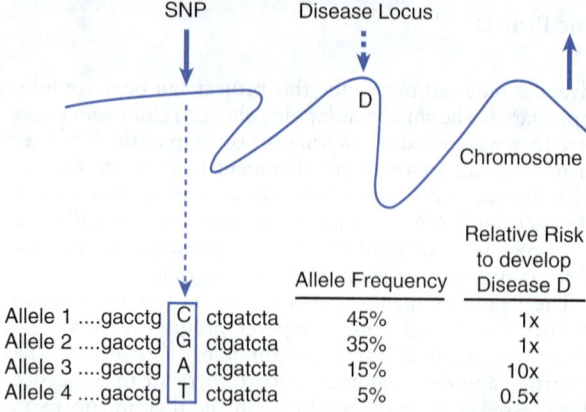

Hypothetical Single Nucleotide Polymorphism Associated with Complex Disease Susceptibilty Locus D

	Allele Frequency	Relative Risk to develop Disease D
Allele 1 ....gacctg C ctgatcta	45%	1x
Allele 2 ....gacctg G ctgatcta	35%	1x
Allele 3 ....gacctg A ctgatcta	15%	10x
Allele 4 ....gacctg T ctgatcta	5%	0.5x

FIGURE 10.6. A hypothetical SNP and its association with a disease susceptibility locus D. This figure depicts a specific DNA change (SNP indicated by the bold arrow) and the association it has with susceptibility locus D. In this example, allele 3 is associated with an increased relative risk and allele 4 a decreased risk.

They occur roughly once per 1,000 base pairs. Approximately 60,000 of these polymorphisms were noted to fall in the coding and untranslated regions of genes; some change the amino acid sequence of constituent genes, generating polymorphism at the protein level. Because these changes are detected easily using methods that are amenable to high throughput analysis, it is possible to study SNPs as functional genetic markers.

Furthermore, because certain combinations of SNPs are preferentially associated together in blocks throughout the genome, they should allow the expedient execution of genetic association studies. Although certain SNP alleles may be associated with increased risks to develop multifactorial diseases, such as diabetes, by virtue of causation or proximity, others may confer protective effects. Figure 10.6 displays what a hypothetical SNP is and how it may be used to make predictions about disease susceptibility. SNP analysis will be important in dissecting the etiology of diseases that exhibit gene–environment interactions and complex inheritance, such as autoimmune, endocrine, behavioral, and developmental disorders. In the future, the simultaneous genetic testing of multiple SNPs might help augment preventive medicine efforts. Several examples of the utility and power of using these genetic markers have appeared; these include their use to identify susceptibility loci for systemic lupus erythematosus, type 2 diabetes, and inflammatory bowel disease.

Gene Organization and Protein Coding Gene Number

The analysis of the human genome sequence has documented that a typical human gene spans ~20 kilobase pairs and contains seven to eight small exons. One area of controversy and debate had been the predictions of human gene number. Earlier estimates had ranged between 50,000 and 100,000 protein coding genes, despite the fact that kinetic reassociation studies of mRNA suggested otherwise. It now appears that the actual number of genes is between 25,000 and 30,000, and the actual protein-coding fraction of the genome is only about 1% to 2%. Figure 10.7 shows the distribution of various protein families in humans encoded by the human genome.

One major difference between human genes and those from lower organisms appears to be that human protein coding genes have evolved new architectures by adding, deleting, and

Predicted Protein Function	Number of Proteins	%
Molecular function unknown	12000	40
Metabolism	3200	13
Transcription/Translation	3100	13
Intracellular signaling	1800	7
Cell-cell communication	1250	5
Transport	1100	5
Protein folding and degradation	900	4
Cytoskeletal/structural	900	4
Defense/Immunity	1050	4
DNA Replication	800	3
Multifunctional proteins	400	2
Cellular processes	500	2

FIGURE 10.7. The function of predicted and known families encoded by the human genome. The approximate number of proteins and percent of the total are indicated. Currently, the largest fraction of genes encode proteins of unknown function.

reordering existing motifs to create new proteins and expand existing families. If one also considers that many genes are alternatively spliced to generate different isoforms, often in a tissue- or developmental-specific fashion, it is possible to envision that the capacity for increased interactions in the human protein set or proteome is much greater than that accounted for by the linear extrapolation of increased gene numbers in humans versus other model organisms, such as *Drosophila* or *Caenorhabditis elegans*. In addition to protein encoding genes, large numbers of non-protein coding RNAs, such as tRNAs, rRNAs, and small nuclear RNAs have been characterized with similar interest. It is likely that many small noncoding regulatory RNAs also exist and have yet to be fully annotated and functionally defined. In fact, in a recent study that compared large genomic sequences from human to several vertebrate species, a substantial number of previously unrecognized, conserved noncoding segments were noted. These findings indicate that a large reservoir of poorly understood but functionally important DNA sequences exist in the human genome and intimate that new insights into human genetic disease will evolve from examining these sequences in health and disease.

The clinical, scientific, and ethical implications of the Human Genome Project are vast and the subject of several reviews. For the general pediatric practitioner, the availability of the human genome sequence should translate to a more precise understanding of the molecular basis of rare and common diseases, the development of tests to define drug response and the potential for adverse reactions, as well as the identification of genetic markers of risk for adult-onset disorders such as hypertension, diabetes, and arteriosclerosis. Drugs have been designed to act on several hundred gene products; the description of 30,000-plus new genes should increase the number of targets available for therapeutic intervention. It may even be feasible in the future to obtain whole genomic sequences for each person, which may enable custom therapies.

DISEASE PRODUCING MUTATIONS

Scientists have known for many years about nucleotide substitutions that produce an amino acid substitution in a protein. The best example of this is the A to T substitution in the sixth codon of the beta-globin gene, which produces a glutamate-to-valine substitution (see Fig. 10.3) and causes sickle cell anemia. A large number of other nucleotide substitutions that produce abnormal hemoglobins have been described. These mutations lead to reduced production of the encoded protein, and they tell us what sequences within and adjacent to the gene are important in expression. Examples of such mutations include the point mutations that produce the beta-thalassemias, which are inherited disorders of globin gene expression.

Molecular Defects in Beta-Thalassemia

The genetic defects in beta-thalassemia are best reviewed within the context of the normal sequence of events in gene expression (see Fig. 10.2). To review, in erythroid cells, the beta-globin gene is transcribed by RNA-polymerase into a globin RNA precursor that contains two intron sequences. Within the nucleus, these introns are excised during RNA processing, and the coding blocks (or exons) are ligated together precisely to form the processed mRNA that is transported to the cytoplasm and translated into beta-globin. Genetic lesions that interrupt the normal sequence of events lead to the decreased beta-globin production that defines beta-thalassemia. We can consider the defined mutations by the phase of the gene expression pathway that is affected. Nearly all thalassemia defects that are known to date involve DNA sequences of the globin gene rather than distant nucleotides in the genome. Mutations in all these classes have been found in beta-thalassemia patients:

- Sizeable deletion of the beta-globin gene
- Transcription mutations (in flanking regions 5' to the gene)
- RNA processing mutations (cap site, RNA cleavage, RNA splicing)
- Translation mutations (frameshift and nonsense codons)
- Post-translation mutations (producing highly unstable globins)

The known molecular defects in beta-thalassemia are displayed in Figure 10.8. At present, about 200 different point mutations and several deletions have been found in various affected ethnic groups. The point mutations are almost all single nucleotide substitutions, about one-half of which affect RNA processing. Each affected ethnic group, whether Mediterranean, Asian Indian, Chinese, or black, has its own battery of beta-thalassemia alleles, usually four to six common ones and a handful of rare ones.

Examples of Mutations in Other Single-Gene Disorders

As mutant genes have been characterized, many examples of the types of mutations observed in the beta-thalassemias and hemoglobinopathies have been found. A common mutation in the phenylalanine hydroxylase gene producing PKU prevents normal RNA splicing at one exon–intron boundary. The mutation in the low-density lipoprotein receptor gene producing a common form a familial hypercholesterolemia in Lebanon is a nonsense mutation that blocks translation. One mutation producing Tay-Sachs disease in Ashkenazi Jews prevents normal RNA splicing of the hexosaminidase A precursor RNA. There are roughly 37,000 characterized point mutations in genes producing single-gene disorders.

MOLECULAR GENETICS OF MALFORMATION SYNDROMES

In many malformation syndromes, the underlying gene mutation(s) has been identified. Selected syndromes and disorders are listed in Tables 10.1 through 10.3 for autosomal dominant, autosomal recessive, and X-linked traits. (For current updates, see the Online Mendelian Inheritance in Man database at http://www3.ncbi.nlm.nih.gov/Omim.) The detection of specific mutations can lead to a more accurate diagnosis and, at times, has led to a reclassification of diagnostic entities and an improved understanding of pathophysiologic mechanisms.

Craniosynostosis Syndromes

Craniosynostosis syndromes represent a group of disorders that illustrate mutational heterogeneity and divergent allelic phenotypes. Craniosynostosis syndromes originally described clinically include Apert, Crouzon, Pfeiffer, and Saethre-Chotzen syndromes, each named after their first clinical reporter. Apert syndrome is caused by one of two adjacent amino acid substitutions (Ser252Trp; Pro253Arg) in a

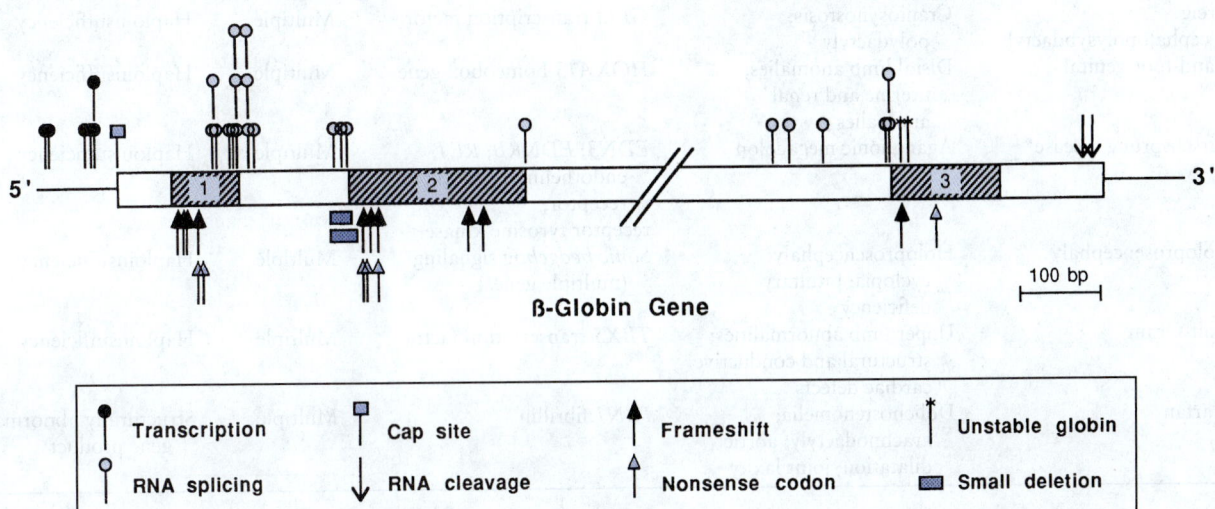

β-Globin Gene

100 bp

● Transcription   ▪ Cap site   ▲ Frameshift   * Unstable globin

○ RNA splicing   ↓ RNA cleavage   △ Nonsense codon   ▦ Small deletion

FIGURE 10.8. Point mutations producing beta-thalassemia. The beta-globin gene is shown with numbered hatched areas representing the coding regions of exons. Boxed open areas between the exons are introns, and boxed open areas at the 5' and 3' ends of the gene are untranslated regions that appear in the messenger RNA. The various types of mutations are denoted by different symbols.

TABLE 10.1

AUTOSOMAL DOMINANT MALFORMATION SYNDROMES AND DISORDERS CAUSED BY IDENTIFIED GENE MUTATIONS

Syndrome	Major Findings	Gene	Mutation	Mechanism of Action
Achondroplasia	Rhizomelic shortening; macrocephaly	FGFR3	Multiple	Gain of function
Apert	Craniosynostosis; syndactyly	FGFR2	Multiple	Gain of function
Alagille	Bile duct paucity; cardiac malformations; butterfly vertebrae	JAG1 ligand for notch receptor	Multiple	Haploinsufficiency
Aniridia	Absent or abnormal iris; cataract; lens dislocation	PAX6	Multiple	Haploinsufficiency
Bannayan-Ruvalcaba-Myhre	Macrocephaly; intestinal hamartomas; speckled penis	PTEN phosphatase	Multiple	Haploinsufficiency
Branchio-oto-renal	Branchial cysts; inner and outer ear malformations; renal malformations	EYA1 homologue of Drosophila, eyes absent	Multiple	Haploinsufficiency
Beals	Dolichostenomelia; arachnodactyly; contractures; "crumpled" external ear	FBN2 fibrillin type 2	Multiple	Structurally abnormal gene product
Campomelic dysplasia	Bowing of long bones; male to female sex reversal; micrognathia	SOX9	Multiple	Haploinsufficiency
Cleidocranial dysplasia	Wide anterior fontanel with delayed closure; hypoplastic clavicles	RUNX2 transcription factor	Multiple	Haploinsufficiency
Coronal synostosis	Craniosynostosis; macrocephaly; brachydactyly	FGFR3	Pro250Arg	Gain of function
Crouzon	Craniosynostosis	FGFR2	Multiple	Gain of function
Currarino	Anorectal malformation; hemisacrum, presacral mass	HLXB9 homeobox 9	Multiple	Haploinsufficiency
Denys-Drash	Wilms tumor; genital malformations; renal insufficiency	WT1 Wilms tumor suppressor gene	Multiple	Haploinsufficiency
Ectrodactyly, ectodermal dysplasia, clefting	Split hand malformation, cleft lip/palate, adontia	p63 p53related protein	Multiple	Dominant-negative or Gain-of-function
Gorlin	Basal cell nevi; macrocephaly; rib abnormalities	PTCH patched trans-membrane receptor	Multiple	Haploinsufficiency
Greig cephalopolysyndactyly	Craniosynostosis; polydactyly	GLI3 transcription factor	Multiple	Haploinsufficiency
Hand-foot-genital	Distal limb anomalies; uterine and renal anomalies	HOXA13 homeobox gene	Multiple	Haploinsufficiency
Hirschsprung disease*	Aganglionic megacolon	EDN3; EDNRB; RET; endothelin 3; endothelin B receptor; receptor tyrosine kinase	Multiple	Haploinsufficiency
Holoprosencephaly	Holoprosencephaly; cyclopia; pituitary deficiency	Sonic hedgehog signaling (multiple genes)	Multiple	Haploinsufficiency
Holt-Oram	Upper limb abnormalities; structural and conductive cardiac defects	TBX5 transcription factor	Multiple	Haploinsufficiency
Marfan	Dolichostenomelia; arachnodactyly; aortic dilatation; joint laxity	FBN1 fibrillin	Multiple	Structurally abnormal gene product

(Continued)

TABLE 10.1
(CONTINUED)

Syndrome	Major Findings	Gene	Mutation	Mechanism of Action
McCune-Albright	Polyostotic fibrous dysplasia; precocious puberty; irregular skin pigmentation	Alpha subunit of G protein	Somatic mosaic (pre-sumed lethal in non-mosaic state)	Gain of function
Milroy	Congenital lymphedema	VEGFR3 vascular endothelial growth factor receptor -3	Multiple	Dominant-negative
Neurofibromatosis type 1	Café-au-lait spots; neurofibromata; axillary freckling	NF1 neurofibromin; tumor suppressor	Multiple	Haploinsufficiency
Neurofibromatosis type 2	Vestibular schwannomas; meningiomas; cataracts	NF2 merlin; tumor suppressor	Multiple	Haploinsufficiency
Noonan	Webbed neck; short stature; pulmonic stenosis cubitus valgus; ptosis; low-set ears	PTPN11, protein-tyrosine phosphatase, nonreceptor-type,11	Multiple	Gain-of-Function
Osteogenesis imperfecta	Multiple fractures; blue sclera; dentinogenesis imperfecta; joint laxity	COL1A1; COL1A2 procollagen molecules	Multiple	Haploinsufficiency or -structurally abnormal gene product
Pallister-Hall	Hypothalamic hamartoma; central polydactyly	GLI3 transcription factor mutations	Protein truncat-ing	(?)Dominant negative
Pfeiffer	Craniosynostosis; broad, medially deviated thumbs and halluces	FGFR1 FGFR2	Pro252Arg Multiple	Gain of function Gain of function
Rieger	Anterior chamber changes; dental hypoplasia; umbilical stump abnormalities	RIEG homeobox gene	Multiple	Haploinsufficiency
Rubinstein-Taybi	Broad thumbs; prominent nose; mental retardation	CBP, CREB binding protein	Multiple	Haploinsufficiency
Saethre-Chotzen	Craniosynostosis; ptosis; syndactyly; hallux valgus	TWIST transcription factor	Multiple	Haploinsufficiency
Sotos	Prenatal overgrowth, macrocephaly variable mental retardation	NSD1 (nuclear receptor binding SET domain)	Multiple	Haploinsufficiency
Stickler	Severe myopia; hearing loss; osteoarthropathy; cleft palate	COL2A1; COL11A1; COL11A2 type 2 procollagen, type 11 procollagen	Multiple	Haploinsufficiency -structurally abnormal gene product
Thanatophoric dysplasia	Lethal neonatal dwarfism; abnormal brain lobulation	FGFR3	Multiple	Gain of function
Townes-Brocks	Preaxial polydactyly; external ear, renal, and anal malformations	SALL1 transcription factor	Multiple	Haploinsufficiency
Treacher-Collins	Malar hypoplasia; malformation of external ear	TCOF1	Multiple	Haploinsufficiency
Tuberous sclerosis	Hamartomas of skin, brain, heart, kidneys; ungual fibromas	TSC1, hamartin; TSC2, tuberin	Multiple	Haploinsufficiency
Ulnar Mammary	Upper limb malformations; apocrine gland/mammary hypoplasia; genital anomalies	TBX3 transcription factor	Multiple	Haploinsufficiency
Van Der Woude	Lip pits and sinuses; cleft lip; cleft lip and palate	IRF6, interferon regulatory Factor-6	Multiple	Haploinsufficiency, Dominant negative

(Continued)

TABLE 10.1
(CONTINUED)

Syndrome	Major Findings	Gene	Mutation	Mechanism of Action
Waardenburg type 1	Deafness; pigmentary changes; dystopia canthorum	*PAX3* homeobox gene	Multiple	Haploinsufficiency
Waardenburg type 2	Deafness; pigmentary changes	*MITF* transcription factor	Multiple	Haploinsufficiency
Waardenburg-Shah	Waardenburg syndrome and Hirschsprung disease	*SOX10* transcription factor *EDN3; EDNRB*	Multiple	Haploinsufficiency

FGFR, fibroblast growth factor receptor.
*Formally considered to be a sex-modified, multigenic trait.

fibroblast growth factor receptor (FGFR2) in practically all cases, and all patients with one of these mutations show the Apert syndrome phenotype. Thus, in Apert syndrome, a strict phenotype–genotype correlation exists. Other mutations in the same gene, giving rise to multiple different amino acid substitutions, have been identified in patients with Crouzon syndrome, making it allelic to Apert syndrome. Pfeiffer syndrome can be caused by either one of multiple mutations in *FGFR2* (some of which are seen also in patients with a Crouzon phenotype, or to a recurrent mutation in *FGFR1*). Thus, Pfeiffer syndrome is heterogeneous.

FGFRs are membrane-bound receptors; their ligands are the fibroblast growth factors. After ligand binding, the FGFRs dimerize, leading to signal transduction through their intracellular tyrosine kinase domains. The previously mentioned mutations are all located within the extracellular and ligand-binding domains of the FGFRs, and they all lead to constitutive activation of the affected receptor. Mutations introducing stop codons or otherwise preventing the gene product from functioning, such as complete gene deletions, cannot lead to this gain-of-function mechanism and thus are not seen in craniosynostosis. Homologous amino acid substitutions in

FGFR1 and *FGFR2* (Pro252Arg and Pro253Arg, respectively) can give rise to gain of function and cause craniosynostosis disorders. *FGFR3* shares high sequence and structural homology with *FGFR1* and *FGFR2*, and a similar mutation (Pro250Arg) has been identified in another type of craniosynostosis. This disorder (coronal synostosis, see Table 10.1) is the first malformation syndrome delineated primarily based on its unique underlying mutation. *FGFR3* mutations have been found in skeletal dysplasias other than the coronal craniosynostosis syndrome. Nearly all cases of achondroplasia are caused by a single "hot spot" mutation in one location in the gene where a CpG dinucleotide resides that produces an amino acid substitution. Hypochondroplasia is caused by either of two base changes causing another amino acid substitution. Thanatophoric dysplasia, a lethal form of skeletal dysplasia presenting with severe craniosynostosis, is caused by several specific *FGFR3* mutations; these mutations occur *de novo* in all cases. Although achondroplasia can be passed on as an autosomal dominant trait, new mutations are relatively frequent and occur almost exclusively during spermatogenesis, as has been shown for the *FGFR2* mutations in Apert syndrome as well.

TABLE 10.2
AUTOSOMAL RECESSIVE MALFORMATION SYNDROMES CAUSED BY IDENTIFIED MUTATIONS*

Syndrome	Major Findings	Gene(s)
Bardet-Biedl Syndrome	Obesity; polydactyly; retinal dystrophy; hypogonadism; learning difficulties	*BBS1-4* (function unknown)
Congenital adrenal hyperplasia	Virilization at birth; salt wasting	*CYP21B* (21-hydroxylase)
Hermansky-Pudlak	Oculocutaneous albinism; lysosomal storage; bleeding tendency	*HPS1-7* (involved in vessicle trafficking)
Leprechaunism	Intrauterine growth retardation; failure to thrive; insulin resistance	*INSR* (insulin receptor)
Male pseudohermaphroditism	Intersex genitalia in genetic male subjects	*17β-HSD* (hydroxysteroid dehydrogenase) or *SRD5A2* (steroid 5δ reductase 2)
McKusick-Kaufman	Hydrometrocolopos, heart defect, polydactyly	*MKKS/BBS6* (chaperonin protein)
Rhizomelic chondrodysplasia punctata	Rhizomelia; epiphyseal stippling; cataracts	*PEX7* (peroxisomal receptor) DHAPAT (dihydroxyacetonephosphate acyltransferase deficiency)
Robinow	"Fetal" facies; mesomelic disproportion with short stature, digital abnormalities hypoplastic genitalia	*ROR2* (receptor tyrosine kinase-like orphan receptor 2)
Smith-Lemli-Opitz	2-3 syndactyly of toes; polydactyly; epicanthus; hypospadia; retardation	*ΔHCR7* (7-dehydrocholesterol-reductase)
Spondylocostal dysostosis	Multiple vertebral segmentation defects	DLL3 (Notch ligand delta-like 3)
Zellweger	Large fontanelle; hypotonia; cryptorchidism; renal cysts	Multiple genes involved in peroxisome biogenesis

*Autosomal recessive traits are caused by the lack of functional gene product; the mutations abolish protein expression or function.

TABLE 10.3

MALFORMATION SYNDROMES CAUSED BY SINGLE-GENE MUTATIONS OF THE X CHROMOSOME

Syndrome	Major Findings	Gene
Aarskog-Scott	Hypertelorism; shawl scrotum	*FGD1*
Anhidrotic ectodermal dysplasia	Sparse hair; hypodontia; lack of sweat glands	*EDA* (transmembrane protein)
CHILD	Congenital Hemidysplasia with Ichthyosiform erythroderma and Limb Defects	*NSDHL* (NAD(P)H steroid dehydrogenase-like protein
Coffin-Lowry	Coarse facies; everted lower lip; retardation; pectus	*RSK2* (protein kinase)
Hydrocephalus; spastic paraplegia	Aqueductal stenosis; retardation, aphasia, shuffling gait; adducted thumbs	*L1CAM* (neural cell adhesion molecule)
Incontinentia pigmenti	Abnormalities of the skin, hair, nails, teeth, eyes, and central nervous system in females, lethal in XY males	*NEMO* (NF-kappa-B essential modulator)
Kallmann	Hypogonadotropic hypogonadism; anosmia	*KAL-X* (neuronal migration factor)
Leri-Weill dyschondrosteosis	Short stature; Madelung deformity	*SHOX* (homeobox gene; in pseudoautosomal region)
Lenz micropthalmia	Micro/anophthalmia, limb anomalies, renal aplasia	*BCOR* (transcriptional repressor)
Lowe	Cataract, renal Fanconi syndrome, metal retardation	*OCRL1* (phosphatidylinositol 4,5 bisphosphate 5-phosphatase)
Male pseudohermaphroditism	Intersex genitalia in genetic male subjects	*AR* (androgen receptor)
Menkes	Kinky hair; neurologic deterioration	*MC1* (copper transporting ATPase)
Opitz	Hypertelorism; cleft lip; hypospadias; imperforate anus	*MID1* (transcription factor)
Simpson-Golabi-Behmel	Overgrowth; heart defects; cryptorchidism; supernumerary nipples; coarse facies	*GPC3* (glypican 3)
Situs inversus	Heteroataxia; cardiac malformations	*ZIC3* (transcription factor)

Contiguous Gene Syndromes and Genomic Disorders

Contiguous gene syndromes represent a group of disorders caused by a dosage imbalance of submicroscopic chromosomal fragments (Table 10.4). This dosage imbalance may be caused by a structural abnormality, such as a deletion or duplication, or it may be functional, as described for uniparental disomy and imprinting (see Chapter 11, Genetics in Pediatric Primary Care). Several genes located in close proximity are affected and, in combination, are responsible for the characteristic phenotype associated with each syndrome. Therefore, single-gene disorders, such as Rubinstein-Taybi or Angelman syndrome, are not included in this definition when caused by a mutation of the respective gene. More than one gene is involved in the findings typical for Williams-Beuren and Langer-Giedion syndrome, and it is most likely that multiple genes are responsible for the phenotypes of Prader-Willi, Smith-Magenis, and DiGeorge/velocardiofacial syndromes.

Genomic disorders are human diseases that are caused by genomic (DNA)-mediated rearrangements, such as deletions, duplications, and inversions that occur at specific locations throughout the genome. Through the study of disease-related genomic rearrangements associated with several different syndromes, including those already mentioned and those to be discussed, a common mechanism for causation has been defined. Dispersed throughout the human genome is a series of recently evolved low-copy repeats (LCRs). These repeats consist of blocks of DNA, 10 to 400 kb in length, that are virtually identical in sequence. Some are specific to certain chromosomes, whereas others are found on more than one chromosome. The large size and chromosomal proximity of these repeats promotes nonallelic recombination, which then leads to deletion, duplication, or inversion on the recombining chromosomes, de-

pending upon the orientation of the repeats and nature of the recombination event. For example, intrachromosomal recombination mediated by LCRs underlies the formation of deletions that cause the Williams-Beuren, Prader-Willi, Angelman, Smith-Magenis, and DiGeorge/velocardiofacial syndromes—hence these contiguous gene syndromes are genomic disorders.

Genomic disorders also can manifest as Mendelian diseases and monogenic traits. Charcot-Marie-Tooth disease type 1A, an autosomal dominant neuropathy, can be caused by duplication of the peripheral myelin protein-22 (*PMP22*). It has been determined that unequal crossing over between directly repeated, homologous DNA sequences that flank the *PMP22* gene, and are 1.5 Mb apart, cause the duplication event. The reciprocal product, a chromosome with a deletion between the same repeats, produces haploinsufficiency for *PMP22*, and causes an entirely different disorder, hereditary neuropathy with liability to pressure palsies. Because these disorders also can be caused by point mutations in *PMP22*, they also may be considered single-gene disorders. Although it remains to be seen if duplications of the regions involved in microdeletion syndromes always account for other clinically recognized disorders in all instances, it does appear to be the case for the Smith-Magenis syndrome region, and other regions are under investigation. Alternatively, these duplications may be lethal at an early stage of embryonal development and therefore will not be seen in live births. Genomic- and LCR-mediated rearrangements underlie the formation of mutant alleles in a variety of disorders, including spinal muscular atrophy, polycystic kidney disease type 1, neurofibromatosis type 1, red–green color blindness, incontinentia pigmenti, hemophilia A, and male infertility. Analysis of the human genome sequence indicates that LCRs may occupy as much as much as 5% of the genome, yet many LCRs have not been associated with clinically recognized disorders to date.

TABLE 10.4

MALFORMATION SYNDROMES CAUSED BY DOSAGE IMBALANCE (SEGMENTAL ANEUSOMY)

Syndrome	Major Findings	Locus	Gene(s)	Disease Caused by
Angelman[a,c]	Retardation; seizures, prominent chin; ataxia; microcephaly	15q11-13	*UBE3A* (ubiqitin protein ligase)	Deletion of maternal allele; paternal UPD; *UBE3A* mutation
Beckwith-Wiedemann	Macroglossia, omphalocele; hypoglycemia; hemihypertrophy; LGA	11p11.5	*p57*[EIP2] (cyclin-dependent kinase inhibitor 1C); *NSD1*; *H19*	*p57*[KIP] and *NSD1* mutations, microdeletions of *H19*; paternal UPD
Charcot Marie Tooth[a,b,c]	Peripheral neuropathy; distal muscle atrophy	17p11.2	*PMP22* (peripheral myelin protein)	Segmental trisomy, point mutations (CMT1A)
HNPP[a,b,c]	Heriditary neuropathy with liability to pressure palsies;	17p11.2	*PMP22* (peripheral myelin protein)	Haploinsufficiency caused by deletion motor neuron swellings
Langer-Giedion (TRP type II)	Trichorhinophalangeal changes; retardation; multiple exostosis	8q24	*EXT1*; *TRPS*	Contiguous gene deletion
Miller-Dieker	Lissencephaly; furrowed forehead; cardiac malformations	17p13.3	*LIS1*	Contiguous gene deletion
Prader-Willi[c]	Hypotonia; hypogonadism; poor suck; hyperphagia Obesity; retardation	15q11-q13		Deletion of paternal allele; maternal UPD
Smith-Magenis[c]	Myopia; behavioral problems; retardation	17p11.2		Contiguous gene deletion
Velocardiofacial[c] (diGeorge; 22 q deletion)	Cleft palate; conotruncal defects; facial changes; hypocalcemia Immune problems	22q11	Multiple	Contiguous gene deletion (?)
Williams[c]	Supravalvular aortic stenosis; facial changes; characteristic behavior	7q11.23	*ELN*; *LIMK1*	Contiguous gene deletion

[a] In addition to the deletion or paternal UPD, Angelman syndrome may be caused by mutation in the *UBE3A* gene; therefore, it also can be considered a single-gene disorder.
[b] CMT1A and HNPP are allelic, as they are caused by duplication or deletion of the region encompassing the *PMP22* gene. In rare instances, point mutations of *PMP22* have been found to cause these disorders; hence, they also may be considered single-gene disorders.
[c] The chromosomal rearrangements seen in Angelman, Prader-Willi, Charcot-Marie-Tooth, HNPP, Smith-Magenis, Velocardiofacial, and Williams-Beuren syndromes are caused by low copy repeat (LCR) mediated recombination.

NONCLASSIC MUTATIONS PRODUCING GENETIC DISEASE

Since the late 1980s, nonclassic types of mutations have been described, some of which lead to unusual nonmendelian inheritance. These types of mutations are (a) unstable repeat sequences, (b) insertion of transposable elements into new genomic sites, (c) uniparental disomy (inheritance of two chromosomal homologues from one parent and none from the other), and (d) imprinting as an explanation for one genotype producing two different phenotypes, depending on which parent provides a defective chromosome.

Unstable Repeat Sequences

The expansion of trinucleotide repeat sequences is responsible for roughly a dozen neurologic diseases, including the fragile X syndrome, myotonic dystrophy, Huntington disease, spinal and bulbar muscular atrophy, and the spinal cerebellar ataxias. Our information on the unstable nature of these sequences is most complete for the fragile X syndrome. This syndrome is one of the most common causes of mental retardation in male subjects (approximately 1 in 1,500 male subjects is affected). When lymphocytes of affected male subjects are grown in folate-deficient medium and their chromosomes are examined, a substantial fraction of X chromosomes contain a break at Xq27 near the distal end of the long arm. This phenotype is associated with the lack of expression of a gene (familial mental retardation-1 or *FMR1*) and the inappropriate methylation of DNA near the 5′ end of the gene. In turn, the inappropriate methylation is a secondary effect of a marked expansion of a trinucleotide repeat (CGG) in the 5′ noncoding region of the *FMR1* gene (Fig. 10.9).

In normal X chromosomes, the repeat number of this trinucleotide is polymorphic, centering around 29, with a normal range of 6 to 45. In some X chromosomes, the repeat number increases to 52 to 200. These chromosomes carry what is termed a *premutation* for the fragile X phenotype. This premutation is associated with normal intelligence, normal methylation of nearby sites, and normal expression of the *FMR1* gene. When a man passes the premutation to a female offspring, it remains essentially unchanged. However, when a female carrier of a premutation passes this X chromosome to her offspring, a significant risk exists for both sons and daughters that the trinucleotide repeat will expand greatly to 200 to 600 copies. This large number of repeats is the full mutation and is associated with inappropriate methylation of nearby DNA and inactivation of the *FMR1* gene. The probability that a premutation will become a full mutation is a function of the size of the repeat in the premutation, being very low if the premutation contains fewer than 60 repeats and approaching 100% if it contains 100 or more repeats. Repeat expansion can occur either in female meiosis or in early mitotic development. In the latter instance, lymphocyte DNA contains the

FRAGILE X: Amplification of (CGG)ₙ in Exon 1 of the FMR-1 Gene

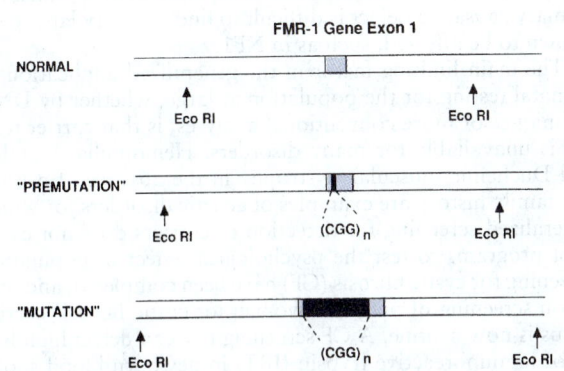

FIGURE 10.9. Expansion of a trinucleotide repeat in the fragile X syndrome. In the normal *FMR1* gene on the long arm of the X chromosome, a CGG repeat sequence is found. When this repeat expands through meiosis from the normal six to 45 repeats to 52 to 200 repeats, the premutation is produced. Offspring of females with the premutation are at high risk of further expansion of the repeat in meiosis or early mitotic development. Massive expansion to 200 to 600 copies of the repeat is the full mutation and leads to inactivation of the *FMR1* gene and to expression of the fragile X syndrome.

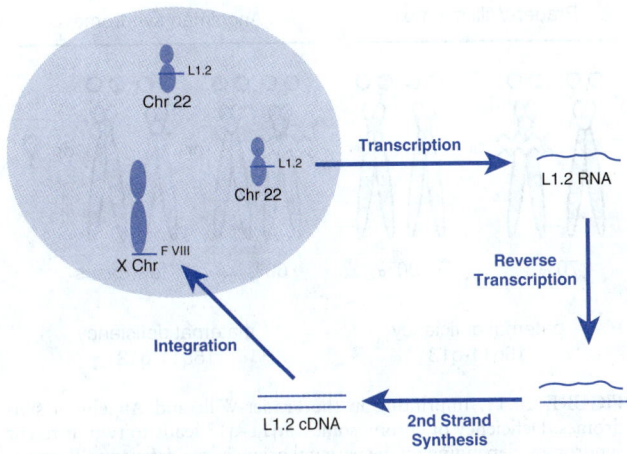

FIGURE 10.10. Retrotransposition of a LINE (long interspersed element) (L1.2) from chromosome 22 in the factor VIII gene on the X chromosome causing *de novo* hemophilia A. A 6-kb LINE element (L1.2) is present as a gene on chromosome 22. In one parent's germ cell, this gene was transcribed into RNA, then reverse transcribed into cDNA, and the double-stranded cDNA was reintegrated back into the genome, disrupting the factor VIII gene at the tip of the X chromosome. Note that the L1.2 genes have not themselves moved but that a new copy of the gene has been placed at a distant location in the patient's genome.

premutation repeat, along with full mutation repeats of various sizes.

Myotonic dystrophy, spinal and bulbar muscular atrophy, and Huntington disease also are caused by expansion of a trinucleotide repeat that inactivates a gene. In these conditions, a polyglutamine track encoded by $(CAG)_n$ in the protein is expanded, causing the protein to form insoluble nuclear aggregates. These disorders are inherited in an autosomal dominant fashion and, like fragile X syndrome, can display anticipation (worsening of the clinical phenotype in subsequent generations) in affected families as well as a propensity for either maternal- or paternal-specific allelic expansion in the premutation state.

Insertion of Transposable Elements

A second nonclassical type of mutation is insertion of a transposable element, either a LINE or an *Alu* element. Descriptions of these larger repeated sequences were presented earlier in this chapter. LINE insertions have been observed in 16 instances of genetic disease, including hemophilia A, Duchenne muscular dystrophy, and retinitis pigmentosa, and in a tumor suppressor gene, APC, in colon cancer. Disease producing *AluI* insertions have been found in over 20 cases, including neurofibromatosis type 1 and hemophilia B. These insertions are rare causes of *de novo* mutation. In the case of LINE insertions, these are derived from roughly 80 to 100 active transposable elements in the average human being. They move through an RNA intermediate using a reverse transcriptase encoded by the element (Fig. 10.10). *Alu* elements are transcribed, but require a reverse transcriptase encoded from an active LINE element to transpose. Although these types of mutations probably have had only a small impact in producing disease, they have had a major impact throughout evolution in modifying our genome.

Uniparental Disomy

Uniparental disomy is an unusual inheritance of two chromosomal homologs from one parent and none from the other.

Rarely, both of the chromosomes of a pair are the identical chromosome inherited from one parent. This is called uniparental isodisomy, and it provides a mechanism to explain the rare occurrence of an autosomal recessive disease when only one parent is a carrier. In two cases of cystic fibrosis, the affected child received two copies of the same chromosome 7 containing a cystic fibrosis mutation from one parent and no chromosome 7 from the other. These children showed other effects of homozygosity for an entire chromosome, such as short stature and developmental delay. Many mechanisms for the phenomenon are possible, but perhaps the most likely is that the fertilized egg was trisomic for chromosome 7 (two copies from parent 1 and one copy from parent 2), but early in embryonic development the copy of chromosome 7 from parent 2 was lost. Cells containing two copies of chromosome 7 (disomic) were then selected over cells containing three copies (trisomic). This is called *trisomy rescue* and has been documented to occur in Prader-Willi syndrome, a disorder that can be caused by uniparental disomy in some cases.

Another example of uniparental disomy is the inheritance in an XY male of both an X chromosome and a Y chromosome from the father and no sex chromosome from the mother. This has been seen in a case of male-to-male transmission of hemophilia A, in which the affected son received a mutant X chromosome (along with a Y chromosome) from his affected father. Uniparental disomy effects have been documented for many human disorders and should be entertained when a recessive disease has an unusual or expanded phenotype in the absence of parental consanguinity.

Imprinting

Imprinting refers to different phenotypes resulting from the same genotype, depending on whether a mutation-marked chromosome is derived from the mother or the father. An example is found in the inheritance of the Prader-Willi and Angelman syndromes, two syndromes in which the affected children have very different clinical manifestations. In Prader-Willi syndrome, paternal deficiency of chromosome 15q11–q13

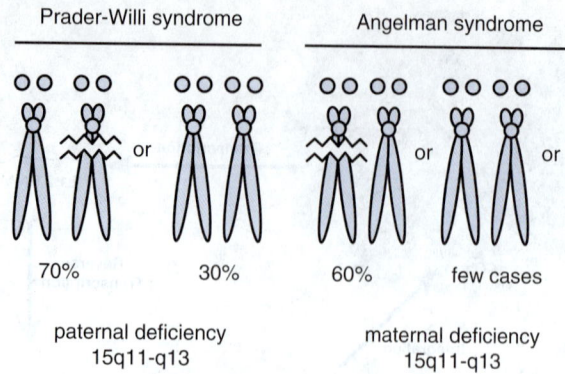

Prader-Willi syndrome   Angelman syndrome

70%   30%   60%   few cases

paternal deficiency   maternal deficiency
15q11-q13   15q11-q13

FIGURE 10.11. Imprinting in the Prader-Willi and Angelman syndromes. Deficiency of chromosome 15q11–q13 leads to two different syndromes, depending on the parental origin of the deficiency. Paternal deficiency of 15q11–q13, either through interstitial deletion or maternal disomy (no chromosome 15 donated by the father), produces the Prader-Willi syndrome. Maternal deficiency of 15q11–13 through interstitial deletion, paternal disomy, mutation in the UBE3 gene, or other unknown mechanisms produces the Angelman syndrome. Filled chromosomes are paternally derived; open chromosomes are maternal in origin.

occurs, whereas in Angelman syndrome, maternal deficiency of the same chromosomal region occurs. Of Prader-Willi cases, 70% have a deletion of the paternal chromosome 15q11–q13 and a normal maternal chromosome 15, whereas 30% have maternal disomy for chromosome 15 and no paternal chromosome 15 (Fig. 10.11). Angelman syndrome may be caused by a microdeletion on the maternal chromosome 15q11–q13, uniparental paternal disomy for chromosome 15, a mutation in the maternally inherited imprinting center, or a mutation in the maternal ubiquitin-protein ligase gene (UBE3A). All these mechanisms lead to compromised expression of UBE3A by the maternal allele, which is thought to be the underlying molecular etiology. The role of methylation in the process of imprinting is thought to be critical, but the true molecular basis of this mysterious process has not been fully explained.

PRENATAL DIAGNOSIS OF SINGLE-GENE DISORDERS BY DNA ANALYSIS

DNA-based tests were first applied on a practical basis to the prenatal diagnosis of sickle cell anemia in 1978; beta-thalassemia in 1980; hemophilia B in 1984; hemophilia A, phenylketonuria, and Duchenne and Becker muscular dystrophies in 1985; cystic fibrosis and Huntington disease in 1986; neurofibromatosis in 1989; and fragile X in 1991. This list should give an indication of the explosion of knowledge and new diagnostic possibilities. The list of disorders that can be diagnosed by such techniques for couples known to be at risk continues to grow and now includes many of the more common inherited disorders and cancer-susceptibility genes. Web-based resources, particularly Online Mendelian Inheritance in Man (www.ncbi.nlm.nih.gov/omim/) and Genetests (www.genetests.org), should allow a rapid assessment of available tests, as clinical or research services.

DNA Analysis: Current Uses and Limitations

Prenatal DNA analysis has been well received for several reasons. First, the fetal samples necessary for diagnosis can be obtained by first-trimester chorion villus sampling or midtrimester amniocentesis. Second, because gene expression

is not required for DNA diagnosis, any nucleated cell type in any stage of differentiation is suitable for analysis. Third, DNA analysis permits the diagnosis of some disorders for which the primary causative defect is difficult to find in a very large gene known to be affected, such as in NF1.

The main limiting factor in the generalized application of prenatal testing for the population at large, whether by DNA techniques or more conventional analyses, is that carrier testing is unavailable for many disorders. Hemophilia A and B and Duchenne muscular dystrophy in the absence of a positive family history are examples of genetic disorders for which generalized screening for detection of carriers does not exist. Pilot programs to test the psychological effect of population screening for cystic fibrosis (CF) have been completed, and mutation screening of pregnant women for cystic fibrosis carrier status is now routine. A CF screening test can detect high levels of immunoreactive trypsin (IRT) in newborn blood spots, and several pilot programs have been undertaken to assess the effectiveness of early diagnosis. On the other hand, effective, inexpensive methods for detecting carriers of globin variants, particularly sickle cell anemia, alpha-thalassemia, and beta-thalassemia, are available through hemoglobin electrophoresis and determination of mean corpuscular volume.

General Methods of DNA Analysis

At present, several methods are used for diagnosis by DNA analysis, including direct detection of the genetic defect and indirect detection using polymorphic sites closely linked to the disease-producing mutation. Direct detection usually can be achieved by various gene screening methods, followed by DNA sequencing of regions that appear altered.

Direct detection can be achieved in three situations: The mutation alters an endonuclease restriction site, as it does in all cases of sickle cell anemia; the mutation is the result of a gene deletion, as in virtually all cases of hydrops fetalis associated with alpha-thalassemia and more than 50% of cases of Duchenne muscular dystrophy; or the mutation is known, and the gene region containing the mutation can be sequenced (beta-thalassemia, alpha-1-antitrypsin deficiency, and cystic fibrosis often are diagnosed in this way).

Direct detection schemes have been aided greatly by the development of the polymerase chain reaction (PCR). This simple technique allows the researcher, in a few hours, to amplify by up to ten million–fold any particular region of the DNA that has been cloned previously or about which at least some sequence is known. For example, a sample of genomic DNA containing two copies of the beta-globin gene per cell (one on

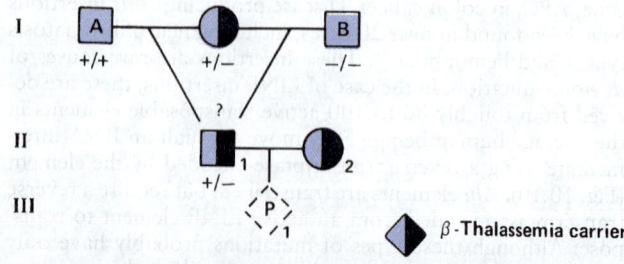

I

II

III

β-Thalassemia carrier

FIGURE 10.12. The problem of mis-stated paternity in prenatal diagnosis by linkage analysis. In the example shown, a mutant beta-globin gene is being tracked using a DNA polymorphism in the beta-globin gene cluster. If the paternity is as shown on the left, the beta-thalassemia gene in the father (II-1) is marked by the positive (+) form of the polymorphism. However, if paternity is as shown on the right, the beta-thalassemia gene in the father (II-1) is marked by the negative (−) form of the polymorphism. It is clear that an error in paternity can lead to an error in the prenatal diagnosis of beta-thalassemia in the case shown.

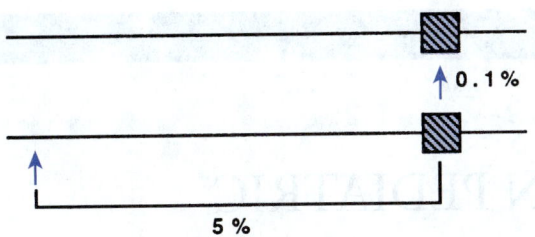

FIGURE 10.13. The problem of meiotic recombination in prenatal diagnosis by linkage analysis. If the polymorphic marker, whether an RFLP, VNTR or SNP, used to track a mutation in the gene shown on the right is within the gene (*top arrow*), the error rate due to meiotic recombination between the polymorphism and the mutation within the gene is very low (0.1%). However, when one uses a polymorphic marker at a 5% meiotic recombination distance from the gene of interest (*bottom arrow*), the error rate for diagnosis due to recombination is 5% for each generation.

each chromosome 11) can be subjected to PCR and, within a few hours, after PCR amplification, the equivalent of one million to ten million copies of the beta-globin gene per cell can be obtained in a test tube. This has led to rapid assays, particularly of direct nucleotide sequencing of the amplified gene, the present method of choice. The PCR technique also has had many applications in research beyond those of gene diagnosis and indeed has revolutionized work in molecular genetics since its introduction in 1985. The accuracy of a diagnosis achieved by a direct detection technique theoretically should be close to 100%. However, in diagnoses achieved by an indirect detection technique using DNA polymorphisms physically close to the gene of interest, false assumptions about paternity may allow a misinterpretation of the inheritance patterns between the marker, whether it is a RFLP, VNTR, or a SNP, and the disease gene (Fig. 10.12). A mistake in diagnosis also can occur if the association between the marker and the defective gene breaks down as a result of interchromosomal DNA exchange at meiosis (meiotic recombination) (Fig. 10.13). The chance of recombination per meiosis is a function of the degree of linkage between the marker and the disease gene. This means that the closer the marker is to the disease gene and the mutation causing the disease, the smaller the chance of a recombination event producing an error in diagnosis. This biologic error rate is determined empirically. Markers within the disease gene are in general more tightly linked to the mutation than extragenic markers and thus are more accurate predictors of inheritance of the disease.

CONCLUSIONS

This chapter has discussed the salient features of gene structure, genomic organization, normal variation, and mutations affecting gene expression. Nonclassical mutations and some examples of unusual inheritance patterns also have been presented. Using gene diagnosis, the prenatal diagnosis and carrier detection of many single-gene disorders, including the most common ones, has become a clinical reality. New lessons have been learned from other disorders, such as those mediated by genomic rearrangements. The striking extent of genetic heterogeneity producing single-gene disorders of man is being illuminated, and the information gleaned from the Human Genome Project will certainly lead to a new generation of molecular diagnostic tools.

GLOSSARY

Allele: An alternative form of a gene; for instance, the beta^s gene is an allele of the beta-gene.

BAC: Bacterial artificial chromosome.

Codon: A group of three nucleotides coding for an amino acid.

Complementary DNA (cDNA): A single-stranded DNA copy of a messenger RNA made with the use of the viral enzyme reverse transcriptase; cDNA contains only the coding sequences of a gene.

Exon: DNA sequences that are transcribed into messenger RNA; most exon sequences also are translated into protein.

5′ and 3′ ends of DNA fragments: By convention, the 5′ end refers to the left end of a DNA fragment, and the 3′ end refers to the right end. Biochemically, 5′ and 3′ refer to the points of attachment of phosphate to ribose on the two ends of the coding strand.

Genomic DNA: DNA contained in the chromosomes in the nucleus of a cell. Mitochondrial, chloroplast, or synthetic DNA are not genomic DNA.

Hybridization: The re-annealing of single-stranded nucleic acid molecules. The formation of double-stranded regions indicates complementary sequences.

Intervening sequences or intron: DNA sequences that interrupt coding sequences of a gene.

Kilobase (kb): One thousand base (nucleotide) pairs of DNA.

Linkage: The close physical association of the specific site in the genome with another on a particular chromosome.

Locus: Any site in the DNA that may contain different sequences when one human genome is compared with another

PCR: Polymerase chain reaction.

Plasmid: A small circular piece of DNA in a bacterium that replicates independently of the bacterial genome.

Probe: Radioactive single-stranded nucleic acid used to locate genomic DNA sequences complementary to it.

Pseudogene: Region of DNA that displays significant homology to a functional gene but has mutations that prevent its expression.

Restriction endonucleases: Bacterial enzymes that recognize and cleave a specific DNA sequence.

SNP: Single nucleotide polymorphism.

Suggested Readings

Cummings CJ, Zoghbi HY. Trinucleotide repeats: mechanisms and pathophysiology. *Ann Rev Genet Hum Genet* 2000;1:281.

Guttmacher AE, Collins FS. Genomic medicine—a primer. *N Engl J Med* 2002;347:1512.

DiLella AG, Marvit J, Lidsky AS, et al. Tight linkage between a splicing mutation and a specific DNA haplotype in phenylketonuria. *Nature* 1986;322:799.

Epstein CJ, Erickson RP, Wynshaw-Boris. *Inborn errors of development: the molecular basis of clinical disorders and morphogenesis.* Oxford Press, 2004.

Lander ES, Linton LM, Birren B, et al. Initial sequencing and analysis of the human genome. *Nature* 2001;409:860.

Maniatis T, Fritsch ER, Lauer J, Lawn RM. The molecular genetics of human hemoglobin. *Ann Rev Genet* 1980;14:145.

Nicholls RD, Knepper JL. Genome organization, function, and imprinting in Prader-Willi and Angelman syndromes. *Ann Rev Genomics Hum Genet* 2001;2:153.

Orkin SH, Kazazian HH Jr. The mutation and polymorphism of the human beta-globin gene and its surrounding DNA. *Ann Rev Genet* 1984;18:131.

Sachidanandam R, Weissman D, Schmidt SC, et al. A map of the human genome containing 1.42 million single nucleotide polymorphisms. *Nature* 2001;409:928.

Saiki RK, Gelfand DH, Stoffel S, et al. Primer-directed enzymatic amplification of DNA with a thermostable DNA polymerase. *Science* 1988;239:487.

Southern EM. Detection of specific sequences among DNA fragments separated by gel electrophoresis. *J Mol Biol* 1975;98:503.

Stalker HJ, Williams CA. Genetic counseling in Angelman syndrome: the challenges of multiple causes. *Am J Med Genet* 1998;77:54.

Stankiewicz P, Lupski JR. Genome architecture, rearrangements, and genomic disorders. *Trends Genet* 2002;18:74.

Thomas JW, Touchman JW, Blakesley RW, et al. Comparative analyses of multi-species sequences from targeted genomic regions. *Nature* 2003;424(6950):788.

Venter JC, Adams MD, Myers EW, et al. The sequence of the human genome. *Science* 2001;292:1838.

CHAPTER 11 ■ GENETICS IN PEDIATRIC PRIMARY CARE

TYLER REIMSCHISEL AND ADA HAMOSH

Many health care professionals consider genetic diseases to be limited to single-gene disorders, such as sickle cell disease, cystic fibrosis (CF), muscular dystrophy (MD), and phenylketonuria. But genes play a much larger role in human disease and health. For example, McCandless et al. have shown that up to 71% of children admitted to a children's hospital have a disorder with a significant genetic component. In fact, all human traits and diseases, including common conditions such as otitis media, are modified by multiple genetic factors. Furthermore, variation in the genetic background of individuals with a given disease or syndrome explains in part the variable clinical manifestations of that disease or syndrome. For example, generalists are well aware of variation in common medical problems such as asthma, attention deficit-hyperactivity disorder, and streptococcal pharyngitis. Just as the environment can influence the severity of these medical problems, host and microbial genes also play a role in the clinical presentation. As the Human Genome Project draws to completion and the entire genetic code of humans is deciphered, we will learn much more about how genes play a role in disease and health. This chapter reviews the current understanding of genetics and its role in the medical problems that the pediatrician may encounter.

GENETIC TERMINOLOGY AND INHERITANCE PATTERNS

A basic understanding of genetic terminology is essential for comprehending genetic principles. A *gene* is the basic unit of genetic information. It is composed of a sequence of nucleotides in DNA within chromosomes. A *codon* is a triplet of three nucleotides or bases, and each codon encodes a single amino acid in a polypeptide. A gene may contain many *exons* and *introns*. *Exons* are sequences of DNA that are transcribed and processed into mature messenger RNA (mRNA), which is the template for translating nucleotide information into polypeptides. *Introns* also are nucleotide sequences of DNA that are transcribed into RNA, but the intronic sequences are spliced out to make mRNA during post-transcriptional processing. Thus, mature mRNA is composed only of RNA that is complementary to the DNA sequences of the exons of a particular gene.

Variability can exist in the DNA sequence at a particular genetic locus. These variants are known as *alleles*. Most genes have a single DNA sequence that is known as the *wild-type allele*. All permanent changes to the DNA sequence of the wild-type allele are known as *mutations*, and alleles that contain mutations are called *mutated* or *variant alleles*. A mutated sequence of DNA that occurs in 1% or more of the population is known as a *polymorphism*. Less common alleles are known as *rare variants*. If a mutation in a gene causes a disease, then the mutation is a *pathogenic* or *deleterious mutation*. Frequently, the term "mutation" is used to denote a change in the DNA

that causes disease, but the term *pathogenic mutation* is preferable. In an individual, the DNA sequence in a gene is the *genotype* of that individual. The *phenotype* in that individual is the biochemical, molecular, and clinical manifestations of the genotype. The *genome* is the entire genetic information of an individual. *Genome* also can refer to the entire genetic information of a population or species.

Many genetic diseases manifest *genetic heterogeneity*, in which more than one pathogenic mutation can lead to the same disease. For example, CF can be caused by more than 1,000 different pathogenic mutations in the CF transmembrane conductance regulator (CFTR) gene. This is an example of a specific type of genetic heterogeneity known as *allelic heterogeneity*, in which different mutations at the same locus or gene lead to the same disease. Another example of genetic heterogeneity is *locus heterogeneity*, in which mutations in different genes lead to the same disease. Locus heterogeneity occurs in a variety of genetic diseases, including Ehlers-Danlos syndrome, tuberous sclerosis, and alpha- and beta-thalassemias.

Alternatively, pathogenic mutations in the same gene can cause distinct clinical phenotypes. This is termed *phenotypic heterogeneity*. For example, many mutations in CFTR cause CF, but some mutations in CFTR cause congenital bilateral absence of the vas deferens without a predilection for pulmonary disease. One of the most striking examples of phenotypic heterogeneity is that different mutations in the gene lamin A/C cause seven distinct diseases, including progeria (premature aging syndrome), a type of dilated cardiomyopathy, early-onset atrial fibrillation, a type of Emery-Dreifuss MD, limb-girdle MD type 1B, Charcot-Marie-Tooth disease type 2B, familial lipodystrophy, mandibuloacral dysplasia, and lipoatrophy with diabetes, hepatic steatosis, hypertrophic cardiomyopathy, and leukomelanodermic papules.

Phenotypic heterogeneity is distinct from *pleiotropy*, another feature that distinguishes many genetic diseases from other etiologies of disease. *Pleiotropy* is the manifestation of multiple, seemingly unrelated, medical problems due to a single gene abnormality. For example, dysfunction of the chloride channel in CF causes recurrent pulmonary infections, pancreatic insufficiency, and infertility in males. Smith-Lemli-Opitz syndrome, a disorder of cholesterol synthesis, causes mental retardation, two- to three-toe syndactyly and other dysmorphic features, urogenital abnormalities, and a low 7-dehydrocholesterol level.

In individuals with a given disease, each feature of the phenotype can present with varying degrees of severity or can be completely absent. This variation in the phenotype of a single disease, termed *variable expressivity*, can occur in individuals with a disease who are from different families and in affected individuals within the same family. The genetic factors that cause the variable expressions of a disease include allelic heterogeneity, locus heterogeneity, and differences in the genes that modify the function and expression of the abnormal gene product. An individual's unique phenotype also is related to his or her environmental exposures and *stochastic* or chance molecular and biochemical events that occur in the individual.

Variable expression of a phenotype should not be confused with penetrance. *Penetrance* is the statistical likelihood that individuals with a particular genotype will have any phenotypic expression, no matter how mild or severe. If a mutation in a gene does not always cause a phenotypic expression, then that gene shows *reduced penetrance*. For example, in some families retinoblastoma does not develop in up to 40% of individuals with a pathogenic mutation in the retinoblastoma susceptibility gene. Unlike expressivity, penetrance is either "full" or "reduced" by a particular percentage; it should not be called "variable." Some diseases show reduced or incomplete penetrance. All diseases have variable expression in their phenotype.

Types of Genetic Alterations

During DNA replication, multiple errors can occur. However, at least 99.9% of these errors are corrected. The efficiency of repairing DNA replication errors ensures the stable transfer of genetic information during multiple generations of cell division. It also minimizes the frequency of genetic diseases due to single-gene defects. Yet, not all errors are corrected, and one error occurs for every 10^{-10} base pairs per cell division. Thus, less than one mutation occurs per cell division.

Some mutations only change a single coding nucleotide base. These *point mutations* can have different molecular effects. For example, a *missense mutation* causes a change in the amino acid that is encoded by that codon. A *nonsense mutation* introduces a base pair that makes the codon a stop codon. The introduction of a premature stop codon causes mRNA degradation in a process called *nonsense mediated decay* (NMD). Other point mutations may disrupt RNA processing by changing a splice site that defines exon–intron boundaries. These mutations lead to frameshift mutations and NMD, or abnormal polypeptide formation. For example, sickle cell disease occurs because a single base substitution (adenine → thymine) at codon 6 changes the sixth amino acid from glutamic acid to valine in the gene that encodes the beta-chain of hemoglobin. This single change causes deoxygenated hemoglobin to polymerize and "sickle."

Some genes normally contain a series of three repeating base pairs or trinucleotides. Pathogenic mutations can occur if a trinucleotide sequence in a gene increases in number during gametogenesis. For example, fragile X syndrome occurs when the trinucleotide cytosine-guanine-guanine in the FMR1 gene increases from the normal repeat length of 6 to 45 repeats to more than 200 repeats. The length of these trinucleotide repeats also can decrease. Thus, expanded trinucleotide repeats are called *dynamic mutations*. Frequently, the repeating trinucleotide encodes a series of glutamines. The current hypothesis for the pathogenesis of many trinucleotide repeat diseases is that polyglutamine aggregates cause abnormal protein folding and function or are toxic to the cells. Because the trinucleotide repeat is a dynamic mutation, trinucleotide repeat diseases manifest *anticipation*, in which the disease can present at a younger age and with a more severe phenotype as the mutation expands in size from one generation to the next. Trinucleotide repeat diseases include Huntington disease, most autosomal dominant spinocerebellar ataxias, Friedreich ataxia, and myotonic dystrophy.

In addition to point mutations, small intragenic deletions, duplications, and insertions can occur. If the number of bases in a deletion, duplication, or insertion is a multiple of three, then there will be a loss or gain of amino acids in the translated protein. However, if the number of bases is not a multiple of three, then the mutation causes a *frameshift* in the DNA sequence that usually leads to mRNA decay because a stop codon occurs prematurely.

Large deletions, duplications, insertions, and inversions also can occur. They can affect many genes and noncoding regions within a chromosome and lead to an abnormal phenotype. Some of these abnormalities can be identified through the microscopic analysis of a high-resolution karyotype. Others are too small to see by light microscopy. These *submicroscopic* abnormalities can be identified by fluorescent *in situ* hybridization (FISH).

Deletions, duplications, insertions, and inversions can alter the number of bases in the DNA sequence. An insertion and deletion can occur if a translocation occurs of a piece of one chromosome into the sequence of a different chromosome. If the translocation occurs without an obvious loss of genetic information on karyotype analysis, then it is a *balanced translocation*. If it appears on the karyotype that genetic material has been lost, then it is an *unbalanced translocation*. Both balanced and unbalanced translocations can cause an abnormal phenotype, because the translocation can disrupt multiple gene sequences, even if no obvious loss of genetic material is present on the karyotype. A translocation can be balanced in a parent and become unbalanced in the offspring. Loci with balanced translocations are prone to errors during mitosis and meiosis because of independent segregation of sister chromatids. An inversion is a mutation in which the orientation of the DNA sequence is reversed. Once again, depending on the size and location of the inversion, this mutation may present as an abnormal phenotype in the individual or the individual's offspring.

Aneuploidy is another chromosomal alteration in which a change occurs in the number of chromosomes. For example, trisomy 21 or Down syndrome is due to an extra copy of chromosome 21. Turner syndrome is due to the loss of an X chromosome in females (45, X).

Inheritance Patterns

Single-gene disorders can be inherited in a variety of Mendelian patterns, including autosomal dominant, autosomal recessive, and X-linked (Fig. 11.1). A *dominantly* inherited disease occurs when only one of the two alleles at a particular gene locus has a pathogenic mutation. A *recessively* inherited disease occurs when both alleles have pathogenic mutations. When one allele has a pathogenic mutation and the other allele has the wild-type base pair sequence, the affected individual is said to be *heterozygous* at that gene locus. If the identical mutation occurs on both alleles, the affected individual is *homozygous* at that locus. In recessively inherited diseases, it is common to have different pathogenic mutations on each allele. In those cases, the affected individual is *compound heterozygous* at that locus. If the gene that has pathogenic mutation(s) is located on one of the 22 autosomes, an *autosomal* dominant or recessive disorder results. In some cases, a disorder can be inherited in an autosomal dominant pattern in one family and in an autosomal recessive pattern in a different family (e.g., osteogenesis imperfecta type 3). This occurs because some mutations are pathogenic if they change only one allele, whereas other mutations are less disruptive to the gene product and must be present in both alleles to cause a particular disease. If the gene that has the pathogenic mutation is located on the X chromosome, the disease is transmitted in an X-linked pattern.

Autosomal Dominant Inheritance

In disorders that are inherited in an autosomal dominant pattern, males and females are affected equally. The disease can

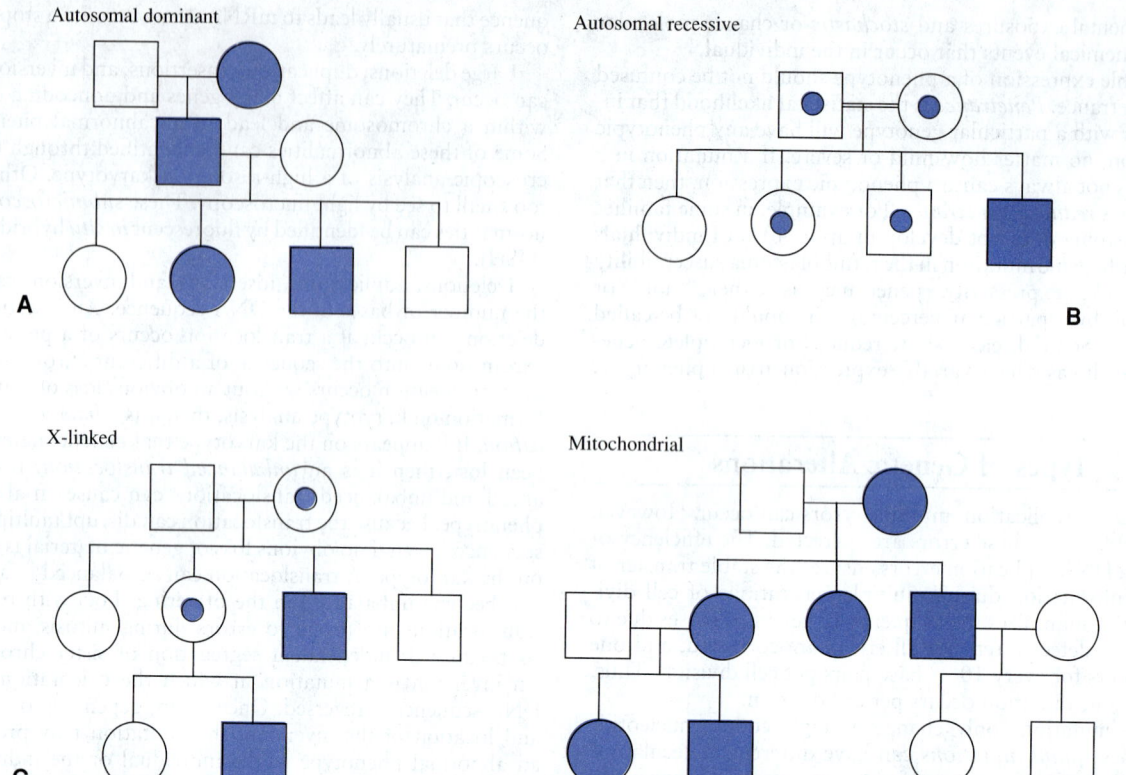

FIGURE 11.1. Typical pedigrees of Mendelian and mitochondrial inheritance patterns. Squares are males; circles are females. Shaded symbols are affected; unshaded are unaffected. Dot in symbol is carrier in autosomal recessive pedigree and obligate heterozygote in X-linked pedigree. Double line denotes consanguinity in the autosomal recessive pedigree.

be inherited from only one parent. Thus, vertical transmission of a disease can be identified in the pedigree of a family with an autosomal dominant condition. Autosomal dominant conditions can also occur *sporadically* when a gene spontaneously mutates in the gamete of an unaffected parent, and the disease presents for the first time in the offspring. Alternatively, some autosomal dominant disorders "skip generations" when the phenotype is expressed minimally or is not expressed at all (*nonpenetrant*) in an individual who has the pathogenic mutation in one of his or her alleles. Offspring of an affected individual have a 50% chance of inheriting the mutation. Unaffected individuals do not pass the disease to their offspring unless the disease is nonpenetrant. Transmission of a disease from a father to a son helps to distinguish autosomal dominant conditions from X-linked disorders (discussed in the section, X-linked Inheritance).

At least three molecular pathophysiologic mechanisms exist for autosomal dominant conditions, including *dominant loss of function* or *haploinsufficiency, dominant gain of function,* and *dominant negative effect*. Dominant loss of function or haploinsufficiency occurs when only 50% of the gene product from the wild-type allele has not enough residual function to prevent disease. This can occur when the gene product is a transcription factor that regulates gene expression or when the product is a structural protein (as in some mutations that cause Marfan syndrome). Dominant gain of function occurs when the pathogenic mutation increases the function of the normal gene product (e.g., achondroplasia) or makes the gene product a toxin to the cell (as in some spinocerebellar ataxia syndromes). A dominant negative effect occurs when the pathogenic mutation encodes for an abnormal protein that interferes with the function of the normal gene product (as in

some mutations that cause osteogenesis imperfecta and Marfan syndrome).

Autosomal Recessive Inheritance

In autosomal recessive disorders, the parents are usually each *carriers* of a mutated allele. As carriers, they are asymptomatic and do not manifest any phenotype of the disease. Each parent has a 50% chance of passing the mutated allele to each offspring, and each offspring has a 25% chance of inheriting both mutated alleles and manifesting the phenotype. Consequently, analysis of a family pedigree may reveal multiple full siblings with a specific disease, but the disease does not affect first-degree relatives (parents and offspring), first cousins, or individuals from other generations unless two affected parents have children. In autosomal recessive diseases, males and females are affected equally. There may be a history of consanguinity in the parents of an affected child, especially if pathogenic mutations in a particular gene are rare in the population. When parents have one child with a given autosomal recessive disease, the risk of those parents having another child with the same disease is 25% for each and every pregnancy. Unaffected siblings of an affected proband have a two-thirds risk of being a carrier of the pathogenic mutation.

Many autosomal recessive diseases are inborn errors of metabolism secondary to defective enzyme function, and almost all inborn errors of metabolism are inherited in an autosomal recessive pattern. The carriers of pathogenic mutations in genes that encode enzymes do not usually manifest the disease phenotype, because most biochemical reactions require less than 25% of the normal enzyme activity. Carriers have 50% of the normal enzyme activity, well above the threshold for dysfunction. Affected individuals develop disease because both alleles carry pathogenic mutations, and the enzyme activity is usually close to 0. Some individuals with a particular metabolic disease may have a milder phenotype. In those cases, the pathogenic mutations encode a protein with some residual enzyme activity, and/or modifier genes in affected individuals minimize the dysfunction of the abnormal gene product.

X-linked Inheritance

If the affected gene is located on the X chromosome, the disorder that results is inherited in an *X-linked* pattern. Although medical literature frequently refers to disorders that are "X-linked recessive" or "X-linked dominant," these terms are not appropriate when discussing X-linked disorders or traits because the X-chromosomes in females undergo *lyonization*, and males have only one X chromosome (*hemizygous*). Lyonization is the mechanism whereby one of the two X chromosomes in females is inactivated. It is a random process that occurs in early embryonic development. At that stage, either the paternal or maternal X chromosome is inactivated in each cell. Disorders that are X-linked can show extreme variation of expression in females, based on the percentage of active X chromosomes that carry a pathogenic mutation. If the X chromosome with the pathogenic mutation is preferentially inactivated, then the inactivation is *skewed*, and the individual has a *favorable lyonization* pattern for that disorder. In those cases, the female may be asymptomatic or show only mild manifestations of the disease. Alternatively, the X chromosome that is not mutated may be preferentially inactivated. This *unfavorable lyonization* will lead to varying degrees of clinical manifestations of the disease. Due to variation in X inactivation, many X-linked disorders have variable expression in females, including color blindness, X-linked mental retardation syndromes, and Duchenne MD.

Males have only one X chromosome. They are said to be *hemizygous* for most genes on the X chromosome; therefore, lyonization does not occur in males. Consequently, any pathogenic mutation on the X chromosome of a male will cause disease. Lyonization in females explains why X-linked diseases in males are more severe than they are in females. Unless an affected female has a pathogenic mutation in the same allele on both X chromosomes, lyonization will usually make some of the X chromosomes without the pathogenic mutation active. The normal allele on this X chromosome will provide a measure of normal gene product that will help diminish the severity of the disease in females. Some X-linked disorders only are manifested in females or are extremely rare in males. These disorders may be lethal in males. Incontinentia pigmenti is one example. However, many X-linked disorders are rare in males because the mutation occurs on the paternal X during gametogenesis. The father passes only the Y chromosome to males (Thomas hypothesis).

Another reason to avoid using the terms "X-linked recessive" and "X-linked dominant" is that female "carriers" of X-linked disorders are not necessarily asymptomatic, as are the carriers of autosomal recessive disorders. Mothers of children with fragile X syndrome can have learning disorders and premature ovarian failure. Mothers of children with ornithine transcarbamylase deficiency (an X-linked disorder of nitrogen metabolism) may avoid protein in their diet and have altered mental status and vomiting episodes when they ingest a high-protein meal. Thus, although X-linked disorders may be more severe in males (including lethality in male fetuses), one should not use the gender of a patient to discredit the possibility of an X-linked disorder when the clinical presentation makes the disease plausible.

The risk of recurrence of X-linked disorders depends on the gender of the proband. Males with an X-linked condition have a 50% chance of passing the pathogenic mutations to their daughters, and no chance of passing the pathogenic mutation to their sons, because sons inherit the Y chromosome from their fathers. If a daughter inherits the pathogenic mutation, the severity of the phenotype will depend on lyonization. On the other hand, females have a 50% chance of passing the pathogenic mutation to their offspring. Once again, if the offspring is a daughter, the severity of the phenotype will depend on lyonization. All sons who inherit from their mother the X chromosome with the pathogenic mutation will manifest the disease phenotype, because males have only one X chromosome.

Not all genes on the X chromosome undergo inactivation. Some genes in the *pseudoautosomal regions* of the X chromosome have matching alleles on the Y chromosome. Like autosomal genes, some genes in the pseudoautosomal regions exchange genetic information during meiosis in a process called *recombination* or *crossing-over*. Other genes on the X chromosome have corresponding alleles on the Y chromosome, but do not cross over. Finally, some genes on the X chromosome are not inactivated and do not have corresponding alleles on the Y chromosome. The gene for the enzyme steroid sulfatase only exists on the X chromosome and does not undergo inactivation. Pathogenic mutations in this gene lead to a form of ichthyosis.

Mitochondrial Inheritance

Mitochondria contain approximately 16.5 kilobases of DNA (mtDNA) that encode 13 proteins that incorporate into oxidative phosphorylation complexes. (Nuclear DNA encodes most of the proteins that comprise the oxidative phosphorylation complexes.) mtDNA also encodes multiple tRNAs and two ribosomal RNAs that are essential for transcription and translation of the mtDNA. Pathogenic mutations in these genes cause many diseases, including Leigh disease; mitochondrial encephalopathy, lactic acidosis, and stroke-like episodes (MELAS); and progressive sensorineural deafness.

Mitochondria are present in every somatic human cell. They are abundant in oocytes, but the few that exist in sperm are not usually viable in the zygote. Thus, offspring inherit all of their mitochondria from their mother, and mitochondrial diseases are inherited only through the maternal lineage. A mother with a mtDNA mutation will pass the mutation to all of her offspring, but a father with a mtDNA mutation will not pass the mutation to any of his offspring. mtDNA has unique properties that make mitochondrial inheritance different from the Mendelian inheritance patterns discussed in the previous sections. Mitochondria are replicated by fission when a cell divides, and mutations can occur any time a cell divides. The mtDNA genome mutates at a rate that is ten times higher than the rate in nuclear DNA. Therefore, mtDNA mutations are much less rare than nuclear mutations, and these mutations can occur throughout the life of an individual.

When a cell divides, mtDNA is distributed randomly among the daughter cells. If a cell has only one type of mtDNA, either normal or mutated, then that cell is *homoplasmic*. Alternatively, a cell may contain both normal and mutated mtDNA, a condition known as *heteroplasmy*. The amount of heteroplasmy can vary between cells in an organ, and among different organs in the same individual. When the percentage of mtDNA with pathogenic mutations within a tissue or organ exceeds a particular *threshold*, a disease phenotype will develop. The threshold for manifesting disease is different for each tissue type. This means that mitochondrial diseases can affect different organ systems in different individuals, even within the same family. Heteroplasmy also affects the inheritance of mitochondrial diseases. Mothers with a higher percentage of mutated mtDNA in their oocytes have a higher rate of disease transmission.

Atypical Inheritance

In single-gene disorders that are inherited in a Mendelian fashion, the disease phenotype does not depend on whether the mutated allele originated in the mother or father. However, some genes in the human genome are imprinted. *Imprinting* is an alteration in the structure of the chromatin, but not in the base-pair sequence, and this alteration marks the gene as being paternal or maternal in origin. Imprinting is one mechanism for regulating gene expression. For example, either a paternally or maternally imprinted gene may be inactivated based on the imprinting. The structural change that occurs in imprinting can be reversed during gametogenesis. For example, when a boy inherits chromosomes from his mother, the maternally inherited imprinted genes are "reimprinted" during gametogenesis as paternal in origin.

In some cases, the phenotype of a particular pathogenic mutation depends on whether the allele with the mutation is imprinted as being paternal or maternal in origin. For example, Prader-Willi syndrome occurs when deletions occur in the paternal chromosome 15q11-q13. But deletions in the same region of the maternally derived chromosome cause Angelman syndrome, a disease that is clinically distinct from Prader-Willi syndrome. Alternatively, Prader-Willi syndrome can occur if a child inherits two copies of a maternal chromosome that contain 15q11-q13 and no paternal copies of the same chromosome region (called *maternal uniparental disomy*). Conversely, Angelman syndrome can develop if a child inherits two copies of the paternal chromosome containing 15q11-q13 and no copies of the maternal chromosome for that region (called *paternal uniparental disomy*). Mutations in imprinted genes and uniparental disomy are probably rare causes of genetic diseases.

Mosaicism

Mosaicism is the presence in one individual of two genetically distinct cell lines that developed from a single zygote. One example of mosaicism that occurs in all normal females is X inactivation, in which one or the other X chromosome is inactivated in each cell. Mosaicism can also occur when pathogenic mutations occur after zygote formation. If the mutation occurs late in development, it may be present in only one organ or only one segment of the body. Mosaicism is a common cause of cancers in which a pathogenic mutation can disrupt cell-cycle regulation and lead to uncontrolled growth of a single cell clone.

Germline mosaicism is the presence of both wild-type alleles and mutated alleles within the parent's germline cells. If the mutation is pathogenic, then an offspring can inherit an autosomal dominant or X-linked disease from an unaffected parent. If the pathogenic mutation occurs early in gonadal formation, multiple oocytes or spermatogonia can carry the mutation. This manifests clinically when more than one child with an autosomal dominant or X-linked disorder is born to unaffected parents. Germline mosaicism can account for up to 15% of cases of a disease (e.g., osteogenesis imperfecta) and should be considered in counseling for recurrence of autosomal dominant, X-linked, and sporadic unidentified syndromes.

Oligogenic Disorders

Bardet-Biedl is a syndrome that causes rod-cone dystrophy and other eye abnormalities, hypogonadism, renal anomalies, polydactyly, learning disabilities, and other neurologic problems. A form of this syndrome is due to two pathogenic mutations in each allele of a single gene and a single pathogenic mutation in another gene. Thus, pathogenic changes in three alleles in two different genes are necessary to cause the syndrome. This is an example of *oligogenic* inheritance.

Complex Inheritance Patterns

As discussed in the first paragraphs, all diseases are influenced by the genome of the patient. For example, some of the most common diseases in the population, including hypertension, diabetes, cancer, heart disease, psychiatric disease, cleft lip and palate, and epilepsy have a heritable component. In a small subset of these diseases, a pathogenic mutation in a single gene may cause the disease. However, in the majority of individuals, multiple genes interact in complex ways to predispose the individuals to disease. In these cases, there may be a family history of the disease, but the pattern does not fit one of the recognized patterns of Mendelian inheritance. Thus, diseases with complex inheritance patterns also are called *nonmendelian* disorders. In other words, single-gene disorders are due to changes in an allele, and alleles always "mendelize." Complex diseases or traits are due to multiple changes in various alleles, and thus complex diseases and traits do not "mendelize."

Complex diseases or traits also are influenced by environmental factors. The environment may cause mutations in a gene that contribute to the disease (radiation exposure may lead to cancer) or may increase the risk of developing a disease (such as dietary factors and their influence on the development of cardiac disease in a person who has a genetic predisposition to the disease). Therefore, the inheritance pattern of complex diseases is sometimes called *multifactorial*, because both genetic and nongenetic factors determine the phenotype. As the Human Genome Project draws to a conclusion, and the role of human genes in health and disease is better understood, the specific alleles that contribute to complex human disease will be better delineated.

THE FAMILY HISTORY

One of the most important steps that every clinician can take in evaluating a patient for a genetic disorder is to obtain a three-generation family history or *pedigree*. Although not all individuals with a genetic disease will have a family history of the disease, taking the time to record this pedigree has many potential benefits. Many physicians perform a family history by asking if anyone else in the patient's family has the same disease or the same symptoms. However, the astute clinician who recognizes that genetic diseases present with variable expression, even within the same family, may be able to narrow the evaluation of a possible genetic disease when only a few features of a disease are present in multiple family members. For example, if a child with mental retardation has a mother with lymphangiomyomatosis and angiomyolipomas, and a family history of renal disease is present, then it is highly probably that the child, mother, and other affected family members have tuberous sclerosis complex. Also, reviewing the pedigree gives the clinician an opportunity to provide anticipatory guidance to the patient and parents about genetic diseases that may be present in their family. For example, a history of breast cancer in a child's maternal grandmother and maternal aunts should prompt the clinician to recommend that the child's mother undergo appropriate screening for breast cancer. Finally, when the health care provider identifies a pattern of inheritance of a constellation of medical problems, it can help the provider provide an estimate of the recurrence risk in the family, even if the specific disease is unidentified.

A short list of issues should be reviewed each time a physician obtains a family history (Box 11.1). The health of the proband's siblings, parents, and grandparents should be reviewed

---

BOX 11.1   **Pertinent Issues to Review in Family History**

- The presence of the same disease or features of the disease in any family members
- Individual symptoms of a specific genetic disorder that is being considered
- History of genetic diseases in the family
- History of recurrent miscarriages, stillbirths, or early childhood deaths
- Neurologic diseases (mental retardation, learning disorders, epilepsy, cerebral palsy)
- Consanguinity

---

in detail. Determine if each sibling is a full- or half-sibling. Ask about half-siblings, because parents may not think that their health is relevant. The age at the time of any death and the cause of the death should be recorded. This is particularly important for death at a young age. If the patient or family cannot provide information about the older members of the family, then the health care provider should ask the patient or family if other members of the family may be able to provide the necessary information. It is also important to ask about miscarriages, stillbirths, and early childhood death, because these can be signs of severe genetic disease in the family.

The physician should ask about other genetic diseases that run in the family, even if they appear to be unrelated to the medical problems that the proband has. If a specific genetic disorder is being considered, each feature of that disorder should be asked about individually. For example, if velocardiofacial syndrome is a possible diagnosis, then the patient and/or family should be asked if other members of the family have only cleft lip or palate, a heart defect, learning disabilities, recurrent infections, or psychiatric problems. If the clinical features of the disease and the pattern of inheritance are consistent with a mitochondrial disorder (see section, Mitochondrial Inheritance), then the myriad features of a mitochondrial disease should be reviewed (Box 11.2). Furthermore, because many genetic diseases affect the nervous system, it also is useful to ask about specific neurologic disorders, including mental retardation, learning disorders, epilepsy, cerebral palsy, movement disorders, and

muscle diseases. As much as possible, the physician should use disease names *and* descriptive words that are clearly understandable by laypersons. For example, one should ask about "recurrent seizures or epilepsy," "school difficulties or a learning disorder," "the need to use a wheelchair or crutches at a young age or cerebral palsy" and "a heart problem that required surgery in a child or childhood heart disease." This will help avoid overlooking a medical problem in the family because the patient or family members do not know the medical term for the condition.

The ethnic origin of the patient's parents should be recorded. Ask the patient or the parents, "Where did your family come from before they lived in the United States?" Finally, ask if the patient's parents are related (*consanguineous*). In many cases, this information will not be volunteered, yet it can be very useful in evaluating a patient for a genetic disease. For example, a union of first cousins doubles the risk of having an autosomal recessive disease (risk increased from 3% to 6%). One can ask about consanguinity by stating, "I ask all my patients this question: Is it possible that your parents are related?" or "Is it possible that you and your spouse are related?"

When obtaining a family history, it is important to emphasize that all sensitive information will be held in confidence. For example, it is not rare for a family member to withhold information about nonpaternity because she is concerned that other family members may learn about it. It may be helpful to explain that, whereas family secrets of this nature can be very important to the health care provider, every effort will be taken to protect the information.

EVALUATION FOR A GENETIC DISEASE

Because genetic diseases can affect any organ system at any age in innumerable ways, a variety of clinical presentations may prompt the primary care provider to consider a genetic etiology to the medical problems. We will review only a few of the more common presentations of a genetic disease, including a family history of similar phenotypes, multiple dysmorphic features, and mental retardation. (Metabolic diseases are a major category of genetic diseases that are diagnosed and treated by geneticists, and they are discussed in Chapters 383 through 393.)

Family History of Similar Phenotypes

Based on the family history, the physician may consider a genetic disorder because multiple family members have similar medical problems or phenotypes. If the physician is able to identify the syndrome or disease based on these features, specific genetic testing can be performed (see section, Genetic Testing). Alternatively, the primary care physician may not be able to diagnose a specific genetic disease based on the constellation of features. In those cases, referral to a geneticist is indicated. If the family is willing, it is preferable that the geneticist evaluates all unaffected and affected family members.

Dysmorphic Features

Genetic syndromes frequently cause dysmorphic features or malformations. Major malformations are defined as those abnormalities that require medical or surgical interventions, including structural brain abnormalities, mental retardation, failure to thrive, cleft lip and palate, congenital heart defects, abnormal secondary sexual development, skeletal

---

BOX 11.2   **Selected Clinical Features of Mitochondrial Diseases**

- Early hearing loss
- Early vision loss from pigmentary retinopathy, optic atrophy, or cataracts
- Cardiomyopathy or dysrhythmias
- Hepatic dysfunction
- Renal disease
- Diabetes or other endocrinopathies
- Mental retardation
- Epilepsy, especially myoclonic epilepsy
- Recurrent strokes
- Ataxia
- Muscle disease
- Psychiatric diseases such as depression and psychosis

dysplasias, severe limb anomalies, and urogenital defects. Multiple examples exist of minor malformations, including abnormally shaped ears or eyes, inverted nipples, birth marks, and abnormal structures of the hands and feet, including clinodactyly, camptodactyly, soft tissue syndactyly, extra digits, and abnormal skin folds or creases (such as a single transverse palmar crease). Isolated malformations are not rare in the general population.

High-resolution karyotype analysis is indicated in every child with two major malformations or one major and two minor malformations. The primary care physician can obtain a karyotype (see section, Genetic Testing) without referral to a geneticist. However, the primary care physician should consider referral to a geneticist before obtaining a karyotype if he or she cannot provide appropriate genetic counseling regarding the indications for a karyotype, its sensitivity and specificity, and the follow-up that will be necessary for any abnormal result. Furthermore, a geneticist can perform a comprehensive physical examination that may lead to the diagnosis of a specific syndrome, can explain the results and implications of a normal or abnormal karyotype, and will discuss the natural history of any identified genetic syndrome. Common syndromes can be diagnosed by many physicians, but less obvious or rare syndromes ought to be evaluated by geneticists who have the most experience with diagnosing dysmorphic syndromes.

Mental Retardation

A significant portion of human genes are expressed in the brain. Therefore, many genetic diseases present with global developmental delay and mental retardation. The genetic evaluation for global developmental delay and mental retardation begins with a complete history and physical examination, because there are many nongenetic causes of global developmental delay and mental retardation, including intrauterine infections, birth asphyxia, and fetal alcohol syndrome (Box 11.3). If the history and physical examination are noncontributory or cannot explain all the clinical features in a particular patient, we recommend that the patient with nonspecific global developmental delay or mental retardation have a basic genetics laboratory evaluation (see Box 11.3). Based on the results of these tests and the history and physical findings, further diagnostic or genetic testing may be indicated. For example, a leukodystrophy identified on a brain MRI will prompt a workup for a leukoencephalopathy. The presence of a cherry red spot on an ophthalmology examination will lead to a workup for a lysosomal storage disease, such as Tay-Sachs disease. Also, carbohydrate-deficient glycoprotein disorders show significant pleiotropy and variable expressivity, including mental retardation, hypotonia, ataxia and pontocerebellar atrophy, inverted nipples, abnormal fat distribution over the buttocks and hips, cardiac anomalies, hepatic failure, endocrine dysfunction, and coagulopathies. However, mild presentations may cause only mental retardation and hypotonia; therefore, we test for these disorders in all children with nonspecific mental retardation and hypotonia. The test for carbohydrate-deficient glycoprotein disorders is the isoelectric focusing of transferrin, a protein that is glycosylated. If these studies are within normal limits, then MeCP2 gene testing should be considered. The basic principle is that nonspecific mental retardation is just that, nonspecific. Therefore, the clinician must look for other associated signs and symptoms that can help guide the evaluation.

In addition to mental retardation, other common medical conditions exist in which a minority of patients with the condition have mutations in a specific gene. They include morbid obesity and mutations in *leptin*, congenital heart defects and microdeletions of 22q11 (velocardiofacial or DiGeorge syndrome), and a type of diabetes, maturity-onset diabetes of the

---

BOX 11.3	Genetic Evaluation of Nonspecific Mental Retardation

Medical History
  Medical history of mother
  Pregnancy
    Exposure to illicit substances and alcohol
    Recurrent infections
    Gestational diabetes
    Gestational hypertension
  Perinatal history
    Delivery course, including gestational age, presence of maternal fever, duration of labor, method of delivery
    Resuscitation after delivery
    Apgar scores
    Growth parameters (weight, length, head circumference)
  Medical problems of child (including epilepsy, movement disorders, other major malformations)
  Presence or absence of neurologic regression
  Complete family history, including presence of mental retardation or other neurologic diseases
Physical examination
  Dysmorphic features (see Appendix B)
  Birth marks
  Organomegaly
  Neurologic examination
Laboratory tests
  Karyotype
    If normal, consider subtelomere FISH analysis
  Fragile X (regardless of gender)
  Plasma amino acids and urine organic acids
  Brain MRI
  Ophthalmology evaluation
  If patient has hypotonia, consider testing for carbohydrate-deficient glycoprotein disorders
  Electroencephalogram only if there are symptoms of recurrent seizures (e.g., staring, automatisms)
  Further studies based on results of above tests
  If above tests are negative, consider testing for MeCP2 mutations

---

young, due to mutations in the glucokinase gene. As our understanding of the pathogenesis of disease increases, more opportunities will arise to perform diagnostic genetic testing for single-gene mutations that lead to a particular phenotype. In addition, as we learn more about the genetic factors that predispose to complex traits, genetic testing will be performed to determine if a particular patient is at risk for developing a complex disease or to determine which genetic factors are influencing the phenotype of the patient's complex disease.

GENETIC TESTING

Multiple genetic tests are available on a clinical basis, and many new techniques that are being developed on a research basis will be available to clinicians in the near future. The tests that are currently available on a clinical basis include cytogenetic tests (such as karyotype, FISH for submicroscopic aberrations, and polymerase chain reaction (PCR) analysis and Southern blotting for fragile X and other trinucleotide repeat diseases), specific biochemical analyte studies [such as serum ammonium; serum and cerebrospinal fluid (CSF) lactate, an acylcarnitine profile, amino acid analysis in plasma, urine, and CSF; and organic acid analysis in urine], specific enzyme assays (such as hexosaminidase testing for Tay-Sachs and Sandhoff syndromes), and direct DNA testing for pathogenic mutations.

The indications for performing a karyotype were discussed in the section, Dysmorphic Features. Chromosomal abnormalities can be inherited in an autosomal dominant pattern. Therefore, if an abnormality is identified in a patient, then the patient's parents should be tested, because one of the parents also may have the abnormality and be asymptomatic or only mildly affected. If the same chromosomal abnormality is identified in one of the parents, then the risk of recurrence in the each of the parent's offspring is 50%, and all children and siblings of the parent should be offered karyotype testing.

In some cases, FISH analysis for a submicroscopic deletion is indicated. FISH can be performed only for a specific chromosomal region. For example, one should consider screening all children with congenital heart defects for velocardiofacial or DiGeorge syndrome, a submicroscopic deletion syndrome on chromosome 22q11. Once again, if a deletion is identified, the parents should be tested, because up to 28% of these parents may also be affected. If the microdeletion is present in a parent, all the parent's children should be tested for the deletion. The recurrence risk for the syndrome is 50% in each subsequent pregnancy. A relatively new FISH technique called *subtelomere FISH* tests the gene-rich subtelomere regions of all 23 pairs of chromosomes for submicroscopic deletions or duplications. This test is sometimes performed in individuals with multiple dysmorphic features. We frequently perform this test in individuals with nonspecific mental retardation, with or without dysmorphic features, if the routine karyotype and other diagnostic tests are unremarkable. For example, submicroscopic deletions at the terminal portion of the long arm of chromosome 22 can present with mental retardation and only minor dysmorphic features. Like other FISH tests, when a chromosomal abnormality is identified, each of the proband's parents should be tested. In a small study using subtelomere FISH, 40% of the children with a deletion had a parent with a related chromosomal anomaly.

Biochemical analyte testing is performed to screen for a variety of metabolic disorders, including amino acidopathies, organic acidurias, urea cycle defects, fatty acid oxidation defects, mitochondrial diseases, and peroxisomal disorders. When one of these screening tests is abnormal, repeat biochemical analysis should be performed to confirm that the abnormality is not a false positive. For example, a serum lactate level or ammonium level is commonly falsely elevated because the sample was difficult to obtain, or it was processed incorrectly. If the analyte is consistently abnormal, appropriate therapeutic interventions should begin and confirmatory testing by enzyme assay or direct DNA testing should be performed.

Enzyme assay testing is performed on a single enzyme of interest. Similarly, DNA testing is performed on only one or a few genes that are associated with a particular disease. Frequently, only a portion of the coding region of a gene or selected exons will be sequenced when those portions of the gene(s) are the areas associated with the greatest percentage of pathogenic mutations. Therefore, just like FISH analysis, the clinician must suspect a specific disease before enzyme analysis or mutation analysis can be performed. Furthermore, each enzyme assay or DNA test has its own sensitivity and specificity, which should be reviewed with the patient or family before testing is performed. For example, the patient or family should be informed that a negative result does not necessarily rule out the disease. Furthermore, the diagnostic laboratory that will perform a DNA-based test usually requires that the patient or guardian sign a specific consent form before the test is completed. These forms usually are available by contacting the laboratory or may be downloaded from the laboratory's web site.

All the genetic testing discussed here can be performed for *diagnostic* purposes. Any physician can perform diagnostic genetic testing if they understand the indications for the genetic test, the features of the disease(s) that may be diagnosed by the test, the sensitivity and specificity of the test, the logistics of obtaining and sending the specimen, and how to interpret the test results. Unlike many laboratory tests, genetic tests can have implications that extend beyond the proband and can affect entire families. Because genetic testing can have economic, social, and emotional implications that may not be obvious, patients and families should receive genetic counseling before the test is performed.

The logistics of obtaining and sending samples for genetic testing can be difficult, especially for physicians who do not perform a specific test frequently. The primary care physician may be able to work with the local geneticist to ensure that the required genetic testing is performed appropriately. For example, each biochemical test must be placed in a specific type of tube, may require special processing (e.g., centrifuged to obtain the plasma, placed on ice, or shipped on dry ice), and may need to be sent to a special laboratory. Frequently, the physician may need to communicate with the hospital or community laboratory personnel to confirm that the sample is packaged appropriately and sent to the correct laboratory. Finally, many genetic tests, especially DNA-based tests, are expensive. In an effort to ensure that a primary physician's office, a hospital laboratory, or the patient does not receive a bill, it is prudent to contact a patient's insurance company by phone or by letter and obtain authorization for the test before sending the sample for analysis. Although this requires extra time and effort, it prevents the health care team or patient from receiving a bill that could cause undue financial hardship.

The genetic tests discussed here also can be performed for prenatal testing, presymptomatic testing, and carrier testing (newborn screening is discussed in Chapter 18). Prenatal testing should be performed only after the pregnant woman or couple has received adequate counseling regarding the risks and indications for prenatal testing, the chorionic villus sampling or amniocentesis procedure, and the implications of the possible test results. In families with a history of a known genetic condition, prenatal testing may be available. For example, some metabolic disorders can be diagnosed prenatally by performing amniocyte or chorionic villus enzyme assay or DNA analysis. Prenatal DNA testing can be performed more efficiently if the mutations in an affected family member have been identified. Although many couples who seek prenatal counseling will consider terminating a pregnancy if the fetus is believed to have a genetic disorder, prenatal counseling and genetic evaluation may be pursued also by couples who want to begin preparing psychologically for a baby with a major medical problem. Furthermore, prenatal diagnosis may help physicians provide appropriate medical interventions following the birth of a baby with a genetic disorder.

Presymptomatic genetic testing in children and adolescents is a complex issue. If presymptomatic testing allows the initiation of a therapeutic intervention that will minimize the severity of the phenotype, then presymptomatic testing can and ought to be performed in the proband's first-degree relatives, regardless of their age. Alternatively, if no effective treatment exists for a disease, presymptomatic testing usually is not appropriate. Before the testing is performed, the physician should have counseling sessions with the patient and family and carefully review the possible benefits and burdens of performing the test. In adolescents or young adults who are sexually active or are considering starting a family, presymptomatic genetic testing may be appropriate and should be discussed as part of a preconceptional counseling session.

Carrier testing usually is performed in individuals of child-bearing age who are planning for a family. For example, some obstetricians are offering women and their partners carrier testing for CF. Typically, the woman is tested first. If she is determined to be a carrier of one of the more common pathogenic mutations for CF, then her partner also can be tested. If he is also a carrier, then they can discuss with a genetic counselor the possibility of having a baby affected with CF. By definition, carriers of a disease-causing mutation will not develop the disease. Therefore, no ethically permissible reason exists to perform carrier testing in children or nonpregnant adolescents.

TREATMENT FOR GENETIC DISEASES

Treatment for genetic diseases falls into five basic categories: patient and family education, special diet regimens, medications, enzyme-replacement therapy, and symptomatic treatment. When a genetic disease is diagnosed, patient and family education is one of the first essential steps for providing comprehensive medical care. Because many genetic diseases are rare, patients and their families usually are unfamiliar with the disease and its manifestations, treatment, and prognosis. Most families have three basic questions: "What is it?" "How do we treat it?" and "Can it happen again?" If the disease is rare, then the physician may need to review the literature about the condition before these questions can be answered. However, taking the time to discuss the diagnosis with patients and their families, answering their questions, and simply listening to them can be very comforting to them and can be a very rewarding aspect of practicing medicine. Many parents will feel guilt about the diagnosis, because it is "their genes" that caused the disorder. Also, parents may want to know if there was something that they did or did not do that caused the disease. The physician should offer continual reassurance that genetic diseases are beyond our control, and that parents should try not to blame themselves, each other, or their families.

Like all serious medical problems, receiving the diagnosis of a genetic disease can be overwhelming to a family. The physician should not feel an obligation to inform the family about every aspect of a disease in a single meeting. Many issues will need to be reviewed on multiple occasions. Disease-specific web sites or family support groups can be very beneficial. It is important to remember that families who have been diagnosed with a genetic disorder are usually experiencing a tragedy, and the physician should make every effort to sit with them, to listen to them, and to comfort them.

For many metabolic diseases due to enzyme deficiencies in intermediary metabolism, a special diet and/or formula is recommended to limit the quantity of specific amino acids or proteins that are upstream from the enzyme defect. For example, in phenylketonuria (PKU), the phenylalanine intake is restricted, and in maple syrup urine disease the quantity of leucine is restricted. Alternatively, other amino acids may need to be supplemented in the diet. For example, in PKU, the patient's diet is supplemented with tyrosine, because the enzyme defect prevents the conversion of phenylalanine to tyrosine. In all cases, adequate calories in the form of carbohydrate and fat are provided to prevent protein catabolism and a secondary rise in the level of the offending amino acid. For glycogen storage diseases and fatty acid oxidation defects, fasting is avoided to prevent increased metabolism through the defective pathways.

Some metabolic diseases are treated with medications. The most dramatic example is the administration of biotin for biotinidase deficiency. Only 10 mg of biotin taken daily will prevent the devastating effects of this disease. Another example is the use of NTBC [2-(2-nitro-4-trifluoromethylbenzoyl)-1, 3-cyclohexanedione] in tyrosinemia type I. Tyrosinemia type I is due to the abnormal function of a protein at the end of the biochemical pathway that metabolizes tyrosine. Toxic metabolites, especially succinylacetone, are formed, and these toxins can cause ocular problems, liver dysfunction, renal Fanconi syndrome, and hepatocellular carcinoma. NTBC blocks an enzyme that is proximal to the enzyme that is defective in tyrosinemia type I. This prevents the synthesis of succinylacetone and other toxic metabolites and prevents the development of the typical clinical features of tyrosinemia type I. Betaine is used to treat homocystinuria and methylene tetrahydrofolate reductase deficiency. Carnitine supplementation is required for many organic acidurias. In organic acidurias, high levels of organic acids bind to acylcarnitine and are excreted in the urine. This depletes the carnitine pool and can lead to a cardiomyopathy or myopathy that is secondary to carnitine deficiency. Beta-blocker or calcium-channel therapy is given to some individuals with Marfan syndrome to help slow dilatation of the aortic root.

An exciting area of treatment for genetic disorders is enzyme replacement therapy for some lysosomal storage diseases. Replacement therapy is currently available for Gaucher disease, Fabry disease, and Hurler disease. Research to develop therapy for Pompe disease and Hunter syndrome is underway. Replacement enzyme usually is given intravenously once a week or once every other week. It can be provided in a genetics clinic, or the geneticist can help local physicians provide the therapy at a facility that is close to the patient. The response to therapy and risk for side effects varies depending on the specific disease, the age of the patient, and the severity of the clinical features at the time that replacement therapy is initiated. Because none of the current enzymes cross the blood–brain barrier, none of them reverses the central nervous system manifestations of the diseases.

Gene therapy is an active area of research for treating CF and severe combined immunodeficiency syndrome (SCID). Unfortunately, early clinical trials in gene therapy have been discouraging. An adolescent with OTC deficiency died from complications of enzyme replacement therapy, and two individuals receiving gene therapy for SCID developed life-threatening leukemias.

Most genetic diseases do not have a specific treatment, including chromosomal abnormalities, skeletal dysplasias, most metabolic diseases, and dysmorphic syndromes. In these cases, only symptomatic treatment is available. Once a genetic disease or syndrome is diagnosed, further diagnostic studies may be necessary to determine if the patient has other medical problems associated with the syndrome. For many genetic diseases, ongoing evaluations are necessary to assess for progression of associated medical problems. If progression in symptoms or signs is identified, early intervention may minimize the severity of the medical problem.

CONCLUSIONS

Genetic knowledge and technology is expanding at a breakneck speed. It is difficult for any physician to stay abreast of the important developments in genetic medicine. Box 11.4 lists excellent resources for reviewing the current understanding of the genetics of specific disorders and diseases. The recommended reading section also contains a list of excellent general genetics textbooks.

Generalists and specialists alike should recognize that good clinical practice does not require an encyclopedic knowledge of diseases and their treatments. Patients and their families expect that their physicians are competent, but they also want their physicians to be compassionate, trustworthy, and honest. Clinicians should be well-informed, but they should not forget the basics of good clinical practice.

BOX 11.4   **Genetic Organizations and Web-Based Resources**

Alliance of Genetic Support Groups
4301 Connecticut Avenue NW, #404
Washington, DC 20008-2304
Telephone: (202) 966-5557
Fax: (202) 966-8553
E-mail: info@geneticalliance.org
Web site: http://www.geneticalliance.org

Gene Tests
Voluntary repository of information on laboratories that perform genetic testing and genetics clinics within the United States and throughout the world. It has links to MEDLINE and OMIM, and has excellent review articles on many genetic disorders. It is supported by the National Institutes of Health and maintained at the University of Washington, Seattle. Web site: http://www.geneclinics.org or http://www.genetests.org.

National Organization of Rare Diseases (NORD)
P.O. Box 8923
New Fairfield, CT 06812
Telephone: (203) 746-6518
Fax: (203) 746-6481
E-mail: orphan@rarediseases.org
Web site: http://www.rarediseases.org

Online Mendelian Inheritance in Man (OMIM)
OMIM is a continuously updated, annotated bibliography of scientific publications on inherited and heritable genetic diseases. It contains a search engine for identifying genetic diseases by clinical phenotype, gene, and OMIM number. It has links to MEDLINE, GeneTests, and additional resources at the National Center for Biotechnology Information. It is supported by the National Institutes of Health and maintained at Johns Hopkins University. Web site: http://www.ncbi.nlm.nih.gov/Omim.

Suggested Readings

Cassidy SB, Allanson JE. *Management of genetic syndromes*. New York: Wiley-Liss, Inc, 2001.

Curry CJ, Stevenson RE, Aughton D, et al. Evaluation of mental retardation: recommendations of a consensus conference. *Am J Med Genet* 1997;72:468.

Jalal SM, Harwood AR, Sekhon GS, et al. Utility of subtelomere fluorescent DNA probes for detection of chromosome anomalies in 425 patients. *Genet Med* 2003;5(1):28.

Korf BR. *Human genetics: a problem-based approach*, 2nd edition. Malden, MS: Blackwell Science, 2000.

McCandless SE, Brunger JW, Cassidy SB. The burden of genetic disease on inpatient care in a children's hospital. *Am J Hum Genet* 2004;74:121.

Nussbaum TL, McInnes RR, Willard HF, eds. *Thompson and Thompson genetics in medicine*, 7th edition. Philadelphia: W. B. Saunders Company, 2004.

Raper SE, Chirmule N, Lee FS, et al. Fatal systemic inflammatory response syndrome in a [sic] ornithine transcarbamylase deficient patient following adenoviral gene transfer. *Mol Genet Metab* 2003;80(1–2):148.

Rimoin DL, Connor JM, Pyertiz RE, eds. *Emery and Rimoin's principles and practice of medical genetics,* 4th edition. Edinburgh: Churchill Livingston, 2002.

Scriver CR, Beaudet AL, Sly WS, Valle D, eds. *The metabolic and molecular basis of inherited disease,* 8th edition. New York: McGraw-Hill, 2001.

Seashore MR, Wappner RS. *Genetics in primary care and clinical medicine*. Stamford: Appleton and Lange, 1996.

Shevell M, Ashwal S, Donley D, et al. Practice parameter: evaluation of the child with global developmental delay. *Neurology* 2003;60:367.

Thomas GH. High male:female ratio of germ-line mutations: an alternative explanation for postulated gestational lethality in males in X-linked dominant disorders. *Am J Hum Genet* 1996;58:1364.

CHAPTER 12 ■ EVALUATING AND USING LABORATORY TESTS

CYNTHIA S. MINKOVITZ AND LAWRENCE S. WISSOW

Health care spending in the United States for clinical laboratory services continues to increase as new and more complex laboratory tests are developed and aggressively marketed. Also increasing is the concern that not all of this spending is in the best interest of good medical care. Laboratory tests can be powerful aids in diagnosis and patient management, but evidence shows that many physicians know little about the tests they commonly order. The result is often extra expense and, at times, avoidable morbidity.

The common use of most laboratory tests has preceded study of how well they perform and in what settings they should be used. This chapter has two goals:

- To list the characteristics of laboratory tests and identify how the clinician can use these characteristics to select the appropriate test
- To describe how laboratory tests fit into the larger process of medical management

DEFINITIONS

In this chapter, the term *test* means a laboratory or clinical procedure, such as a determination of serum sodium concentration or a urinalysis. The concepts discussed here apply equally to most other procedures used to gather clinical information. For example, questions in a medical history or maneuvers in a physical examination can be considered tests for which performance characteristics can be defined and measured.

Test characteristics also can be incorporated into a technique called *decision analysis*. Decision analysis can be used to outline variations in the process and outcome of care for a particular condition. It can facilitate understanding how patient signs and symptoms, tests, patient preferences, and alternative outcomes contribute to diagnosis or treatment decisions. This technique also prompts decision makers to incorporate the probabilities that particular events will occur and to quantify the value placed on each outcome.

CHARACTERISTICS OF TESTS

Practical Considerations

One major class of decisions involved in choosing a test is practicality. Sometimes little choice exists; only one test or method offers the possibility of obtaining the needed information. Alternatively, choices may be guided by the existence of practice guidelines or critical pathways at institutions in which the provider practices. Most of the time, however, a variety of tests are possible, and they vary in cost, availability, risk to the patient, and speed of obtaining results.

Equipment

The skill or equipment required to perform the tests may vary, requiring the clinician to choose carefully which laboratory or machine to entrust with the analysis. Economic incentives often play a major role in this decision. For example, clinicians may help control costs, generate revenue for themselves, and obtain quicker answers by installing relatively simple laboratory equipment in their offices. These machines may measure the same parameters (e.g., hemoglobin, blood protoporphyrin) as more complicated central laboratory equipment, but they may use different methods that do not always yield parallel results over the entire range of clinically important values. They also require constant upkeep and testing using standard specimens, a task usually taken for granted when tests are performed in organized laboratories. Even simple office laboratory equipment such as centrifuges, timers, and incubators must be monitored consistently to ensure proper functioning.

Quality-Control Issues

Most texts on clinical laboratory methods suggest quality-control measures and programs suitable for office laboratories. The importance of quality control and method-to-method variation cannot be overemphasized. In 1985, for example, the American College of Pathologists sent aliquots from a standardized blood sample for serum cholesterol determination to more than 5,000 clinical laboratories. Reported results ranged from 197 to 379 mg/dL compared with a reference laboratory determination of 263 mg/dL. Wide variations, even among laboratories using identical autoanalyzers, suggested that uneven quality-control procedures rather than methodologic differences were responsible for most of the discrepancies. Physicians should determine whether the laboratory to which they regularly send specimens participates in externally run quality-

control programs and how closely quality is monitored internally.

Concerns about quality control led to the Clinical Laboratory Improvement Amendments of 1988 (CLIA). This federal legislation was enacted in an effort to improve patient care by ensuring the accuracy of laboratory tests performed in physician offices and other sites. Under CLIA, all facilities performing laboratory tests on human specimens must receive a CLIA certificate indicating which tests the laboratory is approved to perform. CLIA regulations initially were thought to have decreased the testing available in practitioners' offices; however, Benjamin suggests that this trend may be reversing because of the growth of waived tests, such as rapid identification of group A streptococcus, tests for detection of pregnancy and ovulation, and spun hematocrit tests. In addition, revisions to CLIA regulations have decreased the burden of inspections for laboratories where the only procedure performed is the provider's own use of a microscope. Technologic advances also have created more accurate testing kits, making it easier to stay in compliance with CLIA standards.

CLIA regulations and site-specific requirements, such as accreditation requirements for hospital laboratories, may limit the availability of on-site laboratory testing. Decisions to pursue laboratory testing increasingly may need to incorporate patient preferences for travel to off-site facilities and provider concerns about the convenience of obtaining results, as well as the usual considerations of the appropriateness of obtaining additional laboratory information.

Performance Characteristics of Tests

How well a test performs can be described by several parameters, each of which is important in determining when the test may be useful. A test's *precision* reflects how much difference to expect if the same specimen was tested repeatedly. For example, a clinician needs to know whether a change from 20% to 30% of neutrophils on a patient's differential white blood cell (WBC) count reflects a resolution of the patient's neutropenia or is likely to be a variation in test performance.

A test's precision is not always related to its *accuracy* (i.e., the relationship of test result to true value of the measured parameter). A machine may measure serum potassium with great precision, but values are meaningless if one does not recognize that hemolysis may render them inaccurate.

Sensitivity and Specificity

Test characteristics derived from the sums and ratios of the four cell values (see Box 12.1) determine how well a test performs a diagnostic task. *Sensitivity* is the likelihood that a test will be positive in the presence of a targeted disease. Sensitivity is defined as $A/(A + C)$ [i.e., the proportion of all individuals with disease X who have a positive result on test 1 (see Fig. 12.1)], or the probability that test 1 will be positive in the presence of disease X. Test sensitivity is critical in screening for asymptomatic disease and ruling out specific diagnoses. When A is large compared to C [i.e., when $A/(A + C)$ is greater than 0.99], relative confidence exists that if the result of test 1 is negative, an individual does not have disease X. As explained below, this alone, however, does not make any claims for what a *positive* test result means.

Specificity is the likelihood of a test to be negative in individuals who do not have the disease. Specificity is defined as $D/(B + D)$ (see Fig. 12.1), the probability of a negative test result in an individual without disease X. Very specific tests often are used to confirm or rule in a suspected diagnosis. When D is very large compared to B [i.e., $D/(B + D)$ is close to 1], a positive result is unlikely to occur in an individual who truly does not have disease X. Specificity alone does not make any claims for what a negative test result means.

BOX 12.1   Two-by-Two Table

The following paragraphs refer to Figure 1, the standard two-by-two cross-tabulation frequently used to describe basic test characteristics. Suppose test 1 is designed to detect disease X. The columns in Figure 1 represent two groups of individuals: Those on the left (+) are known to have disease X; those on the right (–) are known to be free of the condition. The rows classify individuals based on results of test 1: The top row (+) counts all those whose test results were positive; the bottom row (–) counts all those whose test results were negative. Each cell (A, B, C, D) divides the group of tested individuals into four categories:

Cell	Have Disease X?	Test Result	Label
A	Yes	Positive	True psoitive
B	No	Positive	False positive
C	Yes	Negative	False negative
D	No	Negative	True negative

If the test worked perfectly, there would be 100% agreement between test results and true presence of disease (cells A and D only). This almost never occurs, which is a reminder

in interpreting test results: A positive (or negative) test result does not guarantee that a disease is (or is not) present. The test helps us estimate how great a chance exists that the disease is present.

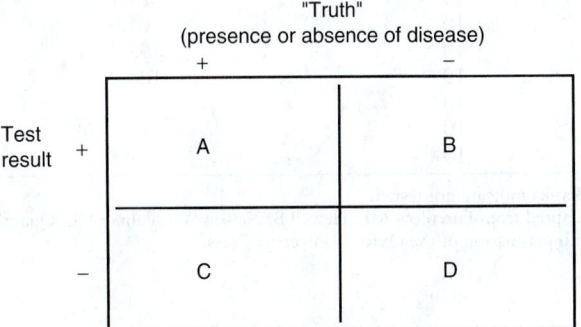

BOX 12.1. FIGURE 1. The two-by-two cross-tabulation used to describe basic test characteristics.

Sensitivity and specificity are further diagrammed in Figure 12.1. The vertical axis corresponds to the columns of the figure in Box 12.1. Counting up the axis represents persons from the (–) column, those without disease X, and counting down represents persons from the (+) column, persons with disease X. The horizontal axis corresponds to the rows of the figure in Box 12.1. Test values considered to be positive are on the right, and test values considered to be negative are on the left. Areas beneath the two curves represent the number of individuals in each cell of the figure in Box 12.1. Two important points about sensitivity and specificity follow.

First, for most tests, some range of results exists that is shared by individuals who have the disease and those who do not. Thus, if the definition of a positive and negative test result

changes, so do the relative sizes of A, B, C, and D and, consequently, the test's sensitivity and specificity. For most tests, a change in definition that benefits sensitivity does so at the expense of specificity, and vice versa. Only changing the test, not the definition, is likely to improve both simultaneously.

Second, how a test is used is determined by where the *cut points* are placed (dotted lines 1 and 2; see Fig. 12.1). Test results below (to the left of) the value of line 1 define a population unlikely to have disease X, whereas results above (to the right of) line 2 indicate near certainty that X is present. The following example is modified from one developed by George Comstock.

During the development of the purified protein derivative (PPD) test for tuberculosis (TB), research was directed toward

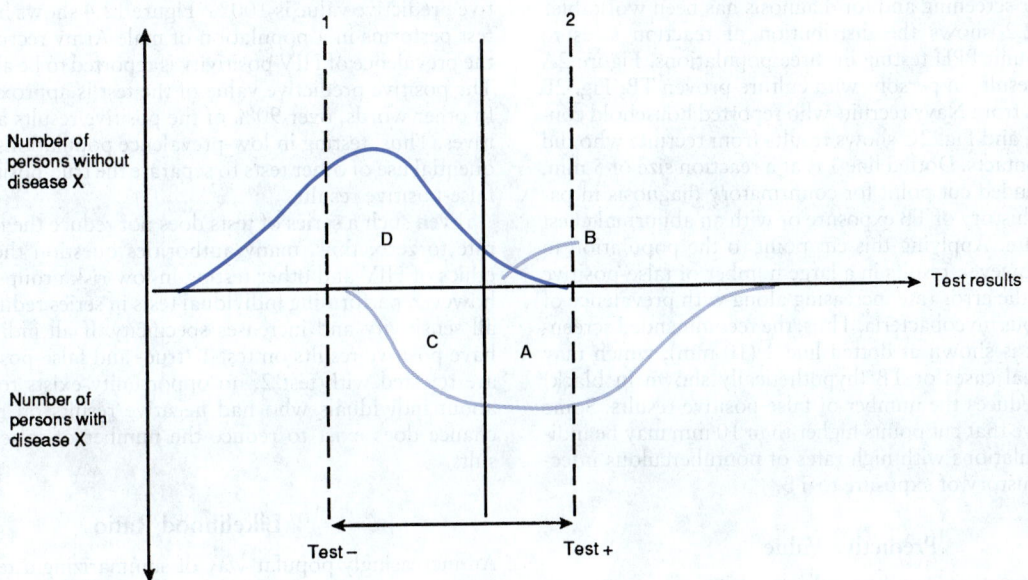

FIGURE 12.1. Sensitivity and specificity of tests (see Box 12.1). Areas enclosed by the curves and lines correspond to the number of individuals in each cell of the figure in Box 12.1.

TABLE 12.1

SENSITIVITY AND SPECIFICITY OF VARYING DOSES OF PURIFIED PROTEIN DERIVATIVE AMONG CHILDREN WITH ACTIVE TUBERCULOSIS AND THOSE WITH NO KNOWN HISTORY OF EXPOSURE

Milligrams per Dose of Purified Protein Derivative	Active Tuberculosis*		Not Exposed to Tuberculosis	
	Percent Positive (Sensitivity)	Percent Negative (False-negative)	Percent Positive (False-positive)	Percent Negative (Specificity)
10^{-9}	3.3	96.7	—	—
10^{-8}	15.0	85.0	0	100
10^{-7}	21.7	78.3	—	—
10^{-6}	65.0	35.0	—	—
10^{-5}	93.3	6.7	6.5	93.5
10^{-4}	100.0	0.0	8.5	91.5
10^{-3}			26.6	73.4
10^{-2}			53.6	46.4
10^{-1}			84.7	15.3

*Blanks indicate not tested.
Adapted from Furcolow ML, Hewell B, Nelson WE, Palmer CE. Quantitative studies of the tuberculin reaction. *Public Health Rep* 1941;56:1082, with permission of the Oxford University Press.

determining the optimal dose needed to detect infected individuals. Furcolow and colleagues tested increasing doses of PPD in known TB patients and in individuals who were presumed to be uninfected. A positive test result was defined as a zone of induration 10 mm in diameter surrounding the site of the PPD intradermal injection.

Table 12.1 shows the proportions of persons in each group testing positive at increasing doses of PPD. A dose of 10^{-4} mg appears to be a good dose for screening purposes; it identifies more than 99% of TB patients, while mistakenly showing positive results for only 8.5% of those who are not infected. This dose is equivalent to the standard 5-tuberculin-unit dose of PPD commonly used for screening today.

TB screening is more complicated, however, because in some parts of the world, false-positive PPD test results come from exposure to nontuberculous mycobacteria. In some parts of the southeastern United States, more than 70% of persons tested have PPD reactions indicating such exposure, which could make diagnosing or screening for TB difficult in such an area. PPD reactions to nontuberculous mycobacteria, however, are usually smaller than reactions to TB. Thus, the use of different cut points for screening and for diagnosis has been workable.

Figure 12.2 shows the distribution of reaction sizes to 5-tuberculin-unit PPD testing in three populations. Figure 2A shows tests results in persons with culture-proven TB; Fig. 2B shows results from Navy recruits who reported household contact with TB; and Fig. 2C shows results from recruits who did not report contacts. Dotted line 1 is at a reaction size of 5 mm, the recommended cut point for confirmatory diagnosis in patients with a history of TB exposure or with an abnormal chest roentgenogram. Applying this cut point to the population in Figure 2C, however, results in a large number of false-positive results, with the error rate increasing along with prevalence of nontuberculous mycobacteria. Thus, the recommended screening cut point is shown at dotted line 2 (10 mm), which may miss some real cases of TB (hypothetically shown in black) but greatly reduces the number of false-positive results. Some experts believe that cut points higher than 10 mm may be indicated in populations with high rates of nontuberculous infection and no history of exposure to TB.

Predictive Value

Usually, it is not enough to know that a test is very sensitive or very specific. What the clinician wants to know is how much confidence there is that a positive test result really means that disease is present or that a negative result really means that disease is absent. The most basic way to express this confidence is with two quantities, the test's positive and negative predictive values. *Positive predictive value* is the proportion of persons who test positive on test 1 and who actually have disease X, or $A/(A + B)$ (see Box 1), or the probability that disease X will be present, given a positive test result. The *negative predictive value* is $D/(C + D)$ (see Box 1), or the probability that disease is not present, given a negative test result.

A test's positive and negative predictive values vary with the prevalence of the target disease in the studied population. This is illustrated by example—the use of enzyme-linked immunosorbent assays (ELISAs) for human immunodeficiency virus (HIV). Although the characteristics of the HIV ELISA vary from manufacturer to manufacturer, in experienced hands the test is believed to have a sensitivity that approaches 100% and a specificity of more than 99%. These statistics are impressive, and the test yields impressive results when used in a high-prevalence population, such as a group of intravenous drug users (Fig. 12.3). With a prevalence of HIV antibodies of about 11%, the positive predictive value is 92% and the negative predictive value is 100%. Figure 12.4 shows how the same test performs in a population of male Army recruits in whom the prevalence of HIV positivity is reported to be about 0.09%. The positive predictive value of the test is approximately 8%. In other words, over 90% of the positive results are false positives. Thus, testing in low-prevalence populations requires sequential use of other tests to separate the true-positive from the false-positive results.

Even such a series of tests does not reduce the false-positive rate to zero; thus, many authorities question the utility and ethics of HIV and other testing in low-risk groups. In general, however, performing individual tests in series reduces the overall sensitivity and increases specificity. If all individuals who have positive results on test 1 (true- and false-positive results) are retested with test 2, no opportunity exists to learn more about individuals who had negative results on test 1, but a chance does exist to reduce the number of false-positive results.

Likelihood Ratio

An increasingly popular way of summarizing a test's capabilities is to state its *positive* or *negative likelihood ratio*. The likelihood ratio is similar to the predictive value in that it helps in assessing the diagnostic benefit of a positive or negative test

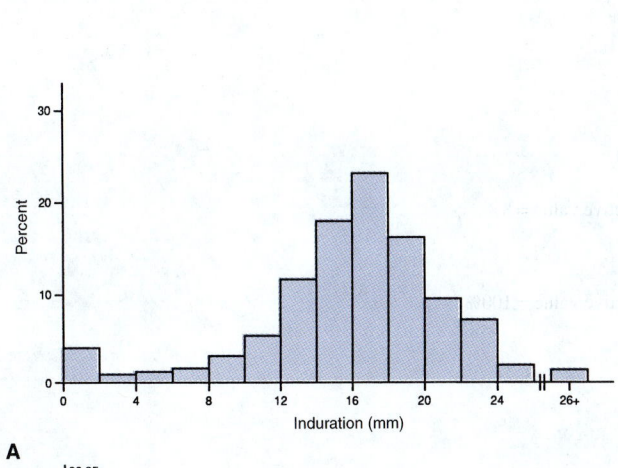

A

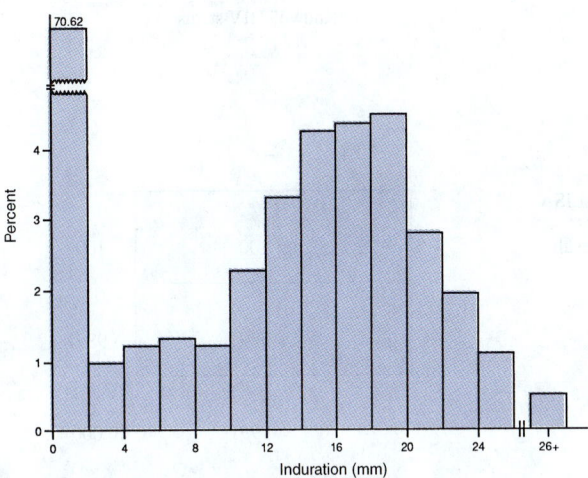

B

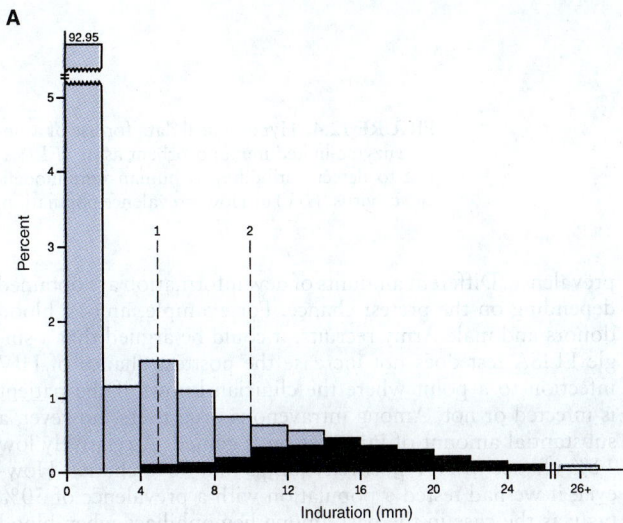

C

FIGURE 12.2. Distribution of reaction sizes to 5-tuberculin-unit purified protein derivative testing in three populations. **A:** Test results in a group of persons with culture-proven tuberculosis. **B:** Results from a group of white male U.S. Navy recruits aged 17 to 21 years who reported household contacts with tuberculosis. **C:** Results from a group of U.S. Navy recruits who did not report contacts, tested from 1961 to 1968. (Reprinted from Rust P, Thomas J. A method for estimating the prevalence of tuberculous infection. *Am J Epidemiol* 1975;101:311, with permission of the Oxford University Press.)

"Known" HIV status

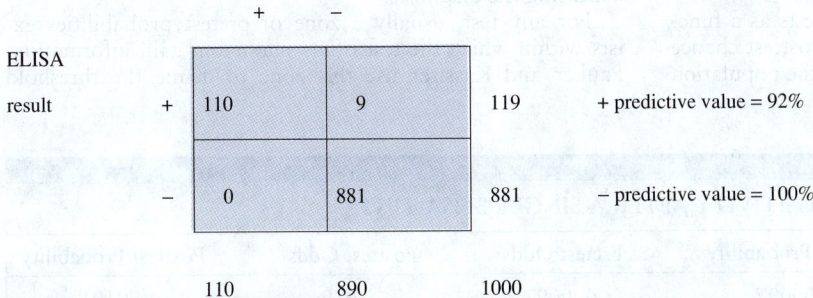

ELISA result

		+	−		
	+	110	9	119	+ predictive value = 92%
	−	0	881	881	− predictive value = 100%
		110	890	1000	

Total hypothetical population = 1000

Prevalence = 11%

False positive rate = 8%

False negative rate = 0%

FIGURE 12.3. Hypothetical data for use of a single enzyme-linked immunosorbent assay (*ELISA*) test to detect antibodies to human immunodeficiency virus (*HIV*) in a high-prevalence population.

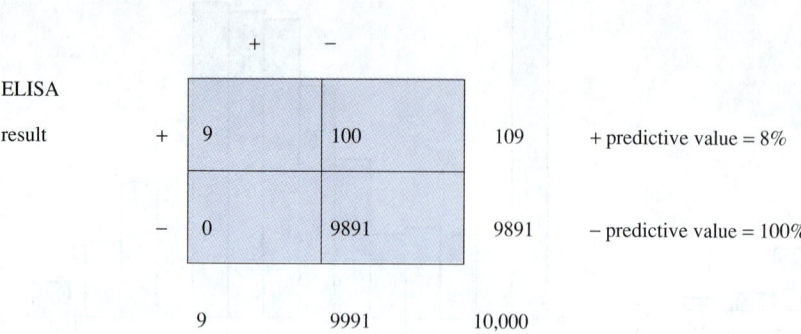

FIGURE 12.4. Hypothetical data for use of a single enzyme-linked immunosorbent assay (*ELISA*) test to detect antibodies to human immunodeficiency virus (*HIV*) in a low-prevalence population.

result. Unlike the predictive value, the likelihood ratio is independent of the prevalence of disease. The likelihood ratio, then, is useful in assessing how well a test will do in different populations or for individuals with higher or lower chances of having a certain disease.

The likelihood ratio is a ratio of probabilities: the probability that the test result is positive in a person who really has the disease compared to the probability that the test result is positive in a person who does not have the disease. For example, a person with disease X is so many times more likely to have a positive result on test 1 than is a person who does not have disease X. The chance that a person with disease X will have a positive test result is the same as A/(A + C) (see Box 1), or the test's sensitivity. The chance that a person without disease X will have a positive test result is B/(B + D) (see Box 1), or 1 minus the test's specificity.

Using a formula known as *Bayes theorem*, the likelihood ratio can be used to calculate, for any level of disease prevalence or pretest chance that a patient has disease, the revised or posttest chance, given the test results, that disease is present or absent.

Table 12.2 shows results of HIV antibody tests as a function of population prevalence of disease. The posttest chance that HIV antibodies are present increases with the population prevalence. Different amounts of new information are obtained depending on the pretest chance. For example, among blood donors and male Army recruits, it could be argued that a single ELISA test does not increase the posttest chance of HIV infection to a point where the clinician knows if the patient is infected or not. Among intravenous drug users, however, a substantial amount of information is gained. A relatively low 11% chance of HIV positivity jumps to a 96% chance. However, if we had tested a population with a prevalence of 50% (as was the case in the past among hemophiliacs when blood products were heavily contaminated with HIV), we would find that the posttest probability still does not reach 100%. This leads to an important general point: When one is relatively certain that a patient does or does not have a disease, performing a diagnostic test adds little extra certainty to the diagnosis. Tests obtained when the diagnosis is fairly certain often confuse the issue rather than help. Not only is little new information gained, but a definite chance exists of getting a contradictory result even with a very good test, which leads to further tests that carry significant morbidity, expense, and risk of further confusing the diagnosis.

For any test, usually a zone of pretest probabilities exists within which the test offers maximum gain information. Pauker and Kassirer use this zone to define the threshold

TABLE 12.2

POSTTEST PROBABILITIES OF HIV SEROPOSITIVITY AFTER A SINGLE ELISA TEST*

Population Group	Pretest Probability	Pretest Odds	Posttest Odds	Posttest Probability
U.S. blood donors 2001[1]	.000097	.000097	.019	.019
Male U.S. military recruits (cumulative 1985–2000)[2]	.00087	.00087	0.17	0.15
Intravenous drug user[3]	.11	.12	24.0	.96

*Based on a sensitivity of 100, a specificity of 99.5, and a likelihood ratio of 200.

Source of pretest probabilities: [1]Dodd RY, Notari EP, Stramer SL. Current prevalence and incidence of infectious disease markers and estimated window-period risk in the American Red Cross blood donor population. *Transfusion* 2002;42:975. [2]Satern WB, Renzullo PO, Carr JK, et al. HIV-1 infection among civilian applicants for US military service, 1985 to 2000: epidemiology and geography. *J AIDS* 2003;32:215. [3]Diaz T, Vlahov D, Greenberg B, et al. Sexual orientation and HIV infection prevalence among young Latino injection drug users in Harlem. *J Womens Health Gender-Based Med* 2001;10:371.

TABLE 12.3

HYPOTHETICAL POSTTEST PROBABILITIES OF DIABETES, GIVEN VARYING PRETEST PROBABILITIES AND DIFFERENT CUT POINTS FOR DEFINING HYPERGLYCEMIA

	Cutoff Glucose Levels (mg/dL)		
	100	130	150
Pretest probabilities			
0.1	0.12	0.35	0.64
0.5	0.56	0.83	0.94
0.9	0.92	0.98	0.99
Hypothetical likelihood ratios			
100 mg/dL—1.3; 130 mg/dL—5.0; 150 mg/dL—16.0			

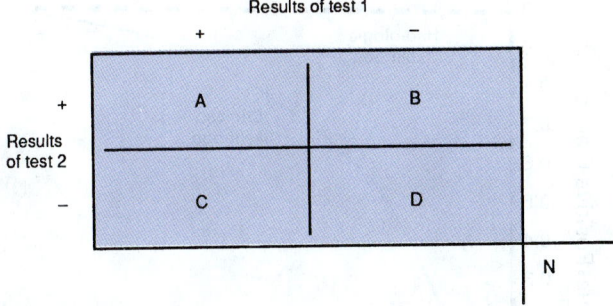

FIGURE 12.5. Two-by-two table for comparison of two tests.

approach to making clinical decisions. At pretest probabilities below the zone of usefulness, one would not test and, if this was a diagnostic test for a treatable condition, would not treat. At pretest probabilities above the zone, one would not test and would proceed as if the test result was positive. Only for pretest probabilities within the zone would one test first before going to the next step in treatment or diagnosis. The test zone is determined by factors beyond sensitivity and specificity. For example, one would be more liberal with a test that was inexpensive and safe or more conservative with a test that had considerable risk or was less accurate.

Sackett and colleagues point out that likelihood ratios may ultimately allow the elimination of single cut points for tests and, instead, provide information about the chances that disease is present at any point in the range of a test's possible results. This idea is appealing because many tested quantities do not lend themselves to yes-or-no dichotomies. For example, hyperglycemia may be defined as a blood glucose level of more than 130 mg/dL, but this definition falsely identifies some people with diabetes as normal. Table 12.3 shows hypothetical posttest probabilities of diabetes for various blood glucose levels and a range of pretest probabilities of disease. Posttest probabilities are calculated as posttest odds/(pretest odds + 1) in which posttest odds are defined as pretest odds × likelihood ratio and pretest odds are calculated as pretest probability/(1 − pretest probability). Table 12.3 shows how a level of 130 mg/dL is more significant for a person with a 50% chance of having diabetes (e.g., someone giving a history of polyuria and polydipsia) than for a person with no symptoms and a low chance of having the disease. On the other hand, a level of 150 mg/dL has clinical significance for someone who is asymptomatic, and even a level of 100 mg/dL might be of concern in someone who had several clinical signs and symptoms and a high pretest chance of illness.

Measures of Agreement

Most evaluations of new tests are based on a comparison with some gold standard, usually a more complicated but more accurate measure considered to be the truth. In many situations, such as the evaluation of new tests for streptococcal pharyngitis discussed in a following section, no readily available measure of truth exists. In these cases, rather than speak of a new test's sensitivity and specificity, we can more correctly speak of how well the new test agrees with the old one.

The simple way to compare *agreement* between two tests is to calculate the proportion of all cases tested in which the two tests give the same result. In Figure 12.5, this is the sum of A (the number of cases in which both test results are positive) plus D (the number of cases in which both test results are negative) divided by N (the total number of cases tested). This method

breaks down, however, when most of the cases are labeled negative (or positive) by both tests. For example, data presented in Figure 12.6 show the agreement between an experienced physician (observer 1) and a new student (observer 2) carrying out auscultation of the heart. The experienced physician labels ten of the 100 children tested as having a murmur; the student, who is not sure how a murmur sounds, labels all the children normal. Agreement between the tests is $(0 + 90)/100 = 0.9$, apparently very high, but it occurs by chance (or a combination of chance plus the fact that most of the children do not have murmurs).

Calculation of the *kappa statistic* separates the component of chance from the observed agreement. The first step in calculating kappa is similar to a chi-square test. The two-by-two table is recreated with the values that would be obtained by chance alone. In the case of agreement, the expected values for A (A') and D (D') should be calculated. The value expected for A, based on chance, is $(A + C)/N \times (A + B)$, whereas the value expected for D is $(B + D)/N \times (C + D)$. The expected degree of agreement based on chance alone is $(A' + D')/N$, which, in this example, is also 0.9.

Kappa is then calculated by taking:

$$\frac{\text{observed agreement} - \text{agreement expected by chance}}{1 - \text{agreement expected by chance}}$$

In the example, kappa is zero. Kappa values of more than 0.75 indicate good agreement beyond what is expected by chance, whereas kappa values of less than 0.40 suggest the two tests show poor agreement.

Receiver Operating Characteristic Curves

Alternative tests may be compared using receiver operating characteristic curves. A receiver operating curve provides a graphic representation of test characteristics using different cutoff points. Sensitivity [or the true-positive rate, or A/(A + C)] is plotted on the y axis, and 1 − specificity [or 1 − the true-negative rate, or B/(B + D)] is plotted on the x axis. A receiver

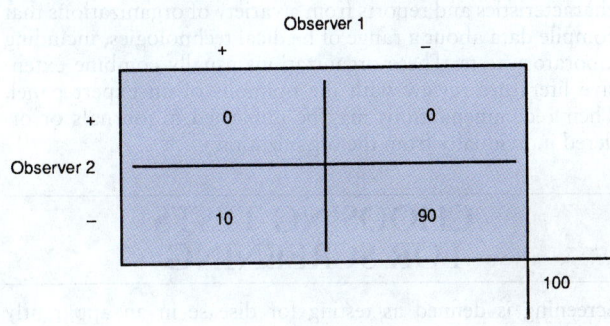

FIGURE 12.6. Hypothetical data for two observers in which observer 2 systematically calls all cases negative.

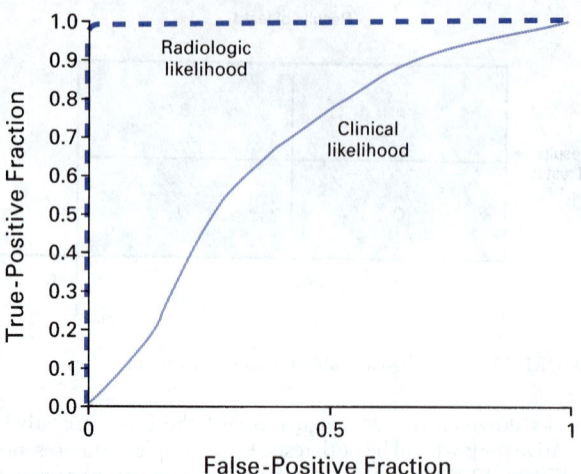

FIGURE 12.7. Correlation between clinical and radiologic likelihood of appendicitis and final outcome. A comparison of receiver operating characteristic curves is shown. (Reprinted with permission from Rao PM, Rhea JT, Novelline RA, et al. Effect of computed tomography of the appendix on treatment of patients and use of hospital resources. *N Engl J Med* 1998;338:141. Copyright © 1998 Massacgesetts Medical Society. All Rights reserved.)

operating curve that extends from the origin through a 45° line signifies a test with no predictive ability, while an ideal curve approaches the upper left corner (perfect sensitivity and specificity). Receiver operating curves have been used to evaluate the diagnostic accuracy of computed tomographic scans for patients with suspected appendicitis (Fig. 12.7). Rao and colleagues demonstrated the superior performance of appendiceal computed tomography over clinical examination in diagnosing acute appendicitis for 100 patients with suspected disease aged 6 to 75 years. Along a given curve, such as for clinical examination, the optimal cut point is where each gain in sensitivity is associated with large decreases in specificity or where the curve "turns the corner" as described by Browner, Newman, and Cummings.

Obtaining Information about Actual Tests

Clinicians often find it difficult to obtain data on the performance characteristics of tests. Laboratory tests, like many other medical technologies, are often put into widespread use before such data are developed or disseminated. Experimental data about laboratory tests may be available in published articles, although often in relatively specialized and technical journals. Haynes and colleagues provide a checklist for reading this type of article and for deciding if a new test is useful.

Other sources of information include journal reviews of test characteristics and reports from a variety of organizations that compile data about a range of medical technologies, including laboratory tests. These organizations usually combine extensive literature review with the opinions of an expert panel. Their recommendations may be published in journals or ordered individually from the organization.

CHOOSING TESTS FOR SCREENING

Screening is defined as testing for disease in an apparently healthy population or individual. Mainly because of test limitations, the goal of screening is not to detect disease in individuals but to identify persons who are at greater risk of having the disease and who warrant further testing. Com-

monly used pediatric screening tests include measurement of hematocrit to detect anemia, perinatal tests to detect inborn errors of metabolism and hemoglobinopathies, and tine tests to detect TB.

First, the clinician must decide whether the target disease is a suitable candidate for detection by screening. Some important considerations follow:

- Is the disease serious enough to warrant the effort and cost?
- Is the disease common enough, relative to its seriousness, to warrant mass testing of persons who show no signs of having it?
- Does the disease have a preclinical phase that allows it to be detected by a screening test?
- Is there any benefit, in terms of improved prognosis, timely genetic counseling, ease of treatment, or risk of transmission to others, in detecting the disease in its preclinical phase?
- Are follow-up mechanisms available so persons who have positive screening results can be counseled and obtain rapid confirmatory testing or treatment?

If a disease is suitable for screening, a test must be identified. Some practical requirements for a screening test follow:

- The test must be easy to perform and interpret, including having relative immunity from subjectivity or minor variations in technique.
- The test should measure something definitely related to the condition under study rather than some epiphenomenon that might not be specific.
- The test must have acceptably low risk, morbidity, and cost to those being tested.

In addition, most screening tests are chosen or designed to be highly sensitive. That is, a negative result ideally indicates a low chance that the tested individual is at risk of having the target disease. A positive result, however, may mean only that the individual is somewhat more likely to have the disease. Further testing is usually required because simple, highly sensitive tests are not often very specific. The best screening tests are both highly sensitive and highly specific. Table 12.4 lists reported values of sensitivity and specificity for some tests commonly used to screen pediatric patients.

ROLE OF LABORATORY TESTS IN MEDICAL DIAGNOSIS

Hypothesis Generation and Testing

History and Physical Examination

As Sackett and colleagues point out, an optimal model of medical decision making involves the sequential formulation and testing of hypotheses about the nature of a patient's illness. The bulk of this process usually takes place during the history and physical examination, only after which laboratory tests are used either to choose among competing hypotheses or to confirm suspicions before initiating treatment.

For example, a 6-month-old female infant is brought to a physician's office with a fever of 39°C and a 12-hour history of irritability. Even before taking the history and performing the physical examination, the physician generates a list of possible problems, then focuses the workup on maneuvers to support or dispute each problem on the list. Has the child been pulling at her ears or is there a previous history of otitis? Has there been a cough or is the respiratory rate increased?

At the end of the history and physical examination, two of the original hypotheses are discarded. The tympanic

TABLE 12.4

SENSITIVITY AND SPECIFICITY FOR SOME LABORATORY TESTS COMMONLY USED IN PEDIATRICS

Test	Target Condition	Sensitivity	Specificity
Guthrie bacterial inhibition assay	Phenylketonuria	Approximately 100%	>99%[a]
Tine (+ >2 mm)	Tuberculosis	32%	99%[b]
(+ >5 mm)		7%	100%
VDRL	Syphilis	86%	97%
Hematocrit	Iron deficiency	79%	93%[c]

VDRL, Venerial Disease Research Laboratories.
[a]Test done at 48 hours of age, infant already feeding on milk; in populations with prevalence of approximately 1 to 12,000, test has positive predictive value of 10% to 20%.
[b]Compared with purified protein derivative; specificity of purified protein derivative varies depending on prevalence of atypical mycobacterial infections.
[c]Derived from study of adult women; gold standard is positive response to trial of iron therapy.

membranes move nicely, the chest is clear, and the respiratory rate and effort are normal, so otitis media and pneumonia are no longer strong possibilities. Although the child is somewhat fussy and prefers being held, she acts alert, smiles briefly, and shows some interest in her bottle of juice. She does not appear toxic; thus, she is relatively unlikely to have a major systemic illness.

Laboratory Test Choice

The next three major hypotheses are a viral syndrome, a urinary tract infection (UTI), and meningitis, with the first two seeming most likely. What laboratory test or tests might the clinician order to differentiate among these conditions? Possibilities include performing a complete blood count, blood culture, urinalysis, lumbar puncture, or no test at all.

One way to approach this problem is to look at the characteristics of the possible tests and determine how quickly these might make it possible to focus on the conditions that are most serious. Ideally, one chooses a single test capable of providing information about all the diagnoses being entertained rather than about just one. Usually, however, a series of disease-specific tests must be performed, often in order of the urgency of the illnesses.

The clinician's first decision might be whether to perform a lumbar puncture. Although the pretest probability of meningitis is fairly low, it is the most serious of the conditions in the differential diagnosis. The lumbar puncture has fairly desirable characteristics for such a situation. Although it is invasive, it has a low complication rate in young patients and can be performed readily by most practitioners. Moreover, it is apparently a very sensitive (although not very specific) test for bacterial meningitis, just the characteristics desired for a screening or rule-out test. Children with no cells in their cerebrospinal fluid are unlikely to have bacterial meningitis, although children with some cells may or may not have the disease. So, if the clinician's pretest concern is high, a lumbar puncture might be performed. Although it may not establish the diagnosis, it is a major aid in assigning the patient to a risk category for urgent serious disease.

Comparing this outcome with the parallel approach of performing a urinalysis to evaluate the presumptive diagnosis of UTI is instructive. Again, even if a catheterized specimen is obtained, the test has a relatively low complication rate and can be performed quickly and reliably by most clinicians. The test's characteristics, however, are different from those of a lumbar puncture.

Observations of white cells or bacteria on urinalysis provide fairly specific (but not very sensitive) indicators of UTI in infancy. These observations are much more reliable in older children. Positive findings are highly suggestive of UTI, but

negative findings, especially from a female patient, probably warrant obtaining a urine culture.

Leukocyte esterase is an enzyme released from white blood cells whose presence in the urine may be caused by infection or inflammation. Testing for leukocyte esterase is felt to be about 80% sensitive and specific, compared to urine culture, for the detection of infection in children under age 2. Certain gram-negative rod bacteria (notably *Escherischia coli*) are able to convert dietary nitrates in the urine to nitrites, which can then be used as a marker of infection. Urine that has not "incubated" in the bladder long enough for the conversion to take place may yield false-negative tests despite the presence of bacteria. Nitrite testing is thought to have a sensitivity to infection of about 50%, but a specificity of nearly 100%.

Another approach is to use a test that, to some degree, provides information about all the possible hypotheses. In this case, the clinician might opt to order a complete blood count, looking especially at the total WBC count. In one series of children with unexplained acute febrile illness, Kupperman and colleagues found that more than 80% of febrile children with bacteremia had a WBC count of greater than 15,000 (sensitivity), whereas approximately two-thirds of children without bacteremia had a WBC count of less than 15,000 (specificity). Thus, the WBC count may be a good test to rule out bacteremia [i.e., if the test result is negative (between 5,000 and 15,000), bacteremia is relatively unlikely]. A positive test result still requires follow-up diagnostic maneuvers to detect bacteremia or specific foci of infection.

USING TESTS TO MONITOR THERAPY

A third major use of laboratory tests is to monitor therapy, either to measure the response of the illness or to check for unwanted side effects. The following are important characteristics of tests used for monitoring:

- Tests must have high precision or reproducibility. Test-to-test variation because of chance must be minimized so clinicians know when a new result reflects true physiologic change. Radiologic studies are particular examples in which variations in technique and interpretation occur from test to test.
- Tests should be noninvasive, atraumatic, and relatively inexpensive so that they can be used as often as necessary.
- Tests must accurately reflect changes in the disease being monitored. Multiple tests or tests from multiple sites may be required to assess adequately all relevant aspects of disease progression. Following the course of treatment for leukemia, for example, may require sampling of multiple sites for evidence of relapse. Alternatively, some disease

markers, such as the sedimentation rate in collagen vascular disease, may be powerful enough that a single test can be used to follow a patient's progress.

- The test procedure or interpretation must control for other factors that could alter the test result. Many serum chemistry determinations, for example, can be altered falsely by hyperglycemia, hyperlipidemia, or hyperbilirubinemia, conditions that also may change during the course of therapy.

ASSESSING INFORMATION ABOUT A TEST

Clinicians frequently must decide if a journal account of a new test warrants its use. The following questions, adapted from Haynes and colleagues, may serve as guides to evaluating an account of a new or old test.

What gold standard did the authors use in their study of the new test? In Box 12.1, it was posited that the individuals in the left column had the disease and those in the right column did not. Usually, no such knowledge exists, and results of the new test are compared with results of another test that has its own degree of uncertainty. A variety of pitfalls can arise:

- The old comparison test may not be performed properly. For example, an account of a new test that differentiates viral from streptococcal sore throats is compared with the gold standard throat culture with its known susceptibility to false-negative results when improperly performed. Were throat swabs performed consistently and meticulously, carried promptly to the laboratory, and plated by a competent technician? Was identification of the organism carried out with an accepted method? This type of problem often surfaces when a new test is put into use while old diagnostic procedures are used, rather than being tested in the context of a deliberate research project. This sort of problem makes it difficult to establish how well the new test really works.
- Even if performed properly, the old test may not be worthy of gold-standard status. Sometimes, no better alternative exists, but often one does. Using the throat swab example again, most research projects involving detection of streptococci in the pharynx use duplicate swabs as a gold standard because a single swab has been found to miss as many as 10% of true-positive cases.
- Those performing the new test should be blind to how the patient is classified by the gold standard. Even relatively objective results can be swayed by biased observation.

What population was used to study the new test? As discussed, the population used to determine a test's characteristics can have a profound influence on parameters such as positive and negative predictive values. Subtle problems also may arise as delineated by Ransohoff and Feinstein, who have related these problems to the spectrum of disease among the studied patients.

- All "disease-positive" patients may be individuals with advanced, unambiguous cases of the disease. It may be unknown how well the test will work in patients with earlier stages of illness or whose diagnosis is more debatable.
- All control patients may be normal. The usual diagnostic task is not to differentiate persons with disease from those who are well but to choose who has a particular disease from among a group of people with similar symptoms. Thus, a test that separates children with rheumatoid

arthritis from normal controls may not differentiate among those with collagen vascular disease, joint trauma secondary to overuse, and toxic synovitis.

How is normal *defined, either for the new test or for the gold standard?* Where a cut point divides normal and abnormal may influence greatly how a test performs and how it can be used. In most cases, the ideal way to define what is abnormal or normal is in terms of the target disease or body function being measured. For example, the best way to define an abnormally low hematocrit for diagnosing iron-deficiency anemia is to pick the point below which most individuals have a response to the administration of iron. Usually, however, cut points are calculated by performing a test on apparently normal individuals, then using statistical methods to define values of the test's results that are outside an expected normal range. In the hematocrit example, a large number of apparently healthy persons would be tested, and the lowest 5% of values would be declared too low. This method has a number of potential problems:

- The population used to define normal may not be representative of all those on whom the test will be used. This is classically the case for tests developed in adult populations and for which normal values in children are not known. Similar problems can occur with race or gender differences.
- The normal population may not be normal. It may contain persons who have the disease in question or other unrelated conditions that change the test's results.
- The use of statistical techniques to define normal and abnormal (i.e., greater than two standard deviations from the mean; less than the fifth percentile) automatically labels a fixed proportion of the tested population as abnormal, regardless of whether this degree of deviation from the average has any physiologic significance.

  Failure to recognize this phenomenon can lead to unnecessary evaluations for problems that do not exist. If a healthy individual undergoes 12 tests, such as on a standard 12-test chemistry panel that uses the rule of plus or minus two standard deviations for normalcy, the chance that all 12 results will be normal is only 54%.

Is it clear how the new test is being used? Whether the new test is used alone or in conjunction with other diagnostic information must be clear. A radiographic film, for example, may be read as is, or the radiologist may be given clinical data to aid in interpretation. Both methods may be valid, depending on the setting in which the test is used, but the latter method may require additional study of the relative weights given to the film and to the clinical information.

Is the new test truly independent of the gold standard? The new test should not incorporate any element of the gold standard. This occurs most often when the proposed test is a symptom complex used to identify a high-risk group of patients. Problems arise, for example, if a new test for UTI requires the presence of fever and dysuria whereas the gold-standard diagnosis was defined as fever and a positive urine culture result. The authors of the new test would then conclude that fever is a useful tool for identifying children at risk for UTI.

Suggested Readings

American Academy of Pediatrics, Committee on Quality Improvement, Subcommittee on Urinary Tract Infection. Practice parameter: the diagnosis, treatment, and evaluation of the initial urinary tract infection in febrile infants and young children. *Pediatrics* 1999;103:843.

American Thoracic Society. The tuberculin skin test. *Am Rev Respir Dis* 1981;123:343.

Benjamin JT. Waiving the office lab back to life. *Contemp Pediatr* 1998;15:38.

Cebul RD, Beck RB. Biochemical profiles: applications in ambulatory screening and preadmission testing of adults. *Ann Intern Med* 1987;106:403.

Diaz T, Vlahov D, Greenberg B, et al. Sexual orientation and HIV infection prevalence among young Latino injection drug users in Harlem. *J Womens Health Gender-Based Med* 2001;10:371.

Dodd RY, Notari EP, Stramer SL. Current prevalence and incidence of infectious disease markers and estimated window-period risk in the American Red Cross blood donor population. *Transfusion* 2002;42:975.

Furcolow ML, Hewell B, Nelson WE, Palmer CE. Quantitative studies of the tuberculin reaction. *Pub Health Rep* 1941;56:1082.

Haynes RB. Department of Clinical Epidemiology and Biostatistics. How to read clinical journals: II. To learn about a diagnostic test. *Can Med Assoc J* 1981;124:703.

Browner WS, Newman TB, Cummings SR. Designing a new study: III. Diagnostic tests. In: Hulley SB, Cummings SR, eds. *Designing clinical research: an epidemiologic approach*. Baltimore, MD: Williams and Wilkins, 1988.

Kuppermann N, Fleisher GR, Jaffe DM. Predictors of occult pneumococcal bacteremia in young febrile children. *Ann Emerg Med* 1998;31:679.

Landis JR, Kock GG. The measurement of observer agreement for categorical data. *Biometrics* 1977;33:159.

Lehmann H. Decision analysis: a language for survival in the era of managed care. *Contemp Pediatr* 1997;14:65.

Pauker SG, Kassirer JP. The threshold approach to clinical decision making. *N Engl J Med* 1980;302:1109.

Ransohoff DF, Feinstein AR. Problems of spectrum and bias in evaluating the efficacy of diagnostic tests. *N Engl J Med* 1978;299:926.

Rao PM, Rhea JT, Novelline RA, et al. Effect of computed tomography of the appendix on treatment of patients and use of hospital resources. *N Engl J Med* 1998;338:141.

Sackett DL, Haynes RB, Guyatt GH, Tugwell P. *Clinical epidemiology: a basic science for clinical medicine*. Boston: Little, Brown and Company, 1991. DISPLAY 15-1. Gene discovery and some definitions.

Satern WB, Renzullo PO, Carr JK, et al. HIV-1 infection among civilian applicants for US military service, 1985 to 2000: epidemiology and geography. *J AIDS* 2003;32:215.

CHAPTER 13 ■ AMBULATORY CARE: PRESENT AND FUTURE

MORRIS GREEN

DEFINITION AND SCOPE OF AMBULATORY CARE

Ambulatory pediatrics encompasses the diagnosis and management of acute disease, developmental problems, and psychosocial illnesses; the continuing care of children with a long-term illness or disability; health promotion; and disease prevention. Approximately one-third of pediatric ambulatory visits are for acute illnesses, usually viral, respiratory, or gastrointestinal; an additional 3% to 10% are for chronic illness or disability; and a further 25% to 30% for health supervision. Psychosocial symptoms or disorders are estimated to affect 20% to 25% of the children and adolescents seen in the pediatric office.

The Institute of Medicine's Committee on the Future of Primary Care has defined primary care as "the provision of integrated, accessible health care services by clinicians who are available for addressing a large majority of personal health needs, developing a sustained partnership with patients, and practicing in the context of family and community."

Ambulatory care, largely synonymous with the primary or general pediatric care given by the pediatrician alone or in partnership with a nurse practitioner, includes health supervision; developmental surveillance; treatment of acute illness and minor trauma; early identification of psychosocial, educational, or biomedical problems; and continuing care of children with chronic illness or disability. In addition to traditional office-based settings, primary care is available in some primary and secondary schools, especially in medically underserved areas. Provided by nurse practitioners or physicians working part-time, with backup by community pediatric and other consultants, school-based services are accessible during school hours, often with arrangements for after-hours emergency care. In addition to treatment for acute illnesses or minor trauma, health clinics in secondary schools may offer early intervention for depression and other psychologic symptoms. The staff also may participate in health education programs to prevent sexually transmitted diseases, unintended pregnancies, substance abuse, risk-taking behaviors, and violence.

PATIENT DEMOGRAPHICS

Except for families living in poverty, in whom illness continues to be overrepresented on a population basis, children in the United States are physically healthier than ever before. The infectious and nutritional problems that were encountered so frequently in the past by the pediatrician have, to some extent, been supplanted by those of a developmental, behavioral, social, or educational nature. The new *Diagnostic and Statistical Manual for Primary Care (DSM-PC), Child and Adolescent Version*, includes diagnostic codes for these disorders.

The American family also has changed dramatically, with an increase in the number of mothers who work outside the home, single-parent households, and the prevalence of parental separations, desertions, divorces, remarriages, live-in partners, and blended families. Children seen by the pediatrician come from much more diverse ethnic, cultural, linguistic, and religious backgrounds than they did a decade ago. In the highly migratory American society, extended family members are also less available than in the past to give child-rearing advice and to provide emotional and physical support; however, the number of grandparents rearing young children has significantly grown. Increasingly, parents invested in the optimal development of their children look to their pediatrician for authoritative guidance concerning child development.

CURRENT TRENDS IN THE DELIVERY OF PEDIATRIC HEALTH SERVICES

The delivery of pediatric health services is in transition from solo to group practice, team care, and the integration of office- with community-based services. Only about one of four pediatricians is in solo practice. Although 75% of pediatricians still practice in communities of more than 100,000 persons, an increasing number work in small or rural towns. A major shift has occurred from inpatient to ambulatory and day hospital care. Day surgery has greatly expanded in scope, and day hospitals or short-stay units are being used for the regulation of diabetes, the treatment of cystic fibrosis, the infusion of blood and chemotherapeutic agents, and the management of acute asthmatic episodes.

Most children in the United States are covered by health insurance for ambulatory care (Box 13.1). Membership in the managed care programs of health maintenance organizations, independent practice associations, preferred provider organizations, and hospital-based health services is steadily increasing. Fee-for-service costs paid directly by the parent are being replaced by reimbursement from third-party payers such as health maintenance organizations. Some pediatric practitioners are salaried or paid on a capitation basis. Primary-care pediatricians serve an average of 3,000 patients each year, including approximately 100 newborns. Because of fewer children per family in the United States, the reduced prevalence of episodic illness in economically secure families, the discovery of new vaccines, and an increased number of pediatricians, many practitioners have more time available to care for adolescents, children with chronic disease, prenatal consultations, sports medicine, and the management of psychosocial, developmental, educational, and genetic problems.

Except in small towns, in which the number of children is not large enough to support more than one pediatrician, or for the physician who prefers solo practice, compelling reasons exist to practice in a pediatric or multidisciplinary group. Advantages include the opportunity to share knowledge as well as call duty; plan family time; participate in continuing pediatric education; develop an area of special interest; work in a community child health program; collaborate in office practice research projects; or teach medical students and residents.

To meet the needs of parents who work outside the home, some pediatric practices have early morning, evening, and weekend hours. Much care continues to be given, however,

in hospital emergency rooms or urgent care centers. Some hospitals and pediatric practices have established satellite offices to increase the geographic access to their services. In rural areas, a pediatrician from a nearby community may hold office hours a few times a week, or the satellite office may be staffed by a nurse practitioner with access to pediatric consultation by phone.

In addition to such primary health care services, ambulatory care may be given by pediatricians with special competence in child development, learning problems, neurodevelopmental disabilities, infectious disease, chronic illness, behavior, allergy, gastroenterology, pulmonology, dermatology, nephrology, rheumatology, adolescent medicine, sports medicine, neurology, cardiology, genetics, hematology/oncology, or endocrinology. Regrettably, some managed-care plans do not authorize consultation with a pediatric subspecialist if an adult subspecialist is on their panel. Referral to a mental health consultant or service frequently is denied.

Psychosocial and developmental problems now require more of the pediatrician's time, including help in promoting adaptation to major family changes or crises such as death, separation, divorce, or remarriage; the care of a child with a long-term illness or disability; developmental delay; and learning disabilities, underachievement, and other school problems. Additional psychosocial symptoms and behavioral complaints include failure to thrive, out-of-control behavior in toddlers, persistent sleep problems, separation anxiety, hyperactivity, chronic headaches, recurrent abdominal pain, poor social skills, and other clinical presentations classified in the *DSM-PC, Child and Adolescent Version*. No aspect of primary pediatric care offers a greater challenge or more promise than the prevention and management of behavioral, social, and learning problems. The major deterrents to its realization are lack of adequate reimbursement by third-party payers and limited training during a pediatric residency.

This aspect of ambulatory care may be delivered jointly by the pediatrician and the nurse practitioner; by the pediatrician and nurse complemented by a part- or full-time psychologist or social worker in the physician's office or school-based program; or through collaboration with these and the behavioral pediatrician, child psychiatrist, child psychologist, occupational or physical therapist, audiologist, nutritionist, speech and language pathologist, educator, and family therapist in the community. Collaboration between primary-care pediatricians and community hospital-based allied health professionals or by traveling consultant teams from an academic health center is another integrated option.

The management of many of the problems and issues encountered in pediatric ambulatory practice is enhanced when office care is complemented or supplemented by such community-based services as nurse home visits; school curricula that promote good health habits, social skills, and conflict resolution or anger control; respite options for parents of children with special health care needs; Supplemental Feeding Program for Women, Infants, and Children nutritional services; child protection services; special education programs; family support agencies; marriage counselors; IDEA Part C programs; developmental child-care centers and preschools; early intervention programs; and parent education classes.

Children who require highly specialized or multidisciplinary ambulatory services usually are referred to academic health centers, regional clinics staffed by traveling teams, or large multidisciplinary group practices. Patients referred for such multidisciplinary or interdisciplinary care include those with myelodysplasia, cerebral palsy, craniofacial anomalies, birth defects, cystic fibrosis, developmental disabilities, learning disorders, behavior problems, seizures, autism, and genetic disorders.

BOX 13.1   Children and Health Insurance

In 2003:
62% of children were insured through private/employer-based health insurance
26.3% were insured by Medicaid/SCHIP
11.7% were uninsured

(Reproduced with permission from American Academy of Pediatrics Fact Sheet: Children's Health Insurance and Medicaid, February 2005.)

PROVIDING CARE FOR CHILDREN WITH LONG-TERM DISORDERS

The care of a child with a long-term disorder requires continuity of care with periodic reassessment, monitoring of the child and family's adaptation to the problem, and reinforcement of a supportive physician–patient alliance. The advocacy of the pediatricians who care for children or adolescents with long-term disorders is critically important, whether through enlisting the most expert help available; communication with the other professionals involved; awareness of family interactions, changes, or crises; coordination of the comprehensive management plan; or gaining public support for additional community services.

When subspecialists are involved in the child's care, consultants generally attend to a specific problem rather than provide primary care. The separate but collaborative roles of the generalist pediatrician and subspecialist must be defined early for each child. Although highly important, the time-consuming participation of the primary-care pediatrician in care coordination, team conferences, counseling, and communication generally is not reimbursed.

By increasing their understanding of an illness or disability and its management, the pediatrician promotes the active participation of the child and parents in ongoing care. Excellent pediatric care of these children and adolescents includes emotional support, anticipatory guidance, promotion of family communication, a focus on the child as a child rather than only on the disorder, an emphasis on family strengths, a caution against social isolation, and enhancement of self-esteem.

HOME CARE

Since the late 1980s, the tremendous growth of medical services outside the hospital makes it possible for children to receive antibiotics, chemotherapy, parenteral nutrition, analgesic agents, and blood products at home. Additional home care services include respiratory therapy, mechanical respiration, oxygen administration, tracheostomy care, apnea monitoring, and respiratory therapy; phototherapy for hyperbilirubinemia; and parenteral nutrition through nasogastric, gastrostomy, or jejunostomy tubes. Home care programs may offer visits by physicians; occupational, physical, developmental, and speech language therapists; social workers; child development specialists; and nurses. Some hospitals support the care of terminally ill children whose parents choose to have them die at home rather than in the hospital. Home visits by a nurse are an important complement to office visits, especially for young, single parents who lack social supports; the family whose infant was born prematurely or with a disability; and the early-discharged mother who hopes to breast-feed successfully.

Early intervention services for children with special needs from birth to 3 years of age authorized by the Individuals with Disabilities Act (IDEA), Part C include occupational and physical therapy, nutrition services, nursing, family training, and counseling.

PEDIATRIC OFFICE: THE CHILD'S MEDICAL HOME

As the child's medical home, the pediatric office has multiple roles, including the following:

- The diagnosis and management of biomedical, developmental, behavioral, and academic problems
- Health promotion and illness prevention

- The care of children and adolescents with a chronic illness or disability
- Telephone advice: In some communities, after-hours calls are answered by nurse practitioners trained in the use of printed protocols
- Family crisis counseling
- Patient education
- Community advocacy
- Services for children in foster care
- Participation in community healthy clinics, adoption services, school health programs, child-care centers, Head Start programs, migrant labor camps, at-risk youth programs, and juvenile justice centers, either in relation to individual children or to program planning and evaluation
- Collaboration with educators concerning a child's learning disorder, behavior, academic underachievement, special health care needs, chronic illness, or technology dependency
- The Pediatric Research in Office Setting (PROS) network consists of over 1,500 pediatric practitioners who participate in research with shared protocols developed by PROS members in their office-based practices

HEALTH SUPERVISION

The present challenge is to increase the effectiveness of health supervision, especially in relation to behavior and development. The American Academy of Pediatrics and other child health advocacy organizations have sought to make health supervision a covered benefit in all health insurance programs.

Health supervision includes an appraisal of the physical, developmental, psychosocial, and educational status of the child; making an effort to view the child in the context of his or her family; the early identification of problems; prompt intervention into problems; anticipatory guidance; the monitoring of parent–child relationships; the fostering good health habits; and the enhancement of family communication. Although the cumulative knowledge base of health supervision has grown substantially in recent years, much additional research is needed to prove the effectiveness of currently recommended practices.

The delivery of personalized care is facilitated by a regularly updated database that includes such demographic information as the composition of the household; ages and health status of the parents and siblings; parental marital status, education, occupation, and workplace; child-care arrangements; the child's school; and the family's religious affiliation.

Because parental strengths are important contributors to health promotion, they should be recognized and reinforced during or at the end of the health supervision consultation by comments such as, "Benjamin is progressing wonderfully, and both of you are doing an excellent job!"

The success of a pediatric visit is measured, in part, by the extent to which the parents' expectations are met. In most cases, these can be inferred from their questions; however, if the pediatrician senses that a significant worry has not been expressed, this can be pursued with a question such as, "Mrs. Black, to be sure that I've answered all the concerns that you had in mind today, what else had you thought about asking me?"

Parents value the reassurance of the pediatrician's examination of their child, authoritative answers to their questions, suggestions for managing perceived problems, and expert anticipatory guidance. Although most parents are comfortable in asking the physician for advice, some are reserved lest they seem inadequate. Others expect doctors to ask about what they need to know. Because some parents do not know exactly what information the pediatrician would find diagnostically useful in relation to a psychosocial or developmental problem, the interview may be enhanced by the selective use of questions such as those included in the publication *Bright Futures: Guidelines to Health Supervision of Infants, Children, and Adolescents*.

Many parents do not think contextually—that is, that the child, family, and community constitute an interactive system. They may not report personal and family stressors such as maternal depression, divorce, alcoholism, a disruptive move, or other discontinuities because they have not appreciated their etiologic relevance to the problems presented by their child. Some topics are, of course, difficult for parents to mention, such as the worry that their child may be mentally handicapped, a secret fear that their child is especially vulnerable to illness or accident, and problems such as parental alcoholism or depression, family violence, marital discord, anger, and financial stress. The completion of a developmental and behavioral screening instrument by the parent and older child or adolescent before the interview may help identify topics that warrant discussion during the present or a later session.

Although 10- to 15-minute sessions are limiting, considerable cumulative time is available if continuity exists over months or years. Unfortunately, this often is lacking with the current frequent changes in health plans. Because complex behavior problems cannot be changed in any major way in a few minutes, their identification during a health supervision visit requires a return pediatric appointment or referral to a mental health center, behavioral pediatrician, child psychiatrist, child psychologist, or social worker. Lengthener sessions also may be indicated during critical periods of family transition, such as divorce, remarriage, death, illness, unemployment, adoption, foster child placement, and other major changes in the family. Although most health supervision services are delivered to an individual patient or family, others must be population based. If the child's environment is unhealthy, the effectiveness of preventive and health-promoting interventions is limited. The trend in health promotion today is toward developing and enhancing supportive environments, rather than concentrating only on attempts to change lifestyles directly. Brief interventions, especially those planned to modify established behaviors, do not work when families are preoccupied with obtaining food, clothing, and shelter. Groups offer shared experiences, mutual support, and social reinforcement in addition to serving as an effective way to present information. Such sessions can be substituted occasionally for or as a supplement to an individual health supervision consultation, especially during the first year of life. Some parents in the group may ask questions that others had not yet considered. Group participants also gain a greater appreciation of the wide range of developmental and behavioral differences among children and learn what has worked for others. Such sessions also are useful in providing anticipatory guidance for the parents of preadolescent children, for older children, and for adolescents, including single teenage parents.

Health Education

Collaboration with the health education programs offered by schools or sponsored by community hospitals, churches, civic organizations, and social agencies may help children and adolescents acquire and maintain such constructive health habits as regular physical activity, good nutrition, and dental health; avoid smoking, obesity, and alcohol or drug abuse; prevent unintended adolescent pregnancies and risk-taking behaviors;

cope with stressors; enhance social skills; help develop a social support network; and train for conflict resolution.

Health supervision consultations also may be supplemented by effective parent handouts, pamphlets, newsletters, reading lists, and other educational materials.

Promoting Successful Outcomes

Health supervision also may contribute to the successful adaptation of parents and children to the changing circumstances of their lives. The ability of parents to adapt is strengthened by their self-confidence and high self-esteem, enjoyment of parenthood, good family communication, awareness of child developmental principles, supportive parent–child and marital relationships, and a willingness to ask for help when needed.

Health developmental outcomes in children include the ability to communicate well, to express feelings, to be optimistic, and to make friends. Other strengths are physical fitness, a positive assessment of personal capacities, good grooming, self-responsibility for health, high self-esteem, and the security of feeling cared for and loved.

Pediatricians play an important role in promoting adaptation through facilitating the mastery of expected and unexpected transitions, events, and crises; by helping children and parents identify their strengths and resources; by suggesting protective strategies; and by early intervention when maladaptive symptoms are identified.

The successful adaptation to expected and unexpected changes and stressors may be promoted by anticipatory guidance, such as preparation for an adoption, a toddler's autonomy, hospitalization, surgery, the changes initiated by puberty, or the remarriage of a parent. Adaptation can be concurrent, as in coping with an infant's difficult temperament, the birth of a baby with a disability, separation, divorce, death, unemployment, suicide, homicide, accidents, sexual assault, serious illness, or a mother's return to work outside the home.

PEDIATRIC EDUCATION

The growing importance of ambulatory care has led to timely changes in the Residency Review Committee Special Requirements for Pediatric Residencies. The required ambulatory care experience has been augmented, and the use of community practices for the continuity of resident experiences is encouraged.

Suggested Readings

American Academy of Pediatrics. *The classification of child and adolescent mental diagnoses in primary care. Diagnostic and statistical manual for primary care. Child and adolescent version*. Elk Grove Village, IL: American Academy of Pediatrics, 1996.

Green M, Haggerty RJ, Weitzman ML, eds. *Ambulatory pediatrics,* 5th ed. Philadelphia: Saunders, 1999.

Green M, Palfrey JS, eds. *Bright futures: guidelines for health supervision of infants, children, and adolescents,* 2nd ed. Arlington, VA: National Center for Education in Maternal and Child Health Publishers, 2002.

Haggerty RJ, Green M. History of academic general and ambulatory pediatrics. *Pediatr Res* 2003;53:188.

Haggerty RJ. Child health 2000: new pediatrics in the changing environment of children's needs in the 21st century. *Pediatrics* 1995;96(Suppl):804.

Palfrey JS. *Community child health*. Westport, CT: Praeger, 1994.

Perrin EC, Stancin T. A continuing dilemma: whether and how to screen for concerns about children's behavior. *Pediatr Rev* 2002;23:264.

CHAPTER 14 ■ FEEDING THE HEALTHY CHILD

LAURENCE FINBERG

Although the feeding of infants and children is a part of the cultural inheritance of all societies, it behooves pediatricians to understand both the underlying nutritional science and to be able to instruct parents in proper techniques, when such instruction is needed.

NUTRITIONAL NEEDS

Energy

Energy is needed to sustain life and to maintain optimal growth and health. In addition, certain macrominerals, trace substances, vitamins, and specific fatty acids also are important. Energy serves as an appropriate denominator for all the other nutrients, when expressed as calories expended to maintain optimal bodily composition and promote growth through infancy, childhood, and adolescence. After cessation of growth, maintenance of optimal composition becomes the goal of good nutrition.

Table 14.1 gives basal or resting expenditures at various ages. Assuming average activity, the basal expenditure should be multiplied by 1.5 to meet the requirement under usual circumstances. Increased body temperature (13% per degree C), ventilating rate, or muscular activity each can increase the expenditure to twice basal; the simultaneous combination of all these may produce a threefold basal expenditure.

The energy requirement is met from protein, fat, and carbohydrate. The only other potential source of calories for humans is ethyl alcohol. The calorie used here, called the kilocalorie, is the nutritionist's unit (1,000 times the calorie of the physicist) and is defined, in heat terms, as the energy required to raise the temperature of a kilogram of water from 15°C to 16°C.

The protein intake, providing approximately 4 cal/kg, is of particular importance. Not all proteins are nutritionally equal for the human diet. A specific group of amino acids, known as the essential amino acids, must be present in the diet because they are not synthesized at all or in sufficient quantities. These are histidine, isoleucine, leucine, lysine, methionine, phenylalanine, threonine, tryptophane, and valine. Arginine, cystine, and probably taurine also are required by low-birth-weight infants. The remaining amino acids can be synthesized from these three for tissue and cellular needs.

The animal protein found in meat, eggs, and milk supply these amino acids requirements in appropriate proportion. Using an optimal dietary protein source requires that a minimum of about 6% of total caloric intake be from protein. (Human milk contains approximately 8% protein.) It is appropriate to have at least 10% of calories from protein after infancy to allow for inefficiencies of digestion and absorption. If the source of calories is only vegetable, a higher percentage of protein (13% to 15%) is needed to include all the essential amino acids without producing toxicity from an excess of some of them. No single vegetable provides all the essential amino acids. Note that, as the expenditure of energy increases, the percentage requirement for protein remains constant. For this reason, giving protein requirements in g/kg at varying ages underestimates the need when the energy expenditure is unusually high (e.g., manual labor, athletic participation).

Fat has an important place in the diet as a provider of energy, yielding approximately 9 cal/g. Two fatty acids, linolenic acid and linoleic acid, are important membrane constituents. These essential dietary components need constitute only 1% to 2% of calories. In infants younger than about 2 years of age, it is important to keep 50% of calories as fat; this keeps the volume of food needed within the range of the infant's capability to ingest and thus assists in normal growth. As the child grows, concern about cholesterol levels and related adult heart disease has led to the recommendation to limit fat to no more than 30% of calories. This aim may be achieved readily by a gradual dietary adjustment between 22 and 30 months of life.

Carbohydrate, the third appropriate source of energy, is required to limit the amounts of protein and fat, either of which may be toxic when ingested in significant excess of the recommended proportions. Small excesses of either protein or fat will be converted to carbohydrate, and the latter may be converted to some fats. Thus, carbohydrate from 40% to 60% of calories is optimal for nutrition and for taste quality in the diet.

Water also is an essential nutrient. Water constitutes 70% of the lean body mass, which is about 60% of the weight when 10% is fat (largely adipose tissue). Normal physiologic processes result in a daily turnover of approximately 10% of weight in the infant and 2% of weight in the older adolescent. This turnover is induced by energy (heat) expended, thus being greater per unit of weight in the more rapidly metabolizing infant with a greater ratio of surface area to weight. The sites of obligatory water loss are evaporation from the skin and lungs (45 mL/100 cal expended), urine formation required to keep a constant composition of extracellular fluid (50 mL/100 cal expended at a concentration of 300 mOsm/Kg), and a small amount in the feces, making the losses 100 mL/100 cal or 1 mL/cal as the obligatory replacement requirement. (The ability to concentrate the urine reduces the requirement, although less so in the early months of life than later.)

TABLE 14.1

BASAL CALORIC EXPENDITURE FOR INFANTS AND CHILDREN*

Age	Weight (kg)	Surface Area (m^2)	Caloric Expenditure (cal/kg)
Newborn	2.5–4.0	0.2–0.23	50
1 wk to 6 mo	3–8	0.2–0.35	65–70
6–12 mo	8–12	0.35–0.45	50–60
1–2 yr	10–15	0.45–0.55	45–50
2–5 yr	15–20	0.6–0.7	45
5–10 yr	20–35	0.7–1.1	40–45
10–16 yr	35–60	1.5–1.7	25–40
Adult	70	1.75	15–20

*Water expenditure equals 1 mL per calorie.

TABLE 14.2

FOOD AND NUTRITION BOARD, NATIONAL ACADEMY OF SCIENCES—INSTITUTE OF MEDICINE DIETARY REFERENCE INTAKES, 1997

Life-Stage Group	Calcium Adequate Intake[a] (mg/d)	Phosphorus RDA[b] (mg/d)	Phosphorus Adequate Intake (mg/d)	Magnesium RDA (mg/d)	Magnesium Adequate Intake (mg/d)	Vitamin D Adequate Intake[c,d] (μg/d)	Fluoride Adequate Intake (mg/d)
Infants							
0–6 mo	210		100		30	5	0.01
7–12 mo	270		275		75	5	0.5
Children							
1–3 yr	500	460		80		5	0.7
4–8 yr	800	500		130		5	1.1
Male							
9–13 yr	1,300	1,250		240		5	2.0
14–18 yr	1,300	1,250		410		5	3.2
19–30 yr	1,000	700		400		5	3.8
31–50 yr	1,000	700		420		5	3.8
51–70 yr	1,200	700		420		10	3.8
>70 yr	1,200	700		420		15	3.8
Female							
9–13 yr	1,300	1,250		240		5	2.0
14–18 yr	1,300	1,250		360		5	2.9
19–30 yr	1,000	700		310		5	3.1
31–50 yr	1,000	700		320		5	3.1
51–70 yr	1,200	700		320		10	3.1
>70 yr	1,200	700		320		15	3.1
Pregnancy							
≤18 yr	1,300	1,250		400		5	2.9
19–30 yr	1,000	700		350		5	3.1
31–50 yr	1,000	700		360		5	3.1
Lactation							
≤18 yr	1,300	1,250		360		5	2.9
19–30 yr	1,000	700		310		5	3.1
31–50 yr	1,000	700		320		5	3.1

RDA, recommended dietary allowance.
[a]Adequate intake: The observed average or experimentally set intake by a defined population or subgroup that appears to sustain a defined nutritional status, such as growth rate, normal circulating nutrient values, or other functional indications of health. For healthy breast-fed infants, adequate intake is the mean intake. All other life-stage groups should be covered at the adequate intake value. The adequate intake is not equivalent to an RDA.
[b]The intake that meets the nutrient need of almost all (97% to 98% individuals in a group.
[c]As cholecalciferol. 1 μg cholecalciferol = 40 IU vitamin D.
[d]In the absence of adequate exposure to sunlight.
(Data used with permission from dietary reference intake data for calcium, phosphorus, magnesium, vitamin D, and fluoride. Washington, DC: National Academy Press, 1997.)

Minerals

Macrominerals

The necessary macrominerals for physiologic functioning and for tissue and bone formation are sodium, chloride, potassium, calcium, magnesium, and phosphorus. Sodium and chloride are the principal ions of the extracellular fluid, and they are needed to determine the volume of that compartment, which includes the subcompartment of the blood plasma. Potassium is the principal cation of cell fluid, and magnesium also is a cell ion. The optimal intake for sodium, potassium, and chloride is approximately 2 meq/100 calories expended, although the permissible range intake for sodium and chloride (from 0.1 to 10 meq/100 cal) is quite large. [A detailed explanation of the role of sodium, chloride, and potassium can be found in Chapter 9, Fluid and Electrolyte Physiology and Therapy.]

Calcium performs many physiologic and biochemical functions in cells and is the principal mineral of the skeleton. Phosphorus (as phosphate) is an essential constituent of all cells and biochemical energy processes, as well as being part of the

mineral skeleton. The recommended daily intake of macrominerals is shown in Table 14.2.

Microminerals (Trace Elements)

The trace minerals also are important for a variety of cell and organ functions. A few deserve particular mention. Table 14.3 describes the major trace mineral requirements necessary for complete function, and Table 14.4 lists their general dietary sources. Those minerals not listed are ingested safely in a general diet that includes the principal food groups.

Iron is a required atom for the heme molecule and for the cytochrome enzymes. It is particularly well conserved by the body, and surplus is stored in the bone marrow and other reticuloendothelial organs.

Copper and zinc also are necessary cell constituents for enzymes, with functions related to blood formulation, insulin production, and other essential metabolic activities.

Iodine is required for thyroid hormone formation.

Chromium is needed for blood cells and other enzymatic needs.

TABLE 14.3

FOOD AND NUTRITION BOARD, NATIONAL ACADEMY OF SCIENCES—NATIONAL RESEARCH COUNCIL RECOMMENDED DIETARY ALLOWANCE,[a] REVISED 1989 (ABRIDGED[b]), DESIGNED FOR THE MAINTENANCE OF GOOD NUTRITION OF PRACTICALLY ALL HEALTHY PEOPLE IN THE UNITED STATES

Category	Age (yr) or Condition	Weight[c] (kg)	(lb)	Height[c] (cm)	(in)	Protein (g)	Fat-soluble vitamins Vitamin A (μg RE)	Vitamin E (mg α-TE)	Vitamin K (μg)	Water-soluble vitamins Vitamin C (mg)	Thiamin (mg)	Riboflavin (mg)	Niacin (mg NE)	Vitamin B_6 (mg)	Folate (μg)	Vitamin B_{12} (μg)	Minerals Iron (mg)	Zinc (mg)	Iodine (μg)	Selenium (μg)
Infant	0.05–0.50	6	13	60	24	13	375	3	5	30	0.3	0.4	5	0.3	25	0.3	6	5	40	10
	0.5–1.0	9	20	71	28	14	375	4	10	35	0.4	0.5	6	0.6	35	0.5	10	5	50	15
Children	1–3	13	29	90	35	16	400	6	15	40	0.7	0.8	9	1.0	50	0.7	10	10	70	20
	4–6	20	44	112	44	24	500	7	20	45	0.9	1.1	12	1.1	75	1.0	10	10	90	20
	7–10	28	62	132	52	28	700	7	30	45	1.0	1.2	13	1.4	100	1.4	10	10	120	30
Male	11–14	45	99	157	62	45	1,000	10	45	50	1.3	1.5	17	1.7	150	2.0	12	15	150	40
	15–18	66	145	176	69	59	1,000	10	65	60	1.5	1.8	20	2.0	200	2.0	12	15	150	50
	19–24	72	160	177	70	58	1,000	10	70	60	1.5	1.7	19	2.0	200	2.0	10	15	150	70
	25–50	79	174	176	70	63	1,000	10	80	60	1.5	1.7	19	2.0	200	2.0	10	15	150	70
	51+	77	170	173	68	63	1,000	10	80	60	1.2	1.4	15	2.0	200	2.0	10	15	150	70
Female	11–14	46	101	157	62	46	800	8	45	50	1.1	1.3	15	1.4	150	2.0	15	12	150	45
	15–18	55	120	163	64	44	800	8	55	60	1.1	1.3	15	1.5	180	2.0	15	12	150	50
	19–24	58	128	164	65	46	800	8	60	60	1.1	1.3	15	1.6	180	2.0	15	12	150	55
	25–50	63	138	163	64	50	800	8	65	60	1.1	1.3	15	1.6	180	2.0	15	12	150	55
	51+	65	143	160	63	50	800	8	65	60	1.0	1.2	13	1.6	180	2.0	10	12	150	55
Pregnant						60	800	10	65	70	1.5	1.6	17	2.2	400	2.2	30	15	175	65
Lactating	First 6 mo					65	1,300	12	65	95	1.6	1.8	20	2.1	280	2.6	15	19	200	75
	Second 6 mo					62	1,200	11	65	90	1.6	1.7	20	2.1	260	2.6	15	16	200	75

[a] The allowances, expressed as average daily intakes over time, are intended to provide variations among most normal persons as they live in the United States under usual environmental stresses. Diets should be based on a variety of common foods to provide other nutrients for which human requirements have been less welf defined. See text for detailed discussion of allowances and of nutrients not tabulated.

[b] This table does not include nutrients for which Dietary Reference intakes have been established (see the National Research Council's *Dietary Reference Intakes for Calcium, Phosphorus, Magnesium, Vitamin D, and Fluoride*, 1997).

[c] Weights and heights of reference adults are actual medians for the U.S. population of the designated age, as reported by the National Health and Nutritional Examination Survey II. The median weights and heights of those younger than 19 years were taken from Hamill PVV, Drizol TA, johnson Cl, et al. Physical growth: National Center for Health Statistics. *Am J Clin Nutr* 1979;32:607. The use of these figures does not imply that the height-to-weight ratios are ideal.

TABLE 14.4

IMPORTANT SOURCES OF TRACE MINERALS IN THE DIET

Mineral	Source
Iron	Liver, meat, fortified infant formula, fortified cereals
Copper	Meats, legumes
Zinc	Meats, nuts, legumes
Chromium	Meats, grains
Iodine	Fish, seafood, vegetables from coastal soils
Manganese	Unrefined grains, nuts, vegetables, fruits
Molybdenum	Legumes, grains, milk
Cobalt or B_{12}	Liver, meats, milk, eggs
Selenium	Meats, eggs, grains

Fluoride, although not required for any vital life process, strengthens the dentine of teeth, making them resistant to caries, and it also may make the skeleton more resistant to osteoporosis. Minute amounts of arsenic, boron, manganese, molybdenum, nickel, selenium, silicon, sulfur, and vanadium also are needed.

Vitamins

Vitamins and a few other organic molecules also are necessary for carrying out biochemical and physiologic functions. Tables 14.5 and 14.6 summarize the sources, requirements, and other features of the vitamins and necessary substances. It is convenient to divide vitamins into those that are fat soluble (vitamins A, D, E, and K), and those that are water-soluble (vitamin B complex and vitamin C). In addition to the major vitamins, healthy diet requires small amounts of choline, carnitine, and inositol.

Vitamin A or retinol is necessary for several functions related to vision and the eye. In addition, it plays a role in respiratory epithelial integrity, adding protection from lung injury in respiratory infections, most notably measles. Excess dosage is toxic and may occur from ingestion of certain foods (such as the livers of polar animals) as well as from an excess intake of supplements.

Vitamin D or cholecalciferol is a precursor molecule for a hormone complex that, together with parathyroid hormone, regulates calcium and phosphorus metabolism. It is formed in the skin by the action of ultraviolet light, but also may be obtained by ingestion from natural sources such as fish liver oils or from fortified milks. The plant sterol ergosterol may be substituted for the animal form, because it undergoes the same transformations in the body to the active hormone calcitriol. A deficiency of vitamin D leads to rickets in children. Excess dosage is toxic.

Vitamin E consists of a group of tocopherols that function as antioxidants, membrane stabilizers, and perhaps others.

Vitamin K consists of a group of naphthoquinones functioning to enable the production of several clotting factors in the liver. Intestinal bacteria produce vitamin K, making its ingestion unnecessary except in circumstances when the bacteria are absent, such as in the newborn or during the prolonged use of antibiotics.

Vitamin C or ascorbic acid is important for the production of intercellular material, vascular integrity, and perhaps other metabolic functions. Deficiency impairs wound healing, and marked deficiency produces scurvy.

Vitamin B_1 or thiamin serves as a cofactor in biochemical reactions involving the oxidative decarboxylation necessary for neural and cardiac function. Deficiency causes beriberi.

Riboflavin, or vitamin B_2, is important in flavoprotein enzymes. Deficiency causes corneal vascularization, cheilosis, and systemic symptoms.

Niacin or nicotinic acid is a constituent of coenzymes, such as NAD and NADP, as well as other dehydrogenase systems. Deficiency causes pellagra.

Folic acid consists of a group of pteridine compounds that are important in many synthetic biochemical functions. Deficiency causes megaloblastic anemia and systemic symptoms.

Vitamin B_{12} or cobalamin is a cobalt-containing molecule necessary for several biochemical functions. Deficiency causes pernicious (megaloblastic) anemia and nervous system disturbances.

Pantothenic acid serves as a constituent of enzymes and as a cofactor in metabolic processes.

Pyridoxine or vitamin B_6 is another constituent of the enzymes involved in decarboxylation. Deficiency produces convulsions and anemia.

Biotin is a part of carboxylase enzymes. Deficiency leads to dermatitis.

Significance of Fiber

Fiber consists of indigestible material from plant cell walls, mostly carbohydrate plus noncarbohydrate polymers. Its role in human nutrition has aroused controversy. On one hand, fiber softens the stool, thereby reducing constipation, and epidemiologic studies associate fiber intake with lower incidence of diverticulitis, cancer, and coronary heart disease in adults. On the other hand, a high fiber intake binds such trace metals as iron and zinc, leading to possible deficiency. A very high fiber intake may lead to premature satiety, excessive reduction of caloric intake and, in some instances, hyperperistalsis. At present, it seems wise to advise a moderate intake of vegetables and of fiber-containing cereals and a concomitant adequate intake of minerals.

FEEDING THE INFANT

In the first few months of life, an infant obtains nutrition from a single liquid source, either from the mother's breast or from a preparation that is usually made from an animal milk source. Historically, breast-feeding was the mode from the time of human origin until the Industrial Revolution in the eighteenth and nineteenth centuries. Modern research confirms that the evolutionary adaptation for infant feeding at the breast remains optimal for the infant and probably for the mother as well in most circumstances.

Breast-feeding

Breast Milk

From a nutritional standpoint, human milk is ideal for infants: it provides a suitable caloric density, contains high-quality proteins in sufficient amount, supplies adequate mineral content for cell and skeletal growth, and it has a low renal solute load that affords plenty of water as protection from dehydration (Table 14.6). These are not the characteristics of other animal milks fed to human infants: each milk is adapted to the specific species that produces it, and it meets the animal's needs in its respective environment.

TABLE 14.5
VITAMIN CHARACTERISTICS, ACTIONS, DISEASE STATES, AND SOURCES

Name	Characteristics	Biochemical Action	Effects of Deficiency	Effects of Excess	Dietary Sources
Vitamin A (retinol) 1 IU = 0.3 μg retinol	Fat soluble, heat stable; bile necessary for absorption, specific binding protein in plasma; stored in liver	Component of visual purple; integrity of epithelial tissues; bone cell function	Night blindness, xerophthalmia, keratomalacia, poor growth, impaired resistance to infection	Hyperostosis, hepatomegaly, alopecia, increased cerebrospinal fluid pressure (also from 13-*cis*-retinoic acid)	Milk fat, egg, liver
Provitamin A (beta-carotene; 1/6 activity of retinol)	Converted to retinol in liver, intestinal mucosa			Carotenemia	Dark green vegetables, yellow fruits and vegetables, tomatoes
Vitamin D (D$_2$-activated calciferol; D$_3$-activated dehydrocholesterol) 1 IU = 0.025 μg	D$_2$ from diet, D$_3$ from action of ultraviolet light on skin; hydroxylated sequentially in liver and kidney to form 1,25-dihydroxycholecalciferol, the active compound: regulated by dietary calcium, parathyroid hormone; anticonvulsant drugs interfere with metabolism	Formation of calcium; transport protein in duodenal mucosa; facilitates bone resorption, phosphorus absorption; synthesis of Ca-binding protein in epithelial cells	Rickets, osteomalacia	Hypercalcemia, azotemia, poor growth, vomiting, nephrocalcinosis	Fortified milk, fish, liver, salmon, sardines, mackerel, egg yolk, sunlight
Vitamin E (1 IU = 1 mg alphatocopherol acetate)	Stored in adipose tissue; transported with beta-lipoproteins: beta absorption depends on pancreatic juice and bile (iron may interfere); requirement increased by large amounts of polyunsaturated fats	Antioxidant, role in erythrocyte fragility; stabilizes biological membranes, prevents peroxidation of unsaturated fatty acids	Hemolytic anemia in premature infants; otherwise, no clearcut deficiency syndrome in humans	Unknown	Cereal seed oils, peanuts, soybeans, milk fat, turnip greens
Ascorbic acid (vitamin C)	Easily oxidized, especially in presence of copper, iron, high pH; absorption by simple diffusion	Exact mechanism unknown; functions in folacin metabolism, collagen biosynthesis, iron absorption and transport, tyrosin metabolism	Scurvy	Massive doses may lead to temporary increase in requirements and may predispose to kidney stones	Citrus fruits, tomatoes, cabbage, potatoes, human milk
Thiamine (vitamin B$_1$)	Heat labile; absorption impaired by alcohol, requirements a function of carbohydrate intake; synthesis by intestinal bacteria	Coenzyme for decarboxylation, other reactions as thiamine pyrophosphate	Beriberi; neuritis, edema, cardiac failure, hoarseness, anorexia, restlessness, aphonia	Unknown	Liver, meat, milk, whole grains, legumes
Riboflavin	Water soluble, light labile, heat stable: synthesis by intestinal bacteria (?)	Cofactor for many enzymes, synthesis flavin adenine dinucleotide, flavin mononucleotide (riboflavin 5'-phosphate)	Photophobia, chellosis, glossitis, corneal vascularization poor growth	Unknown	Meat, milk, egg, green vegetables, whole grains

(Continued)

TABLE 14.5
(CONTINUED)

Name	Characteristics	Biochemical Action	Effects of Deficiency	Effects of Excess	Dietary Sources
Niacin (nicotinic acid, amide)	Water soluble, heat and light stable; availability from corn enhanced by alkali; synthesized in the body from tryptophan (60:1), some by intestinal bacteria	Component of coenzymes I and II (nicotinamide-adenine dinucleotide, nicotinamideadenine dinucleotide phosphate), many enzymatic reactions	Pellagra; dermatitis, diarrhea, dementia	Nicotinic acid (not the amide) causes flushing pruritus	Meat, fish, whole grains, green vegetables
Pyridoxine (vitamin B_6); also pyridoxal, pyridoxamine	Water soluble, heat and light labile, interference from isoniazid; pyridoxal is the active form	Cofactor for many enzymes (e.g., transaminases, decarboxylases)	Dermatitis, glossitis, cheilosis, peripheral neuritis; in infants, irritability, convulsions, anemia	Unknown	Liver, meat, whole grains, corn, soybeans
Folacin group of compounds containing pteridine ring, p-aminobenzoic, and glutamic acids	Slightly soluble in water, light sensitive, heat stable; some production by intestinal bacteria; ascorbic acid involved in interconversions; interference from oral contraceptives, anticonvulsants	Tetrahydrofolic acid is the active form; synthesis of purines, pyrimidines, methylation reactions, one-carbon acceptor	Megaloblastic anemia, impaired cellular immunity	Only in patients with pernicious anemia not receiving cobalamin	Liver, green vegetables, cereals, oranges
Cobalamin (vitamin B_{12})	Slightly soluble in water, heat stable only at neutral pH, light sensitivity; absorption (ileum) depends on gastric intrinsic factor; CoA part of the molecule	Coenzyme component; erythrocyte maturation, central nervous system metabolism, methylmalonyl CoA mutase	Pernicious anemia, neurologic deterioration methylmalonic acidemia	Unknown	Animal foods only: meat, milk, eggs
Pantothenic acid	Water soluble, heat stable; daily requirement unknown but estimated at 5–10 mg	Component only CoA; many enzymatic reactions	Observed only with use of antagonists: depression, hypotension, muscle weakness, abdominal pain	Unknown	Most foods
Biotin	Water soluble; synthesized by intestinal bacteria; deficiency only with large intake of egg whites, TPN	Coenzyme: acetyl CoA carboxylase	Dermatitis, anorexia, muscle pain, pallor, alopecia	Unknown	Liver, egg yolk, peanuts
Vitamin K (naphthoquinones)	Fat soluble; bile necessary for absorption; synthesis of intestinal bacteria	Blood coagulation; factors II, VII, IX, X	Hemorrhagic manifestations	Water-soluble analogues only: hyperbilirubinemia	Cow's milk, green leafy vegetables, pork, liver

CoA, coenzyme A; TPN, total parenteral nutrition.
Reprinted with permission from Committee on Nutrition, American Academy of Pediatrics. Pediatric nutrition handbook, 3rd. ed. Elk Grove Village, IL: American Academy of Pediatrics. 1998: 136.

TABLE 14.6
CONTENT OF INFANT FEEDINGS[a]

| Name | Percent of Calories | | | Cal/mL | Sodium | | Chloride | | Potassium | | Calcium | | Phosphate | | Renal Solute |
	P	Fat	CHO		mEq/L	mEq/100 cal	mEq/L	mEq/100 cal	mEq/L	mEq/100 cal	mEq/L	mEq/100 cal	mEq/L	mEq/100 cal	(mOsm/100 cal)
Human milk	8	51	41	0.67	6	0.9	10	1.4	12	1.8	340	51	150	22.4	12
Whole cow's milk	22	49	29	0.67	22	3.3	30	4.5	37	5.5	1,200	180	930	139	33
Skim cow's milk	40	5	55	0.34	22	6.6	30	9.0	37	4.1	1,200	133	930	103	24
Evaporated cow's milk: H$_2$O 1:1 + 5 g CHO/dL	17	37	46	0.9	22	2.4	30	3.3	37	41	1,200	133	930	103	24
Evaporated milk: H$_2$O 1:1 + 10 g CHO/dL	11	33	56	1.1	22	2	30	2.7	37	3.4	1,200	109	930	85	20
Infant formula[b]	10	50	40	0.67	8	1.2	12	1.8	15	2.4	520	73	400	60	16
Infant formula + 5 g CHO/dL	8	42	50	0.87	8	0.9	12	1.4	15	1.7	520	60	400	46	12
Pregestimil[c] protein hydrolysate no lactose	13	36	51	0.67	13	1.9	16	2.4	18	2.7	600	90	400	60	19
PM 60–40[c] low mineral milk	9	50	41	0.67	7	1	13	1.7	15	2.2	400	56	200	28	14

CHO, carbohydrate; P, protein.

[a]The infant feedings illustrate the problem in trying to reduce sodium and other renal solute while maintaining an adequate protein intake. The practical minimum of protein is approximately 8% of total daily calories when from a high-quality animal source (12% to 15% from vegetable sources). When cow's milk or other protein is used (as contrasted to human), it is wiser to use a higher minimum because digestion and absorption may be inefficient, although theoretically an even lower protein percentage intake may be successful. The usual modifier for feedings is carbohydrate, which produces no renal solute. Renal solute comes from protein, primarily as urea, and from minerals primarily sodium salts. Note that when the sodium load is reduced by carbohydrate dilution so is the phosphorus load; which also may be important in other conditions. Not also that skim milk, when a major portion of the diet is a particularly poor feeding providing a maximum stress to water balance.

[b]Representative of the major commercial infant formulas.

[c]Commercial preparations; product composition as of 1994.

Reprinted with permission from Finberg L, Kravath RE, Hellerstein S. Water and electrolytes in pediatrics. *Philadelphia: Saunders, 1993.*

Human milk also contains antibodies and macrophages that help protect the infant from gastrointestinal pathogens and possibly other deleterious organisms. As important, a psychological bonding effect occurs during breast-feeding that helps ensure nurturing. Moreover, the mother–infant dyad also ensures a proper caloric supply, because vigorous sucking by the infant determines maternal milk production, which in turn leads to infant satiety, reducing the vigor of sucking.

The nutrient content of human milk serves the complete needs of the infant for the first 4 to 5 months of life, with the exception of vitamin D. That substance, cholecalciferol, is produced in the skin from 7-dehydrocholesterol by the action of ultraviolet light. In modern urban environments in the temperate zone, the breast-fed infant should receive a supplement of vitamin D, at least 200 units in aqueous form daily. The iron content of human milk is low but very well absorbed. The infant is born with excess hemoglobin in the blood for the oxygen environment outside the uterus; therefore, the breakdown of red cells provides excess iron, which is stored in the reticuloendothelial system. Rapid growth with an increasing blood volume reclaims this iron for optimal hemoglobin concentration in 3 to 4 months. The iron derived from breast milk adds another month or so, and by the time they are 5 months of age, most infants require more iron than breast-feeding supplies to meet the needs of their increasing blood volume. At this time, swallowing has matured sufficiently to accept the solid foods that should be offered to supply the needed iron.

Feeding Process

The technique of feeding is important for early success. An optimal time and place to start nursing is shortly after birth. The mother should support her breast either with the thumb and forefinger above the areola with the other fingers below (scissor grip) or with all of the fingers under the breast with only the thumb above (palmer grip). The nipple should be placed squarely into the infant's mouth so that he may latch on securely with a tight seal. The infant should initially be allowed about 5 minutes on one breast, and then allowed about 5 minutes or so on the other. The first fluid received is colostrum, which has fewer nutrients, but more immune factors than the milk produced a few days later. Once an optimal nursing encounter has occurred over the first 2 days, the act of suckling causes a release of oxytocin and produces the "let-down" phenomenon of spontaneous lactation. In time, this reflex occurs when the mother hears the infant cry or sees the infant receptive to feeding. The very occurrence of let-down signifies the establishment of a good early nursing relationship. Emptying of the breast by suckling or pumping stimulates prolactin release and completes the mechanical–endocrine cycle.

The starting breast should be the alternated with each feeding. Usually, the infant will nurse about eight times a day. It is wise to allow the infant's hunger to determine the schedule, taking care not to let prolonged nursing on an empty breast cause soreness and inflammation.

The breast-fed infant may exhibit a wide range of stooling patterns, ranging from a stool with each feeding to as few as one every 2 days. The stools produced by the infant during breast-feeding lack a foul odor and will persist for as long as no other food is supplemented.

Problems Associated With Breast-feeding

Jaundice in excess of the usual neonatal "physiologic" bilirubin levels in plasma occurs in infants who are breast-fed because of caloric deprivation, slow stool evacuation, or both. Supplying supplemental glucose water feedings aggravates this increase. As the milk supply comes in and more rapid stooling begins, this breast-feeding phenomenon resolves. One must make sure that no concomitant pathologic cause exists for the jaundice.

In about 0.5% of infants, breast-feeding is associated with an increase in the unconjugated bilirubin level in plasma between the fourth and ninth day of life. This is attributed to an inhibiting substance, possibly by a fatty acid in the milk, which suppresses glucuronidation in the infant liver. The bilirubin level decreases if breast-feeding is suspended, but this is rarely necessary, because no consequence of this type of hyperbilirubinemia occurs. If the cause of jaundice is uncertain, one day of pumping the breast while giving formula to the infant leads to a significant decline in bilirubin levels, and feeding should be resumed.

If the mother does not get the infant to suckle because of inexperience or other problems in the early days, starvation and water deprivation leading to hypernatremic dehydration occurs. Any low-volume output state results in an increased concentration of all the solutes in the milk. Colostrum also has a higher concentration of minerals and protein when the volume is low. This increased concentration of sodium and chloride (usually as much as 40 to 50 mEq/L) is not sufficient to cause hypernatremia if the volume is sufficient for the minimal water requirement. Thus, water deprivation, not increased solute, is causal and should be remedied by appropriate fluid therapy while an effort is made to increase milk production by the mother.

Contraindications to breast-feeding are few. In general, they include in the mother the presence of chronic infection not quickly reversible (e.g., active pulmonary tuberculosis, HIV) and the use of certain drugs. In most cases, the agents are antineoplastic or antithyroid drugs, but also include illicit drugs such as cocaine and heroin. The *AAP Nutrition Handbook* provides a more complete list. Obviously, drugs that suppress lactation, such as bromocriptine, are contraindicated for the mother. Virtually everything that appears in either the maternal plasma or her lipid tissue appears in the milk. Water-soluble molecules come from the plasma, at plasma concentrations, and usually produce insignificant effects. However, lipid-soluble molecules may become concentrated in the milk because of its high fat content.

Formula Feeding

Every effort should be made to encourage breast-feeding, but such efforts should not include intimidation or the provocation of guilt. Some women find the process unattractive or even repugnant. The feeding of infant formula also will satisfy completely the nutritional needs of the infant for growth. Adequate affection and bonding also are achievable easily.

On the other hand, the necessity of the mother's working does not necessarily interdict nursing. The use of a breast pump and a refrigerator at the work site readily accommodates nursing when direct breast-feeding is not possible.

Cow's Milk Preparations

To make cow's milk suitable for infants, it must be modified. The important differences between unmodified whole cow's milk and human milk are shown in Table 14.6. In the United States, a number of manufacturers supply infant formula that conforms to mandatory U.S. Food and Drug Administration (FDA) specifications, which in turn have been based on advice from the Committee on Nutrition of the Academy of Pediatrics. Protein and lactose are extracted from cow's milk, the protein is modified and reduced in amount, and both it and lactose are returned to the formula. Vegetable fat is substituted for butter fat, with some variance in composition by differing manufacturers. Vitamin and accessory substances are added, and the mineral composition is adjusted toward that of human milk. The addition of vitamin C, which is lacking in cow's milk, and the addition of vitamin D, which is not adequate in human milk, make the formula nutritionally complete and obviate the need for supplementation. The addition of iron to the infant formula takes care of the need for the entire first year of life, if the formula is fed for that period. The amount of iron present does not cause either diarrhea or constipation, as has occasionally been alleged. No need ever exists to use the so-called "low iron" formulas.

Formula also may be made from mixing evaporated milk, water, and a carbohydrate source such as sucrose, corn syrup, or dextromaltose. At one time, these mixtures served as the formula for most infants in the United States. Since 1998, less than 1% of American infants are fed using this formula. The reason to use such mixtures is to reduce monetary expense at the cost of increased labor and some risk from inappropriate mixing and from contamination. The carbohydrate is added to dilute the high mineral content of cow's milk, especially the phosphate, and then water is added to bring the caloric density back to that of human or cow's milk, 0.67 cal/mL or 670 cal/L. The previously recommended mixture of 13 oz evaporated milk (EM), 17 oz water, and 2 tablespoons of sugar or corn syrup can no longer be conveniently accomplished, because EM is now available in a 12-oz can. However, 12 oz EM, 18 oz water, plus 2 tablespoons of sugar or corn syrup is quite satisfactory, although the phosphate is a bit high for the first week of life. EM has added vitamin D but not vitamin C, and to avoid deficiency, vitamin C must be supplemented either through drops or orange juice.

Soy Milk Preparations

Soy "milk" products and special formulas in which the protein is hydrolyzed to amino acids also are available. The soy products use glucose and corn syrup for carbohydrate instead of lactose. They are often prescribed for cow's milk intolerance or cow's milk allergy, although such conditions are uncommon. If an infant has true allergy to cow's milk protein, then amino acid hydrolysate mixtures, although expensive, are better choices, because soy protein is as likely to cause allergic reaction as cow's milk protein. Lactase deficiency in infancy is very rare, although it has become increasingly common in African American, Asian, and some white children older than 2 years.

Use of Formulas

The prepared infant formulas are sold in three forms of decreasing expense: ready to feed, concentrated liquid that requires dilution with an equal amount of water, and a powdered form that requires preparation by mixing. Care must be taken with the latter two to keep the mixing accurate, so that feedings are neither overconcentrated nor dilute. If the bottle is prepared fresh for each feeding, sterilization is not required. Partially consumed, used formula should not be kept longer than 1 hour. Unused formula may be stored in a refrigerator for up to about 8 hours. If longer storage is required for prepared formula, terminal sterilization (placing bottles in boiling water for 20 minutes) should be used.

FEEDING THE OLDER CHILD

Six Months to One Year of Age

By 6 months to 1 year, the infant's swallowing mechanisms have matured, and she is ready for solid foods. Of course, juices may be offered sooner. For the breast-fed infant, foods containing iron, such as fortified cereals and vegetable–meat mixtures, are important. Although cereal has become a traditional first solid, many infants accept the slightly sweet pureed vegetables or fruits more readily. Each new food should be introduced one at a time, with a day or two between. After a few weeks, the diet can be quite varied, with two to three solids (1 or 2 tablespoons each) offered two or three times daily. The same program should be offered to formula-fed infants. Unless an adverse reaction occurs (uncommon) to a food, the entire diet of properly prepared food may be offered, as long as it is initially pureed and then increasingly textured as teeth appear.

Near the end of the first year is the customary weaning period from breast or bottle in present-day Western society, although other cultures wean infants either earlier or even much later. Breast-fed infants usually may be weaned directly to the cup if weaning occurs during this period.

Second Year

At about the second year, the period of very rapid growth has passed, and the infant's previously robust appetite has slackened. Social interactions also have become complex, and parents often are puzzled by periods of food refusal. Such behavior is usual at this age, and is interspersed with periods of eating more avidly. The weight gain during the second year may be only 3 to 4 lbs (1½ to 2½ kg), whereas the growth curve for length is normal. Failure to grow normally is the only cause for nutritional concern.

Two to Five Years of Age

During this time, the diet expands to that of the adult range. Emphasis should be on variety, with adequate protein, some of it from an animal source (milk, eggs, meat, including fish and poultry) and sufficient calories. Because of concern about the harmful effects of saturated fat in later years, many believe it prudent to restrict fat to not more than 30% of calories, and saturated fat to 10% or less. This may be done in a common-sense way, without compulsive attention, such as supplying skim milk and a minimum of butter and trans-fat margarines. If parents insist for cultural or religious reasons on a completely vegetarian diet, then vegetables, grains (rice, corn), and beans should be matched for their complementary amino acid deficiencies. As long as milk and or eggs are included, such a diet is safe. However, a total absence of all animal protein causes deficiency of vitamin B_{12}, and if the vegetables are not matched properly, even more serious malnutrition will result. Occasional binges for a single food occur from time to time during this period and are usually self limited and harmless.

Six to Thirteen Years of Age

During this period, the diet becomes that of the adult in range, although sophistication in spicing nuance is usually deferred by taste choice. Good nutrition supports school performance. In inner-city children, who commonly may have nutritional problems, the school breakfast program and the school lunch program should be encouraged. As the pubertal period approaches, the caloric consumption increases markedly.

Adolescence

Particular attention to iron and calcium intake, especially in girls, is important at this time of accelerated growth in general and of the skeleton in particular. The eating of fast food becomes common; this is not necessarily harmful if balanced

Anatomy of MyPyramid

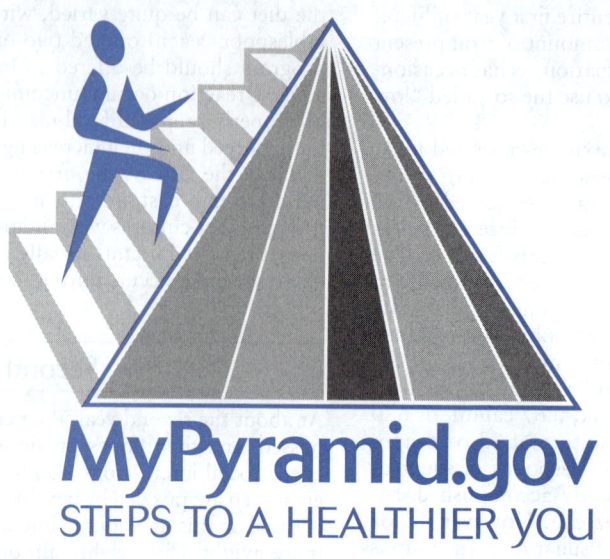

| GRAINS | VEGETABLES | FRUITS | OILS | MILK | MEAT& BEANS |

FIGURE 14.1. U.S. Department of Agriculture "My Pyramid" recommendations for overall healthy eating. (Reproduced with permission from U.S. Department of Agriculture Center for Nutrition Policy and Promotion.)

over intervals of a couple of weeks with other items. High fat intake, particularly of saturated fat, should not exceed the advised limits, although occasional individual meals may do so.

Society's fascination with leanness in women has produced a special problem for adolescent girls, which parents and physicians need to combat. [For more information on problematic eating behaviors, please see Chapter 108, Eating Disorders.] For an overall healthy diet, Figure 14.1 shows the U.S. Department of Agriculture's recommendations, which are applicable to anyone older than 2 years.

Suggested Readings

Finberg L, Kravath RE, Hellerstein S. *Water and electrolytes in pediatrics,* 2nd ed. Philadelphia: W.B. Saunders, 1993.

Foman SJ. *Nutrition of normal infants.* St. Louis: CV Mosby Co., 1993.

Kleinman RE, ed. *Pediatric nutrition handbook,* 5th ed. Elks Grove Village, IL: American Academy of Pediatrics, 2003–2004.

Lawrence RA. *Breast-feeding,* 3rd ed. St. Louis: CV Mosby Co., 1989.

National Research Council. *Recommended Dietary Allowances,* 10th ed. Washington, D.C.: National Academy Press, 1989.

American Academy of Pediatrics Nutrition Handbook, 5th edition. 2004.

CHAPTER 15 ■ IMMUNIZATION

NEAL A. HALSEY

Immunizations are among the most efficacious and cost-effective interventions available to improve the health and well-being of children. In the second half of the twentieth century, smallpox has been eradicated, wild-type poliomyelitis viruses have been eliminated from all but a few countries, and the global efforts to eradicate wild-type polioviruses from the world should be completed by the time this book is published. Measles, mumps, rubella, tetanus, diphtheria, and *Haemophilus influenzae* type b (Hib) infections have been reduced to levels that are 99% or more lower than the prevaccination era in the United States.

Several vaccines have been added to the routine immunization schedule in recent years, including hepatitis B, varicella, and pneumococcal conjugate vaccines that have already had an impact on childhood disease; other vaccines in development will prevent additional infectious diseases and cancers, further reducing the burden of disease in children and adults.

ROUTINE IMMUNIZATION SCHEDULE

The American Academy of Pediatrics (AAP), the American Academy of Family Physicians, and the Advisory Committee on Immunization Practices (ACIP) of the Centers for Disease Control and Prevention (CDC) jointly prepare an updated immunization schedule every January, which is published in the *Pediatrics*, *Morbidity and Mortality Weekly Report* and in *Family Physician* (Fig. 15.1).

Locations of Current Immunization Information

The schedule and other valuable information about recommended vaccines can be found on the CDC's Web site (www.cdc.gov/nip). Readers are encouraged to obtain updated schedules every year and familiarize themselves with the changes. Specific information regarding each vaccine and details regarding the immunization process are available in the *Red Book* (Report of the Committee on Infectious Diseases), which is published every 3 years. The CDC also publishes a document entitled "General Guidelines on Immunization" (www.cdc.gov/nip/publications/acip-list.htm), which summarizes key recommendations and is updated periodically.

The annual updating of the Recommended Childhood and Adolescent Immunization Schedule reflects the rapidly changing field of immunizations and the need for physicians to have access to this information in a timely manner.

Web sites with the most recent guidelines are maintained by the CDC's ACIP (www.cdc.gov/nip/acip) and the AAP's Committee on Infectious Diseases (www.aap.org). The Food and Drug Administration (FDA) also maintains a detailed Web site with valuable information on vaccines, additives, recalls, the approval process, and recent recommendations of advisory committees (www.fda.gov/cber/vaccines.htm). Additional general information on immunization is available on the Immunization Action Coalition's Web site (www.immunize.org). Information on vaccine safety is available on the Institute for Vaccine Safety's (www.vaccinesafety.edu), the FDA's, and the CDC's Web sites.

Vaccine Information Statements and Record Keeping

Health care providers are required to provide specific information to parents before administering vaccines. Vaccine information statements are updated periodically by the CDC and are available from health departments, the CDC's Web site, and the AAP. Physicians are required by law to maintain careful immunization records on all children under their care, including the type of vaccine administered, lot number, manufacturer, date of immunization, and clinic or office where the vaccine was administered. Assistance with record keeping is available from both the AAP and the CDC; efforts are under way to label every vaccine vial with bar codes to simplify the data-collecting process for physicians.

Additional information is available on package inserts included with each vaccine. At times, the guidelines from advisory committees are in conflict with information in the package insert. Advisory committees take into account societal factors and incorporate knowledge from other vaccines to provide guidelines when data are limited. Vaccine companies are permitted to seek approval for indications supported by data specific to their product, and the companies often add cautions

or contraindications to circulars to protect themselves from possible litigation in areas of uncertainty.

Catch-Up Immunization Schedules

For children who are behind in the immunization schedule, including recent adoptees without evidence of previous immunizations, an accelerated immunization schedule is recommended (Tables 15.1a and 15.1b).

Schedule for Adoptees

The World Health Organization (WHO) recommends the immunization schedule presented in Table 15.2. In general, vaccines produced in other countries meet WHO standards, and written immunization records from a reliable source indicating receipt of these vaccines should suffice for adequate evidence of protection against the diseases. Although the intervals for administering the first three doses of the diphtheria, tetanus, and pertussis (DTP) vaccine and oral poliovirus (OPV) vaccine are shorter than routinely recommended in the United States, these schedules have been shown to be effective and are acceptable for DTP and OPV. Recent data generated in the United Kingdom indicate that the Hib vaccine administered at 2, 3, and 4 months of age may not have provided optimal protection against disease when no booster dose was given. Verbal immunization histories for adopted children generally should not be accepted. In most developing countries, several vaccines that are routinely administered to children in the United States are often not available, including rubella, mumps, varicella, and Hib vaccines. The use of the hepatitis B vaccine has increased in developing countries, with more than 100 countries administering the vaccine in programs to all infants. When doubt exists regarding the accuracy of immunization records, children should be reimmunized in accordance with the catch-up immunization schedule (see Tables 15.1a and 15.1b).

Lapsed or Delayed Immunizations

Intervals longer than recommended for routine immunization are commonly encountered in children who do not have regular health care providers or who have lived overseas. Intervals longer than recommended are not an indication for restarting the immunization schedule at any age. Immunologic memory is induced by one or two doses of vaccine, which appears to be long lasting. Even if a sufficient response was not induced to provide long-term protective levels of antibody, subsequent doses administered years later induce a secondary antibody response to tetanus, diphtheria, hepatitis B, and other vaccines. For live viral vaccines, the purpose of the second (or third) dose is to induce immunity in children who did not respond to the first vaccine. Therefore, intervals are not an important variable to consider when administering vaccines to children with delayed or lapsed immunization. The appropriate number of doses needed to complete the series should be administered.

Immunization Tracking

Physicians are actively encouraged to maintain a formal tracking system to identify infants and young children who are deficient in immunizations. Special software is available through the CDC to assist with tracking and assessing the immunization status of all children in a pediatric practice.

Recommended Childhood and Adolescent Immunization Schedule UNITED STATES • 2006

Vaccine ▼ Age ▶	Birth	1 month	2 months	4 months	6 months	12 months	15 months	18 months	24 months	4–6 years	11–12 years	13–14 years	15 years	16–18 years
Hepatitis B[1]	HepB	HepB		HepB[1]		HepB					HepB Series			
Diphtheria, Tetanus, Pertussis[2]			DTaP	DTaP	DTaP		DTaP			DTaP	Tdap		Tdap	
Haemophilus influenzae type b[3]			Hib	Hib	Hib[3]	Hib								
Inactivated Poliovirus			IPV	IPV		IPV				IPV				
Measles, Mumps, Rubella[4]						MMR				MMR		MMR		
Varicella[5]						Varicella					Varicella			
Meningococcal[6]							Vaccines within broken line are for selected populations		MPSV4		MCV4		MCV4	MCV4
Pneumococcal[7]			PCV	PCV	PCV	PCV			PCV		PPV			
Influenza[8]					Influenza (Yearly)					Influenza (Yearly)				
Hepatitis A[9]									HepA Series					

Legend: ▨ Range of recommended ages   ▮ Catch-up immunization   ▮ 11–12 year old assessment

This schedule indicates the recommended ages for routine administration of currently licensed childhood vaccines, as of December 1, 2005, for children through age 18 years. Any dose not administered at the recommended age should be administered at any subsequent visit when indicated and feasible. ▮ Indicates age groups that warrant special effort to administer those vaccines not previously administered. Additional vaccines may be licensed and recommended during the year. Licensed combination vaccines may be used whenever any components of the combination are indicated and other components of the vaccine are not contraindicated and if approved by the Food and Drug Administration for that dose of the series. Providers should consult the respective ACIP statement for detailed recommendations. Clinically significant adverse events that follow immunization should be reported to the Vaccine Adverse Event Reporting System (VAERS). Guidance about how to obtain and complete a VAERS form is available at www.vaers.hhs.gov or by telephone, 800-822-7967.

FIGURE 15.1. Recommended childhood and adolescent immunization schedule, United States, January to December 2004. Approved by the Advisory Committee on Immunization Practices (ACIP), the American Academy of Pediatrics (AAP), and the American Academy of Family Physicians (AAFP).

1. **Hepatitis B vaccine (HepB).** *AT BIRTH:* All newborns should receive monovalent HepB soon after birth and before hospital discharge. **Infants born to mothers who are HBsAg-positive** should receive HepB and 0.5 mL of hepatitis B immune globulin (HBIG) within 12 hours of birth. **Infants born to mothers whose HBsAg status is unknown** should receive HepB within 12 hours of birth. The mother should have blood drawn as soon as possible to determine her HBsAg status; if HBsAg-positive, the infant should receive HBIG as soon as possible (no later than age 1 week). **For infants born to HBsAg-negative mothers**, the birth dose can be delayed in rare circumstances but only if a physician's order to withhold the vaccine and a copy of the mother's original HBsAg-negative laboratory report are documented in the infant's medical record. *FOLLOWING THE BIRTHDOSE:* The HepB series should be completed with either monovalent HepB or a combination vaccine containing HepB. The second dose should be administered at age 1–2 months. The final dose should be administered at age ≥24 weeks. It is permissible to administer 4 doses of HepB (e.g., when combination vaccines are given after the birth dose); however, if monovalent HepB is used, a dose at age 4 months is not needed. **Infants born to HBsAg-positive mothers** should be tested for HBsAg and antibody to HBsAg after completion of the HepB series, at age 9–18 months (generally at the next well-child visit after completion of the vaccine series).

2. **Diphtheria and tetanus toxoids and acellular pertussis vaccine (DTaP).** The fourth dose of DTaP may be administered as early as age 12 months, provided 6 months have elapsed since the third dose and the child is unlikely to return at age 15–18 months. The final dose in the series should be given at age ≥4 years. **Tetanus and diphtheria toxoids and acellular pertussis vaccine (Tdap—adolescent preparation)** is recommended at age 11–12 years for those who have completed the recommended childhood DTP/DTaP vaccination series and have not received a Td booster dose. Adolescents 13–18 years who missed the 11–12-year Td/Tdap booster dose should also receive a single dose of Tdap if they have completed the recommended childhood DTP/DTaP vaccination series. Subsequent **tetanus and diphtheria toxoids (Td)** are recommended every 10 years.

3. *Haemophilus influenzae* **type b conjugate vaccine (Hib).** Three Hib conjugate vaccines are licensed for infant use. If PRP-OMP (PedvaxHIB® or ComVax® [Merck]) is administered at ages 2 and 4 months, a dose at age 6 months is not required. DTaP/Hib combination products should not be used for primary immunization in infants at ages 2, 4 or 6 months but can be used as boosters after any Hib vaccine. The final dose in the series should be administered at age ≥12 months.

4. **Measles, mumps, and rubella vaccine (MMR).** The second dose of MMR is recommended routinely at age 4–6 years but may be administered during any visit, provided at least 4 weeks have elapsed since the first dose and both doses are administered beginning at or after age 12 months. Those who have not previously received the second dose should complete the schedule by age 11–12 years.

5. **Varicella vaccine.** Varicella vaccine is recommended at any visit at or after age 12 months for susceptible children (i.e., those who lack a reliable history of chickenpox). Susceptible persons aged ≥13 years should receive 2 doses administered at least 4 weeks apart.

6. **Meningococcal vaccine (MCV4).** Meningococcal conjugate vaccine (MCV4) should be given to all children at the 11–12 year old visit as well as to unvaccinated adolescents at high school entry (15 years of age). Other adolescents who wish to decrease their risk for meningococcal disease may also be vaccinated. All college fresh men living in dormitories should also be vaccinated, preferably with MCV4, although **meningococcal polysaccharide vaccine (MPSV4)** is an acceptable alternative. Vaccination against invasive meningococcal disease is recommended for children and adolescents aged ≥2 years with terminal complement deficiencies or anatomic

(Continued)

TABLE 15.1a

FOR CHILDREN AND ADOLESCENTS WHO START LATE OR WHO ARE MORE THAN 1 MONTH BEHIND UNITED STATES, 2006

Catch up Schedule for Children Aged 4 Months to 6 Years Dose 1 (Minimum Age)	Minimum Interval Between Doses			
	Dose 1 to Dose 2	Dose 2 to Dose 3	Dose 3 to Dose 4	Dose 4 to Dose 5
DTaP (6 weeks)	4 weeks	4 weeks	6 months	6 months[1]
IPV (6 weeks)	4 weeks	4 weeks	4 weeks[2]	
Hep B[3] (birth)	4 weeks	8 weeks (and 16 weeks after first dose)		
MMR (12 months)	4 weeks[4]			
Varicella (12 months)				
Hib[5] (6 weeks)	4 weeks: if first dose given at age <12 months 8 weeks (as final dose): if first dose given at age 12–14 months No further doses needed: if first dose given at age ≥15 months	4 weeks[6]: if current age <12 months 8 weeks (as final dose)[6]: if current age ≥12 months and second dose given at age <15 months No further doses needed: if previous dose given at age ≥15 months	8 weeks (as final dose): this dose only necessary for children age 12 months–5 years who received three doses before age 12 months	
PCV[7]: (6 weeks)	4 weeks: if first dose given at age <12 months and current age <24 months 8 weeks (as final dose): if first dose given at age ≥12 months or current age 24–59 months No further doses needed: for healthy children if first dose given at age ≥24 months	4 weeks: if current age <12 months 8 weeks (as final dose): if current age ≥12 months No further doses needed: for healthy children if previous dose given at age ≥24 months	8 weeks (as final dose): this dose only necessary for children age 12 months–5 years who received three doses before age 12 months	

DTaP, diphtheria, tetanus, and acellular pertussis; IPV, inactivated poliovirus; Hep B, hepatitis B; MMR, measles, mumps, and rubella; Hib, *Haemophilus influenzae* type b; PCV, pneumococcal conjugate vaccine.

This table gives catch-up schedules and minimum intervals between doses for children who have delayed immunizations. There is no need to restart a vaccine series regardless of the time that has elapsed between doses. Use the chart appropriate for the child's age.

1. DTaP: The fifth dose is not necessary if the fourth dose was given after the fourth birthday.
2. IPV: For children who received an all-IPV or all-oral poliovirus (OPV) series, a fourth dose is not necessary if third dose was given at an age older than 4 years. If both OPV and IPV were given as part of a series, a total of four doses should be given, regardless of the child's current age.
3. Hep B: Administer the 3-dose series to all children and adolescents younger than 19 years of age if they were not previously vaccinated.
4. MMR: The second dose of MMR is recommended routinely at age 4 to 6 years but may be given earlier if desired.
5. Hib: Vaccine is not generally recommended for children aged older than 5 years.
6. Hib: If current age is younger than 12 months and the first two doses were PRP-OMP (PedvaxHIB or ComVax [Merck]), the third (and final) dose should be given at age 12 to 15 months and at least 8 weeks after the second dose.
7. PCV: Vaccine is not generally recommended for children aged older than 5 years.

Source: National Immunization Program—Centers for Disease Control and Prevention. www.cdc.gov/nip/recs/child-catchup.pdf

FIGURE 15.1. (Continued) or functional asplenia and certain other high risk groups (see *MMWR* 2005;54 [RR-7]:1-21); use MPSV4 for children aged 2–10 years and MCV4 for older children, although MPSV4 is an acceptable alternative.

7. **Pneumococcal vaccine.** The heptavalent **pneumococcal conjugate vaccine (PCV)** is recommended for all children aged 2–23 months and for certain children aged 24–59 months. The final dose in the series should be given at age ≥12 months. **Pneumococcal polysaccharide vaccine (PPV)** is recommended in addition to PCV for certain high-risk groups. See *MMWR* 2000;49(RR-9):1-35.

8. **Influenza vaccine.** Influenza vaccine is recommended annually for children aged ≥6 months with certain risk factors (including, but not limited to, asthma, cardiac disease, sickle cell disease, human immunodeficiency virus [HIV], diabetes, and conditions that can compromise respiratory function or handling of respiratory secretions or that can increase the risk for aspiration), healthcare workers, and other persons (including household members) in close contact with persons in groups at high risk (see *MMWR* 2005;54[RR-8]:1-55). In addition, healthy children aged 6–23 months and close contacts of healthy children aged 0–5 months are recommended to receive influenza vaccine because children in this age group are at substantially increased risk for influenza-related hospitalizations. For healthy persons aged 5–49 years, the intranasally administered, live, attenuated influenza vaccine (LAIV) is an acceptable alternative to the intramuscular trivalent inactivated influenza vaccine (TIV). See *MMWR* 2005;54(RR-8):1-55. Children receiving TIV should be administered a dosage appropriate for their age (0.25 mL if aged 6–35 months or 0.5 mL if aged ≥3 years). Children aged ≤8 years who are receiving influenza vaccine for the first time should receive 2 doses (separated by at least 4 weeks for TIV and at least 6 weeks for LAIV).

9. **Hepatitis A vaccine (HepA).** HepA is recommended for all children at 1 year of age (i.e., 12–23 months). The 2 doses in the series should be administered at least 6 months apart. States, counties, and communities with existing HepA vaccination programs for children 2–18 years of age are encouraged to maintain these programs. In these areas, new efforts focused on routine vaccination of 1-year-old children should enhance, not replace, ongoing programs directed at a broader population of children. HepA is also recommended for certain high risk groups (see *MMWR* 1999;48[RR-12]:1-37).

TABLE 15.1b

FOR CHILDREN AND ADOLESCENTS WHO START LATE OR WHO ARE MORE THAN 1 MONTH BEHIND UNITED STATES, 2006

Catch-up Schedule for Children Age 7 through 18 Years	Minimum Interval Between Doses		
	Dose 1 to Dose 2	Dose 2 to Dose 3	Dose 3 to Booster Dose
Td[1]	4 weeks	6 months	6 months: if first dose given at age <12 months and current age <11 years 5 years: if first dose given at age >12 months and third dose given at age <7 years and current age >11 years 10 years: if third dose given at age >7 years
IPV[2]	4 weeks	4 weeks	IPV[2]
Hep B	4 weeks	8 weeks (and 16 weeks after first dose)	
MMR	4 weeks		
Varicella[3]	4 weeks		

IPV, inactivated poliovirus; Hep B, hepatitis B; MMR, measles, mumps, and rubella; Td, diphtheria toxoid.

This table gives catch-up schedules and minimum intervals between doses for children who have delayed immunizations. There is no need to restart a vaccine series regardless of the time that has elapsed between doses. Use the chart appropriate for the child's age.)

1. Td: Adolescent tetanus, diphtheria, and pertussis vaccine (Tdap) may be substituted for any dose in a primary catch-up series or as a booster if age appropriate for Tdap. A five-year interval from the last Td dose is encouraged when Tdap is used as a booster dose. See ACIP recommendations for further information.
2. IPV: For children who received an all-IPV or all-oral poliovirus (OPV) series, a fourth dose is not necessary if third dose was given at an age older than 4 years. If both OPV and IPV were given as part of a series, a total of four doses should be given, regardless of the child's current age. Vaccine is not generally recommended for persons aged older than 18 years.
3. Varicella: Give two-dose series to all susceptible adolescents aged older than 13 years.

Source: National Immunization Program—Centers for Disease Control and Prevention. www.cdc.gov/nip/recs/child-catchup.pdf

GENERAL OVERVIEW OF IMMUNIZATION

Vaccines

Vaccines act by stimulating specific immune responses that prevent either infection or disease from the naturally occurring organisms. Several methods have been used to produce the vaccines that are in use today (Table 15.3).

Passive Immunization

Passive immunization involves the administration of preformed antibody in the form of intramuscular immunoglobulin, intravenous immunoglobulin (IGIV), or concentrated monoclonal antibodies. Specific immunoglobulin preparations and their indications are shown in Table 15.4.

Most passive immunization is administered after high-risk exposure to individuals who have not been immunized against the disease in question and to those at high risk of severe complications, such as children born to women who are chronic carriers of hepatitis B surface antigen. Preexposure prophylaxis occurs in patients with underlying immune deficiency disorders who are incapable of developing protective levels of antibody after immunization or in persons who are at increased risk of exposure and cannot receive a vaccine, such as children under 2 years of age who need to be protected against hepatitis A infections. Replacement immune globulin therapy for patients with immune deficiency disorders requires monthly infusions of IGIV.

Adverse reactions have occurred after administration of all immunoglobulin preparations, but these reactions are usually mild and self-limited. Fever and chills occur at times during infusion of IGIV. Aseptic meningitis occurs in less than 1% of IGIV recipients, but headache, myalgia, light-headedness, nausea, and vomiting occur somewhat more commonly. Flushing, hypertension, and tachycardia can occur from vasomotor instability or volume overload. Hypersensitivity reactions occur rarely, but selective IgA-deficient individuals develop antibodies to IgA after infusions of IGIV. Therefore, IgA-deficient individuals normally do not receive replacement immunoglobulin therapy. In rare instances when therapy is needed, IgA-depleted IGIV is indicated.

All human immunoglobulin and other blood-derived preparations carry a theoretical risk of transmission of infectious agents. Multiple procedures are required in the preparation of the products to ensure the inactivation of all known transmissible agents, but the potential exists for unknown agents to be transmitted, as occurred before identification of the hepatitis C virus.

TABLE 15.2

IMMUNIZATION SCHEDULE OF THE EXPANDED PROGRAM ON IMMUNIZATION OF THE WORLD HEALTH ORGANIZATION[a]

Age	Vaccines	Hepatitis B	
		Schedule A	Schedule B
Birth	BCG, OPV	HBV	—
6 weeks	DTP, OPV	HBV	HBV
10 weeks	DTP, OPV	—	HBV
14 weeks	DTP, OPV	HBV	HBV
9 months[b]	Measles, yellow fever[c]	—	—

BCG, bacille Calmette-Guérin; DTP, diphtheria, tetanus, and pertussis vaccine; HBV, hepatitis B vaccine; OPV, oral poliovirus vaccine.
[a]OPV is also administered to all children on the same day in national immunization day campaigns conducted in regions where polio has recently been endemic.
[b]In Latin America, the Pan American Health Organization recommends the measles vaccine at 12 months of age and periodic campaigns to administer supplemental doses.
[c]For endemic areas only.

Vaccine Handling and Storage

Most vaccines should be maintained at refrigerator temperature (2°C to 8°C, 36°F to 46°F). Some vaccines, however,

TABLE 15.3
TYPES OF IMMUNIZING AGENTS

Agent	Examples
Immunoglobulins	
Immune globulin intravenous	Immune globulin intravenous (IGIV)
Purified antibody from human plasma	Immune globulin human (IG)
	Tetanus immune globulin (TIG)
	Rabies hyperimmune plasma immune globulin (RIG)
Monoclonal antibodies	Palivizumab (respiratory syncytial virus monoclonal antibody)
Vaccines	
Inactivated whole organism	Whole-cell pertussis, some influenza vaccines
Purified polysaccharides	Meningococcal vaccine, pneumococcal polysaccharide
Protein subunit	Influenza, hepatitis A
Polysaccharide conjugate	*Haemophilus influenzae, Streptococcus pneumoniae,* or *Neisseria meningitidis* polysaccharides chemically linked with carrier proteins
Toxoids	Tetanus and diphtheria toxoids
Recombinant antigen	Hepatitis B surface antigen
Live viral (attenuated)	Measles, mumps, rubella, varicella, live cold adapted intranasal influenza
Reassortant	Live cold-adapted influenza vaccine

require maintenance at freezer temperatures (e.g., OPV, varicella vaccine), and the temperature requirements for the varicella vaccine are more stringent than for OPV. Lyophilized vaccines can be frozen without harm, but several liquid vaccines (e.g., DTP, inactivated poliovirus [IPV], and hepatitis B) lose potency with freezing because of disruption of bonding with adjuvants, chemical separation, or disruption of antigens. Specific guidelines are available in package inserts.

Sites of Administration

Sites of administration are listed in Box 15.1. The preferred site for intramuscular administration of vaccines is the anterolateral thigh or the deltoid muscle. The anterolateral thigh is usually chosen for infants and toddlers, but some physicians prefer to administer intramuscular injections in the deltoid after 15 months of age to minimize the effect of local reactions on ambulation. The buttocks generally should not be used for immunization because of possible inadvertent damage to the sciatic nerve and the possibility of decreased immunogenicity. The ventrolateral gluteal site is preferred when it is necessary to use the buttocks for injection of large volumes of immunoglobulins. Administration of all vaccines in the recommended schedule may require multiple injections per visit. More than one injection can be given into the same extremity as long as the injections are separated by enough distance to differentiate local reactions, generally 1 to 2 inches.

Recommendations for needle length vary. For subcutaneous injections, 3/8- to 5/8-inch needles are adequate at any site.

TABLE 15.4
PASSIVE IMMUNIZATION PRODUCTS

Product	Use
Rabies immune globulin	Postexposure prophylaxis after high-risk animal exposures
Tetanus immune globulin	Treatment of persons with tetanus, prophylaxis after high-risk injuries in unimmunized persons, and infants born to unimmunized women
Diphtheria antitoxin (horse serum derived)	Treatment of persons with diphtheria
Hepatitis B immune globulin	Infants born to HBsAg-positive mothers and after blood or percutaneous exposure
	Postexposure prophylaxis after high-risk bites
Cytomegalovirus immune globulin intravenous	Posttransplant exposure to high-risk tissues
Respiratory syncytial virus immune globulin intravenous or palivizumab (monoclonal antibody)	Infants and children younger than 2 years at increased risk of severe respiratory syncytial virus infections
Varicella-zoster immune globulin	Postexposure prophylaxis in unimmunized children with underlying immune deficiency disorders
Intravenous immune globulin	Prevention of infection in immunodeficient individuals
	Treatment of chronic parvovirus B19 or persistent enterovirus infection
Botulism immune globulin intravenous (human)	Treatment of infant botulism caused by type A or type B *Clostridium botulinum*
Immune globulin	Prevention of hepatitis A in unimmunized individuals after exposure

Source: U.S. Food and Drug Administration/Center for Biologics Evaluation and Research. www.fda.gov/cber/efoi/approve.htm

---

BOX 15.1   Sites of Administration

Intranasal
  Cold-adapted influenza vaccine
Oral
  Oral poliovirus (OPV) vaccine
Intramuscular
  Diphtheria, tetanus, and acellular pertussis (DTaP)
    vaccines
  Hepatitis B
  Haemophilus influenzae type b (Hib) vaccine
  Inactivated influenza vaccine
  Inactivated poliovirus (IPV) vaccine
Subcutaneous
  Measles, mumps, and rubella (MMR)/measles/rubella
    vaccines
  Meningococcal polysaccharide vaccine
  Pneumococcal conjugate vaccines
  Varicella vaccine

The depth of subcutaneous fat tissue varies by site, age, and nutritional status. For intramuscular injections, the technique used can affect the depth to muscle tissues. The best general advice is to be certain that the needle is long enough to penetrate the middle of the muscle mass and to use the technique that is most appropriate for the size of the individual receiving the intramuscular injection. When the muscle is bunched up, the depth of subcutaneous fat is increased. When the muscle is bunched and the needle is inserted at a 45-degree angle, a 7/8- to 1-inch needle is appropriate for intramuscular injections in infants and most children. However, 5/8-inch needles are appropriate for newborns and have been used successfully in infants younger than 6 months when the injection technique involves flattening of the subcutaneous tissue and injecting at a 90-degree angle. For administration of intramuscular injections in the deltoid muscle, needles of 7/8- to 1-inch in length usually are sufficient in children from 4 to 18 years of age. For females weighing more than 80 kg, a $1^1/_2$-inch needle is needed, and for females weighing more than 120 kg, a 2-inch needle may be necessary.

The needle gauge should be sufficient to allow easy administration of the vaccine. A 25-gauge needle has been used successfully for many vaccines, but for vaccines of a high viscosity, a 23- or 22-gauge needle may be indicated.

Intradermal immunization is uncommon and usually not recommended for primary immunization at any age, with the exception of special formulations of rabies vaccine. A 25- or 27-gauge needle is sufficient.

All injections should be made with a separate needle and syringe. Needles and syringes should be disposed of in proper, safe containers. Needles should not be recapped, because this is a common source of inadvertent needlestick injuries and potential transmission of blood-borne pathogens.

After insertion of the needle to the muscle or subcutaneous tissue, many experts recommend aspiration to be certain that the injection is not intravascular. If a blood return is observed, then the needle should be removed and injected at an alternative site. However, evidence from large-scale immunization clinics where aspiration had not been performed revealed no evidence of increased adverse events and some experts have questioned the need for aspiration. Brief pressure on the injection site is usually sufficient to prevent bleeding. Bandages are not necessary but sometimes are applied for psychological purposes.

Standards on Immunization

To enhance the delivery of immunizations to children, the AAP, the National Vaccine Advisory Committee, and the U.S. Public Health Service have endorsed a set of standards for health care providers who administer vaccines. The detailed recommendations that go with these standards are available through the AAP or the CDC (Table 15.5).

CONTRAINDICATIONS, NONCONTRAINDICATIONS, AND CAUTIONS

Contraindications to Immunizations (CDC 2002)

For children with intact immune systems, there are few absolute contraindications to receiving the first dose of any vaccine. The following general rules apply to all vaccines.

Immediate Hypersensitivity Reactions

Anaphylaxis or angioedema after a previous dose of vaccine or a vaccine component, diluent, or preservative is usually a contraindication to giving subsequent doses of the same vaccine or component unless the person is at high risk of serious complications from the target disease. Vaccines produced in chick embryo tissue cultures, including measles and mumps vaccines, do not contain detectable amounts of egg protein, and children with egg allergy can safely receive these vaccines without skin testing. However, inactivated influenza and yellow fever vaccines are produced in eggs, and true hypersensitivity to egg protein is usually a contraindication to these vaccines. Some hypersensitivity reactions to vaccines are caused by components added to vaccines, such as the gel stabilizer in measles vaccines. Mild allergic reactions are not contraindications to receiving subsequent doses, but may require special investigations. Children who have mild allergic reactions following a dose of vaccine should consult with an allergist or vaccine safety specialist prior to receiving subsequent doses of vaccines.

Encephalopathy or Encephalitis

Encephalopathy or encephalitis within a few days after DTP or diphtheria, tetanus, and acellular pertussis (DTaP) vaccine administration is a contraindication to receipt of subsequent doses. A febrile seizure following any vaccine is not a contraindication to receipt of subsequent doses of the vaccine were other vaccines that might induce fever. Children who have had encephalitis or encephalopathy of unknown cause unrelated to immunizations can safely receive all recommended vaccines if the neurologic condition is stable. Children with progressive neurologic disorders characterized by developmental delay or neurologic findings, such as infantile spasms, should defer the DTaP vaccine until the condition has been diagnosed and the child is stable.

Immune Deficiency Disorder

Inactivated or subcomponent vaccines pose no additional risk to patients with immune deficiency disorders, but some patients may not be protected from the target disease. Live vaccines can cause serious adverse events in patients with immune deficiency disorders, but some patients can safely receive live vaccines. In the absence of an effective host immune system, the live viral or bacterial agents can replicate unchecked

TABLE 15.5

STANDARDS FOR CHILD AND ADOLESCENT IMMUNIZATION

Availability of Vaccines

Standard 1	Vaccination Services Are Readily Available
Standard 2	Vaccinations Are Coordinated with Other Health Care Services and Provided in a Medical Home When Possible
Standard 3	Barriers to Vaccination Are Identified and Minimized
Standard 4	Patient Costs Are Minimized

Assessment of Vaccination Status

Standard 5	Health Care Professionals Review the Vaccination and Health Status of Patients at Every Encounter to Determine Which Vaccines Are Indicated
Standard 6	Health Care Professionals Assess for and Follow Only Medically Accepted Contraindications

Effective Communication About Vaccine Benefits and Risks

Standard 7	Parents/Guardians and Patients Are Educated About the Benefits and Risks of Vaccination in a Culturally Appropriate Manner and in Easy-to-Understand Language

Proper Storage and Administration of Vaccines and Documentation of Vaccinations

Standard 8	Health Care Professionals Follow Appropriate Procedures for Vaccine Storage and Handling
Standard 9	Up-to-Date, Written Vaccination Protocols Are Accessible at All Locations Where Vaccines Are Administered
Standard 10	People Who Administer Vaccines and Staff Who Manage or Support Vaccine Administration Are Knowledgeable and Receive Ongoing Education
Standard 11	Health Care Professionals Simultaneously Administer as Many Indicated Vaccine Doses as Possible
Standard 12	Vaccination Records for Patients Are Accurate, Complete, and Easily Accessible
Standard 13	Health Care Professionals Report Adverse Events After Vaccination Promptly and Accurately to the Vaccine Adverse Events Reporting System (VAERS) and Are Aware of a Separate Program, the National Vaccine Injury Compensation Program (VICP)
Standard 14	All Personnel Who Have Contact with Patients Are Appropriately Vaccinated

Implementation of Strategies to Improve Vaccination Coverage

Standard 15	Systems Are Used to Remind Parents/Guardians, Patients, and Health Care Professionals When Vaccinations Are Due and to Recall Those Who Are Overdue
Standard 16	Office- or Clinic-Based Patient Record Reviews and Vaccination Coverage Assessments Are Performed Annually
Standard 17	Health Care Professionals Practice Community-Based Approaches

Source: Centers for Disease Control and Prevention. *Epidemiology and prevention of vaccine-preventable diseases: the pink book*, 8th ed. 2004. www.cdc.gov/nip/publications/pink/default.htm

and cause serious systemic disease. For example, the risk of vaccine-associated paralysis after the OPV vaccine is increased by at least 1,000-fold in persons with agammaglobulinemia. Some exceptions may be made after consultation with experts in immunology or infectious diseases. Patients with inherited (primary) or acquired immune deficiency disorders should receive specific advice regarding which vaccines they should receive from immunologists or vaccine specialists. Patients with HIV infection can receive live measles, mumps, and rubella (MMR) or varicella vaccines if their CD4 count is greater than 15%. Other patients with primary or acquired deficiency of T cells generally should not receive live viral vaccines. Patients who have been successfully treated for cancer can usually be successfully immunized with both live and inactivated vaccines, but specific waiting times are recommended after completion of chemotherapy and assurance that patients are in remission. Many mild immune deficiency disorders, such as subclass IgG deficiency disorders, have been identified that are not associated with adverse events following immunization. Patients with disorders of white blood cell function, such as chronic granulomatous disease, can receive all inactivated varicella and live viral vaccines.

Pregnancy and Live Vaccines

Pregnancy is generally a contraindication for administering live vaccines unless there is a serious threat from the target disease and vaccination is the only alternative. A pregnant woman or a nursing mother living in the household is not a contraindication to administering OPV, MMR, or varicella vaccines. The

MMR vaccine viruses are not transmitted from the vaccinated child to household contacts. Although one instance of varicella vaccine virus transmission from a child to his pregnant mother has been documented, no evidence of infection was observed after an elective abortion was performed for other reasons. Some experts have advised waiting until the second trimester to immunize children with varicella vaccines if a susceptible pregnant woman is in the household and there is no evidence of a local outbreak of chickenpox.

Noncontraindications and Misconceptions

Children with mild upper respiratory infections or gastroenteritis can receive routine immunizations as there is no evidence of any increased risk from vaccination of children with these infections. Vaccines should be administered to children with these mild illnesses if the vaccines are recommended, especially in circumstances in which uncertainty exists regarding return for completion of the immunization series. The presence of mild illnesses has not interfered with the immune response to vaccines. Low-grade fever (less than 39°C) is not a contraindication to immunization. If children have other manifestations of illness or the cause of the fever is undetermined, a febrile response to the vaccine could be confused with signs of progression or exacerbation of the intercurrent illness. A judgment should be made regarding the feasibility of the child's returning within a few days to be immunized if uncertainty exists regarding the cause of the concurrent illness. Children who are deficient in immunizations should be immunized regardless of

TABLE 15.6

REPORTABLE EVENTS AFTER VACCINATION (EFFECTIVE AUGUST 26, 2002)

Vaccine/Toxoid	Event	Interval From Vaccination
Tetanus in any combination: DTaP, DTP, DTP-HiB, DT, Td, or TT	A. Anaphylaxis or anaphylactic shock	7 days
	B. Brachial neuritis	28 days
	C. Any sequela (including death) of above events	NA
	D. Events described in manufacturer's package insert as contraindications to additional doses of vaccine	See package insert
Pertussis in any combination: DTaP, DTP, DTP-HiB, P	A. Anaphylaxis or anaphylactic shock	7 days
	B. Encephalopathy (or encephalitis)	7 days
	C. Any sequela (including death) of above events	NA
	D. Events described in manufacturer's package insert as contraindications to additional doses of vaccine	See package insert
Measles, mumps, and rubella in any combination: MMR, MR, M, or R	A. Anaphylaxis or anaphylactic shock	7 days
	B. Encephalopathy (or encephalitis)	15 days
	C. Any sequela (including death) of above events	NA
	D. Events described in manufacturer's package insert as contraindications to additional doses of vaccine	See package insert
Rubella in any combination: MMR, MR, R	A. Chronic arthritis	42 days
	B. Any sequela (including death) of above event	NA
	C. Events described in manufacturer's package insert as contraindications to additional doses of vaccine	See package insert
Measles in any combination: MMR, MR, M	A. Thrombocytopenic purpura	7–30 days
	B. Vaccine-strain measles viral infection in an immunodeficient recipient	6 months
	C. Any sequela (including death) of above event	NA
	D. Events described in manufacturer's package insert as contraindications to additional doses of vaccine	See package insert
OPV	A. Paralytic polio	30 days/6 months
	B. Vaccine-strain polio viral infection	30 days/6 months
	C. Any sequela (including death) of above events	NA
	D. Events described in manufacturer's package insert as contraindications to additional doses of vaccine	See package insert
IPV	A. Anaphylaxis or anaphylactic shock	7 days
	B. Any sequela (including death) of the above event	NA
	C. Events described in manufacturer's package insert as contraindications to additional doses of vaccine	See package insert
Hepatitis B	A. Anaphylaxis or anaphylactic shock	7 days
	B. Any sequela (including death) of the above event	NA
	C. Events described in manufacturer's package insert as contraindications to additional doses of vaccine	See package insert
Haemophilus influenzae, Type b, (conjugate)	A. Events described in manufacturer's package insert as contraindications to additional doses of vaccine	See package insert
Varicella	A. Events described in manufacturer's package insert as contraindications to additional doses of vaccine	See package insert
Rotavirus	A. Intussusception	30 days
	B. Any sequela (including death) of the above event	NA
	C. Events described in manufacturer's package insert as contraindications to additional doses of vaccine	See package insert
Pneumococcal conjugate	A. Events described in manufacturer's package insert as contraindications to additional doses of vaccine	See package insert

DT, diphtheria toxoid; DTaP, diphtheria, tetanus, and acellular pertussis vaccine; DTP, diphtheria, tetanus, and pertussis vaccine; DTP-Hib, diphtheria, tetanus, and pertussis vaccine and *H. influenzae* type b vaccine; IPV, inactivated poliovirus; M, measles vaccine; MMR, measles, mumps, and rubella vaccine; MR, measles and rubella vaccine; OPV, oral poliovirus; P, pertussis vaccine; R, rubella vaccine; Td, diphtheria toxoid; TT, tetanus toxoid.
Source: VAERS www.vaers.hhs.gov/reportable.htm

the presence of mild to moderate disease to avoid making them further deficient in immunization schedules.

Reporting Vaccine-Preventable Diseases and Adverse Events

The reporting of all cases of disease preventable through the administration of vaccines recommended for routine use in all children is required in most states. The information is transmitted to the CDC, and up-to-date information regarding the incidence of vaccine-preventable diseases is available through the

CDC's Web site. All serious and unexpected adverse events that occur following vaccinations should be reported to the Vaccine Adverse Events Reporting System (VAERS) (Table 15.6).

Compensation for Vaccine-Associated Injuries

The National Vaccine Injury Compensation Program was established to provide appropriate compensation for families when injuries caused by vaccines have led to permanent sequelae or death. A table of compensable events has been established (Table 15.7) and is updated periodically. Children or

TABLE 15.7

NATIONAL VACCINE INJURY COMPENSATION PROGRAM (EFFECTIVE APRIL 26, 2002)*

Vaccine	Illness, Disability, Injury, or Condition Covered	Time Period for First Symptom or Manifestation of Onset or of Significant Aggravation After Vaccine Administration
I. Tetanus toxoid–containing vaccines (e.g., DTaP, DTP-Hib, DT, Td, TT)	A. Anaphylaxis or anaphylactic shock[1]	0–4 hours
	B. Brachial neuritis[6]	2–28 days
	C. Any acute complication or sequela (including death) of above events[4]	NA
II. Pertussis antigen–containing vaccines (e.g., DTaP, DTP, P, DTP-Hib)	A. Anaphylaxis or anaphylactic shock[1]	0–4 hours
	B. Encephalopathy (or encephalitis)[2]	0–72 hours
	C. Any acute complication or sequela (including death) of above events[4]	NA
III. Measles, mumps, and rubella virus–containing vaccines in any combination (e.g., MMR, MR, M, R)	A. Anaphylaxis or anaphylactic shock[1]	0–4 hours
	B. Encephalopathy (or encephalitis)[2]	5–15 days
	C. Any acute complication or sequela (including death) of above events[4]	NA
IV. Rubella virus–containing vaccines (e.g., MMR, MR, R)	A. Chronic arthritis[5]	7–42 days
	B. Any acute complication or sequela (including death) of above event[4]	NA
V. Measles virus–containing vaccines (e.g., MMR, MR, M)	A. Thrombocytopenic purpura[7]	7–30 days
	B. Vaccine-strain measles viral infection in an immunodeficient recipient[8]	0–6 months
	C. Any acute complication or sequela (including death) of above events[4]	NA
VI. Polio live virus–containing vaccines (OPV)	A. Paralytic polio	
	— in a nonimmunodeficient recipient	0–30 days
	— in an immunodeficient recipient	0–6 months
	— in a vaccine-associated community case	NA
	B. Vaccine-strain polio viral infection[9]	
	— in a nonimmunodeficient recipient	0–30 days
	— in an immunodeficient recipient	0–6 months
	— in a vaccine-associated community case	NA
	C. Any acute complication or sequela (including death) of above events[4]	NA
VII. Polio inactivated virus–containing vaccines (e.g., IPV)	A. Anaphylaxis or anaphylactic shock[1]	0–4 hours
	B. Any acute complication or sequela (including death) of above event[4]	NA
VIII. Hepatitis B antigen–containing vaccines	A. Anaphylaxis or anaphylactic shock[1]	0–4 hours
	B. Any acute complication or sequela (including death) of above event[4]	NA
IX. *Haemophilus influenzae* type b polysaccharide conjugate vaccines	A. No condition specified for compensation	NA
X. Varicella vaccine	A. No condition specified for compensation	NA
XI. Rotavirus vaccine	A. No condition specified for compensation	NA
XII. Vaccines containing live, oral, rhesus-based rotavirus	A. Intussusception	0–30 days
	B. Any acute complication or sequela (including death) of above event[4]	NA
XIII. Pneumococcal conjugate vaccines	A. No condition specified for compensation	NA
XIV. Any new vaccine recommended by the Centers for Disease Control and Prevention for routine administration to children, after publication by Secretary of the U.S. Department of Health and Human Services of a notice of coverage	A. No condition specified for compensation	NA

DT, diphtheria toxoid; DTaP, diphtheria, tetanus, and acellular pertussis vaccine; DTP, diphtheria, tetanus, and pertussis vaccine; DTP-Hib, diphtheria, tetanus, and pertussis vaccine and *H. influenzae* type b vaccine; M, measles vaccine; MMR, measles, mumps, and rubella vaccine; MR, measles and rubella vaccine; P, pertussis vaccine; PRP, polyribosylribitol phosphate; R, rubella vaccine; Td, diphtheria toxoid; TT, tetanus toxoid.

*Qualifications and Aids to Interpretation

1. Anaphylaxis and anaphylactic shock mean an acute, severe, and potentially lethal systemic allergic reaction. Most cases resolve without sequelae. Signs and symptoms begin minutes to a few hours after exposure. Death, if it occurs, usually results from airway obstruction caused by laryngeal edema or bronchospasm and may be associated with cardiovascular collapse. Other significant clinical signs and symptoms may include the following: cyanosis, hypotension, bradycardia, tachycardia, arrhythmia, edema of the pharynx and/or trachea and/or larynx with stridor, and dyspnea. Autopsy findings may include acute emphysema, which results from lower respiratory tract obstruction; edema of the hypopharynx, epiglottis, larynx, or trachea; and minimal findings of eosinophilia in the liver, spleen, and lungs. When death occurs within minutes of exposure and without signs of respiratory distress, there may not be significant pathologic findings. (Continued)

TABLE 15.7

(CONTINUED)

2. Encephalopathy: For purposes of the Vaccine Injury Table, a vaccine recipient shall be considered to have suffered an encephalopathy only if such recipient manifests, within the applicable period, an injury meeting the description below of an acute encephalopathy, and then a chronic encephalopathy persists in such person for more than 6 months beyond the date of vaccination.
    I. An acute encephalopathy is one that is sufficiently severe so as to require hospitalization (whether or not hospitalization occurred).
        A. For children less than 18 months of age who present without an associated seizure event, an acute encephalopathy is indicated by a "significantly decreased level of consciousness" (see "D" below) lasting for at least 24 hours. Those children less than 18 months of age who present following a seizure shall be viewed as having an acute encephalopathy if their significantly decreased level of consciousness persists beyond 24 hours and cannot be attributed to a postictal state (seizure) or medication.
        B. For adults and children 18 months of age or older, an acute encephalopathy is one that persists for at least 24 hours and is characterized by at least two of the following:
            (1) A significant change in mental status that is not medication related, specifically a confusional state, or a delirium, or a psychosis;
            (2) A significantly decreased level of consciousness, which is independent of a seizure and cannot be attributed to the effects of medication; and
            (3) A seizure associated with loss of consciousness.
        C. Increased intracranial pressure may be a clinical feature of acute encephalopathy in any age group.
        D. A "significantly decreased level of consciousness" is indicated by the presence of at least one of the following clinical signs for at least 24 hours or greater (see paragraphs (2)(I)(A) and (2)(I)(B) of this section for applicable timeframes):
            (1) Decreased or absent response to environment (responds, if at all, only to loud voice or painful stimuli);
            (2) Decreased or absent eye contact (does not fix gaze upon family members or other individuals); or
            (3) Inconsistent or absent responses to external stimuli (does not recognize familiar people or things).
        E. The following clinical features alone, or in combination, do not demonstrate an acute encephalopathy or a significant change in either mental status or level of consciousness as described above: sleepiness, irritability (fussiness), high-pitched and unusual screaming, persistent inconsolable crying, and bulging fontanelle. Seizures in themselves are not sufficient to constitute a diagnosis of encephalopathy. In the absence of other evidence of an acute encephalopathy, seizures shall not be viewed as the first symptom or manifestation of the onset of an acute encephalopathy.
    II. Chronic encephalopathy occurs when a change in mental or neurologic status, first manifested during the applicable time period, persists for a period of at least 6 months from the date of vaccination. Individuals who return to a normal neurologic state after the acute encephalopathy shall not be presumed to have suffered residual neurologic damage from that event; any subsequent chronic encephalopathy shall not be presumed to be a sequela of the acute encephalopathy. If a preponderance of the evidence indicates that a child's chronic encephalopathy is secondary to genetic, prenatal, or perinatal factors, that chronic encephalopathy shall not be considered to be a condition set forth in the table.
    III. An encephalopathy shall not be considered to be a condition set forth in the table if in a proceeding on a petition, it is shown by a preponderance of the evidence that the encephalopathy was caused by an infection, a toxin, a metabolic disturbance, a structural lesion, a genetic disorder, or trauma (without regard to whether the cause of the infection, toxin, trauma, metabolic disturbance, structural lesion, or genetic disorder is known). If at the time a decision is made on a petition filed under section 2111(b) of the Act for a vaccine-related injury or death that it is not possible to determine the cause by a preponderance of the evidence of an encephalopathy, the encephalopathy shall be considered to be a condition set forth in the table.
    IV. In determining whether or not an encephalopathy is a condition set forth in the table, the Court shall consider the entire medical record.
3. Seizure and convulsion: For purposes of paragraphs (b)(2) of this section, the terms "seizure" and "convulsion" include myoclonic, generalized tonic–clonic (grand mal), and simple and complex partial seizures. Absence (petit mal) seizures shall not be considered to be a condition set forth in the table. Jerking movements or staring episodes alone are not necessarily an indication of seizure activity.
4. Sequela: The term "sequela" means a condition or event that was actually caused by a condition listed in the Vaccine Injury Table.
5. Chronic arthritis: For purposes of the Vaccine Injury Table, chronic arthritis may be found in a person with no history in the 3 years prior to vaccination of arthropathy (joint disease) on the basis of:
    A. Medical documentation, recorded within 30 days after the onset, of objective signs of acute arthritis (joint swelling) that occurred between 7 and 42 days after a rubella vaccination;
    B. Medical documentation (recorded within 3 years after the onset) of the persistence of objective signs of intermittent or continuous arthritis for more than 6 months following vaccination; or
    C. Medical documentation of an antibody response to the rubella virus.
    For purposes of the Vaccine Injury Table, the following shall not be considered as chronic arthritis: musculoskeletal disorders such as diffuse connective tissue diseases (including but not limited to rheumatoid arthritis, juvenile rheumatoid arthritis, systemic lupus erythematosus, systemic sclerosis, mixed connective tissue disease, polymyositis/dermatomyositis, fibromyalgia, necrotizing vasculitis and vasculopathies, and Sjögren's syndrome), degenerative joint disease, infectious agents other than rubella (whether by direct invasion or as an immune reaction), metabolic and endocrine diseases, trauma, neoplasms, neuropathic disorders, bone and cartilage disorders, and arthritis associated with ankylosing spondylitis, psoriasis, inflammatory bowel disease, Reiter's syndrome, or blood disorders.
    Arthralgia (joint pain) or stiffness without joint swelling shall not be viewed as chronic arthritis for purposes of the Vaccine Injury Table.
6. Brachial neuritis is defined as dysfunction limited to the upper extremity nerve plexus (i.e., its trunks, divisions, or cords) without involvement of other peripheral (e.g., nerve roots or a single peripheral nerve) or central (e.g., spinal cord) nervous system structures. A deep, steady, often severe aching pain in the shoulder and upper arm usually heralds onset of the condition. The pain is followed in days or weeks by weakness and atrophy in upper extremity muscle groups. Sensory loss may accompany the motor deficits, but is generally a less notable clinical feature. The neuritis, or plexopathy, may be present on the same side as or the opposite side of the injection; it is sometimes bilateral, affecting both upper extremities. Weakness is required before the diagnosis can be made. Motor, sensory, and reflex findings on physical examination and the results of nerve conduction and electromyographic studies must be consistent in confirming that dysfunction is attributable to the brachial plexus. The condition should thereby be distinguishable from conditions that may give rise to dysfunction of nerve roots (i.e., radiculopathies) and peripheral nerves (i.e., including multiple mononeuropathies), as well as other peripheral and central nervous system structures (e.g., cranial neuropathies and myelopathies).
7. Thrombocytopenic purpura is defined by a serum platelet count less than 50,000/mm^3. Thrombocytopenic purpura does not include cases of thrombocytopenia associated with other causes such as hypersplenism, autoimmune disorders (including alloantibodies from previous transfusions), myelodysplasias, lymphoproliferative disorders, congenital thrombocytopenia, or hemolytic uremic syndrome. This does not include cases of immune (formerly called idiopathic) thrombocytopenic purpura (ITP) that are mediated, for example, by viral or fungal infections, toxins, or drugs. Thrombocytopenic purpura does not include cases of thrombocytopenia associated with disseminated intravascular coagulation, as observed with bacterial and viral infections. Viral infections include, for example, those infections secondary to Epstein-Barr virus, cytomegalovirus, hepatitis A and B, rhinovirus, human immunodeficiency virus (HIV), adenovirus, and dengue virus. An antecedent viral infection may be demonstrated by clinical signs and symptoms and need not be confirmed by culture or serologic testing. Bone marrow examination, if performed, must reveal a normal or an increased number of megakaryocytes in an otherwise normal marrow.
8. Vaccine-strain measles viral infection is defined as a disease caused by the vaccine strain that should be determined by vaccine-specific monoclonal antibody or polymerase chain reaction tests.
9. Vaccine-strain polio viral infection is defined as a disease caused by poliovirus that is isolated from the affected tissue and should be determined to be the vaccine strain by oligonucleotide or polymerase chain reaction. Isolation of poliovirus from the stool is not sufficient to establish a tissue-specific infection or disease caused by vaccine-strain poliovirus.

Source: Health Resources and Services Administration, U.S. Department of Health and Human Services. www.hrsa.gov/osp/vicp/table.htm

adults who develop a complication from vaccines included in the table are automatically compensated and do not have to go through formal litigation proceedings. Information on how to apply for compensation can be obtained from the National Vaccine Injury Compensation Program (Health Resources and Services Administration, U.S. Department of Health and Human Services, Parklawn Building, Room 8A-35, 5600 Fishers Lane, Rockville, MD 20857; telephone: 800-338-2382; Web site: www.hrsa.gov/osp/vicp).

Establishment of the Vaccine Injury Compensation Program has effectively reduced litigation against health care providers and vaccine manufacturers and provided appropriate and timely compensation to families that have been adversely affected by rare, serious adverse events after immunization.

SPECIFIC IMMUNIZING AGENTS

Hepatitis B Vaccine

Hepatitis B vaccines currently available in the United States are made by recombinant technology in yeast. The first vaccines were plasma derived from patients who were chronic carriers of hepatitis B surface antigen; similar vaccines are in use in some other countries. All of the vaccines are highly (more than 95%) effective at inducing immunity and protecting against the chronic carrier state and other hepatitis B–associated diseases. In the United States and more than 100 other countries, the hepatitis B vaccine is recommended for routine administration to all infants. Catch-up immunization is indicated for all children through 18 years of age. Preference is given for starting immunization at birth, with the second dose administered 1 or 2 months later; the third dose is given at least 4 months after the first dose, but preferably at 6 months of age. For children born to women known to be hepatitis B surface antigen negative, the first dose of vaccine may be deferred until 1 to 2 months of age. If children are receiving a combination vaccine that includes hepatitis B at 2, 4, and 6 months of age, administration of an extra dose at birth is acceptable and not associated with any increased risk of adverse events. The hepatitis B vaccine alone has been shown to be highly effective in reducing the risk of maternal–infant transmission from chronic carrier mothers. However, additional administration of hepatitis B immune globulin shortly after birth further reduces the risk of transmission to approximately 5%. In developing countries where the cost of hepatitis B immune globulin is prohibitive, routine immunization with vaccine alone is the usual practice. Immunization schedules for older children and adults are usually at time 0, 1 to 2 months later, and 4 to 6 months after the first dose. Immunization at intervals of up to 1 year between doses have been shown to be highly effective in simplifying the catch-up immunization of older children who are routinely seen only at annual intervals. Routine administration of the hepatitis B vaccine to all children, adolescents, and high-risk adults has contributed to the marked decline in the incidence of hepatitis B in the United States. The target is elimination of transmission, but this will take 20 to 40 years because of the large number of chronic carriers in this country.

Diphtheria and Tetanus Toxoids and Pertussis Vaccine

The combined DTaP vaccine is recommended for routine administration at 2 months, 4 months, 6 months, 12 to 18 months, and 4 to 6 years of age. Similar products containing the whole cell pertussis (DTwP) vaccine are no longer available in the United States, but are widely used in developing countries. DTaP is associated with lower rates of fever, local redness and swelling, grand mal seizures, hypertensive hyporesponsive episodes, malaise, and decreased appetite than DTwP.

Diphtheria and tetanus toxoids are highly effective, and their routine use has led to almost complete elimination of diphtheria and tetanus in the United States. Only a few cases of diphtheria occur each year in the United States, most in inadequately immunized immigrants. Toxin-producing *Corynebacterium diphtheriae* have been eliminated in most areas of the United States, but isolates were obtained in South Dakota during the 1990s in a population that was previously known to have circulation of the organism. These data indicate the continued circulation of toxin-producing strains and emphasize the need for complete and timely immunization of all children. Immunity from diphtheria and tetanus toxoids wanes with time. Booster doses are recommended at 11 to 12 years of age with a preparation containing a reduced concentration of diphtheria toxoid to reduce the risk of local adverse events. Although tetanus toxoid alone is available, it is not recommended for use because of the need to maintain diphtheria immunity. Seroprevalence surveys have been conducted in many countries and indicate that a high proportion (30% to 50%) of individuals 40 years of age or older do not have protective levels (0.01 IU/mL) of diphtheria antitoxin in their blood, raising concerns about the potential for widespread diphtheria epidemics. Epidemics with 30,000 to 50,000 cases a year occurred in Russia and other former Soviet Union countries in the mid-1990s; fortunately, little spread occurred in the United States and other areas. The epidemic appears to have been caused by inadequate immunization and failure to administer booster doses to adolescents and adults.

Most tetanus cases in the United States have occurred in individuals 40 or 50 years and older who were never completely immunized in infancy or who had received no booster doses beyond early childhood. The majority of cases have occurred in individuals who had fewer than three doses for primary immunization.

The occasional cases of neonatal tetanus in this country usually have occurred in infants born to women who were pregnant when they entered the United States or who became pregnant shortly after entering the United States. In many developing countries, only 25% to 50% of women of childbearing age have been adequately immunized against tetanus. Immunized women have protective levels of antibody that are transmitted across the placenta and protect the infant against tetanus even though the umbilical stump may become colonized with tetanus spores because of unclean deliveries. Pediatricians caring for families recently immigrating to the United States should verify the immunization status of women of childbearing age and ensure complete immunization, including the administration of two doses of tetanus toxoid in pregnancy (separated by at least 1 month) for women with uncertain or inadequate past immunization records.

Pertussis vaccines have provided 70% to 90% protection against pertussis in most studies. In European efficacy studies, lower estimates of efficacy were observed with one whole-cell vaccine produced in the United States. In these studies, children received only three injections without a booster dose at 12 to 18 months of age, as has been the practice in the United States. DTaP preparations licensed in the United States have induced 83% to 90% efficacy in clinical trials conducted in European studies.

Although whole-cell DTP preparations were considered interchangeable, some uncertainty exists as to the interchangeability of DTaP products because of the varying concentrations of different antigens and different methods of preparation

TABLE 15.8

DIPHTHERIA, TETANUS TOXOIDS, AND ACELLULAR PERTUSSIS PRODUCTS AVAILABLE FOR USE IN INFANCY OR ADOLESCENCE (UNITED STATES)

Manufacturer	Product Name	Components in μg per Dose			
		PT	FHA	PN	Fim
Aventis Pasteur	Tripedia	23.4	23.4	0	0
Aventis Pasteur	Daptacel	10	5	3	5
Glaxo SmithKline	Infanrix	25	25	8	—
Glaxo SmithKline	Pediarix	25	25	8	—

FHA, filamentous hemagglutinin; Fim, fimbriae (agglutinogens); PN, pertactin; PT, pertussis toxoid.

(Table 15.8). Therefore, the AAP and ACIP have recommended that, when feasible, the same DTaP preparations should be used for the primary series. However, if the preparation used previously is unknown or unavailable at the time a child presents for immunization, then any DTaP should be used to ensure timely completion of immunization. All DTaP preparations contain pertussis toxoid, which is believed to be the most important antigen for prevention of serious disease. Also, studies have demonstrated that two doses of some DTaP preparations produce high levels of protection.

Because pertussis in infants younger than 6 months is a severe and life-threatening illness, efforts are being made to prevent transmission of *Bordetella pertussis* from adolescents and adults to young infants. Special preparations of acellular pertussis vaccines combined with tetanus for administration to adolescents or young adults and diphtheria toxoids (CTdap) have been licensed and are recommended. In Canada, routine immunization of adolescents against pertussis with the special preparations has become standard practice because immunity wanes after either immunization or natural infection. Efforts are under way to obtain approval from the FDA for use of these preparations in the United States to reduce the risk of clinical disease in adults and decrease the likelihood of transmitting *B. pertussis* to young infants.

Poliomyelitis Immunization

IPV vaccines have replaced live OPV in the United States because OPV vaccines cause vaccine-associated paralytic polio in the recipient or a contact at a rate of approximately 1 in 780,000 children who receive their first dose of vaccine. IPV vaccine was first licensed in 1955, and widespread use led to a rapid termination of the large-scale epidemics that were affecting 30,000 to 50,000 children every year in the United States. The original IPV was of lower potency than the cur-

rent enhanced-potency IPV, which became available in 1987. IPV alone induces approximately 95% reduction in intestinal virus replication after a challenge with OPV, as compared with 99% reduction after a three-dose series of OPV or infection with wild-type virus. The global efforts to eradicate polio from the world are anticipated to be successful by 2006. Immunization with IPV vaccine in developed countries will continue for at least several more years to ensure the lack of circulation of wild-type polio viruses. In developing countries, the OPV will be discontinued after eradication of wild-type virus because OPV can revert to wild-type virus and cause community outbreaks of paralytic disease. Developing countries' program managers will need to decide if they should switch to the more expensive IPV vaccine or if immunization against polio should be discontinued altogether. The WHO will coordinate a global strategy to discontinue OPV simultaneously throughout the world.

Haemophilus influenzae Type b Vaccine

Hib vaccines consist of the outer polysaccharide coat from type b strains of *H. influenzae* chemically linked to protein carriers. The conjugation of the polysaccharide to a protein alters the way the host immune system processes the antigen. Plain polysaccharide vaccines were ineffective in children younger than 18 months, but the conjugated polysaccharide vaccines have been highly effective in infants as young as 6 weeks of age. Four polysaccharide conjugate vaccines are available (Table 15.9).

The vaccines approved for primary immunization of infants are considered equivalent and interchangeable if three doses are administered. PRP-OMP (polyribosylribitol phosphate conjugated to the outer membrane protein of *Neisseria meningitidis*) has been successfully combined with the hepatitis B vaccine and can be administered in a two-dose series rather than a

TABLE 15.9

HAEMOPHILUS INFLUENZAE TYPE B CONJUGATE VACCINES

Manufacturer	Abbreviation	Trade Name	Carrier Protein
Aventis Pasteur	PRP-T	ActHIB, OmniHIB	Tetanus toxoid
Wyeth-Lederle Vaccines	HbOC	HibTITER	CRM$_{197}$ (a nontoxic mutant diphtheria toxin)
Merck & Co.	PRP-OMP	PedvaxHIB	OMP (an outer membrane protein complex of *Neisseria meningitidis*)
Merck & Co.	PRP-OMP/Hep B	Comvax	OMP
Glaxo SmithKline		PEDIARIX	Tetanus toxoid

three-dose primary series. A single dose of this vaccine induces protection rapidly and therefore has been preferred in settings where a high incidence of invasive Hib disease occurs in young infants, such as in the Native American population. PRP-T (PRP conjugated to tetanus toxoid) and HbOC (PRP conjugated to a mutant diphtheria toxoid) have been successfully combined with whole-cell DTP preparations, and one preparation of PRP-T combined with DTaP is available for administration on the fourth and fifth doses but not for primary immunization of infants.

Measles, Mumps, and Rubella Vaccines

Measles, Mumps and Rubella vaccines are usually administered as a combined product (MMR).

Measles Vaccine

The MMR vaccine is routinely administered at 12 to 15 months of age, and a second dose is given at 4 to 6 years of age. The second dose can be administered at any time as long as at least 1 month has elapsed after the first dose. The first dose of the measles vaccine may be given as early as 6 months of age in settings where a measles outbreak occurs in the community. If this occurs, then a dose of the MMR vaccine is given at the usual 12 to 15 months of age and a third dose at 4 to 6 years of age. The response to the measles vaccine at less than 12 months of age is suboptimal because of interference by passively acquired maternal antibodies that disappear at a variable and unpredictable rate. Some infants receive little or no antibodies from their mothers and respond adequately as early as 6 months of age. Others receive much higher concentrations of maternal antibodies and still have trace amounts of passive antibodies to blunt the replication of the live virus vaccine as late as 12 months of age. Advisory committees recommend that all children receive two doses of the MMR vaccine; the first dose induces protection in nearly 95% of vaccines and the second dose ensures close to 100% immunity. The very high infectivity of measles has resulted in continuing outbreaks of disease despite populations in which 98% to 100% of children have received one dose of vaccine. Intensive efforts have been made to ensure that all children receive measles-containing vaccines at the recommended age. This enhanced program has resulted in elimination of endemic measles transmission in the United States and the entire Western Hemisphere, although periodic outbreaks still occur. Major efforts have been introduced to administer second doses of measles vaccines to children in Africa through national campaigns, which dramatically interrupts the transmission of and reduces the incidence of measles and measles-related mortality. Within a few years, a global effort to eradicate measles should be initiated.

Approximately 5% to 15% of children receiving the first dose of the MMR vaccine develop a fever of 39.4°C or higher, a rash lasting 1 to 3 days, or both. Other complications include rare cases of transient thrombocytopenia and encephalitis in less than 1 per million vaccinees. The rates of adverse events are lower in children receiving the second dose of vaccine because only approximately 5% are susceptible. Hypersensitivity reactions have been demonstrated to be caused by allergy to the gelatin stabilizer or neomycin. Studies have demonstrated that skin testing for egg allergy or tests using the vaccine were not predictive of which children would develop allergic reactions to the vaccine. Current guidelines call for routine administration of MMR vaccines to children, even if they have severe egg hypersensitivity, because no significant amount of egg protein is present in these vaccines.

Children who have received blood or blood products, including IGIV, need to be assessed individually to determine the length of time after blood product administration that vaccines can be effectively administered. Administration of washed red blood cells delivers only a small amount of passive antibodies, and virtually no delay in administration of the measles vaccine is necessary. However, children who receive large doses (1,600 to 2,000 mg/kg) of IGIV need to defer immunization for 11 months. Specific guidelines can be found in the references from the AAP and the CDC listed at the end of this chapter. Measles and other live virus vaccines should not be administered to children with underlying immune deficiency, with the exception of children who have asymptomatic human immunodeficiency virus (HIV) infection and whose CD4 counts reveal that they are not severely immunocompromised. Children who have received high doses (greater than or equal to 2 mg/kg/day) of corticosteroids for 2 or more weeks should wait at least 1 month before measles-containing vaccines are administered.

Rubella Vaccine

Following a single dose of the rubella vaccine, approximately 95% of individuals are protected; nearly 100% are protected after two doses. The rubella vaccine produces a transient rash and lymphadenopathy in a small percentage of children, but the rate is not increased when given with the measles vaccine. Joint pains develop in approximately 0.5% children but occur more commonly in postpubertal girls, 25% of whom report such symptoms. Transient arthritis develops in 10%. Studies now indicate that the rubella vaccine is not associated with increased risk of persistent arthritis, although some earlier studies suggested that this might be the case. Transient paresthesias and pains in the arms and legs have been reported rarely. The widespread use of the rubella vaccine in the United States has led to the almost complete elimination of congenital rubella syndrome and prevented the 6- to 9-year cycle of epidemics that occurred before vaccine licensure in 1969. Endemic transmission of rubella in the United States was interrupted in recent years. The only cases occurring are imported or linked to import cases.

Mumps Vaccine

Before licensure of the mumps vaccine, mumps was the most common cause of encephalitis in the United States. Now, occurrence of mumps is at an all-time low and is rarely the cause of encephalitis. The mumps vaccine is produced in chick embryo tissue cultures in a method similar to measles vaccines. The guidelines for mumps vaccines are similar to those for measles and rubella because the vaccines are usually combined. Few adverse events occur from the mumps vaccine, although isolated incidences of nerve deafness, febrile seizures, orchitis, and parotitis have been documented. In most of these cases, a causal relationship has not been demonstrated and the disorders have been transient. Contrary to some myths, the vaccine has never been associated with sterility.

Varicella Vaccine

The varicella vaccine became available in the United States in 1995 and is recommended for universal immunization of all children 12 months to 18 years of age who have not had chickenpox. A single dose is considered sufficient for those through

12 years of age, but two doses are recommended for children 13 years of age and older. One dose provides approximately 95% protection against severe disease and 70% to 80% protection against any illness in most studies. Most vaccinated children who have developed signs of varicella after close exposures (usually in households) have modified or very mild cases with an average of only 40 small skin lesions, many of them papules rather than vesicles. Some physicians and parents have been apprehensive about accepting the vaccine because of concern about long-term protection; they point out that subclinical boosts in immunity from exposure to varicella may have occurred. The vaccine has been shown to induce long-lasting immunity in Japan, where it has been in use for more than 20 years. In the United States, studies of children followed for up to 10 years have shown lasting protection. Advisory committees have not recommended a second dose of the vaccine, in part because of its relatively high cost. In time, perhaps with other manufacturers entering the market with a combination varicella–MMR vaccine, a second dose of the varicella vaccine may be administered, which would help allay concerns regarding the breakthrough cases. All parents should be strongly encouraged to vaccinate their children. Approximately 100 deaths per year occurred from varicella in the United States prior to the introduction of the vaccine, almost all of which could have been prevented if immunization was universal. More than 80% of the children who died from varicella had no underlying immune deficiency disorder or other factors that would allow for prediction of severe disease. The varicella vaccine may be administered simultaneously with the MMR vaccine at separate sites.

Side effects from varicella vaccine include mild vaccine-associated macular, papular, or vesicular rash in 7% to 8% of children and adolescents. The median number of skin lesions is less than five in most studies, and most of the lesions were macular or papular and resembled mosquito bites. In approximately 4% of cases, one or two varicella-like lesions developed at the site of injection, presumably from tracking of the virus along the needle. Rare cases of zoster have occurred in vaccinated children, and the vaccine virus has been isolated from a zoster lesion, indicating the potential for persistence of the vaccine virus as well as wild-type virus in the dorsal route ganglion. However, the rate of zoster developing after vaccination appears to be much lower than after wild-type virus infection. Thus, the vaccine protects against zoster as well as wild-type disease. Formulations of the varicella vaccine must be stored at –15°C or colder. Efforts are under way to improve the stabilizers so that the vaccine can be kept at routine refrigerator temperatures. Children 13 years and older should receive two doses of the vaccine and all health care workers should be immunized. Children with underlying immune-compromising conditions should not receive the vaccine with the exception of HIV-infected children who have CD4 lymphocytes of greater than 25%. Children who cannot receive the vaccine should receive varicella-zoster immunoglobulin after exposures, and extra efforts should be made to ensure that all household contacts are immune through immunization or a past history of natural disease to prevent the introduction of varicella into the household. New high potency formulation of a varicella vaccine has been shown to protect against zoster in adults and should be licenced in 2006. No serious complications from the vaccine have been identified.

Meningococcal Vaccine

Two types of meningococcal vaccines are now in use. A plain polysaccharide vaccine is available in the United States to pro-

tect against *Neisseria meningitidis* types A, C, Y, and W135 in children 2 or more years of age. This vaccine is not administered routinely to children because the risk of disease is relatively low, the vaccine does not induce lasting immunity, and response in children 2 to 5 years of age is lower than in adults. The plain polysaccharide vaccine is recommended for children at increased risk of disease, including those with esplenia or complement difficiency.

A polysaccharide-protein conjugate vaccine containing types A, C, Y, and W135 was approved in 2005, and is recommended for all children 11–12 years of age, for previously unvaccinated 15–16 yr olds, college freshman living in dorms, and others at high risk of disease. Conjugate meningococcal group C vaccines are now in routine use in the United Kingdom and Canada, and these vaccines are effective as early as 6 to 8 weeks of age. The A, C, Y and W135 conjugate meningococcal vaccine is likely to be licensed in the United States for use in younger children soon, and advisory groups will determine the appropriate use. No serious complications to this vaccine have been identified.

Pneumococcal Vaccines

Two types of pneumococcal vaccines are licensed in the United States: a plain polysaccharide vaccine that protects against 23 pneumococcal types and a conjugate vaccine that protects against seven pneumococcal types (PCV7). The pneumococcal conjugate vaccine contains polysaccharides from seven common pneumococcal types conjugated to a modified diphtheria toxoid and has been shown to induce high levels of protection in infants. Three doses of this vaccine are usually recommended for all infants, although advisory committees have had to scale this back to two doses at times of severe shortage. The vaccine is recommended for children up to 5 years of age who are at high risk for pneumococcal infections. If vaccination is started after 12 months of age, two doses are recommended 6 to 8 weeks apart. For immunocompetent children greater than 24 months of age, only one dose is recommended, and two doses are recommended for high-risk children 12 through 59 months of age. Efforts are under way to increase the number of pneumococcal serotypes in the vaccine. These vaccines will have increased effectiveness for children, especially in developing countries where the serotypes' distribution differs from that in the United States.

The pneumococcal polysaccharide vaccine is recommended for children 2 years or older who are at increased risk for developing severe complications from *Streptococcus pneumoniae* infections, including children with sickle cell disease, asplenia, nephrotic syndrome, chronic renal failure, immunosuppression including organ transplantation or cancer chemotherapy, HIV infection, leaks of cerebrospinal fluid, or chronic cardiovascular or pulmonary disease. High-risk children who have received the pneumococcal conjugate vaccine should receive a single dose of the plain polysaccharide vaccine at 24 months of age to increase the number of serotypes that they are protected against.

Influenza Vaccine

Two types influenza vaccines are available: a cold-adapted, live, intranasal vaccine and an inactivated subunit vaccine. Both types of vaccines effectively prevent severe disease caused by influenza in children. The effectiveness depends on the ability of vaccine manufacturers to match the current circulating influenza strains. The overall efficacy for inactivated influenza

TABLE 15.10

SCHEDULE FOR INFLUENZA IMMUNIZATION[a]

Age	Dose (mL)[c]	Number of Doses
6–35 months	0.25	1–2[d]
3–8 years	0.5	1–2[d]
9–12 years	0.5	1
>12 years	0.5	1
5–50 yr[e]	0.5	1

[a] Vaccine is administered intramuscularly.
[b] Split-virus vaccine may be termed *split, subvirion,* or *purified surface-antigen* vaccine. Only split virus vaccines are marketed in the United States.
[c] Dosages are those recommended in recent years. Physicians should refer to the product circular each year to ensure that the appropriate dosage is given.
[d] Two doses administered at least 1 month apart are recommended for children who are receiving the influenza vaccine for the first time.
[e] Intranasal vaccine.

vaccines has been 70% to 80% for prevention of influenza-related illness. These studies have been conducted primarily in older adults for whom the vaccine is routinely recommended. However, these individuals have decreased responses to vaccines of all types, and the true efficacy in younger children may be higher if the match is correct. Inactivated influenza vaccine is recommended on an annual basis for all children 6 to 23 months of age and for children of all ages who are at increased risk of complications from influenza. In the first year that children younger than 9 years receive the inactivated influenza vaccine, they should receive two doses (Table 15.10) at least 1 month apart. Subsequently, a single dose administered every year just before the influenza season (usually in October or early November) is indicated. Children over 23 months of age for whom the vaccine is routinely recommended include those with chronic pulmonary disease such as asthma, significant cardiac disease, immunosuppressive disorders or therapy, HIV infection, sickle cell anemia, or other hemoglobinopathies, and children who require long-term aspirin therapy for treatment of rheumatoid arthritis or Kawasaki disease. Children receiving aspirin therapy may be at increased risk for development of Reye syndrome after wild-type influenza infection. Advisory groups recommend that other children who are potentially at increased risk of complications also may benefit from vaccination, including those with diabetes mellitus, chronic renal disease, chronic metabolic disease, or any other condition that may compromise children. In addi-

tion, the ACIP has recommended that women who are pregnant during the influenza season be immunized. Also, household and other close contacts of high-risk patients should be immunized to decrease the risk of introduction of wild-type influenza into the home. The AAP has indicated that vaccination should be considered for individuals whose group activities could be significantly disrupted by outbreaks of influenza, including students, athletes, and those living in residential institutions. Pediatricians are advised that any healthy child or adolescent who requests immunization should be immunized.

Inactivated influenza vaccine is associated with low-grade fever and malaise in a small percentage of children, usually 6 to 24 hours after vaccination. In children 13 years of age and older, approximately 10% develop local reactions. Studies in adults have indicated a small increased risk of Guillain-Barré syndrome, approximately one to two per million vaccinees. The data are from adults only because insufficient numbers of children have been immunized to determine accurately if there is any increased risk. The risks of serious consequences from influenza are several hundred–fold higher than from vaccine.

A live cold-adapted influenza vaccine has been approved for persons 5 to 50 years of age. This vaccine also contains three different influenza viruses and is updated annually in an effort to match the influenza strains that are currently circulating. This vaccine is administered through an intranasal spray device; one-half the dose is given in each nostril. Data from two efficacy trials have revealed high levels of protection against clinical influenza, and the protection may be greater than with inactivated vaccines. One study found that the protection from live intranasal vaccine may persist for a second influenza season if the viruses are closely related.

Hepatitis A

Two hepatitis A vaccines are available in the United States; both are inactivated subcomponent viral vaccines. The antigen content is determined by two methods that are not directly comparable (Table 15.11). Both vaccines are administered in a two-dose series separated by 6 to 12 months. Recent data demonstrate that intervals longer than 12 months are equally effective. Both vaccines are approved only for use in children 2 years and older, and available evidence indicates that the two-dose series should produce long-lasting immunity. Studies are in progress to determine if vaccination as early as 12 months of age is effective, but immunization of children less than 12 months of age has revealed suboptimal immune responses. Side effects are relatively mild.

TABLE 15.11

HEPATITIS A VACCINE DOSES[a]

Age (years)	Vaccine	Antigen Dose	Volume per Dose (mL)
2–18	Havrix (SmithKline Beecham)	720 EL.U.[b]	0.5
	Vaqta (Merck)	25 U[c]	0.5
19 and older	Havrix (SmithKline Beecham)	1,440 EL.U.	1.0
	Vaqta (Merck)	50 U	1.0

[a] Both vaccines are administered in a 0-, 6-, to 12-month schedule.
[b] EL.U. indicates enzyme-linked immunoassay units.
[c] Antigen units (each unit is equivalent to approximately 1 mg of viral protein).
A combination hepatitis A/hepatitis B vaccine (Twinrix) is available for persons 18 years of age and older.

Suggested Readings

American Academy of Pediatrics Committee on Infectious Diseases. Recommended childhood and adolescent immunization schedule—United States, January-June 2004. *Pediatrics* 2004;113(1 Pt 1):142.

Centers for Disease Control and Prevention. Recommended childhood and adolescent immunization schedule—United States. *MMWR* 2005;53(51): Q1-3.

Centers for Disease Control and Prevention. General recommendations on immunization: recommendations of the Advisory Committee on Immunization Practices and the American Academy of Family Physicians. *MMWR* 2002;51:No.RR-2.

Pickering LK, ed. *Red Book: 2003 Report of the Committee on Infectious Diseases,* 26th ed. Elk Grove Village, IL: American Academy of Pediatrics, 2003.

Plotkin SA, Orenstein WA, eds. *Vaccines,* 4th ed. Philadelphia: Elsevier, 2004.

Web sites with Up-to-Date Vaccine Information:
American Academy of Pediatrics—www.aap.org
Centers for Disease Control and Prevention—www.cdc.gov
Health Canada—www.hc-sc.gc.ca
Immunization Action Coalition—www.immunize.org
Institute for Vaccine Safety—www.vaccinesafety.edu

CHAPTER 16 ■ INJURY PREVENTION AND CONTROL

MODENA HOOVER WILSON AND REBECCA LEVIN-GOODMAN

In the United States and many other countries, injury is the leading cause of death for pediatric patients who survive the perils of the first few days and months of life. Injury also is a prominent cause of morbidity and disability. It precipitates numerous emergency department visits and hospitalizations and adds substantially to health care costs. To say that injury is now the most important health problem of childhood is not an exaggeration.

Injury is a disease that is neither inherited nor congenital. An agent outside of the child is always involved, and injury therefore can be prevented. After injury occurs, prompt and appropriate medical care is needed to minimize the consequences.

Injury control includes preventing events that may cause injury; preventing or modifying the transfer of energy, which eliminates or minimizes the injury if the event occurs; and ensuring timely and age-appropriate field care, transport, treatment, and rehabilitation for the injured child if injury occurs.

The subset of injuries that are often labeled "intentional" (e.g., homicide and suicide) accounts for a significant proportion of injury deaths, even in childhood (Table 16.1). These receive special attention in Chapter 105. This chapter is directed toward the prevention of unintentional injury.

EPIDEMIOLOGY OF INJURY IN CHILDHOOD AND ADOLESCENCE

Motor vehicle–related events claim more children's lives than any other event (Table 16.1), but other numerically important causes of unintentional injury deaths during childhood and adolescence include drowning, pedestrian events, suffocation, fires and burns, poisonings, pedalcyclist events, unintentional firearm injuries, and falls (Table 16.1).

Although during early infancy the number of injury deaths is exceeded by other causes, the importance of injury should not be overlooked. Injury death rates during the first year of life are high when compared with injury death rates in other preadolescent age groups. Unintentional injury causes approximately 45% of all childhood deaths occurring after infancy (Table 16.2).

The events leading to injury death vary by age, because children differ in vulnerability, ability, and exposure to hazards by age. Compare the toddler who inadvertently hangs in the drapery cord with the intoxicated adolescent driver who crashes into a tree after the graduation party.

Death from injury is tragic and all too common, but it is only a portion of the injury problem. According to the Centers for Disease Control and Prevention, for every childhood death caused by injury, there are approximately 34 injury-related hospitalizations and 1,000 emergency department visits. Every year 20% to 25% of children are injured severely enough to need medical attention, miss school, and/or be confined to bed rest. Other data, inclusive of persons of all ages and injury events of all types, show that approximately 150,000 injury deaths occur in the United States each year. Confirming the scope of the problem are the estimates that for every one of those deaths there are approximately 18 injury-related hospitalizations, 250 emergency department visits for injury, and 400 episodes of injury.

PRINCIPLES OF INJURY CONTROL

The enormous number of unintentional injuries has prompted an increasingly organized effort to understand and control the problem. Several key principles have emerged.

TABLE 16.1

NUMBER OF INJURY DEATHS FOR CHILDREN AND ADOLESCENTS, BY AGE GROUP, UNITED STATES, 2000

	Age Group (in Years)					Total Number of Deaths
	<1	1–4	5–9	10–14	15–19	
All deaths	28,035	4,979	3,253	4,160	13,563	53,990
All injuries	1,295	2,221	1,556	2,164	10,437	17,673
Unintentional injuries	881	1,826	1,391	1,588	6,755	12,441
Motor vehicle occupant	88	201	284	375	2,623	3,571
Drowning	75	493	201	174	371	1,314
Pedestrian	16	269	222	199	332	1,038
Suffocation	526	151	45	72	70	864
Fires and burns	39	297	183	84	79	682
Poisoning	14	32	17	28	351	442
Pedalcyclist	—	4	57	107	59	227
Firearm, unintentional	1	18	18	49	107	193
Motorcyclist	—	—	4	22	158	184
Falls	8	36	16	21	99	180
Other unintentional	114	325	344	457	2506	3,746
Homicide	349	356	140	231	1914	2,990
Firearm	12	28	50	137	1549	1,776
Suicide	—	—	7	300	1621	1,928
Firearm	—	—	—	110	897	1,007

Source: Centers for Disease Control and Prevention. Web-based Injury Statistics Query and Reporting System (WISQARS) [National Center for Injury Prevention and Control, Centers for Disease Control and Prevention Web site] 2002. Available at: www.cdc.gov/ncipc/wisqars. Accessed October 1, 2003.

Injury control is more than accident prevention. An injury is not the same as an accident. The focus for the health professional should be on controlling the disease (i.e., the injury). Although unintended, most accidents and the injuries they produce are predictable. For example, it is easy to foresee that a child riding a walker may fall down an unguarded stairway or off a porch and be injured on the hard surface below. These injury-producing events can be predicted and avoided. Injuries can be prevented even though accidents occur. To illustrate, seat belts do not prevent car crashes, but they do decrease injuries sustained in a car crash. While the word "accident" is commonly used by the public to refer to events that result in injury, many injury control specialists propose avoiding the word entirely because it may connote that injuries are unavoidable.

Injury can be viewed in the same epidemiologic framework as infectious disease. Energy is the agent of injury. Although the full list includes chemical, radiation, and electrical energy, most pediatric injury is caused by mechanical or thermal energy. The injury occurs when energy impinges on the host at a level the host cannot resist. Like the microbial agents of infectious diseases, the agents of injury can be conveyed to the host by an inanimate object (e.g., vehicle) or an animal (e.g., vector). The agent and host interact in an environment that is subject to biologic, social, and economic influences, all of which may influence the result. Injury can be controlled by influencing one or more of these factors: agent, vehicle, vector, host, or environment.

Injury-control strategies can be grouped by their temporal relation to the injury event. Some strategies are preevent phase; they reduce the likelihood that an event with injury-producing potential will occur. Some are event phase in that they reduce injury during the event. Postevent phase strategies reduce the resulting damage after the injury has occurred.

Reducing injury requires preventing or reducing the interaction between the agent and host, and a complete approach to injury control requires attention to all three phases of the injury event. Haddon has provided an organizing framework for understanding the relationship of variables and interventions to the potential for injury. Table 16.3 provides examples of how the Haddon Matrix can be applied to various types of unintentional injury.

To be effective, a strategy must decrease injury if it is used, and it must be used. These are separate considerations. Many strategies have never been adequately evaluated. The Harborview Injury Prevention and Research Center provides systematic reviews of the effectiveness of childhood injury prevention interventions on the World Wide Web. Strategies are sometimes recommended by advocates before evidence of effectiveness has accumulated because they make scientific sense or because they are similar to other successful strategies. If strategies are retained despite demonstrated lack of efficacy, resources are diverted from developing or promoting effective alternatives.

Efficacious strategies may fail because people fail to use them. Unfastened seat belts do not reduce injury. A prime role for health professionals is to educate and motivate families to use strategies known to prevent or reduce injury.

The most desirable injury control strategies are automatic. Automatic, or *passive*, strategies are those that protect persons without individual action, or they are built in. For example, if all passenger cars are factory equipped with driver-side airbags, male adolescent drivers, a group at extremely high risk for car-crash injuries and death, benefit without any change in their knowledge or behavior.

By contrast, strategies that require frequent individual action, such as buckling a seat belt, are called *active*. These strategies are likely to be omitted by some people all of the time and by many people at least some of the time. Achieving widespread use of new active strategies (e.g., car safety seats) appears to require the addition of incentives and removal of disincentives and may only occur after a gradual change in cultural attitudes. Some persons, often those at highest risk, are unprotected because they fail to comply.

TABLE 16.2

AGE-BASED INJURY PREVENTION COUNSELING TOPICS

Infants and Preschoolers	
Traffic safety	Appropriate use of child safety restraints
	Seat belt use by parents
Burn prevention	Smoke detectors in home
	Hot water temperature between 120°F and 130°F
	Matches and lighters out of reach
Fall prevention	Window guards/stairway gates
	Avoidance of infant walkers
	Not leaving infant alone in high places
Poison prevention	Safe storage of medicine and household products
Drowning prevention	Elimination of water hazards
	Constant supervision in bath and around water
	Complete fencing of pools/spas
	Personal flotation devices while boating
Choking prevention	Small objects and solid foods as choking hazards
Firearm safety	Removal of guns from places children live and play
Emergency preparation	Training in infant cardiopulmonary resuscitation for adults
School-Age Children	
Traffic safety	Appropriate use of booster seats and seat belts
	No all-terrain vehicle (ATV) use by children younger than 16
	Safe pedestrian practices
	Bicycle helmets
	Protective equipment for in-line skating and skateboarding
Water safety	Swimming lessons/no swimming alone
	Personal flotation devices while boating
Sports safety	Safety equipment and physical conditioning
Firearm safety	No handguns in the home
	Safe storage of guns
Adolescents	
Traffic safety	Seat belt use
	Alcohol and motor vehicle crashes
	Motorcycle and bicycle helmets
	Protective equipment for in-line skating and skateboarding
Water safety	Avoidance of alcohol use in water-related activities
	Personal flotation devices while boating
Sports safety	Safety equipment and physical conditioning
Firearm safety	No handguns in the home
	Safe storage of guns

Adapted from The Injury Prevention Program (TIPP) of the American Academy of Pediatrics.

Many strategies fall between the two extremes of active or passive. For example, a parent may take action once to protect family members over time by turning down the water heater to prevent scald burns or by installing an automatic sprinkler system to reduce the possibility of fire. Purchasing, installing, and maintaining a smoke alarm powered by batteries requires periodic action.

Passive strategies are usually preferable to active strategies because they avoid the issue of compliance and are therefore more effective. Unfortunately, passive strategies are not available to prevent all types of injuries. Health care providers must continue to encourage the use of active strategies that are known to be efficacious.

Strategies that prevent unintentional injuries may also prevent some inflicted injuries: abuse, homicide, and suicide. For instance, if water heaters do not heat water to a temperature that will burn skin, tap water scalding is prevented no matter what the intent of the caregiver. Reduction in the availability of handguns can be expected to prevent unintentional childhood and adolescent firearm deaths and many homicides and suicides.

AVENUES OF INJURY CONTROL

Education and Health Promotion

Health professionals traditionally try to change behaviors that affect health by counseling patients and their families. Understanding of successful physician communication and counseling techniques continues to grow. Certainly, anticipatory guidance for injury prevention must go beyond the simple delivery of information. Increased knowledge about an injury problem and prevention strategies does not lead reliably to action. Counseling for behavior change requires soliciting information (finding out what the parent or patient knows, is doing, and intends to do); providing sensitive and sensible advice; focusing on parental or patient perceptions of risks, benefits, and barriers to change; and encouraging change through time.

An increasing number of injury issues are being added to the list of possible subjects for anticipatory guidance. They compete for the limited time available during a health supervision visit. The health provider must have a strategy for setting

TABLE 16.3

HADDON MATRIX

Phase of Event	Examples of Injury Control Variables and Interventions			
	Human	Agent or Vehicle	Physical	Socioeconomic
Pre-event	Sobriety	Child-resistant caps on medications	Weather conditions	Reduced production of handguns and bullets
	Adult supervision	Child-resistant cigarette lighters	Four-sided fencing surrounding swimming pools	Urban crowding
Event	Bicycle helmet use	Air bags	Traffic-calming measures	Seat belt laws
	Car safety seat use	Loose-fill surface materials on playgrounds	Smoke detectors	Affordability of protective equipment
Post-event	Age	Fuel system integrity	Distance to and quality of emergency medical systems	Training of emergency medical service personnel
	Physical condition	Flame-resistant sleepwear	Rehabilitation programs	National Poison Help Line

Source: Adapted from Pedialink continuing medical education course. Moving Kids Safely: Introduction to Car Safety Seats [Pedialink Web site]. Available at: www.pedialink.org. Accessed October 7, 2003; and Widome MD, ed. *Injury prevention and control for children and youth,* 3rd ed. Elk Grove Village, IL: American Academy of Pediatrics, 1997.

priorities among injury-prevention topics. An implicit and an increasingly more explicitly stated approach is to base choices on the child's developmental age, features of the preventable injury (severity, frequency), and features of the recommended prevention strategy (e.g., demonstrated effectiveness, availability, and cost).

Gains have been made with a health promotion approach that delivers the message from many respected sources and provides rewards for demonstrating the desirable behavior. Schools, community groups, agencies, and the popular media all can have roles in modifying beliefs and behaviors that affect injury and injury prevention. Informed health care providers can stimulate and advise on these efforts by providing leadership or consultation.

Educating persons in power, whose decisions determine the risk of injury for many, may produce the best results. These people include leaders in schools and child-care centers, health care providers, leaders of public agencies, legislators and regulators, law enforcement professionals, leaders of voluntary organizations, designers, architects, builders, engineers, leaders of business and industry, and those controlling the mass media.

Legislation, Regulation, and Enforcement

Legislative and regulatory efforts to bring about injury control can occur at the local, state, or federal level. Little uniformity exists among local jurisdictions or states with regard to measures affecting injury. Illustrating this is motor vehicle occupant safety. Although an increasing number of states require seat belt use by front-seat car occupants and all require car safety seat use for particular categories of young passengers, the specific legislation varies widely. Some states allow *primary enforcement,* which means that noncompliance is sufficient reason to stop the driver. Others allow only *secondary enforcement,* meaning that the citation can be made only if another offense has prompted action. Passenger ages and positions, vehicle types, and penalties under the law also vary, leaving many persons unprotected even by full compliance with the law. The

level of enforcement is not uniform and often is so spotty that it negates the intention of the measure. Nevertheless, the impact of such legislation on injury can be documented. States with long-standing car safety seat laws have experienced decreased infant motor vehicle occupant death rates. Specifically designed legislation has been shown to be an effective strategy for injury control. Health professionals should be advocates for children in the legislative arena.

Legislative authority or specific legislation must precede agency action in many cases. Agencies that control personal practices and the environment (e.g., boards of parks and recreation, health departments, schools, athletic associations, traffic authorities, regulators of consumer products) can promulgate within their authority regulations that decrease the likelihood of childhood and adolescent injury. Smoke alarm and sprinkler system requirements can be set for building construction, specific pool fencing requirements can be mandated, children transported in private cars on school trips can be required to wear seat belts, and fireworks can be prohibited within city limits. The success of well-designed regulations depends on enforcement or the perception of enforcement. Unenforced regulations, like knowledge without behavior change, cannot prevent injury.

Legislation enacted for other reasons may also have injury-reduction potential. The Emergency Highway Energy Conservation Act (1974) reduced the speed limit to 55 miles per hour to conserve gasoline. The highway death rate fell. When many states revoked this conservative limit, deaths increased with speeds. A bill requiring a deposit on glass bottles, promulgated for environmental reasons, resulted in fewer pediatric emergency department treatments of lacerations. The activity of the Consumer Product Safety Commission (CPSC), created by the Consumer Product Safety Act of 1972, is the centerpiece of federal efforts to eliminate unreasonable hazards associated with consumer products. In this role and as administrator of several earlier acts (the Flammable Fabrics Act, 1953; the Refrigerator Safety Act, 1956; the Federal Hazardous Substances Act, 1960; and the Poison Prevention Packaging Act, 1970), the CPSC has had a special role in injury control for children. It reacts to petitions, complaints, or clues from its surveillance systems, including the National Electronic Injury Surveillance System, which collects injury data from approximately 100 hospital emergency departments nationally. The CPSC can negotiate voluntary product changes, and it can regulate sales and force product recalls. There has been significant public concern over the safety of children's products and furniture, which often are not subject to stringent testing standards, and the effectiveness of the product recall system. Health professionals can advocate for voluntary product testing by manufacturers and encourage parents and child care providers to be aware of product recalls announced by the CPSC. Health professionals should bring product-related injuries to the attention of the CPSC and CPSC findings to the attention of their patients and communities.

Litigation

Where educational, legislative, and regulatory options have failed to bring about injury control, litigation may succeed. Pertinent to the protection of adolescent drivers, for instance, is the facilitating role that litigation against automobile makers has played in expediting the provision of airbags in automobiles. More recently, various municipalities have pursued lawsuits against gun manufacturers, modeled on successful litigation against the tobacco industry, in hopes of encouraging manufacturers to take steps to limit children's access to firearms.

INJURY CONTROL AND PERSONAL FREEDOM

Objections to the implementation of injury control strategies are often framed as defenses of personal freedom. For younger children, the argument is sometimes made that injuries are a necessary part of the trial and error learning process of growing up. However, automatic strategies—those that protect the child without constant action—can be viewed as freeing the child to explore with less restriction in an inherently safer environment. Protection of the young child is generally accepted with less tension than measures addressing any other segment of the population. Many precedents exist for societal intrusion to ensure the health and welfare of children.

The argument against restricting adolescents to protect them from injury is made also on behalf of adults: The informed person has a right to take risks. Unfortunately, the injuries and psychological and financial burden are not always confined to the person taking the risk.

INJURY RISK

Injury is a common problem. No child or adolescent can be considered free from risk. However, some patterns may be helpful in designing programs or counseling individual patients.

Demographic Issues

Throughout the lifespan, male subjects have higher injury death rates than female subjects. This increased risk is apparent even before the age of 1 year; the total injury death rate for infant boys is approximately 1.3 times the rate for girls. In adolescence, the differential is even more striking, with a male-to-female ratio of approximately 2.8:1.0. The differences appear to reflect differences in likelihood of involvement in hazardous activities. Whether these differences in male behavior are entirely because of socialization (i.e., role expectations) or reflect innate behavioral characteristics specific to boys and men is not clear. Gender differences are greatest for fatal and other severe injuries.

If the full spectrum of injury is considered, rates are highest for both genders during adolescence. The adolescent injury death rate is exceeded only by that for the most elderly segments of the population.

Injury death rates vary with ethnicity and economic status. Native Americans have the highest injury rates of population groups in the United States. Blacks are a second group at particularly high risk. Asian Americans have the lowest rates. Some of the differences by race can be explained by differences in socioeconomic status. Considerable evidence suggests that unintentional injury rates are highest in the lowest-income areas. Unintentional injury death rates fall markedly as the per capita income increases. Whites and blacks of the same income level have approximately the same death rates from unintentional injury.

There are unique injury concerns in children with special health care needs. For example, children with behavior disorders such as attention deficit hyperactivity disorder (ADHD) have been found to have 1.5 times the odds of sustaining injuries than children without behavior disorders. Targeted injury prevention measures can address the increased risk of children with special needs. For instance, children with seizure disorders are at greater risk for drowning and should be supervised closely while taking a bath or swimming; showers should be used instead of baths if privacy concerns prevent direct supervision.

Although homicide rates are highest where the population is most dense, unintentional injury rates are highest in the most remote rural areas. Unlike differences in injury rates by race, disparities by population density do not narrow when adjustments are made for differences in per capita income.

Demographic associations, although they provide interesting clues to the complexity of injury causation and are helpful in program development, do not significantly narrow the task for health care providers. Persons who belong to the higher-risk demographic categories may require extended counseling time and effort, but patients who do not fall into the demographic categories of highest risk cannot be excluded from counseling, because no group is free from all injury risk. Although the concept of the accident-prone person has been popular, evidence has provided no easy rubric for limiting injury control counseling to a small subset of patients. Injury appears to be far too evenly spread across the population to allow any narrow definition of the subpopulation at risk.

Developmental Issues

The types of injuries to which a child is most vulnerable varies with personal circumstance and with age. Age is a rough correlate of size, developmental ability, and lifestyle, all of which influence exposure.

Infants

After adolescents, infants are the pediatric age group with the highest injury death rate. The small size of infants may be the first of their developmental disadvantages predisposing to injury. With small body size comes a small airway that is easily occluded. A small body slips through small spaces that do not always permit the relatively large head to follow, resulting in entrapment injury. Tests with anthropomorphic dummies suggest that unrestrained infants become missiles during car crashes or are crushed between the car interior and the body of the adult who was holding them. Infants, completely dependent on their caregivers, are handled on elevated surfaces for the caregiver's convenience, precipitating falls. The motor skills of infants are primitive, precluding easy escape from danger, which results in a relatively high rate of drownings, suffocations, and deaths from fires and burns.

Infants spend most of their time in their own homes or in the homes of substitute caregivers, and most injuries in infancy occur in the home. Making the home a safe (i.e., childproof) environment is worthwhile.

Toddlers

After babies develop motor skills that allow them to get around on their own by creeping or crawling and especially by walking, their injury profile changes. Toddlers are busy pushing, pulling, finding, poking, mouthing, climbing, and exploring. An active toddler can exhaust even the most vigilant parent. The toddler may run into the street, tumble down stairs, or disappear in crowds. Even the most passive toddler occasionally escapes a distracted parent. Toddlers have no impulse control. They do not understand cause and effect. Making the indoor environment a safe area for exploration is worthwhile. Although the injury death rate for the toddler does not stand out, the rate of nonlethal injuries is quite high.

Preschoolers

Increasingly sophisticated motor and intellectual skills combined with the desire to imitate the behavior of older children and adults bring the preschooler in contact with a whole new group of injury risks. For example, the child in this age group becomes a tricyclist and then a tentative bicyclist. Curiosity about matches and fires burgeons. Although skills are becoming sophisticated, judgment is not. The child of this age cannot be relied on to recognize danger. Thinking is magical: "If superheroes can fly, so can I."

Elementary School–Aged Children

The grammar school age group is quite healthy. Persons of this age boast the lowest injury death rate of the lifespan, but over 35% of deaths that occur are caused by unintentional injury, as are many urgent medical visits and hospitalizations.

Often for the first time, the child is coping independently with the traffic environment. More children this age die as pedestrians than as motor vehicle occupants, and bicycling injuries begin to take their toll. Children of this age are still not capable of making accurate judgments about speed and distance. Their decisions begin to be heavily influenced by the actions and opinions of their peers. Their motor skills and knowledge (e.g., for lighting a fire, firing a gun, mowing a lawn, or starting a motor vehicle) far outstrip their judgment.

Early Adolescents

As they approach adolescence, children are given more freedom, spend more time without adult supervision, and range farther from home. Peer pressure exerts its most profound influence. Helmets and seat belts may be eschewed by the group. Risk taking becomes more conscious. The traffic environment poses the biggest hazard, particularly for those who ride with older adolescent friends who drive, who operate any kind of motorized vehicle themselves, or who ride a bicycle in traffic.

Older Adolescents

Adult privileges and practices are attained by older adolescents without adult experience, ability, and responsibility. The assumption of the adult behaviors of drug and alcohol use and use of weapons play an important but incompletely understood role in this age group, in which injury, if both unintentional and intentional are included, accounts for approximately 75% of all deaths. The older adolescent has the highest risk of any age group for motor vehicle occupant death. Many younger adolescents and most older adolescents work, so workplace injuries become important. The most serious are motor vehicle related, homicides, or from falls or fires. Older adolescents have a significantly higher risk of work-related injuries than the general working population. Intentional injuries (i.e., suicide, homicide) also take a striking toll.

MAJOR INJURIES

More than 12,000 persons younger than 20 years lost their lives in unintentional injury events in the United States in 2000. Motor vehicle traffic injuries alone were responsible for approximately 7,500 deaths in this age group, about 60% of all unintentional injury deaths. Not all potential causes of serious injury can be presented in this chapter. The rest of this section concentrates on the most severe unintentional injury events as reflected in mortality statistics. Selected sources of data on childhood and adolescent injury are listed in the resources at the end of this chapter.

Motor Vehicle–Related Injuries

Not surprisingly, most children and adolescents who die of transportation-related injuries were motor vehicle occupants. Pedestrians struck by motor vehicles in traffic make up the second largest group. A significant number of deaths also is attributed to motorcycle and bicycle incidents. Because of their impressive numbers and severity, prevention of motor vehicle occupant deaths has served as the flagship effort of the field of injury control, but the protection of child passengers needs continuing attention. Of particular concern are the injuries related to the improper use and placement of car safety seats.

Injuries from motor vehicle crashes are a leading cause of death well into adulthood, and they are an important cause of permanent disability. Motor vehicle injuries account for a large proportion of brain and spinal cord injuries and of disfiguring facial injuries. Sources of motor vehicle–related injury, the prevention of which is not discussed in this chapter, include trains, aircraft, school buses, farm machinery, and riding lawn mowers.

Among the pediatric age groups, adolescents are at highest risk for motor vehicle–related injury, but the number of deaths related to motor vehicles is significant throughout the age span. The male-to-female ratio, which portrays an increased risk for male subjects at every age after 1 year, is especially high during adolescence. The fatality rate for motor vehicle injury is particularly high for unrestrained infants involved in crashes. For children aged 1 to 4 years, the number of pedestrian deaths exceeds the number of motor vehicle occupant deaths. For all other age groups except the very elderly, motor vehicle occupant injuries outstrip pedestrian injuries as a cause of death.

Although motor vehicle travel increases with income, motor vehicle injury and death rates decrease, for several likely reasons: differences in urbanization, local road conditions, vehicle types, driving behavior, seat belt use, and quality of medical care. The motor vehicle death rate in rural areas is higher than in urban areas, a difference accounted for almost entirely by motor vehicle occupant deaths.

Motor Vehicle Occupants

Incidence. Approximately 3,600 children and adolescents younger than 20 years were killed as motor vehicle occupants in the United States in 2000. Injury and death rates peak during adolescence for both girls and boys, although adolescents travel fewer vehicle miles than adults. Male teenage drivers have higher fatal crash rates than any other group.

Motor vehicle occupant death rates have been declining since the 1960s, a fortunate fact attributed to changes in roads and vehicles as well as to seat belts, car safety seats, and more recently, airbags. In a substantial but decreasing proportion of crashes with fatalities, a driver's blood alcohol level is found to be elevated.

Because of adolescents' risk-taking behavior and lack of driving experience, young drivers are at greatly increased risk of crashing. Teenagers' motor vehicle fatality rate is higher than that of any other group, and on a per-mile-drive basis, 16-year-old drivers are more than 20 times as likely to have a crash as the general driving public. Young drivers, aged 15 to 20 years, make up 6.6% of licensed drivers in the United States, but 14% of drivers involved in fatal crashes and 16% of drivers involved in police-reported crashes.

Prevention. Motor vehicle occupant injuries can be reduced by preventing crashes or by reducing the forces that impinge on the body during crashes. In addition to modifying vehicles and reducing speed, forces can be reduced by spreading them over a wider area of the body and by increasing the distance over which the body decelerates. This is accomplished by restraint systems and by airbags. Most safety equipment in vehicles is designed to be protective for adults; additional measures must be taken to afford children adequate protection. Topics of specific interest to health professionals caring for children include counseling and advocacy issues.

Counseling Points. Injury can be prevented by the use of appropriate restraint systems for age and size, as shown in Table 16.4. Each year the American Academy of Pediatrics publishes "Car Safety Seats: A Guide for Families," which includes a list of car safety seats currently on the market. At least 80% of car safety seats are used improperly, so counseling should include information about the correct use of car safety seats; patients can be referred to a local Child Passenger Safety Technician for additional assistance. (A list of certified technicians is available from the National Highway Traffic Safety Administration's Web site at http://www.nhtsa.dot.gov/CPS/Contacts/index.cfm.) Be-

cause infants restrained in car safety seats in the front passenger seats of automobiles with passenger-side airbags and young children out of position in the front seat have been killed when airbags deployed, it is particularly important to counsel families that infants and young children should always ride properly restrained in the back seat.

Special attention should be paid to use of booster seats for school-age children. Children aged 4 to 8 are more likely to be improperly restrained, usually with the lap/shoulder belt before it fits, than other age groups; these children would be much safer properly restrained in belt-positioning booster seats. Clinicians can suggest that a child ride in a booster seat until the seat belt fits properly, usually at about 4'9" in height and between 8 to 12 years old. Parents should be encouraged to make the transition to the lap/shoulder belt once it fits properly, to continue to insist on the use of seat belts through adolescence and into adulthood, and to set the standard by using their own seat belts. The advantage of airbags plus seat belts for adolescents and adults should be stressed.

Parents should be reminded that teenagers are only beginning to learn the complex task of driving and should provide a low-risk, supervised environment to do so. Parents can be encouraged to limit the number and age of passengers, nighttime driving, and unsupervised driving for teenage drivers, and they should impose penalties for breaking these rules. Drinking and driving should be discouraged, and parents should be encouraged to provide adolescents with a safe ride home.

Parents of very small premature infants, children with severe developmental disabilities, and children in casts that preclude using a standard safety seat need special guidance. In particular, infants born at less than 37 weeks' gestation should be observed in a car safety seat before hospital discharge to monitor for possible apnea, bradycardia, or oxygen desaturation. Infants with desaturation, apnea, or bradycardia in a semiupright position should travel in a supine or prone position in a car bed, an alternative safety device designed for this purpose.

Advocacy Issues. Advocacy issues include providing restraint devices for children with special needs, extending persons and vehicles covered under state safety seat and seat belt laws,

TABLE 16.4

RECOMMENDATIONS FOR CAR SAFETY SEAT USE

Type of Restraint	Appropriate Use	Typical Age for Use
Car bed	Use for infants under 21 lb. if medically indicated (usually premature or low-birth-weight infants with documented oxygen desaturation, apnea, or bradycardia in a semiupright position)	Premature infants
Infant-only seat (always used rear-facing)	From minimum weight allowed by seat to 20–22 lb.	Birth to <1 year
Convertible safety seat (rear-facing)	Until child is at least 1 year of age and at least 20 lb., preferably to maximum rear-facing weight and height allowed by seat	Birth to 1–2 years
Convertible safety seat (forward-facing)	Child must be at least 1 year of age and at least 20 lb.; use forward-facing to maximum weight and height allowed by seat	1–2 to 4 years
Combination seat with internal harness; forward-facing seat with internal harness; integrated child seat	Child must be at least 1 year of age and at least 20 lb.; use with harness to maximum weight and height allowed by seat; children who weigh <40 lb. are best protected in a seat with an internal harness	1–2 to 4 years
Belt-positioning booster seat	Use after child has outgrown seat with internal harness, until lap/shoulder belt fits the child	4 to 8–12 years
Lap/shoulder belt	Use when shoulder belt fits across midchest and shoulder, lap belt lies low and snug across thighs, and child can sit all the way back against vehicle seat with knees bent at edge of vehicle seat	Beginning at 8–12 years

Source: American Academy of Pediatrics, Committee on Injury and Poison Prevention. Selecting and using the most appropriate car safety seats for growing children: guidelines for counseling parents. *Pediatrics* 2002;109:550.

enforcing safety seat and seat belt laws, increasing the minimum licensing age or the provisional licensing period or extending the curfew (i.e., limitation on nighttime driving) associated with provisional licenses, and maintaining lower speed limits.

Pedestrians

Incidence. The second-largest category of vehicle-related deaths is that of persons on foot killed by motor vehicles. In such crashes, the pedestrian is completely unshielded and is at a great disadvantage. The overall trend in pedestrian death rates has been downward despite the fact that evidence for effective countermeasures is sparse. Improvement in the childhood pedestrian injury rate may be related more to declining rates of walking rather than to injury prevention campaigns or counseling.

In the year 2000, 1,038 child pedestrians were killed in the United States. During the pediatric years, the pedestrian death rates are highest for those between 15 and 19 years, and boys are overrepresented. Pedestrian deaths are an urban disease, with two-thirds of the deaths and even more of the injuries occurring in urban areas. Although less frequent than urban pedestrian injury events, rural events are much more likely to result in death, probably because of higher vehicle speeds.

Most childhood pedestrian injuries occur when children run into the street in the middle of a block or attempt to cross between intersections. Some deaths occur when motor vehicles invade the pedestrian's space on a sidewalk or median strip. The weight of the vehicle and the speed at which it is traveling are important determinants of the severity of injury. The death-to-injury ratio is approximately three times higher for heavy trucks than for cars, and it increases as the posted speed limit increases. Most often, the front of a motor vehicle strikes the pedestrian, but children are also killed when they run into the side of the moving vehicle, are struck by the vehicle's protruding hardware (e.g., mirror), or are run over by the rear wheels of a truck or bus. More pedestrians are killed walking along a roadway in the same direction as traffic than against traffic. Allowing motorists to make a right turn after stopping at a red light has increased pedestrian injuries in urban areas, because as drivers look left for oncoming traffic, they do not always see pedestrians approaching from the right. Although most pedestrian injuries and deaths do occur in traffic, during the first few years of life a sizable proportion of pedestrian deaths occur in nontraffic areas (e.g., driveways, lanes), often with the driver backing over a toddler playing in the area. Nontraffic pedestrian deaths are particularly high in rural areas.

Prevention. Not surprisingly, child pedestrian injuries increase with traffic volume, speed, curbside parking, and a dearth of protected play areas. Unfortunately, educational programs to improve child pedestrian behavior appear to have modest effects at best and are particularly disappointing when fielded in the absence of other measures. The most successful strategies to date appear to be changes in vehicle design and traffic "calming" measures (i.e., measures that decrease the number of motor vehicles on a roadway and their speed). Wherever and whenever possible, motor vehicle traffic and child pedestrians should be physically separated with barriers or space.

Counseling Points. Counseling might include advice on street-crossing timing and training, using barriers between play areas and traffic, planning the route to school, and avoiding walking in or along streets or roads, especially at night.

Advocacy Issues. Advocacy issues include slowing motor vehicle speeds in residential areas, diverting traffic from residential areas and around schools, prohibiting parking where children are likely to cross, loading and unloading school buses and cars away from traffic, developing safe off-street play areas, and building sidewalks and convenient walkways where pedestrian traffic is heavy or making other modifications of high-risk sites.

Motorcycles and Other Motorized Vehicles

Incidence. The rate of injuries associated with vehicles that travel at high rates of speed, especially on roads and highways, and provide no external protection for riders is high. Although children and adolescents may be physically capable of operating vehicles such as motorcycles, minibikes, mopeds, trail bikes, all-terrain vehicles, and snowmobiles, the risk under many conditions, including off-road driving, is excessive. Use by children and young adolescents should be strongly discouraged.

The per mile death rate, the number of deaths per registered vehicle, and the death-to-injury ratio for motorcycles are all higher than for passenger cars. In the year 2000, 184 people younger than 20 years were killed in the United States while riding a motorcycle. The disparity between death rates by gender is extreme, with many more young men dying than young women. Crashes and injuries increase with increasing vehicle power. Alcohol abuse plays a part, particularly in nighttime, single-vehicle crashes. Helmets clearly decrease severe injury and death rates among motorcyclists. Deaths decrease when laws requiring riders to wear helmets are in place, although perfect compliance with the laws does not occur.

Minibikes, minicycles, and trail bikes are all motorized two-wheeled cycles that range from little more than a bicycle to almost a motorcycle. They vary in speed and other capabilities. Because they are marketed for off-road use, they do not fall under federal safety standards for road vehicles or the usual licensing procedures for vehicle and driver. The size and marketing of many are clearly targeted at children and adolescents, and they account for a number of pediatric deaths and injuries.

In 2001, over 33,000 children under 16 years of age were injured riding all-terrain vehicles (ATVs), a 56.5% increase since 1997. ATVs come in three- or four-wheel versions and are marketed for use on rugged terrain. The three-wheeled version is notably unstable, with overturns on slopes leading to catastrophic injury. A ban on the sale of three-wheeled ATVs in the United States went into effect in December 1987, but many are still in use. Manufacturers have agreed that high-powered ATVs should not be marketed to children younger than 16 years, but dealer compliance is thought to be less than perfect. High speeds; lack of differential on the rear wheels, which makes turning difficult, especially for children; and vehicle weight all contribute to the high risk. ATV-related injuries tend to be more severe than those related to bicycles or other sports, and some studies suggest that children suffer more severe injuries than adults.

Snowmobiles, capable of reaching high speeds, also take a heavy toll among the pediatric age groups. Of the 10,000 injuries in 1 year, 10% were to children 14 years or younger, with persons between 15 and 24 years of age incurring one-quarter of all injuries. Given the seasonal and regional limitations on snowmobile use, the injury rate appears quite high. Many states require registration of snowmobiles and some require a driver's license to operate on public lands or roads, but few put restrictions on driver age. A few require child operators to wear helmets. Head injuries from crashes and rollovers cause most of the deaths.

Prevention. The vehicles discussed in this section, especially the heavy and powerful ones, carry a very high injury risk. They are not toys. Operation of motorized vehicles by persons under the legal driving age should be deemed inappropriate and strongly discouraged. Careful instruction by an experienced and mature operator should precede operation at any age, and helmets and protective clothing should be worn. Adults should be discouraged from carrying children as passengers on these vehicles, but if they do, they should be experienced drivers, sober, and willing to drive slowly.

Counseling Points. Counseling, although unstudied for this subject, might include information about avoiding motorcycles and off-road vehicles for children younger than driving age, discouraging the use of motorcycles and off-road vehicles by adolescents because of the high rate of serious injury, using helmets and other protective clothing for operators and passengers, and avoiding use of off-road vehicles on public roads because other motor vehicles may be encountered.

Advocacy Issues. Advocacy issues include equipment modifications to make these motorized vehicles safer; regulating the marketing and sales of the products to children, licensing of operators, and minimum age requirements; prohibiting the use of off-road vehicles on public roads; and promulgating and enforcing helmet laws.

Bicycles

Incidence. Children and adolescents are disproportionately represented among the bicyclists killed in the United States. In 2000, 227 bicycle-related deaths occurred among people younger than 20 in the United States, and there were many more injuries. The death rate is highest for children between the ages of 10 and 14 years. Most bicycling deaths involve collision of the bicyclist with a motor vehicle, and most involve head or neck injury. Male riders have higher injury rates and much higher death rates than female riders.

Most injuries and deaths occur during warm months and in the afternoon or early evening. The weekend is not a particularly vulnerable time, as it is for other motor vehicle deaths, probably because alcohol abuse does not play as large a part. Rates also vary less with urbanization, socioeconomic status, and region.

Children are often seriously injured when they ride out of a driveway, side street, or alley into the path of a motor vehicle. Cyclist error can be identified as a precipitating factor in many crashes, although this is unlikely to be the most fruitful area for prevention. Collisions during street riding occur most often at intersections or when the cyclist is riding against traffic.

Although collisions with motor vehicles are more likely to result in severe injury or death, falls from bicycles are much more common, with some resulting in serious head injuries or fractures of the extremities. The quality of the riding surface affects the likelihood of a fall. Also contributing to injury are mechanical failure, clothing entanglement, stunt riding, and double riding. Infants and young children carried on the back of an adult's bicycle are a special case of double riding. The extra weight of the passenger makes the bicycle more difficult to maneuver and to stop. Without a special carrier that shields and restrains the child, the child may fall from the bicycle or get feet or legs caught in bicycle spokes. The infant passenger is vulnerable during any crash.

The pressure of the handlebars or seat can cause neuropathy or perineal irritation. Falls on the top bar of the boys'-style bike cause straddle injuries, and abdominal injuries result from falls on the handlebars.

Prevention. All cyclists should wear helmets, because most serious injuries and deaths are caused by head injury. Helmets can reduce the likelihood of brain injury in a crash or fall by as much as 88%. Legislation plus community-wide education campaigns appear to be the combination most likely to increase helmet use. Helmets, as well as other protective gear, are also recommended for other recreational activities involving wheels (e.g., in-line skating and skate-boarding).

Skills-based bicycle safety programs for children, when evaluated, have not consistently decreased injuries. Whenever and wherever possible, bicyclists, especially child bicyclists, should be separated from motor vehicle traffic.

Counseling Points. Counseling should include as the highest priority the proven strategy of always wearing a helmet. Additional counseling points might include carrying infants in a special protective seat, preventing young children from riding in the street or on the road, stressing the importance to older children and adolescents of obeying traffic rules—especially riding with rather than against traffic—when riding on the road, and avoiding riding after dark.

Advocacy Issues. Advocacy issues include implementing bicycle helmet laws, separating bicycle and motor vehicle traffic, decreasing the speed of motor vehicles on shared roadways, and improving the riding surface.

Injuries Not Involving Motor Vehicles

Injuries occur wherever children are—at home, at school, and in places of recreation. Causes and kinds of injury are so numerous that no discussion can be exhaustive. The clinician and parent must be alert for injury potential when viewing the child's whole lifestyle and milieu. Injuries incurred in homes are particularly prevalent among infants and toddlers. Among the most common or important events are drowning, suffocation, fires and burns, poisoning, falls, and unintentional firearm injuries. Demanding particular attention at an older age are the injury risks children and adolescents may face during recreational (e.g., sports-related injuries) or occupational (e.g., farm injuries, burns and lacerations in fast-food jobs) activities. The principles of prevention are sufficiently generic to permit wise choices when hazards are identified. The most common unintentional injury events resulting in death but not involving motor vehicles are discussed in the following sections.

Drowning

Incidence. Drowning (i.e., death from submersion) is second only to transportation injuries as a cause of unintentional injury death for children and adolescents, accounting for approximately 1,300 deaths each year. Drowning death rates peak at 1 to 2 years of age and rise again in adolescence. The increased drowning risk experienced by boys is apparent at a very early age, but it becomes even more exaggerated in adolescence. In 2000, 79% of drowning victims were male.

Most toddler and preschooler drownings occur when a child is briefly unattended and falls into a body of water. Over half of these drownings take place in swimming pools, often at home. The increasing popularity of home whirlpools, hot tubs, and spas is providing new places for young children to drown. Infants and toddlers can drown in any amount of water that is sufficiently deep to cover the nose and mouth; diaper pail, toilet bowl, large bucket, and bathtub drownings occur. Older children, adolescents, and adults also inadvertently fall into water and drown, and approximately one-third of unintentional drowning deaths occur that way. Only one-fourth of the drowning victims were swimming before death. Of those, most were not swimming in designated areas but in unsupervised rivers, creeks, or quarries. Drownings while scuba diving, skin diving, or surfing make up only a small fraction of all cases. Most boating-related drownings are associated with small recreational boats. Drowning follows a boat's capsize or a fall overboard. Personal flotation devices often were not available or were not in use.

Drownings are more likely to occur on weekends and during the warm months. Alcohol is involved in many adolescent drownings. The number of boating drownings has decreased modestly and other drownings more dramatically, with the largest decrease for those between 5 and 19 years of age.

Water is associated with additional injury hazards. For instance, diving where the water depth is inadequate accounts for a significant proportion of spinal cord injuries. Body surfing also is associated with spinal cord injuries. Hair can become trapped or body parts affixed by the suction developed by improperly grated pool and spa drains, resulting in submersion injury.

Prevention. Home water hazards should be eliminated. An adult should never leave the room with an infant in the bathtub, even for a few seconds. When infants and toddlers are in or around water, an adult should be within arm's length, providing "touch supervision." Wherever possible, fixed physical barriers should prevent children from accessing water hazards. Particularly important is the requirement for unbreachable fencing around all four sides of swimming pools. For home pools, this separates the pool from the house and yard. Swimming and boating should be permitted only in designated areas, after adequate training, and with supervision by an adult who has not been drinking alcohol. All persons in boats should wear personal flotation devices.

Counseling Points. Counseling includes adult monitoring of infants and young children during bathing, maintaining constant close supervision by an adult of young children in and around water, having isolation fencing around pools, decreasing water hazards in a young child's environment, swimming and boating in designated areas only, wearing personal flotation devices, avoiding use of alcohol during water-related recreation, and training pool owners in cardiopulmonary resuscitation. Swimming lessons should be discouraged until a child turns 4, as younger children are generally not developmentally ready for formal swimming lessons, and parents should be reminded that swimming lessons at any age will not make children "drown-proof."

Advocacy Issues. Advocacy issues include requiring four-sided pool fencing, draining or fencing quarries and other sites where water may pool over hidden hazards, decreasing alcohol consumption during water-related activities, and enforcing requirements for use of personal flotation devices.

Fires and Burns

Incidence. Deaths from fires and burns have decreased dramatically in the past decade. Still, there were 682 child and adolescent deaths in the United States in the year 2000. House fires cause most deaths. Most persons who die in house fires die of smoke inhalation and are dead before rescue and medical attention arrive. House fire death rates are highest for young children and for the elderly. Both groups are disadvantaged in at least two ways: They are less able to escape after fire breaks out, and they have high fatality rates with burn injury. Although male subjects have higher fire and burn death rates, the disparity between the genders is not so great as for some other injuries.

Only a small proportion of house fires are attributed to children playing with matches or other ignition sources. Cigarettes are a much more common cause. Typically, a cigarette falls onto upholstery or a bed during the evening hours and smolders there until conflagration breaks out in the early morning while the residents sleep. Heating equipment (e.g., portable heaters, chimney fires, wood sparks) is the next most prominent cause of residential fires. Improperly installed or maintained heaters also cause deaths from carbon monoxide poisoning.

Racial differences in death rates are particularly pronounced for young children, with black and Native American death rates especially high. These rates are partially explained by socioeconomic differences, because the disparity decreases in high-income areas. House fires occur more commonly in the winter and on the weekend, the latter perhaps reflecting a period of increased alcohol use.

Clothing ignition burns, once relatively common for young girls, are now rare in children. Gasoline and automotive burns are important in adolescence. Although decreasing, fire and burn injury is still of significance because of the proportion of injury fatalities for which it is responsible and because of the terrible toll of pain, prolonged medical treatment, and permanent disfigurement it exacts.

Scald and contact burns are an important cause of injury morbidity in childhood. Hot liquids, often coffee or the liquid from a tipped-over cooking pot, cause most childhood burn hospitalizations. Another major source of scald burns is hot water from the tap. Burns from contact with a hot object, including the iron, stove, oven, hot comb, grill, cooking pot, heater grate, lighted cigarette, and fireworks, are common in childhood. Although occasionally severe or permanently damaging, these burns usually affect a more limited skin area and are therefore more easily treated than scalds. Burns to the face, eyes, hands, and genitals are particularly likely to result in long-term problems.

Some contact burns and hot water scalds are inflicted by the caregiver or result from willful neglect. Often, however, the circumstances of injury remain in doubt. Some prevention strategies may protect without regard to intent. If water from the tap is not hot enough to burn infant skin, the injury would be prevented no matter what the intent.

Prevention. The greatest gains in preventing fire and burn injuries can be made by the elimination and early detection of house fires. Working smoke detectors should be on every floor of every home. Self-extinguishing cigarettes, child-resistant cigarette lighters, decreasing use of space heaters, and elimination of substandard heating and wiring all are helpful. Although it has a smaller effect on mortality statistics, decreasing hot water temperature can decrease morbidity, as can measures that redesign products (e.g., wide-based cups, coffee pots that do not tip) to reduce other sources of scald and contact burns.

The severity of burns can be decreased by immediately cooling the burned skin by immersing it in cool water or applying a cool wet pack.

Counseling Points. Counseling includes advice on having smoke detectors, adjusting hot tap water temperature to between 120°F and 130°F, avoiding cigarette-initiated fires, planning escape routes in case of fire, placing home fire extinguishers near locations where fires are likely to start (e.g., kitchen), keeping ignition sources away from children, using safe home heating, avoiding private use of fireworks, learning "drop and roll" in case of clothing ignition, and cooling a burn.

Advocacy Issues. Advocacy issues include smoke detector requirements, fire-safe cigarettes, childproof cigarette lighters, automatic sprinkler systems in buildings, building codes that prevent house fire deaths, and firework bans except for community displays.

Suffocation

Incidence. A major cause of injury death during infancy is asphyxiation by choking or by mechanical blockage or compression of the airway. Asphyxiation can occur when the child is trapped in an airtight space or when the child's airway is constricted from the outside, as in hanging. Suffocation (or asphyxiation) claimed the lives of 864 children and adolescents in the United States in the year 2000. Crib strangulations occur when the baby's relatively small body slips between the bars, and the head, too large to follow, is trapped. Current CPSC regulations for slat spacing for new cribs (2-3/8 inches or less) prevent such events, but old cribs may still be in use. Child suffocation fatalities are concentrated among children younger than 4 years, with the peak occurring in the first year. Round, firm food products (e.g., pieces of hot dog, candy, nuts, raw vegetables, grapes) are the most common airway-blocking agents in early childhood. Also choked on are small objects like round or pliable toys (e.g., small balls, uninflated balloons), pop tops, safety pins, coins, and pieces of makeshift pacifiers, bottle nipples, or plastic-lined disposable diapers. Older children and adults usually choke on meat.

Children are also asphyxiated in inadvertent hangings in drapery, pacifier, clothing, or toy cords; when lids fall on them as they peer inside a toy chest; when they are trapped between the frame and mattress of a bed or in the folds of a mesh playpen; when their nose and mouth are covered by a soft basket, pillow, beanbag, or waterbed; when, unattended, they slip out of a high chair; inside plastic bags; in old refrigerators; in excavations that collapse; or when inadvertently covered by materials such as grain in the farm environment. The likely events vary with age.

Prevention. Parents can be taught what to do if a child chokes and can be cautioned about household choking and suffocation hazards such as foods that may block the airway of a young child and unsafe crib designs. The most promising prevention strategies, however, probably are those that involve redesign and regulation of hazardous products.

Counseling Points. Counseling includes advice on avoiding foods and nonfood objects on which infants and toddlers are likely to choke; avoiding cords in children's clothing or environments in which they may hang; purchasing age-appropriate toys so that toys for young children do not have small parts; ensuring a safe sleeping environment for infants (e.g., crib slat space no more than 2-3/8 inches; no soft enveloping surfaces); avoiding entrapment hazards; being aware of the danger of earthen caves, tunnels, and excavations; and knowing rescue techniques for choking.

Advocacy Issues. Advocacy issues include regulation of hazardous toys and children's furniture, building and playground codes and regulations, clothing designs that eliminate cords, and fencing of construction sites and excavations.

Unintentional Firearm Injuries

Incidence. Children in the United States have a uniquely high risk of being shot. As with burn injuries, intent is not always easy to judge. Guns in this culture are widely available and over all age groups are responsible for 2% of all unintentional injury deaths, approximately two-thirds of homicides, and more than one-half of suicides. Children can be the victims of all three. Unintentional shootings kill several hundred and severely injure many additional children and adolescents each year. Even more children and adolescents are murdered with guns. Suicide, most often accomplished with a gun, is the third leading cause of death in male adolescents, exceeded only by unintentional injuries and homicide. Nonwhite adolescent boys are more likely to be murdered with a gun than to die in any other way. High household handgun prevalence is strongly correlated with high firearm suicide rate, and the homicide mortality rate is four times higher in states with the highest gun ownership than it is in states with the lowest gun ownership.

No other type of injury shows such a strong inverse association with socioeconomic status. Rates for unintentional firearm deaths are ten times higher in low-income areas than in high-income areas and are highest in rural and remote areas. Boys and men are at highest risk, with a male-to-female ratio of 6:1 for unintentional shootings.

Boys between the ages of 13 and 17 years have the highest rates of unintentional shooting death. The most common

scenario for unintentional shootings is for one child to shoot another at home with a gun kept by an adult, ostensibly for the family's safety. Although unintentional firearm deaths have been decreasing, suicides and homicides have increased for adolescents and children, respectively. The presence of a gun in the home increases the risk of adolescent suicide.

Although some fiercely assert the right of the individual to keep a gun for protection, the fact remains that a gun in the home is much more likely to kill a family member than an intruder. Children cannot be trusted to handle a gun safely, even though they quickly acquire the mechanical skill and strength to fire one. No amount of exhortation is enough to ensure that they will not make a deadly error. What effect television or toy gun play has on the number of gun injuries in this country is not clear. Nonpowder firearms, often provided to children as toys, clearly are associated with high injury rates.

Prevention. Children should never have access to firearms. If parents choose to own guns, the unloaded guns should be locked away and kept in a separate location from ammunition. Trigger locks, lock boxes, personalized safety mechanisms, and trigger pressures that are too high for young children to achieve are possible design options that could reduce the chance of unintentional firearm injury. If parents allow older children to learn to shoot, such training should be under the strictest supervision.

Counseling Points. Counseling includes advice about the danger of guns in the home, safe storage of firearms, removal of firearms from the homes of suicidal adolescents, and the danger of nonpowder firearms as toys. Parents can be encouraged to ask about the presence of firearms in homes their children visit; they may find this easier if they ask along with other safety-related questions such as those concerning pets or allergies.

Advocacy Issues. Advocacy issues include laws that prohibit access to firearms by minors and control the manufacture, sale, and use of handguns. The sale and use of nonpowder firearms can also be addressed. The American Academy of Pediatrics states that the most effective way to reduce firearm injuries is regulation, including bans on handguns and assault weapons.

Acute Poisoning

Incidence. Most deaths from acute poisoning are among adults. Two pediatric age groups incur most of the childhood poisoning events: children between the ages of 1 and 4 years (fewer than 50 deaths per year) and adolescents between the ages of 15 and 19 (approximately 300 unintentional deaths per year). The American Association of Poison Control Centers reported more than 1.2 million ingestions of a potential poison by children younger than 6 years in 2001. More than one-half of poison exposures are in children, but children younger than 5 years comprise less than 1% of poisoning fatalities. The most common poison exposures for children are ingestion of household products such as cosmetics, cleaning products, pain relievers, foreign bodies, and plants.

A satisfying decrease in the number of early childhood unintentional poisoning deaths has occurred, from 500 per year in the 1940s to 25 in 1997, in part caused by the vigorous efforts of many health care professionals and a combination of strategies. The sharpest decline followed the introduction of child-resistant packaging in 1970, after legislation required that toxic substances accessible to children be sold in containers difficult for a young child to open. The replacement of more toxic medications with less hazardous ones (e.g., acetaminophen for aspirin) has also been instrumental. Effort is required to sustain and extend this success, and acute poisoning still results in many hospital admissions and emergency department visits for children. Adolescent intentional poisoning deaths (i.e., suicides) are covered in Chapter 129.

Children and adolescents are not exempt from carbon monoxide poisoning from car exhaust and faulty heating systems. For all ages taken together, carbon monoxide from motor vehicle exhaust is the most common agent in poisoning deaths. Many unintentional deaths result from motor vehicle exhaust each year. Deaths peak in adolescence for girls and women and early adulthood for boys and men. Rates are higher in low-income and rural areas and during the coldest months. Suicidal deaths from carbon monoxide are much more common than unintentional deaths.

Prevention. The key to preventing unintentional and intentional poisonings is to prevent access to lethal quantities of chemicals. This can be done in several ways, but the more automatic the approach is (i.e., the less it depends on a caregiver's watchfulness), the better it is.

Counseling Points. Counseling includes advice on keeping potential poisons out of sight and out of reach in a locked cabinet, buying medications in modest amounts, keeping products in their original containers, always replacing child-resistant caps immediately after use, knowing when and how to call the Poison Control Center (the national number in the United States is 800-222-1222), safely disposing of all unused and no longer needed medications, not referring to medicines as candy, maintaining the home heating system and car exhaust system, and eliminating hazardous chemicals (e.g., kerosene, caustics) from the home environment. Syrup of ipecac was traditionally recommended to induce emesis in the home, but research has shown that the risks of this treatment outweigh the benefits; parents should be advised to discard syrup of ipecac by flushing it down the toilet. Activated charcoal is not recommended for home use either.

Advocacy Issues. Advocacy issues include maintaining and extending requirements for child-resistant packaging, continuing the practice of packaging antipyretics for children in sublethal total doses, and supporting regionalized Poison Control Centers.

Falls

Incidence. In the year 2000, 180 children and adolescents suffered fatal falls in the United States. The highest pediatric fall death rates are among adolescent males. Most of these fatal falls are from extreme heights. Children in the 0- to 4-year age group are more likely to suffer fatal falls than are other preadolescents.

Falls are an extremely common cause of nonfatal injury, are an important cause of brain injury, and are the leading cause of unintentional injury emergency department visits for children. Falls are also a prominent cause of hospitalization and an important cause of brain injury.

Falls can occur on the same level (e.g., slipping while walking on an icy sidewalk), from one surface to another (e.g., off a bed or changing table to the floor, down stairs), from a vehicle (e.g., a car, pickup truck, bike), or from a height (e.g., out of an upper-story window, off the slide). Most severe injuries and fatalities result from falls of two stories or more.

Little variation is seen between high- and low-income areas or between urban and rural areas in overall morbidity and mortality from falls, but the specific events vary. Illustrating the special risks of the environment and the success of intervention is the decrease in fatal falls of children from New York City high-rise apartment windows after the Board of Health's program to install guards on the windows of apartments with young children.

The majority of the more than 200,000 annual playground injuries result from falls. Fractures are common. Many falls involve stairways. Baby walkers appear to be associated with a high risk, particularly because of their propensity for being ridden down unguarded stairways or off porches. Falls from shopping carts are a problem in the youngest age groups. Falls from vehicles (e.g., from the back of a pickup truck) and falls that occur while playing on roofs, in trees, on bridges, or in other elevated structures affect older children and adolescents and are likely to be severe. Falls associated with recreation are common in childhood and adolescence (e.g., from a skateboard, bicycle, horse, or playground equipment). Falls on and from trampolines are a particularly important source of injury to the central nervous system. Work-related falls, such as from scaffolding or ladders, also occur in adolescence. The health provider must remember that many inflicted injuries are falsely attributed to falls.

The forces that cause injury in a fall depend on velocity at impact, which is determined by the height of the fall, and the stopping distance. A fall from a greater height is more serious. Although not so intuitively obvious, it is better to stop slowly (i.e., to decelerate over a greater distance). The compressibility of the surface and of the presenting body part is important. Contrast the head of a toddler landing on cement with the buttocks landing on a thick carpet; the laws of physics and clinical experience predict much less damage in the latter situation. Surfaces that allow increased distance for deceleration are referred to as "forgiving" and are greatly preferred where children are likely to fall.

Prevention. Environmental redesign has much to offer in protecting all segments of the population from falls. Studies show, for example, that fall injuries are reduced when playground equipment height does not exceed 5 feet. Falls from a height should be prevented by barriers. Where falls are predictable, forgiving surfaces should be in place to cushion the fall. Wood chips or sand to a depth of 9 to 12 inches reduce playground fall injuries.

Counseling Points. Counseling includes advice on not using a baby walker or carrying a child in a shopping cart, timing of the move from crib to a low bed, guarding stairways with special gates in homes with toddlers, using restraining belts on baby furniture (e.g., high chairs, changing tables) and constantly attending babies on high surfaces, installing guards on all openable windows above the first story, choosing safe home playground equipment and installing it over a forgiving surface, avoiding informal use of trampolines, using protective equipment and helmets where appropriate for recreational activities, using safely designed side rails on bunk beds, and not allowing children to ride in a vehicle in which they cannot ride restrained (e.g., the back of a pickup truck).

Advocacy Issues. Advocacy issues include baby walker design and regulations, the design and use of furniture for children, window guard regulations, code specifications of guard rails small children cannot climb over or fall through, playground design and regulations, provision of forgiving surfaces where children are likely to fall, and building codes that reduce falls on steps.

HEALTH CARE PROVIDER'S ROLE IN INJURY CONTROL

Anticipatory Guidance

Health care providers cannot ignore in their professional encounters with children and adolescents the primary cause of morbidity and mortality. Discussion of every possible event and safety measure, however, would overwhelm both the practitioner and the patient. Although specific research on the subject has not been done, injury control experts think it is doubtful that counseling on more than three or four issues at a single visit can be effective. Issues must be chosen for emphasis. When the practitioner follows a child through time, advice can be staged in an age-appropriate schedule. Counseling topics can be chosen for a particular child because they meet one or more of the following criteria:

- The injuries are severe (i.e., likely to result in death or permanent disability).
- The injuries are quite common for the age group.
- Effective prevention strategies are known and practical.
- The child is at special risk because of developmental age, medical condition, or exposure.

If more than one of these criteria are met for a child during one visit, the impetus for anticipatory guidance is hard to ignore. The more a clinician knows about the patient and the patient's milieu, the more focused the anticipatory guidance can be.

To aid the practitioner, counseling schedules have been prepared that suggest the most important topics to be covered for most children of specific ages. Table 16.2 suggests age-based injury prevention counseling topics. Additional discussion of precautions for parents and children can be found in the American Academy of Pediatrics' *Injury Control for Children and Youth*. The American Academy of Pediatrics also provides an educational package called *The Injury Prevention Program (TIPP)*, which is composed of age-appropriate surveys and instructional sheets in Spanish and in English that outline the major causes of childhood injuries and their prevention, a schedule, and a physician's guide. Regional Injury Prevention Centers funded by the Centers for Disease Control and Prevention and the Division of Injury Control at the Centers for Disease Control and Prevention are valuable resources.

Office-based anticipatory guidance as usually provided, no matter how well intentioned, falls short of accomplishing injury control. The word of the physician is not enough to protect children from injury. Clinicians must take the advice of the educational experts about how to maximize these limited moments with families. Group well-child care, for example, seems to be a more successful format for anticipatory guidance about injury prevention than individual counseling.

Advocacy

If all health providers do to prevent injury is to admonish patients and families during regularly scheduled health care visits, the problem will not be conquered. Physicians have an obligation to advocate about issues directly affecting the health of their patients. Clinicians can be advocates for individual patients; for example, a clinician can help a low-income family obtain a specialized child restraint for a child with special health care needs through Medicaid. Health care providers also can be very effective community advocates for injury control. When health care providers remain silent on injury issues, the community may mistakenly assume that injury is not a matter of health. The National SAFE KIDS Campaign, based at the Children's National Medical Center in Washington, DC, provides materials for community advocacy; local SAFE KIDS coalitions in all 50 states offer valuable opportunities for health care providers to get involved in injury prevention at the grassroots level.

Clinicians can be pivotal in the community approach to injury control by providing consultation, urging design changes, testifying for legislation, informing on regulations, and ensuring that the trauma system serves children well. Many of the gains recorded in injury control have resulted from such open advocacy on the part of health care workers for their patients.

Suggested Readings

American Academy of Pediatrics, Committee on Injury and Poison Prevention. *TIPP (The Injury Prevention Program): a guide to safety counseling in office practice*. Elk Grove Village, IL: American Academy of Pediatrics, 1994.

American Academy of Pediatrics, Committee on Injury and Poison Prevention. Office-based counseling for injury prevention. *Pediatrics* 1994;94:566.

Baker SP. Childhood injuries: the community approach to prevention. *J Public Health Policy* 1981;2:235.

Bass JL, Christoffel KK, Widome M, et al. Childhood injury prevention counseling in primary care settings: a critical review of the literature. *Pediatrics* 1993;92:544.

Centers for Disease Control and Prevention. Medical expenditures attributable to injuries—United States, 2000. *MMWR* 2004;53:1.

Centers for Disease Control and Prevention. Web-based Injury Statistics Query and Reporting System (WISQARS) [National Center for Injury Prevention and Control, Centers for Disease Control and Prevention Web site]. 2002. Available at: www.cdc.gov/ncipc/wisqars

Cohen LR, Runyan CW, Downs SM, Bowling MJ. Pediatric injury prevention counseling priorities. *Pediatrics* 1997;99:704.

Committee on Injury Prevention and Control, Division of Health Promotion and Disease Prevention, Institute of Medicine. *Reducing the burden of injury: advancing prevention and treatment*. Washington, DC: National Academy Press, 1999.

Haddon W. Advances in the epidemiology of injuries as a basis for public policy. *Public Health Rep* 1980;95:411.

Harborview Injury Prevention and Research Center. Systematic reviews of childhood injury prevention interventions. Available at: http://weber.u.washington.edu/~hiprc/childinjury/menu.html.

Rivara FP, Grossman DC. Prevention of traumatic deaths to children in the United States: how far have we come and where do we need to go? *Pediatrics* 1996;97:791.

Runyan CW, Gerken EA. Epidemiology and prevention of adolescent injury: a review and research agenda. *JAMA* 1989;262:2273.

Widome MD, ed. *Injury prevention and control for children and youth*, 3rd ed. Elk Grove Village, IL: American Academy of Pediatrics, 1997.

Wilson MH, Baker SP, Teret SP, et al. *Saving children: a guide to injury prevention*. New York: Oxford University Press, 1991.

CHAPTER 17 ■ CHILD MALTREATMENT

ROBERT M. REECE

EPIDEMIOLOGY OF CHILD MALTREATMENT

In the United States in 2003, approximately 2.9 million children were reported to Children's Protective Service (CPS) agencies for abuse and/or neglect. Approximately one-third of the reported cases (906,000) were substantiated as abuse or neglect after investigation, representing a rate of 12.4 per 1,000 U.S. children. Approximately 60% suffered neglect, 19% were physically abused, 10% were sexually abused, and 5% were emotionally maltreated. In addition, 17% were associated with other types of abuse. (These numbers add up to over 100% because many children are victims of more than one type of maltreatment.) The highest victimization rates were for the 0- to 3-year age group, and girls were slightly more likely to be victims than were boys. Pacific Islander children, American Indian or Alaska Native children, and African-American children had the highest rates of victimization. The rate of white victims of child abuse or neglect was 11.0 per 1,000 children of the same race or ethnicity; the rate for Pacific Islanders was 21.4 per 1,000 children; for American Indian or Alaska Natives, 21.3 per 1,000 children; and for African-American children, 20.4 per 1,000 children.

Approximately 1,500 children died from child abuse and neglect in 2003, a rate of 2 deaths per 100,000. More than 75% of these deaths occurred in children under 4 years of age; 10% were 4 to 7 years old; 5% were 8 to 11 years old; and 6% were 12 to 17 years old.

Almost 60% of all perpetrators were female because the most common pattern of maltreatment was a child neglected by a female parent. Victims of physical or sexual abuse were more likely to be maltreated by a male parent, a male relative, or other males. Parents were the perpetrators of maltreatment in 80% of cases.

DEFINITIONS OF CHILD MALTREATMENT

The definition of physical abuse in Public Law 93-247 is "the physical or mental injury, sexual abuse, negligent treatment, or maltreatment of a child under the age of eighteen by a person who is responsible for the child's welfare under circumstances which indicate the child's health or welfare is harmed or threatened thereby." *Neglect* occurs when a caretaker responsible for a child either deliberately or by extraordinary inattentiveness permits a child to suffer or fails to provide one or more of the conditions generally deemed essential for developing a person's physical, intellectual, or emotional capacities.

PHYSICAL ABUSE

Bruises

Several studies of bruises in random populations of children have shown that the locations of nonintentional bruises are related to the developmental stage of the child. Bruises anywhere on the body are extremely uncommon in infants less than 6 months old but are more commonly seen as the child becomes increasingly mobile. Infants who do not yet "cruise" bruise only rarely. In Sugar's study bruising was rare in normal children on the hands, buttocks, cheeks, nose, forearms, or chest. Bruises on the lower legs were found to be uncommon in children less than 18 months of age in Roberton's study, but in Sugar's series nearly one in five of the "cruisers" (10 to 18 months of age) and half of the "walkers" had bruises, most frequently on the shins and knees. In Roberton's study, head and facial injuries were common in the 10- to 18-month-old age group and uncommon over the age of 4 years. Less than 1% of children below 3 years of age had lumbar bruises, but lumbar bruises occurred in 14% of the children of school age.

"Aging" of Bruises

The color changes that occur in bruises are quite variable in relationship to the age of the bruise. The difficulties inherent in assessing the age of bruises include variability in the depth, the location, the vascularity of the underlying tissue, and the age and skin complexion of the child. Superficial bruises occur almost immediately, while deep bruises may take days to appear. The color of the bruise also depends on the depth of the bruise, with yellowish tinges appearing in 3 days in superficial bruises, while in deeper bruises the yellow color may not be appreciated until 7 to 10 days. Blood is seen sooner in loose tissues (such as around the eyes). In one study of 369 photographs of bruises, the authors concluded that (a) a bruise with any yellow must be older than 18 hours; (b) red, blue, and purple or black may occur anytime from 1 hour to resolution; (c) red color has no bearing on the age of the bruise because red color can be present in bruises no matter what the age is; and (d) bruises of identical ages and cause on the same person may not appear as the same color and may not change at the same rate. Visual aging of bruises is an inexact science and should not be relied upon to ascertain that a particular bruise is consistent with a specific age. As in all injuries, the history of the injury is important, along with an appraisal of the biomechanics required to produce the tissue damage in question.

Distinguishing between Inflicted and Nonintentional Bruises

Inflicted bruises often have characteristic locations, patterns, or shapes that can help differentiate them from nonintentional

TABLE 17.1

RELATIONSHIP OF LOCATION AND CAUSE OF BRUISES

Inflicted	Nonintentional
Upper arms	Shins
Trunk	Bony prominences
Upper anterior legs	Lower arms
Sides of face	Forehead
Ears and neck	Under chin
Genitalia, buttocks	

injuries (Table 17.1). Bruises located over bony prominences are more likely to be nonintentional, whereas bruises on the dorsal surface of the body are more likely to be inflicted. Certain patterns of bruising help identify the inflicting agent (Box 17.1).

Differential Diagnosis

Both common and rare skin conditions need to be considered when diagnosing skin bruises (Box 17.2). Other more rare causes of bruising, petechiae, or purpura, but less likely to be confused with child abuse, include Rocky Mountain spotted fever, disseminated intravascular coagulopathy, meningococcemia, vitamin K deficiency secondary to cystic fibrosis, head lice with maculae caeruleae (linear bruises), capillary hemangiomas, eczema, purpura fulminans, spider bites, and calcium chloride cutaneous necrosis.

BOX 17.1   Shape/Size/Patterns of Inflicted Bruises

Pinch marks appear as small double bruises.

Open-handed slap produces clear skin mark where fingers hit (negative image), with fingers outlined by linear stress petechiae. This happens with high-velocity injuries; with high velocity and large forces, bruising is seen as a positive image outlined by petechiae.

Belts, ropes, strings, cords, shoes, hairbrushes, coat hangers, extension cords, kitchen utensils, and many other instruments can leave identifiable imprints.

Vertical bruises on the buttocks at the margin of the gluteal cleft can be due to whipping, paddling, or spanking. The mechanics of this injury involve a crimping of the skin at the gluteal cleft margins.

Bruises under the fingernails (subungual hematomas)

Bilateral black eyes in a child are almost always of inflicted origin. Attribution of this injury to another child by the caretakers is common, but children under 10 years of age have neither the motivation nor the power to inflict this degree of injury.

Petechiae on the face and neck, and subconjunctival hemorrhages from strangulation injuries.

Bruises on the pinna of the ear from "boxing" the ears with both open hands, or by pinch injuries while pulling the child by the ear.

Tattooing

Factitious dermatitis (Munchausen by proxy)

BOX 17.2   Differential Diagnosis of Cutaneous Lesions in Child Abuse

"Mongolian spots": More accurately termed slate blue nevi, these bluish-gray discolorations of the skin occur in many children of African, Asian, or Mediterranean origin. They are present at birth, may be extensive, involve multiple areas, and may be seen on any part of the body. They are most commonly seen on the buttocks or lower back.

Ehlers-Danlos syndrome: This inherited connective tissue disorder is characterized by skin fragility (easy bruisability), joint hypermobility, and skin hyperelasticity.

Erythema multiforme: Intradermal hemorrhage and petechiae, with purpura usually starting at the palms, soles, hands, feet, and leg extensor surfaces, and extending to the trunk and face is typical. Target lesions are flat macules with small papular centers.

Coagulopathies: Idiopathic thrombocytopenic purpura, leukemia, hemophilia, von Willebrand's disease.

Henoch–Schönlein purpura: This is thought to be an IgA-mediated vasculitis in small vessels of involved organs. Seventy-five percent of all cases occur in children 2–11 years of age, with younger children rarely affected.

Secondary syphilis: Purpuric lesions sometimes on the palms and soles.

Allergic shiners: Dark areas under eyes often seen in children with hayfever or other allergic rhinitis.

Cultural rituals: Cao gio (coining), cupping, quat shat (spooning).

Phytophotodermatitis: Lime, lemon, or other citrus fruit juice on skin followed by exposure to sunlight produces hand print patterns.

The approach to the evaluation of suspected abusive cutaneous injuries is shown in Box 17.3.

Burns

Burns are defined as a chemical and physical insult to tissue resulting from thermal, electrical, chemical, or radiation mechanisms.

Epidemiology

Approximately 40,000 children under the age of 15 years are hospitalized each year because of burns and more than 2,000 children die from burn injury each year. Most studies show that 20% of burns in young children are abusive. Burns represent 10% of all physical abuse cases. Scald burns comprise 85% of all burns in childhood, with the greatest prevalence in children less than 4 years of age. Flame burns account for 13% of the total, with chemical and electrical burns representing the remainder. Boys are burned more often than girls. As in most maltreatment, burns of inflicted origin are seen more often in younger children than accidental burns.

Types of Burns

Thermal Burns

Scald Burns. Forced immersion scalds are usually uniform in depth, with sharply demarcated borders, and flexion creases are relatively spared. When a child's hands or feet are held

of wood and coal fires, have been implicated in dry contact burns.

Chemical Burns. Strong acids and alkalis (lye, calcium chloride) can cause cutaneous burns or the burns can be internal if the chemical agent is ingested or placed into a body cavity.

Electrical Burns. The combination of heat and direct action of electrical forces on polarized molecules in tissue causes electrical burns. The evolution of electrical burns occurs over a longer period of time than scalding or dry contact burns. Microwave burns cause a preferential burning of tissues with high water content, such as skin and muscle. Cutaneous burns from "stun guns" have been reported, consisting of a pair of small (0.5 cm) superficial circular burns.

Bites

Human bites may be seen as a manifestation of abuse. This form of abuse, when perpetrated by an adult, is a primitive behavior and is a critical red flag when deciding about the future safety of the child in an environment where this has happened. Certain characteristics of human bites help to determine whether they are from a child or an adult. Adult bite marks usually only reach from one canine tooth to the other and only one dental arch is represented. A child's bite usually involves both arches and the distance between the canines is usually less than 2.5 cm using dental rulers. Photographs of bite marks with a dental ruler in the picture can be extremely helpful. Dental impressions can be taken from the victim and perpetrator to match the bite marks on the skin. Saline swabs can be used to pick up saliva for ABO grouping or DNA.

Head Injuries

More fatalities and long-term morbidity are due to abusive head injury than from any other form of physical abuse. The types of abusive head injuries range from asymptomatic scalp swelling, mild to moderate bruising, and skull fracture, to intracranial bleeding, axonal injury, and brain swelling resulting in stupor, coma, and death. When a child under 3 years of age comes for medical care with a serious head injury without a readily apparent major trauma history (motor vehicle accident, falls from heights over 10 feet), the chances are high that this is an inflicted injury.

When a seriously head-injured child is being evaluated and treated medically, it is crucial that a detailed, analytical—but not challenging or accusatory—history be obtained from the caretakers. Parents who have inflicted an injury will often invent an explanation as to how the injury occurred. Thus, the skill of interviewing becomes an important foundation on which to build the diagnostic formulation. The person collecting the history should ideally be someone with experience in child abuse cases and one who does not have immediate responsibility for the medical treatment required by the child. Gentle probing, with inquiries and request for clarification on questionable portions of the history, often will reveal discrepancies between the history of the injury and the actual findings on examination. The failure to suspect inflicted neurotrauma as the cause of nonspecific signs such as irritability, lethargy, poor feeding, or vomiting may result in a missed diagnosis and risk of further trauma to the child. In one recent study, the diagnosis of abusive head trauma had been missed in nearly one-third of cases, as evidenced by the presence of old subdural collections in cases in which there was acute bleeding due to subsequent episodes of abuse.

The history of the pregnancy, labor and delivery, and neonatal course and a history of family diseases are important, with

---

<table>
<tr><td>BOX 17.3</td><td>Approach to Evaluation
of Cutaneous Injuries</td></tr>
</table>

Detailed history including mechanism of injury, identification of discrepancies between history and injuries, prior accidents, past medical history, developmental history, and family history

Complete skin examination noting location, size, shape, pattern, and color of bruises; photodocumentation

Complete physical examination including measurements for height, weight, and head circumference

Developmental history

Observation of the parent–child interaction

Appropriate laboratory examinations: May include hematocrit, hemoglobin, blood smear, and bleeding and clotting studies (platelet count, prothrombin time, partial thromboplastin time, factor V analysis)

Skeletal survey in any child under the age of 3 years in which the possibility of child abuse is being considered

---

forcibly in hot water, the burns take on a stocking or glove appearance, and the burns are often bilateral. Buttocks, lower back, and perineum burns occur when a child's middle body is forcibly held under hot water. In some cases, areas are spared from scalding if these areas of skin are in contact with a relatively cooler surface such as the bottom of a tub (donut burns). In other cases, body creases are spared because apposing surfaces of skin are not exposed to the scalding agent. All these signs suggest restricted motion and significant exposure time. Essential in the evaluation of scalding burns is an understanding of the time and temperature relationships of water. It is self-evident that longer durations of exposure and higher water temperatures exert the most effect on the extent of damage to tissues. This relationship is shown in Table 17.2.

Dry Contact Burns. Objects of all kinds, especially household appliances, are responsible for the lesions seen with this type of burn. The most frequent appliances are irons, hair dryers, hair curlers, cigarette lighters, light bulbs, grills from stoves or heaters, and cigarettes. Often the burn can be identified by the unique imprint of the burning agent. Cigarette burns are circular and blister early; when healed, they appear craterlike, with hyperpigmented edges. They are most frequently seen on the hands or feet, but are reported in all areas of the body. Accidental cigarette burns do occur but appear to be "brushed lesions" that are ovoid, and the resultant burns are more superficial. Nonintentional burns from the metal frames of car seats, seatbelt buckles, baby carriers, strollers, playpens, and other baby equipment, as well as burns from ashes and embers

TABLE 17.2

TIME-TEMPERATURE SCALE (AFTER MORITZ): EXPOSURE TIME (IN SECONDS) TO CAUSE SECOND-DEGREE BURN

Temperature (°F)	Adult's Skin	Child's Skin
127	60	
130	30	10
140	5	1
150	2	<1
158	1	<1

BOX 17.4   **Injuries to the Scalp**

Bruises (visible externally)
Bruises (intra- and subcutaneous; not visible externally)
Lacerations
Abrasions
Subgaleal hematomas
Alopecia (hair loss secondary to hair-pulling)

---

particular attention to bleeding and clotting disorders, neurologic diseases, metabolic and bone disease, or other genetic conditions of the family. The past medical history of the child, including previous injuries and serious illnesses or hospitalizations, and a review of systems should be obtained. The social milieu with attention to the living arrangements and the relationships of household members should be explored.

Because head injuries are of such serious consequence, the general physical examination of the child with a head injury may overlook less urgently compromised organ systems. Bleeding visceral organs are the most glaring and potentially disastrous omissions, but overlooking cutaneous injuries can deprive the diagnostician of important clinical data because of the fleeting nature of these injuries. Likewise, inspection of the oral cavity for intraoral lesions and a search for hidden surface head lesions under the hair are important. The neck should be carefully inspected for signs of injury (strangulation, hand or finger bruising). The presence of bruises on the back, on the thighs, or in the perineum should also be noted. Photo documentation of such injuries is highly desirable.

The examination of the retina is of utmost importance. This should be carried out ideally by pupillary dilation and indirect ophthalmoscopy, but in lieu of that, by direct ophthalmoscopy. When possible, this should be done by a pediatric ophthalmologist and pictures should be taken of the retina.

The types of injuries in serious abusive head injury include trauma to the scalp (Box 17.4), skull fractures (Table 17.3), subdural or subarachnoid bleeding, cerebral edema, axonal injuries, parenchymal tears and contusions, and injuries to the cervical spinal cord.

Bleeding in the epidural space is usually arterial and occurs because of trauma to the overlying skull, resulting often in a skull fracture of the temporoparietal bone that tears a branch of the middle meningeal artery. The bleeding in the epidural space appears as an elliptical density on computerized tomography (CT) scan. It can accumulate rapidly and can, if not diagnosed and treated promptly, lead to coma and death. An epidural hematoma is more often nonintentional than abusive in origin, but can be seen as a consequence of abuse. Prompt medical attention and, in some cases, evacuation of the hematoma, usually results in the rapid resolution of symptoms and signs.

Bleeding in the subdural and/or the subarachnoid spaces is due to the stretching and breaking of the veins bridging from the surface of the brain to the dural sinuses. These veins are fixed to the brain and to the dural membrane. With motion of the brain, these veins break and bleed.

Bleeding within the brain substance (parenchyma) is primarily due to trauma, a vascular or hypoxic insult to the brain itself.

Shaken Baby/Shaken Impact Syndrome

The term *shaken baby syndrome* has been criticized because it ascribes a clinical condition to an unwitnessed act that may or may not include impact. The arguments for and against this term are beyond the scope of this chapter, but the term is so widely used that it will be used here.

There are no reliable statistics regarding the incidence of shaken baby/shaken impact syndrome (SBS/SIS) since there are no central reporting registries to collect these data. Estimates range from 600 to 1,400 cases per year. SBS/SIS occurs in babies, usually under 1 year of age, but is also described in children considerably older. There is considerable support—clinical, confessional, and experimental—for the concept that shaking and, in many cases, impact by throwing the child against a surface and resultant deceleration are the responsible mechanical forces producing the subdural hematoma, brain injury, and consequent cerebral edema leading to raised intracranial pressure. There has been much discussion about shaking versus shaking plus impact as the mechanism for the production of the lesions seen in SBS/SIS. This began with Duhaime's 1987 article in which she described a retrospective study of 48 cases of shaken baby syndrome seen at her institution. Of these, 62% had clinical evidence of blunt trauma to the head (bruising, skull fracture), and postmortem evidence of blunt trauma was present in all of the fatal cases. In this report, she also studied the forces generated when three types of dolls were shaken. Using a strain gauge measuring forces during shaking, she was unable to demonstrate enough force from shaking to account for the extent of damage seen in clinical cases. She concluded that impact with rapid deceleration of the intracranial contents was necessary for these lesions. This discussion has continued, with some investigators citing the absence of evidence of impact in a substantial number of their reported cases. The criticism of the theory that impact is required cites the crudeness of the doll models used in Duhaime's study and the fact that no good data exist to inform us about what magnitude of forces are required to injure the infant brain. There are currently ongoing biomechanical studies to try to determine the required forces to produce the classic clinical, radiographic, and pathologic changes due to inflicted childhood neurotrauma. The absence of factual information about the characteristics of all of the structures in the live infant's head inhibits this effort, but attempts are being made, through biomechanical and animal models, to learn more.

Interviews with confessed perpetrators indicate that the usual trigger for these assaults is inconsolable crying by the infant. Frustrated by attempts to stop the crying, the perpetrator loses control and seizes the infant, either by the chest, under the arms, by the arms, or by the neck, and violently shakes the baby, followed by throwing the baby onto a hard or soft surface. The time of the shaking varies, usually ranging from around 5 seconds to 15 or 20 seconds. It has been estimated by video recordings of a person shaking a doll that the number of shakes ranges between two to four per second. During the

---

TABLE 17.3

FRACTURES OF THE SKULL

Simple	Linear—not crossing suture lines
	Temporoparietal constitute the vast majority
	Less than 2 mm separation
Complex	Linear—crossing suture lines
	Linear—>2 mm separation
	Branching or stellate
	Comminuted (isolated fragments of bone)
	Depressed (comminuted with bone fragments impinging on the brain)
	Compound (overlying laceration)
	Diastatic (growing)

shaking, the head rotates wildly on the axis of the neck, creating multiple forces within the head. The infant stops crying and stops breathing during the shaking, causing decreased oxygen supply to the body, particularly the brain. Recent reports that the respiratory center may be damaged during these traumatic events, leading to dysfunctional respiratory efforts after the shaking has stopped, would partially explain the hypoxic changes seen in the brains of infants who succumb. The infant brain, with much higher water content than the adult brain, is much softer than an adult brain, having the consistency of gelatin. The absence of myelination contributes to the relative softness. These factors make the brain more easily distorted and compressed within the skull. Shaking and the sudden deceleration of the head at the time of impact do several things:

1. The veins that bridge from the brain to the dura, which is fixed to the inside of the skull, tear open and bleed, creating the subdural hematoma or subarachnoid hemorrhages so characteristic of the syndrome.
2. There is internal commotion in the brain as well as movement of the brain within the skull, causing direct trauma to the brain substance itself.
3. Axons are injured, shearing off during the commotion to the brain.
4. The lack of oxygen during and after the assault causes further irreversible damage to the brain substance.
5. Damaged neurons release excitatory amines that cause vasospasm, adding to the oxygen deprivation in the brain and destruction of adjacent neurons.

The combined effect is massive destruction of the brain tissue, causing immediate brain swelling and enormous increases in intracranial pressure. This causes compression of the blood vessels, thereby decreasing the oxygen supply to the brain even further. It is these insults to the brain, not the subdural or subarachnoid bleeding, that cause the signs, symptoms, clinical and radiographic findings, and course of SBS/SIS.

Associated Injuries in Shaken Baby Syndrome—Retinal Hemorrhages. There are several theories about the cause of retinal hemorrhages (RHs). The first holds that increased intracranial pressure causes RHs. The chief argument against this theory is that RHs occur much less frequently in nonintentional head injuries than in those resulting from shaking despite the fact that both have increased intracranial pressure. In a recent study of head injuries from a variety of causes, both abusive and accidental, RHs were seen in only 2% of a group of 233 accidentally head-injured children under the age of 6 years and in 33% of the children with inflicted head injury.

The second theory postulates that RHs are due to a disruption of the layers of the retina. There are ten layers in the retina, all richly supplied with blood vessels. Proponents of this theory state that when these layers are subjected to the lines of force associated with shaking, they slide across one another, shearing these vessels so that they bleed. This would explain why the RHs unique to SBS/SIS are flame-shaped or dot/blot as the blood tracks between the layers of the retina. RHs seen in SBS/SIS are usually extensive in distribution in the retina, are not confined to the posterior pole, are numerous, and involve multiple layers of the retina. RHs seen in other conditions are usually closer to the surface, so-called preretinal hemorrhages, and resolve quickly (Box 17.5).

Although retinal hemorrhages are the most commonly found ocular lesion in SBS/SIS, other lesions may also be seen. These include retinal detachment, optic nerve injury, retinal folds, and cupping of the optic nerve secondary to raised intracranial pressure. Although RHs are not pathognomonic of inflicted head trauma, they are present in a high percentage of abuse cases and are not present in most accidental traumas, after cardiopulmonary resuscitation, or after seizures. Other

---

BOX 17.5 **Differential Diagnosis of Retinal Hemorrhages**

Vaginal delivery: Occurring in 40% of children delivered vaginally, these fine petechial preretinal hemorrhages usually resolve within 10–14 days of delivery and resolve spontaneously, leaving no residuals.
Bleeding disorders: Isolated retinal hemorrhages in coagulopathies have not been described. When they occur, they are in association with other sites of bleeding.
Arteriovenous malformations: Extremely rare in infancy
Increased intracranial pressure: Present in most cases of serious childhood neurotrauma, both from nonintentional and inflicted injuries
Bacterial meningitis: Even when bacterial meningitis was common (before vaccines made this a rare disease), the incidence of retinal hemorrhage in meningitis was only seen in 1% of cases. With the rarity of bacterial meningitis in clinical pediatrics in this era, this cause for retinal hemorrhage would be extraordinarily rare. It is also not likely that meningitis would not be diagnosed by clinical assessment and culturing and examination of cerebrospinal fluid.
Accidental head trauma: Recent literature on the incidence of retinal hemorrhages in nonintentional head trauma indicates their rarity in these cases.

---

associated injuries may include bruising and/or skeletal injuries such as posterior rib fractures and classic metaphyseal lesions of the long bones. These should be sought by skeletal survey.

Clinical Manifestations of Shaken Baby Syndrome. Symptoms and physical findings are variable depending on the length and severity of the shaking and whether the infant was thrown onto a surface. The syndrome can be seen as a continuum from a short duration of shaking with little or no impact, to severe, prolonged shaking and major impact (Fig. 17.1). All of the symptoms are caused by axonal damage from trauma and/or hypoxia, diffuse or focal cerebral edema, and resultant increased intracranial pressure. In moderate to severe cases, the signs and symptoms begin almost immediately after the shaking and reach their peak within 4 to 6 hours.

Diagnosis of Abusive Head Trauma

Laboratory Studies. Children with head trauma severe enough to be admitted to the hospital should also have laboratory studies to support diagnoses of associated trauma in other organ systems, to anticipate hematologic and biochemical alterations sometimes attendant to head trauma, and also to seek for the manifestations of their neurologic status. These studies are displayed in Box 17.6.

One study examining coagulopathy in pediatric abusive head trauma found that there were prothrombin time prolongations in 54% of patients with parenchymal damage and in 20% of those without demonstrable parenchymal damage. Other coagulation markers (partial thromboplastin time, platelet counts, and fibrinogen levels) were also altered. The authors hypothesize that these abnormalities in coagulation elements are due to tissue factor release from damaged parenchymal cells, which, when complexed with factor VII, activate coagulation via the extrinsic pathway, leading to disseminated intravascular coagulation.

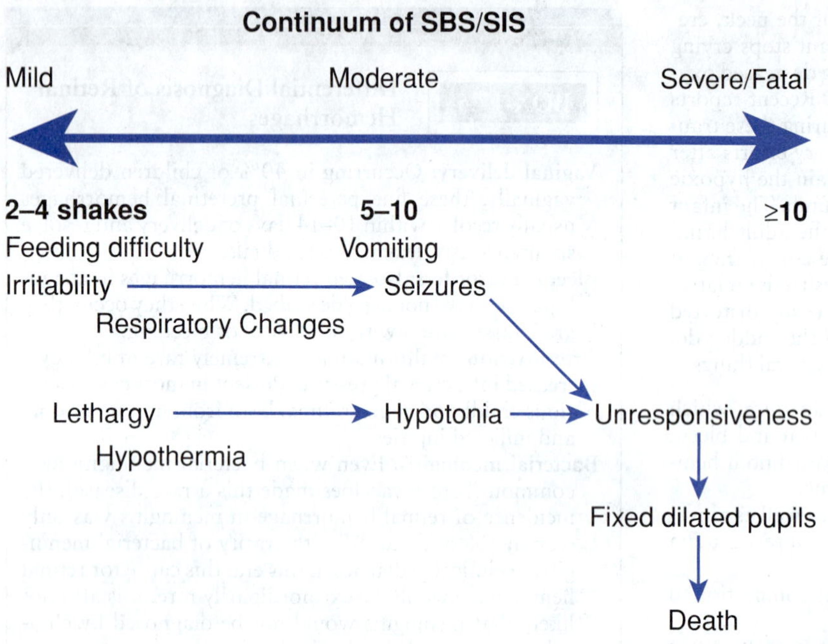

Continuum of SBS/SIS

Mild   Moderate   Severe/Fatal

2–4 shakes   **5–10**   **≥10**

Feeding difficulty   Vomiting

Irritability ⟶ Seizures

    Respiratory Changes

Lethargy ⟶ Hypotonia ⟶ Unresponsiveness

    Hypothermia

Fixed dilated pupils

Death

FIGURE 17.1. Conceptual model of the "dose response" in shaken baby/shaken impact syndrome (SBS/SIS).

Imaging Studies. In most instances of moderate to severe head injury, the first imaging modality should be CT head scans without contrast for evaluation of the intracranial structures. It is readily available in most hospitals and can be performed safely with life support systems operating during the procedure. Bone windows should be employed along with the standard scan. Plain radiographs of the skull will usually show existing skull fractures better than CT will. Magnetic resonance imaging (MRI) is ordinarily used as a confirmatory test rather than an initial one due to the longer scan times and need for life support, but MRI gives superior detail in showing parenchymal changes and smaller subdural hematomata.

Skeletal surveys are recommended in serious head trauma since the diagnosis of abuse may be made or supported if unsuspected or occult traumatic injuries are found in other parts of the appendicular skeleton. Such accompanying skeletal fractures are seen in roughly half of the cases of abusive head injury. Posterior rib fractures are present in some cases of shaken infants and may be seen acutely with bone scintigraphy or by follow-up thoracic films in 10 to 14 days to see callus formation at the site of these fractures.

Prognosis of Patients with Abusive Head Trauma. There are few long-term outcome studies and these have small numbers of subjects followed over relatively short periods of time. These studies show an early mortality rate of 15% to 25%, and 80% to 90% of the survivors are left with varying degrees of compromise ranging from severe learning disabilities to persistent vegetative state. In some studies, a significant proportion of early survivors later died.

Abdominal Injuries

The second most common cause of fatality in child physical abuse, abdominal injuries account for between 6% and 8% of all physical abuse. Reported fatality rates are between 40% and 50%.

Distinguishing between Accidental and Inflicted Abdominal Injuries

Features distinguishing accidental abdominal injuries from abusive ones were reported by Ledbetter (Table 17.4). Injuries to hollow viscera (the intestinal tract) were the most common

---

BOX 17.6

Laboratory Examinations in Inflicted Childhood Neurotrauma

Complete blood count with morphology
Serial hematocrits
Serum electrolytes, BUN, creatinine, serum and urine
    osmolality
Urinalysis
AST, ALT, alkaline phosphatase
Creatine phosphokinase (CPK)
Cultures of blood, urine, cerebrospinal fluid (if safe to
    perform lumbar puncture)
PT, PTT, TT, platelet count, fibrinogen, and FDP
Stool for blood
Arterial blood gases

ALT, alanine transaminase; AST, aspartate aminotransferase; BUN, blood urea nitrogen; FDP, fibrin degradation products; PT, prothrombin time; PTT, partial thromboplastin time; TT, thrombin time.

TABLE 17.4

ACCIDENTAL VERSUS ABUSIVE ABDOMINAL INJURIES

	Abuse	Accidental
Median Age	2.6 years	7.8 years
History	Discrepant	Motor vehicle crash
Medical attention	Delayed	Prompt
Organ involved	Hollow viscus	Solid organ
Mortality rate	53%	21%

in Ledbetter's series. However, Price reported that in his study of 33 fatal cases of abusive abdominal blunt trauma, liver lacerations were the most common finding (52%), followed by small bowel injuries (30%), pancreatic injury (15%), mesenteric damage (33%), adrenal (6%), and great vessel injury (3%). When the small bowel is injured, the distribution of injuries is 30% duodenum, 60% jejunum, and 10% terminal ileum.

Gastric rupture is rare, although it has been reported as an inflicted injury. The second most common organ for abusive injury is the liver, particularly the more midline portion, and the third most common is the pancreas. The pancreas may be injured secondary to blunt trauma to the upper abdomen, usually as the result of a fist, a foot, or another implement (broomstick, plunger handle) being forcefully thrust into the epigastrium. In some cases, the pancreas is divided in two by the applied force against the spine. Pancreatitis develops because of the disruption of the acinar and ductal integrity, the seepage of enzymes into tissue spaces, and the activation of proteolytic and lipolytic enzymes. Pancreatic pseudocysts develop later as a result of the body's response to the enzymatic inflammation.

Chylous ascites and chylothorax have been reported as a consequence of child abuse. This disruption of lymphatic drainage in the abdomen results in an accumulation of chylous fluid within the peritoneal cavity.

The kidney and urinary tract are uncommon sites for abusive injuries. The most common genitourinary site for abuse is the scrotum. Scrotal hematoma may be the result of direct trauma to this area or be the extravasation of blood from intraabdominal bleeding.

Signs and symptoms of traumatic abdominal injuries are shown in Box 17.7. Recommended laboratory studies are shown in Box 17.6.

Diagnosis: Imaging Studies

The preferred initial study to diagnose abdominal or thoracic injury is the plain radiograph. Two frontal views of the abdomen, one supine and one erect, are recommended. If the child is too ill to obtain an erect view, a horizontal beam cross-table lateral can be used. If obstruction, perforation, pneumoperitoneum, hemoperitoneum, or ascites are present, this technique will usually identify them. If there is obstruction, contrast media can be used to localize the lesion. Barium is the preferred contrast medium unless perforation is suspected, in which case a water-soluble contrast medium should be used. A frontal view of the chest is recommended for possible thoracic injuries, including rib fractures. A skeletal survey should also be obtained at the earliest possible opportunity, especially in severely injured children, since future opportunities may not occur and important forensic evidence may be lost. Obviously, the clinical

condition of the child must determine the performance of the studies. Contrast studies for the genitourinary tract are rarely indicated since the advent of CT scanning, but a voiding cystourethrogram (VCUG) may be needed if lower urinary tract ruptures need delineation.

The CT scan is the most useful imaging technique for evaluation of solid organ injuries by demonstrating alteration in the architecture of these organs. Contrast studies are better for showing hollow organ lesions, and the CT depends in these cases on the presence of extravasation of contrast material, which is usually an indication for surgical exploration. Most intramural hematomata without perforation do not require intervention but resolve with supportive care unless there are bleeding complications.

Thoracic Injuries

Pharyngeal, hypopharyngeal, and esophageal perforations are infrequently reported as manifestations of child abuse. The presenting signs and symptoms include hematemesis, coughing, gagging, poor feeding, respiratory distress, cyanosis, and fever. Radiographic features include retropharyngeal and subcutaneous emphysema, pneumomediastinum, and retropharyngeal swelling. In approximately half of the reported cases, chest radiography revealed multiple healing rib fractures. Laryngoscopy may show lacerations or abrasions of the soft and hard palate and will locate perforation of the pharynx, hypopharynx, or esophagus. Mediastinitis may result from infection of oral or nasal organisms.

Cardiac Injuries

Inflicted injury to the heart is rare. Cohle and associates reported six fatal cases of abusive cardiac lacerations in children ranging from 9 weeks to 21/2 years of age. Another entity, commotio cordis, has been described in abuse. This results from a direct blow to the chest over the heart at a particular point in the cardiac cycle when the electrical impulse for heartbeat is interrupted and cardiac standstill occurs.

A summary of visceral injuries is shown in Table 17.5.

Skeletal Injuries

The true prevalence of skeletal injuries in child abuse is unknown. Reported frequency varies from 11% to 55%, although estimates of fractures in abused children under 1 year of age is as high as 70%. Nearly half of these are unsuspected clinically, and almost half involve more than one bone. The vast majority (80%) of abuse fractures are seen in children under 18 months and only 2% of fractures in this age group are of accidental origin. Leventhal et al. reported that 24% of 350 fractures in children less than 3 years of age from emergency room logs were categorized as abuse. Twenty-five percent were skull fractures, 16% humeral fractures, 11% femoral fractures, 17% tibial or fibular fractures, 14% rib fractures, and all others comprised 17%. They concluded from their study that the fractures were most likely to have been inflicted where there was no history of injury, fractures of the long bones of the upper and lower extremities in children less than 1 year of age, and midshaft or metaphyseal fractures of the humerus.

The "Classic Metaphyseal Lesion"

Although extremity fractures are the most common abusive fractures in children, certain types of fractures are more specific for abuse than are others. The "classic metaphyseal lesion"

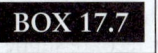

BOX 17.7   **Signs and Symptoms of Abdominal Injuries**

Abdominal tenderness
Distention
External bruising (rare)
Absent bowel sounds
Blood in nasogastric aspirate or in the rectum
Neurologic impairment
Low hematocrit
Hematuria

TABLE 17.5

SUMMARY OF VISCERAL INJURIES: ABDOMINAL AND THORACIC

Organ	Injury	Signs/Symptoms/ Findings
Hypopharynx, esophagus	Traumatic perforation	Feeding difficulty Coughing, bloody sputum Palatal abrasions Sloughing lesions Interstitial emphysema Mediastinitis Rib fractures on radiographs
Stomach	Traumatic perforation	Shock and collapse Distended abdomen Free peritoneal air on radiograph
Duodenum	Blunt abdominal trauma	High intestinal obstruction Gastric dilation Vomiting
Jejunum, ileum	Blunt trauma	Possible peritonitis Intramural hematoma Perforation secondary to obstruction
Colon, rectum	Anal penetration	Lower abdominal pain Constipation Rectal bleeding
Genitourinary tract	Sexual abuse Sadistic abuse	Bruising, abrasions Tears of external genitalia Rupture of bladder
Liver	Blunt upper abdominal trauma	Abdominal distention Shock, collapse Elevated transaminases (AST, ALT) CT evidence of injury
Spleen	Blunt upper abdominal trauma	Peritoneal irritation Blood loss, shock Associated rib fractures CT evidence of injury
Pancreas	Deep blunt epigastric trauma	Abdominal distention, tenderness Elevated amylase, lipase CT evidence of injury

ALT, alanine transaminase; AST, aspartate aminotransferase; CT, computerized tomography.

(CML) of long bones is the most specific fracture of inflicted injury, considered pathognomonic for abuse. This so-called "corner fracture," "bucket handle fracture," "metaphyseal flag," or "metaphyseal fragmentation fracture" has been studied and shown to be a series of planar microfractures through the most immature portion of the primary spongiosa region of the end of the long bones, producing a disclike fragment at this site. This fractured portion of the bone, depending on the projection of the x-ray beam, will appear as a fragment (corner fracture) or a semilunar loop (bucket handle). The torsional force required to produce these lesions are those associated with the shaken baby syndrome or the application of rotational vectors to the long bones.

Fractures of the Long Bones

The femur, humerus, and tibia are the long bones most often affected by transverse or oblique/spiral fractures, but there are no specific types or locations for abusive fractures, emphasizing the need for careful history taking, attention to the age of the child, and use of the skeletal survey for children under 2 years of age.

Fractures of the Lower Extremities. Twenty to thirty percent of fractures of abuse involve the femur. Although common in abuse, femoral fractures have a low specificity for abuse in the ambulatory child. Oblique or spiral fractures are no more specific for an abusive origin than an accidental one. They result from torsional forces applied to the extremity that can occur due to manual torsion with abuse or a twisting against a planted foot with a fall.

Between 7% and 18% of all fractures in abused children involve the *tibia*. The CML is more common in the tibia than at any other site. A wide variety of tibial shaft fractures occur, and none is specific for abuse. Toddler fractures are accidental oblique fractures of the tibia in the 9-month to 3-year-old child. They can occur without the knowledge of caretakers and produce symptoms of limp, disinclination to bear weight on the affected leg, or pain on standing. These are often due to unobserved trivial incidents and can cause localized tenderness with no swelling. In many cases of toddler fractures, the initial radiographs are negative, and only on follow-up films 2 or more weeks after the injury is the fracture apparent owing to the callus formation at the fracture site. Uncommon in abuse, fibular fractures usually are accompanied by tibial shaft fractures. Fractures of the bones of the feet are rare in abuse and when present usually involve the metatarsals.

Fractures of the Upper Extremities. Fractures of the humerus are the second most common long bone involved in abuse. In this long bone, spiral and oblique fractures are more common abusive injuries and occur as the result of torsional forces as the arm is twisted. Supracondylar fractures have a low specificity for abuse, but in the study by Strait and colleagues, 20% of all supracondylar fractures in their series of children under 3 years of age were diagnosed as inflicted in origin.

The incidence of abusive fractures of the forearm ranges from 4% to 20% among all skeletal injuries. More common in the distal radius and midshaft, they can be buckle or transverse and are indistinguishable from accidental injuries. Taking into account the age of the patient, however, the history of the injury and the social context will help elucidate the likelihood of abuse or accident as the cause. The prevalence of hand fractures is between 0% and 3% and can involve the metacarpals or the phalanges. Fractures of the hands or feet are subtle but important injuries in abused infants. When they are seen, child abuse should be considered.

Rib fractures, often unsuspected clinically and only discovered by skeletal surveys, comprise up to a quarter of fractures seen in abuse. Most of these are posterior fractures followed by lateral fractures in the midaxillary line. Overlying bruises of the thoracic wall may be observed, but often are absent. Unless the fractures have been present long enough to produce callus, they may not be discernible on plain radiography, and it is in these cases that bone scintigraphy may be useful.

BOX 17.8   Elements of the Skeletal Survey

BOX 17.8   Elements of the Skeletal Survey

Skull: Frontal and lateral (lateral to include the cervical spine)
Spine: Frontal and lateral thoracolumbar spine
Chest: Frontal (for rib and spinal detail)
Upper extremities: Frontal (to include shoulder and hands)
Lower extremities: Frontal (to include lower lumbar spine, pelvis, and feet)

BOX 17.9   Differential Diagnosis of Childhood Fractures

Accidental trauma
Obstetric trauma
Prematurity, leading to osteopenia
Nutritional deficiencies, such as rickets, scurvy
Metabolic disorders, such as Menkes syndrome, secondary hypoparathyroidism, T-cell disease
Drug toxicity, such as methotrexate, prostaglandin therapy, hypervitaminosis A
Infection, such as osteomyelitis, syphilis
Neuromuscular disorders
Skeletal dysplasias
Neoplasms

Posterior rib fractures are frequently multiple and bilateral. Most involve the rib head at the costovertebral articulation or the rib neck near the costotransverse process articulation. Kleinman and colleagues have demonstrated that levering of the rib neck over the fulcrum of the transverse process of the vertebral body accounts for the heavy preponderance (87%) of posterior rib fractures in the area of the rib head and neck. The fracture site is primarily on the inner (visceral) surface of the rib in posterior rib fractures and on the outer (parietal) surface of lateral rib fractures, reflecting the points of strain during chest compression.

Attribution of rib fractures to cardiopulmonary resuscitation (CPR) has no foundation in the literature. No rib fractures have been seen in studies of this phenomenon in large populations of children undergoing CPR.

Vertebral body fractures are anterior vertebral body compression fractures and are caused from hyperflexion during shaking or other violent handling.

Clavicular fractures are reported in 3% to 10% of abused children but lack specificity for abuse. Scapular fractures are uncommon fractures, both from intentional and nonintentional origins.

Diagnosis: Imaging Techniques

The skeletal survey is the preferred diagnostic technique for imaging the skeleton in suspected child abuse. Although radionuclide scintigraphy has certain useful applications (acute subtle fractures, rib fractures), it is not without inherent technical shortcomings and is dependent upon the level of competence of the radiologist interpreting it. Box 17.8 details the views recommended for the skeletal survey. An estimate of the age of fractures can be made using the healing times for soft tissue and long bones displayed in Table 17.6. The differential diagnosis of childhood fractures is shown in Box 17.9, the specificity of radiologic findings is contained in Box 17.10,

and a guide to suspecting abuse in fracture cases is seen in Box 17.11.

Differential Diagnosis: Osteogenesis Imperfecta

Osteogenesis imperfecta (OI) is a generalized disorder of connective tissue with a broad spectrum of clinical expression. One classification of the disease is based on the clinical expression and has four types. When the disorder is confused with inflicted skeletal trauma, it almost always involves types I and IV. When multiple fractures are seen in infants or young children, OI needs to be considered and ruled out. In nearly all cases, careful history of the child and family and good clinical evaluations, including physical examination, thorough radiographic assessment, and consultation with a pediatric radiologist and, where possible, with a geneticist, will resolve the diagnostic question. In only extremely rare cases is it necessary to obtain biopsies for collagen culture. These are confirmatory in about three-quarters of the cases and as such are not completely reliable. The characteristics of the four types of OI are shown in Box 17.12.

BOX 17.10   Specificity of Radiologic Findings

High specificity
Classic metaphyseal lesion
Rib fractures, especially posterior
Scapular fractures
Spinous process fractures
Sternal fractures

Moderate specificity
Multiple fractures, especially bilateral
Fractures of different ages
Epiphyseal separations
Vertebral body fractures and subluxations
Digital fractures
Complex skull fractures

Common, but low specificity
Subperiosteal new bone formation
Clavicular fractures
Long bone shaft fractures
Linear skull fractures

TABLE 17.6
DATING OF SKELETAL AND SOFT TISSUE INJURIES

Resolution of soft tissues	2–5 Days	4–10 Days	10–21 Days
Periosteal new bone	4–10 days	10–14 days	14–21 days
Loss of fracture line definition	10–14 days	14–21 days	
Soft callus	10–14 days	14–21 days	
Hard callus	14–21 days	21–42 days	42–90 days
Remodeling	3 months	1 year	2 years

(From: O'Connor JF, Cohen J. Dating fractures. In: Kleinman P, ed. *Diagnostic imaging in child abuse*. St Louis: Mosby, 1998.)

BOX 17.11   **When to Suspect Abuse**

Metaphyseal fractures in children <2 years of age
Posterior rib fractures
Scapular fractures
Spine fractures
Sternal fractures
Multiple, especially bilateral, fractures
Fractures to hands or feet
Fractures in infants or very young children
Fractures seen in children in poverty
Fractures seen in former prematurely born children
Fractures seen in children with developmental handicaps
Fractures seen with associated other injuries not attributable to accidents

---

Paterson described 39 patients over 10 years of age who had multiple fractures in infancy. The fractures occurred at home in 32 cases and in the hospital in 7 cases. Paterson believed these cases to represent a form of self-limiting OI. He coined the term "temporary brittle bone disease" to describe this situation. Since his description, no other credible reports of this condition have been reported, and Paterson has been unable to demonstrate that these cases have some underlying defect to explain the fractures. There is no evidence in the medical literature to establish this as a valid entity, and it is not accepted as a plausible explanation for otherwise unexplained multiple fractures in infancy.

Munchausen Syndrome by Proxy

Munchausen syndrome by proxy (MBP) or pediatric condition falsification (PCF) is a bizarre form of child abuse in which the child is the victim of a form of the mother's mental illness, the psychodynamics of which are poorly understood. It is defined as a circumstance in which (a) illness is simulated or produced by a parent (almost invariably the mother) or someone who is in loco parentis; (b) the child comes for medical assessment and care, usually persistently, often resulting in multiple medical procedures; (c) knowledge about the cause of the child's illness is denied by the perpetrator; and (d) acute symptoms and signs in the child abate when the child is separated from the perpetrator.

Rosenberg tabulated the presenting complaints and the methods of fabrication in reported cases up to 1986. As of this writing, the types of presentations have reached over 100. The goal of the diagnostic process continues to be the gathering of evidence to prove that the condition in the child is either produced or simulated (faked). Once MBP is being considered as a possible diagnosis, a strategy for the meticulous collection of data about the child and his or her surroundings must be developed. The team of hospital staff caring for the child and interacting with the mother should meet regularly in team conferences to discuss the evolving information. Extremely careful notes in the chart (or alternate record) are essential because the details are the most important elements in the formulation of the diagnosis. It is often prudent to inform the child protection agency, law enforcement, and the prosecuting attorney's office that such a case is being investigated. Child psychiatry, child psychology, hospital social work services, hospital legal counsel, or risk management representatives should be part of the team. Pediatric subspecialists who are familiar with diseases exhibiting the signs and symptoms shown by the child should be consulted to investigate the possibility of a disease within their realm of expertise. For example, hematologists should be involved where there is unexplained bleeding, and infectious disease consultants should contribute their input if the condition in question involves a possible infectious component. The goal is to collect evidence either to support the diagnosis of pediatric disease falsification or to refute it. Covert video surveillance is sometimes employed in these cases; this should be done with the full understanding of the ward team, hospital administration, and legal department. There are arguments about the use of covert video surveillance; those who favor its

---

BOX 17.12   **Characteristics of Four Types of Osteogenesis Imperfecta (OI)**

OI type I
Comprises 70% of all cases
Autosomal dominant inheritance or spontaneous
    mutation
Fragility mild to moderate
Osteoporosis present
Sclerae blue
Hearing loss common
Wormian bones seen in the skull
Fractures generally occur before age 5 years
Bowing of the long bones seen
May have dental abnormalities (dentogenesis imperfecta)
Easy bruising seen

OI type II
10% of all cases
Always lethal in fetus
Autosomal dominant inheritance
Severe osteoporosis, bone fragility

Intrauterine growth restriction
Sclerae blue-black

OI type III
Comprises 15% of cases
Sporadic autosomal dominant new mutation
Severe osteopenia and fragility
Multiple fractures and deformity that is progressive
Two-thirds have fractures at birth

OI type IV
Rare, comprising 5% of cases
Autosomal dominant or spontaneous mutation
Osteoporosis generally present
Degree of fragility variable
Variable number of fractures
Sclerae normal
May have fracture-free periods
Bones may appear normal at time of first fracture
Frequent wormian bones

use argue that the goal of the hospital should be to diagnose and protect children and there are sometimes no other options than to collect data in this fashion. When the cases come before a court, it is essential that all involved with that proceeding are prepared to present their information and are sure of their facts. The ultimate outcome of the child's well-being will rest on this. Seldom does an opportunity to diagnose MBP on a subsequent admission occur. The long-term outcome of cases of MBP is poorly researched because of the difficulty following such families due to their disappearance after being exposed, but those studies that have been done have demonstrated almost uniformly dismal outcomes, including child fatalities and long-term disability.

OTHER FORMS OF ABUSE

Childhood Sexual Abuse

Kempe defined sexual abuse as "the involvement of children and adolescents in sexual activities they do not understand, to which they cannot give informed consent or that violate social taboos." The keywords in all useful definitions of child sexual abuse "emphasize the unwanted, manipulative and exploitative factors while recognizing the importance of age or developmental level differences between participants."

Diagnosis

The diagnosis of childhood sexual abuse depends on information derived from three domains: disclosure of the event(s) by the victimized child; sexually specific behaviors exhibited by the child, described by the nonoffending parent or caretaker and in some cases observed by the health care professional consulting on the case; and the results of a specialized medical examination performed by a qualified physician, physician's assistant, or pediatric nurse practitioner, including the obtaining of appropriate cultures for sexually transmitted diseases (STDs) and forensic evidence when indicated. Of these, the disclosure is of greatest importance.

Disclosure. Disclosure interviews should be conducted with the child's comfort and well-being as the first and foremost consideration. The setting for the interview should be in a multidisciplinary child-friendly setting, where all who need the information of the interview can watch, either through a one-way mirror or by closed-circuit video recording. Ideally, a single interview should be conducted so that the child does not need to be interviewed repeatedly. There should be meticulous documentation of the interview and the method of documenting will depend on legal jurisdictions. Well-trained and skilled personnel should conduct these interviews, allowing the child to tell his or her story about alleged sexual encounters. The interviewer must guard against overinterpretation of statements made by the child and avoid using leading questions or implied rewards for answering questions in certain ways.

Behavioral assessments should be developmentally and age-appropriate. They should be performed by pediatricians with a subspecialty in child development, or by doctoral-level psychologists or child psychiatrists with special training in child development and child sexual abuse.

Distinguishing between sexual behaviors that are abnormal and those that are developmentally appropriate has been clarified in recent years by the studies of Friedrich and others. There is considerable sexual curiosity as well as stimulative and masturbatory activity in young children that is considered normal because of how commonly it is seen in studies of normative sexual activity in large cohorts of children. Not seen in large percentages of children in these studies were such things as

asking others to do sexual acts, trying to have intercourse, and orally contacting the genitalia of other children; these sexualized activities are considered good evidence of having been sexually exposed and/or abused. Developmentally appropriate behaviors, such as masturbation, become inappropriate when done frequently or compulsively to the exclusion of other normal play activity, or when done in public. When a child does sexually intrusive or coercive behaviors, these are also evidence of abnormal sexual development and imply abnormal sexual exposure.

Physical Examination. All children in whom an allegation of sexual abuse has been made should have complete physical examinations, including a specialized anogenital examination. Without such an examination, the child will not have had a complete evaluation. More importantly, after the examination the child needs to be assured that he or she is physically normal. Up to 10% of children proven to have been sexually abused have tissue markers of injury. Ideally, video colposcopy should be available and operated by qualified examiners, but the examination is not completely dependent on the availability of colposcopic equipment. Most important in the examination is preparation of the child and parent for the examination. This utilizes familiar pediatric skills of rapport building, explaining the examination to the child, gaining the cooperation of the child in the performance of the examination, and respecting the child's wishes if the examination needs to be terminated. Reassurance during the examination will allow the examination to proceed in most cases. Ideally, the examination should be done in both the supine, frog-leg position and in the knee–chest position. The important structures to be examined in the female are the labia majora and minora, the hymen, the posterior fourchette, the fossa navicularis, the perineal region posterior to the genitalia, and the anus. Professionals who perform these examinations should appreciate the wide variety of normal variants as well as the abnormal tissue markers for sexual abuse, since so much depends on accurate interpretation of these examinations. Most children's hospitals have consultants who have expertise in this field, and there are now textbooks with details on the nuances of such examinations.

Certain principles of examination for sexual abuse should be observed:

- Examinations should never be forced on a child.
- Examinations can be done under anesthesia when required.
- Forensic kits should only be used when indicated.
- Cultures for STDs should only be done when indicated.
- Unless there is an urgent need for examination, these examinations should not be done in emergency departments or in clinical settings that do not specialize in sexual abuse examinations.

One of the great advantages of using colposcopy for these examinations is the opportunity for peer review of the findings. Since most physicians have had little or no training in the interpretation of anogenital anatomic findings, it is important that experts who do have sufficient experience are available to help.

The diagnosis of child sexual abuse must be based on a combination of what the child says happened, the corroborated sexualized behaviors of the child, and the results of the physical examination. The ideal setting for this process is in a child-friendly site where a multidisciplinary group of competent interviewers, mental health professionals, and physicians with pediatric and sexual abuse evaluation training can work as a team to reach the most accurate assessment of the child's condition.

Child Neglect

Definitional problems abound in child neglect. Helfer and Dubowitz have proposed broad definitions that incorporate not only caregiver acts and omissions, but also societal and institutional conditions (hunger, lack of health insurance) that adversely affect children. They suggest that child neglect be defined as "a condition in which a child's basic needs are not met, regardless of cause. Child neglect is a phenomenon that varies in type, severity and chronicity. Both actual and potential harm are of concern and the more serious the harm or risk, the more severe the neglect."

More often, neglect has been narrowly defined as acts of omissions by those responsible for the child's health and well-being. Some have found it convenient to divide neglect into categories: physical neglect, emotional neglect, medical neglect, and educational neglect, each of these with subcategories. Clear and identifiable harm or injury is central to laws governing neglect in most jurisdictions. A pattern of omissions in care has been an important criterion of neglect, but a single act of omission can be catastrophic. Taking all these factors into account, neglect can be considered a failure to meet a child's needs in terms of food, clothing, shelter, health care, education, supervision, and nurturance. The etiologies of neglect are multifactorial and can be attributed to factors in the parents, child, family unit, and community. Some of these factors are shown in Box 17.13.

Many cases of neglect are not reported. The National Child Abuse and Neglect Data System (NCANDS) report in 2001 indicated that 57% of the 903,000 substantiated cases of child maltreatment reported to CPS agencies were victims of neglect. Added to this are another 12% who were victims of psychological abuse and medical neglect. Physical neglect is the most common form. Nearly half of all child fatalities due to child maltreatment are from some form of neglect. The manifestations of child neglect are shown in Box 17.14.

BOX 17.13   Causes of Child Neglect

Parental characteristics
Maternal depression
Maternal drug use during pregnancy

Child characteristics
Temperamentally difficult children ("high annoyance potential")
Chronically disabled children
Low birth weight or prematurity

Family characteristics
Attachment disorders
Unrealistic expectations
Chaotic families with impulsive mothers
Social isolation
Stress (illness, unemployment, eviction, arrest)

Community and societal characteristics
Communities with few social services have higher incidence.
Inadequate education and poverty are correlated with neglect.

BOX 17.14   Manifestations of Child Neglect

Physical child neglect
Inappropriate nutrition, shelter, clothing, or hygiene; failure to thrive

Medical neglect
Refusal or delay of health care

Supervisory neglect
Drowning, poisoning, house fires, "accidents," failure to use seat belts, exposure to domestic violence, exposure to guns
Abandonment or expulsion of a child from the home or other custody issues (leaving child with others for long periods of time)

Emotional neglect
Inadequate nurturance/affection
Chronic/extreme spouse abuse
Permitted drug/alcohol abuse, maladaptive behavior (chronic delinquency)
Refusal or delay of psychological care
Unrealistic expectations for developmental stage

Educational neglect
Failure to provide education as prescribed by law

Types of Neglect

Inappropriate Nutrition and Failure to Thrive. Obesity can produce cardiovascular problems, hypertension, diabetes, psychosocial problems, and premature mortality. Family habitus needs to be considered, but often overfeeding is a shared family problem, often deriving from maternal depression or other psychological aberrations. Documentation of persistently exceeding the normal weight parameters on standard growth charts helps make the diagnosis.

On the other end of the nutritional spectrum, failure to thrive (FTT) is defined as a condition in which a child's growth is below the norms for the child's age and sex. The proximate cause of this growth failure is malnutrition, either primary or secondary. Medical conditions responsible for growth failure are numerous, but the most common categories are those that interfere with caloric intake or retention. These include, but are not restricted to, infections (urinary tract infection, untreated dental problems, large tonsils, recurring otitis media, sinusitis), gastrointestinal conditions (chronic nonspecific diarrhea, gluten-sensitive enteropathy, gastroesophageal reflux, cystic fibrosis, lactose intolerance), parasitic infestations, human immunodeficiency virus, and lead poisoning.

The diagnosis of failure to thrive, from all causes, rests on nutritional evaluation and treatment, anthropometric assessment, psychological assessment, and assessment of the family environment. Children with FTT who are referred to child protective agencies fall into two broad categories: those whose safety requires placement and those in less severe jeopardy whose caretakers require protective monitoring and support to comply with the treatment plan. When placement is carried out, the foster parents must be selected carefully, and assurance must be obtained that they can carry out the treatment plan. The medical issues to be taken into account when evaluating a child for FTT are shown in Box 17.15.

BOX 17.15   Medical Issues in the Evaluation of Failure to Thrive

Familial factors
Consanguinity
Developmental delay
Potentially growth-retarding familial illnesses such as cystic fibrosis, lactose intolerance
Short height of both parents, patterns of familial short stature with the possibility of malnutrition or deprivation in their backgrounds
Identification of psychosocial stressors, such as illness in a family member, serious mental illness, substance abuse, history of eating disorders, or developmental impairment
Perinatal factors
Prematurity or low birth weight
Intrauterine growth restriction
Prenatal exposure to legal psychoactive drugs (caffeine, nicotine, alcohol)
Prenatal exposure to illegal psychoactive drugs (marijuana, cocaine, opiates)
Exposure to sexually transmitted diseases, including human immunodeficiency virus
Exposure to other maternal infections during pregnancy
Postnatal medical factors
Almost all severe and chronic childhood illnesses can cause growth failure. The mechanisms for this growth failure may be due to enzymatic, endocrine, and metabolic reasons, but include nutritional and psychosocial reasons.

Medical Neglect. It can be a daunting task to diagnose medical neglect with any degree of certitude in this era of alternative lifestyles and alternative medicine. It is helpful to utilize a set of questions to weigh the evidence (Box 17.16).

Supervisory Neglect. Failure to provide safe environments for children may constitute supervisory neglect. Children who are left alone in bathtubs or around water buckets and drown as a result are victims of supervisory neglect. Likewise, being left home alone and perishing in a house fire; failure to make secure toxic substances, with subsequent poisonings of a child; and failure to use automobile restraints, window locks, smoke detectors, and stairway gates are all examples of supervisory neglect.

Intervention in Neglect

The following are basic principles of intervention in neglect:

1. Determination that the child is neglected and the risk of future harm
2. Development of understanding of all the factors in the neglect
3. Interdisciplinary approach

Specific steps in intervention are listed in Box 17.17.

The Effects of Witnessing Violence

Most conceptualizations of child maltreatment involve acts of commission or omission, but in the recent past the effect of a child witnessing violence, either within the family or within his or her environment, has come to the attention of pediatric

---

BOX 17.16   Questions to Ask about Neglect

1. Is there risk of substantial harm as a result of the action (inaction)?
2. Is there evidence of substantial harm as a result of the action (inaction)?
3. Why did the parents (caretakers) not seek care or "comply" with the advice?
4. How did the medical system attempt to engage the caretakers (parents) in providing for the child's medical needs?
5. What are the potential benefits of medical care/advice?
6. What are the potential risks of medical care/advice?
7. What was the expected outcome (by the parents) without medical care?
8. What was the expected outcome (by the caretakers) without medical care?
9. Were the parents aware of that expected outcome? Did they believe that to be the outcome?
10. Was the poor outcome related to the parental omission, or were there intervening factors involved in that outcome?

---

professionals. As we have seen the attitude of society change regarding tolerance for intimate partner violence, we have also begun to appreciate the toll on the child of witnessing such violence. Groves has pioneered this field and offers some lessons she has learned from her observations. Witnessing violence "changes the emotional landscape for children by distorting their emerging view of the world and their place in it. This change can become a fixed worldview. Young children's understanding of events is shaped by their cognitive development and they create their own meanings of the events" unless explanations by adults can change this formulation. The child's sense of safety is dependent on absence of violent events. After having a traumatic experience, many children have a sense of "pervasive pessimism" or "a sense of foreshortened future. Children's exposure to violence exacts emotional, social, cognitive and physiological costs." These traumatic exposures are thought to have effects on the developing brain, bringing about both structural and functional changes. The limbic system—especially

---

BOX 17.17   Specific Steps in Intervention in Neglect

1. Interventions should be based on existing knowledge and theory.
2. Maternal mental health problems should be addressed.
3. Target underlying contributory factors in the neglect.
4. Use family's natural and informal supports.
5. Begin with the least intrusive approach.
6. Enlist the services of the local child protective services.
7. Outline the structure of intervention for both professional staff and family.
8. Use home health visitors in the implementation of interventions.
9. Understand that intervention is long term.

the amygdala and hippocampus—is thought to be vulnerable to harm. The hippocampus is concerned with the formation and retrieval of verbal and emotional memories. The amygdala creates the emotional content of those memories.

Teicher has hypothesized that "early stress generates molecular and neurobiological effects that alter neural development in an adaptive way that prepares the adult brain to survive...in a dangerous world.... Stress sculpts the brain to exhibit various antisocial, though adaptive, behaviors."

Witnessing violence is a stressor in childhood that has effects in several domains. Emotional development and social functioning are shaped by these observations. The child's ability to learn and moral development are affected. The child's ability to negotiate intimate relationships as adolescents and adults reflects early experiences in observing the significant adults in his or her life negatively modeling those negotiations. It is toxic because the child perceives himself or herself to be in danger, and further, the child is robbed of both parents—one the aggressor, one the victim. There is no safe refuge.

Pediatricians and other child health care professionals can help by assuring the child that he or she is loved, that the parental fighting has nothing to do with him or her, by giving permission for the child to talk, and by providing a safe environment for the child and nonabusing parent. In therapy, overcoming the child's denial and shame and establishing a sense of safety are the underpinning for healing.

ADULT CONSEQUENCES OF CHILDHOOD MALTREATMENT

Psychoanalysts have asserted for years that adverse childhood experiences influence people throughout the lifespan. Now, evidence from the fields of epidemiology, psychology, and neuroscience is supporting those claims. Studies of the health harms in both psychological and medical domains are increasingly showing both correlations and direct links to adverse experiences in childhood.

Post-traumatic Stress Disorder

Since World War I we have known about "shell-shock" as a cause for extreme delayed psychological distress in combat veterans. More recently the phenomenon of reliving past traumatic experiences has been broadened to include a wide range of traumatic events and has been designated as post-traumatic stress disorder (PTSD) consisting of four components:

1. A stressor that "would be markedly distressing to almost anyone"
2. Reliving of the experience (flashback, or intrusive memory happening in the present)
3. Detachment symptoms—used to avoid the memory
4. Presence of physiologic symptoms secondary to flashbacks. Examples include gagging, tachycardia, rapid breathing, numbness in fingers and toes, and chronic tension headaches.

In addition to PTSD, other mental health disorders have been linked to adverse childhood experiences. These include severe depression, anxiety disorders, substance abuse, dissociative identity disorder, somatization, and eating disorders such as bulimia nervosa.

Medical Consequences

There is increasing evidence that maltreatment is correlated with medical problems in adulthood. Felitti and colleagues, in their retrospective studies of the effects of adverse childhood

experiences (ACEs) on 13,494 adults whose average age was 57 years, present sound epidemiologic data to show the connection between childhood abuse and later health harms. The adverse childhood experiences in this survey included physical abuse (11%), sexual abuse (22%), emotional abuse, violence against the mother, substance abuse in the household (26%), mental illness, and criminal behaviors of members of the household. Fifty-two percent of those surveyed reported one form or another adverse experience. Those who had experienced four or more forms (6%) had 4- to 12-fold rates of alcoholism, drug abuse, depression, and suicide attempts; two- to fourfold rates of smoking, "poor health," 50 or more sexual partners, and sexually transmitted diseases; risk for teenage pregnancy; and 1.5-fold rates of physical inactivity and obesity when compared with those with no adverse experiences. A positive correlation was also found between adverse experiences in childhood and rates of ischemic heart disease, cancer, chronic lung disease, skeletal fractures, and liver disease. Low academic achievement, teen pregnancy, juvenile delinquency, and adult criminality have also been reported.

ECONOMIC COSTS OF CHILD MALTREATMENT

The costs to society of child abuse and neglect are both indirect and direct. In addition to the personal tragedy of the medical and mental health consequences cited above, the costs to society increase because of the rising need for mental health and substance abuse treatment programs, police and judicial involvement, prisons, and public assistance programs. In 1998, federal expenditures to the states for child welfare programs exceeded $4.5 billion. In a study in Missouri, the direct economic costs of shaken baby cases that occurred over a 10-year period was $6.9 million, or approximately $32,500 for each case. Fifteen years ago, Daro estimated that lost productivity alone could account for the loss of $1.3 billion annually. In the current economy it could be double that amount.

There is cost benefit to providing effective prevention programs. In one study in 1992, Caldwell concluded that providing either comprehensive parent education or home visitation services for every Michigan family expecting its first child would amount to only 5% of the estimated total state cost of combating maltreatment after it has occurred. We don't lack the knowledge to reduce child maltreatment, but we lack the will to do it. It is up to governmental leaders to decide to put prevention efforts in place to offset both the economic and the humanitarian costs of child maltreatment.

Suggested Readings

Ablin DS. Osteogenesis imperfecta: a review. *Can Assoc Radiol J* 1998;49:110.

Ablin DS, Sane SM. Non-accidental injury: confusion with temporary brittle bone disease and mild osteogenesis imperfecta. *Pediatr Radiol* 1997;27:111.

Alexander RC, Levitt CJ, Smith WL. Abusive head trauma. In: Reece RM, Ludwig S, eds. *Child abuse: medical diagnosis and management.* Baltimore: Lippincott Williams & Wilkins, 2001:47.

Alexander RC, Sato Y, Smith W, et al. Incidence of impact trauma with cranial injuries ascribed to shaking. *Am J Dis Child* 1990;144:724.

Alexander RC, Surrell JA, Cohle SD. Microwave oven burns to children: an unusual manifestation of child abuse. *Pediatrics* 1987;79:255.

Anda RF, Chapman DP, Felitti VJ, et al. Adverse childhood experiences and risk of paternity in teen pregnancy. *Obstet Gynecol* 2002;100:37.

Anda RF, Croft JB, Felitti VJ, et al. Adverse childhood experiences and smoking during adolescence and adulthood. *JAMA* 1999;282:1652.

Anda RF, Felitti VJ, Chapman DP, et al. Abused boys, battered mothers, and male involvement in teen pregnancy. *Pediatrics* 2001;107:e19.

Anda RF, Whitfield CL, Felitti VJ, et al. Adverse childhood experiences, alcoholic parents, and later risk of alcoholism and depression. *Psychiatr Serv* 2002;53:1001.

Andronicus M, Oates RK, Peat J, et al. Non-accidental burns in children. *Burns* 1998;24:552.

Bays J. Conditions mistaken for child physical abuse. In: Reece RM, Ludwig S, eds. *Child abuse: medical diagnosis and management*. Philadelphia: Lippincott Williams & Wilkins, 2001:177.

Benhaim P, Strear C, Knudson M, et al. Post-traumatic chylous ascites in a child: recognition and management of an unusual condition. *J Trauma* 1995;39:1175.

Betz P, Liebhardt E. Rib fractures in children—resuscitation or child abuse? *Int J Legal Med* 1994;106:215.

Billmire ME, Myers PA. Serious head injury in infants: accident or abuse? *Pediatrics* 1985;75:340.

Bonnier C, Nassagne MC, Evrard P. Outcome and prognosis of whiplash shaken infant syndrome: late consequences after a symptom-free interval. *Dev Med Child Neurol* 1995;37:943.

Bush CM, Jones JS, Cohle SD, Johnson H. Pediatric injuries from cardiopulmonary resuscitation. *Ann Emerg Med* 1996;28:40.

Caldwell RA. *The costs of child abuse vs. child abuse prevention: Michigan's experience*. East Lansing, MI: Michigan Children's Trust Fund, 1992.

Case MES, Nanduri R. Laceration of the stomach by blunt trauma in a child: a case of child abuse. *J Forens Sci* 1983;28:496.

Cohle SD, Hawley DA, Berg KK, et al. Homicidal cardiac lacerations in children. *J Forens Sci* 1995;40:212.

Cooper A, Floyd T, Barlow B, et al. Major blunt abdominal trauma due to child abuse. *J Trauma* 1988;28:1483.

Dalton HJ, Slovis T, Helfer RE, et al. Undiagnosed abuse in children younger than 3 years of age with femoral fracture. *Am J Dis Child* 1990;144:875.

Daro D. *Confronting child abuse: research for effective program design*. New York: The Free press, Macmillan, Inc., 1988.

Defining child maltreatment: a multidisciplinary overview. *Child Welfare* 1984;58:497.

Denton JS, Kalelkar MB. Homicidal commotio cordis in 2 children. *J Forens Sci* 2000;45:734.

Department of Health and Human Services, Office of Human Development Services. CFRS1340.2. Definitions. Washington, DC: U.S. Government, 1987.

Dube SR, Felitti VJ, Dong M, et al. Childhood abuse, neglect and household dysfunction and the risk of illicit drug use: the adverse childhood experience study. *Pediatrics* 2003;111:564.

Dubowitz H, Black M. Child neglect. In: Reece R, ed. *Treatment of child abuse: common ground for mental health, medical and legal professionals*. Baltimore: Johns Hopkins University Press, 2000.

Dubowitz H, Black M, Starr RSZ. A conceptual definition of child neglect. *Crim Justice Psychol* 1993;20:8.

Duhaime AC, Gennarelli TA, Thibault LE, et al. The shaken baby syndrome: a clinical, pathological and biomechanical study. *J Neurosurg* 1987;66:409.

Feldman KW, Brewer DK. Child abuse, cardiopulmonary resuscitation and rib fractures. *Pediatrics* 1984;73:339.

Felitti VJ. Childhood sexual abuse, depression and family dysfunction in adult obese patients: a case control study. *South Med J* 1993;86:732.

Felitti VJ, Anda RF, Nordenberg D, et al. Relationship of childhood abuse and household dysfunction to many of the leading causes of death in adults: the adverse childhood experiences (ACE) study. *Am J Prev Med* 1998;14:245.

Finkel MA, DeJong AR. Medical findings in sexual abuse. In: Reece RM, Ludwig S, eds. *Child abuse: medical diagnosis and management*. Baltimore: Lippincott Williams & Wilkins, 2001:208.

Friedrich WN. Behavioral manifestations of child sexual abuse. *Child Abuse Negl* 1998;22:523.

Friedrich WN. Clinical considerations of empirical treatment studies of abused children. *Child Maltreat* 1996;1:343.

Friedrich WN, Fisher J, Brougton D, et al. Normative sexual behavior in children: a contemporary sample. *Pediatrics* 1998;101:e9.

Friedrich WN, Grambsch P, Broughton D, et al. Normative sexual behavior in children. *Pediatrics* 1991;88:456.

Geddes JF, Hackshaw AK, Vowles GH, et al. Neuropathology of inflicted head injury in children I. Patterns of brain damage. *Brain* 2001;124:1290.

Gelles R. Problems in defining and labeling of child abuse. In: Starr R, ed. *Child abuse prediction: policy implications*. Cambridge, MA: Ballenger Publishing Company, 1982.

Gilliland MGF. Interval duration between injury and severe symptoms in non-accidental head trauma in infants and young children. *J Forens Sci* 1998;43:723.

Gilliland MGF, Folberg R. Shaken babies—some have no impact. *J Forens Sci* 1996;41:114.

Gilliland MGF, Luchenbach M. Are retinal hemorrhages found after resuscitation attempts? A study of the eyes of 169 children. *Am J Forens Med Pathol* 1993;14:187.

Groves BM.Boston: Beacon Press, 2002.

Haviland J, Russell RIR. Outcome after severe non-accidental head injury. *Arch Dis Child* 1997;77:505.

Helfer R. The neglect of our children. *Pediatr Clin North Am* 1990;37:923.

Hymel K, Abshire T, Luckey D, Jenny C. Coagulopathy in pediatric abusive head trauma. *Pediatrics* 1997;99:371.

Jenny C, Hymel KP, Ritzen A, et al. Analysis of missed cases of abusive head trauma. *JAMA* 1999;281:621.

Kelly BT, Thornberry TP, Smith CA. *In the wake of childhood violence*. Washington, DC: National Institute of Justice, 1997.

Kempe CH. Sexual abuse, another hidden pediatric problem: the 1977 C. Anderson Aldrich Lecture. *Pediatrics* 1978;62:382.

Kleinman PK. *Diagnostic imaging in child abuse*, 2nd ed. St. Louis: CV Mosby, 1998.

Kleinman PK, Blackbourne BD, Marks SC Jr, et al. Radiologic contributions to the investigation and prosecution of fatal infant abuse. *N Engl J Med* 1989;320:507.

Langlois NEI, Bresham GA. The aging of bruises: a review and study of the color changes with time. *Forens Sci Int* 1991;50:227.

Ledbetter DJ, Hatch EI, Feldman KW, et al. Diagnostic and surgical implications of child abuse. *Arch Surg* 1988;123:1101.

Leone RJ, Krasna IH. Spontaneous neonatal gastric perforation: is it really spontaneous? *J Pediatr Surg* 2000;35:1066.

Leventhal JM, Thomas SA, Rosenfeld NS, Markowitz RI. Fractures in young children. Distinguishing child abuse from unintentional injuries. *Am J Dis Child* 1993;147:87.

Levin AV. Ocular manifestations of child abuse. In: Reece RM, Ludwig S, eds. *Child abuse: medical diagnosis and management*. Baltimore: Lippincott Williams & Wilkins, 2001.

Ludwig S. Visceral injury manifestations of child abuse. In: Reece RM, Ludwig S, eds. *Child abuse: medical diagnosis and management*. Baltimore: Lippincott Williams & Wilkins, 2001:157.

Missouri Children's Trust Fund. *The economic costs of shaken baby syndrome survivors in Missouri*. Jefferson City, MO: Missouri Children's Trust Fund, 1997.

Mortimer PE, Friedrich M. Are facial bruises in babies ever accidental? *Arch Dis Child* 1983;58:75.

National Child Abuse and Neglect Data Systems. Responses from the States on child maltreatment incidence. Washington, D.C.: US Government Printing Office, 2001.

Odum A, Christ E, Kerr N, et al. Prevalence of retinal hemorrhages in pediatric patients after in-hospital cardio-pulmonary resuscitation: a prospective study. *Pediatrics* 1997;99:e3.

Paterson CR, Burns J, McAllion WJ. Osteogenesis imperfecta: the distinction from child abuse and the recognition of a variant form. *Am J Med Genet* 1995;45:187.

Price EA, Rush LR, Perper JA, Bell MD. Cardiopulmonary resuscitation-related injuries and homicidal blunt abdominal trauma in children. *Am J Forens Med Pathol* 2000;21:307.

Reece RM, Arnold J, Splain J. Pharyngeal perforation as a manifestation of child abuse. *Child Maltreat* 1996;1:364.

Reece RM, Sege R. Childhood head injury: accidental or inflicted? *Arch Ped Adol Med* 2000;154:11.

Roberton DM, Barbor P, Hull D. Unusual injury? Recent injury in normal children and children with suspected non-accidental injury. *BMJ* 1982;285:1399.

Rosenberg DA. Web of deceit: a literature review of Munchausen syndrome by proxy. *Child Abuse Negl* 1987;11:547.

Rosenberg NM. Frequency of suspected abuse/neglect in burn patients. *Pediatr Emerg Care* 1989;5:219.

Sandramouli S, Robinson R, Tsaloumas M, Willshaw HI. Retinal haemorrhages and convulsions. *Arch Dis Child* 1997;76:449.

Sheridan RL, Ryan CM, Petras LM, et al. Burns in children younger than 2 years of age: an experience with 200 consecutive admissions. *Pediatrics* 1997;100:721.

Simon P, Baron R. Age as a risk factor for burn injury requiring hospitalization during early childhood. *Arch Pediatr Adolesc Med* 1994;148:394.

Spevak MR, Kleinman PK, Belanger PI, et al. Cardiopulmonary resuscitation and rib fractures in infants. *JAMA* 1994;272:617–618.

Strait RT, Siegel RM, Shapiro RA. Humeral fractures without obvious etiologies in children less than 3 years of age: when is it abuse? *Pediatrics* 1995;96:667.

Sugar NF, Taylor JA, Feldman KW. Bruises in infants and toddlers: those who don't cruise rarely bruise. *Arch Pediatr Adolesc Med* 1999;153:399.

Teicher M. Scars that won't heal: the neurobiology of child abuse. *Sci Am* 2002:68.

Touloukian RJ. Abdominal trauma in childhood. *Surg Gynecol Obstet* 1968;127:561.

Tzioumi C, Oates RK. Subdural hematomas in children under two years. Accident or abuse? A 10-year experience. *Child Abuse Negl* 1998;22:1105.

Widom CS. Child abuse, neglect, and violent criminal behavior. *Criminology* 1989;27:251.

Widom CS. The cycle of violence. *Science* 1989;244:160.

Widom CS. Understanding the consequences of childhood victimization. In: Reece RM, ed. *Treatment of child abuse: common ground for mental health, medical and legal professionals*. Baltimore: Johns Hopkins University Press, 2000.

Willman KY, Bank DE, Senac M, Chadwick DL. Restricting the time of injury in fatal inflicted head injury. *Child Abuse Negl* 1997;21:929.

SECTION II ■ THE FETUS AND THE NEWBORN

a: GENERAL PRINCIPLES OF GROWTH AND DEVELOPMENT

CHAPTER 18 ■ NEWBORN SCREENING

STEPHEN G. KAHLER

The newborn screening of infants for metabolic disorders began more than 40 years ago, for phenylketonuria (PKU), following the discovery of children with mental retardation, eczema, and microcephaly who had a peculiar odor to their urine. An identification of the odoriferous compound, discovery of the enzyme deficiency, creation of a synthetic diet devoid of phenylalanine, and the invention of a simple method for measuring phenylalanine in large numbers of samples led to the development of newborn screening. It became apparent that rapid diagnosis and institution of the diet could minimize toxicity from phenylalanine, and that the blood sample could be used for other tests. What follows is a discussion of the history and basis of newborn screening, the current status, especially as practiced in the United States, and possibilities for the future. Incidence figures are approximate. Details of the diagnosis and management of conditions discussed are presented in other chapters.

HISTORY

Newborn screening became practical with the development of a rapid, inexpensive test that could be done in batch format. Robert Guthrie, a microbiologist at the State University of New York at Buffalo, developed a bacterial assay for phenylalanine quantitation in blood dried on filter paper. This test is known as the Guthrie test, and the filter paper cards often are called Guthrie cards. From this beginning in the early 1960s, major strides have been made by public health institutions in preventing mental retardation, death, and disability. All states in the United States have their own or shared newborn screening programs, and private firms also offer primary or supplemental screening tests. A newborn screening program comprises screening and follow-up tests, diagnosis, management, education, and evaluation of these components. Increasing interest is voiced for a national screening policy for the United States, to define minimum standards for all programs.

Screening programs have developed according to criteria set forth in the 1960s, which propose that screening is appropriate if a test is available, feasible, and affordable, and the disorder is difficult to recognize clinically, sufficiently prevalent, and treatable (Box 18.1). Because prevalence varies depending on the disorder and the population, adapting these principles to specific local situations has led to great variation among programs. Phenylketonuria, hypothyroidism, galactosemia, and sickle-cell disease and hemoglobinopathies are tested in all U.S. screening programs. Congenital adrenal hyperplasia and biotinidase are tested in many programs (Box 18.2), and cystic fibrosis (CF) in a few. Required tests are called *mandated* tests.

BOX 18.1 **Screening Criteria for Genetic Conditions***

A test is available.
Testing is feasible and affordable.
The disorder is difficult to recognize clinically.
The disorder is "sufficiently" preventable.
The disorder is treatable.

---

*Criteria formulated by the World Health Organization in 1968.

Expanded newborn screening refers to the use of tandem mass spectrometry (see section, Expanded Newborn Screening Using Tandem Mass Spectrometry and Box 18.3). It is used in about 30 state programs, and several other states are considering it. Maple syrup urine disease, homocystinuria, and tyrosinemia, formerly tested in some states by other methods, are part of most expanded newborn screening programs. For those tests not mandated in a particular jurisdiction, supplemental screening is available on a voluntary basis or through private laboratories. All developed countries have screening programs, and many developing countries have programs available in some locations or hospitals. The current situation for the United States can be found at http://genes-r-us.uthscsa.edu/. Screening programs also exist for congenital hearing loss and some infections.

BOX 18.2 **Standard Screening Test Conditions in Many States**

Phenylketonuria
Hypothyroidism
Hemoglobinopathies (e.g., sickle-cell disease)
Galactosemia
Biotinidase deficiency
Maple syrup urine disease
Homocystinuria
Cystic fibrosis
Congenital adrenal hyperplasia

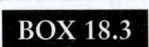

Disorders Detected by Expanded Newborn Screening Using Tandem Mass Spectrometry

BOX 18.3

Acylcarnitine profile
Organic acid disorders
  2-Methylbutyryl-CoA dehydrogenase deficiency
  3-Methylglutaconyl-CoA hydratase deficiency
  *3-Hydroxy-3-methylglutaryl-CoA lyase deficiency (HMG)
  *Glutaric acidemia-type I (GA 1)
  Isobutyryl-CoA dehydrogenase deficiency
  *Isovaleric acidemia (IVA)
  *3-Methylcrotonyl-CoA carboxylase deficiency (3MCC deficiency)
  3-Methylglutaconyl-CoA hydratase deficiency
  *Methylmalonic acidemias (MMA)
  *Vitamin B_{12} deficiency (due to maternal deficiency)
  Malonic aciduria
  *Mitochondrial acetoacetyl-CoA thiolase deficiency (3-Ketothiolase deficiency)
  *Multiple carboxylase deficiency
  *Propionic acidemia (PA)

Fatty acid oxidation disorders
  *Carnitine deficiency, including transporter defect
  *Carnitine palmityl transferase deficiency-type I (CPT-I)
  *Carnitine/acylcarnitine translocase deficiency (TRANSLOCASE)
  *Carnitine palmityl transferase deficiency-type II (CPT-II)
  *Very long-chain acyl-CoA dehydrogenase deficiency (VLCAD)
  *Trifunctional protein deficiency (TFP deficiency)
  *3-Hydroxy long-chain acyl-CoA dehydrogenase deficiency (LCHAD)
  Long-chain acyl-CoA dehydrogenase deficiency (LCAD)
  *Medium-chain acyl-CoA dehydrogenase deficiency (MCAD)
  *Short-chain acyl-CoA dehydrogenase deficiency (SCAD)
  Short-chain hydroxy acyl-CoA dehydrogenase deficiency (SCHAD)
  2,4-Dienoyl-CoA reductase deficiency
  *Multiple acyl-CoA dehydrogenase deficiency (MADD or glutaric aciduria type II)
  *Ethylmalonic encephalopathy

Amino acid disorders
  *Phenylketonuria (PKU)
  *Disorders of biopterin metabolism
  *Tyrosinemia (type I is not reliably detectable in the newborn period)
  *Citrullinemia (ASA synthetase deficiency)
  Citrullinemia type II (citrin deficiency)
  *Argininosuccinic aciduria (ASA lyase deficiency)
  *Argininemia
  Hyperammonemia, hyperornithinemia, homocitrullinuria (HHH) syndrome
  Hypermethioninemia
  *Homocystinuria (cystathionine-beta synthase deficiency)
  *Maple syrup urine disease (MSUD)
  *Nonketotic hyperglycinemia-5-oxoprolinuria

_____
*Included on the March of Dimes list of major disorders to be targeted by newborn screening programs.

CONSENT AND LEGAL ISSUES

All U.S. jurisdictions require that newborn screening be offered. Some states specify the tests and methods to be used; in others, these are decided by the laboratory or health department, guided by its advisory committee. The number of conditions tested for ranges from four to over 50, if one counts mild and severe forms of several disorders separately. Newborn screening for metabolic diseases and hemoglobinopathies requires a blood sample obtained by heel stick or sometimes by venipuncture. Blood sampling for screening tests has been regarded as within the scope of ordinary neonatal care, but increasingly it is regarded as requiring active informed consent from the parent. Consent should be obtained at a prenatal visit. Some states require a signature for the test to be performed ("opt in"); others require the test, and signature is required to refuse it ("opt out" or "informed dissent"). Refusal of the test must be carefully documented. Funding for newborn screening testing occurs through state legislatures, charges to hospitals, federal block grants to states, and sometimes through direct charges to patients.

DETAILS

Collection of Blood

The Guthrie card should be filled out before the sample is obtained and checked against the baby's identification. The blood spots usually are obtained by heel prick after warming the heel and pricking with a sharp lancet on the medial or lateral segment of the side of the heel. The heel may be squeezed gently to express the blood. Blood is sometimes drawn into capillary tubes and then applied to the card. Blood also may be obtained by venipuncture, as long as an anticoagulant is not used.

The blood is applied to one side of the Guthrie card, spotting until all circles are completely filled. Repeated spotting, especially if the card has become partially dried, will lead to over-saturation of the card and abnormal results. Contamination of the card with any other fluid will invalidate the results. Samples should be dried at room temperature, and not stacked until completely dry.

Samples should be obtained in accordance with the local program's policy, usually 48 to 72 hours after birth, assuming no unusual circumstances. If the infant is to be discharged before then, a sample must be obtained at the time of discharge, and a second sample obtained by 2 weeks after birth. A few programs require a second sample at 2 weeks, regardless of the time of discharge. If the infant is older than 1 week, the normal ranges commonly used may not be appropriate. Samples should be sent to the lab daily by the most expeditious method (courier or postal service).

Ideally, the most important tests will be completed within 24 hours of arrival (but most labs do not operate on a 7-day basis), and the other tests soon after. Depending on the test, an abnormal result will be reported or followed by a second-tier test on the same sample. Abnormal results must be reported promptly, and the family should be contacted by the physician, follow-up program, or laboratory for follow-up testing or urgent referral to a specialist, depending on the disorder and degree of danger. Urgency varies with the condition—highly urgent for congenital adrenal hyperplasia, galactosemia, organic acidurias, and urea cycle disorders, less so for hypothyroidism and most hemoglobinopathies. Sensitivity and specificity vary considerably among the different tests, and a differential diagnosis must be considered for nearly every abnormal result. Normal results are typically reported to the birth hospital and physician. Computerized data tracking and reporting are standard practice. The card may be kept by the laboratory for a few years or indefinitely, or may be discarded quickly, depending on state law and storage facilities.

Follow-up and Treatment

Newborn screening is commonly integrated with the follow-up program, but this connection depends on the state or program. Communication among primary care providers and parents, medical specialists, nutritionists, and social workers is part of a comprehensive program. Special infant formulas and medical foods may come directly from the state program or may have to be obtained from local or hospital pharmacies. Insurance reimbursement for formulas and foods, which can be quite costly, is variable. Lifelong therapy involves life-long expense, and there is always the possibility of loss of affordable insurance coverage.

FAMILY IMPLICATIONS

When a patient with a heritable condition is identified through newborn screening, an evaluation of other family members, especially siblings, should be considered. Most metabolic disorders are inherited in an autosomal recessive manner. In some instances, testing of healthy older siblings not is needed; ascertaining their clinical status or the results of their newborn screening will suffice, but testing may be offered for reassurance. In conditions with variable age of presentation, or if screening for a condition has been recently added (e.g., medium-chain acyl-CoA dehydrogenase, or MCAD deficiency), it is imperative to test siblings. Parents should receive genetic counseling regarding the implications and options for future pregnancies and a rapid evaluation of subsequent children.

When a recessive disorder is diagnosed, the recurrence risk is 25% for the same set of parents. It is important to be aware of the issues surrounding possible or apparent nonpaternity. This is especially important if parents already have been tested for carrier status; for example, in carrier screening programs for sickle cell disease and CF. Carrier screening programs themselves can be a source of error, leading to results inconsistent with newborn screening results.

ETHICAL ISSUES

Laboratory testing is only one part of a comprehensive newborn screening program. Issues of equitable and affordable access to testing, follow-up treatment, and medical care must be confronted before a public health program can be implemented. For many conditions, the treatment is life-long and expensive; however, those screening tests that lead to early diagnosis and therapy can result in better outcomes and thus savings in lives, intelligence, disability, and the costs of medical care, compared with the course that follows diagnosis after the onset of clinical illness. A sophisticated cost–benefit analysis of screening for medium-chain acyl-CoA dehydrogenase (MCAD) deficiency has been conducted by Venditti et al. and can be extended to other conditions.

HAZARDS

Errors and missed treatment in newborn screening can occur because of clerical mistakes (wrong name or address, wrong card), or failure of the parent to provide an accurate home address or name of physician. If the infant is extremely premature, has not yet been fed or is receiving total parenteral nutrition, or has a major illness, the results must be interpreted with that knowledge. Transfusion can alter the result of many tests, especially hemoglobin, biotinidase, and the enzyme assay for galactosemia. Some babies are not screened because of home birth, failure of communication of screening status between hospitals at time of transfer, or because of parental refusal. Careful record keeping can minimize the chance of an infant being overlooked. If screening is not universal, but based on ethnic classification (as some states have done for selective screening of hemoglobinopathies), opportunities arise for missing cases because of erroneous classification or clerical error. It is simpler to screen all infants.

Errors can occur in the screening process. If a screened disorder is suspected on clinical grounds, one should always do the appropriate definitive test, even if a written copy of the initial negative report is available.

Ensuring that all infants have been screened is the responsibility of all who care for them. Missed cases are more often due to inadequate follow-up or lack of screening than to laboratory error or "false-negative" results.

TESTS AND DISORDERS

Standard Tests

Phenylketonuria

PKU and its milder variants occur in 1 in 10,000 to 25,000 infants. Untreated PKU leads to irreversible mental retardation, with the greatest damage occurring in the first year. The institution of a restricted diet in the first month and strict adherence prevents nearly all problems. The original Guthrie test uses a bacterial inhibition assay (BIA), in which blood spots are applied to agar plates seeded with *Bacillus subtilis*. The plates are impregnated with 2-thienylalanine, which inhibits growth unless a high concentration of phenylalanine is present in the blood spot. The original Guthrie test is being replaced by tandem mass spectrometry (see section, Expanded Newborn Screening Using Tandem Mass Spectrometry). An automated fluorometric test has been used in some states. Antibiotics can interfere with the Guthrie test (which is based on bacterial growth), but not with the two other methods.

A positive result requires repeat testing for confirmation. Confirmed high values then must be validated, and the specific defect ascertained. Severe phenylalanine hydroxylase (PAH) deficiency is the cause of classical PKU. Several hundred mutations in the PAH gene are known. Milder mutations result in mild PKU or benign hyperphenylalaninemia.

The treatment of classical PKU involves significant restriction of dietary phenylalanine, accomplished by limiting natural protein (i.e., in mother's milk or standard infant formula) to the amount tolerated. A synthetic formula provides the remainder of calories and other nutrients, together with protein in a safe form (devoid of phenylalanine, and with supplemental tyrosine, the product of the impaired enzyme). With frequent careful monitoring, even infants with severe PKU can be safely and successfully breast-fed, using the synthetic formula first at each feeding, followed by the breast.

Dietary restriction is critical for optimal infant development and must be maintained throughout childhood. Growing consensus affirms that "diet for life" is the best approach for many patients. It is essential that women with PKU be on the diet and in good control before becoming pregnant, because poor control during the pregnancy will expose the fetus to high levels of PHE, causing microcephaly and mental retardation and sometimes heart malformations.

In 1% to 2% of cases, elevated phenylalanine is due to a variety of problems with the synthesis or metabolism of the tetrahydrobiopterin cofactor of PAH. Other biopterin enzymes (tyrosine hydroxylase, tryptophan hydroxylase) also will be affected, and the treatment of this disorder (malignant hyperphenylalaninemia) is quite difficult. All infants identified as having elevated PHE should be tested for these defects by urine analysis of pterins. (More detailed information on PKU can be found in Chapter 385.)

Hypothyroidism

Congenital hypothyroidism (CH) usually is due to dysgenesis of the thyroid gland. Unlike most other screened disorders, hypothyroidism does not have a strong familial component and is quite unlikely to occur in siblings. The incidence is roughly 1 in 4,000 infants. No major ethnic predilection is noted.

CH is screened for either by first measuring thyroid hormone (T4) or thyroid-stimulating hormone (TSH), and using the other as a secondary test. If T4 is the primary test, typically the lowest 10% of samples will be subject to secondary TSH screening. If the TSH is elevated, the infant will require follow-up investigation. Programs that use TSH as the primary or initial analyte may miss secondary forms of hypothyroidism; an argument can be made that thyroid screening using both analytes will have the best chance of detecting all cases of hypothyroidism in infants. Therapy for primary hypothyroidism is the simple provision of thyroid hormone, once the diagnosis has been established with certainty. Iodide-deficiency hypothyroidism and its congenital form, cretinism, is rare in the United States because of adequate iodide in most of the water supply and widespread use of iodized salt. (More detailed information on hypothyroidism can be found in Chapter 380, Thyroid Gland.)

Hemoglobinopathies

In the 1980s, screening for hemoglobinopathies was prompted by the demonstration that significant morbidity and mortality in sickle cell disease occurred in the first 6 months, primarily due to bacterial infection, and that early intervention to prevent pneumococcal sepsis was effective. Sickle cell disease accounts for about 65% of all cases of hemoglobinopathies in the United States. Newborn screening detects many other hemoglobinopathies, such as thalassemias, as well as heterozygotes (carriers) of mutant hemoglobins.

Primary screening of hemoglobin is usually done by isoelectric focusing of hemoglobin eluted from the Guthrie card; high performance liquid chromatography (HPLC) or electrophoresis on cellulose acetate has been used by a few programs. Positive results are referred for secondary (confirmatory) testing by a different method, including DNA-based assays or immunologic tests. Hemoglobin results usually are presented as the series of hemoglobins detected: for example, FAS for a sickle-cell heterozygote (who has the usual high infantile level of Hgb F). Positive results should prompt a rapid evaluation of the infant by an experienced physician. (More detailed information on hemoglobinopathies can be found in Chapter 290, Hemoglobinopathies and Thalassemias.)

Galactosemia

Galactosemia due to deficiency of galactose-1-phosphate uridyltransferase (GALT) is an important cause of hepatic dysfunction and jaundice in the newborn period. The hyperbilirubinemia is a mixture of conjugated and unconjugated fractions, unlike the usual unconjugated hyperbilirubinemia of the newborn. Cataracts, cerebral edema, renal tubular dysfunction, and sepsis with gram-negative organisms may occur. Screening is based on either determination of enzyme activity, or measurement of accumulating metabolites (galactose, galactose-1-phosphate). The former is a more expensive assay, and the latter depends on adequate milk intake (24 hours is desirable). The enzyme may lose activity if the blood spot is not dried and handled properly, thus leading to a high number of low values (false-positive results). The incidence of classical galactosemia is 1 in 60,000 infants.

The infant with galactosemia may be quite ill at the time of diagnosis, or may be doing well. Breast feeding or lactose- and galactose-containing formula must be stopped immediately. Many excellent infant formulas are devoid of lactose (a glucose-galactose disaccharide) and galactose. The infant must be evaluated and confirmatory testing arranged. Urine reducing substances will disappear within a day of withdrawal of galactose, whereas the erythrocyte galactose-1-phosphate level will be elevated for weeks. Scrupulous avoidance of galactose is essential for the first several years; some patients with mild galactosemia may be able to tolerate some milk products when they are older; infants with the mildest variants may not need galactose restriction.

In addition to classical galactosemia and its variants, galactokinase deficiency and epimerase deficiency also can be detected by metabolite accumulation. (More detailed information on galactosemia can be found in Chapter 387.)

Biotinidase Deficiency

Biotinidase deficiency leads to a failure of recycling of biotin, a vitamin essential for the function of four carboxylases (for propionyl-CoA, 2-methylcrotonyl-CoA, acetyl-CoA, and pyruvate). Unlike most vitamin cofactors, biotin is covalently bound (to lysine) in the enzyme, so this bond must be broken when the enzyme is recycled, before the biotin is again available. The consequences of deficiency include developmental delay, seizures, ataxia, deafness, and dermatitis; biochemical manifestations include lactic acidosis and organic aciduria reflecting the impaired carboxylases. Treatment is the simple provision of supplemental biotin daily. The incidence of biotinidase deficiency is roughly 1 in 90,000 infants. Screening is performed by enzyme assay. Confirmatory testing is done by quantitative serum assay. Biotinidase deficiency was originally called late-onset multiple carboxylase deficiency. The early-onset form, due to holocarboxylase synthase deficiency, uncommonly responds to biotin. (More information on biotinidase deficiency can be found in Chapter 385.)

Maple Syrup Urine Disease

A deficiency of branched-chain ketoacid dehydrogenase activity impairs the catabolism of leucine, isoleucine, and valine. Manifestations of maple syrup urine disease (MSUD) include vomiting and feeding aversion, followed by severe ketoacidosis and cerebral edema. Intercurrent infections aggravate an already unstable metabolic state. Restriction of the toxic but essential amino acids requires careful management and meticulous attention to infections. Early diagnosis can lessen the catastrophic illness that may occur at presentation. Some programs have used a BIA test in the past; MSUD screening now is part of most expanded programs using tandem mass spectrometry (MS/MS). The overall incidence is perhaps 1 in 200,000 infants, but in a population at high risk because of founder effect, such as Mennonites in the United States, the incidence can be a thousand times greater, and DNA-based carrier screening programs may be appropriate. (More information on maple syrup urine disease can be found in Chapter 385.)

Homocystinuria

The most common cause of major homocysteine accumulation is cystathionine-beta-synthase deficiency. Untreated homocystinuria can cause coagulation defects and vascular occlusions leading to mental retardation and stroke, lens dislocation, a slender Marfanoid phenotype (without aortic dilatation), and osteoporosis. Treatment with pyridoxine supplementation effectively lowers the homocysteine level in about half of patients. Dietary management also may be necessary. Homocysteine concentration in the blood in homocystinuria is massively elevated, compared to the mild elevations seen with folate insufficiency and disorders of folate metabolism. For technical reasons, however, screening is based on measuring the methionine level, which may be normal in the newborn period. The role of other coagulopathies contributing to the pathology seen in homocystinuria is not understood. Homocystinuria occurs in 1 in 100,000 to 1 in 200,000 births. (More information on homocystinuria can be found in Chapter 385.)

Cystic Fibrosis

Newborn screening for CF is not done in most U.S. jurisdictions, but it is well-established in some. A recent advisory panel (2004) has recommended adding CF testing to all screening programs. The incidence is 1 in 2,000 infants in the high-risk population originating in northern Europe, and less in other parts of the world. Screening is based on an analysis of immunoreactive trypsinogen (IRT) activity. Increased activity can reflect pancreatic dysfunction, often due to CF. Secondary testing can be done using DNA analysis for the commonest mutation (△F508), or a panel of mutations. If two mutations are found, the diagnosis is confirmed; if one mutation is found, a second undetected mutation may be present or, more likely, the infant is heterozygous (and clinically unaffected). The infant's status can be established by sweat chloride measurement, commonly done at 1 month of age. Infants with severe CF manifesting as meconium ileus will be recognized clinically in the first week. CF testing may not be performed on the newborn sample until the end of the first month, so that, if the lab finds a positive result requiring further action, the infant will be old enough for a sweat chloride test, and the parents do not have to wait in a state of high anxiety.

CF is present worldwide, with the most common allele originating in northern Europe. This one allele accounts for about 70% of the CF alleles in that population. Finding a heterozygous infant means that at least one of the parents also carries that mutation; if the other parent is also heterozygous, the couple is at risk for a child with CF. The identification of a heterozygous infant should lead to an offer of carrier testing for both parents, analogous to the situation for sickle-cell trait and other hemoglobin variants. The recent advent of carrier testing for CF of pregnant couples in the United States means that an increasing number of adults will know their carrier status within the limits of detection. Because several hundred mutations are known, carrier screening programs will have a false-negative rate of a few percent due to the presence of untested mutations. This situation is in contrast to that for hemoglobinopathies, in which the presence of the normal allele is positively verified by its product (Hgb A), resulting in a lower false-negative rate. (More information on CF can be found in Chapter 236, Cystic Fibrosis.)

Congenital Adrenal Hyperplasia

Congenital adrenal hyperplasia (CAH) is a group of disorders of impaired steroid synthesis and compensatory adrenal hyperplasia. Incidence of the severe form is 1 in 10,000 to 1 in 15,000 infants, but the very mildest forms can be a hundred times more common in certain populations. The commonest form by far is deficiency of 21-hydroxylase, with a resulting deficiency of glucocorticoids and mineralocorticoids and the excess production of androgens. The result is a variable degree of adrenal insufficiency and virilization, with the two contrasting phenotypes called salt-wasting and simple virilizing forms. Even milder forms have been recognized recently.

The most severe form of classical CAH is characterized by urinary salt-wasting and cardiovascular collapse with septic shock in the first weeks of life. Girls may have complete labial fusion and clitoromegaly, creating an apparent male phenotype with undescended testes, and even boys may be obviously virilized. Severe adrenal insufficiency is a medical emergency. Milder forms of CAH without salt-wasting or notable virilization occur and lead to advanced bone age followed by early cessation of growth.

Many forms of impaired adrenal steroid synthesis lead to accumulation of 17-hydroxyprogesterone (17-OHP), making this the preferred analyte for newborn screening. It is detected by fluoroimmunoassay or liquid chromatography-tandem mass spectrometry (LC-MS/MS). Second-tier molecular testing (DNA) may help simplify the difficult problem of borderline 17-OHP elevations. 17-OHP levels change rapidly after birth and are elevated in premature infants, so interpretation of results is difficult and many false-positive results can occur. A stratification of cut-off levels based on gestational age (not necessarily birth weight), age at testing, and other factors can increase the test precision. A positive result can be a metabolic emergency; thus, infants must be evaluated immediately and the blood electrolytes checked. Gender assignment for infants with ambiguous genitalia requires careful evaluation and consultation. (More information on congenital adrenal hyperplasia can be found in Chapter 381.)

Tyrosinemia

Tyrosine elevations can occur as part of generalized liver dysfunction, transient tyrosinemia, or due to specific enzyme dysfunction. Type I tyrosinemia due to fumarylacetoacetate hydrolase deficiency leads to hepatic and renal dysfunction, and a high risk of hepatocellular carcinoma is present. Type II tyrosinemia due to tyrosine aminotransferase deficiency leads to palmoplantar keratosis and corneal ulcerations, with a risk of mental retardation. Each of these conditions has a specific treatment. Tyrosine can be measured by BIA, fluorometric assay, or as part of expanded newborn screening by MS/MS. However, sensitivity is relatively low (infants with tyrosinemia may have a normal tyrosine level in the newborn period); therefore, some labs do not measure tyrosine as part of the newborn panel. (More information on tyrosinemia can be found in Chapter 385.)

EXPANDED NEWBORN SCREENING USING TANDEM MASS SPECTROMETRY

MS/MS, an instrument with two mass spectrometers coupled in tandem, has enormous analytical power. It is well-suited to characterize acylcarnitines, a class of compounds reflecting the cellular production and use of various acyl-CoA compounds. The acyl-CoAs are intermediates in much of organic acid and fatty acid metabolism. Carnitine is the carrier molecule that brings long-chain fatty acids into the mitochondria. The fatty acids are transferred to Coenzyme A (CoA) for beta-oxidation. If fatty acid oxidation is impaired, the accumulated metabolite coupled to CoA can be transferred back to carnitine, then exported from the mitochondria and the cell. Many organic acids, derived from amino acids, undergo a similar metabolic process. MS/MS separates a mixture of molecules that share a common molecular feature—in this case, carnitine—and identifies them. Those components of the mix are then reported as an acylcarnitine profile. Normal values and ratios are known for many species. Several amino acids also can be reliably analyzed by MS/MS using the same butyl derivatization as is used for acylcarnitine analysis. Total analysis time for acylcarnitines and amino acids is about 2 minutes, and the preparation and analysis procedures can be automated.

The most common disorder detected by acylcarnitine analysis is MCAD deficiency, with its characteristic elevation of octanoylcarnitine [See Chapters 386 and 409.] Patients with MCAD deficiency may have hypoglycemia or encephalopathy triggered by fasting and infection. Symptoms or even death may result in the newborn period before feeding is established. MCAD deficiency occurs in about 1 in 10,000 to 1 in 15,000 infants, and is especially common in patients with ancestors from Northern Europe and the British Isles. Many other fatty-acid and organic-acid disorders are characterized by severe and progressive acidosis, with liver, muscle, heart, and brain involvement. Early diagnosis can minimize the injury that occurs in the newborn period and optimize outcome.

The amino acids detected by MS/MS include phenylalanine, tyrosine, methionine, leucine, and isoleucine (which have the same mass), and the urea cycle metabolites arginine and citrulline. Thus, the disorders of phenylalanine, tyrosine, homocystine and methionine metabolism; maple syrup urine disease; and the urea cycle disorders citrullinemia (CIT), argininosuccinic aciduria (ASA), and argininemia can be detected by this method. CIT and ASA lead to hyperammonemia, with vomiting and coma; argininemia causes progressive brain injury without hyperammonemia.

OTHER TESTS

Hearing Loss

Congenital hearing loss has a multitude of causes, including genetic and structural factors and prenatal infection. The incidence of severe hearing loss (greater than 35 dB) occurs in 1 to 3 of every 1,000 infants. Congenital hearing loss has numerous genetic causes, some with associated malformations, and many nongenetic causes. Early recognition leads to early treatment using amplification, the early introduction of signing, and other modalities, as indicated. U.S. federal aid is available to support state programs, so most states are establishing hearing screening.

Screening is done by auditory brainstem response (ABR) or oto-acoustic emission (OAE) testing. Those abnormalities detected in screening programs require confirmation using ABR testing. Hearing screening is the most expensive component of newborn screening.

Infections

Human Immunodeficiency Virus (See also Chapters 137, 138, and 139)

Two states currently screen newborns for human immunodeficiency virus (HIV). The benefits of early diagnosis and therapy are well-established. Screening pregnant women allows for earlier diagnosis (of the mother), earlier therapy for both her and the infant, and the opportunity to minimize the chance of vertical transmission during pregnancy, at delivery, or via breast feeding. Screening infants using an ELISA assay for IgM antibodies allows the identification of those at-risk infants not found by maternal testing during pregnancy. The incidence of HIV in the United States is about 3 in 1,000 infants, but it is much higher in some populations; the risk of transmission during pregnancy or childbirth can be reduced from about 30% to 40% to less than 5% if infected mothers and their newborns are treated with antiretroviral medications. The treatment of HIV and preventing its transmission to infants is one of the most important public health problems worldwide. (More information on HIV can be found in Chapters 139 through 141; information on immunodeficiency can be found in Chapters 362 and 427.)

Toxoplasmosis

Two states currently screen for congenital toxoplasmosis, which occurs in 1 in 10,000 pregnancies in the United States. Early recognition allows for earlier therapy; screening identifies infants in whom clinical diagnosis would be delayed because the classic triad of microcephaly, retinopathy, and cerebral calcifications is not present. Some countries screen and monitor antibody-negative women during pregnancy, because seroconversion will indicate recent infection and greater risk to the fetus. (More information on toxoplasmosis can be found in Chapter 83, Neonatal Toxoplasmosis and Chapter 222, Toxoplasmosis.)

Neuroblastoma

Urine screening for catecholamine metabolites had been used in Japan for two decades. The program was started on the premises that neuroblastoma is relatively common, and early detection would lead to improved outcome. However, neuroblastomas present at birth usually regress, whereas those that exhibit malignant potential usually arise later. A careful review showed that the newborn screening program did not provide any advantage, therefore it was discontinued in 2004. (More information on neuroblastoma can be found in Chapter 308, Neuroblastoma.)

FUTURE DEVELOPMENTS

Glucose-6-Phosphate Dehydrogenase Deficiency

Several hundred alleles of glucose-6-phosphate dehydrogenase (G6PD) produce deficient activity. These alleles generally are derived from the malarial areas of Europe, Africa, and Asia. The commonest form of G6PD deficiency in the United States is the A–allele in African Americans. The A–allele is not a major source of chronic symptoms or pathology, but, like many variants, it can be associated with hemolysis triggered by certain types of drugs or infections. The Mediterranean allele has similar properties, as well as a susceptibility to fava beans. Rarer forms of G6PD deficiency are associated with ongoing hemolysis or congenital nonspherocytic hemolytic disease. G6PD activity can be measured using the Guthrie blood spot. Only a few programs in the United States offer this test presently. G6PD is carried on the X chromosome, so deficiency is more common in males, but females can be affected because of nonrandom X inactivation (lyonization) or homozygosity (inheriting a deficient allele from each parent). (More information on G6PD deficiency can be found in Chapter 291.)

Lysosomal Storage Disorders

Over forty lysosomal storage disorders exist, in which the progressive accumulation of material leads to cell death and organ dysfunction. Overall, the incidence of lysosomal storage diseases is greater than 1 in 10,000 births. In the Ashkenazi Jewish population, non-neuronopathic Gaucher disease, an exceedingly variable disorder, much more common. Intravenous enzyme therapy for this condition has been available for more than a decade. Stem-cell transplantation and enzyme replacement are realistic options for therapy in many of the other disorders. Enzyme is now available for mucopolysaccharidosis I (MPS I) (Hurler, Scheie, and intermediate forms), and Fabry disease, and will be available soon for other disorders, including Pompe disease and Maroteaux-Lamy syndrome (MPS VI). These advances in treatment are an impetus to find a generic marker or a panel of enzyme assays for lysosomal dysfunction, before symptoms and damage occur. (More information on lysosomal storage disorders can be found in Chapter 389, Lysosomal Storage Disorders.)

Duchenne Muscular Dystrophy

Duchenne muscular dystrophy, an X-linked disorder that occurs in 1 in 3,000 boys, can be suspected by finding a major elevation of creatine kinase (CK or CPK). Some laboratories have included screening for this disorder, although it is not currently treatable, because early diagnosis allows for better management and genetic counseling regarding recurrence. When treatment is available, early diagnosis will be essential. (More information on Duchenne muscular dystrophy can be found in Chapter 409.)

Fragile X Syndrome

Fragile X syndrome is the commonest single-gene cause of mental retardation. Although X-linked, it can cause mental retardation in girls as well as boys. The fundamental defect is an expansion of a trinucleotide repeat region of DNA in the FMR1 gene. The incidence of large expansions ("full mutation"), which invariably cause mental retardation, is 1 in 2,500 boys. Girls, having two X chromosomes, are variably affected when heterozygous, and the incidence is 1 in 5,000. The incidence of smaller expansions ("premutations"), which are generally asymptomatic, is as high as 1 in 250 females and 1 in 800 males. Some older men carrying premutations will have a parkinsonian disorder. Premutation expansions carried by females may lead to full mutation in the next generation. The risk of expansion occurring is related to the size of the premutation expansion. Newborn screening using a DNA technique has been proposed as a means for early identification;

this would allow for close tracking, earlier intervention, and genetic counseling regarding risks for other pregnancies and relatives. Pre-pregnancy or prenatal screening also has been suggested.

PHARMACOGENETIC SCREENING

The role that genetic polymorphisms play in nonallergic drug reactions raises the possibility that such reactions could be avoided by screening patients before drugs are given, and perhaps the best drug for a situation could be determined in advance. The cytochrome P-450 enzymes are a major site of variation, as are the enzymes involved in glucuronidation. The use of nonsteroidal antiinflammatory drugs, anesthetics (including muscle relaxants and depolarizing agents), antibiotics, cancer chemotherapeutic agents, lipid-lowering agents, and mood stabilizers are all candidates for improvement. Screening for differences in drug metabolism might be done using DNA techniques, once sufficiently broad panels have been developed. Deciding which screening might be appropriate for newborns, and which should be offered later, will be an evolving process.

CONCLUSIONS

Newborn screening has developed over 40 years. Each new test initially has led to anxiety for parents and physicians,

---

BOX 18.4   Internet Resources

Comprehensive up-to-date information on U.S. screening programs is available from the National Newborn Screening and Genetics Resource Center web site, maintained at the University of Texas Health Sciences Center in San Antonio. The web site is called GeNeS-R-US, [Genetic and Newborn Screening Resource Center of the United States] and is accessed at http://genes-r-us.uthscsa.edu/. Links also are provided to the various state screening program web sites.
The March of Dimes [http://www.modimes.org/]
Save Babies through Newborn Screening Foundation [http://www.savebabies.org]
AboutNewbornScreening.com [http://www.aboutnewbornscreening.com/default.htm]
University of Utah [http://gslc.genetics.utah.edu/]
Exceptional Parent magazine [http://www.eparent.com/healthcare/birthDisorders.htm]

International Sites
United Kingdom [http://www.newbornscreening-bloodspot.org.uk/]
Geneva Foundation for Medical Education and Research [http://www.gfmer.ch/Guidelines/Neonatology/Neonatal_screening.htm]
Australia [New Children's Hospital at Westmead (Sydney, New South Wales); http://www.chw.edu.au/prof/services/newborn/]

followed by increasing comfort and confidence for both. Minimizing false-positive results minimizes the number of parents and physicians alarmed unnecessarily. Education and support for physicians and other health care providers is essential, so that they can act confidently when notified by the screening program that an abnormal result has occurred. (For available Internet resources see Box 18.4.) As with earlier screening programs, expanded screening will generate some positive results found in children who might remain asymptomatic for life. Prior to expanded newborn screening, only the screening test for hemoglobinopathies covered a class of compounds representing many disorders. The expanded screening program, using tandem mass spectrometry, therefore is unprecedented in terms of the number of disorders being added simultaneously to newborn screening programs. The experience gained with this approach will undoubtedly be beneficial as we enter the era of population screening for molecular traits that confer risk or protection for chronic or catastrophic conditions throughout the human lifespan.

ACKNOWLEDGMENTS

I wish to thank Susan Panny, M.D., of the Maryland Department of Health and Mental Hygiene, and Henry N. Kirkman, M.D., Emeritus Professor of Pediatrics, University of North Carolina, for their careful review and contributions to this chapter.

Suggested Readings

Hoffmann G, Nyhan WL, Zschocke J, et al. Newborn Screening. In: *Inherited metabolic diseases*. Philadelphia: Lippincott Williams and Wilkins, 2002.
Holtzman NA, Watson MS, eds. Promoting safe and effective genetic testing in the United States. Final report of the task force on genetic testing. (National Institutes of Health-Department of Energy Working Group on Ethical, Legal and Social Implications of Human Genome Research.) Baltimore: Johns Hopkins University Press, 1998.
Venditti LN, Venditti CP, Berry GT, et al. Newborn screening by tandem mass spectrometry for medium chain Acyl CoA dehydrogenase deficiency: a cost effectiveness analysis. *Pediatrics* 2003;112:1005.

CHAPTER 19 ■ CONGENITAL MALFORMATIONS

LEWIS B. HOLMES

FREQUENCY OF MAJOR AND MINOR ANOMALIES

A major malformation is usually defined as a structural abnormality that has surgical, medical, or cosmetic importance. Major malformations are more common in spontaneously aborted fetuses than in term infants. Approximately 2% of infants of at least 20 weeks' gestational age have a major malformation (Table 19.1). The frequency of malformations is higher among older children, because hidden abnormalities, such as kidney malformations and mild heart defects, have been detected. Having a single major malformation is much more common than having multiple malformations.

Minor anomalies are much more common than major malformations. A minor malformation is an abnormality that has no surgical or cosmetic significance (Fig. 19.1). These malformations occur in fewer than 4% of all newborns of the same race and gender. Minor physical features that occur in more than 4% of infants are considered normal variations. The frequencies of specific minor physical features vary among racial groups. For example, preauricular sinus and accessory nipples are more common among black than among white infants (Table 19.2). The pediatrician examining newborn infants should expect to find a few minor anomalies and normal variations. Finding three or more minor anomalies should prompt a careful assessment for the presence of a major malformation, because they are present in approximately 20% of these infants. Finding some specific minor anomalies may necessi-

tate further diagnostic study. For example, an infant found to have a branchial sinus and a preauricular tag or sinus may have the branchio-oto-renal syndrome, a hereditary disorder in which serious kidney malformations occur. A capillary hemangioma and lipoma over the lumbar spine can be a sign of a lipomeningocele, in which tethering of the spinal cord can occur.

RECOGNIZED ETIOLOGIES OF MALFORMATIONS

The causes are known for about 60% of major malformations. Chromosome abnormalities include trisomy, deletion, unbalanced translocations, and uniparental disomy. Deletions should be tested for with fluorescent *in situ* hybridization (FISH) techniques for special malformations, such as chromosome 22q11.2 deletion in infants with heart defects and chromosome 17p13.3 deletion in infants witth lissencephaly. Subtelomeric deletion studies identify subtle chromosome deletions in about 5% of children with anomalies and developmental delay. Thousands of malformations attributed to autosomal dominant, autosomal recessive, and X-linked etiologies have been cataloged and are usually diagnosed by clinical comparisons (http://www.ncbi.nlm.nih.gov/omim/). Molecular testing may be available to confirm the diagnosis. The laboratories providing molecular testing for specific malformations can be identified from GeneTests (www.genetests.org).

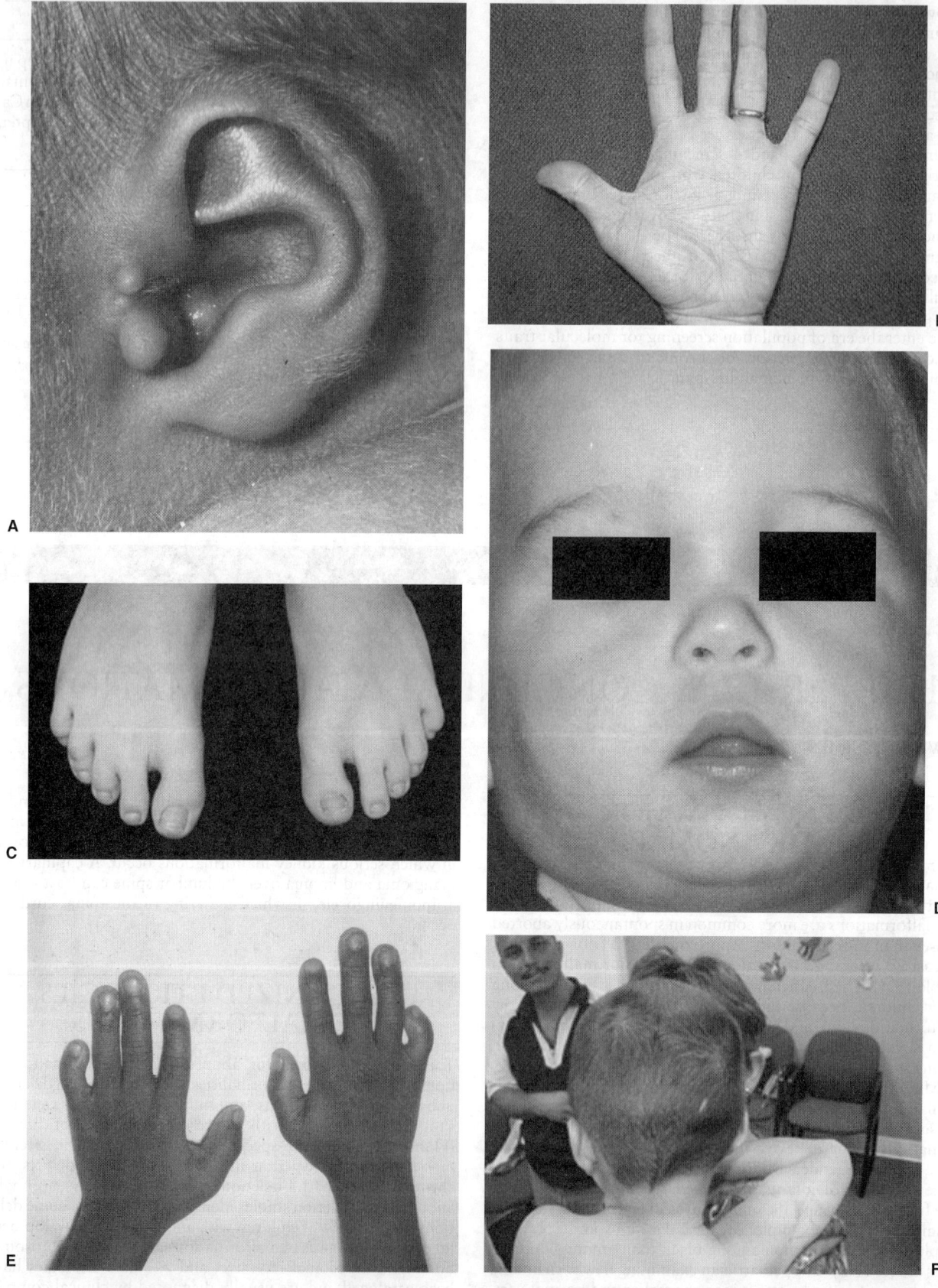

FIGURE 19.1. Examples of minor anomalies. **A:** Preauricular tag. **B:** Simian crease, left hand. **C:** Syndactyly, toes 2 to 3. **D:** Anteverted nostrils. **E:** Bilateral clinodactyly, finger 5. **F:** Double hair whorl (Continued)

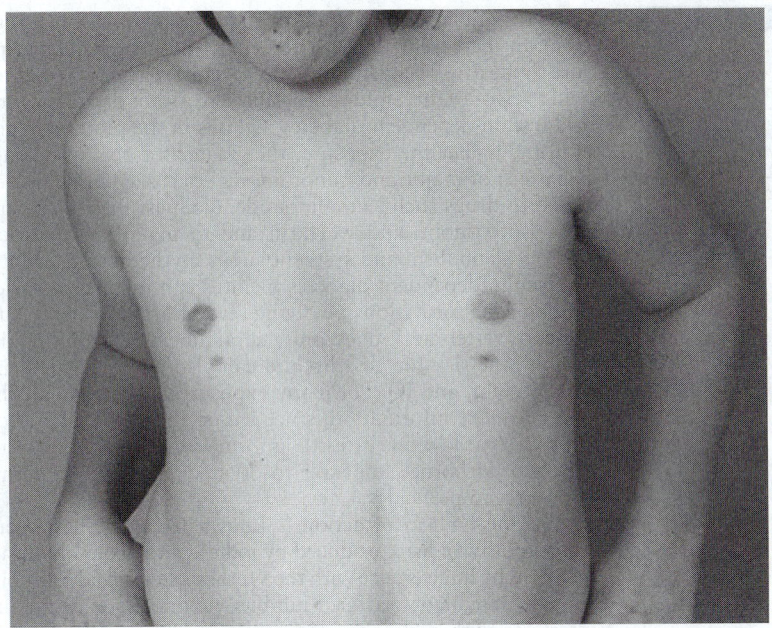
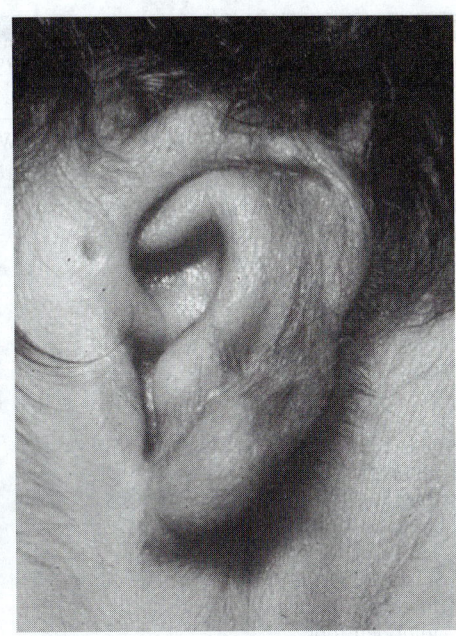

FIGURE 19.1. (Continued) **G:** Bilateral extra nipple. **H:** Preauricular sinus. (All photos courtesy of the Greenwood Genetic Center, Greenwood, South Carolina.)

Malformations Caused by Multifactorial Inheritance

The most common malformations (e.g., heart defects and spina bifida) are attributed to multifactorial inheritance, a process in which mutant genes and environmental factors are presumably involved. For all malformations attributed to multifactorial inheritance, the likelihood that a subsequent sibling (or the offspring of an affected parent) will be affected is 10 to 20 times greater than the risk in the general population (Table 19.3) but less than in instances involving autosomal recessive and autosomal dominant genes with complete penetrance. As an example of an environmental factor, periconceptional supplementation with folic acid decreases significantly the occurrence of anencephaly or spina bifida and heart defects. Several genetic abnormalities have been identified that are associated with the occurrence of spina bifida as well as Hirschsprung disease. Some studies have shown a strong interrelationship between maternal cigarette smoking, the presence of specific genetic markers, and the occurrence of either orofacial clefts or low birth weight.

Malformations Caused by Teratogens

The teratogenic exposures during pregnancy that cause malformations include maternal conditions or diseases, maternal infections, drugs taken during pregnancy, exposures to heavy

TABLE 19.1

CONGENITAL MALFORMATIONS IN NEWBORN INFANTS: RECOGNIZED ETIOLOGIES*

	Percent	Number[†] of Total Genetic causes	Example
Genetic causes			
Chromosome abnormalities	157 (45)	10.1	Trisomies, deletions
Single mutant genes	48	3.1	Chondrodystrophies
Familial	225 (3)	14.5	Renal agenesis
Multifactorial inheritance	356 (23)	23.0	Anencephaly, some heart defects
Teratogens	49	3.2	Infants of diabetic mothers
Uterine factors	39 (5)	2.5	Breech presentation
Twinning	6 (2)	0.4	Acardia, conjoinings
Unknown cause	669 (24)	43.2	Gastroschisis
Subtotals	1,549 (102)	100.0	
Overall total births	69,227		

*Total frequency 2.2%.
[†]Parentheses indicate elective terminations.
(Reproduced with permission from Nelson K, Holmes L. Malformation due to presumed spontaneous mutations in newborn infants. *N Engl J Med* 1989;320:19.)

TABLE 19.2

MINOR ABNORMAL PHYSICAL FEATURES: RACIAL DIFFERENCES

	Black Infants (%) (N = 871)	White Infants (%) (N = 4,125)
Palpable metopic suture	42.4	64.5
Double hair whorl	6.1	7.2
Overfolded helix, left ear	51.1	37.9
Epicanthal fold, left	1.3	2.5
Anteverted nostrils	2.0	2.6
Preauricular sinus, left ear	2.6	0.3
Preauricular tag, left ear	0.7	0.3
Extra nipple, left or right side	2.2	0.2
Simian crease, left hand	1.3	2.2
Both hands	0.7	0.5
Sydney line, left hand	8.5	14.0
Clinodactyly, fifth finger, left hand	7.2	8.1
Syndactyly, toes 2 to 3 to first interphalangeal joint, left foot	0.5	0.6

metals, and the prenatal diagnostic procedure chorionic villus sampling (Box 19.1). The first trimester of the pregnancy is the period of exposure most likely to produce malformations. Exposures in the second and third trimester also are of concern, because they could be related to the occurrence of renal tubular dysplasia (from angiotensin-converting enzyme inhibitors), microcephaly, growth retardation, and cognitive dysfunction. The risk that the exposed fetus will be damaged is typically expressed relative to the frequency of similar problems in the general population. The rate of major malformations ranges from an increase of at least ten- to 20-fold from fetal exposure to the drugs isotretinoin (13-*cis*-retinoic acid) and valproic acid to two- to threefold for the anticonvulsant drug phenytoin and insulin-dependent diabetes mellitus in the mother. In general, the higher the exposure, the greater the risk of damage. A pattern of major and minor anomalies is seen in infants exposed to drugs such as thalidomide, diethylstilbestrol, phenytoin, isotretinoin, and warfarin and to maternal conditions such as alcoholism and systemic lupus erythematosus. Maternal insulin-dependent diabetes mellitus can produce a variety of major malformations involving several organ systems, such as heart, vertebrae, kidney, and neural tube. Cigarette smoking doubles the risk for cleft lip and can also decrease head size, birth weight, and IQ. For many exposures, such as to alcohol or lead, more information is needed on the risk, if any, from exposures to low levels. Little information is available on the effects of airborne exposures to organic solvents and dermal exposures to pesticides.

The mechanism of action is known for some teratogens. The hypothyroidism produced by iodides and propylthiouracil is caused by interference with the synthesis of thyroid hormone. The anticoagulant warfarin inhibits vitamin K reductase and interferes with early chondrogenesis. Animal models suggest that exposure to valproate alters HOX gene expression and can cause, by homeotic transformations, vertebral malformations. Predictive testing to identify women with genetic predispositions and at increased greater risk for fetal damage has not been developed.

Malformations Caused by Uterine Factors

Uterine factors that cause fetal abnormalities are crowding, breech presentation, and vascular disruption. Breech presentation can cause hip dislocation and clubfoot deformity because

TABLE 19.3

MALFORMATIONS ATTRIBUTED TO MULTIFACTORIAL INHERITANCE

Malformation	Race/Nationality	Prevalence in Newborn Infants (Rate per 100)	Recurrence Risk	
			Affected sib, Normal Parents (%)	One Affected Parent, No Affected sibs (%)
Anencephaly	White	0.01	2–3	NA
	Black	0.005	?	?
Spina bifida	White	0.01	2–3	2–3
	Black	0.005	?	?
Cleft palate	White	0.03	4.3	6.2
	Black	0.01	?	?
	Japanese	0.05	2.3	?
Club foot (talipes equinovarus)	White	0.08	2.9	1.4
	Japanese	0.08	?	?
	Polynesian	0.8	?	?
Hypospadias	White	0.08	7.0	7.0
Intestinal agangliosis (Hirschsprung disease)	White	0.02		2.0
	Short segment		2.6, affected brother; 1.0, affected sister	
	Long segment		7.9, affected brother; 7.0, affected sister	
Ventricular septal defect	White	0.2	1.5–4.2	6–10, affected mother; 2, affected father

---

BOX 19.1   Recognized Human Teratogens

Drugs
Aminopterin/amethopterin
Androgenic hormones
Angiotensin converting enzyme (ACE) inhibitors
Busulfan
Carbamazepine
Chlorobiphenyls
Cocaine
Cyclophosphamide
Cyclosporin
Diethylstilbestrol
Etretinate
Fluconazole
Heroin/methadone
Iodide
Isotretinoin (13-*cis*-retinoic acid)
Lithium
Methimazole
Phenobarbital
Phenytoin
Propylthiouracil
Prostaglandin
Tetracycline
Thalidomide
Trimethadione/paramethadione
Valproic acid
Warfarin

Heavy metals
Lead
Mercury

Radiation
Cancer therapy

Maternal conditions
Alcohol
Insulin-dependent diabetes mellitus
Iodide deficiency
Maternal phenylketonuria
Myasthenia gravis
Obesity, severe
Smoking cigarettes/marijuana
Systemic lupus erythematosus
Vitamin A deficiency

Intrauterine infections
Cytomegalovirus
Herpes simplex
Parvovirus
Rubella
Syphilis
Toxoplasmosis
Varicella
Venezuelan equine encephalitis virus
West Vile Virus

Other exposures
Chorionic villus sampling (CVS)
Dilation and curettage (D&C)
Gasoline fumes (excessive)
Heat
Hypoxia
Intracytoplasmic sperm injection (ICSI)
Methyl isocyanate
Methylene blue
Polychlorinated biphenyls
Toluene (excessive; glue sniffing)
Trauma, blunt

---

of continued fetal growth within the confines of the mother's pelvis. These are positional deformities, not structural abnormalities. Likewise, crowding in a septate uterus or in multiple gestations can produce positional deformities.

Vascular disruption is caused by a sequence of events that includes hypoxia, hemorrhage, and tissue loss. The result is referred to as *amniotic band syndrome*. Postulated causes include early amnion rupture, placental injury from abdominal trauma, chorionic villus sampling, and intense uterine contractions at 6 to 8 weeks produced by the prostaglandin E$_1$ (misoprostol).

Malformations Caused by Twinning

Monozygous twins are more likely to have major malformations than are singletons. Some of these abnormalities (e.g., acardiac fetus, conjoined twins, and embolization of material from a deceased co-twin) occur only in monozygous twins. Other conditions, such as cloacal exstrophy and sirenomelia, are more common among twins than singletons.

Suggested Readings

Brackley KJ, Kilby MD, Morton J, et al. A case of recurrent fetal anomalies associated with a familial subtelomeric translocation. *Prenatal Diagnosis* 1999;19:570.

Faiella, A, Wernig M, Consalez GG, et al. A mouse model for valproate teratogenicity: parental effects, homeotic transformations and altered HOX expression. *Hum Mol Gen* 2002;9:227.

Friedman JM, Polifka JE. *Teratogenic effects of drugs: a resource for clinicians (TERIS)*, 2nd ed. Baltimore: Johns Hopkins University Press, 2000.

Golden CM, Ryan RM, Holmes LB. Chorionic villus sampling: a distinctive teratogenic effect on fingers? *Birth Defects Research (Part A): Clinical and Molecular Teratology* 2003;67:557.

Leppig KA, Werler MM, Cann CI, et al. Predictive value of minor anomalies. I. Association with major malformations. *J Pediatr* 1987;110:531.

Mastroiacovo P, Castilla EE, Arpino C, et al. Congenital malformations in twins: an international study. *Amr J Med Gen* 1999;83:117.

McKusick VA. *Mendelian inheritance in man: catalog of autosomal-dominant, autosomal-recessive, and X-linked phenotypes*, 12th ed. Baltimore: Johns Hopkins University Press, 1990. (www.ncbi.nlm.nih.gov/Omim)

Morrison K, Papapetrou C, Hol FA, et al. Susceptibility to spina bifida: an association study of five candidate genes. *Ann Hum Genet* 1998;62:379.

Passarge E. Dissecting Hirschsprung disease. *Nat Genet* 2002;31:11.

Wang X, Zuckerman B, Pearson C, et al. Maternal cigarette smoking, metabolic gene polymorphism, and infant birth weight. *JAMA* 2002;287:195.

CHAPTER 20 ■ GROWTH AND METABOLIC ADAPTATION OF THE FETUS AND NEWBORN

RICARDO UAUY, PATRICIA MENA, AND JOSEPH B. WARSHAW

Recent developments in understanding the fetal origins of adult health demonstrate the importance and complexity of the interaction of genetic and epigenetic factors with nutrients, hormones, substrates and toxicants in determining health and disease throughout life. The task of pediatricians is not limited to childhood. It is increasingly to promote health and prevent disease from the moment of conception onward (Fig. 20.1).

GENETIC AND ENVIRONMENTAL INFLUENCES ON FETAL GROWTH

Genetic Influences

Genetic composition has a profound influence on fetal growth. This is perhaps most clearly demonstrated by the effects of an abnormal number of chromosomes (aneuploidy). Turner syndrome (45 X0), trisomy 21, trisomies 13 and 18, triploidy, and polyploidy are all associated with poor fetal growth, and experimental studies have shown slow cell division in trisomic or triploid cell lines. Aberrant fetal growth also accompanies nonaneuploid disorders. Hereditary gigantism (Sotos syndrome) and the genetic forms of dwarfism represent extremes. Uniparental disomy (abnormal parent-of-origin genetic expression) of chromosome 7 is associated with poor growth in Silver-Russell syndrome, whereas a similar abnormality of chromosome 11 leads to fetal overgrowth in Beckwith-Wiedemann syndrome.

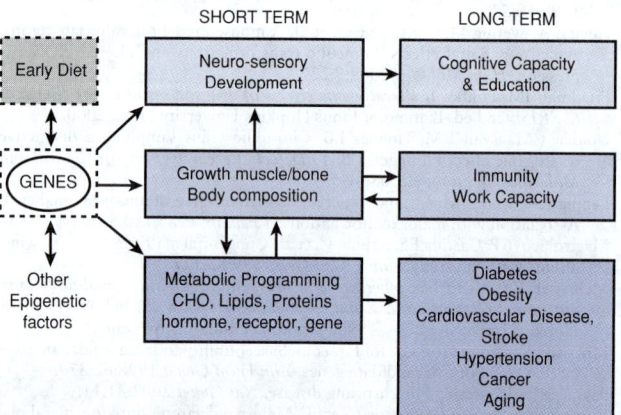

SHORT TERM   LONG TERM

FIGURE 20.1. Interaction between early diet and genotype in defining relevant health and quality of life outcomes. Early nutrition affects not only brain development, growth, and body composition but also metabolic programming that impacts occurrence of diet-related adult chronic disease, immunity, capacity for physical work, and cognitive and educational performance.

Genetic influences play a role in the birth weight variability observed among ethnic groups, ranging from a mean birth weight of 2,400 g in pygmies to a mean of 3,500 g or greater in affluent subpopulations of industrialized countries (Box 20.1). The effect of genotype also is evident in the greater birth weight among males, averaging 150 g more than females at term.

Uterine and Placental Influences

Environmental influences on fetal growth include uterine blood flow, placental function, and local uterine, placental, and umbilical circulation. Taken together, these determine the substrate and gas flux available to the fetus. In general, the placenta and baby grow proportionately; large babies have large placentas and small babies, small placentas, with the placenta weighing about 20% of the baby's weight. Conditions that compromise placental size and function, such as abnormal uterine anatomy, ectopic placental insertion, placental abruptio or

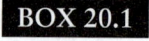

BOX 20.1 — Genetic, Hormonal, and Environmental Influences on Fetal Growth

A. Genetic and fetal factors
   1. Species, race, gender
   2. Congenital anomalies
   3. Chromosomal disorders
   4. Fetal hormones (insulin, corticosteroids, thyroid hormone, androgens)
   5. Growth factors (IGF I and IGF II, EGF and TGF-1)
B. Maternal uterine environment
   1. Uterine and placental anatomy
   2. Utero-placental function
   3. Human placental lactogen
   4. Substrate fluxes and transfer
   5. Uterine blood flow
   6. Maternal systemic disease
C. Macroenvironment
   1. Infectious agents (STORCH[a])
   2. Diet and nutrition
   3. Social and emotional stress
   4. Drugs and smoking
   5. Teratogens and toxins
   6. Altitude and temperature
   7. Ionizing radiation

───────────
[a]STORCH, syphilis, toxoplasmosis, rubella, cytomegalovirus, herpesvirus.

infarction, placental hemangioma or arteriovenous fistulae, congenital infections, and abnormal cord insertion may adversely affect fetal growth. Decreased placental blood flow measured with Doppler ultrasound undoubtedly plays a role in the intrauterine growth retardation associated with maternal toxemia, severe diabetes and/or long standing hypertension, and tobacco smoking.

Placental influences in addition to blood flow and placental surface area include placental hormones and growth factors. Their effects may be mediated indirectly through modification of blood and substrate flow or directly by regulation of cell replication and differentiation.

Maternal Nutrition

The maternal nutritional environment is critical for fetal growth. Although the mother tends to buffer the effect of adverse environmental conditions on the fetus, maternal weight gain during pregnancy is positively correlated with infant birth weight. The classic studies of the Dutch famine during World War II showed a mean birth weight reduction of 300 g among infants whose mothers suffered severe caloric deprivation during the last trimester of gestation. In previously well nourished mothers, caloric deprivation must be extreme before fetal growth is compromised. However, in women from developing countries, where malnutrition is entrenched over generations, a moderate energy deficit will have an adverse effect. In this regard, studies have shown that maternal height, in part the result of early nutritional influences, has a positive association with birth weight. After 2 years of age, the growth of the infant correlates better with mean parental height rather than maternal height alone; genetic factors contributed by both parents are important in determining final size, whereas early maternal nutrition, reflected in maternal height, is the major determinant of fetal growth. The effects of maternal size may be multigenerational. Mothers who were small for gestational age (SGA) at birth are at greater risk of having an SGA or preterm baby. These effects may be mediated through the size of the uterus and its capacity to hypertrophy and increased blood flow in response to pregnancy.

First-born infants on average weigh less than subsequent infants. Mothers less than 15 and over 35 years of age have a higher incidence of low-birth-weight babies, only partially explained by parity and socioeconomic risk factors. Maternal nutrition, especially in adolescents, and uterine and placental factors, are thought to play a role.

The practical consequence of these findings is that the evaluation of fetal growth should consider infant sex, maternal height, and birth order in addition to gestational age.

Micronutrients

Micronutrient minerals and vitamins are increasingly recognized as agents that affect embryogenesis and the incidence of congenital malformations.

Folate intake before and during early embryogenesis alters the incidence of neural tube defects (NTDs). The involvement of a genetic component for NTDs is evident in the high rate of recurrence in families and individual mothers. NTDs are also more frequent in certain ethnic groups. If NTDs were solely genetic, prevalence should not vary over time, yet NTDs are more frequent in periods of nutritional deprivation, such as during the 1945 Dutch famine. These observations led to the discovery of the striking benefit of maternal administration of doses of 400 μg of folic acid. Folic acid from food sources must be reduced to tetrahydrofolic acid before it is metabolically active. Genetically determined defects in the responsible enzyme, methylenetetrahydrofolate reductase, have been found in 35% to 50% of mothers bearing children with NTDs, thus accounting for the protective effect of folate supplementation. Heterogeneity in receptor-mediated folate transport may explain susceptibility to NTDs unrelated to reductase activity.

Retinoic acid, derived from retinol (vitamin A), is a regulator of gene expression and a teratogen early in embryonic development. Of interest, retinoic acid decreases the risk of spina bifida in animals. The folate receptor gene is a target for retinoic acid transcriptional regulation, providing a possible explanation for folate-retinol interaction. The regulation of folate receptors may explain the occurrence of NTDs in association with low vitamin A intake.

Maternal zinc deficiency has been implicated in abnormal fetal growth and enhanced susceptibility to such teratogens as alcohol, valproic acid, and arsenic.

Interaction of Genes and Diet

The beneficial effect of folic acid is only one example of the relationship between genetic composition and diet. The interaction of genes and the early diet not only determines brain development, growth, and body composition but also the later prevalence of nutrition-related chronic disease and some types of cancers. Genes are differentially expressed depending on the exposure to the epigenetic nutrients and toxicants. Thus, a similar genotype may define multiple phenotypes. The regulation of gene expression can occur at multiple levels. Nutrients can bind to specific or nonspecific ligands that interact with response elements in DNA. Nutrients may change the phosphorylation status of a protein and thus its activity. At the post-transcriptional level, nutrients may modify native RNA processing, messenger RNA (mRNA) transport and stability, and breakdown rates. Nutrients may modify the rate of mRNA translation. Finally, nutrients can modify the turnover rates of enzymes and other proteins, thus affecting their activity level.

Maternal Medical Disorders

Preeclampsia, chronic hypertension, collagen vascular disease, and renal disease all affect fetal growth by compromising maternal nutritional status and interfering with uterine and placental perfusion. Severe maternal anemia and diminished cardiac output secondary to heart disease and/or cyanotic congenital heart disease affect fetal growth by decreasing oxygen availability to the maternal uterine compartment. Early abnormalities in embryonic fuel metabolism in prediabetic or diabetic mothers may play a role in determining abnormal fetal growth and may also be teratogenic; later, maternal hyperglycemia induces fetal hyperinsulinism and macrosomia with enhanced growth of peripheral adipose tissue, muscle hypertrophy, and increased liver glycogen stores. The goal of health care and nutrition before and during pregnancy must be to prevent both intrauterine growth restriction (IUGR) and macrosomia.

Intrauterine infections, including rubella and cytomegalovirus infections, can impair fetal growth. Toxoplasmosis, syphilis, and herpes infections, although less frequent during the first trimester, may affect fetal growth by arresting cell replication during critical stages of development, causing typical patterns of malformations and severely compromised growth.

Other Influences on Fetal Growth

Altitude is associated with diminished fetal growth due to lower ambient oxygen tension. Radiation exposure has been associated with microcephaly and abnormal fetal growth. Organic solvents and heavy metals, especially mercury and cadmium, have been associated with malformation and compromised fetal growth. Smoking, especially in the last trimester of pregnancy, reduces birth weight and length; the effect is proportional to the number of cigarettes smoked. Pre- and postnatal growth failure and microcephaly characterize the fetal alcohol syndrome. Growth restriction occurs in infants born to mothers addicted to heroin, cocaine, or methadone. Other drugs with adverse affects include anticonvulsants (phenytoin [Dilantin], phenobarbital, and carbamazepine [Tegretol]), antifolates (methotrexate), warfarin (Coumadin), and prednisone.

INTERACTION OF NUTRIENTS, HORMONES, AND GROWTH FACTORS DURING PERINATAL GROWTH

Fetal growth depends on adequate nutritional substrates and on the action of insulin and growth factors such as epidermal growth factor and IGF-I and -II. Insulin regulates fetal lipogenic activity and has a permissive role in protein synthesis and hepatic glycogen deposition. Fetuses with insulin deficiency secondary to pancreatic agenesis or with a defective insulin receptor have marked IUGR with decreased adipose tissue and little weight gain during the last trimester of pregnancy (leprechaun syndrome). Conversely, fetal hyperinsulinism results in increased adiposity in human infants of diabetic mothers.

Protein feeding, as well administration of several essential and nonessential amino acids, stimulates insulin secretion in the fetus and neonate. Increasing arginine levels during parenteral infusion also has been shown to increase serum insulin levels. The correlation of urinary excretion of the insulin precursor C-peptide with weight gain suggests that insulin may be a growth-promoting factor for infants on high-protein diets. Preliminary evidence from controlled clinical studies in extremely small preterm infants has shown increased tolerance to glucose and higher weight gain in infants infused with insulin during their initial postnatal days.

Peptide growth factors that influence fetal growth and maturation include the insulin-like growth factors (IGF-I and -II). In the fetus, these act independently of growth hormone. IGF-I influences terminal differentiation of a number of tissues, including brain astrocytes, neural outgrowth, and myogenesis; and, although the influences of IGF-I appear to be local, serum concentrations of IGF-I correlate with birth weight. Both IGF-I and -II are complexed to binding proteins that modulate their biological activity. After birth, higher levels of IGF-I are observed in IUGR infants during catch-up growth, especially in association to gain in length. Epidermal growth factor (EGF) and transforming growth factor-1 (TGF-1) influence the growth and differentiation of epithelial cells in lung and gut. Receptors for EGF are present throughout development and are increased in number in the placenta and lung in fetuses with growth restriction induced by uterine artery ligation, thus suggesting a role for EGF in fetal growth retardation. Leptin is a circulating polypeptide hormone expressed by adipocytes and placenta. A positive relationship exists between fetal leptin concentrations and both gestational age and fetal weight.

Thyroxin and glucocorticosteroids have important influences on specific organ development and functional and metabolic adaptation, but relatively little influence on fetal somatic growth.

PLACENTAL TRANSPORT AND METABOLISM

The placenta transfers metabolic substrates and other nutrients from the mother to the rapidly growing fetus. In addition, the placenta allows for the excretion of fetal waste products and performs important metabolic and hormonal functions.

Anatomy

In the human placenta, the fetal villi are directly bathed by maternal blood; therefore, the fetal capillary circulation is separated from maternal blood by fetal connective tissue and the placental epithelium, composed of the cytotrophoblast and the syncytiotrophoblast. A clear understanding of placental ultrastructure is necessary in order to discuss the functional correlates. As shown in Figure 20.1, the uppermost layer of fetal tissues, the syncytiotrophoblast, is in direct contact with maternal blood. Microvilli increase the surface area necessary for transport. Syncytial vacuoles are responsible for the transport of macromolecules and may be specifically targeted by cell surface receptors. The extensive endoplasmic reticulum and the high density of mitochondria provide the anatomic basis for both synthetic activities and transport through the cytoplasm of the trophoblast. The multinucleated syncytiotrophoblast is derived from the actively replicating cytotrophoblast. The trophoblast represents the only uninterrupted cell layer interposed between the fetal capillary and maternal circulations.

The placenta grows at a very rapid rate during the initial stages of pregnancy. Placental growth is characterized by both increased numbers of villi and microvilli and proliferation of fetal capillary vessels. In this way, the surface area available for maternal–fetal exchange is greatly enhanced. Nutrients in maternal blood must cross the trophoblast cell layer and the basement membrane to reach the loose connective tissue surrounding the fetal capillaries (Fig. 20.2).

Placental Transfer Mechanisms

Placental transfer occurs through several mechanisms. Transfer through diffusion is determined by the concentration gradient between fetal and maternal blood. Most small molecules appear to be transferred by simple diffusion; these include water, sodium, urea, oxygen, and carbon dioxide. A special case is the transport of glucose, the major energy substrate of the fetus. Glucose diffusion is selective and facilitated. Glucose transporter proteins (see section, Transfer of Specific Nutrients) have been described in the microvilli of the trophoblasts facing the maternal decidua and the fetal capillary. The transporters are not responsive to insulin; they bind hexoses solely and have the highest affinity for glucose.

Another mode of transfer is active transport. This requires energy and can occur against a concentration gradient. Such is the case for calcium, magnesium, and L-amino acids. For many of these nutrients, and for water-soluble vitamins, specific transport proteins have been identified. The transfer of intact proteins or other hydrophobic macromolecules probably is mediated by pinocytosis or, more specifically, receptor-mediated endocytosis. The latter process requires a specific cell surface receptor and was initially described for the low-density lipoproteins (LDLs). It has now been characterized for iron, folate, vitamin B_{12}, insulin and other macromolecules. This mechanism probably accounts for the transfer of IgG during the last half of pregnancy. Transplacental transfer of IgG is highly specific and occurs at a faster rate than the transport of smaller proteins.

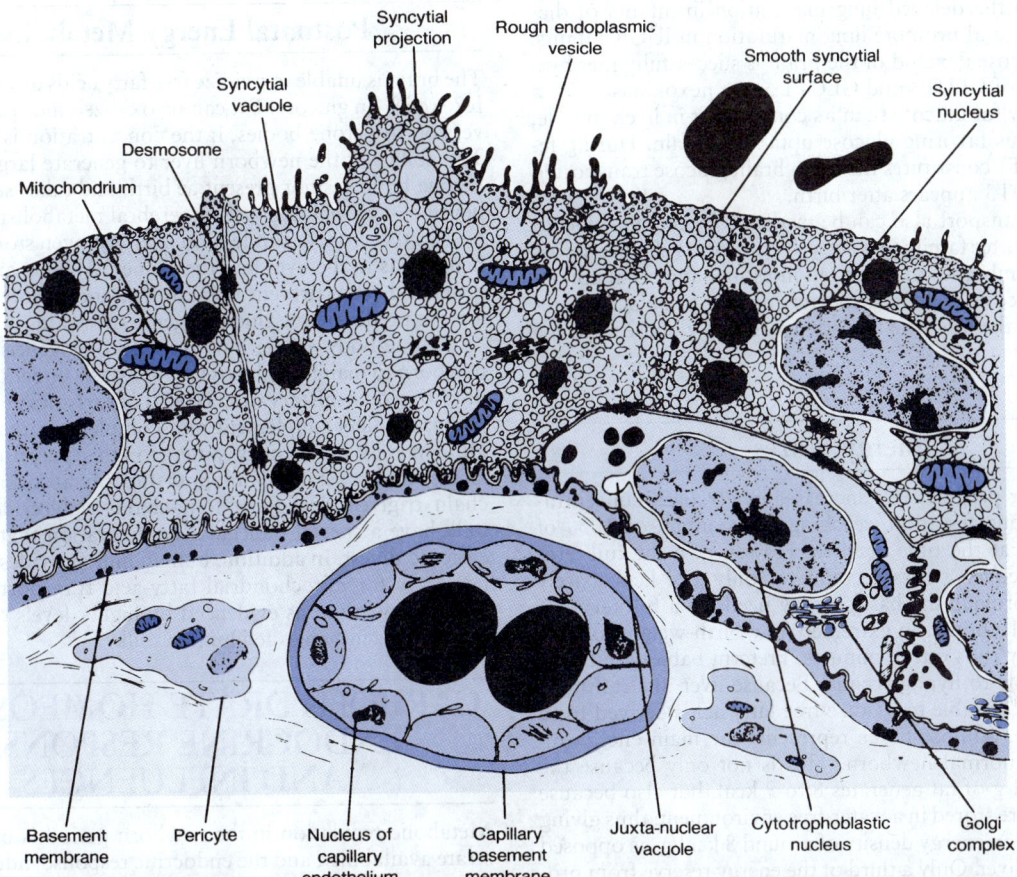

FIGURE 20.2. Diagram of structure of a placental membrane (seen by electron microscope). The syncytial trophoblast (upper portion of the figure) is exposed to maternal blood. Microvilli increase the area for transfer. Syncytial vacuoles may be part of the pinocytotic process for protein transfer. The rich mitochondrial and endoplasmic systems provide the machinery for intense synthetic activity. The syncytiotrophoblast, which is incapable of cell division, derives from the cytotrophoblast. (Reprinted with permission from Boyd JD, Hamilton WJ. *The human placenta*. Cambridge: Heffer & Sons, 1970.)

Transfer of Specific Nutrients

The fetus is totally dependent on the intraplacental circulation for the provision of substrate. Fetal swallowing of amniotic fluid represents a nonsignificant additional transfer mechanism. As mentioned, glucose is transferred by selective facilitated diffusion. Of interest, the placenta metabolizes large amounts of glucose to lactate, and lactate, rather than glucose, may be the major precursor for fetal hepatic glycogen and fatty-acid synthesis. Thus, the major sources of energy for the fetus, glucose and lactate, are transferred through diffusion. Gas exchange and fetal urea excretion occurs through the same mechanism.

In contrast, the transfer of amino acids occurs against a concentration gradient and is energy dependent. Amino acid levels in the fetal circulation are 30% higher than in the mother. In addition, the L-isomer form of amino acids is transferred more rapidly than the D-isomers. With few exceptions, such as IgG (see section, Placental Transfer Mechanisms), intact proteins are not transferred across the placenta.

The placental transport of lipids occurs mainly in the form of free fatty acids. Intact very-low-density lipoproteins (VLDLs) or LDLs do not cross the placenta. During the last trimester of pregnancy, some of the increase in the fetal requirement for fatty acids is met by increased transport across the placenta. However, most fatty acid accretion is a product of fetal lipogenesis from nonlipid precursors. Essential fatty acid needs of the fetus are met solely by transplacental transport and reflect maternal dietary supply.

ENERGY METABOLISM

Glucose Transport

Glucose is the major energy substrate for the fetus and the newborn, although the fetus is capable of utilizing lactate, free fatty acids, or ketone bodies under special conditions. Glucose is able to induce its own non–energy dependent transporters, appropriately named the GLUT1 to -7 family. The variation in GLUT isoform expression during development is time and tissue specific. GLUT1, expressed in virtually every fetal cell except neurons, accounts for most basal glucose uptake. GLUT3 is a high-affinity transporter found in placenta. In situations of maternal glucose scarcity, this transporter may be capable of scavenging maternal glucose for placenta and fetal needs. The expression of insulin-sensitive GLUT4 appears late in gestation in cardiac and skeletal muscles, and in adipocytes. GLUT1 is more highly expressed in fetal than in adult lung. Normal insulin–cortisol ratios stimulate glucose transport, whereas high insulin–cortisol ratios inhibit glucose uptake. This may contribute to the delayed lung maturation in infants of diabetic mothers and promote lung maturation in IUGR infants. The high glucose demand of the brain is successfully met by a combination of GLUT3 and GLUT1 and a hexokinase with a higher affinity for glucose than its counterpart in liver, muscle, or kidney, thus favoring glucose uptake by brain. During fetal life, GLUT1 constitutes the main brain glucose transporter, whereas GLUT3 appears after birth.

Glucose transport also can be mediated by the Na–glucose linked transporter family that actively transports glucose across the apical membranes of polarized intestinal and renal epithelial cells. Glucose–Na cotransporters appear to be active prenatally; thus, the intestine is ready to absorb glucose with the first feed.

Energy Stores

The fetal liver progressively increases its glycogen concentration throughout gestation, reaching a maximum of 10% of organ weight at the time of birth. However, in the full-term newborn, glycogen stores account for only 100 kcal, barely sufficient to provide the basal energy needs of a full-term infant for 8 to 10 hours. In extremely low-birth-weight infants, glucose supply runs out in minutes. Preterm babies are therefore susceptible to hypoglycemia. Because liver, skeletal muscle, and heart are able to oxidize free fatty acids derived from adipose tissue, adipose tissue represents the main energy reserve for the normal newborn. This is not only because the oxidation of 1 g of fat generates 8 to 9 kcal, but also because triglycerides are stored in a water-free environment, thus giving adipose tissue an energy density of around 8 kcal/g, as opposed to 1 kcal/g of liver. Only a third of the energy reserve from protein is available as an energy source; lean body mass losses in excess of one-third are associated with adverse functional consequences.

This information allows for a quantitative assessment of energy reserves for the fetus and has been linked to the survival potential under conditions of semistarvation. A full-term infant has enough energy reserve to support its needs for several weeks. An infant with a birth weight under 1,000 g has reserves for only a few days.

Lipid Metabolism

Most fetal triglycerides are derived from fatty acids produced in the fetal liver and placenta, because fatty acid transport is meager and lipoprotein transfer from the mother is insignificant or nonexistent. Of interest, the fetal brain and lung also are capable of lipogenesis to produce the unique lipids important for their function. As fetal plasma fatty acids enter adipocytes and are re-esterified to triglycerides, adipose tissue exhibits dramatic growth during the last trimester of pregnancy. A 27-week fetus has only 1% of its body weight as fat, whereas the figure is 16% in the normal full-term infant.

Substantial quantities of fetal body fat, especially that located in the vicinity of the major large vessels, is metabolically active. This fat is rich in heme-containing cytochromes and mitochondria and hence is brown in color. Its function is to produce heat. Lipid vesicles provide the fatty acids for oxidation, and the mitochondria possess a specific protein that uncouples aerobic fuel oxidation from ATP formation, producing heat. Activation of this nonshivering thermogenesis is triggered by sympathetic stimulation of lipolysis. With advancing postnatal age, shivering thermogenesis is established. Most brown fat involutes or becomes white fat.

Postnatal Energy Metabolism

The brain is unable to oxidize free fatty acids directly and therefore relies on glucose. Fat can be oxidized indirectly, after conversion to ketone bodies, if the concentration is high enough. The ability of the newborn liver to generate large amounts of ketone bodies is not present at birth and takes several days to develop. The maintenance of cerebral metabolism on an acute basis is therefore dependent on liver glycogen stores and gluconeogenesis in the liver and the kidney. Alanine and glutamine, generated from protein breakdown, and lactate and glycerol are the predominant gluconeogenic substrate.

Ketone-body oxidation and gluconeogenesis enable the newborn to maintain glucose homeostasis under the conditions of fasting or semistarvation typical of early postnatal life. Early postnatal diets supplement and complement these responses. Human milk is uniquely suited for this purpose. It contains lactose and substantial amounts of easily absorbable medium-chain triglycerides. Even long-chain triglycerides in human milk have a special molecular configuration that makes them easier to digest. In addition, human milk provides the carnitine necessary for mitochondrial fatty-acid transport and ketone-body production, as evidenced by higher levels of plasma ketone bodies in babies fed human milk.

CARBOHYDRATE HOMEOSTASIS: ENDOCRINE RESPONSES AND INFLUENCES

Metabolic regulation in the newborn period is based on substrate availability, and the endocrine response induced by these substrates. During fetal life, after the twentieth week of gestation, the fetal pancreas produces insulin. This hormone regulates the accumulation of glycogen in liver, muscle, and lung. At the same time, it promotes lipogenesis and triglyceride storage within adipose tissue. Insulin also enhances protein synthesis in muscle. The action of insulin is modulated by glucocorticoids, which regulate gene expression and induce various enzymes related to glycogen and lipid synthesis. Steroid hormones are responsible for the induction of glycogen synthetase type I, which is activated by insulin and responsible for glycogen synthesis. Fetal steroid hormone concentrations are low throughout much of gestation. This explains why, despite detectable circulating insulin after 13 weeks gestation, glycogen accumulation does not occur until the twenty-seventh week.

At the time of birth, the constant supply of maternal glucose is interrupted, and the infant's blood glucose concentrations decrease. As a result, insulin levels fall and glucagon increases. The ratio between insulin and glucagon is essential in the regulation of gluconeogenesis and glycogenolysis. The hepatic intracellular signaling cascade induced by glucagon responds exponentially, such that small changes in glucagon induce large changes in glycogenolysis and glucose availability. Glycogen synthesis and degradation and gluconeogenesis are summarized in Figure 20.3.

Glucagon and cortisol promote gluconeogenesis. Glucagon and catecholamines, in addition to activating the glycogenolytic pathway, promote lipolysis (generating glycerol, a gluconeogenic precursor) and free fatty acids. Free fatty acids directly and indirectly provide an alternative to glucose as oxidative fuel (see section, Postnatal Energy Metabolism). High glucagon and cortisol levels and low insulin levels favor protein catabolism, especially skeletal muscle protein breakdown, thus yielding amino acids for gluconeogenesis.

The postnatal changes in respiratory quotient (Table 20.1), defined as the ratio between carbon dioxide production and

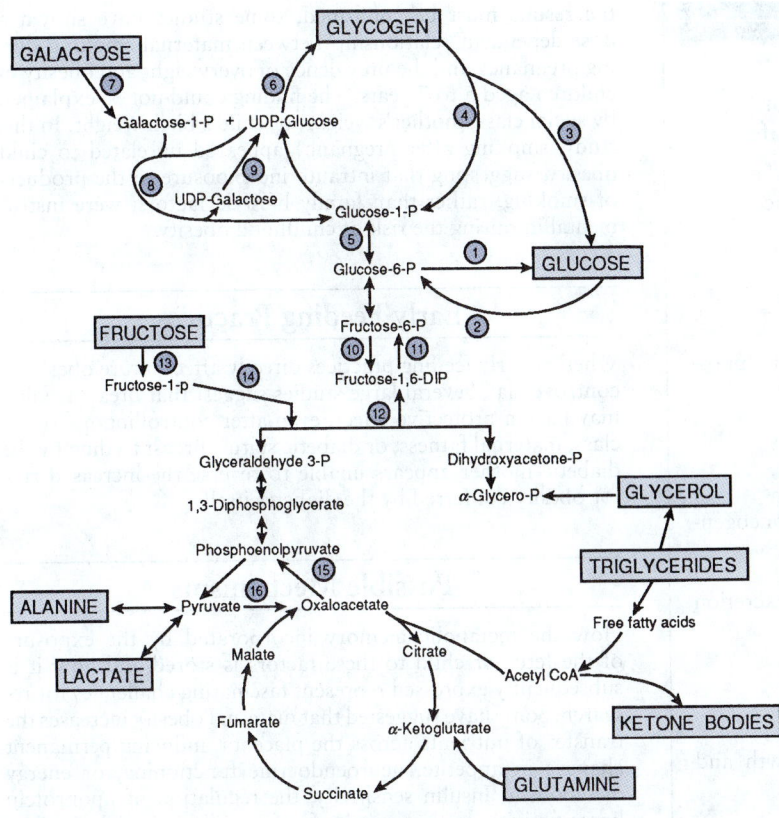

FIGURE 20.3. Metabolic pathways involved in glycogen synthesis and degradation and gluconeogenesis. Key enzymes are designated by number: (1) glucose-6-phosphatase; (2) glucokinase; (3) amylo-1,6-glucosidase; (4) phosphorylase; (5) phosphoglucomutase; (6) glycogen synthetase; (7) galactokinase; (8) galactose-1-phosphate uridylyl transferase; (9) uridine diphosphogalactose-4-epimerase; (10) phosphofructokinase; (11) fructose-1,6-diphosphatase; (12) fructose-1,6-diphosphate aldolase; (13) fructokinase; (14) fructose-1-phosphate aldolase; (15) phosphoenolpyruvate carboxykinase; (16) pyruvate carboxylase; DIP, diisopropyl phosphate; UDP, uridine diphosphate.

oxygen consumption, reflect the postnatal fuel transition from glucose to a mixture of glucose and fat. A respiratory quotient of 1.0 corresponds to the predominant use of glucose as a fuel for oxidation. A value of 0.7 corresponds to exclusive fatty-acid oxidation.

Thyroxine and growth hormone promote lipolysis and further potentiate gluconeogenesis. Arginine vasopressin (AVP) also has been shown to induce a hyperglycemic response in the fetus. AVP is released during fetal stress and may represent a major modulator of fetal metabolism, in addition to regulating cardiovascular responses.

In summary, the goal of neonatal glucose homeostasis is to provide the brain and other vital organs with sufficient glucose as a key energy source. Virtually all hormones except insulin will increase glucose, which is then taken up preferentially by the brain. The sequence described in this section constitutes

the basis for perinatal glucose adaptation and can be verified in virtually all mammalian species.

LONG-TERM HEALTH EFFECTS OF FETAL GROWTH: OBESITY AND DIABETES

Long-term Consequences of Birth Weight

Evidence accumulated in recent decades reveals that nutrition early in development may have permanent and long-term effects on the risk of future obesity. This "metabolic program" interacts with genetic factors to create a "set point" that affects an individual's body weight throughout the lifespan. The earliest data are derived from the Dutch famine in World War II. The cohort exposed to famine in the last trimester of gestation was found to have a reduced prevalence of obesity at age 18 years, the age of recruitment by the Dutch army. In contrast, an increased prevalence was noted in those exposed to famine during early and mid gestation. Other studies have examined the effect of birth weight, a proxy for fetal growth, on weight during adolescence and adulthood. Virtually all of these studies demonstrate a clear association of birth weight with subsequent adiposity. Large-scale epidemiologic studies have suggested that adult body mass index (BMI) is linked to weight at birth through a nonlinear relationship, with the higher adult BMI associated with both the lowest and the highest weights at birth. These studies suggest that fetal undernutrition and low birth weight may be linked to a future susceptibility to develop cardiovascular disease, diabetes, and obesity. Strong evidence supports the notion that the heaviest babies are at risk of becoming heavy adults.

TABLE 20.1

ENERGY RESERVES OF THE NEWBORN AT VARIOUS BIRTH WEIGHTS AND GESTATIONAL AGES

Weight (g)	Gestational Age (wk)	Energy Reserve (kcl)			
		Glycogen	Protein	Fat	Total
200	18	0	65	9	74
1,000	27	4	416	90	510
2,000	33	16	960	1,080	2,056
3,500	40	70	1,694	5,040	6,804
2,200	40	26	871	1,108	2,005

Adapted from Sharad DV, Ivengam L. Composition of the human fetus. *Br J Nutr* 1972;27:305; Widdowson EM, Dickerson JWT. Composition of the body. In: Diem K, Lentner C, eds. 1973 Scientific tables. Basel, Switzerland: Ciba-Geigy, 1973:517.

BOX 20.2

Immediate Neonatal Adaptations Necessary for Successful Extrauterine Life

A. Cardiovascular
   1. Reduction pulmonary vasculature resistance
   2. Increase lung blood flow
   3. Closure of ductus arteriosus
   4. Separate right and left cardiac pumps
B. Pulmonary
   1. Maturation of alveoli and capillary network
   2. Development of the surfactant system (phosphatidylcholine and phosphatidylglycerol)
   3. Rhythmic respiration
   4. Maturation of antioxidant enzyme systems
C. Metabolic-Endocrine
   1. Thermogenesis and temperature regulation
   2. Glucose homeostasis (glycogenolysis, gluconeogenesis)
   3. Neuroendocrine responsiveness
   4. Enzymatic maturation for detoxification, excretion and metabolism of fuels and substrate.
D. Nutritional
   1. Intermittent rather than continuous feeds
   2. Digestion and absorption of nutrients
   3. Excretion of acid, nitrogen, and electrolytes
   4. Maintenance of nutrient supply for growth and development
E. Neurodevelopmental
   1. Integrated responses to environmental stimuli
   2. Maintenance of autonomic regulation under new conditions
   3. Activation of sensory input and processing necessary for learning
   4. Operation of reflexes and behaviors needed for survival

---

Consequences of Maternal Diabetes

Maternal diabetes during pregnancy results in offspring with higher birth weight and higher risk of subsequent obesity, although only after 4 to 5 years of age. In this case, the risk of obesity seems to be independent of birth weight and maternal weight, suggesting an independent effect of the intrauterine environment. A study examining 7-year-old children born to mothers with gestational diabetes found an increased prevalence of obesity in children of mothers who required insulin, but not in children of mothers who had glucose intolerance or gestational diabetes, but did not require insulin. In the Bogalusa Heart Study, children (average age 15 years) of diabetic mothers showed greater body fatness, higher blood pressure, and raised fasting levels of blood glucose, insulin, glucagon, and triglycerides. The latter measures remained significantly raised after adjusting for higher BMI. Similarly, the weights of Pima Indian children and adolescents exposed to diabetes during gestation were dramatically increased when compared with infants whose mothers were prediabetic or infants whose mothers did not have and did not develop diabetes.

Consequences of Tobacco Use

Smoking during pregnancy adversely affects fetal linear growth and may promote obesity in children and adults. Although the results must be confirmed, some studies have shown a dose-dependent relationship between maternal smoking during pregnancy and the prevalence of overweight and obesity in children aged 5 to 7 years. The finding could not be explained by social class, mother's weight, or child's birth weight. In this study, smoking after pregnancy appeared unrelated to child obesity, suggesting that intrauterine exposure to the products of smoking, rather than family lifestyle factors, were instrumental in raising the risk of childhood obesity.

Early Feeding Practices

Whether early feeding practices directly affect future obesity is controversial. Several large studies suggest that breast feeding may have a protective effect, even after controlling for social class, maternal fatness, or diabetic status. Breast feeding by the diabetic mother appears unable to reverse the increased risk for obesity conferred by the diabetes itself.

Possible Mechanisms

How the metabolic memory incorporated by the exposure of the fetus or child to these factors is stored and how it is subsequently expressed represent fascinating challenges for research. Some have suggested that maternal obesity increases the transfer of nutrients across the placenta, inducing permanent changes in appetite, neuroendocrine functioning, or energy metabolism. Insulin sensitivity, the regulation of lipoprotein lipase activity, or the capacity for fat oxidation might be programmed *in utero*. The relative contributions of shared maternal genes and intrauterine factors must be carefully isolated as the metabolic determinants of body weight are explored. If maternal obesity increases the risk for subsequent obesity, the obesity epidemic could accelerate through successive generations. Meanwhile, because undernutrition at early or middle gestation also can induce permanent physiologic changes that result in obesity, as indicated by an analysis of the Dutch famine cohort, it is possible that populations experiencing both extremes of nutrition are at risk. This may explain the observation that stunted children in developing nations are at particularly high risk of obesity as diet and physical activity undergo a rapid "nutrition transition" to more Westernized patterns.

An important role for growth during early development was first suggested by Barker. He found higher risk of cardiovascular diseases, hypertension, and type 2 diabetes mellitus in adults with low birth weights. It is not clear whether these "programmed effects" can be modified. It is interesting that preterm infants fed human milk during the first month of life have a significantly lower arterial pressure during adolescence. This and other data suggest that "fetal programming" might be modifiable by dietary interventions after birth.

NUTRITION AND GROWTH OF PREMATURE INFANTS

Providing adequate nutrition is one of the great challenges in caring for preterm newborns. Very low-birth-weight (VLBW) infants often lose 12% to 15% body weight over the initial 10 days of life. Even with parenteral and enteral nutrition, they may take 15 to 20 days to regain birth weight. The catch-up growth of VLBW infants may last 3 to 8 weeks, during which time they grow at rates of 15 to 25 g/kg/day. Nutritional practices have shortened hospital stays and have likely contributed to the improved survival and long-term outcome of VLBW infants. Parenteral nutrition with glucose, amino acids, and lipids has been key to the improved survival of VLBW infants. The benefits of aggressive nutritional support include better glucose control, decreased loss of lean body mass, and improved provision of protein and micronutrients. Present clinical practice includes early introduction of parenteral nutrition, with introduction of amino acids within the first 24 hours and the initiation of parenteral lipids within the first 72 hours. Parenteral nutrition has proved to be lifesaving for neonates with significant gastrointestinal malformations or postnatally acquired disease, such as necrotizing enterocolitis or short bowel syndrome.

Enteral Nutrition: Recommended Intakes

Human milk, even in small volumes (10 to 20 mL), promotes gut maturation and prevents the intestinal atrophy induced by the lack of enteral feeding. Preterm human milk has a higher protein and sodium content than mature milk but has insufficient calcium, phosphorus, and protein to support catch-up growth in VLBW infants, even if volumes of 150 to 200 mL/kg are given. Human milk fortifiers are used to increase the nutrient content of human milk. Human milk also contains a variety of nutritional and non-nutritional factors that may modulate postnatal growth and development. Recommended energy and protein intakes for low-birth-weight infants vary from 110 to 150 kcal/kg for energy and from 2.5 to 4.2 g/kg daily for protein. The variability results from differences in estimated fecal losses and energy allowance for growth. In most studies, the resting metabolic rate of preterm infants, including postprandial thermogenesis, is 50 to 60 kcal/kg/day. The energy expenditure related to minor thermal stress despite a controlled environment is 10 kcal/kg. An additional 10 kcal/kg is provided for activity; fecal losses vary from 10 to 40 kcal/kg, depending on what is fed. The allowance for synthesis and storage (growth) is 35 to 60 kcal/kg; thus, the energy cost of weight gain has been estimated to be 4 to 5 kcal/g of weight gain. If the weight gain is predominantly lean, the cost is somewhat lower (2 to 3 kcal/g). For adipose tissue, however, the energy cost may be as high as 8 to 9 kcal/g. The American Academy of Pediatrics recommendations of 120 kcal/kg for energy and 3.0 to 3.5 g/kg of protein for the nutrition of low-birth-weight infants remain essentially valid.

Present efforts are directed at defining the needs of the extremely low-birth-weight infant (i.e., birth weight less than 800 g). The goal in providing calories for VLBW and low-birth-weight infants is that they attain, as early as possible, a body weight approximating that of a normal fetus of the same conceptional age. A second goal, often unspecified, is that the quality of the tissue gain be similar to that which would have been accreted *in utero* at the equivalent gestation. The first goal is achievable with presently available commercial formulates specifically designed for preterm infants or by feeding fortified human milk. Most studies also show that the fat-to-lean ratio of tissue gained *ex utero* is higher than what is normally accreted *in utero*. The higher fat-to-lean ratio of weight gain of VLBW infants during catch-up can be interpreted as an unavoidable consequence of postnatal nutrition and growth regulation. Alternatively, it may be interpreted as resulting from an inadequate supply of key nutrients for optimal lean-tissue accretion. Evidence suggests that this problem may be the result of the high energy supplied and the insufficient protein relative to energy in most commercial formulas; others have suggested that zinc or other micronutrients may be deficient relative to the needs for optimal lean tissue accretion.

Present neonatal nutritional practices make it feasible not only to attain *in utero* growth rates, but also to accrete sufficient lean tissue to reach close to normal weight and body composition by 40 weeks or term birth. This requires a high energy intake, closer to 120 to 140 kcal/kg/day (rather than the traditional 100 kcal/kg/day) and a protein intake of 3.5 to 4.5 g/kg/day. This high energy intake is needed to optimize protein use for optimal catch-up. The high-energy, high-protein feeding induces higher insulin levels, as measured by urinary excretion of C-peptide. Fat accretion is initially higher than the expected *in utero* gain, but because the normal fetus progressively increases in fat content, the projected relative excess fat decreases with advancing age. Rate and composition of weight gain of low-birth-weight infants can be manipulated by protein and energy intake; however, the extent of the dietary effects is dependent on biologic variables that are not fully understood.

Recent experience with the use of recombinant growth hormone is of interest in terms of promoting growth in very low-birth-weight infants who fail to recover with nutrition alone. The potential for efficacy may be real, but the long-term effects should continue to be assessed, because the immediate gains may be offset by unknown consequences that cannot be fully discarded based on present knowledge.

Suggested Readings

Barker DJP. Fetal origins of coronary heart disease. *Br Med J* 1995;311:171–174.

Barker DJP, Osmond C, Golding J, et al. Growth in utero, blood pressure in childhood and adult life, and mortality from cardiovascular disease. *Br Med J* 1989;298:564.

Brosnan PG. The hypothalamic pituitary axis in the fetus and newborn. *Semin Perinatol* 2001;25:371.

Eriksonn JG, Försen T, Tuomilehto J, et al. Catch-up growth in childhood and death from coronary heart disease: longitudinal study. *Br Med J* 1999;318:427.

Fant ME, Weisoly D. Insulin and insulin-like growth factors in human development: Implications for the perinatal period. *Semin Perinatol* 2001;25:426.

Gewolb IH, Warshaw JB. Influences on fetal growth. In: Warshaw JB, ed. *The biological basis of reproduction and developmental medicine.* New York: Elsevier, 1983;365.

Glazier JD, Cetin I, Perugino G, et al. Association between the activity of the system A amino acid transporter in the microvillous plasma membrane of the human placenta and severity of fetal compromise in intrauterine growth restriction. *Pediatr Res* 1997;42:514.

Gluckman PD, Pinal CS. Regulation of fetal growth by the somatotrophic axis. *J Nutr* 2003;133:1741S.

Hassink SG, Lancey E, Sheslow DV, et al. Placental leptin: an important new growth factor in intrauterine and neonatal development? *Pediatrics* 1997;100:1.

Hofman PL, Cutfield WS, Robinson EM, et al. Insulin resistance in short children with intrauterine growth retardation. *J Clin Endocrinol Metab* 1997;82:402.

Kashap S, Schulze KF, Ramakrishnan R, et al. Evaluation of a mathematical model for predicting the relationship between protein and energy intakes of low birth weight infants and the rate and composition of weight gain. *Pediatr Res* 1994;35:704.

Kimura RE, Warshaw JB. Metabolism during development. In: Warshaw JB, ed. *The biological basis of reproduction and developmental medicine.* New York: Elsevier, 1983;337.

Klein CJ. Nutrition requirements for preterm infant formulas. *J Nutr* 2002; 132:1395S.

Leger J, Oury F, Noel M, et al. Growth factors and intrauterine growth retardation. I. Serum growth hormone, insulin-like growth factor (IGF)-I, IGF-II, and IGF binding protein 3 levels in normally grown and growth-retarded human fetuses during second half of gestation. *Pediatr Res* 1996;40:94.

McClellan R, Novak D. Fetal nutrition: how we become what we are. *J Pediatr Gastroenterol Nutr* 2001;33:233.

Mena P, Llanos A, Uauy R. Insulin homeostasis in the extremely low birth weight infant. *Sem Perinat* 2001;25:436.

Ozkan H, Aydin A, Demir N, et al. Associations of IGF-I, IGFBP-1 and IGFBP-3 on intrauterine growth and early catch-up growth. *Biol Neonate* 1999;76:274.

Sadiq HF, Das UG, Tracy TF, Devaskar SU. Intrauterine growth restriction differentially regulates perinatal brain and skeletal muscle glucose transporters. *Brain Res* 1999;823:96.

Shingal A, Cole TJ, Lucas A. Early nutrition in preterm infants and later blood pressure: two cohort after randomised trials. *Lancet* 2001;357:413.

Shingal A, Fewtrell M, Cole TJ, Lucas A. Low nutrient intake and early growth for later insulin resistance in adolescents born preterm. *Lancet* 2003;361:1089.

Tanner JM. Physical growth from conception to maturity. In: *Foetus into man,* 2nd ed. Ware, U.K.: Castlemead Publications, 1989.

Widdowson E. Chemical composition of newly born animals. *Nature* 1950; 166:626.

Ziegler EE, Thureen PJ, Carlson SJ. Aggressive nutrition of the very low birth-weight infant. *Clin Perinatol* 2002;29:225.

CHAPTER 21 ■ GENERAL OBSTETRIC CARE

ALEXANDRA C. SPADOLA AND MARY E. D'ALTON

The goal of obstetric care is to support a woman, healthy or otherwise, through pregnancy with minimal risk to her own health and maximal benefit to the fetus. The challenge of modern obstetrics is to manage pregnancy, a normal physiologic process, with as little interference as possible, while identifying and treating complications that may arise. Risk factor screening and early recognition of complications allow for timely intervention, consultation with appropriate specialists, and, as indicated, transfer to tertiary centers with expert perinatology and neonatology staff. It must be stressed, however, that in obstetrics high-risk scenarios can develop rapidly and unexpectedly in the context of an otherwise normal labor and delivery. Every hospital delivering babies must be equipped to give adequate intrapartum care and must be prepared to perform a cesarean delivery within 30 minutes.

The broad spectrum of perinatal problems requires the full consideration of the medical and social factors that can affect the mother, fetus, and neonate. This awareness can be achieved by cooperative interaction between the mother, the obstetrician, the pediatrician, medical consultants, nurses, and social workers involved in perinatal care, as well as between the community and regional medical centers providing these services. Such collaborations afford the best opportunities for the goal of achieving healthy mothers and infants.

PRENATAL CARE

Prenatal care is an essential part of general obstetric care. Prenatal care ideally begins before conception with an assessment of obstetric risk factors and optimization of maternal health status. As recommended by the American College of Obstetrics and Gynecology (ACOG), women and their partners should be offered screening for genetic disorders specific to their ethnic background, such as the mutations for Tay-Sachs and cystic fibrosis. Common maternal diseases such as diabetes mellitus and chronic hypertension should be well controlled. Patients who require pharmacologic management of their medical conditions should be transitioned to regimens that are the least teratogenic. Women with severe medical problems such as heart disease or renal failure should be counseled as to their potential risks during pregnancy as well as the possible fetal complications. For example, a woman with pulmonary hypertension may face as high as 50% mortality with pregnancy; women with severe renal failure have high rates of preeclampsia and prematurity.

An important goal of prenatal care is the prevention of adverse fetal outcomes. Alcohol abuse in pregnancy is a leading cause of preventable developmental delay in the United States. Drinking has not clearly been demonstrated safe in any quantities and should be avoided. Tobacco and illicit drug use should cease. Proper nutrition and vitamin supplementation have been shown to reduce the incidence of congenital diseases. Women

at high risk for having a fetus with a neural tube defect should be placed on high doses of folic acid even before conception. Similarly, the prenatal identification of women infected with human immunodeficiency virus (HIV) allows for the administration of antiretroviral agents that have been shown to reduce the transmission of HIV to the fetus from 25% to 8%.

Prematurity continues to be the largest contributor to neonatal morbidity and mortality; prevention of preterm labor remains one of the most challenging aspects of obstetric care. Despite extensive research, history of prior preterm delivery remains the most powerful risk factor for premature birth, and minimal advances have been made in the management of preterm labor once it occurs. Over the last two decades the rise in the incidence of multiple gestations due to assisted reproductive techniques has contributed to the increase in low-birth-weight infants.

Perinatal mortality ranges from a low of 3 in 1,000 live births born to low-risk women with apparently normal fetuses to 145 in 1,000 live births born to women with high-risk pregnancies such as those with type 1 diabetes mellitus. Box 21.1

BOX 21.1   **Identification of Perinatal Risk Situations**

Maternal conditions
Maternal medical disease (e.g., hypertension, diabetes, cardiac disease)
Poor obstetric history (e.g., prior stillbirth)
Antepartum hemorrhage
Postterm gestation (greater than 42 weeks)
Prolonged rupture of membranes
Rhesus incompatibility
Low socioeconomic status
Maternal age younger than 16 years or older than 35 years
Maternal drug or alcohol abuse

Fetal conditions
Abnormal fetal presentation (e.g., breech)
Fetal growth retardation
Multiple pregnancy
Polyhydramnios
Oligohydramnios
Malformation

Conditions of labor and delivery
Preterm labor
Prolonged labor
Operative delivery (e.g., forceps delivery, vacuum extraction)
Prolapsed umbilical cord

BOX 21.2 — Fetal Anomalies and Genetic Syndromes Amenable to Prenatal Diagnosis

Structural anomalies
Congenital heart disease
Ventral wall defects
Neural tube defects
Skeletal dysplasias
Renal agenesis
Gastrointestinal atresias
Diaphragmatic hernias
Cleft lip/palate
Genetic syndromes
Aneuploidy
Tay-Sachs disease
Cystic fibrosis
Sickle cell anemia
Gaucher disease
Niemann-Pick disease
Galactosemia
Homocystinuria
Maple syrup urine disease
Smith-Lemli-Opitz syndrome

This list is by no means complete. Advances in ultrasound and molecular genetics have allowed for an ever-growing number of genetic syndromes that can be diagnosed antenatally.

---

lists various high-risk perinatal conditions. The expanding field of prenatal diagnosis has lead to advances in the recognition of fetal disease. Box 21.2 lists some of the detectable pathologic conditions. The list of treatable diseases that can be diagnosed and managed *in utero* is much shorter (Box 21.3). For further discussion of prenatal diagnosis see Chapter 22. Consultation with or transfer of patient care to a specialist in maternal fetal medicine, also known as a perinatologist, can be invaluable in many high-risk pregnancies. The challenge of obstetric care is to properly identify those women with risk factors in a timely fashion so that interventions can be made to minimize potential adverse maternal and fetal effects.

BOX 21.3 — Potentially Treatable Fetal Conditions

Fetal anemia: red blood cell isoimmunization; parvovirus infection
Fetal thrombocytopenia: alloimmune thrombocytopenia
Fetal cardiac arrhythmias
Aqueductal stenosis
Bladder outlet obstruction
Twin–twin transfusion syndrome
Toxoplasmosis
Congenital adrenal hyperplasia
Sacrococcygeal teratoma
Congenital diaphragmatic hernia
Congenital cystic adenomatoid malformation of the lung
Fetal chylothorax
Smith-Lemli-Opitz syndrome

MATERNAL ADAPTATIONS TO PREGNANCY

Pregnancy is a normal physiologic condition, not an illness. However, the metabolic changes that occur during pregnancy affect every organ system. Not only can these alterations mimic symptoms of disease, but they can also significantly impact the assessment and management of illness during pregnancy. Understanding and recognizing these changes is crucial to the proper care of all pregnant patients.

The cardiovascular adaptations to pregnancy are profound. To provide sufficient blood flow to the uterus, and thus an adequate supply of nutrients to the growing fetus, uteroplacental blood flow reaches an astounding 500 to 700 mL/minute at term. The maternal cardiac output must increase by almost 50% to accommodate this added circulatory loop, and the maternal blood volume increases accordingly by 1.5 L (Fig. 21.1). This increased blood volume is accompanied by a similar, though slightly smaller, increase in the circulating red blood cell mass, leading to what is referred to as the physiologic anemia of pregnancy. The iron requirements for this degree of red blood cell production are substantial— approximately 1 g of elemental iron for an entire pregnancy— and make pregnant women prone to iron deficiency. Supplemental iron is recommended, especially during the third trimester.

Maternal renal function is augmented as early as the first trimester with increases in the glomerular filtration rate and renal plasma flow that parallel the increases in cardiac output. A resulting decrease in serum creatinine and urea nitrogen levels can be observed. This can lead to increased dosage requirements to achieve therapeutic drug levels for medications excreted via the kidneys.

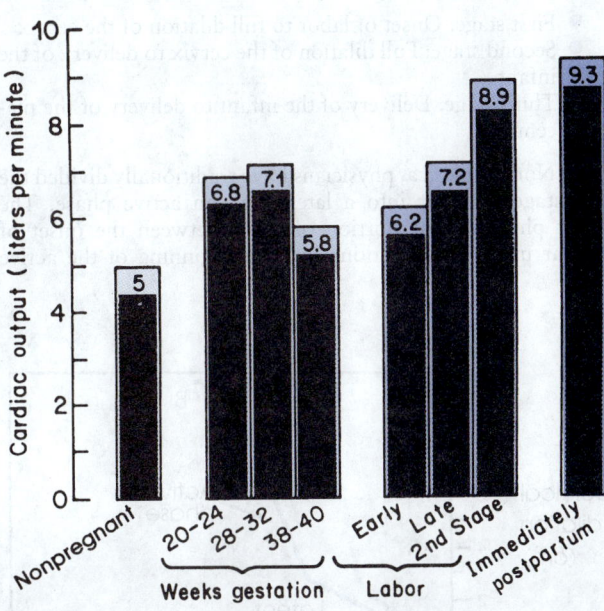

FIGURE 21.1. Cardiac outputs during three stages of gestation, labor, and immediately postpartum are compared with values of nonpregnant women. All values were determined with women in the lateral recumbent position. (Adapted from Ueland K, Metcalfe J. Circulatory changes in pregnancy. *Clin Obstet Gynecol* 1975;18:41; presented by Hankins GDV, Cuningham FG, Pritchard JA. Cardiopulmonary consequences of hypertension during pregnancy and puerperium. Williams Supplement No. 8, 1986.)

The production of high levels of progesterone by the placenta leads to changes in the gastrointestinal, pulmonary, and renal systems. Progesterone causes relaxation of smooth muscle, which induces slowing of the entire gastrointestinal tract, increasing gastric emptying times, symptomatic reflux, and constipation. The ureters become physiologically dilated, leading to urinary stasis and an increased risk of urinary tract infection. Central stimulation of the respiratory center by progesterone is responsible for the slight respiratory alkalosis and compensatory metabolic acidosis observed in pregnant women. In addition to mechanical changes of the thorax and an increase in intra-abdominal contents, this hormonal effect contributes to the mild dyspnea many pregnant women experience.

The placenta also produces human placental lactogen, a polypeptide homologous to human growth hormone. Its metabolic effects include an increase in lipolysis and the release of free fatty acids as well as the induction of a relatively "diabetogenic" state, with insulin resistance in the maternal tissues ensuring a continuous supply of glucose to the developing fetus. Women who are at baseline elevated risk for type 2 diabetes due to ethnic background, age, or body mass index may not be able to compensate for these changes and will develop gestational diabetes during the latter half of pregnancy.

LABOR AND DELIVERY

Normal Labor and Delivery

The intelligent management of labor rests on an understanding of its mechanics and normal progression. Labor is defined as the onset of regular uterine contractions accompanied by progressive dilation and effacement of the cervix and descent of the fetal presenting part. In the 1950s, Friedman began to study the labors of large numbers of women and published his now famous curve, which graphs cervical dilation as a function of time (Fig. 21.2). It has been the convention to divide this curve into three parts, or stages:

- First stage: Onset of labor to full dilation of the cervix
- Second stage: Full dilation of the cervix to delivery of the infant
- Third stage: Delivery of the infant to delivery of the placenta

In North America, physicians have traditionally divided the first stage of labor into a latent and an active phase. The latent phase is that portion of labor between the onset of regular uterine contractions and the beginning of the active

phase, when the relatively flat portion of the Friedman labor curve gains slope; this represents the phase of maximal cervical dilation. The average duration of labor is approximately 9 hours for a nulliparous patient and 5 hours for a multiparous patient.

Induction of Labor

Induction of labor is the stimulation of labor before its natural onset and is indicated for a number of medical–obstetric or fetal complications of pregnancy. Elective inductions, which are performed for the convenience of the patient or the professional staff, are rarely appropriate. Indicated induction of labor is initiated when prolongation of the pregnancy increases the risks for either the mother or the fetus over the perceived benefit of further maturation. ACOG's list of maternal indications for labor induction includes preeclampsia, fetal demise, abruptio placentae, and chorioamnionitis. Deterioration in fetal status by antenatal fetal testing often prompts induction in various high-risk situations such as pregnancies complicated by diabetes mellitus, hypertensive disorders, and intrauterine growth retardation, as well as postterm pregnancies. The decision to induce labor can be greatly influenced by estimated gestational age, as is the case of preterm premature rupture of membranes without evidence of intrauterine infection.

Contraindications to vaginal delivery include nonvertex fetal presentation, placenta previa, and a previous uterine incision or surgery such as a classic cesarean section or myomectomy in which the full thickness of the uterine wall was incised. An elective cesarean section may be performed when antenatal testing indicates fetal intolerance of labor or contraindications exist to uterine contractions. A prior low transverse cesarean delivery is not considered a contraindication for induction; however, the patient should be advised of her decreased probability of success and a slightly increased risk of uterine rupture. ACOG recommends that prostaglandin induction agents not be administered to patients with a history of prior cesarean delivery given the evidence suggesting significantly higher rates of uterine rupture.

Pain Relief in Labor

As women enjoy greater access to education about the birth process, pain relief in labor remains a major concern to obstetric patients. While two main forms of analgesia exist for patients—parenteral narcotics and regional anesthesia—some 60% of women in the United States choose either epidural or combined spinal–epidural analgesia during labor. The choice of analgesic or anesthetic technique depends on the experience and knowledge of the anesthesia team and obstetrician, the clinical context, and increasingly the personal preference of the patient herself.

Regional anesthesia can provide safe, effective analgesia for laboring patients. The major maternal and fetal risk is hypotension related to sympathetic blockade. Fetal bradycardias seen following the administration of regional anesthesia may be a result of decreased uterine perfusion or an increase in uterine activity causing hyperstimulation. A recent meta-analysis comparing parenteral opioids to epidural anesthesia reported an increase by 42 minutes of the first stage of labor and 14 minutes of the second stage of labor. Additionally, much of the published data suggest that epidural anesthesia is not associated with an increased risk of cesarean section as was previously suspected. Overall, the advantages of regional anesthesia for both vaginal and cesarean deliveries are that the patient is awake and her infant has little if any risk of drug depression.

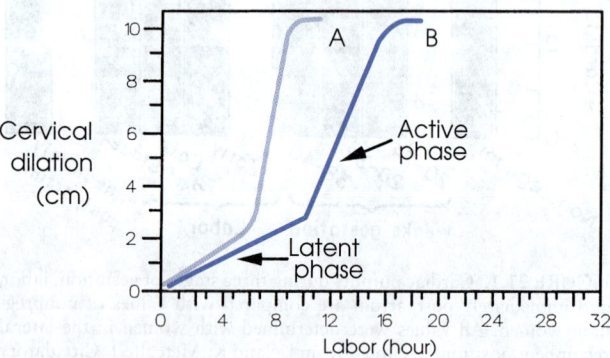

FIGURE 21.2. Normal labor during the first stage. A: Average multipara. B: Average primigravida.

If given in appropriate doses and repeated only if necessary, narcotics ease the pain of contractions, are easy to administer (intravenously or intramuscularly), and only rarely cause fetal depression. Meperidine, nalbuphine, and butorphanol are some of the common opiate derivatives used. Though rarely needed, an opiate antagonist such as naloxone should be easily available for treatment of the neonate.

For routine cesarean deliveries the risks of general anesthesia to both mother and fetus generally outweigh any benefit; most often spinal block is used. Anesthesia-related deaths rank sixth in the causes of maternal mortality in the United States and are 17 times higher with general anesthesia. For the fetus, transplacental passage of the anesthetic agents can result in neonatal depression. This effect is related to the anesthetic agents used and the length of time between induction and delivery of the infant. Currently, general anesthesia may be indicated in the setting of a cesarean delivery so emergent as to preclude spinal anesthesia, unanticipated cesarean hysterectomy, or when relative or absolute contraindications to regional anesthesia exist (e.g., severe maternal thrombocytopenia).

EVALUATION OF FETAL WELL-BEING

Obstetricians have a number of tools for evaluating the status of the fetus. Noninvasive techniques are by far the most commonly used and include ultrasound and electronic fetal monitoring. In select situations, invasive monitoring of the fetus with fetal heart rate electrodes, fetal scalp pH assessment, and even fetal blood analysis through percutaneous umbilical blood sampling can provide necessary information about fetal status.

Ultrasound provides indirect evidence of adequate fetal oxygenation and a normal fetal acid–base status by documenting adequate fetal growth, normal amniotic fluid levels, and normal fetal behavior (fetal movement, tone, and breathing motions) as measured in the biophysical profile. Doppler studies of arterial blood flow provide information on the status of the fetoplacental unit. They have been validated as a means of predicting outcomes. Specifically, the evaluation of flow in the umbilical artery has proved most valuable in pregnancies complicated by intrauterine growth restriction with absence or reversal of end-diastolic flow correlating with adverse fetal and neonatal outcomes. Increased fetal middle cerebral artery flow

has been studied as a marker for fetal anemia and is used in the evaluation of pregnancies at risk for hydrops fetalis.

Electronic fetal monitoring, now routine in many labor and delivery suites, uses Doppler ultrasound technology to trace the fetal heart rate and its variations over time while simultaneously recording uterine activity. The nonstress test is so named because it is merely a tracing of the fetal heart rate over time, with no external stressors (e.g., contractions) on the uterine environment. A reassuring or reactive test result is one that displays accelerations of the heart rate to 15 beats per minute above the baseline, occurring twice in a 20-minute test period. The contraction stress test is the same examination performed with spontaneous or induced contractions; a reassuring or negative test result is one in which no heart rate decelerations occur in response to the uterine contractions. The nonstress test and contraction stress test have proved to be reliable indicators of a well-oxygenated and nonacidotic fetus. When reassuring, the tests can predict a very low rate of perinatal mortality with a high degree of sensitivity. The major drawback to the tests is a high rate of false-positive test results, especially in low-risk populations. The contraction stress test, for example, has a 50% false-positive rate (i.e., one-half of the fetuses with a nonreassuring result are not acidotic).

The use of fetal heart rate monitors in labor remains controversial. Although some studies have reported a decrease in neonatal morbidity in continuously monitored labors (as evidenced by a decrease in neonatal seizure rates), little evidence exists that long-term morbidity or mortality is avoided in low-risk women. Indeed, many studies report an increased cesarean section rate with external monitoring in labor without a concomitant decrease in neonatal morbidity or mortality. Because of this, ACOG allows that low-risk labors may be safely monitored with intermittent auscultation of the fetal heart rate after an initial evaluation of fetal well-being. High-risk groups such as women with medical problems like diabetes, hypertension, or systemic lupus, or whose pregnancies are complicated by fetal growth restriction or meconium-stained fluid, should still be monitored with continuous fetal heart rate tracing during labor.

An example of a normal intrapartum fetal heart rate tracing is shown in Fig. 21.3. The presence of heart rate accelerations and the absence of decelerations are reassuring. It should be noted, however, that fetal heart rate decelerations during labor are common and usually benign. Variable decelerations, so named for their temporal relationship to the uterine contraction, have a typical V-shaped morphology and are the most common deceleration seen in labor. Variable decelerations,

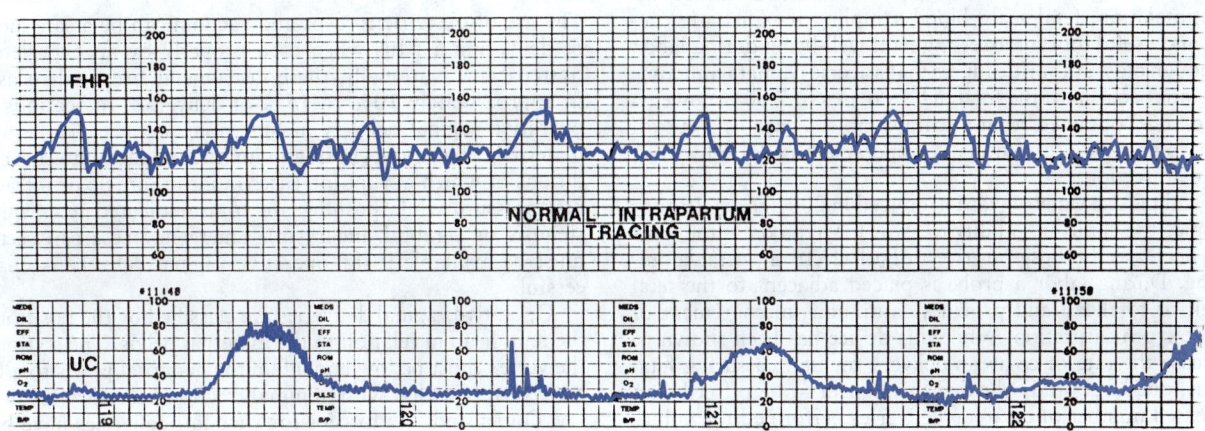

FIGURE 21.3. A normal intrapartum fetal heart rate (FHR) tracing with uterine contractions (UC). No decelerations are seen. Variability and FHR accelerations are normal.

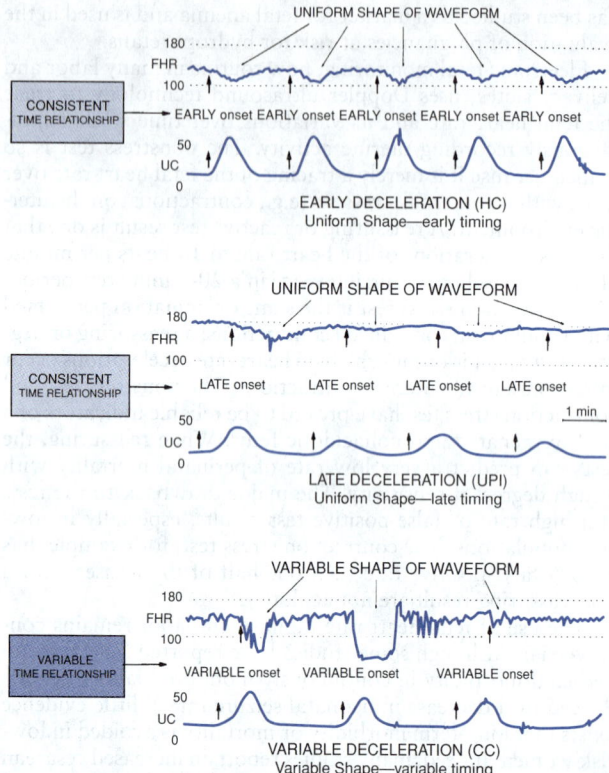

FIGURE 21.4. Fetal heart rate (FHR) decelerations in relation to the time of onset of uterine contractions (UC). CC, cord compression; HC, head compression; UPI, uteroplacental insufficiency. (Reprinted with permission from Hon EH. *An atlas of fetal heart rate patterns.* New Haven, CT: Harty, 1968.)

unless deep, repetitive, or prolonged, are not associated with adverse fetal outcomes. Similarly, early decelerations (smooth, shallow decelerations occurring with contractions) are always benign and associated with fetal head compression. Late decelerations, if repetitive, may be indicative of placental insufficiency and a hypoxic fetus and should prompt *in utero* fetal resuscitation, further investigation with fetal scalp pH determination, delivery, or all three actions (Fig. 21.4).

Fetal scalp blood sampling for pH analysis is used as an adjunct to fetal heart rate monitoring to confirm or exclude fetal acidosis implied by a fetal heart rate tracing. Although increasingly replaced by other, less invasive means of confirming fetal well-being such as fetal scalp stimulation and vibroacoustic stimulation, fetal scalp blood sampling remains an accurate and useful tool for assessing fetal well-being during labor. Although most authorities agree that adverse neonatal outcome does not occur until the fetal pH decreases to 7.00 or lower, a pH of 7.20 obtained from a scalp sample is used as a cut-off point to prompt intervention (i.e., operative vaginal delivery or cesarean section).

Fetal pulse oximetry was introduced in 2001 as an effort to enhance the clinician's ability to asess for hypoxia in the fetus and decrease the false-positive rate of electronic fetal monitoring. During labor a probe is placed adjacent to the fetal cheek or forehead and provides continuous measurement of fetal oxygen saturation. While this device has been shown to decrease the rate of cesarean delivery for nonreassuring fetal status, one large study showed this benefit to be offset by an increased number of cesarean deliveries performed for failure to progress. At this time ACOG cautions against widespread adoption of this new method of fetal monitoring until more studies have demonstrated its utility.

OPERATIVE DELIVERY

Cesarean Delivery

The cesarean delivery rate in the United States has increased from 5.5% to more than 22% since 1970. Initially a procedure performed for maternal indications (placenta previa, radiographically documented cephalopelvic disproportion, failed induction, or severe preeclampsia), cesarean delivery has become one of the most common surgical procedures performed in the United States. Explanations for this increase include a widespread cessation of vaginal breech deliveries for singletons, an increase in the number of repeat cesareans and inductions, an increase in deliveries for nonreassuring fetal status (perhaps because of the use of intrapartum monitors), and a climate increasingly attuned to medicolegal concerns. Efforts to decrease the cesarean delivery rate have mainly been directed toward reducing the number of primary sections for dystocia via a more judicious use of labor augmentation and encouraging vaginal births after cesareans when appropriate to reduce the repeat section rate.

Although cesarean delivery can be regarded as a reasonably safe surgical procedure, it is associated with a higher risk of morbidity and mortality than that routinely associated with vaginal delivery. Acute maternal complications of cesarean delivery include anesthesia accidents, aspiration pneumonitis, hemorrhage, injury to the bowel or bladder, and (rarely) amniotic fluid embolism. Patients undergoing cesarean section have febrile puerperal complications at a rate that is 5- to 20-fold higher than the vaginal route. Often noted by the opponents of routine elective cesarean delivery are the cumulative risks to the patient with each repeat cesarean delivery. Risk of abnormal placentation with its greater potential for life-threatening hemorrhage and need for hysterectomy and blood transfusion increases over multiple cesarean deliveries.

Neonatal risks also exist in cesarean delivery. Across all gestational ages, neonatal respiratory morbidity increases, although the cause and pathophysiology of this complication are matters of dispute; it often is seen when the cesarean delivery is performed in the absence of labor. Some cases of respiratory morbidity after cesarean delivery are caused by true iatrogenic prematurity, in which inaccurate gestational dates result unexpectedly in a premature infant.

Operative Vaginal Delivery (Vacuum and Forceps)

The use of obstetric forceps and vacuum can be a safe means of delivering a fetus when used properly by an experienced obstetrician. Nationally, these instruments are used to assist in approximately 10% to 15% of deliveries. Indications for operative vaginal delivery include nonreassuring fetal status, maternal exhaustion, chorioamnionitis, and rare maternal conditions in which abrupt increases in intrathoracic or intracranial pressure while pushing are contraindicated (e.g., mitral stenosis or cerebral aneurysm). Emergency cesarean section must be available if the operative vaginal delivery is unsuccessful.

Operative vaginal deliveries are classified by the position of the fetal head in relation to the maternal pelvis. The station of the vertex must be low enough in the maternal pelvis to allow an easy application with minimal traction necessary for delivery. Outlet and low-forceps (or vacuum) deliveries have been shown to be safe for both mother and fetus and are characterized by a fetal head that has descended in the pelvis so that the leading point of the fetal skull is at least 2 cm beyond the ischial spines. High-forceps deliveries have been abandoned in the United States and have no place in modern obstetrics.

Forceps have been shown to have higher potential for maternal trauma to the perineum. When used properly they carry minimal risk to the fetus. The incidence of cephalohematomas is higher in vacuum deliveries (14% to 16%) than in forceps deliveries (2%). Rarely the bleeding occurs in the subgaleal space and the bleeding can be severe enough to cause hemodynamic changes in the fetus. Serial use of both operative methods on a single patient has also been abandoned due to its association with increased fetal risk. Failure of one method should prompt cesarean delivery. A pediatrician should be available for all operative deliveries.

PRETERM LABOR AND DELIVERY

Labor is preterm when it occurs before 37 completed weeks from the first day of the woman's last menstrual period. Menstrual dates are often uncertain and first-trimester ultrasound is considered the gold standard in pregnancy dating. In later trimesters the clinical examination and ultrasound are less accurate and may be in error by as much as 2 to 3 weeks. Distinguishing between labor and preterm contractions presents another challenge. Pharmacologic inhibition of labor must be instituted early if it is to be effective; yet, if therapy is withheld until strong evidence of labor exists such as progressive cervical dilation, the process may be advanced to a point at which tocolysis is unlikely to be effective. Conversely, if only marginal evidence of preterm labor exists, unnecessary drug therapy can introduce potentially harmful effects to the mother or fetus.

Four major classes of tocolytic medications are used in the United States. Although its efficacy in preventing long-term morbidity and neonatal mortality has been challenged, tocolysis is routinely employed to delay delivery for timing of administration of steroids. Intravenous magnesium sulfate is the most commonly used tocolytic and is well studied due to its administration for seizure prophylaxis in preeclamptic patients. Fetal adverse affects can include central nervous system and motor depression. Its protective affect on the development of cerebral palsy is currently being studied. Calcium channel blockers and nonsteroidal antiinflammatory drugs have also been shown to be efficacious as first-line agents. Indomethacin is associated with premature closure of the ductus arteriosus and is not recommended for use after 32 weeks or for longer than 48 hours. Beta-sympathomimetics are an additional class of tocolytic agents. Terbutaline is an effective acute agent to effect uterine muscle relaxation, but it is associated with significant side effects such as maternal and fetal tachycardia, chest discomfort, anxiety, and pulmonary edema, with no demonstrated significant reduction in perinatal morbidity and mortality.

While the efficacy of tocolytic agents to prevent preterm delivery is low, the use of antenatal corticosteroids in patients at risk for preterm delivery has proven to be the single most important intervention obstetricians can perform to prevent neonatal morbidity and mortality. The use of corticosteroids in patients with preterm labor has been studied extensively, and the preponderance of evidence suggests that their use in patients less than 34 weeks estimated gestational age is associated with a decrease in neonatal mortality, respiratory distress syndrome, intraventricular hemorrhage, and long-term respiratory and neurologic morbidity. One of the primary benefits to treating preterm premature rupture of the membranes without evidence of intrauterine infection with prophylactic broad-spectrum antibiotics is to prolong the latency period and allow time for the administration of corticosteroids.

Despite advances in the treatment of preterm labor, prematurity is responsible for more neonatal deaths than any other single cause except congenital malformations. The management of these labors in facilities with both expert obstetric care and a neonatal intensive care unit capable of caring for premature infants is crucial and often necessitates the transfer of pregnant women from an outlying community hospital to a tertiary center. This is especially true for extremely premature and very low-birth-weight infants for whom the initial resuscitative efforts and management greatly affect survival.

The delivery of extremely premature infants (23 to 25 weeks) is complicated by a paucity of data indicating that routine cesarean delivery is beneficial to these infants and by the poor short-term and long-term survival data at these gestational ages. For these reasons, patients are often faced with difficult decisions regarding the level of obstetric intervention desired (e.g., fetal monitoring and/or cesarean delivery for nonreassuring fetal status). Similar conflicts occur in determining which newborns should be aggressively resuscitated. Frank discussions among the patients and their families, the obstetric staff, and the neonatology team can be difficult when an unexpected delivery is imminent. However, informed decisions are essential to the creation of an appropriate and thoughtful management plan.

MECONIUM

Meconium staining of the amniotic fluid occurs in 8% to 16% of pregnancies and was historically thought to represent evidence of fetal distress or hypoxia. In many cases, however, its presence in the amniotic fluid is a result of the normal function of the maturing fetal gastrointestinal tract. Moreover, when meconium passage is associated with fetal insult, the timing of the hypoxia is not always evident and may not be ongoing (i.e., it may have occurred hours or days before the discovery of meconium in the amniotic fluid). In the presence of reassuring fetal testing expedient delivery is not indicated on the basis of meconium staining alone. Meconium aspiration syndrome with its morbid effects on neonatal oxygenation affects 2% of infants found to have meconium-stained fluid. Appropriate intrapartum management is described in Chapter 24.

Suggested Readings

American College of Obstetricians and Gynecologists. Fetal heart rate patterns: monitoring, interpretation, and management. ACOG Technical Bulletin No. 207. Washington, DC: ACOG, 1995.

American College of Obstetricians and Gynecologists. Fetal pulse oximetry. ACOG Committee Opinion No. 258. Washington, DC: ACOG, 2001.

American College of Obstetricians and Gynecologists. Induction of labor. ACOG Practice Bulletin No. 10. Washington, DC: ACOG, 1999.

American College of Obstetricians and Gynecologists. Operative vaginal delivery. ACOG Practice Bulletin No. 17. Washington, DC: ACOG, 2000.

Brown BL, Gleicher N. Intrauterine meconium aspiration. *Obstet Gynecol* 1981;57:26.

Connor EM, Sperling RS, Gelber R, et al. Reduction of maternal-infant transmission of human immunodeficiency virus type 1 with zidovudine treatment. Pediatric AIDS Clinical Trials Group Protocol 076 Study Group. *N Engl J Med* 1994;331:1173.

Eltzschig HK, Lieberman ES, Camann WR. Medical progress: regional anesthesia and analgesia for labor and delivery. *N Engl J Med* 2003;319.

Ewigman BG, Crane JP, Frigoletto FD, et al. Effect of prenatal ultrasound screening on perinatal outcome. *N Engl J Med* 1993;329:821.

Freinkel N, Dooley SL, Metzger BE. Care of the pregnant woman with insulin-dependent diabetes mellitus. *N Engl J Med* 1985;313:96.

Friedman EA. *Labor: clinical evaluation and management*, 2nd ed. New York: Appleton-Century-Crofts, 1978.

Gyetvai K, Hannah ME, Hodnett ED, Ohlsson A. Tocolytics for preterm labor: a systematic review. *Obstet Gynecol* 1999 Nov;94:869.

Halliday HL, Sweet D. Endotracheal intubation at birth for preventing morbidity and mortality in vigorous, meconium-stained infants born at term. Cochrane Neonatal Group. *Cochrane Database of Systematic Reviews 3, 2005.*

Halpern SH, Leighton BL, Ohlsson A, et al. Effect of epidural vs. parenteral opioid analgesia on the progress of labor: a meta-analysis. *JAMA* 1998;280:2105.

Hawkins JL, Beaty BR, Gibbs CP. Update on U.S. OB anesthesia practice. *Anesthesiology* 1999;91(Suppl):A1060.

Herbst A, Ingemarsson I. Intermittent versus continuous electronic monitoring in labour: a randomised study. *Br J Obstet Gynecol* 1994;101:663.

Hobel CV, Hyvarinen MD, Okader DM, et al. Prenatal and intrapartum high-risk screening. I. Prediction of the high-risk neonate. *Am J Obstet Gynecol* 1973;117:1.

Konte JM, Holbrook RHJ, Larons RK Jr, Creasy RK. Short-term neonatal morbidity associated with prematurity and the effect of a prematurity prevention program on expected incidence of morbidity. *Am J Perinatol* 1986;3:283.

Leveno KJ, Cunningham FG, Nelson S, et al. A prospective comparison of selective and universal electronic fetal monitoring in 34,995 pregnancies. *N Engl J Med* 1986;315:615.

Macones GA, Marder SJ, Clothier B, Stamilio DM. The controversy surrounding indomethacin for tocolysis. *Am J Obstet Gynecol* 2001;184:264.

Martin JA, Hamilton BE, Ventura SJ, et al. *Births: final data for 2000. National vital statistics reports. Vol. 50, No. 5.* Hyattsville, MD.: National Center for Health Statistics, 2002:1.

McDonald D, Grant A, Sheridan-Pereira M, et al. The Dublin randomized controlled trial of intrapartum fetal heart-rate monitoring. *Am J Obstet Gynecol* 1985;152:524.

Menacher F, Curtin SC. Trends in cesarean birth and vaginal birth after previous cesarean, 1991–1999. NVSR Vol. 49, No. 13. 15 2002-1120.

National Institutes of Health. Effect of corticosteroids for fetal maturation on perinatal outcome. NIH Consensus Statement 12, 1994:1.

Nelson KB, Dambrosia JM, Ting TY, Grether JK. Uncertain value of electronic fetal monitoring in predicting cerebral palsy. *N Engl J Med* 1996;334:613.

Pierce J, Gaudier FL, Sanchez-Ramos L. Intrapartum amnioinfusion for meconium-stained fluid: meta-analysis of prospective clinical trials. *Obstet Gynecol* 2000;95:1051.

Sadovsky Y, Amon E, Bade ME, Petrie RH. Prophylactic amnioinfusion during labor complicated by meconium: a preliminary report. *Am J Obstet Gynecol* 1989;163:613.

Schieve LA, Meikle SF, Ferre C, et al. Low and very low birth weight in infants conceived with use of assisted reproductive technology. *N Engl J Med* 2002;341:731.

Smaill F, Hofmeyr GJ. *Antibiotic prophylaxis for cesarean section (Cochrane Review). The Cochrane Library, Issue 4, 2003.* Chichester, UK: John Wiley & Sons, Ltd.

Thacker SB, Stroup DF, Peterson HB. Efficacy and safety of intrapartum electronic fetal monitoring: an update. *Obstet Gynecol* 1995;86:613.

Towner D, Castro MA, Eby-Wilkens E, Gilbert WM. Effect of mode of delivery in nulliparous women on neonatal intracranial injury. *N Engl J Med* 1999;341:1709.

Weber K. National Task Force on Fetal Alcohol Syndrome and Fetal Alcohol Effect: defining the national agenda for FAS and other prenatal alcohol related effects. *MMWR* 2002;51:9.

Yancey MK, Herpolsheimer A, Jordan GD, et al. Maternal and neonatal effects of outlet forceps delivery compared with spontaneous vaginal delivery in term pregnancies. *Obstet Gynecol* 1991;78:646.

CHAPTER 22 ■ FETAL EVALUATION AND PRENATAL DIAGNOSIS

ANDREW J. HEALY, TRACY SHEVELL, AND MARY E. D'ALTON

Serious birth defects, often genetically determined, complicate the lives of 3% of newborns and their respective families. These disorders account for 20% of deaths during the newborn period, surpassing prematurity as the leading cause of neonatal mortality and contributing to an even higher percentage of the serious morbidity in infancy and childhood. The cost of neonatal intensive care is staggering; higher still are the costs of rehabilitation programs for the severely handicapped. The impact on an affected family is perhaps immeasurable.

With growing recognition of the frequency and importance of congenital disorders as well as social trends toward delayed parenthood and smaller family sizes, prenatal diagnosis plays an important role in the management of many pregnancies. The goal of prenatal diagnosis is to provide anatomic, genetic, physiologic, and biochemical information about the fetus, thereby facilitating maximum reproductive choices for the parents.

able fetal disorder. The American College of Obstetricians and Gynecologists (ACOG) recommends the use of a questionnaire to elicit genetic information that may help elucidate these factors. Counseling before prenatal diagnosis is of critical importance. The central issue is balancing the risk of an abnormal child against the risk associated with an investigative or interventional procedure. Prospective parents must understand the concept of excluding or establishing a specific diagnosis with a high reliability but without complete certainty. One of the most important goals in genetic counseling is to help patients understand the reproductive options that are available. A person's previous experience, ethnicity, cultural background, and religious beliefs may affect his or her acceptance of prenatal diagnosis and the choices made following the diagnosis of an abnormality. Counseling should be nondirective and concentrate on the accurate presentation of all the facts and options available. Common indications for prenatal counseling and diagnosis are summarized in Box 22.1.

INDICATIONS FOR PRENATAL DIAGNOSIS

Both general and specific risk factors must be ascertained to determine if a pregnancy has an increased risk of a diagnos-

General Factors

Numeric chromosomal abnormalities occur with increased frequency with advancing maternal age (Table 22.1). Standard

---

BOX 22.1   **Indications for Prenatal Testing**

General factors
Maternal age greater than or equal to 35 at time of delivery
Maternal serum alpha-fetoprotein concentration
Triple screening (maternal serum alpha-fetoprotein, human chorionic gonadotropin, and unconjugated estriol)

Specific factors
Previous child with structural defect or chromosomal abnormality
Stillbirths, neonatal deaths
Parent with structural abnormality
Parent with balanced translocation
Inherited disorders (cystic fibrosis, metabolic disorders, sex-linked recessive disorders)
Maternal medical disease (diabetes, phenylketonuria)
Teratogen exposure (ionizing radiation, anticonvulsant medicines, lithium, isotretinoin, alcohol)
Infections (rubella, toxoplasmosis, cytomegalovirus)

Ethnic factors

Disorder	Ethnic Group	Screening Test
Tay-Sachs disease	Ashkenazi Jews, French Canadians	Decreased serum, hexosaminidase A
Sickle cell anemia	Black Africans, Mediterraneans, Arabs, Indo-Pakistanis	Presence of sickling in hemolysate followed by confirmatory hemoglobin electrophoresis
Thalassemia	Mediterraneans, Southern and Southeast Asians, Chinese	Mean corpuscular volume less than 80 fL (alpha and beta) followed by confirmatory hemoglobin electrophoresis

---

TABLE 22.1

MATERNAL AGE AND ESTIMATED RATES OF CHROMOSOMAL ABNORMALITIES AT TIME OF EXPECTED LIVE BIRTH

Maternal Age	Risk for Down Syndrome	Total Risk for Chromosomal Abnormalities
20	1/1,667	1/526
25	1/1,250	1/476
30	1/952	1/385
35	1/385	1/202
36	1/295	1/162
37	1/227	1/129
38	1/175	1/102
39	1/137	1/82
40	1/106	1/65
41	1/82	1/51
42	1/64	1/40
43	1/50	1/32
44	1/38	1/25
45	1/30	1/20
46	1/23	1/16
47	1/18	1/13
48	1/14	1/10
49	1/11	1/7

Modified from Hook EB. Rates of chromosome abnormalities at different gestational ages. *Obstet Gynecol* 1981;58:282; Hook EB, Cross PK, Schreinemacher MS. Chromosomal, abnormality rates at amniocentesis and in live-born infants. *JAMA* 1983;249:2034.

---

practice is to offer prenatal cytogenetic diagnosis to all women who will be 35 years or older at their delivery date. Testing for biochemical markers in maternal serum identifies patients at risk for certain cytogenetic and structural abnormalities. Alpha-fetoprotein, the major protein of early fetal life, is synthesized in the fetal liver and yolk sac. Open neural tube and ventral wall defects are associated with exposed fetal membrane and blood vessel surfaces, which increase the level of alpha-fetoprotein in amniotic fluid and maternal serum. Low levels of maternal serum alpha-fetoprotein and unconjugated estriol are associated with trisomies 21 and 18.

The single marker that yields the highest detection rate for Down syndrome is human chorionic gonadotropin, which is significantly elevated in this syndrome. The combined use of the markers human chorionic gonadotropin, unconjugated estriol, maternal serum alpha-fetoprotein, and maternal age leads to detection of approximately 60% of cases of Down syndrome, with a false-positive rate of 6.6%. The use of ultrasonography to verify gestational age reduces the false-positive rate to 3.8%.

Maternal serum alpha-fetoprotein screening should be offered to women at 16 to 20 completed weeks of pregnancy. Careful evaluation of gestational age is of critical importance because maternal serum alpha-fetoprotein values increase steadily throughout the second trimester. Because of population

differences in median maternal serum alpha-fetoprotein values, laboratories must take into account variables such as race, multiple gestations, diabetes mellitus, and maternal weight when determining results. Most centers in the United States utilize a cutoff of 2.0 to 2.5 times the median for the general population screened for neural tube defects. Invasive procedures such as amniocentesis may give rise to maternal alpha-fetoprotein elevations; therefore, blood samples for screening markers should be obtained before amniocentesis is performed.

Dimeric inhibin A represents an additional serum analyte consistently reported to enhance the detection rate of Down syndrome when included in second-trimester screening. In a large prospective study assessing 1,256 patients, inhibin A performed extremely well; with a fixed false-positive rate, up to 23% more cases of Down syndrome were detected than with the traditional multiple-marker screening test. Using alpha-fetoprotein, estriol, total human chorionic gonadotropin, and inhibin A, along with maternal age, 70% of cases of Down syndrome were detected for a 5% false-positive rate. Using this "quad-screen" could lead to fewer genetic amniocenteses than the traditional triple screen; therefore, measuring this analyte may lower the cost per Down syndrome pregnancy identified.

Specific Factors

Following the birth of a child with trisomy 21, the likelihood that a subsequent child will have a similar chromosomal abnormality is approximately 1%. The recurrence rate for neural tube defects is 2% to 5%, compared with a general population risk of 1 to 2 per 1,000 births. The general recurrence risk of a cardiac defect is 2% to 4%, compared with the general population risk of 4 to 8 per 1,000 live births. If a parent has spina bifida, congenital heart disease, or a known chromosome translocation or inversion, an increased chance exists that a child will have a related defect. Antenatal diagnosis is possible for many inborn errors of metabolism, almost all of which are transmitted in an autosomal recessive fashion. Maternal diabetes and maternal phenylketonuria are associated with an increased risk of fetal malformations. Other known teratogens include ionizing radiation, drugs, and maternal infections.

Ethnic Factors

The gene frequencies of various genetic disorders differ among geographic population groups. Carrier detection programs can be applied to different ethnic groups at risk for specific diseases (e.g., for Tay-Sachs disease in Ashkenazi Jewish populations, hemoglobinopathies in African Americans, and thalassemia in people of Mediterranean origin). The populations involved and the methods of screening are listed in Box 22.1.

Multifetal Gestations

Multifetal gestations have increased dramatically over the past generation, mainly resulting from advancements in artificial reproductive techniques (ARTs). These pregnancies are at greater risk for preterm delivery, and as a result contribute significantly to perinatal morbidity and mortality. In an effort to improve neonatal outcome, mainly through prolonging gestational age of delivery, select hospitals throughout the country offer multifetal reduction. This procedure involves the termination of one or more fetuses in a multifetal pregnancy in the effort to optimize outcome for the remaining fetus(es). Occasionally a multifetal pregnancy may include an aneuploid or anomalous fetus. Under these conditions, a selective termination is performed in which a particular fetus is targeted for termination.

PRENATAL DIAGNOSIS PROCEDURES

Amniocentesis

Amniotic fluid contains viable cells of fetal origin in addition to dissolved proteins and other chemicals. The first diagnosis of a chromosomal abnormality by amniotic fluid analysis was reported in 1967, and by the mid-1970s the safety and accuracy of midtrimester amniocentesis were well established. Midtrimester amniocentesis helped create the field of prenatal diagnosis and has become the gold standard to which other procedures for prenatal diagnosis are compared. Midtrimester amniocentesis is usually performed under ultrasound guidance at 16 weeks' gestation in an outpatient setting. Chromosome studies can be obtained by culturing the few viable cells present in amniotic fluid, and the results are generally available in 10 to 14 days. However, rapid karyotype analysis may be performed using fluorescent *in situ* hybridization (FISH) to determine the status of chromosomes 21, 18, 13, X, and Y in uncultured amniotic cells. This enables preliminary results to be given to the patient in 2 to 5 days and may be extremely helpful in patients with newly diagnosed fetal anomalies. Amniocentesis carries an estimated risk of fetal loss of 0.5% to 1.0%. Culture failure occurs in less than 1% of cases.

Chorionic Villus Sampling

The success of midtrimester amniocentesis initially led to a reduction in the emphasis placed on first-trimester diagnosis, but because of the inherent advantages of first-trimester fetal diagnosis, a few investigators continued to explore this approach. Moreover, the development of molecular methods of gene analysis focused more attention on first-trimester fetal tissue sampling.

Ultrasound guidance has been key to the success of chorionic villus sampling (CVS), and this sampling procedure is now done with a high success rate. Chorionic villi may be obtained by aspiration via a transcervical catheter or transabdominal needle using ultrasound guidance. The choice is based on placental location and operator preference and experience.

The main advantage of CVS over amniocentesis is the earlier availability of results, because the procedure is generally performed between 10 and 12 weeks' gestation. Performing amniocentesis at this gestational age is discouraged because of concerning data regarding fetal outcomes, specifically a high fetal loss rate and an increased risk of talipes equinovarus. An additional advantage of CVS is the increased amount of tissue obtained when compared with amniocentesis; this increased tissue mass is beneficial when DNA or enzymatic diagnosis is necessary. Results based on a direct preparation of spontaneously dividing cells are usually available in 24 to 48 hours, and final results from cultured cells in 10 to 14 days. However, amniocentesis must be used at the appropriate gestational age for assays in which amniotic fluid is essential (e.g., alpha-fetoprotein concentration).

Limb-reduction defects have been reported to occur with increased frequency in some series of CVS performed at 56 to 66 menstrual days. The proposed mechanism of the defects is a form of vascular insult leading to hypoperfusion of the fetus. However, this has not been a consistent finding. Although a time-sensitive relationship for limb defects is possible, and operator experience may be a factor, a causal relationship between CVS and limb defects is not firmly established.

Percutaneous Umbilical Blood Sampling

Fetal blood can be obtained from approximately 18 weeks' gestation with a 20- or 22-gauge spinal needle directed with ultrasound guidance into the umbilical cord. Access to the fetal circulation permits prenatal evaluation of many fetal hematologic abnormalities, including isoimmunization, hemoglobinopathies, thrombocytopenia, and coagulation factor abnormalities. Fetal blood can be used for the prenatal diagnosis of some inborn errors of metabolism and permits assessment of viral, bacterial, and parasitic infection by serology and culture. Fetal blood sampling may clarify chromosome mosaicism detected by cytogenetic analysis of amniotic fluid cells or chorionic villi.

Rapid karyotyping for congenital abnormalities is the most common indication for fetal blood sampling in the United States. Cytogenetic results usually are available from short-term fetal lymphocyte cultures within 48 to 72 hours.

The perinatal loss rate from percutaneous umbilical blood sampling (PUBS) is approximately 2% over the background risk to a particular fetus. Because many of the fetuses studied have severe congenital malformations, the background loss rate is high in comparison to the population undergoing amniocentesis or CVS. Because PUBS carries a substantially greater risk of pregnancy loss than amniocentesis, it should be reserved for those situations in which diagnostic information cannot be achieved by safer means.

Fetal Biopsy

Fetal biopsy was initially performed by fetoscopy but is now performed using ultrasound guidance. Certain genetic skin disorders, such as epidermolysis bullosa, that, at present, cannot be diagnosed by DNA analysis may be diagnosed with fetal skin sampling. Fetal muscle biopsy has been reported to diagnose Duchenne muscular dystrophy in a family that had uninformative DNA study results.

Assessing the safety and accuracy of fetal biopsy is difficult because experience is limited. Patients should be made aware of the investigational nature of the procedure. Rapid advances in DNA technology will delineate the molecular basis of many diseases that currently require fetal biopsy, and as this occurs, the need for these procedures will decline.

Ultrasound

Ultrasound is an important aid in assessing gestational age, monitoring fetal growth and health, confirming placental site, detecting multiple gestation, and diagnosing major fetal anomalies. Some teratogens and infections produce structural abnormalities that are potentially detectable with ultrasound but not with other prenatal diagnostic approaches. Visualization of fetal anatomy is essential in diagnosing anatomic defects inherited in a polygenic, multifactorial fashion. Individual centers report excellent results in ultrasound diagnosis of renal and bladder anomalies, hydrocephaly, and neural tube and ventral wall defects. Ultrasound is also useful in diagnosing mendelian disorders characterized by anatomic defects such as skeletal dysplasia, and common chromosomal abnormalities with associated phenotypic abnormalities (Box 22.2).

The most common major congenital abnormalities are cardiovascular malformations, which are among the major malformations most frequently missed by prenatal ultrasound. A

BOX 22.2   Sonographic Findings in Chromosomal Abnormalities

Trisomy 21
Duodenal atresia, tracheoesophageal fistula, esophageal atresia; polyhydramnios is used if these gastrointestinal lesions are present
Cardiac abnormalities (atrioventricular canal defects, ventricular septal defects, artrial septal defects)
Hypoplasia of middle quadrant of the fifth digit
Second-trimester findings: thickened nuchal fold greater than 5 mm; ratio of actual-to-expected femur length, 0.91

Trisomy 18
Intrauterine growth retardation
Polyhydramnios
Clenched hands with overlapping digits
Clubfeet, rocket-bottom feet
Cardiac abnormalities (ventricular septal defect)
Omphalocele diaphragmatic hernia
Choroid plexus cysts

Trisomy 13
Holoprosencephaly
Cleft lip and palate
Cardiac abnormalities (venticular septal defect)
Polydactyly
Omphalocele
Polycystic kidneys

---

four-chamber view of the fetal heart is suggested for ultrasound examination in pregnancy. The use of a four-chamber view in obstetric sonography has resulted in a significant increase in referrals to perinatal centers, which permits the delivery to take place at a center capable of caring for the newborn with congenital heart disease. When this image is obtained, approximately 60% of congenital heart defects can be diagnosed. The sensitivity is increased when outflow tracts are evaluated. Additionally, the role of nuchal translucency measurement in identifying fetuses at risk for congenital heart disease is under investigation.

When a fetal anomaly is diagnosed with ultrasound, echocardiography should be performed because fetuses with an extracardiac anomaly have a 23% risk of having a cardiac defect. Conversely, fetuses with a cardiac defect have a 25% to 45% risk of having another anatomic defect. Karyotype analysis should be offered in most cases of cardiac and extracardiac malformations, because approximately one-third will have a chromosomal disorder. Knowledge of abnormal karyotypes may significantly affect perinatal management and may also influence mode of delivery. Several of the aneuploid chromosomal defects exhibit characteristic ultrasonographic patterns (see Box 22.2). Karyotyping may not be necessary for all malformations detected with ultrasound (e.g., congenital adenomatoid degeneration of the lung or isolated pyelectasis).

Prenatal diagnosis often enables antenatal consultations with subspecialists, which can affect management decisions, in addition to influencing the timing, route, and location of delivery in an effort to maximize neonatal outcome. Occasionally, *in utero* treatment has been undertaken. Intrauterine shunts have been placed for bladder outlet obstruction and isolated pleural effusions. Open fetal surgery has been performed to manage congenital diaphragmatic hernia, open neural tube defects, and complete bladder obstruction. All of these interventions are investigational and their effects on outcome are unproven.

One of the most promising ultrasound techniques for early prenatal diagnosis currently being evaluated in the United States is nuchal translucency (NT). Nuchal translucency is the measurement of soft tissue in the posterior aspect of the fetus between the cervical spine and skin. An increased NT has been associated with Down syndrome. Although studies have varied regarding the ability to detect Down syndrome using NT, in general, using age and NT can detect approximately 80% of Down syndrome pregnancies. This noninvasive screening method is promising; however, the technique used to obtain the measurement is very specific, and without proper training, the sensitivity for detection appears to decrease significantly. In addition to Down syndrome, other congenital anomalies have also been found to be associated with an increased NT. These include other trisomies (13 and 18), Turner syndrome, sex chromosome aneuploidy, triploidy, cardiac anomalies, and genetic syndromes such as Noonan, Jarcho-Levin, and Smith-Lemli-Opitz.

Prenatal ultrasound also has a vital role in the monitoring of fetal well-being, especially after a condition with high likelihood of adverse outcome or a fetal abnormality has been diagnosed. Biophysical profile (BPP), which measures movement, tone, amniotic fluid volume, and breathing, along with Doppler studies assessing arterial and venous systems of the fetus may help identify those neonates with diminished reserve that may benefit either from increased surveillance or iatrogenic preterm delivery. More specifically, Doppler flow studies of the umbilical arteries are employed to monitor fetuses with intrauterine growth restriction. Doppler flow studies of the middle cerebral artery (MCA) are utilized to monitor the degree of anemia in fetuses with Rh isoimmunization, often assisting with timing of more invasive procedures such as PUBS.

Screening ultrasounds in low-risk pregnancies are commonly performed in the United States. Nevertheless, the data supporting the utility of anatomic surveys in this population are limited. In 1997, ACOG published its most recent guidelines on routine ultrasounds in low-risk pregnancies. These guidelines were generated following a review of studies published in the English language after 1985, including the well-known Helsinki study and the Routine Antenatal Diagnostic Imaging with Ultrasound (RADIUS) study. Although the specificity of an anatomic survey was found to exceed 99%, the sensitivity was highly dependent on the sonologist and the population surveyed (practice based versus hospital based). Both the Helsinki and RADIUS studies demonstrated detection rates that were more than twofold higher in the university-based hospitals compared with the nontertiary centers. Excluding elective terminations, routine ultrasound screening in low-risk populations has not been shown to significantly improve perinatal morbidity and mortality. Therefore, ACOG currently recommends that low-risk pregnancies undergo ultrasound only for specific indications.

Three-Dimensional Ultrasound

Three-dimensional (3-D) ultrasound uses multiplanar imaging and allows the examiner to move between different planes of interest. The technology complements ultrasound imaging by providing views traditionally seen only with magnetic resonance (MR) and computerized tomography (CT) scans. Although the images produced are considerably more enjoyable to expectant parents than their 2-D counterparts, the proper use of this technology is currently under investigation. Presently, 3-D ultrasound is utilized in the evaluation of fetal long bones, reducing the interference from signals generated by soft tissues. These images are also helpful in further defining anomalies detected on traditional sonograms. Moreover, 3-D ultrasound may expand the screening and diagnostic abilities of first-trimester ultrasound by allowing the examiner to view the fetus in optimal positions that are not always possible to obtain in real time, such as for NT measurements. As this technology continues to develop and sonographers and sonologists become more experienced, the role of 3-D ultrasound will likely expand.

Magnetic Resonance Imaging

Magnetic resonance imaging (MRI), a modality known as much for its ability to contrast soft tissue as for its lack of use of ionizing radiation, represents a recent addition to the techniques used in prenatal diagnosis. Initially, the application of MRI had been limited due to fetal motion; however, during the 1990s ultra-fast MRI sequences were developed. This eliminated many of these motion artifacts, allowing for better-quality studies. MRI can now be performed with images obtained in approximately 400 milliseconds, allowing fetal imaging to be accomplished without maternal or fetal sedation.

MRI is being used with greater frequency to confirm suspected clinical diagnoses and to provide additional information that may optimize prenatal counseling. The benefits of MRI include the ability to view a large field and use multiple planes for reconstruction of fetal structures, making complicated anomalies easier to visualize. Although fetal MRI is not currently indicated as a primary imaging method for any particular fetal anomaly, there are instances in which the information obtained may complement what is obtained with prenatal ultrasound examination. MRI has been extremely helpful in further clarifying abnormalities of the fetal central nervous system, neck, chest, abdomen, and pelvis, and in examination of the placenta. Among the diagnoses in which the imaging modality has been found useful are agenesis of the corpus callosum, congenital diaphragmatic hernia, congenital cystic adenomatoid malformation of the lung (CCAM), persistent cloaca, and placenta accreta. MRI is also especially useful when ultrasound examination of the fetus may be limited as a result of oligohydramnios.

Although there is no evidence MRI can produce harmful effects to the fetus, its safety has not been definitively proven by the Food and Drug Administration. Therefore, centers that use this modality as an adjunct to prenatal diagnosis limit its use until completion of the first trimester, avoiding exposure of rapidly dividing cells to possible teratogens.

Amniocentesis for Assessment of Fetal Lung Maturity

Iatrogenic preterm delivery still represents an important and preventable cause of respiratory distress syndrome. Fetal pulmonary maturity should be documented by some method before elective delivery, and this applies equally to the low- and high-risk patient. Certain clinical situations such as diabetes mellitus are known to be associated with delayed pulmonary maturation. When the lecithin-to-sphingomyelin ratio exceeds 2:1 and phosphatidyl glycerol is present, the chance of respiratory distress syndrome in the newborn of a diabetic patient is remarkably low.

The assessment of fetal lung maturity is important in determining the timing of a repeat cesarean delivery. For patients being considered for elective repeat cesarean deliveries, if one of the following criteria is met, fetal maturity may be assumed and amniocenteses need not be performed:

- Fetal heart tones have been documented for 20 weeks by fetoscope or for 30 weeks by Doppler.
- Thirty-six weeks have elapsed since a pregnancy test with a positive serum or urine human chorionic gonadotropin result was performed by a reliable laboratory.
- An ultrasound measurement of the fetal crown–rump length obtained at 6 to 11 weeks supports a gestational age of 39 weeks or more.
- An ultrasound obtained at 12 to 20 weeks confirms the gestational age of greater than 39 weeks determined by clinical history and physical examination.

Current Efficacy of Screening Methods

Chromosome analysis for the prenatal diagnosis of fetal aneuploidy is currently offered to women who will be 35 years or older at the time of delivery. Nearly all genetic procedures performed in the United States are performed in the 5% of women who are older than 35 years. This approach detects only 20% of cases of Down syndrome; the use of maternal serum alpha-fetoprotein screening in women of all ages identifies an additional 25% of cases. Use of maternal serum alpha-fetoprotein, human chorionic gonadotropin, unconjugated estriol, and maternal age identifies approximately 60% of cases of Down syndrome. Clinicians using a maternal serum alpha-fetoprotein screening program can expect to detect 80% to 90% of fetuses with neural tube defects, almost all cases of gastroschisis, and 70% to 80% of cases of omphalocele. The use of routine ultrasound screening, including a four-chamber view of the heart, potentially can diagnose approximately half of major cardiac, kidney, and bladder anomalies that would not be detected with maternal serum alpha-fetoprotein screening. When a targeted ultrasound examination is done to detect malformations suspected by history or screening ultrasonography in referral centers with skilled ultrasonologists, the sensitivity and specificity exceed 90%.

THE FUTURE

Noninvasive genetic testing is clearly the ideal alternative to invasive methods of diagnosis, which possess an inherent loss rate. First-trimester screening techniques will complement and perhaps even replace the current second-trimester tests, permitting women and families to exercise their reproductive choices earlier, reducing the risk of complications.

A novel technique for isolating fetal cells from maternal blood is currently under investigation in an effort to achieve this goal. This technique separates fetal cells from maternal blood through the identification of specific fetal cell surface antigens. It is hoped that further research in the methods of cell separation will allow noninvasive testing to replace its invasive counterparts.

With the completion of the mapping of the human genome, molecular genetic techniques may be available for the detection of many common monogenic disorders. Cost-effective screening will be the next goal for many new disorders. Preimplantation genetic diagnosis is a novel technique that provides results of genetic testing even before an embryo is placed in the uterus. In most cases, single cells or blastomeres are biopsied from embryos generated using assisted reproductive techniques and then analyzed for chromosomal abnormalities or single gene disorders. In addition, polar bodies can be biopsied from oocytes and subjected to similar analyses. These techniques can be offered to patients with significant family histories or to women of advanced maternal age undergoing fertility treatment to prevent abnormal offspring and increase implantation rates. The future of prenatal diagnosis will likely employ various techniques directed at preventing congenital disease rather than simply diagnosing it.

Suggested Readings

American College of Obstetricians and Gynecologists. Routine ultrasound in low-risk pregnancy. ACOG Practice Pattern No. 5. Washington, DC: ACOG, 1997.

Bianchi DW, Flint AF, Pizzimenfi MF, et al. Isolation of fetal DNA from nucleated erythrocytes in maternal blood. *Proc Natl Acad Sci USA* 1990;87:3279.

Bush MC, Eddleman KA. Multifetal pregnancy reduction and selective termination. *Clin Perinatol* 2003:623.

The Canadian Early and Midtrimester Amniocentesis Trial (CEMAT) Group. Randomized trial to assess safety and fetal outcome of early and midtrimester amniocentesis. *Lancet* 1998;351:242.

D'Alton ME, Caigo S, Biancho DW. Prenatal diagnosis. *Curr Probl Obstet Gynecol Fertil* 1994;March/April:41.

Firth HV, Boyd PA, Chamberlain P, et al. Severe limb abnormalities after chorion villus sampling at 56–66 days' gestation. *Lancet* 1991;337:762.

Froster UG, Baird PA. Limb-reduction defects and chorionic villus sampling. *Lancet* 1992;339:66.

Haddow JE, Palomaki GE, Knight GJ, et al. Prenatal screening for Down's syndrome with use of maternal serum markers. *N Engl J Med* 1992;327:588.

Hook EB, Cross PK, Schreinemacher MS. Chromosomal abnormality rates at amniocentesis and in live-born infants. *JAMA* 1983;249:2034.

Hyett JA, Clayton PT, Moscoso G, Nicolaides KH. Increased first trimester nuchal translucency as a prenatal manifestation of Smith-Lemli-Opitz syndrome. *Am J Med Genet* 1995;58:374.

Hyett JA, Perdu M, Sharland GK, et al. Increased nuchal translucency at 10–14 weeks of gestation as a marker for major cardiac defects. *Ultrasound Obstet Gynecol* 1997;10:242.

Levine D. Magnetic resonance imaging in prenatal diagnosis. *Curr Opin Pediatr* 2001;13:572.

Lockwood CJ, D'Alton ME, Platt LD, Bahado-Singh, R. New developments in OB ultrasound. *Contemp ob/gyn* 2001;46:12.

Merkatz IR, Nitowsky HM, Macri JN, Johnson WE. An association between low maternal serum alpha-fetoprotein and fetal chromosomal abnormalities. *Am J Obstet Gynecol* 1984;14:886.

Pretorius DH, Nelson TR. Three-dimensional ultrasound imaging in patient diagnosis and management: the future. *Ultrasound Obstet Gynecol* 1991;1:381.

Rhoads GG, Jackson LG, Schlesseiman SE, et al. The safety and efficacy of chorionic villus sampling for early prenatal diagnosis of cytogenetic abnormalities. *N Engl J Med* 1989;320:609.

Saari-Kemppainen A, Karjalainen O, Ylostalo P, Heinonen OP. Ultrasound screening and perinatal mortality: controlled trial of systematic one-stage screening in pregnancy. *Lancet* 1990;336:387.

U.S. Food and Drug Administration. Guidance for content and review of a magnetic resonance device 510 (k) application. Washington D.C.: U.S. FDA, Aug. 2, 1988.

Wald NJ, Cuckle HS. Maternal serum alpha-fetoprotein measurement in antenatal screening for anencephaly and spina bifida in early pregnancy. Report of the U.K. Collaborative Study on alpha-fetoprotein in relation to neural-tube defects. *Lancet* 1977;1:1323.

Watson JD. The Human Genome Project: past, present and future. *Science* 1990; 248:44.

Wenstrom KD, Owen J, Chu DC, Boots L. Prospective evaluation of free (beta)-subunit of human chorionic gonadotropin and dimeric inhibin-A for aneuploidy detection. *Am J Obstet Gynecol* 1999;181:887.

CHAPTER 23 ■ MANAGEMENT OF THE NORMAL NEWBORN

REGINA REYNOLDS, ELIZABETH H. THILO, AND ADAM A. ROSENBERG

The care and evaluation of the normal newborn infant includes an assessment of the mother's past and current pregnancy history, delivery care of the newborn, and a complete physical assessment of the newborn. Elements of normal newborn care involve a risk assessment for potential medical and social problems, monitoring of feeding and elimination during a 24- to 72-hour hospital stay, performance of routine screening tests, and the transition to home with adequate outpatient follow-up. The environment should promote maternal–infant bonding and be sensitive to the needs of both mother and infant.

HISTORY

The newborn infant history, no matter how brief, is always important. The history of this pregnancy, previous pregnancies, and the mother's and father's medical and genetic history are relevant. In the review of the current pregnancy, both antepartum and intrapartum events should be included, as well as the mother's medical history: age, gravidity, parity, chronic medical conditions, medications, diet, tobacco use, and acute illnesses during pregnancy. The results of the prenatal screening laboratory tests (Box 23.1), ultrasound examinations, amniocentesis information, and tests of fetal well-being (nonstress tests, fetal biophysical profiles, and Doppler assessment of fetal blood flow patterns) are important. These will help to assess the risk of asphyxia, congenital and genetic abnormalities, hyperbilirubinemia, hypoglycemia, and bacterial and viral infections. The social history will identify the mother's support system and readiness to care for a newborn infant. The family history may reveal an increased risk for genetic diseases and hyperbilirubinemia.

Preexisting diseases (e.g., asthma and diabetes mellitus) and pregnancy-specific conditions (e.g., pregnancy-induced hypertension, preeclampsia/eclampsia, preterm labor, vaginal bleeding, premature rupture of membranes, gestational diabetes, and acute infections) may alter fetal outcome. Maternal fever, fetal distress, meconium-stained fluid, type of delivery, and the infant's condition after delivery, including the need for resuscitation, are important.

DELIVERY ROOM MANAGEMENT

The infant should be dried under a radiant heat source. The nose and mouth should be suctioned as needed. The heart rate, respirations, and color should be evaluated. A cap should be placed to avoid heat loss. Resuscitation should be initiated if indicated. Apgar scores should be assigned. A stable infant can be bundled and given to the mother. Depending on the condition, the infant can either be left with the mother or taken to the nursery for closer observation and monitoring.

GROWTH AND GESTATIONAL AGE ASSESSMENT

Weight, length, and occipitofrontal circumference should be measured and plotted on an appropriate growth chart to determine the infant's growth percentiles for gestational age. Infants can be categorized as small for gestational age (SGA; less than or equal to 10% for weight), appropriate for gestational age (AGA), or large for gestational age (LGA; greater than or equal to 90% for weight). Categorization depends on the accuracy of the last menstrual period supported by an early obstetric ultrasound, if available. A postnatal examination can also be used to assess gestational age, because fetal physical characteristics and neurodevelopment progress in a predictable fashion (Fig. 23.1). Postnatal assignment of gestational age is generally within 2 weeks of the infant's actual gestational age.

If weight, length, and head circumference are all less than or equal to 10% in an SGA infant, the infant is symmetrically growth restricted. This implies a causative factor from early pregnancy such as a constitutionally small infant or a chromosomal disorder, drug or alcohol abuse, or viral infection. Asymmetric growth restriction (only the weight less than or equal to 10%) implies a causative factor later in pregnancy, such as pregnancy-induced hypertension or placental insufficiency. Asymmetric growth restriction tends to be associated with better later growth and developmental outcome.

Infants that are SGA or LGA are at increased risk for neonatal problems. SGA infants are at increased risk for fetal distress, hypoglycemia secondary to decreased glycogen stores, and polycythemia. LGA infants are at risk for birth trauma due to shoulder dystocia, hypoglycemia secondary to hyperinsulinemia, cardiomyopathy, and polycythemia.

INITIAL NEWBORN EXAMINATION

Much of a newborn's initial examination can be performed by inspection. For example, an infant breathing without chest wall retractions or grunting respirations with good skin color is unlikely to have underlying lung pathology. Much of the neurologic examination can also be accomplished by observation. Any previously unknown abnormalities should be pointed out to the parents at the time of discovery.

Cardiovascular

The cardiovascular examination should be performed first, ideally with the infant sleeping. Observation will show central cyanosis, the presence of which suggests congenital heart disease. Cyanosis of the hands and feet, or acrocyanosis, is normal in a newborn infant. Mild cyanosis around the mouth, or circumoral cyanosis, is normal if the tongue is pink. Next, the heart rate should be measured. A newborn heart rate can vary between 100 and 160 beats per minute while the infant is awake and quiet and may be as low as 75 to 80 beats per minute during sleep. Irregularities of rhythm are not uncommon; they usually result from premature atrial or ventricular contractions. The irregularity usually disappears when the infant becomes active and the heart rate increases. Heart murmurs in the first day of life are common and usually benign. On the other hand, congenital heart disease can be present without a murmur. Pulses should be palpated in both the upper and lower extremities. Diminished pulses in all extremities may be indicative of left ventricular dysfunction or critical aortic stenosis. Diminished femoral pulses when compared to brachial pulses suggest coarctation of the aorta or an interrupted aortic arch.

Chest and Lungs

The respiratory examination is also best accomplished when the infant is quiet. Again, observation of the chest and its movements can reveal much about the infant's status. One should

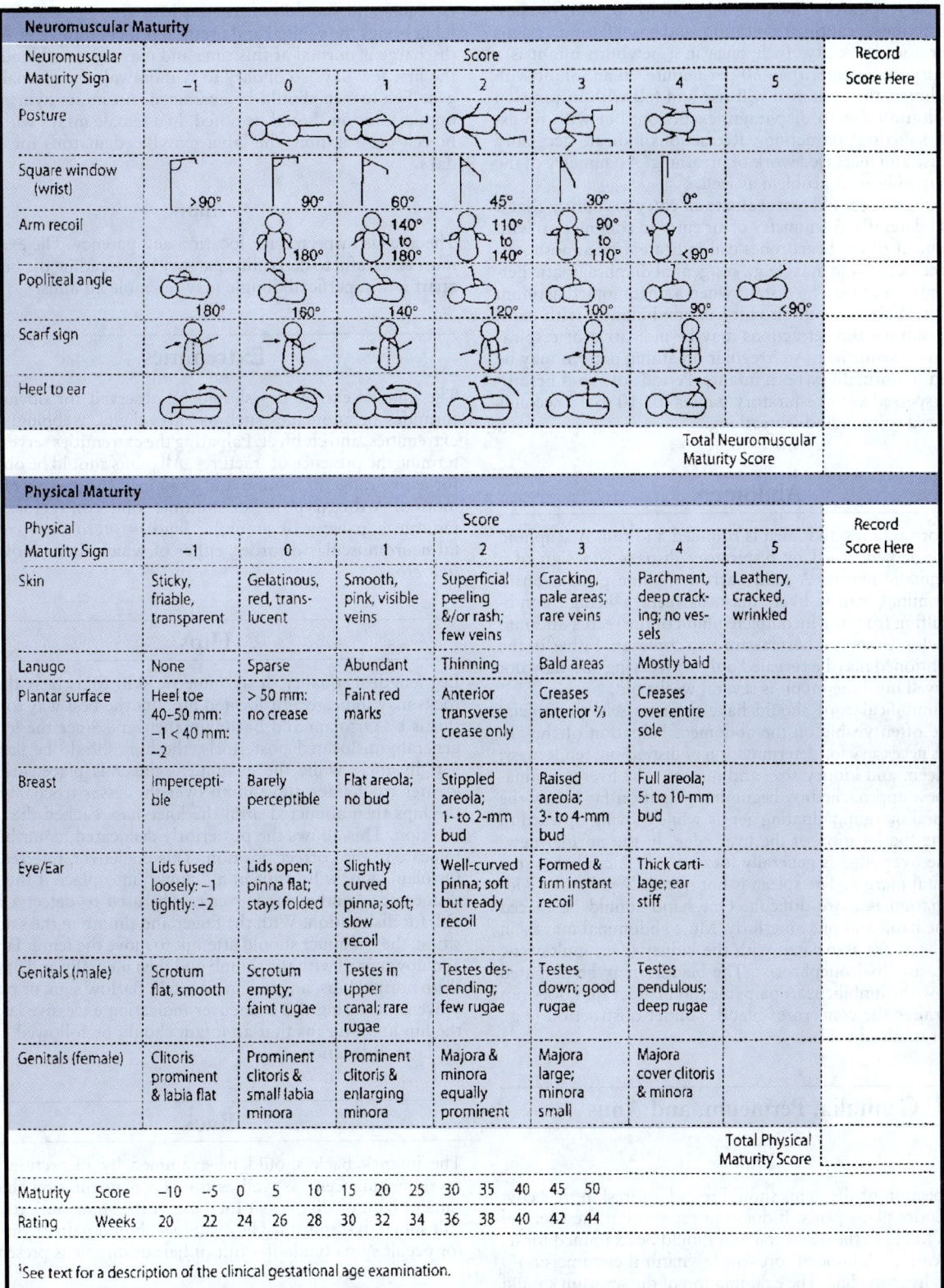

Neuromuscular Maturity

Neuromuscular Maturity Sign	Score							Record Score Here
	−1	0	1	2	3	4	5	
Posture								
Square window (wrist)	>90°	90°	60°	45°	30°	0°		
Arm recoil		180°	140° to 180°	110° to 140°	90° to 110°	<90°		
Popliteal angle	180°	160°	140°	120°	100°	90°	<90°	
Scarf sign								
Heel to ear								

Total Neuromuscular Maturity Score

Physical Maturity

Physical Maturity Sign	Score							Record Score Here
	−1	0	1	2	3	4	5	
Skin	Sticky, friable, transparent	Gelatinous, red, translucent	Smooth, pink, visible veins	Superficial peeling &/or rash; few veins	Cracking, pale areas; rare veins	Parchment, deep cracking; no vessels	Leathery, cracked, wrinkled	
Lanugo	None	Sparse	Abundant	Thinning	Bald areas	Mostly bald		
Plantar surface	Heel toe 40–50 mm: −1 < 40 mm: −2	> 50 mm: no crease	Faint red marks	Anterior transverse crease only	Creases anterior ⅔	Creases over entire sole		
Breast	Imperceptible	Barely perceptible	Flat areola; no bud	Stippled areola; 1- to 2-mm bud	Raised areola; 3- to 4-mm bud	Full areola; 5- to 10-mm bud		
Eye/Ear	Lids fused loosely: −1 tightly: −2	Lids open; pinna flat; stays folded	Slightly curved pinna; soft; slow recoil	Well-curved pinna; soft but ready recoil	Formed & firm instant recoil	Thick cartilage; ear stiff		
Genitals (male)	Scrotum flat, smooth	Scrotum empty; faint rugae	Testes in upper canal; rare rugae	Testes descending; few rugae	Testes down; good rugae	Testes pendulous; deep rugae		
Genitals (female)	Clitoris prominent & labia flat	Prominent clitoris & small labia minora	Prominent clitoris & enlarging minora	Majora & minora equally prominent	Majora large; minora small	Majora cover clitoris & minora		

Total Physical Maturity Score

Maturity	Score	−10	−5	0	5	10	15	20	25	30	35	40	45	50
Rating	Weeks	20	22	24	26	28	30	32	34	36	38	40	42	44

¹See text for a description of the clinical gestational age examination.

FIGURE 23.1. New Ballard score for assessment of fetal maturation of newly born infants. (From Ballard JL, Khoury JC, Wedig K et al. New Ballard score, expanded to included extremely premature infants. *J Pediatr* 1991;1119:417.)

observe for respiratory rate (normal = 30 to 60) and for chest wall retractions, grunting respiration, and nasal flaring as signs of respiratory difficulty. Tachypnea in a newborn infant is a respiratory rate greater than 60 per minute. In an infant with normal lungs, the abdomen will rise and fall with inspiration and expiration due to diaphragm excursion, but with no associated subcostal retractions. Retractions indicate accessory muscle use and increased work of breathing. Asymmetry of the chest may indicate a problem as well.

Auscultation should first evaluate air entry to confirm that it is equal bilaterally. Asymmetry of air entry in conjunction with displacement of the heart tones can indicate a pneumothorax or a space-occupying mass (e.g., congenital diaphragmatic hernia). Heart tones may be distant when a pneumomediastinum is present. A decrease in air entry in combination with expiratory grunting and retractions may be indicative of respiratory distress syndrome. An irregular breathing pattern may be observed in normal newborn infants. Periods of rapid breathing interspersed with respiratory pauses for 10 to 15 seconds are referred to as periodic breathing.

Abdomen

A newborn infant's abdomen is rounded and full. A scaphoid abdomen accompanied by respiratory distress is a sign of a diaphragmatic hernia. A mild narrow midline protrusion of the abdominal wall is likely diastasis recti, a benign condition resulting from the incomplete union of the rectus abdominus muscles. Umbilical hernias are also common. Either of the aforementioned may be revealed only with crying and may not be observed until the infant is several weeks old.

The umbilical cord should have three vessels. Superficial veins are often visible on the abdomen. Palpation of the abdomen is necessary for determination of distention; tenderness; liver, spleen, and kidney size; and masses. The liver examination is best approached by beginning palpation far below the right costal margin, palpating gently while moving upward to determine the location of the liver edge. In the normal newborn, the liver edge is generally located 1 to 2 cm below the right costal margin. The spleen is not normally palpable. Kidney palpation is more difficult. One hand should be placed under the flank and one anteriorly. Most abdominal masses in the newborn are associated with the kidney (e.g., multicystic or dysplastic, hydronephrosis). The bladder may be palpated just below the umbilicus. A palpable full bladder that does not resolve raises the concern of bladder outlet obstruction (e.g., posterior urethral valves).

Genitalia, Perineum, and Anus

Male

The inspection of the penis should reveal a foreskin that covers the entire glans penis. It does not retract, but the urethral orifice is found at the distal end and should be examined for its exact location. A hooded foreskin (a "natural circumcision") indicates hypospadias. The examination of the scrotum should include size and degree of rugation. Palpation of the testes notes their location and size. The size of the penis and scrotum, the degree of scrotal rugation, and the location of the testes change with gestational age (Fig. 23.1).

Female

Inspection of the female external genitalia is best accomplished with the legs in frog-leg position. The labia majora usually cover the labia minora completely in a term infant. The clitoris is visible and should be examined for size. Separation of the labia brings the vaginal and urethral orifices into view. A white discharge is normal at this time and may become bloody over the first few days secondary to withdrawal of maternal estrogen. The hymen should be examined. An intact hymen without perforation should be noted. In a female infant with frank breech presentation, the labia may be edematous for several days.

Anus

The anus is inspected for location and patency. The examiner must be careful to determine patency by spreading the buttocks apart as a superficial dimple may resemble an anus.

Extremities

The infant's extremities should be observed for obvious deformities or anomalies such as extra digits, webbing, absent extremities, and clubfeet. Palpating the extremities serves to determine the presence of fractures. All joints should be observed for active range of motion and examined for passive range of motion. Arthrogryposis, or multiple joint contractures, may indicate a paucity of amniotic fluid *in utero* or a congenital neuromuscular disorder, either of which limits movement *in utero*.

Hips

Leg length inequality or asymmetric skin folds near the buttocks may indicate a dislocated hip, but the best way to assess this is by Ortolani and Barlow maneuvers. Since the femur is generally dislocated posteriorly, the hips should be flexed to a right angle while the examiner's finger is placed over the greater trochanter and thumb over the lesser trochanter and the hips then abducted until the knee has reached the lateral position. This allows the posteriorly dislocated femur head to relocate to the correct position. This maneuver, referred to as Ortolani sign, will result in a "clunk" into place if the hip is dislocated. Another maneuver can be used to detect a hip at risk for dislocation. With the finger and thumb in the same position, the examiner should attempt to move the femur laterally and downward with the thumb and then medially and upward. With normal hips, no movement is felt. Barlow sign, or positive movement during this maneuver indicating excessive laxity in the hip joint, means that an infant should be followed closely for later dislocation.

Back

The infant's back should be examined by inspection for a myelomeningocele, as well as for skin pigmentation changes, tufts of hair, or dimples at the base of the spine indicating occult spinal dysraphism. The examiner should palpate the spine for occult spina bifida if a tuft of hair or dimple is present.

Neck

The neck should be inspected for fistulas or cysts. Palpation can reveal the position of the trachea and lymph nodes or masses. The clavicles should be palpated for crepitus indicating a fracture. The examiner should be sure the neck is supple with full range of motion. Neck masses anterior to the sternocleidomastoid muscle represent branchial cleft remnants; posterior to the muscle, cystic hygromas; and within the muscle, a hematoma.

Redundant skin or webbing of the neck may be seen in Turner syndrome.

Head

Molding may be caused by the pressure of the birth canal on the infant's skull. This will resolve with time, but should be distinguished from other birth injuries involving the skull. Caput succedaneum is edema that crosses suture lines, while a cephalohematoma is bleeding contained by suture lines because it is under the periosteum. A subgaleal hemorrhage is fluctuant and results in blood accumulation beneath the scalp in a large space. The fontanelles should be examined for presence and size. The anterior fontanelle can range in size from 1 to 4 cm. The posterior fontanelle is generally closed to less than 1 cm in a term infant. A third fontanelle may be palpated as a bony defect in the sagittal suture of the parietal bones and can be associated with trisomy 21. Sutures should be palpated to confirm they are freely mobile.

Eyes

A newborn infant's eyelids may be edematous, making the eye examination difficult. A complete examination can be done after the edema resolves. Turning off an overhead light and holding the infant upright to face the examiner may provoke an infant to open his or her eyes. The infant's eyes should have full range of motion when the head is turned from side to side. Dysconjugate eye movements may be present but should not persist. Subconjunctival hemorrhages may be present. Pupils should react to light, and the red reflexes should be symmetrical. If asymmetry, dark spots, or a white reflex is noted, the infant should be examined by an ophthalmologist. The iris should be examined for Brushfield spots and colobomas.

Nose

The nose is subject to trauma from passage through the birth canal; therefore, the size, shape, and any deformities (e.g., deviated septum) should be noted. Patency of the nares is assessed by placing a chilled metal surface underneath the nares and observing fog on the metal surface. Bilateral choanal atresia results in respiratory distress and cyanosis that resolves with crying.

Ears

Ears should be inspected for form, size, position, and rotation. Malformation and malposition may be associated with chromosomal and syndromic variants. Preauricular pits and tags should alert the examiner to the possibility of hearing loss and renal anomalies. The ear canal should be examined for patency and the tympanic membrane visualized if possible.

Mouth

The palate should be inspected and palpated for the presence of a submucous cleft. Ebstein pearls are small white cysts located medially at the junction of the hard and soft palate. Natal teeth are occasionally found. Some infants have a short frenulum and the tongue does not protrude well, but the infant should be observed while feeding before intervention is warranted. The mouth may be asymmetric from facial nerve palsy or an absent angularis oris muscle.

Skin

At birth, the newborn infant is often covered in white-yellow vernix caseosa, and may have fine lanugo hair over the shoulders and upper back. Dry, cracked, or peeling skin is seen with postterm pregnancy. Bruising and petechiae over the presenting part can result from the birth process, but petechiae over the entire body warrant further investigation. Generalized cyanosis merits immediate evaluation and is discussed in the cardiovascular examination section. Pallor indicates blood loss, either acute or chronic, or shock. Generalized redness of the skin, plethora, is associated with polycythemia. Jaundice presenting in the first 24 hours is abnormal and merits evaluation. Other skin abnormalities are discussed in Chapter 68.

Neurologic Examination

As stated previously, much of the neurologic examination can be obtained from observation and from the infant's responses during the rest of the physical examination. The infant should be moving all extremities and the facial movements should be symmetric. Tone, cry, and alertness are easily defined as well. The normal newborn is born with a set of reflexes that diminish over the first few months of life. The reflexes, listed in Box 23.2, are indicative of the peripheral nervous system. Central nervous system damage, systemic disease, or congenital neuromuscular

---

BOX 23.2   Newborn Reflexes

- Sucking reflex—a response to a nipple or gloved finger being placed in mouth. This reflex develops by 14 weeks' gestation.
- Rooting reflex—the turning of the head to the side of a facial stimulus. This reflex develops by 28 weeks' gestation.
- Palmar and plantar grasp—the grasp that occurs in response to something being placed in the infant's hand or touching the underside of the foot. This reflex develops by 28 weeks' gestation and disappears by 4 months of age.
- Traction response—as the infant is pulled upright to a sitting position, the head initially lags, and then active flexion brings the head into midline position.
- Placing response—the infant's foot is placed under a surface such as a table edge. The infant will respond by lifting the leg to place the foot on the surface when the top of the foot is touched.
- Moro reflex—this reflex is elicited by lifting the infant's arms off the examining surface and then releasing them simultaneously and quickly. The infant should respond with extension and abduction of the upper extremities and flexion and mild abduction of the lower extremities, followed by adduction of the upper extremities.
- Tonic neck reflex—turning the infants head to one side will cause the arm and leg on that side to extend while the contralateral arm and leg flex, giving the appearance of a fencing position.
- Deep tendon reflexes—a Babinski response is normal until 18 months of age, and clonus is often elicited but should not be sustained.

disorders may not be reflected by the presence or absence of these reflexes alone.

CARE OF THE WELL NEWBORN INFANT

The goals of the newborn nursery are to create an environment to promote mother–infant bonding, establish feeding, and teach techniques of newborn care. All of these goals are facilitated by combined mother–baby care that is prevalent in most institutions. Surveillance of the infant by the staff is also an important facet of newborn care. The staff must be vigilant for signs and symptoms of illness, including temperature instability, change in activity, refusal to feed, pallor, cyanosis, early or excessive jaundice, tachypnea and respiratory distress, delayed (beyond 24 hours) passage of the first stool or urine, and bilious vomiting. Other elements of routine care include eye prophylaxis for gonococcal ophthalmia with erythromycin ointment and administration of 1 mg of vitamin K intramuscularly to prevent hemorrhagic disease. All infants should be vaccinated against hepatitis B as described in Chapter 77. Cord blood is collected in all infants and used for blood typing and Coombs testing in infants born to type O or Rh-negative mothers.

Rapid glucose testing should be done in at-risk infants (e.g., infants of diabetic mothers; slightly preterm, SGA, LGA, or stressed infants). Values less than 45 mg/dL should be confirmed with a laboratory determination of blood glucose. In infants with clinical signs of anemia or polycythemia, a hematocrit should be measured at 3 to 6 hours of age. State-mandated newborn genetic screening is done prior to discharge. Screening protocols vary from state to state. Many screen for phenylketonuria (PKU), galactosemia, sickle cell disease, cystic fibrosis, hypothyroidism, and congenital adrenal hyperplasia. In many states a second screen is done at 8 to 14 days because a screening test for PKU prior to 48 hours of age may be falsely negative. Hearing testing is also performed prior to discharge.

Standard teaching for newborn care includes advice for umbilical cord care. This may include application of alcohol to promote drying of the cord or simply leaving the umbilical stump open to air. Parents should be counseled about recognition of a fever and other signs of illness and avoidance of contagious illnesses. They should understand normal feeding and elimination patterns, diaper care, foreskin and circumcision care, crying and normal sleep–wake cycles, sleeping in the supine position, bathing techniques, and skin care. They should be taught to use a bulb syringe to clear the nose and cautioned about exposure to the sun and avoidance of tobacco smoke. They also should be counseled about automobile safety.

FEEDING THE WELL NEWBORN INFANT

The healthy term infant will feed every 2 to 5 hours on demand. The first feeding will usually occur by 3 hours of age. Breast milk is the diet of choice, but a standard 20 cal/oz infant formula is adequate. Intake gradually increases over the first 3 days to about 100 mL/kg/day. Table 23.1 provides the normal expected patterns of feeding and elimination of the breast-fed infant. The benefits of breast-feeding are shown in Box 23.3.

Contraindications to breast-feeding are maternal human immunodeficiency virus (HIV) infection, active herpes breast infection, active maternal tuberculosis, infant galactosemia, and certain maternal drug exposures (e.g., amphetamines, chemotherapy agents, cocaine, and heroin). Hospital practices that facilitate successful breast-feeding include joint mother-baby care, avoiding the use of pacifiers and supplemental formula, and providing lactation consultation. It is important that an experienced professional observe and assist with at least one feeding to prevent problems such as sore nipples, unsatisfied babies, engorgement, and poor milk supply.

COMMON PROBLEMS IN THE TERM NEWBORN

There are a number of common medical problems in the normal newborn. These are discussed in other chapters but merit brief mention here. The most common problem is jaundice. This can be seen related to bruising or cephalohematomas, polycythemia, poor enteral intake such as "lack of breast milk" jaundice, and hemolysis. Blood typing and a Coombs test are justified in all newborns born to mothers with either type O blood or who are Rh negative. Infants who develop jaundice in the first 24 hours of life should have a serum bilirubin determination and should be evaluated for causation (see Chapter 26). Jaundice in the second 24 hours of life should be evaluated and the serum bilirubin charted by hour of age to assess the need for later intervention and the timing of outpatient follow-up (Fig. 23.2). Phototherapy can be considered for infants in the greater than 95th percentile for serum bilirubin on the hour-specific nomogram (8 mg/dL at 24 hours, 13 mg/dL at 48 hours, and 16 mg/dL at 72 hours).

Screening for hypoglycemia is based on risk or clinical signs. SGA and LGA infants as well as those who have had a difficult delivery or other physiologic stress should have a blood glucose determination. Whole blood glucose values less than 45 mg % or 45 mg/dl after a feeding will require intravenous glucose. Hematocrit measurement should only be done in infants likely to have anemia (based on a history of blood loss, hemolysis, or clinical signs such as pallor and hypotension) or polycythemia (based on risk factors such as intrauterine growth restriction or maternal diabetes or clinical signs such as plethora or tachypnea).

Respiratory problems in the newborn nursery are usually due to transient tachypnea (retained lung fluid), aspiration syndromes, pneumothorax, and pneumonia (see Chapter 41). Any infant with persisting tachypnea or with respiratory distress and cyanosis in room air should be transferred to an intensive care unit. Pneumonia should be suspected in an infant born to a mother with chorioamnionitis or who has a positive vaginal culture for group B streptococcus and has not been treated with appropriate antibiotics for more than 4 hours prior to the birth of the infant. Congenital heart disease in the newborn may present with either cyanosis not responsive to supplemental oxygen or poor perfusion and respiratory distress with poor pulses (see Chapter 53). Heart murmurs in the first days of life rarely indicate a structural heart problem. If the infant is pink and well perfused and has no respiratory distress and palpable, symmetric pulses, the murmur is most likely transitional. Transitional murmurs are soft (grade 1 to 2 of 6), heard at the upper left to midsternal border, and generally loudest in the first 24 hours after birth. If the murmur is more prominent than grade 2 of 6 or persists beyond 24 hours, if blood pressures in the right arm and leg differ by greater than 15 mm Hg, or if the pulses in the lower extremities are difficult to palpate, a cardiology consultation should be arranged.

The initial evaluation of birth trauma after a difficult delivery will occur in the newborn nursery. The most common injuries are soft tissue bruising, fractures (clavicle, humerus, or femur), and cervical plexus palsies. Cranial injuries include

TABLE 23.1

GUIDELINES FOR SUCCESSFUL BREAST FEEDING[1]

	First 8 Hours	8–24 Hours	Day 2	Day 3	Day 4	Day 5	Day 6 Onward
Milk supply	You may be able to express a few drops of milk.		Milk should come in between the second and fourth days.			Milk should be in. Breasts may be firm or leak milk.	Breasts should feel softer after feedings.
Baby's activity	Baby is usually wide-awake in the first hour of life. Put baby to breast within 30 minutes after birth.	Wake up your baby. Babies may not wake up on their own to feed.	Baby should be more cooperative and less sleepy.	Look for early feeding cues such as rooting, lip smacking, and hands to face.			Baby should appear satisfied after feedings.
Feeding routine	Baby may go into a deep sleep 2–4 hours after birth.	Feed your baby every 1–4 hours or as often as wanted—at least 8–12 times a day.	Use chart to write down time of each feeding.			May go one longer interval (up to 5 hours between feeds) in a 24-hour period.	
Breast-feeding	Baby will wake up and be alert and responsive for several more hours after initial deep sleep.	As long as you are comfortable, nurse at both breasts as long as baby is actively sucking.	Try to nurse both sides each feeding, aiming at 10 minutes per side. Expect some nipple tenderness.	Consider hand expressing or pumping a few drops of milk to soften the nipple if the breast is too firm for the baby to latch on.	Nurse a minimum of 10–30 minutes per side every feeding for the first few weeks of life. Once your supply is well established, allow your baby to finish the first breast before offering the second.		Nipple tenderness is improving or is gone.
Baby's urine output		Baby must have a minimum of one wet diaper in first 24 hours.	Baby must have at least one wet diaper every 8–11 hours.	You should see an increase in wet diapers (up to four to six) in 24 hours.	Baby's urine should be light yellow.	Baby should have six to eight wet diapers per day of colorless or light yellow urine.	
Baby's stool		Baby should have a black-green (meconium) stool.	Baby may have a second very dark (meconium) stool.	Baby's stools should be in transition from black-green to yellow.		Baby should have three or four yellow, seedy stools a day.	The number of stools may decrease gradually after 4–6 weeks of life.

[1] Modified, with permission from L. Gabrielski, RN MSN IBCLC, Lactation Support Services, The Children's Hospital, Denver, 1999.

BOX 23.3 — Benefits of Breast-feeding

Is a natural, easily digested milk optimal for infant growth and development
Enhances mother–infant interaction
Protects against infant illnesses
Enhances cognitive development

---

cephalohematoma and subgaleal hemorrhage. Bleeding into the large subgaleal space is associated with difficult operative vaginal deliveries and repeated attempts at vacuum extraction. It can lead to hypovolemic shock and death. Any infant with freely moving fluid under the scalp needs close observation to monitor for an increase in the fluid collection and the need for replacement of blood volume and clotting factors.

Drug-exposed infants are evaluated and managed in the newborn nursery. The drugs most commonly abused are tobacco, alcohol, marijuana, cocaine, methamphetamine and narcotics. An infant with clinical signs consistent with drug withdrawal should have a urine and meconium toxicology screen sent. Suspicious clinical history includes placental abruption, poor prenatal care, and intrauterine growth restriction. Clinical signs include irritability, hyperactivity, incessant hunger, diarrhea, and jitteriness or seizures. These infants should be swaddled in a quiet, low-light environment. Exces-

sive irritability can be managed with phenobarbital (15 to 20 mg/kg loading dose, followed by 3 to 5 mg/kg/day). If diarrhea and weight loss are prominent in the narcotic-addicted infant, tincture of opium (25-fold dilution to 0.4 mg/mL morphine equivalent; 0.1 mg/kg every 4 hours to start) titrated to improvement in symptoms measured by a withdrawal score, or methadone 0.05 to 0.1 mg/kg every 6 hours can be used. Treatment is tapered over several days to weeks depending on severity.

DISCHARGE OF THE NEWBORN INFANT

Discharge at 24 to 48 hours is safe if there are no contraindications (Box 23.4) and a follow-up visit at 48 to 72 hours after discharge is arranged. Most infants with severe cardiorespiratory disorders, infections, and other transitional problems are identified in the first 6 hours of life. Problems such as breast-feeding difficulties and jaundice can be anticipated and handled with close outpatient follow-up plans.

CIRCUMCISION

Circumcision is an elective procedure performed in healthy, stable infants. Potential medical benefits include prevention of phimosis, paraphimosis, balanoposthitis, and urinary tract infections. Later benefits include decreased incidence of cancer of the penis and sexually transmitted diseases. Most parents elect to have a circumcision for nonmedical reasons. The procedural

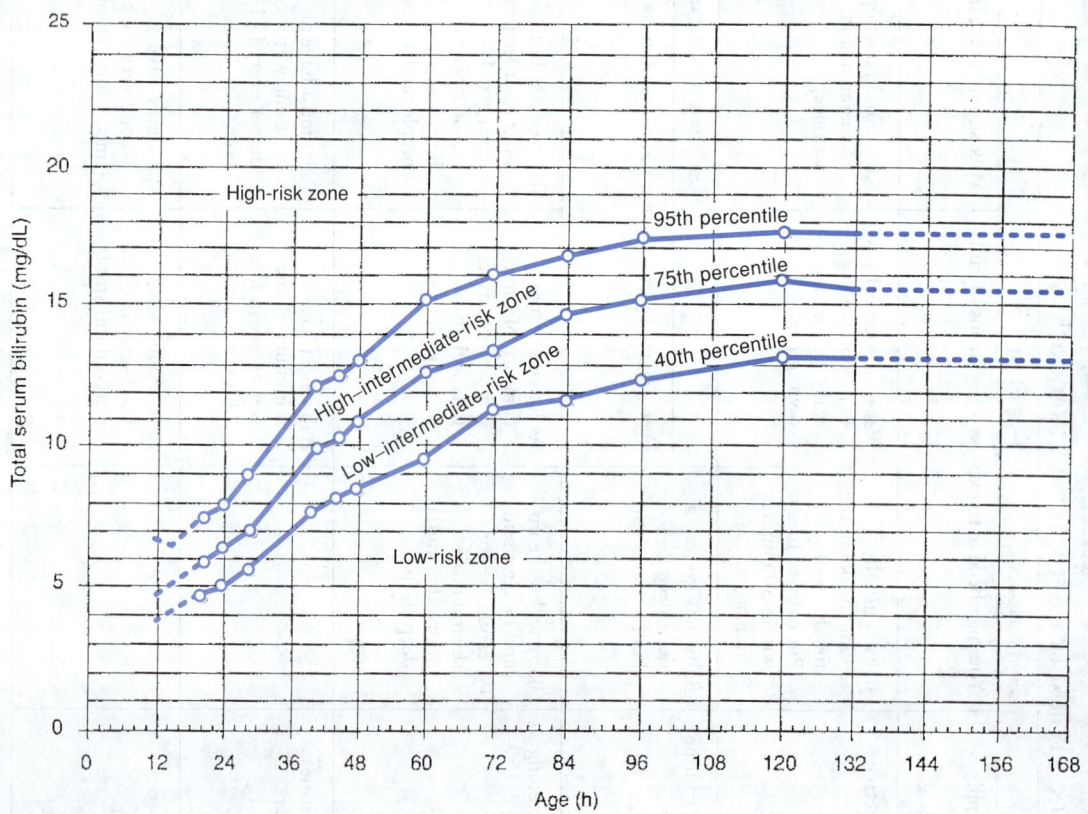

FIGURE 23.2. Risk designation of term and near-term newborns based on their hour-specific bilirubin values. (Reproduced from Bhutani VK, Johnson L, and Silvieri EM. Predictive ability of a predischarge hour-specific serum bilirubin test for subsequent significant hyperbilirubinemia in health term and near-term newborns. *Pediatrics* 1999;103:61.)

BOX 23.4	Criteria for Discharge at Less Than 48 Hours

Contraindications
Jaundice at less than 24 hours
High risk for infection (maternal chorioamnionitis or inadequate group B streptococcus prophylaxis)*
Known or suspected narcotic addiction or withdrawal
Physical defects requiring evaluation
Oral defects impairing feeding

Relative contraindications (infants at risk for feeding problems or excessive jaundice)
Prematurity or borderline prematurity (less than 38 weeks' gestation)
Birth weight less than 2,700 g
Baby not arousing for feeds; not demanding regularly
Medical or neurologic problems
Twins or higher multiples
ABO blood group incompatibility or severe jaundice in a previous child
Mother with breast-feeding problems with a prior infant
Breast-feeding mother with breast surgery involving periareolar areas

---

*Discharge may be allowed at 24–36 hours with a completely normal transition.

BOX 23.5	Take-home Points

Growth for gestational age should be obtained in all newborns to assess risks for certain newborn problems (e.g., hypoglycemia).
A careful and complete physical examination should be done in all newborn infants.
All newborns should undergo certain screening tests: newborn genetic diseases screen, hearing screen, and blood typing with Coombs testing in babies born to mothers with type O or Rh-negative blood.
Newborns should be carefully monitored for jaundice and clinical signs of infection (especially with maternal chorioamnionitis or with positive group B streptococcus cultures).
Feeding needs to be carefully assessed, especially in the breast-fed infant.
A 48-hour follow-up visit should be scheduled after discharge to reassess feeding and degree of jaundice.

CONCLUSION

A list of important points from the chapter are highlighted in Box 23.5.

Suggested Readings

American Academy of Pediatrics. Group B streptococcal infections. In: *RedBook 2003 Report of the Committee on Infectious Diseases,* 26th ed. Elk Grove Village, IL: American Academy of Pediatrics, 2003:584.
American Academy of Pediatrics, Subcommittee on Hyperbilirubinemia. Management of hyperbilirubinemia in the newborn infant 35 or more weeks of gestation. *Pediatrics* 2004;114:297.
Thureen PJ, Deacon J, Hernandez JA, et al., eds. *Assessment and care of the well newborn,* 2nd ed. Philadelphia: Elsevier, 2005.

risks include infection, bleeding, removal of too much skin, and urethral injury. The combined incidence of these complications is less than 1%. Local anesthesia with a dorsal penile nerve block or circumferential ring block should be done with 1% lidocaine. Techniques that allow visualization of the glans (e.g., Plastibell or Gomco) are preferred to blind techniques (e.g., Mogan clamp). Circumcision is contraindicated in infants with hypospadias, epispadius, and chordee.

---

d: NEWBORN INTENSIVE CARE

CHAPTER 24 ■ THE NEWBORN INTENSIVE CARE UNIT

RICHARD A. EHRENKRANZ

Newborn intensive care developed from the concept that a more intensive approach to neonates who require special care (both preterm infants and full-term infants with medical or surgical problems) would result in a significant decrease in neonatal morbidity and mortality. The first newborn special care unit was established at Yale–New Haven Hospital (YNHH) in 1960, and the subspecialty of neonatology evolved during the following years. Remarkable advances have been made in the care of neonates, and about 900 newborn special care units or newborn intensive care units (NICUs) have been established; each provides essentially everything necessary for the life support of a preterm or sick neonate. Many of the advances in neonatal care have been based on research in developmental physiology, biochemistry, pharmacology, and nutrition, which has increased manyfold the understanding of the uniqueness of neonates, particularly of the very low-birth-weight infant. In addition, advances in medical technology have led to the development and neonatal application of life-support systems, monitors, equipment, and techniques such as ultrasound, computed tomography, and magnetic resonance imaging.

In many university and large community hospitals today, newborn intensive care is just one component of a perinatal center. Such a center also includes facilities for prenatal evaluation, observation, and care of the fetus and mother both before and during labor; facilities for observation of neonates at risk of difficulties during their adaptation to the extrauterine environment; and facilities for continuing and rehabilitative care of growing preterm infants and of infants recovering from acute problems. In some perinatal centers, observation of high-risk neonates is done within the NICU; in others, within a transitional nursery. In addition, the perinatal center has become a regional resource, accepting transfers of women in premature labor, with toxemia, or with other risk factors that indicate the probable need of maternal or neonatal special care or observation, and accepting transfers of neonates who are preterm or have other medical or surgical problems.

Finally, a NICU may exist in a hospital without an obstetric service (e.g., a free-standing children's hospital) and then provides care only for transferred neonates.

CHARACTERISTICS OF NEWBORN INTENSIVE CARE UNIT PATIENTS

A large percentage of neonates admitted to NICUs are preterm infants. However, any infant who requires or may require the special attention available within a NICU is an appropriate admission. Because many neonatal problems can be anticipated before delivery, communication between the obstetric and pediatric members of the perinatal center (the perinatologists and the neonatologists, respectively) is essential to optimize management plans.

Factors associated with high-risk pregnancies and infants are listed in Tables 24.1 and 24.2. High-risk pregnancy is associated with social and lifestyle characteristics of the pregnant woman, such as her socioeconomic status, and with her prior obstetric and medical history, such as a history of premature labor or delivery or diabetes mellitus. Some of these factors have been shown to adversely affect maternal well-being with increasing gestation and necessitate a preterm delivery for maternal indications. Other factors develop during the pregnancy or are recognized during the process of labor and delivery, such as oligohydramnios, polyhydramnios, preeclampsia and eclampsia, or meconium staining of the amniotic fluid. The prevalence of second-trimester ultrasound examinations has led to the antenatal diagnosis of many congenital malformations, including diaphragmatic hernia, omphalocele, gastroschisis, and cardiac defects such as hypoplastic left heart syndrome and transposition of the great vessels. However, unexpected medical or surgical problems may be recognized in the immediate neonatal period. Because these risk factors and problems correlate with an increased incidence of fetal and neonatal problems and account for a substantial percentage of perinatal mortality and morbidity, most of these high-risk infants are admitted to a NICU for observation, diagnosis, and management.

TABLE 24.1

FACTORS ASSOCIATED WITH HIGH-RISK PREGNANCIES AND INFANTS: SOCIAL AND HISTORICAL

Maternal social and lifestyle characteristics
Age less than 16 or greater than 40 years
Alcohol or substance abuse
Low socioeconomic status
Noncompliance with health care system(s)
Obesity
Poor diet
Poor physical fitness
Single parent
Smoking

Obstetric history
Infertility
Multiparity, especially grand multiparity (more than six pregnancies lasting beyond 20 weeks)
Rh or other blood group sensitization
Previous pregnancies with
    Abnormal presentation
    Antepartum bleeding after first trimester
    Cephalopelvic disproportion
    Cesarean section delivery or instrumented delivery other than elective low-forceps
    Gestational diabetes mellitus
    Poor pregnancy outcome, including multiple spontaneous abortions, fetal or neonatal death
    Postterm delivery
Preeclampsia/eclampsia
Premature labor or delivery
Premature rupture of fetal membranes
Prolonged labor
Previous infant with congenital malformation, genetic disorder, mental retardation, cerebral palsy
Primary or recurrent genital herpes simplex infection

Medical history
Anemia, nutritional (e.g., iron, folate, or vitamin B_{12} deficiency), or hemoglobinopathy
Cardiovascular disease, congenital or acquired
Collagen vascular disease
Diabetes mellitus, insulin-dependent or diet-controlled
Epilepsy
Hereditary disorders
Hypertension
Hyperthyroidism
Hyperparathyroidism and hypoparathyroidism
Idiopathic thrombocytopenic purpura
Myasthenia gravis
Neoplasia
Pulmonary disorders, especially if associated with frequent episodes of hypoxemia or hypercapnia
Renal disease
Other chronic diseases or disorders requiring continued pharmacologic therapy

Regional Organization of Perinatal Care

Table 24.3 correlates neonatal patient types with the level of perinatal services to be provided by a hospital. Such categorization of perinatal care levels was designated by the first Committee on Perinatal Health in a 1976 publication, *Toward Improving the Outcome of Pregnancy,* and was useful in the development and organization of coordinated regional perinatal

TABLE 24.2

FACTORS ASSOCIATED WITH HIGH-RISK PREGNANCIES AND INFANTS: CURRENT PREGNANCY LABOR AND DELIVERY AND NEONATAL

Current pregnancy
Abnormal biophysical profile
Abnormal fetal growth, intrauterine growth retardation, or
    macrosomia
Age less than 16 or greater than 40 years
Alcohol or substance abuse
Decreased fetal movement
Exacerbation of preexisting medical disorder
Fetal arrhythmia or spontaneous decelerations
Infection: bacterial (gonorrhea, syphilis, tuberculosis), viral
    (rubella, cytomegalovirus, varicella-zoster), parasitic
    (toxoplasmosis)
Intrauterine diagnosis or suspicion of anomaly or genetic
    disorder
Multiple gestation
Oligohydramnios
Polyhydramnios
Rh or other blood group sensitization
Smoking
Surgery and anesthesia
Vaginal bleeding from abruptio placentae or placenta previa
Vaginal colonization with chlamydia, *Ureaplasma*, or group B
    betahemolytic streptococci

Labor and delivery
Abnormal presentation
Acute blood loss at delivery
Amnionitis
Cesarean section delivery (especially if not elective repeat)
Fetal heart rate abnormalities
Fetal pulmonic immaturity
Fetal scalp pH <7.2
Instrumented delivery other than elective low-forceps
Meconium staining of amniotic fluid
Preeclampsia/eclampsia
Premature or prolonged rupture of the fetal membranes
Premature labor
Prolapsed umbilical cord
Prolonged labor

Neonatal
Apgar score at 5 minutes <3, or lack of spontaneous
    respiratory activity for longer than 5 minutes
Birth weight <2,500 g (especially <1,500 g) or >4,000 g
Birth weight-gestational age discrepancy (small for gestational
    age, large for gestational age)
Hemodynamic instability
Major congenital malformations, such as abdominal wall
    defects, cardiac defects, central nervous system defects,
    diaphragmatic, hernia, tracheoesophageal fistula with
    esophageal atresia
Metabolic instability such as hypoglycemia, hypocalcemia
Nonimmune hydrops fetalis
Postterm birth, gestational age >42 weeks
Preterm birth, gestational age <37 weeks
Respiratory distress
Temperature instability

TABLE 24.3

NEONATAL PATIENT TYPES AND LEVEL OF PERINATAL SERVICES

Level I
Immediate resuscitation of depressed neonates
Management of high-risk infant until transfer to level II or III
    center
Nursery care of large premature neonates (>2,000 g) without
    risk factors
Management of physiologic jaundice
Normal newborn care

Level II
Level I, plus management of selected neonatal problems,
    including
    Prematurity at <32 weeks
    Mild to moderate respiratory distress syndrome
    Suspected neonatal sepsis
    Hypoglycemia
    Infants of diabetic mothers
    Hypoxia/ischemia without life-threatening sequelae

Level III
Levels I and II, plus management of all neonatal problems,
    including
    Prematurity at <32 weeks or with very low birth weight
        (<1,500 g)
    Severe respiratory distress syndrome
    Persistent pulmonary hypertension
    Sepsis
    Severe postasphyxia sequelae
    Major congenital malformations
    Complex problems requiring subspecialty consultation

Adapted from American Academy of Pediatrics, American College of
Obstericians and Gynecologists. *Guidelines for perinatal care*, 3rd ed.
Elk Grove Village, IL: American Academy of Pediatrics, 1992:236.

basic, specialty, and subspecialty levels of care by the second Committee on Perinatal Health in a 1993 publication, *Toward Improving the Outcome of Pregnancy: The 90s and Beyond.* Although the individual needs of the mother and neonate might require different levels of care, maintenance of the mother–infant dyad was urged. Table 24.4 lists the responsibilities of in-hospital perinatal services designated by basic, specialty, and subspecialty care levels. Recommended standards for NICU design have also been proposed; the recommendations reflect the severity of illness and types of patients treated at a hospital.

A reclassification of level II and level III NICU services has been recently considered by the American Academy of Pediatrics Committee on Fetus and Newborn. It has been proposed that level II units be divided into IIa and IIb units and that level III units be divided into IIIa, IIIb, and IIIc units. Level IIa units would care for physiologically immature, moderately ill, or convalescing infants over 1,500-g birth weight or 32 weeks' gestation, while IIb units could also provide brief periods of mechanical ventilation or continuous positive airway pressure (CPAP) to these infants. Level IIIa units would provide sustained life support (i.e., conventional mechanical ventilation) for infants over 1,000-g birth weight or 28 weeks' gestation and might perform minor surgical procedures. Level IIIb units would provide comprehensive care for infants under 1,000-g birth weight or less than 28 weeks' gestation. Those NICUs would also provide such therapies as high-frequency oscillatory ventilation and inhaled nitric oxide, and have prompt on-site access to a full range of pediatric subspecialty and surgical consultants. Hospitals with level IIIc NICUs would provide extracorporeal membrane oxygenation (ECMO) and surgical repair of complex cardiac anomalies.

services. Health care economic pressures since then have tended to undo regionally coordinated perinatal systems by encouraging hospitals to raise their level of obstetric, neonatal, or both types of services. In an effort to respond to this changing environment, functional descriptions were used to define

TABLE 24.4

RESPONSIBILITIES OF IN-HOSPITAL PERINATAL SERVICES

Basic care

Surveillance and care of all patients admitted to the obstetric service, with an established triage system for identifying high-risk patients who require transfer for specialty or subspecialty care

Proper detection and supportive care of unanticipated maternal–fetal problems that occur during labor and delivery

Capability to begin an emergency cesarean delivery within 30 minutes of the decision to do so

Availability of blood and fresh-frozen plasma for transfusion

Availability of anesthesia, diagnostic imaging, and laboratory services on a 24-hour basis

Care of postpartum conditions

Resuscitation and stabilization of all neonates born in hospital

Normal newborn care, including evaluation of the condition of healthy neonates and continuing care of those neonates until their discharge

Stabilization of small or ill neonates before transfer for specialty or subspecialty care

Consultation and transfer arrangements

Parent–sibling–neonate visitation

Data collection and retrieval

Specialty care

Performance of basic care services listed previously

Care of high-risk mothers and fetuses, both admitted and transferred from other facilities

Stabilization of ill newborns before transfer to a subspecialty care facility

Care of preterm infants with a birth weight ≥1,500 g or gestation ≥32 weeks

Care of moderately ill newborns who have problems that are expected to resolve rapidly

Subspecialty care

Provision of comprehensive perinatal care services for both admitted and transferred mothers and neonates of all risk categories, including basic and specialty care services listed previously

Care of mothers with preterm labor and impending delivery at <32 weeks' gestation, and with such problems as severe intrauterine growth restriction with oligohydramnios, severe preeclampsia, chorioamnionitis, or complex medical or surgical problems

Care of neonates with birth weights <1,500 g or <32 weeks' gestation, and with complex medical or surgical problems such as severe immune or nonimmune hydrops fetalis, congenital heart disease, open neural tube defects, abdominal wall defects, or diaphragmatic hernia

Research and educational support

Analysis and evaluation of regional data, including data regarding perinatal complications

Initial evaluation of new high-risk technologies

Adapted from American Academy of Pediatrics, American College of Obstetricians and Gynecologists. *Guidelines for perinatal care*, 5th ed. Elk Grove Village, IL: American Academy of Pediatrics, 2002:10.

Related to this discussion of NICU level, several recent studies have reported an association between NICU patient volume and NICU level of care at the hospital of birth on neonatal mortality. Although delivery at a hospital with a large NICU does not guarantee a good outcome, level IIIb and IIIc units with a patient census of at least 15 patients tend to have the best outcomes. This relationship appears to be due to structural and organizational aspects of care that are possible at hospitals with large delivery services and NICUs.

Local Organization of Newborn Care

Newborn nursery services are often divided between the normal newborn nursery and a NICU. Medical staff assigned to the NICU are called to be present at the delivery of any infant believed to be at risk for developing neonatal problems because of the presence of factors associated with high-risk pregnancies (see Tables 24.1 and 24.2). Many of these infants, as well as other infants in whom high-risk clinical findings (see Table 24.2) are observed postnatally, are admitted to the NICU for observation, diagnosis, or management. Most of these infants are transferred to the normal nursery within 12 hours of birth or admission and are considered short-term admissions.

Survival Trends

Survival of very low-birth-weight infants improved steadily until the mid-1990s and then tended to plateau. Figure 24.1 graphs survival data for infants born at YNHH in 1971, 1977, 1982, 1986, 1991, 1997, and 2002 with birth weights between 501 and 750 g, 751 and 1,000 g, and 1,001 and 1,500 g. Although survival of infants with birth weights of 1,001 to 1,500 g has ranged from 92% to 96% since 1986, survival of infants with birth weights of 751 to 1,000 g rose from about 76% to 87%, and survival of infants with birth weights of 501 to 750 g almost doubled, increasing from about 35% to 61%. The improved survival for infants with birth weights of 501 to 1,000 g most likely reflects continued refinement in the management of extremely low-birth-weight infants, the widespread use of surfactant replacement therapy since 1991, and antenatal corticosteroids since 1994. Survival of infants with birth weights less than 500 g has, however, remained at less than 20%. Surfactant replacement therapy is discussed in Chapter 42.

Birth weight–specific survival statistics and percentage of survival without severe intraventricular hemorrhage, necrotizing enterocolitis, or bronchopulmonary dysplasia are shown in Table 24.6 for a recent 4-year period from 15 centers participating in the National Institute of Child Health and Human Development (NICHD) Neonatal Research Network. This table also displays the intercenter differences in birth weight–adjusted survival; variation is most evident in the lowest birth-weight groups. Differences in the philosophy of care and management policies most likely account for much of the intercenter variability in survival and suggest that, as Hack put it, "the practice of neonatal medicine remains in part an art rather than an exact science." Network data shown in Table 24.7 demonstrate an increasing trend of survival without an increase in morbidity until the mid-1990s, but a leveling off of those outcomes since that time.

Figure 24.2 displays survival plots by gender for infants 501- to 800-g birth weight cared for at NICHD Neonatal Research Network centers from 1997 to 2000. For each 100-g birth weight interval, females have higher survival rates. Although the majority of deaths occurred within the first 7 days following birth, this graph demonstrates the continued mortality beyond the first month of life.

Surviving preterm infants with birth weights of less than 1,000 g remain patients within NICUs or intermediate care units for an average of 2 to 4 months. The length of hospitalization tends to be inversely related to birth weight and may be prolonged if complications develop. Therefore, although they may account for a minority of the admissions to a NICU, the

TABLE 24.5

ADMISSIONS TO THE NEWBORN SPECIAL CARE UNIT, YALE–NEW HAVEN CHILDREN'S HOSPITAL, 1997 TO 2002

	1997	1998	1999	2000	2001	2002
YNHH live births	4,912	4,910	4,786	4,749	4,606	4,718
Total NBSCU admissions	1,468	1450	1360	1,380	1,295	1,308
Short-term admissions	583	544	487	503	459	448
% NBSCU admissions	39.7	37.5	35.8	36.5	35.4	34.3
% YNHH live births	11.9	11.1	10.2	10.6	10.0	9.5
Neonatal transfer	131	123	106	120	107	110
% NBSCU admissions	8.9	8.5	7.8	8.7	8.3	8.4
Long-term admissions, inborn	754	783	767	757	729	750
% NBSCU admissions	51.4	54.0	56.4	54.9	56.3	45.4
% YNHH live births	15.4	16.0	16.0	15.9	15.8	15.4

NBSCU, Newborn Special Care Unit; YNHH, Yale-New Haven Hospital.

majority of infants found on any day within an intensive care nursery may be very low-birth-weight (1,500 g or less) infants at various points in their hospitalization.

NEWBORN INTENSIVE CARE UNIT STAFF

The size and composition of the medical staff varies according to the size of the NICU; the type of perinatal and neonatal services offered at the hospital (see Tables 24.3 and 24.4); whether the NICU is part of a university medical center, a large community hospital, or a moderate-sized community hospital; and the role that the NICU plays within the regional perinatal system. Most NICUs are directed by full-time physicians who are board-certified pediatricians with subspecialty training and usually certification in perinatal–neonatal medicine.

The size of the NICU nursing staff, particularly the number of nurses assigned per shift, is also a function of the size of the NICU, the level of neonatal care provided, and the case mix. Most NICUs employ only registered nurses. Nurse-to-patient ratios of 1:1 for the sickest infants, 1:2 for intermediate-care patients, and 1:4 for healthier infants who require little extra care have often been used to determine the number of nurses needed per shift. However, patient classification scoring systems that more accurately reflect the actual number of nursing care hours needed by the patients each shift have become common.

Expanded nursing roles are common in the NICU. Neonatal nurse transport teams have been trained at many centers. Using

management protocols, they have assumed the responsibility of performing most neonatal transfers.

In addition to medical and nursing staffs, respiratory therapists and social workers play essential roles in the NICU. Because respiratory distress is one of the most common medical problems of NICU patients, respiratory therapists are often assigned to the NICU around the clock. The respiratory therapist ensures that all respiratory equipment is functioning, assists in giving chest physiotherapy, and assists in monitoring the response to various respiratory treatments, such as bronchodilator therapy in infants with bronchopulmonary dysplasia. The respiratory therapist may also perform pulmonary function tests on intubated NICU patients, obtaining data about the infant's need for continued ventilatory assistance or response to medical therapies. It is common for a respiratory therapist to participate in a neonatal transport. Furthermore, respiratory therapists have become part of the DR resuscitation team since mechanical ventilation or nasal CPAP has been increasingly initiated in the delivery room with extremely low-gestational-age neonates.

Having an infant admitted to a NICU, even for short-term observation, produces stress and anxiety in the parents. For parents whose infants are very small or very sick or have multiple problems, such stress is often overwhelming. Social workers assigned to NICUs work with parents during this emotionally and psychologically draining time. They ensure that the parents understand the information being told to them by the medical team so that they can play an active role in selecting management options. If necessary, the social worker helps the parents begin the grieving process. Often, the social worker continues to counsel parents long after an infant's discharge or death.

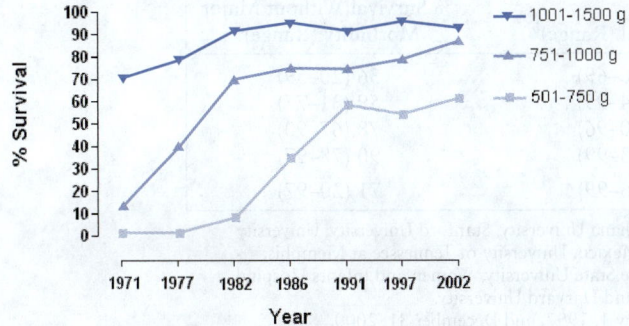

FIGURE 24.1. Survival data for infants born at Yale-New Haven Hospital in 1971, 1977, 1982, 1986, 1991, 1997, and 2002 with birth weights between 501 and 750 g, 751 and 1,000 g, and 1,001 and 1,500 g.

NEONATAL TRANSPORT

Although the best transport isolette is the uterus, maternal transfer of a woman who develops a risk factor during labor (see Table 24.2) is not always possible. In addition, because many neonatal problems (see Table 24.2) are not predicted before delivery, regional neonatal transport systems have been developed. Maternal and neonatal transfers should be performed as soon as possible after a potential problem appears likely. If the medical and nursing staffs at referring hospitals can identify and stabilize high-risk neonates quickly while awaiting the transfer team, the birth weight–adjusted mortality of outborn infants will be similar to that of inborn infants.

Transport back to the referring hospital once an infant no longer requires the special services available at the NICU is

TABLE 24.6

ADMISSIONS BY BIRTH WEIGHT, NEWBORN SPECIAL CARE UNIT, YALE-NEW HAVEN CHILDREN'S HOSPITAL, 1997 TO 2002

Birth Weight (g)	1997	1998	1999	2000	2001	2002	Total	Percent of Long-Term Inborn Admissions*
<500	5	18	11	7	8	10	59	1.3
500–749	24	34	29	27	30	37	181	4.0
750–999	37	34	32	22	27	31	183	4.0
1,000–1,249	21	36	39	29	29	26	180	4.0
1,250–1,499	29	32	32	28	38	30	189	4.2
1,500–1,999	90	118	98	93	103	109	611	13.5
2,000–2,499	108	105	108	119	126	132	698	15.4
≥2,500	440	406	418	432	368	375	2,439	53.7
Total	754	783	767	757	729	750	4,540	100.0

*Long-term admissions, Yale-New Haven Children's Hospital (YNHCH).

an essential component of a regional perinatal system. Back-transfer helps to ensure the availability and efficient use of NICU beds for the care of critically ill neonates. Therefore, parents should be informed about this policy during discussions after maternal and neonatal transfer.

Parents

The parents of a neonate admitted to a NICU must be encouraged to visit their infant regularly. Unlimited visiting privileges for parents are the rule in most NICUs. Provisions are usually made for visiting by grandparents, siblings, other family members, and friends. The NICU staff should explain to the parents the reason for admission, initial management plan, expected hospital course with the more common difficulties, and standard NICU routines. The NICU staff should be prepared to repeat and augment this information so that each infant's parents understand it. Before an infant's discharge home, especially after a prolonged hospitalization, parents should be encouraged to become actively involved in daily care, such as feeding, diaper changing, and bathing. If the infant will continue to receive medications after discharge, the parents must also learn to

measure the dose and administer it. Finally, although the medical staff must direct medical care, parental input and guidance should be sought and considered when medical care becomes extraordinary and possibly futile.

COST-EFFECTIVENESS OF NEWBORN INTENSIVE CARE UNIT CARE

In the United States and other developed countries, continued advances in neonatal–perinatal medicine have improved markedly the chance of survival and the quality of outcome for very low-birth-weight infants. As shown in Fig. 24.1 and Tables 24.7 and 24.8 approximately 50% of infants with birth weights of 501 to 750 g now survive. These infants, however, especially those with birth weights below 600 g, are at high risk for significant morbidities during their initial neonatal hospitalization, for significant long-term neurodevelopmental sequelae, and for continued health problems requiring ongoing care and often rehospitalization. Because hospital charges for the initial hospitalization may exceed $2,000 per day, the smallest, sickest infants commonly incur initial hospital charges well in excess

TABLE 24.7

SURVIVAL AND MORBIDITY STATISTICS 1997–2000, NATIONAL INSTITUTE OF CHILD HEALTH AND HUMAN DEVELOPMENT, NEONATAL RESEARCH NETWORK[a]

Birth Weight (g)	N	% Survival (Range)[b]	% Survival Without Major Morbidity (Range)[c]
501–750	2,527	56 (36–69)	36 (20–59)
751–1,000	2,787	88 (74–95)	59 (31–77)
1,001–1,250	2,942	94 (90–96)	78 (67–90)
1,251–1,500	3,477	96 (93–99)	90 (78–97)
Totals	11,733	85 (36–99)	71 (20–97)

[a]Case Western Reserve University, Emory University, Indiana University, Stanford University, University of Cincinnati, University of Miami, University of New Mexico, University of Tennessee at Memphis, University of Texas Southwestern Medical Center, Wayne State University, Women and Infants Hospital, Yale University, University of Alabama at Birmingham, and Harvard University.
[b]% Inborn survivors (intercenter ranges) between January 1, 1997, and December 31, 2000.
[c]Major morbidity defined as an oxygen requirement at 36 weeks postmenstrual age, proven necrotizing enterocolitis, and grade III to IV intraventricular hemorrhage.
Adapted from Fanaroff AA, Stoll BJ, Wright LL, et al. Very-low-birth-weight (VLBW) outcomes of the NICHD Neonatal Research Network, January 1997 through December 2000: a plateau: is further imrovement feasible? Submitted for publication.

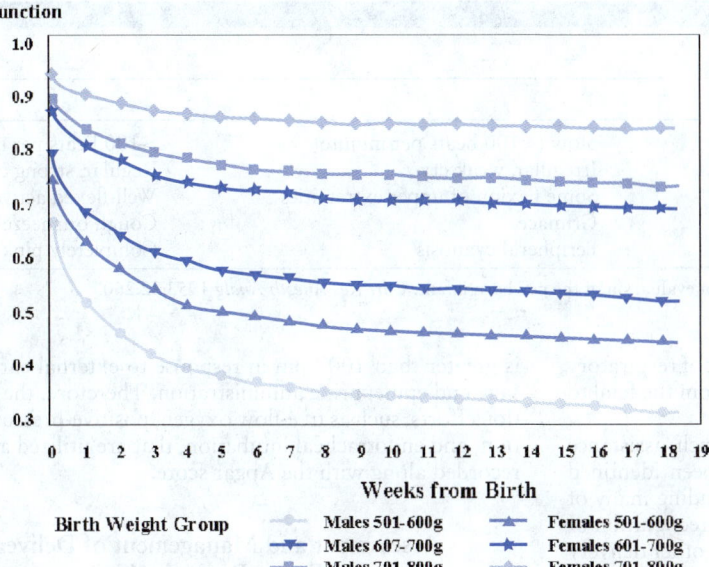

Survival Function

Weeks from Birth

Birth Weight Group
- ○ Males 501-600g
- ▼ Males 607-700g
- ■ Males 701-800g
- ▲ Females 501-600g
- ★ Females 601-700g
- ◆ Females 701-800g

FIGURE 24.2. Survival plots by gender for infants with birth weights of 501 to 800 g at National Institute of Child Health and Human Development Neonatal Research Network Centers, 1997 to 2000.

of $150,000. In addition, many incur significant posthospitalization costs. Therefore, the cost-effectiveness of NICU care for infants with birth weights of less than 600 g or less than 24 weeks' gestation has been questioned.

Neonatal intensive care is costly not only to the individual family, but also to society. These costs increase with decreasing birth weight and gestational age. However, any attempt to limit neonatal intensive care to those extremely low-birth-weight infants least likely to benefit raises important ethical questions. In addition, neonatologists are usually unable to determine at birth which extremely low-birth-weight preterm infant will survive intact and which will survive with significant health or neurodevelopmental problems. Thus, as survival rates have steadily improved, the absolute number of handicapped survivors has increased with the number of normal survivors. Therefore, neonatologists must include parents in any discussion about whether to continue the extreme measures being provided to their extremely low-birth-weight preterm infants.

pendent existence. Such adaptation demands major physiologic changes in several organ systems as well as a reorganization of overall metabolic processes. For example, *in utero* the human fetus is totally dependent on the mother for respiratory gas exchange, nutrient supply, waste product removal, and thermoregulation. After delivery, the neonate's lungs must replace the placenta as the site of respiratory gas exchange; stored glycogen and absorption of nutrients by the gastrointestinal tract provide for metabolic homeostasis and growth; the task of waste elimination is taken over by the gastrointestinal tract and kidneys, with the latter also responsible for the maintenance of water and electrolyte balance; and the neonate must be prepared to supply energy to maintain body temperature. In most newborn infants (approximately 85% to 90%), these changes proceed smoothly, and the infants require little or no assistance after delivery. However, a few require help and close observation until they complete the transition successfully, and the occasional infant fails completely to adapt.

NEWBORN RESUSCITATION

Birth is a transition from the intrauterine to the extrauterine environment. It encompasses a series of complex events through which every infant must pass to achieve successfully an inde-

Delivery Room Resuscitation

Resuscitation of an infant in the delivery room provides the assistance that a newborn needs as he or she begins the transition from intrauterine to extrauterine existence. The main goals of

TABLE 24.8

MORBIDITY AND MORTALITY DATA, 1988 TO 2000, NATIONAL INSTITUTE OF CHILD HEALTH AND HUMAN DEVELOPMENT, NEONATAL RESEARCH NETWORK

	% Survival		% Survival w/o Major Morbidity*	
Year	501–1,000 g	1,001–1,500 g	501–1,000 g	1,001–1,500 g
1988	64	90	44	81
1991–92	63	94	60	85
1993–94	68	94	51	83
1995–96	71	96	51	84
1997–98	73	95	51	84
1999–2000	72	95	50	95

*Major morbidity defined as an oxygen requirement at 36 weeks postmenstrual age, proven necrotizing enterocolitis, and grade III to IV intraventricular hemorrhage.
Adapted from Ehrekranz RA, Wright LL. NICHD Neonatal Research Network: contributions and future challenges. *Semin Perinatol* 2003;27:264.

TABLE 24.9

APGAR SCORE

Sign	0	1	2
Heart rate	Absent	Slow (<100 beats per minute)	>100 beats per minute
Respiratory effort	Absent	Irregular, weak cry	Regular, strong cry
Muscle tone	Flaccid	Some flexion of upper extremities	Well-flexed active motion
Reflex irritability	No response	Grimace	Cough or sneeze
Color	Central cyanosis	Peripheral cyanosis	Completely pink

Adapted from Apgar V. A proposal for a new method of evaluation of the newborn infant. *Curr Res Anesth Analg* 1953;32:260.

delivery room resuscitation are the establishment of respiratory activity with gas exchange and the conversion from the fetal to the neonatal circulation.

Although most neonates do not require much assistance in the delivery room, several conditions have been identified that increase the risk of perinatal asphyxia, including many of the factors listed in Tables 24.1 and 24.2. Early recognition of these conditions by obstetricians, midwives, and other delivery room attendants is one of the most important steps in ensuring prompt neonatal resuscitation. Many of these conditions are known before delivery, and a pediatrician or other appropriate person experienced in newborn resuscitation should be available to evaluate and resuscitate the infant. However, because many intrapartum problems cannot be anticipated, appropriate equipment and drugs must be available, all delivery room attendants must understand the principles of neonatal resuscitation, and at least one must be skilled at resuscitating a neonate.

Apgar Score

In 1953, Dr. Virginia Apgar proposed a method of evaluating the newborn infant in the delivery room based on five easily determined signs. This evaluation, known as the *Apgar score* (Table 24.9), gives a rating of 0, 1, or 2 to each sign. A score of 10 indicates that the infant is in the best possible condition, whereas a score of less than 3 implies moderate to severe birth depression. Currently, a score is assigned at 1 and 5 minutes. The 1-minute score is a guide to the infant's well-being. It indicates the degree of depression and previously had been used to suggest appropriate resuscitative measures. Although the 5-minute score had been thought to correlate with neonatal morbidity, it more accurately indicates the response to resuscitative efforts. If the Apgar score at 5 minutes is still less than 7, additional scores every 5 minutes for a total of 20 minutes have been recommended to assess response and the appropriateness of continued resuscitative measures.

In practice, the infant's respiratory activity, heart rate, and color are the best indicators of the need for resuscitation, not the 1-minute Apgar score. Bradycardia in a newborn is most often related to inadequate respiratory activity. Therefore, attention should be directed to ensuring airway patency and then to assisting breathing. Because cardiac output depends primarily on the heart rate, restoring the heart rate improves circulation, resulting in improved color. In addition, color, tone, and reflex irritability are partially related to the infant's gestational age and physiologic maturity. The more preterm an infant is, the more likely that the completely pink body and the diminished tone and minimal reflex irritability are a function of immaturity and not asphyxia.

Furthermore, although the Apgar score at 5 minutes may indicate an infant's response to resuscitative efforts, it makes no clear distinction between the infant whose heart rate is greater than 100 beats per minute (bpm) after vigorous stimulation, the infant whose heart rate is greater than 100 bpm after initiation of positive-pressure ventilation, and the infant whose heart rate

is greater than 100 bpm in response to external cardiac massage and epinephrine administration. Therefore, the resuscitation efforts, such as free-flow oxygen, positive-pressure ventilation, and endotracheal intubation, that are utilized are usually recorded along with the Apgar score.

Assessment and Management of Delivery Room Resuscitation

Figure 24.3 is an algorithm of the delivery room management and assessment recommended by the American Academy of Pediatrics and the American Heart Association. This overview is briefly discussed; it is based not on the Apgar score, but on evaluation of respiratory activity, heart rate, and color. Table 24.10 lists equipment and drugs that should be available for delivery room resuscitation.

As soon as the infant's head is delivered, the mouth, nose, and pharynx are gently suctioned with a bulb syringe or suction catheter connected to mechanical suction. After the rest of the infant is delivered and the umbilical cord is clamped and cut, the infant is transferred in a head-down position and placed under a radiant heater on a resuscitation table. Most infants begin to cry between the time the body is delivered and the cord is cut.

The neonate should be quickly and thoroughly dried and not left in contact with or covered by wet towels or blankets. This should minimize evaporative heat loss, while placement under a preheated radiant warmer should minimize radiant and convective heat loss. Then the infant is positioned on his or her back with the neck slightly extended; elevating the infant's shoulders approximately 2 cm off the mattress with a rolled blanket or towel may help to maintain this position. Once correctly positioned, the mouth and nose are gently suctioned with a bulb syringe or a suction catheter. The mouth is suctioned first, so that nothing is in the mouth for the infant to aspirate. Blind, deep, or vigorous nasopharyngeal suctioning with a suction catheter can be hazardous if performed within the first minutes of life, because it can result in laryngeal spasm and increased vagal tone with apnea and bradycardia. For this reason, unless meconium staining of the amniotic fluid exists, deep suctioning of the oropharynx should be delayed for several minutes until normal ventilation has been established. The delivery room management of infants delivered with meconium staining of the amniotic fluid is discussed separately.

The neonate's respiratory activity, heart rate, and color should then be evaluated simultaneously. Auscultation of the chest permits an assessment of respiratory activity and heart rate, while visual observation permits a concurrent assessment of color. Heart rate can also be determined by palpation of the umbilical cord or of the brachial artery. Both drying and suctioning provide stimulation that promotes breathing and stimulates heart rate. If respiratory activity is inadequate additional tactile stimulation should be provided by flicking the heel or slapping the sole of the infant's foot or by rubbing the infant's back. Free-flow oxygen should be given to the

Algorithm for Delivery Room Resuscitation

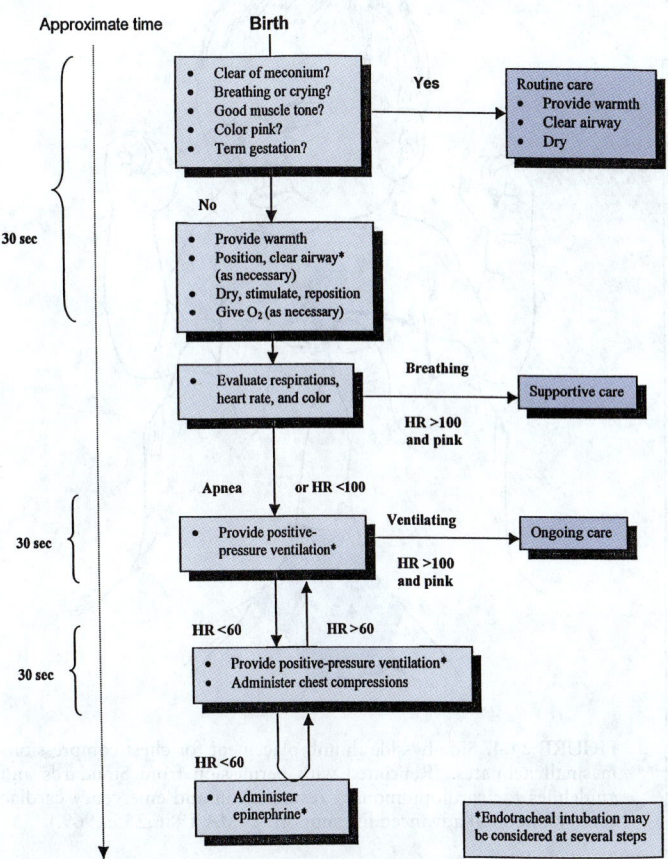

FIGURE 24.3. Algorithm for resuscitation of the newly born infant.

infant with central cyanosis who is breathing spontaneously and has a heart rate of more than 100 bpm. Free-flow oxygen is unnecessary for infants with only peripheral cyanosis (acrocyanosis). The activities performed up to this point—drying the infant, suctioning the airway, and providing tactile stimulation—should be completed within 30 seconds. These infants should be observed to ensure that adaptation to extrauterine life is progressing satisfactorily.

If the infant is apneic or if the infant's respiratory effort is insufficient to maintain a heart rate of more than 100 bpm, positive-pressure bag and mask ventilation with oxygen should be initiated promptly. After a 30-second period of ventilation at a rate of 40 to 60 breaths per minute, the infant's heart rate should be evaluated. If the heart rate is more than 100 bpm and if the infant displays spontaneous breathing activity, positive-pressure ventilation can be discontinued; free-flow oxygen should be provided until the infant remains pink. If spontaneous respirations remain inadequate or if the heart rate remains below 100 bpm, positive-pressure bag and mask ventilation should be continued. If the heart rate is less than 60 bpm, positive-pressure ventilation should be continued and chest compressions should be initiated. Alternatively, if an individual skilled at endotracheal intubation is present in the delivery room, the infant can be intubated and the heart rate response to positive-pressure ventilation by bag and endotracheal tube can be used to determine the need for chest compressions.

Ventilation by bag and mask or by bag and endotracheal tube should be confirmed by movement of the chest and auscultatory evidence of equal, bilateral aeration. A ventilatory rate of 40 to 60 breaths per minute should be maintained. If chest compressions are required, positive-pressure ventilations must be interposed between compressions. Currently, a venti-

lation is recommended to follow every third compression, and 90 compressions and 30 ventilations should occur each minute.

Chest compressions can be performed with either of two techniques. With one method, both thumbs are placed over the middle third of the sternum, and the other fingers encircle and support the back, while the sternum is compressed approximately 1 to 2 cm (Fig. 24.4). The thumbs are positioned on the sternum just below the imaginary line drawn between the nipples; thumbs may have to be superimposed with very low-birth-weight infants. Alternatively, compressions could be administered with the tip of the middle finger and either the index or ring finger of one hand placed on the sternum approximately one fingerbreadth below the nipple line; the other hand could be used to support the infant's back. The lower sternum should not be compressed, because abdominal organs might be injured.

If the heart rate improves and climbs to more than 60 bpm after approximately 30 seconds of chest compressions and ventilation, chest compressions can be discontinued. In most cases, positive-pressure ventilatory assistance should be continued until the infant has been transferred to the NICU, where blood pressure, perfusion, arterial blood gases, and acid–base status can be evaluated. If the infant's heart rate does not improve and remains less than 60 bpm after a 30- to 60-second period of adequate positive-pressure ventilation with oxygen and chest compressions, epinephrine should be given. Although epinephrine can be given intravenously, administration via the endotracheal tube is easier (0.1 to 0.3 mL/kg of a 1:10,000 solution, intravenously or endotracheally). Doses of epinephrine may be repeated every 5 minutes if required.

In addition to epinephrine, the neonatal resuscitation program developed jointly by the American Academy of Pediatrics and the American Heart Association recommends the

TABLE 24.10

EQUIPMENT AND DRUGS NECESSARY FOR DELIVERY ROOM RESUSCITATION

Equipment

Resuscitation table with radiant heat source
Oxygen with flow meter
Mechanical suction regulator
Ventilation bag with pressure manometer
Face masks with sizes for premature and term infants
Oral airways, sizes 0 and 00
Endotracheal tubes and adapters with stylets and without
    cuffs or shoulders (internal diameters of 2.5, 3.0, and
    3.5 mm)
Laryngoscope with blade sizes for premature and term infants
Suction catheters, 6 and 8 Fr., with thumb suction control
Meconium aspirators, with thumb suction control port
Bulb syringes
Syringes: 1, 3, 5, 10, and 20 mL
Needles: 19- to 25-gauge, 5/8 to 1.5 in, long
Styletted small vein catheters, 16- to 24-gauge
Umbilical catheters: 3.5 and 5 Fr. vessel catheters; 5 Fr.
    feeding tubes
Three-way stopcocks
Scissors
Adhesive tape
Povidone-iodine Solution

Drugs and fluids

Epinephrine, 1:10,000 (0.1 mg/mL) preparation, 10-mL
    ampules
Naloxone, 1.0 mg/mL preparation, 2-mL ampules
Normal saline (or Ringer's lactate)
Sodium bicarbonate, 4.2% (0.5 mEq/mL) solution, 10-mL
    ampules
Sterile water, 10-mL ampules

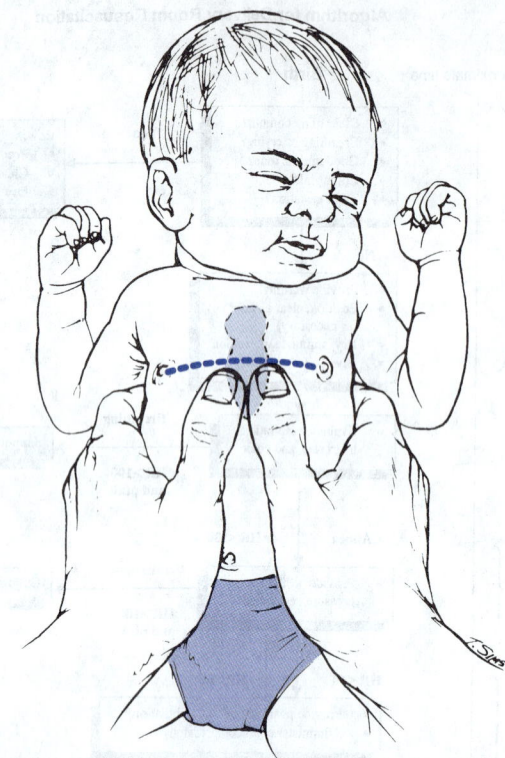

FIGURE 24.4. Side-by-side thumb placement for chest compressions in small neonates. (Reprinted with permission from Standards and guidelines for cardiopulmonary resuscitation and emergency cardiac care. VI: neonatal advanced life support. *JAMA* 1986;255:2969.)

use of naloxone hydrochloride (Narcan) to reverse respiratory depression associated with a history of maternal narcotic administration within the 4 hours immediately preceding delivery, sodium bicarbonate to restore acid–base balance, and volume expanders to improve tissue perfusion.

Infants who demonstrate respiratory depression secondary to maternal narcotic administration usually have adequate heart rates or respond readily to positive-pressure bag and mask ventilation. Naloxone, a competitive narcotic antagonist with a duration of action of 1 to 4 hours, can be administered (0.1 mg/kg per dose) intravenously, endotracheally, intramuscularly, or subcutaneously. Therefore, infants who are treated must be monitored closely for recurrent respiratory depression; repeated doses may be given. Administering naloxone to the infant of a narcotic-addicted mother may precipitate seizures.

Sodium bicarbonate should be given when a significant metabolic acidosis has been documented or is assumed to be present. Therefore, demonstration of a severe metabolic acidosis by arterial blood gas analysis is the best indication for treatment with sodium bicarbonate. Its use is not recommended after short periods of asphyxia that respond quickly to positive-pressure ventilation with oxygen. Sodium bicarbonate should not be given unless the infant is being adequately ventilated, because it causes the arterial Pco_2 to increase. The increased Pco_2 results from the spontaneous conversion of bicarbonate to water and carbon dioxide following its addition to a closed acidotic system, which is analogous to a poorly ventilated patient. Furthermore, in view of the association of rapid, undiluted sodium bicarbonate administration and intracranial hemorrhage in neonates, it should be used

cautiously and should never be given by rapid push (2 mEq/kg of a 0.5 mEq/mL solution, infused over at least 2 minutes, is recommended).

A volume expander should be considered when evidence exists of acute bleeding with signs of hypovolemia in an infant requiring resuscitation. Although losses of 10% to 15% of total blood volume may not produce signs in the delivery room, a loss of 20% or more of total blood volume is often associated with pallor persisting after oxygenation; weak, thready pulses with a good heart rate; a poor response to resuscitative efforts; and a decreased blood pressure (if measured). A volume of 10 mL/kg of normal saline, or Ringer's lactate can be infused over approximately 10 minutes; O-negative whole blood or packed red blood cells may also be given, but these may not be as readily available as the other fluids.

During a neonatal resuscitation in the delivery room, vascular access is most readily achieved by inserting a fluid-filled umbilical catheter (or feeding tube) into the umbilical vein. The tip of the catheter should lie 2 to 3 cm below the surface of the abdominal wall, at a location at which free flow of blood is present. Inserting the catheter farther into the umbilical vein might position the catheter tip within a branch of the portal vein, and infusing resuscitative solutions into that vessel might result in liver damage. The catheter should be secured with a tape bridge. As described in a following section, this catheter must be kept filled with fluid and closed to air at all times, because an air embolus might result if a large negative intrathoracic pressure was suddenly generated. Because emergency catheterization of the umbilical vein usually is not performed aseptically, the catheter should be removed after better vascular access has been established following transfer to the NICU. Consideration should also be given to the use of prophylactic antibiotic coverage. Umbilical vessel catheterization is described later in this chapter.

In summary, delivery room resuscitation involves the same "ABCD" sequence used during any cardiopulmonary resuscitation: The airway is established, breathing is initiated, circulation is supported, and then, if necessary, drugs are given.

Meconium Staining of the Amniotic Fluid

Meconium staining of the amniotic fluid occurs in 0.5% to 20.0% of all deliveries. Although the presence of meconium in the amniotic fluid may indicate fetal distress that might result in the birth of an asphyxiated or stillborn infant, numerous instances exist of fetal distress and asphyxia without meconium-stained amniotic fluid, as well as numerous instances of meconium staining without evidence of fetal distress. However, several studies have demonstrated increased rates of neonatal morbidity and mortality in association with meconium staining of the amniotic fluid, usually secondary to meconium aspiration pneumonia.

Because the development of meconium aspiration pneumonia requires the combination of meconium in the posterior pharynx and trachea and respiratory activity, the optimal management would be to remove any meconium from the trachea before the infant breathes, and thus prevent movement of meconium into the lower bronchial tree. Because several studies have demonstrated that this approach is effective in decreasing the incidence and severity of meconium aspiration pneumonia, management plans that have coordinated obstetric and pediatric efforts in the delivery room have been developed. First, the infant's mouth, pharynx, and nose are suctioned by the obstetrician with a suction catheter connected to mechanical suction as soon as the infant's head appears on the perineum, and before the delivery of the infant's shoulders and the onset of respirations. With a cesarean section, the infant is suctioned as soon as the head is delivered through the uterine incision and before the delivery of the thorax. Some obstetricians also aspirate gastric contents before the delivery of the thorax. After delivery, additional suctioning or stimulation is not performed by the obstetrician. The infant is brought immediately to the resuscitation table, and additional suctioning of the airway is performed, if indicated, before the infant is dried.

The infant's respiratory status directs the pediatric management. If the infant vigorously cries, spontaneously begins regular respiratory activity following delivery, and has a heart rate greater than 100 bpm, tracheal suctioning is not recommended and may cause airway injury. However, prompt tracheal suctioning is performed via a meconium aspirator or an endotracheal tube affixed with a suction adapter connected to mechanical suction (maximum pressure of 100 mm Hg) if the infant does not cry and begin regular respiratory activity spontaneously, cries and then demonstrates respiratory distress (e.g., retractions or cyanosis), or has a heart rate less than 100 bpm. The duration of suction can be regulated via the thumb control port on the meconium aspirator. The meconium aspirator or endotracheal tube is withdrawn as suction is applied. Suction catheters inserted through the endotracheal tube may be inadequate to remove thick, tenacious meconium and therefore are not recommended. Furthermore, because meconium has been found in the trachea of some infants in the absence of meconium in the mouth or larynx during direct laryngoscopy, a decision to perform tracheal suctioning should not be solely based on the findings at direct laryngoscopy. *When possible, initiation of ventilatory stimulation or positive-pressure ventilation should be delayed until meconium is no longer removed by tracheal suction.* However, if the infant's heart rate is severely depressed, it may be necessary to initiate positive-pressure ventilation sooner. Mechanical suction should be used so as to minimize the risk of exposure to potentially infectious body fluids. In addition, performing tracheobronchial lavage

---

BOX 24.1	Conditions Associated with Neonatal Respiratory Distress

Central nervous system damage or depression
Cervical spinal cord injury
Maternal analgesics and anesthetics
Very low birth weight
Spontaneous pneumothorax or pneumomediastinum
Diaphragmatic hernia
Obstructive malformations of the epiglottis, larynx, or
   trachea
Pulmonary hypoplasia
Nonimmune hydrops fetalis
Acute intrapartum blood loss

in the delivery room is not recommended and may increase morbidity.

Special Problems Interfering with Delivery Room Resuscitation

In addition to central nervous system damage or depression from intrauterine or intrapartum asphyxia, cervical spinal cord injury, and maternal analgesics and anesthetics, several other reasons explain why a neonate might experience difficulty in establishing and sustaining effective respiratory activity. Pediatricians and other delivery room personnel who manage delivery room resuscitation should always be alert to such possibilities (Box 24.1).

Very low-birth-weight preterm infants may lack the strength to maintain adequate respiratory effort and may require respiratory assistance in the delivery room to sustain gas exchange. Some of these infants may be further depressed by sepsis or pneumonia caused by clinical amnionitis or by maternal therapies such as magnesium sulfate used to treat preterm labor or preeclampsia or eclampsia. Because the incidence of respiratory distress syndrome is substantial in infants less than 30 weeks' gestation, some clinicians will prophylactically administer surfactant to them in the delivery room.

As many as 3% of full-term infants develop a spontaneous pneumothorax or pneumomediastinum after a normal spontaneous vaginal delivery. This air leak appears to develop as a complication of the intrathoracic pressure generated by the infant during the initial respiratory efforts. Although a pneumomediastinum may produce tachypnea, it rarely results in significant respiratory difficulty. A pneumothorax interferes with the establishment of respiratory activity only if it is large and under tension, producing mediastinal shift and compromising circulation and the contralateral lung. Breath sounds are diminished or absent on the side with the pneumothorax, but also may be decreased over the other side of the chest. Transillumination of the chest may facilitate diagnosis of a pneumothorax by "lighting up" the affected hemithorax. Although some of these infants may require intubation and respiratory support, prompt aspiration of the free air is essential to permit the collapsed lung to reexpand. If a tension pneumothorax is suspected and the infant's condition is deteriorating, with increasing cyanosis and worsening respiratory distress, aspiration of the chest should be performed in the delivery room. This technique is described in the following section.

The presence of a scaphoid abdomen, immediate cyanosis, and respiratory distress suggests the presence of a diaphragmatic hernia. Diaphragmatic hernias usually occur on the left side of the thorax, inhibiting the normal growth and development of the left lung and often inhibiting the growth and development of the right lung because of displacement of the mediastinum and the heart to the right. Breath sounds are diminished or absent on the left, and the heart sounds are heard in the right chest. Endotracheal intubation should be performed quickly, because respiratory activity and cardiac function will be further compromised as the bowel fills with gas. An infant with a diaphragmatic hernia diagnosed by antenatal ultrasound should be delivered at a tertiary level hospital so that the delivery and immediate postnatal care can be coordinated by the obstetrician, neonatologist, and pediatric surgeon. The delivery room team should intubate the infant promptly and insert a nasogastric tube so as to minimize distention of the bowel by swallowed air. The pathophysiology and management of diaphragmatic hernia are discussed in Chapter 30.

Congenital anomalies such as bilateral choanal atresia, laryngeal webs, and other obstructive malformations of the epiglottis, larynx, or trachea prevent air exchange. If respiratory movements are observed but no air movement occurs when the infant's mouth is closed, the mouth and posterior pharynx should be cleared of secretions, an oral airway should be established, and the patency of each choana should be determined by attempting to pass a suction catheter through each nostril into the posterior oropharynx. If effective air exchange is not achieved, laryngoscopy and endotracheal intubation should be performed. The endotracheal tube should bypass any upper respiratory tract obstruction and permit air movement during respiratory activity. The management of these problems is discussed in Chapter 30.

Pulmonary hypoplasia may occur in association with renal agenesis or dysplasia and other congenital anomalies as part of Potter syndrome. It also may occur secondary to prolonged rupture of the fetal membranes. These infants require immediate endotracheal intubation and very high peak inspiratory pressures to achieve chest expansion and air movement into the lungs. Multiple pneumothoraces may develop during these resuscitative efforts.

Nonimmune hydrops fetalis, a condition implying an excess of total body water that is not associated with a circulating antibody against a red blood cell, may hinder the establishment of effective respiratory activity. The excessive accumulation of extracellular fluid includes subcutaneous edema, pleural and pericardial effusions, ascites, polyhydramnios, and placental thickening. A pleural effusion interferes with expansion of the lungs by occupying intrathoracic volume; ascites interferes with expansion of the lungs by pushing the diaphragm up, disrupting its normal activity and decreasing effective intrathoracic volume. Therefore, once an airway has been established and positive-pressure ventilation initiated, it may be necessary to perform bilateral thoracentesis and abdominal paracentesis in the delivery room, so that pleural and ascitic fluid can be removed. Because polyhydramnios is often seen in conjunction with nonimmune hydrops, many affected infants are identified antenatally during a diagnostic obstetric ultrasound evaluation. Other infants may have been diagnosed prenatally during evaluation of a fetal tachyarrhythmia. Additional ultrasound examinations of these infants before delivery will alert the delivery room team about the presence, size, and location of pleural fluid and ascites, ensuring prompt action if necessary. In addition, ultrasound-guided aspiration of pleural and/or abdominal fluid by the obstetrician prior to a cesarean section delivery may facilitate delivery room resuscitation of these infants.

The pathophysiologic causes predisposing to the excessive extracellular fluid accumulation associated with nonimmune hydrops are unknown. Table 24.11 lists reported causes of nonimmune hydrops.

Occasionally, an infant presents with pallor and shock at the time of delivery. This clinical picture results from an acute, significant intrapartum blood loss that may be associated with such problems as abruptio placenta; ruptured umbilical or placental vessels; fetal–placental, fetal–maternal, or fetal–fetal hemorrhage or transfusion; cesarean section incision through an anterior placenta; or intraabdominal hemorrhage secondary to laceration of the liver or splenic rupture because of a difficult

TABLE 24.11

CONDITIONS ASSOCIATED WITH NONIMMUNE HYDROPS FETALIS

Category	Conditions
Hematologic	Homozygous alpha-thalassemia, chronic fetomaternal transfusion, twin-to-twin transfusion, acardius, atrioventricular shunts, hemorrhage or thrombosis, maternal drugs (e.g., chloramphenicol)
Cardiovascular	Severe congenital heart disease (e.g., complex congenital heart defects, atrioventricular septal defects, premature closure of the foramen ovale, hypoplastic left and right heart), arrythmias or congenital heart block, myocardial and endocardial disease, cardiac tumors (e.g., rhabdomyomas)
Respiratory	Cystic adenomatoid malformation of lung, diaphragmatic hernia, pulmonary lymphangiectasia, pulmonary sequestration, intrathoracic mass
Gastrointestinal	Bowel atresias, volvulus, duplications of the gut, peritonitis
Urinary/renal	Urethral and ureteral atresia, bladder neck obstruction, posterior urethral valves, cloacal malformation, congenital nephrosis
Chromosomal	Turner syndrome; trisomies 13, 18, and 21; triploidy; miscellaneous aneuploidy
Placental	Umbilical vein thrombosis, torsion of cord, chorioangioma
Intrauterine infection (with or without hemolysis)	Cytomegalovirus, toxoplasmosis, syphilis, parvovirus, parasitic diseases
Recognized syndromes	Dwarfing syndromes (e.g., thanatophoric, Jeune, hypophosphatasia, achondrogenesis), arthrogryposis, Neu-Laxova syndrome, Pena-Shokeir syndrome, Noonan syndrome, multiple pterygium syndromes, Meckel syndrome
Metabolic disorders	Lysosomal storage disorders (including mucopolysaccharidoses), Gaucher disease, gangliosidoses, sialidosis
Miscellaneous	Amniotic band syndrome, fetal tumors (e.g., teratoma, neuroblastomas, Wilms, angiomas)

Adapted from McGillivary BC, Hall JG. Nonimmune hydrops fetalis. *Pediatr Rev* 1987;9:197.

or breech delivery. As described previously, volume should be administered if, after adequate ventilation with oxygen, there is a poor response to resuscitation, and the infant remains pale and tachycardiac, with weak pulse and poor capillary refill. In the delivery room, 10 mL/kg of estimated body weight of normal saline, or Ringer's lactate can be infused over approximately 10 minutes via a catheter (or feeding tube) inserted into the umbilical vein. After transfer to the NICU, 10 mL/kg of packed red blood cells can be given over approximately 30 minutes, and the need for additional volume expansion or pharmacologic support of blood pressure can be determined.

Discontinuation of Resuscitative Measures

The decision to stop resuscitation remains difficult. The decision is based on personal experience of the resuscitator with respect to the immediate and long-term success of the resuscitative efforts; consideration of the parents' feelings, understanding, and expectations; and the resources available for continued management and support of the infant. In most cases, a delivery room resuscitation should be as vigorous and aggressive as possible. After transfer to the nursery, the status of the infant can be evaluated and discussed with the parents. If continued care is futile, it is appropriate to discontinue extraordinary support.

Transfer from the Delivery Room

As noted previously, the aim of delivery room management of the newborn is to ensure the satisfactory transition from intrauterine to extrauterine existence. In addition to performing appropriate resuscitative efforts, personnel also should examine the infant for the presence of congenital malformations or other conditions that might require prompt medical or surgical intervention. If congenital malformations are noted, they should be shown and described to the parents in the delivery room. Heat loss should be minimized by drying infants with a warmed towel, caring for them beneath a radiant heat source, and wrapping them in a warm blanket.

Because most infants have 1-minute Apgar scores of greater than 7 and adapt well to the extrauterine environment, they should spend time with their mothers in the delivery or postpartum recovery room. If a mother intends to breast-feed, her child should be put to breast at that time. The infant then should be transferred to the nursery for routine admission procedures.

Most infants who require more than just tactile stimulation and facial oxygen in the delivery room should be transferred to a NICU or transitional nursery for observation, evaluation, and initial care. In addition, many infants who have a factor or problem associated with high risk (see Table 24.2) should be transferred to a NICU for initial evaluation and care. Transfer from the delivery room should not occur until oxygenation, ventilation, and heart rate have been adequately established, but the transfer should be expedited so that management can be continued and optimized.

NEWBORN INTENSIVE CARE UNIT ADMISSION ROUTINES, MONITORING, AND PROCEDURES

On admission to the NICU, every infant should be weighed; vital signs, including an apical pulse, respiratory rate, blood pressure, and axillary temperature, should be obtained; and

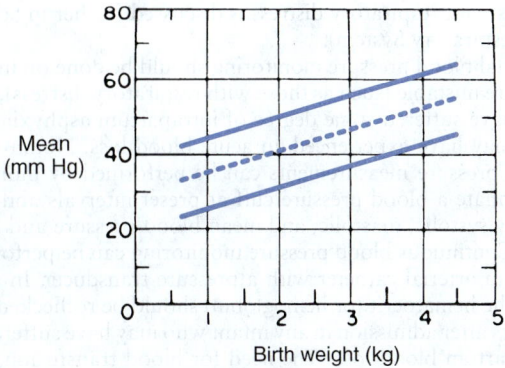

FIGURE 24.5. Linear regression (*broken line*) and 95% confidence limits (*solid lines*) of mean arterial blood pressure on birth weight in 61 healthy newborn infants during the first 12 hours after birth; $y = 5.16 \times +29.80$, n = 443, r = 0.80; $p < .001$. (Reproduced with permission from Versmold HT, Kitterman JA, Phibbs RH, et al. Aortic blood pressure during the first 12 hours of life in infants with birth weight 610 to 4,220 grams. Pediatrics 1981;67:607–613.)

a capillary hematocrit (or hemoglobin) and blood sugar (e.g., with glucose oxidase–impregnated reagent strips) should be measured. Vitamin K_1 (0.5 to 1.0 mg) should be given intramuscularly and ophthalmic prophylaxis should be given (0.5% erythromycin ointment, 1% tetracycline ophthalmic ointment, or 2.5% povidone–iodine ophthalmic solution). Surface electrodes should be placed, and monitoring of cardiac function should be initiated, with simultaneous display of rate and electrocardiographic pattern. Proper placement of the surface electrodes permits some monitors to display a respiratory pattern based on thoracic impedance.

The normal heart rate and respiratory rate for neonates range from 120 to 160 bpm and 40 to 60 breaths per minute, respectively. Arterial blood pressure is directly related to birth weight; Fig. 24.5 displays the normal range for mean arterial blood pressure during the first 12 hours of life. Adequate mean blood pressure can also be estimated from the infant's birth weight in kilograms: 40 mm Hg at 1 kg, 50 mm Hg at 2 kg, and 60 mm Hg at 3 kg. After axillary temperature is determined on admission, body temperature can be monitored continuously with a skin temperature probe (or thermistor) or with serial axillary temperature measurements. Environmental temperature should be adjusted to maintain the skin or axillary temperature between 36.0° and 36.5°C. Oxygen consumption has been shown to be minimized with such an environmental temperature (neutral thermal environment).

The hemoglobin concentration at birth is a function of the infant's gestational age, averaging 16.8 g% at term, 15 g% at 34 weeks, and 14.5 g% at 28 weeks. Infants with blood sugar measurements of less than 45 to 50 mg/dL should receive intravenous glucose or, if possible, should be fed.

Any infant who has respiratory distress or who requires supplemental inspiratory oxygen after delivery should be monitored expectantly with a pulse oximeter. Pulse oximeters measure oxygen saturation by detecting differences in the absorption of a red light and an infrared light signal by a pulsating arteriolar vascular bed. Depending on the severity of the respiratory distress, an arterial blood gas measurement should be considered, and the need for mechanical ventilatory assistance and placement of an umbilical (or peripheral) arterial catheter for serial arterial blood gas measurements evaluated. Although capillary blood gas measurements satisfactorily estimate arterial pH and P_{CO_2} during the first 24 hours of life, estimates of arterial P_{O_2} are inaccurate and unreliable. Fortunately, pulse oximetry provides an easily obtained, accurate assessment of inspiratory oxygen needs. The evaluation and management of infants with respiratory distress is discussed further in Section IIf (Respiratory System).

Serial blood pressure monitoring should be done on infants who are unstable (such as those with respiratory distress), who may have suffered some degree of intrapartum asphyxia, and who may have experienced an acute blood loss. Noninvasive blood pressure measurements can be performed by monitors that inflate a blood pressure cuff at preset intervals and then display systolic, diastolic, and mean blood pressure and heart rate. Continuous blood pressure monitoring can be performed from an arterial catheter with a pressure transducer. In addition, the hematocrit (or hemoglobin) should be rechecked 4 to 6 hours after admission in any infant who may have suffered an intrapartum blood loss. The need for blood transfusion, volume expansion, or pharmacologic support of blood pressure is made in response to the infant's evolving clinical status and the presence or absence of hypotension, poor capillary refill, a decrease in hematocrit (or hemoglobin), metabolic acidosis, and decreased urine output.

These initial assessments, plus a physical examination and gestational age assessment, are often performed while the infant lies under a radiant warmer. If stable, the neonate is moved to a heated Plexiglas isolette, which permits observation and easy maintenance of body temperature. If unstable, the neonate is often managed on the warmer to facilitate access by medical and nursing staff. For example, neonates requiring mechanical ventilatory assistance may be initially cared for on an open warmer, where such procedures as administration of surfactant replacement therapy, reintubation, placement of umbilical vessel catheters, chest tube placement, suctioning, and chest radiologic studies are more easily performed. As soon as possible, however, the infant should be moved into an isolette, because an infant's insensible water loss is greater when cared for under a radiant warmer.

The age at which enteral feedings are initiated depends on such factors as the infant's birth weight and gestational age, a history of fetal distress, and the presence and severity of respiratory distress. Intravenous fluids and parenteral nutrition solutions should be provided until enteral feedings are well established so as to maintain normal fluid and electrolyte status and to optimize protein and calorie intake. At YNHCH, enteral feedings in infants weighing less than 1,250 g at birth are delayed for at least 24 hours; then small volumes are offered by nasogastric tube if the infant's condition is stable. Enteral feedings are delayed in infants with birth weights between 1,250 and 1,500 g for at least 12 hours. Then, if the infant is stable, feedings are advanced as described previously while parenteral nutrition is tapered. Finally, with larger infants, enteral feedings are initiated within 6 hours of birth if the infant is stable. However, feedings are delayed for at least 24 hours for any infant with a birth weight of more than 1,250 g with a history of fetal distress or with respiratory distress.

Initial Medical Management of Infants with Severe Perinatal Asphyxia

Infants who have suffered severe perinatal asphyxia may develop hypoxic-ischemic encephalopathy and may demonstrate a spectrum of multiorgan injury; therefore, they must be managed expectantly. Their level of consciousness and neurologic examination, including neurovital signs and level of arousal, must be followed carefully. If clinical signs of increased intracranial pressure develop, a cranial ultrasound should be performed to look for evidence of intraventricular or parenchymal hemorrhage, mass effect, generalized edema, or shift of the midline. A head computed tomographic scan should be done if subdural hemorrhage is suspected or if the cranial ultrasound

study produces questionable findings. Although performing a lumbar puncture to document increased intracranial pressure or monitoring intracranial pressure noninvasively is not routine, many neonatologists attempt to minimize cerebral edema during the first 48 to 72 hours of life by restricting fluid intake and maintaining serum osmolality between 290 and 300 mOsm/L. A more detailed discussion of the neurologic evaluation and management of infants with hypoxic-ischemic encephalopathy is found in Chapter 34.

Severely asphyxiated infants usually require mechanical ventilatory assistance with correction and stabilization of arterial pH, Po_2, and Pco_2. Some may require treatment for meconium aspiration pneumonia or persistent pulmonary hypertension; the management of these problems is discussed in Chapters 47 and 48. Because treatment of those infants with medications that produce neuromuscular blockade or sedation may interfere with observation of seizure activity, serial electroencephalographic monitoring has been suggested.

Cardiac activity may be depressed by severe asphyxia, and inotropic support may be required. Assessment of myocardial injury with echocardiography, electrocardiography, and serial cardiac enzyme study has been advocated. Central venous pressure monitoring also may be helpful in managing infants with severe myocardial dysfunction, impaired renal status, and uncertain volume status.

Acute renal failure also is seen commonly in severe asphyxia. Renal function should be monitored closely by determining urine output (oliguria is less than 0.5 mL/kg/hour) and performing serial laboratory measurements of blood urea nitrogen, serum creatinine, serum and urine electrolytes, and fractional excretion of sodium. Also, body weight should be measured at least once a day.

Asphyxia may predispose the gastrointestinal tract to the development of necrotizing enterocolitis caused by intestinal ischemia. Therefore, these infants are usually observed without enteral feedings for the first several days of life, and then feedings are initiated and cautiously advanced when the infant has active bowel sounds and is considered stable.

In addition, severe asphyxia may produce hepatic damage and a coagulopathy. Hepatic injury is usually followed with serial serum bilirubin measurements; determination of liver enzyme [i.e., alanine aminotransferase (serum glutamic-pyruvic transaminase), aspartate aminotransferase (serum glutamic-oxaloacetic transaminase)] activity would be performed if the direct (or conjugated) bilirubin level is elevated. Coagulation status is often evaluated clinically and by measuring the platelet count. If there is evidence of clinical bleeding or thrombocytopenia, then coagulation studies should be performed.

Ventilatory Equipment for Resuscitation

Two standard types of ventilation bags exist, a self-inflating bag and an anesthesia bag. The self-inflating bag refills itself because of its elasticity, independently of gas flow. An intake valve or a series of valves at one end of the bag allows it to be rapidly reinflated. However, unless this type of bag is fitted with an oxygen reservoir that surrounds the intake valve(s), oxygen flowing into the bag is diluted by the air that is reinflating the bag, and high concentrations of oxygen cannot be delivered. Although the self-inflating feature makes this bag easier to use, some self-inflating bags deliver oxygen only when they are compressed. Self-inflating bags that permit free-flow oxygen are preferable. Finally, even though many self-inflating bags are equipped with a pressure-limited pop-off valve that is preset at 30 to 40 cm of water, a pressure manometer is recommended during any positive-pressure ventilation. Since the end-expiratory pressure returns to zero after each breath with most types of self-inflating bags, CPAP/positive end-expiratory pressure (PEEP) valves that can be attached to self-inflating bags are now available. Very low-birth-weight infants may require peak inspiratory pressures of only 15 to 20 cm of water to achieve adequate chest expansion, whereas asphyxiated term infants initially may require peak inspiratory pressures as high as 60 cm of water.

The anesthesia bag is reinflated by a continuous flow of air or oxygen from a compressed gas source. Delivery of an adequate ventilatory volume requires that the bag be refilled sufficiently between breaths. This is a function of the rate of air/oxygen gas flow into the intake port, adjustment of a flow control or exit valve, and the soundness of the seal between the infant and the face mask or endotracheal tube. If ventilation is interrupted and the mask is removed from the infant's face or the bag is disconnected from the endotracheal tube, the bag promptly deflates; it must be allowed to reinflate before positive-pressure ventilation can be restarted. However, this is a flow-through system, and facial oxygen can be provided by directing the ventilation port (with or without a mask) toward the infant's face. The anesthesia bag can deliver very high inspiratory pressures, so a pressure gauge must be included within the respiratory circuit so that peak inspiratory pressures can be monitored. In addition, the flow control or exit valve permits this type of ventilatory bag to maintain PEEP during positive-pressure ventilation; in contrast, unless a self-inflating bag includes a CPAP/PEEP valve, the end-expiratory pressure returns to zero after each breath. Although the ability to deliver a high inspiratory pressure and maintain a PEEP are advantages of this ventilation bag, it is often considered more difficult to use properly.

Face masks, oral airways, and endotracheal tubes should be available in sizes appropriate for preterm and term neonates. Face masks should conform to the infant's facial features and should form a tight seal while covering the nose and mouth. The masks should have a low dead space. Transparent masks and masks with cushioned rims are available. Such masks help the resuscitator position the mask and form a tight facial seal.

An oral airway may be helpful when an infant is ventilated with a bag and mask. Oral airways push the tongue down and forward into the floor of the mouth and ensure a patent airway.

Most of the endotracheal tubes used today are made of siliconized polyvinyl chloride, which is nonirritating and malleable and conforms to the trachea after being warmed to body temperature. The largest endotracheal tube that fits easily into the trachea should be used during intubation: the smaller the tube, the greater the airway resistance and the more difficulty in suctioning during pulmonary toilet. The tube should be noncuffed, and a small gas leak should be present around the tube during positive-pressure ventilation. Cuffed tubes have been associated with subglottic and tracheal necrosis in neonates. Appropriate endotracheal tube size (internal diameter) is a function of body weight: body weight less than 1,000 g, 2.5 mm; 1,000 to 2,000 g, 3.0 mm; 2,000 to 3,500 g, 3.5 mm; and more than 3,500 g, 4.0 mm. In addition, many endotracheal tubes have a black line above the tip of the tube, ranging from approximately 2 cm with 2.5-mm tubes to approximately 3.5 cm with 4.0-mm tubes. If this line is placed at the level of the vocal cords, the tip of the tube should be above the carina and in the midtrachea. In the delivery room, the tip-to-lip measurement can also be used to estimate if the tube is in the midtrachea; adding 6 to the infant's estimated weight in kilograms provides a rough estimate of the correct distance between the tube tip and the vermillion border of the upper lip. Therefore, 7 cm is the appropriate tube length for infants estimated to be about 1,000 g, 8 cm for infants about 2,000 g, and 9 cm for infants about 3,000 g; for extremely low-gestational-age infants with birth weights less than 750 g, tube lengths of about 6 cm are often adequate.

The endotracheal tube should have a uniform internal diameter over its entire length. Tubes such as Cole-type tubes, which decrease their diameter at the tracheal end to produce a short, narrow segment that extends into the trachea while the tapered area or shoulder rests on the vocal cords, should not be used if positive-pressure ventilatory support will be continued. Although these tubes may be easier to insert during an emergency, they have been associated with significant damage to the glottis and they increase airway resistance and dead space.

Laryngoscopy and Endotracheal Intubation

To facilitate endotracheal intubation, the infant should be lying supine under the radiant warmer of the resuscitation table with a rolled or folded towel under the shoulders to produce slight neck extension (Fig. 24.6). In this position, the infant's chin is slightly extended as if sniffing the air. Hyperextending the infant's neck usually obstructs visualization of the glottic opening and the vocal cords. The infant's head is steadied by the operator's right hand or by an assistant. The laryngoscope is held between the thumb and first finger of the operator's left hand and the infant's chin is grasped firmly with the second and third fingers of that hand. During intubation, the infant's heart rate is monitored by auscultation or with a cardiac monitor. The appropriate-sized blade of a lighted laryngoscope is inserted near the right corner of the infant's mouth and advanced between the tongue and palate for approximately 2 cm. As the blade advances, it should be moved to the left side of the mouth. This maneuver moves the tongue to the left of the blade and permits visualization of the base of the tongue and epiglottis.

The blade is advanced into the vallecula, the space between the base of the tongue and the anterior surface of the epiglottis. Gentle elevation of the tip of the blade lifts the epiglottis anteriorly, revealing the glottic opening. In addition, the fourth or small finger of the left hand can press on the hyoid bone to move the larynx posteriorly and expose the glottis. Then, under direct visualization, the endotracheal tube is inserted along the right side of the blade into the trachea, approximately 2 to 3 cm below the level of the vocal cords (when applicable, the black line on the tube should be at the level of the vocal cords). The laryngoscope blade is then removed while the position of the tube is maintained by the right hand on the infant's face.

The laryngoscope blade should not be advanced below the epiglottis to "pick it up," or to elevate it, because it is easily traumatized. Also, placing the blade below the epiglottis obscures visualization of the glottic opening. However, this might not be possible with extremely low-birth-weight infants in whom the hypopharynx is quite small. The endotracheal tube should not be passed through the grooved opening of the laryngoscope blade, because that also obscures visualization.

When intubation is complete, the lungs should be expanded with a ventilation bag. Tube placement should be confirmed by auscultatory evidence of equal, bilateral breath sounds over the axillary regions and symmetric chest movement. Unequal breath sounds and chest excursions suggest that the tube is probably in the mainstem bronchus of the lung producing the louder breath sounds. In that case, the tube should be withdrawn until breath sounds improve and become equal. Esophageal intubation results in poor breath sounds and chest movement, but loud sounds over the stomach. The tube should be immediately removed and then tracheal intubation reattempted after a brief period of bag and mask ventilation with oxygen. Colorimetric CO_2 detectors connected to the endotracheal tube have been shown to provide confirmatory evidence that the tube is in the trachea rather then the esophagus. Once

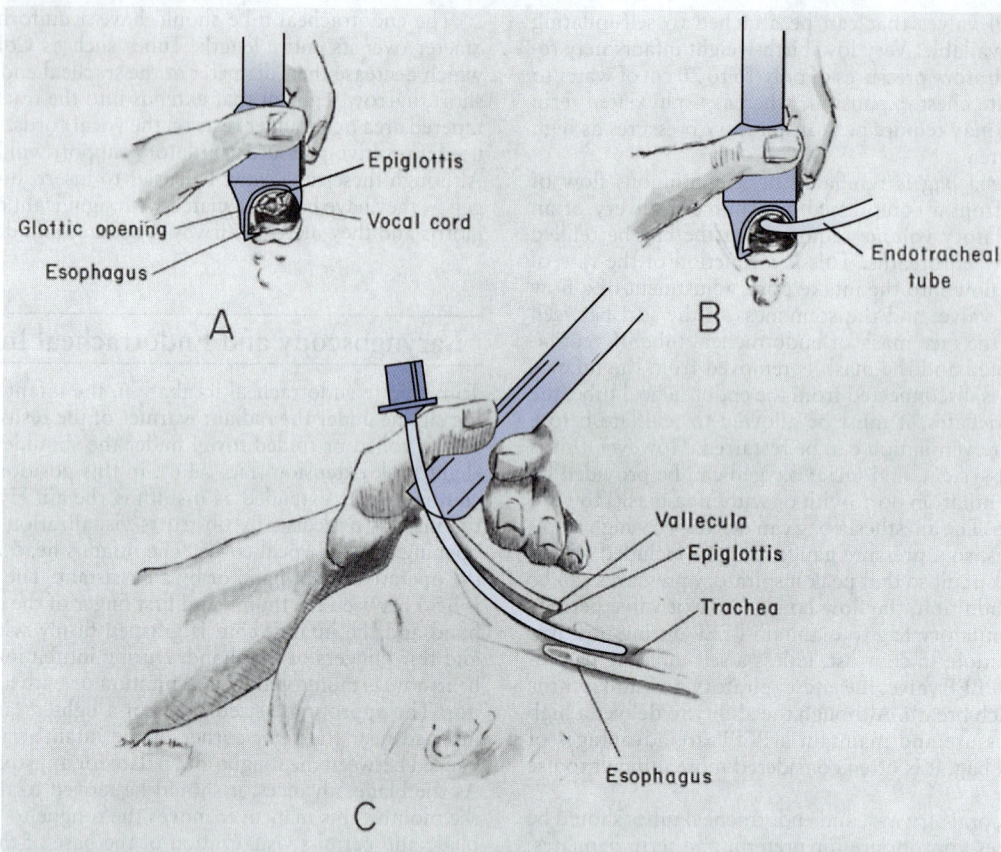

FIGURE 24.6. Technique of endotracheal intubation. **A:** Direct laryngoscopy. Note the glottic opening below the epiglottis and between the vocal cords. The esophagus is below the glottis. **B:** Insersion of the endotracheal tube through the glottic opening from the right corner of the mouth. **C:** The endotracheal tube is within the trachea. Note that the tip of the laryngoscope blade is in the vallecula, above the anterior surface of the epiglottis, and that the esophagus is below the trachea. (Reprinted with permission from Ehrenkranz RA. Delivery room emergencies and resuscitation. In: Warshaw JB, Hobbins JC, eds. *Principles and practice of perinatal medicine: maternal-fetal and newborn care.* Menlo Park, CA: Addison-Wesley, 1983:209.)

the tube is secured, a chest roentgenograph should be obtained to confirm tube position.

Umbilical Vessel Catheterization

An umbilical arterial catheter is most often used for monitoring arterial blood gases, arterial blood pressure, and vascular access. An umbilical venous catheter is most often used for monitoring central venous pressure, performing exchange transfusions, and providing vascular access in very low-birth-weight infants. Radiopaque, single- or multilumen end-hole catheters may be used for pressure monitoring, blood sampling, and vascular access; 3.5 Fr. catheters are often used with infants less than 1,500 g and 5 Fr. catheters for larger infants. A catheter with end and side holes may be used when the umbilical vein is being catheterized for an exchange transfusion; 5 and 8 Fr. sizes are available. The catheters are usually marked at centimeter intervals. A syringe filled with a heparinized solution (5% or 10% dextrose and water or normal saline, with 0.5 to 1.0 U of heparin per milliliter) is attached to the sterile three-way stopcock that has been inserted into each port at the distal end of the catheter. Each lumen of the catheter is filled with the heparinized solution and the stopcock turned off to that lumen.

The infant is placed on an infant warmer with the head at the open or distal end to allow resuscitation if necessary. The heart rate is monitored with a cardiac monitor during the procedure, and the infant should receive supplemental oxygen or ventilatory assistance as indicated. The distance that the catheter should be inserted from the abdominal wall is estimated from the infant's crown–heel length or the shoulder–umbilicus distance (Table 24.12). Umbilical vessel catheterization is done aseptically. Therefore, after adequately restraining the infant's extremities and grasping the end of the umbilical cord by the cord clamp or with a Kelly clamp, the umbilical cord, umbilicus, and periumbilical area are prepared with a povidone–iodine solution and then draped so that only the cord is exposed. Umbilical cord tape is tied loosely around the cord, as close to the abdomen as possible, and should be tightened if bleeding occurs. The umbilical cord is then cleanly cut approximately 1.0 to 1.5 cm from the umbilicus with a scalpel blade or large scissors. The length of cord remaining must be added to the estimated catheter length.

The side of the umbilical cord stump is then grasped with nontoothed forceps or a hemostat, the cut surface is blotted, and the umbilical vessels are isolated. The single, large, thin-walled oval vein should be readily distinguished from the two smaller thick-walled arteries, which are usually constricted and appear pinpoint in size. With arterial catheterization, one of the arteries is gently dilated by placing the closed tips of a small nontoothed forceps into the lumen and allowing the spring of the forceps to spread the tips apart. A blunt probe may also be used to dilate the vessel lumen. Once dilated, the opposite walls of the artery can be grasped with small nontoothed forceps

TABLE 24.12

ESTIMATION OF VESSEL CATHETER LENGTH

Crown-Heel Length (cm)	Length of Umbilical Artery Catheter (cm)		Length of Umbilical Vein Catheter (cm)[c]	Shoulder-Umbilicus Length (cm)[d]
	Low Placement[a]	High Placement[b]		
34	5.0	10.0	5.5	10.0
38	6.0	11.5	6.5	11.5
42	7.0	13.0	7.5	12.5
46	8.0	14.5	8.0	13.5
50	9.0	16.0	9.0	15.0
54	10.0	18.5	10.0	16.5

[a]Length of catheter from abdominal wall to bifurcation of the aorta.
[b]Length of catheter from abdominal wall to the diaphragm within the aorta.
[c]Length of catheter from abdominal wall to reach the inferior vena cava just above the diaphragm.
[d]Length from above the lateral end of the clavicle to the umbilicus.
Adapted from Dunn PM Localization of the umbilical catheter by postmortem measurement. *Arch Dis Child* 1966;41:69.

by an assistant. While the catheter is held approximately 1 cm from its tip with small curved forceps, it is inserted in the lumen of the artery. If the artery is well dilated, an assistant may not be needed to hold the lumen walls apart. The catheter is then slowly advanced to the estimated length.

Obstruction to umbilical arterial catheter insertion may be encountered at either the level of the anterior abdominal wall or farther on at approximately the bladder level. Obstruction may be relieved by gentle caudad traction on the umbilical stump accompanied by 30 to 60 seconds of steady pressure. The other umbilical artery should be tried if it is impossible to catheterize the first vessel. Obstruction to catheter insertion may be related to dissection of the catheter out of the vessel lumen. Successful catheterization occasionally can be accomplished if the obstructed catheter is left in place while a second catheter is slid alongside it within the same vessel. If the first catheter is occupying a false track, it may permit the second

catheter to remain within the umbilical artery as it is advanced into the abdominal aorta.

If the stopcock is open to air while the catheter is being inserted, blood will enter the catheter, indicating successful catheterization. Arterial pulsations can also be noted with blood in the catheter and with the stopcock closed to the infant. If any question exists about whether the artery or vein is being catheterized, however, the stopcock should not be open to air during catheter insertion. If an umbilical venous catheter were opened to atmospheric pressure at a time when the infant generated a large negative intrathoracic pressure such as with crying, a large volume of air could be sucked into the right side of the heart and cause an air embolus.

Catheter placement should be confirmed by abdominal radiographs. Although an anteroposterior view of the abdomen is usually adequate for this purpose (Fig. 24.7), if any question exists, a lateral view demonstrates the location of the catheter

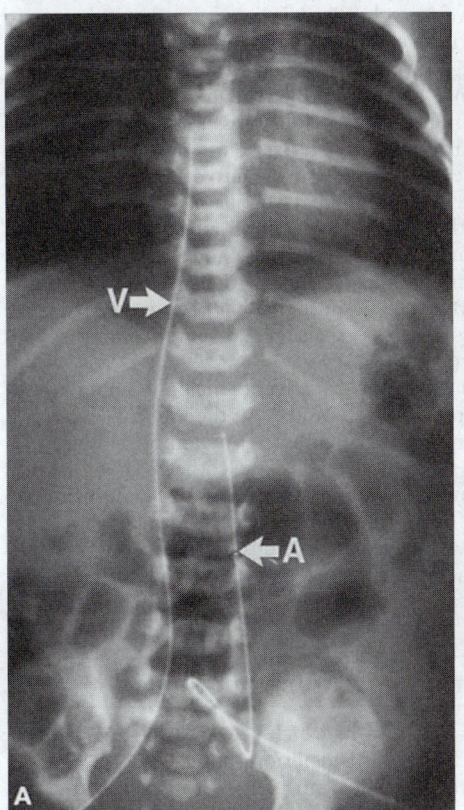
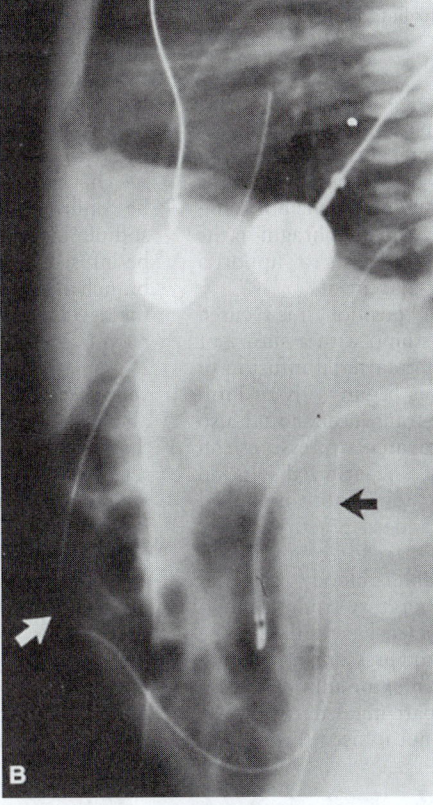

FIGURE 24.7. Umbilical vessel catheterization. A: Anteroposterior radiograph demonstrating an umbilical arterial catheter (A) in the abdominal aorta overlying the L1 and L2 interspace and an umbilical venous catheter (V) in the right atrium. Note the characteristic V-shaped appearance of the arterial catheter compared with the linear appearance of the venous catheter. B: Lateral radiograph of the same neonate demonstrating catheters entering umbilical vessels at the abdominal wall (*white arrow*). The umbilical venous catheter proceeds cephalad as it passes via the ductus venosus into the inferior vena cava and then into the right atrium, whereas the umbilical arterial catheter (*black arrow*) initially proceeds caudally via the umbilical artery, then loops cephalad via the hypogastric artery, and iliac artery into the abdominal aorta, lying over the spine.

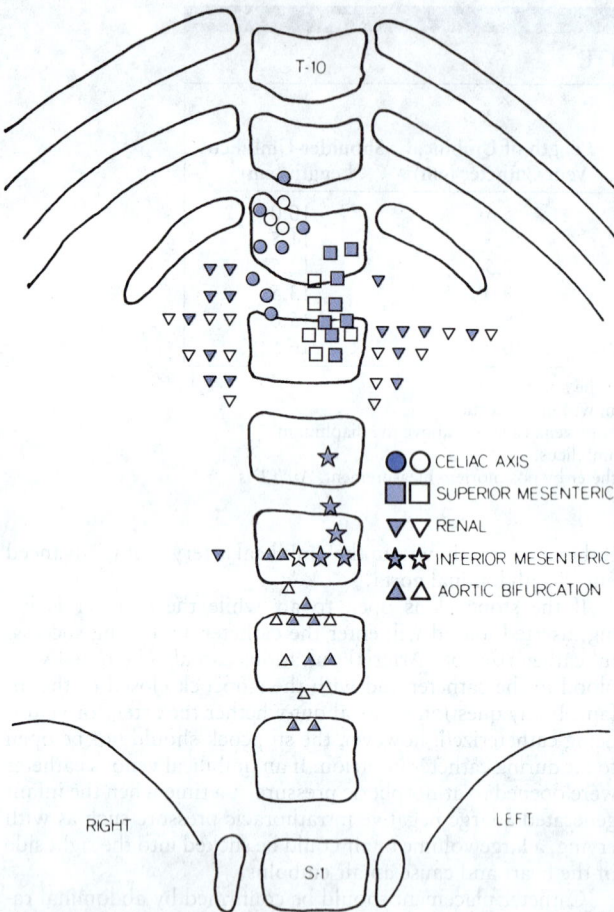

FIGURE 24.8. Distribution of the major aortic branches found in 15 infants. Filled symbols represent infants with, and open symbols represent infants without, cardiac, renal, or both anomalies. (Reprinted with permission from Phelps DL, Lachman RS, Leake RD, Oh W. The radiologic localization of the major aortic tributaries in the newborn infant. *J Pediatr* 1972;81:336.)

tip and confirms that an umbilical artery has been catheterized. Two preferred locations exist for the tip of the umbilical artery catheter: lying within the lower abdominal aorta over the third or fourth lumbar vertebra, so that it is below the origin of the renal and inferior mesenteric arteries and above the aortic bifurcation (Fig. 24.8); or lying just above the diaphragm in the thoracic aorta. However, little information exists to support a preference for low versus high catheter placement.

Once the catheter tip is in satisfactory position, it is secured to the Wharton jelly of the umbilical stump with a suture or taped to the abdominal wall, and an intraarterial infusion of a dextrose and/or electrolyte solution is begun with an infusion pump. An arterial blood pressure transducer should also be attached to the catheter so that intravascular pressures can be continuously monitored. Infusion of a heparinized solution (0.5 to 1.0 U of heparin per milliliter) through an umbilical artery catheter is common but not standard practice. Many clinicians have used umbilical arterial catheters primarily for monitoring blood pressure and for obtaining blood for arterial blood gas measurements and other laboratory studies. However, the availability of multilumen catheters has resulted in the use of one of the catheter lumens for blood pressure monitoring and blood sampling and the other lumen(s) for administration of medications, blood products, and parenteral nutrition. At YNHCH, vasoactive medications are not infused through an umbilical arterial catheter.

Blanching or cyanosis of a lower extremity is commonly observed following placement of an umbilical arterial catheter. Blanching or cyanosis is thought to represent vasospasm produced by the catheter's presence within the arterial system extending between the umbilical artery and the bifurcation of the aorta. This problem should be treated by warming the opposite leg; the warmth should increase blood flow to the affected leg because of reflex vasodilation. Warming the leg that is blanched or cyanotic is contraindicated, because the warmth increases oxygen consumption in tissue that is already compromised, potentiating the problem. The catheter should be removed if no improvement occurs. Infusion of lidocaine through an umbilical arterial catheter to diminish vasospasm is not recommended. Several clinicians have recently reported successful reversal of persistent peripheral tissue ischemia following removal of the umbilical arterial catheter with application of topical nitroglycerin ointment (2%) over the femoral artery and at several other locations of the affected leg.

To monitor central venous pressure, a catheter may be placed via the umbilical vein into the inferior vena cava just above the diaphragm near the right atrium (see Fig. 24.7). Before catheterizing the umbilical vein, any visible clot is removed with a forceps. Then, a catheter filled with a heparinized solution is introduced into the lumen of the vein. This catheter should always be closed to air, for the reasons noted previously. The catheter is slowly advanced the estimated distance (see Table 24.10) from the abdominal wall through the ductus venosus into the inferior vena cava. Because of the orientation of the heart within the chest, an umbilical venous catheter commonly passes from the inferior vena cava through the right atrium and foramen ovale into the left atrium. In a well-oxygenated infant, this location can be easily discerned from the color of the blood within the catheter; in sicker patients, a blood gas or a chest radiograph is necessary. Leaving this catheter in the left atrium is not recommended.

Obstruction to umbilical venous catheter insertion indicates that it has entered the portal system and is probably wedged within a small vein in the liver. Reinserting the catheter after withdrawing it several centimeters and rotating it often results in its passage through the ductus venosus. Occasionally, the catheter cannot be inserted into the inferior vena cava via the umbilical vein. If central venous pressure monitoring is required, another route of catheterization is necessary, such as by a catheter inserted percutaneously into a femoral vein.

The location of an umbilical venous catheter tip should be confirmed with radiography. Hypertonic solutions, such as sodium bicarbonate and 25% dextrose and water, should not be infused into an umbilical venous catheter located within a branch of the portal vein, because that has been associated with the development of liver necrosis, portal vein thrombosis, and necrotizing enterocolitis.

To perform an exchange transfusion, the tip of an umbilical venous catheter preferably should be in the inferior vena cava above the diaphragm. If the catheter tip cannot be placed in that location via the umbilical vein, the catheter should be inserted into the umbilical vein to a depth of 2 to 3 cm from the abdominal wall. Then, an umbilical arterial catheter should be inserted and the exchange performed by simultaneous removal of blood from the arterial catheter and infusion of the blood into the venous catheter.

Aspiration of a Pneumothorax

In an emergency situation in which a tension pneumothorax is suspected and the infant is deteriorating, a 16- or 18-gauge styletted, small vein catheter can be used to evacuate the air from within the thorax. The appropriate anterior hemithorax is cleaned with an antiseptic preparation. The styletted cannula is inserted at a 45-degree angle to the skin between the anterior axillary and the midclavicular line, just above the fifth or sixth rib, but caudal to the breast. The cannula is directed cephalad. When the stylet enters the pleural space, the cannula is advanced several centimeters at approximately a 15-degree angle to the skin as the stylet is withdrawn. A 20-mL syringe attached to a three-way stopcock is quickly connected to the adapter of the catheter. Air is aspirated into the syringe and then evacuated from the syringe when the stopcock is closed to the infant and open to air. If the infant is receiving positive-pressure ventilation, positive intrathoracic pressure is produced and air will

not enter the pleural space if the cannula is left open. If possible, emergency aspiration of a pneumothorax should not be done with a needle that is left within the pleural space, because the needlepoint can penetrate and damage lung tissue after the air is evacuated and the lung reexpands. Furthermore, after emergency aspiration of a tension pneumothorax, a thoracostomy tube is often inserted to prevent reaccumulation of the air. The cannula may be left in place until insertion of the thoracostomy tube is completed.

Tube thoracostomy can be performed without prior aspiration of the pneumothorax if the infant is more stable and can withstand the extra time required for this procedure. Insertion of a tube thoracostomy is performed aseptically (Fig. 24.9).

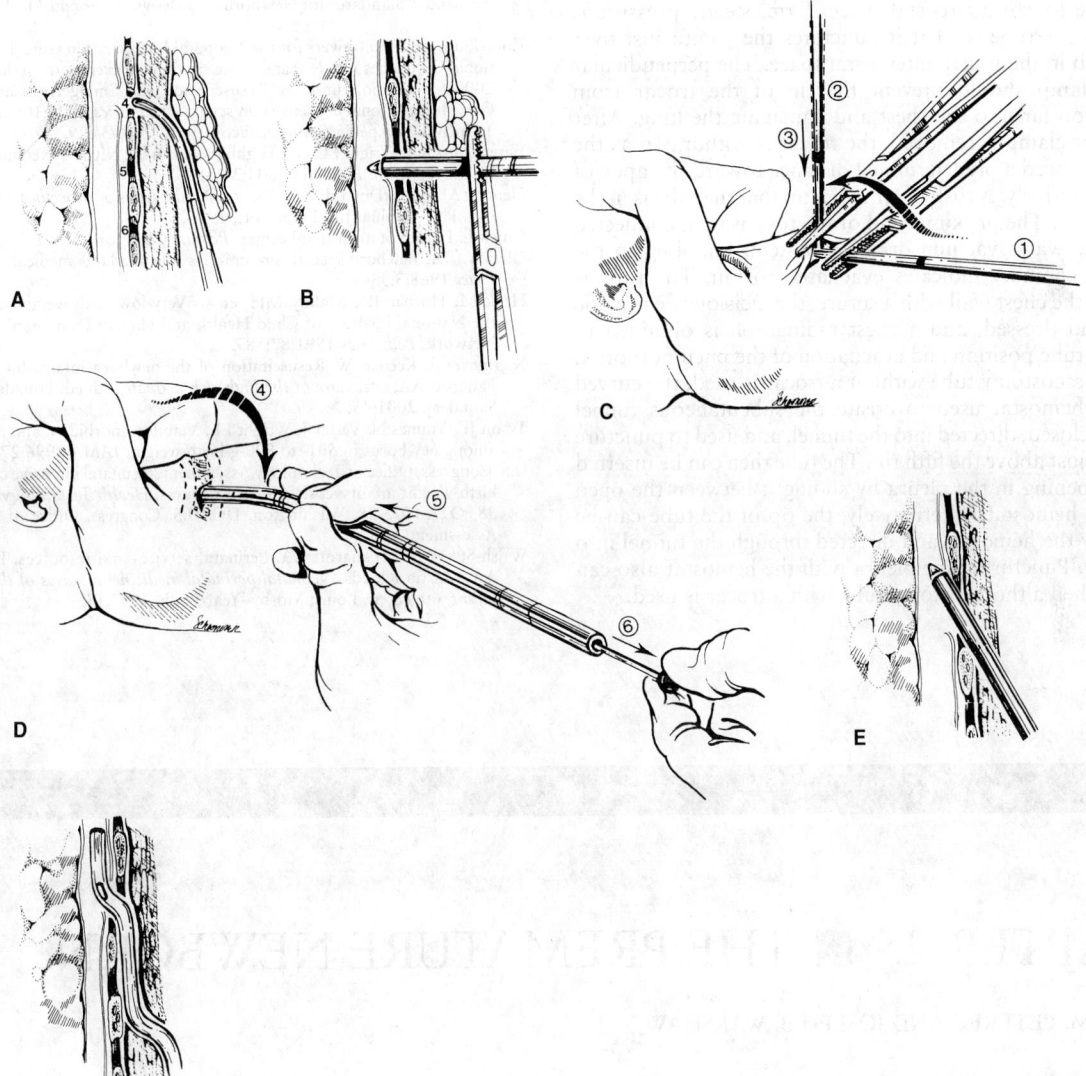

FIGURE 24.9. Insertion of a thoracostomy tube with a trocar. (A) Tunnel from the sixth to the fourth intercostal space (ICS) with a curved mosquito hemostat. (B) Place a straight clamp perpendicularly across the tube and pass the tube along the tunnel to the entry site in the fourth ICS. (C) (1) Rotate the tube perpendicular to the chest wall. (2) Holding the clamp, apply firm, steady pressure so that the trocar punctures the pleura. (3) The clamp should prevent the tip of the trocar from entering too deeply into the pleural cavity. (D) (4) Rotate the tube so that it is parallel to the chest wall. After removing the clamp, advance the tube anteriorly toward the apex of the lung (5) while withdrawing the trocar (6). (E) Tube is directed anterior cephalad into the pleural space. (F) Path of the tube is through the subcutaneous tunnel into the pleural space. (Reprinted with permission from Fletcher MA, Eichelberger MR. Thoracostomy tubes. In: Fletcher MA, MacDonald MG, Avery GB, eds. *Atlas of procedures in neonatology.* Philadelphia: JB Lippincott Company, 1983:272.)

The infant is positioned with the affected side of the chest raised approximately 60% off the bed and the arm on that side restrained, without external rotation over the head. The lateral aspect of the chest is prepared with a povidone–iodine solution and then draped. After administering a local anesthetic over the sixth or seventh intercostal space between the midaxillary and the anterior axillary line, a horizontal incision approximately 1 cm long is made. Then, with a curved mosquito hemostat, a subcutaneous tunnel is made by spreading the tissue from the incision site to the fourth intercostal space. If a thoracostomy tube with a trocar is used, the distal portion (approximately 2 to 3 cm from the tip) is bent to create approximately a 135-degree angle, and a straight clamp is placed perpendicularly across the tube, approximately 1.5 cm from the tip. The thoracostomy tube is directed through the subcutaneous tunnel toward the fourth intercostal space. Firm, steady pressure is applied to the tube so that it punctures the pleura just over the fifth rib in the fourth intercostal space. The perpendicular straight clamp should prevent the tip of the trocar from plunging too far into the chest and damaging the lung. After the straight clamp is removed, the trocar is withdrawn as the tube is advanced a predetermined distance toward the apex of the lung anteriorly. A rush of air indicates that the tube is in the pleural space. The proximal end of the tube is then connected to an underwater vacuum drainage system; bubbling in the water-seal chamber indicates evacuation of air. The tube is secured to the chest wall with a suture, the incision site is made airtight and dressed, and a chest radiograph is obtained to document tube position and evacuation of the pneumothorax.

If a thoracostomy tube without a trocar is used, the curved mosquito hemostat used to create the subcutaneous tunnel should be closed, directed into the tunnel, and used to puncture the pleura just above the fifth rib. The tube then can be inserted into the opening in the pleura by sliding it between the open tips of the hemostat. Alternatively, the tip of the tube can be grasped by the hemostat and directed through the tunnel into the thorax. Puncturing the pleura with the hemostat also can be done when a thoracostomy tube with a trocar is used.

Suggested Readings

American Academy of Pediatrics, American College of Obstetricians and Gynecologists. *Guidelines for perinatal care,* 5th ed. Elk Grove Village, IL: American Academy of Pediatrics, 2002.

American Academy of Pediatrics, American Heart Association. *Textbook of neonatal resuscitation,* 4th ed. Elk Grove Village, IL: American Academy of Pediatrics, 2000.

Avery GB. Part one: general considerations. In: Avery GB, Fletcher MA, MacDonald MG, eds. *Neonatology: pathophysiology and management of the newborn,* 5th ed. Philadelphia: Lippincott Williams & Wilkins, 1999:3.

Cifuentes J, Bronstein J, Phibbs CS, et al. Mortality in low birth weight infants according to level of neonatal care at hospital of birth. *Pediatrics* 2002;109:745.

Committee on Perinatal Health. *Toward improving the outcome of pregnancy. The 90s and beyond.* White Plains, NY: March of Dimes Birth Defects Foundation, 1993.

Committee to Establish Recommended Standards for Newborn ICU Design. Recommended Standards for Newborn ICU Design. *J Perinatol* 1999;19(Part 2):S1.

Contributors and Reviewers for the Neonatal Resuscitation Guidelines. International Guidelines for Neonatal Resuscitation: an excerpt from the Guidelines 2000 for Cardiopulmonary Resuscitation and Emergency Cardiovascular Care: International consensus on science. *Pediatrics* 2000;106(3). Available at: http://www.pediatrics.org/cgi/content/full/106/3/e29.

Ehrenkranz RA, Wright LL, eds. Highlights from the NICHD Neonatal Research Network. *Semin Perinatol* 2003;23(4).

Fletcher MA, MacDonald MG, Avery GB, eds. *Atlas of procedures in neonatology.* Philadelphia: J.B. Lippincott, 1983.

Gluck L. Design of a perinatal center. *Pediatr Clin North Am* 1970;17:777.

Gluck L. The newborn special care unit. Its role in a large medical center. *Hosp Pract* 1968;3:33.

Hack M, Horbar JD, Malloy MH, et al. Very-low-birth-weight outcomes of the National Institute of Child Health and Human Development Neonatal Network. *Pediatrics* 1991;87:587.

Niermeyer S, Keenan W. Resuscitation of the newborn infant. In: Klaus MH, Fanaroff AA, eds. *Care of the high-risk neonate,* 5th ed. Philadelphia: W.B. Saunders, 2001:45.

Tyson JE, Younes N, Verter J, Wright LL. Viability, morbidity, and resource use among newborns of 501- to 800-g birth weight. *JAMA* 1996;276:1645.

U.S. Congress, Office of Technology Assessment. Neonatal intensive care for low-birth-weight infants: costs and effectiveness. *Health Technology Case Study 38,* OTA-HCS-38. Washington, DC: U.S. Congress, Office of Technology Assessment, 1987.

Walsh-Sukys MC, Fanaroff AA. Perinatal services and resources. In: Fanaroff AA, Martin RJ, eds. *Neonatal-perinatal medicine: diseases of the fetus and infant,* 6th ed. St. Louis: Mosby–Year Book, 1997:13.

CHAPTER 25 ■ THE PREMATURE NEWBORN

STEVEN M. PETEREC AND JOSEPH B. WARSHAW

Preterm delivery is probably the most important problem in obstetrics and neonatology today. Over 400,000 preterm births occur each year in the United States. It is the leading cause of perinatal, neonatal, and infant mortality. Approximately two-third of infant deaths in the United States occur in the 7% to 8% of infants born with a birth weight of less than 2,500 g. A higher rate of preterm delivery is a major reason that the United States has one of the highest infant mortality rates among developed nations. Preterm births also are responsible for a large proportion of long-term neurodevelopmental handicaps in children. It is estimated that preterm births account for approximately one-third of all health care spending for infants and a tenth of all health care spending for children in the United States.

DEFINITIONS AND TERMINOLOGY

The fetus or newborn infant is defined as *term* during the interval between 37 and 42 weeks after the onset of the mother's last menstrual period. A preterm newborn is defined as an infant delivered before completion of 37 weeks of gestation. The word *premature* often is used synonymously with *preterm,* although for any given pregnancy, maturation may lag behind or forge ahead of gestational age. This chapter focuses on the problems of prematurity, which for the most part are those of preterm infants.

Other important terms are *low birth weight* (LBW), which describes infants with birth weights less than 2,500 g, *very low birth weight* (VLBW), which describes infants with birth weights less than 1,500 g, and *extremely low birth weight* (ELBW), which describes infants with birth weights less than 1,000 g. Just as the degree of maturation does not always parallel gestational age, birth weight may be small or large for gestational age. Thus, some preterm infants are not LBW, and some LBW infants are not preterm. Disorders of growth rate and particular problems associated with infants who are small for gestational age are discussed in Chapter 20, Growth and Metabolic Adaptation of the Fetus and Newborn and Chapter 27, Intrauterine Growth Retardation.

EPIDEMIOLOGY

Incidence

The preterm birth rate in the United States was 9.4% in 1981, and over the next two decades rose steadily to a rate of 12.0% in 2002 (Fig. 25.1). The increase in the preterm birth rate can be explained by a failure to combat medical and social conditions associated with preterm birth, as well as an increase in the frequency of multiple births (many due to infertility treatments), an increase in obstetrical interventions, and an increase in ascertainment. The rate of very preterm birth (less than 32 weeks' gestation) is approximately 2%.

The rate of LBW rose in parallel with the preterm birth rate. The LBW and VLBW rates were 7.8% and 1.45%, respectively, in 2002 (see Fig. 25.1). Significant disparities in these rates exist between races. For example, in 2002, the preterm birth rate for non-Hispanic whites was 11.0%, for Hispanics, 11.6%, and for blacks, 17.5%.

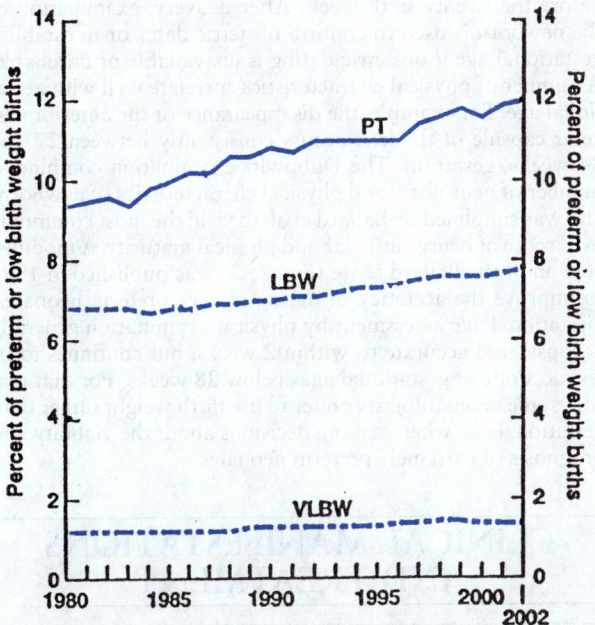

FIGURE 25.1. Percent of births that were preterm (PT), low birth weight (LBW), and very low birth weight (VLBW) in the United States, 1980–2002. (Modified with permission from Arias E, MacDorman MF, Strobino DM, et al. Annual summary of vital statistics–2002. *Pediatrics* 2003;112:1215.)

TABLE 25.1

MATERNAL FACTORS PREDISPOSING TO SPONTANEOUS PRETERM LABOR AND DELIVERY

Demographics
  Age less than 17 years or greater than 35 years
  Low pre-pregnancy weight
  Short stature
  Low socioeconomic status
  Black race
Lifestyle
  Poor prenatal care
  Poor weight gain during pregnancy
  Alcohol, tobacco, or cocaine use
  Occupational factors
  Psychological stress
Medical conditions
  Multiple gestation
  Polyhydramnios
  Genital tract colonization or infection
  Periodontal disease
  Uterine anomalies or fibroids
  Placenta previa
  Vaginal bleeding
  Spontaneous rupture of membranes
  Cervical incompetence
  Trauma or surgery
  Coitus and orgasm
  Antiphospholipid antibody syndrome
Previous preterm delivery
Genetic factors

Risk Factors

Most preterm births are spontaneous, due to preterm labor, premature rupture of membranes, or cervical incompetence. Approximately 20% to 30% of preterm births are elective deliveries for maternal or fetal indications. These include maternal preeclampsia, placental abruption, fetal growth restriction, and fetal distress.

Preterm labor is the major cause of preterm delivery. Risk factors for preterm labor include maternal demographic characteristics, maternal lifestyle factors, and medical conditions (Table 25.1). As noted, race is a strong demographic risk factor. Important maternal lifestyle factors include poor prenatal care, poor nutrition, smoking, cocaine use, and possibly psychologic stress. Maternal medical conditions include causes of uterine overdistension such as polyhydramnios and multiple gestation. The twin birth rate was 3.0% in the year 2001, and about half of all twins are born preterm. The rate of VLBW in twin gestations is approximately ten times that in singleton pregnancies. Triplets and higher-order multiple gestations account for approximately 0.2% of births. Ninety percent of triplets are born preterm, at a mean gestational age of 33.5 weeks. Between 1980 and 2000, the rate of twin births increased approximately 50% and that of higher-order multiples by 400%; fortunately, the rate of higher-order multiple births appears to have plateaued.

Preterm delivery has been associated with leukocytosis of the amniotic fluid or chorioamnion, and bacteria have been cultured from the amniotic fluid of women in preterm labor with intact membranes. Genital tract colonization or infection (with such organisms as *Ureaplasma urealyticum, Mycoplasma hominis, Trichomonas vaginalis, Gardnerella vaginalis,* peptostreptococci, and bacteroides species) thus may be important

TABLE 25.2

RISK OF RECURRENT PRETERM DELIVERY*

	Whites				Blacks		
	Second Pregnancy				**Second Pregnancy**		
First Pregnancy	20 to 31 Weeks	32 to 36 Weeks	≥37 Weeks	**First Pregnancy**	20 to 31 Weeks	32 to 36 Weeks	≥37 Weeks
20 to 31 weeks	8	20	72	20 to 31 weeks	13	23	63
32 to 36 weeks	2	15	83	32 to 36 weeks	4	21	76
≥37 weeks	0.5	5	94	≥37 weeks	2	11	87

*Data expressed as percentages. Includes 122,722 white and 56,174 black women whose first and second pregnancies ended in singleton stillbirths or live births of newborns weighing at least 500 g, or delivered at 20 weeks of gestation or more, if birth weight unknown.
(Adapted from Adams MM, Elam-Evans LD, Wilson HG, et al. Rates of and factors associated with recurrence of preterm delivery. *JAMA* 2000;283:1591.)

causes of preterm labor and delivery. Bacterial vaginosis is present in 10% to 25% of patients in general gynecologic and obstetric clinics, occurs more frequently in black women than in white women, and appears to increase the risk of preterm delivery more than twofold.

Several population-based studies have demonstrated that one of the strongest risk factors for preterm delivery is a history of a previous preterm delivery. Women who deliver at earlier gestational ages are at a greater risk of subsequent preterm birth. For example, in one study, white women whose first birth occurred between 32 and 36 weeks' gestation had a rate of preterm delivery of 17% in the subsequent pregnancy, whereas those whose first birth occurred before 32 weeks' gestation had a rate of preterm delivery of 28% in the subsequent pregnancy. The rate of recurrent preterm delivery was higher in blacks than in whites (Table 25.2).

The tendency for preterm delivery to recur may be due to the persistence of medical or lifestyle factors associated with preterm birth. A genetic predisposition to preterm delivery also may be present. Preterm delivery and LBW both have been shown to have a strong familial aggregation in the United States. The risk of preterm delivery is higher in mothers who were born preterm than in mothers who were born at term. A specific genetic locus associated with preterm delivery has not been identified, however.

PATHOGENESIS

Although many risk factors for preterm labor have been identified, the pathophysiologic events leading to preterm delivery are largely unknown. Many findings associated with preterm labor, such as the presence of inflammatory cytokines in the amniotic fluid, fetal fibronectin expression in cervicovaginal mucus, and an elevation in maternal salivary estriol, occur weeks or months before preterm birth, suggesting a chronic pathophysiologic process. Decidual hemorrhage, hormonal changes, mechanical factors, and infection all may be important triggers to preterm labor. Mechanical factors and infection can lead to injury or inflammation at the decidua–chorioamnion interface. This may explain the presence of fetal fibronectin (a basement membrane protein produced by the fetal membranes that helps adhere the placenta and membranes to the decidua) in the cervicovaginal mucus of women who deliver preterm. Bacterial infections, in part through the release of endotoxins and exotoxins, stimulate the production of cytokines and lead to prostaglandin release, neutrophil activation, and the release of other bioactive substances, such as metalloproteases. Prostaglandins stimulate uterine contractions, and metalloproteases both attack the chorioamnionic membranes (causing rupture) and remodel collagen in the cervix (causing softening). The relative role of infection in initiating preterm labor,

and the possibility of treating infection and inflammation to prevent preterm delivery, are areas of active investigation. Recent studies showing that progesterone treatment can prevent preterm delivery emphasize the possible role of hormonal imbalances in the pathogenesis of preterm labor.

DIAGNOSIS: GESTATIONAL AGE ASSESSMENT

As noted above, a preterm infant is defined as one delivered before completing 37 weeks of gestation. An accurate assessment of gestational age is not only necessary to diagnose preterm delivery but also influences several aspects of the care of preterm infants. The gestational age affects decisions regarding interventions at the limits of viability, influences caregivers' expectations of problems related to organ system immaturity, influences pharmacokinetics of certain drugs, affects the anticipated schedule of resolution of a number of problems of prematurity, and influences the timing of hospital discharge.

Obstetric dating is determined by the timing of the last menstrual period and by measurements of fetal size by ultrasound before the twenty-sixth week. After delivery, examination of the newborn is used to confirm obstetric dates or to establish gestational age if obstetric dating is unavailable or unreliable. A number of physical characteristics correlate well with gestational age. For example, the disappearance of the anterior vascular capsule of the lens occurs consistently between 27 and 34 weeks' gestation. The Dubowitz examination combines a number of neurologic and physical characteristics of newborns and was simplified by Ballard et al. to yield the most commonly used score of neuromuscular and physical maturity. A modified version of the Ballard score (Fig. 25.2) was published in 1991 to improve the accuracy of dating of very preterm neonates. Gestational age assessment by physical examination generally is considered accurate to within 2 weeks, but continues to be less accurate at gestational ages below 28 weeks. For that reason, some neonatologists prefer to use birth weight rather than gestational age when making decisions about the viability and prognosis of extremely preterm neonates.

CLINICAL MANIFESTATIONS AND TREATMENT

Transition from Intrauterine to Extrauterine Life

The resuscitation and stabilization of neonates immediately after delivery are discussed in Chapter 24, The Newborn

Neuromuscular maturity

	−1	0	1	2	3	4	5
Posture							
Square window (wrist)	>90°	90°	60°	45°	30°	0°	
Arm recoil		180°	140–180°	110–140°	90–110°	<90°	
Popliteal angle	180°	160°	140°	120°	100°	90°	<90°
Scarf sign							
Heel to ear							

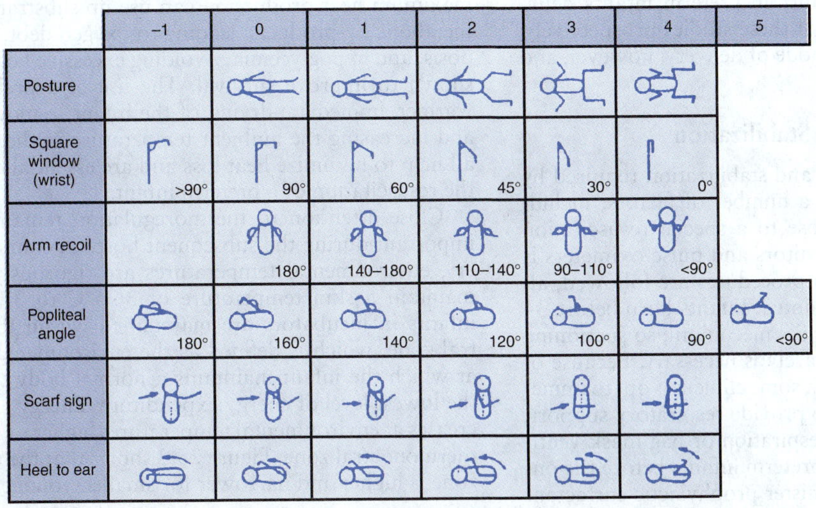

Physical maturity

Skin	Sticky, friable, transparent	Gelatinous, red, translucent	Smooth, pink; visible veins	Superficial peeling and/or rash, few veins	Cracking pale areas, rare veins	Parchment, deep cracking, no vessels	Leathery, cracked, wrinkled
Lanugo	None	Sparse	Abundant	Thinning	Bald areas	Mostly bald	
Plantar surface	Heel–toe 40–50 mm: −1 <40 mm: −2	>50 mm No crease	Faint red marks	Anterior transverse crease only	Creases anterior 2/3	Creases over entire sole	
Breast	Imperceptible	Barely perceptible	Flat areola, no bud	Stippled areola 1–2 mm bud	Raised areola 3–4 mm bud	Full areola 5–10 mm bud	
Eye/ear	Lids fused loosely: −1 tightly: −2	Lids open; pinna flat, stays folded	Slightly curved pinna; soft; slow recoil	Well-curved pinna; soft but ready recoil	Formed and firm, instant recoil	Thick cartilage, ear stiff	
Genitals: male	Scrotum flat, smooth	Scrotum empty, faint rugae	Testes in upper canal, rare rugae	Testes descending, few rugae	Testes down, good rugae	Testes pendulous, deep rugae	
Genitals: female	Clitoris prominent, labia flat	Prominent clitoris, small labia minora	Prominent clitoris, enlarging minora	Majora and minora equally prominent	Majora large, minora small	Majora cover clitoris and minora	

Maturity rating

Score	Weeks
−10	20
−5	22
0	24
5	26
10	28
15	30
20	32
25	34
30	36
35	38
40	40
45	42
50	44

FIGURE 25.2. Expanded New Ballard Score for determining gestational age by assessments of physical and neuromuscular maturity. (Reprinted with permission from Ballard JL, Khoury JC, Wedig K, et al. New Ballard Score, expanded to include extremely premature infants. *J Pediatr* 1991;119:417.)

Intensive Care Unit. The transition from intrauterine to extrauterine life is more difficult for the preterm infant than the term infant because of the functional immaturity of many organ systems. For example, many preterm neonates have underdeveloped lungs and immature respiratory drive, and they develop respiratory insufficiency immediately after delivery. Transition also is made more difficult by impaired thermoregulation, immunoincompetence, fragility of the germinal matrix of the brain, and renal and hepatic immaturity of the preterm infant.

Prenatal Support

Many pregnancies that result in preterm delivery benefit from maternal referral to a high-risk obstetric service. It also is helpful for a neonatologist to meet with the parents before delivery. During this consultation, the neonatologist can become familiar with the details of the obstetric history, let the parents know what to expect after delivery, and answer questions. When delivery is anticipated at the limits of viability, they may discuss the choice between limited or aggressive intervention.

Antenatal interventions used for the treatment of preterm labor include monitoring of fetal well-being, attempts at tocolysis, and pharmacotherapy aimed at minimizing subsequent neonatal morbidity. Antibiotics are used after preterm rupture of membranes to prolong gestation and possibly decrease neonatal morbidity. Antibiotics also are used intrapartum for preterm neonates to try to prevent the vertical transmission of group B streptococcal disease. Antenatal corticosteroid therapy has been proven to improve survival, decrease the incidence and severity of respiratory distress syndrome, and decrease the incidence of intraventricular hemorrhage in preterm infants. Other benefits, and risks, of prenatal corticosteroid therapy (including possible adverse neurodevelopmental affects) continue to be evaluated.

The mode of delivery may affect the outcome of preterm deliveries. Neonates with birth weights between 600 and 1,250 g delivered by cesarean section have a lower incidence of early intraventricular hemorrhage than those delivered vaginally. Others have noted lower mortality in preterm infants delivered by cesarean section. None of these studies prospectively, randomly assigned mothers to mode of delivery, however, and further evaluation is needed.

Delivery Room Stabilization

The delivery room resuscitation and stabilization required by a preterm newborn depends on a number of factors, including gestational age. Delivery close to a special resuscitation room with cardiorespiratory monitors and pulse oximeters is desirable. Standard resuscitation procedures are followed, although several points should be noted. Infants born before 34 weeks' gestation do not usually pass meconium, so suctioning of meconium from the trachea rarely is necessary. Because of anticipated functional immaturity, some clinicians opt to immediately intubate ELBW infants to provide respiratory support, without a trial of spontaneous respiration or bag mask ventilatory support. Others intubate preterm infants before the onset of respiratory effort to administer prophylactic surfactant therapy. Finally, the first steps in neonatal resuscitation—the provision of a heat source and drying of the infant to minimize evaporative heat loss—are of exceptional importance in preterm neonates and are discussed in the following section.

Thermoregulation

In utero, the fetus is warmer than the mother and has a body temperature of 37.6°C to 37.8°C. At delivery, the wet, naked infant is exposed to delivery room air temperatures of 22°C to 25°C. Significant heat loss can occur in the first few minutes after birth, through each of the four mechanisms of heat transfer—conduction, convection, radiation, and evaporation. Heat loss after delivery can result in a decrease in body temperature of 1°C to 3°C in just minutes.

Newborns behave as homeotherms and try to maintain body temperature within a narrow range. They respond to environmental cold stress by utilizing subcutaneous fat as an insulating medium, vasoconstricting peripheral vessels to shunt blood away from the body surface, assuming a posture of flexion to minimize skin surface area, and, most importantly, increasing heat production. Unlike adults who shiver to produce heat, neonates increase their metabolic rate to produce heat, an adaptation known as *nonshivering thermogenesis*. This increase in metabolic rate is achieved primarily through the breakdown of brown fat. Brown adipose tissue differentiates from reticular cells at approximately 26 weeks of gestation. At term, it constitutes 6% of the body weight and 40% of the body fat stores. The lipolysis of brown fat is induced by the release of norepinephrine and thyroid hormones, which are stimulated by cold stress.

Preterm neonates have an impaired response to cold stress. They have less insulating subcutaneous fat, have an impaired ability to peripherally vasoconstrict, have a relatively greater surface area from which to lose heat, and cannot assume a flexion posture to decrease surface area. Finally, their ability to generate heat by nonshivering thermogenesis is markedly impaired. In LBW preterm infants, brown adipose tissue may be markedly diminished or even functionally absent. In addition, VLBW infants may not exhibit a thermogenic response to lowered skin temperatures. Thus, they may be functionally poikilothermic for days after birth, dependent on the thermal environment for the maintenance of optimal body temperature. The ability to thermoregulate improves with advancing postnatal age, and VLBW infants have been demonstrated to have increased subcutaneous body fat deposits and increased thermogenic potential by 3 weeks of age.

Although some decrease in body temperature may facilitate the transition from intrauterine to extrauterine life, excessive heat loss is detrimental to the newborn. Prolonged and maximum heat production can use up substrate and increase metabolic by-products, leading to oxygen debt, metabolic acidosis, and hypoglycemia. Avoiding excessive heat loss has been shown to improve survival. The use of a preheated radiant warmer, immediate drying of the infant, removing wet linen, and increasing the ambient temperature in the delivery room all help to minimize heat loss and are essential components of the resuscitation of a preterm infant.

Close attention to thermoregulation remains exceedingly important during the subsequent hospital course. In the nursery, environmental temperatures are rigorously regulated to maintain a skin temperature of 36.5°C to 37.0°C. Preterm infants in incubators are maintained within the thermoneutral zone, which is defined as the environmental temperature at which the infant maintains a normal body temperature at the lowest level of energy expenditure. Energy expenditure increases at environmental temperatures higher or lower than the thermoneutral zone. Figure 25.3 shows that the thermoneutral zone is higher and narrower for smaller, younger infants.

Problems of Prematurity

Problems experienced by preterm infants are caused primarily by the functional immaturity of multiple organ systems. The degree of functional immaturity, and thus the frequency and severity of neonatal morbidities, is inversely related to gestational age and birth weight. Table 25.3 demonstrates this relationship for selected neonatal morbidities. Several points about the problems of prematurity can be made. First, virtually every organ system is involved to some degree. Second, many of the problems of preterm infants are partially iatrogenic. Almost all the therapies currently used in the neonatal intensive care unit have side effects that can add to the morbidity, and in some cases mortality, of preterm neonates. Perhaps the most obvious example is the role of ventilator-induced barotrauma, volutrauma, and oxygen toxicity in the development of chronic lung disease or bronchopulmonary dysplasia. Other examples are presented in Table 25.4. The care of the preterm neonate requires careful consideration and a balancing of the benefits and risks of every therapeutic intervention.

Finally, most of the problems of prematurity resolve with growth and maturation. (Exceptions, such as long-term growth restriction and neurodevelopmental and pulmonary sequelae, are discussed in subsequent chapters.) The rate of resolution of these problems is extremely variable. For example, indirect hyperbilirubinemia usually resolves within several days of birth, even in the most preterm neonate, whereas apnea of prematurity can persist for weeks or months. The duration of many problems is influenced by both the degree of initial immaturity and complicating factors, including iatrogenic injury. For example, the duration and severity of chronic lung disease is much greater in a 24-week-gestation neonate who, in addition to respiratory distress syndrome, develops pulmonary edema from a patent ductus arteriosus (PDA), pulmonary interstitial emphysema from ventilator-induced barotrauma, or nosocomial sepsis and pneumonia.

Respiratory Function

Impaired respiratory function is usually the most serious problem after the delivery of a preterm newborn. At the limits of viability (22 to 23 weeks' gestation), the fetal lungs frequently cannot sustain extrauterine life because of inadequate surface area for gas exchange, inadequate thinning of the air–blood barrier, surfactant deficiency, and several other maturational deficiencies. As the lungs grow and mature in the third trimester, these deficiencies disappear. Maternal corticosteroid

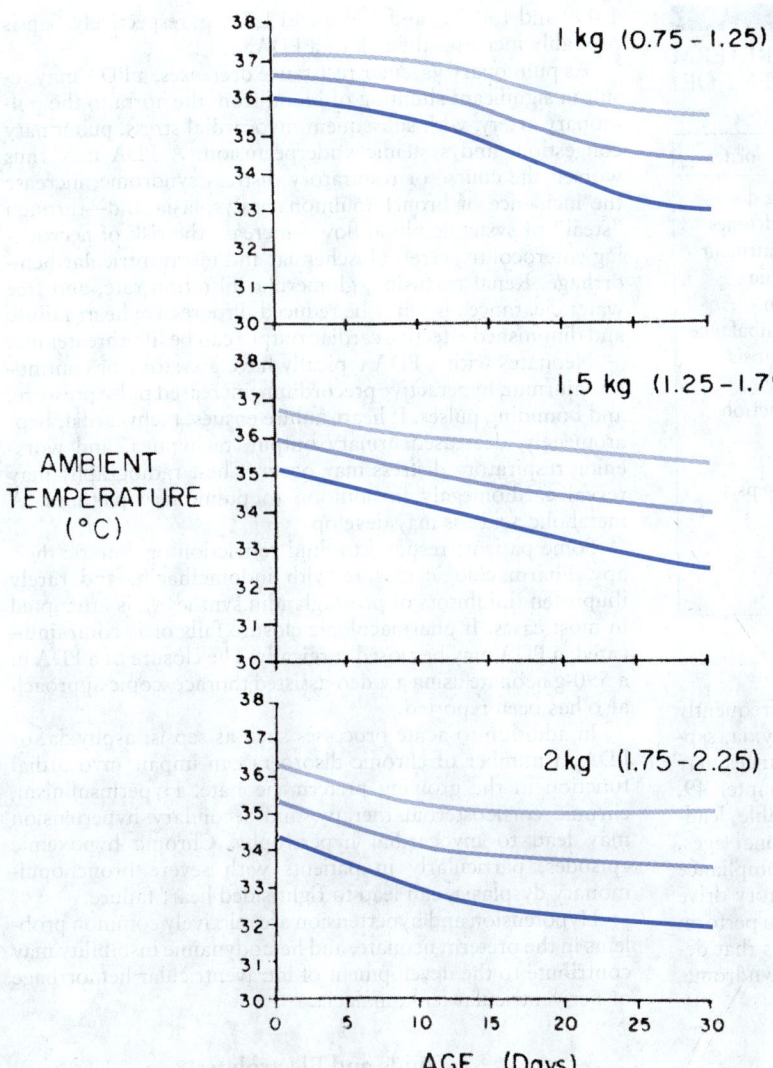

AMBIENT TEMPERATURE (°C)

1 kg (0.75 – 1.25)

1.5 kg (1.25 – 1.75)

2 kg (1.75 – 2.25)

AGE (Days)

FIGURE 25.3. Range of ambient temperatures defining a thermoneutral environment in infants with birth weights of less than 1,250 g (*upper panel*), 1,250 to 1,749 g (*middle panel*), and 1,750 to 2,250 g (*lower panel*). (Reprinted with permission from Bell EF, Gray JC, Weinstein MR, et al. The effects of thermal environment on heat balance and insensible water loss in low-birth-weight infants. *J Pediatr* 1980;96:452.)

treatment before delivery accelerates lung maturation and decreases the incidence of respiratory distress syndrome. Exogenous surfactant therapy corrects surfactant deficiency, but has no effect on the other problems of the premature lung. Surfactant deficiency and neonatal respiratory distress syndrome are discussed in depth in Chapter 42, Respiratory Distress Syn-

drome, and chronic lung disease or bronchopulmonary dysplasia is discussed in Chapter 50, Bronchopulmonary Dysplasia.

Immaturity of other respiratory system components besides the lungs frequently causes problems for preterm infants. Preterm infants may have decreased central respiratory drive, particularly if born before 30 to 32 weeks of gestation. In

TABLE 25.3

NEONATAL MORBIDITY BY BIRTH WEIGHT*

	Birth Weight (g)		
	501–750	751–1,000	1,001–1,500
Respiratory distress syndrome	69	53	27
Chronic lung disease	46	33	10
Patent ductus arteriosus	50	37	17
Late-onset septicemia	45	31	12
Necrotizing enterocolitis	10	8	4
Grade III or IV intraventricular hemorrhage	23	13	5
Periventricular leukomalacia	3	2	1

*Data expressed as percentages. Data are from 5,848 infants born in 1999 and 2000 at centers participating in the National Institute of Child Health and Human Development (NICHD) Neonatal Research Network. (Adapted from Fanaroff AA, Hack M, Walsh MC. The NICHD Neonatal Research Network: changes in practice and outcomes during the first 15 years. *Semin Perinatol* 2003;27:281.)

TABLE 25.4

EXAMPLES OF SECONDARY DISORDERS OF PRETERM INFANTS THAT RESULT FROM THE TREATMENT OF PRIMARY DISORDERS

Primary Disorder	Intervention	Secondary Disorder
Respiratory distress syndrome	Mechanical ventilation	Chronic lung disease Air leak syndromes
Chronic lung disease	Corticosteroid therapy	Growth impairment Hyperglycemia Hypertension
	Diuretic therapy	Electrolyte imbalance Nephrocalcinosis Osteopenia
Patent ductus arteriosus	Indomethacin	Renal dysfunction
Gastrointestinal immaturity	Parenteral hyperalimentation	Cholestasis
	Central venous catheter	Bacteremia, sepsis
Multiple organ dysfunction	Laboratory tests	Anemia

infants delivered at 24 to 28 weeks' gestation, apnea frequently persists beyond 38 weeks' postmenstrual age. Asphyxia, sepsis, intracranial hemorrhage, and metabolic disturbances may exacerbate this problem. (Apnea is discussed in Chapter 49, Apnea.) The preterm neonate's airway also is less stable, leading to obstructive apnea. Finally, at earlier gestational ages, less ventilatory muscle mass and greater chest wall compliance is present. Thus, even with adequate central ventilatory drive and a patent airway, VLBW infants may not be able to perform the work necessary for effective ventilation. Diseases that decrease lung compliance, such as respiratory distress syndrome, compound this problem.

Cardiovascular Function

Unlike the lungs, which are not involved in gas exchange *in utero,* the fetal heart must function throughout most of gestation. Problems of the cardiovascular system in the preterm neonate are thus rarely caused by functional immaturity. Rather, cardiac insufficiency usually is caused by the persistence of a PDA, myocardial dysfunction secondary to other acute problems such as sepsis or asphyxia, or congenital heart disease.

In utero, the ductus arteriosus is patent, under the influence of prostaglandins and the low oxygen tension of fetal blood. It carries 55% to 60% of the combined cardiac output and allows the majority of the right ventricular output to bypass the pulmonary circulation by shunting blood from the pulmonary artery to the descending aorta. After birth, the plasma oxygen tension increases sharply, effecting a reactive vasoconstriction of the ductus arteriosus. In addition, because the lung is a major site of prostaglandin catabolism, postnatal increases in pulmonary blood flow result in a higher rate of prostaglandin degradation.

The ductus arteriosus is functionally closed within 10 to 15 hours of birth in most term neonates, and by 2 days in almost all term neonates. Closure of the ductus arteriosus is delayed in preterm neonates, possibly because of an impaired vasoconstrictor response to the increase in oxygen tension. The incidence of a persistently PDA depends on gestational age and postnatal age. In a large national collaborative study, a symptomatic PDA was noted during hospitalization in 42%, 21%, and 7% of neonates with birth weights between 500 and 999 g,

1,000 and 1,499 g, and 1,500 and 1,750 g, respectively. Sepsis probably increases the risk of a PDA.

As pulmonary vascular resistance decreases, a PDA may result in significant shunting of blood from the aorta to the pulmonary artery, with subsequent myocardial stress, pulmonary congestion, and systemic underperfusion. A PDA may thus worsen the course of respiratory distress syndrome, increase the incidence of bronchopulmonary dysplasia and—through "steal" of systemic blood flow—increase the risk of necrotizing enterocolitis, cerebral ischemia, and intraventricular hemorrhage. Renal perfusion, glomerular filtration rate, and free water clearance also may be reduced. Progressive heart failure and diminished effective cardiac output can be life-threatening.

Neonates with a PDA typically have a systolic or continuous murmur, hyperactive precordium, increased pulse pressure, and bounding pulses. If heart failure ensues, tachycardia, hepatomegaly, decreased urinary output, tachypnea, and worsening respiratory distress may occur. Chest radiography may reveal cardiomegaly in addition to pulmonary plethora. A metabolic acidosis may develop.

Some patients respond to fluid restriction or diuretic therapy. Pharmacologic closure with indomethacin, and rarely ibuprofen (inhibitors of prostaglandin synthesis), is attempted in most cases. If pharmacologic closure fails or is contraindicated, a PDA may be closed surgically. The closure of a PDA in a 590-g neonate using a video-assisted thoracoscopic approach also has been reported.

In addition to acute processes such as sepsis, asphyxia, or PDA, a number of chronic disorders can impair myocardial function in the growing preterm neonate. Hyperinsulinism, chronic corticosteroid therapy, and secondary hypertension may lead to myocardial hypertrophy. Chronic hypoxemic episodes, particularly in patients with severe bronchopulmonary dysplasia, can lead to right-sided heart failure.

Hypotension and hypertension are relatively common problems in the preterm neonate, and hemodynamic instability may contribute to the development of intraventricular hemorrhage or periventricular leukomalacia.

Fluids and Electrolytes

After birth, neonates lose body weight because of a loss of body water, primarily from the extracellular compartment. This physiologic weight loss represents an isotonic contraction of body fluids, is associated with a diuretic phase, and is part of the normal adaptation to extrauterine life. VLBW infants have a higher body-water content and a higher ratio of extracellular to intracellular water. Because of their different body composition, neonates with lower birth weights lose a greater proportion of their body weight after birth. For example, the mean maximum postnatal weight loss is approximately 10% of birth weight for infants weighing 1,000 to 1,500 g compared to 5% to 7% for those weighing 2,500 g. The administration of excessive fluids to prevent this contraction has been associated with a higher incidence of symptomatic PDA, necrotizing enterocolitis, and bronchopulmonary dysplasia.

Fluid and electrolyte requirements in the newborn are related to net fluid expenditures, normal changes in body composition, and the integrity of renal regulatory functions. Water expenditures include insensible water loss from the skin and respiratory tract, water used to excrete renal solute loads, and water lost in stool. Electrolytes are lost predominantly in urine and stool. Both water and electrolytes must be accreted for normal growth.

The calculation of maintenance fluid requirements for preterm neonates is complicated by the extremely wide variation in insensible fluid losses. Respiratory water loss generally accounts for approximately 33% of insensible water loss, but can be reduced to nearly zero for infants breathing humidified

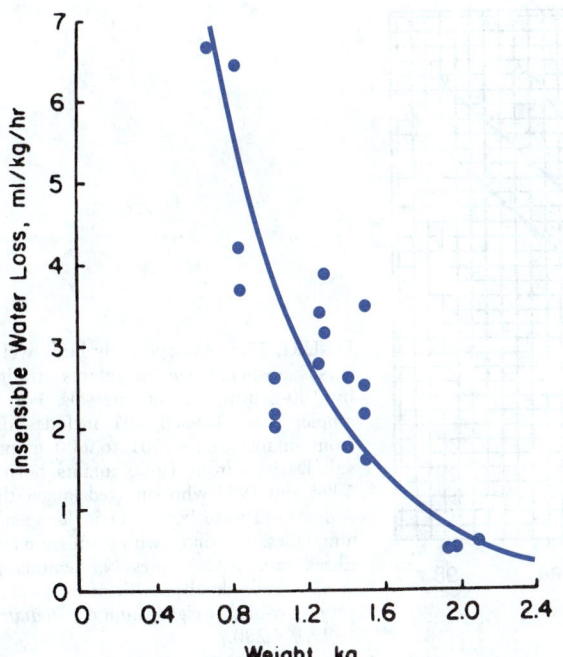

FIGURE 25.4. Insensible water loss as a function of birth weight in premature infants nursed under radiant warmers. (Reprinted with permission from Costarino AT, Baumgart S. Controversies in fluid and electrolyte therapy for the premature infant. *Clin Perinatol* 1988;15:863.)

air from mechanical ventilators or oxygen hoods. Transepidermal water loss is substantially higher for smaller, less mature infants because of their thin, poorly developed skin, low subcutaneous body fat deposits, and high surface area–to–body mass ratios. In Figure 25.4, it can be seen that the smallest neonates supported under a radiant warmer can have insensible water losses as high as 6 to 7 mL/kg/hour, or 144 to 168 mL/kg/day. By the end of the first week of life, the skin becomes less permeable and transepidermal water losses can be reduced by 50%. Insensible fluid losses increase with phototherapy, radiant warming, hyperthermia, and activity. Transepidermal fluid losses can be limited by increasing ambient humidity or through the use of heat shields, membranes, dressings, or topical agents.

Urine output also can vary tremendously in the first several days after preterm delivery. An early oliguric phase persists in some infants, particularly if they are septic, asphyxiated, or on nephrotoxic medications such as indomethacin. Some preterm infants experience diuretic phases in which urine output exceeds 5 to 6 mL/kg/hour, or 120 to 140 mL/kg/day.

The provision of maintenance fluids to the preterm infant must thus be individually tailored and requires careful, prolonged attention. After selecting a particular fluid infusion rate, adjustments must be made based on serial weights, electrolytes, and urine output. Weight loss greater or less than that expected from normal contraction of the extracellular fluid compartment mandates compensatory decreases or increases in fluid infusion. After adjusting for sodium intake and output, hyponatremia may reflect relative free-water overload and the need to decrease fluid intake, whereas hypernatremia may reflect relative free-water depletion and the need for increased fluid intake.

Maintenance electrolyte requirements are generally 2 to 3 mEq/kg/day of sodium and 1 to 3 mEq/kg/day of potassium, starting at 1 to 2 days of life. Abnormalities and immaturity of renal function may significantly alter these requirements

in preterm infants. Infants born at less than 34 weeks' gestational age have a glomerulotubular imbalance that results in decreased free water clearance and increased urinary losses of sodium, bicarbonate, and glucose. In addition, the capacity to acidify the urine and excrete ammonia is limited. Sodium losses may be as high as 8 to 10 mEq/kg/day, although the typical range is 2 to 3 mEq/kg/day. Bicarbonate loss may result in a metabolic acidosis unless adequate replacement is given.

Overall, the basic goals of early fluid management are to maintain an appropriate intravascular volume, allow the normal contraction in the extracellular water compartment, and to prevent pathologic electrolyte imbalances.

Nutrition and Growth

At delivery, nutritional support from the mother ends and the infant's energy expenditure increases. Achieving a positive energy balance adequate to promote growth depends on the level of nutritional support relative to energy expenditure. Energy requirements in the neonatal period are partitioned into several components, including basal metabolism, thermic effects of feeding, thermoregulation, fecal calorie losses, physical activity, and growth, which includes the energy necessary for synthetic processes and the energy stored in new tissues. Growth of 10 to 15 g/kg/day can usually be achieved by providing 100 to 120 kcal/kg/day to preterm infants. Some infants, especially those with chronic lung disease, need a greater number of calories. Slightly fewer calories are required for growth when they are provided parenterally rather than enterally.

Parenteral nutrition is generally begun within 24 to 48 hours of birth. It is important to provide adequate nitrogen for protein synthesis. Net protein accretion will not occur unless positive nitrogen and caloric balance is achieved. Generally, protein intakes of 2.5 to 4.0 g/kg/day meet the needs of preterm infants and are not toxic. Carbohydrates should account for 50% to 70% of the nonprotein calories. Glucose infusions are started at approximately 5 to 6 mg/kg/minute and are advanced to approximately 12 to 14 mg/kg/minute. Essential fatty acid deficiency may occur within 72 hours in preterm infants receiving no fat intake. Minimal essential fatty acid provision is generally achieved with 0.5 g/kg/day of intravenous lipid emulsion. Lipid infusions are typically begun within 48 to 72 hours of birth and steadily increased to provide approximately 3 g/kg/day. Hyperlipidemia is rare, and lipids are better tolerated when prepared as 20% solutions. Enteral nutrition is usually started within a week of delivery, depending on the infant's medical condition. Most VLBW infants are advanced to full enteral feeds slowly over several days, and are given special preterm formulas or fortified breast milk to provide additional calories, protein, calcium, and phosphate.

Ideally, the growth of the infant would approximate fetal growth, which is approximately 10 g/day from 20 to 22 weeks' gestation, 20 g/day from 28 to 30 weeks' gestation, and 30 g/day from 34 to 36 weeks' gestation. This is rarely the case. Of more than 1,400 ELBW infants born at National Institute of Child Health and Human Development (NICHD) Neonatal Research Network centers in 2000 and 2001, 89% had growth failure at 36 weeks' corrected age. Of infants born at 34 weeks' gestation or less, the incidence of growth restriction (lower than the 10th percentile) at hospital discharge is approximately 28%, 34%, and 10% for weight, length, and head circumference, respectively. Poor postnatal growth may be associated with worse neurodevelopmental outcome.

The rate of neonatal weight gain usually is plotted against postnatal growth curves, such as those shown in Figure 25.5. These curves include data from sick infants, and thus do not necessarily reflect optimal growth. Growth curves for length and head circumference also have been generated. Growth

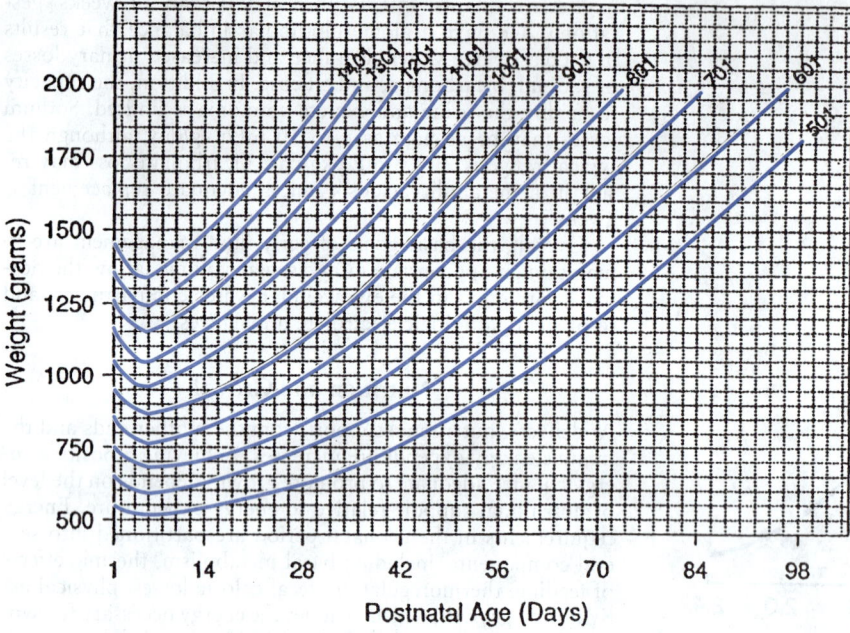

FIGURE 25.5. Average daily body weight versus postnatal age for infants stratified by 100-g birth weight intervals. For example, curve labeled 501 includes data from infants in the 501 to 600 g interval. Derived from 1,660 infants born in 1994 and 1995 who survived longer than 7 days and were free of major congenital anomalies. (Reprinted with permission from Ehrenkranz RA, Younes N, Lemons JA, et al. Longitudinal growth of hospitalized very low-birth-weight infants. *Pediatrics* 1999;104:280.)

in head circumference reflects brain growth, and growth in length reflects skeletal growth, both of which are important to follow.

Issues related to growth and metabolic adaptation of the fetus and newborn are discussed in greater depth in Chapter 20, Growth and Metabolic Adaptation of the Fetus and Newborn.

Renal Function

The development of renal function is described in Chapter 61, Renal and Genitourinary Diseases. The close relationship between immaturity of renal function and fluid and electrolyte balance in the preterm neonate was described previously. Impairment or immaturity of renal function affects the clearance of many drugs used in preterm neonates, and dosage and dosing intervals must be based on chronologic and gestational age.

Endocrine and Metabolic Function

The regulation of blood glucose concentrations can be a particular problem for the preterm newborn. *In utero,* glucose is transported across the placenta at a rate of approximately 4 to 6 mg/kg/minute, and fetal glucose levels are approximately 20% lower than maternal levels. At delivery, preterm neonates have limited glycogen stores, impaired gluconeogenesis, and limited alternative fuels. Common problems such as respiratory distress, sepsis, asphyxia, and hypothermia increase metabolic demands and hasten the depletion of energy stores. Unless early feeding is anticipated, preterm infants usually are started on intravenous glucose infusions shortly after delivery to avoid hypoglycemia. An infusion of 10% dextrose at 80 mL/kg/day provides 5.6 mg/kg/minute of glucose, which usually maintains euglycemia.

Hyperglycemia is less frequent in preterm infants, but can occur with stress or as carbohydrate intake is increased for nutritional support. After the first week of life, insulin therapy is used occasionally to treat hyperglycemia in these settings, particularly if high serum glucose levels are limiting nutritional support or leading to glucosuria and an osmotic diuresis.

Hypocalcemia also is a common problem in preterm infants, particularly those who are septic, asphyxiated, or growth restricted. Metabolic bone disease (including osteopenia, rickets,

and fractures) may appear after several weeks of intensive care, especially in VLBW infants with chronic lung disease.

Abnormal function of the hypothalamic-pituitary-adrenal axis is common in premature neonates, especially during the first week of life. The adrenal gland shows a blunted response to adrenocorticotropic hormone stimulation or other stressors, and increased levels of cortisol precursors and corticotropin-releasing factor are found in premature infants during the first week of life. Some VLBW infants thus do not increase their cortisol levels despite respiratory failure, and many preterm infants with hydrocortisone-responsive hypotension have been described. Premature neonates with adrenal insufficiency may be at increased risk of adverse outcomes, such as chronic lung disease.

The endocrine problems of the neonate are discussed in more depth in Chapter 62, Neonatal Endocrinology.

Hematologic Function

The normal fetal hematocrit increases from approximately 40% at 22 to 25 weeks' gestation to 50% at term. The development of anemia is a frequent problem in the preterm neonate and occurs for a number of reasons. These include phlebotomy losses, a shorter red blood cell life span (approximately 35 to 50 days, in contrast to 60 to 70 days in the term infant), rapid growth and increase in blood volume, and diminished erythropoietin output in response to anemia. Preterm neonates thus experience an earlier and deeper nadir in hemoglobin and hematocrit than do term neonates.

VLBW infants commonly receive transfusions of packed red blood cells for anemia. At the University of Iowa, between 1993 and 1994, 69% of infants weighing less than 1,500 g were transfused, and transfused infants received an average of 4.5 transfusions. The indications for transfusion in the preterm neonate are complicated and include not only the hemoglobin or hematocrit, but also the infant's clinical condition, growth rate, anticipated phlebotomy losses, and potential for erythropoiesis.

An intense effort has been made to decrease the number of transfusions received by sick preterm newborns. To minimize phlebotomy losses, nurseries try to limit the number of blood draws, and clinical laboratories try to minimize the amount of blood required for a given assay (using so-called micromethods). Exogenous erythropoietin therapy has been shown to stimulate erythropoiesis and decrease transfusion requirements, and current studies are investigating ways to optimize its efficacy. Finally, many blood banks assign a unit of matched blood to a specific VLBW infant, and then draw aliquots of blood from that unit over the next 30 to 40 days to meet transfusion requirements. These dedicated units substantially limit the number of blood donors an infant is exposed to if he or she requires multiple transfusions.

Other hematologic problems such as thrombocytopenia, disseminated intravascular coagulation, thrombosis, and neutropenia are more common in preterm infants. Indirect hyperbilirubinemia is also extremely common in the preterm neonate and is discussed at length in Chapter 26, Neonatal Hyperbilirubinemia.

Immunologic and Infectious Diseases

The potential role of infection in preterm labor was discussed previously. Infection is a major cause of morbidity and mortality in preterm infants. NICHD data regarding VLBW infants show that approximately 2% have culture-proven early-onset sepsis, and the incidence of undiagnosed early-onset sepsis is certainly much higher. In addition, 25% of VLBW infants have late-onset sepsis, and approximately 17% of their deaths are due to proven or suspected infection.

Intrapartum antibiotic therapy for women delivering before term may decrease the risk of vertically transmitted infection. It also may be responsible for a recent shift from gram-positive to gram-negative organisms as the most common cause of early-onset sepsis in VLBW infants. Among VLBW infants born at NICHD centers between 1998 and 2000, *Escherichia coli* was the most common pathogen, followed by group B streptococcus and *Haemophilus influenzae*.

Approximately 50% of late-onset sepsis in VLBW infants is caused by coagulase-negative staphylococci. This organism and fungi are particularly important pathogens in infants with percutaneous central venous catheters. Congenital and postnatally acquired viral infections also contribute to infectious morbidity and mortality in preterm infants. Specific neonatal infections are discussed in Chapters 71 to 88.

Preterm neonates are deficient in almost all aspects of cellular and humoral immunologic function. Preterm infants are immunized according to their postnatal age, on the same schedule as term neonates. Killed polio vaccine is substituted for attenuated live virus vaccine. The use of pooled intravenous IgG to prevent or treat bacterial sepsis in the preterm neonate remains controversial. Selected preterm infants, especially those with bronchopulmonary dysplasia, are treated with monthly parenteral respiratory syncytial virus (RSV) immune globulin during RSV season to decrease the morbidity and mortality associated with this virus.

Neurologic Function

The preterm newborn is at higher risk of a number of neurologic problems, including intraventricular-periventricular hemorrhage, periventricular leukomalacia, retinopathy of prematurity, hearing loss, hydrocephaly, and seizures (see Table 25.3). The incidence of intraventricular hemorrhage among VLBW infants is approximately 30%, and it is an important cause of morbidity and mortality. This subject is discussed in depth in Chapter 32, Intraventricular Hemorrhage of the Preterm Neonate. Even preterm infants without identifiable neuroimaging abnormalities may have subsequent neurodevelopmental problems, as discussed in the section, Neurodevelopmental Outcome. Recent data, including some derived from magnetic resonance imaging (MRI), suggest that diffuse white-matter injury is relatively common in very preterm infants and often is not detected by cranial ultrasonography.

Gastrointestinal Function

Developmental disorders of gastrointestinal function are discussed in Chapter 55, Developmental Disorders of Gastrointestinal Function. Because of functional immaturity, as well as other concurrent illnesses, feeding the very preterm infant often is quite difficult. Feeds are initially given in small volumes, and tolerance is assessed by monitoring gastric residuals, the abdominal examination, the stooling pattern, and the stool for visible or occult blood. The potentially fatal gastrointestinal disease, necrotizing enterocolitis is discussed in Chapter 59, Necrotizing Enterocolitis. Infants who do not tolerate enteral feeds and receive prolonged parenteral nutritional support are at risk of developing cholestasis.

For preterm infants unable to tolerate nutritive feeds, small nonnutritive feeds may reduce the severity of cholestasis, stimulate intestinal maturation, reduce the amount of time to subsequently tolerate full enteral feeds, and improve growth.

Gastroesophageal reflux is more common in preterm infants, and may lead to aspiration, poor growth, or poor feeding. Its association with apnea, bradycardia, or desaturation episodes is controversial. Desaturation episodes during feedings can be due to uncoordinated sucking, swallowing, and breathing. The pattern of breathing during oral feedings usually matures by 35 to 38 weeks postconceptional age.

The time of first stool passage is delayed in preterm infants. In a series of infants with birth weights of 1,000 g or less, the median age at passage of the first stool was 3 days. Thirty percent of infants had not passed their first stool by 7 days of life.

Vascular Access

Umbilical vessel catheterization is discussed in Chapter 24, The Newborn Intensive Care Unit. Umbilical arterial catheterization is almost routine in VLBW infants shortly after delivery because of the difficulty in establishing alternative vascular access, the need for careful monitoring, and the need for frequent blood draws for laboratory tests. In some cases, an umbilical venous catheter is placed for additional access, with the tip of the catheter passing through the ductus venosus and positioned in between inferior vena cava just below the right atrium. After several days, umbilical catheters are removed, and in many cases percutaneous central venous catheters are placed.

Although often essential for monitoring, intravenous access, and nutritional support of the very preterm infant, these catheters are a source of iatrogenic morbidity and, in rare cases, mortality. Careful monitoring must be paid to thrombotic, ischemic, hemorrhagic, and infectious complications.

Discharge Criteria

The problems of prematurity outlined previously may lead to neonatal mortality or long-term morbidity. With the exception of pulmonary and neurologic sequelae, however, most problems steadily improve and disappear with time and growth of the preterm infant. Many neonatal intensive care units (NICUs) transfer "feeding and growing" infants who weigh more than approximately 1,000 g and are on minimal respiratory support from an intensive care room to a step-down room or unit. A number of milestones must then be reached before a preterm neonate is considered ready for discharge home. Although most preterm infants are not ready for discharge until approximately 35 weeks postmenstrual age and weighing 1,800 g, these are not rigid discharge criteria. Criteria for discharge are outlined in Table 25.5. Communication with the infant's pediatrician

TABLE 25.5

GUIDELINES FOR DISCHARGE OF PRETERM NEONATES

Thermoregulation
    Maintaining normal body temperature in an open crib
Feeding/Nutrition
    Growing at an appropriate rate
    Taking all of feedings by mouth
    If unable to feed by mouth, arrangements made for tube feedings
Cardiorespiratory Function
    Stable cardiorespiratory status at rest
        If born less than 35 weeks' gestation
            Monitored at least 7 days .
            Off methylxanthines and free of significant events* at least 7 days
        If born at 34–35 weeks' gestation and never on methylxanthines, monitored 2–7 days
    No significant cardiorespiratory events during feeds
    Passed a car seat test if less than 37 weeks' gestation
Family Readiness
    Discharge teaching completed
    CPR training performed in selected cases
Community Readiness
    Primary care provider identified and received information, and follow-up arranged
    Specialty services arranged as needed
Miscellaneous
    State-mandated screening tests completed
    ROP screening completed per American Academy of Pediatrics (AAP) guidelines
    Hearing screening completed
    Immunizations completed per AAP guidelines
    RSV prophylaxis completed per AAP guidelines

*A "significant event" is defined as apnea of 20 seconds or more or apnea of less than 20 seconds with HR of less than 80 for more than 10 seconds, saturation of less than 80%, cyanosis, pallor, or need for intervention to restore breathing and oxygenation.
(Adapted from Herson V, Ehrenkranz R. Neonatal Intensive Care Unit (NICU) discharge guidelines. Connecticut Chapter of the American Academy of Pediatrics, 2001, and American Academy of Pediatrics Committee on Fetus and Newborn. Hospital discharge of the high-risk neonate-proposed guidelines. *Pediatrics* 1998;102:411.)

is particularly important, given the complicated histories and possible special needs after the discharge of these infants.

Length of Stay

Obviously, the more premature an infant is, the longer his or her hospitalization will be. Most neonates are observed until a postmenstrual age of at least 35 weeks. Many ELBW infants require hospitalization until their estimated date of confinement or beyond. In Figure 25.6, the length of hospital stay of 1,262 surviving LBW infants without congenital anomalies is plotted against birth weight and gestational age. When performing a prenatal consultation with a family about to deliver a preterm infant, it is helpful to let them know the possible length of stay in the hospital of their child.

PROGNOSIS

Survival

The survival of preterm infants has improved steadily since the 1970s. Data from the NICHD Neonatal Research Network show that survival to discharge of infants with birth weights of 501 to 1,500 g has increased from 74% in 1988 to 80% in 1991 to 84% in 1995 and 1996. The greatest improvement in survival has been for infants with birth weights between 500 and 750 g. This increase in survival is due to improvements in obstetric care and in the neonatal care of problems of prematurity. For example, in the 1990s, the widespread use of sur-

factant replacement therapy for respiratory distress syndrome was probably the most important factor in improving survival of preterm infants.

The survival of preterm infants increases with increasing birth weight and gestational age. Table 25.6 shows the survival of infants born at Yale–New Haven Children's Hospital between 1993 and 2002 by birth weight and gestational age. By approximately 27 weeks and 800 to 900 g, survival is 90%; and by approximately 31 weeks and 1,250 to 1,500 g, survival is very close to that of term infants.

Many centers prefer to report mortality (and morbidity) based on birth weight, because it can be measured relatively accurately. Gestational age, although generally less accurate, is a better predictor of maturation and chance of survival, however. A growth-restricted infant of a more advanced gestational age has a better chance of survival than an appropriately grown baby of the same weight but earlier gestational age. A Web site registry (www.medicine.uiowa.edu/tiniestbabies) documents to date the survival of over 70 infants with a birth weight less than 400 g, and seven infants with a birth weight less than 300 g, most of whom were of more advanced gestational age than their weight would suggest. For example, survival and normal neurodevelopmental outcome of a small-for-gestational-age, 26 6/7 weeks' gestation infant with a birth weight of only 280 g has been reported.

The chance of survival is also influenced by race and by gender, with blacks and females having a survival advantage. Survival at a given gestational age also varies widely by medical center. This may be due to differences in patient populations, but also, for very premature infants, by the aggressiveness of caregivers. The survival rates for very preterm infants by gestational age in two recently published series also appear in

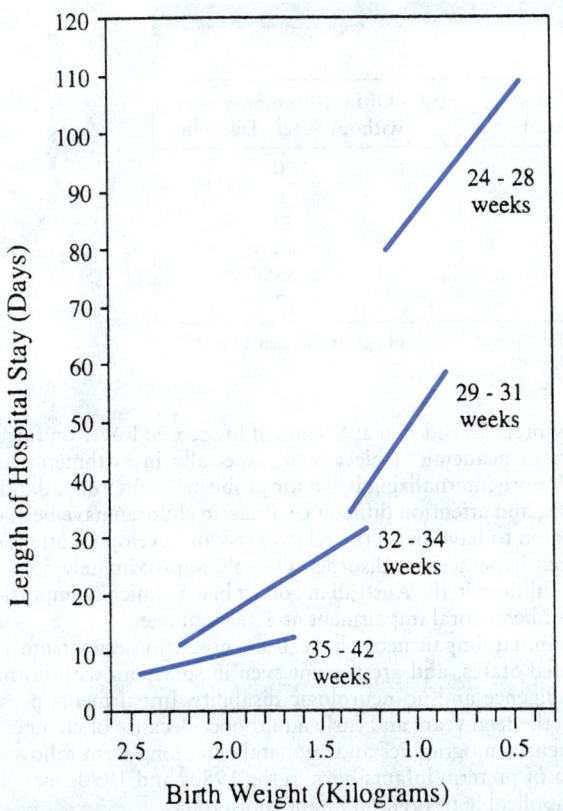

FIGURE 25.6. Mean length of hospital stay versus birth weight within gestational age groups for surviving, nonanomalous, low-birth-weight, neonatal intensive care unit patients. (Reprinted with permission from Rawlings JS, Smith FR, Garcia J. Expected duration of hospital stay of low birth weight infants: graphic depiction in relation to birth weight and gestational age. *J Pediatr* 1993;123:307.)

Table 25.6. A significantly lower survival rate is reported in the United Kingdom/Ireland and Australia series than in the United States. For example, at 23 weeks' gestation, survival was 11% in the United Kingdom/Ireland, 10% in Australia, and 30% at the NICHD Neonatal Research Network centers. At this gestational age, 51% of United Kingdom/Ireland deaths occurred in the delivery room without admission to a newborn intensive care unit, and 77% of deaths in Australia occurred without intensive care. By contrast, in many United States series, less than 10% of deaths at 23 weeks' gestation occur without the provision of intensive care. In addition, population- or regional-based series (such as those from the United Kingdom/Ireland and Australia), which include all births, may demonstrate lower survival than hospital-based series such as the NICHD.

Table 25.6 shows that no infant with a gestational age of 22 weeks or less has survived at Yale–New Haven Children's Hospital. Occasional reports surface of survivors at 22 weeks' gestation, and in NICHD Neonatal Research Network centers 12 of 56 (21%) of infants born at 22 weeks' gestation in 1995 and 1996 survived. There also exist rare reports of survival at 21 weeks' gestation. The gestational age of some of these infants may be inaccurate, and most neonatologists consider 22 or 23 weeks' gestation to be the lower limit of viability.

Neurodevelopmental Outcome

Surviving premature infants are at increased risk of neurodevelopmental problems. VLBW infants, in particular, are at risk of surviving with a severe disability or impairment, such as cerebral palsy, blindness, deafness, or decreased cognitive functioning. The rate of disability generally increases with decreasing gestational age and birth weight, and also is affected by survival selection, associated medical problems, and sociodemographic factors. Perinatal asphyxia, intraventricular hemorrhage, periventricular leukomalacia, chronic lung disease, necrotizing enterocolitis, and late-onset sepsis are medical

TABLE 25.6

SURVIVAL BY GESTATIONAL AGE AND BIRTH WEIGHT*

| | Gestational Age | | | Birth Weight | |
Weeks	Yale 1993–2002 $n = 7,119$	UK/Ireland 1995 $n = 1,185$	Australia 1991–1992 $n = 438$	Weight (g)	Yale 1993–2002 $n = 7,119$
22	0	1	0	≤499	9
23	26	11	10	500–599	41
24	52	26	33	600–699	63
25	75	44	58	700–799	78
26	86		73	800–899	90
27	89		78	900–999	91
28	92			1,000–1,249	93
29	90			1,250–1,499	97
30	95			1,500–1,749	98
31	97			1,750–1,999	97
32	98			2,000–2,499	98
33	99			≥2,500	99
34	99				
35	98				
36	98				
≥37	99				

*Data expressed as percentages. Survival is to discharge of live born infants. Years are years of birth. Yale data are for inborn infants and include 626 infants born at a gestational age of 27 weeks or less. (Other data adapted from Costeloe KC, Hennessey E, Gibson AT, et al. The EPICure Study: outcomes to discharge from hospital for infants born at the threshold of viability. *Pediatrics* 2000;106:659, and Doyle LW. Outcome at 5 years of age of children 23 to 27 weeks' gestation: refining the prognosis. *Pediatrics* 2001;108:134.)

TABLE 25.7

DISABILITY BY GESTATIONAL AGE*

Gestational Age (Weeks)	Survival to 5 Years	Of Survivors, Severe Disability	Of Live-born Survivors without Severe Disability
22	0	—	0
23	10	40	6
24	33	33	22
25	58	25	43
26	72	24	55
27	77	6	72

*Data expressed as percentages. (Adapted from Doyle LW. Outcome at 5 years of age of children 23 to 27 weeks' gestation: refining the prognosis. *Pediatrics* 2001;108:134.)

problems that have been associated with adverse neurodevelopmental outcomes, such as cerebral palsy and impaired cognitive function.

The incidence of moderate or severe neurodevelopmental disability at 18 to 30 months in surviving children whose birth weight was less than 750 g or gestational age was less than 25 weeks is approximately 30% to 50%. Table 25.7 shows the percentage of survivors with severe disability by gestational age in Australia. The percentage of live-born infants who survived without severe disability was only 6% to 7% at 23 weeks and approximately 20% at 24 weeks' gestation. As noted above, this series was population-based, and a significant proportion of babies born at these gestational ages were not offered intensive care. For infants born in 1997 and 1998 at NICHD Neonatal Research Network centers, the frequency of cerebral palsy, Bayley Mental Developmental Index of less than 70, and Bayley Psychomotor Developmental Index of less than 70 at 18 to 22 months corrected age was 18%, 36%, and 25%, respectively, for infants born at 22 to 26 weeks' gestation, and 11%, 22%, and 15%, respectively, for infants born at 27 to 32 weeks' gestation.

Table 25.8 shows the frequency of several specific neurodevelopmental deficits by birth weight in infants born in the United States.

Although some deficits may improve over time, a number of studies have shown that preterm infants have an increased incidence of cognitive, behavioral, and educational impairments at school age. More than 50% of surviving children with birth weights of less than 1,000 g require special education or repeat a grade of school by 8 to 11 years of age. In the Australian regional cohort, ELBW or less than 28 weeks' gestation children born in the 1990s had a full-scale IQ almost 10 points lower than normal birth weight controls at 8 years of life. ELBW or

very preterm children at 8 years of life scored lower on formal tests of academic achievement, especially in arithmetic, and had more internalizing behavior problems, immature adaptive skills, and attention difficulties. Preterm children have been estimated to have twice the relative risk of developing attention deficit hyperactivity disorder. Overall, approximately 55% of the children in the Australian cohort had a clinically important neurobehavioral impairment at 8 years of age.

Similar impairments have been noted in series from the United States, and are present even in survivors with normal intelligence and no neurologic disability. Impairments persist into the teen years and early adulthood. Because of changes in patient demographics and neonatal care, long-term follow-up data of preterm infants born in the 1980s and 1990s may not be applicable to preterm infants born today.

Other Long-term Problems

By school age, VLBW infants have had a greater number of medical problems (including respiratory conditions), poorer growth, more surgical procedures, and more hospitalizations than matched children born at term. Even asymptomatic teenagers without apparent pulmonary disability who were VLBW at birth have a higher frequency of pulmonary function abnormalities consistent with obstructive lung disease. Rehospitalizations are most often related to chronic conditions associated with prematurity (such as bronchopulmonary dysplasia, posthemorrhagic hydrocephalus, or failure to thrive), infections, and the need for herniorrhaphy.

The follow-up of infants discharged from the NICU is described in greater depth in Chapter 28, Follow-up of Infants Discharged from Newborn Intensive Care.

TABLE 25.8

DISABILITY BY BIRTH WEIGHT*

	Birth Weight (g)					
	401–500	501–600	601–700	701–800	801–900	901–1000
Number of survivors	15	94	208	237	290	307
Cerebral palsy	29	17	21	17	15	15
Seizure disorder	0	4	5	6	6	5
Blindness (uni- or bilateral)	21	3	5	5	8	5
Hearing impairment	7	11	14	9	9	7
Bayley MDI <70	31	45	41	42	35	31
Bayley PDI <70	36	34	35	31	25	25
Any major deficit	43	63	59	55	52	44

*Data expressed as percentages, except for number of survivors evaluated. Evaluation performed at 18 to 22 months corrected age. Twenty-two percent of survivors were lost to follow-up. MDI, mental development index; PDI, psychomotor development index. (Adapted from Vohr BR, Wright LL, Dusick AM, et al. Neurodevelopmental and functional outcomes of extremely low birth weight infants in the National Institute of Child Health and Human Development Neonatal Research Network, 1993–1994. *Pediatrics* 2000;105:1216.)

SPECIAL ISSUES

Parental Support

Even the delivery of a relatively stable preterm infant may be one of the most anxiety-provoking events that the parents have ever faced. Parents also must deal with a lack of control over the situation in the intensive care nursery. Caregivers should attempt to provide structure and predictability to disordered circumstances, anticipate questions and concerns, and be willing to offer the same messages repeatedly. Timely communication of both normal and abnormal findings helps alleviate parental anxiety.

Occasionally, parents need to make end-of-life decisions. Preterm neonates, especially those born near the limits of viability, may develop irreversible lung disease, sepsis, or necrotizing enterocolitis or sustain a profound central nervous system insult, such that continued medical care becomes futile. Rather than continuing medical care until death occurs on full support, many neonatologists recommend withdrawal of medical support. Withdrawal of support is the most common mode of death in the NICU. Approximately 80% of ELBW infant deaths occur after withdrawal or withholding of support. Around the time of withdrawing support, effective and compassionate communication with the family is essential. Extended family members, clergy, and social workers can provide support in addition to that provided by the nurses and doctors involved in the child's care.

Ethical Issues

Many ethical issues must be addressed in the NICU, especially when caring for VLBW infants. As noted earlier, 22 to 23 weeks' gestation is considered the limits of viability. When an infant is born around this gestational age, decisions must be made regarding how aggressively to intervene. These decisions are complicated by the different religious and personal beliefs of parents and by uncertainties regarding outcome. As noted earlier, caregivers in the United States may provide more aggressive care to infants born extremely prematurely than caregivers in other parts of the world. Ethical questions about the use and distribution of limited resources can be raised. A recent population-based study contrasted the care of infants born at 23 to 26 weeks' gestation in New Jersey, where there was nearly universal initiation of intensive care (95% of infants received assisted ventilation, and only 10% of deaths occurred without it) and the Netherlands, where there was selective initiation of intensive care (only 64% of infants received assisted ventilation, and 45% of deaths occurred without it). Although baseline population characteristics were not identical, compared to the Netherlands, survival to age 2 was significantly higher in New Jersey (46% versus 22%), but the incidence of disabling cerebral palsy among survivors was also significantly higher (17% versus 3%). Compared to the Netherlands, more aggressive care in New Jersey was associated with 24 additional survivors, 7 additional cases of disabling cerebral palsy, and a cost of 1,372 additional ventilator days, per 100 live births.

The withdrawal of support from critically ill neonates, especially when done because of anticipated survival with a "poor quality of life," also raises many difficult ethical issues. A more in-depth discussion of these and other ethical issues in neonatology appears in Chapter 29 Ethical Issues in Neonatology.

Economics

The cost of care for infants born preterm is high, due to the relative frequency of preterm delivery, the intensity of care in the NICU, including the need for many ancillary services, and the increased survival rates of LBW infants. In addition, long-term health costs of survivors are often significantly greater than those of term newborns. In 1988, the estimated cost of health care, education, and child care for the 3.5 to 4 million children between 0 and 15 years old who were born at LBW was $5.5 to $6 billion more than if they were born at normal birth weight. The annual initial care alone of preterm infants born between 1989 and 1992 was estimated at $5.8 billion.

Cost is inversely related to birth weight and gestational age. The estimated mean neonatal hospital costs for surviving singleton infants born in California, in 1996, with birth weights 500 to 749, 750 to 999, 1,000 to 1,249, and 1,250 to 1,499 g were $224,400, $144,000, $92,700, and $51,900, respectively. Although individual survivors from the smallest birth-weight categories accrue the highest costs, the care of these infants as a whole consumes only a small portion of total NICU resources, because they make up a relatively small proportion of NICU admissions, their mortality is high, and the interval from birth to death of nonsurvivors is short. The long-term costs of care of survivors from these birth weight categories are higher if a disability is present. The 2-year costs for ELBW infants who were born in Helsinki from 1991 to 1997, who were normally developed, mildly disabled, and severely disabled, were 25-, 33-, and 68-fold greater than those of normal birth weight controls, respectively.

The allocation of extensive resources to preterm neonates, especially those born near the limits of viability, remains controversial, and controlling costs is difficult. Quality improvement initiatives of hospitals in the Vermont Oxford Network aimed at decreasing nosocomial infection and chronic lung disease in LBW infants have resulted in decreases in the cost of care. Prenatal care that improves neonatal outcome may demonstrate the greatest cost effectiveness. In 1985, it was estimated that for every dollar spent on prenatal care, $3 was saved in the first year after delivery and an additional $10 was saved over a lifetime. As an example of an avoidable source of expense, the cost of neonatal care attributable to maternal smoking in 1996 was estimated at $367 million. Continued attempts must be made to make the neonatal care of preterm infants cost effective.

PREVENTION AND FUTURE IMPROVEMENTS IN OUTCOME

Prevention of Preterm Delivery

Attempts to prevent preterm delivery have been hampered by the limited understanding of its causes and by the failure to reverse many of the maternal demographic and lifestyle risk factors for preterm labor. As noted earlier, the incidence of preterm delivery has in fact increased for most of the last two decades. Interventions to prevent teen pregnancies, prevent unplanned pregnancies, improve access to prenatal care, prevent sexually transmitted diseases, decrease smoking and other drug use during pregnancy, relieve stress, and improve the work environment of pregnant women either have not been attempted or have met with limited success. The rate of smoking during pregnancy (as reported on birth certificates) has declined from approximately 20% in 1989 to 12% in 2000. A change in smoking habit after a preterm delivery also has been shown to influence the risk of recurrent preterm delivery.

Although reduced activity, bed rest, and sexual abstinence have been recommended to prevent preterm births, no data support their efficacy. Some evidence supports prophylactic cervical cerclage for women with cervical incompetence, to prolong gestation. As noted earlier, the rate of higher-order multiple gestations has plateaued recently, and changes in obstetrical practice aimed at decreasing that rate clearly would decrease the preterm birth rate.

Despite the important role infection is believed to play in the development of preterm labor and premature rupture of membranes, studies on the use of antibiotics to prevent preterm delivery have shown generally disappointing results. A number of randomized trials have looked at the role of antibiotic treatment in women with infection-related risk factors. For example, a recent study of metronidazole in 1,953 pregnant women with asymptomatic bacterial vaginosis failed to show a decrease in the rate of preterm delivery in the treatment group. Treatment with metronidazole also has failed to prevent preterm delivery in pregnant women with asymptomatic *Trichomonas vaginalis* infection. In a third recent trial, the antibiotic treatment of pregnant women who were fetal fibronectin–positive between 21 and 26 weeks' gestation did not decrease the incidence of spontaneous preterm birth. Finally, a study of 400 women with periodontal disease showed that periodontal treatment significantly reduced the rate of preterm low birth weight.

In 2003, The American College of Obstetricians and Gynecologists recommended against treating women in preterm labor with antibiotics for the sole purpose of preventing preterm delivery because of negative clinical trials and meta-analyses. In women with preterm rupture of membranes between 24 and 32 weeks' gestation, however, antibiotic treatment increases the interval to delivery and decreases neonatal morbidity. The use of antibiotics in selected settings to prevent preterm birth remains an area of active interest.

In 2003, a randomized study of 463 pregnant women with a history of spontaneous preterm delivery showed that treatment with weekly injections of 17 alpha-hydroxyprogesterone, starting at 16 to 20 weeks' gestation, decreased the rate of preterm delivery in the current pregnancy from 55% to 36%, and the rate of delivery at less than 32 weeks' gestation from 20% to 11%. Another study showed that progesterone vaginal suppositories decreased the incidence of preterm delivery. The reproducibility and generalizability of these encouraging studies must be determined.

Prediction of Preterm Delivery

Preventing spontaneous preterm birth may be more successful if one could predict which women are at highest risk of this problem. Researchers have identified a positive cervical-vaginal fetal fibronectin test, shortened cervical length, elevated levels of maternal serum alpha-fetoprotein, alkaline phosphatase, granulocyte colony-stimulating factor, and other markers as predictors of preterm delivery. The utility of these markers is limited by relatively low positive predictive values. For example, the rate of spontaneous preterm birth at less than 30 weeks' gestation is 0.3% for women with negative fetal fibronectin tests at 24 and 26 weeks, but only 16% for women with positive tests at 24 and 26 weeks. Using a combination of these markers may enhance the prediction of preterm delivery. Even if preterm delivery cannot be prevented, the accurate prediction of those at high or low risk of preterm delivery may be helpful in making decisions about maternal transfer to tertiary centers, and about interventions such as antenatal corticosteroid therapy.

Improving the Outcome of Preterm Neonates

Clinical Trials and Benchmarking

Given the frequency of preterm delivery and the attendant morbidities and costs, it is not surprising that great effort is directed at improving the care of preterm neonates. The limitations of small, single-institution clinical trials have been overcome in part by multicentered trials, which can enroll larger numbers of patients. For example, a multicenter study that enrolled 807 ELBW infants has demonstrated that vitamin A supplementation decreases the risk of chronic lung disease. Although the reduction is modest (death or chronic lung disease occurred in 55% of treated infants compared to 62% of controls), the large number of patients enrolled allowed the beneficial effect to be demonstrated with a high degree of statistical certainty. Formal associations of neonatal units, such as the Vermont Oxford Network and the NICHD, have performed many powerful observational and interventional studies aimed at improving the care of preterm neonates.

Meta-analyses of similar clinical trials also help determine the overall efficacy of interventions. The Cochrane Database of Systematic Reviews periodically publishes meta-analyses of a wide range of maternal and postnatal interventions for preterm infants.

Another approach to improving care is based on interinstitutional collaboration. A wide range exists in the frequency of mortality and morbidities at different institutions. For example, among NICHD Neonatal Research Network centers, in 1999 and 2000, the incidence of chronic lung disease in VLBW infants ranged from 2% to 81%. The incidence of late-onset septicemia ranged from 3% to 59%. Although some of these differences are due to differences in patient populations, much is probably due to differences in care. The Vermont Oxford Network's Neonatal Intensive Care Collaborative Quality Project has focused on identifying "potentially better practices" through an analysis of the process of care, literature review, and benchmarking visits to "superior performing units" in the network. Participating NICUs have been able to decrease the rates of overall nosocomial infection, coagulase-negative staphylococcus infection, and chronic lung disease.

The Neonatal Intensive Care Unit Environment

The outcome of preterm infants also may be improved by optimizing their physical environment. Exposure to noise in the NICU may result in cochlear damage and disrupt the normal growth and development of preterm infants. In 1997, the American Academy of Pediatrics issued a statement that encouraged strategies to reduce noise in the nursery and suggested avoiding noise levels of more than 45 dB. Excessive ambient light also may be detrimental to the preterm infant, although a clinical trial of continuous reduced light showed no beneficial effect on medical outcomes. The importance of day–night cycles in newborns is unknown, but infants born at less than 31 weeks' gestation have been shown to grow better in cycled light. Finally, the optimal amount of stimulation of preterm infants also is poorly defined. Although tactile and kinesthetic stimulation of stable, growing preterm neonates may facilitate growth and behavioral organization, excessive stimulation may result in autonomic responses that are detrimental to the sick neonate.

Mounting evidence suggests that increased physical contact between the preterm infant and his or her parents is beneficial. "Kangaroo care" of preterm infants, in which they are held directly against one of their parent's naked chest for periods of time, may decrease the frequency of apnea, decrease nosocomial infection, enhance breast-feeding, and lead to improvement in other physiologic parameters.

Increasing attention is being paid to the negative effects of pain in the preterm neonate. Appropriate analgesia for painful procedures is indicated, as for term neonates and older children.

"Developmental care" or "developmentally supportive care" is thus purported to include such interventions as decreasing ambient light, cycling light, reducing environmental noise, positioning infants, clustering care-giving to allow periods of uninterrupted sleep, promoting non-nutritive sucking and grasping, encouraging oral feeding, and maximizing the involvement of parents in their infant's care. Whether such interventions truly support development and improve outcome has yet to be determined.

Post-Discharge Interventions

Optimizing the outcome of preterm infants logically would include continued special services after discharge from the NICU. Unfortunately, early intervention in the first 3 years after neonatal discharge (including frequent home visits and parental education) has resulted in little long-term improvement in full-scale IQ, behavior, or health at 5 years of life, particularly for infants with birth weights of less than 2,000 g.

CONCLUSION

Future improvements in the care of preterm infants hopefully will reduce morbidities, minimize iatrogenic injury, and improve survival and long-term outcome. Although some improvements in survival rates may occur, especially at 22 to 26 weeks' gestation, they will be limited by maturational constraints. Advances in the care of preterm infants must continue to address ethical issues and cost-to-benefit analyses. Ultimately, the most cost-effective, ethical, and desirable advances will be those directed at preventing preterm delivery itself.

Suggested Readings

Allen MC, Donohue PK, Dusman AE. The limit of viability—neonatal outcome of infants born at 22 to 25 weeks' gestation. *N Engl J Med* 1993;329:1597.

Anderson P, Doyle LW. Neurobehavioral outcomes of school-age children born extremely low birth weight or very preterm in the 1990s. *JAMA* 2003;289:3264.

Assessment of risk factors for preterm birth. ACOG Practice Bulletin No. 31. American College of Obstetricians and Gynecologists. *Obstet Gynecol* 2001; 98:709.

Bruck K. Neonatal thermal regulation. In: Polin RA, Fox WW, eds. *Fetal and neonatal physiology*, 2nd ed. Philadelphia: W.B. Saunders, 1998:676.

Butte NF. Meeting energy needs. In: Tsang RC, Zlotkin SH, Nichols BL, Hansen JW, eds. *Nutrition during infancy*, 2nd ed. Cincinnati: Digital Educational Publishing, 1997:57.

Cowett RM. Hypoglycemia and hyperglycemia in the newborn. In: Polin RA, Fox WW, eds. *Fetal and neonatal physiology*, 2nd ed. Philadelphia: W.B. Saunders, 1998:596.

Doyle LW and the Victorian Infant Collaborative Study Group. Evaluation of neonatal intensive care for extremely low birth weight infants in Victoria over two decades: I. Effectiveness. *Pediatrics* 2004;113:505.

Dubowitz LMS, Dubowitz V, Goldberg C. Clinical assessment of gestational age in the newborn infant. *J Pediatr* 1970;77:1.

Fanaroff AA, Hack M, Walsh MC. The NICHD Neonatal Research Network: changes in practice and outcomes during the first 15 years. *Semin Perinatol* 2003;27:281.

Ferrara TB, Hoekstra RE, Couser RJ, et al. Survival and follow-up of infants born at 23 to 26 weeks of gestational age: effects of surfactant therapy. *J Pediatr* 1994;124:119.

Gerdes JS. Clinicopathologic approach to the diagnosis of neonatal sepsis. *Clin Perinatol* 1991;18:361.

Gilbert WM, Nesbitt TS, Danielsen B. The cost of prematurity: Quantification by gestational age and birth weight. *Obstet Gynecol* 2003;102:488.

Ginsberg HG, Goldsmith JP, Stedman CM. Survival of a 380-g infant. *N Engl J Med* 1990;322:1753.

Goldenberg RL, Hauth JC, Andrews WA. Intrauterine infection and preterm delivery. *N Engl J Med* 2000;342:1500.

Hack M, Fanaroff AA. Outcomes of children of extremely low birthweight and gestational age in the 1990s. *Semin Neonatol* 2000;5:89.

Hack M, Flannery DJ, Schluchter M, et al. Outcomes in young adulthood for very-low-birth-weight infants. *N Engl J Med* 2002;346:149.

Hay WW, Lucas A, Heird WC, et al. Workshop summary: nutrition of the extremely low birth weight infant. *Pediatrics* 1999;104:1360.

Horbar JD, Rogowski J, Plsek PE, et al. Collaborative quality improvement for neonatal intensive care. *Pediatrics* 2001;107:14.

Lemons JA, Bauer CR, Oh W, et al. Very low birth weight outcomes of the National Institute of Child Health and Human Development Neonatal Research Network, January 1995 through December 1996. *Pediatrics* 2001;107:e1.

Lorenz JM, Paneth N, Jetton JR, et al. Comparison of management strategies for extreme prematurity in New Jersey and the Netherlands: outcomes and resource expenditure. *Pediatrics* 2001;108:1269.

Martin RJ, Miller MJ, Carlo WA. Pathogenesis of apnea in preterm infants. *J Pediatr* 1986;109:733.

Meis PJ, Klebanoff M, Thom E, et al. Prevention of recurrent preterm delivery by 17 alpha-hydroxyprogesterone caproate. *N Engl J Med* 2003;348:2379.

Shaffer SG, Weisman DN. Fluid requirements in the preterm infant. *Clin Perinatol* 1992;19:233.

Stoll BJ, Hansen N, Fanaroff AA, et al. Changes in pathogens causing early-onset sepsis in very-low-birth-weight infants. *N Engl J Med* 2002;347:240.

Strauss RG. Red blood cell transfusion practices in the neonate. *Clin Perinatol* 1995;22:641.

Van Marter LJ, Pagano M, Allred EN, et al. Rate of bronchopulmonary dysplasia as a function of neonatal intensive care practices. *J Pediatr* 1992;120:938.

Vohr BR, Wright LL, Dusik AM, et al. Center differences and outcomes of extremely low birth weight infants. *Pediatrics* 2004;113:781.

Wall SN, Partridge JC. Death in the intensive care nursery: physician practice of withdrawing and withholding life support. *Pediatrics* 1997;99:64.

Wood NS, Marlow N, Costeloe K, et al. Neurologic and developmental disability after extremely preterm birth. *New Engl J Med* 2000;343:378.

CHAPTER 26 ■ NEONATAL HYPERBILIRUBINEMIA

WILLIAM J. CASHORE

Jaundice is one of the most common conditions found in newborn infants, and the measurement of the serum bilirubin concentration is probably the diagnostic laboratory test most often performed in the newborn nursery. Although most neonatal jaundice is caused by a maturational delay in bilirubin conjugation and excretion, the outcome is nearly always benign. However, physicians must be alert for the minority of cases in which the cause of hyperbilirubinemia is pathologic or the clinical course is atypical, with exaggerated and possibly harmful levels of hyperbilirubinemia. The observation and follow-up of the newborn infant must be planned and arranged to identify such cases early enough in the clinical course to ensure timely evaluation and treatment.

DEFINITION

The term *hyperbilirubinemia* implies an excessive level of serum bilirubin, potentially associated with a pathologic cause or outcome. During their first few days of postnatal life, most newborns have maximum serum bilirubin levels that exceed the upper limits of normal for adults, even when no disease is present. The reason for this "physiologic" hyperbilirubinemia is a developmental delay in the conjugation and excretion of bilirubin as the infant achieves a postnatal transition from dependence on placental clearance of fetal bilirubin to the maturation of self-contained hepatic uptake and enzymatic and excretory pathways for bilirubin conjugation and elimination.

Because mild, transient jaundice is part of the normal physiologic transition for many newborns, we prefer to reserve the term "neonatal hyperbilirubinemia" for cases in which jaundice appears earlier, persists longer, or reaches higher bilirubin levels than expected for age during the neonatal and postnatal periods. Some cases of neonatal hyperbilirubinemia represent an exaggeration of the physiologic pattern, whereas others have detectable causes, usually increased red-cell breakdown leading to increased bilirubin production or an exaggerated delay or inhibition of conjugating enzyme (glucuronyl transferase) activity. Typical neonatal hyperbilirubinemia is predominantly unconjugated or indirect-reacting. A minority of infants present with conjugated (direct-reacting) hyperbilirubinemia, a condition with a different pathogenesis than the more common indirect hyperbilirubinemia.

EPIDEMIOLOGY

In 2,416 well, term infants at 3 to 4 days of age, Maisels and Gifford (1986) found peak bilirubin levels (mean $\pm$ S.D.) of 5.7 ± 3.3 mg/dL in formula-fed and 7.3 ± 3.9 mg/dL in breast-fed newborns, respectively. In most babies, bilirubin levels spontaneously declined after day 4. Of their patients, 6.1% had peak bilirubin values of greater than or equal to 13.0 mg/dL, with more breast-fed babies in the upper percentiles (9% of breast-fed versus 2.2% of formula-fed babies). Other surveys have shown similar differences between breast- and formula-fed newborns. Bhutani et al. found a 95th percentile value of 17 mg/dL and a 40th percentile value of 11.5 mg/dL at age 4 days in a largely breast-fed newborn population. In several large surveys of jaundiced infants without prior treatment, approximately 1 in 100 had peak bilirubin levels of greater than or equal to 20 mg/dL, and about 1 in 700 had levels of greater than or equal to 25 mg/dL at readmission.

Mean postnatal bilirubin levels and the incidence of "severe" hyperbilirubinemia vary with race and ethnicity. Within the population of the United States, newborns of Asian Pacific and Central American ethnic origin have average bilirubin levels which are slightly higher, and newborns of African-American origin slightly lower, than those of white newborns. Within-group variation is generally larger than between-group differences. The extent to which these intergroup differences reflect differences in diet, environment, and genetic control of bilirubin production and excretion is undetermined.

Because visible cutaneous and scleral jaundice in newborns is usually noted only when the serum bilirubin level exceeds 7 to 8 mg/dL, most self-limited developmental jaundice with a maximum bilirubin level at or below the mean value for newborns remains undetected. Visible jaundice develops in about 25% to 40% of newborns with bilirubin levels in the range of 10 to 12 mg/dL or greater. Many term newborns have a length of nursery stay less than or equal to 48 hours, so that some infants not visibly jaundiced in the nursery may become severely jaundiced by 4 to 5 days of age. The early identification and differential diagnosis of jaundice (Table 26.1) in these infants may be assisted by a system-based approach of regular visual or instrumental screening for jaundice before discharge, noting the age of onset and the progression of the baby's jaundice by age in hours. Other helpful observations include evidence of maternal–fetal major or minor blood group incompatibility; family history; associated findings, such as hematomas or evidence of infection; the method of feeding; and the duration, intensity, and clinical course of the jaundice beyond the third day.

CAUSES

Bilirubin is the breakdown product of heme, derived via heme oxygenase and biliverdin reductase, with release of 1 mole of carbon monoxide for each mole of heme metabolized. Circulating bilirubin is transported on albumin to receptor sites in the liver, and then is conjugated by bilirubin uridine disphosphate-glucuronyl transferase to its water-soluble form, also called "conjugated" or "direct-reacting" bilirubin. The products of conjugation include bilirubin monoglucuronide and diglucuronide, the latter being the predominant conjugated form in humans.

Bilirubin conjugates enter the small bowel via canalicular transport and bile excretion. In the course of normal metabolism, they are oxidized further by the intestinal brush border and bacterial enzymes (mainly the latter) and excreted in the stool. Because the bowel is not colonized and does not fully function during fetal life, the hepatic conjugation and transport system is relatively inactive in the fetus, so that bilirubin produced from fetal red cells *in utero* mostly circulates in the unconjugated form.

This unconjugated or "indirect reacting" bilirubin is albumin-bound, relatively lipophilic, and can be transferred across the placenta again to the maternal circulation for conjugation and excretion by the maternal liver. At birth, as the maternal excretory pathway is removed, the development of normal conjugating capacity, canalicular transport, and metabolism and excretion of conjugated bilirubin in the small and large bowel require several days before this disposal pathway becomes adequate for the quantitative conjugation and excretion of bilirubin. Associated with the gradual maturation of bilirubin conjugation and excretion is the accumulation of unconjugated or indirect-reacting bilirubin in the plasma until the pathways mature.

Factors Associated with Hyperbiliruinemia

Classically, neonatal unconjugated hyperbilirubinemia has been attributed primarily to low levels of bilirubin glucuronyl transferase activity in the fetal and neonatal liver. The specific roles of inhibitors of glucuronyl transferase activity, such as maternal steroids, as well as postulated activators of enzyme expression, remain unclear. Other factors in the genesis of physiologic jaundice (unconjugated hyperbilirubinemia) include:

1. Discontinuation of placental mechanisms for fetal bilirubin transfer and detoxification.
2. Persistent patency of the ductus venosus, which diverts some blood flow away from the hepatic sinusoidal bed, shunting some unconjugated bilirubin past the loci of uptake and conjugation in the hepatocytes.
3. A greater rate of bilirubin production in the infant (6 to 8 mg/kg every 24 hours) than in the adult, secondary to a larger red blood cell mass and shortened survival time of fetal red cells.
4. Diminished binding of unconjugated bilirubin to neonatal serum albumin.

TABLE 26.1

DIFFERENTIAL DIAGNOSIS OF NEONATAL HYPERBILIRUBINEMIA

Cause	Associated Findings
Unconjugated ("Indirect") Hyperbilirubinemia	
Hemolytic Disease (Isoimmune)	
ABO incompatibility	Positive Coombs' antiglobulin test (anti-A or anti-B); microspherocytes
Rh incompatibility	Maternal anti-Rh titer; positive Coombs' test; nucleated RBCs
Other minor blood group incompatibility	Positive Coombs' test; RBC morphology variable
Structural or Metabolic Abnormalities of RBCs*	
Hereditary spherocytosis	Family history; splenomegaly; microspherocytes
Glucose-6-phosphate dehydrogenase (G6PD) deficiency	Family history; recent exposure to an oxidant in food or drug; with or without splenomegaly
Hereditary Defects in Bilirubin Conjugation	
Crigler-Najjar syndrome–Type I	Complete lack of glucuronyl transferase; severe, lifelong, unconjugated hyperbilirubinemia
Crigler-Najjar syndrome–Type II	Defective glucuronyl transferase with recurrent or chronic moderate hyperbilirubinemia; phenobarbital usually increases conjugating enzyme activity
Gilbert disease (Arias syndrome)	Family history; mild, recurrent hyperbilirubinemia due to a promoter region defect or structural polymorphism in glucuronyl transferase; usually responds to phenobarbital
Bacterial sepsis	History and findings compatible with neonatal infection; often an increase in direct bilirubin as well
Breast-milk jaundice	Mild to moderate, but persistent, hyperbilirubinemia; usually improves when breast milk is discontinued
Physiologic jaundice	Usually mild to moderate; no predisposing factors; self-limited (duration <1 week)
Conjugated (direct) hyperbilirubinemia	
Congenital biliary atresia	Dilated intrahepatic ducts; no bile excretion
Extrahepatic biliary obstruction	Extrahepatic cyst or mass; dilated main or common bile ducts
Neonatal Hepatitis	
Bacterial	Findings compatible with neonatal sepsis
Viral	Inflammatory changes; other systemic signs of specific viral infection
Nonspecific	Inflammatory changes without a specific infectious etiology
TPN-related	Hepatocellular cholestasis with variable fatty and inflammatory changes; usually reversible, but occasionally progresses to cirrhosis
Short-bowel related	Hepatocellular inflammation and small bile duct proliferation due to bile acid recirculation and bacterial overgrowth in the small bowel
Inspissated bile syndrome	Persistent direct hyperbilirubinemia associated with isoimmune hemolytic disease
Post-asphyxia	Compatible history, plus increased hepatocellular enzyme concentrations
Alpha$_1$-antitrypsin deficiency	Decreased alpha$_1$-antitrypsin levels; recurrent or "chronic" lung disease
Neonatal hemosiderosis	Hemosiderin-filled macrophages on biopsy

RBCs, red blood cells.
*Only the two most common disorders are listed, as examples.

5. Diminished levels of intracellular bilirubin binding (Y) protein.
6. Impaired canalicular excretion of organic anions in the developing liver.

In addition, bilirubin appears to undergo a significant entero-hepatic circulation in the newborn. Conjugated bilirubin in the adult intestinal tract is reduced by (predominantly) anaerobic intestinal flora to poorly absorbable urobilinogen. These flora are not all present in the fetal and neonatal intestine. Instead, beta-glucuronidase present in the neonatal intestine hydrolyzes bilirubin mono-or diglucuronide back to unconjugated bilirubin, which is subsequently reabsorbed into the portal circulation, thus contributing to the "bilirubin overload" and further taxing already stressed metabolic and excretory pathways. Thus, the delayed passage of meconium can cause an elevation in the serum bilirubin level.

Some newborns who show an unusually early onset, exaggerated and sustained level, or uncommonly long duration of hyperbilirubinemia may require medical attention. In Maisels and Gifford's patients, noted above, and in similar large series, a definite cause for exaggerated hyperbilirubinemia was found in only 45% to 50% of the infants evaluated. Therefore, about 3% of term newborns may have exaggerated or sustained hyperbilirubinemia as part of their "normal" development, whereas another 3% to 5% may have clinically significant hyperbilirubinemia associated with some other identifiable cause. Therefore, although hyperbilirubinemia is a frequent observation in the nursery, the term by itself indicates only that the level of jaundice observed is greater than expected for a normal healthy infant of the same age. Further observation and diagnostic studies are needed to establish a cause for the hyperbilirubinemia.

Associated Conditions

Infants of Diabetic Mothers

The infants of diabetic mothers often have polycythemia, with an increased red cell mass that leads to an increased daily rate of bilirubin formation. They may have some acquired structural or metabolic instability of their red cells (e.g., increased glycohemoglobin) related to their glucose metabolism. In general, they follow a less mature pattern of physiologic development (including bilirubin conjugation) than do term infants of similar birth weight, whose mothers are not diabetic.

Immaturity

Delay in the conjugation and excretion of bilirubin varies between individuals, but some infants may have predisposing factors to delayed excretion. The most common underlying condition is immaturity. Otherwise healthy preterm infants (<37 weeks gestation) tend to have maximum serum bilirubin levels 30% to 50% higher than their term counterparts, with increasing serum unconjugated bilirubin continuing until as late as the sixth or seventh postnatal day, and sometimes persisting into the second week. If heavier and physiologically stable preterm infants are cared for and discharged from well-baby nurseries, their pediatricians must keep in mind the possibility of prolonged or late jaundice.

Breast-fed Infants

Breast-fed infants can have a combined inefficiency of hepatic conjugation and gastrointestinal excretion of bilirubin, mediated by factors in breast milk that may suppress hepatic function, increase reabsorption of bilirubin from the small bowel, or both. As noted earlier, their mean bilirubin concentration is slightly higher, duration of jaundice somewhat longer, and the incidence of clinically detectable hyperbilirubinemia during the first week is more frequent in breast-fed than in formula-fed infants.

About 2% of breast-fed infants have a longer (2- to 8-week) course of moderate hyperbilirubinemia, usually in the range of 10 to 15 mg/dL, while feeding adequately on breast milk and gaining weight, with no other abnormal clinical findings. Arias et al. showed that high levels of 3-alpha, 20-beta-pregnanediol in mothers' milk were associated with decreased bilirubin conjugation and persistent hyperbilirubinemia. However, subsequent studies have not found the association to be consistent. Multiple hormonal or enzymatic factors may be involved in suppressing the hepatic conjugation of bilirubin or cleaving bilirubin conjugates in the neonatal small bowel in certain mother–baby pairs, thereby promoting the reabsorption and enterohepatic recirculation of unconjugated bilirubin. Although the pathogenesis of breast-milk jaundice is controversial, most babies have only mild hyperbilirubinemia. Refractory, severe cases usually respond to cessation of breast-feeding for 36 to 48 hours, with a prompt decrease in serum bilirubin.

Hospital feeding schedules and practices may abet jaundice in breast-fed infants by delaying the initial breast feedings during a prescribed observation period and by adherence to feeding intervals of once every 4 hours, rather than early nursing patterns of 8 to 10 times daily. Delay in feeding and suboptimal intake also delay and decrease meconium output and delay the transition to normal stools rich in bile pigments.

Delayed Intestinal Transit

Infants who are not fed or have high intestinal obstructions (e.g., pyloric stenosis or duodenal atresia) may have exaggerated levels of jaundice from the combined effects of lack of nutritional substrate for conjugation, lack of peristalsis for excretion, and consequent reabsorption of bilirubin from an obstructed or nonfunctioning bowel.

Genetic Variations in Conjugation

Genetic variations in the conjugating enzyme, bilirubin glucuronyl transferase, may act independently to impair and delay conjugation or may act in concert with other genetic or environmental influences to cause early or severe persistent neonatal hyperbilirubinemia. To date, more than 50 mutations or polymorphisms in UDPGT-A1, the gene encoding hepatic bilirubin glucuronyl transferase, have been identified. With substantial individual variation, several clinical phenotypes have been associated with specific classes of mutations (see Table 26.1).

Crigler-Najjar Syndrome, Type I, is caused by an absence of glucuronyl transferase activity with severe, persistent unconjugated hyperbilirubinemia. An autosomal recessive nonsense or "stop" mutation terminates protein synthesis proximal to the C-terminal of the enzyme, precluding glucuronidation of any substrates that enter this pathway. Patients with this disorder have severe, persistent hyperbilirubinemia of 20 to 35 mg/dL or higher, beginning in the newborn period. Liver histology is normal, and usually no other findings of liver disease or hemolytic anemia are present.

Nearly all patients with Type I Crigler-Najjar syndrome eventually develop bilirubin-related neurologic impairment, even if early recognition and aggressive treatment with exchange transfusion and phototherapy averts (or postpones) neonatal kernicterus. Patients treated with daily phototherapy, oral administration of bilirubin binding or solubilizing agents, or suppression of bilirubin formation via inhibition of heme oxygenase (experimental at present) often "escape" from control. This may occur during an intercurrent illness (e.g., a viral infection), with an abrupt increase in unconjugated bilirubin years or decades after neonatal survival. Hepatic transplantation, which provides the missing enzyme, is curative and should be attempted before irreversible neurologic damage occurs.

Type II Crigler-Najjar Syndrome is caused by substitution mutations in UDPGT-A1, generally autosomal recessive, with variable penetrance. Neonatal jaundice may be severe and lead to kernicterus. Subsequent unconjugated bilirubin levels may vary from 6 to 20 mg/dL, sometimes increasing during acute illnesses. In Type II Crigler-Najjar Syndrome, increased enzyme activity can be induced with low-dose phenobarbital (3 to 5 mg/kg/day), sometimes with clinical resolution of the hyperbilirubinemia. The clinical course is generally milder than Type I, and amenable to pharmacologic treatment as noted for Type I.

Gilbert disease is characterized by a mild elevation in serum bilirubin levels, typically of 2 to 6 mg/dL. Liver function and histology are normal, except for minor changes noted on electron microscopy. This disorder usually results from a mutation in the promoter region of UDPGT-A1. A different mutation in several Japanese kindreds is a single amino acid substitution (Arg 71 → Gly) in the enzyme protein. Mutations for Gilbert disease have a frequency of 2% to 10% in various human populations. Heterozygous individuals are sometimes mildly affected. Newborns can have more severe jaundice than older children or adults, sometimes exceeding 20 mg/dL. In newborns either homozygous or heterozygous for genes causing Gilbert disease, early jaundice is more severe in breast-fed infants or in those who also carry gene mutations for red cell G6-PD deficiency. Intercurrent illness or caloric deprivation may increase serum bilirubin levels two- to threefold in this disorder. Low-dose phenobarbital increases bilirubin conjugation and excretion in patients with mild, chronic jaundice or acute flare-ups of Gilbert disease.

Hypothyroidism

Hypothyroidism may cause persistent unconjugated hyperbilirubinemia, which is sometimes a presenting sign of neonatal thyroid hormone deficiency. Jaundice noted in newborns with hypopituitarism is presumably secondary to hypothyroidism. The typical presentation would be a newborn with nonhemolytic hyperbilirubinemia unresponsive to standard therapy, and with a low T_4 and high thyroid stimulating hormone (TSH) level on neonatal metabolic screening tests.

Lucey-Driscoll Syndrome

Lucey-Driscoll syndrome, a condition of severe neonatal hyperbilirubinemia capable of causing kernicterus, is thought to be caused by the inhibition of glucuronyl transferase in the neonatal liver by an unidentified factor present in maternal serum and urine. After initial treatment with exchange transfusions, infants with this rare disorder have shown normal development without further episodes of jaundice.

Intravascular and Extravascular Hemolysis

Hemolysis or, more rarely, ineffective erythropoiesis, increases bilirubin production. The principal causes of hemolysis in newborns are antibody-mediated hemolytic anemias (e.g., Rh or ABO incompatibility); enclosed hemorrhage (e.g., cephalohematoma, intracranial hemorrhage, or skin bruising); hemolysis associated with group B streptococcal or *Escherichia coli* septicemia; or an abnormality of red-cell structure or metabolism (e.g., hereditary spherocytosis or glucose-6-phosphate dehydrogenase deficiency). Increased bilirubin production associated with hemolysis can be detected as an increase in pulmonary carbon monoxide excretion using sensitive equipment to detect small amounts of carbon monoxide in expired air. Jaundice from enclosed hemorrhage is generally evident by 3 to 5 days of postnatal life, because extravasated hemoglobin is metabolized slowly.

The most common causes of hemolysis in term infants are isoantibody-mediated hemolytic anemias resulting from maternal–fetal ABO or Rh incompatibility. Although not all susceptible infants are affected, 25% of normal pregnancies are ABO incompatible, and about 12% are Rh(D) incompatible.

Neonatal polycythemia (central hematocrit of greater than 65%) can be seen in infants of diabetic mothers, infants with adrenal hyperplasia, placental insufficiency, twin-to-twin transfusion, or aggressive "stripping" of the umbilical cord. When combined with shortened fetal red-cell survival time, polycythemia may increase the infant's bilirubin load. Postnatal hemoconcentration and red-cell breakdown may be gradual, with hyperbilirubinemia becoming clinically evident after 48 hours. Partial exchange transfusion for symptomatic polycythemia/hyperviscosity will decrease the bilirubin load by lowering the hematocrit.

Drug-Associated Jaundice

Some drugs, such as vitamin K in excessive amounts, also may cause hemolysis. Maternal oxytocin has been associated with neonatal hyperbilirubinemia, but this appears to be secondary to osmotic changes in the fetal/neonatal circulation.

BILIRUBIN TOXICITY

High concentrations of bilirubin are toxic to the central nervous system, with the basal ganglia being the most vulnerable areas and cortical damage occurring relatively infrequently. The reason for this susceptibility of the basal ganglia is not known. Clinical manifestations of bilirubin toxicity most frequently affect the basal ganglia and cranial nerve nuclei. The most characteristic findings are opisthotonos, extensor rigidity, tremors, ataxic gait, oculomotor paralysis, and hearing loss. Fatal cases in the newborn period often are characterized by loss of the suck response and lethargy, followed by hyperirritability, then seizures and death. The acute phases of bilirubin toxicity in severely affected infants sometimes are accompanied as well by gastric and pulmonary hemorrhages.

In fatal cases, the meninges and cortical surface may be lightly stained, but dense regional bilirubin staining is found in the basal ganglia, globus pallidus, hippocampus, and sometimes, cerebellum. In later deaths, scarring and gliosis may be found in these or adjacent areas that presumably were sites of bilirubin deposition. Neurologic damage in survivors corresponds to injury in the areas found to be stained in many autopsies. Intelligence and higher cortical functions are relatively spared, whereas ataxia, choreoathetosis, tremors, oculomotor palsy, and central hearing loss persist.

In general, the serum unconjugated bilirubin concentrations that are associated with overt bilirubin encephalopathy (or kernicterus, the pathologic term for nuclear staining with bilirubin) are substantially higher than the levels seen in ordinary clinical practice. Bilirubin levels generally associated with clinical signs of kernicterus in term infants tend to be in the range of 25 to 30 mg/dL or higher. In epidemiologic surveys of bilirubin encephalopathy associated with Rh hemolytic disease, basal ganglia staining or clinical signs of bilirubin encephalopathy were seen occasionally when the serum indirect bilirubin level reached or exceeded 20 mg/dL. In most proven cases, however, the bilirubin levels were considerably higher, often approaching 30 mg/dL. On the other hand, well-documented cases exist of patients with indirect bilirubin levels in the range of 30 to 35 mg/dL who did not experience serious long-term sequelae. Therefore, no precise bilirubin level has been clearly established at which either safety or permanent harm can be guaranteed.

Premature infants, especially those with birth weights of less than 1,500 g, and some infants with sepsis or metabolic complications of asphyxia or respiratory distress may be vulnerable to bilirubin toxicity at lower indirect bilirubin concentrations. During the 1960s and 1970s, cases of basal ganglion staining at maximum bilirubin levels of 10 to 15 mg/dL, along with other cases of more generalized cortical and subcortical bilirubin staining, were reported in preterm infants and sometimes even in term infants, with postnatal complications often marked by sepsis or asphyxia. A few such patients had overt neurologic findings of bilirubin encephalopathy, but in many cases "low bilirubin kernicterus" was an incidental finding at autopsy, unsuspected from the clinical course. The clinical significance of low bilirubin kernicterus and its developmental implications for the follow-up of jaundiced preterm infants are uncertain, but the incidence of bilirubin staining in the central nervous system discovered only at autopsy seems to have decreased since the 1980s.

At present, moderate hyperbilirubinemia in the range of 15 to 20 mg/dL appears to pose little or no acute or long-term developmental risk to otherwise normal infants. Term infants with hyperbilirubinemia in this range show, at most, only subtle and short-term behavioral changes, without detectable long-term neurodevelopmental sequelae on follow-up. In the range of 20 to 25 mg/dL, some term infants become less active and responsive, and also show reversible increases in conduction time and occasional decreases in wave amplitude on determination of auditory brainstem evoked potentials. The long-term significance of abnormalities in brainstem evoked potentials is not clear, but auditory conduction generally returns to normal as bilirubin concentrations fall back into the normal range or respond to treatment.

In summary, uncontrolled levels of severe hyperbilirubinemia produce a characteristic pattern of damage in the basal ganglia, manifested by basal ganglion staining at autopsy or by subcortical neurologic deficits in survivors. In the range of 20 to 25 mg/dL of indirect bilirubin, some term infants show subtle but reversible sensory and behavioral changes of uncertain prognostic significance. Low bilirubin kernicterus in preterm infants remains a diagnostic and developmental puzzle, with a definitive solution becoming less likely as the incidence of low-bilirubin kernicterus declines in this high-risk group.

Bilirubin neurotoxicity is probably mediated by the entry of free unconjugated bilirubin into susceptible areas of the central nervous system. Possible mechanisms for bilirubin entry include diffusion of unconjugated bilirubin, a somewhat lipophilic small molecule, across an intact blood–brain barrier or damage to the blood–brain barrier with significant entry of plasma contents into the brain. Nearly all the bilirubin in the circulation is tightly bound to albumin, but at very high levels, the bilirubin concentration may exceed the albumin concentration available to bind it, resulting in increased diffusion of "free" bilirubin across the blood–brain barrier into the brain's extravascular space. In most cell models of bilirubin toxicity, free bilirubin (i.e., not bound to plasma albumin) produces adverse effects not seen when the same concentration is bound to an equimolar concentration of albumin. Therefore, it is a plausible, although unproved, hypothesis that the free fraction of unconjugated bilirubin is the species responsible for bilirubin neurotoxicity. In very immature or high-risk infants, however, especially those with kernicterus as an incidental or autopsy finding, it is also plausible that injury to tight-junction or transport sites in the blood–brain barrier allows entry of albumin-bound bilirubin, with incidental staining at autopsy. Controversy regarding the relative contributions of "free" bilirubin and antecedent central nervous system injury in neonatal kernicterus remains unresolved.

DIAGNOSIS

The decision to measure the serum bilirubin concentration in newborns is based on the infant's age at onset of visible jaundice, presence of neonatal or perinatal conditions that might increase the risk of severe jaundice, expected age at discharge, and plans and resources for short-term follow-up. Sometimes, prenatal or delivery room screening procedures establish the likelihood of an antibody-mediated hemolytic anemia with a need for early neonatal assessment to predict the postnatal course and initiate treatment. Babies without evidence of hemolytic disease should be screened at regular intervals for neonatal jaundice. Inspection of the baby, undressed and in adequate light, several times a day when diapers are changed or vital signs are taken, allows early recognition of cutaneous or scleral jaundice in many cases. For nonwhite infants, part of the examination can include brief compression with the examiner's thumb over a firm surface such as the forehead, sternum, or upper thigh; briefly blanching the skin may help to reveal an underlying yellow color.

Transcutaneous skin reflectance with a suitably calibrated photometer is an instrumental aid to the early recognition of jaundice and estimation of the level of clinically evident jaundice. The reflectance of jaundiced skin correlates well enough with serum bilirubin levels to be used as a screening test. Some nurseries also perform hour-specific bilirubin levels in the blood samples drawn for metabolic screening before discharge.

Observation alone does not guarantee the identification of early or mild jaundice, or a reliable estimation of the serum bilirubin level. Despite these limitations, the art of observing newborns for jaundice should be taught and encouraged, because occasions may arise when inspection is the only tool available.

Both clinical observation and skin reflectance document that cutaneous jaundice progresses from the face downward in term infants. Scleral and facial jaundice become visible at bilirubin levels of 6 to 8 mg/dL, jaundice of the shoulders and trunk becomes apparent at 8 to 10 mg/dL, jaundice of the lower body is noticeable at 10 to 12 mg/dL, and generally distributed jaundice can be seen at 12 to 15 mg/dL. Because of differences between observers, patients, and settings, the bilirubin values at which jaundice is recognized can vary considerably from the numbers above. Although the distribution and intensity of jaundice provide only semi-quantitative information, documented regular observation can provide an early recognition of evolving hyperbilirubinemia, with the advantages that early detection may provide for timely diagnosis, intervention, and follow-up. Often, nurses are the first to note jaundice in the clinical record, and nurses' notes or messages should be followed up by re-examination of the infant and the performance of appropriate laboratory studies as indicated.

The time when jaundice is first noted, and quantitative estimates of bilirubin level by transcutaneous or laboratory measurement, should be interpreted according to the infant's age *in hours*. Visible jaundice on the first day should never be considered normal, and it requires further evaluation and follow-up. Faint jaundice, first appearing only on the third or fourth hospital day (or barely detectable at a 48-hour discharge) is more likely to be consistent with the average bilirubin levels expected in well, term infants. Jaundice appearing early on hospital day 2, and progressing throughout that day until the time of discharge, is likely to peak even higher during the subsequent 2 to 4 days and merits at least a short-term follow-up examination 24 to 48 hours after discharge, or even an in-hospital evaluation to determine the hour-specific bilirubin level before discharge.

In addition to a laboratory request to determine total and direct (conjugated) bilirubin, the early clinical detection of hyperbilirubinemia should prompt a thorough examination of the abdomen, with palpation of the liver and spleen, and a review of maternal and neonatal records for evidence of blood group incompatibility, a direct antiglobulin test and positive antibody titer, and a family history of neonatal or childhood jaundice in siblings or other relations. All women receiving prenatal care or admitted to a hospital for delivery should have ABO and Rh(D) types determined. Rh(D) negative mothers also should have their titers for anti-Rh(D) antibodies determined during prenatal care and again at delivery. At birth, a cord or peripheral blood specimen should be obtained from each newborn. If the mother is Rh(D) negative, the infant's blood group should be determined, and an antibody screen performed if the infant is Rh(D) positive. If the mother is O positive, determination of the newborn's blood group and antibody status need not be routine, but should be readily available on blood collected at birth if the infant shows early signs of jaundice or anemia.

Although 25% of pregnancies potentially are ABO incompatible, only a minority (10% to 15%) of these have hemolytic disease as documented by anemia, microspherocytosis, hepatosplenomegaly, and a positive antibody test. Group A or B newborns of group O mothers may have positive tests resulting from passive placental transfer of naturally acquired maternal anti-A or anti-B antibodies, but without evidence of accelerated RBC destruction. Conversely, some newborns with clinical signs of ABO hemolytic disease do not have positive antibody (Coombs') tests despite other signs of hemolytic anemia and jaundice. Therefore, the routine use of cord blood type and direct antiglobulin test for anti-A or anti-B antibodies is not a sensitive or specific "screen" for neonatal ABO hemolytic disease. If an antibody-mediated hemolytic anemia is suspected because of family history, splenomegaly, or early jaundice, in addition to serum bilirubin and antibody identification by indirect antiglobulin test (with or without elution of antibodies from the newborn red cell), determination of hemoglobin, hematocrit, red-cell indices, reticulocyte count, and red-cell morphology should be performed. For the more common instance of benign, self-limited developmental hyperbilirubinemia, a complete blood count is not necessary unless there is strong reason to suspect hemolysis or infection as the source of the hyperbilirubinemia. For known cases of Rh sensitization, perform hemoglobin, hematocrit, and bilirubin determinations on cord blood as well as on subsequent postnatal specimens. For most cases of suspected ABO hemolytic disease, cord blood determinations are not necessary because ABO incompatibility usually does not cause significant jaundice or anemia at birth.

The age at first presentation of clinical jaundice and the subsequent rate of increase in bilirubin levels sometimes will help the physician to infer the clinical course and likely outcome of an infant with hyperbilirubinemia. The rate of increase in the serum bilirubin level can be estimated by dividing the first bilirubin level by the patient's age at the time, and subsequent changes in bilirubin level by the change in age between determinations. This allows the physician to estimate whether the rate of increase is normal or abnormal, and whether the increase in bilirubin over time is sustained or declining. For example, the expected maximum rate of increase in bilirubin for otherwise normal infants with nonhemolytic jaundice is about 5mg/dL/day, or 0.2 mg/dL/hour. Visible jaundice on the first day, or a bilirubin concentration greater than 10 mg/dL within the second 24 hours, therefore, is outside the normal range for rate of increase in bilirubin and potentially results from a pathologic cause.

Estimating the rate of increase during the interval between bilirubin determinations also allows the physician to estimate the change in bilirubin that is likely to occur over the next 12 to 24 hours, and to plan subsequent bilirubin determinations accordingly. If an infant has significant early jaundice (i.e., serum bilirubin level of 10 mg/dL or higher on the first day), and the calculated rate of increase exceeds 0.2 mg/dL/hour, repeat determinations should be followed about every 12 hours until bilirubin levels stabilize or there is a clear indication for treatment. In the meantime, the clinician can use the initial rate of bilirubin accumulation and the subsequent rate of increase as a guideline to further diagnostic efforts to determine the underlying cause of the jaundice, if it is not clearly physiologic.

Physiologic jaundice and hemolytic hyperbilirubinemia are of the indirect-reacting variety. Because obstructive liver disease from various causes also may present with neonatal hyperbilirubinemia, the initial evaluation of a jaundiced infant requires a determination of the direct, as well as the total, serum bilirubin concentration. Rapid methods that report only total bilirubin (or its equivalent as skin reflectance) are acceptable as early screens for hour-specific bilirubin, prior to more detailed evaluation, or for short-term follow-up of established unconjugated hyperbilirubinemia during its treatment and resolution. For persistent or recurrent jaundice or follow-up of obstructive jaundice, confirmatory measurements of direct bilirubin also should be performed at suitable intervals. Direct bilirubin concentrations persistently above the range of 1.0 to 1.5mg/dL require a separate diagnostic evaluation, especially if the direct fraction continues to rise.

MANAGEMENT

The clinical course in most cases of neonatal jaundice defines the problem as benign and self-limited. Unless the infant has clear evidence of a hemolytic anemia or some other significant perinatal or postnatal abnormality, most cases of "physiologic hyperbilirubinemia" can be managed with observation, serial bilirubin measurements, and reassurance. Despite an extensive differential diagnosis for neonatal jaundice, the majority of cases are attributable to a small number of causes that are usually detectable by serial bilirubin determinations, examination of the patient, and review of maternal and neonatal blood type and antibody studies.

The benign and self-limited course of most cases of neonatal jaundice makes it unnecessary to pursue extensive diagnostic studies in the first few days. However, assessment for early jaundice before hospital discharge is appropriate to identify patients

needing early follow-up for the onset of jaundice during a short hospital stay (see Figure 23.2). Urgent readmission for unanticipated severe hyperbilirubinemia, and sometimes kernicterus, is more likely in patients lacking close and early follow-up.

Management of Rh Incompatibility

Until recently, Rh isoimmunization was a common cause of neonatal anemia and hyperbilirubinemia, and was the underlying cause for most cases of kernicterus in term infants. Sixteen percent of North American women are Rh-negative—in most cases negative for the Rh D antigen. At delivery of her first Rh-positive child, or sometimes because of a placental hemorrhage or spontaneous abortion of an Rh-positive fetus, the Rh-negative mother receives a small transfusion of Rh-positive fetal red cells. When Rh-positive fetal cells enter the circulation of an Rh-negative recipient, the maternal immune system develops an antibody response to foreign Rh-positive red-cell antigen.

Later exposure to Rh-positive fetal red cells, either during a subsequent Rh-positive pregnancy or sometimes by later transplacental passage of fetal red cells during the same pregnancy, increases maternal IgG antibody against the red cells of her fetus. Maternal anti-Rh IgG then recrosses the placenta to the fetal side, attacking and destroying fetal Rh-positive red cells. As maternal antibody production increases, fetal cells are hemolyzed extravascularly as well as intravascularly, as soon as they become sufficiently antigenic to be recognized by the antibody. During the second half of a sensitized pregnancy, the fetus has progressive hemolytic anemia and intrauterine hyperbilirubinemia. In the most severely sensitized cases, intrauterine anemia becomes so profound that high-output heart failure, anasarca, and hydrops fetalis develop. Many infants with profound anemia and hydrops are stillborn or survive only a short time after birth.

The course of an Rh-sensitized pregnancy may be monitored by the measurement of maternal anti-Rh antibody titer; serial ultrasound examinations to detect fetal hepatomegaly, splenomegaly, or peripheral edema; and transabdominal sampling of amniotic fluid for bilirubin pigments or of placental blood for fetal hemoglobin, hematocrit, and bilirubin level. An increase in amniotic fluid bilirubin or a steady decrease in fetal hematocrit, especially when combined with ultrasonographic evidence of evolving hepatosplenomegaly or edema, indicates a worsening prognosis and need for fetal rescue through transabdominal red-cell transfusion or an emergency delivery if the fetus is near term.

Before the effective prevention of Rh sensitization, Rh hemolytic disease caused many of the most severe cases of neonatal hyperbilirubinemia and was an important cause of kernicterus. With proper maternal screening, all present-day cases of Rh sensitization should be detected prenatally and the pediatrician forewarned.

At birth, maternally cross-matched packed O negative red cells should be available. Cord blood should be sent to the laboratory for immediate determination of serum total and direct bilirubin, hemoglobin, hematocrit, and red-cell indices and morphology. The characteristic abnormality of the red-cell count in a newborn with Rh hemolytic disease is the presence in large numbers of nucleated red cells (erythroblasts), hence the name *erythroblastosis fetalis*. The nucleated red cells are the survivors of the hematopoietic system's efforts to match the rate of Rh-positive red-cell destruction by the circulating antibody.

Immediate postnatal management of severely affected infants may require replacement of red cells, diuresis, aggressive treatment of high-output heart failure, and ventilatory support. Less severely affected infants are viable and may even appear

TABLE 26.2

EXCHANGE TRANSFUSION

Criteria
Cord indirect Br >5 mg/dL
Cord Hgb <10 g/dL
Postnatal increase in Br >1 mg/dL/hour
Anemia (Hgb 10–12 mg/dL) plus postnatal increase in
    Br >0.5 mg /dL /hour
Postnatal increase in Br >20 mg/dL

Technique
Use citrate phosphate dextrose (CPD) blood, 160–170 mL/kg
Umbilical vein catheter (or continuous vein–artery technique)
Aliquots: withdraw/infuse 5 mL/kg/minute
Operating time: 60–90 minutes
Ca^{2+} replacement: monitor heart rate continuously
Hgb, Hcrit, and Br before and after exchange
No oral intake 1 hour before and 5 to 6 hours after procedure

Results
Decrease in plasma Br to 50% to 55% of pre-exchange value
    (30% rebound in 1 hour)
Decrease in tissue Br: re-equilibration with plasma
Decrease in circulating antibody
Replacement of susceptible RBCs
Partial correction of blood volume and decreased RBC mass

Complications
Embolism
Unstable cardiac output and blood pressure
Ruptured spleen/liver
Hyperkalemia
Hypocalcemia
Hyperglycemia or hypoglycemia
Metabolic acidosis
Infection
Transfusion reaction

Br, bilirubin; Hgb, hemoglobin; Hcrit, hematocrit.

well at birth, but may have progressive postnatal anemia and hyperbilirubinemia. Without treatment, hemoglobin may fall by more than 1 gm/dL/day to a profoundly anemic level, and bilirubin may progress from cord levels of 5 to 10 mg/dL to extremely high unconjugated bilirubin levels at a rate of increase greater than 1 mg/dL/hour.

Postnatal management of Rh disease is a model for aggressive intervention in severe neonatal anemia or hyperbilirubinemia. Prompt correction of the circulating hemoglobin level with packed red cells is indicated if the hemoglobin concentration at birth is 8 to 10 mg/dL or less, especially if the newborn also has respiratory distress or difficulty with the normally expected fetal-to-neonatal transition. The volume transfused, usually 25 to 50 mL/kg of packed red cells by partial exchange, is calculated to correct the hemoglobin level to 11 to 13 mg/dL. If the cord indirect bilirubin concentration exceeds 5 mg/dL, or if the early postnatal rate of increase is 1 mg/dL/hour or faster, a double-volume whole blood exchange transfusion should be performed as soon as possible. This procedure, outlined in Table 26.2, stabilizes the red-cell mass by replacing most of the infant's circulating and vulnerable Rh-positive cells with Rh-negative donor cells compatible with the major blood groups and not susceptible to the circulating anti-Rh antibody. Replacement of plasma lowers the bilirubin concentration and somewhat lowers the circulating antibody level, although the latter effect on antibody levels is generally less efficient than removing most of the antibody-coated red cells. The nonjaundiced donor plasma also provides adult albumin not yet satu-

rated with bilirubin, allowing re-equilibration of bilirubin from the tissues with a fresh supply of plasma albumin.

After initial postnatal management of Rh disease, serial bilirubin determinations are performed as often as every 4 hours, but not less often than every 8 to 12 hours, depending on the rate of bilirubin increase after transfusion. The initial exchange transfusion should reduce the serum bilirubin concentration by about 50%. Extravascular bilirubin then equilibrates rapidly with the plasma, causing a short-term 30% rebound increase in plasma bilirubin. For example, if the initial bilirubin concentration is 20 mg/dL and the exchange transfusion lowers it to 10 mg/dL, within 1 to 2 hours after the procedure, the bilirubin concentration will rebound to about 13 mg/dL. If the rate of increase in bilirubin remains greater than 0.5 mg/dL /hour over the next 10 to 12 hours and 2 or 3 successive bilirubin determinations, a repeat exchange transfusion is advisable before the serum bilirubin reaches 20 mg/dL. A second exchange transfusion also is appropriate if postnatal anemia continues to progress rapidly. After the first postnatal day, if the rate of increase in bilirubin is less than 0.5 mg/dL/hour, and if the hemoglobin is stable, the infant should be followed with serial bilirubin determinations. Jaundice at this stage can sometimes be controlled by phototherapy, but a repeat exchange transfusion should be planned if the serum indirect bilirubin reaches or exceeds 20 mg/dL. During the early, acute period of rapid hemolysis with progressive anemia and hyperbilirubinemia, commonly used approaches to neonatal jaundice, such as phototherapy and intravenous hydration, are not contraindicated, but may be insufficient by themselves to modify the clinical course of jaundice and anemia (especially the latter) until hemolysis is better controlled through the replacement of damaged red cells and removal of antibodies.

Fortunately, maternal screening and widespread use of anti-Rh immunoglobulin during the third trimester and immediately after delivery have reduced the incidence of maternal Rh sensitization and neonatal hemolytic disease until they are now comparatively rare in the developed world. Continued screening and immunization will be needed to maintain this therapeutic success. Breakthrough cases may continue to occur on occasion, related to undetected placental hemorrhage, missed spontaneous abortions, or other reproductive accidents.

Management of ABO Incompatibility

ABO hemolytic disease is more common than Rh hemolytic disease, but is more benign. In nearly all cases, the mother's blood type is group O (the major blood type in 40% of the North American population) and the infant's blood type is group A or B. Prenatal detection of ABO incompatibility is not feasible and generally not necessary. Instead of sensitization during pregnancy, preformed maternal anti-A or anti-B proteins of the IgG class are transferred passively to the infant late in the pregnancy or at parturition. Rapid early hemolysis of fetal cells occurs, with splenic recognition and removal of antigen–antibody complexes. Because fetal red blood cells have only about 7,500 to 8,000 A or B antigen sites per cell (versus 15,000 to 20,000 in the adult), the fetal cells do not agglutinate and may not be destroyed completely. Splenic removal of the antibody may damage the cell membrane, which then repairs itself and re-enters the circulation as a microspherocyte. Likewise, the low number of antigen–antibody sites on fetal cells may give a weakly positive or even a negative direct Coombs' reaction. The antibody may be identified correctly by incubation of the neonatal serum with incompatible adult red cells and performance of an *indirect* Coombs' test. Because not all ABO-incompatible pregnancies result in neonatal hemolysis, clinical and laboratory confirmation of a neonatal hemolytic disorder is necessary to confirm the diagnosis.

ABO incompatibility seldom presents with severe jaundice or severe anemia at birth, but the rate of increase in bilirubin on the first postnatal day may lead to preparations for an exchange transfusion in some cases. If the initial rate of increase exceeds 1/mg/dL/hour, if the newborn is significantly anemic (hemoglobin 10 g/dL or less), or if serum bilirubin reaches 15 to 20 mg/dL within the first 24 hours, a double-volume exchange transfusion is indicated after the indirect bilirubin level has exceeded 18 to 20 mg/dL and before it exceeds 25 mg/dL.

Exchange Transfusion

As a general approach, exchange transfusion should be considered for any newborn with a serum bilirubin level in the range of 20 to 25 mg/dL from any cause. Sustained hyperbilirubinemia in this range is potentially hazardous, as evidenced by changes in brainstem conduction time, changes in feeding and responsiveness as noted anecdotally by many observers, and occasional cases of overt kernicterus at these bilirubin levels. It also may be significant that, after prolonged exposure to unconjugated bilirubin at 25 mg/dL, extravascular bilirubin may constitute 30% to 50% of the body's total bilirubin stores. After an initial double-volume exchange transfusion at 25 mg/dL, a short-term decline in serum bilirubin to 12 to 13 mg/dL is followed rapidly by a rebound to the range of 16 to 17 mg/dL. If the source of the hyperbilirubinemia remains untreated or if failure of bilirubin excretion persists at these levels, within a few hours the serum bilirubin may rise again to its pre-exchange level, making a second exchange transfusion necessary. If an infant with hemolysis is treated with earlier exchange transfusions to maintain the post-exchange bilirubin between 10 to 20 mg/dL, the risk of needing a second exchange transfusion is diminished somewhat, and the duration of exposure to extreme levels of hyperbilirubinemia is shortened.

Phototherapy

Just as bilirubin is probably the most common laboratory determination performed in the newborn nursery, phototherapy probably is the most common treatment performed. The systematic use of fluorescent light to lower bilirubin levels followed the observations of Cremer, Perryman, and Richards, in 1958, that jaundice was less frequent in a well-lighted nursery in a new wing of their hospital than in a dimly lighted nursery in an older wing. The mechanism of phototherapy was initially thought to involve the degradation of bilirubin to smaller molecules and excretion of the degradation products. More detailed biochemical studies showed that light in the spectral range of 400 to 500 nm (blue-green) induces configurational and structural isomers of unconjugated bilirubin. The bilirubin isomers are more water-soluble than their parent compound, bilirubin IX-alpha, and are therefore transported through the liver more rapidly than the predominant form of unconjugated bilirubin. Blue-green light on the skin at 5 to 20 $\mu W/cm^2/nm$ rapidly converts unconjugated bilirubin (UCB) to its more soluble isomers in a dose-dependent fashion. Doses below 3 to 4 $\mu W/cm^2/nm$ produce inefficient photo conversion, whereas "intensive" light doses of 20 to 30 $\mu W/cm^2/nm$ or more, achievable with narrow-spectrum or LED light sources designed for phototherapy, can convert a higher percentage of bilirubin in the skin to its isomers and lower serum bilirubin more rapidly than "conventional" fluorescent light sources. Photoconversion to isomers is rapid and quantitatively related to light intensity and the area of skin exposed. Initial photoconversion is followed by slower distribution of the isomers from the skin into the circulation and their subsequent excretion by the liver.

Studies of bilirubin photoconversion and excretion indicate that the excretion of photoisomers via the biliary tract into the duodenum may be rate-limiting for the dose response to phototherapy in newborns. In addition, once isomerized bilirubin reaches the bowel, it may reconvert to the normal form of UCB, because it is no longer exposed to light. Unless photobilirubin entering the small bowel is converted rapidly to other water-soluble products or quickly excreted, some entero-hepatic recirculation of photobilirubin via reconversion to bilirubin IX-alpha may occur. Therefore, even with a rapid conversion of bilirubin to its photo products, a rapid decline in serum bilirubin may not always follow. Rather, the bilirubin concentration in the plasma may stabilize in equilibrium with its photo products, the rate of hepatic excretion, and its rate of recirculation from the bowel to the blood if, in the small bowel, it merely enters a "third space" without being excreted. Perhaps, then, an apparent delay in the bilirubin response to phototherapy is not surprising, given the balance to be achieved between rates of bilirubin production, turnover by photoconversion, excretion, and reabsorption in a complex system.

A potential advantage of phototherapy, even without a marked decline in the serum bilirubin level, is the conversion of 10% to 30% of the circulating bilirubin to water-soluble isomers that should be less likely to cross the blood–brain barrier than the more lipophilic parent compound. Photoconversion of part of the circulating bilirubin, with the liberal use of early phototherapy in high-risk newborns, may be part of the reason for a decline in low bilirubin kernicterus among such newborns, even though early phototherapy produces little or no change in eventual total serum bilirubin levels. Because the mechanism of phototherapy seems unrelated to the underlying cause of jaundice, and because photoconversion of bilirubin in the circulation may be somewhat neuroprotective, no strict contraindication exists to using phototherapy to control hyperbilirubinemia of hemolytic origin, provided the initial problems of hemolysis and rapid onset of hyperbilirubinemia have been treated adequately. Regardless of whether a newborn receives phototherapy, the criteria for an exchange transfusion should remain the same in these circumstances until a neuroprotective effect of bilirubin isomerization is proven clearly.

Phototherapy as an anticipatory or preventive treatment can be started at about 5 mg/dL lower than the level of bilirubin indicated for an exchange transfusion; for example, at about 15 to 18 mg/dL for jaundice with a hemolytic component and an "exchange level" of 20 to 22 mg/dL, or about 18 to 20 mg/dL for nonhemolytic jaundice with an "exchange level" of 22 to 25 mg/dL. "Intensive" treatment may sometimes be effective in babies who have already reached an exchange transfusion threshold. For best results, the areas of skin exposed and the therapeutic levels of light employed should be maximized and continued unchanged throughout the course of treatment. The practice of reducing light intensity as the bilirubin falls is not evidence-based and may prolong treatment. A post-treatment "rebound" of 1 to 2 mg/dL is expected from the re-equilibration of bilirubin photo products with their parent compound, and is inconsequential if successful phototherapy lowered the plasma bilirubin by 30% to 50%. A follow-up bilirubin level check within 1 to 2 days may be requested to verify the treatment effect.

Extrapolation of treatment criteria for term infants to lower threshold levels for preterm infants is not evidence-based. Because preterm infants have lower albumin levels, a presumably less mature blood–brain barrier, and greater clinical instability than term infants, starting phototherapy at lower bilirubin levels appears prudent and safe. However, the weight-based algorithms for phototherapy used in many nurseries have not been validated. "Prophylactic" phototherapy in bruised, extremely low-birth-weight (ELBW) infants will not treat jaundice effectively until enough bilirubin is present in the skin for adequate photoconversion of bilirubin. Until the results of suitably conducted clinical trials are available, a prudent recommendation would be to maintain serum bilirubin at less than 10 mg/dL in ELBW infants (<1,000 g) and at less than 15 mg/dL in VLBW infants of 1,000 to 1,500 g.

Other Therapeutic Considerations

Feeding promotes peristalsis and colonization of the bowel. Peristalsis increases bile flow and the rate of bilirubin excretion as the stools change from meconium to transitional to the bilirubin-rich, yellowish-brown stools that appear at several days of life. Simultaneously, bowel colonization with normal flora promotes the enzymatic conversion of bilirubin to products that are not reabsorbed or reconverted to UCB. Unfed or underfed newborns tend to have persistent jaundice. An underfed nursing infant may show improvement of jaundice with increased frequency of nursing and an increase in milk intake within the first few days. The enterohepatic circulation of bilirubin can be reduced by feeding agar or charcoal to the newborn, but these approaches have not gained popularity. Phenobarbital in low doses stimulates the hepatic excretory system for bilirubin and increases activity of the conjugating enzyme. Infants with a family history of severe hyperbilirubinemia suggesting a conjugation defect or those with contraindications to exchange transfusion (e.g., for religious reasons) may benefit from maternal or early neonatal administration of phenobarbital in low doses, generally much lower than would be required for seizure therapy. This approach can be used selectively for enzyme induction in patients with certain genetic defects in bilirubin conjugation, for example, Gilbert disease.

A potential treatment for hemolytic hyperbilirubinemia, perhaps also useful for the longer-term management of patients with Type I Crigler-Najjar syndrome, would be the inhibition of heme oxygenase to decrease the rate of bilirubin formation from its heme precursor. Synthetic heme analogues, such as tin protoporphyrin and tin mesoporphyrin, are competitive inhibitors of heme oxygenase, the rate-limiting enzyme in the degradation of hemoglobin to bilirubin. Animal models and preliminary clinical studies have shown that the administration of metalloporphyrin heme analogues results in decreased bilirubin formation and excretion of heme pigments into bile and urine. In addition, metalloporphyrin given to neonatal animals or human newborns shortly after birth can prevent or ameliorate hyperbilirubinemia. With further drug development and documentation of safety and efficacy, heme oxygenase inhibitors may offer specific therapy for unconjugated hyperbilirubinemia, especially of hemolytic origin.

Breast-milk Jaundice

Most breast-fed infants have normal postnatal serum bilirubin levels that do not require specific diagnosis or treatment. Early hyperbilirubinemia in breast-fed newborns may be associated with suboptimal milk intake, excessive weight loss, infrequent stools, and inadequate excretion of bilirubin. No fixed interval between birth and the first breast feeding is necessary if the mother and baby are in good condition after delivery. During the first several days postpartum, nursing on demand at intervals more frequent than every 4 hours may help to stimulate lactation, avoid excessive weight loss, and aid the transition from meconium to normal stools. Routine supplementation of breast feeding with bottled water is counterproductive, diminishing the thirst response between nursing periods while providing inadequate substrate for hepatic function and inadequate bulk for peristalsis. Supplementation should be reserved

for those infants in whom milk intake and hydration are clearly inadequate and weight loss is excessive.

Preterm infants of 35 to 37 weeks gestation and weighing 2,500 to 3,000 g may appear healthy at birth, but may not nurse as well as full-term infants and still may have immature liver function. This includes some infants delivered by cesarean section before term, with the smooth initiation of nursing complicated further by the mother's postoperative condition. Hepatic immaturity and inadequate intake may increase the likelihood of hyperbilirubinemia. Supplementation of feeding may be needed for adequate hydration and nutrition until lactation is well established. Phototherapy for hyperbilirubinemia in the range of 15 to 20 mg/dL may be used during the first several days, until hepatic function matures and adequate excretion of bilirubin begins.

The discontinuation of breast feeding in a well baby with persistent hyperbilirubinemia requires the careful use of clinical judgment and ongoing family support. Many cases of breast-milk jaundice are mild and require no intervention except for bilirubin determinations once or twice in the first several weeks after discharge, to follow the resolution of the problem. More severe cases, which often appear toward the end of the first week and then fail to resolve or progress toward even higher bilirubin levels, may benefit from discontinuing breast feeding for 36 to 48 hours. In the first few postnatal days, however, discontinuation of nursing may not lower the bilirubin level or establish the probability of a breast-milk inhibitor of hepatic function. The hormonal or enzymatic factors associated with persistent breast-feeding jaundice may not become operative until nursing is well established.

Hyperbilirubinemia caused by breast-milk factors usually responds to the temporary cessation of nursing, with a short-term decline of serum bilirubin by 2 to 4 mg/dL, after which nursing can usually be resumed with little or no further increase in bilirubin. Only rarely is hyperbilirubinemia severe and persistent enough to require complete discontinuation of breast feeding. Phototherapy is indicated for a minority of breast-fed infants with hyperbilirubinemia that persists above 15 to 20 mg/dL and is unresponsive to temporary discontinuation of breast feeding.

Some authorities suggest that full-term breast-fed infants without other risk factors require no treatment until the serum bilirubin level reaches or exceeds 20 mg/dL, and that exchange transfusion is not indicated in these otherwise "low-risk" infants until serum bilirubin reaches or exceeds 25 mg/dL. Medical supervision and even daily follow-up of infants with borderline but still increasing bilirubin levels is important. Predischarge identification of infants at risk for high levels of hyperbilirubinemia, either by family history or by a nursery screening procedure for early jaundice, can help to identify newborns who may need early and close follow-up for hyperbilirubinemia. Undetected, unsupervised hyperbilirubinemia in breast-fed infants thought to be at little or no risk occasionally may progress to levels of 25 to 30 mg/dL or greater. Besides the uncertain risk of neurologic damage from prolonged, extremely high bilirubin levels, some infants with extreme hyperbilirubinemia are later found to have risk factors, not recognized at birth, that increase the risk of developing bilirubin encephalopathy.

Direct (Conjugated) Hyperbilirubinemia

Direct hyperbilirubinemia resulting from intrinsic liver disease or hepatobiliary obstruction may first appear in the newborn. Early in the course, these conditions may present with predominantly indirect or unconjugated hyperbilirubinemia, but in most cases the direct or conjugated fraction of bilirubin quickly rises to levels in excess of 2 mg/dL and remains elevated.

Conjugated bilirubin appears not to be toxic to the central nervous system, but the persistence of conjugated hyperbilirubinemia requires diagnostic evaluation to determine the nature of the hepatic abnormality.

In high-risk or low-birth-weight infants requiring prolonged intravenous fluid and nutritional support, cholestasis related to parenteral nutrition is the most common cause of persistent direct hyperbilirubinemia. In most cases related to prolonged parenteral nutrition, direct bilirubin remains elevated for several weeks after the initiation of gastric feedings, and then gradually declines to normal values. A minority of total parenteral nutrition (TPN)-dependent infants develop progressive hepatocellular injury and signs of hepatic failure, especially if their need for prolonged TPN is associated with a medical or surgical short-bowel syndrome.

Medical therapies to ameliorate the hepatic injury from prolonged intravenous nutrition (e.g., cycling of TPN, cholecystokinin, ursodeoxycholate) are currently undergoing clinical trials, especially for surgical short-bowel syndrome.

Other causes of persistent conjugated (direct) hyperbilirubinemia include bacterial or viral infection, nonspecific neonatal hepatitis, and persistent direct hyperbilirubinemia with inspissation of bile after an episode of severe hemolysis (sometimes seen in Rh disease), or congenital intrahepatic or extrahepatic biliary obstruction. Mixed or obstructive hyperbilirubinemia generally represents diseases that that persist well beyond the neonatal period, with different implications for health and development than unconjugated hyperbilirubinemia. Infants with cholestatic or obstructive jaundice presenting in but persisting beyond the newborn period should be referred for diagnosis and treatment to a pediatric center where the staff have specific expertise in pediatric gastroenterology or liver disease.

Should the conjugated bilirubin be subtracted from total bilirubin for the evaluation of unconjugated hyperbilirubinemia? This author agrees with others that unconjugated bilirubin is more likely to be toxic to the central nervous system than conjugated bilirubin, and conjugated bilirubin may not be toxic to the brain at all. Infants presenting with cholestatic or obstructive jaundice are more likely to benefit from evaluation and management of their underlying liver disease than from phototherapy and exchange transfusion. However, recent expert consensus supports the use of total rather than indirect bilirubin concentrations for evaluation and management when neonatal unconjugated hyperbilirubinemia presents in the usual way and the direct fraction is low in proportion to the total bilirubin.

CONCLUSIONS

In summary, most cases of neonatal hyperbilirubinemia are developmental, benign, and self-limited. Significant and potentially dangerous hyperbilirubinemia may occur in a minority of otherwise normal bottle-fed infants, in a larger number of breast-fed infants, and in many infants with hemolytic disorders. Nursery-based screening procedures are recommended for the prospective identification of infants who may be at increased risk of severe hyperbilirubinemia after discharge. "Typical" cases of physiologic jaundice may be managed with serial bilirubin determinations, close observation, and reassurance. For more severe or complicated cases, after initial neonatal stabilization and specific diagnosis, exchange transfusion is the treatment of choice for indirect hyperbilirubinemia in excess of 20 mg/dL or bilirubin levels rising rapidly in association with hemolysis. Phototherapy can be used to stabilize indirect hyperbilirubinemia from any cause, and potentially may offer the brain additional protection by isomerization of UCB. Early follow-up is recommended for newborns with jaundice before

TABLE 26.3

ANTICIPATORY MANAGEMENT OF NEONATAL JAUNDICE

1. Know maternal blood type
2. Know baby's blood type if mother is Rh-negative; if mother is
   Group O, determine baby's blood type if:
   a. The baby has early jaundice or
   b. A previous baby had ABO hemolytic disease
3. Screen all newborns to identify early jaundice
4. Identify risk factors present by hour-specific bilirubin level and/or
   Coombs' test, G-6PD screen, Hgb, Hcrit, RBC indices and morphology
5. Observe, repeat, and discharge if jaundice is nonprogressive and no risk factor is present; arrange early postdischarge follow-up (24 to 72 hours)
   or
6. Start therapy as described below, if indicated by
   a. Approaching threshold
   b. Risk factors present
7. Start phototherapy when bilirubin is below expected exchange transfusion level
8. Exchange Transfusion
   a. Early, if conditions are met
   b. Later, if phototherapy fails to control serum BR

discharge from the nursery; longer follow-up is needed for a minority of infants who have prolonged jaundice associated with breast-feeding. Table 26.3 outlines a suggested approach to the anticipatory management of neonatal jaundice.

Suggested Readings

Ahdab-Barmada M, Moosy J. The neuropathology of kernicterus in the premature neonate: diagnostic problems. *J Neuropathol Exp Neurol* 1984; 43:45.

American Academy of Pediatrics, Subcommittee on Hyperbilirubinemia. Clinical practice guideline: management of hyperbilirubinemia in the newborn infant 35 or more weeks of gestation. *Pediatrics* 2004;297.

Arias IM, Gartner LM, Seifter S, Furman M. Prolonged neonatal unconjugated hyperbilirubinemia associated with breast feeding and a steroid, pregnane-3(alpha), 20(beta)-diol, in maternal milk that inhibits glucuronide formation in vitro. *J Clin Invest* 1964;43:2037.

Bowman JW. Immune hemolytic disease. In: Nathan DG, Orkin SH, eds. *Nathan and Oski's hematology of infancy and childhood*, 5th Ed. Philadelphia: W.B. Saunders Co, 1998:53.

Cashore WJ. Bilirubin metabolism and toxicity in the newborn. In: Polin RA, Fox WW, Abram SH, eds. *Fetal and neonatal physiology*, 3rd ed. Philadelphia: W.B. Saunders Co., 2004:1199.

Cremer RJ, Perryman PW, Richards DH. Influence of light on the hyperbilirubinemia of infants. *Lancet*. 1958;1:1094.

Gourley GR. Pathophysiology of breast-milk jaundice. In: Polin RA, Fox WW, eds. *Fetal and neonatal physiology*, 2nd ed. Philadelphia: W.B. Saunders Co, 1998:1499.

Johnson LH, Bhutani VK, Brown AK. System-based approach to management of neonatal jaundice and prevention of kernicterus. *J Pediatr* 2002;140:396.

Maisels MJ, Gifford K. Normal serum bilirubin levels in the newborn and the effect of breast-feeding. *Pediatrics* 1986;78:837.

Maisels MJ. Jaundice. In: Avery GB, Fletcher MA, MacDonald MG, eds. *Neonatology: pathophysiology and management of the newborn*, 5th ed. Philadelphia: Lippincott Williams & Wilkins, 1999:765.

Maisels MJ, Ostrea EM Jr., Touch S, et al. Evaluation of a new transcutaneous bilirubinometer. *Pediatrics* 2004;113:1628.

McDonagh AF, Lightner DA. 'Like a shriveled blood orange'—bilirubin, jaundice, and phototherapy. *Pediatrics* 1985;75:443.

Nakamura H, Takada S, Shimabuku R, et al. Auditory nerve and brainstem responses in newborn infants with hyperbilirubinemia. *Pediatrics* 1985;75: 703.

Ritter DA, Kenny JD, Norton HJ, Rudolph AJ. A prospective study of free bilirubin and other risk factors in the development of kernicterus in premature infants. *Pediatrics* 1982;69:260.

CHAPTER 27 ■ INTRAUTERINE GROWTH RESTRICTION

JOSEPH B. WARSHAW

Intrauterine growth restriction (IUGR), formerly referred to as intrauterine growth retardation, represents a final common pathway by which genetic and environmental influences result in low birth weight for gestational age. IUGR has been defined most commonly in the United States as a birth weight of less than the tenth percentile for gestational age. This definition probably overestimates the incidence of IUGR, because it is unreasonable to consider that 10% of all births have a pathologic restriction of growth. Small infants with no evidence of adverse genetic or environmental influences should be spared the IUGR label, which connotes pathology, and should be defined as small for gestational age (SGA). The term *SGA* should be applied to all infants less than the tenth percentile, and *IUGR* generally should be reserved for infants less than the third percentile, recognizing that some infants with growth restriction will fall out of this range if an insult occurs late in gestation. Thus, although all infants with IUGR also are SGA, not all SGA infants have IUGR.

Confusion about definitions is increased further by significant differences in the tenth percentile birth weights at each gestational age that have been published. Differences in published standards of growth have been influenced by racial composition, socioeconomic status of the population, and altitude above sea level when the standards were developed. What is necessary for an effective comparison between populations is the adoption of a single standard for fetal growth (e.g., the standards developed by Brenner from 30,772 deliveries from 21 to 44 weeks' gestational age in Cleveland). The Brenner standards include correction factors for poverty, race, and gender.

ETIOLOGY OF IUGR

Recognition and treatment of IUGR require an understanding of the diverse etiologies that result in restricted fetal growth. The growth pattern of the infant with IUGR often reflects the underlying condition that has resulted in growth restriction. The terms *proportionate* and *disproportionate* have been used to distinguish newborns with decreased growth potential from those with restricted growth because of fetal malnutrition. There may be intergenerational risks for IUGR. Mothers who were SGA at birth have twice the risk of having an infant with IUGR.

Newborns with decreased growth potential caused by conditions such as chromosomal disorders, congenital infections, or exposure to environmental toxins characteristically have body proportions that are proportionate or symmetric (i.e., the head, length, and weight generally occur within similar percentile grids), or the head is small relative to the body, as in microcephaly. Obstetric monitoring of the fetus with decreased growth potential characteristically demonstrates decreased body growth, including that of the head, from midgestation or earlier. Fetuses with decreased growth potential are at high risk for major malformations or congenital infection.

Newborns with fetal malnutrition have reduced weight out of proportion to length or head circumference and may exhibit a sparing of head growth during late gestation. These infants are disproportionate, with the head circumference and length closer to the expected percentiles for gestational age than those for weight. Nutritional constraints on growth are unusual before 24 to 25 weeks' gestation except in a multiple pregnancy. In most cases, only after that time will restriction in blood supply to the fetus result in IUGR. In mild to moderate degrees of IUGR, head growth may proceed along normal percentile grids, with a decrease in body fat and restriction in length and weight (disproportionate growth). This sparing of head growth is thought to result from circulatory changes in the fetus that favor a redistribution of blood flow to the heart and brain. Doppler blood flow measurements of the fetus have shown increased carotid and decreased visceral blood flow in fetuses with IUGR as compared to those with normal growth. These changes may be mediated by release of vasopressin from the fetal hypothalamus or by prostaglandins. Exceptions to this general pattern may be seen. In instances of extreme nutritional restriction in the fetus with class D diabetes or other conditions that result in severely compromised uterine blood flow, even head growth may be decreased.

Infants with either proportionate or disproportionate IUGR should be evaluated carefully for conditions causing hydrocephalus or microcephaly that also may confound the measurements. Figure 27.1 summarizes the etiology of IUGR. The importance of environmental exposures such as cigarette smoking cannot be overestimated. In the developed countries of the world, cigarette smoking remains an important determinant of low birth weight. Cigarette smoking among women in the developing world is increasing, and remains a concern about teenagers in the United States.

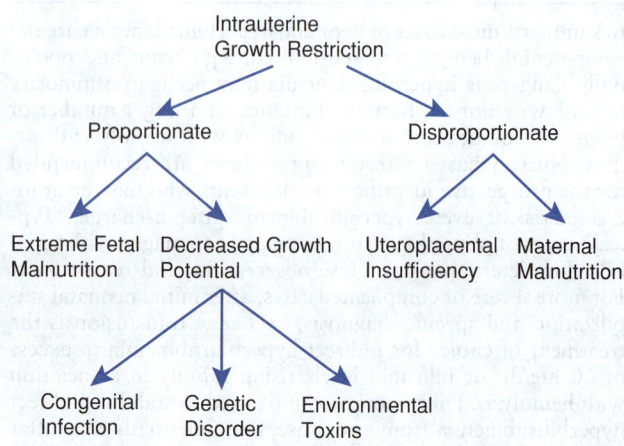

FIGURE 27.1. Classification of intrauterine growth restriction.

The pattern of postnatal growth is also important to record and follow. As a consequence of decreased growth potential, infants with proportionate growth restriction may exhibit sluggish postnatal growth even with adequate nutrition. A slow rate of postnatal growth may be seen in genetic disorders, congenital infections, or fetal alcohol syndrome. Infants with growth restriction secondary to fetal malnutrition often exhibit rapid growth when adequate nutrients are provided in the postnatal period, which is a good prognostic finding. Approximately 30% of nutritionally induced newborns with IUGR are still below the third percentile at 2 years of age.

MANAGEMENT

Optimal management of IUGR should begin with recognition of the problem *in utero* so that informed decisions can be made concerning the appropriate time and method of delivery. This includes consideration of the options of cesarean section versus vaginal delivery. If biophysical data obtained during fetal monitoring show fetal distress, cesarean section may be the preferred mode of delivery. Decreased maternal weight gain or very low prepregnancy weight should alert the obstetrician to the likelihood of fetal growth restriction. Measurement of fundal growth and ultrasonography can confirm the diagnosis by monitoring such parameters of fetal growth as the biparietal diameter, the relationship of head size to body size, femur length, and fetal abdominal circumference.

Strategies to treat fetal growth restriction have included therapies to decrease platelet aggregation and abnormalities in uteroplacental circulation seen in toxemia of pregnancy as well as maternal nutritional supplementation and oxygen therapy. These potential therapies require further investigation.

Maternal parenteral nutritional supplementation is controversial. An adverse influence was observed when short-term administration of glucose to normal patients before delivery resulted in a significant increase in lactic acid and a decrease in pH. When the fetus is adapted to a decreased nutrient supply, a potential risk may be associated with increasing nutritional intake without a corresponding increase in fetal oxygenation. Indeed, several of the changes seen in IUGR can be considered adaptations to an adverse intrauterine nutritional environment: sparing of brain growth, increased red cell mass, and small size itself, in which the size of the fetus may be appropriate to the availability of nutrients. Even early lung maturation can be considered an adaptation that improves the opportunity for a good postnatal outcome. There is also some evidence that the calorically restricted fetus can regulate its own growth. In animal studies, nutritionally deprived fetuses have decreased levels of insulin-like growth factors (IGF) and an increased level of IGF binding protein. This effectively modulates fetal growth by decreasing the growth-promoting effect of the IGF. A smaller fetus with IUGR would have decreased caloric requirements, which can be advantageous for the fetus. Similar data have been observed in stressed newborns.

Important problems of the infant with IUGR secondary to intrauterine malnutrition are summarized in Box 27.1. Appropriate management can prevent many of these problems (Box 27.2). If birth asphyxia occurs, support measures should be instituted immediately, including the establishment of an effective airway and the management of meconium if present. Suctioning and clearing the meconium from the airway before delivery of the thorax and the infant taking the first breath, together with tracheal suction if meconium is present at the level of the cords, have greatly reduced problems associated with meconium aspiration. Meconium aspiration is rarely seen in infants of less than 35 weeks' gestation; therefore, hypoxia per se is the major problem in those infants. An estimate of the degree of acidosis can be obtained from the cord blood pH.

BOX 27.1   **Problems of the Newborn with Intrauterine Growth Restriction**

Birth asphyxia
Meconium aspiration
Persistent fetal circulation
Hypothermia
Hypoglycemia
Hypocalcemia
Polycythemia
Congenital malformation

Hyaline membrane disease is generally less of a problem in infants with disproportionate IUGR because of the accelerated lung maturation commonly seen in these infants. Some asphyxiated newborns exhibit significant right-to-left cardiac shunting, making systemic oxygenation difficult to achieve. This is a consequence of chronic intrauterine hypoxia, which results in abnormal thickening of the smooth muscle of small pulmonary arterioles, thereby reducing pulmonary blood flow and increasing right-to-left blood flow at the atrial level or through the ductus arteriosus. Diagnosis is suggested by pulse oximetry and in most cases can be confirmed by Doppler flow measurements of right-to-left shunting. Diagnosis can also be confirmed by measuring the disparity between preductal (right radial) and postductal (umbilical arterial) Po_2. Because acidosis and hypoxia modulate pulmonary arteriolar vasomotor tone, therapeutic efforts should be directed toward reversing these conditions. Some infants appear to improve with an induced respiratory alkalosis (pH 7.45 to 7.55). Treatment of persistent pulmonary hypertension has been revolutionized by nitric oxide therapy, which is effective in reversing pulmonary hypertension in most cases. Extracorporeal membrane oxygenation had a surge in popularity in the treatment of this condition, but the efficacy of this expensive and complex intervention has not been clearly established and has, in most cases, been superceded by nitric oxide therapy.

Apgar scores should be assigned in the delivery room, and the infant should be dried rapidly and warmed to prevent hypothermia. As soon as the infant is stable, anthropometric measurements should be taken and plotted on standard growth grids. Accurate measurements determine whether a newborn with IUGR follows the disproportionate or proportionate pattern of growth. Measurements include the standard growth parameters of weight, height, and head circumference. The ponderal index ([weight in grams × 100]/[length in cubic

---

BOX 27.2   **Management of the Infant with Intrauterine Growth Restriction**

Assess gestational age and take careful history for drugs and other information
Prevent hypothermia
Check central hematocrit
Monitor blood sugar within first 45 minutes
Evaluate for congenital infections and congenital malformations
Evaluate chromosomal and genetic factors as indicated
Follow up carefully

centimeters]) also has been used to identify infants with decreased weight relative to length; however, applications of standard measurements of length, weight, and head circumference to standard growth grids are generally more useful.

A careful assessment of gestational age should be done in all infants with IUGR. The examination most commonly used is a modification of a scale developed by Dubowitz that includes physical signs involving skin color and texture, hair, breast size, plantar creases, ear form and firmness, external genitalia, and neuromuscular assessment, which measures tone, posture, and reflexes. Scores are assigned for these measures, with a total score being used to assign gestational age. This examination can be completed in approximately 10 minutes and has a predictive error of plus or minus 2 weeks in infants weighing more than 1,000 g. The examination is most accurate when performed within the first 6 hours of life and by two observers.

Newborns with IUGR secondary to fetal malnutrition (e.g., those with decreased uteroplacental blood flow) are disproportionate, with the head and length generally in higher percentiles than the weight. These infants frequently appear scrawny as a result of their marked decrease in subcutaneous fat. They have an alert appearance and have higher Dubowitz ratings than do premature infants with similar weights.

Infants should be examined for genetic causes of IUGR, including the presence of congenital malformations. They also should be evaluated for any signs of congenital infection. The examination should include weighing and examining the placenta to determine whether structural or vascular abnormalities are contributing to IUGR. A small placenta is common in pregnancies complicated by fetal nutritional failure or hypoxemia.

Many of the problems of newborns with IUGR relate to their markedly decreased metabolic reserves. A risk of perinatal asphyxia exists when oxygen and metabolic demands exceed the oxygen provided by the uteroplacental circulation. This underscores the need for careful biophysical monitoring of the at-risk fetus to alert the obstetrician to the presence of uteroplacental insufficiency. Hypoglycemia is found frequently in the immediate postnatal period of the nutritionally deprived fetus. Hypothermia may increase oxygen and glucose requirements. Blood glucose should be measured, and a central hematocrit should be measured to detect polycythemia. Hyperviscosity and hypoglycemia are primarily problems of the nutritionally growth-restricted newborn. Those with IUGR secondary to congenital infection, genetic disorders, or environmental insults are less likely to experience these complications.

Hypoglycemia is best treated by early recognition and prevention. All infants with IUGR should have blood sugar screened within the first 30 to 45 minutes of life. These infants are at risk for hypoglycemia because of decreased fuel stores secondary to their fetal malnourished state, decreased gluconeogenesis, and an increase in the peripheral use of glucose because of polycythemia and cold stress. The best treatment for hypoglycemia is prevention by early feeding. Treatment of hypoglycemia is discussed in Chapter 63, Infant of the Diabetic Mother.

Hypocalcemia also may occur in the newborn with IUGR, generally in association with neonatal stress. Only rarely do infants require a regimen of parenteral calcium, which should be given with constant monitoring and with good venous access to avoid skin sloughing.

Hyperviscosity secondary to polycythemia in infants with IUGR can result in venous thrombosis and central nervous system injury and also can contribute to hypoglycemia. Polycythemia results from increased erythropoietin levels secondary to fetal hypoxemia. Because blood viscosity sharply increases when the central hematocrit exceeds 65%, partial exchange transfusion should be considered in infants with IUGR when the hematocrit exceeds that level.

Some controversy exists concerning whether partial exchange transfusion should be done in polycythemic infants who are asymptomatic. Infants treated with partial exchange transfusion may have fewer neurologic problems than those not transfused. The symptoms of hyperviscosity include respiratory distress, plethora, cardiac failure, and neurologic signs, including jitters and seizures. Partial exchange transfusion is done using normal saline or 5% salt-poor albumin to replace blood that is removed, which is preferable to plasma because of the high viscosity of adult fibrinogen in plasma. The formula used to calculate the amount of blood to be withdrawn (V) in a partial exchange transfusion is as follows:

$$V = \text{estimated blood volume} \times [(\text{actual hematocrit} - \text{the desired hematocrit})/(\text{the actual hematocrit})]$$

PROGNOSIS

Newborn Outcomes

The most important aspect of IUGR is neurodevelopmental outcome, and this depends in large part on the cause. Infants with IUGR secondary to environmental insult or decreased growth potential generally have outcomes that are poor and reflect the underlying neuropathology of conditions caused by the environmental or genetic insult.

Generally, infants with growth restriction that spares head growth relative to weight and length have more favorable outcomes. Even those infants in whom there has been a decrease in intrauterine brain growth may show substantial postnatal catch-up. The vast majority of full-term infants with IUGR are of normal intelligence. Outcome is more difficult to predict in preterm infants with IUGR, who appear to have a higher incidence of handicap, including cerebral palsy, than that of the general population. More extensive follow-up with these infants is required when they reach school age. The performance levels they achieve may be influenced by social class, with children from higher social classes scoring better on standard IQ tests and school achievement evaluations. In an important study of IUGR outcome in a lower socioeconomic class population, it was shown that infants with IUGR had a twofold greater risk for developmental delay as compared with the controls. Of real concern was the high rate of developmental delay in controls in this population, highlighting the importance of poverty in developmental outcome. Nevertheless, the outlook for most infants with nutritional IUGR is favorable if the postnatal environment is adequate. Most infants with IUGR, whether premature or full-term, achieve normal intelligence by 5 to 6 years of age, although there may be a risk for subtle deficits such as school problems and learning disabilities. Modern neonatal care has prevented death and much of the morbidity historically associated with IUGR.

Infants with IUGR with major genetic or chromosomal disorders (e.g., trisomy 18 or 13) have virtually a 100% incidence of severe handicap and death, whereas outcome in those with congenital infection appears to be more variable. More than 75% of infants with congenital rubella infection have a mental handicap requiring special education. They also may have learning deficits and disturbances associated with hearing loss or blindness. Infants with cytomegalovirus infection may have only minor or no sequelae, whereas those who present with microcephaly or significant growth restriction generally have poor outcomes, with handicap rates generally exceeding 50%. Testing for hearing loss is important in all infants diagnosed with congenital infection.

When evaluating outcome of newborns exposed to pharmacologic agents, it may be difficult to dissociate the effect of the primary disease state from that of the medication. Clearly, however, many drugs are associated with poor outcomes. Fetal alcohol syndrome, for example, is associated with slow postnatal growth and poor developmental outcome. Prenatal cocaine exposure has been associated with IUGR and microcephaly. Exposure to therapeutic agents such as phenytoin, warfarin sodium, and narcotics may result in IUGR, slow postnatal growth, and a spectrum of developmental disabilities. Infants with these conditions require thorough evaluation, including appropriate counseling with the family.

Non-neurologic Long-term Consequences

Much recent attention has been given to the Fetal Origins Hypothesis, that is, the increased risk of diabetes and heart disease in adults who were low-birth-weight newborns. This higher incidence of hypertension, glucose intolerance, and hyperlipidemia in the fifth and sixth decades has been termed *syndrome X*. The reported impact on adult health may be significant. The incidence of glucose intolerance among individuals weighing less than 2,500 g at birth was 40% at age 50. For another example, individuals who were exposed *in utero* to the Dutch famine at the end of World War II have demonstrated decreased glucose tolerance at age 50 as compared with those conceived in the year after the famine. Fetal growth restriction may imprint an endocrine dysfunction, perhaps by altering hypothalamic function and metabolic regulation. For example, there is some evidence that adults born with

low birth weight have an exaggerated response to adrenocorticotropic hormone. The mechanisms responsible for the impact of IUGR on health status in later life, however, require further investigation.

Suggested Readings

Allen MC. Developmental outcome and follow-up of the small-for-gestational-age infant. *Semin Perinatol* 1984;8:123.

Barker DJP. The malnourished baby and infant. *Brit Med Bull* 2001;60:69.

Black VD, Lubchenco LO, Koops BL, et al. Neonatal hyperviscosity: randomized study of effect of partial plasma exchange transfusion on long-term outcome. *Pediatrics* 1985;75:1048.

Brenner WE, Edelman DA, Hendricks CH. A standard for fetal growth for the United States of America. *Am J Obstet Gynecol* 1976;126:555.

Diamond FB. Fetal growth programs future health: causes and consequences of intrauterine growth retardation. *Adv Pediatr* 2001;48:245.

Dubowitz LM, Dubowitz V, Goldberg C. Clinical assessment of gestational age in the newborn infant. *J Pediatr* 1970;77:1.

Ehrenkranz RA. The Neonatal Inhaled Nitric Oxide Study Group. *N Engl J Med* 1997;336:599.

Kramer, MS. The epidemiology of adverse pregnancy outcomes: an overview. *J Nutr* 2003;133:1592S.

Lubchenco LO, Hansman C, Dressler M, et al. Intrauterine growth as estimated from liveborn birth-weight data at 24 to 42 weeks of gestation. *Pediatrics* 1963;32:793.

Ravelli ACJ, Vander Muelen IHP, Michels RPJ, et al. Glucose tolerance in adults after prenatal exposure to famine. *Lancet* 1998;351:173.

Resnik, R. Intrauterine growth restriction. *Obstet Gynecol* 2002;99:490.

Stein ZA, Susser M. Intrauterine growth retardation: epidemiological issues and public health significance. *Semin Perinatol* 1984;8:5.

Warshaw JB. Intrauterine growth restriction revisited. *Growth Genet Horm* 1992;8:5.

CHAPTER 28 ■ FOLLOW-UP OF INFANTS DISCHARGED FROM NEWBORN INTENSIVE CARE

DAVID T. SCOTT AND JON E. TYSON

Some of the first follow-up programs for premature infants were questionnaire surveys undertaken in Europe in the second decade of the twentieth century. Not surprisingly, these surveys did little to clarify the long-term prognosis of premature infants. By the 1950s and 1960s, some significant methodologic advances had occurred: population-based samples and standardized assessments. With the advent of newborn intensive care units in the early 1960s, the population of low-birth-weight survivors began to grow, and by the late 1970s, newborn follow-up programs had begun to proliferate.

The need for follow-up programs for high-risk newborns has now been widely accepted. However, there has been little discussion of their multiple (and sometimes competing) purposes, which have included providing comprehensive and specialized care for high-risk survivors, monitoring rates of handicap among infants discharged from intensive care units, and answering specific research questions.

In designing a follow-up program, a careful delineation of its specific purposes is key. This delineation will inform decisions

about issues such as patient selection, frequency of visits, evaluation methods used, interventions used, communication with parents and community physicians, duration of follow-up, and program funding.

Two contrasting approaches to follow-up care are outlined in Table 28.1. The *clinical service model* is designed to provide individualized medical care to high-risk survivors. This approach has the advantages of flexibility, efficiency, and orientation to patient needs. Although widely used, this approach is unlikely to provide unbiased estimates of the prevalence of health and development problems in surviving high-risk infants, or an assessment of the effects of perinatal problems on and therapies for various outcomes. Such information has considerable relevance for health policy and perinatal care. The *epidemiologic model* is designed to address these additional needs. However, the epidemiologic model entails considerable effort and expense to identify and recruit all high-risk patients in a defined region, to train staff, and to ensure unbiased, valid, and well-calibrated assessments of outcome.

TABLE 28.1

CONTRASTING APPROACHES IN NEWBORN FOLLOW-UP PROGRAMS

Domain	Clinical Service Model	Epidemiologic Model
Initial identification of cases	"Convenience" samples (e.g., all cases from one institution)	Population-based samples
Case selection	Composite clinical judgment of degree of risk	Fixed, objective criteria (e.g., birth weight)
Recruitment	Samples often shaped by access factors (e.g., distance from institution, access to telephone)	Great effort made to control differential loss of hard-to-follow patients in population
Frequency of visits	Often adjusted to fit severity of history or findings	Usually a fixed schedule of required visits with provision for extra visits if clinically indicated
Control/comparison groups	Only cases followed	Controls or some other comparison group also followed
Blinding of assessors	Assessor knowledgeable about neonatal course and prior follow-up findings	Assessor deliberately blinded to neonatal history and prior follow-up findings
Assessment reliability	Less attention to standardizing assessments and verifying reliability	Considerable attention to standardizing assessments and verifying reliability
Staffing	Clinician often serving as caregiver and evaluator; ideally, the same clinician for serial visits to facilitate rapport and familiarity	Ideally, a different evaluator at each visit to avoid examiner bias
Surveillance procedures	Procedures adapted to patient's clinical history and current clinical problems	Typically, a fixed battery of assessment procedures, focused on outcomes of greatest interest
Treatments/interventions	Variable treatments based on clinical judgment	Restricted treatment options to avoid altering phenomena under study
Communication with parents	Unrestricted and designed to increase understanding	Restricted to avoid self-fulfilling prophecies, "teaching to test," loss of "blindness," and so forth
Duration of follow-up	Patients often discharged when considered healthy or normal	Special efforts made to retain all patients throughout predefined evaluation period
Financial arrangements	Typically, fee-for-service; patient provides own transportation	Patients often reimbursed for expenses or paid for time; transportation often provided

For most follow-up programs, some synthesis of the clinical service and epidemiologic approaches is needed to ensure that both follow-up care and outcome assessments are of high quality. Some outcome measures (e.g., developmental assessments at specific age points) should be assessed by personnel carefully trained and blinded to previous findings. To reduce the likelihood that examiner expectations for high-risk infants would influence the evaluations (and to provide a full-term frame of reference), the examiners should know that some control infants (e.g., healthy infants born at term) will be included. At the same time, health care should be given on a schedule determined by patient needs, and it should be provided by personnel who are familiar with perinatal and follow-up findings and who have a good rapport with the family. Whenever feasible, follow-up should be provided for infants with any of the neonatal problems listed in Box 28.1.

For infants who have primary pediatricians skilled in managing disorders such as bronchopulmonary dysplasia, short-gut syndrome, and the sequelae of intracranial hemorrhage and hypoxic-ischemic encephalopathy, follow-up clinics may need to provide no more than standardized neurodevelopmental assessments. However, indigent populations have the most limited access to health care and the highest prevalence of neurodevelopmental morbidity. For other infants, the provision of comprehensive medical care in the follow-up clinic may be important, both to manage health problems and to reduce loss to follow-up. If more than 10% to 20% of patients are lost to follow-up, only imprecise and possibly biased estimates of the prevalence of handicap will be obtained. The fact that tradi-

tional follow-up programs are not designed to provide comprehensive health care partly accounts for the uncertainty about the outcome of high-risk infants from economically disadvantaged families. Broyles et al. conducted one program of comprehensive care for high-risk inner-city infants. In that program,

---

BOX 28.1   **Some Indications for Newborn Follow-up Referral**

Birth weight of 1,250 g or less
Treatment with mechanical ventilation for 12 hours or longer
Bronchopulmonary dysplasia
Recurrent apneic episodes at or beyond 38 weeks postconceptional age
Grades 2 to 4 intraventricular hemorrhage, intracerebral lesions, or ventriculomegaly by sonogram or computed tomography
Seizures or persistent neurologic abnormality
Meningitis
Cystic white-matter disease
One or more major congenital anomalies
Any problem requiring major surgery in the neonatal period

the addition of comprehensive primary care (instead of conventional follow-up care only) yielded reductions in three areas: loss to follow-up; total health care costs; and, most important, the incidence of life-threatening illnesses (death or admission for pediatric intensive care).

MEDICAL EVALUATION AND CARE

Routine medical care for high-risk infants includes administration of immunizations and evaluation of growth, vision, and hearing. Immunizations for preterm infants should be given at the same postnatal age as for term infants. Growth is assessed in much the same manner as for full-term infants, except that more stable growth trajectories and better predictions of later growth status are generally obtained by plotting growth measures on a postterm (corrected) age scale. Vision examinations may be indicated for many premature infants who received oxygen therapy. If no retinopathy has been identified, periodic eye examinations should be performed until the retina is mature (usually by 2 to 3 months after term); if retinopathy has been identified, eye examinations should continue until the disease process is stable or resolving. Several indications exist for routine hearing screening in this population (Box 28.2). Screening for hearing loss may be based on behavioral or electrophysiologic responses to sound. Methods to assess behavioral responses to sound are relatively inexpensive, but electrophysiologic methods are often required during the first year after birth.

At discharge, high-risk infants may have multiple unresolved medical problems. Methods of treatment or management that have been recommended for these problems include various anticonvulsant regimens for infants with recurrent seizures; a variety of specialized programs for infants with sensory or motor handicaps; bronchodilators, diuretics, physiotherapy, high-calorie feedings, and oxygen for infants with bronchopulmonary dysplasia; apnea monitors and theophylline for infants who have recurrent apneic episodes before nursery discharge; concentrated feedings or nutritional supplements for infants with growth failure; special formulas and parenteral nutrition at home for infants with severe short-gut syndrome; and medications or placation for infants with gastroesophageal reflux.

The pathophysiology and treatment of the difficult ongoing problems of high-risk survivors are complex, and a detailed discussion is beyond the scope of this chapter. All the treatment methods noted previously have potential hazards; few have been evaluated in randomized trials of discharged preterm infants. Thus, the indications for these treatments remain con-

troversial. Whenever possible, their use should be carefully monitored by physicians with specialized experience.

NEUROLOGIC ASSESSMENTS

Several methods of neurologic assessment have been described, both for the neonatal period and for the ensuing months. The method most familiar to practicing physicians focuses on infant reflexes and posture. However, this method may not be adequate for early identification of subtle findings. The method of Milani-Comparetti and Gidoni emphasizes vestibular function and body posture. This method includes 27 assessments that are relatively time consuming; many of these items are more familiar to physical therapists than to physicians. A method based on primitive reflexes also has been advocated.

Amiel-Tison has described a method for assessing neurologic status during the first year that is an extension of the neurologic items used in assessing gestational age in the neonatal period (e.g., assessment of heel-to-ear maneuver, popliteal angle, dorsiflexion angle of the foot) (Fig. 28.1). Like other methods of neurologic assessment, however, this method has not been demonstrated to have high accuracy in predicting later handicap.

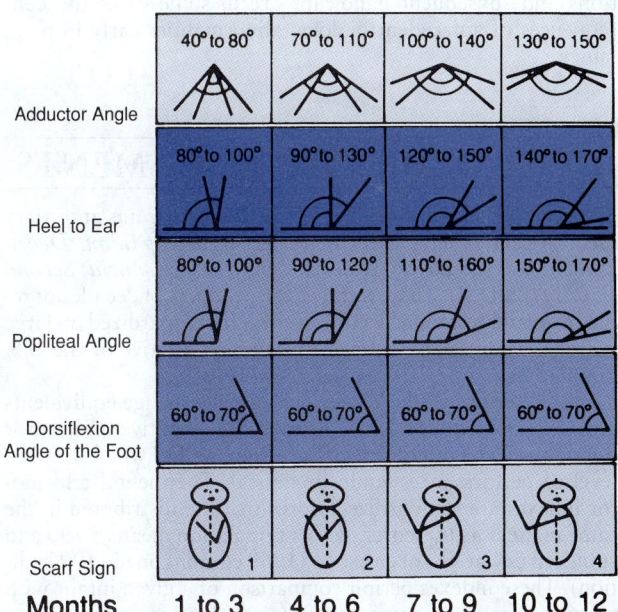

FIGURE 28.1. Normal pattern of passive tone within first year of life. *Adductor angle:* The infant is supine. The legs are opened as far as possible by the examiner. The angle formed by the legs is measured. *Heel to ear:* The infant is supine. The buttocks are kept on the table. The legs are kept straight and the feet moved toward the ears. When there is resistance to the movement, the angle formed from the table surface to the legs is measured. *Popliteal angle:* The infant is supine. The buttocks are kept on the table. The legs are flexed to either side of the abdomen until there is resistance. Then the legs are extended. When there is resistance to this movement, the angle formed between the lower and uppper leg is measured. *Dorsiflexion angle of the foot:* The foot is flexed, and the angle between the foot and leg is measured. *Scarf sign:* The infant is supine. The examiner takes one of the infant's hands and pulls the arm across the infant's chest until there is resistance. The position of the elbow is noted. (Reprinted from Ellison P. Neurologic development of the high-risk infant. *Clin Perinatol* 1984; 11:45. Adapted from Amiel-Tison C. A method for neurologic evaluation within the first year of life. *Curr Probl Pediatr* 1976;7:1.)

BOX 28.2	**Some Indications for Audiologic Evaluation**

Birth weight of less than 1,500 g
Potentially toxic levels of bilirubin
Congenital malformations involving the external ear, palate, face, or skull
Congenital nonbacterial infections
Meningitis
Prolonged administration of aminoglycosides or other ototoxic drugs
Family history of hearing loss

A low predictive accuracy for classic neurologic assessments in infancy was noted in the National Collaborative Perinatal Project. The neurologic findings at 4 months were reported for children who had cerebral palsy at 7 years. At 4 months of age, only 33% of children with cerebral palsy were classified as having an abnormal neurologic examination result; 31% were regarded as neurologically suspect and 36% as normal at 4 months. Conversely, many infants with suspect or mild neurologic findings (e.g., mild hypotonia, mild hypertonia of the legs) subsequently become normal. This fact has led some follow-up investigators to describe a transient dystonia that appears and then resolves spontaneously during the first year. In the National Collaborative Perinatal Project sample, however, 84% of infants with moderate or severe quadriplegia at 1 year and 87% of those with moderate or severe hemiparesis at 1 year were classified as having cerebral palsy at 7 years.

In Britain, Evans et al. have developed a standard form for describing childhood motor deficits of central origin, in part to "allow comparisons between areas and countries where registers of children with cerebral palsy are kept and to permit the grouping of children with similar deficits for research into etiology and effectiveness of interventions."

The causes of handicaps in childhood are often difficult to determine with certainty. They often have been assumed to result from perinatal complications. However, some investigators have reported an increased incidence of minor congenital anomalies and other dysmorphic features among handicapped children. Such findings suggest that both perinatal complications and subsequent handicaps are in some cases the consequences of antecedent biologic abnormalities early in pregnancy.

DEVELOPMENTAL ASSESSMENTS

Since the 1970s, most newborn follow-up programs at tertiary medical centers have used the *Bayley Scales of Infant Development* and the *Bayley Scales of Infant Development, Second Edition* (BSID-II). These tests are the products of decades of refinement and restandardization and were standardized on large national samples constructed to be representative of the U.S. population.

Both editions of the Bayley Scales generate age equivalents and developmental indexes, in both the cognitive and motor domains. The age equivalents are the age for which a given level of performance would be typical. The mental and motor indexes are standardized scores that are distributed in the same manner as IQ scores, with a population mean of 100 and standard deviations of either 16 (1969 edition) or 15 (1993 edition). These indexes permit comparison of a given infant with other infants of the same age. When evaluating premature infants during the first years of life, most developmental clinicians now use the infant's postterm or corrected age (i.e., the age computed from the child's due date), so that the comparison will be with other infants of the same biologic (postconceptional) age.

Interpreting the Bayley index requires caution. Pairwise differences smaller than 7 or 8 points may well arise from measurement error. In a large, multisite cohort of low-birth-weight infants from the Infant Health and Development Program, the correlation between the Bayley Mental Index and IQ at age 8 ranged from 0.44 (Bayley at 12 months vs. Wechsler IQ at age 8) to 0.66 (Bayley at 24 months vs. Wechsler IQ at age 8). Consequently, about 20% to 40% of the variance in age-8 IQ is shared with the variance in the Bayley Mental Index. Some variation exists among clinicians in the descriptive labels used to describe Bayley scores. An example of such labels is provided in Table 28.2.

TABLE 28.2

EXAMPLES OF DESCRIPTIVE LABELS FOR THE BAYLEY INDEX

Bayley Index	Descriptive Label
≥110	Above average; ahead of schedule
90–109	Average; on schedule
80–89	Low normal
70–79	Borderline; gray zone
60–69	Developmental delay: mild to moderate
<60	Developmental delay: moderate to severe

Experience with BSID-II has raised questions about its suitability for use with atypically developing children. As Washington and her colleagues discovered, the item-set format of the BSID-II can prove problematic in children with uneven development or in those with large developmental delays, both of which categories are encountered with increased frequency in newborn follow-up programs. For such children, at least, the 1969 edition of the Bayley Scales may still prove useful at times.

A third edition of the Bayley Scales is due to be released in late 2005. Its technical strengths and limitations remain to be determined.

ADDITIONAL METHODOLOGIC ISSUES

Several methodologic issues should be considered in designing a follow-up program.

Demographic Issues

Follow-up studies often have been more careful in describing their samples' medical characteristics than their demographic characteristics. However, vast literature documents the sensitivity of many of the commonly used outcome measures to environmental influences. Some evidence exists that the sequelae of neonatal events are ordinarily more easily documented in the first or second year after discharge, after which time the effects of postnatal environmental factors may begin to obscure the effects of mild to moderate neonatal insults.

Blinded Assessments

Many ambiguities are inherent in standardized developmental assessments, particularly in the first years after birth. The best way to ensure that outcome assessments are not contaminated by self-fulfilling prophecies (and other biases) is to keep certain follow-up personnel deliberately uninformed about the child's medical and social history.

Calibration of Standardized Assessments

It is sometimes difficult to compare Bayley data from different institutions, in part because of growing evidence that interexaminer calibration is surprisingly difficult to achieve and maintain. In some multisite studies, calibration errors of more than half a standard deviation have been encountered during reliability training, even with experienced examiners. Ongoing reliability training is necessary to ensure that the standardized data remain well calibrated.

Developmental Instrumentation

Despite some additions to the array of neurodevelopmental instruments, the array of options remains relatively constrained for the first 3 years of life. Some methods that rely on visual attention or on habituation paradigms seem better suited for the laboratory than for the clinic, because a substantial minority of infants may fail to meet the behavioral requirements of the procedure.

Several clinical assessment packages are being used in "birth to three" programs developed in response to federal legislation. Some of these clinical instruments attempt to evaluate the child's developmental status in as many as a dozen subdomains (e.g., fine motor, social, receptive language). However, cognitive development during the first 3 years may be too undifferentiated to permit reliable and valid assessment in numerous subdomains; in reality, subdomain scores in the first years of life may be only unreliable estimates of some broader common factor.

Age Range

Some early newborn follow-up programs followed children only until they were 6 months or 1 year old. Moderate to severe disabilities often can be detected in the first year of life, but subtle and mild conditions sometimes do not become apparent until later. We recommend that follow-up assessments continue *at least* until 18 months' postterm age, both to allow some opportunity to assess early language and to permit reasonable screening for subtler cases of cerebral palsy. Learning disabilities, attention disorders, and executive-function disorders usually cannot be identified until later in childhood.

Choice of an Age Scale

Early follow-up studies often calculated the age of premature children from the date of their premature birth. Thus, premature children were compared with full-term children who were the same postnatal age but a more advanced postconceptional age. Not surprisingly, the full-term children were almost always taller, heavier, and more advanced developmentally. It was unclear whether the putative delays among the premature children were genuine sequelae of prematurity and its complications, or only the consequences of their younger postconceptional age. Other studies have attempted to put premature children on the same biologic footing as full-term controls by using the child's postterm or corrected age.

Although the use of the postterm age for premature children has gained ever-wider acceptance, the age range over which it should be used is controversial. In some early studies in which the degree of prematurity was modest and the samples were small, the use of postterm age did not seem to make a significant difference after 1 or 2 years, and the investigators thus changed from the corrected-age scale to the chronologic-age scale after that point. However, as more survivors with greater and greater degrees of prematurity were studied, the effects of using the corrected versus the chronologic age could be seen at progressively later ages. For this reason, some investigators (including the authors) now use the postterm age indefinitely.

Issues Under Investigation

The contribution of follow-up clinics may be enhanced by greater emphasis on relating obstetric and neonatal care to outcome, which is best assessed in randomized trials to determine the effect of new or unproven methods of care on outcome through at least 18 months. Follow-up clinics have not ordinarily undertaken assessments of the effects of neonatal outcome and newborn intensive care on parents or other family members. However, a better understanding of these effects on parents whose infants died, as well as on parents whose infants survived, is needed; this information would be particularly salient for neonatologists confronted with determining when a prognosis is so bleak that intensive care is unwarranted. Follow-up studies would also be more useful for parental counseling in the neonatal period if the reported findings included the percentage of *all births* of a particular birth weight (or gestational age) who survived without impairment. (Most follow-up studies report only the percentage of those *discharged home* in these categories who survived without impairment.)

NEUROLOGIC AND DEVELOPMENTAL INTERVENTIONS

Therapies such as early physical therapy have been used in an attempt to prevent or ameliorate neurologic handicaps, but the few clinical trials in this area to date have not found convincing evidence that these interventions are effective.

Since the early 1960s, several early-intervention programs have been developed in an effort to promote normal development, particularly for socioeconomically disadvantaged children. However, there has been less evidence of benefit for children who are biologically at risk, largely because most of the early studies in this area had methodologic limitations (e.g., nonrandomized designs).

One well-controlled, multisite, randomized clinical trial was the Infant Health and Development Program (IHDP). Additional information about the IHDP is presented in Box 28.3.

RESULTS OF FOLLOW-UP STUDIES OF VERY LOW-BIRTH-WEIGHT INFANTS

Parents, physicians, health economists, and others have worried that the increased survival of ever-smaller premature infants may increase the number of handicapped children. Many early studies compared recent survivors with those during the late 1940s to mid-1960s. However, neonatal outcome during those earlier years was compromised by iatrogenic disease due to a variety of causes, such as misuse of oxygen, chloramphenicol, sulfonamide, and vitamin K. Some evidence exists that before these years, low-birth-weight infants who did survive had a low incidence of handicap that is unlikely to be equaled with the improved survival rates—at lower and lower birth weights—in modern neonatal units. In the study of the 1946 British national cohort (all legitimate single births with a birth weight of less than 2,000 g born in England during the first week of March 1946), the average IQ and the proportion of survivors who were handicapped at age 15 years were similar to those of matched children born at term. However, no infants with birth weights below 1,000 g had survived, compared with survival rates of 20% to 50% in more recent population-based studies.

The incidence of handicaps reported in recent years, although not so low as noted for the 1946 cohort, has been lower

---

BOX 28.3   Infant Health and Development Program (IHDP)

At each of eight clinical sites, premature, low-birth-weight children were randomly assigned either to a follow-up group or to an intervention group. Children in the follow-up group received medical follow-up care and blinded developmental evaluations; children in the intervention group received the same follow-up services, with the addition of a broad-spectrum early-intervention program for them and their families.

At 3 years postterm age, differences were found in each of the three IHDP outcome domains. In the cognitive domain, large IQ effects were noted: among children with birth weights between 2,001 and 2,500 g, intervention children exhibited a cognitive advantage of 13.2 IQ points; among intervention children with birth weights of 2,000 g or less, the IQ advantage was 6.6 points. Secondary analyses suggested that the IQ effects were largest for children from disadvantaged families. In the behavior domain, there was a small but significant tendency for mothers of intervention children to report fewer behavior problems than mothers of follow-up children. In the health domain, mothers of children with birth weights of 2,000 g or less reported more

illnesses and health conditions for intervention children than for follow-up children; no differences were found on a measure of serious health conditions, however.

The IHDP sample was reassessed in two follow-up studies beyond age 3 years (the age at which the intervention ended). At age 5 (2 years after the intervention ended), no significant differences were found in the behavior or health domains. In the cognitive domain, no significant differences remained in the lighter birth-weight stratum (less than 2,000 g), although modest but significant residual differences were found in the heavier birth-weight stratum. At age 8 (5 years after the end of the intervention program), there were, again, no significant differences in the behavior or health domains. In the cognitive domain, however, the heavier birth-weight stratum showed a significant 4.4-point IQ advantage in the intervention group; a somewhat larger treatment effect was found on a standardized vocabulary test. Thus, early-intervention programs appear to enhance the developmental progress of many low-birth-weight, premature infants, but the treatment effects may diminish over time once the intervention is withdrawn.

---

than incidence figures reported in most follow-up studies before the introduction of intensive care. Most of these studies are based on unblinded assessments of populations treated in referral centers and followed in follow-up clinics based on a clinical service model. Thus, their findings are difficult to interpret. The best follow-up studies have assessed geographically defined populations, and the findings from these studies indicate that the increasing survival of small premature infants has not been accompanied by an increase in the proportion of survivors who have disabilities. With advances in perinatal care, such as the use of antenatal corticosteroids and postnatal surfactant therapy, the proportion of survivors with disabilities has remained stable or even declined. This is no small achievement. However, the substantial increase in survivors appears to be accompanied by some increase in the absolute number of disabled survivors.

The proportion of survivors born at less than 750- to 1,000-g birth weight who have disabilities has been reported at approximately 20% to 25%, and the proportion with disabling cerebral palsy is approximately 10%, a problem particularly associated with neonatal brain hemorrhage or ischemia. Considerable concern has been expressed about the high proportion (approximately 50%) of extremely low-birth-weight survivors who have neurobehavioral dysfunction and school problems, and about the effect of such problems on the quality of life for these children and their families. Some reassurance has been provided by a controlled study of self-assessed quality of life among a cohort of Canadian adolescents who weighed less than 1,000 g at birth. The great majority of these long-term survivors and their parents rated their quality of life as quite satisfactory. This finding and the methods to assess quality of life deserve further study and evaluation in U.S. populations.

Suggested Readings

Bennett FC. Developmental outcome. In: *Neonatology: pathophysiology and management of the newborn,* 6th ed. Philadelphia: Lippincott Williams and Wilkins, 2005.

Bernbaum JC, Hoffman-Williamson M. *Primary care of the preterm infant.* Philadelphia: Mosby-Year Book, 1991.

Broyles RS, Tyson JE, Heyne ET, et al. Comprehensive follow-up care and life-threatening illnesses among high-risk infants: a randomized clinical trial. *JAMA* 2000;284:2070.

Drillien CM, Drummond MB. *Neurodevelopmental problems in early childhood.* Oxford: Blackwell, 1977.

Ellison P. Neurologic development of the high-risk infant. *Clin Perinatol* 1984;11:41.

Evans P, Johnson A, Mutch L, Alberman E. A standard form for recording clinical findings in children with a motor deficit of central origin. *Dev Med Child Neurol* 1989;31:119.

Hack M, Fanaroff AA. Outcomes of extremely low birthweight and gestational age in the 1990s. *Semin Neonatol* 2000;5:89.

Hack M, Youngstrom EA, Carter L, et al. Behavioral outcomes and evidence of psychopathology among very low birth weight infants at age 20 years. *Pediatrics* 2004;114:932.

Hakansson S, Farooqi A, Holmgren PA, et al. Proactive management promotes outcome in extremely preterm infants: a population-based comparison of two perinatal management strategies. *Pediatrics* 2004;114:58.

Lorenz JM, Wooliever DE, Jetton JR, Paneth N. A quantitative review of mortality and developmental disability in extremely premature newborns. *Arch Pediatr Adolesc Med* 1998;152:425.

Marlow N, Wolke D, Bracewell MA, Samara M, for the EPICure Study Group. Neurologic and developmental disability at six years of age after extremely premature birth. *N Engl J Med* 2005;352:9.

McCarton CM, Brooks-Gunn J, Wallace IF, et al. Results at 8 years of early intervention for low-birth-weight premature infants. The Infant Health and Development Program. *JAMA* 1997;277:126.

O'Shea TM, Goldstein DJ. Follow-up data and their use in evidence-based decision-making. *Clin Perinatol* 2003;30:217.

Palmer FB, Shapiro BK, Wachtel RC, et al. The effects of physical therapy on cerebral palsy: a controlled trial in infants with spastic diplegia. *N Engl J Med* 1988;318:803.

Saigal S, Pinelli J, Hoult L, et al. Psychopathology and social competencies of adolescents who were extremely low birth weight. *Pediatrics* 2003;111:969.

Schmidt B, Aszatolos EV, Roberts R, et al. Impact of bronchopulmonary dysplasia, brain injury, and severe retinopathy on the outcome of extremely low-birth-weight infants at 18 months: result from the trial of indomethacin prophylaxis in preterms. *JAMA* 2003;289:1124.

Tyson JE, Stoll BJ. Evidence-based ethics and the care and outcome of extremely premature infants. *Clin Perinatol* 2003;30:363.

Vohr BR, Wright LL, Dusick AM, et al. Center differences and outcomes of extremely low birth weight infants. *Pediatrics* 2004:781.

Washington K, Scott DT, Johnson KA, et al. The Bayley Scales of Infant Development-II and children with developmental delays: a clinical perspective. *Dev Behav Pediatr* 1998;19:26.

CHAPTER 29 ■ ETHICAL ISSUES IN NEONATOLOGY

ALAN R. FLEISCHMAN

Scientific and technologic developments over the last several decades have made substantial advances in the care of neonates and have made it possible to save the lives of the majority of even the sickest and smallest babies. Newborns as young as 23 to 24 weeks gestational age and weighing about 500 g survive at a rate of greater than 30% in most neonatal centers in the United States. Infants of 1,000 g and 28 weeks of gestation, thought to be at the threshold of viability in the 1960s and 1970s, have a consistently greater than 95% survival rate. In addition, surgical techniques have been developed to correct or ameliorate congenital anomalies of the heart, kidney, intestine, liver, and brain. Intravenous parenteral nutrition allows infants to grow and gain weight with normal development for weeks, months, or even years without oral intake. These advances in neonatal medicine have enhanced the lives of countless children, yet at the same time, they also have resulted in saving the lives of some children who are left with severely disabling and handicapping conditions.

Severe disability has been reported in approximately one-third of the surviving infants born at less than 25 completed weeks of gestation. Such major morbidities include cerebral palsy, mental retardation, blindness, or deafness. Even infants born at 26 to 28 weeks' gestation have a significant risk of poor outcomes. It is clear that, despite a major decrease in mortality in premature infants of very low birth weights, no concomitant decrease in percent morbidity has been achieved.

Clinicians are unable to predict with any degree of certainty the long-term outcome of individual infants who are critically ill. Caring for neonates having the potential for survival, but with a poor future quality of life, creates major ethical dilemmas for clinicians and parents alike. An awareness of these ethical dilemmas or value conflicts is not new to those responsible for the care of infants. Historically, physicians felt obligated to make treatment decisions based on their personal beliefs about the future quality of life for their patient. At times, professionals shared this decision making with the family, but often it was thought to be part of the doctor's job to make such choices. These decisions usually were made within the privacy of the delivery room, nursery, or pediatric unit. Rarely discussed openly, most members of society did not realize that value-laden decisions were being made and rationalized as medical judgments. To a large extent, families and society wished these decisions to be private matters, because they were far too complex and personal for public involvement and debate.

However, another sort of revolution has occurred concomitant with the evolution of new technology in neonatal intensive care. The role of the American physician has changed from that of the highly respected and rarely questioned paternalistic decision-maker into a collaborator who provides recommendations for health care decisions that are made in conjunction with the patient and family, rather than by the physician alone. This changing physician's role is consistent with an increasing desire for autonomy reflected in many parts of American society. Patients and families expect to be fully informed and increasingly responsible for decisions about their own health care. In the pediatric context, family-centered care has emerged as the operationalization of increasing respect for the importance of the family in ensuring the health and well-being of children. Family-centered care in neonatology is grounded in collaboration among the family and health professionals responsible for the care of a sick infant; it may involve the family in all aspects of care and in shared decision making in the best interests of the child.

PATIENT AUTONOMY AND THE BEST INTERESTS OF THE CHILD

In ethics, the principle of respect for persons argues for a patient's fundamental right to self-determination. This right to autonomous choice for adults with capacity empowers them to consent to or refuse recommended treatments, even when the physician perceives those treatments to be in the patient's best interest. A second conviction of the principle of respect for persons requires that those individuals who lack the ability to make choices for themselves are entitled to special protections. Neonates clearly are not autonomous and are unable to participate in decision making about their own care.

Respect for a person's right of self-determination is operationalized in medicine in the doctrine of *informed consent*. This doctrine assumes that the patient can understand the risks and benefits of alternative treatments and can make an informed choice. The process of informed consent, when it relates to young children or to any individuals who lack the capacity to decide for themselves, invokes the use of a *proxy* or *surrogate*. A proxy consent is not based on an individual's choice, but rather on another's perception of the appropriate choice.

Many have argued that the respect for a person's fundamental right of self-determination should be extended to respect for the family as an autonomous unit making substituted judgments for members who cannot participate in decision making. This extension of the principle of respect for persons occasionally may be problematic when applied to neonates. The principle of informed consent for autonomous adults is extremely powerful in that it allows capable adults to refuse treatments, despite negative consequences. However, parental refusal of treatments that are deemed to be beneficial for their infant does not hold the same weight as refusals by competent adults for treatments on themselves. Parental refusal of a needed therapy does not relieve the physician or other health care provider from an ethical duty to the child, particularly if the refusal of such treatment puts the child at significant risk.

To preserve the child's future right to autonomous decision making, guardians of pediatric patients are charged with the responsibility of asking what best promotes the child's interests. This child-centered "best interest" standard emphasizes that children ought to be valued as individuals, and it protects children in situations involving conflict between what is best for the child and what is best for others. This principle supports making a decision solely for the benefit of the infant, sometimes, although rarely, even in conflict with parental beliefs.

Determinations of best interest often are made in the presence of significant medical uncertainty about the outcome of the proposed treatment. In general, physicians have a great deal of difficulty in admitting their lack of certainty about the benefits of continued treatment or the initiation of new interventions. Jeff Lyon, in his book *Playing God in the Nursery*, graphically portrays the dilemma of uncertainty: "If it is hard to justify creating blind paraplegics to obtain a number of healthy survivors, it is equally hard to explain to the ghosts of the potentially healthy that they had to die in order to avoid creating blind paraplegics."

American neonatologists tend to deal with this uncertainty by considering it far worse to let an infant die who could have lived a reasonable life than to save an infant who becomes devastatingly disabled. Both outcomes are tragic. What is clear is that the value-laden decision about what is in the best interest of an individual infant often is uncertain. Many have argued that those who will bear the burden of the decision—namely, the family—ought to have the major role in making it. When faced with a lack of certainty about what is in an infant's best interest, the physician's obligation is to share with the family a clear understanding of the various treatment options and make a recommendation consistent with what the treatment team believes is in the child's best interest. Ultimately, however, in these difficult cases, family discretion should prevail. The physician's values should not be imposed inappropriately, and continued treatment should not be forced, when hope for benefit is unlikely.

Decisions should be collaborative, with the child's interests at the center of the analysis, but with parents responsible for the choice, unless they are making a decision clearly against the best interest of the child. Prolonging an infant's life should not be viewed as an end in itself, but should be weighed against the probable quality of that future life.

MAKING DECISIONS FOR CHILDREN WITH DISABLING CONDITIONS

At the core of all discussions concerning the appropriate process for making decisions for seriously ill neonates is the question of how much we value members of our society who have disabling and handicapping conditions. A distinct tension remains between the ostensible societal valuing of the disabled, as represented by legal initiatives and public policy, and the deeply held personal feelings of many individuals. In general, however, the last several decades have shown an increasing respect for the retarded and disabled in our society. Concomitantly, there has been an increasing public awareness that decisions are being made by physicians and parents in neonatal intensive care units to withhold or withdraw treatments from neonates who are at risk for disabilities and handicapping conditions. This knowledge resulted in several efforts during the 1980s by the U.S. Department of Health and Human Services to promulgate regulations concerning appropriate standards for foregoing of life-sustaining treatment for neonates. At the same time, the President's Commission for the Study of Ethical Problems in Medicine and Biomedical and Behavioral Research issued its report "Deciding to Forego Life Sustaining Treatment," and the Bioethics Committee of the American Academy of Pediatrics developed guidelines for the establishment and operation of bioethics committees, which would prospectively review cases

in which the foregoing of life-sustaining treatment was under consideration. It was hoped that these committees would provide consultation and decision review to assist families and health care providers in the process of decision making, as well as to protect the interests of the infants in neonatal intensive care units.

Federal regulations, currently in effect, do not mandate unnecessary or inappropriate treatments. They allow physicians to use reasonable medical judgment in making treatment recommendations and allow physicians to involve parents in the decision-making process. The regulations give the responsibility for protecting neonates with potentially handicapping conditions to the individual states; federal involvement is severely limited. Furthermore, the federal regulations strongly urge the formation of infant care review committees (which the American Academy of Pediatrics calls infant bioethical review committees) to facilitate decision review and to assist in the interaction among physicians, the family, the hospital, and the child protective services agency of the state.

Many fear that the parental authority for decision making for infants might be circumvented or supplanted by bioethics consultation or committee review. Some have argued that these judgments are best made by the treating physician at the bedside, who is most familiar with the medical facts as well as with the infant's interests and the family's wishes. However, infant bioethics committees can enhance the process of decision making by reviewing the medical facts, and they can protect the infant's interests by invoking ethical principles and not merely intuition in decision making. Such committees can increase the role of parents in decision making and can provide ethical comfort to both families and health care professionals who are ultimately responsible for these difficult decisions.

CONCEPT OF FUTILITY

Increasingly, a new type of ethical dilemma is occurring in neonatal intensive care units. Physicians who have become comfortable with the concept of families having the discretion to choose to withhold or withdraw life-sustaining treatments from critically ill newborns are becoming concerned about families who insist on their infant's receiving life-sustaining treatments that are deemed by the professionals to have minimal, if any, benefit to the child. Physicians are invoking the concept of "futility" in an attempt to limit parental discretion to demand marginally beneficial or inappropriate treatment. This invoking of the concept of futility reflects one of the consequences of involving parents more deeply in the decision-making process: health care professionals sometime disagree with the parents' choice. Based on the physician's independent obligation to the child, society has developed procedural mechanisms to override parental refusal of those treatments thought to be in the child's best interests. This process can be done through infant bioethics committee involvement or, ultimately, through the courts. Similarly, physicians have an obligation not to provide parent-requested treatments to infants that will only inflict pain and increase suffering and have no potential benefit for the child. Such treatments appropriately can be labeled futile. However, when parents request a treatment that offers a low likelihood of benefit, even in the face of significant burden, health care professionals ought not arrogate to themselves the right to preclude treatment by calling the treatment futile. When caring, concerned parents request continued attempts to save the life of their child, if such treatments are possibly helpful, the physician should not use the language of futility in an attempt to impose her view of the interest of the child over the values of the family.

Parental discretion should be given broad latitude in choices for children when honest uncertainty exists about the benefits-to-burdens ratio of continued treatment. However, parental discretion to demand treatment ought not to be unlimited. Physicians and other health care providers, based on their own strongly held personal beliefs, have the right to opt out of the care of an individual child for whom they believe the benefits of treatment do not outweigh the burdens. In addition, society has the right, through its laws, regulations, and institutions, to limit individual resource allocation for patients unlikely or unable to benefit from continued treatment.

EXPERIMENTATION IN THE NEONATAL INTENSIVE CARE UNIT

An ethical dilemma of a different type is evident in the initiation of clinical interventions and experimentation in the neonatal intensive care unit. Numerous therapeutic misadventures exist that are the hallmark of the early years of neonatology. These have included the excessive use of oxygen and resultant retrolental fibroplasia; the unexpected complications of the use of various antibiotics; and the use of rapid infusions of sodium bicarbonate to buffer metabolic acidosis, which increased the incidence of intraventricular hemorrhage. All these therapeutic modalities were instituted by well-intentioned clinicians whose motivation was based on a desire to help patients who would otherwise die or be severely impaired.

Physicians often are reluctant to subject innovative therapies to the discipline of a true experiment (i.e., a randomized clinical trial) to ensure that the proposed therapy is not only effective but has few risks and negative consequences. Innovative clinicians are often self-deluding when they attempt to explain away a treatment failure or a complication from a new therapy that seems to have positive results. Galen, the famous physician of ancient Greece, reported the following analysis of his innovative therapeutic cocktail: "All who drink of this remedy recover in a short time, except those whom it does not help, who all die; therefore, it is obvious that it fails only in incurable cases." Neonatology has had many clinical interventions that have not been subject to careful experimental scrutiny.

The clinical research scientist is certainly motivated by a desire to create new interventions that will ultimately benefit many patients. However, the motivating principle in clinical research, as distinct from clinical practice, is not beneficence but rather the generation of new knowledge and the seeking of truth. The subjects of a clinical research study should not believe that the experimental intervention is deemed effective by the clinician; rather, the clinician must maintain a healthy skepticism that allows the honest randomization of patients to an intervention or control group. Informed consent from the family is mandatory, and withdrawal from the research must be allowed at any time during the course of treatment. This experimental approach to innovative therapies, including such diverse treatments as extracorporeal membrane oxygenation, nitric oxide ventilation, intestinal transplantation, and the initiation of a new antibiotic, is mandatory to protect the interests of present and future infants, so that therapies become standard practice only after appropriate scrutiny.

DEATH IN THE NEONATAL INTENSIVE CARE UNIT

Although the neonatal intensive care unit is a place for aggressive and innovative treatment as well as experimental clinical research, it is also the site of the death of many critically ill infants. Each neonatal intensive care unit must develop an environment that allows for the humane care of the dying infant and the family. When a decision is made that continued therapeutic intervention is no longer in the child's interests, or that the child is in the inexorable downhill spiral that will result in death, all technologic intervention should be withdrawn from the baby, and supportive care and caring should be the therapeutic modality used. Infants should not have to die attached to electronic machines and invasive technology. Neonatal intensive care units should have quiet, private areas where families can be together and interact with their child at the end of life. This sensitive approach to the actual dying process is an important first step toward the resolution of this life crisis within the family. Appropriate counseling and bereavement services should be available both around the time of death and afterward.

CONCLUSIONS

Awareness of and concern for the value conflicts inherent in the field of neonatal intensive care are an important part of the practice of neonatology. Being sensitive to these issues and developing practices that are both in the best interests of infants and respectful of their parents are critical to the continued development of the field.

Suggested Readings

American Academy of Pediatrics. Guidelines for infant bioethics committees. *Pediatrics* 1984;74:306.

American Academy of Pediatrics. Family-centered care and the pediatrician's role. *Pediatrics* 2003;112:691.

Campbell DE, Fleischman AR. Limits of viability: dilemmas, decisions, and decision makers. *Am J Perinatol* 2001;18:117.

Department of Health and Human Services. Nondiscrimination on the basis of handicap. *Fed Reg* 1983;48:9630.

Department of Health and Human Services. Child abuse and neglect prevention and treatment program and services and treatment for disabled infants: model guidelines for health care providers to establish infant care review committees. *Fed Reg* 1985;50:14878.

Fleischman AR. Bioethical review committees in perinatology. *Clin Perinatol* 1987;14:379.

Fleischman AR, Nolan K, Dubler NN, et al. Caring for gravely ill children. *Pediatrics* 1994;94:433.

Hack M, Fanaroff A. Outcomes of children of extremely low birthweight and gestational age in the 1990s. *Early Hum Dev* 1999;53:193.

Kliegman RM, Mahowald MB, Youngner SJ. In our best interests: experience and workings of an ethics review committee. *J Pediatr* 1986;108:178.

Lorenz JM. Survival of the extremely preterm infant in North America in the 1990s. *Clin Perinatol* 2000;27:255.

Lyon J. *Playing God in the nursery.* New York: Norton, 1985.

President's Commission for the Study of Ethical Problems in Medicine and Biomedical and Behavioral Research. *Deciding to forego life-sustaining treatment.* Washington, DC: United States Government Printing Office, 1983.

Silverman WA. Human experimentation in perinatology. *Clin Perinatol* 1987;14:403.

Truog RD, Brett AS, Frader J. The problem with futility. *N Engl J Med* 1992; 326:1560.

Wood NS, Marlow N, Costeloe K, et al. Neurologic and developmental disability after extremely preterm birth. *N Engl J Med* 2000;343:378.

CHAPTER 30 ■ SURGICAL CONSIDERATIONS AND POSTOPERATIVE CARE OF THE NEWBORN

ROBERT J. TOULOUKIAN

Major advances in the care of the newborn have improved the survival and quality of life dramatically for babies born with a major congenital anomaly or acquired condition requiring emergency surgery during the first month of life. In most centers, the overall survival rate approaches 85% to 90%. The modern era of neonatal surgery can be traced to the early 1960s, with the establishment of tertiary-care neonatal special-care units, innovative surgical techniques, modern ventilatory management, intravenous nutrition, and the multimodal treatment of sepsis and shock.

Perinatology, with its emphasis on the diagnosis and treatment of high-risk fetuses having congenital anomalies, has paralleled the development of the high-risk obstetric service, thereby reducing the need for infant transport from community to tertiary-care centers. Improved radiologic modalities, including ultrasonography, computed tomography (CT), and magnetic resonance imaging (MRI), have revolutionized our ability to perform a noninvasive evaluation of a sick newborn. Certain fetal intervention procedures have become safe, and even hysterotomy with open corrective operation has resulted in fetal salvage.

Most surgical procedures in newborns are carried out by pediatric surgeons who are general surgeons with an additional 2 years of training obtained in one of 36 approved training centers in the United States and Canada (2003). This training encompasses the fields of neonatal and general surgery, head and neck trauma, transplantation, burns, endoscopy, gynecology, and urology. Diaphragmatic hernia, esophageal atresia, Hirschsprung disease, intestinal atresia, imperforate anus, omphalocele, and gastroschisis are certain "index" neonatal conditions for which exceptional technical skill and judgment must be learned by pediatric surgical trainees. Because each condition occurs no more than once per 3,000 live births, regionalization of care is required to achieve sufficient surgical expertise within the limited period of training. Currently, more than 600 active board-certified pediatric surgeons practice in

the United States and Canada, the majority of whom are affiliated with a tertiary-care neonatal center.

The interface between neonatology and pediatric surgery begins with an initial evaluation of the infant and continues through the postoperative period. As in all other fields of pediatrics, good communication is needed. Because an infant's condition must be monitored closely, neonatologists and primary nurses are essential partners of the surgeon. Surgeons, however, remain the responsible physicians for the overall care of surgical patients, determining the timing of operation, the need for supplementary evaluations, the progression of feeding schedules, antibiotic usage, and the like. That this relationship must be both collaborative and collegial is essential.

PRENATAL DIAGNOSIS

Prenatal diagnosis has revolutionized the surgical care of the newborn with a correctable anomaly (Table 30.1). Screening ultrasonographic examination and determination of the maternal serum alpha$_1$-fetoprotein provide the first level of evaluation by the obstetrician, who then refers the mother for perinatology and pediatric surgical consultation at a center for high-risk patients. At this time, the surgeon and parents discuss the diagnosis and proposed treatment, further diagnostic testing (e.g., amniocentesis for chromosome analysis), and the corrective surgery required, along with its risks and potential benefits. Furthermore, the family should have a clear understanding of the potential for long-term physical disability or neurologic impairment in their infant. Hand-drawn illustrations, the use of medical textbooks, and clinical examples taken from the surgeon's own experience may help to clarify many important questions about the fate of the fetus. More recently, the Internet has been the source of information for many parents.

The advisability of terminating a pregnancy sometimes is raised if the diagnosis of a noncorrectable anomaly is made

TABLE 30.1

PRENATAL DETECTION AND OVERALL SURVIVAL OF COMMON NEONATAL SURGICAL CONDITIONS

	Incidence (Live Births)	Prenatal Detection Rate (%)	Diagnostic Markers	Overall Survival (%)
Esophageal atresia	1:2,000	20	Polyhydramnios	90
Intestinal atresia	1:2,500	75	Polyhydramnios	95
Abdominal wall defects (with normal chromosomes)	1:3,000	90	Elevated MSAFP	95
Cysts and tumors	1:3,000	90	Elevated MSAFP	95
Neural tube defects	1:400	90	Elevated MSAFP	Variable
Diaphragmatic hernia	1:2,500	90	Elevated MSAFP	50
Urinary tract obstruction	1:3,000	95	Oligohydramnios	90

MSAFP, maternal serum alpha, fetoprotein.

before the twenty-fourth week of gestation. Specific indications for termination would include chromosome abnormalities incompatible with normal life (omphalocele with trisomy 13 or 18), severe neurologic impairment (e.g., encephalocele or anencephaly), or hazards to maternal health, but the need for corrective surgery alone is not deemed an appropriate reason to terminate a pregnancy. Delivery in a tertiary-care center obviates the need for infant transport and shortens the time from birth to surgical correction. This is mandatory for babies with congenital diaphragmatic hernia, abdominal wall defects, or intestinal obstruction when emergency surgery is required within hours of birth. Recent reports have cautioned against unnecessary cesarean section in the absence of evidence of fetal distress.

INFANT TRANSPORT

Surgical conditions that are diagnosed postnatally require emergency transport of the neonate to a tertiary-care center. Esophageal atresia, Hirschsprung disease, and other forms of lower intestinal obstruction, including anorectal anomalies, are not detected routinely by prenatal ultrasonography but are potentially life-threatening within the first 12 to 24 hours of life. Despite the increasing number of babies with congenital diaphragmatic hernia diagnosed by routine prenatal screening, some of these infants' disorders are not detected until respiratory distress develops shortly after birth. The indication encountered most frequently for emergency transport (from a level 2 nursery) is the baby who has "suspect" necrotizing enterocolitis and develops peritonitis after medical management is begun. For these reasons, a tertiary-care center must provide the capability for prompt transport by ambulance, helicopter, or other aircraft, depending on the distance from the referring hospital to the neonatal center.

The transport team consists of a cadre of neonatal nurses with advanced training in resuscitation, endotracheal intubation, institution of a peripheral intravenous line, umbilical artery catheterization, and insertion of a nasogastric or chest tube. The risks associated with specific anomalies and the means by which to prevent further injury or clinical deterioration should be understood. Babies born with a gastroschisis have rapid conductive heat and evaporative fluid loss. The exposed viscera must be covered with warm, moist saline sponges and plastic wrap to prevent additional fluid loss and inadvertent twisting of the mesentery or bowel. Early intervention with intravenous glucose solution is life-saving for a newborn who has omphalocele and macroglossia (Beckwith syndrome), becomes hypoglycemic, and could have brain-damaging seizures.

PREOPERATIVE PREPARATION

Several special considerations render the surgical care of the neonate unique. Box 30.1 lists general concerns in the surgical care of newborns.

Temperature Regulation

The premature neonate's ratio of skin surface area to lean body mass is higher than that in an older infant or child. In the neonate, increased metabolic demands and the absence of a normal thermogenic shivering mechanism produce peripheral vasodilatation, resulting in rapid surface cooling and systemic hypothermia. This concern is particularly valid both in the stressed preterm infant, whose nutritional reserves are minimal, and when body cooling also leads to increased metabolism, which raises oxygen requirements. As heat loss continues, peripheral vasoconstriction occurs, with shunting of arterialized

---

BOX 30.1 General Considerations in the Surgical Care of the Newborn

Temperature regulation
Respiratory support
Cardiovascular status
Radiographic evaluation
Vascular access, fluid replacement
Antibiotic management
Catheters
Additional diagnostic tests
Informed consent

---

blood, increased lactic acid load, and eventually a profound metabolic acidosis.

Hypothermia is minimized by examining the infant under a radiant heat warmer and by exposing the infant only for short periods when it is essential. Particularly concerning is the infant with gastroschisis or omphalocele, because evaporative fluid loss compounds the hypothermia. The use of a warming mattress and supplementary radiant heating lamps are additional helpful measures to prevent hypothermia. Once the initial evaluation of the infant is complete, a humidified and warmed isolation incubator (Isolette) provides the best substitute for the uterus.

Respiratory Support

Careful attention must be given to the airway and lungs because hypoxemia, hypercapnia, and oxygen desaturation often occur in the face the of extrinsic compression of the airway or because of the pulmonary aspiration of salivary or gastrointestinal secretions. This complication may develop rapidly in babies with cervical cystic hygroma involving the floor of the mouth and paratracheal tissues, those with such thoracic problems as congenital diaphragmatic hernia, or those with esophageal atresia with tracheoesophageal fistula. Abdominal distention and upward displacement of the diaphragm also may restrict ventilation in babies with neonatal intestinal obstruction. This problem is particularly common with more distal obstruction, such as meconium ileus, and in babies with a large ovarian or duplication cyst or hydronephrotic kidney. Careful monitoring of respiratory status is essential to detect apneic spells. These risks are magnified in a preterm infant because of the intrinsic tendency to irregular respiratory patterns. Any tendency toward desaturation mandates continuous monitoring, use of supplementary oxygen, and (often) institution of nasal continuous positive pressure or placement of an endotracheal tube with intermittent mandatory ventilation. A primary example of the importance of careful respiratory monitoring is seen in a newborn with congenital diaphragmatic hernia with adequate ventilation at birth. Because of the tendency toward an accumulation of air in the herniated intrathoracic stomach or bowel, the contralateral lung rapidly becomes compromised. In these patients, a combination of peripheral oxygen saturation and arterial blood gas determinations is important to detect hypoxia or a rising carbon dioxide level. A mixed respiratory and metabolic acidosis is a common occurrence.

Cardiovascular Status

Many infants with cyanotic congenital heart disease, such as aortic stenosis or hypoplastic left heart syndrome, appear to be perfectly stable at birth and begin to show evidence of deoxygenation after the ductus arteriosus closes 24 to 48 hours after birth. Increased resistance in the pulmonary vascular bed, such as occurs in infants with pulmonary hypoplasia and congenital diaphragmatic hernia, tends to keep the ductus patent and cause right-to-left shunting of deoxygenated blood into the systemic circulation. The infant with a noncardiac anomaly also may have increased pulmonary vascular resistance secondary to hypoxia, acidosis, hypothermia, and hypovolemia. Unnecessary delays in treating newborns with intestinal obstruction predispose such infants to pulmonary aspiration that will aggravate any underlying tendency to increased pulmonary vascular resistance.

Radiographic Evaluation

At least one set of radiographic studies is obtained in any baby needing an abdominal or thoracic operation. Additional studies, including ultrasonography, CT, and MRI also may be useful.

The plain chest roentgenogram is diagnostic of the great majority of surgically correctable thoracic problems, including diaphragmatic hernia (Fig. 30.1), tension disturbances secondary to pneumothorax or hydrothorax, and even those lesions intrinsic to the lungs, such as lobar emphysema or congenital adenomatoid malformation. Caution must be exercised in distinguishing suspected congenital pulmonary cysts from a diaphragmatic hernia by obtaining an ultrasonography of the diaphragm or even by gastrointestinal contrast studies. Ventilation perfusion scans will give valuable information about the possibility of pulmonary hypoplasia in patients with diaphragmatic eventration, a condition that may be either congenital or secondary to brachial plexus birth injury.

Plain abdominal roentgenograms obtained in multiple views (i.e., supine, prone, and oblique) remain the gold standard in evaluating babies for intestinal obstruction, perforation, or a mass lesion. The oblique view is our choice for detecting free air with necrotizing enterocolitis. When such roentgenograms are repeated at 6-hour intervals, perforation with free air over the liver may be recognized before peritonitis is established and the baby becomes septic. Visualizing the number, distribution, and size of the dilated intestinal loops is very helpful in determining the site of obstruction. A diagnosis of duodenal stenosis can be facilitated by having the radiologist inject 30 or 40 cc of air through the nasogastric tube and then obtaining a prone view of the abdomen to best visualize a "double bubble." When the etiology of duodenal obstruction remains uncertain, barium is introduced through the nasogastric tube to assess the location of the duodenum and thereby rule out malrotation, which can be associated with midgut volvulus. With more distal obstruction, the differential diagnosis among meconium ileus, ileal stenosis, meconium plug syndrome, and Hirschsprung disease can be confusing. Because plain films are nondiagnostic, a barium (or water-soluble contrast) enema should be carried out on an emergency basis. In many instances, the enema is therapeutic, but a submucosal biopsy must be obtained if Hirschsprung disease remains a diagnostic possibility.

Bulky external masses, such as cystic hygroma or sacrococcygeal teratoma, often are complex lesions in which vital structures, including major vessels or nerves, are involved. High-resolution ultrasonography with color Doppler clearly will distinguish arterial and venous supply and is helpful in guiding the surgeon at the time of excision. Intraabdominal or thoracic tumors and cysts can be evaluated similarly and, in the case of a flank mass, ultrasonography immediately distinguishes a cystic lesion, such as a hydronephrotic or multicystic kidney, from a solid mass, such as a mesoblastic nephroma, for which prompt excision should be carried out. More complex lesions containing both solid and cystic components, such as a neuroblastoma, will require further evaluation by CT or MRI. Urinary catecholamines and bone marrow aspiration and biopsy may be necessary before attempts are made at resection. Any paraspinal tumor is assessed best by MRI.

Vascular Access and Fluid Replacement

Prompt venous cannulation is essential, and often a combination of venous and arterial access is required in a neonate who is undergoing surgery. A peripheral venous line in the hand or foot, and an umbilical arterial catheter situated above the renal vessels, provide access for both the maintenance and replacement crystalloid fluids or blood and the means to monitor arterial blood gases and systemic blood pressure. Arterial cannulation is important for the newborn with a congenital diaphragmatic hernia or in similar circumstances when major fluctuations in oxygen or carbon dioxide concentrations are anticipated. However, it is needed less often in stable infants whose oxygen saturation is determined satisfactorily by a cutaneous oxygen saturation monitor. If the baby has an enlarged abdomen because of an intraabdominal mass, obstructed intestine, or an abdominal wall defect, venous cannulation in the upper extremity is preferred strongly to avoid impedance of antegrade flow in the inferior vena cava once corrective surgery has been carried out. Rarely, if ever, is a peripheral intravenous cutdown procedure required, but central venous catheter placement has become very useful, either by cannulation of the internal or external jugular vein under direct vision (Broviac 2.7 Fr., Davol, Inc., Providence, RI), or by percutaneous insertion of the catheter in the upper or lower extremity, from which it is then passed to the cavoatrial site. Percutaneous catheters and venous catheters may be inserted under fluoroscopic surveillance in the operating room or in the neonatal intensive care unit after the primary operation has been carried out.

The composition and volume of maintenance and replacement crystalloid fluid will vary from case to case, depending principally on the estimate of dehydration. Although the normal fluid requirement during the first 24 to 48 hours of life is perhaps one-half of usual maintenance, both extrinsic and internal losses may occur; these losses cause hypovolemia and increase the fluid requirement. The following formula, based on clinical assessment, has proved to be very useful in estimating the degree of dehydration or hypovolemia: 5% (just detectable; dry mucous membranes, poor skin turgor); 10% (skin tenting, sunken fontanelle, oliguria); 15% (shock, anuria).

Initially, salt-containing solutions may be given to reverse so-called third-space loss in infants with intestinal obstruction or vomiting. Fluid deficits in excess of 5% of body weight can be corrected by giving boluses of 10 mL/kg normal saline fluid until the urine specific gravity is less than 1.010. Infants with gastroschisis and omphalocele also have a significant evaporative loss of fluid that must be replaced before operation. Infants who are dehydrated severely, unstable, or hypotensive should be given bolus replacement of 1% to 3% of body weight. Even babies with a large cystic hygroma or sacrococcygeal teratoma may sustain sudden internal hemorrhage or fluid retention, which may cause clinical signs of hypovolemia.

Extensive preoperative laboratory evaluation of the newborn with an acute surgical problem usually is not needed. The necessity of obtaining certain basic studies, however, including a complete blood count with platelet determination, is obvious. Such additional tests as serum electrolyte, blood urea nitrogen (BUN), and creatinine determinations; liver function tests; or coagulation studies are required only under specific circumstances. Blood is sent routinely to the blood bank for typing and cross-matching at a time early enough for the results to be available in the operating room. A so-called split unit of 50 mL

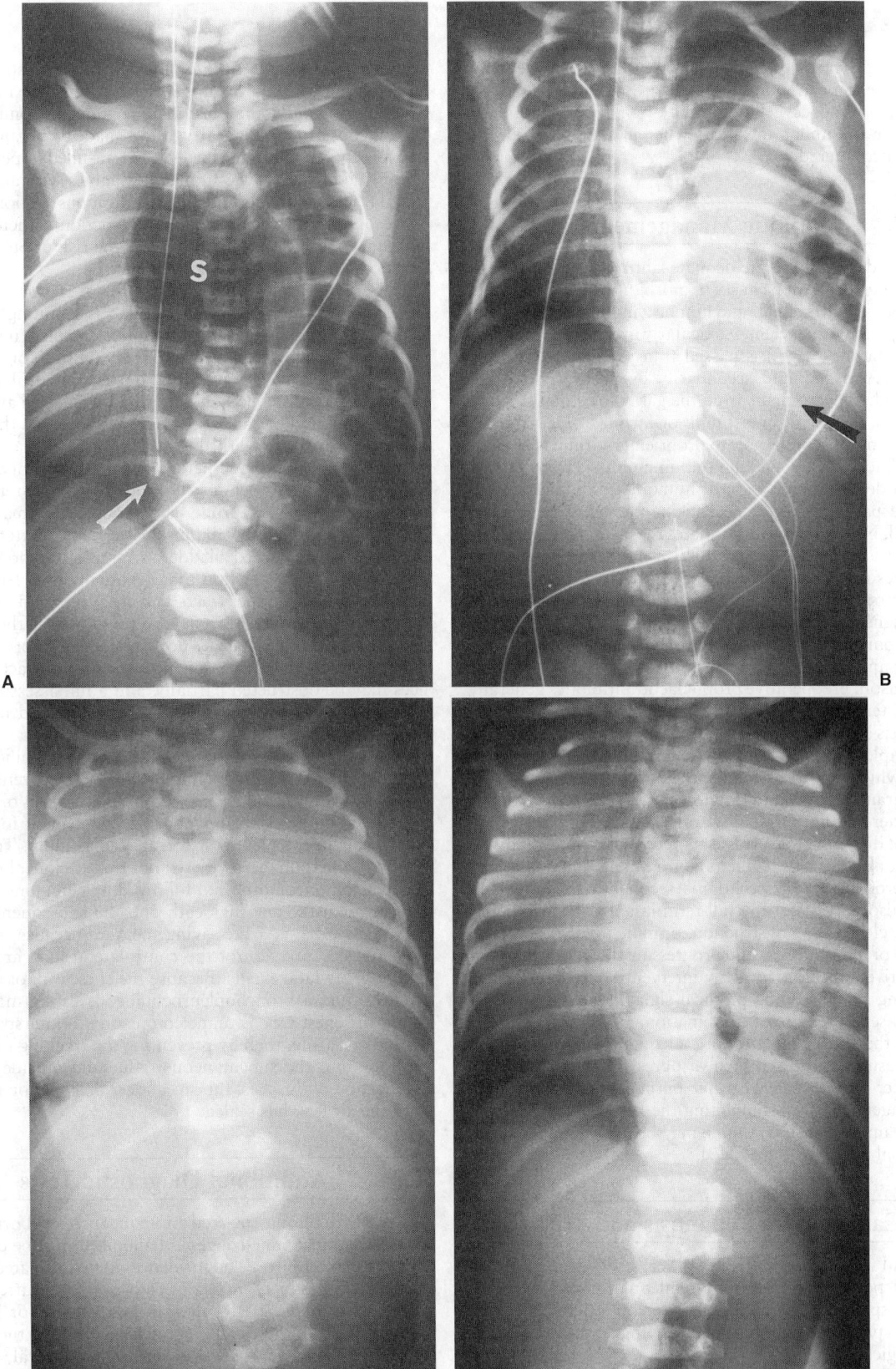

FIGURE 30.1. Left diaphragmatic hernia. **A:** Note numerous loops of air-filled intestine and the air-filled stomach (S) in the left hemithorax. Marked contralateral shift of the mediastinal structures is apparent. The tip of the nasogastric tube is in the distal esophagus (*arrow*). **B:** Later, with the nasogastric tube now advanced into the stomach (*arrow*), note how the stomach has been decompressed and the intestines partially decompressed. Much less mediastinal shift is noted. Note paucity of gas in the abdomen. **C:** Another infant with an early film demonstrating an airless diaphragmatic hernia in the left hemithorax. Note the position of the stomach. A marked contralateral shift of the mediastinal structures is present. **D:** A little later, some air is seen in the loops of the intestine in the left hemothorax. (Reprinted with permission from Swischuk LE. *Imaging of the newborn, infant, and young child,* 5th edition. Philadelphia: Lippincott Williams & Wilkins, 2004:69.)

of packed red blood cells is sufficient for almost all neonatal procedures, except in unusual instances, such as in an infant with a large sacrococcygeal teratoma or an abdominal neuroblastoma or in similar instances wherein major blood loss might be encountered.

Antibiotic Management

Unrecognized sepsis and inadequate antibiotic coverage are among the most common causes of morbidity and death in surgical neonates. Both cellular and humoral immune mechanisms may be impaired or deficient, particularly in the preterm infant. Immunoglobulin G (IgG) is passed transplacentally, whereas secretory IgA is acquired secondarily by absorption of the antibody-laden macrophage from the gastrointestinal tract. In most centers, the use of breast milk or fortified breast milk in the preterm infant is preferable to proprietary formulas because of the likelihood that some humoral immunity is transferable. Whether a delayed acquisition of humoral antibodies plays a role in the pathogenesis of necrotizing enterocolitis remains conjectural. No evidence substantiates the claim that a preterm infant who is fed fresh breast milk or colostrum-containing lymphocytes enriched with secretory IgA has a lower risk of having necrotizing enterocolitis.

Early signs of sepsis in the newborn are subtle and include the development of hypothermia, bradycardia, and lethargy; seizures or apneic respiratory arrest usually are later sequelae. For this reason, preoperative prophylactic antibiotics generally are administered to babies undergoing major surgery or for suspected sepsis after appropriate cultures are obtained. The standard is a triple combination of ampicillin, gentamicin, and clindamycin, which provides broad-spectrum coverage against the common gram-positive and gram-negative organisms, including the anaerobic flora. Usually, gram-negative organisms are the cause of disseminated intravascular coagulation. This disorder most commonly affects the preterm infant who has necrotizing enterocolitis from peritonitis secondary to perforated bowel; it also may affect the full-term infant with meconium peritonitis, closed-loop obstruction, or midgut volvulus. A deterioration of the vital signs and progressing thrombocytopenia are adjunctive indicators for early intervention in the presence of confusing or misleading physical signs alone. Reversal of established sepsis requires a combination of prompt operation to remove the source of infection, adequate antibiotic coverage, fluid resuscitation, and such vasopressors as dopamine or dobutamine. They improve cardiac output, both by acting as inotropic agents and by stimulating the beta receptors of the heart. Dopamine and dobutamine may be used together when conventional measures have failed.

Use of Catheters for Diagnosis and Treatment

The careful placement of a small catheter in the upper esophageal pouch, the gastrointestinal or urinary tract, and the pleural space may be appropriate for both diagnostic and therapeutic purposes and may play an important role in the care of surgical neonates.

A feeding tube (8 Fr.) tests the patency of the choanae and upper esophagus. Passing the tube through each choana will rule out the possibility of membranous or bony choanal atresia in babies with upper-airway obstruction. Nasal discharge may be the only sign of unilateral choanal obstruction, but bilateral obstruction causes acute respiratory distress in newborns who are obligate nasal breathers. The diagnosis of esophageal atresia must be considered in babies with drooling or mucous oral secretions and episodes of coughing, choking, and cyanosis. This impression can be confirmed by gently passing a feeding catheter through the nose or mouth into the esophagus and meeting resistance in the upper thorax. The tube must be firm enough to avoid coiling in the upper pouch. Confirmation of the diagnosis of esophageal atresia is made by obtaining a plain chest roentgenogram that reveals the air-filled upper pouch accompanied by air in the stomach of babies with an associated distal tracheoesophageal fistula. Continuous suction of the upper esophageal pouch with a sump suction catheter prevents pooling of secretions and minimizes the risk of pulmonary aspiration.

Emptying the stomach with a nasogastric tube is useful in determining whether a newborn who is vomiting at birth or is not tolerating feedings has partial or complete intestinal obstruction. Residual volumes that are bile-tinged or in excess of 25 mL strongly suggest intestinal obstruction or ileus, and nasogastric decompression and intermittent suction are required. The tube should be taped to the upper lip or (in the case of a preterm infant) passed through the mouth.

A 5 or 8 FR. feeding catheter also can be used for decompression of the urinary tract obstructed by posterior urethral valves or in babies who have prune-belly syndrome with a congenital absence of abdominal wall musculature. Intermittent catheterization of the enlarged bladder is essential to prevent reflux and urinary tract infection that eventually may lead to a deterioration of the upper tracts and renal function. The careful placement of a catheter in a urogenital sinus or in the single orifice of a baby with a cloaca is done best under fluoroscopy so as to delineate the full anatomy. In some cases, the accessory orifices may be obstructed partially, and a full assessment of the underlying anatomy will require cystoscopy and (eventually) operative intervention.

The risk of a pneumothorax has decreased significantly with the advent of the pressure-limited, time-cycled ventilator, but any baby with unexplained oxygen desaturation or abnormal arterial blood gases requires prompt assessment for the presence of air in the pleural space or mediastinum. Transillumination of the thoracic cavity to confirm the clinical impression of a tension pneumothorax, followed by percutaneous aspiration of air using an Angiocath and the subsequent insertion of a chest tube, is a life-saving measure because mediastinal shift and compression of the contralateral lung are dramatic and possibly fatal events. Because the chest wall of a newborn is fairly thin, a bronchopleurocutaneous fistula may develop unless the chest tube is tunneled one or two interspaces above the insertion site, thereby preventing the tracking of air along the tube into the subcutaneous tissue and outside the body. Connection of the chest tube to underwater suction is required until the air leak has sealed.

Additional Diagnostic Tests

The evaluation for associated anomalies in a newborn with one major life-threatening congenital anomaly must be carried out within hours of birth. The incidence of an associated anomaly may be as high as 50% in babies with esophageal atresia or omphalocele or may be fairly low in gastroschisis or jejunoileal atresia. Well known in the surgical neonate is the so-called VACTERL syndrome (an association of vertebral, anorectal, cardiac, tracheoesophageal, and renal and limb anomalies). The cardiac anomalies in this condition may not be life-threatening (e.g., small ventricular septal defect), but they may be more complex, as in a baby with multiple intracardiac defects, and they require preoperative echocardiography for full assessment. In general, this procedure is carried out before the first operation in a baby with esophageal atresia or an anorectal anomaly, whereas urologic evaluation for associated renal abnormalities may be conducted by ultrasonography in the early postoperative period. Some prioritization of the additional diagnostic tests is important to avoid delaying the operation. The importance of chromosome analysis as part of the prenatal diagnosis has been discussed, but rarely should it interfere with the timing of surgery. In an emergency, a rapid assessment of the chromosome status may be achieved by harvesting cells from the bone marrow. One instance in which operation may be delayed is to determine the chromosome status of a baby with an omphalocele and presumed trisomy 13 or 18. If such is confirmed, we have preferred nonoperative treatment by simply covering the omphalocele sac with allograft or amniotic membrane. The graft protects the sac and prevents rupture with evisceration, rendering surgery unnecessary in patients with severe neurologic impairment and no hope for survival. On the other hand, infants born with duodenal atresia and Down syndrome should undergo surgical correction. In unusual instances, a court order may be required to carry out the surgery at an opportune time.

Informed Consent

Obtaining written operative consent should be viewed as the final extension of the preparation of the parents for an infant's surgery. Informed consent also should include a thorough understanding of the underlying condition, and the potential risks and benefits of the operation must be understood clearly by the parents before their signatures are obtained. Pertinent information should be given in each of the following categories: the diagnosis, the nature and purpose of the proposed treatment, the prognosis if the proposed treatment is carried out, the risks associated with the proposed treatment, the feasible treatment alternatives, and the prognosis if the treatment is refused. A written summary of what was told to the family by the surgeon also should be included on the operative consent form and in the hospital record, both for further clarification and as an indication that these subjects were discussed if litigation ever is raised in the future.

POSTOPERATIVE CARE

Certain general considerations and special issues regarding the postoperative care of newborns should be emphasized. Box 30.2 lists both general considerations and special issues in such postoperative care.

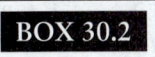

BOX 30.2 **Postoperative Care of the Newborn**

General Considerations
Maintenance and replacement of intravenous fluids
Core body temperature
Ventilatory support
Vascular access
Antibiotic coverage
Nasogastric decompression
Pain control

Special Issues
Total parenteral nutrition
Extracorporeal membrane oxygenation
Stomal care
Family support
Discharge home

The postoperative care of newborns is largely a continuum of the many steps already described as part of the preoperative preparation. The surgeon summarizes these concerns in a list of steps known as the *postoperative orders*. Several important issues should be reemphasized.

Maintaining a normal core body temperature in the operating room is difficult because of the large skin surface area and the tendency for the viscera to be exposed to a cooler environment during an abdominal or thoracic operation. For that reason, returning infants to the servocontrolled isolation incubator (Isolette) or radiant warmer immediately after the procedure is imperative, and core body temperature must be monitored carefully. In most cases, a 1°C to 2°C fluctuation can be reversed by rewarming within the first few hours after return to the newborn intensive care unit (NICU).

Some infants will require postoperative endotracheal ventilation until they are fully reactive and sustaining a normal respiratory pattern. With appropriate weaning of the intermittent mandatory ventilation rate and inspired oxygen content, elective extubation is possible under controlled circumstances, with the full staff available if the respiratory status falters. Preterm infants younger than 46 to 60 weeks' postconceptional age are at higher risk to develop apnea and bradycardia after general anesthesia. This issue is particularly relevant after elective procedures, such as inguinal herniorrhaphy in babies having a history of previous mechanical ventilation, bronchopulmonary dysplasia, or a patent ductus arteriosus.

Adequate vascular access should have been achieved before beginning the operative procedure. The position of the central venous line and the function of any peripheral line should, again, be assessed on returning infants to the nursery. In most instances, a plain chest roentgenogram will provide information about the position of the tip of the endotracheal tube, a central venous catheter, the status of the lungs, and even the location of the nasogastric tube. If an umbilical venous or arterial catheter has been inserted, an abdominal film also should be obtained to ascertain the position of the tip of the catheter. Umbilical artery catheters should be positioned clearly above the level of the renal vessels superimposed on the T11 and T12 vertebrae or just above the bifurcation of the aorta at the L2 or L3 level, but never at the presumed orifices of the renal or mesenteric arteries.

Appropriate antibiotic coverage should be continued for a minimum of 48 hours when any hollow viscus has been entered or for as long as 2 weeks when established peritonitis or intraabdominal abscess is being treated. In high-risk patients, such as preterm infants requiring inguinal herniorrhaphy, our usual practice has been to give a single dose of prophylactic antibiotics before commencing the operative procedure. In these patients, postoperative antibiotics are not required.

Maintaining adequate decompression of any hollow viscus entered during the course of the operative procedure is essential. Paramount to this end is the use of nasogastric decompression for gastrointestinal surgery. The smallest catheter that is effective at preventing distention is an 8 Fr. feeding tube. Smaller catheters are appropriate only for gavage feedings. Urinary tract drainage using a feeding catheter also may be indicated in selected instances, such as the need to monitor hourly urinary output or in cases of suspected bladder outlet obstruction. Bagging the perineum and performing a simple Credé maneuver will enable the quantitation of total urinary output and the determination of urine specific gravity.

Achieving adequate pain control has been a highly publicized, emotionally charged issue in the matter of newborns. Pain-induced wincing and cries, splinted ventilation, and tachycardia are recognized sequelae of inadequate pain control in babies undergoing major surgery. The placement of an epidural catheter for continuous and bolus infusion of hydromorphone in the epidural space is preferable to intravenous morphine for major thoracic and abdominal procedures. This approach has reduced the need for prolonged postoperative endotracheal ventilation and the risk of respiratory depression.

Special Issues

Achieving long-term venous access for the purpose of administering total parenteral nutrition, antibiotics, or blood and blood products has been a lifesaving measure in babies requiring major surgery. The majority of these patients have had multistage closure of omphalocele or gastroschisis, necrotizing enterocolitis with a proximal ileostomy, or short bowel syndrome after resection for midgut volvulus, intestinal atresia, or meconium ileus with meconium peritonitis. As indicated previously, a Broviac catheter or subclavian central venous line can be placed before leaving the operating room or by the fourth or fifth postoperative day, when sepsis no longer is a contraindication. When parenteral nutrition is needed, the glucose concentration should be increased to provide over several days a caloric intake adequate to prevent glycosuria. In preterm infants with a low renal threshold for the tubular excretion of glucose, supplementary insulin may be required to prevent glycosuria. Successful total parenteral nutrition is judged by the achievement of weight gain without catheter sepsis or metabolic complications.

Extracorporeal membrane oxygenation (ECMO) has progressed from a clinical research project to a recognized practice in the management of severe neonatal respiratory failure. The 1999 Neonatal Extra-Corporeal Life Support Organization Registry (Ann Arbor, MI) reported a survival rate in excess of 80% for 13,138 babies treated in 117 active centers. Indications included pulmonary immaturity, meconium aspiration syndrome, congenital diaphragmatic hernia, and persistent pulmonary hypertension rather than pulmonary parenchymal disease. Survival ranged from 59% for congenital diaphragmatic hernia to 94% of babies with meconium aspiration. ECMO is performed in a specially dedicated area within the neonatal special care unit; it entails the cannulation of the carotid artery and jugular vein in the neck under local anesthesia. A modified heart-lung machine (Fig. 30.2) is used to take over part or all of cardiac and lung function for a period as long as 3 weeks, although the usual time on ECMO is 5 to 7 days. Vital to the success of this procedure is the experience and training of the ECMO team, which includes the pediatric surgeon supervising the procedure and the assisting neonatologist, nurse, perfusionist, and respiratory therapist. Proper patient selection also increases the likelihood for success by excluding babies with severe bilateral pulmonary hypoplasia, intracranial hemorrhage, structural cardiac defects, preterm infants younger than 34 weeks' gestation, and patients with irreversible lung disease, such as those with severe bronchopulmonary dysplasia.

Congenital diaphragmatic hernia in babies who have failed to respond to "gentle" mechanical ventilation for persistent fetal circulation remains the principal indication for ECMO, both before operation and postoperatively. The potential for eventual survival after repair generally is heralded by a "honeymoon period," during which time reasonably normal oxygenation can be achieved. The extended use of hyperventilation and pulmonary arterial vasodilators, such as tolazoline, tends to aggravate underlying pulmonary disease by introducing an element of barotrauma. High-frequency oscillatory ventilation, inhaled nitric oxide, and liquid ventilation are currently used in high-risk congenital diaphragmatic hernia patients before ECMO, but improved outcome with these modalities has not been documented.

The creation of an intestinal stoma is necessary in most babies with necrotizing enterocolitis and in selected patients with meconium ileus and anorectal anomalies. A centrally located

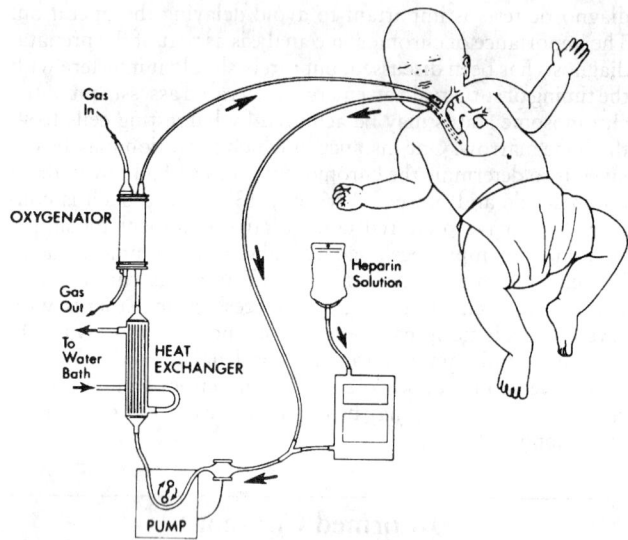

FIGURE 30.2. Extracorporeal membrane oxygenation perfusion system. (Reprinted with permission from Krummel TM, Greenfield LJ, Kirkpatrick BV, et al. Clinical use of an extra-corporeal oxygenator in neonatal pulmonary failure. *J Pediatr Surg* 1982;17:526.)

single stoma, to a large extent, will ease postoperative care. When the stoma begins to function by evacuating liquid meconium, effluent is captured with a collecting bag. Occasionally, the functional stoma will be accompanied by a second, more distal stoma known as a *mucus fistula*. The stomas should be separated by space sufficient to prevent spillover of intestinal contents. A 3% bismuth tribromophenate/petrolatum blend (Xeroform) or petroleum jelly dressing of the second stoma is more than sufficient to prevent mucosal ulceration and bleeding. In almost all patients, except those with long-segment Hirschsprung disease and anorectal malformations, intestinal tract continuity is restored before they are discharged from the unit. Several weeks may pass, however, during which time adequate weight gain is achieved by a combination of parenteral and oral nutrition. Nonnutritive feedings of small aliquots of an elemental diet may minimize the risk of cholestatic jaundice and the subsequent development of sludge or calculi in the biliary tract. When preterm babies reach the approximate weight of 2.0 kg, contrast studies of the unused (distal) portion of the gastrointestinal tract are indicated, either via the rectum or the mucus fistula, to rule out the presence of an intrinsic obstruction or stricture. Then reconstitution of the gastrointestinal tract can be carried out, and the risk of intercurrent salt and water imbalance from diarrheal illness will be avoided. Bile–acid diarrhea continues to be a problem in certain patients, even after the stomas have been closed. Both cholestyramine, a bile salt resin that prevents choleretic enteropathy, and bismuth subsalicylate (Pepto Bismol) have been used successfully in our nursery to prevent this complication.

Perhaps the single most important role of surgeons in the postoperative period is dealing with the family's anxiety and providing emotional support. Although much of this duty is shared naturally by neonatologists, primary nurses, and social workers, those surgeons who performed the operative procedure must remain in close, even daily, contact with the family and be ready to explain clearly the steps and measures that are being used in the recovery period. Because untimely events or even reoperation is common, early discussions of any trend are important to prepare the patient's family appropriately. The day of discharge home is one of great celebration for both the natural and extended family of a baby who has required prolonged hospitalization in the newborn special care unit.

Suggested Readings

Barlow B, Santulli TV, Heird WC, et al. An experimental study of acute neonatal enterocolitis—the importance of breast milk. *J Pediatr Surg* 1974;9:587.

Bartlett RH, Toomasian J, Roloff D, et al. Extracorporeal membrane oxygenation (ECMO) in neonatal respiratory failure. *Ann Surg* 1986;204:236.

Bethel CAI, Seashore JH, Touloukian RJ. Cesarean section does not improve outcome in gastroschisis. *J Pediatr Surg* 1989;24:1.

Chervenak FA, Isaacson G, Touloukian RJ, et al. Diagnosis and management of fetal teratomas. *Obstet Gynecol* 1985;66:666.

Dudrick SJ, Wilmore DW, Vars HM, et al. Long-term parenteral nutrition with growth development and positive nitrogen balance. *Surgery* 1968;64:134.

Fonkalsrud EW. Pediatric surgery—a specialty come of age. *J Pediatr Surg* 1991;26:239.

Gertler JP, Seashore JH, Touloukian RJ. Early ileostomy closure in necrotizing enterocolitis. *J Pediatr Surg* 1987;22:140.

Gollin G, Bell C, Dubose R, et al. Predictors of postoperative respiratory complications in premature infants and inguinal herniorrhaphy. *J Pediatr Surg* 1993;28:244.

Harrison MR, Golbus MS, Filly RA. *The unborn patient. Management of the fetus with a correctable defect.* San Diego: Grune & Stratton, 1984.

Henry MC. Moss RL. Current issues in the management of necrotizing enterocolitis. *Sem Perinatol* 2004;28:221.

Pletcher BA, Friedes JS, Breg WR, Touloukian RJ. Familial occurrence of esophageal atresia with and without tracheoesophageal fistula: report of two unusual kindred. *Am J Med Genet* 1991;39:380.

Quan L, Smith DW. The VATER association: vertebral defects, anal atresia, TE fistula with esophageal atresia, radial and renal dysplasia. *J Pediatr* 1973; 83:104.

Smith NP. Jesudason EC. Featherstone NC. Corbett HJ. Losty PD. Recent advances in congenital diaphragmatic hernia. *Arch Dis Childhood* 2005; 90:426.

Touloukian RJ, Hobbins J. Maternal ultrasound in the antenatal diagnosis of surgically correctable fetal abnormalities. *J Pediatr Surg* 1980;15: 373.

Touloukian RJ, Keller MS. High proximal pouch esophageal atresia with vertebral, rib, and sternal anomalies: an additional component of the VATER association. *J Pediatr Surg* 1988;23:76.

Touloukian RJ, Markowitz RI. A preoperative x-ray scoring system for risk assessment of newborns with congenital diaphragmatic hernia. *J Pediatr Surg* 1984;19:252.

Touloukian RJ, Weiss RM. The obstructed bladder syndrome in the neonate. *Surg Gynecol Obstet* 1976;143:965.

e: NEONATAL NERVOUS SYSTEM

CHAPTER 31 ■ NEUROEMBRYOLOGY

LAURA R. MENT AND BARBARA R. POBER

Congenital malformations of the central nervous system represent a major cause of infantile mortality and morbidity and result in neuroanatomic abnormalities that range from the structural to the cellular levels. The basis for some of the more common central nervous system malformations is discussed in this chapter within the context of development of the fetal neuraxis.

NEURAL TUBE DEFECTS

Neural tube defects (NTDs) are among the most common congenital malformations and occur in more than 1 per 1,000 live births. For this reason, they are also among the best studied. The fetal nervous system begins development on the eighteenth day of gestation. The primordial neural tube is derived from the ectodermal layer, and the ectoderm on the dorsal portion of the embryo, along with the underlying notochord and chordal mesoderm, induces the formation of the neural plate. Closure of the neuroectoderm begins on the twenty-second day of gestation and is accomplished by invagination of the lateral margins of the neural plate. Experimental animal data and empirical human data suggest that closure of the neural tube begins independently in several different sites along the tube; bidirectional "zippering" between closure sites then follows. The anterior neuropore closes by day 25 or 26 and the posterior neuropore closes 2 to 3 days later to form a closed, continuous cavity that constitutes the primitive ventricular system and central canal of the cord.

Disruption of the neural tube closure process at any of the primary closure sites produces variable-sized defects in different anatomic locations, resulting in the recognized conditions of anencephaly, spina bifida, encephalocele, and spinal dysraphism. In the majority of cases, the NTD is the only malformation present in the affected child; however, a significant fraction of patients have additional congenital malformations, an underlying genetic condition, or both.

Anencephaly, the presence of an exposed rostral mass of neural tissue, is produced by the early failure of anterior neural tube closure and has an incidence of approximately .3 to .35 in 1,000 births. Approximately 15% of these infants are stillborn, and the rest die shortly after birth.

Encephalocele, an insult thought to occur on approximately the twenty-sixth gestational day, can be a less severe malformation involving defective closure of a portion of the neural tube in association with a bony skull defect. Although 75% to 80% of these lesions occur in the occipital region, similar abnormalities have been noted in the frontal and parietal regions. Frontal and nasal encephaloceles are more common in infants of Asian ancestry and frequently present in the newborn period. In this condition, a soft sac of varying size protrudes through a bony defect and may contain only cranial meninges or meninges and neural tissue. Communication usually is present between the ventricular cavity and the encephalocele, and hydrocephalus may be noted. Encephaloceles are the least frequent of the NTDs and occur in 1 in 5,000 to 1 in 10,000 live births. Compared with anencephaly and spina bifida, however, encephaloceles are more commonly associated with other birth defects or occur as part of genetic syndromes.

The most common form of spina bifida, myelomeningocele, is a restricted failure of posterior caudal neural tube closure believed to occur before 26 days' gestation. The majority of these lesions occur in the lumbar and lumbosacral regions, and the incidence is said to be between .4 and .5 per 1,000, with one of the highest incidences found in the northern regions of the British Isles. Pathologically, the majority of lesions result in a dorsal displacement of neural tissue such that a sac or an open placode remains on the infant's back. Skeletal anomalies, including absence of the vertebral arches, lateral displacement of the pedicles, and a widened spinal canal, are present uniformly, and an incomplete, although variable, dermal covering is present. Clinical features relate to the level of the spinal cord that is involved and to the extent of the lesion. Generally, disturbances in lower extremity motor function, sphincter function, and bladder function are noted. Secondary orthopedic problems of the lower extremities (dislocated hips, clubfeet, and congenital contractures known as *arthrogryposis*) can occur *in utero* because of lack of fetal movement. Hydrocephalus is seen in almost 75% of cases and is associated nearly always with a type II Chiari malformation or kinking and elongation of brainstem structures. The morbidity and mortality seen in this disorder are dictated by the level of the lesion. High lesions (above T11) are associated with higher morbidity, lower intelligence, and greater disability, whereas the outcome for individuals with lower lesions (below L3) is considerably better. Other factors influencing outcome include complications of meningitis (from the open sac), hydrocephalus, and renal involvement. In addition, delivery by cesarean section has been advocated to preserve lower extremity function to the fullest extent.

Other dysraphic states include meningocele and diastematomyelia. Meningocele is herniation of the meninges unaccompanied by neural tissue and covered by skin or a thin-walled membrane. Similar to myelomeningocele, these lesions are most common in the lumbosacral region, and defects in the vertebral arches may be present. Some patients have abnormalities of gait, particularly during periods of rapid growth, or loss of previously acquired bladder control. Meningoceles generally are not associated with hydrocephalus.

Spina bifida occulta usually refers to a vertebral defect without herniation of the contents of the spinal canal. This condition is found most commonly in the lumbosacral region and has been noted radiographically in as many as 15% of the general population. Occasionally, spina bifida occulta may be suspected by the presence of hairy tufts or birthmarks at the base of the spine. Rarely, a sinus tract may lead into an intraspinal cyst or epidermoid structure. All infants with recurrent gram-negative bacterial meningitis should be examined carefully for sinus tracts, because these may act as a source of infection.

In diastematomyelia, the spinal cord is divided by a bony or cartilaginous spur extending from the dorsal surface of the vertebral body. This is associated with an NTD in more than 50% of cases and may cause neurologic deficits by producing traction on the cord. Lipomas are hamartomatous lesions associated with dysraphic states and are located most commonly in the region of the filum terminale.

Although the occult dysraphic states may go undetected in early childhood, 80% are associated with dermal lesions and vertebral defects. Later in childhood, as the spinal cord ascends to its position in adult life, patients may have gait disturbances, foot deformities, sphincter dysfunction, and scoliosis. The failure of the spinal cord to ascend, as a result of either primary malformation or secondary tumor, is known as *tethering of the cord.*

The cause, or causes, of NTDs are currently under investigation. Candidate genes involved in NTDs include many genes in the folate metabolism pathway as well as those responsible for folate transport. Genes in this pathway have been the focus of intense research effort since convincing proof that periconceptual vitamin supplementation with folic acid reduces NTD occurrence by approximately 70%. Although variations in several genes, such as 5,10-methylenetetrahydrofolate reductase, appear to confer risk of NTDs in selected populations, no single gene has been identified as causal of NTDs in humans. Research in model organisms, such as the recent discovery that mutations in the gene Scrb1 cause NTDs in mice, suggest that gene identification in humans will be shortly forthcoming.

The majority of NTDs occur as isolated birth defects but as many as 20% occur in association with other birth defects, chromosome abnormalities, or specific genetic syndromes; recognition of the latter subgroups is important, as the recurrence risk could be high. Another group at high risk for NTDs is the children of women receiving anticonvulsants such as valproic acid or carbamazepine; the incidence of spina bifida is as high as 1% to 2% in exposed fetuses. However, most cases of NTDs are isolated and are attributed to "multifactorial inheritance," meaning a combination of unidentified genes and environmental factors that interact to interfere with normal neural tube closure. Once a couple has given birth to a child with a multifactorially caused NTD, the chance of a second child being affected is approximately 3% to 4%. If a couple has two children with NTDs, the recurrence risk rises to 10% to 15% for subsequent children. Prenatal diagnosis of NTDs is widely available and is strongly recommended for mothers at higher than baseline population risk. Maternal serum alpha-fetoprotein tests performed during the fifteenth to eighteenth weeks of pregnancy detect 88% to 100% of cases of anencephaly and 80% of cases of open spina bifida. False-positive test results are related to twin gestation, underestimation of gestational age, other open body defects, or threatened or missed abortion. When the serum alpha-fetoprotein level is elevated, ultrasonographic examination to evaluate for gestational age, multiple pregnancy, or congenital malformations is indicated. If sonographic examination fails to identify the cause of the elevated serum alpha-fetoprotein, an amniocentesis and amniotic fluid alpha-fetoprotein determination should be performed.

Data from numerous studies have demonstrated that periconceptual vitamin supplementation with folic acid significantly reduces the occurrence of NTDs in all couples, whether or not a family history of this problem exists. The biologic basis for this effect is as yet unknown but presumably is attributable to correction of an underlying genetic defect with high-dose folate supplementation.

DISORDERS OF VENTRAL INDUCTION

The concept of ventral induction refers to the developmental events that occur under the primary influence of the prechordal mesoderm. The major inductive relationship between the prechordal mesoderm and the developing cerebrum occurs ventrally at the rostral end of the fetus and influences the development of the forebrain and facial structures.

Holoprosencephaly

Malformations of the forebrain generally have been attributed to failure of normal segmentation and cleavage of the prosencephalon into paired cerebral hemispheres. In holoprosencephaly (HPE), there are varying degrees of failure of the primordial forebrain to divide into separate cerebral hemispheres. At the most severe end of the spectrum, the cerebral hemispheres remain as a single-sphered structure having a large central ventricle with abnormalities of the basal ganglia, thalami,

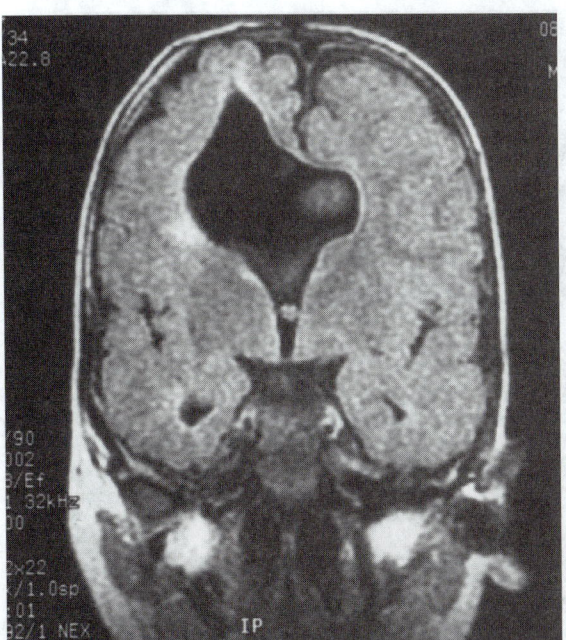

FIGURE 31.1. This magnetic resonance imaging scan of a young infant with a large head (greater than 95% for age) demonstrates holoprosencephaly. Note the single large frontal ventricle with failure of division of the single frontal hemisphere.

and hypothalamus. A magnetic resonance imaging scan of a patient with holoprosencephaly is provided in Figure 31.1; note the presence of the large, single, frontal ventricle in this young child with macrocephaly and motor delay. HPE may also result in abnormalities of the optic and facial structures.

HPE is thought to be the most common disorder of neural development during embryogenesis, but has been reported to occur in only 1 in 13,000 live births because of the high incidence of fetal demise among affected embryos. Although the occurrence of this condition is usually sporadic, approximately 20% of cases of holoprosencephaly have an identifiable genetic cause. Several different genes responsible for HPE have been reported. One form of autosomal dominant familial HPE is caused by mutations in the sonic hedgehog gene (SHH) located on chromosome 7; a small percentage of sporadic cases are also caused by mutations in this gene. The protein product of the SHH gene is thought to function as one of the midline signals responsible for cleavage of the cerebral hemispheres. Mutations in the SHH gene are associated with a broad range of problems, from seemingly asymptomatic mutation carriers to cyclopia and holoprosencephaly. Additional genes responsible for HPE include TGIF, ZIC2, SIX3, PTCH, and CRIPTO. TGIF and ZIC2 are located on chromosomes 18 and 13, respectively, which is not surprising given the presence of numerous reports of cytogenetic abnormalities involving these chromosomes. Interestingly, approximately 4% of patients with Smith-Lemli-Opitz syndrome, an autosomal recessive disorder caused by a block in cholesterol synthesis, have HPE, suggesting an important role for cholesterol in normal forebrain development.

Facial anomalies in children with HPE range from a single median eye and rudimentary nasal structures to ocular hypotelorism or hypertelorism and median cleft lip and cleft palate. The majority of affected infants are reported to have severe neurologic impairment and die shortly after birth. A small fraction of children with milder forms of HPE associated with less severe forebrain defects survive, and some become ambulatory and sufficiently verbal to attend special schools.

Agenesis of the Corpus Callosum

Development of the corpus callosum is associated with migrational events in the divided cerebrum. The earliest fibers appear at 11 weeks of gestation and formation is complete at 20 weeks. Agenesis of the corpus callosum (ACC), either partial or complete, is therefore a marker of migrational dysgenesis, and ACC may be either an isolated, primary event or secondary to metabolic, structural, or chromosomal abnormalities of corticogenesis.

Not surprisingly, the clinical features vary from the incidental finding of callosal agenesis on magnetic resonance imaging, computed tomographic (CT) scan, or autopsy examination to developmental delay, seizures, and motor abnormalities. A characteristic CT scan is shown in Figure 31.2; complete ACC can be accurately diagnosed by prenatal ultrasonography after 20 to 22 weeks of gestation.

ACC frequently occurs as an isolated malformation without other central nervous system or systemic defects. Although most of these cases appear to be sporadic and are therefore associated with a low recurrence risk, families with X-linked, autosomal dominant, and autosomal recessive ACC have been reported. The underlying genetic mutations in these families have yet to be identified.

ACC can also occur with additional central nervous system and systemic malformations. Many of these more complex associations represent chromosomal, genetic, or metabolic syndromes. Chromosomal abnormalities associated with ACC include trisomies 13 and 18; the metabolic disorders associated with ACC include glutaric aciduria type 2, nonketotic hyperglycinemia (Fig. 31.3), pyruvate dehydrogenase deficiency, and Zellweger syndrome. Finally, several specific genetic syndromes are associated with ACC. Two well-recognized X-linked genetic conditions are Aicardi syndrome (ACC, infantile spasms, and chorioretinal lacunae) and hydrocephalus with stenosis of the aqueduct of Sylvius. The latter has been shown to be caused by mutations in the L1 cell adhesion molecule, L1CAM, a protein involved in neuronal migration and growth.

DISORDERS OF NERVE CELL PROLIFERATION

During the second through fourth gestational months, cells of the developing brain proliferate and migrate. Most of the developing neurons and glial cells arise from the primordial cells found in the periventricular germinal matrix, or subventricular zone. Within this region, the cells migrate back and forth, dividing at the ventricular surface to enter the pool of progenitors. In response to signals that are not yet known, a fraction of the postmitotic cells exit the cell cycle to become neurons or glia, and migrate outward toward the newly formed cortical plate. Primary neuronal migrations occur in the second through fourth gestational months, whereas glial precursors that arise in the germinal zone may continue to proliferate in postnatal life.

Microcephaly

Primary microcephaly is often a genetic condition. The most common forms of primary microcephaly are autosomal recessive disorders characterized by severe microcephaly (greater than two standard deviations below the mean for age, sex, and gestation), intellectual impairment, and poor speech. This abnormality is thought to derive from a neuronal cell proliferation abnormality that occurs before the fourth month of gestation. Neuropathologic defects in gyral pattern and cortical

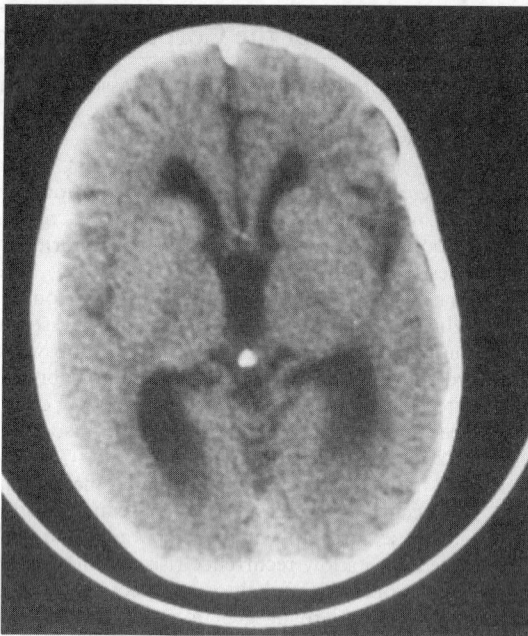
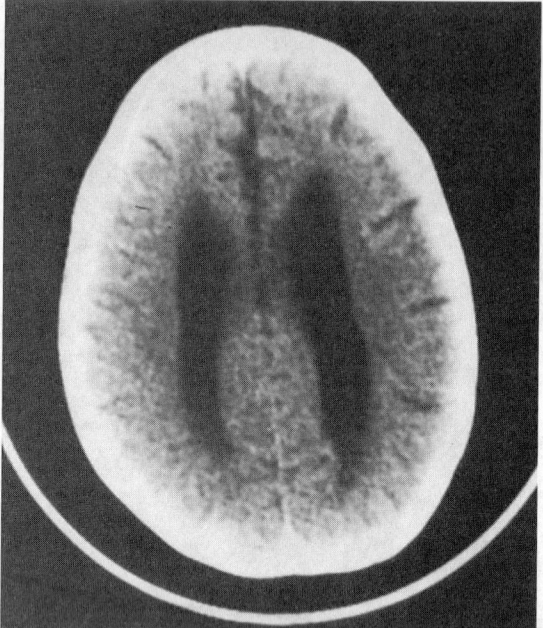

FIGURE 31.2. In these computed tomographic scans of an infant with seizures and agenesis of the corpus callosum, the lateral ventricles appear parallel and closer in position than might be expected. The third ventricle is enlarged and occupies a relatively superior position in this study. Finally, the interhemispheric fissure can be traced dorsally to the third ventricle.

lamination, as well as heterotopias, have been reported. Several different genetic loci have been mapped for autosomal recessive microcephalies, and four responsible genes have been identified. The gene for microcephaly type 1 encodes for the protein microcephalin and mutations result in premature chromosome condensation which may be detected on routine chromosome analysis.

Autosomal dominant microcephaly has also been observed in numerous families; intelligence is generally normal or only mildly impaired.

Primary microcephaly can be a feature of numerous genetic syndromes such as Rubinstein-Taybi, Cornelia de Lange, and Dubowitz syndromes, as well as a finding in most children with chromosomal abnormalities such as trisomies 21, 18, and 13.

Secondary microcephaly usually refers to a small head circumference and, thus, a small brain as a result of some insult occurring during the latter half of pregnancy or in the perinatal period. Secondary microcephaly is found in association with maternal drug ingestion, maternal phenylketonuria, fetal alcohol syndrome, radiation before 20 weeks' gestation, and congenital infections, including rubella, cytomegalovirus, coxsackievirus, and toxoplasmosis. Suspected other causes include intrauterine or perinatal anoxia or trauma and metabolic disorders.

Macrencephaly

Macrencephaly is observed in a heterogenous group of disorders and refers to the presence of a large or "heavy" brain. Although macrencephaly is not well described neuropathologically, it is found in association with a number of genetic syndromes, some of which are diagnosable by specific genetic testing, including Sotos syndrome (cerebral gigantism), Beckwith-Wiedemann syndrome, achondroplasia, neurofibromatosis, multiple hemangiomatosis, and familial isolated macrencephaly. The alterations in corticogenesis resulting in macrencephaly may be unique for each of these conditions.

Hemimegalencephaly

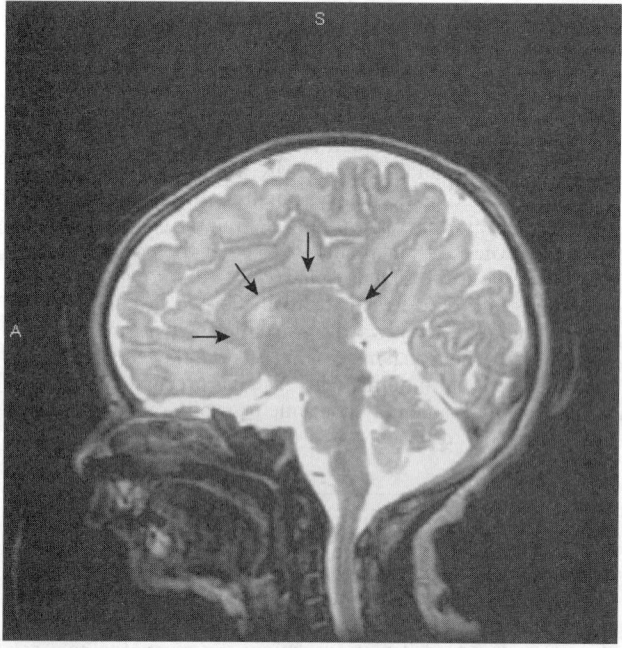

FIGURE 31.3. This T1 magnetic resonance imaging scan of a neonate with hypotonia and seizures demonstrates agenesis of the corpus callosum; metabolic testing revealed a diagnosis of nonketotic hyperglycinemia.

Hemimegalencephaly, or unilateral megalencephaly (Fig. 31.4), is a rare hamartomatous malformation of the brain. Hemimegalencephaly is considered to be a primary disturbance in

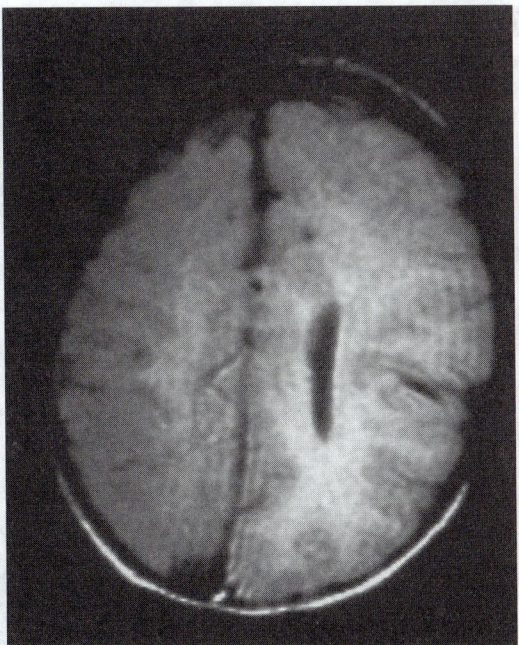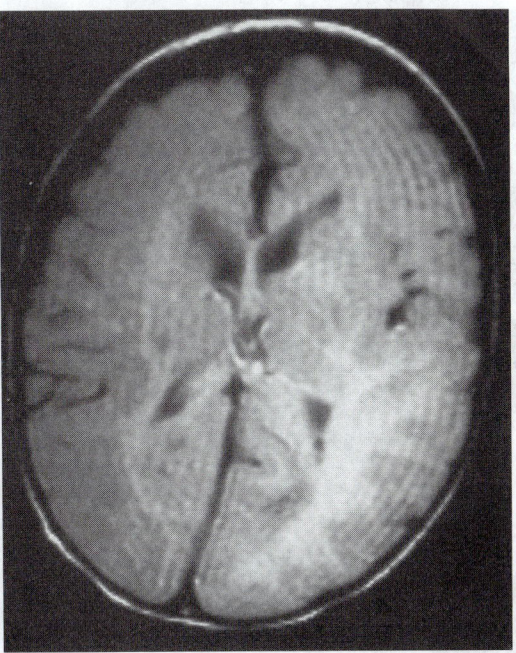

FIGURE 31.4. This magnetic resonance imaging scan of hemimegalencephaly shows a larger hemisphere on the right with posterior pachygyria. This condition is associated with the clinical triad of intractable seizures, profound developmental delay, and progressive hemiparesis.

cellular lineage, differentiation, and proliferation, and results in cortical overgrowth characterized by significant increases in the number of cortical synapses and secondary pachygyria of one cerebral hemisphere. This condition may be diagnosed by prenatal ultrasonography; postnatally, symptoms include a triad of clinical findings characterized by intractable seizures, profound developmental delay, and progressive hemiparesis. Patients with hemimegalencephaly may require epilepsy surgery to achieve adequate seizure control.

DISORDERS OF NERVE CELL MIGRATION

Lissencephaly

During the third to fifth months of gestation, abnormalities of the migrating neuroblasts and glioblasts may result in abnormal gyral development. Lissencephaly, or "smooth" brain with little or no gyral pattern, includes a spectrum of gyral malformations ranging from complete agyria (absent gyri) to regional pachygyria (broad gyri). An abnormally thick cortex, reduced or abnormal lamination, and diffuse neuronal heterotopias are the hallmarks of lissencephaly. To date, five genes have been discovered that cause lissencephaly in humans: LIS1 (platelet-activating factor acetylhydrolase), 14-3-3-epsilon, DCX, RELN, and ARX. Mutations in DCX, a gene on the X chromosome, causes subcortical band heterotopias in female carriers but severe lissencephaly in affected males.

Classical (previously known as type I) lissencephaly is associated with brain abnormalities ranging from generalized agyria–pachygyria to subcortical band heterotopias. Classical lissencephaly is recognized most commonly in two genetically related disorders, Miller-Diecker syndrome and isolated lissencephaly sequence. Patients with either disorder have profound neurologic problems, including seizures, mental retardation, hypotonia, and feeding abnormalities, but those with Miller-Diecker syndrome have, in addition, characteristic dysmorphic facial features. Both of these disorders are caused by alterations in the gene LIS1, located on chromosome 17p13.3; specifically, mutations in the LIS1 gene cause isolated lissencephaly sequence, whereas patients with Miller-Diecker syndrome have a deletion-producing loss of the LIS1 gene plus several adjacent genes including 14-3-3-epsilon. X-linked lissencephaly with abnormal genitalia is a form of lissencephaly associated with absent corpus callosum, neonatal seizures, temperature instability likely due to hypothalamic dysfunction, and abnormal genitalia with micropenis and cryptorchidism. ARX is the causative gene for this condition. Although the genetic alterations causing lissencephaly are usually sporadic *de novo* mutations, every effort should be made to confirm the presence of a mutation or deletion so recurrence risk counseling and prenatal diagnostic testing can be offered. Recurrence can be particularly high for the X-linked disorders, DCX and ARX, if the mother is a mutation carrier.

Cobblestone (previously type II) lissencephaly is associated with agyria, pachygyria, and polymicrogyria with a "pebbled" cortical surface; additional defects such as hydrocephalus, brainstem and cerebellar hypoplasia, and retinal abnormalities are frequent, and congenital muscular dystrophy may be present as well. The type II lissencephaly syndromes, Walker-Warburg syndrome and Fukuyama muscular dystrophy, are related autosomal recessive disorders caused by mutations in the genes FCMD and POMT1.

The neuroimaging studies of infants with this condition are characterized by a paucity of periventricular white matter, a squared configuration of the lateral ventricles, and abnormal gyral patterns, as shown in Figure 31.5. Similarly, the brains of infants with pachygyria demonstrate relatively few broad gyri with an abnormally thick cortical plate. Like children with lissencephaly, those with pachygyria suffer profound neurodevelopmental disability, seizures, and shortened lifespan.

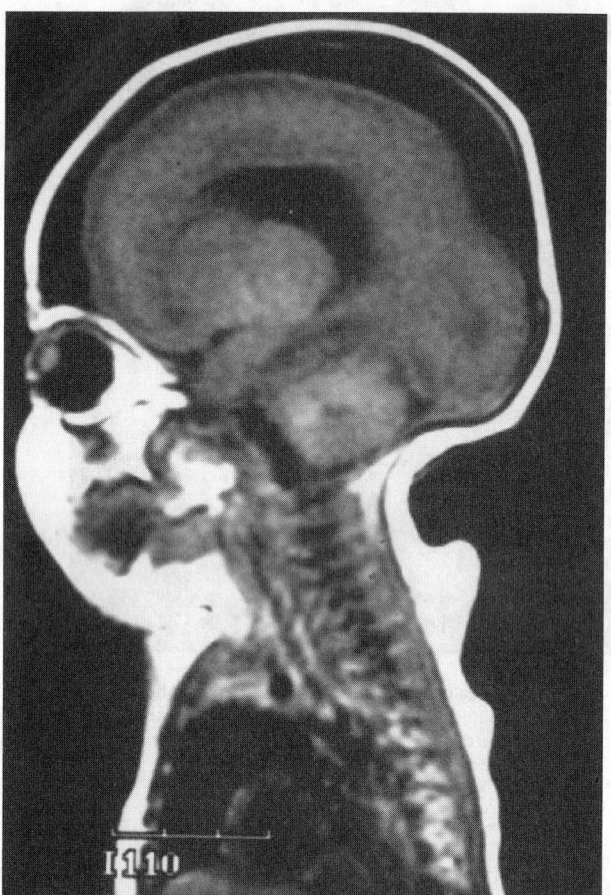
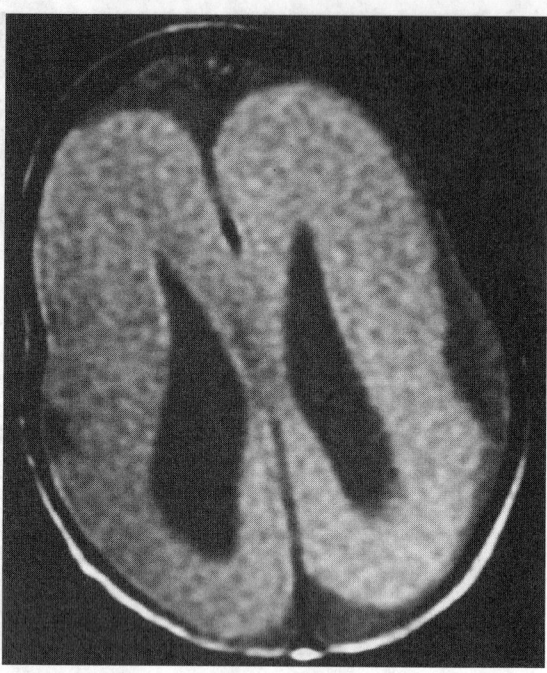

FIGURE 31.5. These magnetic resonance imaging scans of an infant with microcephaly and seizures demonstrate the enlarged configuration of the lateral ventricles, paucity of periventricular white matter, and abnormal gyral pattern characteristic of lissencephaly.

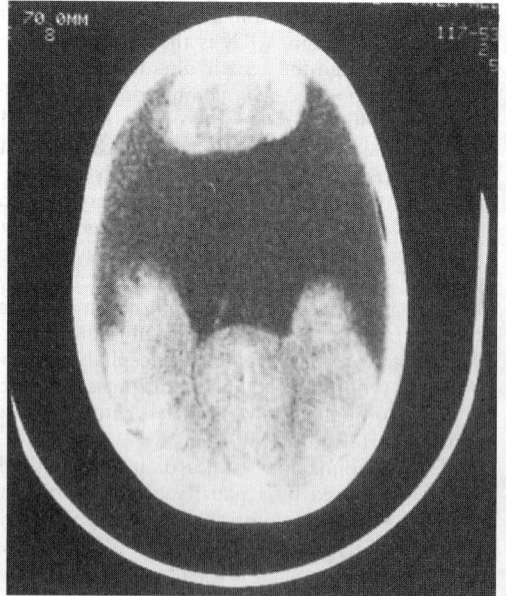
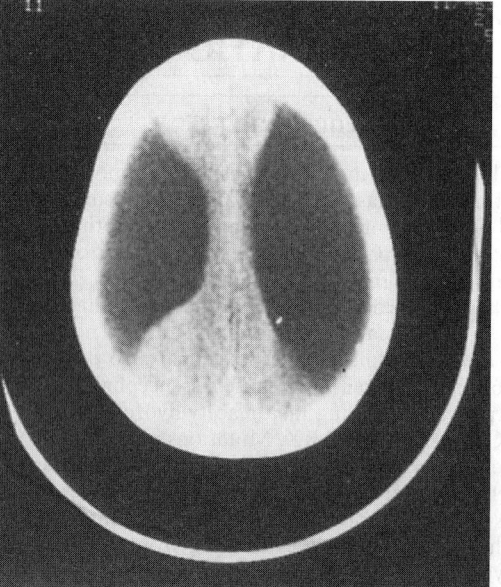

FIGURE 31.6. These computed tomographic scans of a 2-year-old boy with schizencephaly, seizures, and profound developmental delay are characterized by large bilaterally symmetric hemispheric clefts that communicate with the ventricular system.

DISORDERS OF LATE NEURONAL MIGRATION

Polymicrogyria

Polymicrogyria is a disorder characterized by the presence of multiple small gyri with abnormal cortical lamination. Although environmental insults including intrauterine hypoxia-ischemia and congenital infections have been reported in some cases of polymicrogyria, several syndromes of bilateral polymicrogyria have recently been described, suggesting a genetic basis for some of these disorders. These include bilateral frontal polymicrogyria, bilateral perisylvian polymicrogyria, and bilateral parasagittal parietooccipital polymicrogyria. The first of these has been mapped to a locus on chromosome 16q12-21 on mutations in the gene GPR56 have recently been identified. In its most severe form, polymicrogyria has been associated with severe developmental delay, seizures, dysconjugate gaze, and bilateral pyramidal and cerebellar signs.

Schizencephaly

Schizencephaly similarly represents a severe form of migrational disturbance, probably also occurring before the third month of gestation. In this disorder, bilateral, symmetric congenital clefts form in the region of the sylvian fissures. Infolding of the cortical gray matter occurs, and a pial–ependymal seam extends from the surface of the brain into the ventricle. Both unilateral and bilateral schizencephaly have been reported, and the etiology of schizencephaly has been attributed to both early vascular events in the developing brain as well as primary cerebral development anomalies, such as the schizencephaly found in patients with mutations in the homeobox gene *EMX2*.

Clinically, most infants are developmentally delayed severely and suffer seizures and spasticity; many also develop hydrocephalus. The CT scan of an infant with schizencephaly (Fig. 31.6) dramatically demonstrates the bilateral symmetric clefts.

Suggested Readings

Barkovich AJ, Kuzniecky RI, Jackson GD, et al. Classification system for malformations of cortical development; update 2001. *Neurology* 2001;57:2168.

Chang BS, Piao X, Bodell A, et al. Bilateral frontoparietal polymicrogyria: clinical and radiological features in 10 families with linkage to chromosome 16. *Ann Neurol* 2003;53:596.

Cohen MM. Malformations of the craniofacial region: evolutionary, embryonic, genetic and clinical perspectives. *Am J Med Gen (Semin Med Genet)* 2002;115:245.

Finnell RH, Gould A, Spiegelstein O. Pathobiology and genetics of neural tube defects. *Epilepsia* 2003;44(Suppl 3):14.

Frey L, Hauser WA. Epidemiology of neural tube defects. *Epilepsia* 2003;44:4.

Hunt GM, Poulton A. Open spina bifida: a complete cohort reviewed 25 years after closure. *Dev Med Child Neurol* 1995;37:19.

Iannetti P, Spalice A, Atzei G, et al. Neuronal migrational disorders in children with epilepsy: MRI, interictal SPECT and EEG comparisons. *Brain Dev* 1996;18:269.

Kato M, Dobyns WB. Lissencephaly and the molecular basis of neuronal migration. *Hum Molec Gen* 2003;12:R89.

Packard AM, Miller VS, Delgado MR. Schizencephaly: correlations of clinical and radiologic features. *Neurology* 1997;48:1427.

Rakic P, Yakovley PI. Development of the corpus callosum and cavum septi in man. *J Comp Neurol* 1968;132:45.

Roessler E, Muenke M. How a hedgehog might see holoprosencephaly. *Hum Molec Gen* 2003;12:R15.

Uyanik G, Aigner L, Martin PR, et al. ARX mutations in X-linked lissencephaly with abnormal genitalia. *Neurology* 2003;61:232.

Yakoyley PI, Wadsworth BC. Schizencephalies: a study of the congenital clefts in the cerebral mantle. I. Clefts with fused lips. *J Neuropathol Exp Neurol* 1946;5:116.

CHAPTER 32 ■ INTRAVENTRICULAR HEMORRHAGE OF THE PRETERM INFANT

LAURA R. MENT

Intraventricular hemorrhage (IVH), or hemorrhage into the germinal matrix tissues with possible rupture into the ventricular system and parenchyma of the developing brain (Fig. 32.1), remains a major problem of preterm neonates. It is believed to be the result of alterations in cerebral blood flow (CBF) to the immature germinal matrix capillary bed. Because the germinal matrix begins to involute after 34 weeks of gestation, germinal matrix hemorrhages (GMHs) and IVH are lesions of preterm infants, and the incidence of GMH/IVH in infants of less than 1,500-g birth weight is now reported to range from 15% to 30%. Seizures, hydrocephalus, periventricular leukomalacia (PVL), and neonatal death are more frequent in infants with GMH/IVH than in those without hemorrhage, when matched for birth weight or gestational age. In addition, although the long-term neurodevelopmental outcome for those infants with lower grades of hemorrhage remains unclear, most observers agree that infants with parenchymal involvement of hemorrhage are at high risk for neurodevelopmental handicap.

Cranial ultrasonography (Fig. 32.2) is the method of choice for diagnosis of GMH/IVH in newborn special care units. A standard grading system, which originally was applied to the computed tomographic scan, has been adapted to cranial ultrasonography examinations. Grade I (or GMH) describes blood in the germinal matrix only, grade II is blood filling the lateral ventricles without distention, grade III is blood filling and distending the ventricular system, and grade IV describes hemorrhages with parenchymal involvement (Table 32.1). The most common site for parenchymal involvement of hemorrhage is the frontal region; many hemorrhages occur bilaterally. Less commonly, the caudate nuclei and occipital periventricular white matter regions are also involved.

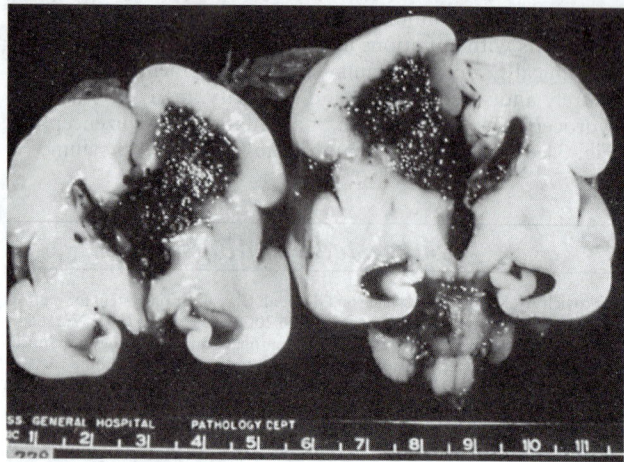

FIGURE 32.1. Coronal sections of the brain of a 28-week gestational age, preterm infant with a large intraventricular and frontoparietal parenchymal hemorrhage.

TABLE 32.1

GRADING SYSTEM FOR NEONATAL INTRAVENTRICULAR HEMORRHAGE

Grade	Description
I	Germinal matrix hemorrhage
II	Blood within but not distending the lateral ventricular system
III	Blood filling and distending the ventricular system
IV	Parenchymal involvement of hemorrhage with or without any of the above

Adapted from Papile LS, Burstein J, Burstein R, et al. Incidence and evolution of the subependymal intraventricular hemorrhage: a study of infants with weights less than 1500 grams. *J Pediatr* 1978;92:529.

PATHOPHYSIOLOGY

IVH is believed to be secondary to alterations in cerebral blood flow to the germinal matrix microvasculature, and the pathogenesis of GMH is most certainly multifactorial.

The germinal matrix, the region of origin of GMH/IVH, is the site of proliferation of neuronal and glial precursors in the developing nervous system that, during the late second and early third trimesters, give rise predominantly to glia and microneurons. By 25 weeks' gestation, almost all the cortical neurons have been generated, axonal and dendritic branching is robust, and synaptic contacts are beginning to form. At this time the capillary bed of the germinal matrix is composed of large, irregular vessels with little evidence for basement membrane proteins or glial supporting structures. In addition, although the blood–brain barrier begins to form during the early third trimester of gestation, the triad of endothelial tight junction formation, basement membrane deposition, and glial investiture does not characterize the microvessels of the germinal matrix zone.

Cerebral blood flow plays a critical role in the pathogenesis of IVH. Although studies in neonatal animals have suggested that the efficiency of cerebral blood flow autoregulation increases with gestational age, cerebral blood flow to the germinal matrix microvessels is largely pressure passive. In this condition, cerebral blood flow varies directly with changes in systemic blood pressure. Thus, if the preterm infant is hypotensive secondary to either *in utero* hypoxia, sepsis, or other postnatal events, CBF may fall and damage to the germinal matrix microvessels may ensue. In addition, respiratory distress syndrome, vigorous resuscitation, hypoxemia, acidosis, pneumothoraces, and seizures have all been shown to increase CBF in preterm neonates, and the association of these risk factors and hemorrhage has been well described.

The relationship among surfactant, respiratory distress syndrome, and the development of GMH/IVH also must be mentioned. Although surfactant has been demonstrated to cause transient increases in CBF, most clinical studies have not noted an increase in GMH/IVH associated with its use. In addition, because surfactant may diminish the acute hypoxemia and hypercapnia associated with respiratory distress syndrome, it actually may contribute to the lower incidence of GMH/IVH that some centers are reporting.

Several authors have suggested that the venous circulation may also predispose the germinal matrix to hemorrhage. At the head of the caudate nucleus, the most common site of IVH, the anteriorly coursing terminal, choroidal, and thalamostriate veins join to form the internal cerebral vein. At that juncture, the internal cerebral vein turns abruptly posteriorly to join the vein of Galen. Elevations in venous pressure resulting from neonatal complications such as respiratory distress syndrome, pneumothoraces, or high-frequency ventilation may increase the potential for venous distension in this fragile venous system and thus permit venous hemorrhagic infarction of the germinal matrix tissues.

Finally, the two other risk factors, the absence of antenatal steroid exposure and neonatal transport, are well-recognized associations with IVH. Steroid exposure accelerates surfactant production and may decrease IVH by decreasing the incidence of respiratory distress syndrome; in addition, steroids are angiostatic and may induce maturation of the germinal matrix microvessels. The risks of neonatal transport have been well described and include hypoxemia, hypercarbia, hypotension, and the need for vigorous resuscitation.

Equally concerning and perhaps more important for the neurodevelopmental outcome of these infants is the observation of markedly diminished CBF after low-grade IVH. Xenon-133 inhalation CBF studies and positron emission tomography have demonstrated prolonged ischemia for more than the first postnatal week in preterm neonates with IVH.

A model for the development of neonatal GMH/IVH is found in Fig. 32.3 and takes into account both the hypotensive–ischemic insults and those clinical events, such as

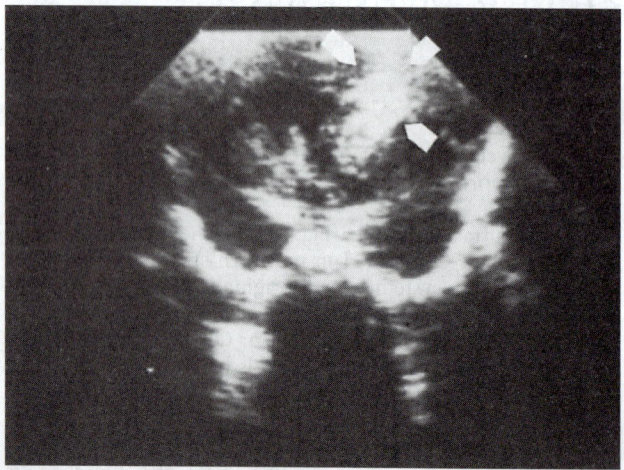

FIGURE 32.2. Coronal ultrasound scan demonstrating a large right parenchymal hemorrhage in a 28-week gestational age, preterm infant with bloody spinal fluid.

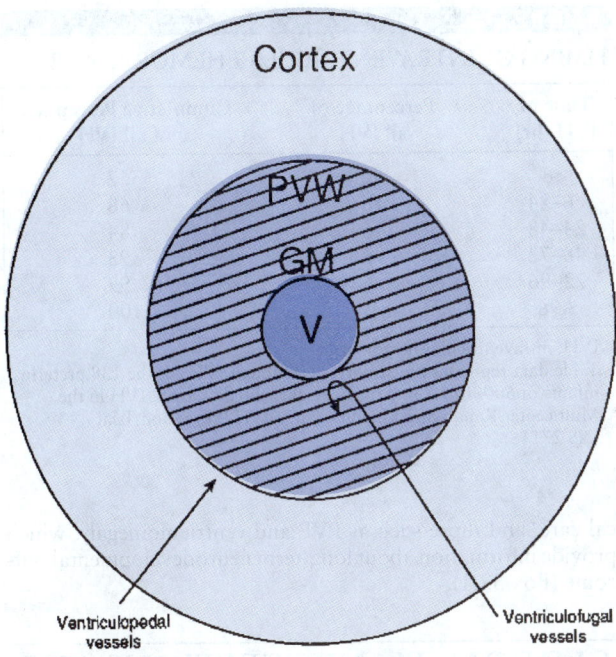

FIGURE 32.3. Model for the development of intraventricular hemorrhage in the preterm infant. BP, blood pressure; CBF, cerebral blood flow; IVH, intraventricular hemorrhage; PVL, periventricular leukomalacia.

pneumothoraces, seizures, and rapid volume resuscitation, to which many tiny and frequently critically ill preterm neonates are exposed.

The neuropathologic consequences of IVH include germinal matrix destruction, periventricular hemorrhagic infarction,

and posthemorrhagic hydrocephalus (PHH). Germinal matrix destruction with secondary cystic formation is a common and expected feature of GMH.

In addition, 10% to 20% of patients with GMH/IVH have periventricular hemorrhagic infarction, also frequently called *hemorrhagic intracerebral involvement*, or grade IV IVH. Some investigators feel that the parenchymal involvement of insult readily visible by cranial ultrasonography (see Fig. 32.2) represents a direct extension of hemorrhage from either the ventricular system or the germinal matrix; others believe that these lesions represent venous infarction of the periventricular white matter. Both proposed mechanisms depend on increased intracranial and (particularly) intraventricular pressure as a primary event. Distinguishing the two lesions *in vivo* is extremely difficult; likely, parenchymal lesions occur secondary to both mechanisms.

The third consequence of IVH is PHH (Fig. 32.4). PHH is more common in those infants with the highest grades of hemorrhage and is less common in those with the youngest gestational ages. It is the result of obliterative arachnoiditis either over the hemispheric convexities, with occlusion of the arachnoid villi, or in the posterior fossa, with obstruction of fourth ventricular outflow through the tentorial notch. Rarely, aqueductal obstruction is caused by an acute blood clot, ependymal disruption, or reactive gliosis.

Periventricular leukomalacia (PVL) is a frequent neuropathologic accompaniment of GMH/IVH but apparently is not caused by it. PVL is the generally symmetric injury of the periventricular white matter demonstrated readily as cystic lesions by cranial ultrasonography (see Chapter 33). In addition, recent studies have suggested that PVL may be detected by diffusion-weighted magnetic resonance imaging prior to changes on ultrasonography. Frequently associated in risk-factor studies with sepsis, chorioamnionitis, apnea, hypotension, and other ischemic events, it has been reported in 25%

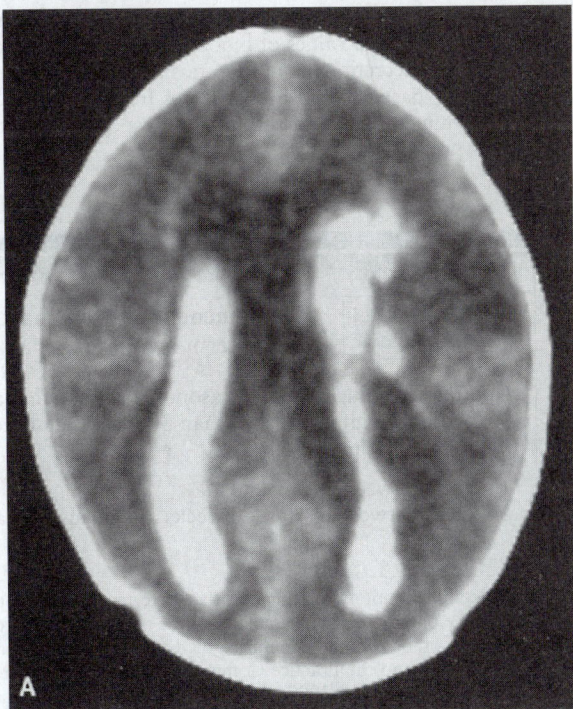

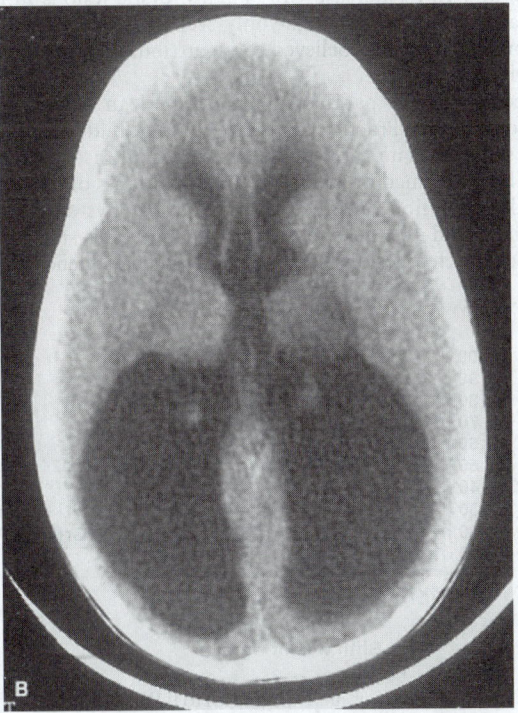

FIGURE 32.4. A: Computed tomographic scan of a preterm infant of 28 weeks' gestational age with bilateral intraventricular hemorrhage. **B:** Repeat computed tomographic scan—performed because of rapidly increasing occipitofrontal head circumference, lethargy, and increasing apneic spells—demonstrates ventriculomegaly. Lumbar puncture revealed an opening pressure of greater than 200 mm of water, consistent with the diagnosis of posthemorrhagic hydrocephalus.

to 50% of infants with GMH/IVH and is believed to represent nonhemorrhagic infarction of the periventricular white matter watershed zone. Although the clinical correlate of PVL is spastic diplegia, only one-half of infants with cranial ultrasound–documented cystic PVL with lesions of 1 cm or greater at term will experience motor handicaps.

EPIDEMIOLOGY

The incidence of GMH/IVH increases as gestational age decreases, and as many as 50% of infants with birth weights of 501 to 750 g have the disorder. In addition, although the overall incidence has been reported to vary between 15% and 30% in large cohorts of infants with birth weights of less than 1,500 g, high-grade hemorrhages are found more commonly in neonates with very low birth weights. Data from the National Institute of Child Health and Human Development (NICHD) Neonatal Research Network for the years 1995–1996 report that 48% of infants of 501- to 750-g birth weight experience IVH. The incidence is 34% for infants of 751- to 1,000-g birth weight, 27% for infants of 1,001- to 1,250-g birth weight, and 20% for those of 1,251- to 1,500-g birth weight. Data from the Yale University School of Medicine are shown in Figure 32.5. Hemorrhages have been reported within the first postnatal hour, and a significant number of hemorrhages occur by the sixth hour. One-half of all preterm infants who will have GMH/IVH demonstrate the disorder on the first postnatal day, and less than 5% have hemorrhage after the fourth to fifth postnatal days. The timing of IVH is shown in Table 32.2.

This risk period for GMH/IVH appears to be independent of gestational age. Some infants, especially those with the earliest onset of GMH/IVH, will have extension of hemorrhage over the first several postnatal days; this progression has been linked to clinical events, such as pneumothoraces and seizures, that are known to increase CBF. Finally, cystic lesions in the germinal matrix, once thought only secondary to congenital infection, are now also believed to be attributable to *in utero* hemorrhages.

A recent Practice parameter of the American Academy of Neurology and the Practice Committee of the Child Neurology Society suggests that routine screening cranial ultrasonography should be performed on all asymptomatic infants of less than 30 weeks' gestation once between 7 and 14 days and again between 36 and 40 weeks' postmenstrual age. This strategy is designed to detect lesions such as IVH, which influence clini-

cal care, and those such as PVL and ventriculomegaly, which provide information about long-term neurodevelopmental outcome (Box 32.1).

CLINICAL MANIFESTATIONS AND COMPLICATIONS

The clinical manifestations of GMH/IVH are varied. In almost 75% of cases, GMH/IVH is thought to be clinically silent, although infants with grade III and grade IV hemorrhages may experience a significant decrease in hematocrit (75% of infants), seizures (10% to 15% of infants), abnormal eye findings (including dilated pupils and loss of eye movements; 33% to 90% of infants), and changes in tone and reflexes (75% to 90% of infants). Persistent bradycardia and apneic spells may be secondary to increased intracranial pressure or to alterations in CBF to brainstem respiratory centers. Infants may have significantly elevated values of blood glucose and evidence of inappropriate secretion of antidiuretic hormone. Finally, patients with large parenchymal hemorrhages frequently experience a persistent metabolic acidosis that is unresponsive to alkali therapy or pressor agents.

TABLE 32.2

TIMING OF INTRAVENTRICULAR HEMORRHAGE

Time of IVH (hr)	Percentage of all IVH	Cumulative Percentage of all IVH
<6	52	52
6–24	16	68
24–48	16	84
48–72	9	93
72–96	6	99
>96	1	100

IVH, intraventricular hemorrhage.
Table data represent time to first detection of IVH for the 138 preterm infants of 600- to 1,250-g birth weight who developed IVH in the Multicenter Randomized Indomethaein IVH Prevention Trial (NS 27116).

BOX 32.1   ### Recommendations for Imaging the Preterm Neonate[1]

Routine screening cranial ultrasonography should be performed on all infants of less than 30 weeks' gestation at the following times:

1. Once between days 7 and 14
2. Again between 36 and 40 weeks' postmenstrual age

---

[1]Recommendations for imaging the preterm neonate from the Practice parameter: neuroimaging of the neonate; Report of the Quality Standards Subcommittee of the American Academy of Neurology and the Practice Committee of the Child Neurology Society. *Neurology*, 2002; this strategy detects lesions such as intraventricular hemorrhage, which influence clinical care, and those such as periventricular leukomalacia and low-pressure ventriculomegaly, which provide information about long-term neurodevelopmental outcome.

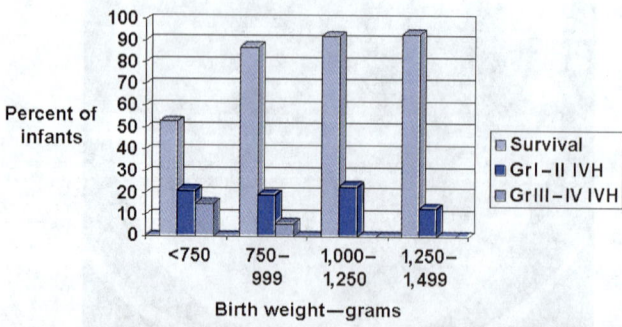

FIGURE 32.5. Incidence of survival, grades I to II IVH and grades III to IV IVH, in the 134 inborn infants with birth weights less than 1,500 g at Yale University School of Medicine, January 1, 2002, to December 31, 2002. For birth weights less than 750 g, n = 47; for 751 to 999 g, n = 31; for 1,000 to 1,249 g, n = 26; and for 1,250 to 1,499 g, n = 30. (Data courtesy of R.A. Ehrenkranz, M.D.)

Infants with GMH/IVH are at risk for the development of PHH and are known to have higher incidences of neonatal seizures, PVL, and low-pressure cerebral ventriculomegaly, as compared with preterm infants without hemorrhage matched for birth weight or gestational age. Finally, most investigators agree that those infants with parenchymal involvement of GMH/IVH are at high risk for neurodevelopmental handicap.

PHH (see Fig. 32.4) is the combination of ventriculomegaly (diagnosed by serial echoencephalography studies) and increased intracranial pressure, defined as an opening pressure of greater than 140 mm H$_2$O on either lumbar puncture or, if indicated, cerebral ventricular tap. PHH generally is a communicating hydrocephalus with a block at the level of the arachnoid villi or, less commonly, at the foramina of Luschka and Magendie in the posterior fossa. Hydrocephalus results when the blood and protein in the cerebrospinal fluid produce a chemical arachnoiditis that may be transient or, less commonly, permanent. A small percentage of infants with IVH will have a noncommunicating hydrocephalus with a block at the level of the aqueduct secondary to an ependymal reaction similar to that of the arachnoid or an acute clot. Infants with the latter type of hydrocephalus will require neurosurgical intervention, whereas the treatment for neonates with communicating PHH (at least initially) is medical.

All infants with intraventricular blood require close ultrasonographic monitoring of ventricular size. These patients should undergo frequent head circumference measurements and cranial ultrasonographic examinations for determination of ventricular size. Because prolonged increased intracranial pressure may result in apnea, vomiting, lethargy, and (ultimately) optic atrophy, the intracranial pressure of infants with head circumferences crossing the expected growth curves and those demonstrating evidence for increasing ventricular size should be checked and, when the diagnosis is confirmed, treatment should be provided. The standard treatment protocol for infants with communicating hydrocephalus includes lumbar punctures with removal of cerebrospinal fluid to normalize intracranial pressure and frequent ultrasound checks of ventricular size. Alternatively, for those infants with evidence of noncommunicating hydrocephalus or intraparenchymal involvement of hemorrhage and shift of the cerebral midline, ventricular taps or the insertion of ventricular catheters with reservoirs performed by neurosurgical personnel are indicated, and the placement of a ventriculoperitoneal shunt ultimately may be necessary.

In many large series of preterm neonates, the incidence of motor handicaps appears to be low. These abnormalities include spastic diplegia, hemiparesis, and (rarely) spastic quadriparesis. Many infants with spastic diplegia have neuroimaging evidence for PVL or low-pressure cerebral ventriculomegaly, but only 50% to 60% of infants with these cranial ultrasonographic findings at term will be found to suffer motor handicap at age 3 years.

Although many investigators doubt the existence of differences in the developmental outcome of infants with grade I, II, or III IVH (as compared with infants with no known evidence of hemorrhage in the neonatal period), data suggest that the rate of cognitive deficits may increase with the grade of IVH in this patient population; data from our own institution are found in Figure 32.6. Infants with parenchymal involvement of hemorrhage, or grade IV IVH, experience a wide range of outcomes; review of the literature suggests that 50% to 85% of all neonates with grade IV IVH will have motor and cognitive handicaps. For many of these children, the development of a porencephalic cyst follows resolution of the parenchymal blood, and this outcome can be demonstrated easily by ultrasound, computed tomography, or magnetic resonance imaging studies (Fig. 32.7).

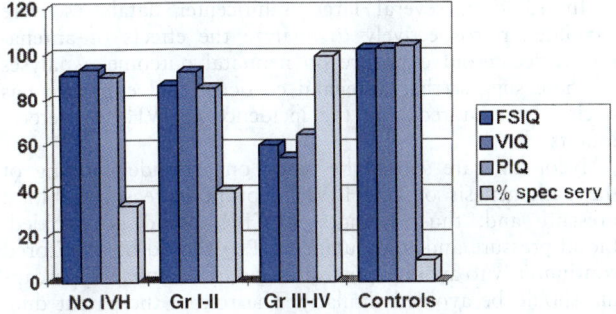

FIGURE 32.6. Cognitive outcome at 12 years corrected age for 206 very low-birth-weight survivors of the Randomized Indomethacin IVH Prevention Trial (NS 27116). One hundred seventy-five children had no IVH, 29 experienced IVH of grades I to II IVH, and three had hemorrhage of grades III to IV IVH. Normal: full-scale IQ greater than 80; borderline: full-scale IQ 70 to 80; mental retardation: full-scale IQ less than 70. IVH, intraventricular hemorrhage.

MANAGEMENT

A variety of measures have been suggested to prevent GMH/IVH. Clearly, the most important way to prevent the disorder is to prevent preterm birth. When that is not possible, the preferable approach is transport of the mother and fetus to a regional perinatal center specializing in high-risk obstetric care; "outborn" infants have consistently higher rates of GMH/IVH than do those who are "inborn."

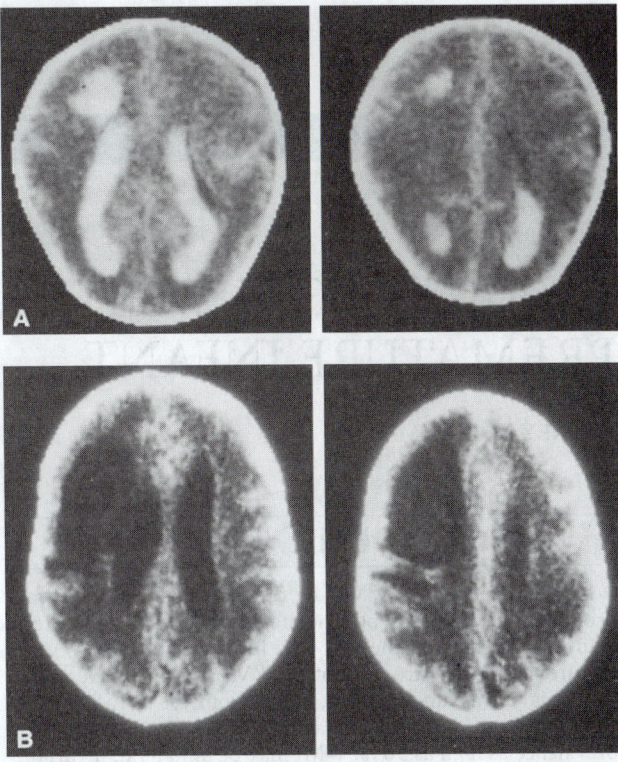

FIGURE 32.7. A: This boy of 27 weeks' gestation initially was found to have a bilateral intraventricular hemorrhage with a right frontal parenchymal component. **B:** Repeat computed tomographic scan 12 weeks later demonstrates a large right porencephalic cyst and moderate ventriculomegaly.

In addition, several large, multicenter databases were evaluated retrospectively to analyze the effects of antenatal corticosteroid exposure on neonatal outcome. Analyses of these suggest that antenatal corticosteroid exposure has a clear role in reducing the incidence of IVH in preterm infants.

Neonatal care should be based on an understanding of the pathogenesis of GMH/IVH. Abrupt increases in blood pressure and, thus, changes in CBF should be avoided. Blood pressure and transcutaneous Po$_2$ should be monitored continuously to avoid hypotension and hypoxemia. Hypercapnia should be avoided similarly. The role of the patent ductus arteriosus and its abrupt closure in the genesis of IVH has long been debated, and it appears that pharmacologic closure promotes smoother changes in blood flow than do surgical procedures.

Finally, multiple pharmacologic intervention trials have sought to prevent GMH/IVH. The drugs used include phenobarbital, indomethacin, ethamsylate, vitamin E, and pancuronium bromide (Pavulon), among others. These agents lower CBF, alter the metabolic rate, scavenge free radicals, stabilize capillary membranes, and prevent fluctuations in CBF, respectively. Although its antenatal administration is discouraged because of significant cardiac, renal, and gastrointestinal sequelae, only low-dose indomethacin (0.1 mg/kg at 6 to 12 postnatal hours by slow intravenous infusion over 20 to 30 minutes and repeated 24 and 48 hours thereafter) has been demonstrated in multiple single-institution studies and a multicenter trial both to lower the incidence and to decrease the severity of IVH. In addition, this agent has not been associated with adverse motor or cognitive outcome in preterm neonates.

Suggested Readings

Allan WC, Vohr B, Makuch RW, Ment LR. Antecedents of cerebral palsy in a multicenter trial of indomethacin for IVH. *Arch Pediatr Adolesc Med* 1997;151:580.

Crowley P, Chalmens I, Keirse MJ. The effects of corticosteroid administration before preterm delivery: an overview of the evidence from controlled trials. *Br J Obstet Gynaecol* 1990;97:11.

Darlow BA, Cust AE, Donoghue DA. Improved outcomes for very low birthweight infants: evidence from New Zealand national population based data. *Arch Dis Child Fetal Neonatal* 2003;88:F23.

Del Toro J, Louis PT, Goddard-Finegold J. Cerebrovascular regulation and neonatal brain injury. *Pediatr Neurol* 1991;7:3.

Huppi PS, Schuknecht B, Boech C, Bossi EA. Structural and neurobehavioral delay in postnatal brain development of preterm infants. *Pediatr Res* 1996;39:895.

Lemons JA, Bauer CR, Oh W, et al. Very low birth weight outcomes of the National Institute of Child Health and Human Development Neonatal Research Network, January 1995 through December 1996. NICHD Neonatal Research Network. *Pediatrics* 2001;107:E1.

Ment LR, Bada HS, Barnes PD, et al. Practice parameter: neuroimaging of the neonate. *Neurology* 2002;58:1726.

Papile LA, Burstein J, Burstein R, et al. Incidence and evolution of the subependymal intraventricular hemorrhage: a study of infants with weights less than 1500 grams. *J Pediatr* 1978;92:529.

Perlman JM, Rollins N. Surveillance protocol for the detection of intracranial abnormalities in premature neonates. *Arch Pediatr Adolesc Med* 2000;154:822.

Shalak L, Perlman JM. Hemorrhagic-ischemic cerebral injury in the preterm infant. Current concepts. *Clin Perinatol* 2002;29:745.

Wells JT, Ment LR. Prevention of intraventricular hemorrhage in preterm infants. *Early Hum Dev* 1995;42:209.

Whitaker AG, Feldman JF, Rossem RV, et al. Neonatal cranial ultrasound abnormalities in low birth weight infants: relation to cognitive outcomes at six years of age. *Pediatrics* 1996;98:719.

Whitelaw A. Intraventricular haemorrhage and posthaemorrhagic hydrocephalus: pathogenesis, prevention and future interventions. *Semin Neonatol* 2001;6:135.

Winter S, Autry A, Boyle CA, Yeargin-Allsopp M. Trends in the prevalence of cerebral palsy in a population-based study. *Pediatrics* 2002;110:1220.

CHAPTER 33 ■ WHITE MATTER INJURY IN THE PREMATURE INFANT

JEFFREY M. PERLMAN

EPIDEMIOLOGY

White matter injury (WMI) represents the most significant problem contributing to both neonatal mortality and long-term neurologic deficits in the very low birth weight (VLBW) premature infant. The true extent of WMI remains unclear and, by cranial ultrasound imaging, ranges from 4% to 15%. Moreover, magnetic resonance imaging (MRI) studies indicate a prevalence as high as 50%. WMI may be unilateral, invariably associated with severe periventricular hemorrhage (IVH) and often termed grade IV IVH; or WMI may be bilateral, usually unassociated with IVH. The latter may evolve to cyst formation, termed periventricular leukomalacia (PVL), or may manifest as a nonprogressive lateral ventriculomegaly. This chapter deals briefly with the different forms of WMI in terms of pathogenesis, prevention, and outcome.

Association with Intraventricular Hemorrhage

The incidence of severe IVH remains substantial in those infants who have the smallest birth weights of the VLBW population. Thus, approximately 26% of infants of birth weight between 501 and 750 g and 12% weighing between 751 and 1,000 g still develop the most severe forms of hemorrhage. The primary lesion is bleeding from small vessels in the subependymal germinal matrix (GM), a transitional gelatinous region providing limited support for the luxurious but very immature capillary bed that courses through it. The genesis of capillary bleeding from within the GM is complex, likely multifactorial, and influenced in part by intravascular, vascular, and extravascular factors. Experimental studies and clinical observations in the sick newborn infant suggest a pressure-passive cerebral circulation relative to systemic vascular changes, a state that increases cerebral vulnerability during episodes of systemic hypo- and/or hypertension. Indeed, experimental and clinical associations have been demonstrated between fluctuations, increases, and/or decreases in systemic blood pressure as well as elevations in venous pressure, that parallel simultaneous changes in the cerebral circulation and subsequent IVH. The bleeding into white matter is invariably related to an ipsilateral GM hemorrhage. This association may reflect an extension of bleeding from the GM into uninjured white matter, or it may represent secondary hemorrhage into an area of already ischemic white matter (i.e., reperfusion injury). Understanding the mechanism(s) contributing to WMI is crucial to preventing this important lesion. Thus, if WMI is directly related to PV-IVH, then prevention of hemorrhage should reduce the occurrence of WMI. However, if PV-IVH and WMI were to occur simultaneously, as a result of a primary ischemic event, with hemorrhage occurring as a secondary phenomenon, then prevention of the IVH is unlikely to effect the primary ischemic process and thus outcome. Indeed indomethacin treatment to prevent IVH in the neonatal period is supportive of this latter concern. Thus, although the incidence of severe IVH is reduced with indomethacin treatment, at 18-month follow-up, neurodevelopmental outcome, including cerebral palsy, remains comparable in treated infants as compared with controls.

Prevention continues to focus on both perinatal and postnatal approaches. Regarding perinatal strategies, the antenatal administration of a single short course of glucocorticoids to augment pulmonary maturation has had the positive, unanticipated benefit of a significant reduction in the incidence of severe IVH. Thus, the unadjusted odds ratio for severe IVH reduction following any antenatal glucocorticoid exposure has ranged from 0.49 to 0.79. A maternal medical condition associated with a lower incidence of IVH is pregnancy-induced hypertension (PIH), an effect that appears to be independent of the administration of magnesium sulfate, a medication often used to treat the condition.

The role of route of delivery and subsequent IVH remains controversial. However, recent data point to an important role of placental inflammation, and in particular fetal vasculitis, in the genesis of severe IVH, which may supersede the influence of route of delivery.

The focus of postnatal strategies should be directed toward the tiniest VLBW infants, that is, those of less than 1,000 g, and in particular those intubated because of respiratory distress syndrome. Postnatal medications evaluated to reduce severe IVH have included phenobarbital, vitamin E, ethamsylate, and indomethacin. Currently, indomethacin appears to hold the most promise, with a significant reduction in the incidence of grade IV IVH observed in infants who received the drug versus controls.

The infant with grade IV IVH is at high risk for delayed neurodevelopment. In particular, when the lesion is large (greater than 1 cm in diameter on head ultrasound scan), the outcome is invariably poor, resulting in both major motor and cognitive deficits. With a smaller lesion (less than 1 cm in diameter), the outcome is less precise, and a small percentage (approximately 20%) may even have a normal outcome.

Periventricular Leukomalacia

Periventricular leukomalacia (PVL) refers to necrosis of white matter adjacent to the external angles of the lateral ventricles,

and it has long been regarded as the principal ischemic lesion of the premature infant. However, recent evidence suggests that the process of WMI is much more complex (see section, Pathogenesis of White Matter Injury). The pathologic features of PVL include both focal and more diffuse white-matter involvement. The focal necrosis is distributed commonly at the level of the occipital radiation at the trigone of the lateral ventricles, and at the level of the cerebral white matter around the foramen of Monro. The typical histologic changes are characterized by coagulation necrosis, microglial infiltration, astrocytic proliferation, and cyst formation. These cavities usually diminish in size over time, with myelin loss and focal ventricular dilation in the region of the trigone as long-term sequelae. The diffuse WMI less frequently undergoes cystic change; however, the ventricular dilation is more prominent.

PATHOGENESIS OF WHITE MATTER INJURY

The pathogenesis of the WMI is complex and likely multifactorial. Two basic factors appear to be important: (a) vascular factors that increase the risk for cerebral hypoperfusion and (b) the intrinsic vulnerability of the differentiating oligodendrocyte within white matter. With regard to vascular factors, immature deep white matter represents an anatomic border zone between the penetrating branches of the anterior, middle, and posterior cerebral arteries. In addition, these arteries appear to have a limited vasodilatory response to $Paco_2$. Finally, under some circumstances, the immature cerebral circulation does not autoregulate; that is, the cerebral blood flow changes passively with changes in systemic blood pressure. These factors in combination (see also Chapter 32) increase the risk for WMI during episodes of systemic hypotension.

The early differentiating oligodendrocyte is vulnerable to injury secondary to release of numerous mediators, including free radicals, excitotoxins, cytokines, as well as lack of growth factors. Studies in newborn animal models subjected to hypoxia-ischemia and/or infection, as well as a recent neuropathologic study in preterm infants, suggest that the mechanism of cell death due to these factors is mediated via apoptosis. Although free radical and excitotoxin release are likely important, accumulating evidence points to a critical role for

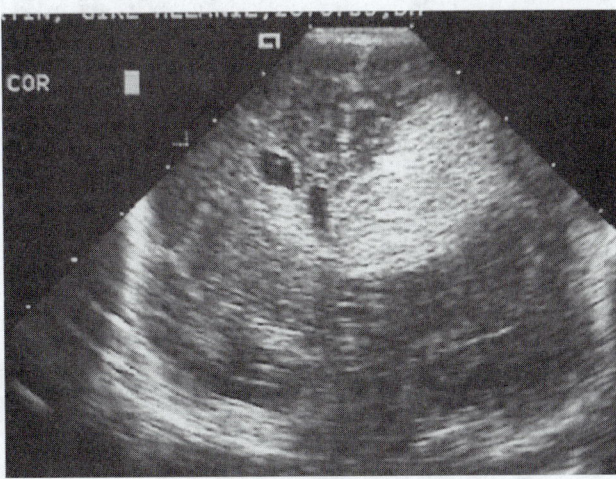

FIGURE 33.1. Coronal section of brain. Note the large intraparenchymal echogenicity within left fronto-parietal white matter (Severe IVH).

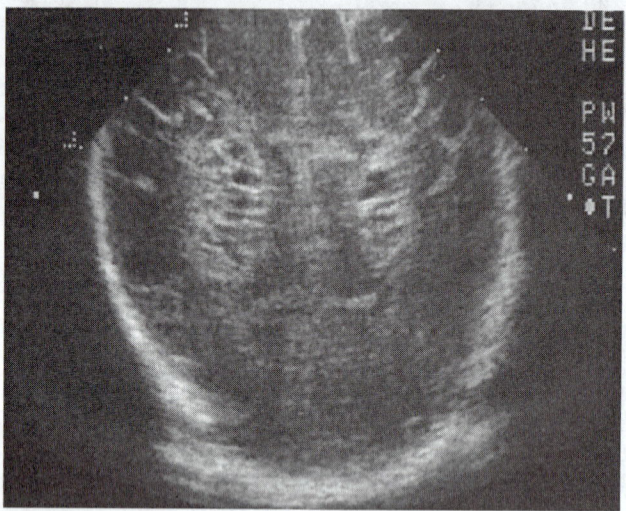

FIGURE 33.2. Coronal section. Note the cysts contained within post white matter.

cytokine release in oligodendroglial precursor cell death. It is well established in animals that ischemia and reperfusion is accompanied by a rapid activation of microglia, secretion of cytokines, and migration of inflammatory cells. Experimental and clinical evidence demonstrates an association between maternal infection and inflammation, including fetal vascular involvement such as funisitis (inflammation of the blood vessels of the umbilical cord) and WMI. For example, intraperitoneal injection of lipopolysaccharides into kittens, and exposure of pregnant rabbits to intrauterine infection, results in white matter injury similar to that seen in humans. Several clinical studies have demonstrated an association between chorioamnionitis, in particular funisitis, and PVL. The link with chorioamnionitis may be mediated via cytokines. Thus, high levels of cytokines have been found in amniotic fluid, cord blood, and neonatal blood of preterm infants who develop PVL or cerebral palsy; microglial expression of TNF-alpha (TNF-α) and interleukin-6 immunoreactivity is found twice as commonly in the white matter of infants with PVL as in the absence of injury.

Perinatal events associated with postnatal cystic PVL include a history of chorioamnionitis, prolonged rupture of membranes, peripartum hemorrhage, asphyxia, hypovolemia, sepsis, hypocarbia, and symptomatic patent ductus arteriosus. Although many of these associations have in common a reduction in systemic blood pressure, clinical studies of infants who developed PVL fail to demonstrate overt postnatal hypotension in most cases. Moreover, postnatal evolution of nonhemorrhagic lateral ventriculomegaly is an insidious process that evolves over weeks.

PREVENTION

The prevention of WMI is likely to be difficult, for several reasons. First, cystic PVL is a relatively uncommon condition; second, the pathogenesis of WMI in general is complex; and third, the presentation is often subtle and only detected by neuroimaging. For example, as noted earlier, increasing evidence points to an association between perinatal infection, such as chorioamnionitis and PVL. However, the mechanism(s) of injury remain unclear; the positive predictive value of a history of chorioamnionitis and subsequent PVL is low and approximates 10%.

PROGNOSIS

Infants with WMI pose significant problems in that the majority have major long-term neurodevelopmental deficits. The most commonly described long-term motor sequelae of PVL has been spastic diplegia. However, recent reports describe a more severe deficit, with involvement of all four extremities as well as visual and cognitive deficits. This severe outcome is consistent with the more diffuse white matter injury noted on magnetic resonance imaging (MRI) as well as from the neuropathology in preterm infants who die with PVL. The genesis of the cognitive deficits remains unclear. It has been speculated that the WMI may secondarily affect neuronal cortical organization due to injury to subplate neurons or late migrating astrocytes.

CONCLUSION

WMI remains a significant problem in the premature infant. The potential mechanisms contributing to injury are complex and involve factors related to blood flow and its regulation, as well as to cellular mediators including cytokines, free radical formation, and excitotoxin release. Long-term neurodevelopmental consequences are substantial, affecting both motor and cognitive function.

Suggested Readings

Leviton A, Paneth N, Reuss L, et al. Maternal infection, fetal inflammatory response and brain damage in very low birthweight infants. *Pediatric Res* 1999;46:566.

Ment LR, Vohr B, Allen W. The etiology and outcome of cerebral ventriculomegaly at term in very low birthweight infants. *Pediatrics* 1999;104:243.

Schmidt B, Davis P, Moddemann D, et al. Long term effects of indomethacin prophylaxis in extremely low birthweight infants. *N Engl J Med* 2001;344:1966.

Shalak L, Perlman JM. Hemorrhagic-ischemic cerebral injury in the preterm infant: current concepts. *Clin Perinatol* 2002;29:745.

Volpe JJ. *Neurology of the newborn*, 4th ed. Philadelphia: W.B. Sanders; 2001.

Wu YW, Colford Jr. JM. Chorioamnionitis as a risk factor of cerebral palsy: a meta-analysis [review]. *JAMA* 2000;2814:1417.

CHAPTER 34 ■ NEONATAL ENCEPHALOPATHIES

DONNA M. FERRIERO

In the twenty-first century, hypoxic-ischemic encephalopathy (HIE) remains the single most important perinatal cause of neurologic morbidity in both the full-term as well as the preterm newborn, occurring in 1 to 3 of 1,000 full-term live births and in an even higher percentage of preterm newborns. The neurodevelopmental sequelae in survivors range from subtle behavioral or language disabilities to more severe problems such as cerebral palsy, mental retardation, pervasive developmental disorders, cortical visual impairment, hearing disorders, sleep disorders, and epilepsy. Previously the terms "perinatal or birth asphyxia" and HIE were used interchangeably to describe this condition, but since many neonates have encephalopathy from a variety of causes other than birth asphyxia, birth asphyxia should be used only for select cases where the insult has been documented by the clinical condition and neuroimaging. This chapter will focus on HIE and its consequences in the preterm and term newborn.

PATHOGENESIS

Etiology and Risk Factors

Term newborns presenting with neonatal encephalopathy have a number of potential causes for their altered neurologic examination (Box 34.1). The most regarded etiology is hypoxia-ischemia, but stroke, traumatic brain injury, infection, toxin exposure, and genetic or metabolic disorders may be equally prevalent. Premature newborns may not show the same signs of encephalopathy as a term newborn, but they can experience injury to the developing brain through the same mechanisms,

resulting in a different pattern of injury due to vulnerability of maturation-dependent populations of neural cells. An understanding of the causes of neonatal encephalopathy is crucial to the concepts of prevention and treatment. Although advances have been made in recognition of the many potential causes, these advances have not led to a reduction in the overall rate of cerebral palsy. Furthermore, the effect of neonatal encephalopathy on cognition has not been adequately studied in large populations.

While many causes of neonatal encephalopathy begin prenatally, the majority of infants with HIE are full-term infants who have had perinatal complications. Recent studies suggest that, although antenatal or genetic factors might predispose some infants to perinatal brain injury, events that occur in the immediate perinatal period are most important in infants presenting with neonatal encephalopathy. Labor imposes both mechanical and hypoxic stress on the fetus and, therefore, if this stress becomes excessive, the newborn is at risk for permanent neurologic sequelae. Intrauterine distress (abnormal fetal heart rate patterns, meconium-stained or infected amniotic fluid, or abnormalities in acid–base balance) or puerperal complications (abruptio placentae, cord prolapse, tight nuchal cord, or mechanically traumatic delivery) can produce the syndrome of HIE. The precise clinical picture and the underlying pathophysiology leading to irreversible neuronal damage vary depending on the severity and duration of the perinatal compromise, as well as on other variables such as gestational age, the presence of maternal factors such as preeclampsia, intrauterine infection, and glycemic status. For example, in acute total asphyxia caused by placental abruption, the clinical picture is that of a severely depressed infant requiring immediate resuscitation. This newborn will remain encephalopathic for many days and have early and refractory seizures and disturbances in multiorgan systems (renal, cardiac, and pulmonary). When the hypoxic-ischemic events occur over a longer duration with less severity, possibly due to an intrauterine inflammatory environment, Apgar scores may be near normal, and severe neurologic depression with multiorgan involvement will not be present. However, the neonate may have poor feeding or subtle abnormalities of the neurologic examination as the only immediate manifestation. Newer technologies such as magnetic resonance spectroscopy (MRS) and diffusion-weighted imaging (DWI), coupled with advanced structural imaging, may be helpful in the early identification of such infants who are at risk for future neurologic handicap.

BOX 34.1 | Neonatal Encephalopathy: Differential Diagnosis

Neonate born at term
Hypoxia-ischemia
Acute infection of the nervous system
Chronic infection of the nervous system
Drug or toxin exposure
Stroke
Inborn error of metabolism
Genetic syndromes

Preterm neonate
Hypoxia-ischemia
Acute or intrauterine infection
Drug or toxin exposure
Inborn error of metabolism
Genetic syndromes
Stroke

Mechanisms Leading to Hypoxic-Ischemic Encephalopathy

In the developing brain, metabolic changes and alterations in cerebral blood flow occur during the injury. There is a shift from oxidative to anaerobic metabolism (glycolysis) with an accumulation of lactic acid and a depletion of high-energy phosphate reserves that can be seen in regions of compromise, especially the basal ganglia (Fig. 34.1). At the same time, failure

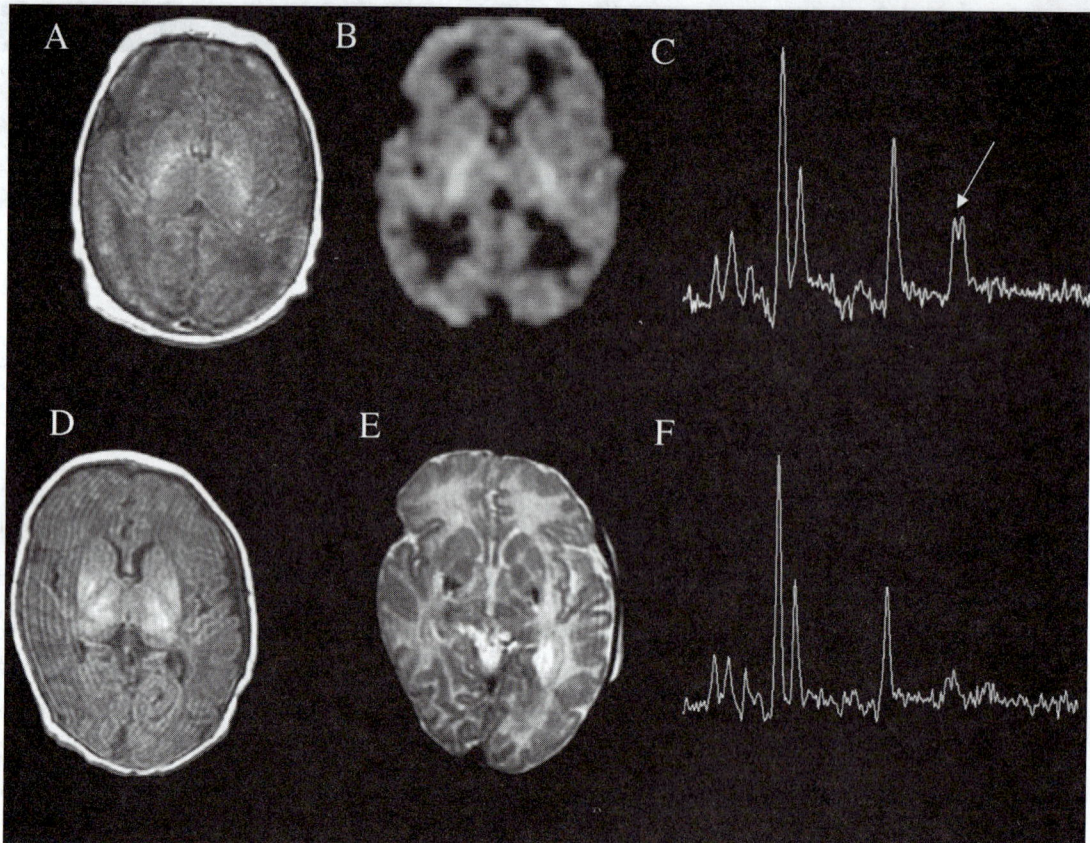

FIGURE 34.1. MR imaging showing characteristic changes on structural imaging, diffusion-weighted imaging and proton spectroscopy in deep grey nuclei. A–C. MR study at 16 hours. Axial Spin Echo (517/8) (SE) image (A) is normal, Diffusion-weighted image (b 700 s/mm^2) (B) shows small areas of reduced diffusion are seen in posterior limbs of internal capsules. Proton MR spectrum (2000/288) (C) from single voxel in thalamus/lentiform nucleus shows markedly elevated Lactate peak (doublet at 1.33 ppm, arrow). D–F. Follow-up at age 15 days. SE (517/8) image (D) shows T1 shortening in lateral putamen and posteromedial lentiform nucleus bilaterally and at the depths of the posterior sylvian cortex. T2-weighted image (E) shows hypointensity in the posterior putamen and abnormal mixed signal intensity in the posterior limb of the internal capsule and lateral thalamus. Proton spectrum (2000/288) from the thalami/lentiform nuclei (F) shows marked diminution in the size of the NAA peak and almost complete disappearance of the lactate peak. (Reprinted with permission from: Barkovich J, Westmark KD, Bedi HS, et al. Proton spectroscopy and diffussion imaging on the 1st day of life after perinatal asphyxia: preliminary report. *AJNR Am J Neuroradiol* 2001;22:1786.)

of energy-dependent ionic pumps results in an early influx of calcium into cells. With alterations in membrane homeostasis, there is a release of the excitatory neurotransmitters, especially glutamate, which activates N-methyl-D-aspartate (NMDA) and non-NMDA receptors that are enriched in particularly vulnerable regions and on targeted cells (neurons and preoligodendrocytes, respectively). This activation results in an increase in the activity of membrane-associated neuronal nitric oxide synthase (NOS) in neurons in the deep gray nuclei, and activation of microglia containing the inducible form of NOS. Increase in NOS activity results in generation of nitric oxide that diffuses over large areas and is both directly and indirectly toxic to vulnerable neurons and preoligodendrocytes with limited antioxidant reserves. These reactive oxygen and nitrogen species will damage membranes, as well as activate injurious genetic programs (transcription factors) that ultimately lead to energy-dependent cell death (Fig. 34.2). The pathologic changes observed in the brain are dependent upon the gestational age at the time of the insult. For example, selective neuronal necrosis of the deep gray nuclei, especially striatum and thalamus, is the most common pathologic finding noted in the term ischemic brain. In the preterm infant, both subplate neurons and preoligodendrocytes are selectively vulnerable, leading to a pattern of early white matter injury, and later diffuse cortical atrophy from disruption of thalamocortical connectivity disturbed by the loss of the subplate population. All of the vulnerable cells are susceptible to oxidative stress; therefore, therapies aimed at reducing the oxidative burden should eventually prove to be neuroprotective.

CLINICAL MANIFESTATIONS

Advances in technology, such as fetal ultrasonography and magnetic resonance imaging (MRI), and certain types of fetal heart rate monitoring can identify fetuses at risk before delivery. Structural lesions of the brain can be seen on ultrasound and distinctively verified by fetal MRI. During the intrapartum period, the evaluation of fetal heart rate and its relationship to uterine contractions has been used to assess fetal status. Investigations indicate that such findings as decelerations in fetal heart rate after a uterine contraction (late decelerations) are related to uteroplacental insufficiency and are influenced considerably by fetal hypoxia. Similarly, decelerations in fetal heart rate beginning with or occurring shortly after the uterine contraction (variable decelerations) appear to be related to umbilical cord compression, which, if continued, can result in reduction in umbilical cord blood flow and fetal hypoxia.

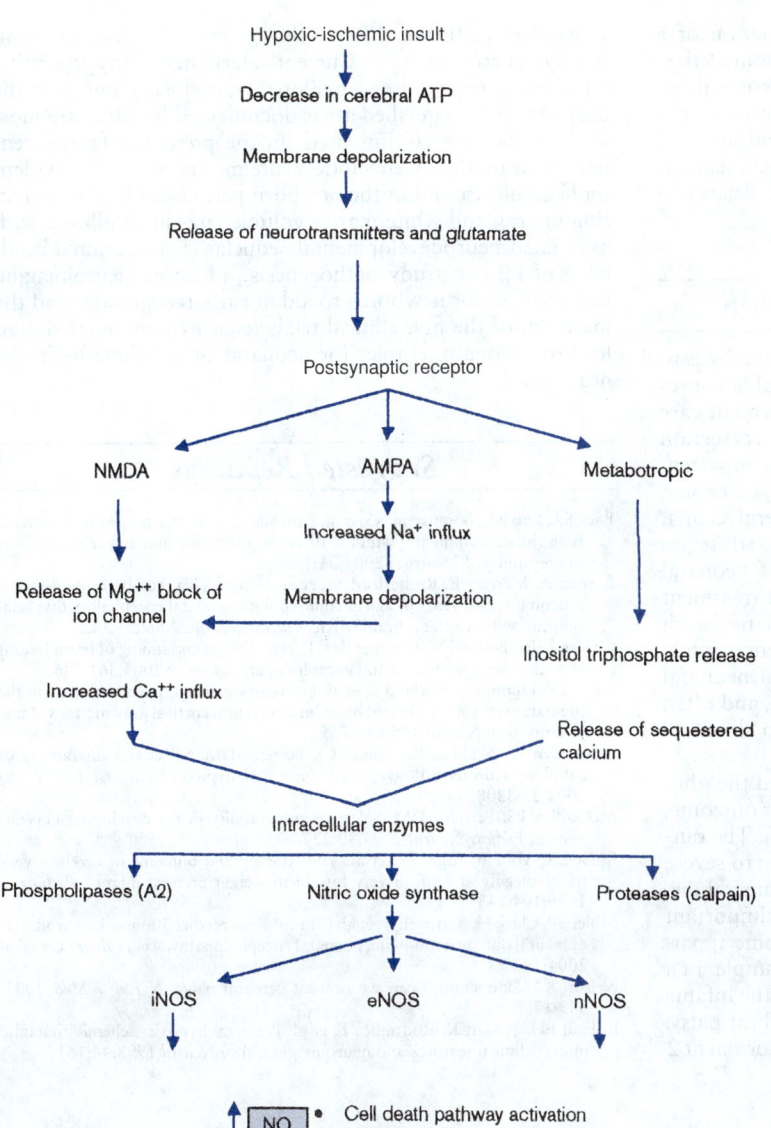

FIGURE 34.2. Flow diagram depicting pathogenetic mechanisms in hypoxic-ischemic encephalopathy. AMPA, (R,S)-alpha-amino-3-hydroxy-5-methylisoxazole-4-propionic acid; eNOS, endothelial nitric oxide synthase; iNOS, inducible nitric oxide synthase; nNOS, neuronal nitric oxide synthase; NMDA, N-methyl-D-aspartate. (Reprinted with permission from *Curr Opin Neurol* 16:147–154, 2003.)

Evaluation of fetal acid–base status by direct fetal blood sampling may provide another index of the oxidative compromise. However, identification of these fetal distress patterns that lead to caesarian delivery do not reduce the incidence of abnormal neurodevelopmental sequelae.

ever, as noted previously, these systemic abnormalities may be absent with less severe but more prolonged hypoxic-ischemic stress. More specialized investigations, such as the use of DWI and MRS imaging of the newborn brain and spinal cord, are providing important information in the newborn period that

DIAGNOSIS

Neonatal encephalopathy is easy to recognize and does not require sophisticated knowledge of the newborn neurologic examination. For any age newborn, the presence of lethargy or coma, altered tone and reflexes, poor or no feeding, and breathing difficulties, especially in the presence of clinically recognizable seizure activity, will uniformly identify neonates at risk (Table 34.1). Although Apgar scores are by far the most widely used index of the physical condition of the infant at birth, relating subsequent neurodevelopmental outcome to the Apgar score is fraught with error. Likewise, umbilical cord pH, PCO$_2$, and PO$_2$ levels are not predictive of future neurologic outcome, but do help to identify the infant at risk in the newborn period. Additional indicators of encephalopathy include the involvement of other organ systems: renal involvement (decreased urinary output), cardiac problems (cardiomyopathy), and liver abnormalities (abnormal liver enzyme levels). How-

TABLE 34.1

SIGNS OF NEONATAL ENCEPHALOPATHY

Encephalopathy Sign	Abnormal
Feeding	Gavage feeds, not tolerating oral feeds
Alertness	Irritable, poorly responsive, comatose
Tone	Hypotonia or hypertonia
Respiratory status	Respiratory distress (needs assisted ventilation: continuous positive airway pressure or mechanical ventilation)
Reflexes	Hyperreflexia, hyporeflexia, or absent primitive reflexes
Seizure	Any *clinical* seizure

will eventually influence management. The association of a profoundly abnormal electroencephalogram (e.g., nonreactive, low-voltage, or burst-suppression pattern) with neonatal encephalopathy carries ominous prognostic implications, but must be interpreted with respect to the gestational age and sleep stage at the time of the examination. In addition, temperature and drug effects (high-dose sedative-hypnotic drugs like phenobarbital) must be considered.

THERAPY AND PROGNOSIS

The first step in management of neonatal encephalopathy is to consider diagnostic possibilities focusing on treatable causes such as infection, toxin exposure, and trauma. Emergent care of the infant at birth includes respiratory support, correction of acid–base abnormalities, and treatment of any organ system failure. It is important to recognize that permissive hypercapnia and avoidance of extreme hyperoxia, hypo- or hyperglycemia, and hyperthermia are critical clinical management strategies that may be neuroprotective. Early recognition of neonatal seizures is critical, and it must be remembered that treatment with phenobarbital will cause electroclinical dissociation such that the neonate may still have electrographic seizures while exhibiting no clinical seizure activity. Treatment of neonatal status epilepticus from hypoxia-ischemia is difficult, and often multiple anticonvulsant medications are required to eliminate electrographic seizure activity.

Recent advances in neuroimaging have increased the ability to determine long-term cognitive and neuromotor outcome, especially when coupled with newborn examination. The outcome following HIE ranges from normal functioning to severe problems, such as cerebral palsy, pervasive developmental disorder, mental retardation, and seizures, to death. It is important to recognize that many of these problems do not become apparent until later in infancy or early childhood. For example, in a recent cohort study in the United Kingdom, 22% of the infants with neonatal encephalopathy died, 36% had cerebral palsy, and of the almost 50% who were considered to be normal at 2

years of age, a further 17% of those went on to develop cognitive dysfunction at age 5. Currently, term newborns presenting with severe neonatal encephalopathy, and early injury to the deep gray and watershed areas documented by MRI, are most likely to be severely impaired. In the preterm infant, recent data indicate that even subtle white matter injury not evident on head ultrasound in the newborn period can lead to reduction in gray and white matter volume later in childhood with associated neurodevelopmental sequelae. Better animal modeling of HIE to study pathogenesis, advanced neuroimaging technologies for newborns to aid in early recognition, and the initiation of the first clinical trials (e.g., hypothermia) should lead to rational therapies for neonatal encephalopathy in the near future.

Suggested Readings

Back SA, Luo NL, Borenstein NS, et al. Late oligodendrocyte progenitors coincide with the developmental window of vulnerability for human perinatal white matter injury. *J Neurosci* 2001;21:1302.

Barnett A, Mercuri E, Rutherford M, et al. Neurological and perceptual-motor outcome at 5–6 years of age in children with neonatal encephalopathy: relationship with neonatal brain MRI. *Neuropediatrics* 2002;33:242.

Cowan F, Rutherford M, Groenendaal F, et al. Origin and timing of brain lesions in term infants with neonatal encephalopathy. *Lancet* 2003;361:736.

Inder TE, Huppi PS, Warfield S, et al. Periventricular white matter injury in the premature infant is followed by reduced cerebral cortical gray matter volume at term. *Ann Neurol* 1999;46:755.

McQuillen PS, Sheldon RA, Shatz CJ, Ferriero DM. Selective vulnerability of subplate neurons following early neonatal hypoxia ischemia. *J Neurosci* 2003;23:3308.

McQuillen PS, Ferriero DM. Selective vulnerability in the developing nervous system. *Pediatr Neurol* 2004;30:227.

Ment LR, Vohr B, Allan W, et al. The etiology and outcome of cerebral ventriculomegaly at term in very low birth weight preterm infants. *Pediatrics* 1999;104:243.

Miller SP, Clark H, Barnwell A, et al. Clinical signs predict 30-month neurodevelopmental outcome following neonatal encephalopathy. *Am J Obstet Gynecol* 2004;190:93.

Nelson K. Commentary: can we prevent cerebral palsy. *N Eng J Med* 2003;349:1765.

Roland EH, Poskitt K, Rodriguez E, et al. Perinatal hypoxic-ischemic thalamic injury: clinical features and neuroimaging. *Ann Neurol* 1998;44:161.

CHAPTER 35 ■ PERINATAL CEREBRAL INFARCTION

LAURA R. MENT AND BARBARA R. POBER

Perinatal cerebral infarction, or stroke, may be defined as the severe disorganization or even complete disruption of the gray and white matter architecture of the developing brain caused by embolic, thrombotic, or ischemic events. Infarcts in early fetal life result in cortical neuronal loss and architectural changes resembling polymicrogyria. Strokes later in gestation are characterized by cavitary changes, or porencephalies, and appear similar to well-defined adult cerebral infarctions. In full-term neonates with stroke, cortical necrosis and hemorrhage into gray and subcortical white matter structures may be apparent.

Although strokes have been reported to occur in approximately 5% of infants coming to postmortem examination, conservative estimates suggest that neonatal stroke is recognized in approximately 1 per 4,000 live births per year, and this diagnosis should be entertained in those infants who have disorders ranging from congenital microcephaly to neonatal seizures to hemiparesis. Findings in an infant with perinatal cerebral infarction depend on both the timing in gestation and the underlying pathophysiology of the insult.

NEONATAL STROKE

Cerebral infarcts in the term neonate may be the result of embolic, thrombotic, thrombocytopenic, infectious, iatrogenic, or ischemic events, and several factors predispose the late-gestation fetus and newborn to stroke. The coagulation pathway in the newborn favors thrombosis, the hematocrit of the term neonate is high, and cerebral blood flow values of infants are low when compared with older children and adults. Finally, the patent foramen ovale permits more than one-half of all blood flow to pass to the brain. Most strokes in full-term neonates occur in the distribution of the middle cerebral arteries, and more than 75% are found in the left hemisphere. This finding may be explained by the relatively straight pathway of the left carotid artery to the developing brain and favors a thromboembolic mechanism for stroke; the right carotid artery follows a more tortuous course. Furthermore, recent data suggest that at least 30% of neonatal strokes are attributable to sinovenous thrombosis.

Pathology

Data from the National Hospital Discharge Survey from 1980 through 1998 demonstrated that the most common causes of neonatal stroke include hematologic disorders, infection, and cardiac anomalies. Less than 5% of infants with stroke had the now well-recognized characteristics of hypoxic-ischemic encephalopathy, suggesting that other etiologies must be considered. The risk factors for neonatal stroke are found in Table 35.1.

Thromboembolic Causes

In many infants, focal stroke is caused by thromboembolism from the placenta, the heart, or intra- or extracranial vessels. Several studies have suggested that coagulation disorders, including the factor V Leiden mutation, and protein C, protein S, and antithrombin III deficiencies are responsible for up to half of all strokes in neonates. Proteins C and S are natural anticoagulants that regulate the cascade of coagulation, inhibit factors Va and VIIIa, and activate fibrinolysis. The factor V Leiden mutation is attributable to a missense mutation of the factor V gene, thereby making it resistant to normal cleavage by activated protein C (APC). Protein C is activated by the thrombin–thrombomodulin complex and degrades factors Va and VIIIa. The factor V Leiden mutation results in increased thrombin generation and thus a shift to hypercoagulability (Fig. 35.1). The prothrombin G20210 and MTHFR (encodes

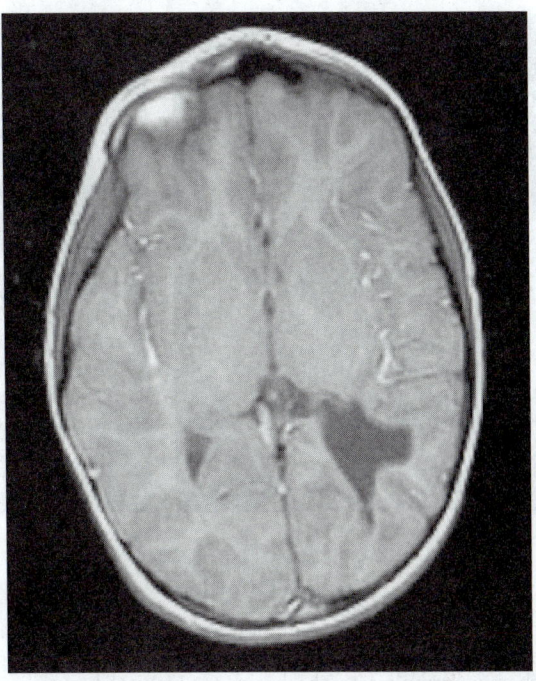

FIGURE 35.1. T1 magnetic resonance imaging (MRI) scans of a full-term infant who developed seizures on the second postnatal day. History revealed that the pregnancy had been complicated by poorly controlled gestational diabetes, and further evaluation revealed that the infant was heterozygous for the factor V Leiden mutation. MRI performed at age 2 years demonstrates focal enlargement of the occipital horn of the left ventricle with almost complete loss of occipital white matter and gray matter atrophy.

NAPDH) 677TT mutations, which also cause a shift toward hypercoagulability, have been implicated in neonatal stroke.

In addition, lipoprotein A is a plasma lipoprotein homologous to plasminogen, and elevated lipoprotein A levels have been found in neonates with focal stroke. Similarly, phospholipids are involved in the activation of protein C, and maternal antiphospholipid antibodies, including anticardiolipin and the lupus anticoagulant, interfere with normal coagulation. Both have also been reported in association with neonatal stroke.

Finally, infection (Fig. 35.2), indwelling catheters, and polycythemia are all associated with a hypercoagulable state, and all have been associated with focal central nervous system lesions in infants.

Sinovenous Thrombosis

Risk factors for sinovenous thrombosis in neonates include perinatal complications and dehydration. Perinatal complications reported with sinovenous thrombosis and stroke include hypoxia, premature rupture of the membranes, maternal infection and neonatal infections of the head and neck. Prothrombotic disorders have also been associated with this cause of neonatal stroke.

Causes of Hemorrhagic Stroke

In contrast, deficiencies of coagulation factors may result in hemorrhagic infarction. These deficits include congenital deficiencies such as factor VIII deficiency (hemophilia A), factor XIII deficiency, severe liver disease, and vitamin K deficiency.

Ischemic Causes

Although significantly less frequent than thromboembolic causes, ischemia may also be associated with neonatal stroke. Ischemic etiologies include severe fetomaternal hemorrhage, and maternal cocaine abuse.

TABLE 35.1

RISK FACTORS FOR NEONATAL STROKE

Thromboembolic stroke	Protein C deficiency
	Protein S deficiency
	Factor V Leiden mutation
	Antithrombin III deficiency
	Increased lipoprotein A
	Polycythemia
	Maternal anticardiolipin antibodies
	Maternal lupus anticoagulant
Hemorrhagic stroke	Factor VIII deficiency
	Factor XIII deficiency
	Vitamin K deficiency
	Severe liver disease
Ischemic stroke	Placental abruption
	Maternal cocaine
Cardiac causes	Cyanotic congenital heart disease
Infectious etiologies	Meningitis, sepsis
Iatrogenic causes	Cardiac catheterization
	Central catheters
	Trauma

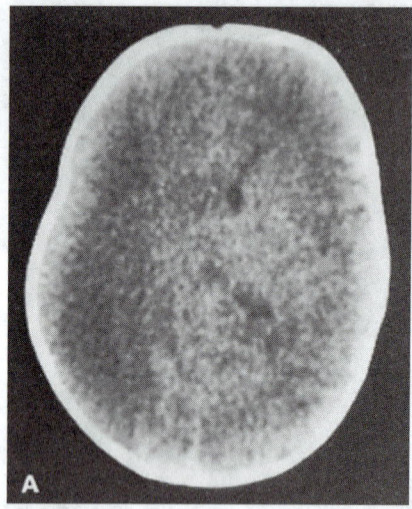
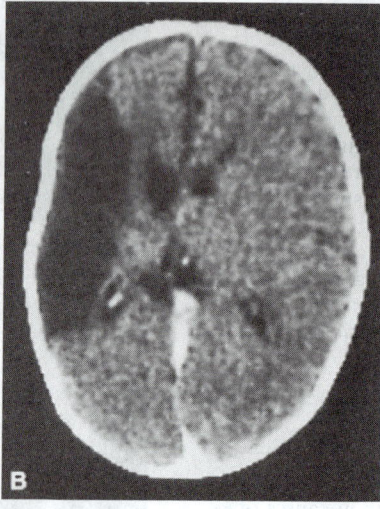

FIGURE 35.2. A: Computed tomographic scan demonstrating left hemispheric low density and effacement of the left lateral ventricle in a full-term infant with right-sided tonic–clonic seizures and meningitis. **B:** Follow-up scan (with contrast) at 1 year of age demonstrates focal tissue loss in the region of the left middle cerebral artery and corresponded to the patient's right spastic hemiparesis.

Cardiac Disorders

Cardiac disorders are a common risk factor for stroke in neonates and can lead to the formation of intracardiac thrombi, which may embolize to the brain. Congenital heart disease, cardiac procedures and surgery, and large vessel dissection have all been reported to be associated with stroke in infants.

Metabolic Causes

Metabolic causes for stroke in the newborn period include homocystinuria, organic acidurias, glutaric aciduria type I, molybdenum cofactor deficiency, and the mitochondrial encephalomyopathies, including MELAS syndrome (mitochondrial encephalopathy, lactic acidosis, and strokelike episodes) and pyruvate carboxylase deficiency.

Iatrogenic Causes

Other origins of stroke in the neonate include iatrogenic causes such as repeated cerebral ventricular taps, cardiac catheterization, and placement of catheters for extracorporeal membrane oxygenation therapy or hyperalimentation.

Additional Triggers for Neonatal Stroke

Stroke in infants may be multifactorial, and several studies have demonstrated that many infants with perinatal cerebral infarction have multiple thrombophilic abnormalities such as factor V Leiden mutation and anticardiolipin antibodies. Additional triggering factors such as asphyxia, sepsis, diffuse intravascular coagulation, and maternal gestational diabetes have been reported in over half of all infants with documented neonatal stroke.

Clinical Manifestations

Although infants with neonatal stroke can have a benign perinatal course, focal seizures are a common presentation and have been reported in 50% to 75% of neonates with stroke. Other common presenting features include hypotonia, hemiparesis, apnea, and respiratory difficulties. The recommended evaluation for neonates with suspected stroke is shown in Table 35.2. Current recommendations for maternal studies are also listed in Table 35.2, but this area is under active investigation.

Diagnosis

The diagnosis of stroke is most often made after neonatal cranial imaging. Although most infants first are studied with cranial sonography or computed tomographic (CT) scans, magnetic resonance imaging (MRI) is the modality of choice for the diagnosis of neonatal stroke. Diffusion-weighted MRI may provide earlier evidence of infarct than traditional MR, CT, or cranial ultrasonography. Further, MR angiography has been demonstrated to be extremely useful in the diagnosis of vascular occlusion or recanalization of vessels in the distribution of the middle cerebral arteries.

Prognosis

Neurodevelopmental Outcomes

The reported neurodevelopmental outcome of children with perinatal cerebral infarction varies widely, although neonatal MRI and electroencephalogram (EEG) studies may provide prognostic information. Recent data suggest, however, that approximately one- to two-thirds of infants with stroke

TABLE 35.2	
EVALUATION OF PERINATAL STROKE	
Imaging Studies	Diffusion-weighted MRI and MRA
	Echocardiogram, cardiac ultrasound
Laboratory Studies	CBC count, platelet count PT/PTT
	Lipoprotein (a)
	Protein C, protein S, antithrombin III
	Factor V Leiden mutation
	Prothrombin 20210 mutation
	MTHFR mutation
	Plasma amino acid analysis
	Lactate, pyruvate
	Urine organic acid analysis
	Urine toxicology screen
Electrophysiology study	EEG
Maternal studies	Anticardiolipin antibodies
	Lupus anticoagulant
	Placental pathology

CBC, complete blood cell; EEG, electroencephalogram; MRA, magnetic resonance angiography; MRI, magnetic resonance imaging; MTHFR, methylenetetrahydrofolate reductase; PT, prothrombin time; PTT, partial thromboplastin time.

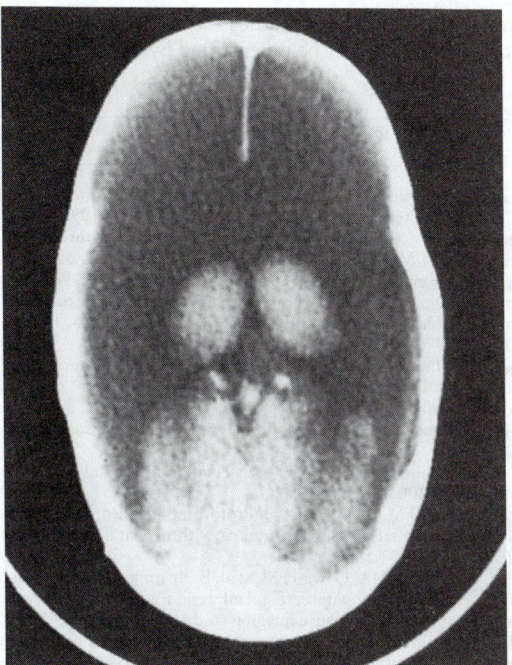

FIGURE 35.3. The computed tomographic scan of a 4-month-old girl with a large head and bulging fontanelle was significant for the diagnosis of hydranencephaly—the presence within an intact cranium of deep gray matter, posterior fossa structures, and brainstem, but nearly complete absence of hemispheric tissue.

documented in the newborn period will experience one or more neurodevelopmental disabilities at preschool age. Three-quarters of infants with abnormal EEG studies during the first postnatal week had motor and/or cognitive handicaps in one large study, and 60% with MRI-documented infarction of the internal capsule, basal ganglia, and posterior limb of the internal capsule developed hemiplegic cerebral palsy in another study.

Recurrent Stroke

Existing data are limited but suggest that the aggregate rate for a 2nd neonatal stroke is 3% to 5%. However, this risk will vary in individual patients according to the specific etiology of the stroke.

FETAL STROKE

The widespread use of fetal ultrasonography and recent advent of fetal MRI studies have permitted both the detection of antenatal stroke and the study of the mechanisms underlying such events. During the mid- to late second and entire third trimesters of gestation, three factors permit the development of cavitary lesions in the fetal cerebrum. The high water content, relatively low myelin concentration, and paucity of active glial response in the developing brain make it susceptible to dissolution and to the secondary formation of such lesions as hydranencephaly (Fig. 35.3) and porencephaly. In hydranencephaly there is almost complete absence of the cerebral hemispheres with intact basal ganglia and brainstem structures. Infants with this condition also experience abnormalities of the cerebellum, olfactory regions, and optic nerves. The normal-appearing cranium is filled with a meningeal sac that contains fluid with a high protein content, thought to be secondary to the primary destructive process. These infants frequently require ventriculoperitoneal shunts and, although many are seen in the newborn period with large heads, in others the hydranencephaly is not detected until the third or fourth postnatal months, when they fail to reach normal milestones. Porencephaly refers to cavitary defects extending from the ventricular space into the cerebral hemisphere.

Clinically, although affected infants may experience increased intracranial pressure from these lesions, the presentation generally depends on the cortical location of the lesion. Finally, insults later in gestation result in regional neuronal cortical loss and areas of focal atrophy that may be accompanied by secondary ventricular system enlargement.

Prenatal imaging reveals hemorrhagic lesions in over 90% of fetuses with stroke, and porencephalies are reported to occur

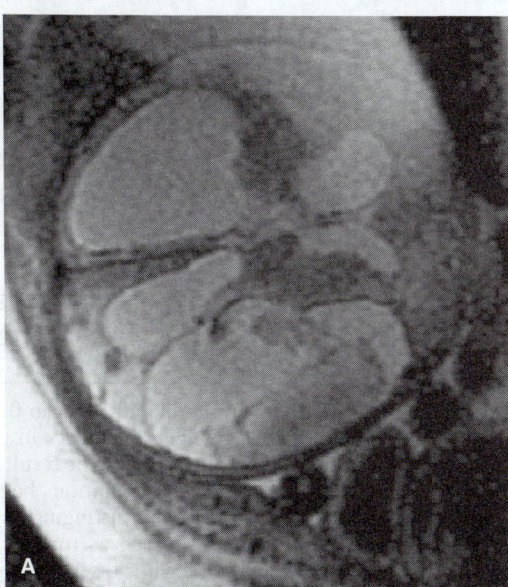
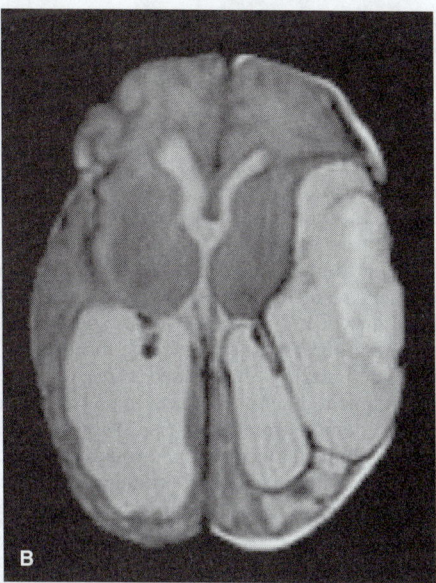

FIGURE 35.4. A: Axial T1 fetal magnetic resonance imaging (MRI) scan of a 34-week fetus with a large left hemorrhagic stroke in the left hemisphere secondary to maternal alloimmune thrombocytopenia. **B:** Follow-up neonatal axial MRI at age 2 days again demonstrates the large left hemisphere hemorrhagic infarct as well as bilateral ventriculomegaly.

in only 13% of lesions detected prior to the onset of labor resulting in delivery.

Pathology

Stroke in the fetus may be caused by hemorrhage, ischemia, thrombosis, or a combination of events. Over one-quarter of reported cases have evidence for hemorrhagic disturbances of coagulation, including maternal alloimmune thrombocytopenia (Fig. 35.4), maternal anticoagulation with warfarin, and fetal von Willebrand disease. Ischemic injury has been postulated as the mechanism for fetal stroke in several cases of significant maternal trauma and placental hemorrhage or abruption; stroke in twins with twin–twin transfusion syndrome is also thought to be secondary to ischemic events. Fetal stroke associated with placental thromboses have been reported in association with maternal viral illnesses and in a single case of fetal protein C deficiency. Finally, fetal disorders such as pyruvate carboxylase deficiency and congenital infections account for approximately one-fifth of all reported cases of fetal stroke.

Prognosis

Prognosis of fetal stroke is difficult to assess but overall appears poorer than for neonatal stroke. Over half of cases reported in the literature resulted in either fetal demise or neonatal death; similarly, half of the surviving infants were found to have cognitive and motor deficits at 1 to 6 years of age.

Similar to neonatal stroke, the risk of recurrent fetal stroke is unknown but will likely be determined by the specific etiology.

Suggested Readings

deVeber GA, Monagle P, Chan A, et al. Prothrombotic disorders in infants and children with cerebral thromboembolism. *Arch Neurol* 1998;55:1539.

deVeber G, Andrew M, Adams C, et al. Cerebral sinovenous thrombosis in children. *N Engl J Med* 2001;345:417–23.

Ferriero DM. Neonatal Brain Injury. *N Engl J Med* 2004;351:1985–1995.

Gunther G, Junker R, Strater R, et al. Symptomatic ischemic stroke in full-term neonates. Role of acquired and genetic prothrombotic risk factors. *Stroke* 2000;31:2437.

Lynch JK, Hirtz DG, deVeber GA, Nelson KB. Report of the National Institute of Neurological Disorders and Stroke Workshop on Perinatal and Childhood Stroke. *Pediatrics* 2002;109:116.

Lynch JK, Nelson KB. Epidemiology of perinatal stroke. *Curr Opin Pediatr* 2001;13:499.

Marret S, Lardennois C, Mercier A, et al. Fetal and neonatal cerebral infarcts. *Biol Neonate* 2001;70:236.

Mercuri E, Cowan FM, Gupte G, et al. Prothrombotic disorders and abnormal neurodevelopmental outcome in infants with neonatal cerebral infarction. *Pediatrics* 2001;107:1400.

Mercuri E, Rutherford MA, Cowan FM, et al. Early prognostic indicators of outcome in infants with neonatal cerebral infarction: a clinical, electroencephalogram, and magnetic resonance imaging study. *Pediatrics* 1999;103:39.

Rutherford MA. What's new in neuroimaging? Magnetic resonance imaging of the immature brain. *Eur J Paediatr Neurol* 2002;6:5.

Scher MS, Wiznitzer M, Bangert BA. Cerebral infarctions in the fetus and neonate: maternal-placental-fetal considerations. *Clin Perinatol* 2002;29:693.

Thorarensen O, Ryan S, Hunter J, Younkin DP. Factor V Leiden mutation: an unrecognized cause of hemiplegic cerebral palsy, neonatal stroke and placental thrombosis. *Ann Neurol* 1997;42:372.

CHAPTER 36 ■ NEONATAL SEIZURES

EDWARD J. NOVOTNY Jr.

Seizures have long been known to be an important sign of neurologic disease in the newborn and accompany neonatal encephalopathies due to a variety of causes. Recent evidence has raised concerns that both seizures and certain medications used in their treatment result in increased risk of neurologic mortality and morbidity. Over the last two decades, bedside video/electroencephalogram (EEG)/polygraphic monitoring in neonates with suspected seizures has raised some important issues regarding the clinical diagnosis of seizures. Two important points have been demonstrated by these studies. First, a significant number of clinical phenomena thought to represent seizures have no accompanying EEG changes on surface recordings. Second, many seizures diagnosed by electroencephalographic criteria have no associated clinical features. This information suggests both that certain types of neonatal seizures may have been overestimated and that the total number of seizures may have been underestimated in the past. These new findings present a diagnostic and therapeutic challenge to clinicians caring for these children and have resulted

in recent changes in the classification, diagnosis, and therapy of seizures in the newborn.

CLASSIFICATION AND CLINICAL MANIFESTATIONS

Neonatal seizures are common and occur in 0.5% to 3.5% of newborns, with a slightly higher incidence in preterm infants. Inconsistency in epidemiologic data is the result of variability in the diagnostic criteria and the populations being studied. The classification is best achieved by distinguishing those infants with primary motor features such as tonic, clonic, and myoclonic activity versus subtle clinical seizure types (Box 36.1).

Generalized tonic–clonic seizures are very rare in the newborn. The behavioral phenomena that most consistently correlate with EEG seizure discharges are partial motor and myoclonic seizures. Clonic seizures involving one limb, one side of

without head deviation and asymmetric posturing of the limbs or trunk are frequently associated with electrographic seizures. The EEG discharges associated with tonic seizures involving the limbs usually consist of rhythmic, high-frequency sharp waves and spikes arising from the frontotemporal regions. The eye deviation is associated with similar discharges arising from the occipital scalp electrodes. Generalized myoclonic seizures are another type, which often have associated electrocortical discharges. The myoclonus occurs sporadically or in a few slow series of jerks. The EEG typically shows high amplitude spike-, sharp-, and slow-wave transients synchronized with the motor activity.

The behavioral phenomena that have a variable association with EEG seizure discharges are the generalized tonic, irregular myoclonic, and subtle neonatal seizures. This last category is also referred to as motor automatism, and specific types may have a greater association with electrographic seizures depending on other clinical features. The subtle neonatal seizure that is the most commonly observed type in several studies has a poor association with EEG seizure discharges in the full-term neonate. However, there is a greater association with electrographic seizures in the premature infant. Their clinical features may further divide subtle seizures into those involving the mouth and tongue, the eyes, and more complex movements such as pedaling, swimming, and stepping. The premature neonates often have simple subtle seizures with eye, mouth, and tongue movements. The electrographic seizures in the premature infants are very distinctive and have a characteristic progression and spread throughout multiple cortical regions with minimal accompanying clinical signs (Fig. 36.1). In the term infant who has more complex motor automatisms, there is often no associated EEG discharge. Myoclonic activity that is irregular, multifocal, and often stimulus-induced is typically not associated with any changes in electrocortical activity. These infants usually have markedly abnormal EEGs for gestational age with suppressed and poorly differentiated background. The infants who have episodes described as generalized tonic seizures rarely have them as a result of an epileptic seizure. Less than 15% of infants with these clinical phenomena had electrographic seizures as a cause. These episodes most

the body, and axial structures such as the tongue and face reliably have accompanying synchronous EEG discharges. These clonic movements are rhythmic and occur at a slow rate of one to four times per second. A feature more commonly observed in neonates is that the clonic activity is multifocal or migratory. This characteristic may cause the seizures to appear generalized. The EEG discharges typically consist of runs of rhythmic sharp–slow wave complexes that spread ipsilaterally over the hemisphere from which they originate. Often the clonic activity is not observed until the EEG discharges spread to the central regions near the motor cortex. At this time the motor activity is synchronized with the EEG activity. Focal tonic seizures in which the infant has sustained deviation of the eyes with or

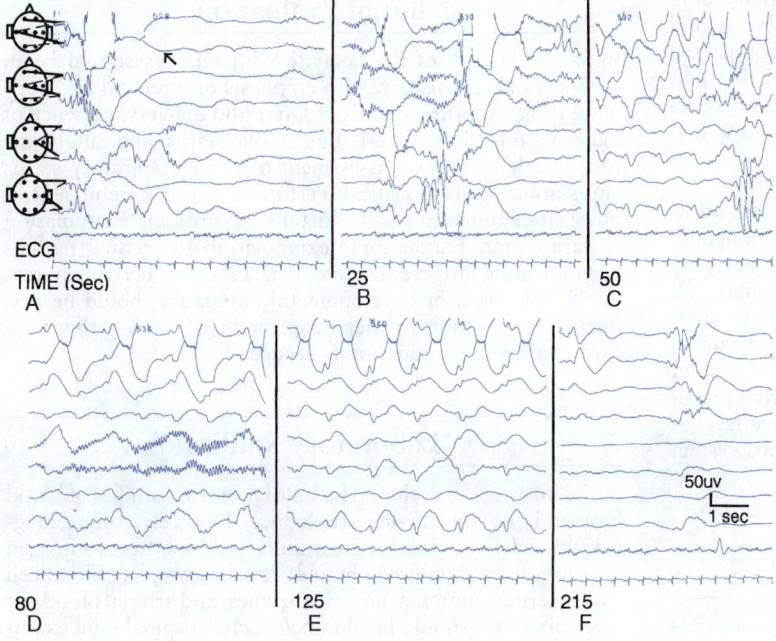

FIGURE 36.1. Subclinical electrographic seizure in a 2-day-old, 29-week estimated gestational age neonate with severe perinatal asphyxia and bilateral intraventricular hemorrhages. The seizure begins with low-amplitude rhythmic alpha activity in the left temporal region (*arrow*). This builds up in amplitude and spreads to the left central region 25 seconds into the ictal event. Fifty seconds into the seizure irregular, sharp–slow waves are observed over the entire left hemisphere, are higher amplitude anteriorly, and spread to the right frontal region. Rhythmic alpha activity is observed to arise from the right central region 80 seconds into the seizure when the infant was noted to open the left eye. The sharp–slow wave activity is maximum over the left temporal region with spread over the entire cortex 125 seconds into the seizure, which ends 215 seconds from its inception.

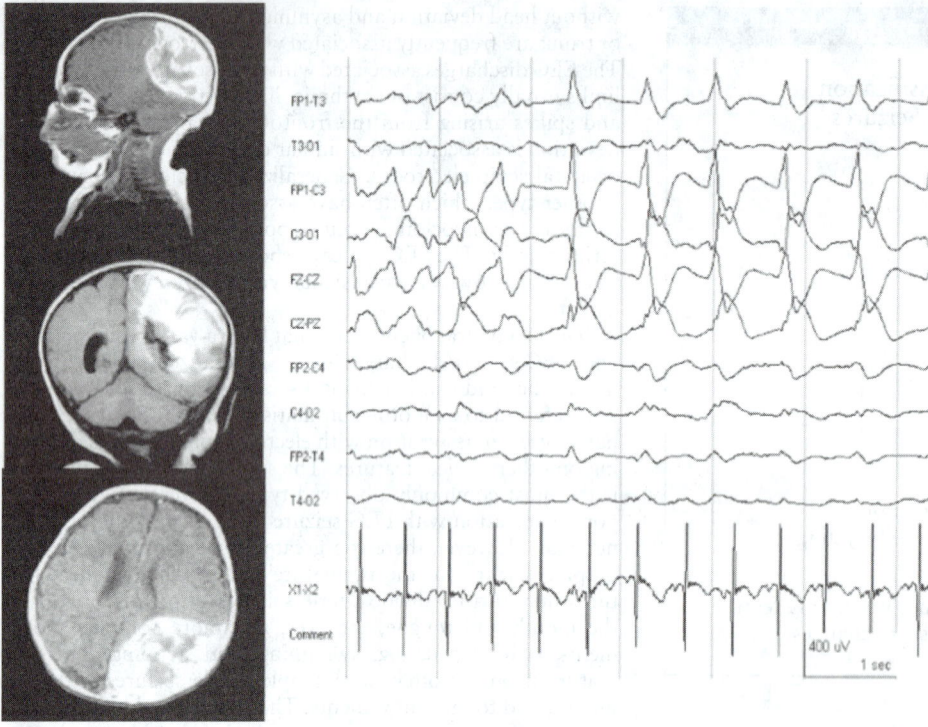

FIGURE 36.2. Magnetic resonance imaging (MRI) scan of the head and electroencephalogram (EEG) of a term infant observed to have clonic activity predominantly involving the right side of the body in the first day of life. The MRI on the left shows sagittal, coronal, and axial T1-weighted images (*from top to bottom*) demonstrating a large hemorrhagic stroke involving the left parietal lobe. The EEG demonstrates nearly continuous epileptic discharges arising from the left hemisphere and midline scalp electrodes. The odd-numbered channels are from the left side of the scalp and even-numbered channels are from the right side. The infant was having nearly continuous right arm and leg motor activity at the time of the EEG.

probably represent decerebrate and decorticate posturing from acute intracranial pathology.

Clinical attributes that differentiate clonic seizures from tremors and clonus are that infants with clonic seizures have slower, more rhythmic motor activity that cannot be restrained, whereas infants with tremors and clonus have rapid, irregular motor activity that ceases with restraint and change in posture. Tremor, clonus, and other nonepileptic motor automatisms are typically induced by various tactile, noxious, and auditory stimuli. Nonepileptic phenomena also demonstrate properties of spatial and temporal summation with increased intensity or frequency of the stimulus. These latter behaviors are abnormal and usually indicate the existence of an encephalopathy, but they do not represent behaviors that warrant treatment with antiepileptic therapy. Another clinical characteristic that aids in distinguishing epileptic from nonepileptic abnormal behavioral phenomena is that epileptic seizures are typically accompanied by changes in heart rate, respiratory pattern, pupil size, and blood pressure. Further video/EEG/polygraphic studies are required in the neonate to better define the temporal and spatial relationships of these autonomic changes with the electroclinical seizure.

As suggested by several investigators, the more recent information on both underestimation and overestimation of neonatal seizures and the past lack of a consensus of what phenomena are truly epileptic seizures in the newborn make all previous investigations of etiology, treatment, and prognosis of limited value. These concerns have the greatest impact on treatment, since prognosis and etiology are interdependent and the seizures are simply a symptom of an underlying neuropathologic process. Recent concerns regarding the effects of antiepileptic drug therapy on the developing nervous system has increased the importance of these issues.

ETIOLOGY AND DIAGNOSIS

The causes of neonatal seizures include perinatal asphyxia, central nervous system infections, intracranial hemorrhages, and cerebral infarcts; these are the most common disorders responsible for neonatal seizures. Developmental anomalies, acute metabolic disorders, and rare inborn errors of metabolism are less common causes. The identification of the latter two categories of causes is crucial since the treatment is management of the underlying disease. Certain types of seizures are observed in infants with specific disorders. Persistent partial motor seizures are typically observed in infants with strokes (Fig. 36.2). Clonic seizures are also commonly seen in infants with hypocalcemia, the incidence of which has decreased dramatically in recent decades. Subtle and tonic seizures are more common in infants with hypoxic-ischemic encephalopathy.

Initial Evaluation

Initial evaluation of the neonate with seizures should begin with a thorough history, with emphasis on prenatal and perinatal drug exposure, details of labor and delivery, presence of maternal infection, maternal metabolic status, and family history of seizures. Early assessment of cardiorespiratory status and stabilization are critical. Performance of a careful general physical examination and a detailed neurologic examination is paramount. Funduscopic examination for retinal pathology indicating intracranial hemorrhage, central nervous system (CNS) infection, or developmental anomalies should be performed. Evaluation for hepatosplenomegaly and a thorough cardiovascular examination is needed.

Laboratory Studies

Initial investigations should include laboratory studies of blood for metabolic abnormalities (Box 36.2). Blood electrolyte, magnesium, calcium, glucose, creatinine, and blood urea nitrogen measurements should be obtained first. A complete blood cell count, serum ammonia, hepatic enzymes, and arterial blood gas determinations should be obtained. Cerebrospinal fluid examination for cell count, protein, bacterial culture, glucose, and

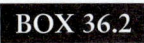

BOX 36.2   **Diagnostic Evaluation of the Neonate with Seizures**

Blood
    Glucose, electrolytes, magnesium, calcium, ammonia, pH, and lactate
Cerebrospinal fluid
    Cell count, protein, glucose, lactate, and culture
Cranial ultrasonography
Clinical neurophysiologic study
    Bedside EEG
    Long-term EEG with pyridoxine infusion (selected cases)
Urine amino acids and organic acids, plasma, and cerebrospinal fluid amino acids (selected cases)
Maternal and newborn titers for congenital infections (selected cases)
Neuroimaging
    CT scan for hemorrhage and calcium deposition
    MRI for cerebral dysgenesis, malformations, and hypoxic-ischemic injury

---

CT, computerized tomography; EEG, electroencephalogram; MRI, magnetic resonance imaging.

---

lactate should be done to exclude CNS infections, hemorrhage, and injury. In selected cases, serum amino and organic acids and cerebrospinal fluid amino acids should be obtained.

Imaging Studies

Head ultrasound is an excellent initial imaging technique that can be useful to exclude major structural anomalies, hemorrhage, and hydrocephalus. However, computed topography or magnetic resonance imaging (MRI) is usually required. MRI studies in the premature and term infant have shown exquisite, high-resolution images of the brain without the use of ionizing radiation. MRI is clearly superior to computed tomography for the identification of cerebral infarcts, cerebral dysgenesis, and brain injury. Magnetic resonance spectroscopy identifies biochemical changes in the brain and can identify rare neurometabolic diseases and provide prognostic information.

Neurophysiologic Studies

Clinical neurophysiologic investigations of the neonate with seizures are best performed during the clinical event thought to be a seizure. This is usually impractical and an EEG should be obtained as soon as possible. The EEG obtained between seizures provides important information about neurologic prognosis that is enhanced with serial recordings. A normal EEG obtained between seizures decreases the probability that a specific behavior thought to be a seizure was an epileptic seizure. The EEG is increasingly being recorded using digital technology, and certain modules can be integrated into the monitors in the intensive care nursery. Many of these systems have technical limitations and require the availability of skilled electroencephalographers familiar with the neonatal EEG. The routine EEG obtained at the bedside in between seizures cannot verify whether a clinical event was an epileptic seizure. Unlike in older children and adults, there are no

specific EEG patterns in the neonatal EEG that have a high association with epileptic seizures. However, there are specific EEG patterns observed in certain CNS infections, such as herpes simplex encephalitis, and neurometabolic disorders, such as nonketotic hyperglycinemia. Persistent asymmetries and focal abnormalities are often highly correlated with structural CNS pathology (Fig. 36.2).

Optimally, continuous EEG monitoring is the method to use to diagnose epileptic seizures and follow response to treatment. Modern digital technology has improved the availability and decreased the size of systems that can be used at the bedside and often be combined with digital video. Alternatively, systems integrated into intensive care monitoring systems have been developed. These systems require varying degrees of technical support and more importantly require clinicians and other personnel familiar with their interpretation and use. Neonates who continue to have persistent clinical seizures after careful clinical assessment and treatment with first-line antiepileptic drugs should have some form of clinical neurophysiologic monitoring. These infants should also have EEG studies with intravenous pyridoxine to exclude this rare treatable neurometabolic disorder.

Certain types of seizures are seen in neonates with specific neurologic disorders. For example, persistent motor seizures are often seen in infants with strokes or congenital anomalies (Fig. 36.2). A newborn with a hemorrhagic stroke possibly associated with a congenital vascular malformation had almost continuous seizures involving primarily the left side of the body. Clonic seizures are seen in infants with hypocalcemia. The incidence of this metabolic disorder causing seizures has decreased significantly because of early recognition and treatment.

Molecular Studies

Over the last decade, several specific epileptic syndromes have been identified to have onset in the neonatal period, and modern molecular studies have identified new causes of these disorders. These disorders include early myoclonic encephalopathy (EME), early infantile epileptic encephalopathy (EIEE), pyridoxine-dependent seizures, and benign familial neonatal convulsions.

EME is characterized by erratic, fragmented motor activity that begins in the first month of life, often in the first week. This myoclonic activity is followed by partial seizures, massive multifocal myoclonus, infantile spasms, and tonic seizures. The EEG shows a burst-suppression pattern with periods of attenuation of the EEG lasting 4 to 20 seconds. The EEG often develops into the hypsarhythmia pattern observed in infantile spasms or a markedly abnormal background with multifocal epileptic discharges. The infants have a severe encephalopathy that is apparent at birth and continue to have delayed milestones and generalized hypotonia and remain unresponsive. Some have microcephaly at birth, and the majority of infants develop a progressive microcephaly associated with cerebral atrophy on neuroimaging. Often the cause is not identified, although some infants are identified to have rare genetic disorders such as glycine encephalopathy, propionic acidemia, D-glyceric acidemia, and other rare recessively inherited diseases.

EIEE, also known as Ohtahara syndrome, has significant overlap with EME. The EEG abnormalities are very similar and the cause may be the same. However, the clinical seizures and course are characterized by tonic seizures in the neonatal period. These seizures are accompanied by an electrodecremental ictal EEG pattern also observed in infantile spasms. The infants have a similar severe encephalopathy, and their epilepsy progresses into infantile spasms, multiple partial seizures with multifocal epileptic abnormalities, and Lennox-Gastaut syndrome with a slow-spike slow-wave EEG pattern. Many of these infants have severe malformations such as lissencephaly and holoprosencephaly. Neuroimaging and molecular studies can identify specifically both X-linked and autosomal disorders that can cause these malformations.

Pyridoxine-dependent seizures are a probable autosomal recessive disorder that has onset in the first 3 months of life, usually in the first week. The disorder is rare, with a prevalence of greater than 1 per 500,000. Despite appropriate treatment with pyridoxine, some children are mentally retarded and develop a leukodystrophy and atrophy that can be seen on MRI. The EEG pattern is nonspecific, but when 50 to 100 mg of pyridoxine is given intravenously, prompt cessation of both clinical and electroencephalographic seizures is observed. The interictal epileptiform activity often disappears and the effect persists for a few hours after treatment. The test should be repeated if results are equivocal or transient. Children with this disorder require lifelong treatment with pyridoxine. Unfortunately, there is currently no molecular diagnostic study available, but biochemical abnormalities such as elevated cerebrospinal fluid (CSF) glutamate and low CSF gamma-hydroxybutyric acid have been identified.

Modern genomic methods have permitted identification of the cause of a group of rare disorders known as benign familial neonatal convulsions (BFNCs), usually with autosomal dominant inheritance with variable penetrance. The family history is a critical part of identifying these infants. They usually begin having seizures by the third day of life. The seizures are often focal clonic and tonic seizures with variable automatisms. Myoclonic seizures are rare. The seizures spontaneously remit in the majority of infants; 10% to 15% later develop another form of epilepsy. The genes for infants with BFNCs encode proteins of ion channels and are part of a group of disorders referred to as channelopathies. Mutations in both sodium and potassium channels have been identified.

THERAPY

The most important aspect of treatment is early and accurate diagnosis of seizures. Modern digital electroencephalographic equipment is able to record signals for long periods of time. The addition of digital video is now almost standard and makes continuous electroencephalographic monitoring more feasible in the neonatal intensive care unit. Recent intensive monitoring studies have identified certain types of seizures that have a high association with epileptic discharges and, as described above, particular clinical features can be used to determine whether an event is an epileptic seizure. Therefore, clonic, partial tonic, and generalized myoclonic seizures can often be treated based on clinical criteria alone. The use of the interictal EEG is limited by the availability of equipment and skilled electroencephalographers in most neonatal intensive care nurseries and the absence of specific EEG patterns that have a high association with seizures in the interictal recording of the newborn. If available, clinical neurophysiologic with video monitoring can be used to identify whether an event is an epileptic seizure, although whether the lack of surface EEG epileptic activity excludes a seizure is controversial. Further clinical studies are required to address this issue.

Another significant issue regarding management brought about by neurophysiologic monitoring is in regard to criteria that should be used for determination of the adequacy of therapy. Should clinical or electrical criteria be used to judge therapeutic efficacy? Several studies have shown that the majority of electrical seizures in the newborn are of short duration and have no accompanying clinical signs. One investigator found that 79% of infants had subclinical electrical seizures and the majority of these newborns were treated with antiepileptic agents. Other studies have shown that electrical seizures persist

TABLE 36.1

ANTIEPILEPTIC DRUGS AND DOSES

Antiepileptic Drug	Loading Dose	Maintenance Dose
Phenobarbital	30–40 mg/kg	3–5 mg/kg/day
Phenytoin	15–20 mg/kg	7–10 mg/kg/day
Fosphenytoin	15–20 mg/kg	7–10 mg/kg/day
Diazepam	0.05–0.15 mg/kg	—

even after treatment. Most animal studies investigating neonatal seizures have demonstrated significant biochemical changes only with prolonged (more than 30 minutes) seizures. Both clinical and electrical seizures in the human neonate typically last less than 3 minutes. Clearly, further information is needed to determine whether brief, subclinical electrical seizures are deleterious to the immature nervous system. In the meantime, therapy should be guided by the response of clinical events that are determined to be epileptic.

The duration of therapy should be guided by the risk of recurrence of seizures and the possible toxicity induced by treatment. Infants with significant structural lesions are at high risk. Infants with hypoxic-ischemic encephalopathy or metabolic causes have a much lower risk. If the neurologic examination and the interictal EEG are normal, the probability of the infant having later seizures is small. The recent concerns of the effects of drugs on the developing nervous system has also dictated that the duration of therapy be kept to a minimum. Antiepileptic therapy is discontinued in most infants prior to discharge from neonatal intensive care, and rarely is treatment continued for greater than 4 to 8 weeks following discharge.

Phenobarbital has been the drug of choice in the treatment of neonatal seizures. This drug is given as a single loading dose of 15 to 20 mg/kg and increased by 5 to 10 mg/kg increments until serum concentrations of 40 mg/L are achieved (Table 36.1). Phenytoin is often a second-line drug and is given at a dosage of 15 to 20 mg/kg at a rate no greater than 1 mg/kg/minute. Fosphenytoin is a newer prodrug of phenytoin that decreases the risk of cardiac arrhythmias and soft tissue injury with extravasation. Both drugs have long half-lives (up to 100 hours) and similar maintenance dosages. Valproic acid, lignocaine, and benzodiazepines (diazepam, lorazepam, and midazolam) have been used in newborns and are available in parenteral forms. There is little to no experience with the use of newer antiepileptic agents, such as vigabatrin, lamotrigine, topiramate, and felbamate, in the newborn. In general, the most efficacious antiepileptic agents should be used and the duration of therapy should be minimized. Further consideration should be given to short-acting agents such as benzodiazepines.

PROGNOSIS

Numerous studies have shown that the prognosis is closely associated with the cause. Studies have shown that mortality may be as high as 30% of newborns and that greater than 50% have significant neurologic and cognitive handicaps. Approximately one-third of infants with neonatal seizures develop epilepsy. The presence of CNS anomalies or structural lesions on neuroimaging studies has a significant impact on the long-term outcome of the infant. For four decades the EEG has been shown to be a valuable tool in determining prognosis in the premature and full-term neonate with various pathologies, including infants with seizures. If specific criteria are used to grade the severity of the background abnormality on the EEG, the degree of abnormality predicts long-term outcome better than the clinical examination. Certain types of seizures determined both clinically and electrographically also permit further refinement of the ability to determine prognosis. Infants with tonic or subtle seizures often have diffuse, severe encephalopathies and a poorer outcome. A unique ictal EEG pattern characterized by bursts of rhythmic 8 to 12 Hz activity are often seen in newborns with severe encephalopathies (Fig. 36.1). These infants often have a poor prognosis. Further investigations combining the clinical examination, the EEG, and neuroimaging are required to refine our ability to determine prognosis.

Research is needed to address many of the issues discussed in this section. Animal studies addressing the molecular mechanisms, biochemistry, and neuroanatomic changes that take place in repetitive seizures in the immature brain are needed. Clinical investigations involving clinical neurophysiology and advanced neuroimaging methods, such as diffusion-weighted MRI and magnetic resonance spectroscopy, are needed. These should be combined with pharmacologic interventions and comprehensive follow-up studies to answer questions critical to the management of this important neurologic disorder.

Suggested Readings

Holmes GL, Khazipov R, Ben-Ari Y. New concepts in neonatal seizures. *Neuroreport* 2002;13:A3.

Levene M. The clinical conundrum of neonatal seizures. *Arch Dis Child Fetal Neonatal Ed* 2002;86:F75.

Mizrahi EM. Consensus and controversy in the clinical management of neonatal seizures. *Clin Perinatol* 1989;16:485.

Mizrahi EM, Clancy RR. Neonatal seizures: early-onset seizure syndromes and their consequences for development. *Mental Retard Dev Disabil Res Rev* 2000;6:229.

Mizrahi EM, Kellaway P. Characterization and classification of neonatal seizures. *Neurology* 1987;37:1837.

Rennie JM, Boylan GB. Neonatal seizures and their treatment. *Curr Opin Neurol* 2003;16:177.

Scher MS. Controversies regarding neonatal seizure recognition. *Epileptic Disord* 2002;4:139.

Scher MS, Alvin J, Gaus L, et al. Uncoupling of EEG-clinical neonatal seizures after antiepileptic drug use. *Pediatr Neurol* 2003;28:277.

Tharp BR. Neonatal seizures and syndromes. *Epilepsia* 2002;43:2.

CHAPTER 37 ■ THE FLOPPY INFANT AND THE LATE WALKER

RICHARD S. K. YOUNG

The pediatrician may occasionally discover that an infant has poor head or truncal tone, and laxity in the arms and legs. This condition is commonly referred to as "The Floppy Infant." The child who is not yet walking independently at 18 months of life is termed a "late walker." Although these terms are not specific, they are useful as interim diagnostic labels until a more conclusive diagnosis is reached. During the past decade, major strides have been made in the understanding of the pathophysiology of these conditions.

HISTORY

In the diagnosis of neurologic disease, the patient's history furnishes clues to the nature of the disorder, and the physical examination and laboratory tests provide confirmation. When the history of an infant with hypotonia is taken, information regarding any family history of neuromuscular disease, the quality of the fetal movements, and the presence of hydramnios should be obtained. The temporal sequence of the disorder is of particular importance (When did it start? Is it progressive or static? Is the child worse today than he or she was one month ago?). The child's pattern of growth and his or her ability to feed should be elicited. Figure 37.1 presents algorithms for general diagnostic approaches to hypotonia.

PHYSICAL EXAMINATION

A general physical examination of any infant with suspected neurologic disease is essential to rule out motor delays caused by systemic disease. It should be determined whether congestive heart failure (dyspnea, edema, organomegaly) may be responsible for weakness or fatigue. The child should be examined for dysmorphic features (suggestive of a chromosomal abnormality) and for signs of endocrinopathy or metabolic disorder (umbilical hernia, dull cry, abnormal hair texture).

Weakness typically manifests in the neck, resulting in poor head control. Weakness in the proximal large muscles of the pectoral and pelvic girdle may result in delay in walking in the older child. The muscles should be inspected for bulk, atrophy, fasciculations, and symmetry. The presence of fasciculations in the tongue muscle is evidence of denervation. The muscle stretch reflexes should be tested, and it should be determined whether sensation is intact. Weakness in the facial or bulbar musculature is prominent in several disorders (myotonic dystrophy, myasthenia gravis, Möbius syndrome).

NEUROLOGIC EVALUATION

Based on the results of the history and physical examination, the physician first should determine whether a problem exists or whether a child simply is at the lower limits of normal. If a neuromuscular disorder is suspected, it should be decided whether the lesion is central (spasticity correlates with upper motor neuron involvement) or peripheral (hyporeflexia correlates with an interruption of the lower motor neuron arc). The pediatrician should think systematically about each element of the motor system, beginning with the cerebral cortex, proceeding to the spinal cord, the anterior horn cells, the peripheral nerves, and the neuromuscular junction (motor end plate) to the muscle fiber. The child's gait should be carefully examined. Toe-walking or hemiplegia may be signs of corticospinal tract disease. An ataxic gait may suggest cerebellar dysfunction, whereas an athetotic gait may implicate the basal ganglia.

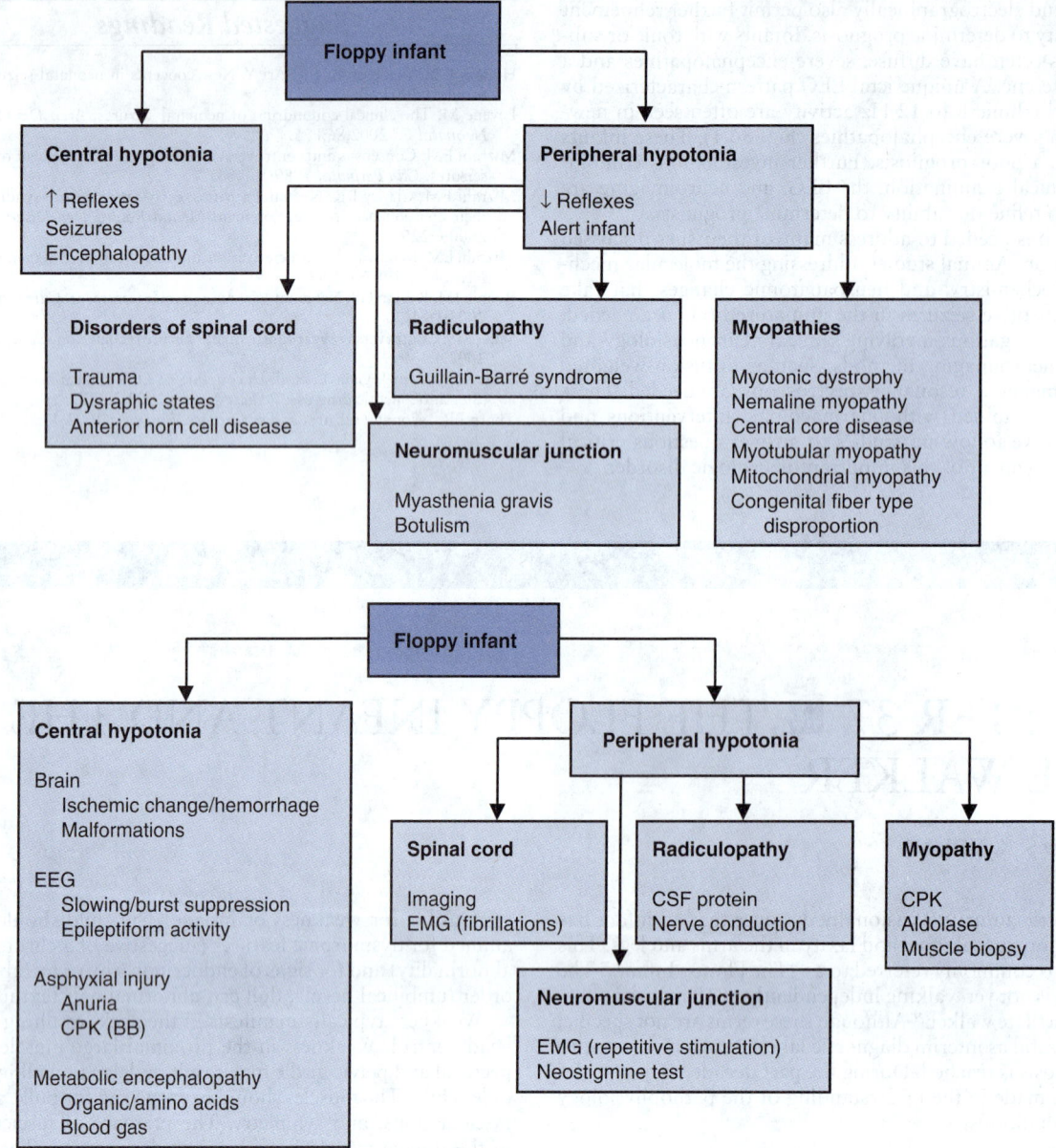

FIGURE 37.1. Algorithms illustrating general diagnostic approaches to hypotonia. CPK (BB), isoenzyme of creatine phosphokinase containing two B subunits; CSF, cerebrospinal fluid; EEG, electroencephalogram; EMG, electromyelogram.

NEURODIAGNOSTIC STUDIES

Cerebral MRI, both imaging and spectroscopy, is a useful method of result for the detection of cerebral causes of the floppy infant. Electromyography often is a helpful adjunct in the diagnosis of Werdnig-Hoffman disease, polyneuropathy, and botulism. Infants with congenital myopathies may require examination of muscle tissue for histologic and biochemical abnormalities.

CAUSES

Central Nervous System Injuries or Malformations

Cerebral injuries or malformations account for approximately one-half of floppy infants (central hypotonia). Cerebral con-

ditions that may result in a floppy infant include hypoxic-ischemic encephalopathy, intracranial infection, cerebral hemorrhage, cerebral trauma, metabolic disorders, cerebral malformations, and chromosomal malformations. Children with these disorders may have seizures or other signs of cerebrocortical dysfunction. Central, as opposed to peripheral, causes of weakness result in spasticity, with ankle clonus, crossed adductor reflex, Babinski sign, and fisting. Strabismus also may suggest central nervous system dysfunction that causes floppiness in an infant.

Spinal Cord Disease

The most common causes of spinal cord disease producing a floppy infant are trauma, dysraphism (myelomeningocele), and degeneration of the anterior horn cells. Cervical spinal cord injury may result from tearing or shearing of the spinal cord during delivery of a large infant. Tumors, infections, or demyelination of the spinal cord are less common. Seesaw respirations

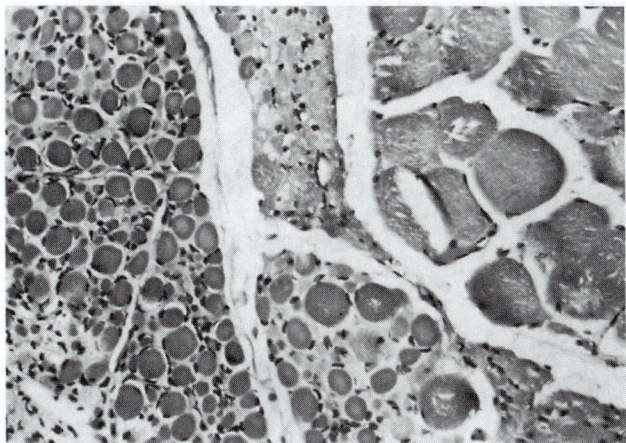

FIGURE 37.2. Muscle biopsy from a patient with Werdnig-Hoffmann disease. Muscle fibers are seen in the far left and lower right areas. They are round and markedly atrophic, whereas those seen in the upper right are either normal in size or hypertrophic. (Hematoxylin and eosin stain; magnification ×130.) (Courtesy of J. Kim, Yale University School of Medicine.)

are a sign of diaphragmatic breathing and indicate that the lesion is above the C4 level (emergence of the phrenic nerve). Widespread degeneration of anterior horn cells also may produce diaphragmatic breathing.

The selective loss of the anterior horn cells may occur during fetal life, in infancy, or during early childhood. If the onset of paralysis occurs *in utero*, the infant may exhibit widespread contractures (arthrogryposis multiplex congenita). One-half of patients with arthrogryposis have either neurogenic or myopathic etiologies, while the other half remains undiagnosed. Virtually all other sensory or association neurons in the nervous system are spared, leaving consciousness unimpaired. The diagnosis is confirmed by the presence of group atrophy on muscle biopsy samples (Fig. 37.2) and by electromyography (EMG). Anterior horn cell disorders (including spinal muscular atrophy) are among the more common autosomal recessive disorders, occurring in 1:10,000 live births, with a carrier frequency of 1 in 50; this disorder maps to a locus at 5q11.2. Anterior horn cell disease (Werdnig-Hoffmann syndrome) accounted for 15 of 41 floppy infants in the study of David and Jones (1994). Genetic testing and counselling for anterior horn disease should be considered in all children with this condition.

The differential diagnosis of anterior horn cell disease also includes enteroviral infections, including polio. In contrast to Werdnig-Hoffmann syndrome, the pattern of involvement in polio is asymmetric, with prominent signs of inflammation in the cerebrospinal fluid (e.g., elevated cerebrospinal fluid cell count, fever). In the United States, poliomyelitis may develop in an immigrant child. The widespread practice of vaccination with a killed poliovirus has reduced the number of cases of vaccine-acquired poliomyelitis.

In some instances, the clinical pattern of Werdnig-Hoffman disease may be mimicked by infant botulism. Infants whose intestinal tracts are colonized by *Clostridium botulinum* develop rapidly progressive or insidious weakness, poor feeding, constipation, and bulbar dysfunction. Both home-canned baby food and honey have been implicated. The annual incidence of infant botulism is two cases per 100,000 live births.

Radiculopathies

Acute inflammatory polyneuropathy (Guillain-Barré syndrome) is an infrequent cause of weakness in the infant and young child. The disorder results from a postinfectious immune attack on the Schwann cells, which produces demyelination of peripheral nerves. Because of the interruption of the lower motor neuron arc, areflexia is present. The diagnosis is established by the presence of elevated protein levels in the cerebrospinal fluid and delay in nerve conduction. Intravenous immunoglobulin has been advocated as a therapy for Guillain-Barré syndrome. Plasmapheresis has not gained wide acceptance because the prognosis of Guillain-Barré syndrome in children is generally benign.

Disorders of the Peripheral Nerves

Peripheral nerve disease, other than Guillain-Barré syndrome, seldom causes weakness in the neonatal period. However, both congenital and acquired (nutritional) neuropathies have been implicated in floppy infants. Electrodiagnostic studies may help to differentiate these individuals. Some disorders of the peripheral nerves occur sporadically (Leigh disease, Riley-Day syndrome or familial dysautonomia, and Möbius syndrome), although Déjérine-Sottas disease is inherited in an autosomal recessive manner.

Disorders Involving the Neuromuscular Junction

Disorders of the neuromuscular junction may cause an infant to be floppy or an older child to be a late walker (Box 37.1). Myasthenia gravis has a unique pattern of muscular involvement with predilection for the face and eyelids. Ptosis is prominent. Weakness of the bulbar musculature may produce dysarthria. Transient myasthenia gravis occurs in 10% to 15% of the infants born to mothers with myasthenia gravis and results from an immune attack on the postsynaptic receptor of the infant muscle. Neonatal myasthenia gravis correlates with high levels of antiacetylcholine receptor antibodies. Mutations within genes encoding the acetylcholine receptor and related proteins of the neuromuscular junction are the cause of the congenital myasthenic syndromes. The diagnosis of neonatal myasthenia may be confirmed by the intramuscular administration of neostigmine, 0.1 mg/kg. Atropine (0.1 mg intramuscularly) should be kept on hand to counteract muscarinic effects such as diarrhea and tracheal secretions. Electromyography using repetitive stimulation is a useful adjunct to diagnosis. Myasthenia in newborns may be genetic and not mediated by antibodies to the acetylcholine receptor. Therapy for the infant with the transient form of neonatal myasthenia is largely supportive. Attention to feeding techniques and respiratory care is needed; tube feedings may be required. Treatment with anticholinesterase may effect dramatic recovery in some cases.

BOX 37.1   **Neonatal Diseases of the Neuromuscular Junction**

Myasthenia gravis
    Transient, congenital
Metabolic disease
    Hypermagnesemia
Toxins
    Kanamycin, gentamicin, neomycin, streptomycin, polymyxin
Infantile botulism

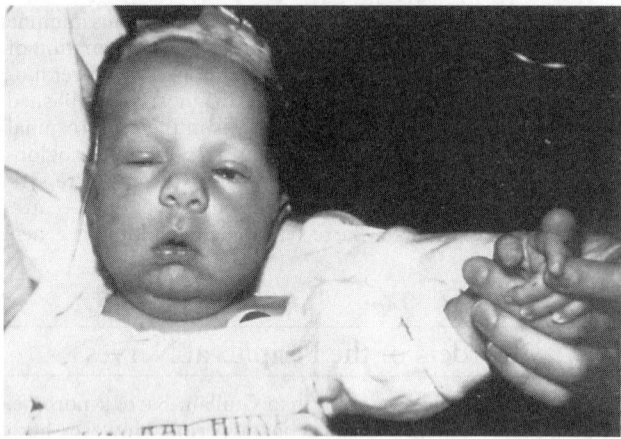

FIGURE 37.3. Myotonic dystrophy. Note the ptosis and "fish mouth" deformity in this infant.

Disorders of Muscle

Myotonic dystrophy is an autosomal dominant disorder and is related to a genetic locus on chromosome 19. The mother with myotonic dystrophy may have a complicated obstetric course, with premature labor, uterine dystocia, and breech presentation. Polyhydramnios may result from inadequate swallowing by the fetus. Myotonic dystrophy should be suspected if the mother exhibits "hatchet" facies, upturned philtrum ("fish mouth" deformity), ptosis, percussion myotonia, or delayed release of grip after shaking hands. Infants with myotonic dystrophy may have ptosis, apnea, or failure to thrive (Fig. 37.3). Electromyography shows "dive bomber" potentials, which consist of repetitive electrical potentials of up to 100 per second that wax and wane in frequency and amplitude. These infants may require ventilatory support but, ultimately, should grow stronger and be able to breathe independently.

Metabolic myopathies are characterized by their histologic appearances. These disorders include central core disease, nemaline myopathy, myotubular myopathy, congenital fiber-type disproportion (Fig. 37.4), and mitochondrial myopathies. Although the specific metabolic defect still may not be clarified, the muscle biopsy sample may show a characteristic histopathologic picture. Patients with central core disease have myocyte cores that are central or somewhat eccentric and

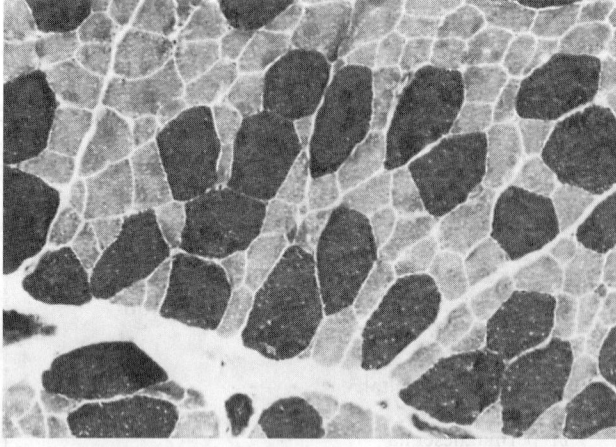

FIGURE 37.4. Muscle biopsy from a patient with congenital muscle fiber-type disproportion. Lightly stained type I fibers are smaller than darkly stained type II fibers. (Adenosine triphosphatase stain, pH 9.4; magnification ×160.) (Courtesy of J. Kim, Yale University School of Medicine.)

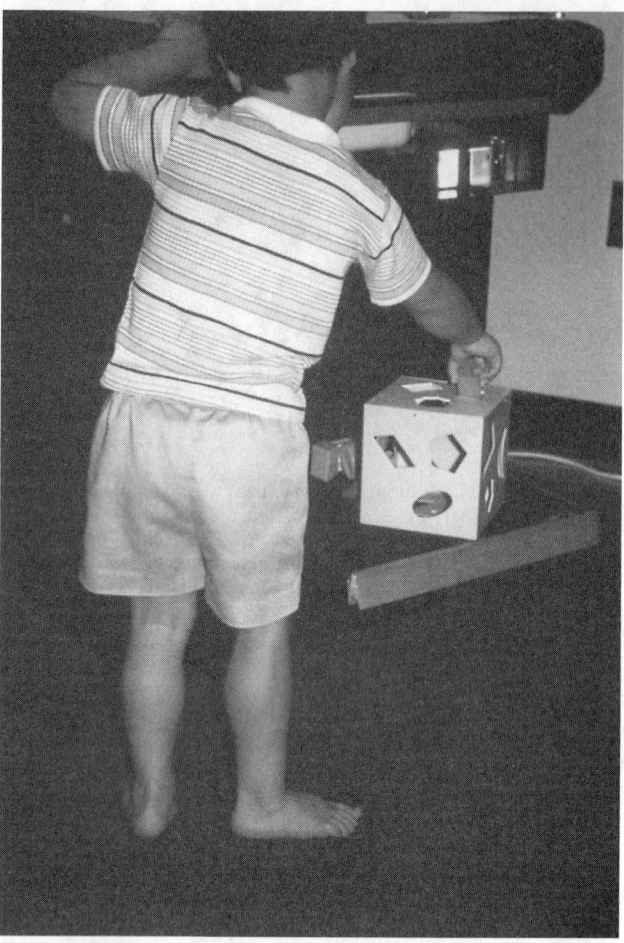

FIGURE 37.5. Duchenne dystrophy. Boys with Duchenne dystrophy are often late walkers. Note the pseudohypertrophy of the calves.

demonstrate well with histochemical stains for oxidative enzymes. The cores are more likely to be found in type 1 (oxidative) fibers. Central core disease is either slowly progressive or nonprogressive.

Nemaline (Greek for rod) myopathies have characteristic broad rods thought to represent abnormal deposition of Z bands of the sarcomere, possibly tropomyosin. Type 1 fibers predominate. Hence, the myopathy represents a defect in the cytoskeleton of the myocyte. Both a fatal infantile form and a more slowly progressive or nonprogressive form of the disease exist.

Muscle fibers in myotubular myopathy resemble fetal myotubes, suggesting maturational arrest. Muscle fibers contain more central nuclei, surrounded by an area that is devoid of myofibrils. Facial weakness, ptosis, ophthalmoplegia, and generalized weakness are suggestive of myotubular myopathy. Mitochondrial myopathies are a group of disorders characterized by the presence of ragged red fibers. Metabolic disturbances in mitochondrial myopathies include defects in substrate transport or use, the electron transport chain, or oxidative phosphorylation. For this reason, plasma lactate levels are elevated as in MELAS syndrome (mitochondrial encephalopathy, lactic acidosis, and strokelike episodes). Other metabolic disorders that produce weakness involve the metabolism of carbohydrates (glycogen storage diseases such as Pompe or McArdle disease), and still others are mitochondrial in origin.

Duchenne dystrophy is the most common X-linked neuromuscular disorder and results from a cytoskeletal defect in dystrophin. Young boys with this disorder are late walkers and have pseudohypertrophy of the calves (Fig. 37.5). When the mother is a carrier, levels of creatine phosphokinase are elevated in proportion to the degree of involvement of the X chromosome.

Suggested Readings

Aydinli N, Baslo B, Caliskan M, et al. Muscle ultrasonography and electromyography correlation for evaluation of floppy infants. *Brain Dev* 2003;25:22.

Bar-Joseph G, Etzioni A, Hemli J, Gershoni Baruch R. Guillain-Barré syndrome in three siblings less than 2 years old. *Arch Dis Child* 1991;66:1078.

Beeson D, Webster R, Ealing J. Structural abnormalities of the AchR caused by mutations underlying congenital myasthenic syndromes. *Ann NY Acad Sci* 2003;998:114.

Bogdanovich S, Perkins KJ, Krag TO, et al. Therapeutics for Duchenne muscular dystrophy: current approaches and future directions. *J Mol Med* 2004; 82:102–115.

Byers RK. Spinal cord injuries during birth. *Dev Med Child Neurol* 1975;17:103.

David WS, Jones HR. Electromyography and biopsy correlation with suggested protocol for evaluation of the floppy infant. *Muscle Nerve* 1994;17:424.

Hoffman EP. Genetic aspects of myopathy. *Curr Opin Rheumatol* 1989;1:419.

Kang PB, Lidov HG, David WS. Diagnostic value of electromyography and biopsy in arthrogryposis multiplex congenita. *Ann Neurol* 2003;54:790.

Kobayashi H, Baumbach L, Matise TC, et al. A gene for a severe lethal form of X-linked arthrogryposis maps to human chromosome Xp11.3–q11.2. *Hum Mol Genet* 1995;4:1213.

Korinthenberg R, Monting JS. Natural history and treatment effects in Guillain-Barré syndrome: a multicentre study. *Arch Dis Child* 1996;74:281.

MMWR. Infant botulism—New York City, 2001–2002. *MMWR Morb Mortal Wkly Rep* 2003;52:21.

Matthes IW, Kenna AP, Fawcett PR. Familial infantile myasthenia: a diagnostic problem. *Dev Med Child Neurol* 1991;33:924.

Morrison KE, Daniels RJ, Suthers GK, et al. High resolution genetic map around the spinal muscular atrophy locus on chromosome 5. *Am J Hum Genet* 1992; 50:520.

Ogino S, Wilson RB. Genetic testing and risk assessment for spinal muscular atrophy (SMA). *Hum Genet* 2002;111:477.

Prasad AN, Prasad C. The floppy infant: contribution of genetic and metabolic disorders. *Brain Dev* 2003;25:457.

Shaw D, Harper PS. Myotonic dystrophy: developments in molecular genetics. *Br Med Bull* 1989;45:745.

Verrijn Stuart AA, Huisman M, van Straaten HL, et al. "Shake hands"; diagnosing a floppy infant—myotonic dystrophy and the congenital subtype: a difficult perinatal diagnosis. *J Perinat Med* 2000;28(6):497–501.

Young RSK, Towfighi I, Marks K. Focal necrosis of cervical spinal cord in utero. *Arch Neurol* 1983;40:654.

CHAPTER 38 ■ NEONATAL ABSTINENCE SYNDROME

ANNE M. JOHNSTON

Neonatal abstinence syndrome (NAS) refers to a constellation of signs and symptoms caused by drug withdrawal in the newborn. In most cases, drug exposure occurs during pregnancy, but it also may describe a syndrome secondary to withdrawal of opioids and sedatives administered postnatally to infants with serious illness. Opioids (naturally occurring, synthetic, and semi-synthetic) are the most frequent drugs that give rise to the typical symptoms. For this reason, the following discussion focuses on the effects of opioid withdrawal on the newborn due to *in utero* exposure.

OPIOID ADDICTION

It is estimated that 1% to 2% of women in the United States use opioids during their pregnancy. Heroin (diacetylmorphine), a semi-synthetic opioid with a rapid onset of action and a short half life, is the most common opioid abused during pregnancy. Although typically it is injected, an increasing number of users are inhaling or smoking heroin. The increasing prevalence of heroin use in adolescents is believed to be partly due to its higher purity, which allows for significant effects through the inhaled route, and also due to its relatively low cost. The use of other opioids, including oxycodone, hydrocodone, and the controlled-release form of oxycodone (OxyContin) has escalated in recent years; many users of these opioid preparations switch to heroin because of its lower cost.

The acute use of heroin and other short-acting opioids stimulates the opiate receptors in the brain, resulting in a constellation of symptoms including euphoria, respiratory depression, analgesia, and nausea. The chronic use of opioids is associated with tolerance; higher doses of the drug are required to obtain the same effect. Tolerance leads to dependence, whereby the

neurochemical balance in the central nervous system is altered and absence of the drug leads to a withdrawal syndrome. Opioid withdrawal is characterized by a constellation of symptoms including agitation, nasal congestion, yawning, diaphoresis, muscle cramps, diarrhea, nausea, vomiting, and depression.

Several mechanisms have been proposed to explain the phenomena of tolerance, dependence, and withdrawal in the setting of chronic opioid exposure. These include (a) increased metabolic breakdown of opioid compounds; (b) decreased neurotransmitter release, resulting in an increased number and sensitivity of postsynaptic receptors; and (c) the down-regulation of opioid receptors, resulting in decreased production of endorphins.

Opioids and Pregnancy

The cycle of opioid use and withdrawal is particularly devastating for the developing fetus. The repetitive pattern of use and withdrawal leads to fetal hypoxia and uteroplacental insufficiency, with a resultant increased risk of prematurity, fetal demise, and low birth weight. Comprehensive prenatal care is essential for these patients.

Medication-assisted treatment has been the standard of care for pregnant opiate addicts. Methadone, a synthetic opioid, has been used with success in opiate addicts. At appropriate dosages, methadone, a synthetic opioid, will eliminate the symptoms and signs of withdrawal, reduce cravings, and block the euphoric effects should supplemental opioids be used. The long half-life and predictable dosing prevents erratic opioid levels in the fetus, and is associated with a longer duration of pregnancy and improved fetal growth. As the pregnancy progresses, methadone is metabolized more rapidly and higher doses are required. Although early reports suggested that the dose of methadone correlated with the incidence and severity of neonatal withdrawal symptoms, recent evidence does not demonstrate such a relationship. It is well accepted that lowering the dose during pregnancy may lead to increased illicit drug use, thus exposing the mother and fetus to more harm. Infants born to women on methadone tend to exhibit more severe and delayed withdrawal symptoms, when compared with those exposed to short-acting opioids, such as heroin. Buprenorphine, a partial opioid agonist, has recently been approved by the United States Food and Drug Administration (FDA) for the treatment of opioid addiction in an outpatient office setting. Although not yet approved for use in pregnancy, early evidence suggests that buprenorphine is associated with a decreased incidence of neonatal withdrawal when compared with methadone.

In addition to the concern regarding withdrawal, the prevalence of hepatitis B, hepatitis C, and human immunodeficiency virus (HIV) is elevated in pregnant addicts, primarily due to needle sharing and unsafe sexual practices. Women should be screened for these infections, and in the case of HIV infection, treatment should be initiated.

The management of addiction in pregnancy is highly complex, and attention must be focused not only on medication, but also on the complicated psychological and social needs of these women. A high number of these women have a history of domestic violence, are poorly educated, financially constrained, and have poor relationships with partners who may also be substance abusers. They have dysfunctional families, with a high prevalence of substance abuse and alcoholism. Many of these women have comorbid psychiatric conditions, most commonly depression and bipolar disorder; all of them suffer from low self-esteem.

Clinical Presentation

The preponderance of cases of neonatal abstinence syndrome is due to *in utero* opioid exposure. The newborn with opioid withdrawal presents with central nervous system excitability, vasomotor signs, and gastrointestinal symptoms (Box 38.1). The timing of onset of symptoms varies; however, infants exposed to heroin or other short-acting opiates typically will present within the first 48 to 72 hours. Those exposed to methadone will often present later, usually within the first 7 days.

The infant is assessed using a standardized scoring system, such as the Finnegan Neonatal Abstinence Scoring System (Fig. 38.1). This tool assesses 21 symptoms and signs. Infants with scores of 8 or greater require more intensive observation and potential pharmacologic treatment. These scores quantify the severity of symptoms and aid in the initiation and tapering of medications. Other scoring systems are available; some of these are simpler to use and may be more applicable to a well baby nursery or outpatient setting.

A thorough maternal history is crucial, including any illicit or prescribed drug intake, tobacco exposure, and alcohol intake. Newborn urine and meconium toxicology screens may aid in the diagnosis. Urine testing generally reflects drug exposure within several days, depending upon the drug. The results of urine testing are rapidly available; however, a high false negative rate is possible, given the rapid clearance of most drugs and the difficulty in obtaining sufficient urine from a newborn in the first day of life. Meconium testing offers the advantage of assessing drug exposure during the previous several months. However, meconium test results frequently are not available for several days, at which time the infant may have been discharged. Testing of human hair for drugs of abuse has the advantage of a wider window for testing, given hair's slow growth

---

BOX 38.1 — Common Clinical Manifestations of Neonatal Opioid Withdrawal

Central Nervous System

- Tremors
- Sleep disturbance
- Irritability
- High-pitched cry
- Hypertonicity
- Seizures

Gastrointestinal

- Poor feeding
- Regurgitation
- Vomiting
- Diarrhea

Other

- Tachypnea
- Nasal congestion
- Fever
- Sweating
- Yawning

---

rate. However, due to the technical complexity of the testing, it has only limited availability and applicability.

The differential diagnosis should include sepsis, hypoglycemia, hypocalcemia, hypomagnesemia, hyperthyroidism, perinatal asphyxia, and intracranial hemorrhage. Recent maternal serologies for hepatitis B, hepatitis C, and HIV should be determined.

Treatment

Approximately 60% to 80% of infants born to women on opioids will require treatment for narcotic withdrawal. At the delivery of a known opioid-dependent woman, naloxone should be avoided in resuscitation of the infant, because it may precipitate seizures.

Supportive care is essential in the management of infants exhibiting signs of withdrawal. Decreased stimulation, swaddling, and frequent feedings on demand are beneficial. Infants may require intravenous fluids to maintain hydration. Caloric expenditure is frequently elevated, and therefore increasing the caloric density of feeds may be indicated.

Pharmacologic therapy is indicated for infants with increasing severity of symptoms (consistent Finnegan score of ≥ 8), in cases of significant vomiting, diarrhea, or seizures (Table 38.1). Short-acting opioid preparations, such as oral morphine or dilute tincture of opium, are the most frequently used medications. Doses are adjusted according to symptoms, with a tapering schedule once the symptoms are under control. Paregoric, a compound containing anhydrous morphine, camphor, ethanol, and benzoic acid, was one of the first opioids to be used in the treatment of neonatal abstinence syndrome. The use of paregoric has declined due to the potentially toxic nature of its constituents. In some centers, oral methadone is used; however, the use of methadone is associated with a longer period of treatment. Phenobarbital is most useful for infants exposed to multiple drugs; however, recent evidence shows that it may reduce the duration of treatment when combined with a short-acting opioid. Diazepam has been used with limited success due to increased sedation and poor sucking, in addition to concerns

Date: _____

Weight: _____

System	Signs and Symptoms	Score	Time								Comments
Central Nervous System Disturbances	Excessive high-pitched cry	2									
	Continuous high-pitched cry	3									
	Sleeps <1 hr after feeding	3									
	Sleeps <2 hr after feeding	2									
	Sleeps <3 hr after feeding	1									
	Hyperactive Moro reflex	2									
	Markedly hyperactive Moro reflex	3									
	Mild tremors disturbed	1									
	Moderate-severe tremors disturbed	2									
	Mild tremors undisturbed	3									
	Moderate-severe tremors undisturbed	4									
	Increased muscle tone	2									
	Excoriation (area) _____	1									
	Myoclonic jerks	3									
	Generalized convulsions	5									
Vasomotor/Respiratory Disturbances	Sweating	1									
	Fever <38.3 (37.2 - 38.2)	1									
	Fever ≥38.3	2									
	Frequent yawning (3-4/interval)	1									
	Mottling	1									
	Nasal stuffiness	1									
	Sneezing (3-4/interval)	1									
	Nasal flaring	2									
	RR >60/min	1									
	RR >60/min with retractions	2									
Gastrointestinal Disturbances	Excessive sucking	1									
	Poor feeding	2									
	Regurgitation	2									
	Projectile Vomiting	3									
	Loose stools	2									
	Watery stools	3									
	Total Score										
	Initials of Scorer										

FIGURE 38.1. Neonatal abstinence scoring system. (Adapted with permission from Finnegan LP. Neonatal Abstinence. In: Nelson NM, ed. *Current therapy in neonatal-perinatal medicine*. Toronto: BC Decker, Inc.; 1985:262.)

TABLE 38.1

PHARMACOLOGIC APPROACHES TO NEONATAL ABSTINENCE SYNDROME

Medication	Dosage
Dilute tincture of opium	■ 0.4 mg/mL morphine equivalent (solution must be diluted) ■ 0.1–0.2 mL/kg PO every 3–4 hours, adjust by 0.1 mL/kg as needed
Morphine	■ 0.4 mg/mL (oral solution must be diluted) ■ 0.1–0.2 mL/kg PO every 3–4 hours, adjust by 0.1 mL/kg as needed
Paregoric	■ 0.4 mg/mL of anhydrous morphine ■ 0.1–0.2 mL/kg PO every 3–4 hours, adjust by 0.1 mL/kg as needed
Methadone	■ 0.05–0.1 mg/kg PO every 6–12 hours, adjust by 0.05 to 0.01 mg/kg as needed; reduce by 5%–10% every 2–7 days as tolerated
Phenobarbital	■ 15–30 mg/kg loading IV, IM, or PO; 2–6 mg/kg/day maintenance; reduce by 10% daily as tolerated
Diazepam	■ 0.3–0.5 mg/kg PO or IM every 8 hours

of late-onset seizures. Clonidine targets the excess adrenergic activity characteristic of opioid withdrawal. Experience with clonidine is limited, although it appears promising in treating most of the symptoms of opioid withdrawal. Chlorpromazine is of limited use, given its multiple side effects, including decreased seizure threshold and cerebellar dysfunction.

Most centers hospitalize the infant for the duration of pharmacologic treatment. This may range from 10 days to 6 weeks, depending upon the symptoms. Some centers have comprehensive outpatient support, enabling them to discharge infants to be managed at home, often in the care of their mother.

In the past, breast-feeding was discouraged for women on methadone doses in excess of 20 mg daily. However, recent evidence suggests that the amount of methadone present in the breast milk is minimal. Therefore, women on methadone maintenance therapy are encouraged to breast-feed their infants, providing they are HIV negative and are not using illicit substances.

Discharge Considerations

The opiate-dependent new mother undergoes an inordinate amount of stress during the postpartum period. Attention to her substance abuse treatment is of paramount importance during this time. Historically, many of the children of these women were placed in foster care, or, in some cases, remained institutionalized. Child protective services vary from state to state in their extent of involvement with these families. Women are assessed for their commitment to substance abuse treatment, their history of child abuse or neglect, and their community support. A comprehensive discharge plan that addresses maternal substance abuse treatment, parenting instruction, and community support will result in better retention in treatment.

Outcome

An evaluation of the outcome of infants born to drug-abusing women is fraught with methodologic difficulties, and results have been conflicting. Drug addicts rarely use only one drug, histories of drug use often are inaccurate, their health and nutritional status are suboptimal, and they often lack prenatal care. Sleeping disturbances and feeding problems have been described in opioid-exposed children during the first year of life. Several studies have described slightly lower scores of infant motor development; others have found no difference when compared with controls.

OTHER SUBSTANCES IMPLICATED IN NEONATAL ABSTINENCE SYNDROME

Alcohol

It is estimated that between 10% and 15% of women in the United States consume alcohol during pregnancy. Fetal alcohol syndrome and fetal alcohol effects are well recognized sequelae of fetal alcohol exposure; they are described in Chapter 27. Infants also may develop signs and symptoms of withdrawal from alcohol in the neonatal period; the clinical presentation is similar to neonatal opioid withdrawal.

Tobacco

It is estimated that between 12% and 18% of women in the United States smoke cigarettes during pregnancy. Infants born to smoking women weigh on average 150 to 250 g less than those born to nonsmoking women. Recent studies have demonstrated changes in neonatal neurobehavior in children born to smoking mothers, with some infants exhibiting a "nicotine withdrawal syndrome."

Marijuana

Approximately 10% of women report marijuana use during pregnancy. Fetal marijuana exposure has not been associated with significant demonstrable sequelae, although recent evidence suggests that newborns may have a slightly lower birth weight. Evaluation of the effect of marijuana alone is complicated by the fact that its use is commonly in conjunction with alcohol and/or tobacco use, both of which have well recognized effects on fetal growth.

Cocaine

Cocaine and crack cocaine use in pregnant women has received much attention, much of it politically driven. It is estimated that from 1% to 5% of women in the United States use cocaine or crack during pregnancy. The effects on the fetus have been conflicting. Reports of impaired fetal growth, congenital anomalies, central nervous system vascular lesions, neonatal behavioral effects, neonatal hypertonia, and language delay have been described in association with cocaine exposure. However, cocaine is seldom used in the absence of alcohol and tobacco; thus, the interpretation of these results is confounded by these exposures. The neonatal abstinence syndrome described in cocaine-exposed infants is more likely due to the effects, not the withdrawal, of the cocaine. It is generally self-limited and of short duration.

Others

Several other medications have been associated with neonatal abstinence. Symptoms of irritability, hypertonia, and tachypnea have been described in infants exposed to selective serotonin reuptake inhibitors (SSRIs). Infants chronically exposed to benzodiazepines and barbiturates have exhibited similar symptoms.

Suggested Readings

Berghella V, Lim PJ, Hill MK, et al. Maternal methadone dose and neonatal withdrawal. *Am J Obstet Gynecol* 2003;189:312.

Chasnoff I. Prenatal substance exposure: maternal screening and neonatal identification and management. *Neoreviews* 2003;9:228.

Coyle MG, Ferguson A, Lagasse L, et al. Diluted tincture of opium (DTO) and phenobarbital versus DTO alone for neonatal opiate withdrawal in term infants. *J Pediatr* 2002;140:561.

Ebrahim SH, Gfroerer J. Pregnancy-related substance use in the United States during 1996–1998. *Obstet Gynecol* 2003;101:374.

Finnegan LP. Neonatal abstinence. In: Nelson NM, ed. *Current therapy in neonatal-perinatal medicine*. Toronto: BC Decker, Inc., 1985:262.

Greene CM, Goodman MH. Neonatal abstinence syndrome: strategies for care of the drug-exposed infant. *Neonatal Netw* 2003;22:15.

Johnson RE, Jones HE, Fischer G. Use of buprenorphine in pregnancy: patient management and effects on the neonate. *Drug Alcohol Depend* 2003;70:S87.

Johnson K, Gerada C, Greenough A. Treatment of neonatal abstinence syndrome. *Arch Dis Child Fetal Neonatal Ed* 2003;88:F2.

Kaltenbach K, Berghella V, Finnegan L. Opioid dependence during pregnancy. Effects and management. *Obstet Gynecol Clin North Am* 1998;25:139.

Kandall SR. Treatment strategies for drug-exposed neonates. *Clin Perinatol* 1999;26:231.

Law KL, Stroud LR, LaGasse LL et al. Smoking during pregnancy and newborn neurobehavior. *Pediatrics* 2003;111:1318.95;149:78.

Osborn DA, Cole MJ, Jeffery HE. Opiate treatment for opiate withdrawal in newborn infants. *Cochrane Database Syst Rev* 2002:CD002059.

Philipp BL, Merewood A, O'Brien S. Methadone and breastfeeding: new horizons. *Pediatrics* 2003;111:1429.

Schindler SD, Eder H, Ortner R, et al. Neonatal outcome following buprenorphine maintenance during conception and throughout pregnancy. *Addiction* 2003;98:103.

Substance Abuse and Mental Health Services Administration. *Overview of Findings from the 2002 National Survey on Drug Use and Health* (Office of Applied Studies, NHSDA Series H-21, DHHS Publication No, SMA 03-3774). 2003. Rockville, MD.

Theis JG, Selby P, Ikizler Y, et al. Current management of the neonatal abstinence syndrome: a critical analysis of the evidence. *Biol Neonate* 1997;71:345.

CHAPTER 39 ■ DEVELOPMENTAL CONSIDERATIONS

IAN GROSS

EMBRYOLOGY

The lung originates as an outpouching from the endodermal tube that gives rise to the gastrointestinal tract. The epithelial lung bud grows anteriorly into mesenchymal tissue, the forerunner of the interstitium and blood vessels of the lung. As the respiratory tract divides and branches, interstitial tissue and blood vessels surround the developing airways. At approximately 28 weeks' gestation in humans, alveolar formation begins. Although this process is active during fetal life, the major increase in the number of alveoli occurs after birth. Approximately 1 million alveoli are present at birth, about 100 million at 1 year, and about 300 million at 6 years, after which the number appears to stabilize. Thus, the capacity of the lung to generate new alveoli continues for a considerable time after birth.

Lung growth itself is regulated, in part, by physical factors. It appears to be stimulated by the distending force of lung fluid in the airways and to be inhibited by the absence of this fluid, as occurs in oligohydramnios. Growth also can be inhibited by external compression, as occurs in diaphragmatic hernia, in which the bowel in the chest compresses the lung. Current research indicates that transcription factors, regulatory genes, and hormones pay a major role in controlling lung growth and budding.

ALVEOLAR MATURATION AND SURFACTANT SYNTHESIS

Because respiratory distress syndrome of the newborn is the result of immaturity of the lung, considerable interest has been expressed in the maturation of the fetal lung and the regulation of this process. During late fetal life, the development of the lung is characterized by an increase in the number and size of the alveoli and by the thinning of the connective tissue septa between them. This development reduces the distance between the alveolar lumen and red blood cells in capillaries in the interstitium, thus facilitating gas exchange. The alveolar lining cells also become flatter in late gestation, further reducing the barrier to gas exchange.

The cuboidal type II alveolar cells are the sites of the synthesis and secretion of pulmonary surfactant, the phospholipid-protein mixture that lines the alveoli of the lung and prevents alveolar collapse due to surface forces. After synthesis, surfactant is stored in the lamellar bodies, which then are secreted onto the surface of the type II cell by a process of exocytosis. In the alveolar lumen, the lamellar body unravels to form a structure known as *tubular myelin* and, ultimately, surfactant lines the surface of the alveolar cells. The onset of the functional maturation of the lung is marked by the appearance of lamellar bodies in the alveolar type II cells.

The major components of surfactant are lipids and proteins. The composition of surfactant obtained from lung lavage (by weight) is as follows:

Lipid (90%):
  Phospholipids (>85%):
    Phosphatidylcholine (75% of phospholipids)
    Phosphatidylglycerol (12% of phospholipids)
  Neutral lipids and cholesterol (3%)
Protein (10%):
  Serum proteins (9%)
  Surfactant-specific proteins (SP) (approximately 1%):
    SP-A (30 to 36 kd)
    SP-B (8 kd)
    SP-C (3.8 kd)
    SP-D (43 kd)

SP-A, a glycosylated protein, was the first SP to be characterized. The gene for human SP-A is on chromosome 10. SP-A is a member of the collectin family, which includes SP-D and mannose-binding protein, and it is related to C1q, the recognition component of complement. The collectins demonstrate lectin activity and function as opsonins, enhancing phagocytosis. *In vitro* studies have shown that SP-A binds gram-positive and gram-negative bacteria, thus facilitating macrophage action. Surfactant derived from homozygous transgenic mice, in which the SP-A gene has been "knocked out," demonstrates decreased association of group B streptococci with macrophages. Also, increased pulmonary infection and dissemination of bacteria to the spleen is demonstrated when these mice are challenged with intratracheal group B streptococci or other bacteria. In animal studies, SP-A also has been shown to protect against viruses such as respiratory syncytial virus and fungi (*Aspergillus* sp.). SP-D, another member of the collectin family, is a lectinlike protein that also may play a role in pulmonary defense mechanisms. The human SP-D gene also is on chromosome 10. These two proteins are components of the innate immune system of the lung. SP-A is decreased in infants with neonatal respiratory distress syndrome.

Although SP-A is an important component of the immune defenses of the lung, its role in surfactant function is uncertain currently. Because SP-A is water soluble, it is not present in surfactants prepared by lipid extraction for clinical use. The other surfactant proteins, SP-B and SP-C, are smaller lipophilic proteins that are present in clinically effective natural surfactant preparations and are thought to be critical for pulmonary surface activity. Homozygous SP-B knockout transgenic mice have been shown to die from respiratory failure at birth with atelectatic lungs. Their type II cells do not have fully formed lamellar bodies, and tubular myelin is lacking. In humans with hereditary SP-B deficiency, lethal respiratory distress also occurs in the neonatal period. The gene for human SP-B is located on chromosome 2, and the gene for SP-C is on chromosome 8.

Although the stimuli for the initiation of surfactant production are not clearly defined, a number of factors are known to accelerate this process. Glucocorticoids, thyroid hormone, cyclic adenosine monophosphate, thyroid transcription factor I, epidermal growth factor, and other agents have been shown to enhance surfactant production in a variety of animal models. In certain circumstances, such as maternal diabetes and male gender, lung maturation and surfactant production may be delayed. (Fetuses in poorly controlled diabetic pregnancies have elevated glucose, insulin, and ketone levels, and it is not currently clear which of these factors is responsible for inhibiting surfactant production.) The secretion of surfactant is stimulated by beta-adrenergic agonists such as terbutaline, purinoceptor agonists such as adenosine, and leukotrienes.

Suggested Readings

Cole FS, Hamvas A, Nogee LM. Genetic disorders of neonatal respiratory function. *Pediatr Res* 2001;50:157.

Hawgood S, Poulain FR. The pulmonary collectins and surfactant metabolism. *Ann Rev Physiol* 2001;63:495.

CHAPTER 40 ■ PHYSIOLOGIC CONSIDERATIONS

IMMANUELA RAVÉ MOSS

Successful transition of the respiratory and pulmonary circulatory system from the fetal to the neonatal state determines postnatal survival. The lungs of the full-term infant do not appear to be ready for postnatal gas exchange. The full complement of airways (but not alveoli) is developed, but the lungs are filled with fetal pulmonary fluid (30 mL/kg body weight).

Although shallow fetal breathing movements occur 30% of the time in the near-term fetus, they are distinctly different from postnatal breathing. As a result of intrauterine P_{O_2} levels of 20 to 30 mm Hg, the fetal pulmonary circulation is constricted, pulmonary vascular resistance is high, and pulmonary blood flow is low. The compliance of the liquid-filled fetal lung at term is low and the compliance of the fetal chest is high.

Thus, major changes must occur rapidly and concurrently following birth so the lung can assume its air-exchanging function. Continuous breathing and ventilation must begin. Pulmonary functional residual capacity must be established. The pulmonary vasculature must dilate to permit an increase in pulmonary blood flow, and fetal pulmonary fluid must be absorbed. These processes are discussed in the following sections.

ONSET OF AIR BREATHING AT BIRTH

The onset of postnatal breathing is associated with an abrupt, birth-related increase in P_{CO_2} and a decrease in P_{O_2}. These chemical inputs, together with a barrage of environmental stimuli including cooling, light, sound, touch, and pressure, promote arousal and powerful breathing efforts. With time, the initial, forceful, deep breaths diminish and are replaced with more moderate tidal breathing. Respiratory frequency shortly after birth is high. The high frequency is attributed to a reflex mediated by J receptors stimulated by the high interstitial pressure created by fetal lung fluid. As the fetal fluid is absorbed into pulmonary capillaries, breathing frequency gradually diminishes. Although the time course varies, stable respiratory function is usually attained by the end of the first postnatal day (Fig. 40.1).

The first breath is critical to the success of the transition from fetal to neonatal life. Forceful contraction of the inspiratory muscles generates the large subatmospheric transpulmonary pressures necessary to overcome surface and viscous forces and open air passages. The first expiration is also active and requires contraction of the expiratory muscles. Because vocal cord adduction occurs at the same time, the first expiration does not proceed to the prenatal lung volume. Instead, the forceful expiration against a partially closed glottis generates positive pressure in the airways and promotes the retention of some air in the lungs, thus initiating the establishment of gaseous functional residual capacity. The active inspiratory–expiratory sequence is repeated over subsequent breaths, so that with time, the air volume remaining in the lung at end-expiration increases until functional residual capacity is established (see Fig. 40.1).

The success of this process depends on adequate secretion of surfactant by alveolar type II cells, and on the establishment of an intraalveolar/acinar film, apparently in the form of stable bubbles, of surfactant-enriched material that lowers the surface tension of the lung.

The newly formed lung air–liquid interface modifies the geometry of the pulmonary vasculature, which, in combination with the increased P_{O_2}, recruits, distends, and opens pulmonary capillaries, dilates pulmonary vessels, and increases pulmonary blood flow. This vascular adaptation is crucial for successful absorption of fetal lung fluid and its removal by the pulmonary circulation.

The absorption of fetal lung fluid is promoted by a perinatal surge in epinephrine that activates beta-adrenoreceptors. These receptors, in turn, activate transepithelial sodium transport utilizing apical sodium channels and a basolateral sodium–potassium–adenosine triphosphatase pump. Of note, this process does not seem to depend on aquaporin-type water channels, although the number of these channels also increases around the time of birth.

Lung fluid absorption (and surfactant synthesis) is enhanced by a synergistic influence of thyroid and steroid hormones triggered by the abrupt increase in P_{O_2} at birth. This absorption

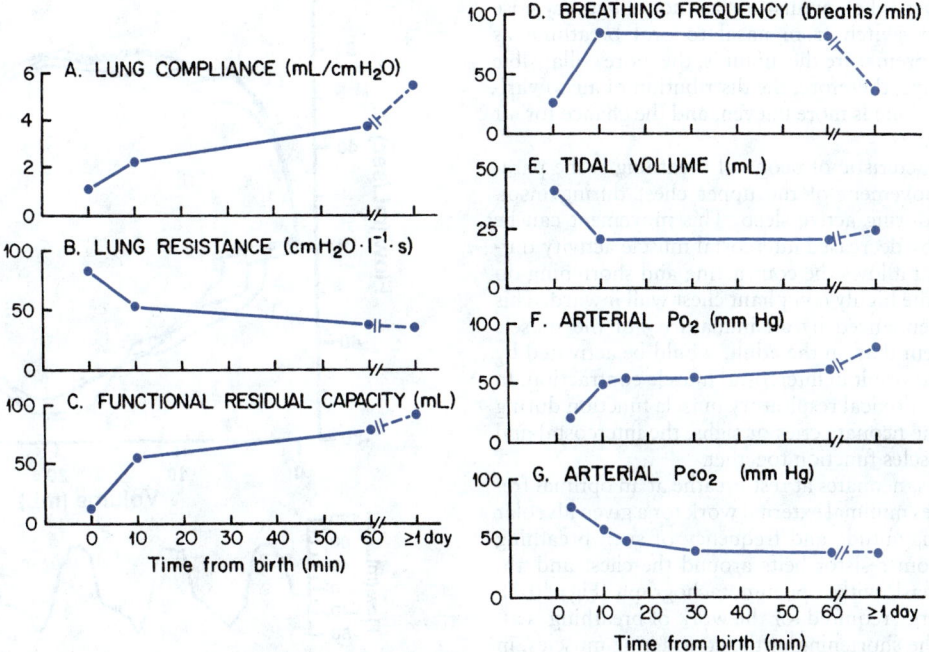

FIGURE 40.1. Respiratory functions of term infants during the first hour after birth and at 1 day of age or older. (Modified from Scarpelli EM, Moss IR. Transition from fetal to neonatal breathing. In: Gootman N, Gootman PM, eds. *Perinatal cardiovascular function.* New York: Marcel Dekker, 1983:43; Mortola JP. Dynamics of breathing in newborn mammals. *Physiol Rev* 1987;67:187; and Nelson NM. Physiology of transition. In: Avery GB, ed. *Neonatology: pathophysiology and management of the newborn,* 4th ed. Philadelphia: Lippincott–Raven, 1994:223.)

is also favored by a pressure gradient from the airspaces to capillaries created by osmotic and hydrostatic forces aided by the positive airway pressure that is created by the expiration against the partially closed glottis. The progressive increase in air and decrease in fetal fluid gradually increase the compliance of the lung and enhance oxygenation. As a consequence, pulmonary resistance decreases further, and the match between lung ventilation and pulmonary perfusion improves (see Fig. 40.1).

RESPIRATORY MECHANICS, BREATHING DYNAMICS, AND GAS EXCHANGE IN THE NEONATE

Pulmonary gas exchange depends in part on the passive mechanical properties of the lung and chest wall. Total respiratory compliance (i.e., the change in lung volume per unit change in transpulmonary pressure) can be assessed *in vivo* with various techniques. Lung compliance can be measured in isolated lungs, and chest wall compliance is the difference between total respiratory compliance and lung compliance.

The chest wall of the neonate is very compliant because of the predominance of thin cartilage and poorly mineralized bone. Therefore, low respiratory total lung compliance in the newborn reflects poor compliance of the lung itself. Lung compliance is lower in the neonate than in the adult, while the stability of the newborn chest and thus its ability to recoil after an exhalation is relatively low. Static resting lung volume is determined by the balance between the tendency of the lung to collapse and the ability of chest wall recoil to prevent collapse. Poor lung compliance and poor chest recoil mean that transpulmonary pressure generated at equilibrium and resting lung volume are smaller, corrected for size, in neonates than in adults.

Dynamic compliance, which is measured during normal breathing and is influenced by the frequency of breathing, is lower, relative to adults, than static compliance. The reasons for the lowered dynamic compliance in the neonate are thought to be (a) the viscous properties of newborn lung tissue and (b) distortion of the pliable newborn chest, resulting in an unbalanced and unequal mechanical function of the chest wall.

During normal breathing, the dynamic functional residual capacity of the neonate is greater than what would be predicted from the passive balance between the inward recoil of the lung and the outward recoil of the chest wall. This variance occurs for two reasons: First, the relatively high breathing frequency in the neonate does not create sufficient time for full expiration. Second, persistent postinspiratory diaphragmatic contraction and laryngeal adduction during expiration hinder complete expiration. The resultant positive airway pressure favors the reabsorption of excess intrapulmonary fluid, helps to keep the airways open, and maintains a relatively large end-expiratory volume, enhancing gas exchange. This situation changes in active sleep, during which laryngeal adductor muscle activity is reduced, so that expiration is more complete and the volume expired is greater. This, in combination with decreased muscle tone and intercostal muscle activity, produces a lower end-expiratory lung volume and, thus, less optimal oxygenation during active sleep.

Airway resistance in neonates per unit of lung weight is greater than in adults, with the most peripheral airways contributing a relatively greater portion of this resistance. The upper airway of the neonate participates in the maintenance of airway patency by the action of dilatory muscles. When these muscles are not operating, the neonatal upper airway is much more pliant than that of the adult and can close at pressures of −4 cm H_2O. Neck extension in the neonate stiffens the upper airway, enhancing its patency, whereas neck flexion enhances its collapse. The total nasal resistance of the neonate is proportionally smaller than that of the adult. Contrary to popular belief, neonates, even when premature, are not obligatory nose breathers and can switch from nasal to oral breathing as needed. The more premature the infant is, the more collapsible are the main airways; therefore, the distribution of air to various portions of the lung is more uneven, and the chance for air trapping is greater.

A striking characteristic of neonatal breathing is the paradoxical inward movement of the upper chest during inspiration, especially during active sleep. This movement can be explained in part by decreased intercostal muscle activity during active sleep that allows the contracting and shortening diaphragm to draw the highly compliant chest wall inward. This might be further enhanced by an immaturity of the muscle spindle reflex system that, in the adult, would be activated by chest distortion and result in intercostal muscle contraction. In contrast to the paradoxical respiratory muscle function during breathing, when the neonate cries or sighs, the intercostal and diaphragmatic muscles function together.

Similar to adults, neonates at rest breathe at an optimal frequency that requires minimal external work for a given alveolar ventilation. The magnitude and frequency of such breathing can be assessed from resistor belts around the chest and abdomen, or via a mask with a pneumotachograph (Fig. 40.2). Whereas some energy required for the work of breathing is always lost during the shortening of the contracting muscles, in the case of the neonate, additional energy is lost because of the chest distortion. Another possible cause for wasted energy is the rounder skeletal contour of the neonatal chest, as contrasted with the flatter, more elongated contour of the adult chest. The rounded chest contour, with a spatial rib arrangement different from that of the adult, precludes an optimal resting length for both the diaphragm and the intercostal muscles, thereby reducing the efficiency of their contraction during inspiration. The final contributor to the reduced efficiency of the neonatal respiratory muscles is their intrinsic mechanical properties. Inspiratory muscles in the newborn, particularly in the preterm infant, have a relatively small mass and are poorly equipped to sustain high work loads because they contain relatively few fatigue-resistant, slow-twitching, highly oxidative fibers, have low glycogen and fat stores, and can easily become hypoxic. Thus, these muscles in the neonate contract less forcefully and may be vulnerable to fatigue.

The match between ventilation and blood perfusion is of paramount importance to gas exchange. In the neonate, pulmonary air distribution is not homogeneous, resulting in increased pulmonary venous admixture. The factors responsible include pliant airways, distortion of the chest wall, and immature respiratory muscles (see previous discussion). As the airways, chest wall, and respiratory muscles mature and as alveoli proliferate, air distribution improves.

The pulmonary circulation changes considerably after birth. The ratio of small pulmonary arteries to alveoli decreases twofold from birth to 6 months of age due to proliferation of alveoli. Vascular walls gradually thin, with a reduction in their elastic tissue. Pulmonary vascular resistance continues to fall, with a consequent increase in pulmonary blood flow (see Chapter 48). Ultimately, alveoli are surrounded by a continuous film of capillary blood. These developmental improvements in ventilatory distribution and pulmonary perfusion and in the match between them result in progressively better gas exchange with increasing postnatal age.

RESPIRATORY CONTROL IN THE NEONATE

Given that neonatal respiration is a continuation of fetal breathing, consideration of the latter is important to the un-

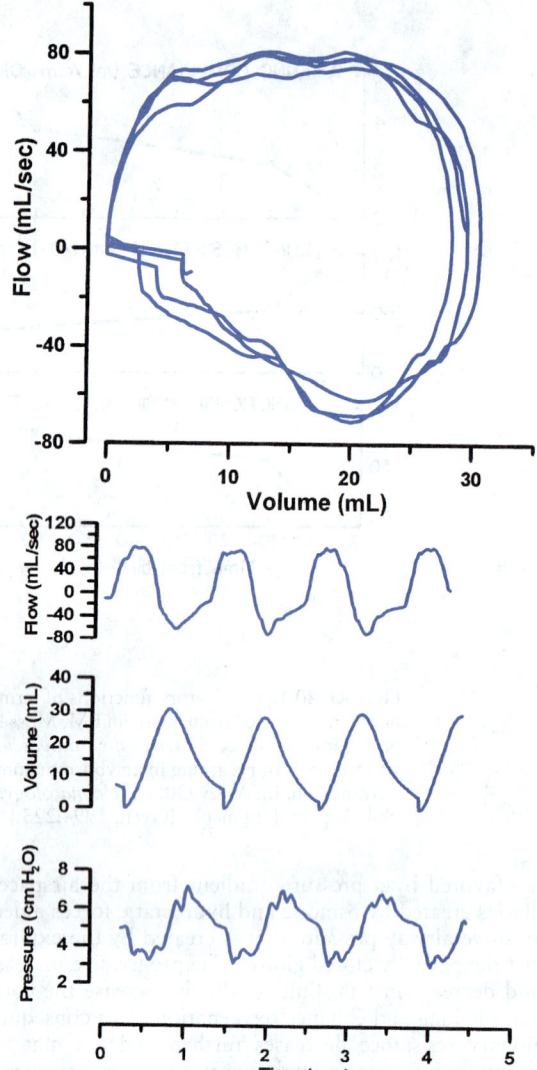

FIGURE 40.2. Spontaneous breathing in a 28-day-old, 4.5-kg body weight, healthy female infant born at term. Breathing was recorded through a fitted face mask and a pneumotachograph during natural sleep. Air flow, measured from pressure differences across a metal screen fixed within a pneumotachograph (second panel, inspiration upward); tidal volume, integrated from the expiratory flow signal (third panel); and transpulmonary pressure, that is, the difference between airway pressure at the mouth and esophageal pressure (fourth panel), are graphed against time. Such recordings can serve to calculate respiratory frequency, minute ventilation, and flow-volume relationships in spontaneously breathing infants. The three-and-one-half breaths shown in the lower three panels served to construct the overlapping flow-volume loops shown in the top panel, in which inspiration commences at zero flow on the left and proceeds upward and to the right, and expiration completes the loop. The flow-volume loops are normal in shape, indicating an absence of airway obstruction. (Courtesy of Ms. Giulia Mesiano, RRT, Respiratory Medicine, Montreal Children's Hospital, McGill University Health Centre, Montreal, Quebec, Canada).

derstanding of normal and abnormal respiratory control in the newborn.

In the near-term human fetus (32 to 40 weeks' gestation), breathing movements are most often associated with periods of body and eye movement and heart rate variability, and least associated with fetal quiescence. Studies in animals confirm that normal fetal breathing is associated with active sleep and wakefulness and not with quiet sleep.

Chemical respiratory reflexes studied in the lamb fetus show that the breathing response to hypercapnia is excitatory and accompanied by arousal, but is greatly blunted when compared with the ventilatory response to CO_2 in mature subjects. In contrast to the CO_2 response, the fetal breathing response to hypoxia is inhibitory, in that breathing movements cease along with a change in behavioral state toward quiet sleep. Because the electrophysiologic activity in the carotid sinus nerve that emanates from the oxygen-sensitive carotid receptors remains intact during fetal hypoxia, the inhibition of breathing during hypoxia is attributed to central mechanisms, as is the blunting of the fetal breathing response to CO_2. Of the various central mechanisms proposed, the importance of arousal has been stressed. The importance of arousal also applies to the effect of somatosensory stimuli, as cooling, the most powerful of these stimuli, produces simultaneous wakefulness and vigorous breathing movements in the near-term fetus.

At birth, respiratory pattern changes abruptly from episodic to continuous breathing. Despite this normal transformation, it is not uncommon for preterm neonates, or even full-term infants, to display spontaneous respiratory pauses; these can be rhythmic (periodic breathing) or not (short central apnea). Periodic breathing and apnea usually occur during sleep and may be considered a continuation of fetal patterns of breathing into postnatal life. The fact that these patterns exist during sleep and disappear with arousal (either natural or induced) underscores the importance of arousal in the maintenance of regular breathing. The frequency of these variations in respiratory rhythm decreases with postnatal maturation as the breathing strategy changes, with an increase in tidal volume and a decrease in respiratory frequency.

The respiratory responses to the chemical stimuli CO_2 and O_2 also change abruptly at birth. The response to CO_2, which involves primarily central chemoreception but also the carotid and aortic chemoreceptors, is heightened at birth, although it does not attain an adultlike sensitivity until several days postnatally. The response to hypoxia gradually becomes biphasic (i.e., an initial hyperventilation through peripheral chemosensory mechanisms followed by respiratory attenuation or even apnea) (Fig. 40.3). The ventilatory responses to these chemosensory stimuli involve both the pump (diaphragmatic and intercostal) and the upper airway (laryngeal) muscles. Behavioral states also play a role in the chemical respiratory reflexes, as these are relatively diminished in sleep, particularly in active sleep. Chemical respiratory stimuli, particularly CO_2, produce wakefulness at the same time that they stimulate ventilation.

Other, nonchemical respiratory reflexes also change during the transition from the early neonatal period to mature life. For example, the response of upper airway muscles to local changes in pressure, the coordination between the upper airway and the main respiratory muscles, and the intercostal–phrenic inhibitory reflex are all less developed in the newborn. Intrapulmonary reflexes are also less developed, including the rapidly adapting (irritant) and the C fiber (J receptor) vagal reflexes.

In contrast, however, some reflexes are more active in the neonate than in the mature subject. An important example involves the behavior of the slowly adapting stretch receptors in the lung that account for the Hering-Breuer lung inflation and deflation reflexes. These reflexes are very important for the newborn, as they adjust respiratory timing to prevent an undue alteration in lung volume. These reflexes are strongest in the youngest infants and weaken with age and maturation. Another striking example is the difference in response shown by the laryngeal/pharyngeal chemical reflex: Whereas stimulation of its chemoreceptors by materials perceived as foreign elicits cough in the adult, in the newborn, it elicits apnea. Apnea can be of central origin and/or associated with severe laryngeal spasm. It can be profound and even irreversible in very young

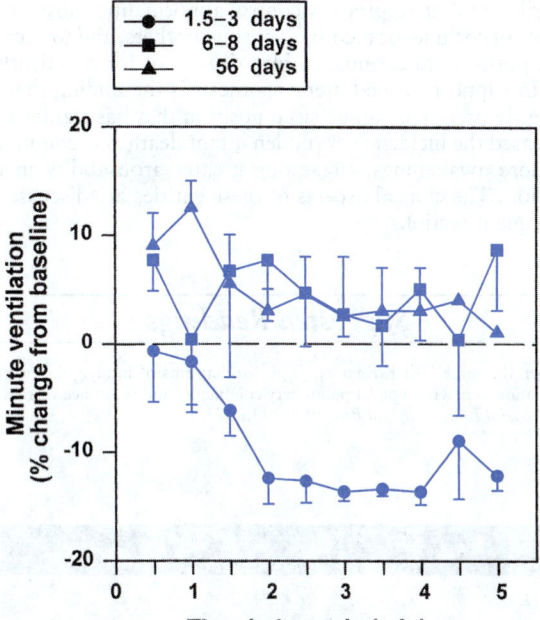

FIGURE 40.3. Ventilatory responses (% change from baseline in normoxia) during 5 minutes of mild hypoxia (15% O_2 in N_2) in four full-term infants studied sequentially at 1.5–3, 6–8, and 56 days of age. Two infants were studied at all three ages, one at the first two, and one at the first and last ages. All infants were unsedated and studied during quiet sleep, in the supine or slightly lateral position, and at an ambient temperature of 23–25°C. Respiratory gases were administered via a nose mask. Air flow, measured from pressure differences across a metal screen fixed within a pneumotachograph, was integrated into tidal volume and the latter was multiplied by respiratory frequency to render minute ventilation. Despite the variability in the data, it is evident that the ventilatory response to hypoxia around birth is primarily depressed and reminiscent of the fetal response to hypoxia, that the response becomes increasingly biphasic with postnatal age, and that the maturation of the response to hypoxia is slower than previously thought. (Redrawn from data presented in Table 2, and including only those infants that were studied at more than one age, from Cohen G, Malcolm G, Henderson-Smart D. Ventilatory responses of the newborn infant to mild hypoxia. *Pediatr Pulmonol* 1997;24:163.)

neonates. The duration of such apnea is inversely proportional to postnatal age.

With the increasing rate of survival among premature infants, special attention must be paid to the development of respiratory-related reflexes in this infant population. For example, in full-term infants, swallowing is fully coordinated with respiration, in that it occurs at end-inspiration and does not interfere with breathing. By contrast, in preterm infants before 32 weeks of postconceptional age, swallowing interferes with normal breathing and produces oxygen desaturation during feeding. As the preterm infant matures, swallowing becomes increasingly linked to end-inspiration.

The tight link between behavioral states and respiration emphasizes the importance of brain processes that control these states. These processes also undergo postnatal development. From the first postnatal day onward, neonates already display ultradian (12-hour) and diurnal (24-hour) sleep–wake cycles. Young neonates spend most of their time asleep, predominantly in active sleep. With time, the total time spent in sleep decreases, and quiet sleep becomes more pronounced. The sleep–wake cycles lengthen gradually, from 30 to 70 minutes in newborns to 75 to 90 minutes in children and adults.

As detailed previously, arousal and wakefulness sustain, accompany, and stimulate respiratory rhythmicity and responsiveness. Indeed, deficient arousal mechanisms are thought to contribute to the respiratory control abnormalities observed in infants of cocaine- or nicotine-abusing mothers, and to account for a portion of near-miss sudden deaths, or for crib death itself. In support of the latter hypothesis is the finding that the currently preferred supine sleep position that has significantly decreased the incidence of sudden infant death is accompanied by more awakenings, suggesting greater arousability in this position. The clinical aspects of these entities are discussed in subsequent sections.

Suggested Readings

Aschner JL, Smith TK, Kovacs N, et al. Mechanisms of bradykinin-mediated dilation in newborn piglet pulmonary conducting and resistance vessels. *Am J Physiol Lung Cell Mol Biol* 2002;283:L373.

Barker PM, Olver RE. Lung edema clearance: 20 years of progress. Invited review: clearance of lung fluid during the perinatal period. *J Appl Physiol* 2002;93:1542.

Davis SD. Neonatal and pediatric respiratory diagnostics. *Respir Care* 2003; 48:367.

Gray PA, Janczewski WA, Mellen N, et al. Normal breathing requires pre-Botzinger complex neurokinin-1 receptor-expressing neurons. *Nature Neurosci* 2001;4:927.

Mellen NM, Janczewski WA, Bocciaro CM, Feldman JL. Opioid-induced quantal slowing reveals dual networks for respiratory rhythm generation. *Neuron* 2003;37:821.

Moss IR. Maturation of respiratory control in the behaving mammal. A Frontiers Review. *Respir Physiol Neurobiol* 2002;132:131.

Moss IR, Laferrière A. Central neuropeptide systems and respiratory control during development. *Respir Physiol Neurobiol* 2002;131:15.

Ramanathan R, Corwin MJ, Hunt CE, et al. Cardiorespiratory events recorded on home monitors. Comparison of healthy infants with those at increased risk for SIDS. *JAMA* 2001;285:2199.

Scarpelli EM. Physiology of the alveolar surface network. *Comp Biochem Physiol Part A* 2003;135:39.

CHAPTER 41 ■ CAUSES OF RESPIRATORY DISTRESS IN THE NEWBORN

IAN GROSS

Respiratory distress is a common presentation of disease in the newborn infant. The term is used to describe a constellation of easily observable physical signs, including rapid breathing (more than 60 breaths per minute), cyanosis, retractions (sucking in of the skin between the ribs, under the ribs, or above the sternum with each breath), flaring of the nostrils, and a grunting sound on expiration. Many clinical causes exist for these signs, and their presence is an indication that further observation or investigation is necessary.

It is important to note, however, that tachypnea may only be a normal or transient condition in the newborn. Babies may breathe rapidly during the first few hours after birth. This phenomenon is related to the clearing of lung fluid from the airways and the cardiopulmonary adjustment to extrauterine life. Tachypnea also may be associated with transient conditions such as hypothermia. Isolated tachypnea, which is not associated with cyanosis, may be managed by observation only during the first few hours of life. If the tachypnea persists or is associated with other evidence of respiratory distress, further investigation is indicated. This analysis usually includes a radiograph of the chest and determination of arterial blood gas levels or of blood oxygen saturation.

The causes of respiratory distress in the newborn include the following:

A. Airway obstruction
  1. Choanal atresia
  2. Congenital stridor (may be caused by congenital defects such as laryngomalacia, vocal cord paralysis, subglottic stenosis, tracheomalacia, laryngeal webs, or aberrant vessels compressing the airways)
  3. Bronchomalacia
B. Pulmonary disorders
  1. Respiratory Distress Syndrome (RDS, hyaline membrane disease) [see Chapter 42]
  2. Transient tachypnea
  3. Pneumonia
  4. Aspiration syndromes
  5. Persistent pulmonary hypertension
  6. Air leak: interstitial emphysema, pneumothorax, or pneumomediastinum
  7. Congenital malformations (e.g., diaphragmatic hernia, pulmonary hypoplasia, congenital lobar emphysema, tracheoesophageal fistula)
  8. Atelectasis
  9. Pulmonary hemorrhage
  10. Chronic lung disease (bronchopulmonary dysplasia)
C. Nonpulmonary causes
  1. Cardiac disease
  2. Metabolic acidosis
  3. Central nervous system disorders
  4. Hypothermia or hyperthermia

Because respiratory distress is caused by many factors that cannot be differentiated by clinical examination alone, a chest radiograph is indicated in any infant who has significant respiratory distress. A sudden deterioration in respiratory status also is an indication for obtaining a chest radiograph to rule out conditions that require urgent treatment, such as pneumothorax. Very early chest films (in the first 2 to 4 hours after birth) may not be helpful in differentiating the various forms of parenchymal lung disease, because the presence of lung fluid tends to produce a hazy appearance or diffuse fine infiltrates. Early radiographs are useful, however, for excluding conditions that require surgical intervention, such as diaphragmatic hernia and air leaks.

If no clear-cut pulmonary cause is present for the respiratory distress, it also will be necessary to exclude the presence of cardiac disease. This usually can be done by chest radiograph, electrocardiogram, and echocardiogram. In some respiratory conditions (e.g., persistent pulmonary hypertension), the echocardiogram is not only useful for excluding heart disease, but also plays a role in the diagnosis and management of the pulmonary disorder. Occasionally, it is useful to determine the response to inhalation of 100% oxygen. In the presence of lung disease, the arterial P_{O_2} should increase after the inhalation of high concentrations of inspired oxygen, whereas with a fixed cardiac right-to-left shunt, there will be little increase in P_{O_2}. This procedure carries the risk of causing closure of a patent ductus arteriosus in some ductal-dependent cardiac lesions.

The following chapters discuss several conditions that cause respiratory distress in the newborn in more detail.

CHAPTER 42 ■ RESPIRATORY DISTRESS SYNDROME

IAN GROSS

Respiratory distress syndrome (RDS) of the newborn, or hyaline membrane disease, is a major cause of illness and death in premature infants. It is the result of immaturity of the lungs at birth and, therefore, with rare exceptions, is seen only in premature infants. Although alveoli first appear at 28 weeks' gestation, lung maturation is usually not adequate to sustain extrauterine life without some form of respiratory support until 32 to 34 weeks' gestation. Babies born earlier than this may have inadequate surfactant, which results in decreased compliance of the lung. Other factors that contribute to lung compliance, such as tissue elasticity, are also believed to be abnormal in these infants. In addition, the anatomic structure of the lung in these infants is not as well suited to gas exchange as that of full-term infants because of the presence of smaller alveoli with larger amounts of interstitial tissue between them. The net result is a lung that is stiff and less well adapted for gas exchange.

EPIDEMIOLOGY

The incidence of RDS varies from country to country throughout the world. It depends on the gestational age of the newborn infant and whether the infant's mother received antenatal glucocorticoid treatment. In general, the incidence of RDS in infants born before 30 weeks' gestation is approximately 60% in those who have not been exposed to antenatal glucocorticoids and about 35% in those who have received an adequate course of glucocorticoid therapy. Between 30 and 34 weeks' gestation, the incidence is approximately 25% in untreated or inadequately glucocorticoid-treated infants, and approximately 10% in those who have received a full course of treatment. In premature infants of more than 34 weeks' gestational age, the incidence is approximately 5%, and RDS is rare in full-term infants.

FACTORS MODIFYING THE RISK OF RESPIRATORY DISTRESS SYNDROME OF THE NEWBORN

The factors associated with an increased risk of RDS include prematurity, maternal diabetes (classes A to C), delivery by cesarean section without antecedent labor, perinatal asphyxia, second twin, and history of a previous infant with RDS. The increased incidence of RDS in infants of diabetic mothers may be related to the hyperglycemia, increased ketones, or hyperinsulinemia that occurs during fetal life. Because labor enhances surfactant production, infants born by cesarean section that is not preceded by labor have an increased incidence of RDS. Acute asphyxia with hypoxia and acidosis appears to inhibit surfactant production. The incidence of RDS is higher in a second-born twin; whether this finding is related to asphyxia is not clear. Finally, there appears to be a familial tendency toward RDS, and a history of a sibling with RDS places a subsequent premature infant at higher risk.

Also, certain conditions decrease the incidence of RDS, such as long-term maternal stress (e.g., toxemia, hypertension), intrauterine growth restriction, maternal infection, maternal heroin exposure, and glucocorticoid treatment. Chronic low-grade maternal stress, as opposed to acute asphyxia, accelerates lung maturation by a mechanism that is not entirely clear. It is possible that hormones such as glucocorticoids are involved.

PATHOGENESIS

Current concepts of the pathogenesis of RDS are illustrated in Figure 42.1. The basic deficit is immaturity of surfactant production and lung structure. This results in a lung that is stiff and prone to atelectasis. Blood continues to perfuse the poorly ventilated areas, resulting in a ventilation-perfusion mismatch hypoxemia. The hypoxemia may in turn cause metabolic acidosis as a result of poor tissue oxygenation. In the presence of hypoxemia, the pulmonary arterioles tend to constrict, producing increased pressure in the pulmonary circulation. Shunting of blood from the right atrium to the left atrium through the foramen ovale may now occur, further aggravating the hypoxemia. Depending on the relative pressures in the pulmonary artery and the aorta, there also may be right-to-left shunting through a patent ductus arteriosus. In most instances, this process is reversible if normal blood gas levels are restored.

Alveolar disruption and necrosis can also occur, resulting in leakage of fluid and fibrin from the pulmonary capillaries into the alveolar space and small airways. This fluid and fibrin

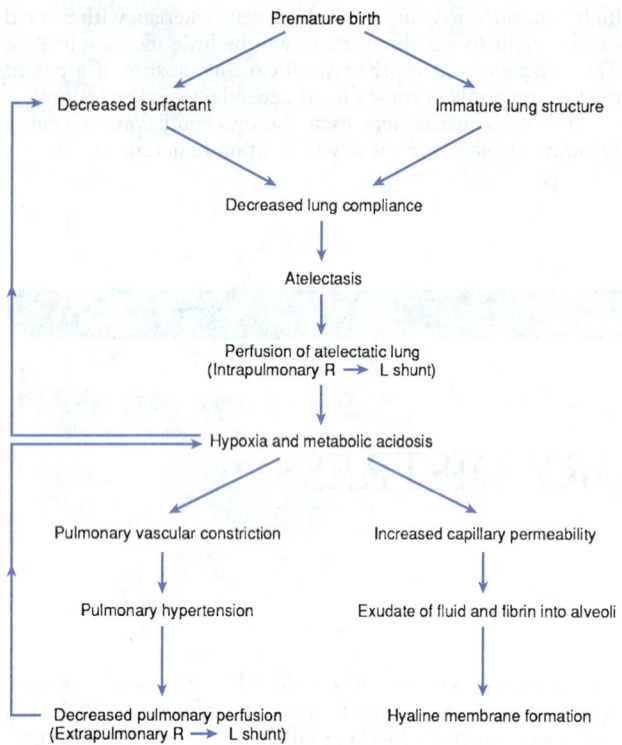

FIGURE 42.1. The pathogenesis of respiratory distress syndrome of the newborn.

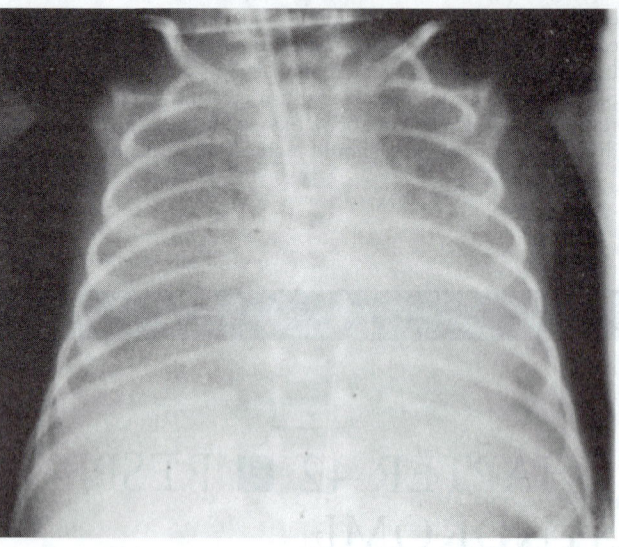

FIGURE 42.2. Roentgenogram of the chest of an infant with respiratory distress syndrome. Note the diffusely opaque lung fields and the indistinct cardiac outline. Radiolucent "air bronchograms" also can be seen.

exudate eventually coalesces to form proteinaceous deposits that, at postmortem examination, are identified as the eosinophilic hyaline membranes characteristic of this disease. It is clear that hyaline membrane formation is a consequence and not a cause of RDS. Hyaline membranes have never been described in stillborn infants; they appear only in infants who have been alive and sick for at least a few hours.

The ductus arteriosus may also play a role in the development of this disorder. If it is patent, as it usually is during the first day after birth in premature infants, blood may flow from right to left, as discussed earlier. If aortic pressure exceeds pulmonary artery pressure, however, flow will be from left to right and overperfusion of the lungs with pulmonary edema may ensue. This complication will further decrease lung compliance.

Finally, because surfactant production is decreased by hypoxia and acidosis, a cycle may be initiated whereby the infant starts off with inadequate surfactant production and becomes hypoxic and acidotic. This, in turn, further inhibits the production of surfactant.

Infants with RDS initially have the classic features of respiratory distress in the newborn (i.e., tachypnea, flaring of the nose, retractions of the chest, cyanosis, and grunting). Radiographs taken at approximately 6 hours after birth reveal evidence of diffuse atelectasis and loss of lung volume (Fig. 42.2). The lung fields, which are relatively opaque, have been described as resembling ground glass or being reticulogranular. Because the lung fields are radiodense, the heart border may be obscured. In addition, air within the bronchi stands out in contrast to the lung fields as "air bronchograms" that may extend down to the diaphragm. This radiographic picture, although characteristic of RDS, may also be seen in neonatal pneumonia in premature infants, and it may be impossible to distinguish RDS from pneumonia on radiographic grounds.

If the infant dies, the characteristic features at postmortem examination are disrupted alveoli and the presence of eosinophilic hyaline membranes. Although these proteinaceous deposits give this syndrome its name, the presence of hyaline membranes is not pathognomonic of "hyaline membrane disease." They also are seen in pneumonia, cardiac failure, and other neonatal conditions characterized by lung injury.

The differential diagnosis of RDS includes other causes of respiratory distress in the premature infant. The condition with which it is most likely to be confused is group B streptococcal pneumonia, which may mimic RDS in almost every respect. At times, it may be possible to differentiate these two disorders only retrospectively, by reviewing the course and pattern of the illness.

CLINICAL MANIFESTATIONS

The clinical course of uncomplicated RDS usually follows a fairly consistent pattern. The infant demonstrates signs of respiratory distress that become worse during the first few hours after birth. In some infants, especially those who are extremely immature, the respiratory distress may be severe from the start. The disease worsens for 48 to 72 hours, reaches a peak, and starts to improve. The onset of recovery is often associated with diuresis. This classic course may not occur, however, in infants with very low birth weights or those who are very sick. With the use of ventilators and high oxygen concentrations, oxidant or mechanical lung injury may induce secondary lung damage, and a prolonged respiratory illness may ensue.

COMPLICATIONS

The major complications of RDS are related to therapy. Air leak is caused by increased airway pressure from mechanical ventilation or continuous positive airway pressure (CPAP). This complication is discussed in more detail in Chapter 46, Pulmonary Air Leaks. Chronic lung disease (bronchopulmonary dysplasia) is believed to result from injury to the lungs by oxygen and ventilation. The fragile lung of the extremely premature infant is particularly susceptible to injury, so the incidence of bronchopulmonary dysplasia is greatly increased in infants with birth weights of less than 1,250 g. Bronchopulmonary dysplasia is reviewed in Chapter 50, Bronchopulmonary Dysplasia.

Catheter complications arise from the insertion of a catheter into the aorta, which can result in thromboembolic complications such as hypertension due to renal arterial thrombosis. Additionally, an increased incidence of intraventricular hemorrhage is seen in infants with RDS. The mechanism may be related to intravascular pressure swings. Because premature infants with RDS are treated with oxygen, they are at particular risk for retinopathy of prematurity. Like bronchopulmonary dysplasia, this complication occurs mainly in infants with birth weights of less than 1,250 g.

THERAPY

Respiratory Care

A major role of neonatal intensive care units is providing respiratory care to infants with RDS. The level of intervention required depends on the severity of the respiratory distress. This is determined primarily by the arterial blood gas levels and by the amount of supplemental oxygen that the infant needs to maintain an adequate arterial oxygen tension (P_aO_2). Generally, the goal of therapy is to keep the P_aO_2 in the range of 45 to 70 mm Hg, the P_aCO_2 between about 45 and 55 mm Hg, and the pH above 7.20.

Although P_aO_2 values of 45 to 70 mm Hg are lower than those observed in healthy full-term infants, they are used, in part, because premature infants are susceptible to oxygen injury to their eyes (retinopathy of prematurity), and this range is generally thought to be safe. In addition, lower P_aO_2 levels permit the administration of lower concentrations of inspired oxygen. High concentrations of inspired oxygen lead to pulmonary oxygen toxicity, an important element in the pathogenesis of bronchopulmonary dysplasia. Low P_aO_2 levels, however, may result in tissue hypoxia and metabolic acidosis. Thus, the P_aO_2 values used are a compromise designed to avoid hypoxia at the low end and oxygen injury to the eyes and lungs at the high end.

The specific indications for, and methods of, respiratory support vary from center to center, but the following guidelines reflect common practice. If the baby requires supplemental oxygen to maintain the P_aO_2 in the 45- to 70-mm Hg range, assisted ventilation is initiated. Depending on the severity of the respiratory distress, this may be by CPAP or intubation and ventilation. If the respiratory distress is judged to be mild (breathing not excessively labored, P_aCO_2 less than 55 mm Hg, inspired oxygen concentration [FIO_2] less than 0.35 to 0.40, no acidosis), usually the first step is to deliver CPAP via nasal prongs, which are small catheters inserted into the nostrils and connected to a source of air and O_2. CPAP is generated by partially occluding expiration so that there is a distending pressure within the airways. This promotes oxygenation by increasing the functional residual capacity and preventing alveolar collapse at the end of expiration. If nasal CPAP is inadequate (e.g., if the infant is laboring to breathe, the P_aCO_2 is greater than 60 mm Hg and rising, respiratory acidosis is developing), or if the FIO_2 required is greater than 0.4 to 0.5, the infant may be intubated and ventilated via an endotracheal tube. At this stage, surfactant therapy also should be initiated. If the respiratory distress is moderate or severe from the start, the infant may be immediately intubated and ventilated, and surfactant is administered soon thereafter. Current practice, however, varies considerably from center to center with some units employing nasal CPAP even in babies with moderate or severe respiratory distress. In the absence of large randomized trials comparing the respiratory and neurologic outcome of babies treated with prolonged CPAP versus early intubation and surfactant administration, it is not possible to recommend

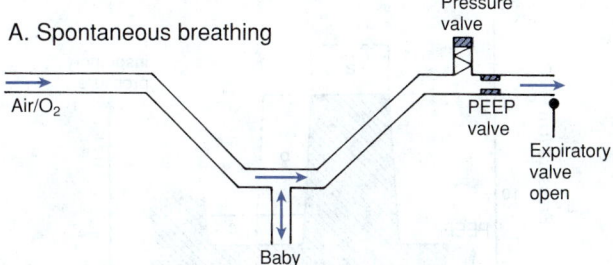

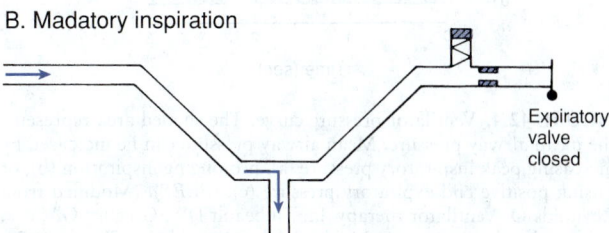

FIGURE 42.3. Time-cycled, pressure-limited infant ventilator with intermittent mandatory ventilation. **A:** When the expiratory valve is open, gas flows through the system. The baby can inhale and exhale spontaneously. The settings of the pressure and positive end-expiratory pressure (*PEEP*) valves are variable. **B:** When the expiratory valve closes, gas is forced into the baby's lungs, producing a mandatory inspiration. The inspiratory rate is determined by the rate at which the valve opens and closes. (Modified from Kirby RR. Design of mechanical ventilators. In: Thibeault DW, Gregory GA, eds. *Neonatal pulmonary care.* Menlo Park, CA: Addison-Wesley, 1979:154.)

one specific approach to the initial management of babies with RDS.

The ventilators most commonly used in neonates are time cycled and pressure limited. The mechanism by which these ventilators operate is illustrated in Figure 42.3. They can be thought of as a T-tube device by means of which gas under pressure is delivered to the infant's lungs when the expiratory valve is occluded. When the expiratory valve is opened, gas flows out of the lungs. The rate of ventilation is determined by the rate at which the expiratory outlet is opened and closed by the valve. At slow ventilation rates, the infant will breathe spontaneously between ventilator cycles. Positive end-expiratory pressure (PEEP) is generated by partially occluding the expiratory port. The peak pressure within the system is regulated by means of a pressure relief valve.

These machines are relatively simple, reliable, and designed to take advantage of the relationship between P_aO_2 and mean airway pressure in infants with RDS. Mean airway pressure is the integrated area under the curve that results when pressure is plotted against time (Fig. 42.4). Experimentally, P_aO_2 in infants with RDS has been shown to vary with mean airway pressure, if oxygen concentration is kept constant. As is shown in Figure 42.4, mean airway pressure may be increased during inspiration by increasing peak inspiratory pressure, or during expiration, by increasing PEEP. It also may be increased by prolonging inspiration at the expense of expiration (inspiratory-to-expiratory ratio). Thus, if the P_aO_2 is too low, it can be elevated by increasing the mean airway pressure or the inspired oxygen concentration. If the P_aCO_2 is too high, more ventilation is required. This is accomplished by increasing the minute volume, which is a function of the rate of respiration and the tidal volume (which is in turn partly determined by the peak inspiratory pressure). If the PEEP is very high, P_aCO_2 may be lowered by decreasing PEEP, thereby increasing tidal volume.

Because the premature lung is extremely fragile and may be injured by inspired oxygen or pressure from the ventilator,

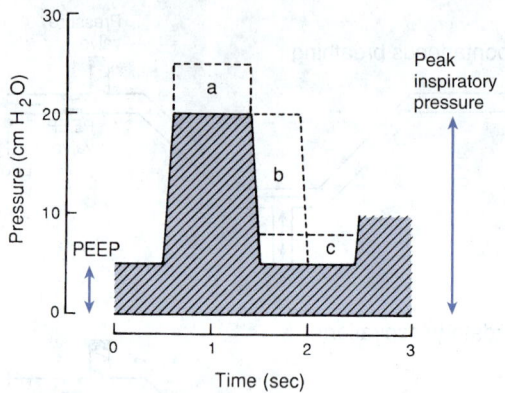

FIGURE 42.4. Ventilator pressure curve. The shaded area represents the mean airway pressure. Mean airway pressure can be increased by increasing peak inspiratory pressure (a), prolonging inspiration (b), or raising positive end-expiratory pressure (c), (*PEEP*). (Modified from Reynolds O. Ventilator therapy. In: Thibeault DW, Gregory GA, eds. *Neonatal pulmonary care.* Menlo Park, CA: Addison-Wesley, 1979: 217.)

the aim of therapy should be to provide adequate oxygenation by use of as gentle a mode of ventilation as possible. Many units accordingly will accept a P_aCO_2 of 50 to 55 mm Hg or higher, as long as the pH is not less than 7.20 to 7.25, rather than increase the peak inspiratory pressure to reduce the P_aCO_2. This approach is known as *permissive hypercapnia*. There is an increasing tendency to accept blood gas levels that might not be considered optimal in the full-term infant or the older child to prevent pressure injury to the lungs.

As the lungs start to recover and compliance improves, usually after 2 to 4 days, respiratory support can be progressively reduced and the infant can be weaned from the ventilator. After extubation, application of CPAP by nasal prongs is usually used in the transition to unsupported breathing.

The role of high-frequency ventilators (primarily oscillators) in the management of RDS is still being evaluated. These ventilators are believed to work by augmented diffusion and provide an extremely high respiratory rate (e.g., 900 to 1,200 breaths per minute) with very low tidal volumes. High PEEP settings are used to produce a mean airway pressure that is sufficient to inflate the lungs adequately. Randomized trials have demonstrated that high-frequency oscillation is an effective rescue therapy for infants with pulmonary interstitial emphysema. In addition, many centers will try high-frequency ventilation if conventional therapy is failing. Studies of the role of high-frequency ventilation in the routine management of RDS have produced conflicting results.

Monitoring

In addition to routine monitoring of temperature and heart rate, assessment of the respiratory status of infants with RDS by means of arterial blood gas determinations is essential. This is usually done by inserting a catheter through the umbilical artery into the aorta or by radial artery catheterization. The catheter can be used to draw arterial samples to determine P_aO_2, P_aCO_2, and pH levels and to record arterial blood pressure continuously via a transducer. Instruments for monitoring oxygenation by noninvasive methods have also been developed. The most widely used device is the pulse oximeter, which records the oxygen saturation of the blood continuously by means of a probe attached to an extremity, such as a fingertip. The oximeter is easy to use, reliable, and safe. In mild cases of RDS, it may be possible to follow oxygenation by means

of a pulse oximeter alone and to avoid arterial catheterization. Capillary blood specimens (e.g., a heelstick) can be used for determination of pH and P_aCO_2 levels; P_aO_2 values obtained in this manner will be unreliable, however.

Surfactant Therapy

The successful use of pulmonary surfactant preparations for the prevention or amelioration of RDS represents one of the major advances in neonatal care. (The composition of surfactant is described in Chapter 39, Developmental Considerations.) Surfactant preparations generally are administered as liquid suspensions that are instilled into the lungs via an endotracheal tube. For this reason, surfactant therapy is confined to infants who are intubated and ventilated. Two approaches to surfactant therapy have evolved. *Prevention therapy* refers to the administration of surfactant immediately after birth in the delivery area to premature infants at risk for RDS. *Rescue* or *treatment therapy* refers to the administration of surfactant to infants with diagnosed RDS; the first dose is usually given within an hour after birth.

The most widely used surfactant preparations are modified natural surfactants. These are extracts of bovine or porcine lung to which selected components, usually phospholipids, are added. The artificial surfactants that are currently available for clinical use are mixtures of synthetic compounds, usually a spreading agent, an emulsifier, and phosphatidylcholine, and are used less frequently because their onset of action is slower than that of the natural surfactants. Artificial surfactant preparations containing synthetic surfactant protein peptides are currently being evaluated in clinical trials.

Large clinical trials have demonstrated the effectiveness of modified natural and artificial surfactants for the prevention or treatment of RDS. These studies have consistently demonstrated a 30% to 40% reduction in mortality from all causes and an even greater decrease in the rate of death from RDS with the use of surfactant therapy. A reduction in mortality was observed with both artificial and natural surfactants, and whether they were given as prevention or as rescue therapy. Other benefits common to all therapies were decreases in the amount of ventilator support needed and in the incidence of pulmonary air leaks (interstitial emphysema and pneumothorax). There also was a lower incidence of RDS in the prevention studies. (Rescue therapy is given only to infants with RDS.) A disappointing finding was the absence of a consistent decrease in bronchopulmonary dysplasia in the surviving infants. This may be due to increased survival of sicker infants who would be at higher risk for this complication.

Subsequent studies have compared the effectiveness of prevention versus rescue therapy. Potential advantages of prevention therapy include better distribution of surfactant in lung fluid that has not yet been absorbed and administration before there is lung injury from ventilation. Potential disadvantages include the fact that many premature infants do not develop RDS and, therefore, would be treated unnecessarily with an expensive agent; the problem of treating a baby who is not yet stabilized, and could be destabilized further; and the inability to check endotracheal tube position carefully before therapy is initiated.

Studies that compared the two modes of treatment directly have reported that prevention tends to be more effective than rescue, in terms of decreased mortality and air leak, in babies of less than about 30 weeks' gestation at birth. However, in these studies, the rescue dose was generally given from 6 to 24 hours after birth, which may be too late to be optimal. There is currently little information on the relative benefit of prevention as opposed to earlier rescue therapy. Prevention therapy does appear to be equally effective whether it is given prior to the first breath or at 10 minutes after birth when the infant has been stabilized. It is now usually recommended that prevention therapy should only be administered to extremely premature infants at high risk of developing RDS and by personnel capable of dealing with the complications of such therapy.

Studies that have addressed the issue of when the first dose of rescue surfactant should be given have generally reported that the effect is greater if surfactant is given prior to 30 minutes to 2 hours after birth. However, many of these studies used artificial surfactants, which tend to have a slower onset of action than natural surfactants. A reasonable approach is to stabilize the infant and initiate surfactant therapy as soon as clinical signs of RDS are apparent—preferably within 30 to 60 minutes. Many centers use this early poststabilization treatment for all infants.

Surfactant therapy has been associated with few complications. There has been no consistent impact on the incidence of infection, severe intraventricular hemorrhage, retinopathy of prematurity (see Chapter 70, Eye Evaluation in the Newborn), patent ductus arteriosus, or necrotizing enterocolitis, although individual studies have reported increases or decreases in some of these conditions. In addition, there is no evidence to suggest that antibodies to surfactant proteins develop in the serum of infants who have received natural surfactant therapy. Long-term follow-up studies have shown benefits in pulmonary function and neurologic status.

Other Aspects of Treatment

Other components of treatment are also important. Body temperature should be maintained by caring for the infant on a radiant warmer or in an incubator. Initially, fluids and nutrients will have to be provided intravenously, as infants who are breathing rapidly do not tolerate oral or nasogastric feedings. Very immature infants may require more prolonged total parenteral nutrition via a central vein. Antibiotics generally are administered, not because RDS is an infectious condition, nor to cover invasive procedures such as catheters, but because in many cases pneumonia cannot be excluded, or because maternal infection is believed to be the cause of premature delivery.

Sodium bicarbonate should be used sparingly. Overuse carries the risk of inducing hypernatremia and may precipitate an intraventricular hemorrhage, particularly if it is given rapidly in bolus form. Acidosis should be treated initially by optimizing ventilation. A persistent metabolic acidosis with a pH of less than 7.20 can be treated with a slow, dilute bicarbonate infusion of 1 to 2 mEq/kg. Persistent acidosis is also an indication to assess general perfusion and to determine if a significant patent ductus arteriosus is present. The latter should be treated by indomethacin therapy or by surgical ligation if indomethacin is not effective.

PREVENTION

There are a number of approaches to prevent RDS in premature infants. These include antenatal prediction of fetal lung maturity, pharmacologic acceleration of fetal lung development, and prevention therapy with surfactant (see previous discussion). The best approach is prevention of prematurity itself.

Antenatal Prediction of Fetal Lung Maturity

Before methods for assessing fetal lung maturity were developed, a significant number of infants born after elective induction of labor or elective cesarean section developed RDS.

In many cases, this outcome was the result of an inaccurate assessment of the duration of gestation.

The fetal lung secretes surfactant into the amniotic fluid. Examination of the amniotic fluid can reveal whether the lung is synthesizing surfactant-associated phospholipids in quantities sufficient to support respiration. This is done most commonly by measuring the lecithin-to-sphingomyelin (LS) ratio and by determining whether phosphatidylglycerol (PG), another surfactant-related phospholipid, is detectable. Lecithin (or phosphatidylcholine) is the most abundant component of surfactant, and the lecithin in amniotic fluid is derived from the fetal lung, whereas the sphingomyelin is derived from nonpulmonary sources. As the lung matures, the LS ratio increases. When this ratio is greater than 2, the fetal lungs are almost invariably mature; a ratio of 1.5 to 2.0 is indeterminate, and a value of less than 1.5 predicts immaturity. The test errs on the side of overpredicting immaturity. If there is no PG in the amniotic fluid and the LS ratio is less than 1.5, an obstetrician considering an elective delivery may decide to delay until such time as the lung is mature.

Measurement of surfactant-specific proteins (SPs; particularly SP-A) in the amniotic fluid has been used experimentally to evaluate lung maturity and appears to be a good indicator. Rapid and relatively simple enzyme-linked immunosorbent assays may increase the clinical use of this test in the future. Determination of gestational age by ultrasound measurements, such as the biparietal diameter of the head, is also useful for preventing inadvertent early elective delivery, with the associated risk of RDS.

Pharmacologic Acceleration of Fetal Lung Maturation

Fetal lung development is known to be controlled by multiple factors. Agents that have been demonstrated to enhance lung maturation include glucocorticoids, thyroid hormones, growth factors (such as epidermal growth factor), transcription factors (such as thyroid transcription factor), and cyclic adenosine monophosphate. Most of this information has come from animal studies, but a substantial body of evidence indicates that glucocorticoids accelerate lung maturation in humans, and these agents have been used clinically since the 1970s for this purpose. Because glucocorticoids act by enhancing RNA transcription and protein synthesis, a process that takes time, they are most effective if the infant is delivered more than 24 hours after the initial dose. The clinical benefits of glucocorticoids decrease if the infant is not delivered within 7 days.

When they are administered appropriately, antenatal glucocorticoids reduce the incidence of RDS by approximately 50%. Other clinically important benefits of antenatal glucocorticoid therapy include decreased early neonatal deaths, intraventricular bleeds and necrotizing enterocolitis, and a tendency to have a better neurologic outcome at follow-up.

It is recommended that antenatal steroids should be used in cases of threatened premature labor before 34 weeks' gestation, if immediate delivery is not anticipated and if there is evidence of pulmonary immaturity, or pulmonary maturity is unknown. The usual regimen is to administer betamethasone, a glucocorticoid that crosses the placenta readily, for a period of 48 hours. If the infant does not deliver within 7 days, one more course of betamethasone may be administered later in the pregnancy if premature labor occurs again. The use of dexamethasone, another synthetic glucocorticoid that crosses the placenta to the fetus, is not recommended due to reports of long-term toxicity to the nervous system. For similar reasons, multiple (more than two) courses of betamethasone should not be given.

Synergy of Antenatal Hormone and Postnatal Surfactant Therapy

Lung compliance and respiratory status are improved by antenatal steroid therapy and postnatal surfactant therapy. Animal and clinical studies also indicate that the effect of both therapies combined is greater than that of either alone. The optimal approach to the management of this condition is the use of antenatal steroids followed by postnatal surfactant, when indicated.

Although these therapies are very effective, it should be noted that one of the most effective means of preventing RDS remains good obstetric care, with the use of pharmacologic agents to inhibit premature labor.

Suggested Readings

Crowley PA. Antenatal corticosteroid therapy: a meta-analysis of the randomized trials, 1972 to 1994. *Am J Obstet Gynecol* 1995;173:322.

Gross I, Ballard PL. Hormonal therapy for prevention of respiratory distress syndrome. In: Polin RA, Fox WW, Abman SH, eds. *Fetal and neonatal physiology*, 3rd ed. Philadelphia: Elsevier, 2003:1069.

Jobe AH. Drug therapy: pulmonary surfactant therapy. *N Engl J Med* 1993; 328:861.

Soll RF, Morley CJ. Prophylactic versus selective use of surfactant in preventing morbidity and mortality in preterm infants (Cochrane Review). In: *The Cochrane Library*, Oxford Update Software, Issue 1, 2003.

Yost CC, Soll RF. Early versus delayed selective surfactant treatment for neonatal respiratory distress syndrome (Cochrane Review). In: *The Cochrane Library*, Oxford Update Software, Issue 1, 2003.

CHAPTER 43 ■ CYSTIC ADENOMATOID MALFORMATION

IAN GROSS

Congenital cystic adenomatoid malformation (CCAM) is believed to be the result of an early focal arrest in lung development. Cystic areas replace the normal bronchi and alveoli in the affected part of the lung. In the majority of cases, the lesion is confined to one lobe and there is a connection, which may be tortuous, to the airway. The blood supply is derived from the pulmonary circulation (and not from an aberrant artery as is the case with pulmonary sequestration). Three types have been described based on the size and number of the cysts:

Type I: Made up of a few large cysts
Type II: Numerous small or medium-sized cysts
Type III: Multiple tiny cysts

CLINICAL MANIFESTATIONS AND COMPLICATIONS

The clinical presentation in the perinatal period varies considerably. The lesion may be diagnosed antenatally by ultrasound; types I and II lesions appear as cystic echolucent masses, whereas type III lesions appear as a large solid mass that may be associated with hydrops due to mediastinal shift and obstruction of the vena cava. Occasionally, the lesion shrinks in size prior to delivery. After birth, infants with symptomatic CCAM present with respiratory distress. The severity varies considerably depending on the size of the lesion and the presence and extent of pulmonary hypoplasia.

DIAGNOSIS

The diagnosis is usually made by radiograph, although in some cases a computed tomographic scan of the chest or a magnetic resonance imaging scan may be needed. The differential diagnosis of thoracic masses includes pulmonary sequestration, diaphragmatic hernia, bronchogenic cysts, and tumors such as neuroblastoma.

THERAPY

Treatment depends on the severity of the presenting symptoms. Antenatal hydrops carries a very poor prognosis, and experimental fetal surgery to drain large cysts or excise affected lobes is currently being evaluated. Babies who present with severe respiratory distress at birth will require mechanical ventilation and management of pulmonary hypertension, if present, before surgical resection. Selective intubation of the unaffected lung has been suggested as a temporizing measure prior to surgery. Extracorporeal membrane oxygenation has been used in selected cases with severe refractory respiratory failure.

Suggested Readings

Adzick NS. Management of fetal lung lesions. *Clin Perinatol* 2003;30:481.

Cortes RA, Farmer DL. Recent advances in fetal surgery. *Semin Perinatol* 2004; 28:199.

Davenport M, Warne SA, Cacciaguerra S, et al. Current outcome of antenatally diagnosed cystic lung disease. *J Pediatr Surg* 2004;39:549.

van Leeuwen K, Teitelbaum DH, Hirschl RB, et al. Prenatal diagnosis of congenital cystic adenomatoid malformation and its postnatal presentation, surgical indications, and natural history. *J Pediatr Surg* 1999;34:794.

CHAPTER 44 ■ TRANSIENT TACHYPNEA OF THE NEWBORN

IAN GROSS

Transient tachypnea of the newborn (also called retained fetal lung fluid, or wet lung) is a benign, self-limited condition seen primarily in full-term infants. It is believed to result from delay in the reabsorption of fetal pulmonary fluid. There is an association between delivery by cesarean section and the development of this condition, possibly because of the compression of the chest during vaginal delivery and the mechanical "wringing out" of fetal lung fluid.

CLINICAL MANIFESTATIONS

Infants with transient tachypnea present with respiratory distress shortly after birth. The features are tachypnea, mild retractions, and sometimes cyanosis. The clinical course usually is transient and mild, with resolution of the problem in 24 to 48 hours. In some infants, the condition is more severe and may persist for 72 hours or longer.

DIAGNOSIS

The diagnosis is made by radiography. The classic appearance is that of a well-aerated lung with streaky markings radiating out from the hila (starburst appearance) and small amounts of fluid in the fissures, particularly the right middle fissure. The major condition from which transient tachypnea must be differentiated is pneumonia. Differentiation can sometimes be difficult in prolonged cases of transient tachypnea, although resolution is usually more rapid than with pneumonia. A chest radiograph showing resolution within 48 hours indicates transient tachypnea.

THERAPY

Treatment is essentially symptomatic. Blood gas levels or oxygen saturation are monitored, and oxygen is administered to maintain an oxygen saturation of 90% to 95%. Occasionally, a brief period of mechanical ventilation may be necessary. If the diagnosis of pneumonia cannot be excluded, antibiotics are given, although transient tachypnea itself does not require antibacterial treatment. This condition is not associated with long-term sequelae such as bronchopulmonary dysplasia, and the prognosis is excellent.

Suggested Readings

Hook B, Kiwi R, Amini SB, et al. Neonatal morbidity after elective repeat cesarean section and trial of labor. *Pediatrics* 1997;100:348–353.

Lewis V, Whitelaw A. Furosemide for transient tachypnea of the newborn. *Cochrane Database of Systematic Reviews* 2002:CD003064.

O'Brodovich HM. Immature epithelial Na$^+$ channel expression is one of the pathogenetic mechanisms leading to human neonatal respiratory distress syndrome. *Proceedings of the Association of American Physicians* 1996;108: 345–355.

CHAPTER 45 ■ PNEUMONIA

IAN GROSS

Pneumonia in the newborn period may arise during the first 2 to 3 days after birth (early onset) or after the first week (late onset). It may occur as an isolated infection or in association with septicemia. Pneumonia that develops shortly after birth is probably acquired *in utero* or intrapartum by hematogenous spread from the mother, by ascending infection from the vagina and cervix, or by aspiration of contaminated secretions immediately after birth. Late-onset pneumonia, similar to other nosocomial infections in the newborn unit, can be transmitted by the infant's caretakers. The most common pathogens are group B streptococci and gram-negative organisms such as *Escherichia coli* and *Klebsiella*, but a wide variety of organisms may be involved. During the 1970s, the group B streptococci emerged as a major cause of pneumonia and septicemia in newborns. Although group B streptococcal infection is still a significant problem, it now occurs with about the same frequency as infection with gram-negative enteric organisms.

CLINICAL MANIFESTATIONS AND COMPLICATIONS

Infants with early-onset pneumonia usually have respiratory distress within the first few hours after birth. If they are premature, the symptoms may be indistinguishable from those of respiratory distress syndrome (RDS). Features that suggest pneumonia rather than RDS include maternal chorioamnionitis, prolonged rupture of the membranes, early onset of apnea, and poor perfusion and shock. The amniotic fluid lecithin-to-sphingomyelin ratio, if available, also is useful in differentiating pneumonia from RDS (a "mature" ratio rules out RDS).

The clinical course of neonatal pneumonia varies considerably. Some infants have fulminant disease with a rapid downhill course and early death. More commonly, moderate respiratory distress develops and assisted ventilation may be required for a few days, after which the baby recovers. The course may be different from that of RDS, which tends to become progressively more severe and to peak at 48 to 72 hours; pneumonia usually follows a more level course. In addition to parenchymal lung disease, some infants also have severe pulmonary hypertension, presumably secondary to pulmonary vasospasm, with right-to-left shunting of blood. These babies may be critically ill and tend to have a labile P_aO_2 with marked hypoxia disproportionate to the severity of their parenchymal lung disease as reflected by the chest radiograph. This complication is associated with significant morbidity and mortality.

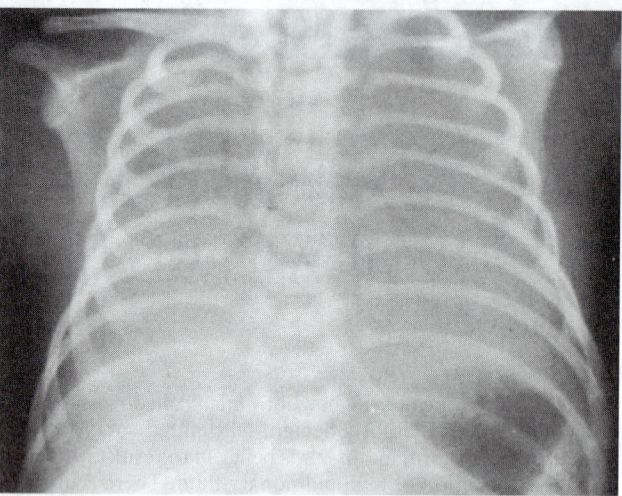

FIGURE 45.2. Respiratory distress syndrome–like pattern in a premature infant with pneumonia. The radiodensity of the lungs is increased greatly, resulting in an opacified appearance.

DIAGNOSIS

Radiographic Appearance

At least four different radiographic appearances have been described in newborn infants with pneumonia and include extensive coarse infiltrates scattered throughout both lungs and lobar consolidation (Fig. 45.1). Also possible is an RDS-like pattern (Fig. 45.2); the radiographic appearance of pneumonia in premature infants, particularly that caused by the group B streptococci, may be indistinguishable from that seen in RDS. It is possible that some of these infants have both RDS and pneumonia. Additionally, scattered small infiltrates may develop in one or both lungs (more commonly in mature than in premature infants).

In the full-term infant with a few scattered lung infiltrates on the chest radiograph, pneumonia must be differentiated from transient tachypnea of the newborn. The respiratory distress of pneumonia usually persists for a few days, whereas transient tachypnea is more likely to resolve within 48 hours. In the pre-

mature infant with a radiographic appearance consistent with RDS, it may not be possible to distinguish the two conditions, at least in the early stages.

Bacteriology

The use of cultures to identify the organism often is not helpful. Unless there is associated septicemia, blood cultures will be negative. If the infant is intubated, tracheal cultures taken through the endotracheal tube can be misleading, particularly if the tube has been in place for some time, as the tube may be colonized with organisms that are not necessarily the same as those that are causing the pneumonia. A tracheal culture taken at the time of initial intubation may be of some value. Surface cultures are not helpful, as the organisms that colonize the skin may not be the pulmonary pathogens. In most cases, the bacteriology of the pneumonia is not established. If the infant dies, hyaline membrane formation may be noted in the lungs; in infants who die of group B streptococcal pneumonia, Gram stain of the lungs may reveal gram-positive cocci enmeshed with the hyaline membranes (Fig. 45.3).

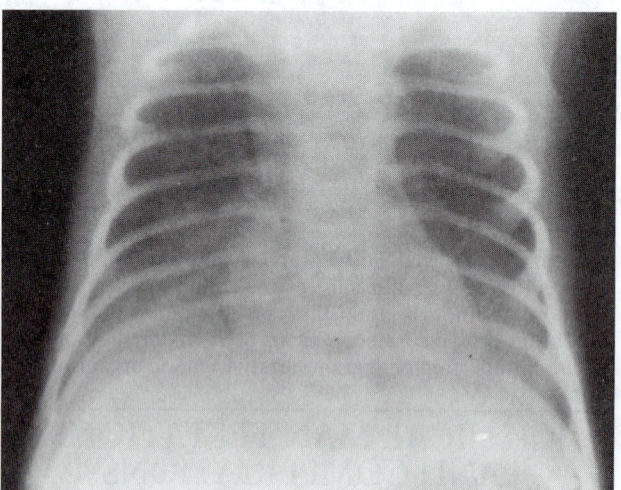

FIGURE 45.1. Bilateral lobar consolidation in an infant with pneumonia.

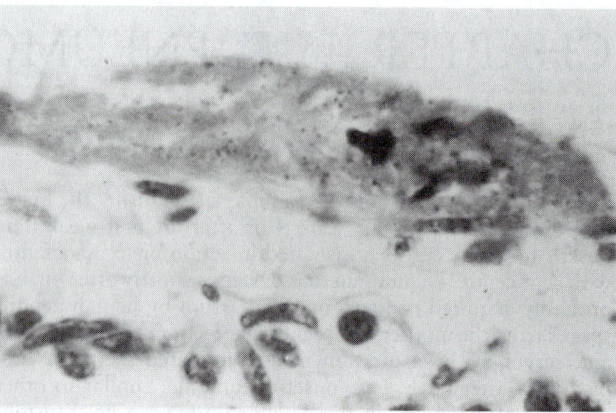

FIGURE 45.3. Gram stain of the lung in group B streptococcal pneumonia. Numerous gram-positive cocci are enmeshed within the proteinaceous hyaline membrane.

THERAPY

The improved survival of infants with serious neonatal infections has been related to advances in supportive techniques as well as antibiotic therapy. Whereas milder cases may be treated with supplemental oxygen only, moderate and severe cases of pneumonia often require ventilator support. The infant's arterial blood gases, blood pressure, peripheral perfusion, and hematocrit should be monitored. If there is evidence of poor perfusion, this should be corrected with infusions of colloids or electrolytes, or inotropic drugs such as dopamine, as indicated. If perfusion is a major problem, evaluation of cardiac filling and contractility will facilitate decisions related to the use of volume expanders or inotropic drugs. Metabolic acidosis may require correction by careful infusion of bicarbonate.

Because a precise bacterial diagnosis is usually not available, broad-spectrum coverage (e.g., with a penicillin and an aminoglycoside) is instituted for 7 to 10 days. If gentamicin is used, peak and trough levels of this antibiotic in the blood should be determined to ensure that the dose and frequency of administration are appropriate.

In those infants who demonstrate evidence of pulmonary hypertension and right-to-left shunting, nitric oxide inhalation can be very effective. (If nitric oxide is not available, infusion of tolazoline may be used by physicians who have experience with this vasodilator and its complications.) In a few infants, the pulmonary hypertension is so severe and intractable that institution of extracorporeal membrane oxygenation (ECMO) is indicated. Nitric oxide, tolazoline, and ECMO therapy are discussed in Chapter 48, Persistent Pulmonary Hypertension.

Most infants with pneumonia do well and survive without long-term sequelae. Patients who require prolonged ventilation with high peak inspiratory pressures and high oxygen concentrations may develop chronic lung disease.

CHAPTER 46 ■ PULMONARY AIR LEAKS

IAN GROSS

Air leak is more common during the newborn period than at any other time of life. This finding probably relates to the facts that assisted ventilation is a relatively common mode of therapy in sick newborn infants, that premature infants have fragile lungs, and that high intrathoracic pressure gradients are generated during the first few breaths. It has been estimated that spontaneous air leak occurs in 1% of all live births, but many of these are asymptomatic. The sites of air leak in the newborn are the pleural cavities (pneumothorax), mediastinum (pneumomediastinum), lung interstitial tissue (interstitial emphysema), and, occasionally, pericardial sac (pneumopericardium) and peritoneal cavity (pneumoperitoneum).

Air leak is a significant problem in infants receiving assisted ventilation. The incidence of pneumothorax and interstitial emphysema in infants with respiratory distress syndrome (RDS) was significantly reduced (from about 25% to about 10%) with the use of surfactant.

TYPES OF AIR LEAK

Pneumothorax

Air leak, particularly pneumothorax, should be suspected in any infant receiving positive airway pressure who suddenly becomes cyanotic. The clinical features suggestive of a tension pneumothorax include shift of the apex beat, decreased breath sounds on the side of the pneumothorax, distention of the chest, and, occasionally, a readily palpable liver and spleen from downward displacement of the diaphragm. In addition, the infant may demonstrate poor circulation or shock.

Diagnosis and appropriate treatment of a tension pneumothorax is a matter of the greatest urgency. The differential diagnosis of an infant who deteriorates suddenly and becomes cyanotic while on a ventilator includes endotracheal tube or large airway obstruction, pneumothorax, and massive pulmonary or intracranial bleed. Once it has been established that the airway is patent, the diagnosis of tension pneumothorax frequently can be made on clinical grounds, assisted by transillumination. This involves shining a bright, focused light on the chest wall after dimming the lights in the room. The part of the chest into which air has leaked may become highly translucent. If the infant is unstable, there usually is not time to obtain a radiograph of the chest; in this situation, the suspected pneumothorax will have to be managed without the benefit of radiographic confirmation. If the infant is stable and there is no acute interference with respiration or circulation, a chest radiograph may be obtained for confirmation of the diagnosis before proceeding to treatment.

The initial step is to insert a needle, preferably a plastic needle with a metal trochar (such as is used for peripheral intravenous infusions), into the chest. The needle should be attached to a syringe by means of a three-way stopcock or, alternatively, to a short length of empty intravenous solution tubing, the end of which is placed under water below the level of the chest. If the baby is lying supine, the air usually will collect in the anterior chest; a suitable site for needle insertion is the anterior axillary line in the fifth or sixth interspace. The diagnosis of pneumothorax is made when insertion of the needle into the pleural cavity results in the release of air under tension, with accompanying improvement in the infant's status. Once the diagnosis has been established, a chest tube should be inserted. The chest tube should be connected to a water seal that is subjected to negative pressure. Drainage should be continued as long as air is evacuated from the chest. When it is clear that air drainage has stopped, the negative pressure should be discontinued, or the chest tube may be clamped. If a chest radiograph, taken after a few hours, shows that the pneumothorax has not recurred, the tube may be removed.

A spontaneous pneumothorax that is not under tension and that is causing little distress may be treated by observation only. Since oxygen is absorbed more readily into the bloodstream than is the nitrogen in air, inspiration of 100% oxygen facilitates resolution of the pneumothorax. This condition is usually benign, however, and breathing 100% oxygen is unnecessary in cases without significant respiratory distress. Resolution occurs satisfactorily if the infant is allowed to breathe room air.

Pneumomediastinum and Pneumopericardium

Pneumomediastinum is generally not treated surgically and resolves spontaneously with time. A pneumopericardium causing significant cardiac tamponade will require drainage. This should be done by a physician who is skilled in this procedure.

Interstitial Emphysema

If air tracks into the interstitial space and stays there, interstitial emphysema results. This problem has become more significant with the increased survival rates of extremely premature infants. Their fragile lungs are particularly prone to interstitial emphysema, which may develop within the first few days after birth when these infants are treated with mechanical ventilation. Interstitial emphysema complicates ventilator management. The free air in the interstitium results in the lungs becoming less compliant so that higher ventilator pressures are required, which in turn facilitates the development of more interstitial emphysema. The resulting barotrauma often results in significant bronchopulmonary dysplasia.

Interstitial emphysema can be difficult to treat. High-frequency ventilation has been shown to be effective for the management of interstitial emphysema in premature infants, and this strategy is usually the first that is tried. Another approach that is sometimes successful is to position the infant so that the side of the chest that is most affected is dependent. The weight on this part of the chest may decrease the movement of the lungs there and assist resolution of the emphysema. Selective intubation may be useful in cases of unilateral interstitial emphysema. The endotracheal tube is inserted down the mainstem bronchus of the unaffected lung, so that only that lung is ventilated. This procedure may result in resolution of the emphysema, but emphysema often recurs when the endotracheal tube is pulled back and both lungs are inflated.

DIAGNOSIS

The definitive diagnosis of all these forms of air leak is made by radiography. A tension pneumothorax appears as a dark, radiolucent area in the pleural cavity (Fig. 46.1). The compressed lung may be seen adjacent to the pleural air accumulation, and the heart is usually shifted away from the pneumothorax. In an infant lying on his or her back, air tends to accumulate anteriorly, so that the free air is in the anterior medial portion of the chest. This appearance can lead to confusion with pneumomediastinum. A lateral film should be taken to further localize the site of air accumulation. In some cases of pneumomediastinum, (Fig. 46.2) the free air compresses the thymus, resulting in the "sail" sign, which is caused by radiolucent air under a triangular thymic shadow. Pneumopericardium is characterized by air that surrounds the heart and adheres closely to its contour (Fig. 46.3). The air crosses the midline underneath the heart as it follows the shape of the pericardial cavity. Interstitial emphysema is apparent as small, round, radiolucent blebs that track through the lung tissue. The air blebs tend to follow a linear pattern.

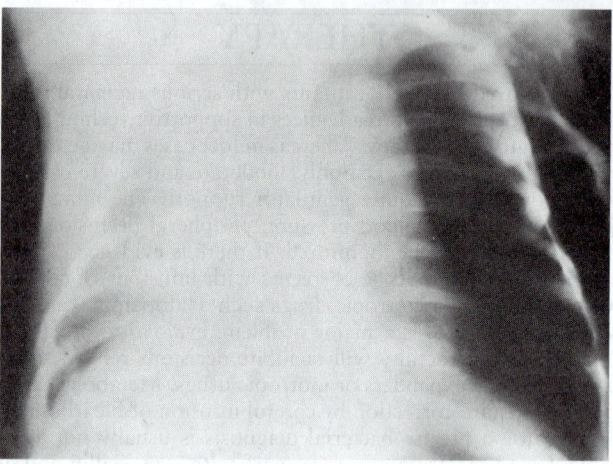

FIGURE 46.1. Tensions pneumothorax. Note the radiolucent air collection in the left chest, compression of the left lung, and shift of the mediastinum to the right.

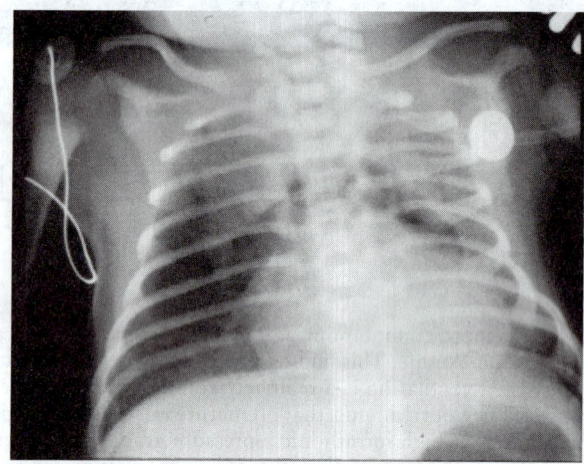

FIGURE 46.2. Pneumomediastinum. Note the medial air collection and the triangular shape of the thymus on the right side ("sail sign").

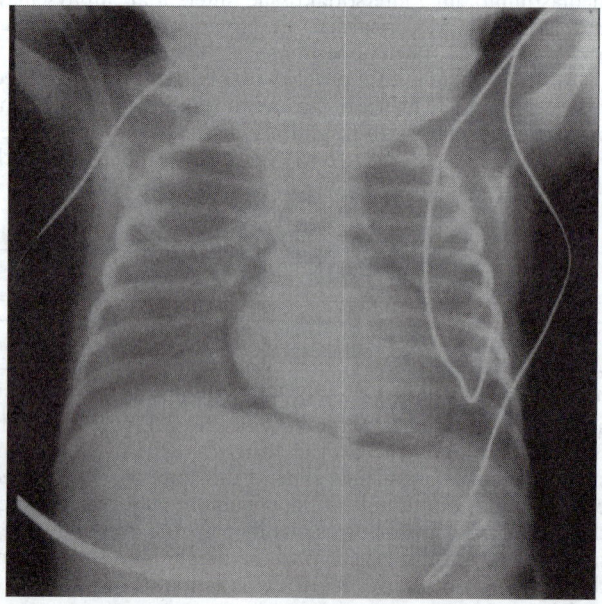

FIGURE 46.3. Pneumopericardium. Note that the air collection crosses the midline and has the same contour as the heart.

CHAPTER 47 ■ MECONIUM ASPIRATION SYNDROME

IAN GROSS

Meconium is passed into the amniotic fluid in approximately 10% of all births. Although passage of meconium may be associated with intrauterine fetal hypoxia, it also occurs in apparently normal deliveries in the absence of asphyxia. It is more common in postmature babies in whom there is evidence of placental insufficiency. Meconium aspiration is not seen in premature infants of less than 34 weeks' gestation, as these infants rarely demonstrate meconium-stained amniotic fluid.

It is currently recommended that if meconium is present in the amniotic fluid or on the baby's skin, and the baby is not vigorous, aspiration of meconium from the pharynx and trachea should be performed immediately after birth. The delivery room management of infants born with meconium is discussed in Chapter 24, The Newborn Intensive Care Unit.

Meconium that has not been cleared from the trachea can migrate peripherally and obstruct the smaller airways. Partial occlusion may result in a one-way valve effect, with distal hyperinflation. Alternatively, the small airways may be blocked completely, leading to atelectasis. In some infants persistent pulmonary hypertension occurs, presumably as a result of intrapartum hypoxia/asphyxia, which cause passage of meconium. The presence of significant pulmonary hypertension considerably complicates the management of these babies.

Infants with meconium aspiration present clinically with respiratory distress and an overdistended chest. Coarse râles may be heard. The chest radiograph reveals hyperinflation of the lungs with patchy infiltrates. Because of the air-trapping effect of meconium in the airways, pneumothorax is common, occurring in 20% to 50% of cases.

Management of these patients is symptomatic. They require oxygen supplementation and, frequently, ventilator therapy. The diffuse small airway obstruction may necessitate the use of relatively high peak inspiratory pressures to maintain adequate ventilation. If conventional ventilator therapy is failing, or if high airway pressure is required, a trial of high-frequency ventilation is indicated. Clinical trials have indicated that administration of surfactant to these infants is beneficial. Trials are in progress to determine whether the benefits of lung lavage with surfactant outweigh the risks, which include destabilizing the baby. The use of antibiotics is controversial; some neonatologists do not use antibiotics in uncomplicated cases of meconium aspiration, whereas others do because of concern for secondary infection. The management of persistent pulmonary hypertension is discussed in Chapter 48, Persistent Pulmonary Hypertension.

Suggested Readings

Finer NN. Surfactant use for neonatal lung injury: beyond respiratory distress syndrome. *Paediatr Respir Rev* 2004;5:S289.
Kinsella JP. Meconium aspiration syndrome. Is surfactant lavage the answer? *Am J Respir Crit Care Med* 2003;168:413.

CHAPTER 48 ■ PERSISTENT PULMONARY HYPERTENSION

IAN GROSS

PATHOGENESIS

During fetal life the tone in the pulmonary arterial system is increased and the pressure on the right side of the heart is greater than that on the left. Consequently, blood is shunted from the right side of the heart to the left through the foramen ovale and the ductus arteriosus (Fig. 48.1). The blood that enters the right atrium via the superior vena cava tends to flow into the right ventricle, whereas blood that enters the right atrium from the inferior vena cava tends to be shunted across the foramen ovale to the left atrium. Much of the flow from the right ventricle is then shunted to the aorta through the ductus arteriosus. After birth and the onset of breathing, pressure in the pulmonary circulation decreases and functional closure of the foramen ovale occurs, followed by anatomic closure of the ductus arteriosus. In some infants, however, pulmonary hypertension develops

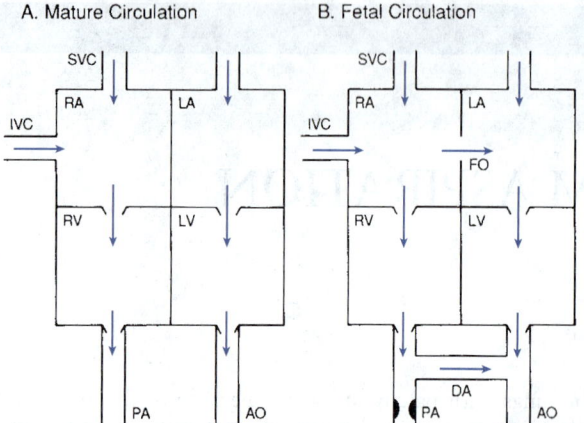

FIGURE 48.1. Comparison of mature and fetal circulations. In fetal life, blood is shunted from the right to the left side of the heart across the foramen ovale and the ductus arteriosus because of the increased pressure in the pulmonary circulation. If pressure in the pulmonary circulation rises again after birth, the shunting recurs. AO, aorta; DA, ductus arteriosus; FO, foramen ovale; IVC, inferior vena cava; LA, left atrium; LV, left ventricle; PA, pulmonary artery; RA, right atrium; RV, right ventricle; SVC, superior vena cava.

again after birth. This results in reestablishment of right-to-left shunting through the foramen ovale or ductus arteriosus; for this reason, this condition is sometimes referred to as *persistent fetal circulation.*

The pulmonary arterioles are sensitive to hypoxia and acidosis and respond to these stimuli by vasospasm. In infants with lung disease or other causes of hypoxia and acidosis, pulmonary hypertension may develop as a consequence of the hypoxia produced by the underlying disease. This secondary type of pulmonary hypertension usually reverses when the underlying problem has been resolved.

In another group of infants, a more persistent form of pulmonary hypertension develops. They are usually full-term or postmature infants with meconium aspiration or with no lung disease, and a history of asphyxia may be present. The underlying lesion in persistent pulmonary hypertension (PPH) is believed to be abnormal muscularization of the small arterioles supplying the distal airways. At birth, the walls of the arterioles supplying the terminal and respiratory bronchioles are usually only partially muscularized. Infants who die of PPH have been shown at autopsy to have extension of this muscularization into the arterioles that supply the alveolar ducts. Resistance to blood flow occurs as the walls of these arterioles are thickened and the vessel lumen is narrow. Asphyxia or other insults occurring after birth may aggravate the situation by triggering spasm of these thickened arterioles, with resulting severe pulmonary hypertension.

It has been suggested that the abnormal muscularization of the pulmonary vasculature is caused by intrauterine hypoxia during late fetal life. *In utero* hypoxia also could account for the association of PPH with meconium aspiration and postmaturity. Infants who are stressed *in utero,* such as postmature infants, are less able to tolerate labor and have a greater tendency to experience intrapartum asphyxia and to pass meconium.

In addition to asphyxia and meconium aspiration, PPH is associated with pulmonary hypoplasia (e.g., diaphragmatic hernia), sepsis, and pneumonia. In diaphragmatic hernia, there is not only pulmonary vasospasm, but also a smaller pulmonary vascular bed in the hypoplastic lung. The hypoxia in these infants may be particularly severe and resistant to therapy. The pulmonary vasospasm in infected infants is thought to be due to vasoactive bacterial toxins.

DIAGNOSIS

The diagnosis of PPH is suggested by the triad of cyanosis, absence of heart disease, and clear lung fields or meconium aspiration. The usual presentation is that of a full-term or postmature infant who may have a history of asphyxia or meconium aspiration. The baby may appear to be well initially, but within the first 24 hours after birth there is progressive cyanosis and tachypnea. A chest radiograph taken at this stage will reveal clear lungs, or scattered infiltrates in the case of meconium aspiration. The lungs may have decreased vascular markings, consistent with diminished pulmonary blood flow. The cyanosis, if untreated, will continue to progress until, eventually, it becomes profound. Shock with decreased peripheral perfusion and hypotension may also develop.

The combination of severe cyanosis with clear lung fields or small infiltrates should raise the suspicion of PPH; the clues are cyanosis that is disproportionate to the radiographic signs of lung disease and a labile (as opposed to a relatively fixed) P_aO_2 or oxygen saturation. The P_aO_2 is labile as the pulmonary arterioles are "twitchy," whereas infants with fixed anatomic heart disease tend to have less variability in the P_aO_2. However, the infant should not be treated for pulmonary hypertension until heart disease has been excluded, preferably by an echocardiogram. Infants with total anamolous pulmonary venous return with obstruction or other causes of cyanotic heart disease may initially have similar clinical features. The echocardiogram will exclude anatomic heart disease and confirm the diagnosis of pulmonary hypertension and right-to-left shunting at the level of the foramen ovale or ductus arteriosus. It may reveal tricuspid regurgitation resulting from the high right-sided pressure. Echocardiography is also useful for assessing right ventricular filling and myocardial contractility, and can be used as a guide for determining intravenous fluid and pressor requirements.

Comparison of right radial (preductal) P_aO_2 to umbilical artery (postductal) P_aO_2 is useful for assessing shunting across the ductus arteriosus. The umbilical P_aO_2 will be lower in the presence of right-to-left ductal shunting. The absence of such a difference, however, does not rule out PPH and right-to-left shunting, because the shunting may occur at the level of the foramen ovale only. Comparison of upper limb (preductal) to lower limb (postductal) oxygen saturation yields similar information.

THERAPY

Infants with PPH present perhaps the most difficult medical management problem in the newborn intensive care unit, and their care draws on all the resources available to modern neonatology. They should be managed by physicians experienced with this problem and in an environment where the appropriate support is available.

Monitoring

Careful monitoring is critical. An umbilical or radial artery catheter should be inserted so that blood gases and blood pressure can be determined. A central venous line may be inserted for fluid administration; it can also be used to monitor central venous pressure, although interpretation of venous pressure may be difficult if there is tricuspid regurgitation. Serial echocardiography is probably more useful for assessing intravascular fluid status. Two pulse oximeters, positioned to register preductal and postductal values (e.g., on the right hand and left foot), are also extremely useful.

Perfusion

Affected infants often have poor cardiovascular perfusion and may require infusions of intravenous fluids or inotropic agents. If peripheral perfusion appears to be diminished, a determination of right-sided ventricular filling should be made. If the echocardiogram or the central venous pressure indicates that an intravenous fluid infusion is required, colloid is probably the agent of choice. If intravascular fluid volume is adequate, but contractility is poor, administration of an inotropic agent is indicated. Most infants with significant disease require both fluid infusions and inotropic agents. Generally, dopamine is the first agent that is used. There is some concern that infusion of dopamine at rates greater than 10 μg/kg/minute may cause pulmonary vasoconstriction, but this does not appear to be borne out by clinical experience. A second agent, such as dobutamine or epinephrine, is often used if perfusion cannot be improved with dopamine alone.

Ventilation

The ventilatory management of infants with PPH varies considerably from center to center. Treatment of this disorder by hyperventilation was common, but this is no longer the case. Hyperoxia and alkalosis are pulmonary vasodilators. The goal of hyperventilation was to reduce the P_aCO_2 to 20 to 25 mm Hg so that a respiratory alkalosis develops and to generate relatively high P_aO_2 levels. Although hyperventilation does increase oxygenation, at least in the short term, there has been increasing concern that this form of therapy significantly damages the lungs, especially when it is prolonged. Pulmonary vasospasm and PPH tend to resolve after a few days, and mortality in some cases appears to be related to lung damage from barotrauma caused by the respirator rather than from the primary problem. For this reason, an increasing number of neonatologists now avoid hyperventilation and use more conservative ventilator management. One approach is to allow the P_aCO_2 to remain at 45 to 55 mm Hg and to accept a P_aO_2 in the range of 45 to 60 mm Hg. The P_aO_2 in many of these infants does respond favorably to an alkaline pH level, however, and the pH can be maintained in the 7.45 to 7.50 range by the intravenous infusion of sodium bicarbonate. Published reports of successful management of infants with pulmonary hypertension, particularly in association with congenital diaphragmatic hernia, have suggested that the need for extracorporeal membrane oxygenation (ECMO) can be substantially diminished if lower oxygen saturation levels (e.g., a preductal saturation as low as 80%) are tolerated. Whereas the lungs are likely to be protected by this approach, there are no published data relating to neurologic outcome after this mode of therapy.

If conventional ventilation, as described above, is not successful, the next step is to try high-frequency ventilation. It is difficult to predict which infants will respond favorably to high-frequency ventilation, but clinical trials have demonstrated that approximately 40% of infants with PPH who fail with conventional ventilation will benefit from high-frequency ventilation.

The labile P_aO_2 and right-to-left shunt usually persist for 4 to 7 days, after which recovery starts to occur. If the lungs have not been damaged by the respirator and oxygen therapy, the infant may be weaned slowly from the ventilator. Some infants become hypoxic when even minor attempts at weaning are made (flip-flop effect), so this must be done slowly and cautiously.

Sedation

Infants with PPH are often very labile and may become hypoxic if they are touched or moved. They may become more stable with adequate sedation. Morphine or other opiates, alone or in combination with benzodiazepine derivatives, are usually effective for this purpose. (Ventilated term infants should always receive some form of sedation.) The question of whether these infants should also be given muscle relaxants such as vecuronium to permit control of ventilation is controversial. Paralysis does facilitate ventilation if the infant is active and fighting the respirator, but the absence of muscular movement decreases venous return and results in significant edema. In addition, paralysis may mask seizures in asphyxiated infants.

Pulmonary Vasodilators

Nitric Oxide

Nitric oxide (NO) is a naturally occurring vasodilator. NO diffuses from endothelial cells into the adjacent vascular smooth muscle cells and dilates both pulmonary and systemic arteries. Its action is associated with cyclic guanosine monophosphate accumulation. Although NO is not a specific pulmonary vasodilator, it acts as such when it is administered by inhalation. Inhaled NO diffuses into the pulmonary vascular bed and relaxes pulmonary arterioles. It then enters the blood, rapidly binds to hemoglobin, and is inactivated so that its effects are limited to the pulmonary vasculature. In addition to reversing pulmonary vasospasm, NO also improves the matching of ventilation to perfusion in the lung. This is because inhaled NO most effectively dilates those blood vessels that are associated with the best ventilated alveoli.

Multicenter randomized trials of the use of inhaled NO in term or near-term infants with PPH have shown a clear and striking benefit, with minimal short-term side effects. If infants with diaphragmatic hernia are excluded, 50% to 60% of babies with PPH have an immediate improvement in oxygenation, which persists. The need for ECMO (see below) is reduced by one-third. Some evidence suggests that inhaled NO may be more effective with high-frequency ventilation, but this finding has not been consistent. Unfortunately, NO is usually not effective in infants with diaphragmatic hernia.

Currently, in the United States inhaled NO is only approved for use for respiratory failure in term or near-term newborn infants. The starting dose is usually 5 to 20 ppm, but this can be increased, if necessary. If there is a positive initial response, NO therapy is continued and attempts are made to wean the infant from the inhaled NO, usually every 12 hours. Therapy is continued until weaning is completed. The usual duration is 5 to 7 days. Administration of inhaled NO may suppress endogenous NO production, and for this reason it has been suggested that the final stages of weaning from NO should be done slowly and the dose of inhaled NO should be maintained at 1 ppm before it is discontinued.

Although NO was previously thought to be toxic to the lungs, animal and clinical studies have indicated that low levels of inhaled NO do not result in pulmonary toxicity. Contamination by nitrogen dioxide (NO_2) may have been responsible for the previously observed toxicity. Inhaled NO can, however, result in elevated levels of methemoglobin. This is usually seen with inhalation of higher concentrations of NO (80 ppm) and resolves rapidly when the NO concentration is decreased. (In this regard, it should be noted that cigarette smoke can contain more than 1,000 ppm of NO.) In addition, NO inhibits platelet aggregation and adhesion *in vitro*, but clinical trials in mature newborn infants have not revealed any problems with bleeding. The incidence of intraventricular hemorrhage will be monitored carefully in future studies of the use of inhaled NO in premature infants. The long-term outcome of term infants who were treated with NO is also being determined.

To monitor for possible toxic effects when inhaled NO is used, methemoglobin should be determined at least daily. The level should be less than 2% to 5%. It is also necessary to check for clinical evidence of bleeding. The levels of NO and NO_2 in the inhaled gas mixture must be monitored. Very little NO_2 is produced by oxidation of NO by the oxygen in the ventilator system. However, checking the NO_2 concentration is particularly important when a new gas tank is opened, as this appears to be the most likely source of contamination with NO_2.

Tolazoline

Before the availability of NO, a variety of agents with limited effectiveness were used to dilate the pulmonary arteries in infants with PPH. The most widely used and probably the most effective pharmacologic agent was tolazoline, a histamine releaser and alpha-adrenergic blocker (no longer available in the U.S.). In approximately one-third of infants with PPH, tolazoline is successful in improving oxygenation. Tolazoline is a general vasodilator and does not act specifically on the pulmonary vasculature; thus, infusion of the drug can cause a drop in systemic blood pressure and aggravate the right-to-left shunt. Because of this systemic vasodilation, it often is advisable to infuse an electrolyte or colloid solution before and during the administration of a test dose of tolazoline. The initial test dose is 1 mg/kg. If there is no response to this, a test dose of 2 mg/kg may be attempted. The blood pressure must be monitored while tolazoline is being infused, and, if it drops significantly, it should be treated with an infusion of colloid, dopamine, or both. If the test dose of tolazoline produces a significant increase in P_aO_2, a constant infusion of 1 to 2 mg/kg/hour can be started. Tolazoline infusion can result in skin flushing, gastric bleeding, oliguria, and other histamine-like effects. It should be discontinued as soon as it is evident that the pulmonary vasculature is no longer labile and the vasospasm has resolved. If inhaled NO is available, there is little reason to use tolazoline.

Extracorporeal Membrane Oxygenation

ECMO, a type of pulmonary bypass, is used for the treatment of refractory cases of PPH. In this procedure, blood is usually diverted from the right side of the heart via a catheter in the jugular vein, anticoagulated, pumped through a membrane oxygenator where oxygen is added and CO_2 removed, and then returned to the baby's arterial system via the carotid artery. This is known as venoarterial ECMO. In venovenous ECMO blood is both removed and returned via the venous system, obviating the need to ligate the carotid artery. ECMO is an effective rescue therapy for selected infants with severe hypoxia who are not responding to conventional medical therapy. With the advent of inhaled NO therapy, the use of ECMO for babies with PPH has decreased markedly. The use of ECMO for neonates with respiratory failure peaked in 1992, when 1,517 cases were reported to the ECMO registry. In 2001, this number had decreased to 773. In the future, it is likely that the majority of newborn infants who receive ECMO therapy will have conditions, such as diaphragmatic hernia, that are less responsive to inhaled NO. Because ECMO involves heparinizing the blood and, in the case of arteriovenous ECMO, ligating the carotid artery, concerns have been expressed about bleeding and neurologic side effects, but follow-up studies of survivors have reported encouragingly good outcomes.

PROGNOSIS

Although the rate of survival for infants with pulmonary hypertension was 50% or less in 1980, survival rates of 80% or better have been reported more recently in association with advances in supportive therapy. Similar survival rates have also been attained in severely ill infants with the use of ECMO. Those infants who survive appear to do fairly well. Significant neurologic problems have been reported in 10% to 20% of the survivors, whether they are treated with conventional therapy or ECMO. Some surviving infants also have residual lung disease as a result of prolonged ventilation and oxygen administration.

Suggested Readings

Boykin AR, Quivers ES, Wagenhoffer KL, et al. Cardiopulmonary outcome of neonatal extracorporeal membrane oxygenation at ages 10–15 years. *Crit Care Med* 2003;31:2380.

Davidson D, Barefield ES, Kattwinkel J, et al. Safety of withdrawing inhaled nitric oxide therapy in persistent pulmonary hypertension of the newborn. *Pediatrics* 1999;104:231.

Elbourne D, Field D, Mugford M. Extracorporeal membrane oxygenation for severe respiratory failure in newborn infants. *The Cochrane Database of Systematic Reviews*, 2002, Issue 1. Art. No.: CD001340. DOI: 10.1002/14651858.CD001340.

Neonatal Inhaled Nitric Oxide Study Group. Inhaled nitric oxide in full-term and nearly full-term infants with hypoxic respiratory failure. *N Engl J Med* 1997;336:597.

Rais-Bahrami K, Wagner AE, Coffman C, et al. Neurodevelopmental outcome in ECMO vs near-miss ECMO patients at 5 years of age. *Clin Pediatr* 2000;39:145.

Roberts JD, Fineman J, Morin FC, et al. Inhaled nitric oxide and persistent pulmonary hypertension of the newborn. *N Engl J Med* 1997;336:605.

CHAPTER 49 ■ APNEA

ROBERT A. HERZLINGER

Apnea of infancy is defined as an unexplained episode of cessation of breathing for 20 seconds or longer, or a shorter respiratory pause associated with bradycardia, cyanosis, pallor, and/or marked hypotonia. Apnea of infancy applies to infants at or beyond 37 weeks' gestation at the onset of apnea. Apnea of prematurity is defined as a sudden cessation of breathing for 20 seconds or longer, or a shorter respiratory pause accompanied by bradycardia or oxygen desaturation in an infant younger than 37 weeks' gestational age, without other identifiable causes. The incidence of apnea of prematurity increases with decreasing gestational age. Apnea occurs in approximately 7% of infants born at 34 to 35 weeks' gestation, 14% of infants born at 32 to 33 weeks' gestation, 50% at 30 to 31 weeks' gestation, and almost all infants of less than 28 weeks' gestation. Apnea decreases with increasing postconceptional age, and usually resolves by 35 weeks' postconceptional age; however, extremely premature infants born at gestational ages of between 24 to 28 weeks may have persistent apnea requiring prolonged hospitalization beyond 40 weeks of postconceptional age.

EPIDEMIOLOGY

Apnea is categorized into three types. Central apnea, which accounts for approximately 40% of episodes, is characterized by an absence of both chest wall movement and nasal air flow; obstructive apnea, accounting for 10% of spells, presents with chest wall movement without nasal air flow; and mixed apnea, accounting for 50% of spells, has both obstructive and central components. The location of the obstruction in obstructive and mixed apnea is usually at the level of the pharynx. Periodic breathing is another manifestation of immature ventilatory control, and is characterized by regular, recurring cycles of breathing of 10 to 15 seconds duration interrupted by pauses of at least 3 seconds in duration. The frequency of periodic breathing decreases with increasing postconceptional age. Periodic breathing is considered to be a normal breathing pattern in preterm and term infants.

PATHOPHYSIOLOGY

The most common cause of apnea during the newborn period is apnea of prematurity, which is attributed to the immaturity of the ventilatory control mechanism. Anatomic correlates of impaired control include decreased synaptic connections, dendritic arborization, and neural myelination. Delayed brainstem auditory evoked responses have been noted in premature infants with apnea, when compared with controls. Chemoreceptor function also is impaired, resulting in a blunted ventilatory response to hypercarbia and hypoxemia. The functional laryngeal obstruction associated with mixed and obstructive apnea has been attributed to discoordination of brainstem control of pharyngeal patency and diaphragmatic contractions. Inhibitory respiratory reflexes and inhibitory neurotransmitters may be more active at an earlier postconceptional age, which may also predispose to apnea. The causes of apnea are outlined in Box 49.1.

The physiologic consequences of severe apnea include hypoxemia, hypercarbia, reflex-induced bradycardia, hypotension, and a decrease in cerebral blood flow. In the face of an immature and unstable ventilatory control mechanism, a wide variety of conditions can induce apnea in premature infants. Full-term infants also may develop apnea as well, as a consequence of these underlying disorders. In contrast to premature infants, a specific etiology is more likely to be identified in the term or near-term newborn with apnea.

The relationship between apnea of prematurity and gastroesophageal reflux remains controversial. Studies have failed to demonstrate a causal relationship between reflux episodes and apnea. In addition, no clear evidence suggests that the pharmacologic treatment of reflux decreases apnea in premature infants. Therefore, it appears that gastroesophageal reflux is rarely the cause for most apneic spells in premature newborns; however, discoordination of suck, swallow, and breathing may present with feeding-associated apnea in premature infants. These episodes also resolve with increasing postconceptional age.

BOX 49.1 Causes of Apnea

Apnea of Prematurity
Central nervous system disorders
Intraventricular/periventricular hemorrhage
Subarachnoid hemorrhage
Infarction
Seizures
Structural anomalies
Central hypoventilation syndrome

Cardiorespiratory disorders
Respiratory distress syndrome
Bronchopulmonary dysplasia
Patent ductus arteriosus

Metabolic disorders
Hypoglycemia
Electrolytic imbalance
Inborn errors of metabolism

Hematologic disorders
Anemia

Infection
Sepsis/meningitis
Respiratory syncytial virus

Gastrointestinal disorders
Necrotizing enterocolitis
Gastroesophageal reflux

Medications
Phenobarbital
General anesthesia
Prostaglandin E

Airway obstruction
Craniofacial anomalies
    Choanal atresia
    Pierre Robin syndrome
    Achondroplasia
Secretions
Neck flexion

Stimulation of inhibitory reflexes
Feeding-associated apnea

Thermoregulatory
Rapid warming

DIAGNOSIS

All infants at risk for apnea of prematurity, that is, those of less than 35 weeks' gestation, require cardiac and thoracic impedance monitoring when admitted to the nursery. This technology may fail to detect significant hypoxemic episodes resulting from obstructive apnea or hypoventilation in premature infants; therefore, pulse oximetry is indicated in these infants as well. Apnea of prematurity is a diagnosis of exclusion. A careful history and physical examination will direct further evaluation. For example, the sudden onset of apnea or an increase in the frequency or severity of apnea in a premature infants mandates an investigation for sepsis and meningitis and the initiation of antibiotic therapy. Apnea presenting in a term infant without explanation is also an indication for evaluation for sepsis and meningitis and antibiotic treatment.

THERAPY

The management of apnea of prematurity is determined by the frequency and severity of the episodes. If these are mild and not associated with cyanosis and bradycardia, they may be treated with gentle stimulation, clearance of secretions from the airway, and avoidance of neck flexion. The prone position has been associated with a decreased frequency of apneic episodes.

If significant apnea persists, methylxanthines are indicated. These medications are effective against mixed, central, and obstructive spells (Box 49.2). Although both theophylline and caffeine are effective in the treatment of apnea, caffeine has emerged as the drug of choice. The advantages of caffeine include its longer half life, allowing once-a-day dosing, and its wider therapeutic index, which reduces side effects, specifically tachycardia and feeding intolerance. Caffeine is administered by mouth or intravenous, as caffeine citrate, with a loading dose of 20 mg/kg/dose, followed within 24 hours by a maintenance dose of 5 to 8 mg/kg/day, administered once a day. The therapeutic trough serum concentration is 5 to 25 μg/mL. Signs of methylxanthine toxicity include tachycardia, cardiac arrhythmias, feeding intolerance, irritability, and seizures. Methylxanthine use has been associated with increased oxygen consumption and decreased weight gain.

Persistent apnea despite methylxanthine therapy is an indication for continuous nasal positive airway pressure (CPAP), which is effective for obstructive and mixed apneic spells. The mechanism of action for CPAP involves the stabilization of the upper airway and chest wall, thus reducing inhibitory respiratory reflexes and increasing functional residual capacity. High-flow nasal cannula also have been used to treat apnea by providing continuous airway pressure. Intubation and mechanical ventilation are indicated if frequent or severe apnea persists despite the above measures. The minimal ventilatory pressure necessary to control apnea should be utilized to reduce barotrauma.

The role of packed red blood cell transfusions in the treatment of premature infants who have apnea and anemia is controversial. Packed cell transfusion (15 mL/kg) should be considered in premature infants with hematocrit levels of less than 30%.

Infants with apnea of prematurity may be discharged home if they are more than 34 weeks' postconceptional age, and have remained apnea free for 7 to 10 days. Premature infants should have pulse oximetry monitoring in car seats prior to discharge, because apnea and desaturation episodes have been associated with the use of these devices. The vulnerability of the respiratory control mechanism persists in premature infants who are at risk for recurrent apnea if exposed to stresses such as respiratory syncytial virus infection, sepsis, or general anesthesia. This risk decreases after 43 weeks' postconceptional age.

PROGNOSIS

The impact of apnea of prematurity on the long-term neurologic outcome of infants has not been clearly defined; however, severe spells associated with bradycardia of less than 80 beat per minute has been associated with a decrease in cerebral blood flow and a risk for hypoxic ischemic brain injury. Although the incidence of sudden infant death syndrome (SIDS) increases with decreasing gestational age, apnea of prematurity is not an independent risk factor for SIDS. Studies have not documented a benefit of home monitoring in reducing the incidence of SIDS; however, home monitoring may be indicated in some premature infants at high risk for recurrent apnea, bradycardia, or desaturation episodes. Predischarge cardiorespiratory recordings have not been shown to be predictive of SIDS. Monitoring can be discontinued after 43 weeks' postconceptional age in most cases. Other infants who are candidates for home monitoring include (a) those who have experienced an apparent life-threatening event (ALTE), (b) infants with tracheotomies or anatomic abnormalities, (c) infants with neurologic or metabolic diseases affecting respiratory control, and (d) infants with chronic lung disease, especially those requiring oxygen, or ventilatory support.

Parents should be informed that monitoring has not been proven to prevent SIDS or sudden death. Pediatricians should emphasize those preventive measures associated with a reduction in the risk of SIDS including supine sleep position; the avoidance of soft sleep surfaces, loose bedding, bed sharing, and overheating; and the elimination of exposure to tobacco smoke.

Suggested Readings

Arad-Cohen N, Cohen A, Tirosh E. The relationship between gastroesophageal reflux and apnea in infants. *J Pediatr* 2000;137:321.

Cheung PY, Barrington KJ, Finer NN, Robertson CM. Early childhood neurodevelopment in very low birth weight infants with predischarge apnea. *Pediatr Pulmonol* 1999;27:14.

Committee on Fetus and Newborn. American Academy of Pediatrics. Apnea, sudden infant death syndrome, and home monitoring. *Pediatrics* 2003;111: 914.

Darnall RA, Kattwinkel J, Nattie C, Robinson M. Margin of safety for discharge after apnea in preterm infants. *Pediatrics* 1997;100:795.

Eichenwald EC, Aina A, Stark AR. Apnea frequently persists beyond term gestation in infants delivered at 24 to 28 weeks. *Pediatrics* 1997;100:354.

Peter CS, Sprodowski N, Bohnhorst B, et al. Gastroesophageal reflux and apnea of prematurity: no temporal relationship. *Pediatrics* 2002;109:8.

Schmidt B. Methylxanthine therapy in premature infants: sound practice, disaster, or fruitless byway? *J Pediatrics* 1999;135:526.

Task Force on Infant Sleep Position and Sudden Infant Death Syndrome. American Academy of Pediatrics. Changing concepts of sudden infant death syndrome: implications for infant sleeping environment and sleep position. *Pediatrics* 2000;105:650.

BOX 49.2   Proposed Mechanisms of Action of Methylxanthines

- Increased minute ventilation
- Increased CO_2 responsiveness
- Enhanced diaphragmatic contractility
- Improved pulmonary mechanics
- Decreased hypoxic ventilatory depression
- Improved pharyngeal muscle tone

CHAPTER 50 ■ BRONCHOPULMONARY DYSPLASIA

KATHLEEN A. KENNEDY AND JOSEPH B. WARSHAW

Most neonates with acute lung disease recover completely within the first week of life. Some of these infants, however, develop chronic respiratory symptoms that persist for weeks to years. In 1967, Northway and colleagues first described the clinical, radiologic, and pathologic manifestations of chronic lung disease in survivors of hyaline membrane disease (HMD) and introduced the term bronchopulmonary dysplasia (BPD). As neonatal intensive care has become more sophisticated over the past three decades, the survival of very low-birth-weight infants has increased dramatically, and chronic lung disease is now seen in very small infants who did not have significant lung disease in the first few days of postnatal life. Although the birth-weight–specific incidence of BPD seems to have remained fairly stable with increasing survival rates, the result of increased survival has been an increase in the absolute numbers of survivors with BPD. In a population-based study of infants born in North Carolina in 1994, chronic lung disease (CLD), defined as either ventilator or oxygen requirement at 30 days postnatal age or 36 weeks postmenstrual age, occurred in 44% and 25% of 500- to 1,500-g survivors, respectively. In the National Institute of Child Health and Human Development (NICHD) Neonatal Research Network, for 501- to 1,500-g infants born in 1995 to 1996, the incidence of CLD (defined as oxygen use at 36 weeks postmenstrual age among 36-week survivors) ranged from 3% to 43% among the centers. The incidence was 52% in 501- to 750-g infants, 34% in 751- to 1,000-g infants, 15% in 1,001- to 1,250-g infants, and 7% in 1,251- to 1,500-g infants. In a variety of study populations, lower birth weight, white race, and male sex have been consistently identified as risk factors for the development of BPD.

DEFINITION

In 1979, Bancalari characterized BPD as tachypnea, retractions, and supplemental oxygen requirement for more than 28 days in infants who had received positive-pressure ventilation for at least 3 days in the first week of life. Associated chest radiograph findings included strandlike densities in both lung fields alternating with areas of normal or increased lucency. The term CLD, usually defined as supplemental oxygen administration at either 28 days of age or 36 weeks adjusted postmenstrual age, has been commonly used in multicenter studies largely for pragmatic reasons. The more stringent diagnostic criterion of oxygen therapy at 36 weeks corrected postmenstrual age has been recommended, because this definition was shown to be a more specific predictor of long-term pulmonary morbidity in very low-birth-weight infants when compared with oxygen therapy at 28 days. Definitions based on oxygen therapy alone have been criticized because many infants have variable requirements for oxygen over time and because the use of supplemental oxygen depends on the oxygen saturation goals chosen by the caregiver. In a recent National Institutes of Health–sponsored workshop on BPD, use of the older term BPD was recommended to maintain a distinction from chronic lung diseases occurring later in life. A new definition of BPD was proposed to distinguish differences in disease severity (mild, moderate, and severe) (see Table 50.1).

ETIOLOGY AND PATHOPHYSIOLOGY

Oxygen toxicity and barotrauma/volutrauma have been implicated in the pathogenesis of BPD, but it is very difficult to isolate these factors from the pulmonary immaturity and acute lung injury for which these treatment modalities are used (see Fig. 50.1). Although BPD initially was described as a complication of HMD [now called respiratory distress syndrome (RDS)], chronic lung disease has become a significant problem in very premature infants without acute lung disease. Conversely, full-term infants who require aggressive oxygen

TABLE 50.1

NICHD/NHLBI WORKSHOP DEFINITION OF BPD

Gestational Age at Birth	Age at Assessment	Mild BPD	Moderate BPD	Severe BPD
<32 weeks	36 weeks postmenstrual age (or discharge if discharged sooner)	Treatment with >21% oxygen for at least 28 days AND		
		Breathing room air at time of assessment	Needing <30% oxygen at time of assessment	Needing >30% oxygen or positive pressure at time of assessment
≥32 weeks	56 days postnatal age (or discharge if discharged sooner)	Treatment with >21% oxygen for at least 28 days AND		
		Breathing room air at time of assessment	Needing <30% oxygen at time of assessment	Needing >30% oxygen or positive pressure at time of assessment

BPD, bronchopulmonary dysplasia; NHLBI, National Heart, Lung, and Blood Institute; NICHD, National Institute of Child Health and Human Development.

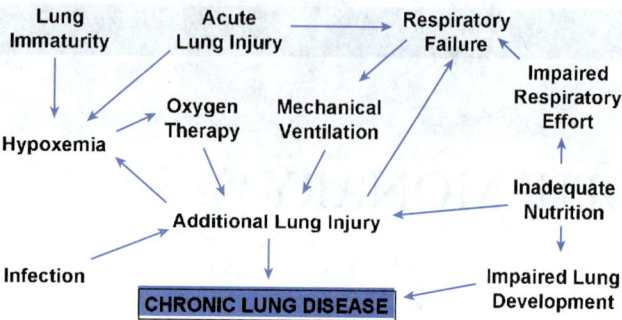

FIGURE 50.1. Complex pathogenesis of BPD.

and ventilator therapy for meconium aspiration, congenital pneumonia, or persistent pulmonary hypertension infrequently develop BPD. Pulmonary air leak, pulmonary edema, patent ductus arteriosus, acquired pneumonia, and poor nutrition also are risk factors for the development of BPD, but these are complications of acute lung injury and prematurity, so their causal role in the pathogenesis of BPD is difficult to establish. For a variety of reasons, the premature lung seems to have an increased susceptibility to iatrogenic lung injury or a decreased capacity to undergo a normal healing process when lung injury occurs. Genetic factors predisposing an infant to develop BPD are suggested by an increased incidence of asthma in first-degree relatives of infants with prolonged BPD.

Pulmonary edema and alveolar necrosis develop within 2 to 3 days in healthy mammals exposed to normobaric hyperoxia. This acute injury is followed by a chronic phase that is pathologically similar to BPD and is characterized by interstitial fibrosis with proliferation of alveolar type II cells and fibroblasts. A causal role of oxygen toxicity is supported by observations in the STOP-ROP study in which infants treated with higher FIO_2 to maintain higher O_2 saturation goals had worse pulmonary outcomes. Protection from the toxic effects of oxygen seems to be related to the ability to prevent or repair cellular damage caused by oxygen free radicals; a variety of enzymatic and nonenzymatic antioxidants are involved in this protection. The premature neonate may be relatively deficient in some of these antioxidants, but there have been relatively few trials of antioxidants in human infants to prevent BPD.

Intratracheally administered superoxide dismutase may decrease the long-term severity of BPD, although it does not appear to affect the incidence of BPD. This finding is provocative and deserves further study. Vitamins A and E are nonenzymatic antioxidants that prevent free radical propagation in cell membranes. Although vitamin E deficiency exacerbates pulmonary oxygen toxicity in laboratory animals, pharmacologic doses of vitamin E do not afford additional protection in nondeficient animals or humans. Neonates have low vitamin E stores at birth and are at risk for deficiency if vitamin E is not provided enterally or parenterally. Deficiency states should be preventable with the use of early parenteral nutrition and fortified human milk or preterm formulas. Premature neonates of less than 36 weeks gestation also have low plasma concentrations and tissue stores of vitamin A. Supplementation with intramuscular vitamin A has been shown to increase the likelihood of survival without CLD in infants less than 1,000 g birth weight requiring supplemental oxygen or mechanical ventilation at 24 hours of age.

Deficiencies of sulfur-containing amino acids and trace minerals such as selenium increase the susceptibility to oxygen-induced lung injury in animals. Such deficiencies are unlikely to occur in infants who are receiving standard enteral formulas for preterm infants. Less is known about the optimal amounts of specific amino acids and trace minerals that should be supplied

in parenteral nutrition solutions. Despite evidence from animal studies that pulmonary oxygen toxicity could be ameliorated by polyunsaturated fatty acid supplementation, preliminary studies in preterm human infants have shown no benefit.

A causal role of barotrauma/volutrauma in the pathogenesis of BPD is supported by the following observations. BPD was seen rarely before positive-pressure ventilators came into use, and some infants develop BPD after mechanical ventilation with low oxygen concentrations. Acute manifestations of barotrauma (pulmonary interstitial emphysema and pneumothorax) are frequent precursors of BPD. Although many investigators have attempted to reduce barotrauma/volutrauma by using different strategies with conventional mechanical ventilators, there have been no large trials to evaluate the impact of particular styles of conventional mechanical ventilation on BPD. Several large trials of synchronized versus nonsynchronized ventilation have shown no effect on BPD. Studies of high frequency oscillatory ventilation to prevent BPD have had variable results; a meta-analysis of all randomized trials showed a modest reduction in CLD that must be balanced against the adverse effects on long-term neurologic outcome shown in the only large trial that assessed long-term outcomes. Permissive hypercapnia (maintaining the P_aCO_2 at greater than 45 to 50) in mechanically ventilated infants has been variably successful in preventing CLD and deserves further study.

A primary causal role for inflammation or infection in the pathogenesis of BPD has not been established but is suggested by the increased incidence of BPD in infants who are colonized with Ureaplasma at the time of birth and in infants whose mothers had chorioamnionitis. Whether early antibiotic treatment would be beneficial has yet to be established. Inflammation is a characteristic finding in the pathology of BPD, and inflammatory mediators have been implicated in the reactive airway disease and pulmonary hypertension that is associated with BPD. Inflammatory mediators, such as eicosanoids, platelet-activating factor, and interleukins 1-beta, 6, and 8, have been found in high concentrations in lung lavage fluid from infants with BPD. Whether this inflammatory response results from infection, oxidant injury, or barotrauma/volutrauma as the primary insult, the inflammation may further exacerbate the primary lung injury and lead to more severe or prolonged lung damage.

PREVENTION

Wide differences in the incidence of BPD among centers (after adjustment for demographic risk factors) have suggested that patient management may alter the risk for BPD. Unfortunately, very few specific strategies for prevention have been evaluated in large clinical trials, and it seems unlikely that a single highly effective preventive measure will be identified for this complex disease process.

Because BPD originally was described as a complication of severe RDS, it might be expected that antenatal steroid treatment and surfactant therapy to prevent or treat RDS would dramatically reduce the incidence of BPD. While antenatal steroids have been shown to reduce the risk of RDS and to reduce the risk of death when given to mothers of preterm infants, the risk of CLD among surviving infants was not reduced. A number of large, multicenter, placebo-controlled surfactant trials have been published. Although most of the large trials have demonstrated a decrease in mortality with surfactant therapy, the incidence of BPD in the survivors generally has not been affected by the administration of surfactant. One explanation for these seemingly disappointing findings is that surfactant deficiency/RDS is only one of multiple factors involved in the pathogenesis of BPD, and it may be relatively less important in infants with extremely low birth weights than in the larger infants described in 1967. Another explanation is that an increase in survivors without BPD was matched by an increase in the number who would have succumbed but survived with BPD as a result of antenatal steroids or surfactant treatment. The end result is no change in the incidence of BPD among survivors, despite a significant increase in the number of infants who survived without BPD.

Retrospective studies have shown strong associations between higher rates of fluid administration and BPD. In a meta-analysis of four randomized trials of restricted fluid administration in the first days or weeks of postnatal life, infants given restricted fluid had reduced mortality and a trend toward reduced BPD among survivors. While these data support judicious administration of fluids in the first few weeks of life, the study designs were too heterogeneous to be able to extract optimal fluid regimens for specific infants. Retrospective studies have also shown a strong association between patent ductus arteriosus (PDA) and BPD. While some have advocated aggressive treatment of PDA to prevent BPD, the observation that prophylactic indomethacin dramatically reduces the incidence of PDA but does not reduce BPD raises doubt about the causal role of PDA in the development of BPD. As discussed above, the risk of BPD can be reduced, although not eliminated, with the administration of supplemental vitamin A to infants of less than 1,000 g birth weight.

Steroids were commonly used in the 1990s to prevent or ameliorate BPD. Early steroid treatment (begun in the first 4 days of life) has been shown to reduce the risk of CLD at 28 days and at 36 weeks postmenstrual age. The increase in gastrointestinal perforations, cerebral palsy, and abnormal neurologic examination at follow-up seen with early steroid treatment has largely curtailed this practice, however. When steroids are administered at 7 to 14 days of age, they significantly reduce CLD and can be used more selectively in infants who remain on the ventilator and are at higher risk of CLD. But the long-term neurologic sequelae are still a serious concern; the benefits and risks for individual patients must be carefully considered. For these reasons, the use of postnatal steroids has decreased dramatically and remains controversial.

DIFFERENTIAL DIAGNOSIS

Two other forms of chronic lung disease in premature infants have been described. Wilson-Mikity syndrome and chronic pulmonary insufficiency of prematurity were described in 1960 and 1975, respectively, as consisting of progressive tachypnea, hypoxemia, and apnea in premature infants who have very mild or no lung disease in the first week of life. Neither of these syndromes has a specific etiology and the clinical course in the first week of life is the main feature distinguishing infants with these syndromes from infants with BPD. This distinction may be somewhat arbitrary. These syndromes may represent different clinical presentations in a spectrum of chronic lung disease related to prematurity, with the clinical manifestations depending on the relative contributions of the various etiologic factors mentioned above.

Cystic fibrosis and alpha-1-antitrypsin deficiency rarely cause pulmonary symptoms in the first weeks of life, but neonates with these genetic disorders who also have acute lung injury shortly after birth may subsequently experience slowly progressive chronic lung disease. Sweat chloride analysis, genetic screening, or determination of serum alpha-1-antitrypsin levels is required to distinguish these disorders from BPD. These evaluations should be considered for infants with progressively worsening BPD.

Viral pneumonia acquired in the early neonatal period can cause progressive hypoxemia and respiratory failure. The diagnosis can be confirmed with nasopharyngeal viral cultures or urine culture for cytomegalovirus.

COMPLICATIONS

Infants with BPD have an increased susceptibility to severe bacterial and viral pneumonia. In the first year after hospital discharge, many infants with BPD are readmitted for pulmonary exacerbations. Respiratory syncytial virus and pertussis infections can be fatal in infants with BPD.

Congestive heart failure with pulmonary and systemic venous congestion frequently complicates the management of infants with BPD, especially during intercurrent infections. The cause of left heart failure in infants with BPD is uncertain. Fluid tolerance varies greatly and must be determined on an individual basis.

Pulmonary hypertension and cor pulmonale can result from many forms of chronic lung disease, including BPD. Mortality is very high in infants with severe BPD and cor pulmonale, and there is no specific therapy for it. Whether cor pulmonale can be prevented by more generous administration of oxygen is unknown; data from two large randomized trials suggest that maintaining higher O_2 saturation goals is of no benefit and might exacerbate the underlying lung disease.

MANAGEMENT

Although exposure to high concentrations of oxygen is thought to be a contributing factor in the pathogenesis of BPD, chronic administration of oxygen is used to prevent hypoxic organ damage in the management of infants with established BPD. Until recently, there were no data from controlled clinical trials to determine optimal ranges for O_2 therapy. A large, multicenter, randomized controlled trial recently compared oxygen saturation targets of 95% to 98% versus 91% to 94% in infants who remained on supplemental oxygen at 32 weeks postmenstrual age. Infants in the higher target group required longer duration of supplemental oxygen and had no improvement in long-term growth or neurologic outcomes. Therefore, there appears to be no benefit of maintaining O_2 saturations at greater than 94%; whether O_2 saturation goals of less than 91% would be safe is unknown, but data from a large observational study suggest that this might be the case.

Pulmonary and systemic edema develop in many infants with BPD when excessive parenteral fluid is administered, and chronic fluid restriction has become common in the management of infants with BPD. Because respiratory infection or hypoxemia predisposes the infant to pulmonary edema, isolated episodes of pulmonary edema do not necessarily warrant chronic restriction of enteral fluid intake. Fluid given enterally is generally tolerated better than fluid given parenterally. Modest fluid (140 to 160 mL/kg/day) and sodium (2 to 3 mEq/kg/day) restriction may decrease oxygen requirements and respiratory work in some infants with BPD. Severe fluid restriction at the expense of adequate nutrition is not indicated.

Although diuretic therapy is used commonly in infants with BPD, the diuretic and nondiuretic cardiopulmonary effects of chronic diuretic therapy in these infants have not been well studied. Diuretic agents have been shown to improve pulmonary mechanics in the short term in infants with BPD. Long-term benefits of diuretic therapy in these infants have not been demonstrated. The efficacy of furosemide versus thiazide diuretics in infants with BPD is unknown, and careful attention must be given to electrolyte balance when either type of diuretic is used in these infants. Replacement of potassium and chloride may be necessary to prevent metabolic alkalosis and hypoventilation during diuretic therapy. Sodium supplementation enhances fluid retention and defeats the purpose of diuretic therapy. Calcium wasting may exacerbate osteopenia of prematurity in infants treated with diuretics.

Infants with BPD have increased airway resistance and increased work of breathing compared with age-matched control infants. Some of these infants have bronchial hyperreactivity that responds favorably to bronchodilator therapy with theophylline, beta-adrenergic agonists, muscarinic antagonists, or ipratropium bromide. There have been no studies evaluating the long-term effects of bronchodilators in these infants. There have been several small randomized trials of inhaled corticosteroids in ventilated infants with BPD. Inhaled steroids appear to increase the short-term likelihood of successful extubation, but there is no information regarding the long-term risks and benefits. Delivery of inhaled medications to non-ventilated preterm infants is problematic and needs further research.

Adequate nutrition is necessary for lung growth and repair, but meeting nutritional needs is often a challenge in infants with BPD. Infants with BPD have tachypnea and increased respiratory effort, and they may require more calories for adequate growth than do infants without respiratory disease. The caloric needs of an individual infant should be determined by the intake required to achieve a sustained appropriate weight gain. Some infants may require as much as 150 kcal/kg/day. If oral or nasogastric feedings are not tolerated, prolonged peripheral parenteral nutrition rarely provides adequate calories and central parenteral nutrition should be considered. Supplemented formulas can be used to increase caloric intake in infants who cannot tolerate increased feeding volumes because of congestive heart failure or gastroesophageal reflux. If standard or preterm infant formulas are supplemented with carbohydrates or fat to increase the caloric density, adequate intake of protein and trace minerals should not be compromised.

Respiratory infections should be prevented, if possible, by avoiding exposure to other patients, hospital personnel, and family members with viral symptoms. When viral respiratory infections occur in infants with BPD, requirements for oxygen, bronchodilator therapy, and diuretics often are increased for at least 1 week. If respiratory failure develops, requiring the reinstitution of ventilator therapy, the mortality is high and recovery may be very prolonged. Palivizumab has been shown to decrease the rate of hospitalizations for respiratory syncytial virus infections in preterm infants. The cost-effectiveness of this therapy has been questioned; it is best justified for very preterm infants (at or below 32 weeks) treated with oxygen for more than 28 days.

PROGNOSIS

Over the past 30 years, there has been a reduction in mortality for infants with BPD, but mortality and morbidity remain high. In a study of infants with less than 1,500-g birth weights (122 with BPD [requiring oxygen for more than 28 days] and 84 infants without BPD), the mortality rate between hospital discharge and 3 years of age was 5.9% in the BPD group compared to 1.2% in the no-BPD group. In another study of infants with less than 1,500-g birth weights with mild CLD (on O_2 at 28 days but not at 36 weeks), severe CLD (on O_2 at 28 days and 36 weeks), or no CLD (58 in each group) born between 1987 and 1991, the postdischarge mortality rate at 1 year adjusted age was low (3%) and not different among the groups. However, the rate of any adverse neurodevelopmental outcome (cerebral palsy, delayed mental or motor development, hearing loss, or severe retinopathy of prematurity) was 3.6%, 21.4%,

and 31.6%, respectively, in the infants with no CLD, mild CLD, and severe CLD. Infants with severe CLD also had shorter length, lighter weight, and a higher rate of hospital readmission. Pulmonary function improves over the first several years of life in infants with BPD, and most survivors have normal exercise tolerance by school age. With formal pulmonary function testing, however, some evidence of increased airway reactivity (attributed to either smaller airways or increased inflammatory mediators) persists into early adulthood.

Suggested Readings

Ambalavanan N, Carlo WA. Hypocapnia and hypercapnia in respiratory management of newborn infants. *Clin Perinatol* 2001;28:517.

Askie LM, Henderson-Smart DJ, Irwig L, Simpson JM. Oxygen-saturation targets and outcomes in extremely preterm infants. *New Engl J Med* 2003;349:959.

Atkinson SA. Special nutritional needs of infants for prevention of and recovery from bronchopulmonary dysplasia. *J Nutr* 2001;131:942S.

Bancalari E, Claure N, Sosenko IRS. Bronchopulmonary dysplasia: changes in pathogenesis, epidemiology and definition. *Semin Neonatol* 2003;8:63.

Barrington KJ, Finer NN. The treatment of bronchopulmonary dysplasia: a review. *Clin Perinatol* 1998;25:177.

Brion LP, Bell EF, Raghuveer TS. Vitamin E supplementation for prevention of morbidity and mortality in preterm infants (Cochrane Review). In: *The Cochrane Library*, Issue 3, 2003. Oxford: Update Software.

Brion LP, Primhak RA, Ambrosio-Perez I. Diuretics acting on the distal renal tubule for preterm infants with (or developing) chronic lung disease (Cochrane Review). In: *The Cochrane Library*, Issue 3, 2003. Oxford: Update Software.

Charafeddine L, D'Angio CT, Phelps DL. Atypical chronic lung disease patterns in neonates. *Pediatrics* 1999;103:759.

Cole CH, Fiascone JM. Strategies for prevention of neonatal chronic lung disease. *Semin Perinatol* 2000;24:445.

Davies PG, Thorpe K, Roberts R, et al. and the Trial of Indomethacin Prophylaxis in Preterms (TIPP) Investigators. Evaluating "old" definitions for the "new" bronchopulmonary dysplasia. *J Pediatr* 2002;140:555.

Davis JM, Parad RB, Michele T, et al. Pulmonary outcome at 1 year corrected age in premature infants treated at birth with recombinant CuZn superoxide dismutase for the North American Recombinant Human CuZnSOD Study Group. *Pediatrics* 2003;111:469.

DeRegnier RA, Roberts D, Ramsey D, et al. Association between the severity of chronic lung disease and first-year outcomes of very low birth weight infants. *J Perinatol* 1997;17:375.

Greenough A, Milner AD, Dimitriou G. Synchronized mechanical ventilation for respiratory support in newborn infants (Cochrane Review). In: *The Cochrane Library*, Issue 3, 2003. Oxford: Update Software.

Henderson-Smart DJ, Bhuta T, Cools F, Offringa M. Elective high frequency oscillatory ventilation versus conventional ventilation for acute pulmonary dysfunction in preterm infants (Cochrane Review). In: *The Cochrane Library*, Issue 3, 2003. Oxford: Update Software.

Jobe AJ. The new BPD: an arrest of lung development. *Pediatr Res* 1999;46:641.

Jobe AJ, Bancalari E. Bronchopulmonary dysplasia. NICHD-NHLBI-ORD Workshop. *Am J Respir Crit Care Med* 2001;163:1723.

Joffe S, Ray GT, Escobar GJ, et al. Cost-effectiveness of respiratory syncytial virus prophylaxis among preterm infants. *Pediatrics* 1999;104:419.

Kennedy KA. Controversies in the use of postnatal steroids. *Semin Perinatol* 2001;25:397.

Lemons JA, Bauer CR, Oh W, et al. for the NICHD Neonatal Research Network. Very low birth weight outcomes of the National Institute of Child Health and Human Development Neonatal Research Network, January 1995 through December 1996. *Pediatrics* 2001;107:e1.

Singer L, Yamashita T, Lilien L, et al. A longitudinal study of developmental outcome of infants with bronchopulmonary dysplasia and very low birth weight. *Pediatrics* 1997;100:987.

The STOP-ROP Multicenter Study Group. Supplemental therapeutic oxygen for prethreshold retinopathy of prematurity (STOP-ROP), a randomized controlled trial: primary outcomes. *Pediatrics* 2000;105:295.

Suresh GK, Soll RF. Current surfactant use in premature infants. *Clin Perinatol* 2001;28:671.

Tyson JE, Wright LL, Oh W, et al. for the NICHD Neonatal Research Network. Vitamin A supplementation for extremely-low-birth-weight infants. *New Engl J Med* 1999;340:1962.

Young TE, Kruyer LS, Marshall DD, Bose CL, and the North Carolina Neonatologists Association. Population-based study of chronic lung disease in very low birth weight infants in North Carolina in 1994 with comparisons with 1984. *Pediatrics* 1999;104:e17.

CHAPTER 51 ■ CARDIOVASCULAR EMBRYOLOGY

LOUIS I. BEZOLD

The development of the cardiovascular system—first organ system to reach functional maturity—is essentially complete by 8 weeks' gestational age in humans. The critical period of heart development occurs between 20 and 50 days' gestation (Fig. 51.1). For some time, anatomic and morphologic studies have formed the major basis of cardiovascular embryology, with recent expansion of our understanding of developmental

mechanisms being gained through advances in molecular biology and experimental embryology.

ORIGINS OF CARDIAC CELL LINES

The mature heart is a composite of several embryonic cell types (Fig. 51.2). Most of the heart, including the endocardium, atrial

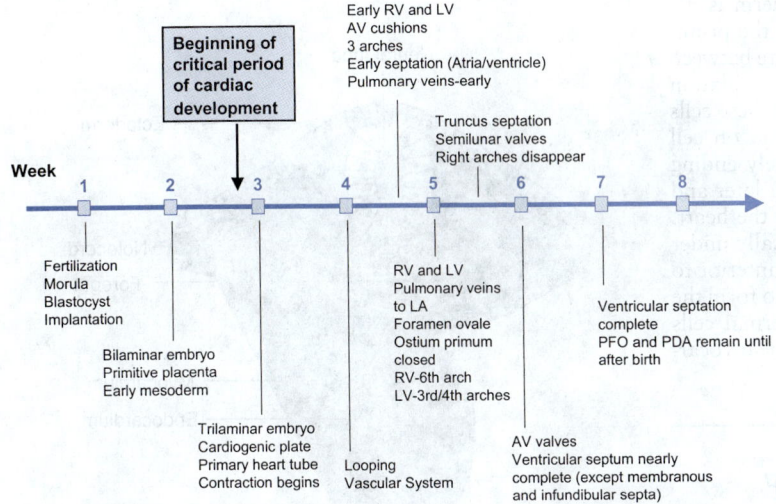

FIGURE 51.1. Timeline of human cardiac development through 8 weeks' gestation.

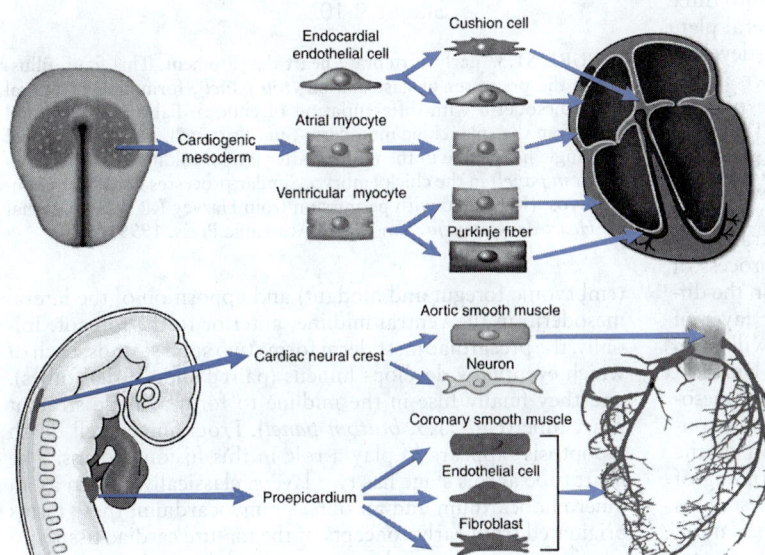

FIGURE 51.2. Cardiac cell lineages. (Reprinted with permission from Harvey RP and Rosenthal N. *Heart development*. San Diego: Academic Press, 1999.)

and ventricular myocardium, and Purkinje cells (specialized conduction systema), are derived from the cardiac mesoderm of the embryo. Cardiac neural crest cell migration contributes to the smooth muscle of the aortic wall, autonomic innervation of the heart, and outlet septation. The proepicardium contributes the epicardium and participates significantly in the development of the coronary arteries.

BASIC EMBRYOGENESIS

After fertilization, the ovum travels down the fallopian tube while undergoing several cellular divisions that result in a multicelled structure called the morula. By the time the morula reaches the uterine cavity on day 4 after fertilization, a cavity develops within it, at which point it is known as a blastocyst. Implantation into the uterine stroma occurs on approximately day 7. By this time, the blastocyst has further differentiated into an inner cell mass, or embryoblast, which ultimately forms the embryo proper, and an outer cell mass, which forms the embryonic membranes and contributes to formation of the placenta and umbilical cord.

The bilaminar germ disk forms during the second week of gestation, with differentiation of the embryoblast into two cell layers: the endoderm (hypoblast) and the ectoderm (epiblast). Late in week 2 of development, a third cell layer, the intraembryonic mesoderm, becomes apparent. The mesoderm is derived from ectodermal cells, which migrate toward the primitive streak in the midline of the embryo and invaginate between the ectoderm and the endoderm, a process called gastrulation (Fig. 51.3, *top panel*). The timing and entry point of these cells through the primitive streak confer some restriction on cell fate, with cells entering early and caudally ultimately ending up in the venous end of the heart and cells entering later and more cranially ending up in the outflow portion of the heart. The mesodermal cells migrate laterally and cephalically under the influence of the underlying endoderm, meeting anterior to the prochordal plate (buccopharyngeal membrane) to form the cardiogenic plate by day 15 of gestation. Mesodermal cells from this region are determined genetically to become myocardial cells by this point.

FORMATION OF THE STRAIGHT HEART TUBE

The intraembryonic mesoderm further differentiates into three portions: the paraaxial, the intermediate, and the lateral plate mesoderm, the last of which contributes to cardiac development. The lateral plate splits to form a cavity known as the intraembryonic coelom, which ultimately forms the pleural, pericardial, and peritoneal cavities. The more medial layer of the lateral plate mesoderm, adjacent to the endoderm, is called the splanchnic or visceral mesoderm (Fig. 51.3, *middle panel*). This layer contains the precardiac mesoderm from which the endocardial and myocardial cells will arise. Multiple transcription factors, anterior endoderm induction, and the process of epithelial-mesenchymal transformation are involved in the differentiation of the precardiac mesoderm. The outer layer of the mesoderm, the somatic or parietal mesoderm, will form the body linings, including the pericardium and the pleura.

In conjunction with cardiogenic plate formation and mesodermal differentiation, the embryo undergoes two major conformational changes. The relatively rapid expansion of the cephalic end of the neural tube results in anterior folding of the cardiogenic area, and accelerated growth of the somites along the longitudinal axis of the body results in the lateral margins of the embryo folding ventrally (Fig. 51.4). The net result of these maneuvers is the formation of an endodermal tube

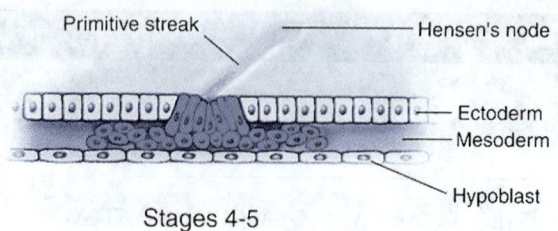

Stages 4-5

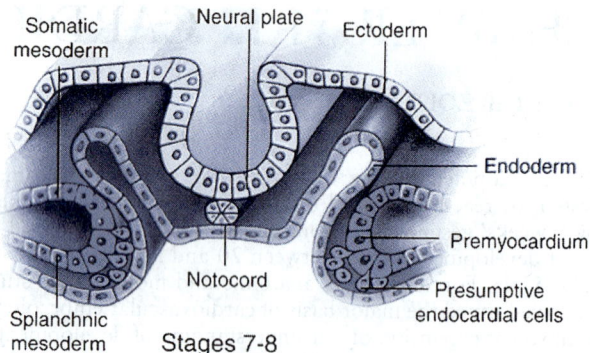

Stages 7-8

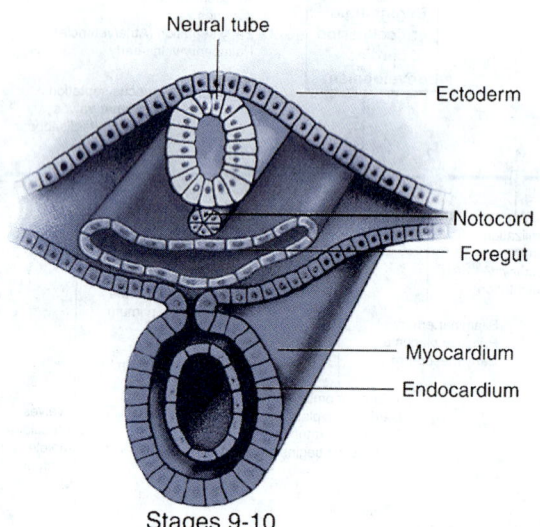

Stages 9-10

FIGURE 51.3. Early vertebrate heart development. This figure illustrates the processes of gastrulation (*top panel*), formation of lateral plate mesoderm with differentiation of endocardial and myocardial cells from the splanchnic mesoderm (*middle panel*), and formation of the single heart tube in the midline after lateral folding of the embryo (*bottom panel*) in the chick embryo. Similar processes occur in human embryos. (Reprinted with permission from Harvey RP and Rosenthal N. *Heart development.* San Diego: Academic Press, 1999.)

(embryonic foregut and hindgut) and apposition of the lateral mesoderm in the ventral midline, anterior to the foregut. Initially, the precardiac mesoderm forms two solid strands, each of which eventually develops lumens (paired endocardial tubes), and they finally fuse in the midline to form a single straight heart tube (Fig. 51.3, *bottom panel*). Programmed cell death (apoptosis) appears to play a role in this fusion process. The heart tube at this stage has two layers, classically known as an inner endocardium and an outer epimyocardium; these terms originated from early concepts of the mature cardiac tissues to which these embryonic layers were thought to give rise. More recent observations have shown that the term epimyocardium

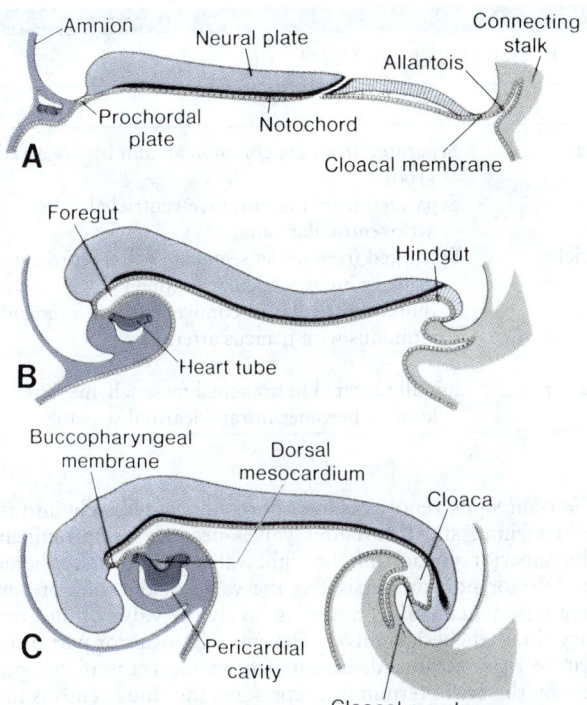

FIGURE 51.4. Cranial caudal midline sections showing anterior rotation of the cardiogenic plate resulting from rapid growth of brain vesicles at **A:** 18 days, **B:** 21 days, and **C:** 22 days. (Reprinted with permission from Langman J. *Medical embryology*, 4th ed. Baltimore: Williams & Wilkins, 1981.)

is inaccurate. This layer actually contains only myocardial cells; the epicardium originates later in development from pericardial villi (proepicardial organ) at the venous end of the heart. Between the two cell layers is a relatively hypocellular material known as cardiac jelly, which also is somewhat of a misnomer because the molecular makeup of this substance is quite complex. Cardiac jelly is thought to contribute significantly to the critical processes of cardiac looping and septation of the atrioventricular canal and conotruncal regions of the heart.

Concurrent with formation of the heart tube, blood islands in the visceral mesoderm form endothelium-lined vessels and blood-forming elements. The primitive heart tube receives the developing systemic veins caudally and connects to the first arterial arches cephalically.

Figure 51.5 shows the primitive straight heart tube. The variability in the interpretation of the segments and the terminology describing them reflects the disagreement that exists in classifying the parts of the primitive heart tube. Table 51.1 outlines the traditional nomenclature of the commonly described embryonic segments, the connecting regions of the primitive heart tube, and the mature heart derivatives to which the segments are thought to give rise. Cellular marking studies suggest that significant portions of both the cephalic and caudal ends of the mature heart are formed during and after cardiac looping, by cells not present in the original heart tube. The molecular processes and precursor cells involved are not well understood but include the migration of extracardiac mesenchymal and neural crest cells.

CARDIAC LOOPING

Cardiac looping, the process by which the straight heart tube normally bends to the right (dextral or D-loop) and slightly ventrally at approximately 23 days' gestation, is a crucial step in cardiac morphogenesis. Looping is the earliest sign of developing left–right asymmetry in vertebrates. Abnormalities of looping are associated with complex congenital heart disease, including abnormalities of ventricular relationships (i.e., ventricular inversion) and heterotaxy syndromes. Complete failure of looping results in embryonic loss. After looping occurs, the external appearance of the heart is similar to the mature organ; however, the heart remains a single tube internally. Looping results in the common atrium being located somewhat posterior and cephalad to the ventricles, and the outlet segment comes to lie in the midline, in a slight depression of the roof of the primitive atria. Looping is critical to the subsequent internal partitioning of the heart tube.

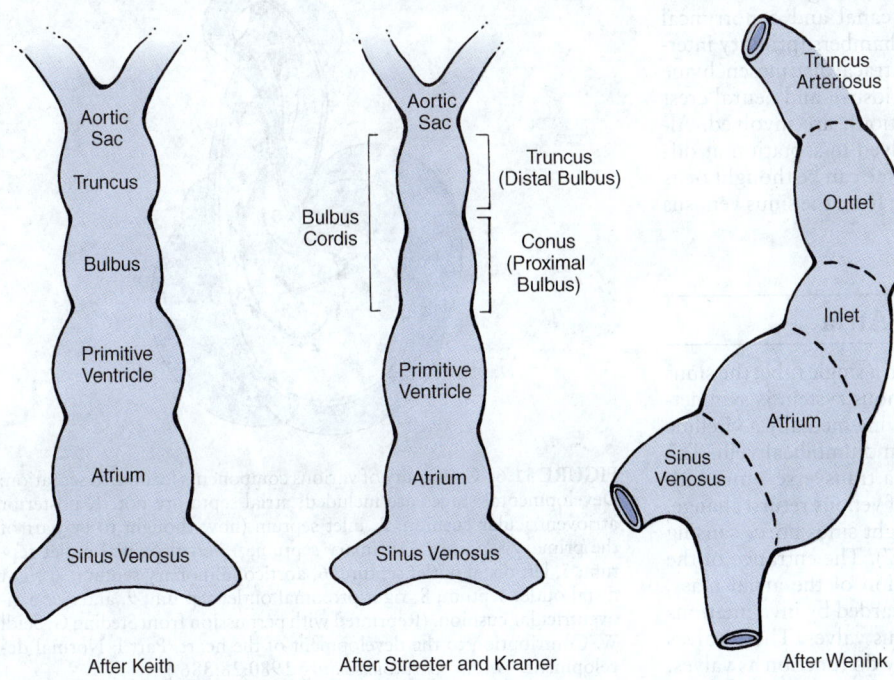

FIGURE 51.5. The primitive straight heart tube as perceived by several different authors. (Reprinted with permission from Anderson RH, Wilkinson JL, Becker AE. The bulbus cordis—a misunderstood region of the developing human heart; its significance to the classifications of congenital cardiac malformations. In: *Birth defects.* Original articles series 1978; XIV(7):1; Wenink ACG. Embryology of the heart. In: Anderson RH, McCartney FJ, Shinebourne EA, Tynan M, eds. *Paediatric cardiology.* Edinburgh: Churchill Livingstone, 1987.)

TABLE 51.1

EMBRYONIC SEGMENTS AND CONNECTING REGIONS OF THE PRIMITIVE HEART TUBE

Segment	Derivative	Notes
Sinus venosus	Smooth venous portions of both atria	Separated from the common atrium by sinoatrial groove
Common atrium	Right and left atrial appendages	Separated from the primitive ventricle by the atrioventricular canal
Inlet segment (primitive ventricle, embryonic ventricle)	Apical and inlet portions of left ventricle	Separated from outlet segment (bulbus cordis) by primary interventricular foramen (bulboventricular or conoventricular foramen)
Outlet segment (bulbus cordis, conus)	Apical and inlet portions of right ventricle, outlets of both ventricles	Continuous with truncus arteriosus
Truncus arteriosus (aortic sac or bulb)	Paired aortic arches, proximal great arteries	Initially located in branchial mesenchyme; after looping becomes intrapericardial structure

The mechanisms that determine left- and right-sidedness and the forces responsible for cardiac looping are not clearly determined, but they are under intensive investigation on the molecular and genetic levels. Currently, the most plausible theory is that cardiac jelly generates a uniform force (caused by changes in the status of hydration within the jelly) that is converted to a directional force by the specific myofibrillar arrangement within the surrounding myocardial cells. Molecular biologic investigations are ongoing using iv/iv and inv/inv mouse models of situs inversus, and molecular biology continues to advance research into the potential roles of signaling molecules and extracellular matrix molecules with asymmetric expression of mRNA at various times in early development.

Internal Partitioning of the Heart

The embryonic heart is a tube within a single closed vascular circuit that must be converted to a four-chambered structure with a second, separate circuit (lungs) for gas exchange. Cardiac septation takes place between days 26 and 37 of gestation. Four concurrent events take place: atrial septation, formation of endocardial cushions and atrioventricular canal septation, ventricular chamber formation and septation, and truncus septation. Multiple cellular mechanisms, including coalescence of hypocellular masses (atrioventricular canal and conotruncal septum), rapid expansion of adjacent chambers (primary interventricular septum), participation by extracardiac mesenchyme (sinus venosus, atria, and truncus arteriosus), and neural crest cell migration (aortopulmonary septation), are involved. Although different mechanisms are involved in septation at different levels, the resulting system of septae can be thought of as a continuous system of ridges extending from the sinus venosus to the truncus arteriosus (Fig. 51.6).

Sinus Venosi and Atria

When the paired heart tubes fuse to form a single tube, the sinus venosi remain paired. The systemic venous system is symmetrical at this point, with each sinus receiving medially a vitelline vein and laterally a common cardinal and umbilical vein. The paired sinuses eventually fuse to form a transverse sinus with right and left sinus horns. As patterns of venous return change, most venous flow comes to enter the right sinus horn, causing it to become more prominent (Fig. 51.7). The entrance of the sinus is shifted to enter the right portion of the atrial mass. This entrance becomes slitlike and is guarded by invaginations of sinus tissue—the right and left venous valves. These valves initially are relatively large and probably do function as valves.

The right sinus venosus is incorporated progressively into the right atrium, and the venous valves become less prominent. The superior portion of the right valve disappears, whereas the inferior portion persists as the valve of the inferior vena cava (eustachian valve) and most likely the valve of the coronary sinus (thebesian valve). The smooth posterior part of the mature right atrium, demarcated from the trabeculated portion by the crista terminalis, represents the sinus venosus that is incorporated into the atrium. The rightward portion of the primitive atrium persists as the right atrial appendage. With growth, the superior and inferior vena cavae separate to enter the right atrium individually. On the left side, the common pulmonary vein grows out and anastomoses with the developing pulmonary venous plexus. The common pulmonary vein is incorporated later into the left atrium, giving origin to its smooth posterior portion. Similar to the right side, the primitive left atrium persists as the left atrial appendage in the mature heart.

Septation of the atria is depicted in Figure 51.8. With looping, the distal heart tube comes to lie anterosuperiorly, creating an external indentation in the roof of the atrium, corresponding

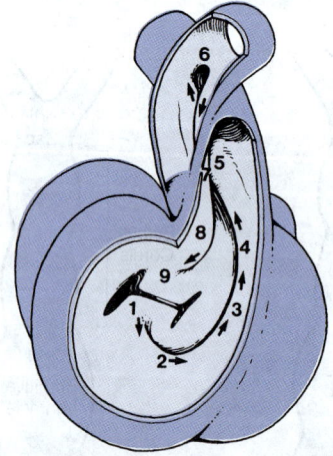

FIGURE 51.6. Continuity of various components leading to septation. Developmental stages are included; atrial septa are not. 1, posterior atrioventricular cushion; 2, inlet septum (now thought to be part of the primary septum); 3, primary septum; 4, left proximal outlet septum; 5, left distal outlet septum; 6, aorticopulmonary septum; 7, right distal outlet septum; 8, right proximal outlet septum; 9, anterior atrioventricular cushion. (Reprinted with permission from Steding G, Seidl W. Contribution to the development of the heart. Part I: Normal development. *Thorac Cardiovasc Surg* 1980;28:386.)

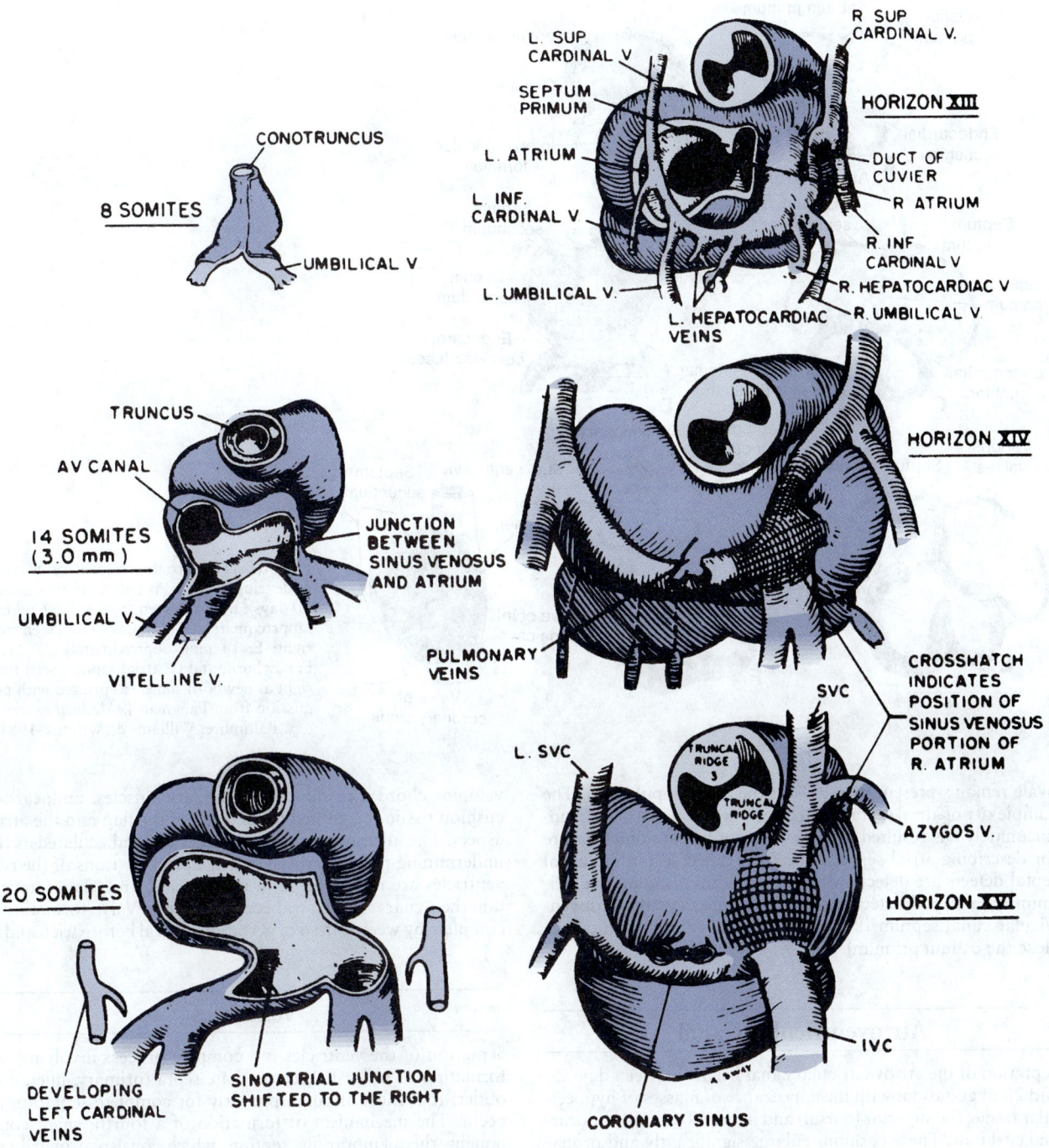

FIGURE 51.7. Dorsal view of changes in the sinus venosus and venous tributaries. AV, atrioventricular; INF, inferior; IVC, inferior vena cava; L, left; R, right; SUP, superior; SVC, superior vena cava; V, vein. (Reprinted with permission from Goor DA, Lillehei CW. *Congenital malformations of the heart*. New York: Grune & Stratton, 1975.)

to an internal structure called the septum primum. The inferior border of the septum primum forms an arc, concave toward the atrioventricular orifice, initially leaving an opening, the ostium primum. The two limbs of this arc become continuous with the developing endocardial cushions of the atrioventricular canal. With fusion of the endocardial cushions, the atrioventricular canal is divided into right and left portions, and the ostium primum closes. Before this closure occurs, a second orifice, the ostium secundum, necessary for continued umbilical venous blood flow into the left atrium, appears in the posterior por-

tion of the septum primum. As the ostium secundum forms, a second septum, the septum secundum, begins to form along the roof of the atrium lying to the right of the septum primum. The inferior rim of this septum also is an arc, with dorsal and ventral limbs extending toward the orifice of the inferior cava. This arc never closes but forms an oval rim, the limbus of the foramen ovale. The septum primum, therefore, forms the flap valve guarding the foramen ovale in utero. After birth, the flap of the foramen (septum primum) closes against the septum secundum, forming the floor of the fossa ovalis (a patent foramen

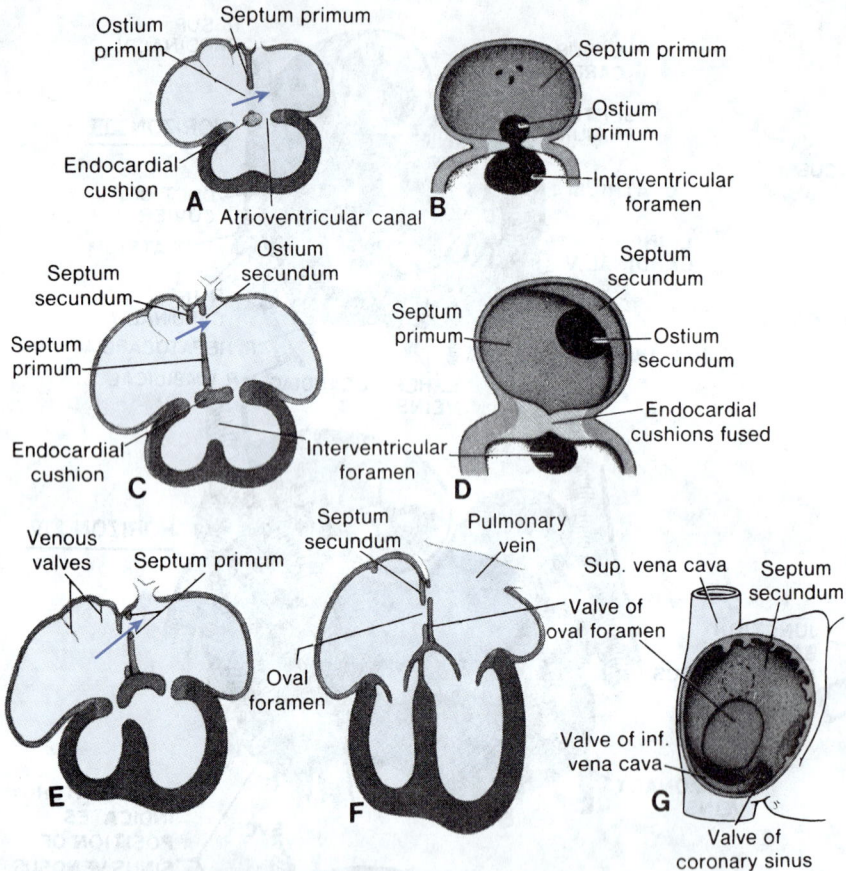

FIGURE 51.8. Atrial septa at various stages of development. **A:** At 6 mm (approximately 30 days); **B:** 6 mm seen from right; **C:** 9 mm (approximately 33 days); **D:** 9 mm seen from right; **E:** 14 mm (approximately 37 days); **F:** newborn; and **G:** atrial septum seen from right at newborn stage. (Reprinted with permission from Langman J. *Medical embryology.* Baltimore: Williams & Wilkins, 1981.)

ovale remains present in ~20% of the adult population). The complexity of atrial septation and foramen ovale formation unfortunately has resulted in somewhat confusing nomenclature for describing atrial septal defects. So-called secundum atrial septal defects are defects within the septum primum, and primum atrial septal defects actually are defects of the atrioventricular canal septum (failure of the endocardial cushions to close the ostium primum).

Atrioventricular Canal

Septation of the atrioventricular canal begins between days 26 and 28 of gestation, with the appearance of masses of hypocellular tissue, the superior (dorsal) and inferior (ventral) endocardial cushions. These cushions enlarge significantly and probably function as valves. Smaller lateral masses, the right and left lateral atrioventricular cushions, appear. By 33 to 34 days' gestation, the superior and inferior cushions have fused, dividing the atrioventricular canal into right and left orifices. In this region, as well as in the conotruncal region, a biphasic process of endothelial (endocardial) cell transformation to mesenchymal cell phenotype, followed by migration into the cardiac jelly, is involved in the process of septation.

Despite their early valvelike function and traditional concepts that they are precursors of the atrioventricular valves, the endocardial cushions now are thought to contribute little to the atrioventricular valve leaflets, based on more recent data. The mitral and tricuspid valves actually are formed by an invagination of sulcus tissue at the atrioventricular groove and a concomitant delamination of ventricular inlet myocardium, leading to the formation of a three-layered flap hanging down into the inlet, attached to the ventricular myocardium by de-

veloping chordae tendinea and papillary muscles. Endocardial cushion tissue is confined to the apex of the flap and the atrial aspect. The inlet myocardium becomes less trabeculated as the undermining process proceeds. The apical portions of the two ventricles are not involved in this process, and, therefore, retain their characteristic trabecular patterns. Valve formation is complete by weeks 5 to 6 of gestation (mitral before tricuspid).

Ventricles

Septation of the ventricles is a complex process involving the formation of at least three separate septa (primary, inlet, and outlet) that must all align properly for complete septation to occur. The mechanism of formation of a fourth, small component, the membranous septum, which consists primarily of endocardial cushion fibrous tissue, is not understood clearly. Abnormal septal formation, malalignment, or both account for the variety of ventricular septal defects that occur.

Concomitant with ventricular septation is the formation and differentiation of the ventricular chambers. The left ventricle begins expanding slightly before the right ventricle does. Initially, the ventricular myocardium is spongiform in nature, with loose trabeculations and sinusoids that allow gas and nutrient exchange to occur before the development of the coronary arteries. Eventually, the myocardium will become compact. Differential expression of transcription factors between the two ventricles during development has been demonstrated. Table 51.1 outlines the embryologic chambers of origin of the mature ventricles.

By 25 to 26 days' gestation, outpockets of the endocardium appear proximal and distal to the primary foramen in the inlet and outlet segments. These segments undergo progressive enlargement by centrifugal growth. Growth of the inlet and outlet segments takes place much faster than does enlargement of the primary foramen. Thus, the anteromedial walls of the two segments appose and fuse, giving rise to the primary interventricular septum. Most accounts describe this structure as extending posteriorly to meet the inferior endocardial cushion, which would require the atrioventricular canal to shift far to the right of its original position, so that the right portion of the canal actually enters the outlet segment.

In other descriptions, the primary septum is confined to the anterior and apical portions of the two segments and does not extend posteriorly to the inferior endocardial cushion. Instead, a second portion of the forming interventricular septum is thought to develop within the inlet segment by a coalescence of trabeculae, developing in continuity with the inferior cushion and dividing the inlet segment such that each ventricle receives a portion of the inlet segment, and the atrial and ventricular septae are aligned. This inlet septum is described as fusing with the left side of the primary septum (Fig. 51.9), which together forms the major portion of the interventricular septum. The site of fusion was said to be obscured on the left ventricular side by subsequent remodeling at the time of mitral valve formation and on the right side by the septomarginal trabecula. This description does not require a rightward shift of the atrioventricular canal and is more consistent with other observations. However, monoclonal antibody studies have demonstrated cells in the region of the atrioventricular canal and primary foramen (between the inlet and outlet segments of the looped heart tube) that are involved in the septation of the inlet portion of the ventricles. The inlet portion of the right ventricle now is thought to be derived from the outlet segment of the primitive ventricular loop (see Table 51.1), and the inlet and apical trabecular parts of the muscular septum are formed by the primary ventricular septum.

The third ventricular septal component is the outlet septum. Within the outlet segment, swellings arise that are histologically similar to the endocardial cushions of the atrioventricular canal. Similarly, endothelial–mesenchymal cell transformation and migration appear to be important processes in normal outlet septum formation. Two pairs of ridges, proximal and distal, fuse to form a spiral septum. In this manner, the anterior and rightward portion of the proximal outlet segment communicates with the pulmonary artery, and the posterior and leftward proximal outlet segment communicates with the aorta. Neural crest cells also participate in outlet septation.

The proximal rightward ridge contacts the right atrioventricular orifice. The proximal leftward ridge comes in contact with the superior rim of the primary septum. Thus, a true interventricular communication with the following boundaries is found: the outlet septum cranially, the primary septum anteriorly and caudally (the caudal portion previously was thought to be a separate inlet septum), and the atrioventricular endocardial cushions posteriorly (see Fig. 51.9). The closure of the interventricular communication occurs by fusion of these structures and the membranous septum.

Aortopulmonary Septum

Embryologists disagree about where the truncus arteriosus begins and ends. The most practical approach is to define the site of the arterial valves as the distal end of the cardiac outlet and to consider the truncus arteriosus as part of the arterial system. The truncus expands asymmetrically into the branchial mesenchyme, with less expansion seen between the origins of the fourth and sixth branchial arch arteries. The extracardiac mesenchyme between these arches grows inward to contribute to the formation of the aortopulmonary septum. Neural crest cells also participate in the septation of the outflow portion

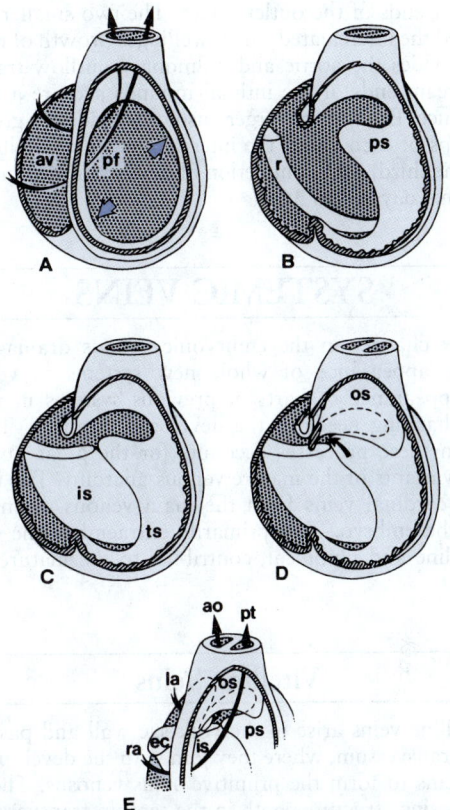

FIGURE 51.9. Development of ventricular septal components, right lateral views. **A:** Before septation. Arrows indicate left and right bloodstreams, which have to pass both the atrioventricular (*av*) and the primary (*open arrows*) junction; pf, primary foramen. **B:** Growth of inlet and outlet segments leads to expansion of the intervening primary fold, resulting in the primary septum (*ps*). At the same time, inlet trabeculations coalesce to form a muscular ridge (*r*) on the posterior wall of the inlet. **C:** Previously, the primary septum was thought to grow out to form a separate inlet septum (*is*), which subsequently fused with the primary septum. The inlet septum now is thought to develop as part of the primary septum. The posterior rim of the latter remains visible as trabecula septomarginalis (*ts*). **D:** Endocardial ridges in the distal part of the outlet fuse to form the outlet septum (*os*). A small interventricular communication (*arrow*) is still present. The left part of the primary fold (*stippled line*) is in the left ventricle, hidden by the outlet septum. **E:** As in D, with the addition of fused atrioventricular endocardial cushions (*ec*), which are present in previous stages (although not depicted). Boundaries of interventricular communication are outlet septum, primary septum, inlet portion of the primary septum, and atrioventricular endocardial cushion. This communication has nothing to do with the primary foramen. Arrows indicate bloodstreams from the right atrium (*ra*) to the pulmonary trunk (*pt*) (through right part of the primary foramen) and from the left atrium (*la*) to the aorta (*ao*) (through left part of the primary foramen). (Reprinted with permission from Wenink ACG. Embryology of the heart. In: Anderson RH, McCartney FJ, Shinebourne EA, Tynan M, eds. *Paediatric cardiology.* Edinburgh: Churchill Livingstone, 1987.)

of the heart, including the aortopulmonary septum. The outlet ridges fuse at the site of arterial valve formation before complete fusion with the aortopulmonary septum takes place.

ARTERIAL VALVES

At the junction of the outlet segment and the truncus arteriosus, an H-shaped outflow channel is formed by four mounds of cushion tissue. The two large mounds of tissue correspond to the upper ends of the outlet ridges. The two smaller mounds are called the intercalated valve swellings. Growth of the larger ridges divides the aortic and pulmonary outflow tracts. The downstream ends of the intimal mounds acquire a valvelike appearance. Each of the larger cushions divides to give rise to two cusps of each valve; the intercalated valve swelling gives rise to the third, with completion of development occurring by gestational days 34 to 36.

SYSTEMIC VEINS

Complex changes in the embryonic venous drainage occur with the appearance of whole new systems of veins and the disappearance of parts of previous systems in response to the changing needs of the developing embryo. The variability in these processes accounts for the great number of normal variants of the mature venous anatomy. The intraembryonic cardinal veins form the main venous drainage system of the embryo. Two primarily extraembryonic systems, the vitelline and umbilical, contribute to the mature venous system.

Vitelline Veins

The vitelline veins arise in the yolk sac wall and pass to the septum transversum, where they join with the developing umbilical veins to form the primitive sinus venosus. They form anastomosing structures both in the septum transversum and around the developing duodenum. Within the septum transversum, the developing liver buds grow into this plexus, breaking it up into developing hepatic sinusoids. With a subsequent shift of the venous drainage to the right sinus venosus, the left hepatocardiac channel regresses, and the right one gives rise to the suprahepatic portion of the inferior vena cava. The duodenal plexus remodels as the duodenal loop forms and gives rise to the portal veins (Fig. 51.10). The growth of the liver buds within the septum transversum spreads laterally.

Umbilical Veins

The umbilical veins are broken up into sinusoids, developing communication with the vitelline sinusoids. The right umbilical vein becomes attenuated, and most of the blood from the placenta passes through the left umbilical vein into the hepatic sinusoids. As the right sinus venosus becomes dominant, an enlargement in the hepatic sinusoids develops between the left umbilical vein and the right hepatocardiac channel. This channel, the ductus venosus, allows blood returning to the heart from the placenta to bypass the hepatic sinusoids.

Cardinal Veins

The anterior cardinal veins, draining the cephalic end of the embryo, are the first intraembryonic veins to appear. The posterior cardinal veins, draining the caudal end of the embryo, appear slightly later. The anterior and posterior cardinal veins join to form the common cardinal vein, which enters the sinus venosus. Anastomoses develop between the right and left anterior cardinal veins. As the venous drainage shifts to enter the right side of the developing heart, the anastomosis enlarges to become the left brachiocephalic vein. The distal

portion of the left common cardinal vein becomes attenuated. The proximal portion of the left sinus horn and the common cardinal vein persist as the coronary sinus. The definitive superior vena cava is derived from the proximal portion of the right anterior cardinal vein and the right common cardinal vein.

The development of the venous drainage of the caudal part of the embryo is much more complex. Several sets of veins appear and then partially regress as the definitive venous drainage is formed. Initially, the caudal portion of the embryo is drained by bilaterally symmetric posterior cardinal veins. A second set of symmetric veins, the subcardinal veins, appears medial to the mesonephros. Transverse anastomoses develop, connecting the posterior cardinal and subcardinal veins. Anastomosis between the two subcardinal veins develops ventral to the developing aorta. A critical anastomosis, the hepatosubcardial junction, develops between the right subcardinal vein and the hepatic sinusoids. This initially small anastomosis eventually enlarges to become the portion of the inferior vena cava between the liver and the entrance of the renal veins. If this anastomosis fails to form normally (so-called interrupted inferior vena cava), the venous return from the lower body bypasses the intrahepatic portion of the inferior vena cava, passing instead through other persistent embryonic pathways, usually as an azygous continuation.

Later, the hepatic sinusoids form a large posterior channel within the liver, which becomes the intrahepatic portion of the inferior vena cava. The portion of the vena cava between the liver and the heart is derived from the right vitelline vein.

The supracardinal veins that appear in the thoracic region participate in the formation of the azygous system. In the lumbar region, they participate in the development of the portion of the inferior vena cava distal to the entrance of the renal veins. The anastomosis between the right subcardinal vein and the veins to the lower extremities enlarges to form the distal portion of the inferior vena cava.

AORTIC ARCH SYSTEM

The embryonic segments of the branchial arterial system are the aortic sac, the six arterial arches, and the paired dorsal aortas. At the time of formation of the single straight heart tube, the distal end bifurcates into the right and left first arterial arches. These arches pass on either side of the foregut to become continuous with a pair of dorsal aortas. The aortic sac is the segment that is just proximal to the arterial arches and just distal to the truncus. The arterial arches are embedded in the branchial arches.

With time, blood flow gradually shifts caudally in the developing arch system. The first and second arch arteries, which initially carry the full flow from the heart, regress. Remnants of the first pair of arteries participate in the formation of the maxillary artery from the mandibular artery and possibly contribute to the external carotid artery. The second-arch arteries contribute to the stapedial and hyoid arteries. The third-arch arteries participate in forming the common carotids and the proximal portions of the internal carotid arteries. The distal portions of the common carotids are derived from the cranial portions of the paired dorsal aortas.

The right and left fourth arterial arches develop differently. The caudal portion of the right dorsal aorta disappears, but the fourth-arch artery persists in continuity with the seventh intersegmental artery to form the distal portion of the right subclavian artery. On the left, the fourth arch gives rise to the portion of the definitive left aortic arch between the takeoff of the left common carotid and the entrance of the ductus

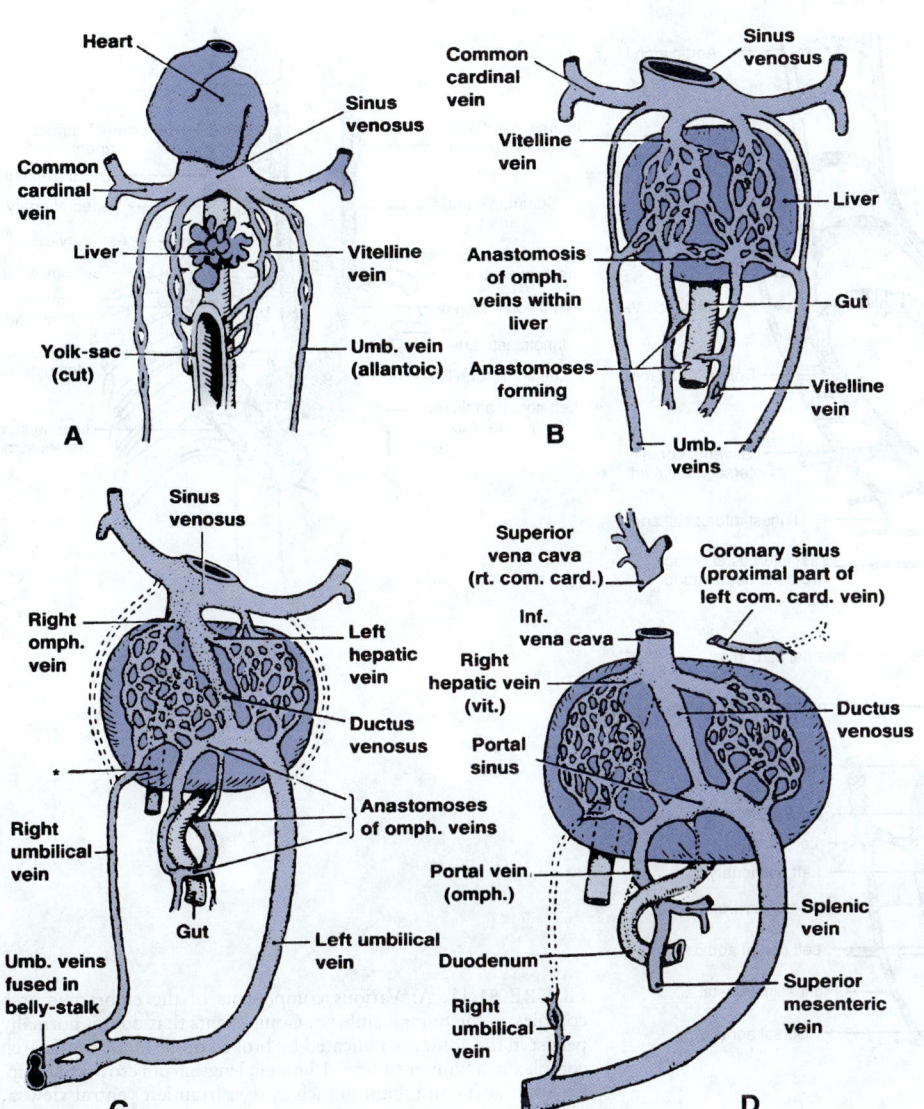

FIGURE 51.10. Changes in the vitelline and umbilical venous systems that lead to the development of the hepatic portal circulation. **A:** Embryos of 3 to 4 mm (fourth week); **B:** embryos of approximately 6 mm (fifth week); **C:** embryos of 8 to 9 mm (sixth week); and **D:** embryos of 20 mm and larger. The asterisk in C indicates the hepatic part of the inferior vena cava. Card, cardinal; com, common; inf, inferior; omph, omphalomesenteric; rt, right; umb, umbilical; vit, vitelline. (Reprinted with permission from Corliss CE. *Patton's human embryology.* New York: McGraw-Hill, 1976.)

arteriosus. The fifth arterial arch is not a precursor of normal adult structures in humans.

The sixth (pulmonary) arches appear during the fourth week of gestation. They are represented by dorsal and ventral portions, which join each other at an angle. The postbranchial pulmonary arteries join the arches at the angle between the dorsal and ventral portions. The ventral portions of these arches gradually merge and, along with the aortic sac, give rise to the main pulmonary artery. The right ventral portion persists as the proximal portion of the right pulmonary artery, whereas the right dorsal sixth arch is interrupted. The left ventral portion is thought to be largely resorbed, contributing little, if at all, to the left pulmonary artery. The left dorsal portion gives rise to the ductus arteriosus (Fig. 51.11).

EPICARDIUM AND CORONARY ARTERIES

The epicardium initially was thought to arise from the same cells that give rise to the myocardium, hence the name epimyocardium. Scanning electron microscopic studies now show that the epicardium migrates radially over the surface of the heart from pericardial villi (proepicardial organ), beginning in the region of the dorsal atrioventricular sulcus and interventricular sulcus. The proepicardial organ is a transitory structure that also contributes some of the nonmyocardial mesenchymal cells of the heart. The epicardium contributes significantly to the development of the coronary arteries. After epicardial migration occurs, the subepicardial space becomes filled by an extracellular matrix populated by mesenchymal cells derived from both the proepicardial organ and the epicardium itself. These cells differentiate into coronary vascular cell lines and contribute to the formation of a subepicardial coronary vascular plexus. This plexus invades the myocardium and continuity is established with the myocardial vascular spaces that are formed by consolidation of intertrabecular spaces lined by endothelium. These spaces form a subendocardial endothelial plexus, which appears to connect to the left horn of the sinus venosus. Later, coronary–aortic continuity is established by the penetration into the aorta from a periaortic vascular plexus, not by the formation of endothelial sprouts from the aortic wall, as previously thought. Cellular adhesion molecules and integrins appear to play critical roles in the formation of the epicardium and coronary arterial system. Parasympathetic ganglia may

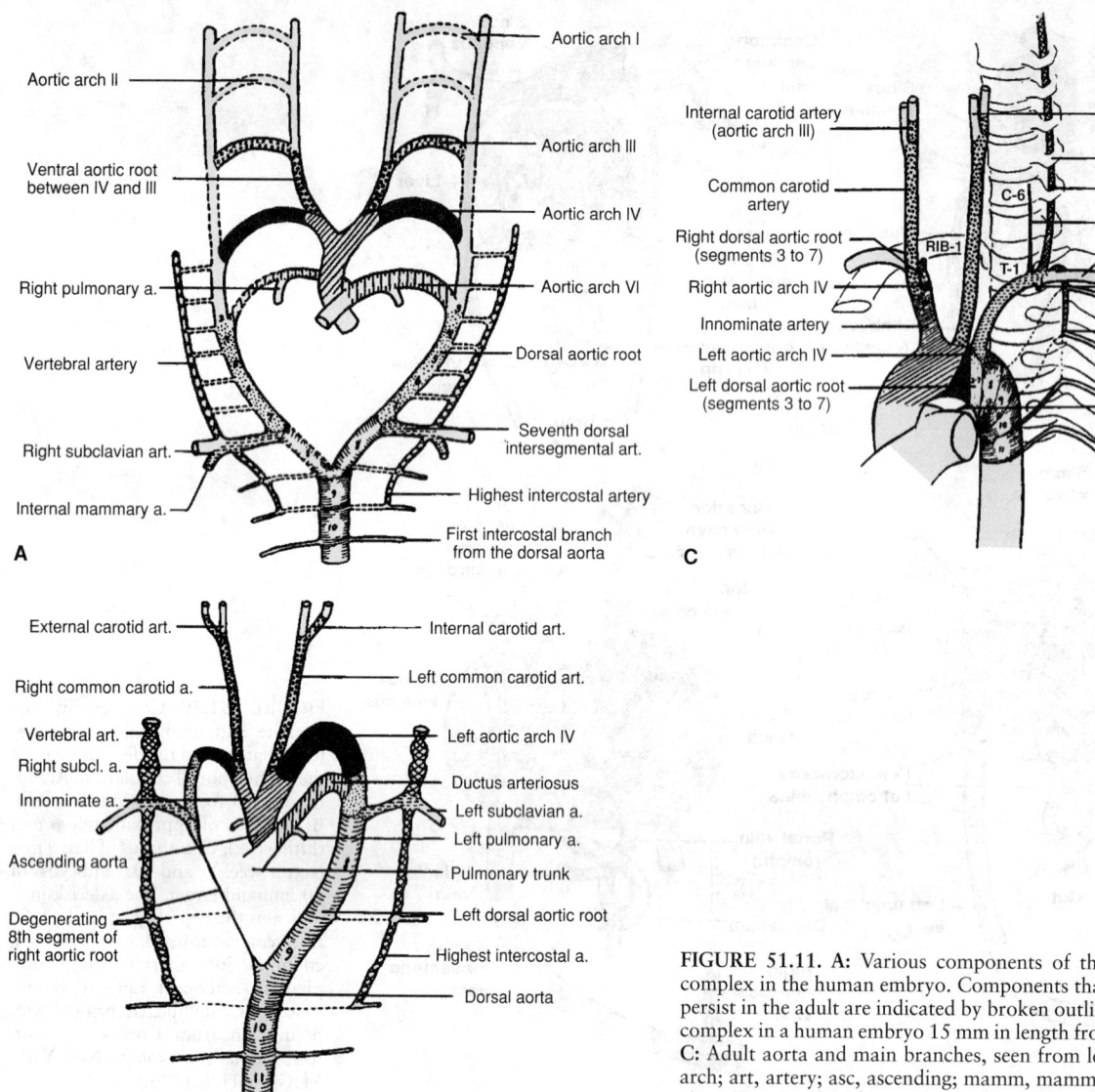

A: Various labels in figure A:
Aortic arch I
Aortic arch II
Ventral aortic root between IV and III
Aortic arch III
Aortic arch IV
Right pulmonary a.
Aortic arch VI
Vertebral artery
Dorsal aortic root
Right subclavian art.
Seventh dorsal intersegmental art.
Internal mammary a.
Highest intercostal artery
First intercostal branch from the dorsal aorta

B: Various labels in figure B:
External carotid art.
Internal carotid art.
Right common carotid a.
Left common carotid art.
Vertebral art.
Left aortic arch IV
Right subcl. a.
Ductus arteriosus
Innominate a.
Left subclavian a.
Left pulmonary a.
Ascending aorta
Pulmonary trunk
Left dorsal aortic root
Degenerating 8th segment of right aortic root
Highest intercostal a.
Dorsal aorta

C: Various labels in figure C:
Internal carotid artery (aortic arch III)
External carotid artery
Common carotid artery
Costal element
Vertebral artery
Right dorsal aortic root (segments 3 to 7)
Asc. cervical art.
Subclavian art.
Right aortic arch IV
Internal Mamm. art.
Innominate artery
Highest intercostal a.
Left aortic arch IV
Left dorsal aortic root (segments 3 to 7)
Ligamentum arteriosum
RIB-1, C-6, T-1

FIGURE 51.11. A: Various components of the embryonic arch complex in the human embryo. Components that do not normally persist in the adult are indicated by broken outlines. **B:** Aortic arch complex in a human embryo 15 mm in length from crown to rump. **C:** Adult aorta and main branches, seen from left ventral view. a, arch; art, artery; asc, ascending; mamm, mammary; subcl, subclavian. (Reprinted with permission from Barry A. The aortic arch derivatives in the human adult. *Anat Rec* 1951;111:221.)

participate in the generation of the definitive coronary artery orifices.

Suggested Readings

Bowers PN, Bruckner M, Yost HJ. Laterality disturbances. *Prog Pediatr Cardiol* 1996;6:53.

Colvin EV. Cardiac embryology. In: Garson AT, Bricker JT, Fisher DJ, Neish SR, eds. *The science and practice of pediatric cardiology,* 2nd ed. Baltimore: Williams & Wilkins, 1997:91.

Ferrans VJ, Rosenquist GC, Weinstein C. *Cardiac morphogenesis.* New York: Elsevier, 1985.

Goor DA, Edwards JE, Lillehei W. The development of the interventricular septum of the human heart. *Chest* 1970;58:453.

Harvey RP, Rosenthal N. *Heart development.* San Diego: Academic Press,1999.

Langman J. *Medical embryology.* Baltimore: Williams & Wilkins, 1981.

McQuinn TC, Takao A. Experimental approaches to cardiac development. In: Garson AT, Bricker JT, Fisher DJ, Neish SR, eds. *The science and practice of pediatric cardiology,* 2nd ed. Baltimore: Williams & Wilkins, 1997:53.

Ruckman RN. Development and maturation of the cardiovascular system. In: Holbrook PR, ed. *Textbook of pediatric critical care.* Philadelphia: Saunders, 1992:242.

CHAPTER 52 ■ EPIDEMIOLOGY OF CONGENITAL HEART DISEASE

DAVID E. FIXLER

Congenital heart disease (CHD) is a leading cause of death during the first year of life. Malformations of the heart occur in about 8:1,000 liveborn infants, resulting in up to 36,000 cases/year in the United States. Children with CHD use between 25% and 30% of the beds in most pediatric intensive care units and therefore consume a large fraction of pediatric health care resources. Because most severe cases now are being managed successfully by surgery, most of these patients are surviving into their reproductive years. Recent studies have shown that the children of women with CHD are at much greater risk of having cardiac malformations. In the next decade, the prevalence of CHD will increase as a result of longer survival and the greater incidence of heart defects in the children of survivors. Pediatric health care providers need to be informed of the prevalence of CHD, the familial risk of CHD recurrence, and risk factors for CHD.

PREVALENCE OF CONGENITAL HEART DISEASE

The prevalence of CHD is the ratio of the number of cases to the number of births in a defined population. Estimating the prevalence accurately requires precise diagnostic criteria for the identification of cases and complete ascertainment of all cases. Diagnostic criteria may include mild cases recognized solely by physical examination, and echocardiography, or it may be restricted to more severe forms diagnosed by cardiac catheterization, surgery, or autopsy. Many types of CHD are not diagnosed until after the neonatal period; therefore, the prevalence rate is affected by the length of the period of observation. In the prospective study by Hoffman and Christianson, data are provided regarding the prevalence of CHD at various age intervals (Table 52.1). These data indicate that fewer than half of the cases were identified during the first week of life.

The reported prevalence of CHD in the United States varies from study to study because of differences in diagnostic cri-

teria, methods of diagnosis, and completeness and length of follow-up (Table 52.2). Important discrepancies among these studies are noted that account for the large differences in reported prevalence rates. The prevalence of CHD among autopsied stillborn infants is 76.9 in 1,000, which is nearly ten times higher than the rate found in liveborn infants. If stillbirths are included in the prevalence figures, the rate increases by about 0.5 in 1,000. The prevalence figure also is influenced by the inclusion of infants born prematurely who have patent ductus arteriosus. Such patients were excluded in most of the recent studies listed in Table 52.2. Which prevalence figure is most correct depends on how the data are to be used. For example, in estimating regional costs of inpatient services, use of the prevalence rates for severe CHD would be most appropriate. In examining the association of heart disease with specific environmental exposures during pregnancy, however, the inclusion of mild cases would be more appropriate.

Prevalence of Specific Types

The frequency of occurrence of various types of CHD among liveborn infants is shown in Table 52.3. This determination is based on 4,390 cases diagnosed in the first year of life from 1981 to 1989 by the Baltimore-Washington Infant Study. These cases included liveborn infants whose condition was diagnosed by echocardiography, cardiac catheterization, surgery, or autopsy. Diagnoses of patent ductus arteriosus in premature infants and mitral valve prolapse were excluded. Isolated ventricular septal defects are by far the most common type of CHD noted, accounting for nearly one-third of all congenital heart defects. Other lesions diagnosed frequently include pulmonic stenosis, atrial septal defect, atrial ventricular septal defect, tetralogy of Fallot, D-transposition of the great arteries, coarctation of the aorta, and hypoplastic left heart syndrome. These eight lesions account for approximately 75% of all cases of CHD. Several other lesions such as cardiomyopathy, pulmonary atresia with intact septum, total anomalous pulmonary venous connection, truncus arteriosus, tricuspid atresia, and interrupted aortic arch are less common but are frequently encountered in critically ill infants in pediatric intensive care units. Therefore, one's impression is biased by the setting of clinical practice.

CLUSTERING OF CONGENITAL HEART DISEASE WITH OTHER CONGENITAL ANOMALIES

Noncardiac congenital anomalies are frequently seen in infants with CHD. Data from the Baltimore-Washington Infant Study indicate that 27.7% of patients with CHD had associated noncardiac defects. This clustering of birth defects is useful for early

TABLE 52.1

CUMULATIVE PREVALENCE OF CONGENITAL HEART DISEASE PER 1,000 LIVEBORN CHILDREN

Age Interval	Cumulative Prevalence
Birth	3.3/1,000
1–6 d	4.0/1,000
7–31 d	5.2/1,000
1–5 mo	7.3/1,000
6–11 mo	7.8/1,000
1–2 y	8.3/1,000
>2–3 y	8.7/1,000
>3–6 y	9.1/1,000

TABLE 52.2

MAJOR US SURVEYS OF CONGENITAL HEART DISEASE

Period	Population	Study Design	Numbers	Prevalence/1,000 Births
1956–1965	12 clinical* centers	Follow-up 1 mo–9 y Mild and severe cases	420	7.7
1959–1966	San Francisco[†] Kaiser Health Plan	Follow-up 5–13 y Mild and severe cases	163	8.8
1969–1977	New England[‡]	Follow-up 1 y Severe cases only, diagnosed by catheterization, surgery, or autopsy	4,065	2.4
1971–1984	Dallas County[§]	Follow-up 2–13 y Mild and severe cases	2,481	6.5
1981–1987	Baltimore-Washington, DC[‖]	Follow-up 1 y Cases diagnosed by echocardiography, catheterization, surgery, or autopsy	4,390	4.8
1985–1992	California[#]	Follow-up 1 y Cases diagnosed by echocardiography, catheterization, surgery or autopsy. Includes stillbirths.	7,012	3.16

*Data from Mitchell et al., 1971.
[†]Data from Hoffman and Christianson, 1978.
[‡]Data from Fyler, 1980.
[§]Data from Fixler et al., 1990.
[‖]Data from Ferencz et al., 1993.
[#]Data from Pradat et al., 2003.

diagnosis of CHD, because the presence of certain anomalies may be the initial indication that a thorough cardiac evaluation is needed. For example, because 50% of infants with Down syndrome have CHD, all infants with trisomy 21 should have complete cardiac evaluations in the first month of life. Other conditions that have a substantial risk of underlying CHD are listed in Table 52.4.

TABLE 52.3

FREQUENCY DISTRIBUTION OF SPECIFIC DEFECTS IN LIVE BIRTHS WITH CONGENITAL HEART DISEASE

Lesion	Percent (%)
Ventricular septal defect	32.1
Pulmonic stenosis	9.0
Atrial septal defect, secundum	7.7
Atrioventricular septal defect	7.4
Tetralogy of Fallot	6.8
D-transposition	4.7
Coarctation of aorta	4.6
Hypoplastic left heart syndrome	3.8
Aortic stenosis	2.9
Patent ductus arteriosus (full-term)	2.4
Heterotaxia	2.3
Double-outlet right ventricle	2.0
Bicuspid aortic valve	1.9
Cardiomyopathy	1.9
Pulmonary atresia with intact septum	1.7
Total anomalous pulmonary venous return	1.4
Common arterial trunk	1.2
L-transposition	1.1
Ebstein anomaly	1.0
Tricuspid atresia	0.7
Interrupted aortic arch	0.7

Modified from Perry LW, et al. Infants with congenital heart disease. In: Ferencz C, Rubin JD, Loffredo CA, Magee CA, eds. *Epidemiology of congenital heart disease*. Mount Kisco, NY: Futura, 1993.

FAMILIAL RISK OF RECURRENCE OF CONGENITAL HEART DISEASE

After the diagnosis of CHD has been made, parents want to know the chance of recurrence. In some cases, the affected child exhibits manifestations of a recognizable syndrome that has specific known genetic risks. CHD in about 8% of children may be explained on the basis of a primary genetic defect. In the majority of cases, however, a specific genetic defect is not recognized. It has been postulated that genetic predisposition interacting with an environmental trigger causes the cardiovascular malformation. In families having a child with CHD, the genetic predisposition already has been expressed, and subsequent pregnancies are associated with a higher risk of cardiac maldevelopment. In a recent study from Britain by Gill and coworkers of 6,640 pregnancies in which a first-degree relative had CHD, the overall recurrence rate was 2.7%. For mothers with CHD, the overall recurrence rate was 2.9%; for fathers

TABLE 52.4

FREQUENCY OF CONGENITAL HEART DISEASE WITH OTHER BIRTH DEFECTS

Defect	Congenital Heart Disease Frequency (%)
Chromosomal Abnormalities	
Trisomy 21	50
Trisomy 18	90
Trisomy 13	50–90
Gastrointestinal Malformations	
Gastroschisis	14
Anorectal anomalies	15
Omphalocoele	20
Duodenal atresia	30
Tracheoesophageal fistula	40
Diaphragmatic hernia	23

TABLE 52.5

ESTIMATED RISK OF CONGENITAL HEART DISEASE RECURRENCE: ONE CHILD WITH CONGENITAL HEART DISEASE

Lesion	Recurrence Risk (%)
Ventricular septal defect	3–6
Patent ductus arteriosus	3–8
Atrial septal defect	3
Tetralogy of Fallot	3
Pulmonic stenosis	2–9
Coarctation	2–8
Aortic stenosis	2
Transposition	2
Endocardial cushion defect	2
Endocardial fibroelastosis	4
Tricuspid atresia	1
Hypoplastic left heart	2–10
Truncus arteriosus	1
Ebstein malformation	1

TABLE 52.6

ESTIMATED RISK OF OCCURRENCE IN CHILDREN: PARENT WITH CONGENITAL HEART DISEASE

Lesion	CHD in Father (%)	CHD in Mother (%)
Aortic stenosis	3–8	13–18
Atrial septal defect	1–7	4–14
Atrioventricular canal	1	14
Coarctation	2–8	4–6
Patent ductus arteriosus	2.5	4–9
Pulmonic stenosis	2	6–15
Tetralogy of Fallot	1.5	2–5
Ventricular septal defect	2	6–17

CHD, congenital heart disease.

In addition, studies have reported higher risks of recurrence than those previously reported for families having left-sided obstructive heart lesions such as coarctation, aortic stenosis, and hypoplastic left heart syndrome.

with CHD, it was 2.2%; and when one child had CHD, it was 2.7%. The recurrence risk when one child has been born with CHD varies with the specific lesion, as shown in Table 52.5. Ranges of risk in the table are listed to indicate differences among studies. When a second case does occur, the infant often has the same type of CHD as the first child; however, this varies according to the defect. Exact concordance for aortic stenosis was 38%, for hypoplastic left heart was 33%, for coarctation was 13%, and for ventricular septal defect was 55% in the recent British study. These data indicate that severe CHD in the sibling does not exclude less severe disease in recurrences and vice versa.

Over the past decade, more information has become available regarding the risk that a child will have CHD when a parent has a specific type of CHD (Table 52.6). The risk of recurrence is greater when the heart disease is in the mother. Estimating the risk for mothers with cyanotic CHD is confounded by their higher rates of spontaneous abortion and interrupted pregnancy. Ranges of risk are shown in Table 52.6 because important discrepancies are found among different studies. Because it has not been feasible for any center to follow all patients with CHD through childbearing age, sampling biases may have occurred that result in underestimates or overestimates of risk.

PRENATAL RISK FACTORS FOR CONGENITAL HEART DISEASE

The embryo is most vulnerable to cardiopathic effects during the developmental period from 20 to 45 days after conception. The first cardiac teratogens identified were those that caused a high frequency of CHD. For example, in 1942, an ophthalmologist first reported a high frequency of congenital cataracts, deafness, and heart disease associated with maternal rubella infection during pregnancy. In that period, prenatal rubella exposure was common, and the virus highly teratogenic when infection did occur. Several other prenatal exposures have been firmly established as cardiac teratogens (Table 52.7).

Maternal alcohol ingestion during pregnancy has been associated with a cluster of cardiac anomalies consisting primarily of ventricular septal defects and atrial septal defects. In children with fetal alcohol syndrome, 42% have been reported to have some form of CHD. From a compilation of 11 exposure studies, the risk of CHD from maternal alcoholism was estimated to be 32%. Because the metabolism of alcohol varies from woman

TABLE 52.7

ESTABLISHED CARDIAC TERATOGENS

Prenatal Exposure	Frequency of Congenital Heart Disease (%)	Most Common Cardiac Defects
Infections		
Rubella	35	Patent ductus arteriosus, pulmonary stenosis, septal defects
Drugs/Substances		
Alcohol	25–30	Septal defects, patent ductus arteriosus
Hydantoins	2–3	Pulmonic/aortic stenosis, coarctation, patent ductus arteriosus
Trimethadione	15–30	Transposition of the great arteries, tetralogy of Fallot, hypoplastic left heart syndrome
Lithium	10	Ebstein anomaly, tricuspid atresia, atrial septal defect
Thalidomide	5–10	Tetralogy of Fallot, septal defects, truncus arteriosus
Maternal Conditions		
Diabetes	3–5	Transposition of the great arteries, septal defects, coarctation
Phenylketonuria	25–50	Tetralogy of Fallot
Systemic lupus	20–40	Heart block

CHD, congenital heart disease.

TABLE 52.8

POTENTIAL CARDIAC TERATOGENS

Prenatal Exposure	Increase in Risk for Specific Cardiac Defects (%)	Defect
Infection		
Influenza	178	Tricuspid atresia
Medications		
Antitussives	790	Atrioventricular septal defect (non-Down)
Benzodiazepines	230	Transposition
Clomiphene	220	Tetralogy of Fallot
Corticosteroids	380	Atrial septal defect
Ibuprofen	310	Bicuspid aortic valve
Nitrofurantoin	570	Coarctation of aorta
Substances		
Marijuana	260	Ebstein anomaly
Cocaine	140	Membranous ventricular septal defect
Hair dyes	270	Pulmonic stenosis
Pesticides	800	Total anomalous pulmonary veins
Degreasing agents	500	Left-sided heart obstructions

Modified from Ferencz C, Correa-Villasenor A, Loffredo CA, Wilson PD. *Genetic and environmental risk factors of major cardiovascular malformation.* Armonk, NY: Futura, 1997.

to woman and toxicity may vary from fetus to fetus, no safe range of maternal alcohol intake has been established.

Several anticonvulsant medications have been shown to be teratogenic. In 2,148 treated epileptic mothers, 20% had children with CHD, the most frequent types being ventricular septal defect, tetralogy of Fallot, and transposition of the great arteries. The risk of CHD after prenatal exposure to barbiturates may be as high as 11%, and that after exposure to phenytoin may be as high as 29%. Other anticonvulsant medications such as phenytoin, valproic acid, and carbamazepine, either alone or in combination, have been associated with substantially increased risk of CHD. Maternal diabetes associated with insulin therapy significantly increases the risk of CHD in an infant. It is difficult to ascertain whether this increased risk is the result of maternal diabetes itself or related to treatment with insulin. In the large Collaborative Perinatal Project, the risk of congenital cardiac defect in children of diabetic mothers was found to be 2.5%. Maternal insulin dependence contributed significantly to the risk, as did poor control of the maternal diabetes.

A hallmark case-control study published by Ferencz and colleagues analyzed prenatal exposures in 4,390 infants born with CHD in the Baltimore-Washington area. The large number of cases allowed the analysis to be stratified by diagnostic groups of CHD. The estimated increase in risk of CHD following maternal exposures 3 months before and 3 months after conception is listed in Table 52.8. Because the analyses involved multiple comparisons, these findings should be interpreted with caution. However, the magnitude of the increases in risk suggests a strong potential for teratogenicity.

Environmental exposures to toxic pollutants have been shown to increase the risk of CHD. Several studies have demonstrated an increased risk in communities with water supplies contaminated with trichloroethane and trichloroethylene. Other studies have shown an association between risk of CHD and living near toxic waste sites or landfills. A study of ambient air pollution and birth defects reported an increased risk for ventricular septal defects with greater carbon monoxide exposures, as well as increased risk for aortic stenosis, pulmonary stenosis, and conotruncal defects with greater ozone exposures. Environmental epidemiology of CHD represents an important area for future investigation that will complement ongoing genetic research.

Suggested Readings

Boughman JA, Kate AB, Astemborski JA, et al. Familial risks of congenital heart defect assessed in a population-based epidemiological study. *Am J Med Genet* 1987;26:839.

Ferencz C, Neill CA. Cardiovascular malformations: prevalence at live-birth. In: Freedom RM, Benson LN, Smallhorn JR, eds. *Neonatal heart disease.* New York: Springer-Verlag, 1991.

Ferencz C, Rubin JD, Loffredo CA, Magee CA. *Epidemiology of congenital heart disease.* Mt. Kisco, NY: Futura, 1993.

Ferencz C, Correa-Villasenor A, Loffredo CA, Wilson PD. *Genetic and environmental risk factors of major cardiovascular malformations.* Armonk NY: Futura, 1997.

Fixler DE, Pastor P, Chamberlin M, et al. Trends in congenital heart disease in Dallas County births, 1971–1984. *Circulation* 1990;81:137.

Fyler DC. Report of the New England Regional Infant Cardiac Program. *Pediatrics* 1980;65:375.

Gill HK, Splitt M, Sharland GK, Simpson JM. Patterns of recurrence of congenital heart disease: an analysis of 6,640 consecutive pregnancies evaluated by detailed fetal echocardiography. *J Am Coll Cardiol* 2003;42:923.

Hoffman JIE, Christianson R. Congenital heart disease in a cohort of 19,502 births with long-term followup. *Am J Cardiol* 1978;42:641.

Mitchell SC, Korones SB, Berendes HW. Congenital heart disease in 56,109 births: incidence and natural history. *Circulation* 1971;43:323.

Nora JJ, Nora AH. Maternal transmission of congenital heart disease: new recurrence risk figures and the questions of cytoplasmic inheritance and vulnerability to teratogens. *Am J Cardiol* 1987;59:549.

Pexieder T. Teratogens. In: Pierpont MEM, Moller JE, eds. *Genetics of cardiovascular disease.* Boston: Martinus Nijhoff, 1987:55.

Pradat P, Francannet C, Harris JA, Robert E. The epidemiology of cardiovascular defects: a study based on data from three large registries of congenital malformations. *Pediatr Cardiol* 2003;24:195.

Ritz B, Yu F, Fruin S, Chapa G, et al. Ambient air pollution and risk of birth defects in Southern California. *Am J Epidemiol* 2002;155:17.

Rose V, Gold RJM, Lindsay G. A possible increase in the incidence of congenital heart defects among the offspring of affected parents. *J Am Coll Cardiol* 1985;6:376.

Whittemore R, Hobbins JC, Engle MA. Pregnancy and its outcome in women with and without surgical treatment of congenital heart disease. *Am J Cardiol* 1982;50:541.

Zierler S. Maternal drugs and congenital heart disease. *Obstet Gynecol* 1985; 65:155.

CHAPTER 53 ■ CARDIOVASCULAR DISEASE IN THE NEWBORN

ANNE MARIE VALENTE, CRAIG E. FLEISHMAN, AND NORMAN S. TALNER

The clinical approach to cardiovascular problems of the newborn must take into account the structural and functional basis of normal and abnormal cardiovascular development. This includes fundamental cardiac embryology, now focused on the molecular events that control cardiac myocyte differentiation and growth; basic ultra structural and functional differences between fetal, neonatal, and adult cardiac muscle; age-related responses to imposed circulatory loads; the transition from the fetal to the neonatal circulation (particularly the role of fetal flow pathways); and the various physiologic types of impaired cardiovascular performance that may be encountered.

This chapter encompasses etiology, the essentials of the development of cardiac structure and function, elements of the fetal and neonatal circulations that may affect disease states, the clinical assessment of cardiovascular performance in the neonate, diagnostic tests that permit the recognition and accurate delineation of a potential cardiac problem, and a functional approach to diagnosis and management that takes into account special clinical problems such as congestive heart failure, impaired systemic perfusion, hypoxemia, and disturbances of cardiac rhythm.

ETIOLOGY

Most cardiovascular diseases encountered in the newborn are congenital and, as such, they represent altered structural development. This can be either abnormal development of a normal structure (aortic or pulmonary atresia, septal defects), failure of a structure(s) to progress beyond a particular embryonic stage (double-outlet right ventricle, truncus arteriosus), or modification of normal flow pathways (coarctation).

In addition to congenital heart lesions, cardiac function in the neonate may be compromised by serious rhythm disturbances (tachycardia, heart block), inflammatory diseases of the myocardium, metabolic defects (e.g., glycogen storage disease, carnitine deficiency), defects of mitochondrial electron transport that interfere with the contractile process, and the adverse effects of intrauterine asphyxia on the myocardium, atrioventricular (AV) valve function, and pulmonary circulation.

Cardiovascular malformations often accompany chromosomal disorders such as trisomy 21, or are observed in the context of certain genetically determined syndromes, metabolic defects, abnormalities of cardiac rhythm, connective tissue disorders, and abnormal tissue growth. The prognosis in many of these syndromes is determined by the cardiovascular status; thus, detailed evaluation during the newborn period is required.

Congenital heart malformations usually result from the interaction between genetic and environmental systems. In certain conditions, a specific etiology has been identified. Maternal rubella during early gestation, for example, produces a syndrome, now largely preventable, in which a patent ductus arteriosus (PDA) and pulmonary artery stenosis are common cardiovascular findings. Cardiac defects, particularly the ventricular septal defect, occur in almost 50% of infants with the fetal alcohol syndrome. The finding of complete heart block in a newborn has been linked to the presence of or subsequent development of a rheumatologic disorder in the mother. Common cardiac findings associated with some specific syndromes are listed in Chapter 52, Epidemiology of Congenital Heart Disease.

Counseling on the incidence and recurrence rates for families of infants with congenital heart disease is extremely important. The availability of fetal cardiac ultrasound studies now permits an accurate determination of the presence or absence of significant structural heart disease in subsequent pregnancies and is recommended for families in which a previous child has been born with a congenital heart defect.

NORMAL CARDIAC DEVELOPMENT

The heart is the first organ to form in vertebrates. At about embryonic day 20 in humans, cells in the anterior lateral plate mesoderm become committed to developing into cardiac cells that form a bilateral cardiogenic field. This cardiogenic field then develops into parallel cardiac primordia that fuse in the midline to form the primitive cardiac tube. The families of signaling molecules, including FGF and BMP, that lead to formation of the primitive heart are expressed by the adjacent endoderm. The myocardium initially forms a trough around the endocardial tube (Fig. 53.1). Between the myocardium and endocardium is the cardiac jelly, which is made up of glycoconjugates. Inductive interactions between the layers is necessary for several steps in heart development. The end result is the formation of a centrally located heart, from cardiac precursors that were bilateral in location. The single cardiac tube has dilatations that constitute the sinus venosus, common atrium, presumptive left ventricle, presumptive right ventricle, and the conus. The truncus is not present in the early heart tube, but is added to the end of the tube from a secondary heart field (Fig. 53.2). A constriction separates each of these regions, and these indentations define the sinoatrial segment, the AV canal, and the bulboventricular canal.

In early development, looping of the bulboventricular region occurs, which tends to move the presumptive right ventricle anteriorly and to the right of the presumptive left ventricle. Cardiac looping is the first indication of right–left asymmetry in the embryo, and it is thought to possibly occur because of differential cell growth or altered cell adhesion. Looping of the heart to the right occurs in all vertebrates, suggesting that this is a critical step in cardiac morphogenesis. Studies of mouse mutants and chick embryos have led to insights into the signals that initiate cardiac looping. At the stage of looping, the embryonic systemic venous return is to the sinus venosus, then to a common atrium and then the presumptive right ventricle via the AV canal, and, finally, to the truncus. The embryonic

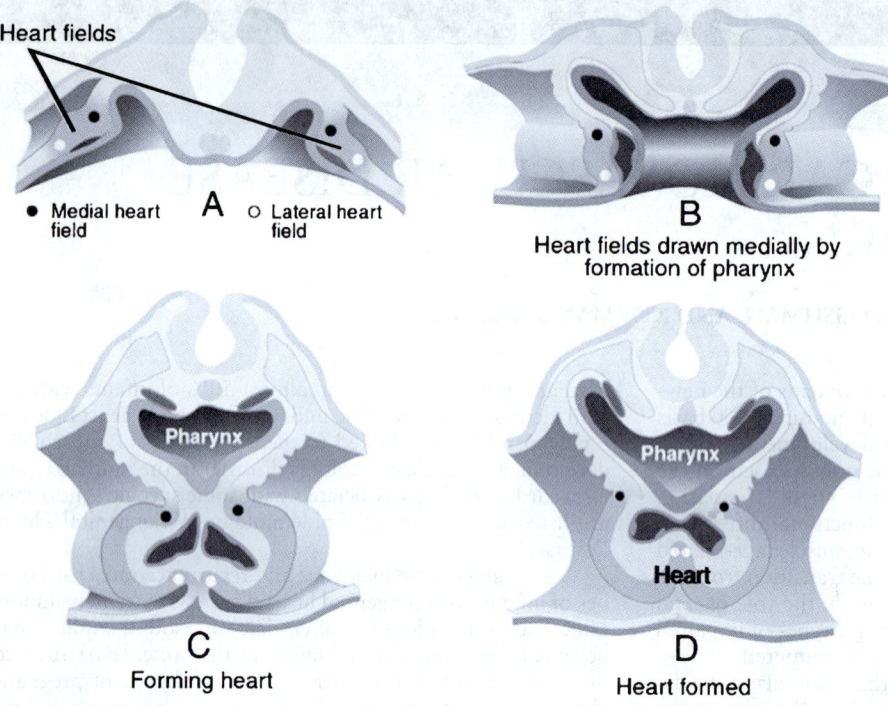

Heart fields

- Medial heart field   A   ○ Lateral heart field

B

Heart fields drawn medially by formation of pharynx

Pharynx

C

Forming heart

Pharynx

Heart

D

Heart formed

FIGURE 53.1. Diagrams showing steps in development of the bilateral primary heart fields in the splanchnic mesoderm into a single midline primary heart tube (A–D). Formation of the midline primary heart tube depends on formation of the foregut pocket, which forms the pharynx. (Reprinted with permission from Kirby ML and Waldo KL. Molecular embryogenesis of the heart. *Pediatr Pathol* 2002:516.)

heart begins to beat concomitantly with the formation of the heart tube and the onset of looping.

The looping process also confers two curvatures to the heart, with the outer curvature being more extensive than the inner. The inner curvature separates the AV canal—the locus for the developing AV valves—from the bulbar-truncal region, where the semilunar valves will originate. The semilunar valves form from endocardial cushions that line the cardiac tube distal to the AV junction. During development, the endocardial cushion tissue divides the heart into separate flow channels that prevents backflow. The remainder of the early developmental

process will result in the partitioning of the atria, ventricles, conus, and truncus, and the establishment of the functioning fetal circulation by the eighth week of gestation. Molecular studies suggest that chamber specification precedes the actual septation of the heart.

The development of the cardiac conduction system occurs prior to septation. The sinoatrial (SA) node, which is the pacemaker of the heart, forms from a caudal region of the straight heart tube. Initially, electrical impulses spread from the SA node throughout the ventricle and across the AV canal region to the ventricles. As the atria and ventricles become electrically isolated, the AV node in a region of the interventricular septum becomes the only pathway of depolarization from the atria to the ventricles. Depolarization of the ventricles continues through specialized conduction tissue. The persistence of conduction pathways around the AV fibrous ring may result in the episodic occurrence of arrhythmias.

HEART TUBE

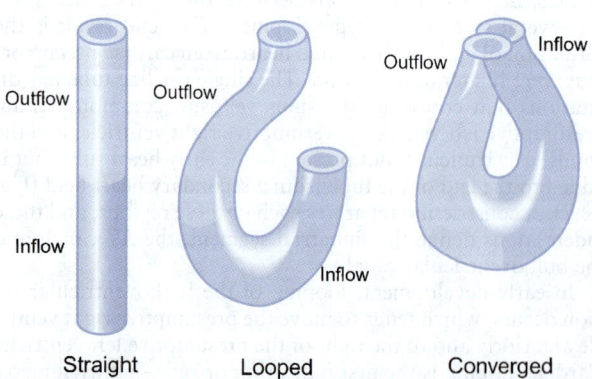

Outflow   Outflow   Outflow   Inflow

Inflow   Inflow   Inflow

Straight   Looped   Converged

FIGURE 53.2. The primary heart tube begins as a straight midline tube with blood entering caudally via the inflow and exiting cranially via the outflow tract. Under normal circumstances, the tube loops to the right, creating an inflow limb and an outflow limb. The distal extremities of the inflow and outflow limbs grow toward each other in a process of convergence that is necessary before septation can create a four-chambered heart. (Reprinted with permission from Kirby ML and Waldo KL. Molecular embryogenesis of the heart. *Pediatr Pathol* 2002:516.)

ABNORMAL CARDIAC DEVELOPMENT

Cardiovascular morphogenesis, as described in the preceding section, involves a number of important developmental mechanisms, including cell growth, migration, death, differentiation, and adhesion. Hemodynamic factors add another component to cardiovascular development. Structural defects found in clinical settings represent those changes in cardiovascular development that are compatible with the fetal circulation. Structural defects may result from various mechanisms. The addition of myocardium from the secondary heart field, which serves to lengthen the primary heart tube, is an essential step in the alignment of the inflow and outflow tracts prior to septation. If this lengthening does not occur normally, ventricular septal defects and dextroposition of the aorta occur. A dextroposed aorta occurs in tetralogy of Fallot and double-outlet right ventricle. The genetic pathogenesis of dextroposed aorta involves proteins such as Nkx2.5, neurotrophin 3, and probably a plethora of others.

Neural crest tissue has been shown to provide ectomesenchyme not only to the pharynx, but also to the outflow tract. The same region of the neural crest provides the postganglionic innervation of the heart. Abnormalities in the migration of ectomesenchymal tissue, as demonstrated by the ablation of the premigratory neural crest in chick embryos and in patients with the 22q11,2 deletion Syndrome (*c*ardiac defects, *a*bnormal facies, *t*hymic hypoplasia, *c*left palate, and *h*ypocalcemia resulting from microdeletions of chromosome 22q11), results in cardiac malformations. Some of these malformations include interruption of the aortic arch, persistence of the truncus arteriosus, and double-outlet right ventricle. Development of the parathyroid gland, thymus, and conotruncal region has been linked to neural crest function, and can account partially for the phenotype in DiGeorge syndrome. Investigations of zebrafish and mouse models seek to better define the genetic basis of many of these malformations.

Abnormalities of intracardiac blood flow can result in left and right heart obstructive defects, such as semilunar valve stenosis, coarctation of the aorta, and hypoplastic left heart syndrome. Abnormal targeted growth can result in anomalous pulmonary venous return. Abnormalities of cell death lead to such lesions as Ebstein malformation of the tricuspid valve and muscular ventricular septal defects. Ventricular growth is particularly sensitive to genetic mutations. In mice models, multiple mutations of genes result in hypoplasia of the ventricular wall and ventricular septal defects.

Extracellular matrix abnormalities are associated with atrioventricular canal defects (AVC) and dysplastic semilunar valves. Investigations into molecular pathways have shown that the normal migration of cells in the extracellular matrix is dependent on the variable expression of certain adhesion molecules throughout the heart (e.g., neural cell adhesion molecule; tenascin). Changes in the normal migration of cells may cause the above-mentioned lesions. The high prevalence of AV canal defects in children with Down syndrome has contributed to the awareness of identifying the critical gene(s) on chromosome 21 that may be linked to the cardiac defects. Down syndrome cell adhesion molecule (DSCAM) is expressed during cardiac development, and increased adhesiveness of mesenchymal cells in the endocardial cushions has been proposed as one of the pathologic mechanisms that contribute to cardiac defects. In addition, the absence of a cofactor essential for the normal expression of myocardial genes will result in a common AVC.

Situs and looping defects result in heterotaxy syndrome, in which a reversal or loss of visceral asymmetry occurs. This syndrome almost always is associated with complex structural defects in the heart. Right–left axis formation is dependent on ciliary movements through a microtubule-dependent motor protein. Activin also plays a role in right–left axis formation. Mice that are deficient in activin receptor IIB display randomized heart looping and malposition of the great arteries.

The normal development of the great arteries involves the transformation from a paired six-aortic-arch system into a definitive vascular pattern, as shown in Figure 53.3. Anomalies of the aortic arch artery derivatives are illustrated in Figure 53.4.

Airway Obstruction with Vascular Malformations

A vascular ring is formed when the trachea and esophagus are completely surrounded by vascular structures. Clinical manifestations of vascular rings range from severe respiratory difficulty to asymptomatic individuals in whom the abnormality is discovered at the time of chest imaging or autopsy. Symptoms

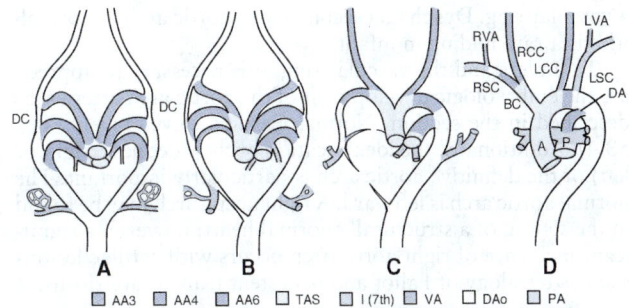

FIGURE 53.3. Schematic summary of the transformation of the symmetrical early human pharyngeal arterial basket into the configuration of the great arteries at birth. **A:** The pattern of paired arch arteries is symmetrical as they branch from the truncoaortic sac and join the dorsal aorta. The first and second arches have disappeared, leaving the third, fourth, and sixth arch arteries. The seventh intersegmental arteries branch from the dorsal aorta cranial to the aortic bifurcation. **B and C:** Transition stages between the early pharyngeal arterial pattern and the final configuration of the great arteries. The right ductus arteriosus narrows and disappears, and the left ductus and the primitive pulmonary arteries enlarge. The dorsal aorta on the left side enlarges, whereas the dorsal aorta on the right remains smaller in diameter. The aortic sac elongates causing the fourth arch arteries to shorten and become transported cranially. **D:** The configuration of the great arteries at birth. (Reprinted with permission from Waldo K and Kirby ML. In: Markwald R, ed. *Living morphogenesis of the heart.* Boston: Birkhauser, 1999.)

depend upon the tightness of the ring. Infants with vascular rings may have significant stridor and hyperextension of their necks. A history of frequent upper respiratory infections, bronchiolitis, or pneumonia is common. Infants who have a history of "noisy breathing since birth" that significantly worsens with upper respiratory tract infections should raise the suspicion of

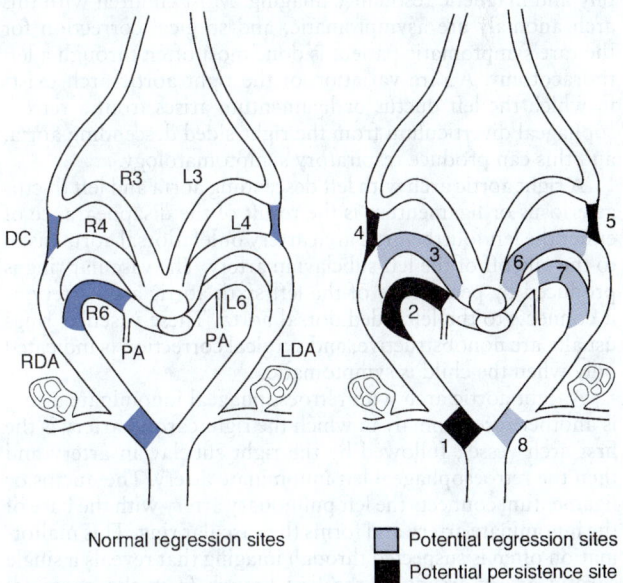

FIGURE 53.4. The drawing on the left illustrates the normal sites of vessel regression to produce normally patterned great arteries and the drawing on the right shows the potential sites of regression that are seen in human malformations involving abnormal patterning of the great arteries (1–8). R3, L3, right and left third arch artery; R4, L4, right and left fourth arch artery; R6, L6, right and left sixth arch artery; PA, pulmonary artery; DC, carotid duct; RDA, LDA, right and left dorsal arch. (Reprinted with permission from Waldo K and Kirby ML. In: Markwald R, ed. *Living morphogenesis of the heart.* Boston: Birkhauser, 1999.)

a vascular ring. Dysphagia secondary to aortic arch abnormalities is a rare finding in infants.

To understand the vascular ring, it is necessary to appreciate the embryologic development of the aortic arch arteries, as described in the section, Normal Cardiac Development (Fig. 53.4). Additionally, the identification of the sidedness (right or left) of the definitive aortic arch is particularly important. The normal aortic arch is leftward. A right aortic arch may be found in the setting of a structurally normal heart; however, a significant incidence of right aortic arch occurs with cardiac lesions such as tetralogy of Fallot and persistent truncus arteriosus.

Double Aortic Arch

Double aortic arch has the presence of both a right and left aortic arch due to persistence of both fourth aortic arch arteries. In this situation, one arch can be either hypoplastic or atretic; this is usually the left arch. Alternatively, both arches may be patent, in which case infants are usually symptomatic with stridor during the first several weeks of life.

Right Aortic Arch Anomalies

A right aortic arch with a diverticulum of Kommerell occurs when there is persistence of the left sixth aortic arch artery (ductus) between the truncoaortic sac and left dorsal aorta, and dissolution of the left fourth aortic arch artery. This results in the left carotid artery as the first branch off the aortic arch, followed by the right carotid artery, and right subclavian artery, and a retroesophageal vessel that gives rise to the left subclavian artery and a left ductus or ligamentum. This particular anomaly can be difficult to distinguish from a right aortic arch with retroesophageal subclavian artery, although the diverticulum of Kommerell is usually a significantly larger vessel than the subclavian artery. Classically, vascular rings were diagnosed by barium swallow esophograms, however these have been largely replaced by ultrasound, computerized tomography and magnetic resonance imaging. Most children with this arch anomaly are asymptomatic, and surgical correction for the rare symptomatic patient is done most often through a left thoracotomy. A rare variation of the right aortic arch exists in which the left ductus or ligamentum arises from a retroesophageal diverticulum from the right-sided descending aorta, and this can produce respiratory symptomatology.

A right aortic arch with left descending aorta and left ductus arteriosus or ligamentum is the result of the disappearance of either the left fourth aortic arch artery or left dorsal aorta distal to the takeoff of the left subclavian artery. The vascular ring is produced by persistence of the left sixth aortic arch artery as it connects to the left-sided dorsal aorta. These vascular rings usually are nonobstructive, and surgical correction is indicated only when the child is symptomatic.

A right aortic arch with retroesophageal innominate artery is another rare anomaly in which the right carotid artery is the first arch vessel, followed by the right subclavian artery and then the retroesophageal left innominate artery. The ductus or ligamentum connects the left pulmonary artery with the base of the innominate artery and forms the vascular ring. This malformation often is suspected through imaging that reveals a single carotid artery arising as the first branch from the proximal aorta.

Left Aortic Arch Anomalies

Left aortic arch with right descending aorta and right ductus or ligamentum is an arch anomaly in which persistence occurs of the right sixth aortic arch artery, which connects to the right pulmonary artery. The surgical approach to this lesion differs from most vascular rings, because a right thoracotomy is preferred to visualize and divide the ligamentum.

Cervical Aortic Arch

A cervical aortic arch is found above the level of the clavicle. A vascular ring exists when an anomalous subclavian artery is present. This usually is associated with a right aortic arch that descends on the right to about the level of the T4 vertebrae, where it crosses behind the esophagus to the left and gives off the left subclavian artery and a ductus or ligamentum. Presentation of cervical arches in infancy may be pulsatile masses in the neck or supraclavicular fossa. Femoral pulses diminish with compression of the mass. Infants have typical symptoms of a vascular ring, including stridor, recurrent respiratory infections, and respiratory distress. Chest roentgenogram may reveal a widened mediastinum without an evident aortic knob.

Pulmonary Artery Slings

In this rare anomaly, the lower portion of the trachea is partially surrounded by vascular structures, with the left pulmonary artery arising from the right pulmonary artery. It is the only instance in which a major vascular structure courses between the trachea and the esophagus. This anomaly often is associated with complete cartilaginous rings in the distal trachea, which can lead to significant tracheal stenosis. Infants present with respiratory distress and stridor. Barium esophagraphy classically reveals anterior indentation of the esophagus. The traditional surgical approach has been a division of the left pulmonary artery from the right pulmonary artery and reanastomosis of the left pulmonary artery in front of the trachea. However, a surgical approach has been described that involves transecting the trachea and reanastomosing it posterior to the pulmonary artery bifurcation, which permits tracheal reconstruction if cartilaginous rings are present.

Innominate Artery Syndrome

An anterior compression of the trachea by the innominate artery may occur, although this is not a form of a vascular ring. Previously, this was thought to be due to a more distal and leftward takeoff of the innominate artery, although imaging studies verifying this are inconsistent. Tracheomalacia often is associated with this situation, and infants present with inspiratory stridor. A lateral chest roentgenogram may reveal anterior indentation of the tracheal air column. Surgical interventions may be required to relieve the compression. These include suspension of the innominate artery from the sternum, or moving the innominate artery more proximal on the aortic arch.

Absent Pulmonary Valve Syndrome

Severe airway problems may occur with tetralogy of Fallot with an absent pulmonary valve. In utero, this lession may result in massive pulmonary regurgitation and the development of significant dilation of the main pulmonary artery and compromise of the large airways and interference with lung development.

DEVELOPMENT OF CARDIOVASCULAR FUNCTION

The primitive embryonic heart initially is a muscle-wrapped contractile tube without valve function, partitions, or a coronary circulation. This circulating system is capable of providing for the oxygen and nutrient needs of the embryo while at the same time removing the end-products of metabolism.

During fetal life, the placenta serves as the site for gas exchange, with almost fully oxygenated blood returning to the fetal body via the umbilical veins. The common umbilical vein enters the porta hepatis, where it is joined by the portal vein. Branches are provided to the left and right lobes of the liver, with the ductus venosus serving as a direct connection to the

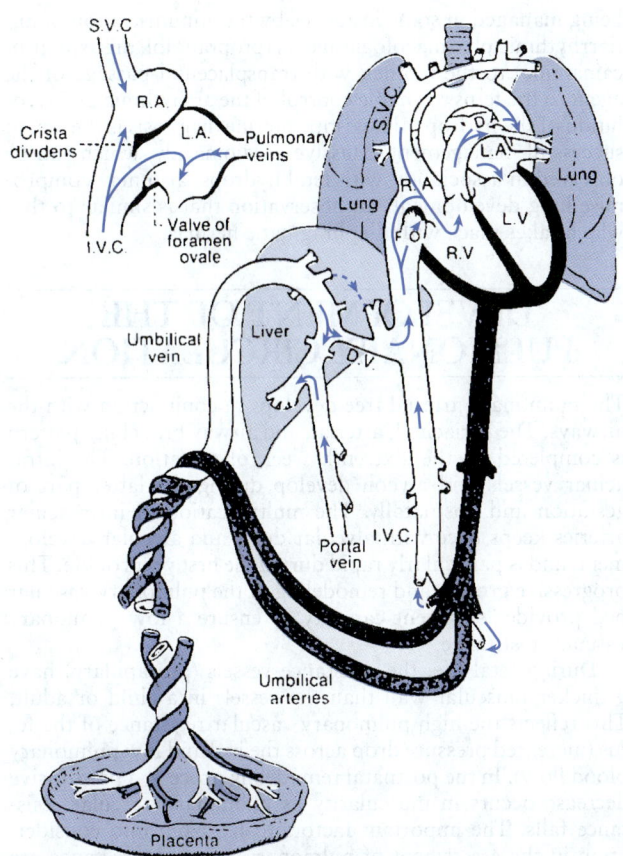

FIGURE 53.5. The fully developed fetal circulation, indicating the fetal flow pathways—foramen ovale, ductus arteriosus, and ductus venosus. The insert shows the direction of flow of the more highly oxygenated placental stream across the foramen ovale. RA, right atrium; LA, let atrium; RV, right ventricle; LV, left ventricle; DA, ductus arteriosus; FO, foramen ovale; DV, ductus venosus; IVC, inferior vena cava; SVC, superior vena cava. (Reproduced with permission from Adams FH, Emmanouilides GC, eds. *Heart disease in infants, children, and adolescents*, 3rd ed. Baltimore: Williams & Wilkins, 1983:12.)

inferior vena cava, thus permitting umbilical venous blood to bypass the hepatic microcirculation. The well-oxygenated umbilical stream is directed across the foramen ovale, allowing blood of the highest O_2 concentration to perfuse the cerebral circulation. The third shunt channel, the ductus arteriosus, allows blood from the right ventricle to enter the descending aorta and essentially bypass the pulmonary circulation. The fetal heart and circulation with functioning flow pathways are shown in Figure 53.5.

The patterns of blood flow in the fetal circulation have been studied in a fetal lamb model, using microsphere techniques. These studies have shown that about 20% of the total systemic venous return is derived from the superior vena caval stream, 3% is derived from the coronary circulation, and 7% is derived from the pulmonary vascular bed. Inferior caval flow accounts for 70% of the systemic venous return, of which 40% derives from umbilical veins, 5% from portal veins, and 25% from the lower fetal body. Fifty-five percent of umbilical venous flow passes through the ductus venosus, whereas 45% flows via the right and left lobes of the liver. Of interest, the left lobe is supplied from the umbilical vein, whereas the majority of the right lobe is perfused with portal venous blood. Under conditions of hypoxemia and flow limitation, a redistribution of venous return occurs, favoring flow through the ductus venosus.

Thus, blood at the level of the entry of the inferior vena cava into the right atrium is derived from four sources: the

ductus venosus (umbilical vein), the distal inferior vena cava, the right hepatic vein, and the left hepatic vein. The most highly oxygenated stream (ductus venosus) is directed preferentially across the foramen ovale, whereas the more distal inferior vena caval blood with a much lower O_2 saturation passes across the tricuspid valve. The higher saturations of left ventricular blood ensure adequate oxygenation of the developing brain as well as provide vital substrates for brain metabolism.

The superior vena caval stream is directed across the tricuspid valve, with only 2% passing from right to left across the foramen ovale. The net effect of the fetal venous return pathways is a lower O_2 saturation on the right side compared with that on the left. The volume of blood in the right and left ventricles also favors the right side in the lamb. Ultrasound and Doppler-derived flow studies across the mitral and tricuspid valves in the developing human fetus, however, indicate that the volume flows on the right and left sides of the heart are almost equal, with only a slight dominance of right ventricular output (55% versus 45%).

The fetal cardiac output represents the combined output of both ventricles. Most of the right ventricular output of the fetus flows into the descending aorta via the ductus arteriosus, whereas the majority of the left ventricular output perfuses the upper body with the aortic isthmus (a segment from the origin of the left subclavian artery to the ductus arteriosus) receiving only 30% of blood from the ascending aorta. The isthmus is the site of the functional separation of the two circuits.

We turn next to an evaluation of fetal and neonatal cardiovascular performance. When compared to the adult heart, the fetal and newborn myocardium is unique with respect to its ultrastructure, mechanical and biochemical properties, metabolism, and autonomic innervation. The developing cardiac myocyte is smaller than the adult cardiac myocyte, and contains relatively more noncontractile mass, with a reduction in cell density. Consequently, force generation and the extent and velocity of shortening are decreased, whereas water content and stiffness are increased. The process of excitation–contraction coupling also differs in the fetus and newborn, when compared with that in the adult. Less development of the sarcoplasmic reticulum and T tubule system is present in the fetus, which may interfere with the movement of calcium ions. Calcium ion increase in the cytosol appears to be provided by trans-sarcolemmal movement rather than by the release of calcium from the sarcoplasmic reticulum, as in the adult. Myofibrillar adenosine triphosphatase levels are low, and age-related differences in contractility also may occur as the result of the decreased activation of the modulatory proteins, troponin and tropomyosin.

Functional integrity exists for the afferent and efferent limbs of the autonomic pathways, although adrenergic innervation is incomplete in the fetus and newborn. This implies that circulating vasoactive agents may play a greater role in cardiovascular adaptation in the more immature individual.

The response of the fetal and newborn myocardium to altered loading conditions reflects diminished cardiovascular reserve, although this point is somewhat controversial. A limited ability may be present to increase cardiac output in response to a volume load, yet the Frank-Starling mechanism is operative. The tension developed during ejection thereby results in a limited increase in stroke volume. In some studies, inotropic interventions produce less of an augmentation in heart rate and cardiac output than is seen in older age groups, whereas decreases in heart rate (to less than 100 beats per minute) appear to be associated with pronounced falls in cardiac output. The fetus and newborn can modify the distribution of cardiac output by increasing vasomotor tone. This is a major adaptive mechanism that permits the perfusion of the myocardium and brain at the expense of the peripheral circulation.

It should be stressed that the overall response of the heart and circulation to a specific stimulus (e.g., volume, afterload increase) is an integrated response. For example, when afterload is increased by increasing systemic vascular resistance, a preload effect occurs as ventricular volume increases. Furthermore, if volume is increased, blood pressure will rise, and thus be associated with a change in afterload. The factors that may be involved in the integrated response of the heart and circulation include: (a) diastolic or filling volume; (b) ejection tension (afterload); (c) vascular impedance; (d) heart rate; (e) contractile state; (f) compliance; and, (g) ventricular interdependence (cross talk). The latter is especially important in the fetus and newborn, in whom volume loading of one ventricle may modify the performance characteristics of the other ventricle. For example, a volume-loaded right ventricle alters the filling characteristics of the left ventricle and vice versa.

Oxygen delivery to the myocardium in the fetus is accomplished through a coronary blood flow per gram that is 90% higher than that in the adult. Myocardial metabolism is maintained via the glycolytic pathway, with nearly 60% of fetal myocardial energy requirements being met by lactate extraction through the tricarboxylic acid cycle. Free fatty acids, the dominant energy source in the adult, are not used as a substrate for the fetal heart. L-Carnitine, a required cofactor for the beta-oxidation of fats, is present in low concentrations in the immediate postnatal period.

As oxygen tension rises after birth, the rate of oxidative metabolism increases and the mass of mitochondria per gram of myocardial tissue doubles. Cytochromes c_1, a_1 and a_3, and cytochrome oxidase rise in concert with the increase in oxygen tension. The myocardial isoenzyme pattern changes from the anaerobic muscle form to the aerobic form, reflecting the transition from the intrauterine to the extrauterine environment.

EFFECTS OF CARDIAC MALFORMATION ON FETAL CIRCULATORY FUNCTION

In most instances, cardiac malformations are tolerated well by the developing fetus because of the presence of the fetal flow pathways (which permit the bypass of obstructive lesions), the existence of the placenta for gas exchange, and the high pulmonary vascular resistance. On occasion, however, the presence of certain malformations interferes with the growth of chamber size, such as when a small foramen ovale compromises left heart development, or when incorporation of the common pulmonary vein into the left atrium fails, resulting in a hypoplastic left atrium (total anomalous pulmonary venous connection). Dominance of one ventricle over the other can modify the size of the great arteries, with the aortic isthmus becoming hypoplastic when flow from the pulmonary artery to the ductus into the descending aorta is the predominant flow pattern. When pulmonary atresia or severe obstruction of right ventricular outflow is present, the preferred pathway is via the aorta, which tends to be enlarged, whereas the pulmonary artery(s) is hypoplastic.

In a few congenital heart defects, the fetal cardiac function is compromised, with cardiac failure arising *in utero*. This occurs when massive AV valve regurgitation, semilunar valve insufficiency, or a large systemic arteriovenous fistula (vein of Galen malformation, giant hemangioma) is present. These share the common hemodynamic theme of right-sided volume overloading, either primarily or secondarily, when left-sided lesions are present. Hydrops fetalis with pericardial and pleural effusions, ascites, and generalized anasarca may occur in the face of these disturbances. This clinical picture also may develop with prolonged fetal tachyarrhythmias. These rhythm disturbances are being managed in some instances by the administration of antiarrhythmic pharmacologic agents (propranolol, digoxin, procainamide) to the mother, with transplacental passage of the agent to the fetus to enable control of the arrhythmia and resolution of the hydrops. Thus, intrauterine diagnosis is the key to successful management. Massive cardiomegaly, which can be observed in association with fetal hydrops, also may compromise lung development, an observation that is similar to that which takes place with diaphragmatic hernias.

DEVELOPMENT OF THE PULMONARY CIRCULATION

The pulmonary arterial tree develops in conjunction with the airways. The periacinal, arterial, and airway branching pattern is completed by the sixteenth week of gestation. The intra-acinar vessels and alveoli develop during the latter part of gestation and postnatally. The multiplication of intra-acinar arteries keeps pace with alveolar ducts and alveolar development, and is particularly rapid during the first years of life. This progressive growth and remodeling of the pulmonary vascular bed provides sufficient capacity to ensure a low pulmonary vascular resistance.

During fetal life, the resistance vessels (precapillary) have a thicker muscular wall than the vessels in a child or adult. This reflects the high pulmonary vascular resistance of the fetus (increased pressure drop across the bed and low pulmonary blood flow). In the postnatal remodeling process, a progressive decrease occurs in muscularity as pulmonary vascular resistance falls. The important factors to be taken into consideration in the assessment of pulmonary vascular resistance are the pressure drop from the pulmonary arteries to the veins, pulmonary blood flow, surface area, muscularity and tone of the resistance vessels, and blood viscosity. The postnatal fall in hematocrit results in a decrease in blood viscosity and contributes to the lowering of pulmonary vascular resistance. The presence of pulmonary hypertension does not necessarily imply an increase in pulmonary vascular resistance if pulmonary blood flow is increased markedly, as occurs with large-volume left-to-right shunts.

In infants with persistent pulmonary hypertension of multiple etiologies, the pulmonary artery pressure is close to or at systemic levels, whereas pulmonary blood flow is decreased (high resistance state). It is imperative, therefore, in the assessment of cardiopulmonary disorders of the infant that the resistance of the pulmonary circulation be taken into consideration. Furthermore, persistent pulmonary hypertension is not in itself a definitive diagnosis. A precise diagnosis is required of the cause of pulmonary hypertension (e.g., lung disease, cardiac problem, primary disorder of pulmonary resistance vessels) so that appropriate management can be carried out. Echocardiography occupies a key role in defining the specific nature of the problem in the pulmonary circulation.

OXYGEN TRANSPORT IN THE FETUS AND NEWBORN

Oxygen transport (delivery) represents the product of the cardiac output and the arterial oxygen content. The arterial oxygen content is determined by the oxygen tension, the affinity of hemoglobin for oxygen, and the absolute hemoglobin level. The hemoglobin concentration is controlled by erythropoietin production. The liver is the site of erythropoietin production in the fetus, as contrasted with erythropoietin production by the kidney in the adult. Because the fetus is exposed to a lower oxygen saturation, the erythropoietin response differs qualitatively or has a different sensitivity to hypoxemia than does the response at later stages of development. The affinity of hemoglobin to oxygen is greater in the fetus and newborn. This is accounted for by the fact that fetal hemoglobin has less affinity for 2,3-DPG (diphosphoglycerate), which competitively decreases hemoglobin–oxygen affinity. This is important for oxygen uptake in the fetus, because placental oxygen transfer occurs at much lower oxygen tension than does alveolar oxygen transfer. The P50 (Po$_2$ at which hemoglobin is 50% saturated with oxygen) is 20 mm Hg for fetal blood and about 28 mm Hg for adult blood. Therefore, postnatally, with an arterial Po$_2$ of 100 mm Hg and a venous Po$_2$ of 40 mm Hg, the amount of oxygen extracted from fetal blood is much less than that extracted from adult blood.

THE TRANSITIONAL CIRCULATION

At birth, the critical event in the transition from the intrauterine to the extrauterine state is the establishment of lung inflation. This initiates a series of events, culminating in a fall in pulmonary vascular resistance and functional closure of the fetal flow pathways. The contact of air containing oxygen with the pulmonary resistance vessels produces vasodilatation, which is accompanied by a marked increase in pulmonary blood flow as pulmonary vascular resistance falls acutely. A continuing search has gone on for the specific mediator of the pulmonary vasodilatation that occurs at birth. Initial focus was on oxygen effect and bradykinin, then on prostaglandins, and, most recently, on the endothelial-derived relaxing factor, nitric oxide (NO). This has important clinical implications in the management of persistent pulmonary hypertension.

While pulmonary vascular resistance is falling, systemic vascular resistance rises consequent to the obliteration of the low-resistance placental circuit. The ductus venosus flow channel also is eliminated at this time.

Left atrial pressure rises as pulmonary venous return increases, and this produces functional closure of the foramen ovale. The postnatal rise in arterial oxygen tension, together with local changes in prostaglandin metabolism, produces a constriction of the ductus arteriosus, with functional obliteration usually complete in a full-term infant by 10 to 15 hours of life. In a preterm infant, however, the mechanisms responsible for ductal constriction are incompletely developed, and closure is delayed.

Any interference with the establishment of ventilatory function (i.e., birth asphyxia) tends to maintain the circulation in the fetal state, with a high pulmonary vascular resistance and right-to-left shunting via the ductus arteriosus and foramen ovale. This can produce the clinical picture associated with persistent pulmonary hypertension, as will be discussed later.

The final obliteration of the fetal flow pathways produces the adult-type circulation that is present in the term infant within a few weeks of birth. The two ventricles now operate in series, with a relatively high cardiac output resulting from the demands of growth and control of body temperature. Pulmonary vascular resistance is almost at adult levels, with resistance vessels characterized by very little medial thickness and increased lumen diameter. Remodeling of the pulmonary vascular bed continues postnatally, however, in concert with airway development.

KEY POINTS IN CLINICAL EVALUATION

As technology advances, pediatricians must continue to attain exceptional skills at taking a history and performing the physi-

cal examination, because this initial assessment often provides invaluable information regarding the functional cardiac diagnosis and leads to a specific etiology and necessary medical and surgical management.

History

The principal points in the history that aid in the clinical evaluation of the potentially critically ill infant with cardiovascular disease include the birth history, the presence of a chromosomal abnormality, a sibling with congenital heart disease, hydrops fetalis and ectopy, intrauterine infections, and other major-organ systemic malformations. A low Apgar score should raise the possibility of the deleterious effects of hypoxemia, hypercarbia, and, acidemia on the myocardial, pulmonary, and systemic circulations. Chronic intrauterine hypoxia is associated with persistent pulmonary hypertension with right-to-left ductal and foraminal shunting. Almost all the chromosomal abnormalities are associated with a high incidence of congenital heart disease, with trisomies 21, 13, and 18 heading the list. Although defects involving the AVC are observed commonly in infants with trisomy 21, other malformations have been seen, such as tetralogy of Fallot and PDA. The American Academy of Pediatrics (AAP) Committee on Genetics recommends all infants with trisomy 21 should undergo a two-dimensional echocardiographic assessment in the routine neonatal evaluation.

Congenital heart disease in a previous child in the family should alert the clinician to possible involvement in a subsequent pregnancy. The use of fetal echocardiography is becoming increasingly important in the prenatal diagnosis of congenital heart disease. Fetal echocardiography should be considered in the following situations: (a) an extracardiac malformation is identified; (b) exposure to a potentially teratogenic agent; (c) family history of congenital heart defects; (d) suspected fetal chromosomal abnormality or genetic disease; (e) maternal disease associated with structural heart defects or fetal cardiac arrhythmia; or (f) suspected cardiac defects based on findings of routine ultrasound.

Intrauterine infections can be associated with life-threatening myocardial dysfunction. Therefore, myocardial structure and function should be assessed in infants suspected of having a septicemic process, particularly if clinical evidence exists of low systemic perfusion.

The presence of malformations that affect multiple organ systems, such as tracheoesophageal fistula, imperforate anus, and cleft palate, should warrant a search for cardiac involvement. Abnormalities of cardiac position (dextrocardia, mesocardia) also demand a cardiac evaluation, whereas a midline liver with or without an abnormality of cardiac position should raise the possibility of atrial isomerism in association with absence of the spleen or polysplenia. The presence of asplenia or polysplenia with a midline liver warrants a radiographic evaluation for malrotation anomalies of the gut. Another important group consists of patients who have aortic arch anomalies, where a strong association exists between the absence of the parathyroid gland and thymus and conotruncal malformations.

Physical Examination

Respiratory Patterns in the Newborn

The pattern of respirations may provide valuable clues to the presence of cardiovascular disease. It is critical to examine the respiratory patterns of an infant because the auscultatory examination may be unremarkable, despite the presence of significant pulmonary edema.

Tachypnea. When lung water is increased, with the accumulation of fluid in the pulmonary interstitial space, tachypnea (rapid, shallow respirations) ensues in response to the stimulation of juxtacapillary volume receptors. This response occurs under any circumstance in which a fluid leak into the pulmonary interstitial space is present (left-to-right shunting, left heart obstructive lesions, inflammatory diseases of the myocardium or lungs, delayed fluid reabsorption). Therefore, tachypnea is a nonspecific finding that demands a careful search for its underlying cause. The diagnosis of transient tachypnea, although descriptive of a breathing pattern, does not provide a precise delineation of etiology. Supporting studies are required to rule in or out cardiovascular or pulmonary problems associated with tachypnea.

Wheezing. Transudation of fluid (water) into peribronchiolar spaces increases small airway resistance and results in wheezing on a cardiovascular basis.

Hyperpnea. When the arterial oxygen tension is extremely low and pulmonary perfusion is decreased or normal, the ventilatory response is that of hyperpnea (rapid, deep respirations), in contrast to the congested lung, in which tachypnea is observed. The hyperpneic response represents hypoxemic stimulation of the arterial chemoreceptors and results in the development of a respiratory alkalosis.

Stridor. An inspiratory stridor in a newborn infant should raise the suspicion of a vascular ring or sling.

Cardiac Evaluation

Perfusion. The status of systemic perfusion must be evaluated carefully. A low output state with any one of a number of causes should be suspected when pulses are difficult to palpate, extremities are cold and pale, and capillary refill is slow. Although this could arise from overwhelming infection, it is common to encounter this clinical picture in newborn infants with critical left heart obstruction or underdevelopment, tachyarrhythmia, or myocardial disease. It should be stressed that palpable femoral pulses in a newborn do not rule out coarctation if the ductus arteriosus is open (see the section on low perfusion states). Bounding peripheral pulses are observed with aortic runoff lesions, notably patent ductus, truncus arteriosus, systemic arteriovenous fistulas, and in the face of severe anemia.

In regard to arteriovenous malformations, reports have been published of diminished femoral pulsations with large cerebral arteriovenous fistulae. In this situation, a steal occurs from the peripheral circulation as blood flows through the low-resistance central nervous system fistula.

Heart Rate. The heart rate should be counted accurately. If it is higher than 220 beats per minute, an electrocardiogram (ECG) must be obtained to define the basis for the increase. Bradycardia (a heart rate of less than 100 beats per minute) may be encountered with hypoxic depression of the myocardium, possible central nervous system disease, or congenital heart block.

Blood Pressure. Many new techniques permit the accurate determination of blood pressure in the newborn. This allows a delineation of infants with serious hypertension and the initiation of a search for the specific basis for the blood pressure elevation. On the other hand, if blood pressure is discovered to be low for developmental age, the causes of hypotension, such as hypovolemia, myoepicardial disease, or left heart obstruction, must be defined quickly and corrected if possible. Blood pressure measurements of both the upper and lower extremity should be a routine part of the newborn examination.

Cyanosis. The presence of a generalized duskiness with involvement of the mucous membranes and nail beds can arise from a number of causes. Diffuse cyanosis requires documentation of the level of arterial oxygen tension and saturation, along with determination of the pH level and the $Paco_2$. Oxygen saturation levels can be derived from these measurements. Oxygen saturation levels also can be determined directly, in a noninvasive fashion, using pulse oximetry. Differential cyanosis, with the lower body being more cyanotic than the upper body, immediately should raise the suspicion of a high pulmonary vascular resistance with right-to-left shunting via the ductus arteriosus. This flow pattern can arise from a number of causes, including coarctation of the aorta, interruption of the aortic arch, and persistent pulmonary hypertension. In the rare situation in which the upper body is cyanotic while the lower body is pink, transposition of the great arteries in association with pulmonary-to-aortic shunting of oxygenated blood via the ductus arteriosus may be present.

Precordial Activity. The activity of the precordium, or lack thereof, provides valuable clinical information regarding cardiac performance. An active precordium is seen in the volume-loaded situation associated with increased ventricular contractility (left-to-right shunt, AV valve regurgitation, hypervolemia). A relatively inactive precordium with signs of compromised systemic perfusion is seen with myoepicardial disease. Patients with hypoplastic left-heart syndrome and coarctation characteristically have a hyperdynamic precordium in addition to decreased system perfusion. This reflects the volume-loaded right heart and pulmonary circulation, whereas systemic perfusion is impaired secondary to constriction of the ductus arteriosus. Precordial activity in the right chest suggests a cardiac malposition.

Aortic and Pulmonary Valve Closure. The examiner should be able to detect normal splitting of the second heart sound, indicating the presence of aortic and pulmonary valve closure. A single second heart sound occurs if one semilunar valve is severely stenotic or atretic, or if the semilunar valves are closing in synchrony (transposition).

Ejection Clicks. Aortic and pulmonary valve ejection clicks are heard just before the onset of turbulent flow. They represent the opening sounds of mobile but thickened semilunar valves. The aortic ejection click is heard at the cardiac apex or in the suprasternal notch. A pulmonary ejection click usually is heard at the left base. Ejection clicks also may be appreciated when an increased volume is flowing into the pulmonary or systemic circulation, although they are heard most commonly when obstructive disease is present.

Gallop Rhythm. A triple rhythm is encountered when increased flow is present across an AV valve or ventricular dilatation is present in association with decreased ventricular contractility or compliance.

Murmurs. Auscultation of the heart should be performed in a fashion similar to ultrasound interrogation during echocardiography. This requires a knowledge of specific anatomic positions, particularly those of the ventricular septum, great arteries, and AV valves. Stethoscopic probing of the cardiac base (second interspace on the right and left) will define outflow tract lesions. The ejection murmur of aortic stenosis is localized to the right base with transmission to the neck, whereas a similar ejection-type murmur, heard best at the second left intercostal space with transmission laterally and to the back, characterizes pulmonic stenosis. Murmurs localized along the lower left sternal border usually reflect defects of the ventricular septum. These murmurs are holosystolic, representing pansystolic flow from the left to the right ventricle. Holosystolic murmurs heard in a similar location occasionally may indicate the presence of tricuspid regurgitation, with some tendency to localize along the lower right sternal margins. An apical holosystolic murmur, usually heard well posteriorly, suggests the presence of mitral valve regurgitation.

The intensity of the murmur does not correlate with the severity of the lesion, and certainly can be influenced by cardiac output and changes in systemic and pulmonary vascular resistance. The total clinical picture must be taken into consideration when attempting to define the severity of a particular lesion.

Systolic ejection murmurs that localize to both axillae and are heard posteriorly are heard with peripheral pulmonary artery stenosis. In the preterm and newborn infant, this may be a normal finding as a result of a discrepancy in size between the main pulmonary artery and its branches. Persistence of this type of murmur beyond 6 months of age should be considered abnormal, and indicates structural narrowing of the pulmonary arterial branches. Another murmur, one that is systolic ejection in timing, is associated with transient left-to-right shunting via the ductus arteriosus in the first 10 to 15 hours after birth, as the pulmonary vascular resistance falls and the ductus arteriosus is undergoing postnatal constriction. Echocardiographic studies in the preterm infant indicate that the ductus arteriosus may remain open for considerably longer periods of time.

Diastolic murmurs are rarely heard in the newborn. An early decrescendo diastolic murmur is heard with pulmonary valve regurgitation, as might be encountered in the absent pulmonary valve syndrome. In the latter instance, significant airway problems may be caused by compression of major bronchi by a massively dilated main pulmonary artery and its branches. Low-pitched, diastolic rumbling murmurs heard along the lower left sternal border or at the cardiac apex, which time with rapid ventricular filling, are associated either with AV valve regurgitation or increased flow across normal tricuspid or mitral valves in the face of a left-to-right shunt lesion (relative stenosis).

The classic auscultatory finding of a PDA is a continuous machinery-like murmur localized under the left clavicle. This represents systolic and diastolic flow into the pulmonary artery via the ductus arteriosus. Recognition of its presence is extremely important in the preterm infant, because a PDA with left-to-right shunting may contribute to continued respirator dependence. The diagnosis should be suspected in any preterm infant with a hyperdynamic precordium and bounding arterial pulsations, even in the absence of significant murmurs. In infants with respiratory distress syndrome, the ductus may be widely patent with no obvious clinical findings. Therefore, diagnosis is dependent on two-dimensional echocardiography with Doppler interrogation, which will demonstrate aortic-to–pulmonary artery shunting. Other causes of continuous murmurs include aorto-pulmonary window, and coronary or systemic AV fistulas.

To-and-fro systolic and diastolic murmurs can be heard in the presence of semilunar valve regurgitation, with the systolic component arising from increased volume flow across a semilunar valve. With anemia, a number of murmurs may be appreciated, all arising from a high cardiac output state with increased flow across semilunar and AV valves.

Hepatomegaly. The size and location of the liver edge provides valuable clinical clues related to cardiac disease and myocardial performance. A liver edge palpated to the left is seen with situs inversus and dextrocardia (mirror-image type), whereas a midline liver raises the possibility of atrial isomerism and splenic abnormalities. Hepatic enlargement accompanies right-sided congestive heart failure. Systolic pulsations are seen with massive tricuspid regurgitation. Presystolic pulsations occur with tricuspid valve obstruction and represent a prominent atrial contraction.

BOX 53.1	Questions to Ask While Reviewing a Chest Film

- What is the cardiac position (levocardia, mesocardia, or dextrocardia)?
- Where is the stomach bubble and liver (situs solitus, inversus, midline liver)? Bronchi (right- or left-sidedness)?
- Is the heart enlarged (age-related normal, influence of thymic shadow)?
- What is the status of lung perfusion (increased pulmonary blood flow, pulmonary venous congestion, diminished pulmonary perfusion)?
- Is the cardiac contour normal? (crescent-like shadow in the right lower lung field, as seen with anomalous connection of the right pulmonary veins to the inferior vena cava)?
- Is there associated lung disease (infection, hypoplasia, diaphragmatic hernia)?
- Is the airway compromised (vascular rings)?

DIAGNOSIS

Chest Film

The chest film provides valuable structural and functional data relative to the underlying cardiac condition. Clinicians should discipline themselves to review the film carefully and attempt to answer the queries listed in Box 53.1.

A careful analysis of these points usually permits a physiologic and, sometimes, a correct anatomic diagnosis, although the presence of open fetal flow channels (ductus arteriosus, foramen ovale) may mask the eventual radiographic picture. Examples of rather typical chest radiographs encountered in critical cardiac disease in the infant are shown in Figure 53.6.

Arterial Blood Gas and pH Levels

Oxygen saturation can be determined noninvasively using a pulse oximeter, which also is a valuable aid in assessing the response to medical or surgical interventions. The data obtained from an analysis of blood gas tensions and pH levels permit the delineation of the severity of hypoxemia if it is present, the metabolic and respiratory consequences of the defect (metabolic and respiratory acidemia), and the degree of ventilatory compensation or decompensation (hypocarbia or hypercarbia). In our experience, the response to the inhalation of high inspired-oxygen concentrations (hyperoxia response) has not proven to be an accurate discriminator between heart, pulmonary vascular, and lung disease, and actually has on occasion been misleading. In situations in which ductal-dependent systemic blood flow occurs (coarctation, aortic atresia), the P_aO_2 may rise significantly, whereas systemic perfusion is compromised further, which results in a severe metabolic acidemia. On the other hand, if ductal-dependent pulmonary blood flow occurs (pulmonary atresia, tricuspid atresia), the arterial oxygen tension will rise only slightly as a result of the increment in dissolved oxygen. Unfortunately, with a fixed high pulmonary vascular resistance or severe lung disease, the increment in oxygen tension or saturation also may be minimal.

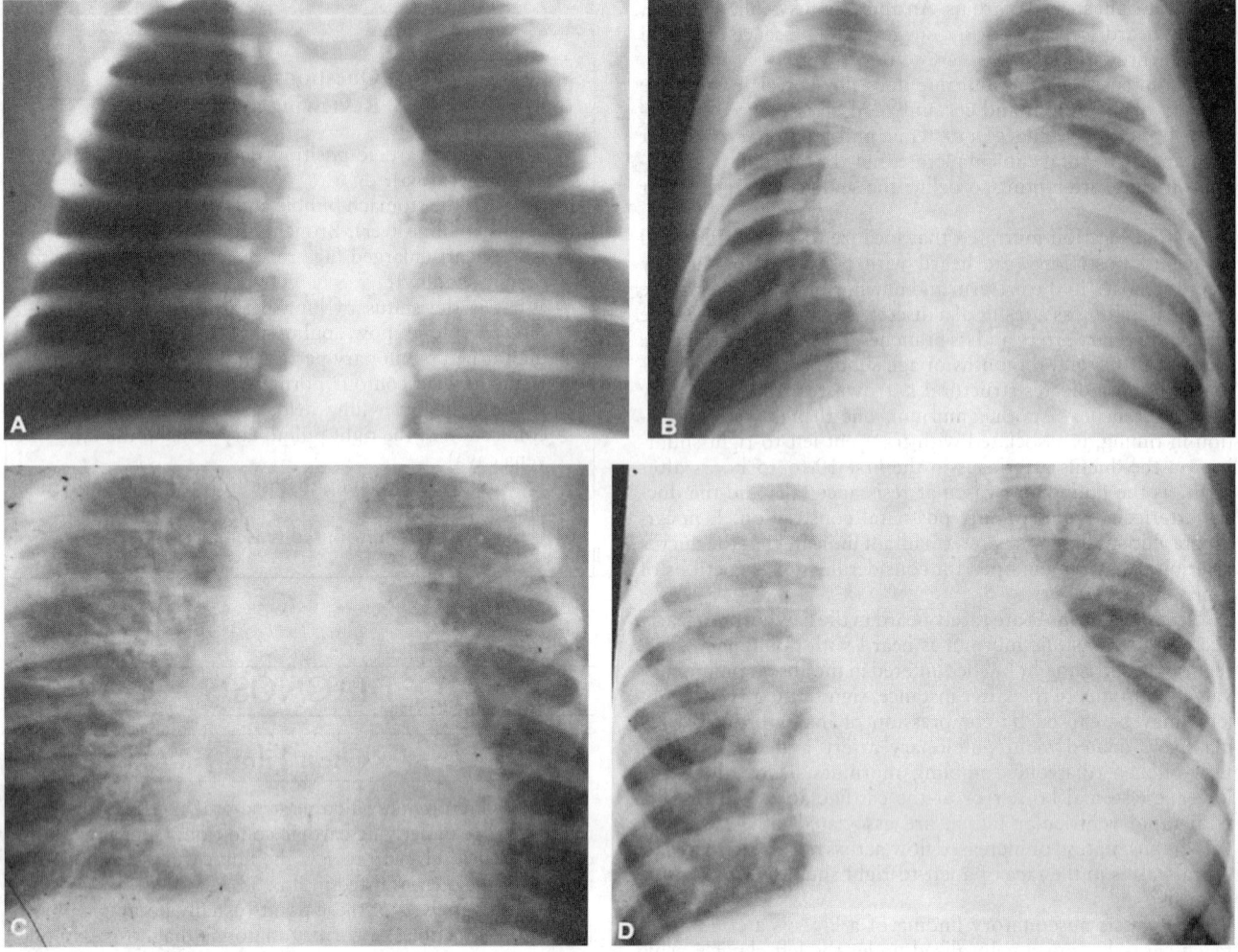

FIGURE 53.6. Chest films illustrating various types of functional impairment observed with critical cardiac disease. **A:** Striking decrease in pulmonary blood flow, as seen with tetralogy of Fallot or hypoplastic right heart syndrome. **B:** Increased pulmonary vascularity in a newborn infant who also was severely cyanotic. This indication suggests the present of transposition of the great arteries. **C:** Marked pulmonary venous congestion of the type seen with severe obstruction to the left heart (coarctation, aortic stenosis) or compromise of pulmonary venous return. **D:** Cardiomegaly and increased pulmonary vascular markings compatible with the finding of a large left-to-right shunt at the level of the ventricle or great artery. (Reproduced with permission from Talner NS. Heart failure. In: Adams FH, Emmanouillides GC, eds. *Heart disease in infants, children, and adolescents.* Baltimore: Williams & Wilkins, 1989:899.)

Hemoglobin and Hematocrit

The packed cell volume and hemoglobin concentration provide clinical clues that aid in the assessment of cardiovascular disease. A hematocrit level elevated above 65% is associated with a high pulmonary vascular resistance (viscosity factor) and right-to-left shunting via fetal flow channels. With significant anemia (a hemoglobin level less than 12 g/dL), a high output state may be present. Infants with large left-to-right shunts evidence signs of congestive heart failure at a time when relative anemia is present (2 to 3 months). The decrease in blood viscosity and postnatal remodeling of the pulmonary vascular bed both contribute to the fall in pulmonary vascular resistance and the resulting large left-to-right shunt.

Blood Glucose and Calcium

Hypoglycemia and hypocalcemia have been implicated in clinical states characterized by low cardiac output. Therefore, these abnormalities should be corrected as part of any attempt to restore normal myocardial contractility.

Myocardial Enzymes

If a suspicion exists of hypoxic myocardial insult, troponin-T and myocardial creatine phosphokinase (CPK) should be obtained to establish the presence of a myocardial injury.

Electrocardiogram of the Newborn

The ECG provides the clinician with valuable data relative to heart rate, potential rhythm disturbances, ventricular and atrial enlargement, myocardial ischemia, and possible electrolyte disturbances. During the newborn period, the ECG must be interpreted in terms of normative values for this age group.

The standard newborn ECG should consist of 12 leads and a rhythm strip. The lead system must be standardized to a known voltage, so that proper interpretation can be made in terms of enlargement. The paper speed should be 25 mm/second, so that rates and intervals can be calculated. Attention should be directed to proper lead placement, particularly of the precordial leads. If electrode paste is smeared, then a common lead usually is traced, which does not permit localization.

Pediatricians must develop a systematic approach for interpreting electrocardiograms, and execute this system every time they evaluate an ECG. First, the ECG must be interpreted in conjunction with the history, physical examination, and other pertinent laboratory findings, electrolyte status, and medications. Second, the heart rhythm must be established. Then, the heart rate and frontal plane QRS axis are determined. The various intervals should be determined, including PR, QRS, and QTc. Heart chamber enlargement should be sought by comparing voltages and patterns to established normal values. Finally, the ST segments and T-waves must be examined carefully for abnormalities that may be suggestive of ischemia.

Determination of Heart Rate

The pediatrician should calculate the heart rate and compare it to age-related normal values. Each major line represents 0.2 seconds when recorded at a paper speed of 25 mm/second. Thus, if one large line separates the RR interval, the rate is 300 beats per minute (one-half beat every 0.2 seconds is equal to 300 beats per minute), which is abnormally rapid. On the other hand, if three large lines separate the R waves, the rate is 100 beats per minute, which is too slow for a newborn.

Electrical Axis

As an approximation, the electrical axis will be perpendicular to the limb lead that adds up to zero (R + S), or parallel to the lead with the highest R-wave voltage. The mean axis of the P wave can be determined in a similar fashion. In the newborn, the normal QRS axis is more to the right than in the older child and the adult. It should be stressed that, although the axis usually correlates with ventricular hypertrophy, this is not necessarily so. Hypertrophy must be assessed from the precordial leads. In the newborn period, the frontal-plane QRS axis is rightward, which is a consequence of the physiologic right ventricular hypertrophy that is present. A superiorly or left-oriented frontal plane QRS axis is suggestive of an AVC defect or tricuspid valve atresia.

Right Ventricular Hypertrophy

At birth, the thickness of the right and left ventricular walls is about equal and, thus, the infant has physiologic right ventricular hypertrophy (RVH). This results in increased rightward and anterior electrical forces, with tall R waves in the right chest and broad S waves over the left precordial leads (Fig. 53.7). This makes the diagnosis of pathologic RVH difficult. Certain patterns are helpful in this regard. A pure R wave or qR pattern in the right precordial leads strongly suggests RVH at any age

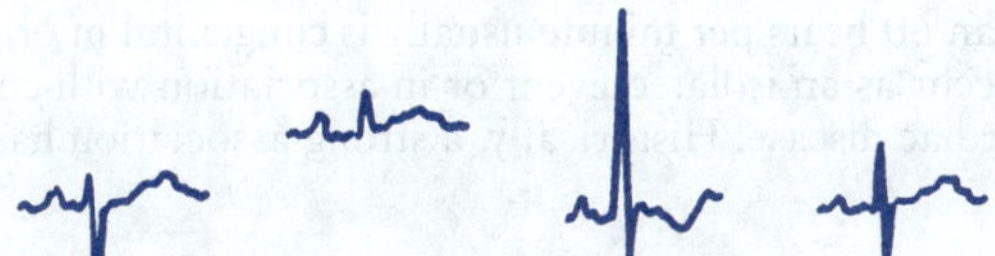

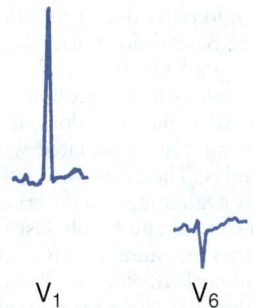

FIGURE 53.8. Significant right ventricular hypertrophy in a newborn infant with severe pulmonary valve stenosis (markedly increased R wave over right precordial lead V_1).

(Fig. 53.8). Additionally, an upright T wave in lead V_1, which persists after one week of age is highly specific for RVH.

Left Ventricular Hypertrophy

The diagnosis of left ventricular hypertrophy in the infant rests on an increase in posterior forces or a decrease in anterior forces (right ventricular) for age. This is reflected by increased left precordial and decreased right precordial voltages (Fig. 53.9). In the newborn, a decrease in anterior forces should suggest the possibility of underdevelopment of the right ventricle (tricuspid, pulmonary atresia). In the face of severe left ventricular hypertrophy, accompanying ST-T wave changes may be present, which indicate the presence of myocardial ischemia. The latter also may be present with critical aortic stenosis.

Atrial Enlargement

Usually, limb lead II is the optimal lead for use in assessing atrial size. Tall, peaked P waves (>2.5 mm) indicate right atrial enlargement, whereas bifid, broad P waves correlate with left atrial enlargement. Because the left atrium depolarizes after the right atrium, the latter part of the P wave may be deformed with any increase in left atrial volume.

ST-T Wave Segment

Primary alterations in the ST-T waves occur with myocardial ischemia, electrolyte disturbances, and pericardial disease. Birth asphyxia has been associated with ECG abnormalities compatible with myocardial ischemia and, in rare instances, a true myocardial infarct pattern has been observed.

Electrolyte Abnormalities

Hypocalcemia is associated with a prolonged QT interval that is heart-rate–dependent (QTc >460 msec in a newborn,

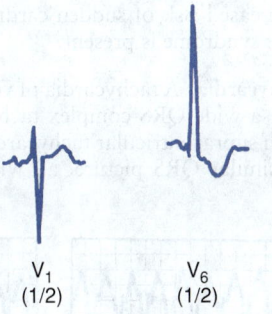

FIGURE 53.9. Left ventricular hypertrophy in a newborn with critical aortic stenosis (decreased forces over right precordial lead V_1 and increased R wave over lead V_6).

FIGURE 53.7. Selective electrocardiographic leads in a normal newborn infant, illustrating right axis deviation and right ventricular dominance.

I   aVF V_1 V_6

V_1 (1/2) V_6 (1/2)

>440 msec in any child older than 1 month of age). The QTc is calculated by using Bazett's formula, which is accomplished by dividing the measured QT interval by the square root of the RR interval. A low serum magnesium level may intensify the findings in hypocalcemia. A prolonged QTc interval also is seen in syndromes that are associated with life-threatening ventricular arrhythmias. The diagnosis of congenital long QT syndrome is made by evaluating specific criteria, which include ECG findings, with clinical and family history.

An elevated serum potassium level is characterized electrocardiographically by peaked, elevated T waves, and indicates serum potassium valves of greater than 7.0 mEq/L. Higher values of serum potassium widen the QRS and decrease the amplitude of the complexes. Decreased serum potassium values lower the T waves and cause the appearance of U waves as serum values become less than 2.5 mEq/L.

Rhythm Disturbances

Paroxysmal Supraventricular Tachycardia. Paroxysmal supraventricular tachycardia in infants is a rhythm disturbance characterized by heart rates of between 240 and 300 beats per minute. Although short bursts of tachyarrhythmia can be tolerated without clinical difficulty, episodes lasting for 24 hours or more can lead to low-output congestive heart failure. If the arrhythmia occurs in an infant with underlying structural heart disease, tolerance for the rapid heart action is decreased. The diagnosis is established by observing a rapid ventricular response with a normal QRS duration (Fig. 53.10). On cessation of the tachycardia, one should look for evidence of preexcitation, involving bridges of muscle between the atria and the ventricles so that impulses can reach the ventricles via two pathways, the normal AV nodal tract and the aberrant pathway. Early but slow excitation of the ventricles occurs, producing a delta wave and the short PR interval. The QRS interval is prolonged as a result of a delay in ventricular activation via the normal and aberrant pathways. Wolff-Parkinson-White syndrome is the most common form of ventricular preexcitation, and although it often is discovered in a structurally normal heart, it does have a higher prevalence in Ebstein anomaly (5% to 15%), and L-loop transposition of the great arteries (up to 5%).

The treatment of the supraventricular tachycardia requires conversion to a sinus rhythm and prevention of further attacks. The patient with a life-threatening tachyarrhythmia should have an indwelling venous line for the administration of drugs and fluids, and the ECG should be monitored continuously during interventions. Adenosine, administered intravenously, is the principal pharmacologic agent used to manage the tachyarrhythmia acutely. If the infant is seriously ill and does not respond to adenosine, synchronized cardioversion should be attempted to restore a normal heart rate quickly. These infants usually require medication to prevent recurrences for at least the first 6 months to 1 year of life, and beta-blockers are the first-line agent of choice. Digoxin has fallen out of favor due to the potential increased risk of sudden cardiac death if Wolff-Parkinson-White syndrome is present.

Ventricular Tachycardia. A tachycardia of ventricular origin is characterized by a wide QRS complex tachyarrhythmia (Fig. 53.11). Although supraventricular tachycardia with aberrancy can produce a similar QRS picture, all wide-QRS tachycar-

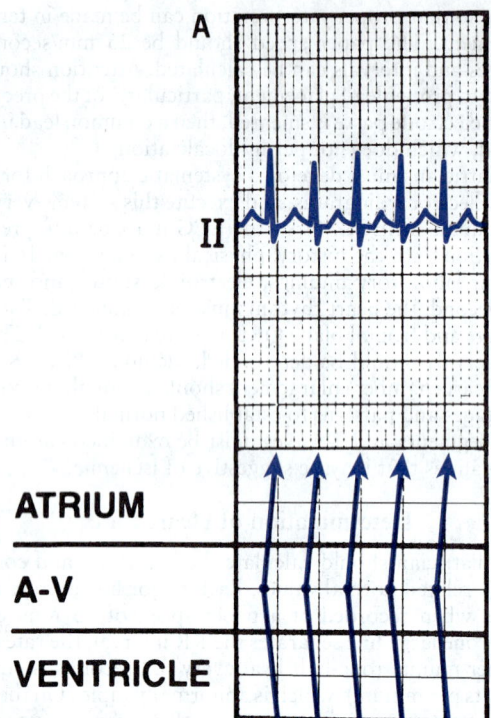

FIGURE 53.10. Supraventricular tachycardia at 290 beats per minute. There are no visible P waves. The P wave probably falls within the QRS complex. In the lower diagram, the dot indicates probable origin of the impulse from the atrioventricular (AV) junction, with retrograde spread to the atrium and antegrade spread through the ventricles. The QRS morphology is normal. This is a reentry-type tachycardia. (Reproduced with permission from Garson A Jr. *The electrocardiogram in infants and children: a systemic approach.* Philadelphia: Lea & Febiger, 1983: 238.)

dias should be considered ventricular in origin until proven otherwise. This tachycardia usually is associated with serious underlying heart disease or overwhelming infection, and it demands prompt therapy. Appropriate management in this situation depends on the infant's clinical status. When perfusion is compromised acutely, direct-current cardioversion is necessary. The initiation of lidocaine or amiodarone infusion should be considered. The diagnosis and management of life-threatening arrhythmias requires prompt consultation with a pediatric cardiologist to provide for both acute and long-term management.

Bradycardia. Regular persistent bradycardia with heart rates of less than 50 beats per minute may be vagally induced. The next most common cause of regular persistent bradycardia is nonconducted atrial bigeminy. Complete AV block also should be considered. If the infant has signs of decreased cardiac output, temporizing measures may include infusions of atropine or isoproterenol or transcutaneous or transvenous pacing.

Third-degree (complete) heart block with a heart rate of less than 60 beats per minute usually is congenital in origin. It may occur as an isolated event or in association with congenital cardiac disease. Historically, a strong association has been

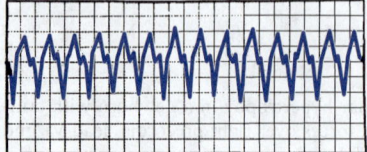
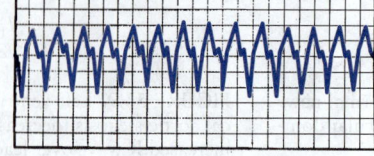

FIGURE 53.11. Wide QRS tachycardia (rate 280) indicative of ventricular origin in a newborn infant.

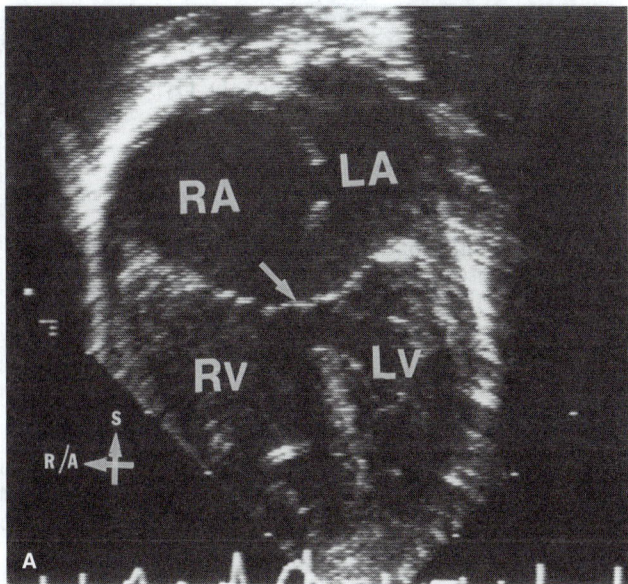 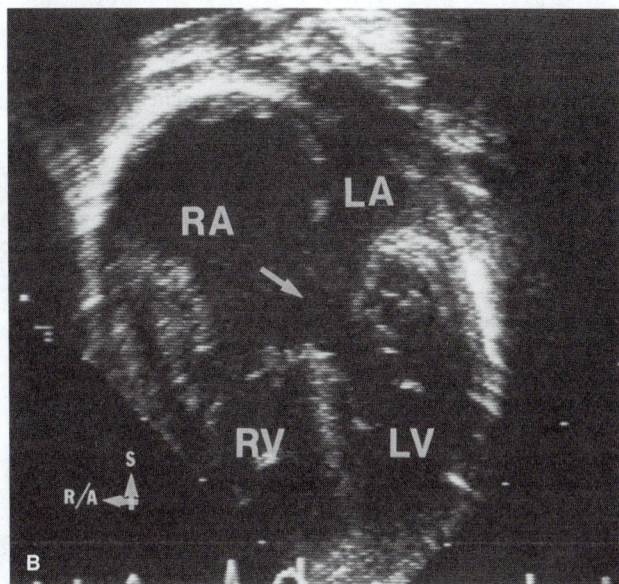

FIGURE 53.12. Four-chamber view in atrioventricular septal defect. **A:** Systole, showing common AV valve (*arrow*) and **B:** diastole, showing complete AV septal defect (*arrow*). LA, left atrium; LV, left ventricle; RA, right atrium; RV, right ventricle; R/A, rightward/anterior; S, superior.

observed between isolated complete heart block and maternal lupus erythematosus. However, recent studies have shown that infants born to mothers of other undifferentiated connective tissue disease and Sjögren's syndrome may have a higher incidence of delivering an infant with complete heart block. Therefore, rheumatologic disorders should be sought in the mother of any infant who presents with complete heart block, even if the mother does not have manifestations of the disease. A significant minority of neonates require ventricular pacing due to signs of low cardiac output. Specific indications for pacing include: (a) resting awake heart rate of less than 50 to 55 beats per minute, (b) wide, complex escape mechanism, (c) ventricular ectopy or (d) signs of congestive heart failure. In the presence of significant congenital heart disease, especially heterotaxy syn-

dromes, pacing is virtually always necessary. Even in the setting of less complex congenital heart defects (atrial septal defects, ventricular septal defects), the additional volume overload in this setting may precipitate congestive heart failure.

ECHOCARDIOGRAPHY

The use of echocardiography, in consultation with an experienced pediatric cardiologist, has had a significant impact on the evaluation and treatment of neonates with suspected cardiac disease. The noninvasive, portable nature of the equipment, along with the anatomic and physiologic information obtained from tomographic and Doppler imaging (Figs. 53.12 and 53.13), results in a rapid, safe, and accurate assessment of the neonatal patient. Through tomographic imaging, the segments of the heart, their connections, and any malformations are identified. The combination of tomographic imaging with Doppler echocardiography provides information on cardiac function and the severity of particular lesions. For example, one can use Doppler echocardiography to estimate the pressure gradient across the aortic valve. In critical aortic stenosis and low cardiac output, however, the left ventricle may not be capable of shortening with enough force to generate a large gradient, despite the severe nature of the lesion.

Echocardiograms should be performed and interpreted by personnel experienced in pediatric echocardiography because of the complexity encountered in congenital heart disease as well as the transitional circulation of the neonate. Under certain circumstances, this may mean transferring the patient to a pediatric cardiology center. An alternative to transferring the patient may be the use of teleconferencing, in which a pediatric cardiologist can supervise and review an echocardiographic study, a physical examination, and other diagnostic studies over large distances through the combination of video, telephone, and computer technology.

In addition to the evaluation of structural heart disease, echocardiography is important in the evaluation of noncardiac diseases. For the neonate with persistent pulmonary hypertension, echocardiography is used to ensure that no primary cardiac basis exists for the clinical presentation, such as obstructed pulmonary venous return or transposition of the great

FIGURE 53.13. Short axis view of D-transposition of the great arteries and ventricular septal defect (*arrow*). Aorta arises from right ventricle, while pulmonary artery arises from left ventricle. A, anterior; AO, aorta; LV, left ventricular; PA, pulmonary artery; RV, right ventricle; S, superior.

arteries. Technologic advances in echocardiography, including three-dimensional echocardiography and contrast echocardiography, will likely increase the importance of ultrasound in the evaluation of the newborn. In addition, magnetic resonance imaging and computerized tomography scanning may reveal additional critical findings in the newborn cardiac evaluation.

CRITICAL CARDIAC DISEASE IN THE INFANT

Life-threatening cardiac disease in the newborn infant occurs in about 3 of 1,000 live births. Of all cardiac conditions capable of producing cardiac failure or severe hypoxemia that were surveyed in New England, eight conditions accounted for about 75% of the total. These included ventricular septal defects, PDA, transposition of the great arteries, tetralogy of Fallot, hypoplastic right-heart syndrome (tricuspid and pulmonary atresia), critical pulmonary stenosis with right-to-left atrial shunting, hypoplastic left-heart syndrome, and coarctation of the aorta. When these lesions are classified on the basis of their fundamental physiologic disturbance, they fall into three major categories; these categories include (a) hypoxemia (transposition, tetralogy, hypoplastic right-heart syndrome, and critical pulmonic stenosis), (b) impaired systemic perfusion (hypoplastic left-heart syndrome and coarctation), and (c) the large-volume left-to-right shunt (ventricular septal defect, PDA). Additional life-threatening situations of importance in the differential diagnosis include common mixing lesions (single ventricle, common atrium, truncus arteriosus), anomalies of pulmonary venous return, and persistent pulmonary hypertension.

Hypoxemic States

Patients with severe hypoxemia represent an exceedingly important group with critical cardiac disease. The clinical focus is

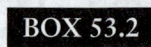

BOX 53.2   **Subgroups of the Hypoxemic Patient Population**

1. Severe outflow obstruction to pulmonary blood flow with intracardiac right-to-left shunting (via a ventricular defect or an atrial communication)
2. Transposition of the great arteries with usually normal to increased pulmonary perfusion
3. Obstruction to pulmonary venous return with pulmonary venous congestion plus obligatory right-to-left atrial shunting
4. Common mixing lesions such as truncus arteriosus, single ventricle, and single atrium. This latter group may have augmented pulmonary blood flow, or diminished pulmonary flow if an element of pulmonary stenosis is present

on the degree of cyanosis, with arterial oxygen tensions usually under 35 mm Hg (saturation <75%). It is extremely important that the clinician recognize the presence of hypoxemia so that safe transportation to a pediatric cardiovascular center can be achieved. The hypoxemic patient population can be categorized further into four major subgroups, listed in Box 53.2.

The chest film, along with the ECG, pulse oximetry, blood gas tensions, and pH level, provide vital data that usually permit physiologic definition of the patient's problem.

Patients whose hypoxemia is the result of severe obstruction to pulmonary blood flow along with a right-to-left intracardiac shunt include those with tetralogy of Fallot (Fig. 53.14A), pulmonary atresia and an intact ventricular septum (right-to-left atrial communication), and tricuspid atresia. The latter two conditions constitute the hypoplastic right-heart

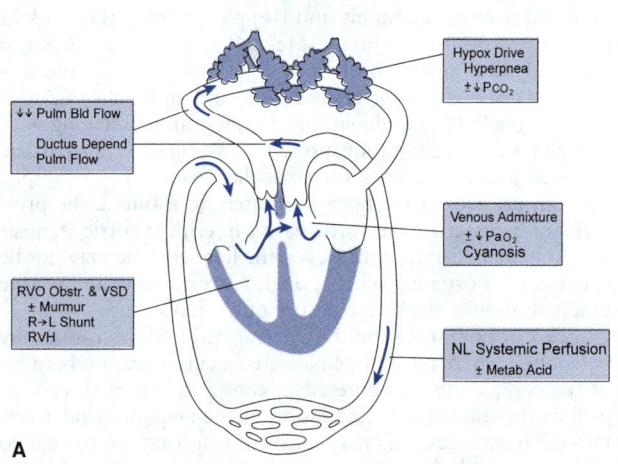

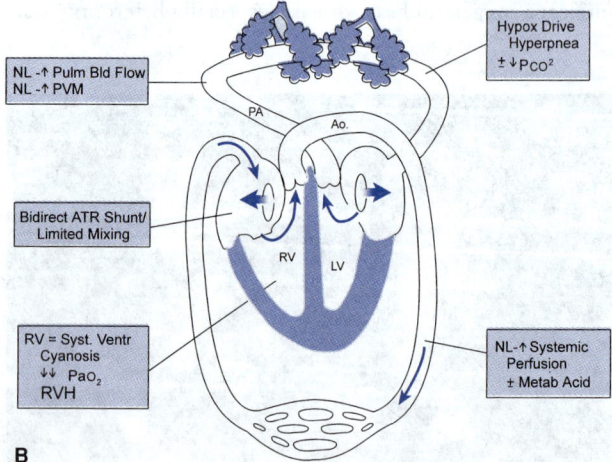

FIGURE 53.14. A-B: Right-to-left shunt. This diagram shows an example of severe right ventricular outflow obstruction (RVO obstr.) and a ventricular septal defect (VSD). There is limited pulmonary blood flow and mixing of oxygenated pulmonary venous blood with systemic venous blood (venous admixture), resulting in hypoxemia. In the newborn, as shown here, some or all of the effects of hypoxemia on respiratory function and systemic perfusion are shown. **B:** Transposition of the great arteries. In the presence of transposed great arteries, most of the systemic venous blood recirculates through the pulmonary circulation with limited mixing into the systemic circulation. The resultant effects of severe hypoxemia on ventilation and systemic perfusion are shown. Hypox, hypoxemic; NL, normal; ventr, ventricle; LV, left ventricle; RV, right ventricle; art, artery; pulm, pulmonary; bld, blood; R, right; L, left; RVH, right ventricular hypertrophy; PVM, pulmonary vascular markings. (Reproduced with permission from Talner NS, Lister G. Recognition of critical cardiac disease in the infant. In: Warshaw JB, Hobbins JC, eds. *Principles and practice of perinatal medicine: maternal, fetal, and newborn care.* Menlo Park, CA: Addison-Wesley, 1983:371.)

syndrome, with a dominant left ventricle. Lung perfusion is via the ductus arteriosus or aorta-pulmonary collaterals in the case of pulmonary atresia, and through a ventricular communication or ductus arteriosus in tricuspid atresia.

When pulmonary perfusion is compromised, and a marked reduction occurs in arterial oxygen tension, the use of prostaglandin E_1 (PGE_1) infusion to dilate the ductus arteriosus can produce striking improvement in the state of oxygenation. This can result in the correction of metabolic acidemia and stabilization of the clinical state, which in turn will permit safe transportation of the infant to a pediatric cardiovascular center. Infants with severe hypoxemia caused by any of these conditions require surgical intervention or balloon valvuloplasty to improve pulmonary blood flow (repair, shunt operations, or relief of outflow obstruction).

The diagnosis of transposition of the great arteries should be suspected in any infant with a low arterial oxygen saturation and a radiographic picture showing normal to slightly increased pulmonary vascularity. With simple transposition, the fundamental problem is impaired intracardiac and extracardiac mixing of the systemic venous and pulmonary venous streams. The result is a systemic circulation of primarily systemic venous blood, while the pulmonary circuit carries the well-oxygenated pulmonary venous return (Fig. 53.14B). What limited mixing occurs usually takes place at the level of the foramen ovale and ductus arteriosus, but is clearly inadequate. Suspicion of the diagnosis demands immediate echocardiographic confirmation. In the past, these infants were palliated by balloon atrial septostomy followed by an atrial switch operation (Mustard, Senning), usually at around 3 to 6 months of age. Over the last 15 years, the arterial switch operation has become the operative procedure of choice. This approach is carried out in the first weeks of life, and relatively long-term follow-up studies indicate excellent results. The pathophysiologic features of the common hypoxemic lesions (obstruction to lung blood flow and transposition) are shown in Figure 53.14.

Anomalies of pulmonary venous return, particularly if they are associated with pulmonary venous obstruction, must be considered in the differential diagnosis of hypoxemic infants with respiratory distress (lung infection, persistent pulmonary hypertension and transposition). These anomalies of pulmonary venous connection result developmentally from failure of incorporation of the common pulmonary vein into the left atrium, with persistence of primitive embryonic connections to system veins (cardinal system), omphalomesenteric veins (portal system), or direct connections to the right atrium. The possibility of pulmonary venous obstruction exists when the abnormal connection is via a long pathway, as in connections to the portal circuit, where two microcirculations must be traversed (pulmonary and hepatic). The possibility of venous obstruction also exists when the connection is supradiaphragmatic as a result of intrinsic pulmonary venous obstruction (stenosis), or when the ascending vertical vein is caught in a hemodynamic vise between the pulmonary artery and the left bronchus.

The only access to the left heart in these conditions of anomalies of pulmonary venous return usually is via the foramen ovale or atrial septal defect. This results in hypoxemia of varying severity. If no pulmonary venous obstruction is present, pulmonary blood flow exceeds systemic flow and arterial desaturation is minimal. Signs of congestive heart failure dominate the clinical picture, and the clinical expression is similar to that encountered in a large-volume left-to-right shunt with a delay in clinical presentation. When pulmonary venous obstruction is present, however, presentation is earlier and hypoxemia is more pronounced. With pulmonary venous obstruction, pulmonary edema is severe, because of the entrapment of blood in the pulmonary circuit. This produces the classic radiographic picture of hazy lung fields (lung edema) with a heart that is

relatively normal in size (reflecting pulmonary venous entrapment outside the heart; see Fig. 53.6C). A slight delay in clinical presentation may occur when the ductus arteriosus remains patent. This will mask the presence of pulmonary venous obstruction, but significant hypoxemia still will be present. This condition can be confused with persistent pulmonary hypertension and transposition of the great arteries, and, therefore, demands early and careful echocardiographic assessment to define the pathway of pulmonary venous return and the position of the great arteries.

When a common mixing chamber exists, the clinical picture is dependent on the status of pulmonary and systemic perfusion. For example, if a single ventricle is the basic underlying lesion, the clinical picture will be dominated by hypoxemia in the presence of obstruction to pulmonary blood flow. Congestive heart failure will develop, however, if pulmonary vascular resistance falls postnatally and a large pulmonary blood flow is present. Infants with truncus arteriosus will have peripheral signs of a runoff into the pulmonary circulation, with bounding arterial pulsations and a wide pulse pressure similar to that seen with a PDA. Unlike in PDA, a significant decrease in arterial oxygen tension will result from the confluence of the well-oxygenated and poorly oxygenated streams at the ventricular and truncal level. The common mixing lesions represent complex malformations and therefore precise diagnosis on purely clinical grounds usually is not possible. Two-dimensional echocardiography using Doppler color flow mapping, however, permits a noninvasive diagnosis. Palliative or corrective surgery is in order, depending on the underlying defect.

Pulmonary hypertension of the newborn or persistence of the fetal circulation is a syndrome of multiple etiologies that produces hypoxemia in the first few days of life. This often is confused with certain congenital heart malformations, particularly transposition and anomalies of pulmonary venous return and right ventricular outflow obstruction. It has been associated with neonatal asphyxia, meconium aspiration, diaphragmatic hernias and lung hypoplasia, hyperviscosity states, pneumonia, and lung hemorrhage. A primary disorder of the pulmonary vascular bed with increased muscularization of the distal pulmonary vessels has been described. The hypoxemia and pulmonary hypertension are linked closely, with right-to-left shunting via the ductus arteriosus, foramen ovale, or intrapulmonary vessels possible. Again, a precise diagnosis is required, because multiple factors may produce these physiologic alterations. Therefore, an echocardiogram to define the status of the pulmonary venous connection and the position of the great arteries is mandatory.

Low Perfusion States

Clinical signs of impaired systemic perfusion dominate in the face of critical obstruction of the left heart (coarctation and interruption of the aortic arch, hypoplastic left-heart syndrome, aortic stenosis), disorders primarily affecting ventricular contractility (myocarditis, cardiomyopathies, birth asphyxia), and situations in which ventricular filling is impaired (tachyarrhythmias, pericardial disease). These signs include diminished pulses, cold extremities, poor capillary refill, and generalized pallor accompanied by a metabolic acidosis. Such observations demand prompt evaluation aimed at defining the nature of the underlying problem and interventions designed to restore cardiac output and systemic perfusion.

Coarctation of the aorta is the most frequently encountered cardiovascular malformation that may produce a life-threatening low perfusion state. The natural history of this malformation has been documented, with the clinical expression dependent on the patency or constriction of the ductus arteriosus. In utero, the basic lesion is a posterior shelf of media and intima that is located opposite the ductus arteriosus. The open ductus permits unobstructed blood flow across the aortic isthmus into the descending aorta. Postnatally, a similar situation exists until the ductus arteriosus undergoes postnatal constriction at its aortic mouth. As long as the aortic mouth of the ductus is open, femoral pulses will be palpable and blood pressure relationships will be normal. Signs of severely compromised systemic perfusion quickly follow ductal obliteration as the left ventricle faces an acute increase in afterload. A similar pathophysiologic picture exists with critical aortic stenosis. The clinical picture is that of an acute shocklike state, often confused with overwhelming infection.

The clinician always must keep in mind that the acute development of a low output state commonly may occur secondary to left heart obstructive lesions such as coarctation, interruption of the aortic arch, and the hypoplastic left heart syndrome. In the latter, all systemic perfusion is dependent on the patency of the ductus arteriosus. When this channel constricts, systemic blood is curtailed and the clinical picture deteriorates rapidly. This occurs despite a rising arterial oxygen tension as the consequence of a high pulmonary–to–systemic blood flow ratio. The use of oxygen inhalation in these infants must be closely monitored, because any increase in oxygen tension will constrict the ductus arteriosus further, adding to the compromise in tissue blood flow in the presence of a ductal-dependent lesion. The use of a ductus arteriosus dilator such as PGE_1 may prove lifesaving, through restoring the perfusion of the systemic circulation. Other therapeutic interventions include the use of the titratable inotropic agents such as dopamine or dobutamine. These improve ventricular contractility, which usually is severely compromised, and provide peripheral vasodilatation as well. After the patient is stabilized, intervention is necessary to remove the mechanical obstruction to the systemic circulation. This may take the form of a surgical repair of a coarctation lesion, balloon valvuloplasty in critical aortic stenosis, or radical palliative surgical procedures or heart transplantation for aortic atresia. The pathophysiology of severe left heart obstructive disease is depicted in Figure 53.15.

The clinical picture of diminished systemic perfusion also may be encountered in neonatal states associated with birth asphyxia, and may be confused with the lesions just described. In addition to the effects on the pulmonary circulation (vasoconstriction), a fall in the pH level, elevation of P_aCO_2, and

a decrease in oxygen tension may impair myocardial contractility. As a result, peripheral perfusion will diminish with the development of a metabolic acidemia. Transient myocardial ischemia secondary to neonatal asphyxial events has been described. This is accompanied by electrocardiographic evidence of myocardial ischemia (ST-T wave changes) and enzymatic changes consisting of elevation of the myocardial CPK and troponin-T levels that are indicative of cardiac muscle damage. On rare occasions, true myocardial infarction may occur, although these infants usually recover without residual myocardial impairment. Echocardiographic assessment of this group of infants has shown diminished systolic function, which improves with the administration of inotropic agents and the use of vasodilators to decrease the afterload on the poorly functioning myocardium. Similar physiologic abnormalities occur with inflammatory diseases of the myocardium, such as viral myocarditis.

Although rare, newborns with inherited disorders of fatty acid utilization (e.g., carnitine deficiency), pyruvate metabolism (e.g., pyruvate dehydrogenase deficiency), and mitochondrial function (e.g., cytochrome deficiencies, X-linked cardiomyopathy) may have a metabolic acidemia and low systemic perfusion. New insights into these diseases have been gained by the application of new methodologies in molecular and cellular biology.

Tachyarrhythmias, either supraventricular or ventricular, are another group of conditions that may present with significant compromise of systemic blood flow. (See section, Rythm Disturbances.) Without underlying heart disease, a heart rate of between 280 and 300 beats per minute can be tolerated for about 24 hours, after which systemic perfusion is impaired critically as a result of inadequate ventricular filling.

Pericardial disease, usually inflammatory or with tumors, also may produce signs of low perfusion secondary to the rapid accumulation of fluid in the pericardial sac that interferes with cardiac filling. Cardiac tamponade can be recognized by a decrease in, or loss of, peripheral pulses with inspiration, with a return of pulse volume on expiration. Diagnosis is confirmed by echocardiography, after which fluid must be evacuated from the pericardial space. The material should be Gram-stained and cultured, and appropriate surgical drainage should be provided. Tumors of the pericardium may produce a similar picture.

EVALUATION ALGORITHMS OF CRITICAL CARDIAC DISEASE IN THE NEWBORN

In an attempt to aid the clinician in detecting and stabilizing the newborn infant who may have critical cardiac disease, we have developed three algorithms that focus on specific, possibly life-threatening clinical problems. These include alterations in heart rate; hypoxemia, as verified by pulse oximetry; and decreased systemic perfusion. If the clinician follows the decision tree pathway outlined in these algorithms, key high-risk situations usually can be diagnosed and appropriate management undertaken.

Heart Rate Abnormalities

Regular persistent bradycardia with heart rates of less than 50 beats per minute may be vagally induced. The next most common cause of regular persistent bradycardia is nonconducted atrial bigeminy. Complete AV block also should be considered. If the infant has signs of decreased cardiac output, temporizing

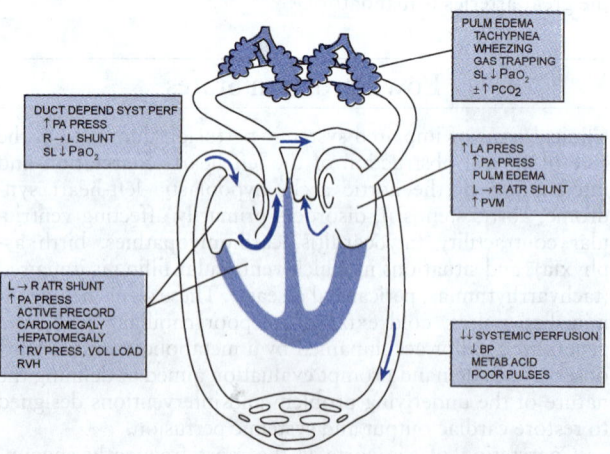

FIGURE 53.15. Pathophysiology of critical left ventricular obstructive disease emphasizing the key roles of the ductus arteriosus and foramen ovale in providing systemic perfusion and decompression of the left heart.

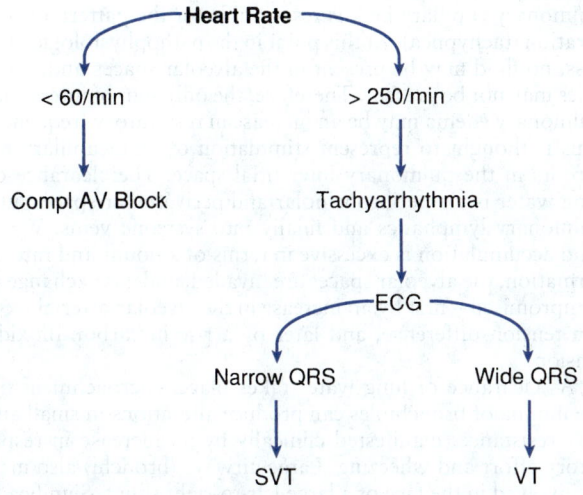

FIGURE 53.16. Decision tree in which heart rate is the entry point. See text for a detailed explanation of management options. SVT, supraventricular tachycardia; VT, ventricular tachycardia; AV, atrioventricular; ECG, electrocardiogram.

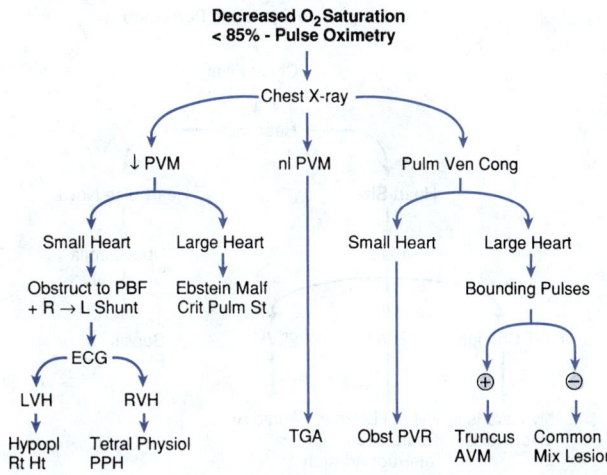

FIGURE 53.17. Decision tree in which a low oxygen saturation as verified by pulse oximetry is the entry point. See text for a detailed explanation of management options. PVM, pulmonary vascular markings; PBF, pulmonary blood flow; pulm ven cong, pulmonary venous congestion; Ebstein malf, Ebstein malformation; crit pulm st, critical pulmonic stenosis; hypopl rt ht, hypoplastic right heart; tetral physiol, tetralogy physiology; PPH, persistent pulonary hypertension; TGA, transposition of the great arteries; obst PVR, obstruction to pulmonary venous return; AVM, arteriovenous malformation; nl, normal; ECG, electrocardiogram; R, right; L, left.

measures may include infusions of atropine or isoproterenol or transcutaneous or transvenous pacing.

With heart rates greater than 240 beats per minute, the most likely diagnosis is supraventricular tachycardia. The QRS duration is normal in this situation. As cited previously, intravenous adenosine is the treatment of choice, followed by a beta-blocker as the agent for preventing recurrences. If a wide-complex tachycardia is present, this must be assumed to be ventricular tachycardia. Appropriate management in this situation depends on the infant's status. When perfusion is compromised acutely, direct-current cardioversion is necessary. The presence of ventricular tachycardia usually is associated with significant underlying heart disease, such as myocarditis; therefore, management is complex and should be performed at a regional cardiovascular center. Rarely, the infant may have no change in circulatory dynamics, despite a persistent ventricular tachycardia. Nevertheless, these infants need precise electrophysiologic evaluation and possibly pharmacologic treatment. The algorithm for heart rate abnormalities is shown in Figure 53.16.

Hypoxemia

When the presenting problem is hypoxemia, as verified by pulse oximetry, a chest film must be obtained to assess pulmonary vascularity. If the pulmonary vascular markings are reduced, the fundamental physiologic abnormality is obstruction to pulmonary blood flow with a right-to-left shunt. An ECG permits the delineation between the hypoplastic right heart, such as pulmonary or tricuspid atresia (left ventricular hypertrophy), and tetralogy physiology with right ventricular dominance. We recognize that some infants have persistent pulmonary hypertension with right-to-left shunting via fetal flow channels. Nevertheless, these infants must be assessed at a regional center, and echocardiography is essential to rule out a cardiac cause for the elevated pulmonary vascular resistance. If the pulmonary vascular markings are decreased in the face of massive cardiac enlargement, then Ebstein malformation of the tricuspid valve or critical pulmonary valve stenosis should be considered.

When the pulmonary vascular markings are normal in association with a low O_2 saturation, transposition of the great arteries must be considered, particularly if the O_2 saturation is less than 65%. On the other hand, if the heart is small, but prominent pulmonary venous congestion is present, then the

diagnosis of obstructed pulmonary venous return with right-to-left atrial shunting should be entertained.

With each of these hypoxemic states, an increase in O_2 saturation may be obtained by the intravenous administration of PGE_1. These infants require ventilation for transport and venous access to administer the pharmacologic agent and to provide volume if the systemic blood pressure falls. Irrespective of the diagnosis, the use of PGE_1 should stabilize the infant, as long as volume is provided as necessary to maintain systemic perfusion and adequate ventilation is maintained. On arrival at a cardiac center, a definitive diagnosis can be made through a review of laboratory and clinical data and through the use of echocardiography.

When cardiac enlargement and prominent pulmonary vascular markings are present in the face of an element of hypoxemia, a common mixing lesion such as truncus arteriosus or single ventricle, or a large arteriovenous malformation should be considered. If the pulses are prominent, truncus arteriosus or an arteriovenous malformation are distinct possibilities. Presentation within the first few hours with a large heart should encourage a search for a cranial or hepatic bruit.

The algorithm for the cyanosis decision pathway is shown in Figure 53.17.

Low Perfusion States

The third high-risk situation concerns those infants with clinical signs of low systemic perfusion. For these patients, the differential diagnosis rests between a primary cardiovascular problem and hypovolemia, perhaps in association with septicemia. The chest film is an extremely helpful clinical aid. If cardiomegaly and lung congestion are present, then left-heart obstructive lesions or myoepicardial disease are likely. When the heart size is normal, hypovolemia is likely, with sepsis being an important consideration.

The ECG provides additional data on which to base a specific diagnosis. Abnormalities in heart rate can lead to decreased systemic perfusion, and must be considered. Primary

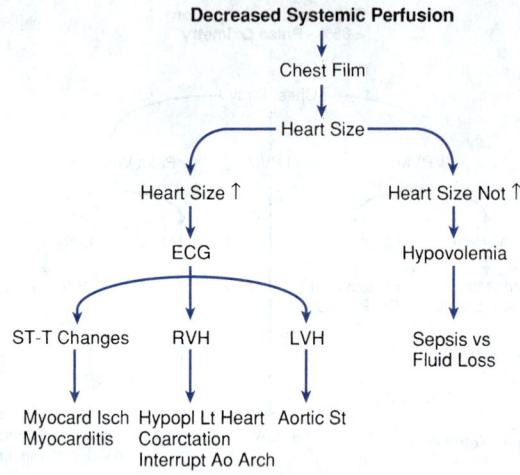

Decreased Systemic Perfusion

↓

Chest Film

↓

Heart Size

Heart Size ↑   Heart Size Not ↑

ECG   Hypovolemia

ST-T Changes   RVH   LVH   Sepsis vs
                                  Fluid Loss

Myocard Isch   Hypopl Lt Heart   Aortic St
Myocarditis   Coarctation
               Interrupt Ao Arch

FIGURE 53.18. Decision tree in which decreased systemic perfusion is the entry point. See text for details of management options. ECG, electrocardiogram; RVH, right ventricular hypertrophy; LVH, left ventricular hypertrophy; myocard isch, myocardial ischemia; hypopl lt heart, hypoplastic left heart; interrupt ao arch, interruption of the aortic arch; aortic st, aortic stenosis.

ST-T wave changes raise the possibility of myocardial ischemia, usually secondary to birth asphyxia. Myocardial enzymes should be determined as verification of myocardial damage. Right ventricular hypertrophy in association with low systemic perfusion is seen with hypoplastic left heart syndrome, coarctation of the aorta, and interruption of the aortic arch. Left ventricular hypertrophy may be seen with critical aortic stenosis, because obstruction took place *in utero* and left ventricular hypertrophy ensued. With hypoplastic left heart, coarctation, and interruption of the aorta, no obstruction takes place until the ductus arteriosus constricts and, therefore, insufficient time has elapsed for ventricular hypertrophy to develop.

The stabilization and transport of this group of infants also requires venous access, withdrawal of blood for blood gas determinations and pH levels, and blood cultures to rule out a septic process. PGE$_1$ can be administered safely via an umbilical venous line to dilate the ductus arteriosus and improve systemic perfusion. As mentioned previously, caution regarding the use of oxygen is in order, because the ductus can be constricted as oxygen tension rises, and this will compromise systemic perfusion further.

Ventilatory support is necessary in this group, because apnea may occur with PGE$_1$ administration. Antibiotic coverage for appropriate gram-positive and -negative organisms is indicated until a septic process has been ruled out. Myocardial support is best provided by an infusion of dopamine or dobutamine. The algorithm for low perfusion states is shown in Figure 53.18.

The Large-Volume Left-to-Right Shunt

In contrast to these acute life-threatening situations, the clinical problems that are secondary to a large communication at the ventricular or great artery level develop gradually over the first months of life as a result of the postnatal fall in pulmonary vascular resistance, which permits a large increase in pulmonary blood flow. This occurs in response to remodeling of the pulmonary vascular bed, with an increase in lumen diameter and a decrease in blood viscosity as hemoglobin levels diminish. As pulmonary blood flow increases, the major clinical manifestations become apparent and reflect altered respiratory function. The accumulation of water in the pulmonary interstitial space, the site of the initial leak of fluid from the

pulmonary capillary bed, is responsible for the pattern of respiration (tachypnea). At this point in the pathophysiologic process, no fluid may be present in the alveolar spaces and, thus, râles may not be present. Therefore, the only sign of interstitial pulmonary edema may be an increase in respiratory frequency. This is thought to represent stimulation of juxtacapillary receptors in the pulmonary interstitial space. The clearance of lung water is via peribronchiolar and perivascular spaces into pulmonary lymphatics and finally into systemic veins. When fluid accumulation is excessive in terms of amount and rate of formation, the alveolar spaces are invaded, and gas exchange is compromised—first by an increase in the alveolar-arterial oxygen tension difference, and later by a rise in carbon dioxide tension.

As clearance of lung water takes place, encroachment on the lumina of bronchioles can produce alterations in small airway resistance, manifested clinically by an increase in respiratory effort and wheezing. Large airways (bronchi) also may be involved in the face of a large left-to-right shunt. Significant bronchial compression by hypertensive, volume-distended pulmonary arteries and an enlarged left atrium and ventricle has been noted. The sites of predilection are the left main stem bronchus and the left upper and right middle lobe bronchi. Lobar atelectasis and obstructive emphysema secondary to these compressive effects may contribute to impairment of gas exchange, which may in turn increase pulmonary vascular resistance. In addition, secondary infection may occur at sites of compromised fluid drainage. The increase in the work of breathing raises oxygen requirements for these infants at the same time that the respiratory problems interfere with feeding. The result is a decrease in intake at a time when metabolic requirements are elevated. All these factors may contribute to the failure of these infants to grow.

Although respiratory signs tend to dominate the clinical picture, major alterations in the performance of the heart and systemic circulation occur as well. Systolic function of the myocardium usually is normal to supranormal. This is the result of increased adrenergic support, as evidenced by an increased heart rate and contractility, and by elevated levels of circulating catecholamines. A high cardiac output state exists, with most of the output, however, flowing from the left-to-right into the pulmonary circulation.

The systemic circulation also is altered by the left-to-right shunt. A redistribution of systemic blood flow occurs, with perfusion of the skin, kidneys, and gastrointestinal tract potentially decreased by regional vasoconstriction. From the clinical standpoint, this manifests as skin pallor and reduced urine formation. The compromise of mesenteric blood flow may result in ischemic gut necrosis, particularly in the preterm infant with a large PDA. Peripheral vasoconstriction occurs as part of the increased adrenergic response that appears to redistribute cardiac output to the more vital organ systems (myocardium, brain).

The overall metabolic response to a large left-to-right shunt is variable. Initially, these infants may be hypermetabolic, creating a situation in which demands are increased in the face of limited supply. In the more chronic stages, oxygen consumption may fall, indicating a severe compromise of oxygen supply.

A number of compensatory mechanisms also operate in the face of the large-volume left-to-right shunt. These include the previously cited increase in adrenergic activity, the renin-angiotensin-aldosterone support mechanism, atrial natriuretic peptide, and alterations in the oxygen affinity of red blood cells. The adrenergic mechanisms result in tachycardia and enhanced contractility (beta$_1$ effect), and the redistribution of cardiac output represents peripheral vasoconstriction (alpha$_1$ effect). The renin-angiotensin-aldosterone system triggered by a decrease in renal perfusion represents an attempt to preserve systemic volume. This decrease in renal perfusion leads

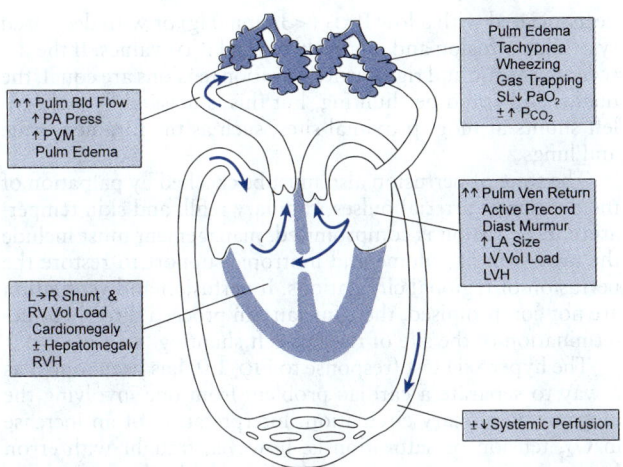

Pulm Bld Flow ↑↑ Pulm Bld Flow / ↑ PA Press / ↑ PVM / Pulm Edema

Pulm Edema / Tachypnea / Wheezing / Gas Trapping / SL↓ PaO_2 / ± ↑ PCO_2

↑↑ Pulm Ven Return / Active Precord / Diast Murmur / ↑ LA Size / LV Vol Load / LVH

L→R Shunt & / RV Vol Load / Cardiomegaly / ± Hepatomegaly / RVH

± ↓ Systemic Perfusion

FIGURE 53.19. Large-volume left-to-right shunt. This figure shows the pathophysiologic consequences of cardiac malformation in the neonate. Flow of blood through the heart and the systemic and pulmonary circulations is shown by the large arrows, and the relative volume of flow is shown by the width of the arrows. This diagram is an example of a large left-to-right shunt at the ventricular level causing excessive pulmonary blood flow and pulmonary venous return. Compromised respiratory function is present, along with extra demands on the ventricles and potentially inadequate systemic perfusion. ↑, increased; ↓, decreased; pulm, pulmonary; bld, blood flow; PA, pulmonary arterial; press, pressure; PVM, pulmonary vascular markings; L → R, left-to-right; RV vol, right ventricular volume; RVH, right ventricular hypertrophy; SL, slightly; ±, occasionally; ven, venous; precord, precordium; diast, diastolic; LA, left atrial; LV vol, left ventricular volume; LVH, left ventricular hypertrophy. (Reproduced with permission from Talner NS, Lister G. The recognition of critical cardiac disease in the infant. In: Warshaw JB, Hobbins JC, eds. *Pathophysiology of cardiac disease in the infant.* Menlo Park, CA: Addison-Wesley, 1983:366.)

to angiotensin formation, which, acting on the renal cortex, results in the production of aldosterone. Salt and water retention occurs in an attempt to preserve intravascular volume. The release of atrial natriuretic factor consequent to atrial distention in these patients may result in diuresis, but the exact function of this substance remains to be delineated. Oxygen delivery can be enhanced by alterations in red blood cell 2,3-diphosphoglycerate (2,3-DPG). This results in increased release of oxygen to the tissues at any given level of oxygen saturation.

Figure 53.19 depicts the pathophysiology of a large-volume left-to-right shunt at the ventricular level (a large PDA would be similar), incorporating the material covered in this section.

SPECIAL PROBLEMS IN MANAGEMENT

Congestive Heart Failure

The treatment of congestive heart failure in the newborn must take into consideration the age-related differences in myocardial performance cited previously (which may influence the adaptation of the cardiovascular system), possible developmental differences in the response to pharmacologic agents, and the potential modulating influences of the fetal flow pathways and the pulmonary circulation. Appropriate management requires a precise anatomic and physiologic diagnosis, and may require support of lung as well as cardiac function. In most instances, reparative or palliative surgical procedures, or an interventional catheterization, will be required to save the infant.

Congestive heart failure in the fetus is manifest as hydrops fetalis. This can arise from regurgitant lesions of the right-sided AV or semilunar valves, large systemic arteriovenous fistulae, myocardial disease, severe anemia, and prolonged tachyarrhythmias. Systemic venous congestion from the elevated right-sided filling pressures and volumes results in hepatomegaly and the accumulation of fluid in serous cavities, and may progress to generalized anasarca. Although the overall prognosis for survival when hydrops develops is poor, some infants have been salvaged by transplacental therapy of life-threatening cardiac arrhythmias with digoxin, propranolol, or procainamide. Intrauterine transfusions also have improved the hemodynamic status of fetuses with severe hemolytic disease.

In preterm infants, particularly those with birth weights of less than 1,500 g, patency of the ductus arteriosus can produce the clinical picture of congestive heart failure and complicate treatment of respiratory distress syndrome. The classic clinical findings (bounding arterial pulsations, continuous murmur) may be absent in these infants, and diagnosis may rest on Doppler-derived flow-velocity determinations demonstrating left-to-right shunting via the ductus into the pulmonary artery. Management of the problem in these infants consists of the intravenous administration of indomethacin, which inhibits prostaglandin synthesis, if platelet counts are adequate and renal function is intact. In instances in which a course of indomethacin therapy does not produce ductal closure (<15%), surgical ligation is necessary.

The overall effectiveness of indomethacin to produce ductal constriction depends on the dose administered and the timing of treatment. Available data does not support routine indomethacin treatment on the first day of life. Although decreasing the incidence of symptomatic PDA and the need for surgical ligation, routine first-day treatment does not appear to significantly decrease morbidity. It has been suggested that infants of less than 1,000 g have the ductus treated when it becomes clinically apparent and before signs of a large shunt are evident. For those infants of over 1,000 grams, the medication is used if a hemodynamically significant left-to-right shunt is present.

When congestive failure accompanies an acute low perfusion state (coarctation, hypoplastic left heart), with systemic blood flow dependent on continued patency of the ductus arteriosus, the administration of PGE_1, which will dilate the ductus arteriosus, may restore tissue perfusion. Restoration of systemic perfusion is the key. In addition to PGE_1, this requires a titratable inotropic agent, such as dopamine or dobutamine, to support myocardial function.

Congestive heart failure is encountered most frequently in infants with large-volume left-to-right shunts (ventricular septal defects, AVC defects, PDA). Treatment of these infants requires interventions to lessen pulmonary and systemic venous congestion while attempts are made to improve systemic blood flow to allow for body growth. Furosemide is the diuretic agent used most widely to promote salt and water loss, and it may be required two to three times a day in the management of severe pulmonary edema. Spironolactone is a valuable adjunct to diuretic therapy, because it tends to reduce potassium loss. Serum electrolyte levels must be monitored when the loop diuretics are used on a frequent basis.

The use of cardiac glycosides in the treatment of the high-output congestive heart failure that accompanies a large-volume left-to-right shunt is somewhat controversial. Because myocardial contractility is not significantly impaired, the need for an inotropic agent has been challenged. Nevertheless, more than 50% of these infants appear to improve clinically. This may be explained on the basis of withdrawal of adrenergic support, thus decreasing oxygen demands. Supporting this hypothesis is the fall in oxygen consumption that is seen in some patients with a favorable clinical response to cardiac glycosides, along with a decrease in the levels of circulating catecholamines.

Vasodilator therapy also has been introduced into the management schema for infants with large ventricular or AV septal defects and dilated congestive cardiomyopathies. With vasodilatation and a lessening of left ventricular afterload, the left-to-right shunt, if present, may diminish, whereas systemic blood flow increases. Angiotensin-converting enzyme inhibitors are the afterload-reducing agents most commonly used. Supportive measures for these infants include oxygen administration, maintenance of a semi-upright position, correction of relative anemia, intravenous hyperalimentation, and the use of a ventilator if respiratory failure is present. A poor clinical response warrants early surgical repair of the defect.

Infants with a dilated cardiomyopathy should be evaluated for the presence of carnitine deficiency (serum, skeletal muscle), because replacement therapy with L-carnitine may be lifesaving by restoring myocardial oxidative function. Some evidence exists for the use of high-dose intravenous immunoglobulin in the setting of acute myocarditis. In other situations, the ultimate management may be heart transplantation.

Persistent Pulmonary Hypertension

Elevation of pulmonary artery pressures and an increase in pulmonary vascular resistance can complicate the management of some of the clinical problems encountered during the newborn period. Persistent pulmonary hypertension may occur rarely as a primary abnormality of the pulmonary vascular bed or be seen accompanying pulmonary disorders (infections, lung hypoplasia, respiratory distress syndrome), diaphragmatic hernias, and certain congenital and acquired cardiac diseases such as large-volume left-to-right shunts, anomalies of pulmonary venous return with pulmonary venous obstruction, and cardiomyopathies. It has become apparent that chronic intrauterine asphyxia can produce structural alterations in the pulmonary vascular bed, which may result in significant postnatal problems in oxygenation resulting from a restricted pulmonary circulation and persistent right-to-left shunting via fetal flow channels. Meconium aspiration at delivery may be only the terminal event in a more chronic intrauterine asphyxial state.

The treatment of these infants rests on establishing the underlying diagnosis and employing therapeutic strategies aimed at increasing oxygen transport, improving ventilatory function, preserving or augmenting cardiac output, and attempting interventions that may lower pulmonary vascular resistance (decreasing blood viscosity, diminishing ventricular filling pressure, surgically relieving pulmonary venous obstruction, and producing vasodilatation).

A rational approach to the diagnosis and management of these patients includes a determination of the arterial blood gas tensions and pH level to define the degree of hypoxemia and the ventilatory status. Next, the clinician should assess the presence or absence of respiratory distress (retractions, grunting, alar flaring, and use of the accessory muscles of respiration). Ventilatory support usually is required if severe hypoxemia dominates the clinical picture; this can be assessed best with an indwelling arterial line (umbilical artery) and simultaneous sampling of arterial blood for P_aO_2 from this site and the right radial artery, with as little disturbance of the infant as possible. Pulse oximetry offers a noninvasive alternative to this approach. When the descending aortic saturation is less than the right radial saturation, right-to-left ductal shunting is present, and pulmonary vascular resistance must exceed systemic vascular resistance. The pH and P_{CO_2} values also aid in patient evaluation. Elevation of P_aCO_2 suggests significant compromise of ventilatory function. A metabolic acidemia can

be associated with a low P_aO_2 (<35 mm Hg) or with decreased systemic perfusion and relatively normal P_aO_2 values. If the descending aortic and right-arm saturation tensions are equal, the ductus still could be shunting, but this is masked by right-to-left shunts at more proximal sites, such as the foramen ovale and lungs.

The state of perfusion also must be checked by palpation of the peripheral arterial pulses, capillary refill, and skin temperature. If perfusion is compromised, management must include the provision of volume and inotropic support to restore the perfusion of regional circulations. If perfusion and ventilation are not compromised, the clinician can proceed directly to determination of the site of right-to-left shunting.

The hyperoxia test (response to F_IO_2 1.0) has been touted as a way to separate a cardiac problem from one involving the lungs or pulmonary circulation. Interpretation of an increase in O_2, tension or saturation is, however, fraught with error. Impressive increments have been observed in the face of cardiac disease, and little or no response in association with severe lung disease. A chest film focused on heart size, lung vascularity, and other malformations (e.g., diaphragmatic hernia) is useful as part of the clinical evaluation. An ECG examined for evidence of myocardial ischemia (ST-T wave changes) and enzyme levels (myocardial CPK) also can aid in establishing a specific diagnosis. It is recommended that part of the assessment include an echocardiogram performed by a cardiologist who is experienced in the evaluation of critically ill newborns.

The treatment of these patients is based on approaches aimed at raising arterial oxygen content and tension. The latter are functions of pulmonary capillary oxygen content, cardiac output, the right-to-left shunt, and oxygen extraction. Each of these variables is capable of being manipulated, given that a change in one of these factors may influence one of the other variables. For example, increasing P_aO_2 by positive-pressure ventilation may impede venous return and diminish cardiac output. On the other hand, raising cardiac output (e.g., with inotropic agents) may increase metabolic demands and intrapulmonary right-to-left shunting.

Raising the inspired oxygen concentration may have a number of beneficial effects. An increase in dissolved oxygen permits about a 10% rise in oxygen saturation, even in the face of a fixed right-to-left shunt. Furthermore, oxygen is capable of dilating constricted pulmonary resistance vessels. The only situation in which oxygen administration may be deleterious is when ductal-dependent systemic blood flow is present (see the section on impaired perfusion). This will *not* take place in conditions such as pulmonary atresia, however, in which ductal-dependent pulmonary perfusion occurs because pulmonary flow is limited, and oxygen saturation will rise only minimally—not enough to compromise the caliber of the ductus.

The hematocrit, by its effect on blood viscosity, is another factor that can alter the response of the pulmonary vascular bed. Hyperviscosity of greater than 65% (a hematocrit of greater than 65%) will raise pulmonary vascular resistance and increase right-to-left shunting. A low hematocrit, on the other hand, limits oxygen-carrying capacity. Therefore, it is appropriate to keep the hematocrit in the range of 40% to 50%. The provision of ventilatory support can lower an elevated P_aCO_2 to normal or low levels, whereas areas of alveolar collapse may be inflated, thereby raising the level of P_aO_2. If the potential deleterious effects of positive-pressure breathing on cardiac output are taken into consideration, and various ventilatory maneuvers are tried while P_aO_2 and P_aCO_2 are monitored, an increase in P_aO_2 can be achieved while circulatory function is maintained.

The provision of adequate cardiac output is essential in the treatment of patients with severe hypoxemia. Hypoxemia usually can be tolerated if cardiac output is maintained, as in the case of infants with congenital heart disease. The combination of low cardiac output and hypoxemia, however, cannot be tolerated.

Cardiac output can be increased by volume infusions of whole blood if blood loss is a problem, or of electrolyte or albumin solutions when hemoglobin does not have to be replaced. If contractility is decreased, as assessed through echocardiographic evaluation, an inotropic agent such as dopamine, dobutamine, or milrinone should be administered. These operate primarily through beta$_1$-receptor function (dopamine and dobutamine) or phosphodiesterase inhibition (milrinone) to increase contractility and decrease afterload.

A reduction in right-to-left shunt flow may be achieved by improving ventilation, particularly in those with impaired ventilation and stiff lungs. Oxygen extraction may be decreased by diminishing oxygen demands or by lessening the work of breathing and decreasing overall metabolic demands.

Conservative management consisting of some, but not a marked degree, of hyperventilation, provision of adequate volume, support of the myocardium, and increased inspired oxygen concentrations appears to result in reasonable survival data. Extracorporeal membrane oxygenation also has yielded encouraging results, but this approach is expensive, requires specialized personnel, and has raised concern relative to the long-term central nervous system effects of ligation of a carotid artery, which is required for the procedure. The introduction of inhaled NO, a potent vasodilator, offers a novel approach to disorders of the pulmonary circulation. Endothelial-derived NO modulates pulmonary vascular smooth muscle tone in experimental animal models of pulmonary hypertension and appears to influence the postnatal decline in pulmonary vascular resistance. Inhaled NO diffuses from the alveolar space to pulmonary vascular smooth muscle, stimulates cyclic guanosine monophosphate (cGMP) production, and induces vasodilation. NO binds to hemoglobin, forming methemoglobin, which is then excreted as urinary nitrite. The successful use of NO offers the possibility of avoiding or at least limiting the use of extracorporeal membrane oxygenation, lessening the requirements for high oxygen concentrations and airway pressures, and thus lowering the risk of acute and chronic lung injury.

Other Cardiac Problems in the Infant

The infant of a diabetic mother may have cardiac involvement, particularly if the diabetes is under poor control. In addition to a higher than normal incidence of congenital heart disease, there may be the development in utero of a hypertrophic cardiomyopathy. This cardiac abnormality can be diagnosed by two-dimensional echocardiography. Of further interest is the fact that the pathologic process is reversible postnatally, usually within 6 months. Therapy with a beta-receptor blocking agent rarely is required unless the infant has significant left ventricular outflow obstruction and compromised systemic perfusion.

Endocrine Disorders with Cardiac Manifestations

Certain endocrinopathies are associated with cardiovascular manifestations. Hypothyroidism may be accompanied by cardiomegaly, decreased contractility, and bradycardia. Signs of cardiac involvement abate when replacement therapy with thyroid hormone is instituted. Tachycardia, increased contractility, bounding pulses, and tachyarrhythmias have been noted in infants of mothers being treated for hyperthyroidism because of high levels of long-acting thyroid-stimulating hormone.

Salt-losing adrenogenital syndrome with high serum potassium levels has been linked to cardiomegaly and decreased

contractility. Myocardial function improves as the endocrine disorder is controlled. In addition, hypocalcemia accompanying parathyroid absence can impair cardiac performance, with contractility increasing as the level of ionized calcium is raised.

Healthy Newborn with a Heart Murmur

The approach to the newborn infant who has a significant cardiac murmur but is entirely asymptomatic, with normal perfusion, respiratory pattern, and oxygenation, still requires additional noninvasive studies until the diagnosis (e.g., a small ventricular defect or mild aortic or pulmonary stenosis) is established firmly. This usually involves obtaining an EKG and an echocardiogram with Doppler assessment. Follow-up with a pediatric cardiologist is recommended to educate the infant's parents regarding the natural history of the defects, including spontaneous closure of some ventricular septal defects and possible progression of any obstruction, as well as the need for subacute bacterial endocarditis prophylaxis for situations that may induce a bacteremia.

Ectopy in the Newborn

Premature supraventricular beats are common. In the absence of underlying heart disease, they usually are benign, disappear during the first weeks of life, and require no therapy. The infant should be monitored for 24 to 48 hours to determine that tachyarrhythmias or bradyarrhythmias are not occurring. All arrhythmias should have ECG documentation, with 24-hour ECG Holter monitoring usually required. Supraventricular premature beats are characterized by a QRS interval of normal duration, with P waves that are distinctly different in shape from the normal P wave. Ventricular ectopy has a wide QRS interval and usually is unifocal. These beats are usually of no consequence in the absence of underlying heart disease. Multifocal premature beats of ventricular origin are associated with underlying myocardial disease and carry a guarded prognosis.

CONCLUSIONS

The approach to the newborn infant with heart disease has taken into consideration the potential influences of the fetal flow pathways, developmental changes in the pulmonary circulation, fundamental differences between developing and mature cardiac muscle, and possible deleterious effects on the transitional circulation of birth asphyxia, altered blood viscosity, and certain cardiovascular malformations. The common high-risk congenital cardiac defects as well as acquired diseases have been classified on the basis of their primary functional abnormality (i.e., hypoxemia, low perfusion state, and large-volume left-to-right shunt). Potential life-threatening disturbances in cardiac rhythm also are considered. Decision trees have been developed for these acute life-threatening situations. Diagnostic tests useful in the evaluation of suspected infants with congenital heart defects have been cited (e.g., chest film, oximetry, blood gas tension and pH levels, ECG, echocardiogram). Finally, special problems that affect patient treatment, such as congestive heart failure and pulmonary hypertension, have been discussed. This pathophysiologic approach should lead the clinician to a prompt recognition of the at-risk infant, a correct functional diagnosis, adequate stabilization and transport, appropriate medical and surgical interventions, and improved long-term outcomes.

Suggested Readings

American Academy of Pediatrics (AAP). Committee on Genetics. Health supervision for children with Down syndrome. *Pediatrics* 2001;107.

American Academy of Pediatrics (AAP). Committee on Genetics. Policy statement. *Prenatal genetic diagnosis for pediatricians. Pediatrics* 1994;93:1010.

Al-Khatib S, Pritchett E. Clinical features of Wolff-Parkinson-White syndrome. *Am Heart J* 1999;138:403.

Anderson PAW. Physiology of the fetal, neonatal, and adult heart. In: Polin RA, Fox WW, eds. *Fetal and neonatal physiology,* vol I. Philadelphia: Saunders, 1992:722.

Brucato A, Frassi M, Franceschini F, et al. risk of congenital complete heart block in newborns of mothers with anti-Ro/SSA antibodies detected by counterimmunoelectrophoresis: a prospective study of 100 women. *Arth Rheum* 2001;44:1832.

Drucker N, Colan S, Lewis A. Congenital heart disease: gamma-globulin treatment of acute myocarditis in the pediatric population. *Circulation* 1994;89:252.

Fretz EB, Rosenberg HC. Diagnostic value of ECG patterns of right ventricular hypertrophy in children. *Can J Cardiol* 1993;9(9):829.

Friedman WF. Physiological properties of the developing heart. In: Marcelletti C, Anderson RH, Becker AE, et al., eds. *Pediatric cardiology,* vol 6. Edinburgh: Churchill Livingstone, 1986:3.

Garson A Jr. *The electrocardiogram in infants and children—a systematic approach.* Philadelphia: Lea & Febiger, 1983.

Kirby M, Waldo K. Molecular embryogenesis of the heart. *Pediatr Dev Pathol* 2002;5:516.

Lister G. Persistent pulmonary hypertension of the newborn. In: Nelson NM, ed. *Current therapy in neonatal-perinatal medicine.* Philadelphia: BC Decker, 1985:278.

Markwald RR, ed. *Living morphogenesis of the heart.* Boston: Birkhauser, 1999.

Olson EN, Srivastava D. Molecular pathways controlling heart development. *Science* 1996;272:671.

Rabinovitch M. Developmental biology of the pulmonary vascular bed. In: Freedom RM, Berson LN, Smallhom JF, eds. *Neonatal heart disease.* London: Springer-Verlag, 1992:45.

Rose V, Clark E. Etiology of congenital heart disease. In: Freedom RM, Benson LN, Smallhom JF, eds. *Neonatal heart disease.* London: Springer-Verlag, 1992:3.

Rudolph AM. *Congenital diseases of the heart.* Clinical-physiologic correlations, 2nd edition. Armonk, New York, Futura Publishing Company, 2001.

Rudolph AM. Distribution and regulation of blood flow in the fetal and neonatal lamb. *Circ Res* 1985;57:81.

Snider AR, Serwer GA, Ritter SB. *Echocardiography in pediatric heart disease,* 2nd ed. St. Louis: Mosby-Year Book, 1997.

Schwartz PJ, et al. Diagnostic criteria for the long QT syndrome: an update. *Circulation* 1993;88:782.

Talner NS, Lister G. The recognition of critical cardiac disease in the infant. In: Warshaw JB, Hobbins JC, eds. *Principles and practice of perinatal medicine: maternal, fetal and newborn care.* Menlo Park, CA: Addison-Wesley, 1983: 363.

Teitel DW. Physiologic development of the cardiovascular system of the fetus. In: Polin RA, Fox WW, eds. *Fetal and neonatal physiology,* vol 1. Philadelphia: Saunders, 1992:609.

CHAPTER 54 ■ CARDIOVASCULAR SURGERY IN THE NEWBORN

GARY S. KOPF AND DENNIS M. MELLO

Congenital heart disease (CHD) occurs in 0.8% to 0.9% of live births. Approximately 30% of these patients will need surgical treatment as a neonate. Table 54.1 lists the most common types of CHD requiring surgical intervention in the neonatal period. Primary cardiac repair or palliation in neonates now is accomplished with reasonably low morbidity and mortality for a variety of complex congenital heart defects in infants as small as 1.5 to 2.0 kg.

Procedures that result in normal physiology are preferred whenever feasible. Reparative operations commonly performed in neonates include the *arterial switch* for transposition of the great arteries, repair of truncus arteriosus, repair of total anomalous pulmonary venous return, closure of ventricular septal defect (VSD), and repair of coarctation. For other complex lesions, repair or palliation are options to be considered depending on individual anatomic substrates and the general condition of the patient. These include pulmonary atresia with VSD, and tetralogy of Fallot. Patients with single-ventricle physiology comprise about 20% of patients with CHD, and can only be palliated, short of transplantation. Palliation consists of a systemic–to–pulmonary artery shunt for most cyanotic patients, or a pulmonary artery (PA) banding for those in congestive heart failure with increased pulmonary blood flow. Neonates with left heart obstruction or hypoplastic left heart syndrome will require more complex palliations such as the Damus-Kaye-Stansel procedure or the Norwood procedure, described in later sections.

Prolonged medical treatment to promote growth often leads to complications with little weight gain and should be used only in mildly symptomatic or asymptomatic patients. Although neonates with CHD can be palliated with prostaglandin E$_1$ (PGE$_1$) infusion for weeks, complications are frequent and the growth seen is often insignificant. Noncardiac malformations, such as gastrointestinal obstruction, tracheoesophageal fistula,

TABLE 54.1

COMMON CARDIOVASCULAR PROCEDURES PERFORMED IN THE NEONATAL PERIOD

Diagnosis	Operation
Transposition of Great Arteries	Arterial Switch
Hypoplastic Left Heart Syndrome	Norwood Procedure or Heart Transplant
Tricuspid Atresia	Blalock-Taussig Shunt
Tetralogy of Fallot	Complete Repair or Blalock-Taussig Shunt
Pulmonary Atresia with VSD	Rastelli Type Procedure or Blalock-Taussig Shunt
Ventricular Septal Defect	VSD Closure or Pulmonary Artery Banding
Truncus Arteriosus	Rastelli Type Procedure
Total Anomalous Pulmonary Venous Drainage	Total Repair
Coarctation	Repair with Extended End-to-end Anastomosis
Patent Ductus Arteriosus	PDA ligation

| BOX 54.1 | Common Uses of Prostaglandins in Congenital Heart Disease |

To Maintain Pulmonary Blood Flow
Transposition of Great
Arteries (if inadequate arterial-venous mixing)
Tricuspid Atresia
Tetralogy of Fallot (rarely necessary in neonates)
Pulmonary Atresia

To Maintain Systemic Blood Flow
Hypoplastic Left Heart Syndrome
Interrupted Aortic Arch
Coarctation of the Aorta

---

or diaphragmatic hernia, usually require surgical repair before the underlying CHD can be addressed, and PGE$_1$ infusion is useful in this group (Box 54.1).

Extreme low-birth-weight neonates (<1,500 g) with CHD are difficult to manage with repair or palliation and remain a challenging problem with high mortality.

GENERAL CONSIDERATIONS

Preoperative Management

Resuscitation and stabilization of cardiac, renal, and respiratory function is critical to optimize surgical outcome. Preoperative shock or renal failure is strongly associated with poor surgical outcome and should be corrected before surgical intervention. Neonates who are dependant on ductal patency for pulmonary blood flow (e.g., pulmonary atresia) or systemic perfusion [e.g., hypoplastic left heart syndrome (HLHS), interrupted aortic arch (IAA)] are treated with PGE$_1$ infusion as early as possible to reverse acidosis, severe cyanosis, or low cardiac output. Inotropic agents, particularly dopamine, dobutamine, and milrinone, are used to increase cardiac output and renal blood flow. Mechanical ventilation is used to ensure adequate gas exchange and oxygenation. Nitrogen balance must be optimized with either enteral or intravenous nutrition if surgery is to be delayed more than a few days.

A diagnosis can be made expeditiously utilizing echocardiography and color flow Doppler. Cardiac catheterization is used only when important physiologic or anatomic questions remain after echocardiographic examination, or if catheter intervention (balloon atrial septostomy, balloon valvuloplasty) is contemplated. Following initial stabilization, surgery should be accomplished as soon as feasible. Additional delay in symptomatic patients for the purpose of weight gain is usually unjustified, because intervening complications usually outweigh the benefits of the often slow and insignificant growth.

Intraoperative Management

Monitoring

Arterial blood pressure is monitored via umbilical, radial, or femoral artery cannulation. Good intravenous access is important, but central venous monitoring is not necessary because transthoracic left and/or right atrial lines can be placed for postoperative monitoring. Urine output is monitored using a bladder catheter. Several electrocardiographic leads are monitored continuously. Temperature monitoring is a critical part of the operative management and is accomplished with tympanic, esophageal, and either bladder or rectal temperature probes.

Intraoperative monitoring using transesophageal echocardiography (TEE) is critically important to reassess anatomy pre-repair, and to check on the anatomic result post-repair. Probes now are available for low-birth-weight neonates.

Incisions

The median sternotomy incision is the standard approach for virtually all open-heart procedures and most palliative procedures in the neonate. The sternum is incised vertically using the sagittal saw. The thymus gland is subtotally resected to facilitate exposure. The pericardium is harvested for use as a vascular patch when necessary. The pericardium is treated with glutaraldehyde solution to increase strength if it will be subject to systemic pressure. Before cannulation for bypass, patients are heparinized with 3 to 4 mg/kg of heparin.

Coarctation repair and ligation of an isolated patent ductus arteriosus (PDA) are approached through the left chest. A left posterior-lateral thoracotomy is made, with entrance through the third or fourth intercostal space. The lung is gently retracted anteriorly to expose the mediastinum.

Cardiopulmonary Bypass

During cardiopulmonary bypass (CPB), venous blood is siphoned into the venous reservoir of the heart–lung apparatus via a single cannula placed in the right atrium, or two smaller cannulae inserted into each vena cava. After traversing a roller pump, membrane oxygenator, heat exchanger, and filter, the blood is returned to the ascending aorta, via an aortic cannula. To provide for the special needs of the neonate, each component of the system is specifically designed to minimize priming volume and blood trauma, and increase the efficiency of gas exchange and heat transfer. The time during which blood is continuously exchanged between the heart–lung apparatus and the patient is referred to as the *total bypass time*.

CPB results in a whole-body inflammatory response, which can lead to generalized edema and an increase in total body water. The priming volume of the heart–lung bypass circuit may be twice that of a neonates' blood volume. The severe and sudden hemodilution decreases oncotic pressure and tends to increase the loss of intravascular fluid into third-space compartments. The inflammatory response to bypass surgery will increase membrane permeability, adding to this third-space effect. The hormonal stress response will result in increased levels of antidiuretic hormone and further contribute to the tendency to accumulate excess fluid. Diuretics, in significant amounts, are almost always needed postoperatively to rid the body of excess total body water. Dilution of clotting factors may contribute to severe coagulopathic states following bypass.

Surgical Strategy

The successful surgical repair of complex lesions requires meticulous attention to every detail. A bloodless, motionless field with a relaxed heart is mandatory. Once bypass is established, the ascending aorta between the root of the aorta and the aortic cannula is clamped. The heart is thereby isolated from the rest of the circulation and a *cardioplegia solution* can be infused selectively into the coronary circulation. Cardioplegia is a cold, hyperkalemic, physiologically balanced crystalloid or crystalloid–blood solution containing glucose, buffer, and electrolytes. With cardioplegia infusion into the coronary circulation, the heart becomes flaccid, and a bloodless, motionless surgical field is produced. A vent suction often is placed into the left ventricle via the right upper pulmonary vein, which returns blood to the heart–lung circuit. This vent helps keep the field dry during cardiac procedures, removes air, and prevents ventricular distension during the rewarming phase after repair is completed. The amount of time during which the ascending aorta is clamped is called the *aortic cross clamp time* and is also the myocardial ischemic time. Current techniques of myocardial protection using cardioplegia, and with topical cooling around the heart as well as systemic cooling, allow for cross clamp times of up to 2 hours or more, with good preservation of myocardial function after bypass. The most complex repairs usually can be accomplished within this time frame.

At the onset of CPB, to protect the heart and other organs, body temperature is lowered using a heat exchanger. A core temperature below 20°C is referred to as *deep hypothermia*. At this temperature, pump flow can be reduced temporarily to as low as 25 to 50 cc/kg/minute, because metabolic demands decrease with hypothermia. This is known as the *low-flow* technique. *Complete circulatory arrest* is another way of creating ideal surgical conditions. Systemic perfusion can be stopped completely once systemic temperatures are below 18°C. The head is packed in ice, because the brain is organ most vulnerable to injury during circulatory arrest. The amount of time during which no systemic flow is present is the *circulatory arrest time*. Arrest times of less than 45 minutes are considered acceptable, but the incidence and severity of neurologic sequelae increase significantly with longer periods. Complete circulatory arrest, even for aortic arch repair, can be avoided by brachiocephalic artery perfusion; however, some surgeons still prefer using total circulatory arrest, which arguably may be just as safe for short periods of time.

Most neonatal procedures can be carried out with exposure through the atria and/or great vessels. A small ventricular incision in the pulmonary ventricle is necessary for some procedures. Incision in the systemic ventricle is poorly tolerated in the neonate and is avoided. Once off bypass, the adequacy of the repair or the existence of residual lesions, and the inotropic state of the heart is evaluated using TEE. Heart rate, volume status, and the contractile state of the ventricles are optimized. Adequate heart rhythm and rate can be adjusted with the use of temporary atrial and ventricular pacing wires, which are routinely inserted in all neonates. Optimum volume status is maintained. Optimal contractility may require an adjustment of inotropic support.

During bypass, extra fluid and electrolytes are partially removed utilizing *ultrafiltration*, a process similar to hemodialysis. After discontinuation of cardiopulmonary bypass, modified ultrafiltration (MUF) can be used to further remove excess fluid and raise the hematocrit. This is done by circulating the patients' blood volume and the bypass circuit volume through the hemoconcentrator while the patient's own heart supports the circulation. This process also may remove inflammatory or myocardial depressant proteins and often improves hemodynamics. After MUF is completed (usually 10 to 15 minutes), the circulating heparin is reversed with protamine.

Two or three chest tubes are inserted for drainage of blood and fluid from the pericardial and pleural spaces. In cases where renal function is questionable, a peritoneal dialysis catheter is placed for drainage of the peritoneum and for dialysis, if necessary. In some CHD centers, this catheter is routinely inserted in neonates.

Delayed Sternal Closure

Infants who have prolonged procedures or who have excessive bleeding in the operating room that requires the transfusion of significant amounts of clotting factors and blood often have generalized edema, which precludes sternal closure without hemodynamic compromise. In such cases, the sternum is left open and the wound closed by sewing a silastic or polytetrafluoroethylene (PTFE) sheet to the skin edges without tension. After 2 to 5 days of diuresis, the sternum usually can be easily closed, a procedure done at the bedside in the ICU. The incremental risk of infection is small.

Postoperative Care

Patients who undergo reparative surgery with a good hemodynamic result can be expected to make a quick recovery within 24 to 72 hours. In patients undergoing palliation, a good balance between systemic and pulmonary flow is the critically important factor. The ventricle should provide systemic flow unimpeded by any obstruction, whereas pulmonary flow is limited by the size of the shunt or by a PA band or other intrinsic obstruction to pulmonary blood flow. In lesions with complete mixing of systemic and pulmonary venous blood, oxygen saturations from 75% to 85% with PO_2 values of about 40 torr are optimal. This generally equates to a pulmonary–to–systemic flow ratio in the range of 2 to 1.

Fluid Balance

Fluid administration is restricted to between one-half and two-thirds of maintenance levels. In the first 24 hours, supplemental red cells, plasma, or albumin may be needed to maintain cardiac output. Overdistension of the heart, with filling pressures above 10 to 12 mm Hg should be avoided, because this is poorly tolerated in the neonate. After the initial 12 to 24 hours following surgery, neonates usually require several days of intense diuresis to rid the body of the excess fluid accumulated perioperatively. Continuous furosemide infusion is effective.

Inotropic Support

Moderate doses of dopamine (3 to 5 μg/kg/minute) and milrinone (0.3 to 0.5 μg/kg/minute) are commonly used. If additional inotropic support is needed, calcium and/or epinephrine may be added. A modest decline in ventricular function often occurs during the first 6 to 18 hours after surgery; this improves the next day. The contractile state can be assessed using transthoracic echocardiography.

Ventilatory Complications

Respiratory problems represent the most common postoperative complications, and frequent blood gas determinations are required to monitor and adjust ventilation. Adequate tidal volume must be maintained, with modest positive end expiratory pressure (PEEP) to prevent progressive atelectasis. Respiratory acidosis and alkalosis are avoided by appropriate changes in ventilator settings. Acidosis will depress cardiac function and increase pulmonary vascular resistance. Alkalosis also can decrease function and impair cerebral blood flow. Sudden, unexpected, severe decompensation in the postoperative patient usually is due to compromised ventilation, including dislodged, malpositioned, or obstructed endotracheal tubes, ventilator malfunction, pleural effusions, and pneumothorax, which must be recognized and treated immediately.

Bleeding

Normal red cell mass with a hematocrit value of 35% to 45%, or higher in cyanotic patients, is maintained to ensure optimum oxygen transport and oncotic pressure. Continuous bleeding, with chest tube outputs of greater than 10% of blood volume per hour, if not due to coagulopathy, may require re-exploration. Postpump coagulopathy is treated using platelets, cryoprecipitate, and fresh frozen plasma and red cells as indicated.

Arrhythmias

Temporary transthoracic bipolar atrial and ventricular pacing wires are placed in the operating room to help manage postoperative arrhythmias. A heart rate in the 120 to 160 beats per minute range is needed to maintain adequate cardiac output, because low neonatal ventricular compliance limits stroke volume expansion. Bradyarrhythmias, including an inappropriate sinus bradycardia or junctional rhythm, can be treated with single or dual chamber pacing. Supraventricular tachycardia is a frequent complication in the immediate postoperative period. The most common of these is junctional ectopic tachycardia. Intravenous amiodarone often is the first line drug treatment for uncontrolled supraventricular and ventricular tachyarrhythmias, and electrolyte disturbances must be treated, particularly low magnesium levels.

Deteriorating hemodynamic status not responding to supportive measures is usually a result of a residual anatomic lesion. The adequacy of surgical repair can be re-evaluated using echocardiographic examination. Cardiac catheterization may be necessary if the echocardiographic examination is not definitive. Once identified, the repair of significant residual lesions should be promptly undertaken, because continued nonoperative treatment usually is futile.

LEFT-TO-RIGHT SHUNTS

Patent Ductus Arteriosus

The ductus arteriosus is a fetal structure connecting the main PA to the descending thoracic aorta. It arises from the superior portion of the bifurcation of the PA, and connects directly to the descending aorta distal and medial to the left subclavian artery. Its length and diameter are variable. In the fetal circulation, over 60% of the cardiac output is directed through the ductus. After birth, when the pulmonary vascular resistance falls and oxygenation increases, the ductus constricts. Spontaneous complete closure occurs in most infants during the first days or weeks of life.

Persistent PDA commonly is seen in extremely low-birth-weight and premature infants. Left-to-right shunt through the ductus causes congestive heart failure, which exacerbates the pulmonary dysfunction of the premature infant. Low systemic output can lead to necrotizing enterocolitis, intracranial hemorrhage, and renal failure. Diagnosis is confirmed using echocardiography. Pulse wave Doppler shows left-to-right shunting and a large left atrium. Medical treatment with indomethacin usually is effective, but may be contraindicated in the presence of compromised renal function or intracranial hemorrhage. Prolonged courses of medical therapy in symptomatic infants can result in further deterioration and should be avoided, because surgical therapy is effective and well tolerated.

Patent Ductus Arteriosus Ligation

Because many of these patients are extreme low-birth-weight neonates weighing between 400 and 1,000 g and having multiple problems, surgery is done at the bedside, or in special procedure rooms in the NICU to avoid the significant hazards of transporting such patients to the operating room. Surgery is performed through a left postero-lateral thoracotomy, with the chest cavity entered through the third or fourth intercostal space. The lung is retracted medially, exposing the aorta and the posterior mediastinum. The ductus and aortic arch are carefully identified. Minimal dissection is carried out between the base of the ductus and the aorta. A small stainless steel clip can be applied to the base of the ductus at the aortic end. Care must be taken to identify and avoid injury to the recurrent laryngeal

and phrenic nerves. A chest drain usually is not needed unless significant bleeding or air leak occurs.

Complications include hemorrhage from a friable ductus, injury to the recurrent laryngeal nerve that loops around the ductus near the area of dissection, and disruption of significant lymphatics, resulting in chylothorax. The latter usually responds to conservative treatment consisting of drainage, dietary therapy, and nutritional support.

Ventricular Septal Defect

VSD is the most common congenital heart anomaly. A large VSD often will produce congestive heart failure after the first 2 weeks of life, as pulmonary vascular resistance falls and left-to-right shunting increases. Symptomatic neonates with congestive heart failure who respond poorly to medical therapy should undergo prompt surgery.

Ventricular Septal Defect Closure

Closure utilizing a pericardial or synthetic patch is the procedure of choice. After CPB is initiated, during cardioplegic cardiac arrest, the VSD is accessed through the right atrium. A perimembranous VSD, the most common type, is found under the septal leaflet of the tricuspid valve. Care is taken to avoid injury to the aortic valve superiorly, or the atrio-ventricular conduction system along the posterior–inferior rim of the defect. Defects located in the outlet septum near the semilunar valve are approached through the PA for patch closure, with sutures attached to the base of the pulmonary leaflets at the superior rim.

Operative mortality (<2%) and morbidity are low for simple VSD closure, even in small neonates. Multiple VSDs can be difficult to close reliably in small infants, and they may require PA banding for palliation. Late pulmonary vascular disease is rare if repair is done in infancy.

CYANOTIC LESIONS

Transposition of the Great Arteries

A D-transposition of the great arteries (D-TGA) is the most common form of cyanotic congenital heart disease presenting in the newborn period. The anteriorly placed aorta arises from the right ventricle and the posterior PA from the left ventricle, producing parallel systemic and pulmonary circuits. Systemic oxygenation is dependent on mixing of oxygenated and deoxygenated blood at the level of an atrial septal defect (ASD), VSD, and/or PDA. PGE_1 infusion or balloon atrial septostomy may be necessary to improve mixing in severely hypoxic neonates. Diagnosis is made using echocardiography, and commonly associated lesions such as VSD (present in about one-third of cases) are evaluated. Cardiac catheterization is not necessary, except to define less common coexisting malformations. The operation usually is performed within the first week of life, before the left ventricle looses significant muscle mass, rendering it unable to support the systemic circulation.

Arterial Switch Procedure

The aorta and PAs are extensively mobilized out to the hilum of the lung. CPB is established, and the PDA is ligated and divided. Operation may be facilitated with the aid of deep hypothermia and low flow or periods of circulatory arrest. The aorta and PA are divided (Fig. 54.1A,B). Buttons of aortic tissue containing the left and right coronary ostia are mobilized to allow for coronary transfer posteriorly to the neo-aorta

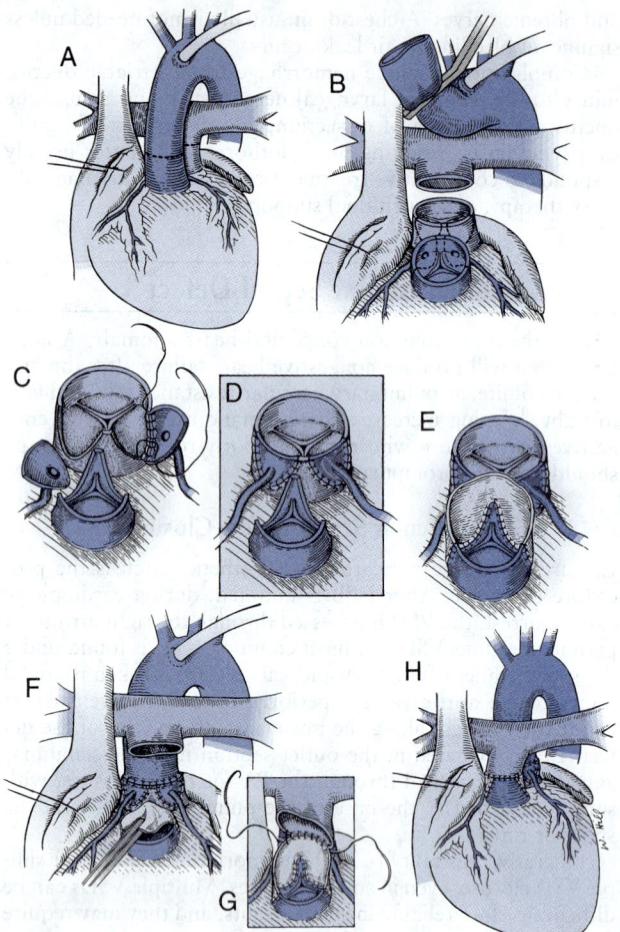

FIGURE 54.1. The arterial switch operation for transposition of the great arteries (TGA). **A:** Aorta and pulmonary artery are transected. **B:** Aorta, which is anterior in TGA, is transposed behind the pulmonary artery; coronary buttons are cut from aortic root. **C,D:** Coronary buttons are sewn to the new aortic root. **E:** Base of new pulmonary artery is repaired with native pericardial patch. **F:** Distal aorta sewn to new aortic root. **G:** Distal pulmonary artery sewn to new pulmonary root. **H:** Completed operation.

(Fig. 54.1C). The coronary buttons are sewn into place, creating the new aortic root (Fig. 54.1D). The *LeCompte maneuver* is then performed, which places the pulmonary bifurcation anterior to the aorta (Fig. 54.1B,F). Anastomosis is carried out between the neo-aortic root and the distal aorta (Fig. 54.1F). The base of the new PA is reconstructed using a pericardial patch (Fig. 54.1E), and the distal PA is anastomosed to the new proximal PA (Fig. 54.1G). The atrial septal defect is closed through the right atrium. If necessary, a VSD can be closed via the right atrium or through the aorta. The final result is a total physiologic and anatomic correction (Fig. 54.1H).

Operative mortality has declined to less than 5%, and primarily is related to technical problems associated with the coronary transfer in patients with difficult coronary variations. The most common late complication has been supravalvar PA stenosis. The PA may be stretched over the neo-aorta, resulting in stricture or compression. Adequate mobilization and reconstruction of the new PA base with generous patches of autologous pericardium (Fig. 54.1E) will help prevent this complication. Intermediate follow-up studies have shown a very low incidence of coronary complications, anastomotic strictures, or aortic valve insufficiency.

The arterial switch operation is currently one of the most common procedures performed in the neonatal period and

has replaced the atrial baffle operations (i.e., Mustard procedure, Senning procedure) as the operation of choice for TGA. Long-term follow-up of atrial switch operations reveals an increasing incidence of arrhythmias and right (systemic) ventricular failure. The arterial switch operation restores normal anatomic and physiologic function and produces excellent late outcomes.

Total Anomalous Pulmonary Venous Drainage

Total anomalous pulmonary venous drainage (TAPVD) is an uncommon anomaly. All pulmonary venous blood drains into a common collecting vein that empties into the systemic venous circulation. The common vein can drain above the heart into the superior vena cava (SVC) system (supracardiac), into the coronary sinus or right atrium (intracardiac), or into the inferior vena cava (IVC) via the ductus venosus and hepatic portal system (infracardiac). The severity of cyanosis, congestive failure, and shock corresponds with the degree of pulmonary venous obstruction, which is most common and most severe in the infracardiac type. All pulmonary and systemic venous return mixes in the right side of the heart. Blood flows to the left side of the heart through an atrial septal defect. Diagnosis is suspected in infants who are suffering from congestive heart failure and have plethoric lungs, but are cyanotic with a small heart. Echocardiography confirms the diagnosis. Severe obstruction with TAPVD is one of the few true cardiovascular surgical emergencies in the newborn for which no effective medical treatment exists.

Repair of TAPVD

All repairs are done using CPB, with moderate or deep hypothermia, with or without total circulatory arrest. The heart is protected using cardioplegia.

Supracardiac Type. The right atrium is entered and the left atrium visualized through the ASD. The common pulmonary vein located directly posterior to the atria is located from the right side of the heart, and the anterior surface is incised to create a wide opening. Incision is then made in the back of the left atrium. Because of the small size of the left atrium, this incision is sometimes extended into the right atrium. A wide side-to-side anastomosis then is created between the back of the atrium and the common pulmonary vein. The ASD is closed primarily or with a patch of pericardium. The ascending vein, which often joins the innominate vein, is usually ligated, care being taken not to damage the phrenic nerve that runs near its lateral surface. The result is a total physiologic repair.

Cardiac Type. When the pulmonary veins drain into the right atrium directly or via the coronary sinus, obstruction is uncommon and patients frequently present after the neonatal period. The repair of the coronary sinus type is the simplest of all the TAPVDs. The right atrium is opened, and the coronary sinus is unroofed, creating a confluence with the left atrium. The atrial septal defect is closed with a pericardial patch so that all coronary sinus blood and pulmonary venous blood drains into the left atrium. Care is taken to avoid the atrio-ventricular node, which is located near the coronary sinus ostium.

Infracardiac Type. These infants often present with severe metabolic acidosis, hypoperfusion, and heart failure because pulmonary venous return is severely obstructed. Immediate surgery is required. Technically, the repair of this type is the most challenging, because the collecting vein lies posterior and inferior to the heart in the extrapericardial space.

The heart is retracted upward and to the right, allowing dissection and the identification of the common pulmonary vein in the retrocardiac space. The connection going below the

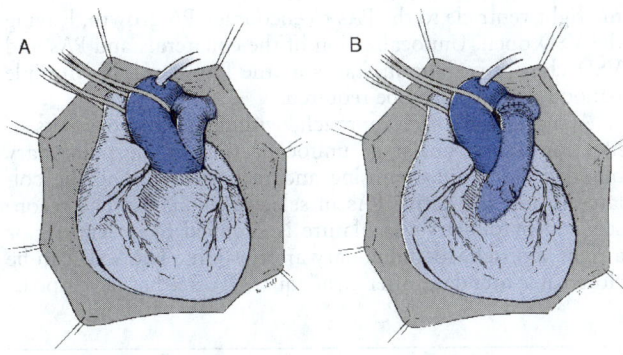

FIGURE 54.2. Rastelli-type repair for truncus arteriosus. **A:** Anatomy of type 1 truncus arteriosus. **B:** Homograft from right ventricle to pulmonary artery. The ventricular septal defect has been closed through the right ventricular incision to route left ventricular blood out of the aorta.

diaphragm often is transected to mobilize the common vein superiorly. Once the veins have been dissected, a direct anastomosis is made to the back of the left atrium, and the ASD is closed through a separate right atriotomy.

Complications associated with the repair of total anomalous pulmonary drainage include anastomotic strictures, and stenoses or hypoplasia of the pulmonary veins. The mortality rate for the group with severe venous obstruction remains significant (20% to 30%) and is related to poor preoperative status and abnormal pulmonary veins.

Truncus Arteriosus

Truncus arteriosus is characterized by the presence of a single arterial trunk (Fig. 54.2A) through which both ventricles eject blood. A VSD below the trunk connects the two ventricles. The PAs arise from this trunk. There may be a short main PA (type 1), or the two main branch PAs may arise near each other directly from the main trunk (type 2). In type 3, the branch PAs arise from different parts of the main trunk. The underlying pathophysiology relates to excessive pulmonary blood flow. Infants with truncus arteriosus develop congestive heart failure when pulmonary vascular resistance drops during the first weeks of life. The treatment of choice is early complete repair.

Truncus Arteriosus Repair

Surgical repair consists of separating the systemic and pulmonary circuits and restoring normal physiology (Fig. 54.2A,B). The operation is performed using CPB, sometimes under deep hypothermia, with periods of low flow. After aortic cross-clamping, the arterial trunk is opened transversely to visualize the origin of the PAs. The PAs then are separated from the aorta with a rim of aortic tissue. The defect in the truncal wall is repaired using a patch. The VSD is closed using a patch through a right ventriculotomy, in such a way as to direct left ventricular blood to the aorta. The right ventricular outflow tract is reconstructed with an 8- to 12-mm diameter valved conduit connecting the right ventricular incision to the PAs, thus restoring normal physiology.

Postoperative pulmonary hypertensive crises marked by sudden pulmonary vasoconstriction and severe right ventricular failure are uncommon when repair is done in the neonatal period. Operative mortality has declined to less than 10%, and is usually related to coexisting anomalies and severe low birth weight. All infants will require reoperation for conduit replacement within 3 to 5 years.

RIGHT SIDED OBSTRUCTIVE LESIONS

General Considerations

Complete or partial obstruction of pulmonary blood flow in the neonate is caused by a variety of conditions, including tricuspid atresia, tetralogy of Fallot (TOF), severe pulmonary stenosis, and pulmonary atresia with or without VSD. When pulmonary blood flow is dependent on a PDA, severe cyanosis and acidosis will develop when the ductus begins to close. Prompt infusion of PGE_1 is imperative. In selected cases with well-formed PAs, a right ventricle of adequate size, and normal coronary anatomy, reparative surgery can be accomplished in the neonate. Low-birth-weight babies or those with univentricular anomalies require palliation consisting of a systemic–to–PA shunt.

Systemic–to–Pulmonary Artery Shunt

The classic Blalock-Taussig shunt (BT shunt), first performed in 1945, consisted of transection of the subclavian artery and end-to-side anastomosis to the PA (Fig. 54.3A). The current approach, a "modified Blalock-Taussig" shunt (Fig. 54.3B), has the advantage of preserving the subclavian artery.

Operation is usually done through a midline sternotomy incision. A 3.0- to 4.5-mm tubular interposition graft of PTFE, depending on the size of the neonate, is anastomosed between the innominate artery and PA (Fig. 54.3B). The shunt often can be accomplished without CPB; however, on occasion, it may be necessary to utilize normothermic CPB to prevent severe desaturation or hemodynamic instability during the procedure. Pulmonary blood flow is determined by the size of the graft. This is critically important, and it must be matched to the size of the neonate. If difficulties are encountered in achieving a balance between systemic and pulmonary blood flow postoperatively, it may indicate inappropriate shunt size, partial occlusion, or thrombosis. When the branch PAs are hypoplastic, a "central shunt" maybe placed between the ascending aorta and main PA (Fig. 54.2C). In selected cases, a graft from the right ventricle to the PA (Sano shunt) also may be used.

Tricuspid Atresia

When the tricuspid valve is atretic, right atrial blood is diverted through an atrial septal defect to the left side of the heart. The right side of the heart is hypoplastic, and pulmonary atresia may coexist. Usually, however, a VSD allows blood to enter the right ventricle and supply pulmonary blood flow. Pulmonary

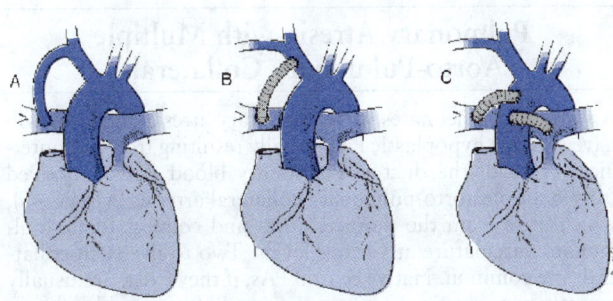

FIGURE 54.3. **A:** Classic Blalock-Taussig shunt. Subclavian artery to pulmonary artery end-to-side anastomosis. **B:** Modified Blalock-Taussig shunt with polytetrafluoroethylene interposition graft between subclavian artery and pulmonary artery. **C:** Central shunt with interposition graft from ascending aorta to main pulmonary artery.

blood flow is often severely limited due to obstruction, but may be balanced or even excessive if the VSD is large. Neonatal palliation because of decreased pulmonary flow consists of a modified BT shunt. If palliation is necessary for excessive pulmonary flow, PA banding or PA ligation along with a modified BT shunt can be used.

Tricuspid atresia may coexist with transposed great arteries (25% to 30%). In such cases, pulmonary blood flow usually is excessive, and subaortic obstruction often is present, because the aorta arises from the hypoplastic right ventricle. Palliation with a Damus-Kaye-Stansel procedure may be necessary to relieve the subaortic obstruction. In this procedure, the main PA is transected and made confluent with the ascending aorta and aortic arch, thus providing an unobstructed outlet from the ventricles. Blood flow is established to the distal PAs via a modified BT shunt.

Tetralogy of Fallot

Although most infants with TOF do not require surgery in the neonatal period, a subgroup with severe right ventricular outflow tract (RVOT) obstruction will present with significant cyanosis. Adequate palliation can be accomplished with a balloon valvotomy or a modified Blalock-Taussig shunt, although primary repair is the procedure of choice in a neonate who has adequate PAs, single VSD, and no major coexisting anomalies.

Repair consists of patch closure of the large malaligned VSD through the right ventricle or right atrium. Right ventricular outflow tract obstruction is relieved by a combination of techniques as indicated: (a) pulmonary valvotomy, (b) right ventricular outlet incision and resection, and (c) pericardial patch reconstruction of the RVOT and/or PA stenosis. If the pulmonary annulus is severely hypoplastic, it is enlarged with a pericardial patch. The majority of symptomatic neonates require the latter type of reconstruction.

Pulmonary Atresia with Ventral Septal Defect

Pulmonary atresia with VSD is characterized by an absence of continuity between the right ventricle and PA. The distal PAs usually are well formed if a patent ductus is present. Palliation consists of constructing a systemic–to–pulmonary artery shunt. Primary neonatal repair is preferable for suitable patients. The VSD is closed through a right ventricular incision. A valved conduit 8 to 12 mm in size is used to connect the right ventricle to the PA. Conduit replacement often will be required at 2 to 5 years, and again later in life. Some patients with an atretic valve but otherwise well-formed RVOT and PAs can be repaired with a transannular patch.

Pulmonary Atresia with Multiple Aorto-Pulmonary Collaterals

A subgroup of neonates with pulmonary atresia and VSD will have severely hypoplastic PAs, usually resulting from intrauterine closure of the ductus. Pulmonary blood flow is derived from multiple aorto-pulmonary collateral arteries (MAPCAS), which arise from the thoracic aorta and connect to the pulmonary vasculature at various levels. Two to five such collaterals are common. Native central PAs, if they exist, are usually severely hypoplastic, 1 to 2 mm in size. Pulmonary blood flow may be increased if the collaterals are large with no obstruction. Patients present with varying degrees of cyanosis.

Various surgical approaches have been undertaken for this complex lesion. Initial palliation may consist of a central shunt from the ascending aorta to the main PA, or alternatively from the right ventricle to the PAs to encourage PA growth, leaving the VSD open. Unifocalization of the collaterals and PAs and VSD closure is done in stages as the PAs develop. Multiple balloon dilations may be required.

A more aggressive approach, within the first 6 weeks of life, consists of one-stage unifocalization of the pulmonary blood flow by anastomosing and reconstructing all the collaterals and the native PAs in selected neonates. The reconstructed pulmonary vasculature is supplied by a central– or a right ventricle–to–pulmonary artery shunt. The VSD can be closed at a later date, after an adequate PA tree has developed.

Pulmonary Atresia and Intact Ventricular Septum

Neonates with pulmonary atresia without VSD will have varying degrees of right ventricular hypoplasia, depending on how early *in utero* the pulmonary obstruction occurred. Blood flows to the left side of the heart through an atrial septal defect. Patients with severely hypoplastic right ventricles may have multiple ventriculo-coronary fistulas, and obstructions in the native coronary circulation can be present. The PAs are usually well developed, with PDA-dependent pulmonary blood flow.

Surgical intervention is required in the neonate to provide pulmonary blood flow. Patients with a severely hypoplastic right ventricle are staged towards a univentricular repair (Fontan operation). Initial palliation consists of a systemic–to–pulmonary artery shunt alone and PDA ligation.

In patients whose right ventricular size is half of normal or more, and significant coronary fistulas are absent, palliation is designed to encourage right ventricular growth by establishing a right ventricular–to–pulmonary artery connection, utilizing balloon or surgical valvotomy, transannular patch, or valved conduit. With growth, the right ventricle may be utilized later in life in a one-and-a-half or two-ventricle repair. A systemic-to–pulmonary artery shunt is added, if it appears that the hypoplastic right ventricle initially may not supply adequate pulmonary blood flow.

Patients with extensive coronary fistula formation and native coronary obstruction have a very poor prognosis. Neonatal heart transplantation has been utilized in an attempt to salvage some of these patients.

LEFT-SIDED OBSTRUCTIVE LESIONS

Aortic Stenosis

Critical aortic stenosis in the neonate can lead to severe left ventricular dysfunction. Supportive measures using inotropic agents and mechanical ventilation may only be partially effective in improving the neonate. Prompt relief of aortic valve obstruction is critical.

Percutaneous transcatheter balloon valvotomy is effective in most cases. Surgical aortic valvotomy is reserved for patients in whom balloon valvuloplasty is not feasible or contraindicated. Surgical valvotomy can be performed precisely under direct vision. A variable degree of left ventricular hypoplasia often is present. Survival correlates with left ventricular size. Survival with a left ventricle size of less than two-thirds normal is rare. Such patients are variants of hypoplastic left-heart syndrome (HLHS), and require a Norwood type reconstruction (see section, Hypoplastic Left Heart Syndrome).

In patients with severe hypoplasia of the aortic annulus with accompanying hypoplastic left ventricular outflow tracts

(LVOT), simple valvotomy will not suffice. In such cases, the neonatal Ross-Konno procedure has been used to reconstruct the entire LVOT. The operation involves replacing the aortic root with a pulmonary autograft and reconstructing the right ventricular outflow tract with a pulmonary homograft.

Coarctation of the Aorta

Neonatal coarctation is a narrowing of the aorta in the periductal area, often accompanied by hypoplasia of the aortic isthmus and arch. A patent ductus arteriosus supplies blood flow to the descending aorta. It is frequently associated with other forms of left-sided obstructive malformations as well as VSD. Patients present with congestive failure and decreased perfusion to the lower body, with diminished lower extremity pulses.

In the neonate, the coarctation becomes more obstructive as the ductus arteriosus closes and the ductal tissue around the coarctation constricts, resulting in severe hypoperfusion of the descending aorta, acidosis, and shock. Infusion of PGE_1 to open the ductus arteriosus will improve the hemodynamic and metabolic state of the patient. Surgery is indicated in all neonates with significant coarctation. Preoperative stabilization, including treatment of metabolic acidosis and renal failure, and often mechanical ventilation, is necessary to ensure good surgical results.

Coarctation Repair

The operation is performed through a left posterior-lateral thoracotomy. The chest cavity is entered through the third or fourth intercostal space. The resection with extended end-to-end anastomosis has become the procedure of choice in the neonate with both coarctation and transverse arch hypoplasia. The operative repair entails ligation and division of the ductus arteriosus, excision of the coarctation, and an extended end-to-end anastomosis between the undersurface of the aortic arch and the descending aorta (Fig. 54.4).

The aorta is mobilized from the ascending to the descending aorta, including the arch branches. Before clamping the aorta, systemic temperature is allowed to drift down to about 34°C to help with organ protection. A modest dose of heparin occasionally is given. Vascular clamps then are placed proximally on the aortic arch, usually occluding the left subclavian and left carotid arteries, but permitting the innominate artery to provide cerebral perfusion. The right radial artery pressure is monitored to ensure adequate innominate artery pressure. The distal clamp is placed well below the coarctation on the descending aorta. The ductus is ligated, and remaining ductal tissue and coarctation is excised. The underside of the aortic arch is opened (Fig. 54.4B). The two vascular clamps are used to approximate the openings, and the extended anastomosis is carried out with fine monofilament suture (Fig. 54.4C). The extended end-to-end anastomosis technique described is par-

ticularly useful to repair infants with hypoplastic isthmus and distal aortic arches. The ischemic time for the distal aorta is less than 25 minutes. (More detailed pictures and text describing the procedure can be seen at http://www.ctsnet.org/doc/6863.)

Those infants who have an accompanying VSD can undergo VSD closure within days or weeks following coarctation repair when indicated. In some cases, complete one-stage repair of VSD and coarctation using an anterior approach and cardiopulmonary bypass may be preferred. Neonates with complex anomalies and coarctation may need combined repair or palliation through a median sternotomy.

Complications include chylothorax and recurrent laryngeal nerve injury. Paraplegia in neonates and infants is extremely uncommon, but has been reported in association with hyperthermia during cross-clamping. Recurrent coarctation occurs in less than 10% using the extended end-to-end anastomosis, and it is adequately treated with transcatheter balloon dilation.

Interrupted Aortic Arch

An interrupted aortic arch (IAA) is defined by a discontinuity of the ascending and descending aorta. It is much less common than coarctation. Descending aortic flow is completely dependent on a PDA, so that survival without treatment is uncommon after the neonatal period. IAA almost always is accompanied by a posterior malaligned VSD with some degree of LVOT narrowing. After stabilization on PGE_1 infusion, neonatal repair is undertaken as soon as feasible.

IAA is classified into three types, depending on the location of the aortic interruption. In type A, the interruption is distal to the left subclavian artery (43%); in type B, the interruption occurs between the left carotid and left subclavian arteries (54%); and in type C, an uncommon form (4%), the interruption is between the innominate and the left carotid artery. Neonates can present in congestive heart failure and profound metabolic acidosis as a result of PDA closure and descending aortic hypoperfusion. Diagnosis is adequately made with echocardiography. Cardiac catheterization is utilized to define unusual variants or associated lesions.

Repair of Interrupted Aortic Arch

The procedure of choice is a single-stage repair via a median sternotomy in which aortic continuity is established and the VSD closed. The aortic arch, ductus, and descending aorta are extensively mobilized. Arch reconstruction can be done utilizing deep hypothermia and circulatory arrest or continuous low-flow perfusion of the brain and body with innominate artery cannulation. The ductus is ligated and, after clamping the descending aorta, residual ductal tissue is removed to avoid recurrent coarctation. Aortic arch repair usually can be done with direct end-to-side anastomosis between the descending aorta and the ascending aorta after suitable mobilization. Occasionally,

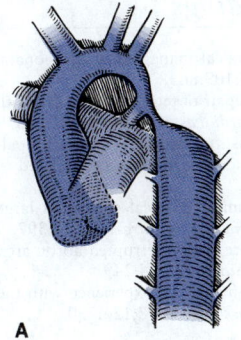
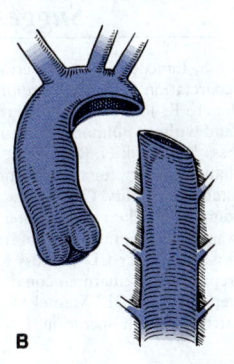
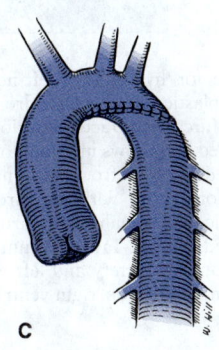

A   **B**   **C**

FIGURE 54.4. A: Severe coarctation of the aorta with hypoplastic isthmus. **B:** Resection of coarctation. **C:** Extended end-to-end anastomosis.

a patch is needed to augment the anastomosis. The VSD is closed through the right atrium or PA, depending on its location. The aortic annulus is often somewhat hypoplastic and the LVOT may be narrowed; care must be taken when placing the VSD patch to avoid further compromise of the LVOT. Operative survival is over 90% and is often related to coexisting severe anomalies, disease in other organ systems, or low birth weight. DiGeorge syndrome is common with type B interrupted aortic arch and other conotruncal abnormalities. LVOT obstruction or aortic narrowing occurs late in 10% to 20% of patients and may require surgical reconstruction or balloon dilation respectively.

Hypoplastic Left Heart Syndrome

Hypoplastic left heart syndrome (HLHS) is a common form of single ventricle, which may include aortic and/or mitral valve atresia and a severely hypoplastic or absent left ventricle (Fig. 54.5A). Systemic blood flow depends on a patent ductus arteriosus, and coronary perfusion is derived from retrograde flow through a severely hypoplastic ascending aorta. Because systemic flow is totally dependant on a PDA, neonatal palliation is essential for survival.

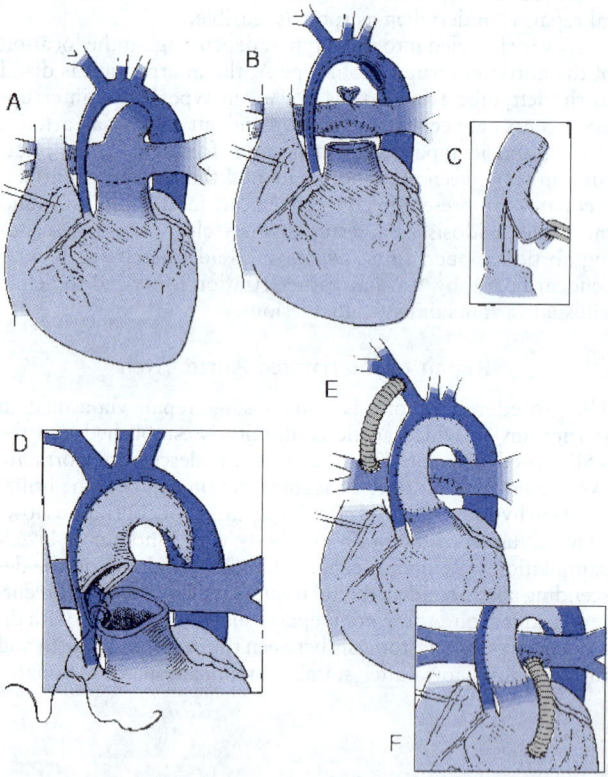

FIGURE 54.5. The Norwood procedure for hypoplastic left-heart syndrome. **A:** Typical anatomy for hypoplastic left-heart syndrome. **B:** Main pulmonary artery transected at bifurcation. Ductus arteriosus ligated and all ductal tissue removed. Dotted line shows incision down to base of ascending aorta. **C:** Wedge-shaped patch cut from pulmonary homograft. **D:** Reconstruction of new aortic root with pericardial patch with side-to-side connection of aortic root to pulmonary artery. **E:** Completed operation showing modified Blalock-Taussig shunt of polytetrafluoroethylene tube between innominate artery and left pulmonary artery. **F:** Sano modification showing shunt from right ventricle to PAs.

Norwood Procedure

The Norwood operation provides palliation and consists of reconstructing the ascending aorta and aortic arch utilizing the main PA, ascending aorta, and an extensive homograft patch (Fig. 54.5B,C,D). The PAs are isolated and pulmonary blood flow is established using either a modified Blalock-Taussig shunt from the innominate artery to the pulmonary trunk (Fig. 54.5E), or a right ventricle–to–pulmonary artery shunt (Sano modification) (Fig. 54.5F). The advantage of the latter is the resultant higher diastolic pressure in the aorta, which produces improved coronary flow. Norwood palliation carries a 10% to 30% operative mortality.

Further surgical palliation includes two subsequent procedures, which is similar for other forms of single ventricle. At 3 to 6 months, the systemic–to–pulmonary artery shunt is taken down and a bidirectional Glenn shunt, consisting of an end-to-side anastomosis between the SVC and the right PA is substituted. This relieves the volume load on the ventricle and provides adequate oxygenation for several years. The Fontan procedure, done at 2 to 4 years, consists of connecting the IVC to the PAs either through an internal atrial tunnel or an external conduit. Following the Fontan operation, the patient should have near-normal oxygen saturations and a modest limitation on exercise capacity. Using this three-stage approach, excellent long-term palliation now is possible for the majority of patients with single-ventricle physiology.

NEONATAL HEART TRANSPLANTATION

Neonatal heart transplants for hypoplastic left heart syndrome or other complex heart disease can be performed with an 80% to 90% operative survival rate, and an actuarial survival rate at 1 year of 75% to 85% and at 3 to 5 years of 70% to 80%. These results compare favorably to those in adult patients. The belief that transplantation in the neonatal period may allow for good long-term results with minimum chronic immunosuppression due to the development of some degree of graft tolerance is supported by data indicating that severe rejection is uncommon, and episodes occurring after 1 year are infrequent on a modest immunosuppression regimen. Initial immunosuppression consists of cyclosporine and azathioprine, with steroids reserved for acute rejection episodes. Of the patients followed for more than a year, most are on cyclosporine monotherapy. Presently, results are encouraging, and continued trials of neonatal heart transplantation appear justified.

The shortage of suitable donors remains a major problem, because 15% to 30% of infants will die awaiting transplantation. Additionally, long-term problems with graft coronary artery disease must be evaluated.

Suggested Readings

Conte S, Lancour-Gayet F, Serraf A, et al. Surgical management of neonatal coarctation. *J Thorac Cardiovasc Surg* 1995;109:663.

DiDonato R, Jonas R, Lang P, et al. Neonatal repair of tetralogy of Fallot with and without pulmonary atresia. *J Thorac Cardiovasc Surg* 1991;101:126.

Forbess JM, Cook N, Roth SJ, et al. Ten-year institutional experience with palliative surgery for hypoplastic left heart syndrome: Risk factors related to stage I mortality. *Circulation* 1995;92:II262.

Hardin JT, Muskett AD, Canter CE, et al. Primary surgical closure of large ventricular septal defects in small infants. *Ann Thorac Surg* 1992;53:397.

Hirooka K, Fraser CD Jr. Ross-Konno procedure with interrupted aortic arch repair in a premature neonate. *Ann Thorac Surg* 1997;64:249.

Hutter PA, Kreb DL, Mantel SF, et al. Twenty-five years' experience with the arterial switch operation. *J Thorac Cardiovasc Surg* 2002;124:790.

Isomatsu Y, Imai Y, Shin'oka T, et al. Coarctation of the aorta and ventricular septal defect: Should we perform a single-stage repair? *J Thorac Cardiovasc Surg* 2001;122:524.

Mair R, Tuer G, Sames E, et al. Right ventricular to pulmonary artery conduit instead of modified Blalock-Taussig shunt improves postoperative hemodynamics in newborns after the Norwood operation. *J Thorac Cardiovasc Surg* 2003;126:1378.

Mello D, Kopf GS. Repair of infantile coarctation and transverse arch hypoplasia with resection and extended end to undersurface of aortic arch anastomosis. Backer CL (ed). CTSNET Experts' Techniques, Congenital Cardiac Experts' Techniques. http://www.ctsnet.org/doc/6863.

Miles RH, DeLeon SY, Muraskas J, et al. Safety of patent ductus arteriosus closure in premature infants without tube thoracostomy. *Ann Thorac Surg* 1995;59:668.

Mitchell MB, Campbell DN, Clarke DR, et al. Infant heart transplantation: Improved intermediate results. *J Thorac Cardiovasc Surg* 1998;116:242.

Razzouk AJ, Chinnock RE, Gundry SR, et al. Transplantation as a primary treatment for hypoplastic left heart syndrome: intermediate-term results. *Ann Thorac Surg* 1996;62:1.

Reddy VM, Petrossian E, McElhinney DB et al. One-stage complete refocalization in infants: when should the ventricular septal defect be closed? *J Thorac Cardiovasc Surg* 1997;113:858.

Rossi AF, Seiden HS, Sadeghi AM, et al. The outcome of cardiac operations in infants weighing two kilograms or less. *J Thorac Cardiovasc Surg* 1998;116:28.

Sandhu SK, Beekman RH, Mosca RS, Bove EL. Single-stage repair of aortic arch obstruction and associated intracardiac defects in the neonate. *Am J Card* 1995;75:370.

Serraf A, Lacour-Gayet F, Robotin M, et al. Repair of interrupted aortic arch: a ten-year experience. *J Thorac Cardiovasc Surg* 1996;112:1150.

Serraf A, Lacour-Gayet F, Bruniaux J, et al. Obstructed total anomalous pulmonary venous return: toward neutralization of a major risk factor. *J Thorac Cardiovasc Surg* 1991;101:601.

Starnes VA, Luciani GB, Wells WJ, et al. Aortic root replacement with the pulmonary autograft in children with complex left heart obstruction. *Ann Thorac Surg* 1996;62:442.

Thompson LD, Doff B, et al. Neonatal repair of truncus arteriosus: continuing improvement in outcomes. *Ann Thorac Surg* 2001;72:391.

Tlaskal T, Chaloupecky V, Marek J, et al. Primary repair of interrupted aortic arch and associated heart lesions in newborns. *J Thorac Cardiovasc Surg* 1997;38:113.

Yoshimura N, Yamaguchi M, Ohashi H, et al. Pulmonary atresia with intact ventricular septum: Strategy based on right ventricular morphology. *J Thorac Cardiovasc Surg* 2003;126:1417.

h: NEONATAL GASTROINTESTINAL SYSTEM

CHAPTER 55 ■ DEVELOPMENTAL DISORDERS OF GASTROINTESTINAL FUNCTION

COLSTON F. McEVOY

Most gastrointestinal disease that presents in the neonatal period can be attributed to congenital anomalies. These defects in gut structure or function result from errors in fetal gastrointestinal development. Appreciation of the normal sequence of gastrointestinal development is key to understanding the abnormalities that can occur.

EMBRYOLOGY

The primitive gut arises during the fourth week of gestation from the yolk sac as a tube extending from mouth to cloaca (Fig. 55.1). This tube consists of three parts, each supplied by a separate artery. Subsequent elongation and division of the primitive gut give rise to all the organs involved in digestion. The foregut develops into the pharynx, esophagus, stomach, proximal duodenum, liver, pancreas, and biliary system. These organs all receive their blood supply from the celiac axis. The midgut develops into the distal duodenum, jejunum, ileum, cecum, appendix, right colon, and part of the transverse colon, which are supplied by the superior mesenteric artery. The hindgut develops into the distal colon, rectum, and superior anal canal, which are supplied by the inferior mesenteric artery. Epithelial cell formation and differentiation begin soon after organogenesis and parallel morphologic development of the digestive system. Digestive, absorptive, secretory, motility,

hormonal, and immune functions develop throughout gestation as well as postnatally.

ESOPHAGEAL ANOMALIES

Esophageal Atresia

Esophageal atresia (EA), with or without an associated tracheoesophageal fistula (TEF), is the most common esophageal malformation, occurring in 1 in 2,000 to 5,000 live births. The defect is thought to result from failed separation of the esophagus and trachea by a septum that forms by the fourth week of gestation.

Five forms of EA with TEF occur (Fig. 55.2). The most common type is a proximal esophageal pouch and fistula connecting the trachea to the distal esophagus. Infants usually present at birth with copious oral secretions, respiratory distress, and aspiration. A history of maternal polyhydramnios is present in approximately 50%. Failure to pass an orogastric or nasogastric tube into the stomach is diagnostic. Roentgenography of the chest and abdomen shows the tube ending or coiled in the proximal pouch (Fig. 55.3A). The presence of gas in the stomach or small bowel is indicative of a coexisting TEF. These infants should be evaluated for other associated congenital anomalies. The origin of the VACTERL or VATER

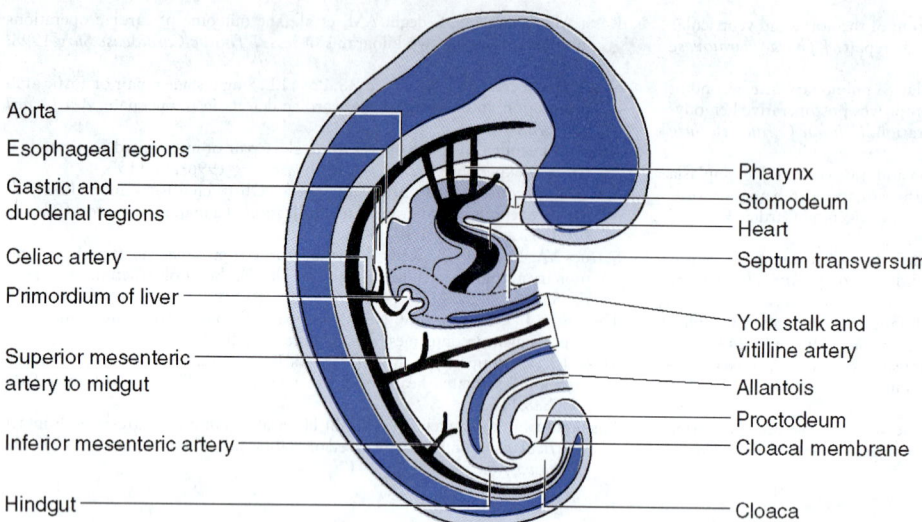

Aorta

Esophageal regions

Gastric and
duodenal regions

Celiac artery

Primordium of liver

Superior mesenteric
artery to midgut

Inferior mesenteric artery

Hindgut

Pharynx

Stomodeum

Heart

Septum transversum

Yolk stalk and
vitilline artery

Allantois

Proctodeum

Cloacal membrane

Cloaca

FIGURE 55.1. Median section of a 4-week embryo showing the primitive gut and its blood supply.

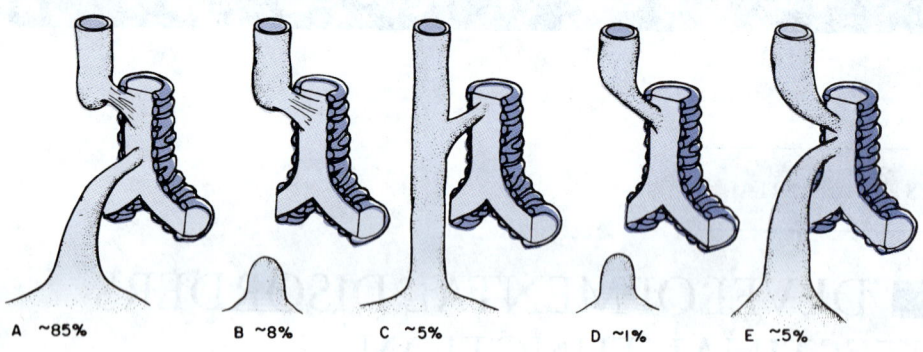

A ~85%   B ~8%   C ~5%   D ~1%   E ~5%

FIGURE 55.2. Esophageal atresia and tracheoesophageal fistula. The most common type of these esophageal anomalies is a proximal atresia with a distal fistula to the trachea. Isolated esophageal atresia is the next most common esophageal anomaly; as indicated, the remaining types are far less common.

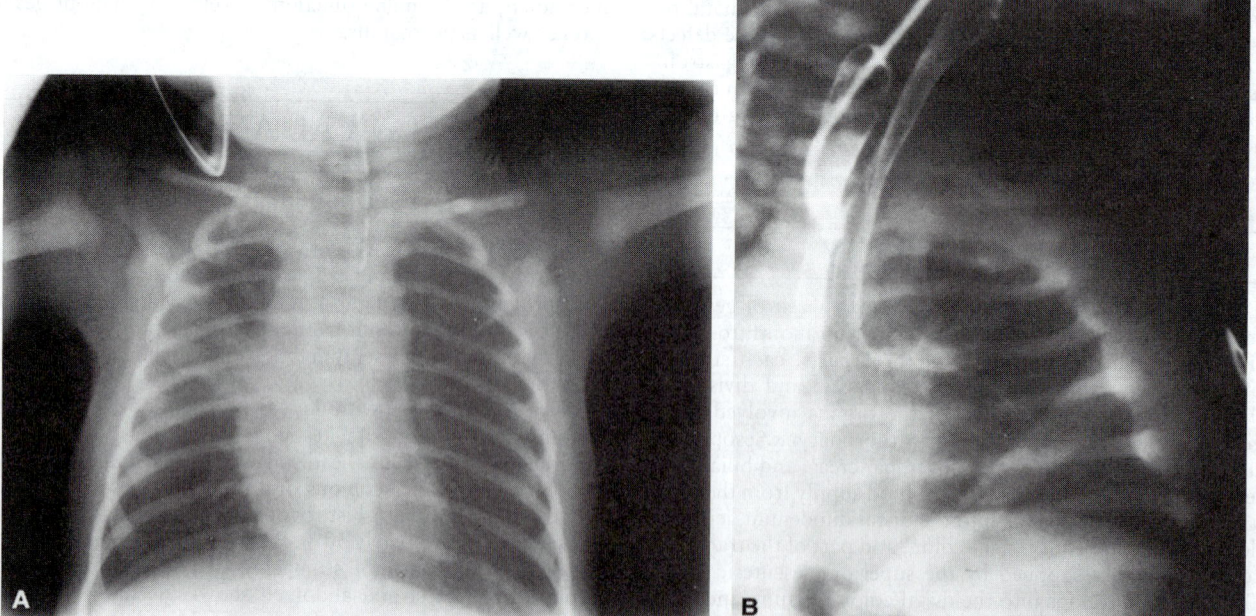

FIGURE 55.3. Radiographic appearance of esophageal atresia and tracheoesophageal fistula (TEF). **A:** A radiopaque catheter that has been placed demonstrates the length of the proximal esophagus in an infant with the most common variety of TEF. **B:** In another patient, contrast material is outlining an H-type variety of TEF.

association (vertebral anomalies, anorectal malformations, cardiac defects, TEFs, renal or radial anomalies, and limb malformations) is unknown. The rarer, H-type TEF, which connects an intact esophagus and trachea, usually presents later in infancy or childhood as feeding difficulties or chronic respiratory disease. This type of fistula requires special pull-back barium esophagraphy to make the diagnosis (Fig. 55.3B).

Surgical treatment of EA and TEF includes identification and ligation of the fistula and, when possible, primary anastomosis of the esophageal remnants. If the gap is too long for end-to-end anastomosis, delayed repair after gradual elongation, colonic interposition, or bringing the stomach up may be performed. Children who have had EA repair often experience chronic problems with gastroesophageal reflux.

Laryngotracheal Clefts

Laryngotracheal clefts also result from incomplete separation of esophagus and trachea. The tracheoesophageal septum fails to complete its cranial growth, thus causing incomplete fusion of the cricoid cartilage and producing a cleft that extends by varying degrees into the larynx and trachea. The presenting symptoms in an infant depend on the extent of the cleft and include choking, aspiration during feeding, stridor, respiratory distress, recurrent pneumonia, and poor cry. Direct endoscopic visualization is the best way to make the diagnosis. Treatment ranges from no treatment in mild cases to intubation, tracheotomy, gastrostomy, or complicated definitive repair in severe cases.

Congenital Esophageal Stenosis and Webs

Congenital esophageal stenosis and webs are associated with EA and TEF. These may be milder variants of incomplete tracheal and esophageal separation or possible failure of recanalization at 10 weeks' gestation. Webs are mucosal membranes that usually occur in the middle portion of the esophagus, typically the proximal end of the distal one-third. Stenosis is narrowing of the more distal esophagus because of tracheobronchial remnants. Neonates with complete webs present with symptoms of obstruction that are similar to those of EA. Stenosis or perforated webs usually present in infants as dysphasia, particularly with solids, as well as with vomiting, poor weight gain, and respiratory symptoms. A contrast study of the esophagus often identifies these lesions. Endoscopy may be helpful in identifying obscure webs and in ruling out strictures secondary to gastroesophageal reflux. A skilled endoscopist also may be able to resect the web. Surgical resection is necessary for complete webs and symptomatic stenoses. Dilation is usually not successful for true congenital esophageal stenosis, which may contain cartilage.

GASTRIC ANOMALIES

Microgastria

Microgastria is a rare malformation resulting from failure of the foregut to dilate. In addition, epithelial cells fail to differentiate, resulting in absent acid secretion. Association with a variety of other anomalies such as asplenia, malrotation, situs inversus, limb abnormalities, spinal deformities, and micrognathia is common. Clinically, infants present with vomiting, diarrhea, poor weight gain, or recurrent pneumonia. A small tubular stomach with incomplete rotation is identified on contrast study, often associated with a dilated esophagus. Opti-

mizing nutrition through small frequent feedings or continuous tube feedings (gastric or jejunal) is the goal of treatment. When necessary, surgical procedures may be attempted to increase gastric capacity.

Gastric Antrum and Pyloric Atresias

Atresias of the gastric antrum or pylorus are rare. Although the embryologic etiology is unclear, segmental defects may result from discontinuation of the endodermal tube before 8 weeks' gestation. An association of pyloric atresia with epidermolysis bullosa inherited as an autosomal recessive disorder has been described. Infants with gastric atresia present within the first day of life with vomiting, upper abdominal distention, and occasional gastric rupture. An abdominal plain film usually shows a large air-filled stomach with no distal gas. An upper gastrointestinal contrast study (UGI) is diagnostic. The absent pyloric muscle may be seen on ultrasound. Surgical therapy, with gastroduodenostomy or gastrojejunostomy, is performed after decompression and suctioning of the stomach with a nasogastric tube and correction of fluid and electrolyte abnormalities.

Antral Web

Antral webs are mucosal membranes that can partially or completely occlude the gastric lumen. Complete obstruction presents shortly after birth as nonbilious vomiting and can progress to catastrophic gastric rupture. These infants may be of low birth weight and have a history of polyhydramnios. Partial obstruction presents later in infancy or childhood as intermittent vomiting, failure to thrive, or postprandial pain or fullness. An incomplete or perforated web may be demonstrated by contrast study or endoscopy. Endoscopic or surgical incision is required if significant obstructive symptoms occur.

Gastric Volvulus

Gastric volvulus occurs when one part of the stomach rotates around another in either an organoaxial (longitudinal) or mesentericoaxial (transverse) direction. Abnormal fixation of the stomach or diaphragmatic abnormalities may contribute to the development of gastric volvulus in children. Associated asplenia and malrotation have been described in infantile cases. In an acute presentation, the symptoms are vomiting, retching, and abdominal pain. Chronic symptoms include postprandial pain, vomiting, and belching. UGI study shows the antrum lying high in the abdomen or in the chest in a mesentericoaxial volvulus. An organoaxial volvulus, seen in the majority of childhood cases, may be more difficult to identify. Surgical treatment to reduce the volvulus and to fix the stomach to the abdominal wall is required. This procedure should be done urgently in acute cases to prevent gastric ischemia and necrosis.

Pyloric Stenosis

Pyloric stenosis develops postnatally in the first weeks of life and results from hypertrophy of the pyloric muscle, which obstructs gastric outflow. The origin is unknown; however, the absence of nitric oxide synthase in the pyloric muscle has been implicated. Nitric oxide is an inhibitory neurotransmitter that mediates smooth muscle relaxation. The incidence of pyloric stenosis is 1 in 250 live births and is three to four times higher in boys than in girls. First-born infants and white infants are

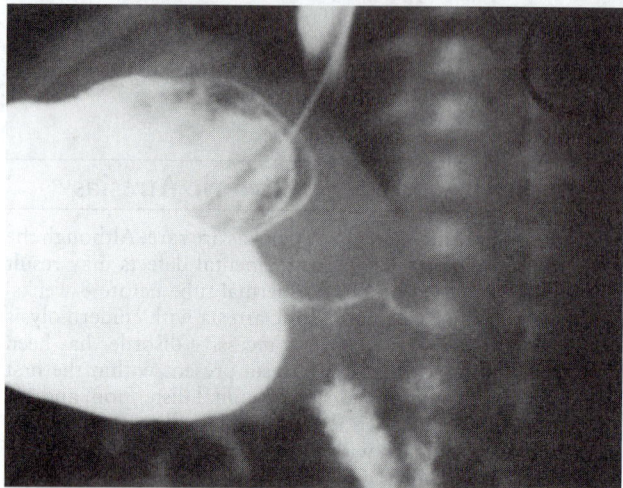

FIGURE 55.4. Pyloric stenosis. This radiograph is a lateral view from a barium study of the upper gastrointestinal tract performed on a vomiting infant. A thin stream of barium is seen exiting from the distended stomach through a markedly narrowed pyloric channel.

affected more commonly. The mode of inheritance appears to be polygenic, with an increased risk in siblings and children.

Pyloric stenosis presents between 1 and 12 weeks of life as nonbilious projectile vomiting. Premature infants may present later. Weight loss and dehydration are seen commonly, as well as hematemesis in 20% and jaundice in 5%. The symptoms begin as regurgitation, which becomes progressively more severe over several days. These infants often appear dehydrated and cachectic. Peristaltic waves may be visualized in the epigastrium. An olive-sized pyloric mass is palpated in the midline or right upper quadrant of the abdomen in up to 80%. Identification of the mass is aided by first decompressing the stomach with a nasogastric tube. Diagnosis is made by ultrasound demonstration of the thickened and elongated pyloric muscle. UGI study characteristically shows a narrow, elongated pyloric channel outlined by a double tract of barium and bulging of the pylorus into the antrum (Fig. 55.4).

Initial therapy should be directed at correction of fluid and electrolyte abnormalities. Classically, infants with pyloric stenosis have hyponatremia, hypochloremia, hypokalemia, and metabolic alkalosis resulting from chronic loss of gastric secretions. Surgical repair is curative. The Ramstedt pyloromyotomy involves incision and division of the pyloric muscle. Persistent gastroesophageal reflux is seen in approximately 15% of patients postoperatively.

INTESTINAL MALFORMATIONS

Nonrotation and Malrotation

After 6 weeks' gestation, the midgut rapidly lengthens while the liver increases in size. The developing bowel exits the abdominal cavity into the umbilical cord, where it undergoes counterclockwise rotation of 270 degrees around the axis of the superior mesenteric artery. At approximately 10 weeks, the jejunum returns into the left side of the abdomen, followed by the ileum and cecum, which fill the right. The dorsal mesentery of the midgut attaches to the posterior abdominal wall from the ligament of Treitz to the ileocecal junction, thus making the duodenum and right colon retroperitoneal. Nonrotation results in abnormal positioning of the small bowel on the right and the cecum and colon on the left. Malrotation, the most common developmental abnormality, occurs when incomplete

rotation places the cecum in the right upper quadrant and fixes the mesentery on a narrow base. The small bowel is at increased risk for twisting on the pedicle of mesentery, a volvulus, which compromises bowel vascularity and may lead to ischemia and necrosis. Another complication of malrotation results when peritoneal bands (Ladd bands) that extend from the cecum to the right upper quadrant obstruct the duodenum.

Midgut volvulus can occur at any age but is most common in infancy. The symptoms are those of upper intestinal obstruction and ischemia: bilious vomiting, abdominal distention, pain, and passage of blood via the rectum. Less severe symptoms may be seen if the volvulus is intermittent or ischemia has not yet developed. These range from episodic vomiting and pain to anorexia, failure to thrive, and chylous ascites from lymphatic obstruction. In the ill-appearing infant, diagnosis and surgical treatment should be prompt to avoid necrosis with loss of bowel or death. Abdominal radiography may show a dilated stomach and duodenum; however, the UGI is diagnostic for both volvulus and uncomplicated malrotation. The volvulus appears as a "corkscrew" narrowing of the distal duodenum. Malrotation is demonstrated by an abnormal position of the ligament of Treitz, normally to the left of the spine, and by visualizing the proximal jejunum on the right side of the abdomen. Duodenal obstruction from bands can also be seen on UGI.

Surgical treatment of malrotation is indicated in symptomatic patients. After reducing the volvulus, if present, the abnormally fixed duodenum, jejunum, and colon are freed (Ladd procedure). In severe cases, ischemic or necrotic portions of bowel may have to be resected, and short gut syndrome may be the consequence if considerable length of bowel is involved. Surgery is recommended for asymptomatic patients, because they are at risk for development of acute volvulus, which is associated with significant morbidity and mortality.

Duplication Abnormalities

Duplication abnormalities of the intestinal tract occur from mouth to anus but are most common in the small bowel, particularly the distal ileum. These cystic or tubular malformations are lined with some type of alimentary mucosa and are located on the mesenteric border of the adjacent bowel with which they share a blood supply and a muscular wall. They may be caused by abnormal recanalization with the formation of two lumen when vacuoles coalesce. Those associated with vertebral or spinal cord anomalies possibly arise from splitting of the notocord during development. Duplications may remain asymptomatic; however, they can present as an obstruction, abdominal mass, perforation, or the lead point for intussusception. Acid secretion from gastric mucosa, present in approximately 20%, may cause ulceration and gastrointestinal bleeding. Most duplications (66%) present during infancy and may be associated with intestinal atresia, other duplications (15%), or spinal or vertebral anomalies. Ultrasound study of the abdomen may demonstrate a cystic structure. A UGI may reveal a duplication if a communication exists with the bowel lumen. Ectopic gastric mucosa will light up on a technetium scan. The diagnosis is confirmed by laparotomy, and treatment is surgical resection or division of the common wall.

Meckel Diverticulum

A Meckel diverticulum is a remnant of the embryonic yolk sac that results from failure of the omphalomesenteric or vitelline duct to involute between the fifth and seventh weeks of gestation. Meckel diverticulum is one of the most common congenital intestinal anomalies, occurring in 1% to 3% of the population, with a male-to-female ratio of 3:1. The diverticulum contains all three intestinal layers and ranges from 2 to 10 cm in length. The diverticulum is located on the antimesenteric border of the distal ileum, usually 40 to 50 cm from the ileocecal valve. More than one-half of these anomalies contain ectopic mucosa, usually of the gastric type. Acid secretion by gastric mucosa may induce ulceration and bleeding of the adjacent intestinal mucosa. Painless intermittent lower gastrointestinal bleeding is the most common presentation of a Meckel diverticulum. These anomalies can be visualized by a technetium scan that labels gastric mucosa. Surgical exploration usually is required to diagnose diverticula that present as intestinal obstruction caused by intussusception, volvulus, or internal herniation. Diverticulitis, which may be complicated by perforation, presents with symptoms similar to acute appendicitis.

Intestinal Atresias

Intestinal atresias are classified into four types. Type I is a membrane made up of mucosa and submucosa that obstructs the lumen. The muscularis and serosa remain intact, and no interruption exists in the continuity of the bowel. Type II consists of a fibrous band connecting interrupted segments of bowel. In type III atresias, the proximal and distal segments of bowel end blindly, with a gap in the mesentery as well. A subtype IIIB, also known as the apple peel type, is proximal atresia with coiling and foreshortening of the distal bowel. The superior mesenteric artery and mesentery distal to the atresia are absent. Type IV atresias are multiple and often occur in families. Most jejunal or ileal atresias are thought to be the result of *in utero* ischemia and necrosis caused by volvulus, intussusception, internal hernias, or interruption of mesenteric blood supply.

The origin of duodenal atresia is different, and this condition is most likely caused by abnormal recanalization of the intestinal lumen during the fifth to eighth week of gestation. Duodenal atresia often is associated with other anomalies such as Down syndrome, congenital heart disease, TEF, malrotation, and renal anomalies. The incidence of duodenal atresia is 0.5 to 1.0 in 10,000. More distal atresias occur in 1 in 20,000 live births, with 5% to 10% having multiple atresias. Thirty-one percent of these anomalies are located in the proximal jejunum, 20% in the distal jejunum, 13% in the proximal ileum, and 36% in the distal ileum. Intestinal atresias sometimes can be diagnosed prenatally because of polyhydramnios and ultrasound evidence of proximal dilatation. Prematurity is associated with both jejunal and ileal atresias.

Clinically, infants present in the neonatal period with bilious vomiting, abdominal distention, and failure to pass meconium. Duodenal atresia can have the classic double-bubble sign on upright abdominal film, with absent gas distally (Fig. 55.5). In other small bowel atresias, plain films are suggestive also of obstruction, showing dilated proximal small bowel with air-fluid levels. Intraperitoneal calcifications indicate prior meconium peritonitis because of intestinal perforation *in utero*. Initial treatment is aimed at stabilization of the patient and includes decompression with nasogastric suctioning and management of fluid and electrolytes. When other life-threatening associated anomalies have been ruled out or identified and treated, surgical resection and reanastomosis can be performed. The prognosis for these infants depends on the amount of remaining small bowel and the severity of coexisting anomalies.

Meconium Ileus

Meconium ileus also causes neonatal intestinal obstruction from occlusion of the intestinal lumen, usually the distal ileum, with abnormally thick meconium secondary to cystic fibrosis. Ten percent to 15% of patients with cystic fibrosis present in this manner. At least one-half of these cases are complicated by

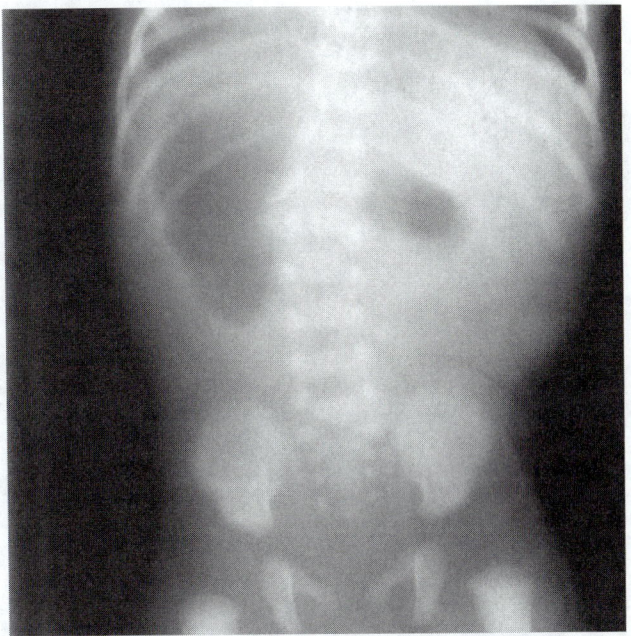

FIGURE 55.5. Duodenal atresia. This abdominal film of a neonate shows gas in the stomach and dilated duodenal bulb, but no air in the distal gastrointestinal tract.

malrotation, volvulus, atresia, and *in utero* perforation. Meconium peritonitis secondary to perforation can lead to ascites, adhesions, and intraabdominal calcifications. In addition to bilious vomiting, distention, and failure to pass meconium, these infants may have palpable bowel loops in the right lower quadrant. Abdominal radiography shows small bubbles indicating meconium and intraperitoneal calcifications if there has been an earlier perforation. Contrast enema demonstrates a microcolon, inspissated meconium in the distal ileum, and proximal bowel dilation (Fig. 55.6). Relief of the obstruction may be attempted with a hypertonic, water-soluble enema (Gastrografin or Hypaque). Surgical treatment includes enterotomy and irrigation with acetylcysteine (Mucomyst), resection of atretic segments, and peritoneal cleansing when necessary. Children with meconium ileus have the same prognosis as any other child with cystic fibrosis.

COLONIC ANOMALIES

Hirschsprung Disease

Hirschsprung disease, or congenital aganglionic megacolon, results from abnormal innervation of the hindgut. Neuronal dysplasia begins at the anus and extends proximally by varying degrees. Histologically, ganglia are absent, and nerve bundles in the submucosa and between the circular and longitudinal muscles are hypertrophied. The distribution of disease most commonly involves the rectosigmoid colon (Table 55.1). The incidence of Hirschsprung disease is 1 in 5,000, with a male-to-female ratio of 3.8:1.0 and an equal distribution in blacks and whites. A familial incidence occurs (10% of cases), often involving the entire colon. Mutations in a tyrosine kinase gene (*RET*) on chromosome 10 and the endothelin receptor-B gene (*ENDR-B*) on chromosome 13 have been linked to the autosomal dominant form of Hirschsprung disease as well as some sporadic cases. These mutations may play a role in maldevelopment of the neural crest–derived cells. Possibly the pathologic features in Hirschsprung disease result when migrating neural

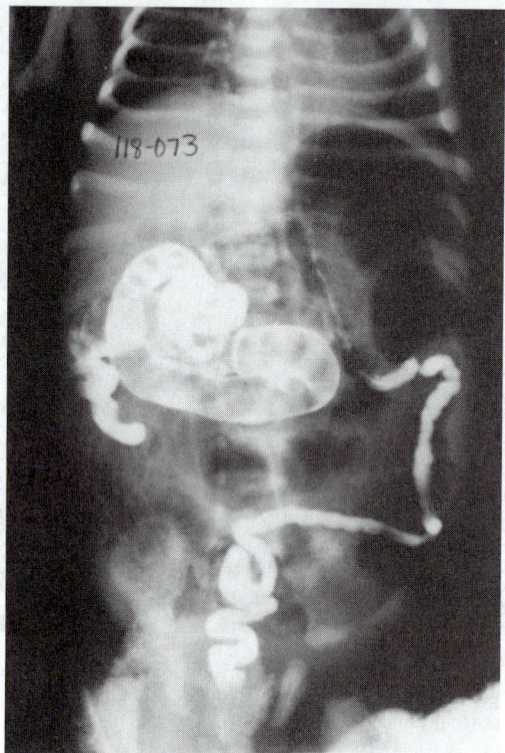

FIGURE 55.6. Meconium ileus. This is an anteroposterior view from a barium enema performed on an infant with intestinal obstruction in the neonatal period. Microcolon, which may occur in both meconium ileus and intestinal atresia, is evident. Unlike in ileal atresia, obstructing plugs of inspissated meconium are present within the lumen of this patient's terminal ileum, a finding suggesting meconium ileus.

crest cells confront an "abnormal microenvironment" in the colon that may be genetically determined.

Clinically, 80% of patients present in the first year of life with failure to pass meconium within the first 48 hours of life and constipation. In some cases, usually those with ultra-short segments of affected colon, the diagnosis may be delayed for years. An association exists between Hirschsprung disease and Down syndrome (3%) and cardiac anomalies (2.5%). On examination, the infant with Hirschsprung disease has a distended abdomen, and rectal examination reveals normal tone with an empty vault. Rapid expulsion of liquid stool following digital examination is characteristic. Enterocolitis, a complication of Hirschsprung disease with significant morbidity and mortality, may result from exposure of mucosa compromised by distention to increased bacteria and toxins because of stasis

TABLE 55.1

EXTENT OF AGANGLIONOSIS IN HIRSCHSPRUNG DISEASE

Area	Percentage (%)
Rectum/rectosigmoid	30
Sigmoid	44
Left colon	11
Splenic flexure	4
Transverse colon	2
Right colon	1
Total colon and above	8

Reprinted with permission from Kleinhaus S, Boley SJ, Sheran M, et al. Hirschsprung's disease: a survey of the members of the surgical section of the American Academy of Pediatrics. *J Pediatr Surg* 1979;14:588.

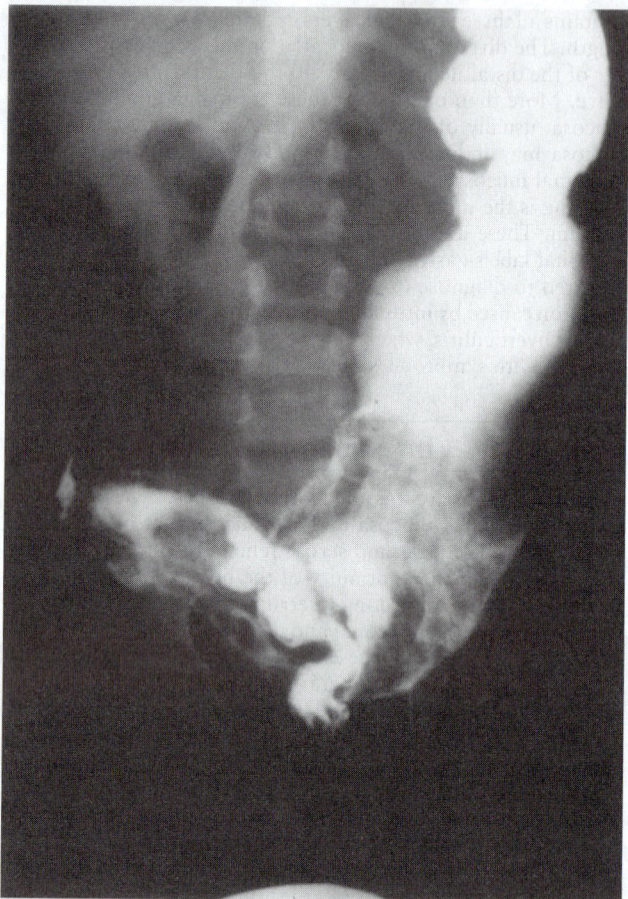

FIGURE 55.7. Hirschsprung disease. A barium enema in an older child shows the transition from normal-caliber aganglionic rectosigmoid to dilated proximal colon.

and overgrowth. These infants develop foul-smelling bloody diarrhea, abdominal distention, and systemic illness with fever and often sepsis. Early diagnosis and surgical treatment of Hirschsprung disease decrease but do not completely eliminate the incidence of enterocolitis.

Suction rectal biopsies and anorectal manometry are the most reliable indicators of Hirschsprung disease. Full-thickness biopsies are diagnostic. A barium enema often demonstrates the transition zone between the aganglionic contracted segment and the dilated proximal bowel. The dilatation of the proximal bowel occurs postnatally as normal colon peristalsis occurs against the functional obstruction of the unrelaxed affected segment (Fig. 55.7). The barium enema therefore may not be diagnostic in the first 2 weeks of life (Fig. 55.8). Delayed emptying of barium on a 24- or 48-hour follow-up film is suggestive of Hirschsprung disease even in the absence of a transition zone, which may not be obvious in short segment disease. Biopsies should be taken at least 2 cm above the dentate line, because the most distal 2 cm of bowel are normally aganglionic. However, biopsies taken much higher may miss ultrashort segment disease. The specimen must be deep enough to contain adequate submucosa to demonstrate the presence or absence of ganglion cells. In addition, staining of the specimen for acetylcholinesterase shows hypertrophied nerve trunks, which, together with absent ganglion cells, are diagnostic for Hirschsprung disease. Manometric findings reveal failure of relaxation of the internal anal sphincter in response to distention by inflation of a rectal balloon.

Surgical management includes definition of the level of abnormal innervation by serial biopsies followed by colostomy to decompress the normal colon and subsequent colonic or ileal

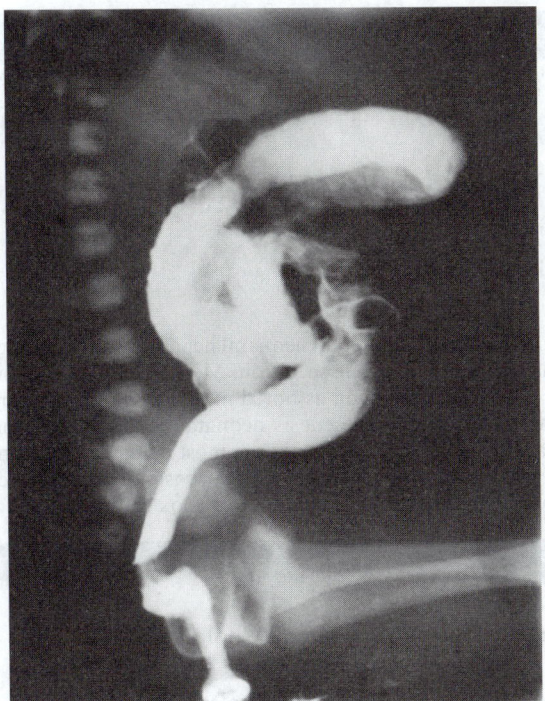

FIGURE 55.8. Hirschsprung disease. This is a lateral view of a barium enema performed on an 8-day-old infant with constipation. The lumen of the rectum is contracted, suggesting congenital segmental aganglionosis; the diagnosis was confirmed later by suction renal biopsy.

pull-through procedures. Ultrashort segment disease may be treated by a myectomy excising a strip of distal rectal muscle.

Imperforate Anus

Abnormal division of the cloaca into urogenital and rectal portions during the fourth to sixth weeks of gestation results in an imperforate anus, which is an invisible opening, usually with a fistula from the distal rectum to the perineum or urogenital tract. The incidence of this malformation is 1 in 5,000, and approximately one-half of cases include other anomalies (often in the VACTERL association). These lesions are categorized as high, low, or intermediate, depending on the level at which the rectum ends in relation to the pelvic muscular sling (Table 55.2). The male-to-female ratio is 2:1 for the high-type

TABLE 55.2
CLASSIFICATION OF ANORECTAL MALFORMATIONS

Boys
  Cutaneous (perineal fistula)
  Rectourethral fistula
    Bulbar
    Prostatic
  Rector—bladderneck fistula
  Imperforate anus without fistula
  Rectal atresia
Girls
  Cutaneous (perineal fistula)
  Vestibular fistula
  Imperforate anus without fistula
  Rectal atresia
  Cloaca
  Complex malformation

Levitt MA, Peña A. Outcomes from the correction of anorectal malformations. *Curr Opin Pediatr*, 2005;17:394.

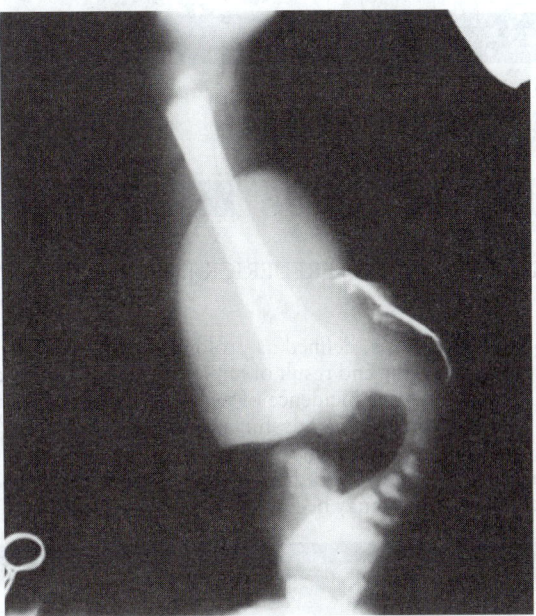

FIGURE 55.9. Imperforate anus. This is a lateral radiograph of the sacrum with the patient upside down. Contrast material is layered on the surface of the perineum; the level of obstruction in the rectum is outlined by bowel gas. The wide gap between the gas-filled distal rectum and the contrast-labeled perineum suggests the diagnosis of imperforate anus.

lesion but equal for low lesions. Infants usually are recognized at birth as having an absent anal opening. Meconium may be seen passing through a fistula on the perineum, coming from the vagina, or in the urine. Treatment depends on identification of the level of the lesion, which is best done with ultrasound or computed tomography rather than traditional upside-down radiography (Fig. 55.9). The spinal cord should be imaged to rule out tethering. The urinary system also should be studied for possible abnormalities. Patients with high or intermediate lesions require diverting colostomies within the first 72 hours of life. The definitive surgery is pull-through of the colon anterior to the puborectalis muscle. Low lesions may require only dilation and have a better prognosis. In contrast to children with high lesions, those with low lesions usually achieve continence.

Suggested Readings

Abel RM. The ontogeny of the peptide innervation of the human pylorus, with special reference to understanding the aetiology and pathogenesis of infantile hypertrophic pyloric stenosis. *J Pediatr Surg* 1996;31:490.

Botto LD, Khoury MJ, Mastroiacovo P, et al. The spectrum of congenital anomalies of the VATER association: an international study. *Am J Med Genet* 1997;71:8.

Kimble RM, Harding J, Kolbe A. Additional congenital anomalies in babies with gut atresia or stenosis: when to investigate, and which investigation. *Pediatr Surg Int* 1997;12:565.

Maxson RT, Franklin PA, Wagner CW. Malrotation in the older child: surgical management, treatment, and outcome. *Am Surg* 1995;61:135.

Moore TC. Omphalomesenteric duct malformations. *Semin Pediatr Surg* 1996;5:116.

Oudshoorn JH, Heij HA. Intestinal obstruction caused by duplication of the caecum. *Eur J Pediatr* 1996;155:338.

Pena A. Current management of anorectal anomalies. *Surg Clin North Am* 1992;72:1393.

Robertson K, Mason I, Hall S. Hirschsprung's disease: genetic mutations in mice and men. *Gut* 1997;41:436.

Sullivan PB. Hirschsprung's disease. *Arch Dis Child* 1996;74:5.

Touloukian RJ. Diagnosis and treatment of jejunoileal atresia. *World J Surg* 1993;17:310.

Walker WA, Durie PR, Hamilton JR, et al., eds. *Pediatric gastrointestinal disease: pathophysiology, diagnosis, management,* 2nd ed. St. Louis: Mosby, 1996.

CHAPTER 56 ■ NEONATAL CHOLESTASIS

DONALD A. NOVAK, FREDERICK J. SUCHY, AND WILLIAM F. BALISTRERI

Neonatal cholestasis, defined as prolonged conjugated hyperbilirubinemia, is the end result of impaired bile flow and excretion. The cumulative incidence of neonatal cholestasis is near 1 in 2,500 live births. Liver dysfunction in the neonate, regardless of the cause, commonly is associated with bile secretory failure and cholestatic jaundice. The potential mechanisms by which bile secretion may be impaired are many. Hepatocellular injury, such as that noted in neonatal hepatitis, may cause functional impairment of bile secretion. Mechanical obstruction to bile flow also may occur, as noted in biliary atresia. Although many disorders can present as neonatal cholestasis, neonatal hepatitis and biliary atresia are the most common syndromes, together accounting for the majority of cases of prolonged conjugated hyperbilirubinemia in infants (Box 56.1).

BOX 56.1   Differential Diagnosis of Conjugated Hyperbilirubinemia (Neonatal Cholestasis)

Bile Duct Obstruction
Cholangiopathies
  Biliary atresia
  Choledochal cyst
  Neonatal sclerosing cholangitis
  Spontaneous perforation of common bile duct
  Bile duct stenosis
  Caroli disease
Other
  Inspissated bile-mucus plug
  Cholelithiasis
  Tumors or masses (intrinsic and extrinsic)

Neonatal Hepatitis
"Idiopathic"
Viral hepatitis
  Cytomegalovirus
  Rubella
  Herpesviruses
    Simplex
    Zoster
    Human herpesvirus type 6
  Adenovirus
  Enteroviruses
  Parvovirus B19
  Hepatitis B
  ? Non-A, non-B, non-C hepatitis
  Human immunodeficiency virus
Bacterial and parasitic hepatitis
  Bacterial sepsis
  Syphilis
  Listeriosis
  Tuberculosis
  Toxoplasmosis

Cholestatic Syndromes
Alagille syndrome
Progressive familial intrahepatic cholestasis
  Type 1: Familial intrahepatic cholestasis 1
  Type 2: BSEP (ATP-dependent bile acid transporter)
  Type 3: *MDR3* deficiency
  Hereditary cholestasis with lymphedema (Aagenaes syndrome)

Benign recurrent intrahepatic cholestasis: Familial intrahepatic cholestasis 1
  Disorders of bile acid synthesis
Peroxisomal disorders
  Zellweger syndrome
Familial cholestasis of North American Indians

Metabolic Diseases
Disorders of amino acid metabolism
  Tyrosinemia
Disorders of lipid metabolism
  Niemann-Pick disease type C
  Gaucher disease
  Wolman disease/cholesteryl ester storage disease
Disorders of the urea cycle
  Arginase deficiency
Disorders of carbohydrate metabolism
  Galactosemia
  Fructosemia
  Type IV glycogenosis
  Carbohydrate deficient glycoprotein syndrome
Disorders of oxidative phosphorylation
Alpha-1-antitrypsin deficiency
Cystic fibrosis
Hypopituitarism (septooptic dysplasia)
Hypothyroidism
Neonatal iron storage disease

Toxic Conditions
Drugs
Parenteral nutrition

Miscellaneous Associations
Shock, hypoperfusion
Langerhans cell histiocytosis
Intestinal obstruction
Erythrophagocytic lymphohistiocytosis
Neonatal lupus erythematosus
Indian childhood cirrhosis
Extracorporeal membrane oxygenation
Autosomal trisomies
Graft-versus-host disease
Venoocclusive disease

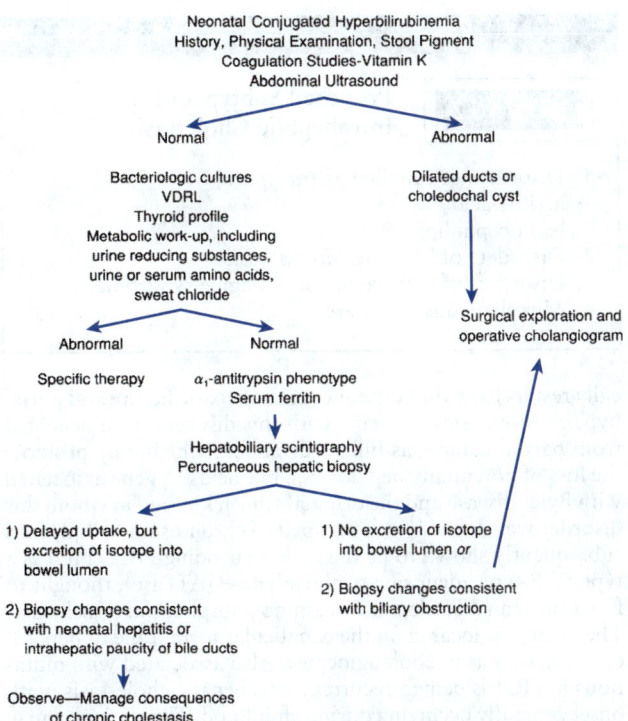

FIGURE 56.1. Flow chart for the workup of neonatal cholestasis.

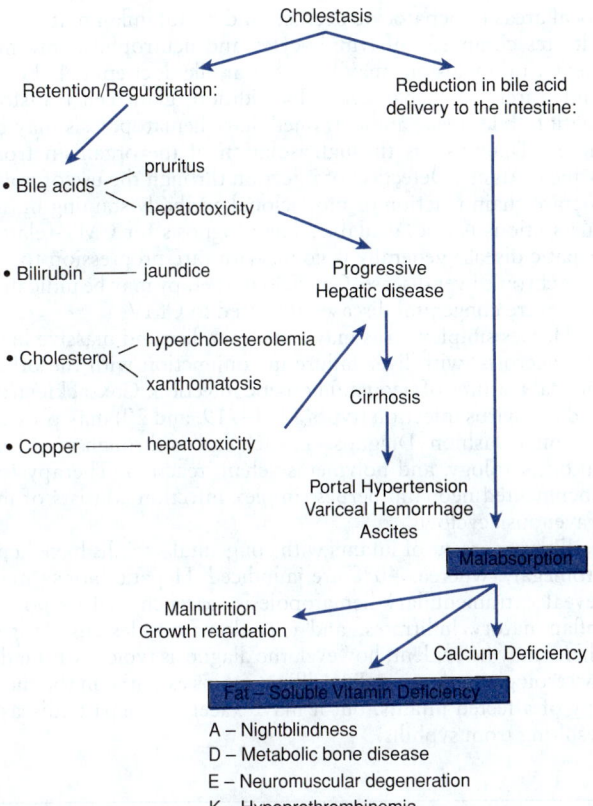

FIGURE 56.2. Consequences of chronic cholestasis.

Identification of the infant with cholestasis begins with measurement of total and conjugated bilirubin fractions (Fig. 56.1). The cholestatic infant will have an elevated conjugated fraction, generally at a level of more than 2 mg/dL and accounting for more than 15% to 20% of the total bilirubin. The possibility of liver or biliary tract disease must be considered in any neonate jaundiced beyond 2 weeks of age. Indeed, jaundice after 11 days in term infants and after 14 days in premature infants is unusual, occurring in only 0.5% of infants in one study. Subsequent efforts must be directed toward rapid diagnosis of and therapy for potentially treatable disorders, such as sepsis, galactosemia, and hypothyroidism or panhypopituitarism, in which delay of diagnosis may have catastrophic consequences. Next, differentiation of biliary atresia from neonatal hepatitis must be accomplished, because the former requires surgical intervention. In all patients with cholestasis, effective management of the consequences of chronic cholestasis is imperative (Fig. 56.2). Early in the workup of any cholestatic infant, vitamin K (2.5 mg) should be given in an effort to prevent life-threatening hemorrhage. Further description of specific diagnostic modalities is included with the discussion of each entity.

INFECTIOUS CAUSES OF CHOLESTASIS

That cholestasis may occur in patients with gram-negative bacterial infection has long been recognized. The incidence of jaundice during episodes of neonatal sepsis has been estimated at 20% to 60%. Urinary tract infections caused by *Escherichia coli* frequently have been associated with jaundice, particularly in male infants. The infants may appear clinically well and may have jaundice as their only symptom. Other bacteria, including gram-negative rods, staphylococci, streptococci, and *Listeria*, have been implicated in cholestasis. Limited autopsy studies have shown centrilobular hepatic necrosis and canalicular bile stasis; these features and direct experimental evidence suggest

that bacterial toxins produce canalicular dysfunction, probably through inhibition of the canalicular multiple organic anion transporter. Jaundice is reversible with successful therapy for the underlying infection. Thus, cultures (blood and urine in particular) are important components of the initial evaluation phase for neonates with cholestasis.

Other unusual infectious causes of neonatal cholestasis include any of the so-called TORCH (toxoplasmosis, other viruses, rubella, cytomegalovirus [CMV], herpes) agents, as well as coxsackieviruses and echoviruses. Parvovirus B19 and human herpesvirus type 6 are associated with cholestatic liver disease. The infant with congenital toxoplasmosis may be noted at birth with hepatomegaly (60%) and hyperbilirubinemia (40%), or these features may develop later in the neonatal period. Although hepatic disease generally is mild, progressive hepatic dysfunction may occur. Hepatic pathologic features are nonspecific and include mononuclear periportal inflammation and canalicular bile stasis. Diagnosis may be made using utilizing serologic assays or through demonstration of the parasite in spinal fluid sediment. Antiparasitic therapy may arrest disease progression.

Congenital rubella may be associated with hepatomegaly in 65% of cases and with jaundice in 15% of cases. The clinical presentation and hepatic pathologic findings are nonspecific. Elevation of aminotransferase values may occur, as may acholic stools. The prognosis for the hepatic disease is good, with progression to hepatic fibrosis and failure uncommon. Diagnosis is through serology and viral isolation. No specific therapy is available.

CMV infection may produce symptoms in the neonate of hepatosplenomegaly and, occasionally, hyperbilirubinemia, in addition to the other well-known stigmata of congenital CMV. In the jaundiced infant with abnormal serum aminotransferase levels, CMV infection is suggested by liver biopsy findings of focal areas of hepatocyte necrosis and portal inflammatory infiltrates composed of lymphocytes and neutrophils. Intranuclear viral inclusions may be noted in bile duct epithelial cells and (rarely) in hepatocytes. In addition, giant cell transformation, bile stasis, and extramedullary hematopoiesis may be noted. Diagnosis is through isolation of the organism from urine or tissue. Detection of infection through the use of polymerase chain reaction or monoclonal antibody staining in tissue sections is also available. The prognosis for CMV-related hepatic disease generally is good, with rare progression to severe chronic liver disease. Ganciclovir therapy may be indicated for severe congenital disease attributed to CMV.

Herpes simplex virus may cause jaundice and massive hepatic necrosis, with liver failure in conjunction with the other clinical features of neonatal herpetic infection. Coxsackievirus and echovirus infection (types 11, 14, 19, and 20) may present in similar fashion. Diagnosis in each case is through viral isolation, serology, and polymerase chain reaction. Therapy for documented neonatal herpes simplex infection consists of intravenous acyclovir.

Eighty percent of infants with congenital syphilis have hepatomegaly, whereas 40% are jaundiced. Hepatic biopsy may reveal extramedullary hematopoiesis, parenchymal or portal inflammatory infiltrates, and granulomatous lesions. Spirochetes may be evident; however, the diagnosis typically is made by serologic evaluation. Penicillin remains essential in the therapy of affected infants, but it may exacerbate hepatic disease resulting from syphilis.

INTRAHEPATIC CHOLESTASIS

Intrahepatic cholestasis is a term that encompasses a diverse group of disorders, some associated with "paucity" of bile ducts, some associated with disordered bile acid metabolism, and others with abnormalities of transport across the hepatocyte membrane. Still others remain undefined. These disorders may present in the neonatal period with jaundice or (later in life) with chronic cholestasis. The term *progressive familial intrahepatic cholestasis* (PFIC) is used to describe a heterogeneous group of autosomal recessive progressive liver disorders in which cholestasis of hepatocellular origin often presents in the neonatal period or the first year of life and leads to death from liver failure at ages ranging from infancy to adolescence. However, it has long been thought, because the clinical, biochemical, and pathologic features and natural progression are variable, that this group has significant heterogeneity. Recent molecular and genetic studies have allowed the identification of genes responsible for three types of PFIC and have shown that these phenotypes are related to mutations in hepatocellular transport systems involved in bile formation. Inherited or acquired dysfunction of the mechanisms involved in the generation of bile flow, especially of canalicular transport proteins, therefore results in substrate retention manifest as cholestasis. A proposed classification of the various disorders comprising intrahepatic cholestasis is depicted in Box 56.2.

Disorders of Canalicular Transport

PFIC 1, or Byler syndrome, is a progressive familial disorder in which jaundice, at first episodic, becomes constant by 1 to 4 years of age. Pathologic study of the liver reveals progressive cholestasis and cirrhosis. Affected children have steatorrhea, failure to thrive, and rickets. Laboratory studies reflect severe cholestasis; serum gamma-glutamyltranspeptidase levels are paradoxically normal. Death occurs in childhood and typi-

---

> **BOX 56.2**   Proposed Subtypes of Intrahepatic Cholestasis
>
> 1. Disorders of canalicular *transport*
>   a. Bile acid
>   b. Phospholipid
> 2. Disorders of bile acid *biosynthesis*
> 3. Disorders of embryogenesis (Alagille syndrome)
> 4. Miscellaneous disorders

cally results from the consequences of hepatic failure and portal hypertension. Some patients with this disorder have benefited from partial cutaneous biliary diversion, which may promote the loss of potentially hepatotoxic bile acids. A gene associated with Byler disease and the original Amish kindred in whom this disorder was defined were mapped to chromosome 18q21 and subsequently shown to be the region encoding FIC1. FIC1 is a type IV P-type adenosine triphosphatase (ATPase), thought to function as an ATP-dependent amino phospholipid translocase. The protein is located on the canalicular membrane of hepatocytes, as well as in cholangiocytes. Also associated with mutations in FIC1 is benign recurrent intrahepatic cholestasis, with onset generally occurring during childhood. The clinical course of this disorder includes recurrent episodes of cholestasis that resolve spontaneously. The mechanism by which alterations in FIC1 cause the phenotype of benign recurrent intrahepatic cholestasis, or those associated with PFIC 1 (see earlier), remain unclear. Although FIC1 does not appear to be a bile acid transporter, mutations in FIC1 are associated with a profound reduction of biliary bile salts.

Non-Amish cases of Byler syndrome (PFIC 2) have been linked to chromosome 2q24 and a mutation in the ATP-dependent bile acid transporter (BSEP), located on the hepatocyte canalicular membrane. This disorder typically presents in infancy with cholestasis and giant cell hepatitis.

Another form of progressive familial cholestasis (PFIC 3) has been linked to mutations in the *MDR3* gene, which encodes a canalicular membrane phospholipid transporter (flippase). Affected infants present in similar fashion to those with PFIC 1 and 2; however, gamma-glutamyl transpeptidase values are elevated in these children. Other syndromes associated with *MDR3* deficiency include later-onset cholestasis in children, cholangiopathies in adults, and cholestasis of pregnancy in heterozygotes.

Dubin-Johnson syndrome may present with cholestasis in the neonatal period. Generally, patients are otherwise asymptomatic, and liver function tests, other than serum bilirubin, remain normal. The disorder has been linked to defective expression of the hepatocyte canalicular membrane multispecific anion transporter.

Disorders of Bile Acid Synthesis

Inborn Errors of Bile Acid Synthesis

Inherited defects in the bile acid biosynthetic pathway can cause cholestasis and progressive liver injury. Novel analytic techniques, including fast atom bombardment ionization with mass spectrometry, have allowed the diagnosis of these disorders; they previously may have been characterized as one of the idiopathic syndromes of cholestasis, such as neonatal hepatitis. The mechanism of cholestasis in these conditions may be twofold, related to a failure to synthesize adequate amounts of primary normal bile acids, which are essential for bile formation, along with the increased production of unusual bile acids with hepatotoxic potential.

Several inborn errors involving the bile acid steroid nucleus have been associated with familial neonatal cholestasis and giant cell hepatitis. The disorders are associated with severe cholestatic jaundice from birth, progressive liver injury and, if untreated, death from hepatic failure early in life. 3-beta-hydroxysteroid dehydrogenase or isomerase deficiency has been confirmed in several patients by the failure to synthesize primary bile acids with the concomitant production and accumulation of increased quantities of 3-beta-hydroxy-D^5-sterol intermediates. delta^4-3-oxosteroid-5-beta-reductase deficiency presents in infants with cholestatic liver disease. The phenotype of this disorder may include infants presenting with NISD. This defect results in markedly reduced primary bile acid synthesis and the accumulation of potentially toxic bile acid precursors, delta^4-3-oxo- and allo-bile acids. 2-methylacyl-coenzyme A racemase deficiency has also been associated with hepatic giant cell formation and the neonatal hepatitis phenotype, as have deficiencies of oxysterol 7-alpha hydroxylase and 25-hydroxylase.

The use of oral bile acid administration to treat inborn errors of bile acid metabolism has been extremely promising. The rationale for this therapeutic approach is that bile acid replacement can provide a stimulus for bile secretion and can inhibit endogenous synthesis and accumulation of potentially toxic bile acids produced in response to the enzyme deficiency. For example, in patients with the delta^4-3-oxosteroid-5-beta-reductase deficiency, combined treatment with cholic acid (to inhibit endogenous bile acid synthesis) and ursodeoxycholic acid (to stimulate bile flow) has been successful in completely suppressing delta^4-3-oxo- and allo-bile acid production and in normalizing or markedly improving liver tests and hepatic histologic features in some patients.

Zellweger Syndrome

Zellweger syndrome (cerebrohepatorenal syndrome) is a fatal autosomal recessive disorder associated with peroxisomal absence. Clinical characteristics include abnormal craniofacial development, severe hypotonia, hyporeflexia, eye abnormalities, hepatomegaly, failure to thrive, psychomotor retardation, calcific stippling of the patella, and renal cysts. Typically, jaundice is present in the first month of life. Death, often secondary to respiratory distress, sepsis, or liver disease, generally occurs within the first year of life. Histologic examination of the liver reveals cholestasis, focal necrosis, and (occasionally) paucity of the bile ducts. Electron microscopic examination is significant for the apparent absence of peroxisomes. Lack of peroxisomal function causes the accumulation of very long-chain fatty acids in the plasma, presumably because of deficient beta-oxidation. Other abnormalities include low levels of plasmalogens, abnormal bile acid and cholesterol metabolism, and elevated levels of pipecolic acid. Apart from the fairly characteristic phenotypic features, diagnosis is aided by measurement of the C26/C22 fatty acid ratio and detection of abnormal bile acid intermediates. Prenatal diagnosis is possible. Other probable "peroxisomal" diseases include Refsum disease, neonatal-type adrenoleukodystrophy, X-linked adrenoleukodystrophy, and chondrodysplasia punctata, rhizomelic type.

Disorders of Embryogenesis

Paucity of the intrahepatic bile ducts, defined as fewer than 0.5 intralobular bile ducts per triad, in the presence of otherwise normal portal areas may represent either a congenital or an acquired disorder, with paucity being the end result of progressive bile duct injury.

Alagille Syndrome

Some children who have hepatic histologic findings demonstrating paucity have, in addition, unique features that suggest a syndrome. The best-studied example is Alagille syndrome (arteriohepatic dysplasia), which denotes a constellation of findings, including the following: abnormal facies (broad forehead, deep-set eyes, hypertelorism, long and straight nose with flat nasal bridge, and underdeveloped mandible), ocular abnormalities (posterior embryotoxon, among other abnormalities), cardiovascular abnormalities (typically peripheral pulmonic stenosis, but intracardiac abnormalites such as tetralogy of Fallot may also be present), vertebral arch defects ("butterfly" vertebrae, hemivertebrae, decreased interpediculate distance), and a variety of renal abnormalities (Box 56.3). Associated findings in patients with Alagille syndrome such as growth retardation, mental retardation, and hypogonadism may be secondary to nutritional deficiencies (e.g., vitamin E). Children with Alagille syndrome may also be predisposed to intracranial hemorrhage and stroke. Patients with this disorder often present in the neonatal period with hepatomegaly and cholestasis. Liver histologic findings early in life may be nonspecific, with portal inflammation, bile duct proliferation, and giant cell infiltration. Biopsy findings later in life (typically by age 6 months) demonstrate the paucity of intrahepatic bile ducts and cholestasis. Generally, the prognosis for this disorder is good, provided careful attention is paid to management of the effects of chronic cholestasis, including fat-soluble vitamin deficiency and pruritus. Cirrhosis develops in 10% to 50% of children in whom hepatic abnormalities are manifest during infancy. Liver transplantation may be required in these patients. Survival may be limited also by accompanying heart disease. Inheritance appears to be autosomal dominant, and several patients with this disorder have been shown to have a partial deletion on the short arm of chromosome 20, now known to be related to deletion or mutation of the *JAGGED1* gene, thought to be important in "cell fate" decisions. *JAG1* mutations are found in approximately 70% of patients with Alagille syndrome. Because multiple mutations have been found, commercial genetic testing is not yet available or practical for this condition.

BOX 56.3 | **Clinical Features of Alagille Syndrome**

1. Chronic cholestasis resulting from bile duct paucity
2. Extrahepatic anomalies (variable expression)
   A. Major Features
      i. Characteristic facies (broad forehead, deeply set, widely-spaced eyes, long straight nose)
      ii. Vertebral arch defects ("butterfly" vertebrae, hemivertebrae)
      iii. Ocular anomalies (posterior embryotoxon)
      iv. Cardiovascular abnormalities
   B. Associated (minor) features
      i. Renal abnormalities
      ii. Exocrine pancreatic insufficiency
      iii. Growth retardation (short stature)
      iv. High-pitched voice
      v. Hypogonadism
   C. Secondary features
      i. Dermatologic (xanthoma)
      ii. Bone disease
      iii. Vitamin deficiency

Nonsyndromic Paucity

Intrahepatic bile duct paucity unrelated to a specific syndrome most likely represents an eclectic variety of liver diseases; the exact nature, however, is unknown. The prognosis for this form, which often recurs within a family, appears to be unfavorable, with frequent progression to biliary cirrhosis and hepatic failure. Bile duct paucity may be seen on hepatic biopsy before 90 days of life, and bile duct destruction may be noted at that time.

Miscellaneous Disorders

Hereditary cholestasis with lymphedema (Aagenaes syndrome), characterized by episodes of recurrent jaundice, associated in later childhood with lymphedema of the lower extremities, is another form of intrahepatic cholestasis. The etiology is unknown; inheritance may be autosomal recessive. Recently, the genetic defect responsible for this defect has been mapped to chromosome 15q. Cirrhosis may occur later in life.

NEONATAL HEPATITIS

Idiopathic Neonatal Hepatitis

Idiopathic neonatal hepatitis is a descriptive term for neonatal cholestatic liver disease for which all other known causes, including metabolic and infectious diseases and extrahepatic obstruction, have been excluded. The incidence of this disorder is approximately 1 in 5,000 births, rendering it the most common cause of neonatal cholestasis and accounting for up to 50% of cases of prolonged neonatal jaundice. This category most likely represents a collection of multiple, as yet undescribed, disorders of hepatic function. Certain areas overlap with the intrahepatic cholestasis category already described.

Clinically, 50% of infants with "idiopathic" neonatal hepatitis have jaundice in the first week of life. Hepatosplenomegaly is common, and some one-third of these infants fail to thrive. Acholic stools may be present, rendering differentiation of this diagnosis from that of extrahepatic biliary atresia difficult. Liver histology varies but typically includes inflammation, hepatocellular unrest, multinucleated giant cells, and extramedullary hematopoiesis. Bile duct proliferation is not usually present. Diagnosis is through exclusion of other causes, including extrahepatic biliary atresia (see Box 56.1). Therapy is directed toward addressing the consequences of chronic cholestasis (see Fig. 56.2). The prognosis varies, but perhaps 80% to 85% of patients will recover, whereas 15% to 20% will have severe, progressive disease. The diseases that demonstrate a pattern of familial recurrence carry the worst prognosis. The fraction of cases of neonatal cholestasis attributable to neonatal hepatitis has diminished and should decline further as additional causes are uncovered (see also Chapter 367). Examples are the recent recognition of the PFIC spectrum, as well as the hepatobiliary consequences of neonatal lupus erythematosus, which may present as neonatal cholestasis or even with neonatal liver failure.

Biliary Atresia

Biliary atresia, which occurs in approximately 1 in 8,000 live births, consists of atresia or hypoplasia of any portion of the extrahepatic biliary system. The obstruction may occur as a discrete distal lesion, allowing surgical drainage of patent portions of bile duct proximal to the atresia. In the most common form, however, the atretic area extends to an area above the level of the porta hepatis and often affects intrahepatic bile ducts, thus rendering surgical drainage difficult.

The clinical presentation (perinatal type) of this disorder is similar to that of neonatal hepatitis. Classically, 65% to 85% of these infants are born at term with normal birth weight. Jaundice develops at 3 to 6 weeks of age in otherwise well-appearing, thriving infants, and the stool eventually becomes acholic. Some 15% of infants (embryonic or fetal type) may have associated defects, including polysplenia, cardiovascular anomalies, and malrotation of the intestine. These infants may also demonstrate earlier age at onset of cholestasis. No genetic predisposition is apparent, and familial recurrence is rare. Hepatic pathologic findings vary with the age of an infant; early biopsy samples may feature the presence of multinucleated giant cells, which decrease in number with age. Classic features of biliary atresia include bile ductular proliferation, bile plugs, and portal or perilobular fibrosis and edema.

Biliary atresia appears to be an evolving lesion with progressive obliteration of bile ducts; this is supported by the finding that several infants with previously documented patent extrahepatic biliary ducts were found, on reexploration, to have biliary atresia. This renders possible the speculation that neonatal hepatitis and extrahepatic biliary atresia represent different manifestations of hepatocyte or biliary tract injury by a single agent, or combination of agents, whether viral, immunologic, or genetic. However, the etiology of the disorder is unknown.

The diagnosis of biliary atresia involves the exclusion of other known causes of neonatal cholestasis. Differentiation of biliary atresia from neonatal hepatitis remains difficult. Clinical features aiding in discrimination include the following: (a) birth weight, because biliary atresia is more common in term infants, whereas infants with neonatal hepatitis are often are born prematurely or are small for gestational age; (b) the presence of associated anomalies or (c) an enlarged, firm liver, both suggestive of biliary atresia; and (d) the consistent absence of stool pigment (associated with biliary atresia). An abdominal ultrasonographic examination permits evaluation for the presence of a gallbladder, which often is absent in biliary atresia. In addition, the ultrasonographic finding of a "triangular cord sign" at the porta hepatis is, in some centers, a sensitive and specific sign of biliary atresia. Further studies should be directed at ruling out endocrine, metabolic, and other miscellaneous causes of cholestasis, as listed in Box 56.1.

Hepatobiliary imaging, using iminodiacetic acid derivatives, may be used. The radionuclide is given intravenously. In patients with biliary atresia, uptake into the liver is rapid, but no excretion into the intestine occurs. Conversely, in patients with neonatal hepatitis, uptake is slow, but excretion does occur. Typically, this study is performed after phenobarbital, 5 mg/kg/day, has been given orally for 3 to 5 days to enhance biliary excretion of the isotope.

Percutaneous hepatic biopsy is highly valuable in the differentiation of neonatal hepatitis and extrahepatic biliary atresia. This procedure may be performed safely using the Menghini technique. Pathologic findings favoring the diagnosis of extrahepatic biliary atresia include bile duct proliferation, bile plugs, and portal and perilobular fibrosis.

If the diagnosis of biliary atresia cannot be ruled out definitively after the described evaluation has been performed, operative exploration (either open or laparoscopic) and cholangiography should be undertaken. This procedure enables recognition of biliary atresia and exclusion of other forms of extrahepatic bile duct disease (stenosis or perforation of the common bile duct). The surgeon should avoid transection of a biliary tree that is patent but small because of biliary hypoplasia or the diminished bile flow associated with intrahepatic cholestasis. Resection is not indicated in these cases. Correctable forms of atresia (distal obstruction), as mentioned, also may be found.

In approximately 80% of cases, however, a "noncorrectable" atresia is found. In patients so affected, further exploration is indicated, and an attempt to establish biliary drainage should be made, using the hepatoportoenterostomy procedure of Kasai. This procedure consists of transection of the porta hepatis, with subsequent apposition of a Roux-en-Y loop of intestine. The rationale is to drain any small, persisting bile duct remnants. Prognosis after this procedure is affected by the age of the patient at the time of operation, with success rates of 90% in infants younger than 2 months decreasing to less than 20% in patients older than 90 days. Also important is the size of the lumina of the residual ducts encountered at surgery; those with diameters of less than 150 μm are associated with a poor prognosis. This operation rarely is definitive in patients with noncorrectable atresia, and most patients will have progressive hepatic disease and repeated episodes of bacterial cholangitis. Management of the patient after the (Kasai) hepatoportoenterostomy operation consists of prompt and vigorous treatment of the episodes of cholangitis and consistent attention to nutritional support. Prophylactic antibiotics are often prescribed, as are perioperative corticosteroids, although definitive evidence supporting these therapies is lacking. Patients in whom bile flow was attained initially after the Kasai operation but in whom drainage subsequently stops probably should undergo reoperation in an effort to establish bile flow again. The use of corticosteroids in this situation also has been advocated. Multiple attempts at reexploration and revision of a nonfunctional conduit should be avoided, however. Regardless of the eventual outcome, one frequent beneficial effect of the Kasai procedure is to provide adequate time for the patient to grow before hepatic transplantation becomes necessary. Biliary atresia without intervention is universally fatal, with the mean age of death being less than 1 year. Liver transplantation now is essential in the treatment of children whose operation is not successful in restoring bile flow and in children in whom liver failure eventually develops despite some degree of bile drainage.

THERAPY

Various aspects of the management of specific disorders are mentioned earlier. The general approach to management of liver disorders is discussed in Chapter 367.

Suggested Readings

Allagille P, Estrada A, Hadchouel M, et al. Syndromic paucity of interlobular bile ducts (Alagille syndrome or arteriohepatic dysplasia): review of 80 cases. *J Pediatr* 1987;110:195.

Balistreri WF. Inborn errors of bile acid biosynthesis and transport: novel form of metabolic liver diseases. *Gastroenterol Clin North Am* 1999;28:145.

Balistreri WF. Intrahepatic cholestasis. *J Pediatr Gastroenterol Nutr* 2002; 35:S17.

Bates MD, Bucuvalas JC, Alonso MH, Ryckman FC. Biliary atresia: pathogenesis and treatment. *Semin Liver Dis* 1998;18:281.

Baumgartner MR, Saudubray JM. Peroxisomal disorders. *Semin Neonatol* 2002;7:1.

Bezerra JA, Balistreri WF. Cholestatic syndromes of infancy and childhood. *Semin Gastrointest Dis* 2001;12:54.

Bezerra JA, Tiao G, Ryckman FC, et al. Genetic induction of proinflammatory immunity in children with biliary atresia. *Lancet* 2003;361:971.

Brosius U, Gartner J. Cellular and molecular aspects of Zellweger syndrome and other peroxisome biogenesis disorders. *Cell Mol Life Sci* 2002;59:1058.

Brucato A, Cimaz R, Stramba-Badiale M. Neonatal lupus. *Clin Rev Allergy Immunol* 2002;23:279.

Buchman MS, Kvittington EA, Nazer H, et al. Lack of 3-beta-hydroxy-delta^5-C27-steroid dehydrogenase/isomerase in fibroblasts from a child with urinary excretion of 3-beta-hydroxy-delta^5-bile acids. *J Clin Invest* 1990;86:2034.

Bull LN, Roche E, Song EJ, et al. Mapping of the locus for cholestasis-lymphedema syndrome (Aagenaes syndrome) to a 6.6-cM interval on chromosome 15q. *Am J Hum Genet* 2000;67:994.

Carlton VE, Knisely AS, Freimer NB. Mapping of a locus for progressive familial intrahepatic cholestasis (Byler disease) to 18q21–q22, the benign recurrent intrahepatic cholestasis region. *Hum Mol Genet* 1995;4:1049.

Clayton PT, Mills KA, Johnson AW, et al. Delta 4-3-oxosteroid 5 beta-reductase deficiency: failure of ursodeoxycholic acid treatment and response to chenodeoxycholic acid plus cholic acid. *Gut* 1996;38:623.

Crosnier C, Lykavieris P, Meunier-Rotival M, Hadchouel M. Alagille syndrome: the widening spectrum of arteriohepatic dysplasia. *Clin Liver Dis* 2000;4:7658.

Davenport M, Kerkar N, Mieli-Vergani G, et al. Biliary atresia: the King's College Hospital experience (1974–1995). *J Pediatr Surg* 1997;32:479.

de Vree JM, Jacquemin E, Sturm E, et al. Mutations in the *MDR3* gene cause progressive familial intrahepatic cholestasis. *Proc Natl Acad Sci USA* 1998;95:282.

Glasova H, Beuers U. Extrahepatic manifestations of cholestasis. *J Gastroenterol Hepatol* 2002;17:938.

Gridley T. Notch signaling and inherited disease syndromes. *Hum Mol Genet* 2003;12:R9.

Jacquemin E. Progressive familial intrahepatic cholestasis: genetic basis and treatment. *Clin Liver Dis* 2000;4:753.

Jansen PL, Strautnieks SS, Jacquemin E, et al. Hepatocanalicular bile salt export pump deficiency in patients with progressive familial intrahepatic cholestasis. *Gastroenterology* 1999;117:1370.

Jansen PLM, Muller M, Sturm E. Genes and cholestasis. *Hepatology* 2001; 34:1067.

Kahn E, Daum F, Marowitz J, et al. Nonsyndromic paucity of interlobular bile ducts: light- and electron-microscopic evaluation of sequential liver biopsies in early childhood. *Hepatology* 1986;6:890.

Kartenbeck J, Leuschner U, Mayer R, Keppler D. Absence of the canalicular isoform of the MRP gene-encoded conjugate export pump from the hepatocytes in Dubin-Johnson syndrome. *Hepatology* 1996;23:1061.

Kaufman SS, Murray ND, Wood P, et al. Nutrition support for the infant with extrahepatic biliary atresia. *J Pediatr* 1987;110:679.

Landing BH. Consideration of the pathogenesis of neonatal hepatitis, biliary atresia, and choledochal cyst: the concept of infantile obstructive cholangiopathy. *Prog Pediatr Surg* 1974;6:113.

Lee LA, Sokol RJ, Buyon JP. Hepatobiliary disease in neonatal lupus: prevalence and clinical characteristics in cases enrolled in a national registry. *Pediatrics* 2002;109:E11.

Li L, Krantz ID, Deng Y, et al. Alagille syndrome is caused by mutations in human *Jagged1*, which encodes a ligand for *Notch1*. *Nat Genet* 1997;16:243.

McKiernan PJ. Neonatal cholestasis. *Semin Neonatol* 2002;7:153.

Narkewicz MR. Biliary atresia: an update on our understanding of the disorder. *Curr Opin Pediatr* 2001;13:4350.

Perlmutter DH, Shepherd RW. Extrahepatic biliary atresia: a disease or a phenotype? *Hepatology* 2002;35:1297.

Petersen C, Ure BM. What's new in biliary atresia? *Eur J Pediatr Surg* 2003;13:1.

Piccoli DA, Spinner NB. Alagille syndrome and the *Jagged1* gene. *Semin Liver Dis* 2001;21:525.

Setchell KD, Suchy FJ, Welsh MB, et al. Delta 4-3-oxosteroid-5-beta-reductase deficiency described in identical twins with neonatal hepatitis. *J Clin Invest* 1988;82:2148.

Shneider BL. Genetic cholestasis syndromes. *J Pediatr Gastroenterol Nutr* 1999;28:124.

Shneider BL, Setchell KD, Whitington PF, et al. Delta 4-3-oxosteroid 5 beta-reductase deficiency causing neonatal liver failure and hemochromatosis. *J Pediatr* 1994;124:234.

Schreiber RA, Kleinman RE. Biliary atresia. *J Pediatr Gastroenterol Nutr* 2002;35:S11.

Smit JJM, Schinkel AH, Oude Elferink RPJ, et al. Homozygous disruption of the murine mdr2 P-glycoprotein gene leads to a complete absence of phospholipid from bile and to liver disease. *Cell* 1993;75:451.

Strautnieks SS, Bull LN, Knisely AS, et al. A gene encoding a liver-specific ABC transporter is mutated in progressive familial intrahepatic cholestasis. *Nat Genet* 1998;20:233.

Strautnieks SS, Kagalwalla AF, Tanner MS, et al. Identification of a locus for progressive familial intrahepatic cholestasis PFIC2 on chromosome 2q24. *Am J Hum Genet* 1997;61:630.

Thompson R, Strautnieks S. BSEP: function and role in progressive familial intrahepatic cholestasis. *Semin Liver Dis* 2001;21:545.

van Mil SW, Klomp LW, Bull LN, Houwen RH. FIC1 disease: a spectrum of intrahepatic cholestatic disorders. *Semin Liver Dis* 2001;21:535.

Wang R, Salem M, Yousef IM, et al. Targeted inactivation of sister of P-glycoprotein gene (spgp) in mice results in nonprogressive but persistent intrahepatic cholestasis. *Proc Natl Acad Sci USA* 2001;98:2011.

Wang L, Soroka CJ, Boyer JL. The role of bile salt export pump mutations in progressive familial intrahepatic cholestasis type II. *J Clin Invest* 2002; 110:965.

CHAPTER 57 ■ SUCKING AND SWALLOWING DISORDERS AND GASTROESOPHAGEAL REFLUX

COLSTON F. McEVOY

Sucking and swallowing begin prenatally, with pharyngeal swallowing observed as early as 10 to 11 weeks' gestation and suckling seen at 18 to 24 weeks. Late-term fetuses swallow amniotic fluid at a rate equal to that of fetal urination. Interruptions in fetal ingestion of amniotic fluid due to gastrointestinal tract obstruction or neurologic abnormalities can upset this balance and result in polyhydramnios.

Nonnutritive sucking is seen in premature infants at 27 to 28 weeks' gestation and in the first 48 hours of life in term infants. This pattern is characterized by short bursts of one to five sucks with long pauses between. The number of sucks increases to 10 to 30 per burst in nutritive sucking, and these bursts become regularly associated with swallowing. In premature infants, a mature sucking pattern sufficient to support total oral intake of calories usually is achieved by 34 weeks' gestation.

Coordination of sucking, swallowing, and breathing is a prerequisite to successful oral feeding. The anatomy of infants is such that a small oral cavity, a relatively large tongue, and an anteriorly and superiorly positioned larynx facilitate nasal breathing and airway protection. Early suckling progresses to true sucking in the older infant, with development of tighter lip approximation around the nipple and a progression from anteroposterior to vertical tongue motions. This progression allows for efficient delivery of liquid to the anterior chamber of the mouth. Swallowing is initiated when the tongue propels a liquid bolus backward into the pharynx. The soft palate closes off the palatopharyngeal isthmus, preventing liquid access to the nasopharynx. The tongue moves posteriorly against the pharyngeal wall while the larynx moves up, closing the epiglottis and preventing access to the airway. The pharyngeal constrictor muscles relax, followed by relaxation of the cricopharyngeus muscle or superior esophageal sphincter, and the bolus enters the upper esophagus. The tongue then moves away from the pharynx, and the epiglottis rises, allowing air into the trachea. Contraction of the cricopharyngeus muscle stimulates peristalsis, which carries the bolus to the distal esophagus. Relaxation of the lower esophageal sphincter permits entry into the stomach.

The causes of dysfunctional sucking and swallowing are varied (Box 57.1) and often result in poor growth due to inadequate oral intake and aspiration. Neuromuscular disease, usually characterized by hypotonia, may cause diminished suck or discoordinated swallow. Structural anomalies or lesions of the mouth, pharynx, or larynx often interfere with the mechanics of sucking and swallowing. At the level of the esophagus, congenital abnormalities, stricture, mucosal inflammation, or extrinsic compression may result in swallowing difficulty.

ACHALASIA

Achalasia is a motility disorder of the esophagus characterized by a functional obstruction of the esophagus. The characteristic findings are absent or nonperistaltic contractions of the esophagus, failure of the lower esophageal sphincter to re-

lax with swallowing, and sometimes a high resting pressure of the lower esophageal sphincter. The estimated incidence in the general population is 1 in 100,000 per year. Only 5% of cases occur in children younger than 5 years of age. Allgrove or Triple A syndrome is an autosomal recessive disorder in which achalasia is associated with alacrima, adrenal insufficiency, and autonomic abnormalities. It often presents in childhood.

Children with achalasia have symptoms of vomiting, regurgitation, or dysphagia. Obstructive symptoms are first precipitated by solids, and as the disease progresses, the ability to swallow liquids may be affected or may be impaired. Affected children may have recurrent pulmonary infections, wheezing, and failure to thrive. An upper gastrointestinal examination may show characteristic "beaking" or tapering of the distal esophagus, with varying degrees of esophageal dilation (more prominent in older children than in the very young). The diagnosis is made by manometry, which shows failure or incomplete relaxation of the lower esophageal sphincter after swallowing, absent or disordered peristalsis, and elevated intraesophageal pressure. Treatment of achalasia consists of balloon dilation or surgical myotomy of the lower esophageal sphincter. Botulinum toxin injected into the lower esophageal sphincter temporarily relieves symptoms of obstruction. Chagas disease causes symptoms similar to those of idiopathic achalasia and is the result of esophageal neuronal damage by the parasite *Trypanosoma cruzi*. After surgical myotomy, gastroesophageal reflux may become a significant problem. Disordered esophageal peristalsis is a lifelong problem and may be the source of chronic symptoms of dysphagia.

GASTROESOPHAGEAL REFLUX

Gastroesophageal reflux (GER) is defined as the spontaneous regurgitation of gastric contents into the esophagus. Reflux occurs physiologically in young infants, the majority of whom have mild symptoms that resolve with age. GER is pathologic (GER disease) in infants who experience complications or in older children and adults. Mechanisms proposed for physiologic reflux include increased transient relaxation of the lower esophageal sphincter (LES), delayed gastric emptying, and an intraabdominal–LES pressure differential. Reduced resting LES pressure and esophageal dysmotility are often secondary results of acid damage to the esophagus in older children and adults but are rarely primary to the condition in infancy. In infants, the short esophagus, large meals in relation to gastric capacity, frequent feeding regimen, supine positioning, frequent Valsalva maneuver during the passage of stool while recumbent, and poorly developed swallowing response are all predisposing factors that improve with age.

The typical clinical presentation of the infant with uncomplicated GER is a "happy spitter" who effortlessly brings up small amounts of milk after feedings but grows well. The symptoms usually begin in the first weeks of life and resolve by 9 to 24 months, often coincident with the introduction of solid foods, with the assumption of the sitting position, and

BOX 57.1 Causes of Abnormal Sucking and Swallowing in the Newborn Period (Birth to 28 Days)

Structural anomalies
General
  Micrognathia
  Cleft palate
  Macroglossia
  Ranula
  Lingual hygroma
  Lingual hemangioma
  Lingual thyroid
  Dermoid cyst (lingual)
  Choanal atresia or stenosis
  Pharyngeal cyst
  Laryngeal cleft
  Esophageal anomalies
Syndromes
  Pierre-Robin
  Trisomy 21
  Trisomies 13–15
  Congenital hypothyroidism
  Glycogen storage disease, type II

Neurologic
Congenital
  Möbius syndrome
  Werdnig-Hoffmann disease
  Neonatal myasthenia gravis
  Familial dysautonomia
Acquired
  Birth asphyxia
  Bulbar palsy
  Palatal paralysis
  Cricopharyngeal achalasia
  Recurrent laryngeal nerve paralysis
  Botulism
  Kernicterus
  Tetanus neonatorum
  Sedation

Muscular
Congenital
  Benign congenital hypotonia
  Myotonic dystrophy
  Muscular dystrophy
  Amyotonia congenita
Acquired
  Hypocalcemia
  Hypomagnesemia
  Hypokalemia
  Hypophosphatemia

Modified from Gyboski J, Walker WA, eds. *Gastrointestinal problems in the infant*, 2nd ed. Philadelphia: Saunders, 1983.

Esophagitis is a complication of GER that, when severe, can lead to bleeding and anemia, stricture formation, or metaplasia (Barrett esophagus). Infants with esophagitis may refuse feedings or have irritability with feedings. Older children report pain or feeling as though food gets stuck when swallowing. Inflammation of the esophageal mucosa from chronic gastric acid exposure causes further esophageal dysmotility, thereby exacerbating regurgitation or vomiting. Rarely, reflux causes failure to thrive in infants who do not retain enough formula to meet their caloric needs or limit their intake secondary to discomfort.

One of the most worrisome yet ambiguous complications of reflux is its association with respiratory disease. Some infants aspirate gastric contents during an episode of reflux. These children often have an underlying neurologic disease that compromises their ability to protect their airway. In addition, they may aspirate oral contents, owing to an uncoordinated swallowing mechanism.

Subclinical reflux may be the cause of refractory asthma or repeated episodes of pneumonia. Conversely, coughing associated with chronic respiratory disease, such as asthma or cystic fibrosis, may induce reflux by increasing intraabdominal pressure.

Apnea or acute life-threatening events in infants have been associated with GER, although proving a cause-and-effect relationship is difficult. Other conditions attributed to GER include recurrent otalgia, dental caries, and Sandifer syndrome, in which the child demonstrates torticollis in response to reflux.

In most infants, the diagnosis of GER can be made on the basis of clinical history and findings. A barium study of the upper gastrointestinal tract can rule out obstruction, hiatal hernia, or esophageal stricture. This radiologic test is not an accurate assessment of reflux because of frequent false-positive and false-negative results. The gold-standard diagnostic test is continuous esophageal pH monitoring to detect the presence of gastric acid in the normally neutral distal esophagus. It enables measurement of the frequency and duration of reflux episodes. This study is most helpful in diagnosing occult GER in patients who present with possible complications or to correlate reflux episodes with symptoms. Esophageal monitoring with equipment that measures impedance rather than pH is under investigation in infants and children. This modality permits evaluation of any fluid movement (acid, alkaline, or neutral) in the esophagus as well as air. Experience with impedance recordings may help clarify whether infant reflux is in fact a pathologic process. At present, impedance studies have already shown that acid blockade neutralizes the refluxate but does not reduce the number of times a fluid bolus enters the esophagus. To determine the relationship of reflux with apnea, a pH study is best performed as part of a multichannel pneumocardiography test. Reflux esophagitis is diagnosed by endoscopy with biopsy. The esophageal mucosa may appear endoscopically normal in mild to moderate esophagitis, but characteristic histologic findings are diagnostic.

Treatment of reflux is conservative in most uncomplicated cases and consists of postural management and modification of feedings. A head-elevated prone position has been shown to decrease reflux in infants, but due to the increased risk of sudden infant death syndrome this position is no longer recommended during sleep. Traditional reflux therapy of semisupine posture in an infant seat or swing is detrimental rather than beneficial. Thickening of the feedings and more frequent smaller volumes may reduce clinical symptoms of GER. A continuous infusion of formula through a nasogastric, gastrostomy, or jejunal tube may be beneficial in treating poor weight gain resulting from severe reflux.

Some infants, particularly those with a family history of atopy, may have worse symptoms with cow or soy milk. They will benefit from a protein hydrolysate formula or from restricting the diet of the breast-feeding mother.

eventually with walking. GER is fairly common in premature infants, especially those with respiratory disease. In infants with more significant regurgitation or frank vomiting, conditions such as obstruction, infection, and metabolic or neurologic disease should be ruled out before the diagnosis of GER is made. Older children and adolescents with GER disease present less frequently with vomiting. As in adults, they more often complain of heartburn, regurgitation, and acid taste. Infants and children with neurologic impairment have a high incidence of chronic reflux.

Pharmacologic therapy is aimed at acid reduction to treat or prevent peptic esophagitis and enhancement of gastric emptying and LES tone with a prokinetic agent. Depending on the severity of GER disease, acid suppression can be achieved with an H_2 antagonist (ranitidine, famotidine, cimetidine) or a proton pump inhibitor (omeprazole, lansoprazole). Antacids can be used for short-term relief of symptoms but are not recommended for chronic therapy. Metoclopramide is currently the only prokinetic used to treat GER in pediatric patients. In infants and children, irritability is a common side effect of this medication. Controlled studies have not shown that prokinetics are effective in controlling symptoms despite improvements in motility and pH studies.

Surgical therapy is reserved for severe reflux disease refractory to medical management or producing life-threatening complications, such as aspiration pneumonia. This procedure, which involves wrapping the gastric fundus around the distal esophagus to prevent reflux, may produce complications such as gas-bloat syndrome, retching, dumping syndrome, breakdown of the wrap, herniation into the thorax, or obstruction secondary to adhesions.

EOSINOPHILIC ESOPHAGITIS

Eosinophilic esophagitis is thought to be an allergic disorder that presents with symptoms similar to GER but is unresponsive to reflux therapy. Children may also have symptoms of dysphagia, odynophagia (severe pain on swallowing), and food impaction. It is more prevalent in adolescent males but can occur at any age. The diagnosis is made by identifying numerous eosinophils (20 or more per high power field) on biopsy specimens of the esophagus. The cause of the esophageal inflammation is thought to be a non–IgE-mediated response to food antigens. Standard allergy tests are not diagnostic for the causative foods in most cases. Treatment includes elimination diet, "swallowed" steroids, or systemic steroids.

Suggested Readings

Derkay CS, Schechter GL. Anatomy and physiology of pediatric swallowing disorders. *Otolaryngol Clin North Am* 1998;31:397.

Gryboski J, Walker WA, eds. *Gastrointestinal problems in the infant,* 2nd ed. Philadelphia: Saunders, 1983.

Hussain SZ, Thomas R, Tolia V. A review of achalasia in 33 children. *Dig Dis Sci* 2002;47:2538.

Kawahara H, Dent J, Davidson G. Mechanisms responsible for gastroesophageal reflux in children. *Gastroenterology* 1997;113:399.

Liacouras CA, Ruchelli E. Eosinophilic esophagitis. *Curr Opin Pediatr* 2004; 16:560.

Rudolph CD, Mazur LJ, Liptak GS, et al. Guidelines for evaluation and treatment of gastroesophageal reflux in infants and children: recommendations of the North American Society for Pediatric Gastroenterology and Nutrition. *J Pediatr Gastroenterol Nutr* 2001;32:1.

Rudolph CD, Link DT. Feeding disorders in infants and children. *Pediatr Clin North Am* 2002;49:97.

CHAPTER 58 ■ DISTENDED ABDOMEN

JOHN H. SEASHORE

Newborn infants normally have protuberant abdomens owing to the relatively large size of their viscera, so judging distention may be more challenging than in older patients. Abdominal distention is a fairly common presenting sign of a variety of congenital anomalies and acquired diseases, however, and its presence or absence should be evaluated during all physical examinations of babies. Abdominal distention may result from abnormal accumulations of air, fluid, or solid tissue. History and physical examination may provide clues as to the likely etiology. For example, an infant who is vomiting bile probably has an intestinal obstruction, one who has severe congenital heart disease and hydrops fetalis most likely has ascites as the cause of distention, and a palpable mass is usually an enlarged organ or a tumor. Plain radiography of the abdomen is most useful for diagnosing conditions resulting from air, whereas ultrasound is the best imaging method for fluid and solid tissue. Many of the conditions that present with distention are covered in other sections of this book. This chapter presents a differential diagnosis and detailed discussion of conditions that are not covered elsewhere.

DISTENTION CAUSED BY AIR

Excessive air is the most common cause of abdominal distention in the neonate (Box 58.1). The distention is uniform throughout the abdomen, which is tympanitic on examination. Air may be within the lumen of the bowel or free in the peritoneal cavity. Intraluminal air is most common and is usually an indication of intestinal obstruction. Adynamic ileus may also cause distention by air-filled loops of bowel. Common causes include necrotizing enterocolitis and sepsis. Plain radiography of the abdomen is the primary means to diagnose these

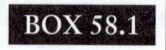

BOX 58.1 **Abdominal Distention Caused by Excess Air**

Air within bowel
Adynamic ileus
Intestinal obstruction
 Atresia
 Meconium ileus
 Hirschsprung disease
 Midgut volvulus

Air in the peritoneal cavity
Perforation of the bowel
 Necrotizing enterocolitis
 Intestinal obstruction
 Spontaneous perforation of the bowel
Dissection from a pneumomediastinum (pulmonary barotrauma)

conditions. Intestinal obstruction is manifested by a few or multiple loops of very dilated bowel with air–fluid levels seen on lateral decubitus views. Air is absent in the region of the distal bowel. Ileus presents a pattern of more diffusely dilated bowel, sometimes very irregular, but not as enlarged as in obstruction. The clinical context often is helpful to distinguish these conditions as well. Infants with an ileus are usually acutely ill and have signs and symptoms of sepsis. Infants with obstruction typically appear well and present with distention, bilious vomiting, and frequently a failure to pass meconium.

Free air in the peritoneal cavity is almost always indicative of perforation of the bowel and is an ominous sign. Infants who have perforated bowel are usually acutely ill with signs of peritonitis and sepsis, but for unknown reasons some babies have a rather bland response to perforation, presenting only with distention. In either case, free air is identified on plain radiography of the abdomen. A round or oblong lucency in the mid- to upper abdomen with a central vertical density (the football sign) seen on a supine film represents free air outlining the falciform ligament. However, the right lateral decubitus view is the most sensitive for seeing free air as a triangular or crescent-shaped radiolucency at the uppermost part of the abdomen or outlining the liver edge.

The most common cause of free air in the neonate is perforation from necrotizing enterocolitis. This is primarily a disease of premature infants but may occur in full-term infants, even after discharge from the hospital. It is discussed in Chapter 59.

Spontaneous perforation of the bowel is an uncommon disorder of uncertain cause. It has been recognized as an entity for many years and occurs in both full-term and premature infants. It has been associated with administration of indomethacin. The onset is sudden, with distention as the primary and sometimes only sign. Free air is present on the initial radiographs, often in massive amounts. At operation, an isolated perforation is found, most commonly in the stomach, colon, or terminal ileum. The hole may be pinpoint or large, but signs of ischemia are lacking in the surrounding bowel, and relatively little evidence of peritonitis exists if the condition is diagnosed and treated promptly. The hole is oversewn, resected, or exteriorized depending on individual findings. Although some of these cases, particularly in infants with known risk factors, may be variants of necrotizing enterocolitis, spontaneous perforation is clearly a discrete entity. The prognosis depends on age, associated conditions, and timeliness of treatment.

In rare cases, free air is not from a bowel perforation but has dissected down from the mediastinum. This can occur in infants who are on ventilators with very high inflation pressure. The resulting barotrauma may cause pneumothorax or pulmonary interstitial emphysema. The key finding, however, is pneumomediastinum, from whence the air may dissect through the various hiatuses of the diaphragm, then into the mesentery, where it ruptures into the free peritoneal cavity. The babies typically have sudden onset of abdominal distention and often have massive amounts of free air in the abdomen. These are obviously very sick infants who are at risk for necrotizing enterocolitis. Therefore, there must be a low threshold to explore these infants unless the air clearly has come from the chest. Measuring the partial pressure of oxygen in the gas aspirated from the abdomen has been suggested as a method to make this distinction.

NEONATAL ASCITES

Serous Fluid

Ascites is an abnormal accumulation of fluid in the peritoneal cavity. The fluid may be serous, urine, an exudate, chyle, blood, or bile (Box 58.2). A fluid wave on physical examination and

---

BOX 58.2 Fluids that Cause Abdominal Distention

Serous fluid
Hydrops fetalis
Hematologic disorders
  Rh isoimmunization
  Thalassemia
  Other congenital hemolytic anemias
Cardiac failure
  Congenital heart disease
  Congenital arrhythmias
Congenital infection
  Cytomegalic inclusion disease
  Syphilis
  Toxoplasmosis
  Rubella
Metabolic disorders
  Lysosomal storage diseases
  Tyrosinemia
  Galactosemia

Urine
Obstructive uropathy
  Posterior urethral valves
  Ureterovesical junction obstruction
  Ureteropelvic junction obstruction

Idiopathic
Inflammatory and infected fluid
Perforation of the bowel
  Necrotizing enterocolitis
  Spontaneous perforation
  Appendicitis
  Hirschsprung disease
  Meconium peritonitis

Chyle
Idiopathic
Mesenteric cyst
Lymphangiectasia
Midgut volvulus

Blood
Ruptured liver or spleen
  Birth trauma
  Other injury
  Child abuse (rare in neonate)
Ruptured liver mass
  Hemangioma
  Mesenchymal hamartoma

Bile
Spontaneous perforation of the bile duct

---

central displacement of bowel gas on plain radiography are suggestive of ascites, but the key to diagnosis is ultrasound examination. The type of fluid is determined by paracentesis with visual and laboratory analysis of the fluid.

The peritoneum, in common with all serous surfaces, constantly secretes and absorbs fluid that is in equilibrium with extracellular fluid and therefore has a similar chemical makeup. Conditions that alter the rate of secretion or absorption may lead to an accumulation of serous fluid in the peritoneal cavity.

Hydrops fetalis is characterized by generalized edema and accumulation of fluid in all the serous cavities and is easily diagnosed by physical examination and ultrasound. Mortality is high in both fetuses and neonates. Rh isoimmunization, which causes profound fetal anemia, is still a common cause of hydrops worldwide, but pretreatment with anti-D antibodies (RhoGAM) has made this condition rare in developed countries.

Nonimmune hydrops may result from a variety of conditions. Congenital heart disease or arrhythmia causing severe heart failure is most common. Thalassemia and other hematologic disorders may cause hemolysis, anemia, and hydrops. Congenital infection, particularly cytomegalovirus and neonatal syphilis, may cause hydrops or isolated ascites. Genetic metabolic disorders that are associated with ascites and occasionally hydrops include lysosomal storage diseases such as Gaucher disease and inborn errors that may cause early liver disease such as galactosemia or tyrosinemia.

Urgent diagnosis of the cause of hydrops to allow treatment where possible is essential to reduce the substantial risk of mortality. Supportive therapy, transfusion, and treatment of heart failure or arrhythmia are provided as appropriate. If the amount of abdominal fluid is massive enough to cause respiratory distress, removal by paracentesis offers temporary relief, but fluid reaccumulation is rapid unless the underlying disorder has been treated adequately.

Urine

Urinary ascites is the next most common cause of increased abdominal fluid. Paracentesis yields a yellow fluid with high levels of urea and other constituents of urine. Most of these patients have obstructive uropathy leading to distention of various portions of the urinary tract and subsequent leakage of urine into the peritoneal cavity. A careful evaluation for posterior urethral valves, ureterovesical junction obstruction, and ureteropelvic junction obstruction is necessary. The actual site of leakage is usually small and hard to find. Hyponatremia is present in approximately 70% of patients, probably due to movement of sodium down its concentration gradient from the higher sodium concentration in extracellular fluid to the lower sodium concentration of urine (autodialysis). Treatment is directed toward the underlying condition, either by definitive repair or diversion of the urinary flow proximal to the obstruction.

Inflammatory and Infected Fluid

Fluid that accumulates in response to inflammation or infection is an *exudate,* characterized by large numbers of white blood cells, increased protein concentration, and the presence of fibrin. The most common cause is perforation of the bowel from necrotizing enterocolitis. Neonatal appendicitis is rare and is usually perforated; the majority of these infants have Hirschsprung disease. Meconium peritonitis is a consequence of antenatal perforation of the bowel from a vascular accident (e.g., volvulus, intussusception) or obstruction (e.g., atresia, meconium ileus). If this occurs long before birth, the peritonitis has usually resolved and the infant presents with obstruction. If it is more recent and ongoing, however, the infant may have signs of peritonitis as well. The inflammatory reaction may be intense despite the absence of bacteria. Calcification of extravasated meconium and the formation of a large pseudocyst are common findings.

The diagnosis of peritonitis in a neonate is subjective and may be subtle but is characterized by tenderness, increased resistance to palpation, and often erythema of the abdominal wall. Muscle spasm or involuntary guarding, which is a key finding in the older patient, is usually absent. The diagnosis is made by a combination of clinical and radiographic findings and is a clear indication for operation to resect ischemic or perforated bowel, to repair the cause of obstruction, or to débride the peritoneal cavity and remove the infected fluid.

Chyle

Chylous ascites is an accumulation of fat-rich lymph, or chyle, in the peritoneal cavity. Fat is primarily absorbed from the bowel and transported via the lacteals to the cisterna chyli at the base of the mesentery and then into the thoracic duct. Chylous ascites presumably results from a leak somewhere in the abdominal lymphatic system. The diagnosis is made by paracentesis, which usually yields a milky fluid if the infant has been fed. Laboratory analysis shows a high lymphocyte count and elevated triglyceride concentration. Known causes of chylous ascites include lymphatic malformations such as mesenteric cyst or lymphangiectasia, and malrotation with midgut volvulus causing lymphatic obstruction but not vascular occlusion. Ultrasound examination of the abdomen and an upper gastrointestinal series should be performed to look for these or other conditions that can be corrected surgically.

Most cases of chylous ascites are idiopathic, presumably owing to a small leak somewhere in the lymphatic system. Because these are difficult to locate, a trial of medical therapy is indicated. Feeding the infant with a low-fat formula in which most of the fat is in the form of medium-chain triglyceride (which is absorbed directly and not transported by the lacteals) should substantially decrease the abdominal lymph flow and allow the leak to heal. Dietary management may be necessary for several months. Repeated or continuous removal of the fluid is not useful; the fluid simply reaccumulates and the removal of large amounts of protein-rich fluid leads to hypoproteinemia. If dietary management is not effective and the infant is symptomatic, a trial of complete bowel rest and total parenteral nutrition may be indicated, although this is expensive and has the potential for complications. If the ascites is intractable, surgical exploration may be necessary. It can be difficult to find the site of leakage. Feeding the infant a lipophilic dye such as Sudan black in cream a few hours before surgery can be helpful. If a leak can be identified and oversewn, the problem should resolve.

Blood

Hemoperitoneum refers to blood in the peritoneal cavity and is rare in neonates. Trauma from a difficult breech delivery is the most common cause. The liver is the most frequent source, followed by spleen and rarely kidney. It occurs mostly in premature infants or infants who are large for gestational age. The blood may initially be contained as a subcapsular hematoma, but the capsule in a baby is flimsy so rupture into the free peritoneal cavity is the rule, either immediately or delayed up to 48 hours. The infant presents a distended, often tense abdomen, sometimes with bluish discoloration. If the bleeding is active and not contained, shock rapidly ensues, and death is likely if the bleeding cannot be controlled surgically. Correction of the known coagulopathy of the neonate by vitamin K prophylaxis may need to be supplemented by transfusions of fresh-frozen plasma. Unfortunately, surgical control of bleeding can be difficult because both the liver and the spleen are very friable in the newborn and do not hold sutures well. Rupture of a liver tumor (see the next section, Distention Due to Enlarged Organs) also presents as shock and massive hemoperitoneum.

Bile

Bile ascites is rare in infants and occurs as a result of spontaneous perforation of the bile duct. This is not related to birth trauma; the cause is unknown, although some cases are related to congenital anomalies or obstruction of the ductal system. The infant has a distended abdomen and jaundice. Other liver function test results are relatively normal. Paracentesis yields deeply bile-stained fluid. If the bile is infected, the patient is acutely ill with bile peritonitis and needs urgent treatment. A detailed ultrasound examination of the pancreaticobiliary region is performed to search for congenital anomalies or evidence of obstruction. Operation is necessary to confirm the diagnosis and to perform operative cholangiography to exclude a correctable cause. In most cases, simple drainage of the area is all that is necessary; the hole in the duct heals spontaneously in 1 or 2 weeks. Attempts to repair or resect the tiny duct usually are not warranted.

DISTENTION DUE TO ENLARGED ORGANS

Hepatic

Enlargement of organs or other solid tissue usually presents as an abdominal mass but may be first noted as distention (Box 58.3). Enlargement due to fluid within an organ also is covered in this section. Physical examination often makes it clear that the distention is in fact a mass, and both history and examination may give clues as to the diagnosis. Ultrasound examination usually identifies the organ involved and clarifies whether the mass is solid or cystic. Computed tomography may be necessary to make a more precise diagnosis, especially for solid masses. Magnetic resonance imaging is occasionally helpful for specific abnormalities.

Diffuse enlargement of the liver may be a manifestation of congenital heart disease and cardiac failure. Congenital infections, such as cytomegalovirus, toxoplasmosis, and syphilis, may cause significant hepatomegaly and distention, with or without ascites as discussed previously. Serologic test results should lead to a correct diagnosis. Genetic metabolic disorders, as discussed earlier, may cause both ascites and liver enlargement. Beckwith-Wiedemann syndrome is characterized by diffuse organomegaly (and therefore abdominal distention), macroglossia, severe neonatal hypoglycemia, and sometimes omphalocele. Urgent neonatal diagnosis is critical to avoid the serious neurologic consequences of untreated hypoglycemia.

Hepatic tumors in the neonate are frequently large and diffuse, presenting as abdominal distention. Vascular lesions are most common. Large, discrete masses involving a single lobe or segment are usually vascular malformations that are not proliferative but also do not involute. They should be resected in case they rupture and cause life-threatening hemorrhage. Diffuse proliferative hemangioendotheliomas are more common, however, and are not amenable to resection. Although these are benign, they frequently present with life-threatening symptoms, including high-output congestive heart failure from extensive arteriovenous shunting and severe thrombocytopenia from intralesional consumption (Kasabach-Merritt syndrome). Abdominal distention and a bruit over the liver are often the key findings leading to a correct diagnosis. The natural history of this lesion is rapid progression in the first months of life, then stabilization and gradual involution and disappearance of the tumor. Cardiac failure is treated with digitalis and diuretics. High-dose corticosteroid treatment is used in symptomatic patients in an attempt to accelerate the natural course of involution. Corticosteroid therapy effectively controls cardiac failure and thrombocytopenia in approximately 50% of patients. Interferon-alpha has shown considerable promise for treatment of life-threatening hemangioendothelioma. If medical therapy fails, radiographic or surgical obliteration of the hepatic artery may control intractable symptoms.

Mesenchymal hamartoma of the liver is a congenital lesion of the liver unique to infants and young children. It may be very large and present as abdominal distention. As the name implies, this is a hamartomatous lesion rather than a neoplasm, typically composed of multiple cysts surrounded by abundant

---

| BOX 58.3 | Enlarged Organs that Cause Abdominal Distention |

Hepatic enlargement
Cardiac failure
  Congenital heart disease
  Arrhythmias
Congenital infection
  Cytomegalic inclusion disease
  Syphilis
  Toxoplasmosis
  Rubella
Metabolic disorders
  Storage diseases
    Lysosomal storage diseases
    Carbohydrate storage diseases
  Tyrosinemia
  Galactosemia
Beckwith-Wiedemann syndrome
Hepatic tumors
  Hemangioma
  Hemangioendothelioma
  Mesenchymal hamartoma
  Metastatic tumors

Renal masses
Hydronephrosis
  Posterior urethral valves
  Ureterovesical junction obstruction
  Ureteropelvic junction obstruction
Multicystic kidney
Polycystic kidney
Renal vein thrombosis
Adrenal masses
Adrenal hemorrhage
Neuroblastoma

Pelvic masses
Ovarian cyst
  Follicular
  Dermoid/teratoma
Hydrocolpos, hydrometrocolpos
  Imperforate hymen
  Vaginal atresia/stenosis
  Cloaca

Retroperitoneal masses
Neuroblastoma
Wilms tumor
Mesoblastic nephroma
Sacrococcygeal teratoma
Lymphangioma

Gastrointestinal masses
Duplication
Mesenteric cyst

---

fibroblasts, collagen, myxoid tissue, and other mesenchymal elements. The only effective treatment is surgical removal, which should be undertaken because of the size of these masses and their tendency to rupture. Hepatoblastoma is an aggressive, often diffuse and bilateral, malignant tumor of the liver. Abdominal distention is usually the presenting sign. Treatment is by combination chemotherapy and surgical resection. This tumor is discussed in more detail in Chapter 67, Malignancy in the Newborn. Massive hepatic metastases from congenital neuroblastoma (see Chapter 67) may occasionally present as abdominal distention.

Renal

Nearly one-half of all abdominal masses in the newborn arise in the kidney, and these are sometimes large enough to cause abdominal distention. Hydronephrosis from various types of congenital obstructions is most common and easily diagnosed by ultrasound. Cystic lesions of the kidney are also common and include multicystic kidney (a dysplastic, nonfunctioning kidney) and polycystic kidney disease, which may be associated with cysts in the liver and other organs. These lesions are discussed in Chapter 61. The urachus is a developmental structure connecting the bladder to the vestigial allantois. If segments of the urachus fail to involute, they may enlarge to form a urachal cyst in the lower abdomen. Occasionally, these can become very large and are prone to infection. Unilateral or bilateral renal vein thrombosis may present as a mass or distention. Known risk factors include prematurity, shock, sepsis, dehydration, and maternal diabetes. Severe renal dysfunction and variable degrees of permanent renal damage are common. Thrombolytic therapy, anticoagulation, or both may be beneficial.

Adrenal hemorrhage in the newborn usually presents as an abdominal mass that may be very large. The lesion is often cystic and may become calcified. It gradually resolves and usually leaves an intact adrenal gland. If the cyst is bilateral, the infant should be monitored for signs of adrenal insufficiency, although this is unusual. The mass should be followed by ultrasound to monitor regression because neuroblastoma may have a similar appearance on imaging studies. Measurement of urinary catecholamine levels is helpful in this differential diagnosis because they are usually elevated in patients with neuroblastoma.

Pelvic

One of the most common abdominal masses in infant girls is an ovarian cyst, which may be large enough to cause abdominal distention. If the cyst is entirely echolucent and free of solid elements on ultrasound examination, a simple follicular cyst is the likely diagnosis, resulting from stimulation by maternal hormones. These resolve in time, but a significant risk of torsion and loss of the ovary and tube exists. The current recommendation is that cysts less than 5 cm in diameter can be followed with serial ultrasound examinations but that larger ones should be excised with preservation of the residual ovary and tube. If the cyst is complex and contains solid elements, it is more likely a dermoid or teratoma, which should be removed. These and other cystic and solid neoplasms of the ovary are discussed in Chapter 61.

Massive enlargement of the vagina (hydrocolpos) or vagina and uterus (hydrometrocolpos) may present as abdominal distention or a pelvic mass. Imperforate hymen can be detected by physical examination and is treated by simple incision of the membrane. Vaginal atresia occurs in a variety of forms that may require complex imaging studies (computed tomography, magnetic resonance imaging) to classify and plan appropriate surgical repair. Female infants with cloacal anomalies may have massive hydrocolpos from urine preferentially entering the vagina. The diagnosis is readily apparent from inspection of the perineum where only a single orifice is found. Urgent decompression of the urinary tract is essential to preserve renal function. The alimentary tract is diverted with a colostomy. Definitive repair includes simultaneous vaginal and rectal pull-through later in the first year of life.

Retroperitoneal

Retroperitoneal tumors are less common in neonates than in infants and young children, but when present may be large enough to cause abdominal distention. Congenital neuroblastoma is most likely to be the 4S stage, with a small primary and large hepatic metastases as noted previously. Wilms tumor is rare in the neonate. The more common congenital renal tumor is mesoblastic nephroma, which shares many histologic features with Wilms tumor but is a distinct clinical entity that almost invariably has a biologically benign course. Surgical removal is usually the only treatment required. Sacrococcygeal teratoma is often massive and usually an exophytic mass projecting out from the lower back and perineum. A significant pelvic component may exist that occasionally is the primary location for the tumor. These are usually mature teratomas in neonates and are cured by excision that includes resection of the coccyx. Lymphangioma of the abdomen or retroperitoneum is a cystic dysplasia of the lymphatic system and may be large enough to cause distention or a palpable mass. Excision is indicated because of the risk of infection or rupture.

Gastrointestinal

Congenital anomalies of the gastrointestinal tract are rarely large enough to cause noticeable abdominal distention in the neonate. Mesenteric cyst is a lymphangioma of the mesenteric lymphatics that may become infected, rupture, or cause intestinal obstruction by direct compression of the bowel or as a focal point for volvulus. Resection is indicated and may require removal of the adjacent segment of bowel. Duplication of the bowel is a cystic or tubular structure that contains all of the layers of bowel but shares a common wall with the adjacent normal bowel. Symptoms may result from compression or obstruction, but many are detected by physical examination. Resection of the duplication requires removal of the involved bowel segment.

Suggested Readings

Brandt ML, Luks FI, Filiatrault D, et al. Surgical indications in antenatally diagnosed ovarian cysts. *J Pediatr Surg* 1991;26:276.

Chung MA, Brandt ML, St-Vil D, et al. Mesenteric cysts in children. *J Pediatr Surg* 1991;26:1306.

Chye J, Lim C, Van der Heuvel M. Neonatal chylous ascites—report of three cases and review of the literature. *Pediatr Surg Int* 1997;12:296.

Clarke H Jr, Mills M, Parres J, et al. The hyponatremia of neonatal urinary ascites: clinical observations, experimental confirmation and proposed mechanism. *J Urol* 1993;150:778.

DeMaioribus CA, Lally KP, Sim K, et al. Mesenchymal hamartoma of the liver. *Arch Surg* 1990;125:598.

Gallagher PG, ed. Nonimmune hydrops fetalis. *Semin Perinatol* 1995;19:435.

Holgersen LO, Subramanian S, Kirpekar M, et al. Spontaneous resolution of antenatally diagnosed adrenal masses. *J Pediatr Surg* 1996;31:153.

Iyer CP, Mahour GH. Duplications of the alimentary tract in infants and children. *J Pediatr Surg* 1995;30:1267.

Keidan I, Lotan D, Gazit G, et al. Early neonatal renal venous thrombosis: long-term outcome. *Acta Paediatr* 1994;83:1225.

Kosir MA, Sonnino RE, Gauderer MWL. Pediatric abdominal lymphangiomas: a plea for early recognition. *J Pediatr Surg* 1991;26:1309.

Merten DF, Kirks DR. Diagnostic imaging of pediatric abdominal masses. *Pediatr Clin North Am* 1985;32:1397.

Nuss R, Hays T, Manco-Johnson M. Efficacy and safety of heparin anticoagulation for neonatal renal vein thrombosis. *Am J Pediatr Hematol/Oncol* 1994;16:127.

Schmidt B, Andrew M. Neonatal thrombosis: report of a prospective Canadian and international registry. *Pediatrics* 1995;96:939.

Selby D, Stocker J, Waclawiw M, et al. Infantile hemangioendothelioma of the liver. *Hepatology* 1994;20:39.

Spigland N, Greco R, Rosenfeld D. Spontaneous biliary perforation: does external drainage constitute adequate therapy? *J Pediatr Surg* 1996;31:782.

Stanley P, Geer GD, Miller JH, et al. Infantile hepatic hemangiomas. *Cancer* 1989;64:936.

Steves M, Ricketts RR. Pneumoperitoneum in the newborn infant. *Am Surg* 1987;53:226.

Touloukian R. Hepatic hemangioendothelioma during infancy: pathology, diagnosis and treatment with prednisone. *Pediatrics* 1970;45:71.

Vanhaesebrouck P, Leroy J, De Praeter C, et al. Simple test to distinguish between surgical and non-surgical pneumoperitoneum in ventilated neonates. *Arch Dis Child* 1989;64:48.

Woltering M, Robben S, Egeler R. Hepatic hemangioendothelioma of infancy: treatment with interferon. *J Pediatr Gastroenterol Nutr* 1997;24:348.

Zamir O, Goldberg M, Udassin R, et al. Idiopathic gastrointestinal perforation in the neonate. *J Pediatr Surg* 1988;23:335.

CHAPTER 59 ■ NECROTIZING ENTEROCOLITIS

KATHLEEN J. MOTIL

Necrotizing enterocolitis (NEC) is the most common gastrointestinal emergency in the infant. This disorder encompasses several distinct disease entities that differ from the most common form of the disease, that is, idiopathic NEC (Box 59.1). Although the etiology of idiopathic NEC is unknown, specific precipitating factors may be implicated in many instances. The clinical manifestations of idiopathic NEC may mimic the symptoms and signs of various neonatal gastrointestinal disorders, and these may be indistinguishable from those of sepsis. NEC has become the single most common surgical emergency in neonatal intensive care units (NICUs). Early recognition and aggressive treatment of this disorder during the last 10 years has led to a markedly improved clinical outcome.

EPIDEMIOLOGY

The overall incidence of NEC is 2.4:1000 live births (range, 0.0:1000 to 7.2:1000) or 2.1% (range, 1.0% to 7.7%) of all admissions to NICUs. The incidence of NEC averages 3% to 4% in infants whose birth weight is less than 2,000 g, and decreases significantly to 1% in infants whose birth weight is greater than 2,000 g. The incidence of NEC in very low-birth-weight infants continues to increase in both absolute and relative terms. Males and females are affected equally. Black and white infants are affected more commonly than are those of Hispanic origin, but the racial patterns reflect the populations served by individual neonatal centers. Seasonal variation does not affect the incidence of NEC. Periodic clusters of cases or epidemics have been reported.

PATHOGENESIS AND ETIOLOGY

The precise etiology of idiopathic NEC is unknown, but it probably is caused by multiple factors in a susceptible host. The features most commonly implicated in the pathogenesis of the disease are ischemic insult to the gut, the presence of bacterial or viral organisms in the intestinal tract, the availability of intraluminal substrate (usually formula or human milk) to promote bacterial proliferation or induce mucosal injury, and altered host defense (Box 59.2). The first two factors (ischemia, infectious agents) are thought to be the predisposing variables that initiate the pathogenesis of NEC. Other factors, such as inflammatory mediators (cytokines), oxygen radicals,

---

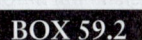

BOX 59.1   Classification of Neonatal Necrotizing Enterocolitis

Neonatal necrotizing enterocolitis (idiopathic)
  Sporadic
  Epidemic
Benign necrotizing enterocolitis (pneumatosis coli)
Neonatal necrotizing enterocolitis associated with precipitating factors
  Exchange transfusions
  Polycythemia
  Congenital heart disease
  Endocrine disorders
  Prolonged diarrhea
  Hypertonic agents (formulas, drugs, contrast media)
  Vitamin E therapy
Neonatal necrotizing enterocolitis associated with primary bowel pathology
  Intestinal obstruction
  Focal intestinal perforation
  Neonatal appendicitis
  Gangrenous colitis
  Hirschsprung disease

BOX 59.2   Pathophysiology of Necrotizing Enterocolitis

Ischemia
  Hypoxia (birth asphyxia, respiratory distress syndrome, apnea, hypotension, hypothermia, patent ductus arteriosus)
  Vascular congestion (congestive heart failure, exchange transfusion, polycythemia)
  Thrombosis (umbilical vessel catheterization)
Intestinal Microflora
  Bacterial organisms and toxins (*Escherichia coli, Klebsiella pneumoniae, Enterobacter cloacae, Enterobacter sakazakii, Pseudomonas, Salmonella, Clostridium difficile, Clostridium perfringens, Clostridium butyricum, Bacteroides fragilis*)
  Viruses (coxsackievirus B_2, rotavirus, coronavirus)
  Fungi (*Torulopsis glabrata*)
Inflammatory Mediators
  Increased cytokine activity (tumor necrosis factor, interleukins, platelet-activating factor)
  Magnesium, copper deficiencies
Intraluminal Agents
  Human milk, commercial formulas (fermentation of fats and carbohydrates)
  Hypertonic solutions (human milk fortifiers, medications, contrast media)
Altered Host Defense
  Developmental immaturity of the intestinal tract (corticosteroids)
  Immaturity of neonatal immune system
  Vitamin E therapy (scavenger of oxygen radicals)

and bacterial fermentation products and toxins, are thought to propagate the disease process. Despite recent advances, the pathogenesis of NEC remains an enigma.

The regulation of mesenteric blood flow to the gut is understood poorly in the infant, but is thought to mimic the "diving reflex" in aquatic animals. During hypoxic conditions, this reflex is a defense mechanism that protects the brain and heart from ischemic damage by shunting blood away from the mesenteric, renal, and peripheral vascular beds. Comparable studies in asphyxiated neonatal piglets have demonstrated that blood flow to the stomach, ileum, and colon is reduced dramatically during a hypoxic episode. With resuscitation, perfusion rebounds, leading to vascular congestion and mucosal hemorrhages secondary to ischemic injury to the blood vessels. These studies support the hypothesis that ischemia contributes to the pathogenesis of NEC in the human infant.

Many perinatal events predispose the neonate to hypoxia. Birth asphyxia, respiratory distress syndrome, apnea, hypotension, hypothermia, patent ductus arteriosus, congestive heart failure, umbilical vessel catheterization, polycythemia, and exchange transfusion have been implicated as ischemic factors in the pathogenesis of neonatal NEC. Nevertheless, some infants with no evidence of these risk factors have the disorder. Moreover, in studies of multiple births in which risk factors such as perinatal asphyxia and respiratory distress are less common in the first-born than in the second-born infant, NEC occurred in the first-born twin in all cases, and in no case did only the second-born twin have NEC. Finally, when infants with NEC are compared with matched controls, few, if any, ischemic risk factors are identified consistently.

The intestinal microflora provides an additional component in the development of ischemic necrosis of the intestinal tract. A number of bacterial, viral, and fungal organisms have been isolated in sporadic and epidemic outbreaks of NEC. Bacterial organisms normally found in the distal gastrointestinal tract, including *Escherichia coli* (56%), *Klebsiella pneumoniae* (28%), *Pseudomonas* (11%), and *Clostridium difficile*, have been recovered from the blood and peritoneal cavities of about one-third of all infants with NEC. Viral particles have been identified concurrently in the feces of infants with NEC and their mothers, the midwives, and the nursing staff involved in treatment of the infants. Fungi also have been isolated from infants born to immunocompromised mothers.

The role of gastrointestinal microorganisms in the pathophysiology of NEC remains unclear. Current hypotheses suggest that either a bacterial invasion of tissue occurs in a passive manner after ischemic damage to the mucosal barrier of the gut, or enteric bacteria and viruses cause the disease directly. Several clostridial species have been implicated causally in the development of NEC because of their production of toxins, their association with pseudomembrane formation, and most important, their ability to produce submucosal and subserosal gas blebs and intestinal gangrene. *Enterobacter sakazakii*, a known contaminant of powdered milk formula, also can contribute to outbreaks of NEC in NICUs. Nevertheless, in many epidemics of NEC, specific pathogens either cannot be identified or, when they are present, are isolated from healthy infants without the disease. Thus, a cautious interpretation of the pathogenicity of specific microorganisms is warranted.

Recent evidence suggests that inflammatory mediators, especially platelet activating factor (PAF), may play a pivotal role in NEC. PAF, an endogenous phospholipid mediator with potent proinflammatory actions associated with hypotension, increased vascular permeability, hemoconcentration, lysozyme enzyme release, and platelet and neutrophil aggregation, induces tissue necrosis. In experimental models of NEC, neutrophil activation and adhesion to intestinal venules initiate a local inflammatory reaction in which PAF triggers tissue injury via tumor necrosis factor (TNF) generation and reactive

radical formation. Xanthine oxidase, the major source of reactive oxygen species, aggravates tissue injury by promoting the peroxidation of unsaturated lipids in cellular and mitochondrial membranes. Subsequent norepinephrine release and mesenteric vasoconstriction result in splanchnic ischemia and reperfusion. Translocation of bacterial endotoxins further amplifies the inflammatory process. Nitric oxide may be a protective modulator of inflammatory injury because it promotes vasodilatation and microvascular integrity, inhibits leukocyte adhesion and activation, and scavenges oxygen radicals. Studies in premature infants with NEC have demonstrated elevated levels of PAF, TNF, and interleukin-6 (IL-6). Magnesium and copper have been implicated in the pathogenesis of NEC, because a deficiency of these minerals may activate the synthesis or activity of cytokines and oxygen free radicals.

Because bacterial involvement in NEC may be associated with usual intestinal flora, topical antibiotics were considered to be potentially useful in the prevention of the disease. The topical administration of aminoglycosides into the gastrointestinal tract either prophylactically or at the time of diagnosis decreases the total colony count of enteric flora. These antibiotics, however, do not provide protection from the development of NEC; do not alter its course, complications, or mortality rate; and may be associated with the emergence of resistant strains of enteric organisms and potentially ototoxic complications in the infant. Therefore, the use of topical aminoglycosides is not recommended for the routine prevention of NEC.

Milk feedings also have been implicated in the pathogenesis of neonatal NEC. About 93% of all infants in whom NEC develops have been fed enterally. Human milk and commercial formulas serve as substrates for bacterial proliferation in the gut. Because neonates partially malabsorb the carbohydrate and fat constituents in milk, reducing substances, organic acids, carbon dioxide, and hydrogen gas may be produced by the bacterial fermentation of these nutrients. When NEC develops, neonates have increased intestinal loss of carbohydrates, leading to reducing substances in the feces and hydrogen-filled cysts within the gut mucosa. Although these observations identify milk feedings as a contributory factor in the development of NEC, the disease may develop in some infants who have never been fed. Additional factors, such as the volume of milk and its rate of administration, may contribute to the development of NEC.

NEC may result from direct mucosal injury induced by hyperosmolar formulas. Although such formulas are used rarely in neonatal nurseries, medications that frequently are administered orally may contain hypertonic additives that irritate the intestinal mucosa and precipitate disease (Table 59.1). Other hyperosmolar agents instilled directly into the bowel for

TABLE 59.1

OSMOLARITY OF DRUGS COMMONLY ADMINISTERED TO NEONATES

Generic Drug	Osmolarity (mOsm/L)	Concentration (mg/mL)
Ampicillin	1,843	50
Nystatin	3,022	100,000*
Multivitamins	6,023	—
Vitamin E	605	36
Ferrous chloride	5,079	157
Calcium gluconate	319	50
Caffeine	90	30
Theophylline	1,012	193
Methyl digoxin	15,250	0.6

*Concentration expressed as units/mL.

diagnostic studies may precipitate NEC, presumably because of fluid shifts, bowel distention, and ischemia. Care should be taken to only use isotonic contrast media to avoid this complication.

Altered host resistance as a result of immunologic and gastrointestinal immaturity in the neonate is believed to play a primary role in the development of NEC. At birth, the human intestinal mucosa has no secretory IgA, the major gastrointestinal immunoprotective antibody. Because human milk contains specific and nonspecific protective factors, such as immunocompetent cells, secretory IgA, lactoferrin, lysozyme, and the *Lactobacillus bifidus* growth factor, it has been fed to neonates to reduce the incidence and severity of NEC. These studies support the protective role of human milk in the prevention of NEC. Despite the presence of these protective factors, NEC has occurred in neonates who were fed refrigerated, pasteurized, or frozen human milk.

The issue of the developmental immaturity of the gastrointestinal tract may be central to the pathogenesis of NEC. One study demonstrated that the risk of developing NEC is diminished significantly in infants whose mothers received antenatal corticosteroids; however, this outcome is not a universal finding. Although their mechanism of action is unclear, corticosteroids may function as nonspecific enzyme inducers, leading to accelerated maturation of the intestinal tract and enhanced protection from disease. Infants who received erythropoietin for anemia of prematurity also had a lower incidence of NEC. Erythropoietin may confer a beneficial effect by protecting against programmed cell death in intestinal epithelium.

The use of vitamin E in the treatment of retinopathy of prematurity has been associated with an increased incidence of NEC. This association was noted primarily in infants whose birth weights were less than 1,500 g, and whose serum tocopherol levels were higher than 3.5 mg/dL. It was hypothesized that the mechanism of excessive scavenging of oxygen radicals, which leads to diminished antimicrobial defenses, increased the risk of developing NEC in these infants. Subsequent trials of vitamin E therapy for the prevention of neonatal intracranial hemorrhage failed to demonstrate an association with NEC, presumably because serum alpha-tocopherol levels were maintained in a range less than 3.5 mg/dL.

Predisposing Factors

Risk factors that predispose the premature infant to NEC have been the subject of controversy (Box 59.3). Risk factors for the development of NEC may be the same in low-birth-weight infants with or without the disease, because the disease affects predominantly low-birth-weight infants who require intensive care. Univariate analysis of a large neonatal database showed that premature infants who developed NEC had lower birth weights and younger gestational ages; were more often African American; had been exposed more often to medications, including pre- and postnatal glucocorticoids, surfactant, caffeine, erythropoietin, and indomethacin; had been exposed more often to invasive procedures such as umbilical vessel catheterization and mechanical ventilatory support, and were less likely to receive human milk than premature infants who did not develop NEC. A multivariate analysis of this same neonatal database showed that the most important risk factor associated with the development of NEC was low birth weight. Other factors independently associated with an increased risk for NEC included being on a ventilator on the first day of life, having received antenatal glucocorticoids, being exposed to both glucocorticoids and indomethacin during the first week of life, and depressed Apgar scores at 5 minutes of life. One additional study suggests that NEC occurred with equal frequency in premature infants who received indomethacin therapy for patent

---

BOX 59.3	Risk Factors Associated with Necrotizing Enterocolitis in Premature and Older Infants

Group I: Preterm infants of less than 2,000 g
  Low birth weight
  On ventilator on first day of life
  Reported to have received antenatal corticosteroids
  Exposed to both glucocorticoids and indomethacin during first week of life
  Depressed Apgar score at five minutes of life
  Duration of morphine exposure
  Treatment for cocaine exposure
Group II: Older infants of more than 2,000 g
  Polycythemia
  Respiratory distress
  Hypoglycemia
  Congenital heart disease and endocrine disorders
  Postoperative repair of abdominal wall defects and gastrointestinal tract lesions

---

ductus arteriosus and those who did not (13% versus 14%, respectively). The analyses of smaller databases suggest that a longer duration of morphine use and treatment for cocaine exposure increase the risk of NEC.

Additional risk factors have been identified for infants who average more than 2,000 g at birth. Polycythemia (peripheral venous hematocrit greater than 65%); respiratory distress, defined by the need for supplemental oxygen for more than 24 hours; and hypoglycemia (serum glucose level less than 30 mg/dL) are the most common clinical features associated with the development of NEC in this group of infants. NEC in term infants, although rare, has been associated with underlying conditions such as congenital heart disease and endocrine disorders, including panhypopituitarism, hypothyroidism, hypoparathyroidism, and congenital adrenal hyperplasia.

Infants who have undergone major abdominal surgery within the first week of life may be at increased risk for the development of NEC. Late-onset NEC may develop in infants with the diagnosis of gastroschisis, omphalocele, jejunal atresia, aganglionosis, and malrotation after surgical repair of the anatomic lesion. These infants have a relentless course, with substantial morbidity (67%) resulting from diarrhea, the short bowel syndrome, and sepsis, and with a mortality rate of 46%. Thus, the presence of abdominal wall defects and other intestinal lesions suggests a possible increased susceptibility to NEC during the postoperative course in these infants.

CLINICAL MANIFESTATIONS AND COMPLICATIONS

Pathologic Findings

Neonatal NEC is a pathologic condition that may be characterized broadly as intestinal infarction. This disorder primarily affects the terminal ileum and colon, although, in severe cases, the entire gastrointestinal tract may be involved. The pathologic findings are variable and reflect the rapidity of disease progression and the presence of underlying pathogenic factors.

On gross examination, the bowel is distended and hemorrhagic. Subserosal collections of gas may or may not be present along the mesenteric border. Gangrenous necrosis, with

TABLE 59.2

GESTATIONAL AGES AND BIRTH WEIGHT OF INFANTS WITH NECROTIZING ENTEROCOLITIS

Gestational Age (wk)	Percentage (%)	Birth Weight (g)	Percentage (%)
<32	33	<1,000	7
32–36	41	1,000–1,500	32
36–40	12	1,500–2,000	32
>40	14	2,000–3,000	19
		>3,000	10

TABLE 59.3

PRESENTING SYMPTOMS AND SIGNS OF NECROTIZING ENTEROCOLITIS

Finding	Incidence (%)
Gastrointestinal findings	
Abdominal distention	89
Hematochezia	
Guaiac-positive stools	80
Grossly bloody stools	43
Fecal reducing substances	71
Gastric residual	
Vomiting	73
Diarrhea	37
Systemic findings	25
Lethargy	84
Temperature instability	81
Apnea	66
Respiratory failure	40
Hypotension	37

or without perforation, may be present on the antimesenteric border. Fibrinous adhesions, thickening of the bowel wall, and areas of stenosis are seen in the healing gut.

The histologic features of bowel ischemia include mucosal edema and hemorrhage, which may progress to transmural bland necrosis. Collections of gas, secondary bacterial infiltration, and acute inflammation may be present. Vascular thrombi are infrequent findings in NEC.

Signs and Symptoms

Nearly three-fourths of all infants with NEC are born prematurely, with a gestational age of less than 37 weeks and a birth weight of less than 2,000 g (Table 59.2). Full-term infants in whom NEC develops generally have congenital heart disease, congestive heart failure, or protracted diarrhea of unknown etiology that is complicated by malnutrition. The onset of symptoms occurs within the first 5 days of life in 44% of infants, although symptoms may occur as late as 12 weeks after birth in 25% of infants. Generally, the postnatal age is related inversely to gestational age at the time of diagnosis.

Significant maternal or perinatal risk factors may be present at the time of diagnosis; many of these factors, however, occur equally in premature infants in whom NEC does not develop. Most infants who are seen in the first week of life are recovering from their initial acute illness at the time of onset of this disorder, and many are considered to be "growing" premature infants.

Feedings with either human milk or commercial formulas have been instituted in 98% of infants in whom NEC develops. The feedings are tolerated poorly, however, and generate gastric retention, the earliest presenting symptom of the disease (Table 59.3). Other gastrointestinal symptoms and signs, including vomiting, abdominal distention, diminished bowel sounds, reducing substances in the stools, and hematochezia (with either guaiac-positive stools or frank blood), follow rapidly. Diarrhea is an infrequent finding. Systemic manifestations of NEC, including temperature instability, lethargy, apnea, respiratory failure, and hypotension, also may be apparent at the onset of the disease.

Subclinical NEC is suspected, but not confirmed, in about 25% of cases, and the symptoms resolve gradually. In 25% to 40% of cases, fulminant progression of the disease occurs, with evidence of perforation and peritonitis that is characterized by abdominal tenderness on palpation; a feeling of fullness or a mass, particularly in the right lower quadrant; and erythema, ecchymosis, or necrosis of the abdominal wall. Lethargy, severe acidosis, sepsis, disseminated intravascular coagulation, and shock may supervene rapidly.

Premorbid risk factors associated with death from NEC have been proposed. Poor prognostic factors include premature rupture of membranes, low Apgar scores at 5 minutes, a prolonged oxygen requirement at birth, abdominal distention,

portal vein gas on radiographic studies, *Klebsiella* septicemia, blood transfusion, and surgical intervention.

DIAGNOSIS

Laboratory studies of infants with NEC may demonstrate a decreased platelet count, increased prothrombin and partial thromboplastin times, and serum factor V concentrations of less than 40%, all of which are consistent with the diagnosis of disseminated intravascular coagulation. Nevertheless, coagulation studies are not obtained routinely. Platelet counts of less than 50,000/mm^3 have been found in 38% of infants with NEC and may lead to significant bleeding complications, such as intracranial hemorrhage. A serial decrease in platelets to levels less than 100,000/mm^3 is thought to correlate closely with gangrenous bowel and impending perforation. A complete blood count and differential are of little assistance in the diagnosis of NEC, but an absolute neutrophil count of less than 1,500/mm^3 or a rapid fall in platelet count is associated with a poor prognosis. Serum biochemical abnormalities are nonspecific. Hyponatremia (serum sodium levels less than 130 mEq/L) and persistent metabolic acidosis suggest the presence of sepsis or necrotic bowel.

The presence of reducing substances, alpha-1-antitrypsin, or blood in the stool may be an early, but nonspecific, presenting sign of NEC. Similarly, levels of C-reactive protein, alpha-1-acid glycoprotein (orosomucoid), lysosomal acid hydrolase, and urinary D-lactate, a metabolite of carbohydrate fermentation produced by enteric microflora, are increased in infants with this disease and may serve as useful markers to discriminate between NEC and other intestinal insults. Elevated breath hydrogen levels may be useful to detect the onset of NEC 24 hours before symptoms appear in a premature infant who is at risk for the development of this disorder. However, most of these tests, with the exception of stool guaiac for blood, are not obtained routinely in the infant with NEC.

Blood cultures may show bacterial growth in one-third of all specimens obtained. Cerebrospinal fluid cultures may be warranted if sepsis or meningitis is suspected. Stool cultures generally show the presence of normal enteric flora. Additional cultures for *Clostridium difficile* and assays for its toxins may be indicated when the history and physical findings support the clinical impression. When abdominal paracentesis is performed in infants with suspected peritonitis, Gram stain and culture of

TABLE 59.4

PRESENTING RADIOGRAPHIC FEATURES OF NECROTIZING ENTEROCOLITIS

Finding	Incidence (%)
Pneumatosis intestinalis	91
Dilatation of bowel loops	83
Persistent "fixed loop"	33
Peritoneal fluid (ascites)	29
Portal venous gas	23
Pneumoperitoneum	17

the peritoneal fluid demonstrate enteric organisms in one-third of the cases. Usually, these organisms are the same as those recovered from blood culture.

Flatplate studies of the abdomen are essential to make the diagnosis of NEC. An abdominal film in the supine, decubitus, or upright position may show the presence of pneumatosis intestinalis, the hallmark of NEC, as well as edema of the bowel wall, dilatation of loops of bowel, ascites, portal vein gas, or free air in the peritoneum. Serial films may reveal the presence of fixed loops of bowel, which is an ominous feature suggesting the presence of intestinal perforation. Radiographic features characteristic of NEC may be seen in 87% of patients at the time a definitive diagnosis is made (Table 59.4). Barium contrast studies are contraindicated if the diagnosis of NEC and its complications are suspected. Further diagnostic imaging studies are of little value.

Abdominal ultrasonography may prove useful to identify gangrenous bowel and impending perforation. The sonographic appearance of the pseudo-kidney sign (i.e., a bowel wall that is characterized by a hypoechoic rim with a central echogenic focus) may serve this purpose. This technique also has been used to demonstrate intermittent hepatic parenchymal and portal venous microbubbles of gas in the absence of the classic radiographic findings of NEC.

The diagnosis of NEC is confirmed when the following triad of clinical features is present: abdominal distention, hematochezia, and pneumatosis intestinalis. Pneumatosis intestinalis may not be identified, however, in nearly 15% of surgically or autopsy-confirmed cases. Similarly, portal vein gas, once thought to be a poor prognostic feature of NEC, may be a transient finding on radiographic examination (Fig. 59.1).

Differential Diagnosis

The differential diagnosis of NEC includes anal fissures, pneumatosis coli, focal intestinal perforation, infectious enterocolitis, neonatal appendicitis, intestinal obstruction, Hirschsprung disease, and spontaneous gastrointestinal perforation.

Anal fissures have been reported in conjunction with NEC, but the significance of the relationship is unknown. Fissures may precipitate the development of the disease by creating a portal of entry for bacteria, or they may be secondary manifestations of the disease entity. Physicians should have a high index of suspicion of NEC when a premature infant has rectal bleeding or guaiac-positive stools in the presence of anal fissures, and the physician should not delay in making a diagnosis or providing treatment.

Pneumatosis coli is a benign form of NEC that is seen primarily in premature infants. Clinical features include gastric residua and vomiting, transient episodes of lethargy and apnea, mild abdominal distention, and frank blood in the stools. Radiographic studies demonstrate intramural intestinal gas limited to the colon and the absence of small-bowel dilatation

and pneumatosis. Recovery is complete within 3 days, and no sequelae are apparent. This entity can be differentiated from classic NEC by its clinical course.

Focal intestinal perforation is an isolated, idiopathic intestinal perforation without gross necrosis. This entity is found primarily in very low-birth-weight infants and is not associated with NEC. The clinical manifestations of focal intestinal perforation differ from those found in NEC; gestational age and birth weight are lower, the incidence of coexistent respiratory distress syndrome is higher, the age of onset is younger, and the rate of survival is higher in infants with focal intestinal perforation. Despite recent controversy, focal intestinal perforation is thought to be a distinct clinical entity.

Infectious enterocolitis may be attributed to a number of pathogenic organisms, including *Salmonella*, *Shigella*, *Campylobacter*, and *Clostridium difficile*, some of which also have been associated with NEC. Stool cultures should be obtained to identify the presence or absence of these organisms. The precise etiology of symptoms may be difficult to determine because of the association between NEC and intestinal organisms, as well as the similarities in the medical management of these two entities.

Neonatal appendicitis may masquerade as NEC. This entity is rare in newborn infants, presumably because of the persistence of the funnel-shaped configuration of the fetal appendix, which is less prone to obstruction. When it occurs, neonatal appendicitis has a predilection for premature male infants and is associated frequently with inguinal hernias. Radiographic features that may assist in the diagnosis of neonatal appendicitis include an abnormal gas pattern and peritoneal fluid in 85% of cases, psoas shadow obliteration in 56%, a thickened abdominal wall in 32%, a fecalith in 32%, and abscess formation in 20%. The findings at laparotomy will distinguish between neonatal appendicitis and NEC.

Gangrenous enterocolitis or perforation may be associated with *intestinal obstruction* resulting from intussusception, meconium ileus, ileal atresia, volvulus, or milk curds. Similarly, *Hirschsprung disease* may present as fulminant enterocolitis with colonic obstruction, diarrhea, and sepsis. Infants with *spontaneous perforation* of the gastrointestinal tract often are more mature than are those with NEC. Perforations occur in the stomach, ileum, and colon. The lesion generally is localized, however, which differentiates this entity from NEC. Bilious vomiting, gastric aspirates, abdominal distention and tenderness, hematochezia, and pneumatosis intestinalis may be seen in any of these entities. A barium enema is of little use in distinguishing among these diagnoses, and generally is contraindicated because it may lead to perforation. Surgical intervention should clarify the dilemma introduced by these clinical conditions.

THERAPY

The treatment of infants with NEC is based on a method of clinical staging at the time of diagnosis (Table 59.5). Infants classified as having stage I or II disease require appropriate diagnostic studies and vigorous medical therapy, whereas those categorized as having stage III disease require surgical intervention.

The medical treatment of NEC primarily is supportive (Box 59.4). When the diagnosis is suspected, oral feedings should be withheld and nasogastric suction and intravenous fluid should be instituted. Initial laboratory studies should include a complete blood count and differential, a platelet count, serum electrolyte and creatinine measurements, blood urea nitrogen, and acid–base studies. Routine cultures of the blood, urine, stool, and cerebrospinal fluid should be obtained. Additional stool specimens should be sent for viral and fungal studies, when

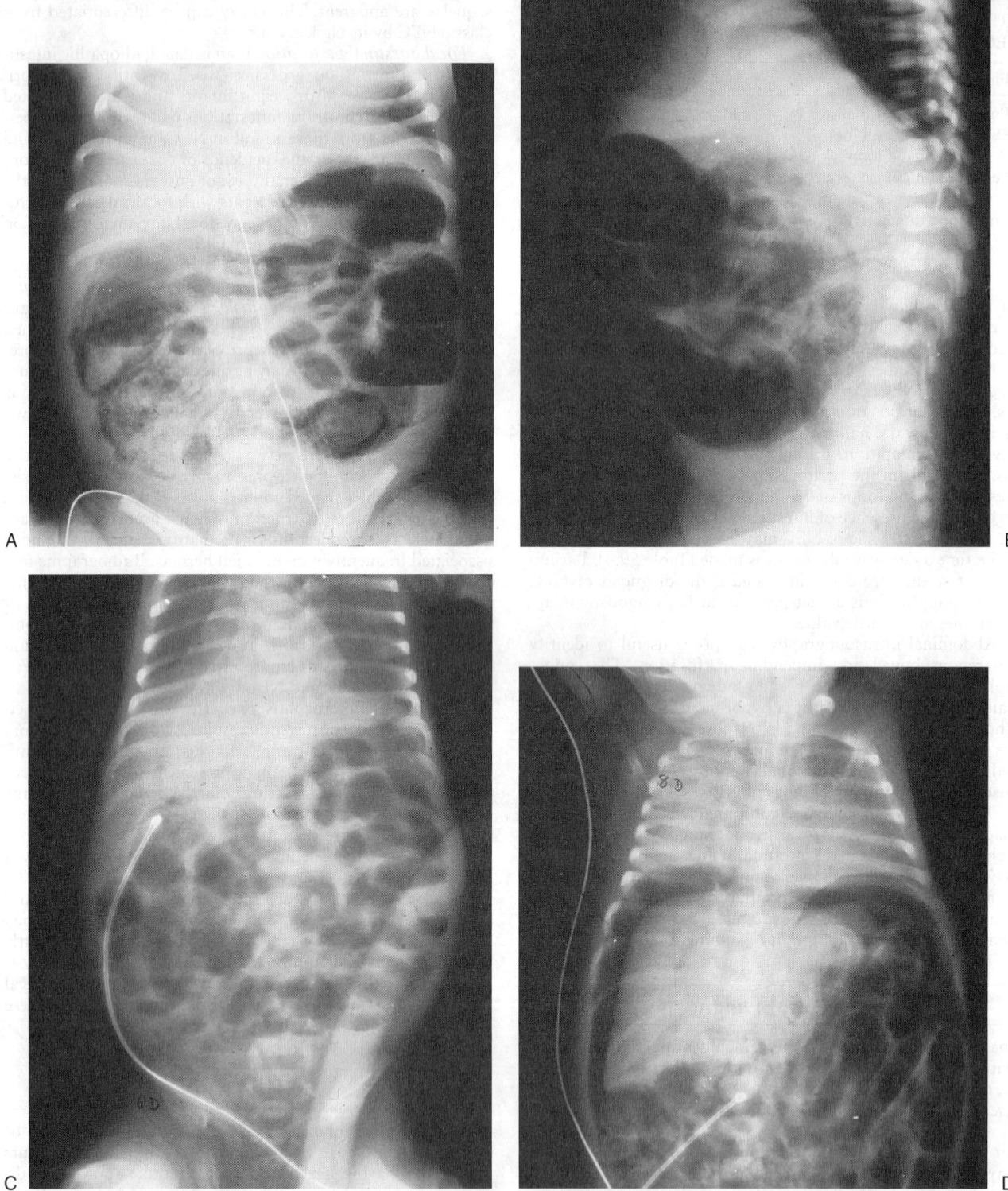

FIGURE 59.1. A–D: Girl with necrotizing enterocolitis. Frontal (A) and lateral (B) radiographs at 2 days of age show dilation of the small and large intestine with extensive intramural gas. Frontal radiograph at 6 days (C) shows generalized small bowel distention and quite extensive gas within the portal veins. There is atelectasis of the right lower lobe. Two days later (D), perforation has occurred, with a large pneumoperitoneum. Gas persists within the portal vein branches within the liver. Aeration of the lungs has deteriorated. (Reprinted with permission from, Elzouki AY, Harfi HA, Nazer H. *Textbook of clinical pediatrics*. Philadelphia: Lippincott Williams & Wilkins, 2000:247.)

TABLE 59.5

STAGING CRITERIA FOR THE TREATMENT OF NECROTIZING ENTEROCOLITIS

Stage	Systemic	Intestinal	Radiologic	Treatment
I. Suspect	Lethargy, temperature instability, apnea, bradycardia	Gastric residual, emesis, abdominal distention, hematochezia	Ileus, intestinal dilation	Parenteral nutrition, nasogastric suction, antibiotics
II. Definite—same features as stage I plus:				
A. Mildly ill	—	Absent bowel sound	Pneumatosis intestinalis	—
B. Moderately ill	Metabolic acidosis, thrombocytopenia	Abdominal tenderness	Portal vein gas	NaHCO$_3$
III. Advanced— same features as stage II plus:				
A. Shock	Respiratory arrest, hypotension, disseminated intravascular coagulation, combined respiratory metabolic acidosis	Peritonitis	Ascites	Intravenous fluids, isotropic agents, paracentesis
B. Bowel perforation	—	—	Pneumoperitoneum	Surgery

appropriate. The stools should be checked routinely for occult blood. Total parenteral nutrition should be provided to maintain the nutritional status of the infant. Parenteral antibiotics that cover a broad spectrum of aerobic and anaerobic organisms should be administered for 10 to 14 days. Although the choice of antibiotic therapy will depend on the resistance patterns of individual institutions, the antibiotics currently recommended include ampicillin, aminoglycosides, clindamycin, and the newer cephalosporins. The administration of topical antibiotics such as gentamicin may reduce the occurrence of NEC and NEC-related deaths; however, this therapy is not recommended because of the increased incidence of colonization of the gut with resistant bacterial strains of significant virulence.

BOX 59.4 Medical Treatment of Necrotizing Enterocolitis

Clinical treatment
  Nothing by mouth
  Intermittent nasogastric suction
  Intravenous fluid replacement
  Total parenteral nutrition
  Broad-spectrum antibiotics
Laboratory treatment
  Hematology
    Complete blood cell count and differential cell count
    Serial (12-hr) platelet counts
  Biochemistry
    Serum electrolytes, blood urea nitrogen, creatinine
  Arterial blood gases
  Fecal occult blood
  Microbiology
    Blood, urine, stool, cerebrospinal fluid cultures
  Radiology
    Serial (6- to 8-hr) abdominal films (supine, decubitus)

Serial abdominal films of the infant in the supine and left lateral decubitus positions (the latter to allow free air to rise over the liver) are recommended every 6 to 8 hours as needed, and serve as the best guide in following the course of the disease. If there is no further progression of illness and the pneumatosis resolves, nasogastric suction may be discontinued. Oral feedings may be resumed gradually within 10 to 14 days after the acute illness.

Surgical intervention is necessary when the disease involves the full thickness of the bowel wall, resulting in gangrene or frank perforation. The decision of when to operate may be difficult; the surgical goal is to stabilize peritoneal infection without sacrificing bowel length. The indications for surgery include rapid clinical deterioration manifested by thermal instability, bradycardia, persistent metabolic acidosis, progressive hyponatremia, and thrombocytopenia; intestinal perforation manifested by pneumoperitoneum on abdominal flat plate; a palpable abdominal mass; intestinal obstruction; or peritonitis manifested as abdominal tenderness and rigidity, progressive erythematous discoloration of the abdominal wall, or the radiographic appearance of a fixed and unchanging collection of intraluminal gas, usually in the right lower quadrant.

Laparotomy, with limited resection and creation of an enterostomy, has been the standard of care for focal perforation in NEC. Although intestinal resection with primary anastomosis may be an alternative approach, this procedure has been associated with lower survival rates compared with infants who underwent intestinal diversion. If an enterostomy has been created, a barium enema should be performed before re-anastomosis to exclude the presence of more distal intestinal strictures. To allow resuscitation and stabilization prior to definitive laparotomy, primary peritoneal drainage or proximal diversion alone may be warranted as a temporizing procedure in very low-birth-weight infants with pan-necrosis involving more than 75% of the intestine. When pan-necrosis is encountered, the operative strategy is to resect only frankly necrotic bowel to prevent short bowel syndrome. To spare final intestinal length, second-look laparotomy and definitive excision within 24 to 48 hours has been proposed as an alternative to initial extensive resection. A novel surgical approach, the "clip and drop-back" technique, ultimately may improve survival outcomes in NEC. In this technique, all portions of nonviable intestine are resected at the initial operation, but enterostomies and anastomoses are not created. The blind-end segments of intestine are returned to the abdomen. Within 24 to 72 hours, laparotomy is performed and bowel continuity is restored. Postoperative wound (infection, dehiscence) and stomal (prolapse, retraction, necrosis, stricture) problems require at least one additional operation in 45% of infants affected with NEC.

Complications

The complications of NEC may occur early or late in the course of the disease, and vary in the frequency of their appearance. The acute complications include sepsis (60%), peritonitis (20% to 30%), meningitis, abscess formation, thrombocytopenia, disseminated intravascular coagulation, and intestinal or extraintestinal bleeding. Antibiotic therapy provides coverage for the treatment of the infectious complications of NEC. Fresh-frozen plasma, platelet concentrates, or an exchange transfusion may be necessary for the hematologic complications. Shock, hypotension, respiratory arrest, hypoglycemia, and metabolic acidosis require aggressive resuscitative efforts in the early stages of advanced disease.

The late complications of NEC include stenosis, stricture formation, intestinal atresia, pericolic abscess, enterocele, enterocolic fistula, and short bowel syndrome. Intestinal stenoses and strictures are the most common complications of NEC, occurring in 14% to 36% of infants treated medically, and less frequently in those treated surgically. The interval during which a stricture may develop ranges from 1 to 20 months; on average, a stricture is detectable by 2 months after the acute episode. About 80% of strictures occur in the colon, predominantly on the left side, but strictures also may be seen in the terminal ileum and jejunum. Multiple strictures may be seen in individual patients. Birth weight, gestational age, disease severity, and the presence of pneumatosis intestinalis do not correlate with the likelihood of stenosis or stricture developing after an episode of NEC. Barium enema studies must be performed before closure of any enterostomy, and may be necessary 4 to 6 weeks after the acute episode of NEC if there are any symptoms of feeding intolerance. About 60% of infants have asymptomatic stenoses, of which one-half may progress to overt symptoms. However, about 20% resolve spontaneously. Strictures are treated surgically. The procedure of choice is resection and primary anastomosis. In rare cases, staged management (i.e., resection and colostomy, followed by closure) may be necessary. The use of a balloon catheter to dilate focal colonic strictures located distal to an enterostomy may be useful in some patients.

Intestinal malabsorption may occur postoperatively in about 9% of patients with NEC when a significant portion of the terminal ileum has been resected or the amount of small bowel remaining after surgery is insufficient to support normal absorptive function. Vitamin B_{12} malabsorption without megaloblastic anemia has been described in children after ileocecal valve and terminal ileal resection has been performed for neonatal NEC. Prolonged vitamin B_{12} therapy may be necessary in these circumstances. In those infants with extensive intestinal resection, prolonged parenteral or enteral nutrition may be required for survival. In a small proportion of children, gastrointestinal function fails to adapt and life-threatening complications such as cirrhosis and end-stage liver failure or recurrent catheter sepsis with subsequent loss of venous access require intestinal, liver, or multiorgan transplantation. Early transplantation results demonstrate an overall 3-year survival rate of 54% with a median follow-up of 29 months.

TABLE 59.6

SURVIVAL RATES OF INFANTS WITH NECROTIZING ENTEROCOLITIS

Birth Weight (g)	Survival Rate (%)
<1,000	43
1,000–1,500	67
1,500–2,000	82
2,000–2,500	44
>2,500	80

PROGNOSIS

The prognosis for NEC has improved considerably as a result of advances in the care of the critically ill infant, earlier diagnosis and treatment, and the institution of a standard aggressive approach in the treatment of this disorder. The overall survival rate currently is 70% to 80%. The prognosis is affected adversely by the degree of prematurity and a higher number of comorbidities (Table 59.6). Late-onset NEC has a better prognosis than the early onset form. Very low-birth-weight infants who have NEC represent a subgroup of infants who generally are more ill, develop NEC later, require surgery with greater frequency than premature infants who weigh more than 1,000 g, and are less likely to survive. Very low-birth-weight infants who survive medical NEC incur hospital charges in excess of $73,000 because of an additional 3-week period of hospitalization, whereas those infants who survive surgical NEC will incur costs in excess of $186,000 because of an additional 2-month hospital stay.

About 50% of the survivors of NEC become normal, healthy children. All are able to meet their daily nutrient requirements orally although they remain below the fiftieth percentile for height and weight. Approximately 93% of survivors are toilet trained, while 10% have more than three bowel movements daily. Nearly 85% of these children are enrolled in school full time, but 28% require special education. Approximately 15% have significant neurodevelopmental morbidity, including mental retardation, which is independent of birth weight or intraventricular hemorrhage. Approximately 21% of these children have speech disturbances that require therapy.

PREVENTION

Preventive measures have been advocated to reduce the frequency or minimize the severity of NEC. These recommendations include avoiding hypertonic formulas, medications, and diagnostic agents in sick newborn infants; performing a phlebotomy and exchange transfusion with plasma when polycythemia becomes critical (hematocrit greater than 70%); placement of arterial umbilical catheters in the aorta distal to the renal arteries; and avoidance of placement of venous umbilical catheters in the portal vein. Human milk may exert a protective effect on the development of NEC because it contains epidermal growth factor and PAF acetylhydrolase, a PAF-degrading enzyme deficient in infants, both of which have been shown to alter the development of NEC in animal models. Feeding schedules that delay by 1 to 2 days the introduction of feeds, provide full-strength human milk or one-half strength formula for 3 days before advancing to full-strength formula, and maintain daily trophic feeds in amounts of 20 mL/kg, particularly with human milk, for 10 days before advancing volume in equal increments, reduce the incidence of NEC.

Polyunsaturated fatty acids, administered as an egg phospholipids preparation in a milk-based formula, lowered the frequency of NEC in premature infants possibly because they modulate the inflammatory cascade via altered PAF metabolism. Arginine supplementation has been shown to reduce the incidence of NEC in premature infants, presumably because it serves as a precursor for the synthesis of endothelial nitric oxide, an important regulator of vascular perfusion in the presence of inflammation and injury. Probiotic therapy using *Lactobacillus GG* and oral immunoglobulin therapy do not reduce significantly the incidence of NEC in premature infants and cannot be recommended. However, daily supplementation with *Bifidus infantis* and *Lactobacillus acidophilus* together may reduce the incidence of NEC by promoting colonization of the intestinal tract with nonpathogenic anaerobic bacteria. Prebiotic therapy using oligofructose confers a protective effect against the development of NEC in experimental animal models by promoting bifidobacteria growth and retarding clostridia colonization of the gut. Epidermal growth factor, a heat-stable peptide trophic to the intestinal mucosa, affects cell proliferation, differentiation, and migration, and may have therapeutic implications for the future prevention and cure of NEC.

Acknowledgments

This work is a publication of the United States Department of Agriculture/Agricultural Research Service (ARS) Children's Nutrition Research Center, Department of Pediatrics, Baylor College of Medicine and Texas Children's Hospital in Houston, Texas. This project has been funded in part with federal funds from the Agricultural Research Service of the United States Department of Agriculture under Cooperative Agreement number 58-7MN1-6-100. The contents of this publication do not necessarily reflect the views or policies of the United States Department of Agriculture, nor does mention of trade names, commercial products, or organizations imply endorsement by the United States government.

Suggested Readings

Amin HJ, Zamora SA, McMillan DD, et al. Arginine supplementation prevents necrotizing enterocolitis in the premature infant. *J Pediatr* 2002;140:425.

Berseth CL, Bisquera JA, Paje VU. Prolonging small feeding volumes early in life decreases the incidence of necrotizing enterocolitis in very low birth weight infants. *Pediatrics* 2003;111:529.

Bisquera JA, Cooper TR, Berseth CL. Impact of necrotizing enterocolitis on length of stay and hospital charges in very low birth weight infants. *Pediatrics* 2002;109:423.

Bolisetty S, Lui K, Oei J, et al. A regional study of underlying congenital diseases in term neonates with necrotizing enterocolitis. *Acta Paediatr* 2000;89:1226.

Bury RG, Tudehope D. Enteral antibiotics for preventing necrotizing enterocolitis in low birthweight or preterm infants (Cochrane Review). In: The Cochrane Library, Issue 2, 2002. Oxford: Update Software.

Butel M-J, Waligora-Dupriet A-J, Szylit O. Oligofructose and experimental model of neonatal necrotizing enterocolitis. *Br J Nutr* 2002;87:S213.

Chandler JC, Hebra A. Necrotizing enterocolitis in infants with very low birth weight. *Semin Pediatr Surg* 2000;9:63.

Dani C, Biadaioli R, Bertini G, et al. Probiotics feeding in prevention of urinary tract infection, bacterial sepsis and necrotizing enterocolitis in preterm infants. *Biol Neonate* 2002;82:103.

Foster J, Cole M. Oral immunoglobulin for preventing necrotizing enterocolitis in preterm and low birth-weight neonates (Cochrane Review). In: *The Cochrane Library*, Issue 3, 2002.Oxford: Update Software.

Guthrie SO, Gordon PV, Thomas V, et al. Necrotizing enterocolitis among neonates in the United States. *J Perinatol* 2003;23:278.

Hallstrom M, Koivisto A-M, Janas M, et al. Frequency of and risk factors for necrotizing enterocolitis in infants born before 33 weeks of gestation. *Acta Paediatr* 2003;92:111.

Hsueh W, Caplan MS, Qu X-W, et al. Neonatal necrotizing enterocolitis: clinical considerations and pathogenetic concepts. *Pediatr Dev Pathol* 2002;6:6.

Hung-Chih L, Bai-Horng S, An-Chyi C, et al. Oral probiotics reduce the incidence and severity of necrotizing enterocolitis in very low birth weight infants. *Pediatrics* 2005;115:1.

Kamitsuka MD, Horton MK, Williams MA. The incidence of necrotizing enterocolitis after introducing standardized feeding schedules for infants between 1,250 and 2,500 grams and less than 35 weeks of gestation. *Pediatrics* 2000;105:379.

Lawrence G, Tudehope D, Baumann K, et al. Enteral human IgG for prevention of necrotizing enterocolitis: a placebo-controlled, randomized trial. *Lancet* 2001;357:2090.

McElhinney DB, Hedrick HL, Bush DM, et al. Necrotizing enterocolitis in neonates with congenital heart disease: risk factors and outcomes. *Pediatrics* 2000;106:1080.

Moss RL, Dimmitt RA, Henry MC, et al. A meta-analysis of peritoneal drainage versus laparotomy for perforated necrotizing enterocolitis. *J Pediatr Surg* 2001;36:1210.

O'Donovan DJ, Baetiong A, Adams K, et al. Necrotizing enterocolitis and gastrointestinal complications after indomethacin therapy and surgical ligation in premature infants with patent ductus arteriosus. *J Perinatol* 2003;23:286.

Okuyama H, Kubota A, Oue T, et al. A comparison of the clinical presentation and outcome of focal intestinal perforation and necrotizing enterocolitis in very-low-birth-weight neonates. *Pediatr Surg Int* 2002;18:704.

Shin CE, Falcone RA, Stuart L, et al. Diminished epidermal growth factor levels in infants with necrotizing enterocolitis. *J Pediatr Surg* 2000;35:173.

Stanford A, Upperman JS, Boyle P, et al. Long-term follow-up of patients with necrotizing enterocolitis. *J Pediatr Surg* 2002;37:1048.

Vennarecci G, Kato T, Misiakos EP, et al. Intestinal transplantation for short gut syndrome attributable to necrotizing enterocolitis. *Pediatrics* 2000;105(2). URL: http://www.pediatrics.org/cgi/content/full/105/2/e25.

Vohr BR, Wright LL, Dusick AM, et al. Neurodevelopmental and functional outcomes of extremely low birth weight infants in the National Institute of Child Health and Human Development Neonatal Research Network, 1993–1994. *Pediatrics* 2000;105:1216.

CHAPTER 60 ■ SHORT BOWEL SYNDROME

JON A. VANDERHOOF

PATHOPHYSIOLOGY

In pediatrics, short bowel syndrome is perhaps the most common indication for the chronic use of parenteral nutrition. In the neonatal period, massive small bowel resection often is necessary because of either congenital anomalies of the gastrointestinal tract or advanced ischemic injury from necrotizing enterocolitis. A smaller number of patients require resection later in life as a result of vascular injury of the small intestine, usually secondary to midgut volvulus, or they have short bowel syndrome as a result of the surgical management of advanced inflammatory bowel disease. Long-term survival without parenteral nutrition depends on the ability of the small intestine to increase its absorptive capacity so that the patient's nutritional needs can be provided through the enteral route.

Adaptation

Many patients with a surprisingly short segment of small intestine eventually develop the ability to live without parenteral nutrition as a result of a compensatory increase in mucosal surface area caused by the adaptive response to massive resection. This compensatory growth is dominated by villus hyperplasia, although some dilatation and lengthening of the remaining small intestine does occur.

As might be expected, increases in villus length and in the number of enterocytes available for absorption per centimeter of bowel are accompanied by a gradual increase in the absorption of nearly all nutrients.

Stimulation of the adaptation process becomes the primary goal of therapy in the treatment of patients with short bowel syndrome. The importance of intraluminal nutrition in stimulating this process has been well documented. The intraluminal nutrients not only are necessary to produce adaptation, but also are essential to maintain the structural and functional integrity of the small intestine.

Nutrients appear to stimulate mucosal adaptation through three independent, but possibly related, mechanisms:

- Direct contact of concentrated nutrients with the mucosal surface appears to stimulate intestinal growth.
- Trophic hormones produced in response to high concentrations of intraluminal nutrients are released both systemically through an endocrine mechanism and locally through a paracrine mechanism to stimulate the production of new enterocytes.
- The release of trophic upper gastrointestinal secretions is stimulated by the presence of intraluminal nutrients.

MANAGEMENT STRATEGIES

The clinical management of short bowel syndrome can be considered best in three phases (Box 60.1). Phase I consists of nutritional repletion with total parenteral nutrition (TPN). Phase II includes the gradual introduction of enteral nutrition, usually by continuous infusion. During phase III, continuous enteral nutrition is reduced incrementally as the patient is weaned gradually to bolus or solid feeding.

Phase I: Stabilization and Nutritional Repletion

During phase I, achieving nutritional repletion and stabilizing fluid and electrolyte balance are the major goals of therapy.

BOX 60.1   Management of Short Bowel Syndrome

Phase I. Stabilization and Nutritional Repletion
 Long-term parenteral nutrition
 Electrolyte replacement
 Monitoring of serum chemistries
Phase II. Gradual Introduction of Enteral Nutrition
 Continuous infusion of enteral formula
 Monitoring of quantity and quality of stool output
Phase III. Reintroduction of Solids
 Weaning to bolus/po diet
 Coordinated introduction of solid foods
 Monitoring for nutrient-deficient states

Home therapy also should be contemplated at this time and, if it is at all possible, organization of and instruction regarding home TPN should be initiated early.

Once it is apparent that the child will require long-term parenteral nutrition venous access with an indwelling catheter or infusion part is required. The decision as to whether TPN will be necessary may be obvious in the case of massive small bowel resection. In questionable patients, failure of adequate growth on a trial of total enteral nutrition is required to make the decision. Parenteral nutrition usually is begun using a 10% dextrose and 2.5% crystalline amino acid solution infused at a rate approximately equal to 1.3 times the maintenance fluid rate for the patient. Incremental increases in dextrose concentration then follow, up to 15% and 20% each day, to allow the patient to achieve total caloric requirements parenterally by the third day. Maintenance quantities of parenteral vitamins and trace metals are added to the parenteral nutrition solution, usually through the use of commercial preparations. In patients with high-output proximal fistulas, additional zinc supplementation may be required. Extra zinc also should be considered in small, preterm infants. Twenty-percent intravenous lipid solution should be administered a minimum of twice weekly to provide at least 8% of the total caloric intake as fat, if substantial enteral feedings are not administered concurrently. Although the primary purpose of intravenous lipid is to prevent the deficiency of essential fatty acids, daily use of the lipid solution may allow additional calories to be provided, if they are needed.

With few exceptions, standard pediatric electrolyte concentrations can be administered with little variation. Routinely, 30 mEq of sodium chloride, 20 mEq of potassium phosphate, 10 mEq of calcium gluconate, and 5 mEq of magnesium sulfate can be added to each liter of TPN solution. Depending on the amino acid solution used, some sodium may need to be administered in the form of acetate to buffer the solution. This will be readily apparent if the patient becomes acidotic while receiving parenteral nutrition. Providing enough calcium phosphate is a problem in some small infants. The addition of L-cysteine, 1,000 mg/L, may allow the provision of additional calcium and phosphorus in the solution without precipitation.

Appropriate monitoring and the replacement of abnormal losses is the key to the use of standard solutions in patients with short bowel syndrome. Patients receiving long-term parenteral nutrition can be managed with infrequent changes in the composition of TPN, provided that abnormal losses are replaced. For example, if a patient has a jejunal fistula or high-volume stool losses, electrolyte concentrations can be measured in the fistula fluid or the stool, and a comparable mixture of fluid and electrolytes can be replaced on a volume-per-volume basis. This prevents excessive loss of fluid and electrolytes, and the patient then can be maintained on standard TPN solutions for prolonged periods. The additional cost of the second infusion pump is more than offset by minimized wastage of parenteral nutrition solution as well as by the relative stability of the patient, which results in a need for fewer serum electrolyte determinations.

Phase II: Gradual Introduction of Enteral Nutrition

During early phases of therapy, electrolyte, blood urea nitrogen (BUN), and glucose levels should be measured daily. After a short period, however, these determinations can be made less frequently. In patients receiving long-term therapy, monitoring is required as infrequently as every 1 to 3 months, once appropriate needs are established. Periodic determination of calcium, magnesium, phosphorus, liver enzymes and, occasionally, trace element and vitamin levels is required.

Once the patient is stabilized on parenteral nutrition, fluid and electrolyte losses are under control, and gastrointestinal motility is returned, phase II begins with a gradual introduction to enteral nutrition, preferably by continuous infusion. This can be accomplished either by using a soft silicone nasogastric tube or, if long-term infusion is planned, through a feeding gastrostomy tube or button device. Initially, 3% to 5% of the total daily caloric intake is often given in the form of an elemental or predigested enteral formula diet such as Pregestimil (Mead Johnson, Evansville, IN) or Alimentum (Ross Laboratories, Columbus, OH). The stool volume, pH level, and reducing substances can be monitored. A marked increase in stool volume or significant malabsorption, as indicated by a persistent stool pH level of less than 5.5, or stools that are positive for reducing substances, contraindicate further advancement of enteral nutrition. Otherwise, the rate of enteral nutrition should be increased gradually and that of TPN should be decreased isocalorically. The rapidity with which the increases can be made depends greatly on the length of the remaining small intestine. The whole process may proceed so rapidly that it is completed in a few weeks. On the other hand, years of TPN may be necessary before total enteral nutrition is tolerated.

The use of continuous infusion offers several advantages to bolus feeding in patients with short bowel syndrome. Because transporters that carry monosaccharides, amino acids, and dipeptides across the small bowel mucosa are saturated continuously, absorption is enhanced. Consequently, a greater percentage of nutrients can be absorbed enterally, decreasing the need for parenteral nutrition. Additionally, short chain fatty acids may be salvaged in the colon and available as a calorie source so re-attachment of bowel segments or re-feeding small bowel contents into the colon remnant may be helpful in weaning the parenteral nutrition.

The selection of an appropriate liquid diet for continuous enteral feeding is controversial. Protein hydrolysates or crystalline amino acids typically are used for a protein source. Protein hydrolysates have the advantage of being absorbed more rapidly than nonhydrolyzed protein. As most protein is absorbed in the form of dipeptides and tripeptides, the use of amino acids may be unnecessary. Although complex diets sometimes are thought to be more trophic than elemental diets, no clear indication exists that an intact protein is better than a protein hydrolysate in inducing mucosal hyperplasia. Carbohydrate generally is provided in the form of either glucose polymers or sucrose. Glucose polymers are hydrolyzed readily by pancreatic and mucosal enzymes and have the advantage of reducing the osmolality of the formula. In the early stages of therapy, lactose generally is poorly tolerated and should be avoided. Many enteral formulations designed for older children have a low fat content. Those that do contain fats often contain a high percentage of medium-chain triglycerides. Contrary to popular belief, high-fat diets usually do not result in increased fluid loss in patients with short bowel syndrome, and dietary fat may be important in stimulating intestinal adaptation as well as slowing gut motility. In older children and adults, intact protein formulas may offer a significant cost advantage and probably are absorbed almost as well as protein hydrolysate formulas. In small infants, however, a significant risk of the development of protein sensitivity or allergy exists and, consequently, protein hydrolysate or even amino acid formulas may offer an advantage in these patients.

Phase III: Reintroduction of Solids

During phase III, solid feedings are begun and the patient is weaned gradually to bolus feedings of an elemental diet to supplement the solid feedings. Solids can be consumed concurrently with the nasogastric or gastrostomy feeding during continuous enteral infusion. During this phase, attention must be paid to potential nutrient-deficient states once the patient no longer is receiving parenteral nutrition. These nutrients specifically include vitamins, minerals, and trace metals. Carbohydrate, protein and, to a lesser extent, fat are relatively well absorbed once parenteral nutrition is discontinued. Poor absorption of fat-soluble vitamins, calcium, magnesium, and zinc is common, however. Poor absorption of vitamin D and calcium may result in rickets or tetany, especially in preterm infants and osteoporosis in order children. Vitamins A, E, and D may be given in aqueous solution, and occasionally parenteral vitamin K is administered. After ileal resection, bile acid and vitamin B_{12} malabsorption are major problems, and bile acid malabsorption may exacerbate further fat-soluble vitamin absorption. If needed, vitamin B_{12} may be administered by injection or nasal inhalation.

Use of Medications in Phase III

In addition to nutrient-deficiency states, the clinician must consider the likelihood that medications administered orally will be absorbed at less than desired levels. This becomes important in the treatment of children with short bowel syndrome who have otitis media or other common pediatric infections. From 10% to 90% of the antibiotics commonly used may be malabsorbed in these infants, resulting in unpredictable therapeutic outcomes in patients treated orally. In these instances, home intravenous antibiotic therapy often is required. Likewise, some oral vaccines may be ineffective.

Some degree of small bowel bacterial overgrowth almost always is present in short bowel syndrome. Pathologic symptoms of excess bacteria depend on the numbers or specific organisms involved (Box 60.2). Chronic bacterial overgrowth may further exacerbate malabsorption. Bacterial overgrowth is likely to occur when the ileocecal valve is absent, when a tight anastomosis or partial obstruction is present, or when a dilated segment of bowel with poor motility exists. Bacterial overgrowth exacerbates malabsorption because of injury of the intestinal mucosa and deconjugation of bile acids, facilitating their reabsorption and reducing bile acid availability for the solubilization of long-chain fats. Such patients may respond to intermittent broad-spectrum antimicrobial therapy. A combination of metronidazole with trimethoprim-sulfamethoxazole may be particularly helpful; clindamycin, because of its efficacy against anaerobic organisms, or oral gentamicin, also may be useful. In some instances, the continuous administration of cyclic antibiotics is required to control bacterial overgrowth. If possible, resecting a tight anastomosis or performing an intestinal tapering procedure is useful in alleviating bacterial overgrowth and often results in marked improvement in absorption.

Metabolic acidoses have developed in some patients as a result of the production of excessive D-lactate by intestinal bacteria. Although both D-lactate and L-lactate are produced by intestinal bacteria, only the L form can be metabolized in humans. D-Lactic acidosis is correctable through the elimination of bacterial overgrowth and should be considered in patients

---

BOX 60.2   **Consequences of Small Bowel Bacterial Overgrowth**

Malabsorption
Intestinal mucosal injury
Deconjugation of bile acids
Frank intestinal mucosal ulceration
D-Lactic acidosis

with short bowel syndrome who have repeated attacks of drowsiness and impaired central nervous system function.

A colitis or ileitis picture similar to that associated with Crohn disease has been described in patients with short bowel syndrome and bacterial overgrowth. Frank ulceration may occur and, if it is unresponsive to antimicrobial therapy, the disorder may respond to anti-inflammatory agents.

Gastric acid hypersecretion is common in infants with short bowel syndrome and many become symptomatic and require acid suppression therapy. Antimotility agents should be used judiciously, because, although they may reduce stool output, they may exacerbate small bowel bacterial overgrowth. Cholestyramine, a bile acid–binding resin, is useful in reducing diarrhea in some patients with ileal resection. Cholestyramine is most effective when used in conjunction with medium-chain triglycerides or low-fat formulas, because cholestyramine may exacerbate fat malabsorption by reducing the functional bile acid pool.

Surgical Management

A number of surgical procedures have been devised to improve absorption in patients with short bowel syndrome. Most involve slowing intestinal transit. The most direct approach is the construction of a valve or sphincter that functions in a manner similar to the ileocecal valve, causing constriction of the lumen and creating a partial mechanical obstruction. The intent also is to prevent retrograde reflux of bacterial contents into the small intestine. Reversed segments of small intestine also have been used, but in children, such procedures usually exacerbate small bowel bacterial overgrowth and, if anything, result in more complications than benefits.

Intestinal lengthening surgery, using either the Bianchi technique or the serial transverse enteroplasty (STEP) procedure occasionally may be helpful. A markedly dilated intestine often develops in patients with short bowel syndrome, secondary to both partial chronic obstruction and adaptation. Tapering dilated segments and/or lengthening reduces stasis and bacterial content, and often improves intestinal function, while preserving or enhancing intestinal length. These procedures have proved to be a valuable adjunct in patients with dilated segments of bowel who respond poorly to antibiotic therapy for bacterial overgrowth.

Small intestinal transplantation should be reserved for a select group of patients who have failed to respond to the above therapies and have life-threatening complications. Improvements in immunosuppression have made long-term survival following intestinal transplantation possible. Long-term survival (greater than 5 years) has ranged around 50%, but newer postoperative therapies are encouraging and suggest that these numbers are improving to around 60% to 70% at major centers.

PROGNOSIS

The prognosis for short bowel syndrome has been altered markedly through the use of parenteral nutrition. Advances in parenteral therapy, including changes in catheter techniques, solutions, understanding of the importance of intraluminal nutrition and, finally, use of parenteral nutrition in the home, have altered markedly the way in which patients with short bowel syndrome are treated. In 1972, the classic paper by Wilmore defined the prognosis for short bowel syndrome in infants. Of 20 infants with a jejunoileal segment length of 38 to 75 cm, 95% survived. Infants with 15 to 38 cm of jejunum and ileum survived 50% of the time, provided the ileocecal valve was intact. Those without an ileocecal valve died, as did infants with less than 15 cm of small intestine, including all those with intact ileocecal valves.

Advances in parenteral and enteral nutrition have significantly changed the statistics regarding short bowel syndrome in the 1980s. Recent studies have demonstrated that survival and normal growth without parenteral nutrition is possible with very little jejunum and ileum with or without an ileocecal valve. Additionally, a recent series has confirmed the improved prognosis of children with short bowel syndrome even without transplantation. Patients with short bowel syndrome now die of the complications of parenteral nutrition, such as severe TPN cholestasis or fulminant septicemia, rather than of malnutrition. Careful attention to details and aggressive enteral nutrition remain the primary focus in the rehabilitative efforts of short bowel syndrome. In patients with no other options, improved immunosuppressive regimes are making intestinal transplantation a viable option.

Suggested Readings

Andorsky DJ, Lund DP, Lillehei CW, et al. Nutritional and other postoperative management of neonates with short bowel syndrome correlates with clinical outcomes. J Pediatr 2001;139:5.

Dorney SFA, Ament ME, Berquist WE, et al. Improved survival in very short small bowel of infancy with use of long-term parenteral nutrition. J Pediatr 1985;107:521.

Goulet O, Baglin-Gobet S, Talbotec C, et al. Outcome and long-term growth after extensive small bowel resection in the neonatal period: a survey of 87 children. Eur J Pediatr Surg 2005;5:95.

Kaufman SS, Loseke CA, Lupo JV, et al. Influence of bacterial overgrowth and intestinal inflammation on duration of parenteral nutrition in children with short bowel syndrome. J Pediatr 1997;131:356.

Kato T, Gaynor JJ, Selvaggi G, et al. Intestinal transplantation in children: a summary of clinical outcomes and prognostic factors in 108 patients from a single center. J Gastrointest Surg 2005;9:75.

Quiros-Tajeira RE, Ament ME, Reyen L, et al. Long-term parenteral nutritional support and intestinal adaptation in children with short bowel syndrome: a 25-year experience. J Pediatr 2004;145:157.

Sondheimer JM, Cadnapaphornshai M, Sontag M, Zerbe GO. Predicting the duration of dependence on parenteral nutrition after neonatal intestinal resection. J Pediatr 1998;132:80.

Spencer AU, Neaga A, West B, et al. Pediatric short bowel syndrome: redefining predictors of success. Ann Surg 2005;242:403.

Sudan D, DiBaise J, Torres C, et al. A multidisciplinary approach to the treatment of intestinal failure. J Gastrointest Surg 2005;9:165.

Sukhotnik I, Siplovich L, Shiloni E, et al. Intestinal adaptation in short-bowel syndrome in infants and children: a collective review. Pediatr Surg Int 2002;18:258.

Thompson JS. Surgical approach to the short bowel syndrome. Procedures to slow intestinal transit. Eur J Ped Surg 1999;9:263.

Vanderhoof JA. Short bowel syndrome and intestinal adaptation. In: Walker WA, Durie PR, Hamilton JR, Walker-Smith JA, Watkins JB, eds. Pediatric gastrointestinal disease, 3rd ed. Hamilton, Ont.: BC Decker, 2000;583.

Weale AR, Edwards AG, Bailey M, et al. Intestinal adaptation after massive intestinal resection. Postgrad Med J 2005;81:178.

CHAPTER 61 ■ RENAL AND GENITOURINARY DISEASES

BILLY S. ARANT, JR.

In most newborns, the kidneys are able to maintain body fluid homeostasis within certain limits. However, these organs may be inadequate to support extraordinary demands placed on them by disease, by the treatment of disease, or by the misinterpretation of normal responses to extrarenal stimuli. This chapter will discuss structural and functional abnormalities of the renal system of neonates.

NORMAL STRUCTURE AND FUNCTION

Embryogenesis and Morphology

Formation of the human metanephric kidney begins during the fifth week of gestation when the ureteric bud, an ectodermal outgrowth of the Wolffian or mesonephric duct that will develop into the renal collecting system, makes direct contact with the caudal mesenchyma of the nephrogenic cord to induce the formation of glomeruli, proximal and distal tubules, and loops of Henle. Failure of these two distinctly different embryonic tissues to establish intimate contact results in failure of the ipsilateral kidney to form normally. All glomeruli are located within the renal cortex. The first ones formed take their final

position in the deep or juxtamedullary region. They contribute most to the function of the developing kidney until nephrogenesis is completed at approximately 34 weeks' gestation. They are nearly equal in size at 40 weeks' gestation to mature glomeruli and have the structures of the renal countercurrent multiplier mechanism—long loops of Henle and *vasa rectae* that extend into the inner medulla and papilla. The final group of glomeruli formed occupies the most superficial position of the subcapsular region of the cortex. They do not exhibit filtration before 34 weeks' gestation and are only 25% or so of the size of juxtamedullary glomeruli at 40 weeks' gestation. In contrast to deeper glomeruli, they have short loops of Henle that extend only into the outer medulla without *vasa rectae* and contribute little to the urinary concentrating mechanism. Nephrogenesis follows a similar pattern after birth if the fetus is born prematurely: The infant born at 26 weeks' gestation may exhibit continued nephrogenesis for approximately 8 weeks after birth. Differences in morphologic arrangement in the developing human renal cortex before and after the completion of nephrogenesis are illustrated in Fig. 61.1.

Cyclooxygenase-2 (COX-2), but not COX-1, is important, especially in the final phase of nephrogenesis, and prostanoids in general seem essential to normal renal development. Angiotensin II is also an important growth factor. Nutrition is also important. If pregnant rats are provided a protein-restricted

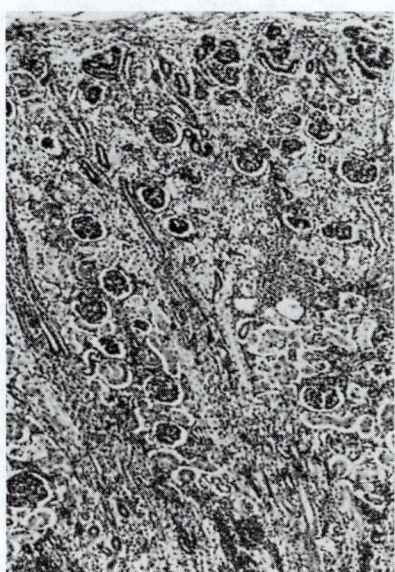
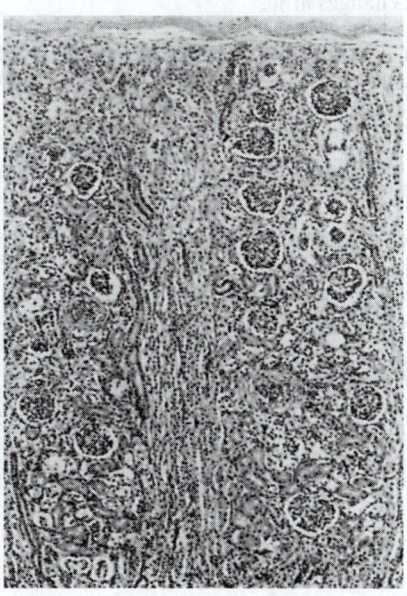

FIGURE 61.1. A comparison of morphology in the developing human renal cortex before and after nephrogenesis is completed. The larger glomeruli in the inner cortex are of similar size at 30 weeks (*left*) and at 40 weeks (*right*). In the superficial cortex, new glomeruli still are being formed at 30 weeks and have very little interposition of tubular structures, whereas at 40 weeks, glomerular size is more homogeneous throughout the cortex, and tubular growth has separated the glomeruli and displaced the most superficial ones away from the capsule. Hematoxylin and eosin stain, ×100. (Photomicrographs courtesy of Dr. J. Bernstein, William Beaumont Hospital, Royal Oak, MI.)

diet, the total complement of nephrons in the offspring's kidneys is reduced. Some have suggested that prematurity alone may result in less than a full complement of 1 million nephrons in each kidney. Alternatively, postnatal management of a high-risk infant may interfere with the completion of nephrogenesis. For example, indomethacin therapy in the preterm infant may imperil nephrogenesis. A reduced number of nephrons may place the individual at later risk of glomerular hyperfiltration, renal insufficiency, or hypertension.

Filtration by newly formed nephrons has been observed as early as 9 weeks' gestation; however, the ureter is patent only from the eleventh week. The transient hydronephrosis during this 2-week interval distends the proximal ureter to give the pelvicaliceal system its characteristic shape. Once the ureter is canalized, urine drains into the urogenital sinus and then into the amniotic sac. The urinary bladder is formed from the lower portion of the allantois and the urogenital sinus. The upper portion of the allantois closes by 32 weeks' gestation to form a fibrous cord. If the bladder outlet is obstructed, the allantois may persist as a patent urachus. The fetal ureter is composed of connective tissue stroma lined by epithelium. The smooth muscle layers that allow the ureter to constrict and shorten during peristalsis and the elastic fibers that permit the ureter to resume its normal caliber and shape are formed between 36 and 48 weeks of gestation. This is complete by the second postnatal month in infants born at term.

The only recognized role of the kidney essential to normal fetal development is its contribution to amniotic fluid volume. Mineral and fluid balance and the excretory functions of the kidney are handled by the placenta and maternal kidney. Failure of urine formation or urinary obstruction results in oligohydramnios and may cause fetal compression. Oligohydramnios before 20 weeks' gestation may be associated with pulmonary hypoplasia.

Glomerular Filtration Rate

The glomerular filtration rate (GFR) has been measured at birth in healthy human neonates at 24 weeks' gestation and has been found to be approximately 0.2 mL/minute, 0.5 mL/minute/kg, or 5 mL/minute/1.73 m^2. Such a low GFR in a child or adult would represent chronic renal insufficiency; therefore, not surprisingly, the neonatal kidney has been mislabeled as functionally immature. Although growth and development of the kidneys continue throughout gestation, the GFR changes little, if at all, before a postmenstrual (gestational plus postnatal) age of 34 weeks, when nephrogenesis is complete. Understanding that the neonate born at 26 weeks' gestation will not exhibit any appreciable change in the GFR until nearly 8 weeks of age (34 weeks after conception) is clinically relevant. In contrast, when birth occurs after 34 weeks' gestation, the GFR increases two- to threefold during the first week of life, just as in full-term infants.

The same developmental pattern determines whether infants are studied at birth at a particular gestational age or are studied after birth at the corresponding postmenstrual age (Fig. 61.2). A similar developmental pattern of GFR has been observed in all mammalian kidneys studied (Box 61.1).

Developmental increases in the GFR continue until the average normal adult GFR of 125 mL/minute is attained during adolescence, when linear growth ceases and the epiphyses close. The adult or mature value of the GFR corrected for body surface area (125 mL/minute/1.73 m^2) is observed rarely before 6 months of age and sometimes only at 12 months of age in infants born at term. During this period the rate of increase in GFR exceeds the rate of body growth.

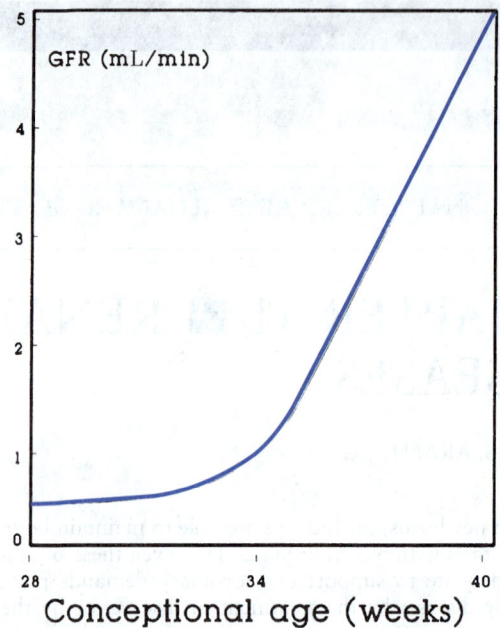

FIGURE 61.2. The pattern of change in the glomerular filtration rate (*GFR*) as compared with the conceptional (gestational plus postnatal) age of healthy human neonates. The line represents the nonlinear relationship calculated from data obtained in healthy neonates during the first 8 weeks of life.

Measuring the GFR in neonates is tedious and difficult when accurately timed and complete collections of urine are required; small errors in collection can produce large errors in calculating the GFR (Box 61.2).

Urinary Volume

Every normal neonate, as well as most with congenital renal abnormalities, will void some urine within 48 hours of birth. Urinary flow rate is, at best, only an indirect measurement of overall renal function. However, because an exact measurement of the GFR in neonates is impractical, clinicians have adopted urinary volume (UV) (mL/hour/kg) as a convenient, although uninformed, indication of "renal function." The volume of urine formed in any given period depends not only

---

BOX 61.1   **Glomerular Filtration Rate in Developing Mammalian Kidneys**

The glomerular filtration rate remains relatively constant until nephrogenesis is complete, before term birth in humans and sheep and after birth in the rat and dog. The biologic regulation of these changes is understood poorly, but because they can occur abruptly, attributing them simply to a process of maturation seems inadequate. More likely, a vasoactive mechanism is responsible; increments in renal blood flow are related inversely to changes in renal vascular resistance, plasma renin activity, circulating levels of angiotensin II, renal synthesis of vasodilator prostaglandins, and, probably, nitric oxide. Renal vascular resistance and cortical blood flow can be changed acutely by one or more of these vasoactive substances.

BOX 61.2	Measuring the Glomerular Filtration Rate in Neonates

Developmental changes in the glomerular filtration rate (GFR) can be monitored satisfactorily in most neonates from serial measurements of serum creatinine concentration (S_{Cr}). For neonates at high risk, S_{Cr} should be measured on the first day of life to allow comparison with subsequent measurements. Creatinine is a product of normal muscle metabolism and is a small molecule that crosses all water-permeable membranes, including the placenta; therefore, S_{Cr} levels in the mother and her fetus are similar. At birth, no correlation exists between S_{Cr} and the gestational age of the infant. Hence, a single measurement of S_{Cr} at birth has no particular value for estimating the GFR. When the GFR increases rapidly in infants born after 34 weeks' gestation, the S_{Cr} is reduced by approximately 50% at the end of the first week of life and usually reaches a stable normal value of 0.25 to 0.40 mg/dL during the second week. In contrast, the GFR does not increase appreciably during the first week of life in infants born before 34 weeks' gestation, and the S_{Cr} actually may increase slightly during the first 48 hours after birth as a result of hemoconcentration and ongoing creatinine production of approximately 8 mg/kg/day. Only minor changes in the S_{Cr} can be expected during the first week of life in normal preterm infants. When a conceptional age of 34 weeks is reached, however, the GFR increases, and the S_{Cr} falls by approximately one-half within a few days, just as in more mature neonates during the first week of life.

GFR corrected for body surface area may also be measured from the formulas derived for premature infants or for full-term infants. The formula for both is GFR (mL/minute/1.73 m^2) = k × body length (cm)/S_{Cr}(mg/dL); for preterm infants, $k = 0.35$, and for full-term infants after the first week of life, $k = 0.45$. Normal values for the GFR for a particular postmenstrual age are available in specialty texts and the literature.

on the GFR but also on tubular reabsorption. The final UV will be minimal and relatively concentrated during hydropenic conditions when the kidney attempts to conserve or restore extracellular fluid volume (ECFV). It is large and dilute when ECFV is excessive or in the presence of tubular dysfunction, failure of the hypothalamus to produce arginine vasopressin (AVP) (central diabetes insipidus), or failure of the collecting duct epithelium to respond to circulating AVP (nephrogenic diabetes insipidus).

For example, the GFR in the fetus is relatively low ($\leq$30 mL/hour/kg), but the UV is high (10 mL/hour/kg). Tubular reabsorption in the fetal kidney is inefficient; it is not necessary for it to be otherwise. Production of amniotic fluid is essential. The positive fluid balance or relative excess of ECFV that is normal for the fetus is assured by placental transfer from the expanded ECFV of the mother. Diuresis in utero is maintained, in part, by altered peritubular forces that reduce proximal tubular reabsorption, by minimal circulating AVP, by fewer aquaporin channels in the principal cells of the collecting duct, and by increased renal synthesis of prostacyclin and prostaglandin E_2 (PGE_2). The diuresis is interrupted briefly during labor with the normal release of AVP, but is resumed after birth as AVP levels

decrease again. The duration of diuresis in a normal neonate is determined by the degree of ECFV excess, by hormonal interactions, and by hemodynamic changes. Because the ECFV in the preterm infant is greater than that in the full-term infant, the postnatal diuresis and relative weight loss after birth is greater.

The normal pattern of changes in urine production begins with a rate of 10 mL/hour/kg in the fetus, at least after 30 weeks' gestation. Output decreases to less than 0.5 mL/hour/kg during parturition and then increases again to 1 to 8 mL/hour/kg, depending on the gestational age of the neonate, until the excess extracellular fluid for that infant is excreted. Thereafter, the UV in the neonate given appropriate fluid intake remains between 0.3 and 2.0 mL/hour/kg, with urinary osmolarity between 50 and 800 mOsm/L or specific gravity of 1.001 to 1.024. AVP acts on specific receptors to increase the number of aquaporin-2 water channels in the apical membrane and aquaporin-4 channels in the basolateral membrane of collecting duct epithelial cells.

High-risk neonates of every gestational age usually are treated from birth with parenteral fluids. Clinical decisions for changing the volume of the fluids given or for prescribing diuretic therapy usually are based on UV instead of changes in body weight, urinary osmolarity, or fractional sodium excretion. Because hemodynamic and hormonal changes may not be the same in every neonate, urine production will vary with factors other than the GFR. For example, before 34 weeks' gestation, the premature neonate excretes approximately 10% of glomerular filtrate as urine. Although the GFR increases after 34 weeks' gestation, tubular reabsorption increases as well, so that by 38 weeks, less than 3% of glomerular filtrate escapes the nephron.

In general, the higher the urinary flow rate (mL/hour/kg) is, the lower the fraction is of glomerular filtrate reabsorbed, not only water but also sodium chloride (NaCl), bicarbonate, amino acids, phosphate, calcium, and glucose. The fractional excretion of glomerular filtrate can be calculated as urinary flow rate (V) divided by GFR (V/GFR) expressed in the same units. In other words, when the urinary flow rate in a very preterm infant weighing 1.0 kg is 3 mL/hour/kg, approximately 10% of glomerular filtrate is not reabsorbed (V/GFR = 0.05 mL/minute $\div$ 0.5 mL/minute = 0.10, or 10%). If this same infant were to excrete only 1% of glomerular filtrate, as does the normal adult, the UV would be only 0.3 mL/hour/kg.

The physiologic basis for or clinical relevance of maintaining UV at 1 mL/hour/kg or greater in every infant has not been documented; however, rarely would any physician delay in prescribing additional fluid therapy or diuretic agents in a neonate whose UV decreases below 1 mL/hour/kg. The importance of maintaining UV is to ensure that sufficient water is present in tubular fluid to permit excretion of the solute load imposed on the kidney. If no solute load is present in infants who are conserving NaCl and are given only dextrose in water to replace insensible water losses immediately after birth, no UV is required. When, in the past, feedings were withheld routinely from preterm infants to prevent aspiration, some infants produced no urine for up to 5 days, with no evidence of renal injury. Moreover, acute renal injury was not obvious in neonates trapped during the Mexico City earthquake who survived longer without fluid than did older victims.

Other factors that may cause a decrease in UV include unrecognized heart failure, shunting of cardiac output away from the renal circulation through a patent ductus arteriosus, and changes in intrathoracic pressure from pneumothorax or mechanical ventilation, either of which can reduce cardiac output and stimulate baroreceptor-mediated release of AVP. In each case, the neonate's condition actually may be worsened by additional fluid therapy or furosemide administration.

Renal Handling of Sodium Chloride

The developing kidney has been characterized as inadequate to maintain NaCl balance, but the developing kidney is limited only when extraordinary demands are imposed on it. Some immature preterm infants have survived (and more will survive in the future) with little or no clinical intervention. They exhibit neither NaCl wasting nor any other tubular dysfunction. Renal tubular function in newborn infants is qualitatively similar to that in adults. When the function of the adult kidney is assessed during chronic expansion of ECFV with saline, it manifests hypotonic saline diuresis, glucosuria, hyperphosphaturia, hypercalciuria, hyperuricuria, and increased excretion of bicarbonate, just as in the human fetus and preterm infant with expanded ECFV. What is interpreted as an inappropriate or immature response by the neonatal kidney is the normal response of the mammalian kidney to changes in effective arterial blood volume (EABV). Baroreceptors in the arterial circulation sense EABV as a combined force of blood volume and blood pressure. When EABV falls because of decreased cardiac output (decreased blood volume) or decreased peripheral resistance (vasodilation), the neonatal kidney responds by conserving volume. The results are oliguria or anuria, NaCl retention, and hypertonic urine. Because this response can follow a change in blood pressure, blood volume, or both, it may be observed when total body water is increased or decreased and when blood pressure is high, normal, or low. Some of the mechanisms that maintain or restore EABV are depicted in Fig. 61.3. Other mechanisms and, in particular, the direct actions of nitric oxide on EABV have not been elucidated fully.

During fetal development, body composition changes dramatically. The content of body water decreases from 96% of body weight at 8 weeks' gestation to less than 80% at 40 weeks' gestation, as the NaCl content decreases from 120 mEq/kg body weight to 80 mEq/kg body weight. This parallel reduction in total body water and NaCl accounts for the decrease in ECFV from 60% to 40% of fetal body weight during the last trimester of pregnancy. After birth, the ECFV is reduced further from 40% to less than 30% of body weight. This developmental decrease in relative ECFV occurs as body tissues expand with an increase in the absolute quantity of ECFV and as a constant hypotonic saline diuresis maintains amniotic fluid volume.

When infants are born prematurely, a variable period of high urinary volume and negative NaCl balance occurs postnatally in an apparent effort by the neonate to reduce its ECFV, as would have occurred had the fetus remained *in utero* until term. However, before the kidney of the preterm neonate can respond by conserving NaCl and water in a manner similar to that of the full-term infant, the maturational differences in ECFV and EABV between premature and mature neonates must be resolved.

Because neonates, regardless of their gestational age at birth, vary somewhat in the exact timing of renal responses to reduced ECFV, each infant must be observed closely to determine when this adaptation has been attained. The best clinical estimate of the timing is provided by changes in urinary volume and excretion of NaCl. The fractional excretion of sodium (FE$_{Na}$) can be calculated from the sodium and creatinine concentrations in random samples of plasma and urine. These values are substituted in the following formula: FE$_{Na}$ (%) = urine sodium concentration × plasma creatinine concentration × 100/urine creatinine concentration × plasma sodium concentration. The relatively large volume of urine produced by the fetal kidney before birth and by the preterm neonate immediately after birth contains higher NaCl concentrations (greater than 50 mEq/L) than that of the full-term infant (less than 20 mEq/L); FE$_{Na}$ is 12% to 15% in the fetus, more than 1% to 7% in the preterm infant, and less than 1% (usually less than 0.5%) in the full-term infant.

The continued hypotonic saline diuresis after birth results in a greater fractional loss of birth weight in preterm infants (10% to 30%) than in full-term infants (3% to 8%). When the excess ECFV has been excreted, further loss of body weight is determined by insensible water losses. This is accompanied by a second period of oliguria or anuria, with urinary volume less than 1 mL/hour/kg, urinary osmolarity greater than 300 mOsm/L, and FE$_{Na}$ less than 1%. This occurs on the first day of life in infants born at term and 3 to 7 days after birth in those born prematurely. If only insensible water losses, not urinary volume, are replaced with dextrose in water before this pivotal point in transitional physiology, subsequent oral or parenteral fluid therapy should replace both urinary volume and insensible water losses. Then, body weight is maintained and weight gain is related to caloric intake and growth.

Although UV increases and urinary osmolarity decreases on this regimen, no increase in urinary NaCl excretion should occur. However, if fluid therapy has replaced urinary volume from birth (greater than or equal to 100 mL/kg/day), the relative excess ECFV of the fetus will be perpetuated, and the hypotonic saline diuresis will continue indefinitely, preventing the creation of a positive NaCl balance, regardless of the amount of NaCl provided. When urinary volume, but not urinary NaCl, is replaced by 5% to 10% dextrose in water, hyponatremia will develop, and clinical evaluation will suggest renal NaCl wasting, the so-called immaturity of neonatal renal tubular function.

The renal handling of NaCl in the neonate can be explained another way. The normal adult produces 180 L of glomerular filtrate daily but excretes less than 1% of that volume as urine. The preterm infant, by comparison, produces approximately 750 mL of glomerular filtrate daily. For a 1,000-g infant to excrete a UV of 1 mL/hour/kg (24 mL every 24 hours), 3.3% of the glomerular filtrate must be rejected along the nephron. If the UV in the same infant were 5 mL/hour/kg, which is not unusual in preterm infants given routinely excessive fluid therapy from birth, 16% of the glomerular filtrate would have been rejected by the tubule. If the sodium concentration of that urine were 75 mEq/L, as is usual in the fetus and in very early premature neonates, 9 mEq/kg/day of sodium would be lost in the urine. If the sodium added to the parenteral fluids provides only the maintenance requirements for older infants

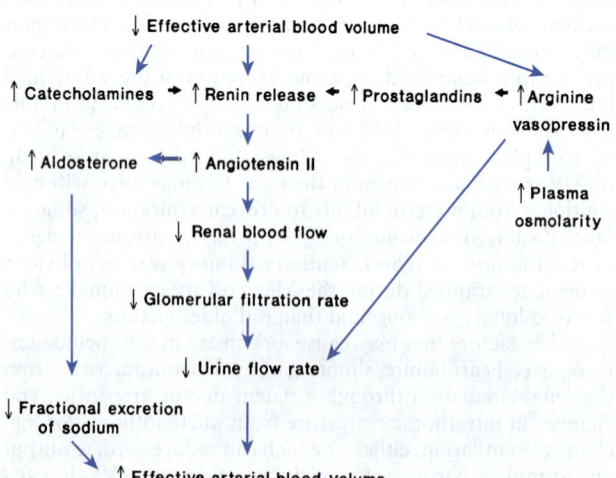

FIGURE 61.3. Schematic representation of the physiologic response to a decrease in effective arterial blood volume.

(2 to 3 mEq/kg/day), many preterm infants will have a negative NaCl balance and hyponatremia. The provision of NaCl in excess of 2 mEq/kg to preterm infants when UV is high (V/GFR less than 3%) is associated with an increase in FE_{Na} and a continued negative NaCl balance. In contrast, when UV is 1 mL/hour/kg or less, urinary sodium concentration rarely is greater than 20 mEq/L. In an infant of the same weight and maturity, less than 0.5 mEq/kg/day of sodium would be lost. Moreover, the infant would exhibit the positive NaCl balance that is essential for growth. Therefore, long-term management of negative NaCl balance does not consist of providing additional NaCl but rather limiting early fluid therapy to replacement of insensible water losses until ECFV normalizes and the second period of oliguria or anuria and reduced FE_{Na} occurs.

Renal Acid–Base Homeostasis

The neonatal kidney once was characterized as being unable to maintain acid–base balance because of its decreased ability to conserve bicarbonate, secrete hydrogen ion, or both. More recently, the kidneys of even premature infants have been demonstrated to excrete an acid load as well as the adult kidney does (approximately 80 mEq/1.73 m^2/day), which is more than adequate to dispose of a normal infant's daily hydrogen ion production. The relative metabolic acidosis commonly observed in preterm infants can be explained, in part, by the lowered renal threshold for bicarbonate—that is, the plasma level above which bicarbonate is wasted along the nephron and appears in the urine. This lower plasma bicarbonate threshold is usually ignored when reported arterial blood gas measurements calculate base deficit by subtracting measured bicarbonate from the normal bicarbonate of the adult. The mistake is compounded, because most blood gas measurements assume a hemoglobin concentration of 12 g/dL when a neonate's hemoglobin is usually higher. Therefore, preterm infants appear to have metabolic acidosis that is clinically inconsequential and may not require correction with sodium bicarbonate. The majority of filtered bicarbonate is reabsorbed in the proximal tubule; therefore, its renal conservation or wasting can be influenced by extrarenal factors, especially changes in ECFV or EABV, regardless of the acid–base status of the infant. When the EABV is perceived by renal baroreceptors to be diminished, the fractional reabsorption of glomerular filtrate (including bicarbonate) along the proximal nephron increases, and the renal threshold for bicarbonate increases; consequently, plasma bicarbonate and arterial blood pH levels increase. Relative metabolic alkalosis develops, but the urine contains no bicarbonate and will have a pH level of less than 6.0, which constitutes renal tubular alkalosis.

In contrast, as EABV is restored, or in the euvolemic neonate is expanded, tubular reabsorption of bicarbonate decreases the renal threshold for bicarbonate. The plasma bicarbonate concentration decreases because of dilution and urinary excretion of bicarbonate, and the arterial blood pH level returns toward normal. If the process continues, relative metabolic acidosis develops in the face of urinary bicarbonate excretion and a pH level greater than 6.0, which constitutes renal tubular acidosis.

Because metabolic acidosis or alkalosis can be produced experimentally in normal animals by altering EABV, the metabolic acidosis of prematurity probably reflects the ECFV excess of the preterm infant as compared to that of the full-term infant. The alkaline urinary pH of normal preterm infants during the first week of life becomes more acidic during the second week as the ECFV is reduced and tubular bicarbonate reabsorption is increased.

Urinary Diluting and Concentrating Mechanisms

The ability of the neonatal kidney to dilute urine maximally to less than 50 mOsm/L in the absence of AVP is identical to that of the adult kidney. The inability of the neonatal kidney to concentrate the urine when the infant is deprived of fluid or loses fluid abnormally is not simply immaturity of kidney function. The fetal kidney has no need to concentrate urine; its essential role is to replenish amniotic fluid volume. The fetal collecting tubule is relatively unresponsive even to very high circulating levels of AVP during normal labor or asphyxia. The physiologic basis for this observation is multifactorial. First, AVP-mediated water movement across the tubular epithelium is antagonized by PGE_2, the renal synthesis of which is increased in the fetus. In addition, PGE_2 inhibits tubular permeability to urea, limiting its contribution to the renal medullary osmotic gradient. The maximum medullary osmotic gradient generated is limited further by PGE_2 inhibition of NaCl reabsorption in the ascending thick limb of Henle. (Furosemide effects a diuresis by stimulating renal synthesis of PGE_2.) The greater synthesis of prostacyclin and PGE_2 by the renal vascular endothelium in the fetus maintains high renal medullary blood flow, which tends to wash out any renal tubule to medullary interstitium osmotic gradient established by active NaCl transport.

Consequently, the maximum urinary concentration possible during adaptation to postnatal life is only slightly hypertonic to plasma, or approximately 350 mOsm/L (specific gravity, 1.011). After birth, the renal synthesis of vasodilator prostaglandins decreases, NaCl reabsorption increases, and tubular permeability to urea increases. Then, the osmolarity of the medullary interstitium can be increased, the collecting duct epithelium can become more responsive to AVP, and urinary osmolarity can increase. The factors responsible for the hypotonic saline diuresis that is physiologic in the fetus interfere with the neonatal kidney's capacity to concentrate the urine and conserve water. When these factors diminish postnatally, the kidney of the very premature infant is the equal of that of a full-term infant. It can concentrate the urine to 600 to 800 mOsm/L. Comparing the maximum concentrating ability of the neonatal kidney to the adult kidney (1,300 mOsm/L) is pointless. Rarely must either the adult or the neonate conserve water to such an extent.

STRUCTURAL ABNORMALITIES OF THE NEONATAL KIDNEY AND URINARY TRACT

Failure in Morphogenesis

Developmental abnormalities of the kidney occur when metanephric induction fails, when normal differentiation and development fail after the metanephros is formed, or when the normal metanephros sustains an insult after nephrogenesis begins. When the ureteric bud does not establish contact with the mesenchyma of the nephrogenic cord, even minimal separation between the tissues of different embryonic origin will prevent induction of the metanephric blastema. Consequently, nephrogenesis does not occur, no urine is produced, and the proximal ureter is not distended to model the pelvicaliceal system. Radionuclide scanning would reveal no renal blood flow; angiography would reveal no renal artery; and retrograde urography would demonstrate that the ureter ends in a blind pouch. This condition, which can be unilateral or bilateral, is termed *renal agenesis.* If it is bilateral and associated with fetal compression, the criteria for *Potter syndrome* are fulfilled.

When the ureteric bud establishes either incomplete contact or contact with only certain regions, the metanephros will have neither a normal complement of nephrons nor a normal gross appearance. The neonatal kidney that is small in size or weight is known as *renal hypoplasia.* If nephrogenesis is relatively uniform throughout the cortex but does not result in the usual 1 million nephrons normal for a human kidney, existing nephrons will hypertrophy. This condition, referred to as *oligomeganephronia,* is recognized only by chance in the neonate. The complication indicating the diagnosis when both kidneys are affected is chronic renal insufficiency, which develops toward the end of the first decade of life.

In some fetuses, whether the induction of metanephric formation is normal or abnormal, further normal differentiation and development are interrupted by some insult, such as exposure to teratogens or infection in the first trimester of pregnancy, by uteroplacental dysfunction, or by urinary tract obstruction at any time during gestation. The term given to this kind of abnormal renal development is *renal dysplasia.* Pathologic findings may include hydronephrosis, parenchymal atrophy, broad or segmental scars, interstitial inflammatory cells in the absence of infection, aglomerular regions of the cortex, tubular atrophy or thyroidization, dilated tubules and collecting ducts (some of which are actual cystic structures), and aberrant structures that are formed also from mesoderm located elsewhere in the body, such as cartilage. Any one of these examples of abnormal renal development may be unilateral or bilateral. In addition, two or more developmental abnormalities may coexist in the same infant. Renal dysplasia may be suspected when the kidney is small by ultrasound examination, but the diagnosis cannot be confirmed by any current imaging technique; only histopathologic evaluation is accurate.

Obstructive Uropathy

Obstructive uropathy, which occurs in 1 in 1,000 live births, is the clinical problem associated most often with *renal dysplasia* in the neonate. Obstruction of urine flow can occur at any point along the urinary tract between the calyx and the urethral meatus; it can be partial or complete; and it can be transient, intermittent, or fixed. If, for example, the proximal ureter fails to canalize completely, *ureteropelvic junction obstruction* will result. This lesion is the most common form of obstructive uropathy; it may be partial or complete.

The most common abdominal mass in the neonate is a hydronephrotic kidney. However, not every kidney thought to be obstructed *in utero* is enlarged at birth. Hydronephrosis occurs only when hydrostatic pressure in the collecting system is increased, and it implies that urine formation continued at least until just before discovery of the enlarged kidney. If obstruction has been long-standing, glomerular filtration and urinary flow cease when the pressure within Bowman's space plus capillary oncotic pressure equals or exceeds glomerular capillary hydrostatic pressure. According to experimental studies of adult mammalian kidneys, normal renal function is not recovered when the complete obstruction persists for more than a week. Moreover, the longer the obstruction continues, the less likely is the return of any renal functions.

Pathophysiology

When the fetal or neonatal ureter is obstructed, its smooth muscle layers are disorganized, and it has few elastic fibers.

Glomerular filtration in the neonate continues longer than in the older child or adult after complete obstruction, because the urinary tract is more easily distended and intraluminal pressures are lower in the neonate. The ureteral wall becomes a dysplastic cylinder of connective tissue with ineffective peristalsis. This causes a relative obstruction to urinary flow and predisposes the infant to urinary tract infection.

When the collecting system is disrupted by increased pressure, urine extravasates into the retroperitoneal space or, occasionally, the peritoneal cavity. The resulting urinary ascites is a welcome sign because the urinary tract has been decompressed and the kidney may be normal despite lower urinary tract obstruction. Another means of decompressing the obstructed fetal urinary tract occurs when the allantois does not close but persists as a urachus or urachal cyst.

Diagnosis

Obstructive uropathy is suggested or identified usually by routine fetal ultrasonography, during the evaluation of an abdominal mass or urinary tract infection in a neonate, and during investigation of intense flank pain after ingestion of a large volume of fluid by a child or adult. If the diagnosis is unclear, an intravenous bolus of fluid given with furosemide will produce a brisk diuresis that will distend the urinary tract proximal to the obstruction. Surgical correction is not always indicated, because up to 70% of uncomplicated lesions resolve spontaneously.

When mucosal folds obstruct the posterior urethra and limit the force or height of the urinary stream in male infants, the diagnosis of *posterior urethral valves* should be suspected and confirmed by voiding cystourethrography. Every male neonate should be screened for this obstructing lesion: At least one experienced observer should note the force or arc of the urinary stream during micturition. If this has not been recorded at the time of discharge from the nursery, parents should be instructed in how to make this observation and to report the finding to the pediatrician during the first week of life. Urethral or lower urinary tract obstruction affects both upper tracts similarly, resulting in bilateral renal and ureteral dysplasia. This is one of the most common causes of chronic renal insufficiency in male infants and children.

Fetal hydronephrosis must be evaluated postnatally by at least renal ultrasonography and voiding cystourethrography. Hydronephrosis from obstruction may not be detected if the ultrasound examination is performed during the oliguric period immediately following birth or from vesicoureteral reflux if the bladder is empty at the time of study.

Therapy

Attempts have been made to intervene during pregnancy to relieve the obstruction as a means of salvaging some renal parenchyma and increasing the volume of amniotic fluid in the hope of preventing pulmonary hypoplasia and fetal compression. However, total destruction of both kidneys from cystic dysplasia has been identified long before the fetus is large enough to undergo such surgery without significant risk. Furthermore, despite anecdotes to the contrary, no identifiable benefit to any fetus ever has been documented as being superior to immediate treatment at birth. The best treatment still is considered to be a well-planned approach for definitive care of the neonate at birth. Unless postobstructive diuresis is anticipated when the urinary tract obstruction is relieved, the patient may rapidly develop volume depletion, hyponatremia with seizures, and hypocalcemia.

Prune-Belly Syndrome

Clinical Manifestations

Prune-belly syndrome is a condition in which the urinary tract findings are nearly identical to those for posterior urethral valves but for one important exception: No obstructing lesion can be found. Convincing evidence implicates the developing prostate as obstructing the fetal urethra transiently. Another similarity between prune-belly syndrome and posterior urethral valves is that both can show abnormalities of muscle tone in the abdominal wall. The classic presentation of prune-belly syndrome is a male neonate with complete absence of abdominal wall musculature. The outlines of bowel loops can be seen, and the abdominal cavity can be examined easily by palpation. In addition, a paucity of smooth muscle is found in the ureters, the urinary bladder, and, sometimes, the gastrointestinal tract.

Therapy

Clinical management involves monitoring the urinary tract for obstruction to urinary flow and its major complication, infection. In addition, GFR should be measured to identify subsequent deterioration. NaCl balance should be determined in an infant who exhibits NaCl wasting and failure to grow normally if replacement is inadequate. Hyperkalemia and metabolic acidosis secondary to decreased distal tubular responsiveness to aldosterone must be corrected. The infant requires an activated form of vitamin D [1,25(OH)$_2$ vitamin D], because he or she, similar to an infant with another form of primary uropathy, has hypocalcemia and renal osteodystrophy even when the GFR is nearly normal. In addition, appropriate counseling for the infant's parents is essential. Although renal function in the infant may seem normal at birth, end-stage renal disease develops in most patients before adolescence.

Renal Cystic Disease

Renal cystic disease occurs in many different forms and nearly defies meaningful classification, at least any that would explain cystogenesis for each type. For instance, a unilateral, single cyst may be discovered incidentally in a neonate with normal renal function. This cyst may persist unchanged throughout life and cause no problem, it may disappear altogether, or it may be the first of many more cysts to form over the next 30 to 40 years in both kidneys. When this diagnostic dilemma is encountered in a neonate, the patient can be observed to document changes in the cyst, in kidney function, and in blood pressure, as has been the practice until very recently. In the absence of a family history of polycystic kidney disease, this option should be exercised only after both parents have had ultrasonographic examination of their kidneys for the presence of cysts. In a more aggressive diagnostic approach, which rarely is warranted, DNA probes can identify the gene PKHD2 that expresses autosomal dominant (adult) polycystic kidney disease when renal tissue is available. The finding of cysts in other organs, particularly the liver, lung, or pancreas, supports the diagnosis of autosomal recessive (infantile) polycystic kidney disease, which occurs in 1 in 20,000 live births in which the PKHD1 gene, located on the short arm of chromosome 6, is implicated. One further clue to the latter condition is the ultrasonographic identification of early hepatic fibrosis which is not always present at birth. Moderate to severe systemic hypertension usually develops in these patients within the first months of life.

Although often referred to as a kidney, *multicystic dysplasia* contains no identifiable renal structure, just cysts, and is usually unilateral. It has no renal artery and does not func-tion. Neonates with this so-called multicystic dysplastic kidney require only casual monitoring for the rare occurrence of enlargement or infection; otherwise, the structure need not be removed. Physicians once were concerned that malignancy might develop, but long-term follow-up has identified no such risk. A voiding cystourethrogram may identify other genitourinary abnormalities, especially contralateral vesicoureteral reflux, in up to 40% of these infants, which pose additional clinical risk of injury to a single kidney.

FUNCTIONAL ABNORMALITIES IN THE NEONATAL KIDNEY

Asphyxia Neonatorum

The kidney develops under conditions of relative hypoxia and is capable of considerable anaerobic metabolism. During the perinatal period, hypoxia alone probably has little, if any, effect on the kidney, but in combination with hypotension and either endogenous release of vasoactive substances or the administration of alpha-adrenergic agonists, hypoxia can cause acute tubular necrosis, cortical necrosis, or medullary necrosis.

By contrast, asphyxia is a combination of severe hypoxia and intense pulmonary vasoconstriction associated with increased AVP. However, the kidney of an infant with asphyxia behaves as if there were increased levels of circulating angiotensin II or decreased nitric oxide synthesis. Acute renal failure with oliguria or anuria is observed commonly in infants with asphyxia, and recovery of renal function usually follows relief of pulmonary vasoconstriction with improvement in lung function.

A possible role for angiotensin II was dismissed after one study in an experimental animal model found no benefit to blocking angiotensin II. However, angiotensin II formation within the kidney is not overcome as easily as it is elsewhere in the body. Possibly, therefore, intrarenal renin release stimulated by AVP and angiotensin II formation causes the intense renal vasoconstriction that is associated with asphyxia. A reduction in the vasodilator prostanoids and nitric oxide may play an important role as well. One future treatment for this often devastating condition may be to inhibit AVP or angiotensin II formation or to administer nitric oxide or its precursor.

Nephrotoxic Drug Therapy

The neonatal kidney once was believed to be more tolerant of drug injury than is the kidney of the child or the adult. This assumption was based on a clinical study in which the assessment of renal function was made inaccurately and then misinterpreted. The newborn kidney always is at risk of toxic injury when proximal tubular reabsorption is maximal, when EABV is decreased, during NaCl or potassium depletion, during hypoxia, and with indomethacin therapy. Oliguria or anuria does not always predispose the kidney to nephrotoxicity. Neonates are not dehydrated with inappropriate secretion of AVP; EABV is increased; total body NaCl and potassium levels are normal; proximal tubular reabsorption is decreased; the GFR is normal; and the drug is diluted in the greater ECFV.

The nephrotoxic effects of antibiotics such as aminoglycosides, vancomycin, and amphotericin B occur with the same frequency in neonates as in older infants, children, and adults. This may not be recognized. For example, aminoglycoside therapy is prescribed for neonates in a higher dosage relative to body size than in adults. Therapy is adjusted according to arbitrarily chosen "effective" peak and trough plasma levels. Because the drug has a large volume of distribution, that is, the

ECFV, more drug must be given to achieve the same peak plasma levels in neonates as compared to adults. Similarly, trough levels are determined by renal clearance, and a much lower trough level will be observed in neonates. The decision to modify or discontinue nephrotoxic antibiotic therapy based only on an increase in plasma trough levels will come several days after the GFR has decreased from the nephrotoxic effects of the drug.

Nephrotoxicity is manifested earlier by a rise in the serum creatinine concentration (S_{Cr}), which in the adult occurs between 4 and 7 days after aminoglycoside therapy is initiated. An increase in S_{Cr} in the neonate may be masked because S_{Cr} is simultaneously falling as maternal creatinine is cleared. Because neither S_{Cr} nor plasma drug levels are ideal for monitoring drug toxicity in the neonate, therapy should be prescribed according to the drug's pharmacokinetics, which vary with postmenstrual rather than postnatal age. For aminoglycosides and vancomycin, the dose interval is every 18 to 24 hours in neonates younger than 34 weeks postmenstrual age and every 12 hours in older infants. The same pattern of change in pharmacokinetics is characteristic of other drugs excreted by the kidney, such as furosemide and indomethacin. The renal effects of indomethacin potentiate the nephrotoxicity of other drugs, especially aminoglycosides.

Urinary Tract Infection

Neonatal urinary tract infections (UTIs) are discovered most commonly when anatomic or functional obstruction to urine flow exists. Uncircumcised males are at greater risk of infection than are circumcised males or females during the first 3 months of life. Even in urinary tracts that are abnormal as a result of myelodysplasia or obstructive uropathy, the urine is sterile at birth. UTI, therefore, is a disease that is acquired in the neonatal period and may be associated with, or be the cause of, septicemia. The urinary tract is the second most common site of origin, after the respiratory tract, for bacterial infections in febrile infants. Whether bacteria originate in the urinary tract or reach the urine as a consequence of bacteremia cannot be determined in every case. Consequently, significant bacteriuria in all neonates, regardless of the etiology, must be treated by evaluating the urinary tract for obstruction once the urine is rendered sterile by effective antibiotic therapy. In the dilated urinary tract without anatomic obstruction, urinary stasis may

occur along dysplastic or hypotonic ureters, and bacteria may grow in urine that fails to drain into the bladder. One characteristic of renal function in a urinary tract that is partially obstructed or one that becomes infected after obstruction is relieved is a clinical picture of *pseudohypoaldosteronism*: hyponatremia, hyperkalemia, and metabolic acidosis.

Although rare in uninfected preterm and full-term infants, vesicoureteral reflux occurs in up to 65% of newborn infants with a first UTI. The growing kidney of the infant is at risk for injury from vesicoureteral reflux and UTI. This is the leading cause of hypertension and chronic renal insufficiency in adolescents and young adults.

Renal Failure

Renal failure should be anticipated in any neonate who is stressed unusually during the perinatal period.

Pathophysiology

The causes of acute renal failure in the newborn are stated in Box 61.3 and can be considered under the broad categories of renal and extrarenal causes. *Renal* causes include anatomic abnormalities and renal injury. If the kidneys are small or cannot be palpated, renal agenesis or hypoplasia or dysplasia should be considered. In contrast, large kidneys are associated with obstructive uropathy, prune-belly syndrome, and renal cystic disease. Unavoidable acute renal injury is associated with asphyxia; significant blood loss at birth (from placental separation, twin transfusion, or cord accident); apnea or bradycardia with difficult or prolonged resuscitation; decreased cardiac output; and renal vein thrombosis. Avoidable causes include thromboses as complications of umbilical artery catheter placement; nephrotoxic effects of contrast medium; combined drug therapy (consisting of tolazoline as a generalized vasodilator and dopamine to raise systemic blood pressure) for pulmonary hypertension; and nephrotoxic drugs such as aminoglycosides, vancomycin, or amphotericin B and indomethacin.

Extrarenal causes of acute renal failure can be considered in two general categories, depending on whether EABV is decreased or increased. EABV can be decreased with decreased total body water, decreased cardiac output, significant left-to-right shunting of blood through a patent ductus arteriosus, low colloid oncotic pressure resulting in decreased circulating blood

---

BOX 61.3   Causes of Renal Failure

Renal causes
Anatomic abnormalities

- Kidneys too small: renal agenesis, hypoplasia, dysplasia
- Kidneys too large: obstructive uropathy, prune-belly syndrome, renal cystic disease

Renal injury

- Asphyxia
- Significant blood loss at birth
- Apnea
- Decreased cardiac output
- Renal vein thrombosis

Thrombosis as complication of umbilical artery catheter placement

Nephrotoxic effects of contrast media
Nephrotoxic drugs

Extrarenal causes
Increased effective arterial blood volume

- Excess fluid administration
- Inappropriate arginine vasopressin secretion

Decreased effective arterial blood volume

- Decreased total body water
- Decreased cardiac output
- Significant left-to-right shunting of blood
- Low colloid oncotic pressure
- Excessive furosemide therapy

volume, or excessive furosemide therapy. Excessive furosemide causes depletion of blood volume and lower peripheral vascular resistance because of displacement of angiotensin II from receptors and vasodilator prostaglandin synthesis. Acute renal failure also can occur in the presence of EABV if EABV is increased by excessive fluid administration or because of inappropriate AVP secretion. Dopamine is often given to raise blood pressure and increase cardiac output. Contrary to a popular notion, dopamine decreases renal cortical blood flow in the neonate, even at the lowest recommended dose, and can cause acute renal failure. Any benefit to renal function with dopamine infusion follows an improvement in EABV. Pancuronium or other paralyzing drugs given to mechanically ventilated infants can produce erratic sympathetic discharges that cause the blood pressure to rise or fall unpredictably, accompanied by changes in EABV and renal function.

The mechanisms through which a decrease in EABV causes oliguria or anuria are represented schematically in Fig. 61.3. A decrease in EABV stimulates the release of catecholamines and AVP; both provoke renin release, which is followed by angiotensin II formation, renal arteriolar vasoconstriction, and a decrease in renal cortical blood flow, GFR, and urinary flow rate. Moreover, AVP release, stimulated either by a decrease in EABV or by a rise in plasma osmolarity, facilitates water reabsorption across the collecting duct epithelium, which reduces the urinary flow rate. Angiotensin II stimulates aldosterone secretion, which promotes tubular Na/K adenosine triphosphatase activity to increase sodium reabsorption. In addition, angiotensin II can stimulate (at low or normal concentrations) or inhibit (at higher concentrations) proximal tubular Na reabsorption. The resulting NaCl and water conservation restores EABV, which then inhibits the compensating mechanisms.

Diagnosis

The diagnosis cannot be supported by a finding of oliguria or anuria alone. One infant at risk of *acute renal failure* may have a transient decrease in urinary volume (less than 1 mL/hour/kg) after birth that is physiologic or functional oliguria, even anuria, when the GFR is normal. Another infant with renal dysplasia or an obstructed urinary tract may have severely impaired renal function with a urinary volume greater than 3 mL/hour/kg. Differentiation between acute renal failure and functional oliguria or anuria by fluid administration or diuretic therapy involves risks. For instance, a fluid challenge in a neonate with excess ECFV from excessive fluid administration or heart failure would aggravate the clinical condition.

The normal hemodynamic response to an acute increase in blood volume in the adult is an increase in cardiac output and a decrease in peripheral resistance, mediated in part by the suppression of vasoconstrictor hormone release and the stimulation of endothelial synthesis of vasodilator prostaglandins and natriuretic peptide, a cardiovascular response to stretch. However, cardiac output in the neonate is already at or near maximal, and peripheral resistance is low. Additional volume in the neonatal circulation can be accommodated only by increasing pulmonary blood volume by shunting of blood through a still patent ductus arteriosus. A mechanism for reducing circulating blood volume is to increase the movement of extracellular fluid into the interstitial space, which accounts for the frequent observation of edema in normal neonates, especially after a large placental transfusion. When pulmonary interstitial water increases, respiratory distress develops or worsens, blood pressure decreases, renal perfusion pressure and the GFR decrease, and, consequently, the urinary flow rate decreases even further. The infant with oliguria or anuria in response to the normal postnatal reduction of ECFV will respond to a fluid challenge with an increase in blood pressure and urinary volume, a decrease in urinary osmolarity, and no appreciable change in

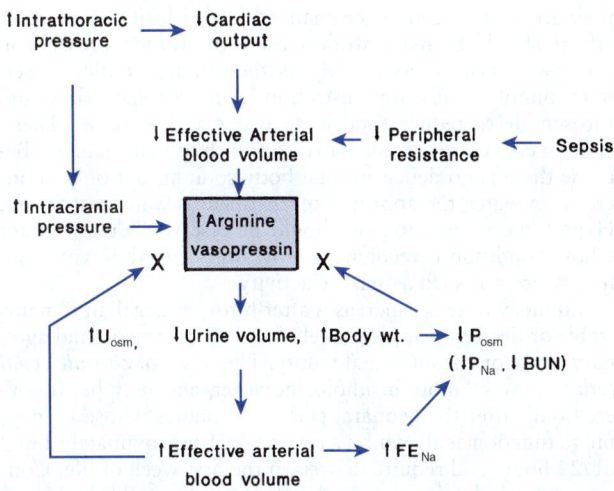

FIGURE 61.4. Pathophysiologic mechanisms that contribute to the consequences of inappropriate arginine vasopressin (AVP) secretion. X indicates a failure of the normal feedback mechanism to reduce hypothalamic release of AVP. BUN, blood urea nitrogen; Wt, weight.

FE_{Na}. A stable FE_{Na} assumes that the infant has not been treated with a diuretic (the half-life of furosemide in preterm infants is greater than or equal to 24 hours). It also assumes that renal injury has not occurred and that EABV or blood pressure is not increased. The diagnosis of renal failure in the newborn, therefore, should not be made without evaluation of urinary osmolarity and FE_{Na}, changes in body weight, perinatal events, and the clinical course of the infant.

The *syndrome of inappropriate AVP secretion* (SIADH) should be suspected in any patient who is mechanically ventilated or in patients with central nervous system infection, intracranial hemorrhage, changes in intracranial pressure, or trauma (surgical or accidental). The pathophysiologic mechanisms involved in inappropriate AVP secretion are depicted in Fig. 61.4. Moreover, any condition that reduces cardiac output or lowers EABV will stimulate baroreceptor-mediated AVP release, and an increase in plasma osmolarity will stimulate osmoreceptor-mediated AVP release. As urinary volume decreases, water being reabsorbed unnecessarily in the distal nephron and collecting duct is added back to body fluids. Plasma osmolarity decreases in proportion to the increase in body weight. Plasma sodium concentration and blood urea nitrogen decrease in proportion to plasma osmolarity. When AVP release is not inhibited (indicated by an X in Fig. 61.4) either by an increase in EABV or by a fall in the tonicity of body fluids, and fluid intake is not restricted to urinary volume only, the increase in body water and weight gain continue. Under normal circumstances, when AVP release is inhibited, urinary osmolarity should be the minimum and urinary dilution the maximum possible (30 to 50 mOsm/L or specific gravity 1.001), just as in diabetes insipidus. Urinary sodium concentration and FE_{Na} may be either increased or decreased, depending on whether EABV is increased or decreased; therefore, urinary sodium excretion is irrelevant to the diagnosis of SIADH. The most important treatment is anticipating the problem in patients who are at risk.

Therapy

When the diagnosis is suspected, but not clinically obvious, fluid therapy should be limited to UV plus an estimate of insensible water losses. Moreover, known stimuli to AVP release should be removed whenever possible. Although ventilator pressure settings cannot be changed just to facilitate diuresis, efforts should be made to decrease intrathoracic pressure in a stepwise fashion as quickly as the infant's condition permits. Simultaneous administration of hypertonic saline and furosemide to reduce total body water and increase plasma sodium concentration is a naive approach to management. Because there is no deficit in total body sodium, but only an increase in water, the appropriate treatment is water restriction. Hypertonic saline infusion should be reserved for the infant whose condition is recognized only after central nervous system symptoms such as seizure activity.

Infants whose S_{Cr} increases after birth, rather than remains stable or decreases appropriately for their postmenstrual ages, have acute or chronic renal failure. The onset of *chronic renal failure* may be more insidious, however, and may be discovered only after the neonatal period. Neonates whose kidneys fail to function at all exhibit a rise in S_{Cr} of approximately 1 mg/dL/24 hours and require dialysis in the first week of life. Continuous ambulatory peritoneal dialysis can be established (even in preterm infants) temporarily for those needing it while waiting for recovery from acute renal failure or longer for those who become candidates for kidney transplantation.

Initial treatment of renal failure should include close attention to correcting and then preventing fluid and electrolyte derangements. If the infant is volume-depleted, euvolemic conditions should be restored. If the infant is overhydrated, fluid intake should be restricted. When necessary, overhydration should be treated by dialysis or continuous arteriovenous hemofiltration. Once euvolemia has been reestablished, further fluid should be restricted to an amount that equals insensible water losses (approximately 30 mL/kg/24 hours) plus the volume of any urine excreted. Because urinary volume is measured more easily than insensible water losses, fluid balance can be assessed only by serial determinations of body weight.

Electrolyte requirements for an infant with renal failure should equal any gastrointestinal and urinary losses plus an amount to ensure positive balance for growth (net sodium balance of +2.2 mmol/day regardless of body weight). In this regard, every infant must be evaluated and treated individually. If hyponatremia develops during treatment and the infant is overhydrated, a normal plasma sodium concentration can be restored by water restriction or, in the euvolemic, asymptomatic infant, by the administration of additional oral NaCl. Hyperkalemia of renal failure may be aggravated further in patients with tubular hyporesponsiveness to aldosterone. Moreover, perinatal stress with hypoxia and metabolic acidosis causes potassium to move out of cells and into the extracellular fluid. The clinical management of hyperkalemia in the neonate is no different from that in older patients.

Hypertension is a problem encountered in association with circulatory or vascular causes of renal injury, such as renal artery or vein thrombosis and cortical or medullary necrosis. Hydronephrosis as a cause of hypertension is less frequent in neonates than in older children and adults. The treatment objectives should be to restore euvolemia by administering appropriate NaCl and fluid therapy and to reduce peripheral vascular resistance by stimulating vascular endothelial synthesis of prostacyclin with hydralazine, diazoxide, or nitroglycerin, or by reducing vasoconstriction with a calcium channel blocker or angiotensin-converting enzyme inhibitor. Cardiovascular stability in newborn infants, especially preterm infants, is dependent on a balance between vasoactive peptides that dilate or constrict. Cyclooxygenase inhibition of prostanoids or a reduction in angiotensin II effects may produce dramatic, even catastrophic, changes in vascular tone.

Systemic acidosis should be treated first with improved ventilation to reduce carbon dioxide tension and increase arterial blood pH and then with alkali therapy (sodium bicarbonate or sodium citrate) to neutralize any remaining excess hydrogen

ion. Hypocalcemia, normally asymptomatic in the first week of life, especially in preterm infants, can become symptomatic in neonates who have renal failure. When renal function is impaired, the ability to excrete phosphate is limited. The hyperphosphatemia normally observed in the neonate will be exaggerated and result in further lowering of the serum calcium concentration. When fed, infants should be given a formula with reduced NaCl and phosphate. However, NaCl may have to be added to the low-phosphate formula for neonates with salt-wasting. Intravenous calcium gluconate and oral calcium carbonate should be combined with activated vitamin D therapy to maintain serum calcium concentrations at a high-normal value to prevent secondary hyperparathyroidism and bone disease.

Too often, adequate nutrition is achieved late in the treatment of neonates with acute renal failure. Attention is focused on the renal failure in the hope that recovery of renal function will occur at any moment. Providing appropriate caloric intake simultaneously makes fluid restriction and electrolyte adjustment more complex. This should not be the case in most neonates when the treatment of renal failure is appropriate and informed, including early peritoneal dialysis. Parenteral amino acids and glucose can be prescribed early in low volumes. Intralipids can increase the caloric intake further. Whenever possible, maximum calories should be provided. Not only will the nutritional status of the infant be improved, but serum potassium and phosphate concentrations also will be controlled more easily.

Dialysis should be used to treat complications of renal failure, *not* during a crisis brought about by a complication of the neonate's previous treatment, but in a planned fashion. Peritoneal dialysis can be initiated after percutaneous placement of a permanent or temporary catheter. Commercially available dialysis solutions with varying concentrations of glucose for altering ultrafiltration can be used; otherwise, special solutions can be formulated.

Suggested Readings

Arant BS Jr. Developmental patterns of renal functional maturation compared in the human neonate. *J Pediatr* 1978;92:705.

Arant BS Jr. Neonatal adjustments of extrauterine life. In: Edelmann CM Jr, ed. *Pediatric kidney disease*, 2nd ed. Boston: Little Brown, 1992:1043.

Arant BS Jr. Sodium, chloride and potassium. In: Tsang RC, Lucas A, Uauy R, Zlotkin S, eds. *Nutritional needs of the preterm infant.* Baltimore: Williams & Wilkins, 1993:157.

Brion LP, Fleischman AR, McCarton C, et al. A simple estimate of glomerular filtration rate in low-birth-weight infants during the first year of life: noninvasive assessment of body composition and growth. *J Pediatr* 1986;109:698.

Chamaa NS, Mosig D, Drukker A, et al. The renal hemodynamic effects of ibuprofen in the newborn rabbit. *Pediatr Res* 2000;48:600.

Chevalier RL. Developmental renal physiology of the low birth weight pre-term newborn. *J Urol* 1996;156:714.

Costarino AT Jr, Gruskay JA, Corcoran L, et al. Sodium restriction versus daily maintenance replacement in very low birth weight premature neonates: a randomized, blind therapeutic trial. *J Pediatr* 1992;120:99.

Lorenz JM, Kleinman LI, Kotagal UR, et al. Water balance in very-low-birth-weight infants: relationship to water and sodium intake and effect on outcome. *J Pediatr* 1982;101:423.

Norwood VF, Morham SG, Smithies O. Postnatal development and progression of renal dysplasia in cyclooxygenase-2 null mice. *Kidney Int* 2000;58:2291.

Rees L, Brook CGD, Shaw JCL, et al. Hyponatraemia in the first week of life in preterm infants. *Arch Dis Child* 1984;59:414.

Seikaly MG, Arant BS Jr. Development of renal hemodynamics: glomerular filtration and renal blood flow. *Clin Perinatol* 1992;19:1.

Simeoni U, Zhu B, Muller C, et al. Postnatal development of vascular resistance of the rabbit isolated perfused kidney: modulation by nitric oxide and angiotensin II. *Pediatr Res* 1997;42:550.

Szefler SJ, Wynn RJ, Clarke DF, et al. Relationship of gentamicin serum concentrations to gestational age in preterm and term neonates. *J Pediatr* 1980;97:312.

Toth-Heyn P, Drukker A, Guignard J-P. The stressed neonatal kidney from pathophysiology to clinical management of neonatal vasomotor nephropathy. *Pediatr Nephrol* 2000;14:227.

Tulassay T, Machay T, Kiszel J, et al. Effects of continuous positive airway pressure on renal function in prematures. *Biol Neonate* 1983;43:152.

Woods LL, Ingelfinger JR, Nyengaard JR, et al. Maternal protein restriction suppresses the newborn renin-angiotensin and programs adult hypertension in rats. *Pediatr Res* 2001;49:460.

Yoo KH, Wolstenholme JT, Chevalier RL. Angiotensin-converting enzyme inhibition decreases growth factor expression in the neonatal rat kidney. *Pediatr Res* 1997;42:588.

Zelenina M, Christensen BM, Palmer J, et al. Prostaglandin E(2) interaction with AVP: effects on AQP2 phosphorylation and distribution. *Am J Physiol Renal Physiol* 2000;278:F388.

CHAPTER 62 ■ NEONATAL ENDOCRINOLOGY

ELIZABETH A. CATLIN AND MARY M. LEE

The transition from an intrauterine to an extrauterine environment at birth requires neonates to make rapid and appropriate homeostatic adaptations for independent living. The hormonal and metabolic responses of infants to stress—be it that of birth, surgery, or infection—at times may be more vigorous than those of adults. These overly robust endocrine–metabolic responses, and the neonate's limited ability to modulate these responses, may be counterproductive in some situations. Alternatively, the neonate may respond inadequately with the rapid development of marked deviations of otherwise carefully protected body constituents. In either case, the clinical manifestations characteristic of older children or adults may be absent, making it difficult to appreciate a perturbation in endocrine function. This chapter covers common endocrine conditions and some of the more unusual endocrine disorders of newborns.

GLUCOSE BALANCE

The transfer of glucose from the placenta to the fetus is a concentration-dependent process driven by fetal glucose levels; this process is mediated by facilitative glucose transporter proteins. The fetus can generate some metabolic responses to nutritional states, although glucose is not produced, thus fetal growth and well-being depend on a maternal supply of glucose. At birth, neonatal plasma glucose values are initially 70% to 80% of maternal values. These values decline briefly before stabilizing by 2 to 3 hours of age. In healthy, term babies receiving enteral feedings by 3 hours of life, plasma glucose concentrations reach their nadir between 1 and 2 hours of life, at mean values of 56 mg/dL (SD +/− 19) (Fig. 62.1).

Intermittent and unpredictable feeding in the early neonatal period stresses the carbohydrate homeostatic capacity of a newborn. Developmental immaturity of two of the three counterregulatory mechanisms—ketogenesis and gluconeogenesis—contributes to the increased risk of hypoglycemia in neonates. Moreover, enteral feeding may be needed to induce the expression of some of the enzymes necessary for ketogenesis. The third mechanism, hepatic gluconeogenesis, often is compromised by peripartum or neonatal stress. In healthy term and preterm neonates, insulin levels are elevated when compared with those of older children and appear to be less closely linked to glucose concentrations. The hepatic suppression of glucose production by insulin during glucose infusion, for example, has been noted to be delayed in newborns relative to that of adults. Extremely low-birth-weight infants (ELBW; infants of less than 1,000 g) have depressed processing of proin-

sulin as well as relative insulin resistance during hyperglycemia. Both relative insulin resistance and defective islet beta-cell processing of proinsulin are responsible for transient hyperglycemia in extremely preterm infants. Therefore, insulin's role in neonatal glucoregulation may differ from its role in later development.

Hypoglycemia

Neonatal hypoglycemia is a common and typically transient problem in newborn infants that has traditionally been defined as a plasma glucose value of 40 mg/dL (2.2 mmol/L) or less. Controversy about the definition of neonatal hypoglycemia exists, however, and operational thresholds have been

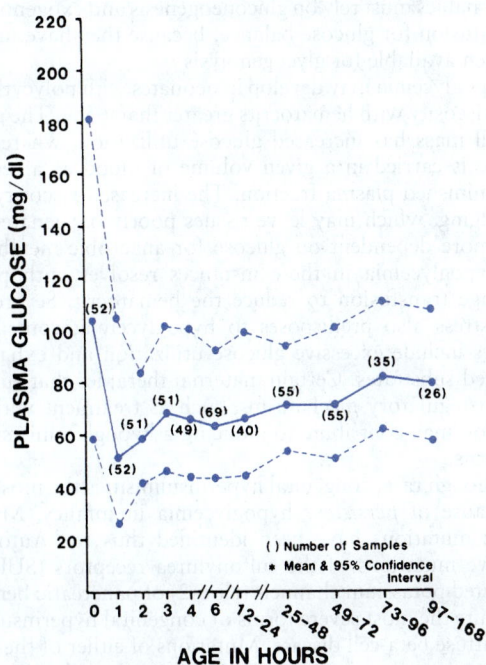

FIGURE 62.1. Predicted plasma glucose values during the first week of life in healthy term neonates with weights appropriate for their gestational age. (Reprinted with permission from Srinivasan G, Pildes RS, Cattamanchi G, et al. Plasma glucose values in normal neonates: a new look. *J Pediatr* 1986;109:114.)

proposed. We contend that, after the initial transient decline at birth, maintaining plasma glucose concentrations greater than 45 mg/dL during the first 24 hours and greater than 50 mg/dL thereafter is a sensible and conservative therapeutic goal, because fetal glucose levels are at least 40 mg/dL, and children and adults may have neuroglycopenic symptoms at glucose levels lower than this (as may neonates). Moreover, infants have an immature ketogenic capacity and are unable to generate ketones adequately as an alternative central nervous system fuel in response to hypoglycemia. Certain infants, including infants of diabetic mothers (IDMs), premature or growth-restricted infants, and perinatally stressed neonates especially are prone to the development of transient neonatal hypoglycemia. Persistent neonatal hypoglycemia is less common and is caused by congenital hyperinsulinism, deficits in counterregulatory hormones, or metabolic disorders that affect fasting adaptation.

Pathophysiology

Persistence of the hyperinsulinemic state after birth in many IDMs who develop elevated insulin secretion *in utero* in response to maternal hyperglycemia causes self-limited hypoglycemia that can be severe but relatively asymptomatic (see Chapter 63, Infant of the Diabetic Mother). Infants with intrauterine growth restriction (IUGR) are at risk for neonatal hypoglycemia; 65% of premature and 25% of full-term IUGR babies become hypoglycemic. Factors contributing to their low plasma glucose levels include decreased glycogen and fat stores, large brain–to–body weight ratio, failure to mobilize alternative fuels adequately, and in some instances, a relative hyperinsulinemia. Premature neonates (less than 37 weeks' gestation) also are at risk for the development of hypoglycemia. They have multiple contributing factors, such as lower total body energy stores, impaired ability to mobilize alternative fuels due to functional immaturity of the metabolic enzymes, and inadequate dietary intake. They also have an increased likelihood of having neonatal distress with sepsis, hypoxia, or perinatal depression, that can further compromise glucose homeostasis. ELBW babies must rely on gluconeogenesis and exogenous glucose infusion for glucose balance, because they have minimal glycogen available for glycogenolysis.

Hypoglycemia may develop in neonates with polycythemia-hyperviscosity with hematocrits greater than 65%. The greater red cell mass has increased glucose utilization, whereas less glucose is carried in a given volume of blood as a result of the diminished plasma fraction. The increased viscosity leads to sludging, which may leave tissues poorly oxygenated and, thus, more dependent on glucose for anaerobic metabolism. The hypoglycemia in these instances resolves with partial-exchange transfusion to reduce the hematocrit. Severe perinatal stress also predisposes to hypoglycemia; contributing features include excessive glucose utilization and exhaustion of stored substrates. Certain maternal therapies that suppress counter-regulatory mechanisms, such as treatment with propranolol, may contribute to inducing a hypoglycemic state in newborns.

Although rare, congenital hyperinsulinism is the most common cause of *persistent* hypoglycemia in infancy. Multiple genetic mutations have been identified thus far. Autosomal recessive mutations of the sulfonylurea receptors (SUR1) or associated potassium channels (Kir6.2) of pancreatic beta cells constitute the most severe forms of congenital hyperinsulinism with diffuse beta-cell disease. Mutations of either of these two adjacent genes on chromosome 11 affect the subunits of the K_{ATP} channel such that insulin secretion is constitutively active and unresponsive to ambient glucose. A sporadic form, due to loss of heterozygosity for the maternal allele and inheritance of an abnormal paternal allele for SUR1, causes focal beta-cell hyperplasia and is clinically indistinguishable from diffuse dis-

ease. These mutations of the ATP-dependent potassium channel are the most common cause of severe neonatal hyperinsulinism with the classic clinical picture of macrosomia, increased insulin/glucose ratios, and a requirement for high glucose infusion rates. Autosomal dominant hyperinsulinism appears to be a milder disease. Although the majority of cases have not been associated with particular mutations, a gain-of-function mutation of the glucokinase gene can cause a mild form of congenital hyperinsulinism that is responsive to diazoxide. Congenital hyperinsulinism with associated hyperammonemia is caused by an activating mutation in the glutamate dehydrogenase gene. These infants typically present later in infancy and have leucine-sensitive hypoglycemia with mild fasting defects.

Neonates with the Beckwith-Wiedemann syndrome (Fig. 62.2) have macroglossia, characteristic ear creases or pits, visceromegaly, omphalocele, and are large for gestational age (LGA). Nearly 50% of reported cases exhibit hyperinsulinemic hypoglycemia caused by diffuse islet cell hyperplasia. Hypoglycemia in such infants may be severe and long-lasting, necessitating pharmacologic management of their hyperinsulinism in addition to glucose supplementation.

Hypopituitarism and isolated growth hormone (GH) deficiency are other endocrine causes of persistent hypoglycemia in infancy. Although growth may remain normal during infancy, associated physical features, such as midline defects or microphallus, are helpful diagnostically. Very infrequently, neonatal hypoglycemia is caused by one of the inborn errors of metabolism in the gluconeogenic or glycogenolysis pathways, such as galactosemia or type I glycogen storage disease (see Chapter 387, Disorders of Carbohydrate Metabolism). Genetic defects of the glucose transporter 1, which transfers glucose across the blood–brain barrier, have been recognized as a cause of central nervous system hypoglycemia and seizures despite normal blood glucose levels.

Diagnosis

Clinicians must have a low threshold for suspecting hypoglycemia in neonates, because the symptoms are subtle.

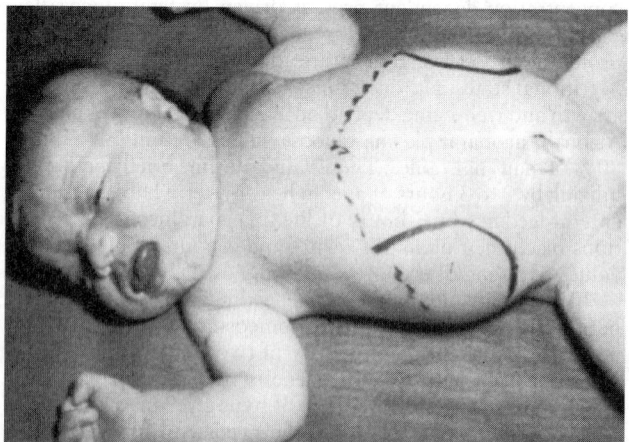

FIGURE 62.2. Neonate with Beckwith-Wiedemann syndrome. This 38 weeks' gestation, 34-cm, 5.218-kg plethoric infant was the third child in this family to be affected with the syndrome. Note, in addition to his large size and abundance of subcutaneous fat, the enlarged tongue and umbilical hernia. The enormously enlarged, multilobular kidneys have been outlined with a skin pencil. The vertical creases on the lobuli of the ears are not shown well. The infant required prolonged infusion of intravenous glucose to prevent hyperinsulinemic hypoglycemia and required a partial glossectomy and repair of the umbilical hernia.

Affected infants may be jittery or manifest such nonspecific symptoms as apnea, seizures, poor feeding, or lethargy, but they may be also essentially asymptomatic. The neurocognitive sequelae of asymptomatic neonatal hypoglycemia are unknown. A careful pregnancy history and physical examination may reveal evidence of growth restriction, visceromegaly, or other clues to the etiology of the hypoglycemia. A plasma glucose level should be obtained; if capillary sampling is used, care must be taken to warm the heel adequately. If the glucose concentration is 40 mg/dL or less in asymptomatic infants or less than 45 mg/dL in infants with symptoms, assessment and possibly treatment should be instituted. Initial screening can be carried out using glucose oxidase strips (e.g., Dextrostix, Chemstrips) or with a bedside glucose analyzer, *but laboratory confirmation of low values is required*. The strips should be fresh or packaged individually, because strips from open bottles may be inaccurate and give erroneously low values.

Therapy

Stable and relatively mature babies may be treated safely with early enteral feedings and careful monitoring of subsequent plasma glucose values. If blood glucose is greater than 45 mg/dL, normal feeding may be started as soon as the infant's condition permits, with capillary glucose monitoring every 1 to 2 hours until blood sugars stabilize in the normal range. If the glucose value is between 25 and 45 mg/dL, a repeat sample is obtained while the baby is given 10 to 15 mL of formula (orally or by gavage feeding) with frequent monitoring of the blood glucose until it is stable (greater than 40 to 45 mg/dL). If the blood glucose is less than 25 mg/dL, parenteral glucose supplementation is required, first administering a "mini-bolus" of 10% glucose, 2 to 3 mL/kg intravenously, followed by a constant infusion of 10% glucose delivered at a rate of 4 to 6 mg/kg/minute, which approximates the basal glucose production rate of the healthy neonate. Glucose values must be monitored closely, with titration of the infusate to maintain normoglycemia.

Infants with transient hypoglycemia or hypoglycemia attributable to one of the self-limited disorders described require supportive therapy to maintain glucose levels in the normal range, but minimal diagnostic evaluation is necessary. Infants with prolonged hypoglycemia, those requiring high glucose infusions (more than 10 to 15 mg/kg/minute), and those with a clinical course suspicious for a pathologic disorder of glucose regulation need further workup. Inappropriately high serum insulin levels (relative to simultaneously obtained plasma glucose levels) without evidence of Beckwith-Wiedemann syndrome or maternal diabetes mellitus suggest hyperinsulinism. Insulin secretion should be suppressed completely during a hypoglycemic episode; thus, the finding of measurable concentrations of insulin and absent ketone production is suspicious for hyperinsulinism. A glucagon stimulation test can help identify a hyperinsulinemic state. In a hypoglycemic infant, the administration of 0.5 mg of glucagon will not raise significantly the plasma glucose, unless glycogen breakdown is being suppressed by insulin (hyperinsulinism) or decreased counter-regulatory hormones (panhypopituitarism). An increase in glucose of more than 30 mg/dL is indicative of glycogen reserve. Therefore, obtaining a blood sample for ketones, free fatty acids, cortisol, and GH, in addition to the insulin level, during hypoglycemia is essential. Evaluation of the gluconeogenic or glycogenolytic pathway may be necessary in rare cases suspicious for these disorders. Fasting studies are at times necessary to assess fasting tolerance and to make a definitive diagnosis.

Infants with hyperinsulinemic hypoglycemia and infants with IUGR may require especially high glucose infusions (15 mg/kg/minute or higher), which usually are delivered via a central venous catheter. Intravenous therapy should be maintained until the glucose level has stabilized. Rebound hypoglycemia in IDMs can be avoided by a slow tapering of the intravenous glucose being administered and the maintenance of the blood glucose in the normal range, avoiding both hypoglycemia and hyperglycemia. If intravenous access is difficult in IDMs, glucagon (0.3 mg/kg to a maximum dose of 1 mg) can be given to override the inhibitory effect of insulin on glycogenolysis and raise an affected infant's blood glucose level within 10 to 15 minutes of the injection. It must be emphasized that glucagon benefits only infants with a large glucose reservoir in the form of glycogen; it is ineffective in low-birth-weight or perinatally depressed infants who have depleted their glycogen stores.

Infants who require very high glucose infusions may need pharmacologic therapy to aid in the treatment of hypoglycemia. Diazoxide suppresses insulin secretion and is the initial choice for hyperinsulinism; the usual dosage is 10 to 15 mg/kg/day. Patients with *SUR1* or Kir6.2 mutations, however, are unlikely to respond adequately to diazoxide and generally require a subtotal 95% to 99% pancreatectomy. Octreotide, a somatostatin analogue, suppresses insulin release and has been useful in conjunction with diazoxide in certain patients for the long-term management of hyperinsulinemia. Glucagon infusions (5 to10 μg/kg/hour) can be helpful as a temporizing measure, particularly preoperatively, but the action of these infusions are not sustained for chronic use. At some centers, focal lesions can be localized intraoperatively and successfully resected. Postoperatively, pharmacologic intervention still may be necessary for optimal glucose control.

Hyperglycemia

Hyperglycemia in neonates is defined as random plasma glucose concentrations greater than 150 mg/dL. The incidence of hyperglycemia has increased in parallel with the increased survival of very premature and high-risk infants. Some studies suggest that hyperglycemia contributes to increased morbidity and mortality in neonates.

Pathophysiology

ELBW infants have a relative insulin insensitivity and delayed processing of proinsulin during hyperglycemia. Other conditions associated with transient hyperglycemia in the newborn period include sepsis, surgical stress, hypoxia, central nervous system insults (including intracranial hemorrhage), and treatment with methylxanthines. Stress-related hyperglycemia results, in part, from elevated catecholamine and cortisol levels. Pancreatic agenesis is a rare cause of neonatal glucose intolerance and is caused by insulin promoter factor 1 mutations; these babies also exhibit significant IUGR. Neonatal diabetes, estimated to occur once in 500,000 births, has a highly variable course. Affected babies may have transient diabetes, with or without periods of remission, or permanent diabetes, and most are small for gestational age. A complete deficiency of glucokinase has been found to cause permanent neonatal diabetes. The small size of these neonates, in contrast to the macrosomia of IDMs, is believed to reflect insulin's important role as an intrauterine growth hormone.

Therapy

In a hyperglycemic neonate (greater than 150 mg/dL), the first measure is to calculate the glucose infusion rate in mg/kg/minute and gradually decrease the rate by 1 to 2 mg/kg/minute every 3 to 4 hours, monitoring glucose levels 30 to 60 minutes after changing the rate. Hypotonic infusates must be avoided. Insulin therapy should be considered if hyperglycemia persists despite the administration of glucose at basal production rates (approximately 4 to 6 mg/kg/minute). Fluid balance, glycosuria, blood pressure, oxygenation, and perfusion should be checked carefully and, if sepsis is suspected, appropriate cultures should be obtained and antibiotics given. In very low-birth-weight infants (of less than 1.5 kg), consider measures to minimize insensible fluid losses, such as transfer from radiant warmers to isolettes. If hyperglycemia persists (greater than 200 mg/dL), therapy may be required using a continuous infusion of regular insulin, starting at 0.01 to 0.02 units/kg/hour, with the aim of maintaining plasma glucose at 100 to 150 mg/dL and taking care to avoid hypoglycemia. ELBW infants often require insulin infused continuously, along with intravenous glucose containing hyperalimentation, to permit the delivery of adequate nutritional substrates for growth. A larger and persistent requirement for insulin generally distinguishes the rare neonate with diabetes mellitus from the infant mounting a vigorous stress response who has transient hyperglycemia that resolves within a few days.

CALCIUM BALANCE

The placenta actively transports calcium to the fetus against a concentration gradient under the regulation of parathyroid hormone–related peptide. The majority of fetal skeletal mineralization takes place during the last trimester. Serum calcium in the newborn, under normal circumstances, decreases for several days after birth, stabilizes, and gradually increases to the concentrations found in older infants and children.

Hypocalcemia

Hypocalcemia occurs commonly in the neonatal period but is generally transient and rarely indicative of a persistent metabolic disorder. Neonatal hypocalcemia is generally subdivided into early and late-onset categories (see Chapter 64, Mineral Metabolism in the Newborn). Early hypocalcemia has been defined as a total serum calcium concentration of less than 8 mg/dL (2.0 mmol/L) in the full-term neonate or less than 7 mg/dL (1.75 mmol/L) in the premature neonate, or, perhaps more precisely, an ionized calcium level of less than 1.0 mmol/L (4 mg/dL) during the first few days of life. Inasmuch as 50% of calcium in serum is bound loosely to protein and varies according to the serum protein concentration, pH, and other factors, the biologically active *ionized* calcium concentration is a better indicator of the calcium status. The postnatal serum calcium nadir at 24 and 48 hours of life normally stimulates the secretion of parathyroid hormone (PTH). The inadequate PTH response of premature neonates, IDMs, and infants with perinatal depression to the decreasing calcium concentrations underlies their susceptibility to early hypocalcemia.

Pathophysiology

Late neonatal hypocalcemia occurs toward the end or after the first week of life and may be caused by congenital hypoparathyroidism, hypomagnesemia, and high-phosphate formula consumption (synonymous with late infantile tetany). Congenital hypoparathyroidism is caused usually by agenesis or dysgenesis of the parathyroid glands, and often is associated with the DiGeorge syndrome or chromosome 22q11 microdeletion syndrome. A transient hypoparathyroidism may be present in infants of women with hyperparathyroidism. Rarely, intrauterine nutritional vitamin D deficiency from severe maternal vitamin D deficiency or hereditary vitamin D–resistant rickets can present with late-onset hypocalcemia. Late-onset hypocalcemia associated with hypomagnesemia may occur in small-for-gestational-age neonates, in those with hepatic disease or small-bowel resections and, very rarely, in infants with mag-

nesium malabsorption or disorders of renal magnesium handling. Hypomagnesemia causes late hypocalcemia via several mechanisms: It inhibits parathyroid hormone (PTH) secretion, induces a relative end-organ insensitivity to PTH, and causes decreased calcium absorption and decreased exchange of magnesium for calcium at the bone surface.

Diagnosis

The diagnosis of neonatal hypocalcemia begins with an assessment of history, clinical signs, and laboratory data. The majority of babies with early neonatal hypocalcemia are asymptomatic and require no treatment except for close follow-up and monitoring. Hypocalcemic neonates may occasionally exhibit seizure activity, tremors, tetany or lethargy, and poor feeding. Monitoring of serum calcium, phosphorus, and magnesium with a careful assessment of intake is indicated in high-risk infants. Late hypocalcemia is more likely to be associated with a chronic condition and, in addition to the laboratory tests mentioned, PTH and vitamin D levels may be helpful diagnostically.

Therapy

Although many neonatal units treat at-risk neonates with early calcium supplementation, the indications for this practice are not clear. Symptomatic early hypocalcemia is usually transient and may require temporary therapy with calcium supplementation. Oral and intravenous calcium supplementation for early hypocalcemia can be achieved with elemental calcium, 75 mg/kg/day as an initial oral dose or 24 to 75 mg/kg/day parenterally, usually given for less than 3 days. The subacute and chronic conditions of late hypocalcemia are treated with calcitriol (1,25-dihydroxyvitamin D), starting with a dose of 0.125 μg once or twice daily and calcium supplementation as described (see Chapter 64). Parathyroid agenesis requires lifelong therapy to prevent hypocalcemia. During the initiation of therapy, serum calcium and phosphorus should be monitored daily to maintain their concentrations in the low-normal range.

Seizures associated with hypocalcemia are treated with intravenous 10% calcium gluconate, 1 to 2 mL/kg, given slowly over 5 to 10 minutes to avoid inducing bradycardia. Care must be taken with the intravenous dosing of calcium-containing solutions to avoid extravasation and associated tissue damage.

Hypercalcemia

Pathophysiology

Neonatal hypercalcemia usually is the result of excessive calcium supplementation, especially in very premature newborns. Babies with Williams syndrome (idiopathic infantile hypercalcemia syndrome with elfin facies and supravalvular aortic stenosis) may have hypercalcemia and nephrocalcinosis, which typically resolves spontaneously by 4 years of age. Primary hyperparathyroidism, although extremely rare, is caused by homozygous mutations of the plasma membrane calcium-sensing receptor (CASR). Heterozygotes for mutations of this receptor have familial hypocalciuric hypercalcemia, which is often asymptomatic, but homozygotes have a severe form of hypercalcemia, which is often lethal.

Therapy

The treatment of neonatal hypercalcemia should be prompt and includes hydration at one-and one-half to two times maintenance using 5% dextrose with 0.5 normal saline and potassium chloride (3 mEq/dL); furosemide given at 1 mg/kg per dose intravenously twice or three times daily to inhibit renal tubular calcium resorption; and phosphate supplementation to maintain normal serum phosphorus values. Vitamin D and calcium intake should be limited, and hydrocortisone may help decrease the intestinal absorption of calcium. Primary hyperparathyroidism often requires surgical resection of the parathyroid glands for definitive management.

MAGNESIUM BALANCE

Critically ill neonates and IDMs in poor glycemic control or substance-abusing mothers are at risk for hypomagnesemia. Maternal nutritional status may contribute to the depressed total serum magnesium levels measured in such neonates, and increased urinary magnesium losses are associated with the diabetic state. A potential problem in the interpretation of magnesium data is that of definition. Whereas magnesium exists in the extracellular compartment in ionized, protein-bound, and miscellaneously bound forms (similar to calcium), hypomagnesemia generally has been defined on the basis of total magnesium levels. Because the ionized fraction of magnesium is considered to be physiologically more relevant, determinations of total magnesium may not represent a valid parameter of neonatal magnesium balance.

Pathophysiology

Neonatal hypomagnesemia may result from inadequate nutritional supplementation in neonates treated with parenteral alimentation or magnesium malabsorption, either associated with surgical short bowel or caused by a rare X-linked defect presenting after the first few weeks of life and requiring lifelong magnesium replacement. Hypomagnesemia caused by renal wasting may be seen as a result of aminoglycoside therapy or as an inherited disorder of renal magnesium handling. IUGR and hepatic disease predispose to neonatal hypomagnesemia. Low magnesium concentrations reduce both the secretory response of the parathyroid gland to hypocalcemia and the end-organ responsiveness to PTH; thus, refractory hypocalcemia may be the first clue to a primary magnesium deficit.

Hypermagnesemia (total serum magnesium levels of greater than 2.1 mEq/L or 1.05 mmol/L) is typically iatrogenic. It can be seen in the babies of mothers being treated with magnesium sulfate or magnesium-containing antacids. Often, a functional ileus is present, and generalized central nervous system depression may result in lethargy, apnea, and diminished responsiveness. Alternatively, parenteral hyperalimentation may provide a relative excess of magnesium.

Diagnosis

Signs of neuromuscular irritability, which may be evident in neonates with hypomagnesemia, may aid in diagnosis. Studies of infants with seizures in the first week after birth revealed that as many as one-half of all neonates with hypocalcemic seizures had coexistent hypomagnesemia.

Therapy

No treatment is needed for transient isolated asymptomatic hypomagnesemia, whereas lifelong oral replacement therapy is needed for magnesium malabsorption and primary hypomagnesemia. The therapy of hypermagnesemia is generally supportive, with intubation and mechanical ventilation as needed for apnea and airway control and parenteral fluid administration during the period of symptomatic ileus. In addition, intravenous calcium may be used as a magnesium antagonist in selected severe instances of symptomatic hypermagnesemia.

When hypocalcemia and hypomagnesemia coexist, the magnesium deficit should be corrected first with intravenous or intramuscular magnesium sulfate, using 5 to 25 mg/kg of elemental magnesium given slowly over 10 minutes. Prophylactic magnesium administration has not been shown to reduce the incidence of associated hypocalcemia in the infants of diabetic women. Chronic magnesium therapy may be initiated with oral doses of elemental magnesium (as magnesium sulfate, gluconate, lactate, citrate, or glycerophosphate), 20 to 40 mg/kg/day.

WATER BALANCE

Neonates are at particular risk for disturbances of water homeostasis, both because turnover is so large compared to body stores and because of the immaturity of the systems that maintain tonicity and fluid volume. These issues are particularly critical in very premature infants, in whom transepidermal water losses may be dramatic. Water balance is achieved by adjustments in intake, prevention of excessive insensible losses, and modulation of urine output. In the newborn period, the sensations of thirst and taste are far less discriminating than they will become with maturity, and the behaviors elicited by thirst are the primitive, nonspecific responses of sucking and crying. When thirsty, neonates will accept hypertonic saline as readily as water and, when they are overhydrated, hunger may supersede the signal to decrease fluid intake. Thus, the regulation of solute intake is dictated primarily by the fluids provided to the infant.

Pathophysiology

Breast milk and commercial formulas that mimic its composition are suited ideally for the maintenance of normal tonicity, with little need for modulation by the antidiuretic hormone system, which regulates output. This system ordinarily operates through the sensing of hypertonicity and the secretion of vasopressin, leading to renal water conservation; this system is functionally immature at birth. In term infants, the maturation of the renal excretory system to the full concentrating capacities characteristic of later life is achieved by approximately age 1 month. Urinary water losses are regulated, not as free water, but relative to the osmotic activity of the solutes being excreted. Systemic hypotonicity is combated maximally when each osmotic solute particle in urine is accompanied by 10 mL of water (dilute urine); hypertonicity is combated when the water loss in urine is reduced to as little as 1 mL/mOsm of solute. This wide range of facultative adjustment of urine tonicity permits the protection of the very narrow range of normal systemic tonicity. The latter is expressed conventionally as 275 to 285 mOsm/kg, but also can be expressed to emphasize the water variable as 3.50 to 3.65 mL of water per milliosmole of solute. Disruption of the normal osmolarity is corrected more slowly in the newborn period, particularly in premature infants, because of their limited capacity to modulate the excretion of solutes or free water.

Disturbances of systemic tonicity in neonates are rarely the result of a malfunction of the endocrine regulatory system and usually can be attributed to the inadequate provision of fluids or the provision of hypotonic or hypertonic fluids, or excessive water losses by diarrhea, heat, or renal dysfunction. Nonetheless, diabetes insipidus (DI)—both the type caused by vasopressin deficiency and the receptor disorder—and conditions of vasopressin overproduction are seen in neonates.

The causes of DI in neonates are the same as those in later life. In the absence of perinatal depression or intracranial hemorrhage, the inherited forms should be considered; in boys, the X-linked nephrogenic type is particularly likely. Infants with central DI and optic nerve hypoplasia or midline defects should be evaluated for anterior pituitary deficiencies.

The syndrome of inappropriate antidiuretic hormone (SIADH) release may be seen transiently after intracranial hemorrhage, severe perinatal depression, or trauma resulting in damage to the neural lobe of the hypophysis and loss of facultative control of vasopressin release. The transient excess vasopressin release may be followed by permanent DI. Occasionally, SIADH is encountered also in neonates with atelectasis or pneumothorax requiring positive-pressure ventilation, presumably as a result of reduced pulmonary blood flow and decreased signals from the stretch receptors of the left atrium. SIADH is a common complication of infantile botulism; venous pooling secondary to the generalized hypotonia may reduce activation of the left atrial stretch receptors.

Diagnosis and Therapy

Diagnosis is difficult, because DI is essentially asymptomatic in breast-fed neonates fed *ad libitum*. With the introduction of solid foods, which yield solute in excess of needs for growth, the formation of concentrated urine begins to be required to prevent systemic hypertonicity. Very frequently, before DI is recognized, mothers and pediatricians have been baffled by unexplained recurrent bouts of fever. Treatment in early life is a continuance of breast milk or dilute formula, with the volumes carefully calculated to maintain satisfactory weight gain and hydration. If the volume of fluids required is such that growth is compromised, a low dose of desmopressin, the long-acting vasopressin analogue, is useful to decrease the daily urine output. In infants, subcutaneous injection rather than intranasal or oral delivery of desmopressin provides the most consistent dosing and accurate dose titration. At initiation of therapy, a close monitoring of serum electrolytes and osmolality, urine output, and weight gain and a careful adjustment of fluid intake to avoid overhydration are essential.

The goal of SIADH treatment is to reduce water intake relative to solutes by limiting intake of hypotonic fluids and replacing insensible losses with 10% dextrose and 0.5 normal saline (NS) or NS. Whereas metabolizable solutes such as glucose and lactate contribute to tonicity in intravenous infusates, these solutes are degraded to CO_2 and water. Hence, their residue is not useful in helping the kidney to correct the water excess of SIADH. If seizures necessitate abruptly returning tonicity to normal, it should be done by the intravenous infusion of hypertonic saline.

AMBIGUOUS GENITALIA

One of the most important decisions clinicians make is that announced in the delivery room: "It's a boy!" or "It's a girl!" Once the announcement is made, a reaction that is reversible only in its earlier stages is set in motion. The way in which parents, relatives, and other child-care providers treat the infant helps cement the process of gender identification in the child. This section deals with those rare situations in which this decision cannot be made with certainty. In this context, it must be remembered that the potential for the development of those structures by which we recognize maleness and femaleness is common to all zygotes, whether 46,XX or 46,XY. For example, should an accident render the gonads nonfunctional in an early embryo with a normal 46,XY constitution, the infant will have

unequivocal female genitalia. On the other hand, female fetuses exposed to androgens, whether endogenous or environmental, will undergo variable degrees of virilization depending on the timing, duration, and severity of the exposure (Figs. 62.3 and 62.4).

The role of genetic or prenatal neuroendocrine influences on gender identity remains controversial, but it is clear that the self-concept of "boy" or "girl" already is established firmly in the toddler. Anything that occurs to threaten gender identification in children's subsequent psychologic development can have serious emotional consequences. These experiences range from children's sensing that the parents are troubled by their gender identity to discoveries in play group or preschool that they are not like others of the same gender. Doubts and questions may arise also during adolescence, when body image and developing sexuality are areas of intense concern. These factors may be precipitated by delayed pubertal maturation or the development of such discordant secondary sexual characteristics as gynecomastia, hirsutism, or clitoromegaly or by the realization that the external genitalia are atypical in appearance. The devastating impact of an inappropriate sex assignment underscores the importance of a careful examination of the genitalia in the delivery room examination. If any doubt exists as to an infant's gender, the physician should make a concerted effort to refrain from an immediate, and perhaps unsuitable, assignment of gender, because this decision will affect the child's rearing.

When gender assignments cannot be made with assurance, an attending pediatrician should immediately mobilize a team of personnel with expertise in the evaluation of intersex disorders. The situation must be explained to the parents so that they understand that further evaluation will be required to determine whether the infant is a male whose genitalia developed incompletely or a female who has undergone virilization. The birth certificate and announcements to family and friends should be put on hold temporarily. The nursery staff and all other health care providers must avoid carefully the personal pronoun in referring to an affected infant. Identification of the genetic constitution, gonadal phenotype, and internal reproductive structures is attained as expeditiously as possible. Ultimately, the decision as to gender assignment is best made jointly by the medical team in conjunction with the parents after all relevant information is available.

Pathophysiology: Types of Ambiguous Genitalia

The best-known, if not the most common, of the disorders giving rise to ambiguous genital development are the congenital adrenal hyperplasia (CAH) syndromes, which account for the majority of infants with female pseudohermaphroditism. These disorders consist of genetic defects in one of the enzymes in the cortisol biosynthetic pathway that results in cortisol deficiency and disturbances in the other steroidogenic pathways (Fig. 62.5). The constellation of clinical findings and laboratory abnormalities depends on the particular enzyme affected (Box 62.1). The most common type, caused by deficient activity of the 21-hydroxylase enzyme (CYP21) gene, results in elevated adrenal androgens that cause variable degrees of virilization, ranging from mild clitoromegaly and posterior labial fusion to almost-normal-appearing male external genitalia with nonpalpable gonads (Fig. 62.6). Male neonates with this syndrome evince no pathognomonic clinical findings until signs of adrenal insufficiency develop. In infants with this and the other steroid biosynthetic deficiencies, the insufficiency of cortisol and aldosterone production mandates that the clinician be alert to the subtle symptoms of feeding intolerance that precede the

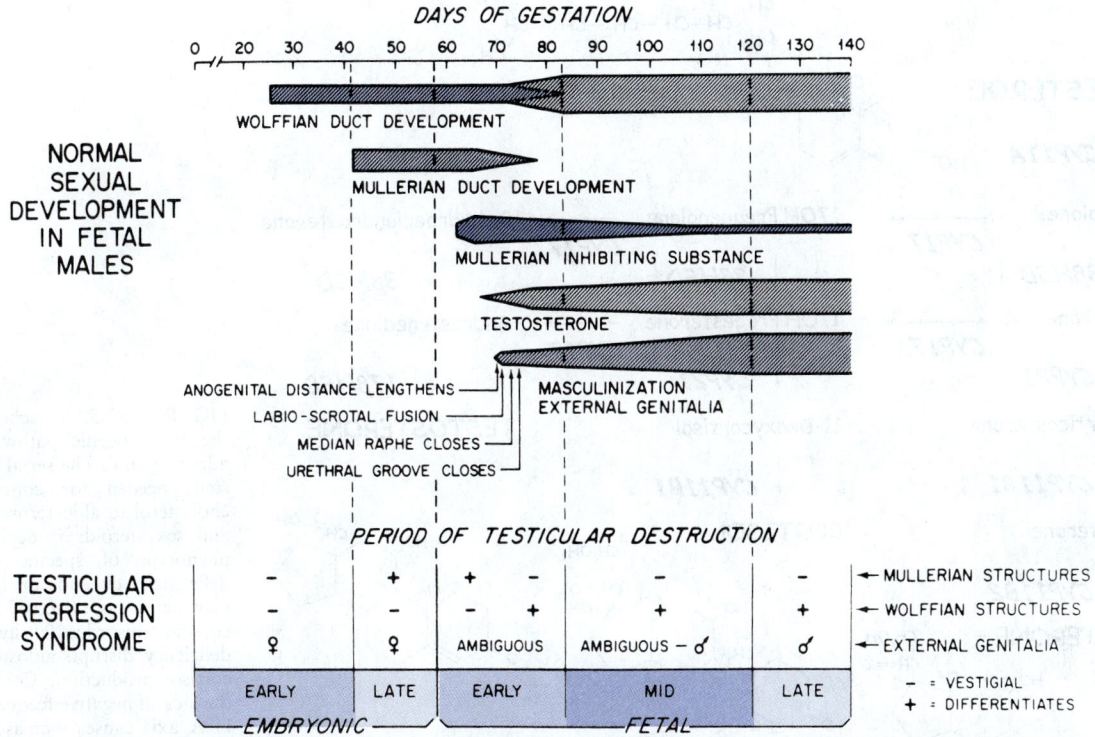

FIGURE 62.3. Timetable of normal genital development and dependence of neonatal appearance on timing in fetal life of loss of testicular function. (Reprinted with permission from Welch WR, Robboy SJ. Abnormal sexual development: a classification with emphasis on pathology and neoplastic conditions. In: Kogan SJ, Hafez ESE, eds. *Pediatric andrology*. The Hague: Martinus Nijhoff, 1981:71.)

rapidly developing hyponatremia and hyperkalemia heralding hypotensive collapse. Occasionally, hypoglycemia may be the first clinical sign of cortisol deficiency. The next most common disorder, 11-hydroxylase deficiency, also causes female genital ambiguity, whereas 3-beta-hydroxysteroid dehydrogenase mutations result in the synthesis of weak androgens that masculinize female fetuses but produce insufficient testosterone concentrations for the full masculinization of male fetuses.

Defects in the steroidogenic acute regulatory protein (a cholesterol transporter) are responsible for lipoid congenital hyperplasia and result in severe cortisol, mineralocorticoid, and androgen deficiency. Rarer causes of the virilization of female fetuses include exposure to environmental androgens from an androgen-secreting tumor in the mother, maternal use of virilizing hormones or drugs, or the rare occurrence of a placental aromatase deficiency.

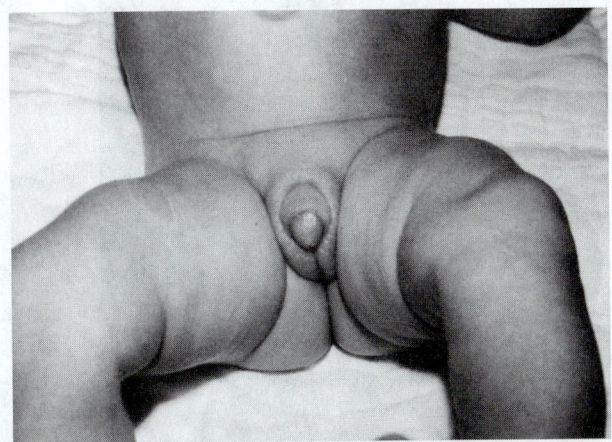
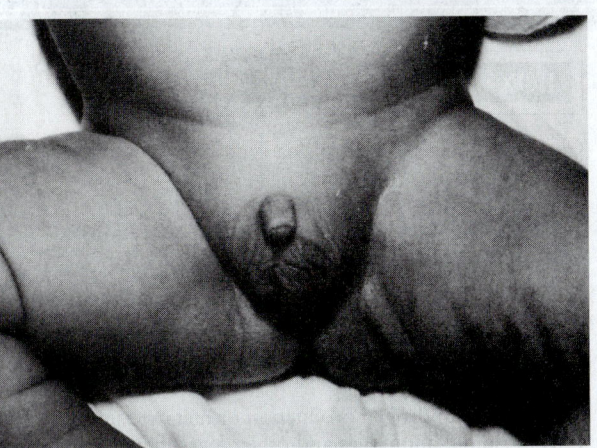

FIGURE 62.4. Two infants with genital ambiguity. These two cases illustrate the difficulty of relying on examination of the external genitalia to determine genetic and gonadal sex. **A:** 46,XX virilized girl with congenital adrenal hyperplasia. The phallus is well developed with perineoscrotal hypospadias, and no gonads are palpable in the labioscrotal folds. **B:** 46,XY boy with microphallus and undescended testicles secondary to hypopituitarism. Normally, the phallus is formed with a penile urethral opening, but the phallus is small, and the scrotum is underdeveloped.

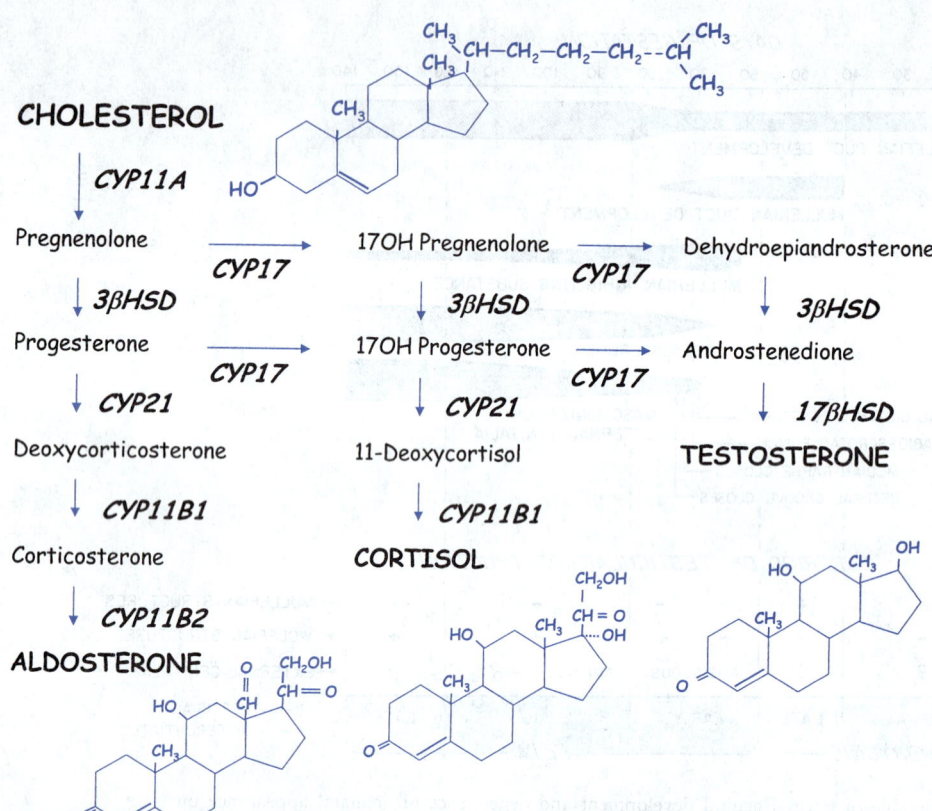

CHOLESTEROL

↓ *CYP11A*

Pregnenolone → 17OH Pregnenolone → Dehydroepiandrosterone

↓ *3βHSD* *CYP17* ↓ *3βHSD* *CYP17* ↓ *3βHSD*

Progesterone → 17OH Progesterone → Androstenedione

↓ *CYP21* *CYP17* ↓ *CYP21* *CYP17* ↓ *17βHSD*

Deoxycorticosterone 11-Deoxycortisol **TESTOSTERONE**

↓ *CYP11B1* ↓ *CYP11B1*

Corticosterone **CORTISOL**

↓ *CYP11B2*

ALDOSTERONE

FIGURE 62.5. A schematic of the steroidogenic pathway in the adrenal gland. The serial enzymatic steps needed for conversion of cholesterol to aldosterone, cortisol, and sex steroids is depicted. The phenotype of specific enzymatic deficiencies depends on the particular pathways affected. The most common disorder, 21 hydroxylase deficiency, disrupts aldosterone and cortisol production. Consequently, the lack of negative feedback on the HPA axis causes increased ACTH stimulation of steroidogenesis and shunting of steroid production to the sex steroid pathway.

A multitude of disorders can disrupt the normal male virilization of the external genitalia and cause male pseudohermaphroditism (Box 62.1). A particularly instructive cause of genital ambiguity in the neonate is the syndrome of testicular regression. Intrapartum testicular infarction is developmentally the "latest" and probably the most familiar of the disorders constituting the spectrum of testicular regression. What might have been diagnosed as bilateral cryptorchidism had the infarc-

tion taken place a few weeks before birth constitutes the late end of a spectrum that extends from early fetal life to birth. The phenotype of an affected neonate depends on the timing of the functional demise of the testis. When this process occurs before the time at which the secretion of müllerian-inhibiting substance (MIS) begins, the phenotype of the conceptus is female both internally and externally. The phenotype of genitalia development in testicular regression undergoes an orderly

---

BOX 62.1	Disorders Giving Rise to Ambiguous Genitalia

Congenital adrenal hyperplasia syndromes
  21-Hydroxylase deficiency
  11-Hydroxylase deficiency
  3-Beta-hydroxysteroid dehydrogenase mutations
Testicular regression (e.g., intrapartum testicular infarction)
Single-gene disorders that compromise testosterone production or bioactivity
Androgen insensitivity disorders (e.g., complete androgen insensitivity syndrome)
Inhibition of androgen production or metabolism
Chromosomal anomalies and other developmental anomalies
Disorders of gonadal determination (e.g., partial gonadal dysgenesis)
Contiguous gene syndromes
Genetic mutations of *SRY* and other autosomal genes in sexual determination pathway

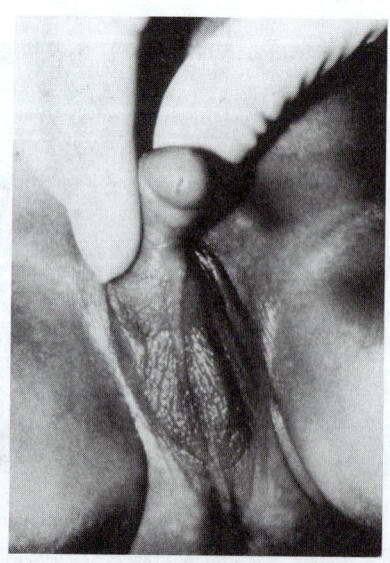

FIGURE 62.6. Infant with 46,XX congenital adrenal hyperplasia. The degree of virilization of this infant resulted in an initial male gender assignment. Note the well-formed phallus, scrotum with rugae, and mild hypospadias. No gonads were palpable.

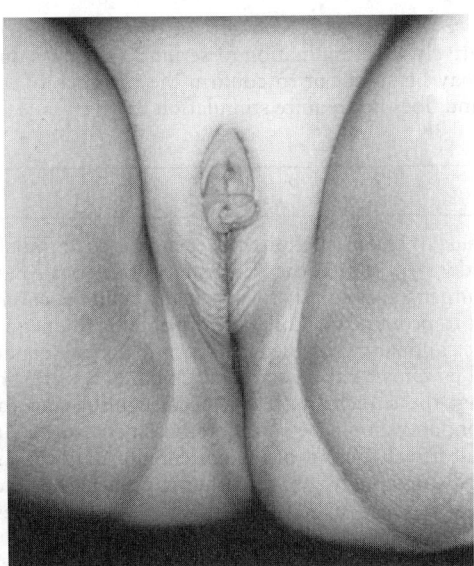

FIGURE 62.7. Infant with early testicular regression syndrome. Severe undervirilization of genitalia in a 46,XY infant with early testicular loss.

transition from being completely female (although lacking ovaries) to being completely male with bilateral anorchidism (Fig. 62.7). The extent of virilization depends on the moment in genital embryogenesis at which testicular function ceased (Fig. 62.3). This result is not always due to mechanical causes, such as twisting of the testicle on its pedicle and subsequent infarction. In certain families, it is programmed as a genetically determined event, and it may occur also secondary to viral infection and as a manifestation of an immunologic disorder. Testicular regression syndrome illustrates—possibly better than any other of the multiple causes of genital ambiguity—that outward neonatal appearance is not indicative of the genetic sex and provides insufficient information to permit a gender designation or even guidance for the parents in gender-role selection.

The genetic causes of male pseudohermaphroditism consist of a number of uncommon heritable single-gene disorders that compromise testosterone production or bioactivity. Single-gene disorders are responsible for the testosterone biosynthetic defects, the androgen insensitivity disorders, and some forms of gonadotropin-releasing hormone deficiency and panhypopituitarism. Of these, a genetic mutation of the androgen receptor is the most common etiology for undervirilization of a genetic male fetus. Complete androgen insensitivity syndrome can be associated with so little ambiguity that a newborn may be unequivocally declared to be a girl, and the diagnosis may not be suspected until the occurrence much later of inguinal hernias or primary amenorrhea. As in the syndrome of testicular regression, the extent of virilization for the testosterone biosynthetic and androgen insensitivity disorders can range from almost completely female genitalia to a normally virilized male with decreased fertility.

Male fetuses can be prevented from full masculine development by inhibitors of androgen production or metabolism. Progesterone exposure has been proposed as having a role in hypospadias, an anomaly that is a feature also of the hydantoin embryopathy seen in the offspring of epileptic mothers taking this inhibitor of 5-alpha-reductase activity. In the majority of infants with male pseudohermaphroditism, the etiology remains unclear even after a thorough evaluation.

Abnormalities in gonadal determination may be associated with major chromosomal anomalies and other developmental anomalies (generally sporadic events), contiguous gene

syndromes, or genetic mutations of *SRY* (testis-determining) and other autosomal genes in the sexual determination pathway. Partial gonadal dysgenesis is the most common disorder of gonadal determination that causes genital ambiguity.

Clinical Manifestations and Diagnosis

Different aspects of sexuality are considered in evaluating an infant with an intersex disorder. *Genetic sex* refers to the XX or XY sex chromosome constitution, and *gonadal sex* refers to whether testes or ovaries are present. The sexual phenotypic gender can be subdivided into the external components and the internal constituents, which may be fairly disparate. Individuals who have a 46,XY karyotype and testes or streak gonads and are undervirilized have *male pseudohermaphroditism*, whereas those with a 46,XX karyotype, genital ambiguity, and ovarian tissue have *female pseudohermaphroditism*. Individuals having both testicular and ovarian tissue and those with dysgenetic or incompletely formed gonads fall into a separate category designated as *abnormal gonadal differentiation*. Given that every conceptus is endowed with the potential for either masculine or feminine phenotypic development (bipotential), the determination of genetic or gonadal sex is impossible on purely clinical grounds. A careful history may bring to light some valuable clues, such as androgen exposure in the mother, or a pedigree exhibiting an excess of infertile females with primary amenorrhea, which would be consistent with classic androgen-insensitivity syndrome.

Physical examination should address such questions as whether the infant has a "chromosomal look" with multiple dysmorphisms or features consistent with a specific syndrome associated with sex reversal or gonadal dysgenesis. Often, such an appearance is evident with sex chromosome anomalies, especially the 45,XO (Turner) and 45,XO/46,XY (mixed gonadal dysgenesis) syndromes. It is even more pronounced in some of the autosomal anomalies—for example, in the genital hypoplasia (micropenis) of trisomy 21 or the chromosome 13q syndrome. Ascertainment of the position of the gonads is important. Mobile, oval masses felt in what apparently are normal labia majora almost certainly will prove to be testes in keeping with "Federman's rule" that a gonad felt below the inguinal ligament will contain testicular tissue. Asymmetry of the external (and internal) genitalia is the hallmark of partial gonadal dysgenesis or true hermaphroditism. In the newborn period, the uterus may be palpable by gentle rectal examination with the fifth digit in virilized females. The female pseudohermaphrodite with CAH may exhibit full masculine development of the phallus with no hypospadias and a roomy, rugate, and often deeply pigmented scrotum, but this always will be empty (Fig. 62.4A). In contrast, male pseudohermaphrodites with decreased testosterone exposure in the third trimester, such as infants with panhypopituitarism, GnRH deficiency, or a testosterone biosynthetic defect, will have a hypoplastic scrotum and small phallus (Fig. 62.4B).

Laboratory studies are used in conjunction with radiologic imaging to complete the evaluation and to assist with gender assignment. In addition to a high-resolution karyotype, cytogenetic testing now includes specific tests for mutations and deletions in the *SRY* gene, and other identified genes in the testis-determining pathway such as steroidogenic factor 1 and the Wilms tumor gene. The functional connotations of the Y chromosome, in terms both of undesirable testosterone secretion in patients raised as girls and of the risk for neoplastic degeneration of the gonads, mandate the identification of Y sequences. Determination of MIS, secreted by the Sertoli cells of the testis, is highly sensitive for identifying testicular tissue in infants with genital ambiguity and nonpalpable gonads and can help delineate abnormal gonadal formation (in which values are low) versus male pseudohermaphroditism (in which values are normal or elevated). Newborn screening for 21-hydroxylase CAH now is available in the majority of states using the filter-paper assay for 17-hydroxyprogesterone. Nevertheless, blood should be obtained for adrenal steroids, testosterone, and gonadotropins in infants with genital ambiguity, and electrolytes should be monitored if CAH is suspected. Testosterone steroid precursors and dihydrotestosterone levels are essential if a defect in the testosterone biosynthetic pathway is in question, although making a definitive diagnosis may require human chorionic gonadotropin stimulation testing to test the pathway adequately.

The help of a pediatric radiologist should be enlisted to ascertain the nature of the pelvic organs and adrenals by use of ultrasonography or retrograde injection of contrast materials. A pediatric surgeon should be involved to perform a cystoscopy to confirm the radiologic findings, to obtain the gonadal biopsy, and for expert guidance in considering the feasibility of surgical reconstruction to give the infant an appearance consonant with the gender assignment being considered. The importance of a clear definition of the internal genital structures cannot be emphasized sufficiently. The vagina tends to be blind (i.e., absence of cervix) and shallow (2 cm) in AIS and long (greater than 6 cm) and topped by a patulous cervix in partial gonadal dysgenesis. In the true hermaphrodite, one gonad may be a normal ovary and the other a normal testis; more commonly, both are ovotestes, but the two types of tissues are both functional and are separated by a cleavage plane. Hence, surgical separation sometimes is possible, with retention of the gonadal tissue appropriate to the gender assigned to the infant.

The laboratory determinations required for gender assignment differ from those that ultimately may be needed for a final diagnosis. Gender-role selection requires cytogenetics and a definition of the internal genital structures by ultrasonography, standard radiography using contrast materials, cystoscopy, or any combination of the three. All babies with genital ambiguity should be monitored for serum sodium, potassium, and glucose concentrations until the CAH syndromes with accompanying cortisol and aldosterone deficiency can be excluded. In patients who have diagnoses of partial gonadal dysgenesis or true hermaphroditism and are raised as males, if the testis is left in place for testosterone synthesis (fertility being unlikely), the parents and, later, the children must be taught to examine the gonad regularly for tumors. Streak gonads, whether unilateral (the classic situation in partial gonadal dysgenesis) or bilateral, always should be removed when the karyotype contains Y material.

In infants who will be reared in the female gender role, any gonadal tissue should be removed that has the potential for androgen secretion at adolescence. In some neonates, addressing the question of whether any such tissue exists is necessary. High levels of gonadotropins (luteinizing hormone and follicle-stimulating hormone of greater than 20 mIU/mL) with negligible serum concentrations of testosterone (less than 20 ng/dL) indicate a negative answer. When this question has gone unaddressed in infants older than 6 months, the postnatal period of hypothalamic-pituitary-testicular activity will have ended. Both the gonadotropins and testosterone will be at nondiagnostically low levels, and a human chorionic gonadotropin stimulation test may be necessary. In response to subcutaneous injections of chorionic gonadotropin (500 IU on two occasions 48 hours apart), the normal testis will increase secretion of serum testosterone to twice the baseline concentration 48 hours after the first dose and will redouble it 72 hours after the second dose. Clearly, in the infant being raised as a girl, any significant rise in testosterone should lead to a search for its source, because of the need for surgical removal of the tissue. Androgen from the adrenal gland is not increased by chorionic gonadotropin but

will be responsive to adrenocorticotropic hormone (ACTH). Alternatively, a determination of serum MIS values during infancy may be sufficient to confirm the presence of testicular tissue and does not require stimulation testing.

Therapy

The timing of reconstruction of the genitalia to harmonize with the gender role selected has become controversial. Early timing of surgery, particularly for especially troubled parents, was thought to promote the ability of the parents to unequivocally raise the child in the assigned gender and improve gender identify and psychosexual satisfaction. Opponents of this have argued that the surgery itself can be disfiguring and can alter sensation, and should be considered cosmetic surgery that requires informed consent of the patient. Currently, insufficient data exists to strongly support either approach, thus each family should be approached individually about their desire for early versus late surgical reconstruction.

In boys with micropenis, treatment with testosterone should not be delayed, because the responsiveness of the phallic tissue may diminish with age. Testosterone in one of the repository forms (testosterone cypionate, or enanthate) can be given once a month, at 15 to 25 mg per dose intramuscularly for 3 to 6 months, until satisfactory phallic growth has been achieved.

ADRENAL DISORDERS

Pathophysiology

The CAH syndromes are the most frequently occurring of neonatal adrenal disorders, but three other conditions deserve mention, despite their rarity (Box 62.2). One is bilateral adrenal hemorrhage as an accident of birth, which leaves the neonate with adrenal insufficiency. The other two are genetic or congenital forms of adrenal hypoplasia.

The cytomegalic type of congenital adrenal hypoplasia is either of X-linked recessive inheritance or part of a contiguous gene syndrome involving Xp21.1–22, in which a mutation or deletion is found in the *DAX1* gene, a recently identified nuclear hormone receptor. In this disorder, the adrenal glands are composed of a fetal zone with large, vacuolated cells but no permanent adrenal cortex. The genitalia are underdeveloped, and surviving males fail to undergo puberty at adolescence because of a deficiency of the hypothalamic gonadotropin-releasing hormone. In the other form, the miniature type, the adrenals resemble those seen in anencephaly and other disorders of hypothalamic and pituitary development and may reflect either pituitary ACTH insufficiency or ACTH unresponsiveness due to mutations in the ACTH receptor.

BOX 62.2   **Important Adrenal Disorders in Neonates**

Congenital adrenal hyperplasia syndromes (most frequent)
Bilateral adrenal hemorrhage, leading to adrenal insufficiency
Genetic adrenal hypoplasia
  Cytomegalic type
   Miniature type

Diagnosis

In infants with congenital adrenal insufficiency, laboratory studies reveal hypoglycemia, hyponatremia, and hyperkalemia. Unlike most the CAH syndromes, low levels of all corticosteroids are evident, including progesterone, cortisol, testosterone, 17-hydroxyprogesterone, and aldosterone, whereas ACTH levels are elevated. During pregnancy, low maternal urinary estriols reflect decreased fetal adrenal steroid production and can be an early diagnostic clue for these disorders.

Therapy

The treatment of adrenal hypoplasia is similar to that for salt-losing CAH, consisting of replacement therapy for the cortisol and aldosterone deficiencies. Large doses of glucocorticoid (three to six times as much as required for maintenance needs) are necessary at diagnosis and in crisis situations. In the newborn period, hydrocortisone, 25 mg, is given as a bolus, then is administered intravenously every 4 to 6 hours. The high doses of hydrocortisone given during stress situations provide adequate mineralocorticoid replacement. Once homeostasis is restored, glucocorticoid replacement is provided with hydrocortisone, 8 to 10 mg/m²/day in two or three doses. Fludrocortisone acetate (Florinef), 0.05 mg daily, is the oral mineralocorticoid of choice. In contrast, treatment of adrenal hyperplasias often requires higher doses of both hydrocortisone (10 to 15 mg/m²/day) and fludrocortisone acetate (0.5 to 0.2 mg daily). Higher doses of glucocorticoids are given during stress, such as febrile illnesses and surgery.

THYROID DISORDERS

Congenital Hypothyroidism

Approximately 1 in 4,000 newborns has congenital hypothyroidism, the most common of the disorders identified through routine newborn screening. The paucity and nonspecificity of clinical symptoms and signs in neonates with hypothyroidism, and the improvement in outcome achieved by the earlier treatment of hypothyroid infants, make this disorder optimal for early diagnosis through newborn screening.

In most states, filter paper samples are assayed initially for thyroxine concentrations; this is followed by a thyrotropin determination in samples below a set cut-off or in those falling within the lowest tenth percentile of the samples assayed that day. If the serum thyroxine concentration is low and the thyrotropin level is elevated (greater than 20 μU/mL), the pediatrician and family are notified immediately by telephone.

Clinical Manifestations

At birth, infants with congenital hypothyroidism are typically asymptomatic, but may be postmature and LGA. Subtle features in the neonate include prolonged jaundice, umbilical hernia, difficulty feeding or sucking, temperature instability, and excessive somnolence. If untreated, clinical findings of a hoarse cry, large tongue, widened fontanels, hypotonia, lethargy, constipation, and mottled, dry skin gradually become evident. Congenital hypothyroidism due to an organification defect can be associated with sensorineural deafness (Pendred syndrome).

Diagnosis and Therapy

On notification of abnormal newborn screen results, the physician should obtain promptly a repeat blood specimen for free T4 and thyroid-stimulating hormone (TSH) to confirm the results of screening. Although the newborn screening programs still measure total T4 values, determination of the free T4 value on the repeat specimen and for future monitoring provides a more accurate index of biologically active thyroid hormone.

While awaiting the results of the repeat determination, levothyroxine (10 to 12 μg/kg/day) should be started and imaging considered to help elucidate the etiology of the hypothyroidism. The initiation of levothyroxine treatment before 14 days of life has been shown to optimize infant neurocognitive development. This approach to screening may miss infants with hypothalamic or pituitary hypothyroidism, a much rarer cause of congenital hypothyroidism (1 in 100,000). In infants with midline defects or those suspected of having mild hypothyroidism or pituitary dysfunction, a low normal free T4 may be indicative of central thyroid disease. Premature infants may have a delayed TSH response to low thyroxine levels, therefore repeat screening every 2 to 4 weeks is recommended for ELBW infants and those older premature infants who have low-normal thyroxine values but normal TSH values until both values clearly are in the normal range. All premature infants in our neonatal intensive care unit are screened at 2 to 3 days, then at 2 weeks, and subsequently monthly until they reach a weight of 1.5 kg.

Even after treatment is started, as long as the TSH values remain elevated, the thyroid tissue can be imaged through scintigraphy, using technetium or ¹²³iodine. Imaging may indicate the complete absence of tissue, thyroid ectopia (the most common anomaly in this group being lingual or sublingual tissue), or a normally positioned gland (dyshormonogenesis). The determination of epiphyseal maturation may be helpful in that the degree of retardation in bone maturation may be related to the duration and severity of the hypothyroidism and may correlate with cognitive outcome. In infants with congenital hypothyroidism, much as in normal neonates, none of the carpal centers or epiphyses of the wrist and hand will be calcified, so such a film has no value. Therefore, the lateral view of a lower extremity from just above the knee to the foot, which can be obtained expeditiously, provides the most information. In this view, the bones of special interest are the calcaneus (which normally ossifies at between 24 and 26 weeks' gestation), the talus (which ossifies at 26 to 28 weeks' gestation), the cuboid (which ossifies at 35 to 40 weeks' gestation), the distal femoral epiphysis (which ossifies at 36 weeks' gestation), and the proximal femoral epiphysis (which ossifies at 38 weeks' gestation).

Neonates found to have low serum thyroxine and high thyrotropin values may not have permanent hypothyroidism. Approximately 5% to 10% of neonates diagnosed with hypothyroidism have transiently abnormal thyroid function tests as a result of the transplacental transfer of maternal blocking antibodies against thyrotropin receptors of the thyroid gland. These antibodies are gamma globulins; with the gradual decline in all maternally inherited gamma globulins that takes place during the first 3 months after birth, the block to normal pituitary–thyroid interrelationships is removed. Nevertheless, treatment for these infants is as essential as for those with athyreosis. Iodine exposure of ill neonates undergoing surgical procedures also may cause transient hypothyroidism that must be treated. With these children in mind, most pediatric endocrinologists advocate a review at age 3 to 4 years of many patients designated as hypothyroid at birth. At this time, in contrast to infancy, a brief period of hypothyroidism is not deleterious to myelinization of the central nervous system. Children in whom a misdiagnosis of permanent congenital hypothyroidism was made, and who have been treated since birth with replacement doses of thyroxine, react in a characteristic fashion when the previously administered levothyroxine dose is halved or discontinued altogether. They will show a slight decline in the thyroxine values, reaching a nadir at approximately 2 weeks, with a rise in thyrotropin peaking at approximately 3 weeks; both values return to normal at 4 to 6 weeks in those with fully competent hypothalamic-pituitary-thyroid systems. Those in whom the diagnosis of permanent thyroid deficiency is confirmed show a much steeper drop in serum thyroxine concentration and a rise in thyrotropin, so that little trouble is experienced at 2 weeks (and almost none at 1 month) in distinguishing between the two types of responses.

Severe acute illness at any time of life is accompanied by a precipitous drop in serum thyroxine concentration, unaccompanied by a rise in thyrotropin. Thus, neonates and preterm infants with respiratory distress syndrome or sepsis account for the majority of "positive" results noted in the neonatal screening programs, with subnormal values for serum thyroxine but normal thyrotropin concentrations. Sometimes, these findings are attributable not to illness but simply to immaturity. These laboratory results may be a manifestation also of a common X-linked trait, deficiency of thyroxine-binding globulin; in male infants, the incidence may be as high as 1 in 5,000 newborns. These infants are euthyroid, with normal levels of free thyroxine despite low total thyroxine, and they do not need extra thyroid hormone. Approximately 1 in 100,000 neonates will have primary hypothalamic or pituitary disease and may need permanent replacement therapy. In the remainder of neonates with low values of thyroxine and normal thyrotropin levels, the thyroxine concentration will be restored to normal relatively rapidly. Box 62.3 discusses the treatment of infants whose screening results are only minimally abnormal.

| BOX 62.3 | Screening Infants for Congenital Hypothyroidism |

In infants whose results are only minimally abnormal, it may be reasonable to obtain a second specimen to verify the results before beginning thyroxine treatment. Just as false-positive screening test results occur, false-negative results also occur (i.e., affected neonates may escape screening or positive results may be misinterpreted as being normal). Furthermore, even well-performed screening is not infallible. On initial screening, approximately 1 in 150,000 newborns (or three of every 100 who ultimately will prove to have congenital hypothyroidism) either will have a thyroxine level sufficiently high that the thyrotropin determination is not performed or will have low thyroxine but normal thyrotropin levels. Such infants will escape detection until a second sample is analyzed or symptoms sufficient for clinical recognition develop. Thus, even in areas where screening is mandated, pediatricians caring for neonates still must be alert to the signs and symptoms of hypothyroidism and must not dismiss the diagnosis as improbable because of a normal newborn test. Screening programs have enabled pediatricians to detect the disorder and initiate treatment within 30 days of birth in perhaps 95% of all affected newborns in the program areas. In New England, most infants now are identified within a week of the screening test. The result has been an enormous improvement in the outlook for such infants. In the large patient cohort of the New England Hypothyroidism Collaborative Study, the affected children in whom treatment was initiated early have been compared with their next-in-age siblings, using a battery of neuropsychologic tests, and have scored equally well.

Congenital Hyperthyroidism

Congenital hyperthyroidism is much less common than is hypothyroidism. Usually, it is a transient disturbance, the result of the transplacental transfer of maternal thyrotropin-stimulating immunoglobulins that stimulate the pituitary thyrotropin receptors. The disorder can be anticipated in infants born of mothers with Graves disease, whether the disorder in the mother is active, suppressed by propylthiouracil or another blocking agent, or asymptomatic as a result of treatment, possibly years earlier, with ablative radioactive iodine or by subtotal thyroidectomy.

Clinical Manifestations and Complications

The characteristics of affected infants are excessive length for gestational age and low weight for length. Hyperthyroid infants are irritable, jittery, sleep poorly, stool frequently, and have feeding difficulties. On examination, these infants appear flushed, wide-eyed, hyper-alert, and emaciated. They may have tachycardia and hypertension with poor weight gain. A goiter may not be appreciated until several days of age.

Diagnosis

The diagnosis of neonatal hyperthyroidism in a neonate is confirmed by a suppressed TSH and elevated free T4 and total T3. If the infant is clinically asymptomatic with stable vital signs and only minimally elevated thyroid function tests, medical intervention may not be necessary. Repeat thyroid function tests should be monitored every few days or upon the development of any symptoms suggestive of thyrotoxicosis.

Therapy

In infants with tachycardia and feeding intolerance, or those with more elevated thyroid function tests, transient therapy is indicated. Treatment is with propranolol (1 mg/kg every 24 hours in three divided doses, increasing daily as necessary to control tachycardia, up to 5 mg/kg every 24 hours), either alone or in combination with propylthiouracil (5 mg/kg every 24 hours in three divided doses, up to 10 mg/kg/day), Lugol's iodine solution 6.3 mg/drop (1 drop every 8 hours), or SSKI 38 mg/drop (1 drop per day). Neonatal thyrotoxicosis may be severe, but usually runs its course in 3 months, in keeping with the elimination of the maternal antibodies responsible for the condition. Frequent examinations, close monitoring of heart rate, weight gain, and growth, and monitoring of thyroid function tests are essential to achieve control of thyroid hormone values in the high normal range or minimally elevated. Caution must be used to avoid inducing a hypothyroid state, because the thyrotoxicosis can resolve rapidly. In rare instances, a dominantly inherited form of permanent Graves disease is encountered, giving the same picture in the neonate as thyrotoxicosis, but persisting and requiring continuing thyroid-suppressive treatment or, ultimately, definitive therapy with either radioactive iodine or subtotal thyroidectomy.

Acknowledgments

We acknowledge Dr. John D. Crawford, Professor Emeritus of Pediatrics, Harvard Medical School and Massachusetts General Hospital, for sharing his extensive experience in the management of infants and children with disorders of the endocrine system.

Suggested Readings

Adrenal Disorders

Migeon CJ, Donohoue PA. Adrenal disorders. In: Kappy MS, Blizzard RM, Migeon CJ, eds. *The diagnosis and treatment of endocrine disorders in childhood and adolescence.* Springfield, IL: Charles C. Thomas, 1994:717.

Seckl JR, Miller WL. How safe is long-term prenatal glucocorticoid treatment? *JAMA* 1997;277:1077.

Speiser PW, White PC. Congenital adrenal hyperplasia. *N Engl J Med* 2003; 349:776.

Speiser PW, White PC. Congenital adrenal hyperplasia due to 21-hydroxylase deficiency (review). *Clin Endocrinol* 1998;49:411.

Speiser PW, Laforgia N, Kato K, et al. First trimester prenatal treatment and molecular genetic diagnosis of congenital adrenal hyperplasia (21-hydroxylase deficiency). *J Clin Endocrinol Metab* 1990;70:838.

Calcium and Magnesium Homeostasis

Cole DE, Quamme GA. Inherited disorders of renal magnesium handling. *J Am Soc Nephrol* 2000;11:1937.

DeMarini S, Tsang RC. Disorders of calcium, phosphorus and magnesium metabolism. In: Fanaroff AA, Martin RJ, eds. *Neonatal-perinatal medicine,* 7th ed. St. Louis, MO: Mosby, Inc., 2002.

Hendy GN, D'Souza-Li L, Yang B, Canaff L, Cole DE. Mutations in the calcium-sensing receptor (CASR) in familial hypocalciuric hypercalcemia, neonatal severe hyperparathyroidism, and autosomal dominant hypocalcemia. *Human Mutation* 2000;16:281.

Kovacs CS, Lanske B, Hunzelman JL, et al. Parathyroid hormone related peptide (PTHrP) regulates fetal-placental calcium transport through a receptor distinct from the PTH/PTHrP receptor. *Proc Natl Acad Sci USA* 1996;93:15233.

Mehta KC, Mimouni F, Khoury J, Tsang RC. Randomized trial of magnesium administration to prevent hypocalcemia in infants of diabetic mothers. *J Perinatol* 1998;18:352.

Munoz R, Khilnani P, Salem M, et al. Ultrafilterable hypomagnesemia in critically ill neonates: prevalence and clinical implications. *Crit Care Med* 1994;22:815.

Salle BL, Delvin E, Glorieux F, David L. Human neonatal hypocalcemia. *Biol Neonate* 1990;58(Suppl 1):22.

Disorders of Genital Ambiguity

Donohoe PK, Crawford JD. Ambiguous genitalia in the newborn. In: Welch KJ, Randolph JG, Ravitch MM, et al., eds. *Pediatric surgery.* St. Louis: Mosby–Year Book, 1986:1363.

Griffin JE. Androgen resistance—the clinical and molecular spectrum. *N Engl J Med* 1992;326:611.

Lee MM, Misra M, Donahoe PK, MacLaughlin DT. MIS/AMH in the assessment of cryptorchidism and intersex conditions. *Mol Cell Endocrinol* 2003;211:91.

MacLaughlin DT, Donahoe PK. Sex determination and differentiation. *N Engl J Med* 2004;350:367.

Misra M, Lee MM. Intersex disorders. In: Moshang T, ed. *Requisites in pediatric endocrinology.* Philadelphia: W. B. Saunders, 2004.

Welch WR, Robboy SJ. Abnormal sexual development: a classification with emphasis on pathology and neoplastic conditions. In: Kogan SJ, Hafez ESE, eds. *Pediatric andrology.* The Hague: Martinus Nijhoff, 1981:71.

Glucose Regulation

Cornblath M, Hawdon JM, Williams AF, et al. Controversies regarding definition of neonatal hypoglycemia: suggested operational thresholds. *Pediatrics* 2000;105:1141.

De Lonlay-Debeney P, Poggi-Travert F, Fournet J-C, et al. Clinical features of 52 neonates with hyperinsulinism. *N Engl J Med* 1999;340:1169.

Farrag HM, Cowett RM. Glucose homeostasis in the micropremie. *Clin Perinatol* 2000;27:1.

Hawdon JM, Aynsley-Green A, Alberti KGMM, Ward Platt MP. The role of pancreatic insulin secretion in neonatal glucoregulation: healthy term and preterm infants. *Arch Dis Child* 1993;68:274.

Hawdon JM, Ward Platt MP, Aynsley-Green A. Patterns of metabolic adaptation for preterm and term infants in the first neonatal week. *Arch Dis Child* 1992;67:357.

Kalhan SC, Parimi P. Gluconeogenesis in the fetus and neonate. *Semin Perinatol* 2000;24:94.

Mitanchez-Mokhtari D, Lahlou N, Kieffer F, et al. Both relative insulin resistance and defective islet beta-cell processing of proinsulin are responsible for transient hyperglycemia in extremely preterm infants. *Pediatrics* 2004;113:537.

Njolstad PR, Sovik O, Cuesta-Munoz A, et al. Neonatal diabetes mellitus due to complete glucokinase deficiency. *N Engl J Med* 2001;344:1588.

Stanley CA, Baker L. The causes of neonatal hypoglycemia. *N Engl J Med* 1999;340:1200.

Schlebusch H, Niesen M, Sorger M, Paffenholz I, Fahnenstich H. Blood glucose determinations in newborns: four instruments compared. *Pediatr Path Lab Med* 1998;18:41.

Srinivasan G, Pildes RS, Cattamanchi G, et al. Plasma glucose values in normal neonates: a new look. *J Pediatr* 1986;109:114.

Stanley CA, Lieu YK, Hsu BYL, et al. Hyperinsulinism and hyperammonemia in infants with regulatory mutations of the glutamate dehydrogenase gene. *N Engl J Med* 1998;338:1352.

Sunehag AL, Haymond MW. Glucose extremes in newborn infants. *Clin Perinatol* 2000;29:245.

Von Muhlendahl KE, Herkenhoff H. Long-term course of neonatal diabetes. *N Engl J Med* 1995;333:704.

Wolfsdorf JI. Hyperinsulinemic hypoglycemia of infancy. *J Pediatr* 1998;132:1.

Thyroid Disorders

Bongers-Schokking JJ, Koot HM, Wiersma D, et al. Influence of timing and dose of thyroid hormone replacement on development in infants with congenital hypothyroidism. *J Pediatr* 2000;136:292.

Fisher DA. Management of congenital hypothyroidism. *J Clin Endocrinol Metab* 1991;72:523.

LaFranchi SH, Snyder DB, Sesser DE, et al. Follow up of newborns with elevated screening T4 concentrations. *J Pediatr* 2003;143:296.

Newborn screening for congenital hypothyroidism: recommended guidelines. *Pediatrics* 1993;91:1203.

Selva KA, Mandel SH, Rien L, et al. Initial treatment dose of L-thyroxine in congenital hypothyroidism. *J Pediatr* 2002;141:786.

CHAPTER 63 ■ INFANT OF THE DIABETIC MOTHER

JOSEPH B. WARSHAW AND WILLIAM W. HAY, JR.

INTRODUCTION AND DEFINITIONS

Diabetes mellitus is the most common medical complication of pregnancy. Diabetes occurs in two forms during pregnancy, overt and gestational. Approximately 1 in 200 pregnancies is complicated by overt diabetes. Overt diabetes refers to clinically apparent diabetes diagnosed prior to or very early in pregnancy. Gestational diabetes develops in an additional 2% to 3% of pregnancies, accounting for 90% of all pregnancies complicated by diabetes of any kind. Gestational diabetes refers to patients in whom diabetes, defined as glucose intolerance of variable severity, develops during later pregnancy and disappears after delivery. Despite advances in perinatal care since the 1970s, diabetes in pregnancy remains a significant cause

TABLE 63.1

CLASSIFICATION OF DIABETES COMPLICATING PREGNANCY

Class	Onset	Fasting Plasma Glucose	2-hour Postprandial Glucose	Therapy
A$_1$	Gestational	<105	<120	Diet and exercise
A$_2$	Gestational	>105	>120	Diet and insulin
A$_2$ (a) Nonobese				
A$_2$ (b) Obese				

Class	Age of Onset (Years)	Duration (Years)	Vascular Disease	Therapy
B	>20	<10	None	Insulin
C	10–19	10–19	None	Insulin
D	<10	>20	Benign retinopathy	Insulin
F	Any	Any	Nephropathy[a]	Insulin
R	Any	Any	Proliferative retinopathy	Insulin
H	Any	Any	Heart	Insulin

[a]When diagnosed during pregnancy: 500 mg or more proteinuria per 24 hours measured before 20 weeks' duration. From the American College of Obstetricians and Gynecologists (1986).

of perinatal morbidity and mortality. Diabetes in pregnancy is classified according to the degree of glycemia (Table 63.1). The term *class A diabetic* often is used interchangeably with *gestational diabetic* or *chemical diabetic* (class A1, fasting blood glucose less than 105 mg/dL), but this use is not totally accurate because women with gestational diabetes with a fasting hyperglycemia of greater than 105 mg/dL may require insulin and are placed into class A2. This classification has been modified slightly over many years, primarily by noting whether the mother is obese, noting whether she simply has impaired gestational glucose tolerance without baseline changes in glycemia, and including other subgroups of women with more chronic complications of diabetes such as kidney disease, advanced stages of retinopathy, and pancreatic disease.

FETAL GLUCOSE SUPPLY AND METABOLISM

Glucose is transported across the placenta from maternal to fetal plasma according to the maternal–fetal arterial plasma glucose concentration gradient. The transport of glucose across the placenta, as with all membranes, follows saturation-limited or Michaelis-Menten kinetics. The K_m for transport is in the high range of normal maternal plasma glucose concentrations, allowing direct control of fetal glucose concentration by that of the mother. Glucose transport across the placenta is facilitated by specific transporter molecules; GLUT 1, a low-affinity transporter, which is the predominant isoform in the placenta; and GLUT 3, a high-affinity transporter that perhaps allows for enhanced transport even with maternal hypoglycemia. As a result of these transport mechanisms in the placenta, fetal plasma glucose concentrations are directly related to, but are about 20% less than those of the mother.

High concentrations of fetal glucose in response to maternal hyperglycemia stimulate the fetal pancreatic islet to secrete insulin. Fetal islet cell volume has been shown to be proportional to maternal glucose concentrations, and fetal macrosomia has been associated with increased plasma insulin and C peptide concentrations in cord blood. Insulin functions as a fetal growth hormone, resulting in the characteristic macrosomia of infants of diabetic mothers (IDMs). This macrosomia is primarily due to increased subcutaneous white fat deposition, the product of excessive glucose, glycerol derived from glucose, and fatty acids and triglycerides from the maternal

plasma that in the presence of insulin are synthesized into fat stores in fetal adipocytes. *In utero*, IDMs are not overgrown until sometime after week 26 or 27; this staging may be related to the development of insulin receptors. Evidence also indicates that insulinlike growth factor–I (IGF-I) contributes to fetal macrosomia. IGF-I may affect muscle mass more than insulin does, although both insulin and IGF-I act to promote cellular hypertrophy and hyperplasia. Insulin also decreases protein breakdown.

The risk of fetal macrosomia is increased when the mean maternal glucose concentration exceeds 130 mg/dL. Infants are the largest when maternal glucose concentrations are episodically increased, particularly following a meal (meal-associated or pulsatile hyperglycemia), as this form of hyperglycemia, when translated into surges of hyperglycemia in the fetus, has the greatest effect on fetal pancreatic insulin secretion.

Measurement of glycosylated hemoglobin (HbA$_{1c}$) provides an important index of longer-term diabetes control. Generally, normal levels of HbA$_{1c}$ are less than 8%. Many studies have demonstrated that elevated HbA$_{1c}$ concentrations are associated with increased perinatal morbidity. The obstetric goal should be maintenance of fasting glucose concentrations at less than 100 mg/dL and other plasma glucose concentrations at less than 130 mg/dL. Triglyceride and free fatty acid concentrations also should be monitored and kept in the normal range, as fetal adiposity is directly related to the maternal plasma concentrations of these substrates as well as glucose. Maternal obesity and subsequent pregnancy weight gain are more important risk factors for fetal macrosomia than either maternal glucose concentration or free fatty acid and triglyceride concentrations alone. All three indices should be monitored frequently in the pregnant woman with diabetes of any kind.

GENERAL CHARACTERISTICS OF INFANTS OF DIABETIC MOTHERS

IDMs have a characteristic appearance, with macrosomia (total body obesity), abundant adipose tissue, and a cherubic facial appearance; their head circumference, however, is similar to that of age-matched normal infants, because insulin does not influence brain growth. A typical IDM is shown in Fig. 63.1. Adipose tissue of IDMs often exceeds the normal 12% to 18% of body weight. The IDM also has an increased glycogen

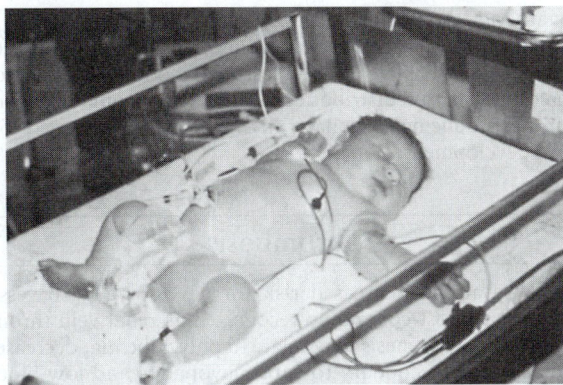

FIGURE 63.1. Infant of a diabetic mother.

content in the liver, kidney, skeletal muscle, and heart. The growth hormone-like effects of insulin result in increased linear growth.

Macrosomia contributes to birth trauma and birth asphyxia. Birth trauma can and should be prevented by frequent ultrasounds of the fetus documenting the degree of macrosomia, pelvic outlet size determinations, and cesarean section delivery. Perinatal asphyxia may occur in 25% of infants of insulin-dependent diabetic mothers. It is more common in macrosomic infants in part because of their size and in part because of the associated metabolic abnormalities. Asphyxia correlates with maternal hyperglycemia before delivery, particularly during labor. Intrapartum maternal and fetal hyperglycemia may result in increased fetal oxygen requirements. This places the fetus at risk of hypoxemia and acidosis during delivery when uterine contractions normally reduce uterine blood flow.

Asphyxia is also more common with maternal nephropathy. Nephropathy is associated with decreased placental blood flow; this association is confounded by the association of nephropathy with more severe maternal hyperglycemia, itself inversely related to placental blood flow.

Finally, changes in hemoglobin in severe diabetes may interfere with oxygen transport. Glycosylation of hemoglobin as with HbA$_{1C}$ increases the affinity of hemoglobin for oxygen, thereby decreasing the uterine venous PO$_2$ and transfer of oxygen to the fetus. Furthermore, decreases in 2,3-diphosphoglycerate (2,3-DPG) seen with recurrent ketoacidosis can add to the decrease in uterine venous PO$_2$. Further potential reduction in oxygen transfer to the fetus may be caused by increased diffusion distance in the thickened basement membranes or edematous trophoblastic villi in diabetic placentas.

OTHER CLINICAL PROBLEMS OF INFANTS OF DIABETIC MOTHERS

Problems of IDMs are summarized in Box 63.1. Despite their large size, IDMs are functionally immature. The risk of surfactant deficiency with respiratory distress syndrome and hyaline membrane disease in these infants is increased six fold until gestational week 38. Fetal hyperglycemia and hyperinsulinism have been associated with pulmonary immaturity and decreased synthesis of surfactant phospholipids and their associated proteins. Hyperbilirubinemia also is an index of immaturity and occurs in some 20% of IDMs. Contributing factors include newborn polycythemia and hepatic immaturity.

BOX 63.1 | **Problems of Infants of Diabetic Mothers**

Birth trauma
Birth asphyxia
Hypoglycemia
Hypocalcemia
Hypomagnesemia
Hyperbilirubinemia
Surfactant deficiency–related respiratory distress syndrome (hyaline membrane disease)
Polycythemia
Renal vein thrombosis
Cardiac septal hypertrophy and myocardiopathy
Congenital malformations

Metabolic Characteristics and Hypoglycemia

At birth, the neonate is separated from the constant supply of maternal glucose. Although IDMs have abundant adipose tissue and glycogen stores, they are less able than normal infants to mobilize these substrate stores. These abnormalities largely are the result of the metabolic effects of insulin, summarized in Box 63.2. Insulin is an anabolic hormone that promotes growth and the movement of glucose, fatty acids, and amino acids into tissues. Normal neonates rapidly mobilize glycogen from the liver and other sites to maintain plasma glucose concentrations. High plasma insulin concentrations inhibit glycogenolysis. Insulin blocks glycogen phosphorylase and inhibits the normal activation of phosphoenolpyruvatecarboxykinase, the rate-limiting enzyme of gluconeogenesis. Fatty acids and ketone bodies are alternative oxidative substrates and therefore help maintain normal glucose concentrations. Insulin increases transport of fatty acids into adipocytes, inhibits fatty acid oxidation, and redirects fatty acids into synthetic pathways. Ketone body production from fatty acids also is decreased. In summary, insulin results in increased glucose use, decreased glucose production, and decreased availability of alternate substrates.

Factors responsible for hypoglycemia in IDMs are summarized in Box 63.3. Blood and/or plasma glucose concentrations should be tested using a glucose monitoring device or a glucose oxidase strip within the first 45 minutes of life in known IDMs. However, infants known to be IDMs, weighing more than 4 kg, or exhibiting the physical characteristics of IDMs should be carefully and frequently monitored for initial and subsequent

---

BOX 63.2 | **Effects of Insulin on Metabolism**

Increase
  Glycogen
  Lipogenesis
  Protein synthesis
Decrease
  Glycogenolysis
  Lipolysis
  Gluconeogenesis

glucose concentrations as if they were IDMs. Hypoglycemia has been variably defined. Current working definitions of the lower limit for plasma glucose concentrations range from 30 to 45 mg/dL (25 to 40 mg/dL in whole blood) in term infants. The best treatment of mild, transient neonatal low glucose concentrations is early feeding, whether the neonate is an IDM or not. A blood or plasma glucose level of less than 20 or 25 mg/dL, respectively, requires intravenous glucose administration unless the infant readily takes a good feeding and remains normoglycemic.

Persistent (more than 30 to 60 minutes following an initial low glucose concentration) hypoglycemia requires intravenous glucose administration. If the infant is asymptomatic, a constant infusion should be started at 4 to 6 mg/kg/minute. If the glucose concentration is extremely low (unmeasurable to less than 10 to 20 mg/dL), especially when accompanied by seizures and/or coma or other symptoms consistent with hypoglycemia, the infant should receive 200 mg/kg of glucose (2 mL of 10% glucose per kilogram of body weight) over 1 minute, followed by a constant infusion of 8 mg/kg/minute (D10W at 115 mL/kg/day). This regimen will rapidly correct the severely low glucose concentration and help minimize the risk of rebound hypoglycemia. Only rarely will more glucose be required.

Hypocalcemia and Hypomagnesemia

Hypocalcemia is more frequent in IDMs. The pathophysiology is discussed in Chapters 62 and 64. Hypocalcemia, defined as a calcium level of less than 7 mg/dL, can contribute to agitation, irritability, and occasionally decreased myocardial contractility. Treatment rarely is necessary, but when indicated, consists of 1 to 2 mL/kg of 10% calcium gluconate given intravenously and 50 to 60 mg/kg/day given orally for maintenance. Maternal magnesium deficiency in diabetics may lead to fetal hypomagnesemia. This can worsen hypocalcemia by impairing parathyroid hormone (PTH) secretion and action because of limited magnesium-dependent adenylate cyclase. Hypomagnesemia (less than 1.5 mg/dL) rarely is of clinical significance. Magnesium treatment should be given with documented clinical signs of hypocalcemia and low plasma calcium and magnesium concentrations.

Polycythemia

IDMs may have symptomatic polycythemia. Fetal hyperglycemia and hyperinsulinism cause increased fetal oxygen consumption, fetal hypoxia, and increased levels of fetal erythropoietin. Increased insulin and insulinlike growth factors also increase red blood cell production. Polycythemia with hyperviscosity can be treated by partial exchange transfusion using saline to decrease the central hematocrit to less than 65% (see Chapter 66). Indications for partial exchange transfusion include respiratory distress, persistent hypoglycemia, and

hematocrits above 70%. The fetal erythropoietic response to hypoxia may occur at the expense of other bone marrow cell lines, particularly platelets. Increased red blood cell production can contribute to redistribution of iron away from developing neurons, producing neuronal iron deficiency and impaired cognitive development.

Thrombosis

IDMs are also at increased risk for developing deep vessel thrombosis, most commonly recognized as renal vein thrombosis. The pathogenesis may relate to polycythemia, decreased cardiac output secondary to cardiomyopathy, and low blood concentrations of the anticoagulant proteins (protein C, protein S, and antithrombin 3). The production of these proteins is decreased by hyperinsulinemia. Treatment of deep vessel thrombosis is supportive, including normalization of oxygenation and blood acid–base balance, but should include heparin when a large thrombus is documented by Doppler flow studies.

Cardiac Disorders

Cardiomegaly is common in IDMs, often associated with thickening of the intraventricular septum and subaortic obstruction. This complication may be one cause of the sudden late gestational deaths and stillbirths that occur occasionally in IDMs. Septal hypertrophy is found by echocardiography in 30% to 40% of patients. Interestingly, this complication is observed also in hyperglycemic low-birth-weight infants receiving parenteral nutrition; it is reversible with normalization of the blood glucose concentration by decreasing intravenous glucose infusion rates.

Congenital Malformations

Congenital malformations are more frequent in the diabetic pregnancy. The incidence of congenital heart disease and other major malformations is two to three times greater than that of the general population (3% to 5%) and has been related to poor control of maternal diabetes during the periconceptional period and the embryonic period that encompasses organogenesis. The incidence of all congenital malformations may be in excess of 10% in poorly controlled diabetic pregnancies. The caudal regression syndrome, characterized by hypoplasia of the sacrum and lower extremities, is found almost exclusively in IDMs (Fig. 63.2). IDMs may exhibit the small left colon

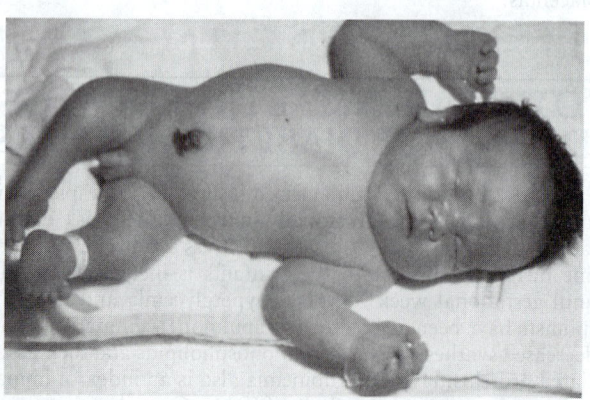

FIGURE 63.2. The caudal regression syndrome.

syndrome, which presents much like Hirschsprung disease (aganglionosis).

Major congenital malformations occur very early in gestation and, therefore, cannot be attributed to fetal hyperinsulinemia. Malformations probably relate to hyperglycemia during critical periods of organogenesis. Other teratogenic factors may include increased concentrations of ketone bodies, triglycerides, and branched-chain amino acids. Optimal control of maternal diabetes should be instituted even before conception to be certain of good control during the period of organogenesis, when congenital malformations occur. Vigorous preconception care of women with diabetes has been shown not only to decrease complications but also to be cost-effective.

Intrauterine Growth Restriction

Intrauterine growth restriction can occur if maternal diabetes is associated with severe vascular disease, particularly when the mother is hypertensive and/or has preeclampsia. Pregnancies thus affected should be monitored carefully and may require early delivery if fetal well-being is jeopardized.

Predisposition to Pathology in Later Life

IDMs may not maintain their macrosomia in early childhood, but they tend to be obese in childhood and adolescence. This has implications for adult obesity and insulin resistance. This is discussed in Chapter 20.

DIAGNOSIS AND MANAGEMENT

Overt diabetes in pregnancy is relatively easily diagnosed when the pregnant mother has high plasma glucose concentrations, glucosuria, polyuria, polydipsia, ketoacidosis, and unexplained weight loss or fasting glucose of 126 mg/dL or higher. Pregnant women with overt diabetes should be managed in a perinatal center by a high-risk pregnancy health care group equipped to monitor the pregnancy and employing staff in a newborn facility capable of caring for newborns in the event of an adverse outcome. Overt diabetes around conception increases the risk of embryopathy (neural tube defects, cardiac defects, caudal regression syndrome, spontaneous abortions). Later in gestation, if not successfully treated, maternal diabetes carries a high risk of fetal death. Overt diabetes in pregnancy also increases the risk of surfactant deficiency and respiratory distress syndrome. The risk of preterm delivery is increased two- to fourfold.

All pregnant women should be screened for gestational diabetes between weeks 24 and 28 of pregnancy. In the two-step procedure, those who have a plasma glucose concentration in excess of 180 to 190 mg/dL 1 hour after the oral administration of 50 g of glucose (and 155 to 165 mg/dL after 2 hours and 140 to 145 mg/dL after 3 hours) should be followed closely and should have a second oral glucose tolerance using 100 g of glucose. If diabetes is suspected based on marked and long-standing obesity, family/ethnic/racial history, or other clinical signs, a one-step procedure using a 100-g oral glucose tolerance test can be done first. Insulin therapy may be required to treat gestational diabetics who have persistent hyperglycemia. Insulin may lead to increased blood pressure, however, better dietary management, especially when combined with exercise, has decreased the need for insulin.

Suggested Readings

Barker DJ. Intrauterine programming of adult disease. *Molecular Medicine Today* 1995;1:418.

Barker DJ, Hales CN, Fall CH, et al. Type 2 (non-insulin-dependent) diabetes mellitus, hypertension and hyperlipidaemia (syndrome X): relation to reduced fetal growth. *Diabetologia* 1993;36:62.

Carrapato MR, Marcelino F. The infant of the diabetic mother: the critical developmental windows. *Early Pregnancy* 2001;5:57.

Coetzee EJ, Levitt NS. Maternal diabetes and neonatal outcome. *Semin Neonatol* 2000;5:221.

Cordero L, Treuer SH, Landon MB, Gabbe SG. Management of infants of diabetic mothers. *Arch Pediatr Adolesc Med* 1998;152:249.

Cowett RM, Farrag HM. Selected principles of perinatal-neonatal glucose metabolism. *Semin Neonatol* 2004;9:37–47.

Cowett RM, Schwartz R. The infant of the diabetic mother. *Pediatr Clin North Am* 1982;29:1213.

Elixhauser A, Weschler JM, Kitzmiller JL, et al. Cost-benefit analysis of preconception care for women with established diabetes mellitus. *Diabetes Care* 1993;16:1146.

Freinkel N, Lews NJ, Akazawa S, et al. The honeybee syndrome: implications of the teratogenicity of mannose in rat-embryo culture. *N Engl J Med* 1984;310:223.

Hay WW Jr. Nutrient delivery and metabolism in the fetus. In: Hod M, Jovanovic L, Di Renzo GC, et al., eds. *Textbook of diabetes and pregnancy*, London: Martin Dunitz, 2003:201.

Jovanovic L. A tincture of time does not turn the tide: type 2 diabetes trends in offspring of type 2 diabetic mothers. *Diabetes Care* 2000;23:1219.

Lindsay RS, Hanson RL, Bennett PH, Knowler WC. Secular trends in birth weight, BMI, and diabetes in the offspring of diabetic mothers. *Diabetes Care* 2000;23:1249.

Manco-Johnson MJ, Carver T, Jacobson LJ, et al. Hyperglycemia-induced hyperinsulinemia decreases maternal and fetal plasma protein C concentration during ovine gestation. *Pediatr Res* 1994;36:293.

Mimouni F, Miodovnik M, Siddiqi T, et al. Perinatal asphyxia in infants of insulin-dependent diabetic mothers. *J Pediatr* 1988;113:345.

Morris MA, Grandis AS, Litton JC. Glycosylated hemoglobin concentration in early gestation associated with neonatal outcome. *Am J Obstet Gynecol* 1985;153:651.

Namgung R, Tsang RC. Factors affecting newborn bone mineral content: in utero effects on newborn bone mineralization. *Proc Nutr Soc* 2000;59:55.

Nelson CA, Wewerka S, Thomas KM, et al. Neurocognitive sequelae of infants of diabetic mothers. *Behav Neurosci* 2000;114:950.

Nold JL, Georgieff MK. Infants of diabetic mothers. *Pediatr Clin North Am* 2004;51:619.

Paisley JE, Hay WW Jr. Infant of the diabetic mother [Pediatric Web site]. Available at: http://www.pediatricweb.com. Accessed January 15, 2000.

Pedersen J. *The pregnant diabetic and her newborn*, 2nd ed. Baltimore: Williams & Wilkins, 1977:15.

Piper JM, Langer D. Does maternal diabetes delay fetal pulmonary maturity? *Am J Obstet Gynecol* 1993;168:783.

Rosenn BM, Miodovnik M. Glycemic control in the diabetic pregnancy: is tighter always better? *J Matern Fetal Med* 2000;9:29.

Schwartz R, Teramo KA. Effects of diabetic pregnancy on the fetus and newborn. *Semin Perinatol* 2000;24:120.

CHAPTER 64 ■ MINERAL METABOLISM IN THE NEWBORN

JOSEPH M. GERTNER

SKELETAL DEVELOPMENT IN THE FETUS AND NEONATE

Histogenesis and Organogenesis of the Skeleton

At the end of a 40-week term of gestation, the neonatal skeleton has reached an organization close to that of the adult. The development of the skeleton depends on the integration of events directing cells derived from primitive mesenchyme to produce bone matrix, mineralize that matrix, and then remodel the resulting bone. This entire process is under complex genetic control and can be distorted by disordered formation of fibrous and nonfibrous matrix proteins, faulty migration of bone-forming cells, the failure to recruit the appropriate cells for bone remodeling, and abnormalities of the hormonal and ionic milieu needed to promote mineralization.

The precursors of bone cells begin to form at approximately 5 weeks' gestation from membranes or rods of mesenchymal cells. Intramembranous bone forms the sides and vault of the skull and the clavicles, whereas endochondral ossification accounts for most of the remaining bones, particularly those of the developing limbs. In both forms of ossification, osteoprogenitor cells condense, mature into alkaline phosphatase–positive osteoblasts, secrete an extracellular ground substance, and begin to mineralize. A network of collagen fibers forms the framework on which the first bony trabecula mineralizes to form the so-called primary spongiosa. Secondary foci of ossification that eventually become epiphyseal centers differentiate from mesenchyme in an analogous manner. Remodeling of the skeleton begins as soon as the primary spongiosa is formed; osteoclasts resorb existing bone, whereas osteoblasts form new bone.

Ionic and Hormonal Effects on the Fetal Skeleton

The mineralization process depends on the controlled delivery of calcium and phosphate to the sites of ossification and on the local effects of the calciotropic hormones (i.e., parathyroid hormone [PTH], calcitriol (1,25-dihydroxyvitamin D), and calcitonin). Calcium and phosphorus are transported across the placenta against a concentration gradient that appears as early as 12 weeks. The quantity transported increases sharply until late in the last trimester, by which time the fetus is accumulating up to 85 mg/kg/day of phosphorus and 150 mg/kg/day of calcium (Fig. 64.1). Placental calcium transport depends on the availability of calcitriol and the PTH-related peptide (PTHrP), but no known intrinsic disorders of the placenta exist that specifically limit calcium and phosphorus accumulation. Mineral deficiency may accompany the general fetal malnutrition characteristic of placental insufficiency. Pathologic consequences can arise from disordered transplacental calcium transport when calcium concentrations in the maternal serum are too high or too low. These disorders are considered in detail in the following section.

PTH is an 84–amino acid peptide secreted by the parathyroid glands that elevates serum ionized calcium by promoting bone resorption. The parathyroid glands are formed from cells of the third and fourth pharyngeal pouches at the sixth to seventh week of gestation and stain positively for PTH by the twelfth week. The parathyroid glands are the principal regulators of extracellular ionized calcium concentration. The chief cells serve both as calcium sensors and effectors of calcium homeostasis. A calcium ion–sensitive G-protein–linked receptor (CaSR) detects ionized calcium concentration in the extracellular fluid and modifies secretion of PTH. Fetal hypoparathyroidism is without effect on the fetus because maternal calcium homeostasis prevails *in utero*. Intrauterine hyperparathyroidism, on the other hand, can lead to pathologic resorption of the fetal skeleton.

The C cells of the thyroid are derived from ultimobranchial (fifth pharyngeal pouch) tissue and also begin to secrete their 22–amino acid peptide, calcitonin, at an early stage of gestation. Acutely, calcitonin lowers the extracellular ionized calcium concentration by inhibiting bone resorption. However, humans of all ages maintain normal calcium homeostasis and bone turnover in the absence of calcitonin (e.g., in athyreotic states) and in the presence of large excesses of the hormone (medullary carcinoma of the thyroid). The physiologic function of calcitonin, both *in utero* and in the neonatal period, is thus obscure. It has been suggested that the neonatal hypercalcitoninemia contributes to neonatal hypercalcemia.

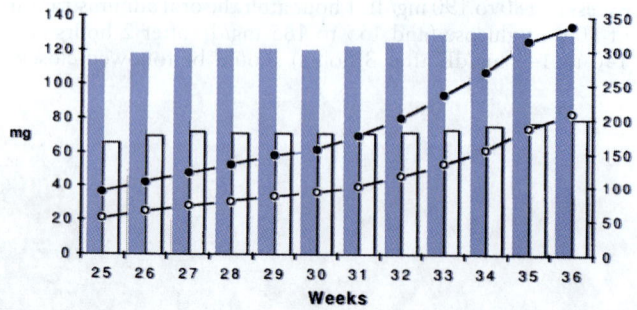

FIGURE 64.1. The intrauterine accumulation of phosphorus and calcium during late pregnancy. White circle, phosphorus (mg/day); black circle, calcium (mg/day).

A third calciotropic hormone, calcitriol, is a lipid-soluble sterol that, unlike the two peptide hormones, can be transported across the placenta. Although clear evidence shows that both the fetal kidneys and the placenta itself can make calcitriol, we do no know what proportion of the hormone is transported from the maternal circulation as opposed to synthesis in the fetus or placenta. However, It has been established that the precursor sterol, calcidiol (25-hydroxyvitamin D), is transported across the placenta. Its concentration in fetal blood is highly correlated with the maternal level, and it is needed for fetal synthesis of calcitriol. The major biologic action of calcitriol, the promotion of intestinal calcium absorption, is, of course, unnecessary during fetal life. The role of fetal vitamin D metabolites in the process of bone development is unclear, but the existence of congenital rickets as a pathologic entity suggests that vitamin D sterols do exert some direct effect on mineralization.

Another substance, discovered more recently than PTH or vitamin D, that may affect prenatal and perinatal bone mineral physiology is PTHrP, which has come under investigation. This 141–amino acid peptide was first characterized in malignant cells derived from patients with the syndrome of hypercalcemia of malignancy. PTHrP shares a region of homology with PTH, encompassing the 13 N-terminal amino acids, and it shares with PTH the power to bind to the type 1 PTH receptor, activating bone resorption and renal tubular phosphate reabsorption. Messenger RNA for PTHrP and the peptide itself are found in the lactating breast, with considerable quantities secreted into the milk, and in placental tissue. The corresponding PTHrP appears to influence the function of the uteroplacental vasculature and to play a part in transplacental calcium transport, but the importance of this role and the effect, if any, of PTHrP on the fetus and infant from the placenta or breast milk remains unclear.

Perinatal Mineral Homeostasis

After delivery, the fetus must adapt to the sudden withdrawal of an abundant placental supply of calcium and phosphate. Mean fetal calcium levels decrease from approximately 11 mg/dL at birth to a nadir of approximately 8.5 mg/dL in full-term and 7.0 mg/dL in premature infants (Fig. 64.2).

These minimum levels of serum calcium occur 1 to 2 days after delivery and give rise to hormonal adjustments that promote the infant's metabolic adaptation to postnatal mineral homeostasis. PTH levels appear to increase postnatally, an appropriate response to the decrease in serum calcium. Serum calcitonin levels are said to be high in the perinatal period, but little information is available concerning changes during the first few days of postnatal life.

Mean serum calcidiol and calcitriol concentrations are lower in neonates than in mothers but do not differ between full-term and premature babies. In full-term and premature infants, serum calcitriol increases from birth to day 5 and decreases again by day 30, but in preterm infants, calcitriol levels are higher than in full-term infants on day 30. The role of calcitriol in calcium homeostasis depends largely on the promotion of gastrointestinal calcium absorption, so it follows that the postnatal increase in calcitriol will be less effective in infants whose oral calcium intake is inadequate or who have disordered intestinal function. Disorders of calcium control in the neonate can arise because of failures of the PTH–vitamin D homeostatic system or because that system is overwhelmed by unfavorable circumstances. These disorders are discussed in the sections on Neonatal Hypercalcemia and Neonatal Hypocalcemia.

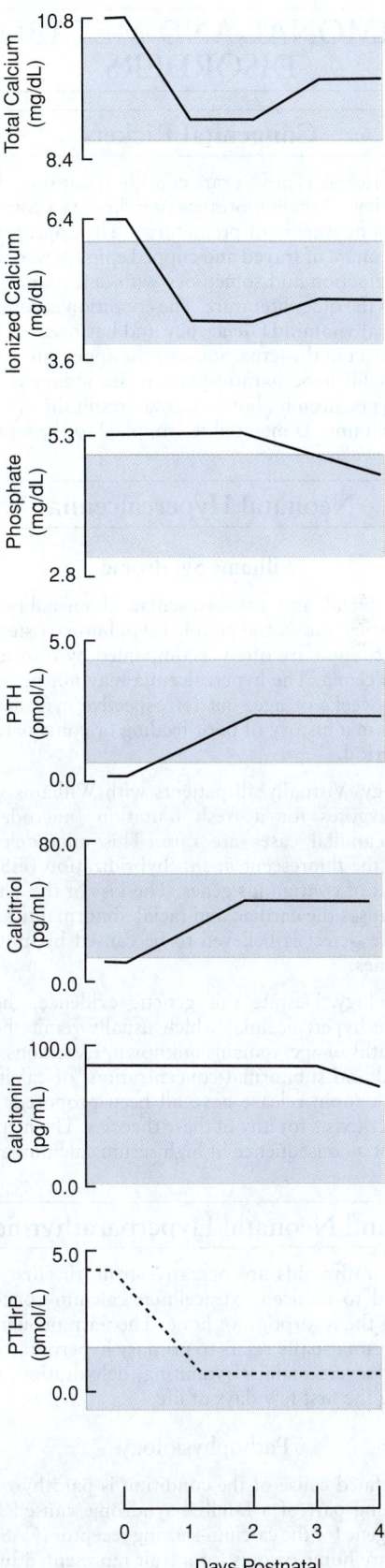

FIGURE 64.2. Changes in biochemical measures in the neonatal period. PTH, parathyroid hormone; PTHrP, parathyroid hormone–related peptide. (Modified from Kovacs CD, Kronenberg HM. Maternal-fetal calcium and bone metabolism during pregnancy, puerperium, and lactation. *Endocr Rev* 1997;18:832.)

HORMONAL AND METABOLIC DISORDERS

Congenital Rickets

Congenital rickets is now a rare condition but is of theoretical interest in view of the importance of rickets as a component of metabolic bone disease of prematurity. The appearance in the full-term neonate of frayed and cupped epiphyses, with general skeletal rarefaction and sometimes with deformities, was well described in the older literature. The condition accompanies severe maternal vitamin D deficiency and has been attributed to the same defect in the fetus. Some of the appearances are likely caused by fetal hyperparathyroidism, secondary to maternal and fetal hypocalcemia, but some may result directly from deficiency of vitamin D metabolites supplied to the fetus.

Neonatal Hypercalcemia

Williams Syndrome

Congenital facial and cardiovascular abnormalities (supravalvular aortic stenosis and peripheral pulmonary stenosis) and mental retardation are often accompanied by transient infantile hypercalcemia. The hypercalcemia may not be recognized until many weeks of age, but retrospective evidence may be obtained from a history of poor feeding or constipation in the neonatal period.

Epidemiology. Virtually all patients with Williams syndrome are heterozygotes for a fresh mutation (microdeletion at 7q11.23). Familial cases are rare. This microdeletion, detectable by the fluorescent *in situ* hybridization (FISH), gives rise to a loss of contiguous genes. The loss of the elastin gene probably causes the cardiac and facial abnormalities, whereas the cognitive defect is believed to be caused by mutations in adjacent genes.

Pathophysiology. Despite this genetic evidence, the precise cause of the hypercalcemia, which usually remits between 9 and 18 months of age, remains unknown. Elevations in calcidiol, elevated and subnormal concentrations of calcitriol, and deficient calcitonin release have all been proposed, but little firm evidence exists for any of these theories. The mental retardation is not a consequence of high serum calcium levels.

Fetal and Neonatal Hyperparathyroidism

The fetal parathyroids are operative from the first trimester and respond to reduced extracellular calcium concentration by inducing the resorption of bone. The term neonatal hyperparathyroidism usually refers to primary hyperparathyroidism detected by severe malaise (vomiting, dehydration, constipation) during the first few days of life.

Pathophysiology

The best-defined cause of the condition is parathyroid hyperplasia forming part of a familial syndrome caused by mutations in the gene for the calcium-sensing receptor (CASR). Most such cases are homozygotes for a trait represented by familial hypocalciuric hypercalcemia (FHH) in the heterozygotes.

A rare condition combining skeletal malformations with some of the biochemical manifestations of hyperparathyroidism is Jansen metaphyseal chondrodysplasia. This rare but theoretically interesting skeletal dysplasia was described in 1934 by Jansen. Recently, gain-of-function mutations in the type 1 PTH receptor gene, which is also the receptor for PTHrP, have been shown to cause the condition. These patients are hypercalcemic with suppressed PTH levels. The embryogenesis of the peripheral skeleton seems to require PTHrP, and it may be disruption of the PTHrP system rather than the activation of PTH receptor signaling that leads to chondrodysplasia in affected individuals.

In secondary hyperparathyroidism, the fetal glands are stimulated by fetal hypocalcemia caused by maternal hypocalcemia. These circumstances can occur in maternal vitamin D deficiency (see previous discussion) and also where the mother has untreated hypoparathyroidism. As in primary hyperparathyroidism, the bones are rarefied and spontaneous fractures may occur. Biochemically the condition evolves from hypocalcemia (present prenatally and responsible for the condition) through normocalcemia to hypercalcemia caused by an autonomous release of PTH even when the neonate is receiving an adequate oral calcium intake. Hypophosphatemia may be caused by PTH-induced phosphaturia. During the first few months of life, the skeletal lesions tend to heal rapidly and the parathyroid glands regress and resume normal function.

Clinical Manifestations and Complications

These infants are always hypercalcemic; soon after delivery they become hypophosphatemic. Immunoreactive PTH levels are high. Aminoaciduria, probably caused by a direct effect of PTH on the renal tubule, is common. Erosion of bone may be seen on skeletal radiographs.

Treatment of Neonatal Hypercalcemia

Hypercalcemia can lead to gastrointestinal dysfunction, failure to thrive, hypercalciuria, and, when severe, dehydration. Treatment should be tailored to fit the severity of the hypercalcemia and its consequences. Emergency treatment is needed for dehydration. Rehydration with 0.9% saline corrects the dehydration of hypercalcemia and induces a kaliuresis. Urinary calcium losses can be further increased by the administration of furosemide 6 mg/kg/day (in divided doses). Calcitonin, given subcutaneously, may be effective for a few days, but tolerance to its action soon develops. In theory, bisphosphonates, which have been used to treat hypercalcemia in older children, might prove useful in this type of emergency. Corticosteroids are not beneficial in hypercalcemia due to hyperparathyroidism, but are effective in Williams syndrome and vitamin D toxicity. Clearly, their chronic use should be avoided because of the many adverse consequences of glucocorticoid administration to young children. In neonatal hyperparathyroidism, emergency parathyroidectomy has been used as a definitive therapy with, in some cases, autotransplantation of some of the parathyroid tissue into an accessible site such as the forearm.

Milder degrees of chronic hypercalcemia can be treated with a low-calcium diet. This should not be undertaken without expert nutritional advice because both calcium depletion and phosphate depletion can result from injudicious use of such diets in growing children. Where hypercalcemia is mild, especially in the aptly named familial benign hypercalcemia (familial hypocalciuric hypercalcemia), no therapy is needed.

Neonatal Hypocalcemia

Neonatal hypocalcemia is generally divided into early and late forms according to the age (in days) of onset. The early form generally begins on the first to third day of life, while the late form becomes evident only after a week or so.

Early Neonatal Hypocalcemia

Hypocalcemia occurs in low-birth-weight and sick infants 1 to 4 days of age. Hypocalcemia may present with jittery movements, convulsions, apnea, or myocardial dysfunction. It may be considered an exaggeration of the physiologic drop in ionized calcium seen at this age.

Pathophysiology. The causes of this hypocalcemia, which is more marked in preterm infants, are unknown. Parathyroid underactivity secondary to the normally high serum calcium of the fetus, diminished bone resorption associated with high calcitonin levels, and poor dietary calcium intake and absorption have all been proposed.

Diagnosis. Direct measurement of ionized calcium has been advocated because unlike measures of total serum calcium, no correction needs to be made for protein concentration or blood pH. Electrocardiography (long QT interval) may also provide a useful clue to the presence of subnormal ionized calcium. An ionized calcium concentration less than 2.5 mg/dL can lead to clinical symptoms. Although theoretically attractive, in practical neonatal intensive care unit settings the ability to measure ionized calcium directly does not seem to bring much clinical advantage over measurement of total calcium.

Late Neonatal Hypocalcemia

This disorder presents clinically at 5 to 10 days of age in full-term, and apparently healthy, neonates. Hypocalcemia is associated with elevated serum phosphate levels. The causes and biochemical findings are summarized in Table 64.1.

Permanent Hypoparathyroidism

Primary hypoparathyroidism may be due to inherited or sporadic isolated absence of the parathyroid glands. In some cases, hypoparathyroidism is combined with some or all of the other features of the DiGeorge syndrome (thymic aplasia, severe congenital heart disease with conotruncal malformations, and certain facial abnormalities). The effect of hypoparathyroidism is to reduce the capacity of affected infants to regulate serum calcium and to excrete phosphate. Symptomatic hypocalcemia may occur within the first day or two after delivery but, more commonly, it appears only as serum phosphate levels rise at 6 to 9 days of age.

Epidemiology

The DiGeorge syndrome is one of a group of overlapping syndromes associated with microdeletions of chromosome 22q and is considered to be a contiguous gene syndrome. Some cases are dominantly inherited. The severity and duration of the hypoparathyroidism are quite variable. It may resolve clinically after the neonatal period, sometimes recurring at times of physical stress such as cardiac catheterization or surgery.

Pathophysiology

A condition commonly classified with hypoparathyroidism is familial hypocalcemia with hypercalciuria. This dominantly inherited condition is due to activating mutations in the CASR gene (see previous discussion), which cause the parathyroid gland to maintain serum ionized calcium at a subnormal setpoint. Thus, serum PTH and phosphate levels are close to normal despite the presence of hypocalcemia with its clinical consequences. Because CASR is localized also in the thick ascending limb of the renal tubule, where activation of the receptor causes a reduction in calcium reabsorption, patients with familial hypocalcemia with hypercalciuria may become severely hypercalciuric as their serum calcium concentration is restored toward normal by treatment.

Diagnosis

The syndrome can readily be diagnosed by examination of a chromosome preparation treated with a fluorescent-labeled DNA probe corresponding to a known sequence in the deleted area (FISH).

Therapy

Treatment is to restore extracellular fluid ionized calcium with oral or intravenous calcium and to restrain the accumulation of phosphate by feeding a low-phosphorus formula such as PM 60-40 (Ross Laboratories, Columbus, OH). If hypocalcemia is severe or if it tends to recur whenever calcium supplements are reduced, a vitamin D metabolite can be added. Permanent therapy may be needed in most cases of primary hypoparathyroidism but some cases, as noted in the discussion on DiGeorge syndrome, seem to recover enough PTH secretory capacity to be able to discontinue treatment after a few months.

Transient (Secondary) Hypoparathyroidism

The parathyroid glands can be suppressed by prolonged intrauterine hypercalcemia, itself secondary to maternal hypercalcemia. Most commonly, the mothers of these babies have primary hyperparathyroidism. The clinical picture is virtually identical to that of primary hypoparathyroidism, but cases due to maternal hypercalcemia remit spontaneously within the first

TABLE 64.1

CAUSES OF LATE NEONATAL HYPOCALCEMIA AND ASSOCIATED BIOCHEMICAL FINDINGS

Condition	Serum Calcium	Phosphorus	Parathyroid Hormone
Hypoparathyroidism			
a. Permanent	↓	↑	↓
b. Hypocalcemia with hypercalciuria	↓	↑ or Nl	Nl
c. Transient (secondary to maternal hypercalcemia)	↓	↑	↓
Excessive phosphorus intake (Unmodified or inadequately modified cow's milk diet)	↓	↑	↑
Renal glomerular failure	↓	↑	↑
Pseudohypoparathyroidism	↓	↑	↑

few weeks of life. A check of maternal serum calcium is a mandatory part of the evaluation of neonatal hypoparathyroidism.

Phosphorus Overload

The ingestion of unmodified cow's milk is no longer seen as a practical problem in developed countries. Cow's milk contains six times as much phosphorus as human milk (950 versus 162 mg/L). Ingestion of a calorically adequate volume of cow's milk overwhelms the capacity of the neonatal kidney to excrete phosphate, consequently causing hyperphosphatemia, which shifts the equilibrium in calcium flow between bone and the extracellular fluid toward bone. It also diminishes calcitriol synthesis. Both of these changes operate to reduce the plasma calcium level. Phosphate accumulation is also a feature of chronic glomerular renal failure, with hypocalcemic tetany as a presenting feature in severely affected babies.

Pseudohypoparathyroidism

Pathophysiology

Resistance to PTH (pseudohypoparathyroidism) is usually caused by a mutation in the gene coding for the guanyl nucleotide subunit of the G-protein–linked PTH receptor (GNAS1).

Clinical Manifestations and Complications

The manifestations of hypoparathyroidism (symptomatic hypocalcemia with hypophosphatemia) may occur in the neonatal period or later in childhood, or they may be absent despite presence of the mutation and other phenotypic manifestations. Because G-protein–linked receptors apart from PTH receptors may also be involved, these children often suffer from hypothyroidism, which may be diagnosed at neonatal screening. Cognitive dysfunction and a characteristic bony phenotype (Albright's hereditary osteodystrophy) are later manifestations, although the characteristic moon facies may be present in affected neonates.

Diagnosis

Biochemically, pseudohypoparathyroidism is distinguished from true hyperparathyroidism by the high serum PTH levels seen in the former. Standard renal function tests can distinguish it from the calcium/phosphorus disturbances of neonatal renal failure.

Treatment of Neonatal Hypocalcemia

Mild hypocalcemia may not require therapy. A neonate with a serum calcium below 7.0 to 7.5 mg/dL (ionized calcium less than 2.8 mg/dL) should be treated to prevent tetany and other symptoms. In severe symptomatic hypocalcemia intravenous therapy is required. Slow parenteral infusions of 20 to 50 mg/kg/day of elemental calcium as the gluconate may be diluted with saline or dextrose infusion fluids and given intravenously. Alternatively, 10 to 20 mg/kg of elemental calcium can be given every 4 to 6 hours. Occasionally, higher doses are needed. Intravenous calcium should be given with great care, because overrapid administration can cause cardiac arrhythmias, whereas the extravasation of calcium salts can lead to local tissue inflammation and even necrosis. Serum calcium should be monitored frequently and the infusion adjusted accordingly. Chronic hypocalcemia is treated by the administration of vitamin D or its metabolites. Calcitriol is the treatment

of choice for chronic hypocalcemia. Circulating calcitriol has a half-life of less than 1 day, greatly enhancing therapeutic safety over earlier vitamin D preparations. Calcitriol dosage in small children is generally higher on a weight-adjusted basis than in the adult dosage (0.25 to 2.0 μg/day, occasionally higher).

Metabolic Bone Disease of Prematurity

Definition and Nomenclature

Metabolic bone disease of prematurity (MBDP) encompasses a spectrum of disturbances in preterm infants, which results in rickets, osteomalacia, and osteoporosis. Milder cases may show only biochemical changes. Rickets and osteomalacia describe undermineralization of normal organic bone matrix (osteoid), while in osteoporosis there is reduced bone mass with a normal ratio of mineral to matrix. Osteopenia describes decreased bone density on imaging. The term does not distinguish between decreased mineralization of quantitatively normal matrix and normal mineralization of diminished quantities of matrix. Little histologic information is available, and it is therefore difficult to assess the relative importance of rickets/osteomalacia versus osteoporosis in MBDP.

Epidemiology

The reported frequency of MBDP varies depending on the diagnostic criteria. The condition affects mainly premature infants, but also those close to term but small for gestational age. In one prospective radiologic survey, fractures were detected in 20% of newborns with a birth weight of less than 1,500 g and gestational age less than 34 weeks. Subclinical disease may be more common, as suggested by the prevalence of elevated serum alkaline phosphatase and decreased bone mineral content.

Pathophysiology

The primary cause of MBDP seems to be a deficiency of phosphate and calcium due to decreased intake. However, mechanical factors, leading to decreased mechanical loading of bone after premature delivery relative to the normal *in utero* state, may also play a part. Initial reports of MBDP involved infants fed human milk and sick neonates, whose illness was usually due to respiratory disease. Human milk is relatively low in calcium and phosphate. Infants with respiratory disease are at risk because of the low mineral concentration in hyperalimentation fluid, fluid restriction when on oral feedings, and increased urinary mineral losses secondary to furosemide therapy. Neonates with other, less common conditions such as hepatobiliary disease are also at risk. From prospective studies, however, it appears that MBDP also affects well preterm infants fed standard formulas.

Although phosphate deficiency is most commonly associated with osteomalacia, it can also lead to osteoporosis. Thus, phosphate-deficient rats show only a modest increase in osteoid, but a marked decrease in trabecular bone volume, indicating osteoporosis. Calcium deficiency also can cause metabolic bone disease, and is implicated in some cases of childhood rickets and in postmenopausal osteoporosis.

Eighty percent of calcium and phosphate accretion for the fetal skeleton occurs during the third trimester, by active transport across the placenta (see Fig 64.1). To maintain an intrauterine growth rate postnatally, comparable quantities must be provided from external sources to premature infants at an equivalent stage of gestation. Provision of adequate phosphorus and calcium is difficult primarily due to the inadequate quantities of these minerals in human milk and standard formulas. Assuming an intake of 150 to 200 mL/kg/day, human milk provides only 25% to 50% of the phosphorus and 35% to

70% of the calcium accumulated in the third trimester. A standard formula provides only 55% to 90% of the phosphorus and 45% to 100% of the calcium. Obviously, human milk and standard formulas provide insufficient amounts of phosphorus and calcium. Furthermore, only a proportion of the minerals absorbed are retained. Retention of phosphorus and calcium depends on the balance between net intestinal absorption and renal excretion. The ability of preterm infants to absorb phosphorus and calcium from the intestine and to reabsorb these minerals in the renal tubule is satisfactory. However, the following dietary factors may influence mineral retention:

1. The calcium-to-phosphorus ratio in the diet, which affects the intestinal and renal handling of both these minerals
2. The influence of the quantity and quality of dietary fat on calcium absorption
3. The use of soy formulas containing phytates, binding both phosphorus and calcium in the gut and decreasing their absorption
4. The effect of the relatively large volumes of intestinal secretions in preterm infants, a consequence of the large food volume needed to satisfy their caloric requirements

Adequate mineral delivery via total parenteral nutrition (TPN) is confounded by the difficulty of maintaining the solubility of concentrated mixtures of calcium and phosphorus. Thus, the amounts of phosphorus and calcium that can be delivered by TPN provide less than 50% of the supply of these minerals delivered to the fetus *in utero*. Whether so-called TPN bone disease or TPN-associated skeletal aluminum toxicity, both described in older children and adults, also play a part in the osteopathy of low-birth-weight infants receiving TPN is not known.

Most preterm infants, including those with bone disease, appear to have normal levels of calcidiol and are able to absorb calcium and phosphorus from the intestine efficiently. Thus, the condition is not caused by vitamin D deficiency. In some cases with MBDP, calcitriol levels are elevated, presumably because of stimulation by hypophosphatemia. Such elevated calcitriol levels may actually contribute to MBDP by stimulating bone resorption. Despite high levels of calcitriol, such infants are not hypercalcemic, possibly because of concomitant dietary calcium deficiency. No evidence exists that abnormalities of PTH or calcitonin production or secretion contribute to bone disease in preterm infants. The role of possible insufficiencies of factors such as trace elements, other nutrients, and growth factors remains to be excluded.

Clinical Manifestations and Complications

MBDP comprises a spectrum extending from overt bone disease (rickets and fractures) (Fig. 64.3) to mild biochemical disturbances. Fractures are usually located at sites (i.e., extremities, ribs) at which the infant may be physically manipulated during diagnostic or therapeutic maneuvers. If one fracture is noted, other fractures are likely. Limb fractures may cause pain, loss of movement, or deformity, whereas rib fractures can exacerbate respiratory distress.

The age at which the bony changes manifest probably depends on growth rate. According to one study, infants who were later to develop rickets had a low serum phosphate by age 2 weeks and an elevated alkaline phosphatase at 4 weeks. Decreased mineralization is evident on dual-energy X-ray absorptiometry (DXA) as early as age 2 weeks. Radiographic changes have been found from 4 to 20 weeks. In one prospective study, 75% of abnormal radiographs were noted by 3 months and all abnormalities by 6 months.

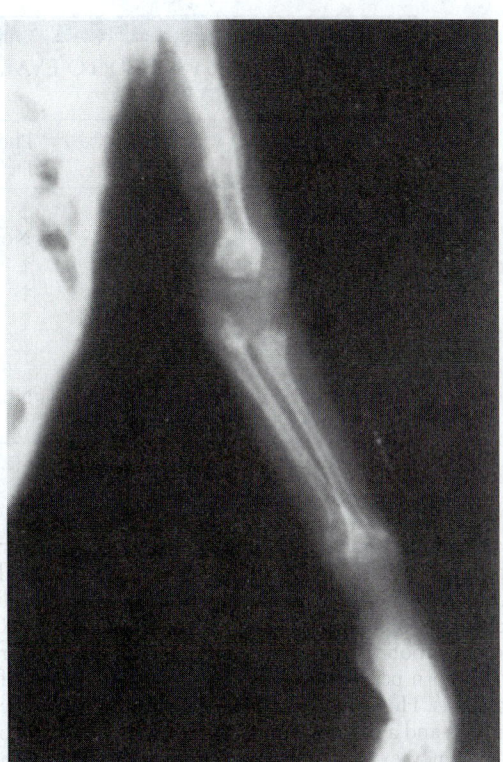

FIGURE 64.3. Osteopenia, rickets, and a healing humeral fracture characteristic of the metabolic bone disease of prematurity. (Courtesy Dr. D. E. Carey.)

Diagnosis

Several methods are used to diagnose MBDP before it manifests clinically. Radiography is unsatisfactory because of the difficulty in standardizing the conditions under which films are taken. In addition, for osteopenia to be detectable by routine radiograph, considerable bone loss must already have taken place. Despite this, the classification outlined in Table 64.2 has been proposed.

DXA has been adapted for use in neonates and has contributed to understanding the prognosis as well as making the diagnoses. In general, the mineral deficiencies of MBDP seem to resolve spontaneously during early childhood.

Biochemical tests may detect early MBDP. Alkaline phosphatase values in subjects with and without radiologic evidence of bone disease overlap. However, an alkaline phosphatase level that is more than five times the maximum adult level may suggest MBDP in a patient who is not on TPN and has no bone disease. A study of urinary pyridinium cross-link excretion (a measure of collagen breakdown) in premature infants revealed weight-adjusted values much higher than those in full-term newborns or older children. Along with the high alkaline phosphatase levels this supports the view that bone turnover is significantly increased in premature infants. Table 64.3

TABLE 64.2

CLASSIFICATION OF METABOLIC BONE DISEASE OF PREMATURITY

Grade 0	Normal bone
Grade I	Bone rarefaction only
Grade II	Metaphyseal changes (fraying, cupping) with subperiosteal new bone formation
Grade III	The previously mentioned changes with fractures

TABLE 64.3

LABORATORY TESTS USED TO EVALUATE INFANTS AT RISK OF METABOLIC BONE DISEASE OF PREMATURITY

	Phosphate Deficiency	Calcium Deficiency	Expected Value for Premature Infant
Serum phosphate	↓	↓	5.0–8.5 mg/dL
Serum calcium	Normal or ↑	Normal or ↓	8.0–11.0 mg/dL
Tubular phosphate reabsorption	↑	↓	85–95%
Alkaline phosphatase	↑	↑	<5% adult upper limit
Urinary calcium	↑	↓*	<4–6 mg/kg/d
Parathyroid hormone	↓	↑	Within adult normal range
Calcidiol (25 OH vitamin D)	Normal	Normal	3.6–10.8 ng/dL
Calcitriol [1,25 (OH)$_2$ vitamin D]	↑	↑	40–80 pg/dL

*Unless caused by excess renal calcium losses (e.g., furosemide).

summarizes the laboratory tests used to evaluate infants at risk of MBDP and indicates findings expected in pure calcium or phosphate deficiency. The mixed picture found in clinical practice leads to correspondingly intermediate results. Other types of metabolic bone disease are very unlikely to present in the newborn period and rarely pose a problem of differential diagnosis. However, vitamin D deficiency produces radiologic rickets and a biochemical picture very close to that of calcium deficiency except for low calcidiol value (less than 5 to 8 ng/mL).

Few reports exist on bone histology in MBDP. The ribs from three preterm infants who died of respiratory distress syndrome (RDS) showed osteomalacia, but to a lesser degree than in classical vitamin D–deficient controls. Osteoporosis, which was not a feature in the vitamin D–deficient controls, was pronounced in the infants with MBDP.

Therapy

A growth rate that approximates the rate *in utero* is a sensible goal and has been endorsed by the Committee on Nutrition of the American Academy of Pediatrics. The amount of phosphorus and calcium retained by the preterm infant must approximate that of the fetus *in utero*. Supplementation of feeds with phosphorus and calcium is difficult because of the formation of insoluble salts when these ions are combined. Some formulas that contain increased quantities of these salts have to be shaken before use. This can be a problem with continuous nasogastrointestinal feeds. Alternating administration of phosphorus or calcium is complicated by high urinary losses of the supplemented mineral. Nevertheless, fortified human milk and some of the special formulas for preterm infants (Similac Special Care, Enfamil Premature) do permit an increase in the absorption and retention of phosphorus and calcium approaching the fetal accretion rate. For example, volumes of 140 to 200 mL/kg/day will provide 185 to 200 mg/kg/day of calcium, 65% of which is retained, approximating the accretion rate of a fetus over 28 weeks (i.e., 120 to 130 mg/kg/day). As for phosphorus, an intake of 100 to 113 mg/kg/day, 71% of which is retained, approximates the accretion rate of a fetus over 28 weeks (i.e., 71 to 80 mg/kg/day).

Prognosis

Although some babies with MBDP may develop fractures and acute biochemical disturbances, little morbidity is noted in most infants with biochemical and radiologic evidence of MBDP. Increasing evidence shows that the condition is self-limiting with recovery of bone mineral content during the first few weeks and months of postnatal life.

Prevention

Increasing phosphorus and calcium retention does not necessarily translate into improved bone structure. Cases have been reported of preterm infants with severe MBDP that resolved after supplementation with phosphorus alone or in combination with calcium. However, the natural course of this condition suggests the possibility that resolution was spontaneous. Several prospective studies investigated whether MBDP could be prevented by increasing the intake (and presumably retention) of phosphorus and calcium. The results and conclusions of these studies have varied, perhaps because mineral retention depends on factors other than the total calcium and phosphorus content of the formula and also because different workers have used different densitometric criteria to evaluate response.

Despite the inconclusive evidence from the supplementation studies, the consensus is that unfortified human milk is not adequate for preterm infants. On the other hand, little overt MBDP has been reported in "healthy" preterm infants fed on standard milk formulas. Therefore, it is recommended that all low-birth-weight infants receive phosphorus and calcium in excess of what is present in breast milk. It has been suggested that such supplementation should continue until the infant's weight reaches 2 kg, but this may have to be modified according to circumstances.

The commercial premature formulas given in the quantities mentioned previously contain maximal allowable intakes for preterm infants of gestational age over 28 weeks. The American Academy of Pediatrics Committee on Nutrition advises a calcium intake of 210 mg/kg/day for preterm infants weighing 800 to 1,200 g. The Committee makes no recommendation for infants beneath or above this range and does not make its own recommendation on phosphorus requirements.

The minimal requirement of phosphorus and calcium for preterm infants on TPN is 30 to 40 mg/kg/day of each element, according to the American Academy of Pediatrics. It may be possible to circumvent the problem of low solubility of ionic mixtures of calcium and phosphorus by lowering the pH of the solution or providing a soluble source of both minerals such as calcium glycerophosphate. This compound has been shown to improve bone mineralization in piglets. Regarding vitamin D, a daily intake of at least 400 IU is recommended in addition to the vitamin D in the feeds. Higher intakes of this vitamin may be necessary where maternal vitamin D deficiency is a consideration.

Potential adverse effects of excessive calcium administration are hypercalcemia, hypercalciuria (with potential for nephrocalcinosis), hypophosphatemia, and decreased fat and phosphorus absorption. Certain calcium preparations such as

TABLE 64.4

MOLECULAR-PATHOGENIC CLASSIFICATION OF GENETIC DISORDERS OF THE SKELETON

Gene or Protein	Inheritance	Clinical Phenotype
Group 1: Defects in Extracellular Structural Proteins		
Group 2: Defects in Metabolic Pathways (Including Enzymes, Ion Channels, and Transporters)		
Tissue nonspecific alkaline phosphatase (TNSALP)	AR, AD	Forms of hypophosphatasia
ANKH (pyrophosphate transporter)	AD	Craniometaphyseal dysplasia
Vacuolar proton pump (TCIR GI)	AR	Infantile osteopetrosis
Cl⁻ channel 7 (CLCN7)	AR	Infantile osteopetrosis
Mutations in carbonic anhydrase II	AR	Osteopetrosis with renal tubular acidosis
Group 3: Defects in Folding or Degradation of Macromolecules		
Cathepsin K (lysosomal proteinase)	AR	Pyknodysostosis
Group 4: Defects in Hormones and Signal Transduction Mechanisms		
PTH/PTHrP, activating mutations	AD	Jansen's metaphyseal dysplasia with hypercalcemia
GNAS1 (stimulatory Gs alpha)	AD	Pseudohypoparathyroidism (Albright hereditary osteodystrophy)
Fibroblast growth factor receptor 3 (FGFR3)	AD	Achondroplasia
TGF-beta-1	AD	Diaphyseal dysplasia (Camurati-Engelmann disease)
SOST (cysteine knot secreted protein)	AR	Van Buchem disease
Group 5: Defects in Nuclear Proteins and Transcription Factors		
NEMO (Nf kappa B essential modulator)	X-linked	Osteopetrosis, lymphedema, and ectodermal dysplasia
Group 6: Defects in Oncogenes and Tumor Suppressor Genes		
Group 7: Defects in RNA and DNA Processing and Metabolism		

From Superti-Furga et al., 2001.
Superti-Furga A, Bonafe L, Rimoin DL. Molecular-pathogenetic classification of genetic disorders of the skeleton. *Am J Med Genet* 2001;106:282.

calcium lactate may result in metabolic acidosis. A potential adverse effect of phosphorus supplementation is hypocalcemia. Vitamin D excess should also be avoided since it can lead to hypercalcemia and hypercalciuria.

Concern that MBDP might also be linked to inadequate mechanical loading of bone has led to proposals that manipulation of the limbs might be helpful. However, the evidence supporting a beneficial effect is scanty.

DISORDERS OF BONE FORMATION

Disorders of Shape

Because the internal structure of a bone critically determines its shape, it is somewhat artificial to distinguish between disorders of morphogenesis and histogenesis. However, some disorders of matrix formation have a striking effect on bone morphology. Many disorders of limb morphogenesis are genetically determined. Such disorders may involve all or most of the skeleton diffusely, in which case a generalized error of histogenesis is likely to be responsible, or may very specifically affect one bone or a defined group of bones. The effort to devise a rational nomenclature for these disorders has led to their classification as dyschondroplasias, which are subdivided into five groups. With advances in genetics, the molecular etiology of many of these syndromes has been discovered.

As can be seen from Table 64.4, the skeletal dysplasias may result not only from abnormalities in structural proteins but also from abnormalities in components of cell signaling systems active in the skeleton. Achondroplasia is one of the more common representatives of the osteochondrodysplasias. Severe forms of this dominantly inherited condition may be recognized at birth or prenatally by ultrasound or radiologically (Fig. 64.4). The disease is due to heterozygosity for an activating mutation in the fibroblast growth factor type 3 receptor. Ho-

mozygosity for the same mutation causes a fatal thanatophoric dwarfism with severe deformities evident at birth. In another example, spondyloepiphyseal dysplasia, a developmental dysplasia of bone has been traced to a mutation in one of the genes coding for proteins of connective tissue (type II collagen).

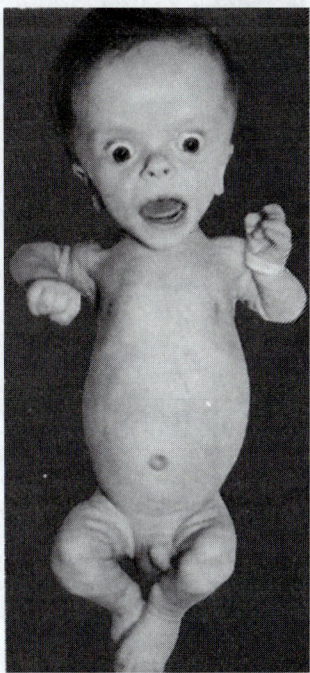

FIGURE 64.4. A three-month old infant with achondroplasia. Note the large head, short limbs, and protruding abdomen. (From Sadler TW. *Langman's medical embryology*, 9th ed. Baltimore: Lippincott Williams & Wilkins, 2003.)

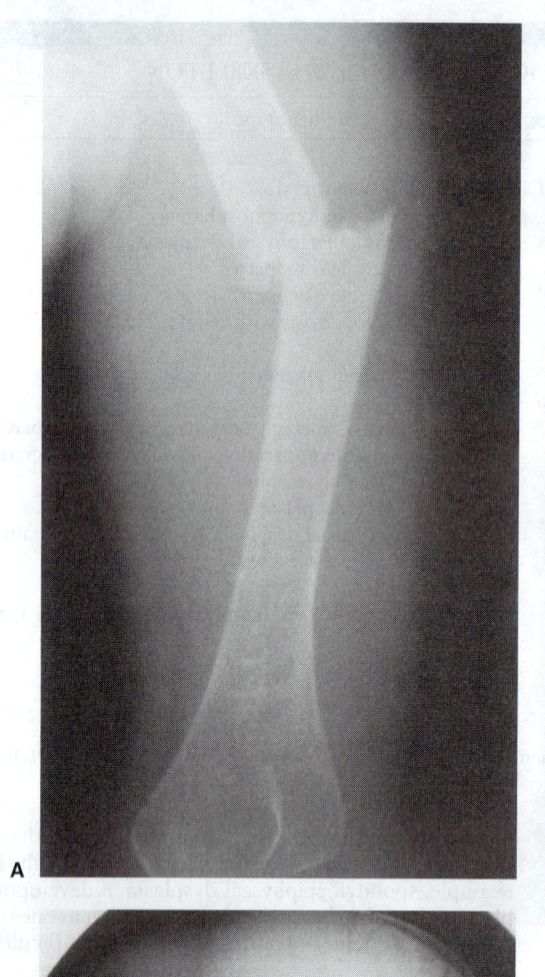

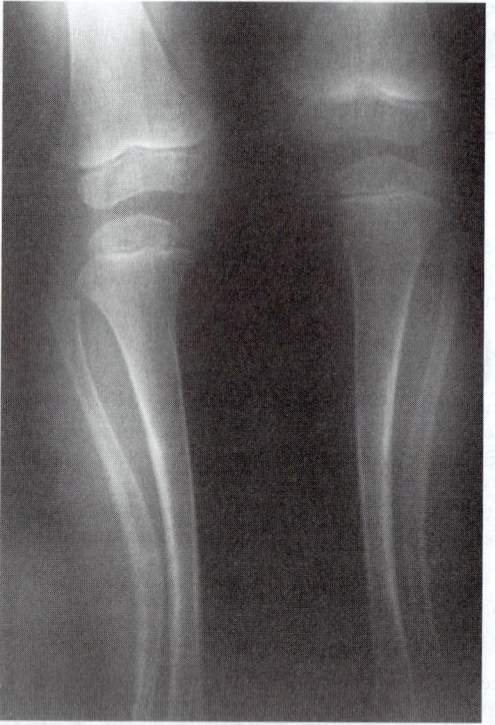

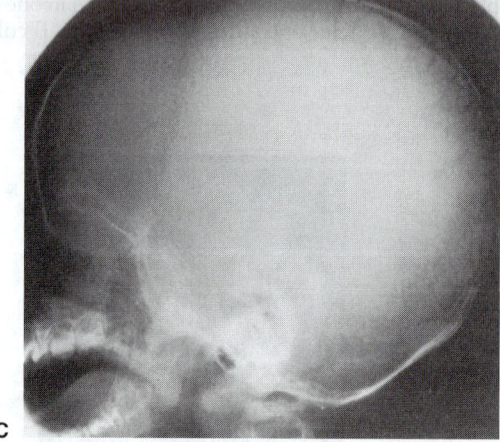

FIGURE 64.5. Osteogenesis imperfecta. **A:** An 18-month-old child (osteogenesis imperfecta) with clinically short stature has a transverse fracture of the left humerus. **B:** Symmetric tibial and fibular bowing. The bones are generally demineralized with thin cortices. **C:** The skull shows multiple sutural (wormian bones). (From Reece RM, Ludwig S. *Child abuse: medical diagnosis and management,* 2nd ed. Philadelphia: Lippincott Williams & Wilkins, 2001:150, with permission.)

DISORDERS OF BONE STRUCTURE

Disorders of bone structure may be due to abnormal bone matrix synthesis or to abnormalities of the ionic or hormonal milieu in which the skeleton develops. In the mucopolysaccharidoses the biochemical defect in the synthesis of cartilaginous matrix is relatively clearly defined. The resulting skeletal dysmorphia is usually mild and is rarely recognized at birth.

Osteogenesis Imperfecta

The term osteogenesis imperfecta (OI) describes a group of inherited diseases in which the bones are unusually brittle and

liable to fracture (Fig. 64.5). The former division into tarda and congenital forms of the disorder has been abandoned in light of more detailed studies of nosology and inheritance and an increasing appreciation of the molecular causes of the various forms. A widely used clinical classification of OI is provided by Sillence (Table 64.5). The forms presenting at birth or during the neonatal period are types II and III of the Sillence classification.

In general, OI is due to any one of a large number of mutations of the genes coding for type I collagen. Babies with type II disease have generally suffered many fractures *in utero;* they are obviously malformed with femoral shortening and often upper limb deformities at birth. The radiologic appearances of the widened, shortened femora, which are due to repetitive fracture and healing with callous formation, are characteristic. The

TABLE 64.5

CLASSIFICATION OF OSTEOGENESIS IMPERFECTA

Type	Fragility	Sclerae	Dental Involvement	Usual Mode of Inheritance	Comments
IA	Present	Blue	Yes	Autosomal dominant	Relatively common
IB	Present	Blue	No	Autosomal dominant	Variable severity
II	Extreme	Blue*	—	? Dominant (germ cell)	Perinatal (see Chapter 433)
III	Severe	Normal	No	? Dominant (germ cell)	Skeletal deformity (see Chapter 433)
IVA	Present	Normal	Yes	Autosomal dominant	Uncommon
IVB	Present	Normal	No	Autosomal dominant	Variable severity

*Blue-appearing sclerae may also be seen in healthy neonates.

disorder was thought to be recessively inherited because more than one affected infant may be born to unaffected parents. However, more recent evidence has accumulated that this type of OI is dominantly inherited with new mutations affecting a parental germ line and being capable of transmission to a number of affected offspring arising from fertilization of affected germ cells. Infants with type I disease pose a much greater diagnostic dilemma. They may not have fractures until during or after birth, raising the possibility that their fractures are the response of a normal skeleton to peri- or postnatal trauma or the effects of nutritional disturbances. In some cases, a positive family history of OI in a parent or sibling leads to the correct diagnosis.

Osteopetrosis

Osteopetrosis is a disorder of bone composition attributable to a dysfunction of the cells that resorb bone. In the most common, recessively inherited form of the condition, the bones consist at birth of dense primary spongiosa since the resorption and remodeling, which normally proceed during intrauterine development, cannot take place. The resistance of the bone to resorption causes "crowding out" of the hematopoietic marrow with consequent anemia and extramedullary hematopoiesis leading to hepatosplenomegaly. In addition, there is failure of bone resorption needed to accommodate structures that must pass through bone. The consequent compression of cranial nerves leads to blindness and deafness at an early age.

Affected babies are recognized by cranial bossing, or by any of the clinical signs mentioned previously, most of which become apparent in the first few weeks of life. Diagnosis is confirmed radiologically by the opaque density of the bones and by the "bone within bone" appearance of some limb bones. Serum biochemistry may be normal, but the failure of bone resorption may negate the skeleton's role as a calcium buffer, leading to intermittent hypocalcemia and consequent secondary hyperparathyroidism and hypophosphatemia.

Because osteopetrosis is the result of failure of a complex system of osteoclastic bone resorption, it might be expected that mutations in any one of several genes might be responsible. Those that may present in the neonatal period include mutations in the vacuolar proton pump, Cl-channel 7 (CLCN7), and the "GL" gene homologous to the gene responsible for osteopetrosis in a strain of mice.

The treatment of infantile osteopetrosis, formerly a uniformly fatal disease, remains unsatisfactory. An important theoretical advance was the discovery by Walker that in an animal model of the disease, the defective cells were of lymphoreticular origin and that bone resorption could be restored by transplantation of spleen or marrow cells from isogeneic unaffected animals. Some excellent results have been obtained using human bone marrow transplantation in affected infants. When this approach is not possible, there has been some success with the use of large doses of calcitriol and interferon gamma.

Suggested Readings

American Academy of Pediatrics, Committee on Nutrition. Nutritional needs of low birth weight infants. *Pediatrics* 1985;75:976.

Bastepe M, Juppner H. Editorial: pseudohypoparathyroidism and mechanisms of resistance toward multiple hormones: molecular evidence to clinical presentation. *J Clin Endocrinol Metab* 2003;88:4055.

Glorieux FH, Bishop NJ, Plotkin H, et al. Cyclic administration of pamidronate in children with severe osteogenesis imperfecta. *N Engl J Med* 1998;339:947.

Hollis BW, Wagner CL. Assessment of dietary vitamin D requirements during pregnancy and lactation. *Am J Clin Nutr* 2004;79:717.

Hsu SC, Levine MA. Perinatal calcium metabolism: physiology and pathophysiology. *Semin Neonatol* 2004;9:23.

Kocher MS, Kasser JR. Osteopetrosis. *Am J Orthop* 2003;32:222.

Markowitz RI, Zackai E. A pragmatic approach to the radiologic diagnosis of pediatric syndromes and skeletal dysplasias. *Radiol Clin North Am* 2001;39:791.

Muenzer J. The mucopolysaccharidoses: a heterogeneous group of disorders with variable pediatric presentations. *J Pediatr* 2004;144:S27.

Pearce SH. Clinical disorders of extracellular calcium-sensing and the molecular biology of the calcium-sensing receptor. *Ann Med* 2002;34:201.

Rauch F, Schoenau E. Skeletal development in premature infants: a review of bone physiology beyond nutritional aspects. *Arch Dis Child Fetal Neonatal Ed* 2002;86:F82.

Silence DO. Osteogenesis imperfecta nosology and genetics. *Ann N Y Acad Sci* 1988;543:1.

Superti-Furga A, Bonafe L, Rimoin DL. Molecular-pathogenetic classification of genetic disorders of the skeleton. *Am J Med Genet* 2001;106:282.

Tassabehji M. Williams-Beuren syndrome: a challenge for genotype-phenotype correlations. *Hum Mol Genet* 2003;12 Spec No 2:R229–R237.

CHAPTER 65 ■ URINARY TRACT INFECTIONS

MARC H. LEBEL

EPIDEMIOLOGY

The incidence of bacteriuria in the neonate is low, ranging from 0.1% to 1.9% in full-term infants and up to 10% in low-birth-weight newborns. In the neonatal period, a preponderance of infection occurs in male infants. In infants less than 2 months of age presenting with fever, urinary tract infection is found in 7.5% of patients. Many studies have reported an increased susceptibility to urinary tract infections in uncircumcised male infants. Other reports suggest that breast-feeding is associated with a lower incidence of infection.

PATHOGENESIS

Urinary tract infections can be acquired by hematogenous infection of the kidney in association with neonatal bacteremia or by the ascending route via the urethra. The short female urethra is thought to allow for ascending infection and explains the higher frequency of infection in girls older than 3 months. In the uncircumcised male infant, accumulation of bacteria in preputial folds with meatal contamination is likely. Specific fimbrial receptors on the foreskin and along the urethra may allow for ascending infection. Malformations of the urinary tract predispose to infection. Between 4% and 20% of infants presenting with urinary tract infection have an underlying malformation of the urinary tract.

Escherichia coli is the most frequent pathogen, causing 75% to 85% of infections. Other gram-negative organisms such as Klebsiella pneumoniae, Enterobacter species, Proteus vulgaris, and Pseudomonas aeruginosa are encountered less often. Gram-positive bacteria (including enterococci, group B streptococci, and Staphylococcus species) are uncommon pathogens in neonates. Candidal infections are seen as part of disseminated candidiasis, in the presence of an indwelling urinary catheter and in newborns requiring intensive care. A few patients have been reported with mixed bacterial infections.

In infants, 50% to 70% of E. coli strains causing urinary infection belong to one of the eight common pyelonephritogenic O serotypes found in older patients; data conflict concerning the frequency of specific polysaccharide K antigens on the surface of E. coli. Furthermore, E. coli can attach to specific receptors on uroepithelial cells. E. coli strains isolated from infants with urinary tract infection show a higher percentage of P and X fimbriation and more type 1 pili than found in matched control patients. Other recognized E. coli virulence factors include hemolysin production, colicin production, resistance to serum bactericidal activity, and the ability to acquire iron. The virulence factors may play a role not only in the localization of the infection (cystitis or pyelonephritis) but also in its severity.

CLINICAL MANIFESTATIONS

Few specific symptoms or signs of urinary tract infection are recognizable in the newborn period. Conversely, clinical mani-

festations vary widely, and many infants are completely asymptomatic. When symptoms are present, they often consist of fever, irritability, decreased feeding, and lethargy. Some patients present with diarrhea, vomiting, or weight loss. Jaundice is seen in approximately 7% of cases and can be accompanied by hepatomegaly and splenomegaly. The genitalia should be carefully inspected and the abdomen palpated gently to detect malformations or enlargement of the kidneys and bladder. Occasionally, an alert caretaker notices crying on urination (i.e., dysuria) or an increased number of wet diapers (i.e., frequency).

DIAGNOSIS

The diagnosis of urinary tract infection is based on examination and culture of an appropriately collected urine specimen. A urine culture should be included in the sepsis workup of all infants older than 72 hours of age. Within the first 3 days of life, urinary tract infection occurs secondary to bacteremia; therefore, such infections can be identified by blood culture. The most reliable test is when urine is obtained by suprapubic bladder puncture. This technique is safe and easy; bleeding or perforation of the bowel occurs rarely. Dehydration, abdominal distention, and a bleeding diathesis are contraindications for suprapubic aspiration. To optimize the yield of a successful tap, the aspiration should be done 30 to 60 minutes after the infant has voided. Any bacterial growth in cultures obtained by a suprapubic puncture is considered significant. Catheterization of the bladder is a valuable and safe procedure when suprapubic aspiration is unsuccessful.

The simplest method, but the least reliable, of collecting a urine culture is by application of a sterile plastic bag after careful disinfection of the perineum; the bag is removed shortly after the child has voided. Results of urine cultures obtained by bagged specimens are helpful when they are sterile, but a positive result is not necessarily indicative of infection because of frequent contamination during the collection process. Therefore, this method of obtaining a urine culture should be considered a screening technique, and the diagnosis must always be confirmed by a better method for urine culture. False-positive rates of 33% and 15% have been reported after obtaining one and two bagged urine specimens, respectively. Before initiation of antibiotics in infants evaluated for possible sepsis, an appropriate urine specimen should be obtained for culture by suprapubic aspiration or catheterization.

Pyuria (more than 10 leukocytes/mm^3) occurs in 75% of infants with proven urinary tract infection. Hematuria and proteinuria may be present. Gram-stained smear of urine sediment reveals bacteria in 80% of cases (including patients without pyuria). Some infants with proven infection, however, have a completely normal urinalysis result. An elevation of blood urea nitrogen and creatinine concentrations and electrolyte abnormalities can be secondary to dehydration or underlying renal abnormalities.

The peripheral leukocyte count is variable, and approximately one-third of patients have a preponderance of polymorphonuclear leukocytes and immature forms. Hemolytic anemia is seen in some patients presenting with jaundice. Bacteremia is present in 20% to 30% of infants; the incidence decreases with postnatal age. Concurrent meningitis is rare but must be ruled out in the septic-appearing newborn. Sterile pleocytosis is seen occasionally. In one study of 260 infants less than 6 months of age who had urinary tract infections, 11.9% had pleocytosis, as defined by more than 35 white blood cells/mm^3 in infants up to 30 days of age and more than 10 white blood cells/mm^3 in infants more than 1 month of age. One of these infants had bacterial meningitis; two had enteroviral meningitis.

In the young infant presenting with jaundice, hepatomegaly, and poor weight gain, biliary atresia or neonatal hepatitis must be excluded. Both conjugated and unconjugated bilirubin concentrations are elevated, whereas other liver function tests such as alanine aminotransferase or aspartate aminotransferase are often only mildly elevated. Urinary tract infection should be included in the differential diagnosis of gastroenteritis in the young infant because both can have similar clinical presentations.

THERAPY

The initial therapy should be given parenterally because of the frequent association with bacteremia in the newborn period. Ampicillin and an aminoglycoside are appropriate before culture and *in vitro* susceptibility results are available. If the patient has renal impairment, a combination of ampicillin plus cefotaxime is an excellent alternative. When a renal abscess with *S. aureus* is suspected, a penicillinase-resistant penicillin (methicillin, oxacillin, nafcillin) or vancomycin should be used. When blood and cerebrospinal fluid (if obtained) culture results are sterile, the usual doses of antibiotics can be reduced. Repeat urine cultures should be done after 48 to 72 hours of therapy to document sterilization. Most patients respond promptly to antimicrobial therapy, by becoming afebrile in 1 to 2 days. If clinical response or urine sterilization is delayed, an immediate evaluation for urologic obstruction or abscess must be made, and the pathogen's *in vitro* susceptibilities must be reviewed. Therapy should be continued for 10 to 14 days in the patient with an uncomplicated case, and a repeat urine culture is performed 1 week after discontinuation of antibiotic therapy. Aminoglycoside drug concentrations should be determined if they are used for more than 2 days or if blood urea nitrogen and creatinine concentrations are elevated.

Radiologic evaluation of the urinary tract is essential for all infants with their first episode of infection to detect underlying anatomic lesions. A renal ultrasound scan is used as an early screening procedure because the imaging does not depend on good renal function and it is a safe and noninvasive procedure. A voiding cystourethrogram is performed within 4 to 6 weeks after treatment. This examination also can be performed before the end of therapy, however, when the patient is afebrile and the urine is sterile. Approximately 50% of infants with urinary tract infection have some abnormalities seen on radiologic evaluation, vesicoureteral reflux being the most common abnormality encountered. Dimercaptosuccinic acid (DMSA) scintigraphy is more sensitive to detect renal involvement and renal cortical scarring and to assess quantitative differential renal function.

PROGNOSIS

The goal of management is to prevent progressive renal damage and its consequences. Children should have regular follow-up examinations, including repeated urine cultures. For infants with reflux, sonography and voiding cystourethrography or radionuclide scan should be repeated 6 to 12 months later, regardless of whether infection occurs in the interim. Chemoprophylaxis with trimethoprim-sulfamethoxazole is provided to all infants with grade 2 or greater reflux and to those with frequent urinary tract infections, regardless of the urologic status. In the first month of life, amoxicillin is used for prophylaxis because of the potential toxicity of sulfonamides in this age group. However, the benefits of prophylaxis have not been clearly demonstrated. The incidence of recurrent infection is 20% to 30%, and almost all recurrences happen during the first year. Minimal to moderate (grades 1, 2, and 3) reflux eventually disappears in most infants at a rate of 13% per year. Medical management should be coordinated with a pediatric urologist for infants with more severe reflux. The role of circumcision in prevention of urinary tract infection in male children should be individualized.

Suggested Readings

Abbott GD. Neonatal bacteriuria: a prospective study in 1,460 infants. *BMJ* 1972;1:267.
Adler-Shohet FC, Cheung MM, Hill M, Lieberman JM. Aseptic meningitis in infants younger than 6 months hospitalized with urinary tract infections. *Pediatr Infect Dis J* 2003;22:1039.
Alanis MC, Lucidi RS. Neonatal circumcision: a review of the world's oldest and most controversial operation. *Obstet Gynecol Surv* 2004;59:379.
Bachur R, Caputo GL. Bacteremia and meningitis among infants with urinary tract infections. *Pediatr Emerg Care* 1995;11:280.
Eliakim A, Dolfin T, Korzets A, et al. Urinary tract infections in premature infants: the role of imaging studies and prophylactic therapy. *J Perinatol* 1997;17:305.
Goldman M, Lahat E, Strauss S, et al. Imaging after urinary tract infection in male neonates. *Pediatrics* 2000;105:1232.
Karlowicz MG. Candidal renal and urinary tract infection in neonates. *Semin Perinatol* 2003;27:393.
Lin DS, Huang SH, Lin CC, et al. Urinary tract infection in febrile infants younger than eight weeks of age. *Pediatrics* 2000;105:E20.
Majd M, Rushton HG, Jantausch B, Wiedermann BL. Relationship among vesico-ureteral reflux, P-fimbriated *Escherichia coli*, and acute pyelonephritis in children with febrile urinary tract infection. *J Pediatr* 1991;119:578.
Marild S, Hansson S, Jodal U, et al. Protective effect of breastfeeding against urinary tract infection. *Acta Paediatr* 2004;93:164.
Schlager TA. Urinary tract infections in children younger than 5 years of age: epidemiology, diagnosis, treatment, outcomes and prevention. *Paediatr Drugs* 2001;3:219.
Schwab CW Jr, Wu HY, Selman H, et al. Spontaneous resolution of vesicoureteral reflux: a 15-year perspective. *J Urol* 2002;168:2594.
Tamin MM, Alesseh H, Aziz H. Analysis of the efficacy of urine culture as part of sepsis evaluation in the premature infant. *Pediatr Infect Dis J* 2003;22:805.
Wald E. Urinary tract infections in infants and children: a comprehensive review. *Curr Opin Pediatr* 2004;16:85.
Wheeler D, Vimalachandra D, Hodson EM, et al. Antibiotics and surgery for vesicoureteral reflux: a meta-analysis of randomized controlled trials. *Arch Dis Child* 2003;88:688.

CHAPTER 66 ■ HEMATOPOIESIS AND HEMATOLOGIC DISEASES

CHARLES T. QUINN AND GEORGE R. BUCHANAN

Hematologic problems are encountered daily by pediatricians caring for sick newborn infants. Alterations in the hematopoietic system most often are reactive, secondary, and even iatrogenic, but they are useful markers of underlying systemic diseases, including infection, asphyxia, and genetic and metabolic disorders. Often, these secondary hematologic problems have serious sequelae, so they must be recognized promptly and must be treated appropriately. Primary hematologic disorders, on the other hand, are rare during the newborn period. Yet, such conditions as hemophilia, immune-mediated thrombocytopenia resulting from transplacental maternal antibody, and inherited hemolytic anemia must be recognized by pediatricians so that they can initiate appropriate management, both acutely and with regard to long-term therapy and genetic counseling.

This chapter reviews the hematopoietic system in fetuses and newborn infants, focusing on common clinical problems that require differential diagnosis and management.

NORMAL DEVELOPMENTAL HEMATOPOIESIS

Hematopoiesis begins in the embryo during the third week of gestation, when blood islands in the yolk sac first produce erythrocytes and leukocytes. By the twelfth week of gestation, the liver and spleen are the predominant sites of hematopoiesis; by 30 weeks' gestation, the bone marrow assumes its ultimate role as the major site of production of the formed elements of the blood. At the time of or shortly after birth, hematopoiesis is restricted to the bone marrow except for the pathologic states described here. At birth, large numbers of pluripotent stem cells also are present in the peripheral blood. Widespread interest has developed in collecting umbilical cord or placental blood for storage to serve as a source of donor stem cells for purposes of transplantation. Umbilical cord blood transplants, using enriched stem cells harvested from placental blood, have been used to reconstitute the bone marrow of human leukocyte antigen–matched siblings or unrelated persons suffering from bone marrow failure, genetic diseases, and leukemia. This area currently is under intense study.

Production of Red Blood Cells

The predominant cellular element in the blood is the erythrocyte, or red blood cell (RBC). The factors controlling erythropoiesis in fetuses and newborns are similar to those of older children. Pluripotent stem cells give rise to morphologically indistinct precursors committed to the erythroid lineage. Under the stimulus of erythropoietin and other humoral factors, these erythroid burst–forming units and colony-forming units give rise to identifiable erythroblasts, which proliferate, begin to synthesize hemoglobin, and mature into differentiated nucleated RBCs. In the final stages of maturation, the nucleus is extruded, and the cell enters the circulation as a young erythrocyte. The major constituent of the erythrocyte is hemoglobin, which binds oxygen in the lungs and transports it to the tissues. Hemoglobin is a tetramer consisting of two pairs of similar polypeptide chains, each attached to a heme molecule, composed of protoporphyrin and ferrous iron, the oxygen-binding site.

The major difference between erythropoiesis in neonates and that in older children and adults is the dynamic but poorly understood "switch" from fetal to adult hemoglobin production. The primary hemoglobin in postnatal life is hemoglobin A, consisting of two alpha chains (whose genes are encoded on chromosome 16) and two beta chains (each of which derives from a 60-kilobase-long gene complex on chromosome 11). As shown in Fig. 66.1, early in fetal life the hemoglobin tetramer contains several types of embryonic globin chains (e.g., epsilon and zeta), the synthesis of which soon declines. During the initial months of gestation, the embryonic polypeptides are replaced by gamma chains, resulting in the predominant fetal hemoglobin or hemoglobin F (alpha$_2$-gamma$_2$). Yet, as early as the fourteenth week of gestation, the "adult" beta globin genes are activated, beta chains are produced, and hemoglobin A (alpha$_2$-beta$_2$) is detectable. Alpha-chain production is sustained at a high level throughout most of fetal life. At the time of birth, gamma- and beta-chain synthesis is approximately equal, and 60% to 80% of the total hemoglobin is hemoglobin F.

Gamma globin synthesis almost ceases during the initial months of life (see Fig. 66.1). By 6 months of age, the percentage of hemoglobin F approximates that of adults (less than 2%). An increased understanding of the gamma-to-beta switch would have an impact on the treatment of a number of diseases (e.g., sickle cell anemia and beta-thalassemia) in which retention of large quantities of hemoglobin F in the erythrocyte is desirable.

Fetal hemoglobin differs from hemoglobin A in a number of ways. Hemoglobin F is resistant to both alkali and dilute acid, forming the basis for two tests for its measurement (the Kleihauer-Betke stain for fetal hemoglobin in individual cells and quantitative measurement of hemoglobin F in a hemolysate). Hemoglobin F can be also differentiated from hemoglobin A by immunologic means. It binds less avidly than does hemoglobin A to 2,3-bisphosphoglycerate, an organic phosphate in the erythrocyte important in modulating oxygen

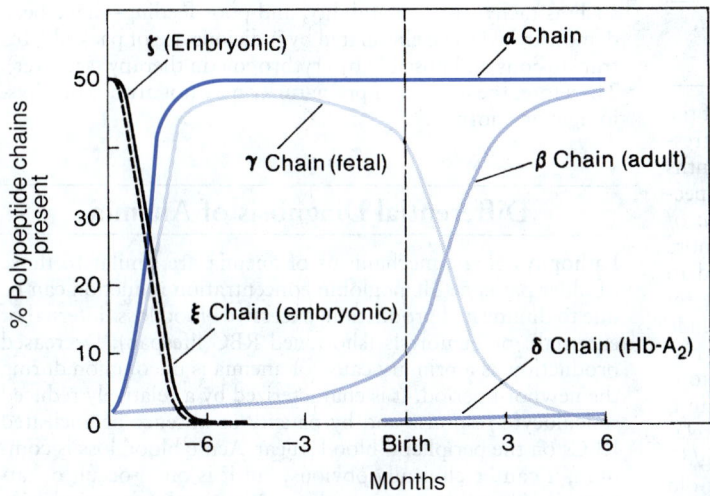

FIGURE 66.1. Changes in human globin synthesis during prenatal and neonatal development. (Reprinted with permission from Bunn HF, Forget GB, Ranney HM. *Human hemoglobins*. Philadelphia: Saunders, 1977:107.)

uptake and release by hemoglobin. Therefore, the affinity of hemoglobin F for oxygen is fairly high, allowing the fetus to extract oxygen from the maternal circulation.

The fetal RBC differs from its adult counterpart in a number of other characteristics. Fetal RBCs are larger and have higher levels of certain glycolytic enzymes, a relative deficiency of key defense mechanisms against excessive oxidation (e.g., glutathione peroxidase, catalase, methemoglobin reductase), diminished deformability, and a shorter lifespan in the circulation.

Leukocyte, Platelet, and Coagulation Protein Production

Like RBCs, granulocytes and platelets are derived from committed precursor cells in the yolk sac, liver, spleen, and then bone marrow. The developmental process and control mechanisms are similar to those noted in older children and adults. Blood coagulation factors and inhibitors, equal in importance to platelets in the fine balance of the hemostatic mechanism, generally are produced in diminished quantities during fetal life. The liver produces most blood coagulation factors and such inhibitors as antithrombin and protein C; the physiologic immaturity of the liver in the fetus and neonate results in reduced levels of most of these factors.

ANEMIA

Normal Values

Because of relative intrauterine hypoxia and the high affinity of hemoglobin F for oxygen (resulting in a shift to the left of the oxygen–hemoglobin dissociation curve), erythropoietin secretion is enhanced during fetal life. Accordingly, during the final months of gestation and at birth, values for hemoglobin and hematocrit are higher than are those for older children. Representative values are shown in Table 66.1. The mean cord blood hemoglobin concentration in term infants is 16.5 g/dL (range, 14 to 22 g/dL). Premature infants have slightly lower values. Values depend on method of delivery, site of blood sampling, postnatal age, and other factors. Capillary specimens are higher (by 1 to 2 g/dL) and generally have a wider range of hemoglobin values than that in samples obtained from the umbilical or peripheral vein. In the performance of serial hemoglobin measurements during the initial hours and days of life, such differences

should be kept in mind; ideally, the same site of sampling is used consistently. Even though venous sampling is technically more difficult, it is preferred because neonatal blood is viscous (owing to the high hematocrit and reduced deformability of individual cells) and peripheral circulation in sick neonates frequently is sluggish.

The blood volume in term infants is 80 to 90 mL/kg at birth (90 to 100 mL/kg in premature infants). During the initial hours of life, a decrease in plasma volume occurs, resulting in an increase in the hemoglobin concentration as compared to cord blood values (see Table 66.1). This alteration is followed by a progressive, slow decline in the hemoglobin concentration termed the *physiologic anemia of infancy*. The lifespan of fetal and neonatal RBCs is approximately 80 days, as compared to 120 days in adults. Reasons for this shortened RBC survival are unclear; it is not due simply to the presence of fetal hemoglobin.

At birth, more RBCs are produced than are in older patients, as shown by the elevated reticulocyte count and the appearance of nucleated RBCs on the peripheral smear. Erythropoiesis can be accelerated further by various causes of fetal hypoxia or anemia. The usual reticulocyte count in cord blood or during the first or second day of life is 2% to 8%, and 3 to 10 nucleated RBCs per 100 leukocytes generally are present. By 3 or 4 days of life, nucleated RBCs disappear, after which their presence is always abnormal, and the reticulocyte count falls (and remains low) until 3 months of age, when recovery from physiologic anemia begins. The erythrocytes of neonates are larger than those of older children. Typically, mean cell volume is 95 to 120 fL, as compared to 70 to 85 fL in children older than several months.

TABLE 66.1

NORMAL HEMOGLOBIN VALUES IN NEWBORN INFANTS

Site and Time of Sampling	Hemoglobin Concentration (g/dL)	
	Mean	Range
Cord blood	16.5	14–22
Venous specimen		
2 days of age	18	14.5–23.0
Capillary specimen		
2 days of age	19	14.5–25.0
7 days of age	16.5	14–22

Physiologic Anemia of Infancy and Anemia of Prematurity

Shortly after birth, erythropoiesis almost ceases because of the oxygen-rich milieu and relative excess of RBCs. The progressive fall in hemoglobin values during the first several months of life in term and premature infants has been named, respectively, the *physiologic anemia of infancy* and the *anemia of prematurity*. In premature infants, the decline occurs more rapidly (with lowest values at 4 to 8 weeks, as opposed to 10 to 12 weeks in term infants), and the anemia is more severe. Factors determining the time course and severity include birth weight, perinatal complications, blood transfusion history (as premature infants who receive multiple transfusions generally exhibit a greater decline), and presence of vitamin E deficiency. Erythropoietin production during this period is relatively decreased. Nadir hemoglobin values may reach 9.5 g/dL at 3 months in term infants and 6 g/dL in 6- to 8-week-old premature infants. Recovery from physiologic anemia is heralded by a slight elevation in the reticulocyte count and a rise in hemoglobin value to levels seen throughout the remainder of infancy. To support erythropoiesis during the recovery stage of physiologic anemia, abundant iron must be available from existing stores, dietary sources, or exogenous supplements, particularly in rapidly growing premature infants, thus necessitating their higher daily iron requirement of 2 mg/kg/day, compared to 1 mg/kg/day for the term infant.

The physiologic anemia of infancy does not respond to iron or folic acid. Healthy term infants and asymptomatic, growing, premature infants require no therapy. However, apneic episodes—as well as other signs and symptoms of hypoxia, such as tachycardia, irritability, and poor feeding—have been demonstrated to be eliminated by judicious use of packed RBC transfusions and possibly by erythropoietin therapy (see later). Therefore, the anemia of prematurity may not always be physiologic or "normal."

Differential Diagnosis of Anemia

Pathophysiologic mechanisms of anemia are similar to those of older patients. Hemoglobin concentration reduction can be due to diminished production, excessive blood loss (internal or external), or hemolysis (shortened RBC lifespan). Decreased production as a primary cause of anemia is uncommon during the newborn period. It is characterized by a relatively reduced reticulocyte response and by paucity or absence of nucleated RBCs on the peripheral blood smear. Acute blood loss is common; it can be clinically obvious, but it is often occult or iatrogenic. Hemolytic anemia during the newborn period may be due either to intrinsic inherited defects in the RBC or to acquired causes. Hemolysis in newborn infants is identified easily by the marked jaundice that usually results from hepatic immaturity. Figure 66.2 depicts an algorithm of the differential diagnosis of anemia during the newborn period.

Anemia Due to Blood Loss

Anemia due to blood loss is more common during the newborn period than at any other time in childhood. Signs and symptoms relate to the duration and amount of blood lost. Acute

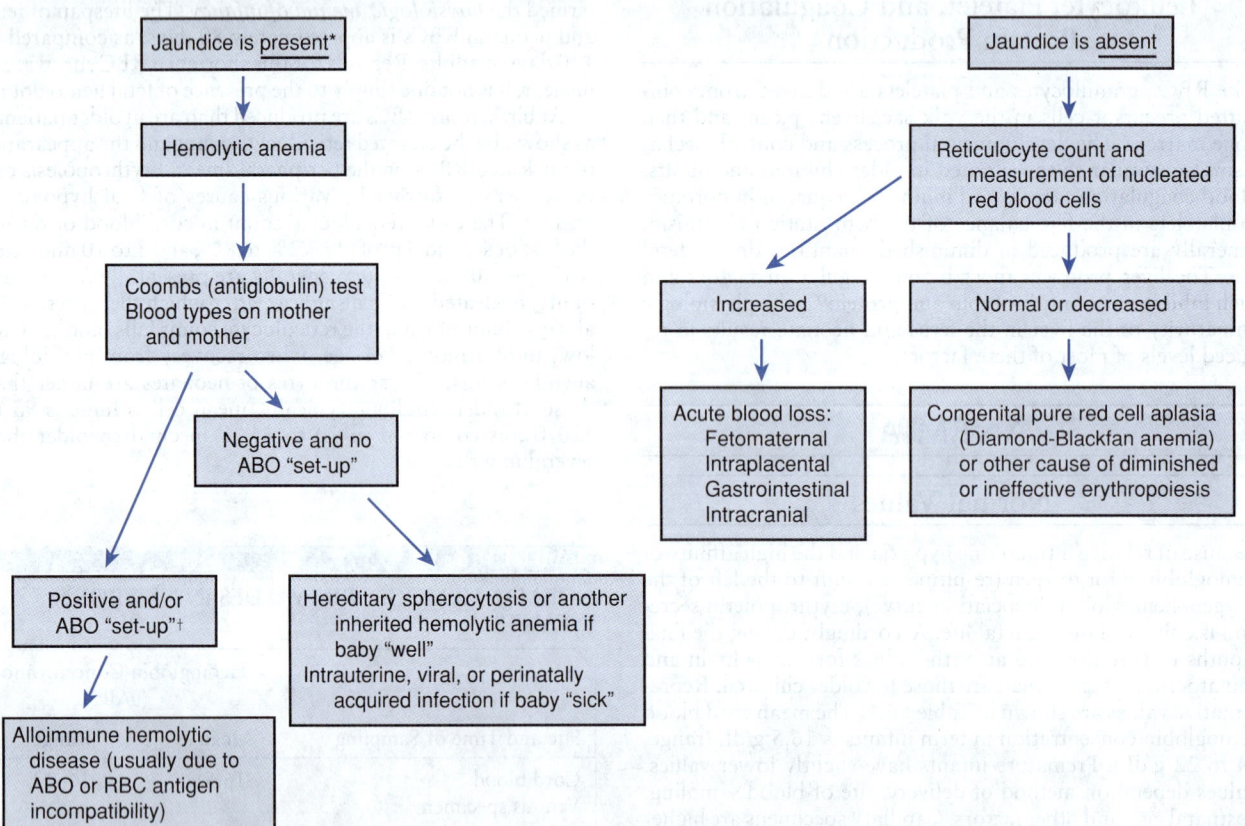

FIGURE 66.2. Diagnostic approach to anemia in the newborn infant (hemoglobin ≤14 g/dL with or without symptoms). The most likely diagnoses are provided in the boxes. In addition, reticulocyte count and number of circulating nucleated red blood cells are nearly always elevated. †Mother group O and baby group A or B.

TABLE 66.2

APT TEST FOR DIFFERENTIATION OF FETAL AND ADULT (MATERNAL) HEMOGLOBIN IN STOOL OR VOMITUS

Mix 1 volume of stool or vomitus with 5 volumes of water.
Centrifuge mixture and remove clear-pink supernatant
   solution containing hemoglobin.
Mix 1 mL of 1% sodium hydroxide with 4 mL supernatant
   and observe color change after 2 minutes.
Remains pink: hemoglobin F
Turns yellow-brown: hemoglobin A (maternal blood)

Adapted from Apt KL, Downey WS. Melena neonatorum: the swallowed blood syndrome. *J Pediatr.* 1955;47:6.

hemorrhage greater than 20% to 30% of the infant's blood volume results in signs and symptoms of shock (pallor, lethargy, tachycardia, hypotension). Jaundice is absent. External blood loss occurs most commonly from the gastrointestinal tract, sometimes from an identifiable anatomic lesion (e.g., ulcer or duplication), but often without apparent cause. In instances of hematemesis or melena, whether the complication is due to swallowed maternal blood or to blood from the baby is determined by the Apt test for fetal hemoglobin (Table 66.2). Hemorrhage may occur from one twin to another or into the umbilical cord, placenta (e.g., abruption, placenta previa, or laceration during cesarean section), or maternal circulation (fetal–maternal hemorrhage). A Kleihauer-Betke or an immunohistochemical stain for fetal hemoglobin-containing RBCs in the mother may allow for an estimate of the amount of transplacental hemorrhage. This complication is not uncommon; in 1 in 100 deliveries, lost blood can be more than 20% of the baby's blood volume, resulting in clinically significant anemia apparent at birth or manifesting later as iron deficiency. Occult blood loss of hemodynamic significance may occur also within the cranial vault of neonates because of their relatively large head size and open sutures. Bleeding in the abdominal cavity, retroperitoneal space, subcutaneous tissues (e.g., scalp), or other internal locations may result in jaundice (because of catabolism of hemoglobin from the resorbed hematomas) in addition to anemia.

In sick premature infants, the most common cause of blood loss is the iatrogenic withdrawal of multiple specimens to monitor blood gases and other laboratory parameters. Such blood sampling can amount to more than 10% to 20% of the tiny infant's blood volume during each 24-hour period and represents the most frequent indication for blood transfusions in such babies.

The treatment of anemia due to acute blood loss depends on the amount and duration of blood loss. Infants with signs of hypovolemia should receive immediate volume replacement (crystalloid, colloid, or packed RBCs). Packed RBC transfusions alone may be indicated for less severe anemia, such as that resulting from repetitive blood sampling.

Hemolytic Anemia during the Newborn Period

Destruction of RBCs intravascularly or by the mononuclear–phagocyte system (primarily spleen and liver) results in production of 32 mg of bilirubin from every 1 g of degraded hemoglobin. The physiologically immature liver of the fetus and newborn is incapable of rapidly conjugating this excess pigment. Therefore, hyperbilirubinemia, usually with clinical jaundice, accompanies all severe hemolytic states during the initial days of life. Hemolysis in the neonate, as in older patients, also is accompanied by reticulocytosis, nucleated RBCs on the peripheral blood smear, and (sometimes) characteristic RBC morphologic changes. Usually, hemolysis during the newborn period is due to RBC injury resulting from antibody binding or mechanical effects.

ABO Incompatibility

Immune-mediated hemolytic anemia results from maternally derived alloantibody directed against antigens on fetal and neonatal RBCs. In current practice, ABO incompatibility is seen most frequently. Generally, a blood group O mother produces IgG anti-A or anti-B alloantibodies that cross the placenta and bind to her infant's type A or B erythrocytes and to other tissues that contain blood group A or B. On the other hand, in women with blood groups A or B, anti-A or anti-B alloantibodies (also called *isohemagglutinins*) generally are of the IgM class and do not cross the placenta. Affected babies present with jaundice during the first several days of life. Usually, anemia is absent or mild, but most patients exhibit an elevated reticulocyte count (usually 5% to 15%) and increased numbers of nucleated RBCs on the blood smear. Also characteristic on the peripheral smear are microspherocytes resulting from partial membrane loss.

Laboratory diagnosis of ABO incompatibility is confirmed by demonstrating the appropriate "ABO set-up" (i.e., type O mother and type A or B baby) and a positive antiglobulin (Coombs) test. In the direct antiglobulin test, IgG antibody on the infant's washed RBCs can be demonstrated. Often, this direct Coombs test is only weakly positive. Anti-A or anti-B alloantibodies often can be eluted from the infant's cells. The indirect antiglobulin test assesses the presence of free anti-A or anti-B alloantibodies in the baby's serum. Such a test is positive in nearly all infants with clinically significant A-O or B-O incompatibility. In general, babies whose jaundice requires phototherapy or exchange transfusion have a stronger antiglobulin reaction and more microspherocytes.

Most babies with ABO incompatibility require no therapy except that directed to the hyperbilirubinemia. Sometimes, symptomatic anemia does not manifest until 4 to 6 weeks after birth.

Rh Incompatibility

Until the late 1960s, the most frequent and severe form of hemolytic anemia in the newborn period was incompatibility between the mother and child in the major antigen of the rhesus or Rh complex (called the *D antigen*), resulting in the syndrome of erythroblastosis fetalis. Unlike ABO incompatibility, in which the offending maternal antibodies are natural (i.e., do not result from sensitization of the mother), Rh-negative women who develop anti-D antibody have been sensitized (immunized) either by a prior blood transfusion of D-positive blood or from that of a previous D-positive fetus. During subsequent pregnancies, anti-D antibody increases in titer, crosses the placenta, coats the fetal D-positive RBCs, and results in severe hemolysis, owing to destruction of these cells in the reticuloendothelial system. Severely anemic infants may die *in utero* or may be born with the syndrome of hydrops fetalis, characterized by anasarca resulting from hypoalbuminemia and congestive heart failure, severe anemia, and massive hepatosplenomegaly (resulting from cardiac failure and extramedullary erythropoiesis). The mortality rate is extremely high. Whether hydropic or not, a large percentage of these Rh-sensitized babies develop extreme jaundice, requiring multiple exchange transfusions.

The problem of Rh hemolytic disease has become less pronounced during the last three decades because of several key research advances. First, anti-D immune globulin now is administered routinely to all Rh-negative women at 28 weeks' gestation and immediately after delivery or after abortion; therefore, few women are sensitized. Those women who do exhibit rising titers of anti-D antibody can be identified early in the pregnancy and can be monitored by amniocentesis, serial amniotic fluid optical density measurements, and estimation of the relative risk of fetal death. Intrauterine transfusions of Rh-negative packed RBCs can be administered to correct the anemia, and planned early induction of labor—followed by vigorous management of the jaundiced, anemic, and often premature infant—has resulted in lower morbidity and mortality rates. Typically, affected babies have a strongly positive direct antiglobulin test; the indirect test usually shows the presence of large amounts of free anti-D antibodies in the baby's and mother's serum. The degree of anemia is variable, but usually hyperbilirubinemia is present. An elevation of the direct fraction of bilirubin is seen in the most severely affected infants, probably resulting from intrahepatic cholestasis (inspissated bile syndrome). The peripheral blood smear shows polychromasia and nucleated RBCs (erythroblastosis) but no microspherocytes, in contrast to ABO incompatibility. Treatment consists of exchange transfusion for marked hyperbilirubinemia or anemia, simple transfusions of Rh-negative packed RBCs for less severe degrees of anemia, and careful follow-up during the first 2 or 3 months of life, when delayed anemia resulting from persisting anti-D antibody or bone marrow suppression may necessitate additional transfusions.

With the diminished frequency and severity of anti-D antibody sensitization, fetal–maternal incompatibility due to minor blood group antigens now has become relatively more common. The pathophysiology and treatment are similar to those of ABO incompatibility and Rh incompatibility disease. The antibodies are directed against another part of the Rh complex (e.g., c and E) or such antigens as Kell, Duffy (Fy), or Kidd (Jk). Immune-mediated hemolysis rarely is observed in babies whose mothers have systemic lupus erythematosus or autoimmune hemolytic anemia.

Mechanical and Toxic Causes of Hemolysis

As in older patients, hemolytic anemia may occur as a result of mechanical factors or of toxins damaging the erythrocyte membrane. Examples include viral and bacterial infection and injury mediated by fibrin strands or altered microvasculature accompanying disseminated intravascular coagulation (DIC). Vitamin E deficiency is now a rare cause of clinically significant hemolysis.

Infantile Pyknocytosis

Occasionally, a hemolytic anemia is seen (especially in premature infants) during the initial weeks of life that is characterized by a predominance of dense spiculated erythrocytes, termed *pyknocytes*, on the peripheral blood film. As expected, the infants often are jaundiced, and the reticulocyte count is elevated. No evidence supports an accompanying vitamin E deficiency, infection, liver disease, or other primary disorder. The anemia and the striking peripheral blood findings resolve spontaneously within 6 or 8 weeks of age. The cause is unknown.

Inherited Hemolytic Anemias

Intrinsic disorders of the RBCs involving the cell membrane, hemoglobin, or enzymatic apparatus also may result in hemolysis during the newborn period. The most common of these disorders is glucose-6-phosphate dehydrogenase (G6PD) deficiency, which occurs most frequently in black, Mediterranean,

and Asian male persons. Protective mechanisms against oxidant injury are inefficient in neonatal RBCs. Hydrogen peroxide or superoxide anion generated during infection or as a consequence of drugs may precipitate hemoglobin, resulting in formation of insoluble Heinz bodies. Inclusion-laden RBCs then are removed by the spleen. Particularly in Chinese and Mediterranean populations, ill-defined oxidant stresses associated with a normal vaginal delivery sometimes result in hemolysis that requires exchange transfusion. Full-term black infants with G6PD deficiency exhibit few problems in the absence of pathologic oxidant stress. Prematurely born black infants deficient in the enzyme, however, may exhibit marked hyperbilirubinemia. The diagnosis of G6PD deficiency is made by widely available screening tests and enzyme assays. False-negative results may occur in affected black infants with reticulocytosis.

In whites of northern European extraction, hereditary spherocytosis is the most common congenital hemolytic anemia. Although this condition is usually inherited as an autosomal dominant trait, the family history is negative for spherocytosis in nearly one-half of cases. Affected babies are jaundiced and have varying degrees of anemia. Typically, the blood smear contains numerous microspherocytes. Evidence of ABO incompatibility (a much more common cause of spherocytes on the neonatal blood smear) is absent. RBC osmotic fragility testing is of limited diagnostic value, because it will only confirm the presence of spherocytes and not distinguish among different causes of spherocytosis.

Another inherited erythrocyte membrane disorder presenting during the neonatal period is hereditary elliptocytosis and its variant, hereditary pyropoikilocytosis. In this dominantly inherited condition seen primarily in blacks, alterations in erythrocyte membrane skeletal proteins may result in a brisk hemolytic anemia shortly after birth. The peripheral blood film shows numerous elliptocytes, many of them small and distorted by surface blebs. As patients grow older, the anemia is less severe, and erythrocyte morphology becomes less striking.

Hemolytic anemia in neonates resulting from other RBC enzymopathies, membrane alterations, or inherited instability of gamma- or alpha-globin chains occurs rarely. Because sickle cell anemia involves the beta-globin chain, and not the fetal gamma-globin chain, affected neonates have no apparent clinical or hematologic abnormalities. Special screening techniques are used for diagnosis of sickle cell disease, which is best made in the newborn period to allow for education, counseling, and prompt initiation of prophylactic penicillin.

Anemia Due to Decreased Production

Anemia resulting from diminished production of RBCs is uncommon at birth. The laboratory hallmark is a diminished or absent reticulocyte count. As in older patients, this deficiency may be due to a bone marrow replaced with malignant cells, absence of marrow precursors, nutritional deficiency, ineffective erythropoiesis, or diminished erythropoietin stimulation. Leukemia and aplastic anemia very rarely occur this early in life. Iron deficiency resulting from chronic fetal–maternal hemorrhage also is uncommon. Hematologic features of iron deficiency (e.g., microcytosis, reduced serum ferritin) are the same as those observed later in life. Recall that a mean corpuscular volume less than 95 fL is microcytic for a newborn. Relative bone marrow suppression occurs commonly during sepsis and may contribute to anemia seen in babies with diverse forms of infection, especially viral.

Diamond-Blackfan anemia (congenital, pure red-cell aplasia) is an uncommon form of hypoproliferative anemia that usually presents at birth or soon thereafter. This disorder results from an absence of erythroid stem cells and is characterized by a macrocytic anemia and absence of reticulocytes, typically with normal values for leukocytes and platelets.

Affected babies may exhibit low birth weight, and physical examination may show thumb anomalies or a phenotype similar to that of Turner syndrome. The disorder occurs equally in both genders.

The major mechanism of anemia in thalassemia syndromes is ineffective erythropoiesis with diminished RBC production, although a hemolytic component exists also. Thalassemia results from reduction in the synthesis of one or more globin chains (usually alpha or beta), resulting in microcytic anemia of variable severity. With the normally diminished expression of the beta-globin gene during fetal and neonatal life, beta-thalassemia (like such qualitative beta-globin hemoglobinopathies as sickle cell disease) does not express itself clinically during the newborn period. Babies with heterozygous forms of alpha-thalassemia, however, do have microcytosis (i.e., mean cell volume less than 95 fL) and an abnormal hemoglobin electrophoresis with 2% to 6% hemoglobin Bart's, a rapidly migrating, unstable tetramer of gamma chains. The alpha-thalassemia trait, resulting from deletion of one or two of the four alpha-globin genes, is common in infants with African or Southeast Asian ancestry. Homozygous alpha-thalassemia causes severe anemia, hydrops fetalis, and even stillbirth. This syndrome, which results from deletion of all four alpha-globin genes, is seen exclusively in Southeast Asians. Several such babies have survived as a result of intrauterine transfusions followed by postnatal chronic blood transfusions or stem cell transplantation.

NEONATAL POLYCYTHEMIA

Polycythemia, a pathologic increase in RBC mass, can cause multiple clinical problems that necessitate acute intervention and may have long-lasting effects. Polycythemia during the newborn period is defined as a venous hematocrit greater than 65%, ideally confirmed on two consecutive specimens. Usually, the etiology is ill-defined (Table 66.3). Maternal–fetal hemorrhage in utero rarely is documented, so the primary mechanisms are placental transfusion at birth (due to delayed clamping of the umbilical cord or elevation of the placenta) or enhanced erythropoiesis associated with elevated erythropoietin production in utero. This condition presumably results from intrauterine hypoxia and often is seen in dysmature or postmature babies or infants of diabetic mothers.

The clinical features result from hyperviscosity in large vessels and in the microcirculation. The problem of excess RBCs can be compounded by their reduced deformability. Clinical features include plethora, tachypnea, irritability, jitteriness, and seizures. Laboratory abnormalities (in addition to high hemoglobin values) may include hypoglycemia, thrombocytopenia, and hyperbilirubinemia resulting from the breakdown of excess RBCs. Cerebral blood flow is reduced, and pulmonary artery pressure usually is increased.

TABLE 66.3

ETIOLOGY OF POLYCYTHEMIA IN NEWBORN INFANTS

Etiology	Relative Frequency
Idiopathic	Most common
Delayed cord clamping	Common
Infant of diabetic mother*	Common
Intrauterine growth retardation*	Common
Down syndrome	Less common
Maternal-to-fetal transfusion	Rare
Twin-to-twin transfusion	Rare
Beckwith-Wiedemann syndrome	Rare

*Demonstrated to be mediated by increased levels of erythropoietin.

Many infants are asymptomatic, and their management and outcome of treatment are controversial. Few would argue that symptomatic infants with polycythemia should be treated by partial-exchange transfusion consisting of removal of the baby's blood and replacement with 3 mL of saline or lactated Ringer's solution for every 1 mL of blood withdrawn. Fresh-frozen plasma as replacement fluid should be avoided, and simple phlebotomy never should be undertaken without concomitant volume replacement. The amount of blood exchanged (in 10- to 20-mL increments) can be calculated by the following formula:

$$\text{Total volume} = \frac{\text{Baby's estimated blood volume (mL)} \times \text{desired reduction in hematocrit (\%)}}{\text{Observed hematocrit (\%)}}$$

Reduction in the venous hematocrit to levels of less than 55% usually results in prompt disappearance of existing signs and symptoms. Most specialists would not recommend a partial-exchange transfusion in asymptomatic infants incidentally found to have polycythemia. Yet, several studies demonstrate subtle long-term motor and psychological effects in young children who had polycythemia during the neonatal period.

BLOOD TRANSFUSIONS DURING THE NEONATAL PERIOD

The most common requirements for blood transfusion in the newborn nursery are sick premature infants in whom frequent blood sampling for monitoring requires replacement therapy. In this and in most other circumstances, packed RBCs (rather than whole blood) are recommended. Efforts must be undertaken to prevent the transmission of viral infection, especially cytomegalovirus (CMV), human immunodeficiency virus (HIV), and hepatitis C. Current blood bank screening practices essentially have eliminated HIV transmission in this setting, and hepatitis B and C also occurs very rarely. To prevent transmission of CMV, either leukocyte-reduced or CMV antibody–negative packed RBCs are indicated. To reduce donor exposure, a single RBC unit can be designated for a sick neonate, and from it multiple aliquots can be transfused as needed over the shelf life of the unit. Other complications of blood transfusion therapy are similar to those observed in older patients.

Under continued study is the use of recombinant human erythropoietin as treatment for the anemia of prematurity. A brisk erythropoietic response to parenterally administered hormone would obviate repetitive RBC transfusions to replace blood withdrawn for studies and to treat apnea of prematurity. Numerous studies have shown that erythropoietin injections several times weekly may raise the hemoglobin concentration and somewhat reduce blood transfusion requirements. Supplemental iron is required to "fuel" the enhanced erythropoiesis, however, and not yet certain is whether the apparent benefits outweigh the cost and potential toxicity of the recombinant hormone. Not surprisingly, erythropoietin has proven of limited value in reducing transfusion requirements resulting from repetitive blood sampling for most premature infants.

Platelet transfusions and granulocyte transfusions are discussed in subsequent paragraphs.

ABNORMALITIES OF LEUKOCYTES

Neutrophils or granulocytes are the predominant form of leukocytes, or white blood cells (WBCs), important in the defense against bacterial infection. The final stages of granulocyte

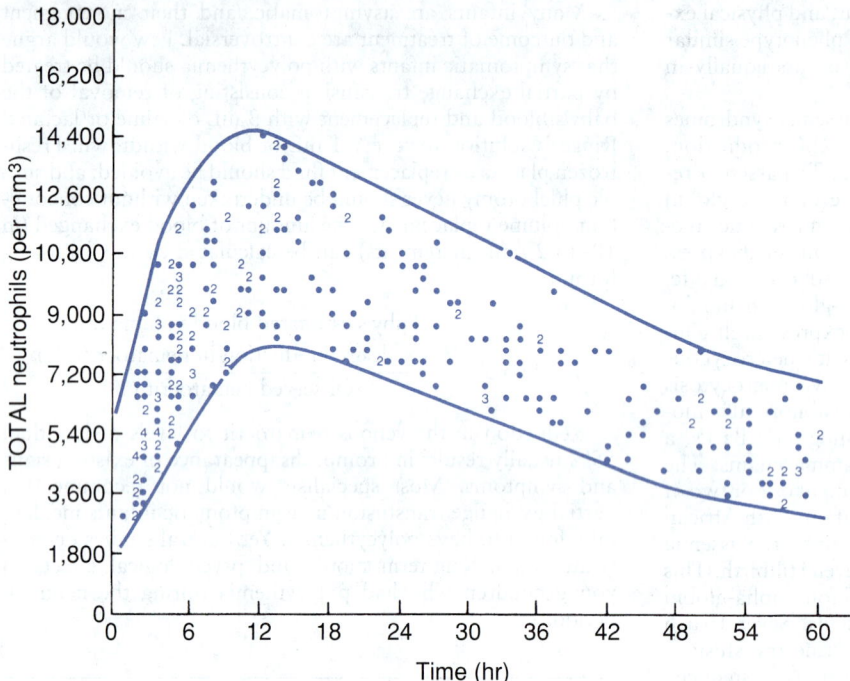

FIGURE 66.3. Total neutrophil count reference range in the first 60 hours of life. Points represent single values; numbers represent the number of values at the same point. (Reprinted with permission from Manroe BL, Weinberg AG, Rosenfeld CR, Browne R. The neonatal blood count in health and disease: I. Reference values for neutrophilic cells. *J Pediatr* 1979;95:89.)

maturation in the bone marrow result in condensation, folding, and segmentation of the nucleus. Normally, only the most differentiated segmented forms are released from the bone marrow. During periods of stress or infection, however, less mature, nonsegmented or band forms enter the circulation.

Varying neutrophil counts [best expressed in absolute terms (i.e., number per cubic millimeter of whole blood) rather than as percentages of total WBC count] depend on postgestational age and other factors. Granulocytes are present early in fetal life and are the predominant form of circulating WBCs during the neonatal period. Numbers of segmented and band forms are normally higher during the first 2 days of life than at any other time during childhood (Fig. 66.3).

The numerous factors affecting granulopoiesis and the circulation and distribution of neutrophils are similar in neonates and older patients. Evidence suggests, however, that the maturation and storage pool (i.e., bone marrow reserves) of neutrophils are reduced in neonates, thus contributing to an impaired neutrophilic response during bacterial infection. Numerous alterations in neutrophil function have been described during the neonatal period, including reduced migration and impaired phagocytic capacity. The clinical relevance of these features with regard to risk of bacterial infection is not well understood.

Neutrophilic responses during bacterial infection are described later. Babies with bacterial infection, particularly septicemia, may have a normal total WBC count, but absolute neutropenia and a relative increase in immature band forms often are observed. This elevated band–to–segmented form ratio is useful in the diagnosis of bacterial septicemia.

Neutropenia

Generally, neutropenia (Table 66.4) during childhood is defined as an absolute neutrophil count of fewer than 1,500 cells per cubic millimeter. Figure 66.3 shows that a different definition applies during the first 3 days of life. The most common cause of severe neutropenia is bacterial sepsis; often, it is accompanied by a relative increase in immature forms, such as bands, metamyelocytes, or even myelocytes. Mild to moderate neutropenia usually is transient, resulting from intrauterine viral infection, maternal hypertension or preeclampsia, birth asphyxia, and certain drugs taken by the mother. Neutropenia

TABLE 66.4

DIFFERENTIAL DIAGNOSIS OF NEUTROPENIA IN NEWBORN INFANTS

Disorder	Relative Frequency	Associated Features
Severe bacterial infection[a]	Common	Relative increase in circulating band and other immature forms
Transient[b] neutropenia related to maternal factors	Common	Maternal hypertension or birth asphyxia
Congenital (intrinsic defect in myelopoiesis)	Uncommon	Sometimes familial; persists indefinitely
Alloimmune (isoimmune) neonatal neutropenia	Rare	Persists up to 3 months; due to maternal antibody against neutrophil antigen

[a]Especially septicemia due to group B streptococci and *Escherichia coli*.
[b]Lasting hours to days.

may be due also to transplacental passage of an antineutrophil antibody resulting from neutrophil antigen incompatibility between the mother and fetus. This condition, termed *alloimmune (isoimmune) neonatal neutropenia*, results in profound neutropenia (usually less than 200 neutrophils per cubic millimeter), with a corresponding increased risk of bacterial infection during the initial weeks of life. The disorder is self-limited. Antineutrophil antibodies, usually directed against the neutrophil-specific NA antigen, can be demonstrated using specialized methods. Rarely, neutropenia is seen on a congenital basis because of inherited defects in myelopoiesis (e.g., severe congenital neutropenia) or accompanying some inherited metabolic disorders (e.g., propionic acidemia and glycogen storage disease type Ib). When neutropenia is a manifestation of hypersplenism, infiltrative disorders, or bone marrow failure, other clinical and hematologic manifestations invariably coexist.

Management of neutropenic neonates is the same as that of older infants and children: treatment of the underlying disorder and vigorous antibiotic management of infectious complications. Granulocyte transfusions may be useful in certain neonates with sepsis and severe neutropenia associated with neutrophil marrow depletion. Recombinant granulocyte colony-stimulating factor, which stimulates production and release of neutrophils from the marrow, also is being explored as a means of raising the neutrophil counts in neutropenic neonates with infection.

Other Leukocyte Disorders

Leukocytosis, usually with a predominance of neutrophilic forms or their precursors, is seen in leukemoid reactions resulting from infection and in inherited neutrophil function disorders, such as leukocyte adhesion protein deficiency. On the other hand, immature myeloid cells predominate in congenital leukemia and the unusual, transient myeloproliferative syndrome observed in neonates with Down syndrome. Marked lymphocytosis is noted occasionally in intrauterine infection.

BLEEDING DISORDERS IN NEONATES

Bleeding and thrombosis are common problems in sick newborn infants, and laboratory alterations in the hemostatic mechanism occur frequently even in the absence of hemorrhage or thrombosis. Because platelet and clotting-factor changes are sensitive measures of many disease processes, they may be thought of as acute-phase reactants.

Normal Hemostatic Values and Pathophysiology

The hemostatic mechanism is a complex process by which blood vessels, platelets, and coagulation proteins interact to prevent excessive bleeding after tissue injury. Pathologic overactivity of this process may result in thrombosis. The initial component in the hemostatic mechanism is the blood vessel wall, which may be more fragile in fetuses and preterm infants than it is later in life. Blood platelets are produced in the bone marrow and interact with injured blood vessel walls to form primary hemostatic plugs, a process requiring a plasma cofactor (von Willebrand factor) and resulting in the generation of prostaglandin intermediates (primarily thromboxane A_2) and in secretion of the platelets' granular contents. The platelet count in fetuses and newborn infants is the same as that in older

patients, with the lower limit of normal at 150,000 per cubic millimeter. Limited studies of platelet life span in neonates suggest a value similar to that in adults: 9 days. *In vitro* studies reveal decreased platelet aggregation in neonates, but the clinical significance of these observations is unclear because the bleeding time—an *in vivo* test of hemostasis—is similar to values in older subjects. Interestingly, the platelet function analyzer test (PFA-100), a clinical laboratory simulation of the bleeding time, often produces shortened closure (bleeding) times in neonates compared to older children and adults.

More than a dozen soluble blood coagulation proteins interact sequentially after tissue injury to produce an insoluble fibrin clot. This blood coagulation mechanism is the second line of defense after the initial formation of the platelet plug. Hepatic synthesis of blood coagulation factors begins early in fetal life. Plasma concentrations of most such proteins are reduced in term infants as compared with those in older children and adults. Levels are lower still in premature infants; plasma concentrations of the vitamin K–dependent factors (II, VII, IX, X) and the contact factors (XI, XII, prekallikrein, and high-molecular-weight kininogen) may be only 10% to 40% of those in adults. However, levels of factors I (fibrinogen), V, VIII, and XIII are similar in neonates and older individuals. Proteins C and S, naturally occurring anticoagulants, guard against excessive thrombosis; their plasma concentrations are approximately one-half of those in adults. Moreover, the fibrinolytic mechanism is impaired in the fetus and neonate. Levels of both procoagulants and inhibitors rise toward adult values at a variable rate during the initial weeks to months of life.

Laboratory Evaluation

As in older patients, the platelet count, prothrombin time (PT), and activated partial thromboplastin time (PTT) are the most useful screening tests of the hemostatic mechanism. Values for these tests in term infants are only slightly higher (i.e., longer) than those in older patients. In preterm infants, however, the PTT is variably prolonged, reflecting physiologic reductions in contact factors and vitamin K–dependent coagulation proteins and possibly heparin effects. Varying PTT values depend on sampling techniques and on laboratory methods and reagents. Other tests useful in evaluating bleeding disorders in neonates are a fibrinogen determination (normal range, 175 to 450 mg/dL) and quantitation of fibrin degradation (split) products (normal value, less than 10 μg/mL) or D-dimer (normal value, less than 0.5 ng/dL). Some laboratories also use the thrombin time as an indirect test of the final stages of coagulation. Measurement of each blood coagulation factor (other than fibrinogen) and assessment of platelet function rarely are necessary.

Obtaining blood specimens for coagulation tests can be difficult because of problems with venous access and babies' small blood volume. In most hospitals, capillary specimens cannot be used for the PT and PTT. If test samples are drawn from a heparinized catheter, the PTT will be spuriously prolonged, even if the catheter is flushed first with a saline solution. Also, the high hemoglobin value of newborn infants may result in an inappropriately increased anticoagulant-to-plasma ratio in the test specimen, resulting in artifactually abnormal values.

General Diagnostic Approach to Bleeding Neonates

As in older patients, the medical history and physical examination are more useful than are myriad laboratory tests in the evaluation of a bleeding or thrombotic disorder. The differential diagnosis of altered hemostasis depends greatly on

TABLE 66.5

BLEEDING DISORDERS IN NEWBORN INFANTS: DIFFERENTIAL DIAGNOSIS BASED ON CHARACTERIZATION OF THE BABY AS WELL OR SICK

Well	Sick
Immune thrombocytopenia (maternal autoantibody or alloantibody)	Mechanical or immune complex–mediated thrombocytopenia
Hemophilia	Disseminated intravascular coagulation
Vitamin K deficiency	Severe liver disease
Local vascular lesion (gastrointestinal tract, abdominal cavity, or retroperitoneal space)	Local vascular lesion (periventricular tissues in premature infant)

whether the infant is "sick" or "well" (Table 66.5). Ill infants, particularly those who are premature, generally have an underlying disorder, such as respiratory distress syndrome, sepsis, birth asphyxia, or a metabolic disorder. The secondary bleeding signs and laboratory alterations generally result from mechanical consumptive thrombocytopenia or DIC. Bleeding infants who are well (i.e., full-term, thriving, and exhibiting no underlying disorder) most frequently have immune-mediated thrombocytopenia, vitamin K deficiency, hemophilia, or a localized anatomic lesion responsible for hemorrhage. An algorithm for the differential diagnosis of thrombocytopenia is provided in Fig. 66.4.

The history should include a family history of excessive bleeding, with careful attention to the mother and her relatives. Presence of an underlying disorder or maternal drug history may be important (e.g., mothers taking anticonvulsants during pregnancy possibly giving birth to babies with vitamin K deficiency). In addition to characterization of whether the baby is sick or well, physical findings of petechiae suggest a platelet

deficiency or fragile vessels. Localized petechiae on the presenting part usually cause no concern. Diffuse petechiae, however, usually result from severe thrombocytopenia. Petechiae are not seen in primary coagulation disorders, such as hemophilia or vitamin K deficiency.

Screening laboratory tests performed on all babies with hemorrhage should include a platelet count, PT, and PTT, with addition of fibrinogen and fibrin degradation product or D-dimer measurements in selected cases.

Treatment approaches for each disorder are discussed later. Because bleeding so often is a secondary phenomenon in sick neonates, treatment should be aimed primarily at the underlying condition. Blood products must be used judiciously. Attention should focus on preventing or stopping hemorrhage rather than on correcting abnormal laboratory tests.

Consumption of Coagulation Factors or Platelets

The most common cause of impaired hemostasis and clinical hemorrhage in neonates is DIC or mechanical consumptive thrombocytopenia. Nearly all sick neonates exhibit multiple mechanisms that may trigger blood coagulation and accelerate platelet aggregation. Often, DIC is observed accompanying respiratory distress syndrome, birth asphyxia, and infection due to multiple pathogens. The problem is compounded by the physiologic diminution of protective anticoagulants, such as antithrombin and protein C.

Infants with DIC usually present clinically with oozing from multiple puncture sites or gastrointestinal bleeding; thrombotic manifestations are noted less frequently. Nearly all babies with clinically significant hemorrhage have striking prolongations of the PT and PTT. The majority also have thrombocytopenia of variable severity (see Fig. 66.3). The PTT alone is not a reliable diagnostic test of DIC in premature infants. Fibrinogen concentration usually is low, and fibrin degradation products and D-dimer are elevated. Some babies with infection or respiratory distress show no laboratory evidence of depleted

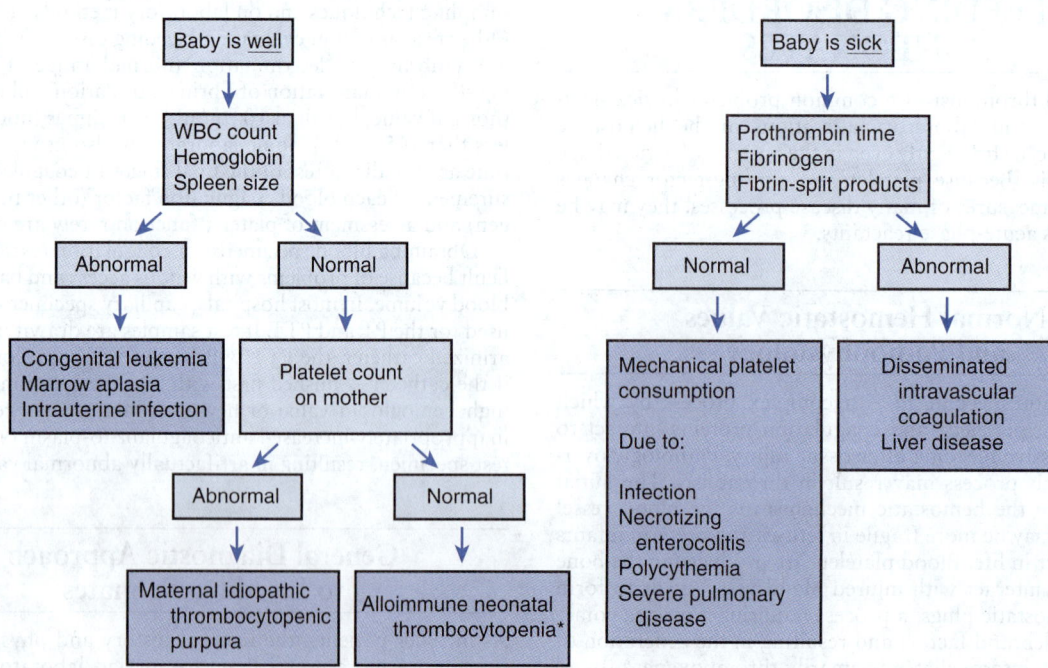

FIGURE 66.4. Diagnostic approach to the newborn infant with thrombocytopenia (platelet count <150,000 per cubic millimeter with or without symptoms). The most likely diagnoses are provided in the shaded boxes.

TABLE 66.6

IMMUNE-MEDIATED THROMBOCYTOPENIA IN NEWBORN INFANTS: DIFFERENCES IN PATHOPHYSIOLOGY, DIAGNOSIS, AND MANAGEMENT

	Maternal Idiopathic Thrombocytopenic Purpura	Alloimmune Neonatal Thrombocytopenia
Usual antigen specificity of offending antibody	"Public" antigens common to all platelets (e.g., glycoprotein IIb-IIIa complex)	Platelet-specific antigen (usually HPA-la) that is absent from the mother's platelets
Maternal platelet count	Usually reduced	Always normal
Therapy with maternal platelets	Not indicated	Treatment of choice for symptomatic infants

clotting factors but manifest only thrombocytopenia (see Fig. 66.4), which is mediated by immune complexes, vasculitis, or endotoxin. Such consumptive thrombocytopenia probably is the most common hematologic abnormality in the newborn nursery. Mechanical injury to platelets also is encountered in babies with renal vein thrombosis, necrotizing enterocolitis, and vascular malformation (Kasabach-Merritt syndrome).

Therapy for DIC or thrombocytopenia accompanying infection is directed primarily toward the underlying disorder. Fresh-frozen plasma and platelet transfusions should be used for overt hemorrhage or grossly abnormal laboratory markers. Ten to 15 mL/kg of apheresis platelet product or one or two units of volume-reduced random donor platelets usually provide a temporary increase in platelet count. Repletion of coagulation proteins with fresh-frozen plasma can be accomplished with a volume of 10 to 15 mL/kg every 12 to 24 hours. Generally, exchange transfusion has not proven useful except in those patients who have coexisting volume overload. At one time, heparin was advocated as treatment for DIC because theoretically it arrests the pathologic overactivity of coagulation; however, no data support its use except in cases of large vessel thrombosis.

Immune-Mediated Thrombocytopenia

Well infants with petechiae, bruising, and moderate to marked thrombocytopenia (but no other abnormal laboratory or physical findings) usually have maternal antibody that has crossed the placenta, coated the platelets, and resulted in their destruction by the mononuclear–phagocyte system. Although bleeding usually is not severe, deaths from intracranial bleeding have been reported. Immune-mediated thrombocytopenia during the newborn period includes two distinct conditions, which differ in the antigenic specificity of the offending antibody: neonatal alloimmune thrombocytopenia and maternal (auto-) immune thrombocytopenic purpura (Table 66.6).

In fetuses and neonates, the degree of immune thrombocytopenia is variable and does not necessarily correlate with the mother's platelet count. In alloimmune (isoimmune) neonatal thrombocytopenia, the mother's platelet count is normal. In this condition, fetal–maternal platelet antigen incompatibility occurs; usually, the antiplatelet antibody is directed against the platelet-specific HPA-1a (PLA1) antigen that is present on the baby's platelets (as a result of inheritance from the father) but not on the mother's. Occasionally, the antibodies can be directed against other platelet membrane proteins. First-born infants may be affected because sensitization of the mother may occur early in gestation. A history of previously affected infants sometimes is obtained.

In both categories of infants affected by passive maternal antibody, the platelet count usually begins to rise by several weeks of age and invariably returns to normal by 3 to 4 months of age. Bleeding signs and symptoms are uncommon after the first 3 or 4 days of life.

Treatment of immune-mediated thrombocytopenia in newborn infants is controversial. Therapeutic considerations begin with the pregnant mother, who often is known to be at risk. Therefore, close cooperation between pediatricians and obstetricians is required in such cases. In maternal immune thrombocytopenic purpura, the risk of hemorrhage in the fetus is fairly small. Thus, therapy should be focused on the mother's bleeding and platelet count. At one time, routine cesarean section was advocated, and platelet counts taken from fetal scalp specimens at the time of delivery were recommended. The risk of hemorrhage at delivery now appears to be low, however, so special intervention is not required. The platelet count in neonates bears little relationship to that in the affected mother.

The situation is different in cases of alloimmune thrombocytopenia. Here exists a substantial risk of intracranial hemorrhage *in utero* and at the time of delivery. Some have recommended that women whose previously affected offspring had intracranial hemorrhage be monitored closely during subsequent pregnancies, with cordocentesis and serial platelet counts performed on the fetus beginning at 20 to 22 weeks' gestation. Severe fetal thrombocytopenia may be treated with infusions of intravenous gamma globulin administered to the mother on a weekly basis until safe delivery by cesarean section is ensured.

Often, the existence of immune-mediated thrombocytopenia is not appreciated until the 1- or 2-day-old baby exhibits petechiae and bruising. Mildly affected infants with platelet counts greater than 20,000 per cubic millimeter need no therapy. More severely thrombocytopenic infants whose mothers have immune thrombocytopenic purpura should probably receive a short course of prednisone or intravenous gamma globulin; usually, platelet transfusions are of no value. Symptomatic babies with alloimmune thrombocytopenia should receive a transfusion of washed maternal platelets (because they lack the antigen to which the antibody is directed), typed HPA-1a negative platelets (not available in most institutions), or an infusion of gamma globulin. Further studies are required to define optimal management strategies for neonates at risk of or demonstrating immune thrombocytopenia.

Vitamin K Deficiency

Newborn infants are at risk of vitamin K deficiency because of inadequate stores in the fetus, reduced bacterial synthesis of the vitamin in the colon (due to absence of endogenous microflora), and limited dietary intake. Human breast milk has relatively little vitamin K in contrast to cow's milk–based formulas. Before the 1950s, hemorrhagic disease of the newborn, resulting from profound depletion of vitamin K–dependent coagulation factors, was a common cause of hemorrhage between the second and fifth days of life. Now, routine practice is for 0.5 to 1.0 mg of vitamin K_1 (phytonadione) to be administered intramuscularly to all neonates. In the developed world, administration of prophylactic vitamin K shortly after birth nearly has eliminated this condition. Some studies show that several oral doses are as effective as an intramuscular injection; the less expensive oral route may be more feasible in underdeveloped countries where breast-fed babies frequently bleed because of vitamin K deficiency. Vitamin K deficiency also may occur in newborns whose mothers have taken anticonvulsants (particularly phenytoin) that have warfarin-like effects. Sometimes, hemorrhagic disease resulting from vitamin K deficiency can be delayed until several months of life, particularly in breast-fed babies who have malabsorption syndromes or have received broad-spectrum antibiotics. Treatment, like prevention, is accomplished by oral or parenteral delivery of vitamin K, which is followed by prompt cessation of hemorrhage and correction of the prolonged PT and PTT within several hours.

Hemophilia

Like vitamin K deficiency, hemophilia generally manifests in well neonates. Male infants at risk of factor VIII or IX deficiency (hemophilia A or B) often are suspected on the basis of the family history. The history may be negative, however, so otherwise well newborn boys who exhibit excessive or prolonged bleeding from circumcision or heel puncture site, intracranial hemorrhage, cephalhematoma, or other unexplained bleeding should be investigated for hemophilia. In both factor VIII and IX deficiency, the PTT is prolonged markedly, but the PT is normal. Factor VIII and IX assays then must be performed to arrive at the specific diagnosis. Therapy consists of prompt intravenous administration of recombinant human factor VIII or IX. Some hematologists recommend that all neonates with hemophilia receive a dose of the appropriate factor within the first day or two of life to prevent intracranial hemorrhage.

During the newborn period, hemorrhage resulting from inherited deficiency of blood coagulation factors other than factors VIII and IX is rare. Classically, factor XIII deficiency presents with hemorrhage from the umbilical stump.

Other Causes of Impaired Hemostasis in the Neonate

Liver Disease

As in older patients, hepatic injury resulting from viruses, metabolic disorders, or hypoxic insults may result in severe bleeding due to profound reduction in the synthesis of multiple clotting factors. DIC and excessive fibrinolysis may contribute to the hemorrhagic state. Other evidence of liver dysfunction usually is apparent; the PT and PTT are prolonged markedly. Treatment, which often is unsatisfactory, consists of administration of fresh-frozen plasma.

Platelet Dysfunction

Although bleeding due to thrombocytopenia is common in neonates, it is uncertain how often qualitative platelet defects predispose to excessive hemorrhage. Infants of mothers who have taken aspirin during the final days of their pregnancies may have a mild bleeding tendency, resulting from impaired platelet aggregation. Also, clinically significant antiplatelet effects of indomethacin have been reported in premature infants receiving this agent to promote closure of the ductus arteriosus.

Thrombocytopenia Due to Diminished Production

Congenital leukemia and other infiltrative disorders, osteopetrosis (marble bone disease), congenital infection, and the thrombocytopenia absent radii syndrome may present with hemorrhage during the first days of life. Other clinical and laboratory features exist in all these conditions.

Local Vascular Lesions

Bleeding from a single anatomic site is not always a consequence of generalized impairment in hemostasis. Most babies with intracranial or abdominal hemorrhage exhibit localized anatomic defects at the site of bleeding. For instance, a congenital malformation, such as duplication, may cause gastrointestinal hemorrhage; birth trauma may cause retroperitoneal or intraabdominal bleeding (e.g., secondary to splenic rupture). In premature infants with respiratory distress syndrome, the most common cause of major morbidity and mortality is intraventricular hemorrhage. Although such babies may exhibit concomitant thrombocytopenia and the expected modest reduction in coagulation proteins, studies in which transfusions of plasma or platelets were administered to such premature infants show no convincing reduction in frequency or severity of intracranial hemorrhage (see Chapter 32, Intraventricular Hemorrhage of the Preterm Infant).

Thrombosis in Neonates

Despite the physiologic reductions in the anticoagulant proteins antithrombin, protein S, and protein C, large-vessel venous or arterial thrombosis is relatively uncommon during the newborn period. It is encountered occasionally in infants with severe dehydration, diabetic mothers, polycythemia, or DIC, especially at sites of catheter placement. Therapy consists of removal of foreign bodies and systemic heparinization. The role of low-molecular-weight heparin preparations given subcutaneously without need for close laboratory monitoring is being explored. Thrombolytic agents to dissolve existing clots (e.g., urokinase, or recombinant tissue plasminogen activator) can be used in select, carefully monitored cases.

Purpura fulminans, a syndrome of diffuse cutaneous thrombotic lesions associated with laboratory manifestations of DIC, is observed occasionally in babies with septicemia. It is encountered also in the rare infant with homozygous congenital protein C or protein S deficiency. Because protein C or S levels are reduced markedly or even are undetectable in these babies, no defense mechanisms allow for the inactivation of factors V and VIII; therefore, uncontrollable thrombosis ensues. Treatment consists of administration of fresh-frozen plasma, prothrombin complex concentrates, and warfarin. Administration of recombinant activated protein C may supplant these therapies in the near future for protein C–deficient neonates.

Some studies have shown that the most common inherited cause of a hypercoagulable state is a mutation involving the factor V molecule, termed *factor V Leiden*, which results in resistance to neutralization of the protein by activated protein C. This mutation affects nearly 5% of the white population (although it is rare in blacks and Asians). Its significance as a contributor to stroke or venous thrombosis during the neonatal period is uncertain.

Suggested Readings

Christensen RD. *Hematologic problems of the neonate.* Philadelphia: W.B. Saunders Company, 2000.

Monagle P, Andrew M. Developmental hemostasis: relevance to newborns and infants. In: Nathan DG, Orkin SH, Ginsburg D, Look TA, eds. *Nathan and Oski's hematology of infancy and childhood,* 6th ed. Philadelphia: Saunders, 2003:121.

O'Brien RT, Pearson HA. Physiologic anemia of the newborn infant. *J Pediatr* 1971;79:132.

Oski FA, Naiman JL, eds. *Hematologic problems in the newborn,* 3rd ed. Philadelphia: Saunders, 1982.

CHAPTER 67 ■ MALIGNANCY IN THE NEWBORN

JACK VAN HOFF

Cancer in neonates is an uncommon problem and one that presents unique challenges to pediatricians regarding both diagnosis and therapy. Many neoplasms discovered at birth or within the first month of life are benign, and others with apparent malignant histology may behave as benign. While this has important implications regarding the possible role of oncogene expression and modulation in embryonal and fetal cells, it complicates the clinician's decisions regarding therapy. Neonates are particularly susceptible to many of the adverse effects of both chemotherapy and radiation therapy, and they may have coexistent problems of prematurity or congenital malformations. Because of these issues, great care must be taken in deciding whether and how to treat neonatal malignancies.

EPIDEMIOLOGY

Few population-based estimates of incidence exist; most reports represent the experience of a single institution. These results are subject to selection bias because of referral patterns and can rarely be used to estimate incidence. Data from a U.S. Surveillance Epidemiology and End Results (SEER) Program study show the incidence of cancer in the first month of life to be 27 per million infants, similar to that seen in several European studies. This number includes cancers that begin in the last month or two of prenatal life, but are not diagnosed until birth. Therefore, the number is probably not significantly different from the incidence of cancer during the rest of the first year of life, which was 18 per million per month in that same study. The incidence of cancer during the first year of life is 223 per million per year, well above the incidence during the rest of the childhood years. Although cancer is uncommon during the newborn period, it can be concluded that it is no less common than it is during later childhood.

The mortality from cancer in the first month of life—six to eight per million per year—is substantially lower than the incidence. The majority of newborns with cancer survive the neonatal period.

Types of tumors seen in the neonatal period are listed in Table 67.1, which presents all neonatal tumors, both benign and malignant, seen at the Children's Hospital of Los Angeles from 1958 to 1985. Hemangiomas, the most common benign lesion of infancy, are generally excluded from discussions of neonatal tumors and are not included here. While teratomas and other soft tissue tumors constitute the majority of all tumors, neuroblastomas, leukemias, and sarcomas account for the majority of cancers in this series.

Table 67.2 compares the distribution of cancers in neonates with that of infants up to 1 year of age and all children less than 15 years of age. Neuroblastoma is the most common cancer in neonates, accounting for over 50% of all cancers. Leukemias (13%), renal tumors (13%), and sarcomas (11%) are the next most common cancers. Overall, the cancers seen in neonates differ substantially from those seen during the rest of childhood when leukemias (31%), brain tumors (18%), and lymphomas (14%) predominate.

TABLE 67.1

NEONATAL TUMORS, CHILDREN'S HOSPITAL OF LOS ANGELES, 1958 TO 1985

Tumor	Total (%)	Malignant (%)
Teratoma	46 (38)	2 (4)
Soft tissue tumor	25 (20)	8 (16)
Neuroblastoma	17 (14)	17 (33)
Leukemia	13 (11)	13 (25)
Renal tumor	7 (6)	3 (6)
Brain tumor	5 (4)	2 (4)
Hepatic tumor	4 (3)	1 (2)
Retinoblastoma	3 (2)	3 (6)
Carcinoma	2 (2)	2 (4)
Total	122 (100)	51 (100)

Adapted wwith permission from Isaacs H. Congenital and neonatal malignant tumors. *Am J Pediatr Hematol Oncol* 1987;9:121.

CLINICAL MANIFESTATIONS

One-half of neonatal malignancies and an even larger percentage of benign tumors are diagnosed on the first day of life; the remainder present over the next month. Numerous lesions have been diagnosed prenatally by ultrasonography, a process that can influence obstetric management and survival of the infant. Neonatal tumors usually present as visible or palpable masses, whether they are malignant or benign (Table 67.3). Visible masses include hemangiomas, teratomas, benign soft tissue

TABLE 67.2

PERCENT DISTRIBUTION OF THE MAJOR TYPES OF CANCER IN NEONATES, INFANTS, AND CHILDREN

Type of Cancer	Neonates <30 Days (%)	Infants <1 Year (%)	Children <15 Years (%)
Leukemia	13	14	31
Central nervous system tumor	3	15	18
Lymphoma	0.3	1	14
Neuroblastoma	54	27	8
Renal	13	11	6
Sarcoma	11	5	11
Hepatic	0	3	1.3
Malignant teratoma	0	6	0.4
Retinoblastoma	0	13	4
Other	5.7	5	6.3

Adapted with permission from Reaman GH, Bleyer A. Infants and adolescents with cancer: special considerations. In Pizzo PA, Poplack DG, eds. *Principles and practice of pediatric oncology.* 4th ed. Philadelphia: Lippincott Williams & Wilkins, 2002:410.

TABLE 67.3

BENIGN AND MALIGNANT TUMORS IN THE NEONATE (BY LOCATION)

Location of Mass	Benign Lesion	Malignancy
Subcutaneous or soft tissue, visible	Hemangioma Teratoma Fibroma Congenital viral infection Branchial or thyroglossal duct cyst Cystic hygroma	Sarcoma Teratoma Neuroblastoma Leukemia
Abdominal or pelvic, palpable	Teratoma Polycystic kidneys Urinary tract obstruction Hepatic hamartoma or hemangioma Gastrointestinal duplication Hepatosplenomegaly	Neuroblastoma Wilms tumor Teratoma Hepatoblastoma Rhabdomyosarcoma Leukemia (hepatosplenomegaly)
Intracranial	Hemorrhage Hydrocephalus Teratoma Vascular malformation	Brain tumor

Adapted with permission from Reaman GH. Special considerations for the infant with cancer. In: Pizzo PA, Poplack DG, eds. *Principles and practice of pediatric oncology*. Philadelphia: JB Lippincott, 1989:265.

tumors or sarcomas, and skin nodules from leukemia, neuroblastoma, or congenital viral infection. Hemangiomas are the most common of all neonatal "tumors," occurring in as many as 2% of all newborns. When subcutaneous, hemangiomas are differentiated from solid tumors by their characteristic appearance. Often, deeper hemangiomas can be differentiated from solid tumors by their blood flow characteristics on magnetic resonance imaging. Though almost all resolve without therapy, some increase rapidly in size and present complex management decisions. Neonatal teratomas occur most commonly in the sacrococcygeal region. Other relatively common locations include the neck and midline of the face. They are usually benign but may contain malignant elements. Sarcomas may present as masses on almost any part of the body including the head, neck, trunk, and extremities. Sarcomas are often clinically indistinguishable from benign soft tissue tumors.

Neonatal solid tumors also may present as palpable abdominal masses. Solid tumors in the upper abdomen are usually neuroblastomas or are renal or hepatic in origin. Common solid tumors in the lower abdomen and pelvis include teratomas, rhabdomyosarcomas of the genitourinary system, and neuroblastomas. They are differentiated from cystic urinary or gastrointestinal malformations by ultrasonography. Solid lesions must be biopsied or resected to differentiate malignancies from benign hamartomas.

Neonatal brain tumors may present with an abnormally large head circumference or bulging fontanelle in addition to the more typical symptoms of increased intracranial pressure such as irritability, decreased responsiveness, or vomiting. Leukemia in newborns usually presents with pallor, petechiae, or purpura. Occasionally, subcutaneous leukemic nodules are seen as dark blue spots on the skin. Retinoblastoma usually presents as leukocoria or strabismus. More advanced lesions may demonstrate signs of local inflammation or heterochromia iridis.

PROGNOSIS

Long-term survival after neonatal cancer is not uncommon. Neuroblastoma, retinoblastoma, germ cell tumor, and kidney tumor all have long-term survival rates better than 50%, whereas long-term survival rates after leukemia or brain tumor are poor.

THERAPY FOR SPECIFIC CANCERS

Solid Tumors

Teratoma

Teratomas are the most frequent perinatal neoplasm, occurring more commonly in females with a female-to-male ratio of 1.5:1. By definition, teratomas contain tissue from more than one of the three main germ layers (ectoderm, mesoderm, endoderm). They are classified as mature (containing only adult-type tissue), immature (containing embryonic-type tissue), or malignant (containing embryonal carcinoma, endodermal sinus tumor, choriocarcinoma, or germinoma).

In the newborn, teratomas are found primarily in the sacrococcygeal region with a large external and relatively small internal or presacral component. Many are now diagnosed prenatally by ultrasonography. Cesarean section is recommended in the case of large tumors, because of the risk of tumor hemorrhage or rupture with vaginal delivery. Approximately 10% of neonatal teratomas contain malignant elements, usually endodermal sinus tumor. In contrast, more than 50% of sacrococcygeal teratomas presenting after 2 months of age are malignant. About 20% of neonatal teratomas contain immature elements. These should be managed initially the same way as mature tumors—by complete surgical resection, including coccygectomy for sacrococcygeal primaries. The incidence of recurrence for both mature and immature tumors appears to be about 10%. These tumors should be followed closely postoperatively with ultrasonography or computed tomography scans for up to 3 years. Malignant teratomas or germ cell tumors in newborns are best treated with aggressive resection. The role of adjuvant chemotherapy is less clear. It appears warranted in light of the beneficial effects of cisplatin-based regimens on germ cell tumors occurring at older ages. The survival of newborns with extragonadal germ cell tumors appears to be excellent, as it is in older children.

Neuroblastoma

Neuroblastoma is the most common form of neonatal cancer, accounting for 30% to 50% of all malignancies in most series. Congenital neuroblastoma is unique in that it may spontaneously regress. Routine postmortem examinations show neuroblastoma *in situ* in the adrenal glands with a frequency 40 times higher than the lifetime incidence of neuroblastoma, implying that the majority of these cases regress without ever becoming symptomatic. A correlate to this is seen clinically in infants with a unique form of metastatic neuroblastoma—stage IV-S (consisting of a localized primary lesion plus liver, bone marrow, or cutaneous involvement)—which often regresses spontaneously. In a recent study, about one-fourth of all newly diagnosed cases of IV-S neuroblastoma regressed without any tumor-directed therapy. Stage IV-S is unique to very young children. It is most common in the neonatal period, where it accounts for 24% of all neuroblastoma cases, less common (15% of cases) between 1 month and 1 year of age, and not seen above 1 year of age.

Most neonatal neuroblastoma is localized (43% stage I+II), regional (24% stage III), or stage IV-S disease. Only a minority (10%) is true stage IV disease with distant metastases, the most common stage (55%) for children over 1 year of age. Because of this stage distribution, the prognosis for neonatal neuroblastoma is much better than the prognosis at older ages. Although the stage at presentation remains a good indicator of the prognosis, the behavior of high-stage neuroblastoma can be most accurately predicted by including histology and biologic factors such as ploidy and oncogene (MYCN) amplification in the analysis. Hyperdiploidy confers a better prognosis and MYCN amplification a decidedly worse prognosis when present. These are currently used to help determine therapy as well as prognosis.

Almost 90% of newborns with neuroblastoma will be long-term survivors, compared to just 50% of children over 1 year of age. Neonates with localized or regional disease have a particularly good prognosis, with long-term survival above 90%. Those with IV-S do only slightly worse; long-term survival estimates are 75%. Only newborns with advanced disease and unfavorable histology or biology do poorly. Recommendations for therapy include surgical resection and observation for neonates with localized disease, and initial chemotherapy followed by delayed resection for those with stage III or IV disease and favorable histology and biology. More aggressive chemotherapy should be reserved for high-stage patients with unfavorable histology or biology. Neonates with IV-S neuroblastoma should be observed without therapy, if possible. Stage IV-S patients who require therapy because of bulky abdominal disease or coagulopathy should be treated with low-dose chemotherapy and followed closely.

Routine screening for all newborns to detect early neuroblastoma by measuring urinary catecholamine levels is feasible and has been studied; however, it is not recommended. The incidence of neuroblastoma has risen in the regions screened, implying detection of tumors that would have regressed without therapy. However, the mortality rate has not decreased in those areas. The aggressive forms of neuroblastoma appear to arise *de novo* after the newborn period and are not detected by early screening.

Renal Tumors

Although renal tumors are one of the more common types of neonatal cancer, solid tumors are a less frequent cause of renal enlargement in the neonate than is hydronephrosis or cystic disease. Furthermore, many of the solid lesions are congenital mesoblastic nephromas, or other variants of the most common malignancy, Wilms tumor. Mesoblastic nephromas are renal hamartomas that are generally considered benign and curable by nephrectomy alone, although more aggressive variants demonstrating local invasion, recurrence, and even distant metastasis have been reported. In North America, neonates with Wilms tumor are treated much the same as older children, with surgery and adjuvant chemotherapy. Recommendations are to give the chemotherapy at reduced (50%) doses to ameliorate toxicity. The prognosis with this approach seems to be as good as that for older ages, in spite of the reduced doses. In Europe, the recommendations are for surgery alone, if the tumor is resectable, a policy that has also yielded excellent survival rates.

Soft Tissue Tumors

In the neonate, benign and malignant soft tissue tumors are second in frequency only to teratomas. Malignant sarcomas are among the most common forms of neonatal cancer (see Tables 67.1 and 67.2). Rhabdomyosarcoma is the most common malignant soft tissue tumor in the newborn, as it is later in childhood. Experience from the Intergroup Rhabdomyosarcoma Studies shows one-half of 14 neonates surviving long term. Recommendations are for multimodal therapy similar to treatment at older ages, with age-related reductions in chemotherapy. The tendency to reduce or eliminate radiation therapy in very young children has led to higher rates of recurrence.

A variety of other sarcomas also occur. Infantile or congenital fibrosarcoma has an excellent prognosis despite its aggressive appearance histologically. Although local recurrence may follow initial resection, congenital fibrosarcomas usually are curable with more extensive surgery, and fewer than 10% metastasize. Unresectable primaries appear to be treatable by chemotherapy. In general, other soft tissue tumors in newborns should be managed with surgery and followed closely for local relapse.

Retinoblastoma

Although rare at older ages, retinoblastoma occurs with greater frequency in neonates. Retinoblastoma has played an important role in the understanding of oncogenesis. Its familial predisposition attracted attention early and placed it in the center of research on the molecular biology of cancer. Retinoblastoma studies led to recognition of an entire new class of oncogenes—the tumor suppressor genes—and identification of the mutant protein product has provided new information on cell cycle regulation. Approximately 40% of all retinoblastomas are familial, related to a germ line mutation on chromosome 13q. Laboratory DNA studies of affected families can identify individuals at risk for developing retinoblastoma.

Familial tumors are almost always bilateral or multifocal, indicating an extreme predisposition to the development of retinoblastoma. Nonfamilial tumors are always unilateral and unifocal. Familial tumors are overrepresented in neonatal series as they present at an earlier age than do nonfamilial tumors. In the largest reported neonatal series, 42 of 46 cases proved to be bilateral, either at presentation or during subsequent follow-up.

In the past, retinoblastoma was treated successfully by enucleation or by radiation therapy, in an attempt to preserve vision for bilateral cases. However, radiation therapy dramatically increases the risk of second cancers, to as much as 50% by 24 years, in these children who are born with a defective tumor suppression mechanism. As a result, children with familial retinoblastoma treated with radiation are more likely to die of a second cancer than of the retinoblastoma, which is highly curable. Recent studies have shown that chemotherapy combined with laser therapy (thermotherapy) or cryotherapy can also successfully treat retinoblastoma, avoiding the second malignancy risk of radiation. It is clear that neonates with retinoblastoma represent a complex problem that extends beyond their initial therapy and that requires careful, lifelong follow-up.

Leukemia

Congenital leukemia is one of the most lethal neonatal malignancies, causing less than 15% of cancers but 30% of all cancer deaths. Acute myeloblastic leukemia (AML) is more common than acute lymphoblastic leukemia (ALL) in newborns, accounting for 64% of cases. During the rest of childhood, 75% of all leukemias are ALL.

Decisions regarding therapy are difficult for several reasons. First, long-term survival is uncommon; only 23% of 109 reported cases were alive at 2 years. Survival is actually better for AML (24%) than for ALL (13%), which is quite different from the prognosis during the rest of childhood. Many neonates have rearrangements of the ALL1/MLL/HRX gene on chromosome 11q23, an event that has been associated with exposure to inhibitors of topoisomerase II. These rearrangements carry a poor prognosis when found at any age.

Second, in spite of the poor overall prognosis, there are repeated reports of spontaneous remission followed by long-term survival in infant AML. In fact, 6 of the 20 known survivors of neonatal leukemia remitted spontaneously and were never treated with chemotherapy. Finally, a benign entity known as the transient myeloproliferative disorder (TMD) or transient leukemia occurs in newborns and can mimic acute leukemia. Unlike leukemia, TMD requires no therapy and usually resolves spontaneously over weeks to months. TMD is seen primarily in infants with Down syndrome and appears to depend on and be unique to trisomy 21. TMD has also been described in phenotypically normal infants; however, in virtually every case the affected child was either a trisomy 21 mosaic or had trisomy 21 in the proliferative bone marrow cells alone. TMD usually can be distinguished from acute leukemia by the presence of a relatively normal hemoglobin and platelet count, and by less than 15% blasts in the bone marrow aspirate, even though both can present with high white blood cell counts and myeloblasts on the peripheral smear.

Therefore, it is recommended that careful evaluation, including a bone marrow aspirate and cytogenetic analysis, precede any decision to treat a newborn with leukemia. Infants with Down syndrome or isolated trisomy 21 on bone marrow cytogenetics should be observed without treatment. Treatment with chemotherapy should be reserved for infants with other cytogenetic abnormalities in their bone marrow cells and either organ involvement or clear progression of disease. Many hematologists offer only supportive care initially, including exchange transfusion to lower a markedly elevated white blood cell count when necessary, while studies are being carried out.

Brain Tumors

Neonatal brain tumors differ from brain tumors in later childhood in histology, location, and prognosis. Teratomas are the most common neonatal brain tumor, accounting for 45% of all lesions. Other relatively common types include gliomas (16%), medulloblastomas (8%), choroid plexus papillomas (7%), and craniopharyngiomas (7%). The large majority of these lesions are supratentorial. Unlike many solid tumors, congenital and neonatal brain tumors have a poorer prognosis than those occurring at older ages. A 2002 review of the world's literature identified 250 infants with perinatal brain tumors, 28% of whom had prolonged survival.

Many of these tumors are very large at diagnosis, and the poor survival is more closely related to the replacement of normal brain tissue by tumor or tumor-related hydrocephalus than it is to the tumor histology. In fact, the percent survival for histologically benign teratomas is worse (12%) than it is for more malignant gliomas (34%), due primarily to the large size of the former. The most common mode of presentation is macrocephaly with or without a bulging fontanelle, and many of the affected neonates suffer dystocia and require special intervention at delivery, secondary to the large fetal skull size. This

is likely the cause of the high incidence of stillbirths (21%) and tumor-related hemorrhage (15%) seen in these patients. Prenatal diagnosis has altered delivery choices and has contributed to prolonged survival in some cases. The prognosis is so poor that some have discouraged an aggressive surgical approach to any of these lesions. Nonetheless, all cases must be considered individually because long-term, disease-free survival has been reported after surgical resection of both low- and high-grade lesions.

Suggested Readings

Abramson DH, Du TT, Beaverson KL. (Neonatal) retinoblastoma in the first month of life. *Arch Ophthalmol* 2002;120:738.

Biondi A, Cimino G, Pieters R, Pui CH. Biological and therapeutic aspects of infant leukemia. *Blood* 2000;96:24.

Bowman LC, Castleberry RP, Cantor A, et al. Genetic staging of unresectable or metastatic neuroblastoma in infants: a Pediatric Oncology Group study. *J Natl Cancer Inst* 1997;89:373.

Brantley MA Jr, Harbour JW. The molecular biology of retinoblastoma. *Ocul Immunol Inflamm* 2001;9:1.

Bresters D, Reus AC, Veerman AJ, et al. Congenital leukaemia: the Dutch experience and review of the literature. *Brit J Haematol* 2002;117:513.

Ferrari A, Casanova M, Bisogno G, et al. Rhabdomyosarcoma in infants younger than one year old: a report from the Italian Cooperative Group. *Cancer* 2003;97:2597.

Gurney JG, Ross JA, Wall DA, et al. Infant cancer in the U.S.: histology-specific incidence and trends, 1973 to 1992. *J Pediatr Hematol Oncol* 1997;19:428.

Gurney JG, Smith MA, Ross JA. Cancer among infants. In: Ries LAG, Smith MA, Gurney JG, et al., eds. *Cancer incidence and survival among children and adolescents: United States SEER program 1975–1995.* NIH Pub No 99-4649. Bethesda, MD: National Institutes of Health, 1999:149.

Isaacs H. Congenital and neonatal malignant tumors. *Am J Pediatr Hematol Oncol* 1987;9:121.

Isaacs H Jr. I. Perinatal brain tumors: a review of 250 cases. *Pediatr Neurol* 2002;27:249.

Isaacs H Jr. II. Perinatal brain tumors: a review of 250 cases. *Pediatr Neurol* 2002;27:333.

Kurkchubasche AG, Halvorson EG, Forman EN, et al. The role of preoperative chemotherapy in the treatment of infantile fibrosarcoma. *J Pediatr Surg* 2000;35:880.

Levie NS, De Kraker J, Bokkerink JP, et al. SIOP treatment guidelines for renal tumors in small infants: fact or fantasy? *Eur J Surg Oncol* 2000;26:567.

Lobe TE, Wiener ES, Hays DM, et al. Neonatal rhabdomyosarcoma: the IRS experience. *J Pediatr Surg* 1994;29:1167.

Low DW. Hemangiomas and vascular malformations. *Semin Pediatr Surg* 1994; 3:40.

Lumbroso L, Doz F, Urbieta M, et al. Chemothermotherapy in the management of retinoblastoma. *Ophthalmology* 2002;109:1130.

Reaman GH, Bleyer A. Infants and adolescents with cancer: special considerations. In: Pizzo PA, Poplack DG, eds. *Principles and practice of pediatric oncology,* 4th ed. Philadelphia: Lippincott Williams and Wilkins, 2002:409.

Rescorla FJ, Sawin RS, Coran AG, et al. Long-term outcome for infants and children with sacrococcygeal teratoma: a report from the Children's Cancer Group. *J Pediatr Surg* 1998;33:171.

Rickert CH. Neuropathology and prognosis of foetal brain tumours. *Acta Neuropathol* 1999;98:567.

Ritchey ML, Azizkhan RG, Beckwith JB, et al. Neonatal Wilms tumor. *J Pediatr Surg* 1995;30:856.

Tsuchida Y, Ikeda H, Iehara T, et al. Neonatal neuroblastoma: incidence and clinical outcome. *Med Pediatr Oncol* 2003;40:391.

Wakai S, Toshimoto A, Nagai M. Congenital brain tumors. *Surg Neurol* 1984; 21:597.

Weitzman S, Grant R. Neonatal oncology: diagnostic and therapeutic dilemmas. *Semin Perinatol* 1997;21:102.

Woods WG, Gao RN, Shuster JJ, et al. Screening of infants and mortality due to neuroblastoma. *N Engl J Med* 2002;346:1041.

Zipursky A, Brown EJ, Christensen H, Doyle J. Transient myeloproliferative disorder (transient leukemia) and hematologic manifestations of Down syndrome. *Clin Lab Med* 1999;19:157.

CHAPTER 68 ■ DERMATOLOGIC DISEASES

TODD E. HOLMES AND PAUL A. KRUSINSKI

BIRTHMARKS

Birthmarks comprise a wide spectrum of common and uncommon congenital disorders, the recognition of which is crucial for predicting the natural course and potential for associated abnormalities. Table 68.1 lists the incidence of common birthmarks.

Pigmented Lesions

Melanocytes are melanin-producing cells that originate in the neural crest and migrate *in utero* to the skin, mucous membranes, eyes, inner ear, and central nervous system (CNS). Tumors of melanocytes in the skin are composed of one of three types of cells: nevus cells, epidermal melanocytes, and dermal melanocytes (Box 68.1). All melanocytic tumors, except freckles, may be present at birth. Freckles are acquired later in childhood. Melanocytic nevi are further classified as junctional, intradermal, or compound when the location of nevus cells is within the epidermis, the dermis, or both, respectively.

Congenital Melanocytic Nevus

Congenital melanocytic nevi (CMN) occur in 1% to 6% of all newborns and are classified according to the size they attain or are predicted to attain in adulthood. Nevi that are less than 1.5 cm in diameter are classified as small, nevi between 1.5 and 19.9 cm in diameter are classified as medium, and nevi that are 20 cm or greater in diameter are classified as large. The very large CMN involving a major portion of the body are often referred to as "giant" or "bathing trunk" nevi. CMN typically present as sharply demarcated, often multicolored and hairy, dark brown patches. In some CMN, especially the larger ones, the overlying skin can be thickened and verrucous, and satellite lesions may be present. CMN are significant because of their increased risk for development of malignant melanoma. The risk for developing melanoma increases with the size of the nevus. The lifetime risk for developing melanoma in patients with CMN less than 20 cm in diameter is estimated to be between 0% and 4.9% with most melanomas developing at or after puberty, whereas the lifetime risk of developing melanoma in patients with CMN greater than 20 cm is estimated to be between 4.5% and 10% with most melanomas arising before puberty. If prophylactic removal is decided, it should be performed early in life for large CMN and any time up to puberty for small and medium CMN. Features that suggest development of melanoma in a CMN include change in color, irregular or scalloped border, change in size or thickness, variation in color within the lesion, bleeding, or ulceration. CMN may have irregular borders and variation in color and thickness from the outset, making it difficult to follow these lesions for early malignant changes (Fig. 68.1). All CMN with atypical or suspicious features should be excised regardless of size.

Patients with large CMN are also at risk for neurocutaneous melanocytosis. The highest risk for melanoma or neurocutaneous melanocytosis is seen in patients with large CMN in a posterior axial location, especially when associated with satellite smaller CMN. Neurocutaneous melanosis can result in seizures, hydrocephalus, or focal neurologic defects. A risk exists of developing a primary malignant melanoma in the leptomeningeal lesions as well as the cutaneous CMN.

Dermal Melanocytosis

Often referred to as Mongolian spots, dermal melanocytosis (DM) is characterized by blue-gray, poorly defined patches

TABLE 68.1

INCIDENCE OF BIRTHMARKS IN NEONATES

Birthmark	Occurrence (%)
Café au lait spot	2.0
Hemangioma	2.6
Melanocytic nevus	1.3
Mongolian spot	25.5
Nevus sebaceous	0.3
Port wine stain	0.3
Nevus flammeus	68.6

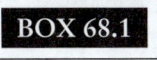

BOX 68.1 **Benign Melanocytic Tumors of the Skin**

Nevus cells
Melanocytic/nevocellular nevus
Epidermal melanocytes
Freckle (ephelis)
Lentigo
Café au lait spot
Dermal melanocytes
Mongolian spot
Blue nevus
Nevus of Ota
Nevus of Ito

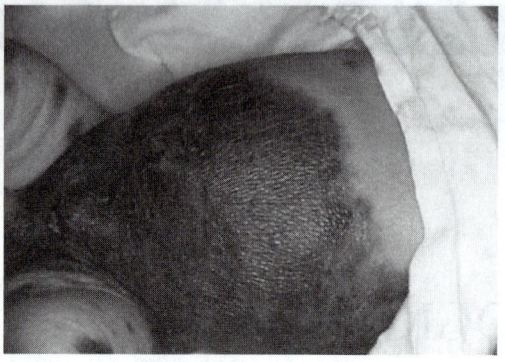

FIGURE 68.1. Giant congenital melanocytic nevus with atypical features, including a scalloped border, irregular pigmentation, and variable thickness. See Color Figure 68.1 in color section.

that are most commonly seen overlying the sacral region of the newborn. It is the most commonly encountered congenital pigmented lesion; however, there are marked racial differences in prevalence. It is seen in 95% of black, 81% of Asian, 46% to 70% of Hispanic, and 10% of white infants. The lesions are due to the delayed disappearance of dermal melanocytes. To help avoid possible confusion with bruising, DM should always be documented when detected on physical examination. DM is benign and usually disappears during the first or second year of life, but may persist in dark-skinned individuals.

Blue Nevus

Blue nevi are uncommon benign tumors composed of dermal melanocytes that may be present at birth. The common blue nevus and the cellular blue nevus cannot be distinguished clinically but differ histologically. Blue nevi are well-circumscribed, slate blue or bluish black papules or nodules with a predilection for the buttocks, face, or dorsum of the hands and feet. Common blue nevi are usually less than 15 mm in diameter and are not a risk for the development of malignant melanoma. Cellular blue nevi are often larger and may rarely undergo malignant transformation into malignant melanoma.

Café au Lait Spot

Café au lait spots (CALSs) are well-circumscribed, homogenously pigmented, light brown macules that range from 1.5

to 15 cm in diameter. They are frequently present at birth, are almost always present by 1 year of age, and may increase in number during early childhood. CALSs are seen in approximately 2% of all newborn infants and up to 25% of the normal adult population. They are more common in darker-pigmented races. The vast majority of patients with CALSs have one or two lesions and have no associated abnormalities. However, the presence of six or more with a diameter of greater than 0.5 cm before puberty and 1.5 cm after puberty is highly suggestive, but not diagnostic, of neurofibromatosis. CALSs are also seen in other disorders, including tuberous sclerosis, McCune Albright syndrome, ataxia-telangiectasia, and Bloom syndrome.

Mastocytosis

Mastocytosis is an uncommon disorder characterized by the abnormal accumulation of mast cells in tissues. Mast cell disease encompasses a spectrum from isolated cutaneous involvement to systemic disease (Table 68.2). The cause for the increase in mast cell numbers is not completely understood. However, mutations of c-kit, the receptor for mast cell growth factor, on mast cells have been demonstrated. Cutaneous lesions appear as red-brown to yellow-brown macules, papules, or nodules that range in size from a few millimeters to several centimeters in diameter. Characteristically, the skin lesions will urticate with rubbing (Darier sign) because of mast cell degranulation and histamine release resulting in increased vascular permeability, edema, and wheal formation. If the edema is marked, blistering may occur. Mastocytomas are present at birth or develop shortly thereafter and appear as reddish-brown plaques or nodules. Single lesions are the rule, although occasionally two or three are present, typically involving the distal extremities, particularly the wrist. Most isolated mastocytomas resolve spontaneously after several years. Generalized cutaneous mastocytosis (urticaria pigmentosa) is characterized by the appearance of multiple red-brown macules, papules, and plaques (Fig. 68.2). The majority of cases occur before puberty, with about half presenting before 9 months of age. Most affected children have significant clearing or complete resolution of the cutaneous lesions by early adulthood. Systemic symptoms may occur because of release of histamine and other mediators from cutaneous lesions and include pruritus, flushing, hypotension, tachycardia, and, less often, diarrhea, dyspnea, and syncope. Systemic mastocytosis with mast cell infiltration of bone, liver, spleen, lymph nodes, skin, and gastrointestinal tract is rare in children.

TABLE 68.2

CLASSIFICATION OF MASTOCYTOSIS

Disease	Age Predominance	Characteristics
Mastocytomas	0–3 months	1–3 reddish-brown nodules or plaques
Urticaria pigmentosa (UP)	Usually presents before 9 months	Multiple reddish-brown macules and papules
Pseudoxanthomatous	Rare variant of UP; mastocytosis	Pale yellow nodules usually present at birth
Diffuse cutaneous mastocytosis	Rare; usually presents before 3 years of age	Reddish-brown, edematous skin with an orange-peel texture; bullae common
Systemic mastocytosis	Adults; rare in children	Cutaneous and systemic mast cell infiltrates
Mast cell leukemia	Adults; rare in children	Mast cells in peripheral blood
Telangiectasia macularis eruptiva perstans (TMEP)	Adults	Multiple reddish-brown telangiectatic macules

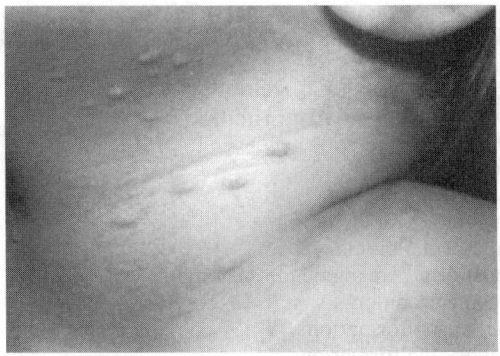

FIGURE 68.2. Multiple pinkish brown papules and nodules of generalized cutaneous mastocytosis. See Color Figure 68.2 in color section.

Epidermal Nevus

Epidermal nevi are benign tumors in which the epidermis is hyperplastic. A variety of names have been given to this lesion, including linear epidermal nevus, nevus unius lateris, ichthyosis hystrix, and systematized epidermal nevus. Most epidermal nevi are present at birth and may become more extensive with age. The lesions are tan, brown, or black verrucous growths arranged in a linear, asymmetric fashion and are more often unilateral than bilateral. The diagnosis of epidermal nevus syndrome is made when epidermal nevi are seen in association with central nervous system, ocular, musculoskeletal, and other organ abnormalities. Inflammatory linear verrucous epidermal nevi (ILVEN) are distinguished from linear epidermal nevi clinically by the presence of pruritus and erythema and histologically by the presence of inflammation and parakeratosis. They are usually present at birth and occur mainly on the extremities in girls.

Nevus Sebaceous

Sebaceous nevi are benign hamartomas of sebaceous and apocrine glands that present at birth on the head or neck. They are well-circumscribed, often linear, yellow-orange, smooth, hairless, verrucous plaques (Fig. 68.3). At puberty, enlargement

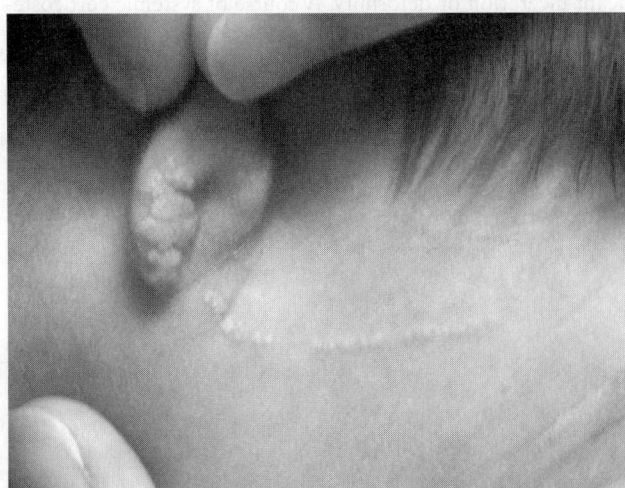

FIGURE 68.3. Linear nevus sebaceous on the neck and posterior ear with typical sharply demarcated, waxy, yellow-orange, pebbly appearance. See Color Figure 68.3 in color section.

occurs as the sebaceous glands become active under androgenic influence. Large sebaceous nevi may be associated with congenital skeletal defects and CNS disease, including mental retardation and seizures, much like those seen in the epidermal nevus syndrome. Small, isolated lesions of sebaceous nevi are not associated with other defects. During adulthood, sebaceous nevi may be complicated by secondary tumor development. Syringocystadenoma papilliferum and trichoblastomas are the most common tumors to arise from sebaceous nevi and occur in approximately 10% of the cases. Basal cell carcinomas (BCCs) were previously believed to be the most common tumors arising from sebaceous nevi. However, retrospective studies have shown that the majority of these cases were actually trichoblastomas. Because most tumors occur in adults older than age 40 and the incidence of BCC is much lower than once believed, prophylactic surgery is of unclear benefit and clinical follow-up is probably sufficient.

Hypopigmented Lesions

Ash Leaf Spot

Ash leaf spots are present in 85% of individuals with tuberous sclerosis and are the only cutaneous manifestation of tuberous sclerosis present at birth or in early infancy. Clinically they are characterized by hypopigmented, leaf-shaped macules with smooth or jagged borders. Linear and confetti-like hypopigmented macules may also be seen. Other skin lesions characteristic of this disorder develop later in childhood or in early adolescence, including adenoma sebaceum (multiple facial angiofibromas), periungual fibromas (Koenen's tumors), shagreen patches, and CALSs. Ash leaf spots persist, and affected individuals may continue to develop new lesions during childhood. Wood's light examination aids in the detection of ash leaf spots in fair-skinned infants.

Nevus Depigmentosus

Nevus depigmentosus (ND), also called achromic nevus, is a congenital hypopigmented macule or patch that is stable in its relative size and shape throughout life. ND should be distinguished from vitiligo. ND is present at birth, whereas vitiligo usually presents later in childhood or adulthood. Lesions of ND are slightly off-white when compared to the milky white lesions of vitiligo. Vitiligo is caused by the complete loss of melanocytes and melanosomes in the skin, whereas the lesional skin of ND is thought to have abnormal melanosomes with a normal complement of melanocytes. ND is usually not associated with other defects.

Piebaldism

Piebaldism is a rare autosomal dominant disorder caused by mutations in the c-kit gene, in which depigmented patches of skin are present at birth. Characteristic features are a white forelock or hypopigmented tuft of hair in the frontal region and the presence of normally pigmented islands of skin within the leukoderma. Some affected individuals have been reported to have cerebellar ataxia, neurosensory deafness, or mental retardation. A white forelock, leukoderma, heterochromic irides and fundi, hypertelorism, congenital deafness, premature graying of hair, confluence of the medial eyebrows, and a broad nasal root are manifestations of Waardenburg syndrome. Also autosomal dominant, there are several genetic variants of this disorder that are caused by mutations of the PAX3, MITF, or ENDRB genes.

Hypomelanosis of Ito

Hypomelanosis of Ito (incontinentia pigmenti achromians) is a rare disorder of irregular, linear, and whorled hypopigmentation on the trunk and extremities. Approximately three-fourths of affected individuals will have associated abnormalities of the CNS, eyes, teeth, nails, hair, musculoskeletal system, or internal organs. In most cases, the pigmentary changes are present at birth or within the first year of life and may become more extensive.

Nevus Anemicus

Nevus anemicus is a congenital developmental anomaly that is characterized by hypopigmented macules of varying size and shape. The involved area is lighter than the normal skin, not because a loss of pigment occurs, but because blood vessels are constricted, producing a permanent blanching of the area. This blanching is a functional rather than a structural abnormality, presumed to be caused by local increased sensitivity to catecholamines. The color difference between the nevus and the normal skin can be accentuated by brisk rubbing; the normal skin becomes red, whereas the nevus does not. A nevus anemicus is not generally associated with other defects and does not change with age.

Vascular Lesions

Normal Variants

Cutis Marmorata. Cutis marmorata is the normal, reticulated, cyanotic mottling of the skin that is a physiologic response to chilling. This change is not normal if it persists after the infant is warmed. Persistent mottling or livedo reticularis implies an obstruction to blood flow such as hyperviscosity or vasculitis.

Harlequin Color Change. The harlequin color change is a benign phenomenon seen in up to 9% of premature infants and is thought to be caused by immature vasomotor control or transient hypothalamic hypoxia with vasospasm. When the infant lies on his or her side, the lower half of the body becomes reddened and the upper half blanches. An episode may last for several seconds or minutes and resolves spontaneously when the infant is placed in the supine position.

Congenital Vascular Abnormalities

Congenital vascular abnormalities can be classified as vascular tumors or vascular malformations (Box 68.2). Vascular tumors are benign neoplasms of vascular endothelium and are characterized by cellular proliferation. Vascular malformations, in contrast, are structural anomalies derived from arteries, veins, or lymphatics and do not have a proliferative phase. These malformations remain stable, with the growth of the lesion correlating with the growth of the child.

Vascular Tumors

Infantile Hemangiomas. Infantile hemangiomas and hemangiomas of infancy are terms now used to describe a group of vascular tumors that have historically been recognized as strawberry hemangiomas or capillary hemangiomas. The most common benign tumor of infancy, infantile hemangiomas occur in up to 2.6% of all neonates and up to 10% of Caucasian children. They are especially common in premature infants, especially those weighing less than 1,500 g, and are two to five times more frequent in females than in males. About half of infantile hemangiomas are present at birth, with the remain-

---

BOX 68.2   Congenital Vascular Abnormalities

Vascular tumors
Infantile hemangioma
Congenital hemangioma
Tufted hemangioma
Kaposiform hemangioendothelioma
Pyogenic granuloma
Vascular malformations
Capillary malformations
Lymphatic malformations
Venous malformations
Arteriovenous malformation

der becoming evident within the first month of life. Infantile hemangiomas may occur anywhere on the skin and mucosal surfaces. Their location in the skin may be superficial, deep, or mixed, which results in a variety of clinical appearances. When fully developed, superficial hemangiomas (50% to 60%) are bright red with a finely lobulated surface. Deep hemangiomas (15%) present as blue-purple masses with minimal to no overlying skin changes. Mixed superficial and deep hemangiomas (25% to 35%) have features of both (Fig. 68.4). If not present at birth, infantile hemangiomas may be preceded by a telangiectatic macule surrounded by an area of pallor, a pink macule, or a bruise-like patch. These early lesions are subtle and are often mistaken for port wine stains (PWSs).

Parents frequently become alarmed when a hemangioma begins to grow, particularly if it becomes eroded or bleeds. The natural history of these lesions must be stressed, because more than 90% resolve spontaneously. Hemangiomas grow rapidly during the first 6 months of life, with most reaching their maximal growth by the time the infant is 18 months old. A general rule is that 30% resolve by 3 years of age, 50% by 5 years, 70% by 7 years, and 90% by 9 years. While most hemangiomas are asymptomatic and can be managed by close observation, up to 20% may have associated complications. Indications for aggressive treatment include compromise of a vital function (sight, respiration, or nutrition), high-output congestive heart failure, consumptive coagulopathy, and significant ulceration or deformity. A course of systemic corticosteroids is the treatment of choice, with a starting dosage of 2 to

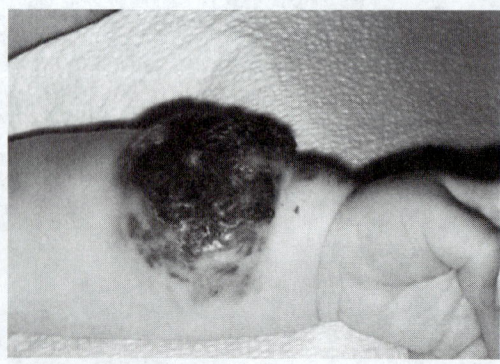

FIGURE 68.4. Mixed superficial and deep infantile hemangioma on the left forearm with ulceration and crusting. The superficial component is bright red; the deep component is blue. See Color Figure 68.4 in color section.

3 mg/kg/day followed by a tapering course over 2 to 4 months. To avoid potential side effects associated with systemic therapy, corticosteroids may be used both intralesionally and topically in selected cases. Pulse dye laser (PDL) surgery is accepted as an effective treatment of ulceration and residual erythema or telangiectasia. PDL treatment of proliferating hemangiomas, however, is more controversial. Interferon alfa is effective, but a significant risk of spastic diplegia has limited its use to those infants with life-threatening or severely function-threatening hemangiomas.

Congenital Hemangiomas. Rarely, infants can present with a fully developed hemangioma at birth. This subset of hemangiomas is distinct from infantile hemangiomas and is characterized by intrauterine growth, little to no growth in the postnatal period, and rapid involution within the first year of life.

Kasabach-Merritt Syndrome. Kasabach-Merritt syndrome, in which platelets are trapped and coagulation factors are consumed locally within a vascular lesion, is a complication of tufted angiomas and kaposiform hemangioendotheliomas. This syndrome is manifested by an enlarging vascular lesion with surrounding ecchymoses and may develop into a full-blown disseminated intravascular coagulation-like picture with thrombocytopenia and a hemorrhagic diathesis.

Diffuse Neonatal Hemangiomatosis. Multiple lesions are seen in approximately 15% of infants with hemangiomas and are an indication of possible visceral involvement. *Diffuse neonatal hemangiomatosis* is a term used to describe infants with multiple visceral and cutaneous hemangiomas. *Benign neonatal hemangiomatosis* is used to describe infants with cutaneous involvement only. The CNS, liver, lungs, and gastrointestinal tract are the most common sites of involvement in diffuse neonatal hemangiomatosis. Affected infants are noted at birth to have small, red to bluish black, papular hemangiomas 0.2 to 2.5 cm in diameter, and they may develop hundreds of similar lesions in infancy (Fig. 68.5). Diffuse neonatal hemangiomatosis is a life-threatening condition with reported mortality rates ranging between 29% and 80%. Treatment with systemic corticosteroids may result in involution of the cutaneous and visceral hemangiomas. If the infants survive, the hemangiomas tend to regress with time, much like typical hemangiomas of infancy.

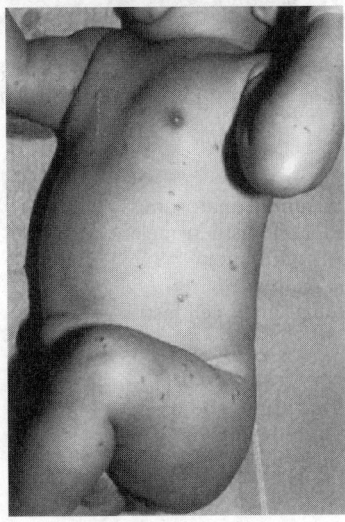

FIGURE 68.5. Newborn with multiple 1- to 4-mm, firm, red, papular cutaneous hemangiomas of the diffuse neonatal hemangiomatosis syndrome. See Color Figure 68.5 in color section.

PHACES Syndrome. Large hemangiomas on the face and neck are seen more frequently in female children (7:1) and are associated with other congenital abnormalities. The acronym PHACES is used to describe these anomalies (posterior fossa brain malformations, hemangiomas, arterial anomalies, coarctation of the aorta and cardiac defects, eye abnormalities, and sternal defects and supraumbilical raphe).

Vascular Malformations

Nevus Flammeus. The most common of all birthmarks, the nevus flammeus is a pink macule found over the glabella, eyelids, nasolabial folds, or nape of the neck. These capillary malformations are often referred to as "salmon patches" or "angel kisses" when they occur on the face and "stork bites" when they occur on the nape of the neck. The facial lesions tend to fade or disappear during childhood, whereas those that occur in the nape area may not.

Port Wine Stain. A variant of nevus flammeus, PWSs present at birth in approximately 3 in 1,000 children. Clinically they are characterized by pink to dark or bluish red macules and patches that are frequently unilateral. Facial lesions are most common and are often distributed in an area supplied by one of the three main branches of the sensory trigeminal nerve. PWSs do not resolve, their growth parallels the growth of the child, and they tend to darken and thicken with age. Soft tissue hypertrophy may produce deformity and dysfunction of the involved area. In addition to this medical indication for treatment, the psychological trauma of a large or disfiguring PWS should not be underestimated. PDL surgery has been shown to be a safe and effective method for removing PWSs with minimal risk for scarring. Several treatments of the entire PWS are necessary for optimal fading or resolution. Beginning laser surgery early in life reduces the number of treatments required for clearing and prevents progression of the PWS.

Sturge-Weber Syndrome. Hallmarks of the Sturge-Weber syndrome include a facial PWS in the distribution of the ophthalmic branch of the trigeminal nerve (V_1), an ipsilateral intracranial vascular anomaly (leptomeningeal angiomatosis), and intracranial calcifications that follow the contours of the cerebral cortex. Between 10% and 15% of patients with a PWS in the distribution of V_1 will develop Sturge-Weber syndrome. The PWS may be bilateral (40%) or involve the trunk and extremities in addition to the face, but no correlation exists between the extent of the cutaneous involvement and the severity of the CNS vascular malformation. Other features of the Sturge-Weber syndrome include seizures (80%), vascular headaches (60%), mental retardation (60%), hemiplegia (30%), hemianopsia (40%), and glaucoma (45%). The highest risk for glaucoma is seen in those individuals with PWS involvement of both the ophthalmic and maxillary divisions of the trigeminal nerve. Studies suggest that all patients with a facial PWS in this distribution are at risk for glaucoma, regardless of the presence of Sturge-Weber syndrome. Therefore, any infant with a PWS involving the V_1 or V_2 divisions of the trigeminal nerve should be followed closely for evidence of glaucoma.

Klippel-Trénaunay-Weber Syndrome. Most commonly observed on an extremity or the trunk, the Klippel-Trénaunay-Weber syndrome is characterized by port wine malformations in association with deep venous malformations, superficial varicosities, and overgrowth of underlying soft tissue and bone. The PWSs are frequently linear and are almost always unilateral. Hypertrophy of the limb or portion of the trunk may be present at birth or develop in infancy. Treatment has been unsatisfactory.

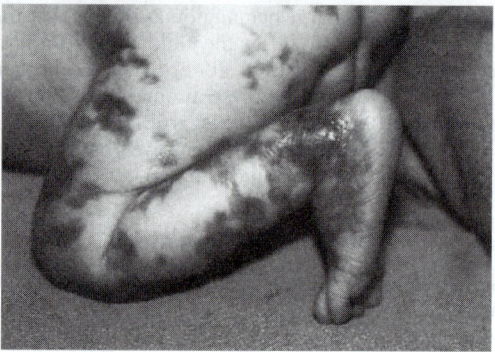

FIGURE 68.6. Reticulated mottling of cutis marmorata telangiectatica congenita with atrophy and telangiectasia of the skin. See Color Figure 68.6 in color section.

Cutis Marmorata Telangiectatica Congenita. Cutis marmorata telangiectatica congenita is a rare congenital vascular malformation characterized by red-purple, reticulated mottling and telangiectasia, with or without ulceration and atrophy of the skin (Fig. 68.6). Unlike cutis marmorata, the reticulated pattern is persistent. One extremity is most commonly affected, but lesions may be bilateral and the trunk may be involved. A variety of associated defects (orthopaedic, ocular, neurologic, and other vascular abnormalities) have been reported in up to 50% of cases. The cutaneous lesions tend to improve with age and may disappear completely.

Angiokeratoma. Angiokeratomas are characterized by dilation of superficial dermal capillaries with hypertrophy and hyperkeratosis of the overlying epidermis. At least six types are recognized, but only one, the angiokeratoma circumscriptum, is present at birth. Lesions are deep red to blue-black, verrucous papules and nodules, and are often arranged in a grouped or linear pattern. Although the lesions remain localized, they do not resolve spontaneously.

Lymphatic Malformation. Lymphatic malformations may be microcystic (aggregates of abnormal microscopic lymphatic channels), macrocystic (aggregates of large interconnected lymphatic cysts), or mixed. The old term for microcystic lymphatic malformations was lymphangioma circumscriptum. Clinically these lesions are characterized by groups of thick-walled, deep-seated, vesicle-like papules resembling frog spawn that appear at birth or early childhood. If purely lymphatic, the vesicles appear clear or translucent, but if a hemangiomatous component is present, they have a red or bluish hue (Fig. 68.7). Macrocystic lymphatic malformations (cystic hygromas) typically present on the neck, axilla, or lateral chest wall as a large translucent soft mass under normal skin. These malformations can be associated with chromosomal or other congenital anomalies. Microcystic lymphatic malformations can be removed by excision. Macrocystic lymphatic malformations are best treated with sclerotherapy. Excision may be attempted when sclerotherapy fails; however, extensive lesions are difficult to remove and often recur.

Blue Rubber Bleb Nevus Syndrome. The blue rubber bleb nevus syndrome is characterized by bluish venous malformations of the skin and viscera. The cutaneous lesions are present at birth but tend to increase in number with age and have a distinctive soft, blue, rubbery, wrinkled appearance. The classic cutaneous lesions are nipple-like lesions that compress easily and refill slowly. Most visceral hemangiomas are found in the small bowel, but they can occur anywhere in the gastrointestinal tract. Other less common sites of visceral involvement in-

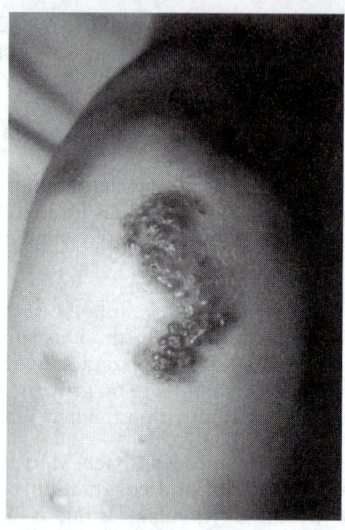

FIGURE 68.7. Lymphangioma circumscriptum with a purple-red hemangiomatous component on the extensor aspect of the elbow. See Color Figure 68.7 in color section.

clude the CNS, lungs, and heart. Affected infants are at significant risk for anemia and serious gastrointestinal bleeding.

VESICULOPUSTULAR AND BULLOUS DISORDERS

Vesicles and Pustules

Box 68.3 and Figure 68.8 present the differential diagnosis of vesicles, pustules, and bullae in the newborn.

Miliaria

Resulting from the occlusion and rupture of sweat ducts in the skin, miliaria occurs in several forms. Miliaria crystallina

---

BOX 68.3   Differential Diagnosis of Vesicles or Pustules in the Newborn

Noninfectious
Miliaria
Erythema toxicum neonatorum
Transient neonatal pustular melanosis
Acropustulosis of infancy
Incontinentia pigmenti
Congenital Langerhans cell histiocytosis
Neonatal acne

Infectious
Congenital cutaneous candidiasis
Staphylococcal folliculitis/impetigo
Congenital herpes simplex
Congenital syphilis
Varicella
Bacterial sepsis
Scabies

Blistering Eruptions

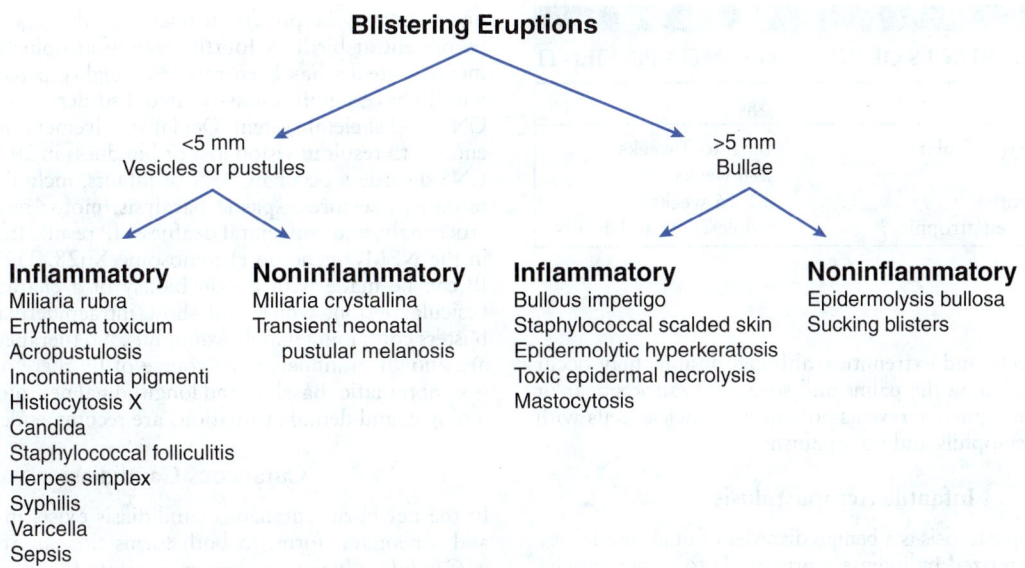

```
Blistering Eruptions
        /                    \
  <5 mm                      >5 mm
Vesicles or pustules          Bullae
    /        \            /          \
```

Inflammatory
Miliaria rubra
Erythema toxicum
Acropustulosis
Incontinentia pigmenti
Histiocytosis X
Candida
Staphylococcal folliculitis
Herpes simplex
Syphilis
Varicella
Sepsis

Noninflammatory
Miliaria crystallina
Transient neonatal
  pustular melanosis

Inflammatory
Bullous impetigo
Staphylococcal scalded skin
Epidermolytic hyperkeratosis
Toxic epidermal necrolysis
Mastocytosis

Noninflammatory
Epidermolysis bullosa
Sucking blisters

FIGURE 68.8. Differential diagnosis for blistering eruptions.

and miliaria rubra (heat rash) are the forms most commonly observed in the neonatal period. Likened to dewdrops on the skin, miliaria crystallina is seen in bundled children or in patients with a high fever. The eccrine sweat ducts rupture superficially in the skin, which results in small, clear, superficial vesicles that have no associated inflammation and are asymptomatic. In miliaria rubra, sweat ducts rupture more deeply within the skin and provoke an inflammatory response resulting in pruritic, erythematous papules that may evolve into vesicles and pustules (miliaria pustulosa). In neonates, the face, neck and trunk are most commonly involved, although a more widespread distribution may occur. Miliaria resolves spontaneously if the infant is kept cool and dry and if topical creams or lotions, which aggravate the condition, are avoided.

Erythema Toxicum Neonatorum

Erythema toxicum neonatorum is a common eruption occurring in approximately one-third of normal newborn infants. It may be present at birth but usually develops on day 2 or 3 of life and is characterized by large, splotchy areas of erythema studded with urticarial papules, vesicles, and pustules (Fig. 68.9). Lesions are found in greatest numbers on the trunk, with fewer on the face and extremities. The palms and soles are not in-

volved. The eruption lasts 7 to 14 days and resolves spontaneously without pigmentary change or scarring. The diagnosis can be confirmed with a Tzanck smear (Giemsa or Wright stain) or Gram stain of the pustule, which will reveal eosinophils with few or no polymorphonuclear cells and no organisms.

Transient Neonatal Pustular Melanosis

Present at birth, transient neonatal pustular melanosis is seen in up to 5% of black infants and 0.3% of white infants. The cutaneous lesions are vesiculopustules without surrounding erythema. The pustules are fragile and rupture quickly, often resolving within 24 hours, leaving a hyperpigmented macule surrounded by a collarette scale (Fig. 68.10). Rarely, pigmented spots without pustules are noted at birth. The pigmented macules resemble freckles and may last for several weeks before resolving. The most common areas of involvement are the lower

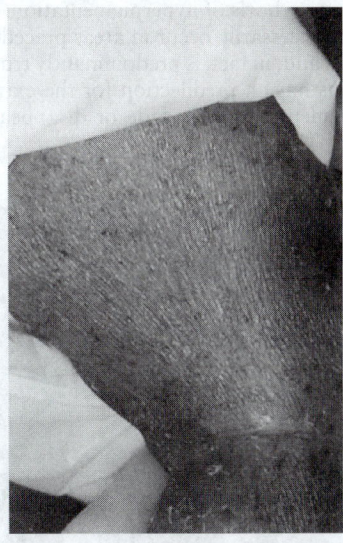

FIGURE 68.9. The hallmark splotchy erythema studded with small papules and pustules of erythema toxicum. See Color Figure 68.9 in color section.

FIGURE 68.10. Hyperpigmented macules of transient neonatal pustular melanosis, many of which are surrounded by a collarette of scale that is the remnant of the roof of the preceding pustule. See Color Figure 68.10 in color section.

TABLE 68.3

CUTANEOUS STAGES OF INCONTINENTIA PIGMENTI

Stage	Age
Inflammatory/vesicular	Birth to 3 weeks
Verrucous	2–6 weeks
Hyperpigmented	12–26 weeks
Hypopigmented/atrophic	Adolescents and adults

face, chin, neck, and extremities, although lesions may occur anywhere, including the palms and soles. A Tzanck smear or Gram stain of a pustule reveals polymorphonuclear cells with few or no eosinophils and no organisms.

Infantile Acropustulosis

Infantile acropustulosis is a benign disorder of unclear etiology that is characterized by intensely pruritic 1- to 3-mm vesicles and pustules on the hands and feet. The scalp, face, and trunk are also occasionally involved. It presents from birth to 1 year of age, recurs in crops, and resolves spontaneously within 2 or 3 years. A Tzanck smear or Gram stain of pustular contents will show numerous neutrophils, occasional eosinophils, and no bacteria. Potent topical corticosteroids and antihistamines may provide symptomatic relief, and intractable cases may be treated successfully with dapsone at 1 to 2 mg/kg/day.

Incontinentia Pigmenti

Also known as Bloch-Sulzberger disease, incontinentia pigmenti (IP) is an uncommon genodermatosis with X-linked dominant inheritance. Ninety-seven percent of affected individuals are females, as this trait is usually antenatally lethal in males. The cutaneous manifestations occur in three distinct stages, not all of which are present in every patient (Table 68.3). The first stage begins at birth or shortly thereafter and is characterized by crops of vesicles in linear streaks or bands on the extremities and trunk (Fig. 68.11). Vesicles continue to develop for 2 to 3 weeks and are followed by the development of warty, hyperkeratotic lesions in a linear array, particularly on the extremities. The third stage tends to begin after age 3 months with linear streaks and whorls of hyperpigmentation. This pigmentation does not necessarily occur in areas preceded by vesicles or warty lesions and, in fact, is predominantly truncal, whereas the early lesions have a predilection for the extremities. Ultimately, the pigmentation may fade or disappear. More than

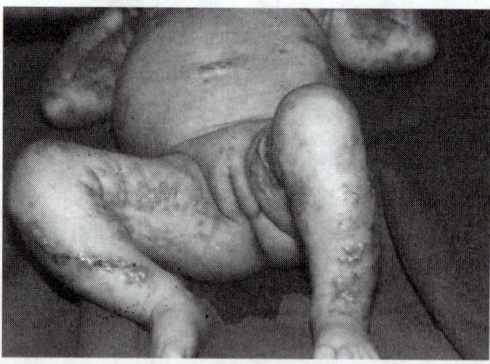

FIGURE 68.11. Vesicular stage of incontinentia pigmenti: linear streaks of vesicles on the extremities with less involvement on the trunk. See Color Figure 64.11 in color section.

one stage may be present at once, and the pigmentation may be present at birth. A fourth stage of atrophic and hypopigmented streaks has been reported. Eighty percent of infants with IP have significant associated disorders of the eyes, teeth, CNS, and skeletal system. Ocular involvement may be serious enough to result in vision loss or blindness in 20% of patients. CNS disorders occur in 30% of infants, including mental retardation, seizures, spastic paralysis, motor retardation, microcephaly, and congenital deafness. IP results from mutations in the NEMO gene on chromosome Xq28. The diagnosis of IP can be made with a skin biopsy of a characteristic early vesicular lesion, which will show intraepidermal, spongiotic blisters containing many eosinophils. No therapeutic measures are known to influence the course of IP; therefore, treatment is symptomatic. Baseline and longitudinal neurologic, ophthalmologic, and dental evaluations are recommended.

Cutaneous Candidiasis

In the newborn, cutaneous candidiasis exists in a congenital and a neonatal form. In both forms the causative organism is *Candida albicans*, a dimorphic yeast found in the vaginal canal in up to 25% of pregnant women. Neonatal candidiasis is manifested as oral thrush or diaper dermatitis and develops after the first week of life. Neonatal candidiasis is presumed to be acquired by the infant during passage through an infected birth canal. Congenital cutaneous candidiasis is an ascending, intrauterine infection. The eruption is noted at birth or within 12 hours after delivery and is characterized by erythematous macules and papules that evolve into vesicles and pustules scattered widely over the body, including the palms and soles. Oral lesions are rare, and the diaper area is relatively spared. After several days, the eruption resolves with desquamation. The diagnosis is established by demonstrating pseudohyphae and budding yeast in a KOH preparation of a pustule or scale. Most infants with congenital cutaneous candidiasis do not have systemic involvement and therefore do well with topical treatment alone. Conversely, systemic congenital candidiasis does not usually present with skin lesions and can lead to death *in utero* or in the immediate neonatal period. The most reliable indicators for predicting the outcome of congenital cutaneous candidiasis are the infant's birth weight and the presence of respiratory distress. Infants with birth weights of less than 1.5 kg or with early onset of respiratory distress are at risk for systemic disease, including candida sepsis or pneumonia.

Neonatal Acne

Neonatal acne (acne neonatorum) is a common condition that occurs in 20% of healthy newborns. Lesions usually present within the first few weeks of life and resolve by 3 months of age. Typically, small, inflammatory papules and pustules are seen on the cheeks and across the nasal bridge (Fig. 68.12). *Malassezia furfur*, a ubiquitous lipophilic yeast, is believed to be chiefly responsible. Stimulation of sebaceous glands by maternal and infant androgens, however, likely contributes. Neonatal acne may be treated topically with 2% ketoconazole cream or benzoyl peroxide lotion, although most cases do not require treatment and parental reassurance is usually adequate.

Folliculitis

Superficial bacterial infections of the pilosebaceous unit are most commonly caused by *Staphylococcus aureus* and should be considered in the differential diagnosis of pustular eruptions in the newborn. Initial lesions are erythematous, folliculocentric papules that evolve into pustules. Lesions remain discrete and do not coalesce. Ruptured pustules eventually heal with hyperpigmentation and rarely scar. Lesions occur most commonly in areas of skin that are either occluded or prone to moisture

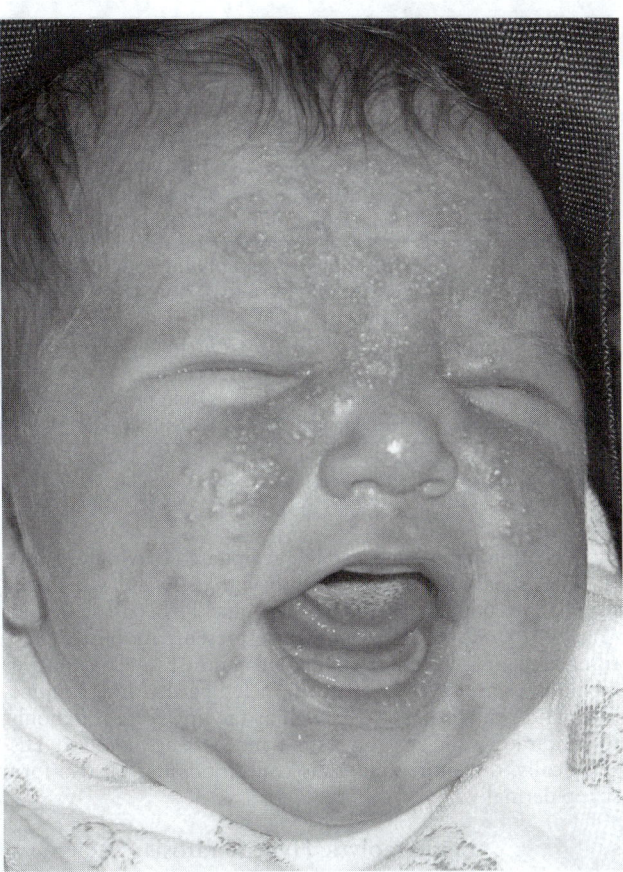

FIGURE 68.12. Inflammatory papules and pustules on the face of an infant with neonatal acne. See Color Figure 68.12 in color section.

and friction such as the buttocks in infants who wear occlusive diapers. The diagnosis may be confirmed with a Gram stain or culture of a pustule. Treatment includes antibacterial soaps such as chlorhexidine and topical antibiotics. Unresponsive or severe cases may require oral antibiotic therapy.

Neonatal Herpes Simplex

Herpes simplex virus (HSV) may be transmitted transplacentally to result in congenital infection (5%) but more commonly produces neonatal infection acquired as a result of passage through an infected birth canal or from an ascending infection associated with prolonged rupture of membranes. According to current estimates there are 1,500 cases of neonatal herpes annually in the United States, which translates to approximately 1 in 3,200 deliveries. Both HSV-1 and HSV-2 may cause neonatal herpes, but most cases are due to HSV-2 (70%). The risk of transmission to a neonate from an infected mother is significantly higher in women who have their first episode of genital herpes around the time of delivery (25% to 57%) than in women with recurrent disease (2%). Affected infants may have localized or disseminated cutaneous lesions as well as mucosal, ocular, CNS, and multiorgan involvement. Cutaneous vesicles may be the first clue to the diagnosis, but they are absent in 20% of affected infants. Skin lesions may be present at birth but usually develop between 4 and 14 days of age and, when few in number, are often on the presenting part of the infant. Typical lesions are grouped vesicles on an erythematous base. Multiple laboratory tests are available to diagnose HSV infection, including viral culture, direct immunofluorescence, polymerase chain reaction (PCR), and serology. The western blot is 99% sensitive and specific for HSV antibodies in the serum;

however, results are confounded by the transplacental transmission of maternal immunoglobulin G. Thus, it plays no role in the diagnosis of neonatal HSV disease. A rapid diagnosis can be made with a Tzanck smear of the base of a vesicle, which reveals multinucleated giant cells in 75% of cases. If left untreated, systemic HSV infection is fatal in most cases. Early antiviral therapy with acyclovir can dramatically reduce mortality. Survivors often have severe developmental and neurologic defects. Antiviral therapy may be considered in women who experience first-episode genital herpes or recurrent genital herpes in the last trimester of gestation.

Congenital Syphilis

Pregnant women who are infected with the spirochete *Treponema pallidum* may transmit the infection to the developing fetus. Congenital syphilis usually results form transplacental infection of the developing fetus but may also be acquired by passage through an infected birth canal. The rates of congenital infection vary depending on the clinical stage of maternal infection, but the highest transmission occurs in untreated pregnant women with primary syphilis. The clinical appearance of infected neonates is highly variable. When symptoms appear within the first 2 years of life the disease is termed early congenital syphilis. Symptoms appearing after that time, often near puberty, constitute late congenital syphilis. Cutaneous findings of early congenital syphilis may resemble or be identical to those seen in secondary syphilis. The most common lesions are round to oval, papulosquamous plaques involving the trunk and extremities, including the palms and soles. Vesicular or pustular lesions are not common but are highly suggestive of the diagnosis, especially when seen on the palms and soles. Oral mucous membrane patches and genital condyloma lata may be present. Similar lesions occur at the mucocutaneous junction of the mouth, which may become fissured and scarred, leading to the formation of rhagades. Other characteristic abnormalities seen in early congenital syphilis include hepatosplenomegaly, lytic bone lesions, and syphilitic rhinitis or snuffles, which usually appear between 2 and 6 weeks of age. Hutchinson triad (Hutchinson teeth, interstitial keratitis, and neural deafness) are components of late congenital syphilis and together are virtually pathognomonic for congenital syphilis.

Bullae

The differential diagnosis of bullae in the newborn is presented in Box 68.4 and Figure 68.8.

Staphylococcal Toxin-Mediated Infections

S. aureus may cause disease by either direct tissue invasion or by release of one of a variety of exotoxins produced by

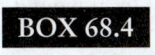

BOX 68.4   **Differential Diagnosis of Bullae in the Newborn**

Bullous impetigo
Staphylococcal scalded skin syndrome
Toxic epidermal necrolysis
Epidermolytic hyperkeratosis
Epidermolysis bullosa
Mastocytosis
Sucking blisters

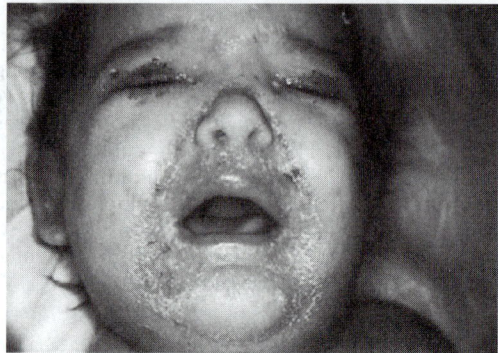

FIGURE 68.13. Characteristic facial appearance of an infant with staphylococcal scalded skin syndrome with purulent drainage and crusting around the eyes, nose, and mouth. See Color Figure 68.13 in color section.

the bacteria. Strains of *S. aureus* that excrete exfoliative toxins are primarily responsible for the skin manifestations of bullous impetigo (BI) and staphylococcal scalded skin syndrome (SSSS).

Staphylococcal Scalded Skin Syndrome. SSSS is primarily a disease of children less than 6 years of age and is occasionally seen in outbreaks in neonatal nurseries. It is preceded by a localized staphylococcal infection, usually a purulent conjunctivitis, omphalitis, rhinitis, pharyngitis, or infected circumcision site. Within a few days of the initial infection, diffuse erythema of the skin develops abruptly with marked skin tenderness and fever. Large, flaccid bullae develop and rupture almost immediately. Large sheets of skin separate and exfoliate, leaving a moist, red surface (Fig. 68.13). The widespread blistering is the result of a circulating exfoliative toxin produced by the staphylococcal organisms at the original site of infection; therefore, organisms cannot be cultured from the bullae but must be recovered from the original site. The toxin cleaves desmoglein 1, a protein component of desmosomes in the upper epidermis, just below the stratum corneum, resulting in superficial blister formation. Desmoglein 1 is not present in the mucosa; therefore, there is no mucous membrane involvement in SSSS. Treatment requires hospitalization for wound care and parental antistaphylococcal antibiotics. With proper treatment, SSSS resolves in 1 to 2 weeks, usually without sequelae. Despite appropriate antibiotic therapy, a 3% mortality is observed due to secondary infections and other complications from the loss of the upper epidermis.

Bullous Impetigo. Akin to a localized form of SSSS, BI is caused by a localized skin infection with exfoliative toxin producing *S. aureus*. BI is most commonly observed in the neonate and may be associated with fever, malaise, and diarrhea. Cutaneous lesions characteristically begin as small, clear vesicles that rapidly enlarge into flaccid, transparent bullae. The bullae are very superficial and rupture easily, forming thin crusts or erosions. In contrast to SSSS, the organisms can be cultured from the blister fluid. Treatment consists of local wound care in combination with either topical or systemic antibiotics.

Toxic Epidermal Necrolysis

SSSS must be differentiated from toxic epidermal necrolysis (TEN) because their causes, courses, treatments, and ultimate prognoses differ (Table 68.4). TEN is presumed to be a hypersensitivity reaction and is a serious disorder with a high morbidity and mortality. It shares clinical and histologic features with, and is thought by some to be the most severe form of, erythema multiforme. Drugs are usually implicated in the etiology

of TEN, although it may also be precipitated by viral or bacterial infections. TEN begins abruptly with fever and widespread macular or papular erythema that quickly becomes bullous (Fig. 68.14). Target lesions may be present. As blisters rupture, large areas become denuded. In contrast to SSSS, mucous membranes are severely affected, including the oral, conjunctival, and genital mucosa, as well as the lips. Less commonly, the respiratory and gastrointestinal mucosae are involved. Histologically, the entire epidermis is necrotic, and blisters form subepidermally.

Epidermolytic Hyperkeratosis

A rare autosomal dominant form of ichthyosis with a 50% spontaneous mutation rate, epidermolytic hyperkeratosis also is referred to as congenital bullous ichthyosiform erythroderma. Heterozygous mutations in the genes encoding for keratin 1 and keratin 10 weaken the structural stability of keratinocytes. Affected infants are born with widespread blistering and red, moist, denuded skin (Fig. 68.15). Within 1 to 2 weeks, generalized blistering resolves and the skin becomes dry, thick, and scaly. During infancy and childhood, crops of localized blisters may occur and heal without scarring. Ultimately,

TABLE 68.4

DIFFERENTIATION OF STAPHYLOCOCCAL SCALDED SKIN SYNDROME AND TOXIC EPIDERMAL NECROLYSIS

	Staphylococcal Scalded Skin Syndrome	Toxic Epidermal Necrolysis
Etiology	Infectious; group II staphylococci	Immunologic; usually drug related
Morbidity/mortality	Low	High
Mucous membrane	Rare	Frequent involvement
Nikolsky sign	Present	Present
Target lesions	Absent	Often present
Level of blister	Subcorneal	Subepidermal

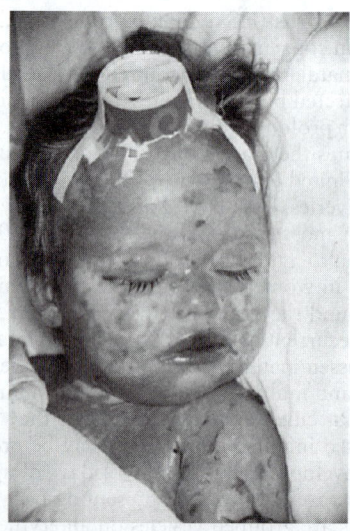

FIGURE 68.14. Maculopapular erythema, with blister formation on the face and extensive denudation on the chest and arm, in an infant with toxic epidermal necrolysis. See Color Figure 68.14 in color section.

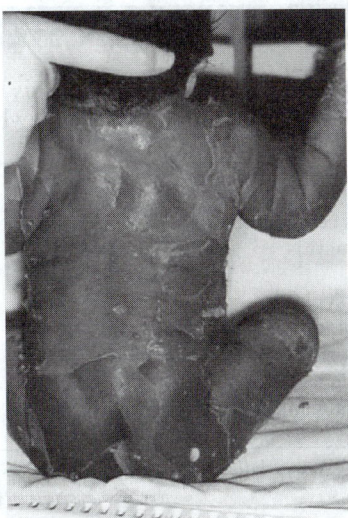

FIGURE 68.15. Newborn with widespread blistering of epidermolytic hyperkeratosis. See Color Figure 68.15 in color section.

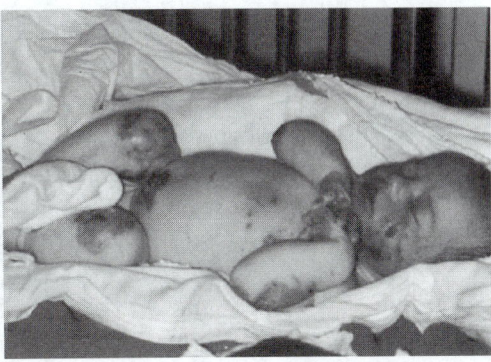

FIGURE 68.16. Generalized epidermolysis bullosa simplex with erosions and bullae on the face, elbows, hands, and knees at sites of trauma. See Color Figure 68.16 in color section.

blisters are replaced by dark, foul-smelling, verrucous, hypertrophic lesions that are most pronounced in body-fold areas.

Epidermolysis Bullosa

Epidermolysis bullosa (EB) is a group of disorders whose primary feature is the formation of blisters after minor trauma to the skin. The inherited forms of EB are generally based on the ultrastructural levels of blister formation within the skin (Table 68.5). All types of EB with primary intraepidermal blisters are classified as *EB simplex*, those with intralamina lucida blisters are *junctional EB*, and those with cleavage in the sublamina densa zone are *dystrophic EB*. There are at least 20 distinctive clinical phenotypes of EB. All types except localized EB simplex begin at birth or early infancy. Bullae arise on normal-appearing skin of the cheeks, chin, elbows, knees, hands, feet, and other easily traumatized sites (Fig. 68.16). Distinguishing among the types of EB clinically may be impossible in early infancy. Specific diagnosis requires sophisticated light and electron microscopical histopathologic studies. There is a high incidence of aggressive squamous cell carcinoma in EB,

which plays a major role in both morbidity and life expectancy, especially in patients with the severe mutilating form of dystrophic EB.

Mastocytosis

Mast cell degranulation with release of histamine in isolated mastocytomas or generalized cutaneous lesions of mastocytosis may result in enough edema to produce grossly visible blisters in the newborn. When blisters predominate, they are frequently mistaken for other disorders such as neonatal herpes or bullous impetigo.

Sucking Blisters

Vigorous sucking by the fetus *in utero* may produce isolated bullae 5 to 15 mm in diameter on the forearm, wrist, hand, fingers, and, rarely, toes. No treatment is necessary for these blisters as spontaneous resolution is the rule.

SCALING DISORDERS

Ichthyoses

Derived from the Greek root *ichthys*, meaning fish, the ichthyoses are a heterogeneous group of diseases that share one common feature: scaly skin. There are five major disorders of cornification: autosomal dominant ichthyosis vulgaris, autosomal recessive lamellar ichthyosis, congenital ichthyosiform erythroderma, X-linked recessive ichthyosis, and autosomal dominant epidermolytic hyperkeratosis. Onset in the neonatal period may occur in all but ichthyosis vulgaris, in which symptoms develop later in childhood. Infants with epidermolytic hyperkeratosis are born with widespread blistering. The collodion baby may be the first manifestation of more than one type of ichthyosis, but it is most commonly seen in infants who subsequently develop lamellar ichthyosis or congenital ichthyosiform erythroderma. Rarely, the skin remains normal in appearance after the collodion membrane is shed. Collodion babies are encased in a tight, shiny membrane that restricts movement and results in ectropion (Fig. 68.17). Fissuring and peeling begin shortly after birth, although complete shedding of the membrane may take weeks to months. Infants should be managed in an isolation incubator with careful temperature control and high humidity, which maximizes flexibility of the skin. Occlusive emollients should be avoided. The harlequin fetus is a severe form of congenital ichthyosis that probably represents a heterogeneous group of disorders. Affected infants are

TABLE 68.5

MAIN TYPES OF EPIDERMIS BULLOSA (EB) AND ASSOCIATED TARGET PROTEINS

EB Type	Protein
EB Simplex	
Weber-Cockayne	Keratins 5/14
Köbner	Keratins 5/14
Dowling-Mera	Keratins 5/14
Mottled pigmentation	Keratin 5
Muscular dystrophy	Plectin
Junctional EB	
Herlitz	Laminin 5
Non-Herlitz	Laminin 5; collagen XVII (BP180)
Pyloric atresia	Integrin alpha$_6$-beta$_4$
Dystrophic EB	
Recessive	Collagen VII
Dominant	Collagen VII

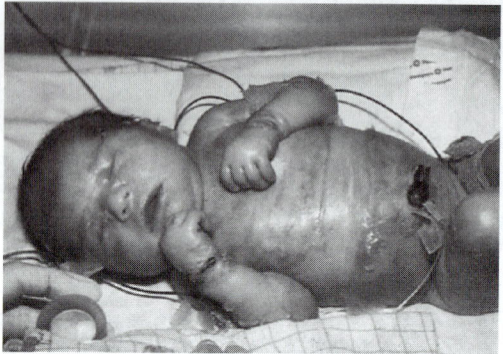

FIGURE 68.17. Collodion baby after partial shedding of the collodion membrane. The hands, arms, legs, and a portion of the abdomen are still encased in a tight, shiny membrane. See Color Figure 68.17 in color section.

> ### BOX 68.5   Differential Diagnosis of Diaper Dermatitis in the Newborn
>
> Seborrheic dermatitis
> Psoriasis
> Langerhans cell histiocytoses
> Atopic dermatitis
> Scabies
> Congenital syphilis
> Contact/irritant dermatitis
> Acrodermatitis enteropathica
> Biotin deficiency
> Streptococcal/candidal intertrigo

born with thick yellow skin that rapidly becomes criss-crossed by deep fissures with moist red bases. Marked ectropion and eclabium are common, as are malformed hands, feet, and ears from restriction of normal development *in utero* by the inflexible skin. Survival beyond infancy is rare.

Seborrheic Dermatitis

Infantile seborrheic dermatitis usually begins about 1 week after birth and may persist for several months. The etiology has been linked to increased sebum production, abnormal sebum composition, and the commensal lipophilic yeast *Malassezia furfur*. Neonates often have an increase in sebum production for several weeks after birth secondary to maternal androgens. Lesions are most commonly found in areas where there is a high concentration of sebaceous glands such as the scalp, face, ears, presternal area, and, less commonly, the intertriginal areas (axillae and inguinal folds). Clinically the lesions appear as well-demarcated, pink to red patches with overlying "greasy" white or yellow flaky scale. Because of its mild and self-limited nature, treatment is not usually indicated. For the more severe or persistent cases, a short course of ketoconazole 2% cream or a low-potency topical corticosteroid may be used.

Atopic Dermatitis

Atopic dermatitis (AD) or eczema is a common skin disease that begins in infancy (although usually not before 2 months of age) in more than half of affected individuals. Usually associated with a family history of atopy (e.g., asthma, allergic rhinitis), AD is characterized by extremely pruritic red papules and thin plaques with overlying scale. In acute lesions, vesicles and serous crusts may be seen. Secondary changes such as excoriations and lichenification are commonly observed in chronic lesions. In neonates, lesions may be found on the scalp, face, extensor surfaces of the extremities, and diaper area. AD is clinically responsive to topical corticosteroids and macrolide immunomodulators (tacrolimus and pimecrolimus).

Psoriasis

Infantile psoriasis is uncommon. The diaper area is the most frequent site of involvement, thus making it difficult to differentiate from other causes of diaper dermatitis (Box 68.5). Typ-

ical psoriatic lesions are sharply demarcated, beefy red plaques with thick, silvery scale (Fig. 68.18). In infants, the scale may be less prominent and may be absent in the diaper area because of the moist environment.

Neonatal Lupus Erythematosus

The hallmarks of neonatal lupus erythematosus are round to oval, erythematous, scaling plaques with varying degrees of atrophy, telangiectasia, and scarring. The face is nearly always involved (Fig. 68.19), and lesions may develop on the trunk and extremities. Affected infants may have systemic disease with congenital heart block, hepatosplenomegaly, pulmonary disease, anemia, neutropenia, or thrombocytopenia. Infants and their mothers have a high incidence of circulating autoantibodies of the Ro/La family, but up to 35% of mothers have no overt signs or symptoms of connective tissue disease and only 1% of women who have these autoantibodies will have a baby with neonatal lupus. Resolution of the skin lesions corresponds with the disappearance of transplacentally acquired maternal Ro/La antibodies between 6 and 12 months of age. Evaluation should include a thorough physical examination, complete blood count, platelet count, antinuclear antibody and Ro/La antibody screen, and electrocardiography. In cases where the

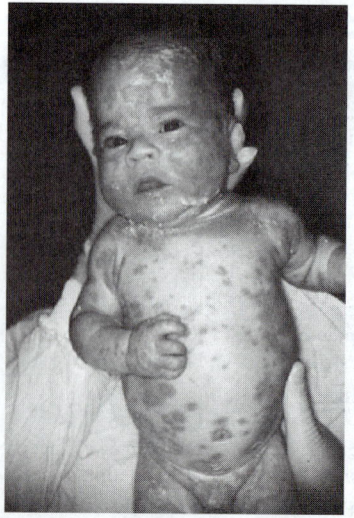

FIGURE 68.18. Beefy red, sharply demarcated, scaling plaques of psoriasis. See Color Figure 68.18 in color section.

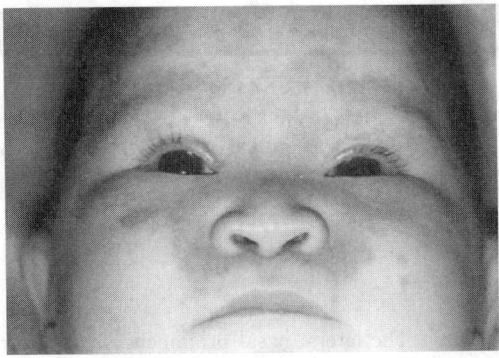

FIGURE 68.19. Characteristic erythematous, scaling plaques over the central face in an infant with neonatal lupus erythematosus. See Color Figure 68.19 in color section.

diagnosis is still in question, a biopsy of a characteristic skin lesion should be performed. Because photosensitivity has been reported, protection from the sun, including the use of sunscreens, is advisable.

Histiocytosis X

Histiocytosis X may mimic seborrheic dermatitis, with an erythematous scaling eruption on the face, scalp, axillae, and diaper area. Discrete, red-brown, scaling papules with petechiae or purpura and failure to respond to topical corticosteroids are features that distinguish histiocytosis X from other similar-appearing disorders. Affected infants may have mucosal erosions or ulcerations, hepatosplenomegaly, and chronically draining ears. The diagnosis can be confirmed with a skin biopsy of a characteristic lesion.

Diaper Dermatitis

A number of disorders may present with or include involvement of the diaper area (Box 68.5). Regardless of the cause, diaper dermatitis persisting longer than 2 or 3 days is usually complicated by a *Candida albicans* infection that should be treated with topical antiyeast preparations. Irritant dermatitis tends to spare the body folds, with accentuation on the convex surfaces exposed to urine and stool. Keeping the skin as dry as possible with frequent diaper changes and protecting with emollients such as petrolatum speed resolution.

Suggested Readings

Birthmarks

Alper JC, Holmes LB. The incidence and significance of birthmarks in a cohort of 4,641 newborns. *Pediatr Dermatol* 1983;1:58.

Berry SA, Peterson C, Mize W, et al. Klippel-Trenaunay syndrome. *Am J Med Genet* 1998;79:319.

Brown TJ, Friedman J, Moise LL. The diagnosis and treatment of common birthmarks. *Clin Plast Surg* 1998;25:509.

Bruckner AL, Frieden IJ. Hemangiomas of infancy. *J Am Acad Dermatol* 2003;48:477.

Ceisler EJ, Santos L, Francine B. Periocular hemangiomas: what every physician should know. *Pediatr Dermatol* 2004;21:1.

Cribier B, Scrivener Y, Grosshans E. Tumors arising in nevus sebaceus: a study of 596 cases. *J Am Acad Dermatol* 2000;42:263.

Frieden IJ, Reese V, Cohen D. PHACE syndrome: the association of posterior fossa brain malformations, hemangiomas, arterial anomalies, coarctation of the aorta and cardiac defects, and eye abnormalities. *Arch Dermatol* 1996;132:307.

Giguere CM, Bauman NM, Smith RJ. New treatment options for lymphangioma in infants and children. *Ann Otol Rhinol Laryngol* 2002;111:1066.

Gurecki PJ, Holden KR, Sahn EE, et al. Developmental neural abnormalities and seizures in epidermal nevus syndrome. *Dev Med Child Neurol* 1996;38:716.

Han-Seung L, Yoo-Sun C, Seung-Kyung H. Nevus depigmentosus: clinical features and histopathologic characteristics in 67 patients. *J Am Acad Dermatol* 1999;40:21.

Heide R, Tank B, Oranje AP. Mastocytosis in childhood. *Pediatr Dermatol* 2002;19:375.

Maguiness S, Guenther L. Kasabach-Merritt syndrome. *J Cutan Med Surg* 2002; 6:335.

Marghoob AA. Congenital melanocytic nevi: evaluation and management. *Dermatol Clin* 2002;20:607.

Metry DW, Hebert AA. Benign vascular tumors of infancy. *Arch Dermatol* 2000;136:905.

Morelli JG. Use of lasers in pediatric dermatology. *Dermatol Clin* 1998;16:489.

Mustafa T, Bodurtha JN, Riccardi VM. Café au lait spots: the pediatrician's perspective. *Pediatr Rev* 2001;22:82.

Nahm WK, Moise S, Eichenfield LF, et al. Venous malformations in blue rubber bleb nevus syndrome: variable onset of presentation. *J Am Acad Dermatol* 2004;50:S101.

Orlow SJ. Congenital disorders of hypopigmentation. *Semin Dermatol* 1995; 14:27.

Papo AS. Melanoma in children and adolescents. *Eur J Cancer* 2003;39:2651.

Santibanez-Gallerani A, Marshall D, Duarte A, et al. Should nevus sebaceus of Jadassohn in children be excised? A study of 757 cases, and literature review. *J Craniofac Surg* 2003;14:658.

Shwayder T. Ichthyosis in a nutshell. *Pediatr Rev* 1999;20:5.

Thomas-Sohl KA, Vaslow DF, Maria BL. Sturge-Weber syndrome: a review. *Pediatr Neurol* 2004;30:303.

Vujevich JJ, Mancini AJ. The epidermal nevus syndromes: multisystem disorders. *J Am Acad Dermatol* 2004;50:957.

Scaling Disorders

Ammirati CT, Mallory SB. The major inherited disorders of cornification. *Pediatr Dermatol* 1998;16:497.

Huang F, Arceci R. The histiocytoses of infancy. *Semin Perinatol* 1999;23:319.

Lee LA. Neonatal lupus. *Pediatr Drugs* 2004;6:71.

Kazaks EL, Lane AT. Diaper dermatitis. *Pediatr Clin North Am* 2000;47:909.

Rothe MJ, Grant-Kels JM. Atopic dermatitis: an update. *J Am Acad Dermatol* 1996;35:1.

Schulz EJ. Genodermatoses. *Dermatol Clin* 1994;12:787.

Vesiculopustular and Bullous Disorders

Feng E, Janniger CK. Miliaria. *Cutis* 1995;55:213.

Francis JS, Sybert VP. Incontinentia pigmenti. *Semin Cutan Med Surg* 1997; 16:54.

Hollier LM, Cox SM. Syphilis. *Semin Perinatol* 1998;22:323.

Lin AN. Management of patients with epidermolysis bullosa. *Dermatol Clin* 1996;14:381.

Plano LRW. Staphylococcus aureus exfoliative toxins: how they cause disease. *JID* 2004;122:1070.

Schwartz RA, Janniger CK. Erythema toxicum neonatorum. *Cutis* 1996;58:153.

Van Praag MCG, Van Rooij RWG, Folkers E, et al. Diagnosis and treatment of pustular disorders in the neonate. *Pediatr Dermatol* 1997;14:131.

Whitley R. Neonatal herpes simplex virus infection. *Curr Opin Infect Dis* 2004;17:243.

CHAPTER 69 ■ CRANIOFACIAL DEFECTS

ROBERT J. GORLIN

EMBRYOLOGY OF THE PRIMARY AND SECONDARY PALATES

The neural crest plays an integral part in facial morphology. When the neural folds fuse to form the neural tube at approximately the fourth week of gestation, ectomesenchymal cells adjacent to the neural plate migrate into the underlying regions. Those in the head and face form essentially all the skeletal and connective tissues of the face: bone, cartilage, fibrous connective tissue, and all dental tissues except enamel. This transformation is effected by induction of these ectomesenchymal cells by the adjacent oral ectoderm and pharyngeal endoderm. Neural crest cells also migrate into the visceral arches, where they surround mesodermal cores.

By the end of the fourth week, the anterior neuropore has closed. What is to be the face consists of a large frontal prominence overlying the first or mandibular arch. If one manually elevates the frontal prominence, one can see into the primary mouth or stomodeum. The primary mouth is separated from the foregut by the buccopharyngeal membrane, which undergoes programmed cell death and ruptures at approximately this time in development. On both sides of the frontal prominence, the nasal placodes are forming. These bilateral structures, located just above the primitive mouth, are represented by local thickening of the surface ectoderm. Rapid proliferation of tissue known as *nasal swelling* occurs both lateral and medial to the nasal placodes. By means of selective cell death and proliferation of tissues, nasal or olfactory pits that extend into the primitive mouth are formed; they are the primitive nostrils.

Extremely active growth occurs during the fifth and sixth weeks (Fig. 69.1). The maxillary swellings, which represent the upper portion of the first pharyngeal arch, enlarge considerably and, by pushing the nasal swellings or prominences medially, cause them to approach each other in the midline. When the two prominences meet, the median nasal prominences and the maxillary swellings merge. Thus, the upper lip is formed laterally by the maxillary prominences and medially by the fused median nasal prominences. This development occurs near the

seventh week. The lateral nasal prominences play no role in formation of the upper lip but form the alae or wings of the nose.

The primary palate consists of the two merged medial nasal processes that form the intermaxillary segment. The intermaxillary segment consists of two portions: a labial component that forms the philtrum of the upper lip (i.e., the indented area flanked by roughly parallel ridges that run from the columella of the nose to the middle of the upper lip) and the triangular palatal component of bone (premaxilla) that includes the four maxillary incisor teeth. The primary palate extends posteriorly to the incisive foramen or, clinically, to the incisive papilla.

The so-called secondary palate forms at least 90% of the hard and soft palates (i.e., all except the anterior portion that holds the incisor teeth). Its development appears to be somewhat more complicated than originally was thought. The palatal shelves originate as swellings or shelflike burgeoning of the medial surfaces of the maxillary prominences. They appear in the sixth week and grow downward, lateral to and somewhat beneath the tongue. Elevation of the palatal processes to a horizontal plane is more "rigorous" anteriorly, nearer the primary palate. Elevation begins during the seventh week.

What promotes the elevation has been called *intrinsic shelf force*, but it has a complex biochemical and physiochemical basis. When the shelves are elevated to the horizontal plane, programmed cell death occurs in the overlying epithelium, permitting flow of ectomesenchyme from each side to close the gap. Complete fusion is effected by the tenth week (Fig. 69.2). In some infants, cystic degeneration of the epithelial remnants occurs, producing evanescent midline palatal microcysts.

CLEFT LIP AND CLEFT PALATE

Epidemiology and Genetics

The degree of cleft formation varies greatly. Minimal degrees of involvement include bifid uvula, linear lip indentations

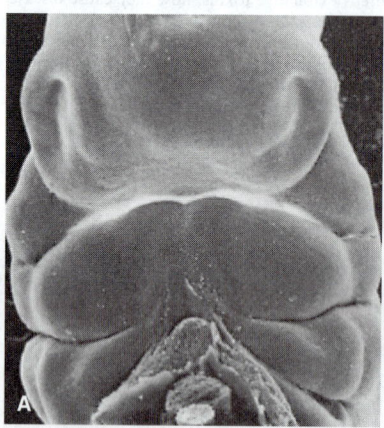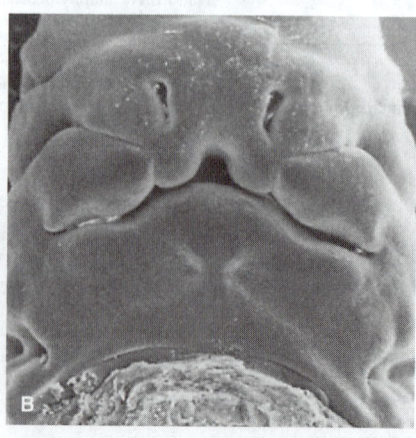

FIGURE 69.1. Embryology of the primary and secondary palates. Scanning electron microscopy of human embryos. A: Early fifth week after fertilization. B: Sixth week after fertilization. Median nasal process is not yet fused with maxillary process of first arch. (Courtesy of K. Sulik, Chapel Hill, NC.)

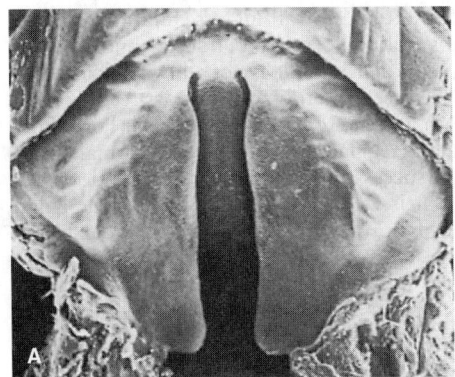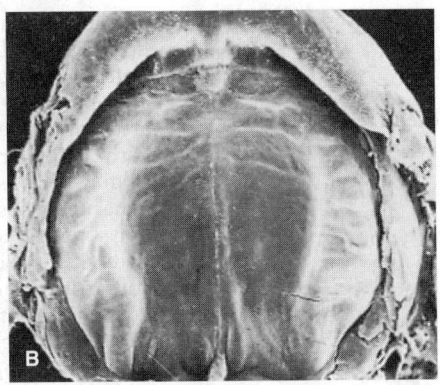

FIGURE 69.2. Scanning electron microscopy view of secondary palate at 8 weeks (**A**) and at 10 weeks (**B**). (Courtesy of K. Sulik, Chapel Hill, NC.)

[so-called intrauterine (incisive foramen)-healed clefts], and submucous palatal cleft. Clefts may involve only the upper lip or may extend to the nostril and may be combined with defects of the hard or soft palate. Isolated palatal clefts may be limited to the uvula or they may be more extensive, cleaving the soft palate or both the soft and hard palates to just behind the incisor teeth.

A combination of cleft lip and cleft palate is more common than isolated occurrences of either. Cleft lip with cleft palate composes approximately 50% of the cases, with cleft lip and isolated cleft palate each constituting perhaps 25%, generally irrespective of race. Cleft lip with or without cleft palate occurs in approximately 1 per 1,000 white births (range, 0.8 to 1.6 per 1,000). Frequency is higher in Native Americans (3.5 per 1,000), Japanese (2.1 per 1,000), and Chinese (1.7 per 1,000); it is lower among African Americans (0.3 per 1,000).

Isolated cleft lip may be unilateral (80%) or bilateral (20%). When unilateral, the cleft more commonly is located on the left side (approximately 70%), but it is no more extensive. Lips are cleft somewhat more frequently bilaterally (approximately 25%) when combined with cleft palate. The cleft lip and palate combination is more common in men than in women. Approximately 85% of cases of bilateral cleft lip and 70% of cases of unilateral cleft lip are associated with cleft palate. Cleft lip is not always complete (i.e., extending into the nostril). In approximately 10% of the cases, the cleft is associated with skin bridges or Simonart bands.

Isolated cleft palate appears to be an entity separate from cleft lip with or without cleft palate. Numerous investigators have determined that siblings of patients with cleft lip with or without cleft palate have an increased frequency of the same anomaly but not of isolated cleft palate, and vice versa. The incidence of isolated cleft palate among both Caucasians and African Americans appears to be 1 per 2,000 to 2,500 births. It occurs somewhat more often in girls, comprising approximately 60% of the cases. Although a 2:1 female-to-male predilection prevails for complete clefts of the hard and soft palate, the ratio approaches 1:1 for clefts of the soft palate only.

Cleft uvula varies in degree of completeness; incomplete clefts are more common. The frequency of cleft uvula (1 in 80 white persons) is much higher than that for cleft palate with no gender predilection. The frequency in parents and siblings of probands ranges from 7% to 15%. Cleft uvula among Native American groups is high, occurring in 1 per 9 to 14 births, depending on tribal group. In African Americans, it is rare. Estimates are 1 per 350 to 400 births.

Congenital velopharyngeal inadequacy, characterized by cleft palate speech (50%) without an overt cleft, is due to a short soft palate (60%), an imperfect muscular union across the soft palate (submucous palatal cleft), or increased depth of the nasal pharynx. Submucous palatal cleft is relatively un-

common, occurring in 1 in 1,200 children. Apparently no gender predilection is demonstrated. Approximately 30% of those with submucous palatal cleft have bifid uvula, with poor mobility demonstrated in 20%. A median deficiency or notch is seen in the bone at the posterior edge of the hard palate. It can be detected digitally or by a light probe placed within the nose. The occult submucous cleft palate can be detected via nasoendoscopy.

Recurrence data do not suggest a simple pattern of inheritance. This finding is bolstered by twin studies indicating the relative roles played by genetic and nongenetic influences. Among twins with cleft lip with or without cleft palate, concordance is far greater in monozygotic (35.0%) than in dizygotic (4.5%) twins. In twins with isolated cleft palate, concordance is not quite as great (monozygotic, 26.0%; dizygotic, 5.8%). This finding suggests a stronger genetic basis for cleft lip with or without cleft palate than for isolated cleft palate. Both cleft lip with or without cleft palate and isolated cleft palate consist of three groups: sporadic (75% to 80%), familial (10% to 15%), and syndromal (1% to 5%). Clefting is heterogeneous. Its variation and liability probably are determined by major genes, minor genes, environmental insults, and a developmental threshold.

Mechanisms of Cleft Production

By definition, cleft lip involves the failure of closure of the primary palate, and cleft palate involves failure of closure of the secondary palate. Knowledge regarding mechanisms involved in regulation of embryonic growth is sparse at best. Growth patterns can be affected also by environmental factors. A long list of teratogenic substances (e.g., corticosteroids, vitamin A, phenytoin, various folic acid antagonists) can produce clefting in rodents. Little evidence, however, suggests that any of these agents plays even a minor role in cleft palate production in humans.

Various genetic and environmental factors may inhibit the flow of neural crest cells or may affect their volume or mass so that contact between prominences is impossible or inadequate. The epithelium covering the ectomesenchyme may not undergo programmed cell death, so fusion cannot take place. Exact timing and exact positioning play critical roles.

Clefts of the primary and secondary palates occur in association in perhaps one-half of cases. A common mechanism of production has been sought. Reduction in size of both the labial maxillary prominence and the palatine process of the maxillary prominences appears to be a reasonable explanation.

Clefts of the secondary palate probably result from either hypoplasia of the shelves or delay in timing of shelf elevation. Experiments carried out on susceptible strains of mice suggest that both mechanisms are operative but at different times in

TABLE 69.1

FACIAL CLEFTS: RISK OF RECURRENCE

Parents	Siblings Normal	Siblings Affected	Cleft Lip Palate (%)	Cleft Palate (%)
Normal	0	1	4.0	3.5
	1	1	4.0	3.0
	0	2	14.0	13.0
One affected	0	0	4.0	3.5
	0	1	12.0	10.0
	1	1	10.0	9.0
	0	2	25.0	24.0
Both affected	0	0	35.0	25.0
	0	1	45.0	35.0
	1	1	40.0	35.0
	0	2	50.0	40.0

Adapted from Tolarová M. Empirical recurrence risk figures for genetic counseling of clefts. *Acta Chir Plast (Praha)* 1972;14:234.

gestation. Large doses of vitamin A given to rodents early in gestation inhibit palatal shelf growth and cortisone given later in gestation inhibits palatal shelf elevation.

Risk of Recurrence

In most cases, the cleft is either isolated or associated with a constellation of anomalies that do not form a recognizable syndrome. Although more than 300 cleft syndromes or associations are recognized, they constitute a low percentage of cases. Efforts must be made to recognize a cleft syndrome, because the pattern of inheritance may be simple, and the genetic risk for future affected children then may be more precise. For example, a parent with or without a cleft and paramedian pits of the lower lip has a 50% chance of having a child with cleft lip or palate.

In the case of isolated clefts, the risk to a first-degree relative of an affected individual is 2% to 4%. This information applies only to risks for similar anomalies (i.e., a parent with isolated cleft palate has no greater risk of having a child with cleft lip with or without cleft palate than anyone else, and vice versa). The risks increase as more individuals are affected. For example, if a parent and a child have clefts, the risk for a future affected sibling increases to approximately 10% to 12%. These and other situations are presented in detail in Table 69.1.

The severity of a facial cleft also affects recurrence risk in the offspring. For example, researchers have found that if a parent has isolated unilateral cleft lip, the recurrence risk is 2.5%. In the presence of unilateral cleft lip *and* palate, the risk increases to 4%, and the risk is more than 5.5% for bilateral cleft lip with cleft palate.

Care of the Infant with Cleft Lip or Cleft Palate

An interdisciplinary team—composed of a surgeon and a maxillofacial surgeon, orthodontist, audiologist, speech-language pathologist, prosthodontist, otolaryngologist, pediatric dentist, and geneticist—is extremely important in helping parents to understand the sequential approach to therapy for the many attendant problems.

Feeding usually requires considerable patience. Those with more severe clefts of the lip or palate should be fed in a sitting position to minimize fluid loss through the nose. Various techniques and equipment are used to feed infants with clefts, but

no single method is optimal for all infants. Infants with cleft lip or cleft palate swallow normally but suck abnormally. A cleft in the lip or palate generally does not allow sufficient negative pressure. In the case of cleft lip only, breast-feeding or an artificial nipple with a large, soft base works well. For infants with cleft lip or palate, regular breast-feeding or normal bottle-feeding often is not successful because they are unable to seal either their lips or their velopharynx. With cleft of the palate only, breast-feeding or normal bottle-feeding usually can be carried out if the cleft is narrow or involves only the soft palate. Soft artificial nipples with large openings are more effective.

Regular bottle nipples do not work well for infants with wider palatal clefts or the Robin malformation sequence. Enlarging the nipple opening in association with a softer nipple with a large base and a long shaft often enables tongue movement to express a greater quantity of milk. One can also deliver milk directly into the mouth with a soft plastic bottle.

It is now well recognized that children with cleft palate will have increased frequency of middle ear infection and fluid resulting in conductive hearing loss. The tensor palatini muscle is the primary muscle that spans the Eustachian tube necessary for adequate ventilation of the middle ear spaces. In children with cleft palate, Eustachian tube dysfunction and subsequent negative pressure in the middle ear space is our ideal environment for fluid buildup and infection. If medication will not resolve chronic infections and fluid accumulation, myringotomies and placement of ventilation tubes are an effective treatment.

Tonsils and adenoids may be helpful in accomplishing adequate velopharyngeal closure for speech. Therefore, caution needs to be taken before considering their removal since velopharyngeal inadequacy and hypernasal speech may result with otoacoustic emission/auditory brainstem response testing.

Assessing auditory function in infants with cleft palates is important and may be carried out more accurately in infants or young children by auditory specialists.

Surgical Repair of Clefts

Closure of the lip usually is carried out between the second and tenth week after birth, depending on the infant's weight and state of health. The primary purposes are to create a seal to allow normal sucking. Various techniques have been used for repair of the lip, depending on the degree and extent of defect. In those cases in which tissue in the two lip segments is insufficient to create an acceptable lip and nose, the surgeon may have to move small flaps of tissue from adjacent areas. For bilateral cleft lip, surgery is more difficult. If the primary palate is not attached to the secondary palate, it may require repositioning. Usually, subsequent surgery is required to correct nasal alar form, to compensate for uneven growth of tissue on the two sides of the lip, or to match evenly the vermilion line on both sides. This secondary surgery may best be performed during the teen years and is dependent upon the child's physical and behavioral growth and development.

Surgical closure of the hard and soft palate often is performed at 9 to 12 months of age, but some surgeons prefer to wait longer. The object is to create airtight and fluid-tight closure of the cleft and to preserve the length and mobility of the soft palate, to accomplish adequate velopharyngeal closure.

Second surgery may be required to achieve adequate closure; sometimes a speech prosthesis may be the best approach.

Associated Anomalies

Cleft lip and palate often occur as isolated anomalies (i.e., thorough examinations conducted over several years have revealed no other primary abnormalities). This statement would

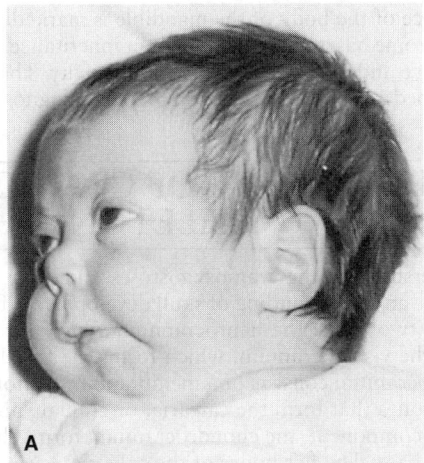 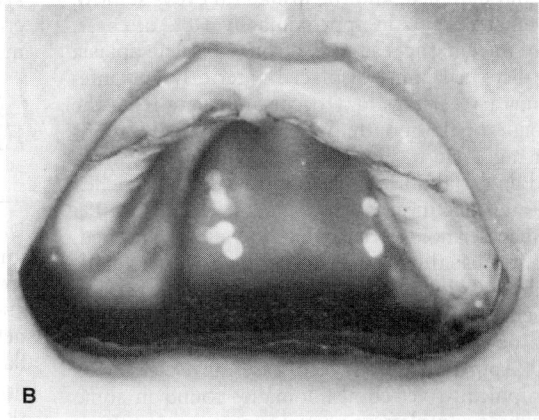

FIGURE 69.3. Robin malformation sequence. **A:** Small retruded lower jaw. **B:** U-shaped palatal cleft.

exclude, for example, the middle-ear infections that occur so frequently secondary to cleft palate.

When data are broken down according to subtype, isolated cleft palate (20% to 50%) generally is acknowledged to be associated more often with other congenital anomalies than are either isolated cleft lip (7% to 13%) or cleft lip with cleft palate (2% to 11%). The frequency with which one or more malformations accompany clefts of all types is almost 28%.

More malformations are found in infants with bilateral cleft lip with or without cleft palate than in those with unilateral cleft lip. The more malformations a child has, the lighter the birth weight is. Congenital velopharyngeal pharyngeal inadequacy has been found to be associated frequently with cervical anomalies. As noted, some of these associated findings form recognizable syndromes. In 1978, 133 such disorders were listed. In 1980, an estimated 204 cleft conditions were recognized: 47 autosomal dominant, 55 autosomal recessive, 6 X-linked, 32 chromosomal, and 64 disorders of unknown nature associated with facial clefting. The current number of "cleft syndromes" is more than 350. Only the Robin malformation sequence, oculoauriculovertebral malformation, and mandibulofacial dysostosis are discussed here.

Robin Malformation Sequence

The Robin malformation sequence consists of micrognathia, glossoptosis, and cleft palate (Fig. 69.3). Approximately 30% of the cases represent Stickler syndrome. The mandible is

small and symmetrically receded. Congenital murmurs or heart anomalies (e.g., ventricular septal defect, atrial septal defect, patent ductus arteriosus) have been observed in 15% to 20% of those who have died in early infancy. Esotropia and congenital glaucoma are relatively common. Approximately 20% exhibit severe mental retardation, but whether this condition is primary or secondary to asphyxia is not known. The palatal defect may vary widely from cleft uvula to clefting that involves two-thirds of the hard palate and is horseshoe shaped. The small mandible often achieves catch-up growth by 4 to 6 years of age, but the angle always is somewhat abnormal. Difficulty in the inspiratory phase of respiration is apparent, with periodic cyanotic attacks, labored breathing, and recession of the sternum and ribs, especially apparent when the child is supine. The respiratory difficulty usually is evident at birth, but it may not be severe for the first week. Immediate airway maintenance is critical. In mild cases, it may be accomplished by keeping the individual prone with the head suspended by a pulley in a stockinette cap. In more severe cases, the tongue tip may be sutured temporarily to the lower lip or anterior mandible. A tracheotomy or surgical advancement of the mandible rarely is required.

Oculoauriculovertebral Malformation

Facial asymmetry due to hypoplasia or displacement of the pinna is common in oculoauriculovertebral malformation (hemifacial microsomia, Goldenhar syndrome; Fig. 69.4). The

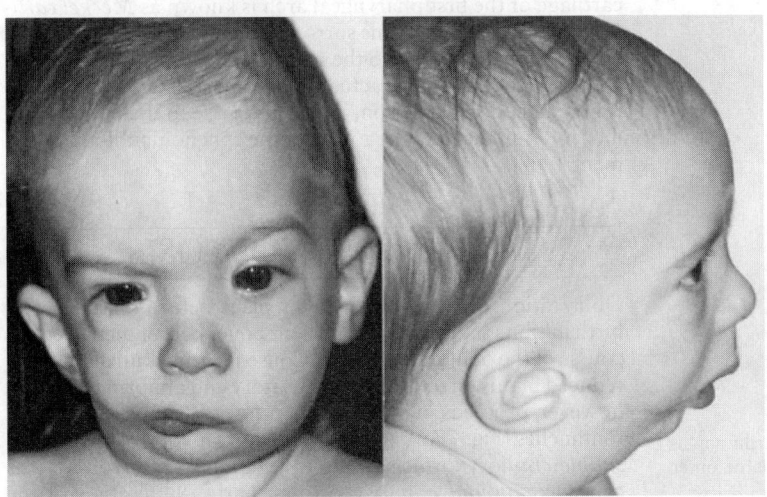

FIGURE 69.4. Oculoauriculovertebral malformation. Note hemifacial microsomia, repaired macrostomia, and low-set, somewhat dysmorphic pinna. Ear tags have been removed. (Courtesy of M. M. Cohen Jr., Halifax, Nova Scotia, Canada.)

maxillary, temporal, and malar bones on the involved side are reduced in size and flattened, and the ipsilateral eye is set low. Bilateral involvement occurs in approximately 10% of cases. Malformation of the external ear varies from complete aplasia to a crumpled, distorted pinna displaced anteriorly and inferiorly. Supernumerary ear tags may occur anywhere from the tragus to the angle of the mouth. When epibulbar dermoids are present, ear tags tend to be bilateral. Conductive hearing loss, due to middle ear abnormalities or absence or deficiency of the external auditory meatus and canal, is found in 40% of cases. Epibulbar dermoid varies: white to yellow, flattened, ellipsoid, solid, and usually located in the lower, outer quadrant at the limbus. Coloboma of the upper lateral eyelid is common in patients with epibulbar dermoids. When unilateral microphthalmia or anophthalmia is present, mental retardation is increased. Approximately 15% of cases have cleft lip or palate. Radiographically, vertebral anomalies found in some 50% of cases include complete or partial synostosis of two or more vertebrae and hemivertebrae. Aplasia or hypoplasia of the mandibular ramus is seen on the ipsilateral side. A small percentage of cases have agenesis of one lung and various renal anomalies (e.g., absent kidney, double ureter). The frequency of the condition is approximately 1 in 3,000 live births. Almost all cases appear to have multifactorial inheritance, with a recurrence risk of approximately 1%. However, in a few families, the disorder appears to be autosomal dominant.

Surgical correction ranges from lengthening the mandible to construction of a new temporomandibular joint and ramus with rib grafts and costochondral junction.

Mandibulofacial Dysostosis

Mandibulofacial dysostosis, or Treacher Collins syndrome, is characterized by downward-slanting palpebral fissures and coloboma of the outer third of the lower lid with deficient cilia medial to the coloboma (Fig. 69.5). The nose appears large because of lack of malar development. A nasofrontal angle commonly is obliterated. Micrognathia is a constant feature. Cleft palate is found in 30%. The external ear frequently is deformed, crumpled forward, or misplaced, with some patients having absence of the external auditory canal or an ossicular defect with conductive hearing loss. Extra ear tags and blind fistulas may be found between the tragus and angle of the mouth. Radiographs show defects in the zygomatic arches. The under-

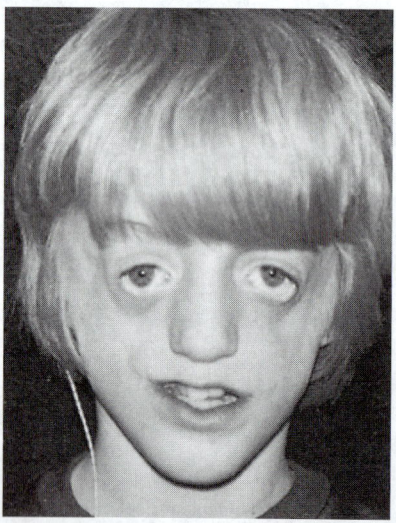

FIGURE 69.5. Mandibulofacial dysostosis. Boy with malar hypoplasia with downward-slanting palpebral fissures. Colobomas of outer third of lower lids. Note hearing aid cord.

surface of the body of the mandible is markedly concave. The syndrome has autosomal dominant inheritance, with high penetrance and markedly variable expressivity. The gene has been mapped to 5q31.3–q33.3, and prenatal diagnosis is possible.

EMBRYOLOGY OF CRANIOFACIAL SKELETON

Understanding the craniosynostoses and their syndromes requires an understanding of skull development. The skull forms from two parts: the neurocranium, which encases the brain, and the viscerocranium, which forms the facial skeleton. The neurocranium consists of a membranous portion composed of flat bones that form the calvaria, or cranial vault. A cartilaginous component, the chondrocranium, forms the bones of the skull base. The flat bones of the calvaria develop by membranous ossification. Several primary ossification centers, consisting of needle-like bone spicules, progressively enlarge and radiate peripherally, forming the frontal, parietal, and occipital bones.

In the newborn, the flat bones of the calvaria are separated by sutures (i.e., narrow bands of connective tissue). Points at which more than two bones meet exhibit wide sutural openings known as *fontanelles*. The largest of these is the anterior fontanelle, at the meeting of the two parietal bones and two frontal bones. The posterior fontanelle is situated at the junction between the two parietal bones and the occipital bone. A third fontanelle occasionally is present in the sagittal suture approximately 1 cm anterior to the posterior fontanelle. Two other embryonal fontanelles are found: the anterolateral (or sphenoidal) fontanelle and the posterolateral (or mastoid) fontanelle. The sutures and fontanelles permit skull bones to overlap during passage of the head through the vaginal canal. After birth, the bones resume their position. The anterior fontanelle usually is clinically closed by 13 months of age (range, 7 to 19 months). The posterior fontanelle, usually clinically inapparent at birth, closes anatomically at approximately 3 months of age. The sutures and fontanelles remain membranous to allow growth of the cranial vault in response to expansion of the brain. Many sutures remain open until adult life. In contrast to the membranous neurocranium, the base of the skull (or chondrocranium) initially consists of several cartilages that fuse and undergo endochondral ossification.

The viscerocranium or facial skeleton is formed mainly from the cartilages of the first two pharyngeal arches. The first pharyngeal arch is divided into a dorsal maxillary process and a ventral mandibular process. The former gives rise to the maxilla, the zygomatic bone, and part of the temporal bone. The cartilage of the first pharyngeal arch is known as *Meckel cartilage*. The ectomesenchyme surrounding the cartilage condenses and ossifies, giving rise to the mandible by membranous ossification. Meckel cartilage actually acts only as a template, except for its most dorsal portion, which gives rise to the malleus and incus. Remnants may be found in the sphenomandibular ligament.

CRANIOSYNOSTOSIS

Obliteration of sutures that takes place before or soon after birth inhibits the growth of adjacent bones perpendicular to the course of the obliterated suture. Consequently, skull diameter is reduced in this direction. Compensatory and abnormal growth, however, proceeds in directions permitted by open sutures and fontanelles (Fig. 69.6). If a single suture is involved, it is termed *simple craniosynostosis*; if multiple sutures are involved, it is called *compound craniosynostosis*. Early obliteration of the

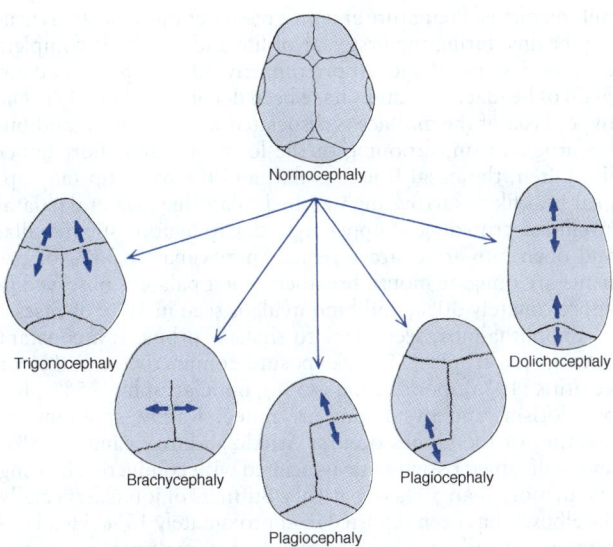

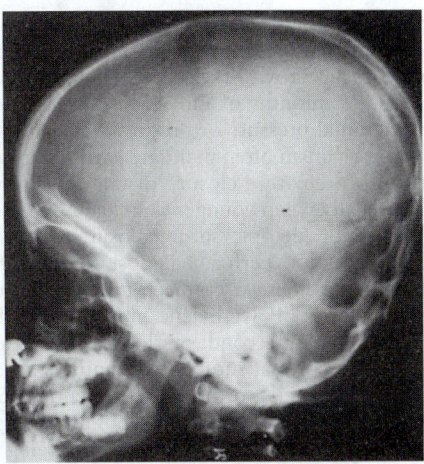

FIGURE 69.8. Brachycephaly.

FIGURE 69.6. Craniosynostosis. Various skull shapes resulting from premature fusion of individual sutures or groups of sutures. (Courtesy of M. M. Cohen, Jr., Halifax, Nova Scotia, Canada.)

sagittal suture results in *scaphocephaly* (*dolichocephaly*; Fig. 69.7). The skull is long and narrow, and the parietal protuberances are absent. As the brain expands, the coronal and lambdoidal sutures are widened, and frontooccipital elongation takes place. In some cases, a bony crest is seen in place of the sagittal suture. In *brachycephaly*, the coronal sutures are fused prematurely, resulting in a short, square-appearing cranial configuration (Fig. 69.8). *Plagiocephaly* refers to skewing of the skull due to premature unilateral fusion of a coronal or lambdoidal suture. *Trigonocephaly* describes a keel-shaped forehead due to premature fusion of the metopic suture. *Acrocephaly* (*turricephaly*) results from multiple suture closures. The highest point on the calvaria usually is near the anterior fontanelle, the head form being short, high, and broad. Chiefly, the coronal suture is affected, although the sagittal and lambdoid sutures frequently are involved. If the anterior fontanelle and metopic suture remain open, the skull expands in abnormal directions, resulting in steep frontal, parietal, and occipital bones and a high, broad, short skull. Often, digital impressions are evident.

Craniosynostosis may be primary, as in simple or compound premature fusion described earlier, or it may be secondary

to a known disorder (e.g., thalassemia, hyperthyroidism, microcephaly, mucopolysaccharidoses, rickets). Little is known about pathogenesis. Transforming growth factor–beta (types 1, 2, and 3), insulinlike growth factor–1, and some fibroblast growth factors and receptors (1, 2, and 3) are expressed at the osteogenic fronts of developing calvarial sutures and play a role in early pathologic closure (i.e., craniosynostosis).

Finally, craniosynostosis may be isolated or syndromic. In 1993, Cohen listed 90 syndromes of craniosynostosis (monogenic, 40; chromosomal, 16; environmentally induced, 4; unknown genesis, 24; miscellaneous, 6). A few more common syndromes are discussed in this chapter: Crouzon disease, Apert syndrome, Saethre-Chotzen syndrome, Pfeiffer syndrome, and Carpenter syndrome.

Epidemiology and Genetics

The frequency of simple or nonsyndromal craniosynostosis is approximately 0.34 to 0.40 per 1,000 newborns. Racial predilection is not apparent. Premature fusion of the sagittal suture is the most common type of simple synostosis, constituting approximately 55% of cases. The male-to-female gender predilection is 3:1. Unilateral or bilateral coronal synostosis comprises approximately 20% to 25% of cases, with a slight predilection for female infants. Metopic synostosis and lambdoidal synostosis each constitute a few percent. Involvement of two or more sutures comprises 15%.

Simple craniosynostosis usually is sporadic. Of patients with coronal synostosis, approximately 10% are familial; of patients with sagittal synostosis, approximately 2% are familial. Among those with familial occurrence, mutations in both fibroblast growth factor receptors 2 and 3 have been demonstrated. In some kindreds, the same suture is subject to synostosis in affected individuals and, in others, different sutures are fused. Sagittal synostosis appears to be most consistent with multifactorial inheritance, the frequency in the general population being approximately 1 in 4,200, with a recurrence risk of approximately 1 in 64 siblings. Twin studies clearly indicated that single-gene inheritance does not play a large role in craniosynostosis because discordance is more frequent than is concordance in monozygotic twins.

Treatment in Infancy

Treatment of craniosynostosis in infancy is controversial. The craniosynostoses represent not only diverse groups, but

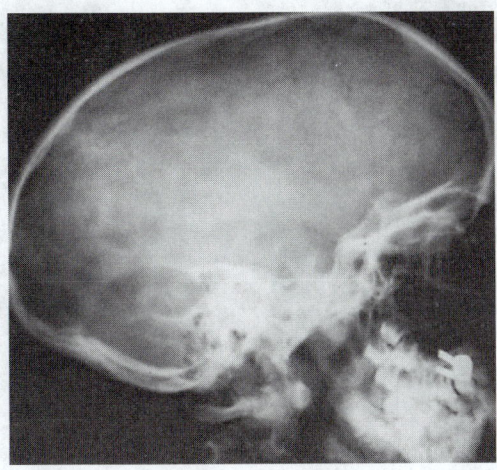

FIGURE 69.7. Scaphocephaly (dolichocephaly).

extreme variability is also found within each group. Opinions regarding treatment vary from conservative observation until completion of facial growth to radical extensive surgical correction in the first months of life. Such complications as increasing intracranial pressure or progressive corneal exposure secondary to exorbitism often mandate early treatment.

Patients with premature closure of cranial sutures should be treated surgically when younger than age 2 years, as should those patients with metopic suture closure younger than 6 months. The operation performed most frequently for simple craniosynostosis is linear craniectomy parallel to the prematurely fused suture. Polyethylene film is inserted over the bony margins to delay secondary closure. Bilateral, premature closure of the coronal sutures frequently is accompanied by anomalies of the facial, orbital, and sphenoid bones, with downward displacement of the orbital roof and overgrowth of the lesser wing of the sphenoid, and the orbits being markedly reduced in size, thus causing exophthalmos. Maximum decompression of the cranial vault rather than orbital decompression is carried out. Canthorrhaphy is performed to avoid dryness of the cornea and prolapse of the globe. Complex plastic surgical treatment of severe facial deformities of craniofacial dysostoses has been described in detail by Tessier. The optimal time for such operations is from 10 to 12 years of age.

Excellent results can be obtained from treating asymmetric synostosis at younger than 1 year of age by unilateral orbital repositioning and forehead remodeling. No further surgery is needed in more than 90% of patients. For bilateral or symmetric synostoses and mild upper-face deformity, orbital advancement and forehead reshaping carried out within the first year of life were less satisfactory, with some 50% of patients needing another major osteotomy. For those with moderate to severe symmetric synostoses (Crouzon disease and Apert syndrome), extensive facial reconstruction is performed at between 7 and 14 years of age. Despite delayed and aggressive treatment, surgical outcome is less satisfactory.

Types of Craniosynostoses

Crouzon Disease

Crouzon disease is characterized by premature craniosynostosis, midface hypoplasia with shallow orbits, and ocular proptosis (Fig. 69.9). Birth prevalence is approximately 16 per 1

million births. Premature and progressive craniosynostosis usually begins during the first year of life and usually is complete by 2 or 3 years of age. Approximately 30% of patients complain of headache; seizures have been documented in 10%. The hypoplasia of the midface is associated with relative mandibular prognathism, drooping of the lower lip, and short upper lip. Often, the nasal bridge is flat, and the nasal tip may appear beaklike. Narrow, high-arched palate due to lateral palatal swellings, crowding of upper teeth due to hypoplastic maxilla, and open bite are characteristic. Approximately 35% of patients are obligate mouth breathers. Cleft palate is observed in approximately 30%, and bifid uvula is seen in 10% of cases.

Exophthalmos, secondary to shallow orbits, is a constant finding. Exotropia (75%), exposure conjunctivitis (50%) or keratitis (10%), poor vision (45%), optic atrophy (25%), hypertelorism, and nystagmus are noted. Rarely, spontaneous luxation of the globes occurs. Atretic auditory canals (15%) and malformed ossicles are associated with conductive hearing loss in more than 50% of patients. Stiffness of joints, especially the elbows, has been reported in approximately 15%. Head circumference and body height generally are smaller than normal.

Radiographically, the coronal and sagittal sutures nearly always are fused, the lambdoidal in 80% of patients. Other findings include digital markings (90%), calcification of stylohyoid ligament (85%), deviation of nasal septum (35%), obstruction of nasal pharynx (30%), and cervical spine anomalies (30%). Cephalometric studies have shown the calvaria to be short, the forehead steep, the occiput flattened, and the cranial base shortened and narrowed, with the clivus especially abbreviated. Inheritance is autosomal dominant, with sporadic cases constituting approximately 50% of cases.

Crouzon disease is due to a mutation in fibroblast growth factor receptor 2 on chromosome 10q25–q26. Many mutation sites have been documented in the third immunoglobulin domain. Crouzon disease with acanthosis nigricans maps to fibroblast growth factor receptor 3 at 4p16.3.

Apert Syndrome

Apert syndrome is characterized by congenital craniosynostosis leading to turribrachycephaly, syndactyly of hands and feet, various ankyloses, and progressive synostoses of the hands, feet, and cervical spine (Figs. 69.10 and 69.11). Most patients are low average. Approximately 25% have pigment dilution of the hair. Facial variability is marked; the orbits are markedly hyperteloric, with the midface usually underdeveloped, lending prominence to the mandible. The skull is malformed, with

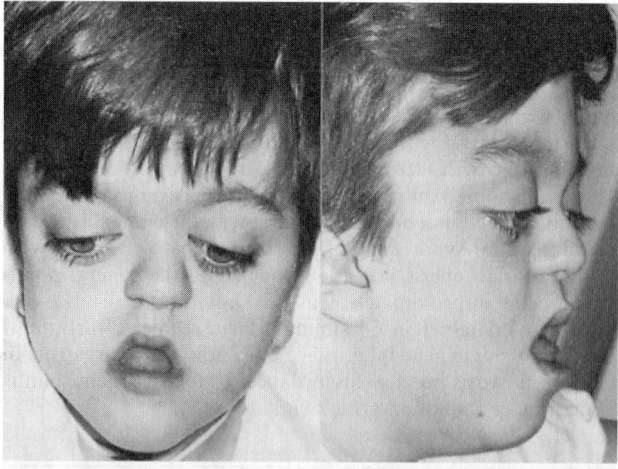

FIGURE 69.9. Crouzon disease. Downward-slanting palpebral fissures, facial asymmetry, hypoplastic midface, exorbitism, relative mandibular prognathism. (Courtesy of M. M. Cohen Jr., Halifax, Nova Scotia, Canada.)

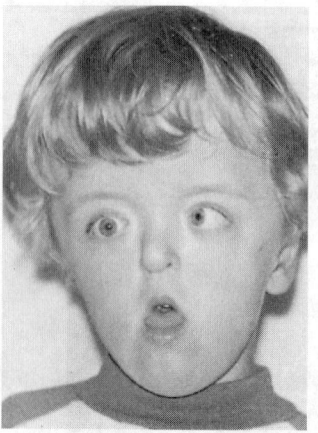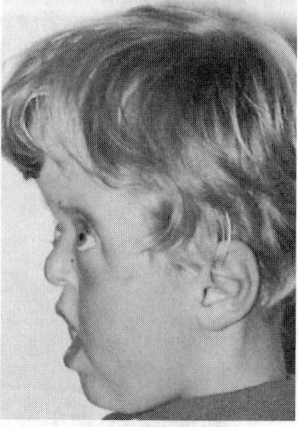

FIGURE 69.10. Apert syndrome. Frontal bossing, brachycephaly, hypertelorism, strabismus, exorbitism, depressed midface. (Courtesy of M. M. Cohen Jr., Halifax, Nova Scotia, Canada.)

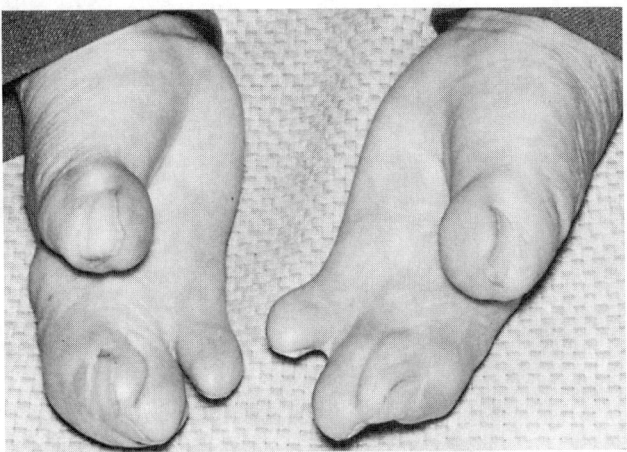

FIGURE 69.11. Apert syndrome. Extensive soft tissue syndactyly of hands. Note middigital hand mass composed of digits 2 to 4 and separate thumb and little finger. (Courtesy of L. Bergstrom, Los Angeles, CA.)

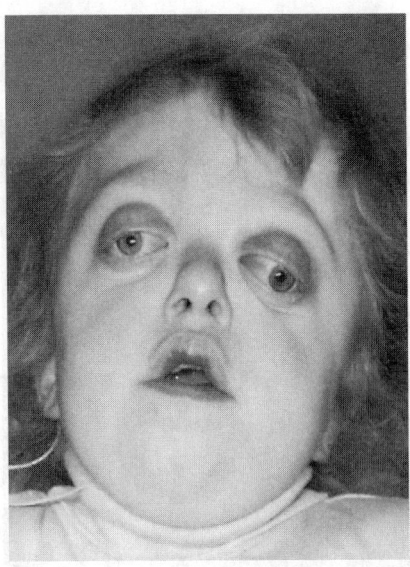

FIGURE 69.12. Pfeiffer syndrome. Exorbitism, downward-slanting palpebral fissures. Note hearing aid cord.

the frontal and occipital bones flattened and the apex of the cranium located near or anterior to the bregma. Cleft of the soft palate has been observed in approximately 35% of cases. Malocclusion is common because of midface hypoplasia. The hands and feet are deformed symmetrically. A middigital hand mass with bony and soft tissue syndactyly of digits 2, 3, and 4 often is found. Often, digits 1 and 5 are attached completely to the middigital hand mass. Frequently, the hallux is separated partially from the rest of the toes, which have complete soft tissue syndactyly and often a common nail. Six metatarsals have been noted in several cases. The upper extremities are shortened, and ankylosis is possible in joints, especially those of the elbow, shoulder, and hip. Acne vulgaris is noted commonly, with extension to the forearms. Apert syndrome occurs in approximately 16 of 1 million births. Inheritance is autosomal dominant, but the number of cases of transmission from parent to child is few because of the mental retardation and physical appearance. The syndrome is due to mutations in the fibroblast growth factor receptor 2 at 10q25–q26, and the mutations are exclusively of paternal origin.

Pfeiffer Syndrome

Pfeiffer syndrome consists of craniosynostosis resulting in turribrachycephaly. Broad thumbs and great toes and partial soft tissue syndactyly of the hands and feet are common. Autosomal dominant inheritance is evident, with complete penetrance and variable expressivity. Pfeiffer syndrome has been shown to be heterogeneous. Pfeiffer syndrome can be divided into three types: type 1 is the classic type, type 2 (constituting approximately 5%) has cloverleaf skull and elbow fusion, and type 3 is similar to type 2 but does not have cloverleaf skull. Various visceral malformations are found in type 3. Both types 2 and 3 are sporadic. The infants usually die within the first few weeks of life.

Most examples map to 10q25–q26 at fibroblast growth factor receptor 2 (*FGFR2*) and, less often, to 8p11.2–p12 (*FGFR1*). Those with cloverleaf skull map to *FGFR2*, whereas those with the milder form generally map to *FGFR1*.

Craniosynostosis, especially involving the coronal suture, results in turribrachycephaly. Increased digital markings may be observed with age. Maxillary hypoplasia, shallow orbits, and depressed nasal bridge also are seen. Orbital hypertelorism, down-slanting palpebral fissures, proptosis, and strabismus have been reported (Fig. 69.12). Intelligence usually is normal,

but severe retardation and various central nervous system defects are observed in survivors of the cloverleaf-skull anomaly.

The thumbs and great toes are broad, usually with varus deformity (Figs. 69.13 and 69.14). Mild soft tissue syndactyly predominantly involves the second and third digits. Occasionally, middle phalanges are absent. The proximal phalanges of both thumbs are trapezoidal but may be triangular. Pollux varus commonly is found. The proximal phalanges of both great toes are trapezoidal, and hallux varus is common. The first metatarsals are broad, with partial reduplication in some cases. Symphalangism of both hands and feet has been reported. Fusion of carpals, tarsals, and the proximal ends of the metatarsals has been noted. Radiohumeral and radioulnar synostoses have been described in types 2 and 3.

Saethre-Chotzen Syndrome

Asymmetric craniosynostosis produces plagiocephaly and facial asymmetry (Fig. 69.15). Acrocephaly and (occasionally) scaphocephaly have been noted. Head circumference frequently is reduced, and often the frontal hairline is low. Strabismus, myopia, hyperopia, ptosis, and hypertelorism are frequent. The ears may be dysplastic, with folded helices, prominent antihelices, and posterior rotation. Some degree of

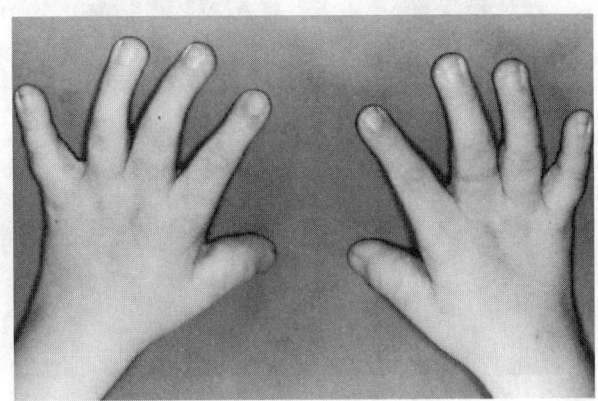

FIGURE 69.13. Wide thumbs of Pfeiffer syndrome.

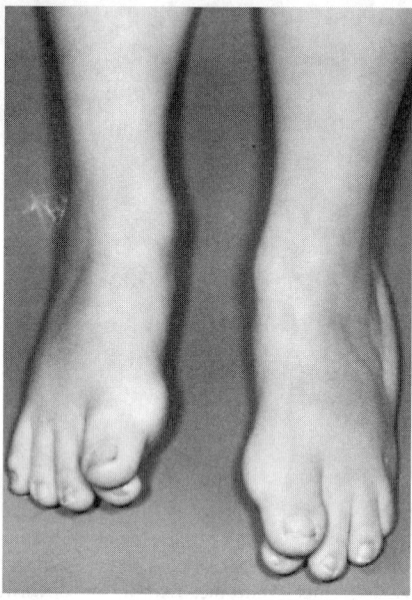

FIGURE 69.14. Wide halluces of Pfeiffer syndrome.

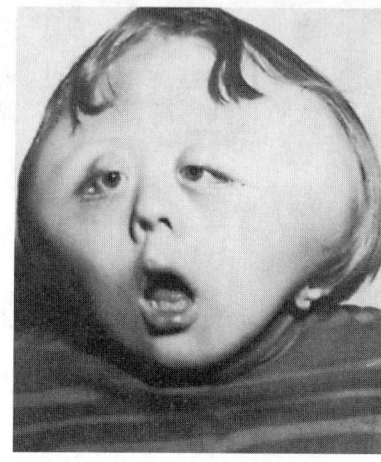

FIGURE 69.16. Carpenter syndrome. Downward-slanting palpebral fissures, hypertelorism, cloverleaf skull.

hearing loss is common. The nose tends to be beaked, with deviation of the nasal septum, and the nasofrontal angle is flattened. Occasional partial cutaneous syndactyly is evident in the second and third fingers. Intelligence usually is normal, but mild to moderate mental retardation has been found occasionally. Inheritance is autosomal dominant, with complete penetrance and variable expressivity. The gene has been mapped to chromosome 7p21.2. Roentgenography usually reveals coronal synostosis, reduced length of posterior cranial base, low position of the sella turcica, reduced facial depth, steep mandibular plane angle, and absence or reduced size of paranasal sinuses.

Carpenter Syndrome

Carpenter syndrome consists of acrocephaly, soft tissue syndactyly (especially involving the third and fourth fingers), brachymesophalangy, preaxial polydactyly and syndactyly of the toes, coxa valga and pes varus, congenital heart disease, mental retardation, hypogenitalism, mild obesity, and hernia. The syndrome has autosomal recessive inheritance.

Height usually is in the low 25% range of normal, but weight often is above average. The obesity mainly involves the trunk, proximal limbs, face, and nape. Usually, the skull is tower-shaped. Although premature fusion may involve all cranial sutures, synostosis often is asymmetric, producing a distorted calvaria, in some cases with cloverleaf skull (Figs. 69.16 and 69.17). On radiography, the sagittal and lambdoidal sutures often are observed to fuse first, the coronals being the last to close.

The hands are short, and the fingers are somewhat stubby, with a simple flexion crease (Fig. 69.18). Soft tissue syndactyly often occurs between the third and fourth fingers, with less pronounced syndactyly between other fingers. Radiography reveals brachymesophalangy of all digits or agenesis of some middle phalanges of the second to fifth digits. Usually present are bilateral varus deformities of the feet and preaxial polydactyly, with duplication of the first or second toe. The toes usually exhibit soft tissue syndactyly. Metatarsus varus and replication of the second toe are frequent. The first metatarsal is short and remarkably broad, with only two phalanges present in each toe. In nearly all cases, genu valgum has occurred, with lateral displacement of the patellae. Congenital heart disease of various types (e.g., ventricular septal defect, atrial septal defect, patent ductus arteriosus, pulmonary stenosis, tetralogy of

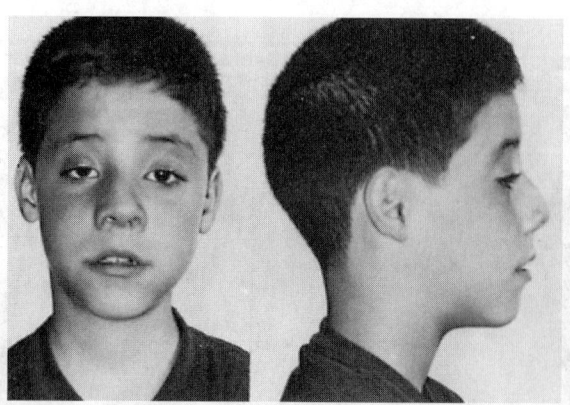

FIGURE 69.15. Saethre-Chotzen syndrome. Note facial asymmetry and ptosis of eyelid.

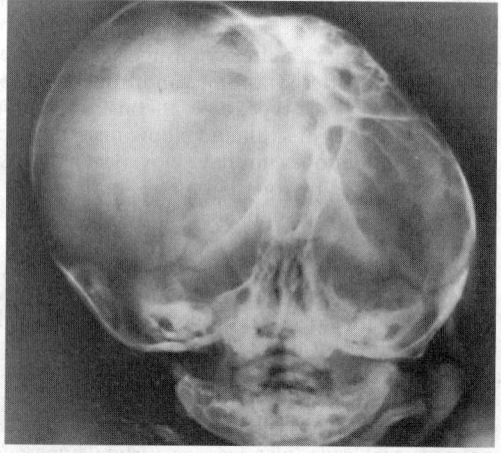

FIGURE 69.17. Asymmetric cloverleaf skull of Carpenter syndrome. (Courtesy of H. Schönenberg, Aachen, Germany.)

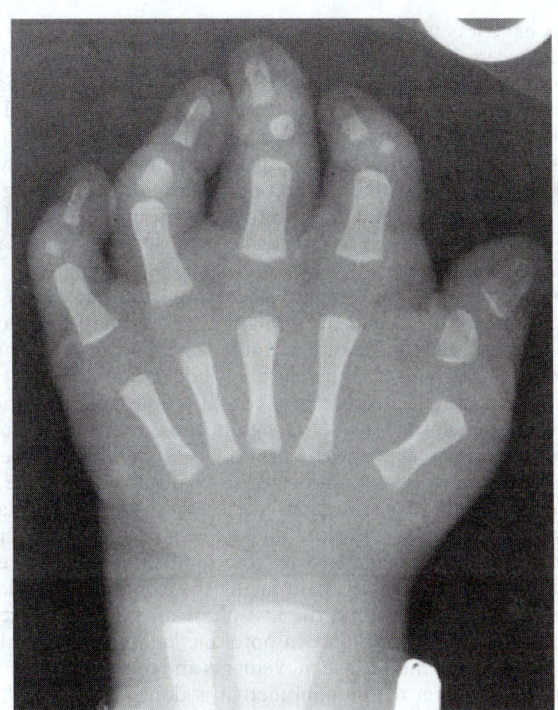

FIGURE 69.18. Hypoplasia of middle phalanges in Carpenter syndrome. (Courtesy of A. Poznanski, Chicago, IL.)

Fallot) have been reported. Most patients are mildly retarded, but some have normal intelligence.

Suggested Readings

Bardach J, Morris HL. *Multidisciplinary management of cleft lip and palate.* Philadelphia: Saunders, 1990.
Bartlett SP, Whitaker LA, Marshac D. The operative treatment of isolated craniofacial dysostosis (plagiocephaly): a comparison of the unilateral and bilateral techniques. *Plast Reconstr Surg* 1990;85:677.

Bellus GA, Gaudenz K, Zackai EH, et al. Identical mutations in three different fibroblast growth factor receptor genes in autosomal dominant craniosynostosis syndrome. *Nat Genet* 1996;13:174.
Bonaiti-Pellie C, Smith C. Risk tables for genetic counseling in some congenital malformations. *J Med Genet* 1974;11:374.
Bruneteau RJ, Mulliken JB. Frontal plagiocephaly: synostotic, compensational, or deformational. *Plast Reconstr Surg* 1992;89:21.
Clarren SK, Anderson B, Wolf LS. Feeding infants with cleft lip, cleft palate, or cleft lip and palate. *Cleft Palate J* 1987;24:244.
Cohen MM Jr. *Craniosynostosis: diagnosis, evaluation and management*, 2nd ed. New York: Oxford University Press, 1999.
Cohen MM Jr. Pfeiffer syndrome update, clinical subtypes, and guidelines for differential diagnosis. *Am J Med Genet* 1993;45:300.
Cohen MM Jr. Syndromes, with cleft lip and cleft palate. *Cleft Palate J* 1978;15:306.
Cohen MM Jr, Rollnick BR, Kaye CI. Oculoauriculovertebral spectrum: an updated critique. *Cleft Palate J* 1989;26:276.
David DJ, Sheen R. Surgical correction of Crouzon syndrome. *Plast Reconstr Surg* 1990;85:344.
Fria TJ, Paradise JL, Sabo DL, et al. Conductive hearing loss—in infants and young children with cleft palate. *J Pediatr* 1987;111:84.
Gorlin RJ. Fibroblast growth factors, their receptors and receptor disorders. *J Craniomaxillofac Surg* 1997;25:69.
Gorlin RJ, Cohen MM Jr, Hennekam RCM. *Syndromes of the head and neck*, 4th ed. New York: Oxford University Press, 2001.
Gorlin RJ, Slavkin HC. Embryology of the face. In: Tewfik TL, Der Kaloustian VM, eds. *Congenital anomalies of the ear, nose, and throat*. New York: Oxford University Press, 1997.
Jones JC. Etiology of facial clefts: prospective evaluation of 428 patients. *Cleft Palate J* 1988;25:16.
Kaban LB, Moses MH, Mulliken JB. Surgical correction of hemifacial microsomia in the growing child. *Plast Reconstr Surg* 1988;82:9.
Marchac D, Renier D. *Craniofacial surgery for craniosynostosis*. Boston: Little, Brown and Company, 1982.
Moller KT, Starr CD, Johnson SA. *A parent's guide to cleft lip and palate*. Minneapolis: University of Minnesota Press, 1989.
Shah CP, Wong D. Management of children with cleft lip and palate. *Can Med Assoc J* 1980;122:19.
Sheffield JA, Reiss K, Strom CJ. A genetic follow-up study of 64 patients with Pierre Robin complex. *Am J Med Genet* 1987;28:25.
Shprintzen RJ, Siegel-Sadewitz YL, Amato J. Anomalies associated with cleft lip, cleft palate, or both. *Am J Med Genet* 1985;20:585.
Tessier P. Craniofacial surgery in syndrome craniosynostosis. In: Cohen MM Jr, ed. *Craniosynostosis: diagnosis, evaluation, and management*. New York: Raven Press, 1986:321.
Vanderas AP. Incidence of cleft lip, cleft palate, and cleft lip and palate among races: a review. *Cleft Palate J* 1987;24:216.
Whitaker LA, Bartlett SP, Schut L, et al. Craniosynostosis: an analysis of the timing, treatment, and complications in 164 consecutive patients. *Plast Reconstr Surg* 1987;80:195.
Wyszynski DF, Beaty TH, Maestri NE. Genetics of nonsyndromic oral clefts revisited. *Cleft Palate Craniofac J* 1996;33:406.

CHAPTER 70 ■ EYE EVALUATION OF THE NEWBORN

DAVID S. WALTON AND GARYFALLIA KATSAVOUNIDOU

Congenital or acquired ocular defects in neonates unfortunately are not rare. In the best interests of both child and family, it is of extreme importance that the neonatologist be well prepared for the eye evaluation of the newborn. The optimum preparation for such an evaluation is acquired through a multiplicity of avenues. Experience is gained from the evaluation of newborns with normal visual systems, and familiarity with

the common neonatal ocular problems and an appreciation for the potential occurrence of unusual problems is helpful. Obtaining a preliminary history of any familial congenital ocular disorders and of adverse prenatal or perinatal conditions (intrauterine problems, prematurity or difficult delivery events) can be very directive and helpful. It is indispensable to perform an informative eye examination, completed as early as possible, to recognize suspected or unexpected neonatal ocular abnormalities.

Following the initial examination, if an ocular abnormality is recognized—or when parents express concerns about the baby's visual system that cannot be explained by normal developmental phenomena—the infant should be promptly examined by an ophthalmologist. Generally, this further evaluation will determine the medical or surgical management of any significant neonatal ocular abnormality. Some conditions, such as infections, glaucoma, or evidence of intraocular abnormalities, are more urgent than others. Communicating the findings of an adverse examination to the child's family, and especially to the mother, must be made attentively to lessen the potential shock and disappointment. Parents may be reassured by learning about their infant's condition and the potential advantages (or not) of early treatment.

OCULAR ASSESSMENT IN THE NEWBORN

The ocular system assessment of the newborn is an essential component of a complete neonatal physical examination. This can be performed quickly. A few specialized pediatric eye examination instruments are helpful and include an ophthalmoscope, a penlight, an optional magnification loupe, and an eyelid speculum. The magnification loupe can be especially helpful for studying anterior segment structures. The use of topical anesthetic and dilating eye drops may be indicated. This examination should be performed while the infant is kept comfortable and warm, and optimally while sleeping or being fed. It is advisable that the least upsetting maneuvers are performed first. The results should all be recorded carefully. The newborn eye examination should include an evaluation of the following:

- Pupillary light responses
- Eyelid position and movement
- Basic tear composition
- Eye position and movements
- Conjunctiva
- Corneal size and transparency
- Iris appearance and symmetry
- Pupillary size, position, and shape
- Lens transparency
- Quality and symmetry of the retinal red reflexes

Vision testing of the newborn lacks precision. Laboratory testing methods reveal that a term newborn possesses a visual acuity of approximately 20/200 and begins to focus (accommodate) by 3 months of age. When presented with an object or light stimulus, the normal newborn may show no response, stare, halt movement of the extremities, or rarely, follow briefly. Blinking or blepharospasm is an expected response to bright light, but its presence is not evidence of intact cortical function. Pupillary constriction to light is the most reliable evidence of neonatal sensory ocular function; it may be present by the postconceptional age of 28 weeks and is consistently present by 32 weeks' gestational age. It increases in amplitude during the last 8 weeks of gestation and is best studied in a somewhat darkened room. The direct pupillary responses of each eye should be compared. The term newborn's pupils are small compared to the larger and variably sized pupils of a preterm neonate of less than 30 weeks' gestational age. A slight difference of pupillary size is present in a small percent of normal newborns. Nystagmus always is a significant observation; it may be secondary to decreased vision, or may be indicative of seizure activity.

The condition of the eyelids and the presence of normal tears can be appraised by observation. Term newborns have basal and reflux tear secretion similar to adults. Preterm infants have less production of tears. This examination may be made uncertain due to postpartum eyelid swelling or irritation caused by silver nitrate prophylaxis. The superior eyelid crease is indicative of levator (elevator) muscle function and should be similar in each lid, but may be absent in the case of congenital ptosis. A slight asymmetry in palpebral fissure width usually is insignificant. Congenital turning out (ectropion) or turning in (entropion) of the eyelid margins towards the cornea should be ruled out because of the risk of corneal exposure and secondary eyelash-related injury.

The extraocular movements and eye position are assessed next. Observe the eye in the straight-ahead primary position. The presence of symmetrical corneal light reflexes is an indication of straight eyes. Whereas an eye deviation during sleep is common, the occurrence of a constant and large deviation when the neonate is awake is significant. Vertical and horizontal conjugate eye movements can be stimulated by head rotation. It is especially important to confirm the presence of abduction (sixth nerve function) in each eye. Vestibular nystagmus, with both fast and slow phases, is expected in the term newborn and is best induced by rotation of the baby and examiner while the infant is held facing the examiner. The slow phase during rotation and the fast phase after rotation occur in the direction of rotation. An optokinetic tape or drum also can be used to stimulate eye movements and to estimate vision.

The inspection of the conjunctiva is done by viewing the white bulbar region of each globe and by everting the eyelids to expose each fornix. Increased redness (injection) and discharge are common indicators of conjunctival inflammation. Familiarity with the normal conjunctiva and its appearance after silver nitrate application can be helpful in assessing a newborn for an infectious conjunctivitis.

The inspection of the anterior segment of the eyes begins with an estimation of the corneal size and transparency. Clarity of the cornea and anterior chamber is suggested by a clear view of the iris and pupils. With practice, the examiner can perform this assessment confidently. A $2\times$ magnification loupe can be used advantageously for this examination. The normal newborn corneal diameters are equal and approximately 10.5 mm in size. Corneas of unequal size, or possessing a measurement 12.5 mm or more, are abnormal. Fluorescein dye may be used topically to help confirm the presence a superficial corneal epithelial defect.

When a total cataract is present, the pupil will appear white, and the normal red reflex obtained by focusing an ophthalmoscope on the pupillary border will be absent. A small lens opacity can be seen as a dark defect against the red reflex background. Diffuse, less dense cataracts will cause the red reflex to be of poor quality and will prevent a clear view of the ocular fundi.

The fundus examination, although not a mandatory part of the examination, should include, when indicated, inspection of the disks, retinal vessels, and macular regions. Small pupils make this evaluation difficult, so it is usually adequate to be reassured by an equal red reflex from each fundus. More pigmented patients possess a darker red reflex. This color variation is proportional to the amount of pigment in the choroid. Neonatal pupils dilate well with the use of mydriatics, which are required when complete funduscopy is indicated.

DISORDERS OF THE EYE IN THE NEWBORN

Abnormal Vision

Congenital disorders associated with poor vision are rarely detected in the newborn period. Even anencephalic infants may exhibit pupillary responses and demonstrate blepharospasm in response to light. Visual behavior develops rapidly, and parents often observe its absence by 1 to 2 months of age. Parental concern that their child "does not see" must be treated attentively and indicates the need for ophthalmologic consultation. A family history of infant blindness, as well as the effects of unfavorable prenatal and perinatal conditions, must be considered. The cause of the visual unresponsiveness may be apparent on inspection of the eyes by the presence of microphthalmos, signs of glaucoma, cataracts, or cloudy corneas. Internal examination of the eyes may detect abnormalities such as vitreous hemorrhage, optic nerve atrophy, or hypoplasia, or may reveal normal findings. Congenital retinal dystrophies may manifest normal fundi and require electroretinography for identification. Poor vision secondary to cortical defects may be associated with minimal eye abnormalities and require neuroimaging for recognition. Delayed visual development and apparent blindness related to abnormal eye movement also must be taken into consideration.

Eyelid Abnormalities

Ptosis is a common eyelid abnormality caused by weakness of the elevator muscle, and it can be unilateral or bilateral. Moderate ptosis may be evidence of Horner syndrome and be associated with homolateral upper-extremity paralysis caused by a birth injury. Widening of the palpebral fissure can be a sign of a congenital facial nerve palsy or be caused by proptosis, which in the newborn can result from a retrobulbar tumor or hemorrhage secondary to birth trauma. A congenital entropion positions the eyelashes against the cornea and requires prompt attention. Colobomatous defects of the eyelids are seen in Goldenhar and Treacher-Collins syndromes.

Tear Abnormalities

The excessive presence of tears suggests common congenital tear duct obstruction; it usually is noticed promptly by parents when it becomes complicated by a discharge. Epiphora (excessive tearing) also may be caused by corneal abnormalities, including corneal ulceration and defects secondary to glaucoma. A deficiency of tears may be isolated or associated with corneal hypesthesia; this places the corneal surface and eyes at jeopardy, as is seen in newborns with familial dysautonomia.

DISORDERS OF EYE POSITION AND MOVEMENT

An intermittent eye deviation in infancy is common and usually observed during periods of drowsiness. A congenital esotropia is seen in approximately 1% of infants; it is typically large and may be associated with impaired abduction of both eyes. Congenital exotropia is unusual. A sixth-nerve palsy may occur with birth, is usually unilateral, and often resolves spontaneously. A congenital fourth-nerve paralysis also can occur, but it is typically recognized after infancy. Congenital third-nerve palsies are rare; they cause ptosis, pupillary abnormalities, external ophthalmoplegia, an exotropia, and are frequently associated with other evidence of central nervous system abnormalities, such as hemiplegia.

Nystagmus always is an important sign of ocular disease. Most infants with congenital nystagmus have ocular or optic nerve defects that adversely affect vision. Tonic defects of eye position of supranuclear origin occur and are associated with tonic downgaze, which may be transient. Eyes also may be

fixed in virtually one position of gaze secondary to hereditary ocular muscle fibrosis. A congenital absence of horizontal gaze caused by a central defect occurs rarely. Hydrocephalus may cause impairment of up gaze.

CONJUNCTIVAL ABNORMALITIES

Ophthalmia neonatorum (conjunctivitis of the newborn) is the most common abnormality of the conjunctiva and is covered in Chapters 85 and 86, Eye Problems. Other conjunctival defects that may be seen are hemorrhage, cysts, and choristomas, including dermoid and lipodermoid cysts.

ANTERIOR SEGMENT ABNORMALITIES

Failure to assess the anterior segment of the newborn may result in delayed recognition of significant abnormalities of the cornea, irides, pupils, and lenses. Corneal opacification occurs with many ocular and systemic conditions. This is an early sign of congenital glaucoma, but also may be caused by primary congenital corneal disease. The possibility of corneal birth trauma also must be considered, especially after a difficult delivery and forceps use (Fig. 70.1). A small cornea may indicate microphthalmos and the increased potential for intraocular anomalies, such as a retinochoroidal coloboma, chorioretinitis, and cataracts.

The irides are ordinarily similar in appearance. The pupils should be small, round, and equal in size. A coloboma of the iris is a congenital defect that gives the inferior pupil a keyhole appearance; it typically is associated with posterior ocular anomalies. Total absence of the iris is seen in aniridia, which produces a large red reflex related to the size of the enlarged pupil (Fig. 70.2). Vascular congestion of the iris vessels may be abnormal and suggests maternal cocaine use. A poor view of the iris can be caused by a neonatal hyphema (blood in the anterior chamber) and by decreased corneal transparency.

CONGENITAL CATARACTS

The most common congenital lens defect is a cataract. This opacification of the lens may be unilateral or bilateral, and is

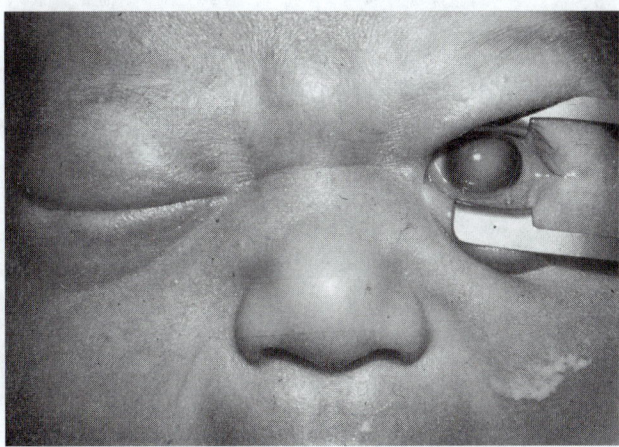

FIGURE 70.1. Newborn with corneal opacification following forceps-related injury. See Color Figure 70.1 in color section.

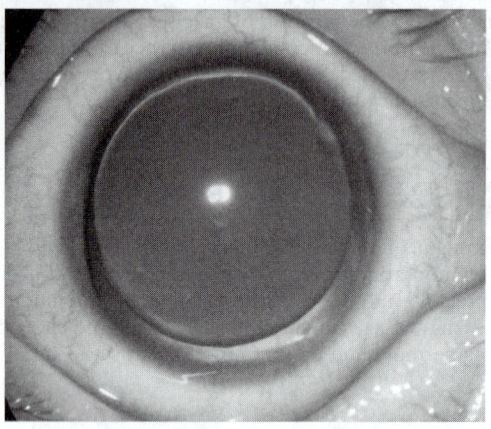

FIGURE 70.2. Enlarged fundus red reflex associated with congenital hereditary aniridia. See Color Figure 70.2 in color section.

detectable with use of a hand light to illuminate the anterior segment (Fig. 70.3) and an ophthalmoscope to produce a red reflex. Suspected cataracts are best studied with a hand-held slit beam. Cataracts may be anterior or posterior in the lens, partial or total, and may be isolated or associated with other ocular and systemic abnormalities. Some cataracts are inherited or inheritable, whereas others are nongenetic. Autosomal dominant inheritance is most common when cataracts are bilateral and genetically determined.

The diverse causes of and associations with congenital cataracts highlights the need for a complete ocular and systemic examination of the young cataract patient to determine the significance of the cataract abnormality (Box 70.1).

The presence of bilateral cataracts in infancy may represent a significant impediment to the development of vision. Greater opacification, irregularity, and posterior location are characteristics of a more visually significant lens defect. Vision develops rapidly in early life, and when this process is impeded during a critical period of approximately 4 months after birth, the potential for developing a higher level of vision is lost. After cataracts are detected, prompt ophthalmologic evaluation is required to consider the infant for cataract removal. When an infant's candidacy and the age for cataract extraction is consid-

ered, both the ocular potential for providing improved vision and the general health and development of the infant should be considered.

RETINAL ABNORMALITIES

Retinal hemorrhages often are present in newborns and are less frequent when delivery is by cesarean section. Vitreous hemorrhage is far less common than retinal hemorrhage. The congenital retinal hemorrhages are usually numerous, occupy the inner layers of the retina, and resolve rapidly. Retinal hemorrhages seen after 3 weeks of age in infancy should, with great reservation, be interpreted as secondary to birth trauma. The probability of a more recent accidental trauma or trauma related to child abuse (shaken baby syndrome) must be considered, even without other evidence of injury.

Infants born prematurely are considered to be at risk for retinopathy of prematurity (ROP). Infants with a birth weight of less than 1,500 g or a gestational age of 28 weeks or less, as well as infants between 1,500 and 2,000 g with a history of an unstable course, are believed to be at risk. Infants weighing less than 1,200 g are considered to be at even greater risk and have an incidence of ROP of approximately 50%. The first examination for ROP should be between 4 and 6 weeks' postnatal age, or between 31 and 33 weeks' postconceptional age. This examination may be done by indirect ophthalmoscopy and requires pupillary dilation. For pupillary dilation, tropicamide 0.5% or cyclopentolate 0.5% and phenylephrine 2.5% are recommended, with the application of a single drop of each to each eye. These agents should be applied carefully to prevent overflow onto the skin, where further systemic absorption can occur. The eyes may be examined individually on different days to lessen the burden on the patient. On examination, the ophthalmologist will look for retinal abnormalities characteristic of ROP. At least two examinations should be performed. The defects are classified using the International Classification of ROP (Box 70.2), a system that defines the retinal defect in respect to location, extent, and severity. Depending on location and severity of the defect, reexamination will be carried out regularly. Each affected infant is evaluated based on the severity, position, and extent of disease, to determine possible candidacy for cryotherapy or laser treatment, which is helpful treatment to halt progressive or active ROP. The Multicenter Trial of Cryotherapy for ROP showed that 44.4% of eyes with the history of advanced ROP achieved 20/200 or worse vision at age 10 years and that only 45.4% of those with better than 20/200 had a acuity of 20/40 or better. ROP is associated with a high incidence of spontaneous regression, especially when normal retinal vascularization has prenatally reached a position anterior to the equator.

CONCLUSIONS

The normal newborn examination record should confirm that each eye has been examined and found healthy, without disease, congenital anomalies, or evidence of injury. Ocular examination of the newborn and recognition of abnormalities require experience that can be acquired best by the repeated examination of neonates. It is advisable that an ophthalmologist be consulted frequently, so that normal variations are learned and diseases are managed promptly. Children born prematurely must be followed carefully for the development of ROP, and the extent of their disease must be monitored carefully to determine their candidacy and need for laser or cryogenic

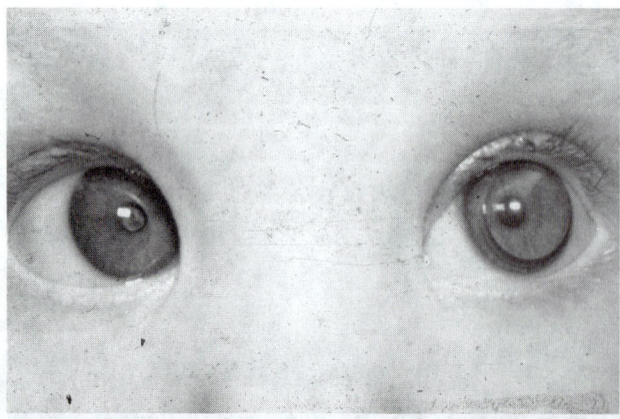

FIGURE 70.3. Infant with leukocoria and related cataract of the right eye and with contact lens in place following cataract removal from the left eye. See Color Figure 70.3 in color section.

BOX 70.1	Etiologic Classification of Congenital Cataracts

Cataracts In Infancy

A. Hereditary Congenital Cataracts
1. Anterior polar cataracts
2. Bilateral lamellar zonular nuclear cataracts (D)
3. Bilateral posterior lenticonus (D)
4. Bilateral greenish blue discoloration anterior capsule (R)
5. Cataracts, microcornea, and microphthalmia (D or XR)
6. Cataracts, microcornea, and dental anomalies (Nance-Horan syndrome) (Xp22.2) (XR)
7. Sutural opacities (carrier of Nance-Horan trait) (XR)
8. Ectopia lentis et pupillae (R)
9. Pulverulent cataract (Coppock cataract) (chromosome 1q,) (D)
10. Pulverulent cataract (Coppock-like), (chromosome 2q33-35, 22q11.2) (D)
11. Anterior polar cataract (D) (chromosome 16q with haptoglobin gene)
12. Aculeiform cataract (chromosome 2q33-35)
13. Congenital central pouchlike cataract, (chromosome 15q21-22)
14. Hyperferritinemia cataract (chromosome 19) (D)
15. Oculocerebrorenal syndrome (Lowe) (Xq26.1) (XR)

B. Idiopathic Congenital Cataracts
1. Unilateral/bilateral cortical cataracts
2. Unilateral sporadic posterior lenticonus cataract
3. Anterior capsule pupillary membrane plaque

C. Embryopathic
1. Maternal rubella syndrome
2. Maternal toxoplasmosis
3. Herpes simplex infection
4. Maternal varicella
5. Cytomegalic inclusion disease

D. Trauma
1. Birth injury
2. Trauma

E. Cataracts of Prematurity
1. Transient cataracts of prematurity
2. Cataracts secondary to ROP laser retinal photocoagulation

F. Congenital Cataracts Associated with Chromosomal Disorders
1. Autosomal dominant cataracts with translocation $[t(3;4)(p^{26.2};p^{15})]$
2. Cri Du Chat ($5p^-$)
3. Aniridia ($11p^-$) nuclear and posterior capsule defects
4. 13 q^- syndrome
5. 13 Trisomy
6. Smith-Magenis syndrome ($17p11^-$)
7. 18 Trisomy
8. 18 p^- syndrome
9. 21 Trisomy
10. Turner syndrome

G. Congenital Cataracts with Systemic Disease
1. Galactosemia
2. Rhizomelic chondrodysplasia punctata
3. Oculocerebrorenal syndrome of Lowe
4. Hallermann-Streiff syndrome
5. Marinesco-Sjögren syndrome (MR, hypotonia, dwarfism, ataxia, cataracts)
6. Syndromes of mental retardation, microcephaly, microphthalmia, cataracts
7. Kniest syndrome (skeletal dysplasia)
8. Incontinentia pigmenti
9. Atopic dermatitis
10. Smith-Lemli-Opitz syndrome
11. Infantile hypoglycemia
12. Congenital cataracts associated with skeletal and cardiac myopathy
13. Mitochondrial complex I deficiency
14. Pearson syndrome: mitochondrial defect syndrome
15. Turner syndrome
16. Rubinstein-Taybi syndrome
17. Blepharophimosis with somatofacial dysmorphism (Schwartz-Aberfeld disease)
18. Trichomegaly, spherocytosis, and bilateral cataracts
19. Schafer syndrome (MR, dwarfism, hyperkeratosis, nail abnormality)
20. Siemens syndrome (cataracts and skin hypoplasia)
21. Maple syrup urine disease
22. Mevalonic aciduria
23. Warburg syndrome
24. Neonatal adrenoleukodystrophy
25. Martsolf syndrome (MR, dwarfism, hypogonadism)
26. CAMFAK syndrome (microcephaly and cataracts)
27. Ellis van Creveld syndrome (chondroectodermal dysplasia)
28. Sotos syndrome (cerebral giantism)
29. CHARGE syndrome
30. Cohen-Holmes-Merhosseini-Walton syndrome
31. DeBarsy syndrome
32. Facial dysmorphism neuropathy syndrome

H. Cataracts Associated with Primary Ocular Anomalies
1. Persistent primary hyperplastic vitreous
2. Congenital aniridia
3. Peters anomaly
4. Ectopia lentis et pupillae (R)
5. Ocular coloboma
6. Congenital retinal disinsertion syndrome
7. Microphthalmos and cataracts with or without other ocular defects
8. Bhaduri syndrome: cataracts, blepharophimosis, iris anomalies (PAX6 abnormality) (D)
9. Familial irido-corneo-goniodysgenesis (D)
10. MICRO syndrome
11. Papillorenal syndrome (PAX2 defect)

retinal therapy. As both neonatology and pediatric ophthalmology progress, information and trained personnel are now more available to help pediatricians and parents in eye care for the newborn.

Suggested Readings

Brodsky MC. *Pediatric neuro-ophthalmology*. New York: Springer-Verlag, 1996.
Isenberg SJ. *The eye in infancy*. Chicago: Year Book, 1987.
Nelson LB, Calhoun JH, Harley RD. *Pediatric ophthalmology*, 4th ed. Philadelphia: Saunders, 1998.
Sira IB, Nissenkorn I, Kremer I. Retinopathy of prematurity (major review). *Surv Ophthalmol* 1988;33:1.
Wright KW. *Pediatric ophthalmology and strabismus*. St. Louis: Mosby, 1995.
Gallin PF. *Pediatric ophthalmology: a clinical guide*. New York: Thieme, 2000.
Cryotherapy for Retinopathy of Prematurity Cooperative Group. Multicenter trial of cryotherapy for retinopathy of prematurity: ophthalmological outcomes at 10 years. *Arch Ophthalmol* 2001;119:1110.
Mets MB. Childhood blindness and visual loss: an assessment at two institutions including a "new" cause. *Tr Am Oph Soc* 1999;77:653.

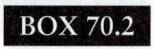

I: NEONATAL BACTERIAL & VIRAL INFECTIONS

CHAPTER 71 ■ SEPSIS NEONATORUM

PATRICK G. GALLAGHER AND ROBERT S. BALTIMORE

Sepsis neonatorum refers to a constellation of clinical and laboratory findings associated with invasive infection during the first 30 days of life. Traditionally, the neonatal sepsis syndrome has been associated with bacteremia, but it may be caused by a variety of pathogens, including bacteria, viruses, and fungi. Neonatal sepsis is an important cause of morbidity and mortality, with case-fatality rates of 15% to 30% even with ideal management. It is important to be familiar with the epidemiology, pathogenesis, etiologic agents, and manifestations of neonatal sepsis so that affected infants receive prompt evaluation and treatment.

EPIDEMIOLOGY

The rate of neonatal sepsis in the United States ranges from 1 to 8 per 1,000 live births, with an average of 2 per 1,000 live births. This rate varies based on socioeconomic factors, availability and utilization of prenatal care, and perinatal risk factors. Worldwide, this rate ranges from 1 to 10 per 1,000 live births, with higher rates in developing countries. Low birth weight and male gender are associated with higher rates of neonatal sepsis. Sepsis rates in preterm infants range from 20 to 30 per 1,000 live births.

Neonatal sepsis usually is classified according to time and mode of onset. *Congenital infection* is acquired *in utero* by transplacental or ascending transmission, with onset before

birth. *Early-onset infection* is acquired by transplacental, ascending, or intrapartum transmission in the perinatal period, shortly before or during the process of birth. *Late-onset infection* is acquired by horizontal transmission, typically in the hospital, at home, or in the community. The appropriate time for dividing early- from late-onset infection is not clear, with opinions ranging from 2 to 7 days of age. Approximately 75% of early-onset group B streptococcal (GBS) infections are symptomatic in the first 24 hours of life, and 80% to 90% are symptomatic by 48 hours of age.

Congenital Infection

The major risk factor for congenital infection is maternal infection (Box 71.1). This is typically a primary maternal infection with a pathogen such as syphilis or human immunodeficiency virus (HIV). Prolonged, premature rupture of membranes also is a risk factor.

Early-Onset Infections

Our knowledge of the epidemiology of perinatally acquired bacterial infections is based on extensive studies of GBS, and to a lesser extent, *Escherichia coli*. The primary risk factor for early-onset GBS disease is the asymptomatic colonization

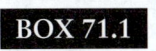

Major Risk Factors for Neonatal Sepsis*

Congenital infection
Maternal infection, usually primary infection
Prolonged, premature rupture of membranes

Early-onset infection
Maternal infection, usually primary infection
Prolonged, premature rupture of membranes
Prematurity
Septic or traumatic delivery
Fetal anoxia
Male sex
Maternal infection (especially urogenital)
Maternal poverty, poor/no prenatal care, preeclampsia, maternal cardiac disease

Late-onset infection
Extreme prematurity
Bronchopulmonary dysplasia
Complex congenital malformations
Short bowel syndrome
Previous broad spectrum antibiotic therapy
Intravascular catheters
Endotracheal intubation
Assisted ventilation
Surgery (including necrotizing enterocolitis)
Contact with hands of personnel colonized with pathogens
Contact with contaminated equipment

*Reproduced with permission from Baltimore RS. Neonatal sepsis: epidemiology and management. *Paediatr Drugs* 2003;5:723.

of the maternal gastrointestinal or genitourinary tracts. GBS colonizes 5% to 40% of pregnant women, with variability in colonization rates attributed to differences in GBS culture techniques and demographic factors. Higher colonization rates are found in African American women and women with diabetes. Lower colonization rates are found in Asian American and Mexican American women, multiparous women, and sexually inexperienced women. GBS colonization throughout pregnancy is inconsistent, even after antibiotic treatment. Mothers not colonized with GBS early in pregnancy may be positive at delivery, and GBS carriers identified early in pregnancy may not be carriers at delivery.

The rate of GBS transmission from colonized mothers to their infants is approximately 40% to 70%. Colonization occurs by transplacental transmission in the presence of maternal bacteremia, ascension from the vagina and cervix through microscopic defects in the amniotic membranes, or through ruptured membranes, surface contamination during passage through the birth canal, and postnatal acquisition in the hospital, at home, or in the community. Despite the high rate of neonatal colonization, only 1% to 2% of colonized infants develop early-onset GBS disease.

The risk factors for early-onset GBS infection (see Box 71.1) include the following: prematurity of less than 37 weeks' gestation; chorioamnionitis; premature rupture of membranes; prolonged rupture of membranes of more than 18 hours, with the risk of sepsis increasing with the duration of rupture prior to delivery; maternal intrapartum temperature of higher than 38°C; sustained fetal tachycardia; and prior delivery of an in-

fant with GBS disease. Similar associations have been observed with other neonatal pathogens. Black race is a risk factor for both early- and late-onset GBS disease. Other factors associated with early-onset GBS sepsis include colonization with a virulent GBS strain, deficient maternal GBS type-specific capsular antibody, maternal colonization at multiple sites, and heavy maternal colonization. Detection of GBS bacteriuria during pregnancy may be a means of identifying the heavily colonized woman whose infant is at increased risk of developing infection. Heavy maternal colonization has been associated with preterm labor, chorioamnionitis, and fetal demise. The twin of an infant infected with GBS is at increased risk, most likely as a result of genetic susceptibility factors, heavy maternal colonization, and/or exposure to virulent strains common for both infants. Maternal diabetes mellitus as a risk factor for neonatal infection is controversial.

Compared to full-term infants, premature infants have a higher risk of neonatal sepsis if the mother has amnionitis or a peripartum infection. Other maternal factors, such as poor prenatal care, low socioeconomic status, and heart disease, are risk factors for both neonatal sepsis and premature birth.

Late-Onset Infections

The risk factors and modes of transmission for late-onset infection in nonhospitalized infants are not well understood. Vertical transmission is responsible for only about 40% to 50% of late-onset GBS disease. The remaining cases are attributed to exposure in the hospital, at home, or in the community.

The epidemiology of late-onset disease in hospitalized infants (see Box 71.1) is discussed in Chapter 88, Nosocomial Infection in the Newborn.

ETIOLOGY

Congenital Infection

Toxoplasma, *Treponema pallidum*, cytomegalovirus (CMV), and HIV are the organisms most frequently associated with congenital infection, usually during a primary maternal infection. Previously, rubella was a frequent cause of congenital infection, but in the United States, congenital rubella has been virtually eliminated by rubella vaccination. Other causes of congenital infection are the same as early-onset infection.

Early-Onset Infection

Prior to the 1970s, staphylococci and gram-negative rod species were the predominant etiologic agents of neonatal sepsis. From the 1970s, persisting into the 1990s, GBS was the predominant pathogen causing early-onset infection in most U.S. nurseries (Table 71.1). Since the institution of intrapartum antibiotic prophylaxis (IAP) for the prevention of GBS disease, the rate of early-onset group B Streptococcal infections has fallen dramatically from 1.7 per 1,000 live births in 1993 to 0.6 per 1,000 live births in 2001 (Fig. 71.1). The CDC has predicted that an 80% drop is possible. Paralleling the decrease in early-onset GBS infection is a relative or absolute increase in early-onset disease due to *E. coli*, in both term and preterm neonates. These two pathogens currently are the major causes of early-onset disease. Other pathogens associated with early-onset sepsis include *Klebsiella pneumoniae* and other enteric gram-negative bacilli, *Enterococcus* species, and *Listeria monocytogenes*. *Streptococcus pneumoniae, Neisseria meningitidis, Haemophilus influenzae* (predominantly nontypeable),

TABLE 71.1

MICROORGANISMS CAUSING NEONATAL SEPSIS

Organism	Yale University*	NICHD Network**	Ohio State University***
	Site and Percent in Each Study		
Years included for each study	1989–2003	1991–1993	1986–1997
Age of infants included in the study	Birth to 30 days	Birth to 3 days	Birth to death or discharge
Gram-positive bacterial species			
Group B *Streptococcus*	12	31	9
Group D *Streptococcus*	9	0	4
Nongrouped and other streptococci	0	7	0
Viridans streptococci	1	9	0
Streptococcus pneumoniae	0	0	<1
Staphylococcus aureus	8	3	4
Coagulase-negative staphylococci	29	7	47
Listeria monocytogenes	<1	0	0
Gram-negative aerobic bacteria			
Escherichia coli	11	16	10
Klebsiella and *Enterobacter*	11	5	8
Pseudomonas aeruginosa	3	0	2
Haemophilus species	1	11	3
Salmonella	0	0	<1
Gram-negative anaerobic bacteria	0	0	0
Fungi	8	1	11
Others	6	10	1
Total number of cases	520	147	433
Mortality rate	12%	26%	12%

*Data from Bizzarro MJ, Raskind C, Baltimore RS, Gallagher PG. Seventy-five years of neonatal sepsis at Yale: 1928–2003. *Pediatrics* 2005;116:59.
**Data from Stoll BJ, Gordon T, Korones SB, et al. Early-onset sepsis in very low birth weight neonates: A report from the National Institute of Child Health and Human Development Neonatal Research Network. *J Pediatr* 1996;129:72.
***Data from Cordero L, Sananes M, Ayers LW. Bloodstream infections in a neonatal intensive-care unit: 12 years experience with an antibiotic control program. *Infect Control Hosp Epidemiol* 1999;20:242.

and groups A, C, and G streptococci are respiratory tract pathogens that occasionally colonize the maternal genital tract and cause early-onset neonatal infection.

Late-Onset Infection

In the 1980s and 1990s, improvements in neonatal intensive care, particularly for the preterm infant, were paralleled by an increase in nosocomial infection by opportunistic

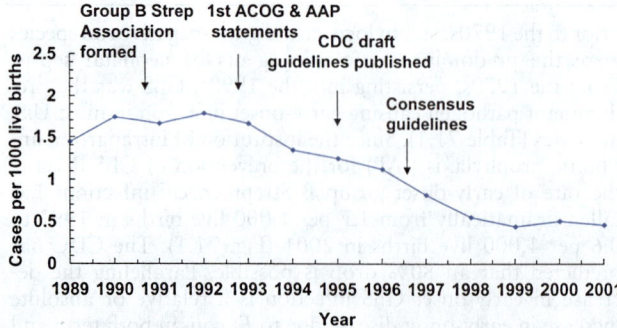

FIGURE 71.1. Incidence of early-onset invasive group B streptococcal disease—selected Active Bacterial Core surveillance areas, 1989–2001, and activities for prevention of group B streptococcal disease. (Reproduced with permission from Schrag S, Gorwitz R, Fultz-Butts K, Schuchat A. Prevention of perinatal group B streptococcal disease. Revised guidelines from CDC. *MMWR Recomm Rep* 2002;51:1.)

organisms such as coagulase-negative staphylococci and *Candida* species in late-onset sepsis. Other organisms associated with nosocomial late-onset disease include *Staphylococcus aureus* (methicillin-sensitive and -resistant), *Enterobacter*, *Serratia*, and *Pseudomonas* species, and *Enterococcus* (vancomycin-sensitive and -resistant) species Nosocomial outbreaks with these species may occur.

In nonhospitalized infants, the etiologic agents of late-onset disease comprise the organisms causing early-onset disease, particularly GBS and *E. coli,* gram-positive organisms including *S. pneumoniae, S. aureus,* and *Enterococcal* species, and gram-negative enteric organisms including *Klebsiella* species and *Salmonella* species. Since the institution of IAP for prevention of GBS disease, unlike the decrease seen in early-onset disease, there has been no change in the rate of late-onset GBS disease. It will be important to monitor whether IAP will influence the etiology of late-onset sepsis.

The significance of anaerobes isolated from blood cultures of neonates remains controversial. Most anaerobic bacteremias are self-limited in the absence of a focal infection. However, *Bacteroides* and *Clostridium* species may be associated with significant disease, especially when peritonitis, fasciitis, or meningitis is present.

PATHOGENESIS

Risk factors for the development of neonatal sepsis include maternal and obstetric factors, virulence factors of the causative organism, and neonatal factors. Factors specific to nosocomial, late-onset infections are reviewed in Chapter 88, Nosocomial Infection in the Newborn.

Maternal and Obstetric Factors

Prior to birth, the placenta and its membranes serve as a barrier to fetal infection, maintaining the fetus in a sterile environment. Acquisition of infection before birth via the maternal bloodstream is rare because of the effectiveness of the placental barrier. Obstetric procedures such as amniocentesis, percutaneous umbilical blood sampling, transcervical chorionic villus sampling, or cervical cerclage may introduce skin or vaginal microorganisms into the sterile uterine cavity, leading to amnionitis and secondary fetal infection.

A common mechanism of fetal colonization and infection is via ascending infection. Organisms from the mother's cervix and vagina invade the amniotic fluid and uterine cavity through microscopic defects or overtly ruptured amniotic membranes. Ingestion and inhalation of these organisms in the amniotic fluid leads to contamination of the respiratory and gastrointestinal tracts, and may lead to bronchopneumonia before birth. Pathogens may adhere to epithelial cells on mucosal surfaces, and then invade the infant's bloodstream. Common entry sites are the conjunctiva, nasopharynx, umbilical cord, and traumatized integument. Delayed clearance from the bloodstream allows pathogens to multiply and cause either disseminated or focal disease. Signs of infection after ascending infection may be present at delivery, within hours of birth, or, less commonly, within several days.

Another common source of neonatal colonization and infection occurs during passage through the birth canal. Contamination with organisms of the mother's cervical, vaginal, or fecal flora occurs by surface contact or aspiration during the process of delivery. How and why colonization, which is common, leads to infection, which is not, is poorly understood.

Virulence Factors

A major bacterial virulence factor is the surface polysaccharide capsule. This capsule determines the specific bacterial serotype and provides many bacteria with the ability to evade killing by providing mechanisms to escape opsonophagocytic killing. The sialic acid–rich polysaccharide surface capsule of GBS has been studied extensively, and all major serotypes of GBS (Ia, Ib, Ia/c, II-VIII) have caused early-onset disease. The GBS capsule acts as a bloodstream survival factor by inhibiting the alternate complement pathway, protecting GBS from opsonization by C3 and subsequent neutrophil killing. Maternal levels of antibodies to type-specific capsular polysaccharides correlate well with protection from GBS.

Other GBS virulence factors include an extracytoplasmic penicillin-binding protein, which promotes resistance to neutrophil killing independent of the polysaccharide capsule; a surface protease that promotes virulence, resistance to opsonophagocytosis, and cleavage of human fibrinogen; and a surface-localized streptococcal beta-protein that resists opsonophagocytosis by down-regulating complement activation.

Bacterial virulence factors that influence the pathogenesis of most types of neonatal meningitis are the surface polysaccharide capsule and/or the production of cytolytic exotoxins. Two virulence factors for GBS meningitis are well characterized: the type III polysaccharide capsule and the beta-hemolysin/cytolysin, a cytolytic exotoxin. The type III GBS polysaccharide capsule is associated with approximately 90% of cases of GBS neonatal meningitis. Its invasiveness is probably due, in part, to poor maternal antibody response to the type III polysaccharide capsule. Similarly, the K1 serotype of *E. coli* and the IVb serotype of *L. monocytogenes* have been associated with neonatal meningitis. Beta-hemolysin/cytolysin

is a pore-forming, membrane-associated cytotoxin that contributes to disease virulence and progression via several mechanisms, including the activation of neutrophil signaling pathways in brain endothelium.

Neonatal Factors

The neonate is a compromised host at risk for invasive infection because of developmental defects in cellular, humoral, and phagocytic immunity. Complement levels are decreased. IgG, an important component of the immune response, is acquired from the mother during the third trimester, resulting in a concentration in the blood of the newborn slightly higher than that of the mother. The specificities of the antibodies and the protection afforded are similar to the mother's. If the infant is premature, the amount of IgG acquired from the mother is decreased, and the neonate is susceptible to those pathogens. In some cases, additional genetically predetermined immune defects or other factors predisposing to infection may be present.

Further impairment to immunity occurs under conditions of prematurity, hypoxia, acidosis, and other metabolic derangements associated with bacterial infection. Infants with galactosemia are particularly susceptible to infection with gram-negative rods, particularly *E. coli*.

Finally, the neonate, particularly the preterm infant, has poor skin and mucosal barriers to infection. These anatomic barriers may be further compromised by trauma before, during, or after delivery, such as those caused by fetal scalp electrode placement, fetal scalp blood sampling, abrasions during delivery, injury from obstetric forceps, umbilical catheterization, and the like.

CLINICAL MANIFESTATIONS AND COMPLICATIONS

The clinical signs of neonatal sepsis are nonspecific (Box 71.2). They may be associated with bacterial, viral, or fungal

---

BOX 71.2   Nonspecific Signs of Sepsis

Lethargy
Apnea
Temperature instability
Tachypnea
Tachycardia
Pallor, poor perfusion
Respiratory distress
Feeding intolerance
Vomiting
Abdominal distention
Diarrhea
Jaundice
Skin rash, petechiae
Hypotension
Irritability
High-pitched cry
Weak suck
Seizures
Bulging or full fontanel

TABLE 71.2

DIFFERENTIAL DIAGNOSIS OF THE SEPTIC-APPEARING INFANT*

Infectious Diseases	Inborn errors of metabolism
Bacterial sepsis	Hypoglycemia
Meningitis	Drugs/toxins—aspirin,
Urinary tract infection	carbon monoxide
Viral infections—Entero-	*Renal Disorders*
virus, respiratory syncytial	Posterior urethral valves
virus, herpes simplex	*Hematologic Disorders*
Pertussis	Severe anemia
Congenital syphilis	Methemoglobinemia
Cardiac Disease	*Gastrointestinal Disorders*
Congenital heart	Gastroenteritis with
disease	dehydration
Supraventricular tachycardia	Pyloric stenosis
Myocardial infarction	Intussusception
Pericarditis	Necrotizing enterocolitis
Myocarditis	Appendicitis
Kawasaki disease	Volvulus
Endocrine Disorders	*Neurologic Disease*
Congenital adrenal	Infant botulism
hyperplasia	Shunt obstruction, infection
Metabolic Disorders	Intracranial hemorrhage
Hyponatremia, hypernatremia	Birth trauma, child abuse
Cystic fibrosis	

*Reproduced with permission from Fleisher GR, Ludwig S, eds. *Textbook of pediatric emergency medicine*. Philadelphia: Lippincott, Williams & Wilkins, 2001.

infection, or with noninfectious disorders including metabolic disorders, intracranial hemorrhage, congenital heart disease, or perinatal asphyxia (Table 71.2). Presentation is variable, from subtle findings such as feeding intolerance, jaundice, and temperature instability to acute onset respiratory failure and septic shock. When pneumonia is present, signs of respiratory distress such as tachypnea, grunting, nasal flaring, retractions, and cyanosis may occur. The clinical course is unpredictable and may be rapidly progressive. The presence of these signs should lead to consideration of a diagnostic sepsis evaluation and prompt initiation of empiric antimicrobial therapy.

Early-Onset Infection

The clinical manifestations of early-onset infection may be present at birth or appear at any time during the first week of life, but approximately 95% of infants with early-onset infection present within the first 72 hours of life. Of the reported patients, approximately 80% are term infants. Onset usually is at or immediately after birth, with symptoms from bacteremia (80%) or pneumonia (7% to 10%). Nonspecific symptoms are most common. In neonates with a pulmonary focus, respiratory symptoms predominate. Persistent pulmonary hypertension may complicate early-onset infection with or without respiratory tract disease. Meningitis, present in only 5% to 10% of early-onset GBS disease cases, typically presents with signs not specific for central nervous system infection.

In the most severe cases, apnea, hypotension, and disseminated intravascular coagulation cause rapid deterioration and death. Even prompt administration of antibiotics and aggressive supportive therapy may be unsuccessful in these overwhelmed infants.

GBS and *E. coli* are associated with most cases of early-onset disease, but many other bacteria can cause an early-onset syndrome, including groups D and G streptococci, nontypable *H. influenzae*, and *L. monocytogenes*.

In other cases of *L. monocytogenes* infection, a flulike illness occurs in the mother prior to delivery, and maternal blood or amniotic fluid cultures may be positive. In the infant, the lung is the primary focus of infection, but hepatosplenomegaly, purulent conjunctivitis, a skin rash consisting of irregular macules and papules or pustules in a truncal distribution, petechiae, and small granulomas on the posterior pharynx may be found.

Rarely, transient GBS bacteremia may occur and produce mild, if any, clinical symptoms. If untreated, however, most bacteremia results in metastatic infection and fulminant disease.

Late-Onset Infection

The clinical manifestations of late-onset infection usually occur in infants 8 to 30 days of age, but may be seen as late as 12 to 16 weeks, particularly in hospitalized premature infants. The onset is most often insidious, and the affected infants present with nonspecific signs of sepsis, sometimes preceded by an upper respiratory tract infection. Fever is frequent. In approximately two-third of cases of late-onset neonatal sepsis syndrome, bacteremia is documented. Unlike early-onset disease, meningitis is common, occurring in 20% to 30% of cases, and seizures may be present. Other manifestations of late-onset disease, particularly due to GBS, include pneumonia, endocarditis, pericarditis, osteomyelitis, septic arthritis, skin and soft tissue lesions, adenitis, peritonitis, omphalitis, and pyelonephritis.

Systemic Inflammatory Response Syndrome

The systemic inflammatory response syndrome (SIRS) to a variety of severe insults, such as infection, trauma, or surgery, is caused by proinflammatory cytokines such as tumor necrosis factor-alpha (TNF-α), IL-6 and IL-8, hormones, and other substances. SIRS is characterized by a combination of alterations in temperature, heart rate, respiratory status, and white blood cell counts. By definition, sepsis is a SIRS-caused by infection. Simple SIRS/sepsis progresses to severe SIRS/sepsis, with acute organ dysfunction, hypotension, or hypoperfusion, and then to SIRS/shock. with hypotension unresponsive to fluid resuscitation. Severe SIRS, hypotension, and multiorgan involvement requiring treatment with cardioactive agents, respiratory support, and in extreme cases, extracorporeal membrane oxygenation (ECMO) support. Congenital, early-onset, and late-onset infection may manifest with SIRS. A systemic fetal inflammatory response syndrome has been associated with preterm labor and significant perinatal morbidity and mortality.

DIAGNOSIS

Laboratory Evaluation

Culture

Whenever bacterial infection of the neonate is suspected, cultures of blood, cerebrospinal fluid (CSF), urine, and infected body fluids that are normally sterile, or an aspirate from an infected soft tissue site or bone, should be obtained before initiating antimicrobial therapy. Many omit urine cultures during the first 48 to 72 hours of life, because bacteria recovered from urine during this period are of hematogenous origin and usually will be isolated from blood cultures.

The optimal amount of blood for culture is 0.5 to 1.0 mL. Sampling from two peripheral sites is more likely to yield a positive result than a single culture. Blood should be drawn from both a peripheral site and from each port of a sterile central vascular catheter when one is in place. Blood cultures usually are not obtained from the umbilical cord or from umbilical catheters beyond the time of initial placement because of high rates of contamination.

Most pathogens in blood cultures are recovered within 48 hours. Common contaminants, such as coagulase-negative staphylococcus or viridans streptococci, are more likely to be pathogens if isolated within 48 hours of incubation and if the same organism is isolated from blood cultures obtained from two separate sites. Obtaining two blood cultures from separate sites from low-birth-weight infants with late-onset disease is essential in some cases to distinguish a contaminant from a true pathogen. Microorganisms isolated only from blood obtained through a catheter when peripheral venous blood cultures are sterile are more likely to represent colonization than septicemia.

Cultures of mucosal surfaces are not helpful in distinguishing the infected from the colonized infant. Similarly, gastric aspirate cultures obtained after birth reflect the maternal environment and do not distinguish the infected from the colonized infant. The polymorphonuclear leukocytes present in the gastric aspirate are of maternal origin and may reflect stress of noninfectious origin. In contrast, culture of the tracheal aspirate obtained at the time of intubation has been useful in identifying the etiologic agent of early-onset neonatal pneumonia. Beyond initial endotracheal tube placement, tracheal aspirates are less helpful, because bacteria frequently colonize the respiratory tract without causing disease.

When a viral etiology is suspected in a case of neonatal sepsis, cultures of blood, urine, stool, and respiratory secretions may be obtained. For some pathogens, rapid viral testing is available. When the diagnosis of herpes simplex virus infection is entertained, cultures from the conjunctiva, pharynx, blood, urine, CSF, stool, and any lesions should be obtained. Rapid testing for herpes simplex virus in CSF and lesions is available in most centers.

Leukocyte Counts

The white blood cell (WBC) and differential count are useful for assessing a neonate who may have sepsis and for evaluating a neonate being treated for proven sepsis. The normal peripheral WBC count of newborns is from 5,000 to 20,000/mm^3, but values outside this range have a poor specificity for predicting sepsis. Leukopenia occurs more commonly than leukocytosis as a sign of overwhelming infection. The absolute neutrophil count, determined by multiplying the WBC count by the fraction of neutrophils, plus bands in the differential, is only a slightly better predictor of sepsis than the total WBC count. Neutropenia is a nonspecific finding, associated with maternal hypertension, asphyxia, and intraventricular hemorrhage, all in the absence of infection. Typically, the neutropenia of infection does not persist for more than 36 hours, whereas the neutropenia observed with noninfectious conditions may persist for several days. Neutrophilia may be associated with maternal fever before delivery or hemolytic disease of the newborn.

The specificity of WBC parameters as an indicator of sepsis is increased by calculating the ratio of the concentration of immature cells of the neutrophilic series (band forms, metamyelocytes, and myelocytes) to total cells of the neutrophil series, known as the I:T ratio. An increased concentration of immature neutrophil series cells and an I:T ratio of greater than 0.2 has moderately increased specificity for sepsis. The I:T ratio takes into consideration the normative values over the first days of life and is less than or equal to 0.12 by the third day of life in noninfected infants. It has only moderate sensitivity, but good negative predictive value if normal.

Other Screening Laboratory Tests

Many infants who do not have infection receive empiric antibiotic therapy for possible neonatal sepsis, leading to growing concerns about the possible deleterious effects of widespread, unnecessary antibiotic use. These concerns have been the impetus for the development of screening tests to identify *asymptomatic* newborns likely to benefit from antibiotic treatment. Acute-phase reactants such as C-reactive protein (CRP), erythrocyte sedimentation rate (ESR), and concentrations of certain cytokines, each have been reported to have moderate positive and negative predictive values. The quantitative CRP test is moderately sensitive for bacteremia if serial determinations are made in the first days of life. A decrease of the CRP during treatment for sepsis is a good determinant of therapy effectiveness and has been used to shorten the length of therapy. Recent studies have shown that IL-6, IL-8, and CD11b, a member of the beta-integrin family of adhesion proteins, are moderately sensitive assays for neonatal bacteremia but have great potential in use as screening tests to exclude bacteremia. Procalcitonin, a prohormone of calcitonin, has been used to differentiate bacterial from viral infections and as an early indicator of neonatal sepsis. Some studies have shown that it has higher specificity for neonatal bacterial sepsis than CRP or IL-6. Clinical studies demonstrating improvement of care using this test are lacking. Although all these tests of acute-phase reactants may be useful, it is not clear which test is the most useful in the first hours after birth, when decisions to begin empiric antibiotic treatment are usually necessary, but their use may allow shortened antibiotic courses.

Combinations of tests have been evaluated for the assessment of asymptomatic newborns with risk factors for sepsis. One combination of screening tests includes blood, urine, and CSF cultures plus a radiograph of the chest, WBC count, I:T ratio, CRP, ESR, and cytokine markers. This panel had a sensitivity of 93%, specificity of 88%, and positive predictive value of 39%. Newborns with a negative screen were at low risk for sepsis and did not need to be empirically treated with antibiotics. Although some physicians use combinations of screening tests to decide upon antibiotic therapy, many others have been unwilling to withhold empiric antibiotic treatment from newborns with risk factors for sepsis such as low birth weight, perinatal asphyxia, or prolonged rupture of the membranes. Currently, no clear standard of practice exists.

Diagnostic Lumbar Puncture

An evaluation of the CSF should be performed in symptomatic infants suspected of having neonatal sepsis. CSF culture, Gram stain, protein, glucose, and cell count should be obtained. Lumbar puncture may be deferred if the infant is clinically too unstable to tolerate the procedure. The CSF evaluation in the infant with meningitis is reviewed in Chapter 72, Meningitis.

Other Laboratory Findings

Diagnostic tests for invasive neonatal bacterial infection, for example, latex particle agglutination tests for GBS disease, have suffered from poor sensitivity and specificity and are not routinely used. Newer tests, under development, may prove helpful in directing clinical management.

A wide variety of nonspecific laboratory findings commonly are associated with the neonatal sepsis syndrome. These include hypoglycemia or hyperglycemia. Metabolic, respiratory, or mixed acidosis may occur. Thrombocytopenia in septic neonates is common, and its etiology complex. Increased

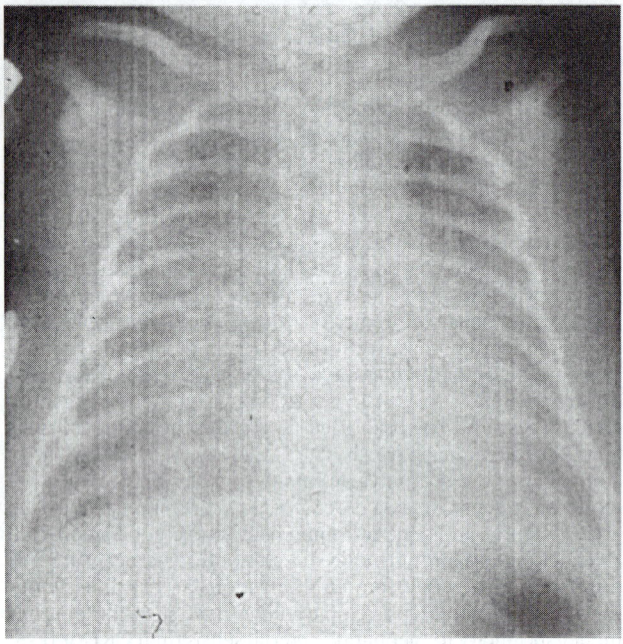

FIGURE 71.2. Chest radiograph of a 1-day-old neonate with bacteremic group B streptococcal pneumonia. A diffuse interstitial infiltrative pattern is seen.

platelet destruction due to the effect of microbial toxins, diffuse endothelial cell injury, increased platelet activation, and disseminated intravascular coagulation, as well as decreased platelet production due to inadequate thrombopoietin response to thrombocytopenia may contribute to thrombocytopenia. Thrombocytopenia is more common in neonatal sepsis due to gram-negative and fungal pathogens, particularly in preterm infants.

Diagnostic Imaging

Chest radiographs should be obtained as part of the diagnostic evaluation of the infant with suspected sepsis and signs of respiratory tract disease. In these cases, chest radiography may demonstrate diffuse or focal infiltrates (Fig. 71.2), pleural thickening, effusion or it may demonstrate air bronchograms indistinguishable from that seen with surfactant-deficient respiratory distress syndrome. Other radiographic studies may be indicated by the specific clinical condition, such as suspected osteomyelitis or necrotizing enterocolitis.

THERAPY

Antibiotic Treatment

The decision to initiate antimicrobial therapy is based on the likelihood that an infant's clinical signs and symptoms are a manifestation of infection or that risk factors suggest a normal-appearing infant is at high risk for developing infection within the first few hours of life. Because of the increased risk of infection and the subtlety of clinical manifestations of infection in premature infants, antimicrobial therapy should be initiated when risk factors or abnormal clinical findings are suggestive of infection.

Many apply the CDC/AAP/ACOG/AAFP algorithm (see Chapter 75) to all asymptomatic infants with obstetric risk factors, for the management of a neonate whose mother re-

ceived intrapartum antimicrobial GBS prophylaxis. The goal of this scheme is to identify and treat all infected infants but to avoid the excessive investigation and treatment of uninfected infants. It must be emphasized that such an approach is applicable only to *asymptomatic term* infants whose mothers *do not* have chorioamnionitis or sepsis in the peripartum period. The omission of a lumbar puncture in asymptomatic term infants with only a single risk factor who are evaluated in the first few hours after delivery is unlikely to jeopardize the diagnosis of meningitis, because term infants with *in utero* meningitis almost always are symptomatic at birth. If the initial blood culture result becomes positive in an infant who did not have a lumbar puncture as part of the initial diagnostic evaluation, the lumbar puncture should be performed as soon as possible to be certain that meningitis has not developed. Lumbar puncture also should be part of the evaluation of infants whose mothers received intrapartum antibiotics and have signs of infection, but who had a sterile blood culture.

Antimicrobial Therapy for Early-Onset Sepsis

The administration of antibiotics for early-onset infections to treat newborns that have risk factors almost always is started before identification of the causative organism, because waiting results in unacceptably high morbidity and mortality. Empiric treatment is designed to provide adequate antimicrobial activity against the likely organisms (Table 71.3). In the absence of focal signs of infection, therapy is directed at the common causes of bacteremia and meningitis, because experience demonstrates that these are the most likely types of infection to present without focal findings. If pneumonia or a urinary tract infection is present, therapy is aimed at the most common causes of these infections.

The recommended treatment of sepsis employs a combination of a broad-spectrum penicillin, usually ampicillin, and an aminoglycoside, usually gentamicin, or a broad-spectrum penicillin and an extended-spectrum (third-generation) cephalosporin (Table 71.3 and Table 71.4). These combinations have been used frequently, they have low toxicity and are low in cost, and they have been associated with relatively low rates of the development of antibiotic resistance. GBS, enterococci, and *Listeria monocytogenes* are susceptible to ampicillin, as are many strains of *E. coli* and *Proteus* species. In nurseries where resistance to the aminoglycosides among gram-negative bacilli is uncommon, gentamicin is active against *E. coli, Klebsiella* species, *Proteus* species, most *Enterobacter* species, and *Pseudomonas aeruginosa*. Species frequently resistant to gentamicin include *Acinetobacter*, many strains of *Enterobacter cloacae*, some strains of *Serratia,* and *Flavobacterium*. If a cluster of sepsis cases caused by these organisms or of antibiotic resistant species occurs, alternative empiric therapy should be considered.

Extended-spectrum cephalosporins provide activity against many of the pathogens, including gram-negative bacilli resistant to gentamicin. The third-generation cephalosporins recommended for neonates, cefotaxime and ceftriaxone, have excellent CNS penetration in the presence of inflammation. However, extended-spectrum cephalosporins are less active than the first- or second-generation cephalosporins against gram-positive cocci, and they are less active against GBS than penicillin or ampicillin. They are inactive against *Enterococcus* species and *L. monocytogenes*, which are not infrequent causes of neonatal sepsis in some large centers. For these reasons, ampicillin is added to a cephalosporin when it is used empirically for neonatal sepsis or meningitis. Ceftriaxone has the potential to displace bilirubin from albumin-binding sites, and should be avoided in infants with hyperbilirubinemia and liver dysfunction.

TABLE 71.3

GUIDELINES FOR EMPIRIC ANTIBIOTIC TREATMENT FOR PRESUMED NEONATAL SEPSIS (WITH OR WITHOUT MENINGITIS) IN THE FIRST MONTH OF LIFE

Clinical Setting	Recommended Antibiotic Regimen	Alternative Regimens
Early-onset sepsis *Late-onset sepsis* (up to 1 month)	Ampicillin plus gentamicin*	Ampicillin plus cefotaxime
Readmission to the hospital from the community	Ampicillin plus cefotaxime (or ceftriaxone†)	Ampicillin plus gentamicin* with or without cefotaxime (or ceftriaxone†)
Occurring in the hospital, with no intravenous catheter(s)	Ampicillin plus gentamicin*	Ampicillin plus cefotaxime (or ceftriaxone†)
Occurring in the hospital, with intravascular catheter(s) in place	Oxacillin or vancomycin plus gentamicin*	Vancomycin plus cefotaxime (or ceftriaxone†)

*Adjust dose according to concentration of the antibiotic in the blood once a steady state has been achieved.
†Ceftriaxone can displace bilirubin from albumin, thus increasing the risk of kernicterus, and may also cause deposition of sludge in the gallbladder; it should be used with caution in newborns, especially those with hyperbilirubinemia and liver dysfunction.

In some cases, the aminoglycoside of choice may not be gentamicin. Some gentamicin-resistant isolates will be susceptible to amikacin. Tobramycin has greater activity against *P. aeruginosa*, a relatively uncommon cause of neonatal infections. Ceftazidime, a third-generation cephalosporin, generally has excellent activity against *P. aeruginosa* and other relatively resistant bacilli, but should be avoided if the organism produces an extended-spectrum beta-lactamase.

Antibiotic resistance may develop in the presence of a high rate of use of broad-spectrum cephalosporins, and resistance to cephalosporins has developed after routine prescription in neonatal intensive care units. Thus, an advantage accrues to using them sparingly, only when they are of proven or theoretical superiority. If a diagnosis of gram-negative bacillary meningitis is based on Gram stain or CSF culture, it is reasonable to use the combination of ampicillin and an extended-spectrum cephalosporin empirically as a first choice.

If isolates of gram-negative rod pathogens are recovered that are resistant to the cephalosporins and the aminoglycosides, the carbapenems imipenem and meropenem may be useful. Of the two, meropenem causes less CNS irritation and fewer seizures. However, a problem with this class of broad-spectrum antibiotics is the high frequency of fungal superinfection that follows its use.

Infants treated with vancomycin or aminoglycosides should have close monitoring of renal function. Aminoglycoside levels are indicated in infants receiving a course of therapy for neonatal sepsis syndrome, infants with rapidly changing renal function, and infants with poor clinical response to aminoglycoside therapy.

Antimicrobial Therapy for Late-Onset Sepsis

Empiric antibiotic therapy for late-onset neonatal sepsis occurring in the neonatal intensive care unit (NICU) should take into consideration the resident flora of the nursery, especially isolates from previously infected neonates, and the risk factors of the individual patient (Table 71.3). The same empiric treatment as for early-onset sepsis, such as ampicillin plus an aminoglycoside, may be used if no intravascular catheters have been in place, if the infant has not been treated for a previous infection, and no isolates of gentamicin-resistant gram-negative aerobic bacilli are present in the unit.

The most common bacterial species causing catheter-associated infections are *S. aureus* and coagulase-negative staphylococci. Although penicillinase-resistant semisynthetic penicillins, such as oxacillin and nafcillin, are usually the agents of choice for treating staphylococci, resistance to this class, commonly referred to as methicillin-resistant *S. aureus* or MRSA, is occurring more commonly in many institutions. Also, coagulase-negative staphylococci more commonly cause symptomatic infection in very low-birth-weight infants, and this species is more likely to have endogenous resistance to the anti-staphylococcal penicillins. The use of vancomycin for the empiric treatment of late-onset infections in institutions with large numbers of methicillin-resistant staphylococci is considered reasonable by many. Generally, an aminoglycoside is added, usually gentamicin, for empiric coverage of gram-negative bacilli while awaiting the results of cultures. Vancomycin is more toxic and less bactericidal compared with the penicillins, and it has activity only against aerobic gram-positive bacteria; thus, it should be continued only when an isolate resistant to other anti-staphylococcal agents is present.

In patients with indwelling intravascular devices, persistent bacteremia usually is due to organisms enmeshed in fibrin adhering to the catheter and is best managed by removing the intravascular catheter. For added antibacterial activity, some practitioners add rifampin to either a semisynthetic penicillin or vancomycin, although there is a lack of data demonstrating effectiveness. Newer antibiotics, such as quinupristin/dalfopristin (Synercid) and linezolid (Zyvox), have activity against methicillin-resistant staphylococci, but data on use in neonates are lacking. Both have significant side effects in older individuals, thus they are not recommended at this time unless conventional antibiotic therapy fails.

Previously healthy neonates who have been discharged and are readmitted to the hospital because of fever for treatment of presumed sepsis or meningitis may be treated empirically with a third-generation cephalosporin (usually cefotaxime or ceftriaxone) plus ampicillin. This combination is active against the usual causes of non–hospital-acquired sepsis such as GBS, enterococci, *Listeria* species, *S. aureus*, and gram-negative bacilli.

The usual duration of treatment for most uncomplicated bacterial infections is 7 to 10 days. Longer courses (14 or 21 days or longer) are indicated for the treatment of meningitis, and septic arthritis and skeletal infections (21 to 28 days). The intravenous route of drug administration is preferred, but similar amounts of drug (area under the curve) may be delivered

TABLE 71.4
DOSAGES AND DOSING INTERVALS OF PARENTERAL ANTIBIOTICS FOR THE TREATMENT OF NEONATAL INFECTIONS

Antibiotic	Dosage (mg/kg/dose)[1]				
	Birth Weight <1200 g	Birth Weight 1200–2000 g		Birth Weight >2000 g	
	Age 0–4 Weeks	Age 0–7 Days	Age >7 Days	Age 0–7 Days	Age >7 Days
Penicillins					
Penicillin G[2]					
Meningitis	50,000 U every 12 hours	50,000 U every 12 hours	50,000 U every 8 hours	50,000 U every 8 hours	50,000 U every 6 hours
Other infections	25,000 U every 12 hours	25,000 U every 12 hours	25,000 U every 8 hours	25,000 U every 8 hours	25,000 U every 6 hours
Ampicillin[2]					
Meningitis	50 every 12 hours	50 every 12 hours	50 every 8 hours	50 every 8 hours	50 every 6 hours
Other infections	25 every 12 hours	25 every 12 hours	25 every 8 hours	25 every 8 hours	25 every 6 hours
Ticarcillin, ticarcillin/clavulanate	75 every 12 hours	75 every 12 hours	75 every 8 hours	75 every 8 hours	75 every 8 hours
Piperacillin,[4] Piperacillin/tazobactam[4]	75 every 12 hours	75 every 12 hours	75 every 8 hours	75 every 8 hours	75 every 8 hours
Penicillinase-resistant penicillins (nafcillin, oxacillin)					
Meningitis, Other infections	50 every 12 hours	50 every 12 hours	50 every 8 hours	50 every 8 hours	50 every 6 hours
Other infections	25 every 12 hours	25 every 12 hours	25 every 8 hours	25 every 8 hours	25 every 6 hours
Cephalosporins					
Cephalothin	20 every 12 hours	20 every 12 hours	20 every 8 hours	20 every 8 hours	20 every 6 hours
Cefazolin	20 every 12 hours	20 every 12 hours	20 every 12 hours	20 every 12 hours	20 every 8 hours
Cefotaxime	50 every 12 hours	50 every 12 hours	50 every 8 hours	50 every 12 hours	50 every 8 hours
Ceftazidime	50 every 12 hours	50 every 12 hours	50 every 8 hours	50 every 12 hours	50 every 8 hours
Ceftriaxone[3]	50 every 24 hours	50 every 24 hours	50 every 24 hours	50 every 24 hours	75 every 24 hours
Other β-lactams					
Aztreonam[5]	30 every 12 hours	30 every 12 hours	30 every 12 hours	30 every 8 hours	30 every 6 hours
Imipenem,[4] Meropenem[4]	20 every 18–24 hours	20 every 12 hours	20 every 12 hours	20 every 12 hours	20 every 8 hours
Aminoglycosides					
Gentamicin[6]	2.5 every 18–24 hours	2.5 every 12–18 hours	2.5 every 8–12 hours	2.5 every 12 hours	2.5 every 8 hours
Tobramycin[6]	2.5 every 18–24 hours	2.5 every 12–18 hours	2.5 every 8–12 hours	2.5 every 12 hours	2.5 every 8 hours
Amikacin[6]	7.5 every 18–24 hours	7.5 every 18–24 hours	7.5 every 8–12 hours	10 every 12 hours	10 every 8 hours
Others					
Clindamycin	5 every 12 hours	5 every 12 hours	5 every 8 hours	5 every 8 hours	5 every 6 hours
Metronidazole[4]	7.5 every 48 hours	7.5 every 24 hours	7.5 every 12 hours	7.5 every 12 hours	15 every 12 hours
Vancomycin	15 every 24 hours	15 every 12–18 hours	15 every 8–12 hours	15 every 12 hours	15 every 8 hours
Chloramphenicol[3,6]	25 every 24 hours	25 every 24 hours	25 every 24 hours	25 every 24 hours	25 every 12 hours
Antifungal Agents					
Amphotericin B	0.5–1.0 mg/kg once daily				
Amphotericin B Liposome and Amphotericin B Lipid Complex	1–5 mg/kg once daily				
Flucytosine[7]	50–150 mg/kg/day PO divided every 6 hours				

[1] Sources of drug doses: Young TE, Mangum B: *Neofax®; A manual of drugs used in neonatal care*. 15th ed. Raleigh, NC, Acorn Publishing, and Baltimore RS: Perinatal bacterial and fungal infections *in* Jenson, H. B., Baltimore, R. S. eds., *Pediatric Infectious Diseases. Principles and Practice*. Second Edition, WB Saunders Co, Philadelphia, 2002. These dosages are for parenteral (intravenous or intramuscular) administration.
[2] Some authorities recommend higher doses, penicillin up to 100,000 U/kg/dose for meningitis, and 50,000 U/kg/dose for other infections, and ampicillin up to 100mg/kg/dose for meningitis and 50 mg/kg/dose for other infections.
[3] Should not be administered to neonates with hyperbilirubinemia or liver dysfunction, especially those born prematurely.
[4] Safety and efficacy in infants have not been established.
[5] Safety and efficacy in infants younger than 9 months of age have not been established.
[6] Dosing should be guided by laboratory determination of serum antibiotic concentrations once a steady state has been reached. These doses are a guideline for beginning therapy.
[7] Safety and efficacy in infants and children younger than 12 years of age have not been established. The dose for older infants is indicated. There are limited data on dosing for neonates.
[8] There are limited data on dosing for neonates.

after intramuscular injections in infants with adequate muscle mass and stable cardiovascular and renal function. Bacterial disease is documented by culture in approximately 10% of infants with suspected sepsis. Therefore, a 7-day course of antimicrobial therapy often is completed in infants whose bacterial cultures are sterile at 48 hours, when no other explanation for the infant's clinical condition exists and an apparent response to therapy has occurred. Appropriate cultures should be repeated after 24 to 48 hours of effective antimicrobial therapy to document the sterilization of the infected body fluid(s). Persistent bacteremia requires further diagnostic evaluation for the identification of a focus of infection, removal of foreign bodies that may be the source of continued seeding of the bloodstream, or further optimization of antibiotic activity against the specific pathogen.

Supportive Care

The provision of supportive care, with particular attention to respiratory, cardiovascular, renal, hematological, fluid and electrolyte, metabolic, and nutritional needs, is of utmost importance in optimizing outcome, particularly in cases accompanied by shock. Respiratory distress is commonly due to a combination of factors, including intraparenchymal abnormalities from infection, decreased respiratory muscle function, and noncardiac pulmonary edema. Ventilatory support, required in some cases, also may improve oxygenation by decreasing the work of breathing. Cardiovascular abnormalities are due to alterations in vascular tone, myocardial dysfunction, and increased oxygen consumption. Ongoing fluid resuscitation to treat capillary leak is necessary. Inotropic and vasoactive agents, such as dopamine and dobutamine, are required in cases unresponsive to fluid resuscitation to increase cardiac output, support the blood pressure, and enhance tissue oxygen delivery. Clinical practice parameters for the hemodynamic support of neonates in septic shock are being developed. Renal support to avoid prolonged oliguria after hypoperfusion is critical, utilizing the careful management of fluids and electrolytes and avoiding nephrotoxic agents. Hematologic support primarily involves replacement therapy, such as packed red blood cells, and fresh-frozen plasma in cases accompanied by disseminated intravascular coagulation. Metabolic support includes the regulation of glucose homeostasis, correction of acidosis, and recognition of liver dysfunction. Early nutritional support may modify the host inflammatory response and improve outcome.

Adjunctive Therapy

Increasing attention has been directed toward the enhancement of the neonate's deficient host responses. Small studies have suggested benefit from various treatment modalities, including exchange transfusion, white blood cell (WBC) transfusion for severe neutropenia and bone marrow failure, intravenous immunoglobulins (IVIG), and specific immune serum globulin preparations in cases of neonatal sepsis. Although WBC transfusions appear to reduce the mortality rate in some studies, the logistics for providing them in a safe and timely manner have been difficult. The use of hematopoietic growth factors, such as G-CSF and GM-CSF, in septic newborns with neutropenia appears potentially promising, but data are limited and results are inconclusive. Insufficient evidence of benefit from G-CSF or GM-CSF exists to recommend either as routine adjunctive treatment for neonates with sepsis, according to a recent review of myeloid colony-stimulating factors in neonatal sepsis. If these agents are indeed beneficial, it will require additional, larger, and well-controlled studies to demonstrate improved survival.

The use of intravenous immune globulin as an adjunct for treating neonatal sepsis also is controversial. Despite lack of response in some studies, a meta-analysis suggests that IVIG (750 mg/kg as a single dose) is beneficial in decreasing the morbidity of neonatal sepsis. Activated protein C is somewhat beneficial in adults and older children with severe sepsis. Recent studies suggest it is not useful or safe in neonates. The use of steroids for reducing death and neurologic sequelae of meningitis has been studied in children and adults, but the results have been inconsistent. Studies to demonstrate whether steroids are either beneficial or associated with an adverse outcome in neonates are not available, and their use for neonatal meningitis cannot be endorsed.

PROGNOSIS

Overall case-fatality rates for neonatal sepsis have decreased from 90% in the 1930s to 15% to 25% in the 1980s, and further to 5% to 20% in recent years. The most recent data from our hospital is that the mortality rate from neonatal sepsis is 3%. This decrease is the result of many factors, including earlier recognition of the nonspecific signs of sepsis, improvements in obstetric and neonatal care, development of improved antimicrobial agents, and significantly, the adoption of IAP for GBS disease. Sepsis-related mortality is higher for early-onset disease and for infants born prematurely. Mortality from early-onset GBS disease has fallen from 55% in the 1970s to 10% to 15% in the 1980s, to a current rate of 3% to 5%. Mortality from late-onset GBS now is only slightly higher than early-onset disease, at 5% to 7%.

Morbidity from GBS meningitis is high despite appropriate diagnosis and antimicrobial therapy (see Chapter 75).

Recurrent GBS infection is uncommon, with an incidence of 1% to 6%. In most instances, recurrent disease represents persistent mucosal colonization and infection with the same GBS strain. In a few cases, a second episode represents infection with a new GBS strain.

PREVENTION

Intrapartum Antibiotic Prophylaxis (IAP)

Studies of prevention of neonatal sepsis have focused on GBS because of its importance in the etiology of neonatal sepsis. This is discussed in Chapter 75, Group B Streptococcal Disease.

CONCLUSIONS

Ongoing, longitudinal monitoring and analyses are needed to address many of the unanswered questions in the evaluation and management of neonatal sepsis. The widespread use of IAP has raised concerns such as the possibility of maternal allergic reactions; increased resistance in GBS, *E. coli*, or other bacteria; and the emergence of other, more virulent pathogens. Important questions still to be answered in the management of neonatal sepsis include:

- What is the optimal antibiotic regimen for IAP?
- How should asymptomatic infants born to high-risk mothers or mothers who have received IAP be evaluated and treated, if at all?
- Are current IAP protocols optimal?
- Would a combined maternal and neonatal chemoprophylactic approach be better?

- How long should initially symptomatic infants with sterile blood cultures be treated?
- What is the appropriate duration of antibiotic therapy for the neonate with proven sepsis?

The application of modern molecular biologic approaches to the problem of neonatal sepsis will hopefully provide many new insights to questions such as:

- What genetic determinants predispose an infant to invasive infection?
- What are the determinants that precipitate the SIRS syndrome?
- Will improvements in diagnostic testing provide rapid, reliable diagnosis?
- Will it be possible to identify the "molecular signature" of invasive pathogens, thus allowing improvements in therapy?
- Can new, more effective antimicrobials and adjunctive agents be developed?

Exciting advances are on the horizon for this common, serious neonatal disease.

Suggested Readings

Ahrens P, Kattner E, Kohler B, et al. Mutations of genes involved in the innate immune system as predictors of sepsis in very low birth weight infants. *Pediatr Res* 2004;55:652.

Areschoug T, Stalhammar-Carlemalm M, Karlsson I, Lindahl G. Streptococcal beta protein has separate binding sites for human factor H and IgA-Fc. *J Biol Chem* 2002;277:12642.

Baker CJ, Edwards MS. Group B streptococcal conjugate vaccines. *Arch Dis Child* 2003;88:375.

Baltimore RS. Neonatal sepsis: epidemiology and management. *Paediatr Drugs* 2003;5:723.

Baltimore RS, Huie SM, Meek JI, et al. Early-onset neonatal sepsis in the era of group B streptococcal prevention. *Pediatrics* 2001;108:1094.

Bernstein HM, Calhoun DA, Christensen RD. Use of myeloid colony-stimulating factors in neonates with septicemia. *Curr Opin Pediatr* 2002;14:91.

Bizzarro MJ, Raskind C, Baltimore RS, et al. Seventy-five years of neonatal sepsis at Yale: 1928–2003. *Pediatrics* 2005;116:59.

Byington CL, Rittichier KK, Bassett KE, et al. Serious bacterial infections in febrile infants younger than 90 days of age: the importance of ampicillin-resistant pathogens. *Pediatrics* 2003;111:964.

Cairo MS, Worcester CC, Rucker RW, et al. Randomized trial of granulocyte transfusions versus intravenous immune globulin therapy for neonatal neutropenia and sepsis. *J Pediatr* 1992;120:281.

Carcillo JA, Fields AI. Clinical practice parameters for hemodynamic support of pediatric and neonatal patients in septic shock. *Crit Care Med* 2002;30:1365.

Centers for Disease Control and Prevention. Prevention of perinatal group B streptococcal disease: a public health perspective. *MMWR Recomm Rep* 1996;45:1.

Cordero L, Sananes M, Ayers LW. Bloodstream infections in a neonatal intensive-care unit: 12 years' experience with an antibiotic control program. *Infect Control Hosp Epidemiol* 1999;20:242.

Davies HD, Adair C, McGeer A, et al. Antibodies to capsular polysaccharides of group B Streptococcus in pregnant Canadian women: relationship to colonization status and infection in the neonate. *J Infect Dis* 2001;184:285.

Despond O, Proulx F, Carcillo JA, Lacroix J. Pediatric sepsis and multiple organ dysfunction syndrome. *Curr Opin Pediatr* 2001;13:247.

Doellner H, Arntzen KJ, Haereid PE, et al. Interleukin-6 concentrations in neonates evaluated for sepsis. *J Pediatr* 1998;132:295.

Doran KS, Liu GY, Nizet V. Group B streptococcal beta-hemolysin/cytolysin activates neutrophil signaling pathways in brain endothelium and contributes to development of meningitis. *J Clin Invest* 2003;112:736.

Franz AR, Steinbach G, Kron M, Pohlandt F. Reduction of unnecessary antibiotic therapy in newborn infants using interleukin-8 and C-reactive protein as markers of bacterial infections. *Pediatrics* 1999;104:447.

Gendrel D, Bohuon C. Procalcitonin as a marker of bacterial infection. *Pediatr Infect Dis J* 2000;19:679; quiz 688.

Giroir BP. Recombinant human activated protein C for the treatment of severe sepsis: is there a role in pediatrics? *Curr Opin Pediatr* 2003;15:92.

Gladstone IM, Ehrenkranz RA, Edberg SC, Baltimore RS. A ten-year review of neonatal sepsis and comparison with the previous fifty-year experience. *Pediatr Infect Dis J* 1990;9:819.

Guida JD, Kunig AM, Leef KH, et al. Platelet count and sepsis in very low birth weight neonates: is there an organism-specific response? *Pediatrics* 2003;111:1411.

Harris TO, Shelver DW, Bohnsack JF, Rubens CE. A novel streptococcal surface protease promotes virulence, resistance to opsonophagocytosis, and cleavage of human fibrinogen. *J Clin Invest* 2003;111:61.

Jenson HB, Pollock BH. Meta-analyses of the effectiveness of intravenous immune globulin for prevention and treatment of neonatal sepsis. *Pediatrics* 1997;99:E2.

Jones AL, Needham RH, Clancy A, et al. Penicillin-binding proteins in *Streptococcus agalactiae*: a novel mechanism for evasion of immune clearance. *Mol Microbiol* 2003;47:247.

Joseph TA, Pyati SP, Jacobs N. Neonatal early-onset *Escherichia coli* disease. The effect of intrapartum ampicillin. *Arch Pediatr Adolesc Med* 1998;152:35.

Manroe BL, Weinberg AG, Rosenfeld CR, Browne R. The neonatal blood count in health and disease. I. Reference values for neutrophilic cells. *J Pediatr* 1979;95:89.

Mehr S, Doyle LW. Cytokines as markers of bacterial sepsis in newborn infants: a review. *Pediatr Infect Dis J* 2000;19:879.

Mittendorf R, Montag AG, MacMillan W, et al. Components of the systemic fetal inflammatory response syndrome as predictors of impaired neurologic outcomes in children. *Am J Obstet Gynecol* 2003;188:1438–4; discussion 1444.

Moore MR, Schrag SJ, Schuchat A. Effects of intrapartum antimicrobial prophylaxis for prevention of group-B-streptococcal disease on the incidence and ecology of early-onset neonatal sepsis. *Lancet Infect Dis* 2003;3:201.

Moylett EH, Fernandez M, Rench MA, et al. A 5-year review of recurrent group B streptococcal disease: lessons from twin infants. *Clin Infect Dis* 2000;30:282.

Paoletti LC, Madoff LC. Vaccines to prevent neonatal GBS infection. *Semin Neonatol* 2002;7:315.

Philip AG, Hewitt JR. Early diagnosis of neonatal sepsis. *Pediatrics* 1980;65:1036.

Schrag S, Gorwitz R, Fultz-Butts K, Schuchat A. Prevention of perinatal group B streptococcal disease. Revised guidelines from CDC. *MMWR Recomm Rep* 2002;51:1.

Schrag SJ, Whitney CG, Schuchat A. Neonatal group B streptococcal disease: how infection control teams can contribute to prevention efforts. *Infect Control Hosp Epidemiol* 2000;21:473.

Schrag SJ, Zell ER, Lynfield R, et al. A population-based comparison of strategies to prevent early-onset group B streptococcal disease in neonates. *N Engl J Med* 2002;347:233.

Stoll BJ, Gordon T, Korones SB, et al. Early-onset sepsis in very low birth weight neonates: a report from the National Institute of Child Health and Human Development Neonatal Research Network. *J Pediatr* 1996;129:72.

Stoll BJ, Hansen N, Fanaroff AA, et al. Changes in pathogens causing early-onset sepsis in very-low-birth-weight infants. *N Engl J Med* 2002;347:240.

Stoll BJ, Holman RC, Schuchat A. Decline in sepsis-associated neonatal and infant deaths in the United States, 1979 through 1994. *Pediatrics* 1998;102:e18.

Towers CV, Briggs GG. Antepartum use of antibiotics and early-onset neonatal sepsis: the next 4 years. *Am J Obstet Gynecol* 2002;187:495.

Velaphi S, Siegel JD, Wendel GD, Jr., et al. Early-onset group B streptococcal infection after a combined maternal and neonatal group B streptococcal chemoprophylaxis strategy. *Pediatrics* 2003;111:541.

von Rosenstiel N, von Rosenstiel I, Adam D. Management of sepsis and septic shock in infants and children. *Paediatr Drugs* 2001;3:9.

Weirich E, Rabin RL, Maldonado Y, et al. Neutrophil CD11b expression as a diagnostic marker for early-onset neonatal infection. *J Pediatr* 1998;132:445.

CHAPTER 72 ■ MENINGITIS

MARC H. LEBEL

EPIDEMIOLOGY

The incidence of neonatal bacterial meningitis is approximately one-fourth of that of neonatal sepsis with a median range of 0.2 to 0.5 cases per 1,000 live births. The rates vary according to nursery and predisposing maternal and infant risk factors. A preponderance of male infants with meningitis caused by gram-negative enteric bacilli exists, but the ratio of male-to-female cases is comparable with that for group B streptococcus. The incidence of meningitis in low-birth-weight infants is approximately three times that of infants with birth weights greater than 2,500 g. Other risk factors associated with an increased incidence of neonatal bacteremia and meningitis include premature or prolonged rupture of membranes, maternal fever or chorioamnionitis, and traumatic delivery. Group B streptococcus and *Listeria monocytogenes* may cause early-onset and late-onset disease. Late-onset infections (after 7 days of life) are more often associated with meningitis.

PATHOGENESIS

Group B streptococci (40% to 55% of cases) and *Escherichia coli* (15% to 20% of cases) are the two most frequent pathogens causing meningitis (Box 72.1). *Listeria monocytogenes* is an important but much less frequently encountered pathogen. In some institutions, nonenterococcal group D streptococci cause a substantial proportion of meningitis cases. *Enterobac-*

| **BOX 72.1** | **Pathogens Causing Neonatal Bacterial Meningitis** |

Most Common
Group B streptococci
Escherichia coli

Less Common
Listeria monocytogenes
Nonenterococcal group D streptococci

Infrequent
Enterobacter sp.
Klebsiella sp.
Salmonella sp.
Other gram-negative bacilli
Streptococcus pneumoniae
Neisseria meningitidis
Haemophilus influenzae type b

Seen in Premature Infants
Staphylococcus sp.
Candida sp.

---

ter species, *Klebsiella* species, *Salmonella* species, and other gram-negative bacilli are infrequently encountered. *Staphylococcus* species and *Candida* species can cause meningitis in premature infants who are subject to invasive supportive management and monitoring devices. Common pathogenic organisms of meningitis in older infants and children (*Streptococcus pneumoniae*, *Neisseria meningitidis*, and *Haemophilus influenzae* type b) are infrequent causes of meningitis in neonates. Group A streptococcus, once a major pathogen of neonatal sepsis and meningitis in the early 20th century, is now only occasionally seen in infants.

Most cases of meningitis result from hematogenous dissemination. Factors that predispose to bacteremia also predispose to meningitis; as many as one-third of infants with bacteremia develop meningitis. Rarely, meningitis is secondary to extension from infected skin through the soft tissues and skull (e.g., infected cephalhematoma). Infants with congenital malformations of the neural tube such as meningomyeloceles can be infected by direct spread from skin surfaces.

The choroid plexus may be the port of entry to the cerebrospinal fluid (CSF) because ventriculitis is present in at least 70% of cases of neonatal gram-negative enteric meningitis; ventricles probably are the initial site of infection and serve as a reservoir for spread of infection throughout the subarachnoid space.

Many organisms causing meningitis in the newborn possess specific surface antigens. The K1 polysaccharide of *E. coli* is present in 75% to 85% of strains isolated from neonates with meningitis. The BIII polysaccharide of group B streptococci is recovered from 30% of early-onset and 90% of late-onset strains causing neonatal meningitis. Type IVb strains of *L. monocytogenes* account for most meningitis cases.

The K1 antigen of *E. coli* confers resistance to phagocytosis and does not activate the alternate complement pathway. Immunochemical similarities exist between glycopeptides of the brain containing sialic acid and the capsular polysaccharide of *E. coli* K1 strains. However, specific antibodies to the K1 antigen appear to be highly protective against sepsis and meningitis. Delayed clearance of *E. coli* because of decreased phagocytosis may allow replication of the organism in the blood to a concentration of 1,000 or more organisms per milliliter, a concentration associated with an increased incidence of meningitis.

The capsular polysaccharide of serotype III of the group B streptococci seems to mediate resistance to phagocytosis; strains expressing this antigen adhere to buccal epithelial cells of neonates better than to those of adults. The presence of type-specific antibodies is necessary for opsonization of type Ia, II, and III strains, and high concentrations appear to confer resistance to the newborn infant. Phagocytosis of the organism is normal in the presence of type III polysaccharide, but chemiluminescence of neutrophils is decreased when exposed to this antigen; however, this decrease in chemiluminescence has also been found with other pathogens.

The pathogenesis of late-onset disease caused by group B streptococci is unclear. In most instances, serotype III is the infecting pathogen. Predisposing risk factors usually are absent. A history of preceding respiratory tract infection is present in many patients. This infection may alter the nasopharyngeal epithelium and facilitate invasion by the streptococci.

Interleukin-1 beta and tumor necrosis factors are detectable in the CSF of almost all infants with bacterial meningitis and are considered important mediators of the inflammation within the central nervous system. High levels of interleukin-1 beta or prolonged persistence of detectable levels of this mediator are associated with a poorer outcome.

Brain abscesses occur in 70% of cases of *Enterobacter sakazakii* meningitis, whereas other gram-negative enteric bacilli cause abscesses in less than 10% of infants. Hematogenous spread is the most likely source of dissemination.

CLINICAL MANIFESTATIONS AND COMPLICATIONS

The clinical manifestations of meningitis in the newborn infant are often nonspecific and indistinguishable from those of sepsis. Meningitis should always be considered when bacteremia is suspected. The cardinal signs of meningitis in older children, such as stiff neck and Kernig and Brudzinski signs, are absent in most infants.

The most frequent signs are temperature instability, respiratory distress, irritability, lethargy, and poor feeding or vomiting. Seizures occur in 40% of newborn infants with meningitis. Other signs include a bulging fontanelle, hyperactivity or hypoactivity, alteration of the level of consciousness, tremor, twitching, apnea, stiff neck or opisthotonos, hemiparesis, and cranial nerve palsy. Some patients present with a severe protracted state of shock. Patients with group B streptococcal infection also may present with hydrocephalus without other signs of infection.

The pathologic findings of meningitis in neonates are similar to those found in older children. A diffuse purulent leptomeningitis is almost always found and is more pronounced at the base of the brain. In the acute phase of the illness, brain edema is frequently present, but cerebral herniation is uncommon. Vasculitis is common with resultant thrombosis and possibly infarct of brain tissue. Brain abscesses can develop in these areas and can involve multiple lobes. Ventriculitis is present in three-fourths of infants, and hydrocephalus develops in approximately one-third. Subdural effusions occur rarely in the neonate. Leukomalacia with porencephaly can develop as a result of tissue anoxia.

DIAGNOSIS

The diagnosis of meningitis is based on examination and culture of the CSF. In most instances, a lumbar puncture should be performed at the time of the sepsis workup. In a recent study, one-third of the very low-birth-weight infants with proven bacterial meningitis had sterile blood cultures, reemphasizing the importance of lumbar puncture in the evaluation of infants with suspected sepsis. However, in a critically ill child, the lumbar puncture can be postponed until the cardiorespiratory condition is stable. Although CSF cultures may be sterile in the infant who has received antibiotics before diagnosis, examination of the CSF for cellular and biochemistry values and for antigen detection is almost always indicative of meningitis.

A gram-stained smear of CSF should be made for all infants, because grossly clear fluid with only a few cells can contain many bacteria. Gram stain or acridine orange smear of CSF reveals bacteria in at least 80% of infants with culture-proven meningitis. Because of the low concentrations of organisms (i.e., 10^3 colony-forming units per mL of CSF), most Gram stain smears of CSF from infants with *L. monocytogenes* meningitis do not reveal the gram-positive bacillus.

TABLE 72.1

NORMAL VALUES FOR CEREBROSPINAL FLUID EXAMINATION IN NEONATES

Value	Term	Preterm[a]
Leukocyte count (per microliter)	7 (0–32)[b]	8 (0–29)
Polymorphonuclear leukocytes (%)	61	57
Protein (mg/dL)	90 (20–170)	115 (65–150)
Glucose (mg/dL)	52 (34–119)	50 (24–63)
Cerebrospinal fluid–to–blood glucose ratio (%)	51 (44–248)	75 (55–105)

[a] Preterm is less than 38 weeks' gestation.
[b] Mean (range).
Adapted from Sarff LD, Platt LH, McCracken GH Jr. Cerebrospinal fluid evaluation in neonates: comparison of high risk infants with and without meningitis. *J Pediatr* 1976;88:273.

The CSF laboratory findings in the neonate differ from those in older children (Table 72.1); this difference may be a result of an increase in the permeability of the blood–brain barrier (i.e., cerebral capillary endothelial cells). By 1 month of age, an infant's leukocyte count should be in the range of 0 to 5 cells per mL. An overlap exists in the different cellular and biochemical characteristics between the infants with and without meningitis. However, fewer than 1% of infants with proven meningitis have an initial CSF examination that is completely normal. Simultaneous concentrations of blood and CSF glucose should be obtained because low CSF glucose can reflect concurrent hypoglycemia, and a CSF–to–blood glucose ratio of less than 0.6 (60%) should be considered suspicious. The CSF leukocyte count is elevated in most newborns with meningitis, and polymorphonuclear leukocytes are preponderant except in some patients with *Listeria* meningitis. The protein concentration may not be elevated at the time of diagnosis. CSF changes characteristic of bacterial meningitis associated with sterile cultures may occur in association with anaerobic infection, most commonly *Bacteroides fragilis*, *E. sakazakii* brain abscesses, or subarachnoid hemorrhage.

Blood culture specimens should be obtained from every patient; 85% of neonates with bacterial meningitis have positive blood culture results at the time of presentation. Latex agglutination for group B streptococci and *E. coli* K1 antigens in CSF and concentrated urine can be performed to facilitate a rapid diagnosis of infection, but false-negative results do occur.

THERAPY

Pharmacologic Therapy

After CSF and blood cultures are obtained, antibiotic therapy should be initiated promptly with ampicillin plus cefotaxime, or with a combination of ampicillin and an aminoglycoside such as gentamicin or amikacin, in meningitis dosages. Therapy should be adjusted depending on results of cultures and susceptibility testing. For group B streptococcal or *L. monocytogenes* infection, 14 days of ampicillin or penicillin therapy is adequate in the patient without complications. The addition of an aminoglycoside to ampicillin for the initial 48 to 72 hours has been suggested by some authors because of synergistic activity against group B streptococci and *Listeria* species, especially if the strain demonstrates *in vitro* tolerance (i.e., a 32-fold difference between the minimal inhibitory concentration and minimal bactericidal concentration). No clinical studies have proven superiority of one regimen over another.

For gram-negative enteric meningitis, ampicillin and gentamicin have been used extensively since the 1970s, but most centers currently use a combination of cefotaxime plus an aminoglycoside. Delayed CSF sterilization for 3 or more days occurs in one-half of infants with meningitis caused by gram-negative pathogens. Because a poor prognosis is correlated directly with duration of positive CSF cultures for more than 3 days, many therapeutic regimens have been evaluated in an effort to improve the rate of bacteriologic response.

Intrathecal aminoglycoside therapy is not associated with improved outcome and is not recommended for neonatal meningitis. Despite higher levels of aminoglycoside achieved in the CSF with intraventricular administration compared with systemic therapy alone, no differences were noted between the two treatment groups in the duration of positive CSF culture results and morbidity. Furthermore, the mortality was 12.5% in the systemic therapy group and 42.9% in the intraventricular therapy group. Three children developed porencephaly along the needle track associated with repeated ventricular taps. From these data, intraventricular administration of aminoglycosides cannot be recommended for routine therapy of neonatal meningitis.

The third-generation cephalosporins offer potential advantages for therapy of meningitis in the neonatal period. They possess extraordinary *in vitro* activity against gram-negative enteric bacilli (including most of the causative pathogens of neonatal meningitis), achieve high serum concentrations, and penetrate well into the CSF. They appear to be safe and well tolerated and lack the nephrotoxicity and ototoxicity associated with the use of aminoglycosides. Third-generation cephalosporins are active against most streptococci but are inactive against *L. monocytogenes* and enterococci. Only ceftazidime provides adequate activity against *Pseudomonas aeruginosa*.

Moxalactam and ampicillin therapy has been compared with amikacin and ampicillin therapy. Moxalactam was comparably effective. The duration of positive CSF culture results was approximately 3 days in each group; no significant differences were noted in the case-fatality rates and subsequent neurologic sequelae. The reasons for the delayed CSF sterilization in some patients in the presence of excellent CSF bactericidal activity (greater than or equal to 1:8) is not fully understood. The CSF space may be considered an area of impaired host resistance. Polymorphonuclear leukocytes have an altered phagocytosis in the subarachnoidal space; opsonic and bactericidal activity is reduced, and the concentrations of immunoglobulins and complement are low. Also, it is possible that an inoculum effect exists that results in decreased activity of the antibiotics in the presence of a high bacterial colony count at initiation of therapy.

Cefotaxime is preferred for therapy of neonatal meningitis over other third-generation cephalosporins because of more extensive experience with this drug in the neonatal period and because it does not alter substantially the bowel flora. However, extensive or exclusive use of a cephalosporin in a closed newborn unit may lead to rapid emergence of resistance. Outbreaks of cefotaxime-resistant *Enterobacter cloacae* infections have been described shortly after beginning routine therapy with cefotaxime for suspected sepsis in two neonatal intensive care units. These agents should be used selectively and as alternatives to the conventional regimen. Because of high biliary excretion and marked alteration of the normal intestinal flora and concern for displacement of bilirubin, ceftriaxone should not be used in the newborn infant.

For gram-negative enteric meningitis, the duration of therapy should be 21 days or longer and should continue for at least 14 days after the first sterile CSF culture result.

For premature infants hospitalized in the nursery for prolonged periods, staphylococci, enterococci, and gentamicin-resistant gram-negative organisms are potential pathogens. An alternative antimicrobial regimen should be considered. A combination of ampicillin and cefotaxime or ceftazidime could be used as initial empiric therapy. When an indwelling vascular catheter or a ventriculoperitoneal shunt is in place or when *S. epidermidis* and methicillin-resistant *S. aureus* are frequent causes of infection, vancomycin plus amikacin or vancomycin plus cefotaxime can be used initially. Metronidazole is indicated for treatment of central nervous system infection caused by *B. fragilis*.

It is suggested that a CSF culture be repeated after 48 to 72 hours of therapy to ensure sterility of the CSF, even though many clinicians prefer to use a more selected approach based on the clinical evolution of the patient. If culture results are positive after 48 hours for group B streptococci and 72 hours for coliform organisms, the susceptibilities of the pathogen should be reviewed. Cranial sonography, computed tomography (CT), or magnetic resonance imaging (MRI) should be considered. In all cases of meningitis caused by *E. sakazakii,* cranial CT or MRI scans should be obtained because of the frequent association with brain abscesses. In patients with an uncomplicated course of gram-negative meningitis, cranial CT or MRI scans should be obtained before discharge. The duration of antibiotic therapy for brain abscess should be at least 4 to 6 weeks, depending on clinical evolution and resolution of the lesion based on repeated tomography. Neurosurgery should be considered early for needle aspiration of the abscess to identify the etiologic agent and to provide drainage or excision of the abscesses. Aminoglycosides are not very effective because of decreased activity in abscess cavities that have a low pH and anaerobic conditions.

Additional Therapy

Only one prospective study evaluated adjunctive therapy with dexamethasone in neonatal bacterial meningitis. There were no differences in mortality and morbidity between the two treatment groups. Dexamethasone cannot be recommended for infants with neonatal meningitis.

Supportive care of the newborn with meningitis is similar to that of the septic infant. Careful neurologic examination should be performed daily and the head circumference measured. Seizures should be controlled with intravenously administered phenobarbital or phenytoin. The serum electrolytes should be followed for detection of hyponatremia as a result of inappropriate secretion of antidiuretic hormone; fluid restriction is instituted if this condition develops. Some newborns with group B streptococcal meningitis develop diabetes insipidus during the course of the illness. Serum concentrations of aminoglycosides in the newborn period are unpredictable, especially for the low-birth-weight premature infant, and should be routinely determined to achieve therapeutic concentrations and avoid toxicity. Every infant should have a brainstem-evoked response audiogram at discharge or within 6 weeks after discharge from the hospital to detect hearing impairment.

PROGNOSIS

Despite improvement in intensive care facilities, meningitis in the neonatal period is still a serious disease. Morbidity remains high, but the case fatality rate has fallen from 15% to 30% in the 1970s to 6% to 15% in the late 1990s. Mortality rates vary depending on the causative pathogen, predisposing risk factors, and availability of intensive care facilities. One study reported lower mortality rates when third-generation cephalosporins were used in the treatment; however, there was no change in the morbidity rates.

Duration of seizures greater than 72 hours, presence of coma, use of inotropes, and leucopenia are the most important predictors of adverse outcome. Poor outcome has also been found in the presence of coma at admission, persistent seizures, low birth weight, ventriculitis, duration of positive CSF culture results, very low or very high CSF leukocyte count, protein concentration higher than 500 mg/dL, and presence of brain abscess. High concentrations of the K1 antigen of *E. coli*, of interleukin-1 beta, and of the polysaccharide of group B streptococci in the initial CSF specimen have been inversely correlated with clinical outcome and with severity of disease.

For group B streptococcus, approximately 15% to 20% of survivors have major sequelae, including spastic quadriplegia, profound mental retardation, hemiparesis, deafness, or blindness. Hydrocephalus develops in 11% of cases, and 13% have a seizure disorder. However, survivors without major sequelae on physical examination seem to function within normal limits and comparably with their siblings.

Sequelae are found in 35% to 50% of survivors of gram-negative meningitis. Ten percent have severe sequelae as defined by failure to develop beyond the age at which the disease occurred or required custodial care. Approximately 25% to 35% have mild to moderate sequelae, which many times do not interfere with adequate, albeit delayed, development. Hydrocephalus develops in one-third of patients. The prognosis of infants with brain abscesses is generally poor.

Suggested Readings

Agarwal R, Emmerson AJB. Should repeat lumbar punctures be routinely done in neonates with bacterial meningitis? Results of a survey into clinical practice. *Arch Dis Child* 2001;84:450.

Chavez-Bueno S, McCraken GH, Jr. Bacterial Meningitis in Children. *Pediatr Clin North Am* 2005;52:795.

Daoud AS, Batieha A, Al-Sheyyab M, et al. Lack of effectiveness of dexamethasone in neonatal bacterial meningitis. *Eur J Pediatr* 1999;158:230.

Heusser MF, Patterson JE, Juritza AP, et al. Emergence of resistance to multiple beta-lactams in *Enterobacter cloacae* during treatment for neonatal meningitis with cefotaxime. *Pediatr Infect Dis J* 1990;9:509.

Holt DE, Halket S, de Louvois J, Harvey D. Neonatal meningitis in England and Wales: 10 years on. *Arch Dis Fetal Neonatal Ed* 2001;84:F85.

Kaplan SL, Patrick CC. Cefotaxime and aminoglycoside treatment of meningitis caused by gram-negative enteric organisms. *Pediatr Infect Dis J* 1990; 9:810.

Kessler SL, Dajani AS. *Listeria* meningitis in infants and children. *Pediatr Infect Dis J* 1990;9:61.

Klinger G, Chin CN, Beyebe J, Perlman M. Predicting outcome of neonatal bacterial meningitis. *Pediatrics* 2000;106:477.

McCracken GH Jr, Mustafa MM, Ramilo O, et al. Cerebrospinal fluid interleukin 1-beta and tumor necrosis factor concentration and outcome from neonatal gram-negative enteric, bacillary meningitis. *Pediatr Infect Dis J* 1989;8:155.

Polin RA, Harris MC. Neonatal bacterial meningitis. *Semin Neonatol* 2001; 6:157.

Scheld WM, Koedel U, Nathan B, Pfister H-S. Pathophysiology of bacterial meningitis: mechanism of neuronal injury. *J Infect Dis* 2002;186:S225.

Stoll BJ, Hansen N, Fanaroff AA, et al. To tap or not to tap: high likelihood of meningitis without sepsis among very low birth weight infants. *Pediatrics* 2004;113:1181.

Stevens JP, Eames M, Kent A, et al. Long term outcome of neonatal meningitis. *Arch Dis Child Fetal Neonatal Ed* 2003;88:F179.

Unhanand M, Mustafa MM, McCracken GH Jr, Nelson JD. Gram-negative bacillary meningitis: a twenty-one year experience. *J Pediatr* 1993;122:15.

CHAPTER 73 ■ OSTEOMYELITIS AND SEPTIC ARTHRITIS

MARC H. LEBEL

EPIDEMIOLOGY

Osteomyelitis and septic arthritis are uncommon diseases in the neonate. When they occur, however, they can cause significant morbidity and permanent disability. The exact incidence of these two diseases is difficult to determine because most centers see only a few cases per year. A preponderance of male infants is affected, and newborns subjected to invasive monitoring are at increased risk.

In most cases, no precipitating factors are noted. Osteomyelitis of the newborn has been reported, however, after heel punctures, umbilical vessel catheterization, exchange transfusion, total parenteral nutrition, fetal monitoring, femoral venipuncture, suprapubic aspiration, and other needle punctures. Osteomyelitis also has been described as a complication of infected cephalohematoma. Broad-spectrum antibiotic therapy, prematurity, central venous catheters, and total parenteral nutrition are risk factors for fungal bone and joint infections.

PATHOGENESIS

Hematogenous dissemination is the most frequent source of suppurative bone and joint infections in the newborn period, but skeletal infection can occur after direct inoculation or as an extension from a contiguous site. The long bones are affected most commonly. The pathogenesis of osteomyelitis differs in the neonate compared with the older child. In the neonatal period, a communication between epiphyseal and metaphyseal vessels exists through sinusoidal vessels that transverse the growth plate. The sluggish flow in the sinusoidal loops of the metaphysis near the growth plate predispose to bacterial sequestration and the development of hematogenous osteomyelitis. The infection can spread through the transphyseal vessels and extend to the epiphysis. Infection of the epiphysis may rupture through the periosteum and enter the joint space, with secondary suppurative arthritis, especially for such joints as the hip and shoulder, where the epiphysis is intraarticular.

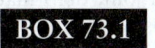

BOX 73.1   Osteomyelitis and Septic Arthritis: Causative Organisms

Staphylococcus aureus
Group B
Streptococcus
Candida species
Neisseria gonorrhoeae
Haemophilus influenzae
Gram-negative bacilli

Another unique feature of neonatal osteomyelitis is the frequency of multiple-bone involvement and contiguous joint involvement. This is particularly true for skeletal infections caused by *Staphylococcus aureus*. The destruction of the hyaline cartilage and the growth plate can lead to long-term sequelae.

The mechanisms of infection secondary to umbilical vessel catheterization may be related to multiple septic embolization through an infected umbilical stump and catheter and to decreased blood flow that might predispose to infection by altering the host defense mechanisms. The infection is generally in the ipsilateral inferior limb, distal to the tip of the catheter.

In group B streptococcal osteomyelitis, the right proximal humerus tends to be affected more frequently. The predilection for this site seems related to minor trauma to the shoulder while passing beneath the pubic bone during delivery.

Osteomyelitis of the os calcii may result from the direct introduction of bacteria at the time of heel puncture for blood sampling; improper site and techniques have been reported as causative events. Osteomyelitis of the skull is associated with the use of fetal scalp monitoring and rarely as a result of extension from an infected cephalhematoma.

Candida species can cause neonatal osteomyelitis and suppurative arthritis in those newborn who require invasive monitoring. Bones and joints are frequent secondary foci of infection in infants with disseminated candidiasis.

The leading pathogen causing osteomyelitis is *S. aureus*; and the group B streptococci, especially serotype III, have been reported with an increased frequency. In some centers, group B streptococcus is the most frequently isolated pathogen in neonatal osteoarticular infections. *Neisseria gonorrhoeae*, as well as gram-negative bacilli such as *Klebsiella pneumoniae*, *Haemophilus influenzae* (type b and nontypable), *Proteus* species, and *Escherichia coli* are infrequent pathogens (Box 73.1).

The pathogens causing suppurative arthritis in the neonate are the same as those causing osteomyelitis; differences in etiology are influenced principally by whether the infection is acquired in the hospital. In a review of 92 cases, Dan reported that the pathogens involved for hospital-acquired infections were *Staphylococcus* species (62%), *Candida* species (17%), gram-negative enteric bacilli (13%), *Streptococcus* species, and *H. influenzae* (4%). For community-acquired infections, the pathogenic organisms were streptococci, mainly group B (52%), *Staphylococcus* species (26%), gonococci (17%), and gram-negative bacilli (4%).

CLINICAL MANIFESTATIONS AND COMPLICATIONS

Skeletal infections in the neonate are difficult to diagnose because of their indolent presentation. Osteomyelitis and suppurative arthritis coexist in many neonates; signs and symptoms can be similar.

Failure to move an extremity spontaneously or apparent pain on movement (when picking up the baby or changing the diaper) may be the first manifestation. Osteomyelitis of the upper extremity occasionally may be misdiagnosed as an Erb palsy. Fever and signs of systemic toxicity are absent in most patients. This lack may cause a delay in diagnosis because parents do not seek medical advice. Irritability and crying at the time of the diaper change can signify involvement of the femur or hip. In the more severe form of osteomyelitis, the initial signs and symptoms can be those of a septic process, with lethargy, fever, and irritability.

On physical examination, a decreased range of motion of the affected extremity may be the only objective sign, but redness and warmth are seen occasionally. Suppurative arthritis of the hip presents with decreased range of motion of the articulation and a tendency to maintain the joint in an abducted, flexed, and externally rotated position.

Osteomyelitis and septic arthritis caused by group B streptococci occur most often in otherwise normal neonates with no predisposing risk factors. These infants have fewer signs of systemic toxicity and frequently are afebrile. Single-bone involvement, particularly of the right proximal humerus, is the most frequent presentation.

Osteomyelitis of the superior maxilla produces a rare but specific syndrome in early infancy that is often misdiagnosed as orbital cellulitis or dacryocystitis. The infant presents with fever, redness and swelling of the cheek, unilateral purulent rhinorrhea, and proptosis if the orbital contents are involved. *S. aureus* is the usual pathogen.

DIAGNOSIS

When the diagnosis of suppurative arthritis and osteomyelitis is suspected, roentgenography of the affected part and the contralateral extremity should be performed. These examinations are frequently abnormal, showing edema of the deep soft tissues, joint space widening, subperiosteal elevation, or lytic lesions. Many patients have multifocal osteomyelitis, with other sites found on roentgenography that do not seem clinically apparent. The roentgenographs can be normal at the onset of disease in infants with osteomyelitis. False-negative results of technetium pertechnetate bone scans in the presence of abnormal roentgenogram results have been reported, but the sensitivity of newer high-resolution cameras has improved diagnostic accuracy significantly. In one study, nuclear bone scans had a sensitivity of 90%. False-positive bone scans may result from calcium extravasation in the soft tissues. Magnetic resonance imaging (MRI) also can be used for the diagnosis of osteomyelitis in infancy. The peripheral leukocyte count usually is not helpful, but the erythrocyte sedimentation rate generally is elevated and is useful in determining duration of therapy. Aspiration of the material from the joint space of the affected bone should be performed, and the contents should be examined for organisms by Gram-stained smears and culture. Blood culture yield the causative pathogen in approximately one-half of patients and always should be obtained.

The differential diagnosis includes Erb palsy, pseudoparalysis of congenital syphilis, and deep cellulitis. Some cases of congenital neuroblastoma or leukemia can produce roentgenographic changes similar to those seen in osteomyelitis.

THERAPY

After specimens have been obtained for culture, an initial empiric therapeutic regimen consisting of a penicillinase-resistant penicillin (nafcillin, oxacillin) and cefotaxime should be initiated, unless the results of the Gram-stained specimens suggest a more specific etiology. In areas where methicillin-resistant *S. aureus* is prevalent, vancomycin should be used instead of the penicillinase-resistant penicillin. The antibiotic therapy is adjusted depending on the results of the cultures and susceptibilities. No indication for intraarticular administration of antibiotics exists, because the penetration of parenterally administered antibiotics in the joint space is adequate.

For hip and shoulder joints, open drainage is an essential part of therapy to prevent vascular compromise and possible subsequent necrosis of the head of the femur or humerus. For other joints, repeated aspirations generally suffice; if pus persistently reaccumulates, open drainage should be performed. For cases of suspected osteomyelitis, aspiration of the site of maximum tenderness or of a positive result of a bone scan should be performed. No consensus exists on the utility of surgical decompression of the subperiosteal space and metaphysis when pus is obtained at the subperiosteal or bone aspiration.

The duration of therapy should be a least 4 weeks. The treatment must be individualized, and based on the resolution of the clinical signs and symptoms and the return of the sedimentation rate to normal. For streptococcal infections, the therapy consists of ampicillin or penicillin, sometimes combined with an aminoglycoside. For staphylococcal infections, nafcillin, oxacillin, or vancomycin (when the strain is methicillin-resistant) should be administered. *Candida* species infections are treated with amphotericin B for at least 4 weeks. In small studies, lipid formulations of amphotericin B have been used in neonates. These preparations may be indicated for infants who develop toxicity or do not tolerate conventional amphotericin B. Fluconazole has been used frequently in neonates with candidal infections, but the data on its effectiveness for the treatment of osteomyelitis is limited. Insufficient data exist on the efficacy and safety of fluconazole in the neonatal period to recommend its use. Physical therapy should be instituted to prevent joint contractures. Although the combination of parenteral and oral regimens is acceptable therapy for older children, insufficient experience exists to recommend that regimen for most neonates with suppurative bone and joint infections.

PROGNOSIS

Effective antimicrobial agents have contributed to the significant decrease in mortality, and death results only occasionally. The degree of residual damage depends on the presence of joint involvement and the duration of illness before diagnosis. As many as 30% to 40% of infants have moderate to severe sequelae, mainly impairment of growth with joint deformation or shortening of limbs. Osteomyelitis or osteoarthritis of the femur, with hip or knee joint involvement, is associated most frequently with sequelae. In contrast, skeletal infections caused by group B streptococci rarely cause long-term sequelae.

Careful clinical and roentgenographic follow-up is essential, because growth retardation with resultant discrepancy in the limb length can occur, and joint dysfunction may not be apparent until many months later. Chronic osteomyelitis is a rare complication of neonatal infections.

Suggested Readings

Aigner RM, Fueger GF, Ritter G. Results of three-phase bone scintigraphy and radiography in 20 cases of neonatal osteomyelitis. *Nucl Med Commun* 1996; 17:20.

Asmar BI. Osteomyelitis in the neonate. *Infect Dis Clin North Am* 1992;6:117.

Bergdahl S, Ekengren K, Eriksson M. Neonatal hematogenous osteomyelitis: risk factors for long-term sequelae. *J Pediatr Orthop* 1985;5:564.

Connoly LP, Connoly SA. Skeletal scintigraphy in the multimodality assessment of young children with acute skeletal symptoms. *Clin Nucl Med* 2003;28:746.

Dan M. Septic arthritis in young infants: clinical and microbiological correlation and therapeutic implications. *Rev Infect Dis* 1984;6:147.

Dobbs MB, Sheridan JJ, Gordon JE, et al. Septic arthritis of the hip in infancy: long-term follow-up. *J Pediatr Orthop* 2003;23:162.

Edwards MS, Baker CJ, Wagner ML, et al. An etiologic shift in infantile osteomyelitis: the emergence of group B streptococcus. *J Pediatr* 1978;93:578.

Fox L, Sprunt K. Neonatal osteomyelitis. *Pediatrics* 1978;62:535.

Ish-Horowicz MR, McIntyre P, Nade S. Bone and joint infections caused by multiply resistant *Staphylococcus aureus* in a neonatal intensive care unit. *Pediatr Infect Dis J* 1992;11:82.

Jaramello D, Treves ST, Kasser JR, et al. Osteomyelitis and septic arthritis in children: appropriate use of imaging to guide treatment. *Am J Roentgenol* 1995;165:399.

Martinez-Aguilar G, Hammerman WA, Mason EO Jr, Kaplan SL. Clindamycin treatment of invasive infections caused by community-acquired, methicillin-resistant and methicillin-susceptible *Staphylococcus aureus* in children. *Pediatr Infect Dis J* 2003;22:593.

Ogden JA, Lister G. The pathology of neonatal osteomyelitis. *Pediatrics* 1975; 55:474.

Pittard WB, Thullen JD, Fanaroff AA. Neonatal septic arthritis. *J Pediatr* 1976; 88:621.

Williamson JB, Galasko CS, Robinson MJ. Outcome after acute osteomyelitis in preterm infants. *Arch Dis Child* 1990;65:1060.

Wong M, Isaacs D, Homan-Giles R, et al. Clinical and diagnostic features of osteomyelitis occurring in the first three months of life. *Pediatr Infect Dis J* 1996;12:1047.

Wopperer JM, White JJ, Gillespie R, et al. Long-term follow-up of infantile hip sepsis. *J Pediatr Orthop* 1988;8:322.

Yousefzadeh DK, Jackson JH. Neonatal and infantile *Candida* arthritis with or without osteomyelitis: a clinical and radiographical review of 21 cases. *Skeletal Radiol* 1980;5:77.

CHAPTER 74 ■ SKIN AND SOFT TISSUE INFECTIONS

MARC H. LEBEL

EPIDEMIOLOGY AND PATHOGENESIS

The most common manifestations of skin and soft tissue bacterial infections are presented in Box 74.1. Initial colonization of the skin occurs during delivery and reflects the organisms present in the birth canal. Subsequently, acquisition of *Staphylococcus aureus* and other bacteria occurs by contamination from the environment, the hands of the parents, and the personnel. The first site of colonization is the umbilical cord. In most infants, this is not followed by an infection.

BOX 74.1	Infections of the Skin and Soft Tissues

Pustular dermatitis and epidemic pustulosis
Bullous impetigo
Staphylococcal scalded skin syndrome (Ritter disease)
Staphylococcal pyoderma
Neonatal folliculitis
Scarlatiniform eruptions
Abscess of skin or scalp
Mastitis or breast abscess
Omphalitis
Cellulitis
Adenitis
Necrotizing fasciitis
Ecthyma gangrenosum

CLINICAL MANIFESTATIONS AND THERAPY

Impetigo

The most frequent skin and soft tissue infection is impetigo neonatorum (see the photo in the color section, Fig. 74.1). This presents with pustular lesions that cluster around the umbilicus and diaper area. It is not usually associated with fever or systemic illness. Risk factors include abrasions of the skin following forceps use, scalp wounds from intrapartum fetal monitoring devices, degeneration of the umbilical cord, intravascular catheter, and circumcision. Gram-positive and polymorphonuclear leukocytes present on Gram-stained smear examination distinguish pustules from erythema toxicum, in which case only eosinophils are seen on the smear. If only a few lesions are present, they are treated effectively by cleansing alone (chlorhexidine solution) or cleansing followed by application of topical antibiotic ointment. More extensive lesions may be treated with oral cephalexin for 5 to 10 days. Bullous impetigo is more likely to spread and should be treated with intravenous antibiotics in the absence of prompt response to local or oral therapy.

Staphylococcal Scalded Skin Syndrome

Staphylococcal scalded skin syndrome, or Ritter disease, is a much more extensive, exfoliative disease caused by phage group II staphylococci (see also Chapter 68, Dematologic Diseases). These organisms elaborate and release a circulating exotoxin that leads to blistering of the upper layer of the skin (stratum granulosum). Infants first present with a tender, sunburn-like erythematous rash. Then bullae develop with desquamation of large areas. Lesions commonly affect the flexures; a large portion of the skin can be affected (Fig. 74.2). The presence of Nikolsky sign (desquamation of the superficial layer of skin after light pressure over areas that appear to be uninvolved) is pathognomonic. The site of toxin production is remote from the area of involvement and is usually the conjunctiva, nasopharynx, umbilicus, or circumcision site. Staphylococcal bacteremia and superinfection are absent. These infants require intravenous therapy to eradicate the source of the toxin.

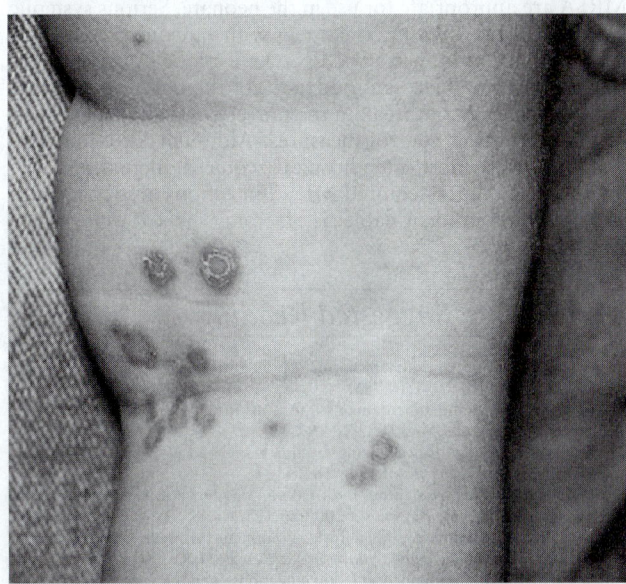

FIGURE 74.1. Impetigo. This photo does not show intact blisters, only the flaccid remains of the lesions. (From Goodheart HP. *Goodheart's photoguide of common skin disorders*, 2nd ed. Philadelphia: Lippincott Williams & Wilkins, 2003.)

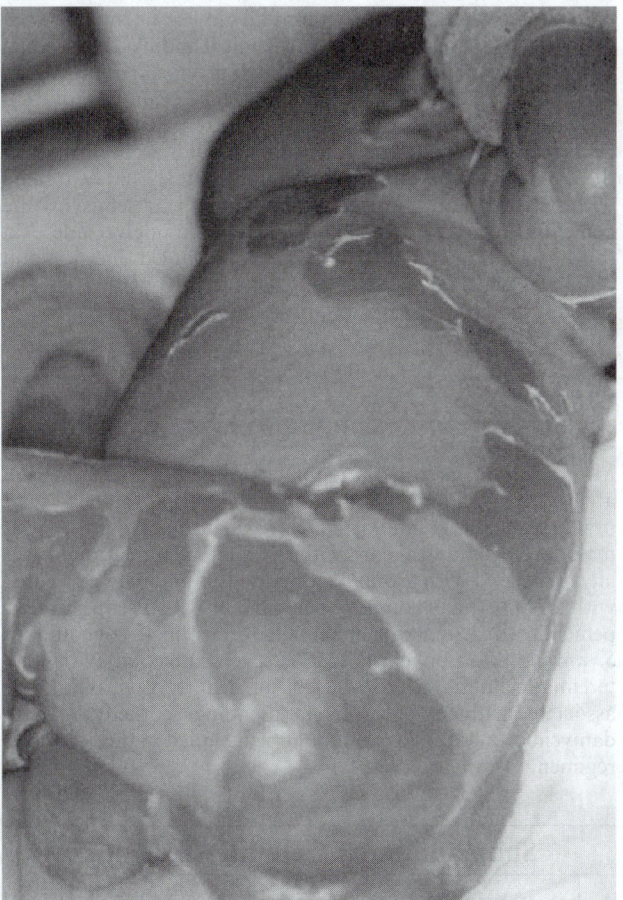

FIGURE 74.2. Scalded skin syndrome. (From Avery GB, Fletcher MA, MacDonald, MG. *Neonatology: pathophysiology and management of the newborn*, 5th ed. Philadelphia: Lippincott Williams & Wilkins, 1999.)

Toxic Shock Syndrome

Toxic shock syndrome is associated with toxins produced by certain strains of *S. aureus*. The focus of infection may not always be apparent. Clinical manifestations in neonates are similar to those seen in older children and adults: sunburn-like rash with mild desquamation occurring in the second week of the illness and multiorgan system involvement with cardiovascular instability. Blood cultures are usually sterile. The toxin-producing staphylococci may be recovered from mucosal surfaces or sites of tissue infection. Intravenous antibiotics and aggressive supportive care are required. Fluid requirements are greater than estimated because of severe capillary leak.

Scalp Abscess

Scalp abscess is a complication of fetal monitoring with scalp electrodes. Any microorganisms present in the birth canal may be implicated. Superficial abscesses are treated with incision, drainage, and cleansing with an antibacterial solution. The presence of cellulitis requires systemic antibiotics. An infected cephalhematoma should be distinguished from a large superficial scalp abscess, and may be complicated by an underlying osteomyelitis.

Mastitis

Mastitis and breast abscess are local lesions that are generally unilateral and present more commonly in female infants, with few, if any, systemic signs. The only clinical findings are swelling with erythema and warmth. Although group B streptococcus and *S. aureus* are the most common agents, gram-negative enteric bacilli have also been isolated. Rarely, bacteremia may be present. A diagnostic aspiration should be performed if there is an area of fluctuation, and the infant should be treated with parenteral antibiotics. A combination of a semisynthetic penicillin (oxacillin or nafcillin) plus an aminoglycoside or a third-generation cephalosporin is recommended. Incision and drainage, when required, should be carried out by a skilled surgeon to avoid damage to normal breast tissue in female infants.

Omphalitis

Minimal drainage from the umbilicus with mild erythema in an afebrile term infant may be treated with local care alone or with oral cephalexin or amoxicillin/clavulanate potassium. A wet, malodorous umbilical cord with minimal inflammation is usually associated with group A streptococcus and may be treated with a 7- to 10-day course of penicillin or with a semisynthetic penicillin (oxacillin or nafcillin) or cefazolin if concomitant *S. aureus* infection exists. More severe infection with bacteremia, cellulitis, necrotizing fasciitis, or peritonitis may be associated with any of the neonatal pathogens; therefore, clindamycin or metronidazole should be included in the antibiotic regimen.

Submandibular Cellulites/Adenitis

A characteristic syndrome of submandibular cellulitis or lymphadenitis has been described in infants with group B streptococcal bacteremia. These infants present at 2 to 10 weeks of age with nonspecific signs of sepsis, fever, and a characteristic swelling with overlying erythema in the submandibular or submental area. Occasionally, the focal cellulitis appears during the first few hours after the patient is admitted to the hospital for treatment of suspected sepsis without a focus. Group B streptococcus is isolated from blood and tissue aspirate. Meningitis is rare. Response to parenteral antibiotic therapy is prompt.

Necrotizing Fasciitis and Ecthyma Gangrenosum

Necrotizing fasciitis and ecthyma gangrenosum are associated with overwhelming sepsis and shock. The initial skin presentation ranges from minimal rash to erythema, induration, or cellulitis. The skin becomes progressively indurated with violaceous discoloration, overlying bullae, and rapid progression to necrosis. The cause may be group B streptococcus alone or mixed bacteria. Most patients have a predisposing condition such as omphalitis, mastitis, balanitis, or use of a fetal scalp electrode. Extensive débridement and broad-spectrum antimicrobials are required in addition to aggressive supportive care. The mortality rate of neonatal necrotizing fasciitis varies from 59% to 85%. Many survivors require skin grafting.

Ecthyma gangrenosum is a manifestation of vasculitis of the cutaneous blood vessels associated with *Pseudomonas aeruginosa* bacteremia, or less commonly, other gram-negative bacilli. The lesion first appears as a vesicle on an erythematous base, then forms a well-demarcated area of induration with a necrotic center surrounded by an erythematous halo. The infecting organism may be isolated from the skin lesion. The septicemia requires parenteral treatment.

Methicillin-resistant *Staphylococcus aureus*

Failure of *S. aureus* skin or soft tissue infections to respond to cephalosporins or semisynthetic penicillins may be caused by methicillin-resistant *S. aureus* (MRSA). Therefore, it is helpful to know whether MRSA is considered endemic locally. Topical mupirocin ointment may be used for superficial MRSA infections. No oral antimicrobial agents that are effective against MRSA are appropriate for use in the neonate. Serious systemic MRSA infections require treatment with vancomycin.

S. aureus, and especially MRSA, infections in the first few weeks of life should be reported to the birth nursery to facilitate recognition of an outbreak in the nursery and implementation of strict infection control measures. Although infections this early in life are most often hospital-acquired, increasing numbers of community-acquired MRSA infections are reported in children without identifiable risk factors.

Suggested Readings

Brook I. The aerobic and anaerobic microbiology of neonatal breast abscess. *Pediatr Infect Dis* 1991;10:785.

Brook I. Cutaneous and subcutaneous infections in newborn due to anaerobic bacteria. *J Perinatal Med* 2002;30:197.

Brook I. Microbiology of necrotizing fasciitis associated with omphalitis in the newborn infant. *J Perinatol* 1998;18:28.

Cimolai N. *Staphylococcus aureus* outbreaks among newborns: new frontiers in an old dilemma. *Am J Perinatol* 2003;20:125.

Conner JM, Soll RF, Edwards WH. Topical ointment for preventing infection in preterm infants. *Cochrane Database Syst Rev* 2004;1:CD001150.

Faden H. Neonatal staphylococcal skin infections. *Pediatr Infect Dis J* 2003; 22:389.

Herold BC, Immergluck LC, Maranan MC, et al. Community-acquired methicillin-resistant *Staphylococcus aureus* in children with no identified predisposing risk. *JAMA* 1998;279:593.

Hsieh WS, Yang PH, Chao HC, et al. Neonatal necrotizing fasciitis: a report of three cases and review of the literature. *Pediatrics* 1999;103:E53.

Jannssen PA, Selwood BL, Dobson SR, et al. To dye or not to dye: a randomized, clinical trial of a triple dye/alcohol regime versus dry cord care. *Pediatrics* 2003;111:15.

Miyairi I, Berlingieri D, Protic J, et al. Neonatal invasive group A streptococcal disease: case report and review of the literature. *Pediatr Infect Dis J* 2004;23:161.

Mullany LC, Darmstadt GL, Tielswch JM. Role of antimicrobial applications to the umbilical cord in neonates to prevent bacterial colonization

and infection: a review of the evidence. *Pediatr Infect Dis J* 2003;22:996.

Nanda S, Reddy BS, Ramji S, et al. Analytic study of pustular eruptions in neonates. *Pediatr Dermatol* 2002;19:210.

Patamasucon P, Siegel JD, McCracken GH Jr. Streptococcal submandibular cellulitis in infants. *Pediatrics* 1981;67:378.

Patel GK, Finlay AY. Staphylococcal scalded skin syndrome: diagnosis and management. *Am J Clin Dermatol* 2003;4:165.

Sawin RS, Schaller RT, Tapper D, et al. Early recognition of neonatal abdominal wall necrotizing fasciitis. *Am J Surg* 1994;167:481.

CHAPTER 75 ■ GROUP B STREPTOCOCCAL DISEASE

CAROL J. BAKER

Lancefield group B *Streptococcus* emerged in the early 1970s as the most frequent cause of neonatal sepsis and meningitis. The reason for this shift in etiologic agents associated with neonatal sepsis remains unknown, despite considerable advances in our understanding of the bacteriologic and immunologic properties of this organism and the pathophysiology, treatment, and prevention of the infections it causes. Group B streptococci also cause pregnancy-related morbidity and invasive infections in infants up to 89 days of age; nonpregnant adults with underlying medical conditions, such as diabetes mellitus, malignancy, immunodeficiency, or neurologic, hepatic, or renal insufficiency; and healthy adults 65 years of age and older. With the implementation of maternal intrapartum antibiotic prophylaxis to prevent early-onset group B streptococcal disease, only one-fifth of the group B streptococcal invasive infections now occur in neonates and young infants.

EPIDEMIOLOGY

Group B streptococci frequently may be recovered from the lower genital and gastrointestinal tracts of pregnant women, but its presence rarely is associated with symptoms before rupture of membranes or labor. Reported carriage rates of group B streptococci in parturients vary from 15% to 40%. Variations are due not only to differences in age, ethnic origin, and geographic location but also to the site and number of culture specimens taken and to differences in bacteriologic methods for the growth and isolation of group B streptococci. Colonization rates are higher in teenagers and black women as compared with white and Hispanic women, and rates are significantly lower in women who are Asian or Native American or Alaskan. When cultures are collected from the lower vagina and rectum (rather than from the cervix or anal orifice) and processed in antibiotic-containing (selective) broth (not solid) media, colonization rates usually are 25% to 40%.

Early-Onset Disease

Clinically and epidemiologically, infant group B streptococcal infection can be divided into two distinct syndromes on the basis of age at onset. Early-onset disease appears within the first 6 days of life and historically had an attack rate of 1.3 to 3.7 per 1,000 live births. The incidence, as of 2003, had fallen to 0.32 per 1,000 live births following the 2002 recommendation for universal group B streptococcal culture screening during pregnancy and intrapartum chemoprophylaxis for all culture-positive women. Nearly 90% of early-onset cases and almost all fatal infections occur during the first day of life. Maternal factors increasing risk for early-onset disease are group B streptococcal bacteriuria during pregnancy, preterm delivery, intrapartum fever, prolonged rupture of membranes is greater than or equal to 18 hours, and African-American ethnicity and perhaps age younger than 20 years. Attack rates are related inversely to birth weight, but most neonates (nearly 80%) with early-onset disease are born at 37 or more weeks of gestation.

Late and Very Late-Onset Disease

Late-onset disease, which occurs at 7 through 89 days of age, has an incidence of 0.4 to 1.7 of 1,000 live births. Except for preterm delivery, the obstetric complications commonly accompanying early-onset disease are not factors associated with the later presentation of infant group B streptococcal infection. Very late-onset disease has been described in very low-birth-weight infants who remain hospitalized and susceptible, presumably through acquisition of colonization at mucous membrane sites and by virtue of immature immune status. Another group of infants with very late-onset infection are those with human immunodeficiency virus (HIV) infection. Very late-onset cases may account for up to 20% of infant group B streptococcal cases. Low levels of maternally derived serum IgG antibody directed against group B streptococcal capsular polysaccharide at delivery also increase the risk for invasive disease, no matter the age at onset.

Serotypes in Early and Late-Onset Disease

The distribution of serotypes has both epidemiologic and clinical significance. In surveys of large numbers of colonized young adults, children, and neonates, five of the nine defined capsular serotypes (Ia, Ib, II, III, and V) are dominant. Colonized neonates reflect the serotype of their mothers in all but the rare infant who acquires group B streptococci from nursery personnel or the community. Serotypes Ia, Ib, II, III, and V account for approximately 35%, 10%, 15%, 30%, and 15%, respectively, of the cases of early-onset disease. Serotype III causes some 85% of cases of group B streptococcal meningitis, regardless of age, and 75% of late-onset disease, irrespective of clinical presentation.

PATHOGENESIS

Streptococcus agalactiae, or group B streptococcus, is a facultative, encapsulated, gram-positive diplococcus that produces a narrow zone of beta-hemolysis on sheep blood agar surrounding flat, grayish white, mucoid colonies. Nonhemolytic and alpha-hemolytic strains have been isolated rarely (approximately 1% to 2%) from humans with invasive infection.

All strains of group B streptococci share the group B–specific cell wall carbohydrate antigen originally defined by Lancefield. The strains may be classified into nine serotypes on the basis of capsular polysaccharides (type-specific antigens) and a surface protein, c, which has two component alpha and beta. The polysaccharide antigens are designated Ia, Ib, II to VII. Strains possessing both the Ia polysaccharide antigen and the c protein antigen now are designated Ia/c (formerly, Ic). The c protein is found on all type Ib, up to 60% type II, and occasional III, IV, and V strains. Surface proteins identified as R and X antigens are found on many strains but have not been associated with virulence. The capsular polysaccharide is the major virulence factor for group B streptococci. Antibodies to these structures are protective for homologous but not heterologous serotypes. The c protein also is a virulence factor, and antibodies to c protein are protective against experimental challenge with strains containing this antigen, but data for humans is lacking. Recent evidence suggests that the extracellular enzyme, beta-hemolysin, also relates to virulence of this organism.

Acquisition of the Organism

The transmission of group B streptococci to the neonate can occur whenever a delivering mother harbors the organism. Exposure may occur by ascending infection through ruptured or (uncommonly) intact amniotic membranes or by aspiration or swallowing of or surface contamination with vaginal fluid as the infant descends through the birth canal. Vertical transmission accounts for asymptomatic infection (or colonization) in approximately 50% of infants born to mothers carrying group B streptococci at delivery. Mothers with "heavy" colonization (more than 10^5 colony-forming units per milliliter) are more likely to transmit the organism to their infants and to deliver a neonate who develops early-onset group B streptococcal disease. Despite the high rate of transmission and colonization in newborns, overall only 1% to 2% of infants born to colonized mothers who don't receive intrapartum chemoprophylaxis develop invasive infection. Initial colonization can persist for weeks to months at various mucous membrane sites. Acquisition of the organism by neonates after hospital discharge has been reported to be uncommon, but few studies have addressed this setting for potential transmission.

Mucosal Colonization and Tissue Invasion

Genital or gastrointestinal colonization in mothers at delivery provides infant exposure that is the necessary prelude of early-onset group B streptococcal infection. The degree of risk correlates directly with the degree (inoculum) of maternal colonization (heavy or light). A direct relationship between length of membrane rupture before delivery and risk of invasive infant disease also has been documented and, because amniotic fluid readily supports the replication of group B streptococci, the longer the interval, the higher is the inoculum. The invasion of respiratory tract epithelium, pulmonary interstitium, endothelium of the pulmonary vessels, and (finally) bacteremia presumably follow aspiration of infected amniotic fluid or birth canal contents. Several case series document that 35% to 65% of infants are symptomatic at birth, indicating that infection often begins *in utero*. In late-onset infection, presumably the first step in pathogenesis is the adherence of group B streptococci to the epithelium in the upper respiratory or gastrointestinal tract, resulting in colonization. Surface proteins, such as adhesins, have been implicated, but their role has been incompletely defined. The mechanisms by which organisms replicating at mucosal surfaces invade are not elucidated, but the presence of capsule is crucial to virulence once the organism reaches the bloodstream. Immaturity of a variety of host defense mechanisms undoubtedly contributes to the age-limited susceptibility of neonates and young infants to invasive group B streptococcal infection.

Bacterial Virulence and Host Defense

The evasion of host defenses is critical to the survival and replication of group B streptococci *in vivo*. When compared to immune effector mechanisms in adults and older infants, neonates (especially preterm infants) are developmentally deficient. Group B streptococci elaborate surface molecules, including capsule, which inhibit host defenses. Pulmonary alveolar macrophages and monocytes [but not polymorphonuclear leukocytes (PMNLs)] are recruited into the alveoli of infants with early-onset infection, but the capsular polysaccharide attenuates this response. This decreased ability to recruit host cells effectively correlates with diminished pulmonary clearance. Once bacteremia ensues, the capsule of the organism, which is necessary for virulence in animal models of lethal bacteremia, inhibits deposition of complement proteins and phagocytosis by PMNLs. In the absence of a sufficient quantity of type-specific antibodies directed against the capsular polysaccharide or of complement, phagocytosis of group B streptococci by PMNLs is minimal.

The role of surface receptors and functional abnormalities in neonatal PMNLs appear important in the pathogenesis and outcome of invasive infection. The development of profound neutropenia in fulminant early-onset sepsis is known to relate to an exhaustion of neutrophil reserves in the bone marrow, and this development occurs rapidly in some infants.

Type-specific immunity also is important in considering the pathogenesis of group B streptococcal infections. One of the earliest observations was that neonates at greatest risk for infection with type III strains were those with low levels of maternally derived type-specific serum antibody to the type III capsular polysaccharide. *In vitro* assays of the functional capacity of this type III–specific group B streptococcal antibody indicate that opsonization, ingestion by PMNLs, and killing of type III group B streptococci require a sufficient amount of type III–specific IgG and complement. Similar observations have been reported for serotypes Ia, Ib, II, and V. The relative deficiency of type-specific group B streptococcal antibodies in cord sera may be related either to very low levels in sera of women of childbearing age (documented in 80% to 90% in most studies) or to failure of placental transport of available maternal antibodies caused by placental abnormalities, delivery before 34 weeks' gestation, or both.

Although the pathogenesis of late-onset group B streptococcal infection is not as well understood, type III strains appear to be uniquely virulent for the healthy term infant older than 6 days. As in those with early-onset infection, infants with late-onset disease exhibit low levels of type-specific antibody in their sera, as do their mothers. The common association of upper respiratory infection with late-onset group B streptococcal meningitis leads to speculation that alteration of the respiratory epithelium by a viral agent favors invasion of epithelium and subsequent bacteremia. Type III strains, the most frequent cause of late-onset disease, elaborate high levels of type-specific polysaccharide into the blood as they multiply, and this contributes to their virulence. The relationship between the terminal sialic acid determinant to the tertiary structure of the type III polysaccharide also allows these organisms to escape several host immune-effector mechanisms.

Presumably, group B streptococci are capable of entering the blood–brain barrier through complex evasive maneuvers. Interactions between type-specific antibodies and serum complement components are important to the opsonization and phagocytosis of type III group B streptococcus and, presumably, bloodstream clearance, but little is known about host–pathogen interactions in the cerebrospinal fluid.

Inflammatory Mediators

Inflammatory mediators play a major role in the pathogenesis of group B streptococcal sepsis. Once invasive infection is established, ongoing replication and degradation of organisms can instigate host inflammatory responses that may be deleterious. Neonates recovering from group B streptococcal disease have circulating immune complexes that may contribute to end-organ damage. These immune complexes also elicit inflammatory mediators, such as leukotriene B$_4$ and interleukin-6 (IL-6). Group B streptococcal cell wall components, particularly peptidoglycan, elicit tumor necrosis factor-alpha (TNF-α), IL-1, IL-6, and granulocyte colony-stimulating factor. TNF-α is found in the acute serum of up to 50% of infants with group B streptococcal sepsis. In animal models of lethal sepsis, pretreatment with either pentoxifylline, which blocks TNF-α, or a monoclonal antibody to TNF-α modestly improves outcome. If pentoxifylline and indomethacin (a blocker of eicosanoid production) are combined in a piglet model of sepsis, however, hypoxemia and pulmonary hypertension are reduced significantly. This suggests that TNF-α and eicosanoids, including thromboxane A$_2$ and prostaglandin I$_2$, have a synergistic effect in sepsis caused by group B streptococcus. In the same model, IL-1 receptor antagonist ameliorates systemic hypotension and prolongs survival. Additional data will be required to characterize fully the inflammatory mechanisms that dictate the clinical consequences of group B streptococcal disease in neonates and young infants.

Pathologic Findings

The pathologic findings in infants with fatal group B streptococcal infection depend on age at onset and clinical syndrome. Histologic findings of congenital pneumonia and atypical hyaline membranes containing these bacteria are characteristic of infants with early-onset group B streptococcal sepsis with pulmonary involvement. In early-onset meningitis, evidence of meningeal inflammation is present in a few infants. Perivascular inflammation with small-vessel thrombosis and parenchymal hemorrhage is found frequently. Some premature infants surviving group B streptococcal sepsis complicated by hypotension develop periventricular leukomalacia, indicating infarction of the white matter around the lateral ventricles. Older infants with fatal group B streptococcal meningitis usually have purulent leptomeningitis and a large number of organisms in the CSF.

CLINICAL MANIFESTATIONS AND COMPLICATIONS

Early-Onset Disease

Early-onset infection usually appears at or within hours of birth (Table 75.1). The highest attack rate is observed in preterm infants born to women with known obstetric factors posing a risk for neonatal sepsis. Clinical syndromes include bacteremia without a focus, pneumonia, and meningitis. Pneumonia and meningitis typically are accompanied by bacteremia. However, it has been estimated before the era of maternal chemoprophylaxis that a single blood culture is sterile in 10% to 15% of cases. Such respiratory signs as tachypnea, grunting, retractions, and cyanosis or an unexpected apneic episode in a previously healthy, term neonate are the first clues of illness in most infants, regardless of the primary focus of infection. Poor perfusion is a presenting finding in some one-fourth of cases and usually is found at birth in infants with *in utero* onset of infection. Nonspecific signs, such as lethargy, poor feeding, tachycardia, and fever, most often occur in term infants without respiratory symptoms. Features predictive of fatal outcome are birth weight of less than 2,500 g, pleural effusion by initial chest radiograph, absolute neutrophil count less than 1,500 per cubic millimeter, apnea, hypotension in the first 12 hours, and initial blood pH of less than 7.25.

Nearly 40% of neonates with early-onset group B streptococcal infection have pulmonary findings. One-third of these infants demonstrate radiographic evidence of congenital pneumonia with distinct infiltrates, and approximately one-half have findings typical of respiratory distress syndrome or transient tachypnea. Among remaining infants, a few exhibit small pleural effusions or pulmonary edema, and in some the initial

TABLE 75.1

COMPARISON OF EARLY- AND LATE-ONSET GROUP B STREPTOCOCCAL INFECTION IN NEONATES

	Early-Onset	Late-Onset	Very Late-Onset
Mean age at onset of symptoms	8 hr	27 d	>3 mo
Incidence	1.3–3.7 per 1,000 live births	0.6–1.7 per 1,000 live births	Unknown
Maternal obstetric risks for sepsis	Common	Uncommon	Common
Common clinical presentations	Pneumonia (40%); meningitis (10%), bacteremia without focus (45%)	Bacteremia without focus (55%); meningitis (35%); osteomyelitis arthritis (5%)	Same as late-onset
Common serotypes	1 (la, lb/c, la/c), III, V	III (75%)	Unknown
Case-fatality rate	5–10%	2–5%	Low

chest radiograph is normal. Reports describe neonates with early-onset group B streptococcal sepsis manifested by respiratory distress, persistent pulmonary hypertension, and a normal chest radiograph. After the development of sepsis, some infants develop hypoxemia and multiorgan failure.

Group B streptococcal meningitis is clinically indistinguishable from bacteremia with or without pulmonary involvement. For this reason, lumbar puncture for cerebrospinal fluid (CSF) studies and culture is always required for accurate diagnosis and appropriate therapy. Reports indicate that meningitis has decreased in frequency from some 25% to less than 10% of cases. Although seizure activity may develop in half of the neonates with group B streptococcal meningitis, rarely is it the presenting symptom. Prolonged seizure activity, focal neurologic signs, or coma are associated with poor outcome, as is the occurrence of shock, neutropenia, or a CSF protein level greater than 300 mg/dL.

Late-Onset Disease

Late-onset group B streptococcal infection occurs in infants at 7 to 89 days of age and has diverse clinical manifestations. The mean age at onset is approximately 24 days, unless the infant was born before 32 weeks' gestation, when presentation may extend until 5 to 7 months of age. The obstetric and early neonatal course usually are uneventful. Although some infants exhibit only fever and mild irritability, others have a few hours of illness culminated by septic shock, neutropenia, and death. As with early-onset infection, infants may present with bacteremia without a focus or may have localization to the central nervous system, skeletal system, soft tissues, or a variety of other foci.

When first described, the most frequent clinical manifestation of late-onset group B streptococcal infection was meningitis. Now, bacteremia without a focus is the most frequent presentation (~65% of cases), perhaps reflecting earlier diagnosis and therapy. Infants with late-onset group B streptococcal disease have comparatively fewer respiratory symptoms than do their early-onset counterparts, but a preceding or concurrent upper respiratory infection is noted in 20% to 30%. In those infants with meningitis (~25% of cases), the course often may be complicated by seizures, diminished perfusion, or apnea, but anticipatory care with timely and appropriate interventions prevent additional morbidity. Meningitis may result in serious intracranial complications, such as focal cerebritis, vascular thrombosis, obstructive ventriculitis, subdural empyema, and communicating hydrocephalus.

Infants with nonmeningeal- focal late-onset infections regularly have accompanying bacteremia. The exception is osteomyelitis. The somewhat older age at onset (mean, 31 days) and the finding of a lytic bone lesion at presentation suggest that osteomyelitis may be acquired during a self-limited early-onset group B streptococcal bacteremia. Group B streptococcal osteomyelitis follows an indolent course with few systemic signs. Decreased use of the involved extremity and pain with passive movement are typical findings. Infants often have a relatively long history before diagnosis (mean, 9 days). Unlike other pathogens causing neonatal osteomyelitis, group B *Streptococcus* has a predilection for the proximal humerus; the femur is the second most common site involved. Rarely is more than a single bone involved. Up to 70% of infants have accompanying pyarthrosis of the adjacent joint. Group B streptococcal septic arthritis without osteomyelitis occurs almost exclusively in the lower extremities and usually involves the hip joint. Onset of illness is acute (mean duration of symptoms before diagnosis, 1.5 days), and concurrent bacteremia is typical.

A variety of foci of late-onset group B streptococcal infection have been reported, but these are uncommon in compar-

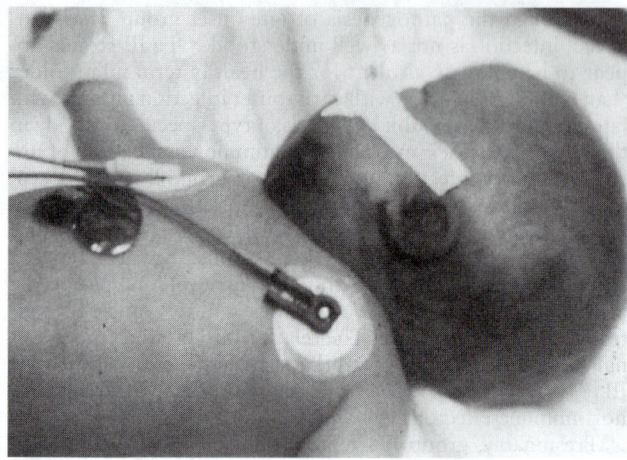

FIGURE 75.1. Necrotizing fascitis of the submandibular area and pinna in a 3-month-old premature infant with late-onset group B streptococcal sepsis. See Color Figure 75.1 in color section.

ison to bacteremia without a focus, meningitis, and bone and joint infection. Infants with facial or submandibular cellulitis due to group B streptococci have been described, as have other soft tissue infections that include adenitis, necrotizing fasciitis, omphalitis, and scalp and breast abscesses (Figs. 75.1 and 75.2). Otitis media alone or in association with facial cellulitis or meningitis also occurs. Endocarditis, pericarditis, myocarditis, endophthalmitis, urinary tract infection, pleural empyema, pneumonia, and peritonitis are rare. Infants with focal infection typically have accompanying bacteremia, and a few also may have meningeal involvement.

DIAGNOSIS

The clinical manifestations of early-onset group B streptococcal infection resemble those of neonatal sepsis resulting from other pathogens. In the preterm infant, the clinical and radiographic distinction between group B streptococcal pneumonia and respiratory distress syndrome or transient tachypnea at onset of illness is impossible. Helpful features suggesting group

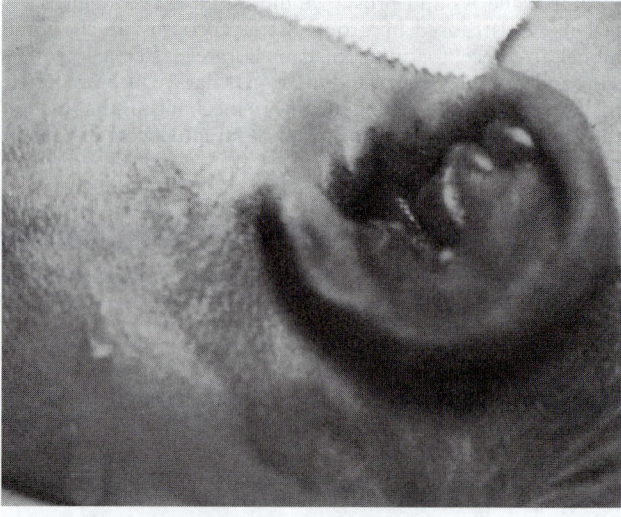

FIGURE 75.2. Close-up of the pinna of the 3-month-old premature infant in Figure 75.1. See Color Figure 75.2 in color section.

B streptococcal pneumonia in this kind of patient are maternal risk factors for sepsis, apnea, and shock within the first 24 hours of life, an Apgar score of less than 5 at 1 minute, neutropenia, and cardiomegaly or pleural effusion on the chest radiograph. None of these features, however, is specific for group B streptococci, and each may be observed with other etiologic agents causing early-onset neonatal pneumonia. Because clinical findings alone cannot identify the 5% of infants with meningeal involvement, each infant with clinical signs of sepsis requires a lumbar puncture as part of the evaluation, unless the clinical condition mandates its deferral until stabilization has been achieved.

The differential diagnosis for late-onset group B streptococcal infection depends somewhat on the focus of infection. Infants who have bacteremia without a focus may present with nonspecific signs and fever, and they may be thought to have a viral illness. Only a high index of suspicion and collection of blood and CSF specimens for culture will lead to a specific diagnosis. The relative lack of systemic findings in an infant of less than 2 months of age with a metaphyseal lytic bone lesion, especially of the humerus, strongly suggests group B streptococcal osteomyelitis. Until group B streptococci are isolated from a bone aspirate or biopsy sample of the affected area, however, other etiologic agents such as *Staphylococcus aureus* and gram-negative enterics must be considered. The diversity of clinical presentations of late-onset group B streptococcal infection requires that it be appreciated as a possible etiologic agent in unknown infection at any site in infants 1 to 12 weeks of age. Isolation of group B streptococci from a normally sterile body site (blood, CSF, bone, synovial fluid, urine) is the only way to prove invasive group B streptococcal infection. Isolation of the organism from skin or mucosal surfaces is not diagnostically significant. Previously, rapid tests that detected the group B streptococcal polysaccharide antigen in urine, serum, or other body fluids were used for diagnosis, but their insufficient sensitivity and poor specificity resulted in discontinuation of their use except for CSF samples.

THERAPY

Penicillin G is the drug of choice for group B streptococcal infections because isolates remain uniformly susceptible. They also are susceptible *in vitro* to first-, second-, and third-generation cephalosporins, semisynthetic penicillins, and vancomycin. Resistance of group B streptococci to the aminoglycosides, colistin, bacitracin, trimethoprim-sulfamethoxazole, and metronidazole is uniform. Susceptibility of group B streptococci to penicillin G is related directly to the inoculum in a body fluid. The high inoculum often found in the CSF of infants with meningitis suggests that these infants may require substantially higher antibiotic concentrations in the CSF to inhibit growth. The combination of an aminoglycoside (usually gentamicin) with penicillin G or ampicillin is synergistic in killing group B streptococci *in vitro* and in experimental animal models. Ampicillin and gentamicin produce rapid killing of group B streptococci and are recommended for initial treatment of group B streptococcal infection and for sepsis of unknown etiology in the infant younger than 1 month. Once group B streptococci are identified in cultures, therapy may be modified to penicillin G alone. Delay in sterilizing CSF (achieved in 95% of patients within 24 to 36 hours) may be related to inadequate antibiotic dose, a high initial CSF inoculum, or an unexpected suppurative focus in the central nervous system. Ampicillin and gentamicin should be continued until sterilization of the CSF has been documented by repeat lumbar puncture (usually at 24 to 48 hours), at which time the regimen may be changed to penicillin G alone.

The optimal dose of penicillin G for treatment of group B streptococcal meningitis has not been investigated, but several facts argue for the use of high-dose therapy. Group B streptococci have relatively high minimal inhibitory concentrations to penicillin G, especially when considering levels achievable in the CSF. Infants with group B streptococcal meningitis often have a high group B streptococcal inoculum in the CSF, which would increase the minimal bactericidal concentration. Reported cases of relapse have been associated primarily with doses of penicillin G of less than 200,000 U/kg/day. Finally, penicillin G is safe in neonates in doses up to 600,000 U/kg/day. For these reasons, penicillin G at a dose of 450,000 to 500,000 U/ kg/day or ampicillin, 300 mg/kg/day, is recommended for treatment of group B streptococcal meningitis. Doses of approximately one-half these amounts are suggested for treatment of non–central nervous system infections. Therapy for 10 days is adequate for pneumonia, bacteremia without a focus, and most soft tissue infections. Two to 3 weeks of treatment are suggested for meningitis, septic arthritis, and severe soft tissue or lymph node infections, and 3 to 4 weeks for osteomyelitis, endocarditis, and ventriculitis (Table 75.2). These recommendations, however, must be tailored to each case. In cases of recurrent infection, eradication of mucosal colonization is desirable. However, administration of oral rifampin given once daily for 4 days (20 mg/kg/day) was not reliably effective, and other antibiotics have not been investigated.

Aggressive supportive measures are responsible for much of the increased survival in infants with invasive group B streptococcal infection. Improved ventilatory care has eased the management of respiratory distress secondary to group B

TABLE 75.2

RECOMMENDED TREATMENT REGIMENS FOR GROUP B STREPTOCOCCAL INFECTIONS IN INFANTS

Clinical Presentation	Antibiotic	Dose (Kilogram Body Weight Per Day)	Duration (d)
Meningitis	Ampicillin plus gentamicin; then penicillin G	300–400 mg plus 7.5 mg;[a] then 400,000–500,000 U	Until cerebrospinal fluid is sterile and strain is known to be susceptible to penicillin G; to complete 14–21[b]
Bacteremia, soft tissue infection, pneumonia	Penicillin G	150,000–200,000 U	10
Septic arthritis	Penicillin G	200,000–300,000 U	14–21
Osteomyelitis	Penicillin G	200,000–300,000 U	21–28
Endocarditis	Penicillin G	300,000–400,000 U[c]	≥28

[a]Antibiotic dose should be modified for low birth weight or age <7 days.
[b]If ventriculitis, extend therapy for 21–28 days.
[c]Plus gentamicin for the first 14 days.

streptococcal pneumonia. Poor perfusion and metabolic acidosis can be treated with both volume expansion and infusion of pressor agents, and seizure activity can be controlled with anticonvulsants. Modern monitoring equipment renders anticipation of these consequences of group B streptococcal infection less problematic. Less conventional adjunctive therapies have been explored in many centers. Granulocyte transfusions in neutropenic infants, infusion of human intravenous immunoglobulin, and extracorporeal membrane oxygenation are among the therapeutic modalities investigated, but none of these is recommended for routine use.

PROGNOSIS

Complications of infant group B streptococcal infection range from negligible functional deficits in infants with septic arthritis to the profound neurologic consequences of severe meningitis. The mortality rate for early-onset infection is estimated to be 5% to 10% (higher in premature infants) and for late-onset disease from 2% to 6%. Factors associated with a fatal outcome in early-onset infection include prematurity, shock, neutropenia, apnea, a 5-minute Apgar score of 6, pleural effusion on the initial chest radiograph, and an initial blood pH of <7.25. Those factors related to death or permanent neurologic sequelae after meningitis are hypotension, neutropenia, coma, status epilepticus, and an initial CSF protein of greater than 300 mg/dL. Three series reported sequelae in survivors of group B streptococcal meningitis up to 8 years after illness. Major neurologic sequelae including global mental retardation, spastic quadriplegia, uncontrolled seizures, cortical blindness, deafness, hydrocephalus, and hypothalamic dysfunction occurred in 17% to 21%. Less severe sequelae, such as spastic or flaccid paresis of one limb, speech and language delay, controlled seizure disorders, unilateral deafness, and mild cortical atrophy seen by computed tomography (CT) of the head, were found in some 20%. The decreasing mortality rate found in many centers may be accompanied also by a lower sequelae rate. Studies published more than two decades ago indicate that at least 70% of the survivors of group B streptococcal meningitis function at or near their age-expected level.

One unusual complication of group B streptococcal sepsis is the unexplained association of early-onset infection with acquired right-sided diaphragmatic hernia. Insufficient diaphragmatic motion has been hypothesized to predispose infected infants to the development of pneumonia, and subsequent respiratory effort leads to herniation.

Relapse or recurrence of infection of both the early- and late-onset type have been reported in an estimated 1% to 2% of cases. In a few cases, however, circumstances (maternal mastitis, undrained abscess, congenital heart disease in an infant with endocarditis and underlying immune deficiency) may predispose infants to recurrence. In the vast majority, however, the reason for recurrence is not apparent. The opportunity for recurrent infection with optimal therapy exists in most patients, because intravenous therapy with beta-lactam antibiotics does not eliminate mucous membrane colonization with group B streptococci. Also, most infants do not develop protective immunity after recovery from sepsis or meningitis. Thus, the opportunity for recurrent bacteremia exists, sometimes with dissemination to focal sites, including the meninges. Molecular techniques have shown that the majority of these recurrent infections are due to the strain implicated in the first episode, suggesting persistent mucosal colonization as the underlying source. Studies attempting to eradicate mucosal colonization in mothers and infants, to date, have been unsuccessful, but an effective method to do this is needed.

PREVENTION

Maternal Intrapartum Prophylaxis

Efforts to prevent neonatal group B streptococcal infection have aimed either to decrease the frequency of group B streptococcal exposure of infants at birth or to alter their immune status. Most widely investigated are attempts to eliminate infant exposure during birth. The first evaluated approach was to attempt to eliminate maternal colonization during pregnancy. Courses of oral ampicillin or penicillin (with or without concurrent treatment of sexual partners) during the third trimester of pregnancy were ineffective in decreasing colonization at delivery. Next, several controlled clinical trials using intravenous ampicillin or penicillin G during labor in women known to carry group B streptococci significantly reduced both vertical transmission of group B streptococci and early-onset disease in neonates.

With the publication of consensus recommendations from the Centers for Disease Control and Prevention, the American College of Obstetricians and Gynecologists, and the American Academy of Pediatrics in 1996 and 1997, maternal intrapartum chemoprophylaxis has become routine. Selection of women initially was based on use of one of two strategies: culture-based screening for group B streptococcal colonization or detection upon admission for delivery of one or more risk factors known to enhance risk for neonatal disease. Active multistate population-based surveillance data now have documented the significant impact of intrapartum antibiotic prophylaxis in the prevention of early-onset infection. The incidence has decreased by 75%, from 1.7 per 1,000 live births in 1993 to 0.35 per 1,000 in 2003. In addition, a multistate retrospective cohort study comparing the effectiveness of the two interventions found that the risk of early-onset disease was significantly lower among the infants of culture-screened women than among those in the risk-based group. The culture screening approach was more than 50% more effective than the risk-based approach in preventing early-onset group B streptococcal disease.

In 2002, revised recommendations from the Centers for Disease Control and Prevention recommend the universal screening of all pregnant women at 35 to 37 weeks' gestation for vaginal and rectal group B streptococcal colonization. Swab specimens should be placed in a transport medium, processed by the microbiology laboratory in selective (antibiotic-containing) broth medium with overnight incubation, and then subcultured onto blood agar medium. The only exceptions to the recommendation for universal screening are women with group B streptococcal bacteriuria during the current pregnancy and those with a previous infant with invasive group B streptococcal disease. These women *always* should receive intrapartum prophylaxis. The risk-based approach should now only be used in situations in which the colonization status is not known at onset of labor or rupture of membranes. In that setting, women with gestations less than 37 weeks, duration of membrane rupture 18 hours or longer, or intrapartum fever of 38°C or more should be given prophylaxis. Women who have group B streptococcal colonization and have a cesarean delivery performed before the rupture of membranes and onset of labor *do not* require intrapartum prophylaxis routinely (Fig. 75.3).

The maternal prophylaxis regimen of choice is intravenous penicillin G at an initial dose of 5 million units, followed by 2.5 million units every 4 hours until delivery. An alternative regimen is intravenous ampicillin at an initial dose of 2 g followed by 1 g every 4 hours until delivery. Because of the increasing prevalence of group B streptococcal resistance to erythromycin (approximately 25%) and clindamycin (approximately 20%), cefazolin at an initial dose of 2 g followed by 1 g every 8 hours is

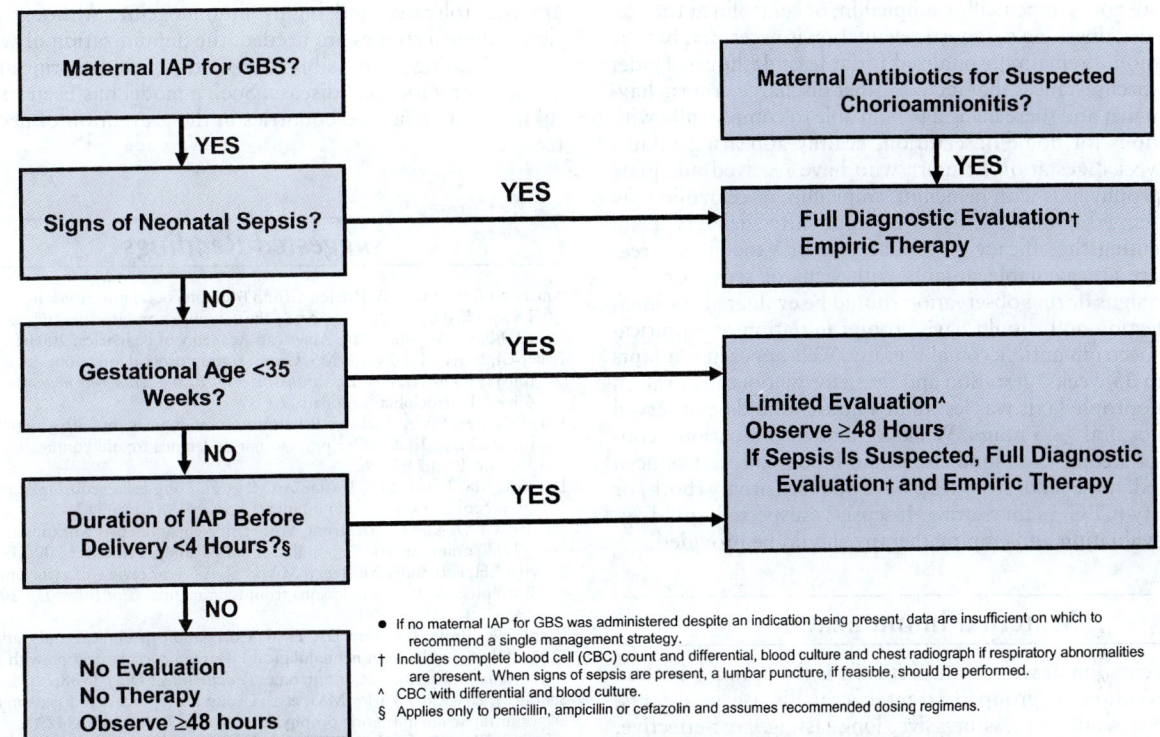

FIGURE 75.3. Algorithm for recommended use of maternal intrapartum antibiotic prophylaxis (IAP) with penicillin, ampicillin, or cefazolin (see text) for the prevention of early-onset GBS disease. (Adapted with permission from Pickering LK, ed. *2003 Red book*. Elk Grove Village, IL: American Academy of Pediatrics, 2003;588.)

recommended for women who are allergic to penicillin but at low risk for anaphylaxis. Clindamycin given every 8 hours may be employed if the colonizing isolate has been tested and found to be clindamycin susceptible. For women at high risk for penicillin anaphylaxis, vancomycin is the antimicrobial of choice, but no data indicate either the duration before delivery that is effective or whether vancomycin penetrates into the amniotic fluid in concentrations sufficient to kill GBS.

Management of Neonates

The management of neonates born to women given chemoprophylaxis depends on clinical status at birth, gestational age, and the duration of antimicrobial prophylaxis before delivery (Fig. 75.4). If the neonate appears healthy, has an estimated gestational age of 35 weeks or more, and has a mother who received

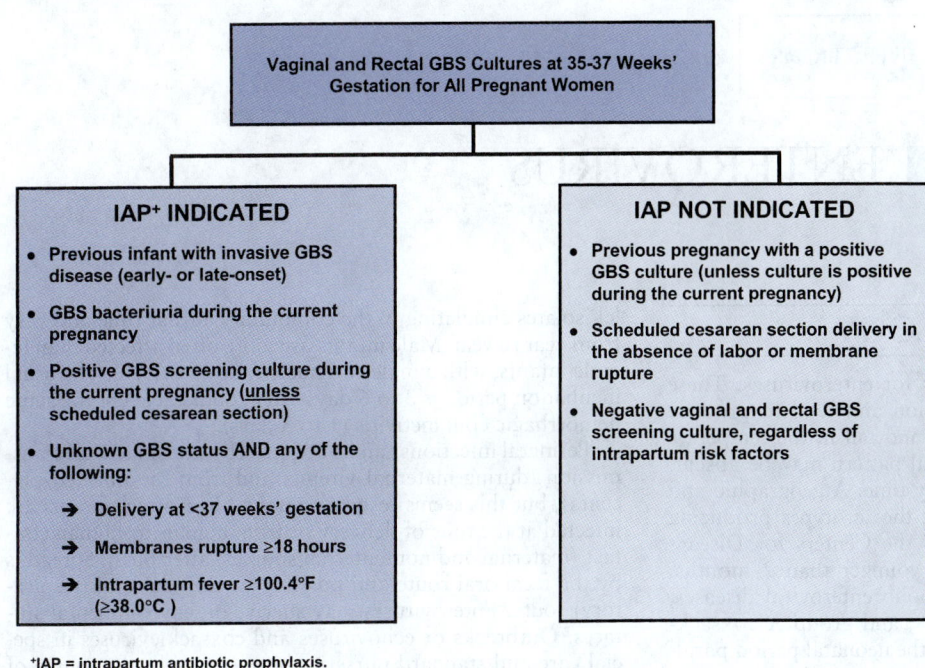

FIGURE 75.4. Algorithm for the management of neonates born to GBS screening culture positive women based on clinical characteristics, gestation and duration of IAP (penicillin, ampicillin or cefazolin) before delivery. (Adapted with permission from Pickering LK, ed. *2003 Red book*. Elk Grove Village, IL: American Academy of Pediatrics, 2003; 590.)

4 or more hours of penicillin, ampicillin, or cefazolin at the recommended doses, no diagnostic evaluation is necessary, but the infant should remain hospitalized for at least 48 hours. Under certain circumstances that include other discharge criteria having been met and there being a person able to comply fully with instructions for home observation, healthy-appearing infants of 38 weeks' gestation or more who have received adequate chemoprophylaxis with penicillin, ampicillin, or cefazolin may be discharged home as early as 24 hours after delivery. Data documenting the efficacy of clindamycin or vancomycin regimens are not available. Infants with signs of sepsis or who develop signs during observation should be evaluated for invasive infection and should have prompt initiation of empirical broad-spectrum antimicrobial therapy. Well-appearing infants less than 35 weeks' gestation and those for whom the duration of chemoprophylaxis was less than 4 hours should be observed in the hospital ≥48 hours. While a "limited evaluation" consisting of a complete blood count and blood culture has been suggested, these laboratory tests have poor sensitivity (both) or specificity (CBC) in this setting. If sepsis is suspected, full diagnostic evaluation and empiric therapy should be provided.

Maternal Immunization

The vaccination of women theoretically is the optimal method for prevention of group B streptococcal disease in infants, because it would be less invasive, long-lasting, cost-effective, and could prevent both early- and late-onset disease. Capsular polysaccharide-protein conjugate vaccines for group B streptococcal types Ia, Ib, II, III, and V have been developed; these are demonstrated to be immunogenic in animals and to induce antibodies that are protective against experimental challenge. Clinical trials to date in nonpregnant adults indicate that they are well tolerated and highly immunogenic. Although additional clinical studies are needed, the immunization of women of childbearing age possibly may protect their offspring against group B streptococcal disease. Such a model has been successful in resource-limited countries in the prevention of neonatal tetanus.

Suggested Readings

American Academy of Pediatrics. Group B streptococcal infections. In: Pickering LK, ed. *Red book: 2003 report of the committee on infectious diseases,* 26th ed. Elk Grove Village, IL: American Academy of Pediatrics; 2003:584.

Baker CJ, Nizet VJ, Edwards MS. Group B streptococcal infections. In: Remington JS, Klein JO, eds. *Infectious diseases of the fetus and newborn infant,* 6th ed. Philadelphia: Saunders, 2005.

Baker CJ, Rench MA, McInnes P. Immunization of pregnant with group B streptococcal type III capsular polysaccharide-tetanus toxoid conjugate vaccine. *Vaccine* 2003;21:3468.

Edwards MS, Rench MA, Haffar AAM, et al. Long-term sequelae of group B streptococcal meningitis in infants. *J Pediatr* 1985;106:717.

Escobar GJ, De-kun L, Armstrong MA, et al. Neonatal sepsis workups in infants ≥2,000 grams at birth: a population-based study. *Pediatrics* 2000;106:256.

Moylett EH, Fernandez M, Rench MA, et al. A 5-year review of recurrent group B streptococcal disease: lessons from twin infants. *Clin Infect Dis* 2000;30:282.

Payne NR, Burke BA, Day DL, et al. Correlation of clinical and pathologic findings in early-onset neonatal group B streptococcal infection with disease severity and prediction of outcome. *Pediatr Infect Dis J* 1988;7:836.

Schrag SJ, Zywicki S, Farley MM, et al. Group B streptococcal disease in the era of intrapartum antibiotic prophylaxis. *N Engl J Med* 2000;342:15.

Schrag SJ, Zell ER, Stat M, et al. A population-based comparison of strategies to prevent early-onset group B streptococcal disease in neonates. *N Engl J Med* 2002;347:233.

Schuchat A. Epidemiology of group B streptococcal disease in the United States: shifting paradigms. *Clin Microbiol Rev* 1998;11:497.

Yagupsky P, Menegus M, Powell KR. The changing spectrum of group B streptococcal disease in infants: an eleven-year experience in a tertiary care hospital. *Pediatr Infect Dis J* 1991;10:801.

---

m: CONGENITAL PERINATAL INFECTIONS

CHAPTER 76 ■ ENTEROVIRUS

MARC H. LEBEL

EPIDEMIOLOGY

Humans are the only natural hosts for enteroviruses. These viruses have a worldwide distribution and tend to produce seasonal outbreaks during summer and fall in the temperate climates; in the tropics, this seasonal pattern may be absent. Sporadic infections can occur at any time. A geographic and year-to-year variation exists among the serotypes producing infections. For isolates reported to the Centers for Disease Control and Prevention in infants younger than 2 months, echoviruses cause 51% of all nonpolio enteroviral diseases, group B coxsackieviruses cause 45%, and group A coxsackieviruses cause 4%. Viral isolates in the neonatal period parallel isolates circulating in the community at that time and vary from year to year. Male infants are more often affected than female infants, with a male-to-female ratio of 1.4:1.0. The usual incubation period is 3 to 6 days after contact, except for acute hemorrhagic conjunctivitis (1 to 3 days).

Perinatal infections can be acquired by transplacental transmission (during maternal viremia and from the infected placenta), but this seems to occur rarely. Most often, infants are infected at the time of delivery or from human-to-human contact (maternal and nonmaternal sources) after birth. Spread is by the fecal-oral route and possibly by the oral-oral (respiratory) route. Enteroviruses may survive on environmental surfaces. Outbreaks or echoviruses and coxsackieviruses in special care and standard nurseries have occurred; the source of infection was either an infected baby or the nursing personnel. The incidence of congenital infection is rare. Some studies reported an increased risk of abortion after maternal infection with an enterovirus, whereas other studies did not. During the peak season of enterovirus activity, the incidence of infection in the first month of life can be as high as 13%. Most of these infections probably are acquired after birth. An increased risk of infection has been associated with lower socioeconomic status, lack of breast-feeding, and absence of passively transferred maternal antibodies. One study reported a possible association between coxsackievirus B infections and severe congenital anatomic defects of the central nervous system.

PATHOGENESIS

Enteroviruses, which are small RNA viruses, are a subgroup of the picornaviruses. Sixty-four enteroviruses are recognized and are divided into different classes: polioviruses (serotypes 1 to 3), coxsackievirus group A (serotypes 1 to 24), coxsackievirus group B (serotypes 1 to 6), echoviruses (serotypes 1 to 34), and enteroviruses (68 to 71). Enteroviruses were originally classified according to their different effects in tissue cultures and animals; however, some strains possess *in vitro* characteristics belonging to more than one class. Newer strains have been assigned only an enterovirus number. More recently, classification of enteroviruses has been based on their genomic characteristics. These viruses have been divided into polioviruses (PV), human enterovirus A (HEV-A), human enterovirus B (HEV-B), human enterovirus C (HEV-C) and human enterovirus D (HEV-D). Echoviruses 22 and 23 have been reclassified in a new genus called Parechovirus.

After initial replication of the virus in the gastrointestinal or respiratory tract, the infection spreads to the lymphoid tissue. From there, a primary viremia occurs with dissemination to other lymphoreticular tissues such as liver, spleen, and bone marrow. In congenital infection, this viremia corresponds to the initiation of the infection. The virus can multiply in these secondary sites, with production of a secondary viremia and appearance of clinical signs and symptoms; the central nervous system, heart, and striated muscle can be seeded during this phase of the illness. With mounting antibody response, the viremia ceases.

Enteroviruses can produce inflammation and tissue necrosis in different organs, depending on the strain involved and the inoculum of the virus. There seems to be an age-related difference in the severity of illness, with very young neonates more severely affected than older infants and children, especially if vertical transmission from the mother to the fetus occurs before or at the time of delivery. Neonates with fatal enterovirus infections have an onset of disease at birth or within a few days of life.

CLINICAL MANIFESTATIONS

The spectrum of infection is wide, ranging from asymptomatic colonization to fulminant disease with myocarditis and death. The percentage of neonates asymptomatically infected is variable according to study, strain involved, presence of transplacentally acquired specific antibody, and time of the year. Many children with enterovirus infections are asymptomatic; some heavily infected children manifest only mild clinical symptoms. However, severe disease seems to be more common in neonates than in older children. In one study of enterovirus infection in children younger than 2 months, Morens reported that 74% of patients had severe disease.

Some infants present only with fever and irritability. The temperature can be as high as 39°C, and the fever lasts an average of 3 days (maximum, 8 days). The most severe manifestation is a sepsis-like illness manifested by fever, lethargy, irritability, abdominal distention, decreased feedings, rash, and hypotonia; this clinical presentation may mimic bacterial sepsis. Disseminated intravascular coagulation, hypotension, hepatitis, and jaundice also may be present.

Viral myocarditis in the newborn period is most often caused by coxsackievirus B infections. The onset is acute with fever, anorexia, listlessness, tachycardia, tachypnea, and cyanosis. Cardiac arrhythmias have been reported, and heart failure can occur. In many instances, a biphasic pattern of fever and symptoms exists. The mortality is elevated for these children, and recovery, if they survive, is slow. Many infants have concomitant involvement of the central nervous system and liver.

Meningoencephalitis is common as part of disseminated disease. The clinical presentation is frequently that of a nonspecific febrile illness, but other symptoms can include lethargy, seizures, vomiting, diarrhea, poor feeding, and tremor. The cerebrospinal fluid (CSF) findings are variable and sometimes can be comparable to those found in bacterial disease. The CSF leukocyte count can vary from a few to several thousand cells, with a predominance of lymphocytes; however, polymorphonuclear leukocytes can be seen early in the disease. The CSF protein and glucose concentrations are usually within normal limits, but the protein concentration can be elevated; hypoglycorrhachia and a CSF-to-blood glucose ratio of less than 0.5 are not uncommon.

Polioviruses can lead to spontaneous abortion, and poliomyelitis is associated with a high rate of paralysis and mortality in the infant, especially if maternal infection occurs late in pregnancy. Enterovirus 71 has been associated with encephalitis and paralysis.

Gastrointestinal infections can be manifested by vomiting, diarrhea, and abdominal distention. Hepatitis with fulminant hepatic failure, jaundice, hepatomegaly, and disseminated intravascular coagulation has been reported with certain echoviruses. Pancreatitis is rare.

Respiratory symptoms frequently are present with other signs or symptoms. Pharyngitis, rhinitis, laryngitis, and interstitial pneumonitis have been associated with enterovirus infections. Cutaneous manifestations include macular, maculopapular, or petechial rashes. Coxsackievirus A16 is associated with hand, foot, and mouth disease, and enterovirus 70 is associated with acute hemorrhagic conjunctivitis.

Outbreaks of enterovirus infections in newborn nurseries have been described in many institutions and tend to occur during the peak incidence of enteroviral activity in the community. An increased risk of infection has been associated with mouth care and gavage feeding. This finding is consistent with a fecal-oral or oral-oral mode of transmission of the virus. The spectrum of disease depends on the infecting serotype.

DIAGNOSIS

A specific etiologic diagnosis of enterovirus infection is based on isolation of the infecting strain and rarely from serology. Polymerase chain reaction for detection of enterovirus RNA can be used for CSF and blood samples; this method is faster and more sensitive than viral cultures. With sterile bacterial culture results in the presence of myocarditis and meningoencephalitis, an enteroviral infection should be suspected. Viral culture results of the nasopharynx, CSF, and stool may be positive in 50% to 70% of patients. Some strains of enteroviruses produce a cytopathic effect on cell line cultures in 3 to 7 days; therefore, viral culture as well as polymerase chain reaction for enteroviruses can help in the clinical management of some patients by allowing discontinuation of antibiotic therapy and earlier discharge from the hospital.

The excretion of enteroviruses in the stool can last for as long as 6 to 12 weeks after the onset of infection. Isolation of a virus from the stool does not necessarily imply that this agent is the infecting strain of the present illness. Isolation of enterovirus from other sites, especially from CSF and tissue specimens, is the best proof of causality. Because of the vast number of serotypes and the absence of a common group antigen for enteroviruses, serologic diagnosis is impractical except when evaluating paired sera for an antibody increase (fourfold or greater increase in neutralizing antibody titer in specimens obtained from 2 to 4 weeks apart) for coxsackieviruses B in cases of myocarditis, if a specific serotype is suspected during an epidemic in the community with a known serotype, or when an enterovirus has been isolated in tissue culture.

Differentiating between viral and bacterial causes can be difficult, but epidemiologic circumstances are helpful. In enteroviral infections, the mother frequently has a history of a febrile illness or gastrointestinal symptoms in the days preceding the delivery. Season of the year and geographic location are two other important considerations. Prolonged rupture of the membranes, prematurity, and low Apgar scores occur less often in enteroviral than in bacterial infections. Herpes simplex infections can present a fulminant course with multisystemic involvement and should be included in the differential diagnosis.

THERAPY

No specific antiviral drug is commercially available for therapy of enteroviral infections, and treatment is supportive. Pleconaril, a newer antipicornaviral agent, was evaluated for therapy of infants with enteroviral meningitis; in a small randomized, controlled trial, it did not demonstrate a benefit over placebo. After appropriate bacterial cultures have been obtained, the decision to give or withhold antibiotic therapy is based on history, clinical status of the patient, and experience of the physician. Supportive care is important, with particular attention to the fluid balance and cardiac and hepatic functions. No evidence suggests that corticosteroids are beneficial in cases of myocarditis, and data from experimental carditis in animals suggest a detrimental effect.

Human immunoglobulins do not alter the course of established enteroviral infections, but they are sometimes used in severe, life-threatening infections. Data are contradictory regarding their efficacy for prevention of clinical disease in exposed newborns in the setting of an outbreak of enteroviral infection in the nursery. Isolation measures, cohorting of patients, and emphasis on hand washing techniques are still the most important measures for limiting spread of infection.

PROGNOSIS

Although most infants with enteroviral infections have a self-limited illness, some develop a fulminant disease with multisystemic involvement. Virulence of the strain and the presence or absence of passively acquired maternal antibodies are thought to alter the outcome. It has been reported that approximately 80% of children with severe hepatic necrosis die, and mortality in infants with myocarditis is as high as 53%. One follow-up study of enteroviral meningoencephalitis showed no neurologic or cognitive defects, but other studies have shown impairment in language and speech skills in some survivors if twitching or seizures occurred during the acute illness. Long-term neurologic follow-up is advisable for those children.

Suggested Readings

Abzug MJ, Cloud G, Bradley J, et al. Double-blind placebo-controlled trial of pleconaril in infants with enterovirus meningitis. *Pediatr Infect Dis J* 2003;22:335.

Abzug MJ. Presentation, diagnosis, and management of enterovirus infections in neonates. *Paediatr Drugs* 2004;6:1.

Amsley MS, Miller RK, Menegus MA, et al. Enterovirus in pregnant women and the perfused placenta. *Am J Obstet Gynecol* 1988;158:755.

Bergman I, Painter MJ, Wald ER, et al. Outcome in children with enterovirus meningitis during the first year of life. *J Pediatr* 1987;110:705.

Byrington CL, Taggart W, Carroll KC, et al. A polymerase chain reaction-based epidemiologic investigation of nonpolio enteroviral infections in febrile and afebrile infants 90 days and younger. *Pediatrics* 1999;103:E27.

Farmer K, MacArthur BA, Clay MM. A follow-up study of 15 cases of neonatal meningoencephalitis due to coxsackievirus B5. *J Pediatr* 1975;87:568.

Gauntt CJ, Gudvangen RJ, Brans YM, et al. Coxsackievirus group B antibodies in the ventricular fluid of infants with severe anatomic defects in the central nervous system. *Pediatrics* 1985;76:64.

Ishiko H, Shimada Y, Yonaha M, et al. Molecular diagnosis of human enteroviruses by phylogeny-based classification by use of the VP4 sequence. *J Infect Dis* 2002;185:744.

Jenista JA, Powell KR, Menegus MA. Epidemiology of neonatal enterovirus infection. *J Pediatr* 1984;104:685.

Johnston JM, Overall JC Jr. Intravenous immunoglobulin in disseminated neonatal echovirus 11 infection. *Pediatr Infect Dis J* 1989;8:254.

Modlin JF. Echovirus infections of newborn infants. *Pediatr Infect Dis* 1988;7:311.

Modlin JF. Perinatal echovirus infections: insights from a literature review of 61 cases of serious infections and 16 outbreaks in nurseries. *Rev Infect Dis* 1986;8:918.

Modlin JF, Polk BF, Horton P, et al. Perinatal echovirus infection: risk of transmission during a community outbreak. *N Engl J Med* 1981;305:368.

Morens DM. Enteroviral disease in early infancy. *J Pediatr* 1978;92:374.

Oberste S, LaMonte A, Khetsuriani N. Enterovirus surveillance: United States 2000–2001. *MMWR Morb Mortal Wkly Rep* 2002;51:1047.

Verboon-Maciolek MA, Nijhuis M, van Loon AM, et al. Diagnosis of enterovirus infection in the first 2 months of life by real-time polymerase chain reaction. *Clin Infect Dis* 2003;37:1.

CHAPTER 77 ■ CYTOMEGALOVIRUS

PABLO J. SÁNCHEZ AND JANE D. SIEGEL

EPIDEMIOLOGY

Cytomegalovirus (CMV) has a worldwide distribution and is the most common cause of congenital infections. CMV occurs in 0.4% to 2.4% of all live births. The acquisition of CMV is usually asymptomatic in the immunocompetent host. Once infected, latent virus persists in leukocytes and tissues. Seroprevalence studies indicate that an inverse relationship exists between socioeconomic status and development of infection. CMV seropositivity in women of childbearing age varies in the United States from 45% in higher socioeconomic groups to 70% in crowded areas with substandard living conditions; this figure increases to nearly 100% in developing countries. Two likely sources of primary CMV infection for pregnant women are infected sexual partners and young children in day-care centers. High rates of infection have been observed among young children in Israeli kibbutzim and in day-care centers in Sweden and the United States, where the rate of viruria may be as high as 70% among children aged 2 to 3 years. Serologic studies demonstrate a 30% seroconversion rate among parents whose children shed CMV as compared with no seroconversions among parents whose children do not excrete the virus.

PATHOGENESIS

The transmission of CMV to a fetus or newborn can occur *in utero*, during delivery, or postnatally. *In utero* infection occurs transplacentally during maternal viremia. Primary CMV infection acquired during pregnancy is associated with a 40% risk of congenital infection, with more severe fetal effects occurring when maternal infection occurs in the first half of pregnancy. However, symptomatic disease is present in only 10% to 15% of these infants. CMV also can be transmitted to the fetus after reactivation of latent infection in the mother. Approximately 0.2% to 2.0% of infants born to women who are seropositive before becoming pregnant are infected *in utero*, but they rarely have clinically apparent disease at birth. Concern exists, however, that maternal coinfection with human immunodeficiency virus (HIV) and CMV may promote perinatal transmission of CMV and result in clinically apparent CMV disease in the newborn, even among those born to mothers with recurrent infection. Recent evidence also suggests that maternal reinfection with a different CMV strain can result in symptomatic congenital disease; the frequency of this occurrence currently is not known.

The transmission of CMV to the newborn infant also may occur intrapartum from contact with infected cervical secretions. In the postpartum period, maternal–infant transmission of CMV occurs during breast-feeding, because 20% to 40% of seropositive women shed CMV into their breast milk. Asymptomatic infection occurs in 60% of infants fed infected breast milk and usually is the result of reactivation of CMV infection in a seropositive mother. Breast-feeding is, therefore, an effective means of providing passive–active immunization of the young infant. In preterm infants who lack maternally derived, transplacental CMV IgG antibodies, the transmission of CMV through breast milk has resulted in symptomatic infection.

An important iatrogenic source of CMV infection is the transfusion of blood that has not been treated to remove viable CMV from a seropositive donor to a seronegative infant. Under such conditions, the incidence is 10% to 30% and usually occurs in infants who weigh less than 1,300 g. The risk of infection is related to the volume of transfused blood, number of donors, and elevated complement fixation titers to CMV in donor blood. Horizontal transmission of CMV in a neonatal intensive care unit has been documented, but is rare.

CLINICAL MANIFESTATIONS AND COMPLICATIONS

Cytomegalic inclusion disease is the most serious but least common manifestation of congenital CMV infection. This syndrome is characterized by multiorgan involvement, with the reticuloendothelial and central nervous systems most frequently affected. Typical clinical features of cytomegalic inclusion disease include intrauterine growth restriction, hepatosplenomegaly, jaundice, petechiae or purpura, microcephaly, chorioretinitis, sensorineural hearing loss, and cerebral calcifications (Table 77.1). These features may occur singly or in combination.

Hepatomegaly with direct hyperbilirubinemia and mild elevation of serum transaminase levels are the most common abnormalities noted in the newborn period. Giant cell transformation, with associated extramedullary hematopoiesis or large inclusion-bearing hepatocytes characteristic of CMV infection is present on pathologic examination of the liver. Hepatitis usually resolves in the first year of life, and development of cirrhosis is rare. Splenomegaly is common and may be the only abnormality present at birth. Thrombocytopenia with petechiae usually is transient but may persist through the first year of life. "Blueberry muffin" spots are palpable, discrete, well-circumscribed, bluish purple lesions on yellow jaundiced skin. These are often mistaken for purpura; they represent dermal erythropoiesis in the more severely affected infants (see Color Fig. 82.1 in color section).

Central nervous system infection with CMV can result in encephalitis and abnormal brain development, with seizures and an elevated protein content in the cerebrospinal fluid (CSF). Cerebral calcifications occur in as many as 50% of newborns with physical examination findings of CMV; their occurrence date the maternal infection to the first trimester of pregnancy. The calcifications typically occur in the periventricular areas (Fig. 77.1), but also may occur within the brain parenchyma and particularly in the basal ganglia (Figs. 77.2 and 77.3). Although these calcifications are best visualized by computed tomography (CT), advances in cranial ultrasonography have provided a readily available and convenient method for their detection. Arrested brain growth results in microcephaly, and obstruction of the fourth ventricle may result in hydrocephalus.

TABLE 77.1

FREQUENCY OF CLINICAL FINDINGS IN INFANTS WITH CONGENITAL INFECTIONS

Clinical Findings	Congenital Infection				
	Rubella	Toxoplasma	CMV	Syphilis	HSV
Intrauterine growth retardation	+++	±	++	++	±
Reticuloendothelial system					
Jaundice	+	++	+++	+++	+
Hepatitis	±	+	+++	+++	+
Hepatosplenomegaly	+++	++	+++	+++	+
Anemia	+	+++	++	+++	−
Thrombocytopenia	++	±	+++	++	+
Disseminated intravascular coagulation	−	−	±	−	++
Adenopathy	++	++	−	++	−
Dermal erythropoiesis	+	−	+	−	−
Skin rash	−	+	−	++	+++
Bone abnormalities	++	−	±	++	−
Eye					
Cataracts	++	±	±	±	−
Retinopathy	++	+++	+	±	+++
Microphthalmia	+	±	±	−	±
Central nervous system					
Microcephaly	+	+	++	−	±
Meningoencephalitis	++	+++	+++	++	+++
Brain calcification	±	++	++	−	+
Hydrocephalus	−	++	±	±	++
Hearing defect	+++	+	+++	+	−
Pneumonitis	++	+	±	+	±
Cardiovascular					
Myocarditis	+	±	±	±	−
Congenital defect	+++	−	−	−	−

±, rare; +, 5% to 20%; ++, 20% to 50%; +++, more than 50%; □, prominent feature of particular infection; CMV, cytomegalovirus; HSV, herpes simplex virus.

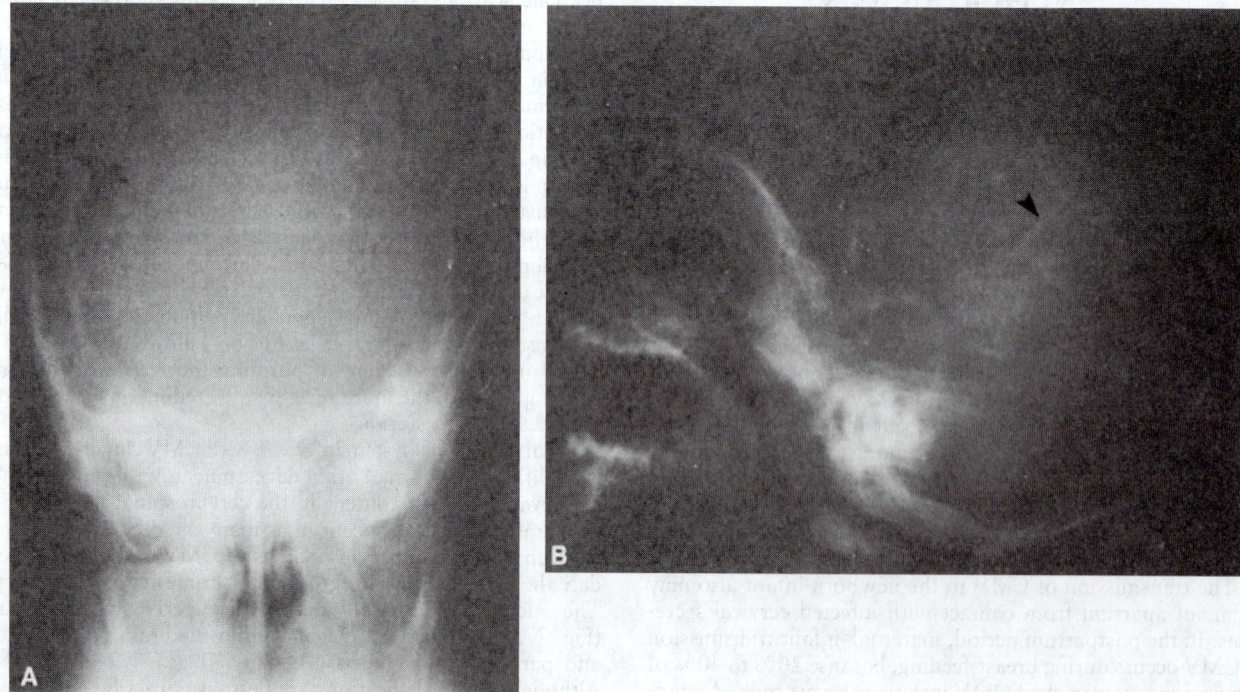

FIGURE 77.1. Anteroposterior (**A**) and lateral (**B**) skull roentgenograms demonstrating cerebral calcifications (*arrow*) lining the ventricles in a neonate with congenital cytomegalovirus infection. (Courtesy of Dr. Guido Currarino, Dallas, TX.)

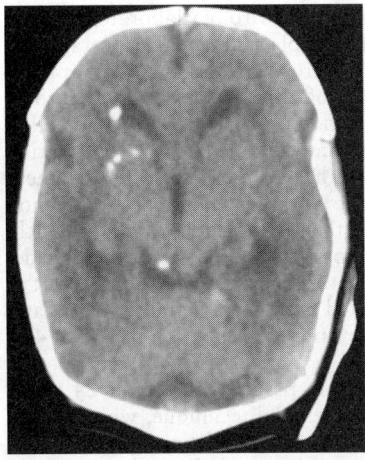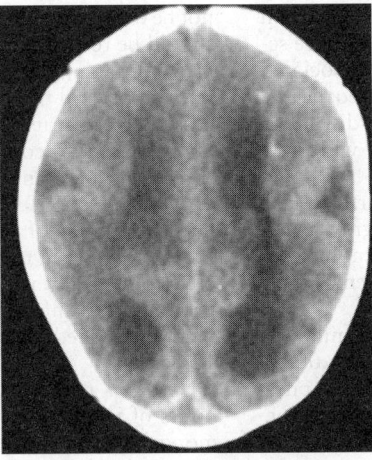

FIGURE 77.2. Computed tomography of brain demonstrating periventricular and posterior fossa dystrophic calcification along with diffuse cortical dysplasia and global paucity of white matter in a newborn with microcephaly and congenital cytomegalovirus infection.

Ocular defects include chorioretinitis (Fig. 77.4), strabismus, optic atrophy, microphthalmia, and cataracts.

The most common manifestation of congenital CMV infection is sensorineural hearing loss resulting from direct viral invasion of the inner ear. It occurs in 50% to 60% of infants with symptomatic congenital infection and in approximately 5% of those with otherwise asymptomatic infection at birth. The hearing loss may be unilateral and unsuspected until early childhood, because the majority of CMV-infected, asymptomatic newborns develop hearing impairment beyond the neonatal period. All infants with congenital CMV infection require periodic evaluation of hearing throughout childhood and adolescence in order to detect progressive hearing loss. Cochlear implantation has been used successfully as early as 1 year of age for those children with profound bilateral hearing loss.

A diffuse interstitial pneumonitis occurs in less than 1% of newborns with cytomegalic inclusion disease. Bone abnormalities in CMV infection consist of longitudinal radiolucent streaks in the metaphysis of long bones ("celery stalk" appearance), particularly the distal femur and proximal tibia (Fig. 77.5). Generalized osteopenia with irregular metaphyseal fragmentation also has been described. Defective enamelization of the deciduous teeth occurs in 40% of symptomatic newborns and in 5% of infants with asymptomatic infection at birth.

Attempts have been made to implicate CMV in congenital cardiovascular, genitourinary, gastrointestinal, and musculoskeletal anomalies. Overall, the teratogenicity of CMV remains in doubt, although CMV has been associated with inguinal hernias in boys.

The type of maternal infection during pregnancy (i.e., primary or recurrent infection) and whether the newborn has clinical manifestations of CMV infection are the two most important factors with respect to prognosis. It was found that 25% of infants born to mothers who had a primary CMV infection during pregnancy manifest some neurodevelopmental sequelae, whereas only 8% of infants born after a maternal recurrent infection have sequelae. Of infants with asymptomatic congenital CMV infection, approximately 90% have no apparent sequelae and only rarely manifest severe neurologic impairment. In contrast, severe intellectual, sensory, and motor deficits are observed consistently in infants and children with chorioretinitis, microcephaly, and intracranial calcifications. Seizures, including infantile spasms, and early death also are seen. Symptomatic infants without central nervous system abnormalities at birth are at less but still significant risk for the development of neurologic and developmental abnormalities.

CMV infection acquired at delivery is manifested by an afebrile pneumonia in 50% of exposed infants or, rarely, hepatitis or encephalitis after an incubation period of 4 to 12 weeks (mean, 8 weeks). In full-term infants, the disease tends to be mild and does not result in late neurologic sequelae. On the

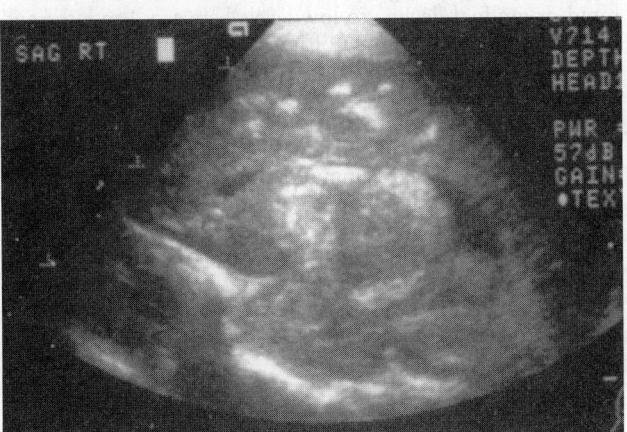

FIGURE 77.3. Cranial ultrasound in a newborn with congenital CMV infection demonstrates extensive and prominent calcifications in thalamus and periventricular regions as well as in the brain parenchyma.

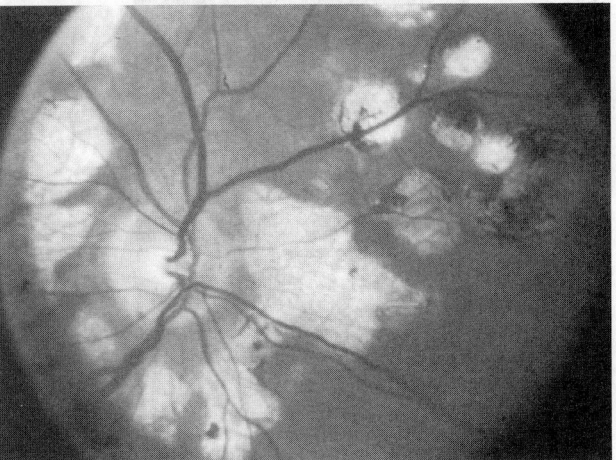

FIGURE 77.4. Patchy, yellow-white lesions of chorioretinitis seen with both congenital cytomegalovirus infection and congenital toxoplasmosis. (See Color Fig. 77.4 in color section.) (Courtesy of Dr. George H. McCracken, Jr., Dallas, TX.)

other hand, in premature infants with birth weight less than 1,500 g, perinatally acquired CMV infection may be more severe. CMV pneumonitis in these infants has been associated with the development of chronic lung disease. Moreover, the administration of dexamethasone for chronic lung disease in CMV-infected preterm infants has been associated with progression of their CMV disease.

Transfusion-acquired CMV infection in low-birth-weight infants may be severe and is characterized by a gray ashen pallor, respiratory distress, pneumonia, hepatosplenomegaly, hepatitis, atypical lymphocytosis, thrombocytopenia, and hemolytic anemia; it has a 10% mortality.

CMV infection acquired through infected breast milk administered to premature infants with birth weights of 1,000 g or less has been associated with a sepsis-like illness with apnea and bradycardia, hepatosplenomegaly, distended bowel, pallor, thrombocytopenia, and elevated liver function tests. It is not known if these infants develop long-term neurologic sequelae.

DIAGNOSIS

The diagnosis of congenital CMV infection is best confirmed by isolation of the virus from urine (Table 77.2). A clean-voided, fresh specimen of urine is preferred. If the sample can-

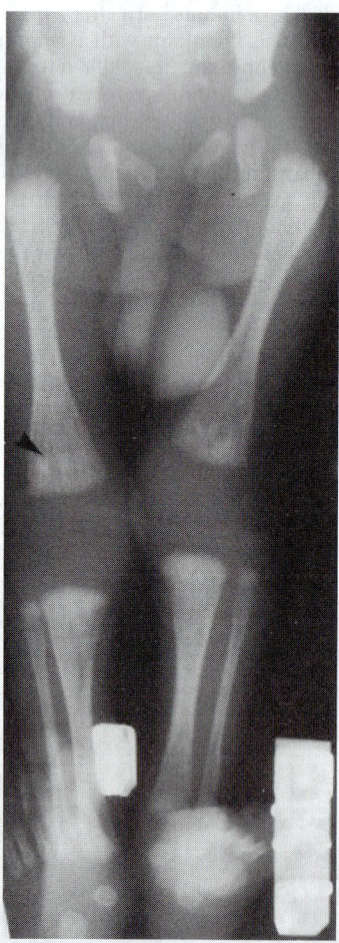

FIGURE 77.5. "Celery stalk" appearance of the femur (*arrow*) and tibia associated with congenital rubella, cytomegalovirus, and syphilis. Alternating bands of longitudinal translucency and relative density represent a disturbance of normal bone metabolism. (Courtesy of Dr. Guido Currarino, Dallas, TX.)

not be transported immediately to a virology laboratory, then it should be refrigerated at 4°C or placed in wet ice. Storage and transport at ambient temperature or freezing result in rapid reduction of viral titer. Culture of saliva has been reported to be as sensitive as urine for detection of congenital CMV infection and represents a convenient and suitable alternative. Isolation of CMV from amniotic fluid has been used also to document *in utero* infection. All infants with congenital CMV infection have high titers of virus in their urine and pharynx at birth. Viral excretion in the urine persists for years, but the titer decreases markedly after 3 months. Pharyngeal shedding is not as prolonged. In infants infected with CMV natally, viruria and pharyngeal shedding appear after an incubation period of 4 to 12 weeks.

CMV is readily identified in tissue culture after 24 to 48 hours of incubation by the shell-vial technique, which uses a monoclonal antibody to detect early CMV antigen. On routine viral culture, characteristic cytopathologic developments occur within 2 weeks of inoculation of the specimen onto a human fibroblast monolayer. To diagnose congenital CMV infection accurately, cultures should be obtained within the first 2 weeks of age. After 3 weeks, viral shedding can occur from either congenital, perinatal, or postnatally acquired infection. Polymerase chain reaction (PCR) performed on such clinical specimens as blood, CSF, and urine has been found to be highly sensitive and specific for the detection of CMV DNA. PCR is the preferred method for detection of CMV in CSF; a positive CMV CSF PCR has been associated with a more severe neurologic outcome. PCR also is preferred for the detection of CMV in blood specimens. The finding of CMV in blood by PCR is supportive of active infection; in neonates, its utility may best lie in the diagnosis of CMV disease acquired natally or postpartum. A positive blood CMV PCR also has been associated with the development of hearing loss in infants with congenital CMV infection. Detection of pp65 antigen in white blood cells has been used to detect active infection in immunocompromised hosts; its requirement for a large quantity of blood has limited its use in neonates. CMV in urine also has been detected by electron microscopy using the pseudoreplica method, which permits the detection of herpesvirus particles within 15 to 30 minutes. This technique detects virus in 95% of specimens with high infectivity titers (greater than or equal to 10^4 per microliter); sensitivity is decreased when specimens are stored at 4°C.

Serologic studies have a limited role in the diagnosis of congenital CMV infection and are not recommended. The presence of CMV-specific IgG antibody denotes passively transferred maternal antibodies. On serial determinations, antibody titers to CMV in most congenitally infected infants show either a rapid or gradual decline to low levels between 4 months and 2 years of age. A minimum of infected infants demonstrate a persistence of the high initial titer. An increase in titer has not been demonstrated in these infants, despite continued shedding of the virus. False-negative antibody levels determined by the complement fixation method have been seen in infected infants. Although the CMV-IgM immunofluorescent test detects 76% of congenitally infected infants, a false-positive rate of as high as 21% has been documented. Commercially available enzyme-linked immunosorbent assays (ELISA) that measure CMV-IgG have excellent reliability, but false-positive test results remain a problem with the CMV-IgM enzyme-linked immunosorbent assays. To interpret test results, the accuracy of the specific kit used must be known.

THERAPY

At present, no antiviral agent is approved for the treatment or prevention of congenital CMV infection. However, ganciclovir

TABLE 77.2

METHODS OF DIAGNOSIS OF CONGENITAL AND PERINATAL INFECTION

	Isolation of Organism	Antigen Detection	Measurement of Antibody	Polymerase Chain Reaction
Cytomegalovirus	++	+	NR	+
Herpes simplex virus	++	+	NR	++
Varicella-zoster	±	±	++	±
Epstein-Barr virus	±	−	++	±
Rubella	±	±	++	−
Toxoplasmosis	±	−	++	++
Syphilis	±[a]	±	++	±
Human Immunodeficiency virus	±	+	NR	++
Hepatitis				
A	−	−	++	
B	−	++	++	±
Delta	−	++	++	−
C	−	−	++	±
Neisseria gonorrhoeae	++	−	−	−
Chlamydia trachomatis	±	++[b]	+[c]	±
Mycoplasmas	++		±	±

−, not available; +, alternative method but usually less helpful; ++, preferred method; ±, possible, but may not be performed routinely by clinical laboratories; NR, not recommended.
[a]Spirochetes visualized by dark-field examination of suspected lesions.
[b]Preferred for conjunctivitis.
[c]Pneumonia only.

has been used to treat some infants with congenital CMV disease. A phase III, multicenter, randomized study of intravenous ganciclovir (6 mg/kg every 12 hours for 6 weeks) for the treatment of infants with gestational age of 32 weeks or older (birth weight of 1,200 g or more) who have congenital CMV infection of the central nervous system was performed by the Collaborative Antiviral Study Group from 1991 to 1999. When compared with infants who received no therapy, those who received ganciclovir were significantly more likely to have either improved or normal hearing at 6 months, and none of the ganciclovir-treated infants had worse hearing. At 1 year or older, those who received ganciclovir also were significantly less likely to have worse hearing than the untreated group. Other beneficial effects of ganciclovir therapy included a significant decrease in median time to normalization of the ALT, as well as improved weight gain and head circumference after 6 weeks of therapy. Long-term neurologic outcome was not assessed.

Ganciclovir also may be useful in other clinical situations. Chorioretinitis involving the macula and possibly affecting vision may respond well to ganciclovir therapy. In premature infants with perinatally acquired CMV infection who develop pneumonia, bronchopulmonary dysplasia, hepatitis, or encephalitis, or those whose CMV infection has been exacerbated by corticosteroid therapy, ganciclovir may be beneficial. However, the appropriate dosing regimen and duration of treatment are not known.

The toxicity of ganciclovir includes neutropenia and thrombocytopenia. In laboratory animals, it is a teratogen and carcinogen, and it causes gonadal atrophy and decreased spermatogenesis.

The efficacy of CMV immune globulin has not been demonstrated in the treatment or prevention of congenital CMV disease. Currently, an ongoing Phase I/II pharmacokinetic evaluation is underway of oral valganciclovir in neonates with symptomatic CMV infection. Such therapy may eliminate the need for prolonged intravenous access and provide a convenient method of delivering long-term oral suppressive therapy.

PREVENTION

Routine serologic screening is not recommended for women of childbearing age because no prophylactic or therapeutic interventions are available during pregnancy. Meticulous adherence to standard precautions, especially hand hygiene after exposure to urine or saliva from young infants and toddlers and immunocompromised patients, is the most effective means of preventing primary CMV infection in pregnant women. Pregnant women are *not* excluded from caring for patients who are known to have CMV infection because of the ubiquity of CMV and the demonstration that health care workers do not have higher rates of seroconversion than control subjects. The greater risk to the pregnant health care worker may be the unidentified infant who is excreting CMV asymptomatically. Adherence to standard precautions for all patients also will prevent nosocomial transmission among patients.

Currently, the routine screening of all newborns for CMV is not recommended. However, because CMV is the most common nongenetic cause of hearing loss, those newborns who do not pass their hearing screen may be screened for CMV. Approximately 5% of these infants will be infected with CMV and will require close audiologic follow-up.

Transfusion-acquired CMV infection is eliminated through the administration of CMV antibody-negative blood products to infants <1,500 g in birth weight. In many neonatal intensive care units, leukofiltration of blood to remove the white blood cell fraction has been used successfully to minimize the risk of CMV acquisition. Frozen deglycerolized red blood cells are also a suitable alternative, because they lack viable leukocytes. Freezing of expressed breast milk at −20°C for 3 to 7 days significantly diminishes CMV titers but does not completely eliminate infectivity. Pasteurization (62.5°C) is required for complete neutralization of the virus.

CMV vaccine ultimately may be the best preventive strategy, but vaccine development remains investigational.

Suggested Readings

Adler SP. Cytomegalovirus transmission among children in day care, their mothers, and caretakers. *Pediatr Infect Dis J* 1988;7:279.

Alpert G, Plotkin SA. A practical guide to the diagnosis of congenital infections in the newborn infant. *Pediatr Clin North Am* 1986;33:465.

Boppana SB, Rivera LB, Fowler KB, et al. Intrauterine transmission of cytomegalovirus to infants of women with preconceptional immunity. *N Engl J Med* 2001;344:1366.

Demmler G. Congenital cytomegalovirus infection treatment. *Pediatr Infect Dis J* 2003;22:1005.

Fowler KB, Stagno S, Pass RF, et al. The outcome of congenital cytomegalovirus infection in relation to maternal antibody status. *N Engl J Med* 1992;326:663.

Fowler KB, McCollister FP, Dahle AJ, et al. Progressive and fluctuating sensorineural hearing loss in children with asymptomatic congenital cytomegalovirus infection. *J Pediatr* 1997;130:624.

Kimberlin DW, Lin C-Y, Sánchez PJ, et al., for the National Institute of Allergy and Infectious Diseases Collaborative Antiviral Study Group. Effect of ganciclovir therapy on hearing in symptomatic congenital cytomegalovirus disease involving the central nervous system: a randomized, controlled trial. *J Pediatr* 2003;143:16.

Litwin CM, Hill HR. Serologic and DNA-based testing for congenital and perinatal infections. *Pediatr Infect Dis J* 1997;16:1166.

Nelson CT, Demmler GJ. Cytomegalovirus infection in the pregnant mother, fetus, and newborn infant. *Clin Perinatol* 1997;24:151.

Rivera LB, Boppana SB, Fowler KB, et al. Predictors of hearing loss in children with symptomatic congenital cytomegalovirus infection. *Pediatr* 2002;110:762.

Stagno S, Pass RF, Dworsky ME, et al. Congenital and perinatal cytomegalovirus infections. *Semin Perinatol* 1983;7:31.

Whitley RJ, Cloud G, Gruber W, et al. Ganciclovir treatment of symptomatic congenital cytomegalovirus infection: results of a phase II study. *J Infect Dis* 1997;175:1080.

Williamson WD, Demmler GJ, Percy AK, et al. Progressive hearing loss in infants with asymptomatic congenital cytomegalovirus infection. *Pediatrics* 1992;90:862.

CHAPTER 78 ■ HERPES SIMPLEX VIRUS

PABLO J. SÁNCHEZ AND JANE D. SIEGEL

EPIDEMIOLOGY

The estimated rate of occurrence of neonatal herpes simplex virus (HSV) infection in the United States is approximately 1 per 3,000 to 20,000 deliveries per year. Most neonatal infections are caused by HSV-2, with some 25% to 30% caused by HSV-1. The seroprevalence of HSV-2 antibodies among American women of childbearing age is 20% to 30%. However, only 5% of these seropositive women have a history of genital HSV infection. It is therefore not surprising that 70% of infants who develop HSV infection are born to women who are asymptomatic for genital infection with HSV at the time of delivery and have neither a history of genital herpes nor a sexual partner with genital HSV infection. The frequency of asymptomatic shedding of HSV at the time of delivery varies from 0.01% to 0.39%. Among women with a past history of genital HSV infection, asymptomatic excretion at delivery is approximately 1% to 2%. Among those who had a primary infection during pregnancy, viral shedding at delivery is 36%. If HSV is diagnosed before the pregnancy, and clinical recurrences have been fewer than six per year, the risk of reactivation at delivery is 10%. If six or more episodes of HSV infection have occurred per year, then the risk of reactivation at delivery increases to 25%. Most important, however, one is unable to reliably predict viral shedding at delivery in any of these women.

PATHOGENESIS

The acquisition of HSV by the infant can occur *in utero*, during delivery, or after birth. *In utero* infection with HSV accounts for approximately 5% of cases. Transmission occurs either transplacentally, during a maternal viremia, or through an ascending route from an infected maternal genital tract. The virus may pass through microscopic tears in the amniotic membranes to produce infection in infants delivered by cesarean section with intact membranes. HSV has been isolated from the blood of a pregnant woman with primary HSV infection, as well as from amniotic fluid, placenta, umbilical cord blood, and fetal tissue obtained at the time of spontaneous abortion. *In utero* acquisition of HSV, presumably from a transplacental route, also is suggested by reports of congenital malformations in infants born to women with genital herpes infection during pregnancy.

The transmission of HSV to the newborn infant usually occurs at delivery (85% of cases). The risk of neonatal infection is higher with primary maternal HSV infection than with recurrent infection (30% to 50% versus 3%) because of the infant's prolonged exposure to large quantities of virus in the absence of protective neutralizing and antibody-dependent cellular cytotoxicity antibodies (Table 78.1). Prematurity, duration of rupture of amniotic membranes greater than 4 to 6 hours, and use of a scalp electrode for fetal heart rate monitoring also increase the risk of HSV infection.

The postnatal transmission of HSV (10% of cases) to the newborn infant may occur after contact with a maternal breast lesion during breast-feeding or from direct contact with other

TABLE 78.1

MATERNAL GENITAL HERPES INFECTION AND RISK OF PERINATAL TRANSMISSION

	Genital Herpes Simplex Virus Infection	
	Primary	Recurrent
Risk of perinatal transmission	30–50%	3%
Site of viral shedding	Cervix	Labia
Duration of viral shedding	3 wk	2–5 d
Quantity of virus shed	Large	Small
Neutralizing antibody	Absent	Present

family members or, rarely, with health care workers who have active herpes labialis lesions. The nosocomial transmission of HSV in newborn nurseries has been documented by restriction endonuclease analysis of viral isolates, but it is rare.

CLINICAL MANIFESTATIONS AND COMPLICATIONS

The clinical manifestations of intrauterine HSV infection are present at birth or within the first 48 hours of delivery. Skin vesicles with scars are common. Seizures, microcephaly, hydranencephaly, porencephaly, intracranial calcifications, microphthalmia, hepatomegaly with or without splenomegaly, and abnormalities on bone roentgenography may be seen. The adrenal gland frequently is involved, and chorioretinitis either is present at birth or develops in the first week of life.

Neonatal HSV infection acquired at birth is categorized by extent of disease: disseminated disease with or without evidence of central nervous system, skin, eye, and mouth involvement; central nervous system disease (encephalitis) with or without skin, eye, and mouth involvement; and localized infection of the skin, eye, mouth, or a combination of the three without visceral organ or central nervous system involvement. Subclinical infection may occur but is uncommon.

Disseminated disease currently accounts for 25% of neonatal HSV infection. Its frequency has decreased from as high as 50% in the years 1973 to 1981. This decrease is probably a result of the prompt diagnosis and treatment of localized infection before dissemination occurs. The average onset of illness is between 10 to 12 days of age, and the principal organs involved are the liver and adrenal glands. Approximately 60% to 75% of infants manifest central nervous system involvement from hematogenous spread of the virus, and 60% to 80% manifest skin, mouth, or eye lesions. The presenting signs and symptoms are nonspecific and include fever, lethargy, irritability, anorexia, vomiting, respiratory distress, apnea, jaundice, seizures and, in the most severe cases, shock with disseminated intravascular coagulation. Elevated transaminase levels and direct hyperbilirubinemia with or without hepatomegaly are common. Splenomegaly often is present. Pneumonitis, pleural effusion, and roentgenographic lesions in long bones also may occur.

Central nervous system disease from axonal transmission of virus accounts for approximately 30% of neonatal HSV infections. Clinical manifestations typically occur at 16 to 19 days of age and include lethargy, irritability, bulging fontanelle, focal or generalized seizures, opisthotonos, decerebrate posturing, and coma. Almost 40% of infants have no skin vesicles. An examination of the cerebrospinal fluid (CSF) reveals an elevated leukocyte count, with a predominance of lymphocytes and an elevated protein content. Red blood cells are occasionally present, indicating hemorrhagic brain involvement. A normal cell count and protein concentration, however, may be found on the initial lumbar puncture.

Localized diseases of skin, eye, mouth, or all three occur in 45% of infants with HSV infection. The hallmark of neonatal HSV infection is the discrete vesicular lesions that occur in 90% of infants with localized infection (see Color Fig. 129.5 in color section). The vesicles usually appear first on the presenting part of the body that was in direct contact with the virus during delivery. Differential diagnosis includes superficial trauma resulting in vesicles on newborn skin. Other vesicular lesions are discussed in Chapter 68. Approximately 70% of untreated infants who present with skin vesicles develop disseminated infection or have progression of disease to involve the eyes or central nervous system. Ulcerative lesions of the mouth, tongue, or palate occur less commonly (10%). Ocular involvement with HSV is manifested by keratoconjunctivitis, uveitis, chorioretinitis, cataracts, and retinal dysplasia. Sequelae of ocular HSV infection include corneal ulceration, microphthalmia, optic atrophy, and blindness. About 2% to 12% of treated infants with a localized infection of the skin, eyes, or oral cavity have subclinical involvement of the central nervous system, as manifested by the development of severe neurologic impairment. About 50% of infants with skin lesions experience one to twelve cutaneous recurrences during the first 6 to 12 months of age.

DIAGNOSIS

The preferred diagnostic method is isolation of HSV from skin vesicles, buffy coat, brain tissue, CSF, stool, urine, throat, nares, or conjunctivae. HSV is isolated from CSF in 5% to 40% of infants with central nervous system involvement. HSV also can be isolated from duodenal aspirate in infants with hepatitis. Typing of HSV should be performed, because evidence suggests that neurologic outcome is significantly worse with neonatal infection caused by HSV-2 as compared with that caused by HSV-1. When mucocutaneous lesions are present, scraping from the base of a vesicle may reveal intranuclear inclusions and multinucleated giant cells by Tzanck test or Wright stain in 60% to 70% of cases; specific HSV antigen may be detected by immunofluorescence in 70% to 80% of cases.

The diagnosis of HSV encephalitis has been improved greatly by the development of the polymerase chain reaction (PCR) for the detection of HSV DNA in CSF. PCR is the currently preferred method for diagnosing central nervous system infection with HSV; it has supplanted biopsy testing of brain tissue. HSV DNA can be detected by PCR in the majority of culture-positive CSF samples even after 1 week of acyclovir therapy. Overall, PCR has a sensitivity of 75% to 100% and a specificity of 71% to 100%. PCR also has been performed on serum for the diagnosis of disseminated disease. Serum HSV PCR ultimately may prove more useful than blood buffy coat culture.

Other tests that aid in the detection of central nervous system abnormalities include electroencephalography, computed tomography (CT), and magnetic resonance imaging (MRI). The characteristic electroencephalographic abnormality is a periodic slow and sharp wave discharge; more commonly, multiple independent foci of periodic activity are present. CT scan may be normal early in the course of the disease, with characteristic abnormalities appearing 3 to 5 days later. The most frequently observed findings in the acute phase are patchy areas of low attenuation in both cerebral hemispheres, or hemorrhage or calcification in the thalamus, insular cortex, periventricular white matter, and along the corticomedullary junction. Late findings include multicystic encephalomalacia and ventriculomegaly, as a result of brain atrophy and destruction. MRI is more sensitive in detecting early abnormalities in the periventricular white matter and in defining the extent of parenchymal lesions. The technetium brain scan is rarely used because of the improved diagnostic yield seen with MRI. When technetium brain-scan results are abnormal, they demonstrate increased perfusion to the abnormal area. Positive findings in any neurodiagnostic study provide enough evidence to initiate and continue antiviral therapy.

In general, serologic tests are not useful for the diagnosis of neonatal HSV infection. Serology is not helpful acutely because antibody may not yet be present with primary or first-episode maternal genital infection and, when present, IgG antibody to HSV in neonates is usually maternal in origin. An increase in antibody titers or seroconversion in the convalescent phase would indicate neonatal infection.

The recent commercial availability of glycoprotein G–based type-specific assays has allowed the identification of individuals with past HSV-1 or -2 infection, with a sensitivity of 80% to 98% and a specificity of greater than 96%. These new assays may help differentiate primary versus recurrent maternal infection, because the test is negative during a primary or first-episode maternal genital infection and positive with recurrent infection. Past serologic methods should not be used, because they did not distinguish reliably between antibodies to HSV-1 and HSV-2.

THERAPY

Two antiviral agents, acyclovir and vidarabine, have decreased the mortality and improved the outcome of neonatal HSV infection. Antiviral therapy is initiated when the characteristic clinical features are present or when a neonate with overwhelming sepsis and negative bacterial culture results does not respond to broad-spectrum antibiotics. HSV may be recovered from brain biopsy specimens even after 24 to 48 hours of antiviral therapy. Acyclovir is preferred over vidarabine (15 to 30 mg/kg over 12 hours) because of its safety and because of the insolubility of vidarabine and the large fluid volume required for vidarabine administration. Although no difference in mortality exists in infants who receive either the 15 or 30 mg/kg /day dosage of vidarabine, a significantly lower percentage of infants who receive the higher dosage have a progression of disease while on therapy. The currently recommended dose of acyclovir for all forms of neonatal HSV infection is 20 mg/kg of body weight administered intravenously every 8 hours. Because of its renal excretion, acyclovir may need to be administered every 12 hours rather than every 8 hours in preterm infants of less than 34 weeks of gestation. This higher dose in neonates has been shown to be safe and more effective in terms of improved morbidity and mortality when compared with a dose of 30 mg /kg /day given to historical controls. The duration of acyclovir therapy is a minimum of 14 days for infants with disease limited to the skin, eye, or mouth, and 21 days for those with disseminated or central nervous system disease. The longer course of therapy is preferred for treatment of encephalitis, because increasing evidence suggests early relapse or recurrence after shorter durations of therapy. Approximately 2% of infants treated with antiviral therapy for 10 to 14 days have recurrence of infection leading to central nervous system disease. Relapse of HSV encephalitis also has been reported after a 10-day course of vidarabine or acyclovir therapy. In addition, in infants with central nervous system disease, a repeat CSF PCR at 21 days of therapy is recommended to assess the need for additional treatment.

Neonatal infections caused by acyclovir-resistant strains of HSV have been reported; foscarnet is the treatment of choice. No data or experience exists on the use of famciclovir or valacyclovir in neonates. Ocular HSV infection requires topical antiviral medication with either 1% or 2% trifluridine, 0.1% iododeoxyuridine, or 3% vidarabine, in addition to parenteral therapy.

PROGNOSIS

The mortality with disseminated disease has been reduced from 85% in untreated infants to 57% in infants treated with either lower-dose acyclovir or vidarabine; 60% of these infants are normal at 1 year of age. With the utilization of a higher dose and longer duration of acyclovir, 12-month mortality has been reduced to about 30%, whereas normal development at 12 months of age is seen in about 80% of survivors. Pneumonitis and disseminated intravascular coagulopathy are associated with an increased risk of death among infants with disseminated infection. The occurrence of seizures before the initiation of antiviral therapy is associated with an increased risk of morbidity.

Mortality among infants with localized central nervous system disease has decreased from as high as 50% in the pre antiviral era, to 15% in the lower-dose acyclovir period, and to 4% with the recent use of higher-dose and longer-duration acyclovir therapy. Prematurity and seizures are associated with mortality. About 30% of infants with central nervous system disease are developing normally at 12 months of age. Most survivors, however, have neurologic sequelae consisting of seizures, spastic quadriplegia, chorioretinitis, microcephaly, hydrocephaly, porencephalic cyst, and psychomotor retardation.

No deaths have occurred among treated infants with localized infection of the skin, eye, or oral cavity, and about 94% of infants are normal at 1-year follow-up examination. Neurologic impairment in these latter infants has been correlated with the presence of three or more skin recurrences caused by HSV-2 in the first 6 months of age. The concern exists that asymptomatic central nervous system invasion may occur either during the acute skin, eye, and mouth infection or at the time of skin recurrences; HSV-DNA has been detected in the CSF of some infants under both of these circumstances. Suppressive acyclovir therapy administered orally at a dose of 300 mg/m^2 every 8 hours has been used to decrease skin recurrences and possibly prevent or ameliorate neurologic morbidity after HSV infection. For similar reasons, acyclovir suppression has been used following HSV encephalitis. However, the evidence for such a practice is lacking. Moreover, chronic acyclovir therapy has resulted in the development of neutropenia and the emergence of an acyclovir-resistant HSV isolate. A multicenter trial is being conducted by the National Institute of Allergy and Infectious Diseases Collaborative Antiviral Study Group to evaluate this treatment; it cannot be recommended for routine use currently.

A beneficial effect of human immunoglobulin that contains a large concentration of anti-HSV antibody has been observed in animal models when administered early in the course of disease. The clinical efficacy of routine intravenous immunoglobulin in humans has not been demonstrated. An IgG monoclonal antibody against HSV has been produced and may ultimately ameliorate or prevent neonatal HSV disease.

PREVENTION

Delivery of the infants of pregnant women with active genital herpes by cesarean section within 4 to 6 hours of rupture of amniotic membranes is the only intervention shown to prevent neonatal HSV infection. Nonetheless, 33% of neonates diagnosed with HSV infection are delivered by cesarean section. The use of fetal scalp electrodes, forceps, and maneuvers that might cause a break in the infant's skin during delivery should be avoided. Acyclovir suppressive therapy provided to women late in pregnancy reduces both clinical and subclinical shedding of HSV-2 in the genital tract. Its use in women following a first episode of genital HSV infection during pregnancy has been shown to prevent a clinical HSV recurrence at delivery, and thereby prevent a cesarean section. Further studies are under way to evaluate the efficacy of acyclovir and valacyclovir and their effect on the newborn. Data from an international Acyclovir Pregnancy Registry (maintained by Glaxo-Wellcome, Inc., in cooperation with the Centers for Disease Control and Prevention) from 1994 to 1999, in which 1,129 pregnancy exposures to acyclovir and 56 valacyclovir exposures occurred, found no increase in birth defects [www.pregnancyregistry.gsk.com/acyclovir.html; tel. (888) 825-5249].

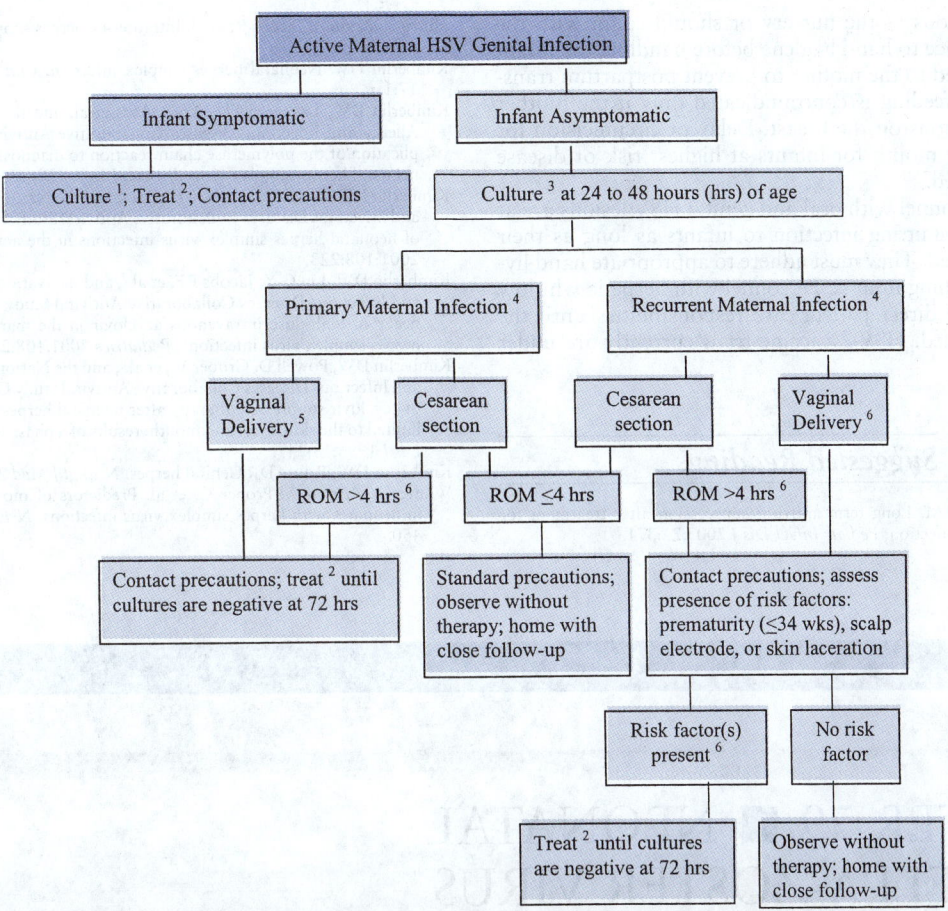

FIGURE 78.1. Management of newborns exposed at delivery to herpes simplex virus (HSV).

HSV, herpes simplex virus; ROM, rupture of membranes; CSF, cerebrospinal fluid; PCR, polymerase chain reaction
1 Culture conjunctiva, nasopharynx/mouth/throat, urine, stool/rectum, cerebrospinal (CSF), blood buffy coat, base of lesion (if present); CSF for HSV PCR; ophthalmologic consult if conjunctival culture is positive or eye examination is abnormal; other tests (liver function tests, complete blood cell count and platelets, magnetic resonance imaging of brain, electroencephalogram) as clinically indicated.
2 Acyclovir (20mg/kg/dose intravenously every 8 hours, or every 12 hours if gestational age <35 weeks); topical eye treatment (1% to 2% trifluridine, 0.1% iododeoxyuridine, or 3% vidarabine) if eye disease is present or conjunctival culture is positive.
3 Culture conjunctiva, nasopharynx/mouth/throat, urine, stool/rectum; if any culture site is positive or infant develops clinical signs of possible HSV infection, complete evaluation[1] and treat[2].
4 Maternal serologic testing with assays that detect type-specific glycoprotein G may be helpful in differentiating between primary or recurrent infection.
5 Some experts recommend empiric acyclovir treatment at birth after HSV cultures are obtained, while others would await positive HSV culture results or clinical manifestations of infection before starting therapy.
6 Some experts would observe infant carefully and not treat unless cultures are positive for HSV or clinical signs of infection are present.

The results of antepartum genital HSV cultures from pregnant women with a history of genital herpes do not predict the infant's risk of exposure to HSV at delivery. Irrespective of method of delivery, all infants born to mothers with active genital herpes lesions should have appropriate cultures performed for HSV. Symptomatic infants are managed as discussed in the section, Therapy, whereas asymptomatic infants should have HSV cultures performed of conjunctiva, mouth/throat or nasopharynx, rectum or stool, and urine at 24 to 48 hours after delivery. Virus present at this time represents active replication and invasive infection, whereas virus isolated from mucous membrane cultures obtained at birth only may reflect surface contamination. HSV isolated from any of these cultures should prompt further evaluation (e.g., CSF analysis for routine studies and HSV PCR, complete blood cell count with differential and platelet count, and liver function tests) for possible dissemination of HSV.

An approach to the management of infants born to mothers with active HSV genital infection at delivery is provided in Figure 78.1. If the mother has primary or first-episode genital herpes, and the infant is born vaginally, by caesarean section following prolonged rupture of membranes, is premature, or has had invasive instrumentation or skin laceration during delivery, prophylactic or anticipatory antiviral therapy is recommended. If the mother has recurrent genital herpes, and the infant is full term and no scalp electrode has been used, antiviral therapy is withheld until culture results are known or clinical signs of disease develop. If the infant is premature or had a scalp electrode, then prophylactic acyclovir therapy is instituted. Antiviral therapy also is initiated if HSV is isolated from any infant culture. This approach is widely recommended, but its efficacy remains unproved.

Infants born to women with active genital herpes, and who are at high risk for being infected, should be managed with contact precautions in the nursery or should room with the mother. Adherence to hand hygiene before handling the infant should be stressed to the mother to prevent postpartum transmission. Breast-feeding is contraindicated only if the mother has vesicular lesions on the breast. Delay of circumcision for approximately 1 month for infants at highest risk of disease may be warranted.

Nursery personnel with oral and genital HSV lesions are at low risk of transmitting infection to infants as long as their lesions are covered. They must adhere to appropriate hand hygiene when handling infants. Personnel with herpetic whitlow should not have direct patient-care responsibilities until the lesions have healed. HSV-2 vaccine trials currently are under investigation.

Suggested Readings

Gutierrez K, Arvin AM. Long term antiviral suppression after treatment for neonatal herpes infection. *Pediatr Infect Dis J* 2003;22:371.

Hutto C, Arvin A, Jacobs R, et al. Intrauterine herpes simplex virus infections. *J Pediatr* 1987;110:97.

Kimberlin DW. Neonatal herpes simplex infection. *Clin Microbiol Rev* 2004; 17:1.

Kimberlin DW, Lakeman FD, Arvin AM, et al. and the National Institute of Allergy and Infectious Diseases Collaborative Antiviral Study Group. Application of the polymerase chain reaction to diagnosis and management of neonatal herpes simplex virus disease. *J Infect Dis* 1996;174:1162.

Kimberlin DW, Lin C-Y, Jacobs RF, et al. , and the National Institute of Allergy and Infectious Diseases Collaborative Antiviral Study Group. Natural history of neonatal herpes simplex virus infections in the acyclovir era. *Pediatrics* 2001;108:223.

Kimberlin DW, Lin C-Y, Jacobs RF, et al. , and the National Institute of Allergy and Infectious Diseases Collaborative Antiviral Study Group. Safety and efficacy of high-dose intravenous acyclovir in the management of neonatal herpes simplex virus infections. *Pediatrics* 2001;108:230.

Kimberlin DW, Powell D, Gruber W, et al. , and the National Institute of Allergy and Infectious Diseases Collaborative Antiviral Study Group. Administration of acyclovir suppressive therapy after neonatal herpes simplex virus disease limited to the skin, eyes, and mouth: results of a phase I/II trial. *Pediatr Infect Dis J* 1996;15:247.

Kimberlin DW, Rouse DJ. Genital herpes. *N Engl J Med* 2004;350:1970.

Whitley RJ, Arvin A, Prober C, et al. Predictors of morbidity and mortality in neonates with herpes simplex virus infections. *N Engl J Med* 1991;324:450.

CHAPTER 79 ■ NEONATAL VARICELLA-ZOSTER VIRUS

WILLIAM V. RASZKA

Varicella-zoster virus (VZV) is one of the eight members of the herpesvirus family. Found worldwide, VZV is an exclusive human pathogen that has the ability to remain latent in the host for decades. Primary infection with VZV—chickenpox—is an exanthematous disease primarily of children. Reactivation of VZV—herpes zoster (zoster or "shingles")—may occur at any time after the primary infection but occurs more often in older individuals. In the pre-vaccine era, almost the entire U.S. birth cohort became infected with VZV during childhood. Since the introduction of an effective vaccine in 1995, however, the incidence rates of VZV infection in the United States have plummeted.

Transplacental VZV infection may occur in as many as 25% of infants whose mothers develop chickenpox during pregnancy. However, very few neonates develop symptomatic congenital infection. Transplacental infection with subsequent clinical sequelae in the fetus has been well described but is very uncommon and dependent on the timing of the infection. In a cohort of women followed prospectively in the United States, the frequency of congenital VZV syndrome was 0.4%. Based on other studies, the incidence rate of embryopathy associated with maternal infection is 2.2% and linked with infection during the first 20 weeks of gestation.

EPIDEMIOLOGY

In the United States, chickenpox is an uncommon infection during pregnancy. Because VZV is not a reportable disease in most parts of the United States, the exact incidence is difficult to know. Large prospective studies completed decades ago calculated the incidence of maternal VZV during pregnancy as 0.8 in 10,000. A more recent study predicted an incidence rate as high as 7 in 10,000. Physicians caring for immigrants from tropical countries may see a higher incidence of disease, because chickenpox is not a universal infection of childhood in countries outside temperate climate zones. Although pregnant women with chickenpox may develop pneumonia and premature labor, a more recent prospective study of approximately 1,400 pregnant European women with chickenpox found no maternal deaths.

PATHOGENESIS

A neonate can acquire VZV infection *in utero* from a mother who is in the viremic stage of chickenpox or postnatally from exposure to infectious respiratory secretions or vesicular fluid in a patient with chickenpox or zoster. After inoculation of the virus onto the surface of the upper respiratory tract or the conjunctivae, the virus replicates locally, before disseminating in 4 to 6 days via an asymptomatic primary viremia. After replication in the liver, spleen, and possibly other sites for another 6 to 8 days, the virus disseminates widely in a high-grade viremia that may be accompanied by typical prodromal signs such as fever, malaise, and anorexia. The characteristic lesions of VZV are vesicles that develop in another 1 to 2 days. Vesicles on the skin are thin walled and filled with a clear fluid, often described as "dewdrops on a rose petal." In chickenpox, the vesicles evolve over several days from macule, to papule,

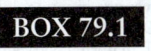

BOX 79.1   Characteristic Features of Fetal Varicella Syndrome

Unilateral cicatricial lesions that correspond to dermatome distribution
Limb paresis/paralysis, hydrocephalus/cortical atrophy, seizures, delayed development, sphincter dysfunction
Chorioretinitis, anisocoria, nystagmus, microphthalmia cataract
Hypoplasia of extremities, digits
Gastrointestinal and genitourinary anomalies
Failure to thrive

---

vesicle, pustule, and crusted lesion and occur in various stages on any mucocutaneous surface. The incubation period for the development of disease is 10 to 21 days, with an average appearance of the rash at 14 days. Patients are infectious for 1 to 2 days before the development of a rash and for 5 days after the last vesicle has crusted. The virus is highly infectious, with attack rates of up to 90% reported in household settings.

In zoster, no viremic stage exists, because the virus reactivates in a single dermatome. The vesicles are infectious until they have crusted.

CLINICAL MANIFESTATIONS AND COMPLICATIONS

The most frequently observed features of congenital VZV syndrome include cutaneous scars (75%); neurologic defects, including paresis (60%); limb hypoplasia or anomalies (50%), and eye lesions including chorioretinitis, micro-ophthalmia, and cataracts (50%). (See Box 79.1). Infants have had microcephaly, hydrocephalus, and other central nervous system manifestation without evidence of a rash. Almost 30% of children with symptomatic congenital varicella die in the first months of life. Rarely, children may develop signs of encephalitis from CNS reactivation of the virus later in infancy.

Infants infected *in utero* more than 5 days before delivery usually appear normal at birth but may go on to develop zoster early in life, without an episode of clinically apparent chickenpox. Maternal zoster is not associated with transplacental infection, because zoster is not associated with a viremic phase except in the severely immunocompromised host.

Infants whose mothers develop chickenpox from 5 days before to 2 days after delivery have a 25% chance of developing chickenpox. Chickenpox in this group of neonates can be severe, because the infants are infected with a large inoculum of virus during maternal viremia and circulating maternal antibody is not present to help ameliorate disease. The incubation period for the development of disease is 1 to 16 days. The clinical features of perinatally acquired VZV infection include severe rash, pneumonia, and hepatitis. Death has occurred in 20% to 30% of untreated infants.

Term neonates born to mothers immune to varicella infrequently develop evidence of chickenpox following exposure to VZV in the neonatal period due to the protective effect of high levels of transplacentally acquired anti-VZV antibody. If chickenpox does develop, it is usually mild. Infants born before 28 weeks gestation to immune mothers have low levels of anti-VZV antibody and should be considered unprotected following exposure.

DIAGNOSIS

The diagnosis of VZV infection can be made clinically in most situations. Several methods of laboratory confirmation are available. A Tzanck smear of scrapings from the base of a vesicle may show multinucleated giant cells, but this is a nonspecific and insensitive way to confirm VZV. Immunofluorescent staining of vesicular scrapings using monoclonal antibodies is the most sensitive and rapid commercially available microbiologic method to confirm VZV and can be used to distinguish VZV from herpes simplex virus (HSV). Although VZV does not grow as well or as fast as HSV, VZV can be recovered from the fluid of vesicles during the first few days of illness. Polymerase chain reaction (PCR) is a very sensitive and specific tool to identify VZV. It is used most often as part of a research protocol and to distinguish wild-type from vaccine-induced varicella. Serologic studies can be used to help confirm or exclude disease. Specific anti-VZV IgG and IgM antibodies can be detected using latex agglutination, enzyme-linked immunosorbent assays (ELISA), or fluorescent antibody-to-membrane antigen tests. In newborns, IgG antibodies are not helpful to confirm infection.

THERAPY

Neonates born with evidence of congenital VZV require no therapy. Neonates with congenital VZV who develop central nervous system manifestations may be treated with acyclovir. Neonates with severe perinatal VZV infection can be treated with acyclovir at a dose of 45 mg/kg/day in three divided doses for 5 to 7 days.

PREVENTION

The most effective way to prevent congenital and perinatal VZV infection is to ensure that all women of childbearing age are immune to VZV. Women who report a history of VZV infection or have been immunized are considered immune. The live, attenuated VZV vaccine induces durable immunity in immunocompetent individuals. Although contraindicated in pregnancy, women given the vaccine inadvertently early in pregnancy have not delivered children with the congenital VZV syndrome. Vaccine-associated virus has been transmitted extremely rarely within households. Hence, a pregnant or breast-feeding woman in the home is not a contraindication to administering the VZV vaccine to susceptible children at the appropriate age. All health care workers should have evidence of immunity either by documented natural infection, appropriate number of vaccine doses, or serologic testing.

Mothers not immune to varicella who develop chickenpox during pregnancy should be given varicella zoster immune globulin (VZIG) intramuscularly within 96 hours of exposure. The dose is 125 U/10 kg of weight, with a maximum of dose of 625 U. Although it is not known whether VZIG will prevent the development of the congenital VZV syndrome, administration does significantly reduce the incidence of congenital infection. VZIG (125 U) should be administered to all neonates whose mothers develop chickenpox within 5 days before or 2 days after delivery. It also is recommended for hospitalized newborns born at less than 28 weeks gestation following exposure, regardless of the maternal immune status. VZIG does not completely prevent infection but does decrease disease severity. Mothers with zoster at the time of delivery should cover the lesions.

Because VZV is so contagious and can be spread by contact with vesicular fluid or airborne respiratory secretions, all patients with active lesions of chickenpox should be placed on both airborne and contact precautions. Hospitalized infants born to mothers who have chickenpox within16 days before delivery and 2 days afterward should be placed in isolation for 21 days. Because VZIG may increase the incubation period of VZV infection, all hospitalized patients administered VZIG should be considered potentially infectious and placed in isolation until 28 days after the exposure.

Although case reports have documented its effectiveness, acyclovir is not generally recommended for postexposure prophylaxis of VZV.

Suggested Readings

Enders G, Miller E, Cradock-Watson J, et al. Consequences of varicella and herpes zoster in pregnancy: prospective study of 1,739 cases. *Lancet* 1994; 343:1548.

Harger JH, Ernest JM, Thurnau GR, et al. Frequency of congenital varicella syndrome in a prospective cohort of 347 pregnant women. *Obstet Gynecol* 2002;100:260.

Huang YC, Lin TY, Lin YJ, et al. Prophylaxis of intravenous immunoglobulin and acyclovir in perinatal varicella. *Eur J Pediatr* 2001;160:91.

Pastuszak AL, Levy M, Schick B, et al. Outcome of maternal varicella infection in the first 20 weeks of pregnancy. *N Engl J Med* 1994;330: 901.

Sauerbrei A, Pawlak J, Luger C, Wutzler P. Intracerebral varicella-zoster virus reactivation in congenital varicella syndrome. *Dev Med Child Neurol* 2003;45:837.

Sauerbrei A, Wutzler P. The congenital varicella syndrome. *J Perinatol* 2000;20: 548.

Seward JF, Watson BM, Peterson CL, et al. Varicella disease after introduction of varicella vaccine in the United States, 1995–2000. *JAMA* 2002;287: 606.

Shields KE, Galil K, Seward J, et al. Varicella vaccine exposure during pregnancy: data from the first 5 years of the pregnancy registry. *Obstet Gynecol* 2001;98:14.

CHAPTER 80 ■ EPSTEIN-BARR VIRUS

WILLIAM V. RASZKA

Epstein-Barr virus (EBV) is perhaps the most ubiquitous member of the herpesviruses family. Similar to herpes simplex virus, EBV infection can lead to a distinct clinical syndrome as well as to asymptomatic shedding of the virus after primary infection. In many parts of the world, infection is universal by age 3 years. In the United States, infection may be postponed until the second or third decade of life. Large prospective studies in the United States and Europe have shown that fewer than 5% of pregnant women are EBV seronegative and that women rarely seroconvert during pregnancy.

Reactivation of EBV during pregnancy could potentially lead to *in utero* infection. However, in a group of pregnant women with evidence of reactivation as evidenced by a rise in EBV early antigen titers, no embryopathy was detected. In most women who have documented EBV during pregnancy, no fetal effects have been observed. Reports of symptomatic congenital EBV infection are exceedingly rare. One child with documented *in utero* EBV infection had micrognathia, cryptorchidism, cataracts, hypotonia, thrombocytopenia, and persistent monocytosis, whereas another had evidence of extrahepatic biliary atresia and onset of jaundice at 5 days of life.

Little is known about the affects of perinatal EBV infection. At least one report suggests that the outcome can be poor.

Neonates born to mothers with EBV infection during pregnancy should be examined carefully. Most of these infants appear normal, and no further investigation is necessary. In neonates with suspected symptomatic congenital EBV infection, acute and convalescent EBV titers, lymphocyte transformation studies, and polymerase chain reaction testing of blood or other tissues may be helpful in confirming the diagnosis.

Suggested Readings

Andronikou S, Kostoula A, Ioachim E, et al. Perinatal Epstein Barr virus infection in a premature infant. *Scand J Infect Dis* 1999;31:96.

Fleisher G, Bolognese R. Persistent Epstein-Barr virus infection and pregnancy. *J Infect Dis* 1983;147:982.

Goldberg GN, Fulginiti VA, Ray CG, et al. In utero Epstein-Barr virus (infectious mononucleosis) infection. *JAMA* 1981;246:1579.

Le CT, Chang RS, Lipson MH. Epstein-Barr virus infections during pregnancy: a prospective study and review of the literature. *Am J Dis Child* 1983;137: 466.

CHAPTER 81 ■ NEONATAL SYPHILIS

PABLO J. SÁNCHEZ AND JANE D. SIEGEL

EPIDEMIOLOGY

Congenital syphilis, a result of fetal infection with *Treponema pallidum,* remains a major public health problem worldwide. In the United States, from 1977 through 1990, a steady increase was seen in the incidence of primary and secondary syphilis among women (Fig. 81.1). This increase was greatest among African Americans and Hispanics of lower socioeconomic status who resided in large urban areas such as Detroit, Houston, Los Angeles, Miami, and New York City. A major contributor to the increase of syphilis in these populations was the exchange of illegal drugs (notably crack cocaine) for sex with multiple partners whose identities were not known. Partner notification, a traditional syphilis-control strategy, was impossible to implement. Moreover, these women rarely sought prenatal care.

Subsequently, the number of cases of early congenital syphilis reported to the Centers for Disease Control and Prevention increased from 108 in 1978 to more than 4,000 cases in 1991 (see Fig. 81.1). This dramatic increase was caused by both an increase in actual cases and the use of revised reporting guidelines. Beginning in 1989, the surveillance definition for congenital syphilis was broadened. The new definition includes not only all infants with clinical evidence of active syphilis, but also asymptomatic infants and stillbirths born to women with untreated or inadequately treated syphilis. Use of the new surveillance case definition increases the number of confirmed or presumptive cases of congenital syphilis by almost fourfold.

During the 1990s, a decrease in early syphilis was noted (see Fig. 81.1); this finding heightened expectations for the eventual control and even elimination of the disease in the United States. Syphilis rates had been at their lowest since reporting began in 1941, having declined 84% during the 1990s. This downward trend was attributed to innovative, community-based programs that identify locations with a high prevalence of syphilis, so-called core environments, such as specific sex-for-drugs locations, as well as core populations at high risk of infection, rather than on a sole reliance on named sexual contacts. Moreover, the awareness of the syphilis epidemic of the late 1980s resulted in wider serologic screening practices in clinics, emergency rooms, and hospitals. Since 2001, however, syphilis has increased among homosexual males, prompting concern for possible cotransmission of the human immunodeficiency virus (HIV). In addition, syphilis continues to occur disproportionately in the rural southern United States.

PATHOGENESIS

Pregnant women with early syphilis are at highest risk of delivering infected infants. Among women with untreated primary, secondary, early latent, or late latent syphilis at delivery, approximately 30%, 60%, 40%, and 7% of infants, respectively, will be infected. Transmission of infection to the fetus usually occurs transplacentally from maternal spirochetemia, but the neonate also can be infected through contact with a genital lesion at the time of delivery. Although congenital infection can occur anytime during gestation, the risk of fetal infection increases as the stage of pregnancy advances. The theory that the Langerhans cell layer of the cytotrophoblast forms a placental barrier against fetal infection before the eighteenth week of pregnancy was disproved by demonstration of spirochetes in fetal tissue from spontaneous abortion at 9 and 10 weeks' gestation and recovery of spirochetes from amniotic fluid at 14 weeks of pregnancy. Electron microscopy findings also disprove this theory by demonstrating the persistence of the Langerhans cell layer throughout pregnancy.

CLINICAL MANIFESTATIONS AND COMPLICATIONS

Syphilis during pregnancy is associated with premature delivery, spontaneous abortion, stillbirth, nonimmune hydrops, perinatal death, and two characteristic syndromes of clinical disease, early and late congenital syphilis. *Early congenital syphilis* refers to those clinical manifestations that appear within the first 2 years of life. Those features that occur after 2 years are designated as *late congenital syphilis*. The clinical manifestations and laboratory findings of early congenital syphilis may be present at birth or may be delayed for several months if the infant remains untreated. The physical signs are a direct result of active infection and inflammation.

Infants with congenital syphilis may be growth restricted at delivery. Hepatitis with hepatosplenomegaly occurs in 50% to 90% of affected infants. Splenomegaly does not occur without liver enlargement. Extramedullary hematopoiesis is seen in both the liver and spleen. Approximately one-third of infants have direct and indirect hyperbilirubinemia and elevated transaminase levels, which may worsen transiently after the initiation of penicillin therapy. Liver abnormalities may require more than 1 year to resolve, but they rarely lead to

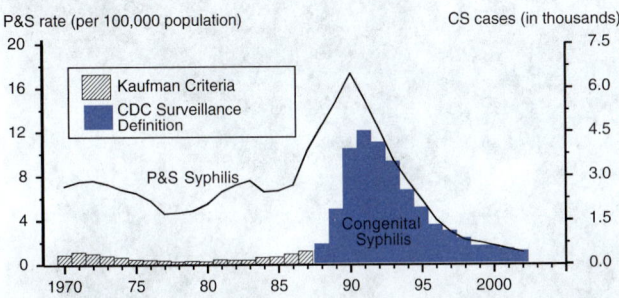

FIGURE 81.1. Case rates of primary and secondary syphilis among women and congenital syphilis cases in the United States, 1970 to 2002. The rate of congenital syphilis increased since 1983, peaked in 1991, and has subsequently decreased. The surveillance case definition for congenital syphilis changed in 1988. (Data used with permission from Centers for Disease Control and Prevention, Atlanta, GA, Public Health Service, 2004.)

cirrhosis. Generalized nontender lymphadenopathy occurs in 20% to 50% of cases, with characteristic involvement of the epitrochlear nodes. Hemolytic anemia with a negative Coombs' test result is common. The peripheral leukocyte count can show either leukopenia or leukemoid reaction. Thrombocytopenia with petechiae and purpura occurs in approximately 30% of infants and may be the sole manifestation of congenital infection.

Mucocutaneous lesions are specific for congenital syphilis and occur in 40% to 60% of affected infants. The rash of congenital syphilis usually is maculopapular and located on the extremities. The lesions are initially oval and pink but then turn coppery brown and desquamate. Desquamation occurs mainly on the palms and soles. A characteristic vesicular bullous eruption known as *pemphigus syphiliticus* may develop with erythema, blister formation, and eventual crusting as healing occurs (see color Fig. 128.8 in color section). Nasal discharge associated with rhinitis or snuffles is initially watery, but it may become thick, purulent, and even tinged with blood (Fig. 81.2). Nasal discharge and vesicular fluid contain large concentrations of spirochetes and are highly infectious. Rarely, mucous patches of the lips, tongue, and palate and condyloma lata in the perioral and perianal areas may occur.

Bone roentgenography shows skeletal abnormalities consisting of osteochondritis, periostitis, and osteitis in 80% to 90% of infants (Figs. 81.3 and 81.4). These abnormalities tend to be multiple and symmetric, with the lower extremities involved more often than the upper extremities. The long bones (tibia, humerus, femur), ribs, and cranium principally are affected. Rarely, bone lesions may be painful or have superimposed fractures resulting in pseudoparalysis of the affected limb (pseudoparalysis of Parrot). Osteochondritis involves the metaphysis and is evident roentgenographically approximately 5 weeks after fetal infection. Typical findings are metaphyseal demineralization and a radiodense band below the epiphyseal

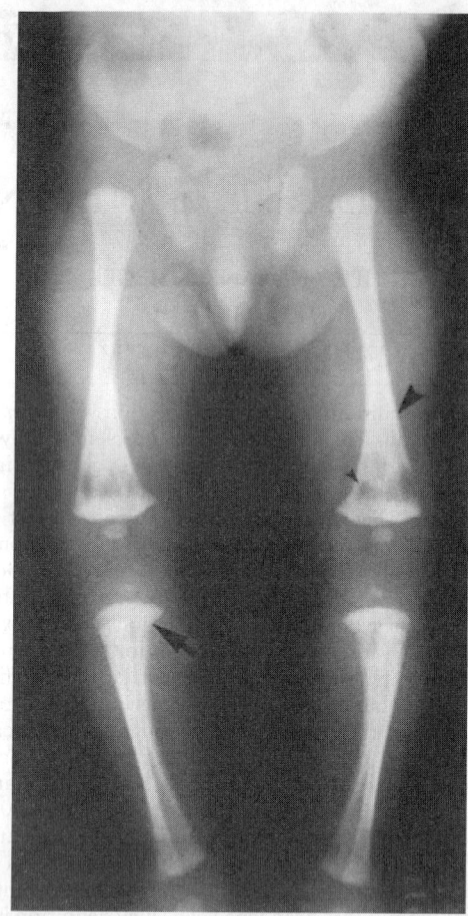

FIGURE 81.3. Bony lesions of early congenital syphilis: symmetric periostitis (*large arrow*); radiolucent metaphyseal area of osteochondritis (*small arrowhead*); bilateral metaphyseal defects on the upper medial aspect of the tibia; and Wimberger sign (*large arrowhead*). Similar changes may occur at the upper ends of the humeri. (Courtesy of Dr. Guido Currarino, Dallas, TX.)

plate that represents a widened and enhanced zone of provisional calcification. An underlying zone of osteoporosis is evident as a radiolucent band. Bilateral demineralization and osseous destruction of the proximal medial tibial metaphysis are referred to as *Wimberger sign* (see Fig. 81.3). The classic transverse saw-toothed appearance of the metaphysis (see Fig. 81.4)

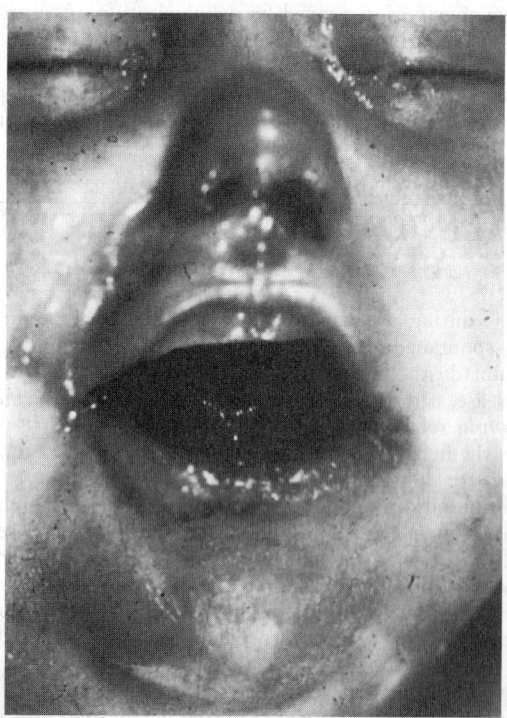

FIGURE 81.2. Sniffles or rhinitis in an infant with early congenital syphilis. This mucous discharge develops after the first week of life. See Figure 81.2 in color section. (Courtesy of Dr. George H. McCracken, Jr., Dallas, TX.)

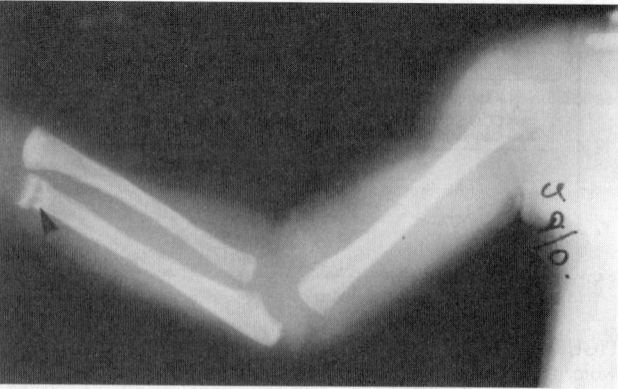

FIGURE 81.4. Saw-toothed appearance of the metaphysis of the distal radius (*arrow*) of an infant with early congenital syphilis. The lucent area represents syphilitic granulation tissue. (Courtesy of Dr. Guido Currarino, Dallas, TX.)

often is not seen on plain roentgenography but is evident on xeroradiography of long bones of stillborn infants with congenital syphilis. Periostitis requires 16 weeks for roentgenographic demonstration and consists of multiple layers of periosteal new bone formation in response to diaphyseal inflammation. Osteitis creates a "celery stalk" appearance in long bones (see Fig. 81.3), resulting from involvement of the medullary canal with resultant diaphysitis. After several months, complete healing of the affected bones occurs, even without antibiotic therapy.

Neurosyphilis occurs in 40% to 60% of infants with congenital syphilis. Two types of central nervous system involvement are described. Acute syphilitic leptomeningitis occurs in early infancy. Chronic meningovascular syphilis with progressive hydrocephalus, cranial nerve palsies, and cerebral infarction secondary to endarteritis usually presents toward the end of the first year of life. Cerebrospinal fluid (CSF) examination reveals pleocytosis with an elevated protein content and a reactive VDRL test result. Hypopituitarism presenting with hypoglycemia also has been reported as a result of treponemal infection of the anterior pituitary gland.

Ocular findings include chorioretinitis, cataract, glaucoma, and uveitis. Nephrosis with generalized edema, ascites, and proteinuria usually occurs at 2 to 3 months of age as a result of immune complex deposition in the renal glomeruli. Other less common manifestations include pneumonitis, pneumonia alba, myocarditis, pancreatitis, and inflammation and fibrosis of the gastrointestinal tract leading to malabsorption and diarrhea.

The clinical manifestations of late congenital syphilis result from ongoing inflammation or from scars caused by an infection of early congenital syphilis. Development of the characteristic lesions is prevented by treatment during pregnancy or within the first 3 months of life. Infants with late congenital syphilis are not infective.

Dental stigmata result from the inflammatory response to *T. pallidum* infection in the developing permanent teeth during late gestation. The affected permanent upper central incisors (Hutchinson teeth) are small, widely spaced, barrel-shaped, and notched, with thinning and discoloration of the enamel (Fig. 81.5). The first 6-year lower molars (mulberry or Moon molars) also may be affected. The top surface has many small cusps instead of the usual four. Enamelization is defective. Infection before the eighteenth week of gestation may result in involvement of deciduous teeth, which then are misshapen, hypoplastic, and prone to dental caries.

The sequela of periostitis of the skull is frontal bossing; of the tibia, saber shins; and of the clavicle, is Higoumenakis sign with sternoclavicular thickening. Clutton joints, or painless synovitis and hydrarthrosis without involvement of the adjacent bones, is rare. Osteochondritis affecting the otic capsule may lead to cochlear degeneration and fibrous adhesions resulting in eighth-nerve deafness, for which corticosteroid treatment may be beneficial.

The sequelae of syphilitic rhinitis include rhagades and short maxilla with a high palatal arch. If the inflammation of the nasal mucosa extends to the underlying cartilage and bone, perforation of the palate and nasal septum occurs, resulting in a "saddle nose" deformity.

Late ocular manifestations include uveitis and interstitial keratitis. Interstitial keratitis usually appears at puberty and is not affected by penicillin therapy. Although corticosteroid treatment may be beneficial, keratitis often has a relapsing course and may lead to corneal clouding and blindness. Possible sequelae of central nervous system infection include mental retardation, hydrocephalus, seizure disorder, cranial nerve palsies, paralysis, and optic nerve atrophy.

DIAGNOSIS

The diagnosis of congenital syphilis is established by the observation of spirochetes in body fluids or tissue and suggested by serologic testing results. *T. pallidum* may be identified by dark-field microscopy, fluorescent antibody, or silver stain of mucocutaneous lesions, nasal discharge, vesicular fluid, amniotic fluid, placenta, umbilical cord, or tissue obtained at autopsy. A diagnosis of congenital syphilis also is suggested by a large, pale, firm placenta, which on microscopic examination reveals acute villitis, villous enlargement, and erythroblastosis. Involvement of the umbilical cord may result in a severe inflammatory reaction within its matrix, which is termed *necrotizing funisitis*.

Serologic tests for syphilis are classified into nontreponemal and treponemal tests. Nontreponemal tests include the VDRL test and the rapid plasma reagin test. The same nontreponemal test should be performed on the mother and infant so that accurate comparisons can be made. A diagnosis of congenital syphilis is supported by an infant's nontreponemal antibody level that is four or more times than that of the mother's serum. The absence of such a finding, however, does not exclude a possible diagnosis of congenital syphilis. Treponemal tests include the fluorescent treponemal antibody-absorption (FTA-ABS) test and a microhemagglutination assay called *T. pallidum* particle agglutination test (TP-PA). These tests are used to confirm the diagnosis of syphilis after a reactive nontreponemal test has been reported. They do not need to be performed in the neonatal period because no comparisons between maternal and infant results can be made; they are qualitative tests and are reported as being reactive or nonreactive. Because these tests detect IgG antibodies that are transferred across the placenta to the infant, all infants born to mothers with a reactive treponemal test also will have a positive test.

A measurement of total cord IgM levels and the results of specific fluorescent treponemal IgM (FTA-ABS-IgM) tests have not proved useful in the diagnosis of congenital syphilis and are therefore not recommended. Elevated cord IgM levels can result from other congenital infections as well as from noninfectious abnormalities. Rheumatoid factor, which occurs frequently in congenital syphilis, interferes with the interpretation of FTA-ABS-IgM test results by producing as many as 35% false-positive results. A 10% false-negative rate also is reported with the use of this test. Similarly, an IgM enzyme-linked immunosorbent assay test (DCL-Syphilis-M test kit, Diagnostic Chemicals Ltd., Oxford, CT) also has suboptimal sensitivity.

Several investigators have used immunoblotting to detect and characterize the specific fetal and neonatal IgM and IgA antibody responses to *T. pallidum*. Specific IgM and IgA reactivity

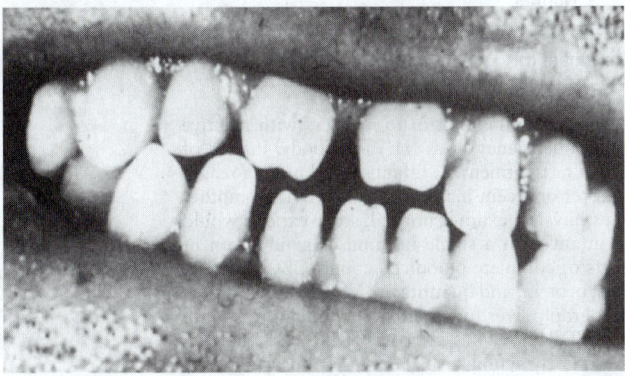

FIGURE 81.5. Hutchinson teeth in a child with late congenital syphilis. The small, widely spaced, notched upper central incisors may be detected by radiography, whereas deciduous teeth are in place. (Courtesy of Dr. George H. McCracken, Jr., Dallas, TX.)

directed against several antigens of *T. pallidum,* and in particular against a membrane lipoprotein with an apparent molecular mass of 47 kd, has been detected in sera from infants with clinical findings of congenital syphilis as well as in those with subclinical infection. Similar IgM reactivity to the 47-kd antigen also has been detected in the CSF of infants with congenital syphilis.

Polymerase chain reaction (PCR) has been used to detect specific *T. pallidum* DNA in tissues and body fluids. Studies with PCR performed on amniotic fluid, neonatal blood, and CSF have yielded sensitivities of 100%, 74%, and 71%, respectively, with excellent specificity. The combined use of IgM immunoblotting and PCR ultimately will aid in the early identification of infected infants, regardless of clinical status.

A practical approach to the evaluation and treatment of infants born to mothers with reactive serologic tests for syphilis is presented in Figure 81.6. Testing of all pregnant women with syphilis for coinfection with the human immunodeficiency virus (HIV) is strongly recommended, because the genital ulcerations seen in syphilis can facilitate the transmission of HIV. All infants born to mothers with reactive serologic test results for syphilis should have a serum quantitative nontreponemal

test performed and be carefully examined for physical signs of congenital syphilis. Infants who have (a) an abnormal physical examination that is consistent with congenital syphilis, (b) a serum quantitative nontreponemal serologic titer that is fourfold or greater than the mother's, or (c) a positive dark-field or fluorescent antibody test result of body fluid should have a complete blood cell count (CBC) and platelet count performed as well as CSF examination for cell count, protein content, and VDRL test. Other tests, such as bone and chest roentgenography, liver function tests, cranial ultrasound, ophthalmologic examination, and auditory brainstem response, should be performed as clinically indicated. These infants are considered to have proved or highly probable disease; spirochetemia with invasion of the central nervous system is likely. Although these infants must receive a full course of penicillin therapy, which treats possible neurosyphilis, it is beneficial for follow-up purposes to establish central nervous system abnormalities at presentation. Nonetheless, the diagnosis of congenital neurosyphilis is difficult to establish. Diagnosis is based on CSF examination that shows a reactive result to the VDRL test, pleocytosis (>25 leukocytes per microliter), and an elevated protein content (>150 mg/dL). The presence of red blood

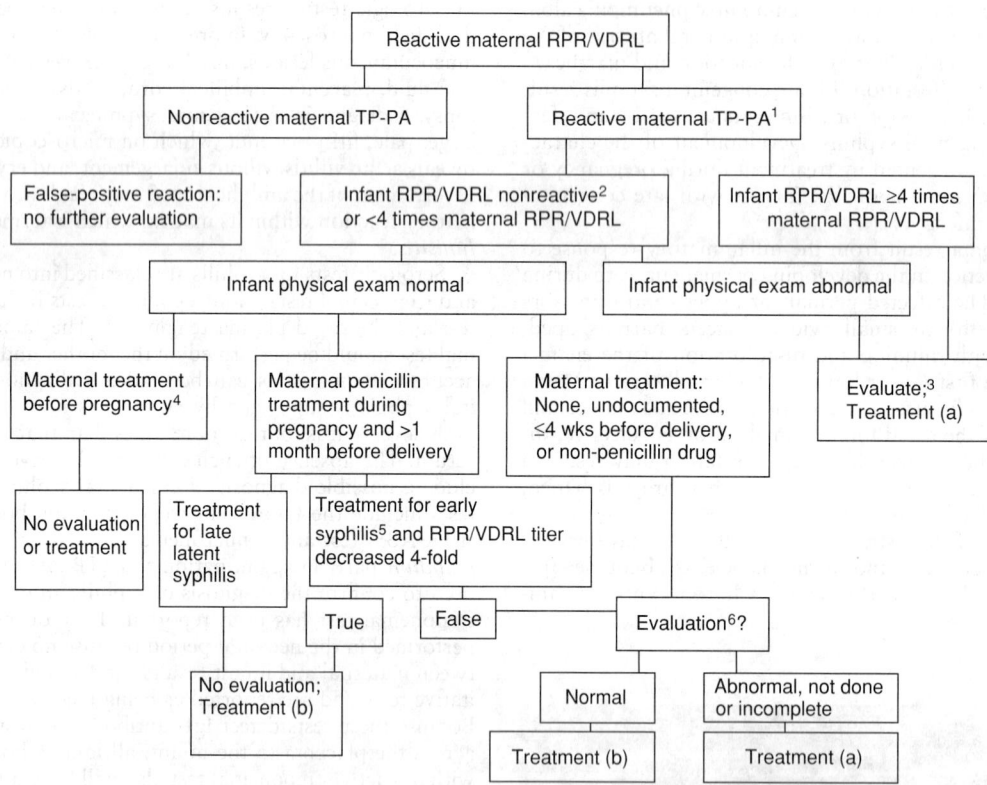

FIGURE 81.6. An approach to the evaluation and treatment of infants born to mothers with reactive serologic test results for syphilis: 1. Test for human immunodeficiency virus (HIV)-antibody. Infants of HIV-Ab positive mothers do not require different evaluation or treatment. 2. Infant's rapid plasma reagin test (*RPR*) may be nonreactive due to low maternal RPR titer or recent maternal infection. If the mother has untreated or inadequately treated syphilis, and infant's physical exam is normal, some experts would not perform diagnostic evaluation but would treat the infant with a single intramuscular injection of benzathine penicillin (50,000 U/kg). 3. Evaluation consists of complete blood cell count (CBC), platelet count; cerebrospinal fluid (CSF) examination for cell count, protein, and quantitative VDRL; other tests as clinically indicated (eye exam, long-bone films; chest radiograph; liver function tests; cranial ultrasound; auditory brainstem response). 4. Women who maintain a VDRL titer of 1:2 or less (RPR ≤1:4) beyond 1 year after successful treatment are considered serofast. 5. Early syphilis is primary, secondary, or early latent infection. 6. CBC, platelet count; CSF examination for cell count, protein, and quantitative VDRL; long-bone films. Treatment: (a) Aqueous penicillin G, 50,000 U/kg intravenously every 12 hours (≤1 week of age) or every 8 hours (>1 week), or procaine penicillin G, 50,000 U/kg intramuscularly in a single daily dose for 10 days. (b) Benzathine penicillin G, 50,000 U/kg intramuscularly in one dose. TP-PA, *Treponema pallidum* particle agglutination assay.

cells in the CSF as a result of a traumatic lumbar puncture can produce a false-positive serologic reaction. Also, a reactive CSF VDRL test may be caused by the passive transfer of nontreponemal IgG antibodies from serum into the CSF. When compared to the isolation of spirochetes from infant CSF by rabbit inoculation, the sensitivity and specificity of a reactive CSF VDRL test, pleocytosis, and elevated protein content are 53% and 90%, 38% and 88%, and 56% and 78%, respectively. Central nervous system infection has been documented in 41% of infants who have any abnormality on clinical, laboratory, or radiographic evaluation, and in 60% of those who have an abnormal physical examination consistent with a diagnosis of congenital syphilis. Spirochetes also have been isolated from CSF by rabbit inoculation in three infants with normal CSF indices and nonreactive CSF VDRL test. These results indicate that central nervous system invasion is common among infected infants, and that once clinical, laboratory, or radiographic evaluation supports a diagnosis of congenital syphilis, then therapy effective against central nervous system disease is warranted.

In infants who have a normal physical examination and a serum quantitative nontreponemal test result that is less than fourfold the maternal titer, further evaluation and treatment depends on the maternal treatment history and stage of infection (see Fig. 81.6). Whether to perform a complete evaluation (lumbar puncture, long-bone radiography, and CBC and platelets) on the infant depends on the planned treatment. Such evaluation must be performed and be completely normal if a single intramuscular dose of benzathine penicillin G therapy is administered.

Infants with reactive serologic test results at delivery should have serial quantitative nontreponemal tests performed until the test results show nonreactivity. Similarly, infants who are seronegative, but whose mothers acquired syphilis late in gestation, should be followed with serial testing after penicillin therapy is instituted. Follow-up for these infants can be incorporated into routine pediatric care at 2, 4, 6, 12, 15, and 24 months. In infants with congenital syphilis, nontreponemal serologic tests become nonreactive within 6 to 12 months after appropriate treatment. Uninfected infants usually become seronegative by 6 months of age. Infants with persistently low, stable titers of nontreponemal tests beyond 1 year of age may require re-treatment. A reactive treponemal test beyond 18 months of age, when the infant has lost all maternal antibody, confirms the diagnosis of congenital syphilis. Infants with abnormal CSF findings should have a repeat lumbar puncture performed at 6 months after therapy. A reactive CSF VDRL test result or an abnormal protein content or cell count at that time is an indication for re-treatment.

THERAPY

The decision to treat an infant for congenital syphilis is based on the clinical presentation, previous serologic test results and treatment of the mother, and the results of serologic testing of the infant and mother at the time of delivery. Treatment at birth is required in the following situations: the infant has clinical, laboratory, radiographic, or a combination of the three findings consistent with a diagnosis of congenital syphilis (symptomatic); maternal treatment was inadequate or unknown; the mother was treated with drugs other than penicillin; the mother was treated within 4 weeks of delivery; maternal treatment cannot be fully evaluated because insufficient time has elapsed

for nontreponemal test titer to decrease fourfold; the mother's sexual partner has not received treatment and the possibility exists of maternal reinfection; or adequate follow-up care of the infant is uncertain. Infants with proved or highly probable disease, or who have a normal physical examination but an abnormal or incomplete evaluation, should be treated with either aqueous crystalline penicillin G (50,000 U/kg intravenously every 12 hours for the first week of life, followed by every 8 hours beyond 7 days of age) or aqueous procaine penicillin G (50,000 U/kg intramuscularly once daily) for 10 days. Infants who have a normal physical examination, CSF studies, CBC and platelet count, and long-bone radiographs can be treated with a single intramuscular injection of benzathine penicillin G at a dose of 50,000 U/kg. If the risk of infection in the these infants is significant, and adequate follow-up cannot be ensured, the 10-day course of aqueous or procaine penicillin is recommended by the Centers for Disease Control and Prevention and American Academy of Pediatrics, regardless of results of the CSF and laboratory examination. Failure of a single injection of benzathine penicillin in the treatment of congenital syphilis has been reported. Treatment failures have been attributed to the inability of penicillin to adequately penetrate and achieve treponemicidal concentrations in certain sites such as the aqueous humor and central nervous system.

PREVENTION

Congenital syphilis is effectively prevented by the prenatal serologic screening of mothers and penicillin treatment of infected women, their sexual partners, and their newborn infants. All pregnant women should have a nontreponemal serologic test for syphilis performed at the first prenatal visit in the first trimester, with the test being repeated at 28 weeks' gestation and at delivery in areas with a high incidence of syphilis. Serologic screening tests should be performed on mothers and not on infants, because the infant may have a nonreactive serologic test result, but the mother's test is reactive at a low level. A newborn should not be discharged home before the result of maternal serologic testing during pregnancy or at delivery is known. All cases of syphilis must be reported to the local public health department, which performs contact investigation and identifies core environments and populations.

Suggested Readings

Centers for Disease Control and Prevention. Sexually transmitted diseases treatment guidelines 2002. *MMWR* 2002;51(No. RR-6):26.

Grimprel E, Sánchez PJ, Wendel GD, et al. Use of polymerase chain reaction and rabbit infectivity testing to detect *Treponema pallidum* in amniotic fluid, fetal and neonatal sera, and cerebrospinal fluid. *J Clin Microbiol* 1991;29:1711.

Ingall D, Sánchez PJ. Syphilis. In: Remington JS, Klein JO, eds. *Infectious diseases of the fetus and newborn infant.* Philadelphia: Saunders, 2001:643.

Larsen SA, Steiner BM, Rudolph AH. Laboratory diagnosis and interpretation of tests for syphilis. *Clin Microbiol Rev* 1995;8:1.

Michelow IC, Wendel GD, Norgard MV, et al. Central nervous system infection in congenital syphilis. *N Engl J Med* 2002;346:1792.

Sánchez PJ. Laboratory tests for congenital syphilis. *Pediatr Infect Dis J* 1998;17:70.

Sánchez PJ, Wendel GD. Syphilis in pregnancy. *Clin Perinatol* 1997;24:71.

Sánchez PJ, Wendel GD, Grimprel E, et al. Evaluation of molecular methodologies and rabbit infectivity testing for the diagnosis of congenital syphilis and neonatal central nervous system invasion by *Treponema pallidum. J Infect Dis* 1993;167:148.

Sheffield JS, Sánchez PJ, Wendel GD Jr. , et al. Placental histopathology of congenital syphilis. *Obstet Gynecol* 2002;100:126.

CHAPTER 82 ■ RUBELLA

WILLIAM V. RASZKA

Rubella, also known as German measles, is characterized by a generalized erythematous maculopapular rash, widespread adenopathy, fever, and in adolescents and adults, transient polyarthralgia. Although the clinical manifestations of rubella have been well described since the nineteenth century, it was not until 1941 that infections in pregnant women were linked to congenital cataracts and other clinical manifestations in neonates now known as the congenital rubella syndrome (CRS). Following licensure of a live, attenuated rubella vaccine in 1969, the incidence of rubella infection has fallen by 99% in the United States. Because rubella is an exclusively human pathogen, one goal of the U.S. immunization strategy is the elimination of indigenous rubella.

EPIDEMIOLOGY

Rubella infection in the United States now is distinctly uncommon. Between 1990 and 1999, the median annual number of reported rubella cases was 232. In only one of the years between 1992 and 1999 were more than 300 cases reported. During this time, the incidence of rubella infection in children younger than 15 years decreased from 0.63 to 0.06 in 100,000 whereas the incidence in adults increased slightly from 0.13 to 0.24 in 100,000. The vast majority of infections have occurred in unvaccinated individuals.

From 1990 through 1999, 117 cases of confirmed or probable CRS have been reported in the U.S. Almost one-third of patients with CRS can be linked to one of two rubella outbreaks in the United States. One outbreak occurred in California in 1989, while the other occurred in a Pennsylvania Amish community in 1991. On average, only six cases of congenital rubella have been reported each year from 1992 through 1999. Since 1993, CRS is seen far more commonly in neonates delivered to immigrants from regions without compulsory rubella immunization.

PATHOGENESIS

The transplacental transmission of rubella occurs during the viremic phase of primary maternal infection, generally a week before the appearance of a rash. Up to 20% of maternal infections occurring in the first 8 weeks of gestation result in miscarriage. Fetal infections occur in 90% of pregnancies when the maternal infection occurred during the first trimester, 25% to 30% during the second trimester, and 53% during the third trimester. The incidence of fetal anomalies varies according to the gestational age at the time of the maternal infection. If rubella infection occurs during gestational weeks 1 to 4, the incidence is 61% compared to 26% for weeks 5 to 8, 8% for weeks 13 to 16, and approximately 1% for subsequent weeks. Most studies report no excess defects in children whose mothers became infected at 18 weeks gestation or later.

Fetal damage is most likely multifactorial and may be secondary to rubella-induced apoptosis, decreased cellular life span, and necrotizing vasculitis. Clinical affects can be seen at the time of delivery or not until years after birth. In contrast to acquired rubella infection, congenital infection results in a persistent, progressive infection. Congenitally infected infants continue to excrete the virus in large quantities for months or even years, despite the presence of circulating antibody.

CLINICAL MANIFESTATIONS AND COMPLICATIONS

Neonates with CRS who were infected early in gestation generally have multisystem involvement and a spectrum of anomalies (Box 82.1 and Table 77.1) Symptomatic infants infected later in gestation may only have focal involvement of the eye or auditory system. Transient findings in the newborn period include generalized lymphadenopathy, hemolytic anemia, pneumonitis, hepatosplenomegaly, thrombocytopenia, and jaundice. "Blueberry muffin" lesions on the skin reflect focal areas of dermal erythropoiesis (see Figure 82.1 and in the color section). Most transient manifestations resolve within weeks of delivery.

The permanent clinical manifestation of CRS can be divided into those seen early (in the newborn) or delayed (in childhood or adolescence). Although almost any organ can be affected, the organ systems most commonly involved include the auditory system, heart, eye, and brain. More than 50% of neonates with clinically apparent CRS have a low birth weight, and persistent growth retardation is common in these children. Hearing loss, often bilateral, occurs in more than 50% and is a major cause of deafness in those parts of the world that do not have a rubella immunization program. More than half of infants have cardiac involvement. The most common lesion is

---

BOX 82.1   Clinical Manifestations of CRS

- *Auditory*. Sensorineural hearing loss of varying degrees is present in nearly all patients. Deafness occurs in 50% of patients as one of several defects or as an isolated defect associated with infection beyond 12 weeks' gestation. All infants with congenital rubella require evaluation of hearing with brainstem auditory-evoked responses
- *Cardiac*. Patent ductus arteriosus with or without pulmonary artery or pulmonic valvular stenosis, aortic stenosis, and ventricular septal defect
- *Ophthalmologic*. Cataract, pigmentary ("salt and pepper") retinopathy, and microphthalmia
- *Neurologic*. Central auditory imperception, delayed development, intellectual deficits, microcephaly, and hypotonia
- *Growth*. Intrauterine and postnatal growth retardation

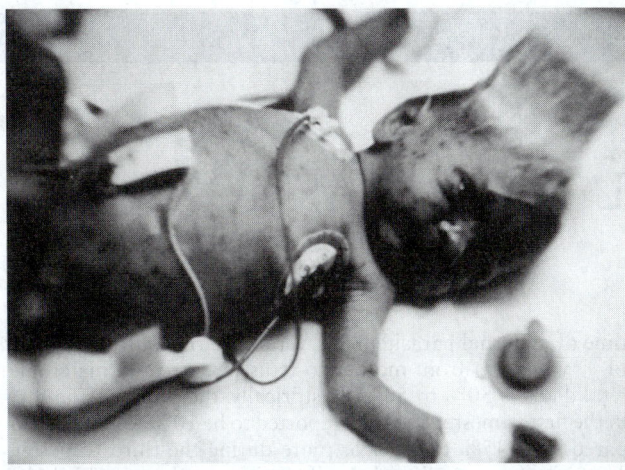

FIGURE 82.1. So-called blueberry-muffin spots. Extramedullary dermal erythropoiesis is observed in the most severely affected infants with congenital cytomegalovirus infection and congenital rubella. See Color Figure 82.1 in color section.

patent ductus arteriosus, which can occur in isolation or in combination with pulmonary valve stenosis, aortic stenosis, or ventricular septal defects. Ocular involvement such as a "salt and pepper" retinopathy, cataracts, and microphthalmia occurs in 20% to 50% of infants with CRS. Central nervous system defects associated with CRS may be present at birth but often become more apparent over time. These include developmental delay, microcephaly, behavioral disturbances, and encephalitis.

Some infants with congenital infection appear normal at birth but develop typical features of CRS syndrome in the first months of life. Late findings that appear more than 2 years after birth include endocrinopathies such as insulin-dependent diabetes mellitus, new or progressive ocular or auditory dysfunction, and central nervous system disease. Overall, permanent manifestations of CRS are seen in approximately 80% of survivors.

DIAGNOSIS

The diagnosis of CRS is confirmed by isolation of virus from neonatal tissues, fluids, or secretions, such as the CSF, nasopharynx, buffy coat, and urine. Although more than 80% of infants excrete the virus at birth, virus isolation is rather challenging in most clinical virology laboratories. Demonstration of rubella-specific IgM antibody at birth in blood or oral secretions and an increase in the infant's IgG titer over 3 to 6 months, with stable or decreasing maternal IgG levels, provides serologic confirmation of the diagnosis (Table 77.2). Although currently used latex agglutination and enzyme-linked immunosorbent assay (ELISA) techniques are more sensitive and specific than older tests, infants with CRS rarely may be born without IgM, and false-positive tests continue to occur. Hence, a negative test for IgM antibody does not definitively exclude the diagnosis, and a positive test must be interpreted

in light of the history and clinical findings. Sensitive PCR tests have been described but are not widely used for assessment.

THERAPY AND PREVENTION

Because no treatment for rubella infection exists, most efforts have focused on prevention. The currently used RA27/3 vaccine strain, grown in human diploid cell cultures, is immunogenic in more than 95% of recipients older than 12 months and provides long-term protective immunity. Rubella immunization is contraindicated in pregnant women. The CDC has followed more than 500 women given rubella vaccine during the first trimester. Vaccine-associated virus can cross the placenta and infect the fetus, because 3% of such exposed neonates excrete the virus immediately following birth. However, vaccine strains of rubella do not cause embryopathy, because no neonates have been identified with any findings suggestive of CRS following immunization of a pregnant woman. Thus, inadvertent vaccine administration at the time of conception or in the first trimester is not an indication to terminate the pregnancy.

The immune status of pregnant women is customarily determined by routine antenatal screening for rubella IgG antibody so that susceptible women can receive postpartum vaccination if they are not rubella-immune. In most pregnant women, the detection of rubella-specific IgG implies immunity from vaccine or from naturally occurring infection well before conception. However, such a result in recently arrived immigrants from countries where rubella is endemic may imply recently acquired infection and potentially serious implications to the fetus.

The routine use of immunoglobulin (Ig) for the postexposure prophylaxis of rubella-susceptible women exposed to rubella early in pregnancy is not recommended currently. The administration of Ig should be considered only if termination of pregnancy is not an option. A dose of 0.55 mL/kg given within 72 hours of exposure to a rubella-susceptible pregnant woman may modify or prevent clinically apparent infection. However, the absence of clinically apparent infection does not preclude fetal infection, because infants with CRS have been born to mothers given Ig shortly after exposure to rubella.

Infants with CRS are considered contagious for the first year of life and should be maintained in contact isolation while hospitalized.

Suggested Readings

Banatvala JE, Brown DWG. Rubella. *Lancet* 2004;363:1127.
Centers for Disease Control and Prevention. Control and prevention of rubella: evaluation and management of suspected outbreaks, rubella in pregnant women, and surveillance for congenital rubella syndrome. *MMWR* 2001; 50(RR12):1.
Litwin CM, Hill HR. Serologic and DNA-based testing for congenital and perinatal infections. *Pediatr Infect Dis J* 1997;16:1166.
Mehta NM, Thomas RM. Antenatal screening for rubella-infection or immunity? *Br Med J* 2002;324:90.
Miller E, Cradock-Watson JE, Pollock TM. Consequence of confirmed maternal rubella at successive stages of pregnancy. *Lancet* 1982;2:781.
Reef SE, Frey TK, Theall K, et al. The changing epidemiology of rubella in the 1990s: on the verge of elimination and new challenges for control and prevention. *JAMA* 2002;287:464.
Sallomi SJ. Rubella in pregnancy. *Obstet Gynecol* 1966;26:252.

CHAPTER 83 ■ NEONATAL TOXOPLASMOSIS

WILLIAM V. RASZKA

Toxoplasma gondii is an obligate intracellular protozoan parasite found in animal species around the world. Although acute infection is usually asymptomatic in normal hosts, congenital infection can result in significant morbidity. Similar to infection with herpesviruses, infection with *Toxoplasma* is generally lifelong. Reactivation, however, generally is uncommon except in immunocompromised individuals.

Members of the cat family are the definitive hosts for *Toxoplasma* and may excrete millions of oocysts daily. Oocytes become infectious after being in the environment for 24 hours or more. Humans, and other mammals, become infected by accidental ingestion of soil or foodstuffs contaminated with oocysts (see Figure 222.1). After ingestion, the oocysts rupture and release sporozoites, which in turn become tachyzoites, the rapidly dividing form characteristic of the acute stage of infection. These tachyzoites disseminate widely via blood and lymph and infect many organs. Once the host develops an effective immune response, the parasite becomes a bradyzoite, the characteristic form of chronic infection, and is localized in tissue cysts. Bradyzoites within intact tissue cysts can survive for the life of the host. Humans, and other carnivores, also may become infected with *Toxoplasma* by consuming animal tissue, such as undercooked pork or mutton, containing infectious cysts. After ingestion, the bradyzoites are released from the tissue cysts in the gut, transform into tachyzoites, and disseminate.

EPIDEMIOLOGY

The prevalence of chronic or latent toxoplasmosis infection varies widely and is dependent upon age, socioeconomic conditions, cat exposure, travel, and eating customs. IgG anti-*Toxoplasma* seroprevalence rates among women of childbearing age in Europe range from approximately 50% in Belgium and France to 10% in Norway. Seroprevalence rates may change over time, because the prevalence in pregnant French women has dropped from 87% in the 1960s to 70% in the mid-1980s. In the United States, the seroprevalence among women of childbearing age has been relatively constant at approximately 15%, with a high of 30% in Birmingham, Alabama and a low of 13% in Minneapolis, Minnesota. The incidence of congenital *Toxoplasma* infection mirrors local or national seroprevalence rates. The estimated incidence of congenital infection in Belgium is 2 per 1,000 and in France 1 per 1,000 live births compared to 1 per 10,000 live births in the United States.

Congenital *T. gondii* infection occurs during maternal parasitemia associated almost exclusively with primary maternal infection. Transmission occurs following asymptomatic (the vast majority) and symptomatic infection. Occasionally, transmission may occur following reactivation of chronic infection among severely immunocompromised women. Very rare case reports have documented congenital infection when primary maternal infection was documented before conception or following maternal reinfection during pregnancy. Generally, the risk of fetal infection increases while the severity of clinical manifestation decreases with advancing gestational age at the time of maternal parasitemia. Overall, the risk of transmission of *Toxoplasma* from mother to fetus in untreated maternal–fetal diads is 30% to 50%. Historically, the transmission rate in the first trimester has been reported to be 10% to 25%, compared with 35% to 60% or more during the third trimester. The risk of severe clinical manifestations apparent at birth decreases from 75% in the first trimester to essentially 0% in the third. The placenta plays a pivotal role in congenital infection, because monozygotic twins have nearly identical congenital toxoplasmosis infection rates but dizygotic twins do not.

CLINICAL MANIFESTATIONS AND COMPLICATIONS

More than 90% of infants with congenital toxoplasmosis are asymptomatic or have no abnormal findings on routine examination at birth. Infants symptomatic at birth are more likely to have been infected early in gestation. First-trimester infection is associated with *in utero* death and severe neurologic and ophthalmic disease. Although no single finding is pathognomic of congenital *T. gondii* infection, concomitant findings of hydrocephalus, chorioretinitis, and intracranial calcifications are highly suggestive of congenital toxoplasmosis infection. Ocular lesions are seen in or develop in almost 90% of symptomatic infants (see Figure 222.1). The most common ocular findings are chorioretinal scars, which frequently involve the macula. Intracranial calcifications are distributed diffusely throughout the brain, in contrast to the periventricular pattern associated with symptomatic congenital cytomegalovirus infection (Figs. 77.2 and 222.2). Other findings include hepatosplenomegaly, lymphadenopathy, fever, and rashes. Abnormal laboratory findings consist of cerebrospinal fluid pleocytosis and elevated protein concentrations, hyperbilirubinemia, and anemia.

Most newborn infants with congenital *T. gondii* infection appear normal at birth. However, careful examination may demonstrate ocular disease or central nervous system (CNS) findings in these apparently normal infants. Fifty of 52 infants born with IgM antibodies to *T. gondii* detected by a New England screening program had normal routine newborn examinations. After the results of the serologic testing were known, 40% of those undergoing additional testing had evidence of CNS or eye abnormalities. Most often, ocular lesions consisted of unilateral macular retinal scars, and CNS lesions were characterized by small, focal cerebral calcifications and mild to moderate elevations of CSF protein. Long-term follow-up studies have shown that as many as 85% of untreated asymptomatic infants go on to develop chorioretinitis, while other significant neurologic sequelae may develop in 10% to 20%. Chorioretinitis or new eye lesions secondary to *T. gondii* infection can occur as late as in the third decade of life and lead to significantly impaired vision.

DIAGNOSIS

Confirming maternal or congenital *T. gondii* infection is challenging, despite the plethora of diagnostic tests available.

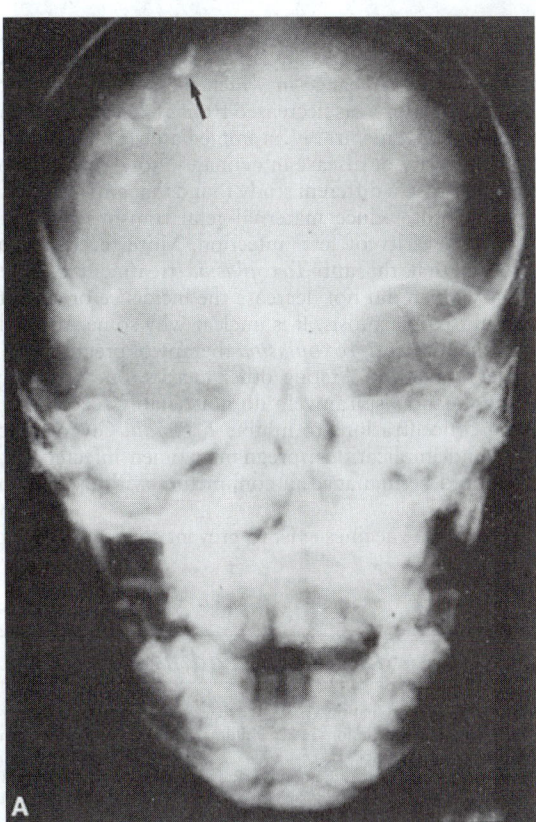
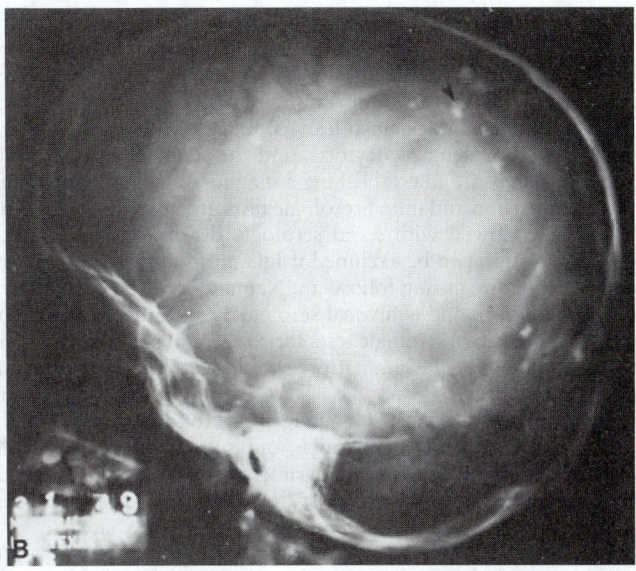

FIGURE 83.1. Anteroposterior (**A**) and lateral (**B**) skull roentgenograms demonstrating diffuse cerebral calcifications (*arrows*) in an infant with congenital toxoplasmosis. (Courtesy of Dr. Guido Currarino, Dallas, TX.)

Methodologies currently available include culture, polymerase chain reaction (PCR), histologic examination of tissues, antigen detection, and serologic tests. However, few laboratories culture for *Toxoplasma*, and results make take weeks to get back. PCR can be used to detect *T. gondii* DNA in amniotic fluid. Examination of the placenta may show tachyzoites and tissue cysts. Antigen tests are insensitive and rarely used. In the United States, the diagnosis of toxoplasmosis most often is made serologically. Given the surfeit of tests with different sensitivities and specificities looking for anti-*Toxoplasma* IgM, IgG, IgA, and IgE antibody (see Table 222.1), practitioners should consult with an infectious disease specialist and rely on a reference laboratory to confirm maternal or congenital infection.

IgG antibodies to *T. gondii* emerge within 1 week of infection, peak in 4 to 9 weeks, and in immunocompetent individuals, usually persist for life. IgG antibodies to *T. gondii* can be detected using the Sabin-Feldman dye test, and enzyme linked immunosorbent assay (ELISA), immunosorbent agglutination assay (ISAGA), or immunofluorescent antibody (IFA) tests. IgM to *T. gondii* also emerge within 1 week of infection and peak in 4 to 5 weeks. However, the persistence of IgM titers is highly variable and dependent on the assay used. Generally speaking, the IgM-ISAGA is the most sensitive IgM test, followed closely by the double sandwich IgM-ELISA. IgM-IFA titers are the least sensitive and specific. Because of the variable sensitivity and specificity of commercially available anti-*Toxoplasma* IgM test kits, in 1997, the U.S. Food and Drug Administration (FDA) published an advisory warning physicians of the limitations of IgM testing. A reference laboratory should confirm all positive IgM tests. All positive IgM tests for *T. gondii* in pregnant women and neonates, even those from a reference laboratory, should be interpreted with caution and confirmed with additional tests. Anti-*Toxoplasma* IgA and IgE emerge early after infection and disappear sooner than IgM antibodies. IgA antibodies, more so than IgE, are helpful in confirming congenital infection.

The interpretation of *T. gondii* antibody tests in pregnant women is dependent on the gestational age at which the testing is performed. Generally, rising anti-*Toxoplasma* IgG antibody titers in conjunction with a positive anti-*Toxoplasma* IgM test is suggestive of acute infection. High-avidity IgG anti-*Toxoplasma* antibody, IgA, and differential agglutination assays performed in reference laboratories may be helpful in confirming acute infection. If maternal infection is confirmed, the fetus should be followed by ultrasound. The best test to confirm fetal infection is PCR sampling of amniotic fluid for evidence of *Toxoplasma* DNA. This can be done as early as 15 weeks' gestational age. The sensitivity of the test ranges from 64% to 97%, with a specificity approaching 100%. Although now rarely done, *Toxoplasma* infection can be confirmed in newborns by isolation of *T. gondii* from the placenta, umbilical cord, or neonatal blood specimens by inoculation into mice. Although PCR can detect *T. gondii* in clinical specimens, congenital infection is most likely to be confirmed serologically on the basis of positive IgM and IgA antibody tests in the first 6 months of life or persistence of anti-*Toxoplasma* IgG antibodies beyond the first 12 months of life. The sensitivity of the IgM-ISAGA and double sandwich IgM-ELISA tests is reported to be 75% to 80%, with high specificity. The IgM-ISAGA is the preferred test to diagnose congenital infection. Indirect immunofluorescent tests should not be used because of their low sensitivity and specificity. Western blot assays comparing the serologic profile of the mother and neonate may be beneficial in some circumstances. Because IgA and IgM antibody can disappear by the time of delivery in an infant infected early in gestation, a negative IgM or IgA anti-*Toxoplasma* antibody test does not exclude infection. An experienced laboratory should perform all serologic tests for *Toxoplasma*. The laboratory with the most experience is the *Toxoplasma* Serology Laboratory in Palo Alto, California.

THERAPY

Infants born to mothers with confirmed *Toxoplasma* infection during pregnancy must be carefully evaluated for clinical manifestation of congenital toxoplasmosis. Infants should undergo an ophthalmic examination and cranial imaging to rule out focal brain lesions or hydrocephalus. A cranial computed tomography (CT) scan is more sensitive than ultrasound at detecting small, calcified lesions. Examination of the CSF for elevated protein, pleocytosis, and the presence of *T. gondii* by PCR may aid in establishing a diagnosis. If both the physical examination and initial serologic tests are normal, the infant can be followed with serial serologic determinations. Congenital infection can be excluded if IgG antibodies disappear without therapy during follow-up. Neonates with abnormal physical findings and equivocal serologic tests, and those with confirmed positive serologic tests for congenital infection, regardless of the physical examination, should be treated with anti-*Toxoplasma* drugs.

The treatment of choice for congenital toxoplasmosis is the combination of pyrimethamine and sulfadiazine (see Table 222.2). The combination of pyrimethamine and sulfadiazine has synergistic activity against the tachyzoite form of *Toxoplasma*. Because pyrimethamine use has been associated with a significant risk of bone marrow suppression, all infants treated for congenital toxoplasmosis also are given folinic acid (leucovorin) to help prevent this occurrence. Even while on folinic acid, the infant's complete blood count should be measured biweekly. If anemia or neutropenia develops, the dose of folinic acid should be increased. Severe bone marrow suppression may necessitate a change in the pyrimethamine dosing. The optimum dosage and duration of anti-*Toxoplasma* therapy is not known, but treatment usually is continued for 1 year.

PROGNOSIS

Treatment has been shown to decrease the incidence of long-term sequelae, particularly new-onset retinal lesions, associated with congenital infection. During therapy, IgM and IgG titers usually fall. After discontinuation of therapy, both may rise again (rebound). The clinical significance of rebound is uncertain, as is the role of retreatment. Infants with congenital infection will need serial ophthalmic examinations through childhood and early adulthood, as well as careful developmental examinations.

PREVENTION

The prevention of maternal *Toxoplasma* infection during pregnancy is the best way to prevent congenital toxoplasmosis. Women either pregnant or hoping to become pregnant should be counseled on general measures to avoid infection. This includes avoidance of undercooked or raw meat products. Bradyzoites in meat can be destroyed by high (160°F) and low (−20°F) temperatures. Seronegative pregnant women should wash their hands well after handling organic matter including raw vegetables. Although indoor cats who do not hunt mice and other animals should theoretically not pose a risk, cat litter should be changed daily by someone else in the household so that oocytes, if excreted, will not become infectious. Counseling and provision of information on the effects of *T. gondii* infection have been shown to decrease seroconversion rates during pregnancy.

Pregnant women with acute *T. gondii* infection often are treated with antimicrobial agents to help prevent or decrease the severity of fetal *Toxoplasma* infection. Currently, pregnant women with acute infection are offered spiramycin help reduce the likelihood of fetal infection. Spiramycin is a macrolide antibiotic only available as an investigational drug in the United States. For confirmed fetal infection beyond the first trimester, many experts recommend the institution of pyrimethamine,

sulfadiazine, and folinic acid. The recommendation to begin spiramycin following seroconversion is based on a prospective controlled study in France in which the overall incidence of congenital infection was decreased from 58% to 23% in mothers who were given spiramycin immediately after seroconversion. The severity of disease in neonates, however, was not altered. In contrast, a different study found that anti-*Toxoplasma* therapy did not reduce maternal–fetal transmission but decreased the severity of fetal infection. More recently, studies have found that the anti-*Toxoplasma* treatment of infected pregnant women did not decrease the incidence or severity of congenital toxoplasmosis. It is unclear why some studies have shown benefit to anti-*Toxoplasma* therapy of pregnant women and others have not. Among other factors, one possibility is that drugs such as spiramycin do not reliably reach adequate placental concentrations to inhibit *T. gondii*. Given the complexities and implications, pregnant women infected with *T. gondii* should be managed in conjunction with experts in the field.

Currently, no vaccines exist to prevent congenital toxoplasmosis.

Suggested Readings

Binquet C, Wallon M, Quantin C, et al. Prognostic factors for the long-term development of ocular lesions in 327 children with congenital toxoplasmosis. *Epidemiol Infect* 2003;131:1157.

Breugelmans M, Naessens A, Foulon W. Prevention of toxoplasmosis during pregnancy—an epidemiologic survey over 22 consecutive years. *J Perinat Med* 2004;32:211.

Foulon W, Villena I, Stray-Pedersen B, et al. Treatment of toxoplasmosis during pregnancy: a multicenter study of impact on fetal transmission and children's sequelae at age 1 year. *Am J Obstet Gynecol* 1999;180:410.

Gilbert R, Dunn D, Wallon M, et al. Ecological comparison of the risks of mother-to-child transmission and clinical manifestations of congenital toxoplasmosis according to prenatal treatment protocol. *Epidemiol Infect* 2001;127:113.

Gilbert R, Gras L, and the European Multicentre Study on Congenital Toxoplasmosis. Effect of timing and type of treatment on the risk of mother to child transmission of *Toxoplasma gondii*. *BJOG* 2003;110:112.

Gratzl R, Sodeck G, Platzer P, et al. Treatment of toxoplasmosis in pregnancy: concentrations of spiramycin and neospiramycin in maternal serum and amniotic fluid. *Eur J Clin Microbiol Infect Dis* 2002;21:12.

Guerina NG, Hsu HW, Meissner HC, et al. Neonatal serological screening and early treatment of congenital *Toxoplasma gondii* infection. *N Engl J Med* 1994;330:1858.

Jara M, Hsu HW, Eaton RB, Demaria A Jr. Epidemiology of congenital toxoplasmosis identified by population-based newborn screening in Massachusetts. *Pediatr Infect Dis J* 2001;20:1132.

Jones JL, Kruszon-Moran D, Wilson D, et al. Toxoplasma gondii infection in the United States: seroprevalence and risk factors. *Am J Epidemiol* 2001;154:352.

Jones JL, Lopez A, Wilson M, et al. Congenital toxoplasmosis: a review. *Obstet Gynecol Surv* 2001;56:296.

McAuley J, Boyer K, Patel D, et al. Early and longitudinal evaluations of treated infants and children and untreated historical patients with congenital toxoplasmosis: the Chicago collaborative treatment trial. *Clin Infect Dis* 1994;18:38.

Mets MB, Holfels E, Boyer KM, et al. Eye manifestations of congenital toxoplasmosis. *Am J Ophthalmol* 1997;123:1.

Mombro M, Perathoner C, Leone A, et al. Congenital toxoplasmosis: assessment of risk to newborns in confirmed and uncertain maternal infection. *Eur J Pediatr* 2003;162:703.

Montoya JG. Laboratory diagnosis of *Toxoplasma gondii* infection and toxoplasmosis. *J Infect Dis* 2002;185:S73.

Pavesio CE, Lightman S. *Toxoplasma gondii* and ocular toxoplasmosis: pathogenesis. *Br J Ophthalmol* 1996;180:1099.

Peyron F, Ateba AB, Wallon M, et al. Congenital toxoplasmosis in twins: a report of fourteen consecutive cases and a comparison with published data. *Pediatr Infect Dis J* 2003;22:695.

Romand S, Wallon M, Franck J, et al. Prenatal diagnosis using polymerase chain reaction on amniotic fluid for congenital toxoplasmosis. *Obstet Gynecol* 2001;97:296.

Wallon M, Cozon G, Ecochard R, et al. Serologic rebound in congenital toxoplasmosis: long-term follow-up of 133 children. *Eur J Pediatr* 2001;160:534.

Wong SY, Remington JS. Toxoplasmosis in pregnancy. *Clin Infect Dis* 1994;18:853.

Zotti C, Charrier L, Giacomuzzi M, et al. Use of IgG avidity test in case definitions of toxoplasmosis in pregnancy. *New Microbiol* 2004;27:17.

CHAPTER 84 ■ HEPATITIS VIRUSES

PABLO J. SÁNCHEZ AND JANE D. SIEGEL

HEPATITIS A

Maternal infection with hepatitis A virus (HAV) in early pregnancy may result, on rare occasions, in prematurity and spontaneous abortion. It has not been associated with increased rates of congenital malformation or intrauterine growth retardation. Pregnant women with HAV hepatitis generally do not transmit the infection to their offspring because the associated viremia is transient and low grade.

These infants, however, are at risk of acquiring infection during delivery if the mother has jaundice or had acute hepatitis within the 2 weeks before and 1 week after delivery. Most infected infants are asymptomatic and exhibit only mild elevations in transaminase levels. Rarely do nausea, vomiting, anorexia, fever, jaundice, and dark urine occur in infancy. The detection of anti-HAV IgM acutely and the persistence of anti-HAV IgG beyond 18 months of age is diagnostic of neonatal infection. Because transmission of hepatitis A to the neonate is rare, routine serologic studies are not recommended for the asymptomatic infant. Exposed infants may receive 0.02 mL/kg of immune globulin intramuscularly as soon as possible after delivery, even though efficacy has not been established. The infant is potentially infectious for 6 weeks and is maintained in contact precautions if hospitalized during this period. Meticulous attention to hand hygiene when handling soiled diapers is stressed.

The nosocomial transmission of hepatitis A within a nursery is rare because of the relatively brief duration and low titer of viral shedding within the stool. However, immunologically immature preterm infants may excrete HAV antigen and RNA for 4 to 5 months after the acute infection. The source infants in reported nursery outbreaks acquired HAV by vertical transmission from the mother in the perinatal period or by transfusion of blood collected from an asymptomatic donor during the brief viremic phase.

Two inactivated HAV vaccines are currently licensed in the United States for use in high-risk individuals 1 year of age or older.

HEPATITIS B

Hepatitis B virus (HBV) is a 42-nm, double-shelled DNA virus. The inner core consists of hepatitis B core antigen, hepatitis Be antigen (HBeAg), DNA, and DNA polymerase. The outer shell is composed of hepatitis B surface antigen (HBsAg).

Epidemiology

In approximately 5% to 10% of adults with acute HBV hepatitis, a chronic HBsAg carrier state develops. HBeAg is found in the serum of some individuals who are HBsAg-positive, and this identifies an infected individual who is at increased risk of transmitting HBV. In the United States, 5% to 8% of the population have been infected with HBV, and 0.2% to 0.9%

have chronic infection. In the absence of prophylaxis, 90% of infants delivered of women who are positive for HBsAg and HBeAg become infected. If the HBsAg-positive mother is HBeAg-negative or has antibody to HBeAg, only 25% or 12% of infants, respectively, become infected.

The vertical transmission of HBV occurs when the mother has acute hepatitis B infection during the third trimester or within the first 2 months postpartum, or if the mother is a chronic HBsAg carrier. Ninety-five percent of neonatal infections occur at the time of delivery from the infant's exposure to infected maternal blood or cervical and vaginal secretions. Approximately 5% of neonatal hepatitis B infections are transmitted transplacentally, presumably as a result of leakage of infected maternal blood into fetal circulation. HBV infection is not associated with congenital defects or fetal malformations. If perinatal infection does not occur, the infant may be at risk for subsequent infection from close contact with household members who are infected or are chronic carriers.

Clinical Manifestations and Complications

Neonatal infection usually is asymptomatic, with only mild elevation of transaminase levels, although chronic hepatitis B infection with or without cirrhosis, chronic persistent hepatitis, and fatal fulminant hepatitis can occur. Infected infants usually do not become HBsAg-positive until several weeks after birth. Approximately 90% of infants infected perinatally become chronic HBV carriers, and one in four infants who become chronic carriers develops cirrhosis or hepatocellular carcinoma. A 275-fold increase in the risk of developing hepatocellular carcinoma occurs during the third and fourth decades in chronic carriers. This risk is greatest for carriers who acquired the infection perinatally. Transmission from infants and young children occurs within households but is rare in child-care centers.

Prevention

Effective prophylaxis of HBV infection has been possible since licensure of the first HBV vaccine in 1982. Both the highly purified vaccine prepared from human plasma (Heptavax B, Merck and Co., West Point, PA; licensed but no longer available in the United States) and the recombinant DNA vaccines (Recombivax-HB, Merck and Co., West Point, PA; Engerix-B, GlaxoSmithKline Biologics, Rixensart, Belgium) are safe, are highly immunogenic (greater than 95%), and have an efficacy of 90% to 95% in neonates. The concentration of HBsAg protein differs in the two vaccines; the pediatric formulation of Recombivax-HB contains 5 μg/0.5 mL, whereas Engerix-B has 10 μg/0.5 mL. The two vaccines are interchangeable within an immunization series. Previously, for high-risk situations (e.g., infant born to HBsAg-positive or HBsAg-unknown mother), 5 μg of Recombivax was given, whereas 2.5 μg was administered to infants born to HBsAg-negative mothers. For ease of administration, the newly recommended dose of Recombivax is 5 μg, irrespective of maternal HBsAg status. Similarly, the dose of Engerix-B in infants is always 10 μg, irrespective of maternal risk factors. Recently, recombinant hepatitis B vaccine has been a component of some combination vaccines with excellent immunogenicity demonstrated. However, only single-antigen hepatitis B vaccine can be used for the birth dose. Single-antigen or combination vaccine containing hepatitis B vaccine may be used to complete the series.

Traditional risk factors of blood exposure, multiple sex partners, and intravenous drug use may identify only 30% to 60% of individuals infected with HBV. Therefore, the Centers for Disease Control and Prevention recommend universal screening for HBsAg early in pregnancy. Testing should be repeated late in pregnancy for women who are negative initially and at high risk for HBV infection or who have had clinical hepatitis since screening was performed.

Perinatal transmission is prevented in greater than 90% of cases by intramuscular administration of 0.5 mL of hepatitis B immune globulin (HBIG) and hepatitis B vaccine to both term and preterm infants of HBsAg-positive mothers as soon as possible, but within 12 hours of birth. In institutions with policies for universal immunization of infants at birth, HBsAg-positive women still should be identified before delivery because of the addition of HBIG to the immunoprophylaxis regimen for their infants. HBV vaccine is administered intramuscularly and concurrently with HBIG but at a separate anatomic site. In infants with birth weight greater than or equal to 2 kg, the administration of HBV is repeated at 1 month and 6 months of chronologic age. In infants with birth weight less than 2 kg, the initial dose of hepatitis B vaccine does not count for the required three-dose schedule. These infants should receive HBV at 1, 2 to 3, and 6 to 7 months of chronologic age. HBsAg may be detected for 1 week or less after a dose of vaccine. An HBsAg-positive result at any other time indicates a prophylaxis failure or *in utero* infection, and the infant should not receive additional doses of HBIG or vaccine. Testing for anti-HBs and HBsAg is recommended at 9 to 15 months of age, but not before 9 months of age to avoid detection of anti-HBs from HBIG administered at birth. The presence of anti-HBs and absence of HBsAg indicates successful prophylaxis and immunization. Infants who are negative for anti-HBs (less than 10 mIU/mL) and HBsAg should receive three additional doses of vaccine at 2-month intervals, followed by retesting for anti-HBs 1 month after the third dose. Alternatively, additional doses of vaccine (one to three) can be administered, and the infant can be tested for anti-HBs 1 month after each dose to determine if subsequent doses are needed. Protection from immunization persists for at least 15 years. Household members and sexual contacts of HBsAg-positive mothers should be screened, and if no evidence exists of previous HBV infection, they also should be immunized.

Infants delivered by HBsAg-positive women are bathed as soon as possible after delivery to remove all maternal blood and secretions. Intramuscular injections should be delayed until bathing is completed; if this is not possible, then meticulous cleaning of the site with alcohol is necessary. These infants require standard precautions. Infants born to HBsAg-positive mothers may breast feed, and there is no need to delay the imitation of breast feeding until after the infant is immunized. Although HBsAG has been detected in breast milk from HBsAg-positive women, breast feeding does not increase significantly the risk of transmission of hepatitis B infection.

Both the American Academy of Pediatrics and the Centers for Disease Control and Prevention recommend universal immunization of all infants with HBV vaccine as the optimal strategy for the prevention of HBV infections. For infants with birth weight greater than or equal to 2 kg and born to mothers who are negative for HBsAg, the first dose of HBV vaccine should be administered to infants preferably at birth but alternatively up to 2 months of age, the second dose at 1 to 4 months of age (at least 4 weeks after the first dose), and the third dose at 6 to 18 months of age (at least 16 weeks after the first dose and at least 8 weeks after the second dose). The third dose should not be given before 6 months chronologic age.

Seroconversion rates in low-birth-weight infants (birth weight of <2,000 g) vaccinated shortly after birth are lower than those in older preterm infants and full-term infants vaccinated at birth. However, all medically stable preterm infants, regardless of birth weight or gestational age, are likely to respond to hepatitis B immunization by the chronologic age of 1 month. For this reason, for premature infants weighing less than 2 kg at birth and born to HBsAg-negative mothers, initiation of the vaccination series is delayed until 30 days of chronologic age if medically stable, or at hospital discharge if before 30 days of age. Alternatively, it could be given at 2 months of age with other routine childhood vaccines. The schedule for follow-up doses is the same as for other infants. Full-term and preterm infants born to HBsAg-negative mothers do not need postimmunization serologic testing for anti-HBs.

Infants with birth weight greater than or equal to 2 kg and born to mothers whose HBsAg status is unknown should receive the first dose of vaccine within 12 hours of birth. Blood should be drawn from the mother at delivery to determine her HBsAg status. If her HBsAg status is positive, then HBIG should be given as soon as possible, but no later than 1 week of age. If the infant's birth weight is less than 2 kg, then HBIG in addition to vaccine should be given within 12 hours of birth. This initial vaccine dose should not be counted as part of the three-dose schedule. The subsequent vaccine schedule is based on the mother's HBsAg status. If this remains unknown, then the infant should be treated as if the mother had been HBsAg-positive.

Infants suspected of having hepatitis B infection should be tested for HBsAg, and if positive, for HBeAg and anti-HBc IgM. The other antibody tests could be positive secondary to the presence of transplacentally acquired maternal antibody. Polymerase chain reaction (PCR) also is available to detect HBV DNA in serum.

HEPATITIS D

Hepatitis D virus (delta virus) is a 35- to 37-nm RNA virus with an internal protein antigen (delta antigen) coated with HBsAg. Because it requires HBV for replication, hepatitis D may occur as a coinfection with acute HBV hepatitis or as a superinfection of an HBsAg carrier. The route of transmission is similar to HBV. Hepatitis D is diagnosed by detection of delta antigen in serum during acute infection and by the appearance of delta antibody. Vertical transmission has been reported and is uncommon, but the exact risk to the infant is undefined. Infants who become HBsAg carriers as a result of perinatal infection are also at risk of delta infection. No product is available to prevent delta infection in HBsAg carriers either before or after exposure.

HEPATITIS C

Hepatitis C virus (HCV) is a small, single-stranded RNA virus belonging to the family of Flaviviridae, which includes the arboviruses of yellow fever and Dengue fever. HCV is the leading cause of infectious chronic liver disease and the most common reason for liver transplantation among adults in the United States. Chronic infection occurs in 85% of patients, and chronic hepatitis with persistent elevation of liver enzymes develops in approximately 70% of infected individuals. Chronic infection leads to cirrhosis in 20% and primary hepatocellular carcinoma in an estimated 1% to 5% within two decades of the onset of infection.

Epidemiology

The seroprevalence of HCV infection in the United States is about 1.8%. Seroprevalence among children younger than 12 years of age is 0.2%; among adolescents 12 to 19 years of age, 0.4%; and among pregnant women, about 1% to 2%. Seroepidemiologic studies show that approximately 1% of volunteer blood donors screen positive for anti-HCV antibody. Before 1986, the receipt of multiple blood transfusions was the most frequent source of HCV infection, with transfusion-associated hepatitis rates of 5% to 13%. New cases of posttransfusion hepatitis C have nearly disappeared since the introduction of multiantigen screening tests for antibody to HCV among blood donors in July 1992, and later by nucleic acid amplification testing of blood units. Other modes of HCV transmission include organ transplantation, intravenous drug use, intranasal cocaine use, sexual activity, occupational injury with blood-contaminated needles, and perinatal exposure. Intrafamilial transmission also has been documented but is infrequent. The rate of seroconversion following exposure to blood from anti-HCV positive patients through accidental needlesticks or cuts with sharp instruments averages 1.8% (range, 0% to 10%).

Perinatal transmission from HCV-infected mothers occurs in approximately 5% (range, 0% to 25%) of their infants. Factors that have been associated with an increased risk of transmission include presence of HCV RNA in the mother at the time of delivery; higher concentrations of plasma HCV RNA; maternal human immunodeficiency virus-1 coinfection, especially advanced stages of acquired immunodeficiency syndrome (AIDS); and specific genotypes of HCV. No differences are apparent in infection rates between infants delivered vaginally and those born by cesarean section. HCV antigen and antibody have been detected in the breast milk of infected women, but transmission by breast milk has never been documented, and HCV infection is not a contraindication for breast feeding. Mothers who are infected with HCV and are breast feeding should consider abstaining if their nipples are cracked and bleeding.

Clinical Manifestations and Complications

Persistent infection with HCV occurs in the majority of infected children. However, most children with chronic infection are asymptomatic, and less than 10% of infected children develop chronic hepatitis, as manifested by mildly elevated liver enzyme levels; fewer than 5% develop cirrhosis. Primary hepatocellular carcinoma secondary to chronic hepatitis C has not been seen in children.

Diagnosis

Infants born to HCV-infected mothers should be tested for anti-HCV IgG after 18 months of age when transplacentally acquired maternal antibody is no longer present. Antibody testing for HCV IgG consists of an initial screening enzyme immunoassay that, if positive, is confirmed by a recombinant immunoblot assay. No HCV IgM assay is available. Nucleic acid testing also is available for the detection of HCV RNA in blood; this test is useful for identifying infected infants before 18 months of age, when maternal HCV IgG antibody is still present. Children who are infected perinatally should have periodic screening of their liver enzymes even if they remain asymptomatic.

Prevention

No chemoprophylaxis or immunoprophylaxis strategies with proven efficacy exist. Immune globulin is not protective, be-

cause blood from anti-HCV-positive donors is excluded from the pool used for preparation, and no neutralizing antibody for HCV has been identified as yet. Interferon treatment at 6 weeks following HCV transmission by accidental needlestick prevented chronic HCV infection in two health-care workers, but further studies are required to determine indications for routine postexposure prophylaxis or use in the HCV-exposed neonate. The combination of interferon plus ribavirin is recommended for treatment of chronic HCV infection in adults, but experience in children is limited.

Routine serologic screening of pregnant women for anti-HCV is not recommended. Screening is recommended for those individuals who inject illicit drugs, received blood or blood products before July 1992, received a solid organ transplant before July 1992, are receiving long-term hemodialysis, received clotting factor concentrates produced before 1987, or have persistently abnormal alanine transaminase concentrations. The U.S. Public Health Service also has recommended that infants who received Gammagard (also called Polygam, Baxter Healthcare Corp., Glendale, CA) between April 1, 1993, and February 23, 1994, be offered screening (alanine aminotransferase and anti-HCV) for HCV infection. This intravenous immunoglobulin product was implicated in an outbreak of HCV infection in 1994.

HEPATITIS E

Hepatitis E virus (HEV) is responsible for water-borne epidemics of non-A, non-B (NANB) hepatitis in several areas of Southeast Asia, North Africa, and Mexico. The viral agent is a spherical, nonenveloped, RNA virus formerly classified in the family Calciviridae, genus *Calicivirus*, but now assigned to a genus of "hepatitis E-like" viruses.

Epidemiology

Transmission occurs by the fecal–oral route, similarly to that of hepatitis A. Epidemic NANB hepatitis occurs more frequently during pregnancy, particularly in the second and third trimesters. The attack rate in the first, second, and third trimesters is reported to be 9%, 19%, and 19%, respectively, with an overall rate of 17% during pregnancy. This statistic compares with a rate of only 2% in similarly exposed men and nonpregnant women of childbearing age. Pregnant women with acute epidemic hepatitis E in the third trimester are also at higher risk for developing fulminant hepatic failure, which is associated with a case fatality rate as high as 75%.

Diagnosis and Prevention

The diagnosis of hepatitis E is based on detection of serum HEV IgM antibody or serum or fecal HEV RNA by PCR. Prophylactic therapy with immune serum globulin has not been shown to be effective. The only preventive measures available are good sanitation and avoiding ingestion of potentially contaminated food and water.

HEPATITIS G

In 1995 and 1996, novel blood-borne viruses were discovered independently by two groups of investigators and are referred to as hepatitis G virus (HGV). These viruses have a genomic organization similar to that of the Flaviviridae and are distantly related to HCV. HGV has been detected in the serum of healthy blood donors and hemodialysis patients, and transmission by transfusion and injection drug use has been reported. HGV also has been detected in patients with community-acquired hepatitis. However, a causal relationship between HGV and hepatitis has not been established; the liver has not been shown to be a site of viral replication. Although persistent infection occurs, it does not lead to chronic disease and does not affect the clinical course in patients with hepatitis A, B, or C. Perinatal transmission of HGV has been documented in three of seven (42.9%) infants delivered by five women who tested positive for HGV RNA in Japan and by an additional infant in a single case report. A carrier state in two of the three infants was demonstrated, but liver function remained normal. In a study from Taiwan, 42 (2%) of 2,046 pregnant women tested positive for HGV RNA. Perinatal transmission was documented in 13 (52%) of 25 infants followed for 12 months. Transmission was facilitated by high maternal HGV RNA levels and vaginal delivery. Viremia was persistent in all infected infants, although transient and mild elevation of serum alanine aminotransferase concentration was noted in only three infants, implying that the hepatic insult is mild and brief. No treatment is available or indicated. The clinical role of HGV remains to be defined.

Suggested Readings

Alter MJ. Epidemiology of hepatitis C in the West. *Semin Liver Dis* 1995;15:5.

Bortolotti F, Resti M, Giacchino R, et al. Hepatitis C virus infection and related liver disease in children of mothers with antibodies to the virus. *J Pediatr* 1997;130:99.

Bradley DW. Hepatitis E: epidemiology, aetiology and molecular biology. *Rev Med Virol* 1992;2:19.

Centers for Disease Control and Prevention. Hepatitis B virus: a comprehensive strategy for eliminating transmission in the United States through universal childhood vaccination: recommendations of the Immunization Practices Advisory Committee (ACIP). *MMWR Morb Mortal Wkly Rep* 1991;40(Rr-13):1.

Centers for Disease Control and Prevention. Prevention of hepatitis A through active or passive immunization. *MMWR Morb Mortal Wkly Rep* 1996;45(Rr-15):1.

Centers for Disease Control and Prevention. Recommendations for prevention and control of hepatitis C virus (HCV) infection and HCV-related chronic disease. *MMWR Morb Mortal Wkly Rep* 1998;47(Rr-19):1.

Centers for Disease Control and Prevention. Guidelines for laboratory testing and result reporting of antibody to hepatitis C virus. *MMWR Recomm Rep* 2003;52(RR-3)1.

American Academy of Pediatrics. Hepatitis B. InPickering LK, ed. *Red Book: 2003 Report of the Committee on Infectious Diseases*, 26th ed. Elk Grove Village, IL: American Academy of Pediatrics, 2003:318.

Granovsky MO, Minkoff HL, Tess BH, et al. Hepatitis C virus infection in the Mothers and Infants Cohort Study. *Pediatrics* 1998;102:355.

Hupertz VF, Wyllie R. Perinatal hepatitis C infection. *Pediatr Infect Dis J* 2003;22:369.

Inaba N, Okajima Y, Kang XS, et al. Maternal-infant transmission of hepatitis G virus. *Am J Obstet Gynecol* 1997;177:1537.

Khuroo MS, Teli MR, Skidmore S, et al. Incidence and severity of viral hepatitis in pregnancy. *Am J Med* 1981;70:252.

Lin HH, Kao JH, Hsu HY, et al. Absence of infection in breast-fed infants born to hepatitis C virus-infected mothers. *J Pediatr* 1995;126:589.

Lin HH, Kao JH, Yeh KY, et al. Mother-to-infant transmission of GB virus C/hepatitis G virus: the role of high titered maternal viremia and mode of delivery. *J Infect Dis* 1998;177:1202.

Noguchi S, Sata M, Suzuki H, et al. Early therapy with interferon for acute hepatitis C acquired through a needlestick. *Clin Infect Dis* 1997;24:992.

Ohto H, Terazawa S, Sasaki N, et al. Transmission of hepatitis C virus from mothers to infants. *N Engl J Med* 1994;330:744.

Rosenblum LS, Villarino ME, Nainan OV, et al. Hepatitis A outbreak in a neonatal intensive care unit: risk factors for transmission and evidence of prolonged viral excretion among preterm infants. *J Infect Dis* 1991;164:476.

Saari TN, and the Committee on Infectious Diseases. Immunization of preterm and low birth weight infants. *Pediatr* 2003;112:193.

Snydman DR. Hepatitis in pregnancy. *N Engl J Med* 1985;313:1398.

Thomas DL, Villano SA, Reister KA, et al. Perinatal transmission of hepatitis C virus from human immunodeficiency virus type 1-infected mothers. *J Infect Dis* 1998;177:1480.

Watson JC, Fleming DW, Borella AJ, et al. Vertical transmission of hepatitis A resulting in an outbreak in a neonatal intensive care unit. *J Infect Dis* 1993;167:567.

Wejstal R, Manson AS, Widell A, Norkrans G. Perinatal transmission of hepatitis G virus (GB virus type C) and hepatitis C virus infections—a comparison. *Clin Infect Dis* 1999;28:816.

Zanetti AR, Tanzi E, Romano L, et al. Multicenter trial on mother-to-infant transmission of GBV-C virus. The Lombardy Study Group on vertical/perinatal hepatitis viruses transmission. *J Med Virol* 1998;54:107.

CHAPTER 85 ■ NEISSERIA GONORRHOEAE

PABLO J. SÁNCHEZ AND JANE D. SIEGEL

The prevalence of gonococcal infection during pregnancy varies from 0.6% to 7.6%. The highest rates are found in single, low-income, nonwhite women younger than 25 years. Gonococcal infection during pregnancy has been associated with septic abortion, chorioamnionitis, premature rupture of membranes, delayed delivery after rupture of membranes, and premature delivery.

EPIDEMIOLOGY

Transmission of *Neisseria gonorrhoeae* to the newborn infant can occur *in utero,* during delivery, or after birth. *In utero* acquisition occurs via an ascending route after rupture of amniotic membranes. More commonly, neonatal infection occurs at delivery from passage through an infected birth canal. Approximately 30% of infants born vaginally to infected mothers become colonized with *N. gonorrhoeae*. Horizontal transmission via fomites, by nursery personnel, and household contacts also is documented. Standard precautions are recommended for hospitalized infants with gonococcal infection. The incubation period is usually 2 to 7 days.

CLINICAL MANIFESTATION AND DIAGNOSIS

Conjunctivitis is the most frequently observed clinical manifestation of gonococcal infection in newborns. Although *Chlamydia trachomatis* is the most common cause of ophthalmia neonatorum, identification and treatment of *N. gonorrhoeae* is especially important because it can cause severe eye damage. Gonococcal conjunctivitis typically appears 2 to 5 days after birth and produces an acute, purulent, bilateral conjunctivitis with lid edema and chemosis. If treatment is delayed, the cornea may ulcerate and scar, resulting in loss of visual acuity. Ultimately, the eye may perforate, resulting in panophthalmitis and loss of the eye. Presumptive diagnosis of gonococcal conjunctivitis may be made by Gram stain of the conjunctival exudate, which demonstrates gram-negative intracellular diplococci. The diagnosis must be confirmed by isolation of the organism on selective media, especially because *Moraxella catarrhalis* and *N. meningitidis* have a similar appearance on Gram stain. Other bacterial pathogens associated with conjunctivitis in the neonate that may be visualized on Gram stain are *Haemophilus* species, *Staphylococcus aureus*, enterococcus, and *Streptococcus pneumoniae*. *Pseudomonas aeruginosa* may cause conjunctivitis with severe complications in debilitated neonates.

Not only the conjunctiva but also the pharynx, umbilicus, urethra, vagina, and rectum can serve as a focus of local or disseminated disease. Disseminated infection usually is manifested by septicemia, meningitis, or septic arthritis that typically involves multiple joints. Cutaneous gonococcal lesions in infants are rare, but gonococcal scalp abscess at the site of previous placement of a scalp electrode has been described.

THERAPY

Infants with gonococcal ophthalmia should be hospitalized, placed on contact precautions for 24 hours after initiation of parenteral antibiotic therapy, and evaluated for signs of disseminated infection. Blood, cerebrospinal fluid, and localized sites should be cultured as clinically indicated. Tests for concomitant infection with *C. trachomatis* also should be performed. Because of the prevalence of both penicillinase-producing and chromosomally mediated resistant strains of *N. gonorrhoeae*, ceftriaxone administered intravenously or intramuscularly at a dosage of 25 to 50 mg/kg/day (maximum, 125 mg) is recommended for empiric therapy of nondisseminated disease. Alternatively, cefotaxime (100 mg/kg intravenously or intramuscularly) can be used and is preferred in the presence of significant jaundice. A single dose of either ceftriaxone or cefotaxime is sufficient for treatment of uncomplicated ophthalmia neonatorum. However, some experts prefer to continue antibiotics until blood and body fluid cultures, if obtained, are sterile at

48 hours. Hourly irrigation of the infected eye with saline until the purulent discharge resolves is an important part of effective therapy. Topical antibiotic treatment alone is inadequate and is unnecessary when the recommended parenteral antibiotic is given. Ceftriaxone (25 to 50 mg/kg intravenously or intramuscularly every day) or cefotaxime (50 to 100 mg/kg/day intravenously or intramuscularly in two divided doses) should be continued for 7 days in the presence of arthritis or septicemia and for 10 to 14 days in the presence of meningitis.

Susceptibility testing is not performed routinely for *N. gonorrhoeae* isolates. Local health departments may be consulted for resistance patterns in a specific community.

PREVENTION

Ophthalmic prophylaxis in the immediate postpartum period with either 1.0% silver nitrate, 0.5% erythromycin ointment, or 1.0% tetracycline ointment is effective in preventing gonococcal ophthalmia. Even with topical prophylaxis, some infants born to mothers with untreated gonococcal infection may develop gonococcal ophthalmia or disseminated disease. Therefore, these infants should receive a single intramuscular injection of ceftriaxone (25 to 50 mg/kg intravenously or intramuscularly; maximum, 125 mg). Alternatively, a single dose of cefotaxime (100 mg/kg intravenously or intramuscularly) can be given. The optimal preventive measure is diagnosis and treatment of maternal gonococcal infection before delivery. Gonococcal infections must be reported to the local health department so that contacts can be traced and treated.

Suggested Readings

American Academy of Pediatrics. Gonococcal Infections. In: Pickering LK, ed. *Red Book: 2003 Report of the Committee on Infectious Diseases*. Elk Grove Village, IL: American Academy of Pediatrics, 2003:285.

Centers for Disease Control and Prevention. Antibiotic-resistant strains of *Neisseria gonorrhoeae*. *MMWR Morb Mortal Wkly Rep* 1987;36(Suppl 5):1.

Centers for Disease Control and Prevention. Sexually transmitted diseases treatment guidelines 2002. *MMWR Morb Mortal Wkly Rep* 2002;51(No. RR-6):36.

Laga M, Naamara W, Brunham RC, et al. Single-dose therapy of gonococcal ophthalmia neonatorum with ceftriaxone. *N Engl J Med* 1986;315:1382.

Sandstrom KI, Bell TA, Chandler JW, et al. Microbial causes of neonatal conjunctivitis. *J Pedia* 1984;5:706.

CHAPTER 86 ■ *CHLAMYDIA TRACHOMATIS*

PABLO J. SÁNCHEZ AND JANE D. SIEGEL

Chlamydiae are bacteria that possess both RNA and DNA but are incapable of producing adenosine triphosphate outside of cells. Therefore, these organisms are obligate intracellular pathogens that require tissue culture cells for growth in the laboratory. Of the two species, *Chlamydia psittaci* and *Chlamydia trachomatis*, only the latter is a genital pathogen associated with neonatal infection. *C. trachomatis* has 18 serologic variants (serovars) divided into two biologic groups (biovars): oculogenital serovars A to K and lymphogranuloma serovars L-1 to L-3. Oculogenital serovars include those that cause trachoma

(serovars A to C), a hyperendemic blinding chronic follicular keratoconjunctivitis that is rare in the United States, while genital and neonatal infections are caused by serovars B and D through K.

The rate of cervical colonization with *C. trachomatis* during pregnancy varies from 2% to 37%. The highest rates are found in young, unmarried, nonwhite women of lower socioeconomic status. Chlamydial infection during pregnancy is usually asymptomatic, although urethritis and mucopurulent cervicitis can occur. Moreover, chlamydial infection can result in pelvic inflammatory disease, ectopic pregnancy, and infertility. Pregnant women with cervical chlamydial infection who have IgM antibody against *C. trachomatis,* however, may be at increased risk for premature rupture of amniotic membranes and delivery of low-birth-weight infants.

EPIDEMIOLOGY

Chlamydial infection of the newborn occurs most often at delivery, secondary to passage through an infected genital tract. Neonatal infection after delivery by cesarean section reflects an ascending route of infection. Transplacental transmission is doubtful because *C. trachomatis* is not associated with abnormalities present at birth that are characteristic of other congenital infections, and IgM antibody directed against *C. trachomatis* has not been detected in umbilical cord blood.

Approximately one-half to two-thirds of infants delivered vaginally by mothers colonized with *C. trachomatis* develop IgM antibody or exhibit a persistence or increase in IgG antibodies to *C. trachomatis* beyond 9 to 12 months of age. Approximately 28% to 66% of exposed infants are colonized in the conjunctivae, 15% to 20% in the nasopharynx or throat, 8% to 14% in the vagina, and 14% to 20% in the rectum. Initial colonization with *C. trachomatis* occurs in the conjunctiva and pharynx, and the rectum and vagina usually become colonized in the second through sixth months of life. Of infants colonized with *C. trachomatis,* 25% to 50% develop conjunctivitis and 5% to 20% develop pneumonia.

CLINICAL MANIFESTATIONS

Conjunctivitis

C. trachomatis is the most common cause of ophthalmia neonatorum in developed countries, where it causes 13% to 74% (mean, 29%) of neonatal conjunctivitis. Onset is usually 5 to 14 days after birth. Clinical illness ranges from a mild mucoid discharge in the medial canthus without significant conjunctival erythema to a profuse, purulent bilateral discharge with lid edema, severe chemosis, and edematous, friable conjunctivae. In the most severe cases, the clinical findings are indistinguishable from those associated with *Neisseria gonorrhoeae.* Subconjunctival lymphoid hypertrophy and follicular conjunctivitis rarely occur in the neonatal period. Some 19% to 83% of infants with conjunctivitis have nasopharyngeal carriage of *C. trachomatis* when first examined.

Gram stain examination of the ocular discharge reveals both polymorphonuclear leukocytes and mononuclear cells. A Giemsa stain examination of a conjunctival scraping that contains a large number of epithelial cells detects chlamydial inclusions in the cytoplasm of the epithelial cells in 50% to 90% of cases.

Untreated chlamydial conjunctivitis resolves spontaneously after several weeks to months. Ocular carriage of the organism may persist for 2.5 years. Rarely, chlamydial conjunctivitis results in mild conjunctival scars with punctate keratitis and micropannus. Normal visual acuity is preserved in most cases.

Pneumonia

C. trachomatis accounts for 15% to 73% of afebrile pneumonia in infants 3 to 11 weeks of age. Often a history of conjunctivitis or mucoid rhinorrhea exists, followed by gradually worsening tachypnea and a characteristic staccato cough.

Most infants are afebrile or have mild temperature elevations. Infants may present with apnea in the absence of other signs of respiratory involvement, or they may develop apnea during the course of the pneumonia. Auscultation of the chest reveals diffuse rales with few wheezes. Hyperexpansion and diffuse bilateral interstitial or alveolar infiltrates are present on chest roentgenography. Lobar consolidation and pleural effusion are unusual. Blood gas values typically show mild hypoxia but not CO_2 retention. Total leukocyte count is usually normal, but 50% to 70% of infants have eosinophil counts greater than 300 per cubic millimeter. Serum levels of IgM, IgG, and IgA usually are elevated. Untreated infants gradually improve after 5 to 7 weeks of illness. Approximately one-half of affected infants have middle ear abnormalities, with *C. trachomatis* isolated from some middle ear aspirates.

Chlamydial pneumonia in premature infants may be severe and require mechanical ventilatory support resulting in bronchopulmonary dysplasia. Children hospitalized for chlamydial pneumonia in early infancy may be at an increased risk of developing long-term pulmonary sequelae such as asthma, chronic cough, and abnormal pulmonary function test results.

The clinical significance of vaginal and rectal colonization with *C. trachomatis* in infancy remains unknown. Nasopharyngeal colonization is associated with rhinitis and nasopharyngitis, with nasal congestion without rhinorrhea lasting for weeks or months. *Chlamydia* is an uncommon cause of myocarditis and otitis media.

DIAGNOSIS

Chlamydial infections in infants must be diagnosed accurately, and clinical findings should not be relied on because of the necessity for treating the mother and her sexual partner. Diagnosis of chlamydial infection is confirmed by inoculation of the clinical specimen onto McCoy cells in tissue culture and by demonstration of the characteristic intracytoplasmic inclusions after several days of incubation. Conjunctivitis can be diagnosed by sampling the inflamed lower conjunctiva, not the purulent drainage, because the organism resides within the epithelial cells of the conjunctiva. Diagnosis of chlamydial pneumonia is best accomplished by isolation of the organism from nasopharyngeal secretions or endotracheal aspirate in a patient with a typical clinical syndrome. *Chlamydia* also may be isolated from lung tissue and pleural fluid.

Rapid detection tests of chlamydial antigen in clinical specimens are available for routine use. A direct fluorescent antibody stain using a monoclonal antibody directed against chlamydial elementary bodies performed on conjunctival scrapings has shown a sensitivity and specificity of 100% in chlamydial conjunctivitis. A second method is an enzyme-linked immunoassay that is semiautomatic and demonstrates a sensitivity of 93% and a specificity of 97% in examination of conjunctival smears. These tests are preferred for diagnosis of chlamydial conjunctivitis because they are accurate and are readily available with quick turn-around time in most clinical laboratories. On the other hand, direct fluorescent antibody staining performed on nasopharyngeal specimens for diagnosis of chlamydial pneumonia has yielded a sensitivity and specificity of only 85% and 75%, respectively. Rapid detection methods also should not be performed on rectal, vaginal, or urethral specimens from infants, because fecal bacteria can cross-react with *C. trachomatis* antisera.

Serologic evaluation is not useful in the diagnosis of chlamydial conjunctivitis because most infants do not develop IgM antibodies, and their antichlamydial IgG antibody is of maternal origin. When pneumonia is present, however, measurement of serum *Chlamydia*-specific IgM titer by microimmunofluorescence has been found to be useful because it is always elevated when clinical disease is apparent. This test is not widely available.

Nucleic acid amplification methods such as polymerase chain reaction and ligase chain reactions are available. These tests are more sensitive than culture and direct detection methods; data are lacking on their usefulness in infancy.

THERAPY

The recommended treatment for both chlamydial conjunctivitis and pneumonia is a 14-day course of either erythromycin estolate (10 mg/kg every 8 hours) or erythromycin ethylsuccinate (10 mg/kg every 6 hours) administered orally. The advantage of orally administered erythromycin over topical antibiotic-containing ophthalmic solutions or ointments is the eradication of C. trachomatis from the nasopharynx, thereby preventing the development of pneumonia. A shorter clinical course with lower relapse rates after oral therapy for conjunctivitis also has been observed. Topical therapy in addition to oral erythromycin is not necessary because therapeutic levels of the drug are achieved in tears after oral administration. The efficacy of oral erythromycin therapy is approximately 80%; a second course may be required. Oral erythromycin has been associated with infantile hypertrophic pyloric stenosis in infants less than 6 weeks of age. The risk of pyloric stenosis following treatment with other macolides such as azithromycin or clarithromycin is not known. Failure of a single oral dose of azithromycin for chlamydial conjunctivitis in infants has been reported; such therapy is not currently recommended. Oral sulfonamides are alternative agents that may be used after the neonatal period.

Treatment of the mother and her sexual partner with azithromycin (1 g orally in a single dose) or doxycycline (100 mg twice a day for 7 days) is recommended at the time of diagnosis of the infant's infection.

PREVENTION

Hammerschlag reports that ophthalmic prophylaxis at birth with 1.0% silver nitrate, 0.5% erythromycin ointment, or 1.0% tetracycline ointment does not prevent chlamydial conjunctivitis. Infants born to mothers with untreated chlamydial infection should be followed closely for development of clinical disease; prophylactic therapy is not currently recommended by the Centers for Disease Control and Prevention or the Committee on Infectious Diseases of the American Academy of Pediatrics. Identification of pregnant women infected with C. trachomatis and treatment with erythromycin or amoxicillin, using azithromycin as an alternative agent (azithromycin or doxycycline for the sexual partner), is currently recommended by the CDC for preventing infection and disease in neonates. C. trachomatis infections in both adults and children must be reported to the local health department for contact identification and treatment.

Suggested Readings

American Academy of Pediatrics. Chlamydia trachomatis. In: Pickering LK, ed. Red Book: 2003 Report of the Committee on Infectious Diseases, 26th ed. Elk Grove Village, IL: American Academy of Pediatrics, 2003;238:778.

Centers for Disease Control and Prevention. Sexually transmitted diseases treatment guidelines 2002. MMWR 2002;51(RR-6):32.

Hammerschlag MR. Efficacy of neonatal ocular prophylaxis for the prevention of chlamydial and gonococcal conjunctivitis. N Engl J Med 1989;320:769.

Hammerschlag MR. Chlamydia trachomatis and Chlamydia pneumoniae infections in children and adolescents. Pediatr in Review 2004;25:43.

Rettig PJ. Chlamydial infections in pediatrics: diagnostic and therapeutic considerations. Pediatr Infect Dis 1986;5:158.

Rettig PJ. Infections due to Chlamydia trachomatis from infancy to adolescence. Pediatr Infect Dis 1986;5:449.

Schachter J, Grossman M, Sweet RL, et al. Prospective study of perinatal transmission of Chlamydia trachomatis. JAMA 1986;255:3374.

CHAPTER 87 ■ GENITAL MYCOPLASMAS

PABLO J. SÁNCHEZ AND JANE D. SIEGEL

The genital mycoplasmas consist of Mycoplasma hominis, M. fermentans, M. genitalium, and Ureaplasma spp. (T-strain mycoplasma; Ureaplasma urealyticum, ureaplasma). Only M. hominis and Ureaplasma spp. have been associated with neonatal infection. Mycoplasmas are pleomorphic organisms that lack a cell wall. Serologic studies demonstrate seven serotypes of M. hominis and at least 16 serotypes of Ureaplasma spp. M. hominis and Ureaplasma spp. are sexually transmitted organisms accounting for female urogenital colonization rates of 20% to 50% and 40% to 80%, respectively. Cervicovaginal colonization is not predictive of such adverse pregnancy outcomes as preterm delivery, low birth weight, and spontaneous abortion. Their role in these events remains controversial. However, both organisms can invade the female upper genital tract and result in endometritis, postpartum fever, and septicemia, as well as in pelvic inflammatory disease (PID). Moreover, Ureaplasma spp. and M. hominis have been associated with histologic chorioamnionitis and surgical wound infection after cesarean delivery, respectively.

EPIDEMIOLOGY

The rate of vertical transmission of Ureaplasma spp. is 45% to 55% in full-term and 58% in preterm infants. Similar data are lacking for M. hominis. Vertical transmission of mycoplasmas occurs in utero or during delivery. In utero transmission occurs either transplacentally or by an ascending route from a colonized maternal genital tract. Mycoplasmas have been isolated from maternal blood at the time of delivery and from amniotic fluid, endometrium, placenta, and aborted fetal tissue. Mycoplasmas also have been isolated from the mucosal surfaces of newborn infants delivered by cesarean section performed before the onset of labor and rupture of amniotic membranes. In utero transmission is thought to be more common among preterm infants, whereas the majority of full-term newborns acquire mycoplasmas at delivery through contact with a colonized birth canal. Colonization of newborn infants is increased in the presence of chorioamnionitis and with decreasing gestational age and birth weight, and it is highest among infants with a birth weight of less than 1,000 g. Postpartum or nosocomial transmission in neonates is not well documented, but probably occurs.

CLINICAL MANIFESTATIONS AND COMPLICATIONS

The role of these organisms in neonatal disease continues to be investigated and defined. Sufficient evidence exists to implicate both organisms as true neonatal pathogens. *Mycoplasma hominis* and *Ureaplasma* spp. have been recovered from the lungs, brain, heart, and viscera of aborted fetuses and stillborn infants with histologic finding of bronchopneumonia. The genital mycoplasmas also have been isolated from blood, urine, cerebrospinal fluid (CSF), and lung tissue of newborn infants with clinical signs of infection. The following clinical associations with *Ureaplasma* spp. have been made: fatal neonatal pneumonia in a term infant documented by isolation of the organism from lung at autopsy and demonstration of elevated serum IgG and IgM titers to *Ureaplasma* spp. in the infant; pneumonia and persistent pulmonary hypertension in five infants from whom *Ureaplasma* spp. was isolated from blood, endotracheal aspirate, pleural fluid, or lung at autopsy; afebrile pneumonitis in infants younger than 3 months; chronic lung disease in low-birth-weight infants whose respiratory tracts were colonized with *Ureaplasma* spp. in the first week of life; chronic lung disease in four infants in whom *Ureaplasma* spp. was recovered from lung biopsy tissue; meningitis in both preterm and full-term infants; osteomyelitis of the femur; nonimmune hydrops fetalis; and scalp abscess at the site of a fetal scalp electrode.

Ureaplasma spp. and *M. hominis* have been recovered from the CSFs of both preterm and full-term infants. In several cases, their isolation has been consistent with a diagnosis of meningitis, with CSF exhibiting pleocytosis consisting of a polymorphonuclear or mononuclear cellular response, hypoglycorrhachia, and elevated protein content. The isolation of *Ureaplasma* spp. from CSF in preterm infants has been associated with severe intraventricular hemorrhage. Waites et al. have reported hemiplegia, hydrocephalus, and developmental delay as sequelae of meningitis caused by *Ureaplasma* spp. and *M. hominis*. In other cases, particularly among full-term infants, isolation of *Ureaplasma* spp. and *M. hominis* has been associated with minimal, if any, CSF abnormalities, and the infants do well without specific antimicrobial therapy. In these circumstances, the pathogenicity of these organisms remains unclear.

Other manifestations of infection with *M. hominis* are brain and scalp abscess, ventriculitis, submandibular adenitis, conjunctivitis, pneumonia, and pericardial effusion. The clinical significance of the isolation of genital mycoplasmas from urine obtained by suprapubic bladder aspiration in infants is not known.

DIAGNOSIS

The diagnosis of mycoplasmal infection is made by isolation of the organism from a normally sterile body fluid or suppurative focus. Because colonization of newborn infants with mycoplasmas occurs frequently, an etiologic role for these agents cannot be supported by isolation from mucosal surfaces only. Certain clinical situations should prompt the performance of mycoplasmal cultures. CSF should be cultured if it has abnormal indices, but routine bacterial cultures are sterile. Consideration also should be given to the culture of blood in infants with sepsis whose routine bacterial, viral, and fungal cultures

have not yielded a pathogen. In neonates with pneumonia who have lung biopsy or bronchoalveolar lavage performed for diagnostic purposes, mycoplasmal cultures should be performed. On the other hand, culture of endotracheal aspirate is problematic, because many infants are colonized with these organisms. If pneumonia is suspected, and the infant is not responding to standard therapy, then the isolation of mycoplasmas from the tracheal secretions may be an indication for the administration of specific therapy (see section, Therapy).

Genital mycoplasmas may be isolated on commercially available special broth and solid media. *M. hominis*, but not *Ureaplasma* spp., may be presumptively identified on blood agar as tiny pinpoint colonies. Serologic tests used to measure antibody to genital mycoplasmas include modified metabolic inhibition test, mycoplasmacidal test, indirect hemagglutination, indirect immunofluorescent test, enzyme-linked immunosorbent assay, and IgM and IgA immunoblotting. Polymerase chain reaction has been developed to detect ureaplasmal DNA in clinical specimens. The use of these tests for the diagnosis of mycoplasmal infection in infants is not well established or available outside of research laboratories.

THERAPY

The decision to treat an infant for possible mycoplasmal infection is based on clinical signs and culture results. No clinical trial data are available on which to base treatment decisions, choice of drug, and duration of therapy. Mycoplasmas are not susceptible to those antimicrobial agents routinely used to treat neonatal infections. Because mycoplasmas lack a cell wall, they are insensitive to penicillins, cephalosporins, polymyxins, and vancomycin. Although they may have moderate sensitivity to aminoglycosides, the minimum inhibitory concentrations of these agents for the genital mycoplasmas are usually too high for therapeutic use. The drugs of choice for the treatment of infection caused by *M. hominis* are chloramphenicol, clindamycin, doxycycline, and tetracycline; for the treatment of ureaplasmal infections, clarithromycin (15 mg/kg per dose every 12 hours), erythromycin, azithromycin, doxycycline, tetracycline, and chloramphenicol are used. Acute cardiorespiratory deterioration, presumably from cardiac arrhythmias, has been reported in neonates treated with intravenous erythromycin lactobionate for presumed ureaplasmal pneumonia. *M. hominis* is resistant to erythromycin, clarithromycin, and azithromycin. Whenever possible, antibiotic susceptibility testing should be performed on all clinically significant isolates, because multiple-drug resistance occurs.

PREVENTION

Erythromycin administered during pregnancy to women colonized with *Ureaplasma* spp. does not prevent preterm delivery or low birth weight. Whether antiureaplasmal antimicrobial agents prevent or ameliorate the chronic lung disease of prematurity in very low-birth-weight infants whose respiratory tracts are colonized with *Ureaplasma* spp. is not known.

Suggested Readings

Cassell GH, Waites KB, Crouse DT. Perinatal mycoplasmal infections. *Clin Perinatol* 1991;18:241.

Cassell GH, Waites KB, Watson HL, et al. *Ureaplasma urealyticum* intrauterine infection: role in prematurity and disease in newborns. *Clin Microbiol Rev* 1993;6:69.

Castro-Alcaraz S, Greenberg EM, Bateman DA, Regan JA. Patterns of colonization with *Ureaplasma urealyticum* during neonatal intensive care unit hospitalizations of very low birth weight infants and the development of chronic lung disease. *Pediatrics* 2002;110:e45.

Sánchez PJ. Perinatal transmission of *Ureaplasma urealyticum:* current concepts based on review of the literature. *Clin Infect Dis* 1993;17:S107.

Wang EEL, Matlow AG, Ohlsson A, et al. Ureaplasma urealyticum infections in the perinatal period. *Clin Perinatol* 1997;24:91.

Wang EEL, Ohlsson A, Kellner JD. Association of *Ureaplasma urealyticum* colonization with chronic lung disease of prematurity: results of a meta-analysis. *J Pediatr* 1995;127:640.

Viscardi RM, Manimtim WM, Sun CC, et al. Lung pathology in premature infants with *Ureaplasma urealyticum* infection. *Pediatr Dev Pathol* 2002; 5:141.

CHAPTER 88 ■ NOSOCOMIAL INFECTION IN THE NEWBORN

ROBERT S. BALTIMORE

Although all infections in newborns born in the hospital are considered to be hospital-acquired (nosocomial), infections manifesting in the first few days of life usually are caused by microorganisms transmitted from mother to infant, whereas infections arising late in the first week of life until discharge from the nursery are considered to be the result of nosocomial transmission. The pathogenesis may not always be clear, because colonization with maternal microorganisms at birth may result in manifest infection weeks later. In addition, many, if not most, infections that manifest after the first 2 days of life are caused by organisms that originate on the neonate's skin or mucous membranes, and a minority can be shown to be transmitted from hospital personnel or inanimate objects. Whereas, in the past, most neonatal infections were caused by maternally transmitted organisms, today, in neonatal intensive care units (NICUs) where most such infections are treated, the majority of infections are considered to be nosocomial. With the survival of an increasing number of very low-birth-weight infants, the hospital stay of infants in NICUs has been longer and susceptibility to infection has been greater than in the past.

EPIDEMIOLOGY

Rates of Nosocomial Bacterial Infections in the Neonate

Nosocomial infections in the normal infant nursery are uncommon (fewer than 1 per 100 discharges), whereas in NICUs rates of approximately 20 to 25 per 100 discharges usually are reported. Because the rate of nosocomial infection is related to length of stay, the number of infections per 100 patient-days may better reflect the overall rate. Rates of 0.5 to 1.5 infections per 100 NICU patient-days have been reported in the past few years. In a 2001 report, the point prevalence of nosocomial infections in NICU patients in a multihospital survey, using standardized National Nosocomial Infections Surveillance methods, was 11.4% of 827 patients surveyed, and in another study by the Pediatric Prevention Network, it was 0.86 per 100 NICU patient-days. The rate of infection is considerably higher in low-birth-weight neonates, and the infection rate in any particular unit may be largely a function of the mean birth weight or gestational age of the neonates in the unit and referral patterns for neonatal surgery. Large multihospital surveillance NICU studies report the most frequent sites of nosocomial

infections are the bloodstream, followed by infections of the lungs, then gastrointestinal tract, eye, ear, and nose and throat sites. The National Institutes of Child Health and Human Development Neonatal Research Network has reported on a cohort of very low-birth-weight infants (401 to 1,500 g birth weight) admitted to participating centers. Among this selected group of infants, 25% developed a nosocomial bloodstream infection (defined as occurring after 3 days of life) in a 1996 report, and 21% in a 2002 report. In the earlier report, 73% of infections were caused by gram-positive bacterial species (55% of which were coagulase-negative staphylococci) and, similar to many other studies, the rate of infection increased with decreasing birth weight or gestational age; these figures change very little in the later report.

Microbiology of Neonatal Bacterial Infections

Table 88.1 shows the major causes of late-onset bloodstream infections in neonates. Focal infections that result from

TABLE 88.1

MICROBIOLOGY OF LATE-ONSET BLOODSTREAM INFECTION: NICHD STUDY 1998–2000. FIRST EPISODES OF SEPSIS

Organism	Percent
Gram-positive organisms	70.2
Staphylococcus-coagulase-negative	47.9
Staphylococcus aureus	7.8
Enterococcus species	3.3
Group B streptococcus	2.3
Other	8.9
Gram-negative organisms	17.6
E. coli	4.9
Klebsiella	4.0
Pseudomonas	2.7
Enterobacter	2.5
Serratia	2.2
Other	1.4
Fungi	12.2
Candida species	9.9
Other	2.3

1313 total episodes (only first episode of sepsis included).

bacteremia (such as meningitis, osteomyelitis, septic and arthritis) and visceral infections usually are caused by the same organisms. Infections that are primarily caused by the spread of organisms from the skin, such as cellulitis, skin abscesses, mastitis, and omphalitis, are likely to be caused by the same organisms. *Staphylococcus aureus* also is a major cause of these infections and is also a cause of osteomyelitis and septic arthritis. Early-onset infections that are usually caused by maternal vaginal flora most likely are due to group B streptococcus, *Escherichia coli*, other enteric gram-negative bacilli and, occasionally, *Enterococcus* species and *Listeria monocytogenes*. In contrast, late-onset nosocomial infections may be caused by any of these species, but are more likely to be caused by coagulase-negative staphylococci, *S. aureus*, enterococci, and *Candida* spp., which are the most common fungi causing infections in the NICU.

The predominate species that cause neonatal nosocomial infections have undergone shifts in the last five decades. In the 1950s, a pandemic of neonatal infections was caused by *S. aureus*, which abated. In the 1960s, gram-negative rod species increased (especially *E. coli*) as a cause of maternally transmitted infections, and *Pseudomonas aeruginosa* was more commonly reported as a cause of hospital-acquired infections. The importance of *P. aeruginosa* appears to be less today, possibly as a consequence of the better hygienic care of medical equipment. In the early 1970s, group B streptococcus became a major threat worldwide, and it is still a threat, although rates are reduced where perinatal prophylaxis with penicillin has been used. Although early-onset group B streptococcal infections have been reduced by 60% to 80%, the rate of late-onset infections has not been affected. Since the 1980s, organisms more associated with late-onset nosocomial infections, such as coagulase-negative staphylococci and *Candida* species, have predominated, and along with this has been a shift in the mode of transmission, from primarily maternally transmitted to primarily hospital-acquired.

In addition to the organisms mentioned, a large number of species are occasional causes of nosocomial infections. These include *P. aeruginosa*, *Citrobacter* species, *Enterobacter* species, *Salmonella* species, *Acinetobacter* species, *Flavobacterium meningosepticum* (which is often multiply antibiotic resistant), as well as group A streptococci. These organisms may appear sporadically, but they also may be responsible for clusters of infections caused by a common source of contamination. Since 2000, NICU infections with methicillin-resistant staphylococci (MRSA) have increased. In addition, the colonization of mucosal and skin surfaces with MRSA has emerged as a major problem in NICUs. MRSA often enter the unit via infants contaminated from their mothers, and it is spread on the hands and objects handled by caregivers.

Nosocomial Viral Infections

Neonatal viral infections of the herpesvirus family, including cytomegalovirus and herpes simplex virus, generally are transmitted from mother to child. This also is true of human immunodeficiency virus type 1 (HIV-1). Rarely, herpes simplex may be transmitted from an adult to a neonate, and cytomegalovirus and HIV-1 have been transmitted via blood transfusion, but these are no longer considered major problems of nosocomial infection in the newborn nursery. Nosocomial viral infections more likely are caused by respiratory viruses, such as respiratory syncytial virus and adenoviruses, or enterically transmitted viruses, such as rotavirus and enteroviruses. These viruses may be transmitted from mother to infant or carried into the nursery by care personnel or visitors. Generally, viral infections in the nursery reflect viral activity in the community. The onset of respiratory viral infection in neonates may be confusing. Periodic breathing, apnea episodes, and lethargy are common presenting signs, but these signs are nonspecific in premature neonates. Enteroviruses (coxsackieviruses and echoviruses) may infect neonates in the NICU or regular nursery and, again, this reflects the community activity of these viruses. The effects on the infant are variable, from nonspecific febrile episodes to aseptic meningitis to overwhelming multiorgan failure.

Nosocomial Fungal Infections

Candida species are the major cause of neonatal fungal infections. In addition to *C. albicans*, the species *C. tropicalis*, *C. parapsilosis*, *C. lusitaniae*, and others also cause neonatal infections. Infections caused by *C. krusei* are uncommon, but are notable because strains of this species are not susceptible to fluconazole. *Candida* species are normal flora of the skin and upper respiratory and gastrointestinal tracts. The elimination of normal bacterial flora by antibiotics allows fungi to proliferate abnormally. Premature infants are at risk because of their relatively poor immunologic function, the frequent use of antibiotics, and the use of corticosteroids. Proliferation of *Candida* on the mucous membranes of the mouth and intertriginous areas is responsible for oral thrush and a common form of diaper dermatitis. It is probably common for infants to become contaminated during birth from a vagina colonized with *Candida*. Transmission to an infant after birth could occur from the skin of the mother or other caretaker.

Intravenous cannulas appear to be a major risk factor for candidemia and disseminated candidiasis in the neonate. Premature infants who receive hyperalimentation fluid containing lipid emulsion appear especially vulnerable to *Candida* as well as to coagulase-negative staphylococcal infections. *Candida* species infections must be suspected in tiny infants (of less than 1,000 g) who have evidence of infection after they have survived the first few weeks of life, and especially those who have been treated with repeated or prolonged courses of broad-spectrum antibiotics for suspected or proven infections.

The clinical manifestations of superficial mucocutaneous candidiasis are characteristic whitish-gray plaques on the mucous membranes of the oral mucosa and the vesicular and pustular lesions of the skin, generally in moist intertriginous areas of the body. The clinical manifestations of candidemia or disseminated candidiasis may include evidence of local infection, such as mucocutaneous lesions or a macular rash, or the symptoms may be nonspecific, such as temperature irregularity, poor feeding, irritability, and changed respiratory pattern. If *Candida* grows from a culture of the blood without evidence of focal infection in any organ, the diagnosis is candidemia. If candidemia and either local infection in visceral organs, the brain, the cerebrospinal fluid, heart valves, lungs, skeletal tissue, or the vitreous of the eye exist, or if pseudohyphae are seen in the urine or in biopsies of tissue, the diagnosis is disseminated candidiasis.

Invasive fungal infections caused by species other than *Candida* are uncommon in neonates, because fungal infections such as aspergillosis, cryptococcosis, coccidioidomycosis, blastomycosis, and histoplasmosis generally are contracted from the environment, and neonates are unlikely to have been exposed. In rare instances, *in utero* exposure may occur. Aspergillus can be present in the hospital environment, often associated with the renovation or construction of a facility, and infants are sufficiently immunocompromised so that invasive infection may occur.

Neonates are subject to superficial cutaneous infection caused by several dermatophytic fungal species such as *Epidermophyton*, *Microsporum*, and *Trichophyton*. When the skin is involved, these species cause ringworm. If treatment is required, griseofulvin can be used. A species from this class, *Malassezia furfur*, has been isolated frequently from the blood

TABLE 88.2

BIRTH WEIGHT–SPECIFIC SEPSIS RATE WITHIN THE FIRST 30 DAYS OF LIFE FOR INFANTS BORN AT YALE NEW HAVEN HOSPITAL, 1978–1988

Birth Weight	Number of Cases of Sepsis per 100 Live Births
600–999 g	8.6
100–1,499 g	4.5
1,500–2,499 g	1.4
>2,500 g	0.1
All infants >600 g	.27

Adapted with permission from Gladstone IM, Ehrenkranz RA, Edberg SC, Baltimore RS. A ten-year review of neonatal sepsis and comparison with the previous fifty-year experience. *Pediatr Infect Dis J* 1990;9:819.

of tiny infants who had indwelling central vascular catheters. This species seems to thrive on lipid and is associated with the use of intravenous fat emulsions. It is unclear whether antifungal agents are at all effective against *M. furfur*, but removal of the intravascular line appears to cure the infection.

Major Risk Factors for Nosocomial Infections

Birth Weight

Birth weight and gestational age are the strongest influences on the nosocomial infection rate. Low-birth-weight infants are predisposed to infection, primarily because of poor immune defenses (relative to the older child), and also as a result of life support systems that breach normal defense barriers. The use of ventilators that bypass the normal lung defenses, catheters that allow the entrance of skin flora organisms to the bloodstream, and medications such as H_2 blockers that reduce the acid in the stomach all contribute to the susceptibility of the low-birth-weight infant to nosocomial infections. By 37 weeks' gestation, the skin is an effective barrier to microbial invasion, but in premature infants with scant stratum corneum, the skin is quite permeable. This defect allows for the easy entry of bacteria, especially in the preterm infant of less than 32 weeks' gestation. After approximately 2 weeks of age, the stratum corneum is well developed, regardless of gestational age. Table 88.2 shows the birth weight–specific bloodstream infection rates in a study at Yale–New Haven Hospital from 1978 to 1988, demonstrating the increased frequency of infections in low-birth-weight infants. Table 88.3 shows more recent data on all nosocomial infections by birth weight from St. Louis Children's Hospital.

TABLE 88.3

BIRTH WEIGHT–SPECIFIC RATES OF INFECTION OF INFANTS TREATED AT ST. LOUIS CHILDREN'S HOSPITAL 1996–1997

Birth Weight	Number of Cases of Infection per 100 Admissions
>750	57
750–999	38
1,000–1,249	24
1,250–1,500	12

Adapted with permission from Zafar N, Wallace CM, Kieffer P, et al. Improving survival of vulnerable infants increases neonatal intensive care unit infection rate. *Arch Pediatr Adolesc Med* 2001;155:1098.

Bloodstream Infections

Bloodstream infections, with or without a recognizable focus of infection, are a major site of nosocomial infections in the NICU. Bacteremia is detected through the use of a blood culture; the only interpretation that is necessary is to determine whether the isolate is a contaminant, either from the skin or in the laboratory. Table 88.1 shows that frequent bloodstream isolates from neonates include such species as coagulase-negative staphylococci and *Candida* species, and these, in addition to such organisms as viridans streptococci and gram-positive rods, may be the cause of symptomatic infections but also commonly may be contaminants. In practice, isolates of bacteria that are recognized neonatal pathogens, and which are not resident on normal skin, are assumed to represent true bacteremias. Isolates of bacteria that may be part of the normal skin flora (commensals) require some interpretation. Multiple isolations of the same strain or species from blood taken by venipuncture rather than through a central catheter, and isolation of an organism when clinical signs of infection exist, increase the probability that the isolate represents a true bacteremia. When doubt exists about the significance of a commensal organism isolated from the blood of a neonate with signs and symptoms suggestive of infection, antimicrobial treatment is usually instituted.

Intravascular Catheters

A strong association exists between the use of intravenous catheters and nosocomial infections. These infections may be manifest as bacteremias or infections at the site of entrance of the catheter through the skin. Any type of catheter is a risk, be it a peripheral catheter, central catheter, peripherally inserted central catheter, umbilical vessel catheter, or radial arterial catheter. The catheter provides a poorly guarded pathway to the vascular system that is associated with intravascular infections, although tunneled Broviac catheters provide more of a barrier to bloodstream invasion. Contamination of the system, leading to infection, also can occur because of contaminated infusate, contaminated medications, and contaminated blood products. The use of lipid emulsions in intravenous hyperalimentation fluids has been associated with an independent increased risk of bacteremia with coagulase-negative staphylococci. Not only staphylococci, but many fungi (including *M. furfur*), appear to use exogenous lipid to enhance their growth rate.

Antibiotic Use

It has not been demonstrated that prophylactic antibiotics administered systemically to uninfected neonates prevent nosocomial infections. In fact, although antimicrobial agents are life-saving in the treatment of infected infants, substantial infection risks exist when antimicrobials are given to neonates; these include superinfections, infections caused by resistant organisms, and drug toxicity.

The prevalence of antibiotic use is so high in NICUs that some of the most convincing data demonstrating that frequent use of antibiotics promotes antibiotic resistance come from these units. In a prevalence and incidence study performed at Yale–New Haven Children's Hospital, it was determined that 92% of infants with a birth weight of less than 1,500 g received antibiotic treatment within the first 48 hours of life. The point prevalence of infants in the NICU receiving antibiotics averaged 33%. In a later study, it was found that exposure to antibiotics in the first week of life predisposes to colonization with organisms prevalent in the NICU and to infections with antibiotic-resistant microorganisms.

Bacteria that normally colonize the skin, mucous membranes, and gastrointestinal tract are an important barrier to colonization by pathogenic microorganisms. These organisms prevent the acquisition of pathogenic organisms from the hospital environment, including antibiotic-resistant bacterial flora and fungi. Because the newborn infant skin is normally sterile at the time of birth and has not yet developed a mature covering of normal flora organisms, antibiotic treatment has an even greater influence on colonization by abnormal flora in infants than it does in older children or adults. With a high prevalence of patients receiving antibiotics at any particular time, antibiotic pressure results in the development of resistance in the resident flora of the unit, and infants are frequently colonized with antibiotic-resistant bacteria and with fungi that proliferate when antibiotics reduce the normal flora. Rapid shifts in the organisms that cause neonatal infections occur when the antibiotics that are used most frequently are changed. This appears to be especially true of the third-generation cephalosporins and agents active against enteric anaerobes; therefore, many infectious-disease specialists recommend that these antibiotics be reserved for the treatment of proven infections caused by susceptible organisms and not for the empiric treatment of ill or stressed neonates.

PATHOGENESIS

Many nosocomial infections are due to endogenous flora (i.e., bacterial flora already present on the skin and mucous membranes invade tissues and the bloodstream because of immature skin and mucosal barriers). Endogenous organisms can cause infections as a consequence of invasive life support machinery. However, exogenous organisms that come from the environment or from other human beings also are an important source of infectious microorganisms. Both routine care and invasive procedures in a nursery provide opportunities for neonates to acquire infections and for infections to be transmitted from infant to infant. Preventing the transmission of exogenous organisms is an important aim of NICU infection control. When clusters of infections caused by the same species are encountered, this strongly suggest a common source and a breakdown of appropriate hygiene, especially when a number of isolates can be shown to be the same strain by immunologic or molecular typing methods. Pulsed-field gel electrophoresis (a very sensitive method of typing organisms by the mobility of their DNA fragments when cut by a restriction endonuclease in an electrical field) is available at many medical centers. This method identifies isolates of the same species that are similar, and therefore probably derivative of the same clone, and it distinguishes them from isolates that are unrelated. Many presumed outbreaks have been shown to be due to multifocal sources of organisms, by showing that organisms of the same species have different gel patterns.

Common source outbreaks of infections in NICUs have been caused by numerous modes of transmission. Scalp electrodes used for peripartum monitoring have caused infection by both bacteria and by herpes simplex virus. Infections entering the infant by the umbilical stump can be caused by colonization of virulent nosocomially acquired organisms. Infections in nurseries have been caused by contaminated eye wash, resuscitation equipment, scrub brushes, hand lotions, various disinfectants, topical ointments, and intravenous fluids. Numerous outbreaks have been traced to contaminated water supply, so any standing water in the unit should be sterile. Sinks that operate improperly, humidifiers, banked human milk, and medical instruments that have been improperly sterilized all have been described as causes of outbreaks.

Personnel delivering care in the unit may be the source of nosocomially transmitted organisms. As already discussed, this is particularly true of infections caused by respiratory and enteric viruses. The prevention of these infections consists of screening visitors for infectious diseases and ensuring that hospital staff seek counsel at the hospital's personnel health office if any symptoms of infection occur. These personnel are usually furloughed until the end of the infectious period if a viral infection is detected. The nasal carriage of streptococci or staphylococci in personnel can be responsible for outbreaks of skin infections in newborns. Group A streptococcal infections can occur in nurseries, as can outbreaks of diarrheal illness caused by enteropathogenic bacteria and viruses. Although group B streptococci generally are transmitted to infants from their mother, horizontal transmission has been reported. Bacterial outbreaks have been traced to personnel with skin infections, and those with either artificial or decorated fingernails.

Although these are all potential risks for spreading infections in nurseries, the hands of nursery personnel remain the most common mode of transmission in outbreaks of infections in neonates. Outbreaks may also be caused by fecal–oral spread via hands of personnel. Coxsackieviruses and toxigenic *Clostridium difficile* infections are spread by the fecal–oral route, but the mode of transmission of rotavirus infection in nurseries is not entirely clear. The lack of specificity of the rotavirus enzyme-linked immunosorbent assay test in neonates has made it difficult to interpret studies of spread in neonates.

Enteroviruses and respiratory syncytial virus are important causes of neonatal infections, and these are spread primarily by the hands of personnel touching contaminating surfaces or clothing; the viruses survive well on hard surfaces in the nursery environment.

Banked breast milk for preterm infants that becomes contaminated during collection or storage has caused infections by *Salmonella* and *Klebsiella*.

Recognition of Clusters of Infections

When a cluster of similar cases occurs within a short time, the situation can be recognized easily. This is the pattern with organisms that have a high disease-to-colonization ratio, such as several infectious diarrheal agents and group A streptococci. More commonly, nosocomial infections are caused by diseases with low disease-to-colonization ratios such as group B streptococci, Enterobacteriaceae, and *S. aureus*. Only one or two cases of overt disease may occur for every 100 infants colonized with the microorganism. Infants colonized with a potential pathogen may not develop disease until after discharge from the nursery.

Routine surveillance, including postdischarge monitoring, is required to demonstrate that an apparent cluster of infections is a significant change from the usual rate of infections in the unit. Although routine culturing of the environment and personnel is not recommended, targeted cultures may be needed when surveillance data suggest an outbreak from a common source. Clusters of infants with either overt infection or colonization with MRSA recently have been reported. Routine surveillance and cohorting of those carrying MRSA has been helpful in controlling these outbreaks.

THERAPY

The treatment of neonatal nosocomial infections is similar to the treatment of neonatal infections in general, and similar antibiotics are used. Empiric antibiotic treatment for older neonates who display new signs and symptoms is similar to that used in newborn infants, but the antimicrobial agents chosen must take into consideration the differences in microbiology between early- and late-onset infections and the possibility of antibiotic resistance. Although coverage for *E. coli*, other Enterobacteriaceae, group B streptococcus, *Listeria*, and *Enterococcus* species is the aim of the empiric treatment of early-onset infections, when nosocomial infection is suspected, coverage is required for *S. aureus*, coagulase-negative staphylococcus, and multiply antibiotic-resistant gram-negative bacterial species. Appropriate coverage may vary depending on the antibiotic susceptibility of organisms in the community. Although ampicillin plus gentamicin may be adequate coverage for early-onset infections in most communities, a penicillinase-resistant penicillin, such as oxacillin or nafcillin, plus an aminoglycoside may be more appropriate for suspected nosocomial infection. Where methicillin-resistant staphylococci are common, vancomycin plus an aminoglycoside may be appropriate empiric therapy for an older neonate, especially if an indwelling central venous catheter is present. If an infant has risk for aminoglycoside-resistant gram-negative rod infections, a third-generation cephalosporin or an aminoglycoside (such as amikacin) resistant to most inactivating enzymes may be indicated. For infections due to organisms resistant to these antibiotics, agents with less safety data in the newborn such as carbapenems, fluoroquinolones, and linezolid may be needed (see Table 77.4). In all cases, evidence of a focal infection and previous culture information should be taken into consideration when designing therapy.

Oral candidiasis (thrush) generally is treated with nystatin solution, 100,000 to 400,000 units orally four to six times a day for 1 week. The higher dose is used if the infection is not cured with the lower dose. Candidiasis of the skin may be treated by exposure to light to dry the skin and aid healing, a drying ointment or powder such as zinc oxide, or nystatin ointment applied three or four times per day.

In the newborn, the treatment of candidemia, with or without evidence of invasive candidiasis, should be with amphotericin B. Management of this antibiotic is discussed in the chapter on sepsis neonatorum (Chapter 71). Only minimal data exist on the use of fluconazole in the neonate, but limited data suggest it is safe and effective in selected cases.

PREVENTION

The prevention of nosocomial infections that are caused by endogenous organisms is difficult. The prevention of such infections usually involves care of the equipment relating to intravenous or intraarterial cannulation, proper insertion, and timely removal. Reducing invasive procedures, protecting skin and mucous membrane surfaces from erosion, and delivering needed nutrition are the major elements in reducing infections caused by a patient's own flora.

The most preventable types of nosocomial infections are those caused by exogenous flora. The aim is to prevent transmission of organisms from people and the environment to the infant. In addition to providing a scrupulously clean environment, caretakers must observe standard precautions. Proper hand washing is necessary to ensure that organisms are not transferred from patient to patient via the hands of medical care personnel or that persons colonized with pathogenic species do not contaminate infants. Appropriate hand washing before and after each patient contact is the most effective and least expensive infection-control practice, yet numerous observational studies have demonstrated that it is not always performed correctly. Gloves should be worn when potentially touching blood or body fluids. Gowning in the nursery has not been shown to lower the infection rate and has been abandoned in most NICUs, except during invasive procedures or caring for infants colonized with organisms requiring contact precautions.

Specific precautions are used for handling infants suspected of having certain infections. Table 88.4 shows the types of isolation recommended for common infections occurring in the NICU. Recommendations for such precautions have undergone some change and simplification since 1996, when the Centers for Disease Control and Prevention recommended standard precautions for all patients and either airborne, droplet, or contact precautions in addition for certain diseases, based on the mode of transmission.

TABLE 88.4

ISOLATION PROCEDURES FOR COMMON NEONATAL NOSOCOMIAL INFECTIONS*

Category of Isolation	Conditions, Organisms
Airborne plus contact	Varicella, varicella in the mother
Contact	Draining abscess
	Enterovirus (coxsackievirus, echovirus)
	Herpes simplex (exposure, disease)
	Multiantibiotic-resistant organisms
	Respiratory syncytial virus
	Rubella (congenital)
Droplet	Adenovirus
	Infection due to *Neisseria meningitidis*, (first 24 hours only)
	Haemophilus influenzae (first 24 hours only)
	Parvovirus B19
	Rubella (acquired)
Standard precautions	*Candida* infections
	Cytomegalovirus infection
	Gonococcal infection
	Human immunodeficiency virus
	Necrotizing enterocolitis
	Nondraining dressed wounds
	Pneumonia
	Syphilis (any)
	Toxoplasmosis

*Standard precautions apply to all patients.
(Data reproduced with permission from Garner JS. Guideline for isolation precautions in hospitals. *Infect Cont Hosp Epidemiol* 1996;17:53.)

In an attempt to reduce nosocomial infections caused by both endogenous and exogenous organisms, investigators have used intravenous immune globulin to prevent infections in low-birth-weight infants. The differences in populations studied, regimens, doses, and intravenous immune globulin formulations make interpretation of these data difficult. Nevertheless, after promising earlier studies, an analysis of current data shows that the addition of intravenous immune globulin to standard therapies is of demonstrable but marginal benefit in preventing sepsis when administered prophylactically, and that this benefit does not justify the expense.

More recent studies have shown that the rate of bacteremia caused by coagulase-negative staphylococci can be reduced if vancomycin (25 μg/μL) is added to the lipid-containing parenteral nutrition fluids of very low-birth-weight infants receiving these fluids via vascular access. This has been demonstrated in three placebo-controlled studies with a total of approximately 180 subjects. Although this number is too low to fully evaluate the effect on the resident bacterial flora in the neonatal units, no untoward effects have been reported. Although little evidence exists that this approach has been adopted in many NICUs, a small high-risk group possibly can be identified that can benefit from such prophylaxis. The potential of this practice to induce resistance to vancomycin causes infectious-disease specialists to hesitate recommending it for routine use.

Suggested Readings

Almuneef MA, Baltimore RS, Farrel PA, et al. Molecular typing demonstrating transmission of gram-negative rods in a neonatal intensive care unit in the absence of a recognized epidemic. *Clin Infect Dis* 2001;32:221.
Baltimore RS. Is it real or is it a contaminant? A guide to the interpretation of blood culture results. *Am J Dis Child* 1987;141:241.
Baltimore RS. Neonatal sepsis: epidemiology and management. *Paediatric Drugs* 2003;5:723.

Baltimore RS. Neonatal nosocomial infections. *Semin Perinatol* 1998;22:25.

Beck-Sague CM, Azimi P, Fonseca SN, Baltimore RS, et al. Bloodstream infections in neonatal intensive care unit patients: results of a multicenter study. *Pediatr Infect Dis J* 1994;13:1110.

Bryan CS, John JF Jr., Pai S, et al. Gentamicin vs. cefotaxime for therapy of neonatal sepsis. Relationship to drug resistance. *Am J Dis Child* 1985;139:1086.

Dent A, Toltzis P. Descriptive and molecular epidemiology of gram-negative bacilli infections in the neonatal intensive care unit. *Curr Opin Infect Dis* 2003;16:279.

Donowitz LG. Failure of the overgown to prevent nosocomial infection in a pediatric intensive care unit. *Pediatrics* 1986;77:35.

Fonseca SNS, Ehrenkranz RA, Baltimore RS. Epidemiology of antibiotic use in a neonatal intensive care unit. *Infect Control Hosp Epidemiol* 1994;15:156.

Freeman J, Goldmann DA, Smith NE, et al. Association of intravenous lipid emulsion and coagulase-negative staphylococcal bacteremia in neonatal intensive care units. *N Engl J Med* 1990;323:301.

Garner JS. Guideline for isolation precautions in hospitals. *Infect Cont Hosp Epidemiol* 1996;17:53.

Gladstone IM, Ehrenkranz RA, Edberg SC, Baltimore RS. A ten-year review of neonatal sepsis and comparison with the previous fifty-year experience. *Pediatr Infect Dis J* 1990;9:819.

Jenson HB, Pollock BH. Meta-analysis of the effectiveness of intravenous immune globulin for prevention and treatment of neonatal sepsis. *Pediatrics* [electronic pages, http://www.pediatrics.org/cgi/content/full/99/2/e2] 1997;99:e2.

Pelke S, Ching D, Easa D, Melish ME. Gowning does not affect colonization or infection rates in a neonatal intensive care unit. *Arch Pediatr Adolesc Med* 1994;148:1016.

Saiman L, Cronquist A, Wu F, et al. An outbreak of methicillin-resistant *Staphylococcus aureus* in a neonatal intensive care unit. *Infect Cont Hosp Epidemiol* 2003;24:317.

Schrag SJ, Zywicki S, Farley MM, et al. Group B streptococcal disease in the era of intrapartum antibiotic prophylaxis. *N Engl J Med* 2000;342:15.

Siegel JD. The newborn nursery. In: Bennett JV, Brachman PS, eds. *Hospital infections*, 4th ed. Philadelphia: Lippincott–Raven, 1998:403.

Sohn AH, Garrett DO, Sinkowitz-Cochran RL, et al. Prevalence of nosocomial infections in neonatal intensive care unit patients: results from the first national point-prevalence survey. *Pediatrics* 2002;139:821.

Stoll BJ, Gordon T, Korones SB, et al. Late-onset sepsis in very low birth weight neonates: a report from the National Institute of Child Health and Human Development Neonatal Research Network. *J Pediatr* 1996;129:63.

Stoll BJ, Hansen N, Fanaroff AA, et al. Late-onset sepsis in very low birth weight neonates: the experience of the NICHD Neonatal Research Network. *Pediatrics* 2002;110:285.

Stover BH, Shulman ST, Bratcher DF, et al. Nosocomial infection rates in U.S. children's hospitals' neonatal and pediatric intensive care units. *Am J Infect Control* 2001;29:152.

Zafar N, Wallace CM, Kieffer P, et al. Improving survival of vulnerable infants increases neonatal intensive care unit nosocomial infection rate. *Arch Pediatr Adolesc Med* 2001;155:1098.

SECTION III ■ ADOLESCENT MEDICINE

CHAPTER 89 ■ INTRODUCTION TO ADOLESCENT MEDICINE

ALAIN JOFFE

Adolescence refers to that stage of human development encompassing the transition from childhood to adulthood. The term *adolescence* (derived from the Latin *adolescere*, to grow into maturity) is broader in scope than the word *puberty*, which usually refers to the physical changes, including sexual maturation, that occur during this transition. Consequently, adolescence has not only physiologic but psychologic and sociocultural dimensions as well. To fully comprehend the significant events and transitions occurring during this period requires knowledge of each of these areas and of their interrelationships.

A thorough understanding of adolescence is important, not only in order to effectively address the health needs of this age group, but also because, in many ways, adolescence sets the foundation for the rest of the adult life-span. For example, virtually no individual begins to smoke cigarettes after age 20 and, conversely, individuals who become or remain obese during adolescence are likely to remain obese as adults. An estimated 65% of adult morbidity or mortality is determined by behaviors with onset or established during the second decade of life.

In 1990, approximately 35 million adolescents aged 10 to 19 years were living in the United States; this number is expected to grow to almost 50 million by 2040. Despite the projected increase in absolute numbers, the percent of the U.S. population comprised of 10- to 19-year-olds is estimated to fall from 14.5% in 2000 to 13% by 2020. Younger adolescents (those 10 to 14 years of age) will make up an increasingly greater proportion of the adolescent population and, by 2040, fewer than 50% of 10- to 19-year-olds will be non-Hispanic Caucasians.

Adolescence is viewed as both the healthiest period of life and the most problematic. For the majority of teenagers, the former is true, and they make the complex transition into adulthood without significant difficulty. In doing so, they accomplish or lay the groundwork for accomplishing several critical developmental tasks: becoming accustomed to a new and markedly changed body, formulating a personal and sexual identity, separating from parents, developing the capacity for intimacy in relationships, establishing a social identity, and preparing the foundation for economic independence.

Many teenagers fail to achieve one or more of these goals and suffer significant morbidity and mortality during this developmental period. Up to one-fourth of 10- to 18-year-old adolescents are at serious risk for school failure or of being injured or killed by various risky behaviors. The remainder are at lower risk but still face significant challenges to their health and optimal growth to adulthood. Mortality rates for 15- to 24-year-old adolescents decreased substantially since the 1950s, but have changed little from 1997 to 2000, the most recent year for which data is currently available.

Age-specific death rates are listed in Table 89.1. Unintentional injuries and homicide are the leading causes of death for young people aged 15 to 24 years. Suicide is the third leading cause of death for 15- to 24-year-old males and the fourth leading cause for young women in the same age range. Homicide is the leading cause of death for 15- to 24-year-old African American males and the second leading cause for 15- to 24-year-old Hispanic males. It is also the second leading cause of death for 15- to 24-year-old female African Americans, and the second or third leading cause of death among 20- to

TABLE 89.1

LEADING CAUSES OF DEATH AMONG YOUTH 10–19 BY RACE, ETHNICITY, AND GENDER (NUMBER OF DEATHS PER 100,000 IN SPECIFIED AGE GROUP) FOR 2000

Caucasian		African-American		Hispanic[1]	
Girls (10–14 years)					
All causes	15.6	All causes	22.1	All causes	14.9
Unintentional injuries	5.7	Unintentional injuries	5.6	Unintentional injuries	5.2
Malignant neoplasms	2.4	Malignant neoplasms	2.1	Malignant neoplasms	2.8
Congenital conditions	0.9	Assault (homicide)	1.8	Assault (homicide)	***
Intentional self-harm (suicide)	0.7	Congenital conditions	1.5	Congenital conditions	***
Assault (homicide)	0.7	Diseases of heart	1.4	Intentional self-harm	***
Boys (10–14 years)					
All causes	23.8	All causes	33.7	All causes	23.5
Unintentional injuries	9.9	Unintentional injuries	12.7	Unintentional injuries	7.1
Malignant neoplasms	3.0	Assault (homicide)	3.5	Malignant neoplasms	5.2
Intentional self-harm (suicide)	2.4	Malignant neoplasms	2.8	Assault (homicide)	2.5
Assault (homicide)	1.1	Intentional self-harm (suicide)	2.2	Intentional self-harm (suicide)	1.4
Congenital conditions	0.9	Chronic lower respiratory diseases	1.8	Diseases of heart	***
Girls (15–19 years)					
All causes	39.7	All causes	44.8	All causes	31.0
Unintentional injuries	22.6	Unintentional injuries	13.0	Unintentional injuries	14.2
Malignant neoplasms	3.0	Assault (homicide)	8.6	Malignant neoplasms	3.6
Intentional self-harm (suicide)	2.9	Malignant neoplasms	3.6	Assault (homicide)	3.1
Assault (homicide)	2.1	Diseases of heart	3.3	Intentional self-harm (suicide)	2.6
Diseases of heart	1.3	Intentional self-harm (suicide)	1.5	Diseases of heart	***
Boys (15–19 years)					
All causes	89.2	All causes	131.6	All causes	103.3
Unintentional injuries	49.3	Assault (homicide)	57.9	Unintentional injuries	46.6
Intentional self-harm (suicide)	13.9	Unintentional injuries	34.9	Assault (homicide)	29.3
Assault (homicide)	8.1	Intentional self-harm (suicide)	9.7	Intentional self-harm (suicide)	9.7
Malignant neoplasms	4.2	Malignant neoplasms	5.3	Malignant neoplasms	4.9
Diseases of heart	2.0	Diseases of heart	4.8	Diseases of heart	2.4

***Figure does not meet standards of reliability or precision.
[1] Youth of Hispanic origin can be of any race.
Data reproduced with permission from Anderson RN. Death: Leading-causes for 2000. *Natl Vital Stet Rep* 2001;50:1.

24-year-old and 15- to 19-year-old female Hispanics, respectively. Over 5,000 young people aged 10 to 24 were homicide victims in 2000; although this number is much higher than in other industrialized countries, it represents a significant decrease (both in terms of absolute numbers and rates) since the third edition of this text was published.

Adolescent morbidity also is associated with risky behaviors and includes such problems as substance abuse (including alcohol and tobacco abuse), mental health problems, school failure and dropout, delinquency, sexually transmitted diseases and their sequelae (pelvic inflammatory disease, ectopic pregnancy, infertility), human immunodeficiency virus (HIV) infection, and adolescent pregnancy.

The rates of substance abuse, which had declined steadily from their peak in the late 1970s and early 1980s, began to climb again in 1992. Lifetime use of any illicit drug peaked in 1996 for eighth graders and in 1997 for tenth and twelfth graders. According to the 2002 Monitoring the Future Survey (www.monitoringthefuture.org/data/02data.html#2002data-drugs), the rates of drug use among eighth graders have declined significantly since then, but have remained relatively stable among tenth and twelfth graders. In 2002, 24.5% of eighth graders, 44.6% of tenth graders, and 53% of twelfth graders reported ever using an illicit drug.

Recent data concerning risky adolescent sexual behaviors are encouraging. According to the 2001 Youth Risk Behavior Surveillance System (YRBSS; www.cdc.gov/mmwr/PDF/SS/SS5104.pdf) conducted by the Centers for Disease Control and Prevention (CDC), the proportion of teenagers who have

ever had sexual intercourse declined from 1991 to 2001. In 1991, almost 51% of high-school girls and 58% of high-school boys reported having intercourse; by 2001, the comparable figures were approximately 43% for high-school girls and 49% for high-school boys. The number of students reporting four or more lifetime sexual partners also decreased. More than 50% of sexually active girls and 65% of sexually active boys reported condom use at last intercourse, a significant increase over the last decade. Pregnancy, birth, and abortion rates among 15- to 19-year-old girls have all substantially declined in the last decade; this is likely due to a decrease in sexual activity coupled with increased access to a wider range of effective contraceptive methods. However, the rates of sexually transmitted infections such as *Chlamydia trachomatis* and *Neisseria gonorrhoeae* continue to be highest among young people age 15 to 24. More ominously, mathematical modeling suggests that 50% of new HIV infections in the United States occur in people under the age of 25, with most acquired sexually.

From a mental health perspective, the 2001 YRBSS indicates that 14.2% of males and 23.6% of females had seriously considered attempting suicide in the 12 months preceding the survey; 6.2% of males and 11.2% of females had actually attempted suicide, with 2% of males and 3% of females surveyed requiring medical attention as a result of their attempt.

Although anorexia nervosa and bulimia nervosa are viewed as the stereotypical nutritional disorders among adolescents, overweight and obesity are far more common. The prevalence of overweight among 12- to 19-year-olds increased from 6%

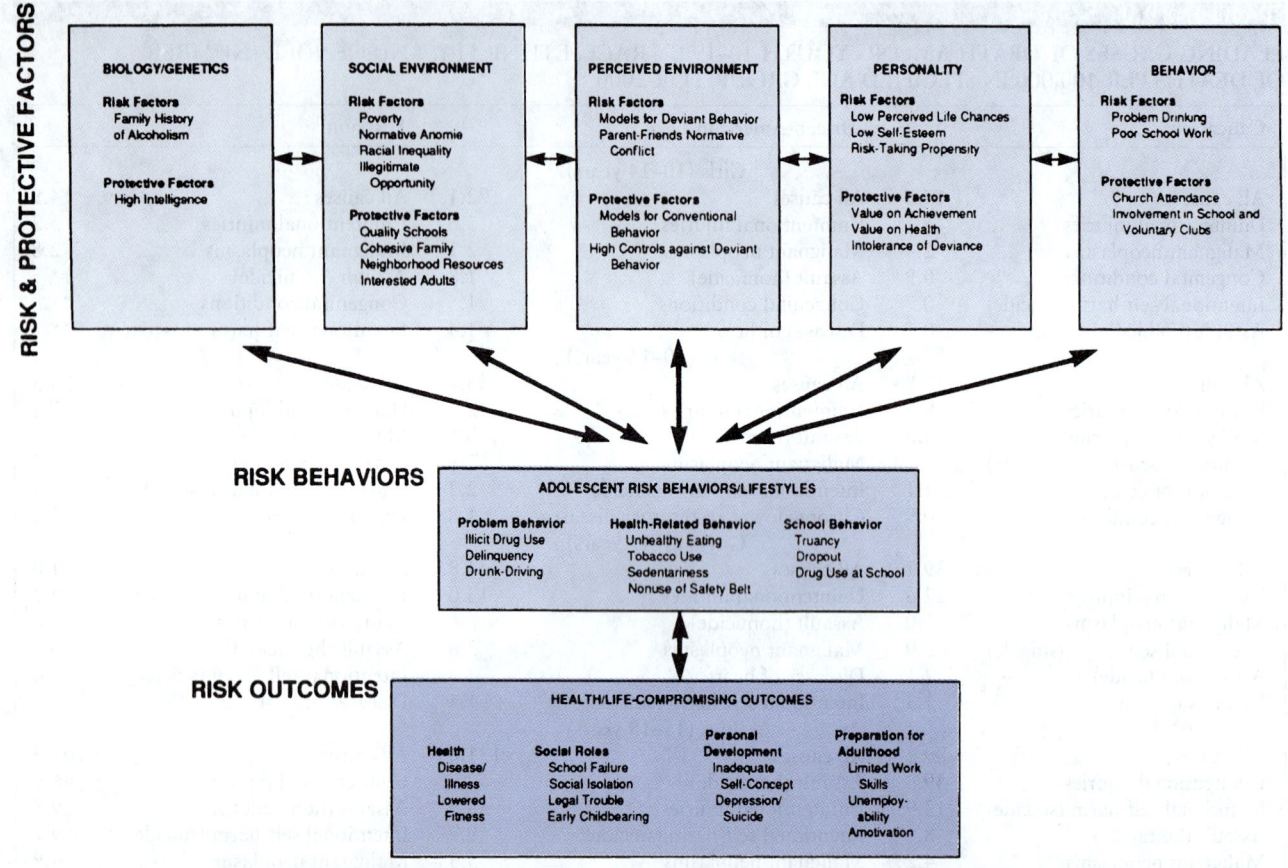

FIGURE 89.1. Interrelated conceptual domains of risk and protective factors. (Reproduced with permission from Jessor R. Risk behavior in adolescence: a psychosocial framework for understanding and action. *J Adolesc Health* 1991;12:597.)

in the early 1970s to 15% by 2000. Although the etiology of overweight is multifactorial, a decline in physical activity and an increase in television viewing and other sedentary behaviors are significant factors.

Since the late 1970s, research examining the etiology of risky behaviors consistently demonstrates that these behaviors are not distributed randomly among adolescents. It is important to recognize that some risky behaviors fulfill the developmental needs of adolescents (e.g., testing the limits of a newly matured body or separating from parents). Others have their roots in the adolescent's individual characteristics (e.g., temperament, sensation-seeking) or in his or her social context (including family, school, community, and socioeconomic status). As a result, some adolescents are at greater risk for adopting risky behaviors than others. Moreover, risky behaviors often coexist within an individual (e.g., a young person who smokes cigarettes is more likely to engage in sexual intercourse and to use other drugs).

Unfortunately, this pattern of risky behaviors has fostered a negative stereotype about adolescents. In contrast, more recent adolescent health research, exploring the related concepts of resiliency and youth development, has cast a much more favorable light on this period of development. Resiliency research focuses on adolescents who live in circumstances that would seem to predict negative outcomes, yet these adolescents survived or even thrived. It identified protective factors such as aspects of the adolescent's temperament, spirituality, feeling connected to family, and/or the ability to seek out a caring extrafamilial adult. Findings from the National Longi-

tudinal Study on Adolescent Health revealed that an adolescent's perception of being connected to family and school were protective against seven of eight risky behaviors assessed in the study. The interplay among resiliency and risk is shown in Figure 89.1.

The youth development framework also assumes a positive view of adolescents. Its basic assumption is that young people have a fundamental need for healthy development that requires a variety of experiences or circumstances that support the youth's development from a child into an adult. These include an environment that provides a sense of personal involvement and belonging and of confidence and security. One proposed list of developmental assets can be found at www.search-institute.org/assets/. Both the resiliency and youth development models have dramatically reshaped the prevailing view of adolescents, from problems that must be fixed or contained to resources that deserve careful and deliberate nuturing.

Thus, the goals of adolescent medicine are twofold: to support adolescents in making a successful transition to adulthood and to encourage healthy lifestyles that promote longevity and well-being for the duration of the human life-cycle. Insight into the nature of the statistics that characterize the dimensions of adolescent health and the potential for improving it comes from a knowledge of the marked biologic and psychologic changes that occur during puberty, as well as from an appreciation of the magnitude of change that has taken place in society. Each of these related areas is discussed separately. A schematic representation of the ensuing discussion is shown in Figure 89.2.

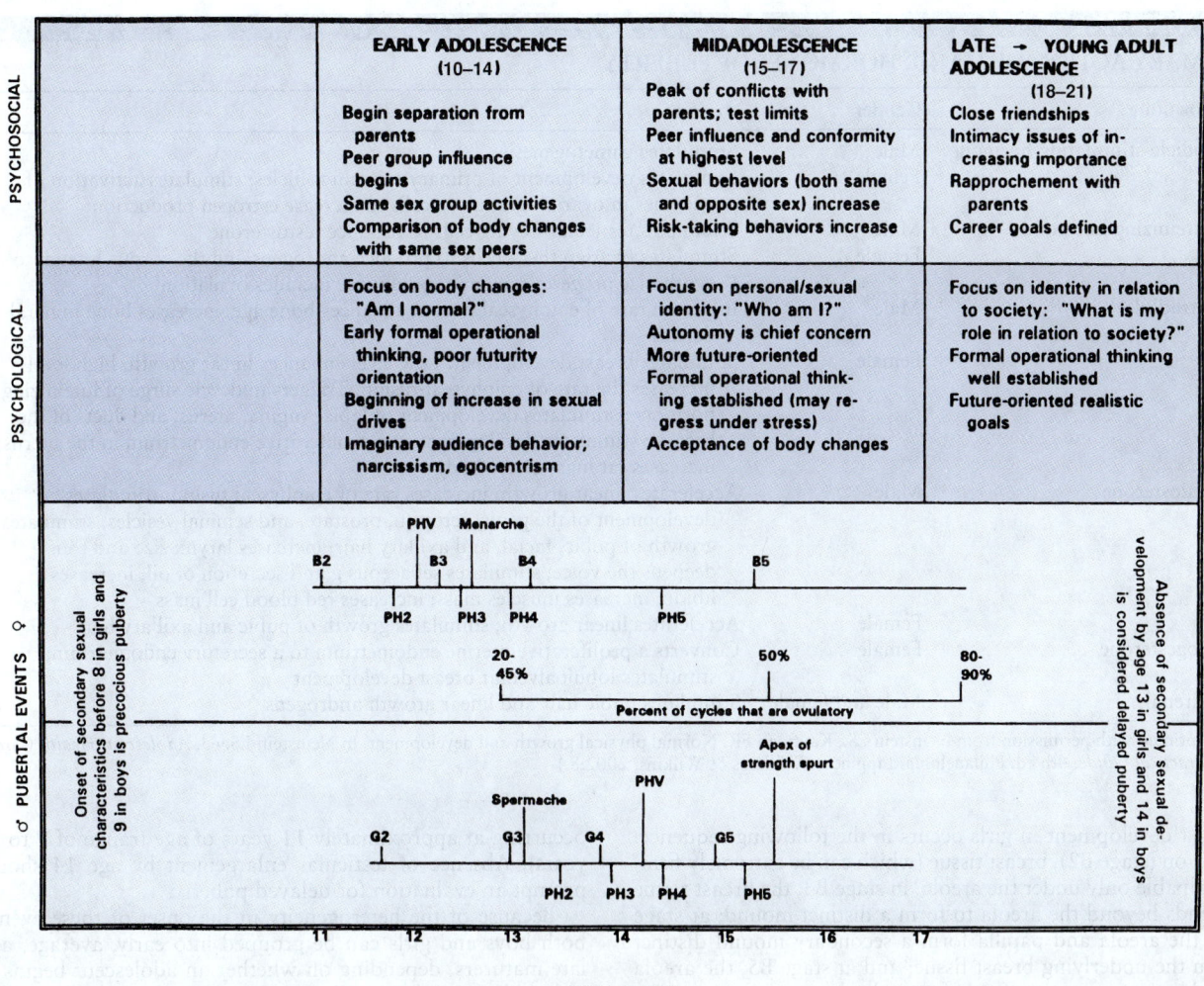

FIGURE 89.2. The temporal relation between the biological, psychologic, and psychosocial events of adolescence. Age limits for the events and stages are approximations and may differ from those used by other authors. The mean age of onset of pubic hair development for boys (13.4 years) is likely too high because of bias in the data collection method. These limits and the points indicating the attainment of individual stages of puberty were chosen for consistency and to reflect the earlier maturation of American versus British adolescents. B2, B3, B4, B5, breast stage 2, 3, and so forth; G2, G3, G4, G5, genital stage 2, 3, and so forth; PH2, PH3, PH4, PH5, pubic hair stage 2, 3, and so forth; PHV, peak height velocity.

BIOLOGIC CHANGES

Hormonal changes associated with sexual maturation begin before any physical signs of puberty are evident. An increased production of adrenal sex steroids (adrenarche) occurs approximately 2 years before maturation of the hypothalamic-pituitary-gonadal axis. Presumably because of a decreased sensitivity to the negative feedback system between the central nervous system and the testes or ovaries, the hypothalamus and pituitary gland begin to secrete increased amounts of gonadotropin-releasing hormone, follicle-stimulating hormone, and luteinizing hormone (LH). This increase is apparent only during sleep in early pubertal adolescents, but by mid puberty it becomes established during the day as well. The sleep-enhanced LH secretion occurs in agonadal patients, indicating that this process results from maturational changes at the level of the central nervous system and hypothalamus, rather than through changes in the gonads.

Secondary to an increased secretion of pituitary hormones, serum levels of testosterone in boys and estrogens (estradiol)

in girls increase progressively during physical maturation. Increased secretion of growth hormone becomes established by mid-puberty. By mid to late puberty, a positive feedback system involving LH and estrogen production leads to an estrogen-induced mid-cycle LH surge and ovulation. The physiologic roles of the various hormones during puberty are shown in Table 89.2.

Tanner's classic studies detailing the growth of adolescents and development of secondary sex characteristics established the foundation for the concept of Tanner stages (or sexual maturity ratings). Boys are assigned separate ratings for both genital and pubic hair development, girls for pubic hair and breast development. Most events occurring during adolescence correlate more closely with sexual maturity rating or skeletal age than with chronologic age.

It is important to note that some pubic hair development can occur through stimulation of hair follicles by adrenal androgens; hence, testicular enlargement and breast development are the more reliable markers of pubertal onset. The various stages of pubic hair development in boys and girls and testicular development in boys is shown in Figures 89.3 and 89.4.

TABLE 89.2

PRIMARY ACTION OF MAJOR HORMONES OF PUBERTY

Hormone	Gender	Action
Follicle-stimulating hormone	Male	Stimulates gametogenesis
	Female	Stimulates development of primary ovarian follicles; stimulates activation of enzymes in ovarian granulosa cells to increase estrogen production
Luteinizing hormone	Male	Stimulates testicular Leydig cells to produce testosterone
	Female	Stimulates ovarian theca cells to produce androgens and the corpus luteum to synthesize progesterone; mid-cycle surge includes ovulation
Estradiol	Male	Increases rate of epiphyseal fusion; advances bone age; increases bone mineral density
	Female	Stimulates breast development. Low level enhances linear growth; high level increases the rate of epiphyseal-fusion. Triggers midcycle surge of luteinizing hormone; stimulates development of labia, vagina, uterus, and ducts of the breasts; stimulates development of a proliferative endometrium in the uterus; increases fat mass of the body
Testosterone	Male	Accelerates linear growth; increases rate of epiphyseal fusion; stimulates development of the penis, scrotum, prostate, and seminal vesicles; stimulates growth of pubic, facial, and axillary hair; increases larynx size and thus deepens the voice; stimulates sebaceous gland secretion of oil; increases libido; increases muscles mass; increases red blood cell mass
	Female	Accelerates linear growth; stimulates growth of pubic and axillary hair
Progesterone	Female	Converts a proliferative uterine endometrium to a secretory endometrium; stimulates lobuloalveolar breast development
Adrenal	Male and female	Stimulates pubic hair and linear growth androgens

(Reprinted with permission from Neinstein LS., Kaufman FR. Normal physical growth and development. In Neinstein LS, ed. *Adolescent Health Care. A Practical Guide.* 4th ed. Philadelphia: Lippincott Williams & Wilkins, 2002;8.)

Breast development in girls occurs in the following sequence: early on (stage B2), breast tissue (which can be extremely firm) is palpable only under the areola; in stage B3, the breast tissue extends beyond the areola to form a distinct mound; at stage B4, the areola and papilla form a secondary mound distinct from the underlying breast tissue; and at stage B5, the areola and breast tissue again form a smooth contour (no separation of areola and breast tissue).

Studies indicate a definite sequence of pubertal events that most adolescents pass through as they mature. Although the sequence is the same, the age at onset of these events and the time interval between events vary. On average, puberty lasts approximately 3 to 4 years, but the range is quite variable. Among girls, full development of breast tissue averages 4 years, but the fifth percentile is 1.5 years and the ninety-fifth percentile is almost 9 years; the average time span for pubic hair development is 2.5 years, with the range being 1.4 (fifth percentile) to 3.10 years (ninety-fifth percentile). Among boys, complete development of the testes can take as little as 1.86 years or as much as 4.7 years (average 3 years); complete development of pubic hair can take less than a year or as long 2.67 years (average just over 1.5 years).

Table 89.3 displays the average ages of onset of puberty in girls and boys and menarche in girls. For girls, the average age of onset of breast budding, the first sign of pubertal development, is approximately 10 years of age, although some African American girls as young as 6 and some Caucasian girls as young as 7 may have breast development. The absence of breast budding by age 13 years should trigger an evaluation for delayed sexual development. Depending on the population studied, as many as 15% of girls develop pubic hair before or concurrently with breast development. Menarche occurs around age 12 to 12.5; girls who have not menstruated by age 15 should be evaluated for primary amenorrhea, as should girls who have failed to menstruate within 4 years of onset of breast budding.

Tanner's longitudinal data indicate that boys enter puberty approximately 1 year after girls, with enlargement of the testes

occurring at approximately 11 years of age (range of 9 to 14 years). Absence of testicular enlargement by age 14 should prompt an evaluation for delayed puberty.

Because of the heterogeneity in the onset of these events, both boys and girls can be grouped into early, average, and late maturers, depending on whether an adolescent begins to mature before, along with, or after the majority of his or her age cohort. Considerable evidence shows these biologic differences correlate with a variety of psychologic and sociocultural advantages and disadvantages, which contribute to a multiplicity of adolescent behaviors. Asynchrony between different aspects of development (e.g., between hormonal levels and age) appears to affect the psychosocial adjustment of boys and girls.

A variety of other somatic changes occur during puberty. Approximately 25% of adult height, 50% of adult weight, and 40% to 50% of bone mass accrue during puberty. During the year when adolescents grow fastest, their growth velocity (centimeters per year) doubles from prepubertal levels. Boys achieve a greater growth velocity than girls. The peak growth spurt in girls occurs approximately 1 year after the onset of puberty, and growth is largely completed by the time girls begin to menstruate. In boys, the growth spurt occurs 2 years after the onset of genital enlargement. Both the legs and trunk grow rapidly, with final adult height caused more by growth of the trunk. Influenced by circulating testosterone, lean body mass as a percentage of body weight in boys increases from 80% or 85% to 90%. This increase is caused by testosterone's effect on muscle development, giving rise to the concept of a strength spurt for boys occurring at Tanner stage 5.

With maturation, girls have increased fat deposition, and their lean body mass decreases from 80% to 75%. The increase in body fat to a critical level of approximately 17% is postulated to trigger the onset of menses. This theory explains the trend for earlier onset of menarche observed in Western countries since 1840, based on improved nutrition among adolescents. Menarche is not synonymous with ovulation. At menarche, only 20% of cycles are ovulatory; it may take an additional 4 years for 80% or more of cycles to be ovulatory.

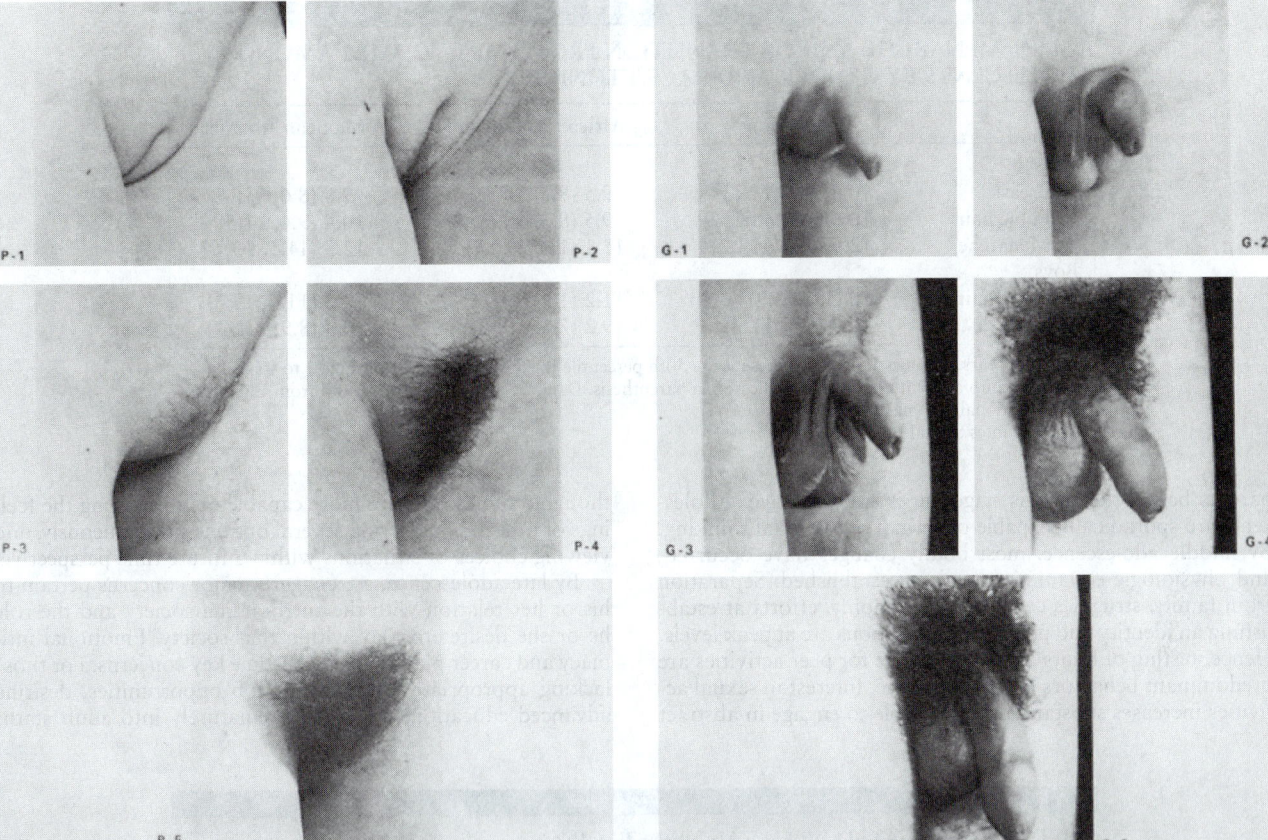

FIGURE 89.3. Stages of pubic hair development in girls. Stage 1: Preadolescent; the vellus over the pubes is not further developed than that over the anterior abdominal wall (i.e., no pubic hair). Stage 2: Sparse growth of long, slightly pigmented, downy hair, straight or only slightly curled, appearing chiefly along the labia. This stage is difficult to see on photographs. Stage 3: Hair is considerably darker, coarser, and curlier. The hair spreads sparsely over the junction of the pubes. Stage 4: Hair is now adult in type, but the area covered is still considerably smaller than in most adults. There is no spread to the medial surface of the thighs. Stage 5: Hair is adult in quantity and type, distributed as an inverse triangle of the classic feminine pattern. The spread is to the medial surface of the thighs but not up the linea alba or elsewhere above the base of the inverse triangle. (Photographs by Van Wieringen et al. Institute for Preventive Medicine, Groningen, The Netherlands. ©Wolters-Noordhoff, The Netherlands.)

FIGURE 89.4. Stages of pubic hair and genital development in boys. Genital—stage 1: Preadolescent; testes, scrotum, and penis are approximately the same size and proportion as in early childhood. Stage 2: The scrotum and testes have enlarged; there is a change in the texture and some reddening of the scrotal skin. Stage 3: Growth of the penis has occurred, at first mainly in length but with some increase in breadth; there is further growth of testes and scrotum. Stage 4: The penis is further enlarged in length and breadth with development of the glans. The testes and scrotum are further enlarged. The scrotal skin has further darkened. Stage 5: Genitalia are adult in size and shape. No further enlargement takes place after stage 5. Pubic hair—stage 1: Preadolescent; the vellus over the pubes is no further developed than that over the abdominal wall (i.e., no pubic hair). Stage 2: Sparse growth of long, slightly pigmented, downy hair, straight or only slightly curled, appearing chiefly at the base of the penis. Stage 3: Hair is considerably darker, coarser, and curlier and spreads sparsely over the junction of the pubes. Stage 4: Hair is now adult in type, but the area covered is still considerably smaller than in most adults. There is no spread to the medial surface of the thighs. Stage 5: Hair is adult in quantity and type, distributed as an inverse triangle. The spread is to the medial surface of the thighs but not up the linea alba or elsewhere above the base of the inverse triangle. Most men will have further spread of pubic hair. (Photographs by Van Wieringen et al. Institute for Preventive Medicine, Groningen, The Netherlands. © Wolters-Noordhoff, The Netherlands.)

The size of the ovaries and uterus of an adolescent increases five- to sevenfold during puberty. The penis doubles in size, and the volume of the testicles increases from approximately 2 mL to 18 mL.

These changes in sexual maturity and body size and composition have significant implications for the health care of adolescents. For example, early maturing adolescent girls are at increased risk for early sexual activity and other risky behaviors, perhaps mediated through friendships with older, rather than same-aged, girls. Gynecomastia occurs commonly at Tanner stage 2 or 3 and may prompt teenage boys to complain of chest pain in the hope that a visit to a clinician will bring reassurance that they are not, in fact, developing breasts. When breast budding is noted in girls, they can be counseled that menarche will likely ensue in approximately 2 years. Certain illnesses are more likely to develop or worsen at one or another stage of pubertal development. For example, scoliosis typically worsens during the time of rapid trunk growth. Other examples are provided in Table 89.4.

STAGES OF ADOLESCENT DEVELOPMENT

Because pubertal and cognitive development vary over a wide range of chronologic ages, characterizing an individual teenager as being in early (10 to14 years), middle (15 to 17 years), or late (18 or above) adolescence is useful. Early adolescence incorporates the period of rapid body change and gives rise to a preoccupation with such changes and the need for reassurance regarding physical normalcy. Initial separation from

TABLE 89.3

AGE OF MENARCHE AND OF TRANSITION FROM SMR1 TO SMR2 AMONG ADOLESCENTS BY GENDER AND RACE/ETHNICITY

	Caucasian	African American	Mexican American
Girls			
Breast	10.4 (9.5, 11.2)[1]	9.5 (8.5, 10.5)	9.8 (8.6, 11)
Pubic hair	10.6 (9.7, 11.5)	9.5 (8.3, 10.6)	10.4 (9.4, 11.5)
Menarche	12.6 (11.9, 13.2)	12.1 (11.3, 12.9)	12.3 (11.5, 13)
Boys			
Pubic hair	10 (11, 12.9)	11.2 (10, 12.4)	12.3 (11.4, 13.3)
Testes	10.0 (8.6, 11.4)	9.2 (7.5, 10.9)	10.3 (8.9, 11.7)

[1]Ages in years. The age indicated represent the 50th percentile for the transition form stage 1 to stage 2 with the 25th and 75th percentiles indicated in parenthesis. Data are adapted from sun and from Chumlea (see additional readings).
SMR denotes Sexual Maturity Rating.

parents begins during this stage but is still tentative. Adolescents are sporadically capable of formal operational thinking. By middle adolescence, most bodily changes have occurred, and physiologic equanimity has been established. Separation from family, struggles concerning autonomy, efforts at establishing an identity and peer group affiliations are at peak levels. Hence, testing of limits and a preference for peer activities are predominant behaviors during this stage. Interest in sexual activities increases substantially. Now able to engage in abstract thought, adolescents are more capable of considering the feelings of others, considering several options simultaneously, and viewing choices or situations within a future time perspective.

By late adolescence, a teenager's major concerns pertain to his or her relation with the surrounding society and the role he or she desires to play within that society. Emotional intimacy and career planning also become key concerns. For those lacking appropriate schooling or job opportunities, desiring advanced education, or forced prematurely into adult status

TABLE 89.4

FACTORS ASSOCIATED WITH TANNER STAGING

Process/Disorder	Tanner Stage
Hematocrit increase (boys)	II–V
Alkaline phosphatase peak (boys)	III
Alkaline phosphatase peak (girls)	II
Adolescent hormonal levels (increase in estrogen for girls and testosterone for boys)	II–V
Peak height velocity (boys)	III–IV
Peak height velocity (girls)	II–III
Short boy with growth potential	II
Short boy with limited growth potential	IV–V
Usual timing of menarche	Late III or early IV
Appearance of menarche	1.0–3.6 years post stage II
Slipped capital femoral epiphysis	(Obese) II or III
Acute worsening of idiopathic adolescent scoliosis (i.e., time for close monitoring)	II–IV
Osgood-Schlatter disease	III
Oral contraceptive prescription	IV
Diaphragm prescription	IV–V
Observe for worsening of straight back syndrome	II–IV
Appearance of "normal" gynecomastia	II or III
Usual appearance of acne vulgaris	II or III
Gonococcal vaginitis	I
Gonococcal cervicitis (with or without pelvic inflammatory disease)	II+
Timing of orchiopexy	I
Decreased incidence in serous otitis media	II or III
Mild regression in virginal hypertrophy	V
Timing of breast reduction	V
Timing of rhinoplasty	V
Strong suspicion for organic disease	II–V (abnormal progression or regression)
Counseling for further breast growth	II
Increased levels of serum uric acid in boys	II–V

Reprinted with permission from Greydanus DE, McAnarney ER. The value of Tanner staging. *J Curr Adolesc Med* 1980;2:21.

because of adolescent parenthood, it can be difficult to resolve these issues and/or the associated concerns regarding prolonged dependence on parents.

PSYCHOLOGIC CHANGES

A variety of authors and theories have outlined the psychologic changes occurring during adolescence. One major change is in cognition. Piaget characterized adolescent thought processes as increasingly sophisticated, with movement from concrete to formal operational, abstract thinking. This maturation encompasses emerging abilities to reflect on concepts lacking concrete representation, to mentally arrange individual pieces into multiple combinations, and as a result, to construct ideals and situations distinct from or in contrast to those existing in reality. Such changes allow increasingly sophisticated concepts and reasoning, making the teenager capable of exploring a broad range of possibilities or solutions when confronted with a new situation or problem. When combined with increased physical maturity, size, and strength, this new cognitive capacity affords the adolescent an increasing sense of mastery over the external world as well as a sense of invulnerability. Many risky behaviors among adolescents can be viewed as an attempt to test the limits and capabilities of newly developed physical and mental prowess.

Preoccupied with bodily changes, early adolescents tend to be extremely concerned with their own needs and, because of their concrete level of reasoning, have difficulty reflecting on another's point of view. As they begin to develop the capacity for formal operational thinking, they become aware of other people's beliefs but are unable to differentiate what is of interest to themselves and to others. They assume that matters of great personal concern must necessarily be of equal significance to others. Adolescents also assume mistakenly that other individuals can read their thoughts. Hence, these young people sometimes act as if they are behaving for an imaginary audience. This notion that others are watching and thinking about them gives rise to the development of a sense of uniqueness and invulnerability (termed the *personal fable* by psychologist David Elkind). The adolescent believes that negative outcomes such as unintended pregnancy, drug addiction, HIV infection, or serious injury happen to others but not to them. This personal fable helps partly to explain why adolescents participate in behaviors adults view as risky.

With the progression of the capacity for formal operational thought, adolescents become capable of considering perspectives other than their own, thereby becoming less egocentric. They also come to realize that other individuals have concerns of their own and are not focused exclusively on the adolescent's needs and desires. These changes do not occur in an all-or-none manner. Adolescents, particularly in early and middle adolescence, may be capable of sophisticated abstract reasoning one day and revert back to more concrete thinking the next, especially during periods of stress. They may appear remarkably self-centered in one situation and altruistic in another. Hence, to adults, adolescents may not always appear to act rationally or consistently with regard to their health care or behavior.

As they mature in their ability to reason abstractly, adolescents also develop a more adult sense of time and futurity orientation. This sense involves the ability to project oneself forward in time to weigh future options and assess the long-term consequences or benefits of various decisions. However, it also presumes a belief that one *has* a future and the capacity to influence it. Adolescents who have repeatedly failed at attempts to make decisions for themselves, have been given little opportunity to develop a sense of control, or who cannot foresee a meaningful future for themselves are likely to feel cynical,

powerless, or unresponsive when confronted with decisions in which a sense of time or concern for the future is critical.

Changes in sexual feelings and sexual relationships during adolescence were key components of Freud's psychosexual theories. An upsurge in sexual feelings and impulses parallels hormonal and genital changes occurring during puberty. At first, such impulses are largely undifferentiated and directed toward persons of the same gender but do not necessarily have implications for future sexual orientation. As the adolescent matures, these impulses generally become directed toward individuals of the opposite sex. However, at least 1.4% of women and 2.8% of men identify themselves as lesbian or gay, respectively, with still others expressing attraction to individuals of both genders.

An important component of the adolescent's maturing sexual identity is the realization that human sexuality involves more than the physical aspects of sex. The meaning of sexuality is influenced by parental beliefs and upbringing and by cultural, religious, and peer-group norms. Given the significant influence of cultural and societal norms in defining acceptable sexual behaviors, those individuals who become aware of their persisting same-sex attraction usually must develop their sexual identity in secret, without the needed support of parents, siblings, or peers. Often stigmatized by the greater society, gay, lesbian, and bisexual youth can derive significant support from a sympathetic pediatrician.

Erik Erikson, another prominent theorist on human development, shifted from the Freudian emphasis on biologic drive states to highlight the critical issue of identity formation. Building on skills achieved earlier in development, adolescents must achieve a sense of who they are. This requires an integration of both bodily and psychologic changes that, because of sexual awareness and maturity, result in a discontinuity with the past. Initial concerns focus on normalcy, then on characteristics of personal identity, and finally on the relationship between one's self and society. Developing a firm sense of identity is a prelude to resolving the young adult challenge of establishing the capacity for intimacy. Failure to do so leads to feelings of personal isolation. Erikson concluded that the development of an individual identity depends on the successful completion of previous developmental tasks. Adolescents who fail to achieve one or more of the preceding tasks during childhood or the various stages of adolescence (e.g., as a consequence of heavy drug use) are at risk for failure to consolidate a sense of identity.

SOCIOCULTURAL CHANGES

Adolescent development takes place within the context of a number of overlapping, interrelated spheres of influence. Families, peers, communities, religions, cultural and ethnic groups, and schools all have values, customs, and taboos that help shape an adolescent's development. Due to broad social changes, families are in a state of flux, with many adolescents being raised by one parent, by a relative other than a parent, or by blended families.

The relationship between the adolescent and each of these socializing influences is complex. Adolescents derive many values from the previously mentioned reference groups. These groups, in turn, may be influenced by personal characteristics of the adolescent. For example, teachers characterize late-maturing boys as above average in intelligence less often than their early- or average-maturing classmates. Similarly, parents have lower expectations for these same individuals to complete college. Sexual activity, largely determined by perceptions of peer norms, also appears to be influenced by an individual's physiologic maturity. Early maturing boys in one study engaged in various sexual behaviors earlier than age-matched counterparts who were on-time or delayed in development. Early maturing girls initiate sexual intercourse at an earlier age than their less physically developed but same-aged peers, perhaps because early maturing girls often have older friends and adopt the norms of that older peer group.

During early and middle adolescence, a gradual separation occurs from parents and parental influence. This distancing occurs, in part, as a consequence of the more complex thought processes of the maturing adolescent, who can now imagine a set of ideal parents to contrast with his or her real ones. Although the peer group becomes increasingly important in an adolescent's life, particularly at middle adolescence, the family does not lose all influence. Families, especially parents, are the primary socializing forces for infants and children up to early adolescence. They continue to be the major source of nurturing and protection for adolescents, who, as a result, enter puberty with values, goals, and beliefs instilled and modeled by parents. This value system is questioned, reanalyzed, and played down during the separation and individuation phase of early and middle adolescence, but it is not entirely abandoned. Rather, the adolescent shifts back and forth between seeking parental support at one moment and appearing to reject it the next. This seeming ambivalence can be frustrating for parents. By late adolescence, a rapprochement is established, and the adolescent usually emerges with a belief system that incorporates, however modified, principles learned largely within the family context.

The challenge for parents or other adult caretakers is to provide adolescents with an environment in which they can continue to develop and refine their emerging physical and cognitive skills. This environment must constantly balance the adolescent's needs for adequate independence (which requires considerable parental flexibility) with legitimate parental expectations regarding respect for parental authority, for other members of the family, and for the orderly functioning of the household.

Such an environment can be best achieved if mutual respect exists among all family members, if household rules are set fairly but flexibly (with input from the adolescent), and if communication is effective. Effective communication is characterized by consistency, clarity regarding expectations for behavior in and out of the family, and a congruence between what family members say and do.

Peer groups serve many important functions for adolescents. While adolescents try to determine who they are and whether they are normal, peer groups provide both social support and a safe way of trying alternative identities. Because they are seeking to separate from parents, adolescents may believe they cannot rely on parental support during the critical period when rapid body changes, increased drive states, and emerging cognitive abilities lead to a period of relative identity diffusion. The peer group provides an alternative support system.

The conformity required for peer group membership can have adverse developmental and health consequences if behaviors such as excessive drinking, cigarette use, or truancy are requirements for membership. As the adolescent becomes more secure in establishing his or her identity, the relationship with the peer group is restructured to a more equitable level.

Much has been written about peer group influence. Although adolescents look to peers for standards governing such things as dress, music, and hairstyles, they continue to respect and rely on parental values in many other areas. It is probably more accurate to say that decisions requiring choices about various aspects of lifestyle activate different referent groups.

CHRONIC ILLNESS

Advances in medical care enable individuals with diseases that once resulted in childhood death to live into the adolescent and young adult years; still others develop a chronic illness during adolescence. As a result, perhaps 10% of adolescents

and their families must confront the challenge of living with a chronic illness as they also confront the developmental tasks of adolescence.

The effect of chronic illness on adolescent development can be significant and complex. At a time when adolescents are concerned about bodily changes and a desire to look like their peers, those aspects of a disease or its treatment that result in altered body size or shape may have an adverse effect on self-esteem and body image. Teenagers with chronic illnesses may be reluctant to take medications that produce visible changes in their bodies and set them apart from their peers. Part of the personal fable implies that the need for medication no longer exists.

Chronic illness can interfere with normal adolescent development and create conflict between teenagers and parents. Anxious parents may be reluctant to grant age-appropriate independence or allow their teenager to make decisions about health care or other aspects of his or her personal life. Chronic illness gives parents justification for holding onto their teenager beyond the point when separation should occur.

Adolescents, in turn, may use their illness to manipulate their parents, avoid responsibility, or justify their unwillingness to meet the difficult challenges of growing to maturity. They also may shun social relationships out of fear of being perceived as different, or, having been protected excessively by parents, may be too immature to engage in appropriate peer activities. Alternatively, feeling the need to establish that they are like other adolescents, those with chronic illness may engage in health-risking behaviors. Such behaviors (e.g., refusal to take insulin) can have serious deleterious effects on their health. Clinicians working with such adolescents and their families must be aware of these underlying dynamics.

LEGAL AND ETHICAL CONSIDERATIONS

Providing health care to adolescents involves a variety of legal and ethical issues. In many health care situations, a conflict exists among adolescents, their parents, physicians, and society about who makes decisions.

As with other areas of medicine, the framework for resolving such dilemmas is based on the patient's best interest, from the patient's perspective and the principles of the doctor–patient relationship. The best interest standard recognizes the primacy of the adolescent's health and well-being and acknowledges the reality that many adolescents will not seek care if they believe parents will be notified, even in circumstances in which lack of treatment poses a threat to their health. Concerning the doctor–patient relationship, the physician should remember that the adolescent, not the adolescent's parents, is his or her patient. Hence, the adolescent should be afforded confidentiality, except when compelling evidence demonstrates the adolescent is not competent to consent or poses a serious threat to himself or herself (i.e., suicidal or seriously involved with drugs) or to others. In some situations, breach of confidentiality is mandated by law (e.g., reporting sexual abuse or incest to social service agencies). Limits of confidentiality should be explained to the adolescent at the beginning of the visit.

No objective standard exists to determine at what age one is competent to give consent for health-care decisions. Some evidence suggests that adolescents as young as 14 years have the same capacity as adults to give consent. Research by Lawrence Kohlberg and Carol Gilligan helps elucidate the manner in which adolescents make such decisions.

All 50 state supreme courts recognize the doctrine of the "mature minor." This concept applies to those at the age of discretion (i.e., age 15 years or older). For these youths, the doctrine applies if the following are true: the minor appears able to understand the procedure and its attendant risks and benefits sufficiently to give genuine informed consent; medical measures are taken for the patient's own benefit; measures are judged as necessary by conservative medical opinion; and a good reason exists, including simple refusal by the minor to request it, why parental consent cannot be obtained.

Competence in making health-care decisions is not an all or none phenomenon. Given the adolescent's desire to be treated as an adult, competence can be presumed in situations in which little risk exists of harm to the adolescent from his or her decision. When situations involve considerable risk (e.g., refusing life-saving treatment) or when dealing with an extremely immature minor, the standard of competency should be more restrictive. Even with a stricter standard, it still may be concluded, as in the case of treatment for sexually transmitted diseases, that treatment without parental consent is warranted.

Rarely does the adolescent refuse any involvement of parents. Initially, out of fear or misunderstanding, adolescents may be reluctant to reveal information to their parents. With careful explanation of the issues involved, and with adequate support by the physician, however, most adolescents eventually do involve their parents.

By recognizing the competence of adolescents to give consent, and based on concern that adolescents might avoid seeking care if confidentiality is not assured, all states have enacted legislation permitting physicians to treat adolescents in a variety of circumstances without parental consent. These include treatment for emergencies, sexually transmitted diseases, mental health problems, drug and alcohol abuse, pregnancy, and contraception (www.agi-usa.org/pubs/journals/gr030404.pdf). Abortion is a more controversial topic, but the U.S. Supreme Court has ruled consistently that a minor may consent to an abortion without parental consent or notification, if she is willing to obtain a judge's consent in lieu of parental consent.

HEALTH ASSESSMENT OF ADOLESCENTS

Health maintenance visits during adolescence are critical. Adolescents undergo a period of enormous physiologic and psychologic change at the same time that they are confronted with a multitude of decisions about various behaviors that can enhance or threaten their well-being. The goals of the health maintenance visit are to reassure and support the adolescent about the normalcy of his or her development, to present information about how lifestyle choices affect health and assist the adolescent in assessing the various choices, and to identify those youth at risk for, or having, adverse health problems as a means of preventing or treating such problems. Both the Bright Futures Project of the Maternal and Child Health Bureau (now headquartered at the American Academy of Pediatrics (http://brightfutures.aap.org/web/healthCareProfessionalstoolsAndResources.asp) and the Department of Adolescent Health of the American Medical Association (www.ama-assn.org/ama/pub/category/1981.html) maintain helpful web sites containing materials for adolescent health visits. The Advisory Committee on Immunization Practices of the CDC recommends a routine visit at age 11 to 12 years to update diphtheria, tetanus, measles, mumps, rubella, and varicella immunizations and to begin hepatitis B immunization for adolescents not previously vaccinated. This visit can serve as the inaugural health maintenance visit for adolescents.

How often such visits should occur is unclear. The American Academy of Pediatrics, as well as many experts in adolescent medicine, recommend yearly visits because of the nature and rapidity of the changes that occur during adolescence are so dramatic. The AMA's Guidelines for Adolescent Preventive Services (www.ama-assn.org/ama/pub/category/1980.html) recommends that a physical examination be performed only once during each period (early, middle, late) of adolescence, but that an assessment of the adolescent's functioning and medically indicated screening tests (such as Papanicolaou smears or screening for *Chlamydia trachomatis*) occur on a yearly basis or more often, as warranted by the adolescent's behavior.

In addition to the standard medical history obtained from patients and their families, certain aspects of the adolescent's level of functioning and lifestyle should be scrutinized. These are outlined in Table 89.5. A useful mnemonic to guide the clinician's systematic evaluation of these areas is HEADSS (*h*ome, *e*ducation, *a*ctivities, *d*rugs, *s*exuality, and *s*uicide/depression). Such information can be gathered by personal interview, paper and pencil or computerized questionnaires, or from a combination of the two. Although some time will be spent with parents, most of the visit should occur alone with the adolescent, unless he or she specifically requests a parental presence.

The direction and content of the interview depend on whether the patient is in early, middle, or late adolescence. Use of an open-ended, nonjudgmental style, interlaced with comments indicating that the intent of the questioning is for information gathering and that such areas are often of concern to adolescents, helps put the adolescent at ease. A good introductory clause is, "Many young people your age are concerned about . . ." In general, it is prudent to ask the least threatening questions first. When asking about such things as illicit drug use or sexual activity, the physician may wish to inquire first about friends' behaviors. Some time needs to be spent with parents to identify their concerns and to round out the picture of the adolescent's level of functioning. Elements of the history appropriate to discuss with the adolescent and parents together includes immunization status, family medical history, history of chronic illness, previous hospitalizations, surgeries, and trauma. Medication use and allergies should also be reviewed.

Especially for adolescents in early puberty, the physical examination is exceptionally important. Concerned with changes in body size, shape, and function, adolescents often seek reassurance about the normalcy of their development. As the physician proceeds through the examination, explaining the procedures and commenting about the results are worthwhile (see Table 89.5 for areas of the physical examination that should be highlighted).

No absolute consensus exists regarding the need for a pelvic examination in teenagers. In general, a sexually nonactive teenager with normal menstrual function does not need a pelvic examination unless she specifically requests one. Examination of her external genitalia, however, should be part of the routine physical examination. Other than sexual activity, indications for a pelvic examination are severe dysmenorrhea unresponsive to nonsteroidal antiinflammatory agents or oral contraceptive pills, vaginal discharge, unexplained vaginal bleeding, amenorrhea or oligomenorrhea, or sexual assault. All sexually active adolescents should be screened for sexually transmitted infections. However, new guidelines concerning Papanicolaou smears recommend that females receive their first Papanicolaou smear within 3 years of the onset of sexual intercourse or by age 21, whichever comes first (see Table 89.5 for recommended laboratory tests and immunization protocols).

COUNSELING

As they mature, adolescents must make numerous decisions with the potential to affect their health. Pressures to behave in a certain manner may be brought to bear by parents, peers, schools, society, and the media (via television, music videos, and movies). Particularly in regards to such behaviors as sexual activity and drug use, adolescents are disproportionately influenced by perceptions of their peers' behaviors, even though

TABLE 89.5

RECOMMENDED CONTENT FOR ROUTINE ADOLESCENT HEALTH VISIT

Medical History
Immunizations: diphtheria, tetanus, polio, measles (two doses after first birthday), mumps, rubella, bacille Calmette-Guérin, varicella, hepatitis B
Chronic illness
Hospitalization
Surgery
Trauma: fractures, burns, head trauma; prior sports injuries; injured in a fight
Medication: over-the-counter, prescribed (include hormonal contraceptives); food supplements; alternative medicines
Family History
Cardiovascular: hypertension; diabetes; obesity; elevated cholesterol/triglycerides; myocardial infarction or angina, peripheral vascular disease, or stroke in family members less than 60 years old
Alcoholism/substance abuse
Psychiatric disorders; suicide
Asthma, tuberculosis
Review of Systems
Dietary habits: typical foods consumed, special diets (e.g., vegetarianism), types and frequency of meals skipped, use of laxatives or other weight loss methods
Recent weight gain or loss
Dental: last dental visit
Eye: last vision check
Gynecologic history (female patients): age of menarche: date of last menstrual period and previous menstrual period
Characterization of menses: amount of bleeding; use of tampons/pads; dysmenorrhea (medications used for treatment); interval between menses; regularity of menses
Psychosocial History (HEADSS)
Home
    Household composition
    Relations with parents (including those not in home)
    Relations with siblings
    Living and sleeping arrangements
    Guns in the home
Education
    School attendance
    Ever failed a grade
    Grades this year compared with last
    Favorite, most difficult, best subjects
    Attitude towards school: sense of belonging; fairness of staff
    Special education needs
    Number of days missed since start of current year
Activities
    Physical activity, regular exercise
    Sports participation, teams
    Work: type of job, hours, wages, satisfaction, safety hazards
    Special interests, hobbies, skills
    Peer relationships, best friends; activities with friends; gang membership
    Weapon carrying; fights
Drugs
    Cigarettes/smokeless tobacco: age at first use, packs or cans per day
    Alcohol (beer, wine coolers): use at school or parties; use by friends, self; Brief screening test for substance abuse (CRAFFT): Have you ever ridden in a *car* driven someone (including yourself) who was "high" or had been using alcohol or other drugs? Do you ever use alcohol or drugs to *relax*, feel better about yourself, or fit in? Do you ever use alcohol or drugs while you are by yourself, *alone*? Do you ever *forget* things you did while using alcohol or drugs? Do your *family* or *friends* ever tell you should cut down on your drinking or drug use? Have you ever gotten into *trouble* while you were using alcohol or drugs? *Two or more yes answers indicates need for further assessment.**
    For any alcohol or other drug use: adverse consequences (driving while under the inflence, accidents, truancy, vandalism; forced sex)
    Concerns about parental alcohol or drug use
Sexuality
Sexual feelings: Opposite or same sex
Sexual intercourse or types of sexual practices; age at first intercourse; gender of sex partner; number of lifetime partners; age of current partner
History of sexually transmitted diseases; last screen; history of pelvic inflammatory disease (women)
Prior pregnancies, abortions; ever gotten a girl pregnant?
Contraception/sexually transmitted disease prevention: use of contraceptives, condoms, consistency of use; use at last intercourse
History of sexual abuse or date rape

(Continued)

TABLE 89.5

(CONTINUED)

Suicide/depression
   Feelings about self: positive and negative
   History of depression or other mental health problems; suicidal thoughts; prior suicide attempts
   Sleep problems: difficulty getting to sleep, early waking
Physical Examination (Most Pertinent Aspects)
Height, weight, body mass index, blood pressue (with percentiles)
General appearance; affect
Skin: acne (type and distribution of lesions); scars; tattoos; body piercing
Dentition
Spine (scoliosis)
Breasts: Tanner stage; masses (females)
   Gynecomastia (males)
External genitalia (all)
   Pubic hair distribution, Tanner stage
   Testicular examination, Tanner stage, masses
Pelvic examination if indicated (see text)
Laboratory Tests
Purified protein derivative only if at risk
Vision and hearing screen
Complete blood count with indices once during adolescence for boys and after menarche for girls. Lipid profile (if positive family
   history)
Sexually active adolescents
   Males: First-part voided urinalysis (FPVU) for white blood cells or leukocyte esterase activity. Detection tests for chlamydia and
      gonorrhea if FPVU positive; serologic test for syphilis
   Females: Detection tests for chlamydia and gonorrhea; serologic test for syphilis; potassium hydroxide/wet preparation mid-
      vaginal pH; Papanicolaou smear (see text)
   Homosexual males: same as above; depending on sexual behaviors, consider testing throat for gonorrhea and rectum for
      gonorrhea and chlamydia; hepatitis B screening if not immunized.
All sexually active adolescents should routinely be offered HIV testing. Informed consent is necessary, and state laws vary as to
   specifics of consent procedure. Thorough, age-appropriate pretest and posttest counseling is essential
Immunizations†
Tetanus and diphtheria (update 10 years or more since last dose)
Measles: two doses of live attenuated vaccine are required after first birthday. Use measles, mumps, and rubella vaccine if not
   previously vaccinated for mumps or rubella. Do not administer rubella vaccine to woman anticipating pregnancy within 30 days
Hepatitis B vaccine: recommended for all adolescents
Hepatitis A vaccine: reccommended for gay/bisexual males
Varicella vaccine: recommended for all adolesscents without history of disease (one dose if younger than 13 years; two doses 4 to 8
   weeks apart if 13 years or older)

*CRAFFT question adapted with permission from the Center for Adolescent Substance Abuse Research at Children's Hospital Boston (see also selected reading).
†For a complete discussion of adolescent immunizations, see *Report of the Committee of Infectious Diseases*, 26th ed. Elk Grove Village, IL: American Academy of Pediatrics, 2003.

these perceptions often overestimate the actual prevalence of these behaviors. The adolescent should be provided with information concerning such areas as sexuality (and, if appropriate, contraception and protection against sexually transmitted diseases); safety (guns, fighting, seat belt and bicycle helmet use); peer pressure; alcohol, tobacco, and illicit drug use; body image concerns; relationships with parents; normal versus abnormal mood states; and coronary artery disease prevention (appropriate nutrition, physical activity). The optimal approach is to collaborate with (rather than lecture to) the adolescent in developing an understanding of the ramifications of various behaviors. This dialogue signals the health care provider's willingness to discuss such matters at future visits. Although the techniques are still of unproven efficacy, most physicians recommend teaching adolescents about breast self-examination; some also advocate teaching young men testicular self-examination.

Parents also should be able to discuss the development of the adolescent and to express concerns. They may need reassurance about the normalcy of their child's development and suggestions regarding setting limits, appropriate and fair discipline, the role of peers, providing positive feedback, and identifying increasing opportunities for independence and re-

sponsibility. Considerable research supports the influence of parents on a wide variety of adolescent behaviors. Because many teenagers model the parental behaviors they observe at home, parents should be made aware of the potential influence of such parental behaviors as use of alcohol, smoking cigarettes, driving after drinking, and use of seat belts. Because of the link between the availability of guns in the home and adolescent suicide, parents should be encouraged not to keep guns in the home or to keep them locked up in an area to which adolescents cannot gain access. The visit should be used also to encourage parents to initiate dialogues with their son or daughter about topics such as sexuality and drug use. Both the Bright Futures and AMA web sites listed earlier contain health education resources for both adolescents and parents.

Suggested Readings

Biehl MC, Park MJ, Brindis C, et al. *The health of America's middle childhood population.* San Francisco: University of California, San Francisco, Public Policy Analysis and Education Center for Middle Childhood and Adolescent Health, 2002.
Chumlea WC, Schubert CM, Roche AF, et al. Age at menarche and racial comparisons in U.S. girls. *Pediatrics* 2003;111:110.

Gilligan C. In A Different Voice. *Psychologic theory and women's development.* Cambridge: Harvard University Press, 1993.

Herman-Giddens ME, Slora EJ, Waserman RC, et al. Secondary sexual characteristics and menses in young girls seen in office practice: a study from the pediatric research in office settings network. *Pediatrics* 1997;99:505.

Jessor R, ed. *New perspectives on adolescent risk behavior.* New York: Cambridge University Press, 1998.

Knight JR, Sherritt L, Shrier LA, et al. Validity of the CRAFFT substance abuse screening test among adolescent clinic patients. *Arch Pediatr Adolesc Med* 2002;156:607.

Millstein S, Petersen AC, Nightingale EO, eds. *Promoting the health of adolescents. New directions for the twenty-first century.* New York: Oxford University Press, 1993.

Muuss RE. *Theories of adolescence,* 6th ed. New York: McGraw-Hill, 1996.

Ozer EM, Park MJ, Paul T, et al. *America's adolescents: are they healthy?* San Francisco: University of California, San Francisco, National Adolescent Health Information Center, 2003.

Rainey DY. Office-based care of adolescents: Part 1. Creating a teen-friendly office. *Adolescent Health Update* 2003;16:1.

Reddy DM, Fleming RF, Swain C. Effect of mandatory parental notification on adolescent girls' use of sexual health care services. *JAMA* 2002;288:710.

Resnick MD, Bearman PS, Blum RW, et al. Protecting adolescents from harm. Findings from the national longitudinal study on adolescent health. *JAMA* 1997;278:823.

Resnick MD. Protective factors, resiliency and healthy youth development. *Adolesc Med* 2000;11:157.

Romer D, ed. *Reducing adolescent risk..* Thousand Oaks, CA: Sage Publications, 2003.

Sun SS, Schubert CM, Chumlea WC, et al. National estimates of the timing of sexual maturation and racial differences among U.S. children. *Pediatrics* 2002;110:911.

Tanner JM. *Growth at adolescence,* 2nd ed. Oxford: Blackwell Scientific, 1982.

CHAPTER 90 ■ BREAST DISORDERS

GINA S. SUCATO

Growth of the breast is usually the first sign of puberty in girls, and it also occurs transiently during normal pubertal development in many boys. Most breast conditions that concern patients and their families are either variants of normal development or benign conditions. Routine breast examination of pediatric patients is important to allow reassurance about these conditions, as well as to detect the less common entities that require further evaluation and management.

BREAST EXAMINATION

Examination of the breast, including inspection and palpation, should occur during routine well-child examinations. During puberty, examination of both the male and female breast affords an opportunity to offer reassurance if indicated. When performing female breast examination, the presence of a chaperone is advisable. The clinician should ask the patient to lie supine and to take one arm out of her gown and place it behind her head. The entire breast should be inspected and then palpated using the flat finger pads of the middle three fingers to make dime-sized circles. A systematic approach, such as following the pattern of the spokes of a wheel or horizontal strips, will ensure thorough breast examination. The sexual maturity rating (Tanner stage) of each breast should be noted. It may put young women at ease to teach breast self-examination simultaneously. However, the primary purpose of teaching self-examination is to promote familiarity and acceptance of the breast, not for early detection of breast cancer, which is exceedingly rare in adolescence. The American Cancer Society now considers breast self-examination an optional component of breast cancer screening for women of all ages.

VARIATIONS OF NORMAL GROWTH AND DEVELOPMENT

Children of either sex can be born with polythelia (supernumerary nipples) or polymastia (extra breast tissue). These variations can be found anywhere from the axilla to the groin in up to 5% of healthy patients. Because polythelia may be as-

sociated with genitourinary abnormalities, a renal ultrasound study may be advisable for infants with this condition if it is accompanied by other congenital anomalies. More than half of both male and female newborns have palpable breast growth, sometimes with bilateral white nipple discharge. This benign condition results from maternal hormonal stimulation and resolves spontaneously, usually by 4 months of age. Although accessory breast tissue is usually asymptomatic, it may become engorged and painful in women during pregnancy or lactation.

Variations of growth and development in girls include breast hypoplasia, asymmetry, and hypertrophy. Amastia (total absence of the breast) is rare and usually unilateral. It is often secondary to chest wall anomalies such as absence of underlying muscle tissue, or Poland syndrome, which is characterized by aplasia of the pectoralis muscles, rib deformities, webbed fingers, and radial nerve palsy. Breast hypoplasia accompanied by signs of androgen excess in a female patient warrants further endocrinologic evaluation. Breast atrophy can be the result of malnutrition or weight loss, as seen with eating disorders or chronic disease.

Breast asymmetry is common, especially during early pubertal breast development. While the breasts are still growing, adolescents can be advised to use bra pads for the smaller breast. Although it frequently corrects by adulthood, visible asymmetry persists in approximately 25% of women, in which case surgical augmentation and reduction mammoplasty are options. Breast hypertrophy, or macromastia, typically begins in adolescence and is associated with obesity. Juvenile, or "virginal," hypertrophy, with massive diffuse enlargement of one or both breasts during puberty, occurs rarely. Corrective surgery is preferably delayed until after breast development is complete.

COMMON CONDITIONS OF THE BREAST

Gynecomastia

Gynecomastia is enlargement of the male breast. During puberty, proliferation of breast tissue in both girls and boys is

TABLE 90.1

DRUGS ASSOCIATED WITH GYNECOMASTIA

Hormones (anabolic steroids, estrogens)
Antiandrogens
Antibiotics (isoniazid, metronidazole, ketoconazole)
Antiulcer drugs (histamine [H_2] blockers, omeprazole)
Cancer chemotherapy agents
Cardiovascular drugs (digitoxin, nifedipine, verapamil)
Psychoactive drugs (diazepam, haloperidol, phenothiazines)
Drugs of abuse (alcohol, marijuana, amphetamines, heroin)
Other (metoclopramide, phenytoin)

Adapted from Braunstein GD, Glassman HA. Gynecomastia. *Curr Ther Endocrinol Metab* 1997:6:401, with permission.

stimulated by estrogen and antagonized by androgens. Early in puberty, adolescent boys may experience a transient imbalance between estrogen and androgen levels resulting in pubertal breast growth. This finding is common in early and middle adolescence and can be found in up to 64% of healthy 14-year-old boys. The majority of estrogen in males is produced outside the male testes, by peripheral aromatization of sex hormones in adipose tissue, muscle, and skin. Significant increase of aromatization, as occurs with obesity, can elevate levels of circulating estrogen and may exacerbate gynecomastia.

Pubertal gynecomastia frequently results in anxiety for boys who nonetheless may be reluctant to voice their concerns. Routine examination of the male breast during puberty offers the opportunity to reassure boys about this common, benign, and self-resolving condition. Only 4% of adolescents will have gynecomastia that persists into adulthood.

Evaluation of the patient with gynecomastia begins with a confidential history to determine use of prescription or other drugs that alter estrogen or androgen activity, some of which are listed in Table 90.1. The history of breast enlargement should include the patient's age and Tanner stage at onset, the progression and duration of breast growth, and the presence of pain. Physical examination should focus on identifying signs of systemic disease, including liver or thyroid disease, assessing Tanner stage of the patient's breasts, genitals, and pubic hair, and ruling out testicular mass or atrophy. Examination of the breast should distinguish gynecomastia from pseudogynecomastia. With the patient supine, place the thumb and forefinger at opposing margins of the breast and gently bring them together toward the nipple. Gynecomastia will be palpable as a disk of rubbery, freely mobile, occasionally tender, breast tissue directly under the areola. With adipose tissue, no discrete mass of breast tissue is present. Masses not consisting of breast tissue are usually not centered directly beneath the areola.

The differential diagnosis of gynecomastia includes pubertal gynecomastia, systemic disease (including malnutrition, liver disease, renal failure, and malignancy), endocrine disease (including primary hypogonadism such as Klinefelter syndrome [47 XXY], secondary hypogonadism, hyperthyroidism, and hormone-secreting tumors), breast masses that do not contain breast tissue (including lipomas, dermoid cysts and lipomas), and pseudogynecomastia related either to prominent musculature or adipose tissue. Breast cancer in male patients of any age is exceptionally rare, accounting for less than 1% of all breast cancers diagnosed in Western countries.

In healthy male adolescents between Tanner stages 2 and 4, pubertal gynecomastia is the most common diagnosis. Unless the history or physical examination suggests systemic disease, hypogonadism, or the use of drugs associated with gynecomastia, further evaluation is not required. Patients with pubertal gynecomastia should be reassured and carefully reexamined at routine physicals. Breast tissue usually regresses in less than 2 years. Medication or drug use implicated in gynecomastia

should be discontinued, and the patient should be reexamined in 2 to 3 months for improvement in symptoms. A more thorough laboratory evaluation is warranted if the onset of gynecomastia occurs before puberty begins or after puberty is completed, if gynecomastia persists for more than 2 years, or if features of the history or physical examination suggest hypogonadism or renal, liver, thyroid, or other systemic disease. In these cases, referral to an endocrinologist or adolescent medicine specialist may be appropriate.

Breast Masses

Breast masses are a common complaint among young women that often provoke great anxiety and fear of malignancy. Fortunately, breast cancer is exceptionally rare among women younger than 20 years old. Adolescents with previous radiation to the chest or with malignant tumors that may metastasize to the breast are at increased risk of malignancy. Clinical findings suggestive of breast cancer include a hard, fixed, irregular mass with overlying skin changes and nipple retraction. In the absence of such findings, adolescents undergoing evaluation of a breast mass can be reassured that cancer is unlikely, because fewer than 1% of all breast tumors in adolescents are cancerous. Most complaints of breast lumps in adolescents are diagnosed as physiologic breast tissue or benign fibrocystic changes.

Fibrocystic, or proliferative, breast changes are found in more than 50% of reproductive-age women, and they manifest as nodularity and diffuse cordlike thickening. In adolescents and young women, this condition typically presents as painless breast masses. Any complaints of associated pain can be treated in the same manner as other mastalgia (see later). As women with fibrocystic changes age, complaints of premenstrual breast tenderness become more common, as does the presence of multiple small cysts. The presence of a single large (greater than 1 cm) cyst is more common in women who are more than 35 years of age, but it can occur in adolescents.

Fibroadenomas are the most common surgically excised breast lesion in adolescents, representing 70% to 90% of benign breast lesions. Common fibroadenomas present as firm, rubbery, mobile, circumscribed lesions that are typically nontender. They are most commonly found in the upper outer quadrant of the breast and have an average size of 2 to 3 cm. Giant (or juvenile) fibroadenomas, those more than 5 cm in size, often grow much more rapidly. Other tumors that are usually benign but should be removed because of malignant potential are cystosarcoma phyllodes, a rare primary tumor with firm, mobile lesions that can grow quickly to more than 13 cm, and intraductal papillomas, abnormal proliferations of cells in mammary ducts that may be associated with bloody nipple discharge.

The history from a patient with a breast mass should include the date of onset of the mass, as well as its location, size, associated symptoms of nipple discharge or pain, and any changes that occur, including those with menses. Patients should be asked about a history of prior breast disease or other malignancy. The clinician should perform a thorough physical examination, including evaluation for hepatosplenomegaly and lymphadenopathy. Complete examination of the breast should be conducted with the patient in the sitting and supine positions.

If a discrete mass is confirmed, the examiner should note the location, consistency, size, mobility, tenderness, warmth, overlying skin changes, presence of nipple discharge, and axillary adenopathy. In the absence of signs suggestive of infection or malignancy, the patient can be observed through at least one complete menstrual cycle. If the mass disappears, it was probably a cyst or fibrocystic breast change. Although many benign breast masses persist for more than 8 weeks, these persistent masses should be evaluated with a combination of physical examination, ultrasound (to assess the dimensions and to distinguish cystic from solid masses), and referral to a gynecologist or breast specialist for fine needle aspiration or core biopsy. Mammography is not useful because of the density of adolescent breasts and because of the low risk for malignancy.

Breast Pain

Mastalgia (breast pain) can be noncyclic, but is more commonly cyclic, with premenstrual worsening. The prevalence in adolescents is unknown, but mastalgia occurs in up to two-thirds of all women. It usually presents as bilateral heaviness or soreness that resolves during menses. The history should document the duration and location of the pain, its relation to menses, and the possibility of pregnancy. The breast examination should exclude the presence of a breast mass. With a normal physical examination and a negative pregnancy test, patients can be reassured that mastalgia is common and usually self-limited. Potential treatments include heat, a well-fitting supportive bra, and over-the-counter analgesics. There are conflicting data about the effectiveness of evening primrose oil and the use of a caffeine-restricted diet; vitamin supplements and diuretics have not been proven beneficial. Experience with pharmacologic treatment of adolescents with medications used in adults such as danazol or bromocriptine is scant.

Infection

Breast infections are seen primarily in newborns and breast-feeding women. Mastitis, infection in lactiferous ducts, and breast cellulitis or abscess may present with pain, induration, and fever. Nonlactating adolescents can develop breast infections related to shaving, piercing, or other trauma. Treatment includes warm compresses and antibiotics directed toward potential responsible organisms which include *Staphylococcus aureus*, *Escherichia coli*, and *Pseudomonas* species. Many appropriate antibiotic treatments such as cephalexin, dicloxacillin, or clindamycin are compatible with breast-feeding, and nursing or breast pumping should be continued. However, if an abscess is present, surgical drainage may be required; breast milk from the affected side should be pumped and discarded.

Nipple Discharge

Nipple discharge in an adolescent is most commonly galactorrhea (inappropriate lactation). Less commonly, nipple discharge can result from a variety of conditions that are nearly always benign in the adolescent patient. The medical history from a patient complaining of nipple discharge should be obtained confidentially. In addition to asking about the character and color of the discharge, the clinician should ascertain prescription and recreational drug use, menstrual history, possibility of recent or current pregnancy, history of nipple stimulation (e.g., during sexual activity), neurologic symptoms including headache and defects in peripheral vision, and constitutional symptoms suggestive of hypothyroidism, renal failure, or other systemic disease. Physical examination should include vital signs, palpation of the thyroid gland, and neurologic assessment including visual fields. On breast examination, nipple discharge can be elicited by either the examiner or the patient by massaging the breast from the outside in toward the nipple.

The examiner should note the color and character of nipple discharge, whether it is unilateral or bilateral, and whether it arises from a single duct or from multiple ducts. Galactorrhea usually arises from multiple ducts of both breasts. Purulent discharge indicates infection. Yellow, brown, or green sticky dis-

TABLE 90.2

DRUGS ASSOCIATED WITH GALACTORRHEA

Drugs of abuse (opiates, cocaine, marijuana, amphetamines)
Anxiolytics (alprazolam, buspirone)
Antidepressants (selective serotonin reuptake inhibitors, tricyclic antidepressants)
Antipsychotics (risperidone, olanzapine)
Antihypertensives (atenolol, verapamil)
Hormonal contraceptives (combined oral contraceptive pills, depot medroxyprogesterone acetate)
Gastrointestinal medications (metoclopramide, cisapride, histamine [H$_2$] blockers)
Herbs used in cooking and as supplements (fenugreek seed, red clover)

Adapted from Pena KS, Rosenfeld JA. Evaluation and treatment of galactorrhea. *Am Fam Physician* 2001;63:1763.

charge may indicate duct ectasia (dilated ducts with stagnant secretions). This may be confused with apocrine chromhidrosis, the secretion of colored sweat by the apocrine glands of the areola. Serous or serosanguineous discharge can be seen with intraductal papilloma, fibrocystic changes, duct ectasia, or cancer. Occasionally, Montgomery tubercles, modified sebaceous glands that look like soft papules around the areola, may secrete a thin, clear to brown discharge. The utility of nipple discharge cytology is limited, and consultation with a gynecologist should be considered for the evaluation of nonmilky discharge.

Galactorrhea can be caused by stimulation of the chest or nipple (including friction from jogging), medication use, pregnancy, chronic renal failure, or endocrine disorders such as pituitary tumors or thyroid disease. Postpartum milk production can occur for months after delivery (even in the absence of nursing) or after pregnancy termination. Galactorrhea associated with amenorrhea or oligomenorrhea usually indicates hyperprolactinemia. Numerous medications, common examples of which are listed in Table 90.2, stimulate prolactin primarily through dopamine blockade or catecholamine depletion.

Initial laboratory evaluation should include a sensitive urine pregnancy test and serum levels of thyroid-stimulating hormone, blood urea nitrogen, creatinine, and prolactin. A prolactin level greater than 100 ng/mL suggests a prolactin-secreting tumor. For the most accurate result, the prolactin level should be obtained between 8 and 10 o'clock in the morning with the patient fasting and several hours after any breast manipulation, including breast examination. Pregnancy and hypothyroidism should be addressed. If it is feasible to discontinue a medication suspected of causing hyperprolactinemia, a repeat prolactin level drawn 2 weeks later should be normal. Patients presenting with galactorrhea associated with unexplained hyperprolactinemia, amenorrhea or oligomenorrhea, or symptoms suggestive of an intracranial mass should be evaluated with neuroimaging to detect a pituitary microadenoma (smaller than 10 mm) or macroadenoma (larger than 10 mm). Magnetic resonance imaging is more sensitive than computed tomography for visualizing the hypothalamus and pituitary.

Patients with galactorrhea who have normal prolactin levels, normal neuroimaging, and regular menses do not require treatment unless they find symptoms bothersome, in which case a dopamine agonist such as bromocriptine or cabergoline can be used. However, patients with hyperprolactinemia are still at risk for amenorrhea, low estrogen levels, and low bone density, even in the absence of a macroadenoma or identifiable microadenoma. Referral to an endocrinologist to evaluate the need for medical treatment may be advisable for these patients.

Suggested Readings

Barton MB, Harris R, Fletcher SW. Does this patient have breast cancer? The screening clinical breast examination. *JAMA* 1999;282:1270.

Braunstein GD, Glassman HA. Gynecomastia. *Curr Ther Endocrinol Metab* 1997;6:401.

Falkenberry SS. Nipple discharge. *Obstet Gynecol Clin North Am* 2002;29:225.

Goldstein DP, Emans SJ, Laufer MR. The breast. In: Emans SJ, Laufer MR, Goldstein DP, eds. *Pediatric and adolescent gynecology,* 4th ed. Philadelphia: Lippincott-Raven, 1998:587.

Neinstein LS. Breast disease in adolescents and young women. *Pediatr Clin North Am* 1999;46:607.

Neinstein LS, Joffe A. Gynecomastia. In: Neinstein LS, ed. *Adolescent health care,* 4th ed. Philadelphia: Lippincott Williams & Wilkins, 2002:264.

Osuch, JR. Breast health and disease over a lifetime. *Clin Obstet Gynecol* 2002;45:1140.

Pena KS, Rosenfeld JA. Evaluation and treatment of galactorrhea. *Am Fam Physician* 2001;63:1763.

Smith RA, Saslow D, Sawyer KA, et al. American cancer society guidelines for breast cancer screening: update 2003. *CA Cancer J Clin* 2003;54:141.

Templeman C, Hertweck SP. Breast disorders in the pediatric and adolescent patient. *Obstet Gynecol Clin North Am* 2000;27:19.

CHAPTER 91 ■ MENSTRUAL DISORDERS

SERGIO R. RUSSO BUZZINI AND MELANIE A. GOLD

Menarche, or the onset of menses, is one of the major milestones of female pubertal development. Although most adolescent girls pass through this transition with relative ease, approximately 50% experience some problem associated with menstruation. This chapter discusses normal menstrual function during adolescence as well as complaints that commonly present to the primary care physician such as amenorrhea, dysfunctional uterine bleeding (DUB), and dysmenorrhea.

NORMAL MENSTRUAL CYCLE

The mean age of menarche in the United States is 12.7 years (12.8 years for caucasian girls and 12.6 for African American girls). In about two-thirds of girls, menarche occurs at sexual maturity rating (SMR) 4 (also called Tanner pubertal stage 4). Menarche begins at about 17% body fat, with 22% body fat required to maintain or restore menstruation. Irregular periods during adolescence are usually related to the lack of regular ovulation. Ovulation is associated with 50% of menstrual periods 1 year after menarche and 80% at 2 years. The later the age of menarche, the longer the interval before cycles become ovulatory. Among adolescents and adults, normal menstrual function is defined broadly as a 21 to 45 day cycle, 2 to 8 days of menstrual blood flow, and 20 to 80 mL of blood loss per menstrual cycle. The wide range of variation of normal menstruation, coupled with the high prevalence of anovulation during the early postmenarchal years, results in much confusion and concern among adolescents and parents. Education about these issues by health care professionals can ease anxiety and circumvent unnecessary evaluations.

AMENORRHEA

Amenorrhea traditionally has been divided into two categories: primary and secondary. Primary amenorrhea is often defined as an absence of menstruation by age 16 years in the presence of normal development of breasts and pubic hair or as lack of menses by age 14 years in the absence of normal development of breasts and pubic hair. The mean time between the onset of breast development and menarche is about 2 years. A lack of menses within 2 to 2.5 years of initiating puberty, especially in a girl who has reached SMR 4 or 5, should raise concern. Secondary amenorrhea is the absence of menstrual periods for a length of time equivalent to at least three of the previous cycle intervals or 6 months of amenorrhea. The definition of secondary amenorrhea should be applied only to those who have already established regular cyclic menstrual periods. It should not be used in cases of amenorrhea presenting in the postmenarchal period when regular ovulatory cycles have not begun. In patients who have taken combined oral contraceptive pills (COCs), 6 months of amenorrhea may pass before initiating evaluation. Patients who have previously received depot medroxyprogesterone acetate injections should be given 12 months for spontaneous return of menses.

Etiology

The same clinical entities can be the cause of either primary or secondary amenorrhea, depending on the relationship between the onset of the particular disease or condition and the timing of pubertal development. Pregnancy should always be considered in the differential diagnosis of primary and secondary amenorrhea. Both hypothyroidism and hyperthyroidism may cause amenorrhea. Amenorrhea may be caused by disorders of hypothalamus, pituitary, ovaries, and outflow tract or by androgen excess. In general, disorders at the level of the hypothalamus or the pituitary gland present with low or normal levels of gonadotropins (follicle-stimulating hormone [FSH] and luteinizing hormone [LH]) (hypogonadotropic hypogonadism), whereas high levels of gonadotropins suggest ovarian failure (hypergonadotropic hypogonadism).

Abnormalities at the level of the hypothalamus include hypothalamic suppression and deficiency in the pulsatile release of gonadotropin-releasing hormone. The most common diagnoses in this category are constitutional delay of puberty, stress, intense exercise, chronic or systemic illnesses (e.g., inflammatory bowel disease, cystic fibrosis, chronic renal failure), drug use (e.g., opiate, phenothiazine, marijuana), obesity, and eating disorders. Less common causes of hypothalamic amenorrhea include space-occupying lesions (e.g., craniopharyngioma, meningioma, glioma) and syndromes associated with hypothalamic dysfunction and pubertal delay such as

Kallmann syndrome (a familial disorder also associated with anosmia), Prader-Willi syndrome, and Laurence-Moon-Biedl syndrome.

Abnormalities at the level of the pituitary include idiopathic hypopituitarism, hyperprolactinemia, infiltrative processes, and infarction. Hyperprolactinemia may be caused by tumors, psychoactive drugs (e.g., haloperidol, phenothiazines, opiates, cocaine), breast stimulation, and renal failure. The most common pituitary tumor is the prolactin-secreting adenoma (prolactinoma). Prolactinomas classically present with galactorrhea, headache, and visual field loss. Although patients who have pituitary adenomas have elevated prolactin levels (usually greater than 100 ng/mL), galactorrhea is not a universal sign, and its absence does not preclude the presence of the tumor. Infiltrative processes may be caused by tuberculosis, sarcoidosis, histiocytosis, syphilis, or hemocromatosis. Infarction of the pituitary may be caused by postpartum hemorrhage (Sheehan syndrome), head trauma, or carotid artery aneurysm.

Abnormalities at the level of the ovaries can be divided into congenital and acquired causes. Among the congenital causes, Turner syndrome (45,XO), occurring in approximately 1 in 2,000 liveborn female infants, is the most common cause of ovarian failure. The classic features associated with this syndrome are short stature, webbed neck, widely spaced nipples, and cubitus valgus. Approximately one-half of patients with gonadal dysgenesis exhibit a mosaic karyotype (e.g., 45,XO/46,XX) or a structural abnormality of the X chromosome. Female adolescents with Turner mosaic or chromosomal incompetence may present with primary amenorrhea, secondary amenorrhea, or regular menstrual cycles. This spectrum is the result of varying amounts of functioning ovarian tissue. They may have none, some, or all of the stigmata of Turner syndrome, depending on what part of the X chromosome is affected. Other less common causes of congenital ovarian failure are pure gonadal dysgenesis, gonadotropin-resistant ovary syndrome, inborn deficiency of 17 alpha-hydroxylase, and galactosemia. Acquired causes of ovarian failure include premature ovarian failure (e.g., autoimmune oophoritis, radiation and/or chemotherapy), trauma, and other disorders (e.g., tuberculosis, sarcoidosis, gonoccocal salpingitis, mumps oophoritis).

Abnormalities at the level of the outflow tract include müllerian agenesis, androgen insensitivity, vaginal septum, imperforate hymen, spontaneous testicular regression, and specific gonadal enzyme deficiencies. Uterine synechiae should be considered in the postpartum or postabortal woman especially if she required vigorous curettage (Asherman syndrome). Other less common causes of uterine synechiae include complications from intrauterine device use and infections (e.g., pelvic inflammatory disease, tuberculosis, schistosomiasis). Müllerian agenesis or Mayer-Rokitansky-Küster-Hauser syndrome is the most common cause of primary amenorrhea resulting from genital tract anomaly. Accounting for as many as 15% of cases of primary amenorrhea, these patients are genetic and phenotypic females presenting with absence of a uterus and an incomplete vaginal pouch. The ovaries, breast, and pubic hair are normal.

The most common diagnosis of androgen excess is functional ovarian hyperandrogenism or polycystic ovary syndrome (PCOS). Associated physical findings such as acne, hirsutism, and obesity may be present, although they tend to be less prominent in adolescents than in adult women. Serum insulin levels may be elevated, and acanthosis nigricans, a cutaneous marker of hyperinsulinemia, may be present. Although polycystic ovaries are often found in adult patients, the appearance of normal ovaries on ultrasonography does not rule out this diagnosis, especially in younger women. Other less common causes of hyperandrogenism include late-onset 21-hydroxylase deficiency, sometimes referred to as nonclassic congenital adrenal hyperplasia, androgen-producing ovarian or adrenal tumors, ovarian stromal hypertrophy (hyperthecho-

---

| **BOX 91.1** | **Causes of Primary and Secondary Amenorrhea** |

Pregnancy
Hypothyroidism and hyperthyroidism
Disorders of the hypothalamus
   Hypothalamic suppression caused by constitutional delay of puberty; stress; intense exercise; chronic or systemic illnesses (e.g., inflammatory bowel disease, cystic fibrosis, chronic renal failure)
   Drug use (e.g., opiate, phenothiazine, marijuana)
   Obesity
   Eating disorders
   Space-occupying lesions (e.g., craniopharyngioma, meningioma, glioma)
   Syndromes associated with hypothalamic dysfunction and pubertal delay (e.g., Kallmann, Prader-Willi, and Laurence-Moon-Biedl syndromes)
Disorders of pituitary
   Idiopathic hypopituitarism
   Hyperprolactinemia (caused by tumors, psychoactive drugs [e.g., haloperidol, phenothiazines, opiates, cocaine], breast stimulation, renal failure, infiltrative processes, or infarction)
Disorders of the ovary
   Congenital causes: Turner syndrome, Turner mosaic or chromosomal incompetence, pure gonadal dysgenesis, gonadotropin resistant ovary syndrome, inborn deficiency of 17alpha-hydroxylase, and galactosemia
   Acquired causes: premature ovarian failure (e.g., autoimmune oophoritis, radiation and/or chemotherapy), trauma, and other disorders (e.g., tuberculosis, sarcoidosis, gonococcal salpingitis, mumps oophoritis)
Disorders of outflow tract
   Müllerian agenesis
   Androgen insensitivity
   Vaginal septum
   Imperforate hymen
   Spontaneous testicular regression and specific gonadal enzyme deficiencies
   Uterine synechiae
Androgen excess
   Functional ovarian hyperandrogenism or polycystic ovary syndrome
   Late-onset 21-hydroxylase deficiency
   Androgen-producing ovarian or adrenal tumors
   Ovarian stromal hypertrophy (hyperthecosis)
   Cushing syndrome
   Use of extraneous androgens

---

sis), and Cushing syndrome, as well as extrinsic sources of androgens, such as anabolic steroid use. Usually, in these cases, virilization is more severe than in PCOS and may include clitoromegaly and deepening of the voice. Box 91.1 summarizes the differential diagnosis of primary and secondary amenorrhea.

History

The patient's history should cover general health including an overview of childhood growth and development, timing and progression of thelarche, adrenarche, menarche, and growth velocity, signs and symptoms of chronic or systemic illnesses, eating habits including any change in weight, emotional stress including physical and sexual abuse, intensity and duration of exercise, sexual activity, hormonal contraceptive and barrier method use, and use of any other drugs or medications. In constitutional delay of puberty, a history in parents or older siblings of delayed menarche, height spurt, or sexual development often exists. Past medical history, including exposure to chemotherapy or pelvic or central nervous system radiation therapy, should be investigated. Review of systems can identify a history of vasomotor symptoms, hot flashes, rapid onset of virilizing symptoms, or thyroid dysfunction. Symptoms of significant headaches and visual disturbance may suggest intracranial tumor.

Physical Examination

General appearance, height and weight including percentiles and body mass index, and vital signs including temperature, pulse, and blood pressure should be documented. Vital signs may be depressed in anorexia nervosa and other starvation states. Skin should be examined for signs of hirsutism, acne, and acanthosis nigricans. Some causes of hyperandrogenicity (e.g., Cushing syndrome, anabolic steroid use) may produce hypertension. SMR should be determined separately for breast and pubic hair development. The breasts should be palpated with attempts to express galactorrhea. Fundoscopy, visual field testing, and cranial nerve assessment serve as initial screens for pituitary tumor and Kallmann syndrome. Teeth and gums should be examined for signs of dental erosion and gingival erythema, whereas parotid glands should be palpated for enlargement from bulimia. The thyroid gland should be palpated for size and nodularity. The abdomen should be examined to identify a pelvic mass, which may indicate pregnancy or imperforate hymen with hematocolpos. On pelvic examination, genital mucosa should be observed for estrogenic effect. Clitoromegaly indicates virilization. In virginal adolescents, a single digit or moistened cotton-tipped swab should be inserted gently into the vagina of patients with primary amenorrhea to ensure patency. Distention or bulging of the external vagina suggests imperforate hymen. A bimanual examination can usually detect the presence of uterus and ovaries. If there is evidence of an obstructed or absent vagina, or if patient anxiety precludes intravaginal examination, a rectoabdominal examination can be done to check for a mass and identify the uterus if present.

Laboratory Evaluation

Laboratory evaluation of primary or secondary amenorrhea begins with a urine pregnancy test, regardless of sexual history. Patients in whom systemic illness is suspected require thorough and prompt evaluation. In addition to complete blood count and sedimentation rate, laboratory evaluation at this point is guided by findings on history and physical examination. If short stature accompanies primary amenorrhea, obtaining a bone age should be considered.

For the adolescent with primary amenorrhea and an unremarkable history, review of systems, general physical examination, and no evidence of vaginal outlet obstruction, the next step is to determine, either by pelvic examination and/or pelvic ultrasound, whether a uterus is present. If not, karyotyping and serum testosterone levels should be determined to screen for müllerian agenesis, androgen insensitivity, gonadal enzyme deficiency, or testicular regression. If the uterus is present with or without complete pubertal development, serum FSH and LH levels will help to distinguish between ovarian failure and problems at the pituitary or hypothalamic levels. It is also recommended to obtain a karyotype on women with premature ovarian failure who are less than 63 inches tall (160 cm) because of the close conjuction of the genes responsible for stature and ovarian function.

The laboratory evaluation of adolescents with secondary amenorrhea and no physical signs of hirsutism or virilization begins with a measurement of thyroid-stimulating hormone, free thyroxine, and prolactin to rule out the possibility of either primary or central hypothyroidism, hyperthyroidysm, and hyperprolactinemia. If the foregoing measurements fail to explain the amenorrhea, a progesterone challenge test should be considered to assess endogenous estrogen production, endometrial responsivity, and outflow tract competency. Within 2 to 7 days after the conclusion of progestational medication, the patient will either have withdrawal bleeding or not. If any amount of bleeding occurs, a diagnosis of anovulation has been reliably and securely established. If no bleeding occurs after progesterone, either the uterus or outflow tract is abnormal or endogenous estrogen production is inadequate or absent. A trial of oral estrogen for 11 days followed by an additional 10 days of both oral estrogen and progestin given together should produce withdrawal bleeding in patients with normal, unobstructed uterus, cervix, and vagina within 2 to 7 days after stopping the medication. A negative response with an otherwise normal evaluation suggests intrauterine scarring or outflow tract obstruction. Once a hypoestrogenic state has been established, laboratory evaluation of amenorrhea continues with measurements of serum FSH and LH levels. Further assessment of hypogonadotropic hypogonadism or hypergonadotropic hypogonaism (ovarian failure) should be conducted according to the clinical suspicion.

Adolescents with secondary amenorrhea and hirsutism or virilization should have measurement of serum testosterone (free and total), dihydroepiandrosterone sulfate (DHEAS), androstenedione, 17-hydroxyprogesterone, FSH, and LH levels. PCOS typically causes normal to moderately elevated levels of DHEAS, androstenedione, or testosterone, and the LH:FSH ratio is often greater than 2.5, which reflects chronic hypothalamic dysfunction but is present in only 50% of patients with PCOS. Total testosterone greater than 200 ng/dL is associated with an androgen-producing tumor, usually of the ovary. DHEA greater than 700 μg/dL is associated with adrenal malignancy, and levels of 500 to 700 μg/dL should prompt evaluation for late-onset congenital hyperplasia. The most common form of this condition is 21-hydroxylase deficiency, which usually produces a high basal level of 17-hydroxyprogesterone. Further workup can include adrenal suppression testing, adrenocorticotropic hormone stimulation test, magnetic resonance imaging, or computed tomography of the abdomen and pelvis.

Management

When a systemic process or endocrinopathy is found to be the cause of amenorrhea, adequate treatment of the underlying disease should result in resumption of ovulatory function. Pituitary adenomas and hyperprolactinemia usually regress in response to bromocriptine or similar agents. Adolescents without müllerian structures and with hypergonadotropic amenorrhea resulting from ovarian absence or failure require estrogen replacement to stimulate pubertal development and to prevent osteoporosis and atherosclerotic heart disease. Adolescents who have endometrial tissue should also get replacement with progestin as well as estrogen, to prevent endometrial hyperplasia. Adolescents with chronic anovulation and subsequent lack of progesterone secretion have an increased risk of endometrial hyperplasia and eventually endometrial cancer. These risks can be eliminated with regular exposure to a progestational agent such as oral medroxyprogesterone, norethindrone, COCs, or depot medroxyprogesterone injections (Depo-Provera). Patients who are hypoestrogenic and anovulatory because of hypothalamic suppression should be given hormonal replacement therapy (e.g., COCs) and should meet daily requirements of calcium and vitamin D to reduce the long-term risks of osteoporosis. The presence of a Y chromosome, as in androgen insensitivity, requires surgical gonadectomy, owing to high neoplastic potential. Adolescents with an imperforate hymen or transverse vaginal septum can undergo surgically repair at the time of diagnosis.

DYSFUNCTIONAL UTERINE BLEEDING

Dysfunctional uterine bleeding (DUB) is a common menstrual problem during adolescence. It is defined as painless abnormal endometrial bleeding in the absence of structural pathologic features or medical illness.

Etiology

Adolescents with DUB have impairments in their normal negative feedback systems caused by an immature hypothalamic-pituitary-ovarian axis. Therefore, rising levels of estrogen do not cause a fall in FSH with simultaneous LH surge and ovulation and subsequent suppression of estrogen secretion. Without this negative feedback, the endometrium becomes excessively thickened. When the endometrium reaches an unstable thickness, uncoordinated sloughing occurs, with the potential for heavy, prolonged bleeding and anemia.

DUB is a diagnosis of exclusion, and other potential causes of bleeding must be investigated (Box 91.2). The differential diagnosis of DUB falls into four general categories: hormonal, pregnancy-related, local pathologic, and related to bleeding diatheses. Hormonal causes are the most common and include PCOS, thyroid dysfunction, hyperprolactinemia, adrenal gland abnormalities and use of hormonal contraception. Bleeding related to pregnancy includes threatened, spontaneous, and elective abortion; molar or ectopic pregnancy; and postabortion endometritis. Other conditions related to an intrauterine pregnancy, such as placenta previa and abruption, may also be associated with vaginal bleeding. Local pathologic features include sexually transmitted disease (e.g., gonorrhea and infection with *Chlamydia* or *Trichomonas*), retained foreign body in the vagina (e.g., retained tampon) or uterus (e.g., intrauterine device), laceration, polyp, uterine arteriovenous malformation, dysplasia, and malignancy. Bleeding diatheses include idiopathic thrombocytopenic purpura, von Willebrand disease, abnormal platelet function resulting from drugs (e.g., aspirin) or systemic illness (e.g., renal failure), bone marrow suppression (e.g., chemotherapy) or infiltration (e.g., leukemia), coagulopathy resulting from inherited clotting factor deficiency, systemic illness (e.g., liver failure), or anticoagulant therapy (e.g., warfarin).

History

The history should include the age of menarche, the menstrual pattern, the severity of blood loss, and the presence of menstrual pain. A complete sexual history should be obtained from the adolescent alone, without the parent or caregiver present and with assurance of confidentiality. The history should include discussion of consensual or forced sexual intercourse,

---

| BOX 91.2 | Differential Diagnoses of Dysfunctional Uterine Bleeding |

Hormonal causes
  Polycystic ovary syndrome
  Thyroid dysfunction
  Hyperprolactinemia
  Adrenal gland abnormalities
  Use of hormonal contraception
Pregnancy-related bleeding
  Threatened, spontaneous, and elective abortion
  Molar or ectopic pregnancy
  Postabortion endometritis
  Placenta previa or abruption
Local pathologic features
  Sexually transmitted disease (e.g., gonorrhea and infection with *Chlamydia* or *Trichomonas*), retained foreign body in the vagina (e.g., retained tampon) or uterus (e.g., intrauterine device)
  Laceration
  Polyp
  Uterine arteriovenous malformation
  Uterine dysplasia or malignancy
Bleeding diatheses
  Idiopathic thrombocytopenic purpura
  von Willebrand disease
  Abnormal platelet function resulting from drugs (e.g., aspirin) or systemic illness (e.g., renal failure)
  Bone marrow suppression (e.g., chemotherapy) or infiltration (e.g., leukemia)
  Coagulopathy resulting from inherited clotting factor deficiency, systemic illness (e.g., liver failure), or anticoagulant therapy (e.g., warfarin)

---

previous pregnancy or abortion, contraception, condom use, number of partners, new partners, past sexually transmitted disease, vaginal discharge, and pelvic pain. A patient's past medical history should be reviewed, as well as any current or recent medications. Asking about easy bruising, epistaxis, gum bleeding, hematuria, rectal bleeding, postoperative bleeding, and family history of clotting or bleeding disorders, especially any history of hysterectomy for heavy or prolonged uterine bleeding, can help to identify patients with bleeding diatheses. All patients with abnormal bleeding should be asked about systemic symptoms suggestive of acute or chronic anemia, including lightheadedness, syncope, fatigue, weakness, and headache.

Physical Examination

In addition to a general physical examination, blood pressure and heart rate in supine, sitting, and standing positions should be performed. Skin, conjunctivae, and mucosa should be examined for pallor, petechiae, and ecchymoses. Evidence of androgen excess (hirsutism, acne, clitoromegaly), acanthosis nigricans, thyroid abnormalities, galactorrhea, hepatosplenomegaly, lymphadenopathy, and any other sign suggesting systemic illness should be noted. Pelvic examination is essential for any adolescent with a history of sexual intercourse. In virginal adolescents, if the hymenal opening is sufficiently wide to admit one finger, then a digital examination can be performed to rule out a foreign body and to palpate the cervix.

If the digital examination is uncomfortable, a rectoabdominal examination may be helpful.

Laboratory Evaluation

Laboratory tests must include a pregnancy test. All sexually active adolescents should have testing for gonorrhea and *Chlamydia* and a wet preparation to rule out *Trichomonas*. Other tests should include a complete blood count with platelet count and thyroid-stimulating hormone level. Coagulation studies (e.g., prothrombin time, partial thromboplastin time, bleeding time, and other more specific studies for von Willebrand disease) are indicated in patients who have a family history of bleeding disorders, have significant blood loss at menarche, or have heavy cyclic menses. Other potential studies for patients with a long history of DUB include determination of FSH (and LH), prolactin, and serum androgens (total and free testosterone, androstenendione, 17-hydroxyprogesterone, and DHEA-S). Other potential diagnostic testing should be individualized according to the history and physical examination, but consideration should be given to assess liver and kidney function. Ultrasonography can be helpful when a pelvic mass is felt or a structural disorder is suspected.

Management

The management of DUB is guided by both the hemoglobin level and the presence of active bleeding. If a patient's hemoglobin level is greater than 12 g/dL and she is not actively bleeding, reassurance and prophylactic iron treatment are suitable. These adolescents should be instructed to keep a menstrual calendar and be reevaluated in 3 months. If a patient's hemoglobin level is between 10 and 12 g/dL with moderate to heavy blood flow, oral estrogen-progestin therapy can be given in the form of COCs in addition to iron supplementation. Any of the low-dose 30- to 35-μg estrogen COC monophasic tablets are useful. One pill every 6 to 12 hours should be taken until the bleeding stops; this usually occurs within 24 to 48 hours. Once the bleeding stops, the dose should be tapered over a week to one pill daily. Placebo pills should be skipped, and COCs should be taken continuously until the patient's hemoglobin is greater than 12 g/dL. Once the hemoglobin is normal, the COCs may be cycled.

If a patient's hemoglobin level is less than 10 g/dL with heavy bleeding, if initial hemoglobin is less than 7 g/dL, or if orthostatic signs are present, the patient should be admitted to the hospital. Transfusion should be considered if there are clinical signs of acute blood loss or the hemoglobin level is extremely low. Conjugated estrogens may be administered initially (25 mg intravenously every 4 hours) until the bleeding slows (usually after two to four doses). At the same time, one COC pill should be taken every 6 hours until the bleeding stops, and then the dose should be tapered to one tablet, three times a day for 3 days, and twice a day for 2 weeks and then down to one tablet a day, skipping the placebo pills until the hemoglobin is greater than 12 g/dL. A progestin (that is in COC) must be added as soon as possible to the intravenous conjugated estrogen regimen to stabilize the endometrium and to prevent heavy estrogen withdrawal bleeding. Nausea is a common side effect of intravenous conjugated estrogen and high-dose COCs; thus, an antiemetic should be given as needed. If there is a medical contraindication to using estrogen, a trial of oral progestin such as norethindrone acetate or medroxyprogesterone may stop the bleeding. Iron supplementation should also be provided. In the rare cases when hemostasis cannot be achieved medically, dilation and curettage are indicated both therapeutically and diagnostically. Bleeding related to pregnancy, infection, and structural disorders requires condition-specific management. Although many of the other differential diagnoses of DUB require specific long-term interventions, their short-term management is similar to that described earlier.

DYSMENORRHEA

Dysmenorrhea is pain with menstruation, usually cramping in nature and centered in the lower abdomen. Dysmenorrhea is the most common menstrual problem in adolescents. It occurs in approximately 60% of 12- to 17-year-old postmenarchal girls and accounts for a large percentage of school absenteeism.

Etiology

Dysmenorrhea is classified as either primary or secondary. Primary dysmenorrhea, a condition associated with ovulatory cycles, is more prevalent in adolescents and is not associated with organic pelvic disease. It results from myometrial contractions induced by the increased production of prostaglandins, especially prostaglandin $F_{2\alpha}$, originating in secretory endometrium. Other symptoms associated with menstrual flow, such as headache, nausea and vomiting, bloating, backache, and diarrhea, can be explained by entry of the prostaglandins and prostaglandins metabolites into the systemic circulation. The symptoms tend to be most severe during the first few days of the menstrual cycle when prostaglandin levels are highest. Secondary dysmenorrhea, which is much less common than the primary disorder in adolescents, is associated with organic disease. Causes of secondary dysmenorrhea include conditions such as endometriosis, pelvic inflammatory disease, uterine fibroids and polyps, presence of an intrauterine device, pelvic adhesions, and ovarian cyst or mass.

History

When a positive history of dysmenorrhea is obtained, questions to differentiate the primary from the secondary form should be asked. Primary dysmenorrhea usually begins when regular ovulatory cycles are established and occurs during the first 2 to 3 days of the cycle. In addition, there is often a positive family history of menstrual pain. Secondary dysmenorrhea should be suspected if the pain is unusually severe, if it began at menarche, if it is increasing in severity, or if it is isolated and related to only one painful period. It is also important to obtain information about exposure to sexually transmitted diseases, previous pregnancies with outcomes, use of hormonal contraceptives, response to analgesic medication, and systemic symptoms. Health care providers can assess the severity of cramps by inquiring about their impact on daily activities such as school and work attendance and participation in social activities.

Physical Examination

A complete pelvic examination may not be necessary in a virginal patient with a history suggestive of primary dysmenorrhea. If the pain is mild and the patient has a normal physical examination including the hymen, a speculum examination is not necessary. A complete pelvic examination is indicated at the initial evaluation if the patient is sexually active or the pain is severe. The examination will help detect a genital tract obstruction, adnexal and/or uterosacral pain suggestive of endometriosis, evidence of sexually transmitted disease or pelvic inflammatory disease, and an adnexal or uterine mass.

Laboratory Evaluation

Generally, no diagnostic tests are needed for the assessment and treatment of primary dysmenorrhea. A complete blood count and a determination of the erythrocyte sedimentation rate should be done if pelvic inflammatory disease is suspected. All sexually active adolescents should have testing for sexually transmitted diseases and pregnancy. When the diagnosis of a congenital anomaly is entertained, pelvic ultrasound or magnetic resonance imaging studies may be helpful. If pain is severe and unresponsive to medical management, diagnostic laparoscopy to rule out endometriosis may be indicated.

Management

The two most effective treatments for primary dysmenorrhea are nonsteroidal antiinflammatory drugs (NSAIDs) and COCs. NSAIDs are the primary modality of therapy and act by inhibiting the synthesis and/or action of prostaglandins, and the most common subgroups are the propionic acid derivatives (e.g., ibuprofen, naproxen) and the fenamates (e.g., mefenamic acid, meclofenamate). When instructing adolescents how to take NSAIDs to prevent dysmenorrhea, advise them to begin taking the medication the day before the menses (if possible) or at the first sign of menses and then continue taking the medication around the clock for the first 2 or 3 days of menses. COCs can be used if the patient wishes contraception or the pain is severe and poorly responsive to NSAIDs. COCs prevent or decrease dysmenorrhea directly by limiting endometrial growth and indirectly by inhibiting ovulation and progesterone secretion. Patients diagnosed with primary dysmenorrhea who do not improve with adequate therapy should be evaluated for causes related to secondary dysmenorrhea. Although data are limited, other hormonal contraceptives may also improve dysmenorrhea.

Suggested Readings

Emans JH, Laufer MR, Goldstein DP. *Pediatric and adolescent gynecology,* 5th ed. Lippincott Williams & Wilkins, 2004.
Joffe A, Blythe M. Handbook of adolescent medicine. *Adolesc Med State Art Rev* 2003;14:289.
Neinstein LS. *Adolescent health care: a practical guide,* 4th ed. Philadelphia: Lippincott Williams & Wilkins, 2002.
Speroff L, Fritz MA. *Clinical gynecology endocrinology and infertility,* 7th ed. Philadelphia: Lippincott Williams & Wilkins, 2004.

CHAPTER 92 ■ ADOLESCENT PREGNANCY AND CONTRACEPTION

MARIA TRENT

Unplanned pregnancy is a major public health problem facing pediatric and adolescent health. In the 2001 Youth Risk Behavior Survey of high school students, 42.9% of girls and 48.5% of boys reported having ever engaged in sexual intercourse. Currently, more than 800,000 pregnancies occur in the United States each year, of which 80% are unplanned, 51% result in a live birth, 35% in abortion, and 14% in miscarriage. These figures represent a significant reduction in adolescent pregnancies over the last few decades. Some of this reduction can be attributed to the finding that fewer adolescents are having sexual intercourse; however, research by the Alan Guttmacher Institute using the 1995 National Survey of Family Growth data demonstrated that the reduction is primarily the result of increased access to and use of highly effective forms of contraception. Despite the finding of no significant differences in sexual behavior among adolescents across industrialized countries, the United States continues to be a leader in this area. Rates of pregnancy and childbearing in the United States are approximately twice that of Great Britain and Canada and are four times higher than Sweden and France. Levels of sexual activity and age of initiation among teenagers in these countries do not differ significantly from those of teenagers in the United States; however, teens in those countries appear to select more reliable methods of contraception. In addition, young people growing up in socially and economically disadvantaged environments are more likely than their less-disadvantaged peers to engage in risky sexual behavior and to bear children during adolescence. The United States, which has the highest per capita income of these countries, also has the greatest proportion of disadvantaged families. European communities have also been able to provide the clear message that childbearing is an adult behavior reserved for persons who have completed their education and vocational training, whereas sexual expression as seen as a normal part of adolescent development. This view appears to foster an expectation of sexual responsibility that is supported by comprehensive sexuality education promoting responsible sexual behavior.

CONSEQUENCES OF ADOLESCENT PREGNANCY

The potential consequences of teenage parenthood include the medical complications of pregnancy, unintended births, physical discomfort and emotional distress associated with abortion, reduced educational attainment, fewer employment opportunities, increased likelihood of welfare reliance, and poorer health and developmental and social outcomes for their children. Experiencing an unplanned pregnancy indicates that a young woman has been involved in sexual contact that has not been protective for sexually transmitted infections (STIs). Central to the adolescent focused goals within the Healthy People 2010 Objectives are the reduction of unplanned pregnancies and STIs in adolescents. The goals of contraceptive management in adolescents are therefore twofold—the prevention of unintended pregnancy and the prevention of STIs and their sequelae. With consistent use, dual methods such as a hormonal method with condoms can prevent unplanned pregnancy as well as the acquisition and spread of STIs.

DIAGNOSIS OF PREGNANCY

Although pregnant adolescents may present for a variety of complaints, late or missed menstrual period is the most common presentation. Other symptomatic presentations include mild abdominal discomfort, constipation, urinary frequency, dizziness, fatigue, nausea, breast tenderness, headaches, or a combination of symptoms. Although some adolescents may express concern about the possibility of pregnancy, many adolescents have not really considered the possibility of pregnancy and believe that their symptoms are representative of another medical problem. Adolescents may also not provide sufficient detail related to sexual activity, and this can further delay diagnosis. For this reason, it is not unusual for adolescents to be diagnosed with pregnancy at an urgent care visit, family planning appointment, or even well physical examination.

Clinical assessment and evaluation of the pregnancy should be initiated at the time of presentation to delay intervention further. Inexpensive urine pregnancy tests can be used to diagnose pregnancy within 7 days of implantation. These tests vary in sensitivity, ranging from 5 to 50 mIU/mL of human chorionic gonadotropin. This is usually sufficient given that most women have human chorionic gonadotropin levels between 50 and 250 mIU/mL at the time of missed period. In general, there is no advantage to use of radioimmunoassay (serum) tests in diagnosing a pregnancy unless a concern exists about threatened abortion and/or ectopic pregnancy.

Pelvic examination, including testing for STI and uterine sizing and dating, is an important aspect of the clinical evaluation. Pregnancies are dated from the first day of the last menstrual period. Given that some adolescents are unsure of date of the last menstrual period, the bimanual examination allows the provider to assess agreement between dates and uterine size. On bimanual examination, the 8-week uterus is the size of an orange, the 12-week uterus is the size of a grapefruit at the level of the pubic symphysis, the 16-week uterus is midway between the pubic symphysis and umbilicus, and the 20-week uterus is at the level of the umbilicus. Testing for *Chlamydia trachomatis* and *Neisseria gonorrhoeae* and a wet preparation for trichomoniasis and bacterial vaginosis are important for the young woman. Infection can threaten the status of the pregnancy of a young woman who plans to continue to term and can complicate a medical abortion. A complete blood count to assess for anemia, syphilis serology, and human immunodeficiency virus (HIV) counseling and testing should also be considered at the time of diagnosis. Quantitative testing and ultrasonography should be considered in women whose uterine size does not correlate with dates or if there are concerns about threatened abortion or ectopic pregnancy.

The approach to counseling the adolescent girl about pregnancy options should be customized depending on the developmental level of the adolescent and the circumstances that resulted in pregnancy. Although the decisions related to the pregnancy rest with the adolescent, she will often need substantial partner and family support. Regardless of the approach used, all options for pregnancy management available to the adolescent should be presented to the adolescent patient for consideration. It is essential that adolescents who present early in pregnancy receive nonjudgmental, accurate, and detailed information about referral options related to prenatal care, adoption, and termination services. Providers who are unable to counsel the pregnant adolescent about all available options should refer her to a provider who can do so. Delaying decision making is commonly seen with younger adolescents who may not have fully grasped the significance of a pregnancy diagnosis or who have real fears related to the availability of parental support. It is important to ascertain the status of the family situation, including her safety at home or potential involvement of a family member in the pregnancy, before assisting the young woman in engaging her family in dialogue. Close follow-up of the pregnant adolescent until a decision is made is important given that the availability of termination is time dependent. The longer that a young woman is undecided about her plans for the pregnancy, the fewer options will remain for her over time.

Adolescents who plan to continue the pregnancy should be referred for prenatal care, prescribed multivitamins with iron, and receive instructions related to use of over-the-counter mediations, avoidance of alcohol and drugs, and common environmental hazards to avoid. Adolescents who opt for abortion should also be counseled regarding self-care before and after the procedure. It is often useful to prepare the young woman before the procedure so she can anticipate how the experience will proceed. Although she will be offered a postprocedure follow-up appointment by the facility providing the procedure, many young girls prefer to be seen by their usual adolescent or gynecologic provider for the follow-up visit. It is important to have a plan in place for long-term contraception before the procedure because hormonal methods can be initiated at the time of termination. Deferring the discussion on family planning until the 2-week postoperative visit will unnecessarily delay initiating an effective contraceptive method, thus potentially making the young woman vulnerable to repeat pregnancy in the coming month when she re-engages in sexual activity.

CONTRACEPTION

General Counseling

Many contraceptive options are available to women in the United States; however, not all options are equal with respect to pregnancy prevention. Obtaining a detailed patient history can often assist in counseling patients on contraceptive options. Important data to obtain during a family planning visit include sexual history, past medical history, family history, and an extensive review of systems. Developmental stage and the availability of parental support related to contraception should also be assessed. Adolescents often select contraception based on their previous experience with a particular method as well as the experiences of relatives and friends. Contraceptive methods are also now advertised in the media, and so this may also drive the selection of a particular type of method or brand. Even if the adolescent has requested a specific type of contraception, it is important to engage the adolescent in a discussion regarding methods the patient has previously used, concerns about a particular method, the experiences of friends and relatives (e.g., sisters and mothers), perceived self-efficacy related to the different methods, and partner involvement and assistance related to using a particular method. Use of the HEADDDS (Home, Education, Activities, Diet, Drugs, Depression, Sexuality) acronym to direct the family planning interview will yield important lifestyle data that can assist providers in guiding patients to select a method that will work best for them. Adolescents should receive routine health care including yearly physical examinations and screening laboratory tests as a part of preventive clinical services, but not as a requirement for initiating contraception. Pelvic examinations are not required before starting contraception. For preventive services, sexually active adolescent girls, whether using hormonal contraception or not, should have STI screening annually or biannually, depending on risk factors. Pap smear screening should be initiated within 3 years of onset of sexual activity or earlier if the girl is immunocompromised or receives only episodic health care. Adolescents who initiate a contraceptive method should be seen every 3 to 6 months so they can solve problems with their health provider regarding side effects or other problems that may arise.

Methods

The failure rates for current contraceptive methods are shown in Table 92.1.

Abstinence

Primary abstinence is the most effective and least expensive form of contraception in the United States. Adolescents who have never had sexual intercourse and who choose to abstain during adolescence avoid the contraceptive and emotional stressors related to maintaining a sexual relationship while navigating other aspects of adolescent development. Although many more adolescents have chosen abstinence as their primary method of contraception in recent years, the fact remains that most adolescents in the United States have had intercourse before their high school graduation.

Secondary abstinence (secondary virginity or celibacy) and periodic abstinence are two additional possibilities that are often overlooked as family planning methods used by adolescents. In secondary abstinence, an adolescent chooses to abstain from intercourse until a desired life point such as being in a long-term, committed monogamous relationship after having previously engaged in intercourse. Periodic abstinence, during which adolescents have periods of sexual inactivity between periods of sexually activity without making a long-term commitment to abstinence, can be more difficult to manage. Adolescents who are not in a relationship may choose not to have sex during that period, but they may re-engage when beginning a new relationship. Re-engaging in sexual intercourse means reestablishing a contraceptive method, which may have been discontinued during the period of inactivity. Many adolescents in this situation will choose to continue a hormonal method during periods of sexual inactivity to reduce the risk of pregnancy associated with an unanticipated unprotected sexual encounter. Condoms should be used in this situation to prevent STI.

Adolescents who choose any form of abstinence should be encouraged and supported regarding their decision. These adolescents should also receive comprehensive sexuality education and should be well informed of the available contraceptive methods, given that making decisions about sex during adolescence is a dynamic process that may result in intercourse regardless of intention.

Outercourse

Many adolescents use outercourse or noncoital intimacy to fulfill sexual desires while reducing pregnancy risk. Given the array of sexual behaviors that adolescents may engage in without actually having vaginal-penile intercourse, it is important that they understand how to prevent STIs, particularly that they avoid contact of ejaculate with the external female genitalia or vagina; barriers should be used to prevent infection through oral or skin lesions from partners infected with herpes, syphilis, or human papillomavirus.

Fertility Awareness

Fertility awareness (or "natural" family planning) relies on the identification of days during the female partner's menstrual cycle during which pregnancy is most likely to occur. Signs and symptoms such as the character of cervical secretions and position of the cervix, menstrual calendar calculations, and/or basal body temperature are used to predict fertile times of the month so couples who do not desire pregnancy can abstain or engage in other methods during fertile periods. Use of this method requires training, record keeping, and excellent communication and cooperation within the couple. The major disadvantages of this method are the high failure rate and the lack of protection against STDs, thereby limiting its use among adolescent populations.

Barrier Methods

Male Condoms. The male condom is the most widely available and used method of contraception.

TABLE 92.1

FIRST-YEAR CONTRACEPTIVE FAILURE RATES

Method	Perfect Use*	Typical Use†
Pill (combined)	0.3	8.0
Tubal sterilization	0.5	0.7
Male condom	2.0	15.0
Vasectomy	0.1	0.2
3-month injectable	0.3	3.0
Withdrawal	4.0	27.0
IUD Copper-T	0.6	1.0
IUD Mirena	0.1	0.1
Periodic abstinence	1.0–9.0‡	25.0
1-month injectable	0.05	3.0
Implant	0.05	1.0
Patch	0.3	8.0
Diaphragm	6.0	16.0
Sponge§	15.0	25.0
Cervical cap¶	18.0	24.0
Female condom	5.0	27.0
Spermicides	18.0	29.0
No method	85.0	85.0

IUD, intrauterine device.
*Most perfect-use rates have been clinically evaluated, but some are based on clinical expertise or "best guesses" (such as some forms of periodic abstinence, withdrawal and no method use).
†Typical-use rates for the implant, the injectable, the pill, the male condom, the diaphragm, periodic abstinence, withdrawal, and spermicides are based on 1991 to 1995 data from the 1995 National survey of Family Growth, as calculated by Fu et al. Typical-use rates for the IUD, sterilization, and the femalec condom are from Hatcher et al. and are adjusted by the ratio of the corrected and standardized failure rate in the first 12 months for all methods (12.9%) to the uncorrected failure rate for all methods (9.9%), as reported in Fu et al. Other typical-use rates are from Hatcher et al.
‡Rates range from 1% for the postovulation regime to 9% for the calendar method.
§Weighted average of the rates for nulliparous and parous women, weighted by the proportion of sponge users who fell into each of those two categories in the 1988 National Survey of Family Growth (41% were nulliparous, 59% were parous). The 1995 and 2002 National Survey of Family Growth had too few sponge users to permit recalculation of this proportion.
¶Simple average of the rates for nulliparous and parous women.
Data from Hatcher RA et al., eds. *Contraceptive technology*, 18th rev. ed., New York: Ardent Media, 2004, Table 9-2 (perfect use); Hatcher RA, Fu H, et al.
Contraceptive failure rates: new estimates from the 1995 National Survey of Family Growth. *Fam Plann Perspect* 1199;31:56 (typical use).
From: Guttmacher Institute, Contraceptive Use, Facts in Brief, New York: Guttmacher, 2005, http://www.guttmacher.org/pubs/fb_contr_use.html.

Male condoms are extremely safe, accessible (because they do not require medical examinations or prescriptions from health care providers to initiate), and inexpensive compared with all available methods aside from abstinence. They are also one of the few contraceptive methods that allow male partners to initiate and become actively engaged in pregnancy and STD prevention efforts with their sexual partners. Users often fear condom breakage or slippage during use; however, several studies have demonstrated that, among experienced users, these events are rare. Consistent and correct condom use among adults is associated with three to four pregnancies per 100 woman-years of use and low STI transmission rates. Unfortunately, many adolescent users are inexperienced, and the failure rate in this population ranges between 10% and 30%.

There are several types of male condom options on the market, including condoms made from latex, polyurethane, and natural membranes. Condoms made of latex have been well demonstrated to protect against STIs. Polyurethane condoms are thinner, more durable, and less constricting than latex condoms. Unlike latex condoms, polyurethane condoms may be used with oil-based lubricants. The United States Food and Drug Administration (FDA) approved polyurethane condoms in 1997 for use by latex-sensitive individuals. Polyurethane condoms are slightly more expensive than latex condoms. Adolescents should be advised to avoid use of condoms made from natural fibers such as lambskin because these condoms are derived from porous materials that may permit passage of herpesvirus, hepatitis virus, and HIV. Spermicides are not recommended because of lack of efficacy against STIs, and they may increase the risk of transmission of HIV in women with multiple daily acts of intercourse.

Despite the many advantages of male condom use, contraceptive negotiation is often required by adolescent girls to promote condom use in the context of sexual relationships with their male partners. Objections to condom use that may be voiced by one party in a relationship include concerns about reduced sensation, availability, trust related to disease-free status and monogamy, and spontaneity. Counseling both male and female adolescents on how to handle these dialogues, while also making condoms available and teaching proper condom placement, will likely increase confidence and adherence to this method. All adolescents who are sexually active should receive instruction and encouragement to use condoms, even if they choose another primary method of contraception. Dual methods, although sometimes more cumbersome for patients, provide enhanced protection against pregnancy in a setting where inexperience increases contraceptive failure.

Female Condom. The female condom is an alternative barrier method affording female adolescents the ability to control both contraception and STD prevention without male cooperation. The female condom is a loose-fitting, double-ringed, polyurethane vaginal sheath measuring 17 cm in length and 7.8 cm in diameter. The internal polyurethane ring is used to insert and to anchor the condom at the level of the cervix. The external ring provides some protection to the external genitalia during intercourse. The inside of the sheath is lubricated with a silicone-based product while additional water-based lubricant is supplied with the condom. Neither the internal nor external lubricant contains spermicide. Although these condoms are more expensive than male condoms and can be slightly more difficult to use, studies of couples have consistently rated the female condom highly acceptable. Additionally, female condoms can be placed in the vagina up to 8 hours in advance, can be purchased without a prescription, and do not require a fitting by a health provider. Some adolescents may complain of a squeaking noise or adherence of the penis to the condom during intercourse. Use of a water-based lubricant can resolve this problem for many couples. Adolescents who choose the female condom should be reminded that male and female condoms should not be used together because adherence may result in displacement of the devices, with resulting contraceptive failure.

Diaphragms and Cervical Caps. Diaphragms and cervical caps provide a physical barrier to conception while the spermicide jelly or foam used with these products affords spermicidal benefits. Both require a prescription from and fitting by a health provider to initiate. These methods are reasonable for short- and long-term contraception among women who cannot realistically rely on their male partner to assist with implementation of contraception, women who need contraception only intermittently, those who are averse to use of hormonal methods, and those who are in a stable, monogamous relationship. Both methods are contraindicated, however, in women who have latex allergies.

Diaphragms are dome-shaped rubber cups with a flexible rim that covers the entire cervix once secured by the anterior and posterior rims. Several types of diaphragms are currently available for fitting: coil spring, arcing spring, and wide seal rim. Before insertion, users apply spermicidal jelly or cream to inside of the dome. After insertion, the diaphragm provides 6 hours of effective contraception. If more than 6 hours elapse or if an additional sex act is anticipated, women are encouraged to reapply spermicide with an applicator without removing the diaphragm. The patient must leave the diaphragm in for at least 6 hours after intercourse. It is recommended that patients not leave the diaphragm in more than 24 hours or use during the menstrual cycle because this may increase the risk for toxic shock syndrome. Women who use the diaphragm for prolong periods may also experience pelvic discomfort, vaginal ulceration from rim pressure, and foul-smelling vaginal odor. The failure rate of diaphragms among perfect users is approximately 6% to 8% and among typical users is 20%. For adolescent users, failure rates have been as high as 35%. Diaphragm users are at increased risk for lower urinary tract infections, and some women experience allergies to the latex materials from which they are derived. Patients should be given detailed written instructions on diaphragm care and use at the time of prescribing. Actual diaphragms should be used during the fitting process so the patient can practice in the clinic with provider assistance.

The cervical cap is a smaller, soft, rubber dome-shaped cup with smooth, firm rim that fits in place around the base of the cervix. As with the diaphragm, spermicide is applied to the dome before insertion. The cap provides 48 hours of contraceptive effects regardless of the number of sexual acts, and reapplication of spermicide is not necessary with each sexual act. The cap should not be worn for more than 48 hours because of the risk of toxic shock syndrome. Women who use the cap for a prolonged period have also reported problems with odor. Failure rates are similar to those of the diaphragm.

Vaginal Spermicides

Vaginal spermicides provide a method that can be initiated by adolescent girls, but condoms are preferred for maximum efficacy against pregnancy and STI prevention. Used alone, spermicides have failure rates as high as 35% among adolescent users. Spermicides can be purchased without prescriptions and are inserted vaginally within 1 hour before intercourse. As noted earlier, multiple daily uses of spermicides have been associated with an increased risk of HIV transmission. Spermicides are also associated with altered vaginal flora and an increased risk of urinary tract infections.

Coitus Interruptus

Coitus interruptus (or the withdrawal method) prevents fertilization of the ovum by preventing contact with the spermatozoa. The couple using this method has vaginal-penile intercourse, but the male partner removes his penis from the vagina and away from the female partner's genitalia before ejaculation. Preejaculate, however, may contain active spermatozoa from a previous ejaculation and/or be infected with STIs. Use of coitus interruptus among adolescents is not recommended given the 19% to 27% failure rate of typical users in the first year, complete reliance on the often inexperienced male partner to predict and withdraw before ejaculation, and the lack of real protection against STI.

Hormonal Methods

Oral Contraceptive Pills

Combined Oral Contraceptive Pills. Estrogen- and progestin-containing combined oral contraceptive pills were introduced to the public after FDA approval in 1960. Numerous changes in the formulations of oral contraceptive pills have been made since that time and have resulted in better side effect profiles and acceptance among women. Currently, there are more than 50 FDA-approved combined oral contraceptive pills on the market. Combined oral contraceptives can be classified by the amount of estrogen and progestin in the various formulations. Progestin potency, however, is considered less often when prescribing oral contraceptive pills because discussions of potency are controversial, and the biologic and clinical effects of the progestin components in the newer formulations of combined pills are similar *in vivo*. Some authors have grouped oral contraceptives by generation, although this terminology is often not helpful. "First-generation" combined pills contain more than 50 μg of ethinyl estradiol or mestranol. "Second-generation" pills contain 30 to -35 μg of ethinyl estradiol with levonorgestrel, norgestimate, and other members of the norethindrone family. "Third-generation" products contain the newer progestins such as desogestrel and gestodene with 20 to 30 μg of ethinyl estradiol. A newer unclassified pill containing drospirenone has also been introduced on the market. Because most of the major side effects associated with combined oral contraceptive pills are the result of the estrogen component, low-dose pills, those containing 20 to 35 μg of ethinyl estradiol, are generally used for contraception in adolescent girls, given the efficacy and improved side effect profiles of these drugs. First-generation pills, however, still have everyday uses such as for emergency contraception (EC) and the treatment of dysfunctional uterine bleeding.

The primary mechanism of action of combined oral contraceptive pills is prevention of ovulation by inhibiting gonadotropin secretion via suppression of the hypothalamic-pituitary axis. Combined pills are available in monophasic (same dose of estrogen and progestin throughout the active pills) and multiphasic (dose of progestin varies throughout the cycle) preparations. The goal of multiphasic (biphasic or triphasic) preparations is to alter the steroid levels to reduce the metabolic effects and clinical side effects without compromising efficacy. Monophasic pills are most often selected for use in young adolescents, because it is easier to manage clinical problems when they occur.

Most clinical problems in adolescents result from missed pills; therefore, a plan for patient management of this issue at the time of prescribing is essential. Other problems may include breakthrough bleeding, amenorrhea, perceived weight gain, headaches, and elevation of blood pressure. Although combined oral contraceptive pills are well studied and safe for use, in rare instances use of pills can result in serious medical problems such as venous thromboses, gallbladder disease, breast tenderness, cardiac or pulmonary disease, strokes, migraines with neurologic problems, hypertension, and vision disturbances associated with hypertension or other systemic disorders. Most providers use the ACHES (Abdominal pain,

Chest pain, Headaches, Eye Problems, or Severe Leg Pain) warning system to assist patients in identifying potential serious complications so they can seek medical care.

Drugs that affect the efficacy of combined oral contraceptive pills include rifampin, phenobarbitol, phenytoin, primidone, and carbamazepine. Ethosuximide, griseofulvin, and troglitazone may also affect the efficacy of these drugs. There is little or no evidence that antibiotics that reduce gastrointestinal flora such as ampicillin, metronidazole, quinolones, and tetracycline affect efficacy; however, patients should be reminded to use condoms. The absolute contraindications to use of combined oral contraceptive pills include untreated hypertension, history or current diagnosis of deep venous thrombosis or pulmonary embolism, liver disease, migraine headaches with focal neurologic symptoms, and major surgery with prolong immobilization. Use of combined oral contraceptive pills in patients with uncomplicated sickle cell disease, smokers less than 35 years of age, and patients who have a history of cholecystectomy is not considered problematic.

The noncontraceptive benefits of oral contraceptive pills include less risk of endometrial and ovarian cancer, fewer ectopic pregnancies, better regulation of menses, less risk of salpingitis, and probably less risk for endometriosis, benign breast disease, rheumatoid arthritis, and ovarian cysts. In addition, oral contraceptive pills can be used in the treatment of dysfunctional uterine bleeding, dysmenorrhea, mittelschmerz, endometriosis, polycystic ovary syndrome, idiopathic hirsutism, acne, bleeding associated with blood dyscrasias, and premenstrual syndrome.

Adolescents who choose combined pills usually start the pill on the first day of their menstrual period, the first Sunday after their menstrual period starts (Sunday Start), or at the time of their clinic visit (Quick Start). Most pill packs are packaged for 28-day cycles. There are 21 days of active hormonal pills and 7 days of inactive reminder pills. Adolescents should anticipate their menstrual period during the first few days of the inactive week. Some young women prefer to reduce the frequency of withdrawal bleeding to four times by taking continuous pills or using a brand with 84-day cycles. Regardless of the combined pill regimen, new and/or young users should be followed-up in 1 to 3 months depending on their level of confidence about method use at the initial consultation to assess weight and blood pressure and to evaluate any potential side effects or concerns the adolescent has related to use of the method. Because this method affords no protection against STIs, condom use is advised.

Progestin-Only Pills. Progestin-only pills (or the minipill) were approved by the FDA in 1973 and are available as an alternative for women who are not able to tolerate the side effects of combined oral contraceptive pills or who have a condition that precludes use of combined pills. Their contraceptive effect is particularly dependent on the effects on endometrial and cervical mucus because ovulation may not be consistently suppressed. The pill must be taken everyday at the same time to have maximum contraceptive protection. The change in cervical mucus takes 2 to 4 hours, and the impermeability to sperm fades 22 hours after administration. The major side effect is irregular bleeding. Given that this method often functions most consistently as a natural barrier method, it is not the preferred regimen for adolescents. Adolescents who use this method should also be asked to commit to regular condom use to provide backup contraception as well as protection against STIs.

Injectables

Depot Medroxyprogesterone Acetate (Depo-Provera). Depot medroxyprogesterone acetate (Depo-Provera; DMPA) is a long-acting injectable contraceptive method approved by the

FDA in 1992. Many adolescent girls select this drug because it is extremely effective and does not require daily, weekly, or monthly reminders to maintain therapeutic contraceptive levels. Each dose of Depo-Provera contains 150 mg of DMPA and is given intramuscularly every 12 weeks. DMPA administration results in increased circulating levels of progestin that are sufficient to suppress the LH surge, thereby preventing ovulation as its primary mechanism of action. Secondary mechanisms include thickening of the cervical mucus and alteration of the uterine environment to prevent pregnancy.

The advantages of DMPA are that young women are able to maintain 3 months of contraceptive effects without significant disruption in lifestyle. This method, however, requires that they receive an injection and seek health care on a quarterly basis. Because many adolescent girls are followed-up as frequently with other methods, the visits do not present a major intrusion. Side effects, however, are the most common reason that women decide to discontinue the method. The most common side effects that affect long-term use are menstrual irregularity and weight gain. Most teen users report amenorrhea by 6 months of use. Some girls experience an increased number of menses while on DMPA. Few women experience heavy bleeding associated with this method; however, if present, other causes of bleeding, such as STI, should be considered. Once other causes of bleeding are ruled out, estrogen-containing pills may temporarily assist with control of bleeding. Weight gain is thought to result from increase appetite and is on average 5 lb in the first year, 8 lb at year 2, and 14 lb at 4 years. DMPA also may result in reduction in bone density problems among young adolescents who initiate this method. Discontinuation rates are on average 30% at 1 year, 50% at 2 years, and 80% by 3 years.

Adolescent girls who select DMPA and who are appropriate candidates for this method are usually started within 5 days of their last menstrual period (or after delivery of an infant or after abortion). Baseline documentation of a negative pregnancy test is also obtained before the first injection. Adolescents return at 11- to 12-week intervals to receive the next injection. DMPA is associated with slower return to fertility than with other methods. On average, noncontracepting women begin to ovulate 9 to 10 months after the last injection. Patients who present more than 15 weeks after the last injection are tested for pregnancy, asked to abstain from sexual intercourse for 2 weeks, and then retested again to ensure the young woman is not pregnant before the next injection. Weight, blood pressure, and side effect profiles should be monitored at follow-up visits. Adolescent patients should be encouraged to use a barrier method such as condoms (male or female) to prevent acquisition of STIs.

This method is ideal for adolescents who need highly effective contraception but who are unable to use daily or weekly contraceptive methods or who have medical problems for which the use of estrogen-containing contraceptives is contraindicated. Caution should be used with women who are taking antiseizure medications or rifampin or who have breast cancer, active liver disease, cardiovascular or cerebrovascular disease, or diabetes with renal, ophthalmologic, or neurologic complications.

Lunelle. Lunelle is a long-acting, combined monthly contraceptive containing 5 mg of estradiol cypionate and 25 mg of medroxyprogesterone acetate in a 0.5-mL solution. Each dose is injected intramuscularly (gluteus maximus or deltoid) every 28 days. The primary mechanism of action is through inhibition of ovulation as with combined oral contraceptive pills. The advantages of this method include excellent efficacy with both perfect and typical use, provision of an entire month of contraception via administration of a single monthly dose, maintenance of menstrual function while using the method, and return to fertility shortly after discontinuing the method. Disadvan-

tages include the injection delivery system, the requirement that the adolescent see a health provider before initiating a method of contraception, and the need for monthly follow-up visits for subsequent injections. Potential side effects are similar to those of oral contraceptive pills and may include menstrual irregularity (breakthrough bleeding, early menses, and/or amenorrhea), weight gain, and breast tenderness. The guidelines for prescribing Lunelle related to contraindications are the same as with combined oral contraceptive pills. Adolescents who opt for this method should be instructed to present within 5 days of starting their menstrual period (or after delivery of an infant or after an abortion). After documenting a negative pregnancy test for menstruating women, the injection is given intramuscularly. The patient should be given an appointment 28 days later at the time of the visit for the next injection.

In October of 2002, the manufacturer voluntarily pulled this method from the market secondary to concerns regarding inadequate dosing. The future availability of this product after further evaluation and/or modification is not clear, despite high acceptability of this method among adolescents. All adolescents who were using this product should have been encouraged to initiate another form of contraceptive use in the interim.

Subdermal Implants. Subdermal implants are a highly effective and reversible method of contraception providing up to 5 years of protection against pregnancy. The first product marketed in the United States contained six silastic rods of levonorgestrel, was recalled for manufacturing problems, and is not currently available for use. This system was also unpopular because of problems associated with removal of the rods. More recently, two-rod and single-rod systems have been developed and approved by the FDA. The two-rod system contains two matchstick-sized Silastic rods, each containing 75 mg levonorgestrel. The implants release 80 μg of levonorgestrel daily in the first month and 50 μg/day at the end of 9 months, and then they level off to 25 to 30 μg/day. Capsules should be removed after 5 years, but they can be removed sooner if desired. Pregnancies rates while on this method are extremely low at 0.24/100 woman-years, and the major side effect associated with use is menstrual irregularity. Other potential side effects include weight gain, mood changes, hair loss, acne, headaches, nausea, and vomiting. Research demonstrated that the two-rod system is well tolerated, and insertion and removal are easier, taking less than 5 minutes for each. Most women in the New York City site of the international trial discontinued the product for nonmedical reasons, the common most being desire for pregnancy. The single-rod implant is 4 cm long and contains 68 mg of etonogestrel, releases 60 μg/day of etonogestrel, and provides 3 years of effective contraception. The advantages of this method are that insertion and removal are less complicated, and it affords users highly effective contraception. Menstrual irregularity, weight gain, and headaches are common side effects noted with this method.

Both these methods are initiated within 5 days of the beginning of the last menstrual period (or after delivery of an infant or after an abortion). Baseline documentation of a negative pregnancy test is also obtained for menstruating women before insertion of the device. The implant(s) are inserted in the upper arm using a minor surgical procedure. Once the device is removed, there is rapid return to fertility. Acceptability of these methods in adolescent populations has yet to be determined.

Women should not use of these implants if they are pregnant, if they are breast-feeding in the first weeks after delivery, or if they have untreated hypertension, acute liver disease, thromboembolic disease, thrombophlebitis, breast cancer, or unexplained vaginal bleeding. Precautions should be used with women who have diabetes, hypertension, lipid abnormalities, gallbladder disease, renal failure, coronary artery disease, or a history of thromboembolic disease.

Contraceptive Patch. The contraceptive patch delivers 20 μg/day of ethinyl estradiol and 150 μg/day of norelgestromin transdermally via the 20-cm^2 patch. The patches have the same mechanism of action as oral contraceptive pills, but they are conveniently dosed, requiring weekly patch changes to maintain effective serum concentrations of hormones to prevent ovulation. The patch is applied for 3 consecutive weeks to one of the designated application sites (upper arm, lower abdomen, upper torso, buttock), followed by a patch-free (hormone-free) week during which menstrual bleeding will occur. Contraindications to use are the same as with combined oral contraceptive pills.

The advantages of this method include weekly dosing compared with daily dosing with oral contraceptive pills, maintenance of serum drug concentrations during the 7-day period of use with each patch, and efficacy comparable to that of oral contraceptive pills without peaks and troughs of serum hormone levels. The patches also remain intact regardless of heat or moisture, a finding suggesting that neither athletic activities nor seasonal changes (temperature) are prohibitive to use of this method. The area of application, however, should be clean and dry, to enhance adherence of the product. Users should be instructed to avoid contact with oily compounds because they may affect adherence for the entire week. The most common potential side effects include headaches, nausea, breakthrough bleeding in the first cycle, nausea, headaches, and hyperpigmented changes at the application site. To avoid hyperpigmentation, patients should be instructed to changes sites with use.

Vaginal Cervical Ring.

The vaginal contraceptive ring was approved by the FDA in 2001 and is a combined hormonal contraceptive in the form of a 5.4-cm diameter flexible ring made of ethylene vinyl acetate polymer. The ring, which is self inserted into the vagina, releases 15 μg of ethinyl estradiol and 120 μg of etonogestrel daily for 3 weeks. Serum hormone levels throughout wear are sufficient to suppress the hypothalamic pituitary axis and thus to prevent ovulation. The ring is then removed after 3 weeks for 1 week for menstruation. At the end of the fourth week, a new ring is inserted. This method has comparable efficacy to that of oral contraceptive pills, with the added advantages of once-monthly self-administration of the method and lower overall hormonal exposure during the course of the month. The ring does not need to be removed during intercourse. If the ring is removed for more than 3 hours, patients should use a backup method for 7 days. Potential side effects include prolonged withdrawal bleeding in 20% to 27% of patients and device-related problems such as vaginal discomfort during intercourse, increased vaginal discharge, and vaginitis in 2% to 5% of patients.

Intrauterine Devices

Two types of intrauterine devices (IUDs) are available for use in the United States. The IUDs are T-shaped devices made of radiopaque polyethylene with two flexible arms for insertion that open to hold the device in place against the fundus. The copper IUD is thought to function primarily as a spermicide, by altering the uterine environment. The levonorgestrel IUD releases 20 μg/day of levonorgestrel/day from a vertical reservoir. The levonorgestrel release results in alteration of the endometrium via thickening of cervical mucus and changes in the uterotubal fluid to prevent fertilization of the ovum. Both these devices provide highly effective contraception with minimal patient effort beyond arranging for insertion, but they are usually not used in adolescents because of increased risk of pelvic inflammatory disease, ectopic pregnancy, and infertility.

Emergency Postcoital Contraception

Emergency Postcoital Contraception (EC) is the only contraceptive method that can be used after unprotected intercourse to prevent pregnancy. Although this method has more recently been widely publicized for use among the general population of women who experience an episode of unprotected intercourse, it has been used since the 1960s to prevent unintended pregnancy in women who were victims of sexual assault. There are two ways to provide EC, through the use of high doses of contraceptive pills and by placement of IUDs. Both combined contraceptive pills and progestin-only pills can be used for this purpose. The Yuzpe method, which uses two large doses with at least 100 μg of ethinyl estradiol and 50 mg of levonorgestrel or 100 mg of norgestrel, is 75% effective in preventing pregnancy. The progesterone-only method utilizes two 75-mg doses of levonorgestrel taken at once or 12 hours apart and is 88% effective at reducing pregnancy. The progestin-only method has better efficacy than the Yuzpe regimen. Although oral contraceptive pill packs can be used to administer EC, dedicated products are now available for patient convenience and adherence. Use of the progestin-only method is preferred, given the higher efficacy and fewer side effects. If the progestin-only product is unavailable, providers can prescribe an over-the-counter emetic such as meclizine taken 30 minutes before the first dose of EC to reduce nausea and vomiting associated with the use of combined pills. Because IUDs are not generally used in adolescents for contraception, placement of an IUD for this purpose is rarely indicated in this population.

CONCLUSION

Many young people initiate sexual intercourse during adolescence, and, fortunately, many contraceptive options are available for their use. Health care providers serving adolescent and young adult populations should be prepared to discuss and develop a plan for pregnancy prevention while also addressing STI prevention. Because the decision to initiate and continue having intercourse is dynamic process, adolescents may vacillate when making decisions about matters affecting their reproductive health. For this reason, abstinence remains the safest choice for adolescents who cannot assume the responsibilities associated with engaging in a sexual relationship. However, adolescents who report using abstinence (primary or secondary) also require comprehensive sexuality education and support. Creating a safe space for open dialogues about the decision to have sex, ongoing sexual behavior, contraception, and STI prevention and ensuring access to a variety of contraceptive options are important aspects of providing comprehensive health care to adolescents and young adults.

Suggested Readings

Alan Guttmacher Institute. *Teen Pregnancy: trends and lesions learned.* Issues in Brief, series 1, 2000.

Audet MC, Moreau M, Koltun WD, et al. Evaluation of contraceptive efficacy and cycle control of a transdermal contraceptive patch vs an oral contraceptive: a randomized controlled trial. *JAMA* 2001;285:2347.

Centers for Disease Control and Prevention. *Tracking the hidden epidemics: trends in the United States 2000.* Atlanta: Centers for Disease Control and Prevention, 2000.

Cromer BA. Bone mineral density in adolescent and young adult women on injectable or oral contraception. *Curr Opin Obstet Gynecol* 2003;15:353.

Cromer BA, Blair JM, Mahan JD, et al. A prospective comparison of bone density in adolescent girls receiving depot medroxyprogesterone acetate (Depo-Provera), levonorgestrel (Norplant), or oral contraceptives. *J Pediatr* 1996;129:671.

Dieben TO, Roumen FJ, Apter D. Efficacy, cycle control, and user acceptability of a novel combined contraceptive vaginal ring. *Obstet Gynecol* 2002;100:585.

Elster AB, Kuznets NJ, eds. *AMA guidelines for adolescent preventive services (GAPS): recommendations and rationale.* Baltimore: Williams & Wilkins, 1994.

Emans SJ, Laufer M, Goldstein. *Pediatric and adolescent gynecology*, 4th ed. Philadelphia: Lippincott-Raven, 1998.

Fraser AM, Brockert JE, Ward RH. Association of young maternal age with adverse reproductive outcomes. *N Engl J Med* 1995;332:1113.

Grunbaum JA, Kann L, Kinchen SA, et al. Youth risk behavior surveillance: United States, 2001. *MMWR CDC Surveill Summ* 2002;51(SS04):1.

Hatcher RA, Trussell J, Stewart F, et al. *Contraceptive technology*. Contraceptive Technology Communications, 2002.

Joffe A, Blythe MJ. Handbook of adolescent medicine. *Adolesc Med State Art Rev* 2003;14:309.

Pettinato A, Emans SJ. New contraceptive methods: update 2003. *Curr Opin Pediatr* 2003;15:362.

Singh S, Darroch JE. Adolescent pregnancy and childbearing: levels and trends in developed countries. *Fam Plann Perspect* 2000;32:14.

Sivin I. Risks and benefits, advantages and disadvantages or levonorgestrel-releasing contraceptive implants. *Drug Saf* 2003;26:303.

Speroff L, Glass RH, Kase KG, eds. *Clinical gynecological endocrinology and infertility*. Baltimore: Lippincott Williams & Wilkins, 1999: 867.

Wan LS, Stiber A, Lam L. The levonorgestrel two-rod implant for long-acting contraception: 10 years of clinical experience. *Obstet Gynecol* 2003; 102:24.

Westhoff C. Emergency contraception. *N Engl J Med* 2003;349:1830.

World Health Organization. *Improving access to and quality of family planning: medical eligibility criteria for contraceptive use*. Geneva: World Health Organization, 2000.

Zieman M, Guillebaud J, Weisberg E, et al. Contraceptive efficacy and cycle control with the OrthoEvra transdermal system: the analysis of pooled data. *Fertil Steril* 2002;77:19.

CHAPTER 93 ■ ADOLESCENT HYPERTENSION

STEPHEN R. DANIELS

Hypertension is a major risk factor for cardiovascular disease in adults. It has been clearly shown in the Framingham Study and other epidemiologic studies that higher levels of systolic and diastolic blood pressure are associated with increased risk of cerebrovascular accidents, myocardial infarction, congestive heart failure, and renal failure.

Blood pressure elevation is also important in adolescents. It has been shown that adolescents with blood pressure elevation are more likely to become adults with hypertension. This phenomenon is often referred to as blood pressure tracking.

Elevated blood pressure in adolescence has been associated with early cardiovascular abnormalities. For example, the Pathobiological Determinants of Atherosclerosis in Youth (PDAY). Study evaluated the effects of nonlipid risk factors on the presence of atherosclerotic lesions in young persons who had died of accidental causes. These investigators found that among persons with normal cholesterol levels, black study subjects with hypertension had more raised lesions in the coronary arteries than black subjects without hypertension. In the Bogalusa Heart Study, the level of blood pressure was associated with the extent of fatty streaks and fibrous plaques in the aorta and coronary arteries. Left ventricular hypertrophy has also been found to be prevalent in children and adolescents with essential hypertension. In one study, 14% of adolescents with hypertension had left ventricular mass index greater than the ninety-ninth percentile for age.

Blood pressure elevation in adolescents is associated with increased risk of adverse effects in the heart and blood vessels. These adverse effects appear to be magnified when hypertension is accompanied by other risk factors such as obesity, dyslipidemia, diabetes mellitus, and cigarette smoking.

Hypertension may also be a presenting feature of important illness. Renal disease, trauma, increased intracranial pressure, and some pharmacologic agents may be associated with blood pressure elevation.

EPIDEMIOLOGY: PREVALENCE OF HYPERTENSION

On an initial measurement of blood pressure, approximately 5% of adolescents will have blood pressure elevation. However, with repeat blood pressure measurements, the prevalence of hypertension is only approximately 2%. The prevalence of primary and secondary forms of hypertension has been somewhat controversial. Although secondary forms of hypertension may be more common in infants and children, in adolescents the prevalence of primary hypertension is probably similar to the 95% prevalence seen in adults. In general, the younger the patient, the higher the blood pressure, and with less family history of hypertension, secondary forms of hypertension are more likely. The common causes of secondary hypertension in adolescents are presented in Box 93.1.

DIAGNOSIS

Blood Pressure Measurement

To recognize hypertension, it is important to measure blood pressure correctly. The National High Blood Pressure Education Program recommends auscultation as the standard approach. However, concerns about mercury toxicity have led some hospitals and clinics to remove mercury column sphygmomanometers and institute use of automated devices. Most automated devices use oscillometric methodology. It is important to review data on validation and reliability before accepting a device for use. Another alternative for blood pressure measurement is to use an aneroid device. However, these devices must be periodically calibrated against a mercury column.

No matter which equipment is used, the selection of an appropriately sized cuff is one of the most important aspects of blood pressure measurement. The recommended approach is to use a cuff with a bladder width that is approximately 40% of the upper arm circumference between the acromion and the olecranon. The length of the cuff bladder should include 80% to 100% of the arm circumference. Manufacturers of cuffs usually have lines on the cuff that indicate the range of arm sizes for which that cuff bladder will be appropriate.

Blood pressure should usually be measured in the right arm with the patient in the sitting position after a period of 3 to 5 minutes of rest. The arm in which the blood pressure is measured should be resting at heart level on a solid surface. The cuff should be inflated approximately 20 mm Hg above the

BOX 93.1	Common Causes of Secondary Hypertension

Renal parenchymal causes
    Glomerulonephritis
    Hemolytic uremic syndrome
    Nephrotic syndrome
Renal vascular causes
    Renal artery stenosis
    Neurofibromatosis
    Fibromuscular dysplasia
    Renal artery thrombosis
Endocrine disorders
    Hyperthyroidism
    Congenital adrenal hyperplasia
    Hyperaldosteronism
    Pheochromocytoma
Vascular causes
    Coarctation of the aorta
    Arteritides
Central nervous system causes
    Increased intracranial pressure
Drugs
    Corticosteroids
    Oral contraceptives
    Nonsteroidal antiinflammatory drugs
    Drugs of abuse
    Anabolic steroids
    Alcohol
    Cocaine
    Amphetamines

point at which the radial pulse disappears. The cuff is deflated at a rate of 2 to 3 mm Hg per second. The first Korotkoff phase (appearance of snapping tones) is used to indicate systolic pressure, and the fifth Korotkoff phase (disappearance of sound) is used to determine the diastolic blood pressure.

Assessment of Blood Pressure

In adults, blood pressure standards are based on the relationship to outcomes. In adolescents, there are no outcome-based standards. Instead, a "distributational" approach is used. In this classification approach, blood pressure percentiles based on the patient's age, sex, and height are used. Blood pressure lower than the ninetieth percentile is considered normal. Systolic or diastolic blood pressure between the ninetieth and ninety-fifth percentiles is considered to be prehypertension. As with adults, adolescents with blood pressure 120/80 mm Hg or higher should also be considered prehypertensive. Blood pressure above the ninety-fifth percentile that remains above the ninety-fifth percentile on three separate occasions is considered to be in the hypertensive range. Those in the hypertensive range should be classified as having either stage 1 or stage 2 hypertension. These cutpoints are presented in Table 93.1. Stage 2 hypertension is when the blood pressure is higher than 5 mm Hg above the ninety-ninth percentile. Stage 2 hypertension often requires immediate evaluation and treatment. The blood pressure percentiles recommended by the National High Blood Pressure Education Program are present in Tables 93.2 and 93.3.

TABLE 93.1

CLASSIFICATION OF BLOOD PRESSURE IN CHILDREN AND ADOLESCENTS

Blood Pressure Level Based on Percentile	Classification
<90th percentile	Normal blood pressure
90th–95th percentile	High normal or borderline blood pressure elevation
>95th percentile	High blood pressure
>95th percentile persistent on at least three separate occasions	Hypertension
95th–99th percentile + 5 mm Hg	Stage 1 hypertension
>99th percentile + 5 mm Hg	Stage 2 hypertension

Clinical Evaluation of Hypertension

Adolescents with suspected hypertension should have a complete history and physical examination. The history and examination may yield clues to whether a secondary form of hypertension is present. For example, a history of abdominal pain, dysuria, frequency, nocturia, and enuresis may suggest the presence of underlying renal disease. The absence of femoral pulses may indicate coarctation of the aorta.

Primary hypertension is rarely accompanied by abnormalities in the history of present illness or the physical examination. Symptoms such as headache, visual disturbance, chest pain, and epistaxis are often attributed to blood pressure elevation, but in fact these features are rarely associated with mild to moderate blood pressure elevation. Adolescent patients with primary hypertension often have a positive family history of hypertension and are more likely to be overweight.

Laboratory Evaluation

The standard approach to laboratory testing at the initial evaluation of adolescents with hypertension includes the urinalysis, blood urea nitrogen, creatinine, electrolytes, and complete blood count. Because cardiovascular risk factors may cluster in patients, particularly when obesity and the metabolic syndrome are present, it is useful to assess the fasting lipid profile. Abnormalities in the history and physical examination may suggest additional laboratory tests to evaluate the possibility of secondary hypertension. Finally, with persistent blood pressure elevation, a renal ultrasound study may provide important information about structural abnormalities of the urinary tract.

Consideration of White Coat Hypertension

Some adolescent patients may have blood pressure elevation only in the physician's office or under other stressful conditions. This is often referred to as *white coat hypertension*. Assessment of possible white coat hypertension can be accomplished by home blood pressure measurement or with 24-hour ambulatory blood pressure monitoring. When home blood pressure measurements are normal or when ambulatory monitoring reveals less than 20% of blood pressures above the ninety-fifth percentile, then the diagnosis of white coat hypertension should be entertained. Conversely, it is not clear that patients with white coat hypertension should be considered to have normal blood pressure. There is evidence to

TABLE 93.2

BP LEVELS FOR BOYS BY AGE AND HEIGHT PERCENTILE

Age, y	BP Percentile	SBP, mm Hg Percentile of Height							DBP, mm Hg Percentile of Height						
		5th	10th	25th	50th	75th	90th	95th	5th	10th	25th	50th	75th	90th	95th
1	50th	80	81	83	85	87	88	89	34	35	36	37	38	39	39
	90th	94	95	97	99	100	102	103	49	50	51	52	53	53	54
	95th	98	99	101	103	104	106	106	54	54	55	56	57	58	58
	99th	105	106	108	110	112	113	114	61	62	63	64	65	66	66
2	50th	84	85	87	88	90	92	92	39	40	41	42	43	44	44
	90th	97	99	100	102	104	105	106	54	55	56	57	58	58	59
	95th	101	102	104	106	108	109	110	59	59	60	61	62	63	63
	99th	109	110	111	113	115	117	117	66	67	68	69	70	71	71
3	50th	86	87	89	91	93	94	95	44	44	45	46	47	48	48
	90th	100	101	103	105	107	108	109	59	59	60	61	62	63	63
	95th	104	105	107	109	110	112	113	63	63	64	65	66	67	67
	99th	111	112	114	116	118	119	120	71	71	72	73	74	75	75
4	50th	88	89	91	93	95	96	97	47	48	49	50	51	51	52
	90th	102	103	105	107	109	110	111	62	63	64	65	66	66	67
	95th	106	107	109	111	112	114	115	66	67	68	69	70	71	71
	99th	113	114	116	118	120	121	122	74	75	76	77	78	78	79
5	50th	90	91	93	95	96	98	98	50	51	52	53	54	55	55
	90th	104	105	106	108	110	111	112	65	66	67	68	69	69	70
	95th	108	109	110	112	114	115	116	69	70	71	72	73	74	74
	99th	115	116	118	120	121	123	123	77	78	79	80	81	81	82
6	50th	91	92	94	96	98	99	100	53	53	54	55	56	57	57
	90th	105	106	108	110	111	113	113	68	68	69	70	71	72	72
	95th	109	110	112	114	115	117	117	72	72	73	74	75	76	76
	99th	116	117	119	121	123	124	125	80	80	81	82	83	84	84
7	50th	92	94	95	97	99	100	101	55	55	56	57	58	59	59
	90th	106	107	109	111	113	114	115	70	70	71	72	73	74	74
	95th	110	111	113	115	117	118	119	74	74	75	76	77	78	78
	99th	117	118	120	122	124	125	126	82	82	83	84	85	86	86
8	50th	94	95	97	99	100	102	102	56	57	58	59	60	60	61
	90th	107	109	110	112	114	115	116	71	72	72	73	74	75	76
	95th	111	112	114	116	118	119	120	75	76	77	78	79	79	80
	99th	119	120	122	123	125	127	127	83	84	85	86	87	87	88
9	50th	95	96	98	100	102	103	104	57	58	59	60	61	61	62
	90th	109	110	112	114	115	117	118	72	73	74	75	76	76	77
	95th	113	114	116	118	119	121	121	76	77	78	79	80	81	81
	99th	120	121	123	125	127	128	129	84	85	86	87	88	88	89
10	50th	97	98	100	102	103	105	106	58	59	60	61	61	62	63
	90th	111	112	114	115	117	119	119	73	73	74	75	76	77	78
	95th	115	116	117	119	121	122	123	77	78	79	80	81	81	82
	99th	122	123	125	127	128	130	130	85	86	86	88	88	89	90
11	50th	99	100	102	104	105	107	107	59	59	60	61	62	63	63
	90th	113	114	115	117	119	120	121	74	74	75	76	77	78	78
	98th	117	118	119	121	123	124	125	78	78	79	80	81	82	82
	99th	124	125	127	129	130	132	132	86	86	87	88	89	90	90
12	50th	101	102	104	106	108	109	110	59	60	61	62	63	63	64
	90th	115	116	118	120	121	123	123	74	75	75	76	77	78	79
	98th	119	120	122	123	125	127	127	78	79	80	81	82	82	83
	99th	126	127	129	131	133	134	135	86	87	88	89	90	90	91
13	50th	104	105	106	108	110	111	112	60	60	61	62	63	64	64
	90th	117	118	120	122	124	125	126	75	75	76	77	78	79	79
	98th	121	122	124	126	128	129	130	79	79	80	81	82	83	83
	99th	128	130	131	133	135	136	137	87	87	88	89	90	91	91
14	50th	106	107	109	111	113	114	115	60	61	62	63	64	65	65
	90th	120	121	123	125	126	128	128	75	76	77	78	79	79	80
	98th	124	125	127	128	130	132	132	80	80	81	82	83	84	84
	99th	131	132	134	136	138	139	140	87	88	89	90	91	92	92
15	50th	109	110	112	113	115	117	117	61	62	63	64	65	66	66
	90th	122	124	125	127	129	130	131	76	77	78	79	80	80	81
	98th	126	127	129	131	133	134	135	81	81	82	83	84	85	85
	99th	134	135	136	138	140	142	142	88	89	90	91	92	93	93
16	50th	111	112	114	116	118	119	120	63	63	64	65	66	67	67
	90th	125	126	128	130	131	133	134	78	78	79	80	81	82	82
	98th	129	130	132	134	135	137	137	82	83	83	84	85	86	87
	99th	136	137	139	141	143	144	145	90	90	91	92	93	94	94
17	50th	114	115	116	118	120	121	122	65	66	66	67	68	69	70
	90th	127	128	130	132	134	135	136	80	80	81	82	83	84	84
	98th	131	132	134	136	138	139	140	84	85	86	87	87	88	89
	99th	139	140	141	143	145	146	147	92	93	93	94	95	96	97

TABLE 93.3

BP LEVELS FOR GIRLS BY AGE AND HEIGHT PERCENTILE

Age, y	BP Percentile	SBP, mm Hg Percentile of Height							DBP, mm Hg Percentile of Height						
		5th	10th	25th	50th	75th	90th	95th	5th	10th	25th	50th	75th	90th	95th
1	50th	83	84	85	86	88	89	90	38	39	39	40	41	41	42
	90th	97	97	98	100	101	102	103	52	53	53	54	55	55	56
	95th	100	101	102	104	105	106	107	56	57	57	58	59	59	60
	99th	108	108	109	111	112	113	114	64	64	65	65	66	67	67
2	50th	85	85	87	88	89	91	91	43	44	44	45	46	46	47
	90th	98	99	100	101	103	104	105	57	58	58	59	60	61	61
	95th	102	103	104	105	107	108	109	61	62	62	63	64	65	65
	99th	109	110	111	112	114	115	116	69	69	70	70	71	72	72
3	50th	86	87	88	89	91	92	93	47	48	48	49	50	50	51
	90th	100	100	102	103	104	106	106	61	62	62	63	64	64	65
	95th	104	104	105	107	108	109	110	65	66	66	67	68	68	69
	99th	111	111	113	114	115	116	117	73	73	74	74	75	76	76
4	50th	88	88	90	91	92	94	94	50	50	51	52	52	53	54
	90th	101	102	103	104	106	107	108	64	64	65	66	67	67	68
	95th	105	106	107	108	110	111	112	68	68	69	70	71	71	72
	99th	112	113	114	115	117	118	119	76	76	76	77	78	79	79
5	50th	89	90	91	93	94	95	96	52	53	53	54	55	55	56
	90th	103	103	105	106	107	109	109	66	67	67	68	69	69	70
	95th	107	107	108	110	111	112	113	70	71	71	72	73	73	74
	99th	114	114	116	117	118	120	120	78	78	79	79	80	81	81
6	50th	91	92	93	94	96	97	98	54	54	55	56	56	57	58
	90th	104	105	106	108	109	110	111	68	68	69	70	70	71	72
	95th	108	109	110	111	113	114	115	72	72	73	74	74	75	76
	99th	115	116	117	119	120	121	122	80	80	80	81	82	83	83
7	50th	93	93	95	96	97	99	99	55	56	56	57	58	58	59
	90th	106	107	108	109	111	112	113	69	70	70	71	72	72	73
	95th	110	111	112	113	115	116	116	73	74	74	75	76	76	77
	99th	117	118	119	120	122	123	124	81	81	82	82	83	84	84
8	50th	95	95	96	98	99	100	101	57	57	57	58	59	60	60
	90th	108	109	110	111	113	114	114	71	71	71	72	73	74	74
	95th	112	112	114	115	116	118	118	75	75	75	76	77	78	78
	99th	119	120	121	122	123	125	125	82	82	83	83	84	85	86
9	50th	96	97	98	100	101	102	103	58	58	58	59	60	61	61
	90th	110	110	112	113	114	116	116	72	72	72	73	74	75	75
	95th	114	114	115	117	118	119	120	76	76	76	77	78	79	79
	99th	121	121	123	124	125	127	127	83	83	84	84	85	86	87
10	50th	98	99	100	102	103	104	105	59	59	59	60	61	62	62
	90th	112	112	114	115	116	118	118	73	73	73	74	75	76	76
	95th	116	116	117	119	120	121	122	77	77	77	78	79	80	80
	99th	123	123	125	126	127	129	129	84	84	85	86	86	87	88
11	50th	100	101	102	103	105	106	107	60	60	60	61	62	63	63
	90th	114	114	116	117	118	119	120	74	74	74	75	76	77	77
	95th	118	118	119	121	122	123	124	78	78	78	79	80	81	81
	99th	125	125	126	128	129	130	131	85	85	86	87	87	88	89
12	50th	102	103	104	105	107	108	109	61	61	61	62	63	64	64
	90th	116	116	117	119	120	121	122	75	75	75	76	77	78	78
	95th	119	120	121	123	124	125	126	79	79	79	80	81	82	82
	99th	127	127	128	130	131	132	133	86	86	87	88	88	89	90
13	50th	104	105	106	107	109	110	110	62	62	62	63	64	65	65
	90th	117	118	119	121	122	123	124	76	76	76	77	78	79	79
	95th	121	122	123	124	126	127	128	80	80	80	81	82	83	83
	99th	128	129	130	132	133	134	135	87	87	88	89	89	90	91
14	50th	106	106	107	109	110	111	112	63	63	63	64	65	66	66
	90th	119	120	121	122	124	125	125	77	77	77	78	79	80	80
	95th	123	123	125	126	127	129	129	81	81	81	82	83	84	84
	99th	130	131	132	133	135	136	136	88	88	89	90	90	91	92
15	50th	107	108	109	110	111	113	113	64	64	64	65	66	67	67
	90th	120	121	122	123	125	126	127	78	78	78	79	80	81	81
	95th	124	125	126	127	129	130	131	82	82	82	83	84	85	85
	99th	131	132	133	134	136	137	138	89	89	90	91	91	92	93
16	50th	108	108	110	111	112	114	114	64	64	65	66	66	67	68
	90th	121	122	123	124	126	127	128	78	78	79	80	81	81	82
	95th	125	126	127	128	130	131	132	82	82	83	84	85	85	86
	99th	132	133	134	135	137	138	139	90	90	90	91	92	93	93
17	50th	108	109	110	111	113	114	115	64	65	65	66	67	67	68
	90th	122	122	123	125	126	127	128	78	79	79	80	81	81	82
	95th	125	126	127	129	130	131	132	82	83	83	84	85	85	86
	99th	133	133	134	136	137	138	139	90	90	91	91	92	93	93

suggest that these patients are at risk for future, persistent hypertension.

Assessment of Target Organ Abnormalities

The most common target organ abnormality in adolescents with hypertension is left ventricular hypertrophy. This is best assessed by echocardiography. When left ventricular mass index is greater than the ninety-fifth percentile, this may be an indication of longer-standing and more severe blood pressure elevation. Patients with blood pressure elevation may also have abnormalities of left ventricular geometry and left atrial enlargement. In addition, funduscopic examination may reveal changes related to hypertension including arteriolar narrowing and arteriovenous nicking. In more severe hypertension hemorrhages, exudates and papilledema may be present.

THERAPY

Nonpharmacologic Management

Many adolescents with blood pressure elevation are overweight. The relationship between overweight and hypertension has been well established both in adults and adolescents. Studies have reported a tripling of the prevalence of overweight from 5% to 15% in adolescents over the last decade. This trend in the prevalence of obesity is probably also leading to a trend toward increasing prevalence of hypertension. Therefore, the first approach to management of the overweight adolescent with hypertension should be weight management. This can be accomplished by improving energy balance with increased energy expenditure through physical activity and decreased energy intake in the diet. It has been clearly demonstrated that weight loss can result in improvement in blood pressure. In adolescents who are still growing and are only mildly overweight, it may be appropriate to stabilize weight rather than to pursue weight loss. However, many adolescents already are at a body mass index greater than 30 kg/m^2, which is a level indicating obesity in adults. Such adolescents are at risk for other adverse health outcomes such as the metabolic syndrome and type 2 diabetes mellitus in addition to blood pressure elevation.

Physical activity has been reported to have a beneficial effect on blood pressure even when weight or body mass index is unchanged. It has been shown that many adolescents have a very low level of physical activity. Physicians and other health care providers should recommend that adolescents engage in 60 minutes/day of vigorous activity. They should also recommend that adolescents reduce their sedentary time, such as by watching television to no more than 2 hours/day.

Another nonpharmacologic approach to blood pressure control is restriction of dietary sodium. Some persons are sensitive to sodium in their diet. This means that as the sodium content in the diet increases, so does their blood pressure. Moderate restriction of dietary sodium appears to have very little risk and will benefit many patients. Patients should be counseled about salt that is "hidden" in foods. Most dietary sodium does not come from salt that is added to food at the table. Patients and their parents should also be counseled that restriction of sodium in the diet may take up to 2 months to have its full effect.

Pharmacologic Management

When blood pressure elevation is persistent despite nonpharmacologic efforts to control it, treatment with medication should be considered. This is particularly true if the elevation of blood pressure is more marked and there is evidence of target organ damage such as the presence of left ventricular hypertrophy. Some adolescents with other disease processes such as renal insufficiency or diabetes should be treated earlier and more aggressively for hypertension. This may help prevent the development of future complications and may preserve renal function in these patients.

There have been few controlled trials of antihypertensive medication use in adolescents. The studies that have been done have tended to be short-term studies. Nevertheless, data on medication use in adults can be extrapolated to adolescents to some extent. There are four major classes of antihypertensive medications to consider in an adolescent patient. These are diuretics, beta-adrenergic blocking agents, angiotensin-converting enzyme inhibitors, and calcium channel blockers. Research in adults has raised concern about the safety and efficacy of long-term treatment of hypertension with calcium channel blockers. Most of this research has focused on shorter-acting calcium channel blockers. Whether this also applies to longer-acting agents currently available is less certain. In addition, research in adults has reemphasized that diuretics can be quite safe and effective in the management of primary hypertension. Each class of antihypertensive agents has issues of risk for certain types of patients that must be considered as a choice of antihypertensive agent is made. For example, beta-adrenergic blocking agents are contraindicated in patients with diabetes mellitus or asthma. Angiotensin-converting enzyme inhibitors may have a teratogenic effect. Therefore, caution should be exercised in their use in adolescent girls who are sexually active and may become pregnant.

Generally, the approach to management is to pick an appropriate agent and start at a low dose. The dose can be titrated upward until blood pressure has been lowered. The National High Blood Pressure Education Program of the National Heart, Lung and Blood Institute has provided more detail on specific doses for specific pharmacologic agents used to treat hypertension in children and adolescents. The goal should be to reduce blood pressure to less than the ninety-fifth percentile. When lowering of blood pressure is not achieved despite increasing the dose, lack of compliance is an important consideration. This issue should be addressed with the patient directly. In some cases, compliance is poor because of a perceived or real side effect of the medication. In other cases, compliance is poor because the patient does not clearly understand the rationale for treatment. In other cases, adolescents require behavioral strategies to improve compliance. It is sometimes necessary to switch to a new class of agents or, when blood pressure elevation is more severe, to combine medications from different classes. Enlisting the assistance of a physician experienced in treating adolescents with hypertension is advisable as the treatment decisions become more complex.

CONCLUSION

The recommended approach to the evaluation and management of hypertension in adolescents is presented in Figure 93.1. This provides a stepwise approach emphasizing that blood pressure elevation may be transient. However, when hypertension is diagnosed, an organized approach to the patient including diagnosis, evaluation, and treatment will result in optimal care.

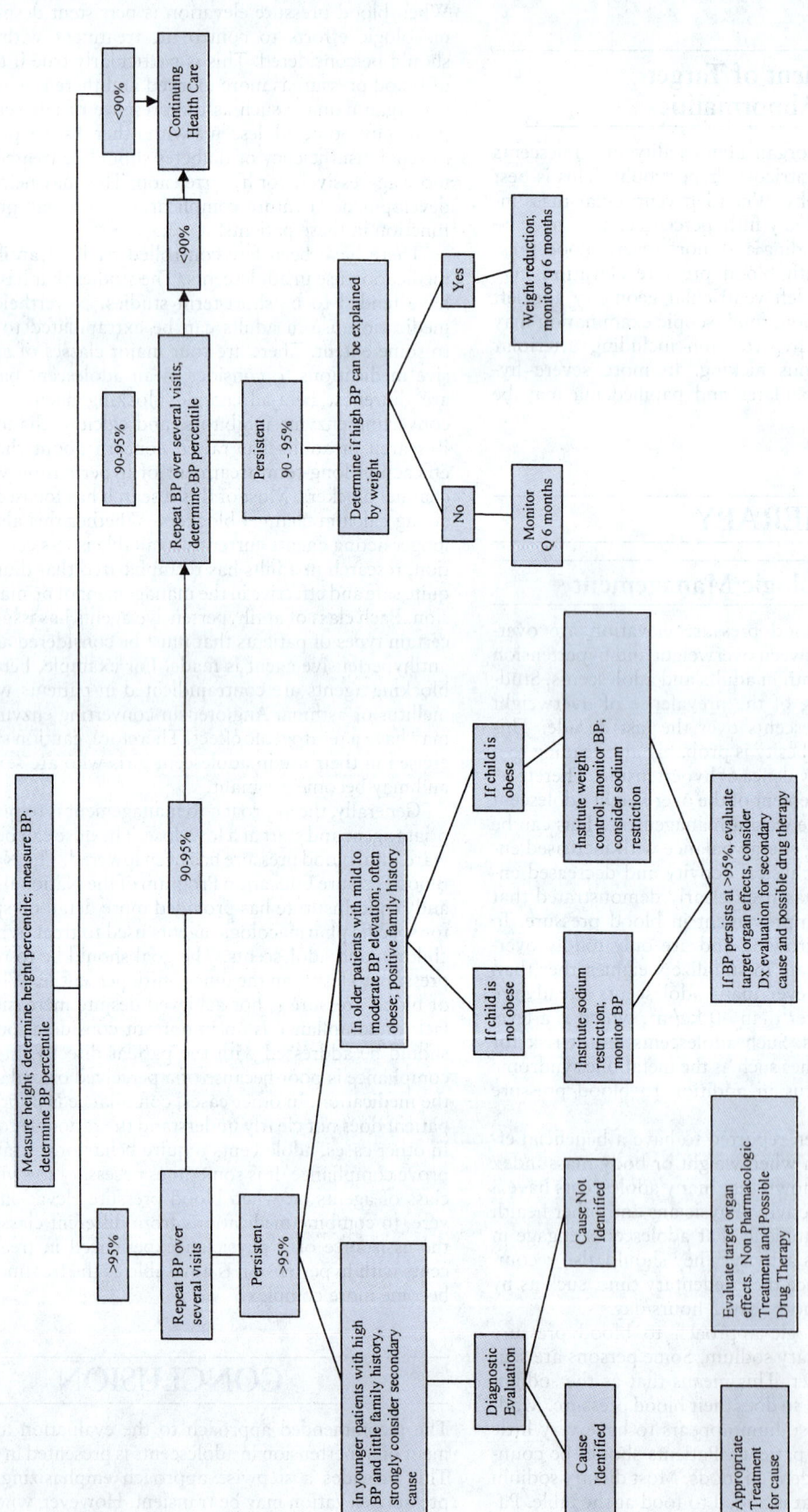

FIGURE 93.1. Flow chart for identifying children with high blood pressure who are in need of diagnostic evaluation and treatment. BP, blood pressure; Dx, diagnosis. From Williams CL, Hayman LL, Daniels SR, et al. Cardiovascular health in childhood: A statement for health professionals from the Committee on Atherosclerosis, Hypertension, and Obesity in the Young (AHOY) of the Council on Cardiovascular Disease in the Young, American Heart Association, Circulation, 2002;106:1178.

Suggested Readings

Berenson GS, Srinivasan SR, Bao W, et al. Association between multiple cardiovascular risk factors and atherosclerosis in children and young adults: the Bogalusa Heart Study. *N Engl J Med* 1998;338:1650.

Daniels SR, Loggie JMH, Khoury P, et al. Left ventricular geometry and severe left ventricular hypertrophy in children and adolescents with essential hypertension. *Circulation* 1998;97:1907.

Falkner B, Daniels SR, Horan MJ, et al. Update on the Task Force report (1987) on high blood pressure in children and adolescents: a Working Group report from the National High Blood Pressure Education Program. *Pediatrics* 1996;98:649.

Falkner B, Daniels SR, Flynn JT, et al. The fourth report on the diagnosis, evaluation, and treatment of high blood pressure in children and adolescents: National High Blood Pressure Education Program Working Group on High Blood Pressure in Children and Adolescents. *Pediatrics* 2004;114:555.

Lauer RM, Clarkn WR. Childhood risk factors for high adult blood pressure: the muscatine study. *Pediatrics* 1989;84:633.

Luepker RV, Jacobs DR, Prineas RJ, Sinaiko AR. Secular trends of blood pressure and body size in a multi-ethnic adolescent population: 1986 to 1996. *J Pediatr* 1999;134:665.

McGill HC Jr, McMahan CA, Zieske AW, et al. Effects of nonlipid risk factors on atherosclerosis in youth with a favorable lipoprotein profile. *Circulation* 2001;103:1546.

Rocchini AP, Katch V, Anderson J, et al. Blood pressure in obese adolescents: effect of weight loss. *Pediatrics* 1988;82:16.

Soergel M, Kirschtein M, Busch C, et al. Oscillometric twenty-four-hour ambulatory blood pressure values in healthy children and adolescents: a multicenter trial including 1141 subjects. *J Pediatr* 1997;130:178.

CHAPTER 94 ■ ADOLESCENT SUBSTANCE ABUSE AND OTHER HIGH-RISK BEHAVIORS

RICHARD B. HEYMAN

Within the inner city and suburbia, among the poor and the affluent, in the white and nonwhite populations, among the educated and illiterate alike, virtually all children are exposed to the influence of tobacco, alcohol, and other drugs (TAOD). "Exposure" takes many forms: one out of four children grows up in a home with an alcoholic relative; the average child is exposed to many forms of protobacco and alcohol media messages on a daily basis (including movies, television and radio, magazines and newspapers, billboards, logo clothing, point-of-sale displays, the World Wide Web), and virtually all movies and 75% of television dramas contain references to TAOD use; drinking is seen as universal in many places frequented by children, including restaurants, sports venues, concerts, festivals, adult parties, and picnics; and, in fact, four out of five students have consumed alcohol by the time they graduate from high school, 80% to the point of intoxication.

Ongoing monitoring of the use of TAOD by children suggests that the youth of the United States will continue to use substances at alarming rates. When asked about usage in the previous 12 months, nearly 40% of high school seniors report marijuana use, 20% report use of other illegal drugs, and one-third are smoking and binge drinking on a regular basis. Actual use is underestimated in studies such as these because they survey only those who are in school. It is thus crucial to consider tobacco, alcohol, and marijuana use to be nearly the norm and to assess every older child and adolescent for this problem.

AT-RISK YOUTH

It is clear that there is a subset of children and adolescents who are at increased risk of substance abuse and for whom extra time should be spent on screening. It is convenient to divide these risk factors into three domains: genetic/family, personal, and community.

Genetic/Family Factors

Numerous studies have documented the role of heredity, especially for so-called type I alcoholism (the kind most common among boys and men and associated with delinquency and antisocial behavior), in which the inheritance from father to son is striking. Genetic evidence is accruing that implicates a role for abnormal dopamine receptors among those who develop alcoholism as well, and researchers continue to find clues to the biologic nature of addictive disorders in general. A family history of alcoholism increases the risk in children by a factor of 4, although fewer than one-third go on to develop the disease. Epidemiologic studies of families also suggest that family structure (disorganized versus organized) and conflict, parenting style (authoritarian or passive versus the authoritative style with its careful limit-setting), family use of TAOD, poverty, lack of religiosity or affinity with organized groups, and significant blocks of unsupervised time ("latchkey" arrangements) all represent risk factors.

Personal Factors

Children with difficult temperaments are at increased risk for the later development of substance use disorders. This is not to say that every irritable and moody child will go on to use TAOD, but children who are aggressive, oppositional, and provocative, as well as those who are risk takers and thrill-seekers, may have inborn susceptibility to drug use and may elicit parental responses that are controlling and negative. Mental health problems, including depression, anxiety, bipolar disorder, and attention deficit-hyperactivity disorder (ADHD), increase the likelihood of subsequent TAOD use. Appropriate treatment may minimize this risk, especially if these problems are identified at an early age. Distorted body image, including the feeling of being overweight or looking older or younger than one's actual age (associated with early or delayed puberty), is a risk factor. Low innate intelligence, disability or poor health, low sense of self-esteem and self-efficacy (the ability to affect and control one's life), and low achievement levels promote a sense of helplessness that may lead to self-medicating with alcohol and other drugs. At the other end of the spectrum, one survey suggested that "more than half of the nation's 12 to 17 year olds are at greater risk of substance abuse because of high stress, frequent boredom, too much spending money, or some combination of these characteristics."

Community Factors

Youth living in neighborhoods where tobacco and alcohol laws are not regularly enforced, where drugs are freely bought and sold, and where users inhabit doorways and parks will be exposed to more opportunities to use as well as the sense that such use is, in fact, normal and acceptable. Where recreational facilities are not available or are not safe, youth will congregate without organized activities. Schools riddled with drugs may not provide appropriate educational and extracurricular opportunities, and the youngster who is not well motivated may founder in such an environment.

ROUTINE SCREENING IN THE OFFICE SETTING

The topic of TAOD use must be addressed as pediatricians interact with families. Prenatal visits should review the impact of maternal TAOD use on the fetus, and visits throughout childhood should stress to the parents the importance of avoiding tobacco smoke exposure, being steadfastly opposed to the use of drugs, and modeling appropriate use of alcohol.

The discussion with children should begin at an early age. The role of media exposure is incontrovertible, and seemingly trivial things such as having a favorite beer commercial or spokesperson (celebrity or animated) and playing with candy cigarettes predict interest in and later use of beer and cigarettes. With the increase in counteradvertising on television, a forum has been opened up through which pediatricians can encourage discussion between parents and their young children.

By the time children reach middle school (age 10 years at the latest), an inventory of personal psychosocial questions should be incorporated into every visit. A discussion of so-called "risk and protective factors" is a useful framework for identifying those youth at risk for substance abuse, and young people and their parents should become accustomed to the care provider's discussing these issues in an open and nonjudgmental way each time they come into the office. Asking about whether the family has discussed sensitive topics such as TAOD use, puberty and sexuality, violence, bullying, and illegal activities and whether the child has had a TAOD prevention program in school may be nonconfrontational ways to begin the discussion of the subject. The issue of confidentiality should be addressed as well, and separate, private discussions with the patient and family should begin at an early age.

Parents should be encouraged to discuss behavioral concerns with the care provider. Questions should be asked about mental health issues such as depression and anxiety, and the signs and symptoms of substance abuse should be reviewed (Box 94.1). Identifying young people with conduct and attentional disorders, as well as "difficult temperaments" (characterized by impulsive, defiant, and antisocial behavior) will allow the clinician to pinpoint another group of patients at increased risk of substance abuse.

BOX 94.1   Signs of Substance Abuse

Early Signs of Substance Abuse

- Mood changes, secretive and erratic behavior, distancing from the family and family activities
- Being away from the home more, spending more time locked away in own room
- Abandoning old friends, associating with new friends, having strangers call and visit
- Change in appearance, dress, hygiene, taste in music, sleep behavior
- Things (perhaps alcohol, prescribed medications, jewelry, electronics) and money missing
- Physical signs, including cough (may request cough medicine), red eyes (may use ocular vasoconstrictor), dermatitis (may use lotions), sniffles and congestion (may use nose spray), bruises, changes in mental/neurologic status (including slurred speech, abnormal pupils)
- Odor of petrochemicals or alcohol on clothes or in room
- Conflicts with teachers, coaches, other young people

Later Signs of Substance Abuse

- Decline in school performance, truancy, loss of interest in extracurricular activities
- No association with old friends, who may, in fact, express concern
- Refusal to participate in family events or even leave own room
- Large blocks of unaccounted-for time, breaking curfews
- Finding drug paraphernalia in the home, including alcohol containers, pipes, rolling papers, empty containers of volatile substances
- Encounters with the police for theft, shoplifting, vagrancy

---

A semistructured interview may be useful for adolescents because it provides a framework for the clinician to use. Among the orally administered screening questionnaires, few are more user-friendly for the busy pediatrician than the HEADSS schema developed by Mackenzie (Box 94.2). This mnemonic allows the clinician to assess quickly a number of critical areas in a young person's life and can be used casually to take inventory even when the patient is being seen for an illness, injury, or sports physical examination. Exploring these domains with particular attention to issues related to substance abuse may reveal information about the following: parental use of TAOD; violence, bullying and drug use in school; sense of self-worth and social competence provided by participation in extracurricular activities (a strong protective factor against TAOD use); use of TAOD by friends and at social gatherings; early or inappropriate sexual behavior; and significant mood alterations that could be triggered or alleviated by TAOD use. Any positive answers relating to TAOD use must be investigated further, as described later. Jessor and Jessor did important work in the area of problem behavior theory and identified the association between early substance use and other negative actions such as youthful initiation of sexual activity, delinquency, truancy, and school failure, as well as other signs of rebellion. Thus, when one identifies a single problem behavior, one must look for others.

BOX 94.2   The HEADSS Schema

Home: Safety, stability, support, responsibilities, privileges
Education: Achievement, skills, strengths, plans, employment
Activities: Pastimes, sports; religious, civic and community involvement
Drugs: Tobacco, alcohol, and other drug use by friends, family; personal use
Sexuality: Satisfaction with body and self, involvement and concerns about sexuality, sexual activity and sexual identity
Suicidality: Symptoms of depression, anxiety, mood disorder, thinking problems

Adapted from Cohen E, MacKenzie RG, Yates GL. HEADSS, a psychosocial risk assessment instrument: implications for designing effective intervention programs for runaway youth. *J Adolesc Health* 1991;12:539.

BOX 94.3   The CRAFFT Questionnaire

Car: "Have you ever ridden in a car driven by someone (including yourself) who was high or had been using alcohol or drugs?"
Relax: "Do you ever use alcohol to relax, feel better about yourself, or just fit in?"
Alone: "Do you ever use alcohol or drugs while you are alone?"
Forget: "Do you ever forget things you did while using alcohol or drugs?"
Friends: "Do your family or friends ever tell you that you should cut down on your drinking or drug use?"
Trouble: "Have you ever gotten in trouble while you were using alcohol or drugs?"

Reprinted with permission from Knight JR, Shrier L, Bravender T, et al. A new brief screen for adolescent substance abuse. *Arch Pediatr Adolesc Med* 1999;153:591.

ADDRESSING THE ISSUE OF THE "POSITIVE SCREEN"

Arguably the greatest barrier to an appropriate assessment for TAOD use is clinician discomfort in knowing what to do when such use is identified. By becoming familiar with the appropriate evaluation and management of substance abuse problems, the physician can initiate appropriate referral and treatment.

When there is suspicion of TAOD use, based on information obtained from parents, the patient, or even a third party, a more comprehensive assessment is appropriate (see Box 94.2). Although dozens of instruments are available to assess adolescent substance abuse (see the excellent review by Winters and colleagues), these are generally too time consuming and complicated for routine use in the primary care office. Knight and associates developed and validated a brief, six-item questionnaire called the CRAFFT (Box 94.3), which can be used easily in the office setting. A young person who admits to *any* use of alcohol or other drugs should be asked the six CRAFFT questions. A single positive answer is of concern, and two positive answers are statistically correlated with significant alcohol or other drug use and identify a patient who should receive a brief intervention and perhaps a more comprehensive assessment.

Comerci has identified some of the important issues to be addressed during such a brief assessment as it is expanded to delineate the level of alcohol and drug abuse. Information should be gathered about what drugs are used and in what combinations, how often and in what venue, and the impact of drug use on family and social life. An assessment of level of use is also important. Macdonald's schema (Box 94.4) has stood the test of time and divides the continuum into five stages. Stage 0 (Curiosity) recognizes that the glorification and normalization of alcohol use are very seductive to naturally curious children, and any child with significant risk factors deserves particularly aggressive prevention services.

Stage I (Learning the Mood Swing) begins with the use of alcohol and tobacco. Tobacco use is a true training ground for subsequent use of other substances. By using tobacco, children become willing and then learn how to obtain and use an illegal (for them) substance, find like-minded people with whom to associate, control and modulate a drug's brain-altering ef-

fects, and hide the use and deceive parents. Alcohol, which is easy to obtain (often cleverly and covertly from the home) and easy to use, is usually the next stage in the continuum. Kandel and Yamaguchi's seminal work from the past 30 years has demonstrated repeatedly that young people proceed through their drug-using careers in somewhat predictable fashion. The use of licit drugs (alcohol and tobacco) invariably precedes the use of illicit ones (generally marijuana first). Boys are more likely to begin with alcohol, whereas girls are just as likely to start with smoking cigarettes. Many girls move from cigarettes to marijuana without using alcohol, whereas many boys move directly from alcohol to marijuana without smoking cigarettes. Furthermore, this research shows conclusively that "two characteristics of an individual's drug history are especially important predictors of progression from a lower to a higher stage of drug use: age of initiation into use of a drug class and extent of use of the drug."

Thus, weekend "partying" may rapidly become the norm, and beginning to associate with a new peer group that can supply drugs is likely to provide positive reinforcement for subsequent experimentation with inhalants, marijuana, and other drugs. At this stage, use is episodic, and there are likely to be few consequences. Schoolwork usually does not suffer because use tends to be restricted to the weekend; participation in activities and family functions usually does not change; and the careful youth can hide use from parents and friends.

In stage II (Seeking the Mood Swing), the now-experienced teen user begins to drink and get high on a more regular basis. Use of alcohol and marijuana become more frequent, and there may be experimentation with other drugs such as amphetamines, club drugs, and prescription medications. The teen develops sources to buy drugs and may dabble in dealing them, and being assured of a regular supply becomes a concern. It is perhaps useful to modify Macdonald's schema slightly here, because many young people can reach stage II (IIa may be a good designation), control their use, and continue to function nearly normally. Grades may be maintained, sports and other activities may not suffer, friend and family relationships may be reasonably healthy, and parents, teachers, and old friends may notice a bit more moodiness and isolation but be unaware that the young person is using drugs. Conversely, many young people progressing to stage II (IIb) begin to deteriorate: grades and

BOX 94.4	Office Interventions for Substance Abuse

Stage 0: Curiosity	Strong message of reinforcement for nonuse, "cognitive-behavioral questions" ("What would tobacco, alcohol, and other drug use do to your life—your plans, family, health, opportunities?"), social competency questions ("What would you do if someone offered . . .? If you saw a friend starting to use?")
Stage I: Experimentation	Careful investigation of use patterns; motivational interview to help patient consider effects of even limited use on self, family, future. Raise issues of brain effects, health, choices, and other risk behaviors. Investigate possibility of co-occurring psychiatric morbidity. Encourage cessation, contract for limited use, review harm reduction strategies, arrange follow-up, identify those patients likely to proceed to further use. Maintain confidentiality.
Stage IIa: Regular use	Intensify in-office assessment, identifying those who are beginning to use on a more regular basis or who are using additional drugs. Reassess patient's "trajectory" and help patient recognize that use has increased despite previous discussions. Reiterate previous concepts of limited use, harm reduction; set limits and carefully outline parameters for when referral and treatment (and loss of confidentiality) will be needed.
Stage IIb: Regular use with consequences	Patient has now violated "contract" and has developed (by definition) "substance abuse disorder" and requires comprehensive assessment, intervention, and probably referral. Breach of confidentiality and referral to a specialist are appropriate at this point.
Stage III/IV: Dependence and addiction	Patients first identified at these stages of substance abuse and require immediate referral for intervention and treatment.

Reprinted with permission from Macdonald DI. *Drugs, drinking and adolescents*. Chicago: Year Book Medical Publishers, 1984.

commitments to activities fall off, behavior and mood become alarmingly erratic, fatigue and indifference become overwhelming, and relationships with family and old nonusing friends suffer. With the need to obtain drugs and get high, there is more absence from the home, and lying and conning behavior become the norm. It can be frustrating for parents and clinicians alike to sort out how much of this kind of behavior is "typical adolescence" and how much may be attributable to drugs. Regardless of the underlying diagnosis, a youngster exhibiting these symptoms is troubled and deserves further evaluation.

By stage III (Preoccupation with the Mood Swing), obtaining and using drugs has become the focal point in life. The pattern of regular use may produce withdrawal or hangover when drugs and alcohol are not available, and stronger drugs such as opioids (including prescription painkillers), hallucinogens, and methamphetamine may become the drugs of choice. Maintaining the habit becomes increasingly expensive, and, if the child works, all proceeds may go to buy drugs. Alternatively, he or she may steal, deal, shoplift, or sell sex for drugs. School, personal hygiene, interpersonal relationships, and normal activities fall by the wayside, and encounters with the law for things such as theft and vagrancy become common.

In stage IV (Using Drugs to Feel Normal), use becomes essentially continuous. Repeated and prolonged exposure has, in many cases, produced major effects on both the drug reward and cognitive areas of the brain. Social functioning may cease to exist, and in many cases the young person becomes destitute and homeless unless a reliable enabler is identified. Overdosing, blackouts, and suicide attempts become common, and the full variety of brain-altering drugs is employed just to maintain a sense of being able to function. The young person who is not rescued from stage IV chemical dependency is at imminent risk for death, and most clinicians would argue that anything and everything must be tried to turn his or her life around at once.

Mention must be made of testing for drugs of abuse. Obtaining urine (or less commonly skin or hair) samples and testing for drugs may provide a snapshot view of a patient's usage. Such tests usually fail to detect alcohol, are subject to rendering false-positive results, are notoriously easy for a savvy teenager to defeat, and, because they measure only "instantaneous use," may provide a false sense of reassurance if results are negative. Drug testing may be useful in confirming a diagnosis and in monitoring abstinence, but in general it should never be used to establish a diagnosis, trick a young person into admitting they use drugs, or provide ammunition for a suspicious parent.

INTERVENTION AND REFERRAL

The appropriate response for the pediatrician who identifies a substance abuse problem in a patient is to provide intervention and/or referral. The concept of intervention (confronting the patient with the problem, frequently in conjunction with family and friends, and challenging him or her to address the issue) has been well studied in the adult population. Although far less has been written about adolescents, Levy and colleagues suggested that pediatricians "should adapt the empirically validated techniques from the adult brief intervention literature, making them developmentally appropriate for adolescents."

The nature of an intervention is logically based on the patient's stage of use. It is important to offer a strong message of encouragement to those choosing not to use TAOD (stage 0), and these patients should be provided with some "what would you do if" role playing to reinforce appropriate refusal techniques if confronted with the choice to use. Pediatricians should be able to address those in stage I and IIa who are experimenting with tobacco, alcohol, and perhaps marijuana, and a caring consultation from the primary care provider who knows the family may, in fact, be all that is needed. Such patients should be counseled about the implications of their choice to use, encouraged to limit exposure, and challenged to practice harm reduction techniques (e.g., only drinking in a safe place, never drinking while driving or riding, avoiding alcohol games, limiting consumption, not experimenting with different and potentially more harmful drugs, and never drinking or using alone). Although lecturing young people is notoriously useless, raising questions about their use, helping them to see inconsistencies in their choices, providing reasons to change behaviors, and listening empathically without confronting are techniques that may help them to change their behavior.

It is important to set realistic goals when working with this unique population of casual, recreational users. These young people may be from solid family backgrounds and may themselves be high achievers. Using scare tactics, "demanding" total abstinence, and forcing them into verbal agreements to change behavior may be counterproductive. Rather, counseling them on limit setting may be more practical and clinically effective. The CRAFFT mnemonic alluded to earlier can be useful as a counseling tool as well, by providing an outline of useful harm reduction goals. Young people should be cautioned not to drive or ride when using drugs or drinking and not to ride in a car with someone who has. Careful advice should be given about using drugs to make themselves feel better, and a brief assessment for depression, anxiety, and suicidality should take place. Caution should be given against using alone or in unsafe places where there is no one to help in an emergency. Drinking should not proceed to the point where it affects level of consciousness, and mention should be made of binge drinking and its dangers. The patient should be asked to call the care provider if anyone—friends, family, teachers, coaches—expresses worry about TAOD use. Parents can be obliquely counseled that all young people are subject to using alcohol and drugs, and that they (the parents) should call if they are concerned about their teen's behavior. Finally, mention should be made of "staying out of trouble," generalizing the phrase to include problems with the law, school, extracurricular activities, family life, and the like.

Educating recreational users about the potential hazards can be useful in helping to create the readiness to change behavior. Because young people are concrete thinkers, it may be most useful to identify immediate consequences of TAOD use (e.g., the expense, breakdown in parental trust, decrease in motivation and physical stamina, odor of tobacco smoke on breath and clothes, problems with school and the law) as against the long-term consequences, which may require more abstract thinking (e.g., loss of independence, impact on future relationships, development of chronic diseases such as cancer, emphysema, cirrhosis, hepatitis, and acquired immunodeficiency syndrome). Some authors suggest preparing a "contract" limiting use or even agreeing to temporary cessation. Regardless of the specific approach, the pediatrician comfortable dealing with these issues can institute brief counseling and should arrange and insist on careful follow-up.

By the time a young person is experiencing consequences of alcohol and other drug use (stage IIb), he or she will require a comprehensive assessment for substance abuse and will in all likelihood require formal intervention and treatment. Pediatricians should be familiar with substance abuse service providers in their community and with the various treatment options available. Consideration must, of course, be given to insurance issues and payment for services. The Substance Abuse and Mental Health Services Administration maintains an excellent Web site (www.samhsa.gov) which is updated frequently and contains information about assessment and treatment programs throughout the country. The methodology of formal intervention and determining treatment and level of care are beyond the scope of this chapter; however, the American Society of Addiction medicine has developed detailed patient placement criteria (the so-called "adolescent crosswalk") to which the interested reader is referred.

CO-OCCURRING PSYCHIATRIC DISORDERS

Young people who use drugs are at increased risk of having a coexisting psychiatric disorder, or so-called "dual diagnosis" or "comorbidity." Studies suggest that between 50% and 80% of drug-using teens suffer concurrently from depression, anxiety, bipolar disorder, ADHD, eating disorder, conduct disorder, and various personality disorders. It is also clear that the earlier the onset of substance abuse, the more likely the teen is to have a coexisting mental health disorder.

Many researchers have studied outcomes of those with dual diagnoses, and the vast body of evidence suggests that neither can be optimally treated unless both issues are addressed. Biederman's studies and reviews, for example, showed that children with ADHD have improved outcomes and lower likelihood of subsequent drug use if the condition is identified and treated early. Patients with depression and anxiety may have primary mental health diagnoses or symptoms caused by their drug use: in either case, such symptoms must be identified and aggressively treated. Many teens with mood disorders self-medicate with drugs, and abuse of amphetamines is common among girls with coexisting eating disorders. Other examples abound, suggesting the crucial nature of Armentano and Solkhah's caveats for any teen being evaluated for substance abuse: a mental status examination and a comprehensive evaluation for coexisting psychiatric symptoms should be performed; those being treated for substance abuse who do not respond should be further evaluated for comorbidity; substance abuse and psychiatric diagnoses must be treated concurrently; and mental health and addiction specialists should work together as needed.

CONFIDENTIALITY

The issue of patient confidentiality surfaces in a number of areas related to adolescent substance abuse as well as other risk behaviors. Portions of the interview with an older child and adolescent must, of course, be conducted in private. To gain the trust and confidence of a young person, some statement of confidentiality should be made. Many authors have written about this topic, and although there is no uniformity of opinion among doctors, lawyers, or ethicists, several principles obtain. The so-called "mature minor doctrine" is generally interpreted to imply that a minor who is not emancipated is capable of consenting to and refusing medical care in most circumstances, as long as he or she is of reasonable intelligence and is able to understand the implications of what is being said or recommended. Furthermore, statutes have uniformly protected physicians providing care for substance abuse services to minors, even without parental consent. Confidentiality must have limits, however, and children or adolescents who are severely ill or in danger of hurting themselves or others must receive help even if confidentiality is breached. Examples would include the adolescent's admitting to driving while intoxicated, using dangerous drugs or using them in a dangerous fashion, or selling and dealing drugs. An older, responsible adolescent who is well grounded and doing well can be given more latitude than a younger adolescent who is struggling. Dubler and Quinn provide a succinct statement that summarizes this issue perfectly: "It would be bad practice for a physician to shield a suicidal patient behind a wall of confidentiality or to report an alcohol experimenter or an inquisitive but responsible sexual beginner. If either of these hypothetical patients developed into an adolescent with a regular pattern of drunk driving or one who was promiscuous . . . it would no longer be acceptable to guard confidentiality . . ." Thus, a young person in stage I or IIa of substance use may be deserving of confidential management and counseling. Anyone who is experiencing consequences of alcohol and other drug use (stages IIb and on) must receive intervention and treatment, and the clinician should feel comfortable revealing the information needed to get the patient into treatment.

Suggested Readings

Armentano ME, Solhkhah R. Co-occurring disorders in adolescents. In: Graham AW, Schultz TK, et al., eds. *Principles of addiction medicine*. Chevy Chase, MD: American Society of Addiction Medicine, 2003.

Belcher HME, Shinitzky HE. Substance abuse in children: prediction, protection and prevention. *Arch Pediatr Adolesc Med* 1998;152:952.

Cohen E, MacKenzie RG, Yates GL. HEADSS, a psychosocial risk assessment instrument: implications for designing effective intervention programs for runaway youth. *J Adolesc Health* 1991;12:539.

Comerci G. Office assessment of substance abuse and addiction. *Adolesc Med State Art Rev* 1993;4:277.

Committee on Substance Abuse, American Academy of Pediatrics. Tobacco, alcohol and other drugs: the role of the pediatrician in prevention and management of substance abuse. *Pediatrics* 1998;101:125.

Graham AW, Schultz TK, et al., eds. *Principles of addiction medicine*. Chevy Chase, MD: American Society of Addiction Medicine, 2003.

Hawkins JD, Fitzgibbon JJ. Risk factors and risk behaviors in prevention of adolescent substance abuse. *Adolesc Med State Art Rev* 1993;4:249.

Jessor R, Jessor SL. *Problem behavior and psychosocial development: a longitudinal study of youth*. New York, NY: Academic Press, 1977.

Johnston LD, O'Malley PM, Bachman JG. *Monitoring the future: national results on adolescent drug use*. NIH publication no. 03-5374. Bethesda, MD: National Institute on Drug Abuse, 2002.

Kandel DB, Yamaguchi K, Chen K. Stages of progression in drug involvement from adolescence to adulthood: further evidence for the gateway theory. *J Stud Alcohol* 1992;53:447.

Knight JR, Shrier L, Bravender T, et al. A new brief screen for adolescent substance abuse. *Arch Pediatr Adolesc Med* 1999;153:591.

Levy S, Vaughan BL, Knight JR. Office-based intervention for adolescent substance abuse. *Pediatr Clin North Am* 2002;49:329.

Macdonald DI. *Drugs, drinking and adolescents*. Chicago: Year Book Medical Publishers, 1984.

Miller W, Rollnick S, eds. *Motivational interviewing: preparing people to change addictive behavior*. New York: Guilford, 1991.

Rogers P, Heyman R, eds. Addiction medicine/adolescent substance abuse. *Pediatr Clin North Am* 2002;49:2.

Schydlower M, ed. *Substance abuse: a guide for health professionals*. 2nd ed. Elk Grove Village, IL: American Academy of Pediatrics, 2002.

Schydlower M, Rogers P, eds. Adolescent substance abuse and addictions. *Adolesc Med State Art Rev* 1993;4:2.

Winters KC, Estroff TW, Anderson N. Adolescent assessment strategies and instruments. In: Graham AW, Schultz TK, et al., eds. *Principles of addiction medicine*. Chevy Chase, MD: American Society of Addiction Medicine, 2003.

CHAPTER 95 ■ SEXUALLY TRANSMITTED DISEASES

DONALD P. ORR AND MARGARET J. BLYTHE

Over the past decade, adolescents in the United States have become increasingly responsible with respect to sexual risk behaviors. The average age of first coitus has risen to about 16 years, the proportions of young people reporting use of effective contraceptive methods and condoms have increased, and pregnancy and birth rates to teens have consistently fallen. However, the number of adolescents with sexually transmitted infections (STIs) remains unacceptably high. Two-thirds of STIs are reported among those less than 25 years of age. The rates of gonorrhea, chlamydia, and human papillomavirus (HPV) are highest in women 15 to 19 years old. Nearly half of the new cases of human immunodeficiency virus (HIV) infections in the United States are estimated to occur in individuals under the age of 25 years. Approximately one out of four sexually active teens is estimated to contract an STI each year.

EPIDEMIOLOGY: RISK FACTORS FOR SEXUALLY TRANSMITTED INFECTIONS AND HUMAN IMMUNODEFICIENCY VIRUS

Limited understanding of STIs and of the consequences of specific sexual behaviors contributes to the risk for infection. Ten to 17% of adolescents who deny vaginal coitus report having tried oral-genital contact, and many adolescents misperceive it as "safe" sex. Fortunately, anal "sex" among younger adolescents (associated with increased risk of transmission for HIV) appears less common than once believed.

Condom practices contributing to the risk for STI include inconsistent use, especially as the length of a relationship increases, and limited intervals between acquiring new sexual partners. Overlapping sexual partnerships (more than one partner during a given time period) are the exception. Exchanging sex for money and gifts (e.g., prostitutes, runaways, the homeless, and "street youth"), incarceration, males having sex with males (MSM), injecting drug use, belonging to a racial/ethnic minority group, living in a neighborhood in which STIs are highly prevalent, and being poor are associated with greater risk for STIs. Lack of immunity, cervical ectopy with increased surface area of columnar epithelium exposure to pathogens, lack of sufficient progesterone (anulovatory cycles), and use of injectable progestins are also thought to confer increased risk for adolescents. Supportive data are limited and conflicting.

Delay in seeking care for symptoms increases the spread of infections. Adolescents are at risk because of stigma associated with STIs, lack of access to health care, and concerns about confidentiality. Many fail to understand that adolescents may consent to their own care for confidential evaluation and treatment of STIs in all states and the District of Columbia. Health care providers should be familiar with local laws because codes governing the age of minor consent and the degree of confidentiality are state specific.

APPROACH TO DIAGNOSIS AND MANAGEMENT OF COMMON SEXUALLY TRANSMITTED INFECTIONS

A sexual history should be obtained on all adolescent patients. (See Chapter 89 on interviewing adolescents.) All sexually active individuals are at risk for acquiring an STI. Screening asymptomatic adolescents should occur according to current recommendations described in the next section.

Evaluation of Symptomatic Individuals

Symptomatic individuals should be evaluated based on both on symptoms and on the prevalence of the most common infections. Serologic screening for HIV and syphilis should be obtained as indicated by history and date of last screen. There are no recommendations to obtain test of cure following treatment for STIs except syphilis.

> *Vaginal discharge:* Inspect external genitals; obtain vaginal secretions for pH, direct microscopy, and potassium hydroxide (KOH) preparation; send appropriate specimen (cervical swab or urine) to detect chlamydia, gonorrhea, or *Trichomonas* (polymerase chain reaction [PCR] or culture if available).
>
> *Urethral discharge/dysuria:* Inspect external genitals; send urethral swab or urine to detect chlamydia, gonorrhea, or, if recurrent symptom, *Trichomonas* (if PCR or culture is available); Gram stain urethral swab/discharge (if available).
>
> *Genital ulcer/genital pain:* Examine for inguinal adenopathy; inspect genitals for lesion(s); swab painful lesions for herpes simplex virus (HSV); swab lesion for darkfield microscopy if available; send blood for syphilis screen; consider chancroid.
>
> *Treatment of sexual partners:* All individuals who have had sexual contact within 60 days with a patient treated for an STI (except HPV or HSV) should be evaluated and empirically treated. Syphilis, gonorrhea, chlamydia, and AIDS are reportable diseases in every state; HIV infection and chancroid are reportable in many states. Because requirements for reporting other STIs differ by state, clinicians must be aware of local requirements.

Patients and partners should be instructed to not have sexual intercourse until therapy is completed and no longer having symptoms or 7 days for those treated with single-dose therapies.

Screening Asymptomatic Adolescents

Most persons infected with STIs are asymptomatic, thus making screening important in management. Nonintrusive testing of urine or vaginal swabs using nucleic acid amplification testing (NAAT) makes screening of asymptomatic adolescents feasible. NAATs are very sensitive and specific, but it is important to remember for this group of tests that the rate of false-positive results increases as the prevalence of infection in the population decreases (Table 95.1). The rates of infection with *Chlamydia trachomatis* have decreased in regions with intensive screening and treatment programs. Screening and treatment for chlamydia of infected women and partners have been shown to reduce pelvic inflammatory disease (PID) significantly and to be cost effective. Current recommendations are to screen annually all sexually active girls and women less

than 25 years of age and pregnant women early in the third trimester.

Recommendations to screen male patients for chlamydia are less clear because no studies on efficacy have been performed. Some clinicians use the presence of leukocyte esterase (LE) in a first-void urine specimen of sexually active male patients as a prescreen to select patients for NAAT testing. Among asymptomatic boys and men, LE has a sensitivity of 59% and specificity of 95% for asymptomatic chlamydia urethritis, thus resulting in a poor positive predictive value (38%) but very good negative predictive value (98%). In one study, screening asymptomatic boys and men for chlamydia was estimated to reduce the risk of PID by 55%. At a prevalence of 5%, the strategy of screening first with LE and then sending only those with positive results for urine-based NAATs was suggested to be the most cost effective.

Although gonorrhea is less prevalent than chlamydia, some recommend screening high-risk sexually active adolescent women annually for *Neisseria gonorrhoeae*. Screening adolescent boys is not recommended because asymptomatic infection is less common.

Although there are no recommendations for screening, the prevalence of *Trichomonas vaginalis* among high-risk sexually active women suggests that annual screening may be useful in this population. Prevalence data are insufficient among male adolescents to recommend screening. It seems prudent to screen sexually active adolescents for infection with *Treponema pallidum* and HIV.

Clinicians should be guided by the prevalence of STIs in their community and knowledge of the adolescent's sexual behaviors, such as multiple sexual partners, failure to use condoms, or previous STIs. More frequent screening (3- to 6-month intervals) of high-risk populations such as adolescents and MSM has been suggested.

SYNDROMES

The causes of common STI syndromes are listed in Box 95.1.

Nongonococcal Urethritis

Urethritis is characterized by mucoid or mucopurulent urethral discharge and is sometimes accompanied by dysuria or urethral pruritis. Asymptomatic infections are common. Nongonococcal urethritis (NGU) is diagnosed if there are more than five polymorphonuclear leukocytes (PMNs)/oil immersion field and gram-negative intracellular diplococci cannot be identified on urethral smears.

Historically, 15% to 50% of NGU cases have been caused by *C. trachomatis*, although other organisms are increasingly identified. Using PCR techniques, *Mycoplasma genitalium* has been found in 18% to 46% of men with NGU; coinfection with chlamydia is common. Culture of *M. genitalium* is difficult and not widely available; PCR techniques are available in some research laboratories. *Trichomonas* may cause NGU and has been identified in 6% to 17% of older men with NGU who are attending STI clinics. The role of *Ureaplasma urealyticum* remains unclear.

Treatment for NGU is the same as chlamydial urethritis. One should suspect *M. genitalium* or *Trichomonas* with treatment failures when reinfection is unlikely. Erythromycin and metronidazole, respectively, are recommended; however, a more recent report has suggested that a 5-day course of azithromycin may be more effective for *M. genitalium* and better tolerated.

TABLE 95.1

SENSITIVITY AND SPECIFICITY OF DIAGNOSTIC TESTS

Diagnostic Method	Sensitivity	Specificity
Tests for Detection of *Chlamydia trachomatis*		
Tissue culture	70–85%	100%
Direct fluorescent antibody (DFA)*,a	80–85%	99%
Enzyme immunoassay (EIA)†	53–76%	95%
Hybridization (DNA-probe)‡	65–83%	99%
NAATs		
Cervical§,‖,#,**	90–94%	98–99%
Urine		
Female§,‖,#	81–95%	98–99%
Male§,‖,#	93–95%	94–98%
Urethra		
Male#	97%	99%
Tests for Detection of *Neisseria gonorrhoeae*		
Culture	80–95%	100%
Gram stain		
Male: symptomatic	90–95%	95–100%
Male: asymptomatic	50–70%	95–100%
Females	50–70%	95–100%
Hybridization‡	92–96%	99%
NAATs		
Cervical§,‖,#,**	92–100%	99–100%
Urine		
Female‖,#(§, not FDA approved)	85–91%	99–100%
Male§,‖,#		
Symptomatic	94–99%	93–100%
Asymptomatic§	79%	100%
Urethra		
Male‖,#	99%	98–100%
Vaginal(§(not FDA approved))	95%	98%

NAATs, nucleic acid amplification tests.
*MicroTrak (Syva).
†Chlamydiazyme EIA (Abbott).
‡Pace2 (Gen-Probe).
§COBAS Amplicor (Roche).
‖ProbeTec (Becton-Dickinson).
#APTIMA Combo 2 (Gen-Probe).
**Digene Hybrid Capture2 (Digene).

BOX 95.1   **Etiology of Common Sexually Transmitted Infection Syndromes**

Discharge Syndromes (Urethritis, Cervicitis, Vaginitis)
- *Chlamydia trachomatis*
- *Neisseria gonorrhoeae*
- *Trichomonas vaginalis*
- *Mycoplasma genitalium*
- *Ureaplasma urealyticum*
- Herpes simplex virus
- *Candida* species

Ulcer Syndromes
- *Treponema pallidum*
- Herpes simplex virus
- *Haemophilus ducreyi*
- *Calymmatobacterium granulomatis* (granuloma inguinale, rare in the United States)
- *Chlamydia trachomatis* serovars L1, L2, or L3 (lymphogranuloma venereum, rare in the United States)

Pelvic Inflammatory Disease
- *Neisseria gonorrhoeae*

- *Chlamydia trachomatis*
- "Normal vaginal flora, e.g., anaerobes, *Gardnerella vaginalis*, *Haemophilus influenzae*, enteric gram-negative rods, and *Streptococcus agalactiae*
- Uncommon: *Mycoplasma genitalium*, cytomegalovirus, *Mycoplasma hominis*, *Ureaplasma urealyticum*

Epididymitis
- *Chlamydia trachomatis*
- *Neisseria gonnorrhoeae*
- Enteric organisms, e.g., *Escherichia coli*

Dermatologic
- *Treponema pallidum*
- *Neisseria gonorrhoeae* (disseminated gonococcal infection)
- Acute human immunodeficiency virus (See Chapter 139)

Mucopurulent Cervicitis

Mucopurulent cervicitis (MPC) is characterized by a purulent or mucopurulent endocervical exudate visible in the endocervical canal or on an endocervical swab specimen; easily induced cervical bleeding (cervical friability) may be present. MPC often is asymptomatic; some women have an abnormal vaginal discharge and vaginal bleeding (e.g., after sexual intercourse). Observation of an increased number of PMNs on endocervical Gram stain has not been standardized as a diagnostic tool and has a low positive predictive value. MPC can be caused by *C. trachomatis* or *N. gonorrhoeae;* however, in most cases no cause is identified. Recent studies have implicated other organisms including *M. genitalium.*

Women with MPC should be evaluated for chlamydial and gonococcal infection and treated accordingly. If the adolescent is at high risk for not returning, empiric treatment for both organisms is indicated. Antibiotic therapy has not been found useful in women with MPC that is not caused by chlamydia or gonorrhea.

Pelvic Inflammatory Disease

Pelvic Inflammatory Disease (PID) refers to a group of infections of the upper genital tract: endometritis, salpingitis, tuboovarian abscess (TOA), and pelvic peritonitis. It is estimated that 10% of untreated gonococcal infections and 20% of untreated chlamydial infections result in PID. PID is associated with significant morbidity including tubal adhesions and increased risk for ectopic pregnancy, infertility, and chronic pelvic pain. One study found that the risk for infertility increased from 11% following one episode of salpingitis to 54% among those with three or more episodes.

Pathology

C. trachomatis or *N. gonorrhoeae* is identified in cervical or tubal specimens in about one-third of cases of acute PID in patients from ambulatory settings and up to two-thirds of women hospitalized for acute PID. Other vaginal flora (anaerobes and *Bacteroides* species, enteric gram-negative rods, coliforms, *Haemophilus influenzae, Gardnerella vaginalis,* and *Streptococcus agalactiae*) have been identified in the endocervix and upper genital tract. Other organisms include *Mycoplasma hominis* and *M. genitalium, U. urealyticum,* and cytomegalovirus. Infection with anaerobes and multiple organisms appears to be common among those with more severe disease and TOA.

Clinical Manifestations and Diagnosis

Because of the spectrum of the sites involved and variability in the amount of inflammation, the symptoms and signs range from minimal (or none) to severe abdominal pain with fever and vomiting. No single historical, physical, laboratory finding, or procedure is both sensitive and specific for the diagnosis of acute PID. For example, laparoscopy, considered the gold standard for the diagnosis salpingitis, will not detect endometritis and may miss mild inflammation of the fallopian tubes. Combinations of historical, physical, and laboratory information may improve either the sensitivity or specificity of diagnosing PID, but not both, and often at the expense of the other. Because it is an upper genital tract infection, pathogenic organisms may not be recovered from the endocervix. Many cases of PID go unrecognized because the symptoms may be subtle (abnormal vaginal bleeding, dyspareunia, vaginal discharge). Thus, PID remains a clinical diagnosis. The clinician should maintain a low threshold for suspecting and diagnosing PID. The risk for impaired fertility increases significantly among those who delay treatment 3 or more days following the onset of symptoms; risk is greatest for those with chlamydial infection believed to cause more subtle symptoms. Empiric treatment should be initiated in sexually active young women and other women at risk for STIs if uterine/adnexal tenderness and cervical motion tenderness are present and no other diagnosis can be identified *at the time of the visit.* Additional signs that may be present and support the diagnosis include temperature elevation (higher than 38.3°C), mucopurulent cervical or vaginal discharge, cervical friability, pyuria, elevated erythrocyte sedimentation rate, and leukocytosis.

Transabdominal and transvaginal pelvic ultrasonography may be useful in the evaluation and management of adolescents diagnosed with or suspected of having PID. High-sensitivity transvaginal examination refines the imaging of tubal and ovarian inflammation and allows specific identification of the degree of tubal involvement and the severity of disease, but it requires insertion of a small vaginal probe. Transabdominal study may define endometritis, focal masses, and total pelvic distortion, but it requires a distended bladder. Both techniques are superior to bimanual examination in detecting TOA.

Therapy

Empiric evidence does not support the hospitalization of all adolescents with acute PID. Research among adults with mild to moderate PID demonstrated no differences in short-term clinical and microbiologic improvement between those managed with inpatient treatment and those given outpatient treatment. Hospitalization is recommended for pregnant adolescents and for those with vomiting, high fever, and TOA (or suspected), as well as for those who fail to respond to outpatient therapy. Treatments are outlined in Table 95.2. Sex partners should be examined and empirically treated for uncomplicated gonococcal/chlamydial urethritis even when these organisms are not identified in the women.

Epididymitis

Sexually active male adolescents are at risk for epididymitis, most often caused by *C. trachomatis* or *N. gonorrhoeae.* Infection with *Escherichia coli* may also occur among those who practice insertive anal intercourse. When this organism is identified in a nonsexually active male patient, one must evaluate the adolescent for anatomic abnormalities of the urinary tract. Adolescents with epididymitis usually present with unilateral testicular pain; swelling and tenderness along with a hydrocele are present on examination. Almost all have asymptomatic or asymptomatic urethritis as demonstrated by more than five PMNs on Gram stain of urethral swab or LE in a first-specimen urine sample. If the diagnosis is unclear, the adolescent must be evaluated for testicular torsion. An endourethral swab should tested for *C. trachomatis* and *N. gonorrhoeae,* or an NAAT may be used to test a first-specimen urine sample. Adolescents should receive empiric therapy for these organisms. Bed rest, scrotal elevation, and analgesics are recommended until symptoms have subsided. Treatments are outlined in Table 95.2.

COMMON PATHOGENS

Chlamydia trachomatis

Genitourinary infections with *C. trachomatis* affect more than 4 million U.S. residents annually. Rates of infection are 4 to 6.5 times higher in female patients than in male patients.

TABLE 95.2

SEXUALLY TRANSMITTED INFECTION TREATMENTS RECOMMENDED BY THE CENTERS FOR DISEASE CONTROL AND PREVENTION*

Uncomplicated Chlamydial Infections of the Cervix, Urethra, and Rectum
Azithromycin[†] 1.0 g PO single dose or
Doxycycline 100 mg bid PO for 7 days

Uncomplicated Gonococcal Infections of the Cervix, Urethra, and Rectum
Cefixime[‡] 400 mg PO in a single dose or
Ceftrixone[‡] 125 mg IM in a single dose or
Ciprofloxacin 500 mg PO in a single dose[§] or
Ofloxacin 400 mg PO in a single dose[§] or
Levofloxacin 250 mg PO in a single dose[§] or
         PLUS if chlamydial infection is not ruled out
Azithromycin 1.0 g PO in a single dose or
Doxycycline 100 mg PO bid for 7 days

Uncomplicated Infections of the Pharynx
Ceftriaxone 125 mg IM in a single dose or
Ciprofloxacin 500 mg in a single dose[§]
         PLUS If chlamydial infection is not ruled out
Azithromycin 1.0 g PO in a single dose of doxycycline 100 mg PO bid for 7 days

Disseminated Gonococcal Infection
Hospitalization is recommended for initial therapy.
Ceftriaxone 1 g IM or IV every 24 hours

Patients allergic to beta-lactam drugs
Ciprofloxacin 400 mg IV every 12 hours or
Ofloxacin 400 mg IV every 12 hours or
Levofloxacin 250 mg IV every 24 hours or
Spectinomycin 2.0 g IM every 12 hours
All regimens continued for 24–48 hours, at which time oral medications may substituted to complete for a 7-day course:
Ciprofloxacin 500 mg PO bid or
Ofloxacin 400 mg PO bid or
Levofloxacin 500 mg PO qd

Urogenital Trichomonal Infection
Metronidazole 2.0 g PO or
Metronidazole 500 mg bid for 7 days

Syphilis
Primary or secondary syphilis or early latent benzathine penicillin G 2.4 million units IM in a single dose. (pregnant: repeat in 1 week)
         Patients with history of allergy to penicillin:
Doxycycline 100 mg PO bid for 2 weeks or
Tetracycline 500 mg qid for 2 weeks or
Erythromycin 500 mg qid for 2 weeks (less effective treatment)
         For allergic pregnant patients:
Skin test to penicillin followed by desensitization if allergic and penicillin treatment

Genital Herpes

First Clinical Episode of Genital Herpes
Acyclovir 400 mg PO tid for 7–10 days or
Acyclovir 200 mg PO five times a day for 7–10 days or

Famciclovir 250 mg PO tid for 7–10 days or
Valacyclovir 1.0 g PO bid for 7–10 days

First Clinical Pharyngeal and Proctitis Infection
Acyclovir 400 mg PO five times a day for 7–10 days

Recurrent Genital Infection with HSV-2
Acyclovir 400 mg PO tid for 5 days (extend to 10 days for HIV infected) or
Acyclovir 200 mg PO five times a day for 5 days (extend to 10 days for HIV positive) or
Acyclovir 800 mg PO bid for 5 days or
Famciclovir 125 mg PO bid for 5 days (500 mg extend to 10 days for HIV positive) or
Valacyclovir 500 mg PO bid for 3–5 days or
Valacyclovir 1.0 g PO bid for 5 days (extend to 10 days for HIV positive)

Suppressive for Recurrent Genital HSV-2
Acyclovir 400 PO bid (may increase to 800 mg bid or tid for HIV positive) or
Famciclovir 250 mg PO bid (500 mg for HIV positive) or
Valacyclovir 500 mg PO bid (bid for HIV positive) or
Valacyclovir 1.0 g PO qd

Severe HSV-2
Acyclovir 5–10 mg/kg body weight IV every 8 hours

Pelvic Inflammatory Disease

Parenteral Treatment
Regimen A
    Cefotetan 2 g IV every 12 hours or
    Cefoxitin 2 g IV every 6 hours
      PLUS
    Doxycycline 100 mg PO or IV every 12 hours
Regimen B
    Clindamycin 900 mg IV every 12 hours
      PLUS
    Gentamycin 2 mg/kg (loading dose), then 1.5 mg/kg every 8 hours

Tuboovarian Abscess
    Add clindamycin or metronidazole to parenteral regimen A

Outpatient Treatment
Ofloxacin 400 mg PO bid for 14 days or
Levofloxacin 500 mg PO qd for 14 days
    With or without metronidazole 500 mg PO bid for 14 days
    OR
Ceftriaxone 250 mg IM or
Cefoxitin 2 g IM PLUS probenecid 1 g PO or
Other parenteral third-generation cephalosporin
    PLUS doxycycline 100 mg PO bid for 14 days
    With or without metronidazole 500 mg PO bid for 14 days

Epididymitis
Ceftriaxone 250 mg IM
    PLUS
Doxycycline 100 mg bid for 10 days

*For alternate treatments see: CDC 2002 Guidelines for treatment of sexually transmitted diseases. MMWR 2002; 51ho.RR06; 1-80. Available at www.cdc.gov/mmwr/preview/mmwrhtml/rrj106al.htm.
[†]Recommended for pregnant women.
[‡]Safe for pregnant women.
[§]Should not be used in areas where quinalone resistance is common (see text).

Adolescent girls and women 15 to 19 years of age are at highest risk of reported infection (2,541/100,000 women); more than two-thirds of all infections are asymptomatic. Rates are highest among African American women, incarcerated youth, homeless/street youth, and those in inner-city schools. Risk fac-

tors include a new sex partner, two or more partners in the prior year, inconsistent use of barrier contraception, prior STI, African American race, and a concurrent STI.

C. trachomatis is associated with the clinical syndromes or symptoms of urethritis, proctitis, and epididymitis in male patients, whereas in female patients, the urethral syndrome, mucopurulent cervicitis, proctitis, and PID are associated with the infection. Important sequelae in women include ectopic pregnancy and infertility. It appears that some women with apparent uncomplicated cervical infection already have subclinical upper reproductive tract infection. Other complications in women include infection of the hepatic capsule (perihepatitis or Fitzhugh-Curtis syndrome) and conjunctivitis and Reiter syndrome (reactive arthritis) for both men and women. Perinatal transmission may lead to neonatal ophthalmologic infection and pneumonia. Infection of the pharynx with *C. trachomatis* is uncommon even in those sexual partnerships practicing oral sex.

Clinical Manifestations

Urethritis and cervicitis are the most common manifestations. When present, symptoms generally appear about 2 weeks after sexual contact, although this is quite variable. Urethritis symptoms are usually mild and include frequency and dysuria. Urethral discharge tends to be mucoid and scant; however, it may mimic the typical purulent discharge of gonorrhea. On examination, there may be meatal erythema. Evidence of inflammation includes more than five PMNs/oil immersion field on Gram stain or positive LE on the first 10 to 20 mL of urine specimen. More than 50% of cervical infections are estimated to be asymptomatic. Symptoms, when present, include odorless vaginal discharge and at times intermenstrual or postcoital spotting. The examination may be normal or may demonstrate cervical friability (bleeding when lightly swabbed with a cotton-tipped applicator) and mucopurulent exudate in the endocervical canal easily detected on an endocervical swab specimen (mucopurulent cervicitis). Increased numbers of leukocytes may be present on an endocervical Gram stain; however, this test has not been standardized, has a low positive predictive value, and is not available in many settings.

Diagnosis

Diagnostic tests are available based on tissue culture, antigen detection, and amplification of nucleic acid sequences of *C. trachomatis* (NAAT). NAATs are of very high sensitivity and specificity and offer many advantages including less invasive sampling (urine, vaginal swabs) and ease of specimen transport (see Table 95.1).

Neisseria gonorrhoeae

Genitourinary infections with *N. gonorrhoeae* (gonorrhea) continue to be a problem and are the second most frequently reported communicable disease in the United States, in which an estimated 600,000 cases occur annually. Rates of gonorrhea have decreased but remain highest among adolescent girls. As with other STIs, African American youth are at higher risk.

Clinical Manifestations and Complications

N. gonorrhoeae is associated with the clinical syndromes or symptoms of urethritis, cervicitis, pharyngitis, proctitis, and conjunctivitis. Complications include epididymitis in boys and men, PID and TOA in girls and women, and disseminated gonococcal infection (DGI) in both. DGI results from gonococcal bacteremia with the entry point mucosal surface(s), causing petechial or pustular acral skin lesions, asymmetric arthralgia/arthritis, tenosynovitis or septic arthritis. DGI may be complicated by perihepatitis or rarely meningitis or endocarditis. Some strains of *N. gonorrhoeae* that cause DGI may be associated with minimal genital inflammation. Patients with a congenital deficiency of the late-acting complement components (C7, C8, and C9) may experience recurrent DGI.

Early symptoms of gonococcal infection are more common among boys and men (more than 90%), appear 3 to 5 days following exposure, and cause most male patients to seek treatment. Gonococcal urethritis may be mild (scant mucoid discharge, dysuria, frequency) or more severe, with intense pain on urination, penile edema, abscess of Cowper (bulbourethral) gland, Tyson glands (sebaceous glands of the prepuce or foreskin), or seminal vesiculitis). Approximately 50% of girls and women with gonococcal genitourinary infection remain asymptomatic. Presentation and findings of uncomplicated infection in girls and women are similar to those caused by *C. trachomatis*.

Diagnosis

Gonococcal urethritis is reliably diagnosed in boys and men by observation of intracellular gram-positive diplococci on Gram stain of the urethral exudate. Culture on Thayer-Martin or Martin-Lewis media and transported and incubated in a carbon dioxide–enriched environment is the method of choice for girls and women and for boys and men when Gram stain is not available. Multiple NAATs are available using urine or urethral, endocervical, or vaginal swab specimens (see Table 95.1).

Therapy

Antibiotic resistance is common in the United States; more than 20% of isolates are resistant. Most strains resistant to tetracycline and penicillin are mediated by chromosomal mechanisms, with plasma-acquired resistance less common. Resistance to fluoroquinolones is increasingly observed in Asia and the Pacific, including the West Coast and Hawaii. Clinicians must take a careful travel history, be aware of local patterns of antibiotic resistance, and remain observant for treatment failures.

Gonococcal infections of the pharynx are more difficult to eradicate than infections at urogenital and anorectal sites. Few antimicrobial regimens can reliably cure more than 90% of pharyngeal infections. Although chlamydial coinfection of the pharynx is unusual, coinfection of gonococcal infections with chlamydia at genital sites sometimes occurs. Therefore, treatment for both gonorrhea and chlamydia is recommended.

Trichomonas vaginalis

The flagellated protozoan *T. vaginalis* is a common cause of vaginal discharge in sexually active women, and it appears to be the most common curable STI among sexually active women, about 5 million cases annually. It is increasing identified as a cause of NGU in older men and accounts for an estimated 5% to 6% of NGU cases in the United States and for up to 17% in sub-Saharan Africa. This infection remains asymptomatic in 10% to 50% of men and women. Infection with this organism has been implicated as a risk factor for transmission of HIV, PID, preterm delivery, and low birth weight.

Clinical Manifestations

The vaginal discharge may be minimal or profuse, malodorous, "frothy," and pruitic. It may result in punctate ectocervical hemorrhages with ulceration (colpitis macularis or strawberry cervix).

Diagnosis

Observing motile, flagellated organisms in a saline preparation of vaginal secretions is diagnostic; the sensitivity is estimated to be 58% to 82%, with a specificity of 99.8%. The pH of vaginal secretions is usually greater than 4.5; addition of 10% KOH may result in an amine (fishy) odor. The sensitivity of Pap smear detection is approximately 57%. Sensitive culture techniques are available using special media and a kit for transport and incubation of urine or urethral/vaginal swabs. A highly sensitive and specific PCR technique is available in a few laboratories but is not yet approved by the Food and Drug Administration. Because this infection may cause an intensive inflammatory response, one should suspect it when observing numerous leukocytes on saline preparation of vaginal secretions even in the absence of motile protozoa when the pH is greater than 4.5.

Therapy

Recent reports have indicated some resistance to the standard antibiotic treatment, metronidazole. Empiric treatment of sexual partners is indicated because asymptomatic infections are common (see Table 95.2).

Treponema pallidum (Syphilis)

Syphilis rates have declined steadily over the past decade, reaching a 30-year nadir in 2000. Only 6,100 cases of primary and secondary syphilis were reported in 2001. However, in 2001, the rate increased slightly among men and was largely accounted for by several outbreaks among MSM in large urban areas. Infection among adolescents is far less frequent than among other age groups. Syphilis increases the risk for HIV transmission.

Primary Syphilis

The first clinical sign of infection is a local lesion that appears approximately 14 to 21 days after sexual contact at the site of inoculation, usually a moist mucous membrane. This progresses to a shallow, painless, clear-based ulcer with indurated margins (chancre). Rubbery, painless regional lymphadenopathy develops approximately 1 week later. Chancres may become secondarily infected with pyogenic bacteria and are painful, with a purulent base. Untreated, the lesion heals in 3 to 6 weeks and progresses to secondary syphilis.

Diagnosis is based on clinical suspicion and a confirmatory laboratory test. Darkfield microscopy of a specimen obtained by abrading the lesion is the test of choice. However, the test is available usually only in specialized laboratories, often associated with departments of public health. A direct fluorescent antibody test (DFA-TP) is also available and useful when darkfield capability is not immediately available and when examining oral lesions. Nontreponemal serologic tests for syphilis (Venereal Disease Research Laboratory test [VDRL], rapid plasma reagin [RPR], automated reagin screen test [ART], unheated serum reagin [USR], or reagin screen [RST]) are important for screening. Because they measure cardiolipin antibodies developed in response to treponemal infection, positive tests must be confirmed by a test specific for *Treponema* (fluorescent antibody absorption test [FTA-ABS], FTA-ABS double staining [DS], or hemagglutination treponemal test for syphilis [HATTS]). About 1% to 2% of the general population has a false-positive nontreponemal test result, with false-positive rates increasing to about 10% of intravenous drug users. Individuals with systemic lupus erythematosus and anticardiolipin antibodies frequently have false-positive VDRL or RPR tests. Nontreponemal serologic tests generally become positive at a relatively low level (RPR less than 1:16) in about 80% of infected individuals at the time they seek medical care; approximately 90% of patients will have a positive treponemal test at the time of clinical presentation.

Secondary Syphilis

Without treatment of the primary syphilis, there is widespread dissemination of *T. pallidum* about 3 to 6 weeks after the appearance of the chancre. An evanescent macular rash is often the initial clinical manifestation of systemic spread. This is followed by symmetric papular eruptions involving the trunk and extremities including the palms and soles. The development of systemic symptoms and the presence of lesions on the palms and soles help differentiate the rash of secondary syphilis from pityriasis rosea, tinea versicolor, and scabies.

Small, superficial, ulcerated mucosal lesions that resemble small aphthous ulcers are common. "Moth-eaten" alopecia may be seen. Condylomata lata (large, raised, whitish-gray lesions) are found in warm, moist genital areas adjacent to the primary site. Other common constitutional symptoms include malaise, sore throat, headaches, weight loss, fever, and myalgia. More than 75% of individuals develop a rash, and 50% to 86% have widespread lymphadenopathy. It is estimated that abnormalities of the cerebrospinal fluid are found in about one-third of patients, but most do not develop symptoms. Nontreponemal tests are almost always strongly positive (RPR greater than 1:32) in secondary syphilis. Positive tests should be confirmed with a treponemal test; a negative treponemal test excludes the diagnosis of syphilis, and causes of false-positive tests, such as systemic lupus erythematosus, must be pursued.

Latent Syphilis

Without treatment, symptoms resolve spontaneously in 3 to 12 weeks, and the patient becomes asymptomatic. During the preantibiotic period, approximately 25% of patients redeveloped active secondary syphilis in the first year. The remaining 75% of patients are considered to have late latent syphilis: one-third become RPR negative, one-third maintain low level RPR activity without signs of the disease, and one-third develop late manifestations of syphilis. These are discussed in standard textbooks and are generally not relevant to adolescents and young adults. Neurosyphilis is poorly understood; the evaluation and management of patients are somewhat controversial and beyond the scope of this text. Readers are referred to the current literature for information.

Referral to public health or infectious disease colleagues experienced with syphilis is strongly encouraged because of the public health implications and the complexity of management. All adolescents diagnosed with syphilis should be tested for HIV.

Herpes Simplex Virus

Infection with HSV types 1 and 2 is common. HSV-2 is most commonly associated with genital infection and HSV-1 with oral infection; however, both organisms may infect either site. The prevalence of HSV-2 infection increased by 30% from 1976 to 1994; rates are higher among women. Analyses of National Health and Nutrition Examination Survey III (1999–2000) data indicate that HSV-1 seroprevalence remains unchanged (59.6%), and the seroprevalence of HSV-2 has decreased 78% (5.8% to 1.5%) among 14 to 19 year olds and by 48% (17.2% to 8.9%) among the 20- to 29-year age group. Most HSV-2–seropositive individuals are unaware that they are infected. Prior infection with HSV-1 is no longer considered protective for HSV-2 infection, but it may decrease the severity of symptoms in first HSV-2 infections.

Pathology

HSV-1 and HSV-2 enter body through the abrasions in the skin or mucous membranes during contact with an infected person. After an average incubation period of 1 week (2 to 12 days), painful, discrete groups of vesicles appear at the site(s) of inoculation and over several days become pustular and erode into small, grouped, shallow ulcers that eventually crust. Virus is shed for at least 10 to 12 days following an initial infection.

The lesions resolve 15 to 20 days after the appearance of the vesicles. Painful lesions develop in more than 95% of boys and men and in 99% of girls and women. Cervical infection is present in 70% to 90% of first episodes and is less common in recurrent disease. All herpes viruses may produce latent infection in sensory ganglia and may be reactivated with recurrence of symptoms and lesions.

Clinical Manifestations and Complications

Initial (primary) infections tend to be associated with more systemic symptoms such as malaise, myalgia, headache, and fever in approximately 40% of boys and men and in 70% of girls and women. Autonomic dysfunction (hyperesthesia or anesthesia of the perineal, lower back, sacral regions, and urinary retention) may occur and is more common among male patients. HSV is rarely associated with transverse myelitis. Local symptoms include dysuria, urethral and cervical discharge, and pain on defecation, tenesmus, or mucoid discharge (proctitis).

More than 90% of those with genital HSV-2 have a recurrence of symptoms within 1 year, during which there is active viral shedding. Most patients develop multiple recurrences. Subclinical reactivation without symptoms is common and is estimated to account for one-third to one-half of all recurrences; virus is shed during subclinical reactivation. Reactivation is less frequent with genital HSV-1; about 60% of individuals with primary HSV-1 genital infection have a recurrence in the first 12 months. The frequency of recurrence decreases over time for HSV-1 and HSV-2. The symptoms associated with recurrences tend to be less severe, more localized to the infected region, and of shorter duration. Nearly 90% of patients with recurrences experience prodromal symptoms, often before the appearance of lesions, ranging mild tingling to shooting pains in the legs, hips, or buttocks.

HSV infections are associated with an approximately twofold increased risk for acquisition of HIV. Conversely, the effect of prior HIV infection on the natural history of HSV-2 is not well understood.

Genital herpes during pregnancy may result in congenital and intrapartum transmission resulting in neonatal herpes. Acquisition of HSV at or around the time of labor carries the highest risk for transmission. Primary HSV is associated with higher risk of complications (chorioamnionitis or premature delivery) because of either the increased likelihood of cervicitis or hematogenous dissemination. Most neonatal herpes results from perinatal transmission at the time of delivery; about 70% of infants with neonatal herpes are born to mothers with symptoms or signs of HSV. The presence of preexisting antibodies to HSV appears to be protective for the infant; the risk for neonatal transmission is less than 1% among women with recurrent HSV-2. The factors associated with risk of infection among infants exposed to herpes are poorly understood. Cesarean section to protect the infant is usually reserved for women with clinical signs of active herpes: cervicitis or genital lesions.

Diagnosis

Highly sensitive and specific diagnostic tests are available. Material should be obtained from unroofed vesicles. Cell culture techniques require about 3 days and can differentiate HSV-1 and HSV-2, but they are dependent on live virus; sensitivity is highest for vesicular lesions (94%) and decreases to 27% for crusted lesions; specificity is greater than 99%. Antigen tests include detection with DFA (more than 90% sensitive, 98% specific) and PCR (95% sensitive, 99% specific).

Identification of HSV-2 specific antibodies in the sera of asymptomatic individuals is useful in demonstrating past infection and indicates risk for asymptomatic viral shedding. Serologic tests are not useful in diagnosing acute infections.

Therapy

Systemic antiviral therapy (nucleotide analogues) is useful in individuals experiencing their first episode and in those with recurrent disease. Several regimens have been demonstrated to decrease the severity and duration of symptoms and the duration and amount of viral shedding. Therapy should be initiated in patients with active lesions and as soon as symptoms begin for those with recurrent infection. Patients with recurrent disease may be given a supply of medication with instructions. Topical preparations are not considered effective and are thus not recommended.

Daily suppressive therapy is useful for individuals with frequent recurrent episodes (four or more annually) and has been shown to reduce the number of recurrences by 70% to 80%. It also reduces, but does not eliminate, subclinical viral shedding; its role in prevention of transmission is unclear. However, one study demonstrated that viral suppression with valacyclovir significantly reduced transmission in infection-discordant heterosexual couples.

Genital Human Papillomavirus

HPVs are small, nonenveloped DNA viruses that infect basal epithelial cells. More than 100 types of HPV have been identified; approximately 40 of these types are transmitted sexually. Most infections are subclinical and asymptomatic. It is estimated that more than 50% of sexually active adults and up to 35% of sexually active adolescent girls have been infected with at least one of the genital HPVs.

Types

HPVs are divided into low-risk and high-risk types, based on their association with clinical sequelae. Common low-risk types associated with exophytic warts include HPV-6 and HPV-11. At least 18 types of HPV are described as high-risk or probable high-risk types because of their link to cervical and other genital malignancies. Five HPV types (16, 18, 31, 33, and 45) are associated with 95% of cervical cancers; other HPV types associated with other 5% of cervical cancers include 26, 35, 39, 51, 52, 53, 56, 58, 59, 66, 68, 73, and 82. More than 90% of women with cervical cancer have also been infected with HPV.

Pathology

Although HPV is common among adolescent girls, it appears that most infections are not persistent. In one study, almost all low-risk HPV infections and two-thirds of high-risk HPV infections were no longer evident by 24 months. Persistence and high-risk types are linked to the risk for abnormal Pap smear and malignancy. However, even among those with low-grade squamous intraepithelial lesions (SILs) on Pap smears, 95% of adolescents had normal cytology at 36 months; only 2.2% progressed to high-grade lesions. Risk for progression was 14 times greater among those with persistent high-risk HPV types. Cofactors linked to progression include HIV infection, smoking, marijuana use, and repeated STIs; progression remains poorly understood. Risk factors for HPV in adolescents are similar to those for other STIs.

Clinical Manifestations and Complications

Exophytic warts of the genitals and anus are common. In the majority of immunocompetent people with anogenital warts, spontaneous regression eventually occurs. As with cervical infections, a few progress to malignancy.

Diagnosis

Most anogenital HPV infections are subclinical and are recognized only if cellular abnormalities are identified on a Pap smear. Newer liquid-medium "thin-preparation" techniques for Pap tests are more sensitive in detecting abnormalities than older methods; they also offer the potential to detect HPV DNA on the same specimen. If high-risk types are detected in girls and women with atypical squamous cells of undetermined signified (ASCUS), referral for colposocopy is indicated. When HPV testing is not available, adolescents with high-grade SILs or persistent low-grade SILs should be referred for colposcopy.

Data support the use of HPV testing on women with ASCUS. The most cost-effective strategy appears to be "reflex testing" in which the sample collected at the time of the Pap smear using liquid-based cytology or a separately obtained swab stored in HPV transport media is sent if ASCUS is identified. Routine screening for HPV is not recommended. The reader is referred to the chapter on gynecology and to recommendations from the American College of Obstetrics and Gynecology and the American Cancer Society for management of patients with abnormal cervical cytology.

Visible warts may resolve without treatment. Removal of symptomatic warts remains the primary goal of treating visible genital warts. Removal does not guarantee eradication of the virus, but it may reduce infectivity. There are no data to indicate that either the presence of genital warts or their treatment is associated with the development of cervical cancer. (See treatment guidelines.) One must exclude high-grade SIL when cervical warts are identified. Referral to a specialist is indicated.

Immunodeficient patients, because of HIV or other reasons, may not respond well to therapy for genital warts. These patients may experience frequent recurrences and are at greater risk for squamous cell carcinoma. Biopsy of lesions is required for diagnosis. Individuals skilled with immunodeficiency states and biopsy should manage these patients.

PREVENTION

Risk-reduction counseling targeting STI risk behaviors leads to increased use of condoms and decreased incidence of STIs for up to 6 months. Research among adults demonstrates that latex condoms can significantly reduce the risk of transmission of HIV, HSV-2 to women, *C. trachomatis*, and *N. gonorrhoeae*. There are no scientific reasons to believe that these findings are not applicable to adolescents. Earlier research on condom effectiveness was frequently methodologically flawed and not easily interpretable. Until additional data are available, it is prudent to recommend condom use for sexually active youth but stress that even 100% correct use is not 100% effective. Use of vaginal spermicides alone containing nonoxynol-9 is not effective in preventing cervical gonorrhea, chlamydia, or HIV infection. Frequent use of spermicides has been associated with genital lesions and an increased risk of HIV transmission. Condoms distributed in the United States no longer contain nonoxynol-9.

Vaccines against the organisms that cause STIs offer the most potential for protection. One large study found that a vaccine against HPV-16 (the HPV associated with 50% of cervical cancers in the United States) was 100% effective in preventing infection for up to 27 months. Tests of multitype HPV vaccines are currently under way. The efficacy of herpes vaccines is unclear, but one study suggests protection for nearly three-fourths of vaccinated women who were seronegative at baseline for both HSV-1 and HSV-2. Immunization against hepatitis B virus is very effective in preventing the disease.

To be most effective, STI vaccines would need to be given to noninfected individuals; reaching children and adolescents before the initiation of sexual intercourse would be critical. Research demonstrates that adolescents express interest in receiving vaccine to "protect against cervical cancer," and it appears that most parents would be willing to have their young adolescents immunized. Higher efficacy of vaccines, physician endorsement, and lower costs have been identified as important vaccine characteristics for acceptance by both parents and teens.

Suggested Readings

Centers for Disease Control and Prevention. *Sexually transmitted disease surveillance, 2001.* Atlanta: U.S. Department of Health and Human Services, 2002.

Centers for Disease Control and Prevention. Sexually transmitted diseases treatment guidelines 2002. *MMWR Morb Mortal Wkly Rep* 2002;51:1.

English A, Kenney KE. *State minor consent laws: a summary,* 2nd ed. Chapel Hill, NC: Center for Adolescent Health and the Law, 2003.

Fortenberry JD, Tu W, Harezlak J, et al. Condom use as a function of time in new and established adolescent sexual relationships. *Am J Public Health* 2002;92:211.

Gates GJ, Sonenstein FL. Heterosexual genital sexual activity among adolescent males: 1988 and 1995. *Fam Plann Perspect* 2000;32:295.

Ginocchio RH, Veenstra DL, Connell FA, Marrazzo JM. The clinical and economic consequences of screening young men for genital chlamydial infection. *Sex Transm Dis* 2003;30:99.

Ho GRF, Bierman R, Beardsley L, et al. Natural history of cervicovaginal papillomavirus infection in young women. *N Engl J Med* 1998;338:423.

Kamb ML, Fishbein M, Douglas JMJ, et al. Efficacy of risk-reduction counseling to prevent human immunodeficiency virus and sexually transmitted diseases: a randomized controlled trial. Project RESPECT Study Group. *JAMA* 1998;280:1161.

Katz BP, Fortenberry JD, Zimet GD, et al. Partner-specific relationship characteristics and condom use among young people with sexually transmitted diseases. *J Sex Res* 2000;37:69.

Koutsky LA, Ault KA, Wheeler CM, et al. A controlled trial of a human papillomavirus type 16 vaccine. *N Engl J Med* 2002;347:1645.

Marrazzo JM, White CL, Krekeler B, et al. Community-based urine screening for *Chlamydia trachomatis* with a ligase chain reaction assay. *Ann Intern Med* 1997;127:796.

McNeeley SG, Hendrix SL, Mazzoni MM, et al. Medically sound, cost-effective treatment for pelvic inflammatory disease and tuboovarian abscess. *Am J Obstet Gynecol* 1998;178:1272.

Moscicki AB, Shiboski S, Broering J, et al. The natural history of human papillomavirus infection as measured by repeated DNA testing in adolescent and young women. *J Pediatr* 1998;132:277.

Munoz N, Bosch FX, de Sanjose S, et al. Epidemiologic classification of human papillomavirus types associated with cervical cancer. *N Engl J Med* 2003;348:518.

Ness RB, Soper DE, Holley RL, et al. Effectiveness of inpatient and outpatient treatment strategies for women with pelvic inflammatory disease: results from the Pelvic Inflammatory Disease Evaluation and Clinical Health (PEACH) Randomized Trial. *Am J Obstet Gynecol* 2002;186:929.

Remez L. Oral sex among adolescents: is it sex or is it abstinence? *Fam Plann Perspect* 2000;32:298.

Romanowski B, Marina RB, Roberts JN, Valtrex HS230017 Study Group. Patients' preference of valacyclovir once-daily suppressive therapy versus twice-daily episodic therapy for recurrent genital herpes: a randomized study. *Sex Transm Dis* 2003;30:226.

Sanders SA, Reinisch JM. Would you say you "had sex" if...? *Lancet* 1999; 281:275.

Schillinger JA, Xu F, Sternberg MR, et al. National seroprevalence and trends in herpes simplex virus type 1 in the United States, 1976–1994. *Sex Transm Dis* 2004;31:753.

Taylor-Robinson D, Horner PJ. The role of *Mycoplasma genitalium* in nongonococcal urethritis. *Sex Transm Infect* 2001;77:229.

Weller S, Davis K. Condom effectiveness in reducing heterosexual HIV transmission. [update of *Cochrane Database Syst Rev* 2001;1:CD003255; PMID: 11687062]. *Cochrane Database Syst Rev* 2002;1:CD003255.

Wald A, Langenberg AG, Link K, et al. Effect of condoms on reducing the transmission of herpes simplex virus type 2 from men to women. *JAMA* 2001;285:3100.

Warner L, Newman DR, Austin HD, et al. Condom effectiveness for reducing transmission of gonorrhea and chlamydia: the importance of assessing partner infection status. *Am J Epidemiol* 2004;159:242.

Zimet G, Mays RM, Strunin L, et al. Parental attitudes about sexually transmitted infection vaccination for their adolescent children. *Arch Pediatr Adolesc Med* 2005;159:132.

Zimet GD, Mays RM, Winston Y, et al. Acceptability of human papillomavirus immunization. *J Womens Health Gender Based Med* 2000;9:47.

SECTION IV ■ DEVELOPMENT AND BEHAVIORAL PEDIATRICS

CHAPTER 96 ■ NORMAL INFANT AND CHILDHOOD DEVELOPMENT

SHARON B. RICHTER, BARBARA J. HOWARD, AND RAYMOND STURNER

A major joy of pediatrics is observing and interpreting the child's changing developmental abilities for the parents. A child's development is based on changes in central nervous system maturation and myelination, modulated by interpersonal and environmental factors. What impacts the family are the continual and often sudden shifts in behavior, cognition, and emotional functioning. These changes result from neurologic readiness and then acclimatization to new experiences in all the child's environments: home, peer groups, and school, as well as the larger macrosystem of the community and culture. Theories about the socioemotional development of children that describe development in terms of achieving different developmental tasks can be very helpful to recognizing what may be motivating a child or confronting a parent. Concepts of neuromaturation can be helpful in making observations of developmental progress and in assisting professionals in remembering typical ages for achieving that progress. Understanding the meaning of the child's behavior is critical to a parent's ability to adapt to or manage it optimally. Successful mastery of normal developmental tasks is considered necessary for the incorporation of new skills to form future developmental competencies. This progression leads to adaptive functioning in later life. This chapter will describe the normal course of development through these tasks as defined by Erikson.

BIRTH TO 18 MONTHS: FROM SURVIVAL TO EXPLORATION

Erik Erikson described the first major developmental task in life as establishing a sense of basic trust rather than remaining in mistrust. This is achieved when the caregiver is responsive to the needs of the baby. He describes this in his book *Childhood and Society*:

> "The infant's first social achievement, then, is his willingness to let the mother out of sight without undue anxiety or rage, because she has become an inner certainty as well as an outer predictability … Mothers create a sense of trust in their children by that kind of administration which in its quality combines sensitive care of the baby's individual needs and a firm sense of personal trustworthiness within the trusted framework of their culture's life style."

The interactions that establish trust also form the basis for attachment. Attachment may be defined as the permanent affective two-way bond that connects people. For parents and infants, this bond develops through interaction over the first 1 to 2 years. Bonding refers to the special initial feelings of affection the caregiver has toward the infant. A sensitive—but not critical—period for the establishment of bonding appears to exist. This period covers the first hours and days of the infant's life and is enhanced by early infant alertness, skin-to-skin contact, and long opportunities to be with the parent, such as when rooming-in after birth. While bonding sets the stage for attachment, it is not essential, as clearly evident in securely attached children who are adopted at later ages. The primary attachment relationship is an important foundation and model for the establishment of trust in others and the understanding of self. Research associates later secure patterns of attachment with repeated early experiences of receiving prompt and sensitive care contingent to the infant's signals of need. When infants experience care unpredictably or care that does not meet their needs, they are more likely to develop a pattern of insecure attachment that, while still considered normal, is associated with less optimal outcomes.

The attachment patterns that develop in infancy have effects into childhood and even into adult life. Secure attachment also leads to a more cooperative relationship between the parent and child. Thus, the degree of attachment has important implications as it affects parental discipline and how the child will conform to family norms. Young children with secure patterns of attachment are more social and more popular during the preschool years and show more joy in mastery of tasks. They have also been shown to have better relationships with other adults and authority figures such as teachers and camp counselors. Apart from relating to others, children who are securely attached develop a better self-concept and emotional maturity than those who are not securely attached. Thus, how a parent responds to an infant sets the stage for how the child sees him- or herself and expects his or her needs to be filled in the future.

These basic needs of infancy that must be consistently and warmly met for a secure attachment pattern to develop are discussed in the following sections.

Need for State Regulation

Within the first 2 to 3 months of life the major developmental tasks are physiologic regulation, state regulation, motor regulation, and interaction. For example, physiologic regulation describes emerging control over the survival functions of regular breathing, bowel motility, temperature control, sucking, and swallowing that mature with time. State regulation refers to the infant's level of alertness and ability to modulate changes from one level of arousal to another. States range from deep sleep, to restless sleep, drowsiness, alertness, fussiness, and restlessness, to full crying.

At birth, infants have the capacity to come to an alert state for brief periods during which they can actively fixate on and search the faces of their caregivers, follow slowly moving targets laterally with their eyes, and localize sounds by turning their heads when human voice range is presented for several seconds. It can be easily recalled that in the first 3 months the major attainments are in the control of the oculomotor system and state (Fig. 96.1; think "eyes"). Over the first few weeks, the periods of alertness increase and attentional/interactive regulation improves with faster and more reproducible fixing and following. At 6 weeks postterm the gaze at the caregiver results in responsive smiling (think "mouth"). By 2 months infants track

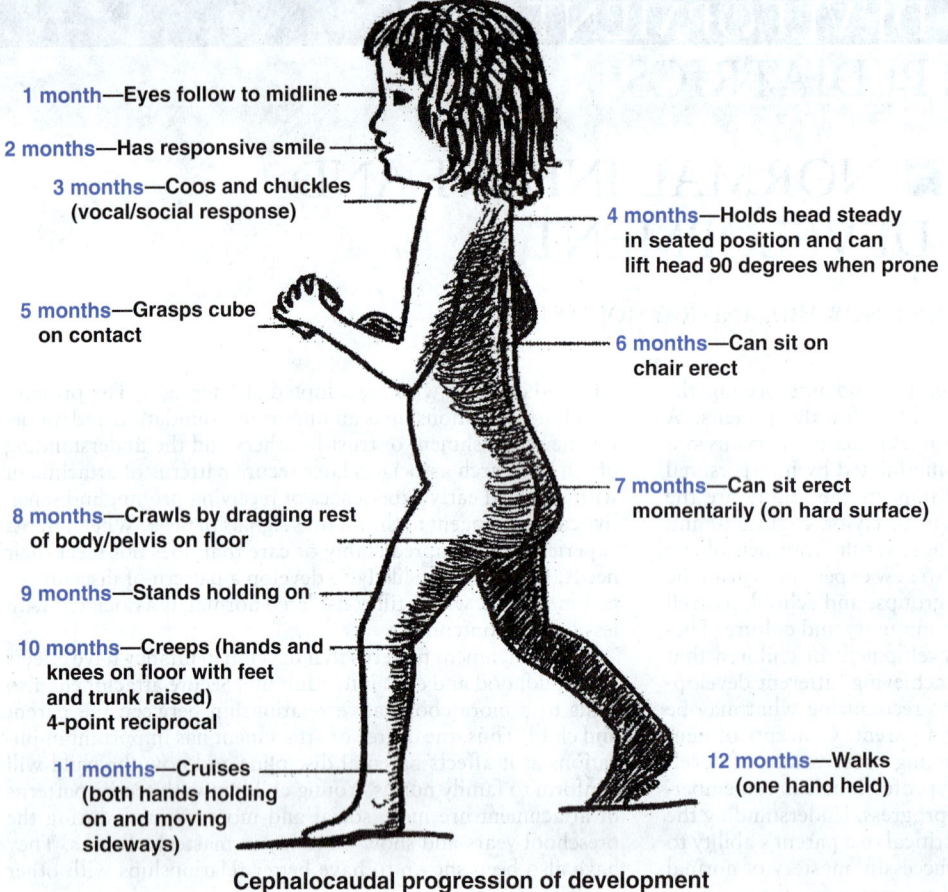

1 month—Eyes follow to midline

2 months—Has responsive smile

3 months—Coos and chuckles (vocal/social response)

4 months—Holds head steady in seated position and can lift head 90 degrees when prone

5 months—Grasps cube on contact

6 months—Can sit on chair erect

7 months—Can sit erect momentarily (on hard surface)

8 months—Crawls by dragging rest of body/pelvis on floor

9 months—Stands holding on

10 months—Creeps (hands and knees on floor with feet and trunk raised) 4-point reciprocal

11 months—Cruises (both hands holding on and moving sideways)

12 months—Walks (one hand held)

Cephalocaudal progression of development

FIGURE 96.1. Cephalocaudal progression. A good way to remember the milestones is to recall the words in quotation marks. Approximate age of attainment: 1 month: "Eyes"—past middle, 2 months: "Mouth"—responsive smile, 3 months: "Vocal Cords"—coo, 4 months: "Neck"—90 degree up prone, 5 months: "Hands"—grasp cube, 6 months: "Upper trunk"—supported sit, 7 months: "Lower trunk"—sit, 8 months: "Pelvis"—drag crawl, 9 months: "Knees"—supported stand, 10 months: "All together"—creep, 11 months: "Ankle"—cruise, 12 months: "Toes"—supported walk.

with their eyes past the midline, and by 4 months tracking is reliable for 180 degrees horizontally and vertical tracking is also possible. State control is more evident in longer bouts of sleep at night, even though total sleep is unchanged, and in more robust alertness during the day. The success of how parents help their infant regulate state cycles by setting routines of eating and sleeping, providing salient visual stimuli (such as faces and high-contrast rounded shiny objects), and avoiding overstimulation (such as excessive noise or handling) contribute to the development of attachment. Assistance with regulation of state is especially important for infants prone to suboptimal state control, such as those who are temperamentally irregular or have trouble adapting and those with neurologic damage, or neurotoxin or neuropharmacologic effects such as lead poisoning, or prenatal substance exposure.

Behavioral concerns parents may have related to state regulation include excessive crying and colic. Normal crying increases at 2 weeks postterm age and peaks around 6 to 8 weeks at $2\frac{3}{4}$ hours per day. It is usually worse at 6 to 11 PM at night. Crying decreases coinciding with increasing capacity to supress responses to sensory stimuli and new neural organization seen by such markers as a more adult-like EEG and visual evoked responses seen by 3 months of age and by the emergence of cooing and more hand-to-mouth movements and sucking. Parents can help reduce crying by swaddling tightly, providing white noise or shushing, vestibularly stimulating in the form of rocking or gentle swinging, or offering a finger or pacifier to suck.

Colic is defined as crying that is greater than or equal to 3 hours per day, 3 or more days per week for at least 3 weeks. Colic researchers usually also require additional signs such as burping, a reddened face, pulling the legs up to the stomach, and inconsolability to fully define colic. Crying reduces to 1 hour per day on its own by 4 months as the baby develops increased control over arousal, but colic-type crying may persist to 6 months. Although medications do not reliably reduce

colic, use of hydrolysate formula in addition to the consoling techniques previously described can help.

Sleep problems are another manifestation of emerging state regulation early in infancy but can easily become learned behavior even in the first 4 months. Initial regulation issues manifest as day–night reversal, but by 4 months postterm infants can have trained night feeding if it is reinforced by feeding and trained night waking if it is reinforced by attention and play. When object permanence is established around 8 to 10 months, night crying that is easily consoled can best be resolved over a 4 to 5 day stretch by allowing the baby to adapt to silent parental company if the infant does not return to sleep on his own. All sleep problems can be complicated by sleep associations after 2 months of age if infants are not helped to learn to fall asleep on their own by being placed in bed awake.

By 12 months of age state regulation problems manifest as temper tantrums, which are common as children's ideas overwhelm their abilities to do or say and their ability to control the resulting feelings. Parents should be advised that providing consistent rules helps reduce frustration and encourages the development of self-regulation. Although parents should not give in to the demands that result in temper tantrums, they can sympathize with and hold their child without reinforcing tantrum behavior. Children's efforts to regulate their own state—thumb sucking, head banging, rocking, masturbating—may be seen as problems by their caregivers (see later).

Need for Positive Emotional Tone and Need for Assistance Regulating Negative Affect

All children have a need for a positive emotional tone from their caregivers and assistance in regulating their negative affect. Positive emotional tone encourages development of secure attachment and enhances resilience under stress, which

TABLE 96.1

NORMAL MILESTONES AT 3 TO 12 MONTHS

	Gross Motor	Fine Motor	Language	Cognitive/Social/Adaptive
3 months	Supports on forearm in prone	Prereach, pointing motions	Cooing (long vowels)	Interacts differently with each parent and strangers, anticipates feeding
4 months	Supports on wrists, rolls prone to supine	Bats at objects, reaches with both arms, plays midline	Laughs, orients to voice	Associates experiences (sound of mother's voice with her face), enjoys looking around at environment
5 months	Sits supported, rolls supine to prone	Reaches more with hand that is closer to object, both arms reach	"Ah-goo," raspberry	
6 months	Sits unsupported, feet to mouth in supine	Unilateral reach, raking with all fingers	Babbles in one consonant syllables	Attached to primary caregiver, follows object trajectory
7 months	Creeps	Transfers objects from one hand to the other	Imitates sounds	Anticipates object trajectory, finger feeds
8 months	Comes to sit, crawls		"Dada" nonspecific	
9 months	Pivots when sitting, pulls to stand, cruises	Rotates hand when grasping an object	"Mama" nonspecific, waves "bye-bye," understands "no"	Uncovers objects hidden, gesture games
10 months	Stands 2 seconds	Picks up small object with pincer movement—thumb opposite several fingers	"Dada" and "mama" specifically	
11 months	Walks alone (ten independent steps)	Points with index finger	One-word, one-step command with gestures	
12 months	Supports on forearm in prone	Index finger opposes thumb in pincer	Two words, immature jargoning	Imitates, comes when called, cooperates with dressing

otherwise can evoke negative affect and aggression. When infants are unable to regulate their own negative emotions, assistance from their caregivers occurs through parental techniques of avoiding stress, distracting, and modeling coping strategies. Caregivers should acknowledge and verbalize the feelings their child is experiencing, thus giving the message that the child is understood and cared about. Excess hostility in the family raises tension and models aggression and may bring about an insecure attachment. Corporal punishment includes pain that can increase aggression and negative affect (Table 96.1).

Need for Mastery

By 9 months of age infants have an increased need for mastery. A common example of conflict from this occurs around feeding, even to the point of failure to thrive when infants are not allowed to exercise mastery over newly developed skills such as feeding themselves. If parents are unable to let them do this—most commonly because they want to avoid a mess or they are afraid that their child is not eating enough—then infants may actually refuse food. The solution is mandating self-feeding. To do this the anxious caregiver may need to read a magazine or do chores nearby to avoid showing concern or taking over the feedings.

Over the first 18 months of life, advances in cognitive, motor, and language development allow the infant to learn about and master the environment through sensory and motor exploration. Some principles about this developmental process are useful to recognize. An infant's response to outside stimuli progresses from generalized reflexes involving entire body movements to localized voluntary actions that are under more control. This allows the infant to develop intentional and pre-

cise movements. As the central nervous system (CNS) matures, afferent nerves undergo myelination before efferent nerves, explaining why sensory perception precedes motor development. For example, ocular combining (i.e., comparing objects visually) occurs before motor grasp (i.e., combining the hand with the object physically). As the efferent nerves are myelinated, development proceeds in a cephalocaudal–proximal–distal direction. This is seen as babies gain head control before trunk control and gain trunk control before they can reach with their hands. Development occurs in a continuous fashion, building on what has gone before; thus, premature infants can be expected to attain milestones at a chronologic age that is adjusted for their weeks of prematurity throughout life (although the adjustment becomes insignificant after about age 2 years). The sequence of attaining milestones of development is always the same in normally developing children, but there is a range in the age at which this occurs. In this chapter all ages should be considered typical of the range rather than defining norms. It is now evident that progress, even including physical growth, normally occurs in spurts with plateaus in progress in between.

Gross Motor Development

Gross motor development from 3 to 6 months extends caudally to include the neck and upper trunk, including the arms, and is characterized by extensor control emerging before control of flexor muscles. Thus, the head is lifted up 90 degrees when prone at 4 months (think "neck") before head lifts forward when supine at 5 months. Increasing abilities caudally in the lower back and legs allow supported sitting by 6 months (think "upper trunk") and unsupported sitting at 7 months (think "lower trunk"). The chest is held off the table and swimming movements occur when prone at 5 months. Development at 6 to 9 months includes distal control of the entire trunk and fingers such that after 6 months the infant can explore his or her world by drag crawling (think "pelvis") and by 9 months can stand with support (think "knees"). Around 10 months the child can creep, often in an odd way (think "put all together") and is soon able to pull to stand and cruise (think "ankle"). At 9 to 12 months distal control is completed, all the way to the feet for walking and fingers for pincering. Learning to stand alone and then walk by 12 months (think "toes") is the most notable gross motor milestone of the first year of life for parents. Once an infant begins to practice walking, the process seems to fuel itself, often replacing all other developmental progress for weeks at a time. Carrying, holding, or diapering an autonomy-driven 12-month-old can be almost impossible and can require jollying, distraction, fast action, and above all a sense of humor.

Fine Motor Development

Advances in fine motor control proceed distally along with inhibition of the opposite extremity to make object exploration possible for the baby. In the concept of continuous development, consider that primitive reflexes may assist this increased control (e.g., the asymmetric tonic neck reflex places the hand in view on the extended arm the baby faces; a parachute response is needed to be safe when learning to walk). Primitive reflexes are often incorporated into subsequent voluntary movements (e.g., the reflex grasp becoming the voluntary grasp). Inhibition of primitive reflexes is often needed for normal movement patterns to proceed (e.g., inhibition of the reflex grasp is needed to acquire a voluntary release; inhibition of the asymmetric tonic neck reflex is needed to roll over). Babies continue to explore by putting their fingers into everything they can, a drive that should not be interpreted as willful hurting or misbehavior. The period between 3 and 6 months is also the time when fine motor capabilities develop rapidly (think "hand"), progressing from barely detectable, prereach movements of the fingers at 3 months, to batting, bilateral reaching, and midline play at 4 months, to the ability to reach with the closer hand at 5 months, to a unilateral reach at 6 months. Fine motor progresses as more precise coordination of the hand makes it possible to pick up small objects. The superior overhand index finger–thumb pincer grasp is perfected by 1 year. At 12 months, children can make stabbing marks on paper with a pencil. By 15 months, they are able to control the pencil enough for scribbling marks, and at 18 months, they can imitate marks on paper. Fundamental manipulative skills reach adult levels by the end of infancy.

Language Development

Language development depends first on visual feedback and later requires auditory feedback to progress. Vocalization in babies begins with reflexive respiratory-type guttural sounds and short vowel sounds in the newborn. The production of long vowel sounds begins at 3 months in response to seeing a social partner (think "vocal cords"). Infants have enough respiratory support and control due to the cephalocaudal progression of trunk support to laugh and squeal at 4 months. Cooing becomes elaborated with razzing sounds by 5 months and simple single consonant babbling by 6 months, even in totally deaf babies who proceed by experimenting with their vocal tools. Further progress, however, requires the infant to hear themselves and others. Infants who can hear can come out with long, loud strings of vocalization by 6 months. At 8 months, "mama" and "dada" are said, at first nonspecifically and by 9 months specifically due to selective reinforcement by their parents. Language continues to progress from simple jargoning (syllables that sound like speech intonation but are not real words) to mature jargoning (which is like immature jargoning but with an actual word). Gesture language starts at 9 months (e.g., bye-bye, pat-a-cake, peek-a-boo). This demonstrates a new ability to imitate from memory combined with the earliest stage of recognizing that symbols can be a means of communication. By 12 months, babies understand a one-step command given with a gesture and can say one word other than "mama" and "dada." At 16 months, vocabulary expands to an average of 40 words, but there is immense individual variability in word production during the second year of life, with some normal children having only a few words by 18 months when the average toddler is already beginning to combine two words. At 15 months, children can begin to follow a one-step command without a gesture.

Cognitive Development

Cognitive development has perhaps best been described by Piaget. He described the first 18 months of cognitive development as the sensorimotor stage. For the first 2 months, the infant's first strategies for organizing experiences are by primitive reflexes such as grasping and rooting. At this stage actions relate only to the immediate environment experienced by the senses and the motor system. Within 3 months, most infants show discrimination by responding differently to their primary caregiver with smoother interactions and more smiling and vocalizing, compared with other people at whom they may simply stare. Between 3 and 6 months, infants continue to refine their mental model of how the world works. By 4 months, the baby has observed and remembered what sounds go with what visual perceptions and show surprise, for example, if the wrong voice comes from a video of a familiar person. By 6 months, infants follow the path of an object dropped in front of them and then look back up as to see whether it will happen again, showing a memory of this type of action. After 6 months, developing infants move on to a stage where they can begin to control at least some aspects of their world, and to know that they are the ones doing this.

The development of object permanence, or the ability to maintain a visual representation in memory of objects when they are hidden or removed, is a major cognitive milestone. Games such as "peek-a-boo" are enjoyed by infants, and eventually they develop games where they want to hide from the parent. This developmental transition extends to infants' ability to remember the primary attachment figures when they are not physically present. This awareness of the primary caregiver's absence often leads to anxiety and distress that is relieved with the reappearance of the caregiver. This is the time of developmental night waking—crying out for the parent they now understand is out there somewhere. During this period infants may also protest the approach of strangers and cling to the primary caregiver in the presence of a stranger—so characteristic as to be called 8-month stranger anxiety even though it may be seen in some infants several months earlier. This period of anxiety is a normal developmental transition that is tied to neurodevelopmental maturation and moderates in a few months; however, anxiety about separation may not be reliably mastered until age 4 years, as seen by the high frequency of normal separation problems for preschool, although its degree is highly related to temperament. By 12 months, infants understand enough about the permanent nature of objects to uncover an object that they have seen hidden and love to practice this through hiding games. They also indicate that they know which functions to expect from various objects and will specifically shake rattles and bang blocks.

In the second year, locomotion increases so that active sensorimotor exploration of the more distant environment is possible. At the same time, expressive vocabulary expands and children learn that they can change their environment through gestures and words; they will show this with demands even for things they really don't want when they get them, much to the frustration of caregivers. Children develop increasingly more complex behaviors to explore the surroundings and wield their influence on the people around them. The relationship with caregivers matures to include reciprocal communication of asking and showing. Children 12 months old practice independence by walking away, demanding what they want, and trying anything but without recognizing that it has consequences. Temper tantrums begin at about 1 year as children confront feelings that are beyond their control, with frustration for not getting what they can now imagine they want as the most common reason. Other reasons include anxiety and difficulty in choosing or doing something. Children with uneven skills (e.g., language delay or poor fine motor control) are particularly prone to tantrums, since they can imagine far more than they can accomplish.

The period from 15 to 18 months is marked by a shift in children's appreciation of their attachment relationship. Having developed some independence, they suddenly realize that they are truly separate from their parents and therefore vulnerable. This often coincides with new motor ability to explore at further distance from their parents. They enter a period of clinging and anxiety known as rapprochement. They want once again to be held, carried, and cared for exclusively by their mother. This is particularly alarming to mothers who are pregnant again as they wonder how they will cope. If mothers resist this clinging it only worsens. A brief hug promptly usually suffices. Self-consoling habits like thumb sucking, masturbating, rocking, head banging, and using transitional objects ("lovies") are prominent during this period of increased awareness of vulnerability and the stress of developmental un-

evenness. If these repetitive habits do not interfere with other activities, they should be allowed as a normal part of development. If they are severe and persistent, further evaluation is needed regarding the child's developmental progress and the adequacy of the caregiving at home and in childcare settings.

The Need to Learn Prosocial Behavior and Empathy

From toddlerhood through adolescence the new needs are in learning how to effectively relate to others. For toddlers this generally means the family. Struggles to cope and be socialized in childcare settings such as biting, pinching, and grabbing reflect the immaturity of these skills for getting along in larger groupings. Although delayed gratification through turn taking is progressively taught and consequences such as "time out" can reduce undesirable behavior from as young an age as 9 months, parental expectations for social skills must often be moderated or the setting adjusted.

18 MONTHS TO 3 YEARS: HOLDING ON AND LETTING GO (TABLE 96.2)

The second developmental task in life according to Erikson is establishing autonomy rather than succumbing to shame and doubt. With newfound gross motor ability and fine motor manipulation, the toddler faces two major conflicting desires: to hold on or let go. That is, toddlers want to both grow up and also stay close to parents. This can be a great source of tension for both the child and the parent. Erikson described this in his book *Childhood and Society*:

TABLE 96.2

NORMAL MILESTONES AT 12 TO 36 MONTHS

	Gross Motor	Fine Motor: Blocks and Drawing	Fine Motor: Feeding and Dressing	Cognitive/Language
12 months	Walks with arms up, in high guard	Stacks two blocks, stabs with a pencil	Uses cup, cooperates briefly in dressing	One to two words, follows one-step command with gesture
15 months	Runs, pivots, walks backwards	Stacks two blocks, scribbles	Uses spoon, removes shoes	Four to six words, immature jargon, follows one-step command without gesture
18 months	Walks up stairs with rail, throws a ball	Stacks three to four blocks, imitates stroke on paper	Uses spoon for solids with little spilling, takes off most clothes	10+ words, combines two words, understands two-part command, names pictures, points to body parts
21 months	Squats during play	Stacks four to five blocks		50 words, names body parts
24 months	Jumps with two feet, stands briefly on one foot, kicks ball, walks downstairs two feet per step	Stacks eight blocks, imitates vertical line	Rotates spoons so that semisolids stay in place, puts on some clothes	300 words, noun–verb sentences, 25% of speech understandable, follows commands with two actions on two objects
30 months	Jumps forward, stands on one foot for 1 second	Imitates horizontal line, draws circle with perseverating lines	Pulls on pants	Uses "I" and other pronouns
36 months	Alternates feet on stairs, can tricycle	Stacks ten blocks, copies circle	Eats neatly, dresses with supervision	900 words, first and last name, age, and sex, colors, three- to four-word sentences, asks "why" incessantly, 75% understandable, understands cold, tired, hungry

"Thus, to hold can become a destructive and cruel retaining or restraining … To let go, too, can turn into an inimical letting loose of destructive forces … From a sense of self-control without loss of self-esteem comes a lasting sense of good will and pride; from a sense of loss of self-control and of foreign overcontrol comes a lasting propensity for doubt and shame."

Toddlers who have secure attachments may be seen running off to explore the environment and then running back to the secure base of the parent. Toddlers have an innate drive to explore and learn about the world and master new skills by repetition. Creating a safe environment for toddlers to explore is important; however, being too protective, preventing the toddler from learning and inhibiting the development of self-confidence. Not being afforded an opportunity to explore signals to the child a lack of confidence by the parent that can increase the likelihood of an attachment pattern characterized by anxiety.

Gross motor capabilities expand with increased strength, balance, and inhibition, allowing unilateral skills so that at 18 months, toddlers can walk up stairs placing the weight on one leg using a hand rail and can throw a ball. By 21 months, they can squat and recover during play. By 24 months, they can jump with two feet and free one leg to kick a ball. They can begin to walk down stairs as well. By 30 months, they can jump and balance on one foot for 1 second as needed to climb out of a crib. At 36 months, they can alternate their feet on the stairs and peddle a tricycle.

Fine motor skills also refine and combine with cognitive abilities so that toddlers have the visual–perceptual–motor skills to manipulate objects with dexterity. At 24 months, toddlers can imitate a vertical line on paper, and by 30 months, they can imitate a horizontal line. By 36 months, they can copy a circle. Fine motor coordination allows them autonomy with dressing. By 18 months, they can undress themselves. At 30 months, they can pull on pants, and by 36 months they are mostly able to dress themselves with supervision, aside from tying shoe laces. Increasing fine motor ability allows an 18-month-old to use a spoon for solids and a 24-month-old to rotate the spoon during feeding. By 36 months, toddlers should have control to eat neatly.

Language skills continue by adding vocabulary and grammatical understanding so that toddlers become more conversational. Two-year-olds can understand simple commands and sentences. While there is large variation in the development of language skills, by 2 years only about 10% of children are not yet combining words or have a vocabulary of less than 50 words. By the end of the second year, they can understand prepositions and opposites, and are able to follow a story with pictures. By 30 months, they understand the concept of "give me one" and some number concepts. Expressive vocabulary expands to an average of 300 words by 2 years to 900 words by 3 years. The average sentence length doubles between 24 and 30 months. They may be able to speak in simple three-part sentences with a subject, adjective, and verb. However, it is not uncommon for there to be a disconnect between comprehension and production causing frustration and associated tantrum behavior in the child who is unable to express what he (usually males) understands. By 36 months, toddlers use pronouns, can ask "what" and "where" questions, and develop rules of grammar such as progressive and past tense and plurals. They can participate in turn taking in conversation and pay attention to the same subject as the adult in a conversation. This is called "joint attention" and is an important part of social language. By 36 months, toddlers are able to tell their name, age, and gender.

Two-year-olds are able to use language to expand on play and put different activities together to make a play sequence. Toddlers begin to have symbolic play. They may feed their dolls or "build" something with toys. Older toddlers use pretend play to learn about things. They may begin to "try on roles" they see in adults. For example, toddlers can pretend to be superheroes or their parents.

After 18 months, children's cognitive abilities are no longer limited to sensorimotor exploration. They enter a new stage that Piaget called "symbolic preoperational thinking." In this stage, they are able to use things to represent other things. Piaget called this "symbolic function." In this preoperational thinking phase, toddlers are still egocentric; that is, they are unable to see things from another person's point of view. Receptive language and cognitive ability generally develop before expressive language. Consequently, toddlers can imagine danger without being able to talk about fear. Emotions may also be overwhelming for the toddler. This imbalance can be expressed by tantrums, as they are toddlers' only way of communicating their distress to their parents. Parents need to modulate their toddlers' environment and help them deal with frustration that does occur by verbalizing it for them, distracting, and comforting rather than seeing all emotional meltdowns as cause for discipline.

Toddlers show interest in gaining independence by asserting their will on others. They may say "no" to everything, or insist on doing everything themselves. They are learning that they have an impact on their environment, but they are unsure how far to push this newfound independence with parents and other caregivers. Toddlers are driven to figure out what the rules are. In trying to master this, they frequently push the limits and test their parents. Parents who provide consistent rules help prepare their toddlers for learning rules outside of the home.

The time between 12 months and 3 years is the period when sexual identification occurs. Gender differences are evident as early as 3 months, with greater activity and greater aggressiveness in boys by 12 months. By 2 years, boys and girls prefer playing with same-sex peers. By 3 years, they have distinctly different toy preferences, can reliably state their gender, imitate their same-gender parent, and begin flirting with the opposite-gender parent.

Children who are rapidly learning to control their motor and language skills soon face the social task of toilet training. When children's normal desire for mastery is respected, learning to use the toilet becomes a source of pride. A child-centered approach is to wait to start training until children are able to give some signal just before they need to void, and then beginning by seating them on a potty chair regularly after meals. Simply waiting until they are 2½ and can be expected to have persistent motivation for desired underpants and imitation of peer models is another option.

At 2 years old, a toddler's drive for autonomy leads to separateness from parents and forming a sense of self. Toddlers develop a sense of self and their place in the world by doing things in their own way, testing their abilities, testing limits, and seeing how adults respond to them. This is an uneven process, however, and toddlers push parents away 1 minute and cling to them the next. This period of growing and separating can be very hard for toddlers and parents alike. They are experiencing a range of moods, emotions, and needs that can be overwhelming. Easily adaptable or even-tempered toddlers may be able to adjust and adapt to these intense experiences with little difficulty. Other children may really struggle with changes in routine, separations, or limit setting. Toddlers need adults to be supportive of their struggle for independence to feel good about themselves. There are some toddlers who may not tolerate the feelings associated with separating from parents and parents who have a difficult time letting go of their babies. These patterns may interfere with autonomy development and lead to problems such as anxiety. The two-year-old's sense of self extends to a strong sense of what they consider to be their property rights (the desired object of the moment). At this age, playing with an object tends to be more interesting than playing with a peer. Their attempts to defend territory makes them more difficult social beings until interest in peers rises in ensuring years.

3 TO 6 YEARS: IMAGINATION AND MASTERY

Erikson's third developmental task is asserting initiative without excessive guilt. He describes the preschool child in this phase in his book *Childhood and Society*:

> "Initiative adds to autonomy the quality of undertaking, planning, and 'attacking' a task for the sake of being active and on the move.... The danger of this stage is a sense of guilt over the goals contemplated and the acts initiated in one's exuberant enjoyment of new locomotor and mental power: acts of aggressive manipulation and coercion which soon go far beyond the executive capacity of organism and mind and therefore call for an energetic halt on one's contemplated initiative."

Three-year-olds are much more capable of problem solving than toddlers, but they still do not think the same way adults do. The hallmark of their cognition at this stage is "magical thinking" because of the ways they try to understand their world. Three-year-olds are still somewhat self-centered and cannot always figure out logical explanations for events (e.g., they often think they are the cause of events). They are still very concrete in their thinking and remain as visual thinkers, only able to pay attention to one aspect of a problem at a time. As a result, preschoolers often come up with very interesting explanations for events (e.g., they may believe that clouds follow them home or that they make rain happen when they are sad). Three-year-olds may think they are going to the doctor when they get into the car because that is where they went the last time. Children's anxieties are eased when caregivers guess at or ask the child what they think is happening and why and address that rather than using nonspecific reassurance or punishment.

Gross motor skills at this age develop to adult capabilities. From 3 to 4 years of age, children can pedal a tricycle and hop on one foot without support. By $4\frac{1}{2}$ years they can skip and make a broad jump. By 5 years old, they can pump a swing. Fine motor skills become refined so that $3\frac{1}{2}$-year-olds can cut with scissors. By 4 years they begin to draw recognizable pictures usually beginning with a tadpole-like person with three body parts. By 5 years old they can begin to print their first name if they have received instruction.

Language development continues to progress based on cognitive advances. From 3 to 4 years of age, children begin to understand and verbalize the concepts of size, numbers, and shapes. They can count to five and identify four colors. Sentence structure matures to combining sentences with conjunctions. From 4 to 5 years old, children can follow a series of three simple instructions. They begin to read a few letters and can tell the meaning of familiar words.

Preschool children continue to learn about the social world through play interactions with peers and siblings. They begin to develop "pretend play," which is representational, consisting of fantasy. This emerges earlier, even at 18 months, when there is play with an older imaginative sibling. Play becomes a way of imitating and practicing events that they are exposed to for the purpose of learning, practicing communication, developing social skills, and enhancing motor and perceptual skills. Play can also serve to ease anxiety. This is seen when children "act" as superheroes to defeat evil villains. Preschool children develop the capacity for "magical thinking" in which irrational but nevertheless magical solutions to problems or events seem possible. For example, children at this age have a perception of death as reversible. Their play may involve "killing" someone and having them come back to life. Thus, "the imaginative play of children serves mental health by keeping the boundaries between fantasy and reality."

At 3 years old, children start becoming less "self-focused" and more of a social being, aware of the needs of others. Preschoolers rapidly learn about rules and ways to behave with others. Three-year-olds love to play with friends and create elaborate games of pretend and make-believe. They are now first able to truly share, not just take turns, as they can see another's point of view. Three-year-olds are more aware of adult roles and have relationships with adults they know. In the third year, they can play cooperatively with other children with minimal conflict and supervision. At 4 years old, they become protective toward younger children. By $4\frac{1}{2}$ years they can play simple board or card games, able to follow the rules. By 5 years, they can establish leadership among other children.

Three-year-olds generally are toilet trained but may need assistance with undressing and hygiene. By $3\frac{1}{2}$ years they can wash their face without help and by 4 years they can dress and undress alone except for shoelaces. In the fourth year, they learn to manipulate buttons. By 5 years, children are able to go to the toilet and wipe without assistance. Although 3-year-olds are still dealing with issues of separation from parents, they may have moved past the intense struggles of the toddler years and are more focused on figuring out their place in the world.

Most normal children go through a phase in development where they develop a love attachment to the parent of the opposite sex, called the "Oedipus complex" as described by Sigmund Freud. During this time, the child imagines the death of their same-sex parent so that they can fulfill that role for the opposite-sex parent. This, of course, leads to contradictory feelings for children as they do not want their parents to die. During the time of the struggle, children may act out more around the same-sex parent as a result of the guilty feelings. Eventually this struggle ends with identification with the same-sex parent and children resolving, "If I cannot take his/her place, I will try to be like him/her." Parents can help their children overcome this struggle by showing affection for each other in front of them and by having the same-sex parent spend more play time with them.

6 TO 12 YEARS OLD: NEED TO SUCCEED

Erikson described the major developmental task of school-aged children as the struggle between showing personal industry rather than succumbing to a sense of inferiority. In *Childhood and Society*, he describes this conflict:

> "The child must forget past hopes and wishes, while his exuberant imagination is tamed and harnessed to the laws of impersonal things—even the three Rs. The child's danger, at this stage, lies in a sense of inadequacy and inferiority."

During this stage, school-aged children have a drive to be successful both academically and socially. If they are unable to be successful, they run the risk of becoming discouraged and "consider themselves doomed to mediocrity or inadequacy."

Cognition changes as the school-aged child enters what Piaget called the "Concrete Operational Stage" in early school age. In this way of thinking, children's representations are connected systematically and logically rather than in the inconsistent way of preschoolers. The world is no longer a magical place, but one of order and predictability. The limit of concrete operations is that children can only operate on things that are present or experienced. New skills acquired in this thought stage are classification, seriation, and conservation. Classification consists of forming vertical and branching hierarchies and seeing the relationships among things. Seriation refers to things being ordered horizontally in lists and rows (e.g., occurring sequentially in time). Conservation means there is an understanding of which transformations change the nature of a thing and which leave its fundamental character intact. For example, at this age children now know that one quart of water poured into a tall thin cylinder and a short fat cylinder is the same amount of water. Preoperational-thinking children would have believed that the water in the taller cylinder was of a greater amount. It is with this better grasp of size and time relationships that children are ready to profit from formal math instruction. As categorizing skills become more refined, some children begin to be fascinated by making collections of objects like stamps and cards, or by having "all" of any set.

Primary developmental tasks during the elementary school years include acquisition of symbol-associative learning, rule-governed play, increased awareness of social expectations, and mastery of more complex cognitive and academic tasks. Elementary-age children typically show great initiative in acquiring new knowledge and skills, and this contributes to their self-esteem. All children want to be successful in the academic arena. "Poor motivation" is not an adequate explanation for school failure. When it seems to be present, an investigation into specific academic weaknesses or mental health difficulties is necessary. A secure parent–child relationship, praising rather than shaming efforts, and consistent and appropriate role modeling of academic interests are the best incentives for achievement.

The ability to succeed in school demands the ability to delay gratification, a skill affected by impulse control, children's experience with having needs met, and the ability to control attention. Typically, attention becomes more focused and sustained during first and second grade. A 6-year-old should be able to focus for about 15 minutes on an appropriate task. A 9-year-old should be able to pay attention for close to an hour. It is important to note that the fact that a child can watch TV or play video games for long periods is not an index of attentional control. TV and video games are more fast paced and stimulating than the normal world that requires attention.

Receptive language skills should expand so that school-aged children are able to understand multistep complex instructions. At 6 years, a child can follow at least three commands in a row; older children can follow five. As children learn to read, they need to understand the rules of grammar and syntax. Children can usually do these things as well as articulate all sounds of the language by the time they are 7. Between 7 and 10 years, mastery of irregular verb forms and tenses should appear. Expressive language continues to develop. At 6 years, children should be able to express feelings and thoughts. Difficulty in expressive language can be subtle and difficult to identify, but children who don't express themselves adequately have more difficulty with emotion regulation and in social situations because they are not able to express themselves verbally and thus break down or act aggressively. They may also have more difficulty academically because they are not as able as their peers to show their teachers how much they know.

Advances in motor development and athletic skills progress to the point that children can function on organized sports teams. The added advantage of group participation is the opportunity to learn rules and practice social interaction. Interaction with peers is important to continued development. Play becomes increasingly complex during this age period as children develop the capacity to play board or card games that involve complex rules.

In the early grades, friendships are usually same sex, but as puberty approaches, friendships extend to the opposite sex. During middle childhood, peer pressure to conform to group standards of appearance, dress, and behavior can be intense as children try to find their place outside the family norms. Cliques may form in which children practice including and excluding. Friends one day may not be friends the next day. Parents may have difficulty in letting their child conform to peer standards. However, some conformity is important to allow children to fit in with their peer group without getting labeled as an outsider. Children begin to form close heterosexual friendships by the time they are 12.

School refusal has two peaks: at first grade and at the start of middle school. Usually, the school refusal in the first grade has to do with separation anxiety in the child and/or the parent. In this case, the child must be required to go to school and family dynamics addressed. When older children don't want to go to school, it is important to explore the cause. These can be learning disabilities, vision or hearing problems, violence at home or school, substance abuse, peer conflicts, testing limits, or mood disorders.

Moral development and empathy continue to progress from a concrete level of rule following toward more independent thinking about right and wrong. As children learn to negotiate the rules of society, they may engage in the behaviors of lying, cheating, or stealing. Children lie, steal, or cheat, among other things, to fulfill fantasies, save face, test limits, or fit in to a peer group. By 6 or 7 years, most children know the difference between reality and what they wish were real, but a few—especially those who have had few successes in the real world—have such great needs that they describe fantasy as if it were real. This is an example of the struggle of industry and inferiority; children want to perceive themselves as successful and may not be able to face the fact that they are not. They may then lie or steal to enhance their image of themselves. In these cases, children may need more opportunities to be successful. Given a situation where admitting guilt ("did you do this?") will incriminate a child or make him or her look stupid or weak, he or she will probably lie. Incriminating questions are best not asked; there are even laws in this country saying that adults do not have to incriminate themselves. Lying to test limits is part of the child's effort to find out what the rules are and how they are enforced. Consistent limit setting with consequences for violations is the best way to manage this. Stealing is also common in the primary grades. Child who steal from a parent, for example, may be feeling rejected or inadequately nurtured. Stealing from a store is designed to test the limits of familial and societal rules and should be handled with clear consequences but without humiliation.

12 TO 17 YEARS: NEED FOR SEPARATION

Erikson described the conflict of adolescence as that of establishing an identity rather than remaining in role confusion. He describes this in *Childhood and Society*:

> "The growing and developing youths, faced with this physiological revolution within them, and with tangible adult tasks ahead of them are now primarily concerned with what they appear to be in the eyes of others as compared with what they feel they are, and with the question of how to connect the roles and skills cultivated earlier with the occupational prototypes of the day. In their search for a new sense of continuity and sameness, adolescents have to refight many of the battles of earlier years, even though to do so they must artificially appoint perfectly well-meaning people to play the roles of adversaries; and they are ever ready to install lasting idols and ideals as guardians of a final identity."

The danger of this stage is continuing role confusion. Adolescents struggle with how they will eventually play a role in society as an adult. They struggle with their self-image and with their sexual identity. To keep themselves together they temporarily overidentify with peer subgroups, to the point of potentially becoming lost within cliques and crowds.

Cognitive development during the adolescent years is characterized by gradually attaining the capacity for abstract thought and hypothetical–deductive reasoning. They can hypothesize about "what could be" and develop the ability to strategize and problem solve. Piaget described this as "formal operational thinking" that forms the basis of logical and scientific thought. Adolescents also have an increased ability to monitor their own thoughts and feelings and report on them, which may appear to adults as an egocentric thinking style. Adolescents may believe and act as though they are "on stage" and their behavior is the focus of interest for everyone else.

Socially, adolescents experience significant changes in their relationships with peers and parents. Their quest for identity occurs through greater autonomy and frequently leads to disagreements with their parents over responsibilities and the extent of their freedom. Adolescents spend most of their time with peers, which offers occasions for further development of social skills and identity formation but also antisocial behavior if that is the norm of their chosen group. There is also a desire for closer intimacy with one partner, the gender choice seeming to be biologically determined. As society prescribes this to be with a member of the opposite sex, homosexual feelings or experiences are a cause for upset in an adolescent and to anyone to whom they reveal these feelings. Homosexual feelings in adolescence should be asked about as they are associated with peer bullying abuse, depression, running way, lesser school achievement, and much greater risk for suicide.

The adolescent develops a set of psychological supports that has been referred to as the "armor of middle adolescence": the helmet of omniscience, which makes them all knowing; the breast plate of omnipotence, which makes them all powerful; and the shield of invincibility, which gives them the ability to defend against and defeat every foe. This psychological armor functions as a double-edged sword. Although it allows adolescents to feel safe enough to separate themselves from their family, it also makes them feel invincible, which may interfere with judgment and result in excessive risk-taking behaviors. Adolescents really believe that they cannot be hurt, get pregnant, flunk out of school, etc. Very commonly, the struggle for autonomy and identity in adolescents is a cause for discord within the family as parents try to keep their child safe or mold their sense of responsibility. A gradual transfer of freedom based on demonstration of responsibility and good judgment should be sought. These struggles may also manifest in other areas such as school or society where adolescents continue to test rules. The peer group replaces the family as a source of values and "norms" and functions to mold the adolescent's self-image during the quest for identity.

Adolescence is a time set aside in our culture for children to learn how to be adults but often without real responsibility and its corresponding rewards. They feel that they must emancipate themselves from the family, establish their sexual identity, establish their intellectual identity, and place themselves within society. In short, they must determine "what they are going to do with the rest of their lives." The end of adolescence ushers in adulthood.

In summary, it is important for physicians caring for children to understand normal child development and psychological theory to translate the meaning of child behavior to the family. By providing anticipatory guidance about stage-related behaviors, many child–parent struggles may be avoided or guided to an optimal outcome.

Suggested Readings

Ainsworth M. The development of infant-mother attachment. In: Caldwell B, Ricciuti H, eds. *Review of child development research*. Chicago: University of Chicago Press, 1973:1.

Bowlby J. *Attachment and loss: Volume 2. Separation*. New York: Basic, 1973.

Bretherton I, Munholland K. Internal working models in attachment relationships. In: Cassidy J, Lewis M, eds. *Handbook of attachment*. New York: Guilford, 1999:89.

Culbertson JE, Newman JE, Willis DJ. Childhood and adolescent psychologic development. *Pediatr Clin North Am* 2003;50:741.

Dixon S, Stein MT. *Encounters with children: pediatric behavior and development*, 3rd ed. Elsevier Science, St. Louis: Mosby, 2000.

Erikson E. Eight ages of man. In: Erikson E, ed. *Childhood and society*. W.W. Norton, 1950:247.

Fraiberg SH. *The magic years*. New York: Charles Scribner's Sons, 1959.

Johnson RL. Adolescent social development. *Pediatr Rev* 1995;16:158.

Piaget J, Inhelder B. *The psychology of the child*. Paris: Presses Universitaires de France, 1969.

Sroufe L, Carlson E, Schulman S. Individuals in relationships: development from infancy through adolescence. In: Funder D, Parke RD, Tomlinson-Keasey C, et al., eds. *Studying lives through time*. Washington, D.C.: American Psychological Association, 1993:315.

Sroufe L, Rutter M. The domain of developmental psychopathology. *Child Dev* 1984;55:17.

Steinberg L. *Adolescence*, 6th ed. Boston: McGraw-Hill College, 2002.

Thompson R. Early attachment and later development. In: Cassidy J, Shaver P, eds. *Handbook of attachment*. New York: Guilford, 1999:265.

Walters E, Kondo-Ikemura K, Posada G, et al. Learning to love: mechanisms and milestones. In: Gunnar M, Sroufe L, eds. *Self processes and development*. Hillsdale, 1991:217.

CHAPTER 97 ■ STREAMS OF DEVELOPMENT: THE KEY TO DEVELOPMENTAL ASSESSMENT

FREDERICK B. PALMER AND ARNOLD J. CAPUTE*

The neurodevelopmental disabilities are diverse but related clinical syndromes of chronic neurologic dysfunction. They can be considered best under the broad and frequently overlapping categories of cerebral palsy, mental retardation, communicative disorders (including the autism spectrum disorders), and neurobehavioral disorders. The syndromes are grouped together because of similarities in presentation, natural history, and traditional treatments, not because of common etiologies. The common thread is the existence of nonprogressive central nervous system (CNS) dysfunction, which results in a functionally significant disruption of the otherwise expected typical sequences of infant and child development.

PEDIATRICIAN'S ROLE IN MANAGING NEURODEVELOPMENTAL DISABILITIES

The pediatrician's role in managing neurodevelopmental disabilities must include but transcend the provision of general

---

*Deceased.

health care. This expanded role includes responsibilities for detection, developmental diagnosis, developmental monitoring, and coordination of developmental services. It requires familiarity with local health, educational, early intervention, social, and other resources. It requires a working knowledge of local intervention program eligibility standards, changing funding options, and other practical issues influencing access to services, especially in a managed-care setting in which the primary-care pediatrician is central in obtaining access to appropriate services. The pediatrician also must recognize family, cultural, and community factors that may influence development or affect efforts to diagnose and treat disability.

The detection or recognition that a child has delayed or atypical development has been a traditional pediatric role because of the almost universal contact with the infant and the family during the first few years of life. Attention to developmental progress should be part of every well-child encounter. Sick-child visits or hospitalizations also offer the opportunity to elicit developmental concerns from caregivers, and these concerns can be explored at later encounters.

The detection of developmental abnormalities can be achieved only partially by a recognition of the risk factors associated with concurrent or subsequent neurodevelopmental disability. Few risk factors have an extremely high likelihood of poor neurodevelopmental outcome. Most factors are unlikely to be associated with disability in an individual child. Moreover, many infants who develop disabilities have no clear history of risk. In most cases, therefore, detection relies on the recognition of neurodevelopmental abnormality—usually a delay in one or more developmental streams.

Developmental screening tests have been used widely in pediatric practice for years. They are not at the same time highly sensitive and specific for neurodevelopmental abnormality, and they do not yield an acceptably small number of false-positive results. That is, a high number of infants with disability, mostly those with milder disabilities, are not detected; some infants without disability are inaccurately designated as having a delay or disability. These are major difficulties, especially when negative screening test results lead to pediatrician complacency and no further efforts at detection, or when frustration with test validity leads to an abandonment of systematic developmental surveillance. The pediatrician should take a broader clinical approach to developmental detection, rather than solely relying on published screening measures.

Developmental diagnosis includes a delineation of the specific neurodevelopmental disability—cerebral palsy, mental retardation, communication disorder, or neurobehavioral disorder—and a quantitation of its severity. A complete developmental diagnosis must recognize the overlaps among these diagnoses. For example, mental retardation and cerebral palsy can coexist, or the child with mental retardation can have an additional expressive language disorder. Other associated disabilities, such as neurobehavioral problems (e.g., deficits in attention), seizures, orthopedic abnormalities, sensory dysfunctions, or growth abnormalities, must be identified. A complete developmental diagnosis usually requires information from other specialists in medical and nonmedical disciplines, which is usually best compiled by and interpreted for the parents by the pediatrician.

Developmental monitoring and coordination of services often can be accomplished by the pediatrician because of his or her orientation as a generalist and experience in dealing with families, schools, and other community agencies. Particularly for younger infants and children, in whom all the manifestations of a neurodevelopmental disability may not yet be clear, the pediatrician must not abdicate this responsibility to other professionals, such as teachers or therapists.

DEVELOPMENTAL STREAMS AND THEIR ASSESSMENT

For the pediatrician to fulfill these roles adequately, a general framework for developmental assessment is necessary. (The framework summarized in this chapter is expanded on in Chapters 98 and 396.) For decades, pediatricians have separated the complex developmental processes into separate developmental streams for easier evaluation. These developmental streams, including language, visuomotor skills, gross and fine motor skills, social development, and self-help, are best analyzed separately. An analysis of each should focus on detecting delay and deviancy.

Developmental delay is best quantitated by the developmental quotient: DQ = developmental age/chronologic age × 100. In children with nonprogressive CNS abnormalities (e.g., static encephalopathies), it represents the rate of development in the measured stream. It provides only a rough guideline for measuring progress. Because it implies a constant rate of development from birth, it should be used with caution after CNS injury acquired during infancy and childhood and when a progressive neurologic process may be present. A language or visuomotor quotient of less than 80 should be seen as frank delay, but a gross motor quotient of less than 50 is generally necessary before ultimate motor disability is likely.

Developmental deviancy, a subtle sign of CNS abnormality, refers to atypical development within a single stream, such as developmental milestones occurring out of normal sequence (e.g., infant who walks before crawling—often associated with mild central hypotonia). Deviancy is useful in detecting mild abnormalities within a given stream if overt delay is not apparent. A recognition of the dissociations between rates of development in different streams is essential for the early diagnosis of atypical development within a specific stream.

COGNITIVE ASSESSMENT

Language

The best single measure of cognitive development in infancy and childhood is language development. Traditional psychologic testing relies heavily on language in its determination of an intelligence quotient, beginning in the preschool years and extending through school age and into adulthood. This is true as early as the third year of life, for which the Stanford-Binet Intelligence Test remains the most commonly used instrument. The Wechsler Scales, the most frequently used intelligence tests in the school years and adulthood, also emphasize the use of language. Infant developmental scales, such as the Bayley Scales of Infant Development and the Cattell Infant Intelligence Test, make less use of language items as measures of developmental progress. However, infant language can be used as an objective tool for early assessment, if professionals are familiar with language markers, their occurrence in typical children, patterns of delay and deviance, and limitations in their use.

The pediatric assessment of early language relies almost entirely on milestones. These prelinguistic and linguistic milestones are related to later cognitive development, and a recognition of early language delay is the most sensitive indicator of subsequent mental retardation or communication disorder. Subtle manifestations of language delay or deviancy indicate the risk for school-aged learning disability and general academic underachievement.

The assessment of infant expressive language development begins in the prelinguistic phase with the sequential occurrence of cooing, babbling, indiscriminate "dada" and "mama," and the discriminate "dada" and "mama," followed by the child's first true word at approximately 1 year of age. With the development of words used spontaneously and with clear meaning, the child enters the linguistic phase. Between 12 and 24 months, an accelerating increase in vocabulary size occurs, which continues through the school years; it is easily measured up to approximately 2 years of age. Similarly, the increase in phrase length occurs with the sole use of single words to approximately 20 months of age, followed by development of two-word phrases, short sentences, and eventually near-normal adult syntax by the late preschool years.

Receptive language development can be traced into the prelinguistic phase of the first several months of life. The earliest receptive language skills are neurosensory. They represent peripheral auditory functioning and the CNS response to sound. The normal newborn alerts to sound by crying, quieting, or otherwise changing state, and by startling, blinking, or by other recognizable responses. By 4 months of age, the child orients to voice by turning to the source of the sound.

Delay in achieving this 4-month skill of auditory orienting may indicate hearing loss, but it may also indicate CNS dysfunction, as seen in mental retardation or communication disorders. It may indicate that the child's receptive language abilities are not yet at the 4-month level. By 9 months of age, the child should indicate his or her understanding of interactive gesture games by participating in them. He should follow a single-step command accompanied by gesture at 12 months and without gesture by 15 months. At 15 months, he should begin to point to body parts on request, and by 2 to 2.5 years of age, the child should be able to follow a series of two independent commands.

The development of the social use of language, or pragmatics, also should be followed. Abnormalities in pragmatic language are a core feature of autism spectrum disorders. Recognizing such abnormalities early is important in the detection of autism spectrum disorders. During the first 2 years of life, children with autism show poor eye contact, poor linking of eye gaze with gesture and vocalization, little or no pointing to objects, and difficulties in shifting their focus of attention based on others' use of eye gaze or gesture. Infants with autism also may show less babbling and less interest in verbal or gestural mimicry.

The pediatrician should be able to detect language delay associated with mild mental retardation or moderate communication disorders (language DQ 50 to 80) by the age of 2 years. Many autism spectrum disorders can be detected by 24 to 30 months. To detect milder communication disorders and subtle delays in language, further assessment by a speech pathologist or psychologist is required, although atypical or deviant language development may have been noticed in the early months of life.

Language delay is best identified by determining the child's level of consistent language performance by milestone criteria, expressing it as a language age, and dividing by the chronologic age to yield a language quotient. A language quotient of less than 80 is regarded as delayed. Previously attained milestones should be converted into language quotients to evaluate the consistency of the rate of development expressed as those quotients. Information can be recorded on graphs, as in Figures 97.1 and 97.2. A "line of best fit" drawn through individual points on this graph represents a developmental rate expressed as the language quotient. This graphic approach allows for the

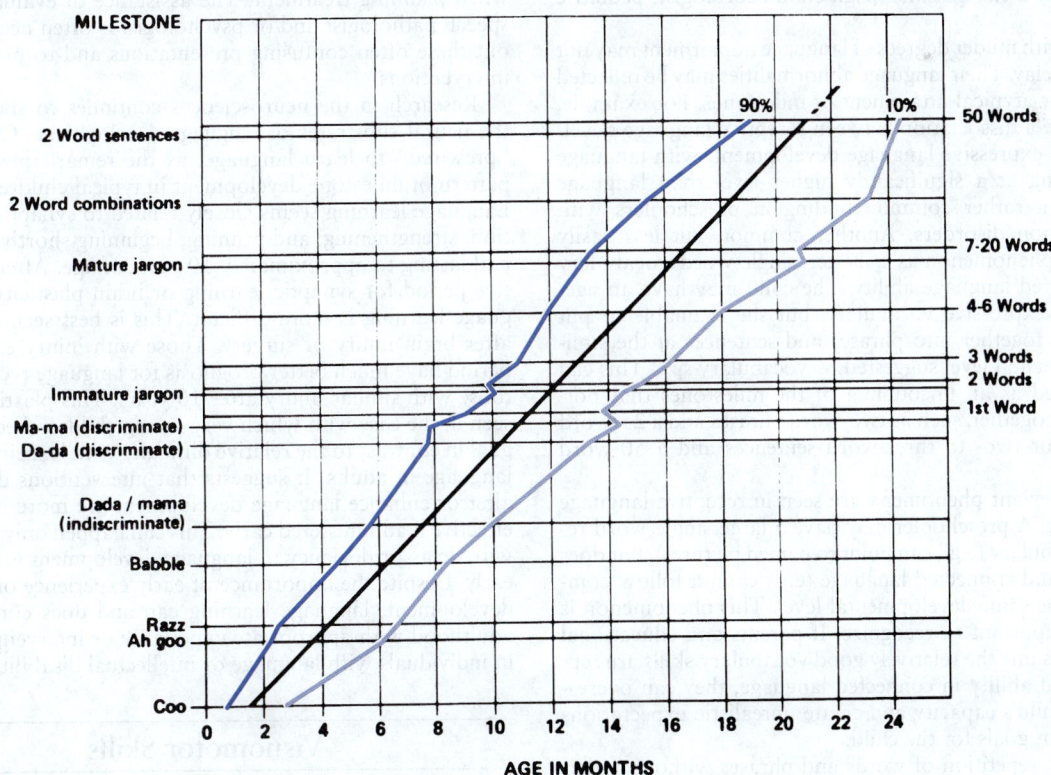

FIGURE 97.1. Expressive language milestones; ninetieth and tenth percentiles for normative population. Infants whose attainment of milestones is consistently later than the tenth percentile are at risk of language and cognitive delay. Slope of the line through the median of each milestone is 1.0 and corresponds to a developmental quotient of 100. Milestone attainment can be plotted on this figure to depict the rate of development, and the plateau or degeneration patterns. (Reproduced with permission from Capute AJ, Palmer AJ, Shapiro BK, et al. Clinical linguistic and auditory milestone scale: prediction of cognition in infancy. *Dev Med Child Neurol* 1986;28:762.)

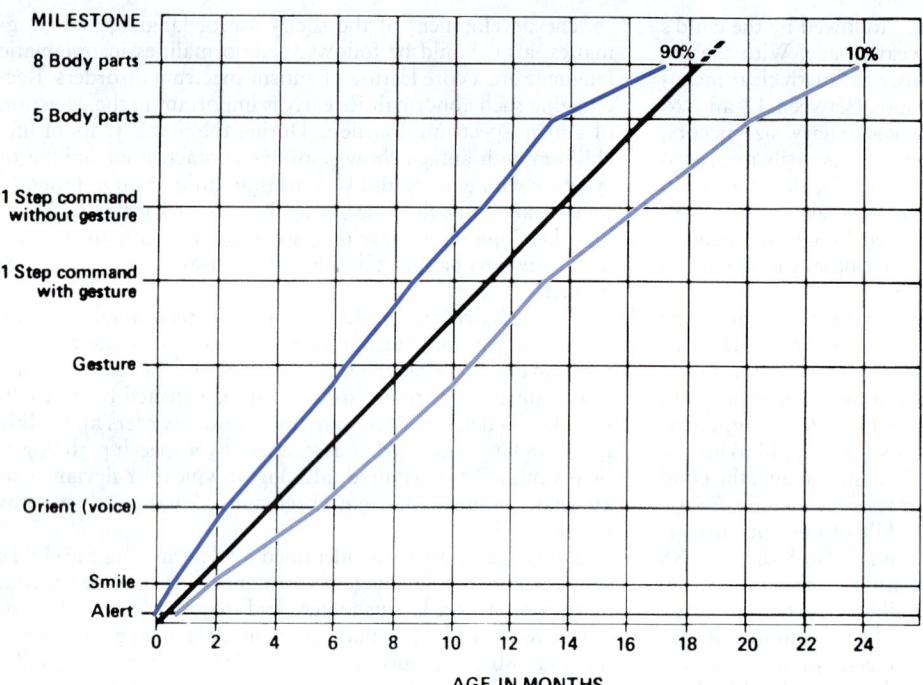

FIGURE 97.2. Receptive language milestones; ninetieth and tenth percentiles for a normative population (see legend for Fig. 97.1). (Reproduced with permission from Capute AJ, Palmer AJ, Shapiro BK, et al. Clinical linguistic and auditory milestone scale: prediction of cognition in infancy. *Dev Med Child Neurol* 1986;28:762.)

easy recognition of changes in the developmental pattern, such as plateauing or loss of skills, which may indicate a progressive neurological disorder or process, and may require systematic evaluation by a subspecialist (e.g., child neurologist, pediatric geneticist).

Infants with milder degrees of language impairment may not have overt delay. Their language abnormalities may be reflected as deviant or atypical attainment of milestones. For example, there may be a dissociation between receptive language development and expressive language development, with language understanding at a significantly higher level than language expression, a rather common finding in preschoolers with communication disorders. Another common but less easily recognized phenomenon is a better single-word vocabulary than connected language ability. The child may have an age-appropriate expressive vocabulary, but she is unable to put these words together into phrases and sentences at the similar developmental level suggested by vocabulary size. This can be manifested as an uncoupling of the milestones that normally occur together, such as two-word phrases and a 25-word vocabulary or two- to three-word sentences and a 50-word vocabulary.

Similar deviant phenomena are seen in receptive language development. A preschooler may have a large single-word receptive vocabulary (e.g., can point to named pictures), but does not understand connected language (e.g., cannot follow commands) at the same developmental level. This phenomenon is especially important to recognize. If parents and educational personnel assume the relatively good vocabulary skills are representative of ability in connected language, they can overestimate the child's capacity and create unrealistic expectations and treatment goals for the child.

Echolalia, repetition of words and phrases without understanding, normally is seen in infants younger than 30 months. Echolalia may be seen in preschoolers with language disorders with good rote memory skills but poor language comprehension. If prominent, it suggests receptive language skills below the level of 30 months. Recognition of such deviancy is key in the early detection of milder disorders. It should prompt a complete evaluation by a speech and language pathologist or psychologist.

Disorders of speech articulation or speech fluency (e.g., stuttering) may occur with or without language disorders. It is important to distinguish them from underlying language delay when planning treatment. The assistance of evaluations by a speech pathologist and/or psychologist is often needed to sort out these often confusing presentations and to plan effective interventions.

Research in the neurosciences continues to shed light on the neural substrates of language development. Children are "prewired" to learn language, as the remarkably consistent pattern of milestone development in typical children suggests. Language learning seems closely related to synaptic organization, strengthening, and pruning, beginning shortly after birth and lasting to approximately 10 years of age. After this sensitive period for synaptic learning or brain plasticity, new language learning is more difficult. This is best seen in children after brain injury or surgery. Those with injury early in this period have much better prognosis for language recovery than those with similar injury after 10 years. This plasticity also is seen in the ease with which very young children become bilingual in contrast to the relative difficulty with learning a second language in adults. It suggests that interventions designed to alter or enhance language development are more likely to be effective if administered early. This can happen only if the child with delay or deviancy in language development is recognized early. Despite the importance of early experience on language development, language learning can and does continue into adulthood with appropriate experience or interventions, even in individuals with language or intellectual disabilities.

Visuomotor Skills

Visuomotor or problem-solving skills make up the other major cognitive stream of development. The purpose for assessing this stream is to quantify the cognitive components of visual and fine motor manipulative tasks. A task may not be achieved because of factors other than cognitive delay. These include visual impairment, gross or fine motor liability, or refusal. However, adequate cognitive abilities frequently overcome mild or moderate upper extremity motor limitations.

The earliest visuomotor tasks are assessable in the first 3 months of life. The visual neurosensory skills include visual fixation before 1 month of age and the development of visual tracking skills and the blink response to visual threat at 3 to 4 months. By this age, basic visual fixation and tracking skills approach full maturity. At the same time, the infant gradually is coming out of the neonatal flexor habitus (with suppression of primitive reflexes) and, by 3 months of age, he should be able to bring his hands to midline and be relatively unfisted. With development of visual tracking abilities and early upper extremity control, eye, head, and upper extremity movements can be used in coordination. This represents the beginning of assessable fine motor problem-solving skills, beginning with the ability to reach, attain, and transfer objects from hand to hand by 5 months of age.

During subsequent months, the infant's abilities become more sophisticated, and the examination draws heavily on tasks demanding the manipulation of blocks, peg boards, form boards, and pencil and paper. Like language development, as the child enters the preschool years, visuomotor abilities become increasingly complex and require the evaluation of a psychologist to describe and quantify. Commonly used infant and preschool psychometric tests include the Bayley Scales of Infant Development, Cattell Infant Intelligence Scale, Stanford-Binet Intelligence Scale, McCarthy Scales of Children's Abilities, and the Wechsler Preschool and Primary Scale of Intelligence.

Although an infant or child may possess the motor ability to carry out certain visuomotor functions, these skills cannot be accomplished unless the necessary cognitive ability exists. This can be exemplified by the 9-month cognitive skill of examining a bell. If the infant is at the 9-month visuomotor level, examination of the bell and manipulation of the clapper are accomplished. If the infant is functioning below this cognitive level, this problem-solving activity is not carried out; the child ignores the bell, mouths it, or pushes it aside.

A valuable sequence of visuomotor pencil and paper tasks are listed in Table 97.1. These tasks range from 12-month random marking through the traditional copying of the Gesell figures and provide information up to a mental age of 12 years. This sequence of tasks should be a component of any visuomotor assessment.

Unlike language milestones, visuomotor tasks do not lend themselves to parental questioning about previously attained skills. The pediatrician usually is limited to determining a current visuomotor age and developmental quotient. Contrasting the rate of visuomotor development with the rate of language development allows the pediatrician to differentiate global

mental retardation from a communication disorder. In the former, broad cognitive delay is manifested in language and visuomotor skills. In language disorders, relative preservation of visuomotor abilities occurs with significantly greater delay observed in language skills (i.e., language/visuomotor dissociation). Before the developmental diagnosis of mental retardation can be made, a valid assessment of both language and problem-solving skills by a psychologist is necessary.

MOTOR ASSESSMENT

Motor, particularly gross motor, development is the stream most familiar to parents and physicians. Motor development is key to the early detection of many disabilities. Significant early motor delay and abnormalities of the neuromotor examination are the hallmarks of cerebral palsy. Most infants with moderate or severe cerebral palsy can be identified in the first 6 to 8 months of life by recognition of delay, abnormalities on neuromotor examination, and perhaps accompanying risk factors.

No useful quantitative association exists between the rates of motor and language development. The degree of motor delay cannot be used to predict the degree of cognitive delay. However, a clear qualitative association exists; infants with motor delay are likely to have other nonmotor developmental abnormalities, including mental retardation and communicative disorders. Mild motor delay is often the first developmental concern expressed for an infant who ultimately is diagnosed as having moderate mental retardation.

The assessment of motor development begins with the determination of motor age by the best performance on milestone criteria, as outlined in Table 97.2. The motor quotient = motor age/chronologic age × 100. A motor quotient less than 50 is likely to be associated with disabling cerebral palsy (e.g., child not sitting without support until after 12 months of age). Motor quotients of more than 70 are generally not associated with motor disability. Infants and children with hemiplegia may be exceptions to this basic rule, because their gross motor skills may be adequate, but they may have significant impairments of the affected extremities that are not easily reflected in an overall gross motor quotient. After a complete motor history and neuromotor examination, it may be helpful to develop motor quotients for each of the four extremities to help establish the topography of the motor disability.

The neuromotor examination offers considerable additional information in establishing topography and in contributing to the early detection of cerebral palsy before outright delay in motor milestones is apparent. The components of the traditional neuromotor examination, such as muscle tone, deep tendon reflexes, involuntary movements, and pathologic reflexes, must be seen in a developmental context. During the first year

TABLE 97.1

VISUOMOTOR SKILLS WITH PENCIL AND PAPER

Skill	Age
Simple marks	12 months
Scribble in imitation	15 months
Scribble spontaneously	18 months
Stroke	24 months
Horizontal and vertical strokes	27 months
Circle in imitation	30 months
Copy circle	36 months
Copy 2-stroke cross	42 months
Copy square	4 years
Copy triangle	5 years
Copy Union jack	5–6 years
Copy horizontal diamond	6 years
Copy vertical diamond	7 years
Copy Greek cross	8 years
Copy cylinder	9 years
Copy cube	12 years

TABLE 97.2

MEAN AGE OF MOTOR MILESTONE ATTAINMENT

Milestone	Mean Age (months)	Standard Deviation
Roll prone to supine	3.6	1.4
Roll supine to prone	4.8	1.4
Sit tripod	5.3	1.0
Sit unsupported	6.3	1.2
Creep	6.7	1.5
Crawl	7.8	1.7
Pull to stand	8.1	1.6
Cruise	8.8	1.7
Walk	11.7	1.9
Walk backward	14.3	2.4
Run	14.8	2.7

TABLE 97.3

CLINICALLY RECOGNIZABLE ABNORMALITIES IN PRIMITIVE REFLEXES

Primitive Reflex	Abnormality
Moro	Moro at any age associated with opisthotonos; visible Moro after 4 months
Asymmetric tonic neck reflex	An obligatory response from which the infant cannot free himself or herself; visible response after 6 months of age
Tonic labyrinthine in supine position	Persistent neck and trunk arching with the child in supine position at any age; visible arching or shoulder retraction after 6 months of age

TABLE 97.4

SELECTED ELICITABLE POSTURAL RESPONSES

Postural Response	Age Of Appearance	Comment
Head righting in supported sitting	6 weeks to 3 months	Must be fully developed before adequate head control and sitting are attained
Landau response	2 months	Early measure of developing trunk control
Derotational righting	4 months	With Landau response, prerequisite to independent rolling from supine to prone positions
Upper extremity protective extension in supported sitting	Anterior, 4 months; lateral, 6 months	Prerequisite to sitting in the tripod position; prerequisite to sitting independently

of life, changes in these parameters occur in normal infants. For example, ankle clonus and other manifestations of lower extremity hyperreflexia are common in infants younger than 4 months. Upper extremity synkinesias and other involuntary movements are frequent in infants younger than 8 months. The extensor plantar response should not be regarded as abnormal in infants younger than 12 months unless it is obviously asymmetric or associated with other abnormal neuromotor signs.

The evolution of primitive reflex activity during the first year of life offers a key to the early recognition of CNS abnormality. Primitive reflexes are subcortical, whole-body motor responses, which develop during gestation, are elicitable at birth, and generally are suppressed during the first 6 months of life with CNS maturation. Abnormally intense primitive reflexes or reflexes that are not suppressed as expected during the first 6 months are signs of neurologic dysfunction. This finding, combined with significant motor delay, suggests cerebral palsy. With minimal or no delay, the primitive reflex abnormalities still reflect CNS dysfunction; abnormalities in other developmental streams should be pursued. Examples of clinically meaningful abnormalities in primitive reflexes are shown in Table 97.3. Asymmetries in primitive reflex activity, such as asymmetric grasps, toe standing, or shoulder retraction, are also clinical signs of abnormality.

Postural responses, unlike primitive reflexes, are maturational motor responses of righting and equilibrium that develop during the first year of life and are necessary antecedents of the more familiar motor milestones. Clinically elicitable postural responses are reflected in Table 97.4. These responses are helpful to the motor therapist in developing realistic short-term treatment goals for the child with cerebral palsy, and they also may be helpful to the pediatrician in recognizing early motor abnormality.

Recently, the objective assessment of spontaneous general movements in the infant has shown considerable promise in detecting cerebral palsy in the first weeks of life, much earlier than previously possible. The neuromotor examination must be seen as complementary to systematic neuroimaging in the infant with or at risk for motor disability. For example, brain ultrasonography or magnetic resonance imaging (MRI) at term age offers considerable help in establishing a motor diagnosis and prognosis.

ASSESSMENT OF ACTIVITIES OF DAILY LIVING

An assessment of self-help abilities or activities of daily living provides useful information. These skills of self-feeding, dress-

ing, and related activities provide information on how the infant integrates the developmental streams into basic daily functioning. Most activities of daily living require a minimal level of motor, language, problem-solving, and attentional maturity to be accomplished. Any problems with attaining these skills further clarify the level of competence in individual streams. For example, the mental age for toileting independently is usually approximately 18 months. A child with mental retardation who is toilet trained by 36 months has a cognitive age of at least 18 months. However, failure to achieve toileting independence does not mean the child does not have the cognitive level of 18 months; it may suggest motor, problem-solving, attentional, or language deficiencies or a lack of opportunity. Delay in the development of adaptive skills, including activities of daily living, is a necessary criterion for the diagnosis of mental retardation. The objective measurement of adaptive skills should be part of the assessment by a psychologist when mental retardation is suspected.

ASSESSMENT OF SOCIAL DEVELOPMENT

Social development, like activities of daily living, should be seen as an amalgamation of development in multiple streams, particularly language. Although environmental influences are important, social dysfunction may be a symptom of neurodevelopmental abnormality. For example, the child who prefers playing with younger children may do so because her communicative abilities are at that level. Certain traditional social milestones, such as play skills, domestic mimicry, parallel play at 24 months, and associative group play at 42 months, are best used as markers of language development. The objective measurement of social development is part of a formal assessment by a psychologist or, when social use of language is the question, a speech pathologist.

TABLE 97.5

BEHAVIORAL SYMPTOMS OF CENTRAL NERVOUS SYSTEM DYSFUNCTION

Common Age of Recognition	Behavioral Symptoms
Prenatal period	Increased, decreased, or late onset of perceived fetal movement
Infancy	Poor feeding, need to awaken for feeding, sustained irritability, abnormal cry, excessive motor activity, excessive rocking or other self-stimulation, decreased social interest
Late infancy through preschool years	Short attention span, distractibility, perseveration, hyperactivity, impulsivity
School age	Hyperactivity, attentional aberrations, impulsivity, fire setting, excessive lying, stealing, cruelty to animals
Adolescence and adulthood	Previously mentioned symptoms plus recurrent misdemeanors, substance abuse, accident proneness, and possibly sociopathy

non-neurological factors may contribute to a child's behavior, but the potential for a neurodevelopmental cause for these abnormalities always should be considered.

The child with more severe neurodevelopmental abnormalities, such as severe or profound mental retardation or severe communication disorder, may demonstrate exaggerated behavioral symptoms. These include marked perseveration or self-stimulatory behavior, self-injury, repeated violent temper tantrums, and dramatically short attention span. Management often requires a combination of pharmacologic means with strict behavior modification techniques. Control of the symptoms often means the difference between institutionalization and supervised community living for the child or adult with retardation.

In addition to the nonspecific neurobehavioral symptoms of neurodevelopmental dysfunction, certain genetic disorders have relatively specific patterns of behavior and/or cognition, often called "behavioral phenotypes." Commonly recognized behavioral/cognitive phenotypes include hyperphagia in Prader-Willi syndrome and stereotypic hand wringing in Rett syndrome. Selected specific behavioral/cognitive phenotypes are summarized in Table 97.6. Attention to this expanding group of characteristic cognitive and behavioral patterns is important for the effective diagnosis and management of neurodevelopmental disabilities. Behavioral management often requires a collaboration between multiple disciplines and community agencies, a task usually best initiated by the child's pediatrician.

BEHAVIORAL ATTRIBUTES OF CENTRAL NERVOUS SYSTEM DEVELOPMENT

Neurologic dysfunction frequently presents as behavioral disturbance, sometimes independent of other obvious neurodevelopmental abnormalities. Commonly recognized examples of behavioral manifestations of CNS dysfunction are listed in Table 97.5. A complete developmental evaluation, whether for the purpose of detection, diagnosis, or development monitoring, evaluates this behavioral stream. As with other streams,

CONCLUSIONS

The expanding pediatric role in neurodevelopmental disabilities requires a practical understanding of developmental assessment, including evaluation of individual developmental streams, recognition and quantification of delay and deviancy, and appreciation of the dissociated rates of development between different streams. Chapters 98 and 396 expand these concepts in the context of mental retardation and cerebral palsy, respectively.

TABLE 97.6

SELECTED BEHAVIORAL/COGNITIVE PHENOTYPES

Disorder	Defect	Reported Behavioral/Cognitive Phenotypes
Angelman syndrome	15q11-13 maternal segment microdeletion; paternal disomy of 15	Severe MR, paroxysmal laughter, ataxia
Fragile X syndrome	X chromosome triplet repeat disorder	MR, gaze avoidance and other autism spectrum disorder features - variable
Klinefelter syndrome	47,xxy	Language-based learning disorders, executive dysfunction
Neurofibromatosis, type 1	Neurofibromin gene mutation	30% learning disability (possibly visuospatial), 10% mild MR
Prader-Willi syndrome	15q11 paternal segment microdeletion; maternal disomy of 15	Intense preoccupation with and seeking of food, lack of satiation
Rett disorder	MeCP2 gene mutation	Loss of developmental skills, characteristic hand wringing movements, hyperpnea
Smith-Lemli-Opitz syndrome	Cholesterol biosynthesis defect	MR, unusual responses to sensory stimuli, irritability, language impairment, sleep cycle disorders, self-injurious behavior, and autism spectrum behaviors
Smith-Magenis syndrome	17p11.2 microdeletion	MR, hyperactivity, self-injury, pulling out nails, inserting foreign bodies into body orifices
Turner syndrome	45,xo	Deficits in visual perceptual abilities, memory, executive function
Williams syndrome	7q11.23 microdeletion	Mild MR, loquacious personality, rich affect, visuospatial skills poorer than language skills

Acknowledgments

Supported in part by grant 90-DD-0578 from the U.S. Department of Health and Human Services, Administration for Children and Families, and by grant 6 T73 MC 00038-10 and 5 T73 MC 00019-10 from the Health Resources and Services Administration's Maternal and Child Health Bureau.

Suggested Readings

Capute AJ, Accardo PJ. Developmental disabilities in infancy and childhood. Baltimore: Paul H. Brookes, 1996.

Capute AJ, Shapiro BK. The motor quotient: a method for the early detection of motor delay. *Am J Dis Child* 1985;139:940.

Committee on Children with Disabilities, American Academy of Pediatrics. The pediatrician's role in the diagnosis and management of autistic spectrum disorder in children. *Pediatrics* 2001;107:1221.

Denckla MB, ed. Specific behavioral/cognitive phenotypes in genetic disorders. *Ment Retard Dev Dis Res Rev* 2000;6:81.

Drillien CM, Drummond MB, eds. *Neurodevelopmental problems in early childhood: assessment and management.* Oxford: Blackwell Scientific, 1977.

Ferrari F, Cioni G, Einspieler C, et al. Cramped synchronized general movements in preterm infants as an early marker for cerebral palsy. *Arch Pediatr Adolesc Med* 2002;156:460.

Gesell AJ, Amatruda CS. *Developmental diagnosis*, 2nd ed. New York: Paul B. Hoeber, 1941.

Hoon AH, Pulsifer MB, Gopalan R, et al. The CAT/CLAMS in early cognitive assessment. *J Pediatr* 1993;123:S1.

Illingworth RS. *The development of the infant and young child*, 8th ed. Edinburgh: Churchill Livingstone, 1983.

Lyle JG. Certain antenatal, perinatal and developmental variables and reading retardation in middle-class boys. *Child Dev* 1970;41:481.

Ment LR, Bada HS, Barnes P, et al. Practice parameter: neuroimaging of the neonate: report of the Quality Standards Subcommittee of the American Academy of Neurology and the Practice Committee of the Child Neurology Society. *Neurology* 2002;58:1726.

Nelson K, Ellenberg J. Antecedents of cerebral palsy, multivariate analysis of risk. *N Engl J Med* 1986;315:81.

Rapin I. Autism. *N Engl J Med* 1997;337:97.

Shonkoff JP, Phillilips DA, eds. *From neurons to neighborhoods: the science of early child development.* Washington: National Research Council and Institute of Medicine, National Academy Press, 2000.

Strauss AA, Lehtinen L. *Psychopathology and education of the brain injured child.* New York: Grune & Stratton, 1947.

Thatcher RW, Lyon GR, Rumsey J, Krasnegor N. *Developmental neuroimaging: mapping the development of brain and behavior.* New York: Academic Press, 1996.

CHAPTER 98 ■ MENTAL RETARDATION

PASQUALE J. ACCARDO, JENNIFER A. ACCARDO, AND ARNOLD J. CAPUTE

In the English-speaking world, the terms *intellectual disability* or *cognitive impairment* are replacing the term older *mental retardation* (see Box 98.1 for an overview of the history of the definition, diagnosis, and treatment of cognitive impairment). *Global learning disability* is preferred in England proper. All these terms characterize serious deficits, predominantly in the cognitive realm, rather than a medical diagnosis. Like cerebral palsy, intellectual disability is best understood as a family of syndromes with similarities that render considering individual clinical presentations separately less helpful to the medical management of the child. Despite much debate among professionals about the model approach to cognitive impairment, the paradigm of the child with brain damage (static encephalopathy) remains the point of departure from which the pediatrician can best pursue diagnosis and counseling.

DEFINITION AND CLASSIFICATION

The definition of intellectual disability (the 317 to 319 codes in the *Diagnostic and Statistical Manual of Mental Disorders, Fourth Edition* [DSM-IV-TR] for mental retardation) has three components:

- Some degree of cognitive delay
- Impaired adaptive behavior
- Onset before 18 years of age

Cognitive delay is delineated by the IQ, with the levels of mental retardation roughly correlating with the number of standard deviations below the mean (Fig. 98.1). It is as imperative in intellectual disability as in other developmental disorders to remember that no child or adult ever can be reduced

to a single number, such as IQ. Human behavior does not admit such simplistic reductionism. The limited utility of IQ scores is further confused by such variables as chronic disease; sensory deficits; prematurity; environmental deprivation; intensive stimulation; the skill and experience of the examiner; the race, gender, and age of the child; the bias of the instruments used; and the interfering presence of behavioral and emotional disorders in the child and the family. These complicating factors need not reduce the IQ score to insignificance; they should instead be viewed as part of the complex clinical circumstances in which children's cognitive behavior is assessed, just as physicians know to interpret quantitative laboratory tests within a broader clinical context. These difficulties also highlight the importance of special competence for the pediatrician attempting to formulate a developmental diagnosis.

The single most important qualification for a diagnosis of intellectual disability remains a validly obtained IQ score of more than two standard deviations below the population mean for the test. Subject to various qualifications, the specific IQ score is the deciding basis for developmental diagnosis, biomedical assessment, parent counseling, educational habilitation, vocational rehabilitation, and disability determination. For using and interpreting the test instruments, the IQ cutoffs for the different levels of retardation (e.g., 70, 50, 35, 20) are more accurately viewed as ranges (e.g., 65 to 75, 45 to 55, 30 to 40, 15 to 25). Using IQ ranges allows a better correlation with cognitive level. In contrast to the more statistically defined field of psychometrics, the measurement of adaptive behavior is less precisely quantified. Clinical judgment of self-help and socialization skills can be aided by instruments such as the Vineland Adaptive Behavior Scales (VABS).

The third criterion, onset before 18 years of age, is least problematic because most cases of intellectual disability are

---

BOX 98.1 History

Cognitive impairment was recognized in the ancient and medieval worlds, but little interest was exhibited in pursuing the problem beyond the bare minimums necessary to resolve questions of property rights. Radical conceptual changes in the philosophy of human nature and significant advances in science had to occur before the right questions could be posed. The requisite progress came together at the time of the French Revolution. Victor, a "feral child" found in the woods at Aveyron, was pronounced an idiot by Pinel, one of the founders of modern psychiatry. Itard received one of the first government research grants to attempt to educate this significantly delayed boy. Over a 5-year period, Itard virtually invented the discipline of special education and pioneered much of behaviorist psychology. His student, Seguin, continued working on habilitation techniques and became an influential leader of the new residential school movement when he emigrated to the United States. With few changes, the special education methodologies these two physicians devised to help persons with mental retardation became the foundation for the early childhood education system popularized in the first half of the twentieth century by a third physician, Maria Montessori.

In the early nineteenth century, Esquirol differentiated "imbeciles" from three classes of more severely limited "idiots" by their functional ability to use language. In 1877, Ireland published the first modern medical textbook on mental retardation, *On Idiocy and Imbecility*, in which he proposed an etiologic classification that would remain valid for most of the next century. Ireland's book also publicized the 1866 description by Down of one of the first specific mental retardation syndromes. However, until 1959 when Le-

jeune identified the specific chromosomal trisomy, difficulty in clinically differentiating Down syndrome from cretinism and other disorders persisted. The pseudoscientific eugenics movement of the later nineteenth and early twentieth centuries precipitated sterilization laws and euthanasia practices and distorted the initial idealism of the educational movement pioneered by Itard and Seguin. The flowering of the age of syndrome identification and molecular genetics in the latter half of the twentieth century somewhat redeemed the contribution of scientific genetics to the study of intellectual disability.

Major progress in the medical and behavioral areas depended heavily on the development of well-designed psychometric instruments for accurate classification. In 1905, the psychologist Binet and the physician Simon published the first standardized intelligence test (later translated into English at Stanford University). This advance ushered in more than half a century of use and abuse of psychometric instrumentation that only partially filled the authors' original intentions of introducing an objective and unbiased measurement device to replace the subjective and sometimes arbitrary opinion of the classroom teacher and untrained professionals. The pediatrician and psychologist Gesell was the first to extend the quantification of development to the period of infancy and early childhood, and his assessment approach avoided some of the major pitfalls of IQ mismeasurement: (a) test scores did not stand alone but acquired meaning only within the broader context of past history, biological risk and repeated assessments, and (b) the dissociation between the various streams of development was used to focus the medical evaluation.

---

congenital, prenatal, or perinatal, and the onset and diagnosis are rarely delayed until adolescence. The rare cases of dementia (i.e., degenerative central nervous system [CNS] disease) and postnatally acquired brain damage are readily recognizable.

EPIDEMIOLOGY

Despite continued medical advances in prenatal maternal care and the prenatal and perinatal treatment of the fetus and new-

born, the overall incidence of intellectual disability has remained relatively stable at approximately 2% to 3% of the population. More than 80% of all persons with intellectual disability are in the mildly delayed range, with twice as many male as female patients. Atypical children with the developmental pattern of normal to borderline intelligence and superimposed language disorders and other deviance or dissociation can be misclassified as intellectually disabled. The recent increase in the occurrence of autism has resulted in large part from a reclassification as autistic of children who previously

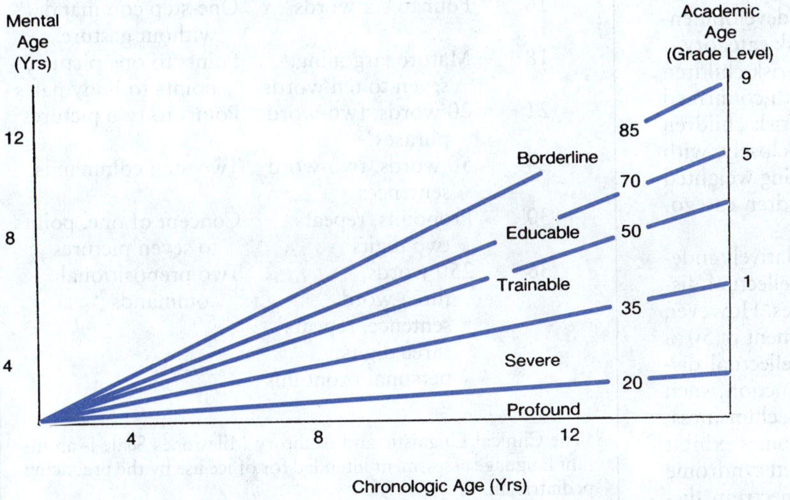

FIGURE 98.1. Levels of academic achievement to be expected with different degrees of intellectual disability at successive ages. The difference between the two ordinal scales reflects the rule of five: mental age level (in years) minus five = grade achievement level (as a grade level). This rule should be used routinely in the office practice of pediatrics. If a child's chronologic age and grade level differ by more than 5 after date of birth, age cut-off for entering school, and current date have been allowed for, further investigation is warranted. Grade retention or failing a grade is almost never an acceptable treatment response for any developmental diagnosis. The neatness of the diagram is artificial since, in life, none of the lines is as straight as suggested in this first-order approximation. The diagram is itself a rule of thumb and not a presentation of statistical data.

would have been called mentally retarded. Careful attention to the pattern of delayed language and socialization skills in the presence of intact to superior nonverbal problem-solving skills should allow the identification of such children as autistic, thus lowering of the incidence of mild intellectual disability.

The effect of technologic innovations in neonatal intensive care units is twofold. First, the mortality and morbidity curves retain the same shape and magnitude but are shifted horizontally (i.e., babies who in the past would have died may now survive with handicaps, and babies who would have survived with handicaps now survive without them). Second, neonatal intensive care unit follow-up and other epidemiologic surveys all suggest a marked increase in the newer morbidity of learning and behavior disorders in children. Some of this latter increase, however, is a product of improvements in diagnostic skills, test sensitivity, and methodologic refinement on the part of the examiners. The further extension of this improved ability to discriminate the finer shades of neurobehavioral dysfunction into the area of mental retardation represents a future research direction for neurodevelopmental pediatrics.

DIAGNOSIS

The early identification of intellectual disability is the responsibility and prerogative of the pediatrician who provides well-child care. Early diagnosis is essential for successful treatment and follow-up of the child.

Screening and Early Diagnosis

Existing screening instruments are far from ideal, and the pediatric practitioner must integrate the specific tests and milestones, neurobehavioral observations, and parental concerns into a larger pattern of specific disability categories. Adequate screening cannot be defined apart from the comfort level of the physician who reaches a specific developmental diagnosis.

No ideal screening or assessment methodology exists for the office pediatrician who must work separate from a range of multidisciplinary diagnostic services. When signs and symptoms of delay were noticed in the past, they were often judged to be temporary phases. Although this occasionally may have been true, they were frequently early markers for mild neurodevelopmental dysfunction, such as the spontaneously resolving early articulation disorder that can later reappear as a reading problem. In some cases, such delays predicted more severe global intellectual disability.

The first step in the pediatric assessment of cognitive impairment is to define the child at risk. Genetic, familial, prenatal, perinatal, and postnatal factors that can affect the developmental rate should be documented. However, an at-risk category is distinct from a developmental diagnosis. Most at-risk children progress normally, while many older children with confirmed developmental diagnoses were never at risk. At-risk children should have their development monitored more closely, with early signs and symptoms of brain dysfunction being weighted more heavily. The treatment of undiagnosed children categorized as at risk remains problematic.

With few exceptions, motor development is relatively independent of cognitive development. Significant intellectual disability is compatible with normal motor milestones. However, cerebral palsy is associated with cognitive impairment in 50% to 75% of patients, and persons with severe intellectual disability often exhibit some degree of motor dysfunction, such as hypotonia, visual motor organization problems, clumsiness, tremor, and ataxia. Some mental retardation syndromes exhibit motor deterioration over time, as occurs early in Rett syndrome and late in cognitive impairment with autistic spectrum disorder.

The most sensitive early marker for intellectual disability is language development. Prelinguistic vocalizations in the first year of life show a clear pattern of delay even in mild cognitive impairment (Box 98.2). However, a significant disorder of language or a learning disability also may present with a distortion of early language milestones, so these delays must be supplemented by an assessment of problem-solving skills. The evaluation can range from an observational description of preferred type of interaction (i.e., 0 to 3 months, visual tracking; 3 to 6 months, reach, grasp, mouthing; 6 to 9 months, grasp, transfer, bang; 9 to 12 months, voluntary casting and release) to the use of formal assessment instruments such as the Bayley Scales of Infant Development (BSID) and the Capute Scales. The pediatrician also may use formal (Box 98.3) or informal lists of developmental milestones or maturational sequences to arrive at one or more developmental quotients (DQs), where DQ = functional age equivalent/chronological age × 100.

BOX 98.2	Clinical Linguistic and Auditory Milestones Scale*	
Age (mo)	Expressive milestone	Receptive milestone
1		Alerts, soothes
2		Social smile
3	Coos	
4	Laughs	Orients to voice
5	"Ah goo," raspberry	Orients (I)
6	Babbles	
7		Orients (II)
8	"Dada" (inappropriately); "Mama" (inappropriately)	
9	Gesture	Orients (III)
10	"Dada" (appropriately); "Mama" (appropriately)	Understands "no"
11	One word	
12	Two words	One-step command with gesture
14	Three words, immature jargoning	
16	Four to six words	One-step command without gesture
18	Mature jargoning, seven to ten words	Points to one picture, points to body parts
21	20 words, two-word phrases	Points to two pictures
24	50 words, two-word sentences	Two-step commands
30	Pronouns, repeats two digits	Concept of one, points to seven pictures
36	250 words, three-word sentence, repeats three digits, personal pronouns	Two prepositional commands

*The Clinical Linguistic and Auditory Milestones Scale is an infant language assessment intended for office use by the practicing pediatrician.

| BOX 98.3 | The Clinical Adaptive Test* |

Age (mo) Skills

1   Visually fixates momentarily, prone I
2   Visually follows horizontally/vertically, prone II
3   Visually follows in circle, prone III, visual threat
4   Unfisted, manipulates fingers, prone IV
5   Pulls down ring, transfers, regards pellet
6   Obtains cube, lifts cup, radial rake
7   Attempts pellet, pulls out peg, inspects ring
8   Pulls ring by string, secures pellet, inspects bell
9   Scissors grasp, rings bell, looks over the edge for toy
10   Combines cube in cup, uncovers bell, fingers pegboard
11   Mature overhand pincer movement, solves cube under cup
12   Releases one cube in cup, marks with crayon
14   Solves glass frustration, out-in with peg, solves pellet in bottle with demonstration
16   Spontaneously solves pellet in bottle, round block in form board, imitates scribble
18   Ten cubes in cup, round hole in reversed form board, spontaneous scribble with crayon, completes pegboard spontaneously
21   Obtains object with stick, square in form board, tower of three
24   Folds paper I, horizontal four-cube train, imitates pencil stroke, completes form board
30   Horizontal and vertical pencil strokes, reversed form board, folds paper II, train with chimney
36   Bridge, copies circle, names one color, draws a person with head and one other part

*The Clinical Adaptive Test is a pediatric clinical observational instrument that measures fine motor, adaptive, and visual perceptual skills in the first 2 years of life and is intended to supplement the Clinical Linguistic and Auditory Milestones Scale in the diagnosis of mental retardation and other developmental disabilities in very young children.

A child with an overall developmental quotient of less than 80 should be followed closely; persistence of a developmental quotient of less than 80 should lead to formal evaluation. A child with a developmental quotient of less than 60 should receive a more detailed biomedical and psychologic assessment. This recommendation is a logical implication of the older two-group theory of retardation, in which organic brain pathology, identifiable causes, and other medical complications increase as the general cognitive level decreases to less than an IQ of 50 (Box 98.1). The milder the delay, the later it comes to the pediatrician's attention. The preschool child with mild intellectual disability often presents with language delay, and the younger school-aged child presents with grade retention.

Certain neurobehavioral symptoms and parental concerns can suggest severe cognitive impairment in infancy, especially if accompanied by CNS irritability (e.g., persistent "colic") and other signs of neurologic disorganization. To various degrees, these behaviors can be considered early nonspecific markers for intellectual disability and other neurodevelopmental disorders:

failure to thrive, prolonged (beyond 3 months) colic, arching, standoffishness and lack of cuddliness, and suspected deafness or blindness. These markers are not to be interpreted in isolation but rather against the background of risk factors and the pattern of milestones yielded by the streams of development discussed in Chapter 97, Streams of Development. Early diagnosis is important for a variety of reasons. Parental concerns about developmental delay often start in infancy and deserve accurate developmental feedback. The biomedical component of the developmental assessment may identify a hereditary or other recurrence risk about which young families should be informed. Supplementary disability income is available for significantly handicapped infants, and with appropriate medical documentation, private health insurance carriers may fund some part of the cost of habilitation programs. Public Law (PL) 99-457 mandates early educational intervention for handicapped infants and preschoolers. The pediatric role in the implementation of this legislation should be as great as that for PL 101-47, the Individuals with Disabilities Education Act, which is an update of PL 94-142, the Education for All Handicapped Children Act. An issue of concern from the medical perspective is the tendency of many early intervention programs to provide services to infants with developmental delays without clearly specifying the degree of the delay. Although most delays eligible for intervention services are too mild to qualify as intellectual disability, some will require a more detailed biomedical assessment.

Medical Evaluation

The pediatric assessment of the child with intellectual disability consists of a careful history to obtain information about familial, genetic, prenatal, perinatal, and postnatal influences on development; a detailed listing of developmental milestones reinforced by records, baby books, photographs, and home movies or videotapes, if appropriate; a neurodevelopmental assessment of the child's abilities, which includes a formal psychometric evaluation by a competent child psychologist skilled in testing children with developmental disabilities; and a physical examination that focuses on the neurologic correlates of organic brain dysfunction and the minor malformations associated with specific syndromes or that nonspecifically reflect prenatal causes (Box 98.4). The goals of this pediatric assessment are to measure functional level; determine the time of onset, duration, and impact of adverse biomedical influences on brain development; delineate associated dysfunctions or other organ system malformations needing treatment; and identify syndromes of genetic importance. Degenerative or progressive conditions often can be ruled out by a careful developmental history.

Probably the single finding that most often confuses the question of developmental regression is the utterance from an otherwise globally delayed child of several words and perhaps even a rote phrase at approximately 1 year of age. This seemingly age-appropriate expressive language is lost before 18 months of age, giving rise to the suspicion of possible CNS deterioration. This benign regression pattern stands in striking contrast to that observed in Rett syndrome, which occurs in girls and may account for as many as one-third to one-fourth of cases of female severe mental retardation. In this condition, girls who appear to be developing normally until 6 to 18 months of age undergo a fairly rapid dementia with a plateauing of head circumference and acquired microcephaly; a loss of purposeful hand movements replaced by stereotypies such as hand wringing reminiscent of those seen in autistic children; ataxia and marked loss of gross motor skills; and later development of seizures and scoliosis. Although the degenerative course is relatively short, the long-term prognosis is one of severe to profound handicap. As one component of "autistic regression" (the other is social withdrawal), the loss

---

BOX 98.4   Minor Dysmorphic Features

Electric hair
Hair whorl abnormality
   Absent
   Poorly defined
   Multiple cowlicks
   Frontal upsweep
   Widow's peak
Head circumference (occipitofrontal circumference)
   greater than 1.5 SD above or below the mean for age
Epicanthal folds
Hypertelorism or increased inner canthal distance
Low-set ears
Absent ear lobules or adherent ear lobes
Other pinnae abnormalities
   Malformed
   Protuberant ("jug handle")
   Flattened
   Rotated
High-arched or steepled palate
Geographic tongue
Clinodactyly of fifth fingers
Palmar crease abnormalities
   Simian, single four-finger transverse crease
   Sydney, proximal four-finger transverse crease
   Hockey stick crease
Sandal gap deformity of toes one and two
Syndactyly of toes two and three
Long middle toe

Minor dysmorphic features may represent components of specific genetic or teratogenic syndromes, but they also are present in many other cases of mental retardation and the entire spectrum of neurodevelopmental disability, including learning disabilities and attention deficit hyperactivity disorder, and they then reflect the influence of a wide variety of factors that can affect the development of the fetal brain in the first trimester. They are nonspecific indicators for the prenatal cause of neurodevelopmental disorders. Conversely, infants with high dysmorphology scores (i.e., weighted or unweighted scores greater than 4) should have their development monitored more closely than usual and probably should be referred for more detailed developmental assessment at the earliest suspicion of delay or deviance.

BOX 98.5   Sample Tests To Be Considered in the Assessment of the Child with Intellectual Disability*

Newborn screening reports
Audiologic assessment
Amino acids studies
Metabolic screening
Cytogenic studies
   Karyotype with high resolution banding
   FMR1 studies
   MECP2 studies
   Molecular screening
      FISH studies for telomeric deletions/rearrangements
      PWS studies
      VCF studies
Computed tomography scan of the head
Magnetic resonance imaging of the head
Electroencephalography
Evoked potentials, auditory and visual
Thyroid function tests
Fibroblast cultures
Titers for infectious agents

---

*None of these procedures is routine. For specific indications, consultations with genetics, neurology, ophthalmology, and dermatology specialists may provide further diagnostic leads.

in pursuit of mythic comprehensiveness. In the earliest stages of the diagnostic process, the family is vulnerable to exaggerated claims by professionals. The eventual failure of implied promises can have serious long-term negative effects on the child with mental retardation, the parents' marriage, and the siblings.

The biomedical data must not be allowed to overrule the most obvious clinical observations. Many of the published data on expected developmental levels in rare and recently described genetic and metabolic disorders are seriously incomplete and potentially misleading. For example, short, dysmorphic, developmentally delayed female subjects with three or four X chromosomes may exhibit significant language disorders instead of mental retardation. Profound microcephaly is compatible with normal nonverbal intelligence.

THERAPY AND PROGNOSIS

The success of early diagnosis depends on a fundamental stability of the rate of intellectual growth. Unfortunately, long-term predictive validity is better with lower IQ scores. A careful assessment of and allowance for complicating factors increases the predictive validity of diagnoses made during infancy. Some children occasionally switch their developmental curves, which can be confusing. In the most common example, some perinatally stressed infants who appear to be developing at a consistently slow rate suddenly accelerate their developmental rate late in the first year of life and then continue to progress at a normal rate. Alternatively, some children function at a mildly delayed rate through the first decade of life but then plateau in skills several years before or after the sixteenth birthday; this can lead to a change in their classification down to the moderately retarded or up to the borderline range. Such transitions appear to be genetically programmed and may be inherent in some of the less common genetic syndromes.

Something similar to this rate alteration occurs in children with the single most common genetic cause of intellectual

of expressive language milestones may reflect other disorders on the autistic spectrum.

Parents should be told whether their child is significantly delayed; how delayed their child is and what that level of delay implies for long-term function; why their child is delayed; with what degree of certainty the cause is known (e.g., definite, probable, possible, unknown); what the recurrence risks are for all family members; what the parents should do in the immediate future to help their child; what the long-term goals are for which they should plan; and what further medical and behavioral assessments can help answer these questions. A multidisciplinary approach is typically necessary to address all these issues.

As with other pediatric problems associated with multiple causes, a shotgun approach to biomedical diagnosis is not warranted. Leads from the history and physical examination should be carefully followed, but no routine workup should occur. Box 98.5 provides a list of diagnostic tests that can be considered. Appropriate consultations should be sought, but the family's energies and resources should not be squandered

TABLE 98.1

TWO-GROUP THEORY OF MENTAL RETARDATION

Level (%)	Early Diagnosis	Long-term Predictability of IQ	Familial Occurrence	Genetic/ Metabolic Syndrome	Seizures and other Neurologic Complications	Behavior Disorder/ Expanded Strauss	Positive Psycho Stimulant Response	Other Organ System Involvement
Sociocultural/residual of mild central nervous system dysfunction								
Mild (80)	Difficult	Fair	Common	Very rare	Less frequent	Infrequent	Infrequent	Rare
Residual of severe central nervous system dysfunction								
Moderate (12)								
Severe (7)								
Profound (1)	Easy	Very good	Rare	Common	Common	Frequent	Rare	Common

The terms used to describe the differences between the mildly retarded (IQ > 50) and the more organically impaired group are meant to indicate a trend that, with exceptions, varies continuously in the same direction as the IQ decreases. Recent advances in the molecular genetics of mild intellectual impairment are tending to lessen the importance of this two-group approach.

disability, Down syndrome. The younger child with Down syndrome in a preschool stimulation program can sometimes function in the borderline intellectual category. The school-aged child with Down typically functions in the range of moderate developmental delay. By late adolescence to young adulthood, IQ scores in the severely delayed range are not uncommon. Part of this deceleration can be explained by the changing correlation between IQ test items at different age levels and the specific profile of skills in patients with Down syndrome. Part of this phenomenon may be related to the early onset of Alzheimer-type changes in trisomy 21. Children with Down syndrome who consistently function at developmental levels significantly lower than expected should be investigated for hearing loss, autism, hypothyroidism, or celiac disease.

Much apparent change in IQ or functional ability may be secondary to the incomplete nature or poor quality of the initial assessment. The halo effect of striking dysmorphic features or marked neuromotor impairment may lead to underestimating a child's abilities. Most children with fetal alcohol syndrome are learning disordered, rather than intellectually disabled. Approximately two-thirds of children with Prader-Willi syndrome are intellectually disabled, but almost all have a superimposed learning disorder that makes an accurate estimate of their functional capacity difficult. Prader-Willi syndrome provides a dual object lesson: the possible coexistence of intellectual disability with learning disability in the same patient and the increasing irrelevance of IQ with age as the major determinant of the level of functioning or independence. Because of the severity of their food-related behavior disorder, for instance, many young adults with Prader-Willi syndrome require group home placements regardless of intelligence levels.

Follow-up of the Child with Intellectual Disability

Follow-up of the child with intellectual disability depends on the nature of the underlying cause and the specific neurobehavioral deficit pattern. For example, among the 14 in 10,000 live births of children with Down syndrome, approximately 35% have congenital heart disease, 20% develop thyroid dysfunction, 15% have cervical spine instability, and 80% may have conductive hearing loss, with a higher-than-normal incidence of cataracts, strabismus, congenital duodenal atresia, Hirschsprung disease, leukemia, and seizures. A structured, multidisciplinary follow-up program can facilitate the provision of coordinated multispecialty care, with the frequency of visits determined in part by the specific organ systems involved. In contrast, what may be the second most common (10 in 10,000 live births) genetic condition with severe mental retardation, fragile X syndrome, has a subtler phenotype without any commonly associated organ system malformations. As an X-linked disorder, it contributes to the higher prevalence of delayed boys over delayed girls.

In the absence of seizures and major organ system malformations, most of the treatment of intellectual disability is carried out through the educational system and other community-based resources. Progressing at a steady rate, the mildly delayed child typically achieves an approximately sixth-grade academic level and is capable of economic independence (see Fig. 98.1). The moderately delayed child does not usually attain a fourth grade academic level with its attendant functional literacy but is capable of supported employment and community living. The education of severe and profoundly delayed children focuses on self-help skills; some can function in group home settings, whereas others will require more institutional residential placements. A few profoundly delayed adults with a functional age less than 18 months do not speak and cannot be toilet trained. Even persons with more severe degrees of intellectual disability increasingly are being integrated into their communities.

In the absence of other major organ system involvement, persons with intellectual disability can be expected to live a normal life span. Failure to achieve independent ambulation and self-feeding are the two developmental milestones associated with decreased longevity.

Regardless of the predicted long-term outcome and placement, the optimal environment for the young child with mental retardation is with his or her family. Parents of children with more severe intellectual disability should be advised early to specify guardianship arrangements in their wills and to finalize legal certification of permanent minority status by middle adolescence.

Managing Behavior Disorders in the Child with Intellectual Disability

Any unexplained deviation from the slow but steady progress along the path predicted for a diagnosed degree of developmental delay demands further investigation. In addition to medical complications, three common profiles should be taken into account. First, despite an accurate overall IQ, the child with intellectual disability may have a superimposed learning disability or sensory-processing impairment that prevents their functioning at the predicted intellectual level. Higher expectations and undue pressures then produce significant acting-out behavior. If behavior problems follow shortly after modifications in class placement or system supports, a careful re-evaluation of these changes is indicated. Behavioral deterioration might then suggest that the supports for inclusion are inadequate.

Second, family stress and dysfunction are more likely with a handicapped child and are much more likely to produce secondary behavioral symptoms in the child with intellectual disability. Such stressors are fairly predictable occurrences at specific critical life stages. Family turmoil reflected in the delayed child's acting-out behavior or school underachievement can be expected at entrance into early childhood special education programs and into kindergarten, puberty or menarche, graduation, workshop or independent living arrangements, and at similar critical events in the lives of other family members. Child physical and sexual abuse at home and in the community probably occur more frequently to children with intellectual disability. The possibility of physical, sexual, and psychologic abuse always should be considered for a sudden or even a long-term behavior disorder unresponsive to routine interventions.

The third and probably most common reason for behavioral problems in persons with intellectual disability is the expanded Strauss syndrome (ESS). Children with ESS can exhibit hyperactivity, inattention, impulsivity, perseveration, aggression, repetitive, self-stimulatory, self-injurious, stereotypic, and sometimes bizarre behaviors. Although the incidence of ESS does seem to correlate inversely with IQ, the syndrome complex can occur in persons with only mild intellectual disability. The treatment of choice is behavior modification and environmental management. In the school setting, this can be accomplished by a Functional Behavioral Assessment (FBA) and the subsequent formulation of a plan for positive behavioral supports.

Psychotropic medication can be a helpful treatment adjunct, but it should not be used alone (Table 98.2). As a rule, such medications should only be used as part of a comprehensive behavioral intervention program after other contributing factors have been carefully addressed or excluded. Pharmacotherapy should target specific behaviors. Drug effects and potential side effects should be monitored closely. After these conditions have been met, the risk-to-benefit ratio might be acceptable. Generally, it would be considered poor medical practice not to consider a trial of medication, if family and school placements are at risk because of the patient's behavior. Stimulant medication is occasionally helpful in persons with mild intellectual disability and attentional problems, and its use should be given special consideration, because the potential side effects of such medication are less than those of other drugs. Neuroleptics may be effective, but their use runs the risk of sedation, dystonic reactions, tardive dyskinesia, and increased cognitive impairment.

A final word of caution is indicated on the use of medication that has direct or indirect effects on the CNS. Any such drug can be anticipated to have unpredictable effects, especially as the degree of mental retardation worsens. As the global percentage of normally functioning brain tissue decreases, fairly atypical responses become the rule. Paradoxic responses to stimulant and sedative drugs may occur; much higher dose of anesthetic may be needed for surgery, while fairly low dosage levels of anesthesia may prove fatal.

PROGNOSIS

In cerebral palsy, the presenting problem is motor abnormality, but the most handicapping aspect of the disorder is the cognitive dysfunction. In intellectual disability, the presenting problem is the cognitive dysfunction, but the most handicapping aspect of the disorder is society's limited ability to accept the limitations of the person with intellectual disability. The ESS often provides the greatest limitation on the ability of the adult with intellectual disability to integrate successfully into the community. With appropriate educational experiences, social competence can exceed the measured cognitive level. However, it is not uncommon to find neurobehavioral symptoms interfering with the achievement of social competence commensurate with mental age level. The issue of social competence assumes increasing importance as deinstitutionalization and normalization principles lead to community integration for persons with increasingly severe degrees of intellectual disability, with marriage and parenting as *de facto* choices currently being made. The children of parents with intellectual disability present pediatricians with a whole new set of challenges.

Idiot is ultimately derived from an ancient Greek word indicating "a private person," a term with increasingly negative connotations, as applied to someone who was not involved in the active political life of the city-state. Pejorative terms such as *idiot, imbecile,* and *moron* have finally disappeared from the medical literature, but the full integration of persons with intellectual disability into modern community structures remains an advocacy objective for all professionals dealing with persons with cognitive impairments.

TABLE 98.2

PSYCHOTROPIC MEDICATION

Class of Drugs	Generic Names	Trade Names
Neuroleptics (major tranquilizers)		
Phenothiazines	Chlorpromazine	Thorazine
	Thioridazine	Mellaril
Butyrophenones	Haloperidol	Haldol
Benzodiazepines (minor tranquilizers)	Diazepam	Valium
Stimulants	Dextroamphet-amine	Dexedrine, Adderall
	Methylphenidate	Ritalin, Concerta
Tricyclic anti-depressants	Desipramine	Norpramin
	Imipramine	Tofranil
Anticonvulsants	Carbamazepine	Tegretol
	Clonazepam	Klonopin
	Diphenylhydantoin	Dilantin
	Phenobarbital	
	Valproic acid	Depakene
Miscellaneous	Busprione	BuSpar
	Clonidine	Catapres
	Naloxone	Narcan
	Propranolol	Inderal
	Risperidone	Risperdal
	Melatonin	

Suggested Readings

Accardo PJ, Capute AJ, eds. Mental retardation. *Ment Retard Dev Dis Res Rev* 1998;4:1.

Aman MG, Collier-Crispin A, Lindsay RL. Pharmacotherapy of disorders in mental retardation. *Eur Child Adoles Psychiatry* 2000;9:I,98.

Battaglia A, Carey JC. Diagnostic evaluation of developmental delay/mental retardation: an overview. *Am J Med Genet* 2003;117C:3.

The Capute Scales: CAT/CLAMS. Baltimore: Kennedy Fellows Association,1996.

Capute AJ, Accardo PJ, eds. *Developmental disabilities in infancy and childhood,* 2 vols. Baltimore: Paul H. Brookes,1996.

Mehes K. *Informative morphogenetic variants in the newborn infant.* Budapest: Akademiai Kiado,1988.

Shevell M, Ashwal S, Donley D, et al. Practice parameter: evaluation of the child with global developmental delay. *Neurology* 2003;60:367.

CHAPTER 99 ■ BIOPSYCHOSOCIAL AND DEVELOPMENTAL APPROACHES IN PEDIATRICS

JAMES C. HARRIS

When parents bring a child to the pediatrician, it is because they are concerned. Their distress and disquietude must be appreciated, as symptoms are elicited and signs are understood so that a sense of confidence can be established. This allows the parents to confidently carry out the recommendations made for the child's care and treatment. The approach to the patient is developmental and biopsychosocial in nature. It is an interactional approach, rather than an exclusively reductionist, biomedical one; it addresses current symptoms and physiologic changes, the meaning of the illness to both child and family, their current psychologic state, their history of adaptation to past illnesses, the family genetic background, and their understanding of this particular illness. To develop an appreciation for this approach, developmental models and the interface of brain and behavior are reviewed in this chapter. See the other chapters in this section for a more detailed discussion of the stress response, resilience to stress, coping with stress, bereavement, and stress-related disorders. Later chapters present the epidemiology, assessment, diagnosis, and treatment of emotional, behavioral, and interpersonal conditions in childhood, reviewed from a biopsychosocial perspective. Guidelines for referral to a child and adolescent psychiatrist are presented in Chapter 115. The inclusion of these disorders is in keeping with a pediatric focus on the "New Morbidity" paradigm, which represents a shift in understanding those areas that impact on the health of children and families.

From a personal developmental perspective, the child is viewed as active and fully engaged in life, using his or her individual genetic and temperamental endowments to master developmental tasks in relation to family, peers, and community, even when the child and the family are faced with illness. Psychologic factors may assume importance in altering individual susceptibility to disease and recovery from illness.

Considering children's behavior more generally, a behavior may be quantitatively different from normal when behaviors that were initially developmentally appropriate persist, as in separation anxiety disorder, or qualitatively different from the average child's adaptation, as in major depression; both of these perspectives are addressed.

THE DEVELOPMENTAL PERSPECTIVE

The developmental perspective is basic to pediatrics. It emphasizes the capacity for change throughout life, an approach now referred to as the *lifespan view* of human development. The child is seen as an active, socially oriented, and developing person, rather than as either a passive respondent to the environment or an individual developing independently of the environmental experiences. Development occurs in phases of progressive change as the child masters new developmental tasks. Early experiences are important in this process, but the child has a remarkable resilience to stress, and as new abilities emerge, the child has new means to master environmental challenges.

Growth refers to changes in the size of the body as a whole, and *development* addresses the differentiation of form (i.e., changes in function shaped by interaction with the external environment). Development is an interactive process and refers, particularly in psychiatry, to emotional and social development. The opportunity to develop one's full biologic and psychologic potential is a result of many interacting factors. Genetic factors are important in establishing the limits of potential, but they are interwoven with environmental experience. Physical trauma, particularly brain injury, affects development and behavior; nutritional factors are critically important.

A developmental perspective has the following characteristics:

- It emphasizes changing contexts and patterns of behavior over time, rather than behavioral stability.
- It recognizes that younger children have considerable developmental plasticity in the nervous system, but that with the pruning of neuronal synapses associated with maturation, the brain's capacity to adapt to injury becomes more circumscribed.
- It acknowledges discontinuity in psychologic development, as well as continuity, connectedness, and the persistence of temperamental traits over time.
- It appreciates that vulnerabilities to some social experiences exist, but that these experiences may be strengthening as they are mastered.
- It appreciates that stressors may have a different effect at one age than at another.
- It asks why certain emotional and behavioral disorders present initially at one age and not at another; why are there differences in age of onset of disorder.
- It suggests an opportunity for prevention by offering interventions within the developmental period.
- It studies how approaches to the interview, diagnosis, and treatment may be better informed by an appreciation of developmental processes, experience, and task mastery.

A developmental perspective also is applied to the study of major mental disorders when they occur during the developmental period. Through the study of developmental psychopathology, the natural history of a major mental illness is studied as it is manifested at different ages and as it influences the mastery of age-appropriate developmental tasks. The capacity to master developmental tasks progresses with age as mental processing becomes more efficient, working memory is enhanced, and thinking becomes more reflective.

From a developmental perspective, the pediatrician considers all the following: the full spectrum of behavior from the molecular level, as seen in enzyme activation in the course of differentiation; the interaction of metabolic and physical changes associated with the development of neurotransmitter and hormonal systems; the development of cognition, intelligence, and the emotions; and individual reciprocal social relationships with family, peers, and community. The last category includes the quality of the interaction of the infant and child with parents, siblings, and others; the child's role in the family system; and the type of child-rearing practices carried out. Child rearing is influenced by the cultural and personal experiences of the parents.

BRAIN MATURATION

The growth of the brain, in contrast to other organ systems, is greatest during the infant and toddler years. By 6 months of age, the brain has reached half of its mature weight, and by 5 years, 90% of its adult weight. The rapid growth of the brain, in contrast to the rest of the body, has important implications from the developmental perspective. This rapid development has been linked to a maturational view of development that argues that abilities are influenced by experience and that they gradually unfold as long as two primary conditions are met: adequate nutrition and an opportunity to interact in a normal, expected environment.

Some parts of the brain mature earlier than others (e.g., the brainstem and limbic system mature before the cerebellum and higher cortical areas). Hearing and vision are present early, but interpretation and understanding of what is heard or seen takes place later. An understanding of the usual sequences of development is relevant in assessing children with developmental delays, but considerable variability in development occurs (e.g., some children normally do not speak until age 3 or 4 years). Delays are more common in boys than girls, indicating possible gender differences in brain development. The association of developmental delay with maturation is hypothetical, and much more must be learned. In intellectual disability, however, the failure of appropriate maturation or interference with normal brain development is an important hypothesis.

Marked individual differences in brain development occur; therefore, although average ages for maturational events exist, to consider a range of months during which development will occur is important and more appropriate (e.g., walking at 10 to 18 months).

Developing parts of the brain are more susceptible to damage from injury, infection, toxins, or malnutrition at times of their most rapid growth. However, the young brain also is more capable of adapting to injury, so that the practical consequences of damage may be less. This is probably because brain functions are not specifically localized but instead involve connections that are present throughout the brain and involve multiple brain regions. In young children who suffer damage to regions vital to function (e.g., the speech area in the left hemisphere), functional changes in the other hemisphere may compensate for the damage. Recovery from brain injury in young children may be more complete than expected because of this neuronal plasticity.

ENVIRONMENTAL INTERFACE

Development is not only a gradual unfolding, but also a process in which experience plays an important role, and learning requires both brain growth and external stimulation. The timing of development is not controlled entirely by genetics, and external environmental stimulation may be needed to facilitate it. The term *plasticity* is used to signify the fact that the organism can be modified by environmental experiences. When behavior in response to a stimulus is measured, plasticity is being measured. For example, if infant kittens are reared with one eyelid sutured closed, vision is impaired in that eye; however, the loss is partially functional, and plasticity is demonstrated, because vision can be substantially restored by administering gamma amino butyric acid (GABA) agonists after the sutures are removed.

The chemistry of brain development also is affected by deprivation, just as in adults the lack of use of an extremity leads to some muscle wasting. Lack of stimulation may retard growth, but extra stimulation does not enhance it if adequate maturation has not occurred. Stimulation may influence particular behaviors at the appropriate time (e.g., babbling in infants is influenced by parents' talking to them and accommodating the prosody or rhythm of their voice to that of the infant). Children who receive specific language training in a day-care center have enhanced abilities compared with those who are involved in free play alone. Stress may interfere with development, as demonstrated by the persistence of enuresis in children with severe burns and the return to bed-wetting in children who have been stressed.

DEVELOPMENTAL TASKS

The development of the person, the *personality*, has been the focus of developmental theorists. Theoretic perspectives have addressed psychosexual development, cognitive development, the development of interpersonal relations, and identity. Psychotherapies have been suggested based on these approaches. Current emphasis is placed on an ethologic model of development that addresses behavior in reference to our biologic background, those patterns of behavior across species that serve the same purpose, the natural selection of behavioral traits, and behavior that is biologically based, such as infant–mother attachment.

Each of the frameworks for development makes assumptions about the capabilities of the infant and young child in regard to recognition and remembrance of past experience, temperamental characteristics, and response to environmental uncertainty. Each of these perspectives suggests an emphasis on socially important features or goals (e.g., self-control, moral development, compassionate interpersonal behavior, and self-awareness are ideal goals). These goals represent developmental tasks to be mastered at different ages.

The child is an active person who masters a series of developmental tasks that meld genetic and temperamental attributes while utilizing psychosocial support (e.g., infants and children are actively involved, capable of interaction, and have individual responses). Infants influence what goes on around them and what happens to them by their behavior; parents respond to their infants' preferences. This is in contrast to an older view that depicted the infant as passive, without individuality, and at the mercy of the environment. The parent–child interaction is one of social reciprocity, as the parents adapt to the child through their individual personalities, past experience with children, and family background. This past interactional history is particularly important to understand in the parents' response to a handicapped or premature child.

DEVELOPMENTAL MODELS OF BEHAVIORAL AND EMOTIONAL DEVELOPMENT

To understand the complex interaction between children and the biologic and environmental influences on them, the child's development can be approached from several perspectives.

Biologic Models

Maturational Model

The maturational view, which was popularized by Gesell, states that development occurs through orderly, nonrandom, patterned sequences determined by biologic and evolutionary history. However, the rate of development is influenced by the individual genetic family history. Although development may be altered by such things as illness, malnutrition, or stressful experiences, fundamental biologic factors direct it. A favorable environment facilitates development; an unfavorable one inhibits development. Neither circumstance changes the basic biologic potential. Gesell sought to describe the form of morphologic or structural growth and psychologic growth. He argued that development has direction (e.g., cephalocaudal and proximodistal), is organized through reciprocal relationships or interweavings (e.g., flexors and extensors develop in a sequence that allows coordinated movement), and may demonstrate functional asymmetry or an unbalanced development that occurs to achieve mastery at a later stage of development (e.g., development of "handedness").

Development is controlled by biologically predetermined patterns that are unvarying, although the rate may vary from one child to another. The environment does not change development, suggesting that environmental influence sometimes is limited. Gesell's investigations focused on normal children living in an average, expectable psychosocial environment that is active and stimulating. Gesell emphasized four areas of development: motor, adaptive, language, and personal and social. In terms of motor development and individual differences in rate of growth and in personality pattern, his investigations often have been replicated. Gesell showed that pushing children excessively during early developmental periods is futile, and thus introduced the concept of the child's readiness for intervention.

Gesell emphasized internal regulation, used age as a marker, provided guidelines for developmental level, noted the sensitivity of responsiveness at certain times in development, observed discontinuity in development, recognized individual differences, and appreciated the effect of the environment as amplifying or reducing behavioral effects. A self-regulatory fluctuation of development finally occurs, with periods of instability followed by stability and consolidation, and cycles of development, with equilibrium following disequilibrium.

Ethologic Model

The ethologic view addresses the roots and mechanisms of behavior in both humans and animals. It addresses classes of behavior that are biologically based: reflexes, taxes, and fixed action patterns. Behaviors that are innate occur without learning (i.e., without practicing) and are species-typical behaviors, such as imprinting in birds. A primitive reflex, such as the tonic neck reflex, is an example of an innate behavior in the human infant. At least 25 such reflexes, including the walking reflex, have been identified in the neonate.

The taxes are locomotor or orienting responses, and include cuddling and other actions involving more than one reflex. The fixed action pattern is a sequence of coordinated motor actions. They are made up of innate releasing mechanisms associated with a signed stimulus (e.g., the mother leaves the room, and that departure is associated with the infant crying). The departure is a signed stimulus leading to an innate releasing mechanism, followed by a fixed action pattern. Another example is the infantile appearance with large head, bulging cheeks, and large eyes, which acts as a signed stimulus for care-eliciting behavior toward the infant. Many parenting behaviors may have an ethologic origin.

Bowlby, using the ethologic approach in the study of infant attachment, has found four separate phases of attachment:

- Preattachment, demonstrated by orienting behavior toward caregivers (e.g., early following with the eyes, smiling, and vocalization)
- Attachment in the making, as the parent responds to the infant's initiative
- Clear-cut attachment, as the toddler walks away and then returns to the caregiver
- Goal-corrected partnership, which occurs at the beginning of the third year of life, as the child begins to understand the adult's behavior and can take the parent's needs into account

The goal of attachment is to anticipate and increase physical proximity with the mother and to gain nurturing. As a consequence of these early experiences, a child increasingly develops internal working models of relationships and secure, insecure, or disrupted patterns of attachment. This model includes an appreciation of genetic and environmental factors.

Sociobiologic Model

The sociobiologic approach, unlike the ethologic approach, places more emphasis on those aspects of development related to and controlled by specific genes, and it gives less importance to the environment. Rather than potentials, the focus is on biologic and psychologic determinism. Sociobiology has been defined by Wilson, its prime proponent, as the "systematic study of the biologic basis of all social behavior." Successful reproduction is emphasized. The theme of sacrifice or altruism is demonstrated in parents of all species in their efforts to preserve the next generation.

Sociobiologists posit several causes for the demonstration of social behavior. One cause is phylogenetic inertia, defined as the organism's tendency to remain unchanged under ecologic pressures. Change is greatest if genetic variability exists in the species. An opportunity to increase the gene pool decreases phylogenetic inertia because, as new genetic material is introduced, the likelihood of change increases.

Antisocial factors that encourage individuals in that species to isolate themselves are also important considerations. Inbreeding of species increases recessive traits and minimizes genetic variability. Another important factor is complexity of behavior, which suggests that complex behaviors, such as parenting, would have higher phylogenetic inertia. The effect of change in behavior on other traits and characteristics is considered, in that the degree to which a change in one system affects another is related to the degree of phylogenetic inertia.

Ecologic pressure represents that part of the environment that encourages the organism to change. This is the nurture side of the nature–nurture equation. The threat of predation provides ecologic pressure in animals to adapt (e.g., ultrasonic separation calls from rodent infants to their mother protect them from predators and maintain social contact). Another pressure is the lack of availability of food, leading to nomadic movement and increased demands to adapt in new environments. Wilson notes that "manipulation of the physical environment is the ultimate adaptation;" therefore, tool use is important in human adaptation.

Demographic characteristics, gene flow, and genetic similarity are important factors in sociobiology. Birth rates, death rates, and population size have important effects on behavior. For example, Calhoun has demonstrated that overcrowding in rats leads to an increase in aberrant social behaviors, increased death rates, and greater susceptibility to disease and stress. Gene flow results from interbreeding with other populations and introduces new genes into that population. Change is faster if new genes enter the population; however, the more genetic similarity in a population, the greater the stability of behavior and the more likely that genetically adaptive behaviors will be maintained. However, inbreeding may increase the risk of maintaining maladaptive traits in the community.

Sociobiologists argue that similar behaviors in humans and animals are genetically related. Research in this area that is pertinent to behavior may be relevant to parenting. An example is the separation cry, which has a similar sonographic frequency in various species of mammals and is a potential model for studies of separation anxiety in children.

Interpersonal Approaches

Sociocultural Model

The sociocultural approach emphasizes the importance of cultural transmission rather than genetic transmission for cognitive development. The major proponent of this approach was Vygotsky, who focused on an interactional view of cognitive development and maintained that higher mental functions (cognitive processes) initially are experienced through interpersonal interaction and subsequently intrapsychically (e.g., the establishment of concrete logic is preceded by the internalization of representational language). Vygotsky emphasized the role of inner speech as a means of problem solving. For instance, a child loses a toy. His mother helps him mentally retrace his activities that day until he becomes aware of its location. Subsequently, the child may use inner language to remember without relying on an adult.

Vygotsky referred to the distance between the actual developmental level, as determined by independent problem solving, and the level of potential development, as determined through problem solving under adult guidance or in collaboration with more capable peers, as the *zone of proximal development*. In the zone of proximal development, self-talk becomes established as an important process in cognitive development and as a means of self-monitoring and self-control. Both cognitive and interpersonal growth occur in the zone of proximal development. Vygotsky's approach has attracted more interest as developmental psychologists begin to study higher cortical functions, particularly regarding perspective taking and social cognition.

Psychodynamic Model

The psychodynamic approach includes psychoanalysis, which was one of the first attempts to offer a systematic theory of development. Freud, the founder of psychoanalysis, described a hypothetical psychic energy, the libido, that was distributed in various ways. His psychoanalytic theory addresses factors outside one's awareness that influence development and included psychodynamic components, a structural system, and a series of progressive psychologic stages. Originally based on studies of conversion symptoms that occurred without a demonstrable organic disorder, the distribution of this libidinal energy was said to depend on the organism's stage of development, experiential history, and current life setting. The primary source of psychic energy was initially suggested to be instinctually expressed through unlearned psychologic drives by which tension was gratified through the infant's or child's behavior. Instincts were seen as psychologic representations of biologic processes. The bulk of psychic energy is outside consciousness in infants and is expressed in seeking pleasure and personal gratification. (However, crying and increased motor activity do serve to bring the infant into contact with the external world.)

The most powerful of the instinctual drives are hunger, the sex drive, and the aggressivon. For example, the hunger drive results in tension, which leads to crying, which is relieved by a parent providing food. The child gradually becomes aware of the relationship to the parent and, by adapting to these responses, develops psychologic structures to mediate future behavior. These psychologic structures are described by Freud in

his structural system under the hypothetical constructs of id, ego, and superego. The first element, the *id energy*, is energy derived from original biologic impulses, and its goal is to obtain instinctual gratification. Part of this id energy is adapted and transformed as conscious associations are made to psychosocial experiences. The second element, the *ego*, is this complex of conscious associations. The ego facilitates adaptation by mediating new conscious behavior, and through the process of identification, begins to discriminate a separate self and to obtain pleasure through adaptation to external reality. The third element, the *superego*, emerges as further psychic energy is transformed into consciousness when the child becomes aware of and incorporates the parents' ethical standards. This ego ideal, or conscience, serves to modulate behavior in relation to parental standards, but it may conflict with the demands of the ego and superego.

The dynamic and structural components interact through a set of defense mechanisms to minimize experienced anxiety. These mechanisms distort reality in the face of potential danger that might threaten ego functioning. They are designed to alleviate the conflicts or stressors that give rise to the anxiety signal. They may be adaptive or maladaptive, depending on the context in which they occur. The most common defense mechanisms are denial, displacement, dissociation, idealization, intellectualization, isolation, passive-aggression, rejection, rationalization, reaction formation, repression, somatization, autistic fantasy, acting out, suppression, splitting, and undoing. Defense mechanisms aid in restructuring the personality as the child experiments with new experiences. They enable psychic energy to remain directed toward a goal rather than being expressed as excessive anxiety. With development, the ego acts as a more effective mediator in modulating anxiety, thereby reducing the need for defense mechanisms in dealing with reality.

Environmental Models

Psychosocial Model

The psychosocial perspective was originated with Erikson, who suggested that psychologic development is the result of an interaction between maturational forces and social forces. This approach emphasizes socialization throughout the lifespan. Erikson suggested a series of eight stages of development that focus on the task of identity formation and introduced the principle of epigenesis, based on an embryologic model, with each psychosocial stage emerging from the previous one. In each stage, a developmental crisis requires resolution, and so the importance of the ego is highlighted (Box 99.1).

At each stage of development, a different conflict has particular significance for the individual. These conflicts are expressed as polarities representing opposite tendencies that, when resolved, lead to a particular virtue. The first five stages deal with the tasks of children and adolescents, the next two address tasks of parents, and the final stage addresses the task for older parents and grandparents. These are all expressed as developmental tasks (e.g., to master an identity crisis in adolescence, the adolescent must address certain questions that require the mastery of earlier developmental stages).

Erikson's major contribution was stressing the importance of the development of a strong ego identity. Erikson said that an immature ego is present at birth and develops through experience. He is referred to as an *ego psychologist*. His formulations are widely used in medicine, psychology, and education.

Behavioral Model

The behavioral model studies only observable behaviors; its theoretic framework emphasizes environmental factors in

BOX 99.1   Erickson's Developmental Stages

- Stage 1: The polarity between trust and mistrust is experienced during the first year of life. If it is resolved with a predominance of trust, the outcome is hope. The question that must be answered with increasing age is, can I trust?
- Stage 2: The polarity between autonomy and shame or doubt is experienced in the second and third years of life. Resolution leads to confidence and a sense of self-control. The question that must be answered with increasing age is, can I be free of self-doubt?
- Stage 3: The polarity between initiative and guilt is introduced at 4 to 5 years of age, when the child is internalizing adult roles and standards. The resolution of the conflict leads to a sense of purposefulness. The question that must be answered is, can I act independently?
- Stage 4: The polarity is between industry and inferiority, and its resolution leads to a sense of competence. This conflict presents itself between ages 6 and 11 years. The question that must be answered with increasing age is, can I be successful in carrying out my goals?
- Stage 5: The polarity relates to establishing a sense of identity and clarifying confusion of roles between ages 12 and 18 years. The questions that are asked are, who am I, what do I believe in, how do I feel about others, and what are my attitudes about myself? Successful resolution leads to fidelity or faithfulness, allegiance, and loyalty toward one's own beliefs.
- Stage 6: With the establishment of fidelity, the young adult is prepared to consider marrying and starting a family. In this stage, the polarity is between intimacy and isolation, and the resolution of this conflict is the experience of love in interpersonal relationships. The question that must be answered is, can I be intimate with another person?
- Stage 7: Following the establishment of intimacy, the next stage presents the polarity between generativity and self-absorption. The resolution of this conflict is the ability to provide loving care to one's own children. The question that must be answered is, can I give of myself to the care of my children?
- Stage 8: The final stage in the life cycle addresses the polarity of integrity and despair. The task of old age is to reflect on having established contentment and satisfaction in one's life. That satisfactory outcome is wisdom. The question the older person asks is, have I found contentment and direction in my life?

developmental outcome. The behaviorist suggests that development is a function of learning; that development is the consequence of different kinds of learning; that differences in individual development are the result of past experiences; that development is the result of the organization of current behavioral patterns; that general limits on behavior come from biologic limitations, that environmental factors determine the choice of behavior; and that the individual's behavior is not a direct consequence of biologic stages. The behaviorist suggests that the behavior is neither biologically determined nor the result of internal biologic processes.

Behaviorists emphasize classical and operant conditioning and study conditioned reflexes (i.e., the reinforcement and extinction of these conditioned responses). Having analyzed behavior, they study generalization of behavior by investigating factors in reinforcement. In the behavioral approach, learning is governed by the responses to environmental stimuli, which are strengthened or weakened by environmental reinforcement. Behaviorists investigate how stimuli are discriminated. They assume that behavior is the function of its consequences; in particular, they study a type of learning called *operant conditioning*. Operant behaviors are controlled by their consequences and not by what precedes them. The emphasis is on the behavior that is emitted, not on the preceding behavior. Factors that affect behavior are studied in terms of positive and negative reinforcers and punishment. Investigations of schedules of reinforcement that are broadly continuous or intermittent are used in behavioral analysis. Techniques of treatment include chaining and shaping of behavior, and attempts to generalize behavior to appropriate environmental settings. In using a behavioral approach, a functional behavioral analysis should be completed, and behavioral enhancement procedures should be emphasized in treatment.

Suggested Readings

Ainsworth MD. Attachments across the life span. *Bull N Y Acad Med* 1985;61:792.

American Academy of Pediatrics. *The classification of child and adolescent mental diagnoses in primary care. diagnostic and statistical manual for primary care (DSM-PC) child and adolescent version.* Wolraich ML, Felice ME, Drotar D, eds. Elk Grove Village, IL: American Academy of Pediatrics, 1996.

American Academy of Pediatrics. Committee on Psychosocial Aspects of Child and Family Health. The New Morbidity revisited: a renewed commitment to the psychosocial aspects of pediatric care. *Pediatrics* 2001;108:1227.

American Psychiatric Association. *Diagnostic and statistical manual of mental disorders DSM-IV-TR,* 4th ed. Text revision. Washington, DC: American Psychiatric Publishing, Inc., 2000.

Bowlby J. Developmental psychiatry comes of age. *Am J Psychiatry* 1988;145:1.

Bowlby J. *A secure base: parent-child attachment and healthy human development.* New York: Basic Books, 1988.

Demetiou A, Spanoudis G, Platsidou M. The development of mental processing: efficacy, working memory, and thinking. *Monogr Soc Res Child Dev* 2002;Serial No. 268, 67:1.

Engel GL. The need for a new medical model: a challenge for biomedicine. *Science* 1977;196:129.

Erikson EH. *Identity and the life cycle.* New York: W. W. Norton & Co., 1994 (reprint ed.).

Erikson E, Coles R, eds. *The Erik Erikson reader.* New York: W. W. Norton & Company, 2000.

Gesell AG. *Gesell and Amatruda's developmental diagnosis; the evaluation and management of normal and abnormal neuropsychologic development in infancy and early childhood,* 3rd ed. New York: Harper Collins, 1974.

Harris JC. *Developmental neuropsychiatry.* Vol I: Fundamentals; vol. II: Assessment, diagnosis, and treatment. New York: Oxford University Press, 1998.

International Classification of Diseases. Classification of mental and behavioral disorders: clinical descriptions and diagnostic guidelines, 10th ed. Geneva: World Health Organization, 1992.

Kazdin AE. Behavior modification. In: Wiener JM, ed. *Textbook of child and adolescent psychiatry,* 2nd ed. Washington, DC: American Psychiatric Press, 1997:821.

Lewis M, ed. *Child and adolescent psychiatry: a comprehensive textbook,* 3rd ed. Philadelphia: Lippincott Williams & Wilkins, 2002.

Magnusson D, ed. *The lifespan development of individuals: behavioral, neurobiological, and psychosocial perspectives.* Cambridge, UK: Cambridge University Press, 1997.

Marans S, Cohen DJ. Child psychoanalytic theories of development. In: Lewis M, ed. *Child and adolescent psychiatry: a comprehensive textbook,* 2nd ed. Philadelphia: Lippincott Williams & Wilkins, 2002:196.

Martin A, Scahill L, Charney DS, Leckman JF. *Pediatric psychopharmacology: principles and practice.* New York: Oxford University Press, 2003.

Rakic P. Genesis of the neocortex in human and nonhuman primates. In: Lewis M, ed. *Child and adolescent psychiatry: a comprehensive textbook,* 3rd ed. Philadelphia: Lippincott Williams & Wilkins, 2002:22.

Rutter M, Rutter M. *Developing minds: challenge and continuity across the life span.* New York: Basic Books, 1993.

Rutter M. Child psychiatric disorders in ICD-10. *J Child Psychol Psychiatry* 1989;30:499.

Volkmar FR, Schwab-Stone M, First M. Classification in child and adolescent psychiatry: principles and issues. In: Lewis M, ed. *Child and adolescent psychiatry: a comprehensive textbook.* Philadelphia: Lippincott Williams & Wilkins, 2002:499.

Salkind NJ. *Theories of human development,* 2nd ed. New York: Wiley, 1985.

Schetky D, Benedek E. *Principles and practice of child and adolescent forensic psychiatry*. Washington D.C.: American Psychiatric Publishing, Inc. 2001.

Smith PK, Cowie H, Blades M. *Understanding children's development*, 4th ed. Malden, MA: Blackwell Publishers, 2003.

Vygotsky LS, Vygotsky S, John-Steiner V, eds. *Mind in society: the development of higher psychologic processes*. Cambridge, MA: Harvard University Press, 1980.

Waters E, Merrick S, Treboux D, et al. Attachment security in infancy and early adulthood: a twenty-year longitudinal study. *Child Dev* 2000;71: 684.

Wiener J, Dulcan M, eds. *Textbook of child and adolescent psychiatry*, 3rd ed. Washington, DC: American Psychiatric Publishing, Inc, 2004.

Wilson EO. *Sociobiology: the new synthesis*. Twenty-fifth anniversary ed. Boston: Harvard University Press, 2000.

CHAPTER 100 ■ PSYCHOSOCIAL INTERVIEW

JAMES C. HARRIS

The goal of the psychosocial interview is to establish a confiding relationship with the child and family. This relationship allows them to develop confidence in the physician.

COMPONENTS OF THE PSYCHOSOCIAL INTERVIEW

The first step is to obtain demographic and other background information from the child and his parents and to determine the reliability of this information. The pediatrician asks the parents and child about their specific concerns, why they are seeking help at this time.

It is important to review precipitating stressful events that may contribute to the behavioral difficulty and address specific concerns; these include academic and school problems, antisocial behavior, emotional conflict, regressive behavior, and interpersonal difficulty. The pediatrician reviews previous treatment and clarifies the effects of the child's current behavior on family function.

The family history is reviewed, to clarify the child's status in regard to foster care, adoption, step-parenting, or other family issues. Questions are asked: Who has custody of the child, whose personality does the child's resemble, and after whom is the child named?

The family background of both parents is reviewed (including *their* childhood), with particular emphasis on the family atmosphere in the parents' childhoods, stresses from emotional or economic causes, and the deaths of or separation from close relatives. Information regarding the grandparents and others closely affiliated with the child is gathered, along with a developmental family history of how the marriage evolved. Also included are the quality of relatedness in the current marriage (e.g., frequency of disagreements and how they are expressed), coping mechanisms dealing with conflict in the family, and the relationship with the family of origin. Siblings are described by age, school placement, history of significant illness, personality, and relationship with family members.

A history of familial diseases should include learning disability, intellectual disability, alcoholism, abnormal personality, suicide, homicide, bipolar disorder, and schizophrenia. In reviewing the child's personal history, one should note the date and place of birth, birth weight, attitude of both parents toward the pregnancy, and whether it was planned or unplanned. If difficulties were encountered during the pregnancy or delivery, the parents' psychological response to that event should be noted.

Developmental milestones should emphasize social responses, including eye contact, social smile, language communication, and interpersonal attachment. The quality of mother–child (dyadic) relationship and the child–mother–father (triadic) relationship requires review. Interpersonal issues that relate to feeding and illness care must be considered. The parents' attitudes toward child rearing, particularly in regard to permissiveness and limit-setting, are assessed.

A behavioral review of symptoms (information regarding temperament, early development, emotional responsiveness, antisocial behavior, attentional difficulties, self-stimulation, and play behavior) is obtained. Assessment of schooling includes the age at beginning school, the current grade, schools attended, type of class placement, and emotional adjustment to beginning school. Separation problems upon the initiation of either preschool or elementary school are reviewed. If absences from school were prolonged, or if school years were repeated, that information—along with specific difficulties in reading, writing, spelling, and mathematics—is noted. Study habits and academic goals are reviewed, and the child's peer relationships are assessed. Whether the child is teased or is a bully is determined, and particular friendships are assessed. Attitudes toward teachers, peers, and schoolwork also are noted.

The child's awareness of sexual identity is assessed by asking questions regarding curiosity about the body and reproduction and about sexual interests and activities. For the adolescent, the interview covers information regarding the mastery of adolescent developmental tasks and the young person's attitude toward entry into adolescence. One looks for mature versus pseudomature behavior and attitudes toward peers, family, and authority. Rebelliousness, drug use, periods of depression or withdrawal, and fantasy life are reviewed. Assessment includes how the young person has responded to puberty, with its accompanying changes in body image (voice changes, hair growth, breast development, menarche), and to sexual concerns.

A mental health history is gathered and should include details of disturbances for which treatment was received and how the treatment was conducted. This is followed by a description of the child's and family's life situation at present, which includes current housing, social situation, parents' work, and financial circumstances. The composition of the household, relationship with neighbors, recent stresses, bereavement, losses or disappointments, and how both parent and child have reacted to these are reviewed. A typical day in the child's life is described, from getting to school, to activities during the school day, the return home, and evening activities.

The physician should consider personality features that are pertinent to the child. These traits include habitual attitudes and patterns of behavior that distinguish the child as an individual. Among personality characteristics are attitudes toward others, with consideration given to the ability to trust others and to make and sustain relationships with them. It must be established whether the child is secure or insecure in interpersonal relationships, is a leader or a follower. The attitude toward interpersonal relationships—whether he or she is friendly, warm, and demonstrative or reserved, cold, or indifferent—is considered. Other characteristics regarding aggressiveness, quarrelsomeness, sensitivity, and suspiciousness are noted. Also considered are attitudes toward the self, including self-dramatizing behavior, egocentric behavior, self-consciousness, and ambition. Attitudes of the child toward personal health and bodily functions are included in assessing whether the child's self-appraisal is realistic or unrealistic.

An assessment of the personality also includes moral and religious attitudes and an evaluation of whether the individual is easygoing, permissive, overconscientious, a perfectionist, or conforming. Mood is considered in regard to lability or persistence and whether the child's attitude toward life is optimistic or pessimistic. Clarification about depression, anxiety, irritability, excessive worrying, and apathy is sought. The ability to express and control feelings of anger, sadness, pleasure, and disappointment is reviewed.

Leisure activities and interests (e.g., books, pictures, music, sports, and creative activities) are noted. How the child spends leisure time, either alone or with others, is assessed.

Finally, the physician asks about daydreams, nightmares, and patterns of reaction to stress. Questions about such reaction patterns should explore the ability to tolerate frustration, loss, and disappointment and should seek a description of circumstances that arouse anger or anxiety and depression. Also investigated is evidence of excessive use of particular psychological defenses, such as denial, rationalization, and projection.

INTERVIEWING THE PARENTS OF AN ILL CHILD

The interview with the parent or parents of an ill child should establish a sense of confidence in them by the physician's careful explanation of the illness and thoughtful responses to their questions. Because parents often must carry out medical and monitoring procedures at home, it is essential that they acknowledge the nature of the child's illness and understand what they are to do. An effective interview facilitates appropriate care. Because the parents are active participants in the child's care, establishing rapport with them is essential, as is remembering that parents are reassured not only by *what* is said but by *how* it is said. Parents are stressed by the child's illness and require psychological support.

To understand the parent's adaptation to the child's illness, the psychological mechanisms normally present in a time of stress must be appreciated. The most common are denial, guilt or self-blame, projection or blaming others, and excessive dependency on others by the parent or the caregiver. Self-awareness by the physician is critical to understanding the parent's adaptation. To determine the degree of the parent's acknowledgment of stress related to the child's illness or developmental disability, the following questions are suggested:

- *To whom do you talk when you are concerned about your child?* This question helps to establish the degree to which the parent is isolated, and whether a confiding relationship with another person exists. It also helps clar-

ify whether the parent is denying the seriousness of the child's illness, thereby putting the child at risk.
- *Who or what do you feel is responsible for causing your child's illness?* This question asks about excessive guilt and self-blame. Self-blaming parents are at risk for developing symptoms of depression.
- *Do you feel that the staff taking care of your child can be trusted?* This question deals with projection and excessive suspiciousness. Parents commonly criticize caregivers as an expression of their projected fear and anxiety.
- *Do you feel adequate to take care of your child, or do you automatically follow directions from others or feel increasingly dependent?* This question deals with dependency and passivity, which may be present in the overwhelmed parent. When this occurs, the physician senses helplessness in the parent, often receives frequent telephone calls, and may be asked to make decisions unrelated to the child's medical care.

Difficulties in dealing with stress result from unresolved feelings of which parents may be unaware. The effectiveness of counseling requires a clarification of the degree of stress and the psychological mechanisms used by parents to adjust to a child's illness. An empathetic approach helps parents to validate their responses and to act with greater confidence.

INTERVIEWING CHILDREN

The pediatrician must take into account both the child's developmental level and the level of communicative understanding. The purpose of the initial meeting is to establish confidence and cooperation as the examination progresses, to get to know the child, and thereby learn the child's response to illness and ability to cooperate with treatment. No matter how benign physicians consider themselves to be, children experience anxiety in encountering a stranger. If the interview is one that deals with behavior and requires an assessment of emotional behavior and interpersonal issues, a more extensive interview is required.

Infants and Toddlers

In examining infants who do not have expressive language, initial observations focus on social milestones. During the first year, the most important of these are the establishment of eye contact, attachment, and the interpersonal use of language through babbling and jargon. The response to newness or change is more intense after 6 months of age, when selective attachments and stranger anxiety emerge as developmental milestones. It is possible to communicate with infants through nonverbal gestures and the language called *motherese*, which involves extending vowel sounds and speaking more slowly. Infants respond to adults' moods and gestures in an active and perceptive way, but only out of their limited experience with familiar caregivers.

The approach to infants, then, is indirect, even casual. Typically, physicians are still and quiet, but close enough to observe. They initially make no direct gesture toward the infant and make no direct eye contact until the infant has "looked them over" from a safe distance. An outstretched hand may prove interesting, and it may encourages an infant to reach out. The best approach is for infants to make the first move. Although dramatic gestures, such as facial contortions and staring, may be soothing to happy children, such gestures may be threatening to anxious children.

Those practitioners holding infants would do well to observe the parents' preferred holding posture and to imitate it. Infants tend to be most secure when they are held in an upright position facing but not directly face-to-face with a stranger. A helpful tactic is for the infant to be able to see the mother over the physician's shoulder.

After the physician has established contact, the examination may proceed as the infant opens up to the examiner. During the examination, talking to the infant, particularly in a soothing tone, may be reassuring. An infant's psychological state must be taken into account.

In toddlers who may be too young to talk, physicians should remember that these children may understand what is said about them. Comprehension precedes verbal expression, and words can be misinterpreted. Also, an anxious tone of voice may have an adverse effect.

Children 2 to 4 Years of Age

In young children who can talk and have a better understanding of what is said to them, the approach is somewhat different. Children at this age may continue to fear the unexpected. Strange procedures and new persons add to that fear, particularly if their earlier experiences have been negative. These fears must be accommodated by using the advantages of better language understanding. In addition, children at this age are very literal in their understanding of the words they use and in those heard from others. Thinking is concrete, and actions are understood in a concrete way; decisions are made on the basis of literal word interpretations. Consequently, descriptions to young children should avoid the use of analogies and generally require that children be asked to repeat what they have been told. For example, children who overhear phrases such as "She has sticky fingers" or "His head is in the clouds" may expect to see clouds and resist being held by the people with "those fingers." Although children gradually understand jokes and abstractions, these elements should be used cautiously when discussing an illness. Learning to speak children's language is enjoyable, and time spent in this way facilitates future visits.

In addition to their literalness, children between 2 and 4 years of age also show a form of transductive reasoning that gives human attributes to inanimate objects. Children attribute feelings and motives to household objects or at least speak as though the objects possess these characteristics. Children may say that a stopped machine has "gone to sleep" and frequently play at putting toys to sleep and waking them. In the office, children may attribute characteristics of life to apparatus and instruments and may fear these things, worrying that the objects may harm the children, cut them, or jump at them. Therefore, a helpful approach is for children to play with instruments before they are used for an examination.

At this age, children tend to be overactive, and pleasing or satisfying them may be difficult. They may delve into everything and act in a destructive and independent manner. It is difficult for them to modulate feelings such as sadness, anger, fearfulness, or jealousy. Children may have difficulty in controlling anger with a younger sibling. Children's behavior demonstrates unpredictability, and directions must be given repeatedly. But the child can be engaged imaginatively through stories that are repeated and cartoons that are watched continuously.

Younger children frequently express fear of physicians. Their fearfulness may represent what they have been told, or what they have experienced in the past. Children also may be influenced by their parents' apprehension before coming for the visit. Parents who trick children into accepting medical treatment by telling them that painful procedures will not be painful or that bad-tasting medications taste good worsen the situation. The best approach is to describe procedures to children accurately, neither exaggerating nor minimizing the effects. This approach should be followed even if the children say that they understand.

The examination should proceed even though children continue to cry after routine precautions have been taken to prevent pain and to relieve anxiety. Step-by-step explanations are important for children who are anxious and for children who are crying and apparently do not seem to be listening. Children may be crying because they are frightened and in pain. This response may be age-appropriate or, if they are ill, appropriate for somewhat younger children. Failure of a child to express fearfulness or suffering may be a greater cause for concern than children's strong reactions.

Children 4 to 7 Years of Age

Fear of medical and surgical procedures is prominent between 4 and 7 years of age. This fear seems to be associated with anxiety about the integrity of the body. Children in this age group demonstrate enhanced bodily awareness and heightened anxiety about potential threats of bodily harm. Concurrent with fear of injury are a sense of pride and a desire to be brave and strong. Children fear anything that might reduce their strength and force them to demonstrate weakness. A new sense of self-esteem accompanies this increased bodily awareness.

Because of these concerns about the body, medical and surgical procedures should be delayed if possible in children with heightened concerns about bodily harm. If the procedure is necessary, the children's feelings must be discussed with them, and they must be prepared carefully, in advance for the procedure. This is particularly true for genital surgery, because children in this age range often are particularly concerned with and aware of their genitals.

In talking to children who do not admit to the presence of an illness, physicians look for ways to reduce fear and anxiety. Emotional warmth and a calm approach can help children feel that they are safe and strong enough, despite concerns about the illness or the recommended treatment. During the examination, an initial period of warming up and talking to a child about his or her successes and interests can alleviate initial anxiety and can form a successful introduction to talking about treatment. By beginning the physical examination with body systems that are functioning well and slowly moving to the problem area, the examiner can cause the examination to go more smoothly. Physicians should not be misled by children's apparent cooperativeness and bravery and should indicate that the procedure may be frightening. The desire to be brave and to conceal fear is acknowledged but, at the same time, children are told that crying is legitimate if they are frightened or if it hurts. Anticipating fearfulness and explaining that most children have fears about an anticipated procedure are a form of psychological immunization. Furthermore, allowing children to play with the examining instruments or, say, a syringe to be used for an injection may relieve anxiety and can stimulate explanations about how healing occurs.

Children 7 to 12 Years of Age

Younger children communicate their feelings through their behavior or through imaginary play. Through play, children clearly may demonstrate their experience of office visits and their experiences at home or in school. During middle childhood (from age 7 on), children can more easily express feelings and fears verbally, but they may be unclear about the reasons for their concerns. Because they may present questions in a veiled fashion, understanding the *meaning* of their questions is important. Frequent and persistent questioning ordinarily indicates a hidden concern.

When children reach middle childhood, they can be interviewed more directly about their behavior, concerns, and their life circumstances. Box 100.1 outlines the questions that may

BOX 100.1   **Interview with an Older Child**

School

1. What grade are you in?
2. What school do you attend?
3. What do you like best about school?
4. How are you doing in school?
5. Is your schoolwork as good as it used to be?
6. Do you have to push yourself to do your work?
7. At school, are you worried or sad about problems when you are trying to work?
8. Do you have trouble with listening to the teacher?
9. Do you have trouble with keeping your mind on your schoolwork?
10. How often are you absent from school?

Friends

1. How many friends do you have in school?
2. How many friends do you have in your neighborhood?
3. How many are good friends?
4. What do you like to do with your friends?
5. Do you wish you had more friends?
6. Do you ever feel shy or hopeless about getting friends?
7. Do you do favors for your friends and not expect to get something back from them?
8. Do you feel bad or guilty if you have done something wrong to a friend?

Activities

1. What do you do when you are by yourself?
2. How do you feel when you are alone?
3. Do you like to spend time by yourself? Is it because it's fun, you are shy, you don't know how to make friends?
4. What are your favorite hobbies?

Family

1. Who lives in your home?
2. Is anyone at your home a troublemaker?
3. To whom are you closest?
4. How do you get along with your mother?
5. How do you get along with your father?
6. What does your mother do that you like? What does she do that you don't like?
7. What does your father do that you like? What does he do that you don't like?
8. Do you have problems with your parents? If so, who is usually to blame?
9. If by magic you could change your family, what would you like to be different?
10. Are you happy in your family?
11. How are your parents getting along with each other?
12. How do you feel when you are away from home?
13. Have you ever thought about running away or leaving home?

Fears and anxieties

1. Most people are afraid of something. What are you afraid of?
2. Do you try to keep away from and feel shy around strangers?
3. Do you feel worried or afraid about school?
4. Do any specific people or situations make you afraid?
5. Do you feel nervous or scared about the future?

Worries and concerns

1. Many children worry about different things. What do you worry about (such as bad things happening or being separated from your family)?
2. Do you worry about these things so much that it interferes with school, friends, or doing things that you like?
3. Do you worry that you make bad things happen?
4. Do you have thoughts that you can't put out of your mind?
5. Sometimes children check on things over and over again. Do you do that?
6. Would you say that you worry a lot or just a little?

Self-image (after the child draws a self-portrait)

1. Do you feel able to overcome your worries or fears?
2. Are you embarrassed about what others think about you? (Do other people make fun of you?)
3. Do you think you're smart, good-looking, and popular?
4. What makes you feel most proud of yourself?
5. Is your family proud of you?
6. If by magic you could change yourself, how would you like to be different?

Mood and behavior

1. People have different feelings and moods. What kind of mood do you usually feel?
2. How often do you feel sad (down, empty, like crying, unhappy, blue)?
3. Do you have less fun recently or have you lost interest in your usual activities?
4. What do you do when you have sad feelings?
5. To whom do you talk when you feel sad?
6. When you're sad, do you feel hopeless?
7. a. Do you ever think of hurting yourself?
   b. (*If answer is yes*) Or even killing yourself?
8. Do you ever think of a way to do it?
9. Do you feel that things will work out for you?

Physical complaints

1. Sleep
   a. Do you have difficulty with falling asleep at night?
   b. Do you have problems with waking up at night or waking up very early in the morning?
   c. Do you ever have nightmares? If you do, what are they about?
2. Eating: During the last month, have you lost your appetite or have you been eating more than usual?
3. Aches and pains: Do you have stomach aches, headaches, or other aches or pains anywhere in your body (especially when you are upset about something)?
4. Bedwetting and fecal soiling
   a. Sometimes, do you wet the bed at night?
   b. When you are upset, have you ever lost control of your bowels and soiled yourself?

Aggressive behavior

1. What do you do when you feel angry?
2. What kinds of things make you feel angry?
3. Do you have trouble with controlling your temper?
4. Do you have trouble with following rules at school or at home?

(Continued)

BOX 100.1   (Continued)

5. Do you argue a lot?
6. Does your family think you are stubborn?
7. Do others think you are stubborn?
8. Have you had to see the principal at school for getting into trouble?

Abnormal mental experiences

1. Do you ever feel that things around you are strange or unusual?
2. Do you ever feel confused or unable to think?

3. Do you feel that people are after you?
4. Do you ever feel afraid of losing your mind or being crazy?
5. Do you ever feel that you have special powers?
6. Do your eyes or ears ever play tricks on you? Do you hear things or see things that other people don't hear or see?

Adapted with permission from Hodges K, McKnew D, Cytryn L, et al. The Children's Assessment Schedule. Durham, NC: Duke University, 1985.

---

be used in an interview with an older child. The interviewer should attempt to cover all the items listed. For some children, a brief warm-up period for chatting or playing may be needed to make them more comfortable before starting the formal interview. Sometimes, to preserve the spontaneity of the interview, asking the questions in an order different from that listed may be appropriate. If one area seems more productive of feelings or pertinent facts, obviously, more time should be spent in that area and additional questions should be asked until the area seems exhausted before proceeding to the next set of questions.

Suggested Readings

Bird B. *Talking with patients,* 2nd ed. Philadelphia: JB Lippincott, 1973:259.

Graham P, Turk J, Verhulst FC. Assessment. In: Graham P, ed. *Child psychiatry: a developmental approach,* 2nd ed. New York: Oxford University Press, 1999.

Harris JC. Assessment, interview and behavior rating scales. In: *Developmental neuropsychiatry.* New York: Oxford University Press, 1998:3.

Kestenbaum CJ. The clinical interview of the child. In: Wiener JM, Dulcan M, eds. *The textbook of child and adolescent psychiatry,* 3rd ed. Washington, DC: American Psychiatric Press, 2004.

CHAPTER 101 ■ MENTAL DISORDERS AND PSYCHOLOGICAL STRESS

JAMES C. HARRIS

Symptoms are signals that something is wrong with the child, and these might indicate a biologic syndrome or disease. On the other hand, symptoms may point to a psychological disorder in the child, or they may be the child's way of responding to an abnormal situation at home or school. Physical or psychological symptoms may interfere with development by preventing a child from participating in age-appropriate activities, and these symptoms may have secondary effects that must be addressed in a comprehensive treatment program.

The concept of a mental disorder indicates an impairment in psychosocial adaptation occasioned by psychological distress and suffering or disability. It is not the expected response to a particular event, but rather the expression of behavioral, psychological, or biologic dysfunction. In assessing a child for a mental disorder, the physician must remember that the presenting symptoms may have multiple meanings to the child and family.

An assessment of symptoms leads to the diagnosis of those problems or syndromes that may be dealt with in pediatric practice or referred for treatment to other professionals. To make this diagnostic assessment, the current psychiatric classification follows a multiaxial system, sequentially addressing the clinical psychiatric syndrome, the presence of intellectual disability or abnormal personality traits, the occurrence of a general medical condition, and psychosocial and environmental problems that may affect diagnosis, treatment, and prognosis. It also provides for a global assessment rating of overall function. The revised *Diagnostic and Statistical Manual of Mental Disorders,* Fourth Edition, Text Revision (DSM-IV-TR), system does not include mixed diagnostic categories (i.e., mixed emotional and behavioral disorder), but *The International Classification of Diseases,* Tenth Edition, does. Both classification systems should be consulted. The *DSM-IV-TR* (2000) classification has a section on disorders usually first diagnosed during infancy, childhood, or adolescence. A primary care version, the *Diagnostic and Statistical Manual for Primary Care* (1996), is available and should be utilized regularly. Because this chapter discusses some of the more severe forms of psychiatric and behavior disorders, the revised *DSM-IV-TR* criteria are reproduced. This chapter considers stress and illness and posttramatic stress disorder.

PSYCHOLOGICAL FACTORS AFFECTING MEDICAL CONDITIONS

Psychological factors contribute to the maintenance, exacerbation, and sometimes the initiation of a general medical condition or illness. The *DSM-IV-TR* uses the diagnostic term "psychological factors affecting medical condition" rather than the terms *psychosomatic* or *somatopsychic* that have been used to emphasize this association in the past. It is more useful to avoid these older terms and to describe specifically the multiple, concurrent conditions or problems with which the child and family present. Psychological factors might include a mental disorder such as anxiety, temperamental attributes, personality traits, or coping style; maladaptive behaviors; stress-related responses; the personal meanings of the illness; and the associated psychosocial circumstances that may influence treatment compliance.

These interacting circumstances, psychological symptoms, and individual responses to illness do not represent a unitary causality or a hypothetical entity called *psychosomatic*. The parents' and child's interpretations and experiences of the illness make each case unique and add to the richness of the encounter between physician and patient. The psychological response to illness can affect the child's motivation to participate in a treatment program designed to facilitate recovery and can affect the parents' attitudes in supporting that recovery. Symptoms may be maintained if the "sick role" has become a habitual one. Although the reasons for the original symptoms may be resolved, the interpersonal response to the illness may continue to maintain the symptoms.

Clinical presentations are affected by general psychological factors related to being acutely ill and to factors related to chronic physical illness. The clinical presentation also is affected by life events, including chronic stress in the family, the parents' attitudes and interpersonal behavior toward the child, attitudes toward hospitalization, and behavior following discharge. Finally, the motivation to recover must be considered. Among the specific disorders that have significant potential for psychological complications are asthma, heart disease, cystic fibrosis, epilepsy, gastrointestinal disease, diabetes mellitus, short stature, and malignancies.

For example, a 7-year-old boy is seen frequently in the emergency department because of asthma. His symptoms respond quickly to symptomatic treatment on each visit, yet his mother returns with her son to the emergency department each week, complaining about his asthma. When she is asked whether his symptoms remind her of any past experience with illness in her life, she begins to talk movingly about her father's death from emphysema that complicated black-lung disease. She had nursed her father through his final illness while pregnant with this boy, who bears a striking physical resemblance to his grandfather and who is named after him. When her son wheezes she becomes terrified, remembering her father's terminal illness, and brings the child to the emergency department. The resolution of her bereavement is the essential ingredient in the treatment of the boy's asthma, and when her bereavement resolves, the frequent emergency department visits end.

Important considerations in treatment are the parents' concerns about the cause of the illness, their need for explanations, their understanding of the meaning of laboratory test results, their rejection or overly protective attitudes toward the child, and their understanding of the use of medication. Each illness has its own psychosocial context. Some issues that may require additional psychological support are anxiety about the child not being able to breathe in asthma, the experience of helplessness about when a seizure will occur, the frustration with encopresis, the fear of coma in diabetes, and the uncertainty about recovery in cystic fibrosis. For the child, excessive restrictions imposed by the parent during illness may influence personality development.

Developmentally, adaptation to the illness is an ongoing saga at home and at school, as the child's psychological experience and comments by others influence day-to-day activities. Yet, most children with acute or chronic illnesses maintain their self-confidence and make full use of psychosocial support.

STRESS AND ILLNESS

This section focuses on those factors that relate to the stress of illness and factors that facilitate recovery. The presence of psychosocial variables and the ways in which they might influence susceptibility, rather than cause disease, are an essential consideration. This approach requires an evaluation of the circumstances that led to the consultation, as well as to the specific presentation of symptoms. The child, in the unique context of his temperament, genetic background, family life, and community experience, is the patient. Both the symptom itself and how it is experienced must be appreciated. The physician should address the external environmental conditions at home and at school, along with the child's response to them, the risk factors that may lead to vulnerability to illness, nutrition and genetic predispositions, the family's and child's perception of the illness and how it affects their views of themselves, the child's temperament, the child's developmental level and the expected behavioral response to illness at that level, and the difficulty of relinquishing the dependence inherent in assuming the role of patient. All these factors are important in an initial assessment aimed at facilitating recovery.

Resilience to Stress

Historically, we have moved from a general emphasis on the effects of adverse life experience on behavior and symptoms to the specific kinds of life experiences that are most likely to lead to disorders. It is important to note that all children do not succumb to illness or become symptomatic when they are subjected to stress. In a study conducted by Rutter, more than half of the children were resilient to the effects of external circumstances on their behavior or somatic symptoms. However, risk factors do interact with developmental stages (e.g., an experience may be stressful and elicit a greater physiologic response in a younger child than in an older one).

In the psychiatric classification system, psychosocial stressors as well as protective factors should be considered. Psychosocial stressors are grouped together on Axis IV in the following categories: problems with primary support group (e.g., death of family member, health problems, divorce); problems related to the social environment (e.g., death of friend, living alone); educational problems (academic problems, peer problems); occupational problems; housing problems; economic problems; problems with access to health care services; problems related to interaction with the legal system and crime; and other psychosocial and environmental problems (e.g., exposure to disasters). To understand vulnerability and resilience to stress, individual differences in how potential stressors are experienced must be taken into account, and it is necessary to note that what is initially stressful may have strengthened the patient for later exposure to similar events. Experiences may be sensitizing or strengthening, depending on a variety of factors. Although the experience may be ultimately strengthening, it is not experienced initially as positive by the child. The effect may be evident as protective only when new exposures to stress occur. For example, individual differences exist in separation experiences in younger children as compared with older ones. To be strengthening, early experience with separation must occur in the context of affectionate support and hopefulness, which may modify the effect of later stressors. On the other hand, early separation may be sensitizing; instead of developing resilience, some children may have exaggerated symptoms when the stress of separation recurs.

An important preventive approach to separation and hospital stress is the hospital-based Child Life program, which provides anticipatory programming to prepare and strengthen the child for hospitalization and provides a normalized setting during the hospital stay. Social support is an important protective factor, and a particularly important element is a *confiding relationship* with one person, usually a parent. The parent's style of interaction; psychological availability; and how, when, and to what degree he or she expresses emotion in the child's presence may be critical factors in the child's psychosocial development.

To understand the child's response to stress, several issues must be considered. The timing of the event, the child's developmental level, and the degree of cognitive development all are important. Young children apparently are not as responsive to separation stress in the first months of life, before developing selective parental attachment. After that time, an interpersonal bond is demonstrated by the child's response to reunion after separation from the parent.

To appraise events cognitively as stressful, the child must attribute personal meaning to them. The child's experience of self-efficacy also influences the response to the stress. The ability to develop strategies for controlling the environment is a psychologicalally protective element. Of importance are the kinds or patterns of stress that are experienced, individual differences in responsiveness, previous interpersonal experiences outside the home, self-esteem and self-efficacy, opportunities to control the situation, availability of intimate relationships, and developmental strategies to cope. The ability to appraise a new situation is a cognitive landmark. A child's ability to act rather than react is important to gauge. A child can respond with feelings of self-esteem and self-efficacy if she is secure in affection and achievement and has had positive experiences appropriate for her temperament. These interpersonal abilities are very important when the child is threatened or alarmed.

Usually a single stressor is not adequate to cause a disorder, even if it persists; disorders ordinarily result from the experience of multiple stressors. Protective factors against stress include positive temperament, gender (school-aged girls are less vulnerable than boys), parental warmth and affection, and the lack of personal criticism. If only one parent is in the home and strife exists, supportive psychosocial measures at school can compensate for lack of support at home.

In a study by Werner and Smith, on infants recovering from illness, those with a history of perinatal stress, poverty, family instability, and limited parental education had worse outcomes. Appropriate rule setting and discipline led to skills in finding relevant models and sources of support from peers, older friends, teachers, and clergy. Other individual protective factors may exist that are not fully appreciated. For example, in contrast to learned helplessness, the child's capacity to help others can be important in promoting development and coping. The ability to show humor in adverse situations has been recognized as important and is associated with social competence in stressful situations.

Reactions to Stress and Adjustment Disorders

When the child fails to master the physiologic consequences of stressful experiences, the presence of severe or continued stressors may lead to impaired social functioning. The resulting anxiety disorders are referred to as *acute stress disorder* and *posttraumatic stress disorder*, or, if severe, a subtype of *adjustment disorder*. The nature of the stress and its severity are designated as acute or enduring.

Acute Stress Disorder

Typically, the individual with an acute stress disorder is dazed, has difficulty in comprehension, and may show initial signs of disorientation and depersonalization. Autonomic symptoms, including sweating, tachycardia, and flushing, are present. Partial or complete amnesia may be present for significant aspect of the event. This period of initial disorientation is followed by a variety of symptoms such as anxiety, sadness, anger, or withdrawal. These symptoms ordinarily resolve within a day or two with supportive management techniques and, if so, do not specifically constitute a disorder. An acute anxiety disorder is diagnosed when dissociative symptoms last a minimum of 2 days and up to 4 weeks (with onset within 4 weeks of the traumatic event) and occur along with persistent re-experiencing of the event and marked avoidance of those stimuli that arouse recollections of the trauma.

Posttraumatic Stress Disorder

Posttraumatic stress disorder is a more protracted or delayed response to a stressful event that is experienced with intense fear or terror and a sense of helplessness. Personal vulnerability may lower the threshold or affect the course, but it does not account for its occurrence. Characteristically, a traumatic event is re-experienced by the child through intrusive memories and dreams. The child avoids situations that are reminiscent of the trauma or shows a lessening of general emotional responsiveness to other persons in his surroundings. Increased arousal, an exaggerated startle, sleep disturbances, headache, and abdominal pain may occur. Younger children exhibit posttraumatic play, wherein they play out the traumatic events over and over in a stereotyped fashion. Examples of trauma that can lead to this disorder include threats to life or physical integrity, destruction of the home or community residence, seeing another person who has been injured or killed in an accident or violent episode, or learning of severe loss or harm to another person. Directly witnessing an event is the most traumatic experience.

Symptoms ordinarily occur immediately after the trauma, but a latency of several months may be present. Avoidance of the situation may occur, including phobic avoidance of similar situations; this may interfere with developmental tasks such as establishing interpersonal relationships or school performance. In some instances, fluctuating moods, anxiety, sadness, and guilt may persist and require treatment. Neuroimaging studies have shown significant neurobiologic changes in posttraumatic stress disorder. Three areas of the brain may be different in patients with posttraumatic stress disorder compared with those in control subjects: the hippocampus, the amygdala, and the medial frontal cortex. The amygdala appears to be hyperreactive to trauma-related stimuli. Exaggerated startle response and flashbacks may be related to a failure of higher brain regions (i.e., the hippocampus and the medial frontal cortex) to dampen the exaggerated symptoms of arousal and distress that are mediated through the amygdala in response to reminders of the traumatic event. The diagnostic criteria for posttraumatic stress disorder are outlined in Box 101.1.

In approaching the child with an acute posttraumatic stress disorder, particularly following physical violence, the child may

---

BOX 101.1   Diagnostic Criteria for Posttraumatic Stress Disorder

A. The person has been exposed to a traumatic event in which both of the following were present:
   1. The person experienced, witnessed, or was confronted with an event or events that involved actual or threatened death or serious injury, or a threat to the physical integrity of self or others.
   2. The person's response involved intense fear, helplessness, or horror. Note: In children, this may be expressed instead by disorganized or agitated behavior.

B. The traumatic event is persistently re-experienced in one (or more) of the following ways:
   1. Recurrent and intrusive distressing recollections of the event, including images, thoughts, or perceptions. Note: In young children, repetitive play may occur, in which themes or aspects of the trauma are expressed.
   2. Recurrent distressing dreams of the event. Note: In children, frightening dreams may occur without recognizable content.
   3. Acting or feeling as if the traumatic event were recurring (includes a sense of reliving the experience, illusions, hallucinations, and dissociative flashback episodes, including those that occur on awakening or when intoxicated). Note: In young children, trauma-specific enactment may occur.
   4. Intense psychological distress at exposure to internal or external cues that symbolize or resemble an aspect of the traumatic event.
   5. Physiologic reactivity on exposure to internal or external cues that symbolize or resemble an aspect of the traumatic event.

C. Persistent avoidance of stimuli associated with the trauma and numbing of general responsiveness (not present before the trauma), as indicated by three (or more) of the following:
   1. Efforts to avoid thoughts, feelings, or conversations associated with the trauma.
   2. Efforts to avoid activities, places, or people that arouse recollections of the trauma.
   3. Inability to recall an important aspect of the trauma.
   4. Markedly diminished interest or participation in significant activities.
   5. Feeling of detachment or estrangement from others.
   6. Restricted range of affect (e.g., unable to have loving feelings).
   7. Sense of a foreshortened future (e.g., does not expect to have a career, marriage, children, or a normal life span).

D. Persistent symptoms of increased arousal (not present before the trauma), as indicated by two (or more) of the following:
   1. Difficulty falling or staying asleep
   2. Irritability or outbursts of anger
   3. Difficulty concentrating
   4. Hypervigilance
   5. Exaggerated startle response

E. Duration of the disturbance (symptoms in criteria B, C, and D) is more than 1 month.

F. The disturbance causes clinically significant distress or impairment in social, occupational, or other important areas of functioning.

Specify if:
   Acute: If duration of symptoms is less than 3 months.
   Chronic: If duration of symptoms is 3 months or more.

Specify if:
   With delayed onset: If onset of symptoms is at least 6 months after the stressor.

Reprinted with permission from American Psychiatric Association. *Diagnostic and statistical manual of mental disorders*, 4th ed. Text revision. Washington, DC: American Psychiatric Association, 2000.

---

be numb or mute, and direct questioning may not be productive. A therapeutic interview that addresses the trauma directly, and indirectly through the use of the imagination, using free drawings and story telling is often an effective approach that tends to alleviate traumatic anxiety. The family, police, or others involved can be consulted about the circumstances, the specific event itself, and the child's subsequent behavior. In the interview with the child, keep in mind that after any stress or loss, a period of strategic emotional withdrawal may occur and should be respected. With severely stressful events, however, intrusive memories of the trauma ordinarily are demonstrated in posttraumatic role-play, stories, or pictures.

The focus of treatment is to provide sufficient support to help the child reenact the event until it is mastered. After the events are reenacted in fantasy, the sequence of emotional release, the reconstruction of the experience, a review of the worst moment, and the direct revelation of the violent events to the therapist can be expected. To help the child cope with the experience, one must establish how it happened and what it meant to the child. Assigning responsibility for the traumatic event and clarifying a plan of action that might have rectified the situation are elements that ordinarily must be addressed.

A review of past trauma, current traumatic dreams, and current stressors also requires discussion. The child is helped to summarize what happened in her own words and to understand how anyone's responses would be similar in the same circumstances. The child should not feel alone, learn to accept support from others, and to appreciate that her own feelings are understandable in these circumstances. The fact that the symptoms may return must be emphasized. At the end of an interview, it often helps for the child to describe what was helpful or distressing about the interview itself. The goal is to relieve symptoms and reestablish trust in others and in the community environment.

Other family members also require support and ongoing preventive interventions. This includes crisis management and the availability of individual and group support networks. The physician's responsibility is to convene a support group and give the family permission to ask for help. The outcome depends on family support, affection, and the child's own efforts. The parents' ability to work through their concerns emotionally must be assessed, and the child's effort at mastery understood and supported.

Adjustment Disorder

Adjustment disorder was previously referred to as *situational* or *adjustment reaction*. It is a maladaptive response to a known stressor. In contrast to posttraumatic stress disorder, the stressor is usually less severe, the precipitating event less overwhelming, and the characteristic re-experiencing of trauma not present. An adjustment disorder is subtyped according to the type of emotional and behavioral symptom (e.g., adjustment disorder with depressed mood, anxiety, mixed anxiety and depressed mood, disturbance of conduct, or mixed disturbance of emotions and conduct). Symptoms are the result of the child's efforts to cope with stress.

Whether the child or adolescent develops a disorder depends on the stress-related factors that have been described previously. Younger children who lack mature coping strategies may be more vulnerable to a disorder, because the impact of a stressor is related to the child's developmental level. Life changes, such as the loss of a caregiver, abuse, divorce, moving, or school changes, vary in their effects according to the child's age, temperament, and the extent of family support.

Adjustment disorder is more problematic to diagnose in adolescents because psychological turmoil may be an aspect of normal adolescent development. Still, psychological symptoms should be taken seriously. When adolescents are interviewed and asked specific diagnostic questions, they often reveal unexpected psychopathology. Although many symptoms prove to be transient, moods often fluctuate, with alternating social withdrawal and expression of good spirits. Frequently, adolescents have concerns about physical development, which is expressed differently in boys and girls.

Conflict over independence is a common concern in adolescence. Certain individuals undergo regression upon exposure to external stressors and they show aggressive behavior, delinquency, anxiety, depression, eating problems, or physiologic disorders. In early adolescence, pubertal changes may be accompanied by rebelliousness and defiance against those in authority and may be manifested by guilt, moody withdrawal, or both. As the adolescent becomes older, heterosexual and homosexual concerns and occupational concerns become more apparent. In the older adolescent approaching the time of leaving home, long-term life goals and a philosophy of life become prominent concerns.

Because current terminology focuses more specifically on the phenomena of psychological experience and behavior, *adjustment disorder* is no longer the catch-all term it was in the past. These changes in definition mean that older studies are difficult to evaluate in regard to their reported outcomes. Adjustment disorders are specifically characterized by their onset as a response to identifiable stressors during the previous 3 months and the absence of specific criteria for other syndromes. The clinical picture of adjustment disorder may suggest other syndromes or specific disorders. For example, the adjustment disorder with depressed mood is a depressive syndrome that may occur in response to psychosocial stress. The outcome of adjustment disorder with depressed mood has been shown to be substantially better than for a major affective disorder.

Adjustment disorders are common, affecting perhaps 2% to 8% of children in community settings and up to 12% of general hospital inpatients. The incidence of the more severe forms is higher in adolescents. The disturbance begins within 3 months of a stressor and lasts no longer than 6 months after an acute stressor. If the stress or adverse circumstances endure, it will take longer to reach a more effective adaptation. If symptoms last more than 6 months, the stressor is considered to be chronic. The etiology of an adjustment disorder may be linked to one or more stressors, with multiple events generally leading to more severe symptomatology. These may be recurrent, occur in the family, or accompany developmental changes.

In an assessment, the types and severity of symptoms and the child's history and personality must be determined and the stressful event, situation, or life crisis must be clarified. The symptoms represent types of adjustment difficulty and are

---

BOX 101.2 — Diagnostic Criteria for Adjustment Disorders

A. The development of emotional or behavioral symptoms in response to an identifiable stressor(s) occurring within 3 months of the onset of the stressor(s).

B. These symptoms or behaviors are clinically significant, as evidenced by either of the following:
   1. Marked distress that is in excess of what would be expected from exposure to the stressors
   2. Significant impairment in social or occupational (academic) functioning

C. The stress-related disturbance does not meet the criteria for another specific Axis I disorder and is not merely an exacerbation of a preexisting Axis I or Axis II disorder.

D. The symptoms do not represent bereavement.

E. Once the stressor (or its consequences) has terminated, the symptoms do not persist for more than an additional 6 months.

   Specify if:

   Acute: If the disturbance lasts less than 6 months

   Chronic: If the disturbance lasts for 6 months or longer

Adjustment disorders are coded based on the subtype, which is selected according to the predominant symptoms. The specific stressor(s) can be specified on Axis IV.

309.0 With Depressed Mood
309.24 With Anxiety
309.28 With Mixed Anxiety and Depressed Mood
309.3 With Disturbance of Conduct
309.4 With Mixed Disturbance of Emotions and Conduct
309.9 Unspecified

Reprinted with permission from American Psychiatric Association. *Diagnostic and statistical manual of mental disorders*, 4th ed. Text revision. Washington, DC: American Psychiatric Association, 2000.

---

described according to the clinical presentation as brief or prolonged anxiety, depressive mood, predominant disturbance of conduct (e.g., antisocial behavior toward others), or mixed disturbances of emotions and conduct.

In diagnosing an adjustment disorder, it should be determined whether impairment in functioning exists. Personality and temperamental traits may be exacerbated by stress. If psychological symptoms accompany physical illness, they are designated separately. The diagnostic criteria for adjustment disorders are outlined in Box 101.2.

Adjustment disorders may resolve without treatment if the stressor is removed. This may not be adequate, however, and symptoms may persist after cessation of the stressor. Certain problems, such as a death or persistent loud disagreements between parents before divorce, are particularly stressful. Short-term counseling or therapy may be indicated on an individual basis for adjustment disorders.

Suggested Readings

Donnelly CL. Pharmacologic treatment approaches for children and adolescents with posttraumatic stress disorder. *Child Adolesc Psychiatr Clin N Am* 2003;12:251.

Engel GL. The psychosomatic approach to individual susceptibility to disease. *Gastroenterology* 1974;67:1085.

Fairbrother G, Stuber J, Galea S, et al. Posttraumatic stress reactions in New York City children after the September 11, 2001, terrorist attacks. *Ambul Pediatr* 2003;3:304.

Kovacs M, Gatsonis C, Pollock M, Parrone PL. A controlled prospective study of DSM-III adjustment disorder in childhood. Short-term prognosis and long-term predictive validity. *Arch Gen Psychiatry* 1994;51:535.

Newcorn JH, Strain J. Adjustment disorder in children and adolescents. *J Am Acad Child Adolesc Psychiatry* 1992;31:318.

Nutt DJ, Malizia AL. Structural and functional brain changes in posttraumatic stress disorder. *J Clin Psychiatry* 2004;65(Suppl 1):11.

Pfefferbaum B. Posttraumatic stress disorder in children: a review of the past 10 years. *J Am Acad Child Adolesc Psychiatry* 1997;36:1503.

Pfefferbaum B, Pfefferbaum RL, Gurwitch RH, et al. Children's response to terrorism: a critical review of the literature. *Curr Psychiatry Rep* 2003;5:95.

Rutter M. Resilience: some conceptual considerations. *J Adolesc Health* 1993; 14:626, 690.

Sandberg S, Rutter M. The role of acute life stresses. In: Rutter M, Taylor E, eds. *Child and adolescent psychiatry: modern approaches,* 4th ed. Oxford: Blackwell, 2002:287.

Steiner H, Carrion V, Plattner B, Koopman C. Dissociative symptoms in posttraumatic stress disorder: diagnosis and treatment. *Child Adolesc Psychiatr Clin N Am* 2003;12:231.

Werner EE, Smith RS. *Vulnerable but invincible: a study of resilient children.* New York: McGraw-Hill, 1982.

Yehuda R. Risk and resilience in posttraumatic stress disorder. *J Clin Psychiatry* 2004;65(Suppl 1):29.

CHAPTER 102 ■ DISRUPTIVE BEHAVIOR DISORDERS

JAMES C. HARRIS

Disruptive behavior disorder is the most recent designation for socially disruptive behavior that is generally more disturbing to others than to the person initiating the behavior. The impairment or disability is in the effects of the behavior on others rather than primarily in distress experienced by the child. This chapter discusses conduct disorder and oppositional defiant disorder. Attention deficit hyperactivity disorder is often associated with disrupted behavior and is discussed in Chapter 113. The co-occurrence of other disorders frequently leads to multiple diagnoses for a disruptive child in the *Diagnostic and Statistical Manual of Mental Disorders,* Fourth Edition (*DSM-IV-TR*), system. It leads to the use of mixed diagnostic categories in *The International Classification of Diseases,* Tenth Edition (*ICD-10*), such as hyperkinetic conduct disorder and mixed disorder of conduct and emotions. In *ICD-10*, oppositional defiant disorder is categorized under conduct disorder. The categories *conduct disorder confined to the family context* and *depressive conduct disorder* are also included in *ICD-10*. The general terms *externalizing symptoms,* such as overactivity and aggression, and *internalizing symptoms,* such as anxiety and depression, have been introduced from factor analytic studies and may be derived from parent rating scales, such as the Achenbach Child Behavior Checklist.

CONDUCT DISORDERS

In both community and university clinics, the broad categories of *conduct and aggressive problem behavior* or of *emotional symptoms* constitute the primary reasons for referral for treatment. The distinction between emotional and conduct disorders is well validated. The conduct symptoms are externalizing symptoms and are of more concern to the parent than to the child. Furthermore, these are often chronic disorders that may, in a small but significant number of cases, be complicated in adolescence by substance abuse, delinquency, and alcoholism or antisocial personality in adulthood. These future risks involve the physician in the effort to intervene and work with other nonmedical professionals to help prevent the frequently poor psychosocial outcome of these conditions.

Disruptive behavior and delinquency have been a particular focus of attention since the initiation of the juvenile court system at the beginning of this century, when psychiatrists, psychologists, and social workers were drawn together to consult in the legal assessment of behaviorally disordered children and adolescents. This early legal concern with the prevention of antisocial behavior was a major factor in the initiation of the child guidance movement in the United States. Following these early efforts in intervention, Hewitt and Jenkins (1946) carried out the first systematic description of aggressive conduct disorder. Their early work suggested the usefulness of distinguishing socialized from unsocialized conduct disorders in children with disruptive behavior. Other investigators have suggested a useful distinction between aggressive and nonaggressive forms and between aggressive and delinquent or antisocial behavior.

In evaluating disruptive behavior, the child's age, gender, and life circumstances must be taken into account. The frequency and persistence of the problems are reviewed, as are specific or generalized situations in which they occur. Symptoms presenting in multiple settings (home, school, community) have a poorer prognosis. An early intervention for conduct problems confined to the home (family context) may prevent subsequent difficulties in other settings.

Conduct disorder is characterized by a repetitive and persistent behavior that violates the basic rights of others or major age-appropriate social norms or rules. As shown in Box 102.1, conduct-disordered behaviors are divided into four main groupings: (a) aggressive threats or behaviors that result in physical harm to people or animals (criteria A1 through A7), (b) nonaggressive behavior that results in property loss or damage (criteria A8 and A9), (c) deceitful behavior or theft (criteria A10 through A12), and (d) serious violation of parental or school rules, such as runaway behavior and truancy (criteria A13 through A15). To establish the diagnosis, at least three of these criteria must be present in the past 12 months, with at least one criterion present in the past 6 months. Moreover, to establish the diagnosis, the behavior leads to clinically significant impairment in social, academic, or occupational functioning and is present in several settings.

BOX 102.1   Diagnostic Criteria for Conduct Disorder

A. A repetitive and persistent pattern of behavior in which the basic rights of others or major age-appropriate societal norms or rules are violated, as manifested by the presence of three (or more) of the following criteria in the past 12 months, with at least one criterion present in the past 6 months:

Aggression to people and animals

1. Often bullies, threatens, or intimidates others.
2. Often initiates physical fights.
3. Has used a weapon that can cause serious physical harm to others (e.g., bat, brick, broken bottle, knife, gun).
4. Has been physically cruel to people.
5. Has been physically cruel to animals.
6. Has stolen while confronting a victim (e.g., mugging, purse snatching, extortion, armed robbery).
7. Has forced someone into sexual activity.

Destruction of property

8. Has deliberately engaged in fire setting with the intention of causing serious damage.
9. Has deliberately destroyed others' property (other than by fire setting).

Deceitfulness or theft

10. Has broken into someone else's house, building, or car.
11. Often lies to obtain goods or favors or to avoid obligations (i.e., "cons" others).
12. Has stolen items of nontrivial value without confronting a victim (e.g., shoplifting, but without breaking or entering; forgery).

Serious violations of rules

13. Often stays out at night despite parental prohibitions, beginning before age 13 years.
14. Has run away from home overnight at least twice while living in parental or parental surrogate home (or once without returning for a lengthy period).
15. Is often truant from school, beginning before age 13 years.

B. The disturbance in behavior causes clinically significant impairment in social, academic, or occupational functioning.
C. If the individual is age 18 years or older, criteria are not met for antisocial personality disorder (see *Diagnostic and Statistical Manual of Mental Disorders*, 4th ed.).

Specify type based on age at onset:

Childhood-onset type: Onset of at least one criterion characteristic of conduct disorder before age 10 years.
Adolescent-onset type: Absence of any criteria characteristic of conduct disorder before age 10 years.

Specify severity:

Mild: Few, if any, conduct problems in excess of those required to make the diagnosis *and* conduct problems cause only minor harm to others.
Moderate: Number of conduct problems and effect on others intermediate between mild and severe.
Severe: Many conduct problems in excess of those required to make the diagnosis *or* conduct problems cause considerable harm to others.

Reprinted with permission from American Psychiatric Association. *Diagnostic and statistical manual of mental disorders*, 4th ed. Text revision. Washington, DC: American Psychiatric Association, 2000.

Childhood-onset and adolescent-onset subtypes are designated, differing in regard to the type of presenting conduct problems, gender ratio, developmental course, and prognosis. As indicated in Box 102.1, these subtypes are rated as mild, moderate, or severe. In the childhood-onset type, at least one criterion presents before 10 years of age. Affected children are more often boys than girls, frequently are aggressive toward others, commonly have disturbed peer relationships, and may have been diagnosed with oppositional-defiant disorder at an earlier age.

Individuals with a childhood onset of behavior problems have a greater likelihood for their disturbed conduct to persist and to have antisocial personality disorder as adults than if the onset occurred during adolescence. Those with the adolescent-onset type are more likely to have adequate peer relationships; however, conduct problems in consort with others are frequent. Adult outcome is better in regard to antisocial behavior, and the male-to-female ratio is lower than for the childhood-onset type.

The solitary aggressive or *unsocialized* form of conduct disorder generally is present in multiple settings and is associated with impairment in interpersonal relationships with other children and lack of close friendships. A lack of integration into a peer group is a key feature, as evidenced by isolation or peer rejection, with unpopularity and lack of empathetic relationships with children of the same age group. Relationships with adults are marked by hostility, argument, and resentment. Close, confiding relationships are absent. Problems range from bullying and excessive fighting to frank destructiveness of property or violent assault. Ordinarily, the problems are pervasive and occur in all settings, but occur predominantly at school or outside the home, in the community.

The group-type or *socialized* conduct disorder applies to conduct disorders occurring in children who are well integrated into their peer group. These individuals participate in antisocial behavior along with others. Relationships tend to be poor with some adults, particularly those in authority, but they may be good with other adults. Stealing, truancy from school, running away from home, and criminal offenses usually occur with a group of companions.

Some children's behavior does not fit into these categories, but their behavior is disturbed severely enough to require treatment. Conduct disorder symptoms may occur in combination with emotional symptoms, such as anxiety and depression. If the diagnostic criteria for depression also are met, both diagnoses are made in *DSM-IV-TR* and both are designated in *ICD-10* (i.e., depressive conduct disorder). The depressive symptoms must be addressed initially in treatment and may be more responsive to intervention.

Epidemiology

Boys are referred more often than girls, and school-aged boys tend to be unsocialized aggressive, whereas older adolescent boys more often present with a socialized conduct problem. Frequently, an association exists with adverse psychosocial environment, difficult family relations, and poor school performance. The onset may be as early as the preschool years, particularly for the solitary aggression occurring outside a social group, with temperamental traits that are associated with aggressive behavior identified in infancy (i.e., the infant with a "difficult temperament"). Inflexibility reported by the mothers of preschoolers, negative parent–child interactions, and high family stress are strongly associated with behavioral adjustment. Boys identified in the first grade with behavioral traits of aggression and social withdrawal were found on follow-up had increased likelihood of being delinquents and substance abusers in adolescence. Associations with alcoholism, antisocial disorders, and somatization disorders in women occur in adult life. Antisocial personalities have been identified in fathers of affected boys. Affected girls reported more somatic complaints without diagnostic confirmation and more often injured themselves than did boys. The postpubertal onset of solitary aggression is more common in girls. Early onset has been associated with attention deficit hyperactivity disorder, articulation problems and, in some studies, perinatal hypoxia.

An estimated 6% to 16% of boys and 2% to 9% of girls younger than 18 years of age present with conduct disorder, making it one of the most frequently diagnosed psychiatric disorders in mental health facilities for older children and adolescents. In Rutter's Isle of Wight study, two-thirds of 10- to 11-year-old children who were disturbed had conduct disorders. Population rates range from 2% to 16%, depending on the setting; rates tend to be higher in socioeconomically deprived areas and more common in boys than in girls by a 4:1 ratio. Boys with conduct disorder make up at least one-third of admissions to child psychiatry services.

Natural History

The course depends on the number and severity of symptoms, their time of onset, the child's personality traits, and family and psychosocial circumstances. Milder cases may resolve; those with more risk factors may become chronic and subsequently may be associated with antisocial personality disorder in adulthood. The type of presentation also makes a difference: The solitary aggressive type may have a worse prognosis than the socialized but aggressive child or adolescent involved in group delinquency. Approximately one-third of those involved in antisocial behavior as preadolescents have difficulty in adulthood.

Symptoms may be severe enough to produce social impairment that leads to a removal from regular school classes or home placement, necessitating foster care or residential settings. Behavior problems often lead to school suspension, legal problems, unwanted pregnancy, and physical injury from accidents, fighting, and self-injury, including suicide and parasuicide. Aggressive and antisocial symptoms, fire-setting, and family deviance are associated with a poor prognosis. Substance abuse is also a commonly associated factor. However, one study showed improvement at 2-year follow-up after intervention.

Family Factors

Children who lack a permanent family are at particular risk. Frequent moves and impersonal home settings lead to particular risks. Children placed outside the home early in life are at greatest risk. The failure of affectionate bonding is a major factor in the genesis of this disorder. Harsh discipline, rejection, lack of nurturing, inconsistent discipline, physical and sexual abuse, and exposure to loud arguments at home without support from either parent are common. Antisocial personality disorder, especially in the father, and alcohol dependence and depressive symptoms in the mother are found more commonly than in the general population, resulting in poor parental models. Single-parent homes without fathers tend to affect boys adversely. Large family size is an issue, as are child-rearing patterns, including lack of self-confidence in a parent, which affects limit-setting by that parent. These risk factors are related to the severity of symptoms, but do not specifically predict the behavior.

From the family systems viewpoint, antisocial behavior in one family member may be the result of a failure in family relationships. If interpersonal communication, effective role modeling, appropriate family organization, and mutual nurturing are established and psychologic disturbances in parents are treated, then the child's symptoms may diminish or resolve. The child's personality and temperament may make him or her more vulnerable to being the family scapegoat. The child's temperament interacts with that of the parent, and this interaction must be carefully considered.

Psychologic Features

Winnicott has suggested that, when children are deprived of essential psychological support at home, antisocial behavior may result. The child may make demands on the personal and material environment, expressed as antisocial behavior, to elicit an interpersonal response. To distinguish it from antisocial personality traits, Winnicott termed this form of antisocial behavior, which draws attention to a child's legitimate emotional needs, the *antisocial tendency*. Having lost hope that others will provide for him, the child may demand a response from the environment. Such behavior includes stealing, lying, and a lack of concern for the rights and feelings of others. Bullying, abuse, and aggressive acts toward others may occur without apparent awareness of the hurt being caused. In some instances, a parent may condone the behavior.

Stealing and associated lying, however, may be expressions of a child's hope that his needs will be satisfied. Those efforts and demands on the environment must be managed, because in some instances, antisocial behavior may be a misguided attempt to demand the care that is a child's right, an aberrant form of reaching out. Another form of antisocial behavior is destructiveness, and this too may be meaningful if it is viewed as an attempt to test the environmental provision for care to see if others can withstand the strain. This formulation is most applicable to children who show remorse and whose stealing, lying, and destruction have a compulsive quality. The child often signals his intention to be disruptive.

If the demand for limits on antisocial behavior cannot be met at home, inpatient hospitalization or a residential setting may be required. The treatment for the antisocial tendency is to provide care, despite the child's provocativeness, allowing the child to find once again the personal care that was withdrawn. Because the failure of the family environment is perceived as a factor in the initiation of the antisocial tendency, reestablishing care is crucial to treatment. For children with antisocial personality traits who steal for gain and lack remorse, behavior treatments rather than psychotherapy are the primary interventions.

Biologic Issues

Changes in social behavior have been documented following physical illness or injuries, particularly those involving the central nervous system. Many children presented with behavior problems after the 1917 encephalitis epidemic. Head trauma, congenital brain dysfunction, and temporal lobe epilepsy are associated with aggressive and antisocial behavior, but they account for only a small proportion of affected children. In children with early onset of severe conduct symptoms and family histories of aggressive behavior in first-degree relatives, genetic factors may increase vulnerability. Efforts are ongoing to identify biologic markers for violent aggressive behavior, including electroencephalography, endocrine, and neurotransmitter investigations.

Diagnosis

Essential to the diagnosis of a conduct disorder is a repetitive and persistent pattern of conduct in which the basic rights and feelings of others, their person, or their property are violated, or major age-appropriate societal norms or rules are violated. At least three of the criteria shown in Box 102.1 must be present in the past 12 months to establish the diagnosis. In addition:

- The patient is not responsive to the effect of his or her behavior on others.
- The behavior causes discomfort not to the perpetrator, but to others who must deal with him or her.
- The problem is a pervasive one, not a single occurrence.
- Antisocial, aggressive, or defiant behavior presents in multiple settings and sometimes with peers.

The most common referral symptoms are fighting, quarrelsomeness, stealing, lying, cruelty, fire-setting, sexual misconduct, and substance abuse severe enough to be distinguished from childhood mischief and adolescent rebellion.

The assessment takes into account the expected behavior for the child's developmental level; for instance, tantrums are common in 2- to 3-year-old children, and a child of 6 or 7 years would rarely be involved in violent crime. Symptoms change with age. Younger children may be more oppositional and defiant, but older children are more directly confrontational with others. The disordered child ordinarily initiates the aggression in fighting with another person. Cruelty to people and animals is characteristic, and destructiveness extends to others' property. Stealing may be aggressive in older children and adolescents and, in severe cases, it may involve confronting a victim physically with a weapon to demand money, take a purse, or initiate extortion. Rape, assault, or suicide may occur in the older individual. Stealing may range from taking without asking to burglary, shoplifting, or forgery. Lying and cheating in games or at school are common, as are school truancy and running away.

Robins suggests that the total number of symptoms and their early onset are of prognostic value, so clarifying the age of onset of each symptom is important. Earlier age of onset has a worse prognosis and is more likely to be associated with aggressive behavior and adult antisocial personality disorder. Early and regular use of tobacco, liquor, or nonprescription psychoactive drugs is common. Of particular concern is the lack of interest in the welfare of others and absence of guilt or remorse after antisocial behavior. The blame for misconduct may be placed on others rather than accepted. Despite an apparent attitude of self-importance and power, self-esteem is generally low. Associated temperamental characteristics often include irritability, poor frustration tolerance, aggressive outbursts of temper, and recklessness, which may have a provocative quality.

Differential Diagnosis

Isolated antisocial behavior does not justify this diagnosis but is designated as childhood or adolescent antisocial behavior, a problem that may require intervention but does not represent a persistent impairment in social and school functioning. Chil-

dren with conduct disorder may have been diagnosed previously as having oppositional defiant disorder. There may be associated diagnoses of attention deficit disorder, manic episode, or symptoms of anxiety and depression that justify a second or underlying primary diagnosis of an emotional disorder. If conduct problems occur in the context of a severe stressor, then adjustment disorder may be the appropriate diagnosis. In the American diagnostic system, multiple diagnoses often are required, particularly when the child is seen in referral at a child psychiatry clinic, where concurrent attention deficit disorder, depressive disorder, or other disorders may be diagnosed. Poor academic achievement, particularly a history of language delay and reading retardation (i.e., 2 years or more below expectation for age and intelligence), may require a second diagnosis.

Therapy

Any child with a conduct disorder requires the care of a psychiatrist or psychologist working in conjunction with the pediatrician. Because family discord and difficult temperament are common, family treatment is needed to effect subsequent change in the child. The prognosis is related to the age of onset, number of symptoms, types of symptoms, family circumstances, prior academic achievement, and whether the behavior represents an antisocial tendency or an antisocial personality trait. Conduct disorder has a poor prognosis, in contrast to the isolated antisocial symptoms that often occur in early adolescence and accompany a search for identity or antisocial tendencies that follow deprivation. The isolated symptom generally responds to a supportive psychosocial environment. The demands that the child or adolescent makes are ordinarily met by a caring and tolerant environment that withstands the demands for autonomy and is a protective factor. A link to poverty is noted, and one study showed that when families moved out of poverty, a major reduction occurred in oppositional disorder and conduct disorder. This is consistent with social causation. The best documented treatment programs involve parent-training programs, such as those described in Patterson's monograph *Living with Children*.

OPPOSITIONAL DEFIANT DISORDER

Children who present with a pattern of hostile, negative, and defiant behavior toward authority figures without serious violations of the basic rights of others are categorized as having oppositional defiant disorder. As shown in Box 102.2, the common complaints are argumentativeness with adults, frequent loss of temper, swearing, defiance of adult requests, and deliberate acts that annoy others. These children or adolescents often blame others for their mistakes or difficulties, rather than accepting blame. This disorder ordinarily occurs at home and may not be present at school. Symptoms are more apparent with adults or peers who know the child well; therefore, symptoms may be minimal during the clinical examination. The child shows lack of insight into his own behavior. Low self-esteem, poor frustration tolerance, mood lability, and temper outbursts are common. Older children and adolescents with this disorder have an increased use of alcohol and other drugs. Onset is usually by age 8 years and no later than early adolescence. The disturbance may evolve into a conduct disorder or mood disorder when the child becomes older.

Oppositional behavior is common in children and adolescents. It may be part of normal adjustment, reactive, or a symptom of another disorder. An epidemiologic study shows negativism to be present in 16% to 22% of a nonreferral population

BOX 102.2 — Diagnostic Criteria for Oppositional Defiant Disorder

A. A pattern of negativistic, hostile, and defiant behavior lasting at least 6 months, during which four (or more) of the following are present:
 1. Often loses temper
 2. Often argues with adults
 3. Often actively defies or refuses to comply with adults' requests or rules
 4. Often deliberately annoys people
 5. Often blames others for his or her mistakes or misbehavior
 6. Is often touchy or easily annoyed by others
 7. Is often angry and resentful
 8. Is often spiteful or vindictive

 Note: Consider a criterion met only if the behavior occurs more frequently than is typically observed in individuals of comparable age and developmental level.

B. The disturbance in behavior causes clinically significant impairment in social, academic, or occupational functioning.

C. The behaviors do not occur exclusively during the course of a psychotic or mood disorder.

D. Criteria are not met for conduct disorder, and, if the individual is age 18 years or older, criteria are not met for antisocial personality disorder (see *Diagnostic and Statistical Manual of Mental Disorders*, 4th ed.).

Reprinted with permission from American Psychiatric Association. *Diagnostic and statistical manual of mental disorders*, 4th ed. Text revision. Washington, DC: American Psychiatric Association, 2000.

at school age. Rates of disorder range from 2% to 16%, depending on the population sampled and whether it is a community or clinic population. To make this diagnosis, evidence of impairment is needed. Criteria for impairment, as shown in Box 102.2, are clinically significant impairment in social, occupational, or academic functioning. Oppositional behavior is seen two to ten times more frequently in boys than in girls. The disorder may be diagnosed as early as age 3 years, but is more commonly seen in school-aged children and adolescents.

The establishment of autonomy is a normal developmental task for children as they begin to develop self-awareness. Oppositional behavior is seen at the end of the first year of life as the child first assumes independence in feeding, but more emphatically between 18 and 36 months. The behavior peaks between 18 and 24 months, when the need to separate and master the environment is strongest. If this developmental phase of oppositional behavior is interpreted by parents as a need to be in control, power struggles may ensue; excessive focusing on the behavior may reinforce it. A normal effort to become independent may become an attempt to be free of external control and perceived overprotection.

A second phase of normal oppositional behavior occurs in adolescence, when the developmental task has to do with becoming separate from the parent and establishing an independent, personal identity. If a perceived risk in expressing aggression overtly exists, it may be expressed in a passive oppositional manner. An appreciation for the need for autonomy is vital at this age, and effective support, although exhausting to provide, is essential for this age group.

Although the onset may be sudden, following acute stress, oppositional behavior more commonly emerges as a prolongation and exaggeration of an earlier developmental stage, becoming increasingly maladaptive. Behavior that is seen as independent and strong-willed in a younger child may be viewed as oppositional and defiant in a school-aged one. The prognosis is best for oppositional behavior that is the outcome of an acute event and poorest for temperamental traits of opposition. Without treatment, passive-aggressive personality may be the adult outcome of a nonaccepting or controlling family environment.

Differential Diagnosis

Children with conduct disorder often have oppositional defiant behaviors, but because of the severity of their behavior, the diagnosis of conduct disorder takes precedence, and oppositional defiant disorder is not diagnosed. Both oppositional defiant disorder and attention deficit disorder often occur together. Oppositional defiant disorder must be distinguished from those problems in following directions that are the consequence of impaired language comprehension (e.g., loss of hearing, mixed receptive/expressive language disorder). In psychotic disorders, such as schizophrenia, oppositional defiant symptoms may be seen early in the course. Oppositional behavior also may be present in major depression, dysthymia, and mania. The diagnosis of oppositional defiant disorder is not made if symptoms occur exclusively in the course of a mood disorder or psychotic disorder.

Therapy

Treatment must address the individual child's need for autonomy and interpersonal relationships within the family. Individual psychotherapy and behavioral methods commonly are used. The child may be seen individually in therapy to develop more appropriate means of expressing autonomy. Family interventions often use treatment approaches based on social learning theory. This requires data-gathering by parents about their child's behavior, including both oppositional behavior and appropriate social interaction. Their cooperation also is necessary in providing appropriate consequences in behavior management. The child with less severe symptoms often is managed in collaboration with a psychologist; however, patients who meet the full criteria for the diagnosis may be referred for psychiatric assessment. Early intervention is essential to prevent progression to conduct disorder.

Suggested Readings

Achenbach TM, Edelbrock CS. Behavioral problems and competencies reported by parents of normal and disturbed children aged four through sixteen. *Monogr Soc Res Child Dev* 1981;46:1.

Bassarath L. Medication strategies in childhood aggression: a review. *Can J Psychiatry* 2003;48:367.

Ben-Amos B. Depression and conduct disorders in children and adolescents: a review of the literature. *Bull Menninger Clin* 1992;56:188.

Bennett KJ, Lipman EL, Brown S, et al. Predicting conduct problems: can high-risk children be identified in kindergarten and grade 1? *J Consult Clin Psychol* 1999;67:470.

Brestan EV, Eyberg SM. Effective psychosocial treatments of conduct-disordered children and adolescents: 29 years, 82 studies, and 5,272 kids. *J Clin Child Psychol* 1998;27:180.

Campbell M, Gonzalez NM, Silva RR. The pharmacologic treatment of conduct disorders and rage outbursts. *Psychiatr Clin North Am* 1992;15:69.

Costello EJ, Compton SN, Keeler G, Angold A. Relationships between poverty and psychopathology: a natural experiment. *JAMA* 2003;290:2023.

Crowley TJ, Riggs PD. Adolescent substance use disorder with conduct disorder and comorbid conditions. *NIDA Res Monogr* 1995;156:49.

Juvonen J, Graham S, Schuster MA. Bullying among young adolescents: the strong, the weak, and the troubled. *Pediatrics* 2003;112(6 Pt 1):1231.

Kazdin AE. Practitioner review: psychosocial treatments for conduct disorder in children. *J Child Psychol Psychiatry* 1997;38:161.

Keller MB, Lavori PW, Beardslee WR, et al. The disruptive behavioral disorder in children and adolescents: comorbidity and clinical course. *J Am Acad Child Adolesc Psychiatry* 1992;31:204.

Kutcher S, Aman M, Brooks SJ, et al. International consensus statement on attention-deficit/hyperactivity disorder (ADHD) and disruptive behaviour disorders (DBDs): clinical implications and treatment practice suggestions. *Eur Neuropsychopharmacol* 2004;14:11.

Lahey BB, Loeber R, Burke J, et al. Waxing and waning in concert: dynamic comorbidity of conduct disorder with other disruptive and emotional problems over 7 years among clinic-referred boys. *J Abnorm Psychol* 2002;111:556.

Loeber R, Lahey BB, Thomas C. Diagnostic conundrum of oppositional defiant disorder and conduct disorder. *J Abnorm Psychol* 1991;100:379.

Lahey BB, Loeber R, Burke J, Rathouz PJ. Adolescent outcomes of childhood conduct disorder among clinic-referred boys: predictors of improvement. *J Abnorm Child Psychol* 2002;30:333.

Patterson GR. *Living with children: new methods for parents and teachers*, Revised edition. Champaign, IL: Research Press, 1976.

Rey JM. Oppositional defiant disorder. *Am J Psychiatry* 1993;150:1769.

Rivara FP, Farrington DP. Prevention of violence. Role of the pediatrician. *Arch Pediatr Adolesc Med* 1995;149:421.

Robins LN. Conduct disorder. *J Child Psychol Psychiatry* 1991;32:193.

Rowe R, Maughan B, Pickles A, et al. The relationship between DSM-IV oppositional defiant disorder and conduct disorder: findings from the Great Smoky Mountains Study. *Child Psychol Psychiatry* 2002;43:365.

Sampson RJ, Raudenbush SW, Earls F. Neighborhoods and violent crime: a multilevel study of collective efficacy. *Science* 1997;77:918.

Shrier LA, Harris SK, Kurland M, Knight JR. Substance use problems and associated psychiatric symptoms among adolescents in primary care. *Pediatrics* 2003;111(6 Pt 1):e699.

Steiner H. Practice parameters for the assessment and treatment of children and adolescents with conduct disorder. *J Am Acad Child Adolesc Psychiatry* 1997;36:122S39S.

Wells KC, Egan J. Social learning and systems family therapy for childhood oppositional disorder: comparative treatment outcome. *Compr Psychiatry* 1988;29:138.

Wiener JM. Oppositional defiant disorder. In: *Textbook of child and adolescent psychiatry*. Washington, DC: American Psychiatric Press, 1997:459.

Winnicott DW. The antisocial tendency. In: *Through pediatrics to psychoanalysis*. New York: Basic Books, 1975:306.

CHAPTER 103 ■ EMOTIONAL DISORDERS WITH CHILDHOOD ONSET

JAMES C. HARRIS

Childhood is a time of considerable developmental plasticity, and research has shown that most children with emotional disorders do not remain symptomatic and do not present as disordered adults. Still, some childhood anxiety disorders can be precursors to continued anxiety and mood disorders in adulthood, especially if there are predisposing temperamental features of behavioral inhibition (social anxiety) in the child and a strong family history of anxiety disorder. Some emotional disorders in childhood appear as quantitative exaggerations of normal developmental trends rather than as qualitatively abnormal behavior. Moreover, symptom complexes beginning in early childhood form less clearly defined entities than adult disorders. From a developmental perspective, the appropriateness of emotional behavior must be gauged in terms of its intensity, frequency, age of onset, duration, and the setting in which it occurs.

Separation anxiety, social phobia, obsessive-compulsive disorder, and generalized anxiety disorder are categorized as anxiety disorders. A child with one anxiety disorder may have other concurrent anxiety disorder diagnoses, so several forms of anxiety disorder may occur simultaneously. Panic attacks accompanying an anxiety disorder ordinarily begin in adolescence, although they may occur in preadolescence.

Children and adolescents may develop fears that are focused on a wide variety of objects or situations. Fears or phobias are not necessarily a part of normal development; some fears, however, do seem specific to a particular developmental phase and may arise in a majority of children (e.g., fear of animals in preschool children). A distinction is made between fearfulness that is qualitatively different from normal behavior and fears that are exaggerations of normal behavior. The developmental age is considered along with the degree of anxiety. Some fears are specific to a particular situation, and others are part of a more generalized anxiety disorder.

In preschool children, transient fears of insects, animals, monsters, and the dark are common. Fears of storms, heights, and bodily harm are common in school-aged children, and fears of entering social situations and concerns about appearance (dysmorphobia) are common in adolescents. If these symptoms persist beyond the developmental period when they are common and are associated with sufficient anxiety to interfere with everyday activities, referral for treatment is recommended.

SEPARATION ANXIETY DISORDER AND SCHOOL REFUSAL

School-related problems, including school refusal as a result of separation anxiety disorder, are a rapidly growing part of pediatric practice. Excessive school absence is a problem of considerable importance nationwide, with both health and social implications. Patterns of absence are established early in the school career; thus, a small proportion of children makes up a large percentage of the absences. Families at high risk for chronic medical and psychosocial problems should be identified by monitoring school absence patterns. School attendance has been suggested as one marker of how well a child is coping with chronic stress. Attending school is the first of many prolonged separations. Eighty percent of preschool children have difficulty adapting to school. By 6 to 8 years of age, symptoms are more common in only children and in those who have been overly dependent.

The child with anxiety causing school refusal was initially described as being truant. However, researchers discovered that these children with school refusal feared that something terrible would happen to their mother, and this fear made them run home for reassurance and relief of anxiety. By 1941, the designation *school phobia* was used to distinguish it from the more common delinquent variety of nonattendance. Phobic tendencies and obsessional symptoms were described, and it was suggested that, if cases were left untreated, a more crippling adult disorder could develop.

Epidemiology

Children with separation anxiety disorder commonly have a second psychiatric diagnosis. Rates are highest during the following periods: at the time of school entry and soon after (5 to 7 years of age), when separation anxiety alone is the most common presentation; at about 11 years of age, when symptoms may be associated with school changes; and at 14 years of age and older, when symptoms begin to differ in type and severity and are associated with more severe psychiatric disorders.

The prevalence of all forms of school refusal is reported to be approximately 4% in young school-aged children; this represents 5% to 8% of referrals to child psychiatry clinics. In 10- to 11-year-old children, the rate is lower (1% to 3%).

Etiology

Most often, school refusal is part of an emotional disturbance; however, the term does not designate one cause. Symptoms may develop in several ways according to the various theories, as follows:

- Psychodynamic theory: Phobic symptoms arise from externalization of frightening impulses and displacement to a neutral object, which is then avoided.
- Learning theory: Maladaptive responses are learned through operant conditioning by adult attention to symptoms.
- Interpersonal or family interaction difficulty (60% to 80% of younger children): An unduly dependent child is affected by maternal anxieties and conflicts and becomes symptomatic when he or she must leave home. An often mutual and hostile dependency in the parent-child relationship exists. Symptoms result from a fear of leaving home.

Precipitating factors may be a minor accident, illness, or operation, leaving home for a new camp or school, the departure or loss of a school friend, or death of or illness in a relative to whom the child was attached. These events are experienced as threats and elicit anxiety. Fear of real situations at school or concerns related to self-esteem make up 50% of cases of school refusal in school-aged children. School refusal has also been reported in children with cancer who have been at home with continuous care over longer periods of time.

In addition, behavioral inhibition may be an early expression of a genetic predisposition to separation anxiety. Animal models suggest that variants of the corticotropin-releasing hormone gene may be associated with being prone to anxiety.

It is also important to determine when there are multiple causes of the child's problem (e.g., when anxiety is related to some aspect of the school situation and the child also has separation anxiety). A depressive disorder must be distinguished from demoralization, especially in the older child and adolescent. A depressive subgroup of school refusers is important to identify, because depressive disorder with suicide has been reported in children and adolescents with school refusal. Eldest and youngest children may be affected more frequently.

Clinical Presentation

The essential feature of a separation anxiety disorder is excessive anxiety concerning separation from the home and from those to whom the child is attached. Separation symptoms are more common in girls than boys and present with the following:

- Vague complaints before school or reluctance to attend school progress to total refusal to go or remain in school despite entreaty, recrimination, and punishment.
- Overt signs of overanxiety and panic when the time comes to leave for school. The child often cannot set out for school or returns after going halfway. When the parent takes the child to school, the separation moment is dramatic, with clinging to the parent and refusal to separate.
- Symptoms may assume a somatic disguise, with loss of appetite, nausea, vomiting, syncope, headache, abdominal pain, vague malaise, diarrhea, limb pains, and tachycardia. Complaints may be expressed in the morning before school or even in school without a clear expression of the fears, which are elicited only on careful inquiry. The child may anticipate the occurrence of symptoms, expecting to be ill, but becomes quickly asymptomatic when allowed to stay home.

Separation anxiety may be manifested as school refusal. The onset may be acute in young children and more gradual in its onset in adolescents and older children, with a decline in peer group activities and activities outside the home. The child may cling to the mother and try to control her, may become stubborn and argumentative in contrast to earlier compliance, and often directs anger toward the mother. There may be no precipitating event other than a change to a more senior school. In this older age group, closer examination may demonstrate depressive symptoms or other behavior problems or, rarely, a psychotic illness. Long-standing family dysfunction may be noted, with a personal history of anxiety when entering social situations. Lack of normal independence and immature sexual identification may be part of the young person's problems in coping with independence.

Diagnosis

Toddlers and preschool children normally show anxiety over real or potential separation from caregivers. A separation anxiety disorder is diagnosed when the fear over separation interferes with developmental tasks and persists, leading to impairment in peer and family relationships. Diagnostic criteria for separation anxiety disorder are described in Box 103.1.

Treatment

Treatment is individualized. Family therapy is recommended to reestablish parent-child boundaries and roles. An immediate goal is to assign family tasks, beginning with immediate return to school after clarifying the child's experience of the school situation.

For those children who fail to respond to psychotherapy or behavioral approaches, pharmacotherapy may be considered for separation anxiety disorder. Treatment studies combining antidepressants with cognitive behavioral therapy for separation anxiety disorder have been effective; however, these medications require careful monitoring for side effects. Serotonin

---

BOX 103.1   Diagnostic Criteria for Separation Anxiety Disorder

A. Developmentally inappropriate and excessive anxiety exists concerning separation from home or from those to whom the individual is attached, as evidenced by three (or more) of the following:
   1. Recurrent excessive distress when separation from home or major attachment figures occurs or is anticipated.
   2. Persistent and excessive worry about losing, or about possible harm befalling, major attachment figures.
   3. Persistent and excessive worry that an untoward event will lead to separation from a major attachment figure (e.g., getting lost or being kidnapped).
   4. Persistent reluctance or refusal to go to school or elsewhere because of fear of separation.
   5. Persistently and excessively fearful or reluctant to be alone or without major attachment figures at home or without significant adults in other settings.
   6. Persistent reluctance or refusal to go to sleep without being near a major attachment figure or to sleep away from home.
   7. Repeated nightmares involving the theme of separation.

8. Repeated complaints of physical symptoms (e.g., headaches, stomachaches, nausea, or vomiting) when separation from major attachment figures occurs or is anticipated.
B. The duration of the disturbance is at least 4 weeks.
C. The onset is before age 18 years.
D. The disturbance causes clinically significant distress or impairment in social, academic (occupational), or other important areas of functioning.
E. The disturbance does not occur exclusively during the course of a pervasive developmental disorder, schizophrenia, or other psychotic disorder and, in adolescents and adults, is not better accounted for by panic disorder with agoraphobia.

Specify if:
   Early onset: if onset occurs before age 6 years.

Reprinted with permission from American Psychiatric Association. *Diagnostic and statistical manual of mental disorders,* 4th ed. Text revision. Washington, DC: American Psychiatric Association, 2000.

---

reuptake inhibitors, such as fluoxetine and fluvoxamine, are preferred for anxiety disorders but are best combined with psychological treatments. Careful monitoring for drug side effects is necessary.

A specific treatment plan includes an early return to school, and the teacher and staff must be fully involved in treatment. The father or both parents should take the child to school in the morning. Regular support and praise for parents in their efforts are essential. Bringing in a school friend to go to school with the affected child may help. Regular interviews, focusing on potential anxiety or stress at home and school, are needed to establish a regular pattern of attendance. A breakdown in attendance after a weekend, after an illness of a day or two, or at the beginning of a new term may be expected. Family illness or bereavement and changes to a new classroom increase the risk of recurrence. The parents must understand that being firm is supportive and is not a rejection of the child's needs, because the child's pleas to stay home can be heartrending. Sometimes an outside person may have to be brought in to take the child to school. Regular office visits and telephone calls are required in the first weeks following the return to school. Family treatment and social work support may be needed, and parental disorders should be treated. The physician must establish a trusting relationship with the family, clarify situations causing anxiety at home, and desensitize, confront, and persist. Hospitalization may be needed if the parent-child bond is strong and outpatient intervention fails.

In most series, two-thirds or more of patients improve. The prognosis is related to the severity of symptoms and the response to psychosocial support.

SPECIFIC PHOBIA

A specific phobia is defined as a marked and persistent fear of a specific object or situation. It is distinguished from a panic attack, in which the fear is of having another panic attack, or from a social phobia, in which the fear is of humiliation or

embarrassment in a social situation. In a specific phobia, exposure to the phobic stimulus ordinarily provokes an immediate response of anxiety, which is associated with a panicky feeling, sweating, tachycardia, and problems with breathing. The more physically distant the patient is from the phobic stimulus, the less severe the symptoms will be. Anticipatory anxiety is generally noted when confrontation with the phobic stimulus is expected.

A diagnosis of specific phobia is made only if avoidance of the phobic stimulus interferes with normal activities or relationships. The anxiety is not relieved by knowing that other people do not regard the situation as threatening. Subtypes include specific phobias of animals and natural events (e.g., heights, thunder) or situations (e.g., being in elevators or enclosed spaces). Diagnostic criteria for specific phobia are described in Box 103.2.

The age of onset of symptoms varies, but certain phobias such as animal phobias almost always start in childhood. These simple phobias beginning in childhood usually disappear without treatment. The degree of social impairment is related to how easily the child can avoid the phobic stimulus. Specific phobias may occur alone or along with another phobic condition, although the reported prevalence varies with the threshold chosen to determine impairment.

Phobias may be learned maladaptive responses. They may represent the persistence of age-related common fears, or they may have unrecognized personal psychological significance.

For phobias considered to be learned responses or developmental in nature, behavior therapy is the appropriate treatment. Methods used include direct exposure to the feared situation with social support or desensitization through systematic presentation of the child's self-generated hierarchy of feared situations while the child is fully relaxed. Operant behavior methods also can be used by providing rewards to the child after planned entry into the feared situation. If the feared situation is social, role rehearsal before entering the situation or observing another child or adult deal with the feared situation is recommended. If the situation has a personal psychodynamic

---

BOX 103.2   Diagnostic Criteria for Specific Phobia

A. Marked and persistent fear that is excessive or unreasonable is cued by the presence or anticipation of a specific object or situation (e.g., flying, heights, animals, receiving an injection, seeing blood).
B. Exposure to the phobic stimulus almost invariably provokes an immediate anxiety response, which may take the form of a situationally bound or situationally predisposed panic attack. Note: In children, the anxiety may be expressed by crying, tantrums, freezing, or clinging.
C. The person recognizes that the fear is excessive or unreasonable. Note: In children, this feature may be absent.
D. The phobic situation is avoided or else is endured with intense anxiety or distress.
E. The avoidance, anxious anticipation, or distress in the feared situation interferes significantly with the person's normal routine, occupational (or academic) functioning, or social activities or relationships, or there is marked distress about having the phobia.
F. In individuals under age 18 years, the duration is at least 6 months.
G. The anxiety, panic attack, or phobic avoidance associated with the specific object or situation is not better accounted for by another mental disorder, such as

obsessive-compulsive disorder (e.g., fear of dirt in someone with an obsession about contamination), posttraumatic stress disorder (e.g., avoidance of stimuli associated with a severe stressor), separation anxiety disorder (e.g., avoidance of school), social phobia (e.g., avoidance of social situations because of fear of embarrassment), panic disorder with agoraphobia, or agoraphobia without history of panic disorder.

Specify type:
Animal type
Natural environment type (e.g., heights, storms, water)
Blood-injection-injury type
Situational type (e.g., airplanes, elevators, enclosed places)
Other type (e.g., phobic avoidance of situations that may lead to choking, vomiting, or contracting an illness; in children, avoidance of loud sounds or costumed characters)

Reprinted with permission from American Psychiatric Association. *Diagnostic and statistical manual of mental disorders,* 4th ed. Text revision. Washington, DC: American Psychiatric Association, 2000.

---

meaning for the child, individual or family treatment approaches may be necessary. Future phobic symptoms can be prevented by teaching the child coping strategies to deal with fearful and unexpected situations.

Specific fears ordinarily resolve over several months. The outcome is generally good for phobias, with remission in approximately two-thirds of the cases over a 3- to 4-year period.

SOCIAL PHOBIA

Social phobia in childhood is manifested by an avoidance of contact with unfamiliar people that is severe enough to interfere with social functioning in peer relationships. Although a desire exists for social contact with peers, family members, and friends, as a consequence of his or her phobic behavior, the child avoids them. The child is likely to seem socially withdrawn or timid when with unfamiliar people and may become anxious when minor requests are made to interact with strangers. The degree of anxiety may result in difficulty in speaking or muteness. These children generally are not assertive and lack confidence. The disorder is more apparent in adolescence, when increased socialization is expected. It usually is associated with another anxiety disorder.

Ordinarily, age of onset is in the early school years, when children have their first opportunity for extensive social contact. However, it may represent a persistence or recurrence of stranger anxiety that typically would have disappeared developmentally. The course of symptoms is variable: Some children have an episodic or even a chronic course, and in others the disorder remits spontaneously. Impairment in social functioning may be quite severe. Children with problems in language development may have increased vulnerability and may avoid situations in which speech would be expected. As a result of this behavior, the child may not form age-appropriate social relationships and may feel isolated or sad. Social phobia of

childhood is more common in girls than in boys and may be more common if the mother had similar symptoms. Children with social phobia should be distinguished, based on severity of symptoms, from children who are reticent or slow to warm up to new people.

Diagnosis

Diagnostic criteria for social phobia are described in Box 103.3. Social phobia may be part of an adjustment disorder; if so, adjustment disorder can be identified because of the presence of a recent psychosocial stressor. In generalized anxiety disorder, the anxiety is persistent and excessive, extending across several settings (e.g., school work, athletics, and social encounters). The anxiety is associated with impaired functioning in these areas and often with somatic symptoms of anxiety. In separation anxiety, the anxiety occurs at separation from the primary caregiver. An avoidant personality trait may be diagnosed if the personality trait persists over several years. In more serious personality disturbances, such as the schizoid traits, the child has difficulty with interpersonal relationships in all settings.

Treatment

After appropriate diagnosis and case formulation, the initial treatment approach addresses the child's individual needs. The focus is on increasing assertiveness in the psychotherapeutic setting and at school. Both child and parents are evaluated to clarify the family's response to the child's behavior and also to assess their ability to support treatment. In some instances, parents have similar personality traits. The parents must understand how the child is controlling interpersonal relationships by his or her anxiety. Families are encouraged to introduce the child to experiences in which anxiety with

---

BOX 103.3   Diagnostic Criteria for Social Phobia

A. A marked and persistent fear exists of one or more social or performance situations in which the person is exposed to unfamiliar people or to possible scrutiny by others. The individual fears that he or she will act in a way (or show anxiety symptoms) that will be humiliating or embarrassing. Note: In children, there must be evidence of the capacity for age-appropriate social relationships with familiar people, and the anxiety must occur in peer settings, not just in interactions with adults.

B. Exposure to the feared social situation almost invariably provokes anxiety, which may take the form of a situationally bound or situationally predisposed panic attack. Note: In children, anxiety may be expressed by crying, tantrums, freezing, or shrinking from social situations with unfamiliar people.

C. The person recognizes that the fear is excessive or unreasonable. Note: In children, this feature may be absent.

D. The feared social or performance situations are avoided or else are endured with intense anxiety or distress.

E. The avoidance, anxious anticipation, or distress in the feared social or performance situations interferes significantly with the person's normal routine, occupational (academic) functioning, or social activities or relationships, or there is marked distress about having the phobia.

F. In individuals under age 18 years, the duration is at least 6 months.

G. The fear or avoidance is not the result of the direct physiologic effects of a substance (e.g., a drug of abuse, a medication) or a general medical condition and is not better accounted for by another mental disorder (e.g., panic disorder with or without agoraphobia, separation anxiety disorder, body dysmorphic disorder, a pervasive developmental disorder, or schizoid personality disorder).

H. If a general medical condition or another mental disorder is present, the fear in criterion A is unrelated to it (e.g., the fear is not of stuttering, trembling in Parkinson disease, or exhibiting abnormal eating behavior in anorexia nervosa or bulimia nervosa).

Specify if:
   Generalized: if the fears include most social situations (also consider the additional diagnosis of avoidant personality disorder).

Reprinted with permission from American Psychiatric Association. *Diagnostic and statistical manual of mental disorders*, 4th ed. Text revision. Washington, DC: American Psychiatric Association, 2000.

---

strangers is manageable. Specific efforts are made to increase self-esteem by establishing new skills such as writing, music, or athletics.

An important issue in treatment is to restructure interpersonal relationships through supportive therapy that assists the child in facing new situations by mastering his or her anxiety. The parents need help in overcoming the child's excessive dependence on them. Often, tightly woven interpersonal relationships are present that are difficult to modify. When the child leaves home and enters a school setting or participates in recreational activities, the opportunity for change is greatest. Selective serotonin reuptake inhibitors have high acute response rates in controlled studies of children with anxiety disorders and are efficacious and well tolerated when these drugs are taken for longer periods.

The persistence of social phobia symptoms may lead to an avoidant personality structure in adulthood, when the treatment outcome is less optimistic than in children. Parents and teachers must appreciate the child's needs and must work together to help the child develop greater autonomy.

OBSESSIVE-COMPULSIVE DISORDER

An obsessive-compulsive disorder is characterized by recurrent obsessional thoughts or compulsive activity that interferes with normal activities and causes psychosocial distress; performance of rituals may last an hour or more. The most common obsessional thoughts focus on fears of contamination (e.g., dirt or feces) and fears of doing something wrong (e.g., stealing or misbehaving). Attempts to resist them may interfere with the normal school routine or interpersonal re-

lationships. The increased tension and anxiety are temporarily reduced by compulsive activity. Common compulsions are hand-washing rituals, having to touch objects in a particular sequence to avoid psychological danger or trouble, and complex bedtime routines. Normal compulsive thoughts are common in middle childhood.

Compulsive behavior is expected to neutralize or prevent discomfort related to a dreaded situation; victims hope to prevent harm to themselves or harm they could cause to others. In older children, the behavior is generally recognized as pointless and ineffective, and attempts are made to resist it. However, younger children may not be as aware of the unreasonableness of their behavior. Anxiety in obsessive-compulsive disorder is secondary rather than primary. Children and adolescents with obsessive symptoms, particularly those with repetitive thoughts, may also develop depressive symptoms as they become frustrated from repeated attempts to resist the thoughts. Individuals with a depressive disorder may develop obsessional thoughts during their episodes of depression. The severity of depressive symptoms and that of obsessional symptoms may parallel each other. Diagnostic criteria for obsessive-compulsive disorder are described in Box 103.4.

Epidemiology and Etiology

Obsessional disorder usually begins in adolescence, but it may begin in childhood. This disorder makes up 1% of child psychiatric referrals. Onset is earlier in boys than in girls, but the disorder is equally common in both genders. Data suggest that this disorder may be more common in children than previously expected. Community studies have estimated a lifetime prevalence of 2.5% and a 1-year prevalence of 1.5% to 2.0%. A report of 5,000 unselected adolescents noted a prevalence

---

BOX 103.4   Diagnostic Criteria for Obsessive-Compulsive Disorder

A. Either obsessions or compulsions exist:
Obsessions as defined by 1, 2, 3, and 4:
1. Recurrent and persistent thoughts, impulses, or images that are experienced, at some time during the disturbance, as intrusive and inappropriate and that cause marked anxiety or distress.
2. Thoughts, impulses, or images that are not simply excessive worries about real-life problems.
3. Attempts to ignore or suppress such thoughts, impulses, or images or to neutralize them with some other thought or action.
4. Recognition that the obsessional thoughts, impulses, or images are a product of his or her own mind (not imposed from without as in thought insertion).

Compulsions as defined by 1 and 2:
1. Repetitive behavior (e.g., hand washing, ordering, checking) or mental acts (e.g., praying, counting, repeating words silently) that the person feels driven to perform in response to an obsession or according to rules that must be applied rigidly.
2. The behaviors or mental acts are aimed at preventing or reducing distress or preventing some dreaded event or situation; however, these behaviors or mental acts either are not connected in a realistic way with what they are designed to neutralize or prevent or are clearly excessive.

B. At some point during the course of the disorder, the person has recognized that the obsessions or compulsions are excessive or unreasonable. Note: This does not apply to children.

C. The obsessions or compulsions cause marked distress, are time consuming (take more than 1 hour a day), or significantly interfere with the person's normal routine, occupational (or academic) functioning, or usual social activities or relationships.

D. If another Axis I disorder is present, the content of the obsessions or compulsions is not restricted to it (e.g., preoccupation with food in the presence of an eating disorder, hair pulling in the presence of trichotillomania, concern with appearance in the presence of body dysmorphic disorder, preoccupation with drugs in the presence of a substance use disorder, preoccupation with having a serious illness in the presence of hypochondriasis, preoccupation with sexual urges or fantasies in the presence of a paraphilia, or guilty ruminations in the presence of major depressive disorder).

E. The disturbance is not the result of the direct physiologic effects of a substance (e.g., a drug of abuse, a medication) or a general medical condition.

Specify if:
With poor insight: if, for most of the time during the current episode, the person does not recognize that the obsessions and compulsions are excessive or unreasonable.

Reprinted with permission from American Psychiatric Association. *Diagnostic and statistical manual of mental disorders*, 4th ed. Text revision. Washington, DC: American Psychiatric Association, 2000.

---

of 2% in whom compulsive thoughts interfered with their daily activities. In reviewing adult cases of obsessional disorder, approximately 20% give a history of their first symptoms before age 10 years, and approximately one-third experienced symptoms by age 15 years.

Symptoms have been reported in children as young as 3 years, but referral is most common in the early teens. In one study, the average age of referral was 14.5 years. Although the disorder is equally common in male and female subjects, the onset in male subjects tends to be earlier. The symptom patterns in children are similar to those seen in adults. In one study, cleaning rituals were most frequent, but counting and checking rituals and repetitive thoughts of violence or sex also were reported. Behavioral symptoms are qualitatively different, rather than an exaggeration of normal development. A sudden onset in adolescence has been reported. Obsessions have been noted following encephalitis, febrile seizures, and temporal lobe seizures.

Some children may become secondarily depressed by their perceived helplessness in dealing with obsessions. These symptoms may also be seen in individuals with severe depressive disorders and in anorexia nervosa. In those instances, the primary disorder is treated.

Treatment

Obsessive-compulsive disorder in children is treated most effectively by using behavioral methods that take into account the child's developmental level. Efforts are also made to help the child find a meaningful context to express his or her symptoms. The alliance between the child and therapist is of considerable importance, as is the family's cooperation in planning treatment. Serotonin reuptake inhibiting drugs have been tested in adults, children, and adolescents for obsessive-compulsive disorder; significant improvements were seen in a group of adolescents, and the effect was independent of an antidepressant action. The long-term effects of this drug treatment remain to be established, but recent studies are encouraging. Resolution of obsessive symptoms leads to concurrent improvement in interpersonal difficulties.

The outcome is variable; however, symptoms tend to persist without treatment. Long-term outcome information is increasingly available using newer treatment approaches. It is proposed that some children with streptococcal infections may develop poststreptococcal autoimmunity resulting in tics and obsessive-compulsive disorder symptoms. The acronym PANDAS (for pediatric autoimmune neuropsychiatric disorders associated with streptococcal infections) has been given to a subgroup who meet five inclusionary criteria: presence of obsessive-compulsive disorder and/or tic disorder, prepubertal symptom onset, sudden onset or episodic course of symptoms, temporal association between streptococcal infections and the emergence of neuropsychiatric symptoms, and associated neurologic findings. Treatment strategies for PANDAS include the use of antibiotic prophylaxis to prevent streptococcal-triggered exacerbations and the use of immunomodulatory interventions (e.g., intravenous gammaglobulin).

GENERALIZED ANXIETY DISORDER

Generalized anxiety disorder in childhood is characterized by excessive or unrealistic anxiety or worry. Children with this condition are extremely self-conscious and worry about the future, particularly about their performance, possible injury, their relationships with peers, and how to meet peer group expectations. Concern may be expressed about tests, completing tasks, and their past behavior. Because of these concerns, the child may spend a great deal of time asking questions about the possible discomfort or the dangers of experiences that are anticipated. These children require considerable reassurance.

Generalized anxiety disorder is equally distributed among male and female subjects and is more common in families in which the mother has an anxiety disorder or another mental disorder. It may be more common in the eldest child in small families, where considerable focus on achievement exists even when the child is apparently doing adequate work in school.

Clinical Presentation

Physical symptoms may include gastrointestinal distress, shortness of breath, nausea, dizziness, headache, or other somatic symptoms. These children may appear tense and may have difficulty falling asleep. Because of anxiety, they may refuse to attend school. Their persistent questions may give a false impression of precocity. Perfectionism, self-doubt, excessive conformity, restlessness, and nervous habits may further complicate the course. A list of diagnostic criteria is presented in Box 103.5.

The onset of symptoms may be gradual or sudden, and worsening may occur with stress. In adult life, symptoms may persist as generalized anxiety disorder or in some instances as social phobia. The age of onset of the earliest symptoms is unknown; however, symptoms of anxiety are observed in infants and preschool children, and physiologic symptoms of anxiety disorder are first reported either in school-aged children or in adolescents.

The major impairment that may result from symptoms is an inability to work effectively in school or to relate appropriately at home. Unnecessary medical evaluations may be generated by the somatic symptoms.

Diagnosis

The differential diagnosis includes mixed anxiety disorders (e.g., combined separation anxiety and social phobia in younger children). In separation anxiety, the focus is on the consequences of personal separation; the child with a generalized anxiety disorder focuses on anticipated future problems. Attention deficit disorder should not be mistaken for this generalized anxiety, because children with this diagnosis, although active, do not usually demonstrate the concurrent anxiety, nor are they overly concerned about the future. However, both conditions may occasionally coexist. Adjustment disorder with anxious mood is demonstrated by the occurrence of a related psychosocial stressor during the previous 6 months. If anxiety is related to a mood disorder or psychotic disorder, anxiety disorder would not be considered as a primary diagnosis.

Treatment

The treatment of a generalized anxiety disorder relies on the establishment of the diagnosis and an individual case formulation. The first issue is whether the anxiety has a symbolic meaning; if so, individual psychodynamic psychotherapy is indicated. Common conflicts that may be out of the child's awareness and need to be understood are sibling rivalry, aggressive or sexual feelings toward parents, and unrecognized conflicts about control. The therapist establishes a consistent setting, acknowledges the patient's emotional needs, establishes appropriate limits, and then initiates therapy. In this setting, a confiding relationship between adult and child may be established and

---

BOX 103.5   Diagnostic Criteria for Generalized Anxiety Disorder

A. Excessive anxiety and worry (apprehensive expectation) occur more days than not for at least 6 months about a number of events or activities (e.g., work or school performance).
B. The person finds it difficult to control the worry.
C. The anxiety and worry are associated with three (or more) of the following six symptoms (with at least some symptoms present for more days than not for the past 6 months). Note: Only one item is required in children.
  1. Restlessness or feeling keyed up or on edge
  2. Being easily fatigued
  3. Difficulty concentrating or mind going blank
  4. Irritability
  5. Muscle tension
  6. Sleep disturbance (difficulty falling or staying asleep or restless unsatisfying sleep)
D. The focus of the anxiety and worry is not confined to features of an Axis I disorder (e.g., the anxiety or worry is not about having a panic attack as in panic disorder, being embarrassed in public as in social phobia, being contaminated as in obsessive-compulsive disorder, being away from home or close relatives as in separation anxiety disorder), gaining weight as in anorexia nervosa, having multiple physical complaints as in somatization disorder, or having a serious illness as in hypochondriasis), and the anxiety and worry do not occur exclusively during posttraumatic stress disorder).
E. The anxiety, worry, or physical symptom complex causes clinically significant distress or impairment in social, occupational, or other important areas of functioning.
F. The disturbance is not the result of the direct physiologic effects of a substance (e.g., a drug of abuse, a medication) or a general medical condition (e.g., hyperthyroidism) and does not occur exclusively during a mood disorder, psychotic disorder, or pervasive developmental disorder.

Reprinted with permission from American Psychiatric Association. *Diagnostic and statistical manual of mental disorders*, 4th ed. Text revision. Washington, DC: American Psychiatric Association, 2000.

specific target symptoms identified. The use of an anxiolytic agent in acute situations may be indicated, especially the use of serotonin reuptake inhibitors. Associated insomnia may require specific intervention for sleep disorder. Family interviews clarify the parents' ability to support the individual therapeutic endeavor with the child and establish the need for concurrent family treatment.

Suggested Readings

American Academy of Child and Adolescent Psychiatry. Practice parameters for the assessment and treatment of children and adolescents with obsessive-compulsive disorder. *J Am Acad Child Adolesc Psychiatry* 1998;37(suppl): 27S.

Bernstein GA, Borchardt CM, Perwien AR, et al. Imipramine plus cognitive-behavioral therapy in the treatment of school refusal. *J Am Acad Child Adolesc Psychiatry* 2000;39:276.

Bowen RC, Offord DR, Boyle MH. The prevalence of overanxious disorder and separation anxiety disorder: results from the Ontario Child Health Study. *J Am Acad Child Adolesc Psychiatry* 1990;29:753.

Broadwin IT. A contribution to the study of truancy. *Am J Orthopsychiatry* 1932;2:253.

Cheer SM, Figgitt DP. Spotlight on fluvoxamine in anxiety disorders in children and adolescents. *CNS Drugs* 2002;16:139.

Eisenberg L. School phobia: a study in the communication of anxiety. *Am J Orthopsychiatry* 1958;114:712.

Fairbanks JM, Pine DS, Tancer NK, et al. Open fluoxetine treatment of mixed anxiety disorders in children and adolescents. *J Child Adolesc Psychopharmacol* 1997;7:17.

Jellinek MS, Kearns ME. Separation anxiety. *Pediatr Rev* 1995;16:57.

Kendall PC, Pimentel SS. On the physiological symptom constellation in youth with generalized anxiety disorder (GAD). *J Anxiety Disord* 2003;17:211.

King NJ, Ollendick TH. Treatment of childhood phobias. *J Child Psychol Psychiatry* 1997;38:389.

King NJ, Bernstein GA. School refusal in children and adolescents: a review of the past 10 years. *J Am Acad Child Adolesc Psychiatry* 2001;40:197.

Last CG, Perrin S, Hersen M, Kazdin AE. A prospective study of childhood anxiety disorders. *J Am Acad Child Adolesc Psychiatry* 1996;35:1502.

Layne AE, Bernstein GA, Egan EA, Kushner MG. Predictors of treatment response in anxious-depressed adolescents with school refusal. *J Am Acad Child Adolesc Psychiatry* 2003;42:319.

Manassis K, Mendlowitz SL, Scapillato D, et al. Group and individual cognitive-behavioral therapy for childhood anxiety disorders: a randomized trial. *J Am Acad Child Adolesc Psychiatry* 2002;41:1423.

Masi G, Mucci M, Millepiedi S. Separation anxiety disorder in children and adolescents: epidemiology, diagnosis and management. *CNS Drugs* 2001;15:93.

McClellan JM, Werry JS. Evidence-based treatments in child and adolescent psychiatry: an inventory. *J Am Acad Child Adolesc Psychiatry* 2003;42:1388.

Ollendick TH, Hirshfeld-Becker DR. The developmental psychopathology of social anxiety disorder. *Biol Psychiatry* 2002;51:44.

Pine DS. Pathophysiology of childhood anxiety disorders. *Biol Psychiatry* 1999; 46:1555.

Rapoport JL, Inoff-Germain G. Treatment of obsessive-compulsive disorder in children and adolescents. *J Child Psychol Psychiatry* 2000;41:419.

Reeve EA, Bernstein GA, Christenson GA. Clinical characteristics and psychiatric comorbidity in children with trichotillomania. *J Am Acad Child Adolesc Psychiatry* 1992;31:132.

Riddle MA, Reeve EA, Yaryura-Tobias JA, et al. Fluvoxamine for children and adolescents with obsessive-compulsive disorder: a randomized, controlled, multicenter trial. *J Am Acad Child Adolesc Psychiatry* 2001;40:222.

Russell A, Cortese B, Lorch E, et al. Localized functional neurochemical marker abnormalities in dorsolateral prefrontal cortex in pediatric obsessive-compulsive disorder. *J Child Adolesc Psychopharmacol* 2003;13(suppl 1): S31.

Schwartz CE, Wright CI, Shin LM, et al. Inhibited and uninhibited infants "grown up:" adult amygdalar response to novelty. *Science* 2003;300:1952.

Smoller JW, Rosenbaum JF, Biederman J, et al. Association of a genetic marker at the corticotropin-releasing hormone locus with behavioral inhibition. *Biol Psychiatry* 2003;54:1376.

Snider LA, Swedo SE. Post-streptococcal autoimmune disorders of the central nervous system. *Curr Opin Neurol* 2003;16:359.

Verduin TL, Kendall PC. Differential occurrence of comorbidity within childhood anxiety disorders. *J Clin Child Adolesc Psychol* 2003;32:290.

CHAPTER 104 ■ DEPRESSION IN CHILDHOOD AND ADOLESCENCE

JAMES C. HARRIS

Depression is a pervasive emotional disorder manifested by negative mood, an inability to obtain pleasure in everyday activities, poor concentration, cognitive complaints of self-blame and worthlessness, reduced personal motivation, and physiologic changes in sleep and appetite. As a symptom or syndrome, depression is not synonymous with sadness or unhappiness. The mood is referred to as *dysphoric* and is one of despair. Irritability, deterioration in school performance, difficulty in peer relationships, and problems in conduct may be the presenting symptoms, which were sometimes referred to in the past as *masked depression*. Without early recognition and effective treatment, depressive episodes can last for months and lead to a continuing deterioration in school performance and already poor peer and family relationships. Adolescent suicide as a consequence of depression is an increasingly significant problem.

Because of children's level of psychological development and the lack of universally accepted diagnostic criteria for depression in children, whether the preadolescent child can be depressed had been a subject of debate. In adolescence, depression often had been ignored and the symptoms attributed to adolescent turmoil. However, it is clear that diagnostic criteria originally developed for use with adults can be used to make the diagnosis in children and adolescents.

Although the same diagnostic criteria for a depressive episode are used for adults and children, as listed in Box 104.1, questions are asked of children based on their developmental level, and parent reports also are used in the diagnosis of children. This approach has led to the recognition of major depressive disorder in children and adolescents. However, the diagnostic lower limit for other forms of depressive subtypes is not established as clearly.

A distinction must be made between the more common reports of sadness seen in pediatric practice, which may be associated with somatic symptoms, unhappiness, bereavement, or demoralization, and a true major depressive disorder (i.e., a constellation of symptoms with a characteristic prognosis). How the child's developmental level affects his presentation is ascertained through structured and semistructured interviews with the child and the parents, self-reports, and self-esteem

---

BOX 104.1   Diagnostic Criteria for Major Depressive Episode

A. Five (or more) of the following symptoms have been present during the same 2-week period and represent a change from previous functioning; at least one of the symptoms is either (1) depressed mood or (2) loss of interest or pleasure. Note: Symptoms that are clearly due to a general medical condition or mood-incongruent delusions or hallucinations should not be included.
1. Depressed mood most of the day, nearly every day, as indicated by either subjective report (e.g., feels sad or empty) or observation made by others (e.g., appears tearful). Note: In children and adolescents, can be irritable mood.
2. Markedly diminished interest or pleasure in all, or almost all, activities most of the day, nearly every day (as indicated by either subjective account or observation made by others).
3. Significant weight loss when not dieting or weight gain (e.g., a change of more than 5% of body weight in a month), or decrease or increase in appetite nearly every day. Note: In children, consider failure to make expected weight gains.
4. Insomnia or hypersomnia nearly every day.
5. Psychomotor agitation or retardation nearly every day (observable by others, not merely subjective feelings of restlessness or being slowed down).
6. Fatigue or loss of energy nearly every day.
7. Feelings of worthlessness or excessive or inappropriate guilt (which may be delusional) nearly every day (not merely self-reproach or guilt about being sick).

8. Diminished ability to think or concentrate, or indecisiveness, nearly every day (either by subjective account or as observed by others).
9. Recurrent thoughts of death (not just fear of dying), recurrent suicidal ideation without a specific plan, or a suicide attempt or a specific plan for committing suicide.
B. The symptoms do not meet criteria for a mixed episode (manic episode and depressive episode).
C. The symptoms cause clinically significant distress or impairment in social, occupational, or other important areas of functioning.
D. The symptoms are not due to the direct physiologic effects of a substance (e.g., a drug of abuse, a medication) or a general medical condition (e.g., hypothyroidism).
E. The symptoms are not better accounted for by bereavement (i.e., after the loss of a loved one); the symptoms persist for longer than 2 months or are characterized by marked functional impairment, morbid preoccupation with worthlessness, suicidal ideation, psychotic symptoms, or psychomotor retardation.

Reprinted with permission from American Psychiatric Association. *Diagnostic and statistical manual of mental disorders*, 4th ed. Text revision. Washington, DC: American Psychiatric Association, 2000.

---

inventories. Interview information from both child and parents is essential to make a diagnosis.

EPIDEMIOLOGY

The earliest indication of depressive symptomatology can appear in a severely neglected infant. This nonorganic failure to thrive may represent a "reactive attachment disorder of infancy and early childhood" and is the result of a dysfunctional parent–child relationship. Information on prevalence is poorly documented, although failure to thrive with no specific etiology has been reported in up to 9% of infants in a rural area. For the preschool child, unhappy mood was reported in 4% to 8% of 3-year-old children in a behavioral survey; girls were affected more frequently than boys.

More than 40% of adolescents interviewed by a psychiatrist reported complaints of misery and sadness. Furthermore, 20% had feelings of self-depreciation, and 7% to 8% had suicidal thoughts. In prepuberty, depressive feelings are much less common. Symptoms were equally divided between boys and girls in prepuberty, but with the onset of puberty, the prevalence increased in girls. In one study, major depressive disorder was found to be rare in 10- to 11-year-old children, with a rate of 3 per 2,000. When the same group was assessed 4 years later, however, the rate had increased threefold, suggesting a potential role of physiologic changes at puberty in the onset of major depression.

Other authors have identified a prevalence of 1.8% of major depressive illness and a 2.5% prevalence of dysthymic disorder (discussed later in this chapter) in an epidemiologic population

survey of 9-year-old children. In adolescence, those authors found a prevalence of 4.7% of major depression and 3.3% of dysthymic disorder, which is similar to the adult prevalence. A review of several studies suggested a rate of 3% to 8% overall in children and adolescents.

Prevalence rates are substantially higher in populations referred to pediatric hospitals or to child psychiatric inpatient and outpatient units. Consecutive admissions on a pediatric ward showed a 7% prevalence of depressive disorder and 38% prevalence of dysphoric moods in children 7 to 12 years old. A psychiatric outpatient study showed that one in nine prepubertal and one in four postpubertal young people seen for evaluation had depressive symptoms. Before puberty, symptoms were twice as frequent in boys, but after puberty, they were twice as frequent in girls.

During the 1980s and 1990s, depression in children was recognized with greater frequency; the greatest prevalence was found in the postpubertal years. Planning based on epidemiologic studies requires agreement on diagnostic criteria for both major depression and other depressive disorders. Achieving agreement is complicated by the recognition of subtypes of depression. Efforts are ongoing to validate assessment criteria and find biologic markers that will improve recognition.

CLINICAL MANIFESTATIONS AND COMPLICATIONS

Depression presents as a biopsychosocial illness. It is a disorder of mood, with symptoms related to neuroendocrine and autonomic dysfunction, along with specific cognitive problems in self-perception. Problems in falling asleep and remaining asleep, anorexia and weight loss, abdominal pain, chest pain, headache, and constipation are associated somatic symptoms. Depression in the parent or child may lead to increased office visits and increased hospitalization for the diagnostic evaluations of ill-defined complaints. How the child presents is influenced by the parent–child relationship; in making the diagnosis, the words that the child has learned to use to describe emotional states must be considered. If the child does not recognize the bodily experience of his or her feelings, his or her vague complaints of not feeling good may be misunderstood. An emotionally healthy child is active, feels good, and has fun in his or her activities.

The child also may have learned to use physical complaints to get attention when experiencing depressed feelings in a household in which emotional expression is discouraged, or the child may have modeled his or her symptoms on a parent's complaints. These patterns may continue in adulthood, so they are best dealt with directly in childhood. Somatic symptoms and vague complaints may be the child's way of expressing the dysphoric feelings associated with grief and minor or major depression.

Complaints of sleep and eating problems are characteristic of depression. In addition, studies of hospitalized children have found headache, fatigue, muscle pain, recurrent vomiting, and abdominal pain to be physical symptoms associated with depression; gastrointestinal symptoms were found to be the most characteristic. Separation anxiety symptoms often accompany depressive symptoms and are classically associated with physical complaints on school mornings. Abdominal pain often is associated with separation anxiety, which may accompany depression. Chest pain also is associated with depression. In one study, 13 of 100 children seen in a cardiac clinic had depressive symptoms; their chest pain had no associated cardiac diagnosis in this population.

Children with severe burns, trauma, or chronic illness are another group at risk for depressive symptoms. Restricted physical activity, sensory isolation, repeated treatment intervention, and sudden and severe loss of health may be factors in their apathy, regression, and withdrawal. Children with chronic handicaps also may be symptomatic. Twenty of 100 handicapped children reporting for orthopedic hospitalization had depressive symptoms.

Although the focus is generally on the child's complaint, attention also must be paid to the parents' problems. In one study, children with recurrent abdominal pain were not different from a control group in their degree of depressive symptomatology; however, 25% of the mothers were mildly to moderately depressed.

DIAGNOSIS

Ordinarily, the parents request help for their distressed or dysfunctional child. Depression can present as a symptom, syndrome, or disorder. As a symptom, it is the expected emotional response to stressful situations; as a syndrome or disorder, it represents an abnormally persistent dysphoric mood. It is essential to differentiate between transient mood changes, which may be normal reactions to stressors, and the despair, irritability, and loss of interest and pleasure that signify depression.

Depression involves not only dysphoria but also changes in self-perception. Those aspects of depression that involve self-blame and worthlessness become evident as the child matures. Thoughts of guilt, helplessness, and hopelessness about the future follow a developmental course, so diagnostic criteria for depression may need to be modified for younger children and children who are mentally retarded. At 4 or 5 years, children are aware of others being proud or ashamed of them, but it is not

until approximately age 8 that they talk meaningfully about being proud or ashamed of themselves. By age 5 or 6 years, the child begins to distinguish accidental from intentional behavior, although earlier in life, bad outcomes are perceived as unintended. Similarly, 5- to 7-year-old children perceive that sadness comes from external events rather than internal feeling states. By approximately age 10 years, the child understands that a personal problem involves psychological distress as well as external stressors. Self-awareness with increased self-consciousness, as well as anxiety about the future, develops in adolescence.

Age and sex are important factors in evaluation. In younger children, assessment is more difficult because of their difficulty in describing their emotions. Younger children do not divorce mood from the context of their experience. Even in adolescence, however, parents and teachers often fail to recognize depression although young people report it. An interview with both the child and parents is essential.

From a diagnostic perspective, the current classification of psychiatric diagnoses lists several emotional disturbances of increasing severity. These range from uncomplicated bereavement and adjustment reaction with depressed or anxious mood to dysthymic disorder and major depression. An adjustment disorder with depressive symptoms following either acute or chronic stress is the most common diagnosis; the next most common is dysthymic disorder. In dysthymic disorder, symptoms have less intensity, are of shorter duration, and occur intermittently, in contrast to a major depressive disorder, which is accompanied by more severe physical symptoms, alterations in perception, and cognitive status. A description of symptom characteristics of a major depressive disorder follows.

Depressed Mood

Depressed mood can be expressed both verbally and nonverbally. Because young children vary in their ability to talk about their depressive symptoms, other informants are needed. For preschool children, teacher and parent reports are particularly important. Irritability and changes in activity, perhaps as a reaction to their dysphoric mood, are seen in preschool children. For these younger children, symptoms vary more with the environmental setting than they do in older children. A parent report helps to distinguish changes in behavior but does not necessarily include the child's specific concerns. The child must be asked specifically about how he feels. The first step is to establish what words the child uses to describe the bad feeling inside (e.g., down, bored, blue, empty, real sad). Nonverbally, a sad expression with downcast eyes and sagging lips is easily recognized; however, changes in facial expression often are more subtle. Adolescents can appropriately label feelings, but they may be guarded in talking about them. They may distort their reports, perhaps because they lack the adult sense of time, and it seems to them that these feelings will never go away. Teenagers may try to hide their feelings from themselves and from adults.

Loss of Interest and Pleasure

A characteristic of depression in children is the loss of a sense of pleasure or fun. The diagnosis of depression requires either this loss of interest or a persistent dysphoric mood. When children have difficulty using words to describe their mood, the demonstration of a loss of pleasure in their usual activities may suffice to make the diagnosis. For example, the child may have friends, but loses interest in playing with them or stares at television but does not watch it and cannot remember or follow the story line. Typical adolescent boredom and apathy must be distinguished from a genuine loss of pleasure in activities. Depression also may occur in teenagers with intellectual disability. For example, a depressed, moderately intellectually disabled young woman with Down syndrome manifested her depression by hiding in a closet at school, refusing to eat, and stopping her regular play with a coloring book after coming home from school.

Preoccupation with Death

A depressed child may have preoccupations about death and persistently talk about the loss of a pet, grandparent, or others who have died. Although the child's concerns may originate in real events, these may be exaggerated in fantasy or spontaneously and unexpectedly be revived.

Suicide, a topic children often know about from the media, should be directly addressed in every depressed child. It does not harm the child to ask about it, but rather offers an opportunity to discuss real concerns. Like adults, children and adolescents who deny their suicidal thoughts are at greater risk for impulsive self-injury. Although completed suicide is uncommon in preadolescents, children in this age group think about suicide and may make plans to carry it out. In adolescence, when suicide is more common, most completed suicides are associated with depression. Suicide attempts are more frequent than completed suicides and often follow arguments with parents or peers in homes where a family history of chronic interpersonal problems exists.

Poor Self-Esteem

Low self-esteem may be difficult to explore in the interview, particularly in younger children. Between the ages of 8 and 10 years, however, the self-concept becomes more firmly established, making the interview more reliable. Younger children can talk about being liked by others, their appearance, and what they would want to have changed in their lives or about themselves. Children may be particularly sensitive about self-concept and refer to themselves as "stupid;" they may reluctantly report derogatory names they are called by others. Their shifts in mood, irritability, and withdrawal adversely affect interpersonal relationships and may result in further reductions in self-approval. Alternatively, to compensate for poor self-image, older children and adolescents may brag unconvincingly about their presumed accomplishments.

Excessive Guilt

Although children or adolescents may experience an overwhelming sense of guilt, it may be difficult to get reliable reports from them. The sensitive parent will say that the child assumes blame unnecessarily or feels overly responsible when things go wrong. A child younger than 8 years of age may not be able to describe guilty feelings or might deny them in an effort to make a good impression. However, guilt may be demonstrated indirectly through behavior (e.g., when a punishment is deliberately sought, or toys are given away or destroyed because the child feels they are undeserved).

Poor Concentration and School Failure

An abrupt change in school performance in a child who was doing well previously may herald the onset of depression. Unlike the learning-disabled child, previous school work would have been at least adequate. Performance may vary in different school subjects because of diurnal mood variability during the day, or may be worse in winter in the occasional child with a seasonal affective disorder. Both lack of interest and diminished ability to concentrate contribute to decreased performance. Unlike the hyperactive child, who is distracted by the environment, the depressed child usually is distracted by his internal emotional state. The teenager may continue to work hard for special teachers, but derives little pleasure from learning and may spend considerable time in completing tasks to the detriment of participation in social activities.

Social Withdrawal

Withdrawal from others commonly occurs with the onset of depression, but unlike the child with a conduct disorder, the depressed child ordinarily has previously demonstrated the capacity to make friends and socialize with them. The child may have talked about having been popular before but no longer does so, now saying that no one likes him or her; the child no longer socializes with peers. The child may set himself or herself up to be rejected by being unavailable or may impose rules on others that they cannot meet. Chronically depressed children require considerable help with reestablishing peer relations as their depression improves.

Altered Psychomotor Activity

Psychomotor retardation is demonstrated by slowness in walking, speaking, eating, and general movement. Questions may be answered slowly and in short phrases with little imaginative elaboration. A depressed hospitalized child may remain relatively immobile during the day. When encouraged to go to the activity room, he or she may be reluctant to go and may require considerable encouragement. On the other hand, the anxiety that frequently accompanies depression in children and adolescents may be demonstrated in increased psychomotor activity. This may be manifested as an agitated depression, with excessive motor activity, or as restlessness.

Fatigue

Increased fatigue as the day progresses is a frequent complaint of both children and parents. In contrast to previous exuberance, the child or adolescent may be too tired to go out with others or participate in family outings that he or she previously enjoyed. The parent may say the child is "just lying around," and the child may want to take afternoon naps.

Sleep Disturbances and Weight Loss

Difficulty falling asleep is the most common sleep complaint, but intermittent nighttime waking and early morning awakening also occur. The parent often is unaware of these symptoms and assumes that the child is sleeping. The child must be asked directly about sleep problems, because often problems are not reported spontaneously.

Weight loss is so characteristic of depression that this diagnosis should always be considered when unexplained weight loss occurs. In one study, depressed children were found to be 10 pounds lighter than a matched comparison group. Children and adolescents ordinarily do not complain about weight loss or changes in appetite. This symptom is often a sensitive topic with parents who have made considerable efforts to get the child to eat. Food refusal or ambivalence about eating is common in children in the hospital setting.

Irritability, Crying without Reason, and Separation Anxiety

Irritability is commonly described by teachers and parents in depressed children and has been found at follow-up in preschool children. It may be a greater concern to adults than the depressed mood. Symptoms of irritability are best elicited from the teacher and parent rather than from the child. Crying for no reason or an unexpected urge to cry is a characteristic more often reported by parents than by children. Separation anxiety may be enhanced, particularly in the younger child.

DIAGNOSTIC CRITERIA FOR DEPRESSIVE DISORDERS

To diagnose a major depressive disorder, the dysphoric mood or loss of interest or pleasure must have lasted at least 2 weeks. Diagnostic criteria for a major depressive episode are shown in Box 104.1.

Dysthymic Disorder

A chronic disturbance of mood or loss of interest or pleasure is present in dysthymic disorder, it but is not as severe or as long in duration as in a major depression. For children and adolescents, the diagnosis requires that symptoms must be present for at least 1 year. The change in mood may be relatively persistent or intermittent, and it may be separated by periods of time when normal mood and interest or pleasure in routine activities last for several weeks. Anxiety disorders and conduct disorders may be present concurrently.

Demoralization

Loss of self-confidence may result from frustration in being unable to accomplish developmental tasks, from inability to meet others' expectations, or as a consequence of negative feedback, negligence, or abuse. Loss of self-confidence is seen in both the learning-disabled and the behaviorally disordered child. These problems in self-esteem may respond to support in the mastery of developmentally appropriate tasks. Persistent failure in school or interpersonal relations may lead from demoralization to an adjustment disorder.

Adjustment Disorder with Depressed Mood

In the past, the most frequently used diagnosis in child psychiatry was adjustment reaction. The term *adjustment disorder* now is used, and specific symptoms are designated. In adjustment disorder, either psychological suffering and distress or an impairment in social functioning must be demonstrated. For example, a child with adjustment disorder might present with depressed mood, anxiety, or a conduct problem. A specific stressor is identifiable as leading to the symptoms, and the usual course is full recovery within 6 months after the removal of the stressor. Emotional or behavioral symptoms in response to an identifiable stressor occur within 3 months of the onset of the stressor. Illness in the family, school changes, and parental separation are common stressors. An adjustment disorder with depressed mood frequently is accompanied by demoralization or loss in personal motivation; however, the symptoms are not of the same magnitude as a major depressive disorder or dysthymic disorder. Symptoms are of short duration and are responsive to environmental changes.

Grief Response

Grief is a normal and expected consequence of personal loss. Immediate grief reactions are milder and of shorter duration in young children than in adolescents or adults. This is perhaps related to their developmental inability to conceptualize past relationships or view death as permanent. After a loss, protest, searching, restlessness, and despair follow a rapid course in the younger child. The child experiences loss at his or her current level of maturation, but may have to deal with the loss again when he or she is older and can reflect on the personal meaning of past experiences in anticipating the future.

Unlike a depressive disorder, grief following bereavement is an adaptive process. After the death of a loved one, the child may strategically withdraw until he or she can cope with or master life events. The intense grief response typically resolves during the first 2 to 3 months following the loss. For example, a 5-year-old boy lost his parents in an automobile accident and went to live with his uncle and aunt. He was withdrawn and initially preoccupied, not talking to adults about the accident and speaking only to his cousins. His readjustment began gradually after he decided in church one Sunday that he now had two sets of parents watching over him, his real parents in heaven and his uncle and aunt in his new home.

The death of a parent may result in increased vulnerability to later depression, particularly when nurturing aftercare is not forthcoming after the loss. Weller notes that 4% of children lose a parent by age 15 years. Unresolved bereavement may place the child at an increased risk for developing psychiatric disorders later in childhood or in adult life. Behavior problems may occur when feelings of grief are not fully expressed and experienced. Although bereaved children usually do cope and make the necessary major readjustments to develop normally, complicated bereavement may occur and may be associated with a depressive syndrome.

To differentiate a normal grief response from a major depressive disorder, the physician should evaluate whether guilt extends beyond actions that were taken or not taken by the surviving person at the time of the loss, persistent thoughts of death, and preoccupation about being unworthy. Siblings may experience survival guilt that may be enhanced if sibling rivalry was present.

In a controlled follow-up study by Black of 105 children and adolescents who lost one parent, dysphoria (sadness, crying, and irritability), falling school performance, and social withdrawal were significantly increased in both genders at a 13-month follow-up visit. Younger children demonstrated temper tantrums, bed-wetting (particularly in girls), and loss of interest in their usual activities. A chronic mood disturbance was noted in 8.5% of the older children and adolescents, but was seen most often in the older girls. The most severe depressive symptoms were found in the postpubertal age group, in which changes in school performance were particularly noteworthy.

A major contributing factor in the child or adolescent's outcome is the surviving parent's adjustment to the loss. A poor outcome may relate to difficulty in the expression of grief, developmental factors associated with understanding the loss, and the surviving parent's difficulty in allowing the child to mourn and to share his own grief. Bereavement or other life events may precipitate depression in some vulnerable individuals, but most children do adapt.

RISK FACTORS

The risk of having a family member affected with mood disorder is 50% for prepubertal children with a major depressive disorder, 35% for adolescents, and 18% to 30% for adults.

Affected children or adolescents are more likely to have a positive family history of depression than adults. Alcoholism and antisocial personality also occur more often in the family members of children with major affective disorders.

Children who are at higher risk of developing a depressive disorder may include those suffering from parental deprivation by separation or death before age 11 years, neglect, abuse, or parental physical or mental illness.

The most common risk factor is loss: of a person, an opportunity, hope about the future, or of one's potential. Despite their illness, most children with chronic illnesses do not become depressed. Temperament, acceptance by parents and others, and capacity to adapt all play a role in this adjustment. The loss of a parent is a major risk factor that may be modified by the substitution of another caregiver; the loss of the same-gender parent seems to be of special importance. The learned helplessness model of depression (Seligman) has been suggested to account for symptoms following unusual stress.

Genetic transmission, social transmission through identification with a depressed parent (in response to altered interpersonal relationships), or both increases the risk for the diagnosis. In a child younger than 18 years with an affected parent, the risk is double that of someone having no parent with affective disorder; the risk increases fourfold if both parents are affected. An increased risk exists in monozygotic over dizygotic twins. Twin studies also suggest a concordance of 76% in monozygotic twins raised together, 67% for those raised apart, and 19% for dizygotic twins.

Ongoing studies of depression diagnosed in adolescence indicate continuity into adulthood. However, longitudinal studies have not yet clarified the full implications of childhood onset. We do not know if childhood and adult forms of depression require different approaches as, for example, may be the case in adult-onset when compared with juvenile-onset diabetes. Because of stronger family loading for the more severe form of depression, childhood onset is most likely related to the genetic form of the disorder.

The type of depressive disorder in the parent is important as well. Major depressive disorder or bipolar disorder (manic-depressive) in a parent has different consequences on a child's behavior. The child must deal with irritability, inconsistency, and erratic affection in a parent with bipolar disorder. Preschool children with a parent who is diagnosed with bipolar disorder have been shown to have more difficulty regulating emotions, greater reactivity to stress, and difficulty in sharing and socializing. On the other hand, if the parent has a major depressive disorder, children may show an increased tendency to suppress emotions and to be less persistent in their play with others.

Biologic Factors

Biologic markers for depression in children and adolescents are being investigated, and such research includes neuroendocrine studies, biochemical investigations, and sleep studies. Studies showing the failure of a growth hormone response to insulin in psychosocial dwarfism have been extended to the study of major depressive disorder in prepubertal children. Growth hormone hyporesponsivity to insulin-induced hypoglycemia and increased growth hormone release during slow-wave (delta) sleep have been reported in children. In the older adolescent, the adult biologic response to depression, exhibiting a reduction in growth hormone release during sleep, has been reported.

Although depressed children have multiple sleep complaints, including difficulty falling asleep and episodes of waking during the night, none of these sleep changes has been demonstrated to be characteristic of prepubertal depression in the sleep laboratory. Sleep changes in adult depression include decreased sleep efficiency, decreased deep (delta) sleep, early onset of dream sleep [shortened rapid eye movement (REM) latency], increased REM density in dream sleep, and abnormal distribution of REM sleep during the night. The failure to demonstrate these abnormalities in children may relate to maturational changes in both slow-wave and REM sleep with age. Some sleep continuity disturbance related to depression becomes evident on entry into adolescence, but REM latency becomes abnormal only in late adolescence. Future studies of sleep in children and adolescents, using more sensitive computerized methods, may help to clarify possible sleep abnormalities.

Biologic markers may exist for major depressive disorder in prepuberty and adolescence, but they have not been convincingly demonstrated. Increased family prevalence and the growth hormone studies are most similar to adult findings. Sleep electroencephalographic studies and abnormality in cortisol secretion have not been demonstrated consistently, which could relate to the degree of biologic maturation. More sensitive methods to elucidate age-related changes in biologic markers are needed.

TREATMENT

Depression may have no specific identifiable single cause: environmental, familial, and physical factors all contribute. Therefore, comprehensive treatment requires multiple therapeutic modalities. Preventive approaches include anticipatory guidance before considering hospitalization and dealing with stressful life crises, such as an impending death in the family. When the stress already has occurred, preventive intervention programs using individual and family approaches to help deal with the effect of the loss have the goal of preventing complications and the progression to a depressive disorder. The convening of a support group is of considerable importance at the time of bereavement. One investigation found that a preventive intervention program of three to six child-oriented bereavement counseling sessions led to fewer behavioral problems, fewer sleep problems, and less depressed mood in children at a 1-year follow-up. Children who received the intervention talked more about the deceased parent. Attending the funeral of the deceased also resulted in improvement in the child's behavior.

Early detection and referral for treatment of suspected cases of depression in children and adolescents is important. When a case is diagnosed, reducing disability and helping the child to achieve maximal function are the primary goals. An educational aspect to treatment involves working with family members. Also, an interpersonal treatment helps the child to deal with the consequences of the depressive illness on his interpersonal relationships with others. Loss of peer relations and secondary family problems are common complications. The prevention or amelioration of poor performance at school, poor social skills, social withdrawal, somatic concerns, and suicide are all targets for intervention and rehabilitation. Early diagnosis may prevent unnecessary medical evaluations. Psychotherapeutic modalities include crisis management, parental counseling, and individual, group, or family therapy.

In the major depressive disorder in which weight loss, sleep disturbance, and cognitive changes are severe, pharmacotherapy with antidepressants frequently is used; definitive studies on the effectiveness of these drugs are now in progress. Selective serotonin reuptake inhibitors (SSRIs), tricyclic antidepressants, and antidepressants with effects on more than one neurotransmitter system, such as venlafaxine, are available. Because a risk of self-poisoning exists, knowledge of drug overdose toxicity, especially for the tricyclic antidepressant group of medications, is essential. A baseline electrocardiogram provides the most sensitive index for assessing later tricyclic toxicity.

Antidepressant dosage should not be increased if the resting heart rate exceeds 130 beats per minute or the PR interval is greater than 0.21 ms, QRS interval is greater than 130% of baseline, systolic blood pressure is greater than 145 mm Hg, or diastolic blood pressure is greater than 95 mm Hg. Tricyclic antidepressants should not be used in children with cardiac conduction defects. Because oral dosage is not well correlated with blood level, plasma levels, when available, must be routinely measured at least 8 hours after a dose. Overall, the SSRIs have been shown to be more effective in children and adolescents than are tricyclic antidepressants, and the SSRIs have a better safety profile. Fluoxetine has been approved by the U.S. Food and Drug Administration (FDA) as safe and effective for the treatment of major depression in children. Wagner et al. reported a pooled analysis of two multicenter randomized trials of depressed 6- to 17-year-olds demonstrating that sertraline is effective and well tolerated. However, the placebo response rate is high in drug treatment trials in youth, suggesting that children are more responsive to nonspecific support than are adults.

An outpatient treatment study by Olson et al. found that more than half (56.9%) of depressed youth were prescribed antidepressant medications. The use of antidepressants has led to concern about risks of abuse, and particularly the relationship of medication use and suicide. The risk for suicide is a major concern in depression, so careful monitoring for suicidal ideation is essential. This monitoring should occur in face to face office visits that ask about suicidal thoughts, irritability, and agitation that may occur after beginning medication, and have been associated with suicidal ideation. However, as Olson et al. found in a community epidemiologic study, appropriate antidepressant treatment may decrease the rate of suicide. These authors reported that a 1% increase in adolescent use of antidepressants was associated with a decrease of 0.23 suicide per 100,000 adolescents per year in youth aged 15 to 19 years.

The most convincing argument for pharmacotherapy is the chronicity and long duration of a major depressive disorder and the depth and extent of psychosocial impairment. Still, pharmacotherapy alone does not ameliorate interpersonal problems with parents and peers; psychotherapy is indicated for these symptoms. A parent's depressive disorder must be considered and recognized, because the parent's symptoms may influence personality development and increase the likelihood of symptom expression in the child.

PROGNOSIS

In one study of a high-risk group of children and adolescents with depressive symptoms, the average duration of a major depressive disorder was 7.5 months. Forty percent of the group went into remission within 6 months, and 90% remitted in 18 months. The younger children had longer episodes than did older ones. Within 5 years of the first episode, the risk of a second episode was 70%. The risk of recurrence of major depressive disorder was greater when an underlying dysthymic disorder was present. The average duration for dysthymic disorder was 3 years, but 6.5 years was the duration of symptoms from diagnosis to recovery for 90% of this group, some of whom later developed major depressive disorder. Adjustment disorder with depressive mood was the most benign of the depressive disorders, usually occurring alone or with an anxiety-related disorder. The average case lasted 5.5 months, and 90% recovery was found within 9 months. None of the children in this group developed major depressive disorders. Prognosis has not been adequately evaluated in children who come from more organized and supportive psychosocial settings.

Although additional studies are critical to characterize further the natural history and to demonstrate the appropriate treatment of depressive disorders in children and adolescents, the evidence to date demonstrates that current diagnostic criteria for major depressive disorder can be meaningfully applied to children and adolescents. Furthermore, depressive disorders diagnosed using these criteria are not transient, but may be acute or chronic conditions. Concurrent anxiety symptoms and conduct problems often are present and may complicate the recognition of the depressive symptomatology. Efforts are under way to determine more effective treatments directed at more rapid recovery and prevention of future episodes. The unmet needs of children and adolescents with depression or bipolar disorder require continuous surveillance, and when diagnosed, evidence-based treatment.

Suggested Readings

Baker KE, Sedney MA, Gross E. Psychologicalal tasks for bereaved children. *Am J Orthopsychiatry* 1992;62:105.

Birmaher B, Ryan ND, Williamson DE, et al. Childhood and adolescent depression: a review of the past 10 years. Part I. *J Am Acad Child Adolesc Psychiatry* 1996;35:1427.

Brent DA, Holder D, Kolko D, et al. A clinical psychotherapy trial for adolescent depression comparing cognitive, family, and supportive therapy. *Arch Gen Psychiatry* 1997;54:877.

Brent DA, Birmaher B. Clinical practice. Adolescent depression. *N Engl J Med* 2002;347:667.

Coyle JT, Pine DS, Charney DS, et al. Depression and bipolar support alliance consensus statement on the unmet needs in diagnosis and treatment of mood disorders in children and adolescents. *J Am Acad Child Adolesc Psychiatry* 2003;42:1494.

Elliott GR, Smiga S. Depression in the child and adolescent. *Pediatr Clin North Am* 2003;50:1093.

Hodges K, Kline JJ, Barbero G, Flanery R. Depressive symptoms in children with recurrent abdominal pain and in their families. *J Pediatr* 1985;107:622.

Kashani JH, Lababidi Z, Jones RJ. Depression in children and adolescents with cardiovascular symptomatology: the significance of chest pain. *J Am Acad Child Psychiatry* 1982;21:187.

Kovacs M, Obrosky DS, Sherrill J. Developmental changes in the phenomenology of depression in girls compared to boys from childhood onward. *J Affect Disord* 2003;74:33.

Nobile M, Cataldo GM, Marino C, Molteni M. Diagnosis and treatment of dysthymia in children and adolescents. *CNS Drugs* 2003;17:927.

Olfson M, Gameroff MJ, Marcus SC, Waslick BD. Outpatient treatment of child and adolescent depression in the United States. *Arch Gen Psychiatry* 2003;60:1236.

Olfson M, Shaffer D, Marcus SC, Greenberg T. Relationship between antidepressant medication treatment and suicide in adolescents. *Arch Gen Psychiatry* 2003;60:978.

Puig-Antich J, Lukens E, Davies M, et al. Psychosocial functioning in prepubertal major depressive disorders. *Arch Gen Psychiatry* 1985;42:511.

Varley CK. Psychopharmacological treatment of major depressive disorder in children and adolescents. *JAMA* 2003;290(8):1091.

Wagner KD, Ambrosini P, Rynn M, et al. Sertraline Pediatric Depression Study Group. Efficacy of sertraline in the treatment of children and adolescents with major depressive disorder: two randomized controlled trials. *JAMA* 2003;290:1033.

Weller EB, Weller RA, Benton T, Wiltsie Pugh, JJ. Grief. In: Lewis M, ed. *Child and adolescent psychiatry: a comprehensive textbook,* 3rd ed. Philadelphia: Lippincott Williams & Wilkins, 2002:470.

Wilens TE, Biederman J, Baldessarini RJ, et al. Cardiovascular effects of therapeutic doses of tricyclic antidepressants in children and adolescents. *J Am Acad Child Adolesc Psychiatry* 1996;35:1491.

Weiss B, Garber J. Developmental differences in the phenomenology of depression. *Dev Psychopathol* 2003;15:403.

CHAPTER 105 ■ SUICIDE

JAMES C. HARRIS

Suicide and parasuicide (suicide attempt) are common among adolescents and common enough among preadolescents to be an important concern. In a child psychiatry clinic, 10% of referrals are made for this reason, and large numbers of adolescents are admitted to inpatient services because of suicide attempts. Suicide was the third leading cause of death in 10- to 14-year-olds and 15- to 19-year-olds in 2000, exceeded only by motor vehicle injuries and homicide. Particularly important is the increase in completed suicides, which has tripled since the 1950s. Each completed suicide represents 30 to 40 (or more) attempted suicides, depending on the age group. In preadolescents, suicide might be overlooked as the cause of death when deaths are recorded as accidental.

EPIDEMIOLOGY

Childhood suicide is described as a self-inflicted death occurring before the fifteenth birthday. It is the only psychiatric condition that is subject to documentation by age, gender, and method in all developed countries. At all ages, the rate in whites is greater than that in nonwhites. In the male population, completed suicides are more common than in the female population, although attempts are more common in the female population. The suicide mortality rate (completed suicide) in 10- to 14-year-olds in 2000 was 1.5 per 100,000; the mortality rate in the 15- to 19-year-old age group was 8.2 per 100,000. Some 4% of high school students have made a suicide attempt in the last year, and 8% have attempted suicide in their lifetime. Estimates hold that only one in eight suicide attempts comes to medical attention.

Apparently, suicide is related to maturation, and younger children may be protected, possibly because planning the event may require abstract reasoning, formulation of a plan, and the development of a poor self-concept. Children attempting suicide also must be able to understand the severity of the situation and understand the means to use to complete the act. The rarity of suicide before puberty also may be lower because two risk factors, depressive disorder and substance abuse, are not common among younger children. Suicide may not be reported fully because of possible stigma, and such underreporting leads to difficulty in interpreting accident statistics that may include suicide in children. For example, if a child deliberately runs into the street, he may do so with suicidal intent. Clarifying the specific means used for suicide is important.

Some have suggested that the increase in completed suicide in the United States for the 15- to 19-year-old group may be explained by the availability of firearms. The most common means for completed suicide is a firearm, followed in descending order of incidence by hanging or suffocation, self-poisoning, and the use of gas. In England, government control of gas in the home led to a significant reduction in suicide, and the control of availability of firearms often has been suggested to bring about a similar effect in the United States.

Suicide attempts occur three times more often in girls than in boys during the adolescent years. However, young men are five times more likely to die by suicide. Young men often use firearms, jump from heights, or inhale carbon monoxide, whereas young women more often use self-poisoning. Often, the word *overdose* is used in emergency room settings to describe such behavior, but the more appropriate designation is *self-poisoning*.

ETIOLOGY

Cognitive maturation is a factor in successful suicide. Children who have higher intellectual ability and higher standards of living may be more prone to deal with failure by blaming themselves. Pressure to admit antisocial behavior after a disciplinary crisis and other interpersonal disagreements may be followed by suicide attempts in vulnerable adolescents. The occurrence of psychiatric illness in families, particularly depression in siblings or parents, is another important risk factor. The best predictor of a suicide attempt is a prior attempt; previous parasuicide has been noted to be as high as 40% in completed suicides. Suicide may occur in the context of psychiatric illness and may be the result of internal conflict. It varies in frequency and intensity with age and often is related to interpersonal difficulties with parents and teachers.

An important etiology of suicide in adolescents is affective disorder, major depression, or bipolar disorder. This condition may be primary, as a response to severe stress, or it may be secondary to another preexisting illness. It is the most significant diagnosis related to completed suicide, and increased risk occurs during the depressed phase or episode. When those with affective disorders are in remission from their depression, the risk of suicide is not increased statistically. The greatest risk occurs during the first year after the diagnosis of the depression.

Two other conditions are associated with completed suicide: drug abuse (particularly alcoholism) and schizophrenia. Suicide associated with schizophrenia is less common than that associated with an affective disorder. For a person with schizophrenia, the history of a previous attempt, the presence of an associated depressive syndrome, or self-destructive hallucinations increase the risk.

In contrast to completed suicide, attempted suicide is more common in individuals who have a hysterical personality style or antisocial personality traits. These personality traits, complicated by the use of drugs, increase the risk for an attempt. An additional risk factor is a family history of suicide. This may be related to the modeling that can occur from knowing that another family member has completed suicide. Family genetic studies provide evidence for familial transmission in suicide; this is confirmed in twin and adoption studies. At a molecular level, serotonin seems to be one of the key neurotransmitters implicated in suicidal behavior. Therefore, genes coding for proteins involved in serotonergic neurotransmission have been extensively studied in case-control association studies on suicide.

CLINICAL MANIFESTATIONS AND COMPLICATIONS

Information about the clinical picture of completed suicide is gathered by techniques termed the *psychological autopsy*, a method initially developed for use with adults but more recently applied to adolescents. Interviews are conducted with those who knew the individual who has committed suicide. The completed-suicide population has a dominance of depression as the primary diagnosis. Few individuals who complete suicide do not have psychiatric symptoms. Suicide assessment takes into account a history of behavioral change before the event: Suicide does not just *happen*. Before an attempt, the most common associated events are communication of suicidal thoughts, history of suicide attempts, and previous contact with a psychiatrist. Most individuals have communicated their intent to others on several occasions (generally by indicating that they wish to die and that others would be better off without them), by comments about methods of suicide, and by predicting that others would find a dead person. Often, these communications are not taken seriously by friends and family members, but taking them seriously is extremely important.

One should look for a family history of suicide, family and peer conflicts, isolation and withdrawal from contacts with others, the impact of recent disappointments, the presence of psychiatric illness, and (particularly) a sense of hopelessness. The following background features are characteristic of the child and family when suicide or a suicide attempt occurs:

- An increased prevalence of psychiatric conditions (e.g., especially depression and personality disorder in parents, a family history of suicide, and difficulties in the parents' marriage)
- Frequent discipline problems (e.g., inconsistent discipline and parental alternation between permissive and restrictive control, leading to conflict)
- Problems in communication among family members, particularly in regard to confiding feelings
- A psychiatric disorder in the child (e.g., a response of hopelessness on an acute basis or a chronic depressive disorder, a history of antisocial behavior, and drug and alcohol abuse)
- Social isolation from peers and family members (e.g., a report by a child who has had limited social support of the loss of that support just before the attempt; a history of running away before the attempt)
- Both pregnancy and chronic physical illness (i.e., potential risk in adolescent sufferers of a chronic long-term physical illness; pregnancy a potential precipitant in teenage girls)

Differential Diagnosis

A completed suicide is a rare event in any pediatrician's practice. However, it is potentially preventable, so the danger signs must be kept in mind. Because suicide is associated so strongly with depression, an awareness of depressive symptoms is paramount. Depressed mood often is recognized, but clarifying whether a depressive syndrome is present is more difficult. Suicidal talk must be taken seriously regardless of whether the would-be suicide's distress makes sense. Individuals who talk about committing suicide may do so; finding out about their concerns is essential. Whenever the question of depression arises, the physician should ask about suicidal thoughts; doing so does not implant them into the patient's mind. If a patient remains depressed, the physician should ask about suicidal thoughts throughout the course of the illness, especially if a plan has been considered. Although most suicidal crises do not result in death, a miscalculation cannot be reversed. When doubt exists, the best choices are consultation with a psychiatrist and hospital admission.

TREATMENT OF UNDERLYING ILLNESS

Because nothing guarantees that suicidal intent will not recur, treating the underlying illness is essential. If that illness is a major affective disorder, antidepressants may be used, prescribed always with the awareness of the risk of overdose or self-poisoning with these agents. Because most individuals communicate their distress, attending to their distress is the most essential intervention.

The profiles of both completed and attempted suicide must be kept in mind. Completed suicides are associated with depressive disorder and schizophrenia. The act is planned carefully, and the method chosen is effective, with plans to be carried out in isolation, often with provisions to prevent interruption of the attempt. The plan is to die. In contrast, those who attempt suicide more often are women than men, they are less likely to be suffering from a major psychiatric illness, and they act impulsively. Often, the means chosen is not thought out carefully and is not rapidly effective. Generally, caution is not taken to prevent rescue, and the act may be carried out in the presence of others, or a means to notify others about the individual's despair may be available. The plan is not to die, but to escape a stressful situation. However, an attempted suicide should not be viewed as a failed suicide, because it might have led to death. The closer the individual's behavior to the pattern of completed suicide, the more concern is indicated. The usual attempt, however, may be a wish to affect another person by the behavior. Consequently, it occurs in a social context and may represent a request for help. The distress is misdirected: The behavior is an act of desperation.

Assessment should be conducted as soon as the child or adolescent can participate in an interview after the appropriate emergency measures. This assessment should take place before discharge from the emergency room or hospital. Ideally, the interview involves a psychiatrist who can help in assessing the risk of recurrence and in other forms of intervention. Both the young person and family members are interviewed. The preferable approach is interviewing the adolescent first, then the parents, and finally the family together. Box 105.1 lists questions to be asked in assessing the risks for suicide.

The first issue to be addressed in the assessment is whether treatment should occur on an inpatient or outpatient basis. Inpatient treatment is essential in the presence of major risk factors (i.e., a serious life-threatening event that was planned and carried out in isolation by a depressed child or adolescent) and of precipitating circumstances: an unsettled and poor support system, continuing suicidal thoughts, and an attitude of hopelessness. Each of these circumstances must be taken into account in developing a treatment plan, which includes treatment of the underlying psychiatric disorder, family intervention in regard to family treatment and psychosocial support, crisis intervention focusing on dealing with precipitating circumstances, and appropriate educational programming.

Ordinarily, the person attempting suicide is admitted to a hospital psychiatric unit for major psychiatric conditions or to a pediatric floor for medical treatment before psychiatric admission. Individual psychotherapy, family therapy, or both may be needed during admission. The impact of a suicide attempt on peers in the neighborhood and at the child's school is another important consideration in community treatment; several instances of multiple suicides in one school have occurred.

BOX 105.1   Assessment for Suicide Risks

1. Establish details of the attempt with specific emphasis on the means used (e.g., self-poisoning, strangulation, self-inflicted wound).
2. What is the expressed intention about death in regard to the attempt?
3. Was anyone informed before or after initiation of the attempt?
4. What were the circumstances that are said to have precipitated the attempt?
5. In what way has the attempt altered these circumstances?
6. Does the child or adolescent have current suicidal intentions and express an attitude of hopelessness?
7. What is the current mental status, with an emphasis on affective symptomatology?
8. Was a history of emotional or behavioral difficulties exhibited in previous weeks or months?
9. Has a physician or a community agency been involved?
10. What is the current support system: friends, family, teachers, religious groups, and other community contacts? How can a confiding relationship be established and a support system be convened?

In summary, recommended interventions include the treatment of psychopathology (especially major depression); amelioration of cognitive distortion and difficulties with social skills, and problem-solving training. Interpersonal treatment must be undertaken to improve affect regulation both individually and in a family context and family education about risk factors. Because of the chronic and recurrent nature of the conditions associated with suicide attempts, a long-term care plan is needed to maintain the child or adolescent's engagement with the treatment team.

PROGNOSIS

The prognosis for those who attempt suicide depends on the ability of child and family to alter the precipitating circumstances, effective treatment of underlying psychiatric conditions, and the availability of psychosocial support. Risk is greatest in those who have made previous attempts, when chronic stress persists, and if underlying psychiatric conditions are not resolved.

Suggested Readings

Allebeck P, Allgulander C, Fisher LD. Predictors of completed suicide in a cohort of 50,465 young men: role of personality and deviant behavior. *Brit Med J* 1988;297:176.

Brent DA. The aftercare of adolescents with deliberate self-harm. *J Child Psychol Psychiatry* 1997;38:277.

Brent DA. Assessment and treatment of the youthful suicidal patient. *Ann N Y Acad Sci* 2001;932:106.

Gould MS, Greenberg T, Velting DM, Shaffer D. Youth suicide risk and preventive interventions: a review of the past 10 years. *J Am Acad Child Adolesc Psychiatry* 2003;42:386.

Gould MS, King R, Greenwald S, et al. Psychopathology associated with suicidal ideation and attempts among children and adolescents. *J Am Acad Child Adolesc Psychiatry* 1998;37:915.

Grunbaum JA, Kann L, Kinchen SA, et al. Youth risk behavior surveillance—United States, 2001. *J Sch Health* 2002;72(8):313.

Johnson JG, Cohen P, Gould MS, et al. Childhood adversities, interpersonal difficulties, and risk for suicide attempts during late adolescence and early adulthood. *Arch Gen Psychiatry* 2002;59:741.

Juon H, Ensminger ME. Childhood, adolescent, and young adult predictors of suicidal behaviors: a prospective study of African Americans. *J Child Psychol Psychiatry* 1997;38:55.

Negron R, Piacentini J, Graae F, et al. Microanalysis of adolescent suicide attempters and ideators during the acute suicidal episode. *J Am Acad Child Adolesc Psychiatry* 1997;36:1512.

Pfeffer CR. Diagnosis of childhood and adolescent suicidal behavior: unmet needs for suicide prevention. *Biol Psychiatry* 2001;49(12):1055.

Purselle DC, Nemeroff CB. Serotonin transporter: a potential substrate in the biology of suicide. *Neuropsychopharmacology* 2003;28(4):613.

Souery D, Oswald P, Linkowski P, Mendlewicz J. Molecular genetics in the analysis of suicide. *Ann Med* 2003;35(3):191.

Shaffer D, Scott M, Wilcox H, et al. The Columbia Suicide Screen: validity and reliability of a screen for youth suicide and depression. *J Am Acad Child Adolesc Psychiatry* 2004;43(1):71.

Shaffer D, Craft L. Methods of adolescent suicide prevention. *J Clin Psychiatry* 1999;60(Suppl 2):70.

CHAPTER 106 ■ SOMATOFORM AND CONVERSION DISORDERS

JAMES C. HARRIS

Somatic symptoms often are associated with anxiety and depressive disorders, and somatic symptoms must be considered as associated with these diagnoses. For example, abdominal pain may accompany separation anxiety and be used as a reason to stay home with the parent. Children with generalized anxiety disorder may be preoccupied with medical illnesses or may present with headache or similar complaints. After bereavement, general pain complaints may be noted, and children with social phobia may feign illness to avoid social interaction.

Children with mood disorders may be preoccupied with sickness and death. However, when severe somatic symptoms are the primary presentation the term *somatoform disorder* is used.

Somatization refers to seeking medical attention for somatic distress and symptoms where no demonstrable pathophysiology is present to account for them. Somatoform disorder refers to severe somatic symptoms that are not based on known psychopathology and that require intervention. The following categories are included: somatization disorder (multiple somatic complaints), conversion disorder (motor or sensory symptoms suggesting a neurologic disorder), pain disorder (pain linked to psychological symptoms), hypochondriasis (excessive preoccupation with being ill), and body dysmorphic disorder (preoccupation with an imaged defect in physical appearance). This chapter focuses on the most commonly encountered of these, conversion disorder. Conversion disorder may present with or without an accompanying general medical condition.

Conversion disorder should be considered when no clear-cut medical reason exists for voluntary motor or sensory symptoms that suggest a neurologic disorder or other general medical condition.

EPIDEMIOLOGY

The diagnostic criteria for conversion disorders are shown in Box 106.1. The prevalence of conversion disorders depends on the clinical setting. Conversion symptoms are reported most often on the general pediatric service, the ophthalmology service, and the neurology service. Child psychiatrists have reported a prevalence of 1% to 3% in referred outpatients. Among new outpatients at a pediatric neurology clinic, the prevalence was about 10% in school-aged referrals. Overall prevalence estimates range from 2% to 10%; the higher number is from a pediatric psychiatry inpatient consultation service. Rates are reported to be higher in children from rural poor populations than in urban children. Conversion disorder most commonly

---

BOX 106.1 — Diagnostic Criteria for Conversion Disorder

A. One or more symptoms or deficits affecting voluntary motor or sensory function that suggest a neurologic or other general medical condition.

B. Psychological factors are judged to be associated with the symptom deficit, because the initiation or exacerbation of the symptom or deficit is preceded by conflicts or other stressors.

C. The symptom or deficit is not produced intentionally or feigned (as in factitious disorder of malingering).

D. The symptom or deficit cannot, after appropriate investigation, be fully explained by a general medical condition, or by the direct effects of a substance, or as a culturally sanctioned behavior or experience.

E. The symptom or deficit causes clinically significant distress or impairment in social, occupational, or other important areas of functioning or warrants medical evaluation.

F. The symptom or deficit is not limited to pain or sexual dysfunction, does not occur exclusively during the course of somatization disorder, and is not better accounted for by another mental disorder.

Specify type of symptom or deficit:
  With motor symptom or deficit
  With sensory symptom or deficit
  With seizures or convulsions
  With mixed presentation

Reprinted with permission from American Psychiatric Association. *Diagnostic and statistical manual of mental disorders*, 4th ed. Text revision. Washington, DC: American Psychiatric Association, 2000.

---

is diagnosed in children and adolescents aged 10 to 15 years. The prevalence tends to be equal for boys and girls in the prepubertal years, but a greater prevalence in girls exists in early adolescence. Symptoms frequently date from a minor illness or surgery. Many children with conversion symptoms have transient symptoms and can be treated as outpatients.

CLINICAL MANIFESTATIONS AND COMPLICATIONS

The most common presentations are neurologic or ocular ones, in which where symptoms and deficits in voluntary motor function or in sensory function suggest a disorder. These include visual or hearing disturbances; localized pains; sensory disturbances such as paresthesias; pain; blindness; problems in gait; weakness; pseudoseizures; and loss of function of an extremity. Such neurologic symptoms do not follow the expected anatomic localization. Emotional unconcern about symptoms may or may not be part of the clinical picture. Symptoms may be preceded by a traumatic life event or personal loss that the child cannot master at his developmental level. Rapid remission is the rule; more than two-thirds of patients improve within a 12-month period. A smaller percentage subsequently are found to have general medical conditions.

ETIOLOGY

A variety of approaches have been taken to understand conversion symptoms. The classic psychodynamic approach suggests that physical symptoms result from conflicts that are outside of personal awareness. The symptom represents punishment for covert, unacceptable wishes. Other authors suggest that children with conversion symptoms find it difficult to put their feelings into words and need help in doing so. If symptoms persist, secondary gain may occur if the patient is allowed to avoid difficult situations or if developmentally appropriate demands are reduced. Learning theorists suggest that imitation of or identification with significant adults is related to symptom formation. For example, a boy who had emotional difficulty dealing with his uncle's stroke identified with the paralyzed uncle and could not use his own arm.

Several authors have found symptoms of mood disorder in parents of children with conversion symptoms. In addition to specific symptoms in family members, stressful interpersonal family crises, threats to the child's dependency, or threatened losses of family members also may be related to etiology. The family may reinforce behavior that is passive, dependent, or even seductive. One must always ask, where did the child learn this symptom?

DIFFERENTIAL DIAGNOSIS

Most children with conversion disorder do not have a histrionic personality style. The diagnosis can occur in children with many psychiatric conditions. Symptoms may vary over time and from one situation to another. The child may or may not show emotional concern about the symptoms.

The physician must remember that some children with conversion disorders are later diagnosed with a general medical condition. Children also may present with undiagnosable conditions that are factitious, or a parent may falsify the medical history (Munchausen syndrome by proxy). A factitious disorder involves the intentional feigning of psychological or physical symptoms and signs to establish "the sick role." These cases are more likely to be confused with other medical illnesses and not conversion disorder. As previously noted, separation anxiety disorder, generalized anxiety disorder, and depressive disorders may have associated physical symptomatology. In addition, children with psychotic disorders may have somatic preoccupations or delusions.

TREATMENT

If a conversion symptom is suspected, the pediatric general medical evaluation should be done rapidly to avoid secondary gain from symptoms. As symptoms resolve, symptom removal generally does not result in the substitution of other symptoms. Interventions with parent and child include reassurance, enhanced verbal expression of feelings, behavioral treatments using suggestion, initiation of rehabilitation methods, relaxation techniques, and pharmacologic management. Basic to the assessment is an understanding of where the child may have learned the symptom and particularly what the child's symptom may mean to the child and the family.

Keep in mind that the symptoms are real to the child, although no specific physical disorder has been diagnosed. Functional deficits have been documented; in one SPECT study of unilateral sensorimotor conversion disorder, blood flow was decreased in specific brain regions (contralateral thalamus and basal ganglia), suggesting a dysfunction of striatothalamic cortical brain circuits. Efforts are made to find a way to allow the child to give up the symptoms honorably. For example, a child was referred for assessment of chest pain. He previously had several neurologic examinations and a hospitalization, all unrevealing. When his history was carefully reviewed, it was learned that symptoms began when a soccer ball hit him in the chest and knocked him to the ground. Later that night, following the chest injury, his grandfather died of a myocardial infarction. The child slept in the same room with the grandfather, and during the terminal illness, his grandfather had suffered

severe angina pectoris. The boy was thought to be sleeping when his grandfather was taken out of the home to the hospital. The boy resembled his grandfather in appearance and did not grieve appropriately at the time of his grandfather's death; his mother also had a complicated bereavement. The chest pain was found to be associated with a complicated bereavement response by the child. After successful bereavement counseling, the chest pain resolved, and the child could return to school.

Collaborative treatment between the pediatrician and child psychiatrist is recommended. Associated depression and anxiety should be diagnosed and treated. The collaborative approach may be more effective than direct referral after assessment, because the family remain concerned about the etiology of physical symptoms. Interventions during the hospital stay that address the child's symptomatology and provide a comprehensive assessment of her psychopathology are integral to the treatment plan. The treatment plan develops mutually agreed-on goals and defines carefully the role of each staff member in facilitating a return to full functioning. A physical therapy program with systems of rewards can be effective.

Suggested Readings

Fritz GK, Campos JV. Somatoform disorders. In: Lewis M, ed. *Child and adolescent psychiatry: a comprehensive textbook,* 3rd ed. Philadelphia: Lippincott Williams & Wilkins, 2002:847.

Goodyear I. Hysterical conversion reactions in childhood. *J Child Psychol Psychiatry* 1981;22:179.

Leslie SA. Diagnosis and treatment of hysterical conversion reactions. *Arch Dis Child* 1988;63:506.

Marshall JC, Halligan PW, Fink GR, et al. The functional anatomy of a hysterical paralysis. *Cognition* 1997;64:B18.

Silver FW. Management of conversion disorder. *Am J Phys Med Rehab* 1996; 75:134.

Vuilleumier P, Chicheri C, Assal F, et al. Functional neuro-anatomical correlates of hysterical sensori-motor loss. *Brain* 2001;124:1077.

CHAPTER 107 ■ PERVASIVE DEVELOPMENTAL DISORDER AND AUTISTIC DISORDER

JAMES C. HARRIS

In 1980, the term *pervasive developmental disorder* (PDD) was introduced into the child psychiatric classification to describe children whose developmental difficulties cross multiple developmental lines (see Box 107.1 for the historical perspective of Autism). This category has been substantially expanded from one specific disorder in the original 1980 classification, autistic disorder, to the inclusion of several other conditions in the *Diagnostic and Statistical Manual of Mental Disorders,* Fourth Edition, Text Revision (*DSM-IV-TR*). The conditions described as PDD in both the *International Classification of Diseases*, Tenth Edition (*ICD-10*), and in *DSM-IV–TR* are autistic disorder, Rett syndrome (see Chapter 98, Mental Retardation), childhood disintegrative disorder, Asperger syndrome, and unspecified forms of PDD. An additional diagnosis, overactivity associated with mental retardation and stereotypical movements, is included in *ICD-10*. Autistic disorder is described here; the *DSM-IV-TR* and *ICD-10* classifications should be consulted for the other conditions.

The syndrome of autistic disorder, in which social, language, cognitive, imaginative and behavioral deficits are apparent, is the prototype of DSM-IV-TR PDD. The relationship between cognitive and language deficits and social abnormalities has been a focus of research. As shown in Box 107.2, diagnostic criteria for autistic disorder have been introduced that focus on qualitative impairments in social interactions and in interpersonal communication, along with a stereotyped restricted pattern of interests and activities. These abnormalities affect functioning in all situations and, in most instances, are present from infancy onward. The disorder is most commonly recognized in the second year of life, but may be recognized up to approximately 30 months of age. The disorder is defined in terms of behavior that is deviant in relation to the child's mental age. The majority of children with this disorder have intellectual disability as a feature of their PDD. Efforts are ongoing to identify additional subgroups within this category.

Confusion sometimes exists about the language disorder in PDD, related to the dual nature and function of language. Language serves the purposes of being a mental tool in thinking and also the primary means of communication with others. Children with PDD have the greatest difficulty with the practical use of language as a communication tool (pragmatic language). The language disorder is in social communication (i.e., in appropriately conversing with others). Difficulty in sharing experiences with others (social reciprocity) is a characteristic feature of PDD, regardless of the child's intellectual level. Communicating feelings poses a particular problem because of the child's difficulty in interpreting the meaning of tone of voice, posture, and facial expression in others in a social context. Additionally, to share the other person's frame of reference requires memories of one's own emotional experience. Remembering and sharing affective experience also is a problem. Deficits exist not only in initiating verbal social communication but also in understanding the nonverbal communication of others.

DIAGNOSTIC ISSUES

Autistic disorder is seen as the most severe form of PDD DSM-IV-TR. Impaired development is manifest before 3 years of age, with characteristic abnormal functioning in social interactions, language (when used in social communication), symbolic or imaginative play, and restricted, repetitive behavior. When the full autistic syndrome is not present, the term *PDD not otherwise specified (atypical autism)* is used in *DSM-VI-TR*. It may be atypical in regard to the age of onset or in not meeting the full diagnostic criteria. Asperger syndrome should be considered in children with no general delay or retardation in language

or cognitive development who show qualitative abnormality in social interaction and demonstrate restricted, stereotyped interests. If the child has a period of normal development followed by a loss of previously acquired developmental skills (including social, communicative, and behavioral functions) that persists over time, the diagnosis *childhood disintegrative disorder* may be used. Overall, the younger the child, the more severe the handicap, and the more problems associated with it.

Associated with PDD are abnormalities in cognitive skills. The specific skill profile is usually uneven regardless of the level of intelligence. In most cases, an association with intellectual disability exists, most commonly in the moderate range (IQ 35 to 49). Abnormalities of posture and motor behavior may occur, including repetitive jumping, hand flapping when excited, walking on tiptoe, and unusual hand or body postures. Motor coordination is variable. Responses to sensory input may be unusual (e.g., insensitivity or excessive sensitivity to pain, cold, or heat; covering the ears in response to some sounds; or resistance to being touched and preoccupations with perceptual sensations, such as lights or odors). Associated abnormalities also may be present in eating, drinking, or sleeping, with diet restricted to a few foods, excessive fluid intake, or recurrent waking at night. Feeling states are difficult to identify in most of the younger children. Lack of fear of realistic dangers is of particular concern. One may see fluctuations in mood for no reason, but absence of emotional reactions is far more common. Self-injury may occur with head-banging or self-biting.

Other major mental disorders may occur with autistic disorder, such as major depressive disorder or schizophreniform disorder, particularly in adolescents. These diagnoses are recognized more easily in higher-functioning individuals whose speech allows them to describe their symptoms more accurately.

EPIDEMIOLOGY

The prevalence for autistic disorder in children is approximately 1 per 1,000. For autistic spectrum disorder in children age 3 to 10 years, the rate was 3.4 per 1,000 in a study conducted by the National Center on Birth Defects and Developmental Disabilities (male–female ratio, 4:1). Overall, the prevalence of autistic spectrum disorder was comparable for African American and white children. Sixty-eight percent of children with IQ or developmental test results had cognitive impairment. As severity of cognitive impairment increased from mild to profound, the male–female ratio decreased from 4.4 to 1.3. An increased prevalence has been shown in siblings of children with autistic disorder, of whom approximately 2% are affected with the full syndrome. A 50-fold risk exists for siblings. The prevalence of learning disability also is increased in siblings of children with autistic disorder. The disorder also has been found more frequently in same-sex twins: 4 of 11 monozygotic twin pairs were concordant for the disorder but it occurred in none of ten dizygotic twin pairs. The presentation varied among the twins. In some instances one twin had autistic disorder and the co-twin was diagnosed with an autistic spectrum disorder (cognitive profile related to learning problems and inherited social cognitive deficits).

PATHOLOGY

Autistic disorder is a neurodevelopmental disorder. Neuropathologic and neuroimaging studies are consistent with brain abnormalities beginning in the prenatal period in early trimesters of pregnancy. Autistic disorder has been associated with several genetic syndromes, such as phenylketonuria and tuberous sclerosis complex. When autistic disorder occurs in specific genetic syndromes, the family genetic background also must be considered. Because the age of recognition, the age when symptoms become apparent, is ordinarily during the second year of life, intercurrent infections and immunizations sometimes have been thought to be causative. However, the National Immunization Program at the Centers for Disease Control and Prevention (CDC) reported similar proportions of autistic and control children were vaccinated by the recommended age or shortly after (i.e., before 18 months) and before the age at which autistic development usually is recognized in children; they found no association with measles-mumps-rubella immunization. Others have proposed that thimerosal (an ethyl mercury containing preservative), which was used in vaccines until 2001, may cause autism. Ethyl mercury is a different molecule than methyl mercury; it is eliminated from the body 7 times faster and is less like to accumulate. More important, it is not actively taken up by the nervous system. No evidence suggests that vaccines containing this compound cause autism. These findings would be expected, because autistic disorder is of prenatal original. The high concordance rate in identical twins and increased risk for autistic spectrum disorder in siblings is consistent with a genetic etiology. Moreover, the twin with the greatest perinatal difficulty has the more severe presentation, thus suggesting the possibility that genetic factors and postpartum stress may interact.

TREATMENT

Treatment in autistic disorder requires a clarification of the diagnosis and the development of an individual treatment plan. Children with autistic disorder have an abnormality in their development that involves socialization, language, and cognition. The children are both delayed and deviant in each of these areas. Most children with autistic disorder (75%) test in the intellectually disabled range on psychological assessments as well; they have an uneven pattern of cognitive abilities, with enhanced factual memory and visuospatial and puzzle-solving abilities, but deficits in symbolic operations, conceptual understanding, and abstract abilities. Language is delayed, and some children do not acquire speech. When language does develop, its development is abnormal, particularly because the children fail to use language for the purpose of social communication in a normal, socially reciprocal fashion characteristic for their age. Using stereotyped phrases and echoing back words are common problems. Finally, socialization itself is deviant, and early milestones in initiating social interaction (e.g., reaching to be picked up, developing selective attachments, nodding yes and shaking one's head no, recognizing the meaning of others' facial expressions, using the eyes to communicate needs, and gesturing to share the reference with others) are delayed or abnormal. As the child with autistic disorder gets older, he or she may want to have friendships, but often does not know how to go about establishing them.

Treatment is further complicated by the child's rigidity and inflexibility in learning new skills. Skills often are learned concretely; therefore, generalizing to new situations is difficult. Applying knowledge to new situations is problematic, and a fear of change may be expressed with a preference for maintaining routines. Play is not imaginative, particularly at the younger ages. Objects are lined up and placed in patterns rather than used in an imaginative way. When imaginative activities do develop, they tend to be stereotyped, and specific rituals may be seen that have a strong compulsive or persevering quality. Object attachment is deviant in that attachment may be to objects such as stones, belts, or cans rather than to soft toys. Additionally, the treatment of associated overactivity, behavioral disruption, tantrums, aggressiveness, and self-injury is required. Some children develop phobias and fears or have difficulty with sleep and with developing toileting routines. Each of these areas must be addressed in any treatment plan.

The overall goals of treatment are to foster normal development and promote specific language development, social interaction, and learning. Treatment requires the establishment of active meaningful experiences, which involves planned periods of interaction, simplified communication, a selection of specific learning tasks, and direct teaching. Individual therapy has the psychoeducational goal to help the child understand social interactions and make appropriate adaptations. Family treatment is needed to help the family understand the nature of the disorder and to resolve guilt. Behavioral approaches are directed toward particular target symptoms, such as aggression or self-injury. Although no pharmacotherapy exists for autism *per se*, symptomatic treatment for aggressive and disruptive behaviors with medications such as risperidone have been beneficial.

Suggested Readings

Bailey A, Phillips W, Rutter M. Autism: towards an integration of clinical, genetic, neuropsychological, and neurobiological perspectives. *J Child Psychol Psychiatry* 1996;37:89.

Bauman ML, Kemper TL. The neuropathology of the autism spectrum disorders: what have we learned? *Novartis Found Symp* 2003;251:112.

Bristol MM, Cohen DJ, Costello EJ, et al. State of the science in autism: report to the National Institutes of Health. *J Autism Dev Disord* 1996;26:121.

DeStefano F, Bhasin TK, Thompson WW, et al. Age at first measles-mumps-rubella vaccination in children with autism and school-matched control subjects: a population-based study in metropolitan Atlanta. *Pediatrics* 2004; 113:259.

Edwardes M, Baltzan M. MMR immunization and autism. *JAMA* 2001;13;285: 2852.

Eisenmajer R, Prior M, Leekam S, et al. Comparison of clinical symptoms in autism and Asperger's disorder. *J Am Acad Child Adolesc Psychiatry* 1996; 35:1523.

Folstein SE, Rutter M. Infantile autism: a genetic study of 21 twin pairs. *J Child Psychol Psychiatry* 1977;18:297.

Frith U. *Autism: explaining the enigma*, 2nd ed. Edinburgh: Blackwell Publishing, 2003.

Frith C. What do imaging studies tell us about the neural basis of autism? *Novartis Found Symp* 2003;251:149.

Frith CD, Frith U. Interacting minds—a biological basis. *Science* 1999;286:1692.

Hill EL, Frith U. Understanding autism: insights from mind and brain. *Philos Trans R Soc Lond B Biol Sci* 2003;358:281.

Filipek PA, Accardo PJ, Ashwal S, et al Practice parameter: screening and diagnosis of autism: report of the Quality Standards Subcommittee of the American Academy of Neurology and the Child Neurology Society. *Neurology* 2000;55:468.

Fombonne E. The prevalence of autism. *JAMA* 2003;289(1):87.

Lainhart JE. Increased rate of head growth during infancy in autism. *JAMA* 2003;290:393.

Kanner L. Autistic disturbances of affective contact. *Nerv Child* 1943;2:217.

McCracken JT, McGough J, Shah B, et al. Risperidone in children with autism and serious behavioral problems. *N Engl J Med* 2002;347(5):314.

Lord C, Leventhal BL, Cook EH Jr. Quantifying the phenotype in autism spectrum disorders. *Am J Med Genet* 2001;105:36.

Rapin I. The autistic-spectrum disorders. *N Engl J Med* 2002;347(5):302.

Rutter M. The treatment of autistic children. *J Child Psychol Psychiatry* 1985;26:193.

Szatmari P, Barttolucci G, Bremner R. Asperger's syndrome and autism: comparison of early history and outcome. *Dev Med Child Neurol* 1989;31:709.

Volkmar FR. Childhood disintegrative disorder: issues for DSM-IV. *J Autism Dev Disord* 1992;22:625.

Yeargin-Allsopp M, Rice C, Karapurkar T, et al. Prevalence of autism in a U.S. metropolitan area. *JAMA* 2003;289:49.

Whitehouse DW, Harris J. Hyperlexia in infantile autism. *J Autism Dev Disord* 1984;11:31.

Wing L. *Autism: a guide for parents and professionals.* New York: Brunner/Mazel, 1985.

CHAPTER 108 ■ EATING DISORDERS

RICHARD E. KREIPE

INTRODUCTION

In 2003, the American Academy of Pediatrics described the role of pediatricians in the identification and management of eating disorders (Box 108.1). Early detection, initial evaluation, and ongoing management in primary care can play a significant role in preventing the illness from progressing and in facilitating referral to interdisciplinary specialists. Within subspecialty care, the management of medical complications, supervision of nutritional rehabilitation, and coordination of the psychosocial and psychiatric aspects of care are often effected by pediatricians, especially those who have experience or expertise in the care of adolescents with eating disorders.

ETIOLOGY AND EPIDEMIOLOGY

The eating disorders anorexia nervosa, bulimia nervosa, and related conditions are best considered final-common pathways that are characterized by body image disturbance that leads to dysfunctional weight control habits and subsequent changes in weight that can result in potentially life-threatening physical and mental health complications. Overestimation of body size or of body parts (generally focused on the abdomen, hips, and thighs) leads to weight control practices intended to either reduce weight or prevent weight gain. Common practices include severely restricting caloric intake (with special attention to the fat content of foods) and behaviors intended to reduce the effect of ingested calories, such as compulsively exercising or purging by inducing vomiting or taking laxatives. Depending on the balance of caloric intake and output, the change in weight may range from extreme loss of weight in anorexia nervosa to fluctuation around a normal to moderately high weight in bulimia nervosa.

Eating disorders have multiple determinants. A combination of biologic, developmental, and sociocultural factors contribute to the predisposition, precipitation, and perpetuation of these disorders, while genetic and twin studies demonstrate a biologic predisposition to both anorexia and bulimia nervosa. Although cultural, social, and environmental factors may play a role, the majority of individuals exposed to these same factors do *not* develop an eating disorder. A family or personal history of substance abuse or depression is common in patients with bulimia nervosa.

The etiologic factor common to all forms of eating disorders is the sense of control or self-efficacy that individuals gain as a result of their weight control habits. In the case of anorexia nervosa, a societal emphasis on thinness, an athlete's attempting to achieve a certain weight to improve performance, or peer pressure to achieve a certain "look" can trigger weight loss in a vulnerable individual. Adolescents who develop bulimia

| BOX 108.1 | Role of the Pediatrician in the Identification and Treatment of Eating Disorders |

Pediatricians:

1. Need to be knowledgeable about the early signs and symptoms of disordered eating and other related behaviors.
2. Should be aware of the careful balance that needs to be in place to decrease the growing prevalence of eating disorders in children and adolescents. When counseling children on risk of obesity and healthy eating, care needs to be taken not to foster overaggressive dieting and to help children and adolescents build self-esteem while still addressing weight concerns.
3. Should be familiar with the screening and counseling guidelines for disordered eating and other related behaviors.
4. Should know when and how to monitor and/or refer patients with eating disorders to best address their medical and nutritional needs, serving as an integral part of a multidisciplinary team.
5. Should be encouraged to calculate and plot weight, height, and body mass index using age- and gender-appropriate graphs at routine annual pediatric visits.
6. Can play a role in primary prevention through office visits and community- or school-based interventions with a focus on screening, education, and advocacy.
7. Need to be aware of the resources in their communities so they can coordinate care of various treating professionals, helping to create a seamless system between inpatient and outpatient management in their communities.

Modified from American Academy of Pediatrics, Committee on Adolescence. Identifying and treating eating disorders (Policy Statement). *Pediatrics* 2003;111(1):204.

nervosa may initially attempt to restrict their caloric intake by skipping meals or reducing the amount of calories ingested to lose weight, only to trigger binge eating that is followed by compensatory vomiting. Although the act of binge eating and vomiting may seem noxious, patients with bulimia nervosa often describe a feeling of getting "high" when they do so.

Eating disorders are not distributed uniformly in the population. More than 90% of patients are adolescent white females from higher-income families, but patients can be of any sex, race, age, or social stratum. As many as 1% of teenage females develop anorexia nervosa, and as many as 5% of older adolescent and young adult females develop symptoms of bulimia nervosa. Less than 10% of patients with eating disorders are male.

Pathogenesis

As previously noted, eating disorders do not have a single pathogenetic mechanism, but most commonly develop in females in relation to various developmental struggles encountered during adolescence. Halmi has noted that eating disorders frequently begin with dieting, which may be transformed into a full-blown disorder by antecedent conditions of biologic vulnerability, premorbid psychological characteristics, family interactions, and social climate. These unhealthy habits serve as a coping mechanism that lessens the negative effects of asso-

ciated psychosocial problems with which the adolescent may be struggling. Researchers are just beginning to understand the biologic basis for how dieting, exercise, amenorrhea, and weight loss may be used to cope with the developmental demands of adolescence.

Factors *predisposing* an individual to develop an eating disorder include (1) being female; (2) possessing traits such as perfectionism, obsessive/compulsiveness, or moodiness; (3) having low self-esteem; (4) engaging in activities that place a high value on thinness, such as classic ballet or modeling, or in which the body is exposed during competition, such as gymnastics, track, or swimming; and (5) being in a weight-conscious environment.

There also appears to be genetically based, biologic vulnerability predisposing individuals to develop an eating disorder. International, multisite studies of families with more than one member having an eating disorder has provided evidence for linkage on chromosome 1 and 10 for anorexia and bulimia, with evidence of candidate genes that may contribute to vulnerabilities for these disorders, including traits such as perfectionism, orderliness, low tolerance for new situations, maturity fears, low self-esteem, and overall anxiety. The clinical relevance of genetic predisposition for an individual is probably similar to that for depression. That is, individuals at high genetic risk, based on possessing one or more relevant genes shared with family members who also have an eating disorder, might never develop an eating disorder themselves, but would be more vulnerable to develop one if they were to diet intensively or to live in an environment that emphasizes dieting and thinness. As is true of most conditions with a genetic component, biology and the environment are both important and interact with each other.

Because eating disorders most commonly appear in the second decade of life, when adolescent developmental issues are prominent, the *precipitating* factors for eating disorders often relate to biologic (sexual maturation), psychological (development of abstract thinking and the emergence of adult psychological traits), and social changes (school transitions, changes in social supports, etc.) of adolescence. In the presence of a predisposed individual, precipitating factors may trigger an eating disorder. Rarely does a single factor give rise to an eating disorder; factors usually accumulate, but the factor most closely related temporally to the appearance of the dysfunctional habits is "blamed" as the "cause" of the eating disorder. However, individuals may engage in weight control habits surreptitiously long before the appearance of the putative causal agent. For example, sexual abuse is commonly identified as a precipitating or causal factor, especially for bulimia nervosa, but sexual abuse generally is associated with a variety of factors that, taken together, create a toxic environment for healthy adolescent development.

Perpetuating factors are those pathogenetic elements that tend to maintain an eating disorder after it develops. Unlike most conditions in pediatrics in which there is a tendency for the patient to want to feel better and comply with treatment, and for healing to occur naturally, eating disorders have a tendency to worsen in the absence of effective treatment. Moreover, patients often resist treatment because accepting it implies losing control as the eating disorder is "taken away" from them. For the pediatric practitioner, the central point is to understand the role that the dysfunctional weight control habits have in perpetuating the dysfunctional cognitive patterns that are associated with eating disorders (dichotomous thinking, overgeneralization, personalization, and magnification). Therefore, the principles of the medical care of the patient, described in greater detail in the section on treatment, needs to focus on improving the physical health of the patient as the foundation upon which effective mental health treatment rests and thereby interrupt the tendency for eating disorders to be self-reinforcing.

CLINICAL MANIFESTATIONS

Anorexia nervosa is characterized by an insufficient and voluntarily restricted caloric intake resulting in weight loss (or failure to gain weight during puberty) that is accompanied by an obsession to be thinner and a delusion of being fat. Patients often restrict intake to less than 1,000 calories per day, are unwilling to accept a body weight greater than 85% of average weight for height, and have a self-concept linked directly to their body weight or image. Weight loss can be extreme. The majority of patients also exercise intensely to accelerate weight loss, but may do so under the guise of sports or dance. Vomiting or laxative use is uncommon, but serious when it occurs.

The key feature of *bulimia nervosa* is repeated episodes of ingesting large amounts (binges) in a brief period. Since perceptions are subjective, patients may consider eating one cookie to be a "binge." Binges are followed by compensatory behaviors intended to rid the body of the effects of food: fasting, exercising, or "purging" through vomiting or laxatives. Patients with bulimia nervosa often feel guilt and shame about both binge eating and the compensatory behaviors that follow. Although "getting rid of food" tends to reduce anxiety, the relief is short-lived, and the cycle of behaviors repeats itself in ways sometimes likened to an addiction.

The symptoms and signs experienced by patients with eating disorders are related to the various habits used to control weight. The major symptoms associated with weight control habits are listed in Boxes 108.2 and 108.3. It is important to note that these findings are closely related to the physiologic effect of the habits themselves and are not diagnostic of an eating disorder, *per se*. The core features that must also be present are *dysfunctional eating habits, body image disturbance,* and *change in weight*.

COMPLICATIONS

No organ is spared the effects of the dysfunctional weight control habits and malnutrition, but certain systems deserve mention in the context of pediatric practice. Among patients with eating disorders, the most concerning acute health problems are *hypothermia* and *cardiovascular instability*; on a long-term basis *amenorrhea* obviously is associated with infertility, but when associated with low weight and calcium intake, it

also predisposes females to *osteoporosis*. Because hypothermia can be profound and uncomfortable, temperature should be measured at each pediatric visit. It can be used both as a marker of hypometabolism and as an incentive to increase intake: understanding that ingesting more energy-containing food/beverage will increase metabolism and helping them feel warmer may induce some patients to increase their caloric intake.

Cardiovascular adaptation to low caloric intake includes weakness, fatigue, dizziness, loss of energy, and fainting, often accompanied by bradycardia and significant orthostatic pulse changes; a pulse increase of more than 30 beats per minute between supine and standing indicates significant compromise and deserves immediate attention. Orthostatic change in pulse is a more sensitive indicator of cardiovascular instability than change in blood pressure. Patients with extreme weight loss, usually over a long period of time, can also experience ventricular tachyarrhythmias; after suicide, this is the most common cause of death. Although described in the lay press, "heart attacks" and "heart failure" are rare among adolescents with eating disorders.

Cardiovascular instability also occurs in bulimia nervosa, but is generally due to volume depletion (also with orthostatic changes) and electrolyte imbalance (hypokalemic, hypochloremic metabolic alkalosis). Erosion of dental enamel due to stomach acid or abrasion of the metacarpophalangeal joint knuckles against the maxillary central incisors when inducing the gag reflex (Russell sign) and enlargement of the salivary glands indicate significant binge eating and vomiting. Monitoring of serum potassium is important when these findings occur.

Hypothalamic amenorrhea can precede significant dieting or weight loss in eating disorders. Because adolescents with bulimia nervosa are less likely to experience amenorrhea and are more likely to be sexually active, testing for pregnancy is appropriate when menses cease in that situation. Amenorrhea is a physiologic adaptation to the physical and psychosocial stressors experienced by females with eating disorders and should not be considered pathologic, *per se*. Nonetheless, some clinicians start sex hormone replacement therapy in an attempt either to induce menses or to protect bones against osteoporosis. However, the monthly blood flow experienced by females taking sex hormones, most often in the form of birth control pills, is merely withdrawal bleeding and *not* a menstrual period, despite the insistence by patients that they are having regular menses. Moreover, in distinction to data regarding the beneficial effect of this treatment for postmenopausal women, there is very little support for any beneficial effect, with respect to bone mineral density, or any other outcome in the use of sex hormone replacement therapy. For both amenorrhea and bone density, the treatment of choice is weight gain through healthy

---

BOX 108.4   Combined *DSM-PC/DSM-IV* Criteria for Eating Disorders: Dieting–Anorexia Nervosa Spectrum

V65.49 Dieting/Body Image Variation

- A significantly overweight child changes eating habits in a realistic, healthy way.
- The child does not completely eliminate any food group, but generally decreases intake of food, especially of sweets and fats, or is eating an appropriate diet.
- The child favors a thin appearance but has a realistic image.
- The individual can stop dieting voluntarily.

V69.1 Dieting/Body Image Problem

- Dieting and voluntary food restrictions are more restrictive and result in weight loss or failure to gain weight as expected during growth but these behaviors are not sufficiently intense to qualify for the diagnosis of anorexia nervosa or eating disorder, not otherwise specified.
- The individual begins to become obsessed with the pursuit of thinness and develops systematic fears of gaining weight.
- The individual also begins to develop a consistent disturbance in body perception and starts to deny that weight loss or dieting is a problem.

307.1 Anorexia Nervosa (from DSM-IV)

- The individual refuses to maintain body weight at or above a minimally normal weight for age and height (e.g.,

weight loss leading to maintenance of body weight less than 85% of that expected; or failure to make expected weight gain during period of growth, leading to body weight less than 85% of that expected).
- Body mass index is less than 17.5 kg/m^2 for older adolescents.
- The individual has an intense fear of gaining weight or becoming fat, even though he or she is underweight.
- There is a disturbance in the way in which one's body weight, shape, or size is experienced, undue influence of body weight or shape on self-evaluation, or denial of the seriousness of the current low body weight.
- In postmenarchal females, there is amenorrhea, that is, the absence of at least three consecutive menstrual cycles. (A female is considered to have amenorrhea if her periods occur only following hormone, for example, estrogen, administration.)

Adapted from Wolraich ML, Felice ME, Drotar D, eds. *The classification of child and adolescent mental diagnoses in primary care, diagnostic and statistical manual for primary care (DSM-PC), child and adolescent version.* Elk Grove Village, IL: American Academy of Pediatrics, 1996; and American Psychiatric Association. *Diagnostic and statistical manual of mental disorders*, 4th ed. Washington, DC: American Psychiatric Association, 1994.

---

eating. Sex hormone treatment may cause some patients to attempt to lose more weight or resist weight gain.

Mental health morbidity in eating disorders is well recognized, both during treatment and following recovery. For the primary care provider, it is important to realize that the focus on abandoning dysfunctional eating habits and gaining weight may actually exacerbate symptoms of depression, anxiety, or obsessive/compulsiveness. Thus, initiation of effective treatment in primary care may precipitate a worsening of the clinical picture, sometimes to the point of requiring crisis intervention. Even in the absence of such situations, patients with eating disorders are at risk of having depression and/or anxiety disorders as adults. As noted previously, the most common cause of death for patients with eating disorders is suicide.

DIAGNOSIS

The American Academy of Pediatrics' *Diagnostic and Statistical Manual for Primary Care* (*DSM-PC*) classification describes a continuum of severity from *variations* (minor deviations from normal that should still be addressed in primary care) to *problems* (more serious manifestations representing subthreshold eating disorders) that are seen much more commonly in the primary care practitioner's office than full-syndrome *eating disorders* that meet the American Psychiatric Association's *Diagnostic and Statistical Manual of Mental Disorders*, Fourth Edition (*DSM-IV*), criteria. Combining these schema, it is useful in primary care practice to consider a dieting–anorexia spectrum and a binge/purge–bulimia spectrum, in which there can be overlap and crossover (Boxes 108.4 and 108.5). Although the focus of

this chapter is on the eating disorders anorexia and bulimia nervosa, variations and problems are more commonly seen in pediatric practice. Armed with knowledge about the disorders, the practitioner can easily address less serious conditions.

Differential Diagnosis

The differential diagnosis for eating disorders includes (1) inflammatory bowel disease, (2) diabetes mellitus, (3) adrenal insufficiency, (4) thyroid disorders, (5) central nervous system tumor, (6) cancer, (7) occult infections, (8) substance abuse, and (9) mood, personality, obsessive-compulsive, or anxiety disorders; these can usually be ruled out through careful history and physical examination. However, there can be overlap. For example, weight loss can lead to mood disturbance that impairs appetite; patients with regional enteritis may note that their abdominal pain worsens when they eat, but when they restrict eating both their physical pain and their sense of self-control improve. Psychiatric comorbidities are common in eating disorders.

Laboratory Findings

Because the diagnosis of an eating disorder is made clinically, there is no confirmatory laboratory test. When found, laboratory abnormalities are due to malnutrition, the weight control habits used, or complications, so that the indicated studies are dictated by the history of weight control methods used and the physical examination. A routine screening battery typically includes (1) complete blood count, (2) erythrocyte sedimentation

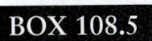

BOX 108.5 Combined *DSM-PC/DSM-IV* Criteria for Eating Disorders: Purging/Binge Eating–Bulimia Nervosa Spectrum

V65.49 *Purging/Binge-Eating Variation*

- Occasional overeating or perception of overeating, either objective or subjective binges, occurs.
- Intermittent concern about body image or getting fat is present in specific situations during which too much food was eaten. Concerns are not pervasive or cross-situational and do not change eating behaviors.
- Normal weight gain is typically present.

V69.19 *Purging/Binge-Eating Problem*

- The individual experiments with vomiting, laxatives, and fasting or exercises to prevent weight gain.
- Isolated episodes are far apart in time.
- The individual has increased episodes of uncontrolled eating, and perceptions of body shape or size become more systematically distorted. Negative self-evaluation is often influenced by weight and body shape.
- The behaviors are not sufficiently intense to qualify for a diagnosis of bulimia nervosa or eating disorder, not otherwise specified.

307.51 *Bulimia Nervosa (from DSM-IV)*

- Recurrent episodes of binge eating occur, characterized by both of the following:

Eating, in a discrete period of time, an amount of food that is definitely larger than most people would eat during a similar period of time and under similar circumstances.

A sense of lack of control over eating during the episode.

- Recurrent inappropriate compensatory behavior occurs in order to prevent weight gain, such as self-induced vomiting; misuse of laxatives, diuretics, enemas, or other medications; fasting; or excessive exercise.
- The binge eating and inappropriate compensatory behaviors both occur, on average, at least twice a week for 3 months.
- Self-evaluation is unduly influenced by body shape and weight.
- The disturbance does not occur exclusively during episodes of anorexia nervosa.

Adapted from Wolraich ML, Felice ME, Drotar D, eds. *The classification of child and adolescent mental diagnoses in primary care, diagnostic and statistical manual for primary care (DSM-PC), child and adolescent version*. Elk Grove Village, IL: American Academy of Pediatrics, 1996; and American Psychiatric Association. *Diagnostic and statistical manual of mental disorders*, 4th ed. Washington, DC: American Psychiatric Association, 1994.

---

rate (should be normal), and (3) biochemical profile. Common abnormalities include (1) low white blood cell count with normal hemoglobin and differential; (2) hypokalemic, hypochloremic metabolic alkalosis with severe vomiting; (3) elevated liver enzymes, cholesterol, and cortisol levels; (4) low gonadotropins and blood glucose with marked weight loss; and (5) generally normal total protein, albumin, and renal function. An electrocardiogram (ECG) may be useful when profound bradycardia or arrhythmia is detected; the ECG usually has low voltage, with nonspecific ST- or T-wave changes. Although prolonged QT$_c$ has been reported, prospective studies have not found an increased risk for this.

THERAPY

In many ways, treatment begins before the patient is ever seen in the clinical setting: a mother may call the primary care provider distraught about having found her daughter inducing vomiting or seeing her son's wasted body when swimming. Or, patients may present for a problem, such as amenorrhea, without suspicion about having an eating disorder. Therefore, the clinician needs an approach that will facilitate the acceptance of the diagnosis, as well as initial treatment recommendations. Clinicians often find a combination of the "nurturant-authoritative" approach described by Levenkron and the "biopsychosocial" model proposed by Engel useful (Box 108.6).

Treatment formally begins with a history and physical examination, including an accurate height and weight measurement. For the examination and measurements, the patient should wear only an examination gown, to minimize the likelihood of putting weights in the underwear. In addition, weigh-ins should occur immediately after voiding, with the urine saved for specific gravity measurement, to minimize the risk of

water loading. Body composition measurement through skin-fold thickness, bioelectrical impedance analysis, or dual energy x-ray absorptiometry is beyond the scope of most primary care practices, and not particularly useful in treatment.

The assessment of an eating disorder should focus on health and the exploration of underlying factors. The first step in assessment is to determine if weight loss is intentional and to detect any unrecognized medical disorders. Direct confrontation about an eating disorder may elicit denial, but questioning about nutritional habits and physical symptoms tend to be less threatening. Pubertal adolescents may fail to increase caloric intake during their growth spurt or may increase their caloric expenditure playing sports and lose weight unintentionally. Older adolescents may lose weight while attempting to "get in shape" or "look better."

The second step in the assessment of a suspected eating disorder is to determine if weight control habits are excessive or unhealthy. This requires determination of (1) symptoms associated with dysfunctional weight control habits; (2) frequency, amount, and type of food and drink ingested; (3) type, duration, and intensity of exercise; and (4) vomiting and laxative or diuretic use. By this step, it should be clear where the patient is falling on the variation–problem–disorder continuum on both the dieting–anorexia and the binge/purge–bulimia spectra. The third step in conducting the nutritional assessment is to determine if the pursuit of thinness is an overriding concern for patients who restrict their intake, or if binge eating and purging is a driving force in the individual's daily activities. It is useful to have the patient identify a desired goal weight, especially if still within a normal weight range.

If the evidence indicates that the adolescent has dysfunctional weight control habits, the fourth step is to determine an immediate plan of action, based on the adolescent's physical health status. For patients who have lost a significant

---

BOX 108.6   Models of Eating Disorders that May Facilitate Diagnosis and Treatment

A pediatrician demonstrates *nurturance* by acknowledging explicitly that the adolescent (1) may be ambivalent about changing any habits, (2) may not agree with the diagnosis or therapeutic recommendations, but (3) will require strength, courage, will power, and determination to recover from the eating disorder. In addition, both patients and parents benefit from recognizing that (1) the patient did *not* "decide" to develop an eating disorder, but *can* decide to recover from it; (2) the eating disorder is a coping mechanism that has both positive and negative aspects; (3) treatment and recovery can be a slow and difficult process; (4) assigning blame, guilt, or fault for the cause of the disorder is counterproductive; and (5) professional help will focus on strengths and restoring health, rather than on deficits in the adolescent or the family.

The *authoritative* aspect of the pediatrician's role comes from his or her expertise in health, growth, and physical development. The primary care treatment goal is the attainment and maintenance of health, and not merely weight gain. In this context, weight gain becomes a means to an end—the goal of wellness—and the role of the pediatrician is that of expert consultant with authoritative knowledge about health, and not a dictatorial authoritarian. Health-focused activities include monitoring the patient's physical status, setting limits on behaviors that threaten the patient's health, involving specialists with expertise in eating disorders on the treatment team, and continuing to provide primary care for health maintenance, acute illness, or injury.

The *biopsychosocial* model employs an ecologic framework with a broad scope, starting with the biologic impairments of physical health related to dysfunctional weight control practices. Although patients often protest, "But there's nothing wrong with me," there are usually symptoms and/or signs that they do not associate with these habits. In addition, there are usually unresolved conflicts in both the intrapersonal (self-esteem, self-efficacy) and interpersonal (with his or her environment at school, at home, with peers, or in the workplace) domains. Weight control practices initiated in an attempt to cope with these issues then become reinforced because of positive feedback (e.g., "external rewards" such as compliments about improved physical appearance, or "internal rewards" such as the perceived mastery over what is eaten or what is done to minimize the effects of overeating through exercise or purging).

---

amount of weight and are exhibiting signs of starvation and hypometabolism, or who have intractable vomiting and electrolyte imbalance, hospitalization should be considered. However, with early recognition, hospitalization can usually be avoided, as long as appropriate outpatient treatment is available.

Physical Examination Findings as a Motivational Tool

Providing feedback regarding abnormalities on physical examination can help motivate patients to change, since they are incontrovertible evidence of not being healthy. For example, the cold, blue hands and feet with slow capillary refill indicate that the body is not getting enough energy from food. Therefore, heat is conserved by lowering the body temperature (cold) and diverting blood flow from the distal extremities; blood that does reach the hands and feet is flowing so slowly (capillary refill) that oxygen is being removed (blue). Likewise, the loss of menstrual periods, fall in blood pressure and pulse, drop in temperature, and growth of lanugo-type hair represent physiologic adaptations to starvation, similar to the changes in a hibernating animal. Recognizing the loss of scalp hair as a complication of semistarvation, or salivary gland enlargement and permanent dental enamel erosion as a complication of vomiting can be an incentive for patients to change. The purpose is not to frighten, but to inform.

Diet and Activity Records

Recording food and drink intake as well as activities and moods aids in both assessment and treatment by identifying dietary patterns, deficiencies, excesses, and strengths; by increasing awareness of habits and behaviors; and by documenting changes during treatment. Weekly journals of intake, purging,

activity, and emotional issues can be used by the pediatrician, the dietitian, and the therapist to monitor progress. Corroborating information from parents regarding the patient's reports should be sought, since this may provide a very different perspective.

Prescribing Daily Structure

Patients with anorexia nervosa tend to have a highly structured day, while those with bulimia often lack structure, resulting in chaotic eating patterns characterized by prolonged intervals of not eating interspersed with binge/purge episodes. For both of these extremes, as well as those with less dysfunctional eating variations and problems, prescribing a daily structure around healthy eating and activity is indicated. The recommended structure should include eating three meals and at least one snack a day, distributed evenly over the day, based on balanced meal planning using the "food pyramid." Eating an adequate breakfast deserves emphasis for all adolescents, but especially those with an eating disorder. Parents should be encouraged to ensure that healthy food is available and that mealtimes are planned into the day.

In addition to structure in meals and snacks, patients should plan structure in the activities. Although exercise is often taken to extremes, completely excluding exercise may lead to further restriction of intake or surreptitious exercise in the middle of the night. The goal is to balance intake and output and to include normal, enjoyable activity as part of a healthy lifestyle.

Prescribing Nutrition

Although a dietitian should be involved in the meal planning and nutritional education of patients, as the most common initial point of contact, the primary care provider generally begins the process of prescribing nutrition. The nutrition prescription should work toward gradually increasing weight at the rate of about $\frac{1}{2}$ to 1 lb per week by increasing energy intake at 100 to 200 kCal increments every few days for patients who need to gain weight toward a target of approximately 90% of average body weight for sex, height, and age. This may require more than 2,500 kCal/day. Stabilizing intake is the goal for patients who are binging/purging. There should be a gradual introduction of "forbidden foods," while also limiting foods that may "trigger" a binge. A standard nutritional balance of 15% to 20% protein, 50% to 55% carbohydrate, and 25% to 30% fat is appropriate. However, the fat content may need to be lowered to 15% to 20% early in the treatment because of continued fat phobia. If refeeding is accomplished with meals and snacks consisting of a variety of foods and beverages (with minimal diet or fat-free products), sufficient nutrients will be provided. Although not necessary, some patients find it easier to take in needed nutrition as canned supplements rather than food. The recommended daily intake of calcium for adolescents 9 to 18 years old is 1,300 mg; if a patient is unwilling or unable to ingest calcium-rich dairy products or calcium-supplemented fruit juices to achieve this intake, supplements containing 500 mg of calcium and 100 IU of vitamin D per dose are appropriate.

Mental Health Treatment

Mental health services can be provided by a psychiatric social worker, psychologist, or psychiatrist. Selective serotonin reuptake inhibitors (SSRIs) have been shown to have no clinical benefit for patients at low weights; fluoxetine is approved for use in bulimia nervosa, even without depression. Evidence-based studies indicate that cognitive-behavioral therapy (CBT), which focuses on restructuring "thinking errors" and establishing adaptive patterns of behavior, is more effective than interpersonal or psychoanalytic approaches. Dialectic behavioral therapy (DBT), in which distorted thoughts are challenged, analyzed, and replaced with healthier ones, requires adult thinking skills and is useful for older patients with bulimia. Group therapy can provide much needed support but requires a skilled clinician, since the convergence of various levels of psychopathology can be challenging as patients may "compete" with each other.

As a general principle, the younger the patient is, the more intimately the parents need to be involved in therapy. Recent studies have shown brief, intensive family therapy to be effective for both anorexia nervosa and bulimia nervosa. The so-called Maudsley Method, described in detail by Lock and colleagues, has two phases. The initial focus is to help parents take control over the patient's eating and weight—in a supportive rather than authoritarian way. Once the patient's weight is under control, responsibility for healthy eating and weight management is transferred to the patient and the treatment focuses on more global family concerns.

PROGNOSIS

Although earlier studies suggested a poor outcome, recent data indicate that 75% to 85% of individuals hospitalized for anorexia nervosa recover fully; for bulimia nervosa, between one-third and one-half of individuals have some form of eating disorder at long-term follow-up. Consistent prognostic factors have not been well delineated, but patients who have significant depression or a history of sexual abuse may be more difficult to treat.

Suggested Readings

Ferguson CP, La Via MC, Crossan PJ, Kaye WH. Are serotonin selective reuptake inhibitors effective in underweight anorexia nervosa? *Int J Eat Dis* 1999; 25:11.

Gordon CM, Dougherty DD, Rauch SL, et al. Neuroanatomy of human appetitive function: a positron emission tomography investigation. *Int J Eating Dis* 2000;27:163.

Grice DE, Halmi KA, Fichter MM, et al. Evidence for a susceptibility gene for anorexia nervosa on chromosome 1. *Am J Hum Genet* 2002;70:787.

Halmi KA. Eating disorders in females: genetics, pathophysiology and treatment. *J Pediatr Endocrinol Metab* 2002;15(Suppl 5):1379.

Katzman DK, Zipursky RB. The impact of the disorder on bones and brain. *Ann N Y Acad Sci* 1997;817:127.

Kreipe RE, Dukarm CP. Outcome of anorexia nervosa related to treatment utilizing an adolescent medicine approach. *J Youth Adolesc* 1996;25:483.

Kreipe RE, Goldstein B, DeKing DE, et al. Heart rate power spectrum analysis of autonomic dysfunction in adolescents with anorexia nervosa. *Int J Eat Dis* 1994;16:159.

Kreipe RE, Harris JP. Myocardial impairment in eating disorders. *Pediatr Ann* 1992;21:760.

Le Grange D, Lock J, Dymek M. Family-based therapy for adolescents with bulimia nervosa. *Am J Psychother* 2003;57:237.

Levenkron S. *Treating and overcoming anorexia nervosa*. New York: Warner Books, 1990.

Lock J. Treating adolescents with eating disorders in the family context: empirical and theoretical considerations. *Child Adolesc Psychiatr Clin N Am* 2002;11:331.

Lock J, Le Grange D, Agras WS, Dare C. *Treatment manual for anorexia nervosa: a family-based approach*. New York: Guilford Press, 2001.

Rock CL, Curran-Celentano J. Nutritional management of eating disorders. *Psychiatr Clin North Am* 1995;19:701.

Rome ES, Ammerman S, Rosen DS, et al. Children and adolescents with eating disorders: the state of the art. *Pediatrics* 2003;111:e98.

Sands R, Tricker J, Sherman C, et al. Disordered eating patterns, body image, self-esteem, and physical activity in preadolescent school children. *Int J Eat Disord* 1997;21:159.

Shebendach JE, Golden NH, Jacobson MS, et al. The metabolic responses to starvation and refeeding in adolescents with anorexia nervosa. *Ann N Y Acad Sci* 1997;817:110.

Strober M, Freeman R, Lampert C, et al. Controlled family study of anorexia nervosa and bulimia nervosa: evidence of shared liability and transmission of partial syndromes. *Am J Psychiatry* 2000;157:393.

CHAPTER 109 ■ SLEEP DISORDERS

JAMES C. HARRIS

Whereas disturbance in sleep is commonly reported in adults, children generally do not complain about sleep difficulties, although their parents might; more often, children's sleep problems go unrecognized and untreated. The usual concern presented by parents is of irregular sleep habits, insufficient or too much sleep, settling for sleep at bedtime, poor sleep, waking during the night, nightmares, night terrors, sleepwalking, bedwetting, and sleepiness during the day. Some disorders are more severe, such as narcolepsy, sleep apnea syndrome (breathing-related sleep disorder), and sudden infant death syndrome (SIDS) associated with apnea. In addition, injuries may occur during sleepwalking. In other instances, sleep problems may be related to disorders such as depression or epilepsy with nighttime seizures.

Sleep is one aspect of the 25-hour circadian sleep–wake cycle that is entrained to a 24-hour clock. Time cues related to bedtime and waking time, mealtime, and school schedules are all considerations in the daily cycle. The sleep cycle is accompanied by particular hormonal rhythms that occur during sleep, such as growth hormone, prolactin, and cortisol release. Growth hormone is released during the initial deep sleep period, and prolactin reaches its peak between 5 and 7 o'clock in the morning. Corticosteroid secretion ordinarily is initiated during the night and may become desynchronized in sleep with changes in the sleep–wake schedule. When the sleep schedule changes, cortisol is initially released at the same time as before, but it gradually adjusts or resynchronizes to the new cycle.

Ordinarily, sleep problems are evaluated on an outpatient basis; more complicated cases, however, may require inpatient sleep laboratory assessment. Developments in classification of sleep problems have provided new information about when these sleep laboratory assessments should be carried out.

EPIDEMIOLOGY

What may seem to be an uninterrupted sleep period is actually made up of a series of 60- to 90-minute cycles, with periods of both non–rapid eye movement (non-REM) and REM sleep. Although these cycles seem uniform and woven together, a child normally experiences five to ten brief, behavioral arousals during the night despite being observed to apparently sleep through the night. In sleep disorders, these underlying patterns may be disrupted with wake-to-sleep transition problems, difficulty in shifting from one sleep stage to another, and failure to return to sleep after a brief arousal. The development of sleep is related to age; the total amount of sleep decreases as children become older, as does the total amount of REM sleep and the total amount of stage 3 to 4 (deep) sleep. Sleep in premature infants is marked by more wakefulness than in full-term infants, with more irregularity and instability in the sleep–wake mechanism. In infancy, the amounts of REM sleep or active sleep are substantially greater than they are later in life, with almost 50% of the infant's time in the first week of life being spent in REM sleep. Gradually, the REM sleep cycles are shifted so that most REM sleep occurs in the second half of the night.

As children grow older, separation anxiety becomes more of an issue for toddlers and young children, and bedtime fears, nightmares, bedwetting, and night terrors emerge. The older group, particularly the adolescent, begins to show sleep patterns similar to those of adults. Difficulty falling asleep, waking during the night, difficulty getting up in the morning, and daytime sleepiness are commonly reported in adolescence. Individual differences in sleep requirements and patterns occur among children, so rigid sleep schedules may complicate bedtime difficulties and sleep problems.

During the first year of life, after the establishment of a full-night sleep pattern, a period of wakefulness occurs at approximately 9 to 11 months of age, followed by the reestablishment of a full-night sleep pattern. In toddlers, the major difficulties are in settling down to sleep and in nighttime waking. In the preschool child, problems with extensive bedtime routines and resisting falling asleep are common. One study found that two-thirds of normal 5-year-old children require more than 30 minutes to fall asleep.

In the grade-school years, parents often note restless sleep. Sleep-related problems are increased when children develop ear, nose, and throat symptoms. Children with emotional and behavioral difficulties have significantly higher numbers of sleep complaints. Achenbach found that clinically referred children had higher rates of nightmares, excessive tiredness, excessive sleep, difficulty with sleeping, and too little sleep compared with normal children. Simeon found, in a sample of 962 normal children and 103 child psychiatry patients, that sleep talking, difficulty falling asleep, night waking, and enuresis, as well as being overtired, were three times higher among patients than in the normal group. Poor or restless sleep was six times as frequent.

Gender differences were not noted among normal children, but large differences were noted between boys and girls in the psychiatric population, with boys having more sleep talking, enuresis, early morning waking, and daytime naps. Girls reported more restless sleep, night waking, and poor sleep. Therefore, both normal and behaviorally disturbed children have a variety of sleep problems. Furthermore, an association exists between frequency of sleep problems and psychological and behavioral disorders.

CLASSIFICATION

The classification system for sleep disorders deals with chronic disorders, not transient disturbances that are part of everyday life. Sleep problems lasting a few nights after a psychosocial stressor are not diagnosed as sleep disorders. Children who are chronically symptomatic for more than a month, however, require further assessment for diagnosis and treatment.

Problems in sleep accompany both mental and physical disorders, particularly conditions involving changes in mood and those causing pain or discomfort. Sleep disturbances may occur at the beginning of an illness and can exacerbate other disorders. If sleep disturbance is the predominant complaint, however, sleep disorder is the primary diagnosis.

The two major groups of sleep disorders are the dyssomnias and the parasomnias. In dyssomnia, the primary difficulty and disturbance is in the quality, timing, or amount of sleep. In parasomnia, the primary disturbance is an abnormal event that occurs during sleep. Other conditions, such as sleep apnea, which is associated with increased daytime sleepiness, and narcolepsy, are classified as hypersomnias related to a known organic factor. Nocturnal enuresis occurring in the first third of the night and associated with sudden arousal from sleep may be regarded as a sleep disorder. A primary sleep condition independent of known mental or physical conditions would be considered a primary insomnia or hypersomnia.

Included among the dyssomnias are insomnias, hypersomnias, and circadian rhythm sleep (sleep–wake schedule) disorders. In insomnia, sleep is deficient in quality or in an amount necessary for normal active daytime functioning. In hypersomnia (excessive daytime sleepiness), the individual feels excessively sleepy during the daytime despite apparently normal sleep length. In circadian rhythm sleep disorders, the person's sleeping and daytime waking pattern is different and is not in keeping with an appropriate day–night routine for the environment.

Insomnia includes a complaint of difficulty in both initiating and maintaining sleep or of not feeling rested after sleep that is apparently adequate. Diagnostic criteria for primary insomnia are shown in Box 109.1. To make the diagnosis, the sleep problem must occur at least three times a week for at least 1 month and must lead to complaints of daytime fatigue or observations by others of symptoms related to sleep, such as irritability. It may be primarily related to a known organic factor or related to a nonorganic mental disorder.

Considerable variation exists in the amount of time it takes for a person to fall asleep or in the amount of sleep that an individual feels is needed to be alert and rested. Ordinarily, sleep begins within 30 minutes after establishing a setting that is appropriate for sleep, although sleep length is variable depending on age. Insomnia may be complicated by treatment with pharmacologic agents such as sedatives or hypnotics. It occurs more often after periods of stress and is related to behavioral or emotional symptoms.

With childhood-onset insomnia, it may take longer to fall asleep, and the sleep may be ill defined and associated with an atypical electroencephalographic (EEG) abnormality. In adolescents, the complaint may be difficulty in falling asleep or premature wakening. In other instances, a delayed sleep phase syndrome may be present in which sleep onset difficulties are associated with difficulty waking in the morning. If the individual is allowed to continue to sleep, however, he or she sleeps a normal number of hours. Price found that normal eleventh- and twelfth-grade students reported a 12.6% incidence of severe sleep disturbance. Those with sleep problems also reported more tension, worries, moodiness, and difficulty with solving personal problems, as well as low self-esteem.

Insomnia may occur in conjunction with other mental disorders such as depressive disorders, anxiety disorders, and adjustment disorder with anxious mood or obsessive-compulsive personality. As noted, insomnia also may occur because of a known organic factor, such as a specific medical condition and the use of psychoactive drugs. These disorders are generally symptomatic when the patient is awake or asleep, as in the case of pain. Some physical disorders seem symptomatic only during sleep, however, as seen in sleep apnea, in which waking respiration is normal. Drugs commonly influencing sleep are amphetamines or other stimulants, corticosteroids, and bronchodilators. Psychoactive drugs and alcohol or amphetamine dependence may disturb sleep as well.

In primary insomnia, the individual frequently worries about not being able to fall asleep at night, and this may become a preoccupation. The individual's worries about unsuccessful attempts to fall asleep increase arousal. However, he or she might be able to fall asleep when not trying to sleep (e.g., while watching television or when away from the usual environment).

HYPERSOMNIA DISORDERS

Children and adolescents with excessive daytime sleepiness or somnolence may be thought to be inattentive and be labeled as lazy or poor learners. These symptoms may be a consequence of insufficient nighttime sleep, sleep quality, or circadian factors. Sleep apnea may be an unrecognized cause of disrupted sleep. Complaints of sleepiness sometimes are minimized by clinicians. The onset of excessive daytime sleepiness often first occurs during adolescence. A careful physical examination and sleep history are important.

Diagnostic criteria for primary hypersomnia are listed in Box 109.2. The primary features are excessive daytime sleepiness or sleep attacks (not accounted for by inadequate amounts of sleep), or prolonged transition into a fully awake state when awakening (sleep drunkenness). The condition occurs every day for at least 1 month or episodically for longer periods of time and is severe enough to interfere with social activities, relationships, and school. Hypersomnia disorders may be primary or related to nonorganic mental factors or organic conditions. Daytime sleepiness is defined as falling asleep easily, often in 5 minutes or less, at any time during the day, even after a normal, prolonged amount of night sleep. Falling asleep is unintentional, making sleep attacks discrete periods of sudden irresistible sleep. Ordinarily, hypersomnia is present every day, most commonly related to sleep apnea or narcolepsy. It may be episodic in the Kleine-Levin syndrome and in atypical forms of depression.

The course of this condition is related to the presence of other associated physical or mental disorders or to the primary

---

BOX 109.1   **Diagnostic Criteria for Primary Insomnia**

A. The predominant complaint is difficulty initiating or maintaining sleep, or nonrestorative sleep, for at least 1 month.

B. The sleep disturbance (or associated daytime fatigue) causes clinically significant distress or impairment in social, occupational, or other important areas of functioning.

C. The sleep disturbance does not occur exclusively during the course of narcolepsy, breathing-related sleep disorder, circadian rhythm sleep disorder, or a parasomnia.

D. The disturbance does not occur exclusively during the course of another mental disorder (e.g., major depressive disorder, generalized anxiety disorder, delirium).

E. The disturbance is not due to the direct physiologic effects of a substance (e.g., a drug of abuse, a medication) or a general medical condition.

BOX 109.2   Diagnostic Criteria for Primary Hypersomnia

A. The predominant complaint is excessive sleepiness for at least 1 month (or less if recurrent) as evidenced by either prolonged sleep episodes or daytime sleep episodes that occur almost daily.

B. The excessive sleepiness causes clinically significant distress or impairment in social, occupational, or other important areas of functioning.

C. The excessive sleepiness is not better accounted for by insomnia and does not occur exclusively during the course of another sleep disorder (e.g., narcolepsy, breathing-related sleep disorder, circadian rhythm sleep disorder, or a parasomnia) and cannot be accounted for by an inadequate amount of sleep.

D. The disturbance does not occur exclusively during the course of another mental disorder.

E. The disturbance is not due to the direct physiologic effects of a substance (e.g., a drug of abuse, a medication) or a general medical condition.

Specify if:

Recurrent: if there are periods of excessive sleepiness that last at least 3 days occurring several times a year for at least 2 years

Reprinted with permission from American Psychiatric Association. *Diagnostic and statistical manual of mental disorders,* 4th ed., text revision. Washington, DC: American Psychiatric Association, 2000.

BOX 109.3   Diagnostic Criteria for Breathing-Related Sleep Disorder

A. Sleep disruption, leading to excessive sleepiness or insomnia, that is judged to be due to a sleep-related breathing condition (e.g., obstructive or central sleep apnea syndrome or central alveolar hypoventilation syndrome)

B. The disturbance is not better accounted for by another mental disorder and is not due to the direct physiologic effects of a substance (e.g., a drug of abuse, a medication) or another general condition (other than a breathing-related disorder).

Reprinted with permission from American Psychiatric Association. *Diagnostic and statistical manual of mental disorders,* 4th ed., text revision. Washington, DC: American Psychiatric Association, 2000.

---

condition. Social and occupational impairment may be mild or severe. Individuals with these problems may become demoralized, and the complications of accidental injury may ensue because of the excessive sleepiness.

Hypersomnia may be related to another mental disorder, particularly mood disorders. Hypersomnia associated with mental disorders occurs more often in adolescence; in contrast, older adults typically complain of insomnia. In other mental disorders, such as somatoform disorder, some personality disorders, or schizophrenia, hypersomnia is uncommon; daytime drowsiness is attributed to nonrestorative sleep.

The majority of cases of hypersomnia or excessive daytime somnolence are related to a known organic factor. Approximately 50% of these are associated with sleep apnea, approximately 25% with narcolepsy, and approximately 10% with sleep-related myoclonus.

When the hypersomnia is related to narcolepsy, cataplexy (episodic loss of muscle tone initiated by strong emotions), hypnagogic or hypnopompic hallucinations, and sleep paralysis (inability to move while falling asleep or on sudden wakening) occur.

Narcolepsy ordinarily begins around puberty. However, obstructive sleep apnea is seen primarily in infants and in older children with large tonsils and adenoids. Both of these conditions lead to impairment. In narcolepsy, the person tries to exert control over his or her emotions, and this may lead to a lack of expressiveness that affects social relations. Individuals with sleep apnea may demonstrate mood changes or irritability, distractibility, and difficulty with attention and memory. On the other hand, primary hypersomnia is not related to another mental disorder or known organic factor.

Sleep Apnea Hypersomnia Syndrome (Breathing-Related Sleep Disorder)

Sleep apnea hypersomnia syndrome may occur in children of any age, but the incidence increases with age and involves boys more often than girls. The diagnostic criteria for breathing-related sleep disorder are shown in Box 109.3. Predisposing factors include enlarged tonsils or adenoids, upper airway or maxillofacial abnormalities, hyperthyroidism, and obesity. Loud snoring is followed by pauses in respiration and brief arousals that are often accompanied by restless movements. Associated symptoms include decreased school performance, excessive daytime sleepiness, recurrence of nocturnal enuresis, morning headaches, changes in mood and personality, changes in weight, and if the condition is persistent and severe, development of pulmonary hypertension. Its effect on intellectual functioning may be greater than that of narcolepsy. Some children may be misdiagnosed as intellectually limited. If symptoms are unrecognized at night, with time, symptoms may become more apparent during the day, particularly if cardiovascular or pulmonary abnormalities develop.

SIDS may be linked to apnea in infants. SIDS is responsible for the death of 2 to 3 infants per 1,000 live births. Children at greater risk are those who have had prior intensive care and whose mothers are addicted to drugs. It occurs more often in boys. Near-miss SIDS is a disorder with various unrelated respiratory, cardiac, or sleep-stage difficulties. Siblings of children with this disorder may have a three- to fourfold increase of SIDS. Some studies have suggested longer intervals between active sleep in the newborn and a decreased tendency to enter short waking periods for 2 to 3 months, suggesting an increased tendency to remain asleep or a problem in arousal from sleep.

More information about sleep apnea and SIDS can be found in Chapter 117B.

Kleine-Levin Syndrome

In Kleine-Levin syndrome, recurrent episodes of excessive sleepiness (hypersomnia) occur that may last days to weeks, taking place in intervals that may be weeks or months apart. It occurs most often in adolescent boys and is associated with excessive binge-eating and frequently with weight gain, hypersexuality, and mood disorders (irritability, aggression). It may represent hypothalamic and diencephalic dysfunction.

Narcolepsy

The prevalence of narcolepsy is thought to be from 0.03% to 0.16% in the general population. Twenty percent of adults with narcolepsy report that they had daytime sleepiness before age 11 years. Family studies indicate a 20 to 40 times increased risk of narcolepsy in first-degree relatives, and twin studies suggest that nongenetic factors also play a role. There are transgenetic mouse models and genetic models in dogs (Dobermans) showing hypocretin dysfunction. The tight association between narcolepsy–cataplexy and the human leukocyte antigen (HLA) allele DQB1*0602 suggests that narcolepsy has an autoimmune etiology in humans.

Children with this disorder are usually referred when teachers complain about napping during class. Unrecognized microsleep may occur, and others may be unaware that naps are taking place. Children with this disorder have been viewed by teachers as poorly motivated and may be thought to have attention deficits or learning problems. The child may become active or apparently overactive as he or she struggles with sleepiness. Hypnagogic, auditory, or visual hallucinations are vivid, often frightening, and may not be reported to parents. Children with this condition may be fearful of going to bed because of their hallucinatory experiences. Unlike those with seizure disorders, children who lose muscle tone with this condition remain aware of their surroundings. Shortened sleep onset with sleep-onset REM are characteristic features. The recent discovery of hypocretin deficiency as the pathophysiologic basis for narcolepsy–cataplexy [neurodegeneration of hypothalamic orexin (hypocretin)-containing neurons] is likely to spur the development of hypocretin analogues for treatment.

CIRCADIAN RHYTHM SLEEP DISORDER

Sleep–Wake Schedule Disorders

The circadian rhythm sleep disorder, as shown in Box 109.4, is characterized by a lack of synchronization between normal sleep–wake schedules demanded by the external environment and the individual's internal circadian rhythm. This results in complaints of either insomnia or hypersomnia, because the individual has difficulty in falling asleep until late at night and also has problems in waking the following day. Children with this condition may have met the criteria for either insomnia or hypersomnia disorder. The recent recognition of genetic influences in the control of circadian rhythms also may spur the development of specific therapies for circadian rhythm disorders.

Delayed Sleep Phase Type

In circadian rhythm sleep disorder, the onset of sleep is advanced or delayed in relation to sleep. If advanced cycles are evident, the individual falls asleep early in the evening and wakes for the day in the middle of the night. In the delayed type, sleep occurs later in the evening and waking occurs in the middle of the day. A disorganized type also exists, in which sleep is generally random in pattern and no major daily sleep period is evident. Finally, the frequently changing type is the

---

BOX 109.4	Diagnostic Criteria for Circadian Rhythm Sleep Disorder

A. A persistent or recurrent pattern of sleep disruption leading to excessive sleepiness or insomnia that is due to a mismatch between the sleep–wake schedule required by a person's environment and his or her circadian sleep–wake pattern.

B. The sleep disturbance causes clinically significant distress or impairment in social, occupational, or other important areas of functioning.

C. The disturbance does not occur exclusively during the course of another sleep disorder or mental disorder.

D. The disturbance is not due to the direct physiologic effects of a substance (e.g., a drug of abuse, a medication) or a general medical condition.

Specify type:

Delayed sleep phase type: a persistent pattern of late sleep onset and late awakening times, with an inability to fall asleep and awaken at a desired earlier time.

Jet lag type: sleepiness and alertness that occur at an inappropriate time of day relative to local time, occurring after repeated travel across more than one time zone.

Shift work type: insomnia during the major sleep period or excessive sleepiness during the major awake period associated with night shift work or frequently changing shift work.

Unspecified type

Reprinted with permission from American Psychiatric Association. *Diagnostic and statistical manual of mental disorders*, 4th ed., text revision. Washington, DC: American Psychiatric Association, 2000.

---

result of frequent changes in sleeping and waking times (e.g., airline travel involving time zone changes).

Associated with the sleep phase type are nonspecific symptoms such as lack of energy and irritability or malaise. Because the circadian rhythm normally lengthens during adolescence, vulnerability to the delayed type increases during this age period. Delayed sleep phase problems are reported in as many as 7% of adolescents. The disorganized type may occur at any age. Impairment in social function is primarily related to the time of day that the sleep disturbance occurs. The condition may be complicated by accidents because of lack of alertness. The *Diagnostic and Statistical Manual of Mental Disorders,* Fourth Edition (*DSM-IV-TR*) diagnostic criteria for circadian rhythm sleep disorder are a mismatch between the normal sleep–wake schedule for a person's environment and his or her circadian sleep–wake pattern, resulting in complaints of either insomnia or hypersomnia.

PARASOMNIAS

In the parasomnias, an abnormal event occurs either during sleep or at the threshold between wakefulness and sleep. This disturbance is the primary complaint and not sleepiness or wakefulness, although symptoms such as sleep apnea (breathing-related sleep disorder) that occur during sleep may lead to a complaint of daytime sleepiness and daytime learning problems. Children with chronic parasomnias may also present with sleep-disordered breathing or, to a lesser extent, restless legs syndrome. The resolution of the parasomnia after the treatment of the sleep-disordered–breathing or restless legs syndrome suggests that the sleep-disordered breathing might trigger the parasomnia.

In a parasomnia such as a nightmare, the child complains about the event, whereas in a night terror, the parent, rather than the child, complains about the event. From the perspective of the sleep disorder classification, enuresis occurring during sleep is a parasomnia. In some instances, nocturnal seizure disorders may mimic the symptoms of parasomnia, thus requiring an overnight EEG to clarify whether the seizures are related to particular sleep stages. Studies of twin cohorts and families with sleep terror and sleepwalking suggest genetic involvement in parasomnias.

Nightmare Disorder

Nightmares are frightening dreams that lead to repeated awakenings from nighttime sleep or daytime naps. The *DSM-IV-TR* criteria for nightmare disorder are shown in Box 109.5. On awakening, the child or adolescent may be tearful or agitated, appear fearful, and seek comfort from the parent. Dream content is best recalled immediately after waking by children with sufficient verbal abilities to describe their experiences. Nightmares occur during REM sleep episodes, and REM sleep occurs primarily in the second half of the night. Therefore, awakenings from nightmares most commonly occur during the second half of the night, being most frequent in the early morning hours. There is tonic motor inhibition in REM sleep, so a child does not appear agitated or talk in sleep during the nightmare. The fearful behavior related to nightmares comes to others' attention only after the child is awakened.

Nightmares occur with equal frequency in boys and girls; the peak age of onset is between ages 3 and 6 years. Nightmares are found in 10% to 50% of preschool children and continue to be experienced, but with less frequency, in older children, adolescents, and adults. Based on behavior after awakening, nightmares also may occur in preverbal children and in children who are intellectually disabled.

The dream is sometimes described by younger children as consisting of pictures that they see at night. The dream consists of vivid mental imagery that is usually visual but may contain auditory, olfactory, or tactile experiences, all of which may be anxiety provoking. During dreaming, it is thought that daily emotional experiences are consolidated into long-term memory. Dreams present a bizarre pattern but generally have a simple narrative structure. Foulkes studied the content of dreams in children at different ages and found that nightmares most commonly concern physical danger to the child by being pursued, attacked, or directly injured. Fears of personal failure or embarrassment are common themes in older children and adolescents. Animals are prominent in the nightmares of preschool children.

The majority of children with nightmares outgrow them. Occasional nightmares are not a reason for concern; however, recurrent or frequent nightmares (several per week) may reflect stressful daytime experiences and require evaluation. Nightmares are not diagnosed if they occur as part of another mental disorder or a particular medical condition, or are secondary to medication or a drug of abuse.

Sleep Terror Disorder (*Pavor Nocturnus*)

Sleep terror disorder is a condition marked by repeated episodes of abrupt awakening from sleep. The episode usually begins with a scream and ordinarily occurs during the first third of the night, in the first interval of non-REM sleep. Sleep terror is accompanied by EEG delta activity (sleep stages 3 and 4) and lasts 1 to 10 minutes. Diagnostic criteria for sleep terror disorder are shown in Box 109.6.

BOX 109.5   Diagnostic Criteria for Nightmare Disorder

A. Repeated awakenings from the major sleep period or naps with detailed recall of extended and extremely frightening dreams, usually involving threats to survival, security, or self-esteem. The awakenings generally occur during the second half of the sleep period.
B. On awakening from the frightening dreams, the person rapidly becomes oriented and alert (in contrast to the confusion and disorientation seen in sleep terror disorder and some forms of epilepsy).
C. The dream experience, or the sleep disturbance resulting from the awakening, causes clinically significant distress or impairment in social, occupational, or other important areas of functioning.
D. The nightmares do not occur exclusively during the course of another mental disorder (e.g., delirium, post-traumatic stress disorder) and are not due to the direct physiologic effects of a substance (e.g., a drug of abuse, a medication) or a general medical condition.

Reprinted with permission from American Psychiatric Association. *Diagnostic and statistical manual of mental disorders*, 4th ed., text revision. Washington, DC: American Psychiatric Association, 2000.

BOX 109.6   Diagnostic Criteria for Sleep Terror Disorder

A. Recurrent episodes of abrupt awakening from sleep, usually occurring during the first third of the major sleep episode and beginning with a panicky scream.
B. Intense fear and signs of autonomic arousal, such as tachycardia, rapid breathing, and sweating, during each episode.
C. Relative unresponsiveness to efforts of others to comfort the person during the episode.
D. No detailed dream is recalled and there is amnesia for the episode.
E. The episodes cause clinically significant distress or impairment in social, occupational, or other important areas of functioning.
F. The disturbance is not due to the direct physiologic effects of a substance (e.g., a drug of abuse, a medication) or a general medical condition.

Reprinted with permission from American Psychiatric Association. *Diagnostic and statistical manual of mental disorders*, 4th ed., text revision. Washington, DC: American Psychiatric Association, 2000.

In a typical episode, the child sits up abruptly in bed, appears frightened, and demonstrates signs of intense anxiety, including dilated pupils, excessive perspiration, piloerection, rapid breathing, and rapid pulse. The child is unresponsive to the efforts of others to comfort him or her until the agitation and confusion subside as the child gradually awakens. There is no memory of the episode the following morning, and behavior may be entirely normal. Occasionally, the child recounts a sense of terror on being aroused from the night terror, but only fragmentary mental images exist, unlike dream recall. These episodes occur more often with fatigue and after stress.

Before a severe episode, EEG delta waves may be higher in amplitude than usual for that phase of sleep, and breathing and heart rate may be slower. The episode itself may be accompanied by a twofold or fourfold increase in heart rate. No psychopathology is associated consistently with night terror in children. The age of onset is ordinarily between 4 and 12 years. The course is variable, usually occurring in intervals of days or weeks, but episodes may occur on consecutive nights. The disorder gradually resolves in children and often disappears by early adolescence. Night terrors are very distressing to parents, and their features must be carefully reviewed. To avoid accidental injury, the child must be protected if he or she gets up during the episode.

Febrile illness has been reported as a predisposing factor. The prevalence is estimated to be 1% to 4% for the full disorder, although a larger percentage of children may have isolated symptoms. This condition is more common in boys than in girls. The disorder is more common among first-degree relatives of people with the disorder than in the general population. Night terrors are arousal disorders and may be followed by sleepwalking as the child grows older.

Treatment consists primarily of educating the family regarding the nature of the parasomnia. In those instances in which symptoms occur quite frequently and are disruptive to the family, pharmacologic treatment with anxiolytic drugs may be indicated.

Sleepwalking Disorder

The diagnostic criteria for sleepwalking disorder are shown in Box 109.7. In sleepwalking, repeated episodes of complex movements lead to leaving bed and walking without the individual's being conscious of the episode or remembering it later. It ordinarily occurs during the first third of the major sleep period, the period of non-REM sleep that contains EEG delta activity (phases 3 and 4). Sleepwalking lasts from a few minutes to approximately half an hour. In a typical episode, the child sits up, makes persevering movements such as picking at a blanket, and then proceeds to semipurposeful movements including walking, opening doors, eating, dressing, or going to the bathroom. The episode may terminate before sleepwalking is accomplished.

When observed, the sleepwalker has a blank face, appears to stare, and is unresponsive to the efforts of others to communicate with him or her or efforts to influence the sleepwalking. Awakening is accomplished only with great difficulty. Coordination is poor during the episode; however, the individual may see and walk around objects. The child may stumble or lose his or her balance and be injured, particularly when taking a hazardous route. If walking terminates spontaneously, the child awakens but is disoriented. In other instances, the child may return to bed without reaching consciousness or may fall asleep in another place away from the bed and be surprised at finding him- or herself there on waking.

On the EEG, slow waves may increase in amplitude in stage 4 sleep just preceding the episode. A flattening of the EEG

BOX 109.7	Diagnostic Criteria for Sleepwalking Disorder

A. Repeated episodes of rising from bed during sleep and walking about, usually occurring during the first third of the major sleep episode.
B. While sleepwalking, the person has a blank, staring face, is relatively unresponsive to the efforts of others to communicate with him or her, and can be awakened only with great difficulty.
C. On awakening (either from the sleepwalking episode or the next morning), the person has amnesia for the episode.
D. Within several minutes after awakening from the sleepwalking episode, there is no impairment of mental activity or behavior (although initially there may be a short period of confusion or disorientation).
E. The sleepwalking causes clinically significant distress or impairment in social, occupational, or other important areas of functioning.
F. The disturbance is not due to the direct physiologic effects of a substance (e.g., a drug of abuse, a medication) or a general medical condition.

Reprinted with permission from American Psychiatric Association. *Diagnostic and statistical manual of mental disorders*, 4th ed., text revision. Washington, DC: American Psychiatric Association, 2000.

---

occurs, indicating arousal before the episode itself. Ordinarily, the high-amplitude slow wave pattern gives way to a mixture of non-REM stages and lower-amplitude EEG activity. This condition is more likely to occur in children who are fatigued or have experienced stress the previous day.

Aggression toward other persons or objects in the environment is infrequent during sleepwalking. If the condition is accompanied by sleep talking, the articulation is poor. Sleepwalkers have an increased incidence of other episodic disorders associated with non-REM sleep, such as sleep terrors. No specific psychopathology, however, has been observed in children with this condition. The onset is ordinarily between 6 and 12 years of age, and it lasts several years. Symptoms usually resolve by the end of the teens or in the early twenties. The primary impairment is the occurrence of injuries during an episode. Febrile illness may occasionally be associated.

Prevalence is estimated at 1% to 6%, but as many as 15% of children may have isolated episodes. It occurs more commonly in boys than in girls. It is also more common among first-degree biologic relatives than in the general population.

Suggested Readings

Chabas D, Taheri S, Renier C, Mignot E. The genetics of narcolepsy. *Ann Rev Genomics Hum Genet* 2003;4:459.
Drake C, Nickel C, Burduvali E, et al. The pediatric daytime sleepiness scale (PDSS): sleep habits and school outcomes in middle-school children. *Sleep* 2003;26:455.
Ferber R. *Solve your child's sleep problem*. New York: Simon and Schuster, 1986.
Guilleminault C, Palombini L, Pelayo R, Chervin RD. Sleepwalking and sleep terrors in prepubertal children: what triggers them? *Pediatrics* 2003;111: e17.

Halbower AC, Marcus CL. Sleep disorders in children. *Curr Opin Pulm Med* 2003;9:471.

Ivanenko A, Tauman R, Gozal D. Modafinil in the treatment of excessive daytime sleepiness in children. *Sleep Med* 2003;4:579.

Kotagal S. Sleep disorders in childhood. *Neurol Clin* 2003;21:961.

Mindell JA, Barrett KM. Nightmares and anxiety in elementary-aged children: is there a relationship. *Child Care Health Dev* 2002;28(4):317.

Mindell JA, Owens JA, Carskadon MA. Developmental features of sleep. *Child Adolesc Psychiatr Clin N Am* 1999;8(4):695.

Nixon GM, Kermack AS, Davis GM, et al. Planning adenotonsillectomy in children with obstructive sleep apnea: the role of overnight oximetry. *Pediatrics* 2004;113(1 Pt 1):e19.

Owens JA, Spirito A, McGuinn M, Nobile C. Sleep habits and sleep disturbance in elementary school-aged children. *J Dev Behav Pediatr* 2000;21.

Rosen CL. Sleep disorders in infancy, childhood, and adolescence. *Curr Opin Pulm Med* 1997;3:449.

Schechter MS. Section on pediatric pulmonology, subcommittee on obstructive sleep apnea syndrome. Technical report: diagnosis and management of childhood obstructive sleep apnea syndrome. *Pediatrics* 2002;109(4):e69.

Stores G. Practitioner review: assessment and treatment of sleep disorders in children and adolescents. *J Child Psychol Psychiatry* 1996;37:907.

Urschitz MS, Guenther A, Eggebrecht E, et al. Snoring, intermittent hypoxia and academic performance in primary school children. *Am J Respir Crit Care Med* 2003;168:464.

Wing YK, Hui SH, Pak WM, et al. A controlled study of sleep related disordered breathing in obese children. *Arch Dis Child* 2003;88:1043.

Wise MS, Lynch J. Narcolepsy in children. *Semin Pediatr Neurol* 2001;8(4):198.

CHAPTER 110 ■ PSYCHOTIC DISORDERS

JAMES C. HARRIS

Psychotic disorders are major mental illnesses that involve abnormalities in thinking, belief systems, and perception. These are demonstrated clinically through incoherence in thinking, delusions, and hallucinations and are associated with major behavioral changes. The psychotic disorders are less common in preadolescence, usually becoming evident for the first time in adolescence and adulthood. Assessment is more difficult in young children and in mentally retarded individuals because the major symptoms are identified through an interview assessment.

The conditions included are schizophrenia, affective and bipolar (manic-depressive) psychoses, organic psychotic states, and atypical psychoses. The last two conditions are not covered here. Autistic disorder and other pervasive developmental disorders are categorized separately because these conditions are neuropsychiatric developmental disorders.

The underlying brain mechanism for schizophrenia has not been identified; however, both genetic and environmental risk factors exist. Neuroimaging studies show reduced cortical gray matter volume in schizophrenia and, in childhood-onset schizophrenia, striking progressive loss of cortical gray matter following the onset of psychosis, more so than in adult onset. There is loss of gray matter in frontal, temporal, and parietal brain regions. Apoptosis (programmed cell death) has been proposed as a contributing pathophysiologic mechanism.

The identification of a chromosomal disorder in some families with bipolar disorder lends further credence to the eventual discovery of a genetic basis for some cases of this disorder. Ongoing investigations in brain imaging may provide additional information about brain dysfunction in each of these conditions.

SCHIZOPHRENIA

Schizophrenia ordinarily presents for the first time in adolescence or young adulthood. It may occur in the prepubertal years, but the diagnostic criteria for adults are difficult to apply in children younger than age 7 years. Whether the condition could be diagnosed before age 7 is a subject of disagreement. The characteristic features include the following:

- **Disorder in thinking:** Thoughts are often incoherent, and the train of thought is lost. This difficulty in thinking is referred to as *derailment* or *loosening of association*.
- **Delusional beliefs:** Delusions are irrational beliefs and may take on a paranoid form in older children. The delusional beliefs arise out of ordinary consciousness and are not secondary to hallucinations or the result of a mood disturbance.
- **Hallucinatory experience:** The hallucination is a false perception that occurs without external sensory stimulation. In schizophrenia, hallucinations are primarily auditory and are described as voices outside the child or adolescent's head that may speak with him or her directly or make reference to him or her in the third person.
- **Disturbance of mobility:** Catatonic behavior refers to motoric immobility or certain types of excessive motor activity (purposeless agitation), extreme negativism (apparently motiveless resistance to instructions or attempts to be moved), abnormal posturing, mutism, echolalia, or echopraxia. Catatonia occurs in both schizophrenia and in affective disorders.

In addition to these classic symptoms, negative symptoms (flat affect, avolition) and, it is increasingly recognized, cognitive deficits are present to varying degrees.

Schizophrenia may have an abrupt or gradual onset. Particularly when the onset is gradual, it may be more difficult for family members to recognize the seriousness of the condition. Children who develop schizophrenia often have a history of developmental delay, although their previous presentation may be normal. When developmental delay is present, language difficulties, clumsiness, social isolation, and muscular hypotonia may be noted. The condition may follow a remitting or chronic course. There may be partial recovery with resolution of acute symptoms, but abnormal motivation and a decreased interest in routine events may follow the initial presentation as residual symptoms.

Epidemiology

In childhood-onset cases the male-to-female ratio is about 2.5:1, but by adolescence the male-to-female ratio is near 1:1. An increased risk exists in first-degree relatives. If a parent or a sibling is schizophrenic, the risk is approximately 12 times that of the general population for the child; the rate of onset in adolescence is approximately 3 per 10,000, compared with 1% in the general population. Children of schizophrenic parents who are raised in foster or adoptive homes maintain the risk for the disorder. Concordance is greater in monozygotic twins.

A schizophrenia-like presentation may occur with stress in children who have brain dysfunction. These are more often brief reactive psychoses, but they may sometimes take on a more chronic picture. Family interactions may contribute to the course of the illness. Family difficulties in adapting to the disorder and strongly expressed, often hostile emotions by family members may precipitate relapse.

Diagnosis

Psychiatric assessment involves clarifying the major symptom picture. The diagnosis is generally straightforward in older adolescents, but in the rare instance that it occurs in a younger child, assessment may be more difficult; unless the specific diagnostic questions are asked, the child may be misdiagnosed as overactive or anxious. Whenever clouding of consciousness occurs, a neurologic disorder should be considered. Epilepsy is an important consideration because confusion and sometimes unusual behavior may follow a seizure. Careful neurologic examination is essential in patient assessment.

Adolescents with a history of autistic disorder have problems in language communication that may be confused with schizophrenia. Brief psychotic episodes may occur after stress in this condition. Both delusions and hallucinations occur in affective psychosis; however, the occurrence of classic manic symptoms and abnormal mental experiences that are congruent with mood, such as the belief that the body is decaying or that one has special powers, can usually differentiate the disorders.

Treatment

A comprehensive treatment program is essential in childhood and adolescence. It should take into account the effect of the illness on the family, the family's response to it, and the need for an appropriate psychoeducational program. The family should be actively involved in the treatment, just as families are involved in other chronic conditions. The physician should help the family to understand that they are not to blame for the disorder.

School programs must be carefully selected, because many programs for the emotionally disturbed inappropriately mix children who have schizophrenia with those who have disruptive behavior disorders. A program that focuses specifically on treating schizophrenia should be sought. During the acute phase of the illness, neuroleptic medication is indicated, and ordinarily this treatment is initiated on an inpatient basis. After hospital discharge, careful psychiatric rehabilitation is required, particularly if a residual lack of motivation and difficulty in adaptation exist. Ongoing family counseling helps to reduce excessive emotional involvement, and supportive psychotherapy is maintained for the child or adolescent. The outcome is variable, but the prognosis is better when a single acute episode occurs in a previously normal child or adolescent. However, overall the prognosis is poor with a chronic course and there is a poor outcome in over 75% of severe cases. New findings linked to the neurodevelopment suggest the importance of neuroprotective strategies that might counteract progressive neuronal loss in childhood-onset cases.

DELIRIUM

Delirium is a syndrome with multiple causes characterized by concurrent disturbances of consciousness and attention, perception, thinking, memory, psychomotor behavior, emotion, and the sleep–wake cycle. It is transient and of fluctuating intensity. Delirium occurs in young children with acute infections and after drug ingestion. Delirium is marked by clouding of consciousness with decreased response to environmental stimuli, misperception, often visual and tactile hallucinations, and disorientation. Treatment is that of the underlying disorder. A supportive environment should be established to provide effective structure for the child.

BIPOLAR (MANIC-DEPRESSIVE) DISORDER

In bipolar disorder, a severe disturbance of mood exists. Abnormalities in thought and perception result from the mood disorder. These conditions may occur as a single episode or as recurrent episodes; if episodes of both depression and hypomania recur, the term *bipolar disorder* is used. Two types of bipolar disorders are described. In bipolar I, classic manic episodes occur. In bipolar II, one or more depressive episodes and at least one hypomanic episode are documented, without a full-blown manic episode ever occurring.

During a manic or hypomanic episode, mood is elevated, and rapid and pressured speech and irritability are observed. The young person is overly energetic, is disinhibited in his or her behavior, and sleeps less than usual. Grandiose ideas about one's capabilities are associated with the episode. Hallucinations may occur but are not common. For example, an affected adolescent may wear flamboyant clothing, drive a car recklessly, distribute gifts, and show inappropriate sexual behavior.

Epidemiology

The onset of bipolar disorder is rare before puberty, but the prevalence increases during the adolescent years. It occurs with equal frequency in boys and girls. A genetic component exists: 12% of first-degree relatives have affective disorders. This is six times the frequency of affective disorder in the general population. Substance abuse is often associated with bipolar disorder.

Diagnosis

If psychotic symptoms are present, a distinction must be made from schizophrenia. Neurologically based mental disorders must be ruled out by examination, and associated suicidal behavior requires careful assessment. Stimulant abuse and some symptoms of attention-deficit hyperactivity disorder may mimic an episode of mania. Clarifying the family history for affective disorders is particularly important.

Treatment

The initial phase of treatment requires ensuring the safety of the patient and those around him or her, and it ordinarily requires hospital admission. Acute treatment with neuroleptic medications to deal with acute symptoms, and initiation of a mood stabilizer (lithium carbonate or sodium valproate) in those with recurrent episodes, constitute the most effective pharmacologic management. Supportive psychotherapy for the child and family is needed to deal with the consequences of the irrational behavior and its effects on family and friends.

Suggested Readings

AACAP Official Action. Practice parameters for the assessment and treatment of children and adolescents with bipolar disorder. *J Am Acad Child Adolesc Psychiatry* 1997;36:138.

Alaghband-Rad J, Hamburger SD, Giedd JN, et al. Childhood-onset schizophrenia: biological markers in relation to clinical characteristics. *Am J Psychiatry* 1997;154:64.

Alessi N, Naylor MW, Ghaziuddin M, Zubieta JK. Update on lithium carbonate therapy in children and adolescents. *J Am Acad Child Adolesc Psychiatry* 1994;33:291.

Asarnow J, Thompson M, Goldstein M. Childhood onset schizophrenia: a follow-up study. *Schizophr Bull* 1994;20:599.

Eggers C, Bunk D. The long-term course of childhood-onset schizophrenia: a 42-year follow-up. *Schizophr Bull* 1997;23:105.

Freedman R. Schizophrenia. *N Engl J Med* 2003;349:1738.

Geller B, Zimerman B, Williams M, et al. DSM-IV mania symptoms in a prepubertal and early adolescent bipolar disorder phenotype compared to attention-deficit hyperactive and normal controls. *J Child Adolesc Psychopharmacol* 2002;12:11.

Harris JC. Schizophrenia: a neurodevelopmental disorder. In: *Developmental neuropsychiatry*, Vol 2. New York: Oxford University Press, 1998:404.

Jarbin H, Ott Y, Von Knorring AL. Adult outcome of social function in adolescent-onset schizophrenia and affective psychosis. *J Am Acad Child Adolesc Psychiatry* 2003;42(2):176.

Kafantaris V. Treatment of bipolar disorder in children and adolescents. *J Am Acad Child Adolesc Psychiatry* 1995;34:732.

Kovacs M, Devlin B, Pollock M, et al. A controlled family history study of childhood-onset depressive disorder. *Arch Gen Psychiatry* 1997;54:613.

Sporn AL, Greenstein DK, Gogtay N, et al. Progressive brain volume loss during adolescence in childhood-onset schizophrenia. *Am J Psychiatry* 2003; 160:2181.

Todd RD, Reich W, Petti TA, et al. Psychiatric diagnoses in the child and adolescent members of extended families identified through adult bipolar affective disorder probands. *J Am Acad Child Adolesc Psychiatry* 1996;35:664.

Weller EB, Weller RA, Fristad MA. Bipolar disorder in children: misdiagnosis, underdiagnosis, and future directions. *J Am Acad Child Adolesc Psychiatry* 1995;34:709.

CHAPTER 111 ■ ENURESIS

NINA SAND-LOUD AND LEONARD A. RAPPAPORT

Enuresis refers to the involuntary discharge of urine beyond the age of expected continence. Daytime wetting, or diurnal enuresis, is considered abnormal after 4 years of age, and nighttime wetting, or nocturnal enuresis, is considered abnormal after 6 years of age. Enuresis can be primary, which refers to having never been dry for a period of 6 months, or secondary, which occurs after a dry interval of at least 6 months. Uncomplicated nocturnal enuresis is primary and monosymptomatic, meaning occurring just at night time, with a normal examination and often a family history of enuresis. Complicated enuresis is more likely to be secondary with diurnal symptoms and a history of constipation and urinary tract infections (UTIs) as well as an abnormal physical examination.

Only 10% of children with enuresis have an underlying disease process causing their enuresis; all the rest remain unexplained. The differential diagnosis of both nocturnal and diurnal enuresis can be divided into four main categories (Table 111.1). When a child initially presents with secondary enuresis, it is always important to consider the possibility of sexual or physical abuse, although this is a very rare cause.

NOCTURNAL ENURESIS

Epidemiology

Although 15% of 5-year-olds have nocturnal enuresis, this number is reduced to 5% of 10-year-olds and then 1% of adolescents, with 15% of children spontaneously resolving per year. The ratio of males to females is 3:2. There are adults who have primary nocturnal enuresis.

Pathology

Hypothesized causes of nocturnal enuresis include high nocturnal urine production, poor arousal from sleep to a full bladder, and a small functional bladder capacity. Family histories and recent genetic studies have also suggested a genetic basis to nocturnal enuresis with linkage on chromosomes 13q, 12q, 22q, and 8q, although heterogeneity exists. However, it has long been observed that nocturnal enuresis tends to cluster in families, with 44% of children wetting the bed if one parent wet the bed and 70% wetting the bed if both parents have a history of

TABLE 111.1

DIFFERENTIAL DIAGNOSIS OF ENURESIS

Diagnostic Categories of Differential Diagnosis	Examples
Increased urinary output	Diabetes mellitus, diabetes insipidus, sickle cell disease, excessive water intake
Increased bladder irritability	Urinary tract infection, constipation, pregnancy, bladder spasm
Structural problems	Ectopic ureter, epispadius (females), partial urethral valves and thickened bladder wall (males)
Abnormal sphincter control	Spinal cord abnormalities, sphincter weakness, neurogenic bladder

TABLE 111.2

BEHAVIORAL INTERVENTIONS

Intervention	Description	Success Rate
Motivational therapies	Include positive reinforcement systems such as placing a sticker on a chart for a dry night or responsibility training, which would include giving children increased age-appropriate responsibility in nonpunitive ways	25% (although a reported 70% of children show some improvement)
Bladder stretching exercises or retention control	Involves practicing to hold urine for progressively longer periods during the day	35%
Fluid intake programs	Restriction of fluid intake in the evenings (important to ensure that not overly restrictive)	15% (close to the spontaneous cure rate)
Hypnotherapy, biofeedback	Similar to such methods when used with other problems	Data unclear but 60% success reported in limited trials
Behavioral conditioning (e.g., alarm/arousal systems)	Association of bedwetting with a consequence (in this case, waking from sleep)	70%–80%

bedwetting. There is also evidence for children with developmental difficulties having an increased incidence of nocturnal enuresis. Lastly, there is no evidence that children with primary nocturnal enuresis have a psychological cause for their bedwetting but rather that bedwetting may cause psychological difficulties for the child.

Diagnosis/Evaluation

A full medical and developmental history along with a family history should be obtained. A problem-specific history is essential and should include the timing and onset as well as the pattern of the enuresis. Daytime symptoms should also be examined such as urgency, frequency, and diurnal continence as well as a history of a slow, intermittent stream. Bowel habits should also be recorded. Important historical information should indicate whether the problem is primary or secondary, whether there are signs of UTIs, and whether there is constipation and/or encopresis. Other important information to obtain would include how this problem affects the child (e.g., sleep-overs) as well as what the parents have done in the past to treat the problem (e.g., positive reinforcement such as rewards; punishment such as loss of privileges; fluid restriction; waking during the night; medications or alarms and specifically how they have been utilized).

A complete physical examination should also be done with special emphasis on the neurologic examination and include deep tendon reflexes and perianal and perineal sensation and reflexes. The back should be carefully observed and palpated for defects such as sacral dimpling and hairy patches. The abdomen should be examined for signs of constipation. Genitalia should always be examined.

Investigations include a urinalysis specifically looking at specific gravity, glucose, and for signs of infection. A urine culture will frequently be done, particularly in females. Other examinations should only be done as directed by history and physical examination.

Treatment

There are two treatment approaches: behavioral interventions and drug therapy (Table 111.2).

As noted in Table 111.2, all behavior modification modalities have some success; however, the alarm is the most successful and longest lasting of treatments. It is reasonable to try motivational therapies as first-line treatment in younger children with primary nocturnal enuresis; however, if therapy is not successful in 2 to 3 months, a different treatment option should be offered, such as behavioral conditioning with an alarm system. The alarm is available in both auditory and vibratory models and conditions the child to awaken before wetting the bed or to contain the bladder contraction while remaining asleep. Initially the waking happens as the child is voiding and eventually before the child voids. An interesting finding is that approximately 50% of successfully treated children sleep through the night rather than waking to void. Alarms are safe, inexpensive, and very effective. Up to 80% of children stay dry after using an alarm system. However, alarms are also time consuming and require motivation on the part of the child and the parent to succeed: the parent must awaken with the child every time the alarm rings since the child needs to go to the bathroom every time he or she wets. Generally the alarm is not recommended in children younger than 7 years old.

Drug therapy includes tricyclic antidepressants (imipramine) as well as desmopressin acetate (DDAVP). Imipramine has been approved by the Food and Drug Administration (FDA) for the treatment of nocturnal enuresis. The exact mechanism of action is unclear but may include increased arousal as well as anticholinergic effects. The appeal of imipramine is that it is easy to administer and is inexpensive. However, it has side effects including headache, abdominal pain, and moodiness as well as significant risks of toxicity. Lastly, it is only 30% to 50% effective, and approximately 60% of children who use imipramine relapse after the medication is stopped. Due to the potential dangers of tricyclic antidepressants, they are rarely used as a treatment for nocturnal enuresis anymore. DDAVP, an analog of antidiuretic hormone (ADH), is also FDA approved for nocturnal enuresis. It works by decreasing urine output for 1 to 7 hours after administration. DDAVP is available in a nasal spray and oral medication and is also easy to administer with minimal side effects and can be used on an as-needed basis. However, DDAVP is only 40% to 60% effective and is expensive. Many children relapse after the use of DDAVP, and there have been reports of hyponatremic seizures probably from overdosage or marked fluid intake after administration.

Overall, every study has shown that alarms have the best outcome in the treatment of nocturnal enuresis and at this point are the best available therapy for nocturnal enuresis.

DIURNAL ENURESIS

Epidemiology

Approximately 3% to 4% of children ages 4 to 12 years have diurnal enuresis. The male to female ratio is 1:2.

Diagnosis/Evaluation

As with nocturnal enuresis, a careful medical and developmental history are important, again examining the timing and pattern of the enuresis as well as any associated symptoms. A complete physical examination is essential, with special emphasis on the neurologic examination and on the abdomen, back, and genitalia.

Investigations once again include urinalysis and urine culture. Depending on any associated symptoms, other investigations may include ultrasound, uroflowmetry, or voiding urethrogram (VCUG), although few children need these additional tests.

Treatment

The most common cause of isolated diurnal enuresis is bladder spasm. Therapies include frequent reminders to use the bathroom in children who hold their urine for too long or a watch that alarms every hour or two to remind the child to use the toilet. Urge containment exercises can be helpful to strengthen sphincter control and increase a child's confidence that he or she can make it to the toilet after a spasm. Exercises are done by having a child go directly to the bathroom when he or she feels the need to urinate and then once at the toilet, to hold the urine for as long as possible. He or she should then stop and start the urine flow several times. This intervention seems to strengthen the sphincter as well as give the child a sense that he or she will be able to make it to the bathroom after a bladder spasm. Medications, such as oxybutynin hydrochloride, are not usually necessary but are helpful for children with an underlying diagnosis such as neurogenic bladder.

Suggested Readings

Harari MD, Moulden A. Personal practice nocturnal enuresis: what is happening? *J Pediatr Child Health* 2000;36:78.

Jalkut MW, Lerman SE, Churchill BM. Enuresis. *Pediatr Clin North Am* 2001;48(6):1461.

Mellon MW, McGrath ML. Empirically supported treatments in pediatric psychology: nocturnal enuresis. *J Pediatr Psych* 2000;25(4):193.

Moffatt M. Nocturnal enuresis: a review of the efficacy of treatments and practical advice for clinicians [Review]. *J Dev Behav Ped* 1997;18(1):49.

Rappaport L. Enuresis—where are we now? What to do? *Pediatrics* 1993;92:465.

Wolfish NM. Sleep/arousal and enuresis subtypes. *J Urol* 2001;166:2444.

CHAPTER 112 ■ ENCOPRESIS

ALISON SCHONWALD AND LEONARD A. RAPPAPORT

Encopresis is defined as repeated passage of stool into inappropriate places in a child over 4 years of age chronologically and developmentally. The behavior is not due exclusively to the direct physiologic effects of a substance (e.g., laxatives) or a general medical condition except through a mechanism involving constipation. As defined by the Academy of Pediatric Gastroenterologists and Nutritionists, constipation is the delay or difficulty in defecation for 2 or more weeks. Reportedly, encopresis affects 2.8% of 4-year-olds, 1.9% of 6-year-olds, and 1.6% of 10- to 11-year-olds. It typically presents in children under 7 years old. More than 90% of encopresis is due to functional constipation, caused when retained stool distends the rectum and leads to the leakage of stool around a stool mass. Stretch receptors in a distended rectum do not seem to signal to the child to defecate until soiling has occurred. Encopresis is not usually caused by underlying psychopathology, but can be associated with emotional distress. No known genetic findings predict encopresis. Rare cases of encopresis are due to damaged corticospinal pathways or anorectal dysfunction after pull-through surgery. Occasionally, a child with encopresis may impulsively pass stool when anxious or suffering from emotional stressors, without underlying constipation.

ASSESSMENT

History begins at birth, with details surrounding bowel function and any treatments used. Past medical and surgical history may identify systemic diseases or medical causes of constipation that require treatments other than laxatives and maintenance of stool regularity. For example, Hirschsprung disease usually presents with difficulty in evacuation from birth, recurrent abdominal distension, and/or emesis. Failure to thrive and enterocolitis may occur in infancy. Encopresis is unusual and rectal examination includes a tight aganglionic bowel around the examining finger.

In taking a history, it is essential to distinguish encopresis from delayed toilet training, where the child never consolidated the ability to stool independently into the toilet. Treatment will depend on whether constipation underlies the stooling accidents, rather than toilet refusal alone; however, toilet refusal is often associated with constipation as well. Developmental history highlights details of toilet training, when and which methods were used, and successes or failures. Most children are toilet trained by 3 years of age in the United States. Children who are not toilet trained until after 4 years of age are outliers in this developmental trajectory.

History must include details of present bowel patterns, such as frequency of stool evacuation into the toilet, stool accidents, stool consistency, and the urge to defecate. Children with functional constipation and consequent encopresis report uncomfortable, often infrequent stooling into the toilet with uncontrolled stool accidents into underwear or pull-ups. More severe, prolonged constipation suggests the need for more aggressive treatment. Any history of abuse or other trauma should be sought as well. Children who have been abused may become incontinent in times of stress or as part of regressive behavior, and are less suitable candidates for rectal suppositories or enemas.

Urinary patterns, diurnal and nocturnal enuresis, and symptoms of urinary infection must be noted, and may reflect neurologic abnormalities or consequent urine contamination. Particularly in females, constipation and encopresis may be associated with urine infections due to poor hygiene. Even without infection, enuresis can be caused by a dilated rectum pushing on and irritating the bladder, causing spasm. History may reveal that increasing stool backup is temporally associated with urine accidents. Charting calendars may illuminate these details.

History taking allows for an essential opportunity to communicate with the child. The child must be a willing and active participant for treatment to be effective, and often children with encopresis are embarrassed when encopresis is discussed. Conveying an understanding of the child's perspective can create a connection between the caregiver and patient, and should include questions about present school and family functioning.

Physical examination of the child with encopresis includes growth parameters, attention to signs of systemic disease, careful neurologic assessment, and examination of the anal opening. Anal fissures can cause ongoing pain with defecation, tags may indicate inflammatory bowel disease, and an absent anal wink may reflect neurologic abnormality. An anteriorly placed anus may be associated with lifelong constipation and deserves referral to a surgeon. Rectal examination can be useful in assessing for Hirschsprung disease and may indicate the degree of rectal impaction to guide treatment. Rectal examination may reveal low anal pressure, reflecting external and/or internal sphincter disease. For most children, a rectal examination performed with the child lying on his or her back in a modified lithotomy position can minimize trauma.

Performing a rectal examination may not be appropriate for the first visit, particularly in a child with a history of sexual abuse or who is overwhelmed with the discussion of this private problem. Often, a digital examination is performed at least once to rule out organic causes of constipation and to prescribe adequate treatment.

Laboratory investigation is necessary only as history or physical examination suggests: rarely labs may include thyroid function tests, electrolytes, calcium, and magnesium. An abdominal radiograph is useful when the history is vague or the child is uncooperative with examination. Lumbosacral spine films or magnetic resonance imaging are advised when lower-extremity neurologic examination is abnormal or sacral abnormalities are visualized.

DIFFERENTIAL DIAGNOSIS

All causes of constipation should be considered in the differential diagnosis of encopresis, although organic conditions are rarely the cause. History and physical examination may suggest Hirschsprung disease, systemic disorders such as inflammatory bowel disease, neurologic causes such as spinal disorders, or anatomic abnormalities such as anal stenosis. Review of systems and growth parameters may contribute to suspicion for hypothyroidism and other endocrinopathies. Careful social history should inquire specifically about sexual or physical abuse that may lead to incontinence as well.

TREATMENT

A limited body of evidence-based data exists to guide the treatment of childhood encopresis. Management includes medication and behavioral interventions, and is geared to the child's developmental stage and degree of constipation. Retention caused by painful fissures requires treatment with lubrication before constipation can be addressed.

A Cochran Database Systematic Review in July 2001 identified 16 randomized or quasi-randomized trials of behavior and/or cognitive interventions (with or without other treatments) for the management of defecation disorders in children. These trials included 843 children. Overall conclusions support behavioral intervention plus laxative therapy, rather than either alone, to improve fecal continence in children with encopresis. Biofeedback was not found effective.

Psychoeducation

When the child first presents with encopresis, the physician should demystify the shame and blame around stool accidents. The child's abdominal radiograph or an illustrated explanation (or both) should be used to explain the process of retained stool that leads to a distended colon, allowing stool to "sneak out" without warning. It should be explained to the patient that retained stool must be cleaned out with medication and that there will be a lot of stool to clean out. The physician should empathize with the child and family's stress and frustration and emphasize the need to break the cycle of impatience that may have developed. The physician should also recognize the role that a child's anxiety plays in exacerbating the symptoms and impairing the treatment and clarify that without treatment, the child truly cannot control the stool leaking out and cannot be blamed.

Initial Clean-out of Retained Stool

Children age 7 years and older without trauma history often succeed with a fast and direct plan: a 14-day cycle of alternating an Adult Fleets enema, bisacodyl suppository, and then bisacodyl pill. Younger children (under age 7), or those who cannot tolerate suppositories or enemas, often do well with polyethylene glycol without electrolytes, starting at one cap in 6 oz. of fluid per day. Impaction present for many months may necessitate higher dosing or the addition of a stimulant (senna or bisacodyl). During the initial clean-out, the child and family should expect a large amount of stool output and be reminded of the radiograph full of stool.

Establishment of Regular Bowel Patterns

After the backed-up stool is evacuated, the child will need a medication and a behavior plan. It makes sense to meet with the child and family after the clean-out is complete to plan this stage of treatment. One option is mineral oil titrated to efficacy, from 2 tablespoons per day to 6 tablespoons twice per day. Polyethylene glycol without electrolytes is also effective, particularly for children who do not tolerate mineral oil's taste or who have oil leakage. Maintenance dose of polyethylene glycol without electrolytes ranges from one-half cap every other day to one cap twice per day. Other options include milk of magnesia, lactulose, and senna-based treatments. Dosing is adjusted to maintain soft, regular stools. As the urge to defecate may not redevelop for 6 to 9 months after constipation is treated, a regular sitting time is necessary. The goal is to stool into the toilet before stool leaks. Sitting after breakfast and dinner for 5 to 10 minutes takes advantage of the body's gastrocolic reflex and can often be incorporated into the daily routine.

The family must work to eliminate any negative associations around toileting that may have developed. Limiting conversation about toileting relieves much stress experienced by the child, and rewarding the child for sitting or taking care of his or her own bodily needs lends a positive aspect to the child's progress. Older children may benefit from having games or activities in the bathroom.

FOLLOW UP

Once impacted stool is evacuated, maintenance of stool regularity typically requires ongoing medication and behavioral

planning. Prescription and over-the-counter laxatives or stimulants (senna or bisacodyl) may be weaned and replaced with mineral oil, increased dietary fiber, or fluid. Children and families should learn to monitor for signs of constipation, such as less frequent, painful, or larger stools, and then to reimplement medication and sitting plans at those times to prevent the recurrence of accidents.

Suggested Readings

Berk LB, Friman PC. Epidemiologic aspects of toilet training. *Clin Pediatr (Phila)* 1990;29(5):278.

Brazzelli M, Griffiths P. Behavioural and cognitive interventions with or without other treatments for defaecation disorders in children. *Cochrane Database Syst Rev* 2001;(4):CD002240.

Levine MD. Children with encopresis: a descriptive analysis. *Pediatrics* 1975; 56(3):412.

Loening-Baucke V. Encopresis. *Curr Opin Pediatr* 2002;14(5):570.

McGrath M, Mellon M, Murphy L. Empirically supported treatments in pediatric psychology: constipation and encopresis. *J Pediatr Psychol* 2000;25(4): 225.

Mikkelsen E. Enuresis and encopresis: ten years of progress. *J Am Acad Child Adolesc Psychiatry* 2001;40(10):1146.

Nurko S, Baker S, Colletti R. Managing constipation: evidence put to practice. *Contemp Pediatr* 2001;(18):56.

CHAPTER 113 ■ SCHOOL DIFFICULTIES

LAURIE E. CUTTING, STEWART H. MOSTOFSKY, AND MARTHA BRIDGE DENCKLA

Difficulties in school are common among children and adolescents. A primary pediatrician will be asked to address problems with school more frequently than many other topics that are emphasized in pediatric training. For example, attention-deficit hyperactivity disorder (ADHD), one of the most common reasons for school underachievement, has an estimated prevalence of 3% to 5% in school-age children, and is therefore more common than many other disorders emphasized in training. It is critical that the pediatrician understand how to address these problems, considering not only their prevalence, but also the major part they may play in a child's life. School failure can have a detrimental effect not only on the acquisition of skills and knowledge, but on self-image and self-esteem as well.

Multiple factors go into a child's success in school. When evaluating children with school difficulties, Occam's Razor, often emphasized in medical training, does not hold true. Comorbidity is common in children with school difficulties, and the clinician must consider the possibility of multiple diagnoses being present simultaneously. Diagnosis is further complicated by the fact that there is often extensive overlap between those diagnoses that are considered in the differential and those diagnoses that occur as comorbidities. For instance, the differential for ADHD includes learning disabilities, anxiety disorders, conduct disorder, and depression; these same disorders may also be present as comorbidities in children with ADHD.

In this chapter, the approach will be to discuss two of the most common complaints that the primary pediatrician will hear related to school difficulties: the child who presents with unexpected reading difficulty and the child who presents with

difficulty staying on task. There will be an in-depth discussion of the approach to these problems. Using these presentations as points of departure, the discussion will then focus on the clinical approach to a child who presents with school difficulties, focusing on differential diagnosis, method of diagnosis (workup), and treatment.

THE CHILD WHO PRESENTS WITH UNEXPECTED READING DIFFICULTY

Reading and other language-based tasks are a large part of the curriculum in early education. After that, reading and language continue to be the foundations upon which most academic subjects are based. Every school subject, even science and math, has a large language component to instruction. It is therefore not surprising that difficulty with language-based tasks, most prominently reading, is a common complaint among children who are having problems in school.

In some children who present with a complaint of difficulty with reading, the problem can be attributed to an isolated reading disability (RD), more commonly referred to as *dyslexia* in the medical and psychological professions. Developmental dyslexia is defined as a chronic disorder characterized by difficulty with acquisition and use of written language that is unexpected on the basis of normal general development and overall cognitive aptitude. Theoretically, other exclusions include emotional problems, educational deprivation, and sensory impairment. Although outside the scope of this discussion, it is important to mention that dyslexia is a lifelong disorder; residual effects, particularly slow reading, are observed in adults with the disorder.

Dyslexia is almost universally viewed as a specific disorder of the phonologic subdivision of the language system. However, pure dyslexia is more the exception than the rule; most children with dyslexia have deficits that are not limited to written language. The border between deficits in reading and deficits in broader aspects of language can be fuzzy, and most children with dyslexia have a broader language deficit that involves aspects of spoken as well as written language (e.g., problems with written composition).

Biomedical research has resulted in a consensus that the underlying deficit in dyslexia is in phonologic skills (or the ability to manipulate the sound structure of the language), which are essential for the development of the ability to decode, or "sound out," words; the difficulty with decoding that children with dyslexia have thus places major constraints on their reading comprehension. However, despite these findings, current educational practice and psychiatry's *Diagnostic and Statistical Manual of Mental Disorders,* Fourth Edition (*DSM-IV*) continue to disregard these findings when defining what constitutes a reading disability. The *DSM-IV* uses the term "reading disorder," which is defined as reading achievement that is "substantially below that expected given the person's chronological age, measured intelligence, and age-appropriate education," but does not make any mention of problems with phonologic deficits. Interestingly, within the realm of "communication disorders," the *DSM-IV* does have a diagnosis of "phonological disorder," which is described as an articulation disorder in which there is a "failure to use developmentally expected speech sounds"; however, there is failure to establish the known connection between problems with certain phonologic skills (e.g., phonologic awareness) and difficulty reading.

Most public school systems define a reading disability on the basis of discrepancy criteria (a discrepancy between full-scale IQ and performance on tests of reading achievement) rather than by the appearance of a subtle neurocognitive deficit in phonologic awareness. Under public law 94-142, the Education for All Handicapped Children Act, passed in 1975, public school systems are required to provide services for children with handicapping conditions, including learning disabilities; however, children with dyslexia often have difficulty with broader aspects of language, which can adversely affect IQ scores (particularly the verbal subtests), making it difficult for children with dyslexia to meet the discrepancy criteria adopted by most public school systems. Their underlying language deficits lower both the aptitude and achievement, precluding a discrepancy. Furthermore, research has shown that the IQ-achievement discrepancy method of defining reading disabilities is not valid: studies have shown that children with IQ-achievement discrepancy and poor readers *without* a discrepancy both show impairments in phonologic skills.

Cognitive assessments of children with reading disability often reveal subtle deficits in inhibitory control and organization consistent with the diagnosis of ADHD. Comorbidity of dyslexia and ADHD is common. Studies from random samples have shown that approximately 36% of children with ADHD have RD and 15% of children with RD have ADHD; however, some researchers have reported comorbidity rates as high as 80%. Although some of these children present with both difficulty reading and difficulty staying on task, others present with reading as the only complaint, and subtle deficits in inhibitory control and organization become apparent only after cognitive testing. (The cognitive deficits associated with ADHD will be discussed in more detail in the section entitled, "The child who presents with difficulty staying on task.")

The cause of developmental dyslexia is presumed to be congenital, with genetic and fetal developmental factors theorized as possible contributors to the development of brain differences that result in ineffective performance of reading and other language-based tasks. Investigations have elicited genetic contributions to dyslexia. Twin studies have pointed to heritability for single word reading and a variety of phonologic skills; recent twin studies have shown that approximately 58% of the deficit in dyslexia is attributable to heritable genetic influences. Linkage studies have implicated possible loci on chromosomes 1, 2, 3, 6, 15, and 18, with a locus on chromosome 6 (6p21.3) the best replicated finding so far.

Analyses of the neuroanatomic basis of acquired difficulty reading in adults (acquired alexia or dyslexia) are consistent with localization to the left angular gyrus. Neurobiologic studies of individuals with developmental dyslexia, including postmortem, electrophysiologic, and imaging studies, have implicated left perisylvian regions, and many theories have focused on postulates of temporal–parietal perisylvian dysfunction. Alternatively, Heilman and others have suggested that the development of phonologic skills may be linked to motor articulatory kinesthesis with localization in more anterior motor speech areas of the brain. More recently, functional magnetic resonance imaging (fMRI) studies have shown that when people with dyslexia are asked to sound out words or perform phonologic tasks, they show reduced activation in left posterior regions and overactivation in anterior and right posterior hemisphere regions. Interestingly, these patterns of activation normalize (i.e., become like normal readers) after people with dyslexia are provided appropriate intervention and are reading at normal levels.

THE CHILD WHO PRESENTS WITH A COMPLAINT OF DIFFICULTY STAYING ON TASK

Another very common school-related problem to which the pediatrician must respond is the child who has difficulty staying on task. This difficulty is often associated with symptoms of impulsivity and hyperactivity. Often, these symptoms will be due to ADHD; however, differential diagnoses, including language/learning disabilities and psychiatric disorders, need to be considered. Often the issue is "in addition to" rather than "instead of" ADHD, as is commonly true for language-based disabilities.

In recent years there has been increased public awareness of ADHD; however, the symptoms that comprise the disorder have been recognized under a variety of names (minimal brain dysfunction, hyperkinetic disorder, attention deficit disorder) for over 30 years. ADHD is common, affecting 3% to 5% of elementary school-age children, leaving little doubt about its impact on school functioning across a large population of children. Studies have revealed a higher incidence of ADHD in males than females, with a ratio of approximately 3:1; however gender-biased diagnostic criteria may account for the size, if not the direction, of the ratio.

ADHD is characterized by symptoms of hyperactivity, impulsivity, and a decreased ability to maintain on-task behavior, particularly during nonpreferred tasks. Currently, the *DSM-IV* uses the term "attention deficit/hyperactivity disorder" and includes three subtypes: "predominantly inattentive," "predominantly hyperactive/impulsive," and a combined type. By definition, signs must be observed prior to 7 years of age. The forms can change over the lifespan; one individual can have the hyperactive/impulsive type as a preschooler, the full syndrome until middle school, and the inattentive type thereafter.

It is children with the inattentive form that will often present with isolated complaints of school difficulty. In children with the hyperactive/impulsive or combined forms of the disorder, signs are typically recognizable at an early age and often include behavioral as well as academic difficulties. In the inattentive form signs may not be evident until the child enters school and begins engaging in nonpreferred activities that require a much greater ability to inhibit off-task behavior. With persistent, focused questioning, however, the clinician can often find a history of off-task behavior during the preschool years. (As is the case for dyslexia, it is important to mention that ADHD is no longer a diagnosis restricted to childhood. It has been reported that approximately 75% of those diagnosed in childhood continue to suffer from residual ADHD in young adulthood.)

The cause of ADHD appears to be heterogeneous. Various adverse environmental factors including infection, toxins such as lead, and prenatal exposure to tobacco or alcohol have been associated with symptoms of ADHD. Genetic factors have also been identified. Several genetic disorders have ADHD as part of the phenotype, and twin studies report heritability rates ranging from .6 to .9. Additionally, siblings of children with ADHD have a three- to fivefold increased risk of having the disorder. Although there is strong evidence for a genetic basis for ADHD, it is not yet clear which genes may be responsible. Most studies that have tried to link candidate genes to ADHD have concentrated on dopaminergic systems; however, there is also some indication that other systems may also be involved (serotonergic and catecholaminergic systems).

Like dyslexia, ADHD is often associated with comorbid conditions. What is more, these comorbid conditions are often differential diagnoses that must be considered in the evaluation of a child who presents with difficulty staying on task. As mentioned in the preceding section, ADHD is often associated with dyslexia and other language-based learning disabilities. These disorders also need to be considered as differential diagnoses, since problems staying on task can result from difficulty understanding verbal and written instructions. In addition, psychiatric disorders such as oppositional defiant disorder, conduct disorder, anxiety disorders, and mood disorders including depression are common comorbidities that must also be considered as possible causes/contributors to difficulty staying on task.

In considering the neurobiologic basis of ADHD, most researchers suggest that the disorder is the result of dysfunction within frontal intentional networks, which are critical for an organism's "preparedness to act." In this model, the core symptoms are thought to be secondary to abnormal selection of motor response to stimuli (difficulty in preparing the response to, rather than attending to, stimuli). The result is unresponsiveness to stimuli that should lead to action and defective inhibition of response to those that should not, with the latter resulting in impulsive and hyperactive behavior.

The neuropsychological profile of patients with ADHD is consistent with signs of insult to the frontal lobes and its interconnected subcortical regions, with most studies identifying deficits in the realm of "executive function," including response inhibition and response preparation. Morphometric studies have consistently shown that children with ADHD have reduced total brain volumes (approximately 5% reduction compared to controls) and show abnormalities in frontal-subcortical regions. Reduction in prefrontal and premotor volumes and abnormalities in the volumes of the caudate and globus pallidus have been reported. In concordance with structural neuroimaging findings, functional neuroimaging studies have also revealed abnormalities in frontostriatal circuitry in individuals with ADHD.

A subgroup of individuals with the inattentive form of ADHD may have a deficit in overfocusing or shifting attention rather than in selection of motor response to stimuli. Two prominent models of attention suggest that parietal lobe dysfunction would be manifest as impairment of stimulus detection, as well as decreased performance on other sensory components of attentional processing including vigilance, selection, disengagement, and shifting. It follows that deficits in the overfocusing subtype are more likely due to pathology in parietal circuits.

EVALUATION OF THE CHILD WHO PRESENTS WITH SCHOOL DIFFICULTIES

Regardless of the chief complaint, the workup of school difficulties needs to take into consideration all possible causes. For instance, in a child who presents with a chief complaint of difficulty staying on task, it would not be appropriate to focus solely on ruling out the presence of ADHD. Several other possibilities that may be the real cause (differential diagnoses) of difficulty staying on task or that may be present in conjunction with ADHD (comorbid diagnoses) need to be considered and ruled out.

The principal components of the evaluation, like all medical evaluations, should include a comprehensive history and examination. Unlike most medical evaluations, however, the examination includes neurocognitive testing that most medical students and residents are not exposed to in their training. This testing will have to be done by a specialist (e.g., a psychologist) to whom a referral is analogous to ordering diagnostic laboratory tests (radiographs, blood work, etc.).

The History

The history should include a comprehensive clinical interview (history of chief complaint ["present illness"], developmental history, past medical history, and family history) as well as standardized questionnaires/rating scales that aid in the diagnosis of ADHD and other neuropsychiatric disorders. The latter should help the primary pediatrician decide whether it is advisable to refer the child to a mental health professional.

In the child with "pure" dyslexia, the history should reveal difficulty specific to tasks involving reading, spelling, and the academic "language arts." Developmentally, problems begin to emerge in preschool and kindergarten when the child is asked to begin naming written letters or associating the letters with their assigned sounds (the most basic reading task), and the child is unable to read words by first grade. Sometimes a useful history of difficulty early on with rhyming or speech "quirks" may be elicited (for example, "It's a froggy day," or "The Madonna is also called the Merchant Mary"); however, it takes a sophisticated parent or teacher to report these malapropisms as anything but "cute" when elicited. Most of these children go on to read; however, they often remain slow readers throughout their lives. There is a continuing impact on any academic task involving reading and written language output and, as the child gets older, there is increased frustration and school failure.

As discussed, dyslexia is a restricted type of language-based disorder (restricted to the phonologic portion of the language domain). Clinically, the division between "pure" dyslexia and a broader language disorder is often unclear, and many children with dyslexia have a history of difficulty with other aspects of language tasks (semantics, syntax). In children presenting with difficulty reading, there may be a history of delay in acquisition of early language milestones. Children with language-based disabilities often have problems with finding the correct sounds (which form words) to express ideas, resulting in imprecise and circumlocutory speech. In contrast to difficulties with one or more aspects of language, there is often a history of strong visual spatial abilities in these children.

The observation of letter reversal while reading is the most well-known and most misunderstood feature of dyslexia. Despite the common perception that these reversals (most commonly "b" and "d") are due to difficulties with visual-spatial processing, research has clearly demonstrated that they are secondary to errors in phonologic awareness. It is more likely that reversals of "b" and "d" are due to the fact that they sound the same and that the oral movements used to produce the sounds are very similar, rather than because they are mirror images of each other.

ADHD is a diagnosis by history; in children presenting with school difficulties the use of multiple techniques for obtaining a history, including clinical interview and rating scales/questionnaires, is critical for accurate diagnosis. The diagnosis of ADHD requires that difficulties be present in at least two settings, so it is important that historical information be obtained from multiple sources that should, at the very least, include parents and teachers. Available school records, including teacher observations, are an important source of information and should be reviewed.

History typically reveals problems with maintaining on-task behavior and impulsivity, associated with inhibitory insufficiencies. In young children difficulty maintaining on-task behavior tends to manifest as hyperactivity and difficulty sitting still; older children more commonly present with problems with focusing on school work. Gender also accounts for differences in phenotype, with boys more commonly showing hyperactivity and impulsivity and girls lack of focus, although it is possible that "motor mouth" hyperactivity and impulsive interruptive speech is more common in younger girls but does not reach threshold for "hyperactivity" or "impulsivity" on existing rating scales. Signs of "inattentiveness" and disinhibition are subject to situational variation and are often dependent upon interest to task; nonpreferred tasks require greater inhibition of off-task behavior and result in greater appearance of "inattentiveness." Independent of interest in task, variability in task performance is a near consistent feature of the disorder.

In understanding the impact of ADHD on school performance, it is important to realize that individuals with the disorder often have difficulties in planning, organizing, and generating strategies for future actions, often collectively referred to as "executive functions" in neuropsychology. The history of a child with ADHD is typically filled with anecdotes about disorganization and poor time management; book bags, desks, and lockers are often in a state of chaos, homework assignments are left at home, books are left at school, and lateness is the "rule." These issues assume greater importance as the child reaches the upper elementary grades, when longer-term assignments are introduced, and reach serious proportions when self-management is assumed to be the norm (the early teenage years). Academically, children with ADHD often have difficulty with the detail aspects of mathematics (e.g., noting plus versus minus signs), as well as organizing and planning out written compositions.

Developmental History

In all children presenting with school difficulties, a comprehensive developmental history should be obtained and care should be taken to ensure that there is no history of developmental regression. If one exists, then a comprehensive laboratory workup to rule out neurodegenerative disorders should be undertaken (discussed later). Psychiatric differential diagnoses need to be considered as well. Historical information, including clinical interview and standardized questionnaires/rating scales, is critical for discerning whether disorders such as depression, generalized anxiety, obsessive-compulsive disorder, or conduct disorder are present.

Past Medical History

Past medical history should focus on history of neurologic signs and conditions that can be associated with school difficulty, including seizures and tics. Birth history should be reviewed, although most children with ADHD and learning disabilities do not have a history of perinatal complications. Family history for dyslexic children is often significant for difficulty with reading, spelling, writing, or learning a foreign language that may be present not only in immediate family members, but in extended family as well; the mother's brothers are the relatives particularly frequently "positive" for school-related problems. Reading disability and characteristics of ADHD often co-occur, so there may be a history of such problems or other behavior problems in children with dyslexia. In children with ADHD, there is often a positive history of impulsivity and off-task behavior in family members; however, because the formal diagnosis of ADHD has existed for only 18 years, a family history of diagnosed ADHD is somewhat uncommon.

Physical Examination

General physical examination, with a focus on particular features, should be conducted. Dysmorphic features can be suggestive of genetic disorders associated with learning disabilities such as Turner syndrome, fragile X syndrome (particularly in females), and Klinefelter syndrome. The skin should be examined to look for stigmata suggestive of neurocutaneous disorders, such as tuberous sclerosis and neurofibromatosis type 1, which are often associated with learning disabilities.

Inattentiveness and off-task behavior can be presenting signs of neurodegenerative disorders such as adrenal leukodystrophy (ALD) or neuronal ceroid-lipofuscinosis (NCL) that need to be considered as differential diagnoses of ADHD (Box 113.1). A history of new onset of signs of distractibility, off-task behavior, and hyperactivity as well as a history of developmental plateau or regression are clues to the possible presence of a neurodegenerative disorder. In these cases, a comprehensive neurologic examination is critical. On general physical examination, abdominal examination to look for organomegaly and funduscopic examination are also important if a neurodegenerative disorder is suspected. It is also important to use history and physical examination to rule out other medical causes of ADHD, particularly endocrine disorders such as hypothyroidism and toxic exposures such as lead toxicity.

Routine aspects of the neurologic examination such as motor strength and deep tendon reflexes are typically unrevealing in children presenting with school difficulties, but if "hard" neuromotor signs are elicited, further laboratory workup to rule out a structural lesion or neurodegenerative process should be undertaken. It is more common for there to be subtle abnormalities on examination of gait and coordination testing including rapid/sequential movements of the hands and feet (finger tapping, hand patting, toe tapping, etc.). A common finding is excessive overflow, including feet-to-hand overflow during stressed gait maneuvers and mirror overflow during rapid/sequential movements. These subtle signs are markers (neurologists refer to them as "neighborhood signs") for behavioral/cognitive abnormalities that may be present in children with school difficulties. For instance, in children with ADHD, excessive overflow movements are often observed as signs of poor inhibitory control, and motor impersistence as a marker for difficulty staying on task. Dyslexic children often have slow and missequenced each-finger-to-thumb touching and slow, awkward tongue wiggling.

BOX 113.1   **Differential Diagnosis of Underlying Causes for Attention-Deficit Hyperactivity Disorder and Learning Disabilities**

Genetic
Fragile X syndrome
Turner syndrome
Klinefelter syndrome
Neurofibromatosis type 1
Tuberous sclerosis
Phenylketonuria

Toxic
Lead
Prescribed medications including antiepileptic
   medications
Malnutrition
Prenatal exposures
Alcohol
Tobacco

Endocrinologic
Hypothyroidism
Congenital adrenal hyperplasia

Neurologic
Adrenoleukodystrophy
Neuronal ceroid lipofuscinosis
Wilson disease
Seizures
Absence epilepsy
Partial complex seizure disorder
Neoplasm

A critical component of the examination of any child presenting with school difficulty is the neurocognitive evaluation, which is performed by an individual, such as a psychologist, whose expertise is administering and interpreting neurocognitive tests in children. In any child presenting with school difficulties, neurocognitive testing should include language-based tests. In children with dyslexia, testing typically reveals variable degrees of language inefficiency with dramatic deficits on tests of phonologic skills (including phoneme segmentation and phoneme blending tasks) and decoding (reading of nonsense words, pronounceable pseudowords, often referred to as "word attack"). Many children with dyslexia have strong visual–spatial abilities; it is important to test this and other visual–perceptual aspects of cognition. This helps establish cognitive strengths that are important for self-esteem and for making recommendations for techniques to accommodate areas of weakness. There is no diagnostic test for ADHD; however, tests of response preparation, inhibition, and organization, such as computerized go-no-go tests, complex figure copying, and visual search, are important in detecting deficits in response to consistency, inhibition, and approach-to-task and can be supportive of the diagnosis made by history.

Laboratory Tests

Currently, there are no laboratory tests that contribute to the diagnosis of ADHD or a learning disability such as dyslexia. Specific laboratory tests, such as electroencephalography (EEG) or

magnetic resonance imaging (MRI) of the brain, should be ordered only when a specific cause is suspected based on history and physical examination.

TREATMENT OF THE CHILD WHO PRESENTS WITH SCHOOL DIFFICULTIES

The approach to the treatment of children presenting with school difficulties is multimodal, involving integration of various components including academic interventions/accommodations, speech/language therapy, behavior modification and other mental health intervention, and pharmacotherapy. The combination of these interventions is aimed at achieving three goals: (1) providing the best possible academic environment in which the child can learn (academic interventions and accommodations), (2) relieving symptoms that may be making it more difficult for the child to function in the school environment (pharmacotherapy), and (3) remediating conditions that may be contributing to or exacerbated by the child's school difficulties (e.g., with speech/language therapy and behavior modification/other mental health interventions).

In the current situation, most interventions are not under direct control of the physician. The primary exception is treatment with medication, and this has perhaps led to an overemphasis in the medical community on pharmacotherapy for the treatment of school difficulties. With other interventions, particularly issues of academic intervention and accommodations, the decisions are primarily in the hands of the school system, unless parents can afford to pay for private speech/language therapy and/or academic tutoring. The physician can play a role in making recommendations with respect to academic placement, needs for in-class or test accommodations, and individualized treatment such as speech/language therapy. The school, however, makes the final decision regarding these interventions. There are often discrepancies between what is recommended and what the school is willing to offer because a public school is obligated to provide "adequate" (not "optimal") opportunities. There is often a gap between the "ideal" education and a "realistic" education. The physician, along with the child's parents, often has to consider whether the academic needs of the child are being adequately met, and if not, consider advocating for the child in the school system.

The physician should play an important role in counseling both parents and children regarding the nature of the diagnosed condition(s); explaining that the presence of a learning disability or ADHD does not necessarily mean that the child is not intelligent. Areas of cognitive and behavioral strengths should be emphasized to communicate that the child is neither "dumb" nor "bad." The physician should also play a role in helping parents to ward off unproven and unnecessary therapies. Disabilities such as dyslexia and ADHD are not easily remedied; educational and behavioral therapies, the standard of treatment, take time and effort to be effective. The field is therefore prone to unproven therapies, such as special tinted optical lenses, special diets, and vitamin therapies, which often steal time and other resources away from parents and children. The time of childhood is precious; physicians need to be careful not to overburden children with too many therapies, particularly unproven ones. This diverts time away not only from more beneficial therapies, but also from socially and emotionally enhancing activities that the child enjoys and in which he or she may excel (such as sports, art, dance, drama, etc.).

The treatment of the child with dyslexia is focused on academic interventions and accommodations and, if there are broader and deeper language issues, speech/language therapy; at this time there are no known medications that address

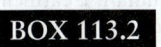

> ### Some Recommended Academic Accommodations for Children with Reading Disability (Dyslexia)
>
> **BOX 113.2**
>
> *Intervention and Therapy*
> Systematic and explicit intervention in phonological awareness and phonics
> Speech and language therapy, if indicated
>
> *Classroom, Coursework, and Accommodations*
> Untimed or extended time tests
> Customized tests to circumvent word retrieval problems (e.g., providing a word bank for fill-in-the-blank tests)
> Reduction in the amount of reading
> Possible exemption from foreign language requirement
> Use of videos and books on tape as adjuncts to texts
> Use of computers with word processing and spelling- and grammar-checking programs
> Use of visual cues and reinforcement

> ### Recommended Academic Accommodations for Children with Attention-Deficit Hyperactivity Disorder
>
> **BOX 113.3**
>
> *Classroom and Course Work*
> Small class size
> Seating that, in context, best accommodates either non-disruptive out-of-seat restlessness or need to keep classmates "out of sight, out of mind"
> Avoiding frequent changes of classes and teachers
> Stimulating course work and classroom setting (explicitly organized, broken into steps that can be reinforced positively)
> Untimed or extended time tests
>
> *Instruction and Therapy*
> Organizational coaching (help with "how" and "when")
> Parent–teacher training in behavior modification, skewed toward the positive ("Catch them being good and reward them")

dyslexia or other learning disabilities. Recommendations regarding educational interventions are, in part, based on age. Younger children (elementary school) should be taught to read using a systematic, explicit, phonologic awareness and phonics-based intervention program. However, while a phonologic and phonics-based approach is the primary intervention needed, care needs to be taken that children *also* receive instruction in reading fluency, vocabulary, and reading comprehension (especially for those who have broader and deeper language issues). Instruction in reading fluency is particularly critical because some children with dyslexia get "stuck on phonics," and many children have residual difficulties of being slow readers.

Although there is limited research available on the nature and course of dyslexia in older children and adolescents, research suggests that they also benefit from the same interventions that younger children do; however, depending on the severity of the reading problem and/or circumstances, older children and adolescents may be better served by a focus on accommodations to "work around" the difficulty with reading (Box 113.2). Accommodations should place an emphasis on the use of visual cues (the visual–perceptual system is often a strength in individuals with dyslexia) to help with learning. Slow reading is often a residual problem and therefore most typically accommodations need to include untimed tests and reductions in the amount of required reading (even with reading fluency intervention, many individuals with dyslexia remain slower-than-average readers). Books on tape or videos can be used as adjuncts to texts. Other accommodations include use of computers with spelling checkers, tutors to help review the content of written material (including spelling), and the use of oral presentations or visual displays (on science or history topics) in place of written tests.

For children with ADHD, treatment involves the use of behavior modification techniques to improve on-task performance maintenance, the use of medications that boost inhibitory control to decrease off-task behavior, and the use of academic accommodations to help create an academic environment in which the child is better able to learn.

Behavior modification utilizes techniques of operant conditioning, stressing positive reinforcement to alter behavior. It is optimal to have a behavioral psychologist involved who would work not only with the child, but also with the parents, teach-

ers, and other supervisory adults. Consistency is extremely important, and the psychologist can help in setting up a coordinated program in which caregivers provide preestablished responses to both positive and negative behavior. For children with ADHD, it is important that consequences be immediate and consistent and that praise and reward for good behavior and performance be emphasized.

Academic accommodations are important for providing a child with ADHD a school setting in which the greatest amount of learning can take place (Box 113.3). Teachers should attempt to provide as much structure and routine as possible. Classrooms should be small in size and the child should be given preferential seating toward the front of the class. Frequent changes of teachers during the day should be avoided. Studies consistently reveal that individuals with ADHD are slow in responding and that untimed tests and limiting the length of homework assignments are essential accommodations. Attempts should also be made at helping to provide organization by using a combination of techniques including keeping an extra set of textbooks at home and using a daily assignment notebook that allows the teacher to communicate directly with parents regarding homework assignments. Alternatively, a buddy system, in which there is a classmate who helps with providing a copy of the assignments and books needed, can be useful, if tactfully arranged.

Much interest or controversy about ADHD is prompted by the most commonly known aspect of its treatment—stimulant medication, often methylphenidate (e.g., Ritalin, Concerta). Amphetamine (e.g., Dexedrine, Adderall) and pemoline (Cylert) are also commonly used to treat ADHD. Although a multimodal approach to ADHD is recommended (combining a stimulant with home and school behavioral management plans as discussed previously), it is the highly publicized stimulant therapy that is frequently the first and sole treatment. The stimulants are reported to be effective in at least 70% of individuals with ADHD, although part of the problem is that many conditions other than ADHD (and normal status as well) can show improvement with stimulant administration. Dose-response relationships may vary with age, intelligence, and the nature of the targeted behavior. While a clear neurotransmitter mechanism remains unclear, the stimulants are thought to affect dopaminergic or noradrenergic motor inhibitory control systems in the brain, thereby reducing impulsive and off-task behavior and potentiating delays between stimuli and responses.

There are concerns that stimulants are being prescribed to make perfectly acceptable students into even better ones ("cosmetic" use) and that stimulant abuse is on the rise. The latter concern, in the general context of substance abuse, is probably more of a psychological than physiologic concern; investigations have found that short-acting stimulants carry relatively low abuse liability due to the brief and mild pleasure experienced with these drugs. A substantial minority of older children and adolescents report a disagreeable feeling of prim sobriety when on stimulant medication. Furthermore, studies have shown that the risk of substance abuse in patients with ADHD is associated with the disorder itself, is increased by the comorbidity of conduct disorder, but is not due to treatment with stimulants.

The other fears surrounding adverse effects of stimulants are (1) stunting of growth after chronic childhood administration and (2) bringing out tics or even Tourette syndrome. Several longitudinal studies have failed to produce evidence of stunted growth in stimulant-treated ADHD, with recent articles suggesting that shorter-than-expected stature may be associated with the disorder itself. The relationship of stimulants to tics raises more complex issues; transient tics (not full blown Tourette syndrome) can be elicited as a side effect, usually subsiding after cessation of treatment. When Tourette syndrome makes its appearance while a child is taking stimulants (because more than half of those with Tourette syndrome also have ADHD and initially present clinically with symptoms/signs of ADHD), it is likely that this would have occurred later, even without using stimulants.

The other side effects of stimulants involve appetite suppression, insomnia, rebound exacerbations of symptoms and signs, and manifestations of "bad mood." Frequently, these side effects are manageable by means of altering dosage or the timing of the doses. Remarkably, the sole non–brain-mediated side effect (liver toxicity) is reported only with pemoline, the least prescribed of the stimulants.

Thus, the major reservations about stimulant treatment for ADHD arise not from what harm it may do but from the limitations of its demonstrated benefits. If the stimulants are not effective or cause unmanageable side effects, alternative medications include the norepinephrine selective reuptake inhibitor atomoxetine (recently released as Strattera); tricyclic antidepressants (desipramine, imipramine, nortriptyline), which have fallen somewhat out of favor due to the known, but uncommon, side effect of cardiac toxicity; clonidine; and bupropion, which has recently been reported to be effective in decreasing symptoms and signs of impulsivity and off-task behavior, particularly in individuals with comorbid depression.

In summary, school problems usually result from complex mixtures of developmental and environmental deficits. Even when "pure," the syndromes of dyslexia and ADHD require long-term, flexible, and multifactorial treatment/support programs.

Suggested Readings

Barkley RA. Behavioral inhibition, sustained attention, and executive functions: constructing a unifying theory of ADHD. *Psychol Bull* 1997;121:65.

Denckla MB. ADHD: topic update. *Brain Dev* 2003;25:383.

Jensen PS, Hinshaw SP, Swanson JM, et al. Findings from the NIMH Multimodal Treatment Study of ADHD (MTA): implications and applications for primary care providers. *J Dev Behav Pediatr* 2001;22:60.

Lyon GR, Fletcher JM, Barnes MC. Learning disabilities. In: Mash EJ, Barkley RA, eds. *Child psychopathology,* 2nd ed. New York: Guilford Press, 2002: 520.

Shaywitz SE. Dyslexia. *N Engl J Med* 1998;338:307.

Torgesen JK. Individual differences in response to early interventions in reading: the lingering problem of treatment resisters. *Learn Disabil Res Practice* 2000;15:55.

Wilens TE, Biederman J, Spencer TJ. Attention deficit/hyperactivity disorder across the lifespan. *Ann Rev Med* 2002;53:113.

Willcutt EG, Pennington BF, Boada R, et al. A comparison of the cognitive deficits in reading disability and attention-deficit/hyperactivity disorder. *J Abnorm Psychol* 2001;110:157.

CHAPTER 114 ■ ADOPTION

LAURIE C. MILLER

Adoption is a positive way to provide children who lack parents with the vital necessities of childhood: a loving home and family. Pediatricians encounter adoption in many ways: preadoption counseling for prospective parents, evaluation of children after adoption, and care and follow-up of adoptees throughout childhood and adolescence. In this chapter, the demographics and medical issues related to domestic and international adoption are reviewed from a pediatric perspective. Special considerations related to international adoption are highlighted.

DEMOGRAPHICS OF ADOPTION

It is estimated that there are somewhere between 5 and 6 million adoptees in the United States today, triple the number just a few years ago. Counting birth parents, adoptive parents, biologic and adoptive siblings, and extended family, tens of millions of Americans are directly connected to adoption. The Evan B. Donaldson Adoption Institute recently found that an amazing six out of ten Americans are personally connected to adoption.

Domestic Adoption

Actual statistics on adoption are not known, because the majority of adoptions in the United States take place informally among relatives and never come under the purview of the legal system. Children may be raised by grandparents, stepparents, or other relatives. The federal government does not keep records of adoption, although some states collect statistics. Domestic adoptions peaked in the 1970s when approximately

TABLE 114.1

TOP TEN COUNTRIES AS SOURCES OF CHILDREN FOR ADOPTION

2002		2001		2000	
China	5,053	China	4,681	China	5,053
Russia	4,939	Russia	4,279	Russia	4,269
Guatemala	2,219	South Korea	1,870	South Korea	1,794
South Korea	1,779	Guatemala	1,609	Guatemala	1,518
Ukraine	1,106	Ukraine	1,246	Romania	1,122
Kazakhstan	809	Romania	782	Vietnam	724
Vietnam	766	Vietnam	737	Ukraine	659
India	466	Kazakhstan	672	India	503
Colombia	334	India	543	Cambodia	402
Bulgaria	260	Colombia	407	Kazakhstan	399
Other	2,358	Other	2,411	Other	1,275
TOTAL	20,099	TOTAL	19,237	TOTAL	17,718

From http://www.travel.state.gov/orphan_numbers.html.

175,000 adoptions per year were legalized. In 1996, the National Council for Adoption Survey recorded 108,463 domestic adoptions. Adoptions were split equally between relatives and nonrelatives. It is estimated that adoption plans are made for fewer than 1% of children born in the United States and only 2% of infants born to single mothers. Of more than 31,000 public adoptions monitored by the Department of Health and Human Services in 1998, nearly one-third crossed racial or cultural lines. Special needs domestic adoptions more than doubled between the 1980s and 1990s (to approximately 20,000 a year). Adoptions from foster care have also increased recently, to about 50,000 in 1998. However, more than 100,000 children in American foster care still await adoption.

International Adoption

The numbers of international adoptions are easier to track because of records maintained by the Department of Immigration and Naturalization Services (INS). The numbers of internationally adopted children fluctuated between 7,000 and 9,000 between 1986 and 1995 but increased to 20,099 in 2002. The sources of these children have changed over time, which reflects political, cultural, and economic changes in the individual countries and the United States (Table 114.1). Nearly 130,000 internationally adopted children have arrived in the United States since 1995, more than 100,000 of them since 1998. Statistics on adoption trends by region, state, and country of origin may be found in Adamec and Pierce and at http://travel.state.gov/int'ladoption.html.

Types of Adoption

Adoptions may be classified in many ways. Adoptions are often described by the amount of information shared between the adoptive and birth parents and the child. These arrangements include traditional or closed adoptions, in which all identifying information remains confidential; semiopen adoptions, in which limited information is shared (directly or through an intermediary) and occasional correspondence may be exchanged; and open adoptions, in which ongoing contact is maintained, including correspondence, phone calls, and visits. Current adoption practices support some degree of openness for the well-being of the child. The constraints of international adoption preclude these practices.

Many types of individuals choose to adopt. Some parents adopt after failed infertility treatment; others with birth children adopt to expand their families. Some gay or lesbian individuals and couples choose to adopt. Single-parent adoption is also increasing; nearly one-third of adoptive parents in the United States in 2002 were single women.

The Internet has greatly expanded availability of adoption resources; for example, a Google search using the key word "adoption" returns over 18 million listings.

WHO ARE THE CHILDREN?

Although children available for adoption may be thought of as orphans, in reality orphans account for only a tiny percentage of potential adoptees. In the United States and other countries, adoptees are born to parents who are young, single, and/or impoverished, or those who suffer from psychiatric disease (especially maternal depression) and/or drug or alcohol abuse. Most internationally adopted children were abandoned—usually by the birth mother after delivery. The unusual situation in China of the one child per family policy, combined with the strong cultural preference for boys, has resulted in the abandonment of hundreds of thousands of infant girls.

The legal steps necessary to ascertain the child's status and availability for adoption vary considerably from country to country, as does attention to the legal rights of the birth parents. Unscrupulous individuals may conspire in abhorrent baby-selling practices. The best defense for prospective adoptive parents is to work with licensed, reputable, experienced agencies, but even then, problems can occur.

Sometimes children available for adoption have been removed from parental custody because of abuse or neglect. In the United States, these children usually reside in foster care prior to adoptive placement. Another group of children available for international adoption may be street children who have come under the protection of government or private child welfare agencies. Again, the prior history of the children is generally not known.

Many children who might potentially be eligible for adoption languish in institutional or foster care because of missing paperwork (e.g., relinquishment documents from the birth father) or legal uncertainties.

Care of the Children Prior to Adoption

Children are cared for in a variety of settings before adoption. In the United States, children adopted after the newborn period often experience multiple foster care placements, with

TABLE 114.2

RECOMMENDED SCREENING TESTS FOR
INTERNATIONAL ADOPTEES

Complete blood count
Urinalysis
Lead level
Hepatitis B sAg, core Ab, and sAb*
Hepatitis C*
Rapid plasma reagin test
Human immunodeficiency virus test*
Thyroid function test
Liver function test
Mantoux test*
Stool for ova and parasites
Newborn screening test
Developmental assessment
Hearing and vision screening
Dental screening
Consider glucose 6-phosphate dehydrogenase and
    hemoglobin electrophoresis

*Repeat in 4 to 6 months.

attendant emotional, psychological, and educational disruptions. Unfortunately, these children also suffer from lack of routine health care, immunizations, dental care, and vision/hearing screening. These deficiencies are especially disturbing as this population has considerable medical needs, including emotional handicaps (33%), serious physical illnesses (13%), mental retardation (19%), and multiple handicaps (15%).

Other countries use different systems to care for abandoned children. In Eastern Europe and China, most children reside in government-run orphanages. Conditions in these facilities vary drastically, but all expose the children to some extent to the risks of institutionalization (Table 114.2). Orphanage caregivers usually try to provide loving, nurturing environments for the children but often are thwarted by financial or other constraints. In some orphanages, children may receive better and more abundant food, clothing, and medical care than poor children living with their parents in the same regions. Nonetheless, these children lack the vital benefits of growing up in a family. In other countries, children may reside in private, often church-run orphanages. Thus, institutionalization is a highly heterogeneous experience for children.

Supervised (usually excellent) foster care is the usual placement for healthy babies awaiting adoption in South Korea. Other countries (Romania, Guatemala) use foster care sporadically. As in our own country, difficulties within the foster care system may occur. Many adoption professionals in Eastern Europe believe that children cannot be adequately supervised in foster care; thus, the institutional approach is preferred.

Most countries evaluate children at different ages to determine the suitability of their placements. This system was the basis of the notorious "switching" centers in Ceauşescu's Romania, where children were "tracked" into different centers based on brief evaluations at age 3 years. In most locations, this periodic reevaluation is done with genuine concern for the well-being of the child. Most countries maintain parallel systems for healthy or handicapped children. Many children assigned to handicapped facilities have conditions that would be readily treatable in the United States; unfortunately, these children may be consigned to institutions with no chance for rehabilitation or education.

Nearly all orphanages are age-restricted, thus requiring children to make multiple transitions from familiar caregivers and environments during childhood. Even within the same facility, children often move to age-specific units every 6 to 12 months.

Sadly, for each child who is adopted, many thousands are left behind in long-term institutional care.

PREPARATION OF THE ADOPTIVE PARENTS

Prospective parents may choose to adopt independently (except in Colorado, Delaware, Connecticut, and Massachusetts) or through an adoption agency. Adoption agencies require a home study that determines the suitability of adoptive parents; independent adoptions require a similar report from the state welfare department or equivalent. The study generally involves several sessions with a social worker and a home visit. The home study addresses the parents' motivation for adoption, moral attitudes, financial status, religious beliefs, employment, educational achievements, marriage, childrearing practices, and housing. Parents also must assemble copies of birth and marriage certificates, letters of recommendation from community leaders, reports of physical and mental health from a physician and a psychiatrist, and financial statements from employers and banks. Police and FBI clearance must also be obtained, including fingerprinting. The documents must be notarized and the notary's seal authenticated by state authorities. For international adoptions, an extract of this document is forwarded to government officials or the affiliated agency in the child's birth country.

Process of International Adoption for Families

The process of international adoption is cumbersome, often stressful, and frequently fraught with bureaucratic delays. The family must accomplish a legal adoption in the child's birth country, followed by a visa investigation supervised by the Bureau of Citizenship and Immigration Services. The process includes an examination by a physician designated by the U.S. embassy in the birth country. The examining physician is instructed to examine the child with attention to "exclusionary conditions" [chancroid, gonorrhea, granuloma inguinale, Hansen disease, lymphogranuloma venereum, syphilis, tuberculosis, human immunodeficiency virus (HIV) infection, mental retardation, sexual deviation, psychopathic personality, mental defect, narcotic addiction, alcoholism, or "one or more attacks of insanity"]. The INS requires HIV and tuberculosis testing only in children older than 15 years or "if risk factors are identified." Until 1997, adoptees, like all immigrants, were required to complete all vaccinations recommended for age before travel; fortunately, a waiver for adoptees was passed. Many prospective parents rely on the visa examination to identify serious problems in their child; however, the examination is often perfunctory. If serious concerns about the health of the child are raised by the referral information, these should be addressed long before the visa examination.

Because of frequent delays in both the birth country and U.S. bureaucracy, the entire process after the prospective parents accept the child referred to them can take as long as 12 to 18 months. Psychologically, most parents feel that at the moment of assignment the child becomes theirs, comparable to the moment in the delivery room when a child is first handed to the parents. This makes the waiting period especially difficult.

Several popular sending countries have recently closed for international adoption (Vietnam, Cambodia, and Romania). The recent passage of the Hague Convention on Inter-Country Adoption is resulting in many changes in adoption practices throughout the world as countries attempt to comply with these new international standards.

Referral and Preadoptive Counseling

The referral is the offer of an individual child to prospective adoptive parents. Most prospective adoptive parents request the advice of a pediatrician when they receive the referral of a child. For both domestic and international adoptions, varying amounts of medical and family history is available. The pediatrician may have the opportunity to request additional information or even testing if indicated. International referrals vary enormously in quality and content. Most sending countries involved in international adoption provide photographs of the child. Referrals of children from Eastern Europe are often accompanied by videotapes of the child. These tapes vary widely in content and quality, but are often helpful in excluding obvious medical or neurologic conditions and can be used to roughly assess development. Most parents are anxious to know if signs of fetal alcohol syndrome are seen. Written reports from Russia and the former Soviet Union have been difficult to interpret because of the system of neurologic diagnosis commonly used there. Virtually all reports from this region include frightening and unusual terms such as perinatal encephalopathy, hypertension-hydrocephalus syndrome, and infringement of the cerebral circulation. These diagnoses are not confirmed when children are examined in the United States. Unusual reports of ultrasound findings also are frequently included (accessory chordae tendinea, cranial deformation of the vascular plexuses). However, useful pedagogic descriptions are often included for older children, as well as comments about the child's language skills, interests, and special abilities.

In general, referrals from South Korea include accurate information about the birth parents' health, education, and occupations; birth data including measurements, Apgar scores, and complications; and records of complete and careful physical and developmental examinations. Parents are often provided with monthly updates, as well as results of routine screening tests and vaccination records. Referrals from China tend to be brief, with the child's name, (assigned) birth date, and a physical examination that nearly always is reported as normal, along with one or two photographs of the child. Weights can best be described as approximations, because the children are rarely weighed unclothed. Usually, results of liver function, hepatitis B, HIV, and syphilis testing also are included. Reports from other Asian countries and South and Central America vary considerably but often include accurate history, physical examination, and laboratory testing. Parents should be cautioned that negative laboratory results on their prospective child are no guarantee of actual health status, because test results may be incorrect or children can become infected (e.g., with hepatitis B) after the test has been done. Laboratory testing in birth countries should be avoided, unless use of sterile needles and syringes and a reputable laboratory can be assured.

Russian law now requires prospective adoptive parents to travel on two separate visits to complete the adoption. Little information about the child is offered prior to the first trip. Parents adopting from Ukraine receive almost no information prior to travel. These parents often seek urgent guidance from their American pediatrician by e-mail (including review of digital photos or videos) after meeting the child.

PEDIATRICIAN'S ROLE

The pediatrician may be consulted at various times during the adoption process. Many parents visit the pediatrician in advance of the adoption, somewhat equivalent to the prenatal visit. This visit allows prospective parents to express their concerns and expectations and to assess the pediatrician's familiarity with adoption-related issues. Pediatricians should be especially sensitive to first-time parents adopting a child beyond the newborn stage. These parents have missed all the anticipatory guidance and parenting and safety advice that are customarily dispensed at routine intervals. Extra attention to these families is essential. For older children, pediatricians are consulted on school readiness and advice on grade placement. Although some older children in institutional care have had educational opportunities, many have never been in a classroom setting. Lack of experience, the challenge of learning a new language, and emotional maturity must all be considered when determining school placement. Pediatricians also are consulted during childhood and adolescence as the children experience adoption-related psychological and emotional issues at different developmental stages.

Medical Issues

The medical issues encountered in adopted children relate to the child's country of origin, age at adoption, and prior life experiences, in addition to genetic, prenatal, and perinatal factors. Inadequate prenatal care; nutritional deficiencies; drug, alcohol, and nicotine exposure; and premature deliveries are more common in women who relinquish their infants in the United States and abroad. In general, medical concerns differ for children adopted domestically and internationally. Domestic adoptions of infants are likely to raise concerns about infection with HIV or possible prenatal drug or alcohol exposure. Although these problems often can be identified in the newborn period, occasionally they manifest only later in infancy. Few statistics are available to indicate the prevalence of these problems. Older children adopted from the foster care system may have suffered prenatal drug or alcohol exposure, neglect, physical or sexual abuse, and multiple placements. Not surprisingly, an increased incidence of learning problems, hyperactivity, and social and emotional problems is found in this group of children.

Family history may or may not be available for domestic or international adoptees. Information about possibly heritable problems as manic-depressive disorder, schizophrenia, or alcoholism should be shared with prospective parents, if available.

These problems, and more, may be found in internationally adopted children. In a survey of 293 international adoptees, 57% were found to have an important medical diagnosis; in 81% of these, the diagnosis was established by screening test results (Table 114.3 lists suggested screening tests for new arrivals). Because these children are rarely placed as newborns, they frequently exhibit some of the medical, developmental, and psychosocial complications of institutionalization. Many of these problems relate to the duration of institutionalization. For example, in a group of Romanian adoptees, the risk of acquiring intestinal parasites increased with the duration of orphanage confinement (Fig. 114.1). Parasites may escape

TABLE 114.3

EFFECTS OF INSTITUTIONALIZATION ON CHILDREN

Exposure to infections
Lack of access to medical diagnosis and treatment
Lack of nurturing physical contact
Poor nutrition and growth
Delayed cognitive development
Physical neglect
Emotional neglect
Vulnerability to physical and sexual abuse
Exposure to poor hygiene

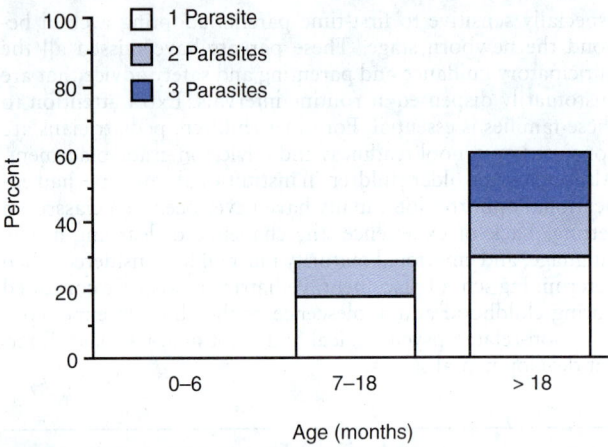

FIGURE 114.1. Risk of parasites related to time in orphanage. Fifty-eight percent of children confined for more than 18 months had a parasite; 45% had multiple parasites.

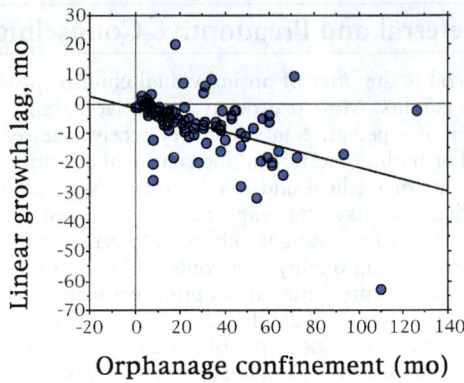

FIGURE 114.2. Linear growth lag in months related to duration of orphanage confinement.

detection on initial screening; children should be retested if poor growth, abdominal pain, or diarrhea present later. Over-all, parasites are found in approximately 60% of international adoptees; *Giardia lamblia* is by far the most frequent isolate.

Viral hepatitis also occurs among international adoptees. Approximately 5% to 7% of international adoptees test positive for hepatitis B surface antigen on arrival in the United States. Hepatitis C is seen infrequently, and HIV is rare, al-though many countries lack sterile disposable needles and sy-ringes, and blood products (immunoglobulin, transfusions) may be used therapeutically for ill children. Because of the pos-sibility that initial screening tests for hepatitis B, hepatitis C, and HIV may be done during a seronegative window, follow-up testing 4 to 6 months after arrival is recommended.

Latent tuberculosis infection is common (approximately 10% of adoptees) despite widespread administration of bacille Calmette-Guérin vaccine. All adoptees should be screened with a Mantoux test, regardless of the presence of a bacille Calmette-Guérin scar (usually found on the left deltoid), unless the vac-cine has been administered recently. Reactions greater than 10 mm should be considered likely evidence of latent tuber-culosis infection in this high-risk population. Children with positive Mantoux reactions should be carefully examined for clinical signs of tuberculosis; treatment with prophylactic isoni-azid is warranted for those with probable latent disease. Man-toux testing should be repeated 4 to 6 months after arrival in those whose test results are negative at entry.

Dietary deficiencies result in anemia and rickets; the latter is exacerbated by indoor confinement of many children during institutionalization. Iron deficiency anemia is found in approxi-mately 70% of international adoptees. Hypothyroidism occurs in areas of endemic iodine deficiency. Lead poisoning may re-sult from industrial pollution, contaminated food or water, or ingestion of lead paint chips from the crib or toys. Lead poi-soning is more common in children adopted from China than in those from other countries.

Other medical problems must be identified by specific screening. For example, syphilis testing is not universal in preg-nant women in many countries, or results may not be available to adoptive parents. Approximately 10% to 15% of the medi-cal reports from Eastern Europe and Russia report a history of maternal syphilis. Generally, these children are given adequate treatment; specific clinical problems have not been detected in this group after adoption.

Newborn screening for phenylketonuria and other meta-bolic disorders is not routinely done as part of screening of newly arrived children, but should be considered especially for infants with developmental delays.

Growth Delays

Growth delays are common in international adoptees. Linear growth lag (in months) has been shown to correlate with the du-ration of orphanage confinement (Fig. 114.2). Each 3 months of orphanage life resulted in a 1-month delay in linear growth. Weight and head circumference delays also are frequent in this population. Although some of the physical delays in this popu-lation undoubtedly result from insufficient caloric intake, some evidence suggests that infants require tactile stimulation to use ingested nutrients. The catch-up physical growth after adop-tion is usually remarkable, particularly in younger children (Fig. 114.3). This pattern is so typical that children who do not show adequate catch-up growth within approximately 6 months after adoption should be carefully evaluated for other causes of short stature or failure to thrive. Recovery from linear growth delays is less complete in older children. Some children have deranged eating habits and require careful evaluation, in-tervention, and supplementation.

Surprising catch-up growth in head circumference is some-times seen as well. The long-term outcome of children with early microcephaly is unknown. Many children appear to do very well developmentally, but may be at increased risk of cog-nitive, learning, and behavior problems in later childhood.

Other Medical Problems

Some studies suggest an increased risk of precocious puberty in international adoptees, presumably caused by dysregulation of hypothalamic hormones in rapid catch-up growth after mal-nutrition.

Many unsuspected medical diagnoses are made in adoptees from institutions after arrival in the United States. Congeni-tal cardiac and orthopedic abnormalities are sometimes found. Undetected hearing loss has been found regularly in this popu-lation, and routine audiograms are recommended. Strabismus is another frequent finding; ophthalmologic evaluation is rec-ommended as well. Older children are likely to have multiple dental caries.

Inadequate vaccination is frequent in international adop-tees. Often, vaccination records are incomplete or simply state "DPT 2." Prospective studies at international adoption clinics reveal that some vaccinated children are not immune. Live virus vaccines that require maintenance of cold chain after manufac-ture may be especially likely to have compromised immuno-genicity. Revaccinating or obtaining titers to verify immunity is therefore advisable.

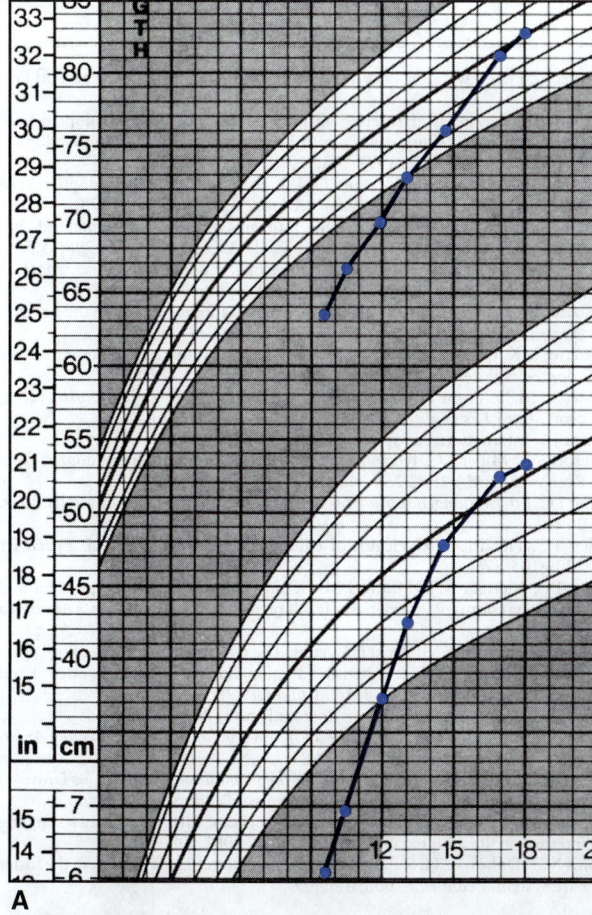

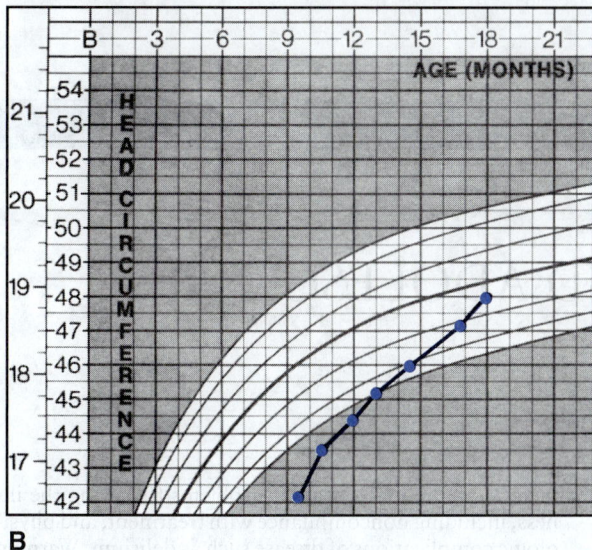

FIGURE 114.3. A: Catch-up growth for weight and height. **B:** Catch-up growth for head circumference.

Uncertain Dates of Birth

Many international adoptees (approximately 15%) have uncertain dates of birth. A child found on the street is assigned an age when entering care. Occasionally, after multiple moves between institutions, birth certificates and other paperwork of abandoned children are lost, or transcription errors occur. Generally, age assignments in the birth country are acceptable. For those few in whom the assigned age seems incorrect, weight, height, head circumference, and developmental, bone, and dental ages should be determined. A period of 6 to 12 months of observation is usually advisable before assigning a definitive legal age assignment. This allows the children to recover from growth and developmental delays and allows determination of the best functional age of the child.

Developmental Delays

Developmental delays are nearly universal in postinstitutionalized children (greater than 90%). Most children show rapid recovery from these delays within the first 6 to 12 months after adoption; however, long-term follow-up suggests that recovery is incomplete in many children. Language delays may be the most problematic and are not adequately addressed by English as a second language programs. In reality, the children have significant delays in their birth languages and require speech therapy rather than simply learning a new language. Early intervention programs and special needs programs within the school system can provide enormous resources to these children and their families.

Behavioral Problems

Behavioral problems are seen in some children after adoption. Some are "orphanage behaviors" such as rocking, head banging, self-mutilation, pain insensitivity, risk taking, and food hoarding. Sensory integration dysfunction may contribute to these behaviors, and therapy specifically addressed to sensory issues may be helpful. Indiscriminate friendliness and lack of stranger anxiety are common and, in some children, may signal attachment problems if persistent. Sleep disturbances are frequent, especially shortly after the adoption. Distractibility, attention-deficit hyperactivity disorder, learning disabilities, auditory processing deficits, depression, and anxiety also are found in this group of children. The frequency of these problems in postinstitutionalized children is unknown. Some postinstitutionalized children who suffered severe deprivation in infancy later exhibit a complex neuropsychiatric behavioral disorder with features of autism, pervasive developmental delay, and posttraumatic stress disorder. A longitudinal study of Romanian children in Canada showed that 4 or more years after adoption approximately one-third of children had no serious problems and were doing well, one-third had a few serious problems but were progressing toward average levels of performance and behavior, and one-third still had several serious problems.

These children remind a new generation of pediatricians about the ill effects of institutionalizing young children, which our predecessors recognized in American orphanages of the 1800s to 1950s (Table 114.3). Optimal treatment for these children is yet to be devised, and the long-term outcome of such children is unknown. Such findings have prompted most adoption professionals to counsel prospective parents that children adopted from institutions should be considered special needs children who likely require a period of rehabilitation, which may be lifelong. Informal surveys of parents who have adopted internationally overwhelmingly indicate that, knowing what they know now, they would make the same decision to adopt. Parent support networks such as Adoptive Families of America and the Parent Network for Post-Institutionalized Children and country-specific organizations such as Families for Russian and Ukrainian Adoption or Families with Children from China can be helpful to families dealing with such challenging children. Adoption agencies also are expanding their role to provide services after placement.

PSYCHOSOCIAL AND EMOTIONAL ISSUES FOR ADOPTEES DURING CHILDHOOD AND ADOLESCENCE

For the adoptee, different issues predominate at different ages. Most adoption professionals counsel parents to be open and honest with their children about adoption and, in the case of international adoption, to celebrate the child's birth heritage. Nonetheless, parents and children must be prepared for comments from strangers, for poorly devised school projects such as drawing family trees, and other, more serious, challenges to personal identity. Although adopted children appear to be overrepresented among populations receiving mental health services, it has never been ascertained whether this is because adoptive families may be more likely to avail themselves of such services or whether it truly reflects an increased incidence of psychosocial difficulties. The process of adoption is likely to make families aware of resources available for themselves or their children.

CONCLUSIONS

Pediatricians can become involved with many aspects of adoption, including preadoption counseling, evaluation of medical referrals provided to prospective parents, and examination of children after placement to ascertain health and developmental status. Adoptive families rely on their pediatrician as a resource and support for medical, behavioral, and developmental issues during the adoption process and throughout childhood and adolescence.

Suggested Readings

Adamec C, Pierce WL. *The encyclopedia of adoption.* New York: Facts on File, 1991.

Albers LH, Johnson DE, Hostetter MK, et al. Health of children adopted from the former Soviet Union and Eastern Europe. Comparison with preadoptive medical records. *JAMA* 1997;278:922.

Benoit TC, Jocelyn LJ, Moddemann DM, Embree JE. Romanian adoption. The Manitoba experience. *Arch Pediatr Adolesc Med* 1996;150:1278.

Cermak S, Groze V. Sensory processing problems in post-institutionalized children: implications for social workers. *Child Adol Soc Work J* 1998;15:5.

Evan B. *Donaldson Adoption Institute. Benchmark adoption survey: report on findings.* New York: Evan B. Donaldson Adoption Institute, 1997.

Hostetter M. Infectious diseases in internationally adopted children: the past five years. *Pediatr Infect Dis J* 1998;17:517.

Hostetter MK, Iverson S, Thomas W, et al. Medical evaluation of internationally adopted children. *N Engl J Med* 1991;325:479.

Hostetter M, Johnson DE. International adoption. An introduction for physicians. *Am J Dis Child* 1989;143:325.

Jenista JA. International adoption. *Pediatr Ann* 2000;29.

Johnson DE, Miller LC, Iverson S, et al. The health of children adopted from Romania. *JAMA* 1992;268:3446.

Miller LC. *International adoption medicine.* New York: Oxford University Press, 2004.

Miller LC, Hendrie NW. Health of children adopted from China. *Pediatrics* 2000;105:E76.

Miller LC, Kiernan MT, Mathers MI, Klein-Gitelman M. Developmental and nutritional status of internationally adopted children. *Arch Pediatr Adol Med* 1995;149:40.

O'Connor TG, Rutter M, Beckett C, et al. The effects of global severe privation on cognitive competence: extension and longitudinal follow-up. English and Romanian Adoptees Study Team. *Child Dev* 2000;71:376.

Pavao JM. *The family of adoption.* Boston: Beacon Press, 1998.

Pertman A. *Adoption nation: how the adoption revolution is transforming America.* New York: Basic Books, 2000.

Pickering LK, ed. *2000 red book: report of the Committee on Infectious Diseases.* Elk Grove Village, IL: American Academy of Pediatrics, 2000.

Saiman L, Aronson JE, Zhou J, et al. Prevalence of infectious diseases among internationally adopted children. *Pediatrics* 2001;108:608.

Simms MD, Dubowitz H, Szilagyi MA. Health care needs of children in the foster care system. *Pediatrics* 2000;106:909.

CHAPTER 115 ■ CHILD AND ADOLESCENT PSYCHIATRIC REFERRAL

JAMES C. HARRIS

Pediatricians should include a child and adolescent psychiatrist on their list of consultants. In considering referral, the pediatrician should remember that a mental disorder represents an impairment in social adaptation. It is accompanied by either painful psychological symptoms or disruptive behavior that is disabling as a result of its effects on others. Referral may be indicated in the following situations:

- Dysfunctional parent–child relationships, particularly involving infants and toddlers, that have not responded to routine parenting strategies: Parent training is particularly important in an era when child abuse and sexual misuse occur far too frequently; these are preventable problems.
- Physiologic, psychological, and behavioral complications of medical illness: These include psychological adjustment to the illness; behavior problems following the illness, including noncompliance with treatment; and physiologic complications of disease such as delirium. Warning signs for adjustment difficulties might be frequent office or emergency department visits, vague complaints that are difficult to ascribe to a physical condition, and continued difficulty adapting to a chronic disease.
- Persistent changes in behavior after stressful experiences: An adjustment disorder or posttraumatic stress disorder may occur after severe stress, such as an accident or loss of a significant family member. Changes in behavior also may accompany marital discord, family violence, psychiatric disorder in a parent, and drug or alcohol abuse by a family member.
- Disruptive behavior disorders and excessive risk-taking behavior: Children with attention-deficit hyperactivity

disorder are vulnerable to both oppositional defiant and conduct disorders. Children with symptoms of stealing, lying, cruelty to animals or other children, drug or alcohol use, or inappropriate sexual behavior are at risk for subsequent delinquency and require early intervention. Risk-taking behavior is frequently seen in adolescents who are struggling with adjustment to a chronic illness or difficult family circumstances.

■ Suicidal behavior (parasuicide) or threats: These behaviors are among the most important reasons to seek consultation.

■ Somatic symptoms associated with a mental disorder: Physical symptoms accompany many of the mental disorders of childhood and adolescence, including separation anxiety disorder, generalized anxiety disorder, social phobia, depressive disorders, anorexia nervosa, schizophrenia, circadian rhythm sleep disorder, and the dyssomnias.

■ Problems related to psychotropic medications: These include self-poisoning, choice of medication, questions regarding side effects, and appropriate dosages. Children with attention-deficit hyperactivity disorder who are receiving more than one medication for their behavior or are taking high doses of medication may require referral.

When using psychotropic medications, it is essential to keep in mind that drug use is only one aspect of the treatment. All children who receive these medications need a multimodality approach to treatment. The modes of treatment include appropriate school placement and individual, family, or group therapy, in addition to the psychotropic agent.

■ Treatment of major mental disorders: The early recognition of affective disorder and schizophrenia in childhood is essential for the child and the family. Suicide is a major complication that may be avoided by early recognition and treatment of depressive disorders. Reluctance by the physician to make these diagnoses because of unrealistic fears about the stigma of having a major mental disorder is unwarranted. The Alliance for the Mentally Ill and other family support groups are effectively advocating to prevent the additional handicap of stigma in the life of mentally ill individuals.

■ Mental disorder in a parent: Psychiatric referral is indicated when personality disturbance and major mental illness, particularly depressive disorder and psychosis, is diagnosed in parents. Substance abuse in parents is of particular concern.

SECTION V ■ PEDIATRIC EMERGENCIES

CHAPTER 116 ■ SELECTED TOPICS IN EMERGENCY MEDICINE

PAULA J. SCHWEICH

Often, visits to the emergency department (ED) are stressful for children and parents. The staff members are strangers to the children, the environment may appear chaotic, and the rooms can be confining and sterile. If the ED is busy, necessitating a wait, children can become tired and restless, and the parents can become impatient. The ED staff should make every effort to ensure that children and parents are as comfortable and calm as possible.

HISTORY TAKING

Chief Complaint

If emergent treatment is needed, a brief history relevant to the problem is obtained so that appropriate therapy can be instituted. After emergent therapy is administered, a more detailed history can be obtained. This detailed history includes a description of the complaint through the length of time of illness, behavior of the affected child during the illness (e.g., interaction and feeding), and associated signs and symptoms. A full review of systems may reveal other important parts of the history.

MEDICAL HISTORY

A short medical history may reveal problems that were not discussed during the initial history. This history should include previous illnesses, including similar symptoms; hospitalizations; allergies to medications; medications past and present; surgeries; and status of immunizations. This information should be included in all ED records.

Physical Examination

The physical examination for all children begins with an assessment of toxicity. Particularly in young children, physicians should have a good idea of how ill an affected child appears before touching the child. Observation of the child should begin during the history-taking portion of the visit. The examination techniques depend on the child's age. In most children, the quiet and nonintrusive parts of the examination are performed first, such as assessment of heart and lungs, and the more threatening parts are examined last, such as assessment of ears and throat. The examination should focus on the system involved with the chief complaint, but a complete physical examination is necessary.

Infants

Assessing the level of toxicity in small infants can be difficult. The history may include poor feeding, lethargy, or excessive sleepiness, and the seriousness of the complaints must be assessed by the physical examination. After observing an affected child in the parent's arms, the physician might hold the infant on his or her lap; this is helpful in assessing the degree of interaction and vigor. If the complaint involves feeding, infant feeding should be observed. During this time, the child's state (e.g., fussiness or irritability) is assessed, and the tone of the extremities is noted. With the baby either on the physician's lap or on the table, the anterior fontanel, heart, and lungs can be assessed, and abdominal examination can proceed. The results of the remainder of the examination, including skin and genitalia, can be noted as the examination proceeds.

Toddlers

Examining a toddler can be a challenge. Often, toddlers are restless and hungry in the ED, and they may react to a physician with stranger anxiety. Initial observation should note whether the child is fussy but calms with a parent, or is irritable and inconsolable. The physician may find that sitting on a stool with wheels is helpful. This approach allows the physician to begin the history taking at a distance from the toddler and to move closer during the discussion. At the end of the history taking, the child might be engaged with an interesting object, such as a beeper or stethoscope toy. If possible, the entire examination should be performed with the toddler in a parent's lap, where the child will feel most comfortable.

In toddlers, starting with an examination of the heart and lungs is crucial. After that phase, the abdomen should be palpated with the child sitting or lying in the parent's lap. This may be the only calm abdominal examination possible. In the presence of concern about the abdomen, further examination is attempted on the table. Examination of the extremities also can be performed on the parent's lap. For an extremity complaint, the parent can palpate and move the child's extremities first, starting with the uninvolved side. This technique should give a sense of whether the child is reacting to pain in the extremity. After the parent examines the limbs, the physician should attempt to examine the extremities in the same order. As in younger infants, the ears and throat should be examined last. This phase also can be performed on the parent's lap, with the child facing forward. The parent places one arm over the child's arms and the other arm over the child's head, firmly holding the head to one side. The throat can be examined with the head held straight forward.

Preschoolers

Because preschool-aged children are developing language skills, they may be able to describe what is bothering them, and the physician can explain calmly what is happening during the examination. The child may be eager to participate with the examination (e.g., holding the stethoscope on the chest). During parts of the examination, the child can be distracted with stories or explanations. For example, in examining the abdomen, if the examiner claims to be trying to feel for what the child ate during the last meal, the child is likely to lie very still and cooperate. Children at this age also feel fear and are imaginative; therefore, it is important to explain often that what is being done will not hurt. However, if a painful procedure is to be performed, such as drawing blood, the physician must be honest and explain what will happen.

School-Aged Children

Examining school-aged children is much easier than examining younger children, because these older children have well-developed language skills, a capacity to reason, and often a basic understanding of why they are in the ED. It is important to tell school-aged children why any treatment procedures are necessary.

Adolescents

Adolescents should be treated as adults with regard to explanations and privacy. Their medical history may be started with a parent in the room, but it is important to examine adolescents in the absence of the parent. More sensitive questions, such as those about sexual activity and drug use, can be asked during this phase of the examination. Also, it is important to address any fears that adolescents may have in regard to their illness.

CARDIOPULMONARY RESUSCITATION IN CHILDREN

Most pediatric cardiopulmonary arrests occur in young, previously healthy children. Every attempt should be made to identify the cause of the arrest, because special considerations may affect treatment. Noncardiac causes predominate; trauma is the leading cause of cardiopulmonary arrest in children 1 to 14 years of age. The most common causes are listed in Box 116.1.

In most patients with out-of-hospital arrest, a progression occurs from hypoxia and hypercarbia, to respiratory arrest and bradycardia, to asystolic cardiac arrest. In the case of acutely ill or injured children, the rescuer may be able to prevent respiratory and circulatory arrest with the correction of hypoxia alone. Because many causes of arrest in children are preventable and because elapsed time until initial resuscitation is such an important factor in survival, special efforts should be made in prevention and prehospital care.

Children who have delayed resuscitation or present in asystole have a poor prognosis, because hypoxemia already will have caused extensive damage to the brain and other vital organs. Survival is more likely if cardiopulmonary resuscitation (CPR) is started immediately, if only respiratory arrest is

---

BOX 116.1 Common Causes of Cardiac Arrest

Cause	Circumstances
Traumatic	Motor vehicle injuries, burns, child abuse, firearm wounds
Pulmonary	Foreign-body aspiration, smoke inhalation, near-drowning, respiratory failure
Infectious	Sepsis, meningitis
Central nervous system	Head trauma, seizures
Cardiac	Congenital heart disease, myocarditis
Other	Sudden infant death syndrome, poisoning, suicide, dehydration, congenital malformations

present, if the arrest is witnessed in the hospital, if the condition is extreme bradycardia rather than asystole, or if only oxygen is necessary.

Basic Life Support

The goals of life support are to optimize cardiac output and to sustain tissue oxygen delivery; most important are the metabolic demands of the myocardium and brain. Because respiratory failure is the most common cause of cardiac arrest in children, basic life support should begin immediately after discovery of the arrest victim. If there is only one rescuer, the cause of the emergency is unknown, and the child is 8 years old or younger, emergency medical services (EMS) should be notified after CPR has been performed for 1 minute ("phone Fast"). In older children, activate EMS first, and then start CPR ("phone First").

When initially approaching the victim, the rescuer should note whether there is any movement, crying or breathing, and color. The first priority is to assess the adequacy of airway, breathing, and circulation. For children who are accident victims and may have a neck injury, the neck should be stabilized with axial traction until a Philadelphia collar can be applied. Gently shaking and calling to the victim help determine degree of response or presence of respiratory difficulty. Affected conscious children should be allowed to position their airway; children automatically assume the best position. Unconscious children should be positioned on a firm surface. When affected children are moved or turned, the head, neck, and torso should be moved as a single unit. If a neck injury is not suspected, the examiner can place one hand on the forehead to tilt the head back to a neutral position. Overextension of the neck should be avoided, because it obstructs the trachea. The fingers of the free hand are placed under the lower jaw at the chin to lift the chin off the airway. For further movement of the jaw, the rescuer's hands are placed on both sides of the victim's head, allowing the palms to tilt the head back. Two or three fingers are placed at each mandibular angle to lift the jaw upward (i.e., jaw thrust). If a neck injury is suspected, the jaw thrust can be used without a head tilt.

After the airway is opened, the rescuer simultaneously should evaluate the chest wall and abdomen for movement, listen over the mouth and nose, and feel with the cheek for air flow. If a child is not breathing, and the airway is in the correct position, the rescuer should deliver two effective slow breaths immediately. The rescuer's mouth can cover the mouth and nose of an infant, or the nose (in older children) can be pinched closed for mouth-to-mouth breathing. In successful mouth-to-mouth breathing, chest movement is visible. If it is unsuccessful, the rescuer should try to reposition the airway and reattempt

ventilation. If still unsuccessful, the rescuer should check for a foreign body in the mouth or pharynx.

A child's airway is obstructed easily by aspiration of liquids and small objects (e.g., mucus, blood, vomitus, the tongue, hard candies, popcorn, nuts, removable parts of toys). Initially, an affected child coughs and gags but, if the obstruction is complete and the airway cannot be cleared, the child loses consciousness. The rescuer should attempt to relieve the obstruction only if the child's cough is weak and ineffective and respiratory difficulty is increasing.

If aspiration is witnessed or strongly suspected, or if an unconscious victim has airway obstruction that cannot be relieved by head-tilting and jaw-thrust maneuvers, the rescuer should attempt to remove the object manually—but only if it is visible on careful inspection. Blind finger sweeps may push a foreign body farther into the airway and should be avoided.

The Heimlich maneuver, a subdiaphragmatic abdominal thrust, produces an artificial cough and is considered safe for children older than 1 year of age. With the child supine, the heel of the rescuer's hand is placed in the midline between the umbilicus and rib cage and is pushed rapidly inward and upward. This maneuver can be repeated five times. It is not performed in a child younger than 1 year of age because of concern for intraabdominal injury. For children younger than 1 year of age, alternating back blows (five blows between the scapulae) and chest thrusts (five compressions, as in CPR) are recommended.

After the two rescue breaths are delivered, the victim is assessed for signs of circulation. Signs of circulation include adequate breathing, coughing, and movement. Health care providers should also perform a pulse check. The brachial pulse is checked in an infant; the carotid pulse in a child. If there are uncertain or no signs of circulation, compressions are started immediately. In small infants, the rescuer can encircle the infant's chest with both hands, support the back with the fingers, and compress the lower half of the sternum with both thumbs. As in adults, children's hearts lie under the lower third of the sternum, and compressions should be performed over this area. The compression phase should be 50% of the cycle. Chest compressions should produce palpable pulses in a central artery.

Chest compressions and ventilation are coordinated at the rate of five compressions to one ventilation (5:1) for infants and children up to 8 years of age. This high ratio of ventilations to compressions is to correct the hypoxia and hypercarbia that is the most common cause of pediatric cardiorespiratory arrest. A ratio of 15 compressions to 2 ventilations (15:2) is recommended for children 8 years of age and older. The compressions are delayed for ventilation. Table 116.1 outlines breathing and circulation requirements for basic life support. Patients should be reassessed 1 minute after resuscitation begins and again every few minutes.

TABLE 116.1

BASIC LIFE SUPPORT

Patient	Respirations/mm	Compressions/mm	Depth	Where to Compress
Infant (<1 yr)	20	100	1/3–1/2 anteroposterior diameter of chest	Place index finger below intermammary line; press with middle and ring fingers
Child (1–8 yr)	20	100	1/3–1/2 anteroposterior diameter of chest	Place middle and index fingers at base of sternum; place heel of hand above that and use for compression
Child (>8 yr)	12	100	1.5–2 inches	Place heel of hand on lower 1/2 of sternum; place other hand on top of first and press with both hands

TABLE 116.2

RESUSCITATION BAGS

Bag	Gas-Filled	Oxygen Concentration	Comments
Self-inflating	Refill independent of gas flow	60%–95% with O_2 reservoir	Easy to use
Flow-inflating	Refill depends on gas flow from source	Same as source	Overfills easily; can transmit high pressure to lungs

Advanced Cardiac Life Support

When children arrive in the ED, basic life support should be in progress. An initial assessment by the emergency physician includes level of consciousness, spontaneous respiratory effort, pulse, blood pressure, cardiac rhythm, temperature, perfusion, and pupillary responses. In advanced life support, as in basic life support, an assessment of airway, breathing, and circulation should begin the rescue.

Airway and Breathing

Children have a higher oxygen demand than adults because they have a higher metabolic rate. Therefore, with apnea or poor ventilation, hypoxemia develops rapidly. Mouth-to-mouth resuscitation provides at most 17% of the fraction of inspired oxygen in advanced cardiac life support. Humidified 100% oxygen should be administered to affected patients immediately on arrival at the hospital (or sooner if possible). The bag, valve, and mask setup (later to be converted to bag, valve, and endotracheal tube) should deliver 100% oxygen and should be equipped with a manometer and pressure-relief valve. Table 116.2 lists the differences between the two types of resuscitation bags. Ventilation bags used for resuscitation should be self-inflating. While equipment for intubation is being prepared (Box 116.2), the bag and valve should be fitted to a clear plastic mask that allows for an airtight seal against the child's face and for a small rebreathing volume. The soft circular masks seal well, and clear masks allow the physician to observe the color of the child and to see any vomitus. An oropharyngeal airway in an unconscious child or a nasopharyngeal airway in a conscious child helps keep the tongue forward during mask ventilation. A shortened tracheal tube can be used as a nasopharyngeal airway. Placing the airway next to the face allows the physician to determine the size of the oropharyngeal airway. With the flange at the central incisors, the tip of the airway should be at the angle of the mandible. The length of a nasopharyngeal airway is determined by the distance from the tip of the nose to the tragus of the ear.

Intubation should be performed as soon as possible if the patient continues without spontaneous respirations or needs prolonged ventilation. Intubation provides better ventilation,

higher oxygen concentration delivery, protection against aspiration, ability to suction secretions from the airways, and the ability to give positive end-expiratory pressure to the patient.

The pediatric airway is more flexible than is the adult airway, the tongue is relatively larger, and an anatomic narrowing exists at the level of the cricoid cartilage, precluding the necessity of using a cuffed endotracheal tube in children younger than 8 to 10 years of age. A cuffed tube with a low-pressure cuff is used for older children. An endotracheal tube of appropriate size is chosen, and one size larger and smaller should be available. If a stylet is used, its tip should be 1 to 2 cm proximal to the end of the endotracheal tube. The formula for determining endotracheal tube sizes is:

$$\text{Inside diameter} = \frac{16 + \text{age (years)}}{4}$$

Newborn, 3.0 to 3.5 Inside diameter (mm).

The depth of insertion from the distal end of the tube to the lip can be estimated by multiplying the internal diameter of the tube by 3. The Broselow tape allows for a length-based determination of endotracheal tube size and drug dosages for cardiac arrest and seizure. Any area that cares for ill children should be equipped with this piece of equipment.

Before intubation, the patient should be preventilated with 100% oxygen by means of a bag, valve, and mask setup, and suction should be easily accessible. During use of the bag, valve, and mask, and during intubation, an assistant should apply pressure to the cricoid cartilage using the thumb and forefinger, to push the esophagus up against the cervical spine. This decreases inflation of the stomach and the risk of aspiration. The mouth and pharynx are suctioned immediately before intubation. The axes of the mouth, pharynx, and trachea must be aligned to directly visualize the glottis. The chin is lifted into a sniffing position. The tip of a straight blade is placed under the epiglottis and is lifted, or a curved blade is placed into the vallecula, the glottic opening is visualized, and the endotracheal tube is placed between the cords. If ventilation is interrupted for more than 20 seconds or the heart rate decreases to less than 60 beats per minute, mask ventilation should be resumed before another intubation attempt. As soon as the endotracheal tube has been placed, the bag and valve are attached for hand ventilation until a ventilator is available. After the clinician checks for symmetric chest movement and bilateral chest sounds, the tube is secured at the mouth, and the position is confirmed by chest radiography. A colorimetric end-tidal carbon dioxide detector may be used as an adjunct to confirm tube placement; however, a negative test (lack of color change) may not indicate esophageal intubation but rather airway obstruction, or poor or absent pulmonary blood flow. The use of an esophageal detector device that confirms endotracheal intubation by the aspiration of air from a correctly placed endotracheal tube also may be useful in older children, but further study is needed in the pediatric age group.

Pulse oximetry is an excellent noninvasive technique for continuously monitoring arterial oxygen saturation before, during, and after intubation. It does not, however, measure the effectiveness of ventilation. Arterial blood gas analysis is still the standard best way to assess the effectiveness of oxygenation, ventilation, and response to therapy.

BOX 116.2   Equipment for Intubation

Oxygen source
Face masks and resuscitation bag
Cardiorespiratory monitor with pulse oximeter
Large-bore suction catheter and suction machine
Tracheal tubes and stylet
Laryngoscope blade and handle
Tape to secure tube
Exhaled CO_2 detector

| BOX 116.3 | Deterioration in an Intubated Patient: "DOPE" |

Displacement of the tube from the trachea
Obstruction of the tube
Pneumothorax
Equipment failure

Adapted with permission from PALS Provider Manual, AHA.

Box 116.3 lists the possible causes of sudden deterioration in an intubated patient. Tracheal tube position is assessed by observation of chest wall movement during manual ventilation, auscultation, and checking tube placement with the laryngoscope. If tube obstruction is suspected, saline is instilled into the tube and suctioned with a catheter. If the tube in occluded, it must be replaced.

Tension pneumothorax is confirmed by decreased breath sounds on the affected side and a radiograph confirming collapsed lung and deviation of the trachea and mediastinal structures away from the affected side. If this is suspected, immediate needle decompression must be performed.

Equipment also should be checked in the presence of patient deterioration. It is essential that the oxygen circuit is uninterrupted and that no leaks are present. The also monitors should be checked.

Circulation

While an airway is being secured, other members of the resuscitation team should be obtaining intravenous access and monitoring pulse and cardiac rhythm. The patient is placed on a hard surface, and chest compressions are performed in the absence of a pulse. Intravenous access is crucial for drug and fluid administration, but achieving it is often difficult in a child with poor circulation. Usually, placing a peripheral intravenous line during an arrest is difficult, and placing a central line in the neck area interferes with resuscitation. The preferred methods for access are femoral vein catheterization, greater saphenous vein cutdown, or intraosseous vascular access. Often, an intraosseous infusion is the easiest and quickest method of access to the circulation and can be used in children of any age. It provides access to the noncollapsible marrow venous plexus, and is a reliable route for administration of drugs, fluids, and blood. The method is outlined in Box 116.4.

The possible causes of the patient's arrest are considered before the administration of intravenous fluids. If a child with prehospital cardiac arrest of unknown cause fails to respond to initial resuscitation measures, consider an initial bolus (20 mL/kg) of a crystalloid. Patients with acute blood loss, shock, or dehydration may require vigorous volume replacement; those with head trauma or hypernatremic dehydration may be harmed further by overzealous fluid administration. Rapid volume expansion is accomplished best with isotonic crystalloid solutions, such as lactated Ringer's solution or normal saline, until such colloid as blood, fresh-frozen plasma, or human serum albumin is available.

Drugs. Various drugs are used to increase the heart rate, to correct hypoxemia, to reverse metabolic acidosis, to improve cardiac contractility, or to increase coronary and cerebral perfusion pressure. The goal is to restore spontaneous circulation and to stabilize an affected child's cardiac rhythm.

| BOX 116.4 | Intraosseous Infusion |

Choose site.
Flat smooth surface of anterior tibia (1–3 cm below tuberosity). Contralateral tibia.
Distal femur (1–2 cm proximal to superior border of patella).
Insert needle.
Use bone marrow needle or 18-gauge spinal needle.
Angle away from joint space.
Use firm twisting motion until decreased resistance.
Check placement.
Remove stylet.
Aspirate marrow if possible.
Flush with saline, even if no aspirate.
Monitor for tissue swelling.
Administer drug.
Use any drug or fluid that can be given intravenously.

Asystole and sinus bradycardia account for 90% of arrhythmias in pediatric patients in arrest. Because primary cardiac disease is a rare cause of cardiac arrest, other ventricular arrhythmias are uncommon. Box 116.5 lists the reversible causes of life-threatening arrhythmias or cardiac arrest.

The preferred route of administration of drugs during resuscitation is intravenous bolus or infusion. In the event of a delay in establishing intravenous access, the lipid-soluble drugs epinephrine, lidocaine, atropine, and naloxone may be given through the endotracheal tube. The tracheal dose of epinephrine is 10 times the intravenous route dose. For endotracheal administration, the drug should be diluted to 5 to 10 mL, pushed in rapidly, and followed by five positive-pressure breaths. All drugs and fluids may be given by intraosseous infusion. Intracardiac injection has serious risks and is not recommended. Figure 116.1 displays protocols for cardiac arrest and arrhythmias. Epinephrine is the key medication used in cardiac arrest. The most important pharmacologic action of epinephrine in cardiac arrest is the alpha-adrenergic–mediated vasoconstriction, which increases aortic diastolic pressure and coronary perfusion pressure. It also increases cardiac automaticity, heart rate, myocardial contractility, and blood pressure. The use of high-dose epinephrine does not improve

---

| BOX 116.5 | Potentially Reversible Causes of Cardiac Arrest: The 4 H's and the 4 T's |

Hypoxemia
Hypovolemia
Hypothermia
Hyperkalemia/Hypokalemia
Tamponade (cardiac)
Tension pneumothorax
Toxins/poisons/drugs
Thromboembolism

Adapted with permission from AHA Guidelines 2000.

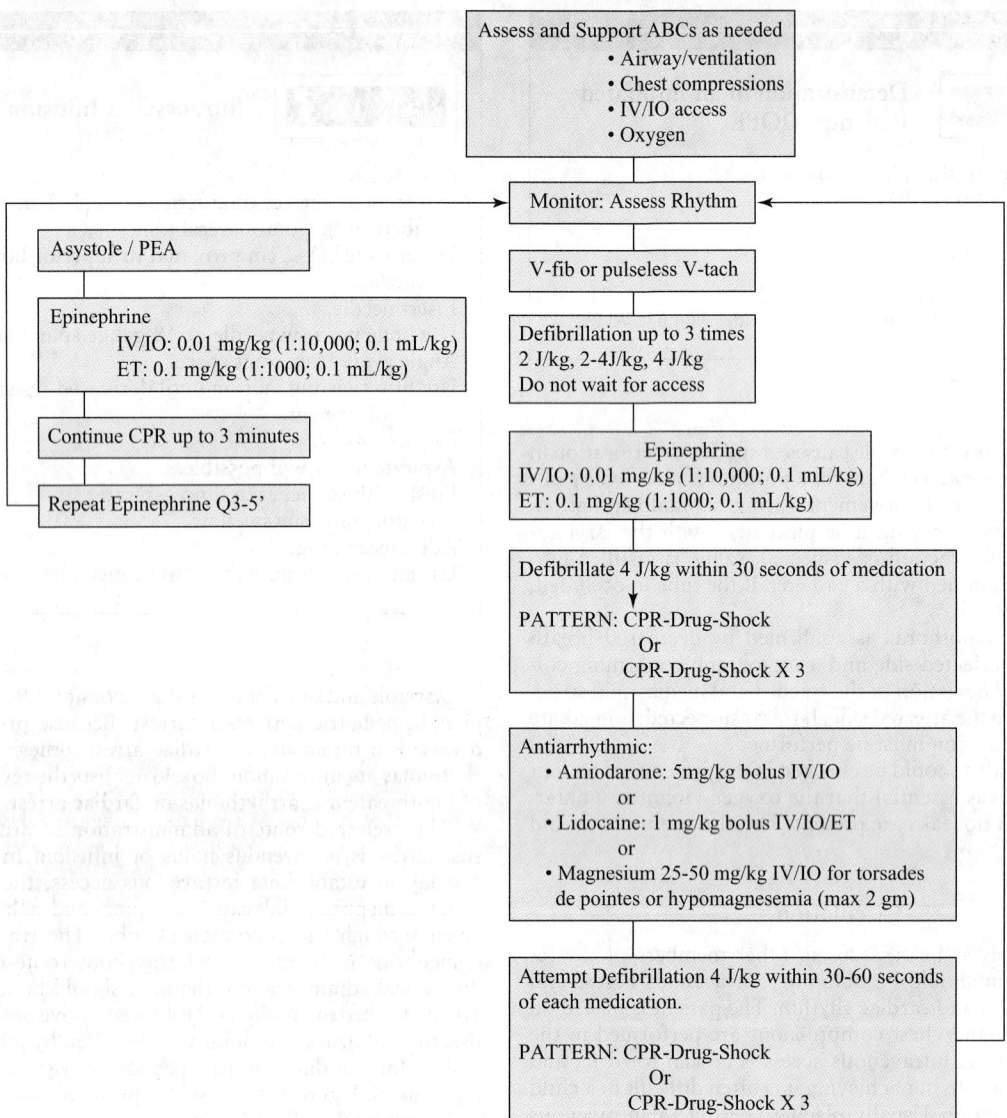

FIGURE 116.1. Protocols for cardiac arrest and arrhythmias. ET, endotracheal tube; IV, intravenous; IO, intraosseous; PEA, pulseless electrical activity; V-fib, ventricular fibrillation; V-tach, ventricular tachycardia. (Adapted with permission from American Heart Association. Guidelines 2000 for Cardiopulmonary Resuscitation and Emergency Cardiovascular Care. *Circulation* 2000;102:I253.)

outcome, and can worsen post-resuscitation cardiac dysfunction. It is not routinely recommended.

The treatment of sinus bradycardia with cardiovascular compromise (heart rate less than 60 beats per minute with poor systemic perfusion) is similar to the treatment of asystole; in addition, atropine, 0.02 mg/kg (minimum, 0.1 mg; maximum, 1.0 mg), should be considered. Because hypoxemia is the most common cause of bradycardia, it is necessary to ensure adequate oxygenation and ventilation.

Ventricular arrhythmias may occur in patients with congenital heart disease, myocardial disease, chest trauma, or drug ingestions. Ventricular fibrillation and pulseless ventricular tachycardia are initially treated with electrical defibrillation, which causes sudden depolarization of the myocardium, to allow intrinsic cardiac automaticity to resume. If defibrillation is not possible immediately, the physician should try to correct hypoxemia and acidosis while setting up the defibrillator.

Pediatric paddles are available in 4.5-cm and 8.0-cm sizes. The correct paddle size is that which allows the entire paddle surface to contact the chest wall. One is placed to the right

of the sternum below the clavicle, and the other is placed on the left anterior axillary line at the level of the nipple (i.e., apex). The electrode–skin interface can be electrode paste or cream; care is taken to apply interface only under the paddles—bridging causes a short circuit. Alcohol pads can cause burns and should never be used as the interface.

The initial dose for defibrillation is 2 J/kg. Subsequent doses are doubled. The procedure must be stopped if the rhythm converts out of ventricular fibrillation. If three shocks do not correct the rhythm, CPR should be resumed with drugs, and the patient should be assessed again for acidosis, hypoxemia, and hypothermia.

If the monitored rhythm is ventricular tachycardia and the patient is symptomatic, the patient undergoes synchronized cardioversion, which is a timed depolarization of myocardial cells and therefore different from defibrillation. The synchronizer circuit must be activated, and the dose is 0.5 to 1 J/kg. If the rhythm is refractory to cardioversion, amiodarone, procainamide, or lidocaine may aid further attempts at cardioversion.

Frequent reassessment, including that of body temperature, is mandatory during any resuscitation.

Parental Presence During Resuscitation. It is common practice in pediatric EDs to have parents present for minor invasive procedures such as venipuncture, intravenous access, urinary catheterization, arterial blood gases, and laceration repair. The vast majority of parents prefer to be present for a procedure on their child; their presence reduces the stress for both the child and the parent(s). The parent may just soothe the child with familiar encouraging words, or in some cases actually help restrain the child for the procedure. Most physicians are comfortable performing even more invasive procedures, such as lumbar puncture, with parents present. Studies show that parental presence does not negatively affect the success of the procedure.

The practice of family member involvement during pediatric resuscitations remains controversial. As with other illnesses and procedures, family members are frequently interested in being present for the resuscitation in order to support their child. It facilitates their understanding of the gravity of the situation and the efforts being made, and the acceptance of the death of their child, if it occurs. Often, the family is present during the pre-hospital resuscitation, but is excluded after arrival at the hospital. It has long been the standard policy in most EDs to exclude family members from the treatment room during the resuscitation of cardiopulmonary arrest and trauma victims. The reluctance of ED staff to permit family involvement may be based on fears that family members will interfere with medical efforts, that observation may reveal apparent weaknesses and failure of medical care, or that the staff may become uneasy and lose concentration and objectivity. It may understandably be more difficult to end the resuscitation efforts with family members present. In addition, many health professionals assume that presence during resuscitation efforts would be an undesirable experience for family members. However, in multiple studies, the responses from relatives who witnessed the resuscitation of their loved one were overwhelmingly positive. The majority of family members who are allowed to be present during resuscitations favor this practice. In fact, in many cases, it helps with the family's grieving process.

If family members are present for a resuscitation, the team should act sensitively to the family's presence, the family should be prepared by the staff for what they will see, a staff member, such as a social worker, should be assigned to the family to act as a liaison, and there should be a seat or space for the family member. If the resuscitation is unsuccessful, the family should be allowed time to say good-bye.

When determining whether family members should be present during a resuscitation, the concerns of both the family and the ED personnel should be addressed. Relatives should not be viewed as an added burden to the staff, but as a part of the medical care and process. Research shows that medical providers who have experienced having family members present during resuscitation favor this practice.

AIRWAY OBSTRUCTION

Airway obstruction may result from processes in the upper or lower airway. Upper airway refers to the level above the secondary bronchi, and lower airway refers to peripheral airways, which usually are less than 3 mm in diameter. Usually, lower airway obstruction involves a diffuse distribution of obstruction. The differentiating characteristics are listed in Table 116.3.

Upper airway obstruction interferes primarily with inspiration. As upper airway obstruction progresses, a small increase occurs in respiratory rate, and a large increase occurs in respiratory effort, leading to dyspnea. The increased respiratory

TABLE 116.3

AIRWAY OBSTRUCTION

	Upper Airway	Lower Airway
Signs and symptoms	Interferes primarily with inspiration Inspiratory stridor Severe retractions Croupy or brassy cough	Interferes primarily with expiration Expiratory wheeze Mild retractions Prolonged expirations Hacking and repetitive cough Patchy areas of atelectasis from areas of complete obstruction
Conditions	Croup Foreign-body aspiration Epiglottitis Retropharyngeal abscess Peritonsillar abscess	Asthma Bronchiolitis

effort causes an increased negative intrathoracic pressure, manifested by retractions. Stridor, a low-pitched respiratory sound, results.

Lower airway obstruction interferes with the expiration of air from the smaller airways, causing the expiratory phase to be prolonged. The turbulent air flow is heard as wheezing. As the obstruction increases, accessory muscles are used. Wheezing increases as the obstruction progresses, and then decreases as air flow becomes limited.

Foreign-body aspiration, croup, epiglottitis, abscesses, asthma, and bronchiolitis are the more common causes of airway obstruction seen in children.

Foreign-Body Aspiration

Foreign-body aspiration is a significant health hazard in young children, particularly those between 6 months and 3 years of age.

Pathophysiology

Most foreign bodies that children aspirate are small and, rather than lodging in the trachea and causing acute obstruction, pass through the trachea to lodge in a main stem bronchus. These small foreign bodies, usually composed of organic matter, are not immediately life-threatening. Peanuts are the most common objects to be aspirated.

Diagnosis

Frequently, the diagnosis of foreign-body aspiration is missed, because children often present with no known history of aspiration, and only subtle signs and symptoms. The diagnosis requires a high index of suspicion and should be considered in any child with unexplained pulmonary complaints. A history of sudden-onset choking or coughing while eating or playing with small objects is helpful but not always obtainable. With delayed diagnosis, affected children may present with recurrent attacks of wheezing diagnosed as asthma, pneumonia, or bronchiectasis.

In most children, a history of the sudden onset of coughing with acute respiratory distress or subsequent coughing, wheezing, or stridor suggests the diagnosis of foreign-body aspiration. The clinical symptoms depend on the location of the

TABLE 116.4

FOREIGN-BODY ASPIRATION

Location of Foreign Body	Common Signs and Symptoms
Trachea	
Total obstruction	Acute asphyxia, marked retractions
High partial obstruction	Decreased air entry, inspiratory and expiratory stridor, retractions
Low partial obstruction	Expiratory wheezing, inspiratory stridor
Main stem bronchus	Cough, expiratory wheezing, blood-tinged sputum[a]
Lobar or segmental bronchus	Decreased breath sounds[b]; wheezing, rhonchi

[a]Usually a later finding.
[b]Localized to area of lung related to affected bronchus.
Adapted from Cotton E, Yasuda K. Foreign body aspiration. *Pediatr Clin North Am* 1984;31:937.

foreign body (Table 116.4). The most frequent physical findings are wheezing, decreased air movement, and rhonchi, all localized over the lung with the involved airway.

In children with foreign-body aspiration, the chest radiographs range from diagnostic to totally unremarkable. The appropriate views include inspiratory and expiratory or bilateral decubitus chest radiographs. Persistent air trapping on an expiratory or lateral decubitus radiograph may be found. Persistent atelectasis or infiltration are other common findings. The foreign body itself rarely is opaque and, therefore, rarely is visible on the radiograph. If initial films appear equivocal or normal, and aspiration is still suspected, fluoroscopy should be performed. Often, the difference in chest wall expansion that may occur with foreign-body aspiration is detected by fluoroscopy.

Therapy

If the child presents to the ED with no air movement, the Heimlich maneuver or back blows are administered (see section Cardiopulmonary Resuscitation in Children). Children with asphyxiating foreign-body aspiration require immediate rigid bronchoscopy for foreign-body removal. However, most aspirations are not life-threatening, and a thorough history and physical examination can be obtained.

If suspicion of foreign-body aspiration is supported by physical examination or radiographs, bronchoscopy is the treatment of choice for foreign-body removal. On radiographic evidence of a radiopaque foreign body or on other strong evidence of a foreign-body aspiration, such as unilaterally decreased breath sounds or obstructive emphysema, rigid bronchoscopy should be performed for foreign-body removal. If the evidence for an aspiration is less convincing, flexible bronchoscopy can be performed first to confirm the diagnosis; then, rigid bronchoscopy can be performed if a foreign body is found. Using flexible bronchoscopy first avoids the risks and expense of general anesthesia in those patients without an aspiration. The degree of urgency depends on the location of the foreign body and the degree of respiratory distress.

Croup

Croup, or laryngotracheobronchitis, is a common syndrome involving inflammation or edema of the subglottic area, causing airway obstruction in the larynx, trachea, or bronchi.

Epidemiology

Usually, croup affects children of 6 months to 4 years of age, with the peak incidence at 1 to 2 years of age. Croup accounts for more than 90% of stridor with fever. It occurs all during the year, but the incidence increases in late fall and winter.

Pathophysiology

Most croup is viral, but it also may be spasmodic (i.e., allergic) or bacterial. As many as 75% of cases of viral croup are caused by parainfluenza viruses; other viruses include respiratory syncytial virus, influenza viruses, and adenovirus. *Mycoplasma pneumoniae* also can cause croup. (See Chapter 189, Parainfluenza Viruses, for more information on croup.)

Viral croup has an insidious onset after a few days of an upper respiratory tract infection. It progresses to hoarseness and the characteristic inspiratory stridor and barking cough. Symptoms wax and wane and usually are worse at night. Oral intake may be decreased.

Spasmodic croup appears as a sudden onset of severe stridor, usually at night, in a well child with no upper respiratory tract infection. The cause is thought to be allergic, but viruses may play a role.

Bacterial croup presents much like viral croup, but with higher fever and with more severe respiratory distress. If an affected child is intubated, pus is found in the trachea. *Staphylococcus aureus* is the most common organism; *Streptococcus pneumoniae*, *Streptococcus pyogenes*, and *Haemophilus influenzae* type b (Hib) also are isolated. Bacterial croup may be a superinfection of viral croup.

Clinical Manifestations and Complications

Usually, children with croup are mildly or moderately ill but rarely appear toxic. Such children demonstrate signs of an upper respiratory tract infection and a low-grade fever. Children with croup have a characteristic barking cough and a hoarse voice. The respiratory examination may show signs of upper respiratory obstruction: inspiratory stridor, suprasternal and intercostal retractions, and an increased respiratory rate.

Diagnosis

Croup is diagnosed on clinical grounds. No diagnostic laboratory tests are available. If the diagnosis is in question, a lateral neck radiograph may be helpful to rule out other causes of upper airway obstruction, such as epiglottitis, foreign-body aspiration, or retropharyngeal abscess. Usually, the lateral neck radiograph in croup shows a normal epiglottis, narrowing of the subglottic trachea, and ballooning of the hypopharynx. A posteroanterior neck view shows tapered narrowing of the subglottic air column, known as the steeple sign.

Children with croup should have oxygen saturation checked, because some with severe disease may be hypoxic due to airway obstruction, parenchymal infection, ventilation-perfusion mismatch or, rarely, pulmonary edema.

Therapy

Children with a barking cough and no respiratory distress can be managed as outpatients with extra fluid intake and a cool mist vaporizer or exposure to outdoor air.

All children with croup should be treated with steroids. The administration of one dose of dexamethasone by the oral or intramuscular route (0.6 mg/kg; maximum, 12 mg) decreases inflammation in the upper airway, reduces severity of symptoms within 6 hours, and may decrease the need for other therapies and later hospitalization. Oral and intramuscular administration have equal efficacy, but the oral route is usually preferable because of ease of administration. Dexamethasone suppresses inflammation for 2 to 3 days after one dose; therefore, further steroid therapy is not necessary. An alternative is to give prednisone initially (2 mg/kg) and to continue the dose daily for 3 days.

Nebulized budesonide, a synthetic glucocorticoid with strong topical antiinflammatory effects, can be used as an alternative or an addition to oral dexamethasone. It has effects similar to intramuscular or oral glucocorticoids. Nebulized dexamethasone is not as effective as the oral or intramuscular routes, and it is not recommended.

In children with stridor at rest, epinephrine, a local vasoconstrictor given by nebulization, temporarily relieves airway obstruction by decreasing edema in the inflamed subglottic region. Although racemic epinephrine has traditionally been the nebulized form of epinephrine used, L-epinephrine works equally as well, is more readily available, and is less expensive. Because the obstruction often returns to pretreatment level in 1 or 2 hours, affected children must be observed carefully for 3 or 4 hours after this treatment, and then may be discharged in the absence of a relapse of significant respiratory distress.

A mixture of helium and oxygen (heliox) has been used in children with severe respiratory distress from various airway problems, but has not been shown to have any advantage over nebulized epinephrine in children with severe croup. Antibiotics are not indicated except on evidence of bacterial disease. Most patients with croup have excellent short- and long-term prognoses; artificial airway intervention rarely is necessary.

Epiglottitis

Epiglottitis, or supraglottitis, is an acute, rapidly progressive, life-threatening airway emergency. Although rare, this condition must be considered in all pediatric patients with an acute febrile illness and symptoms of upper airway obstruction. Cellulitis and edema of the epiglottis, aryepiglottic folds, and hypopharynx narrow the glottic opening. During inhalation, when the structures are pulled inward, stridor and difficulty in breathing occur. During expiration, the airway structures are pushed away, and the glottis is opened. If the edema progresses, the airway may become obstructed completely, and an artificial airway must be established immediately. Pulmonary edema may lead to ventilation-perfusion mismatch and hypoxia.

Pathophysiology

In the past, epiglottitis was an infection caused almost exclusively by Hib, and it affected children most commonly at approximately 3 years of age (range, 2 to 7 years). Since conjugate vaccines for Hib have been developed and widely distributed, the incidence of epiglottitis has decreased by more than 90%. The disease is affecting older children and adults, and the causative organism most commonly is group A beta-hemolytic streptococci. Other organisms include *Moraxella catarrhalis* and *S. pneumoniae*. Since 1990, only approximately one-fourth to one-third of cases of epiglottitis have been caused by Hib. Although the age of onset and the organism causing epiglottitis have changed, the clinical presentation, laboratory, and radiographic findings have remained consistent. The incidence peaks during spring and late fall.

Clinical Manifestations and Complications

Typically, children who are older than 2 years of age with epiglottitis present with an acute febrile illness of less than 24 hours' duration. They may complain of a sore throat and show progressive respiratory distress. On physical examination, often the fever is in excess of 39°C, and the child appears anxious and toxic. If the airway is compromised, the patient sits for-

ward with the neck extended and chin thrust out. Such patients may have difficulty in swallowing and may be drooling. Respiratory signs include a hoarse cough, tachypnea, inspiratory stridor, retractions, and cyanosis. If epiglottitis is suspected, the throat should not be examined, and the child should be left undisturbed. The clinical presentation of epiglottitis in children younger than 2 years of age is more variable and may mimic viral croup. Such young children may have low-grade fever, a history of upper respiratory tract symptoms, and a croupy cough.

Diagnosis

Laboratory and radiographic results may be helpful in the diagnosis of epiglottitis but are not essential early diagnostic tools. A lateral neck radiograph is necessary only if the clinical presentation is not straightforward and the patient is stable. If radiography is indicated, a physician experienced in difficult airway management should accompany the child. Classically, the lateral neck radiograph shows a thumb-shaped epiglottis and narrowing of the posterior airway. Frequently, a complete blood count reveals an increased leukocyte count with a shift to the left. Cultures of the blood and epiglottis, performed in the operating room, often reveal the causative organism.

Occasionally, croup may be confused with epiglottitis and vice versa. Table 116.5 shows the main differentiating characteristics of these two diseases. Croup is diagnosed much more frequently than is epiglottitis.

Therapy

Epiglottitis can be managed with few complications after early suspicion and rapid treatment. Physicians who first see affected children must act quickly to prevent complete airway obstruction. If such children are seen at a tertiary-care center, immediate involvement of ED physicians, an anesthesiologist, an otolaryngologist, and the pediatric intensive care staff is essential. If affected children first are seen by a private pediatrician in an office or clinic, available support staff should be contacted, and arrangements should be made for transport. Children should not be transferred without an accompanying physician prepared to manage the airway.

Affected children should be allowed to assume the most comfortable position, and oxygen is supplied by mask or is blown by the face. The physician or staff must not agitate patients by restraining them, examining the throat, drawing blood, or starting an intravenous line. As soon as possible, children are transported to the operating room, are anesthetized, and are intubated. Usually, the supraglottic structures are inflamed, and culture specimens are taken. Blood can be drawn

TABLE 116.5

DIFFERENTIATION BETWEEN CROUP AND EPIGLOTTITIS

Characteristic	Croup	Epiglottitis
Age	6 mo to 4 yr	2–10 yr
Site	Subglottic	Supraglottic
Onset	Gradual history of upper respiratory infection	Rapid, usually <24 hr
Presentation	Inspiratory stridor; hoarse, barking cough	Inspiratory stridor; high fever, toxic appearance; sits forward
Etiology	Viral	Bacterial

for culture and complete blood count, and intravenous antibiotics are given. If the airway is obstructed completely at any time and intubation is not possible, an emergency cricothyrotomy is performed.

Studies have indicated that some older children with epiglottitis may be more successful at managing their secretions and may not require intubation. Children with minimal respiratory distress and little or no drooling may be able to be managed with careful observation in a pediatric intensive care unit.

Most cases of sudden death from epiglottitis can be avoided with rapid diagnosis and management. However, some deaths from epiglottitis occur in patients if the disease follows a rapid course and respiratory obstruction occurs before medical care can be obtained or in patients with secondary complications, such as septic shock.

Retropharyngeal Abscess

Retropharyngeal abscess (RTA) is a potentially lethal infection of the deep-neck space, anterior to the prevertebral layer of the deep cervical fascia. Often, the process starts with cellulitis of the posterior pharyngeal wall and progresses to abscess formation. It is most common in children younger than 5 years of age, when the retropharyngeal space contains multiple lymph nodes that drain the nasal cavity, nasopharynx, and sinuses.

Pathophysiology

Although RTA in children usually is a result of the lymphatic spread of infection from the respiratory tract, it also can result from a penetrating foreign body or other trauma, or from contiguous spread from vertebral osteomyelitis. Often, the RTA is polymicrobial, with aerobes and anaerobes. The predominant organisms are *S. pyogenes*, *S. aureus*, and oropharyngeal anaerobic bacteria. The differential diagnosis includes epiglottitis, foreign-body aspiration, vertebral osteomyelitis, and lymphoma.

Clinical Manifestations and Complications

Usually, children with RTA have histories of pharyngitis or upper respiratory infection and a sudden onset of high fever. Such patients may have sore throat or difficulty in swallowing; small children may refuse to eat. Breathing may be noisy and, if the abscess impinges on the larynx, affected children will have stridor. Such children may be drooling and have a toxic appearance with the neck extended. Torticollis or meningismus may be present. Usually, cervical lymphadenopathy is evident. On direct examination, a bulge may be seen in the posterior pharyngeal wall, often unilaterally.

The most common complication of RTA is airway obstruction, and affected children must be observed carefully during treatment. Because the retropharyngeal space is contiguous with the mediastinum, direct extension of infection can ensue downward into the mediastinum, causing mediastinitis. The abscess also can rupture, with aspiration that causes respiratory distress or pneumonia.

Diagnosis

If children are seen early in the process of cellulitis and abscess formation, the diagnosis can be difficult. If RTA is suspected, and the child is stable, a lateral neck radiograph is obtained. The optimal film is obtained in the inspiratory phase and in moderate cervical extension. This view shows widening of the prevertebral space at C2; it also may show loss of the normal cervical lordosis and presence of air in the soft tissues. Because obtaining optimal films is difficult in a young child and the retropharyngeal soft space changes appearance rapidly with

respiration and crying, interpreting measurements of the space width is difficult. If the diagnosis is questionable or if surgery is planned, a computed tomographic (CT) scan is obtained.

CT with contrast can be used to differentiate between retropharyngeal cellulitis and abscess. It also provides accurate information about the exact location and extent of the abscess and its relation to the great vessels. Color-flow Doppler ultrasonography also may be helpful in evaluating abscess formation.

Therapy

In the event of significant respiratory distress, emergent airway management is essential. Most children with RTA are stable and can be managed with intravenous antibiotics. Antibiotics are chosen to cover normal oropharyngeal flora, penicillinase-producing *S. aureus*, and *Bacteroides* species. For a fluctuant abscess, surgical drainage is performed by percutaneous aspiration or by incision.

Peritonsillar Abscess

Peritonsillar abscess (PTA) is an acute accumulation of purulent material between the tonsillar capsule and the superior constrictor muscle of the pharynx.

Epidemiology

The most common deep-space infection of the head and neck, PTA is the most common sequela of acute tonsillitis. Although it can be seen in the first decade of life, it occurs most commonly in adolescents and adults.

Pathophysiology

Antibiotic treatment of tonsillitis does not always prevent the development of PTA, and affected children may be receiving antibiotics when the abscess forms. Usually, cultures of aspirates from the abscess are polymicrobial, including aerobes and anaerobes. The most common organisms are group A beta-hemolytic streptococcus, *S. aureus*, *H. influenzae*, and such anaerobes as *Bacteroides* species, viridans streptococci, and *Fusobacterium necrophorum*. The differential diagnosis includes epiglottitis, peritonsillar cellulitis, foreign-body aspiration, dental infections, and neoplasms.

Clinical Manifestations and Complications

Usually, children or adolescents with PTA complain of severe unilateral throat pain and have a history of preceding or current pharyngitis. Affected individuals may have difficulty in speaking, swallowing, or opening their mouths, and they speak with a "hot potato" voice.

On physical examination, affected patients may appear toxic, may exhibit a high fever, and may be drooling because of difficulty in swallowing; often, torticollis or trismus is evident. Markedly tender cervical adenopathy is present. The involved tonsil is markedly inflamed and edematous and usually is bulging inferiorly and medially. The uvula may be pushed toward the opposite side. Affected children may be dehydrated from inability to take fluids.

The most common complication of PTA is airway obstruction. In the event of respiratory compromise, the abscess can be drained in the ED with a needle and syringe. Other complications include rupture and aspiration, ulceration of the large submaxillary arteries, sepsis, and mediastinitis.

Diagnosis

If differentiation between peritonsillar cellulitis and abscess is difficult, ultrasonography or contrast CT studies are helpful. Ultrasonography, either externally on the neck or intraorally, can distinguish reliably the early stage of peritonsillitis from well-established abscess formation and can locate the abscess accurately. If PTA is suspected in young, uncooperative children with fever and drooling, or in patients with severe trismus, CT with contrast also is helpful in localizing and defining an abscess.

Therapy

The most important part of the management of PTA is drainage of the abscess. Usually, needle aspiration is the initial drainage procedure. After appropriate sedation and local anesthesia, aspiration is performed by an otolaryngologist. This procedure cures more than 90% of cases of PTA. If the abscess does not resolve, the otolaryngologist may choose to perform an intra-oral incision and drainage or acute tonsillectomy. In children with a history of recurrent tonsillitis and an increased risk of recurrence of PTA, the otolaryngologist may choose to perform a tonsillectomy.

The medical management of PTA, along with drainage, includes hydration, pain relief, and antibiotic treatment. Usually, culturing the aspirate is not necessary, and antibiotics are chosen to cover the aforementioned organisms. After abscess drainage, cooperative adolescents often can be treated as outpatients with antibiotics and pain medication. In younger children, usually intravenous hydration and antibiotics are necessary.

Asthma

Asthma, or reactive airway disease, is a chronic condition with acute exacerbations of inflammation, bronchospasm, mucosal edema, and mucus production, all of which contribute to widespread airway narrowing and various degrees of airway obstruction. Children have status asthmaticus if they are unresponsive to initial treatment or have a significant chance of suffering from respiratory failure without vigorous further treatment.

Epidemiology

Asthma affects 4% to 6% of children in the United States, and children with asthma account for a large percentage of urgent ED visits. The prevalence of and mortality from asthma have increased since the 1980s.

Pathophysiology

Initial symptoms result primarily from bronchoconstriction; as symptoms persist for several days, airway inflammation and edema become more prominent. The airway obstruction is diffuse and distributed unevenly, causing some alveoli to be overventilated while others are underventilated. This uneven distribution of ventilation creates ventilation-perfusion mismatch and subsequent hypoxemia.

Diagnosis

The assessment of children with an asthmatic attack includes history, physical examination, pulmonary function tests, and, rarely, laboratory tests. The history assesses the current episode and the patient's predisposition to severe exacerbations. The objective of the initial history is to obtain information important for the immediate treatment of a child in distress. It should include the precipitating factors and duration of the attack, most recent times and doses of current medications (including steroids), the course of previous attacks (including intensive care admissions, oral intake, vomiting), and other medical problems. A more detailed history can be obtained later in a more relaxed fashion.

The physical examination focuses on general appearance, mental status, respiratory status, and hydration. Alteration in mental status may be a sign of both hypoxia and hypercarbia. The physician should note an affected patient's position of comfort, ability to speak in sentences, severity of retractions, and quality of air movement. The respiratory examination includes respiratory rate, assessment of air movement, use of accessory muscles, wheezing, and cough. Younger children become tachypneic to increase their vital capacity. If such children have moderate or severe respiratory distress with wheezing, sufficient air movement is present to cause turbulence and at least some ventilation; if such patients are in distress and are not wheezing, they likely are in respiratory failure.

Many scores have been devised to assess the severity of an asthmatic episode. Although a score may not be accurate in assessing the degree of hypoxemia, it is helpful for initial assessment of the severity of the episode and for continuing reassessment in a disease in which clinical status changes rapidly. Table 116.6 shows an example of an asthma scoring system. A statistically significant positive correlation exists between the score and the P_{CO_2}.

When evaluating a child with asthma, the vast majority of important information is in the history and physical examination. The pulse oximeter and peak flow meter are the most helpful instruments in evaluating patients with asthma. A decrease in oxygen saturation is an early sign of airway obstruction, and the pulse oximeter gives an accurate and continuous reading of the oxygen saturation. However, it does not evaluate ventilation and is not meant to replace careful and frequent clinical reassessment. Conflicting studies exist on the value of pulse oximetry for predicting exacerbation outcome.

The pulmonary function test usually available in an ED is the peak expiratory flow rate using a hand-held peak flow meter. This test is effort-dependent and is not as accurate as measurement of forced expiratory volume in 1 second (FEV_1), but it is useful for assessing initial and post-treatment airway obstruction in cooperative children.

An arterial blood gas level rarely is necessary in assessing patients with asthma. Clinical signs such as fatigue or worsening mental status should alert the physician to a deteriorating respiratory status. The arterial blood gas level is only supporting

TABLE 116.6

ASTHMA SCORE*

Scored Items	0	1	2
P_{O_2} or cyanosis	70–100 (RA) None	<70 (RA) In air	≤70 (40% F_{IO_2}) In 40% F_{IO_2}
Inspiratory breath sounds	Normal	Unequal	Decreased to absent
Accessory muscles used	None	Moderate	Maximal
Expiratory wheezing	None	Moderate	Marked
Cerebral function	Normal	Depressed or agitated	Coma

RA, room air.
*Score: ≥5 indicates impending respiratory failure; ≥7 and P_{CO_2} = 65 indicates respiratory failure.
Wood DW, et al. A clinical scoring system for the diagnosis of respiratory failure. *Am J Dis Child* 1972;123:227.

evidence for respiratory failure. The moderate asthmatic exacerbation is characterized by compensatory hyperventilation, causing hypocapnia and respiratory alkalosis. If the attack becomes more severe and an affected patient cannot maintain adequate ventilation, the Pco_2 level increases and pH level decreases, resulting in respiratory acidosis. A normal or high Pco_2 level in the face of hyperventilation or fatigue indicates that a child's respiratory efforts no longer are able to compensate for the airway obstruction. If repeated arterial sampling is anticipated, such as in the intubated patient, an arterial line should be inserted.

Other than arterial blood gas measurements, laboratory studies are of limited use in evaluating asthmatic patients. Leukocytosis may be caused by asthma, adrenergic drugs, and steroids. Urinalysis may show ketones from poor oral intake and dehydration. Chest radiography typically shows hyperinflation, indicated by flattened diaphragms, increased anteroposterior diameter, hyperlucent lungs, peribronchial thickening, and areas of atelectasis that may be misinterpreted as pneumonia. Because the results of the chest radiograph rarely alter management, the study should be reserved for specific indications, such as deteriorating clinical condition, chest pain, subcutaneous emphysema, suspected pneumothorax, or high fever. In rare instances, an entire lobe or lung collapses or pneumothorax exists. Fever alone is not an indication for chest radiography in children with asthma, because viral respiratory infections are one of the most common triggers for asthmatic exacerbations.

Therapy

Hypoxemia is an important and early component of asthma, and oxygen should be given to every patient. Further oxygen therapy is guided by the results of pulse oximetry.

The initial management of an acute asthmatic episode consists of the administration of aerosolized beta$_2$ agonist drugs. Beta-adrenergic receptors act on airway smooth muscle to produce bronchodilation; stimulation of these receptors results in increased mucus clearance, vasodilation, and inhibition of mast cell degranulation. Compared to the subcutaneously administered beta agonists, the nebulized agents act faster, have a prolonged duration of action, and produce fewer side effects. The beta$_2$-selective medication most commonly used is racemic albuterol, repeated every 20 minutes (Table 116.7). Levalbuterol, the pure R isomer of albuterol, may be used in lower doses than racemic albuterol (R + S isomers) to produce the same degree of bronchodilation. In patients with severe respiratory distress, albuterol can be given by continuous nebulization. Because the administration of inhaled beta$_2$-adrenergic medications may cause a temporary decrease in oxygen saturation, these drugs may be delivered with oxygen.

The traditional method to deliver aerosolized albuterol has been nebulization with saline in a small-volume nebulizer. This method of delivery allows the use of oxygen but results in inefficient drug delivery to the lungs, requires a power source, and takes at least 10 minutes for each treatment. Studies show equal efficacy in delivery by metered-dose inhaler with an attached spacer device (MDI-S), even in children younger than 2 years of age. The MDI-S has several advantages, including a reservoir of aerosol that can be inhaled slowly after actuation, increased drug deposition in the lower airways, portability, easy dose titration, and short time of treatment. Children should take at least five breaths after each puff of drug is delivered into the spacer device. For young children, a face mask rather than a mouthpiece can be used. Use of a metered-dose inhaler allows an easy transition to home therapy with the same device.

The recognition of the importance of the parasympathetic nervous system in the pathogenesis of asthma has led to the use of anticholinergic drugs in the treatment of asthma (see Table 116.7). Ipratropium bromide is a synthetic cholinergic antagonist with a prolonged action of bronchodilation. It blocks airway acetylcholine receptors, preventing reflex bronchoconstriction; with little systemic absorption, it has no systemic anticholinergic effects. Ipratropium should always be given in combination with beta$_2$-agonists. Well-designed studies show that ipratropium and albuterol given together are more effective than albuterol alone, especially in moderate to severe asthma exacerbations. It should be given along with at least the first 3 albuterol treatments; it has an effect in approximately 30 to 90 minutes. The use of ipratropium bromide may decrease hospitalization in the group of patients with more severe bronchoconstriction.

Steroids are an important part of the initial and ongoing treatment of asthma (see Table 116.7). Steroids are effective against the inflammatory part of the disease process and also may have effects on the beta-adrenergic receptors, through enhancing the responsiveness to the beta-adrenergic agents. Corticosteroids should be started in all children with moderate to severe asthma exacerbations. Steroid use may produce a positive effect within 3 to 4 hours. The oral and intravenous routes are equally as efficacious, and oral prednisone given early in the ED visit has been shown to reduce the need for hospitalization within 4 hours of administration. Recent studies show that two doses of oral dexamethasone 24 hours apart are as effective as a 5-day course of prednisone. The first dose is given in the ED. It has the advantage of reduced dosing, less vomiting and

---

TABLE 116.7

ASTHMA DRUG DOSES

Drug	Route	Dose
Albuterol	Nebulized	0.15 mg/kg; maximum 5 mg (1 ml)
		Continuous: 0.5 mg/kg/hr; max 15 mg/hr
Albuterol	MDI-S	0.5 puffs/kg (90 mcg/puff); max 10 puffs
Levalbuterol	Nebulized	0.075 mg/kg; max 2.5 mg
Ipratropium bromide	Nebulized	<20 kg: 250 meg/dose
		>20 kg: 500 meg/dose
Prednisone	Oral	2 mg/kg/day; maximum 60 mg
Dexamethasone	Oral	0.6 mg/kg; maximum 16 mg
Methylprednisolone	IV	2 mg/kg loading dose; max 80 mg
Terbutaline	SQ	0.01 cc/kg; max 0.4 cc
Terbutaline	IV	Bolus 10 meg/kg; max 500 meg
		Drip 0.1 meg/kg/mm

IV, intravenous; SQ, subcutaneous; PO, oral.

improved compliance. If affected patients require an intravenous line for another reason and the intravenous route for steroid is chosen, methylprednisolone is used, because of its limited mineralocorticoid effects. If the patient is discharged home from the ED, oral prednisone or dexamethasone is prescribed.

Many new, aggressive therapies are available for wheezing children with severe respiratory distress, after initial treatment with beta agonists and steroids. Albuterol can be given as a continuous nebulization rather than as distinct treatments. Terbutaline, a beta$_2$-specific agonist, can be given subcutaneously or intravenously in children with severe respiratory distress. It is given intravenously as a bolus followed by a continuous infusion (see Table 116.7). Indications include faint or absent breath sounds, increasing P_{CO_2} with respiratory distress or fatigue, and failure to respond to previous appropriate therapy. Other agents used in asthmatic patients with impending or actual respiratory failure include magnesium sulfate and ketamine. Several studies in the adult literature (but few in the pediatric literature) confirm that intravenous magnesium sulfate can relieve bronchoconstriction in severe asthma exacerbations. Ketamine appears to increase catecholamine levels and to directly relax bronchial smooth muscle. It can be used as the sedative for the intubation of asthmatic patients or to improve bronchodilation after intubation in children with intractable bronchospasm.

Other than drug therapy, general supportive measures are important in the care of asthmatic children. Many children with asthma are at least mildly dehydrated, and hydration therapy proceeds as in any dehydrated children. No evidence suggests that large amounts of fluid have a beneficial effect in well-hydrated asthmatic children, and vigorous fluid administration may be contraindicated. Affected children should be in as quiet and restful an environment as possible.

Antibiotics are used in asthmatic patients only on good clinical evidence for pneumonia or other infection. A chest radiograph with atelectasis may be misinterpreted as pneumonia because the radiologic appearances often are indistinguishable. Assessing the febrile asthmatic patient for pneumonia is easier after the wheezing has cleared. No support for the use of expectorants exists, and sedatives are strongly contraindicated.

With the use of oral steroids and the ability to deliver beta$_2$-adrenergic agents at home by nebulization or metered-dose inhaler, fewer children are admitted to the hospital for asthma exacerbations. Many studies have looked at clinical variables, such as peak flow rate, length of wheezing episode, and response to initial adrenergic treatment, in attempting to predict the outcome of a particular asthmatic episode. No particular variable or set of variables accurately predicts outcome. Admission to the hospital is indicated if affected patients have ongoing respiratory distress or hypoxia, or exhibit a history of severe and poorly responsive exacerbations. The inability to maintain adequate hydration orally, or familial inability to deal with the necessary ongoing treatment at home are other factors to be considered.

Bronchiolitis

Bronchiolitis is the most common acute viral infection of the lower respiratory tract in infants, and it causes mild to severe respiratory distress.

Epidemiology

Bronchiolitis most commonly affects infants 2 to 8 months of age, but it can be seen in children as old as 2 years of age. It is the most frequent cause of infant hospitalizations during yearly winter outbreaks.

Pathophysiology

In most cases, the causal organism is respiratory syncytial virus. Other pathogens include parainfluenza viruses, adenovirus, influenza viruses, and *M. pneumoniae*. The organism invades the epithelial cells of the bronchioles, causing mucosal inflammation with sloughing of cells, edema, and increased mucus secretion. The resultant narrowing of the small airways causes uneven air trapping and overdistention of the lungs; ventilation-perfusion mismatch can lead to hypoxemia or hypercarbia.

Clinical Manifestations and Complications

The diagnosis of bronchiolitis is made on the basis of clinical presentation, age of the child, and season. After a few days of an upper respiratory infection, the child has an acute onset of cough and tachypnea. The chest examination reveals wheezing and rales bilaterally; these findings may change on subsequent examinations. If moderate or severe respiratory distress is present, the child may eat poorly, be dehydrated from poor oral intake, and be irritable. Increased respiratory rate and, in severe disease, nasal flaring and retractions are seen.

Infants who are younger than 2 months of age or who have a history of prematurity, congenital heart disease, bronchopulmonary dysplasia, or other underlying pulmonary disease are at increased risk of apnea, severe illness, and respiratory failure requiring ventilatory support. Findings consistent with more severe disease include low oxygen saturation, respiratory rate greater than 70 breaths per minute, ill or toxic appearance, history of apnea, or consolidation on chest radiograph.

Diagnosis

No routine laboratory tests exist for bronchiolitis. RSV antigen testing is not necessary for outpatient management. A chest radiograph shows nonspecific changes; it may show diffuse hyperinflation with patchy areas of infiltration or atelectasis. An arterial blood gas determination may be necessary for more severely ill infants. Young infants with bronchiolitis and fever are unlikely to have serious bacterial infection, and most do not need a routine sepsis evaluation. However, young infants with bronchiolitis are not protected from serious bacterial infection, and if any concern exists, they should be evaluated to rule out a bacterial infection as well.

Therapy

In addition to supportive care, such as oral fluids, antipyretics, and oxygen for hypoxia, the treatment for bronchiolitis remains controversial. Bronchiolitis is a lower respiratory bronchospastic illness presenting similarly to asthma; therefore, treatment with both nebulized beta$_2$-agonists and steroids has been studied extensively. However, bronchiolitis does not have uniform bronchoconstriction, and direct damage occurs to the respiratory endothelium. Because bronchiolitis is a viral illness, antibiotics are not useful.

Conclusive evidence for the overall efficacy of beta$_2$-agonists such as albuterol is unavailable, but many children with bronchiolitis have a reversible component to their airway obstruction and benefit from a nebulized bronchodilator. Nebulized epinephrine, with its alpha and beta activity, is a more efficacious medication than albuterol (3 ml of 1:100 L-epinephrine). Racemic epinephrine has no advantage over isomeric (L) epinephrine. If clinical improvement is noted with a trial of nebulized epinephrine or albuterol, further treatment is warranted. This can be accomplished at home with a portable nebulization machine or a metered dose inhaler.

Although numerous trials have not proven any benefit from systemic steroids in acute bronchiolitis, recent studies show some clinical improvement and decreased hospitalization rate from the early use of oral (1 mg/kg dexamethasone) or intramuscular steroids. The routine use of steroids is not recommended at this time.

The child with bronchiolitis should be hospitalized for hypoxia or severe respiratory distress, or if poor oral intake or dehydration are concerns. Infants younger than 2 months of age have a significant risk of apnea. If the child is an outpatient, and is displaying high respiratory rate, fatigue, or poor oral intake, close follow-up is necessary. The parent should be advised that the disease might worsen, especially at night, before it improves. Most children are completely well in 2 to 3 weeks.

Prognosis

The prognosis for a child with bronchiolitis is excellent, and the complications of persistent wheezing, apnea, or superimposed bacterial pneumonia are rare. When an infant presents with a first episode of wheezing with an upper respiratory tract infection, it is impossible to differentiate bronchiolitis from reactive airway disease triggered by a viral infection. If the patient has other signs of atopy or a family history of allergies or reactive airway disease, the diagnosis of reactive airway disease is more likely. The association between bronchiolitis and the later development of reactive airway disease also is unclear. Many interacting family and environmental factors determine the risk of reactive airway disease, such as a family history of reactive airway disease and atopy, and exposure to allergens and tobacco smoke.

ANAPHYLAXIS

Anaphylaxis is an extreme systemic allergic reaction involving multiple organ systems. It is the clinical manifestation of a type I hypersensitivity reaction mediated by immunoglobulin E (IgE) or IgG.

Pathophysiology

Anaphylaxis is caused by hypersensitivity to a foreign substance, and it usually occurs within a few hours of oral or parenteral exposure to the antigen. Preformed active mediators, including histamine and secondary mediators, are released from mast cells and basophils. The onset is unpredictable, and the organ systems involved, symptoms, and severity vary.

Common triggers of anaphylactic reactions include *Hymenoptera* stings, primarily bees and wasps; latex; drugs, such as penicillins and local anesthetics; foods, such as nuts, seafood, and eggs; iodinated contrast media for radiologic studies; blood products; and hormones, such as insulin.

Clinical Manifestations and Complications

The most common clinical features of anaphylactic reactions are listed in Box 116.6. Skin and respiratory manifestations are present in more than 90% of all anaphylactic reactions. Anaphylaxis may progress slowly or rapidly. Most commonly, manifestations are limited to the first few hours after exposure to the allergen, but the initial reaction may be delayed for hours or may recur up to 72 hours after initial recovery. The most severe reactions usually begin within 5 to 10 minutes of exposure. If a secondary wave of symptoms occurs, their severity correlates to the intensity of the initial reaction. Urticaria may be localized to the exposed area or may be generalized; often, it is accompanied by angioedema, a swelling of the lower dermis and subcutaneous tissues. Cardiovascular collapse is the most

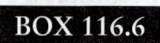

| BOX 116.6 | Clinical Features of an Anaphylactic Reaction |

Cutaneous: pruritus, urticaria, angioedema
Respiratory: bronchospasm, laryngeal edema, stridor
Circulatory: hypotension, cardiac arrhythmias, tachycardia
Gastrointestinal: diarrhea, abdominal pain
Neurologic: lethargy, disorientation, syncope

common life-threatening event. In the presence of clinical signs of respiratory distress, such as voice change or dyspnea, difficulty in swallowing, or circulatory collapse, treatment must proceed immediately.

Diagnosis

In evaluating anaphylaxis, an affected patient's history focuses on the time immediately preceding the reaction in an effort to determine exposure to an antigen. The physical examination focuses on vital signs; airway, including swelling and bronchospasm; circulation, including heart rate and rhythm; skin changes, such as urticaria and angioedema; and central nervous system changes.

Therapy

Treatment begins with monitoring and support of the airway, breathing, circulation, and cardiac rhythm. Initial treatment includes oxygen and intravenous fluids. Epinephrine, given subcutaneously or intramuscularly, is the drug of choice in most systemic reactions (0.01 mL/kg of 1:1,000 concentration; maximum, 0.4 mL). This dose can be repeated as often as every 5 minutes if necessary. A delay in treatment with epinephrine is reported as the principal reason for poor outcome in patients with anaphylaxis. Intravenous epinephrine (0.1 mL/kg; 1:10,000 solution) should be used only in severe cases in monitored patients. Intravenous or intramuscular antihistamines, such as diphenhydramine, also should be given to all children with anaphylaxis. They play a secondary, but important, role.

Many patients, including those with a history of asthma, develop bronchospasm during anaphylaxis. This condition is treated with 100% oxygen, subcutaneous or intramuscular epinephrine, a nebulized bronchodilator (e.g., albuterol), and steroids. Signs of upper airway obstruction are treated with nebulized racemic epinephrine (0.5 mL). If severe airway obstruction cannot be relieved, intubation or tracheotomy may be necessary.

Anaphylaxis may include vasodilation and a rapid decrease in plasma volume, requiring intravenous fluid boluses for support of blood pressure. Colloid or crystalloid infusion, such as lactated Ringer's solution or normal saline, is given in boluses of 20 mL/kg of body weight and is repeated as often as necessary. If an affected patient remains hypotensive, the Trendelenburg position and a 1:10,000 epinephrine infusion, starting at 0.1 μg/kg/minute, may be used. Occasionally, other vasopressors, such as dopamine, may be necessary for severe hypotension.

Intravenous corticosteroids should be given to every child with anaphylaxis to help prevent late-onset reactions. For extensive allergic reactions without anaphylaxis, a 3- to 5-day course of oral steroids may help alleviate symptoms. Minor allergic reactions are not treated with steroids.

Generalized cutaneous reactions, such as urticaria or angioedema, may be treated with intravenous, intramuscular, or oral diphenhydramine at the dose of 1 mg/kg administered every 4 to 6 hours. In patients with persistent allergic urticaria, intravenous cimetidine (5 mg/kg; maximum, 300 mg) may be beneficial.

The acute symptoms of anaphylaxis should subside within 1 to 2 hours. After initial treatment, the patient should be observed for several hours to ensure that a late response does not occur. Children with severe symptoms involving the respiratory and cardiovascular systems should be observed and monitored for 24 hours.

After treatment of the acute reaction, careful follow-up is essential. If at all possible, the cause of the reaction should be determined. Affected patients should see their physician for possible allergy testing, counseling about allergens, and preventive therapy. Children with more severe symptoms should be treated with oral antihistamines and steroids for 2 to 3 days, and should have a preloaded injectable dose of epinephrine (Epi-Pen) available for emergencies.

FEVER IN YOUNG INFANTS

Fever is a common complaint of patients in a pediatric ED. It can signify a range of illness from minor viral processes to serious bacterial infection. The average normal core temperature of a young infant is $37.5° \pm 0.3°C$, with fever defined as a temperature in excess of $38.0°C$. This temperature can be influenced by illness, age, metabolic rate, environmental temperature, and excessive bundling. Infants with a history of a documented fever, but who are afebrile at time of evaluation, should be considered to be febrile.

The standard method of determining the core temperature in an infant is rectal measurement. As compared to rectal measurements, axillary methods detect fever in approximately one-half of febrile infants, and often skin measurements also are inaccurate. The tympanic thermometer has limited use in infants; it is not reliable in detecting the presence and height of fever.

Pathophysiology

Infants with elevated temperature have an increased risk of serious bacterial infection (SBI), including bacteremia, meningitis, urinary tract infection, gastroenteritis, pneumonia, and bone and soft tissue infections. Very young infants have immature immune systems and also may not be able to localize infection well, increasing the risk of SBI. The risk of SBI in infants who are younger than 3 months and have temperature in excess of $38.0°C$ is between 5% and 10%. In one large meta-analysis, 8.6% of nontoxic infants younger than 3 months had SBI, 2% had bacteremia, and 1% had meningitis. The predominant organisms are listed in Box 116.7.

Young infants with infection from herpes simplex virus type 2 also may present with fever. Infected mothers are asymptomatic at delivery in as many as 75% of cases. Primary infection has a 30% transmission rate to the baby; recurrent infection has a 3% transmission rate. In the presence of a positive maternal history for infection or any lesions on the child, appropriate cultures should be obtained and treatment should be started with intravenous acyclovir.

Diagnosis

The dilemma in the evaluation and treatment of infants with fever stems from the difficulty in determining those infants who

---

| BOX 116.7 | Serious Bacterial Infections in Infants: Common Organisms |

Bacteremia-meningitis
<30 days
  Group B streptococcus
  Escherichia coli
  Listeria monocytogenes
>30 days
  Group B streptococcus
  E. coli
  Salmonella species
  Streptococcus pneumoniae
  Haemophilus influenzae type b
  Neisseria meningitidis

Gastroenteritis
Salmonella species
Shigella species
Yersinia enterolytica
Campylobacter

Urinary tract infection
E. coli
Klebsiella pneumoniae
Group B streptococcus
Enterococcus

Osteomyelitis
Group B streptococcus
E. coli
Staphylococcus aureus

---

are at highest risk of SBI. A very thorough history and physical is performed. However, even the best clinical judgment is limited, because well-appearing infants may have SBI. In large studies, more than 10% of infants with bacteremia look well to the examining physician. Many signs and symptoms of illness in these infants are subtle, such as decreased eye contact or alertness, poor feeding, mild tachypnea, or increased sleeping.

The traditional workup and treatment for febrile infants includes a chest radiograph; blood for complete blood cell count and culture; urine for urinalysis and culture; spinal fluid for chemistries, cell counts, and culture; and admission for intravenous antibiotics until cultures are negative. This traditional conservative approach has been challenged by many researchers and clinicians.

Therapy

Management strategies have been developed for febrile infants younger than 90 days of age. As with any guidelines, they allow great flexibility for options, taking into account the experience of the treating physician, the place of evaluation (ED versus office), the reliability of the caregivers, and the parental preference after a discussion of risks and benefits of the treatment options. No universal consensus exists for the evaluation and treatment of these young infants.

Several approaches have been developed for infants who fit into a "low-risk" category for SBI. One set of criteria to define "low risk," the Philadelphia criteria, apply to term, well-appearing infants 29 to 60 days of age who have been previously healthy, have received no recent antibiotics, and have no focal bacterial infection on physical examination (except otitis media). The criteria include the following laboratory test results: peripheral white blood cell count less than 15,000 cells per cubic millimeter with a band-to-neutrophil ratio of less than 0.2; urinalysis with fewer than ten white blood cells per high-power field on a spun urine and no bacteria on Gram stain; fewer than five white blood cells per high-power field on stool (if diarrhea), and cerebrospinal fluid (CSF) with fewer than eight white blood cells per high powered field and no bacteria on Gram stain. A chest radiograph is obtained only if there are respiratory symptoms or a low oxygen saturation on pulse oximetry. The negative predictive value for SBI in these infants is 99%. Increasing evidence suggests that hospitalization or antibiotics may not be necessary in such low-risk infants, thus avoiding the risk of iatrogenic complications (including infiltrated intravenous lines, contaminated cultures, and drug reactions) and the high cost of hospitalization. The options for these low-risk infants include hospitalization without antibiotic treatment, home observation with intramuscular ceftriaxone (50 mg/kg), or home observation without antibiotic treatment.

Considerable controversy still surrounds the management of febrile infants younger than 30 days of age. Even though most studies do not find a significantly increased risk of SBI in these infants, as compared to those 30 to 60 days of age, most physicians are uncomfortable with outpatient management of such infants. Most physicians would perform a complete workup, including CSF, and would admit them for intravenous antibiotics.

In infants between 30 and 60 days of age, with a complete diagnostic evaluation that is entirely negative, it is safe to discharge the baby home without antibiotic treatment. If home observation is planned, crucial factors are having a reliable caregiver to observe the child, a telephone at home, transportation, and the ability to return for follow-up care within 24 hours. Affected children should be reevaluated in 24 hours, or sooner in the presence of any new concerns by the caregiver. On follow-up, in the event of a positive blood or urine culture in a child who still is febrile, the child is admitted to hospital for intravenous antibiotics after a full sepsis evaluation. If the urine culture is positive, and the child appears well and is afebrile, he can be treated with outpatient antibiotics.

Infants who are ill-appearing or who do not meet the Philadelphia criteria are admitted for parenteral antibiotics, pending culture results. If such children appear to have a specific problem, such as potential respiratory syncytial viral illness, they may need only a focused evaluation and treatment rather than a full workup.

Many physicians are more comfortable with outpatient observation without antibiotics in infants 60 to 90 days of age. These infants are treated according to the preceding guidelines, with more physicians choosing fewer tests and simple observation. (For febrile children 3 to 24 months of age, see Chapter 403, Febrile Seizures.)

SEIZURES

Many children who have a seizure are otherwise healthy; in others, it is a symptom of serious underlying illness.

Epidemiology

Seizures are a common neurologic emergency. Approximately 5% of children have at least one seizure by 16 years of age, and 1% to 2% of ED visits are related to seizures.

Pathophysiology

A seizure is a paroxysmal electrical discharge of neurons in the brain, causing a transient change in the level of consciousness or an involuntary alteration of motor activity, sensation, or behavior. A partial seizure from a localized focus in the brain has a focal onset and can be motor, sensory, or psychomotor. A generalized seizure involving both cerebral hemispheres can be tonic, clonic, tonic-clonic, myoclonic, or absence. A convulsion is a seizure that manifests primarily as repetitive motor activity. Absence seizures consist of brief staring spells lasting less than 10 seconds, with no postictal period. Epilepsy, or seizure disorder, connotes recurrent seizures. Most seizures are brief, lasting less than 2 minutes; if a convulsion is persistent, or if repetitive seizures ensue without intercurrent regaining of consciousness for an hour or longer, an affected patient is in status epilepticus, a medical emergency.

The more common causes of seizures are listed in Box 116.8. It is important to determine whether a seizure actually has occurred. Certain conditions easily may be mistaken for seizures, including breath-holding spells, syncopal attacks, movement disorders such as tics and tremors, cardiac dysrhythmias, pseudoseizures, shaking chills, and hyperventilation. True seizures have abrupt onset, are usually brief, have impairment of consciousness (except simple partial seizures), have simple purposeless motor activity, have a postictal period, and the patient cannot recall the event. Generalized tonic-clonic seizures (grand mal) are the most common form of status epilepticus and will be discussed in more detail.

BOX 116.8   Common Causes of Seizures in Children

Simple febrile seizures
Infections
Intracranial infections—bacterial or aseptic meningitis, encephalitis
Shigellosis

Head trauma
Direct trauma
Shaking injury

Metabolic abnormalities
Hypoxia
Hypoglycemia—insulin reaction in diabetics, alcohol ingestion
Electrolyte disturbances or dehydration
Hypocalcemia
Pyridoxine deficiency
Renal failure
Hepatic failure
Inherited metabolic disorders

Toxic ingestions (rule out suicide attempt)
Alcohol
Theophylline
Cocaine

Withdrawal of anticonvulsant medications
Miscellaneous
Hypertensive encephalopathy
Brain tumor
Intracranial hemorrhage
Idiopathic

Diagnosis

For diagnostic purposes, seizure patients can be divided into four groups: febrile patients, patients with known seizure disorders, traumatized patients, and others (idiopathic seizures). After affected children are stable, a complete history and physical examination help determine the cause of the seizure and guide ongoing management. It is essential to check conditions that need immediate therapy. The history should include questions about the current seizure (including how it started, loss of consciousness, type, and duration); features and frequency of previous seizures; underlying medical conditions; fever; abnormal behavior; development; pica; head injury; possible ingestion of toxins; birth history; and current medications, including anticonvulsants.

The patient should be completely undressed to assess cutaneous signs of systemic disease and infection. The physical examination includes assessment of vital signs, level of consciousness, evidence of trauma or infection, and signs of underlying systemic disease. Abnormal neurologic signs, such as pupillary changes, increased or decreased muscle tone, or Babinski sign, are common during and after a seizure. Serious neurologic abnormalities, such as asymmetric pupils, signs of increased intracranial pressure, focal deficits, and posturing, may indicate a serious neurologic problem that needs immediate further assessment and treatment by a neurologist.

The selection of laboratory studies is determined by a patient's age, history, and physical examination. The traditional tests of electrolytes, calcium, and magnesium rarely are abnormal in children after infancy and are required only on suspicion of a relevant abnormality. A complete blood count with differential is obtained only on suspicion of infection. Other studies, such as lumbar puncture, urinalysis, toxicology screens of serum and urine, blood cultures, liver function, ammonia, and lead levels, are obtained only if indicated by history and physical examination. Patients with known seizures, who have a typical seizure while on medications and have returned to normal, usually only require a measurement of available anticonvulsant levels.

Neuroimaging, such as CT scan, is considered for patients with persistent alteration in consciousness, history of head trauma, evidence of increased intracranial pressure, or suspicion of a mass lesion. A lumbar puncture is indicated for children with a febrile seizure and meningeal signs; it is very unusual for meningitis to present solely as a simple febrile seizure. If concern exists about increased intracranial pressure, a CT scan should be performed before a lumbar puncture.

Therapy

The management of seizures in the ED includes stabilization of such patients, identification and treatment of any acute underlying medical conditions, and provision of good follow-up care.

Initial Management

Patients in status epilepticus need immediate treatment to prevent significant hemodynamic and metabolic complications such as hypoxia, tachycardia, hypertension, hyperthermia, and acidosis. Treatment starts with assessment of airway, breathing, and circulation. A comprehensive approach includes a relevant history, physical examination, and initiation of oxygenation, intravenous access, initial diagnostic studies, pharmacologic intervention, and treatment of the precipitating cause. Monitoring of vital signs, including pulse oximetry, is essential. To assess respiratory compromise, an arterial blood gas analysis is obtained if the seizure is prolonged. In addition to poten-

TABLE 116.8

DRUGS USED IN TREATING STATUS EPILEPTICUS

Drug	Dose and Route
Lorazepam	0.1 mg/kg IV; maximum, 10 mg; maximum rate, 2 mg/min. May repeat once in 5–10 min
Diazepam	0.2 mg/kg IV; maximum, 20 mg; maximum rate, 5 mg/min. May repeat once in 5–10 min
Phenytoin	15–20 mg/kg IV; maximum, 1 g; maximum rate, 1 mg/kg/min. For persistent seizures, possible additional doses, up to total of 30 mg/kg
Phenobarbital	15–20 mg/kg IV; maximum, 30 mg/kg; maximum rate, 1 mg/kg/min
Pentobarbital	5 mg/kg IV plus infusion 1–4 mg/kg/hr
Lidocaine	1–2 mg/kg IV plus infusion 6 mg/kg/hr
Chloral hydrate	30 mg/kg PR
Paraldehyde	5–10 ml PR

IV, intravenous; PR, per rectum.

tial hypercapnia and hypoxemia, the blood gas may show an anion gap metabolic acidosis secondary to lactic acidosis. For poor ventilation, the patient needs rapid-sequence intubation with a short-acting paralytic agent and intracranial pressure precautions. Before intubation, a nasogastric tube is inserted to prevent vomiting and aspiration.

An intravenous line is placed in patients with ongoing seizure activity or exhibiting compromised mental status. Blood is drawn at this time for relevant diagnostic studies, and a bedside glucose determination is obtained. If the blood glucose is low, 2 mL/kg of 25% solution of dextrose is given.

As soon as intravenous access is established, the ongoing seizure is treated with intravenous anticonvulsant medication. Affected patients should be monitored while these medications are given, because they have significant hemodynamic and respiratory-depressant side effects. Physicians should be familiar with the potential problems and be prepared to intubate or support the circulation if necessary.

Benzodiazepines are considered the best first-line drugs for status epilepticus, because they are potent and rapidly-acting (Table 116.8). Intravenous lorazepam is preferable to diazepam, because it is less likely to cause respiratory depression and has a longer duration of action. Diazepam also can be used rectally in the prehospital phase of treatment. Midazolam, a benzodiazepine with a very rapid onset of action and short half-life, can be used initially or in refractory cases. Midazolam has many routes of administration, including intravenous, intramuscular, rectal, intranasal, and buccal. Intravenous phenytoin, a longer acting medication, should be administered as soon as possible. Fosphenytoin is a prodrug of phenytoin that does not have the cardiac side effects of phenytoin and therefore can be administered more quickly. It is dosed in "phenytoin equivalents (PE)." It also can be given intramuscularly in the absence of intravenous access.

If the seizure persists, more intravenous phenytoin can be administered, or phenobarbital can be added. The respiratory status must be closely monitored, because phenobarbital causes significant respiratory depression, especially when given after a benzodiazepine. Refractory seizures can be treated with infusions of midazolam or lorazepam, or through the induction of a barbiturate coma using pentobarbital. Other medications that have been used for refractory status epilepticus include lidocaine, propofol, chloral hydrate, paraldehyde, and isoflurane anesthetic.

Terminating a seizure may be difficult in the presence of an uncorrected underlying disorder, such as hypoxemia, hypoglycemia, or an electrolyte disturbance. These conditions should be detected and treated as soon as possible. Isotonic fluids containing glucose are given at a slow rate that will not exacerbate cerebral edema. Ceftriaxone (100 mg/kg) is given if serious infection, such as meningitis, is suspected. With cessation of the seizure, airway patency and adequate ventilation often return.

Patients having a seizure must be protected from physical harm. Affected children are placed on a soft surface and are restrained as necessary. Fever control is part of supportive care. Body temperature may be elevated from infection or from the seizure itself, and fever increases metabolic demands.

After a seizure has been stopped in the ED, any underlying conditions that may have caused the seizure must be treated. A neurologist should be consulted concerning ongoing seizure management.

If a seizure cannot be controlled, if cardiovascular signs are unstable, or if neurologic examination results are abnormal after the seizure and immediate postictal period, an affected patient should be hospitalized for further observation and management. (The nonemergent care of children with seizures is discussed in Chapter 401, Epilepsy.)

Further Management

Simple Febrile Seizure. Febrile seizures are a common occurrence in young children. For a diagnosis of simple febrile seizure, several criteria must be met: 6 months to 6 years of age, generalized tonic-clonic seizure of less than 20 minutes' duration, occurrence within 24 hours of onset of the fever, normal development and neurologic examination results, and no personal or family history of afebrile seizures. A family history of febrile seizures often is noted. If an affected child and the seizure meet these criteria, and the child looks well after an antipyretic and observation, the diagnosis is a simple febrile seizure. Routine laboratory and imaging studies are not indicated. No further treatment for the seizure is necessary, and the child is evaluated and treated as any child with a fever of that degree. Antipyretics are used to control fever. Prophylaxis with antiepileptic medication is not indicated.

A child with a simple febrile seizure has an approximately 30% risk of recurrence of a febrile seizure, usually within 1 year. Factors that increase the chance of a recurrence include age less than 18 months, less than 1 hour between start of fever and occurrence of seizure, family history of febrile seizures, and low-grade fever at the time of seizure. An electroencephalograph (EEG) is not indicated for children with febrile seizures. The family should be counseled on emergency management of further seizures, such as lying the child on her side, and reassured that no increased risk of neurologic damage occurs.

If the criteria for simple febrile seizure are not met, an affected child is currently receiving antibiotics, or if such a child has other signs of illness (e.g., photophobia, nuchal rigidity, or positive Kernig sign), a lumbar puncture may be necessary to rule out meningitis. Central nervous system infections rarely are found, even in children with "atypical" or complex febrile seizures. Other laboratory studies are performed as necessary. Children with febrile seizures have the same risk for bacteremia and urinary tract infection as febrile children without a seizure.

Known Seizure Disorder. Many children presenting with seizures have chronic seizure disorders and already are taking anticonvulsant medication. Often, the seizures in such children are due to inadequate anticonvulsant drug levels in the blood. The child also may have an intercurrent illness that lowers the seizure threshold. An important factor is to ask whether this seizure is typical for this patient (or whether an affected child needs further evaluation), how often the seizures usually occur (if at all), and whether the child is taking the anticonvulsant medication. Often, patients have not been given the medication, have exhausted the supply, or are vomiting the medication. Management involves checking serum drug levels and loading an affected patient intravenously or orally. Follow-up care should be arranged with the patient's usual provider.

Trauma and Seizure. Seizures may be secondary to head trauma. Such trauma may be obvious, with external bruising, or occult, as in a shaking injury. Posttraumatic seizures are classified by time after injury: immediate (less than 24 hours), early (during the first week), or late (after the first week). The sooner after the injury the seizure occurs, the better is the prognosis. Immediate seizures require no treatment, and the prognosis is excellent. Early seizures indicate a focal injury with a 25% incidence of further seizures. Late seizures indicate focal scarring and are associated with a high risk of additional seizures. Emergency studies to be considered include CT scan, subdural tap, and lumbar puncture. A neurologist should be consulted concerning treatment. In the case of major head trauma and evidence of increased intracranial pressure, treatment for these problems should start immediately.

Idiopathic Seizure. Many patients have seizures from an unknown or idiopathic cause; 70% of afebrile seizures are idiopathic. Well-appearing children and adolescents with a first unprovoked afebrile seizure do not need laboratory studies, lumbar puncture, or routine neuroimaging. Children with new-onset neurologic deficit or long-lasting changes in mental status, or with predisposing factors such as bleeding disorders, head injury, or malignancy, may need a CT or magnetic resonance imaging (MRI). Young children with a focal seizure can have a nonurgent MRI at a later date. Most first-time seizures do not need ongoing outpatient treatment, unless abnormal CT or other test results are found. The decision about whether to treat affected patients prophylactically with anticonvulsants should be made with the primary-care doctor or neurologist. Anticonvulsant drugs do not offer full protection against further seizures, and they all have potential side effects ranging from minor to severe. Such patients need close follow-up, including an outpatient EEG to diagnose certain seizure syndromes and provide information on risk of recurrence.

CHEST PAIN

Chest pain is a common complaint of children, a condition affecting a wide range of patients but exhibiting no gender predominance. This complaint elicits particular anxiety in children and their parents, who often equate chest pain with cardiac disease. However, cardiac disease is rare in children, and usually the origin of the pain is benign. All patients deserve to be evaluated carefully and thoroughly.

Epidemiology

Children younger than 12 years of age account for approximately one-half of children with chest pain and are more likely to have a cardiorespiratory cause of pain, such as pneumonia, cough, asthma, or cardiac disease; adolescent patients are more likely to have musculoskeletal, psychogenic, or idiopathic causes.

Pathophysiology

The causes of chest pain in children are listed in Box 116.9. An organic cause is found more often on acute onset of pain, abnormal findings on physical examination, pain that awakens

| BOX 116.9 | Possible Causes of Chest Pain |

Idiopathic
Musculoskeletal
Chest wall strain
Trauma
Rib fracture
Costochondritis

Respiratory
Severe cough
Asthma
Pneumonia
Pneumothorax
Pulmonary embolus

Psychological
Anxiety
Conversion disorder
Depression

Cardiac
Coronary artery disease (ischemia)
Dysrhythmias (supraventricular tachycardia, ventricular tachycardia)
Structural abnormalities
Infection (pericarditis, myocarditis)

Gastrointestinal
Reflux esophagitis
Esophageal foreign body

Miscellaneous
Sickle cell anemia
Abdominal aortic aneurysm
Shingles
Cocaine ingestion
Breast tenderness

a child from sleep, or fever. Nonorganic causes are found more often with a family history of heart disease or chest pain (raising concerns in a child or the family) or a history of chronic chest pain in the child. A large prospective study from an inner-city pediatric ED evaluated more than 400 patients with chest pain. The most common diagnosis in the study (21%) was "idiopathic." A follow-up study of these patients showed that most of the chest pain had nonorganic causes.

Respiratory disorders, such as persistent cough, asthma, or pneumonia, cause 20% of chest pain, usually from overuse of chest wall muscles. Less common respiratory disorders causing chest pain are spontaneous pneumothorax, pulmonary embolus, and cocaine ingestion.

Other common identifiable causes of chest pain found in the aforementioned study were musculoskeletal disorders (15%), costochondritis (9%), and direct trauma (5%). Musculoskeletal pain results from vigorous activity or sports causing strain to the chest wall muscles, whereas costochondritis may follow a viral illness or minor trauma.

A significant number of children, particularly those older than 12 years of age, have chest pain from psychogenic causes (9%). This malady affects both girls and boys, and it may result from stress (e.g., problems with friends, family, or school) or from depression.

Although rare, cardiac causes of chest pain do exist in children. Unknown cardiac disease is an unusual cause of chest

pain in children, but should be considered more seriously if the pain is exercise-induced or if an abnormal cardiac examination occurs. Some children have chronic or previous conditions that render them prone to exertional chest pain, such as Kawasaki disease, diabetes mellitus, chronic anemia, or anomalous coronary arteries. Toxic exposure, particularly cocaine use, can cause chest pain that ranges from mild pain from minor barotrauma to the severe pain of a myocardial infarction.

Gastrointestinal disorders also can cause chest pain. Reflux esophagitis can cause burning substernal pain. Ingestion of foreign bodies or caustic substances also can cause chest pain, possibly with respiratory distress.

Diagnosis

A thorough history and physical examination should reveal the etiology of chest pain in most patients. Laboratory studies rarely are helpful; their use will be dictated by the history and physical examination.

History

The history focuses on the character of the chest pain. Considerations include the frequency and severity of the pain; whether it interrupts daily activity, such as school attendance; and whether it awakens the child at night. Constant or severe pain is more distressing to such children but may not imply a serious etiology. The location of the pain is only occasionally helpful in the diagnosis, such as burning pain in esophagitis.

Patients with chronic chest pain are unlikely to exhibit a serious organic cause. However, acute pain is more likely to be organic (although not necessarily serious).

Pain induced by exercise is more likely to have a cardiac or respiratory origin. Asthma is a common cause of exercise-induced chest pain. Other important historical precipitating factors include trauma, muscle strain, and foreign-body ingestion. Any current psychologic stresses also should be investigated.

A history should evaluate for more serious associated symptoms, such as palpitations, syncope, or fever. Chest pain may be part of an underlying illness, such as asthma or pneumonia. If cough is present, its character, chronicity, and timing should be investigated.

The examiner should ascertain whether any previous factors in an affected patient predispose to chest pain. These factors include trauma, asthma, heart disease, Kawasaki disease, collagen vascular disorders, sickle cell disease, chronic anemia, diabetes mellitus, cigarette smoking, and shingles.

Substance abuse is an equally important consideration. An examiner should determine whether the child has any history of substance abuse, particularly cocaine.

Rare disorders, such as hypertrophic obstructive cardiomyopathy, are familial. Most children with a family history of heart disease or chest pain, however, are more likely to exhibit a nonorganic cause of chest pain.

Physical Examination

A strong correlation exists between an abnormal physical examination and the presence of organic disease. Particular attention should be paid to vital signs, including blood pressure. Assess for any acute emergency and follow with a system-by-system approach. For severe distress, immediate treatment is begun.

Patients with pain from psychogenic causes may be in acute distress with hyperventilation or may be calm, rendering the anxiety and stress less apparent. Hyperventilating patients do not demonstrate cyanosis or accessory muscle use.

BOX 116.10   Chest Examination

Chest wall
Tenderness
Bruising
Asymmetry
Breast masses
Subcutaneous air

Lungs
Breath sounds
Rales
Wheezes
Retractions

Cardiac
Heart sounds
Murmurs
Arrhythmias

After a general examination, the investigation should focus on the chest examination (Box 116.10). A respiratory etiology should evince some respiratory signs or symptoms, such as cough, respiratory distress, decreased breath sounds, rales, wheezes, or tachypnea.

Chest wall tenderness is the most common finding in children experiencing chest pain, and it may be indicative of trauma or costochondritis. Costochondritis produces tenderness over the costochondral junctions; it may be sharp or radiating, unilateral or bilateral, and it may last for months. It can be exacerbated by deep breathing, activity, or change in position. Inspection and palpation of the chest wall may reveal evidence of trauma, such as bruising.

If the child exhibits respiratory distress, fever, stabbing chest pain, and a cardiac examination with friction rub, distant heart tones, and neck vein distention, pericarditis is the likely diagnosis. The symptoms of myocarditis are more subtle, with mild pain, fever, muffled heart tones, tachycardia and, possibly, orthostatic changes. The heart would appear enlarged on a chest radiograph.

Cocaine use should be considered in adolescents who present with anxiety, severe chest pain, hypertension, and tachycardia.

Laboratory Tests

Generally, laboratory studies are not helpful in establishing a specific diagnosis, but they may confirm what is suspected from history and physical examination. Certain findings in the history and physical examination warrant further studies: history of acute onset of pain or pain on exertion; history of heart disease or related serious medical conditions; history of drug use; serious associated symptoms, such as syncope, shortness of breath, or palpitations; foreign-body ingestion; fever; or history of trauma. Further studies should be obtained also for abnormal findings on the examination, such as respiratory distress, subcutaneous air, or other heart or lung abnormalities.

In the event of severe respiratory distress, an arterial blood gas analysis and a chest radiograph should be obtained. A chest radiograph is indicated also in children with fever or abnormal breath sounds. An electrocardiogram (ECG) is indicated on any evidence of cardiac involvement, such as severe tachycardia, palpitations, arrhythmia, murmur, or rub. A screen for toxicology may be indicated in adolescents with acute chest

pain, hypertension, and tachycardia, looking for the possibility of cocaine ingestion. Patients with chest pain and syncope need referral for a Holter monitor to detect arrhythmias and structural heart disease. A complete blood count and a sedimentation rate test have very limited value except for suspected infection or collagen vascular disease.

Not every patient presenting with chest pain requires a chest radiograph and ECG. If affected patients have chronic chest pain and a normal history and physical examination, they need only reassurance and follow-up care.

Therapy

Children with chest pain and severe distress need immediate treatment, possibly including blood gas analysis to determine respiratory status, chest radiograph, ECG, and administration of oxygen. However, the majority of patients need no immediate therapy.

Children with specific disorders are treated appropriately. For pneumonia, antibiotics and close follow-up are appropriate. For an esophageal foreign body, the appropriate specialist should be consulted. If esophagitis is suspected, a trial of antacids is initiated. If the final assessment is musculoskeletal pain, analgesics and rest are recommended. If pain is thought to be psychogenic or idiopathic, reassurance is given, and appropriate follow-up is arranged.

If a concern exists about cardiac disease, patients should be referred to a cardiologist. Patients with known cardiac disease, and those with new findings suspicious for cardiac disease, such as chest pain with exertion or accompanied by syncope, dizziness, or palpitations, should seek further medical advice.

Chest pain is often a chronic symptom. All patients should be offered follow-up if symptoms persist. A study of patients receiving long-term follow-up for chest pain showed that finding serious disease over time is unlikely if it is not found initially.

PAIN AND SEDATION

A significant number of children presenting to the ED experience pain. This pain can be the result of such medical illnesses as headache, abdominal pain, or sickle cell disease, or can result from traumatic injury, such as broken bones. In addition, many of the diagnostic and therapeutic procedures performed in the ED are painful. Undertreatment of pain makes children frightened and anxious, with possible physiologic and psychologic consequences.

Pain Management

The treatment of pain in children is often inadequate, due to failure of the medical professional to appreciate the pain, fear of causing complications or obscuring the diagnosis, or lack of training in pain control. In recent years, the treatment of pain in the ED has become a priority. The armamentarium of the emergency physician for the treatment of pain has increased dramatically. Still, many patients are not given adequate medication to manage their pain, or procedures are performed without adequate pain control.

Clinical Manifestations and Complications

Multiple studies have confirmed that even the smallest infants experience and remember pain. A number of methods can be used to assess pain in infants and children. The assessment tool needs to be age-appropriate, easy to administer, reliable, and cross-cultural. Observation of behavior, physiologic parameters, parental and patient reporting, and mechanism of disease or injury all give important clues to the degree of pain.

Physiologic parameters, such as heart rate, blood pressure, and respiratory rate are especially useful in preverbal children. Infant pain scales combine these physiologic parameters with behavioral observation, such as facial expression and motor activity.

Toddlers and preschoolers are more able to use words to express feelings of pain, and may be able to point to the most painful spot, but will have difficulty describing intensity or quality of pain. A facial expression scale for pain, showing a range of faces from "no hurt" to "most hurt" is appropriate and reliable for children 3 to 5 years of age.

Older children can use numeric rating scales for assessing level of pain, such as a scale from 1 to 10. The Children's Hospital of Eastern Ontario Pain Scale (CHEOPS), which evaluates expression and behaviors, has been validated in children older than 5 years of age.

Therapy

The type of pain management used should be individualized to the patient's condition and to the level of pain experienced.

Patients with a minor injury or medical illness may be treated with oral analgesics (e.g., acetaminophen) or nonsteroidal antiinflammatory drugs (NSAIDs) (e.g., ibuprofen) (Table 116.9). Non-narcotic analgesics are the most commonly used pain medications in the ED. They are safe and have no CNS or respiratory depression. Just as antipyretics are given to patients with fever, patients who present with conditions amenable to these medications, such as musculoskeletal injuries, headaches, or small burns, should receive them while treated in the ED. Children with moderate pain can be treated with acetaminophen or NSAIDs with added codeine or oxycodone. Codeine can cause nausea and constipation, and therefore oxycodone is preferred for some children.

Children in severe pain usually require parenterally delivered narcotics to achieve pain relief. The intravenous route allows for rapid drug delivery and also allows for a medication to be titrated to effect. In the ED, morphine is the standard opioid for the management of severe pain, whether the pain derives from a femur fracture or from a vasoocclusive crisis in patients with sickle cell disease. Initially, morphine should be delivered at a dose of 0.1 mg/kg in opioid-naive patients, although significantly more may be necessary in patients with recurrent acute pain (see Table 116.9). In either class of patients, the dose should be titrated to relieve their pain. Fentanyl is a more potent and shorter-acting synthetic opioid that can be used for treating pain or as part of a regimen for treating procedural pain, such as fracture reduction or burn débridement. It causes less cardiovascular instability and histamine release than morphine does. The other advantages of fentanyl include its rapid onset (2 to 3 minutes) and its short duration of action (20 to 40 minutes). Fentanyl also is available for delivery in a transmucosal Oralet form (fentanyl lollipop) that obviates the need for intravenous placement in some patients. However, this form of fentanyl has been associated with a high incidence of vomiting, which limits its use for procedural pain management and sedation.

The side effects of opioids include nausea, vomiting, respiratory depression, hypotension, pruritus, and decreased gastrointestinal motility. Pain relief usually is achieved at levels that do not cause respiratory depression. Naloxone, an opioid antagonist, should be on hand for the reversal of severe opioid side effects.

Ketorolac is a parenteral nonsteroidal antiinflammatory drug useful in the treatment of pain associated with musculoskeletal injuries, vaso-occlusive episodes and migraine headaches, and conditions in which narcotic medication may be undesirable. It can also be used as an adjunct to opiates in other painful conditions.

In some cases, behavioral or mind–body methods can be used to decrease stress and anxiety and help alleviate pain. These techniques can be complex hypnotic or imagery techniques, or simple distractions such as bubble blowing, music, or play. Often, these distractions can be used in conjunction with pharmacologic relief. In addition, the surroundings should be as calm and relaxing as possible. Parents should be present whenever possible, and they should be informed how they can be most helpful. The physician or nurse should be honest about the pain associated with any procedures, and they should explain this to the child at a level that the child can understand.

TABLE 116.9

AGENTS ADMINISTERED FOR PAIN AND SEDATION

Drug	Dose	Use
Ibuprofen	10 mg/kg Q6–8 h PO	Mild pain such as musculoskeletal injuries
Acetaminophen with codeine	1 mg/kg codeine PO	Injuries, burns, minor procedures
Ketorolac	0.5–1.0 mg/kg IV (max. 30 mg)	Injuries, migraines, vaso-occlusive crisis
Morphine	0.1 mg/kg IV	Severe pain (vaso-occlusive crisis, fracture)
Fentanyl	1–3 mcg/kg IV	Pain, painful procedure (fracture reduction, burn debridement)
Ketamine	0.5–2.0 mg/kg IV 2–4 mg/kg IM	Procedural pain, sedation (fracture reduction, laceration repair)
Propofol	2 mg/kg IV, induction	Procedural sedation (fracture reduction, laceration repair)
Nitrous Oxide	50%	Procedural pain, sedation (laceration repair, fracture reduction)
Toradol	1 mg/kg IV	Pain (migraine headache, vaso-occlusive crisis)
Midazolam	0.1–0.2 mg/kg IV 0.25–0.75 mg/kg PO 0.2 mg/kg Intranasal	Anxiolytic for painful procedures (laceration repair with local anesthetic, fracture reduction with fentanyl-ketamine)
Pentobarbital	1–3 mg/kg PO/PR/IM	Painless procedures (CT scan)
Chloral hydrate	50–100 mg/kg PO/PR	Painless procedures (CT scan)

CT, computed tomography; IM, intramuscular; PO, oral; PR, per rectum.

Sedation

Children undergoing painful procedures in the ED require appropriate sedation and analgesia both for pain control and the alleviation of anxiety. The most common procedures in the pediatric ED requiring sedation are complex laceration repair and fracture reduction. Effective and safe sedation improves cooperation, outcomes, and patient and parent satisfaction. Several short-acting agents are available to provide the necessary level of sedation required for the procedure. The physician responsible for the sedation must have the appropriate required training and capability of airway management, and the staff must be trained in monitoring and documentation. The sedation team must anticipate and be prepared for such events as loss of protective airway reflexes, hypotension, hypoventilation, and hypoxemia.

Before any planned procedure, the options for sedation and the risks involved are discussed with the patient and parent(s). Patients at increased risk for complications should be identified. A full history and physical examination is performed, focusing on relevant medical problems, allergies, previous sedations, medications, and time since last eating. Required fasting time before sedation is controversial, and it may be that no advantage accrues to waiting longer than 2 hours. Physical examination should focus on cardiorespiratory status and any head and neck abnormalities that could complicate airway management. If the patient is considered to be at high risk for complications, sedation should not be performed in the ED.

Appropriate monitoring is essential and required for all patients undergoing sedation. It is best to have a nurse or physician dedicated to the monitoring. Visual inspection of respiration and color is supplemented by pulse oximetry, cardiorespiratory monitoring, and intermittent blood pressure evaluation. Appropriate precautionary equipment should be available (Box 116.11). Specific guidelines are outlined by the American Academy of Pediatrics and in institutional policies.

When the procedure has been completed, and the child is less stimulated, ongoing effects of the sedative medication may persist, such as cardiorespiratory compromise or vomiting. It is essential to continue full monitoring until the child returns to presedation activity, using guidelines for a systematic postsedation assessment.

BOX 116.11 — Equipment Available for Sedation and Pain Management

Supplies
Suction apparatus
Oral and nasal airways
Bag valve mask
Laryngoscope and endotracheal tubes
Oxygen tubing and masks

Monitors
Cardiorespiratory monitor
Sphygmomanometer
Pulse oximeter

Medications
Oxygen
Epinephrine
Atropine
Lidocaine
Naloxone
Flumazenil

Agent(s) are selected with consideration for the appropriate level of sedation and analgesia required for the procedure, duration of sedation needed, and patient and parental concerns. The intravenous route allows more reliable administration and titration of the drug(s) and is safer should any complications arise requiring further treatment. Intramuscular administration is unpredictable.

Specific Agents

Pentobarbital. Barbiturates depress the reticular activating system; they are sedatives with no analgesic effects. The barbiturate pentobarbital can provide effective sedation for nonpainful procedures such as radiologic imaging. It has a slower onset and longer duration of action than barbiturates such as thiopental (see Table 116.9).

Midazolam. Benzodiazepines often are used for sedation during pediatric procedures; they do not provide analgesia. Intravenous midazolam often is preferred over diazepam, because it is more potent, faster acting, and has a short duration of action (see Table 116.9). It also provides amnesia for the event. It can be used alone or in conjunction with opioids or ketamine for sedation before a procedure such as lumbar puncture or fracture reduction. The administration of midazolam with strong opiates such as fentanyl increases the risk of hypoventilation.

Midazolam can be given orally for sedation and anxiolysis before wound repair and other minor procedures. Onset of sedation with orally administered midazolam is 20 to 30 minutes. Nasal midazolam spray also has been used successfully to relieve pain and anxiety during minor procedures. Midazolam must be used in conjunction with systemic analgesia or local anesthesia for painful procedures.

Ketamine. Ketamine is a widely used dissociative agent that has sedative, analgesic, and amnestic effects. Despite producing deep sedation, respiration and airway reflexes are unaffected. It is especially useful for complex laceration repair or fracture reduction. It is the only sedative that can be effectively and reliably used through the intramuscular route, although the length of sedation is less predictable.

The side effects of ketamine include bad dreams and hallucinations, which can be reduced by the concurrent use of a benzodiazepine. Hypersalivation should be treated with a concurrent dose of atropine or glycopyrrolate. Other rare side effects include laryngospasm, hypertension, and increased intracranial pressure. It should not be used in patients with head injuries, young babies, and children with upper respiratory infections.

Propofol. Propofol is a very short-acting intravenous sedative. It is a favored agent for painful procedures, with onset of less than 60 seconds and fast emergence. After an initial dose, further doses are titrated for sedation during the procedure, with quick return to baseline after the procedure is completed. Propofol can cause transient hypotension and respiratory depression, and it requires careful monitoring. For painful procedures, it can be combined with fentanyl or local anesthetics. Compared to ketamine, propofol has a more rapid and comfortable recovery, with minimal side effects.

Nitrous Oxide. Nitrous oxide is an inhaled sedative for older children; it is given by a demand-valve face mask in a 50:50 mixture with oxygen. It has rapid onset and is short acting. It has an amnestic and dissociative effect, and is noninvasive. Nitrous oxide can be used for the management of procedural pain and sedation. A scavenging system should be in place to prevent health care worker exposure to the gas. Nitrous oxide is not universally effective, so other methods of analgesia may be necessary.

TABLE 116.10
LOCAL ANESTHETICS

Drug	Dose	Use
Lidocaine 1%	4 mg/kg (max.)	Wound anesthesia, local
	7 mg/kg (max.	dermal anesthesia
	with epi.)	
Bupivacaine	2 mg/kg (max.)	Peripheral nerve blocks;
		prolonged anesthesia
LET	3 ml	Wound anesthesia
EMLA	2.5–5.0 g	Local dermal anesthesia

LET, lidocaine, 4%; epinephrine, 0.1%; tetracaine, 0.5%. EMLA: lidocaine (2.5%) and prilocaine (2.5%).

Local Anesthesia

Often, local anesthesia is necessary before wound repair, incision and drainage, lumbar puncture, and intravenous cannulation in the ED. Lidocaine is the local anesthetic used most commonly (Table 116.10). It is effective, inexpensive, and has minimal toxicity. A 1% solution (10 mg/mL) is infiltrated locally to provide anesthesia. Its peak analgesic effect is approximately 5 minutes after injection, and can last up to 2 hours. Lidocaine without epinephrine added can be used for wounds on any area of the body, including mucosal surfaces. Lidocaine with epinephrine can be used for areas that are not end organs or mucous membranes; epinephrine, a vasoconstrictor, limits removal of the analgesic by local blood flow, thus increasing its duration and potency.

Techniques used to minimize the pain of lidocaine infiltration include slow infiltration, buffering with sodium bicarbonate (1 mL $NaHCO_3$ to 9 mL lidocaine), injection of the solution into the open wound instead of through the epidermis, and warming the lidocaine solution to body temperature before infiltration.

The use of topical anesthetic agents is an important advance in analgesia for wound repair. They are easy to apply, painless, and do not distort wound edges. There is improved patient cooperation and less need for sedation and physical restraint, and less emotional trauma for the child. Topical anesthetics are most effective for small wounds less than 5 to 6 cm in length, and on the face or scalp, where high vascularity allows for greater diffusion of the agent. The efficacy is considerably less in extremity lacerations; thus, supplemental lidocaine should be used for patients with those lacerations.

TAC (tetracaine, 0.5%; adrenaline, 1:2,000; cocaine, 11.8%) is a widely used topical anesthetic agent. Because of concerns of toxicity from cocaine and cost, TAC has been largely replaced by LET (lidocaine, 4%; epinephrine, 0.1%; and tetracaine, 0.5%). LET is used as a solution or is mixed with cellulose to form a gel applied to the wound for 20 to 30 minutes to allow for anesthesia. The gel form keeps the anesthetic more contained and is therefore easier to use. Topical agents are not indicated for use on mucus membranes.

EMLA cream (eutectic mixture of local anesthetics) is a combination of lidocaine (2.5%) and prilocaine (2.5%); it provides transdermal anesthesia before painful procedures, such as venipuncture, intravenous catheter placement, lumbar puncture, and drainage of abscesses. EMLA takes at least 1 hour of application to achieve a 3-mm depth of anesthesia, which limits its use in the ED.

Vapocoolant sprays, such as ethyl chloride, or a similar product, dichlorodifluoromethane-trichloromonofluoromethane (Fluori-methane), can be sprayed onto the skin just before injection. The chemical is allowed to evaporate for a few seconds, the skin is cooled, and the injection is given.

BITES

Epidemiology

Human and nonhuman animal bites are common among children. More than one-half of such bites are minor, but certain initially innocuous-appearing bites can lead to serious infectious complications. Most often, animal bites affect the extremities; however, nearly two-thirds of bites to children younger than age 4 involve the head and neck. Human bites account for 1% to 3% of mammalian bites. They range from minor abrasions in young children to deep fist wounds during fights. Dog bites account for approximately 90% of nonhuman bites that require medical attention, but are often lacerations with a low incidence of infection. If they are punctures or crush injuries, they have a higher infection risk. Cat bites account for approximately 10% of mammalian bites and are more often deep punctures with an increased risk of infection. Factors that increase the risk of infection in bite wounds include poor local wound care, location on the hand or over a joint, puncture or crush injury, treatment delay of more than 12 hours, and patient immunosuppression.

Pathophysiology

Most wounds are colonized by mixed aerobic and anaerobic organisms obtained from the skin of the victim and the oral cavity of the biter. An average infected bite wound yields three to five organisms on culture, including aerobes and anaerobes, with the highest estimate of organisms emanating from human bites. *Pasteurella multocida* is the most common aerobic pathogen in cat bite infections; *Pasteurella canis* predominates in dog bites. Clinical infection with *Pasteurella* is characterized by rapid development of an intense inflammatory response with significant pain, erythema, and swelling within 24 to 48 hours. Other common aerobic organisms found in infected dog and cat bite wounds are *Staphylococcus* species, *Streptococcus* species, and *Corynebacterium* species. The most common anaerobes in dog and cat bite infections are *Bacteroides fragilis*, *Prevotella*, *Porphyromonas*, and *Fusobacterium* species. Approximately 50% of the wounds have at least one organism with beta-lactamase activity. The predominant aerobic organisms isolated from human bites are alpha- and beta-hemolytic streptococci, *S. aureus*, *Staphylococcus epidermidis*, and *Eikenella corrodens*. *E. corrodens* can cause severe bite wound infections. The anaerobic bacteria isolated most frequently are *Bacteroides*, *Fusobacterium*, and *Peptostreptococcus*. Human bites also can transmit hepatitis viruses B and C, herpes simplex virus, and primary syphilis.

Diagnosis

The history and examination of a bite indicate how serious the injury and potential complications are. The history begins with determining the type of offending animal, its immunization status, and whether it was provoked. Most human bites in young children are inflicted by other children and are superficial. Adolescents may sustain hand bite injuries, such as deep lacerations and avulsions, from striking another person on the teeth. Dogs have strong jaws and are capable of producing large tear and crush injuries. Cats have small, sharp teeth that can penetrate into deeper tissues, increasing the chance of infection. The mechanism of injury, whether the injury is a puncture or crush, and the lapse of time since the injury are other factors influencing treatment. Wounds more than 12 to 24 hours old are more likely to become infected. Further important questions include other specific complaints, general medical history, allergies to antibiotics, and immunization and tetanus status.

On physical examination, the location, extent, and depth of the wound should be noted carefully, and any signs of infection should be sought. Attention should be paid to nerve and tendon function and to the possibility of underlying joint penetration.

Therapy

Cleansing, copious irrigation, and careful débridement of devitalized tissue reduce the incidence of infection. Some children may require sedation for adequate care of the wound. The area around the wound should be cleansed with povidone-iodine solution, which has a wide antibacterial and antiviral spectrum. This treatment is followed by forceful irrigation with normal saline through a 19-gauge needle attached to a large syringe. This high-pressure irrigation is more effective in reducing bacterial counts than is soaking. After local anesthesia, all visible devitalized tissue is débrided, and the wound is checked for foreign matter and injuries to tendons, joints, and bones. Debridement of puncture wounds is not recommended. After debridement, irrigation is repeated. If fracture or foreign body is suspected, radiographs are obtained.

The closure of bite wounds is controversial. If a wound is uninfected and is examined within 24 hours of injury, usually it can be closed primarily. Facial wounds should be closed for cosmetic reasons. Primary closure of bite wounds does not increase the incidence of infection unless closure is more than 24 hours old or the wound is clinically infected, is a hand wound, or is a deep puncture wound. All wounds that are infected or are more than 24 hours old initially are left open. These wounds can heal by granulation or delayed primary closure.

Human and cat wounds in high-risk locations can be packed with gauze soaked in an antibacterial agent and can be sutured in 4 to 7 days in the absence of signs of infection. If the bite is small and in a cosmetically acceptable area, it is left to heal by granulation and secondary intention. Wound cultures for aerobic and anaerobic organisms should be obtained only if the wound appears infected. The face is an area of rich vascularity with decreased risk of infection. Most bites to the face are closed in a single layer to minimize scarring.

The use of prophylactic antibiotics is a complex and controversial issue for which no large prospective randomized studies have provided substantiation. Minor bite wounds, including low-risk dog bites, have a low risk of infection and generally do not require antibiotic prophylaxis. Initial cultures of wounds do not predict subsequent infection.

Prophylactic antibiotics for 3 to 5 days probably are useful for patients with wounds at high risk of infection. These wounds include bites to the hand, bites more than 12 hours old, deep puncture wounds or severe injuries, and most cat bites. For high-risk dog bites, dicloxacillin or cephalexin will cover the majority of pathogens. Amoxicillin-clavulanic acid is a good alternative, and has good coverage against *Pasteurella*. Cat bites are at high risk of infection because they are usually on the hand and are puncture wounds. The recommended antibiotics include amoxicillin-clavulanic acid or cefuroxime axetil. The same antibiotics are recommended for high-risk human bites, such as clenched fist injuries. In penicillin-allergic patients, erythromycin, azithromycin, or ciprofloxacin (in the adolescent patient) can be used. If the wound has evidence of infection, it should be cultured aerobically and anaerobically. Broad-spectrum antibiotics, such as ampicillin-sulbactam, cefoxitin, or ceftriaxone cover the most common organisms in severe infections, they and are reasonable choices before the pathogen is known. Additional therapy of infected wounds is guided by Gram stain and culture results.

After initial care, most children with bite wounds can be managed as outpatients with careful follow-up. Affected patients are asked to return within 48 hours for a check of the wound, at which time any infection should be apparent, with redness, swelling, tenderness, or drainage. Patients with high-risk wounds should be rechecked within 48 hours, and then daily for 2 to 3 days.

Larger injured areas on extremities and wounds over joints are immobilized and elevated. Tetanus toxoid is given if indicated, and rabies prophylaxis is considered, depending on the animal species and area. In the United States, the animals infected most commonly with rabies are skunks, raccoons, and bats, but other animals, including dogs and cats, may be infected. A final decision about whether to treat a potentially exposed patient can be made in conjunction with a local health department. Treatment consists of thorough local wound care (irrigation with iodine solution and débridement) and passive and active immunoprophylaxis. Human rabies immune globulin is given as soon as possible to cover the time during which the patient has insufficient active antibody production. The dose is 20 IU/kg; as much of the full dose as possible is infiltrated into the wound; the rest is given as an intramuscular injection. At the same time, active immunization is begun with one of the three available rabies vaccines; 1 mL is given intramuscularly on days 1, 3, 7, 14, and 28. If the offending animal is found to be uninfected, treatment is stopped.

Bite wounds that have a high incidence of complications and should be seen by a consultant include nonsuperficial or hand wounds older than 8 hours, wounds with extensive infections, severe disfigurement or tissue loss potentially requiring grafting, and wounds suggesting the possibility of tendon, joint, or cartilage injury. Most of these patients require hospital admission. Patients with systemic signs of infection or failure of outpatient management should be admitted for intravenous antibiotics.

WOUND CARE

The goals of wound care are to avoid infection and achieve a good cosmetic appearance. Wound care begins with a careful history of when, where, and how an injury occurred. The type of wound, the amount of contamination, and the delay until treatment determine the management. Other important history includes tetanus immunization status, allergies (especially to latex and local anesthetics), bleeding disorders, other relevant medical conditions, and medications. The initial examination includes the extent and severity of the visible lesion, where it is located, and the pulse and sensation distal to the injury. Any obvious associated injuries to nerves, muscles, tendons, vessels, or bones at the wound site or elsewhere should be sought.

Anesthesia and Sedation

In young children, especially those younger than 3 years of age, sedation may be necessary for proper examination and repair of a wound. The child can be wrapped in a sheet for restraint. A variety of available sedatives and analgesics can decrease the anxiety and discomfort associated with wound repair in young children. Sedatives, analgesics, and their doses are listed in Table 116.9.

The wound and surrounding area should be washed gently with soap and water or dilute iodine solution before the injection of local anesthetic. Buffered lidocaine (1:10 mixture of sodium bicarbonate and lidocaine) or bupivacaine (0.25% or 0.50%) is injected slowly through the wound margins with a small-gauge needle (27-gauge; see Table 116.10). Bupivacaine allows longer duration of anesthesia. If the wound is in a highly vascular area (excluding the digits, nose, ears, or genitalia), lidocaine with epinephrine can be used. Topical anesthesia with LET is an excellent alternative for head and face lacerations in children. Topical anesthetics must be kept away from the eyes and mouth. Fingers and toes are anesthetized most easily with a digital block.

Decontamination

For minimizing wound infection, the removal of contaminating bacteria, devitalized tissue, and any foreign bodies is crucial. When the wound is anesthetized, it can be irrigated using a large blunt needle and a 20- to 30-mL syringe. The volume used depends on the suspected contamination of the wound. Normal saline is an effective irrigant. A 1% povidone-iodine solution does not have any significant benefit over saline. Detergent-containing products can cause local tissue injury and should not be used for irrigation. Wounds also may be scrubbed with a soft brush to remove any gross contamination. After irrigation, any devitalized tissue must be débrided, and irregular edges should be excised.

The wound should be explored thoroughly for injuries to deep tissues and structures, for joint penetration, and for foreign bodies. Foreign bodies are more likely in wounds with a mechanism of injury suggesting foreign body, severe pain, joint tenderness, or signs of infection. Examining a wound correctly requires proper hemostasis, a cooperative or properly restrained and sedated patient, and a direct and close light source. After inspection, the wound should be probed using a blunt instrument. On doubt about the presence of a foreign body, particularly glass, metal, or gravel, appropriate radiographs should be obtained. Ultrasonography also may be used in certain circumstances. If a foreign body is found in a wound, and it is not removed easily, appropriate consultation is obtained.

Wound Repair

Most lacerations can be closed primarily with simple interrupted skin sutures using nonabsorbable suture material, such as nylon or polypropylene. An absorbable material, such as mild chromic gut, can be used for small lacerations to avoid the necessity of removing the sutures. Sutures should be placed just tightly enough to approximate and evert the edges; the ensuing wound edema after the closure may cause ischemia if the sutures are too tight.

Subcutaneous sutures with an absorbable suture material, such as Vicryl or chromic gut, are placed for a deep wound or significant tension. Extensive wounds to the face, hand, perineum, or genitals, or a wound in combination with a fracture, should be seen in consultation with a surgeon.

Wounds with high risk of infection, such as heavily contaminated wounds, animal bites, and deep punctures, should not be sutured immediately; delayed primary closure may be possible after 4 or 5 days.

A dressing is applied to absorb blood and to protect, compress, and immobilize the area. The first layer of the dressing should be nonadherent, with an absorbent material overlying it, and wrapped with a bulky immobilizing dressing. Extremities should be elevated and ice should be applied during the first 24 hours.

Topical antibiotic ointment (bacitracin or Neosporin) should be applied to the wound for 2 days after repair. Most patients do not need systemic antibiotics. Parents should receive instructions to watch for signs of infection, such as erythema, warmth, swelling, or draining, and return if any of those concerns arise. If the wound is more than 18 hours old before treatment, has high risk of infection, or already shows signs of infection, antibiotics should be prescribed for a short course. Affected patients are seen again in 24 to 48 hours to check the wound for healing and signs of infection. Sutures are removed from the face in 3 to 5 days, from the scalp in 7 days, from the extremities in 7 to 10 days, and from the joints in 10 to 14 days.

The development of tissue adhesives, cyanoacrylates, has provided an important alternative for the repair of selected lacerations. They are painless to apply, easy to use, decrease time of treatment, and do not need to be removed. Tissue adhesives are best for low-tension wounds of less than 4 to 6 cm in size. The initial strength of a wound closed with adhesive is not as strong as one closed with sutures but has equal strength within a week. They should not be used for animal bites or puncture wounds, heavily contaminated or infected wounds, wounds in areas with high skin tension (joints) or thick hair, on mucosal surfaces, or in areas with repetitive friction (hands and feet). Adhesives are most useful on face and scalp wounds.

As in wounds to be sutured, a topical anesthetic is applied, and the wound is thorough irrigated. The surface of the wound should be placed as flat as possible, to avoid running of the adhesive. If tissue adhesives are used around the eyes, ointment should be applied to the lashes and lids to prevent unintended bonding of the lashes and lids. Wound edges are approximated by hand or with Steri-strips, the wound is wiped dry, and the adhesive is applied lengthwise along the wound. Several more layers are then applied. A film forms over the wound and creates a bond, under which healing can occur. Several studies show that the final cosmetic results are as good or better than the result with suture repairs, and there is no increased risk of infection.

Staples are another alternative for wound closure, primarily on the scalp. They have low tissue reactivity, do not increase rates of infection, and need to be removed. The wound should be irrigated well before placement.

Surgical tape may be used on wounds partially through the dermis if no stress is evident on the edges; this tape is not to be used over joints or on any area in which wound edges will be pulled apart. It also can be used after suture removal to decrease wound tension.

BURNS

Burns are a common injury in children, exacting a large toll in loss of function, deformity, pain, and psychologic stress. Most children with burns are younger than 6 years of age, and the majority of these injuries are from scalds from hot liquids, or contact burns. Nonaccidental trauma should be suspected if unusual burns are present, such as cigarette or iron burns, or if the history is inconsistent with the burn noted.

Pathophysiology

Burn wounds have traditionally been classified as first, second, or third degree. This classification is being replaced by the terms superficial, superficial partial-thickness, deep partial-thickness, and full-thickness (Table 116.11).

The presence of complicating injuries, and the depth and extent of the burn, determines the level of care required. The

TABLE 116.11

ASSESSMENT OF DEPTH OF BURN

Full	Characteristic	Superficial Partial-Thickness	Superficial Thickness	Deep Partial Thickness
Example of injury	Sunburn	Scald	Grease	Immersion
Appearance	Dry, red	Moist, blisters, red	Wet or waxy, blisters, variable color	Waxy, white to leathery gray
Sensation	Painful	Painful	Perception of pressure	Perception of deep pressure

extent of the burn is expressed as a percentage of total body surface area (TBSA); the "rule of nines" is one method used to assess this (Fig. 116.2). A helpful rule for estimating the extent of scattered, irregular burns is that the surface area of the patient's palm represents approximately 1% of body surface area. Superficial burns are not included in this assessment. Children with other injuries such as smoke inhalation, TBSA burn greater than 10%, or full thickness burns greater than 5% are among those who need to be admitted or referred to a burn center for intravenous hydration and surgical care (Box 116.12).

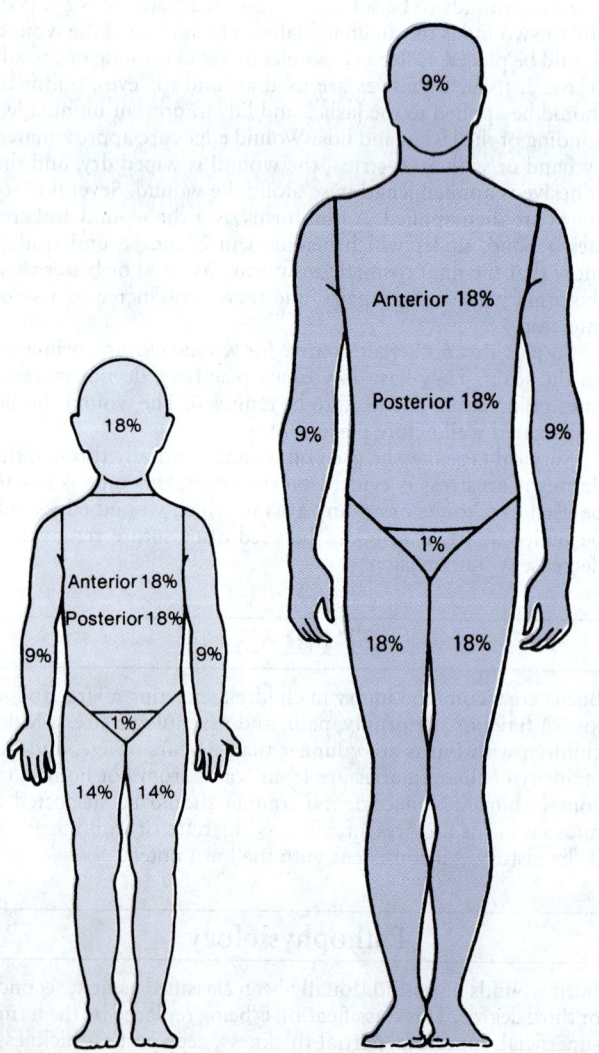

FIGURE 116.2. Rule of nines for child (left) and adult (right). (Adapted with permission from Scherer JC. *Introductory medical-surgical nursing*, 4th ed. Philadelphia: Lippincott, 1986:687.)

Therapy

A patient with burn wounds should have a full history and physical examination to assess for evidence of further injury, such as respiratory distress from smoke or chemical inhalation, unstable cardiovascular status, and other trauma related to the event.

Any cardiovascular or respiratory compromise should be evaluated and treated immediately with oxygen and supportive treatment as needed. If inhalation of smoke or gases has occurred, the likelihood of respiratory deterioration should be anticipated; upper airway edema from smoke-inhalation burns or soft tissue edema of the neck and face may compromise airway patency and breathing. The child should be intubated prophylactically if airway or pulmonary injury is suspected. Carbon monoxide poisoning should be assessed with a CO level.

Intravenous crystalloid fluids are administered to patients with moderate to severe burns, to counteract the fluid losses from increased capillary permeability. Normal saline or lactated Ringer's solution is given, at an initial rate of 4 mL/kg of body weight per 24 hours for each percent of TBSA burned. Maintenance fluids are added. Half of this fluid is given in the first 8 hours.

All burned or hot clothing should be removed immediately, and the burned area covered with cool saline-soaked dressings. Necrotic tissue and embedded pieces of clothing or debris are removed by copious irrigation with a large gauge syringe. Small bullae are left intact, but bullae greater than 2 cm should be débrided, as they are easily ruptured, and the fluid may become infected. The wound is washed with mild soap and water. Disinfectants can inhibit wound healing. The burn is dressed with silver sulfadiazine or bacitracin and a fine mesh gauze. A bulky absorbent material should be used to prevent contamination. Dressing changes are generally daily to every other day, or more frequently if the dressing becomes soaked.

Pain from a burn can be treated with acetaminophen or NSAIDs, with opioids as needed. Local anesthesia may be necessary during burn care.

If the child is discharged, careful follow-up should be arranged to watch for signs of infection or other complications.

BOX 116.12   **Criteria for Admission of Burn Victims**

More than 5% body surface area of full-thickness burn
More than 10% body surface area of partial-thickness burn
Serious burns of hands, feet, groin, face, joints
Inhalation injury
Other significant injuries or medical problems
Chemical or electrical burns
Suspected child abuse

Suggested Readings

Resuscitation

American Heart Association. Guidelines 2000 for Cardiopulmonary Resuscitation and Emergency Cardiovascular Care. *Circulation* 2000;102(Suppl I): I 253.

Luten RC, Wears RL, Broselow J, et al. Length-based endotracheal tube and emergency equipment in pediatrics. *Ann Emerg Med* 1992;21:900.

Mondolfi AA, Grenier GM, Thompson JE, et al. Comparison of self-inflating bags with anesthesia bags for bag-mask ventilation in the pediatric emergency department. *Pediatr Emerg Care* 1997;13:312.

Young KD, Seidel JS. Pediatric Cardiopulmonary resuscitation: a collective review. *Ann Emerg Med* 1999;33:195.

Zaritsky AL, Nadkarni VM, Hickey RW, et al, eds. PALS Provider Manual. American Heart Association, 2002.

Parental Presence during Resuscitation

Bauchner H, Vinci R, Bak S, et al. Parents and procedures: a randomized controlled trial. *Pediatrics* 1996;98:861.

Boie ET, Moore GP. Brummett C, et al. Do Parents want to be present during invasive procedures performed on their children in the emergency department? A survey of 400 parents. *Ann Emerg Med* 1999;34:70.

Sacchetti A, Lichenstein R, Carraccio CA, et al. Family member presence during pediatric emergency department procedures. *Pediatr Emerg Care* 1996; 12:268.

Croup

Johnson DW, Jacobson S, Edney PC, et al. A comparison of nebulized budesonide, intramuscular dexamethasone, and placebo for moderately severe croup. *N Engl J Med* 1998;339:498.

Luria JW, Gonzalez-del-Rey JA, DiGiulio GA, et al. Effectiveness of oral or nebulized dexamethasone for children with mild croup. *Arch Pediatr Adolesc Med* 2001;155:1340.

Rittichier KK, Ledwith CA. Outpatient treatment of moderate croup with dexamethasone: intramuscular versus oral dosing. *Pediatrics* 2000;106:1344.

Waisman Y, Klein BL, Boenning DA, et al. Prospective randomized double-blind study comparing L-epinephrine and racemic epinephrine aerosols in the treatment of laryngotracheitis. *Pediatrics* 1992;89:302.

Weber JE, Chudnofsky CR, Younger JG, et al. Abstract. A randomized comparison of helium-oxygen mixture (Heliox) and racemic epinephrine for the treatment of moderate to severe croup. *Pediatrics* 2001:107(6).

Foreign Body Aspiration

Baharloo F, Veyckemans F, Francis C, et al. Tracheobronchial foreign bodies. Presentation and management in children and adults. *Chest* 1999;115:1357.

Epiglottitis

Garpenholt O, Hugosson S, Fredlund H, et al. Epiglottitis in Sweden before and after introduction of vaccination against *Haemophilus influenza* type b. *Pediatr Infect Dis J* 1999;18:490.

McCollough M. Progress toward eliminating *Haemophilus influenza* type b among infants and children. *Ann Emerg Med* 1999;34:110.

Valdepena HG, Wald ER, Rose E, et al. Epiglottitis and *Haemophilus influenzae* immunization: the Pittsburgh experience—a five-year review. *Pediatrics* 1995;96:424.

Abscesses

Ahmed K, Jones AS, Shah K, et al. The role of ultrasound in the management of peritonsillar abscess. *J Laryngol Otol* 1994;108:610.

Lee SS, Schwartz RH, Babadori RS. Retropharyngeal abscess: epiglottitis of the new millennium. *J Pediatr* 2001;138:435.

Stever TE. Peritonsillar abscess: diagnosis and treatment. *Am Fam Physician* 2002;65:93.

Asthma

Anderson AB, Zwerdling RG, Dewitt TG. The clinical utility of pulse oximetry in the pediatric emergency department setting. *Pediatr Emerg Care* 1991;7:263.

Barnett PLJ, Caputo GL, Baskin M, et al. Intravenous versus oral corticosteroids in the management of acute asthma in children. *Ann Emerg Med* 1997;29:212.

Ciarallo L, Brousseau D, Reinert S. Higher-dose intravenous magnesium therapy for children with moderate to severe acute asthma. *Arch Pediatr Adolesc Med* 2000;154:979.

Fuglsang G, Pederson S, Borgstrom L. Dose-response relationships of intravenously administered terbutaline in children with asthma. *J Pediatr* 1989;114:315.

Khinett H, Fuchs SM, Saville AL. Continuous vs. intermittent nebulized albuterol for emergency department management of asthma. *Acad Emerg Med* 1996;3:1019.

Milgrom H, Skoner D, Bensch G, et al. Low-dose levalbuterol in children with asthma: safety and efficacy in comparison with placebo and racemic albuterol. *J Allerg Clin Immunol* 2001;108:938.

Qureshi F, Zaritsky A, Lakkis H. Efficacy of nebulized ipratropium in severely asthmatic children. *Ann Emerg Med* 1997;29:205.

Qureshi F, Zaritsky A, Poirier MP. Comparative efficacy of oral dexamethasone versus oral prednisone in acute pediatric asthma. *J Pediatr* 2001;139:20.

Schuh S, Johnson D, Stephens D, et al. Comparison of albuterol delivered by a metered dose inhaler with spacer versus a nebulizer in children with mild acute asthma. *J Peds* 1999;135:22.

Bronchiolitis

Antonow JA, Hansen K, McKinstry CA, et al. Sepsis evaluations in hospitalized infants with bronchiolitis. *Pediatr Infect Dis J* 1998;17:231.

Flores G, Horwitz R. Efficacy of beta₂-agonists in bronchiolitis: a reappraisal and meta-analysis. *Pediatrics* 1997;100:233.

Garrison MM, Christakis DA, Harvey E, et al. Systemic corticosteroids in infant bronchiolitis: a meta-analysis. *Pediatrics* 2000;105:E44.

Kellner JD, Ohlsson A, Gadomski AM, et al. Efficacy of bronchodilator therapy in bronchiolitis: a meta-analysis. *Arch Pediatr Adolesc Med* 1996;150:1166.

Kupperman N, Bank DE, Walton EA, et al. Risks for bacteremia and urinary tract infections in young febrile children with bronchiolitis. *Arch Pediatr Adolesc Med* 1997;151:1207.

Menon K, Sutcliffe T, Klassen T. Clinical and laboratory observations: a randomized trial comparing the efficacy of epinephrine with salbutamol in the treatment of acute bronchiolitis. *J Pediatr* 1995;126:1004.

Schuh S, Coates AL, Binnie R, et al. Efficacy of oral dexamethasone in outpatients with acute bronchiolitis. *J Pediatr* 2002;140:27.

Anaphylaxis

Dibs SD, Baker MD. Anaphylaxis in children: a 5-year experience. *Pediatrics* 1997;99;e1.

Lee JM, Greenes DS. Biphasic anaphylactic reactions in *pediatrics*. *Pediatrics* 2000;106:762.

Reisman RE. Insect stings. *N Engl J Med* 1994;331:523.

Fever

Bachur RG, Harper MB. Predictive model for serious bacterial infections among infants younger than 3 months of age. *Pediatrics* 2001;108:311.

Baker MD, Bell LM, Avner JR. The efficacy of routine outpatient management without antibiotics of fever in selected infants. *Pediatrics* 1999;103:627.

Baraff LJ. Management of fever without source in infants and children. *Ann Emerg Med* 2000;36:602.

Herzog LW, Coyne LJ. What is fever? Normal temperature in infants less than 3 months old. *Clin Pediatr* 1993;32:142.

Seizures

Sharma S, Riviello JJ, Harper MB, et al. The role of emergent neuroimaging in children with new-onset afebrile seizures. *Pediatrics* 2003;111:1.

Gold CR, Pierog J. A rational approach to pediatric seizures. *Pediatr Emerg Med Rep* 2000;5:121.

Chest Pain

Kocis KC. Chest pain in pediatrics. *Pediatr Clin North Am* 1999;46(2):189.

Selbst SM, Ruddy R, Clark BJ. Chest pain in children. Follow-up of patients previously reported. *Clin Pediatr* 1990;29:374.

Pain and Sedation

American Academy of Pediatrics. Guidelines for monitoring and management of pediatric patients during and after sedation for diagnostic and therapeutic procedures: addendum. *Pediatrics* 2002;110:836.

Bishop-Kurylo D. Pediatric pain management in the emergency department. *Top Emerg Med* 2002;24(1):19.

Dachs RJ, Innes GM. Intravenous ketamine sedation of pediatric patients in the emergency department. *Ann Emerg Med* 1997;29:146.

Ho K, Spence J, Murphy MF. Review of Pain-measurement tools. *Ann Emerg Med* 1996;27:427.

Koren G. Use of eutectic mixture of local anesthetics in young children for procedure-related pain. *J Pediatr* 1993;122:S30.

Krauss B. Management of acute pain and anxiety in children undergoing procedures in the emergency department. *Pediatr Emerg Care* 2001;17:115.

Ljungman G, Kreuger A, Andreasson S. Midazolam nasal spray reduces procedural anxiety in children. *Pediatrics* 2000;105:73.

Resch K, Schilling C, Borchert B, et al. Topical anesthesia for pediatric lacerations: a randomized trial of lidocaine-epinephrine-tetracaine solution versus gel. *Ann Emerg Med* 1998;32:693.

Seikel K, Smith K. The safety and efficacy of propofol for procedures and imaging in the pediatric emergency department. *Pediatrics* 1999;104(S):691.

Vardi A, Salem Y, Padeh S, et al. Is propofol safe for procedural sedation in children? A prospective evaluation of propofol versus ketamine in pediatric critical care. *Crit Care Med* 2002;30:1231.

Bites

Cummings P. Antibiotics to prevent infection in patients with dog bite wounds: a meta-analysis of randomized trials. *Ann Emerg Med* 1994;23:535.

Fleisher GR. The management of bite wounds. *N Engl J Med* 1999;340:138.

Smith PF, Meadowcroft AM, May DB. Treating mammalian bite wounds. *J Clin Pharm Therap* 2000;25:85.

Wounds

Cumming P, Del Beccaro MA. Antibiotics to prevent infection of simple wounds: a meta-analysis of randomized trials. *Am J Emerg Med* 1995;13:396.

Hollander JE, Singer AJ. Laceration management. *Ann Emerg Med* 1999;34:356.

Khan A, Dayan PS, Miller S, et al. Cosmetic outcome of scalp wound closure with staples in the pediatric emergency department: a prospective, randomized trial. *Pediatr Emerg Care* 2002;18:171.

Quinn J, Wells G, Sutcliffe TJ, et al. tissue adhesive versus suture wound repair at 1 year: randomized clinical trial correlating early, 3-month, and 1-year cosmetic outcome. *Ann Emerg Med* 1998;32:645.

Trott AT. Cyanoacrylate tissue adhesives. *JAMA* 1997;277:1559.

Burns

Clayton MC, Solem LD. No ice, no butter. Advice on management of burns for primary care physicians. *Postgrad Med* 1995;97:151.

Mlcak R, Cortiella J, Desai MH, et al. Emergency management of pediatric burn victims. *Pediatr Emerg Care* 1998;14:51.

Monafo WW. Initial management of burns. *N Engl J Med* 1996;335:1581.

Peate WF. Outpatient management of burns. *Am Fam Physician* 1992;45:1321.

CHAPTER 117A ■ APPARENT LIFE-THREATENING EVENTS

GERALD M. LOUGHLIN AND JOHN L. CARROLL

An apparent life-threatening event (ALTE) describes a complex of observations and events that are perceived by the child's caregiver to be life-threatening (Table 117A.1). In 1986, a National Institutes of Health (NIH) Consensus Conference defined ALTE as "an episode that is frightening to the observer and that is characterized by some combination of apnea (central or occasionally obstructive), color change (usually cyanotic or pallid, but occasionally erythematous or plethoric), marked change in muscle tone (usually marked limpness), choking, or gagging." In some cases, the observer fears that the infant has died."

Older descriptive terms for this condition [aborted sudden infant death syndrome (SIDS), near-miss SIDS] are a source of confusion and should not be used; the persistence of such terms reflects a misunderstanding of the epidemiology and prognostic implications of an ALTE. Two observations serve to illustrate

this point. Because an ALTE must, by definition, be observed, any cause of death that was truly quiet, such as a sudden cardiac arrhythmia, would be less likely to appear as an ALTE and more likely to result in quiet unexpected death. Likewise, because observation is required, an ALTE is most likely to be observed and reported when the parent or caretaker is awake, which biases the reporting of events to times when the parent is more likely to be awake. Because it is impossible to ascertain whether an episode was actually life-threatening, the incidence of ALTE is unknown or, at best, crudely estimated. In New Zealand, the average annual hospital admission rate for ALTE was reported to be 9.4 in 1,000 live births, which probably underestimates the incidence, because it excludes milder cases not admitted to the hospital.

Whatever the cause, the pediatrician faced with one of these infants is presented with a frustrating management problem. Despite the absence of definitive information on the etiology and exact nature of the event, evaluation and therapeutic decisions must be made. This chapter focuses on how these children should be evaluated and treated.

TABLE 117A.1

HISTORY OF INFANTS WITH UNEXPLAINED APPARENT LIFE-THREATENING EVENTS

Symptom	Percent of Infants
Apnea	82
Pallor	70
Limpness	60
Cyanosis	48
Pallor and limpness	47
"Lifelessness"	41
Coldness	16
Not clear if breathing	14
Stiffness	11
Staring/rolling eyes	10
Shallow breathing	4

Modified from Dunne KP, Matthew TG. Near-miss sudden infant death syndrome: clinical findings and management. *Pediatrics* 1987;79:889.

ETIOLOGY

ALTE is not a diagnosis. The term merely describes a common manner of presentation for many different disorders (Table 117A.2). In most studies of ALTE, a possible or likely cause of the event is discovered in approximately half of cases. The occurrence of an ALTE often reflects developmental immaturity in cardiorespiratory responses; these infants appear to experience an exaggerated response to commonly occurring stressors in an infant's life. However, ALTE also may represent signs of sepsis, meningitis, poisoning, and other potentially life-threatening conditions. Thus, anything that can cause the appearance described in the NIH's definition may be an underlying cause of ALTE.

Previously, an ALTE with no definable etiology was termed *apnea of infancy*. We find this term confusing, and prefer the designation *ALTE of unknown etiology*. In both term and

TABLE 117A.2

SOME CAUSES OF APPARENT LIFE-THREATENING EVENTS

Cardiac
Congestive heart failure
Arrhythmia

Respiratory
Infection, pneumonia, respiratory syncytial virus
Respiratory failure

Sepsis

Gastrointestinal
Gastroesophageal reflux
Dysfunctional swallowing

Central nervous system
Seizures
Brainstem neoplasm or compression
Infection
Central hypoventilation syndromes

Metabolic disorders
Hypoglycemia
Medium-chain acyl-CoA dehydrogenase deficiency

Prematurity
Apnea of prematurity
Anemia

Child abuse

Poisoning

preterm infants, approximately 90% of unexplained ALTEs occur before the infant is 16 weeks old. Although apnea may be one component of an ALTE, central apnea is a normal finding at all ages; not all episodes of apnea, even if abnormal, are life-threatening; and not all ALTEs involve apnea. The role of apnea in the pathophysiology of ALTE is further complicated because some apnea is a component of the normal variability of breathing in nearly all infants. The absence of airflow, termed apnea, may be the result of absence of respiratory effort (central), obstruction of the airway (obstructive), or a combination of both mechanisms (mixed). Occasional short central apnea, typically of less than 20 seconds and usually preceded by a sigh, may be a normal finding at any age. When it is prolonged longer than 20 to 25 seconds, or is accompanied by bradycardia, cardiac arrhythmia, pallor, hypotonia, or cyanosis, it is termed *pathologic apnea* and warrants further investigation. *Periodic breathing*, recognized as alternating periods of apnea and regular breathing, is defined as three or more breathing pauses of more than 3 seconds' duration, with less than 20 seconds of breathing between pauses. Short-duration episodes of periodic breathing occur normally during infancy. Central apnea events (of less than 20 seconds) often are misinterpreted by anxious parents as being dangerous, thus adding to the dilemma. Physicians caring for infants with an ALTE must be aware that variability in respiratory pattern, and even short central apnea, is common in otherwise perfectly healthy infants.

APPROACH TO THE INFANT AFTER AN APPARENT LIFE-THREATENING EVENT

Our lack of understanding of the pathogenesis of SIDS, coupled with our inability to predict who is at risk for a sudden unexplained death, places the physician responsible for infants who experience an ALTE in a difficult position. Unfortunately, the limitations of our knowledge have resulted in confusion and controversy surrounding the management of infants who are perceived as being at risk of sudden death. This discussion focuses on a practical approach to the diagnosis and management of infants with ALTE, based on available data. As new information is added and clinical experience expands, these recommendations will undoubtedly change.

Although the European Society for the Study and Prevention of Infant Death (ESPID) published recommendations for evaluation of infants with ALTE in 2004 (see Suggested Readings), no comprehensive official guidelines exist for the evaluation and management of ALTE in the United States. General guidelines from U.S. sources may be pieced together from general statements in Consensus Conference Statement from the 1986 NIH Consensus Conference on Infantile Apnea and Home Monitoring and the 2003 Policy Statement from the American Academy of Pediatrics on Apnea, Sudden Infant Death Syndrome, and Home Monitoring (see Suggested Readings).

The first steps in evaluating these patients should focus both on ruling out treatable causes of life-threatening events and on determining if a life-threatening or dangerous event actually occurred. In many instances, parents have witnessed a normal physiologic variation that appears to be life-threatening to the inexperienced layperson. Normal infants can experience respiratory pauses lasting for up to 20 seconds during sleep. Many of these are not associated with color change or desaturation, and frequently they are preceded by a sigh. To a parent waiting for a baby to start breathing again, however, even 10 seconds can seem like an eternity. Thus, this infant may be brought to medical attention in an urgent fashion and labeled as abnormal. The physician is confronted by an anxious parent or caretaker who believes that he has witnessed an event that has endangered the child's life. Somehow, the physician caring for this child must identify the infant at true risk.

A detailed history of the event is essential. Table 117A.3 summarizes the important features of this history. A description of the circumstances preceding the event is key. Was the patient awake or asleep? Events that occur when the child is awake are often found to be secondary to gastroesophageal reflux or a seizure. Was the event associated with body movements or unusual posturing? Again, this suggests a seizure disorder or gastroesophageal reflux. Was the child struggling to breathe (suggestive of airway obstruction), or were respiratory efforts absent?

An accurate description of the intervention required to reestablish normal breathing is important, because the need for vigorous resuscitation appears to correlate with increased risk of recurrent severe spells and even death. Recovery spontaneously or with minimal intervention (i.e., touching the infant) is reassuring and may suggest that what was witnessed was most likely a normal physiologic event. Information about the time required to reverse the event and the infant's mental and physical status after the event also is important in planning subsequent evaluation and therapy.

Was the infant premature? Was the delivery difficult? Was respiration initiated in normal fashion at birth? Was there evidence of prior respiratory difficulties? Has the child's growth and development been appropriate? These questions help to establish a predisposition to abnormalities in control of respiration and also help to identify a chronic condition.

A history of how the infant handles feeding is important. Dysfunctional swallowing is more common in preterm infants and can trigger reflex apnea and bradycardia by direct aspiration, stimulation of laryngeal chemoreceptors, or by reflux of formula into the nasopharynx. Apnea may be central or obstructive, and often occurs during feeding in preterm infants. However, if reflux occurs, apnea may occur at varying intervals after feeding.

TABLE 117A.3

APPARENT LIFE-THREATENING EVENTS DIAGNOSTIC EVALUATION

History
Detailed description of the event from all observers: was the infant asleep or awake; position infant found in; duration of event; action required to terminate event; association with feeding, choking, formula in nose, body movement; infant's state after event
Perinatal history: labor and delivery, neonatal respiratory problems
Review of systems: Infection, feeding, weight gain, vomitting, diarrhea, diet

Physical examination
Vital signs
General appearance, growth parameters
HEENT (head, ears, eyes, nose, mouth, and throat)
Neck: masses, rigidity
Chest: respiratory rate, respiratory noises, signs of upper airway obstruction
Cardiac: rate, rhythm, murmurs
Abdomen
Neurologic examination: developmental milestone, tone, reflexes, strength, sensorium, affect
Feeding and sleep patterns

Laboratory screening at the time of first medical contact
Hemoglobin and hematocrit
Acid–base status
Blood glucose, if not fed for several hours
Electrocardiogram to check for prolonged QT interval

Is there a family history of sudden unexplained death in other siblings or relatives? Multiple deaths in a family should make one suspicious about the potential for child abuse or an inherited metabolic disorder. Is there a family history of snoring or obstructive sleep apnea? This information suggests a possible familial predisposition to respiratory control disorders. Table 117A.3 highlights the essential components of the physical examination. An assessment of growth and development, along with a focus on cardiac, neurologic, and respiratory systems, is necessary to identify the subtle signs of chronic conditions that may predispose to life-threatening events. Similarly, evidence of an acute infection (sepsis, central nervous system, respiratory) should be sought so that appropriate therapy can be initiated.

Laboratory Studies

A comprehensive laboratory evaluation should be reserved for those infants whose history and physical examination suggest that a significant event took place. This can be a challenge, because the observer's report often does not help the physician to make these decisions. When the infant is brought to medical attention, a measure of acid–base status and either an arterial blood gas or a measurement of serum bicarbonate and a measurement of blood glucose (if the child has not eaten in several hours), should be obtained as soon as possible. Obviously, the longer the interval between the event and obtaining the sample lessens the value of the data, but it is still worth doing. A serum bicarbonate level is a particularly useful test. A low value suggests that the event may have been severe enough to result in a metabolic acidosis, or may suggest the presence of an underlying metabolic disorder. On the other hand, an elevation of serum bicarbonate is consistent with chronic compensation for

TABLE 117A.4

OTHER STUDIES POSSIBLY INDICATED IN CHILDREN WITH APPARENT LIFE-THREATENING EVENTS

Study	Possible Diagnosis
Chest radiography	Pneumonia, bronchiolitis, screen for cardiac disease
Barium swallow	Dysfunctional swallowing, gastroesophageal reflux, upper airway obstruction
Electroencephalography	Seizure disorder
Electrocardiography and echocardiography	Rule out cardiac disease or cor pulmonale
pH probe	Suspicion of gastroesophageal reflux
Documented cardiorespiratory monitoring	Unusual apnea, recurrent events or alarms, concerns about compliance, suspected child abuse
Polysomnography	Unusual apnea, need to assess oxygenation and ventilation, rule out obstructive apnea

respiratory acidosis. Hypoglycemia may indicate an underlying metabolic disorder, such as medium-chain acyl-CoA dehydrogenase deficiency as the cause of the ALTE. A complete blood count with differential, looking for anemia, polycythemia, and signs of acute infection, also should be a part of this initial screening approach. An elevated hematocrit suggests underlying chronic hypoxemia. On the other hand, low hematocrit values have been associated with apnea in the preterm infant. The white blood cell count is a window on infection. Long QTc syndromes and other rhythm disturbances may be detected by electrocardiogram.

Based on results of the initial screening tests, the history and physical examination, or subsequent observations, other studies may be indicated (Table 117A.4). These tests are not necessary for all infants with ALTEs, however, because their yield without specific indications is generally low. For example, events temporarily related to feedings or associated with choking and obstructive breathing, particularly when the infant is awake, require a study of both swallowing and esophageal function. Apnea with feeding is best evaluated with a videofluorographic swallowing study (VFSS) using barium of various consistencies. Esophageal pH monitoring to document abnormal gastroesophageal reflux, or an association between a reflux episode and clinical symptoms, may be helpful in defining a potential relationship. If an initial workup result is negative, and the infant is stable, additional testing can be deferred pending the child's subsequent clinical course.

Assessment of Cardiorespiratory Patterns

Stimulated by the hypothesis that some aberration of cardiorespiratory control is involved in a significant number of ALTEs, attempts have been made to record heart rate and respiratory rate over extended periods in these infants, to identify underlying abnormalities in cardiorespiratory control that may identify a cause or predict recurrences.

Pneumography

Previously, cardiac rate and rhythms, as well as respiratory movements, were monitored by transthoracic impedance, and the data from 24 hours was recorded on a hard copy for review (a pneumogram). It was hoped that these data could identify infants who were at risk for repeat ALTEs. Many centers still obtain pneumograms before, during, and at the completion of monitoring. However, clinical experience has demonstrated that these studies have no predictive value with respect to starting, continuing, or stopping home monitoring.

Cardiorespiratory monitors with data storage capabilities (commonly termed "documented monitoring") have been the standard of care since the late 1990s. The monitors are programmed to record electrocardiogram (EKG) information, respiratory pattern, and heart rate when triggered by apnea or bradycardia. The data can be downloaded and later reviewed to determine whether cardiorespiratory events were real ("true") or artifactual ("false") alarms. At present, pneumograms should not be considered a routine part of the evaluation of an ALTE, and they are not required either to initiate or discontinue home monitoring. Both these decisions can be made on clinical grounds alone, and documented monitoring has replaced the traditional 24-hour pneumogram. The advantages of documented monitoring are that it records all the events that trigger alarms, provides invaluable data on compliance with use of the monitor, and provides a longer window of recorded monitoring than the standard pneumogram. Monitoring is minimally invasive and can be performed at home, without disrupting the infant's routine or introducing extraneous stimuli.

Unfortunately, limitations to documented cardiorespiratory monitoring also exist. It does not predict the risk for SIDS or recurrent ALTE. Obstructive apnea cannot be identified. No behavioral information is provided other than a parental diary. The sleep state either must be assessed from the diary provided by the parents or inferred from heart and respiratory patterns. The impedance monitoring can detect prolonged central apnea and bradycardia, but it cannot provide data on the physiologic significance of less dramatic events, such as periodic breathing or brief apneas. In spite of these limitations, documented monitoring may be quite helpful and has been found to be useful in situations in which parents report recurrent alarms. Extended home recording may provide both extremely useful information about the nature of the recurrent alarms and corroboration of the parents' reports. The American Academy of Pediatrics recently published new guidelines for the use of home cardiorespiratory monitoring (see Table 117A.6).

Polysomnography

Alternatively, cardiorespiratory patterns can be studied using standard nocturnal polysomnography in a sleep laboratory. Table 117A.5 presents the variables typically recorded. These studies are generally performed overnight, in a dedicated sleep laboratory, but also have been obtained in young infants during daytime naps. Some concern has been expressed that nap studies may miss abnormal events that occur only at night; thus, clinical decision making based on a normal nap study should be approached with caution.

Polysomnography provides extensive physiologic information. Not only can obstructive apnea be identified, but the physiologic consequences of events such as periodic breathing, hypopnea, and short apnea spells can be identified, because oxygenation and end-tidal CO_2 are monitored. Significant gas exchange abnormalities can occur in some infants during episodes of periodic breathing or short apneas (Fig. 117A.1). Neither the duration nor the frequency of these short central apneas would distinguish these infants from those who

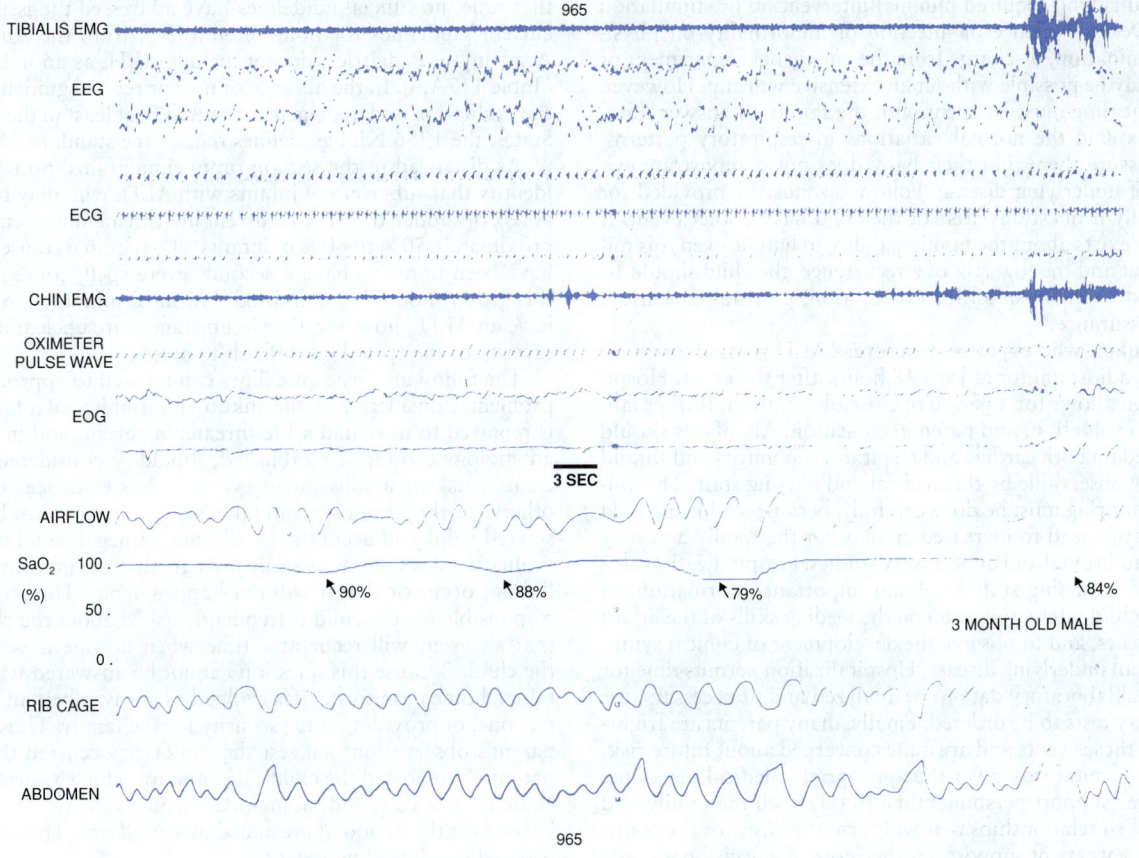

FIGURE 117A.1. A polysomnography tracing from a 3-month-old infant with a history of recurrent spells (see Table 117A.5 for a description of the parameters measured). Note the dramatic decreases in oxygen saturation associated with brief (3-second) apnea.

experience no change in oxygenation. Polysomnography also provides important information on the relationship between breathing patterns and sleep states. Because a technician is present and the study is frequently videotaped, behavioral events can be correlated with physiologic recordings. This is especially useful if seizures are considered as a cause of the apnea. In addition, if gastroesophageal reflux is a concern, esophageal pH levels also can be monitored and the physiologic consequences of a reflux episode recorded. The limitations of polysomnography include more disruption to usual routines, studies performed in strange surroundings, and many more wires attached to the infant than in the home setting. These studies also are more expensive. Unfortunately, as with pneumograms, polysomnography has not been shown to be predictive of subsequent risk for SIDS or ALTE. However, only a few studies have used polysomnography in a large number of infants with ALTE. Obstructive and central apneas have been identified in some infants thought to be at risk for SIDS. These obstructive spells would not have been detected by pneumograms.

In summary, studies of cardiorespiratory patterns cannot be used to predict subsequent risk for death from SIDS. However, if used judiciously, these studies can provide important diagnostic information useful in the management of selected infants who have severe or recurrent ALTE or recurrent alarms while on home monitoring. They also can provide important physiologic data on events that may appear benign in terms of duration.

THERAPY

For infants who required minimal intervention or stimulation and have no evidence of infection or abnormality on physical examination, discharge from the emergency department or clinic may be possible without an extensive workup. However, sufficient time must be spent with the family to answer questions, explain the normal variations in respiratory patterns, and reassure them that their baby does not demonstrate evidence of underlying disease. Follow-up must be provided for the family if questions arise or the child has another event. If concern exists about the family's ability to handle even this minor event and the low risk of a recurrence, the child should be admitted to the hospital for observation, parental education, and reassurance.

An infant who experiences a severe ALTE should be monitored in a hospital for at least 48 hours after the event. Hospitalization allows for a period of close observation, further laboratory evaluation, and parental education. All infants should be placed on both cardiac and respiratory monitors and should be easily observable by the medical and nursing staff. This initial monitoring must be done carefully, because undocumented false alarms lead to increased anxiety for the family and may lead to additional and unnecessary studies. Hospitalization also allows the nursing staff to obtain important information on parent–child interactions and on the feeding skills of the infant and parents, and to observe the development of clinical symptoms of an underlying disease. Hospitalization permits time for the initial laboratory data to be analyzed and, if necessary, for secondary tests to be ordered. Finally, many parents are frightened by these events and are quite concerned about future risk. A brief hospital stay gives the appropriate medical personnel and other support personnel time to talk with the family and to establish relationships that will form the basis for the continuity of outpatient support. Furthermore, if a decision is made to initiate cardiorespiratory monitoring, enough time will be available to train the family in the use of the monitor and in infant CPR.

TABLE 117A.5

PARAMETERS MONITORED IN POLYSOMNOGRAPHY IN CHILDREN

Parameters	Description
Electroencephalography	Stage sleep, identify seizure activity
Electrooculography	Records extraocular movements for staging sleep
Electromyography	Sleep stage, records muscle tone and movements
Electrocardiography	Cardiac rate and rhythms
Inductive plythesmography	Respiratory movements, impedance
Magnetometers	Respiratory movements, impedance
Nasal/oral thermistors	Air flow
End-tidal CO_2	Ventilation
Pulse oximetry	Oxygenation
Videotaping	Records noises, sleep behaviors, and activity

Home Monitoring

Although technically not a treatment, home cardiorespiratory monitoring has emerged as the most widely used approach to the problem of ALTEs. The use of monitoring following ALTE was recommended by the 1986 NIH Consensus Development Conference on Infantile Apnea and Home Monitoring. Since that time, no official guidelines have addressed the issue, and current guidelines for home monitoring, from the American Academy of Pediatrics, do not include ALTE as an indication (Table 117A.6). In the absence of new or revised guidelines for the evaluation and management of ALTE, at least in the United States, the 1986 NIH guidelines remain the standard of care.

As discussed in the section on pneumograms, no tests can identify that subgroup of infants with ALTE who may be truly at risk of sudden death or recurrent life-threatening events. Approximately 50% to 60% of infants who required resuscitation have been noted to have a second severe spell; consequently, this group should be monitored. For most infants reported to have an ALTE, however, the circumstances are unclear and the severity of the episode is difficult to assess.

The following basic guidelines can be used to approach the problem. Considering all the unknown variables, an infant who is reported to have had a life-threatening event, and in whom an etiology cannot be established, should be considered at increased risk of a subsequent event. Unless evidence suggests otherwise, the parent's or caretaker's observations must be considered valid and accurate. In addition, a negative laboratory evaluation does not necessarily indicate that a significant event did not occur or that it will not happen again. The physician responsible for the child is frequently asked about the chances that an event will recur at a time when no one is watching the child. Because this question cannot be answered with certainty, home monitoring has evolved as a way, albeit an imperfect one, of providing some security for the family. Thus, if the parent's observations suggest that an event occurred that apparently threatened the child's life, and for which a correctable cause cannot be found, home-documented monitoring should be used for the period of presumed increased risk. This decision is based on *clinical judgment*.

Instituting home monitoring is a medical recommendation with advantages and disadvantages that must be discussed in detail with the family. Home monitoring should be instituted

TABLE 117A.6

CURRENT RECOMMENDATIONS FOR HOME CARDIORESPIRATORY MONITORING*

1. Home cardiorespiratory monitoring should not be prescribed to prevent SIDS.
2. Home cardiorespiratory monitoring may be warrented for premature infants who are at high risk of recurrent episodes of apnea, bradycardia, and hypoxemia after hospital discharge. The use of home cardiorespiratory monitoring in this population should be limited to approximately 43 weeks' postmenstrual age or after the cessation of extreme episodes, whichever comes last.
3. Home cardiorespiratory monitoring may be warrented for infants who are technology dependent (tracheostomy, continuous positive airway pressure), have unstable airways, have rare medical conditions affecting regulation of breathing, or have symptomatic chronic lung disease.
4. If home cardiorespiratory monitoring is prescribed, the monitor should be equipped with an event recorder.
5. Parents should be advised that home cardiorespiratory monitoring has not been proven to prevent sudden unexpected deaths in infants.
6. Pediatricians should continue to promote proven practices that decrease the risk of SIDS—supine sleep position, safe sleeping enviroments, and elimination of prenatal and postnatal exposure to tobacco smoke.

*From: Committee on Fetus and Newborn. American Academy of Pediatrics Policy Statement: Apnea, Sudden Infant Death Syndrome, and Home Monitoring. Pediatrics Vol. 111 No. 4 April 2003.

TABLE 117A.7

CHARACTERISTICS OF AN ACCEPTABLE HOME CARDIORESPIRATORY MONITOR

- Ability to detect central apnea
- Ability to detect bradycardia and tachycardia
- Ability to record waveforms for chest-wall motion and EKG when triggered
- Ability to identify what type of event triggered the alarm
- Ability to minimize motion and other types of artifact
- Ability to record and display times of usage so that adherence can be assessed
- Simplicity of operation
- Safety of leads/wires
- Portability
- Battery backup
- Ability to detect unauthorized changes in settings

only after a careful assessment of the home environment, including the skills and abilities of those responsible for the infant. The individuals responsible for the infant must be instructed in the use of the monitor and in infant CPR. The family should be prepared to recognize and deal with subsequent spells, including making provisions for contacting emergency services.

Follow-up for the infant and access to support systems are essential to the success of any home monitoring program. These infants should be referred to centers with resources dedicated to the management of infants on home monitoring. These centers, in conjunction with primary-care physicians, can provide the appropriate level of support for these families. Contact with the family should be frequent initially, and then can be tapered as the family settles into the routine.

Home monitoring is not without problems. False alarms are a significant nuisance. Despite attempts on the part of manufacturers to minimize them, they are still an unavoidable problem. Monitoring systems must be sensitive to disturbances in normal cardiorespiratory patterns. As a result, shallow breathing episodes, which are a regular occurrence during deep sleep, are frequently interpreted by the monitor as apnea, and alarms are triggered. The monitor cannot distinguish between these events and pathologic events; thus, the monitor software should be programmed to alarm in all ambiguous situations. In addition, heart-rate norms are not clearly established and, as the infant matures, isolated bradycardia alarms may increase in frequency. After the alarm, parents usually find the infant sound asleep and breathing normally. Readjusting the low–heart-rate alarm often alleviates this problem, but these spells must be distinguished from bradycardia associated with obstructive apnea or hypoxemia. The characteristics required for a basic monitor for home use are summarized in Table 117A.7. Many monitors in use today have these characteristics, but none of the commercially available home monitors can detect obstructive apnea. State-of-the-art monitors should be able to recognize

central pauses of varied duration as well as bradycardia and tachycardia. The monitor also should be able to tell when the monitor is not working or when a lead is loose. Because parents are asked to provide information about what triggered alarms, the monitor should indicate what initiated the alarm.

The home monitor should not require an engineering degree to be used safely. It should have a simple operating manual, and the supplier must be able to provide troubleshooting services and personal instruction in the use of the monitor. Infants at risk for life-threatening events frequently must be monitored in settings other than the home. Events have been reported in car seats, for example, and therefore the monitor must be portable and operate from a reliable battery source.

Safety is an additional factor. Reports of infants who have been electrocuted because a monitor lead was inadvertently plugged into an AC outlet by a sibling and of infants who have become entangled in monitor wires demonstrate the need to minimize these electrical and mechanical hazards. Active and inquisitive siblings pose a particular problem. Monitors can be turned off and alarm settings changed by curious siblings, so the monitor alarm should sound if the power is turned off or the settings are changed inadvertently. Many monitors have been "child-proofed," by requiring that any change must occur in a certain sequence or while a second button is depressed, essentially preventing the average inquisitive toddler from making unauthorized and unrecognized changes in the monitoring status.

The expertise and reliability of the home care company that supplies the monitor are as important as the equipment itself. No real controls or standards exist for the companies that supply and service home cardiorespiratory monitors. The physician prescribing the machine must monitor the supplier to ensure the quality of the equipment delivered and the adequacy of training and company responsiveness to families' requests and needs. Although monitor use is not without its downsides, most families are relieved to have something to fall back on, especially if the initial event occurred during a nap or at night, times when infants usually are unobserved. Occasionally, after a thorough discussion of the risks and benefits, some parents may choose not to initiate monitoring. This is not unreasonable, because monitoring has not been clearly shown to prevent death or subsequent severe events. The one instance in which this noninterventionist position is not appropriate is in the case of an infant who required vigorous resuscitation to overcome the first event. These infants appear to be at significant risk for subsequent life-threatening spells and should be monitored.

When a treatable cause of the event has been identified, appropriate therapy initiated, and the problem controlled, home monitoring should not be necessary. Exceptions to this recommendation can be made if the treatment efficacy is questionable or if compliance with drug therapy may be a problem. In these instances, temporary use of the monitor may be helpful. Also, if the cause of a life-threatening spell is not readily amenable to therapy, home monitoring may be used to protect the child until a therapeutic plan can be developed. Home monitoring should not be necessary for infants who have had spells associated with an acute infection, once treatment or time has resulted in a resolution of the acute illness.

An area of particular concern and confusion is that of the risk for siblings of documented SIDS victims. Previous data suggest that these infants are at increased risk for SIDS, but more recent studies have indicated that this risk is minimally increased, if at all, over that in the general population. Based on these data, the recommendation of a National Institutes of Health Consensus Conference was that siblings should not be monitored automatically, until two deaths have occurred in the family. This conference recommendation may be the most controversial and difficult to follow. Considering the uncertainty surrounding SIDS, and the effects on family function from fear of losing a second child to this unknown syndrome, monitoring an infant through the first several months of life may reduce stress in the family. If the second child should have a life-threatening episode, the presence of a system in the home that may detect the problem and may prevent a death will undoubtedly reduce anxiety about such an occurrence in the home. Our recommendation for subsequent siblings of SIDS victims is that home monitoring should be considered, and the pros and cons should be discussed with the family. However, counseling the family about crib safety, sleeping environment safety, back sleeping position, environmental tobacco smoke exposure, and other risk-reduction measures is likely to be far more important and effective than home monitoring.

Home monitoring also has been recommended for infants who have experienced apnea of prematurity (AOP) and for infants with bronchopulmonary dysplasia. The available data, as well as the recommendation of the National Instituted of Health Consensus Conference, suggest that a history of AOP does not increase the risk of SIDS beyond that of prematurity itself. Thus, home monitoring generally is not indicated for infants with AOP, unless apnea persists at the time of anticipated discharge or the infant continues on theophylline or caffeine therapy at home (Table 117A.6). Monitoring in either the home or hospital should be continued for several weeks after theophylline or caffeine is discontinued. On the other hand, infants with bronchopulmonary dysplasia who require supplemental oxygen have an increased risk of sudden unexplained death. Whether these children should be considered at high risk for SIDS is irrelevant; because the increased risk of untoward events in these infants appears real, these children should be monitored until several weeks after oxygen therapy has been stopped. The best monitoring approach for infants on home oxygen is controversial, with recent trends moving towards the use of home pulse oximetry instead of cardiorespiratory monitoring for this group.

Home monitoring is not a panacea. The extensive use of home monitoring has had no effect on the incidence of SIDS overall. However, home monitoring has had some influence on the outcome for infants who were observed to have had a life-threatening event requiring vigorous intervention. Several studies have demonstrated a reduction in subsequent deaths in this high-risk population. Monitoring also is a mixed blessing for the family. The frequent false alarms are a particular problem, because no way exists to know that the alarm is false until the infant is checked by an adult. Monitors change the family's lifestyle. The mother often bears the major burden of responsibility for the child. Routine daily procedures like vacuuming and showering must be scheduled around times when someone is available to monitor the infant. Locating baby-sitters is

a problem, because the idea of caring for a child who is at risk for a life-threatening event generally frightens away caretakers. Many baby-sitters are not CPR-certified. Thus, families often find themselves isolated. Respite care or help in identifying and training alternate caretakers is an important component of any comprehensive monitoring program. Parent support groups often are helpful. However, the stress imposed by this invasion of technology is less than that created by the lack of a diagnosis and the fear of repeat events that might not be detected until it is too late. In general, monitors provide a sense of security for families and, despite the limitations and nuisance, many families would prefer to have the monitor.

The decision to discontinue monitoring is influenced by a variety of factors. If monitoring was initiated for an ALTE, it should be continued for at approximately 2 months beyond the last event or real alarm. Bradycardia caused by inappropriate alarm setting or shallow breathing interpreted as apnea by the monitor should not be counted. Cessation of monitoring for other conditions is based on the natural course of the disease and the response to therapy. If drug therapy (methylxanthine, anti-reflux, or seizure medication) has been used, monitoring usually should be continued for at least 1 month after the drug therapy has been stopped. This guideline is somewhat arbitrary, and decisions must be individualized. Monitoring for a sibling of a SIDS victim often is continued until several weeks beyond the age at which the other child died, mainly for reasons of parental anxiety. As discussed above, this is a controversial indication for home monitoring, and no official guidelines exist. Discontinuing the monitor may be difficult for some parents. Many families become dependent on it, so that the physician and support team frequently must increase their involvement with the family to support them through the weaning process. Families anxious about stopping the monitor should start by not monitoring the infant during naps to facilitate the transition to no monitoring.

MANAGEMENT OF SPECIFIC CONDITIONS ASSOCIATED WITH APPARENT LIFE-THREATENING EVENTS

If a particular condition is identified as the probable cause of the event, therapy should be directed at the underlying disease process, recognizing that the life-threatening event is merely a consequence of this disorder. In that context, the more common conditions associated with apnea or life-threatening events are discussed individually. It is important to note that official guidelines do not address most of these specific conditions and the decision to use home monitoring is an individualized clinical decision in most cases.

Apnea of Prematurity

Apnea with periodic breathing is common in infants born before 37 weeks' gestation and is termed AOP when a treatable cause cannot be found. It has been estimated that one-half of premature infants exhibit periodic breathing, and that at least one-half of those infants develop AOP. AOP should resolve by 37 to 38 weeks' gestational age and usually does not recur. Results from a recent, large, multicenter study on the natural history of prolonged apnea and severe bradycardia revealed that such events are rare, in both term and preterm infants, after approximately 43 weeks' postconceptional age.

Occasionally, AOP may not resolve, even by the time the infant is otherwise ready to be discharged to home. Such persistent AOP may warrant treatment or continued monitoring at home. Because it generally resolves by 37 to 38 weeks after conception, it was formerly a problem almost exclusively encountered in the newborn nursery. However, the move toward the earlier discharge of these infants may result in increasing numbers of preterm infants who are at home while still vulnerable to this disorder. Most neonatologists require an apnea-free interval before discharge, typically approximately 5 to 8 days. Although work by Darnall et al. has demonstrated that this approach should reduce the risk of subsequent apnea events, these data also show that infants born before 28 weeks' gestation are still at risk for apnea, even at ages past term. The pediatrician must be aware of this entity, because episodes of AOP may occur after the infant has been discharged and thus might be considered an ALTE. In general, methylxanthine therapy is stopped before discharge, and the primary therapy for persistent AOP is home monitoring. If a decision is made to use methylxanthines in the outpatient setting, monitoring is indicated and should be continued for 2 to 4 weeks after the medication has been stopped. Similarly, an apnea-free period of at least 1 month should be required before monitoring is stopped in infants who were not discharged on drug therapy. Although approximately 18% of SIDS victims are preterm infants, no evidence exists that a history of AOP *per se* increases the risk for SIDS.

Acute Infections

In general, infections, including meningitis, sepsis, and pneumonia, should be treated as in routine practice. Bronchiolitis caused by respiratory syncytial virus is frequently associated with apnea early in the course of the illness, often before the usual manifestations of bronchiolitis are apparent. Therapy is supportive. Occasionally, ventilatory support is required. The pathogenesis of the apnea associated with acute infection is unknown, but it is thought to be self-limited, and it typically resolves within 1 month. Treatment of the apnea with respiratory stimulants is usually not indicated or needed. Limited data exist on the indications for home monitoring in this population. Because the condition appears to be self-limited, monitoring is generally unnecessary. If significant concern exists about subsequent events, then the recommendations for an ALTE with no definable etiology should be used.

Gastroesophageal Reflux

If an association between the ALTE and gastroesophageal reflux is established, either through laboratory studies or by clinical observation, simple standard medical management should be initiated. Persistence of spells after the institution of therapy, or an initial spell that results in a need for vigorous resuscitation, is an indication for anti-reflux medications including prokinetic agents and an acid-blocker. Only limited clinical research data support their use, but experience has documented a positive response to these agents in terms of a reduction in episodes in some patients. If the ALTE was severe, or concern exists about the effectiveness of therapy, home apnea and bradycardia monitoring also could be instituted. Although fundoplication generally is not needed, some infants have persistent spells and documented reflux despite medical management. Surgery is indicated if it can be established that the control of reflux through the use of continuous low-volume nasogastric feeding results in cessation of the episodes and that these spells are severe enough to represent a continued threat to the child's life. Because gastroesophageal reflux generally is a self-limited condition, a conservative approach usually is justified.

The maturation of gastroesophageal sphincter function generally results in a cessation of ALTE in these children.

Seizures

Seizures can present as apnea spells, especially apnea during wakefulness. Frequently, the diagnosis of seizure is not readily apparent because these infants may not have tonic-dome movements. Electroencephalography is required for diagnosis. Therapy should focus on seizure control. Home monitoring may be indicated for a limited time, until seizure control can be ensured.

Dysphagia

Events related to feeding are most common in premature infants and represent a maturational delay in the integration of breathing and the suck–swallow mechanism. Improvement is predicated on the assumption that substantial central nervous system injury has not occurred. In the most severe cases, avoidance of oral feedings is necessary until maturation occurs. Occasionally, apnea during feeding is associated with marked gastroesophageal reflux. Monitoring generally is not required for apnea exclusively associated with feeding, because the events occur during feeding, a time when the infant is being observed. A safe feeding strategy must be instituted for these infants, however, and concerns regarding gastroesophageal reflux must be addressed. Therapy is based on the results of the modified barium swallow, the response to manipulations of feeding, as well as the presence of underlying central nervous system injury.

Disorders of Respiratory Control

Infants with respiratory control disorders most often experience episodes during sleep. Central apnea with secondary bradycardia can occur and, if recurrent, can result in marked hypoventilation and hypoxia. Occasionally, obstructive or mixed apnea occurs. The effectiveness of therapy using medications (e.g., respiratory stimulants) is quite limited. In more severe cases, assisted ventilation during sleep, either with noninvasive nasal ventilation or traditional mechanical ventilation via a tracheostomy, may be necessary. These infants require nocturnal cardiorespiratory monitoring.

Child Abuse

Data from Southall et al. have raised concerns about the role of child abuse as a cause of ALTE, especially recurrent events. This diagnosis can be quite difficult to establish, because the parents involved in this behavior can often be quite convincing. The events described seem real, and the parents can appear to be traumatized by the ALTE. This situation is complicated by the physician's attitude toward the parents of children who are reported to have had an ALTE. Frequently, the doctor accepts the parents' concern and observations as being valid and never thinks in terms of child abuse. Sadly, child abuse is not uncommon, and physicians caring for these infants must not lose sight of its role in infants who present with an ALTE. Establishing a diagnosis can be quite challenging, and places the physician in the role of a detective. As described by Southall et al., covert surveillance may be necessary to establish the diagnosis.

APPARENT LIFE-THREATENING EVENTS WITH NO DEFINABLE CAUSE

Infants who have ALTE with no definable cause are a major management dilemma for the practitioner. The data on the risks of subsequent spells and possible death are limited and somewhat biased by interventions. The physician has, at best, three therapeutic options: no intervention, the use of respiratory stimulants, or home monitoring. Doing nothing often is not a choice because of parental anxiety surrounding the risk of subsequent events. Because monitoring has not been demonstrated to reduce the incidence of SIDS, some have recommended a nonintervention approach once treatable or diagnosable conditions are eliminated. This choice is not popular with many families, but it is an option, assuming the family can be reassured and the physician is comfortable that the event is not severe or likely to recur. Unfortunately, many families and physicians are extremely uncomfortable with doing nothing. In general, an ALTE of unknown cause is handled best with judicious use of home monitoring in selected cases.

PREVENTION

Much work remains to be done in improving our understanding of the pathogenesis of life-threatening events. This work must include studies of respiratory control during both sleep and wakefulness, better methods of identifying the population at true risk and, if it remains a cornerstone of management, improved monitoring.

Suggested Readings

Brazy JE, Kinney HC, Oakes WJ. Central nervous system structural lesions causing apnea at birth. *Pediatrics* 1987;111:163.
Carbone T, Ostfeld BM, Gutter D, Hegyi T. Parental compliance with home cardiorespiratory monitoring. *Arch Dis Child* 2001;84(3):270.
Committee on Fetus and Newborn. American Academy of Pediatrics. Apnea, sudden infant death syndrome, and home monitoring. *Pediatrics* 2003;111(4 pt 1):914.
Darnall RA, Kattwinkel J, Nattie C, Robinson M. Discharge after apnea in preterm infants. *Pediatrics* 1997;100:795.
Dunne KP, Matthews TC. Near-miss SIDS: clinical findings and management. *Pediatrics* 1987;79:889.
Farrell PA, Weiner GM, Lemons JA. SIDS, ALTE, apnea, and the use of home monitors. *Pediatr Rev* 2002;23(1):3.
Fleming PJ, Blair PS. Sudden unexpected deaths after discharge from the neonatal intensive care unit. *Semin Neonatol* 2003;8(2):159.
Garg M, Kurzner SI, Bautista DB, Keens TG. Clinically unsuspected hypoxia during sleep and feeding in bronchopulmonary dysplasia. *Pediatrics* 1988;81:635.
Gray PH, Rogers Y. Are infants with bronchopulmonary dysplasia at risk for sudden infant death syndrome? *Pediatrics* 1994;93(5):774.
Guilleminault C, Pelayo R, Leger D, Philip P. Apparent life-threatening events, facial dysmorphia and sleep-disordered breathing. *Eur J Pediatr* 2000;159(6):444.
Harrington C, Kirjavainen T, Teng A, Sullivan CE. Altered autonomic function and reduced arousability in apparent life-threatening event infants with obstructive sleep apnea. *Am J Respir Crit Care Med* 2002;165(8):1048.
Kahn A, for the European Society for the Study and Prevention of Infant Death. Recommended clinical evaluation of infants with an apparent life-threatening event. Consensus document of the European Society for the Study and Prevention of Infant Death, 2003. *Eur J Pediatr* 2004;163(2):108.
Keens TG, Davidson-Ward SL. Apparent life-threatening events. In: Loughlin GM, Eigen H, eds. *Respiratory disease in children: diagnosis and management.* Baltimore: Williams & Wilkins, 1994.
NIH Consensus Development Conference Proceedings. Infantile apnea and home monitoring. NIH publication No. 87-2905. U.S. Department of Health and Human Services, National Institutes of Health, 1986. [http://consensus. nih.gov/cons/058/058-intro.htm.]
National Institutes of Health Consensus Development Conference on Infantile Apnea and Home Monitoring, Sept 29 to Oct 1, 1986. *Pediatrics* 1987;79: 292.
Oren J, Kelly D, Shannon DC. Identification of a high-risk group for SIDS among infants who were resuscitated for sleep apnea. *Pediatrics* 1986;77:495.
Page M, Jeffery H. The role of gastro-oesophageal reflux in the aetiology of SIDS. *Early Hum Dev* 2000;59(2):127.
Petersen DR, Sabotta EE, Daling JR. Infant mortality among subsequent siblings of infants who died of SIDS. *Pediatrics* 1986;108:911.
Ramanathan R, Corwin MJ, Hunt CE, et al., for the Collaborative Home Infant Monitoring Evaluation (CHIME) Study Group. Cardiorespiratory events recorded on home monitors: comparison of healthy infants with those at increased risk for SIDS. *JAMA* 2001;285(17):2199.
Southall DP. Home monitoring and its role in SIDS. *Pediatrics* 1983;72:133.
Southall DP, Plunkett MCB, Banks MW, et al. Covert video surveillance for life-threatening child abuse. *Pediatrics* 1997;100:735.
Weese-Mayer DB, Brouillette RT, Morrow AS, et al. Assessing validity of infant monitoring alarms with event recording. *Pediatrics* 1989;115:702.
Werthammer J, et al. SIDS in infants with bronchopulmonary dysplasia. *Pediatrics* 1982;60:301.

CHAPTER 117B ■ SUDDEN INFANT DEATH SYNDROME (SIDS)

JOHN L. CARROLL AND GERALD M. LOUGHLIN

The sudden unexpected death of a baby is a devastating event, both for the family and for the infant's pediatrician. When postmortem examination, clinical history, and a death scene investigation fail to reveal an adequate cause of death in an infant who has unexpectedly died, it is called sudden infant death syndrome (SIDS).

SIDS is a common cause of death in infants during the first year of life. It is not a diagnosis, but rather descriptive of a syndrome based on not finding a diagnosis. Despite over 5,500 published articles on the subject, with over 3,500 addressing etiology, no definitive cause has been identified. However, epidemiologic studies have clearly demonstrated that SIDS is strongly linked to the prone sleeping position for infants and exposure to cigarette smoke. In many countries, including the United States, public education campaigns targeting sleeping position and smoke exposure have resulted in a dramatic decline in the SIDS rate. Thus, through risk-reduction approaches, the incidence of SIDS can be reduced substantially, even if the cause or causes are not fully understood.

Whatever the cause or causes may be, the pediatrician in practice is faced with frustrating practical management dilemmas. These include trying to understand why one of his infant patients has suddenly and unexpectedly died, helping the surviving parents and siblings, and counseling the parents about SIDS risk in subsequent siblings. In addition, because the definition of SIDS requires a death scene investigation (see below), parents must cope with police or other authorities coming into their home to interrogate them and investigate the scene where the death occurred. Pediatricians can play a major role in helping parents through this extremely difficult and trying period.

New insights into the paramount importance of risk factors, such as the prone or side sleeping positions and cigarette smoke exposure, indicate the potential for major reductions in the SIDS rate. By educating parents about risk-reduction and thus minimizing the proportion of infants sleeping prone or on their side, decreasing maternal smoking and postnatal environmental tobacco smoke exposure, and improving prenatal care, pediatricians can have a major impact on child health (Table 117B.2).

DEFINITION

SIDS is the default "cause of death" after a thorough postmortem investigation fails to reveal a cause of an infant's unexpected death; in other words, it is a diagnosis of exclusion. SIDS is currently defined as "The sudden death of an infant less than 1 year of age, which remains unexplained after a thorough investigation, including a performance of complete autopsy, examination of the death scene, and review of the clinical history." This definition restricts the age to infants of less than 1 year of age and requires a thorough investigation; it explicitly states that if no death scene investigation is performed, a diagnosis of SIDS cannot be made. This definition is now widely accepted, and the U.S. Centers for Disease Control (CDC) has published detailed guidelines for the death scene investigation of sudden, unexplained infant deaths. It is noteworthy that, although rare, sudden unexpected deaths do occur in infants of older than 1 year of age. Unexplained death in older infants should prompt additional investigation for unusual disorders such as metabolic or cardiac defects.

EPIDEMIOLOGY

Most deaths caused by congenital anomalies occur during the first week of life, leaving SIDS as the most common single cause of death between 7 days and 365 days of age. At the time of this writing, approximately 2,500 to 3,000 infants each year die of SIDS in the United States, making the overall incidence about 0.7 to 0.8 SIDS deaths per 1,000 live births. However, the rate of SIDS among American Indians (1.5 per 1,000) and African Americans (1.4 per 1,000) is still more than double that of Caucasians (0.6 per 1,000), in spite of a large overall reduction in the incidence of SIDS.

The epidemiology of SIDS changed dramatically between 1988 and 2004, due largely to successful risk-reduction campaigns in many countries. The SIDS rates in some countries have declined more than 80% and reductions of greater than 50% are common, all brought about through risk-reduction strategies, mainly decreasing the proportion of infants sleeping in the prone or side sleeping positions. In the United States, between 1992 and 1996, the proportion of infants sleeping prone decreased from about 75% to approximately 20%, accompanied by an approximately 40% decline in the SIDS rate over the same period. A further decline in the SIDS rate would be anticipated if the pre- and postnatal exposure of infants to tobacco smoke could be substantially reduced.

SIDS has a very striking and characteristic age distribution, with most deaths occurring between 1 and 5 months, peaking at 2 to 4 months postnatal age. The apparently unimodal age distribution of SIDS, with a single peak at about 12 weeks, does not mean that SIDS is due to a single cause; indeed, evidence suggests that the likely causes of SIDS vary with age at death. SIDS appears to be more common in males, for reasons that are not understood. It is also seasonal, being more common in winter. Most SIDS deaths occur during sleep (or at least when the infant was supposed to have been asleep), but deaths are reported to have occurred in awake infants.

Risk Factors

Environmental Risk Factors

Infant Sleeping Position. Apparently, due to fear of vomiting and aspiration, it became standard practice in many countries to place babies to sleep in the prone position. Without any scientific evidence to support the practice, so-called baby experts have been strongly recommending the prone infant sleeping position for decades. However, numerous studies from many countries, including the United States, clearly show that the prone sleeping position for infants is associated with the highest risk for SIDS, the supine sleeping position with the lowest risk, with the side-lying position conferring an intermediate risk for SIDS. The side sleeping position is associated with an increased SIDS risk because it is unstable, allowing infants to roll into the prone position. In 1992, the American Academy of Pediatrics (AAP) issued a policy statement recommending that healthy infants, when being put down for sleep, be positioned on their side or back. In 1996, in response to new evidence that the side position conferred an increased risk for SIDS, the AAP issued a new policy statement recommending that healthy infants should sleep on their backs. In the 4 years following the 1992 AAP statement, the proportion of infants sleeping prone in the U.S. declined from about 75% to about 20%, and the SIDS rate dropped approximately 40%.

How is sleeping position related to SIDS? Several investigators believe that it is related to developmental vulnerability, allowing a baby sleeping prone, with his face in contact with blankets or other porous bedding material, to rebreathe exhaled air, leading to asphyxia and suffocation. After about 6 months of age, when an infant can spontaneously change head, face, and body position and the cardiorespiratory control system is more mature, he is likely to be past the vulnerable period. Other possible contributing mechanisms include widespread alveolar collapse with hypoxemia and bronchoconstriction, impaired body heat loss and hyperthermia, or upper airway obstruction. Some evidence suggests brainstem abnormalities in areas that mediate ventilatory responses to elevated CO_2, blood pressure, and arousal responses during sleep. However, the relationship between subtle brainstem abnormalities and SIDS remains unknown.

No scientific evidence shows, at least with respect to SIDS, that there is any advantage to the prone sleeping position for healthy infants. Nor does any scientific evidence exist, despite "common sense" fears of aspiration, that the supine sleeping position is harmful to a healthy infant. Since the recommendation of the supine sleeping position for healthy infants, several studies have looked for important adverse effects of the supine sleeping position for infants and found none. Therefore, it is clear from numerous studies that the prone sleeping position is dangerous and that the supine sleeping position is safe for healthy infants. Evidence also is mounting that the prone sleeping position is particularly dangerous for low-birth-weight and premature infants. For these infants, sleeping position recommendations should be individualized, keeping in mind the risk of asphyxia associated with the prone sleeping position. Similarly, in certain medical conditions, such as gastroesophageal reflux, recommendations concerning sleeping position must be individualized. It should also be noted that the supine position recommendation applies only to sleep. When infants are awake, there appears to be some benefit from spending time in the prone position.

Recent research indicates that infants who are unaccustomed to sleeping in the prone position, who are placed prone to sleep, are a much greater risk of SIDS than infants who are "used to" or accustomed to sleeping prone. The typical scenario is an infant who sleeps on her back at home, but at several months of age is placed prone for sleep at a day-care center or other alternative caregiver setting. Thus, the prone sleeping position is of particularly high-risk for infants unaccustomed to sleeping in this position.

Maternal Smoking and Fetal Hypoxia. Maternal cigarette smoking is a major risk factor for SIDS. One large study found that 70% of mothers in the SIDS group smoked during pregnancy. A cigarette consumption–SIDS dose–response curve was demonstrated more than 20 years ago. After controlling for other risk factors, maternal smoking at least doubles the risk of SIDS. According to the National Institute of Child Health and Human Development (NICHD) SIDS study, if a mother smokes during pregnancy, the SIDS risk is 3.4 times higher than for controls. Numerous studies have demonstrated that maternal smoking increases the risk of SIDS in a dose-dependent fashion. The more a mother smokes during pregnancy, the greater the risk for SIDS.

In addition, numerous studies demonstrate that environmental tobacco smoke (ETS) exposure increases the risk of SIDS, also in a dose-dependent fashion. Whether expressed as number of smokers in household, number of cigarettes exposed to per day, or hours of smoke exposure per day, study results agree that the risk of SIDS increases many-fold with increasing ETS exposure. When family members smoke in the same room with the baby, the risk of SIDS may be increased 20-fold or more. In countries where the rate of prone sleeping position has been reduced to below 20%, it is estimated that tobacco smoke exposure accounts for approximately 50% to 60% of the remaining SIDS rate. In these countries, where the proportion of infants sleeping prone has been minimized, smoke exposure has become the number-one modifiable risk factor for SIDS.

Pre- and postnatal smoke exposure is particularly dangerous for low-birth-weight and premature infants. Studies demonstrate that smoke exposure dramatically increases SIDS risk in low-birth-weight or premature infants, as much as 60- to 80-fold compared to matched controls not exposed to tobacco smoke. A similar interaction occurs between smoke exposure and the prone sleeping position. Although the prone sleeping position is dangerous for all infants, the risk of SIDS from sleeping prone is magnified when the infant is also smoke-exposed.

Another interesting interaction suggests a role for fetal hypoxia. Maternal anemia greatly enhances the SIDS risk for infants of smoking mothers. An anemic smoking mother appears to be about four times more likely to have an infant die of SIDS than a nonanemic, nonsmoking mother. Such a strong interaction with anemia and smoking during pregnancy suggests that fetal hypoxemia, prenatal nutrition, or other toxicity may play a role in SIDS.

Unsafe Sleeping Environments. Unsafe sleeping environments, especially soft mattresses or other porous bedding material, increase the risk of rebreathing exhaled gases and therefore the risk of accidental asphyxia and suffocation. The U.S. Consumer Product Safety Commission (CPSC) has reported that as many as 30% of deaths diagnosed as SIDS may have been due to unsafe bedding material. The CPSC has issued specific recommendations concerning crib construction, crib mattress specifications, and bedding materials appropriate for infants. Infants should sleep in an environment that meets CPSC safety guidelines, on a CPSC-approved mattress, without soft or porous bedding material (including stuffed animals, pillows, fluffy bumpers, etc.) that could pose a danger of rebreathing.

Bed Sharing and Infant–Parent Co-Sleeping. Infant–parent co-sleeping may have numerous benefits both for parent and child. However, sleeping in a bed designed for adults may expose the infant to hazardous bedding material such as thick quilts, pillows, or comforters. In addition, infant–parent co-sleeping, when one or both of the parents are smokers, may be associated with increased SIDS risk due to smoke exposure. If parents elect to co-sleep with their infant, every effort should be made to minimize the dangers of having an infant sleeping in a bed designed for adults with bedding material designed for adults.

Breastfeeding. Several studies have suggested that lack of breastfeeding is a risk factor for SIDS, whereas others have not shown an effect of breastfeeding on SIDS risk. Although breastfeeding clearly has many benefits, its relationship to SIDS remains to be demonstrated.

Infection. The role of infection as a risk factor remains in dispute. A variety of bacteria and viruses have been identified from SIDS victims, but no consistent association has been found between SIDS and infection with any particular organism. Parents often report that the infant showed "cold symptoms" just before a SIDS death, giving a general impression that infection is associated with SIDS. However, the NICHD SIDS Cooperative Epidemiological Study analyzed 800 SIDS cases with respect to matched control infants. They found that 29% of SIDS cases had a cold on the day of death, but so did about the same proportion of control infants. Numerous studies have made exhaustive attempts to implicate infection in SIDS, but so far the association between infection and SIDS is unclear.

Nutrition. Serum prealbumin levels, which reflect recent poor nutrition, and the mineral content of bone, an indicator of chronic poor nutrition, have been reported to be normal in SIDS infants. Many studies have tried to identify nutritional deficiencies in SIDS victims; so far, none have been found.

Family, Home, and Child-Care Practices. The most potent modifiable risk factors for SIDS are clearly the prone and side sleeping positions and tobacco smoke exposure. In addition, numerous studies have shown an association between SIDS and other maternal and socioeconomic factors such as young maternal age, mother unmarried, less than high school education, low income, inadequate or infrequent prenatal care, crowded living conditions, multigravidity, lack of breast-feeding, and parental drug use. Studies from England have found a strong association between SIDS and such factors as "housing in poor repair," parents unemployed, poor financial circumstances, and the family not owning their house or not having a telephone. Such associations suggest that, in addition to sleeping position and smoke exposure, other parental or environmental factors are important.

Illicit Drugs. Cocaine exposure may affect neurologic development, possibly leading to postnatal abnormalities of cardiorespiratory control, sleep, and arousal. Several studies to date indicate that the SIDS risk is higher in the infants of substance-abusing mothers; the incidence figures range between nine and 150 deaths per 1,000 live births. Another study, however, found no difference in the SIDS rate between cocaine-exposed and nonexposed infants. Although drug-exposed infants may exhibit disordered sleep, respiratory control abnormalities, and an increased risk of sudden unexpected death, no study has shown that these factors are causally related to SIDS, and no study has shown that death is related to drug exposure *per se*.

Over-the-Counter Medications. In the NICHD SIDS study, 43% of SIDS victims had a history of a cold within 2 weeks before death, and 29% of parents reported cold symptoms within 24 hours before death. Sick infants are likely to be treated with over-the-counter medications containing antihistamines, phenothiazines, or other powerful sedatives. One study found that SIDS victims and matched controls had the same incidence of cold symptoms, but infants dying of SIDS were much more likely to have received cold medicine before death. About 25% of SIDS infants had been given phenothiazine-containing cold remedies within 48 hours of death, compared with only 2% of control babies.

Immunization. Several controlled studies have shown that DPT immunization does not increase the risk of SIDS. However, the possibility of a relationship between SIDS and immunizations is still being actively studied.

Infant Risk Factors

Race. African Americans and Native Americans have the highest rates of SIDS in the United States; babies of Asian origin have the lowest. However, no study has been able to sort out an increased SIDS risk due to race per se, as opposed to differences in environmental factors.

Birth Weight and Prematurity. Birth weight and prematurity are two of the strongest risk factors for SIDS. The NICHD SIDS study found that infants with birth weights below 2,500 g and below 1,500 g were about 5 and 18 times, respectively, more likely than controls to die of SIDS. Similarly, infants with preterm birth at less than 37 weeks' postconceptional age and less than 33 weeks' postconceptional age were 5 and 16 times, respectively, more likely to die of SIDS than controls. Several other studies have confirmed these results. An increased SIDS risk also has been reported in small-for-gestational-age full-term infants.

Neonatal Risk Factors

Apnea. Despite widespread beliefs about infant apnea and SIDS, to date, no controlled study has shown that apnea of prematurity is a risk factor for SIDS. The NICHD SIDS study found that other neonatal factors such as hypothermia, tachypnea, poor feeding, cyanosis, irritability, fever, and respiratory distress were statistically more likely to have occurred in SIDS infants but were not of predictive value. For decades, the medical literature has erroneously linked prolonged infant apnea strongly with SIDS. However, several studies now have shown that infant apnea does not correlate with subsequent SIDS death.

PATHOLOGY

Autopsy

For many years, pathologists have searched unsuccessfully for pathologic markers that would positively identify these infants. SIDS remains a pathologic diagnosis of exclusion. Table 117B.1 lists several proposed subtle pathologic findings in SIDS, but many of these so-called "subtle" pathologic findings of SIDS are matters of great debate. No pathologic finding has been found to be diagnostic of SIDS.

TABLE 117B.1

REPORTED PATHOLOGIC FINDINGS IN SUDDEN INFANT DEATH SYNDROME

Main finding
No pathology that explains death

Currently accepted "subtle" findings[a]
Brainstem gliosis[b]
Frothy secretions at nose or mouth[b]
Hepatic erythropoiesis[b]
Intrathoracic petechiae
Minor inflammatory changes (respiratory tract)
Periventricular leukomalacia[b]
Persistence of dendritic spines in "respiratory centers" of brainstem[b]
Pulmonary congestion[b]
Pulmonary edema[b]
Retention of periadrenal brown fat
Unclotted blood in left ventricle[b]

Unconfirmed to date
Abnormal development of vagus nerve
Abnormal pulmonary surfactant
Abnormalities of carotid body
Decreased laryngeal cross-sectional area
Escherichia coli toxin
Elevated hypoxanthine levels in vitreous humor
Increased immunoglobulin levels in lung washings

Validity seriously in question
Clostridium difficile toxin (not different from controls)
Retained hemoglobin F (conflicting results from different studies)

[a]Agreement between several investigators.
[b]Some investigators question whether these differ significantly from deaths due to other causes.

Death Scene Investigation

The unexpected death of an infant always raises the question "Why?" Such a question cannot be answered fully without all available information concerning the circumstances of death. Clinical history from caretakers is important but insufficient. A variety of environmental factors would not be recognized by untrained observers and are likely to be missed even by a physician taking a thorough history. Despite disagreement about the proportion of SIDS cases that are due to nonaccidental injury or neglect, most investigators would agree that at least some deaths are non-natural. A recent policy statement from the American Academy of Pediatrics Committee on Child Abuse and Neglect estimated that 2% to 5% of deaths diagnosed as SIDS may involve intentional injury.

Past beliefs that SIDS has nothing to do with environmental factors, child-care practices, accidents, neglect, or intentional injury were not based on scientific data. Recent reports suggest that if a more complete death circumstances inquiry were conducted, some SIDS deaths could be explained. The death scene investigation may be more important than autopsy in some cases. Without a thorough death scene investigation as part of every SIDS investigation, we will never be able to determine the proportion of SIDS cases that are related to modifiable or avoidable risk factors.

PATHOGENESIS

The cause or causes of SIDS are unknown. The search for the causes of SIDS has been further complicated by the study of so-called infants at risk or high-risk infants, since identification of groups that are at risk is a matter of dispute. Much of the scientific data that have been proposed or assumed to describe infants at risk may or may not actually apply to most SIDS victims.

Apnea Hypothesis

Early reports associating SIDS with prolonged apnea led to the so-called "apnea hypothesis" of SIDS, which dominated the field for over 15 years, from about 1972 to 1987. However, several large studies, involving many thousands of infants, have failed to demonstrate any relationship between infant apnea and the risk of SIDS.

The Triple-Risk Model of SIDS

In 1994, the "triple-risk" model of SIDS was introduced, proposing that SIDS resulted from the "intersection" of three overlapping factors: (a) a vulnerable infant; (b) a critical developmental period in homeostatic control, and (c) an exogenous stressor(s). According to Filiano and Kinney, the originators of the "triple-risk" model of SIDS, "An infant will die of SIDS only if he/she possesses all three factors." Thus, an underlying "vulnerability" (e.g., neurophysiological defect) was required. In other words, according to the "triple-risk" model, normal infants do not die of SIDS. However, although this model has been widely quoted, no evidence suggests that an underlying defect or "vulnerability" is necessary in order for SIDS to occur. Others have argued that normal developmental vulnerability due to the immaturity of cardiorespiratory control, combined with a variety of possible exogenous stressors, is sufficient to result in expected death.

Respiratory Control and Developmental Vulnerability

Many investigators believe that cardiorespiratory control is involved in the etiology of most SIDS cases. One "cardiorespiratory control hypothesis" proposes that SIDS could result from developmental abnormalities in cardiorespiratory control, including the brainstem control centers, chemoreceptor responses, autonomic control, autoresuscitative gasping mechanisms, arousal from sleep, and upper airway control. Several large prospective studies have reported that, in general, subtle findings o occur concerning respiratory and cardiac variability, higher mean heart rates, and other findings suggestive of subtle autonomic nervous system abnormalities. However, no study to date has found predictive respiratory control abnormalities in babies destined to die of SIDS.

After birth, the infant does not simply grow larger; rather, many (if not all) systems show continued structural and morphologic maturation. The lungs are not fully developed until about 8 years of age. The central nervous system continues to undergo significant structural modification for years. Just as motor skills and reflexes are primitive in the newborn and develop slowly in the infant, many physiologic responses are incompletely developed at birth. These include the major changes in cardiorespiratory control that occur during the first 6 months of life. The infant's ability to "defend" herself against hypoxia or asphyxia changes during the first 6 months of life. In this sense, all infants are vulnerable to a variety of postnatal insults at certain times. Vulnerability could be increased in some infants due to prenatal insults (smoking, substance abuse, poor nutrition, anemia during pregnancy), abnormal development

(e.g., delayed central nervous system maturation), or postnatal factors (e.g., illness or medication with sedative drugs).

The "developmental vulnerability" hypothesis proposes that SIDS may result from a variety of insults (e.g., prone sleeping with rebreathing of exhaled air, thermal stress, infection) to a vulnerable infant. Any one factor, occurring in isolation, may not lead to death, but particular combinations of stresses or a particular insult at a vulnerable time may be lethal for 0.7 per 1,000 infants. Thus, there would be no single cause of SIDS. SIDS could result from a variety of stresses and multiple causes of vulnerability that vary with age. Such an etiology would be consistent with variable pathologic findings, multiple risk factors, parental and environmental factors that appear to play a variable role, and risk factors that vary depending on the age at death.

The normal vulnerability associated with immature cardiorespiratory control, combined with a severe asphyxial challenge due to sleeping in the prone position (for example), may be sufficient to cause SIDS. Recent studies have shown abnormalities of neurotransmitter receptor binding in a brainstem area that may be important in mediating ventilatory responses to hypercapnia. However, whether brainstem abnormalities are necessary for SIDS to occur remains unknown.

Unsafe Sleeping Environments

Multiple studies show that unsafe sleeping environments are associated with a high-risk of unexpected, sudden death. A study of unexpected infant deaths in St. Louis showed that the vast majority of infants who died were not sleeping in a crib. Most were found dead in unsafe sleeping environments, such as makeshift beds, sofas, or adult beds. Other studies have demonstrated that an infant need not be sleeping prone in order to experience "asphyxial" conditions; even seemingly light bedcovers near or over an infant's face may result in CO_2 buildup and hypoxia. Many investigators now believe that most deaths previously classified as SIDS were actually due to accidental or nonintentional asphyxia in unsafe sleeping environments.

The day-care sleeping environment presents several dangers that increase the risk of SIDS. Infants are often placed to sleep in unsafe sleeping environments (e.g., sofas, comforters, soft mattresses, adult beds) in the day-care setting. Day-care providers may be unaware of the current sleeping position recommendations for infants and often are not aware of an individual infant's usual sleeping position.

Upper Airway and Small Airways Occlusion

It has been suggested that SIDS may sometimes be caused by nasal/oral occlusion and airway obstruction in an infant with the face pressed into a pillow or mattress. Several studies have suggested that pulmonary surfactant was abnormal in SIDS victims, compared with control infants who died of non-SIDS, nonpulmonary causes. Abnormal surfactant may lead to widespread alveolar collapse, causing hypoxia and death. More study is needed in this area before a conclusion is possible.

Cardiovascular Causes

The long QT syndrome and hypersensitivity to vagal stimulation both have been suggested as causes, but neither has been proved to be associated with SIDS. Tachycardia and decreased heart rate variability have been found in infants who later die of SIDS, but the meaning of these findings is unknown. Fatal autonomic control abnormalities, resulting in sudden hypotension and a "shock-like" condition, have been proposed to play a role in SIDS. Although arguments along these lines are promising, research data are inconclusive at this time.

Defects of Metabolism

Underlying metabolic abnormalities such as medium-chain acyl-CoA dehydrogenase deficiency, ethylmalonic-adipic aciduria, multiple acyl-CoA dehydrogenase deficiency, long-chain acyl-CoA dehydrogenase deficiency, and systemic carnitine deficiency may cause sudden unexpected death during infancy. However, the proportion of SIDS cases that may be attributable to metabolic disorders is probably very small. An underlying metabolic disorder may be more likely in cases of apparent SIDS in older infants (older than 12 months).

Infection

Acute bacterial and viral infections, intrauterine and perinatally acquired chronic infections, and various toxins elaborated by infectious organisms all have been proposed as possible causes or predisposing factors for SIDS. Although infection may play an indirect role, to date no evidence links SIDS to any specific infectious etiology.

Delayed Neural Development

A hypothesis involving abnormal neural maturation is attractive, because it could at least partially explain the developmental vulnerability to SIDS. Abnormalities described so far include delayed central nervous system myelination, astrogliosis, periventricular and subcortical leukomalacia, detailed dendritic pruning, and other suggestions of abnormal nervous system development. However, no neuropathologic finding has been causally linked with SIDS.

Impaired Arousal Responses During Illness

It is well known that children and adults tend to sleep more when sick. This is not simply a matter of feeling bad, but involves infection-related increased levels of somnogenic substances that exaggerate the tendency to sleep and may impair arousal. Such somnogenic substances include muramyl peptides, the lipid-A moiety of endotoxin, poly (I C), interleukin-1, and others. It has been suggested that infection leads to increased levels of somnogenic substances, increased sleep, impaired arousal, and an increased vulnerability in the infant to airway obstruction or other causes of asphyxia. This is a promising area in need of further exploration.

GROUPS PROPOSED TO BE AT INCREASED RISK OF SIDS

Traditional groups said to be at increased risk include premature infants, subsequent siblings of SIDS victims, survivors of apparent life-threatening events (ALTEs) and, recently, infants of substance-abusing mothers. Prematurity and low birth weight are potent risk factors for SIDS and are not in dispute.

Siblings of SIDS Victims

If a predisposing physiologic abnormality is operative in SIDS, it could be hereditary (e.g., defects in metabolism). If family factors, child-care practices, or environmental factors play a role, these would probably be similar for subsequent siblings of a SIDS victim. Finally, if intentional injury is a factor in a particular SIDS case, subsequent siblings in the same family are likely to be at increased risk. A family in which multiple SIDS death occur should be investigated for all these possibilities.

Several studies show an increased risk of SIDS, as well as other causes of death, in families that have had one SIDS death. The literature on the risk to a subsequent sibling after one SIDS death is unclear at present.

Apparent Life-Threatening Event

ALTE is the appropriate term currently used for what used to be called "near-miss" for SIDS. ALTE applies to infants who have been observed to have pallor, cyanosis, apnea, choking, or other signs that they might be in danger of dying. Are infants who experience an ALTE at higher risk of SIDS? The NICHD SIDS study found that 7% of mothers of SIDS victims recalled a previous episode of "baby turned blue or stopped breathing," compared with 3% of matched controls. Although this was statistically significant, the most important finding was that 93% of mothers of SIDS infants recalled no ALTE. Available data suggest that ALTE infants constitute only a small number of SIDS cases, and that most infants dying of SIDS do not experience a prior, clinically apparent ALTE.

PREDICTION

The probability of SIDS cannot be predicted for an individual infant. No test, including a pneumogram or polysomnography (sleep study), is useful for determining SIDS risk. No test can predict SIDS risk for a family or a subsequent sibling. No test can determine which infants should use home apnea monitoring or when a home monitor can be appropriately discontinued. However, we can predict increased risk for premature infants, low-birth-weight infants, infants placed to sleep prone or on their side, infants exposed to pre- or postnatal tobacco smoke, and so forth, opening the door for a variety of risk-reduction approaches.

MANAGEMENT

As Mandell et al. have described in several articles, the management of SIDS is the management of the surviving parents and the extended family, surviving siblings, and subsequent siblings. The parents and siblings have no warning and are frequently in a state of shock when they come into contact with the medical system. Parents often cannot believe what has happened. They may become angry, guilty, and self-blaming.

The pediatrician's role varies as the case evolves. Immediately after the death, the pediatrician can help the family cope with the initial shock and arrangements for death scene investigation and autopsy. The pediatrician should be an advocate for the proper investigation, as discussed above. Parents will ask, "What did we do wrong?" Because, in most cases, the parents did nothing wrong, appropriate counseling during this time can be of tremendous benefit to confused, self-blaming, self-questioning families. When death scene investigation results and autopsy results are available, the pediatrician should review these in detail with the family. Most often, these results will reassure the family that the death was not their fault. If some evidence of accident or injury is found, then disclosure of such information, as painful as it may be, could only be in the best interest of future children.

In addition to self-blaming, parents often have their own beliefs about SIDS, perhaps expressing concerns about environmental factors and risk to their other children. The father's reaction may be quite different from the mother's and may require a different counseling approach. All parents will be concerned about hereditary factors and the risk to subsequent children, and the pediatrician will be called on to counsel parents on these issues.

The pediatrician also experiences grief and anxiety when a patient dies of SIDS. It is natural to wonder what serious medical problem she might have missed. Fear of being held responsible may lead to intense self-questioning. One study of pediatricians' reactions to SIDS revealed sadness, shock, frustration, anger, guilt, regret, hurt, and feelings of inadequacy.

The reaction of a surviving sibling to SIDS in the family should not be overlooked. Young children do not understand. Older siblings are suddenly deprived of the role of older brother or older sister, often with devastating results. Surviving siblings may feel responsible, thinking that something they did caused the baby's death. Others deny their feelings. The pediatrician should anticipate these problems, inform parents, and if necessary counsel the children. Professional counseling may be necessary.

The pediatrician's role extends to when the parents decide to have subsequent children. One should anticipate that the birth of a subsequent child will raise many concerns and questions. A danger for the subsequent sibling is overprotection or the "vulnerable child" syndrome. The pediatrician can evaluate any actual risk and advise the parents appropriately. The articles by Mandell et al. provide a wealth of useful information concerning SIDS and the family.

HOME MONITORING

Home cardiorespiratory monitoring, as currently used in the United States, is intended to improve the outcome of any infant perceived to be at increased risk of sudden death. However, after decades, home monitoring has not decreased the incidence of SIDS. In 1986, the Consensus Development Conference on Infantile Apnea and Home Monitoring found that there were no reports of scientifically designed studies of the effectiveness of home monitoring on ALTE, subsequent siblings of SIDS victims, premature infants, or other pathologic conditions and, in 2004, this remains true. Current recommendations are summarized in Chapter 117A, Apparent Life-Threatening Events, Table 117A-6. The first recommendation of the 2003 American Academy of Pediatrics Policy Statement on Apnea, Sudden Infant Death Syndrome, and Home Monitoring states that "Home cardiorespiratory monitoring should not be prescribed to prevent SIDS." Therefore, at least according to current official guidelines, "SIDS prevention" is not an indication for home monitoring.

Pediatricians often have questions concerning when to discontinue home monitoring. No tests, including pneumograms or polysomnography, will answer this question. Discontinuing monitoring is a clinical decision based on the overall clinical picture. In general, monitoring can be discontinued when no significant abnormal cardiorespiratory events have occurred for several consecutive months.

Memory monitors, which provide a hard-copy printout of all alarm events, are in common use today. Although the monthly cost is higher than that for conventional cardiorespiratory monitoring, the overall cost is often lower because most alarm events are false (artifact). Much of the guesswork is taken out of monitor decision-making because the physician and parents can review the hard copy, be reassured that serious cardiorespiratory events did not occur, and discontinue the monitor sooner than it would have been using conventional monitoring.

PREVENTION

Pediatricians and family practitioners can have a major impact on SIDS through parent and caregiver education. In 2005, the question is not "Can the rate of SIDS be reduced by risk-reduction measures?" The question today is "How much more can SIDS be reduced by reducing risk exposure?" Since 1988 and 1989, in many countries, the rate of SIDS already has been reduced more than 50%, and by as much as 80% in some. Although progress has been made in the area of sleeping position, there has been very little, if any, impact on smoking during pregnancy or on postnatal ETS exposure. If current risk estimates are correct, by further reducing the rate of prone sleeping and reducing pre- and postnatal smoke exposure, it should be possible to reduce the U.S. SIDS rate by 80%, from the 1990 SIDS rate. Recommended and suggested risk reduction measures are shown in Table 117B.2.

TABLE 117B.2

SIDS RISK REDUCTION THROUGH CAREGIVER EDUCATION

1. **Recommend the supine sleeping position for healthy infants**
   The prone sleeping position is dangerous for infants. Side sleeping confers an intermediate risk of SIDS. The prone sleeping position is particularly dangerous for low birthweight and premature infants.
2. **Educate parents about the dangers of smoking during pregnancy and exposing the baby to tobacco smoke after birth**
   Smoke exposure increases the risk of SIDS and is particularly dangerous for low birthweight and premature infants.
3. **Recommend the use of a firm crib matterss, preferably CPSC approved**
   Any mattress design or material that interfaces with air circulation around the baby's face increases the potential for rebreathing exhaled air, increasing the risk of asphyxia and suffocation. Babies should not sleep on surfaces not approved for infants (e.g., sofas, bean-bag chairs, pillows).
4. **Inform parents that some bedding materials can be dangerous**
   Comforters, thick blankets, sheepskins, pillows, and some stuffed toys can cause an infant to rebreathe and asphyxiate. Parents should be informed to avoid these and other items, such as fluffy bumper pads, that increase the risk of suffocation.
5. **Educate parents about bed-sharing**
   Bed-sharing may have benefits for parent and child. However, bed-sharing also exposes the infant to adult bedding material which may be hazardous. In addition, infant bed-sharing with parents who smoke may increase smoke exposure. The pediatrician can help parents who wish to bed-share with their infant minimize risks and miximize benefits.
6. **Help parents be "informed consumers" of organized day care services**
   Day care providers may be unaware of the relationship between SIDS and sleeping position, hazardous sleeping environments, or smoke exposure. Parents can reduce the risk of SIDS at day care by being 'informed consumers' and giving specific instruction concerning the care of their infant at day care.
7. **Teach parents to avoid overheating**
   SIDS may be related to thermal stress due to overdressing the baby and/or overheating the room in some cases.

Suggested Readings

Aligne CA, Stoddard JJ. Tobacco and children. An economic evaluation of the medical effects of parental smoking. *Arch Pediatr Adolesc Med* 1997 Jul;151(7):648.

American Academy of Pediatrics—Task Force on Infant Positioning and SIDS: 1992. *Pediatrics* 1992;90:1120.

American Academy of Pediatrics—Committee on Child Abuse and Neglect and Committee on Community Health Services. Investigation and review of unexpected infant and child deaths. *Pediatrics* 1993;92(5):734.

American Academy of Pediatrics—Committee on Child Abuse and Neglect. Distinguishing sudden infant death syndrome from child abuse fatalities. *Pediatrics* 1994;94(1):124.

American Academy of Pediatrics—Task Force on Infant Positioning and SIDS. Positioning and sudden infant death syndrome (SIDS): update. *Pediatrics* 1996;98(6):1216.

American Academy of Pediatrics—Task Force on Infant Positioning and SIDS. Does bed sharing affect the risk of SIDS? *Pediatrics* 1997;100(2):272.

American Academy of Pediatrics—Committee on Environmental Health. Environmental tobacco smoke: a hazard to children. *Pediatrics* 1997;99(4):639.

Blair PS, Fleming PJ, Bensley D, et al. Smoking and the sudden infant death syndrome: results from 1993–1995 case-control study for confidential inquiry into stillbirths and deaths in infancy. Confidential Enquiry into Stillbirths and Deaths Regional Coordinators and Researchers. *Br Med J* 1996;313 (7051):195.

Bulterys MG, Greenland S, Krauss JF. Chronic fetal hypoxia and SIDS: interaction between maternal smoking and low hematocrit during pregnancy. *Pediatrics* 1990;86:535.

Centers for Disease Control—Guidelines for death scene investigation of sudden, unexplained infant deaths: recommendations of the interagency panel on sudden infant death syndrome. *June* 1996;45:RR-10.

Cnattingius S, Nordstrom ML. Maternal smoking and feto-infant mortality: biological pathways and public health significance. *Acta Paediat* 1996;85(12):1400.

Committee on Fetus and Newborn. American Academy of Pediatrics. Apnea, sudden infant death syndrome, and home monitoring. *Pediatrics* 2003;111(4 Pt 1):914.

Cote A, Gerez T, Brouillette RT, Laplante S. Circumstances leading to a change to prone sleeping in sudden infant death syndrome victims. *Pediatrics* 2000;106(6):E86.

DiFranza JR, Aligne CA, Weitzman M. Prenatal and postnatal environmental tobacco smoke exposure and children's health. *Pediatrics* 2004;113(4 Suppl):1007.

Fleming PJ, Blair PS, Bacon C, et al. Environment of infants during sleep and risk of the sudden infant death syndrome: results of 1993–1995 case-control study for confidential inquiry into stillbirths and deaths in infancy. Confidential Enquiry into Stillbirths and Deaths Regional Coordinators and Researchers. *Br Med J* 1996;313(7051):191.

Fleming PJ, Blair PS. Sudden unexpected deaths after discharge from the neonatal intensive care unit. *Semin Neonatol* 2003;8(2):159.

Filiano JJ, Kinney HC. A perspective on neuropathologic findings in victims of the sudden infant death syndrome: the triple-risk model. *Biol Neonate* 1994;65(3-4):194.

Goldwater PN. Sudden infant death syndrome: a critical review of approaches to research. *Arch Dis Child* 2003;88(12):1095.

Guntheroth WG, Lehmann R, Spiers PS. Risk of SIDS in subsequent siblings. *J Pediatr* 1990;116:520.

Guntheroth WG, Spiers PS. The triple risk hypotheses in sudden infant death syndrome. *Pediatrics* 2002;110(5):e64.

Hoffman H, Damus K, Hillman L, Krongrad E. Risk factors for SIDS: results of the National Institute of Child Health and Human Development SIDS cooperative epidemiological study. *Ann NY Acad Sci* 1988;533:13.

Hunt L, Fleming PJ, Golding J. Does the supine sleeping position have any adverse effects on the child? I. Health in the first six months. *Pediatrics* 1997;100(1):e11.

Klonoff-Cohen HS, Edelstein SL, Lefkowitz ES, et al. The effect of passive smoking and tobacco exposure through breast milk on sudden infant death syndrome. *JAMA* 1995;273(10):795.

Kraus JF, Greenland S, Bulterys M. Risk factors for SIDS in the U.S. Collaborative Perinatal Project. *Int J Epidemiol* 1989;18:113.

MacDorman MF, Cnattingius S, Hoffman HJ, et al. Sudden infant death syndrome and smoking in the United States and Sweden. *Am J Epidemiol* 1997;146(3):249.

Mandell F, Dirks-Smith T, Smith MF. The surviving child in the SIDS family. *Pediatrician* 1988;15:217.

Mandell F, McClain M. Supporting the SIDS family. *Pediatrician* 1988;15:179.

Mandell F, McClain M, Reece RM. Sudden and unexpected death: the pediatrician's response. *Am J Dis Child* 1987;141:748.

Mitchell EA. The changing epidemiology of SIDS following the national risk reduction campaigns. *Pediatr Pulmonol Suppl* 1997;16:117.

Mitchell EA, Tuohy PG, Brunt JM, et al. Risk factors for sudden infant death syndrome following the prevention campaign in New Zealand: a prospective study. *Pediatrics* 1997;100(5):835.

Moon RY, Patel KM, Shaefer SJ. Sudden infant death syndrome in child care settings. *Pediatrics* 2000;106(2 Pt 1):295.

Moon RY, Biliter WM. Infant sleep position policies in licensed child care centers after back to sleep campaign. *Pediatrics* 2000;106(3):576.

Moon RY, Biliter WM, Croskell SE. Examination of state regulations regarding infants and sleep in licensed child care centers and family child care settings. *Pediatrics* 2001;107(5):1029.

Moon RY, Oden RP. Back to sleep: can we influence child care providers? *Pediatrics* 2003;112(4):878.

Nicholl JP, O'Cathain A. Epidemiology of babies dying at different ages from SIDS. *J Epidemiol Community Health* 1989;43:13.

NIH Consensus Development Conference Proceedings. Infantile apnea and home monitoring. NIH publication no. 87-2905. U.S. Department of Health and Human Services, National Institutes of Health, 1986. [http://consensus.nih.gov/cons/058/058_intro.htm].

National Institutes of Health Consensus Development Conference on Infantile Apnea and Home Monitoring, Sept 29 to Oct 1, 1986. *Pediatrics* 1987; 79:292.

Oyen N, Markestad T, Skaerven R, et al. Combined effects of sleeping position and prenatal risk factors in sudden infant death syndrome: the Nordic Epidemiological SIDS Study. *Pediatrics* 1997;100:613.

Wennergren G. Combined effects of sleeping position and prenatal risk factors in sudden infant death syndrome: the Nordic Epidemiological SIDS Study. *Pediatrics* 1997;100(4):613.

Ramanathan R, Corwin MJ, Hunt CE, et al. ; for the Collaborative Home Infant Monitoring Evaluation (CHIME) Study Group. Cardiorespiratory events recorded on home monitors: comparison of healthy infants with those at increased risk for SIDS. *JAMA* 2001;285(17):2199.

Schellscheidt J, Oyen N, Jorch G. Interactions between maternal smoking and other prenatal risk factors for sudden infant death syndrome (SIDS). *Acta Paediat* 1997;86(8):857.

Shoemaker M, Ellis M, Meadows S, Gannons M. Should home apnea monitoring be recommended to prevents SIDS? *J Fam Pract* 2004;53(5):418.

Sundell HW. SIDS prevention—good progress, but now we need to focus on avoiding nicotine. *Acta Paediat* 2004;93(4):450.

Taylor JA, Krieger JW, Reay DT, et al. Prone sleep position and the sudden infant death syndrome in King County, Washington: a case-control study. *J Pediatr* 1996;128(5 Pt 1):626.

Taylor JA, Davis RL. Risk factors for the infant prone sleep position. *Arch Pediatr Adolesc Med* 1996;150(8):834.

Waters KA, Gonzalez A, Jean C, et al. Face-straight-down and face-near-straight-down positions in healthy, prone-sleeping infants. *J Pediatr* 1996;128(5 Pt 1):616.

Wennergren G, Alm B, Oyen N, et al. The decline in the incidence of SIDS in Scandinavia and its relation to risk-intervention campaigns. Nordic Epidemiological SIDS Study. *Acta Paediat* 1997;86(9):963.

CHAPTER 118 ■ ACUTE HEAD TRAUMA

N. PAUL ROSMAN

Throughout the world, trauma continues to be the leading cause of death and disabilities, with most of the deaths and almost all of the severe, prolonged disabilities being caused by traumatic damage to the nervous system. Pediatric head injuries are an important contributor to this morbidity and mortality; in the United States, 2 to 5 million children sustain some degree of head trauma each year. The frequency is greater in children 5 years of age and younger than in those who are older, with head injury being the most common neurologic cause of death and disability in young children. Such injuries, occurring twice as frequently in boys as in girls, have many different causes, including falls; bicycling, skateboarding, snowboarding, and other recreational activities; competitive sports (e.g., football, ice hockey, and boxing); motor vehicle accidents; hand gun injury; and physical assault, including child abuse (with 25% of cases of head trauma in children younger than 2 years of age being due to nonaccidental trauma).

Every year in the United States, approximately 200,000 children are hospitalized with head injuries, and approximately 5,000 children die as a result of such trauma. Of these 5,000 deaths, approximately 1,500 occur from child abuse. Mortality from pediatric head injuries has been estimated to be as high as 10 per 100,000 per year. The worldwide incidence of brain injury may be as high as 500 million cases per year.

Each year in the United States, almost 30,000 persons age 19 years or younger suffer permanent disability from moderate or severe head trauma. These disabilities include posttraumatic epilepsy, cognitive impairment, learning difficulties, and behavioral and emotional problems.

In this chapter, we review the anatomic and pathophysiologic basis of head injuries in children. An approach to the diagnosis and management of acute head injuries in children is given, and the clinical disorders observed in such children are described. The prognosis in acute brain injuries and their long-term effects are discussed.

PHYSIOLOGY

The scalp, skull, and brain all can suffer injury as a result of head trauma. Figure 118.1 depicts the brain, surrounding structures, and major associated pathologies that can complicate head trauma. The scalp, a highly vascular structure, is outermost; its inner surface is formed by the galea aponeurotica, a tendinous sheath connected anteriorly to the frontalis muscle and posteriorly to the occipitalis muscle. Beneath the galea is the subgaleal compartment, a potential space containing loose connective tissues. Next lies the skull, the outermost portion of which is the pericranium, or external periosteum. The outer and inner tables of the skull are separated by the diploic space, which is crossed by small veins. The dura lies immediately below the inner table of the skull and is relatively avascular when contrasted with the leptomeninges, which are applied closely to the brain and extend into the sulci for varying distances. Small-caliber veins within the leptomeninges cross the subdural space to drain into dural sinuses. The brain is bathed in and protected

by cerebrospinal fluid (CSF), the pathways of which include the cerebral subarachnoid spaces, cisterns at the base of the brain, ventricular cavities, interconnecting channels, and foramina. The intracranial vascular system includes large vessels (e.g., internal carotid arteries and dural sinuses), intermediate-sized vessels (e.g., middle cerebral arteries and veins), and small capillaries.

Intracranial pressure (ICP) is the sum total of pressures exerted by structures within the cranium. Brain tissue, the intracranial vascular tree, and CSF play roles in determining ICP, as does the bony cranium. The skull of the newborn or older infant is not a rigid box, but rather consists of several membranous bones, with fontanelles and unfused bony structures providing outlets for the increases in ICP that commonly occur in the head-injured child. By contrast, once the cranial sutures have fused, the foramen magnum provides the only major outlet through which increases in ICP can be accommodated.

DIAGNOSIS

Patient History

Children of different ages sustain various types of head traumas. The specific circumstances of head trauma must be determined, and the predisposing factors must be identified. Such information should be sought directly from an injured child whenever possible and also from observers, such as playmates, teachers, parents, ambulance attendants, or others at the scene of the accident. Under emergency circumstances, such as posttraumatic status epilepticus or acute intracranial hemorrhage,

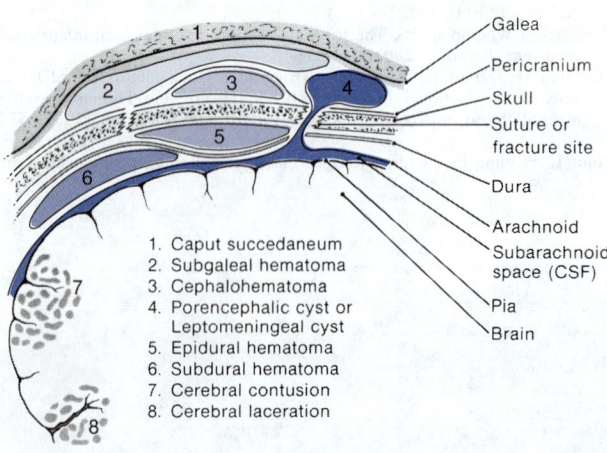

1. Caput succedaneum
2. Subgaleal hematoma
3. Cephalohematoma
4. Porencephalic cyst or Leptomeningeal cyst
5. Epidural hematoma
6. Subdural hematoma
7. Cerebral contusion
8. Cerebral laceration

Galea
Pericranium
Skull
Suture or fracture site
Dura
Arachnoid
Subarachnoid space (CSF)
Pia
Brain

FIGURE 118.1. The brain, surrounding structures, and major types of pathology after acute head injury. CSF, cerebrospinal fluid. (Reprinted with permission from Rosman NP, Herskovitz J, Carter AP, et al. Acute head trauma in infancy and childhood. *Pediatr Clin North Am* 1979;26:708.)

someone other than the person treating the injured child may be needed to obtain the history. Details of the accident should be supplemented by observations of memory loss, repetitive questioning, confusion, visual disturbance, and symptoms of increased ICP, such as altered consciousness, vomiting, severe headache, and changes in vital signs. A history of previous immunizations, drug allergies, current medications, and possible drug intoxication also should be obtained.

The principal mechanisms of head injury are contact and acceleration-deceleration. Lesions caused by an object striking the head, or vice versa, include scalp laceration, skull fracture, epidural hematoma, brain contusion, and intracerebral hemorrhage. By contrast, acceleration-deceleration, which results from head movement immediately after the injury, leads to intracranial and intracerebral pressure gradients and to shear, tensile, and compressive strains. Such inertial (nonimpact) lesions are responsible for cerebral concussion, diffuse axonal injury, and acute subdural hematoma.

General Physical Examination

Vital signs demand immediate diagnostic study and sometimes mandate emergency treatment. Characteristic changes in pulse, blood pressure, and respirations may indicate shock (i.e., decreased blood pressure and increased pulse) or increased ICP (i.e., increased blood pressure, decreased or increased pulse, slowed or irregular respirations). Usually, a decrease in blood pressure in the head-injured child is caused by an injury in another location, such as thoracic, intraabdominal, or retroperitoneal hemorrhage or bleeding into soft tissues surrounding a long-bone fracture. Occasionally, however, bleeding into the scalp may be sufficient to produce shock (as with subgaleal hematoma) or bleeding inside the skull (as with epidural hematoma). Other causes for hypotension in the head-injured child are spinal cord injury, cardiac contusion or tamponade, and tension pneumothorax.

The entire body should be scrutinized for signs of trauma. Physical examination should include a search for injury to the neck, chest, abdomen, and long bones and a careful inspection of the skin. Long-bone fractures, which occur in one-third of patients with severe head injuries, may be complicated by fat embolism. The neck should be examined with care, because of possible injury. In cases of suspected neck trauma, the neck should not be moved; the neck is immobilized by sandbags and adhesive tape or a firm collar. Such injury is suggested by cervical abrasions or cervical spine tenderness. Meningismus can result from cervical trauma, subarachnoid blood, or herniation of the cerebellar tonsils.

The head must be examined carefully. The scalp should be inspected and palpated for tenderness or depression. All scalp lacerations should be probed with a sterile-gloved finger in search of a foreign body or an underlying skull fracture. Tension of the anterior fontanelle should be assessed in young infants. Transillumination of the skull in infants and young children may detect abnormal accumulations of fluid, including blood, outside or inside the skull. Cranial ultrasound examination may be helpful when the anterior fontanelle is open. Periorbital hemorrhage (raccoon-eyes sign), ecchymosis behind the ear (Battle sign), blood behind the eardrum (hemotympanum), and bleeding from the ears or nose should be noted. These signs, along with CSF otorrhea or rhinorrhea, indicate a basilar skull fracture.

Neurologic Examination

The neurologic examination should include an assessment of the child's alertness, orientation, and memory; a neuro-

ophthalmologic examination; and testing of motor and sensory functions, reflexes, and coordination. When possible, testing of orientation and memory should include the child's account of the episode that caused the head trauma. The presence and extent of any retrograde and anterograde (posttraumatic) amnesia should be determined. Additional assessment of memory should include testing of the child's digit span and recall of several items after 5 minutes. A child's repeated asking of the same question is reminiscent of Korsakoff psychosis, a posttraumatic, anterograde-type memory disturbance.

The level of consciousness may range widely. The Glasgow Coma Scale (GCS) (Table 118.1A), with scores ranging from 3 (worst) to 15 (best), provides a useful and reproducible scoring system for quantifying the level of consciousness and for systematically following a head-injured child's clinical course. The child's best motor response (score, 6 to 1), best verbal response (score, 5 to 1), and eye opening (score, 4 to 1) are assessed. In the young, nonverbal child, modifications in the GCS must be made. Although a variety of coma scales have been proposed for pediatric practice, a modification of the GCS that has been particularly useful is seen in Table 118.1B. In the child younger than 1 year, with eye opening, the verbal stimulus used is a shout rather than a command and for the best motor response, spontaneous movements rather than those in response to commands are assessed. With verbal response in children 5 years or younger, a score of 5 is given for appropriate words and phrases (2 to 5 years) or babbling and cooing (0 to 2 years); a 4 is given for inappropriate words (2 to 5 years) or consolable crying (0 to 2 years); a 3 is given for persistent crying or screaming to pain (0 to 5 years); a 2 is given for grunting or moaning to pain (0 to 5 years); otherwise, the same criteria as in the older child are used in scoring the younger child's responses. Although most studies have reported a correlation between a low GCS score and severe neurologic morbidity and substantial mortality rates, children with a low GCS score (3 to 5) sometimes do surprisingly well if the head injury has not been complicated by a hypoxic-ischemic insult. Numerous factors, including intubation, orbital swelling, sedation, and neuromuscular blockade, interfere with accurate scoring with the GCS, thus limiting its predictive value.

TABLE 118.1A

GLASGOW COMA SCALE

Response	Score
Eye opening	
Spontaneous	4
To speech	3
To pain	2
Nil	1
Best motor response	
Obeys	6
Localizes	5
Withdraws	4
Abnormal flexion	3
Extends	2
Nil	1
Verbal response	
Oriented	5
Confused conversation	4
Inappropriate words	3
Incomprehensible sounds	2
Nil	1

Reprinted with permission from Jennett B, Teasdale G. Aspects of coma after severe head injury, *Lancet* 1977;1:878.

TABLE 118.1B

GLASGOW COMA SCALE MODIFIED FOR PEDIATRIC PATIENTS

Eye response

Score	*>1 yr*	*<1 yr*	
4	Spontaneous	Spontaneous	
3	To verbal command	To shout	
2	To pain	To pain	
1	None	None	

Motor response

Score	*>1 yr*	*<1 yr*	
6	Obeys commands	Spontaneous	
5	Localizes pain	Localizes pain	
4	Withdraws to pain	Withdraws to pain	
3	Abnormal flexion to pain (decorticate)	Abnormal flexion to pain (decorticate)	
2	Abnormal extension to pain (decerebrate)	Abnormal extension to pain (decerebrate)	
1	None	None	

Verbal response

Score	*>5 yr*	*2–5 yr*	*0–2 yr*
5	Oriented and converses	Appropriate words and phrases	Babbles, coos
4	Confused conversation	Inappropriate words	Cries but is consolable
3	Inappropriate words	Persistent crying or screaming to pain	Persistent crying or screaming to pain
2	Incomprehensible sounds	Grunts or moans to pain	Grunts or moans to pain
1	None	None	None

Scoring: Severe, <9; moderate, 9–12; mild, 13–15.

Neuro-ophthalmologic evaluation should include a measurement of pupillary size and reactivity. Small pupils are seen with diencephalic and pontine injuries; a unilateral dilated pupil suggests temporal lobe herniation on the same side. The fundi should be examined carefully, with evidence of retinal and preretinal (subhyaloid) hemorrhages and papilledema specifically sought. Abnormalities of ocular gaze and position may include roving eye movements, limited lateral and vertical gaze, and skew deviation. When clearly no neck injury has occurred, the oculocephalic (doll's-eye) maneuver can be used to assess any apparent limitation of eye movements. This procedure is performed with the child supine by rotating the head to one side and then the other. When the head is moved to the left, the eyes should deviate to the right (and vice versa) if brainstem pathways controlling eye movements are functioning normally. Lateral gaze can be tested also in the comatose patient by caloric stimulation: The child's head is elevated 30 degrees above horizontal, and one external auditory canal is irrigated with ice water. If brainstem function is normal, the eyes should turn toward the ear being irrigated. An important precaution is ascertaining that the auditory canal is clear and that the eardrum is intact before performing this test. In an alert child, testing of visual acuity, visual fields, and optikokinetic nystagmus also should be performed.

The extent of examination of the motor system will depend on the child's alertness. When the child is comatose, abnormal posturing (e.g., decorticate, decerebrate) should be sought. Noxious stimulation, such as a sternal rub, may be required to produce such posturing. Muscle tone may be reduced (hypotonia) or increased (spasticity or rigidity) in a hemiparetic or paraparetic distribution. In a responsive child, motor impairment can be detected by testing individual muscles, examining conventional gait and stressed gait, and observing the outstretched arms for evidence of a drift. Also, performing sensory testing may be possible. The neurologic examination is completed by testing for abnormal reflexes, such as a palmar grasp, suck, or root; by eliciting deep-tendon reflexes; and by checking for plantar responses.

Investigative Studies

Plain Radiography

The need for radiologic examination of the child with a head injury is determined by the severity of the head trauma as reflected by alterations in consciousness and by the presence or absence of focal neurologic signs. Enthusiasm for eliminating unnecessary and expensive radiologic examinations in children with minor head trauma is increasing, because of the infrequency with which abnormalities are found. Although many physicians recommend that plain skull radiography be abandoned in favor of performing immediate cranial computed tomography (CT), which is a wise approach in a severely head-injured child who needs immediate care, many fractures (e.g., linear, basilar, and facial fractures; focal depressions) are visualized better on skull radiographs than with CT. Awareness of the presence of such fractures is important; for example, a fracture of the squamous temporal bone may overlie an acute epidural hematoma, and a parietal fracture may be the site of a fracture that later begins to grow.

Severe head injury with significant loss of consciousness and focal neurologic signs (GCS score, 3 to 8) requires plain radiography and further radiologic study in most patients, after blood loss is controlled and cardiorespiratory stability is established. The initial examination in severe head trauma should include anteroposterior and lateral views of the cervical spine. It also should include anteroposterior, inclined anteroposterior (Towne), and both lateral views of the skull. At least one lateral view should be taken with a horizontal beam (cross-table) to demonstrate any air–fluid levels in the cranial cavity or in the paranasal sinuses (indicative of compound or basal fracture). If a depressed skull fracture is suspected, both standard views and tangential views of the area should be obtained. With extensive head or facial trauma, radiography should include a Waters projection of the facial bones and films of the orbits. In moderate head trauma with localizing neurologic signs or a history of loss of consciousness (GCS score 9 to 12), routine skull radiography alone usually will suffice. When the patient has no history of neck injury, obtaining cervical spine films probably is unnecessary. In mild head trauma without focal neurologic signs or loss of consciousness (GCS score 13 to 15), usually skull and spine films are not needed. Aside from skull and spine films, additional radiography (i.e., chest, pelvis, long bones) frequently is indicated, depending on clinical circumstances.

Cranial Computed Tomography and Magnetic Resonance Imaging

In the presence of more severe head trauma or localizing neurologic signs, many imaging modalities are available, but the most helpful and least invasive is cranial CT. A cranial CT scan probably should be done also in anyone who has lost consciousness after a head injury, is amnestic for the injury, or has signs of a basilar or calvarial fracture. With persistent or progressing neurologic signs, a CT scan should be done as soon as possible, the child's clinical state permitting. Cranial magnetic resonance imaging (MRI) has had an increasing role in the evaluation of head-injured children. Advantages of MRI include safety (no known biologic hazards and no reported side effects), the ability to image in any plane, excellent depiction of normal and pathologic anatomy, the ability to identify vessels without contrast injection (magnetic resonance angiography), and superiority to cranial CT in demonstrating the posterior fossa, where bone artifacts interfere with CT imaging. Further, MRI often will show parenchymal abnormalities in head-injured patients in whom no abnormalities are seen on CT. However, substantial limitations in using MRI with critically ill patients exist, particularly the inability to monitor such patients while they are being imaged. Thus, with acute head injuries, CT almost always is the imaging procedure of choice, whereas MRI is of greatest assistance in evaluating subacute and chronic injuries.

Usually, unilateral intracranial hemorrhage is readily evident on CT as a relatively dense mass during the immediate posttraumatic period, when the study should be performed without the infusion of a contrast medium. Recognizing acute bleeding (bleeding present within the first 1 to 3 days after injury), both extra-axial (as with subdural hemorrhage) and intra-axial (as with cerebral contusion), frequently is more difficult with MRI than with CT. This limitation arises because the deoxyhemoglobin in such lesions causes a signal that is isointense with brain on T1-weighted images and is hypointense on T2-weighted images. By contrast, edema surrounding areas of acute parenchymal hemorrhage is well-visualized with MRI because T2-weighted images of edema show high signal intensity. Because of the ease of obtaining sections in multiple planes with MRI and because no MRI signal is transmitted by bone, small collections of blood (e.g., a thin convexity extra-axial hematoma) may be visualized more easily with MRI than with CT. For this reason, MRI is more useful than is CT in imaging the posterior fossa. The sensitivity of MRI was illustrated in a series of 50 head-injured patients studied radiologically within 1 week of sustaining injury. Abnormalities indicating primary brain damage were found twice as often with MRI as with cranial CT.

After several days, blood that is broken down incompletely may be of the same density as contiguous brain; thus, if a CT scan (rather than MRI) is performed at that time, it should be done with and without intravenous iodinated contrast material. Vital signs and neurologic status should be monitored carefully because the potential for reactions to iodinated contrast is the same regardless of whether it is used for intravenous pyelography, angiography, or CT. Provision should be made for the management of these reactions at the time of injection and for several hours thereafter. When contrast is not used, and intracranial hemorrhage is not apparent, a hemorrhage still may be suspected if a deformation of ventricular structures or a shift of the midline is present. With bilateral lesions, such as acute subdural hematomas of infancy, a shift of midline structures may not occur. Bilateral intracranial hemorrhages also may produce ventricular enlargement through the blockage of the cerebral subarachnoid spaces or may cause reduction in ventricular size through compression of brain tissue. CT also can show brain edema with reduced ventricular size, loss of brain tissue with ventricular enlargement, and most skull fractures.

MRI is especially useful for detecting lesions that are isodense on CT, such as subacute extra-axial hematomas (3 to 14 days) and chronic extra-axial hematomas (greater than 14 days). Such lesions disclose high signal intensity on both T1- and T2-weighted images because of the formation of methemoglobin in subacute hematomas and increased protein content in hematomas that have become chronic. Diffuse white-matter shearing injuries are visualized very well with MRI because these lesions disclose increased signal intensity on T2-weighted images.

A great value of both CT and MRI is their use in documenting an intracranial process over the course of time. Although initial studies performed within a few hours of injury may be negative or may disclose only minor changes, follow-up studies may document changes in the size of a lesion, appearance of new lesions, brain swelling, deformation of the ventricular system, shift of midline structures, or brain herniation. Later studies also can show chronic sequelae of head injury, such as hydrocephalus and brain atrophy.

Ultrasonography

In newborns or young infants with open fontanelles and sutures, real-time cranial ultrasonography may be very useful in demonstrating intracranial blood (i.e., intraventricular, parenchymal, subarachnoid), displacement of the ventricular system, hydrocephalus, encephalomalacia, and brain calcifications.

Magnetic Resonance Angiography

In some cases of head trauma, magnetic resonance angiography may be needed to demonstrate injuries to major vessels of the head and neck. Additionally, it is helpful in providing supportive evidence for the determination of brain death.

Lumbar Puncture

Lumbar puncture (LP) should not be performed in a head-injured child unless complicating central nervous system (CNS) infection is suspected. Usually, an LP is contraindicated when significantly increased ICP is present, and one is absolutely contraindicated when evidence of an intracranial mass exists. LP may yield evidence of infection, as with meningitis complicating a basilar skull fracture; of recent subarachnoid bleeding, as with cerebral contusion; of older subarachnoid bleeding, as with xanthochromic CSF accompanying a chronic subdural hematoma; and of increased ICP, which can complicate several types of head injuries.

Subdural Taps

Subdural taps may be indicated as a diagnostic measure, as a therapeutic measure, or both. A maximum of 15 mL of fluid is removed from each subdural space without aspiration; within 1 to 2 days, the taps can be repeated.

Other Studies

In moderately and severely injured children and in those in whom the cause or circumstances of the injury are unknown, additional studies may be indicated. They include complete blood cell count; serum amylase; urinalysis; platelet and clotting studies; toxic screen on blood, urine, and gastric aspirate; and skeletal survey for old and recent fractures.

TREATMENT

General Support

The management of the child with head injury must be directed to the entire patient. The head and neck must be stabilized; with suspected neck trauma, a firm cervical collar (Philadelphia type) or sandbags or tape and Velcro straps attached to a backboard should be used. Life-threatening obstruction of the airway may result from blood, vomiting, secretions, a foreign object, or the tongue (the last especially with severe mandibular fractures). Accessible foreign objects should be removed, and patency of the airway maximized by proper positioning. Usually, a chin lift will relieve upper airway obstruction. If any concern about an accompanying cervical spine injury exists, a jaw thrust, not a chin lift, with the head kept in a neutral position, should be used to open the airway.

Ventilatory management is assisted by inserting an oral airway into the oropharynx; if needed, ventilatory support should be provided. Suctioning should be performed without touching the carina. In comatose children and in others with airway obstruction or ineffective respiratory effort with a diminished gag and cough, and in patients with a GCS of less than 8, orotracheal or nasotracheal intubation usually is needed. Nasotracheal intubation should not be used if a basal skull fracture is suspected. Intubation diminishes the risk of aspiration (of oropharyngeal secretions, blood, or vomitus) and the risk of airway obstruction, assists in tracheal suctioning, and is mandatory for controlled ventilation. The head and neck should be moved with great care, so any associated neck injury is not exacerbated. Optimal conditions for intubation are provided by rapid induction of intravenous anesthesia with propofol 1 to 2 mg/kg or etomidate 1.5 to 3 mg/kg; with any hemodynamic instability, however, a combination of fentanyl, 1 to 5 μg/kg, and midazolam, 0.1 mg/kg, could be given intravenously instead. Intravenous lidocaine, 1 to 1.5 mg/kg, should be given 1 to 2 minutes before intubation, with neuromuscular blockade accomplished with intravenous high-dose vecuronium, 0.2 to 0.3 mg/kg, or vecuronium, 0.01 mg, followed by succinyl choline, 1.5 mg/kg. Oxygen (100%) should be given at 3 to 10 L/minute by bag and mask or by nasal prongs, with the P_aO_2 maintained at 90 to 100 mm Hg. Cardiac rate and rhythm should be monitored.

An intravenous line should be established; blood testing should include hematocrit, type and cross-match, and amylase (for evidence of pancreatic injury). Sites of hemorrhage must be controlled, and blood volume must be maintained. With infrequent exceptions, shock is not a sign of head injury in children. It usually is caused by associated injury, such as rupture of an abdominal organ (e.g., liver); bleeding into extracranial soft tissues (as with a pelvic fracture); peritonitis (after spillage of contents from a ruptured intestine); traumatic pancreatitis; or associated spinal cord injury ("spinal shock"). Occasionally, however, rapid intracranial bleeding into the epidural space or even into the scalp can cause shock. In all children with severe head injury, a central venous line to monitor central venous pressure should be placed, and an arterial line should be inserted to monitor arterial blood pressure, assess cerebral perfusion pressure, and facilitate blood gas measurements. Normal systolic blood pressure varies with age: 50 to 60 mm Hg in neonates; 70 to 80 in toddlers; 80 to 90 in school-aged children; and 90 to 100 in adolescents. Mean systemic arterial blood pressure should be maintained at 65 mm Hg at least to ensure adequate cerebral circulation. Hypovolemia (greater than 20% blood volume loss) is corrected by intravenous crystalloid (such as lactated Ringer solution or normal saline) or colloid (hydroxyethyl starch or 5% albumin in a bolus of 10 to 20 mL/kg, repeated as necessary to establish adequate perfusion).

A slowing in pulse rate may indicate an encouraging response to treatment for circulatory insufficiency, but it also can be a danger signal, reflecting increased ICP. Circulatory failure with a fall in blood pressure is treated with volume replacement, after which epinephrine, 0.1 to 0.5 μg/kg/minute, or norepinephrine, 0.05 to 0.2 μg/kg/minute, can be given. With cardiac arrest, in addition to ventilation and chest compressions, the child should be treated in accordance with the Pediatric Advanced Life Support (PALS) recommendations.

Accompanying injuries, such as those to the scalp, chest (especially pneumothorax), great vessels, abdominal viscera, pelvis, limbs, or spine, may require specific treatment. Chest films aimed at looking for rib fractures, hemopneumothorax, and mediastinal widening should be obtained. With suspected abdominal bleeding or intestinal perforation, abdominal ultrasonography, CT scanning, or diagnostic peritoneal lavage should be performed.

Pseudosubluxations of the cervical spine, especially at C2 to C3 and C3 to C4, found normally in approximately 20% of children in the first decade of life, may be sources of unnecessary concern. Fractured limbs should be splinted. The stomach should be emptied by nasogastric intubation (to prevent vomiting, aspiration, and pressure on the diaphragm, causing secondary respiratory compromise), and the bladder should be catheterized. Fever should be controlled by sponging and antipyretics. When circulatory status is adequate, the intake of iso-osmolar fluids should be given at or slightly above normal maintenance. Electrolyte abnormalities and coagulation defects should be corrected. Vital signs should be followed with care. An elevation of systolic blood pressure, a slowing or speeding of the pulse, and slowed or irregular respirations are indicative of intracranial hypertension (see section, Raised Intracranial Pressure). When seizures occur, anticonvulsants should be given (see section, Posttraumatic Seizures).

Emergency Room Management of a Child with Mild Head Trauma

Children, adolescents, and young adults frequently are evaluated in emergency departments after sustaining minor head trauma. Useful data concerning the management of such children are few in number and not uncommonly conflicting. Thus, the American Academy of Pediatrics (AAP) and the American Academy of Family Practice (AAFP) have developed a Clinical Practice Guideline to assist in managing patients between 2 and 20 years of age who have sustained an isolated, minor, closed head injury. By definition, such patients show a normal mental status on initial examination, have no focal or otherwise abnormal findings on neurologic examination, and have no physical evidence of skull fracture. Additionally, they may or may not have sustained a brief (less than a minute) loss of consciousness, they may have had a seizure immediately after their head injury, they may have vomited, and they may have developed headache and lethargy.

When no loss of consciousness has occurred in such children, following a thorough history and physical and neurologic examinations, the child should be observed for at least 24 hours in the clinic, office, emergency department, and/or at home under the care of a competent adult; careful observation should continue for the next several days, watching for any change in the patient's clinical status. CT scanning, skull radiographs, or MRI rarely are needed. When a brief loss of consciousness has occurred following such head injury, a slightly increased risk of an intracranial injury (1% to 5% versus less than 1% with no loss of consciousness) exists. Again, following a thorough history and physical and neurologic examinations, the child should be observed in any of the above settings and/or at home under the care of a competent adult. Because of its sensitivity and specificity, cranial CT scanning may be useful in identifying the small number of such patients in whom some intracranial abnormality is present, although only rarely are medical, neurosurgical, or other interventions needed. Factors that may indicate a clearer need for CT scanning include a delay from the time of injury until the time when the patient is first seen, a scalp hematoma overlying the course of the middle meningeal artery, and those few patients with minor head trauma in whom clinical worsening occurs. Skull radiographs or MRI are almost never needed. If imaging seems desirable, cranial CT scanning is the best modality to use; if the CT scan is normal, an adverse outcome is very unlikely.

In children younger than 2 years of age who have had a minor head injury, the risk for skull fracture and intracranial injury is higher than in older patients. Additionally, clinical assessment is more difficult in very young children, and their risk for nonaccidental injury is higher. Thus, based on the assessed risk for intracranial injury, four guidelines have been suggested for the evaluation and management of children younger than 2 years old following a minor head injury:

- In those determined to be of high risk for intracranial injury, a cranial CT scan should be done.
- In those who show symptoms indicating possible intracranial injury, a CT scan should be done or the child should be observed for at least 4 to 6 hours post-injury, watching for any new symptoms or signs. If any develop, a CT scan should be done. If none develop, the child can be discharged home under the watchful eye of a competent adult.
- When some risk for skull fracture or intracranial injury is apparent, a CT scan and/or skull radiographs should be done or, alternatively, the child should be observed for 4 to 6 hours post-injury and then discharged home if no change has occurred.
- Finally, when the risk of intracranial injury appears to be very low, skull radiographs are not needed, but the child must be observed carefully in the manner described above.

It is important to stress that, whereas all the above guidelines are reasonable suggestions, proposed by health professionals knowledgeable about pediatric head injuries, these guidelines are not supported by large numbers of controlled clinical studies. In some cases, clinical judgment should take precedence, and if the clinician is concerned, even if the child looks well, CT scanning should be performed.

Hospitalization

Many factors influence the decision concerning whether to hospitalize head-injured children. Hospitalization is indicated or should be considered seriously with changing vital signs; posttraumatic seizures; altered mental status, particularly prolonged unconsciousness; persisting memory deficit; focal neurologic signs; depressed skull fracture; basilar skull fracture; enlarging scalp swelling; persisting severe headache, especially with neck stiffness; recurrent vomiting; unexplained fever; neuroradiologic abnormalities of concern; and an unexplained injury raising the question of possible child abuse.

Posttraumatic Seizures

Early posttraumatic seizures or early posttraumatic epilepsy, which occurs within the first week after head injury, develops in approximately 5% of children hospitalized after encurring a head trauma. Of these children, 20% to 30% will have additional seizures beyond the first week. Infants and young children are at greater risk for the development of early posttraumatic seizures than are older children and adults. The incidence of early posttraumatic seizures that occur after severe traumatic brain injury in children varies from 20% to 40%. The risk is greater with lower GCS scores. After adjustment for the GCS and the duration of coma, the risk of early posttraumatic seizures occurring after severe head injury is three times greater in infants than in older children to age 12 years.

The management of posttraumatic seizures in children is essentially the same as that of nontraumatic seizures. Phenytoin (Dilantin) is the drug of choice because of its rapid entry into the brain and its lack of a prominent sedative effect. It should be administered intravenously in a dose of 18 to 20 mg/kg (rate, 25 to 50 mg/minute) while the pulse and electrocardiogram are monitored for bradycardia, arrhythmias, and hypotension. The maximum dosage is 1,000 mg. Phenytoin, given intravenously, must be administered with care; if it should infiltrate into the skin and subcutaneous tissues, it can cause severe tissue necrosis. As an alternative to phenytoin, fosphenytoin can be given. Although it is much more expensive than is phenytoin, it has several clinical advantages. It not only can be given intravenously, it can be given at three times the rate of phenytoin; it also can be given intramuscularly, which is of great assistance when intravenous access is a problem; additionally, it is much less irritating than is phenytoin at the injection site. Fosphenytoin is rapidly converted to phenytoin after administration. The usual loading dose is 15 to 20 mg/kg. If seizure activity continues, intravenous diazepam (Valium) can be administered in a dose of 0.2 to 0.5 mg/kg (maximum rate, 1 to 2 mg/minute), with a total dosage not greater than 2 to 4 mg in infants or 5 to 10 mg in older children. The same dose of diazepam can be repeated every 10 to 30 minutes, for a total of three doses if necessary. Lorazepam (Ativan) is a benzodiazepine, structurally similar to diazepam but with a longer duration of action. It is given intravenously in a dose of 0.05 to 0.1 mg/kg (maximum rate, 1 mg/minute), for a maximum total dosage of 4 mg. If needed, an additional 0.05 mg/kg can be given 10 minutes later.

Phenobarbital is another drug that can be given for seizures complicating acute head injuries. It should be administered intravenously in a dose of 15 to 20 mg/kg (rate, 30 to 100 mg/minute). If necessary, one-half of the initial dose can be repeated after 1 hour and every 4 to 6 hours thereafter (maximum dosage, 300 mg).

Any of these drugs, given individually or in combination, can cause respiratory depression; thus, the treating physician must be prepared to manage the airway and/or to intubate.

In the head-injured patient who has not had a seizure, prophylactic antiepileptic drugs have not proved to be beneficial in preventing later epilepsy. At least ten well-controlled studies of seizure prophylaxis after head injury have been reported.

All these studies have enrolled patients at high risk for the development of posttraumatic seizures, usually those with severe head injuries, and have compared one or two active drugs to placebo or to no drug; in most of these studies, treatment was begun within 24 hours. Both carbamazepine and less consistently, phenytoin have been shown to be effective in preventing early posttraumatic seizures, but neither of these drugs (nor phenobarbital) has been shown to be effective in preventing late posttraumatic seizures in head-injured patients.

Increased Intracranial Pressure

ICP, the summation of pressures derived from structures within the cranium, is determined by pressures exerted by brain, cerebral blood vessels, and CSF. ICP is elevated if it measures more than 20 to 25 mm Hg in adults, more than 15 mm Hg in older children and adolescents, more than 5 mm Hg in children 1 to 5 years, or more than 3 mm Hg in newborns. In acute head trauma, causes of increased ICP include bleeding (into the epidural, subdural, or subarachnoid spaces or into the brain), brain hyperemia with diffuse brain swelling (days 2 to 3 after injury), brain edema accompanying brain contusion or hematoma (days 3 to 5), acute hydrocephalus from subarachnoid bleeding and impaired resorption of CSF (days 7 to 10), and pseudotumor cerebri.

The brain can adapt temporarily to increased ICP by displacing CSF through the foramen magnum into the distensible lumbar subarachnoid space; some adaptation also is accomplished by compressing the low-pressure intracranial venous system. The major adaptive mechanism, however, is an increase in the rate of CSF resorption, which can increase to as much as 2 mL/minute or to six times its rate of formation. When these mechanisms no longer can compensate adequately for the rise in ICP, clinical signs of increased ICP become evident. The clinical symptoms and signs of acutely increased ICP are demonstrated in Table 118.2. No single treatment for increased ICP exists. Therapeutic modalities used include supportive measures and medical and surgical treatments.

Supportive Measures

When ICP is increased, respiratory support must be provided. Sedative and paralytic agents (noted in the section, General Support), which do not increase (and which may decrease) ICP, should be given. Circulatory support also should be provided (as described in General Support). With worsening intracranial hypertension and impending herniation, rapid-sequence intubation and monitoring of blood gases are essential. The head should be elevated to 30 degrees above horizontal and should be stabilized in the midline. Seizures must be arrested with intravenous anticonvulsants. Sufficient fluid should be given to maintain the patient in a state of isotonic normovolemia. The maintenance of an adequate blood volume is essential to ensure a satisfactory cerebral perfusion pressure (CPP) to help to control intracranial hypertension. Efforts should be made to maintain a CPP of at least 70 mm Hg in adults, 60 mm Hg in adolescents, and 40 mm Hg in children. Sometimes crystalloid, colloid, or vasopressors are required. Under normal circumstances, one should try to maintain serum osmolality between 300 and 320 mOsm/L. Fever should be treated aggressively with antipyretics and a cooling blanket if needed.

Intracranial Pressure Monitoring

Continuous monitoring of ICP has been especially valuable in poorly responsive head-injured patients because following such patients by clinical parameters alone is difficult. Although the criteria for ICP monitoring in head trauma have not been established firmly, most physicians would advocate its use in head injuries when a patient's GCS score is 5 or less, or is 8 or less with CT evidence of a mass lesion or brain injury (such as contusion, shearing, or diffuse cerebral swelling). Such monitoring also is indicated in head-injured children who are unconscious or in shock, who have a deteriorating neurologic examination, or whose CT scan shows distortion or displacement of brain. Patients whose ICP is being monitored also should have arterial and central venous lines placed, and vital signs should be monitored continuously. Such patients should be managed in an intensive care unit.

The advantages of monitoring ICP are the ability to measure a patient's ICP and to assess the need for treatment, its efficacy, and the duration of treatment to maintain (when possible) a CSF pressure of less than 20 mm Hg. Also, although elevations in ICP may be accompanied by signs of acute brainstem dysfunction, sometimes no clinical change is observed. Thus, intracranial monitoring can be highly valuable in providing early recognition of damaging (and potentially lethal) elevations of ICP.

Monitors for ICP can be classified into those using fluid to couple the ICP to an external transducer (e.g., ventricular catheter) and those that are not fluid-coupled (e.g., intraparenchymal fiberoptic pressure monitor; external anterior fontanelle monitor, using a counter balancing pressure system). Fluid-coupled monitors include those placed in the subarachnoid space or, more often, those placed into the ventricular system. Recordings from ventricular catheters are accurate and reliable, and ventricular access allows drainage of CSF to lower ICP, although occasionally, when such withdrawal is excessive, epidural or subdural hematomas develop. Also, brain penetration is required, and infections occur in 2% to 12% of cases, although most such infections are not clinically significant. Rarely, seizures may develop.

Intraparenchymal fiberoptic pressure devices have a small diameter that allows recording from virtually any intracranial space and from brain parenchyma, and they are more accurate than are external anterior fontanelle monitors. Although intraparenchymal catheters have been used for as long as several weeks without complicating infection, and although the risk of hemorrhage is less than 0.5%, difficulties with calibration and fractures of the fiberoptic elements can contribute to spurious ICP recordings.

TABLE 118.2

CLINICAL SYMPTOMS AND SIGNS OF ACUTELY RAISED INTRACRANIAL PRESSURE

Infants
Full fontanelle
Separated sutures
(Macrocrania)
(Papilledema)

Children
Headache
Papilledema

Both
Altered mental state
Vomiting
Strabismus [cranial nerve VI, (III) palsies]; "setting sun" sign
Altered vital signs (increased blood pressure, decreased or increased pulse rate, decreased or irregular respirations)
(Signs of herniation)

Rosman NP, Oppenheimer EY, O'Connor JF. Emergency management of pediatric head injuries. *Emerg Med Clin North Am* 1983;1:149.

Although the many advantages provided by ICP monitoring are undeniable, in some situations, the monitoring can be falsely reassuring. For instance, temporal lobe or posterior fossa lesions can cause local increases in pressure that are undetected by conventionally placed monitoring devices; also, placing the monitor contralateral to the side of a supratentorial mass tends to give a lower ICP reading than does placing the monitor ipsilateral to the mass. ICP monitoring has had its greatest impact in managing severe brain injuries, in which elevations of ICP occur commonly, and numerous studies have shown that the control of such elevations improves clinical outcome.

Medical Management

In the absence of ventricular drainage, or as an adjunct to ventricular drainage, which can be intermittent or continuous, several medical measures are useful in managing acutely elevated ICP with head trauma. These treatments are summarized in Table 118.3. An important consideration in choosing therapeutic alternatives is to remember that, although brain swelling sometimes will occur during the first 2 to 3 days after a head injury because of an increase in cerebral blood volume, cerebral blood flow can be diminished markedly during the first day. Between days 3 to 5, increases in ICP usually are the result of cerebral edema. A further elevation of ICP often is seen on days 7 to 10, probably secondary to communicating hydrocephalus, with an increase in CSF volume caused by interference in its reabsorption.

Osmolar Therapies

Two osmolar therapies (mannitol, hypertonic saline) are very useful in the management of raised ICP. Brain capillaries (the site of the blood brain barrier) are nearly impenetrable to both mannitol and saline. Mannitol is the cornerstone in the management of raised ICP in pediatric and adult traumatic brain injury. It reduces ICP by two distinct mechanisms. First, it produces a rapid reduction in ICP by lowering blood viscosity, resulting in reflex cerebral vasoconstriction and a decrease in cerebral blood volume. This effect is transient, lasting less than 75 minutes. Later, an increase in cerebral blood volume sometimes is seen. The second mechanism by which mannitol reduces ICP is by an osmotic effect. Because no transport carrier for mannitol exists in brain capillaries, mannitol given intravenously remains in plasma and creates an osmotic gradient, causing water to move from the brain through capillary walls into their lumina, thereby reducing ICP. This effect develops more slowly, in 15 to 30 minutes, and persists for 1 to 6 hours. It is dependent on an intact blood brain barrier. When mannitol is administered repeatedly, fluid and electrolyte imbalances (particularly hypokalemia), dehydration, and hypotension may result. Euvolemia should be maintained by fluid replacement, and the serum osmolality should be kept below 320 mOsm/L. It is essential that serum (and urine) electrolytes be monitored regularly. Above these levels, mannitol loses its effectiveness, and acute renal failure may occur. Mannitol may accumulate in injured brain regions, and a reverse osmotic shift may occur, with fluid moving from the circulation into the brain parenchyma, which can exacerbate intracranial hypertension ("rebound"). This effect is most marked when mannitol is in the circulation for extended periods of time, which supports the use of intermittent boluses. Fluid and electrolyte problems and the development of "rebound" intracranial hypertension limit mannitol's long-term use. Effective bolus doses range from 0.25 g/kg to 1.0 g/kg of body weight.

A resurgence in the use of hypertonic saline in the treatment of increased ICP has developed recently. Like mannitol, it reduces elevated ICP by an osmotic effect. Additionally, like mannitol, it reduces blood viscosity, resulting in vasoconstriction and reduced cerebral blood volume. It also has a dehydrating effect on the endothelium of cerebral blood vessels, causing an increase in vascular diameter, which in turn, causes an increase in regional cerebral blood flow. A continuous infusion of 3% saline, between 0.1 to 1.0 mL/kg of body weight/hour, is given, using the minimum dose needed to maintain ICP at less than 15 mm Hg. In contrast with mannitol, with the use of hypertonic saline, a serum osmolarity of up to 365 mOsm/L can be tolerated, even when used in combination with mannitol. As with mannitol, electrolytes must be monitored regularly. Potential side effects include a "rebound" increase in ICP, subarachnoid hemorrhage, and renal failure.

Hyperventilation can produce a rapid reduction in ICP. It induces hypocapnia, which leads to vasoconstriction and a

TABLE 118.3

MEDICAL TREATMENT OF ACUTELY ELEVATED INTRACRANIAL PRESSURE IN PATIENTS WITH HEAD TRAUMA

Agent	Dose	Administration	Onset of Action	Peak Action	Advantages	Side Effects or Limitations
Mannitol	0.25–1.0 g/kg	Every 1–4 hr IV	5–30 min	15–90 min	Prompt action	Fluid—electrolyte imbalances; renal failure; intracranial bleeding; rebound
Hypertonic saline (3%)	0.1–1.0 mL/kg	Every hr	10 min	Approximately 3 hr	Prompt action	Renal failure; subarachnoid hemorrhage; rebound
Hyperventilation	Reduce $PaCO_2$ to between 35 and 30 mm Hg	Continuous	Seconds to minutes	2–30 min	Very prompt action	Effect may not be sustained; cerebral ischemia
Pentobarbital	Loading: 5–10 mg/kg Infusion: 1–3 mg/kg/hr	Continuous	1–2 min	Minutes	Prompt action; no rebound	Hypotension; renal failure; need for careful monitoring
Hypothermia	32–33°C	Continuous	Approximately 1 hr	2–3 hr	No rebound	Cardiac arrhythmias; need for careful monitoring

reduction in cerebral blood flow. This condition is accompanied by a reduction in cerebral blood volume, resulting in a decrease in ICP. Hyperventilation, however, is associated with a risk of developing iatrogenic ischemia. As a result, physicians have moved away from using aggressive hyperventilation (P_aCO_2 less than 30 mm Hg) in the management of severe traumatic brain injury to minimize the risk of complicating cerebral ischemia. Brief use of aggressive hyperventilation can be very effective, however, and in the setting of acute neurologic deterioration and/or impending herniation, it can be life-saving. Hyperventilation works quickly, and it does not potentiate intracranial bleeding or lead to a secondary increase in ICP (i.e., "rebound"). An acute reduction in arterial P_aCO_2 of 5 to 10 mm Hg will lower ICP by 25% to 30% in most patients. Because hyperventilation lowers ICP by inducing vasoconstriction, it probably should not be used during the first 24 hours after a head injury because cerebral blood flow often is decreased at that time. The duration of the reduction in ICP varies but usually lasts only hours as the CSF alkalosis normalizes. Although this alkalosis can be prolonged with the addition of the buffer tromethamine (THAM), hyperventilation should be used as a temporizing measure only, until more definitive, longer-lasting treatments can be initiated. On occasion, mild hyperventilation (P_aCO_2 of 30 to 35 mm Hg) may be considered for longer periods to treat intracranial hypertension refractory to other interventions. The inability to reduce ICP in head-injured patients through hyperventilation usually indicates a grave prognosis.

Induction of coma with barbiturates sometimes has been helpful in the management of intracranial hypertension in hemodynamically stable patients with salvageable severe head injuries in whom other measures have failed. Pentobarbital has been the barbiturate most often used. Barbiturates reduce increased ICP by reducing cerebral metabolism and can do so by as much as 50%. Also, barbiturates reduce intracranial hypertension by causing cerebral vasoconstriction, thereby lowering cerebral blood flow and ICP. Serum pentobarbital levels sufficient to achieve electrical silence or burst suppression on EEG should be maintained. A loading dose of 5 to 10 mg/kg is given, following which a continuous infusion of 1 to 3 mg/kg/hour is given. The advantages of barbiturate coma include rapidity of action and absence of rebound; it also does not potentiate intracranial bleeding. The patient must be monitored carefully in an intensive care facility. The barbiturate doses needed to reduce ICP often depress cardiac output, and thereby blood pressure, necessitating inotropic support with epinephrine. The reduction of ICP with barbiturates has not been demonstrated convincingly to improve neurologic outcome in head-injured children. In the management of head-injured patients, failure of barbiturate coma therapy to reduce ICP usually is an ominous sign.

Hypothermia is an additional means of treating increased ICP. The cerebral metabolic rate is decreased by almost 50% when body temperature is lowered to 30°C. The target temperature usually is 32°C to 33°C, moderate hypothermia. The mechanisms of action and the advantages and limitations of hypothermia are very similar to those of barbiturate coma, with approximately a 6% reduction in cerebral blood flow for each degree Centigrade that the temperature is lowered. Reduction in ICP is more rapid with pentobarbital than with hypothermia. Hypothermia probably is never adequate as the sole method of managing intracranial hypertension and should be considered only in selected cases of increased ICP refractory to other interventions.

Steroids such as dexamethasone (Decadron) act more slowly than do hyperosmolar agents in reducing increased ICP. Their mode of action is not known. They may stabilize the blood–brain barrier, enhance brain energy supplies, promote excretion of electrolytes and water, reduce CSF formation, stabilize lysosomal and other cell membranes, and facilitate CSF absorption impaired by inflammatory changes in the subarachnoid space or arachnoid villi. Steroids do not produce rebound and do not potentiate intracranial bleeding, although complicating infection, gastrointestinal hemorrhage, and the suppression of endogenous cortisol may occur. Despite their widespread use in managing head injuries, steroids have not proved to be helpful in controlled clinical trials, in reducing increased ICP or improving functional outcome in children with severe traumatic brain injuries.

Diuretics reduce brain water and decrease the formation of CSF and, therefore, have been used in treating increased ICP. These agents include acetazolamide (Diamox), ethacrynic acid (Edecrin), and furosemide (Lasix), with the last seemingly the most potent of the three. The dose of furosemide is 0.5 to 1.0 mg/kg. It induces potassium loss and can result in significant dehydration; also, it is potentially ototoxic, particularly when given in rapidly repeated high doses. Diuretics alone are not very effective in rapidly reducing major elevations in ICP, but they may be effective in chronic treatment when only a moderate reduction in pressure is needed. Acetazolamide probably should not be used in patients with head injuries because its central vasodilator effect may transiently exacerbate intracranial hypertension.

Surgical Management

On occasion, elevations in ICP cannot be reversed adequately by specific interventions or by the medical means discussed. Surgical management may be indicated in such circumstances. Aspiration of the subdural spaces (as discussed) may be therapeutically helpful. For marked elevation in ICP with signs of impending or evolving brain herniation, a ventricular tap with slow withdrawal of CSF may be lifesaving. If the increased ICP continues unremittingly, decompressive craniotomy may be needed.

Although no definite evidence supports that controlling ICP alters the outcome in head-injured children, anyone who has seen a substantial number of such patients can remember children in whom control of intracranial hypertension has been lifesaving.

CLINICAL SYNDROMES IN ACUTELY HEAD-INJURED CHILDREN

Scalp Injuries and Swellings

Contusion and laceration probably are the most frequent complications of head injury. Lacerations should be cleaned thoroughly and sutured, if necessary. An underlying skull fracture should be sought.

If the child's tetanus immunization status is known not to be up-to-date or is unknown and the possibility of tetanus cannot be excluded, tetanus immune globulin is recommended, with a single dose of 3,000 to 6,000 units given intramuscularly to children or adults. Some authorities recommend that part of the dose be infiltrated locally around the wound. The wound should be cleaned thoroughly and débrided. Further details regarding recommendations for tetanus prophylaxis depend on the patient's previous immunization status and the nature of the scalp wound and are provided in the *Red Book: 2003 Report of the Committee on Infectious Disease*, American Academy of Pediatrics.

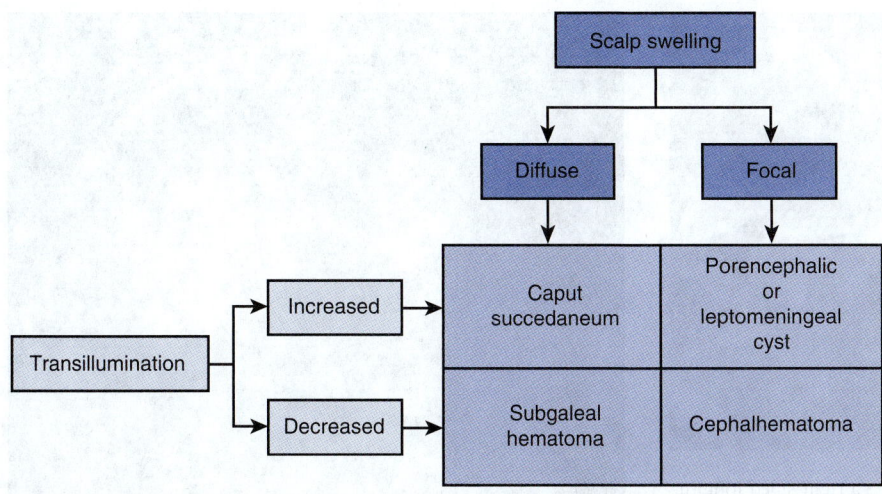

FIGURE 118.2. Clinical approach to the diagnosis of scalp swellings in childhood. (Reprinted with permission from Rosman NP. Managing acute head trauma. *Contemp Pediatr* 1986;3:34.)

In older children, most scalp swellings that occur after head trauma are the result of subgaleal hematomas, but other possibilities must be considered, particularly in newborns. In neonates, diffuse scalp swelling with decreased transillumination suggests a subgaleal hematoma, whereas diffuse scalp swelling with increased transillumination indicates a caput succedaneum. When the scalp swelling is focal, the newborn very likely has a cephalhematoma (subperiosteal hemorrhage), particularly when the swelling is parietal in location and transillumination is decreased. In approximately 5% to 25% of such patients, an accompanying skull fracture is present. When the swelling is focal and transillumination is increased, a porencephalic or leptomeningeal cyst with an associated growing skull fracture is suggested. The approach to the clinical diagnosis of posttraumatic scalp swellings in childhood is summarized in Figure 118.2.

No treatment is required for a subgaleal hematoma, caput succedaneum, or cephalhematoma; in fact, aspiration of fluid from the scalp is contraindicated because of possible complicating infection. Cephalhematomas commonly calcify and are reabsorbed into the underlying bony calvarium. A leptomeningeal cyst must be treated surgically, however, with removal or replacement of the protruding arachnoid and repair of the dural tear.

Skull Fractures

Six major varieties of skull fractures can occur in childhood: linear, depressed, compound, basal, diastatic, and growing. Linear skull fractures constitute approximately 75% of pediatric skull fractures; they are especially frequent occurrences in children younger than 2 years of age, and most are temporoparietal in location. Although they need not be treated themselves, such fractures may overlie serious intracranial pathologic conditions, such as an epidural hemorrhage, for which treatment is urgently required. Thus, if a linear fracture involves the squamous temporal bone or the sagittal suture, a CT scan should be performed promptly. Linear fractures heal within 1 to 2 months. When found in infants or young children, the possibility of neglect or inflicted injury always must be considered.

In depressed skull fractures, either continuity of the bony calvaria is disrupted or the skull may simply be indented, resulting in a ping-pong or pond fracture unaccompanied by a break in the cranial vault. Pond fractures occur in normal infants only in the newborn period, when the cranium is not as well mineralized and is more easily distorted than those in older children.

Focally depressed skull fractures may remain undiagnosed if a clinician fails to obtain tangential skull radiographs, which usually demonstrate a characteristic double density (bone-on-bone) appearance. Although depressed skull fractures are visualized best with plain radiography, many can be seen also on CT, particularly when a bone fragment is displaced. Skull fractures, when depressed, are of particular concern because the underlying brain may have been contused or lacerated by the depressed fragments. Although surgical elevation of depressed fractures has been advised when the depression is more than 5 mm in depth or when the depressed fragment extends below the inner table of the skull, such elevation appears not to reduce the risk of development of posttraumatic epilepsy, presumably because brain injury is sustained at impact.

Compound, or open-skull, fractures have a direct communication between a scalp laceration and the fracture site. These fractures are called penetrating if a tear in the dura also is present. Such fractures are of urgent concern because of the danger of complicating infection. Treatment involves meticulous débridement of the wound, search for a foreign body, copious irrigation with a sterile solution before closure, administration of parenteral antibiotics, and, if needed, tetanus prophylaxis. When a compound depressed fracture is found, the fracture should be elevated promptly to minimize the risk of complicating infection developing.

The two main varieties of basal fractures are frontobasal and petrous. Because of the anatomic complexity of the base of the skull, only approximately 20% of basal skull fractures can be recognized on standard skull radiography. Although the addition of multiplanar tomography and thin-section CT substantially increases the frequency with which such fractures can be demonstrated radiographically, the firm diagnosis of basal skull fracture usually depends on the recognition of coexisting signs. This diagnosis often can be inferred, if not confirmed, by coexisting signs that include hemorrhage in the nose, nasopharynx, or middle ear; overlying the mastoid bone (Battle sign); or around the eyes (raccoon-eyes). Sometimes, cranial nerve palsies occur, most frequently affecting cranial nerves I, VII, and VIII. Usually, petrous fractures of the skull base occur in one of two directions, the more common of which is longitudinal. Longitudinal petrous fractures may result in loss of blood or CSF from the ear, a conductive hearing loss (from injury to the tympanic membrane or middle-ear structures) that usually resolves, and facial palsy that is delayed in onset for 5 to 7 days and that usually disappears completely (Fig. 118.3). The less common petrous fracture is transverse. With this type of fracture, hemotympanum and CSF otorrhea are seen less

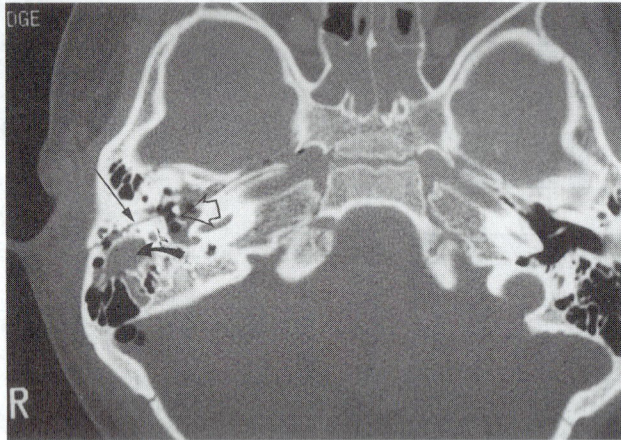

FIGURE 118.3. CT scan of skull base showing a right-sided longitudinal fracture extending through the mastoid air cells into the middle ear (*straight arrow*) causing disruption of the middle ear ossicles (*open broad arrow*). There is partial ossification of the mastoid air cells from blood (*curved arrow*).

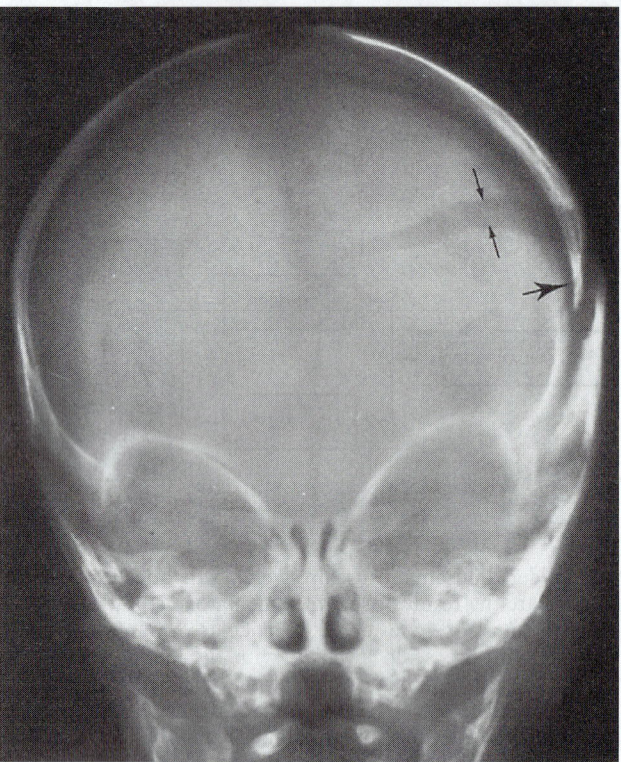

FIGURE 118.4. Posteroanterior radiograph of the skull shows a "growing" parietal skull fracture (*small arrows*) in a 9-week-old infant with an adjacent depressed parietal fracture; the depressed fragment (*large arrow*) lies beneath the squamous temporal bone.

commonly, accompanying severe sensorineural hearing loss usually is permanent, and facial palsy tends to appear earlier and to have poorer recovery than that with longitudinal fractures.

CSF rhinorrhea and otorrhea, reflecting fractures of the cribriform plate or petrous temporal bone, respectively, are worrisome signs of basal fracture because of the risk of development of complicating bacterial meningitis. The longer the duration of the CSF leak, the greater the risk of development of complicating bacterial meningitis. The causative organism usually is *Streptococcus pneumoniae*, with *Haemophilus influenzae*, *Streptococcus pyogenes*, and *Neisseria meningitidis* less frequently being the cause. Results from several studies, including a meta-analysis of 1,241 patients with basilar skull fracture, suggest that antibiotic prophylaxis does not prevent meningitis. If signs of meningitis are present, empiric coverage against most organisms can be achieved using vancomycin in combination with either ceftriaxone or cefotaxime. Ninety percent of CSF leaks close within 7 to 10 days. With a persisting leak for which a surgical repair may be needed, particularly in fractures of the cribriform plate, metrizamide CT cisternography or a high-resolution CT scan with the injection of water-soluble contrast into the CSF can be very useful in identifying the site of the leak.

Hemorrhage into the cranial sinuses can cause a radiographic appearance simulating sinusitis. Skull films may demonstrate intracranial air (pneumocephalus), indicating continuity between a paranasal or mastoid sinus and the inside of the skull. Occipital fractures involving the foramen magnum may be accompanied by tachycardia, hypotension, and irregular respirations secondary to brainstem dysfunction.

Diastatic skull fractures are traumatic separations of cranial bones at one or more suture sites. Most frequently, they affect the lambdoid suture and occur in the first 4 years of life. Such fractures should be followed closely in children younger than 3 years of age because they can become sites of so-called growing fractures.

Growing skull fractures are caused by the herniation of tissue through torn dura and an accompanying fracture (linear or diastatic) into the overlying scalp. Such fractures occur most often in the parietal region (Fig. 118.4). The herniating tissue is either solid brain parenchyma or cystic in nature, usually a porencephalic cyst (communicating with a lateral ventricle) or (less often) a leptomeningeal cyst. The pulsating herniat-

ing tissue and associated scarring prevent fusion of the fracture margins and cause the fracture line to widen. Although occasionally such fractures evolve acutely, more often they develop from several weeks to 6 months after head injury. The great majority occur in children younger than 3 years of age and mainly during the first year of life. They require surgical repair.

ACUTE INJURY TO BRAIN

Pathophysiology

Mechanical forces acting on the skull may expose the brain to the effects of acceleration, deceleration, or rotation. Acceleration occurs when a stationary head is hit by a moving object, such as a baseball bat. Deceleration (negative acceleration) occurs when a moving head meets a relatively fixed object, such as a concrete sidewalk. A blow delivered to the head in an asymmetric fashion, the usual circumstance, imparts movement to the head that is predominantly rotational. Traumatic lesions produced by linear acceleration tend to be limited to subdural hematomas and superficial contusions. By contrast, brain lesions from rotationally induced injuries typically are widespread, can occur remote from the site of impact, and may be superficial or deep. Typically, such shear–strain injuries occur at one of three topographic levels: the cortical surface of the brain (contusions), cerebral white matter [diffuse axonal injury (DAI)], or brainstem and deep gray matter nuclei.

The physical qualities of the skull play a role in the pathogenesis of accompanying brain injury. Compression of the partially elastic cranium may cause it to impact directly on the underlying brain and produce a crushing injury. The region of brain opposite the point of impact is the site of suddenly increased negative pressure, which is thought to contribute to contrecoup injury.

Diffuse Axonal Injury

The shearing forces induced by rotational acceleration-deceleration of the head act on white matter to cause mechanical disruption of nerve fibers and subsequent focal white-matter lesions. Such lesions, seen very often on MRI in acutely head-injured children, are a consequence of DAI caused by differential movement of brain regions with different densities. Most of the injuries occur in lobar white matter, particularly at the cortical white matter junction of the frontal and temporal lobes. DAI is seen also in the corpus callosum, especially in the posterior one-half of the body and the splenium, and in the rostral dorsolateral brainstem, although lesions in the latter regions rarely occur without accompanying lesions in lobar white matter. The fourth most common site of these injuries is the basal ganglia. These neuropathologic events follow a centripetal sequence. Thus, in milder injuries, damage typically is restricted to the cortex, but with increasing severity, the diencephalon and then the mesencephalon can be affected as well. Thus, when lesions are found in the brainstem, diffuse damage also is found elsewhere. Most of the damage is microscopic, and only 10% of patients have demonstrable abnormalities on CT scan; hemorrhagic tissue-tear lesions of more than a few millimeters can be seen, whereas nonhemorrhagic lesions cannot be detected on CT unless they are large enough to show tissue hypodensity, probably from edema. The lesions of DAI are better visualized on T2-weighted and fluid attenuation inversion recovery (FLAIR) sequences with MRI because those sequences show white-matter pathology particularly well (Fig. 118.5). DAI occurs in almost 50% of patients with severe head injury, causes 35% of all head injury deaths, and is the most common cause of the vegetative state and severe disability until death.

Secondary effects of brain trauma are not uncommon occurrences. Of these, brain swelling, mainly of subcortical white matter and the centrum semiovale, is of particular concern. In infants and young children particularly, such swelling can be massive. When diffuse cerebral swelling is accompanied by DAI and intraventricular hemorrhage, uncontrollable intracranial hypertension often results. Brain herniation may follow.

Cerebral Concussion

Concussion is a functional neuronal disturbance causing an alteration in mental state, with or without loss of consciousness, that occurs immediately after a head injury. The causative trauma usually is direct and blunt. The force of injury needed to produce a concussion generally is somewhat less than that required to produce a skull fracture. Concussion is much more likely to occur when the head moves freely after impact (acceleration-deceleration) than when the head is firmly in place (compression). Concussion also can occur in the absence of direct head trauma if sufficient whiplash-type force is applied to the brain. Concussive injuries cause an increase in ICP, followed by a temporary shear strain on the upper brainstem, resulting in an altered mental state. The brain that has received a concussive injury does not show any consistent morphologic abnormality. Physicians continue to debate, however, whether concussion has a permanent pathologic accompaniment—the absence of proof of pathology is not proof of its absence—The clinical state would appear to be caused by the suddenly increased and unmet energy demands of the brain.

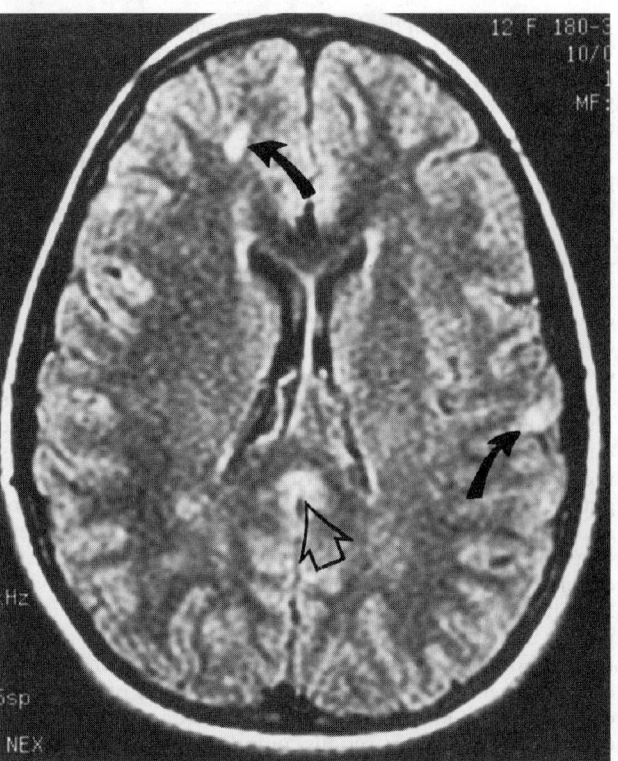

FIGURE 118.5. Cranial magnetic resonance imaging (FLAIR sequence) in a 12-year-old girl 9 days after she was struck on the left side of the head while riding unrestrained in the front seat of a car that collided with another vehicle. Multiple areas of shearing injury are seen, both superficial at the cortical white matter junction (*curved black arrows*) and deeper in the splenium of the corpus callosum (*open arrow*).

Confusion and amnesia are the hallmarks of concussion. Early symptoms of concussion (minutes to hours) include headache, dizziness, lack of awareness of surroundings, nausea, and vomiting. Concussion, when accompanied by loss of consciousness, commonly is associated with three types of amnesia: (a) temporary retrograde that antedates the head injury, sometimes by 2 years; (b) permanent retrograde that encompasses the few seconds to minutes immediately before the injury; and (c) temporary posttraumatic (anterograde) characterized by impaired ability to form new memories, usually lasting for some hours after the injury. Late symptoms of concussion (days to weeks) include headache, lightheadedness, inattention, memory disturbance, fatigability, irritability, low frustration threshold, photophobia, impaired visual focus, sonophobia, tinnitus, anxiety, depression, and sleep disturbance.

Concussion and Contact Sports

Sports injuries in children 7 to 13 years of age occur in 1 to 2 of every 100 athletic events. One percent of these injuries are concussions, with 300,000 sports-related concussions occurring each year in the United States. The severity of concussion must be considered in deciding whether and when an injured player can return to athletic competition. Grade 1 concussion is characterized by transient confusion, no loss of consciousness, and clearing of mental status in less than 15 minutes. The characteristics of grade 2 concussion are the same as those for grade 1, except that mental status changes last longer than 15 minutes. In grade 3 concussion, a period of unconsciousness occurs. On the basis of the severity of the concussion and the sideline evaluation of the athlete with a concussive injury (mental status testing, neurologic tests, provocative exercise tests), recommendations have been put forth by the Quality Standards Subcommittee of the American Academy of Neurology to help in deciding when such players might be permitted to return to competitive play. With a grade 1 concussion, if the player seems fully back to normal within 15 minutes, he may return to the contest, but with a second grade 1 concussion in the same competition, he is eliminated from competition for the next week; he then may return to competition only if he is fully asymptomatic. With a grade 2 concussion, he is removed from competition for a week; if he is then fully back to baseline, he can return to competition, but if he sustains a second grade 2 concussion, he is removed from play for at least two additional symptom-free weeks. With a grade 3 concussion, the player is removed from competition for 1 or 2 weeks, depending on the duration of unconsciousness (seconds versus minutes); if he is then fully back to normal, returns to play, and suffers a second grade 3 concussion, he is withheld from competition for a minimum of 1 symptom-free month. These recommendations were based on expert opinion but have received only weak general endorsement. This lack of endorsement is further supported by a study in which severity of concussion, assessed in 21 rugby players using three grading scales (American Academy of Neurology, Colorado Medical Society, Robert Cantu), showed no clear relationship to the presence or persistence of neuropsychologic test abnormalities found 2 and 10 days after the concussion. Thus, once any serious complications of a head injury can be excluded (e.g., intracranial hemorrhage), one might ask whether a decision to withhold such athletes from participation in competition is warranted. Yet, studies have shown that athletes with a history of previous concussion are more likely to sustain future concussions. Studies also have shown that after three or more concussions, with yet another concussion, the immediate sequelae are greater and recovery is slower.

In the United States, 20% of high school football players and 10% of college football players sustain a cerebral concussion, with the risk of sustaining a concussion in football being four to six times greater for a player with a previous concussion than for those with no such history. Repeated concussions have been shown to cause cumulative neuropsychologic and neuroanatomic damage, even when the incidents are separated by months or years. The so-called second-impact syndrome is the result of a second concussion while an affected individual still is symptomatic from an earlier event. One postulation is that the first insult disturbs the brain's autoregulatory mechanisms, with consequent vascular congestion and poor brain compliance. Because of this presumed poor compliance, malignant brain swelling after a relatively minor second impact can result in a marked increase in ICP, followed by rapid deterioration. Such swelling is seen more commonly in children than in adults. The results of such second-impact injuries can be catastrophic, with permanent disability or death.

Postconcussive Syndrome

Although children with concussions should be followed closely for at least 24 hours, with particular attention given to alertness, responsiveness, and vital signs, most children who suffer an uncomplicated cerebral concussion recover uneventfully. Some children, however, can be fairly disabled if they develop a postconcussion syndrome. Actually, two pediatric postconcussion syndromes can be seen: one in adolescents, the other in younger children. Symptoms in adolescents, which include headache, dizziness, irritability, and impaired concentration, usually are relatively mild and self-limited. By contrast, younger children show behavioral changes that can include aggression, disobedience, behavioral regression, inattention, and anxiety. The duration of such symptoms can vary from several days to several months and, on occasion, can persist.

The pathogenesis of the postconcussion syndrome is unsettled. Organic, environmental, and emotional factors all have been cited. Evidence for an organic basis for this disorder is mounting, however, with minor physiologic and anatomic alterations of axons, primarily in brainstem, thought to be important in causation. The occurrence of attentional difficulties as a prominent feature of the postconcussion syndrome suggests persisting dysfunction of deep subcortical structures, including the medial temporal lobes and upper brainstem. Because partial complex seizures, usually of temporal lobe origin, may occur after head trauma, their presence always must be considered in a child with a posttraumatic behavioral change. Also, anticonvulsants, particularly phenobarbital, may affect a child's personality and behavior adversely.

A common triad of symptoms that often develops after minor head injuries in young children includes lethargy, irritability, and vomiting, unaccompanied by loss of consciousness. These symptoms, attributed to torsion of the brainstem, usually subside within 48 to 72 hours.

Cerebral Contusion and Laceration and Posttraumatic Epilepsy

In contrast to concussion, a bruising (contusion) or tearing (laceration) of brain tissue occurs in cerebral contusion and laceration. A blunt head injury predisposes to contusion, a penetrating injury or a depressed skull fracture to laceration, although laceration can occur in the absence of both (especially in young children, whose skulls can undergo substantial deformation at injury). In addition to being caused by direct brain injury (e.g., laceration associated with a penetrating injury), contusion and laceration can be caused by forceful impact against the dural septa or irregular bony projections of the skull, particularly in the anterior and middle cranial fossae. Brain lesions can occur immediately beneath the site of impact (site of compression, causing a coup injury) or more remotely beneath the skull surface opposite the impact (site of low pressure or rarefaction, causing a contrecoup injury). The frontal poles, orbital gyri, cortex above and below the sylvian fissures, temporal poles, and lateral and inferior temporal lobes are the most vulnerable regions.

The diagnosis of contusion or laceration is established clinically by the presence of focal neurologic signs, including seizures, known (or presumed) to be absent before head injury. Frequently, cranial CT or MRI will provide important radiologic confirmation. Because both contusion and laceration cause some hemorrhage within the brain, additional support to either diagnosis is provided by finding red blood cells in CSF obtained by lumbar puncture. Lumbar puncture usually is not indicated in the management of pediatric head injuries, however, and may be contraindicated, except in patients with suspected complicating meningitis.

One complication of concern in cerebral contusion and laceration is posttraumatic epilepsy. The areas of the brain most important in the genesis of posttraumatic epilepsy are the mediotemporal, posterofrontal, and anteroparietal lobes. Posttraumatic epilepsy occurs more often with laceration than with contusion. When skull fracture occurs, posttraumatic epilepsy is more likely to occur with a depressed than with a linear fracture (Fig. 118.6). When concussion with loss of consciousness has accompanied a contusion or laceration, posttraumatic epilepsy is more likely to occur when the duration of unconsciousness is longer than 1 hour and when the period of

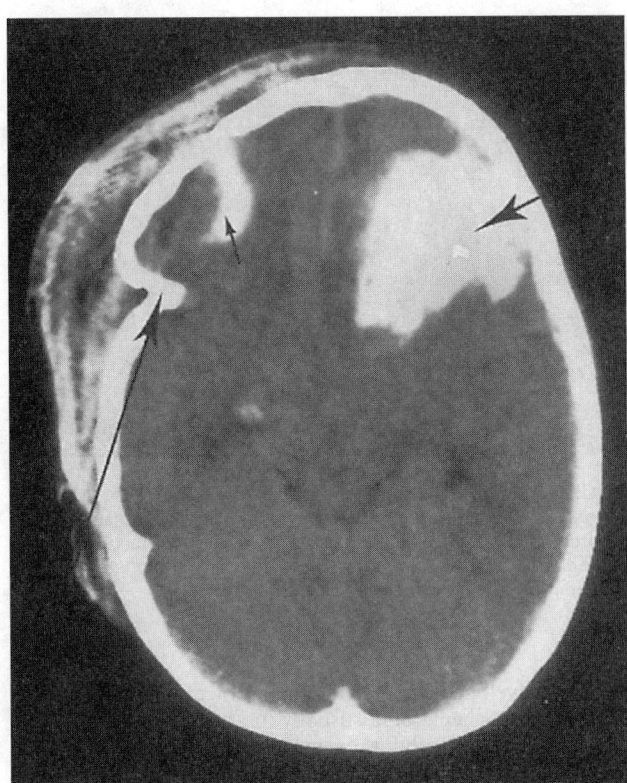

FIGURE 118.6. Cranial computed tomographic scan shows a depressed skull fracture (*long arrow*) in a 4-year-old child with overlying subgaleal hematoma and an underlying cerebral contusion (*small arrow*) with a contralateral cerebral hematoma (*large arrow*).

posttraumatic amnesia lasts longer than 24 hours. Electroencephalography has been unhelpful in predicting the occurrence of posttraumatic epilepsy in head-injured children.

Approximately 5% of children hospitalized because of head trauma will suffer a seizure within the first week after injury (i.e., early posttraumatic epilepsy). Of these, one-third occur in the first hour after injury, one-third between 1 and 24 hours, and one-third between 1 and 7 days. Focal seizures, with or without secondary generalization, occur in 60% to 80% of persons, particularly children with early posttraumatic seizures; generalized tonic-clonic seizures occur in most of the remainder. Early posttraumatic seizures occur most often in children younger than 5 years of age, especially those younger than 2 years, and in such children, the causative trauma can be quite mild. Two-thirds of these patients have more than one seizure, and approximately 10% (especially young children) have status epilepticus. Findings associated with an increased risk of development of early posttraumatic epilepsy include skull fracture, acute intracranial hemorrhage, focal neurologic signs, and more than 24 hours of either unconsciousness or posttraumatic amnesia. Such early posttraumatic seizures are followed by seizures beyond the first week in 20% to 30% of patients.

Late posttraumatic seizures, or late posttraumatic epilepsy (i.e., occurring beyond the first week of head injury), also occur in approximately 5% of patients hospitalized for head trauma. Unlike early posttraumatic seizures, late posttraumatic seizures occur more often in adults than in children; 60% to 70% are generalized, although some of those are of focal onset (i.e., with secondary generalization). More than one-half of the patients who develop late posttraumatic epilepsy have their first seizure within a year of sustaining the head injury, but in more than one-fourth, seizures develop more than 4 years later. Factors increasing the risk of development of late posttraumatic

epilepsy include posttraumatic amnesia lasting longer than 24 hours, acute intracranial hemorrhage, depressed skull fracture, dural penetration, and antecedent early posttraumatic epilepsy. Approximately 75% of such children will develop additional seizures. Of these patients, approximately 50% will cease having attacks regardless of the nature of the injury or the therapy used, approximately 25% will experience infrequent or rare seizures, and approximately 25% will continue to experience 10 to 15 seizures per year (usually resistant to treatment). A long latency period between the time of injury and the onset of seizures and a high seizure frequency render the recurrence of seizures more likely.

The management of acute posttraumatic seizures in the head-injured child was discussed earlier. Maintenance antiepileptic drug therapy clearly is indicated in patients with late posttraumatic epilepsy and probably should be given to children with early posttraumatic epilepsy as well.

Nonaccidental Head Injury in Children

One quarter of all cases of head trauma in children younger than 2 years of age are due to nonaccidental trauma; most such cases are caused by child abuse, with inflicted head injury being the most common cause of traumatic death in infancy. Nonaccidental head trauma in young children with accompanying intracranial hemorrhage (subdural; subarachnoid) and ocular hemorrhage (preretinal or subhyaloid; retinal), often with minimal external evidence of trauma, strongly suggests the diagnosis of "shaken baby syndrome." Such injuries have been attributed to repetitive whiplash motions at the relatively hyperextensible neck of the young child. Direct trauma often is inflicted as well, however, and most abused infants also show evidence of blunt impact to the head. Thus, the term "shaking-impact syndrome" probably reflects more accurately than does "shaken baby syndrome" the pathogenesis of these injuries. With nonaccidental head trauma, evidence of external injury is seen less often in young infants than in older infants and children. In a neuropathologic study of 53 fatal pediatric cases of inflicted head injury (37: 9 months or younger; 16: 10 months to 8 years), diffuse axonal injury was rare, found in only 6% of cases, whereas vascular axonal injury was much more common, found in 40%. In infants 9 months of age or younger, focal axonal injury often was seen in the lower brainstem and cervical spinal roots; by contrast, in older infants and children, axonal damage, presumably vascular, was seen most often in hemispheric white matter. In 77% of the 53 cases, severe hypoxic encephalopathy occurred. Many children with nonaccidental head injury have a history of apnea at the time of the shaking. Shaking of a young infant probably can cause brainstem stretch injury from cervical hyperextension/flexion, leading to apnea and resultant hypoxic brain injury. However, in some such cases, the caretakers of these children shake them vigorously, thinking the children have stopped breathing.

Acute Epidural and Subdural Hematomas

The clinical points that aid in the diagnosis of and differentiation between acute epidural and subdural intracranial hematomas are outlined in Table 118.4. Both types of hematomas are located much more frequently above the tentorium than in the posterior fossa. Above the tentorium, subdural hematoma occurs five to ten times more often than does epidural hematoma. Acute epidural hematoma usually is temporoparietal in location and is associated with a fracture of the squamous portion of the temporal bone in approximately 70% of patients. Epidural hematoma often is caused by laceration of the underlying middle meningeal artery, but this cause

TABLE 118.4

CLINICAL FEATURES OF ACUTE EPIDURAL AND SUBDURAL HEMATOMAS

Clinical Feature	Epidural Hematoma	Subdural Hematoma
Supratentorial		
Frequency	Less than subdural	5–10 times greater than epidural
Skull fracture	70%	30%
Source of hemorrhage	Arterial or venous	Almost always venous
Age	Usually >2 yr	Usually <1 yr
Location	Usually temporoparietal	Usually frontoparietal
Laterality	Usually unilateral	75% bilateral
Seizures	<25%	75%
Preretinal and retinal hemorrhages	Uncommon	Very frequent
Increased intracranial pressure	Present	Present
Cranial computed tomographic configuration	Usually lenticular	Curvilinar or crescentic
Mortality	Relatively high	Usually lower than epidural
Morbidity	Low	High
Infratentorial		
Frequency	2–3 times greater than subdural	Less than epidural
Skull fracture	Almost always	Frequent
Source of hemorrhage	Venous	Venous
Impaired consciousness	Frequent	Frequent
Acute hydrocephalus/ medullary compression	Variable	Variable
Other posterior fossa signs	Variable	Variable

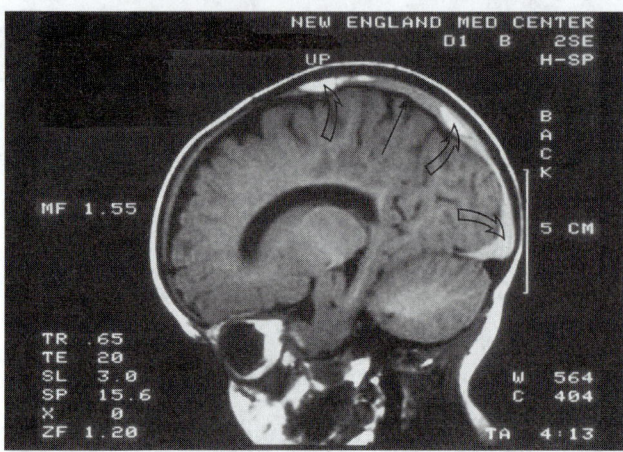

FIGURE 118.7. Cranial magnetic resonance imaging (T-1 weighted image) in a 6-month-old "shaken" boy with progressive macrocrania, vomiting, decreased feeding, anemia, and healing rib fractures. There are hematomas in the subdural space, both acute (*straight arrow*) and subacute (*curved open arrows*).

occurs more often in adults than in children, in whom up to 50% of epidural hematomas are of venous origin, originating from dural sinuses, middle meningeal veins, and emissary and diploic veins. Acute subdural hematomas usually are caused by tearing of bridging veins that pass from the cerebral cortex across the subdural space to the dural sinuses beneath the skull. Occasionally, they are of arterial origin. An accompanying skull fracture is present in only 30% of patients. Splitting of the cranial sutures may be observed when an acute subdural hematoma is sufficiently large to elevate ICP. Frequently, the brain underlying the hematoma is contused. Shaking injury without direct trauma to the head also can cause subdural hemorrhage.

Acute subdural hemorrhages are seen most often in infants, with a peak frequency occurring at age 6 months; acute epidural hematomas usually occur in older children, in whom the dura adheres less firmly to the inner table of the skull. In both types of hematomas, the degree of antecedent head trauma may be fairly mild. This fact was highlighted in a prospective study of 610 adolescents and adults examined after apparently sustaining minor head injuries; several of the patients developed life-threatening intracranial hematomas. Acute epidural hematomas usually are unilateral, whereas at least 75% of acute subdural hematomas are bilateral. The latter hematomas, in contrast with the epidural type, usually are frontoparietal in location. Seizures occur in fewer than 25% of children with acute epidural hematomas but are seen in 60% to 90% of those with acute subdural hematomas. Retinal and preretinal hemorrhages are very frequent findings with acute subdural hematomas but are uncommon with acute epidural hematomas. A biphasic course (impaired consciousness, alertness, impaired consciousness), said to be characteristic of acute epidural hematoma in adults, rarely occurs in children.

The relatively large volumes of extravasated blood in epidural and subdural hematomas typically produce symptoms and signs of increased ICP. These signs or symptoms summarized in Table 118.2, include irritability or lethargy, vomiting, fullness of the anterior fontanelle, headache and papilledema, and elevation of systolic blood pressure, with a decreased or increased pulse rate and slowed irregular respirations. With sufficient elevation of pressure in the supratentorial compartment, unilateral transtentorial herniation may occur.

Cranial CT is particularly valuable in differentiating between acute epidural and subdural hematomas. The former usually assumes a lens-like (biconvex) configuration, contrasting with the curvilinear or crescentic shape of the latter (Fig. 118.7); however, exceptions are common. Both types of hematomas may coexist in the same patient. The mortality rate in children with acute epidural hematoma has varied from 9% to 17%, but survivors tend to be relatively free of neurologic residua. Although mortality from acute subdural hematoma occurs less frequently than from acute epidural hematoma, in some series, the rate has been as high as 17% to 20%. Further, the incidence of morbidity (i.e., motor deficits, seizures, cognitive impairment) is greater with acute subdural hematomas because of the frequency of accompanying injury to the underlying brain.

Although they can occur also in the posterior fossa after head injury, epidural and subdural hematomas occur much less frequently in this infratentorial location than above the tentorium. In contrast to their relative frequencies above the tentorium, acute epidural hematomas occur two to three times more frequently than do acute subdural hematomas below the tentorium. Occipital skull fractures are common findings with both types of hematomas, particularly the epidural ones, with which they are an almost invariable accompaniment. Bleeding is of venous origin in both types of hematomas in the posterior fossa. Clinical signs include impairment of consciousness, headache, vomiting, and altered respirations. Only one-half of affected children have posterior fossa signs, such as ataxia, nystagmus, and cranial nerve palsies. These posterior fossa hematomas may be complicated by upward herniation of the cerebellum through the tentorial notch or, more often, by downward displacement of the cerebellar tonsils through the foramen magnum.

When epidural hemorrhage is suspected clinically, usually the diagnosis should be confirmed by cranial CT; such hematomas may progress very rapidly, however, with signs of acutely elevated ICP and progressive hemiparesis, necessitating immediate neurosurgical treatment [i.e., craniotomy, surgical removal of blood clot, and identification (if possible) of the bleeding source].

When subdural hemorrhage is suspected clinically, neurosurgical intervention rarely is needed before confirmation of the diagnosis by cranial CT. Occasionally, however, with acutely elevated ICP in infants in whom a subdural hematoma is suspected, the subdural space should be tapped as a combined diagnostic and therapeutic measure.

Subacute and Chronic Subdural Hematomas

In addition to acute subdural hematomas, in which symptoms appear during the first 48 hours, such hematomas can be subacute (symptoms appearing between 3 and 21 days) or chronic (symptoms appearing after 21 days). Unlike acute subdural hematomas, which occur most frequently in infants, most chronic subdural hematomas occur in older children and adolescents. In these less acute hematomas, as in the acute ones, recurrent vomiting from intracranial hypertension can occur. Macrocrania, reflecting a longer-standing increase in ICP, often is present; additionally, the head may have a boxlike appearance.

Transillumination of the skull characteristically demonstrates a diffuse increase in the spread of light. The anterior fontanelle may be excessively large or full. Funduscopy may show papilledema. Seizures occur frequently; motor deficits, including hypertonicity and jitteriness, can be found; and systemic signs, including irritability, vomiting, fever, anemia, and poor weight gain, are common occurrences. The skin and other body areas may show signs of previous injury.

MRI is the ideal imaging modality to demonstrate these lesions. The MRI findings depend on the predominant type of hemoglobin found in the hematoma, which varies with age. Initially, the hematoma is composed primarily of oxyhemoglobin and has a signal intensity that is isointense with brain on T1-weighted images and either isointense or hypointense with brain on T2-weighted images. During the first few hours, oxyhemoglobin is converted to deoxyhemoglobin, with a signal intensity that continues to be isointense on T1-weighted images but hypointense on T2-weighted images. Starting 2 to 4 days after the trauma occurs, deoxyhemoglobin then is converted to methemoglobin, which shows increased signal intensity on T1-weighted images and low or increased signal intensity on T2-weighted images. Eventually, the red blood cells in the hematoma break down, and the clot becomes composed of extracellular methemoglobin, which is hyperintense on T1- and T2-weighted images. As subdural hematomas become chronic, a thick outer membrane and a thin inner membrane begin to develop at 1 and 3 weeks, respectively.

The methods of treating these hematomas include (a) subdural taps with aspiration of subdural fluid; (b) external drainage with shunting of fluid from the subdural space to the peritoneum or to a pleural cavity; and (c) burr holes (or occa-sionally craniotomy), with aspiration or surgical removal of subdural clots.

PROGNOSIS IN ACUTE BRAIN INJURIES

Most children hospitalized after sustaining a head injury with an accompanying concussion, skull fracture, or cerebral contusion will recover completely, usually within 1 to several days; a small number of such children, however, develop a postconcussion syndrome or posttraumatic seizures. An even smaller number will have sustained a severe head injury, with prolonged coma followed by persisting cognitive, behavioral, or motor deficits.

Severe head injuries in children younger than 4 years of age and in adolescents produce a higher mortality rate than do those in school-aged children. Similarly, morbidity is greater in preschool children than in those who are older. These differences can be explained, at least in large measure, by differences in the types of traumas sustained most often by children of different ages. In infants, toddlers, and young children, diffuse injuries and multiple insults (e.g., falls, child abuse) are common occurrences. In school-aged children, injuries often are focal and less severe (e.g., bicycle accidents, sports injuries). Older children and adolescents, on the other hand, tend to suffer more impact injuries (e.g., motor vehicle accidents).

Severe Head Injuries and Neurologic Outcome

In 1975, a Glasgow Outcome Scale (GOS) was developed to assist in the assessment of neurobehavioral sequelae and neurologic deficits in head-injured patients. The original GOS had five categories: death; persistent vegetative state (no meaningful responsiveness with the environment); severe disability (conscious but disabled and dependent on others for some daily support); moderate disability (disabled but independent in daily activities); and good recovery (resumption of normal occupational and social activities).

Of patients severely disabled at 3 months after injury, 23% made a good recovery, 43% became moderately disabled, and only 31% remained severely disabled at 12 months. Among vegetative patients, 6% improved to moderate disability, 47% became severely disabled, and the remaining patients either remained vegetative or died. These substantial improvements in severely injured patients between 3 and 12 months after sustaining the injury had not been anticipated. The validity of the GOS is supported by its strong correlations with length of coma, initial GCS score, type of intracranial lesion, and length of posttraumatic amnesia. The primary criticism of the GOS is its relative insensitivity to clinically significant improvements, particularly beyond 6 months after injury.

The GCS has proved useful in assisting with the prediction of mortality and neurologic morbidity after head injuries. Using this scale, head injuries can be classified as mild (score 13 to 15), moderate (9 to 12), or severe (3 to 8). With regard to mortality, in the absence of accompanying systemic injury, severely head-injured children with GCS scores from 6 to 8 rarely, if ever, die. With a GCS score of 4 or 5, death is still unlikely. In patients with a GCS score of 3, however, the mortality rate is between 50% and 100%, often within the first 2 to 3 days after injury, with a high probability of substantial cognitive and other neurologic residua in the survivors. In most instances, the child's cognitive dysfunction, personality change, emotional upset, and difficulties in social adjustment are more disabling than are any residual motor deficits. With a GCS score of 4 or 5, cognitive, academic, and other neurologic deficits are found in 50% to 60%. If the GCS score is 6 or better, however, a head-injured child has an 80% to 90% chance of recovering independent function with only minimal neurologic disability. Perceptual motor skills frequently are impaired in severely head-injured children, and those difficulties tend to persist. By contrast, persisting speech deficits are relatively uncommon sequelae. Although the mortality rate clearly is lower with a higher initial GCS, even with an initial GCS of 7, mortality rates range from 15% to 25%.

Duration of Posttraumatic Coma and Neurologic Outcome

Posttraumatic coma of less than 24 hours rarely is associated with permanent neurologic or neuropsychologic sequelae in the head-injured child. In severely head-injured children aged 10 years or younger, the average length of coma for those returning to normal intelligence was 1.7 weeks; for borderline intelligence, 3 weeks; for mild retardation, 8 weeks; and for severe retardation, 11 weeks. Children older than age 10 years usually had a longer duration of coma and a similar relationship between duration of coma and cognitive outcome. Such benchmarks notwithstanding, children and adolescents have a greater capacity than do adults for recovering from severe head injuries and can show improvement in cognitive and social skills for more than 3 years.

The GCS score obtained 12 months after a head injury has occurred is the outcome statistic compared most frequently in different series. Of those who, by 12 months, had made a good recovery or who by then were moderately disabled, almost two-thirds already had reached this level within 3 months of the injury, and 90% had done so by 6 months. Only 10% of those who were severely or moderately disabled at 6 months were in the next better category by 1 year. Only 5% improved sufficiently after 12 months to reach a better category.

Neurologic Outcome in Mild Head Injuries

Mild head injuries are those caused by blunt trauma or sudden acceleration-deceleration, with periods of unconsciousness for 20 minutes or less, a GCS score of 13 to 15, no intracranial complications, and cranial CT findings limited to skull fracture. Most children with these types of injuries appear to recover quickly and completely, although later neurologic deficits, often quite subtle, sometimes are found. These deficits include symptoms of postconcussion syndrome, temporary cognitive difficulties, behavioral changes, and occasional posttraumatic seizures. Many authors feel that diffuse axonal injury (as discussed previously) is the brain pathology most likely to underlie neurologic morbidity after mild head injuries, in addition to that following a number of more severe head injuries.

Age as a Factor in Neurologic Outcome

Of the many factors influencing outcome after head injury, the severity of the injury is most important. The patient's age is the second most important factor influencing outcome. Many reports have shown that children usually recover more fully than do adults after head injuries of comparable severity. A 1-year rate of good outcome was found in 55% of patients 19 years of age or younger, but in only 21% of older patients, despite similar post-resuscitation GCS scores in both groups.

Pupillary Response as a Predictor of Neurologic Outcome

The absence of bilateral pupillary responses after a severe head injury has been sustained is correlated with mortality rates of 90% to 100%.

Intracranial Pressure as a Factor in Neurologic Outcome

The proportion of ICP measurements greater than 20 mm Hg is the fifth most powerful predictor of outcome in head injury, after patient age, admission GCS score, motor score, and admission pupillary examination.

Suggested Readings

American Academy of Neurology. Report of the Quality Standards Subcommittee: Practice Parameter: the management of concussion in sports [summary statement]. *Neurology* 1997;48:581.

American Academy of Pediatrics. Report of the Committee on Quality Improvement, American Academy of Pediatrics and the Commission on Clinical Policies on Research, American Academy of Family Physicians: Clinical Practice Guidelines: the management of minor closed head injury in children. *Pediatrics* 1999;104:1407.

Bullock MRR, Alves OL, Gilman CB, Ward JD. Advanced neuromonitoring for brain injury. In: Randolph AG, ed. *Current concepts in pediatric critical care—2003.* Society of Critical Care Medicine. 32nd Critical Care Congress. San Antonio, TX, 2003.

Carney NA, Chesnut R, Kochanek PM. Guidelines for the acute medical management of severe traumatic brain injury in infants, children, and adolescents. *Pediatr Crit Care Med* 2003;4:S1.

Cooper PR, ed. *Head injury,* 3rd ed. Baltimore: Williams & Wilkins, 1993.

Crowe W. Aspects of neuroradiology of head injury. *Neurosurg Clin North Am* 1991;2:321.

Duhaime A-C, Christian CW, Rorke LB, Zimmerman RA. Nonaccidental head injury in infants—the "shaken-baby syndrome." *N Engl J Med* 1998;338:1822.

Geddes JF, Hackshaw AK, Vowles GH, et al. Neuropathology of inflicted head injury in children. I. Patterns of brain damage. *Brain* 2001;124:1290.

Geddes JF, Hackshaw AK, Vowles GH, et al. Neuropathology of inflicted head injury in children. II Microscopic brain injury in infants. *Brain* 2001;124:1299.

Gentry LR. Imaging of closed head injury. *Radiology* 1994;191:1.

Guskiewicz KM, McCrea M, Marshall SW, et al. Cumulative effects associated with recurrent concussion in collegiate football players. The NCAA concussion study. *JAMA* 2003;290:2549.

Hinton-Bayre AD, Geffen G. Severity of sports-related concussion and neuropsychological test performance. *Neurology* 2002;59:1068.

Kochanek PM. Therapeutic options in the management of traumatic brain injury in children. In: Randolph AG, ed. *Current concepts in pediatric critical care—2003.* Society of Critical Care Medicine. 32nd Critical Care Congress. San Antonio, TX, 2003.

Narayan RK, Wilberger JE, Povlishock JT, eds. *Neurotrauma.* New York: McGraw-Hill, 1996.

Rosman NP, Oppenheimer EY. Post-traumatic epilepsy. *Pediatr Rev* 1982;3:221.

Rosman NP, Oppenheimer EY, O'Connor JF. Emergency management of pediatric head injuries. *Emerg Med Clin North Am* 1983;1:141.

Rosman NP. Acute head trauma. In: McMillan JA, DeAngelis CD, Feigin RD, Warshaw JB, eds. *Oski's pediatrics: principles and practice,* 3rd ed. Philadelphia: Lippincott Williams & Wilkins, 1999.

Rosman NP. Traumatic brain injury in children. In: Swaiman KF, Ashwal S, eds. *Pediatric neurology: principles and practice,* 3rd ed. St. Louis: Mosby Inc., 1999.

Schutzman SA, Barnes P, Duhaime A-C, et al. Evaluation and management of children younger than two years old with apparently minor head trauma: proposed guidelines. *Pediatrics* 2001;107:983.

Suarez JI. Hypertonic saline for cerebral edema and elevated intracranial pressure. *Clev Clin J Med* 2004;71(Suppl 1):S9.

Vinken PJ, Bruyn GW, Klawans HL, Braakman R, eds. Head injury. *Handbook of clinical neurology,* Vol 57 (RS 13). Amsterdam: Elsevier, 1990.

CHAPTER 119 ■ GENERAL PRINCIPLES OF POISONING MANAGEMENT

JAMES D. FORTENBERRY AND M. MICHELE MARISCALCO

Intensive educational and treatment efforts by health care providers and poison control centers have significantly reduced morbidity and mortality from childhood poisoning. As a result, deaths from poisoning in the United States have decreased to less than 25 annually in children less than 6 years old and to approximately 100 in those less than 19 years old. In the young child, fatalities have shifted from unintentional household exposures to therapeutic errors, environmental exposures, and adverse drug reactions. Of approximately 2.3 million annual poisoning episodes, however, the majority (66%) still occur in children from less than 18 years of age.

Accidental poisonings make up 80% to 85% of all poisoning exposures. Usually, accidental intoxication in young children is caused by the ingestion of a single product, but suicidal older children or adolescents often ingest multiple drugs. Ingestions should be considered intentional in any affected child older than age 5 years, but suicidal ideation should particularly be considered in adolescent patients. Further discussions with an affected patient should be held to ascertain a cause, including any psychosocial stressors. In most cases, psychiatric consultation should be used to determine whether patients at risk remain likely to harm themselves or need further crisis intervention.

DIAGNOSIS

The diagnosis of poisoning may not be obvious. Often, the diagnosis is not considered because of purposeful falsification by older patients or because young or confused patients are unable to provide an adequate history. Poisoning should be considered strongly in children who exhibit acutely developed disturbed consciousness, abnormal behavior, seizures, coma, respiratory distress, shock, arrhythmias, metabolic acidosis, severe vomiting and diarrhea, or other puzzling multisystem disorders without another known etiology. Underlying drug or ethanol intoxication also should be considered in adolescent and adult victims of accidental trauma. At a later time, issues of family stressors and environmental factors predisposing to an accidental ingestion also should be addressed.

History

During stabilization, information should be obtained from family members, friends, or paramedics who have transported the patient to the hospital about the possible agent, the mode of intoxication, the maximum potential dose, and the time since exposure. If poisoning is suspected, but the history is not confirmatory, information regarding different drugs in the home should be obtained by inquiring about illnesses of the patient and other family members. A determination that an ingested compound is nontoxic (Box 119.1) can enable the provider to avoid subjecting the child to invasive therapies and even admis-

sion. Alternatively, a determination of the specific compound early in the course of treatment can help focus treatment. In particular, determination that a compound highly toxic to a child in small quantities (Box 119.2) can heighten concern and the intensity of intervention. The products listed in Box 119.2 have the potential to be fatal in children less than 2 years of age with as little as 1 to tablets or 1 to tablespoons of liquid ingested. Determining the amount of a toxin ingested can be difficult, although estimates of pills ingested from those remaining can be helpful as a starting point. For an estimation of liquid ingestion, the volume of a swallow has been calculated to be approximately 0.27 cc/kg body weight.

Physical Examination

The physical examination can be particularly helpful in the case of a questionable exposure to a toxic agent. Certain constellations of symptoms and physical findings may suggest a specific ingestion (Table 119.1). However, children who arrive in the emergency department with a diagnosis of poisoning frequently are asymptomatic. Of those who do present with clinical findings, gastrointestinal tract symptoms (e.g., nausea, vomiting, diarrhea, cramps) and central nervous system depression (e.g., drowsiness, coma) are most common. Other common findings are referable to the respiratory tract (e.g., cough, dyspnea, respiratory depression), cerebellum (e.g., ataxia, nystagmus), central nervous system (e.g., hyperactivity, tremor, convulsions, confusion, delirium, hallucinations), and cardiovascular system (e.g., heart rate, cardiac arrest).

Laboratory and Toxicology Tests

Routine laboratory tests also can aid in the diagnosis and management of poisoned patients. Decreased hemoglobin saturation with a normal or increased arterial oxygen partial pressure is found in patients with carbon monoxide poisoning or in methemoglobinemia. Serum metabolic acidosis with an increased anion gap suggests the ingestion of methanol, ethylene glycol, paraldehyde, toluene, iron, isoniazid, or salicylates. An elevated measured serum osmolarity compared with a calculated osmolarity indicates the presence of low-molecular-weight and osmotically active compounds, such as methanol, isopropyl alcohol, and ethylene glycol. Hypoglycemia can be seen in patients intoxicated by ethanol, methanol, isopropyl alcohol, isoniazid, acetaminophen, salicylates, and oral hypoglycemic agents. Serum pregnancy testing also should be obtained in pubertal females as a possible etiology for intentional ingestion.

Toxicology testing may be helpful in confirming the clinical diagnosis of drug intoxication. However, identifying all available drugs with a high degree of specificity and sensitivity is impossible because of time limitations. Instead, a drug screen

BOX 119.1   Commonly Ingested Substances of Low Toxicity

Adhesives
Antacids
Baby product cosmetics
Ball-point pen inks
Bathtub float toys
Bath oil (castor oil and perfume)
Bleach (<6% sodium hypochlorite)
Body conditioners
Bubble bath soap
Candles (beeswax or paraffin)
Caps (toy pistols, potassium chlorate)
Chalk (calcium carbonate)
Clay (modeling)
Cosmetics
Crayons (marked A.P., C.P.)
Dehumidifying packets (silica or charcoal)
Detergents (phosphate only)
Deodorants
Deodorizers (spray and refrigerator)
Elmer's Glue
Etch-A-Sketch
Eye makeup
Fabric softeners
Grease
Hair products (dyes may be caustic; sprays, tonics)
Hand lotions and creams
Hydrogen peroxide (medicinal, 3%)
Incense
Indelible markers
Ink (black, blue; nonpermanent)
Laxatives
Lipstick
Lubricant
Magic markers
Makeup (eye, liquid facial)

Matches
Newspaper (possible lead poisoning from chronic ingestion)
Paint (indoor: latex)
Pencil (lead-graphite, coloring)
Perfumes
Petroleum jelly (Vaseline)
Phenolphthalein laxatives (Ex-Lax)
Play-Doh
Polaroid picture-coating fluid
Porous-tip ink marking pens
Putty (less than 2 oz.)
Rouge
Rubber cement
Sachets (essential oils, powder, talc aspiration)
School pastes
Shampoos (liquid)
Shaving creams and lotions
Soap and soap products
Spackles
Suntan preparation
Sweetening agents (saccharin, cyclamates)
Teething rings (water sterility)
Thermometers (mercury)
Toothpaste (with and without fluoride)
Vaseline
Vitamins (with or without fluoride)
Water-color paints
Zinc oxide

Modified with permission from Committee on Accident and Poison Prevention, American Academy of Pediatrics. The non-toxic ingestion. In: Aronow R, ed. *Handbook of common poisonings in children*, 2nd ed. Evanston, IL: American Academy of Pediatrics, 1983:16.

BOX 119.2   Products with Lethal Potential in Small Doses for Very Young Patients

Acetonitrile	Hyoscyamine sulfate
Ammonium fluoride	Imidazoline products
Benzocaine	Lindane
Brodifacoum (others)	Methadone
Butyrolactone	Methanol
Camphor	Methyl salicylate
Chloroquine	Pennyroyal oil
Chlorpromazine (others)	Quinine
Clozapine	Salt
Desipramine (others)	Senenious acid
Diphenoxylate	Theophylline
Hydrocarbons	

Modified with permission from Emery, Singer J. Highly toxic ingestions for toddlers: when a pill can kill. *Pediatr Emerg Med Rep* 1998;3:111.

is performed. Because drug screens vary among institutions, the physician should know exactly which drugs can be detected. Generally, toxicology screening tests detect a wide range of narcotics, analgesics, barbiturates, antidepressants, tranquilizers, sedative-hypnotics, and various other drugs and abused substances. Ethylene glycol, lithium, iron, cyanide, lead, and other heavy metals usually are not included in drug screening tests. Some centers have access to rapid, comprehensive drug screening using high-performance liquid chromatography methodology. In general, the history and physical examination are more important in the acute management of drug overdose than is a comprehensive drug screen. Positive drug screen findings merely confirm exposure to that substance, and such an exposure should not be assumed to be responsible for the clinical findings of the moment.

THERAPY

The three goals of poisoning treatment are:

1. Preventing further drug absorption
2. Providing antidotal therapy
3. Hastening the elimination of an absorbed poison

TABLE 119.1

TOXIDROMES: PROMINENT CLINICAL FINDINGS AS AN AID TO DIAGNOSIS OF THE UNKNOWN INGESTION

Drug Involved	Clinical Manifestations
Anticholinergics (atropine, scopolamine, tricyclic antidepressants, phenothiazines, anti-histamines, mushrooms)	Agitation, hallucinations, coma, extrapyramidal movements, mydriasis, dry mouth, tachycardia, arrhythmias, hypotension, decreased bowel sounds, urinary retention; flushed, warm, dry skin
Cholinergics (organophosphates and carbamate insecticides)	SLUDGE syndrome (salivation, lacrimation, urination, defecation, gastrointestinal cramping, emesis), sweating, meiosis, bronchorrhea, rales and wheezes, weakness, paralysis, confusion and coma, muscle fasciculations
Opiates	Slow respirations, bradycardia, hypotension, hypothermia, coma, meiosis, pulmonary edema, seizures
Sedatives and hypnotics	Coma, hypothermia, central nervous system depression, slow respirations, hypotension, tachycardia
Tricyclic antidepressants	Coma, convulsions, arrhythmias, anticholinergic manifestations
Salicylates	Vomiting, hyperpnea, fever, lethargy, coma
Phenothiazines	Hypotension, tachycardia, torsion of head and neck, oculogyric crisis, trismus, ataxia, anticholinergic manifestations
Sympathomimetics (amphetamines, phenylpropanolamine, ephedrine, caffeine, cocaine)	Tachycardia, arrhythmias, psychosis, hallucinations, delirium, nausea, vomiting, abdominal pain, piloerection
Alcohols, glycols (methanol, ethylene glycol; also salicylates, paraldehyde, toluene)	Elevated anion gap, metabolic acidosis
Serotonin syndrome—usually multiple psychoactive agents (selective serotonin reuptake inhibitors, tricyclic antidepressants, buspirone, lithium, fenfluramine)	Confusion, agitation, myoclonus, diaphoresis, hyperreflexia, diarrhea

Modified with permission from Mofenson NC, Greensher J. The unknown poison. *Pediatrics* 1974;54:337 and Chu J et al. Update in clinical toxicology. *Am J Respir Crit Care Med* 2002;166:9.

Several methods may be used to terminate the patient's exposure to a toxic substance or to mitigate its effects. For respiratory exposure, removal of the victim from the toxic environment is usually all that is necessary, with careful observation for latent effects of exposures to pulmonary irritants. Involved eyes should be washed with water for at least 10 to 15 minutes. For dermal exposure, the skin should be flushed immediately with water and then should be washed with copious amounts of water and soap. All contaminated clothing should be removed.

Basic Life Support

Attention to basic life support and emergency cardiorespiratory support must precede any diagnostic studies in the poisoned child. Respiratory failure can result from upper airway obstruction, central nervous system depression, continuous convulsions, neuromuscular blockade, increased oral and airway secretions, aspiration, and pulmonary edema. An adequate airway is the first priority. Airway patency can be accomplished by jaw-thrust or chin-lift maneuvers or by the placement of an oral or nasopharyngeal airway or an endotracheal tube. Only endotracheal intubation protects from the hazards of aspiration in the airway of a comatose patient lacking a gag reflex.

Usually, hypotension in poisoned children is associated with hypovolemia from excessive volume losses or is considered secondary to vasodilation or capillary leak with third-space losses. Guidelines for fluid resuscitation in hypotensive patients can be applied (see Chapter 453, Shock). The insertion of a central venous line or pulmonary arterial catheter to measure cardiac output and left ventricular filling pressure may be necessary, if hypotension continues despite aggressive fluid administration and inotropic agents.

Direct myocardial depression and arrhythmias are less frequent contributors to hypotension. The detection of arrhythmias depends on continuous electrocardiographic monitoring. All drugs used to treat arrhythmias can be dangerous and must be used with great care. The use of short-acting drugs is best. The frequency and recurrence of arrhythmias are increased by hypoxia, acidosis, and electrolyte abnormalities. The specific treatment of complicating arrhythmias is accomplished best if the intoxicating agent is known, but emergency therapy may be needed before a specific poison is diagnosed. The most common arrhythmias are ventricular ectopic beats and ventricular tachycardia. Usually, these arrhythmias are treated with lidocaine, procainamide, or amiodarone. In the case of membrane-depressant drugs such as tricyclic antidepressants (TCAs), some conventional antiarrhythmic agents, such as quinidine or procainamide, are contraindicated. Lidocaine remains the drug of choice. Sinus or junctional bradycardia may respond to intravenous atropine. If available, intravenous isoproterenol should be considered for unresponsive sinus, junctional, or ventricular bradycardia. Complete atrioventricular block should be treated with an isoproterenol infusion and possibly a transvenous pacemaker.

The control of convulsions is a common problem. Seizures can result from direct toxicity or indirectly from hypoxia, hypoglycemia, and electrolyte disturbances. Anticonvulsant drugs may be ineffective in many ingestions. Potentially useful agents are diazepam, lorazepam, phenobarbital, and phenytoin or fosphenytoin. Hyperthermia should be treated with cooling blankets rather than with antipyretic drugs. Hypothermia is treated or prevented with warming devices. Coagulopathy may occur in certain ingestions, and blood or factor replacement therapy may be indicated.

Gastrointestinal Decontamination

The traditional principles of gastrointestinal decontamination once considered standard have undergone scrutiny in recent years. Previously, dilution was recommended as an initial step in the management of toxic ingestions. However, several studies demonstrated that dilution actually enhances the absorption of ingested toxins; therefore, it should not be used.

Gastric Lavage and Emesis

Standard approaches to management have included gastric emptying by emesis or gastric lavage. Evidence suggests that these techniques may not improve toxin retrieval significantly when used in the emergency department and, in the case of ipecac, may delay the effective use of more beneficial agents such as activated charcoal and N-acetylcysteine. Ipecac was long considered effective if given within 30 minutes after an ingestion, rendering it valuable for home use. However, recent studies have questioned its benefit. The American Academy of Pediatrics has recommended that ipecac no longer be used routinely as a home treatment strategy, and that existing ipecac in the home be disposed of safely.

Gastric lavage has more potential efficacy, but is likely beneficial only with drugs that delay gastric emptying, such as narcotics or tricyclic antidepressants (TCAs), or with drugs that form concretions. Lavage is contraindicated in alkali ingestions because of the increased risk for esophageal perforation. It should be used cautiously in patients at risk for developing mental status changes, and endotracheal intubation should be performed first, to protect children with absent or compromised airway reflexes. Given the uncertain benefits of gastric lavage, patients who are otherwise asymptomatic should not be sedated and intubated for the sole purpose of performing lavage. Lavage should be performed with an affected patient in a left-side-down, head-down position and is accomplished best with use of a large orogastric hose. A 28 Fr. (9-mm) Ewald tube is the smallest that can be used effectively, because pills and fragments may not pass through smaller bores. This problem limits the benefits of lavage in small children. A 36 Fr. (12-mm) tube is optimal for adolescents and adults. The most significant retrieval may result from aspirating gastric contents before instilling lavage fluid. Warm physiologic saline should be used in aliquots of 10 mL/kg in pediatric patients (200 to 400 mL in adolescents) and should be continued until the lavage return is clear.

Activated Charcoal

Activated charcoal effectively minimizes the gastrointestinal absorption of toxins by adsorbing them onto its large surface area. The use of activated charcoal has risen significantly as studies have demonstrated that activated charcoal produces better toxin recovery and fewer complications than do emesis or gastric lavage techniques. It should be considered as the

---

BOX 119.3 **Toxins Not Effectively Adsorbed by Activated Charcoal**

Ethanol
Methanol
Hydrocarbons
Cyanide
Iron
Ethylene glycol
Acids
Alkalis
Lithium

---

primary means of gastrointestinal decontamination in most ingestions, with the exception of a few compounds in which its use is not effective or recommended (Box 119.3). Activated charcoal is most effective if administered during the first hour after ingestion. Approximately 5 to 10 g of charcoal is required for each 1 g of drug ingested. The treatment for ingestions of unknown amounts of toxin should be achieved by standard charcoal doses of 1 g/kg (50 to 100 g for adolescents).

Activated charcoal is odorless and tasteless, but its appearance often renders oral acceptance difficult, and the addition of cola or chocolate milk can improve tolerance. Nasogastric tube administration should be performed without delay if an affected child refuses oral intake. Charcoal aspiration can occur, causing bronchospasm and pneumonitis, and thus emphasizes the need for adequate airway protection before administration in the obtunded patient.

Activated charcoal in multiple doses increases the serum clearance of certain medications. Multiple-dose activated charcoal uses "gastrointestinal dialysis" to adsorb drugs available across the gastrointestinal mucosa and to take advantage of the enterohepatic recirculation of certain medications. This method has proved effective in oral and intravenous theophylline overdoses and is beneficial for other selected compounds (Box 119.4). A standard dose of activated charcoal should be given initially; then 0.5 g/kg should be administered orally every 4 hours until serum drug levels are nontoxic or clinical symptoms of ingestion have resolved. Some patients tolerate repeated doses poorly. The histamine$_2$ receptor antagonists, such as ranitidine, may decrease vomiting, and administering charcoal as a continuous drip in saline through a syringe pump can be helpful.

BOX 119.4 **Toxins with Improved Clearance by Multiple-Dose Activated Charcoal**

Theophylline or aminophylline
Phenobarbital
Carbamazepine
Benzodiazepines
Salicylates
Tricyclic antidepressants
Phenothiazines
Phenytoin

Whole-Bowel Irrigation

Whole-bowel irrigation can be considered for use with the ingestions of medications with sustained release and delayed absorption, such as some calcium channel antagonists and enteric-coated aspirin. Whole bowel irrigation also can aid in the clearance of whole pill fragments, such as iron tablets or the other toxins not well adsorbed by activated charcoal. Polyethylene glycol electrolyte solutions prescribed at continuous rates have been successfully employed for irrigation.

Given the uncertain benefits of these techniques, decontamination procedures should only be used in the child who has ingested a potentially life-threatening amount of a toxin and in whom the procedures can be performed without undue risk.

Other Methods of Drug Elimination

For enhancing the elimination of an absorbed poison, the available procedures that have the greatest value are diuresis, dialysis, and hemoperfusion. These methods should be used only in exceptional circumstances, in which the danger of the persisting poison probably exceeds that of removing it, and if the physical and pharmacologic properties of the poison suggest that the method would be effective.

Several criteria favor forced diuresis with pH alteration as an effective therapeutic modality in hastening elimination. The drug must be excreted primarily by the kidneys; drugs that are highly lipid-soluble, highly protein-bound, or are excreted primarily by the liver are removed poorly using this method. The pK of the drug (i.e., the pH at which the proportion of the ionized and unionized forms of that drug are equal) must be such that, by altering urinary pH, enough ionization can occur to ensure adequate trapping of the drug in the tubule lumen, which inhibits reabsorption. Alkaline diuresis enhances the excretion of drugs with pK values of 3.0 to 7.2, such as salicylate and barbiturates. Less commonly, drugs with pK values in the range of 7.2 to 9.5 [e.g., quinidine, phenylcyclidine (PCP), fenfluramine, amphetamine] can be enhanced by acid diuresis.

Forced diuresis is achieved by the administration of intravenous fluids at a volume of at least twice the maintenance requirements, to establish urine output of 2 to 5 mL/kg/hour. Such diuretics as mannitol and furosemide can be used to maintain high urine output. Alkalinization of the urine (pH of 7.0 or higher) is accomplished by adding sodium bicarbonate in concentrations of 50 to 75 mEq/L to the intravenous fluids, while proportionally decreasing fluid sodium chloride content. Often, hypokalemia complicates this therapy, and aggressive potassium supplementation may be required. Acetazolamide, a carbonic anhydrase inhibitor, achieves urinary alkalinization through its ability to enhance urinary bicarbonate excretion. However, systemic acidosis is induced and may worsen salicylate toxicity by increasing the proportion of nonionized, lipid-soluble serum salicylate, enhancing its penetration into the central nervous system. Acidification of the urine to a pH of 4.0 to 5.0, using ammonium chloride or hydrochloric acid, promotes the excretion of poisons that are weak bases. The potential complications of forced diuresis include fluid overload with cerebral edema, pulmonary edema, hyponatremia, and water intoxication. Alkalemia and hypokalemia may complicate bicarbonate use. Hyperammonemia may complicate ammonium chloride use, particularly with underlying renal or liver disease.

Although indications for using the techniques in children are not well defined, hemoperfusion and hemodialysis to enhance actively the removal of intoxicating compounds can be useful with severe or progressive clinical intoxication in patients unresponsive to aggressive medical therapy, with ingestion and absorption of a potentially lethal dose of a toxin, with impaired

normal route of excretion, and with development of complications of coma.

In adults, hemoperfusion over resins or charcoal has been shown to be the most effective method of extracting some poisons, including barbiturates, methaqualone, glutethimide, TCAs, theophylline, and acetylsalicylic acid. Blood from a venovenous shunt is passed, with the help of a pump, over a "bed" of resin or activated charcoal. The facilities and skills necessary are the same as those needed to perform hemodialysis. With the use of continuous hemofiltration devices, the practice of this technique in children has become more common. Complications include thrombocytopenia, hypotension, hypothermia, and hypocalcemia.

Dialysis may effectively remove drugs that are poorly protein-bound, are highly water-soluble, have a low volume of distribution, and have molecular structures and physical characteristics that enable rapid diffusion across dialysis membranes. Such molecules as methanol, ethanol, ethylene glycol, and procainamide hydrochloride are removed by dialysis. Consultation with a toxicologist and/or local poison control center, as well as a renal specialist, should be employed in any decision regarding use of hemodialysis techniques.

MANAGEMENT OF SPECIFIC TOXINS

The preceding principles may be applied to most ingestions. An effective pharmacologic antagonist or chelating agent is available for fewer than 5% of ingestions. Table 119.2 provides basic information regarding specific antidotes for selected ingestions. Consultation with a local poison control center or a toxicologist can provide invaluable advice regarding the management of specific ingestions. Specific management of acetaminophen and salicylate ingestion are discussed in Chapters 120 and 121, respectively, but the management of several other common toxins is reviewed here.

Iron Ingestion

Since 1984, iron has accounted for an average of 2% of all exposures in children younger than 6 years. Usually, overdoses in young children occur as accidental ingestions rather than as intentional overdoses. Most fatalities occur after the ingestion of adult iron supplements, with fewer cases related to adult vitamins with iron.

Ingested iron increases capillary permeability, intravascular permeability, and vasodilation upon overwhelming the intestinal barrier and entering the circulation. When available free iron exceeds circulating transferrin-binding levels, toxicity of the liver and other parenchymal organs ensues. Typically, iron intoxication follows four clinical stages, although the presence, duration, and order of these stages may vary. The initial phase, occurring shortly after ingestion, is produced by direct effects on gastric and ileal mucosa, and induces abdominal pain and vomiting. Gastrointestinal hemorrhage may occur. Fever, leukocytosis, and hyperglycemia are associated findings. In severe intoxications, shock and encephalopathy may occur in this early stage. In the second phase, a deceptively stable period of ameliorated symptoms and subtle physical findings may follow for 6 to 72 hours. However, some patients advance to a third phase, with return of gastrointestinal symptoms, metabolic acidosis, coagulopathy and overt shock, and liver dysfunction, rarely progressing to hepatic necrosis. Survivors may develop a fourth phase of gastrointestinal scarring and acute obstruction 4 to 6 weeks after ingestion.

The prediction of potential iron toxicity determines treatment. Estimation of the total dose ingested is helpful but often

TABLE 119.2

SELECTED PEDIATRIC ANTIDOTES FOR ACUTE INTOXICATIONS

Toxin	Trigger for Use	Antidote	Administration
Acetaminophen	Toxic level at 4 hours based on nomogram or suspected toxic level based on ingestion history prior to level	N-acetylcysteine	Oral, NG (IV pending FDA approval), 140 mg/kg; then 70 mg/kg q4h, at least 36 h (17 doses recommended)
Anticholinergics	Confirm cause of altered mental status	Physostigmine	IV, 0.02 mg/kg (adult 2 mg, child 0.5 mg) over 5–10 min
Benzodiazepines	Confirm cause of altered mental status	Flumazenil	IV, 0.005–0.01 mg/kg at 0.2 mg/min rate; maximum 1 mg
Beta-blockers	Cardiovascular toxicity	Glucagon	IV, 0.15 mg/kg bolus; 0.1 mg/kg/h maintenance
Calcium channel blockers	Cardiovascular toxicity	10% Calcium chloride solution	1–2 cc/kg over 5 min; repeat every 10–20 min
Cyanide	Any manifestations	3% Sodium nitrite solution and	IV, 0.2–0.3 cc/kg over 5 mins; maximum 10 cc
		25% Sodium thiosulfate solution	IV, 1–2 cc/kg over 1–2 min
Ethylene glycol, methanol	Acidemia; >20 mg/dL ethylene glycol level	Fomepizole (preferred) or 10% ethanol	IV, 15 mg/kg bolus; 10 mg/kg q12h × 4, 15 mg/kg q12h thereafter IV, 10 cc/kg: continuous 1.5 cc/kg/h
Iron	Serum iron >TIBC, or 350–500 mcg/dL	Deferoxamine	IM, 90 mg/kg; maximum 1 g, or IV, 10–15 mg/kg/h
Isoniazid	Neurotoxicity; >40 mg/kg ingestion	Pyridoxine	IV, 75 mg/kg bolus; maximum 5 g
Opioids	CNS depression	Naloxone	0.1–0.4 mg/kg bolus; 0.16 mg/kg/h continuous
Organophosphate	Nicotinic, muscarinic or CNS manifestations	Atropine and pralidoxime	IV, 0.05–0.1 mg/kg bolus; repeat as necessary 25–50 mg/kg over 15–30 min; continuous 10–20 mg/kg/h up to 500 mg/h
Oxidants	Methemoglobinemia, >20%–30%	1% Methylene blue solution	1–2 mg/kg over 5 min; repeat 1 mg/kg
Sulfonylureas	Hypoglycemia	Octreotide	Subcutaneous 1 mcg/kg every 12 h; IV, 15 ng/kg/min

Modified with permission from Bryant S, Singer J. Management of toxic exposure in children. *Emerg Med Clin North Amer* 2003;21:101, and Wolf AD, Berkowitz ID, Liebelt E, Rogers MC. Poisoning and the critically ill child. In: Rogers MC, ed. *Textbook of pediatric intensive care*. Baltimore: Williams & Wilkins, 1996:1315.

unreliable. A conservative estimate of 60 mg/kg elemental iron warrants physician evaluation. Serum iron levels should be obtained 2 to 4 hours after ingestion; after 6 hours, the liver has cleared most free iron, and levels may be misleading. Mild toxicity may occur with iron levels of 100 to 300 μg/dL, and moderate toxicity occurs at levels of 300 to 500 μg/dL. Generally, severe toxicity is associated with serum iron levels greater than 500 μg/dL. However, treatment should not be withheld in symptomatic patients, because considerable overlap in levels has been reported (Chyka et al.). Total iron-binding capacity lower than serum iron levels suggests a risk for toxicity, but a measured level above the serum iron level does not preclude toxicity. Empiric deferoxamine challenge with 40 mg/kg (maximum dose, 1 g) administered intramuscularly can be used to demonstrate excess circulating free iron, which is chelated and excreted in the urine with a classic pink-orange "vin rose" color. Significant symptoms should encourage aggressive treatment, and abdominal radiographs should be obtained to look for tablet concretions.

Gastric emptying procedures, including lavage with bicarbonate and deferoxamine, have been attempted but have not been shown to be effective. Activated charcoal does not adsorb iron and is not recommended. Whole-bowel irrigation has been found useful to hasten the passage of undissolved iron tablets. Use can be based on abdominal radiographic evidence of ra-

diopaque material, with irrigation for at least 4 to 6 hours (or until rectal effluent is clear), if the patient's condition permits. Deferoxamine, an avid iron chelator, should be initiated in cases of moderate or severe iron poisoning (serum iron level of greater than 500 μg/dL, or greater than 350 μg/dL with significant symptoms). Doses may be given intramuscularly or as a continuous intravenous infusion (15 mg/kg/hour, maximum daily dose 360 mg/kg). Adverse effects from deferoxamine are unusual, but hypotension or pulmonary edema may occur with high doses or rapid infusion rates. The end point for discontinuing deferoxamine is uncertain, but use should be considered for 8 to 12 hours with moderate toxicity and for 24 hours with severe toxicity. Close monitoring and supportive therapy for shock are essential.

Organophosphate Poisoning

Organophosphate poisoning is a leading cause of nonpharmaceutical ingestion fatality in children. Such organophosphates as parathion, malathion, and diazinon are common components of agricultural and domestic insecticides. They are absorbed across skin and mucous membranes by means of topical contamination, ingestion, inhalation, and they bind irreversibly to neuronal and erythrocyte cholinesterase and to liver pseudocholinesterase. This process results in failure to terminate the effects of acetylcholine centrally at cortical, respiratory, and cardiac centers and peripherally at nicotinic and muscarinic receptor sites. Symptoms include muscle fasciculations, weakness, paralysis (i.e., nicotinic effect), miosis, salivation, lacrimation, diarrhea, bradycardia (i.e., muscarinic effect), obtundation, seizures, and apnea (i.e., central effect). Symptoms are evidence of a more than 50% reduction in enzyme activity. The onset of symptoms may be immediate or delayed for up to 24 hours.

The measurement of decreased serum pseudocholinesterase and erythrocyte cholinesterase confirms the diagnosis, but treatment should be based on suspicion when these symptoms are present, even without documented organophosphate exposure. Gastric emptying by lavage should be considered, using adequate airway protection. Atropine given in high doses (0.05 mg/kg) antagonizes central and muscarinic effects, but it does not decrease the muscle weakness and paralysis induced by nicotinic blockade. Repeated doses are given until cholinergic signs resolve. A continuous infusion may be necessary, because recrudescence can occur for at least 24 hours. The patient should be monitored for anticholinergic toxicity. Pralidoxime, a cholinesterase-reactivating oxime, is indicated for patients with significant muscle weakness, particularly those requiring mechanical ventilation for respiratory muscle dysfunction. Pralidoxime should be initiated early, owing to the rapid development of resistance by organophosphate-cholinesterase complexes, and doses may have to be repeated over the first 24 hours of treatment.

Hydrocarbon Ingestion

Hydrocarbon ingestion typically involves common household products, most often furniture polish or gasoline. Substances with low viscosity and high volatility, such as gasoline and kerosene, present the greatest risk for aspiration, which is the major danger from hydrocarbon ingestion. The determination of the exact formulation ingested is important, because some mixtures may include aromatic compounds, such as benzene, that produce central nervous system toxicity. Fluorinated hydrocarbons, can induce seizures and cardiac dysrhythmias if inhaled. Children rapidly develop coughing, gagging, choking, and vomiting, which limit the volume of ingestion but may increase the likelihood of aspiration. Typically, dyspnea, cyanosis, and respiratory failure ensue over the first 24 hours. Roentgenographic changes are seen in most cases within 12 hours after exposure, and patients with these changes almost always are symptomatic on initial presentation.

The management of hydrocarbon ingestion is primarily symptomatic. Gastric emptying procedures should be used only following the ingestions of aromatic substances, if the hydrocarbon is mixed with another toxin, or in very high-volume ingestions; otherwise, the risk of aspiration may increase. Activated charcoal is ineffective in hydrocarbon ingestion. Patients with asymptomatic ingestion should be observed for approximately 6 hours and can be discharged if no symptoms or hypoxemia develop. Symptomatic patients should be hospitalized for observation, pulse oximetry monitoring, and serial roentgenograms. Neither prophylactic antibiotics nor corticosteroids have proved beneficial, and these agents may increase the risk for superinfection. Patients who develop respiratory failure require intubation and mechanical ventilation, often requiring high levels of positive end-expiratory pressure and other interventions for adequate oxygen delivery.

Tricyclic Antidepressant Ingestion

The ingestion of TCAs, including imipramine, amitriptyline, and the secondary amine desipramine, has been a major cause

---

BOX 119.5 — Treatment of Tricyclic Antidepressant Overdose

Support of vital functions
Maintain patent airway and adequate ventilation.
Monitor blood pressure, vital signs, level of consciousness.
Evaluate electrocardiographic width of QRS interval.
Maintain or induce alkalemia with sodium bicarbonate bolus or infusion (pH 7.45–7.55).

Drug removal
Consider gastric lavage because of delayed gastricx emptying.
Administer activated charcoal; repeat every 4–6 hours.
    Dialysis and hemoperfusion are ineffective.

Seizures
Differentiate true seizures from pseudoseizures.
Rule out metabolic causes.
Benzodiazepines are initial treatment choice.
    Phenytoin or phenobarbital are used for ongoing seizures.

Cardiac effects
Hypotension
    Provide intravascular volume (10–20 mL/kg), maintain alkalemia.
If persistent, supply alpha agonists (norepinephrine, phenylephrine).

Arrhythmias
    Supraventricular tachycardia is most common.
Seek other causes.
Maintain alkalemia and supplement volume; consider beta blocker if ineffective.
Bradycardia
    Look for other sources.
Maintain alkalemia; give beta agonists if no response (norepinephrine, isoproterenol). Use electrical pacing if other measures are ineffective.
Ventricular ectopy
    Administer lidocaine (be aware of myocardial depression, seizures); use phenytoin if this is ineffective.
Avoid quinidine, procainamide.

Other illnesses and follow-up
Perform pregnancy test in all pubertal females.
Conduct a social and mental health evaluation.
Limit access to tricyclic antidepressants and other medications.

Modified with permission from Braden NJ, Jackson JE, Walson PD. Tricyclic antidepressant overdose. *Pediatr Clin North Am* 1986; 33:287.

of ingestion-related fatalities, responsible for up to 25% of all serious overdoses in children and adults and up to 20% of pediatric deaths. Cases of TCA ingestion are likely decreasing because of the increased use of serotonin reuptake inhibitors, such as fluoxetine (Prozac) and sertraline (Zoloft), for treatment of depression. This class has proved safer in overdose than TCAs, with less potential central nervous system and cardiovascular toxicity.

TCAs have very narrow therapeutic windows; therapeutic imipramine doses are 1 to 3 mg/kg, whereas 10 to 20 mg/kg produces moderate to severe toxicity, and 30 to 40 mg/kg may be fatal. TCAs block the presynaptic uptake of neurotransmitters norepinephrine and serotonin. In addition, TCAs block sympathetic alpha-adrenergic receptor and parasympathetic muscarinic (cholinergic) receptor response, thus producing a variety of hemodynamic effects in toxic doses. TCA absorption may be delayed, owing to its anticholinergic effects. TCAs have quinidine-like activity at therapeutic doses, prolonging conduction times that predispose to wide-complex tachycardias at toxic levels. They are highly protein-bound and lipid-soluble and may have significant enterohepatic recirculation. Although total dose correlates with toxicity, quantitative TCA levels are not helpful in determining management, which should be based on clinical presentation. Decreased cardiac conduction rate, as seen by widened QRS interval (greater than 100 ms) is a helpful clinical correlate of severe toxicity but may be normal in children, even in the presence of serious overdose. TCA toxicity should be suspected in patients presenting with signs of anticholinergic poisoning, coma, or hypotension.

Most TCA ingestions that require treatment (Box 119.5) will necessitate intensive care monitoring, owing to the potential for respiratory difficulties, life-threatening arrhythmias and hypotension, and seizures. No specific antidotes are yet available, although Fab fragment antibodies are in development. Use of flumazenil specifically should be avoided, because it can enhance seizure potential. General therapeutic measures include gastric decontamination and the use of multiple-dose activated charcoal, because of delayed gastric emptying and high enterohepatic recirculation seen with TCAs. Hemoperfusion and dialysis are ineffective removal techniques. Strict attention should be paid to monitoring vital signs and to intervening early with an artificial airway and mechanical ventilation. The induction of alkalemia has been shown to be one of the best specific TCA therapies due to its potential stabilization of cardiac membranes and consequent reduction of arrhythmias. Hypotension can occur from alpha-adrenergic blockade and is treated with fluids and alpha-agonist vasopressors as needed. Both arrhythmias and seizures can occur, and treatment often is difficult. Pseudoseizures (myoclonus, tremor, chorea) can occur in up to 50% of patients with TCA overdose and must be differentiated from true seizure activity. Metabolic acidosis and hypokalemia also are seen in the first 24 hours.

Suggested Readings

Banner W, Tong TG. Iron poisoning. *Pediatr Clin North Am* 1987;33:393.

Braden NJ, Jackson JE, Walson PD. Tricyclic antidepressant overdose. *Pediatr Clin North Am* 1986;33:287.

Bryant S, Singer J. Management of toxic exposure in children. *Emerg Med Clin North Am* 2003;21:101.

Chyka PA, Butler AY, Holley JE. Serum iron concentrations and symptoms of acute iron poisoning in children. *Pharmacotherapy* 1996;16:1053.

Committee on Accident and Poison Prevention, American Academy of Pediatrics. The non-toxic ingestion. In: Aronow R, ed. *Handbook of common poisonings in children,* 2nd ed. Evanston, IL: American Academy of Pediatrics, 1983:16.

Committee on Injury, Violence, and Poison Prevention, American Academy of Pediatrics. Poison treatment in the home. *Pediatrics* 2003;112:1182.

Kirk M, Pace S. Pearls, pitfalls and updates in toxicology. *Emerg Clin North Am* 1997;15:427.

Kulig K. Initial management of ingestions of toxic substances. *N Engl J Med* 1992;326:1677.

Lewander WJ, Lacoutre PG. Office management of acute pediatric poisonings. *Pediatr Emerg Care* 1989;5:262.

Litovitz T, Manoguerra A. Comparison of pediatric poisoning hazards: an analysis of 3.8 million exposure incidents. *Pediatrics* 1992;89:999.

Manoguerra AS. Gastrointestinal decontamination after poisoning: where is the science? *Pediatr Clin North Am* 1997;13:709.

McGuigan MA. Acute iron poisoning. *Pediatr Ann* 1996;25:33.

Mokhlesi B, Leikin J, et al. Adult toxicology in critical care: specific poisonings. *Chest* 2003;123:897.

Osterhoudt K, Shannon M, Henretig FM. Toxicologic emergencies. In: Fleisher GR, Ludwig S, eds. *Textbook of pediatric emergency medicine,* 4th ed. Baltimore: Williams & Wilkins, 2000:887.

Vernon DD, Gleich MC. Poisoning and drug overdose. *Crit Care Clin North Am* 1997;13:647.

Watson W, Litovitz T, et al. 2002 annual report of the American association of poison control centers toxic exposure surveillance system. *Am J Emerg Med* 2003;21:353.

Woolf AD, Berkowitz ID, Liebelt E, Rogers MC. Poisoning and the critically ill child. In: Rogers MC, ed. *Textbook of pediatric intensive care.* Baltimore: Williams & Wilkins, 1996:1315.

CHAPTER 120 ■ SALICYLISM

M. MICHELE MARISCALCO

The frequency of salicylism in U.S. children peaked in the 1960s at 25% of all ingestions. Because of changes in product packaging and the introduction of child-resistant closures, the incidence of aspirin ingestion, and the death rate associated with it, have declined. Based on over 20,000 salicylate exposures reported to the American Association of Poison Control Centers (ASPC) Toxic Exposure Surveillance System (TESS) during 2003, 17% of exposures occurred in children younger than 6 years of age, no fatalities occurred, and only 0.1% of exposures resulted in major morbidity. Thus, salicylate exposures are rarely fatal in those most vulnerable to poisonings—children younger than 6 years of age. Intentional overdose or therapeutic errors account for the higher morbidity and mortality in adolescents and adults. In the 2003 TESS, 36 fatalities occurred among those older than 6 years of age. Combined major morbidity or death occurred in 1.5% of all those with salicylate exposures in this age group.

Chronic salicylism appears to produce greater morbidity than acute salicylate poisoning in the pediatric and geriatric age group. Chronic salicylism can occur because of therapeutic errors, the administration of several salicylate-containing preparations simultaneously, or normal dosing in a dehydrated child. The diagnosis of chronic salicylism may be delayed because its symptoms of fever, vomiting, and tachypnea resemble the disease process for which the salicylate is being used therapeutically.

Aspirin and salicylic acid products are the active ingredients of hundreds of therapeutic prescription and over-the-counter products. Particularly problematic are oil of wintergreen and bismuth subsalicylate. Oil of wintergreen (methyl salicylate) is a common ingredient of liniments, ointments, and essential oils used in the treatment of musculoskeletal pain. Its pleasant smell encourages its "sampling" by children. Its high content of salicylate makes it extremely toxic. One teaspoon is approximately equivalent to 7,000 mg of salicylate, or about 22 adult aspirins. As little as 4 mL can be fatal to a child. Its use in topical agents can also be a source of chronic intoxication, particularly in the elderly. Bismuth subsalicylate (Pepto-Bismol), an anti-diarrheal medication, contains 262 mg of bismuth subsalicylate per 15 mL, or about 130 mg total subsalicylate. An 8-ounce dose contains the equivalent of six to seven 325-mg tablets of adult aspirin.

TOXICOKINETICS

In therapeutic doses, aspirin is absorbed rapidly from the upper small intestine. With overdosage, however, absorption may occur more slowly. Thus, blood salicylate concentrations can continue to increase for as long as 24 hours after ingestion. Salicylates are distributed unevenly throughout the body fluids and tissues. The low apparent volume of distribution suggests that salicylate remains largely in the central compartment. At therapeutic doses, salicylate is significantly bound to plasma proteins (possibly as high as 80% to 90%). Albumin is the major protein responsible for the extensive protein binding. The degree of protein binding is dependent on both the concentration of salicylic acid and the amount of albumin. As protein-binding sites become saturated in overdosed patients, the amount of non-protein-bound salicylic acid increases, which increases the potential for significant toxicity. Conditions that deplete albumin and other proteins predispose the patient to a disproportionate risk of severe salicylism at a given plasma concentration.

If acid–base status is normal, salicylates are highly ionized. Thus, diffusion of salicylates across the blood–brain barrier and into the central nervous system (CNS) are reduced. Patients with salicylism may develop metabolic acidosis, which increases the fraction of nonionized salicylate. A higher nonionized fraction results in a greater CNS penetration, increased CNS concentration, and elevated cerebral spinal fluid (CSF) concentration. High CSF concentrations are associated with CNS toxicity and greater morbidity.

Initially, the hydrolysis of salicylate salt or aspirin results in the formation of salicylic acid. Salicylic acid undergoes further biotransformation and elimination via first-order processes. As higher doses of salicylate are ingested, biotransformation pathways become saturated, and elimination converts from a dose-dependent first-order process (rate proportional to the dose) to a zero-order process (i.e., a fixed amount of salicylic acid is metabolized per unit of time, regardless of the dose). These toxicokinetics of salicylic acid account for the prolonged elimination half-life, which approximates 20 to 30 hours. In contrast, no reduction occurs in the initial hydrolysis of acetylsalicylic acid (aspirin) to salicylic acid.

Renal clearance accounts for most of the elimination of salicylates and is enhanced from 2% to more than 80% as pH and ionization increase. The kidneys eliminate salicylate by both glomerular filtration and tubule secretion. Salicylate also is reabsorbed, however, in the renal tubule. Reabsorption is affected by urinary pH and urine flow rate. Only nonionized molecules are reabsorbed. Because salicylate is a weak acid (pKa 3.5), the nonionized fraction increases as pH level decreases. Under normal conditions, that is, in the presence of an acidic urine, reabsorption is favored. However, as the urine becomes more alkaline, the amount of ionized salicylate increases, and the proportion that is reabsorbed by the renal tubule decreases.

Neonates absorb salicylate as rapidly as any other age group, but they metabolize it more slowly. Renal elimination is slower in children than in adults, and they have reduced albumin concentrations, which increases plasma salicylate concentrations. The volume of distribution increases in proportion to the dose, suggesting that children may have higher tissue concentrations than are inferred by the plasma concentration.

PATHOPHYSIOLOGY

The toxic effects of salicylate are complex and multifactorial. The acute ingestion of large quantities, particularly in children, may produce nausea and vomiting as a result of local gastric irritation and the stimulation of chemoreceptor trigger zones; this results in dehydration. Table 120.1 summarizes the mechanisms, metabolic consequences, and clinical pathophysiology of acute aspirin toxicity. The primary effects of toxic levels of salicylate include the direct stimulation of the CNS respiratory center and is independent of increased oxygen consumption or carbon dioxide production. Metabolic acidosis is the result of the collective effects of elevated lactic acid and pyruvic acid secondary to Krebs cycle enzyme inhibition, increased ketone body formation from accelerated lipid metabolism, and amino acidemia from inhibition of aminotransferases. In younger children, in chronic salicylate toxicity, and in large-dose poisoning in older children, metabolic acidosis appears early and clinically predominates. Older children with moderate- or small-dose poisoning and most adults are able to compensate the metabolic acidosis by hyperventilation, resulting in respiratory alkalosis. Hypoglycemia is uncommon but quite severe when it occurs. Hyperglycemia is more common. Significant CNS hypoglycemia can occur with normal blood glucose levels.

Severe fluid and electrolyte loss can occur with salicylate toxicity. Increased heat production, because of the uncoupling of oxidative phosphorylation, hyperpnea, and tachypnea, all lead to an increase in insensible water loss. Decreased oral intake and vomiting, and the increase in obligatory water and electrolyte loss necessitated by the enhanced renal solute load of organic acids, further aggravates the water, sodium, and potassium loss. The renal excretion of bicarbonate is increased, contributing to the metabolic acidosis.

ACUTE SALICYLATE POISONING

Diagnosis

The usual symptoms of acute toxicity include disorientation, nausea, vomiting, dehydration, hyperpnea, hyperpyrexia, oliguria, tinnitus, coma, and convulsions. Other less common findings include bleeding, respiratory depression, pulmonary edema, acute tubular necrosis, hepatotoxicity, nephropathy, bronchospasm, anaphylaxis, hemolysis, and electroencephalographic abnormalities. Ototoxicity is directly related to unbound serum salicylate concentration. It is reversible. Tinnitus can occur with salicylate levels of 200 mg/L, and hearing loss reaches its maximum of 40 decibels at levels exceeding 400 mg/L.

The onset of symptoms usually occurs within 1 to 2 hours, but may be delayed 4 to 6 hours due to absorption of

TABLE 120.1

MECHANISMS OF SALICYLATE TOXICITY AND PATHOLOGIC RESPONSE

Toxicity Mechanism	Pathologic Response	Metabolic Compensation	Signs and Symptoms
Elevated salicylate concentration (acidic substance)	Decrease in serum pH	Contributes to metabolic acidosis; alters platelet function (hypoprothrombinemia)	Increase bleeding time
Stimulation of medullary respiratory center	Hyperventilation	Decreases in plasma P_aCO_2 with respiratory alkalosis	Tachypnea, tachycardia, dehydration
Renal compensation for respiratory alkalosis	Increased excretion of HCO_3^-; retain H^+	Contributes to compensatory metabolic acidosis; CNS toxicity	Irritability, restlessness, tinnitus, dehydration, seizures, coma
Renal vascular injury	Increased permeability to plasma proteins		Proteinuria
Direct effects on gastric mucosa	Local gastric irritation and stimulation of chemoreceptor trigger zones	Dehydration, contributes to acidosis	Gastric irritation, nausea, vomiting
Inhibition of Krebs cycle enzymes	Accumulation of organic acids	Contributes to metabolic acidosis and lactic acidosis	Gastric irritation, nausea, vomiting
Oxidative uncoupling of electron transport chain	Prevents combination of phosphate with ADP	Decreased formation of ATP, enhanced glycolysis, lactic acid, pyruvic acid; contributes to metabolic acidosis	Hyperthermia, tachycardia, dehydration, cardiovascular collapse, hypoglycemia
	Increases peripheral demand for glucose	Stimulates lipid metabolism, releases fatty acids, contributes to metabolic acidosis	
Injury to alveolar capillary membrane	Increased permeability to fluid and protein	Hypoxemia, hyperpnea	Pulmonary edema

sustained-release preparations or the formation of gastric concretions. Severity of symptoms peaks between 12 and 24 hours. The estimated amount of drug ingested may potentially predict the severity of the clinical syndrome; however, clinical presentation and *serial* serum levels determines the degree of toxicity. *Salicylate poisoning is a dynamic process and regular assessments and an ongoing reappraisal of management strategies are required.* Table 120.2 demonstrates the degree of poisoning based upon the symptoms. Note that salicylate levels reflect the peak level, and that children and elderly patients have more severe symptoms at lower salicylate levels than non-elderly adults.

Salicylate levels should be measured in any patient who has a history of potentially serious ingestion (greater than 125 mg/kg). Plasma levels measured before 4 hours after ingestion are difficult to interpret. Specific care should be taken when reviewing these plasma levels as instances of errors have occurred when caregivers misread the concentrations in mg/dL rather mg/L. Laboratory values may be reported either way. Serum levels should be followed every 3 to 4 hours until they peak, which may be as late as 12 to 24 hours following ingestion, particularly with enteric-coated aspirin.

The Done nomogram was created to assist in clarifying the level of intoxication that should prompt investigation (Fig. 120.1). However, much controversy surrounds its use because it was derived from only 24 patients with acute ingestions (one-third of whom were adults) and never has been subjected to rigorous study as a diagnostic or screening tool. It frequently over- and underestimates the severity of the intoxication. It is not useful if ingestion has occurred over hours or days, ingestion was of enteric-coated or sustained-release compounds, the compound is oil of wintergreen, the patient has renal insufficiency, the patient is acidemic, or if the time of ingestion is unknown. Note that the Done nomogram serum concentration

is in *mg/dL*. Many toxicologists do not recommend the use of the Done nomogram.

Therapy

As with all ingestions, therapy initially is directed toward ensuring adequate ventilation, oxygenation, and cardiovascular stability. There is no antidote to salicylate poisoning, and management is directed towards preventing further absorption and increasing elimination in those with moderate or severe intoxication.

Activated charcoal effectively absorbs aspirin. An initial dose of 1 to 2 g/kg (50 g in adults) is recommended if ingestion is 125 mg/kg or higher, or the dose is unknown. As always, ensure that the airway is protected before the administration of activated charcoal. The use of repeated doses of activated charcoal is controversial, with conflicting interpretations of limited the data. Aspirin does form concretions in the stomach, and it may be important to recoat the surfaces of such concretions with charcoal to reduce ongoing absorption. The administration of a second dose may be particularly valuable in adults who have ingested substantial quantities of an enteric-coated or sustained-release preparation. The suggested repeated doses of activated charcoal are 0.25 to 0.5 g/kg (25 g in adults), depending on the dose and dosage form of the drug ingested, every 4 to 6 hours until the salicylate level peaks.

Fluid therapy is aimed at promoting renal salicylate excretion and restoring hydration and electrolyte balance. Large volumes of isotonic solution such as lactated Ringer's solution may be necessary to restore the circulating blood volume, correct hypotension, and improve peripheral perfusion and urine flow. Subsequent fluid replacement depends on the degree of dehydration. The fluid should contain dextrose with

TABLE 120.2

CLINICAL FEATURES AND TREATMENT OF ACUTE SALICYLATE OVERDOSE

Level of Intoxication	Peak Salicylate Level*	Clinical Features	Usual Dose Ingested**	Treatment
Asymptomatic	Adults: <300 mg/L Children/elderly: <200 mg/L	Asymptomatic	<125 mg/kg	Hydrate with oral fluids. Close observation may occur as outpatient.
Mild	Adults: 300–600 mg/L Children/elderly: <200–450 mg/L	Lethargy, nausea, vomiting, tinnitus, dizziness	>125 mg/kg	Rehydrate with intravenous fluids, oral fluids may be used. Monitor urine output and fluid balance carefully. Measure glucose, urea, electrolytes, blood gases.
Moderate	Adults: 600–800 mg/L Children/elderly: 450–700 mg/L	Mild feature + tachypnea, hyperpyrexia, sweating, dehydration, loss of coordination, restlessness	>300 mg/kg	IV hydration and monitoring of biochemical parameters. Urinary alkalinization. Minimize hypernatremia, correct hypokalemia. Initial bolus of 2 mEq/kg of sodium bicarbonate followed by infusion of 150 mEq of sodium bicarbonate in 1 L of D5W. Adult rate: 150–200 mL/hour, Child rate: twice maintenance fluid rate. Titrate alkalinization to keep urine pH >7.5, and serum pH ≤7.55. Keep urine output 1–2 mL/kg/h minimum.
Severe	Adults: >800 mg/L Children/elderly: >700 mg/L	Hypotension; significant metabolic acidosis after rehydration; renal failure (oliguria); CNS: coma, convulsions, hallucinations, stupor	>500 mg/kg	Alkalinize urine, fluid administration should be based upon urine output. Hemodialysis should. Increased monitoring of electrolytes, blood gases, glucose usually required.

*First level after 4 hours, and repeat salicylate level every 3 hours until a peak concentration is reached.
**Note that treatment strategies should be based upon *symptoms* and *serial levels*, and not on dose ingested.

saline (0.45%) because CNS glucose concentrations can be depressed even with mild blood hyperglycemia. The addition of potassium is necessary to correct hypokalemia after the urine output is established. Hyperpyrexia is managed by external cooling with a cooling blanket. Because the patient with serious poisoning is at risk of developing pulmonary edema, fluid retention, or both, aggressive fluid replacement may be counterproductive. Urine output and renal function must be carefully monitored.

The therapy of acidosis is critical in the management of salicylate intoxication. Acidosis enhances the passage of salicylate (nonionized form) from the extracellular space into the cells, including the blood–brain barrier, where it disrupts mitochondrial function. Sodium bicarbonate's alkalinization effect occurs solely in the extracellular space and increases the level of ionized drug in the extracellular plasma. The intracellular-to-extracellular gradient of diffusible, nonionized drug is increased, thus enhancing the trapping of salicylate in the extracellular plasma.

Alkalinization of the urine is indicated for any patient with moderate to severe toxicity. Baseline biochemical assessment should include plasma creatinine and electrolytes, glucose, and arterial acid–base status. An intravenous line should be established, and/or a central line if appropriate. A bladder catheter should be inserted. Fluid deficit must be corrected. Alkalinization should *not* be delayed to achieve normokalemia. Refer to Table 120.2 for a treatment schema. The period of administration of the loading dose of sodium bicarbonate may be

shortened and/or the dose increased if preexisting acidemia is present. An 8.4% solution (1 mEq/mL) of sodium bicarbonate is a vesicant and can cause tissue necrosis if it extravasates. Titrate the sodium bicarbonate–containing fluids or give additional boluses of intravenous sodium bicarbonate to achieve and maintain a urine pH of greater than 7.5. Monitor urine pH every 15 to 30 minutes until urine pH is in the range 7.5 to 8.5, then hourly. Sodium bicarbonate administration may aggravate hypernatremia and hypokalemia, and it may precipitate hypocalcemia and seizures. In the moderately and severely intoxicated patient, hourly measurements should be considered for plasma potassium and sodium, central venous pressure, acid–base status (arterial pH should not exceed 7.55), plasma salicylate concentrations (until peak), and urine output. Urine alkalinization should be discontinued when the concentrations fall below 350 mg/L in an adult or 250 mg/L in a child. No indications exist for "forcing" diuresis with diuretics, such as furosemide or mannitol. Acetazolamide used to alkalinize the urine is contraindicated, because it leads to metabolic acidosis through the inhibition of bicarbonate reabsorption in the proximal tubules.

Frequent clinical evaluation for brain–blood disequilibrium is mandatory in any patient with salicylate intoxication. CNS status may improve as the plasma pH increases, because of a shift of salicylate equilibrium from brain to blood despite a lack of urine alkalinization.

Hemodialysis should be used for severe clinical features including coma, convulsion, acute renal failure, pulmonary

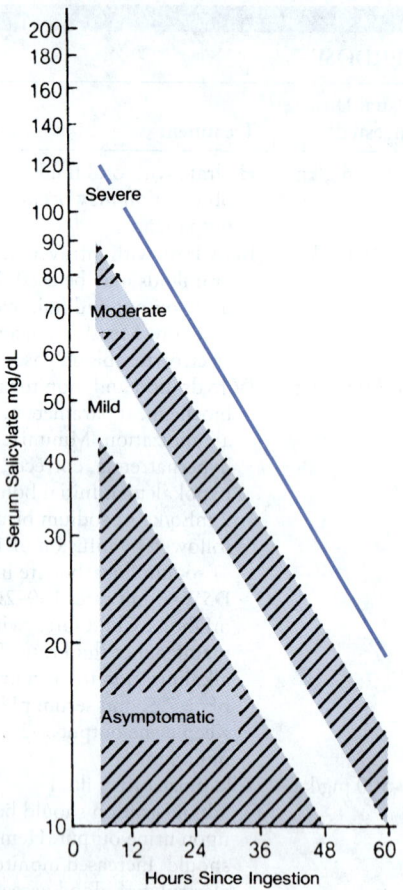

FIGURE 120.1. Done nomogram for estimating the severity of acute, single ingestion of non–enteric-coated aspirin. (Reprinted with permission from Temple AR. Acute and chronic effects of aspirin toxicity and their treatment. *Arch Intern Med* 1981;141:364.)

edema, or severe acidosis not responding to hydration and alkalinization. It should be considered when plasma levels exceed 800 mg/L. In the 2003 annual report of the AAPCC Toxic Exposure Surveillance System, 14 of 23 deaths occurred in patients with a salicylic acid level less than 800 mg/L. Thus, determining the need for dialysis should not be based solely on levels. Alkalinization should not be delayed while instituting dialysis, and evidence supports doing both concomitantly. Hemodialysis is the treatment of choice, although continuous venovenous hemofiltration with dialysis has been used successfully.

CHRONIC SALICYLATE POISONING

Chronic salicylate poisoning (the repeated administration of therapeutic or excessive doses of salicylate for a period longer than 12 hours) is associated with more severe symptoms than acute intoxication, particularly the development of acidosis and disturbances of the CNS. Children and elderly adults are at increased risk of chronic salicylate poisoning. How much salicylate is required to cause chronic salicylate poisoning, and over what period, is not known. Although daily doses as low as 32 mg/kg have been associated with this complication, Temple

estimated that a daily dose of 100 mg/kg for at least 2 days is needed. Severe chronic poisoning occurs at lower plasma levels than with acute intoxication, and clinical features correlate poorly with levels. Chronic salicylate intoxication has been erroneously diagnosed as numerous conditions including systemic inflammatory response syndrome, acute abdomen, impending myocardial infarction, encephalopathy, sepsis, diabetic ketoacidosis, viral encephalitis, and organic psychosis. Salicylate toxicity should be considered in patients with unexplained acid–base disturbances, hyperventilation, or confusion. The diagnosis is confirmed with biochemical evidence of ingestion. Supportive measures and the use of urinary alkalinization are the same as indicated for acute toxicity. The use of activated charcoal is probably of no benefit, because the absorption has already occurred in most patients. The threshold to institute extracorporeal techniques to enhance elimination is much lower than that for acutely poisoned patients.

REYE SYNDROME

The Reye syndrome phenotype has been associated with the use of salicylates, in particular during influenza or varicella outbreaks. It is not associated with acute intoxication. The incidence of Reye syndrome has fallen dramatically during the years from 1980 to 1989. The clinical picture in adults and children is similar, although the association with salicylate is less strong in adults than in children. Vomiting, followed shortly afterward by encephalopathy, develops after an acute illness. The diagnosis is best confirmed by percutaneous liver biopsy (microvesicular fatty change within the hepatocytes with little or no inflammatory infiltrate or necrosis and with evidence of ultrastructural changes in the mitochondria on electron microscopy). In both adults and children, mortality is about 30%. Many drugs, in addition to salicylates, are associated with this syndrome, including tetracyclines, valproic acid, acetaminophen, and phenformin.

Suggested Readings

American Academy of Clinical Toxicology; European Association of Poison Centres and Clinical Toxicologists. Position Statement and Practice Guidelines on the Use of Multi-dose Activated Charcoal in the Treatment of Acute Poisoning. *Clinical Toxicology* 1999;37(6):731.

Barile FA. Acetaminophen, salicylates, and non-steroidal anti-inflammatory drugs. In: Barile FA. *Clinical toxicology: principles and mechanisms.* Boca Rotan: CRC Press, 2004:191.

Borkan SC. Extracorporeal therapies for acute intoxications. *Critical Care Clinics* 2004;18:393.

Curry SC. Salicylate. In: Reisdorff EJ, Roberts MR, Wiegenstein JG, eds. *Pediatric emergency medicine.* Philadelphia: Saunders, 1993:667.

Dargan PI, Wallace CI, Jones AL. An evidence based flowchart to guide the management of acute salicylate (aspirin) overdose. *Emerg Med J* 2002;19:206.

Ellenhorn MJ, Schonwald S, Ordog G, Wasserberger J, eds. *Ellenhorn's medical toxicology: diagnosis and treatment of human poisoning,* 2nd ed. Baltimore: Williams & Wilkins, 1997.

Gaudreault P, Temple A, Lovejoy F. The relative severity of acute versus chronic salicylate poisoning in children: a clinical comparison. *Pediatrics* 1982;70:566.

Krenzelok EP, Kerr F, Proudfoot AT. Salicylate toxicity. In: Haddad LM, Shannon MW, Winchester JF, eds. *Clinical management of poisoning and drug overdose,* 3rd ed. Philadelphia: Saunders, 1998:675.

Proudfoot AT, Krenzelok EP, Vale JA. Position paper on urine alkalinization. *J Toxicol Clin Toxicol* 2004;42(1):1.

Temple A. Acute and chronic effects of aspirin toxicity and their treatment. *Arch Intern Med* 1981;141:364.

Yip L. Salicylates. In: Dart RC. *Medical toxicology,* 3rd ed. Philadelphia: Lippincott Williams & Wilkins, 2004:739.

CHAPTER 121 ■ ACETAMINOPHEN OVERDOSE

M. MICHELE MARISCALCO

EPIDEMIOLOGY

Acetaminophen is the most common pharmaceutical involved in overdose. As reported by the American Association of Poison Control Centers Toxic Exposure Surveillance System in 2003, acetaminophen overdose accounted for 10% of more than 1.3 million pharmaceutical exposures. Of the 350,000 exposures to pharmaceutical agents that resulted in some degree of toxicity, acetaminophen was involved in 21% of these cases. Of the 2,054 deaths resulting from pharmaceutical substances, 327 (16%) were attributed to acetaminophen either singly or in combination with at least one other substance. This is in contrast to 225 deaths from all stimulants and street drugs and 213 deaths from opioids reported during that same year. Children less than 6 years old accounted for 31% of all exposures to acetaminophen, and those from 6 to 19 years old accounted for 21%. However, of the 327 deaths associated with acetaminophen, only six were in children less than 6 years of age and seven were in those aged 6 to 19 years. Of those less than 6 years old, three deaths were the result of chronic therapeutic error, the cause of one was unknown, and one was the result of malicious intent. The final child died of an unintentional ingestion of acetaminophen, diphenhydramine, and iron. Of the seven children older than 6 years who died, all were older than 14 years; five had intended suicide, one cause was unknown, and one died as a result of a chronic therapeutic error. Of the 313 adults who died of acetaminophen overdose, 17 were more than 65 years old. Nine adults died as a result of therapeutic errors with the ingestion of acetaminophen alone or in combination with other products. Of these, six were older than 65 years of age.

These data emphasize the following key points: (a) acetaminophen is by far the single most common agent resulting in the highest number of pharmaceutical exposures; (b) despite its wide therapeutic index, acetaminophen exposure results in a disproportionate share of toxicity; (c) although children less than 6 years of age are overrepresented in the number of exposures to toxicity, nonetheless little major toxicity, including death, result; (d) most exposures in individuals greater than 6 years of age are the result of intended suicide; (e) the number of deaths caused by the ingestion of acetaminophen as a result of therapeutic error is disproportionately represented by those less than 6 and greater than 65 years of age; and (f) specific antidotal therapy (i.e. N-acetylcysteine [NAC]) improves the outcome of those who have experienced significant acute exposures.

TOXICOKINETICS AND TOXICODYNAMICS

The maximum adult therapeutic dose of acetaminophen is 1 g, four times a day at 4-hour intervals. The pediatric dose is 10 to 15 mg/kg, four to five times a day (total of 75 mg/kg/day). An acute overdosage of approximately 15 g is thought to be the threshold for production of toxicity in adults. For more than 25 years, the reported threshold dose for acute ingestion in children has been 150 mg/kg. However, this dose is empiric and extrapolated from adult data. More recent investigations and consideration of pharmacokinetic features unique to children suggest raising the level to 200 mg/kg. In single-dose ingestions, children younger than 6 years ingest less drug than adolescents. In adolescents, the overdose is either a suicide attempt or a manipulative episode, and handfuls of tablets typically are consumed. It has been difficult to define a "toxic" dose in those patients with prolonged supratherapeutic dosing. In adults, it is hypothesized that repeated supratherapeutic ingestion of 10 g/day for 2 days is associated with liver injury. In children, 150 mg/kg/day for 2 or more days is believed to be the threshold level that will produce toxicity.

Acetaminophen is absorbed rapidly after an oral therapeutic dose, producing a peak plasma level between 30 and 60 minutes after ingestion. This absorption may be delayed in overdose, so peak plasma levels may not occur until 4 hours after ingestion. Approximately 94% of the drug is metabolized to the glucuronide or sulfate conjugate; 2% is excreted unchanged in the urine. Neither the conjugated forms nor the unchanged forms are hepatotoxic. The remaining 4% is metabolized through the cytochrome P-450 mixed-function oxidase system, primarily CYP2E1 and, to a much less extent, CYP3A4, to form a toxic, electrophilic metabolite, N-acetyl-p-benzoquinone imine (NAPQI). After therapeutic dosing, any NAPQI formed is conjugated with glutathione (GSH) to produce mercapturic acid, which is excreted in the urine.

With a significant overdose, the CYP2E1 enzyme system becomes increasingly important for metabolizing acetaminophen, and large amounts of NAPQI are formed. Hepatic GSH is the primary antioxidant that conjugates and neutralizes NAPQI. Liver GSH stores can be depleted with an acute or chronic overdose. When the liver GSH stores are sufficiently depleted, usually to approximately 70% of normal, NAPQI quickly accumulates. Although short-lived, NAPQI forms adducts with more than 40 cellular components, including deoxyribonucleic acid, lipids, enzymes, and cellular organelles. Because the CYP2E1 is primarily located in centrilobular hepatocytes (i.e., those around the central vein), injury initially is confined to this region. Oxidative stress, lipid peroxidation, and mitochondrial damage all play a role in the centrilobular necrosis. A second stage of injury then occurs involving Kupffer cells, cytokine release, and various reactive oxygen species that propagates injury beyond the centrilobular areas. These substances also signal hepatocyte proliferation and regeneration. If injury is limited, and hepatic regeneration is sufficient, liver recovery can be complete.

Organ systems other than the liver can be affected immediately after overdose, including the kidney (about 5% to 10% in one series) and central nervous system. Rarely, a renal defect occurs without concomitant hepatic damage. Elevation of pancreatic enzyme levels has been reported in as many as 22% of unselected patients.

Drug induction and disease interactions have been proposed to increase vulnerability to acetaminophen. The issue in each case is whether the acetaminophen increases the production of NAPQI or impairs defences to the reactive metabolite (e.g., reduces GSH). Liver disease including hepatitis and cirrhosis and "starvation" were thought to result in reduced GSH levels, thus increasing the risk of NAPQI formation with overdose. Subsequent studies have proven that these assumptions were not correct. Phenytoin and phenobarbital, which increase total cellular P-450, were also thought to increase the toxic effects of acetaminophen. Neither phenobarbital nor any of the barbiturates increases CYP2E1; thus, these drugs do not affect acetaminophen metabolism. Phenytoin has no effect on CYP2E1 but does induce glucuronyl transferase, so it may potentially be hepatoprotective by increasing glucuronidation. Ethanol enhancement of acetaminophen toxicity has also been misunderstood. Ethanol consumption on a long-term basis may maximally induce CYP2E1 about twofold, and there is some depletion of GSH in alcoholic patients. Long-term heavy abusers of alcohol are therefore probably at greater risk for toxicity from an overdose of acetaminophen, but not from therapeutic doses. In contrast, the acute coingestion of alcohol and acetaminophen in children and adults appears to be hepatoprotective. This is likely because the alcohol competes with acetaminophen at the CYP2E1-binding site.

As stated earlier, children younger than 6 years have different patterns of toxicity and are half as likely to develop acetaminophen plasma levels in the toxic range compared with adolescents and adults. Several mechanisms for decreased toxicity in children less than 6 years old have been postulated, including (a) higher turnover rates of GSH, resulting in more glutathione available for detoxification; (b) increased rates of sulfatization; (c) spontaneous vomiting after ingestion; and (d) increased ratio of liver to body weight, in effect providing increased ability to detoxify acetaminophen.

of prothrombin time may appear as early as 8 hours after overdose, and more than one-half of all patients with liver injury develop some elevation of these values within 24 hours. Lethargy is rarely seen during this stage. If lethargy develops, some other agent should be considered in addition to or instead of the acetaminophen. During the second stage, most patients begin to feel better. If no treatment was received or treatment was unsuccessful, the levels of AST, ALT, international normalized ratio (INR), and/or partial thromboplastin time (PTT) rise. Patients who have elevations of AST or ALT levels greater than 1,000 IU/L commonly demonstrate other evidence of liver dysfunction by 24 to 72 hours after overdose, including elevations in bilirubin.

During the third stage, from 72 to 96 hours after ingestion and as early as 48 hours, transaminase levels as high as 50,000 IU/L may be seen in patients with severe acetaminophen overdoses. Examination of the liver at this point demonstrates centrilobular necrosis. In the final stage, within 14 days of ingestion, hepatic abnormalities should return to normal. Follow-up evaluations of patients who experienced significant hepatotoxicity and survived reveal no sequelae clinically or on hepatic biopsy. Patients who ultimately die or who require liver transplantation progress to hepatic necrosis, including jaundice, coagulation defects, hepatorenal syndrome, and hepatic encephalopathy. Some degree of renal injury develops in almost 50% of patients with severe liver injury. However, renal failure is reversible if the patient survives.

Coma with metabolic acidosis is an unusual but well-documented presentation of acute severe acetominophen poisoning. There have been several reports of comatose patients presenting with metabolic acidosis and a very high acetaminophen level (greater than 800 mg/L), with very little evidence of liver injury. Prompt treatment with NAC can prevent liver injury in these patients.

CLINICAL MANIFESTATIONS

The manifestations of acute acetaminophen poisoning are well described, and the clinical course of acetaminophen toxicity has four stages (Table 121.1). In the first stage (i.e., first 24 hours), adult and adolescent patients develop nausea, vomiting, diaphoresis, and general malaise. Children younger than 6 years show little diaphoresis and vomit earlier. Young children often develop vomiting regardless of the acetaminophen level and may have no other symptoms unless the blood level is in the toxic range. Symptoms usually develop within 12 hours in patients with toxic levels of acetaminophen. Evidence of liver injury as reflected by elevations in aspartate aminotransferase (AST) and alanine aminotransferase (ALT) and prolongation

DIAGNOSIS

After acute and subacute overdosage of acetaminophen, one must determine the need for treatment with the antidote for acetaminophen, NAC. The Rumack-Matthew nomogram uses a timed plasma acetaminophen level drawn at least 4 hours after ingestion to establish the likelihood of liver injury (Fig. 121.1). This nomogram was empirically derived from 64 patients with untreated acetaminophen poisoning at the Edinburgh poison treatment center. A line connecting a point at 200 μg/mL at 4 hours after ingestion and 50 μg/mL at 12 hours after ingestion was found to separate all patients with liver injury from those in whom liver injury did not develop. As shown in Figure 121.1,

TABLE 121.1

STAGES OF ACUTE ACETAMINOPHEN TOXICITY

Stage	Time after Ingestion	Signs and Symptoms	Laboratory Findings
1	4–12 hours	Nausea and vomiting possible	Normal or mildly elevated AST, ALT
1a	12–24 hours	Anorexia, nausea vomiting, pallor, diaphoresis, malaise, confusion, hypotension arrhythmias	ALT, AST rising
2	24–72 hours	Clinical improvement, right upper quadrant pain increased	ALT and AST peaking; bilirubin and INR and/or PTT rising
3	72–96 hours	Centrilobular necrosis; jaundice, coagulopathy, encephalopathy; nausea and vomiting, arrhythmias, renal failure, death	Peak levels of ALT, AST, bilirubin, PTT
4	4–14 days	Resolution of hepatic injury if reversible	Return to baseline levels

AST, aspartate aminotransferase; ALT, alanine aminotransferase; INR, international normalized ratio; PTT partial thromboplastin time.

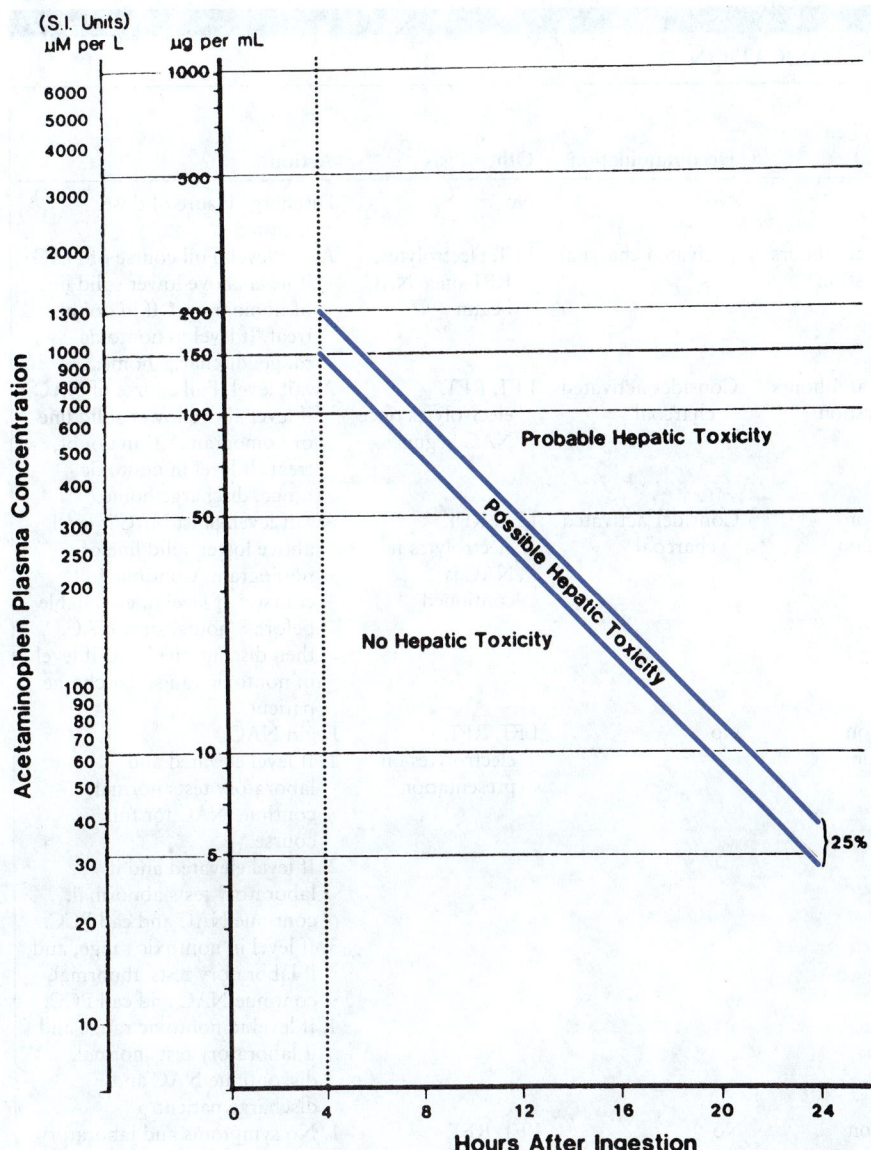

FIGURE 121.1. Semilogarithmic plot of plasma acetaminophen levels over time. Levels drawn less than 4 hours after ingestion will not represent peak levels. The lower solid line 25% below the standard nomogram is included to allow for possible errors in acetaminophen plasma assays and estimated time from ingestion of an overdose. (Reprinted with permission from Rumack BH, Matthew H. Acetaminophen poisoning and toxicity. *Pediatrics* 1975;55:871.)

there is a second line created 25% below the original line as the "possible hepatic toxicity" line. This modification of the nomogram was requested by the Food and Drug Administration, to allow for possible errors in either the measurement of acetaminophen plasma levels or the estimated time from ingestion. In the United States, NAC administration is begun if the acetaminophen level falls above the lower 4-hour line (i.e., 150 μg/mL). In patients who have acute ingestion of extended-release formulations of acetaminophen, it is recommended that at least two serial acetaminophen levels be performed at least 4 to 6 hours apart. The nomogram is not useful in suspected toxicity with long-term or prolonged ingestion of therapeutic doses.

The definition of hepatotoxicity after acetaminophen overdose has been an AST (or ALT) level of 1,000 IU/L or greater. Severity of liver injury is monitored using repeated laboratory testing. Tests include serum electrolytes, ALT, AST, INR, PTT, platelet count, and renal function tests. Patients may become acidotic, and if bicarbonate ion is depressed, blood gases should be followed. In patients in whom toxicity develops, continued close monitoring of liver synthetic function is critical including INR, PTT, and serum glucose levels, because glycogen depletion will occur and gluconeogenesis may be impaired.

Many pitfalls are encountered in the assessment of the patient with acute overdose. The most common is basing critical decisions on the patient's history. Often, the dose is underreported, and the time from ingestion is particularly difficult to obtain (Table 121.2). The first acetaminophen level should not be obtained before 4 hours after ingestion. Patients with suspected or known repeated supratherapeutic ingestion should have an acetaminophen level drawn at presentation along with a serum AST or ALT. If the liver enzymes are normal and the acetaminophen level is less than 10 μg/mL, the patient can be discharged. If the acetaminophen level is greater than 10 μg/mL or the AST is greater than 50 IU/L, the patient should be treated with NAC. Because acetaminophen poisoning can present acutely as central nervous system depression, shock, hypothermia, and metabolic acidosis, or later with hepatic dysfunction, the diagnosis should be considered in any patient with these constellation of symptoms.

THERAPY

NAC is the antidote for acetaminophen poisoning. In its conversion to cysteine, NAC restores GSH reserves by providing

TABLE 121.2

TREATMENT OF ACETAMINOPHEN INTOXICATION

Amount of Ingestion	Time of Ingestion	Draw Acetaminophen Level	Decontamination	Other Tests	Action
<150 mg/kg		No	No	No	Discharge if sure of dose ingested
≥150 mg/kg OR unknown amount	<2 hours	Draw level at 4 hours after ingestion	Activated charcoal	LFT, electrolytes, RFT once NAC begun	Await level. Full course of NAC if level above lower solid line of nomogram.* If in doubt, treat. If level in nontoxic range, discharge home.
≥150 mg/kg OR unknown amount	2–4 hours	Draw level at 4 hours after ingestion	Consider activated charcoal	LFT, RFT, electrolytes once NAC begun	Await level. Full course of NAC if level above lower solid line of nomogram.* If in doubt, treat. If level in nontoxic range, discharge home.
≥150 mg/kg OR unknown amount	4–8 hours	Draw level on presentation	Consider activated charcoal	LFT, RFT, electrolytes if NAC is continued	Await level. Start NAC if level above lower solid line of nomogram. Continue full course.* If level not available before 8 hours, start NAC, then discontinue NAC if level in nontoxic range. Discharge patient.
≥150 mg/kg OR unknown amount	8–24 hours or unknown	Draw level on presentation	No	LFT, RFT, electrolytes on presentation	Begin NAC. 1. If level elevated and laboratory tests normal, continue NAC for full course.* 2. If level elevated and if laboratory tests abnormal, continue NAC and call PCC. 3. If level in nontoxic range, and if laboratory tests abnormal, continue NAC and call PCC. 4. If level in nontoxic range and if laboratory tests normal, discontinue NAC and discharge patient.
≥150 mg/kg OR unknown amount	>24 hours	Draw level on presentation	No	LFT, RFT, electrolytes on presentation	1. No symptoms and laboratory tests normal, then discharge home. 2. If symptoms or abnormal laboratory tests, start NAC and call PCC.
Overdose by therapeutic intent		Draw level on presentation	No	LFT, RFT, electrolytes on presentation	Start NAC 1. Level >10 μg/mL. Continue NAC.* 2. AST >50 IU/L. Continue NAC. Call PCC.

LFT, liver function testing; NAC, N-acetylcysteine; PCC, poison control center; RFT, renal function testing; for nomogram see Figure 121.1;.
*If at the completion of NAC, patient is asymptomatic and laboratory tests are normal, patient may be discharged. If, however, the patient is symptomatic OR laboratory tests are abnormal, then continue NAC at 150 mg/kg intravenously over 24 hours OR 4 hourly dose 70 mg/kg orally and call PCC.
Adapted from Wallace CI, Dargon PI, Jones AL. Paracetamol overdose: an evidence based flowchart to guide management. *Emerg Med J* 2002;19:202.

sulfhydril donors for the eventual detoxification of NAPQI. In addition, NAC increases sulfate conjugation, thereby preventing NAPQI production. Finally, NAC acts as an antioxidant and thus potentially provides some beneficial effect in the second stage of toxicity, as outlined earlier.

As always, treatment of acetaminophen begins with the consideration of decontamination. Activated charcoal (50 g for

adults or 1 g/kg in children) should be administered to all who have ingested acetaminophen if the treatment can be given within 1 to 2 hours of ingestion (see Table 121.2). Whether to administer activated charcoal after this period remains controversial, though the American Academy of Pediatrics recommends the use of activated charcoal within 6 to 8 hours of drug ingestion. Activated charcoal is not recommended for use after

TABLE 121.3

DOSAGE OF N-ACETYLCYSTEINE

Route	Age	Regimen	Total Dose (mg/kg)	Length of Treatment (Hours)
Oral	Adult or child	140 mg/kg, followed 4 hours later by 70 mg/kg at four hourly doses for 17 doses*	1,300	72
Intravenous†	Adult	1. 150 mg/kg NAC in 200 mL 5% dextrose over 15 minutes followed by 2. 50 mg/kg NAC in 500 mL 5% dextrose over 4 hours followed by 3. 100 mg/kg NAC in 1,000 mL 5% dextrose over 16 hours	300	20.25
Intravenous	Child	1. 150 mg/kg in 3 mL/kg 5% dextrose over 15 minutes followed by 2. 50 mg/kg in 7 mL/kg 5% dextrose over 4 hours followed by 3. 100 mg/kg NAC in 14 mL/kg 5% dextrose over 16 hours	300	20.25

NAC, N-acetylcysteine.
*May have shortened course under some circumstances. See text for details.
†NAC can cause anaphylactoid type response including flushing, itching, rashes, angioedema, broncospasm, and hypertension. This risk is greater with intravenous NAC than with oral administration. If such a response occurs, NAC should be stopped, and if necessary an intravenous antihistamine should be administered. Once adverse effects have settled, the NAC can be restarted at a rate of 50 mg/kg over 4 hours.

8 hours of ingestion, unless a second toxin is ingested. Ipecac should not be used in the emergency department setting, because its use delays the use of activated charcoal. Although ipecac is no longer available without a prescription, nontheless home use of ipecac may be useful. One study suggested that ipecac may be of value and concluded that children who ingest between 140 and 200 mg/kg of acetaminophen and demonstrate ipecac-induced emesis within 60 minutes can be safely managed at home.

Acetaminophen plasma levels should be tested no sooner than 4 hours after ingestion (see Table 121.2). A significant change in sensorium necessitates investigation into ingestion of other substances. Laboratory evaluation on arrival at a health care facility includes an acetaminophen level obtained 4 or more hours after ingestion, baseline AST level, ALT level, bilirubin level, prothrombin time, creatinine level, pregnancy test for women of childbearing age, and toxicologic screen. Because aspirin is a frequent coingestant, a salicylate level should be considered.

For individuals who present less than 8 hours after an overdose of 7.5 g or 150 mg/kg or more (or when the amount of acetaminophen ingested is unknown), the decision to initiate NAC therapy may be delayed until an acetaminophen level is available (see Table 121.2). NAC is the most efficacious if administered within 8 hours of drug ingestion. However, NAC should be administered as late as 24 hours after ingestion. NAC can be administered either orally/intragastrically or intravenously. The dosage and the length of treatment vary depending on the route (Table 121.3). No studies have demonstrated the superiority of one treatment regimen over the other, although in the United States, until recently only an oral preparation was available. The intravenous route of NAC may be preferable for those patients who are unable to tolerate the intragastric route, that is, those who have gastric dysmotility

or repeated vomiting. However intravenous NAC can cause adverse effects including flushing, itching, rashes, angioedema, bronchospasm, and hypertension. In those patients with an adverse event, NAC should be stopped, and, if necessary, should be given an antihistamine before restarting the infusion.

If oral NAC is instituted, treatment continues for 72 hours (see Table 121.3). The initial oral dose is 140 mg/kg, with subsequent doses at 4-hour intervals of 70 mg/kg for an additional 17 doses. The dose must be repeated if the patient vomits within 1 hour of administration. Aggressive antiemetic therapy is critical to successful treatment with oral preparations of NAC. These drugs include metoclopramide (0.5 to 1.0 mg/kg intravenously). Diphenhydramine should be considered for coadministration to decrease the risk of metoclopramide-induced dystonic reaction. If emesis persists, ondansetron (0.15 mg/kg intravenously) or droperidol (0.05 to 0.06 mg/kg per dose) may be useful. If emesis still persists, insertion of a nasogastric tube or duodenal tube and infusion of the NAC over 30 minutes can be instituted. The 72-hour NAC protocol may be unnecessary in many cases in which acetaminophen is eliminated before the oral regimen is complete. Stopping treatment earlier may mean that some patients will have a relatively asymptomatic and possibly, but not assuredly, modest rise in enzymes. One retrospective study terminated NAC treatment when the acetaminophen level became zero. Of the 33 patients who received the truncated protocol and subsequent AST determinations, about 10% demonstrated a minor increase in the AST level.

For a patient who has ingested a potentially toxic amount of acetaminophen (or if an unknown amount is ingested) and in whom an acetaminophen level cannot be obtained within 8 hours after the ingestion, a loading dose of NAC should be administered immediately. If the acetaminophen level then returns in the nontoxic range, the NAC is stopped. A pregnant woman should be administered a loading dose of NAC as soon as possible, regardless of time since overdose, because a potential exists for fetal toxicity after maternal overdose, and fetal wastage has been correlated with treatment delay. If the acetaminophen level is then found to be nontoxic, further doses of NAC will be unnecessary. Even after 24 hours of ingestion, late administration of NAC has been shown to be of some benefit and should not be withheld if there is evidence of hepatic injury or if the acetaminophen level is above the treatment line (see Table 121.2).

Monitoring should continue throughout the observation period. Physical findings are nonspecific during stages 1 and 2, and patients may demonstrate only abdominal tenderness. As stage 3 begins, an enlarged liver may be palpated, and scleral icterus can be seen. Mental status may deteriorate. Constructional dyspraxia is an easy and sensitive way to follow mental status changes. The patient is asked to draw a house with a door, window, chimney, and walkway. The test is repeated at intervals, and deterioration of the drawing is consistent with worsening of hepatic function. Laboratory monitoring should occur as outlined earlier. There is no indication for repeated measurement of acetaminophen levels except for those patients with potential ingestion of extended-release preparations or if early termination of NAC is being considered. Indicators of severe acetaminophen poisoning with referral to a specialized liver center for consideration of transplantation include the following: (a) progressive coagulopathy or INR greater than 2 at 24 hours, INR greater than 4 at 48 hours, or INR greater than 6 at 72 hours; (b) renal impairment; (c) hypoglycemia; (d) metabolic acidosis (pH less than 7.3, bicarbonate less than 18) despite rehydration; (e) hypotension despite fluid resuscitation; or (f) encephalopathy.

Once NAC treatment is complete, if the patient is asymptomatic and the laboratory test results are normal, then the patient can be discharged home. Before discharge, a review of the circumstances of the poisoning should be reviewed, and the patient and family should be counseled. Any patient older than the age of 6 years who has an acute toxic ingestion should have a psychiatric evaluation for a potential suicide attempt. This recommendation is based on the observation that by the age of 6 years, a child should recognize the risks of taking harmful substances.

If after treatment with NAC the patient remains symptomatic or the laboratory test results remain abnormal, then NAC should be continued, and the regional poison control center be consulted (see Table 121.2). If an unknown amount of acetaminophen is ingested or the length of time from ingestion is known, and laboratory test results are abnormal, then the regional poison control center should be consulted, even as NAC is instituted.

OVERDOSE WITH THERAPEUTIC INTENT

In an 1998 report of 47 children who developed hepatotoxicity after sustained supratherapeutic acetaminophen administration, almost 50% involved children younger than 2 years, 88%

had received acetaminophen for 1 to 5 days, and six (15%) had received daily doses ranging from 50 to 75 mg/kg/day. More than half had been given adult-strength acetaminophen. In those children in whom a serum acetaminophen concentration was available and the last dose of acetaminophen could be discerned with accuracy, 73% had serum concentrations that were in the potentially toxic range. In marked contrast to children with acute intoxication, 54% of the patients died. Three potential therapeutic variables could contribute to iatrogenic therapeutic acetaminophen poisoning in infants and children: (a) confusion by the caretaker in the interpretation of dosing information; (b) administration of adult-strength preparations; and (c) observation that pediatric-strength preparations are not working and therefore stronger adult preparations are administered to improve the desired effect.

In patients who present with a history of chronic acetaminophen excess or factors that may contribute to increased toxicity (fasting and repeated administration, ingestion of other drugs, and so forth), a modified treatment approach is necessary. On presentation, baseline values of acetaminophen, AST, ALT, bilirubin, and prothrombin time should be obtained, and a loading dose of NAC should be administered pending results (See Table 121.2). The nomogram cannot be used to determine which patients will benefit from treatment. If AST or ALT is greater than 50 IU/L or the serum acetaminophen level is greater than 10 μg/mL, then NAC is begun. It is unclear how long to treat such patients, and information from the regional poison control center could provide further insight. Current recommendations are that treatment continue until the acetaminophen level is close to zero and liver functions have improved to near normal.

Suggested Readings

American Academy of Pediatrics Committee on Drugs 1991–2000. Acetaminophen toxicity in children. *Pediatrics* 2001;108:1020.

Barile FA. Acetaminophen, salicylates, and non-steroidal anti-inflammatory drugs. In: Barile FA, ed. *Clinical toxicology: principles and mechanisms.* Boca Rotan, FL: CRC Press, 2004:191.

Buckley NA, Whyte IM, O'Connell DL, et al. Activated charcoal reduces the need for N-acetylcysteine treatment after acetaminophen (paracetamol) overdose. *Clin Toxicol* 1999;37:753.

Dart RC, Rumack BH. Acetminophen (paracetamol). In: Dart RC, ed. *Medical toxicology,* 3rd ed. Philadelphia: Lippincott Williams & Wilkins, 2004:723.

Heubi JE, Barbacci MB, Zimmerman HJ. Therapeutic misadventures with acetaminophen: hepatotoxicity after multiple doses in children. *J Pediatr* 1998; 132:22.

Kociancic T, Reed MD. Acetaminophen intoxication and length of treatment: how long is long enough. *Pharmacotherapy* 2003;23:1052.

Mohler CR, Nordt SP, Williams SR, et al. Prospective evaluation of mild to moderate pediatric acetaminophen exposures. *Ann Emerg Med* 2000;35:239.

Perry H, Shannon MW. Efficacy of oral versus intravenous N-acetylcysteine in acetaminophen overdose: results of an open-label, clinical trial. *J Pediatr* 1998;132:149.

Rivera-Pinera T, Gugig R, Davis J, et al. Outcome of acetaminophen overdose in pediatric patients and factors contributing to hepatotoxicity. *J Pediatr* 1997; 130:300.

Tenenbein M. Acetaminophen: the 150 mg/kg myth. *J Toxicol Clin Toxicol* 2004; 42:145.

Wallace CI, Dargan PI, Jones AL. Paracetamol overdose: an evidence based flowchart to guide management. *Emerg Med J* 2002;19:202.

Watson WA, Litovize TL, Klein-Scwhartz W, et al. 2003 annual report of the American Association of Poison Control Centers Toxic Exposure Surveillance System. *Am J Emerg Med* 2004;22:335.

CHAPTER 122 ■ PLANT POISONING

M. MICHELE MARISCALCO

Plants are among the most common category of accidental ingestions reported by poison centers. In the United States, plant ingestions account for 10% of all calls. In the industrialized world, most ingestions involve house and garden plants, only a small fraction of which pose a serious toxic threat. Most pediatric cases involve either "nibbling events," which rarely produce more than temporary discomfort, or exposure to nontoxic house plants. However, significant morbidity and mortality have occurred in children who have ingested plant substances that were stored in the home for other than decorative purposes. Such cases frequently involve hallucinogenic plants and mushrooms, products made from plants than contain belladonna alkaloids (jimson weed), or teas and other concoctions produced for "herbal highs" (morning glory seeds, wild lettuce, yohimbine, catnip).

Proper identification of the plant that the child has ingested is crucial for effective therapy and management; however, identification may be problematic, especially over the telephone. Relatives or friends can bring in specimens of the consumed plant when questions exist about the identity of the plant. However, identification may remain difficult without familiarity of poisonous and nonpoisonous plants in a particular locale.

INITIAL MANAGEMENT OF POISONING

As outlined in previous chapters, syrup of ipecac is no longer recommended for use at home by the American Academy of Pediatrics. In addition, emesis may be hazardous when large amounts of leafy plant products have been ingested, owing to possible glottic obstruction. Dilution is also not routinely recommended after ingestion of a medication. However, dilution by having the child drink 100 to 200 mL of water or another drink is a routine recommendation for the ingestion of a nonpharmaceutical agent. It is unclear whether this recommendation should be routinely followed in plant poisoning. Referral to the local poison control center may be helpful in making the determination of potential toxicity. Parents should be reminded to have the number of the poison control center easily accessible. As with any ingestion, symptomatic cases or those with toxic potential should be referred to the emergency department.

On presentation to the emergency department, the child should be evaluated and treatment begun unless the plant can be identified and is known to be nontoxic. The use of activated charcoal may be indicated because many of the toxins delay gastric absorption. Because the use of multiple oral doses of activated charcoal in plant ingestions has not been studied sufficiently, this approach cannot be routinely recommended. The child should be observed for a short period. If the plant is identified and is thought to be nontoxic or if it cannot be recognized and the child remains asymptomatic, the child may be discharged. If the child ingested a potentially toxic species or is symptomatic, he or she should be admitted for further observation and supportive treatment. Plant poisonings may be complex and not well delineated in the existing literature, and multisystem problems should be anticipated, even though the plant may be in a specific toxin category.

PLANT TOXINS

Most of the symptomatic plant poisonings in the United States are from a large heterogenous group that causes gastrointestinal irritation. The following is a description of the most common plant toxins, along with clinical manifestations of poisoning and recommended therapies.

Calcium Oxalate Crystals

Philodendron and dieffenbachia are the most common plant exposures in developed countries. Elephant ear plants are the most common plant exposures in other less developed countries. These three plants belong to the Araceae family, which contains more than 1,800 known species. These family members contain calcium oxalate crystals, which, when the plant is chewed, are ejected from specialized explosive "ejector cells." These crystals then become lodged in the lining of the mouth, tonge, and throat and thus lead to local inflammatory reactions, which include burning, irritation, edema of the buccal cavity, hypersalivation, and aphonia. Chewing of the leaves cause minor mouth and throat burning. However, ingestion of the leaves from these plants can result occasionally in severe oropharyngeal injury with airway compromise. There is no indication for the use of antibiotics, atropine, or antihistamines. Antacids as demulcents and neutralizing agents have been recommended.

Toxins Causing Severe Gastoenteritis

Severe vomiting, colicky abdominal pain, and diarrhea can result from ingestion of pokeweed roots and stems, wisteria seeds, buttercup leaves, daffodil bulbs, and seeds and pods from the bird of paradise. Twenty to 30 of the bright red or black berries of the holly tree are estimated to be a fatal dose for a small child. Holly contains ilicin and several unidentified toxins that cause diarrhea, vomiting, nausea, and abdominal pains. Boxwood contains a toxic alkaloid that can cause severe gastroenteritis if a moderate quantity of leaves is eaten.

The rosary pea (i.e., jequirty bean or Indian bean) and castor beans are attractive seeds and are used extensively in inexpensive beadwork and jewelry. They contain a toxalbumin that is released when chewed, causing violent hemorrhagic gastroenteritis that leads to profound dehydration and circulatory collapse. Therapy consists of fluid and electrolyte management. Alkalinization of the urine with sodium bicarbonate may prevent precipitation of hemoglobin and its products in the kidney tubules.

Cardiac Glycosides

The leaves of common foxglove, oleander, and lily of the valley and the berries of mistletoe contain cardiac glycosides. Soon after ingestion, the child may complain of mouth irritation, vomiting, and diarrhea. As the digitalis is absorbed, acute digitalis effects ensue as evidenced by bradycardia with progressive heart block and hyperkalemia. A randomized control trial in Sri Lanka demonstrated that the use of digoxin-specific Fab antibody was highly effective in treating oleander-induced dysrhythmias and electrolyte disturbances. Anecdotal reports indicate that digoxin-specific Fab antibody may be efficacious in reversing acute effects with other cardiac glycoside–containing plants. Mistletoe also contains sympathomimetic agents that may cause seizures and hypertension.

Nicotine and Nicotine Alkaloids

Nicotine and nicotinelike alkaloids are found in wild tobacco leaves, golden chain tree seeds, all parts of yellow jasmine, and poison hemlock seeds and leaves. Ingestion leads to spontaneous vomiting within 1 hour. Salivation, headache, fever, mental confusion, and muscular weakness may follow, and the child's condition may deteriorate, with convulsions, coma, and death caused by respiratory failure.

Water hemlock has been labeled the most violent plant toxin known. Rapid-onset seizure activity has been reported after its ingestion. Ingestion is also characterized by tremors and muscle rigidity. Charcoal is especially useful in adsorbing these nicotinic alkaloids. Additional treatment consists of intensive supportive care with control of seizures and ventilatory assistance.

Solanine

Other members of the nightshade family, such as the blue and black nightshade, Jerusalem cherry, and wild tomato, contain the toxic alkaloid solanine. Symptoms of solanine ingestion include vomiting, nausea, diarrhea, convulsions, and respiratory and central nervous system depression. Therapy consists of support of respiration and symptomatic treatment.

Belladonna Alkaloids

Jimson weed, belladonna (i.e., deadly nightshade), and angel's trumpet contain belladonna alkaloids, with atropine as a major constituent. Symptoms include visual blurring, dilated pupils, dryness of the mouth, hot and dry skin, fever, tachycardia, absent bowel sounds, urinary retention, delirium, and psychosis. Convulsions and coma may follow. Treatment consists of supportive care. Physostigmine may be used cautiously for severe sequelae. Anticholinergic poisoning has also been reported with a large number of tea constituents including burdock root, jimson tea, lobelia, mandrake, and thornapple. In 1993, 959 incidents of anticholinergic poisoning associated with consumption of plants containing belladonna alkaloids were reported to poison control centers; 15 patients had symptoms requiring hospitalization.

Teas

A tea popular in Mexico and the southwestern and western United States called *gordolobos* has caused several deaths in children and adults. Teas may also include the alkaloids tansy, ragwort, comfrey, fat wolf herb, groundsel, or mullein. The alkaloids in the tea are responsible for the acute and chronic liver disease that occurs after overdose. Other tea constituents such as chamomile can result in anaphylaxis in those patients sensitive to ragweed, asters, and chrysanthemum.

Cyanide

Cyanide is an integral part of the chemical structure of amygdalin and prunasin, which are found in a surprising number of plants. Some examples of cyanide-containing plants include peach, apricot, plum, apple, chokeberry, lima bean, and hydrangea. Cyanide usually is concentrated in traditionally nonedible parts of commercial fruits, such as apricot kernels and apple seeds. Serious illness and deaths have been reported among children who ate large amounts of raw apricot kernels. Gut hydrolysis is required for release of free cyanide, and intestinal decontamination using available cyanide kits may be lifesaving.

MUSHROOM POISONING

Mushrooms cause an estimated 50% of all deaths from plant poisoning in the United States. Susceptibility to mushroom toxins varies greatly among species and persons. The severity of poisoning by a particular toxic mushroom also may depend on the season, the degree of maturity of the specimen, and the quantity of mushrooms consumed by the individual.

Classification: Early and Late Symptom Onset

Two main groups of mushrooms can be characterized on the basis of the interval between ingestion and symptom onset. Toxins that give rise to self-limited neurologic or gastrointestinal tract illness cause symptoms within 15 minutes to 2 hours after ingestion. More potent toxins capable of causing fatal poisonings do not generally produce symptoms until 6 to 18 hours after ingestion. Regardless of the type of mushroom, the initial management for all suspected mushroom poisonings includes supportive measures and administration of activated charcoal.

Mushrooms with early-onset symptoms fall into three groups. Those with muscarinic effects produce cholinergic symptoms within 1 hour, such as sweating, lacrimation, blurred vision, miosis, watery diarrhea, abdominal cramps, and bradycardia. Other mushrooms affect principally the central nervous system, causing dizziness, incoordination, ataxia, muscle twitching, hyperkinetic activity, and hallucinations within 2 to 3 hours of ingestion. Another group exerts its effect solely on the gastrointestinal tract, by causing nausea, vomiting, diarrhea, and abdominal cramps. Management of patients with early-onset symptoms of mushroom ingestion requires careful attention to fluid and electrolytes. The use of barbiturates and benzodiazepines should be avoided, because they may exacerbate symptoms.

Mushrooms causing symptoms that are delayed 6 to 24 hours after ingestion usually produce serious and potentially fatal poisoning. Two groups are recognized, both of which contain toxins causing cellular destruction. The first group, predominated by *Gyromitra esculenta* ("false morel"), produces nausea and vomiting followed by muscle cramps, abdominal pain, and severe watery or bloody diarrhea. In more serious poisonings, fever, liver failure, and central nervous system symptoms may supervene, sometimes followed by convulsions, coma, and death. The second group of poisonous mushrooms, *Amanita phalloides,* is responsible for 95% of fatal mushroom poisonings. The latent period of onset is 6 to 24 hours. The toxic effects are caused by phallotoxins that act first, causing gastrointestinal symptoms including nausea, vomiting, abdominal pain, and diarrhea, and the amatoxins, which are responsible for cellular destruction, particularly renal and hepatic, through inhibition of protein synthesis.

Therapy

The initial step in the treatment of any case of mushroom poisoning is rapid identification of the mushroom species. A mycologist with experience in mushroom identification is essential for this task. Attention is paid to the latency period between consumption and symptom onset. Therapy should be geared to close monitoring of electrolyte and circulating volume status, hydration, and general supportive care. If more than 6 hours have elapsed between ingestion and onset of symptoms, potentially fatal poisoning from amatoxin should be anticipated. Gastric emptying often is delayed after ingestion. Some toxins, especially the amatoxin, undergo enterohepatic circulation, making repeated doses of charcoal useful for the first 48 hours.

Patients may present with renal or hepatic failure. Appropriate laboratory tests such as blood urea nitrogen, creatinine, serum alanine aminotransferase, serum aspartate aminotransferase, coagulation profiles, and bilirubin should be undertaken in any suspected amatoxin poisoning. Hypoglycemia, gastrointestinal hemorrhage, coagulopathy, and encephalopathy may occur in patients with liver failure. Therapies such as thioctic acid, pyridoxine, high-dose penicillin, and corticosteroids have not been proven to be effective in controlled studies. In cases of potentially severe ingestions, contact should be made with toxicologists at a regional poison center to determine the current recommendations on management of these patients. Liver transplantation has been successful in patients with liver failure.

Orellanine-containing mushrooms are founds within the family of Cortinariaceae. These mushrooms are found in deciduous forests in continental Europe and North America. Ingestion of the toxin orellanine results in no or mild gastrointestinal symptoms. Therefore, most patients present 2 or more days after ingestion, when they are already suffering from renal damage. Treatment if the patient is presented early enough should include activated charcoal. No specific treatment is available, but management includes supportive care with renal replacement therapy.

Suggested Readings

Anticholinergic poisoning associated with herbal tea: New York City, 1994. *MMWR Morb Mortal Wkly Rep* 1995;44:193.

Bond GR. The role of activated charcoal and gastric emptying in gastrointestinal decontamination: a state of the art review. *Ann Emerg Med* 2002;39:272.

Brent J, Kulig K. Mushrooms. In: Haddad LM, Shannon MW, Winchester JF, eds. *Clinical management of poisoning and drug overdose,* 3rd ed. Philadelphia: WB Saunders, 1998: 365.

Committee on Injury and Poison Prevention of the American Academy of Pediatrics. Biological toxins. In: Rodgers GC, Matyunas NJ, eds. *Handbook of common poisonings in children.* Elk Grove Village, IL: American Academy of Pediatrics, 1994:237.

Committee on Injury, Violence and Poison 2002–2003, American Academy of Pediatrics. Policy statement: poison treatment in the home. *Pediatrics* 2003; 112:1182.

Eddleston M, Persson H. Acute plant poisoning and antitoxin antibodies. *J Toxicol Clin Toxicol* 2003;41:309.

Francis PD, Clarke CFR. Angel trumpet lily poisoning in five adolescents: clinical findings and management. *J Pediatr Child Health* 1999;35:93.

Fung F, Clark RF. Health effects of mycotoxins: a toxicological overview. *J Toxicol Clin Toxicol* 2004;42:217.

Karlson-Stiber C, Persson H. Cytotoxic fungi: an overview. *Toxicon* 2003; 42:339.

Kunkel DB, Braitberg G. Poisonous plants. In: Haddad LM, Shannon MW, Winchester JF, eds. *Clinical management of poisoning and drug overdose,* 3rd ed. Philadelphia: WB Saunders, 1998:375.

Riordan M, Rylance G, Berry K. Poisoning in children. Part 4: household products, plants and mushrooms. *Arch Dis Child* 2002;87:403.

Tagwireyi D, Ball DE. The management of elephant's ear poisoning. *Hum Exp Toxicol* 2001;20:189.

CHAPTER 123 ■ LEAD POISONING

HERBERT L. NEEDLEMAN

The clinical picture of childhood lead poisoning (plumbism) has changed dramatically over the past 20 years. Acute symptomatic lead poisoning, once a common problem, now is a rare event. Lead encephalopathy is even rarer. Most pediatric residents will not see a case of acute plumbism during their training; few will encounter the problem in their career. At the same time, epidemiologic studies from around the world on the effects of lead in children have demonstrated behavioral and cognitive deficits in the absence of symptoms, at levels of blood lead once considered harmless. Traditional treatments using chelating agents are ineffective at these levels of lead in blood. As a result, the principal domain of lead toxicity has shifted from the clinic and hospital to the public health arena, where the effects of lead at clinically silent doses on child development remains a major issue.

Lead poisoning, unlike most of the illnesses examined in this textbook, is a manmade disease. The metal's neurotoxic properties were recognized as least as far back as the second century B.C., when Dioscerides, the author of *Materia Medica*, wrote that "Lead makes the mind give way." For centuries, plumbism was thought to be exclusively a disease of workers and drinkers of adulterated wine. (Despite being aware of lead's toxic properties, ancient Romans used it to counteract the astringent flavor of tannic acid in grapes and thus sweeten wine.) The decrease in fecundity and simultaneous rise in madness in upper class Romans has attracted speculation that the metal played a role in the downfall of the Empire.

Childhood lead poisoning was first reported in 1892, at the Brisbane Children's Hospital in Australia. In 1914, the first American report of a poisoned child was published. For decades thereafter, acute childhood lead poisoning was believed to have only two outcomes: death or complete recovery without any residua. The first follow-up study of children who had recovered from acute poisoning was published in 1943, and reported that 19 of 20 recovered cases had severe school problems, behavior disorders, and impaired cognition. This paper established the long- term consequences of acute intoxication, and speculated that undiagnosed lead exposure was among the prominent causes of school and behavior problems.

For six decades between 1920 and 1980, symptomatic childhood lead poisoning was relatively frequent, particularly in the eastern United States. Eighty-nine cases were treated at the Boston Infants and Children's Hospital between 1924 and 1933; 45 of these had encephalopathy, and 11 died. In Baltimore, between 1950 and 1960, 611 cases with 48 deaths were reported. Between 1955 and 1960, in Philadelphia, 223 cases with 41 fatalities were reported. Chicago reported 429 cases and 67 deaths between 1959 and 1961.

The removal of lead from gasoline in the United States, begun in the 1970s and completed by 1991, resulted in a dramatic lowering of blood levels. The mean blood lead level in 1975 was 15.5 μg/dL. At the time of writing, the mean blood lead level is 2 μg/dL, robust testimony to the benefits of sound public health policy. Current data indicates that 2.2% of children under 6 years of age have blood lead levels greater than 10 μg/dL.

The definition of the toxic level of lead in blood, set at 60 μg/dL in the 1960s and 1970s, has, as a result of epidemiologic studies of lead-related cognitive deficits in asymptomatic children, been reduced in steps to 40, 35, and 25 μg/dL. It currently has been set at 10 μg/dL. Recent studies have demonstrated effects on children's cognition at levels below 10 μg/dL. As a result, modern pediatric attention has shifted from treating symptomatic acute poisoning to finding and preventing effects in asymptomatic children exposed at lower doses.

SOURCES OF LEAD

The major sources of lead for children are old paint, dust, water, and air. Removing lead from gasoline has markedly reduced airborne lead, and blood lead concentrations have correspondingly declined. Airborne emissions from stationery sources such as smelters or battery manufacturing continue to present risks for nearby residents.

Clinicians must consider many less frequent sources of lead when evaluating a poisoned child. Hobbies in the home, such as stained glass making, handloading of ammunition, or ceramics, may introduce lead into household air and dust and raise the body burdens of resident children and adults. Some cosmetics, particularly surma, used by Hindus, and kohl, used by Muslims as eye makeup, have extremely high concentrations of lead. Many folk remedies, such as greta and azarcon, used by Mexicans to treat gastrointestinal disorders, contain large amounts of lead. In some cases, ceramic tableware from foreign countries may release lead into food; some imported toys may be painted with lead-based paints; and some imported plastic Venetian blinds may release substantial amounts of lead after exposure to sunlight.

The concentration of lead in standing water (reservoirs and aquifers) is low. Lead enters drinking water somewhere between the street main and the kitchen tap. Although the use of lead solder in household plumbing has been banned, many older houses have lead solder joints. This can be a hazard if the water supply is soft (of low mineral content) and corrosive. Some brass plumbing fixtures contain lead.

The single greatest contemporary source of lead exposure is household paint. Although lead began to be supplanted by titanium oxide as a pigment in the 1950s, and was banned from household paint in the 1970s, many houses inhabited today were built before 1950 and have leaded surfaces. Many of these surfaces chalk and powder. This liberates lead into household dust and makes it available to the exploring fingers of children. Windowsills and frames are particularly rich sources of lead. Approximately 18 million children under 5 years of age are reported to live in houses built before 1950.

Lead paint has a sweet flavor. Because paint in use before 1950 may contain as much as 50% lead by weight, the ingestion of paint chips is dangerous behavior. Many young children display mouthing behavior, but the seeking and persistent ingestion of nonfood substances (pica) is abnormal and is a strong risk for lead toxicity. The current World Health Organization (WHO) standard for the permissible intake of lead is 25 μg/kg/week. A single 1 gm flake of paint can have as much as 500,000 μg of lead.

Lead dust is a major source of lead for children. It is not necessary for paint to be flaking to contribute to household dust. When paint chalks or powders, or when airborne lead settles, the particles become part of the composite of finely ground, powdered earth and organic material that makes up household dust. A recent pooled analysis of 12 epidemiologic studies found a strong relationship between interior lead-dust loadings and blood lead levels in resident children. Consequently, the Environmental Protection Agency has reduced the household lead-dust standard to 40 μg/ft^2, 250 μg/ft^2 for windowsills, and 250 μg/ft^2 for window troughs.

EPIDEMIOLOGY

The prevalences of blood lead levels above 10 μg/dL over the past 27 years obtained by the National Health and Examination Survey are summarized in Table 123.1. With the removal of lead from gasoline, the prevalence of blood leads above 10 μg/dL declined from 88.2% to 2.2%. The number of children exceeding 10 μg/dL has declined from 13,500,000 in 1976 to 1980 to 434,000 in 1999 to 2000.

Lead is not distributed evenly throughout the population: Low-income families, African American and Hispanic children, and inner city residents have substantially higher blood lead levels. This should not be taken to mean that middle-class white children are spared. The widely held belief that lead exposure does not happen to middle-class white children has obstructed the screening of children in this group, and as a result, many cases of toxicity have been missed. A prevalence of 2.2% has led many to dismiss the problem of lead exposure as solved; however, this prevalence means that in each 1-year cohort of children, 88,000 have unacceptable levels of lead exposure, and that in a clinical practice of 3,000 children, 66 have elevated blood lead levels. Newer data, summarized here, show the effects of lead at serum levels below 10 μg/dL. This increases markedly the number of children now recognized at risk.

TABLE 123.1

BLOOD LEAD LEVELS IN AMERICAN CHILDREN FROM 1976 TO 1999

Year	Geometric Mean Blood Lead Levels	Prevalence of BLL $\geq$10 μg/dL (%)	Estimated Number of Children with BLL $\geq$10 μg/dL
1976–1980	14.9	88.2	13,500,000
1988–1991	3.6	8.6	1,700,777
1991–1994	2.7	4.4	890,000
1999–2000	2.2	2.2	434,000

Absorption, Distribution, and Excretion

Lead is taken into the body through the lungs and the gastrointestinal tract. The absorption of inorganic lead through the skin is negligible: Children absorb more lead from the gut (40% to 50%) than adults (20% to 24%). The absorption of respired lead is a function of particle size and respiratory rate. Lead particles of less that $0.5\ \mu M$ penetrate deeply into the lung, where between 30% and 50% are absorbed directly into the bloodstream. Larger particles are trapped in the upper respiratory tract, migrate up into the pharynx, and are swallowed and absorbed from the gut. Because children are more active and have a higher respiratory rate, they tend to respire and absorb more airborne lead.

Deficiencies of iron, zinc, or calcium increase the amount of lead absorbed from the gut. After absorption, lead enters the bloodstream and is distributed to soft tissues and bone. The residence time of lead differs in these organs. The half-life of lead in blood is 35 days, whereas the half-life in adult bone is approximately 27 years. The half-life of lead in children's bones has not been measured, but, given the rapid remodeling during childhood, is unquestionably shorter. Lead in soft tissues and the brain has a longer half-life than that in the blood. Most lead in blood is contained within the red blood cell; the concentration of lead in plasma, the transport medium, is generally lower. The largest amount of lead in the body is contained within bone. The various pools of lead within blood, bone, and soft tissue are in active communication and maintain a stasis of lead levels within the entire body. If a child has an elevated blood lead concentration, treatment by chelation will reduce the serum concentration abruptly; however, after treatment has ended, blood lead levels gradually rise as a transfer occurs from the lead pools in soft tissue and bone pools back into the blood.

Lead is excreted primarily through the gut and kidney. Chelating agents enhance urinary excretion by altering the solubility of lead. Small amounts of lead also are excreted in the bile, hair, nails, and sweat. Ninety-five percent of the adult body burden of lead is in bone, where it is relatively biologically inactive. Under certain conditions, bone lead is remobilized. These include fractures with immobilization and hyperthyroidism. Lead is mobilized from bone during pregnancy and is transferred across the placenta to the fetus. With aging, the demineralization of bone takes place, thus releasing lead into the bloodstream. Postmenopausal women have higher blood lead levels than premenopausal women, and lower cognitive test scores in postmenopausal women have been reported in association with blood lead levels. The question of the role of lead in cognitive impairment and dementia in older subjects is intriguing but unstudied.

PATHOLOGY

Lead is a powerful and versatile toxin. It affects the central and peripheral nervous systems, bone marrow, kidney, and myocardium, and the endocrine and immune systems. Lead is a reactive divalent cation with particular affinity for the sulfhydryl groups on proteins. It also catalytically cleaves tRNA phosphoribose at specific sites, and it binds to phosphokinase C more avidly than intracellular calcium. Its potential toxic mechanisms extend, but are not limited to, disturbances in mitochondrial structure and function; competition with other divalent cations for binding sites; disturbances in membrane function; inhibition of enzyme activity; increased vascular permeability; disturbances in dendritic arborization, synaptogenesis, and pruning back of dendrites; effects on myelin function; disturbances in neurotransmitter release and function; disturbances in calcium metabolism; interference with the development of the endogenous opioid system; and interference with cell adhesion.

Lead is picked up avidly by mitochondria, and it produces swelling and distortion of the mitochondrial christae. Uncoupled energy metabolism, inhibited cellular respiration, and altered calcium kinetics are associated with these changes. Lead competes with calcium for transport across the cell membrane and within the cell. This alters the release of neurotransmitters in the synapse. Although attention has focused on the inhibition of enzymes in the heme pathway, a large and diverse number of enzymes are affected by lead. These include brain adenyl cyclase, sodium-potassium adenosine triphosphatase (ATPase), 1,25-dihydroxy vitamin-D hydroxylase, $5'$ pyrimidine nucleotidase, guanine hydroxylase, and phosphokinase C. In the heme pathway, delta-aminolevulinic acid dehydratase (ALA-D) is extremely sensitive to lead. The inhibition of ALA-D results in increased aminolevulinic acid (ALA). ALA is a weak gamma-aminobenzoic acid (GABA) agonist, and through presynaptic inhibition, may produce a decreased release of GABA. This effect may be responsible for the excitatory symptoms seen in porphyria, and may account in part for the disordered behavior that accompanies lead poisoning. The effects of lead on the N-methyl-D-aspartate (NMDA) receptor and its long-term potentiation also have been reported. This may have important implications in the learning abilities of lead-exposed children.

At high levels of exposure, children's kidneys can be affected, and a reversible Fanconi syndrome has been observed. The most important target of lead in children is the central nervous system (CNS), and the most significant expression of CNS disturbance is behavioral. Severe acute lead poisoning can produce swelling and hemorrhage in the brain. This picture of acute encephalopathy, while once a common expression of lead intoxication, now is quite rare. The screening of children and the consequent early detection is one reason for this change. Other reasons include an increased awareness of the disease, improvement of the housing stock, removal of lead from food cans, and reduction of lead in the atmosphere and dust.

CLINICAL MANIFESTATIONS AND COMPLICATIONS

Our understanding of the fundamental principles of the diagnosis and management of childhood lead poisoning is owed almost entirely to the work of a single person, the author of the preceding version of this chapter, the late Dr. J. Julian Chisolm.

Clinical lead poisoning often is insidious in onset, and may take place over a period of weeks. It may be precipitated by an infection, such as otitis media. The earliest signs are nonspecific behavioral changes: listlessness, altered mood, irritability, anorexia, and sleep disturbances. Abdominal pain, constipation, arthralgia, headaches, and vomiting may present as the disease progresses. Headache, vomiting, clumsiness, staggering, and drowsiness may presage the onset of encephalopathy, which is ushered in by stupor, coma, and convulsions.

Symptoms may be observed at blood lead levels of 40 μg/dL, although some children with much higher blood levels may display no apparent signs. Because of this phenomenon, a prudent rule that should be followed is that any child with anemia, behavioral change, hyperactivity, weight loss, abdominal pain, or the symptoms listed above should have a blood lead test.

THERAPY

The cornerstone of lead toxicity treatment is identifying the source of lead and terminating exposure to that source. In the absence of this, other remedies are futile. A careful history should inquire into sources other than paint. Where available, local health authorities should be involved in inspecting residences. If a source in the home is found, residents should optimally relocate while abatement takes place. If this is not possible, the areas being abated should be sealed until the work has been done and thorough clean-up has occurred. Abatement can be dangerous to workers and residents if not done properly. Only contractors trained and licensed for lead abatement should be employed. After abatement and cleanup has been finished, dust samples from the treated areas should be obtained to ensure a lead-free environment.

The three major chelating agents for lead toxicity are ethylenediaminetetraacetic acid (EDTA), dimercaptosuccinic acid (DMSA or succimer), and 2.3 dimercaptopropanol (British Antilewisite or BAL). The introduction of chelating agents in the 1950s radically changed the outcome from acute lead encephalopathy, lowering the mortality rate from over 60% to 5%. The efficacy of chelating agents such as EDTA in severe acute plumbism with encephalopathy is well established. The effectiveness has never been evaluated rigorously in children with less severe disease, and to this day remains unclear.

Because it possesses equal efficacy and can be given orally, succimer has largely replaced EDTA. After succimer was introduced as an oral chelating agent, the National Institute of Environmental Health Sciences (NIEHS), to evaluate its efficacy at lower exposures, funded a large multicenter study of children with blood lead levels between 20 and 44 μg/dL. Seven hundred forty-one subjects between 13 and 30 months of age were randomized to succimer and placebo groups. The succimer-treated subjects initially had lower blood lead levels than controls, but after treatment was concluded, blood lead levels in both groups did not differ. IQ scores in the succimer-treated group were 1 point lower and parent behavioral ratings slightly worse than controls at the conclusion of the trial. A re-analysis of the data, looking at IQ scores and lead levels within treatment groups, found no change in IQ in the succimer group, whereas the placebo group had a 4 point increase for every 10 points decrease in blood lead. The reason for this apparent therapeutic paradox is unclear. A possibility is that succimer, at lower blood lead levels, may increase the transport of lead across the blood–brain barrier. Succimer is as effective as EDTA for high lead levels, but is not effective at blood lead levels below 45 μg/dL.

For children with blood lead levels of greater than 45 μg/dL, a 19-day course of succimer is the preferred treatment. After exposure has been controlled, the child is given succimer in a dose of 1,050 mg/m^2 in three divided doses for 3 days, and 700 mg/m^2 for 16 days. Succimer is supplied in 350 mg capsules, has an unpleasant odor, and should be given mixed with applesauce, peanut butter, or ice cream. Admission to a hospital is important to complete home evaluation, begin source control, and train the mother in administering the drug. She should watch it being mixed and given to the child, and then give it under supervision. Without this training, compliance can suffer.

EDTA and BAL continue to have a place in treatment. For patients who cannot take oral medicine, or who have an allergic reaction to succimer, EDTA becomes the drug of choice. The dose of EDTA is 1,500 mg/m^2 divided into 4 doses, given intravenously or by deep intramuscular injection. BAL is reserved for children with blood lead levels greater than 70 μg/dL or with signs of encephalopathy. Encephalopathic patients should be given BAL 500 mg/m^3, divided into four doses, by deep intramuscular injection for 5 days, with EDTA given either IM or IV for 5 days. Patients with CNS signs should have fluids administered with caution to avoid a further rise of intracranial pressure.

THE CHANGING PICTURE OF LEAD TOXICITY

Neurotoxic Effects of Lead Toxicity

Cognitive deficits in children with no visible signs of lead toxicity first were reported in the 1970s. Since then, over 30 studies of children, conducted around the world, have demonstrated deficits in cognition as measured in IQ tests. As blood lead levels have declined, the effects of lead on the CNS have been demonstrated at lesser doses. In the 1970s, when the mean blood lead level was 15 μg/dL, the lack of a true low-lead referent group prevented the detection of effects at the lowest concentrations. The general reduction of blood lead levels now has permitted contrasts with subjects bearing very low amounts of lead in blood and tissues. The application of more sensitive measures of outcome, more sensitive and precise analytical methods for measuring lead in body tissues, and better epidemiologic and biostatistical techniques have combined to demonstrate the effects of lead at lower and lower concentrations. Investigators now can compare children to referent groups with blood lead levels as low as 1 μg/dL. When forward studies of children from birth onward showed effects on IQ at blood lead levels between 10 and 25 μg/dL, and one study showed effects below 10 μgdl, the Centers for Disease Control (CDC) reset the defined toxic threshold at 10 μg/dL. Many hints surfaced that lesser levels were neurotoxic, and recently (2002 and 2003) two studies have shown deficits in subjects with lead levels below 10 μg/dL. The slope of the inverse lead–IQ association is steeper at levels below 7 μg/dL, raising interesting speculations about the underlying mechanism. The evidence that no threshold exists for lead is becoming more persuasive as more sensitive studies are published. Unlike most metals, lead has no function in human metabolism, and interference with biochemical and physiologic mechanisms has been demonstrated at micromolar concentrations. A recent study (September 15, 2003) examining neurite growth in rodent brain cell cultures showed decrease in neurite length at lead concentrations of 0.2 μg/dL (.01 μM).

Deficits in speech and language, attention, and classroom behavior also have been reported in relation to low level lead exposure (Fig. 123.1). Early studies were cross-sectional in nature, but later, forward studies from birth onward confirmed the association between lead and deficit, and supported the causal nature of the association. A follow-up of lead-exposed but asymptomatic subjects into young adulthood found that the high-lead group had a sevenfold increase in high school graduation failure and a sixfold increase in reading disabilities. This indicates that the effects of childhood lead exposure are permanent, and affect life success and adjustment (Fig. 123.2).

Most studies of lead at low doses have concentrated on IQ. However, behavioral dyscontrol is among the more important and largely ignored expressions of lead neurotoxicity. The parents of lead-poisoned children have frequently reported behavioral changes after recovery, and complained that previously placid children became fidgety, irritable, oppositional, and aggressive. The first follow-up study of lead poisoning, conducted by Byers in 1943, was triggered by the observation that two children referred to his clinic for violent behavior had been patients treated earlier for lead poisoning.

This question of lead and antisocial behavior only recently has received attention. Four studies of children report associations between lead exposure and delinquent behavior. In Philadelphia, among children formerly enrolled in the Collaborative Perinatal study, the most influential predictor of arrest in adolescence was a prior history of lead poisoning. A cohort

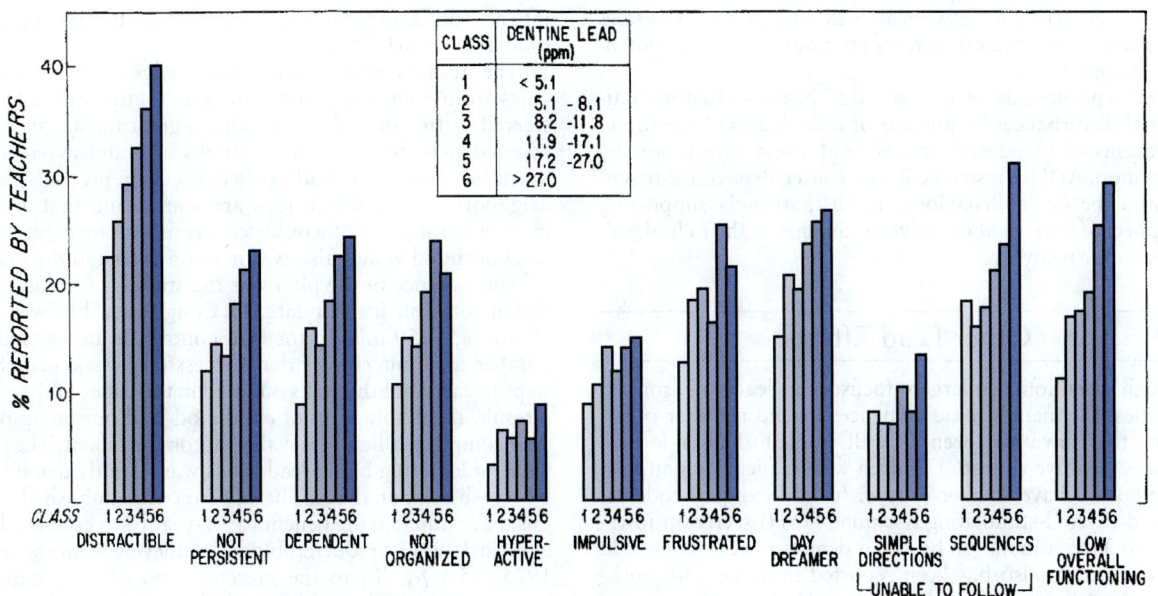

FIGURE 123.1. Deficits in psychologic and classroom performance of children with elevated dentine lead levels. Ratings of 2,146 primary school children by teachers of 11 classroom behaviors using a forced-choice questionnaire. Subjects were grouped according to ascending dentine lead level from less than 5.1 ppm to greater than 27 ppm. The height of the bars indicates the proportion of negative ratings. (Reproduced with permission from Needleman HL, Gunnoe C, Leviton A, et al. Deficits in psychological and classroom performance of children with elevated dentine lead levels. *N Engl J Med* 1979;300:689.)

study of children with elevated bone lead levels measured by x-ray fluorescence found higher scores for aggression, attentional disorders, and delinquent behavior. Another study, using self reports of delinquency, found elevated scores to be associated with cumulative blood lead levels. A case-control study

of arrested and adjudicated delinquents found that delinquents had significantly higher bone lead levels, and the odds ratio for elevated bone lead levels was 4:1. The population-attributable risk estimated for this sample ranged between 11% and 38%. These findings are supported by a number of ecologic studies

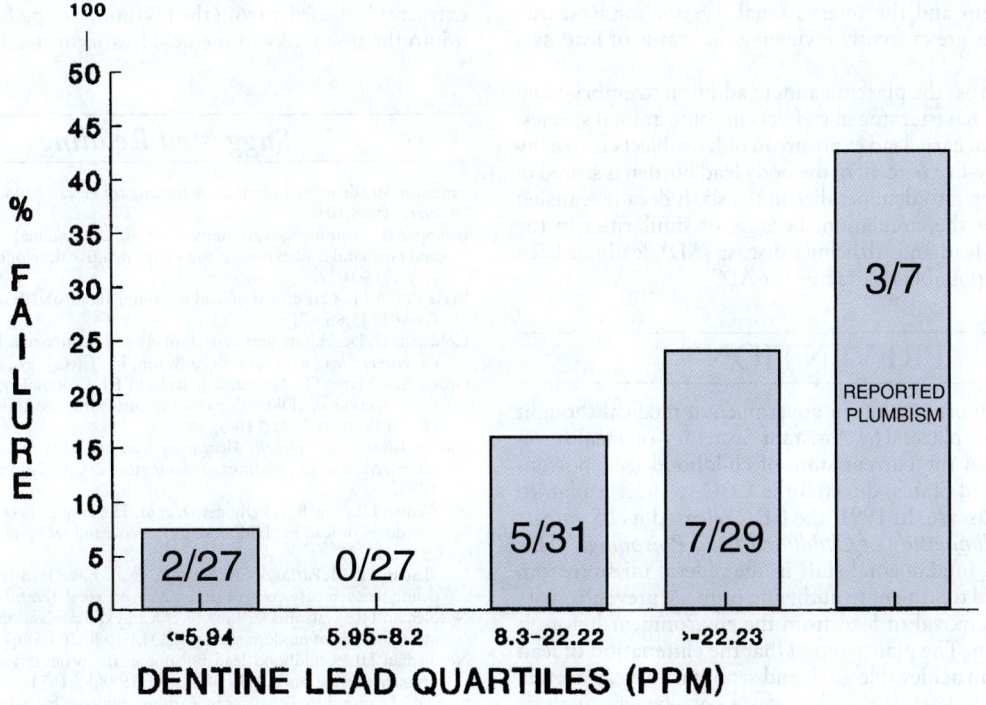

FIGURE 123.2. The rate of failure to graduate from high school in subjects according to their dentine lead levels 12 years earlier. Subjects were grouped in quartiles according to dentine lead concentration. (Reproduced with permission from Needleman HL, Schell A, Bellinger D, et al. The long-term effects of exposure to low doses of lead in childhood: an 11-year follow-up report. *N Engl J Med* 1990;322:83.)

that report correlations between air lead concentrations or sales of leaded gasoline and crime rates after adjustment for potential confounders.

Lead exposure has been reported to be associated with attentional disturbances. A number of investigators have found associations of blood and dentine lead levels with scores on the Connors ADHD instrument, the Rutter Behavioral Inventory, and the Child Behavior Checklist, strongly supporting the reports of parents about adverse changes in their children's conduct after recovery.

Other Lead Effects

Although attention has largely focused on lead's neurotoxic properties, the metal's toxic influences extend to other organ systems that have not been as well studied. The endocrine system is sensitive to lead. Children with clinically significant lead exposure have smaller stature. In lead-exposed rodents, impaired thyroid-stimulating hormone (TSH) secretion in response to TRF stimulation has been demonstrated. Depressed thyroid function also has been reported in adult lead workers and those lead-poisoned by drinking home-distilled liquor. Lead workers also have been reported to display defects in spermatogenesis. Lead-poisoned rats had lower levels of testosterone and luteinizing hormone. Maternal bone and infant blood lead levels recently were shown to be inversely associated with birth weight and weight gain at 1 month of age. A recent study using National Health and Nutrition Examination Study (NHANES III) data found that girls with blood lead levels of 3 μg/dL had significant delays in pubic hair and breast development, compared with those with blood lead levels of 1 μg/dL.

The carcinogenic property of lead is an understudied issue. Workplace lead exposure is associated with increased risks for kidney, lung, and brain tumors. This association is supported by experimental findings in rodents. Both the National Toxicology Program and the International Agency for Research on Carcinogens are currently reviewing the status of lead as a carcinogen.

Lead salts cross the placenta and, in addition to embryo and fetal mortality, have teratogenic effects in some animal species.

The effects of early lead exposure in older subjects is worthy of study. Ninety-five percent of the body lead burden is stored in bone. Bones begin to demineralize in the sixth decade, causing lead to re-enter the circulation. Because of similarities in the distribution of lead and Alzheimer disease (AD), lead has been suggested as a possible risk factor for AD.

PREVENTION

In 1991, an important shift in governmental medical thought and policy took place. The Assistant Secretary of Health, on being briefed on the current state of childhood lead poisoning in the United States, directed the CDC to draft a plan to eliminate the disease. In 1991, the CDC released its *"Strategic Plan for the Elimination of Childhood Lead Poisoning."* This plan marked a fundamental shift in the federal mission from case finding and treatment to authentic primary prevention; its goal was the removal of lead from the environment before it entered children. The plan asserted that the elimination of lead exposure was an achievable goal, and set out a 15-year agenda to accomplish it. Part of the plan was a cost–benefit analysis of complete elimination. The cost of deleading the 23 million houses built before 1950 and containing lead was estimated at $33.7 billion. The monetized benefits from deleading, taking

into account avoided medical and special education costs, were estimated at $61.7 billion.

The authors of the plan acknowledge that the calculated gains from complete abatement were conservative. Not considered in the analysis were other significant health benefits: avoided hypertension and heart disease, and avoided delinquent behavior. That lead exists in excess in precisely the same neighborhoods in which jobs are scarce, and that an investment in full abatement would decrease unemployment and raise neighborhood values also was not considered in the plan.

The issuance of the plan was the stimulus for considerable action to fulfill its mandate. In Congress, a bill was passed allocating $250 million for lead control. It also stimulated a number of counterforces that successfully weakened effective steps to carry out the tasks outlined in the pages of the plan. As a result, the elimination of childhood lead poisoning remains an incomplete, albeit achievable, accomplishment. The societal value of lowering blood lead levels was recently demonstrated by cost–benefit analyses. The CDC recently published an analysis that estimated the benefit to a 1-year birth cohort (children born in 1998) of reducing blood lead levels from the mean in 1975 (15.5 μg/dL) to the present mean of 2.2 μg/dL to be between $119 billion and $319 billion.

In 1991, the American Academy of Pediatrics (AAP), in the service of primary prevention, recommended universal screening except where data showed that children were not at risk of exposure. In 1993, the AAP recommended that every child have a blood lead test between 9 and 12 months of age, and if possible, again at 2 years of age. In 1998, the AAP replaced the recommendation for universal screening with screening targeted at high prevalence areas. Some public-health specialists, including this author, believe that this curtailment was a mistake, and that universal screening remains a cost-effective public health response. Universal screening is a provisional stratagem. The real task is to take lead out of the environment before it enters children's bodies. Lead poisoning is a man-made disease; therefore, given the proper motivation, man should be able to extract this disorder from the textbooks of pediatrics and enter it into the textbooks of medical history instead.

Suggested Readings

American Academy of Pediatrics. Screening for elevated blood lead levels. *Pediatrics* 1998;101.

Bellinger D, Leviton A, Waternaux C, et al. Longitudinal analyses of prenatal and postnatal lead exposure and early cognitive development. *N Engl J Med* 1987;316:1037.

Byers R, Lord E. Late effects of lead poisoning on mental development. *Am J Dis Child* 1943;66:471.

Goldstein G. Developmental neurobiology of lead toxicity. In: HL Needleman, ed. *Human lead exposure.* Boca Raton, FL: CRC Press, 1992.

Grosse SD, Matte TD, Schwartz J, Jackson RJ. Economic gains resulting from the reduction in children's exposure to lead in the United States. *Environ Health Perspect* 2002;110(6):563.

National Research Council. Measuring lead exposure in infants, children and other sensitive populations. Washington D.C.: National Academy Press, 1993.

Needleman HL, Schell A, Bellinger D, et al. The long-term effects of exposure to low doses of lead in childhood: an 11-year follow-up report. *N Engl J Med* 1990;322:83.

Needleman H, McFarland CE, Ness R, et al. Bone lead levels in adjudicated delinquency: a case-control study. *Neurotoxicol Teratol* 2002;24:711.

Needleman HL, Gatsonis C. Low level lead exposure and the IQ of children: a meta-analysis of modern studies. *JAMA* 1990;263(5):673.

Needleman HL. Childhood lead poisoning: the promise and abandonment of primary prevention. *Am J Pub Health* 1998;88:1871.

Rice DC. Lead-induced changes in learning: evidence for behavioral mechanisms from experimental animal studies. *Neurotoxicol* 1993;14:167.

Schwartz J, Pitcher H, Levin R, et al. Costs and benefits of reducing lead in gasoline: final regulatory analysis. Washington D.C.: USEPS/OPA, 1985.

CHAPTER 124 ■ MINOR BURNS

PENELOPE TERHUNE LOUIS

Approximately 2 million burn injuries occur every year in the United States. Of these, about 30,000 are treated in an inpatient setting. There are 1,000 to 5,000 pediatric deaths per year secondary to burn injury. Minor burns, which constitute approximately 95% of all burns treated in the United States, are generally superficial and do not exceed 10% of the total body surface area. They have no significant involvement of the hands, feet, face, or perineum, and they rarely require hospitalization. No full-thickness component and no other complications exist. In the management of minor burns, survival is not the issue; most of these burns heal regardless of therapy. Undertreatment and overtreatment are common and may result in infection or delayed healing, with discomfort and prolonged morbidity. The goals of minor burn management include wound healing, patient comfort, and rapid rehabilitation.

BURN ASSESSMENT

The seriousness of a burn injury can be defined by its depth, its location, the surface area involved, and patient's age and general health. Even in minor burns, accurate estimation of the surface area is mandatory. The Lund and Browder chart should be used to adjust for the smaller surface area of the lower extremities of children (Fig. 124.1).

Burn Classification

The four-level burn classification is based on the depth of the injury: first-, second-, third-, and fourth-degree burns (Fig. 124.2). In first-degree burns, tissue destruction is superficial,

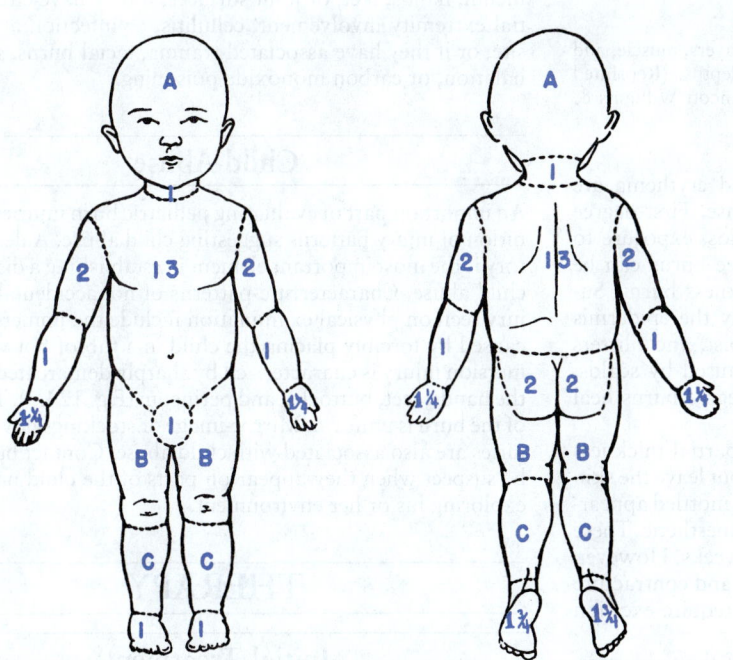

RELATIVE PERCENTAGES OF AREAS AFFECTED BY GROWTH

Area	Age 0	1	5
A = ½ of Head	9½	8½	6½
B = ½ of One Thigh	2¾	3¼	4
C = ½ of One Leg	2½	2½	2¾

% BURN BY AREAS

Probable 3rd° Burn	Head_____ Neck_____ Body_____ Up. Arm_____ Forearm_____ Hands_____
	Genitals_____ Buttocks_____ Thighs_____ Legs_____ Feet_____

Total Burn	Head_____ Neck_____ Body_____ Up. Arm_____ Forearm_____ Hands_____
	Genitals_____ Buttocks_____ Thighs_____ Legs_____ Feet_____

Sum of All Areas_____   Probably 3rd°_____   Total Burn_____

FIGURE 124.1. Modified Lund and Browder chart. This chart is used to determine the extent of burns in children because it is based on age, thus compensating for changes in growth. (Reprinted from Harwood-Nuss A. *The clinical practice of emergency medicine*, 3rd ed. Philadelphia: Lippincott Williams & Wilkins, 2001.)

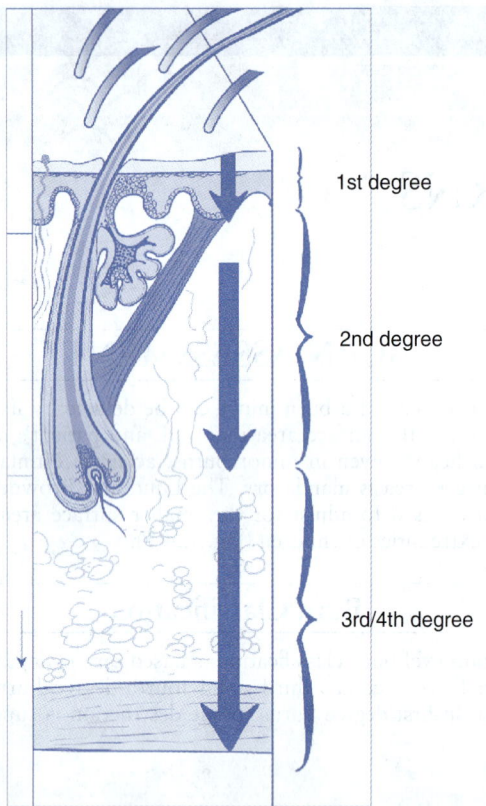

FIGURE 124.2. Burn depth. Cross-section of skin layers, muscle, and bone, with corresponding classification of burn depths. (Reprinted from Life ART Pediatrics Collection. © 2005 Lippincott Williams & Wilkins. All rights reserved.)

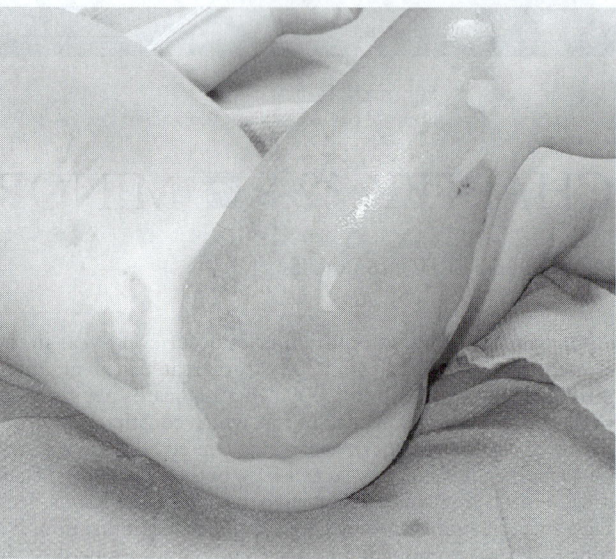

FIGURE 124.3. Hot water burn in an immersion pattern. (Reprinted from Reece RM, Ludwig S. *Child abuse: medical diagnosis and management,* 2nd ed. Philadelphia: Lippincott Williams & Wilkins, 2001.)

involving only the epidermis. Local pain and erythema are present without blistering or systemic response. First-degree burns are the result of contact with hot liquids, exposure to ultraviolet light, or flash burns. Second-degree burns can be divided into superficial and deep partial-thickness burns. Superficial partial-thickness injuries involve only the epidermis and dermis. The wounds appear red and moist, and blisters form. Tactile and pain sensors are intact. Caused by scalds, flash, and contact with hot objects, second-degree burns heal with minimal scarring.

The second-degree burns classified as deep partial-thickness burns involve the entire epidermis and dermis but leave the skin appendages intact. These deeper injuries have a mottled appearance, with areas of pale injury that are dry and anesthetic. These wounds usually heal spontaneously in 4 to 6 weeks. However, they may heal with late hypertrophic scarring and contracture formation. Deep partial-thickness burns may require excision and grafting.

Third-degree burns involve destruction of the epidermis, dermis, and subcutaneous tissue. The area appears white, red, or black and contains deep blisters or thrombosed blood vessels. The elasticity of the burned dermis is destroyed, resulting in a dry, leathery texture. These full-thickness burns require skin grafting if they are larger than 2 or 3 cm in diameter or are in an area of cosmetic importance.

Fourth-degree burns involve deep injury to bone, joint, or muscle, usually resulting from high-voltage electrical injury.

Factors Affecting the Severity of Burns

The location of the burn is important. Critical areas include the eyes, ears, face, hands, feet, and perineum. Other factors that are important are the age of the patient, associated trauma, in-

halation injury, and preexisting health problems. Patients must be hospitalized for their injuries if they have severe burns, if they require fluid therapy, if they have involvement of the perineum, hands, feet, or joint surfaces, if they have circumferential extremity involvement, cellulitis, or infection at the burn site, or if they have associated trauma, facial burns, smoke inhalation, or carbon monoxide poisoning.

Child Abuse

An important part of evaluating pediatric burn injuries is recognition of injury patterns suggesting child abuse. A detailed history is the most important element in establishing a diagnosis of child abuse. Characteristic patterns of nonaccidental burn injury seen on physical examination include the immersion burn caused by forcibly placing the child in a tub of hot water. Immersion injury is characterized by sharply demarcated burns of the hands, feet, buttocks, and perineum (Fig. 124.3). The depth of the burn is uniform. Mirror-image or stocking-glove burn injuries are also associated with child abuse. Contact burns must be suspect when they appear on parts of the child not used in exploring his or her environment.

THERAPY

Initial Treatment

Treatment of the burn begins at the scene of the accident, with elimination of the heat source, and the areas of minor burn are placed in tepid rather than ice water. The burn area is wrapped in a clean towel, and the victim is taken to an emergency facility. The potential benefits of cooling the burned area are controversial. At best, these benefits last only through the first minutes after the injury. After this period, application of cold water may result in prolonged edema, may impair healing, and may convert a partial-thickness to a full-thickness injury.

Chemical burns should be irrigated with copious amounts of water. Adhered tar should be cooled with water, but the tar should not be removed at the scene of the accident.

An accurate history should be obtained, including when and where the accident occurred and the burn-causing agent. The history should help determine whether smoke inhalation or associated injuries occurred. Pertinent medical history, including drug allergies, medication record, and systemic illness, must be obtained at this time.

Tetanus prophylaxis is the same for minor burns as it is for other injuries. In the management of clean wounds in patients who have completed the primary series of tetanus toxoid or who have received a booster within 5 years, a dose of tetanus toxoid is not required. In patients with burn wounds, a booster dose should be given if the primary series was not completed or if a booster has not been received in the past 5 years.

Burn wounds initially may be covered with saline-soaked sponges, which decrease the pain during patient evaluation. The wounds are then washed with mild soap and water, excess debris is removed, and hair is shaved from the margins of the burn.

During evaluation of the burn, tar and asphalt are removed by a petroleum distillate with a hydrocarbon structure. Mineral oil and petroleum ointment, such as bacitracin or Neosporin, may also be used. Tar and asphalt should not be peeled off because of the additional damage to hair and skin that may result.

Chemical burns should be irrigated for 20 minutes. A neutralizing agent usually should not be administered because the resulting reaction may produce heat, causing a more severe injury.

Controversy exists about débriding blisters. Blisters may be left intact, fluid can be evacuated leaving the overlying skin intact, or the blister may be débrided. If the blister is left intact, the wound heals in the blister fluid environment. If the fluid is evacuated, the remaining skin acts as a protective layer covering the wound. The technique used depends on the burn's location and size and on the reliability of the patient's caretaker to care for the wound.

Follow-Up Care

Except for large burns of infants, first-degree burns generally require no treatment. However, various antiseptic and anesthetic ointments may be used and may protect the burned area from the air and provide relief. Use of anesthetic agents in the ointment is not recommended, because large areas may be involved and absorption of the anesthetic agent may cause toxic effects.

Minor burn injury is not associated with immunosuppression, hypermetabolism, or increased susceptibility to infection. Topical chemotherapeutic agents, such as mafenide acetate (Sulfamylon), silver sulfadiazine (Silvadene), silver nitrate, and providone-iodine (Betadine), are used in major burn injuries to prevent burn wound sepsis. These agents should not be used in minor burns, because they delay wound healing. Systemic antibiotics are not indicated in minor burns, because they may predispose the wound to infection with resistant organisms.

Basic wound care consists of keeping the wound clean and moist while it heals. The wound should be washed with mild soap and water and dried lightly. An ointment such as bacitracin or Neosporin should be applied and the wound covered with nonstick porous gauze. Wound care may initially need to be performed daily if any question remains about the extent or depth of the wound or about patient reliability. Each caretaker must be instructed in a program of range-of-motion exercises. Adequate physical therapy prevents prolonged edema that may impair wound healing.

The burn wound should have total epithelial coverage in 2 or 3 weeks. A patient with superficial partial-thickness injury must be followed until epithelial coverage occurs and then examined at 6 weeks for hypertrophic scarring. Recently healed partial-thickness burn wounds become dry. A mild lanolin lotion may be used until natural skin lubrication mechanisms

return. The patient should avoid sun exposure during the period of wound healing. Sunscreen probably should be used even on healed areas when exposure to direct sunlight is expected. Pruritus is a common complaint in maturing burn wounds.

Many methods are available for managing outpatient burn wounds. Some physicians recommend bulky dressings for 2 weeks. Although bulky dressings prevent painful trauma to the burn area, they may encourage bacterial overgrowth in the warm, moist environment. Range-of-motion exercises are difficult with bulky dressings in place. The ideal dressing for burn wounds have adherence, flexibility, permeability, transparency, lack of antigenicity, sterility, ease of application, and low cost. Materials used that have these characteristics include Tegaderm, Opsite, and Biobrane. The use of prosthetic skin substitutes in the treatment of partial-thickness burns has become popular, but expertise in the use of this therapy is necessary.

Management of critical areas including the face, ears, eyes, hands, feet, and perineum often requires hospitalization. Superficial burns of the face are treated by exposure. The face is washed with mild soap and water. A thin layer of ointment may be applied to the open wounds to prevent drying. Superficial burns of the ears are treated with ointment. Deeper injuries are treated with topical chemotherapy and, to avoid chondritis, avoidance of excessive pressure to the area. Suspected corneal burns should be confirmed with fluorescein. Superficial corneal burns are treated with vigorous irrigation, ophthalmic antibiotic ointment, and eye patching. More serious injuries should be evaluated by an ophthalmologist.

To minimize swelling in superficial burns of the hands and feet, the extremity should be elevated. Range-of-motion exercises and instructions for the exercise program are an important part of initial management. Patients with circumferential burns require hospitalization to observe for adequate circulation. Patients with perineal burns require hospitalization for observation of urinary obstruction secondary to edema.

COMPLICATIONS

Most complications in small burn injuries result from overtreatment, with too vigorous dressing changes pulling off newly formed epithelium, or the use of topical and systemic antibiotics resulting in infection with resistant organisms or pseudomembrane formation requiring débridement. Minor burns, which comprise most burns requiring treatment, are best managed with a simple protocol. These injuries are not associated with the severe complications of major burn injuries and do not require the same aggressive interventions in wound care.

Suggested Readings

Andronicus M, Oates RK, Peat J, et al. Nonaccidental burns in children. *Burns* 1998;24:552.

Banco L, Lapidus G, Zavoski R, et al. Burn injuries among children in an urban emergency department. *Pediatr Emerg Care* 1994;10:98.

Carvajal HF. Fluid resuscitation of pediatric burn victims: a critical appraisal. *Pediatr Nephrol* 1994;8:357.

Cockington RA. Ambulatory management of burns in children. *Burns* 1989;15:271.

Finkelstein JL, Schwartz SB, Madden MR, et al. Pediatric burns: an overview. *Pediatr Clin North Am* 1992;39:1145.

Palmeri TL, Greenhalgh DG. Topical treatment of pediatric patients with burns. *Am J Clin Dermatol* 2002;3:529.

Passaretti D, Billmire DA. Management of pediatric burns. *Craniofac Surg* 2003;14:713.

Sheridan RL, Remensnyder JP, Schitzer JJ, et al. Current expectations for survival in pediatric burns. *Arch Pediatr Adolesc Med* 2000;154:245.

Smith ML. Pediatric burns: management of thermal, electrical, and chemical burns and burn-like dermatologic conditions. *Pediatr Ann* 2000;29:367.

Warden GD. Outpatient care of thermal injuries. *Surg Clin North Am* 1987;67:147.

CHAPTER 125 ■ RESPIRATORY COMPLICATIONS OF BURNS AND SMOKE INHALATION (RESPIRATORY BURNS)

MARIANNA M. SOCKRIDER

Respiratory complications are a major source of morbidity and mortality from fires. Overall, nearly one-third of all victims of major burns suffer from various degrees of smoke inhalation injury. Smoke inhalation is responsible for approximately 75% of deaths from structural fires in the United States. The mortality rate is greater among patients who have both cutaneous burns and inhalation injury. Severe injury to the respiratory tract can occur in the absence of surface burns. Several factors are associated with greater risk of incurring respiratory injury: trapping of victims in confined spaces, unconsciousness of victims, fires involving plastics or steam, and victims who are small children or elderly individuals. The likelihood of suffering asphyxia or respiratory inhalation injury is increased in the presence of cutaneous burns. Unconscious victims are at higher risk of incurring injury caused by loss of the protective mechanisms of holding one's breath and laryngospasm. Injuries of the respiratory tract are distributed as follows: 60% upper airway, 30% major lower airway, and 10% parenchymal. Injuries may occur at several levels simultaneously.

The time course of clinical symptoms depends on the type and severity of injury. Carbon monoxide (CO) intoxication, upper airway tract injury, and tracheobronchial obstruction develop in the first 24 hours. Late pulmonary injury likely is attributable to metabolic, infectious, or circulatory derangements complicating the surface burns. During the next 2 to 5 days, noncardiogenic pulmonary edema may develop, particularly in the presence of superimposed sepsis. Nosocomial pneumonia and pulmonary embolism usually occur late, more than 5 days after the event.

TYPES OF DIRECT RESPIRATORY INJURIES

Direct respiratory injuries are classified as asphyxial, thermal, and chemical or toxic (Table 125.1).

Asphyxial Injuries

Hypoxemia may occur as a consequence of CO intoxication, low inspired oxygen tension at the fire site, or ventilation-perfusion mismatch as a result of airway obstruction, atelectasis, and/or fluid overload.

Thermal Injuries

Thermal injury may result from exposure to direct flames, inhalation of hot gases, or inhalation of steam. The normal function of the upper airway as a heat exchanger limits the exposure of the lower airway to thermal injury. Direct thermal damage, then, affects primarily the supraglottic airways. Immediate injury to the oropharyngeal area with edema, erythema, and ulceration may lead to life-threatening upper airway obstruction. Steam produces the most serious burns because of its higher heat-carrying capacity. Only with steam, which is a very unusual occurrence in most fires, or with prolonged exposure to high ambient temperatures does thermal injury occur to the intrathoracic airways.

Chemical/Toxic Injuries

Chemical or toxic injury occurs from exposure to a variety of noxious gases. Chemical injury occurs more frequently than does heat injury. The site of injury depends on the duration of exposure, the size of soot particles, and the solubility of the gases. Damage to the airways results mainly from chemicals that are present in smoke. Particulate matter carried in the smoke (soot) probably does not itself produce injury; toxic gases may be absorbed on the surface of the particles and

TABLE 125.1

TYPES OF RESPIRATORY INJURIES SEEN WITH FIRE OR SMOKE EXPOSURE (MAY BE CONCURRENT)

Direct Injury Type	Mechanisms of Injury
Asphyxial/hypoxemia	Carbon monoxide intoxication
	Low inspired oxygen tension
	Ventilation-perfusion mismatch
Thermal	Exposure to direct flames
	Inhalation of hot gases
	Inhalation of steam
Chemical/toxic	Inhalation of noxious gases
	Direct irritant effects on airways
	Pulmonary edema
	Systemic effects with absorption of toxins
	Reflex bronchoconstriction (soot)
Indirect Injury Type	**Mechanisms of Injury**
Hypoventilation	Chest wall burn/eschar
	Chest wall edema
	Pain
	Medication effect: sedation
Aspiration	Gastric aspiration
Atelectasis	Hypoventilation
	Airway obstruction
Pulmonary edema	Fluid overload
	Sepsis
Infection	Pneumonia

carried into the lungs. The soot particles may be responsible for inducing reflex bronchoconstriction. The inhaled gases may act as airway irritants, or they may be absorbed and become systemic toxins. Irritant gases, such as hydrogen chloride and oxides of nitrogen and sulfur, combine with water in the lung to form corrosive acids or alkalis. Aldehyde gases lead to the denaturation of surface proteins, resulting in pulmonary edema. The two principal systemic toxins are hydrogen cyanide and CO.

Hydrogen Cyanide

Cyanide exposure resulting from the incomplete combustion of products such as plastics and acrylics may be a significant, often hidden, cause of comorbidity in smoke inhalation. Hydrogen cyanide gas causes systemic cyanide poisoning by inhibiting cellular oxidation. Studies of fire victims have revealed concentrations of toxic cyanide, with significantly higher levels found in those who die than in those who survive. Blood cyanide levels correlate with levels of CO. Plasma lactate levels are better correlated with cyanide levels, and a plasma lactate concentration greater than 10 mmol/L is a sensitive indicator of cyanide poisoning. All patients who are obtunded and have significant acidosis should have their levels of plasma lactate and cyanide measured.

Carbon Monoxide

CO is the gas most commonly produced in fire. CO intoxication and hypoxia may account for as many as 80% of smoke inhalation fatalities, particularly deaths that occur at the scene of the fire. CO produces its toxic effects by three mechanisms:

- It has a higher affinity for hemoglobin and displaces oxygen.
- It alters the ability of hemoglobin to release oxygen to the tissues.
- It impairs the ability of tissue cells to use oxygen.

Although the oxygen content in the blood is reduced, arterial oxygen tension (P_aO_2) is normal. Because the carotid body is thought to respond to the P_aO_2, ventilation may not be stimulated until acidosis develops, which, together with the fact that carboxyhemoglobin (COHb) is bright red, renders the clinical diagnosis very difficult to establish. The bright red color of the blood also renders the currently available oximeters unreliable. The clinical manifestations of CO poisoning vary with the level of COHb. Mild intoxication (level less than or equal to 20%) may lead to headache, dyspnea, decreased visual acuity, and alteration of higher cerebral function. Moderate intoxication (level of 20% to 40%) may lead to irritability, nausea, dim vision, impaired judgment, and rapid fatigue. Severe intoxication (level of 40% to 60%) may lead to confusion, hallucinations, ataxia, shock, and coma. Concentrations higher than 60% usually are fatal.

TYPES OF INDIRECT RESPIRATORY INJURIES

Indirect mechanisms also contribute to pulmonary pathophysiology in fire victims (see Table 125.1). Mechanical interference with breathing may occur with restricted chest wall movement caused by chest burns, eschar formation, or chest wall edema. Pain, as well as the use of narcotics to control pain, may increase the risk of hypoventilation. Airway obstruction may be caused by gastric aspiration. Atelectasis may result from hypoventilation or airway obstruction. Secondary lung injury may result from sepsis and fluid overload. The large amounts of intravenous fluids usually given to counteract ongoing surface

and "third-space" losses in the tissues can result in pulmonary vascular engorgement with diminished myocardial function and increased vascular permeability caused by diffuse airway inflammation. The postburn lung is at risk for development of pneumonia. A review of 4,451 consecutive children with thermal injuries noted secondary pneumonia in 41.5% of children with fire burns and in 55% with hot water burns. Organisms may enter the body through the skin at the burn site.

CLINICAL ASSESSMENT

The initial clinical assessment of fire victims should include evaluation for upper airway tract obstruction, central nervous system impairment, and cardiac arrhythmias. Respiratory symptoms such as tachypnea, cough, hoarseness, stridor, and chest retractions may be delayed, rendering them insensitive early indicators of injury. Second- and third-degree burns involving the respiratory area between the nose and lips have been associated with both upper airway tract edema and late-onset pulmonary problems, and they indicate a need for providing more aggressive early intervention. Carbonaceous sputum serves only as a marker of exposure, with little diagnostic or prognostic import. The pulmonary examination may reveal diminished breath sounds, wheezes, crackles, and hoarseness. Both physical findings and symptoms may be delayed for as long as 15 hours after the injury.

The laboratory evaluation should include determination of the COHb level, a complete blood count, and an arterial blood gas analysis. If COHb is greater than 10%, inhalation injury can be suspected. An abnormal P_{O_2} in relation to the fraction of inspired oxygen ($F_{I_{O_2}}$) is another early indicator of smoke inhalation and a strong indication for hospital admission; however, this reading initially may be normal. Soft tissue radiography of the neck may demonstrate upper airway tract edema. A chest radiograph should be obtained. Although the initial chest radiograph may appear normal or may show only hyperinflation, subsequent radiography may demonstrate pneumonitis, atelectasis, or pulmonary edema. Peribronchial infiltrates may persist for weeks. The negative predictive values of normal chest radiographs (38% to 59%) and arterial blood gas measurements (40% to 74%) are low. Normal findings do not exclude inhalation injury. A xenon-133 lung scan or spirometry may demonstrate early obstructive ventilatory defects that imply the presence of airway injury. These defects may have an early onset, antedating radiographic and arterial blood gas abnormalities; however, obtaining these studies may not be practical in young pediatric patients. For patients with surface burns, the reductions in forced vital capacity and forced expiratory volume in 1 second (FEV_1) correlate with the extent of surface burns and reflect restriction of the chest and perhaps increased lung water.

Fiberoptic endoscopy allows immediate direct visualization of the airway injury. Early laryngoscopy is recommended to evaluate compromising intraoral edema, especially in patients with facial burns and those who have had significant exposure. Endoscopic findings such as laryngeal or tracheal edema, ulceration or inflammation of airway mucosa, and soot deposits confirm the presence of respiratory tract injury and may antedate radiographic and arterial blood gas abnormalities. The negative predictive value of fiberoptic bronchoscopy is 88% to 100%. It may be most helpful in victims in whom the results of initial studies are normal or equivocal.

THERAPY

The basic tenets of therapy are maintenance of an adequate airway, correction of hypoxia, reversal of ventilation-perfusion abnormalities, clearance of airway debris and secretions, and prompt recognition and treatment of bacterial infection. At the scene, 100% oxygen should be administered, and airway patency should be established. Fire victims with any risk of having inhalation injury should be observed for at least 24 hours for the development of respiratory symptoms. The American Burn Association has established specific criteria for referral to a burn center that include patients with burns involving the face and inhalation injury.

Indications for endotracheal intubation include severe burns to the face, laryngeal obstruction, difficulty in handling secretions, and progressive respiratory insufficiency. Swelling increases during the first 8 to 24 hours, and worsening should be anticipated if any degree of laryngeal obstruction is present on early examination. Pressure-controlled ventilation in combination with permissive hypercapnia is very useful in the management of most patients. Several studies suggest that high-frequency ventilation may be safer and more effective than is conventional ventilation because it decreases ventilator-associated barotrauma and mechanically mobilizes retained secretions. Extubation usually can be accomplished within 2 to 5 days. Tracheostomy commonly is reserved for situations in which acute respiratory distress occurs in a child who cannot undergo endotracheal intubation or who fails to tolerate extubation. A randomized study of patients at high risk for developing prolonged ventilator dependence found no difference in ventilator support, length of stay, incidence of pneumonia, or survival with early tracheostomy. Use of extracorporeal membrane oxygenation has been reported in victims who are poorly responsive to maximal ventilatory support.

Pulmonary toilet may be facilitated by use of bronchodilators, humidification, and chest physical therapy to enhance the removal of necrotic material, minimize bronchoconstriction, and avoid atelectasis. Bronchoalveolar lavage may need to be performed to clear inspissated secretions. Use of aerosolized heparin and N-acetylcysteine also has been reported to reduce bronchial plugging and cast formation. Cautious use of resuscitative fluids is encouraged because overhydration is associated with a marked increase in pulmonary edema.

Corticosteroids have no established benefit and actually may increase the risk of development of infection. Prophylactic antibiotics offer no benefit and may lead to the development of resistant organisms. Daily surveillance of sputum Gram stain may be helpful to detect potential pathogenic organisms should clinical deterioration occur. Treatment should be based on the results of Gram stain and culture of lower respiratory tract secretions. Aseptic care of the trachea and humidifying equipment are essential in the prevention of infection.

CO is excreted primarily through the lungs. Treatment of CO intoxication with 100% oxygen leads to reduction of the COHb level by one-half in 40 to 60 minutes. The role of using 2 to 3 atm of oxygen is controversial. Although hyperbaric oxygen does lower COHb levels more rapidly, whether it provides a significant advantage over the administration of an inspired concentration of oxygen of 1.0 or whether it affects the incidence of delayed neurologic complications in patients whose COHb level already is less than 30 on arrival at the hospital is questionable.

Although the diagnosis of cyanide poisoning is difficult to establish, it should be suspected in victims of fires in which plastics or chemicals are fuel and in patients who remain comatose after COHb levels decrease to less than 30. Cyanide poisoning is treated with sodium nitrite to induce methemoglobinemia, followed by a slow intravenous infusion of sodium thiosulfate.

PROGNOSIS

Most patients who sustain smoke inhalation and survive regain nearly normal function. Few follow-up studies exist; however, airway hyperreactivity, bronchiectasis, bronchiolitis obliterans, tracheal stenosis, and airway granulation tissue formation have been reported.

PREVENTION

The United States has one of the highest fire fatality rates in the developed world, and three-fourths of these deaths are in residential fires. Homes should be equiped with functioning smoke detectors, which can significantly lower the risk of death. Almost half of the nation's fire deaths occur in the 6% of homes that do not have smoke detectors. The average adult will wake up within 27 seconds of the alarm's sounding, and research indicates that a home can be evacuated safely in 3 minutes. However, children may not wake up with a fire alarm. It is also not uncommon for children to hide in the closet or under their beds. An adult who can reliably wake up to a smoke alarm should be around sleeping children. Adults who are sleep deprived, who have been drinking alcohol, or who are taking certain medications may or may not be awakened by the alarm themselves. Parents need to recognize the need to assist children and adolescents in waking up and exiting their homes. Families should develop a home fire escape plan and practice it. The general rule is "First Up, Last Out." The first person to awaken makes sure that everyone else in the home is awake and exiting. Children need to be taught safe exit procedures during a fire, what to do if their clothes catch on fire, and to recognize fire hazards in the home.

Suggested Readings

American Burn Association. Burn unit referral criteria, 1999. Accessed at 12/17/04 http://www.ameriburn.org/BurnUnitReferral.pdf

Bruck D. Non-awakening in children in response to a smoke detector alarm. *Fire Safety J* 1999;32:369.

Bye MR, Mellins RB. Lung injury from hydrocarbon aspiration and smoke inhalation. In: Chernick V, Boat TF, eds. *Kendig's disorders of the respiratory tract in children*, 6th ed. Philadelphia: WB Saunders, 1998:566.

Carman B, Cahill T, Warden G, et al. A prospective, randomized comparison of the volume diffusive respirator vs. conventional ventilation of burned children. *J Burn Care Rehabil* 2002;23:444.

Desai MH, Micak R, Richardson J, et al. Reduction in mortality in pediatric patients with inhalation injury with aerosolized heparin/acetylcystine [correction of acetylcysteine] therapy. *J Burn Care Rehabil* 1998;19:210.

Herndon DN, Spies M. Modern burn care. *Semin Pediatr Surg* 2001;10:28.

Liebelt EL. Hyperbaric oxygen therapy in childhood carbon monoxide poisoning. *Curr Opin Pediatr* 1999;11:259.

Marshall SW, Runyan CW, Bangdiwala SI, et al. Fatal residential fires: who dies and who survives? *JAMA* 1998;279:1633.

Ruddy RM. Smoke inhalation injury. *Pediatr Clin North Am* 1994;41:317.

Saffle JR, Morris SE, Edelman L. Early tracheostomy does not improve outcome in burn patients. *J Burn Care Rehabil* 2002;23:431.

Warda L, Tenenbein M, Moffatt MEK. House fire injury prevention update. Part I: a review of risk factors for fatal and non-fatal house fire injury. *Injury Prev* 1999;5:145.

Warda L, Tenenbein M, Moffatt MEK. House fire injury prevention update. Part II: a review of the effectiveness of preventive interventions. *Injury Prev* 1999;5:217.

Whitelock-Jones L, Bass DH, Millar AJ, et al. Inhalation burns in children. *Pediatr Surg Int* 1999;15:50.

Wolf SE, Debroy M, Herndon DN. The cornerstones and directions of pediatric burn care. *Pediatr Surg Int* 1997;12:312.

CHAPTER 126 ■ FOREIGN BODIES

MARTIN I. LORIN

From the nose to the distal airways, the respiratory tree has been the recipient of a wide range of unnatural, exogenous materials. Aspiration of foreign bodies is a significant cause of morbidity and mortality in children.

NOSE

Nasal foreign bodies usually are more of an annoyance than a threat to life. Most of them are inserted by toddlers or preschoolers themselves. Occasionally, a piece of tissue placed in the nose to stop a nosebleed inadvertently stays in place for days to weeks. The classic finding of an intranasal foreign body is persistent, unilateral, purulent nasal discharge that may be tinged with blood. Foul odor is a common finding. Occasionally, nasal foreign bodies have dislodged posteriorly and have been aspirated, either spontaneously or during an attempt at removal. Although the diagnosis should be readily apparent, copious or dried secretions can obscure the foreign body. Alternatively, the foreign object may be misinterpreted as a nasal polyp.

Removal of most nasal foreign bodies is accomplished readily in the office without use of general anesthesia. Sedation may be required but usually is not necessary.

Soft or irregularly shaped objects that can be grasped easily by forceps are best removed in this way. Retrieval of a round, hard object, such as a bead, is accomplished best by inserting an ear curet past the foreign body and then applying gentle forward pressure.

UPPER AIRWAY (LARYNX AND TRACHEA)

Aspiration of foreign material into the larynx and trachea can be lethal, and aspiration of foreign bodies into the upper airway is estimated to be the second leading cause of accidental death in the home among children younger than 5 years of age. In most cases, the diagnosis is evident immediately. Sometimes, however, a child may aspirate while alone or asleep, and sudden unexpected death or sudden onset of severe respiratory distress may occur. Although the aspirated material usually is a piece of food or candy, various other objects have been recovered from the larynx and trachea. The plastic cap of a water pistol, a fragment of a balloon, and a piece of bubble gum are examples of objects that have been recovered at autopsy.

Very small foreign objects in the trachea generally are not life-threatening. Although one would imagine that such objects would be either coughed out promptly or aspirated more deeply, this is not always the case; foreign bodies may remain in the trachea for days or even weeks, often becoming embedded in granulation tissue. Although the predominant clinical feature is inspiratory stridor, associated expiratory wheezing is present in approximately 25% to 50% of cases. Cases have been misdiagnosed as croup or tumors. Eggshells, plastic toys or parts of toys, and watermelon seeds are examples of objects that have remained in the trachea for extended periods.

Signs and symptoms of an upper airway foreign body may be mimicked by an esophageal foreign body that is pressing on the posterior trachea. Remarkably, in some cases, esophageal foreign bodies cause stridor or wheezing without pain and without difficulty in swallowing.

Most patients with acute life-threatening upper airway obstruction caused by a foreign body are treated in the field, usually by someone who is not a physician. By the very nature of the condition, few patients requiring urgent treatment reach the hospital before intervention occurs. Consequently, most physicians have had little direct personal experience in treating patients with life-threatening upper airway foreign bodies. Obviously, controlled studies in humans cannot be performed. Available data are from anecdotal case reports, studies in anesthetized animals (some of which had an endotracheal tube in place during the experiment), mechanical models, and theoretic considerations.

Maneuvers used in treating acute, severe upper airway foreign bodies include (a) abdominal thrust (Heimlich maneuver) for patients older than 1 year of age, (b) back blows and chest thrusts for patients younger than 1 year of age, and (c) finger sweeps of the oropharynx.

To perform the abdominal thrust with the victim sitting or standing, the rescuer stands behind the patient with his or her arms wrapped around the victim's abdomen and one fist grabbed by the other hand, slightly above the navel and well below the xiphoid process. The rescuer then forces the fist into the abdomen with a quick upward thrust. If the patient is supine, the rescuer places the heel of one hand, with the other hand on top, on the abdomen in the location described and exerts a sudden upward pressure in the midline. Back blows are applied with the heel of the hand high between the scapulae. Chest thrusts are similar to external cardiac compressions, delivered quickly in a series of four thrusts.

The Heimlich maneuver is potentially dangerous to abdominal viscera, especially the liver in infants, and back blows can drive the foreign body further into the airway. As a compromise, the former is used for patients older than 1 year of age and the latter for infants younger than 1 year old.

Recommendations for emergency management of an upper airway foreign body are as follows: If the victim can speak, breathe, or cough, all interfering maneuvers are unnecessary and dangerous. The patient should be permitted to try to clear the obstructing object by spontaneous cough while preparations are made for emergency transportation to the nearest medical facility.

If intervention is required for a choking child older than 1 year of age, the first maneuver should be a series of abdominal thrusts (Heimlich maneuver). If the Heimlich maneuver fails to relieve the obstruction and the patient loses consciousness, direct removal of the obstructing object is attempted. Blind finger sweeps of the hypopharynx are used only for patients older than 8 years of age. For younger patients, the oropharynx should be inspected, and finger-sweep removal of a foreign body should be attempted only if the object can be seen. If airway patency and breathing are not achieved by these maneuvers, mouth-to-mouth resuscitation is attempted. If this approach fails, abdominal thrusts are repeated.

For an infant who is 1 year of age or younger, abdominal thrusts are not recommended. The child is positioned on his or her abdomen, in a head-down position at approximately 60 degrees, supported on the rescuer's thigh or forearm. A series of five back blows is delivered rapidly. If this fails to relieve the obstruction, the child is turned over, face up, and five chest thrusts are administered. If this fails and the patient loses consciousness, the pharynx should be visualized. If the foreign body cannot be seen and removed, mouth-to-mouth resuscitation is attempted. If obstruction persists, the sequence of back blows and chest thrusts is repeated.

LOWER AIRWAYS (BRONCHI)

Most aspirated foreign bodies are either promptly coughed out or lodge beyond the carina, in a major bronchus or in a more distal airway. The peak incidence of pulmonary aspiration of foreign bodies in children is between the first and second birthdays, more often in boys than in girls. More than 90% of foreign body aspiration occurs before the child's fifth birthday. The variety of foreign bodies that have been aspirated is impressive. Food is the object most commonly aspirated and varies with regional and ethnic dietary customs. The peanut is the most common object to be aspirated by young children in the United States; it accounts for almost 50% of cases in some series, whereas watermelon seeds head the list in Turkey. Other items commonly aspirated include sunflower seeds, pieces of apple (including the stem and pits), teeth, and toys. Unfortunately, most aspirated foreign bodies are radiolucent. In the series of Black and colleagues, only 12% of pulmonary foreign bodies were radiopaque. Some objects, such as eggshell and the aluminum pull tabs from soft-drink containers, are barely radiopaque. These objects can be seen on chest roentgenography, but they often are missed if the film is not scrutinized closely.

In the classic case (which, of course, is seen only occasionally), a previously well toddler suddenly starts to choke and cough while eating, playing with a toy, or crawling on a carpet. The coughing and choking subside, only to be followed by wheezing. Often, however, the child has no history to suggest aspiration, or the episode is recalled only in retrospect, after the foreign body has been removed and identified. The onset of symptoms may be gradual. Occasionally, the onset may coincide with an upper respiratory tract infection and fever, rendering diagnosis especially difficult to establish.

If the foreign body is relatively large and impacts in a major or lobar bronchus, symptoms generally are acute, with wheezing and respiratory distress. If the foreign body is relatively small and lodges in a segmental bronchus, symptoms are more likely to be chronic, with persistent cough, wheezing, and signs of pulmonary infection.

Although wheezing is one of the most common signs associated with a pulmonary foreign body, it is far from being invariably present. In one study of children with bronchial foreign bodies, wheezing was exhibited in only 60% and stridor in only 13%.

To a large extent, the clinical picture is determined by whether the foreign body causes partial or total obstruction of the bronchus in which it is trapped. Partial obstruction results in wheezing that is predominantly expiratory and may be either unilateral or bilateral. In some cases of bilateral wheezing, the expiratory wheeze clearly is louder over the involved hemithorax. Whether the contralateral wheezing in these cases represents a generalized reflex bronchoconstriction or merely transmission of the wheezing sound is not clear. Partial obstruction results in a check-valve mechanism in the airway, with progressive air trapping in the involved lung, lobe, or segment. On physical examination, breath sounds may be decreased over the involved lung, and the trachea and cardiac impulse may be shifted *away* from the involved lung. Tachypnea and retractions are common findings. Cyanosis generally is seen in only severe cases, usually when the foreign body is obstructing a major bronchus. Radiographically, obstructive emphysema involving a lung, lobe, or segment is the hallmark of a foreign body that is partially occluding an airway. In some cases, the overexpansion of the involved lung is mild and is not discernible on a plain roentgenogram of the chest. In such situations, fluoroscopy or inspiratory and expiratory roentgenograms may show an apparent shift of the mediastinum *away* from the involved lung during expiration because the uninvolved lung is able to empty and, therefore, becomes smaller during expiration, whereas the involved lung is obstructed and remains hyperinflated. Visually, the mediastinum appears to be moving *away* from the involved lung during expiration.

When the foreign body occludes the involved airway completely, the result is atelectasis rather than hyperaeration. Clinically, this condition is evident by decreased breath sounds, with or without rales. Although the trachea and cardiac impulses usually are unchanged, in severe cases, they may be shifted *toward* the involved lung. Chest roentgenography reveals atelectasis of the affected area.

Fever, rales, purulent sputum, and radiographic evidence of pneumonia can occur with either partial or complete occlusion. Pneumonia may be noted in 15% to 20% of cases.

The mainstay of management of foreign bodies in the lower airways is endoscopic removal. If the presence of a foreign body is uncertain, endoscopy can be diagnostic as well as therapeutic.

The procedure should be performed in the operating room or in a suitably equipped endoscopy suite, and the endoscopist should be experienced in caring for the pediatric patient. The highest-quality, most current endoscopic equipment should be available. Optimal treatment includes management by an anesthetist skilled in the care of young children. These ideal conditions often are not available locally, and, if the patient's condition is stable, the best approach may be to transfer the child to a facility where skillful pediatric endoscopic treatment is available. Efforts to dislodge the foreign body by chest physical therapy ("postural drainage") are dangerous and should not be attempted. After the child has undergone endoscopy, edema of the airway, as well as parenchymal changes in the lung from which the foreign body was removed, may take days to subside. With proper treatment, the mortality rate for aspiration of foreign bodies into the lower airways should be exceedingly low.

Suggested Readings

American Heart Association in collaboration with the International Liaison Committee on Resuscitation. Guidelines 2000 for cardiopulmonary resuscitation and emergency cardiovascular care. Part 9: pediatric basic life support. *Circulation* 2000;102(suppl):I253.

Baker DM. Foreign bodies of the ears and nose in childhood. *Pediatr Emerg Care* 1987;3:67.

Black RE, Johnson DG, Matlak ME. Bronchoscopic removal of aspirated foreign bodies in children. *J Pediatr Surg* 1994;29:682.

Blazer S, Naveh Y, Friedman A. Foreign body in the airway: a review of 200 cases. *Am J Dis Child* 1980;134:68.

Burton EM, Brick WG, Hall JD, et al. Tracheobronchial foreign body aspiration in children. *South Med J* 1996;89:195.

Cotton E, Yosuda K. Foreign body aspiration. *Pediatr Clin North Am* 1984;31:937.

Eren S, Balci AE, Dikici B, et al. Foreign body aspiration in children: experience of 1160 cases. *Ann Trop Pediatr* 2003;23:31.

Esclamado RM, Richardson MA. Laryngotracheal foreign bodies in children: a comparison with bronchial foreign bodies. *Am J Dis Child* 1987;141:259.

Greensher J, Mofenson HC. Emergency treatment of the choking child. *Pediatrics* 1982;70:110.

Halroyd HJ, Aron WR, Greensher J, et al. First aid for the choking child: Committee on Accident and Poison Prevention, American Academy of Pediatrics. *Pediatrics* 1981;67:744.

Heimlich HJ. First aid for choking children: back blows and chest thrusts cause complications and death. *Pediatrics* 1982;70:120.

Kosloske AM. Bronchoscopic extraction of aspirated foreign bodies in children. *Am J Dis Child* 1982;136:924.

Pediatric basic life support. *JAMA* 1986;255:2954.

SECTION VI ■ CLINICAL OVERVIEWS

CHAPTER 127 ■ ORAL PROBLEMS

KATHERINE S. KULA AND STUART D. JOSELL

Oral health is a necessary part of a child's total physical and emotional health and requires a multidisciplinary approach from all health providers. Recognition and prevention of oral problems reduces the cost and risk of dental care, particularly in medically or physically compromised patients. Although most problems in the oral cavity are traditionally considered to be in the realm of dentistry, a physician examines a child earlier and more frequently than a dentist and can provide early education and dental referral to prevent or minimize oral problems. The physician should be able to identify oral problems that, left untreated, could contribute to growth abnormalities or to systemic disturbances. However, accurate diagnosis and correct treatment of abnormalities frequently require dental referral for additional diagnostic tests.

Knowledge of normal facial and oral structures, processes, and timing and sequence of events helps a clinician diagnose various local and systemic problems. Some of the most common pediatric dental problems and their treatment are discussed in this chapter.

EXAMINATION

The oral structures should be examined routinely at birth and at well-child visits. Early examinations can reveal abnormalities that require treatment or serve as a baseline against which to compare later development. Factors to consider during an oral examination are support of the child's head, access, visibility, timing, systematic approach, and protection of the clinician's fingers. Observant parents can provide good information about changes in a child's head and neck areas that can be overlooked by a clinician.

Extraoral Examination

Extraoral structures are the easiest to examine because they can be observed with the child on the parent's lap or against the parent's shoulder. The proportions of the face, the profile, and the integrity of the lips should be evaluated. Children should exhibit relative symmetry of the soft tissue, hard tissue, and dentition. The face and neck should be palpated gently to determine if swollen nodes or other abnormalities are present.

Intraoral Examination

An intraoral examination can be conducted with the child in any one of a number of positions, depending on the child's age and willingness to cooperate. In most cases, the mouth of a young child can be examined while the child is lying on the examination table. Alternatively, the parent and the clinician can sit knee to knee, with the child lying with his head on the clinician's lap and his arms and legs held on the parent's lap.

The physician should start the intraoral examination by performing a sweeping palpation of the areas between the lips and cheeks and the alveolar ridges, across the roof of the mouth, and on top of and under the tongue to determine the presence of abnormal structures. If the sucking reflex of an infant is intact, the infant usually reacts to the examining finger as if it were a nipple. In examining older children, the physician must take care to avoid being bitten.

A visual examination should follow the palpation. Using the thumb and forefinger of each hand, the physician should slightly extend the lips in an apical direction for better visualization of the area between the ridges and the lips. The cheeks should be slightly distended with a tongue blade or with a forefinger, preferably with the patient's mouth open, allowing the buccal vestibules, Stensen duct, buccal mucosa, ridges, and teeth, if present, to be examined.

If the child is cooperative, he or she should be asked to open the mouth widely and extend the tongue so that the top of the tongue can be examined. The child should then raise the tongue to the roof of the mouth so that the ventral surface of the tongue, floor of the mouth, and lower teeth can be seen. The physician can hold the tip of the tongue with a piece of cotton gauze and then extend the tongue slightly to view its sides. If no small intraoral mirror is available for viewing the palate, the child's head, which may be rested on the examination table, in the crook of a parent's arm, or on the clinician's lap, can be tipped backward for viewing the palate and upper teeth. A pen light permits better visualization of the oral cavity.

NORMAL ANATOMY

Intraoral Soft Tissue

The mouth of the newborn is characterized by toothless alveolar pads or ridges in the maxilla and mandible. The ridges vary considerably in shape and frequently have small bumps or protrusions under which lie the developing primary teeth. Teeth are usually not erupted in the newborn. The maxillary alveolar ridge is typically demarcated from the rest of the palate by a palatal alveolar groove that disappears with time. In the child with teeth, healthy gingiva surrounding the teeth is normally light pink and firm. It should not bleed spontaneously or on slight pressure.

Bands of tissue that extend from the lip or cheek to, over, or through the alveolar ridge are called *frena*. With development, the frena usually move apically toward the vestibule.

Numerous filiform and fungiform papillae should cover the dorsum of the tongue, which is normally light pink. Circumvallate papillae appear as circular raised bumps on the dorsum of the tongue and separate the anterior portion of the tongue from the posterior portion. The lingual surface of the tongue and the floor of the mouth should be well vascularized. Raised structures, which represent salivary gland ducts, are usually visible in the floor of the mouth.

The mouth should be moist from saliva secreted from three major salivary glands and minor glands. Normally these glands are not palpable. The parotid gland, the largest of the major glands, lies within the cheek with its opening (Stensen duct) surrounded by a slight mass of tissue on the buccal mucosa approximately adjacent to the maxillary permanent molars. The superior border of the submandibular gland lies in the floor of the mouth and its ducts (Wharton ducts) pass under the anterior portion of the tongue, where they appear as long, raised areas, and open into the sublingual caruncula, which lies at the midline of the tongue. The sublingual gland lies in the floor of the mouth. This gland can open directly under the tongue through multiple small excretory ducts or can unite with the submandibular duct through the sublingual Bartholin duct. Minor salivary glands are present in the circumvallate papillae on the dorsum of the tongue, along the lingual frenum on the ventral surface of the tongue, and in the palate.

Salivary function is extremely important to the health of the oral cavity. Saliva is a multicomponent substance that serves numerous functions. Saliva lubricates food and facilitates swallowing. Lubrication of the occluding surfaces of the teeth helps minimize tooth abrasion. Salivary amylase breaks down starch primarily in the mouth. Immunoglobulin A and other proteins in the saliva are thought to prevent bacterial attachment. Numerous salivary proteins such as lysozyme, lactoferrin, and lactoperoxidase appear to be bacteriocidal or bacteriostatic. Fluid from the tissues around the teeth contributes antibodies, phagocytic cells, and antibacterial products. Multiple ions and other components in the saliva help maintain the oral tissues.

An important function of saliva is its ability to neutralize and clear foodstuffs from the mouth. Saliva contains bicarbonate ions that buffer acidic, potentially destructive substances. Bicarbonate ions increase in concentration with increased salivary flow and increase the buffering capacity of the saliva. Various salivary proteins also buffer acids. Salivary flow also clears oral debris. The greater the flow rate is, the more frequently swallowing occurs, and the faster debris is cleared from the mouth. However, debris clears from various areas of the mouth at different rates because of the compartmentalization of the mouth. The differences in clearance rates make teeth in some areas of the mouth more susceptible to caries than teeth in other areas.

The flow rate of saliva from all areas of the mouth appears to increase with age up to 15 years, when it reaches that of an adult. The average stimulated salivary flow rate for 5-year-old children is approximately 0.5 mL/minute, slightly more than 1.0 mL/minute for 10-year-old children, and approximately 2.0 mL/minute for 15-year-old adolescents. Considerable variability in stimulated salivary flow rates exists. Unstimulated flow rates (e.g., during sleep) are almost negligible and minimally clear food (e.g., sugar in antibiotics or from the baby bottle) from the mouth or neutralize acids. The increased time that these sugars and their acidic byproducts spend in the mouth increases the susceptibility of teeth to caries. Factors such as head–neck radiation and some drugs can damage salivary glands, decreasing the salivary flow rate and causing ram-

pant decay, difficulty in swallowing, and inability to lubricate the oral tissues.

The extraoral palpation often can be used as a screening for intraoral infections, particularly when nodes are palpable. The submental nodes drain the mandibular anterior teeth, their surrounding labial gingiva, and the lower lip. The submandibular nodes receive lymphatic drainage from the submental nodes, maxillary structures, mandibular posterior teeth and surrounding structures, tongue, and nasal cavity. The parotid gland drains into the preauricular nodes. The cervical nodes receive lymphatic drainage from the base of the tongue, the sublingual area, the posterior palate, and the preauricular, submandibular, and submental nodes. Thus, swollen nodes can indicate abscessed teeth or other intraoral infections or diseases.

Dentition

Dental Stages

Primary Dentition. The dental stage in which only primary (baby) teeth are present is called *primary dentition*. Twenty primary teeth normally erupt between the ages of approximately 4 and 30 months (Table 127.1). The timing of eruption varies among ethnic and racial groups (e.g., African Americans tend to have an earlier eruption and exfoliation pattern than American Caucasians), but, in general, if 20 primary teeth are not present by 36 months of age, the child should be referred to a pediatric dentist for evaluation.

Eruption is usually symmetric from side to side. Eruption tends to occur slightly earlier in the mandibular arch than in the maxillary arch. The sequence of eruption is usually the central incisor, lateral incisor, first molar, canine, and second molar. All primary teeth are usually into occlusion (touching) by the age of 3 years (Fig. 127.1).

Upon biting, all of the maxillary teeth should touch the mandibular teeth vertically and overhang the mandibular teeth horizontally about a half a tooth. The midlines of the dentition should coincide with each other and the face. Spacing in the primary dentition is normal and allows a better chance for the larger permanent teeth to erupt into normal position. Variations of normal occlusion include lack of spacing, but there might not be as much room for the permanent teeth. The lips should touch each other easily with no muscle strain when the child touches the teeth together and the tip of the chin and the lips should be on the same line as the nose. In general, this simplistic description of a normal occlusion remains through adulthood.

Mixed Dentition. Mixed dentition is a dental stage in which the roots of the primary teeth resorb, the primary teeth exfoliate and are replaced by the permanent teeth, and the first permanent molars erupt behind the primary molars. The mixed dentition stage begins at approximately 6 years of age, when the first permanent molars or the permanent incisors erupt, and continues until approximately 13 years of age, when the last primary tooth is replaced by a permanent tooth. Usually, a 3- to 4-year span occurs between the eruption of the permanent incisors and first molars and the eruption of the permanent canines and premolars. The sequence of eruption varies among children and between the dental arches, but in general, either the first permanent molar or the mandibular central incisors erupt first. The timing and sequence of eruption and exfoliation of contralateral teeth are usually symmetric, but might vary as much as 6 months. Abnormalities of sequence (Fig. 127.2), timing, or position should be evaluated by a dentist.

Occasionally, a permanent tooth erupts before exfoliation of the primary tooth (Fig. 127.3). This does not present a problem if the primary tooth is mobile; the permanent tooth usually moves into proper position within the arch. However, the child

TABLE 127.1
CHRONOLOGY OF HUMAN DENTITION*

Tooth	Hard Tissue Formation Apparent on Radiographs	Amount of Enamel Formed at Birth	Enamel Completed	Eruption	Root Completed
Deciduous dentition					
Maxillary					
Central incisor	4 months *in utero*	Five-sixths	1.5 months	7.5 months	1.5 years
Lateral incisor	4.5 months *in utero*	Two-thirds	2.5 months	9 months	2 years
Cuspid	5 months *in utero*	One-third	9 months	18 months	3.25 years
First molar	5 months *in utero*	Cusps united	6 months	14 months	2.5 years
Second molar	6 months *in utero*	Cusp tips still isolated	11 months	24 months	3 years
Mandibular					
Central incisor	4.5 months *in utero*	Three-fifths	2.5 months	6 months	1.5 years
Lateral incisor	4.5 months *in utero*	Three-fifths	3 months	7 months	1.5 years
Cuspid	5 months *in utero*	One-third	9 months	16 months	3.25 years
First molar	5 months *in utero*	Cusps united	5.5 months	12 months	2.25 years
Second molar	6 months *in utero*	Cusp tips still isolated	10 months	20 months	3 years
Permanent dentition					
Maxillary					
Central incisor	3–4 months	—	4–5 years	7–8 years	10 years
Lateral incisor	10–12 months	—	4–5 years	8–9 years	11 years
Cuspid	4–5 months	—	6–7 years	11–12 years	13–15 years
First bicuspid	1.5–1.75 year	—	5–6 years	10–11 years	12–13 years
Second bicuspid	2–2.25 years	—	6–7 years	10–12 years	12–14 years
Second molar	2.5–3 years	—	7–8 years	12–13 years	14–16 years
Third molar	7–9 years	—	12–16 years	17–21 years	18–25 years
Mandibular					
Central incisor	3–4 months	—	4–5 years	6–7 years	9 years
Lateral incisor	3–4 months	—	4–5 years	7–8 years	10 years
Cuspid	4–5 months	—	6–7 years	9–10 years	12–14 years
First bicuspid	1.75–2 years	—	5–6 years	10–12 years	12–13 years
Second bicuspid	2.25–2.5 years	—	6–7 years	11–12 years	13–14 years
Second molar	2.5–3 years	—	7–8 years	11–13 years	14–15 years
Third molar	8–10 years	—	12–16 years	17–21 years	18–25 years

*Mean ages.
Reprinted with permission from McCall I, Schour M. Studies of tooth development: the growth pattern of human teeth, part II. *J Am Dent Assoc* 1940;27:1918.

should be encouraged to extract the primary tooth as soon as possible. If the primary tooth is firmly attached, the child should be referred to a dentist for evaluation of the primary tooth, because it may prevent the permanent tooth from coming into good arch alignment.

Permanent Dentition. Permanent dentition is the stage that follows replacement of the last remaining primary tooth with a permanent tooth. The second molar should erupt within a year of the loss of the last primary tooth (Table 127.1). The third

molar varies in its eruption time but usually does not erupt before the age of 17 years. The normal complement of permanent teeth is 32, with 16 in the maxilla and 16 in the mandible.

Normal Occlusion and Malocclusion

Occlusion refers to the manner in which the teeth fit together when biting and in the variety of tooth contacts that occur during mastication, swallowing, clenching, grinding, and other normal and abnormal mandibular movements. Occlusion is affected by the relative positions of the skeletal bases (the maxilla

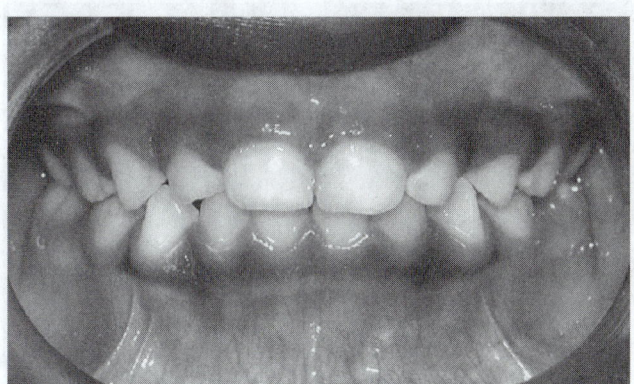

FIGURE 127.1. Normal nonspaced primary dentition with coincident midlines and overlap of maxillary teeth over the mandibular teeth.

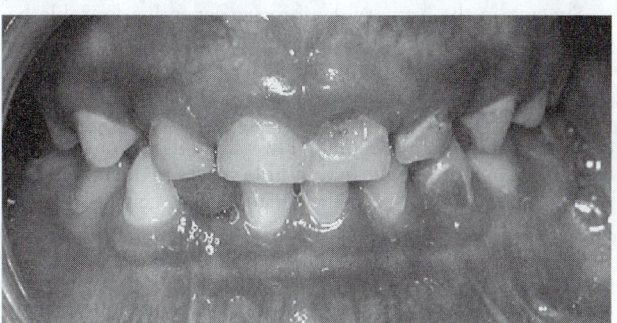

FIGURE 127.2. Primary dentition with white spot lesions, cavitated dental caries, and asymmetric, atypical loss of mandibular incisor.

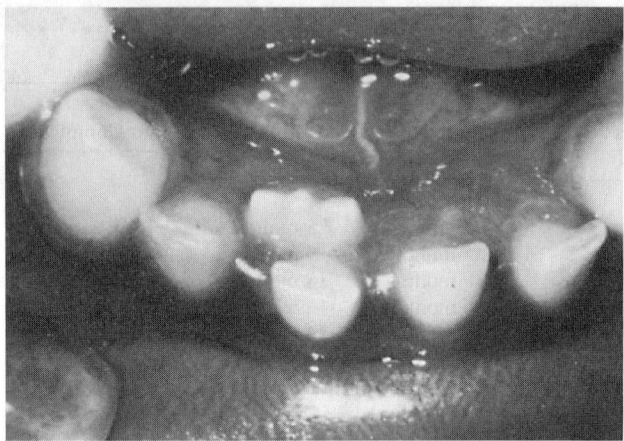

FIGURE 127.3. Double row of teeth in which a permanent incisor has erupted before primary tooth exfoliation. (Courtesy of Dr. Mark Wagner, University of Maryland Dental School.)

and the mandible), by the position of the alveolar bone around the teeth, and by the relative positions of the teeth within the alveolar bone.

In dentistry, every bite that differs from ideal occlusion is considered malocclusion. Malocclusion can be caused by skeletal or dental imbalance or by a combination of the two. Various degrees of malocclusion occur. Some malocclusion is considered within the normal range and is compatible with good dental health and function. Between 75% and 90% of children younger than 18 years in the United States have some degree of malocclusion. Approximately 15% to 30% have a handicapping condition requiring orthodontic treatment.

The significance of malocclusion is that it can interfere with chewing coarse or tough foods. It might not be aesthetically appealing, an important factor that causes psychological problems for some children. Malocclusion can cause trauma of soft tissues so severe that the tissue is stripped from the bone around teeth and the teeth are lost. Whereas some malocclusions can be corrected with early growth modification and some at a later age with orthodontics alone, some malocclusions are so severe that orthognathic surgery is required in addition to orthodontics.

The occlusal form of each dental arch should be smooth, symmetric, and without crowding or undesirable spacing. Lack of symmetry can indicate skeletal growth discrepancy, space loss due to trauma or caries, excessive rotation of teeth, or a congenitally missing tooth.

The dental midlines of the mandibular and maxillary arches should coincide with each other in occlusion (see Fig. 127.1) and should coincide with the midline of the face. Midline discrepancies greater than 1 mm indicate skeletal or dental problems that require dental referral.

Spacing in the primary dentition is generally desirable because the permanent teeth replacing the primary teeth are usually larger and require more space. Maxillary anterior spacing in the mixed dentition can be caused by pressure from the unerupted permanent canines on the incisor roots and may close on eruption of the canines. However, missing or impacted teeth or trauma can cause undesirable spaces in the mixed dentition. Spacing in the permanent dentition is generally not as desirable.

Spacing in the permanent dentition can be caused by generalized or localized smaller tooth structure than arch space, supernumerary teeth, a large fibrous frenum, congenitally missing (Fig. 127.4) or extracted teeth, cysts, and abnormal and unbalanced forces on the dentition such as those seen with thumb sucking. In some cases, adjacent teeth drift into the

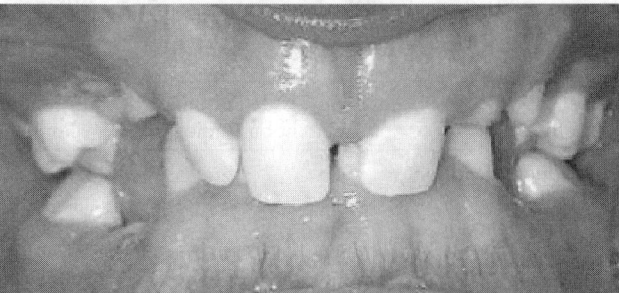

FIGURE 127.4. Multiple congenitally missing teeth and deep overbite in the mixed dentition of patient with ectodermal dysplasia.

spaces through rotation and tipping, contributing to malocclusion.

Crowding in the primary dentition is usually an indication that crowding will become worse with age. Slight crowding in the mixed dentition might be alleviated later.

The vertical relation between the permanent front teeth (i.e., overbite) is considered ideal when the maxillary incisors overlap the mandibular incisors about 1 to 2 mm (about 20% overlap). An overbite is considered severe if 5 to 7 mm of the mandibular incisors are covered; it is considered extreme if greater than 7 mm of the mandibular incisors are covered (Fig. 127.4). Approximately 15% to 20% of the children in the United States have severe to extreme overbites.

Teeth in the maxillary arch should hang outside those in the mandibular arch by approximately one-half of a tooth width. A crossbite exists if one or more maxillary teeth lie inside the mandibular teeth or completely outside the lower teeth (Fig. 127.5). Approximately 3% to 9% of the children in the United States have crossbites. Crossbites can be the result of dental positioning or skeletal discrepancies in the maxilla or the mandible. Small dental or skeletal discrepancies can cause the cusp tips of the teeth of both arches to meet and deflect to one side, resulting in a functional unilateral crossbite. Whereas small discrepancies are often difficult to detect, large discrepancies can result in noticeable facial asymmetry. Many patients with a unilateral crossbite exhibit facial asymmetry. Functional crossbites should be corrected as soon as possible to prevent increased asymmetry with age. Anterior crossbites in which the front maxillary teeth lie inside the mandibular teeth are frequently seen in children with concave or very straight faces, indicating skeletal imbalances.

A vertical open bite (Fig. 127.6) exists when the maxillary incisors do not touch the opposing incisors. Approximately 4% to 8% of adolescents in the United States have open bites. The

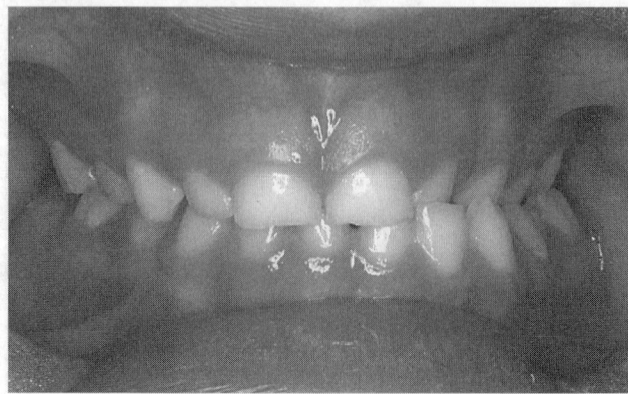

FIGURE 127.5. Functional unilateral crossbite with noncoincident midlines in the primary dentition.

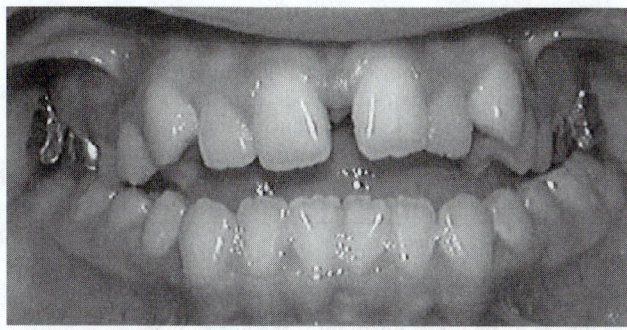

FIGURE 127.6. Vertical open bite and posterior crossbite in the permanent dentition.

severity of the open bite can vary in the vertical height and in the number of teeth involved. Some children have an open bite that extends to their molars. For these children, chewing, such as biting through a sandwich, can be a problem. Open bites can be caused by digit sucking, excessive tooth mass for the jaw, trauma, and severe skeletal discrepancies. Children with skeletal open bites can have excessively long lower faces.

Normally, the backs of the maxillary incisors should touch the front of the mandibular incisors. If a horizontal open bite exists between the maxillary and mandibular incisors, it is called an *overjet*. An overjet can result from problems such as a discrepancy in the lengths of the maxilla and mandible or digit habits. A child with a large overjet can have an excessively convex profile because of a relatively deficient mandible as compared with the maxilla.

All posterior maxillary teeth should touch the mandibular teeth unless the patient is at a normal dental developmental stage in which primary teeth are exfoliating and permanent teeth are erupting. The lack of occlusion or the presence of vertical space may indicate a growth discrepancy in the area. Eruption proceeds at approximately 1 mm a month, and a space caused by a normal exfoliation and eruption of teeth should be closed or almost closed within approximately 6 months. Occasionally, teeth are partially visible but impacted because of lack of arch space.

In general, a child with crowding, a crossbite, an open bite, midline discrepancies, a deep bite, or a large overjet should be referred to an orthodontist for evaluation.

Determining the anteroposterior relation of the maxillary teeth to the mandibular teeth can be difficult. The key to screening a patient for gross occlusal problems is that the profile frequently reflects the relation of the maxilla to the mandible. A young child normally has a slightly convex facial profile that becomes straighter with growth of the mandible. Teenagers who have a maxilla and a mandible that are in good relation to each other tend to have straight profiles. A profile that is definitely convex or concave indicates skeletal imbalances, and orthodontic referral is recommended for those patients. Early intervention in the growth processes of the maxilla or mandible may prevent future surgical procedures to position the jaws better. However, mandibular growth can be difficult to predict. Mandibular growth can continue into adulthood, requiring surgery to correct the facial deformity and related malocclusion.

HABITS THAT CONTRIBUTE TO ORAL PROBLEMS

Habits such as digit sucking and lip sucking can contribute to malocclusions and, in the case of mouth breathing, to gin-

gival inflammation. Other habits, such as bruxism and self-mutilation, cause destruction of oral tissues. However, some oral habits are little more than nuisances.

Digit Sucking

Digit sucking, which usually begins during the first year of life or before weaning, is the most common oral habit. Although the habit usually diminishes in frequency with age, some adults continue to suck their digits. A wide range exists in the reported prevalence, reaching a level as high as 86% of children between 1 and 10 years of age.

Possible causes of digit sucking include the rooting reflex, lack of sucking satisfaction during eating, peer modeling, and psychological problems. Although the habit is considered normal during infancy, the older child who continues to suck may have an emotional problem. Peer pressure and highly critical parents often compound the problem.

Digit sucking is a dental and social concern when it detrimentally affects occlusion. Many children discontinue the habit early or do not suck frequently or with great intensity. However, when the habit is frequent and intense, a greater chance exists that significant dental and skeletal deformities will be present. The deformities include anterior open bite, flaring maxillary incisors, retruded and crowded mandibular incisors, increased overjet, posterior crossbite, anteriorly displaced maxilla, and retruded mandible.

The critical age at which digit sucking should be stopped to minimize the effect on the permanent dentition is controversial. Many open bites self-correct if a child stops sucking before eruption of the maxillary permanent anterior teeth. Self-correction of the malocclusion depends on its severity, the flaccidity of the perioral soft tissue, and the presence of other oral habits, such as tongue position, mouth breathing, and lip habits. Severe oral problems require early intervention by the dentist.

Digit sucking can involve the thumb or one or more fingers. A variety of positions for the digits are assumed during sucking and appear to cause different occlusal changes. For example, a child who sucks only a digit on one side may exhibit a one-sided open bite. In contrast, a two-thumb sucker usually exhibits a wide and more symmetric open bite.

Even if the clinician does not see the child sucking and the parents do not report the habit, digit sucking should be considered if an open bite or overjet is observed during oral examination. If the incisors involved in the overjet are spaced and have no lingual support from the mandibular incisors, the clinician should suspect a digit-sucking habit. Children frequently do not respond or are untruthful to direct questions about sucking. Instead of asking directly, the hands of the child should be examined for extra clean, wrinkled, or red digits and calluses, which are diagnostic of frequent, intense sucking. The physician can then ask less threatening questions: "Are these the fingers that you suck the most?" "Do these fingers taste the best?" In the absence of signs on the hands, the examiner can ask, "Which fingers do you like to suck the most?" to elicit more truthful answers.

A simple explanation of the effects of the habit on the teeth may help some children stop their habit. Before deciding on any definitive treatment, however, the physician should determine the child's desire to stop. If the child is motivated, positive reinforcement programs with the parents' cooperation can be established. A reward system or a reminder such as an adhesive bandage on the digit can be used. If the habit is too deeply established to stop by positive reinforcement alone, the dentist can insert an intraoral habit appliance to serve as a reminder. This is usually effective. Additional orthodontics may be required in some children.

If the child is not motivated to stop the habit, appliances should not be used. The child may continue to suck, embedding the appliance into the soft tissue or causing orthopedic movement of the maxilla or intrusion of abutment teeth. Alternatively, the child may cause tissue damage by removing the fixed appliance. Counseling should be suggested to determine the reason for the child's lack of motivation.

If digit sucking is associated with an emotional problem, counseling should be encouraged. Counseling should be considered for parents or families who cannot cope with the child's habit. Negative reinforcement of the habit causes some children to become more adamant about sucking.

Pacifier Sucking

Prolonged and intense sucking of a pacifier can cause malocclusions similar to those produced by digit sucking. The problems are usually minimal and tend to self-correct after the habit is discontinued.

Pacifiers are used to satisfy an infant's nonnutritive sucking needs and delay an infant's feeding time when nursing or bottle-feeding is inconvenient. Prevalence studies report that as many as 45% of infants use pacifiers. The habit is discontinued in most children by 3 years of age, but it should be discontinued by 1 year. The simplest form of treatment is to discard the pacifier so that the child cannot find it. Parents should be cautioned not to dip pacifiers in honey or other sweet liquids, a practice associated with rampant caries.

Lip Habits

The two major lip habits involve wedging the lips between prominent upper incisors and the lower incisors and licking, sucking, or biting the lips. Forcefully wedging the lower lip between the teeth can cause additional protrusion of the upper incisors. Puckering of the skin over the chin occurs during this activity, because the mentalis muscle inserts into the soft tissue of the chin. An intraoral appliance can be used to minimize the action, but it does not correct the malocclusion.

Licking, sucking, or biting the lips is not associated with malocclusion but may result in chapping or drying of the lips and surrounding skin. Lip balm, face cream, or other lubricating material is recommended for palliative treatment.

Bruxism

Bruxism refers to the grinding of the teeth. The maxillary and mandibular teeth normally contact only during chewing and swallowing. During most of the day, they assume a rest position with as much as 5 mm of interocclusal space between the two arches. However, some children clench or grind their teeth.

The clinical signs vary from small wear facets to extensive wear of the teeth. The abrasion appears to stimulate cells within the pulp to form additional (sclerotic) dentin to protect the pulp. In some cases, the rate of abrasion is so great that the pulp can be seen through clear sclerotic dentin. In severe cases, the rate of abrasion exceeds the rate of dentin formation, exposing the pulp and resulting in a dental abscess. Bruxism can contribute to fracture of the teeth, muscle fatigue, and temporomandibular joint dysfunction and discomfort.

Bruxism is usually a subconscious activity and may occur during waking or sleeping periods. Parents usually report that the child grits his or her teeth together, particularly at night. Children with neurologic disorders are reported to engage in bruxism with the same intensity day and night.

If crossbites are observed, orthodontic treatment is indicated. If psychological stress is contributing to the bruxism, parental and child counseling and psychiatric referral may be necessary. Bite guards can provide palliative treatment when worn at night and, if necessary, during the day.

Mouth Breathing

Mouth breathing is associated with excessive drying of the anterior gingiva with a concomitant increase in chronic gingivitis. This effect is seen in patients who cannot close their lips easily or whose normal rest position of the lips is open.

The causal association between mouth breathing and a facial type characterized by a long, narrow face, short, flaccid lips, a narrow nose, and an expressionless face is controversial. It would be logical to expect factors such as adenoidal hypertrophy and allergy to affect a child with narrow nasal passages more than a child with wide passages, but some children with open-mouth posture and a mouth-breathing habit have no history of significant nasal obstruction. In addition, some children whose nasal obstruction is eliminated continue to mouth breathe.

Orthodontic treatment can eliminate the malocclusion and minimize some factors involved in not being able to close the lips properly. Evaluation by an otolaryngologist and an allergist may be necessary. If the mouth breathing continues despite a patent nasal airway, a program of positive reinforcement or the use of an oral shield over the lips may be effective.

Tongue Thrust

Tongue thrust is an infantile pattern of swallowing in which the tongue flattens and moves forward between the anterior teeth. Approximately 97% of newborns exhibit tongue thrust. Tongue thrust decreases with age; 3% of 12-year-old children exhibit the habit.

Tongue thrust is associated with open bite, incisor protrusion, and mandibular retrusion. However, the relation is uncertain. Three-fourths of children with tongue thrust who exhibit malocclusion in the primary teeth do not develop malocclusion of the permanent teeth. The swallowing pattern appears to mature in most children by 8 or 9 years of age, the time in which the permanent incisors are completely erupted. The efficacy of intraoral appliances is documented, but not always permanent. Treatment is contraindicated if no malocclusion or speech problem exists.

The cause of tongue thrust is controversial. Functionally, it appears that the tongue compensates for a small jaw and large lymphoid tissue by anterior thrust during swallowing. Growth of the mandible and reduction of lymphoid tissue appear to correspond with decreased thrust.

Intraoral and Perioral Piercings

Placing jewelry into a pierced tongue or lip is associated with tooth fractures, scarring, metal hypersensitivities, and infections. Piercings should be discouraged.

ORAL ANOMALIES

Various oral anomalies associated with developmental disturbances such as clefts can be detected at birth, within a few weeks of birth, or at the time of tooth eruption, whereas others such as ectodermal dysplasia are usually diagnosed much later. The categorization of oral anomalies into discrete entities is difficult since some are manifestations of an entire tissue

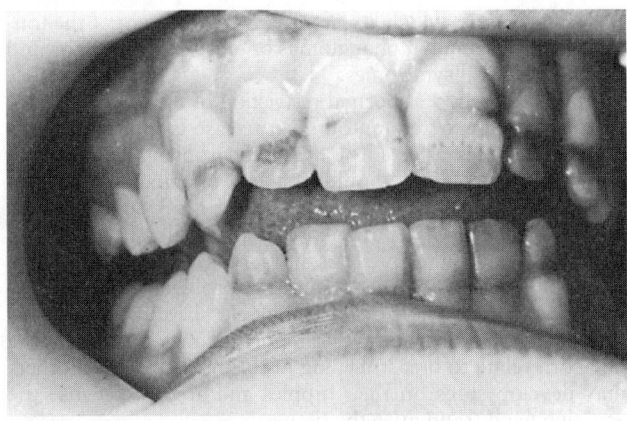

FIGURE 127.7. Linear hypoplasia resulting from tetracycline treatment at approximately 2 to 3 years of age.

dysfunction, such as ectodermal dysplasia, whereas others are nonspecific. Disorders involving mineralization, such as vitamin D–resistant rickets, can affect bone and tooth formation. Although abnormalities of the teeth can be differentiated simplistically on the basis of tooth color, shape, number, position, and eruption, this method of categorization has its pitfalls, and frequently overlaps exist. Understanding of the genetic and environmental basis of numerous conditions (e.g., congenitally missing teeth) is increasing, but is often rudimentary.

The pediatrician should know that different tooth types undergo formation at different times and that crown formation starts at different times for the permanent teeth compared with the primary teeth. The crowns of primary teeth and the first permanent molars begin formation *in utero*, whereas the other permanent teeth usually mineralize after birth. Knowledge of the effects of genetic disorders such as ectodermal dysplasia (see Fig. 127.4), drugs such as tetracycline (Fig. 127.7), and treatments such as head and neck irradiation (Fig. 127.8) on tooth formation allows the clinician to counsel parents about their children's future dental development and to assess the risks and benefits of treatment. More than 200 syndromes are associated with dental or head and neck anomalies. However, only clefts will be discussed because of the lack of space.

Clefts

Incomplete or total lack of fusion of the various facial processes during the fifth to seventh week *in utero* can result in various forms of clefting. Clefting in the maxillary area is far more common than clefting of the lower lip or jaw and can involve

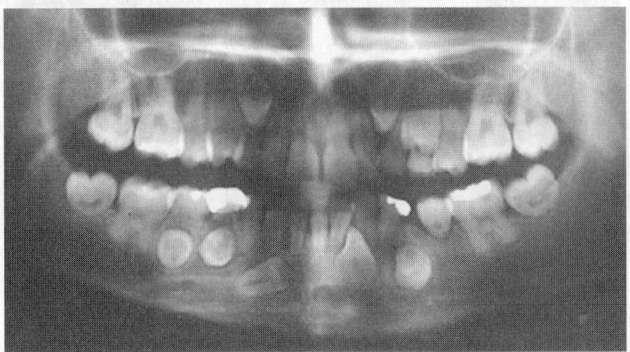

FIGURE 127.8. Panoramic radiograph showing lack of permanent mandibular tooth root formation and tooth impaction caused by two bouts of radiation treatment before the age of 5 years.

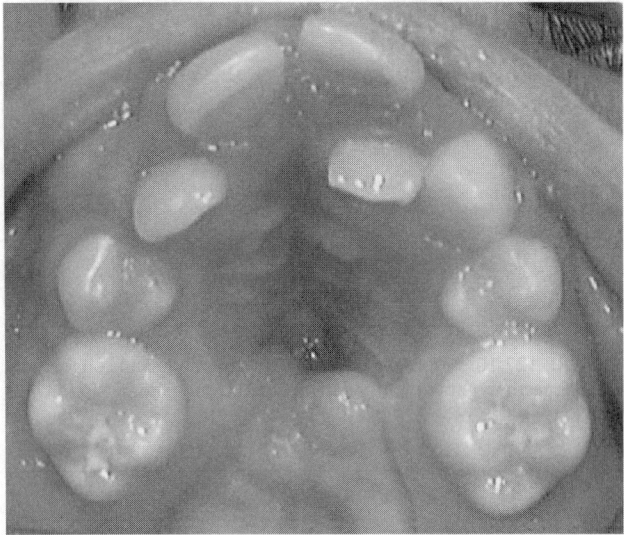

FIGURE 127.9. Maxillary arch of patient with a partially repaired isolated cleft palate showing malocclusion with severe crowding, congenitally missing teeth, and malalignment.

different structures. Approximately 1 in every 600 newborn babies worldwide is affected by cleft lip with or without cleft palate (CL/P) or isolated cleft palate (CP). The prevalence of CL/P reportedly varies depending on the ethnic group and the manner of reporting.

The severity of the cleft and its associated oral problems varies from an incomplete cleft lip with only a small notching in the vermillion border to a complete cleft lip, either unilateral or bilateral, that extends through the alveolar process affecting the dentition and the dental arch form. Isolated CP can involve only the uvula or extend through the hard palate (Fig. 127.9).

Clefting can be manifested as part of a syndrome caused by single mutant genes or by chromosomal defects such as trisomy 13. Environmental factors such as maternal anticonvulsant drugs and smoking are implicated in some cases.

The patient with clefts may have numerous problems in addition to the cosmetic appearance. Palatal clefting may affect an infant's ability to feed because of interference with sucking. Palatal clefting also affects the child's speech.

Abnormalities in tooth number, structure, and appearance frequently occur in the area of clefting. Missing teeth, supernumerary teeth, and malformed teeth are common in the areas surrounding the cleft. Supernumerary and malformed teeth will need to be evaluated for extraction or restoration. Radiographs are necessary to determine the status of these teeth prior to alveolar grafting. The alveolar bone in the area of the cleft is often inadequate to support adjacent erupting teeth.

Dental malocclusions are common and often severe (Fig. 127.10), requiring orthodontic correction of crossbites prior to alveolar grafting. When the growth of the maxilla and the mandible is not coordinate as with Pierre Robin anomalad, orthodontic treatment can be required at least three times (correction of crossbites prior to alveolar grafting, when all the permanent teeth erupt, and when growth is completed and orthognathic surgery is required to correct the jaw relations).

Surgical repair of the cleft lip and palate with orthodontic treatment can produce reasonable aesthetics and function. However, these patients have multiple problems and should be treated by a team including a surgeon, speech pathologist, orthodontist, and pediatric dentist as well as others for maximum benefit. Timing of various procedures and the skill of the specialists is important in producing the best aesthetic and functional result with the least financial and time commitments.

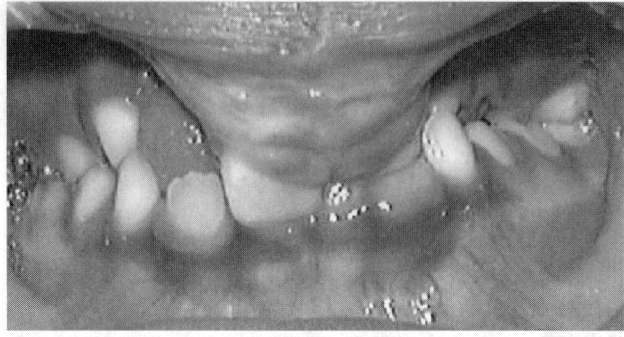

FIGURE 127.10. Severe malocclusion with crossbite and congenitally missing teeth in patient with bilateral cleft lip and palate.

Cysts

Newborn infants may exhibit several types of dental cysts related to vestigial embryonic structures. The literature is confusing concerning some of their names and embryonic sources. Two cysts, Epstein pearls and Bohn nodules, occur in approximately 80% of newborns. Epstein pearls are white-yellow cysts occurring along the median palatal raphes or at the junction of the hard and soft palates. They result from remnants of epithelial tissue entrapped during palatal fusion.

Bohn nodules are white-yellow cysts occurring along the lateral aspects of the alveolar ridges and along the periphery of the palate. They may develop from heterotrophic salivary gland tissue or from remnants of the dental lamina. No treatment is necessary.

Dental lamina cysts, named after their potential source, are fluid-filled cystic formations found on the crest of the alveolar ridges. In most cases, they are asymptomatic and regress spontaneously; however, if they interfere with eating, surgical intervention may be indicated.

Neonatal alveolar lymphangiomas are fluid-filled lesions occurring on the lingual alveolar process in the molar region of the mandible. Spontaneous regression is observed in some cases, but the progression of these lesions is unknown.

Tumors

Congenital epulis, which consists of granular cells, most often is seen at birth in the anterior maxillary region. The epulis usually is pedunculated and varies from a few millimeters to several centimeters in diameter. Simple excision is the treatment of choice, and recurrence is rare. The origin of this tumor is unknown.

The neuroectodermal tumor of infancy is most often found in infants younger than 6 months. Usually occurring in the maxilla, it is a smooth-surfaced, rapidly expanding lesion of the alveolus that may or may not be pigmented. Radiographs of the lesion show a radiolucency with displaced primary teeth. The treatment of choice is simple surgical excision. Recurrence has been reported.

Tongue and Stoma Anomalies

Microglossia, a rare anomaly, is manifested as a small or vestigial tongue and is most frequently associated with defects involving the limbs and digit reductions. Deformities of the arch and mandible are usually present and require correction. Speech is relatively unaffected.

Macroglossia, which is also rare, is enlargement of the tongue resulting from lymphangiomas or muscle hypertrophy and occurs in several syndromes.

Ankyloglossia is abnormal restriction of the tongue caused by a tight lingual frenum. Surgical release is indicated if the gingival tissue is affected or if speech problems exist. However, speech problems should first be evaluated by a speech pathologist. Most children adapt well to ankyloglossia and require no surgery. Reports exist of ankyloglossia associated with deviation of the epiglottis and larynx. These patients can develop dyspnea and other respiratory problems that are minimized with correction of the ankyloglossia and positions of the epiglottis and larynx. Other reports of ankyloglossia in the newborn relate to breast-feeding problems. Lactating mothers may develop sores on their nipples and areolas because the erupting teeth traumatize the tissues.

A cleft tongue may result from incomplete fusion of the lateral embryologic swellings. A bifid tongue results from complete lack of fusion of the lateral embryologic swellings.

Microstomia, a small mouth opening, is a rare disorder associated with various syndromes, such as whistling face syndrome. Aesthetics, normal oral hygiene, and normal ambulatory dental care can be compromised by the restrictive oral opening.

Tooth Anomalies

Shape

Enamel hypoplasia, which can range from pits or furrows in the enamel surface to complete absence of enamel, results from disturbances in tooth formation or mineralization. Hypoplastic teeth can be extremely unaesthetic, sensitive to thermal changes, and prone to caries and abrasion. Morbidity can be as high as with trichodentoosseous syndrome, in which many patients develop multiple abscesses and become edentulous before they reach 20 years of age.

The etiology of hypoplasia can be genetic or environmental. Hereditary enamel defects frequently affect all the teeth. The extent of hypoplasia caused by an environmental factor depends on the length of time the insult was present, the systemic versus local nature of the insult, and the toxicity of the insult. Environmental factors such as excess fluoride supplementation, vitamin D deficiency, tetracycline therapy (see Fig. 127.7), hypothyroidism, head and neck radiation (see Fig. 127.8), maternal infections while *in utero*, measles, other infections, and trauma (Fig. 127.11) can cause disturbances in enamel

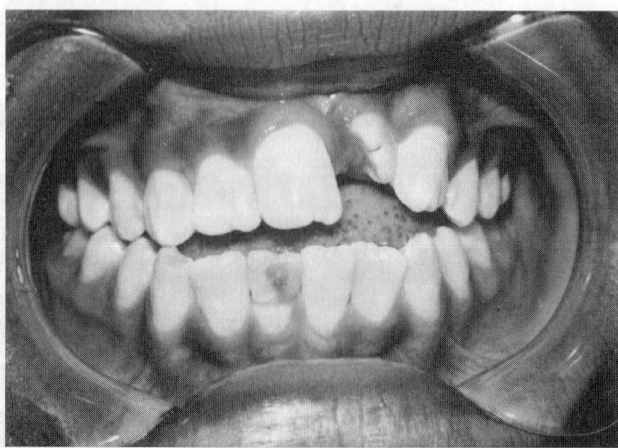

FIGURE 127.11. Hypoplastic and discolored lower front permanent tooth resulting from trauma to primary incisors. Trauma also affected the eruption of the upper front teeth.

formation that permanently affect the structure of the teeth. As a result of the systemic nature of these disturbances, all teeth in which enamel was forming at the time of the insult may show permanent deformation in the particular segment of forming enamel or the root.

Localized hypoplasia affecting one or a few adjacent teeth is caused by factors such as trauma or a dental abscess. Generalized hypoplasia is obvious in certain hereditary disorders such as amelogenesis imperfecta or trichodentoosseous syndrome. Congenital syphilis is manifested by permanent incisors that are shaped like screwdrivers and by first permanent molars that have irregular occlusal surfaces with multiple enamel blebs (i.e., mulberry molars). Patients showing generalized enamel hypoplasia may also have other anomalies present and should be referred for diagnostic tests and possible genetic counseling.

Enamel hypoplasia, besides being unaesthetic, can contribute to dental sensitivity, caries, and increased wear of the teeth. Restorative procedures such as composite resins or crowns may be indicated.

Number

Congenital abnormalities such as absence or overproduction of teeth usually occur because of problems with initiation or proliferation. These abnormalities cause problems with function, dental arch spacing, and aesthetics.

Single supernumerary teeth occur most frequently in the area of the maxillary incisors; multiple supernumerary teeth are associated with various genetic syndromes, such as cleidocranial dysplasia and Gardner syndrome. These supernumeraries can block the eruption of normal teeth.

The congenital absence of one or several teeth is called hypodontia (see Fig. 127.4), whereas absence of all teeth is termed anodontia. Missing lateral incisors and premolars occur frequently in the general population and have been associated with mutations of the *PAX9* and *MXS1* genes. Missing teeth tend to run in families due to their genetic cause. Anodontia can be related to generalized defects of tissue involved in tooth formation, such as ectodermal dysplasia. Patients with ectodermal dysplasia may display hypodontia or anodontia.

Size

Abnormalities of tooth size, shape, or number may occur separately or together. Many supernumerary teeth have abnormal shapes or sizes. Similarly, the teeth of patients with hypodontia may be abnormally shaped. Patients with such abnormalities may benefit from orthodontics or restorative dentistry.

Microdontia, smaller than normal tooth size, may be confined to a single tooth or may be generalized. Microdontia of the maxillary laterals is a frequent form of microdontia that appears to be genetically controlled and has been associated with impacted canine teeth. The contralateral incisor is often congenitally missing. Generalized microdontia, although rare, is exhibited in some cases of pituitary dwarfism.

Macrodontia, larger than normal tooth size, may be localized or generalized. Patients with hemifacial hypertrophy exhibit unilateral macrodontia; persons with pituitary gigantism may have generalized macrodontia.

Color

Color is an important diagnostic indicator of tooth anomalies (Table 127.2). Bluish brown or opalescent teeth that exhibit extreme wear and fractures are usually caused by an autosomal dominant defect in dentin formation called *dentinogenesis imperfecta*. In this condition, dentin formation continues after eruption, obliterating the dental pulp and causing the unusual color changes. This abnormality can occur concurrently with

TABLE 127.2

ETIOLOGY OF COMMON TOOTH DISCOLORATIONS

Color	Cause
Generalized	
Bluish brown	Dentinogenesis imperfecta
Yellow	Amelogenesis imperfecta; tetracycline ingestion
Reddish brown	Porphyria; fluorosis
Blue/bluish green	Rh incompatibility
Brown	Tetracycline ingestion
Gray	Tetracycline ingestion
Localized	
Yellow	Trauma; chromogenic bacteria; caries
Gray	Trauma
Black/blackish brown	Trauma; liquid iron supplements; tobacco; tea or other foods; chromogenic bacteria; caries
Pink	Internal resorption

osteogenesis imperfecta, a group of collagen disorders associated with bone fragility.

A generalized yellow color can indicate a form of amelogenesis imperfecta, in which the enamel is defective. This disorder is hereditary and two types are associated with abnormal facial forms.

In addition to causing enamel hypoplasia, tetracycline administration while teeth are forming can cause an unaesthetic generalized or linear pattern of yellow or brown, which may subsequently change to gray as a result of oxidation by sunlight (see Fig. 127.7). The severity of discoloration varies with the type of tetracycline, dosage, and timing of administration during tooth formation. Doxycycline appears to cause little or no discoloration; oxytetracycline causes a light yellow color; and chlortetracycline, demethylchlortetracycline, and tetracycline cause stronger yellow or gray-brown discolorations.

Generalized reddish brown teeth are associated with porphyria. Teeth with a generalized blue or bluish green tinge are associated with Rh incompatibility, in which hemosiderin is incorporated into the dentin. Symmetric reddish brown discoloration of teeth superimposed onto white hypocalcified or hypoplastic areas is associated with moderate to severe fluorosis. A history of greater than optimal fluoride concentration in the water supply or improper fluoride supplementation dosage is necessary to substantiate the diagnosis.

Color localized to one or two teeth usually indicates trauma (e.g., yellow, gray, or black) or internal resorption (e.g., pink). Green, gold, or black generalized to the gingival borders of the tooth is usually caused by accumulations of chromogenic bacteria on the teeth or staining from liquid iron supplements, coffee, tea, or chewing tobacco.

Eruption

The time of tooth eruption is highly variable between and within populations, making it difficult to diagnose some eruption problems until they are blatant. Generalized delayed eruption is associated with hormonal abnormalities (e.g., hypothyroidism, hypopituitarism) and syndromes (e.g., Gardner syndrome, Down syndrome, progeria). Delayed eruption that is more localized is associated with former trauma or impacted teeth.

Premature eruption of primary teeth occurs in the United States in approximately 1 in 2,000 to 3,500 live births. Teeth present at birth are called *natal teeth*; teeth that erupt within 30 days after birth are called *neonatal teeth* (Fig. 127.12). Natal

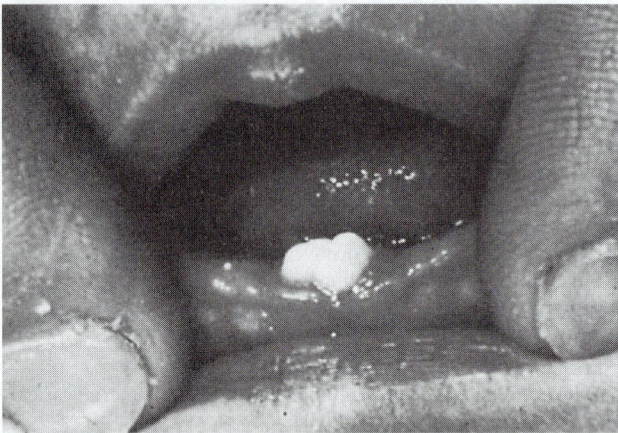

FIGURE 127.12. Neonatal teeth. (Courtesy of Dr. Mark Wagner, University of Maryland Dental School.)

and neonatal teeth are usually part of the normal complement of primary teeth and may result from vertical displacement of the tooth follicle. In approximately 15% of reported cases, a family history of premature eruption exists, which may be associated with endocrine problems. Neonatal teeth erupt most frequently in the area of the mandibular central incisor. The crowns may appear well formed or yellow with an irregular surface. Although the gingival growth may eventually obscure them, the enamel portions that are clinically obvious do not continue to develop and remain hypoplastic. Crown and root formation is incomplete, and the teeth are frequently mobile, making aspiration of tooth shells a risk. Abrasion against these teeth can produce lesions called *Riga-Fede disease* on the tongue or the opposing ridge. Breast-feeding may produce maternal discomfort. Extraction is recommended if these teeth are excessively mobile or cause lesions; otherwise, they should be allowed to remain. Generalized premature eruption of teeth can be associated with hyperthyroidism and precocious puberty.

Premature exfoliation of teeth can be attributed to disorders such as periodontitis, acrodynia, Papillon-Lèfevre syndrome, and Ehlers-Danlos syndrome. Localized problems of eruption (i.e., eruption or exfoliation) may be caused by dental caries, localized periodontitis, trauma, cysts, and supernumerary teeth.

If problems with eruption are identified, the patients should be referred for a dental examination.

ORAL LESIONS AND INFECTIONS

Soft or hard tissue lesions occurring in the areas of the face, neck, or mouth (Table 127.3) may be localized or may be manifestations of systemic disease. The physician should document the history, locality, lymph node involvement, number, texture, size, color, and pain or tenderness. Associative factors such as edentulous areas, caries, other lesions, and systemic diseases should be assessed to determine the potential source as localized or systemic.

Pigmented Lesions

Pigmentation or melanotic perioral or intraoral lesions in the mouth can occur for quite a few reasons. Some are relatively benign, whereas others can indicate acute or chronic diseases or disorders that can be life-threatening. A few of the more common lesions are discussed. For example, oral freckles frequently occur on the lips of children exposed to sunlight. These

---

TABLE 127.3

ORAL LESIONS

Pigmented Lesions	Raised Lesions	Swellings
Oral freckles	Papilloma	Eruption cyst
Peutz-Jeghers syndrome	Pyogenic granuloma	Eruption hematoma
Blue nevus	Fibroma	Dentigerous cyst
Vascular lesions	Ulcers	Primordial cyst
Hemangioma	Aphthae	Odontogenic keratocyst
Telangiectasia	Periadenitis mucosa	Branchial cleft cyst
Angiomas	Necrotica recurrens	Thyroglossal duct cyst
Petechiae	Behçet syndrome	Periapical abscess
Lymphangioma	Trauma	Fibrosarcoma
	Mucositis	Ewing sarcoma
		Eosinophilia granuloma
		Fibrous dysplasia
		Cherubism
		Central giant cell granuloma
		Mucocele
		Ranula
		Torus

are usually considered benign unless they are seen intraorally, in which case they should be biopsied.

Multiple pigmented lesions seen in the oral cavity and on the lips, face, and possibly the fingers suggest Peutz-Jeghers syndrome. Dominantly inherited, this syndrome is characterized by intestinal polyps, which may cause abdominal cramping and can lead to gastrointestinal carcinoma. Although skin spots fade with age, oral pigmentation remains throughout life.

A blue nevus may occur at any intraoral site but is most commonly found in the anterior region. It is a characteristic blue and is usually flat or dome shaped in children. It should be biopsied because of a tendency for malignant transformation.

Racial or ethnic pigmentation (see Fig. 127.1) is usually generalized over the gingiva and is considered normal. Wide variation in intensity of color occurs. Heavy metal poisoning can also cause melanotic areas in the gingiva that can look similar to ethnic pigmentation.

Amalgam tattoos or a bluish black discoloration can be present in the tissue around teeth if the amalgam was not cleaned from the tissue after a restoration was placed. Sometimes, the amalgam-impregnated tissue can be identified and the diagnosis confirmed by taking a radiograph.

Drug therapy, melanoma, and Kaposi sarcoma should be considered in the differential diagnosis.

Vascular Lesions

The most common intraoral locations of hemangiomas or blood vessel proliferations are the lips, tongue, and buccal mucosa. If removal is indicated, cryosurgery may be the method of choice.

Oral vascular lesions are seen in various systemic disorders such as hereditary hemorrhagic telangiectasia. Telangiectasias, multiple capillary and venous dilation of the skin and mucous membranes, vary in size from pinpoint to nodular, and in color from bright red to purple. Oral telangiectasias are most frequently seen on the lips and tongue, but they also occur on the palate, gingiva, buccal mucosa, and mucocutaneous junctions.

Bleeding occurs from oral lesions in approximately 20% of patients.

Angiomatous lesions (e.g., port wine nevi) may occur on the gingiva and buccal mucosa of patients with encephalotrigeminal angiomatosis. Petechiae may occur as a result of continual trauma, such as digit sucking or sexual abuse, or as a result of streptococcal infection. Lymphangiomas can occur anywhere in the mouth. Macroglossia may result from large lymphangiomas on the tongue. Small lesions can be removed surgically; large asymptomatic lesions are usually not removed.

Arteriovenous malformations also occur in the head–neck region and can be bilateral. They are considered congenital and appear to increase in size around the time of puberty when they are frequently diagnosed. Abnormal bluish areas around mobile teeth can be indications of such a lesion. They become apparent when either trauma occurs, baby teeth are exfoliated, or permanent teeth are extracted. An unexpected event can result in mortality, significant scarring, or loss of structure.

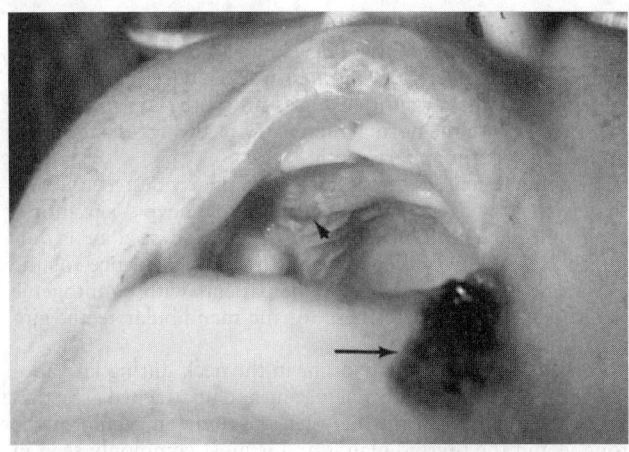

FIGURE 127.13. Extraoral lesion (*arrow*) and oral mucositis (*arrowhead*) in a patient receiving chemotherapy.

Raised Lesions

Papillomas are benign neoplasms that are usually pedunculated and have finger-like projections. They occur anywhere on the soft tissue of the oral cavity and range in size from a few millimeters to more than 1 cm in diameter. The treatment of choice is simple excision at the base of the lesion.

Pyogenic granulomas usually occur on the gingiva in response to an irritant (e.g., calculus, minor trauma). They are especially common in pregnant women. They are usually red, elevated, and ulcerated in their early stages; later they may become fibrotic, appearing similar to fibromas. The treatment of choice is removal of the irritant, simple excision of the lesion, and good oral hygiene.

Fibromas are sessile, smooth lesions up to 1 cm in diameter. They may become ulcerated or ossified. The treatment of choice is simple surgical excision.

Ulcers

Aphthous ulcers are painful, yellowish depressions of necrotic tissue surrounded by erythema. Usually fewer than six lesions occur during an outbreak. These ulcers range in size from a few millimeters to 1 cm in diameter and occur only on buccal or labial mucosa and other unbound oral tissue. Their onset can occur in childhood, and each recurrence can last as long as 14 days. Recurrent aphthous ulcers appear to be familial. Some investigators suggest that the causative factor is *Streptococcus sanguis*. Others suggest autoimmune factors; deficiencies of vitamin B_{12}, folate, iron, and zinc; and gluten sensitivity. Cases of aphthous ulcers in which scarring occurs are called *periadenitis mucosa necrotica recurrens*. These lesions can persist for as long as 6 weeks and occur so frequently that the patient is rarely free of aphthae. Treatment for aphthous ulcers usually is empiric; however, for children older than 8 years, a tetracycline mouth rinse (125 mg/5 mL) used four times daily produces good results and prevents secondary infection. Corticosteroid treatment can be helpful and should be considered in severe debilitating cases of major recurrent aphthous ulcers.

Patients with ulcers similar to aphthae who have skin, ocular, and genital lesions may have Behçet syndrome, which is discussed in Chapter 434 (Rheumatic Diseases of Childhood).

Traumatic ulcers, which occur relatively frequently, are associated with a history of trauma, such as tooth brushing, or with an obvious associative factor, such as a fractured tooth. Saltwater rinses or correction of the causative factor usually is adequate treatment. Viscous benzocaine should be used with caution because of the potential for seizures in very young patients who use it excessively.

Oral mucositis (Fig. 127.13) is one of the major oral complications of cancer treatment and can be caused by head or neck irradiation or by chemotherapy. The mucositis produced by head or neck irradiation is painful at rest and particularly when eating hard or spicy foods. Chemotherapeutic treatment of leukemia produces stomatitis more frequently than chemotherapy for solid tumors because of the higher doses of drugs and greater immunologic suppression. Interference with DNA, RNA, or protein synthesis by the drugs results in a thinning of the oral mucosa, which may ulcerate and allow life-threatening bacterial, fungal, or viral infections to occur. Because indigenous oral florae are associated with many of these infections, cancer patients must establish and maintain good oral hygiene.

Before cancer treatment, all patients must have dental examinations to identify and remove or minimize potential sources of irritation and infection, including orthodontic and prosthetic appliances, broken restorations, and broken or carious teeth.

A high proportion of mucositis in immunologically suppressed patients is associated with herpes simplex virus (HSV). Diagnosis based on clinical impressions is inadequate and must be based on viral cultures or immunologic test results. Prophylactic regimens are suggested if a patient is seropositive for HSV. Mouthwashes such as chlorhexidine and allopurinol may reduce the severity of mucositis.

Swellings

A swelling on the gingiva of a young patient with an edentulous area where teeth are expected to erupt may be an eruption cyst. Occasionally, blood fills the cystic area, making the swelling appear bluish like a hematoma; this kind of cyst is called an *eruption hematoma*. Observation alone usually is the treatment of choice. However, simple incision into the crestal portion of the swelling may be necessary. This can cause bleeding, but it can be controlled easily.

The oral epithelial invaginations or ducts of epithelial processes (e.g., palatine processes) are possible areas of cyst formation during fetal development. Whether all oral areas of embryonic fusion are involved in cyst formation is an unanswered question.

Hard tissue swelling in the area of an unerupted tooth may be caused by any number of cysts. For example, dentigerous cysts, which are associated with developing teeth, most commonly occur around third molars, maxillary canines, and mandibular premolars. The epithelial lining of a dentigerous cyst has a high probability of developing metaplasms and neoplasms. Alternatively, a primordial cyst can develop from a degenerated enamel organ that forms no tooth. Cyst formation in a person with the normal number of teeth suggests degeneration of a supernumerary tooth.

An odontogenic keratocyst is a particularly destructive cyst that is sometimes associated with multiple nevoid carcinoma syndrome. The peak incidence for the keratocyst alone is during the second decade of life, and the peak incidence for the syndrome is the first decade. Some patients with odontogenic keratocysts exhibit paresthesia of the mandibular teeth, gingiva, and lips.

Brachial cleft cysts may occur in the neck during late adolescence. They are usually fluctuating and unattached. The thyroglossal tract cyst forms between the foramen cecum of the tongue and the thyroid glands and is most commonly seen in young people. Its growth is usually slow and asymptomatic unless it is near the tongue.

Swelling and fever can occur with dental abscessing of teeth caused by dental caries, trauma, or periodontal disease. Usually, a carious or fractured tooth is associated with this lesion. The swelling usually is rapid and may have been preceded by a parulis (i.e., gum boil) on the gingiva. The teeth may be mobile, and the child may report spontaneous or elicited pain. However, many young children may not report pain. The abscess can develop into cellulitis with the infection threatening either the airway (Fig. 127.14) or the eye. The gingiva of some children with periodontal disease may actually flap away from the roots if severe bone loss exists.

A fibrosarcoma may cause swelling and pain. Hard or soft tissue swelling with pain, facial neuralgia, and lip paresthesia is manifested in Ewing sarcoma. Patients with eosinophilia granuloma, which also is manifested by oral swelling, usually have an inflamed gingiva, mobile teeth, and pain. Some of these patients may exhibit bone lesions, exophthalmos, and diabetes insipidus.

Cherubism is a bilateral hard tissue swelling affecting the maxilla and mandible. This fibroosseous condition, inherited as an autosomal dominant trait, becomes clinically apparent when the child is 2 to 4 years of age. Growth usually becomes static by 10 years of age. Tooth displacement and impaction are frequently observed. A radiograph of the jaw reveals large multilocular lesions.

Fibrous dysplasia of the bone may occur in the jaws in monostotic form, in polyostotic form, or as a part of Albright syndrome. The rate of expansion of a monostotic form, involving a single bone, is surprisingly rapid during the active growth phase. This form usually completes its active growth phase during childhood. The polyostotic form is associated with lesions in multiple bones. If endocrine disturbances are producing precocious growth, sexual development, and large café au lait spots, the clinician should consider the diagnosis of Albright syndrome. Jaw lesions are hard, nonpainful, slowly enlarging masses that can interfere with tooth eruption and usually produce facial asymmetry. Nasal obstruction and proptosis or exophthalmos can result if the lesions occur in the maxilla. Radiographically, lesions can look like ground glass.

Central giant cell granulomas occur in children. These lesions rarely involve pain, although they may aggressively expand and erode through the cortical bones of the mandible or maxilla.

Mucoceles (i.e., mucous retention cysts) appear primarily on the lower lip but may occur elsewhere in the mouth. Superficial mucoceles are usually translucent and round, and deeper ones appear blue and manifest swelling, particularly if traumatized frequently. Mucoceles are generally painful and tend to recur even when ruptured. The treatment of choice is simple excision.

Ranulas are large mucoceles that occur under the tongue. They usually are unilateral, painless, and soft and can appear bluish. Continued growth of a ranula can cause respiratory distress. The treatment of choice is marsupialization. Recurrence requires excision of the lesion and the adjacent salivary gland.

Tori are benign, slowly expanding bone growths that frequently occur at the midline of the palate or along the lingual aspects of the mandible. Large growths may be traumatized during eating. They are rarely a problem in childhood.

Candidiasis

Oral candidiasis (i.e., thrush) can appear anywhere on the soft tissue of the mouth. It ranges in appearance from mild erythema to small, white plaques to an extensively white mouth. The plaques are easily removed, leaving a raw-appearing surface. Severe ulcerative or necrotic lesions indicate invasive infection of underlying tissues and are therefore associated with a poorer prognosis than are superficial lesions. Newborns can be infected during passage through the vagina of a mother with a *Candida albicans* infection, and infants can contract it from mothers with breast infections. Persons with angular cheilosis of the commissures of the mouth, which appears as a symmetric cracking of tissue, are susceptible to *Candida* infection. Immunosuppressed patients and patients on long-term, broad-spectrum antibiotics and oral contraceptives are susceptible to infection. Nystatin is used successfully in the treatment of infants. For older patients, removal of the primary problem in addition to nystatin rinses is necessary. Clotrimazole troches are recommended.

Herpetic Gingivostomatitis

Herpetic gingivostomatitis is an HSV infection in which the primary attack is characterized by fever, malaise, dysphagia, sialorrhea, pain, and lymphadenitis. Vesicles may occur on the lips and throughout the entire mouth. They usually rupture within 24 hours, leaving shallow yellow ulcers surrounded by

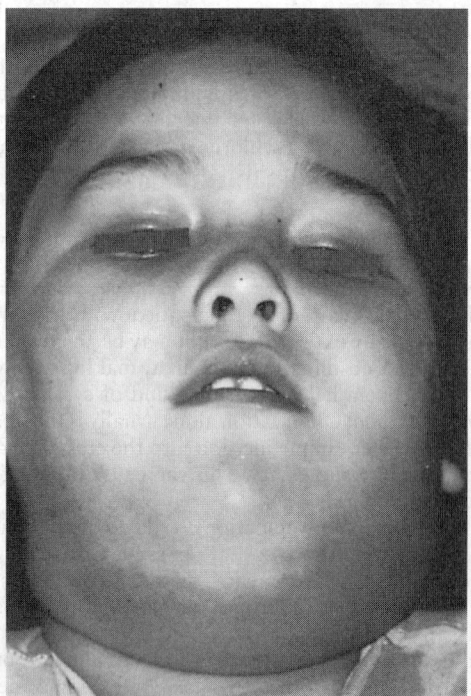

FIGURE 127.14. Cellulitis resulting from a dental abscess.

erythema. Onset is usually in early childhood. Recurrent infections produce small vesicles or ulcers surrounded by erythema on tissue bound to bone (e.g., attached gingiva and palate). Exfoliative cytology within 4 days of lesion formation is diagnostic. Treatment is primarily palliative and includes administration of nonacidic fluids. Prevention of dehydration is important. Lesions heal within 7 to 14 days.

Geographic tongue represents a benign reduction in the filiform papillae in patches that may migrate periodically. The cause is unknown, but psychosomatic factors have been suggested.

The effects of teething on infants are questionable. Although disturbances such as diarrhea, drooling, and fever have been reported during teething, the cause–effect association is questionable. The 2-year period during which the primary teeth are erupting happens to be a period during which a child's immunologic capabilities are relatively low and infections are frequent. Hard or cold teething rings have variable effects, depending on the child. Acetaminophen liquid can help relieve an irritable child.

Dental Caries

Despite advances in prevention, dental caries remains endemic in the United States. The average child between the age of 6 and 14 years has approximately three decayed, missing, or filled primary or permanent teeth as a result of dental caries. Approximately 80% of children in the United States by 17 years of age have one or more permanent teeth with dental caries. Approximately 25% of children aged 5 to 17 years have most of the dental caries.

The number of caries increases with age as more permanent teeth erupt into the mouth. The rate of attack on permanent teeth appears to be the greatest during adolescence, when the posterior teeth with the most grooves and fissures erupt. In addition, the interproximal smooth surfaces of the teeth contact each other for long periods, making them more susceptible to caries.

Dental Caries Development

Dental caries result over time from a multifactorial interaction among a susceptible tooth (i.e., host), microorganisms, and a cariogenic diet. A tenacious deposit of plaque, which is composed of salivary glycoproteins, bacteria, and bacterial products, forms on the teeth. Cariogenic bacteria metabolize dietary carbohydrates, particularly sucrose, and produce acids, such as lactic acid, which demineralize enamel and dentin, producing dental caries (cavities). *Streptococcus mutans* and lactobacilli are the major bacteria in the caries process. The earlier the colonization of *S. mutans* occurs in an infant's mouth, the greater is the child's risk of caries. Studies have shown that *S. mutans* has colonized 30% of babies 3 months of age. Transmission is often from the mother, which means that mothers with apparent dental caries and neglect should be referred for treatment as soon as possible. Dental anatomy such as grooves and fissures, exposure to fluoride ions, and the amount of salivary flow influence the susceptibility of teeth to dental caries.

Frequent contacts with food, particularly food that is sticky and contains sucrose, expose teeth to prolonged decreases in the pH of the plaque and potentially long demineralization times. Physical or chemical disruption of plaque, such as occurs with tooth brushing, flossing, or use of chlorhexidine rinses or gels, minimizes and can actually reverse the colonization of the cariogenic bacteria and decrease plaque pH. Although numerous methods are used to detect caries for research projects and clinically, a clinician should be able to visualize white-spot lesions (see Fig. 127.2) on the flat surfaces of the teeth as well

as cavitations on the exposed surfaces of the teeth. However, incipient caries or even large cavitated lesions may exist on interproximal surfaces or other surfaces that cannot be seen. In fact, large carious lesions may exist below the enamel surface with only a visibly small opening present in the enamel surface.

Although caries may attack any surface of a tooth, the most susceptible surfaces appear to be those with pits or grooves. These areas may become carious within 6 to 12 months after eruption of the tooth. The smooth (i.e., interproximal, buccal, lingual) surfaces of the teeth usually develop caries more slowly than the pits and fissures. A patient is considered to have rampant caries if the caries occur in typically less susceptible areas, such as between the lower incisors and on the lingual surfaces of the mandibular molars. Although root caries are common in adults, developing as the periodontium recedes apically from the crown of the tooth, they may occur in children, in whom they may appear as orange-brown softenings below the cervical bulge of the teeth. A child who exhibits root caries should be evaluated for periodontal disease or other systemic complications that allow the periodontium to recede.

The dynamic processes of demineralization and remineralization are continuously occurring on the enamel surfaces. If the rate of demineralization is slower or the same as the rate of remineralization, clinically apparent caries do not form. However, an area of remineralized byproducts of demineralization can form what clinically appears to be an intact surface but microscopically is porous. Approximately 5% of the mineral in this surface zone has been lost. As a result of the mineral loss below the surface, the surface reflects light differently and appears to be whiter than the surrounding noncarious areas. When enough mineral is lost that the surface cannot be supported, the surface cavitates and shows visually obvious caries.

Dental caries still in the white-spot stages with clinically intact surfaces can remain static or be remineralized by an increase in the factors (e.g., fluoride) that contribute to remineralization. This can be accomplished to varying degrees, depending on the extent of compliance by the patient, but it usually requires a multifactorial approach. Dental caries are best controlled through increased frequency of exposure to topical fluoride through fluoridated water, toothpastes, rinses, or gels; diet, with the emphasis on decreasing the number of sweets contacting the teeth throughout the day; and increased oral hygiene. Caries on the buccal and lingual surfaces are more easily controlled in this manner than interproximal caries or caries in the pits and fissures, because the former are detected visually at early, surface stages, when they are most accessible to fluorides and plaque removal. Caries in the pits and fissures are less accessible to such treatment and therefore not as easily controlled.

Dental caries in pits and fissures can be minimized by the placement of sealant materials that adhere to the surface of the enamel, by the creation of micropores in the enamel surface into which tags of sealant physically lock, or by chelation. These materials are most effective when introduced as soon as possible after eruption of a susceptible tooth. Sealants stop incipient caries and significantly reduce the number of vital bacteria in a groove. The effectiveness of sealants is related to their retention, which depends on patient cooperation during placement, saliva control, and the eruptive status of the tooth. A median reduction of 60% of caries can occur with school-based sealant programs. Alternatively, children with erupting teeth should be referred to dentists to have sealants placed.

In the case of carious lesions that have a broken surface, the tooth cannot be remineralized to the extent that the surface can be reformed. Although fluoride can allow remineralization of the outermost surfaces and slow demineralization processes interiorly, demineralization can continue into the pulp before it can be stopped, particularly if a cariogenic diet and poor oral hygiene are continued. Dental restoration is usually indicated to restore the surface and function of such a tooth, to prevent further deterioration of the tooth, to eliminate the foci of infection for caries or periodontal disease in the oral cavity, and to prevent loss of space within the dental arch. A child can be placed on a topical fluoride therapy to promote remineralization and inhibit demineralization throughout the mouth while dental restoration is completed.

Caries frequently progress through the enamel as wedge-shaped lesions that spread laterally at the dentinoenamel interface when they reach the dentin and undermine the enamel. By the time the enamel surface fractures under masticatory forces (e.g., chewing on ice), the lesion is usually large and has progressed as far as the pulp, requiring removal of the pulp or extraction of the tooth.

As caries progress toward the pulp, inflammation can cause the pulp to form more dentin, which acts as a barrier to the carious process. However, if demineralization is taking place faster than dentin formation, caries can proceed into the pulp, causing more inflammation. The edema that occurs within the closed pulp chamber can cause dental pain.

A necrotic tooth can drain through the carious coronal tissue, causing the patient no pain. If coronal drainage is not available, necrosis can extend beyond the pulp chambers of the tooth to the root apices of the anterior primary teeth or to the area between the roots of the primary molars, possibly affecting permanent tooth structure. Although the inflammation can localize around the tooth, it can cause bone expansion and pain. Fistulization through bone can occur, so that the tooth drains into the periodontal sulcus next to it or through the alveolus toward the tongue or the face. The alveolus can exhibit a fistula through the gingiva or mucosa or a parulis (i.e., gum boil) that is not open to drainage. A fistula in the soft tissue usually is not associated with dental pain. The parulis can be chronic or acute, depending on the amount of drainage from it. Radiographically, the abscess can be diagnosed as a widening of the periodontal membrane or as a radiolucency in the alveolar bone at the root apices or in the furcation of the primary molars.

Cellulitis (see Fig. 127.14) is the most serious consequence of infection spreading into the soft tissues. If the infection involves the submandibular, sublingual, and submental spaces, elevation of the tongue and floor of the mouth may obstruct the patient's airway. Trismus (i.e., inability to open the mouth) may occur. The child might not present with pain if the infection is in the primary dentition, even with cellulitis. High fever, malaise, and lethargy are frequently associated with acute dental infection. The patient might not eat properly as a result of pain on mastication or sensitivity to hot or cold.

Children exhibiting pain and swelling caused by a dental abscess should be referred immediately to a dentist for extraction or pulpal treatment to save the tooth. The patient should be placed on antibiotics for 7 to 10 days. The antibiotic of choice is penicillin; erythromycin is the second choice. Recalcitrant infections should be cultured for antibiotic sensitivity. Analgesics can be given for pain, but aspirin should be avoided in case tooth extraction is required.

Medically compromised patients who are placed at increased risk by dental infections include those with immunosuppression, sickle cell disease, heart disease, liver disease, kidney disease, diabetes mellitus, and leukemia. Patients in whom systemic risk is increased by dental treatment include those with hemophilia, heart defects, connective tissue disorders, and osteogenesis imperfecta; in these patients, local anesthetic injections and other dental manipulations might increase the risk of bleeding or cause tissue sloughing, which may compromise airways or increase the chances of infection, scarring, or bone fracture. Dental treatment is not contraindicated in these patients, but special precautions must be taken, including antibiotic coverage, availability of plasma substitutes, and coagulation tests.

It is critical that children who are beginning, who are currently receiving, or who have received chemotherapy, a bone marrow transplant, and/or radiation receive a dental examination and treatment as a part of both precancer and cancer treatment because of the high risk of septicemia due to oral infections. Multidisciplinary cooperation is required in the treatment of such patients.

Systemic Conditions Contributing to Dental Caries

Various systemic illnesses or conditions place children at increased risk for dental caries and, in some cases, can complicate dental treatment. A team approach to prevent caries and provide necessary dental treatment is required for total patient care. At the time of diagnosis, a dental consultation should be obtained, with recommendations reinforced at each clinic visit.

In patients with the recessive dystrophic form of epidermolysis bullosa, intraoral and circumoral bullae form at sites of pressure or trauma and result in severe and extensive scarring. Scarring can result in loss of oral vestibules, loss of mobility of the tongue, and microstomia. Tooth brushing can cause significant bullae formation, which contributes to scarring. The lack of oral hygiene, prolonged oral clearance, and soft cariogenic diets probably contribute to the high caries rate. Routine dental treatment is complicated by the microstomia and by the potential for significant bullae formation as a result of oral manipulation.

Chlorhexidine and fluoride rinses are recommended. However, the chlorhexidine rinse or gel might have to be applied with cotton-tip applicators to minimize the burning sensation that may result in poor compliance. Fluoride rinses that are unflavored and contain low concentrations of alcohol are accepted better for the same reasons.

Patients with mental retardation are at increased risk for dental caries if they do not receive routine and thorough oral hygiene and a relatively noncariogenic diet. Patients who ruminate can exhibit generalized decalcification of their teeth as a result of prolonged contact with acid from the stomach. Other patients can require frequent feedings, which contribute to frequent acid exposure from plaque on their teeth. Ideally, a dental program for these patients should involve routine oral hygiene carried out by a well-trained and motivated dental hygienist and a dental examination with preventive treatment at each routine checkup. In addition, the daily caregivers should be trained to provide oral hygiene care for the children. Training should include proper positioning of a child's head for access, visibility, stability, and comfort for the child and the care provider. Training should include various methods of obtaining access to the mouth of an uncooperative child. Modified toothbrushes and flossing implements can be helpful for children who can handle some aspects of their oral hygiene themselves.

In some patients with behavioral or muscle control problems, such as patients with spastic cerebral palsy or mental retardation, dental prostheses to replace extracted teeth may be contraindicated, and malocclusion may result. Placement of orthodontic appliances is discouraged in many of these patients because of the need to place, maintain, and adjust appliances on a relatively quiet individual. If a child has to be taken to general anesthesia to place orthodontic appliances, routine adjustments will be difficult without sedation or general anesthesia, and cleaning is extremely difficult. The cost-to-benefit ratio definitely contraindicates the placement of orthodontic appliances in these cases. The key to maintaining health in these patients is the prevention of dental diseases such as caries.

Dental treatment can sometimes be accomplished only with behavioral management or sedation techniques. Physical restraints may be required to prevent patients from hurting themselves or the clinicians. General anesthesia is required for some children who have extensive dental needs, severe behavioral problems, or medical problems.

Gastrointestinal reflux and bulimia may cause decalcification of teeth because of frequent acid exposure. Repeated intake of various forms of medication, such as aspirin and antibiotics, is associated with high caries rates in some children, possibly as a result of a high sucrose content in the medication in conjunction with poor salivary clearance. Because of the dental problems seen in children who go to bed with sugary fluids in baby bottles, parents should be told not to administer oral medications with a high sugar content to a child just before bedtime unless the teeth are cleaned after ingestion.

Salivary gland dysfunction caused by head and neck irradiation, disease, or drugs contributes significantly to caries risk. Decreased salivary flow rate prevents buffering of acids and oral clearance of sugar. Daily applications of a fluoride gel, scrupulous oral hygiene, and diet modifications to minimize the ingestion of cariogenic foods minimize the caries rate in children with diminished salivary flow.

Systemic Conditions Contributing to a Decrease in Caries

Children whose diets have been altered for systemic reasons (e.g., fructose intolerance, diabetes) to exclude cariogenic foods appear to have a lower caries rate than do other children their age.

Nursing Caries

Dental caries can be particularly destructive in children older than 1 year who continue to nurse (Fig. 127.15). Frequent contact with sweetened liquids from the bottle throughout the day and particularly during sleep, when the salivary flow rate is minimal, exposes the child to multiple and prolonged decreases in salivary pH. Because the salivary flow rate is minimal during sleep, a child who nurses just before or periodically during sleep is particularly susceptible to caries. Decalcification is rapid in the newly erupting and partially mineralized primary teeth, and pulpal involvement occurs rapidly because the primary tooth enamel is relatively thin.

Continued and frequent breast-feeding also is implicated as a causal factor in nursing caries. Mothers should be informed that nursing on demand past the age of 1 year can result in dental caries. Sweetened pacifiers are also sources of dental caries. The number of teeth and severity of caries involved in nursing caries probably depend on the eruption sequence of the primary teeth, the length of time nursing continues, the frequency of nursing throughout the day, the types of fluids

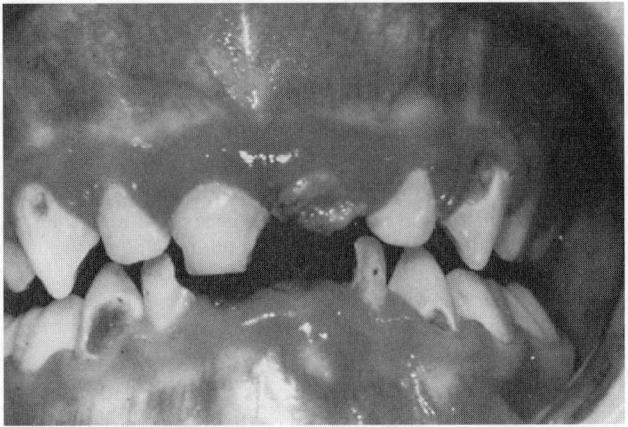

FIGURE 127.15. Nursing caries.

given in the bottle, and whether nursing occurs just before or periodically during sleep.

Nursing caries are first noticeable as a white-spot lesion, usually on the buccal or lingual side of the tooth. The white-spot lesion does not always to appear at the gingival border of the tooth, because primary teeth are continuing to erupt in the infant. Depending on the rate of demineralization, the lesion can cavitate and proceed to the pulp. If the rate of demineralization is rapid, the root of the tooth might not develop fully before the tooth abscesses. If this occurs, the tooth is usually extracted.

The maxillary incisors are most frequently and extensively involved, with the primary molars being the next most frequently and severely involved. The mandibular incisors are not as commonly involved, although they erupt at approximately the same time as the maxillary incisors. The position of the tongue during nursing and the saliva released from under the tongue appear to protect the mandibular incisors. Mandibular incisor involvement usually indicates frequent and probably continued nursing; in the case of patients who continue to nurse until 4 years of age, the destruction can be devastating.

In particularly advanced cases, extraction of primary incisors has been necessary at 14 months of age. Early extraction of primary incisors before eruption of the canines (at approximately 18 months) may result in loss of arch space and create future orthodontic problems; extraction of primary incisors at a later age usually does not compromise arch space.

Water is the only safe fluid in a baby bottle for children older than 1 year. Sugar water, commercial sodas, sweetened tea, fruit juices, fruit drinks, and milk contribute to nursing caries.

If nursing caries are identified, the parent should be informed of the cause and of the potential results of lack of treatment and should be referred to a dentist who treats young children. Parents should be told to completely discontinue bottle-feedings or, if necessary, to gradually dilute the contents with water until the child is taking only water in the bottle or discontinues use of the bottle completely. Although not all children who nurse for prolonged periods develop dental caries, it is currently not possible to determine which children will have problems.

A complete diet history should be obtained from the parents to determine whether the total diet is adequate. A child who is ingesting only the contents of the bottle might be malnourished. Extensive nutritional counseling should be performed. Other members of the family should be involved if they provide care for the child.

Although most children with nursing caries do well with simple ambulatory dental care, some require sedation or general anesthesia. The treatment options depend on the extent of disease, the extent of patient and parent cooperation, and the existence of compromising medical conditions.

Restorative procedures and tooth extraction for nursing caries are often carried out in same-day surgery units, although some patients might require overnight hospitalization because of medical problems. If the cost of same-day surgery or overnight hospital care is prohibitive for the parents, the procedures might be carried out in the dentist's office with sedation. Office treatment with sedation can be used in cases in which treatment is not extensive, the patient is amenable to ambulatory care, and parent cooperation is good.

Periodontal Diseases

Gingivitis

Gingivitis, the most common periodontal disease, is an inflammation of the gingival tissues usually caused by a bacterial infection. The amount of edema and the tendency for gingival bleeding increases with the severity of the gingivitis. The causative factor most commonly associated with gingivitis is poor oral hygiene, but other factors, such as mouth breathing, fractured or decayed teeth, and use of birth control pills, can contribute to an increased inflammatory response.

Bacterial colonization of the teeth and gingiva is normal. The pathogenicity of the organisms in the dental plaque is the key determinant in gingivitis. As gingivitis progresses, the bacterial population within dental plaque exhibits a characteristic shift from low to high numbers of organisms, from gram-positive cocci to rods and gram-negative anaerobes, filamentous organisms, and spirochetes. No conclusive evidence exists that gingivitis in children develops into periodontitis, a more progressive form of periodontal disease that involves loss of alveolar bone.

Calculus, which is calcified plaque, forms when plaque remains undisturbed on the teeth. This process is influenced by the ratio of calcium to phosphate in the saliva and by the pH of the saliva. Calculus can occur above or below the gingiva and is associated with varying degrees of gingivitis. Calculus is occasionally seen on the teeth of children with prepubertal periodontitis. Apparently heavy unilateral deposits of calculus may indicate that the child has pain on chewing as a result of a carious or periodontally involved tooth and therefore limits chewing to one side, allowing calculus formation on the other. Unilateral calculus deposits can indicate a unilateral salivary gland dysfunction or unilateral pain preventing chewing on that side.

Although an increased incidence of gingivitis has been associated with puberty, the relation between hormonal fluctuations and degree of gingivitis is unclear. Increased gingival metabolism of estrogen and increased prostaglandin production have been implicated in the increased severity of gingivitis during pregnancy. Gingivitis is associated with the eruption of primary and permanent teeth and appears to decrease in severity after the teeth erupt fully. Orthodontic and prosthetic appliances increase susceptibility to gingivitis as a result of the decreased accessibility for cleaning.

In most cases, a professional dental cleaning followed by good home care, including tooth brushing and flossing, decreases the incidence and severity of gingivitis. In some cases, restoration of fractured or carious teeth decreases the severity of localized inflammation.

A physician should recognize that the inflammation, bleeding, and openings through the epithelial layers around the tooth associated with gingivitis can contribute to profound systemic problems in compromised patients. In hemophiliacs who do not practice good oral hygiene, areas around the teeth may bleed spontaneously or with eating. Ulcerated gingiva is a source of bacterial infection in children who are susceptible to subacute bacterial endocarditis infection, children who are immunosuppressed, and children with uncontrolled diabetes mellitus, kidney disease, or organ transplants. Children with leukemia who are undergoing chemotherapy are at risk for septicemia if they develop pericoronitis or periodontitis.

Fibrotic hyperplastic gingiva often occurs in children receiving phenytoin (Dilantin) for seizure control. Careful titration of the dosage of Dilantin and excellent oral hygiene can control the severity of the gingival overgrowth. However, surgical removal of the overgrowth can be required in some cases.

Mucogingival Problems

Recession of gingiva apically from the cementoenamel junction of the tooth can result in loss of support for the tooth, exposure of pulpal canals, and entrapment of bacteria in an area normally not cleaned by routine brushing. Recession can involve one or more teeth and could be the result of periodontal disease causing bone loss. Alternatively, a tooth may be so abnormally positioned that a thin layer of alveolar bone covers the root. Lack of adequate oral hygiene can cause inflammation, which destroys friable tissues covering the root, or vigorous scrubbing of the area can cause tissue destruction and root exposure.

Abnormal frenum placement can cause recession or clefting. A frenum may interfere with proper placement of a toothbrush, or muscle movement may pull the tissue from the root surface. Frenum problems can occur from the buccal or the lingual sides of the alveolus.

Periodontitis

Periodontitis is the inflammatory destruction of the alveolar bone. Pain, abscessing, tooth loss, and loss of masticatory ability and aesthetics can result. Juvenile periodontitis occurs around the permanent teeth of adolescents, especially the incisors and first molars. Bone loss is usually detected during or after puberty. Some children exhibit an apparent lack of dental plaque or calculus and mildness of gingivitis that masks severe bone loss. The bone loss may be localized to first permanent molars and incisors or may be generalized. Periodontitis should be suspected in children who have teeth with exposed roots.

There are reports of periodontitis around the primary teeth of otherwise healthy children. Little is known about this prepubertal periodontitis, but some children have a mild form of neutrophil chemotactic defect. Progression varies, with tooth exfoliation occurring close to the normal exfoliation time or so rapidly that almost all primary teeth are lost by 5 years of age. These patients have mild to severe gingivitis.

Periodontitis has been reported in children with various systemic diseases or syndromes associated with neutrophil dysfunction or neutropenia. Children with Down syndrome have greater than normal susceptibility to periodontal disease, which may be associated with impaired neutrophil function. Periodontitis has been reported in conjunction with various kinds of neutropenia. Significantly, not all patients with familial neutropenia exhibit periodontal bone loss. The differences have been attributed to various degrees of oral hygiene, suggesting that the susceptibility to periodontal disease is inherited but that bacteria may be the causative factor. Numerous bacteria are associated with juvenile periodontitis, but *Haemophilus actinomycetem comitans, Bacteroides gingivalis, Bacteroides forsythus,* and spirochetes appear to be the most likely pathogenic organisms involved.

Periodontal disease and early exfoliation of primary teeth are associated with hypophosphatemia, diabetes mellitus, Papillon-Lèfevre syndrome, Chédiak-Higashi syndrome, scleroderma, leukemia, fibrous dysplasia, acrodynia, acatalasia, and histiocytosis X. Signs and symptoms of periodontitis include abnormal timing and sequencing of tooth exfoliation, recession, abnormal mobility of teeth, pain on occlusion, and gingival condition ranging from almost healthy to edematous with spontaneous bleeding.

Although a genetic tendency toward periodontitis seems likely, the immediate causative factor seems to be dental plaque. This suggests that treatment should consist of antibiotic therapy, but bacteria that invade the gingiva are not readily susceptible to antibiotics. The most successful treatment of juvenile periodontitis consists of scaling of the teeth, surgery, and tetracycline administration over a 3-week period. Although tetracycline is usually contraindicated for children younger than 8 years, it is the drug of choice if *Haemophilus* infection is confirmed. Little is known about effective treatment of prepubertal periodontitis; extraction of selected teeth with scaling and antibiotic coverage is suggested.

Pericoronitis

An acute infection called *pericoronitis* can occur around erupting molar teeth as a result of the accumulation of bacteria under a flap of tissue called an *operculum* or as a result of abrasion from an opposing tooth. Pericoronitis is most commonly seen around permanent third molars but may occur around first or second permanent or primary molars. The tissue around the tooth becomes erythematous, edematous, and sensitive. Tissue swelling results in additional trauma from the opposing tooth. Cellulitis, fever, lymphadenopathy, pain (possibly radiating to the ear, throat, or floor of the mouth), trismus, and malaise may accompany the infection. The child may not be able to occlude properly if the swelling is extensive.

Treatment consists of irrigation under the tissue flap with a blunt-end needle and syringe and administration of antibiotics. Extraction of the opposing tooth in the case of third molars or excision of the operculum may be required. Incision and drainage are indicated in some cases.

Acute Necrotizing Ulcerative Gingivitis

Acute necrotizing ulcerative gingivitis is a gingival infection caused by spirochetes. The disease is associated with stress, poor oral hygiene, and local tissue trauma. Severe bone loss and gingival recontouring can result.

The usual manifestations of acute necrotizing ulcerative gingivitis are pain, a foul mouth odor, and crater-like destruction of the interdental papillae. The lesions can extend beyond the papillae and are covered by a pseudomembrane. Lymphadenopathy, fever, and malaise can occur.

Treatment consists of a professional dental cleaning and irrigation. Administration of antibiotics such as penicillin is suggested. Gingival surgery might be required after the acute phase of infection if significant tissue damage has occurred. Patients with acute necrotizing ulcerative gingivitis should be evaluated for neutropenia.

Hereditary Gingival Fibromatosis

Hereditary gingival fibromatosis is a nonpainful, generalized growth of firm, fibrotic gingival tissue. Onset is usually reported at the time of eruption of the primary teeth, and the condition usually ceases after all the permanent teeth have erupted. Proliferative gingival growth can cover the crowns of all the teeth, move teeth, and prevent eruption.

The cause of fibromatosis is unknown, although an autosomal dominant pattern of inheritance is seen in some cases. The condition has been reported in patients with mental retardation, epilepsy, and hypertrichosis.

The treatment of choice is surgical excision of the gingival tissue and increased oral hygiene, but recurrence is common even with meticulous hygiene. Tissue enlargement usually resolves after tooth extraction, a treatment alternative.

TRAUMA

Epidemiology

A child's attempts to walk initiate a traumatic period for the child and parents. Falls caused by lack of coordination and physical timing can result in numerous traumatic injuries to the face and oral structures. The incidence of these injuries peaks at approximately 2 to 4 years of age. Trauma to the permanent dentition tends to peak at approximately 8 to 10 years of age. Boys appear to be twice as prone to facial trauma as girls.

Falls, sports injuries, vehicular accidents, and physically handicapping conditions contribute to facial trauma, particularly in older children. Approximately 20% of head–neck trauma and one-third of dental trauma is related to sports. Facial trauma is evident in approximately one-half of all children who are physically abused. Depending on the population, as many as 30% of 7-year-old children exhibit trauma to the primary dentition, and as many as 25% of 14-year-old adolescents exhibit trauma to the permanent dentition. Most injuries involve the anterior teeth, particularly the maxillary central incisors.

Evaluation

Examination of a child who has sustained trauma should include several basic components: medical history; tetanus immunization history; description of cause, place, and time of accident; history of loss of consciousness; systemic conditions and symptoms; and extraoral and intraoral examinations. Factors such as acute bleeding, compromised airways, and level of consciousness take precedence over dental treatment. In most other cases, however, immediate referral to a dentist is required for additional evaluation and treatment. The success of treatment frequently depends on the rapidity with which it is provided.

Discussion of trauma in this chapter is limited to ambulatory patients, but the physician should realize that any child suffering from a blow to the head may have facial bone fractures, tooth injuries, and intraoral soft tissue lacerations or contusions, all of which can contribute to blood loss, compromised airways, infection, pain, lack of healing, and future deformity (see Fig. 127.10). An intraoral examination should be performed as soon as possible, with the timing of dental treatment determined on an individual basis, depending on the severity of the child's condition and what other kinds of treatment are required.

Physical examination should include inspection of the ears for blood, which can indicate condylar fracture of the mandible. The nose should be checked for cerebrospinal fluid or blood. The face, lips, and oral soft tissue should be examined for lacerations or ecchymosis. Acute bleeding should be controlled immediately. Lacerations should be gently cleansed and examined for extent of damage and presence of foreign bodies. Lacerated lips and tongues should be carefully inspected for pieces of teeth or other foreign bodies, particularly if teeth are fractured. Radiographs are required to check for foreign bodies before any suturing is done. Ecchymosis around the eye can indicate fracture of the nose or malar bone; ecchymosis in the upper buccal vestibules can indicate fracture of the sinus, malar bone, or alveolar bone; and ecchymosis in the lower buccal vestibules or floor of the mouth indicates possible mandibular fracture. The facial bones, alveoli, and jaws should be palpated for step fractures or point pain that would indicate fractures. Limitation or deviation on opening and closing of the mouth may indicate fracture of the mandible or other facial bones.

The occlusion should be examined for abnormalities and, if possible, the child's subjective evaluation of the occlusion should be elicited to determine whether alveolar fractures, jaw fractures, or tooth displacements have occurred. Parents can be asked to compare the child's occlusion before and after the trauma. Maxillary mobility should be determined as a screen for maxillary fracture. Teeth should be examined to detect fracture, mobility, displacement, gingival bleeding, pain, and loss.

Trauma can extend to more than one structure. More than one type of injury can occur as a result of one event, and injuries can be caused by a combination of numerous accidents. Although extensive classifications of trauma to the teeth and their supporting structures exist, the best method of handling tooth trauma is to refer the patient immediately to a dentist for necessary data collection, diagnosis, and treatment. Trauma can cause injury that is not visually apparent and will require a radiograph to diagnose. Lack of timely treatment can result in necrosis, with possible abscessing and loss of the tooth. The prognosis for teeth with various injuries depends on the type of treatment and the amount of time elapsed before treatment. Thus, timely referral to a dentist is necessary.

Traumatic Injuries

Dental Fractures

Fracture of the tooth can result in severe pain, particularly when it exposes the pulp. Color is a good criterion for determining tooth fracture that exposes the pulp. Enamel is relatively white, dentin is more yellow, and pulp is red. Therefore, an enamel fracture alone should be white, a fracture into dentin should exhibit yellow surrounded by white, and a fracture into the pulp should appear as red surrounded by yellow and white.

Approximately 20% to 65% of reported dental trauma is crown fracture without pulp exposure; approximately 5% to 8% is crown fracture with pulp exposure. Immediate dental referral is the treatment of choice. Root fractures are not always visually apparent and require dental radiographs. The prognosis of the tooth depends on the area of the fracture.

Trauma to the primary teeth may cause injury to the underlying permanent teeth, which may be in various stages of development. The extent of injury to the permanent teeth may include one or all of the following: discoloration, malformation, hypomineralization, and eruption problems. The severity of each problem varies. Some of the problems may occur as an immediate result of the trauma; others may occur as a result of continued inflammation in the area of a traumatized tooth.

An intruded primary tooth may be allowed to reerupt by itself over a few months if it appears that it will cause no additional damage to the permanent tooth, whereas a displaced primary tooth with an exposed root should be extracted because of the potential damage to the permanent teeth. Because inflammation occurs when primary teeth are allowed to erupt on their own, the medical history of the patient influences treatment. For example, in patients with susceptibility to subacute bacterial endocarditis or systemic immune deficiency, the affected primary teeth should usually be extracted if the prognosis is poor. If inflammation is severe when a tooth is allowed to reerupt, additional evaluation is necessary, and extraction may be indicated. Use of a relative benefits and problems list during treatment planning is recommended.

Intruded permanent teeth require repositioning and splinting if it appears that the tooth will not erupt or will not erupt into an ideal position. Orthodontic repositioning of the teeth may be required if immediate ideal positioning is not possible.

An extruded tooth usually is longer than the crowns of the adjacent teeth. Treatment of extruded permanent teeth involves immediate intrusive force followed by splinting. The physician should force the tooth into the socket, have the child bite on gauze, and then immediately refer the child to a dentist. If the teeth cannot be repositioned fully into the sockets, the child should be referred immediately to a dentist. Local anesthesia might be required to eliminate pain during treatment.

Extruded primary teeth should be extracted since injury to the forming permanent tooth follicles can occur if primary teeth are forced back into the alveolus.

Teeth can be displaced laterally in any direction, with or without alveolar bone fracture. Displaced segments of alveolar bone usually contain the teeth within them. The bone and teeth should be repositioned by application of opposite-finger pressure at the area of obvious fracture and at the incisal tips of the teeth. Splinting is required in many cases to retain the position of the fragment, and occlusal reduction may be required to avoid occlusal contacts. Occasionally, primary root tips project through the gingiva, and extraction is necessary.

Avulsion is the total displacement of a tooth from its socket. The frequency of avulsion caused by trauma ranges from 7% to 15% in the primary dentition and from 0.5% to 15.0% in the permanent dentition. The maxillary central incisors are avulsed most frequently because of their single conical tapering roots and their potential prominence. A bleeding hole appears where a tooth should appear. However, the clinician should never assume that a tooth has been totally avulsed unless a radiograph shows no evidence of tooth structure or the child presents the entire tooth. Partial avulsion or total intrusion can occur.

In the case of avulsed permanent teeth, treatment should be instituted as soon as possible. The parent or guardian should quickly wash the tooth in saliva or saline solution and reinsert the tooth as far as possible into the alveolus. If the tooth cannot be reimplanted by the parent or physician immediately, it could be stored in the buccal vestibule of an adult's or the child's mouth, depending on the child's age and cooperation. An alternate storage medium is saline solution. Keeping the tooth moist is of greatest concern. The child should be seen by a dentist immediately. Splinting and possibly root canal therapy are required. The prognosis depends on the time elapsed between avulsion and treatment and the conditions under which the tooth has been stored. A 95% long-term failure can be predicted when reimplantation has not occurred within 2 hours. Reimplantation of primary teeth is not indicated because of potential damage to the underlying permanent teeth.

Fracture of the Supporting Bones

Discussion of treatment of fractures of the alveolus, mandible, or maxilla requires more detail than allowed in this chapter. However, the physician should be aware of the possibility of fracture of any of these structures. Fractures to these areas are infrequent, occurring most often in automobile injuries, fights, and bicycle accidents, but any fall or injury that involves a direct blow to the chin or the face can result in bony fractures.

Bruising, point tenderness, atypical occlusion, atypical mobility, percussion sounds, and step defects can be used to diagnose alveolar or jaw fractures. Radiographs must be taken that visualize these areas well. However, clinical or radiographic evidence of fracture may not be obvious at the time of the initial examination.

Alveolar fractures occur more frequently in permanent than in primary dentition, but the alveolus supporting newly erupted primary incisors without other erupted teeth is susceptible. Alveolar fractures are frequently associated with tooth dislocation.

Treatment of alveolar fractures of the permanent dentition involves reduction and splinting of the affected area with local anesthesia. Alveolar fractures of the primary dentition may not require splinting but do require a soft diet for several weeks.

The prognosis depends on the time elapsed between injury and treatment. Teeth splinted within 1 hour after alveolar fracture develop pulp necrosis less frequently than teeth splinted after longer intervals do. Alveolar fractures involving permanent teeth usually heal. However, delayed complications of alveolar fractures, including pulpal necrosis, canal obliteration, root resorption, and loss of alveolar bone, are frequent. Root development of primary teeth may be arrested. Immediate and extended dental attention is required.

In the mandible, the region of the mandibular angle, the neck of the condyle, and the area of the canine are the most common sites of fracture. The developing cuspid is positioned close to the mandibular border and provides a weak area for fracture to occur. Radiographs of the condyles are indicated for a child who has been hit in the chin.

Fracture of the maxilla is often through tooth-bearing areas. Another area of maxillary fracture involves separation of the palate from the body of the maxilla such that the fracture line occurs above the root apices and travels through the floor of the nose and the tuberosity. Another area of fracture involves the maxilla and frontal process and the nasal bones on both sides of the face but not the zygomatic bones, which remain intact. This fracture virtually separates the midface from the cranium. The third area involves complete separation of the entire facial skeleton from the cranial bones and passes through the sutures of the temporal and zygomatic bones, frontal and zygomatic bones, frontal bones and maxilla, and frontal and nasal bones.

Treatment of jaw fractures in children with developing teeth involves exact repositioning and usually intermaxillary fixation. However, reports indicate that condylar fractures require mobilization as soon as possible to prevent ankylosis of the condyle. The short bulbous primary dentition and the edentulous areas of mixed dentition can present problems of stabilization. Antibiotics are required if inflammation involves the fracture line. Fractures involving the follicles of developing teeth and fractures in which permanent erupted teeth are preserved require special attention to infection control. Swelling and abscess formation occur in 10% to 18% of children with developing permanent teeth. If possible, the developing or erupted permanent teeth should be preserved.

Fewer inflammatory complications of fractured jaws occur if the jaws are immobilized within 48 hours after injury than if immobilization is delayed. Delayed complications are similar to those of alveolar fractures and require dental follow-up.

Prevention

The unexpected nature of injuries makes prevention of trauma difficult. The physician can identify high-risk children and make recommendations to minimize trauma. Dental factors such as increased overjet, flaring incisors, and insufficient lip closure contribute significantly to the risk of dental trauma. For example, children with overjets exceeding 6 mm have triple the number of traumatic dental injuries of children with normal occlusion. They should be referred to a dentist or orthodontist for orthodontic evaluation and treatment.

Sports injuries can be minimized by the use of intraoral mouth guards. In addition to protecting the teeth and soft tissue, mouth guards effectively minimize concussion, condylar fractures, and neck injuries and the complications ensuing from these injuries. Well-fitting mouth guards can be made by a dentist from a dental cast or can be formed from stock guards that are purchased in a store, heated, and molded intraorally to the player. Commercial guards that are not molded to the individual player usually do not fit as well and are not as comfortable as custom-made guards. In general, custom-made guards provide better retention, comfort, speech pattern, and tear resistance than the other form of mouth guards; they are, however, more expensive than commercial guards, particularly if a child requires replacements as a result of loss or eruption of teeth. Children in orthodontic treatment require special mouth guards because of the braces. Mouth guards are mandatory in many organized football leagues and highly recommended for soccer, lacrosse, and ice hockey. The responsibility of the team physician or a physician evaluating a player's fitness is to recommend a mouth guard for any child participating in contact sports.

Players should be told to wear mouth guards into the shower after playing and to clean them, dry them thoroughly, and store them in a perforated tray. The guards should be rinsed with a mouthwash or antiseptic before use. Unfortunately, many sports injuries do not occur during organized sports, where the use of mouth guards can be controlled; many occur in yards, alleys, empty lots, and streets where children play informally.

Children with disorders such as epilepsy, cerebral palsy, chronic vertigo, self-mutilation, and other psychomotor conditions that contribute to loss of balance should be evaluated for protective headgear or a mouth guard to prevent orofacial trauma. Children with cerebral palsy, epilepsy, chorea, and other psychomotor disturbances who exhibit grinding of teeth may need a mouth guard to prevent severe abrasion to their teeth, but lack of patient compliance is a contraindication. Frequent reevaluation of the mouth guard may be necessary to determine its condition. The oral trauma or severe abrasion of teeth that results from grinding in some comatose and decerebrate patients can be minimized by use of mouth guards. Intraoral fixation may be required in some patients to prevent choking or removal of the guard.

The use of normal safety precautions, such as seat belts for children on child bicycle seats and car seats or safety belts in cars, minimizes injuries.

BURNS

Electrical Burns

Oral electrical burns occur most frequently in preschool children, usually when the children place the female portion of live extension or appliance cords into the mouth or bite into exposed or poorly insulated live wires. The electrolytic saliva forms a short circuit between the cord and the oral tissues.

The severity of injury ranges from superficial burns to extensive third-degree burns that can involve portions of the lips, commissures of the mouth, tongue, and other oral tissues. The extent of tissue destruction may not be immediately obvious, and the child may not experience pain, because nerves are frequently damaged.

The edema and drooling that might occur within a few hours usually subside within 1 week. The lesion generally consists of an erythematous band of tissue surrounding a mass of grayish or yellowish tissue. The necrotic tissue gradually forms an eschar, which is shed in 1 to 3 weeks. Although hemorrhage is not an immediate problem, it may occur from 3 days to 3 weeks after the burn, when the necrotic tissue sloughs, exposing granulation tissue, or when the weakened arterial walls rupture. As healing occurs during the next 2 to 3 months, fibrous tissue forms in the wound, causing it to become indurated. Within 6 months, the immature scar tissue that forms might cause defects ranging from minor scarring to significant unaesthetic and crippling deformations or microstomia and crowding of teeth. Potential contraction of the scar tissue is decreased within 1 year after trauma as the scar tissue softens.

Treatment depends on the severity of the burn and the physical status of the patient. The patient's tetanus immunization history should be updated if necessary. Conservative tissue débridement is suggested, and parents should be given instruction about cleansing and potential hemorrhage control. Antibiotics should be prescribed if signs of secondary infection exist. Small, superficial burns may require only observation, but extensive burns should be managed with an interdisciplinary approach. Within the first 10 days after the burn, the child should be seen by a dentist for construction of a burn appliance. Although required in some cases, surgery can be avoided or minimized by the appropriate selection, proper fit, and compliant use of a burn appliance. The purpose of the appliance is to limit scar contracture and prevent microstomia by applying pressure evenly to both commissures of the mouth. The design of the appliance depends on presence of teeth, the extent of the burn, and the extent of cooperation of the patient.

Parents should be taught to clean and replace the burn appliance after meals. Parents should be informed that the success of treatment depends on compliance with instructions. Repeat visits should be spaced frequently at the beginning of treatment (e.g., 2 days, 1 week, and 3 weeks) and then once every 4 to 6 weeks for a year to reinforce patient compliance and to modify the appliance as necessary. At the end of 1 year, the patient should be reevaluated to determine the need for surgical intervention.

If surgical intervention is required, a burn appliance should be inserted when the sutures are removed. The appliance should be worn 24 hours a day until the clinician determines that it is no longer needed.

Chemical Burns

Patients should not hold an aspirin over the area of a toothache to reduce the pain; the aspirin can cause oral chemical burns by the salicylic acid. The burn is an irregular, whitish lesion that usually approximates an abscess or carious tooth.

If a child complains of dental pain, parents should call a dentist, maintain proper oral hygiene, and administer acetaminophen systematically for pain. They should be informed of the potential tissue damage associated with improper use of aspirin. Parents should be informed that, if extraction is required, aspirin may contribute to bleeding.

PARENTAL COUNSELING AND REFERRAL

A physician should inform parents about the importance of good dental care to the overall health and future dentition of their children. Mothers with apparent dental neglect and caries should be referred for dental treatment to decrease the risk of transmitting S. mutans to their babies. Nursing by bottle should be stopped when the child is 12 months of age, and the child should never go to bed with a bottle filled with anything but water. A well-balanced diet containing few refined carbohydrates, particularly sticky sugars, should be emphasized. Between-meal snacks should consist of cheeses, fresh fruits and vegetables, and other nonsweet foods.

The importance of good oral hygiene should be stressed, and parents should be advised that they should clean their children's teeth because young children generally are not capable of cleaning their teeth adequately. Children's teeth should be cleaned after breakfast and at night before sleep. Tooth cleaning should be started with the eruption of the first primary tooth, when it can be accomplished with a soft gauze or cloth. A small, soft toothbrush can be used when the child is older and accepts it. Parents do not need to floss their children's teeth until tight contacts exist between adjacent teeth. The lack of fine motor skills prevents most children from learning to floss their own teeth adequately until approximately 8 to 10 years of age. A floss holder is helpful for both the parent and the child to provide them easier access to the teeth.

Children should be referred by 1 year of age to a pediatric dentist who is concerned about primary prevention. This is particularly important for children who have medical, physical, or mental handicaps. The focus should be on preventing dental disease. Physicians are strongly encouraged to refer patients to dentists willing to work with young children.

The physician should inform parents of the importance of fluoride in controlling dental caries. Water fluoridation is the most effective and economic means of controlling caries and generally does not require patient compliance. In areas that have suboptimal fluoride concentrations in the drinking water (less than 0.7 ppm), fluoride supplements should be prescribed.

The current dosage schedule (see Chapter 14, Feeding the Healthy Child) for fluoride supplements is based on the age of the child and the fluoride concentration in the drinking water. Too great a dose of fluoride can result in dental fluorosis, a condition that may range in severity from thin, opaque areas on the teeth to large, discolored areas and hypoplasia. Fluoride supplementation should begin within a few months after birth. Mild fluorosis might occur in low-weight children, but the average person probably will not notice it.

Prescribing fluoride supplements to breast-fed infants living in fluoridated areas requires caution. Mothers frequently supplement breast-feeding with tap water or liquids mixed with tap water and often discontinue breast-feeding earlier than they had originally expected. The infant could be exposed to higher than optimal doses of fluoride. Mothers living in an area with water fluoridation should be advised to discontinue fluoride supplements as soon as the infant is not exclusively breast-fed. Fluoride supplements ingested by a nursing mother result in little or no increase in the fluoride levels of her milk and are not recommended as a substitute for direct supplementation of the child.

The efficacy of prenatal fluoride supplementation is controversial. Although clinical studies tend to support the efficacy of prenatal fluoride supplementation, many of these studies suffer from flaws of design and interpretation. The Food and Drug Administration does not currently approve the marketing of prenatal fluoride supplements, but physicians and dentists are not restricted from prescribing them. The reader is referred to Chan, Wyborny, and Kula for a more detailed review of fluoride metabolism and supplementation.

Children should use fluoride toothpastes that are approved by the American Dental Association. Toddlers should use no more than required to color the bristle tips of the toothbrush.

Suggested Readings

Abrams RG, Kula KS, Josell SD. Early childhood prevention programs. In: Hardin JF, ed. *Clinical dentistry*. Philadelphia: Lippincott-Raven, 1988.

Andreasen JO, Andreasen FM. *Textbook and color atlas of traumatic injuries to the teeth*, 3rd ed. Copenhagen: Munksgaard, 1994.

Chan JT, Wyborny LE, Kula KS. Clinical applications of fluorides. In: Hardin JF, ed. *Clinical dentistry*. Philadelphia: Lippincott-Raven, 1990.

Hartsfeld JK. Premature exfoliation of teeth in childhood and adolescence. *Adv Pediatr* 1994;41:453.

National Institutes of Health Consensus Development Conference on Oral Complications of Cancer Therapies. Diagnosis, prevention, and treatment. *National Cancer Institute Monograph* No. 9, 1990.

Proffit WR, Fields HW. *Contemporary orthodontics*. St. Louis: Mosby, 2000: 742.

Reference Manual 2001–2002. *Pediatr Dent* 23:1.

Scully C, Flint SR, Porter SF. *Oral diseases*. St. Louis: Mosby, 1996:371.

Seow W, Cheng E, Wan V. Effects of oral health education and tooth-brushing on mutant streptococci infection in young children. *Pediatr Dent* 2003;25:223.

Taylor LB. A review of selected microstomia prevention appliances. *Pediatr Dent* 1997;19:413.

Truman BI, Gooch BF, Evans CA. The guide to community preventive series: interventions to prevent dental caries, oral and pharyngeal caners, and sports-related craniofacial injuries. *Am J Prev Med* 2002;Suppl:84.

Vargas CM, Crall JJ, Schneider DA. Sociodemographic distribution of pediatric dental caries: NHANES III, 1988–1994. *J Am Dent Assoc* 1998;129:1229.

Wan A, Seow W, Purdie D, et al. The effects of chlorhexidine gel on *Streptococcus mutans* infection in 10-month-old infants: a longitudinal, placebo-controlled, double-blind trial. *Pediatr Dent* 2003;25:215.

Wyszynski D. *Cleft lip & palate from origin to treatment*. Hong Kong: Oxford University Press, 2002:518.

CHAPTER 128 ■ PEDIATRIC OPHTHALMOLOGY

ELIAS I. TRABOULSI

NORMAL DEVELOPMENT OF THE EYE

Ocular and orbital structures are derived from two populations of cells: mesodermal and ectodermal. The vascular endothelium, extraocular muscles, and part of the temporal sclera are derived from mesoderm. The three types of ectodermal cells that contribute to the remaining ocular structures are neural ectoderm, neural crest cells, and surface ectoderm. Most mesenchymal tissues of the eye and orbit are derived from the neural crest.

At the end of the second week of gestation, through adjacent mesodermal induction, the ocular primordia arise from the neural plate. The optic vesicles form from neuroectoderm and approach surface ectoderm to induce the lens placode. At 4 weeks' gestation, the optic vesicle and lens placode invaginate, and vessels of the hyaloid system are incorporated into the globe through this formed embryonic fissure, located inferiorly in the developing globe. At the beginning of the fifth week, the embryonic fissure closes, and by the sixth week, the entire double-layered optic cup is formed. The inner neuroectodermal cell layer becomes the multilayered sensory retina, and the outer layer becomes the retinal pigment epithelium. The neuroectodermal layers induce the surrounding mesenchyme to produce the stroma of the choroid and the melanocytes of the uveal tract. The collagenous coats of the eye, the bones, and soft tissues of the orbit and the sheaths of the optic nerve are derived from the neural crest. A number of developmental genes, the best studied of which being the *PAX6* gene, play an essential role in normal ocular development. These genes are expressed in the embryonic eye structures and are mutated in some ocular malformations such as aniridia.

Normal Milestones

A normal pupillary response indicates functioning afferent and efferent visual pathways. This response is usually present by 31 weeks' gestation. The blink response to light occurs by 30 weeks' gestation. A blink response to threat is not observed until 5 months of age. Estimates of visual acuity in young infants are based on the ability to fixate and follow targets, on the presence or absence of nystagmus, and on the indifference to occlusion of either eye. The infant would fuss if a seeing eye is closed and a poorly seeing eye is left uncovered. In older infants, good vision allows normal play behavior and interaction with parents and provides the children with the ability to notice and find small objects and distant visual targets. Human faces are seen by infants as young as a few hours of age. Questioning a mother about her child's response to her face and smile is a useful clue to the child's ability to see in the absence of major neurologic and developmental impairment. The presence of an optokinetic response to a rotating drum with vertical or horizontal stripes is also used to rule

out blindness in infants with suspected total visual loss (vide infra).

Acuity Measurement in Infancy

Objective techniques of visual acuity assessment in infancy include optokinetic nystagmus (OKN), visual-evoked potentials (VEPs), and forced-choice preferential looking (FCPL) techniques. In the OKN technique, a drum with black and white stripes is rotated so that the stripes are moved in an arc across 180° of the infant's visual field. This results in an involuntary horizontal jerk nystagmus in the seeing infant. The fast phase of the nystagmus is in the direction opposite that of the moving stripes. OKN response to a smaller stripe width indicates better visual acuity.

Analysis of the latency and amplitude of VEPs elicited by phase-alternated checkerboards of variable size or square-wave gratings can also be used to determine visual acuity in infants. The level of acuity is directly proportional to the amplitude of the VEP and inversely proportional to the latency of the evoked response. VEPs are not affected by acoustic stimuli, movements of the observer's limbs, or some eye movements.

FCPL techniques are based on the observation that infants prefer to look at a patterned stimulus than on a field of homogeneous gray color of equal overall luminance. The Teller Acuity Cards II are probably the most frequently used and reliable instruments that rely on this technique. In this examination, the infant is presented simultaneously with a patterned stimulus consisting of black and white stripes on one side, and with a gray screen of space-average luminance equal to the patterned stimulus on the other side. The observer, who is peeping at the infant through a hole between the two stimuli, is masked to the relative position of the striped or checkered stimulus and the gray screen. The observer records the visual response of the child by noting which side the child's eyes are pointed to as patterns with decreasing stripe widths are presented. Acuity is estimated from the smallest stripe width the child prefers over the homogeneous field. Although tedious, this is a useful behavioral technique for assessing visual acuity and diagnosing a variety of ocular diseases. Its most common application is the determination of the response amblyopia to treatment in the preverbal child.

Table 128.1 summarizes estimates of normal visual acuity during the first year of life based on the three methods described. Each of these methods has its limitations and inconsistencies, but all have proven useful in the objective assessment of visual acuity in infants. Occasionally, infants have a maturational delay in visual development in the absence of structural ocular abnormalities or nystagmus. There is frequently a concomitant delay in motor skill development. This condition should only be diagnosed if organic causes of reduced vision such as media opacities, optic atrophy, and retinal dystrophies such as Leber congenital amaurosis are excluded. An ocular examination and a normal or only slightly reduced

TABLE 128.1

DEVELOPMENT OF VISUAL ACUITY IN INFANCY AS ASSESSED BY VARIOUS TECHNIQUES

Method	Full-Term Newborn	2 Months	4 Months	5 Months	1 Year	Age at Which 20/20 is Detectable
Optokinetic nystagmus	20/400	20/400	20/200	20/100	20/60	—
Visual-evoked potential	20/100–20/200	20/80	20/80	20/20–20/40	20/20	6–12 months
Forced choice preferential looking	20/200–20/200	—	—	20/100	20/50	18–24 months

electroretinogram differentiate delayed visual maturation from the other conditions.

Acuity Measurement in Older Children

Allen pictures or Lea symbols are most commonly used to assess vision in 2- to 3-year-old children. The pictures or symbols are either projected in decreasing sizes at a fixed distance or are presented to the child on cards of a fixed size at increasing distances. In the Sheridan-Gardiner test, the child is shown geometric shapes, letters, or patterns of decreasing sizes and asked to point to identical patterns on a chart held at reading distance. The E game can be used for the child who is older than 3 years of age but cannot yet read letters. The child is asked to point his or her fingers or hand in the direction of the open end of the horizontal lines of E's of decreasing sizes on a chart or on cards. It may be necessary to teach the child to play the E game or to recognize Allen pictures at home before the examination.

Caution must be used in interpreting the visual acuity of children tested by a method that involves the recognition of letters. Children will not admit that they do not know the letters and can mislead the examiner. Children with unilateral visual loss may also "peak" from the better eye if it is not adequately occluded.

OPHTHALMOLOGIC EXAMINATION

The recommendations of the American Academy of Ophthalmology and the American Association for Pediatric Ophthalmology and Strabismus are that an ophthalmologic examination be performed whenever questions arise about the health of the visual system of a child of any age. The recommendations also include the following:

1. A pediatrician, family physician, nurse practitioner, or physician assistant should examine a newborn's eyes for general eye health including a red reflex test in the nursery. An ophthalmologist should be asked to examine all high risk infants, that is, those at risk to develop retinopathy of prematurity (ROP); those with a family history of retinoblastoma, glaucoma, or cataracts in childhood; those with retinal dystrophy/degeneration or systemic diseases associated with eye problems; or when any opacity of the ocular media or nystagmus (purposeless rhythmic movement of the eyes) is seen. Infants with neurodevelopmental delay should also be examined by an ophthalmologist.
2. All infants by 6 months to 1 year of age should be screened for ocular health including a red reflex test by a properly trained health care provider such as an ophthalmologist, pediatrician, family physician, nurse, or physician assistant during routine well-baby follow-up visits.

3. Vision screening should also be performed between 3 and $3\frac{1}{2}$ years of age. Vision and alignment should be assessed by a pediatrician, family practitioner, ophthalmologist, optometrist, orthoptist, or individual trained in vision assessment of preschool children. Emphasis should be placed on checking visual acuity as soon as a child is cooperative enough to complete the examination. Generally, this occurs between ages $2\frac{1}{2}$ and $3\frac{1}{2}$. It is essential that a formal testing of visual acuity be performed by the age of 5 years.
4. Some evidence currently exists to suggest that photoscreening may be a valuable adjunct to the traditional screening process, particularly in preliterate children.
5. Further screening examinations should be done at routine school checks or after the appearance of symptoms. Routine comprehensive professional eye examination of the normal asymptomatic child has no proven medical benefit.
6. School-aged children who pass standard vision screening tests but who demonstrate difficulties learning to read should be referred to reading specialists such as educational psychologists for evaluation for language processing disorders such as dyslexia. There is not adequate scientific evidence to suggest that "defective eye teaming" and "accommodative disorders" are common causes of educational impairment. Hence, routine screening for these conditions is not recommended.

Visual acuity can be assessed in the pediatrician's office with Allen cards or Sheridan-Gardiner cards for children 3 to 5 years of age, and with Snellen acuity charts for older children who know the alphabet well. The E chart may also be used. In preverbal or retarded children, symmetry of visual acuity between the two eyes can be determined by the pattern of fixation. In the latter, vision is recorded as being central or eccentric, steady or interrupted by abnormal or involuntary movements, and maintained or preferred to one eye or the other.

The primary health care provider can check ocular alignment using the cover test, the cover-uncover test, or the Hirschberg corneal light reflex test. The light reflexes should be symmetrically located in the corneas. The cover and cover-uncover tests are based on the observation that children with strabismus use one eye for fixation while the other eye is deviated. When the fixating eye is covered, the deviated eye moves in or out to pick up fixation. If the eye moves from the nasal side to the temporal side, it is esotropic; if it moves from the temporal side toward the nose, it is exotropic. Pupillary responses are checked with a bright light source, and the direct (i.e., stimulated pupil constricts) and consensual (i.e., other pupil constricts when light is shined in one eye) light reflexes are recorded. An afferent pupillary defect during the swinging light test (i.e., pupil dilates instead of constricting as light is moved from the other eye back to the one with the dilating pupil) usually indicates an optic nerve problem such as atrophy or neuritis on the side of the afferent defect.

The direct ophthalmoscope can be used to check for the presence of cataracts or other ocular media opacities. A +10 diopter lens is dialed into the ophthalmoscope, and the ophthalmoscope light is shined into the pupil from a distance of about 1 m while the observer is looking into the ophthalmoscope; cataracts appear as black shadows over a red background. Direct ophthalmoscopy allows examination of the disc, macula, and blood vessels in the posterior pole area. Dimming the light of the ophthalmoscope and shining the light into the pupil from a distance of less than an inch while the child is looking at a distance with the other eye maximizes the chance of having a good view of the disc and posterior pole.

Children with strabismus or those with evident or suspected ocular abnormalities should be immediately examined by an ophthalmologist, as should infants suspected to have impaired vision. Children with syndromes or diseases known to involve the eye, those with a family history of early onset of ocular disease, or those with developmental delay or suspicion of visual handicap should also be examined immediately. Visual handicaps need to be ruled out in children with scholastic failure or learning disabilities.

To evaluate a child with an ocular problem, the ophthalmologist obtains detailed pertinent ocular, developmental, and systemic histories; gestational, natal, and neonatal histories; and any family history of similar or other systemic and ocular diseases. The following examinations should be routinely performed in the pediatric ophthalmologist's office: (1) estimate of visual acuity in infants and toddlers and exact visual acuity in older children; (2) examination of ocular motility and determination of binocularity of vision; (3) a good anterior segment examination, preferably using the slit lamp; (4) examination of pupillary responses; (5) a dilated fundus inspection using the indirect ophthalmoscope; and (6) a cycloplegic refraction.

DISORDERS APPARENT AT BIRTH OR SHORTLY THEREAFTER

Congenital malformations may be observed at any age. We will only discuss the most common ones and those requiring medical attention or screening for associated systemic abnormalities. Children with any of the following conditions should be referred to the pediatric ophthalmologist.

Birth Trauma

Although birth trauma is not a congenital anomaly *per se*, it is discussed here because it is evident soon after birth. Forceps injuries to the eye are unilateral and most frequently involve the left eye, probably because the most common position of the infant's head is left occiput anterior. In these injuries, lid swelling and corneal opacification are apparent soon after birth. Characteristic vertical or oblique breaks in Descemet membrane are observed on slit-lamp examination, in contrast to the horizontal breaks or Haab striae of congenital glaucoma. Myopia, astigmatism, and amblyopia may subsequently develop. More severe injuries can lead to intraocular hemorrhage, breaks in Bruch membrane of the retina, or even rupture of the globe. Prolonged labor and anatomic crowding are predisposing factors.

Adnexal Disorders

In cryptophthalmos, the upper and lower lids are completely fused, although the underlying eyeball may be completely normal. Surgical incision in the area of the palpebral fissure may open directly into the anterior segment of the eye. The cryptophthalmos or Fraser syndrome includes lid fusion, hyper-

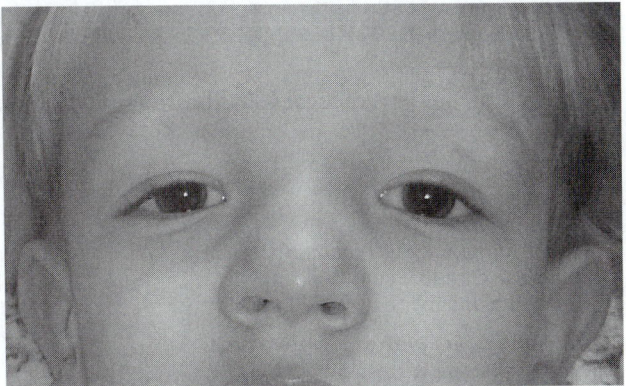

FIGURE 128.1. Midface of patient with Waardenburg syndrome. Note telecanthus and white forelock.

telorism, and cardiac and genital anomalies; it is inherited as an autosomal recessive disorder and results from mutations in the *FRAS1* gene, which appears to be important in signal transduction in the extracellular matrix.

Upper lid colobomas (i.e., full-thickness defects in lid tissue involving the lid margin) are seen in Goldenhar syndrome, a variant of the oculoauriculovertebral sequence, in conjunction with epibulbar dermoids and preauricular skin tags. Lower lid colobomas are more characteristic of the Treacher Collins syndrome, a form of mandibulofacial dysostosis.

Distichiasis is the growth of true cilia in ectopic locations and in extra rows along the lid margin and out of the orifices of meibomian glands. The distichiasis–lymphedema syndrome is inherited in an autosomal dominant fashion and results from mutations in the *FOXC2* gene.

Hypertelorism is a radiologic diagnosis that refers to an increased distance between the two orbits. Telecanthus refers to an unusually long distance between the inner canthi; the ratio between the inter-inner canthal distance and the inter-outer canthal distance is normally about 1:3. Telecanthus and outer displacement of the inferior lacrimal puncti are seen in Type I Waardenburg syndrome (Fig. 128.1), other features of which include heterochromia, deafness, and a white forelock; this syndrome is classified with the neurocristopathies and results from mutations in the *PAX3* gene. Hypertelorism occurs in many dysmorphic syndromes, discussed in Chapter 166.

Anterior Segment Disorders

In microcornea, the corneal diameter is 10 mm or less. Microphthalmos may or may not be present.

In microphthalmos, the anteroposterior diameter of the eye is short (normally 18 mm at birth). High hyperopia or myopia is often present. Chorioretinal or iris colobomas and other ocular anomalies may also exist. Microphthalmos may be unilateral, bilateral, isolated, or part of a multisystem dysmorphic syndrome (Box 128.1). Nanophthalmos (i.e., pure microphthalmos) is an autosomal recessive condition involving high hyperopia and a predisposition to narrow-angle glaucoma and spontaneous choroidal effusion.

In megalocornea, the corneal diameter is increased to more than 12.5 mm. The intraocular pressure and endothelial cell count are normal. Megalocornea is usually X-linked recessive and may be rarely seen in Marfan syndrome. Congenital glaucoma should be ruled out in infants with enlarged corneal diameter. Table 128.2 lists the differences between congenital glaucoma and megalocornea.

BOX 128.1   Practical Classification of Microphthalmia/Coloboma

Isolated

Microphthalmia (AD, AR, XR)
  Colobomatous
  Noncolobomatous (nanophthalmos)
Isolated uveoretinal coloboma
Microphthalmia with cyst

Microphthalmia with ocular anomalies

Microphthalmia with cataract (AD, AR)
Microphthalmia with myopia and corectopia (AD)
Microphthalmia with ectopia lentis
Microphthalmia with congenital retinal detachment
  (AR)
Persistent hyperplastic primary vitreous (sporadic)
Aicardi syndrome

Microphthalmia with mental retardation

Microphthalmia with mental retardation
  (AD, AR, XR)
Microphthalmia with mental retardation and congenital
  spastic diplegia (Sjögren-Larsson syndrome)

Microphthalmia with craniofacial malformations

Facioauriculovertebral sequence
Hallermann-Streiff syndrome
Amniotic band syndrome
Transverse facial cleft
Microphthalmia with cleft lip/palate
Microphthalmia with microcephaly
Microphthalmia with microcephaly and retinal folds
  (XR, AR)
Microphthalmia with hydrocephalus and congenital
  retinal nonattachment (Warburg syndrome)

*Microphthalmia with malformations of the hands
  and feet*

Microphthalmia with polydactyly
Waardenburg anophthalmia syndrome (AR)
Subgroup of CHARGE association (bifid thumbs)

*Microphthalmia with multiple congenital anomalies
  (syndromes)*

CHARGE association
Duker syndrome
Lenz microphthalmia syndrome (XR)
Oculodentoosseous dysplasia (AD, AR)
Cryptophthalmos syndrome (AR)
Cerebrooculofacial syndrome (AR)
Goltz syndrome or focal dermal hypoplasia (XD)
Lowe syndrome (XR)
Meckel-Gruber syndrome (AR)
Basal cell nevus syndrome of Gorlin-Goltz (AD)
Congenital contractural arachnodactyly (AD)
Rubinstein-Taybi syndrome
Cross syndrome (AR)
Fanconi syndrome (AR)
Diamond-Blackfan syndrome (AR)
Epidermal nevus syndrome

Microphthalmia in chromosomal anomalies

T-13 (Patau syndrome)
4p- (Wolf-Hirschhorn syndrome)
18q-
18r
T-18 (Edward syndrome)
Cat-eye syndrome (marker 22)
Other chromosomal aberrations

Microphthalmia and intrauterine insults

Maternal drug intake: thalidomide, alcohol, isotretinoin
Maternal vitamin A deficiency
Maternal fever or radiation exposure
Maternal uncontrolled phenylketonuria
Intrauterine infections: cytomegalovirus, Epstein-Barr virus,
  varicella, herpes simplex, rubella, toxoplasmosis

AD, autosomal dominant; AR, autosomal recessive; XD, X-linked
dominant; XR, X-linked recessive.

In sclerocornea, there is loss of transparency of the cornea. This results from irregular arrangement of the collagen fibrils, which are normally arranged in a hexagonal fashion in the transparent cornea. Other ocular abnormalities such as aniridia, cataracts, and coloboma may coexist with sclerocornea. Patients may also have systemic birth defects.

TABLE 128.2

DIFFERENCES BETWEEN MEGALOCORNEA AND CONGENITAL GLAUCOMA

	Megalocornea	Congenital Glaucoma
Corneal size	Enlarged	Enlarged
Corneal clarity	Clear	Opaque, steamy
Endothelium	Normal	Reduced endothelial density
Descemet membrane	Normal	Horizontal breaks
Symptoms	None	Photophobia; tearing
Inheritance	X-linked	Autosomal recessive

Anterior segment dysgenesis is a term that encompasses a variety of developmental defects of the anterior chamber angle and iris. These malformations are most commonly caused by abnormal neural crest differentiation into corneal endothelial cells, anterior chamber angle, and anterior iris. In the mildest form called posterior embryotoxon, there is a prominent anteriorly displaced Schwalbe line (i.e., peripheral end of Descemet membrane). In the Axenfeld anomaly, iris strands are attached to the anteriorly displaced Schwalbe line. The Rieger anomaly involves hypoplasia of the anterior stroma of the iris in addition to the abnormalities already described. Anterior segment dysgenesis is inherited in an autosomal dominant fashion. At least three genetic loci have been assigned to syndromes featuring a Rieger ocular phenotype. Developmental of adult open-angle glaucoma occurs in 50% of these patients over the course of their lifetime. The Rieger syndrome combines anterior segment dysgenesis with hypodontia and redundant umbilical skin. It is inherited in an autosomal dominant fashion and its gene, *PITX2*, has been mapped to 4q23. *PITX2* is a homeobox-containing gene and is important in neural crest development.

Peters anomaly involves a central defect in Descemet membrane, with various degrees of adhesion of the iris and lens

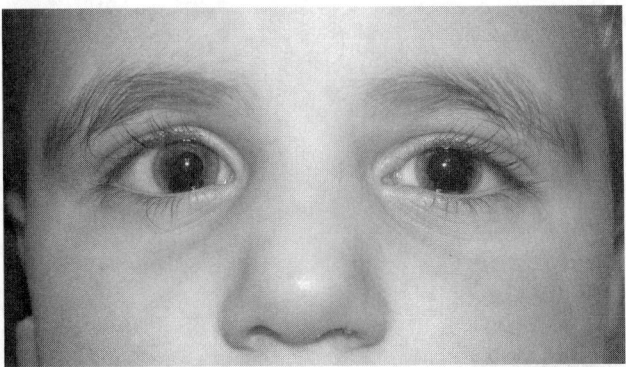

FIGURE 128.2. Patient with aniridia. Note the presence of iris remnants in both eyes, right more than left.

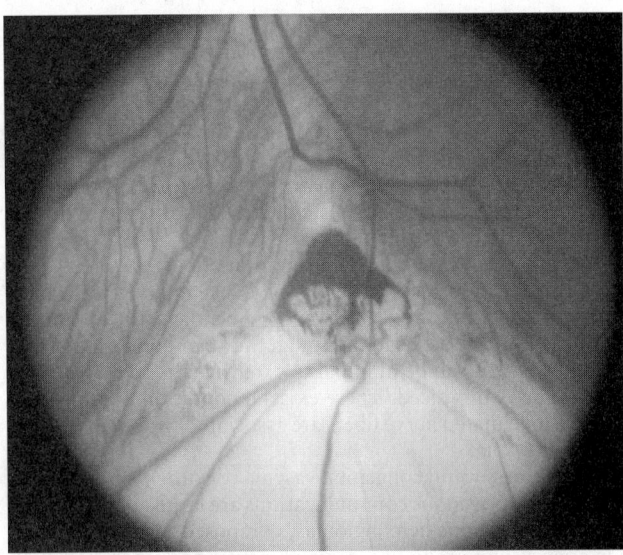

FIGURE 128.3. Typical inferior chorioretinal coloboma along the line of closure of the embryonic fissure. The optic nerve is at the upper edge of the figure.

capsule to the central cornea; these presumably develop from failure of separation of the lens from the surface ectoderm as the cornea is forming. Cataracts may be present. Combined cataract extraction and penetrating keratoplasty are required in severe cases. Most instances are sporadic, although autosomal recessive and autosomal dominant forms have been observed. Glaucoma is common and is a leading cause of visual loss in these patients. One-quarter to one-fourth of patients with Peters anomaly have other ocular malformations and a similar proportion of patients have other birth defects of the brain, heart, kidneys, and extremities.

mal irregular dominant with reduced penetrance), or they may be part of a complex malformation syndrome of known or unknown cause. Box 128.1 presents an etiologic classification of ocular colobomas and of microphthalmia.

Uveal Tract Disorders

In aniridia (Fig. 128.2), a rim of rudimentary iris is always present at the iris root. The associated ocular features include cataracts, ectopia lentis, developmental glaucoma, corneal pannus, persistence of the retina over pars plana, and foveal hypoplasia leading to decreased visual acuity and nystagmus. Aniridia can be sporadic or hereditary with autosomal dominant transmission. Sporadically affected family members may have atypical iris defects and pseudopolycoria. Wilms tumor has been associated only with sporadic aniridia, and the Wilms tumor, aniridia, genitourinary abnormalities, and mental retardation (WAGR) syndrome has been associated with a deletion of the short arm of chromosome 11. Aniridia results from mutations of the *PAX6* gene located on 11p13.

In ocular melanocytosis or melanosis oculi, there is hyperpigmentation of the uveal tract from increased numbers of normal melanocytes. Uveal malignant melanoma develops in less than 1% of patients. In oculodermal melanocytosis or nevus of Ota, ocular melanocytosis is associated with congenital hyperpigmentation of the skin in the distribution of the trigeminal nerve. Oculodermal melanocytosis is more common in African Americans and in Asians than in Caucasians, but malignant melanoma is less frequent in the former than in the latter.

Persistent strands of the pupillary membrane are commonly seen and result from failure of regression of the embryonic tunica vasculosa lentis that obliterates the pupil *in utero*. The strands seldom interfere with vision.

Chorioretinal colobomas are defects in the retina and uveal tract caused by failure of the embryonic ocular fissure to close. Typical colobomas are located inferiorly because the embryonic fissure is located inferonasally. The iris, ciliary body, inferior choroid, or optic nerve head may be involved singly or in combination (Fig. 128.3). Eyes with colobomas may be of normal size but are generally microphthalmic. Large colobomas may produce a white reflex from the pupil and have been confused with eyes that harbor retinoblastoma. Colobomas may be isolated, sporadic, or hereditary (most commonly autoso-

Vitreous Disorders

Persistence of hyaloid vessels and vascular loops at the optic disc results from incomplete regression of the hyaloid system of blood vessels. Vision is normal. Rarely, retinal vascular occlusive disease has resulted from twisted prepapillary loops.

Mittendorf dot and Bergmeister papilla are glial remnants of the regressed hyaloid system at the posterior lens capsule and optic disc, respectively. No patent blood vessels are found within these fibrous remnants.

Persistent hyperplastic primary vitreous (PHPV) or persistent fetal vasculature (PFV) is the most severe developmental anomaly that involves the vitreous and the globe. The affected eye is microphthalmic, the ciliary processes are elongated, and there is some degree of anterior or posterior hyperplasia of the fibrous and glial tissue surrounding the hyaloid blood vessels. There may be an associated cataract. PHPV is a unilateral condition affecting male and female patients equally. Visual prognosis depends on the severity of the microphthalmia and the associated retinal traction and dysplasia. The younger the patient is, the more likely it is that surgical intervention to remove the cataract and clear the visual pathways can improve visual potential. After a lensectomy and vitrectomy procedure, immediate aphakic correction and aggressive amblyopia therapy are necessary to produce useful vision. Surgery should be performed before 2 months of age, and parents should be informed about the guarded prognosis. Surgery prevents the later occurrence of angle-closure glaucoma, which otherwise develops in many patients with PHPV. Because it causes a white pupil, PHPV should be differentiated from retinoblastoma on the basis of clinical clues and ultrasonography or computed tomography.

Retinal Disorders

Retinal dysplasia is a pathologic term describing abnormal, disorderly acinar, tubular, and rosette-like formations in the retina. It is a prominent feature in trisomy 13 and can be produced by intrauterine insults or infection. Retinal dysplasia can lead to the appearance of a white pupil and should therefore be differentiated from retinoblastoma. Retinal dysplasia is also present in patients with Norrie disease, an X-linked condition characterized by congenital blindness, deafness in about 25% of patients, and a progressive neuropsychiatric illness. The gene has been cloned and can be tested for mutations in individuals suspected to have this condition.

Myelinated nerve fibers are found in about 1% of autopsy eyes. These are present at birth, have a feathery appearance, and are usually found in the nerve fiber layer in contiguity with the optic nerve head, although they can be separate from it. Involvement can be minimal to extensive. In extensive cases a scotoma is produced. There exists a condition in which extensive myelinated nerve fibers are associated with high myopia and amblyopia.

There are several congenital vascular disorders of the retina. Retinal arteriovenous communications are large, dilated retinal vessels. Cavernous hemangiomas, composed of dilated saccular aneurysmal grape-like compartments, are associated with similar central nervous system and cutaneous hemangiomas. These vascular tumors may be inherited in a dominant fashion, and result from mutations in the *KRIT1* gene. Coats disease (i.e., congenital retinal telangiectasia) is discussed later in this chapter, in the section on retinoblastoma. Von Hippel-Lindau disease is an autosomal dominant condition characterized by retinal capillary hemangiomas (Fig. 128.4); cerebellar, medullary, and spinal cord hemangioblastomas; and a variety of other cystic and neoplastic lesions throughout the body. The lesions include cysts of the pancreas, kidney, lungs, and ovaries; adenomas of the liver, epididymis, and adrenals; hypernephromas; pheochromocytomas; and familial islet cell tumors. Retinal lesions may be complicated by exudative retinopathy and retinal detachment and have been treated with various degrees of success by laser photocoagulation and cryotherapy. The disease is caused by mutations in the tumor-suppressor *VHL* gene.

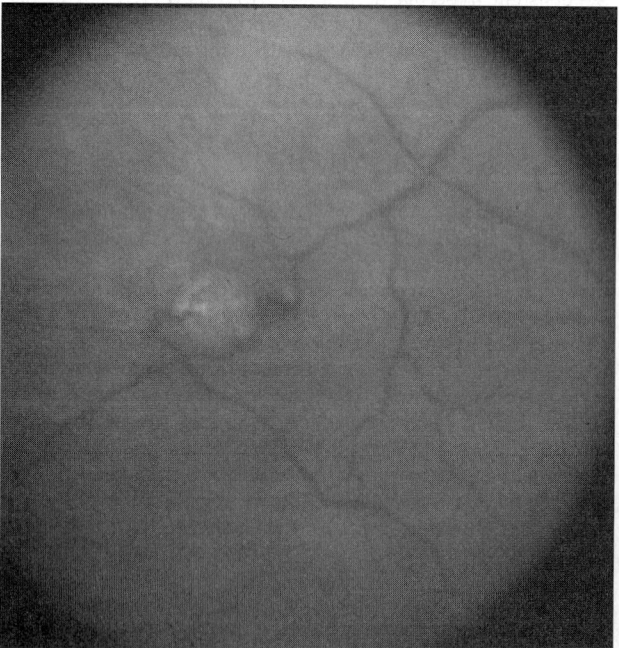

FIGURE 128.4. Small retinal capillary hemangiomas in a patient with von Hippel-Lindau disease.

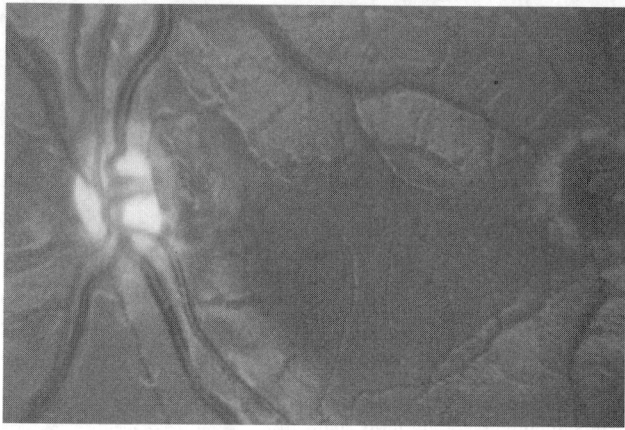

FIGURE 128.5. Very small optic nerve head characteristic of optic nerve hypoplasia. Note increased distance between nerve head on the left and fovea on the right. In normal conditions, one can fit about two optic discs in the area between the disc and the fovea.

Optic Nerve Disorders

Optic nerve hypoplasia is probably the most common ocular developmental anomaly. It is nonprogressive and characterized by a subnormal number of axons in the affected nerve with normal mesodermal and glial supporting tissues. Subtle, segmental, and severe forms are seen. Classically, the nerve head is one-half to one-third of the normal size, pale to gray, and surrounded by a yellowish halo bordered on either side by a darker ring of pigment, the so-called double ring sign (Fig. 128.5). The retinal vessels are frequently tortuous. Bilateral cases are more frequent than unilateral cases, with variable asymmetry. Visual acuity ranges from poor light perception to normal, and visual field defects are common. Severe bilateral cases are manifested in infancy with poor visual development and nystagmus; less severe and more subtle forms are detected only later in life. Optic nerve hypoplasia has been reported with porencephaly, isolated cerebral atrophy, basal encephaloceles, congenital suprasellar tumors, colpocephaly, and anencephaly. Neuroradiologic abnormalities and hypopituitarism with growth restriction and hypothyroidism appear to be most common in patients with bilateral, severe involvement. Although most cases are sporadic, dominant inheritance has been reported. Maternal diabetes has been associated with an increased incidence of mild optic nerve hypoplasia and good visual acuity. Other rare associations include maternal viral infections and maternal ingestion of quinine and anticonvulsants. Optic nerve hypoplasia may be a common feature of the fetal alcohol syndrome. Other ocular features of the fetal alcohol syndrome are strabismus and a typical configuration of the lids with mild bilateral ptosis and down-slanted and horizontally shortened fissures.

In septooptic dysplasia (De Morsier syndrome), bilateral optic nerve hypoplasia is associated with lack of a septum pellucidum, partial or complete agenesis of the corpus callosum, and dysplasia of the anterior third ventricle. Hypopituitarism may be present. All children with optic nerve hypoplasia should undergo magnetic resonance imaging (MRI) of the brain and pituitary and should have pediatric neurologic and endocrinologic evaluations.

The morning glory disc anomaly (MGDA) is a congenital malformation in which the optic nerve head is excavated, with white tissue at its center and a raised annulus of pigmentary chorioretinal change at its edge (Fig. 128.6). Its appearance and the degree of dysplasia vary. Most cases are unilateral, and visual impairment varies greatly, with vision ranging

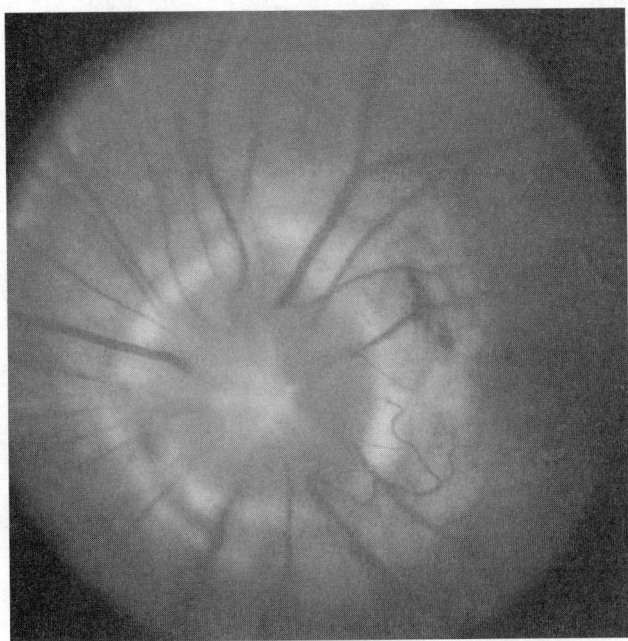

FIGURE 128.6. Morning glory disc anomaly. There is a large opening of the posterior sclera with radial vessels, peripapillary ring of tissue, and central tuft of glial tissue.

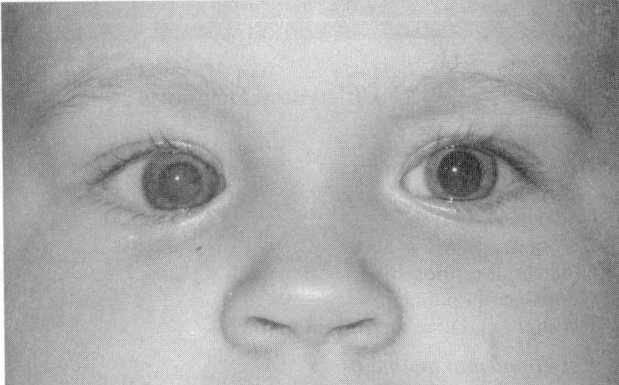

FIGURE 128.7. Dimmer, light orange or tan reflex from right eye as opposed to red reflex from left eye. See Color Figure 128.7 in color section.

from 20/30 to light perception only. Several ocular anomalies may coexist with the disc anomaly. Associated systemic abnormalities include basal encephaloceles, Moyamoya disease, and rare kidney malformations. Infants and children with MGDA should undergo magnetic resonance angiography (MRA) of the carotid circulation to specifically look for vascular abnormalities and Moyamoya vessels. Nonrhegmatogenous retinal detachment occurs in about one-third of cases and is thought to be due to the accumulation of fluid from between the subarachnoid space into the subretinal space through the malformed optic papilla.

Corneal Opacities

The five categories of disease leading to corneal opacification at birth or in the first few months of life are congenital anomalies, intrauterine and perinatal infections, birth trauma, glaucoma, and corneal dystrophies. Metabolic conditions such as the mucopolysaccharidoses and the mucolipidoses do not give rise to corneal opacification before a few months of age. All children with corneal opacification should be referred to an ophthalmologist.

Leukocoria

Leukocoria (white pupil) is a white or tan reflex in the normally black pupillary area (Fig. 128.7). The reflex, which may be observed in certain ambient lighting conditions or only in certain directions of gaze, could theoretically result from opacification or tumefaction of any structure behind the iris (e.g., lens, vitreous, retina, choroid). Box 128.2 lists conditions that may be associated with leukocoria. The exact cause of the white reflex should be determined as soon as possible so that treatment for the underlying disease can be started. Retinoblastoma, discussed elsewhere in this chapter and in Chapter 101, is a major concern for children with leukocoria.

Retinopathy of Prematurity

Retinopathy of prematurity (ROP) is a vasoproliferative retinal disease that occurs in premature infants exposed to high concentrations of oxygen for prolonged periods. Two phases are observed: an acute proliferative phase and a cicatricial phase in which scarring and traction retinal detachment occur. More than 90% of patients with acute disease undergo spontaneous regression, and fewer than 10% of eyes develop significant cicatrization. It is estimated that about 40,000 premature infants are born annually in the United States, and that about 5% of these babies develop some degree of cicatricial ocular damage. Of the latter group, only 5% are totally blind or have severe permanent visual impairment. The most important risk factor in the development of ROP is low birth weight. The disease is rare in infants who weigh more than 2000 g at birth. ROP develops in 2% to 20% of babies weighing between 1,000 g and 1,500 g, and in 30% to 40% of those weighing less than 1,000 g. Other risk factors include gestational age, duration and concentration of oxygen exposure, shift of the oxygen dissociation curve by transfused adult hemoglobin, sepsis, high light intensity, hypoxia, and hypothermia.

Retinal vessels start growing at the nerve head from hyaloid vessels at 4 months' gestation and progress centrifugally to reach the nasal retina by 8 months and the temporal retinal periphery by 9 months or shortly after birth. ROP results from incomplete vascularization and sprouting of new vessels from the demarcation line between vascularized and nonvascularized retina. The pathogenic mechanisms of new vessel formation and the roles of the various agents implicated in ROP have not been fully elucidated; hypoxemia and hyperoxic damage to growing retinal vessels seem to be important factors. Fibrovascular proliferation results in traction on the normal retina, dragging of the macula and disc, and in partial or total retinal detachment in severe cases. In progressive ROP, the iris is involved, and dilated iris vessels can be seen on anterior segment examination.

An international committee developed a staging classification of ROP. In stage I, there is a demarcation line between vascular and avascular retina. In stage II, there is thickening of the demarcation line and formation of an intraretinal ridge. In stage III, new vessels arise from the ridge, and hemorrhages may be seen on or adjacent to the ridge. In stage IV, subtotal retinal detachment occurs posterior to the ridge, possibly involving one or more quadrants with traction and/or exudative components; the detachment is extrafoveal in stage IV-A and involves the fovea in stage IV-B. In stage V, there is total funnel-shaped retinal detachment, the funnel taking on one of various

BOX 128.2   Differential Diagnosis of a White Pupillary Reflex (Leukocoria)

Hereditary conditions
Norrie disease
Congenital cataract
Coloboma
Congenital retinoschisis
Incontinentia pigmenti
Familial exudative vitreoretinopathy

Developmental anomalies
Posterior hyperplastic primary vitreous
Cataract
Coloboma
Retinal dysplasia
Congenital retinal fold
Myelinated nerve fibers
Morning glory disc anomaly
Congenital corneal opacities

Inflammatory conditions
Nematode endophthalmitis (toxocariasis)
Congenital toxoplasmosis
Congenital cytomegalovirus retinitis
Herpes simplex retinitis
Peripheral uveoretinitis

Metastatic endophthalmitis
Orbital cellulitis

Tumors
Retinoblastoma
Retinal astrocytoma
Medulloepithelioma
Glioneuroma
Choroidal hemangioma
Retinal capillary hemangioma
Combined retinal hamartoma

Miscellaneous conditions
Retinal telangiectasia with exudation (Coats disease)
Retinopathy of prematurity
Rhegmatogenous retinal detachment
Vitreous hemorrhage
Perforating ocular injuries
Battered child syndrome

Modified from Shields JA, Augsburger JJ. Current approaches to the diagnosis and management of retinoblastoma. *Surv Ophthalmol* 1981;25:347.

configurations. Dilated posterior pole vessels place the disease level at the "plus" level, and the disease becomes more likely to progress to more advanced stages. The various stages can be localized to one of three zones of posteroanterior involvement. Neovascularization in stage III is quantified by clock hours of circumferential involvement. The more posterior the separation between vascularized and nonvascularized retina is, the lower the zone is. The more clock hours of neovascularization there are and the lower (or more posterior) the zone of the disease process is, the more likely is the progression to a poor visual outcome.

Newborns at risk for ROP should be examined by an ophthalmologist after discontinuation of oxygen therapy and before hospital discharge. If ROP is discovered, examinations should be repeated frequently. Significant changes may occur within days in patients with stage III disease, and laser therapy may be indicated. Most retina specialists have abandoned cryotherapy and favor the use of laser ablation in ROP. If regression is documented, examinations are done less frequently. The optimal time for examination is 6 to 10 weeks postpartum because this is when most cases of ROP are detected. Long-term complications of regressed ROP include high myopia and angle-closure glaucoma.

Current treatment of ROP consists of laser surgery to the avascular retina to arrest progression of the disease. A large multicenter trial has documented the value of this therapy. ROP has to reach, in general, a threshold of "plus" disease with 5 contiguous clock hours of neovascularization or 8 noncontiguous clock hours of neovascularization before treatment is initiated. However, more recent studies suggest that earlier treatment may be beneficial to selected patients, especially those with zone 1 and plus disease. Laser treatment appears to be better tolerated by infants and achieves similar favorable outcome as compared to the more invasive and less–well-tolerated cryotherapy. Vitrectomy and scleral buckling are performed in stages IV and V of the disease; visual results are variable but some patients achieve ambulatory or better vision. Intra-

venous vitamin E supplementation is not helpful in the prevention of ROP in premature infants and may be associated with a higher than normal risk of intraventricular hemorrhage and other complications of prematurity.

COMMON EYE PROBLEMS

Errors of Refraction

The most common cause of poor vision in childhood and adolescence is an error of refraction, the presence of which can be determined accurately by retinoscopy. The indications for prescribing glasses in children include significant visual impairment that interferes with the child's activity or the presence of asthenopia (ocular strain), strabismus, anisometropia (unequal error of refraction between the two eyes), or high astigmatism. The latter three conditions all predispose to amblyopia.

Visual Impairment

The pediatrician or ophthalmologist may be faced with the very delicate situation of parents observing poor visual responsiveness in their baby; the situation is even more complex in the case of a concomitant developmental delay or associated systemic disease. Before any statement is made about the infant's visual status or prognosis, a pediatric ophthalmologist should be consulted to perform a thorough evaluation. The clinical assessment includes observing the infant's general responsiveness to visual stimuli, recording abnormal ocular movements, and documenting wandering conjugate eye movements, which in blind children are usually horizontal and roving with or without tonic spasms and vertical jerky movements. Strabismus may or may not be present, and pupillary responses to a bright light stimulus may be reduced from normal levels. A careful search for organic eye disease and developmental anomalies is made, and refraction is tested. Optokinetic testing and cortical visual-evoked responses are helpful in documenting the presence of vision. Electroretinography should be performed for children in whom blindness is strongly suspected but who have a normal ocular examination and no evidence of cortical visual impairment. This test allows the detection of Leber congenital amaurosis, an autosomal recessive retinal dystrophy with onset at birth and in which visible retinal abnormalities may be absent or minimal.

Unilateral visual loss is more difficult to detect. Affected infants or children usually present with strabismus or with leukocoria, or the condition may be discovered on routine examination. Causes of unilateral blindness include unilateral high errors of refraction; various congenital abnormalities of the eye, especially optic nerve hypoplasia; trauma; and rarely retinoblastoma. All efforts should be made to uncover the cause of severe visual impairment in infants and children so that appropriate therapy can be instituted early and so that prognosis and genetic counseling can be offered in cases of inherited diseases with ocular involvement.

Leber congenital amaurosis is characterized by moderately to severely reduced vision before the age of 1 year, poor pupillary reaction, retinal degeneration, and markedly reduced or extinguished electroretinographic waveform. The disease is autosomal recessive, but there is genetic heterogeneity and several genetic defects have been identified to date. The ophthalmoscopic appearance is variable, ranging from normal to a typical retinitis pigmentosa-like picture with bone spicule formation, attenuation of retinal vessels, and waxy optic atrophy. Associated retinal changes include a salt-and-pepper appearance, chorioretinal atrophy, macular colobomas, retinitis punctata albescens, disc edema, and a nummular pigmentary pattern with round to oval pigmented lesions. Affected eyes may develop cataracts or keratoconus when the affected person is in his or her teens or 20s. Congenital cataracts are rare. Infants with Leber congenital amaurosis are usually examined in the first year of life because of poor vision, wandering eye movements, photophobia, and the oculodigital sign (i.e., the infant rubs the blind eyes, probably in an attempt to elicit some visual images through mechanical excitation of the retina). Although ophthalmoscopic findings change with age, visual acuity remains stable except in a subgroup of patients with macular "colobomas," in whom vision deteriorates. Associated systemic abnormalities include polycystic kidney disease, osteopetrosis, and skeletal anomalies. Neuropsychiatric disorders and mental retardation may coexist in patients with Leber congenital amaurosis and may be associated with concomitant central nervous system malformations or disease. The electroretinogram is essential to the diagnosis of this condition. Other causes of poor vision in infancy include bilateral optic nerve hypoplasia, achromatopsia, albinism, aniridia, congenital stationary night blindness, macular coloboma, and infectious chorioretinitis. Systemic diseases with retinal findings similar to those of Leber congenital amaurosis include Senior syndrome (familial nephronophthisis and tapetoretinal degeneration); Saldino-Mainzer syndrome (Senior syndrome plus cone-shaped epiphyses of the hands); Bassen-Kornzweig syndrome (abetalipoproteinemia); several peroxisomal disorders such as neonatal adrenoleukodystrophy, Zellweger syndrome, and infantile phytanic storage disease; and neurodegenerative disorders such as infantile neuronal ceroid lipofuscinosis. Peroxisomal disorders should be suspected in infants with pigmentary retinopathy, cataracts, hypotonia, and a Zellweger phenotype. Recent therapeutic interventions in animal RPE65 models of Leber congenital amaurosis promise effective intervention in some patients with this devastating disease.

Retinitis pigmentosa is a group of hereditary diseases characterized by progressive degeneration of the retina, retinal pig-

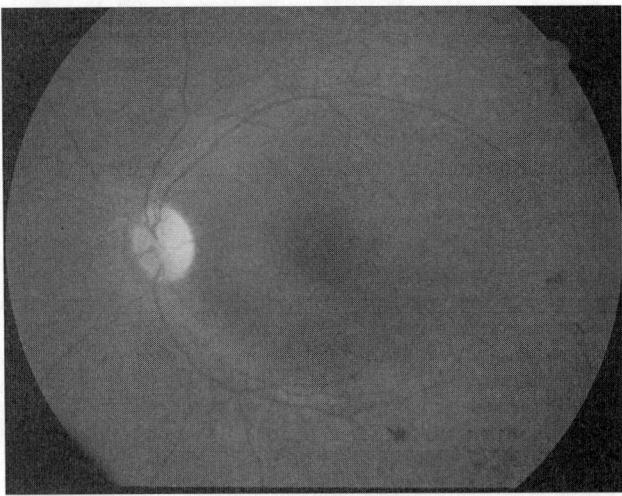

FIGURE 128.8. Fundus of patient with retinitis pigmentosa. The optic nerve head is pale, the blood vessels are attenuated, and there is mild atrophy and bony black spicule formation in the periphery.

ment epithelium, and choroid, with resultant loss of visual field and acuity. Ophthalmoscopy characteristically shows thinning of retinal vessels, waxy pallor of the optic disc, and peripheral bone corpuscle pigmentary changes, first in the equatorial area (Fig. 128.8). Choroidal sclerosis is a late feature of the disease. As the condition progresses, a peripheral scotoma appears, enlarges, and eventually reduces the visual field to a central area where acuity may be well preserved. Night blindness is a universal finding. Diagnosis is made clinically and confirmed on electroretinography. The electroretinographic response is markedly subnormal or nonrecordable, even in the absence of subjective visual symptoms. Other ocular findings include posterior subcapsular cataracts, myopia, keratoconus, and vitreous degeneration with a cellular response. About 25% of families with autosomal dominant retinitis pigmentosa have mutations in the rhodopsin gene. Others have mutations in the peripherin gene or other molecules involved in the process of phototransduction. Three modes of inheritance are recognized. X-linked recessive and autosomal recessive retinitis pigmentosa are more severe, start earlier, and result in earlier blindness than the autosomal dominant form. Nongenetic cases exist, confounding determination of the cause.

The Usher syndromes combine autosomal recessive retinitis pigmentosa with congenital deafness. Several types exist and show genetic heterogeneity. Box 128.3 lists some conditions associated with a retinitis pigmentosa-like fundus picture and symptoms.

Obstruction of the Lacrimal System

The majority (61%) of lacrimal drainage obstructions in children are developmental; others are caused by infections (24%), trauma (12%), and dysfunction (3%). Nasolacrimal duct (NLD) obstruction, most commonly caused by a failure of the distal membranous end of the NLD to open, occurs in 1.75% to 6.1% of infants and is bilateral in as many as one-third of cases. NLD obstruction may be caused by blockage elsewhere in the lacrimal system or by absence of the puncti or canaliculi, hence interfering with the normal drainage of tears. Rarely, lacrimal obstruction occurs as part of the facial clefting syndromes and the Goldenhar syndrome.

Infants with lacrimal obstruction present with a "wet-eyed" appearance, persistent or intermittent tearing, and various

Syndromes and Metabolic Diseases Involving Retinal Dystrophy

Usher syndrome
Alström syndrome
Kearns-Sayre syndrome
Bardet-Biedl syndrome
Cockayne syndrome
Retinitis pigmentosa with nephronophthisis
Abetalipoproteinemia
Mucopolysaccharidosis I, II, and III
Mucolipidosis IV
Neuronal ceroid lipofuscinosis
Cystinosis
Hyperornithinemia with gyrate atrophy of the choroid
    and retina
Methylmalonic aciduria with homocystinuria
Myotonic dystrophy
Olivopontocerebellar atrophy with macular degeneration
Sjögren-Larsson syndrome
Alagille syndrome

degrees of mucopurulent discharge over the medial canthal area and lids. Pressure over the lacrimal sac area expresses whitish material from the lacrimal puncti. Superimposed dacryocystitis may exist, and dacryocystoceles (Fig. 128.9) or fistulas may develop.

Most obstructions (90%) resolve spontaneously by 18 months of age, and lid hygiene alone is the indicated treatment in most cases. Fingertip or cotton-tip applicator massage over the lacrimal sac area, with massage directed inferiorly while the upper end of the lacrimal system is blocked, may be tried for a short period of time; this results in increased pressure inside the system, possibly causing the distal membrane to rupture into the nose. Chronic antibiotic therapy should be avoided. Some pediatric ophthalmologists prefer early probing after a short trial of conservative management for 2 to 4 weeks; this results in early patency of the system and avoids potential infections and continuous cosmetic annoyance. Patients are probed in the operating room under inhalation anesthesia. The surgery is successful in more than 90% of patients. If it fails, it may be repeated with or without silicone intubation of the lacrimal system. Silicone stents are left in place for 3 to 6 months. If probing and silicone intubation fail to maintain a patent sys-

tem, a dacryocystorhinostomy is performed. This procedure provides direct drainage of tears from the lacrimal sac into the nose. Complex microsurgical procedures can be performed for agenesis of the lacrimal puncti or canaliculi, for lacrimal fistulas, and for strictures of the lacrimal system. Dacryocystitis should be treated with systemic antibiotics and may resolve only after nasolacrimal probing.

Infections

Congenital Infections

The growing fetus acquires toxoplasmosis transplacentally in the third trimester of gestation from the often clinically healthy mother. At birth, affected infants have hydrocephalus, although intracranial calcifications may not yet be seen. Prematurity, low birth weight, microcephaly, and failure to thrive are frequent. The typical ocular lesions are large, healed chorioretinal scars with pigmented borders, usually in the macular area. Chorioretinal scars may be unilateral or bilateral. Occasionally, a newborn exhibits active lesions. Areas of active retinitis have a whitish, fluffy appearance and are associated with vitreous inflammatory cells. Strabismus and nystagmus may develop later. The diagnosis is made on clinical grounds and is confirmed serologically through complement fixation, indirect hemagglutination, and fluorescent-tagged antibody determinations.

Toxoplasma retinitis in older children, mostly around puberty, is usually due to reactivation of dormant organism at the edges of old congenital scarring. There is growing evidence that primary infection from the ingestion of organisms in raw meat can lead to new, nonreactivated retinitis. Toxoplasma retinochoroiditis may be associated with various degrees of vitreous and anterior segment inflammation. Small peripheral lesions without vitreous inflammation can be observed. Larger lesions warrant antimicrobial therapy; sulfadiazine, pyrimethamine, clindamycin, trimethoprim-sulfadoxine, and tetracycline have been used in various combinations. Some physicians use a 24-month course of pyrimethamine-sulfadoxine combined with folinic acid in all patients with congenital toxoplasmosis. The mother is also treated if prenatal testing is positive. This treatment regimen appears to offer satisfactory compliance, adequate serum concentrations, and good preventive efficacy.

Topical corticosteroids and cycloplegics should be given if ocular inflammation is mild. Severe inflammation and lesions impinging on the macula and optic nerve should be treated with systemic corticosteroids to minimize the damaging effects of necrotizing inflammation.

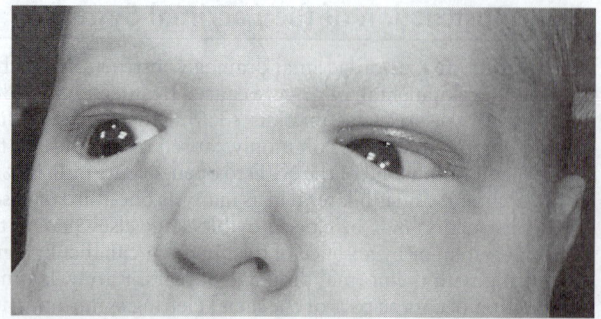
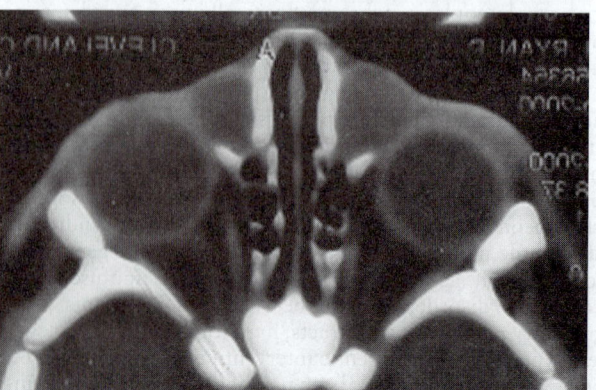

FIGURE 128.9. A: Clinical appearance with bilateral bluish bulges in area of lacrimal sac. See Color Figure 128.9A in color section. **B:** CT scan reveals cystic lesions in areas of lacrimal sac.

One of the main features of rubella embryopathy is the accompanying ophthalmopathy. Cataracts develop in more than half of patients with ocular rubella and are most likely to follow maternal infection between the second and eleventh weeks of gestation. The cataracts have a distinctive appearance, with a dense central opacity surrounded by a rim of more normal, although liquefied, cortex and a normal capsule. The lens may be swollen, and a total cataract may develop. Live virus in the lens may complicate surgical management, in which the lens has to be totally aspirated and preoperative steroids administered to minimize postoperative inflammation.

Because of associated ocular abnormalities, the visual outcome of cataract surgery in congenital rubella remains grim despite early intervention and aggressive occlusion therapy. Corneal edema may exist at birth, and keratoconus and corneal decompensation may develop later. The developing iris and ciliary body may be affected by the viral infection, and iris atrophy, lack of a dilator muscle, and focal necrosis of the iris pigment epithelium may occur. The anterior chamber angle may fail to develop adequately, possibly causing cleavage abnormalities. Rubella retinopathy, which gives the fundus a salt-and-pepper appearance, is most obvious in the posterior pole. The abnormal pigmentation is due to irregularities in distribution, hypoplasia, and hyperplasia of the retinal pigment epithelium. The retinopathy is progressive, and although vision is usually unaffected, visual acuity levels of 20/60 and less have been observed in the absence of cataracts or glaucoma. Ten percent of infants with congenital rubella have congenital glaucoma, which develops early in embryonic life and is therefore associated with a poor visual prognosis. Corneal clouding due to glaucoma should be differentiated from corneal clouding due to corneal involvement by the virus. Microphthalmos or microcornea may occur because of interference of the virus with normal ocular development. Oculomotor disorders such as strabismus, nystagmus, and ocular torticollis occur in 20% of children with congenital rubella syndrome. Strabismus is most often due to underlying amblyogenic factors such as cataracts, glaucoma, cortical blindness, optic atrophy, and high refractive errors.

Most cytomegalovirus infections at birth are clinically insignificant. Symptomatic babies are usually quite ill with hepatosplenomegaly, jaundice, petechiae, microcephaly, intracranial calcification, optic atrophy, and retinitis (Fig. 128.10). Mortality is high. Long-term effects of congenital infection are deafness and slow development. The typical ocular feature is a retinitis similar to that of adults, with hemorrhages and exudates usually along blood vessels. Ocular disease is seen in 20% of symptomatic newborns who have other affected organs, and occurs only if the infection is intrauterine. Associated ocular abnormalities include anophthalmia, optic nerve hypoplasia and colobomas, Peters anomaly, and iridocyclitis. Cytomegalovirus retinitis has been observed in infants with acquired immunodeficiency syndrome and may lead to blindness if the macula is involved.

Congenital syphilis is rare in developed countries because of the widespread use of antibiotics, screening for the disease before marriage, and maternal screening at the onset of pregnancy. Infants with congenital syphilis have fever, skin rash, pneumonitis, and hepatosplenomegaly. Active choroiditis may be seen, but most affected babies have only peripheral pigmentary changes. Active keratitis is rare.

Neonatal herpes simplex virus (HSV) ocular infection is transmitted to the newborn in the mother's infected birth canal during delivery or shortly before though ruptured membranes. Twenty percent of neonates with HSV infection have ocular involvement, which can take the form, in order of decreasing frequency, of conjunctivitis, keratitis, retinitis, cataracts, and microphthalmia. Most cases are associated with cutaneous herpetic vesicles. Neonatal HSV conjunctivitis and keratitis are seen in the first 2 weeks and must be differentiated

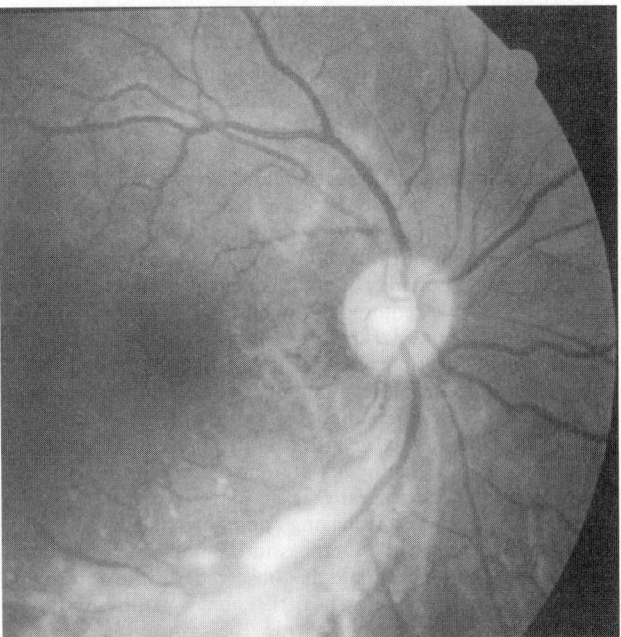

FIGURE 128.10. Cytomegalovirus retinitis. The exudation and hemorrhages occur along blood vessels, shown here along the superotemporal arcade.

from other causes of ophthalmia neonatorum. Cataracts associated with neonatal HSV infection may be unilateral or bilateral. They may be secondary to uveitis or to direct viral invasion of the lens. Retinitis is usually diagnosed between 3 weeks and 3 months of age but may be detected earlier. Retinal findings range in severity from small peripheral chorioretinal scars to blinding necrotizing retinitis. Active retinitis is marked by patches of yellow-white intraretinal exudates, intraretinal hemorrhages, vascular sheathing, vitreitis, and anterior chamber pleocytosis. Retinal detachment may occur in severe cases. Other causes of infantile retinitis include cytomegalovirus, syphilis, rubella, *Toxoplasma* infection, *Candida* infection, tuberculosis, and histoplasmosis.

Ophthalmia Neonatorum

Conjunctivitis is the most common ocular disease of newborns, occurring in 1.6% to 12% of neonates. The cause and incidence of neonatal conjunctivitis have been altered by the routine use of silver nitrate and antibiotic prophylaxis. Silver nitrate is effective in preventing gonococcal conjunctivitis, but it has no effect on *Chlamydia trachomatis*. The 1980s were marked by a dramatic increase in the prevalence of chlamydial neonatal conjunctivitis due to maternal genital chlamydial disease. The use of 1% tetracycline ointment and of erythromycin ointment, instead of silver nitrate drops, has reduced the incidence of gonococcal and chlamydial ophthalmia neonatorum. Direct immunofluorescent monoclonal antibody staining has proved useful in the diagnosis of neonatal chlamydial conjunctivitis. Of 100 neonates with conjunctivitis in one study, 43 were found to have chlamydial disease. Rates as high as 73% have been reported. Other causal agents in ophthalmia neonatorum include *Staphylococcus aureus*, *Haemophilus influenzae*, *Streptococcus pneumoniae*, *Escherichia coli*, *Proteus mirabilis*, *Klebsiella pneumoniae*, *Branhamella catarrhalis*, *Neisseria gonorrhoeae*, *Pseudomonas aeruginosa*, *Staphylococcus epidermidis*, *Streptococcus viridans*, and coxsackievirus A9.

The external appearance of the eye is generally the same, regardless of the causative agent. In addition to swelling of the lids and conjunctiva, there is profuse and sometimes bloody discharge, especially if pseudomembranes are formed. The timing of the infection in relation to birth is helpful, although not diagnostic, in the determination of the causative agent. Chemical and mechanical conjunctivitis occur in the first day of life and are due to birth trauma and manipulation or to silver nitrate prophylaxis itself. Gonococcal conjunctivitis, which is acquired in the birth canal, usually becomes manifest between days 2 and 4. The remaining organisms cause conjunctivitis at various time intervals after birth. Pseudomonas conjunctivitis is particularly aggressive and may be complicated by corneal ulceration and blindness. It is acquired in the hospital and should be suspected in infants on mechanical ventilation with other foci of *Pseudomonas* infection. Treatment consists of frequent instillation of fortified topical aminoglycoside or fluoroquinolone eye drops and systemic aminoglycosides or other appropriate antibiotics if other foci of infection are present. Gonococcal conjunctivitis and chlamydial conjunctivitis require systemic and topical antibiotic therapy.

An infant suspected of having conjunctivitis should be immediately isolated. If the infant is in the nursery, strict handwashing precautions should be observed. If the mother is found to be free of gonorrhea, the nursery staff should be checked for the disease, which may be transmitted through hand contact. Conjunctival scrapings for Gram and Giemsa stains and for a direct immunofluorescent monoclonal antibody stain for *Chlamydia* should be obtained. Aerobic, anaerobic, and chlamydial cultures should all be done. Therapy is initiated based on the results of the staining, with definitive culture pending. Patients suspected of having chlamydial disease should be given oral erythromycin ethylsuccinate (50 mg/kg/day in four divided doses) for 2 weeks. If erythromycin fails to clear chlamydial conjunctivitis, a 2-week course of oral trimethoprim-sulfamethoxazole and a concurrent 1-week course of topical tetracycline usually result in the eradication of the infection. If gonococcal conjunctivitis is suspected, the infant is admitted to the hospital and started on intravenous aqueous penicillin G potassium (50,000 U/kg/day; 20,000 units/kg/day if the infant is premature; in four divided doses) and saline lavage of the eyes. Parents and their sexual partners should be treated for chlamydial and gonococcal infection in the usual manner. Gram-negative bacilli indicate treatment with gentamicin sulfate ophthalmic ointment, using one application four times per day for 1 week. If gram-positive cocci or inflammatory cells without organisms are found, erythromycin ophthalmic ointment should be given four times per day for 1 week.

Bacteria may be cultured from the conjunctivae of infants with chlamydial conjunctivitis. The child with recurrent conjunctivitis should be suspected of having nasolacrimal duct obstruction, and patency of the lacrimal system should be tested. The management of obstruction of the lacrimal system was discussed earlier in this chapter.

Hordeolum and Chalazion

A hordeolum results from acute infection of the meibomian glands that are located in the tarsal plates in the lid and that secrete the mucinous component of the tear film. A hordeolum is characterized by swelling, redness, and pain near the lid margin. The inflammatory process leads to the formation of a small abscess that points and ruptures to the outside within a few days. Treatment consists of the frequent application of warm water compresses and the application of antibiotic ointment three to four times per day.

Granulomatous inflammation of the meibomian glands leads to the formation of chalazia that appear as small bumps within the lid tissues over the tarsal plates (Fig. 128.11). Treatment consisting of warm compresses and combination

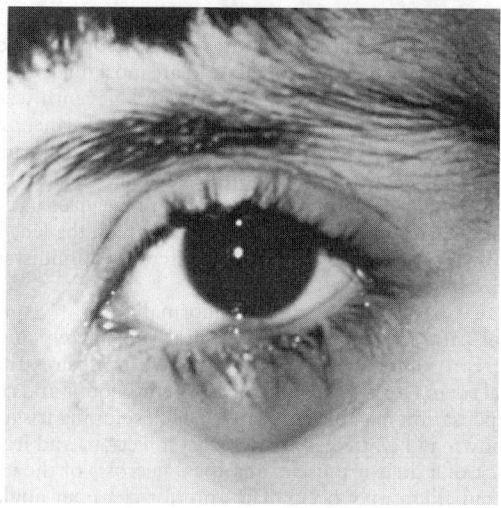

FIGURE 128.11. An unusually large chalazion of the lower lid. Chalazia are usually much smaller than hordeola and can be detected by palpation.

antibiotic–steroid ointment should be tried for 2 to 4 weeks. If the chalazion fails to resolve and is cosmetically blemishing, it can be excised through a conjunctival approach. Intralesional Celestone injections have been tried with some success.

Conjunctivitis

Three major categories of conjunctivitis are recognized: infectious, allergic, and traumatic or chemical. Ocular conditions that should be differentiated from simple conjunctivitis include iritis (i.e., inflammation of the iris, a form of anterior uveitis), acute glaucoma, traumatic corneal abrasions, and infectious corneal ulceration. Table 128.3 lists the differentiating features of these various conditions.

In bacterial conjunctivitis, conjunctival hyperemia is marked, and there is a moderate to copious purulent discharge (Fig. 128.12). The patient is usually in pain and has a foreign body sensation in the eye. Vision, pupillary reflexes, intraocular pressure, and corneal clarity are all normal. Staphylococcal blepharitis or chronic infection or inflammation at the lid margins is a common associated finding. Cultures may be obtained, and bilateral antibiotic eye drops or ointment should be started. Antibiotic choices keep changing, but broad-spectrum antibiotic drops or ointment should be used initially; they may be changed later, depending on the results of culture and antimicrobial sensitivity. Antibiotics may prevent recurrences and shorten the course of the disease somewhat, but bacterial conjunctivitis usually improves within 4 to 5 days irrespective of treatment.

Viral conjunctivitis may lead to a mild purulent discharge, but tearing and lid swelling, with or without preauricular lymphadenopathy, are the prominent features. Photophobia and blepharospasm with squeezing of the lids, usually in response to light, occur if the cornea is involved. Adenoviruses are common causative agents. Primary herpetic conjunctivitis is not easily recognized unless it is accompanied by herpetic lesions on the lids (Fig. 128.13). Treatment of viral conjunctivitis (except for herpes simplex type 1) is symptomatic; mild steroid drops may be given if inflammation and swelling are severe. Cold compresses and lubricants can be used.

The hallmark of allergic conjunctivitis is itching. There is usually a stringy mucoid discharge. Allergic conjunctivitis may be seasonal or be associated with hay fever. The patient frequently has a history of allergic disorders. Mild vasoconstrictor,

DIFFERENTIAL DIAGNOSIS OF CONJUNCTIVITIS

Finding	Acute Conjunctivitis	Allergy	Iritis	Acute Glaucoma	Corneal Abrasion/Ulcer
Pain	Mild	None	Moderate	Moderate	Severe
Tearing	Mild to moderate	Moderate	Moderate	None	Severe
Discharge	Moderate to copious	Moderate	None	None	Watery/purulent
Incidence	Very common	Very common	Uncommon	Uncommon	Common/uncommon
Vision	Normal	Normal	Mildly decreased	Decreased	Decreased
Injection	Diffuse	Diffuse	Perilimbal	Perilimbal	Diffuse
Cornea	Clear	Clear	Clear	Clear to cloudy	Clear/hazy
Intraocular pressure	Normal	Normal	Normal	Increased	Normal
Pupil size	Normal	Normal	Small	Middilated	Normal
Pupillary reaction	Normal	Normal	Poor	Very poor	Normal
Culture	Causative organism	Normal	Normal	Normal	Normal/causative agent

Modified from DeAngelis C. The eye. In: DeAngelis C, ed. *Pediatric primary care,* 3rd ed. Boston: Little, Brown, 1984:221.

decongestant drops are usually sufficient to improve symptoms in mild cases; mild steroid drops may be necessary in more severe cases. In vernal conjunctivitis, a seasonal, rather severe allergic ocular condition characterized by large palpebral conjunctival papillae and perilimbal infiltrates, 4% Cromolyn sodium drops have decreased recurrence rates and shortened the course of the disease if administered frequently and prophylactically. Several new agents are available for the treatment of ocular allergy and include the antihistamines Patanol and Livostin and the mast cell stabilizer Alomide.

Although rarely encountered with current modes of practice, the classic example of a chemical conjunctivitis is that induced by silver nitrate prophylaxis or Credé procedure in newborns. Any chemical that reaches the ocular surface is potentially toxic. The most serious of the chemical conjunctivitises are those caused by alkali. Many common household detergents are strong alkali that can cause serious ocular injuries if they come in contact with the eye. An ophthalmologist should be immediately consulted in case of suspected ocular alkali burns. Pending the ophthalmologist's arrival, topical anesthetic drops should be instilled and the eye copiously irrigated for as long as possible with at least 2 L of normal saline solution or until a litmus paper test reveals a normal pH. Any debris or foreign bodies should be washed out of the conjunctival fornices. Because the bulk of the ocular damage occurs within the first few minutes of exposure, irrigation should be done immediately. The ophthalmologist treats the patient for the ocular surface, cornea, and lid problems that are produced by these potentially severe injuries.

Periorbital and Orbital Cellulitis

Periorbital and orbital cellulitis are bacterial infections of the eyelids and orbital area. In preseptal or periorbital cellulitis, the infection remains anterior to the orbital septum, a fibrous structure located in the lids and separating the orbit proper from the subcutaneous lid structures. In orbital cellulitis, the infection involves the orbit proper and may affect all orbital structures, including extraocular muscles, sensory and motor nerves, and the optic nerve. The two types may coexist, and one may lead to the other.

Bacterial organisms may gain access to the preseptal or orbital space through the lid skin secondary to insect bites, pustules, or trauma. They may also gain access through adjacent infected paranasal sinuses, upper respiratory tract, or teeth. *S. aureus* is the most common cause of disease acquired through the lids. With the increasing prevalence of methicillin-resistant *S. aureus* (MRSA), appropriate cultures and sensitivities should be obtained and empiric initial antimicrobial therapy should take into account the possibility that MRSA is the responsible organism.

Other causative organisms are *Streptococcus pyogenes, Peptostreptococcus, Bacteroides,* and others. *H. influenzae* gains access to the orbit from upper respiratory tract infections, bacteremia, or sinusitis. It is a leading cause of periorbital and orbital cellulitis in children. Children younger than 5 years of age are immunologically most susceptible to *H. influenzae,* especially to the b serotype. Fungal orbital cellulitis

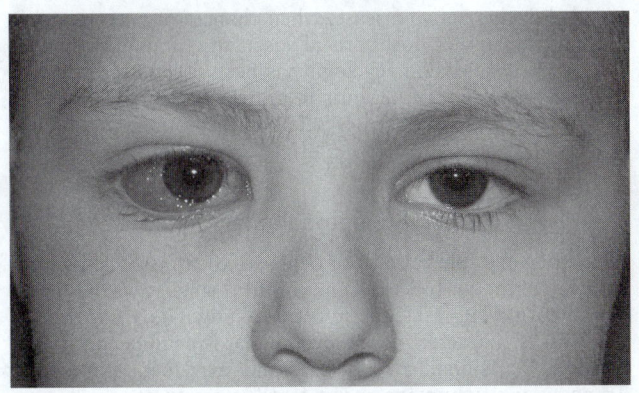

FIGURE 128.12. Right conjunctivitis. Note conjunctival chemosis, redness, and discharge. See Color Figure 128.12 in color section.

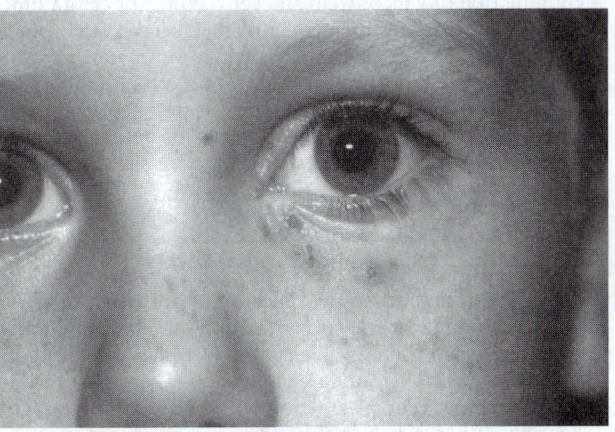

FIGURE 128.13. Periocular vesicular lesions of herpetic blepharoconjunctivitis. The recognition of the skin lesions allows the diagnosis of herpes simplex disease.

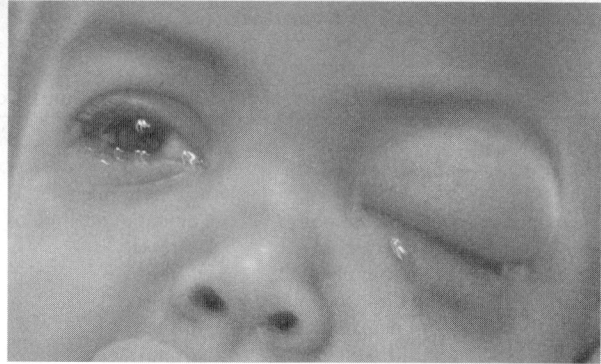

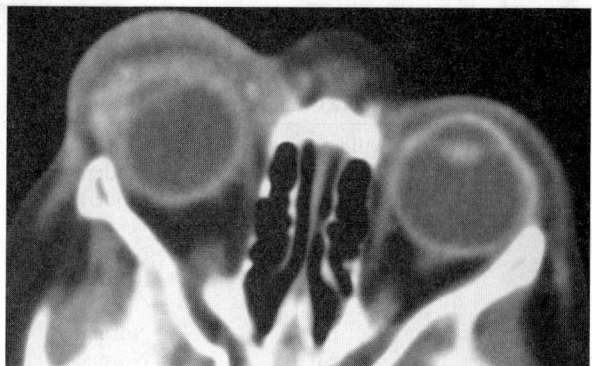

FIGURE 128.14. A: Severe swelling in left lids in this child with preseptal cellulites. **B:** CT scan reveals that inflammation is restricted to preseptal area.

such as phycomycosis or aspergillosis is rare, usually occurring only in immunocompromised or ketoacidotic persons; the orbit is involved through extension of the disease from infected paranasal sinuses.

Proptosis and limitation of ocular motility differentiate orbital from preseptal cellulitis. Fever, lid swelling, redness, and hotness occur in both (Fig. 128.14A). Computed tomography is helpful in documenting orbital involvement and delineating orbital and subperiosteal abscesses, as well as revealing any evidence of sinusitis (Fig. 128.14B). Tomography is used to exclude the diagnosis of rhabdomyosarcoma. Complications of orbital cellulitis include orbital abscess, subperiosteal abscess, cavernous sinus thrombosis, meningitis, brain abscess, and orbital apex syndrome.

Orbital cellulitis is a medical emergency, and early diagnosis and treatment are imperative. Children with this condition should be admitted to the hospital. A complete blood count and cultures of any skin lesion around the eye or nasopharynx, blood, and subcutaneous aspirate should be obtained. Computed tomographic films of the orbits are mandatory. An ophthalmologist should be consulted. Periorbital cellulitis is treated with intravenous antibiotics until the periorbital induration and redness decrease. Oral antibiotics are then substituted for intravenous therapy for an additional 7 to 10 days. If a skin infection is documented in the cause of the condition, penicillinase-resistant penicillin such as methicillin or cloxacillin, or other antibiotics that would be effective against the suspected bacterial agent should be administered. With the emergence of beta-lactamase–producing strains of *H. influenzae*, cephalosporins have become the mainstay of treatment. A combination of vancomycin and ceftriaxone (or cefotaxime) is appropriate empiric therapy until the specific organism is identified.

For orbital cellulitis, intravenous antibiotics are given for 2 weeks, followed by oral antibiotics in the recovery phase. Surgical drainage of orbital abscesses may be necessary if they are localized. More extensive surgery is necessary in the rare instance of mucormycosis.

Keratitis and Corneal Ulcers

Bacterial keratitis and corneal ulceration are unusual in the absence of trauma or use of contact lenses. The conjunctiva is hyperemic, and there is a central or peripheral corneal epithelial defect with surrounding infiltration. There usually is an anterior chamber cellular reaction with or without hypopyon formation. When a bacterial ulcer is suspected, scrapings of the ulcer margins should be obtained for Gram stain, and routine cultures should be taken. If no organisms are identified on the slide smear, broad-spectrum antibiotics are started with a

combination of tobramycin (14 mg/mL) one drop every hour alternating with fortified cefazolin (50 mg/mL) one drop every hour. If the corneal ulcer is small, peripheral, and superficial, intensive monotherapy with fluoroquinolones is an alternative treatment. Other antimicrobials can be used, depending on the clinical progress and laboratory findings. The most common organisms to spread after trauma are staphylococci. For wearers of soft contact lenses with rapidly progressing central corneal ulceration and melting, *Pseudomonas aeruginosa* should be considered to be the causative agent until proved otherwise. Fungal and amebic ulcers are rarely seen in the pediatric population but should be suspected in the case of chronic ulcers that are not responding to antibiotic therapy.

Herpes simplex keratitis is one of the leading causes of loss of vision in young adults. Primary infection occurs in childhood in the form of a conjunctivitis or keratoconjunctivitis with or without the formation of classic epithelial dendritic lesions. After the primary infection, the virus remains latent in the trigeminal or other ganglia. In recurrences, the virus travels to the cornea by way of the sensory nerves, causing dendritic or geographic lesions. Treatment in such cases consists of débridement of the ulcer margin and frequent administration of topical antiviral agents such as idoxuridine, adenosine arabinoside, or trifluorothymidine until healing occurs. Stromal keratitis is characterized by corneal stromal necrosis, thinning, and neovascularization. Because immunologic factors play a role in stromal disease, treatment involves use of steroids in conjunction with antiviral medications. Disciform keratitis develops in patients with previous dendritic disease owing to an immunologic stromal reaction to herpes antigens. Treatment consists of cautious use of mild steroids. Corneal transplantation may be necessary in patients with recurrent disease that has resulted in opaque vascularized corneas. Surgery is to be avoided during active disease, when chances of graft rejection are high because of host corneal vascularization and reactivation of the virus. Oral acyclovir has been used successfully to prevent recurrence of keratitis in grafted patients. The use of oral acyclovir in primary herpetic keratoconjunctivitis is controversial.

Endophthalmitis

Nematode endophthalmitis or ocular toxocariasis results from invasion of the eye by the second- or third-stage larva of the dog roundworm. This systemic infection, known as visceral larva migrans, is characterized by fever, hepatosplenomegaly, pneumonitis, occasional encephalitis, and extreme eosinophilia. Transmission to humans occurs from ingestion of roundworm eggs in soil contaminated by feces from infected dogs, or from contaminated hands or fomites. A history of geophagia or pica should be obtained in children suspected of having ocular toxocariasis.

In the United States, visceral larva migrans is most prevalent in the south-central and southeastern regions. Children with visceral larva migrans are most often boys between 6 months and 3 years of age at the onset of symptoms. There usually is a history of contact with puppies, and many children are reported by parents to be geophagic. Leukocyte counts range from 30,000 to 90,000 with 50% to 90% eosinophils, and the eosinophil count may remain elevated for months or years. Granulomas form in infected tissues after the acute stage of eosinophilic abscesses subsides.

Severe cases of nematode endophthalmitis are treated with steroids. Anthelmintics such as diethylcarbamazine or thiabendazole relieve symptoms and shorten convalescence time. For most patients, prognosis is excellent, and in many, the disease is self-limited and subclinical. However, associated encephalitis and myocarditis may be lethal. Ocular involvement may occur after a clear-cut episode of previous visceral larva migrans, concurrently with the systemic disease, or without any previously manifested disease. It is usually manifested as endophthalmitis with a solitary chorioretinal granuloma with or without retinal traction. The granuloma may be in the posterior pole or in the fundus periphery. The disease is most often unilateral in children, although bilateral occurrences have been reported in adults. There is no pathognomonic presentation. Children are seen because of uveitis or endophthalmitis, strabismus, or poor vision. Ocular toxocariasis has commonly been confused with retinoblastoma, and the eyes of many children with toxocariasis have been unnecessarily enucleated in the past. Ultrasonography differentiates the granulomas of ocular toxocariasis from retinoblastoma by the absence of high peaks due to calcifications in retinoblastoma. An enzyme-linked immunosorbent assay (ELISA) for *Toxocara canis* is positive at a 1:8 dilution in about 90% of patients with ocular toxocariasis, but it is uniformly negative in patients with retinoblastoma. Cytology of aqueous humor is likely to reveal eosinophils in toxocariasis and tumor cells in seeded retinoblastoma. Severe ocular toxocariasis can lead to numerous complications and even loss of the eye. Systemic and topical steroids should be administered to reduce ocular inflammation and its sequelae, and anthelmintics should be given to destroy the larvae. Intraocular surgery and laser treatment are performed in selected cases.

Bacterial endophthalmitis is rare in the pediatric age group. It may occur after intraocular surgery such as cataract extraction or filtering surgery for glaucoma, after trauma, or secondary to bacterial embolization from endocarditis or disseminated infection. It can be a blinding condition if the intraocular contents are destroyed by necrotizing inflammation. Vitreous cultures and intravitreal injection of antibiotics should be performed early, and the patient should be started on systemic antibiotics and concentrated topical antibiotic eye drops. A therapeutic vitrectomy may also be helpful and serves to empty the globe from the white cells that are causing the destruction of the ocular layers. The visual prognosis is guarded.

Pinguicula and Pterygium

Pingueculae are elevated conjunctival lesions that usually occur near the nasal or temporal corneoscleral limbus in the area of the interpalpebral fissure. When these growths impinge on the cornea, they are called pterygia (Fig. 128.15). Histopathologically, the lesions consist of degenerated collagen that looks like elastin but is not digested by elastase. Ultraviolet radiation is thought to play an important role in the pathogenesis of pterygia. No treatment is required except in cases of recurrent inflammation of a pinguecula, for which mild steroid drops are given. If a pterygium grows toward the central corneal area,

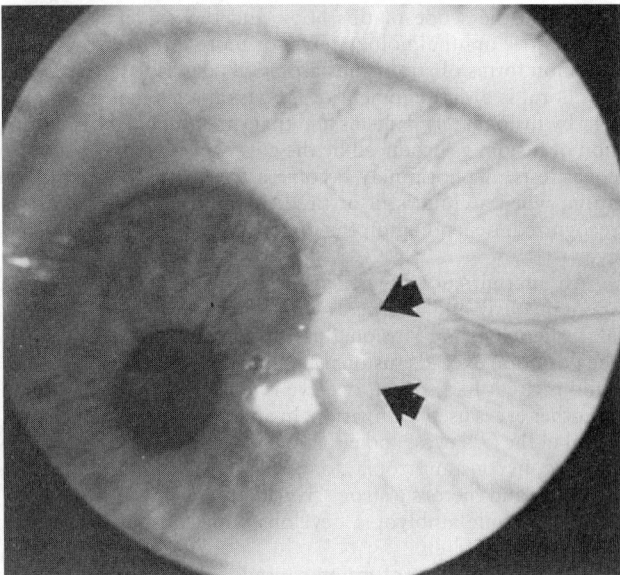

FIGURE 128.15. Anterior-segment photograph showing a small pterygium (*arrows*).

surgical excision may be indicated. There is a 30% to 40% rate of recurrence after excision.

Strabismus and Amblyopia

The pediatrician often has reason to suspect ocular misalignment in an infant or child. Pseudostrabismus is the false impression of ocular misalignment as a result of a prominence of epicanthal folds or variations in orbital alignment in a young child. Pseudostrabismus may simulate esotropia (inward deviation of an eye) or, less frequently, exotropia (outward deviation of an eye). Well-centered corneal light reflexes in both eyes and normal fixation patterns are usually sufficient to rule out true constant strabismus (Fig. 128.16). Parents can be reassured that epicanthal folds will decrease as the child grows and the nasal bridge becomes more prominent, pulling the skin away from the globe and uncovering more of the sclera. A positive family history of strabismus should raise suspicion of true strabismus, in which case a detailed ophthalmologic assessment is always mandatory. A detailed discussion of all types of strabismus

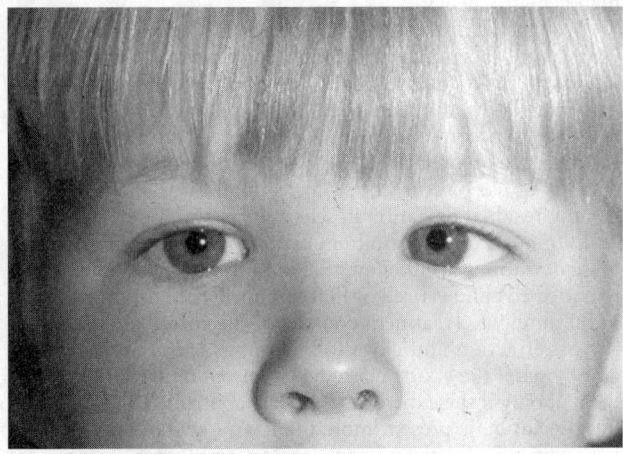

FIGURE 128.16. Hirschberg test. Corneal light reflex falls on temporal edge of pupil in the left eye indicating the presence of esotropia.

is beyond the scope of this book and the reader is referred to pediatric ophthalmology texts for more information. Some common forms of strabismus are briefly described hereafter.

Phoria is a misalignment of the visual axes that is kept latent by fusional mechanisms and that can be elicited by disruption of fusion, as produced by the cover-uncover and alternate cover tests. A phoria may become a tropia, or constant deviation, when a child is ill or tired. Exophoria or esophoria is recognized, depending on the direction of drift of the covered eye.

An intermittent tropia exists if ocular misalignment occurs spontaneously and alternates with longer periods of good ocular alignment and fusion. Intermittent tropias occur when the deviation exceeds fusional capabilities, especially when the child is tired. In a tropia, one eye is constantly deviated while the other eye is used for fixation. In alternating tropias, vision is equal in the two eyes, and either one deviates when the other is fixating. In constant tropias, one eye is always in the abnormal position, and there is a strong fixation preference for the other eye. Strabismic amblyopia develops with constant tropias in very young children.

Amblyopia is loss of vision caused not by an organic ocular or visual pathway lesion, but rather by disuse of one eye and predominant use of the other. The mechanism of vision loss is thought to be of central nervous system origin. This is a reversible process in younger children, and one major aim of strabismus treatment is the prevention or reversal of amblyopia, in addition to the restoration of good ocular alignment and of binocular vision. Amblyopia therapy consists of patching of the better eye to allow stimulation of the central visual centers from the deviated eye. The younger the child is, the faster and more dramatic is the response to short periods of occlusion therapy. Longer periods of patching are required in older children. There is some debate about the upper limit of age at which amblyopia is still reversible; it may be around 10 years of age. Pharmacologic penalization using atropine cycloplegia of the better seeing eye has been shown to be as effective as patching in patients with moderate (20/40 to 20/80) amblyopia.

Congenital or infantile esotropia is not present at birth but is diagnosed in the first 6 months of life. The angle of ocular deviation is usually large, and there is little refractive error. Associated conditions include overacting inferior oblique muscles and dissociated vertical deviations, which may manifest later in childhood despite initial surgical therapy and good ocular alignment (Fig. 128.17). Surgery should be performed before 2 years of age, and preferably around 6 months of age, if binocular vision is to be achieved. There is frequently a positive family history for this likely autosomal recessive disease with high gene frequency.

Accommodative esotropia becomes evident in the first few years of life. It is probably the most common type of strabismus in clinical practice. It is due to an inordinate amount of convergence followed by unilateral inward deviation of the eye in response to accommodative efforts to focus a retinal image in the presence of a relatively large degree of hyperopia. Therapy consists of use of corrective glasses in all cases and of surgery for any residual deviation in selected cases.

Exophoria and intermittent exotropia are intermittent outward deviations of either eye that initially become evident when the affected child is tired or ill. Exophoric patients often squint in the sunlight. Treatment consists of the correction of any error of refraction and close follow-up. There is no associated amblyopia if the exotropia remains intermittent. Surgery is indicated only if the exotropia is poorly controlled and the manifest deviation is present more than 50% of the time. Patients with constant exotropia can develop amblyopia. Congenital exotropia is much less common than congenital or infantile esotropia and is treated surgically.

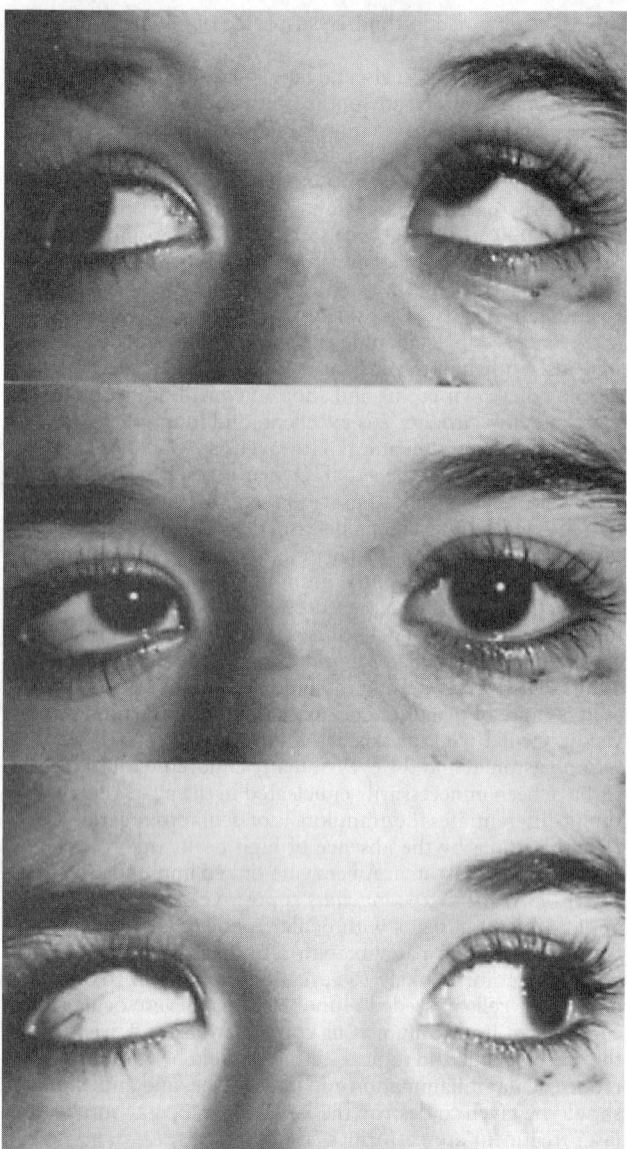

FIGURE 128.17. Right esotropia with overaction of the inferior oblique muscles. Notice the elevation of the abducted eye (toward the nose) in right and left gazes, indicating overaction of the inferior oblique muscles.

Duane syndrome type I is characterized by esotropia, limited abduction of the eye, and retraction of the globe with palpebral fissure narrowing on attempted adduction (Fig. 128.18). Girls are affected more commonly than boys and left eyes more than right. Duane syndrome type I results from innervation of the lateral rectus muscle by a branch of the oculomotor nerve and absence of the sixth nerve nucleus and its fasciculus and nerve to the lateral rectus; this abnormal congenital cranial dyseinnervation leads to co-contraction of the medial and lateral rectus muscles on attempted adduction. Other less common types of Duane syndrome include Duane type II, in which there is limitation of adduction of the involved eye, and type III, which is characterized by limited adduction and abduction. Some patients with Duane type I have ipsilateral hearing loss. Others have associated Goldenhar syndrome or radial ray skeletal defects. Some cases have occurred in patients with the fetal alcohol syndrome.

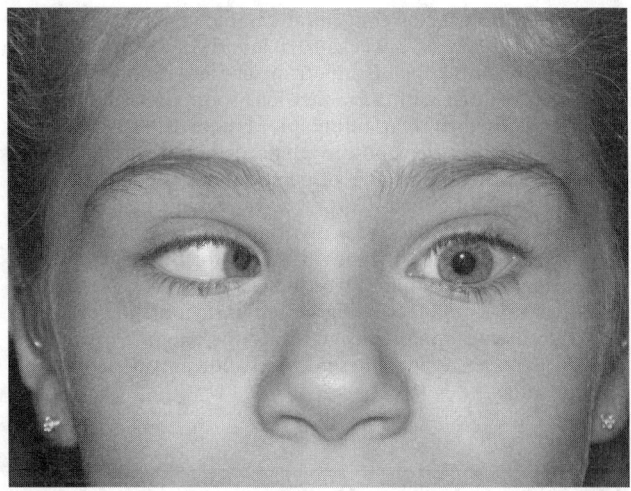

FIGURE 128.18. Patient with left Duane syndrome attempting to look to the left. Left eye does not abduct beyond midline.

In Brown superior oblique tendon sheath syndrome there is an inability to elevate the eye in adduction (Fig. 128.19). Most cases are congenital, although acquired cases have been documented. The treatment results in elongating the superior oblique tendon using a silicone spacer.

Möbius syndrome is characterized by unilateral or bilateral sixth- and seventh-nerve palsies. Affected children usually demonstrate esotropia and an expressionless face. Babies with this condition have difficulties breast-feeding and sucking their bottles. Associated anomalies include the Poland anomaly (absence of the pectoralis muscle and radial defects) and terminal limb defects.

Extraocular muscle palsies in children result in incomitant strabismus where different measurements are obtained in different directions of gaze; the largest deviation is measured in the field of action of the affected muscle. Children with acquired palsies may not verbalize a complaint of diplopia, but they may squint, cover one eye with a hand, or assume a compensatory head posture to avoid diplopia.

Third-nerve palsies are most commonly due to trauma or to increased intracranial pressure, and they may be complete or incomplete. Other causes include inflammation, infectious and parainfectious processes, vascular lesions, tumors, and degenerative and demyelinating disease involving the nerve. Diabetes is not a cause of third-nerve palsy in the pediatric population. Associated neurologic defects are good clues to the location

of the lesion causing the nerve palsy. Like third-nerve palsies, fourth-nerve palsies are commonly due to trauma or tumor, but many are idiopathic and present at birth. Examination of old photographs reveal the characteristic head tilt and provide a good clue to the chronic and benign nature of congenital fourth-nerve palsies. Surgery is indicated to relieve the torticollis that may lead to chronic neck pain and to scoliosis.

Sixth-nerve palsies are common in children. They may indicate neurologic disease, but many are transitory and benign and follow viral infections. A sixth-nerve palsy may be the result of increased intracranial pressure from hydrocephalus, tumor, intracranial hemorrhage, or cerebral edema. It may be due to trauma, inflammatory conditions such as meningitis, and degenerative or demyelinating conditions. Benign sixth-nerve palsy in children develops 1 to 3 weeks after a febrile illness and usually subsides within 6 months. The child with cranial nerve palsy should undergo a complete neurologic evaluation, including computed tomography or magnetic resonance imaging of the head. A history of recent viral disease should be obtained, and the child should receive care from an ophthalmologist and a neurologist.

Nystagmus refers to rhythmic oscillations of the eyes that occur independently of normal movements. In pendular nystagmus, the velocity of movement is equal in the two directions. In contrast, jerk nystagmus has slow and fast components. The different kinds of nystagmus are named according to the refixation and the direction in which the nystagmus occurs (e.g., in right-beating jerk nystagmus, the fast refixation component is to the right). In conjugate nystagmus, binocular oscillations are in phase, unlike disjugate or dissociated nystagmus, which can be monocular or binocular with a slow component that is out of phase. Latent nystagmus is elicited by interruption of binocular vision such as occlusion of one eye. Congenital nystagmus is present at birth and may be associated with abnormal head movements and positions. Visual acuity is usually decreased. Albinism is probably the most common cause of nystagmus in childhood. Tyrosinase-positive oculocutaneous albinism may be difficult to diagnose except using the slit lamp. Retroillumination reveals total iris transillumination in patients with any type of albinism. In addition, patients with albinism have foveal hypoplasia and misrouting of optic nerve fibers.

Strabismus may be superimposed on congenital nystagmus, which can be inherited as an autosomal dominant, recessive, or X-linked recessive trait. Sensory defect nystagmus is due to defects in the afferent visual system. Any abnormality of the eye that interferes with good image formation and transmission from the retina can result in nystagmus. Motor defect nystagmus is due to a defect in the efferent motor system, possibly at the level of centers or pathways for conjugate motor control.

Spasmus nutans is characterized by small-amplitude and very-fast-velocity nystagmus accompanied by head nodding and sometimes torticollis. Spasmus nutans starts between 4 and 12 months of age and usually subsides spontaneously after 3 years of age. Intracranial tumors have been rarely associated with this type of nystagmus. Neuroimaging studies are indicated. Any child with abnormal eye movements should be promptly evaluated by an ophthalmologist.

Cataracts

Cataracts are opacities of the crystalline lens (Fig. 128.20). Hereditary cataracts are most often transmitted in an autosomal dominant fashion. Developmental cataracts may be associated with chromosomal abnormalities, intrauterine infections, and certain metabolic diseases. Ocular disorders associated with cataracts include chronic uveitis, retinal detachment, microphthalmos, Peters anomaly, and aniridia. Ocular trauma may result in the development of lens opacities. Chronic steroid

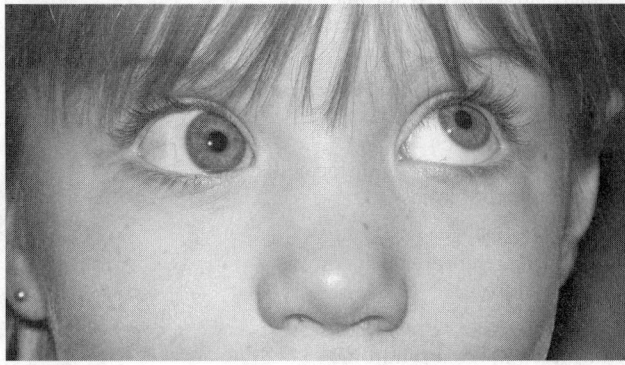

FIGURE 128.19. Patient with right Brown syndrome. Right eye cannot elevate in adduction because of tight right superior oblique tendon.

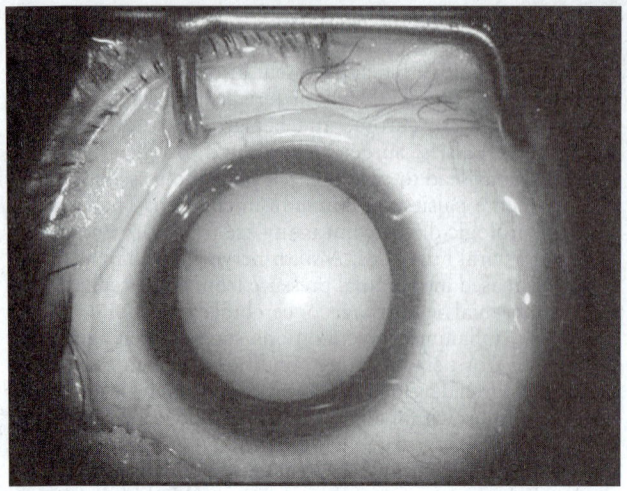

FIGURE 128.20. Total cataract. The pupil is pharmacologically dilated.

disease. In the case of congenital cataracts, surgery is generally done as early as 2 weeks to 1 month of age to avoid severe sensory amblyopia. If an intraocular lens is not implanted, the infant is fitted with a contact lens soon after surgery, and patching is used to treat amblyopia. Frequent refractions and changes of contact lens power are needed, and parents should be aware of the importance of perseverance if good visual results are to be obtained. Conservative management of partial cataracts includes the use of mydriatics if the opacity is central, and patching of the uninvolved eye for the treatment and prevention of amblyopia. Over the last few years, intraocular lenses have become increasingly used in the optical correction of children with aphakia, even under the age of 2 years. The current experience with these devices indicates an acceptable level of safety.

Ptosis

Congenital ptosis, the most common cause of upper-lid drooping in children and young adults, is due to faulty development of the levator palpebrae muscle. Most cases are unilateral, and the degree of severity varies. Superior rectus palsy may coexist. Familial cases are inherited as an autosomal dominant trait, and there is a dominant syndrome of congenital ptosis, phimosis, and epicanthus inversus. Infants with severe ptosis usually assume a chin-up head posture and look with both eyes in downgaze. Amblyopia is uncommon, and cosmetic surgery is usually delayed until the child attends school. Exceptions include instances where the lid covers the pupil and the child, once with a chin posture, gives it up for monocular vision and is at high risk for amblyopia.

Acquired ptosis in childhood demands special attention because it usually indicates potentially serious neurologic disease. Paralytic ptosis is seen in third-nerve palsy, and the differential diagnosis of acquired paralytic ptosis is the same as that of acquired third-nerve palsy. Neuromuscular ptosis is seen in myasthenia gravis and in myopathies such as myotonic dystrophy and congenital myotonia. Lid trauma can result in transient or permanent ptosis. Inflammation, swelling,

and other drug ingestion may lead to the development of cataracts, as may exposure to therapeutic irradiation for the treatment of orbital or ocular tumors. Box 128.4 lists various conditions associated with congenital or developmental cataracts.

Evaluation of the infant or child with cataracts includes a full ophthalmologic examination to exclude associated ocular disease and to assess visual status. Ocular ultrasonography should be performed in eyes with totally opaque lenses. The child should be evaluated by the pediatrician for associated systemic conditions as listed in Box 128.4. A family history of congenital cataracts in a parent or grandparent suggests dominant isolated cataracts. Both parents have to be examined with a slit lamp and after pupillary dilation for the presence of subclinical lens opacities. The presence of lens opacities in one parent establishes the diagnosis of hereditary cataracts.

Bilateral complete cataracts should be extracted early, and visual prognosis is generally good if there is no other ocular

---

BOX 128.4   Chromosomal and Hereditary Conditions Associated with Cataracts

Chromosomal disorders
Trisomy 13
Trisomy 18
Trisomy 21

Metabolic disorders
Galactosemia
Galactokinase deficiency
Albright pseudohypoparathyroidism
Wilson disease
Fabry disease
Refsum disease
Homocystinuria
Myotonic dystrophy

Skin diseases
Incontinentia pigmenti
Ectodermal dysplasia

Rothmund-Thompson syndrome
Werner syndrome

Mandibulofacial syndromes
Hallermann-Streiff syndrome
Stickler syndrome with Pierre Robin sequence
Rubinstein-Taybi syndrome

Connective tissue and skeletal syndromes
Conradi syndrome
Marfan syndrome
All syndromes involving dislocated lenses
Other bone dysplasias

Renal diseases
Lowe oculocerebrorenal syndrome
Alport syndrome

Central nervous system diseases
Marinesco-Sjögren syndrome
Sjögren syndrome

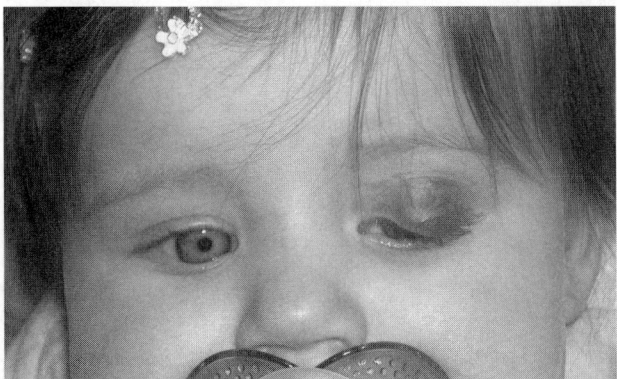

FIGURE 128.21. Significant ptosis of left upper lid secondary to a capillary hemangioma.

scar tissue, and tumors of the lids can lead to acquired ptosis (Fig. 128.21).

Pseudoptosis may be due to hypotropia of the ipsilateral eye or to lid retraction or proptosis of the contralateral eye.

In Horner syndrome, sympathetic denervation leads to mild ptosis, miosis, and anhydrosis of the ipsilateral face. Heterochromia, with a lighter iris on the affected side, may be present in congenital Horner syndrome. Ptosis is due to denervation of the Müller muscle, which is supplied by the sympathetic nerves and inserts on the upper tarsal plate.

Infantile Glaucoma

Primary infantile glaucoma, with an incidence of about 1 in 100,000 births, is due to an abnormal development of the trabecular meshwork (i.e., trabeculodysgenesis), resulting in reduced outflow of aqueous humor from the developing eye and increased intraocular pressure. All ocular layers are stretched, leading to buphthalmos (i.e., large, prominent eye) and optic nerve head damage with an abnormally large cup-to-disc ratio. Primary infantile glaucoma is inherited in an autosomal recessive fashion and is most common in populations with high rates of consanguineous marriages. At least two genes have been mapped for this genetically heterogeneous disease, one of which (*CYP1B1*) has been identified as a cause of more than 75% of cases. About 80% of patients are detected by 6 months of age. Symptoms and signs include corneal enlargement and clouding, tearing, photophobia, and blepharospasm. Thirty percent of cases are unilateral and the male-to-female ratio is 3:2, suggesting the possible existence of an X-linked variant. Intraocular pressure measurements vary from 20 to 50 mm Hg or more. Corneal diameter is usually enlarged but may be normal early. Corneal epithelial edema and stromal clouding result from failure of the endothelial cell pump, which normally dehydrates the cornea. Horizontal breaks in Descemet membrane (i.e., Haab striae) are diagnostic (Fig. 128.22). The corneal enlargement in congenital glaucoma should be differentiated from megalocornea, which is discussed in the section on anterior segment disorders in this chapter.

The treatment of infantile glaucoma is surgical. Goniotomy and trabeculotomy open the Schlemm canal to the anterior chamber. In trabeculotomy, the approach is through a sclerotomy site, but in goniotomy, it is through a directed incision at the opposite limbus by way of the anterior chamber. Multiple surgeries may be necessary to achieve optimal control of the intraocular pressure, but results appear to be equal for the two approaches. Oral acetazolamide (10 to 15 mg/kg/day) and topical timolol maleate (0.25%) or other drops may be given while the child awaits surgery. Optic nerve cupping is reversible

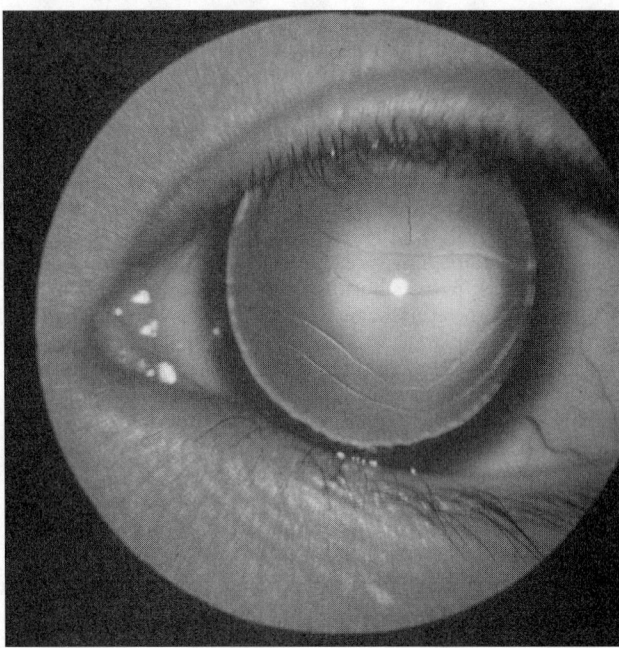

FIGURE 128.22. Haab striae. Linear opacities in the cornea are areas of discontinuity in the Descemet membrane that represent breaks in this rigid structure when the globe was exposed to high pressure in early infancy.

in infants after normalization of intraocular pressure. High myopia and astigmatism are generally present because of ocular axial elongation and corneal deformity. Any error of refraction should be corrected postoperatively to prevent anisometropic amblyopia.

Infantile glaucoma is associated with several other conditions, including anterior segment dysgenesis, congenital rubella, neurofibromatosis 1, mucopolysaccharidosis I, Lowe oculocerebrorenal syndrome, Sturge-Weber syndrome, and several chromosomal abnormalities. In diseases manifested by microspherophakic or dislocated lenses, such as Weill-Marchesani syndrome, homocystinuria, and Marfan syndrome, pupillary block by the dislocated lens and secondary glaucoma may develop. Other causes of secondary glaucoma in children include trauma, inflammation, ROP with secondary angle-closure glaucoma, lens-induced glaucoma, steroid-induced glaucoma, and glaucoma secondary to intraocular tumors, such as retinoblastoma, juvenile xanthogranuloma, and medulloepithelioma.

Uveitis

The uveal tract comprises the iris, ciliary body, and choroid. Iritis, cyclitis, iridocyclitis, choroiditis, and panuveitis refer to inflammation of the different parts of the uveal tract singly or in combination. Peripheral uveitis refers to inflammation of the extreme fundus periphery. Endogenous or nonpurulent uveitis is rare in children. As in the adult population, males are affected twice as frequently as females. About half of the cases have binocular involvement. The younger the affected child is, the more diffuse is the inflammation. Uveitis can be classified as granulomatous or nongranulomatous, depending on the type of cellular reaction involved.

Iritis produces exudation of protein into the anterior chamber with the production of flare or diffraction of a light beam. Inflammatory cells, seen floating in the anterior chamber, can form keratic precipitates on the posterior surface of the cornea.

A hypopyon is the accumulation of inflammatory cells in the anterior chamber, forming a visible whitish fluid level inferiorly. Hypopyon may be seen in retinoblastoma, in which the malignant cells accumulate in the anterior chamber.

Inflammation of the posterior uveal tract produces a cellular reaction in the anterior or posterior vitreous. Prolonged inflammation results in peripheral anterior synechiae or adhesions between the peripheral iris and cornea, or posterior synechiae or adhesions between the iris and the lens. Cataracts may develop. Choroiditis may spread to overlying retina, producing a chorioretinitis. Active chorioretinal lesions are white; inactive lesions or chorioretinal scars have black areas of hyperpigmentation and white areas of scarring. A particular complication of chronic uveitis in children is the deposition of calcium in a band-shaped pattern in the superficial layers of the cornea, mostly in the interpalpebral fissure area, producing band keratopathy. This complication is seen predominantly in conjunction with juvenile rheumatoid arthritis (JRA).

Children with uveitis may complain of pain, photophobia, lacrimation, and blepharospasm, and if they are old enough, they may notice disturbances in vision. Other children may be completely asymptomatic.

The most common cause of posterior uveitis in children is toxoplasmosis. Anterior uveitis is seen in JRA, Still disease, herpes simplex, and sarcoidosis. Many cases are of undetermined cause. Because symptoms may be lacking altogether in children with JRA and uveitis, frequent routine examinations are indicated to rule out asymptomatic inflammation. These examinations are done at intervals of 2 to 4 months, especially in subtypes of JRA where uveitis is more commonly present. Untreated uveitis results in adhesions between the iris and lens (posterior synechiae), cataracts, glaucoma, and cystoid macular edema. The increasing use of methotrexate in the treatment of JRA has resulted in a significant drop in the frequency and an easier control of uveitis in these patients. Any patient with JRA who develops uveitis and is not receiving methotrexate should probably start taking it. About 15% to 25% of cases of uveitis in children are of the peripheral variety, also called pars planitis. This disease is usually bilateral and can start as early as 7 years of age. Its onset is insidious; redness, photophobia, and tearing are usually absent. Progressive visual impairment occurs secondary to macular edema and posterior subcapsular cataracts. Characteristic "snowball" inflammatory deposits may be seen in the pars plana area, but they are not a universal finding. The cause of this disease is unknown. Therapy consists of administration of topical and systemic steroids. The disease runs a variable course, with exacerbations and remissions over several years. Other causes of uveitis in children include sarcoidosis, syphilis, tuberculosis, sympathetic ophthalmia, Behçet disease, Vogt-Koyanagi-Harada disease, histoplasmosis, and ankylosing spondylitis.

Trauma can induce an iridocyclitis, with cells and flare in the anterior chamber and symptoms of pain, photophobia, lacrimation, and blepharospasm. Treatment consists of administration of cycloplegic drops with or without mild steroid drops for a few days.

TUMORS

Orbital Tumors

After orbital infiltration with inflammatory cells, the two most common tumors in the pediatric population are dermoid cysts and capillary or infantile hemangiomas, which together make up more than 50% of all orbital tumors. Other orbital tumors, in order of decreasing frequency, are rhabdomyosarcoma, optic nerve glioma, neurofibroma, lymphangioma, metastatic neuroblastoma, inflammatory pseudotumor, lipoma, leukemia,

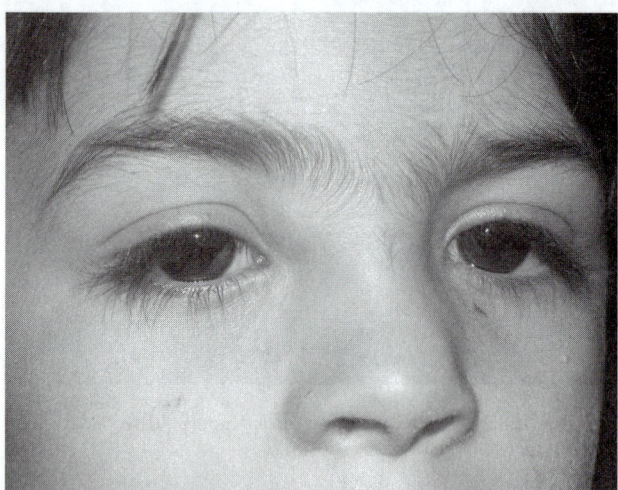

FIGURE 128.23. Right orbital dermoid at the base of the nose.

lymphoma, meningioma, and other rarer tumors, including teratoma, orbital extension of retinoblastoma, schwannoma, and other even rarer conditions. The more common lesions are discussed in the following sections.

Dermoid Cyst

Dermoid cysts account for about 40% of orbital tumors of childhood. They are choristomatous lesions that arise from retained ectodermal tissue along the lines of closure of fetal bone fissures. They can be present in the lid, brow, or orbit (Fig. 128.23). Deep orbital cysts arise within diploë of orbital bones and may have an hourglass appearance. Although these are congenital tumors, less than 25% are evident at birth. Their delayed appearance in most cases is probably due to postnatal growth. The tumors are nontender, well circumscribed, and of a rubbery or doughy consistency. More than one-half are located in the upper outer orbital quadrant. Less than 3% arise deep within the orbit. Diagnosis is made on clinical grounds and with the assistance of ultrasonography and computed tomography. Orbital bony structures may be compressed by the tumor, and well-circumscribed bony defects may be present. Deep cystic orbital lesions are harder to diagnose, and other orbital cystic tumors may be confused with dermoids. Anteriorly located tumors are easily excised, although care should be taken not to rupture the cyst wall, because the cyst contents may elicit a severe local inflammatory response. Deep orbital cysts are more difficult to excise.

Capillary Hemangioma

Capillary hemangiomas of infancy are vascular orbital tumors composed of proliferating capillaries. The bulk of the tumor consists of proliferating plump endothelial cells. More than 90% of these tumors have a visible superficial component, allowing diagnosis on the basis of clinical inspection alone. There may be a bluish discoloration of the overlying skin, a tangled vascular mass, or the classic strawberry mark (Fig. 128.24). The tumor swells when the child cries. One-third of tumors are present at birth, and 95% are diagnosed by 6 months of age. The lesion continues to grow after birth but eventually regresses spontaneously. Regression is complete in about 75% of patients by 7 or 8 years of age. Girls are affected more frequently than boys.

Local complications include ptosis, occlusion of the visual axis, ulceration and bleeding from the tumor surface,

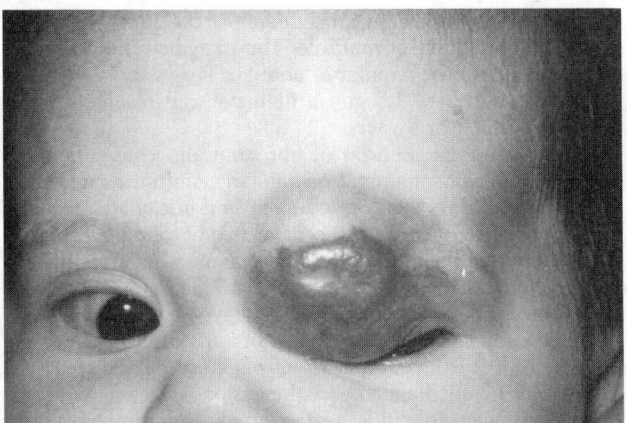

FIGURE 128.24. Capillary hemangioma of the left upper lid causing an S-shaped deformity and occluding the visual axis. The patient also had significant astigmatism, presumably from compression of the globe by the tumor.

and infection. One rare complication in large hemangiomas is platelet sequestration. Amblyopia may result from occlusion of the eye by the tumor and the droopy lid. The tumor may also compress the globe and lead to high degrees of astigmatism, anisometropia, and amblyopia. One-fourth of patients have one or more cutaneous capillary hemangiomas elsewhere on their body.

Treatment consists of observation if the visual axis is clear and there is no astigmatism. Systemic steroids and intralesional injections of Celestone are the mainstay of therapy in vision-threatening capillary hemangioma. One or more injections induce rapid regression of the tumors in most cases. Other modes of therapy include surgery and low-dose radiotherapy, but these are not commonly used.

Idiopathic Inflammatory Pseudotumor

The diagnosis of idiopathic orbital pseudotumor requires exclusion of several inflammatory, tumorous, infectious, and traumatic orbital conditions that may have an inflammatory component. These latter disorders include Graves disease, systemic vasculitis, Wegener granulomatosis, juvenile xanthogranuloma, sinus histiocytosis with massive lymphadenopathy, angioneurotic edema, bacterial orbital cellulitis, mucocele, orbital mucormycosis, parasitic infestations, trauma with retained foreign body, inflammatory reactions around primary benign tumors, and malignant orbital tumors. About 5% of patients with idiopathic inflammatory pseudotumor are in the pediatric age group, and only 2% of biopsied orbital masses in children fall in this disease category.

Pain differentiates this condition from other orbital mass lesions that cause proptosis. Most cases are unilateral. Bilateral cases are likely to be associated with a poorer prognosis or with the subsequent diagnosis of systemic disease, such as Wegener granulomatosis. Iritis occurs in about 25% of cases. The erythrocyte sedimentation rate and eosinophil count may be elevated.

Pathologically, there is a localized or diffuse aggregation of inflammatory cells that may form well-defined lymphoid follicles. There may be an aggregation of plasma cells, lymphocytes, or eosinophils, and a granulomatous inflammatory response. In some cases, proliferation of connective tissue predominates, while in others, the inflammatory infiltrate is predominantly perivascular. Ultrasonography and computed tomography are helpful in diagnosing idiopathic inflammatory pseudotumor if components of inflammatory edema and an inflammatory mass lesion can be identified. A trial of systemic steroids is often used to confirm the diagnosis and initiate treatment. Response to treatment may be dramatic and about 75% of patients respond well to this modality. Low-dose irradiation has been used in refractory cases.

Rhabdomyosarcoma

Rhabdomyosarcoma, the most common primary malignant orbital tumor of childhood, accounts for 9% of orbital masses in children. Because it is lethal if untreated, it should always be suspected in the child with acquired ptosis or a lid, epibulbar, or orbital mass. This tumor arises from mesenchymal precursors of muscle cells and forms three pathologic types: embryonal (78%), alveolar (14%), and differentiated (8%). Over 90% of orbital rhabdomyosarcomas occur in children younger than 16 years of age. The main presenting sign of rhabdomyosarcoma is unilateral, often fulminant proptosis. There may be ptosis or a palpable orbital or lid mass. Occasionally, the tumor presents as a lid or a conjunctival mass. The two keys to diagnosis are a high index of suspicion and an early biopsy. Computed tomography is helpful in delineating the extent of the disease.

The major prognostic factor in this condition is the extent of disease at the time of institution of therapy. Metastases occur most frequently to lungs and bone marrow, and the tumor may extend locally to the intracranial cavity and paranasal sinuses. Excellent survival rates are obtained with combined radiotherapy and chemotherapy, although many eyes are ultimately enucleated because of the complications of radiation therapy. Exenteration, once the mainstay of treatment, is reserved for cases in which medical treatment fails, for cases with orbital recurrences, and for cases in which megavoltage radiotherapy is not available.

Metastatic Neuroblastoma

Neuroblastoma is a tumor of the embryonic sympathetic neuroblasts. It is the third most common malignant tumor in children after leukemia and brain tumors. Forty percent to 50% of neuroblastomas arise in the adrenal glands, 25% in other retroperitoneal sites, 10% in the mediastinum, and 2% to 5% in the neck. Primary intraspinous, intracranial, and soft tissue tumors have also been described. In some cases the primary site cannot be identified. Metastases spread by way of the bloodstream to distant sites, particularly the skull and orbit. Metastases also occur by way of lymphatics to adjacent and distant lymph nodes, and by direct extension from the right adrenal gland into the liver. Metastatic neuroblastoma accounts for about 3% of orbital tumors in children. Orbital involvement may precede, concur with, or follow diagnosis of the primary tumor.

Patients most commonly present with proptosis and may have periorbital swelling and lid ecchymosis. Ptosis and miosis are seen in neck tumors because of compression of sympathetic fibers leading to an ipsilateral Horner syndrome. Severe proptosis results in anterior segment complications, such as conjunctival necrosis and corneal exposure, and in restriction of ocular motility. Intracranial metastases produce papilledema and optic atrophy. Orbital metastases indicate stage IV neuroblastoma and are associated with a poor prognosis.

Ocular Tumors

Retinoblastoma

Retinoblastoma is covered in depth in Chapter 101, and the discussion here is restricted to some general diagnostic considerations. Retinoblastoma is the most common intraocular malignancy in childhood. It occurs in about 1 in 15,000 live births and is responsible for about 1% of deaths in the pediatric population. The hereditary and sporadic cases of retinoblastoma are caused by deletion or mutation of both alleles of the *RB1* gene on chromosome 13. Most cases are diagnosed before the age of 4 years. Boys and girls are equally affected. Mortality is low if treatment is instituted before metastases occur, with 5-year survival rates of 90% in unilateral and 80% in bilateral cases. It is vital that this condition be diagnosed and treated as early as possible.

The average age at diagnosis is about 1 year for bilateral disease and 2 years for unilateral disease. Disease in infants with a positive family history is discovered earlier because of examination shortly after birth. The most common manifestation of retinoblastoma is a white reflex from the pupil (i.e., leukocoria), most often observed by parents when the child is looking in a direction that puts the tumor in the path of the incident light. Other manifestations include convergent or divergent strabismus, pseudohypopyon, hyphema, periorbital swelling, and red eye.

Accurate and prompt diagnosis is invaluable if adequate therapy is to be instituted and enucleation for simulating conditions is to be avoided. Pediatricians should suspect the tumor in any patient with leukocoria, especially if any other family member has had an eye enucleated in infancy or childhood. Strabismus is the next most common sign of retinoblastoma, and a search for retinal pathology or tumor should be routinely carried out in infants and children with ocular misalignment.

Age at presentation, sex, laterality of ocular involvement, and family history are good clues to the differential diagnosis of retinoblastoma, because the various simulating conditions appear in characteristic age groups and may show male predominance or predominantly uniocular or binocular involvement. More than 90% of retinoblastomas can be easily diagnosed by ophthalmologists using indirect ophthalmoscopy and ultrasonography or computed tomography. About 50% of patients referred to tertiary specialized ophthalmic oncology centers to rule out retinoblastoma turn out to have the tumor; the rest have one of the several simulating conditions listed in Box 128.2.

Coats disease or idiopathic retinal telangiectasia is usually a unilateral retinal disease of boys that is most often diagnosed in the first decade of life. However, bilateral cases, cases in girls, and cases with onset in adulthood can occur. Coats disease is characterized by telangiectasias, aneurysms, and focal bulb-like dilations of the retinal vessels. The dilated vessels leak fluids, proteins, and lipids into the retina and subretinal space, resulting in retinal edema, circinate exudates, and serous retinal detachment. The accumulation of mounds of yellow-white subretinal exudates, especially in the macular area, leads to common confusion of Coats disease with retinoblastoma. Patients may be completely asymptomatic or may present with decreased vision, strabismus, or leukocoria. The ophthalmoscopic detection of the characteristic telangiectasias is diagnostic. Fluorescein angiography can also be performed. Visual prognosis is poor in patients with diffuse and posterior pole retinal involvement. Cryotherapy or laser surgery may be used to obliterate leaky vessels. Patients with mild peripheral disease may be observed.

Juvenile Xanthogranuloma

This benign tumor affects the skin and eyes of children younger than 5 years of age. Eighty-five percent of patients are younger than 1 year of age. The eyelid is most frequently affected, followed by the epibulbar area and orbit. Intraocular lesions are located in the iris and ciliary body and are discovered as iris nodules, spontaneous hyphema, unilateral glaucoma, or heterochromia iridis.

Skin lesions, which appear suddenly on the upper part of the body, can be solitary or multiple. They may be yellow, orange, or brown, or may be papular or nodular. They vary in size from a few millimeters to 1.5 cm in diameter and resolve spontaneously within 2 or 3 years.

Histopathologic sections of fibroxanthomatous tumor tissue reveal chronic inflammation and large multinucleated cells, called Touton giant cells, in which several nuclei are arranged in a circular fashion around a central area of foamy cytoplasm. The differential diagnosis of these iris tumors includes medulloepithelioma, primary iris cysts, melanoma, leiomyoma, and neurofibroma. The severity of ocular involvement is variable. If large or clinically aggressive tumors are left untreated, the eye may be lost from complications of glaucoma and recurrent intraocular hemorrhage. Surgical excision, systemic and topical steroids, acetazolamide, and external irradiation have been used with various degrees of success.

Medulloepithelioma

Medulloepithelioma is a rare congenital tumor that arises from the nonpigmented ciliary epithelium. Cell type and arrangement are extremely variable because of the pluripotentiality of the cell of origin. If cartilage, brain, striated muscle, or other heterotopic cells are present, the tumor is called teratoid medulloepithelioma. Both simple and teratoid tumors may exhibit histologic evidence of malignancy. These tumors become evident in the first decade of life, with an average age at enucleation of 5 years. The tumor is invariably unilateral, and the family history is negative for similar tumors.

Presenting signs include a visible iris tumor or iris distortion, secondary glaucoma, a white pupillary reflex, spontaneous and posttraumatic hyphema, and reduced visual acuity or strabismus. The differential diagnosis includes retinoblastoma, persistent hyperplastic primary vitreous, primary iris cyst, melanoma, leiomyoma, and neurofibroma of the ciliary body. Treatment consists of early enucleation, before the tumor extends into the orbit. Prognosis after early enucleation is excellent. Excision of localized tumors is associated with good long-term survival. This tumor is not radiosensitive.

OPHTHALMOLOGIC MANIFESTATIONS OF SYSTEMIC DISEASE

It is impossible to cover the ophthalmologic manifestations of all pediatric systemic diseases, and only selected common ones with major ocular findings are discussed here.

Marfan Syndrome

Marfan syndrome is an autosomal dominant condition characterized by skeletal abnormalities with excessive length of the distal limbs, loose jointedness, scoliosis, and anterior chest deformities. The affected person is usually taller than the rest of his family. Cardiovascular abnormalities in the form of aortic root dilation, dissecting aortic aneurysm, and mitral valve prolapse are common. Complications of aortic dilation have been the major cause of death, which occurs at an average age of 45 years. With the recent advances in cardiothoracic surgery, survival has improved significantly.

Ocular abnormalities in Marfan syndrome include subluxation of the lens, usually but not invariably in an upward and outward direction (Fig. 128.25), moderate to severe myopia, tremulousness of the iris or iridodonesis, megalocornea, an unusually deep anterior chamber angle, presenile cataracts,

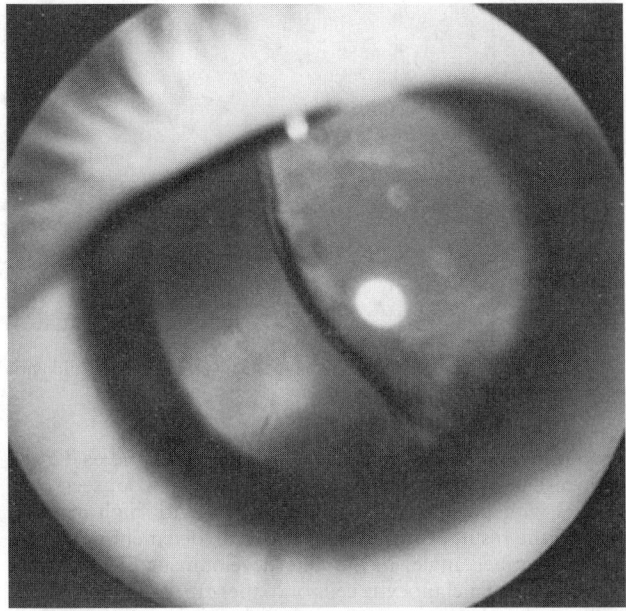

FIGURE 128.25. Subluxated lens in a patient with Marfan syndrome.

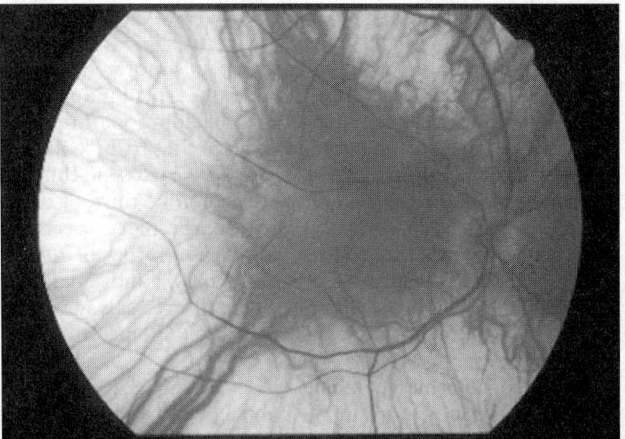

FIGURE 128.26. Fundus of patient with albinism. Note the total absence of pigment, the prominence of the choroidal vasculature, and the absence of a foveal reflex indicating foveal hypoplasia.

and retinal detachment. Retinal detachment may occur spontaneously in eyes with axial myopia or after cataract extraction. The lens does not usually dislocate into the anterior chamber in Marfan syndrome. Patients presenting with lenses in the anterior chambers and a marfanoid habitus should be considered to have homocystinuria until proven otherwise. A negative test for homocystinuria is required for the diagnosis of Marfan syndrome. Marfan syndrome is due to mutations in the fibrillin gene on chromosome 15. Fibrillin is a major component of connective tissue and serves as a scaffold for the deposition of elastin. Fibrillin is abundant in the lens zonules and in the peripheral parts of the lens capsule. It is also found in all ocular layers.

Other diseases associated with lens subluxation include the Weill-Marchesani syndrome, hyperlysinemia, sulfite oxidase deficiency, Kniest syndrome, and Stickler syndrome. Dislocated lenses in the absence of systemic abnormalities are features of an autosomal recessive condition called *ectopia lentis et pupillae*. In *ectopia lentis et pupillae* there is mild anterior segment dysgenesis and often an abnormal position of the pupil on the nasal aspect of the iris.

Patients suspected of having Marfan syndrome should undergo ocular examinations immediately to look for lens subluxation, which is present in about 50% to 60% of patients. The management of subluxated lenses includes optical correction of the myopic and astigmatic errors and of lens extraction in selected cases. Patients with Marfan syndrome are predisposed to amblyopia and strabismus that can be present in up to 15% of cases, and care should be taken to detect these two problems and to manage them appropriately.

Albinism

Albinism refers to the absence or scarcity of melanin in the skin, eye, or both. All conditions featuring albinism are genetically determined and involve defects in the normal process of melanogenesis. There are several forms of oculocutaneous albinism, all of which are inherited in an autosomal recessive fashion. Ocular albinism is X-linked recessive. A number of disorders have dermal hypopigmentation without ocular al-

binism. The general aspects of albinism are discussed elsewhere in this textbook.

All types of oculocutaneous and ocular albinism are characterized by nystagmus, strabismus, decreased foveal reflex, absence of pigment in the retinal pigment epithelium and uveal tract (Fig. 128.26) with iris transillumination, prominence of choroidal vessels, and high astigmatic refractive errors. Visual acuity is reduced, most often to the 20/100 to 20/200 range, but vision can be as good as 20/30 in certain forms of tyrosinase-positive oculocutaneous albinism. Although photophobia is generally believed to be a major symptom in albinism, it is not universal, and sunglasses may further compromise already decreased visual acuity. As patients get older the intensity and frequency of their nystagmus improves. Abnormal decussation of temporal optic nerve fibers in the optic chiasm occurs in all forms of albinism and in all genera and species with albinism.

Errors of refraction should be fully corrected in all patients with albinism to maximize visual acuity and to prevent additional amblyopia. Strabismus is corrected surgically, although patients never achieve binocular vision. Referrals for special education and low-vision aids are necessary.

Monocular telescopes are prescribed at 5 or 6 years of age. Like all children with poor vision, albino children should be allowed to hold their reading material as close to their eyes as they like. They should be seated in the front row in class. Professional genetic counseling is advisable in families with an albino child. The tyrosinase gene has been cloned and numerous mutations have been detected. Patients with tyrosinase-positive oculocutaneous albinism have mutations in the P gene that codes for a membrane protein, or they may have mutations in the tyrosinase gene, which do not inhibit its function completely. One should remember the association of albinism with the Chediak-Higashi syndrome and the Hermansky-Pudlak syndrome, both of which are associated with significant systemic morbidity.

Juvenile Diabetes Mellitus

Ocular complications of juvenile diabetes mellitus most often involve the retina but may affect the conjunctiva, cornea, iris, lens, optic nerve, and extraocular muscles. Transitory refractive changes causing transitory blurring of vision are due to swelling and detumescence of the lens secondary to changes in blood sugar levels. Diabetic cataracts are relatively rare in well-controlled juvenile diabetics. Transient lens opacities can be seen in poorly controlled patients. Cranial nerve palsy is occasionally seen in juvenile diabetics who have had the disease for more than 10 years.

Retinopathy in juvenile diabetes depends more on the duration than on the control of the disease. No retinopathy is detected by fluorescein angiography if the duration of the diabetes is less than 4 years, but the incidence rises to 25% after 5 to 9 years and to more than 70% after 10 years. One-third of patients have proliferative retinopathy, and one-third of those are legally blind. These figures can be expected to decrease with better blood sugar control, closer monitoring of retinal changes, and early institution of laser therapy, if indicated. Vitreoretinal microsurgical techniques have allowed salvage of the eyes of many patients who would have been doomed to blindness in the past.

Several syndromes combine diabetes and various ocular findings. Alström syndrome is characterized by diabetes, severe retinal degeneration with blindness and cataracts, obesity, and severe nerve deafness. Wolfram syndrome features diabetes mellitus, diabetes insipidus, optic atrophy, and sensorineural deafness. Other diseases with occasional diabetes mellitus and ocular manifestations include Bardet-Biedl syndrome, Cockayne syndrome, Friedreich ataxia, Prader-Willi syndrome, and Werner syndrome.

Tuberous Sclerosis

Tuberous sclerosis (Bourneville disease) is characterized by multiple central nervous tumors, epilepsy, cutaneous lesions in the form of adenoma sebaceum of the face that develop during puberty, subungual fibromas, shagreen patches of the skin, and sometimes café au lait spots and nevi. Mental deficiency is seen in 50% of patients. The major ocular abnormalities are hamartomas of the optic nerve and retina. Long-standing tumors have a refractile multinodular appearance and have been likened to mulberries, clumps of tapioca, or frog's eggs. Retinal tumors may have a flat contour and appear as spots in the fundus that range from smooth to fluffy and from milky white to yellowish. Central nervous system tumors may cause papilledema and optic atrophy, usually the main cause of visual loss. The size and location of the various tumors determine their effect on visual acuity. Secondary glaucoma, inflammation, and intraocular hemorrhage are rare complications.

Neurofibromatosis

There are two types of neurofibromatosis. The peripheral type, neurofibromatosis 1 or von Recklinghausen disease (*NF1* gene), is assigned to chromosome 17, and the central type or neurofibromatosis 2 (*NF2* gene) to chromosome 22. The central type is characterized by tumors of the pontine angle (acoustic neuromas) with no ocular involvement, except for the occurrence of combined hamartomas of the retina and retinal pigment epithelium in some patients and cataracts in late childhood and early adulthood. The peripheral type is characterized by neurofibromatous tumors in many parts of the body. The principal cutaneous lesions are café au lait spots and diffuse and plexiform neurofibromas (Fig. 128.27). Neurofibromas, gliomas, and meningiomas occur in the central nervous system, and ependymomas of the spinal cord have been described. Patients may have neurofibromas of the peripheral and autonomic nervous systems. Pheochromocytomas occur in less than 1% of patients.

About 80% of patients with peripheral neurofibromatosis who are older than 6 years have pigmented iris nodules, also known as Lisch nodules (Fig. 128.28). These nodules are composed solely of cells of melanocytic origin and do not correlate with the extent or severity of other manifestations. They ap-

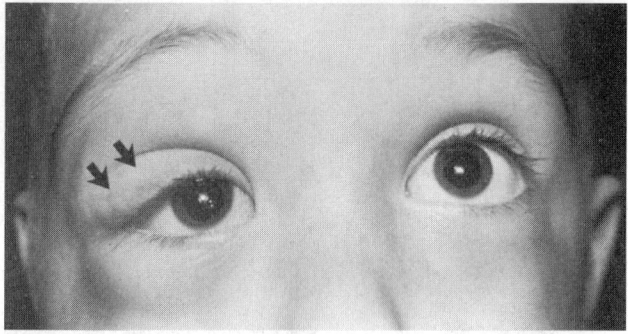

FIGURE 128.27. Plexiform neuroma of the lid (*arrows*) in a child with neurofibromatosis.

pear as lighter tan-colored lesions in dark irides and as darker, brownish lesions in light-colored irides. Glaucoma, seen only in eyes with neurofibroma of the lid and with high myopia, may be the result of neurofibromatous involvement of the anterior chamber angle, incomplete development of the angle, overgrowth of melanocytic cells onto the trabecular meshwork, and peripheral anterior synechiae. Rubeosis iridis may or may not be present. Trabeculotomy is the procedure of choice for glaucoma in children with neurofibromatosis 1.

Patients with neurofibromatosis may develop gliomas of the optic pathways, most commonly in the orbital portion of the optic nerve, with or without posterior extension into the optic chiasm. The clinical manifestations of optic nerve gliomas include proptosis, usually preceded by unilateral visual loss. An afferent pupillary defect and color vision defects usually exist, and there may be strabismus. Ophthalmoscopy may reveal disc pallor or papilledema. Retinal striae and hyperopia may occur secondary to direct pressure from the tumor on the globe. Radiographic studies are diagnostic and may reveal enlargement of the optic canal. Computed tomography of the orbits helps differentiate this tumor from optic nerve meningioma and delineates its posterior extension. Chiasmal gliomas may affect hypothalamic and pituitary function and may produce nystagmus and a variety of nonspecific visual field defects. If intracranial pressure is elevated, there may be bilateral papilledema. Bitemporal hemianopia may not develop.

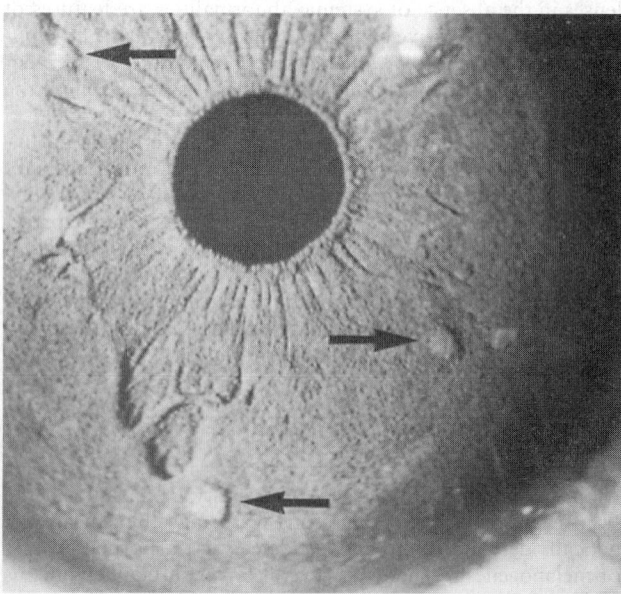

FIGURE 128.28. Hamartomas (i.e., Lisch nodules) of the iris (*arrows*) in a patient with neurofibromatosis.

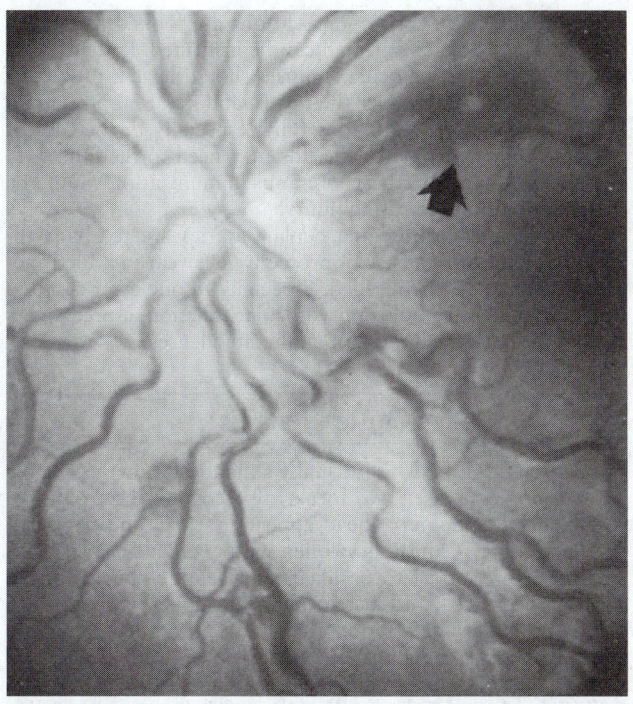

FIGURE 128.29. Retinal findings in a 7-year-old girl with acute lymphocytic leukemia. Notice the vascular tortuosity, optic nerve head swelling, blot hemorrhages, and white-centered hemorrhage (*arrow*).

Most optic nerve gliomas are diagnosed clinically on the basis of signs, symptoms, associated systemic findings of neurofibromatosis, and computed tomographic studies. Because these tumors are histologically benign, conservative management of those lesions that do not extend intracranially is recommended. Tumor resection in blind, severely proptotic eyes is accepted.

Leukemia

Ten percent of children with acute leukemia have clinically detectable ocular manifestations. Retinopathy is most common in patients with profound anemia and thrombocytopenia. Intraretinal blood in the form of nerve fiber layer hemorrhages, dot and blot hemorrhages, and white-centered hemorrhages is usually seen (Fig. 128.29). Retinal and nerve head infiltration by leukemic cells is a sign of central nervous system involvement in more than 90% of patients. Histopathologically, the uveal tract is the ocular structure that is most commonly infiltrated by leukemic cells. Choroidal infiltrates, which may appear as round, pale areas, are common, but they are difficult to detect clinically. Orbital involvement, which occurs less frequently, is manifested by the formation of chloromas, periorbital swelling, and exophthalmos.

The different types of leukemias are discussed in Chapter 96.

OPHTHALMOLOGIC MANIFESTATIONS OF HEADACHES

Migraine

The main clinical manifestations of migraine are paroxysms of headache and abnormal visual sensations. The headache is usually unilateral and intense and lasts hours or days. Accompanying symptoms include photophobia, irritability, nausea, vomiting, and other gastrointestinal symptoms. Prodromal symptoms may occur. Onset of migraine may be in childhood, at puberty, or later in life. Characteristic visual sensations of migraine are scintillating scotomas, which usually start in the macular area of the hemifield, progress to the periphery, and are outlined by scintillations. The edges of the scotomas may be shimmering or take on the appearance of fortification figures. Scotomas may be transient, accompany or precede headaches, or be the only manifestation of migraine. They are caused by a focal disturbance in the occipital cortex. Other sensory and motor disturbances can occur in migraine. Extracerebral ocular manifestations of migraine include unilateral visual loss, retinal arteriolar constriction, retinal and vitreous hemorrhage, and ischemic papillitis. Transient ophthalmoplegia is a well-recognized manifestation of migraine that usually has its onset before the age of 10 years. Most commonly, it takes the form of a third-nerve palsy with pupillary involvement; less commonly, the fourth and sixth nerves are involved. Treatment of migraine is discussed in Chapter 162.

Errors of Refraction and Strabismus

Uncorrected astigmatism and hyperopia may give rise to headaches and ocular fatigue (i.e., asthenopia) in children; corrective glasses should be prescribed in such cases. Myopia does not result in asthenopic symptoms. Phorias and intermittent tropias may result in headaches due to continued efforts to maintain ocular alignment and binocular vision.

Ocular problems are generally uncommon causes of headaches in children, and other possible causes should be investigated.

LEARNING DISABILITIES, DYSLEXIA, AND VISION

In a position paper by the Committee on Children with Disabilities, the American Academy of Pediatrics (AAP), the American Academy of Ophthalmology (AAO), and the American Association for Pediatric Ophthalmology and Strabismus (AAPOS) is the following statement about learning disabilities and vision problems: "Learning disabilities are common conditions in pediatric patients. The etiology of these difficulties is multifactorial, reflecting genetic influences and abnormalities of brain structure and function. Early recognition and referral to qualified educational professionals is critical for the best possible outcome. Visual problems are rarely responsible for learning difficulties. No scientific evidence exists for the efficacy of eye exercises ("vision therapy") or the use of special tinted lenses in the remediation of these complex pediatric developmental and neurologic conditions." Pediatricians should understand the general issues related to dyslexia and should consult with pediatric psychologists and psychiatrists with expertise in this subject for more detailed information. Comprehensive ocular examinations by a pediatric ophthalmologist are recommended as part of the evaluation of a child with learning difficulties to rule out treatable vision and ocular problems such as refractive errors, strabismus, and amblyopia.

EMERGENT EYE PROBLEMS

Emergent eye problems are often seen in the emergency room or clinic and require immediate consultation with an ophthalmologist.

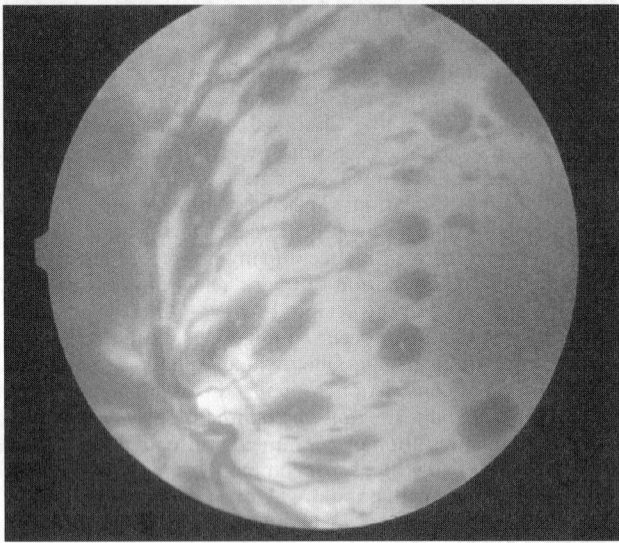

FIGURE 128.30. Numerous retinal hemorrhages in an abused infant. (Courtesy of Dr. F. James Ellis.)

Battered Child

The ophthalmologic manifestations of physical child abuse have received much attention in the literature, as have the social and medical manifestations. The spectrum of ocular problems seen in battered children is broad, and findings may be due to delayed complications of acute injuries. General physical and social findings in physically abused children are discussed in Chapter 26. The incidence of ocular involvement in abused children is about 30% to 40%. Most commonly, intraocular hemorrhages are seen in the retina (Fig. 128.30), vitreous, or anterior chamber. Less common findings include periorbital edema and ecchymosis, retinal detachment or dialysis, cataracts, chorioretinal atrophy, subluxated lenses, traumatic mydriasis, papilledema, subconjunctival hemorrhage, esotropia, corneal opacity, and optic atrophy. Bleeding into the optic nerve sheath may be the only finding in shaken babies. A detailed ophthalmologic examination should be part of the routine evaluation of children suspected of being physically abused.

Trauma

Ophthalmologic trauma may be divided into blunt injuries, penetrating injuries, and injuries involving the globe, orbit, adnexa, or any combination of these three. Nonpenetrating injuries to the globe include thermal, ultraviolet, electrical, and chemical burns, corneal abrasions, and contusions.

Contusions to the eyeball may result in subconjunctival hemorrhage, hyphema, iritis, iridodialysis and iris sphincter tears, subluxated lenses that may become cataractous, angle recession with delayed glaucoma, ghost cell glaucoma, vitreous hemorrhage, retinal and choroidal tears, detachment and rupture, and optic nerve injury with edema or avulsion. Penetrating injuries to the globe may produce corneal lacerations, corneoscleral lacerations, scleral lacerations, or double-penetrating injuries. An intraocular foreign body may be retained. Lid lacerations may involve the lacrimal drainage system and may result in traumatic ptosis. Extraocular muscles may become entrapped in blow-out orbital fractures, leading to restrictive strabismus.

A detailed ophthalmologic examination by an ophthalmologist is mandatory in all cases of periocular and ocular injuries,

and all of the described complications are looked for so the appropriate management plan can be instituted. Patients with suspected penetrating ocular injuries should have a protective metallic shield placed over their eyes, and no attempts should be made to open the lids forcefully; especially in the case of a young child, opening of the lids may need to be done with the patient under anesthesia. Tetanus immunization should be given, as in any penetrating injury.

Sports- and work-related ocular injuries are receiving increased attention. The use of protective eyewear in athletic activities should be encouraged, especially in one-eyed children and children with compromised ocular function, a predisposition to retinal detachment, or subluxated lenses.

Optic Neuritis

In children, optic neuritis is usually a manifestation of systemic or neurologic disease. Two forms are recognized: retrobulbar, in which the optic nerve head appears normal, and papillitis, in which the nerve head is swollen with nerve fiber layer hemorrhages. In contrast to papilledema, in optic neuritis visual acuity is decreased, and there is abnormal color perception, an afferent pupillary defect, and always a central scotoma. There may or may not be pain on moving the eye. If the retina is inflamed, the condition is called neuroretinitis. In children, optic neuritis may occur as a complication of the encephalomyelitis that follows an exanthem, or it may develop as part of acute meningitis. Multiple sclerosis may develop years later. A number of toxins, including lead, and drugs, including ethambutol and isoniazid, can cause optic neuritis. An ophthalmologist should be consulted in the case of any child with optic neuritis.

Papilledema

Papilledema is optic disc swelling due to increased intracranial pressure (Fig. 128.31). Several stages are differentiated ophthalmoscopically. In the early stages there is hyperemia and blurring of the disc margins with mild disc swelling. In fully developed papilledema, there is more disc swelling, venous

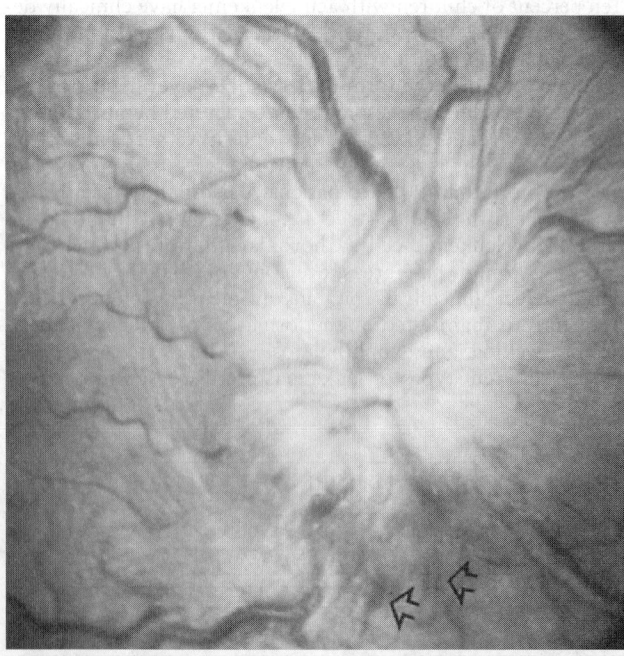

FIGURE 128.31. Notice the elevated disc, folds in the peripapillary retina, and the flame-shaped hemorrhages (*arrows*).

engorgement, splinter hemorrhages at the disc margins, and various amounts of exudate into the macular area. The chronic stage is characterized by persistence of disc elevation, resolution of hemorrhages, and the appearance of grayish exudates on the surface of the rounded disc. In the late stage there is postpapilledema atrophy, in which the disc becomes flat and atrophic and retinal vessels are attenuated.

Papilledema may be simulated by several conditions, including high hyperopia, buried optic disc drusen, optic disc infiltration by tumor (e.g., leukemia) or inflammation (e.g., sarcoid), and primary optic disc tumors (e.g., glioma, hamartoma, hemangioma). Neovascularization at the optic disc margin may be confused with papilledema. Papilledema in children may be accompanied by headaches and nausea that are due to increased intracranial pressure. Vision is usually unimpaired, and visual fields show only an enlarged blind spot. There is no color vision defect and usually no afferent pupillary defect. Chronic papilledema may be associated with visual field and acuity loss. Causes of papilledema include intracranial tumors, such as infratentorial lesions, subdural hematomas, brain abscesses, arteriovenous malformations, subarachnoid hemorrhage, and meningoencephalitis; rarely, papilledema is caused by a spinal cord tumor. Optic disc swelling is seen in the mucopolysaccharidoses, the craniostenoses, juvenile diabetes, and, rarely, Guillain-Barré syndrome.

Papilledema in benign intracranial hypertension (i.e., pseudotumor cerebri) is associated with increased intracranial pressure, normal or small ventricles, and normal cerebrospinal fluid. Symptoms of this condition include headache, disturbances of visual acuity, diplopia, nausea, dizziness, alterations of consciousness, and tinnitus. Pseudotumor cerebri is an isolated phenomenon in 50% of cases but may be associated with obstruction of cerebral venous drainage, endocrine and metabolic dysfunction, ingestion of certain drugs and toxins, and several systemic illnesses. Although this condition was considered benign by many, progressive visual field and acuity loss may result. Patients with intractable headaches or those with evidence of optic neuropathy have been treated with various degrees of success by repeated lumbar punctures, acetazolamide, steroids, ventriculoperitoneal shunting, and optic nerve sheath decompression.

Retinal Detachment

Retinal detachment is rare in the pediatric population. Hereditary conditions featuring vitreoretinal degeneration and high myopia are associated with early onset of retinal detachment in some cases. These conditions include familial high myopia, the Stickler syndrome, Kniest dysplasia, spondyloepiphyseal dysplasia congenita, Ehlers-Danlos syndrome, and Marfan syndrome. Retinal detachment may complicate congenital ocular abnormalities, such as the morning glory disc anomaly, optic pits, and chorioretinal colobomas.

Symptoms of retinal detachment include sudden onset of floaters, flashes of light, and the appearance of a black veil in parts of the visual field. Early diagnosis and surgical correction are imperative, and patients with predisposing conditions should be examined at frequent intervals. Retinal breaks may be treated prophylactically. All children with signs or symptoms consistent with retinal detachment should be referred to an ophthalmologist.

Suggested Readings

Committee on Children with Disabilities. Learning disabilities, dyslexia, and vision: a subject review. *Pediatrics* 1998;102:1217. Updated online at http://www.pediatrics.org/cgi/content/full/102/5/1217

Committee on Practice and Ambulatory Medicine, Section on Ophthalmology. Eye examination and vision screening in infants, children and young adults. *Pediatrics* 1996;98:153.

Early Treatment for Retinopathy of Prematurity Cooperative Group. Revised indications for the treatment of retinopathy of prematurity: results of the early treatment for retinopathy of prematurity randomized trial. *Arch Ophthalmol* 2003;121:1684; Comment in *Arch Ophthalmol* 2003;121:1769.

Taylor D, Hoyt C, eds. *Pediatric ophthalmology and strabismus*, 3rd ed. Philadelphia, W.B. Saunders, 2005.

Teller, DY. First glances: the vision of infants. *Investigative Ophthalmol Visual Sci* 1997;38:2184.

Traboulsi EI, ed. *Genetic diseases of the eye*. New York: Oxford University Press, 1998.

Wright KW. *Pediatric ophthalmology for pediatricians*. Philadelphia: Williams and Wilkins, 1999.

Wright KW, Spiegel P, eds. *Pediatric ophthalmology and strabismus*, 2nd ed. Springer, 2002.

CHAPTER 129 ■ PEDIATRIC DERMATOLOGY

DANIEL P. KROWCHUK AND WALTER W. TUNNESSEN, JR.

Complaints involving the skin are common reasons why parents seek medical care for their children. Data from the 2003 National Ambulatory Medical Care Survey showed that in approximately 8% of visits to primary care providers for children, a cutaneous diagnosis was recorded. The volume of skin-related problems makes it necessary for physicians who care for children to gain some facility in recognizing and managing the most common cutaneous disorders.

Dermatology is a visual specialty. With experience, most common problems affecting children's skin can be recognized, including the subtle variations in presentation. For uncommon cutaneous problems, atlases (including electronic atlases [see Resources at the conclusion of this chapter]), texts, or other sources can be used to aid in identification. As in most medical specialties, an organized approach to the problem is most helpful in leading to the correct diagnosis.

TERMINOLOGY

This chapter is designed to assist the reader in the diagnosis of skin problems. The approach is based on morphologic appearance. If clinicians can describe what they see, they already may have conquered a major obstacle to diagnosis. Describing cutaneous lesions is not as easy as it may sound. Practice in using descriptive terminology is the key to success. The sections of this chapter are based primarily on lesion morphology. The first step in an organized approach to skin lesions is to define the descriptors.

A *macule* is a circumscribed area of change in skin color without elevation or depression of the skin surface; macules generally are less than 1 cm in diameter. A *patch* is a large macule, greater than 1 cm in diameter. *Papules* are solid, elevated, palpable lesions less than 0.5 cm in diameter; *nodules* are larger papules that can lie in the epidermis or in the dermis or subcutaneous tissues. *Plaques* are elevated, plateau-like lesions formed most frequently by the confluence of papules.

A *vesicle* is a fluid-filled blister less than 0.5 cm in diameter; a *bulla* is a blister that is 0.5 cm or greater in diameter. A *pustule* is a blister filled with cellular debris, generally white blood cells, which gives the lesion a white or yellowish color. A *wheal* is the result of localized edema in the skin. It is pink or pale and usually is rounded or flat-topped, sometimes with irregularly shaped margins. Wheals are evanescent, lasting less than 24 hours in any one place. They are associated almost invariably with pruritus.

Telangiectases are permanent superficial dilations of venules, capillaries, or arterioles that may or may not blanch with pressure. *Lichenification* is a thickening of the skin in which the normal skin markings usually are accentuated; prolonged rubbing or scratching of the skin is necessary to produce this change. *Crusts* are accumulations of dried serum, blood, pus, or other exudative materials on the surface of the skin. *Scales* are flakes of skin, either loose or adherent, that are composed of compact keratin. An area of *sclerosis* is one that feels indurated or thickened and has lost its normal elasticity. The surface coloration may show hyperpigmentation, hypopigmentation, or both. Normal skin appendages (i.e., hair and sweat glands) are absent from the sclerotic area.

An *erosion* is a superficial epidermal loss that has a moist base; an *ulcer* is a deeper lesion, extending into the dermis and sometimes below it. *Atrophy* of the skin produces a depression in the skin surface. If the epidermis is atrophic, the skin appears thin and translucent, and it wrinkles when the edges of the affected area are pinched.

In addition to the foregoing types of morphologic changes described, the pattern formed by the lesions on the skin should be noted. Lesions may be arranged in lines, as are the linear vesicles seen in allergic contact dermatitis due to poison ivy; they also may be grouped, as are the vesicles observed in herpes simplex, or dermatomal, as in herpes zoster. The distribution of the lesions also should be noted. For instance, seborrheic dermatitis commonly involves not only the scalp but the eyebrows and nasolabial folds as well. Psoriasis often affects traumatized areas, such as the elbows and knees. Pityriasis rosea presents as ovoid, slightly scaly thin plaques arranged along lines of skin stress, particularly on the back where they mimic the appearance of the branches of a fir tree. Acne occurs almost exclusively on the face, shoulders, back, and chest.

The headings of most of the sections that follow are morphologic descriptors of cutaneous lesions. The most common dermatologic conditions are covered in these sections, with the emphasis placed on clinical appearance, differentiation from other lesions, and suggestions for management. Some conditions can have different clinical presentations. In these cases, the condition is presented in each pertinent section. Therefore, discussions about contact dermatitis can be found under Vesicles, Scaling and Dry Lesions, and Pruritic Lesions.

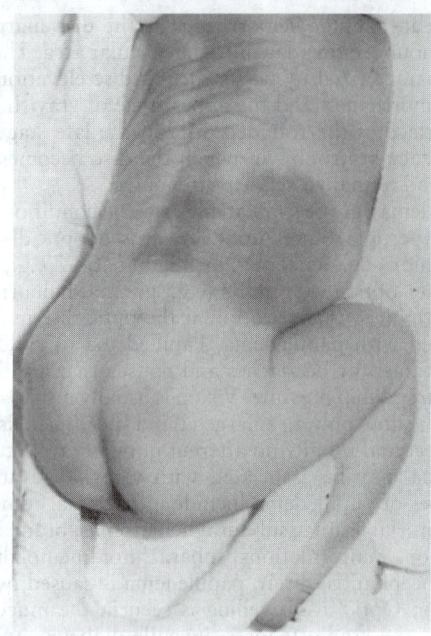

FIGURE 129.1. The blue-gray hyperpigmentation of mongolian spots is most common over the buttocks and back.

SKIN LESIONS IN THE NEONATAL PERIOD

Macules and Patches

Hyperpigmented

Mongolian Spots. Present at birth, mongolian spots are blue-gray or blue-green and represent areas of dermal melanosis. They occur most frequently in the lumbosacral area (Fig. 129.1) and over the shoulders. Occasionally, they are found on the anterior trunk and extremities; only rarely are they seen on the face. More than 90% of African Americans, 80% of Asians, and 46% of Hispanics have mongolian spots, whereas fewer than 10% of Caucasians have them.

Although these lesions tend to disappear with time (usually by the ages of 4 to 5 years), the color change persists in 5% of children. Because mongolian spots have been mistaken for bruises associated with child abuse, educating parents and nursery or day-care workers regarding the congenital nature of the patches is important. Mongolian spots are believed to result from arrested migration of melanocytes from the neural crest. Because the spots are benign, no therapy is necessary. Malignant degeneration has not been reported.

Café au Lait Macules. Café au lait macules (CALMs) are light to dark brown in color, well defined, and range in size from a few millimeters to many centimeters. In a cohort of 4,641 newborns, 12% of African American and 0.3% of Caucasian infants had at least one of these lesions. African American infants were more likely to have more than one lesion: 4.4% had two, and 1.8% had three or more. None of the Caucasian infants had more than one lesion. The incidence of CALMs increases with age; among children under the age of 10 years, 13% of Caucasian and 27% of African American children have at least one CALM. Multiple CALMs are associated with neurofibromatosis type 1; they also can be seen in other syndromes. (See Hyperpigmented Macules in the section Skin Lesions in Infancy, Childhood, and Adolescence, later.)

Linear and Whorled Nevoid Hypermelanosis. Linear and whorled nevoid hypermelanosis is the term used to describe linear, streak-like, or swirling patterns of hyperpigmentation that follow the lines of Blaschko, the lines that reflect the pattern of migration of embryonic cells from the neural crest. Pigmentation is present at birth or within the first few weeks of age. Over time, it becomes more prominent and then stabilizes. Linear and whorled nevoid hypermelanosis most often is a disorder limited to the skin, although occasional infants will have skeletal or developmental abnormalities. The condition is believed to result from mosaicism of neuroectodermal cells prior to migration. The differing skin colors represent two separate cell populations.

Nevus of Ota. A nevus of Ota is an uncommon, bluish or gray-brown patch of pigmentation that occurs on the skin of the face, usually in the distribution of the first and second branches of the trigeminal nerve. Perhaps two-thirds of affected infants have an associated ipsilateral bluish discoloration of the sclera. Although they are most common in Asians, the lesions may occur in deeply pigmented individuals. Approximately one-half are congenital; the rest appear later, often during the second decade of life. Histologically, a nevus of Ota is identical to a mongolian spot and likely results from errors in migration of melanocytes from the neural crest. Unlike the mongolian spot, however, the nevus of Ota does not undergo spontaneous regression. If scleral pigmentation is present, glaucoma may occur. Malignant degeneration occurring within a nevus of Ota is rare. Management options for the nevus include the use of a covering cosmetic or treatment with a pigmented lesion laser.

Nevus of Ito. A patch of hyperpigmentation similar to the nevus of Ota but occurring over the shoulders, in the supraclavicular areas, and on the sides of the neck, the upper arms, and the scapulae is known as the *nevus of Ito*. These lesions persist throughout life. Treatment options are analogous to those for the nevus of Ota.

Congenital Melanocytic Nevi. Congenital melanocytic nevi (CMN) are present in 1% of newborns (color Fig. 68.1 in color section). Most of the nevi are small, well defined, and flat or minimally elevated. When compared with normal surrounding skin, CMN are at increased risk for the development of malignant melanoma. For small lesions (e.g., those less than 1.5 to 2 cm) and those of intermediate size, this risk is low (likely less than 1% to 2%) and malignant transformation is highly unlikely before puberty. However, the lifetime risk of melanoma developing in a large lesion (e.g., greater than or equal to 20 cm) is as high as 6% to 7% and this change may occur early in life (Fig. 129.2).

Infants with small or intermediate-sized lesions may be managed with observation during childhood. Surgical intervention may be considered in the unlikely event that lesions change in size or appearance. Although controversial, some experts advise elective excision of these lesions at puberty depending on their location and the anticipated cosmetic outcome of the procedure. The management of large CMN also is controversial. Owing to the risk of malignant change, many experts advise excision, although the size and distribution of the nevus may render removal difficult and disfiguring. Thus, the management of CMN must be individualized based on the nature of the lesion and the family's preference. Finally, infants with large CMN overlying the head or posterior trunk may have underlying neurocutaneous melanosis, a benign or malignant melanocytic infiltration of the leptomeninges. Infants with such lesions may benefit from magnetic resonance imaging of the head or spine.

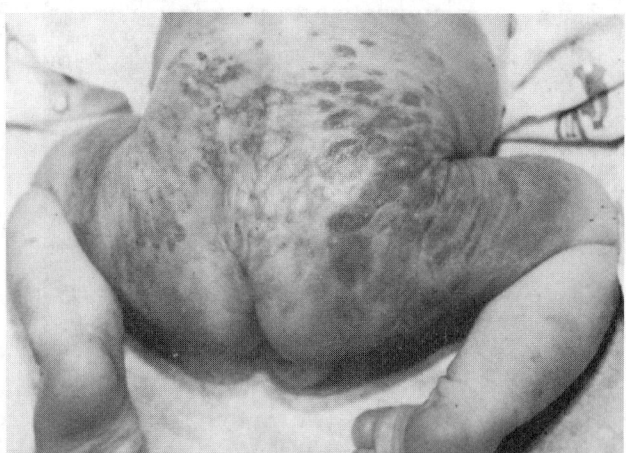

FIGURE 129.2. Extensive hyperpigmentation and nodules in a large congenital melanocytic nevus.

Hypopigmented

Ash Leaf Macules. Hypopigmented macules are present in 0.4% to 0.6% of newborn infants. A single lesion in an otherwise healthy infant likely represents an isolated cutaneous finding. However, multiple hypopigmented macules should raise concern that the lesions represent ash leaf macules associated with tuberous sclerosis, an autosomal dominant disorder characterized classically by the triad of seizures, mental retardation, and adenoma sebaceum. Ash leaf macules are the earliest sign of tuberous sclerosis and often are present at birth. They are oval-shaped hypopigmented macules measuring 2 to 12 mm that typically are located on the trunk or extremities. In lightly pigmented individuals, they may be recognized more easily by the use of a Wood lamp in a darkened room.

Hypomelanosis of Ito. Linear or streaked hypopigmentation following the lines of Blaschko is termed *hypomelanosis of Ito*. As with linear and whorled hypermelanosis (discussed earlier), hypomelanosis of Ito likely reflects cutaneous mosaicism. Most affected infants are well; rarely, the disorder may be associated with seizures, mental retardation, or skeletal or ocular abnormalities.

Nevus Depigmentosus. The name *nevus depigmentosus* is a misnomer since lesions are hypopigmented, not depigmented. Lesions usually are solitary, large, irregularly shaped patches that are present at birth and located on the trunk or extremities. A nevus depigmentosus usually represents an isolated cutaneous abnormality that will persist throughout life.

Papules

White

Milia. Single or multiple 1- to 2-mm yellowish white papules, known as *milia*, occur in some 40% of newborns. These lesions are found most commonly over the cheeks, forehead, nose, and nasolabial folds (Fig. 129.3). Much less commonly, they may be found on the trunk or extremities. Histologically, they represent cysts composed of keratin and are similar to Epstein pearls, the whitish papules noted on the palates of many newborns. Treatment is unnecessary; the cysts disappear in the first few weeks of life.

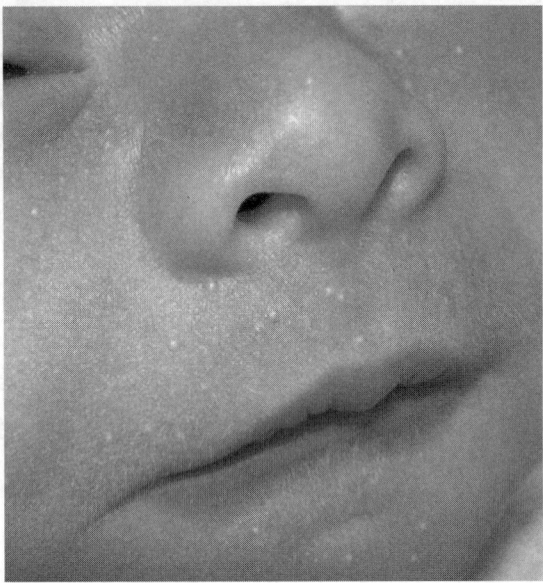

FIGURE 129.3. Milia on the face of a newborn. (Courtesy of P. Sagerman)

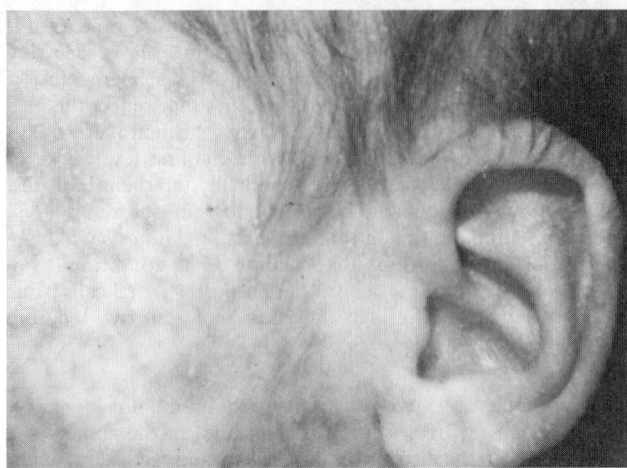

FIGURE 129.4. Diffuse, pinpoint papules and pustules of miliaria on the face of an infant.

Yellow

Sebaceous Gland Hypertrophy. Stimulation of the sebaceous glands (which lie at the base of the pilosebaceous units) by androgens often leads to the appearance of tiny, yellowish papules over the nose and, occasionally, other parts of the face. Because androgen levels decline over time, the appearance of these papules is transient, and clearing occurs in a few weeks. No therapy is necessary.

Erythematous

Erythema Toxicum. The erythematous macules, papules, and (sometimes) vesicles of erythema toxicum (color Fig. 68.9 in color section) occur in at least one-half of term newborns; they are less common in premature infants. Generally, the lesions appear between the first 24 and 48 hours of life and are described best as resembling flea bites. The individual lesions tend to last less than 24 hours, but new lesions can appear during the first 2 weeks of life and, occasionally, later. Clinical difficulty may arise in separating the lesions of erythema toxicum from those of more ominous conditions, such as staphylococcal pustulosis or herpes simplex virus infection. Identification of large patches of macular erythema surrounding the lesions is one way to recognize erythema toxicum. If uncertainty exists, a vesicle or pustule may be opened and the contents placed on a glass slide and stained with a Wright stain. In erythema toxicum, microscopic examination will reveal the predominance of eosinophils. A peripheral eosinophilia often is present as well. To exclude the possibility of staphylococcal pustulosis, a Gram stain and bacterial culture may be performed. If herpes simplex virus infection is a concern, a Tzanck smear, direct fluorescent antibody test, polymerase chain reaction, or viral culture may be obtained. The cause of erythema toxicum has not been elucidated. No treatment is necessary for this benign condition.

Neonatal Acne. Comedones, erythematous papules, and pustules—all resembling the acne of adolescence—may occur in the neonatal period, generally at 2 to 4 weeks of life. Male infants are affected primarily, and the lesions generally occur on the cheeks and almost never are seen on the chest and back. Androgenic stimulation of the sebaceous glands is responsible for the appearance of the lesions. Generally, the eruption

disappears in weeks or months, and no therapy is required. Occasionally, in severe or prolonged cases, topical erythromycin or 2.5% benzoyl peroxide can be prescribed. Pustules suggesting neonatal acne may be caused by *Malassezia furfur* or *M. sympodialis* yeasts in a condition called *neonatal cephalic pustulosis* (see Vesicles and Pustules, later). A potassium hydroxide scraping may differentiate this condition from acne.

Miliaria. Miliaria is the term applied to lesions that occur as the result of sweat duct obstruction and rupture. Three forms exist: miliaria crystallina, miliaria rubra (the most common type), and miliaria pustulosa. Miliaria crystallina is a tiny, teardrop-like, clear, fragile vesicle caused by the superficial plugging of sweat ducts. The lesions appear shortly after birth (particularly on the forehead), have no surrounding erythema, and disappear rapidly without intervention. Miliaria rubra, in contrast, is associated with surrounding erythema as a result of extravasation of sweat into the epidermis, causing localized inflammation (Fig. 129.4). In miliaria pustulosa, more intense inflammation results in the formation of pustules. Young infants seem particularly prone to miliaria, perhaps in part because of parental concern about keeping them warm. The areas most likely to be affected are the face, skin folds of the neck, shoulders, and diaper area. Therapy consists of removing excessive clothing, avoiding the application of thick emollients (that may obstruct sweat ducts), and maintaining a comfortable environmental temperature.

Vesicles and Pustules

Transient Neonatal Pustular Melanosis

Transient neonatal pustular melanosis presents as pustules, ruptured pustules with a collarette of scale (that represents the remnants of the pustule roofs), and small hyperpigmented macules (in the sites of previous pustules). It occurs in 4% to 5% of African American infants and in fewer than 1% of Caucasian infants. The face, chin, neck, and shoulders are the areas most commonly affected. If vesiculopustules are present, they disappear within 1 to 2 days. In contrast, the pigmented macules may take weeks or even months to fade. The pustules are 1 to 3 mm in diameter, usually are flaccid, and have no surrounding erythema (see color Fig. 68.10 in color section). Most have very little content on rupturing, including perhaps a few neutrophils. The cause of this disorder is unknown, but it appears to be an entirely benign condition. A Gram stain of the contents of a pustular lesion should prove most helpful in differentiating transient neonatal pustular melanosis from bacterial pustulosis. No therapy is necessary.

Neonatal Cephalic Pustulosis

A condition that may mimic neonatal acne is neonatal cephalic pustulosis caused by infection with the yeasts *Malassezia furfur* or *M. sympodialis*. At 2 to 3 weeks of age, inflammatory papules and pustules appear. Unlike neonatal acne, however, neonatal cephalic pustulosis is not characterized by comedones and lesions are distributed more widely, involving the scalp and trunk, as well as the face. To confirm the diagnosis, a potassium hydroxide preparation performed on a scraping of a lesion will reveal yeast spores. Neonatal cephalic pustulosis resolves without treatment but a topical antiyeast preparation may be applied to hasten its disappearance.

Congenital Candidiasis

Congenital cutaneous candidiasis is an uncommon disorder that is acquired *in utero*. Lesions are present at birth or develop shortly thereafter. The newborn's skin often is diffusely erythematous and scaly. Tiny papules, vesicles, and pustules also are present. Examination of a scraping of the lesions should reveal the budding hyphae and pseudohyphae of *Candida*. Congenital candidiasis typically is limited to the skin, although premature infants may develop systemic involvement with pneumonia or sepsis. Cutaneous lesions are treated with a topical antiyeast preparation (e.g., nystatin).

Herpes Simplex Virus Infection

Vesicular lesions, whether grouped (as is typical) or scattered (as sometimes occurs in the neonatal period), always should suggest the possibility of herpes simplex virus (HSV) infection. The majority of infants in whom herpes infections develop are born to mothers who are unaware of their own infection with the virus. Infection usually is acquired during passage through the infected birth canal, although ascending infection, particularly in association with premature rupture of the amniotic membranes, also is recognized. Neonatal HSV infection usually has its onset during the second or third week of life, but it may appear at birth or as late as 4 weeks of age.

Three forms of infection are recognized, each accounting for approximately one-third of all cases. Skin, eye, and mouth (SEM) infection begins at a mean of 11 days of age. Classically, infants present with clustered vesicles on an erythematous base. Lesions are concentrated on the head, particularly in areas of trauma, such as the site of placement of a scalp electrode (Fig. 129.5). Over several days, the vesicles become pustules, rupture, and form crusts. Occasionally, lesions will be widespread or in a distribution mimicking that of herpes zoster. Involvement of the mucous membranes produces shallow ulcers. If untreated, as many as 70% of infants with SEM infection develop disseminated disease.

Disseminated HSV infection has its onset at a mean of 11 days of age producing symptoms and signs suggestive of bacterial sepsis. Multiple organ systems are involved, including the liver, lungs, brain, and adrenal glands. Approximately 60% of affected infants also have skin lesions. The mortality rate associated with disseminated disease is high, even with effective treatment. Central nervous system infection begins at a mean of 17 days of age and is heralded by fever, altered sensorium, seizures, and coma. Sixty percent of affected infants have associated skin lesions.

The importance of immediate diagnosis of HSV infection cannot be overemphasized. Suspicious lesions should be tested

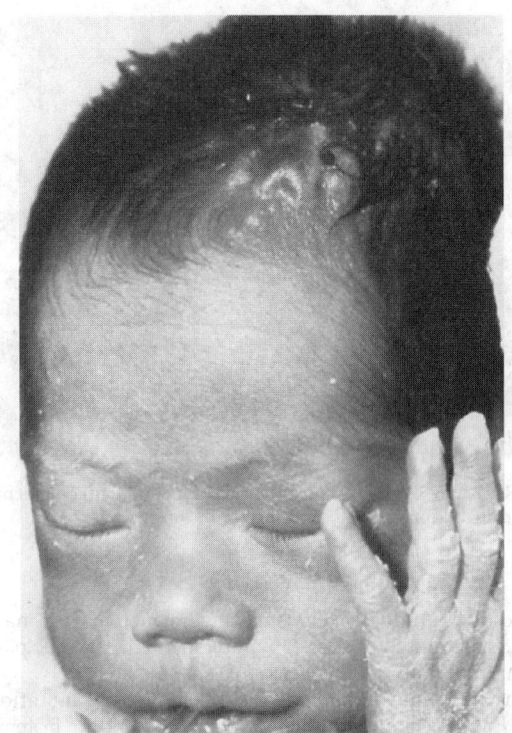

FIGURE 129.5. Clustered vesicles of neonatal herpes simplex virus infection that developed at the site of a scalp electrode. See Color Figure 129.5 in color section. (Courtesy of Alec Wittek, MD.)

by viral culture or polymerase chain reaction. In experienced hands, rapid diagnosis may be obtained via the performance of a Tzanck preparation. Parenteral acyclovir therapy should be administered without delay.

Neonatal Varicella

Neonatal varicella is an uncommon condition resulting from *in utero* infection in the 2 to 3 weeks before delivery. The lesions in neonates are similar to those seen in older infants and children, with crops of macules and papules developing into teardrop-like vesicles. The diagnosis is suspected by a maternal history. A Tzanck preparation will reveal multinucleated giant cells, but this finding does not differentiate between varicella and herpes simplex virus infection. Because disease may be severe, it is recommended that newborns whose mothers develop varicella 5 days before to 2 days after delivery receive varicella-zoster immune globulin.

Incontinentia Pigmenti

Incontinentia pigmenti (IP) is a rare genodermatosis with cutaneous abnormalities that occur in four stages. The earliest lesions are vesicles on erythematous bases that are arranged in a linear pattern on the trunk or extremities (Fig. 129.6; color Fig. 68.11 in color section). The lesions are present at birth or appear within the first 2 weeks of life. Individual lesions last 1 to 2 weeks but new lesions may appear for months. In this stage, IP often is confused with herpes simplex virus infection or impetigo. The second stage, which may overlap with the first, is characterized by verrucous (wart-like) papules located primarily on the extremities, but not necessarily at the sites previously affected by vesicles. This stage peaks at 12 to 26 weeks of age and resolves within 1 to 2 years. The third stage is one of tan to slate-gray hyperpigmentation that is arranged in a linear or whorled pattern on the trunk and extremities. This stage

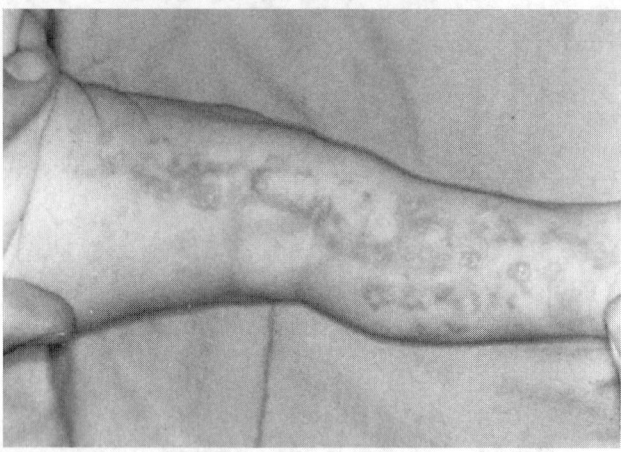

FIGURE 129.6. Papulovesicular lesions of incontinentia pigmenti in a linear distribution on the flexor surface of one leg.

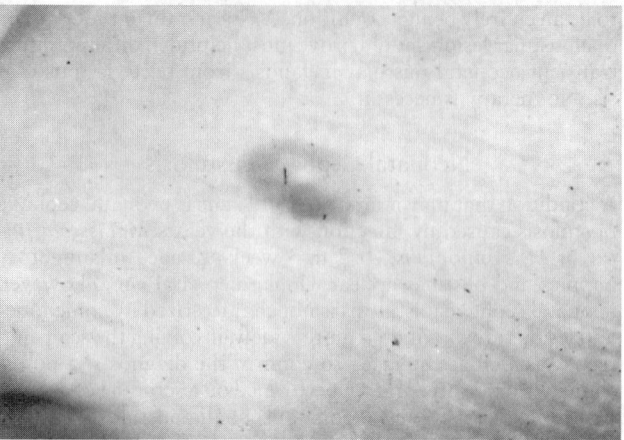

FIGURE 129.7. A solitary bullous lesion, due to sucking *in utero*, on the dorsum of a newborn's hand.

also resolves gradually. The final stage, which may or may not occur, is composed of subtle, hypopigmented, atrophic patches of skin, especially on the legs.

IP is an X-linked dominant disorder caused by mutations in the *NEMO* gene. More than 97% of cases occur in females, suggesting that the condition is lethal for males *in utero*. It is a multisystem disorder affecting tissues derived from the neural crest. The majority of patients have extracutaneous disease involving the central nervous system (e.g., seizures, spastic paresis, microcephaly, or mental retardation), eye (e.g., strabismus, blindness, cataracts, or optic nerve atrophy), teeth (e.g., cone-shaped or irregularly shaped teeth), hair (e.g., alopecia), and bones (e.g., hemivertebrae, extra ribs, or syndactyly). Thus, children with IP require a multidisciplinary approach to management.

Eosinophilic Pustular Folliculitis

Eosinophilic pustular folliculitis is an uncommon disorder that usually occurs in neonates. However, a more widespread and persistent form has been described in children with human immunodeficiency virus infection. The disease is characterized by recurrent crops of pruritic, follicular, papulopustular lesions. The lesions tend to coalesce into plaques and occur most commonly on the scalp, face, chest, and back. Smears from the pustules show eosinophils, and peripheral eosinophilia is common. The lesions are sterile. The cause of the lesions is not known and the course varies. Treatment with topical corticosteroids of moderate potency has met with modest success.

Bullae

Sucking Blisters

Infants commonly suck their hands or fingers *in utero*. Occasionally, a thick-walled bulla on the dorsum of the hand, fingers, or forearm will result (Fig. 129.7). Their characteristic appearance and location and the observation of the infant sucking the affected area are helpful clues to this diagnosis. Treatment is supportive; a topical antibiotic and dressing may be applied as needed.

Bullous Impetigo

Bullous impetigo is caused by infection with strains of *Staphylococcus aureus* that elaborate toxins (exfoliative toxins A and

B) that damage intercellular adherence resulting in the formation of bullae. It may occur at a few days of age, but generally it begins during the second or third week. Individual lesions are bullae that have a small rim of erythema. The bullae rupture easily, leaving an eroded, moist base that forms a crust and is surrounded by a rim of scale, the remnant of the blister roof. To confirm the diagnosis, the contents of a bulla may be cultured and a Gram stain performed.

Infants who appear well and have limited disease may be treated with an oral antistaphylococcal antibiotic. If signs of systemic infection are present, however, the infant should be evaluated appropriately and treated parenterally.

Elaboration of exfoliative toxins also may lead to staphylococcal scalded skin syndrome, characterized by generalized erythema and the appearance of bullae, particularly in areas of trauma. There may be widespread loss of skin resulting in fluid loss and thermal instability. (See Bullae in the section Skin Lesions in Infancy, Childhood, and Adolescence, later.)

Epidermolysis Bullosa

Epidermolysis bullosa (EB) represents a group of rare hereditary diseases. The disorders result from defects in proteins involved in anchoring the epidermis to underlying structures. This, in turn, causes skin fragility with vesicles, bullae, and erosions. Depending on the disease type, involvement of the mucosae of the mouth or gastrointestinal or respiratory tracts may be present. Some forms of EB present at or shortly following birth with blisters and erosions resulting from delivery or handling (see color Fig. 68.16 in color section). The diagnosis of EB is based on family history, clinical findings, and cutaneous biopsy. Treatment is supportive, including gentle handling and bathing; the use of a soft nipple for feeding and loose-fitting diapers and clothing; and the application of a topical antibiotic to erosions. EB is discussed more completely later in this chapter (see Bullae in the section Skin Lesions in Infancy, Childhood, and Adolescence, later).

Congenital Syphilis

Bullae and vesicles are an unusual presentation of congenital syphilis (Fig. 129.8). Most common on the extremities, they rupture rapidly, leaving an eroded surface. More commonly, flat-topped papules and plaques are seen that affect the mucocutaneous junctions, including the angles of the mouth and perineum (e.g., condyloma lata). Ovoid, slightly scaly, salmon-colored macules may also be present on the trunk and extremities (Fig. 129.9).

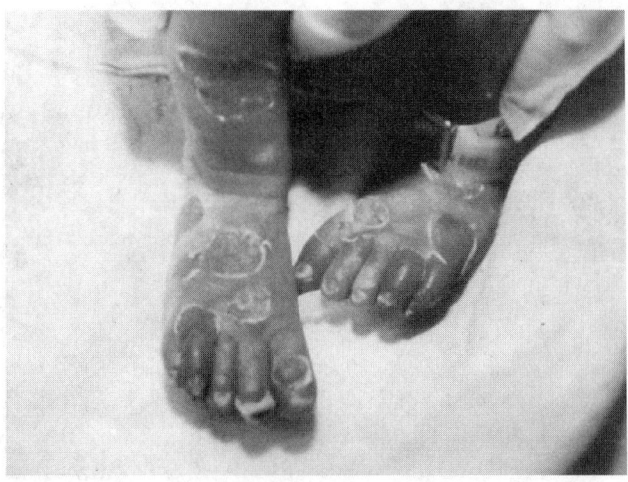

FIGURE 129.8. Pemphigus syphiliticus, a widely disseminated vesiculobullous eruption in an infant with early congenital syphilis. See Color Figure 129.8 in color section. (Courtesy of Charles Ginsburg, MD.)

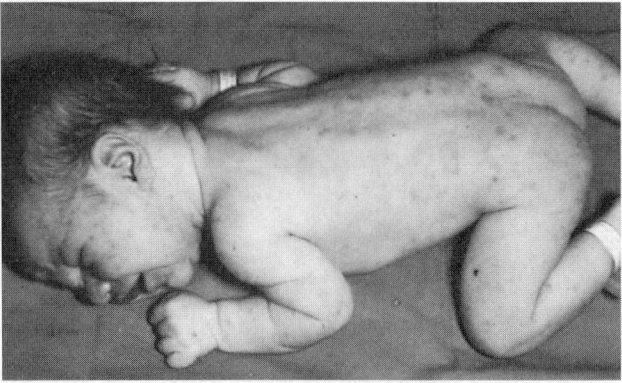

FIGURE 129.10. Diffuse, purplish papules and nodules create a blueberry-muffin appearence in an infant with congenital rubella.

Purpura

Hemorrhagic lesions may occur on the skin of newborns for a variety of reasons. Infectious causes always should be considered, including bacterial and congenitally acquired infections.

Congenital Rubella

Purpuric lesions of infants infected with rubella virus *in utero* are caused most commonly by thrombocytopenia. On occasion, the purpuric lesions take on an infiltrative or nodular quality, producing a blueberry-muffin appearance (Fig. 129.10). The lesions actually are areas of extramedullary hematopoiesis rather than true cutaneous hemorrhage.

Congenital Cytomegalovirus Infection

Petechiae in conjunction with intrauterine growth restriction, hepatosplenomegaly, and hyperbilirubinemia always should raise the question of congenital infection. Cytomegalovirus is the most prevalent of these infections. Most of the purpuric lesions are the result of thrombocytopenia. Blueberry muffin–like lesions also have been documented.

Plaques and Nodules

Subcutaneous Fat Necrosis

Subcutaneous fat necrosis is a disorder of unknown cause that often occurs in association with birth trauma. Lesions typically are not present at birth but appear within the first weeks of age. The areas most commonly affected are the cheeks, buttocks, back, arms, and thighs. Lesions are irregular, hard, erythematous, or violaceous nodules that seem nontender. The size of the nodules varies. Occasionally, the lesions may become calcified, but generally they resolve spontaneously in 1 to 2 months without scarring. Some infants may develop symptomatic hypercalcemia that must be treated appropriately. No therapy of the skin lesions is necessary.

Nevus Sebaceus

The nevus sebaceus (of Jadassohn) is present at birth and usually is found on the scalp (color Fig. 68.3 in color section). The area is devoid of hair, slightly raised, smooth or with a velvety texture, and yellow to yellow-orange. Lesions vary in size and can be found on the face as well (Fig. 129.11). Sebaceous nevi represent benign hamartomas containing an increased number of sebaceous glands. Most represent isolated cutaneous

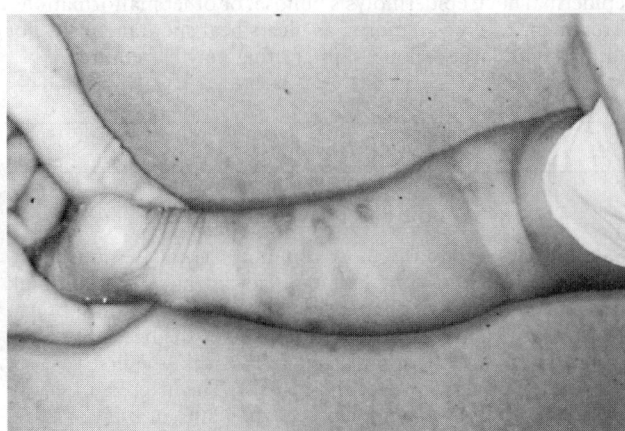

FIGURE 129.9. Ovoid, brownish lesions with a fine scale on the leg of a neonate with congenital syphilis.

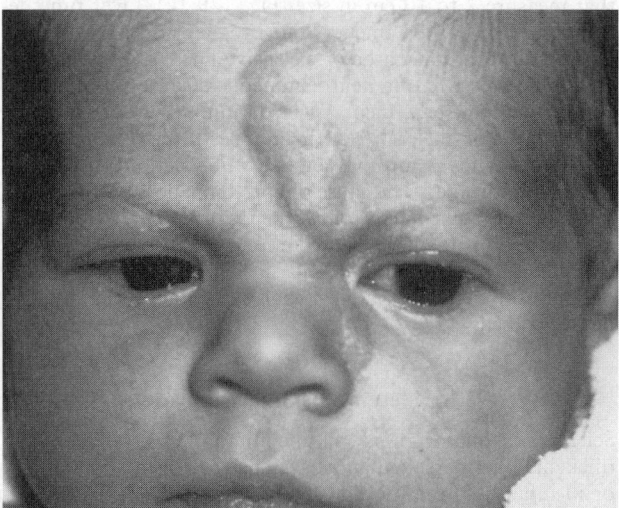

FIGURE 129.11. A tan-yellow plaque of a sebaceus nevus on the forehead. (Courtesy of P. J. Honig, MD.)

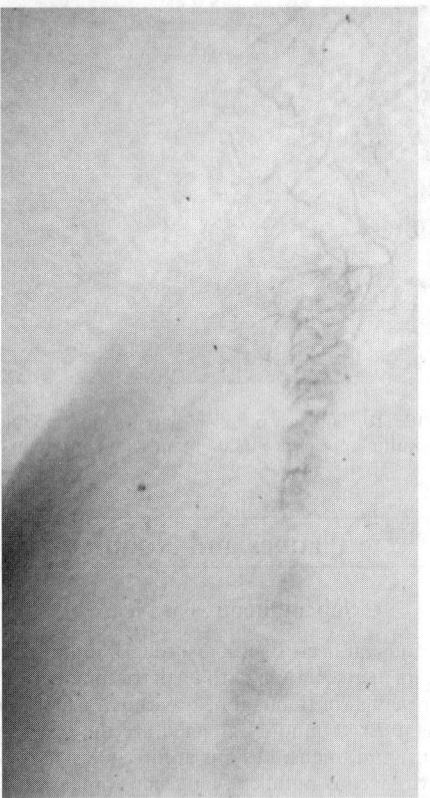

FIGURE 129.12. Linear epidermal nevi in the axillary area.

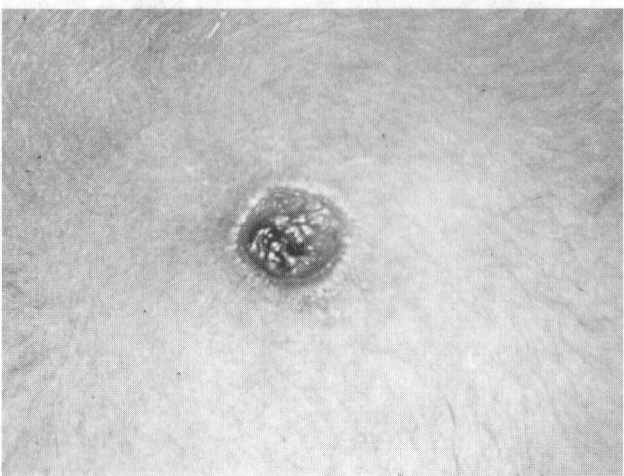

FIGURE 129.13. An ulcer of aplasia cutis congenita on the scalp of a newborn.

abnormalities but large or extensive lesions may be associated with mental retardation, seizures, or ophthalmic or skeletal malformations. Due to a small risk of malignant transformation (e.g., to a basal cell carcinoma) after puberty, elective excision may be considered at adolescence.

Epidermal Nevi

Epidermal nevi usually are present at birth but may appear during childhood or adolescence. They are verrucous-appearing, skin-colored or somewhat hyperpigmented papules or plaques that measure 2 to 10 cm in size (Fig. 129.12). Over time, lesions become darker, thicker, and rougher and may develop an unpleasant odor. Large or extensive linear lesions may indicate the presence of a neurocutaneous disorder with central nervous system (e.g., mental retardation, seizures), eye (e.g., strabismus), or skeletal (e.g., hemihypertrophy, kyphoscoliosis) abnormalities, and may be a feature of the Proteus and CHILD syndromes. The cause of epidermal nevi is not known but they represent hamartomas (benign tumors composed of normal but disorganized skin components). There is no risk of malignant transformation. If treatment is desired, application of a keratolytic agent, surgical excision, or laser therapy may be considered.

Sclerema Neonatorum

Sclerema neonatorum is an uncommon, rapidly spreading thickening of the subcutaneous tissue that occurs in preterm or ill infants during the first few weeks of life. The skin becomes tight, shiny, and nonpitting. Affected infants usually are seriously ill with other problems and rarely survive once this condition appears.

Dermoid Cysts

The small, rubbery, smooth subcutaneous nodules characteristic of dermoid cysts occur most frequently on the head and neck. Congenital lesions formed from embryonic ectoderm, they are lined by stratified squamous epithelium. Almost 40% are periorbital, and approximately 30% occur in the eyebrows. The lesions usually are solitary and asymptomatic, and they are managed by surgical excision. Lesions in the midline of the scalp or forehead or at the glabella may have an intracranial extension. Therefore, imaging of the bone and central nervous system should be conducted prior to excision.

Ulcers

Aplasia Cutis Congenita

Aplasia cutis congenita is characterized by a congenital absence of the skin. Affected infants usually exhibit a single lesion that may be a round or oval ulcer or atrophic scar that is located on the scalp at or near the vertex (Fig. 129.13). Individual lesions range in size from 1 to 3 cm. Occasionally, there is an associated defect in the cranium. Although aplasia cutis congenita most often represents an isolated cutaneous abnormality, it may be associated with limb abnormalities, sebaceous or epidermal nevi, epidermolysis bullosa, or other malformations. Treatment rarely is required as ulcers heal spontaneously. For infants with large lesions, skin grafting may be required.

Vascular Lesions

Salmon Patch (Nevus Simplex)

Salmon patches are the most common vascular lesions in infancy, seen in almost one-half of all newborns. These dull-pink macules composed of dilated dermal capillaries are most prevalent over the glabella, eyelids, and nape of the neck. Facial lesions tend to fade with time, generally within the first years of life. Neck lesions, however, may persist. The macules often are called *stork bites* (when located at the nape) or *angels' kisses* (when located on the face). During crying, older infants and children may demonstrate flushing in areas of previous lesions that have faded.

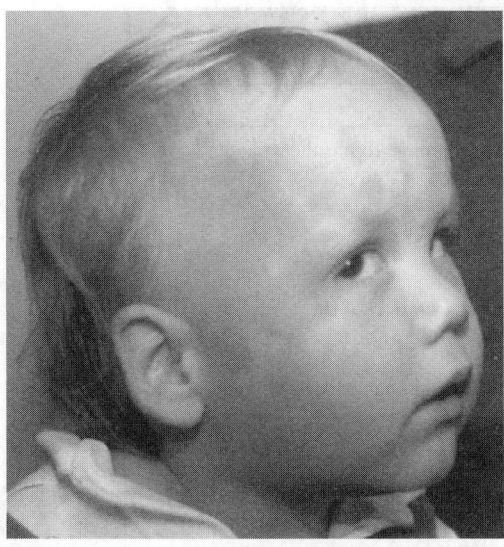

FIGURE 129.14. A port wine stain involving the right frontotemporal area.

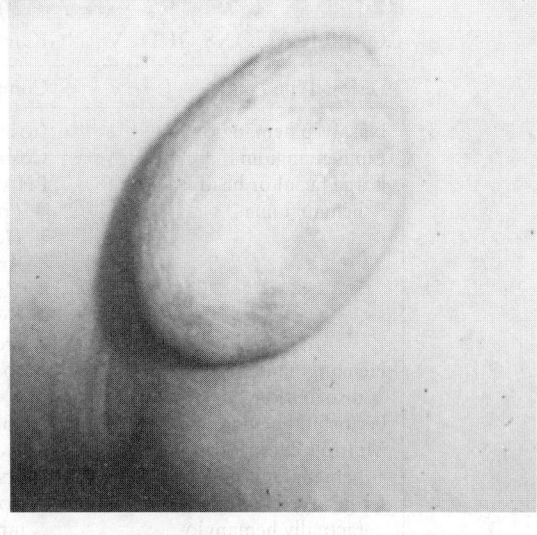

FIGURE 129.15. A large superficial hemangioma shows whitening of the surface, indicating the start of resolution.

Port Wine Stains

The benign salmon patch must be differentiated from the port wine stain, which is a congenital, permanent vascular malformation composed of mature vessels. Port wine stains (PWSs) are reddish or reddish purple and typically are darker than salmon patches (Fig. 129.14). They may occur anywhere on the body, although they are seen most commonly on the face. Infants with PWSs involving the distribution of the first and second branches of the trigeminal nerve (upper and lower eyelids, respectively), all three branches of the trigeminal nerve, or both sides of the face are at risk for Sturge-Weber syndrome. In this sporadic disorder, the vascular malformation involves not only the skin, but also the ipsilateral leptomeningeal vessels, particularly those in the parietooccipital region. Slow flow through these vessels causes hypoxic injury that, in turn, may result in seizures or contralateral hemiparesis. The vascular malformation also may affect the ipsilateral eye. Abnormalities of the choroid and episcleral vessels may lead to retinal detachment or glaucoma, respectively. PWSs on the extremities usually represent an isolated abnormality and only rarely are associated with overgrowth of the extremity (Klippel-Trenaunay syndrome). Because PWSs tend to become darker and thicker with time and may develop surface bleeding, children with significant facial PWSs should be referred for consideration of pulsed dye laser therapy early in life.

Harlequin Color Change

Harlequin color change is a curious phenomenon usually noted in the first few days of life in low-birth-weight infants. When such infants are placed on their sides, a sharp midline demarcation develops in the color of their bodies, with the upper one-half turning pale and the lower one-half turning deep red. A change in position results in resolution of the color change. The phenomenon can last for a few weeks and is attributed to a temporary imbalance in the regulatory mechanisms of the autonomic nervous system.

Hemangiomas

Hemangiomas are benign vascular tumors that proliferate during the first 6 to 9 months of age and then begin to involute, resulting in complete regression in most children. Hemangiomas may be present at birth but typically appear at 2 to 4 weeks of age. They are observed in as many as 10% of 1-year-olds. In some newborns, a hypopigmented macule, within which are telangiectatic vessels (a *prehemangioma*), heralds the appearance of a hemangioma. Superficial hemangiomas (often called strawberry hemangiomas) occur in the upper dermis. Deep hemangiomas appear as nodules with normal overlying skin and a bluish discoloration. Lesions with superficial and deep components are termed mixed hemangiomas (color Fig. 68.4 in color section).

Hemangiomas grow rapidly during the first 6 months of life, reach a quiescent stage when the patient is 6 to 12 months old, and then begin to regress when the child is between 12 and 18 months old. Signs of regression include patches of gray on the surface of the lesion (Fig. 129.15). By the time the patient is 5 years old, 50% of lesions will have regressed; by age 9, 90% will have done so. After regression, an area of atrophy, telangiectases, or hypopigmentation may remain. With large lesions, redundant skin may be the major cosmetic defect. Deep hemangiomas may not show complete regression.

Complications of hemangiomas are infrequent. Erosions are the most common complication, particularly for lesions in the diaper area (Fig. 129.16, color Fig. 68.4 in color section).

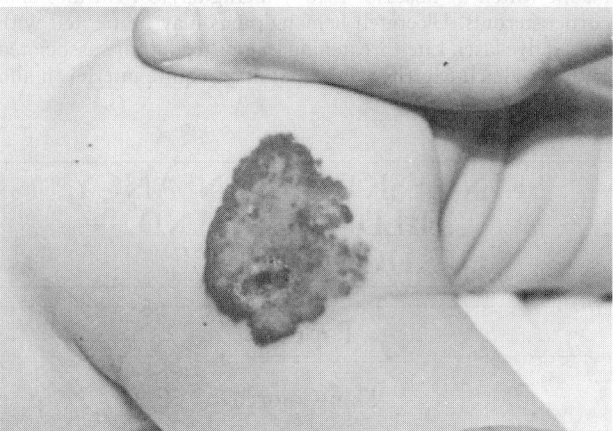

FIGURE 129.16. The surface of this superficial hemangioma has become ulcerated.

TABLE 129.1

COMPLICATIONS OF HEMANGIOMAS

Lesion Type	Complication
Nasal tip hemangioma	Cosmetic disfigurement, damage to nasal cartilage
Lip hemangioma	Cosmetic disfigurement
Large facial or head hemangioma	PHACES syndrome ■ *Posterior fossa abnormalities* ■ *Hemangiomas* ■ *Arterial abnormalities* ■ *Cardiac defects and coarctation of the aorta* ■ *Eye abnormalities* ■ *Sternal clefting*
Hemangioma in the "beard" distribution	Associated laryngeal hemangiomas or airway compression
Periorbital hemangioma	Amblyopia, glaucoma
Multiple cutaneous hemangiomas	May have associated visceral lesions (e.g., central nervous system, lungs, hepatic, gastrointestinal)
Large atypical hemangiomas (actually hemangio-endotheliomas or tufted angiomas)	Lesions may trap platelets, resulting in localized intravascular coagulation

Hemangiomas that become eroded are painful, may become infected, and are prone to scar. They should be treated with a barrier cream and, if infected, an oral antibiotic. If they fail to heal within 1 to 2 weeks, consultation with a pediatric dermatologist is indicated. Bleeding occurs rarely and usually responds well to the application of direct pressure. Infants with multiple cutaneous hemangiomas (color Fig. 68.5 in color section) occasionally have associated visceral lesions in the central nervous system, lungs, liver, or intestines. If present, visceral lesions may result in high-output cardiac failure or hemorrhage. Most infants with systemic involvement present by 2 months of age with respiratory distress, hepatomegaly, a heart murmur, or anemia. The presence of multiple cutaneous hemangiomas should prompt the conduct of a careful history and physical examination. If suspicion exists about visceral involvement, initial screening studies might include a complete blood count, chest radiograph, abdominal ultrasonography, and stool for occult blood. Other potential complications of hemangiomas are presented in Table 129.1.

Since most hemangiomas are small and do not threaten vital structures, no therapy is needed. Complicated hemangiomas should be managed in conjunction with a pediatric dermatologist and other specialists as appropriate. Depending on the lesion type and location, therapeutic options include oral prednisone (often at doses of 2 to 4 mg/kg/day) or intralesional corticosteroids. Ulcerated hemangiomas may be treated with pulsed dye laser. Life-threatening lesions (e.g., those associated with Kasabach-Merritt syndrome) may require interferon alfa or other agents.

SKIN LESIONS IN INFANCY, CHILDHOOD, AND ADOLESCENCE

Papules

Skin-Colored

Warts. Warts are among the most common skin lesions affecting children; they also are among the most frustrating, because treating them often is difficult. Warts are caused by infections with human papillomaviruses (HPVs), DNA viruses of which more than 70 different types have been described. HPV types usually can be related to a specific clinical presentation of the wart; for example, types 1, 2, 4, and 7 cause common warts on the hands and feet. Untreated warts generally have a life span of a few months to 5 years or more. Approximately two-thirds disappear within 2 years, but self-inoculation and spread to other persons may occur. Several types of warts are recognized:

■ Common warts (verrucae vulgaris) are rough skin-colored papules that often are located on the hands. The lesions usually are round, and tiny dark specks frequently can be seen through the surface. These dots represent thrombosed capillaries in the warty tissue. Occasional lesions, particularly those on the face and scalp, may appear as finger-like projections (i.e., filiform warts).

■ Plantar warts occur on the plantar surface of the foot where pressure forces their growth inward, resulting in deep, painful lesions. Plantar warts may be single or grouped in clusters (i.e., mosaic warts). The black specks of thrombosed capillaries help to distinguish warts from corns, which are localized areas of hyperkeratosis over pressure points.

■ Flat warts are tiny, flat-topped, skin-colored papules that occur primarily on the face and dorsa of the extremities. Their surface is smooth, and they may number in the hundreds. At times, they seem to form plaques as they coalesce.

■ Genital warts (condylomata acuminata) tend to be soft, flesh-colored to slightly pigmented papules that may be pedunculated (Fig. 129.17). The occurrence of genital warts in children always should raise the suspicion of sexual abuse. However, in children younger than 2 to 3 years, the condition often results from infection acquired during vaginal delivery.

The response of individual warts to any therapy is variable. Because most warts resolve spontaneously, no intervention is a reasonable choice for some patients. However, parents and older children often desire treatment. For common warts, such keratolytic agents as salicylic and lactic acids in flexible collodion offer painless and effective, albeit slow-acting, therapy. Each day, the warts are soaked in warm water, dried, and

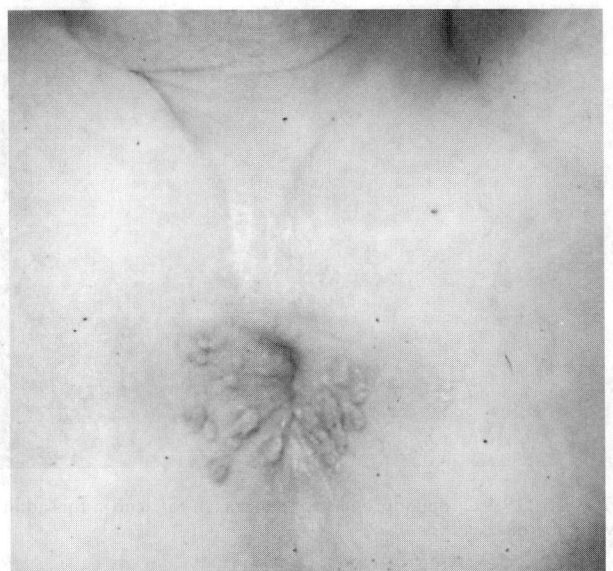

FIGURE 129.17. Skin-colored papules of condylomata acuminata in the anal verge.

débrided with a pumice stone or an emery board; thereafter, the keratolytic agent is applied. Covering the wart with tape may increase the effectiveness of the treatment. The application of liquid nitrogen or other cryogen is similarly effective but is painful and poorly tolerated by young children. To prevent regrowth of remaining wart tissue, keratolytic therapy should be used in the interval between freezing treatments. Imiquimod, a topical immune response enhancer, also may be effective in the treatment of common warts. The options for treating plantar warts are analogous to those described for common warts. However, a higher potency keratolytic agent may be selected. For resistant warts, cantharidin, a blistering agent, may be applied carefully by the clinician in the office. Alternately, patients may be referred for consideration of immunotherapy, laser therapy, or surgical excision.

Options for treating flat warts include topical tretinoin applied daily or the modalities described for managing common warts. Genital warts often respond to the application of podophyllin 25% in tincture of benzoin applied at intervals of 1 to 3 weeks. Patients are advised to remove the medication 4 to 6 hours later by washing. Options for home therapy of these lesions include podofilox and imiquimod. For recalcitrant lesions, laser therapy may be required.

Keratosis Pilaris. Keratosis pilaris is a common, benign skin condition characterized by follicular papules distributed most commonly on the extensor surfaces of the upper arms, thighs, or face. Lesions possess a central plug of keratinaceous material and occasionally have surrounding erythema. They appear most commonly in the second decade of life and, when present on the face, can be mistaken for acne. The cause of keratosis pilaris is unknown but it occurs most often in individuals with atopic dermatitis or ichthyosis vulgaris. For patients who are distressed by the appearance of the lesions, mild keratolytics, such as emollients containing ammonium lactate, urea, or lactic acid, can be used to reduce their prominence. Tretinoin also may prove effective, although it may prove irritating, particularly when used on the face in young children. Patients should be counseled that treatment rarely is completely successful and that lesions may persist.

Id Reaction. Dermatophyte infections, particularly tinea capitis, may induce an immune or "autosensitization" phenomenon

called the id reaction. Lesions are numerous, tiny, skin-colored papules (or occasionally vesicles) that are concentrated on the trunk and extremities. The id reaction often appears after systemic antifungal therapy is begun and should not be mistaken for a drug reaction. The presence of papules, vesicles, and other lesions of the palms and fingers may suggest an id reaction caused by tinea pedis. No specific therapy of the id reaction is required.

Lichen Spinulosus. The key clinical feature of lichen spinulosus is round patches of grouped follicular papules, each possessing a spine of keratinaceous material. The lesions are skin-colored or slightly hypopigmented but usually stand out from unaffected skin. They generally are asymptomatic. The lesions may appear in crops relatively rapidly and are found most commonly on the neck, abdomen, buttocks, lateral thighs, and extensor surfaces of the extremities.

The cause of lichen spinulosus is unknown. The histologic picture is one of hair follicles dilated with a keratinaceous plug. Children with atopic dermatitis seem to be most prone to these lesions. The course is variable; the condition may last indefinitely, although affected sites can change over a period of months without therapy. Treatment with a keratolytic agent, such as an emollient containing ammonium lactate or lactic acid, may improve the appearance of lesions.

Syringomas. Syringomas are firm papules that typically appear skin-colored, but may be yellow or brown. They are found most commonly on the lower eyelids and neck, and generally measure 1 to 3 mm. Females are affected twice as frequently as are males, and the lesions appear most often at puberty. Pathologically, the lesions are benign tumors of eccrine glands. Syringomas persist and may increase in number over time. The lesions appear commonly in individuals with Down syndrome. For patients who desire treatment, laser therapy may be effective.

Eruptive Vellus Hair Cysts. Eruptive vellus hair cysts are skin-colored, red-brown or brown-black, 1- to 4-mm, soft, smooth-surfaced papules. The lesions may be scattered or grouped, and typically occur over the anterior chest and extremities. The onset of lesions occurs in the first decade of life. Although lesions usually occur sporadically, an autosomal dominant mode of inheritance has been documented in some cases. The condition may resolve spontaneously or it may persist, and it usually is asymptomatic. If treatment is desired, tretinoin or lactic acid may be applied topically or individual lesions curetted.

White or Hypopigmented

Molluscum Contagiosum. Lesions of molluscum contagiosum, caused by a DNA poxvirus, are described best as pearly papules. Their size may vary from that of a pinhead to more than 1 cm in diameter. The top of the lesion is almost translucent, often revealing a whitish core known as the *molluscum body*. Larger lesions may have a central umbilication (Fig. 129.18). The number of papules present may vary from few to hundreds. Spread by autoinoculation is common; other members of the family can become infected through contact with the affected person. Individuals with atopic dermatitis are prone to the development of widespread lesions.

Although some physicians recommend no treatment, the condition may last months to years, and parents frequently ask that something be done. In the presence of only a few lesions, in a willing patient, they can be removed with a curet or the surface opened with a needle and the contents expressed. Cantharidin, applied carefully by the clinician in small amounts to each lesion, is painless and effective in causing blistering and extrusion of the central core. Liquid nitrogen, imiquimod, keratolytics, and podophyllin also have been used. Tretinoin also

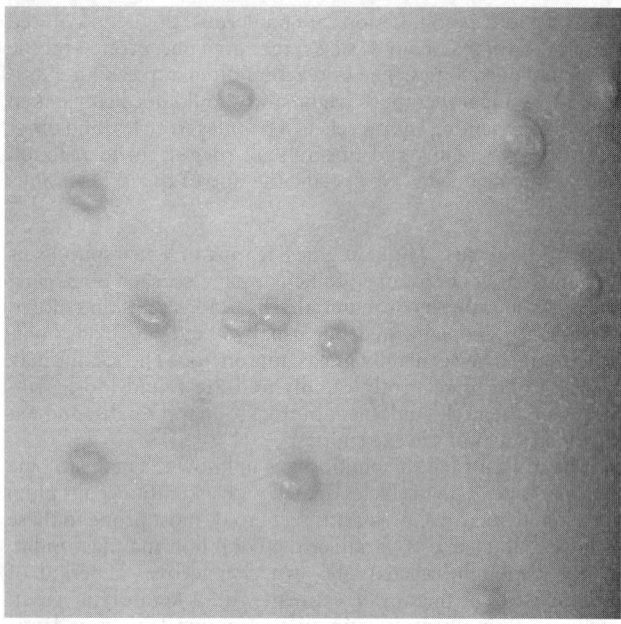

FIGURE 129.18. Translucent papules of molluscum contagiosum. Note the central umbilication of the larger lesions.

may be effective, but irritation of surrounding normal skin may preclude its continued use.

Milia. Milia are discussed in the section Skin Lesions in the Neonatal Period. They commonly are present in newborns but may appear in suture lines, in healed abrasions, at sites of chronic skin erosions in children with epidermolysis bullosa, and at damaged and subsequently healed sites in children with porphyria. Although seldom necessary, incision and expression of the cyst may be performed.

Lichen Nitidus. The tiny (less than 2 mm) papules in lichen nitidus are skin-colored (although they may be hypopigmented in those who are more deeply pigmented) and have a smooth and somewhat shiny surface. The trunk, genitalia, abdomen, and forearms are affected most frequently. Lesions often are numerous and may appear in a linear arrangement at sites of trauma, known as the *Koebner phenomenon*. The cause is unknown, and the pinhead- to pinpoint-sized lesions have a variable course, lasting months to years. No therapy has been demonstrated to be effective, although the application of a topical corticosteroid may be employed for the minority of patients for whom pruritus is a problem.

Erythematous

Miliaria. Miliaria rubra or *prickly heat* is a common condition caused by sweat retention. Obstruction in eccrine ducts leads to their rupture with release of sweat into surrounding tissues. Most commonly, this leads to the formation of tiny erythematous papules located in body folds or on the neck and forehead. Miliaria rubra and the related disorders, miliaria crystallina and pustulosa, are discussed in the section, Skin Lesions in the Neonatal Period, earlier.

Angiofibromas. Angiofibromas are hamartomatous papules and nodules composed of fibrous and vascular tissues. They are solid, are pink or skin-colored, and generally appear after the ages of 2 to 3 years, most commonly on the face. Their key significance is their association with tuberous sclerosis, a neurocutaneous, autosomal dominantly inherited disorder with central nervous system and systemic involvement. Sometimes, the

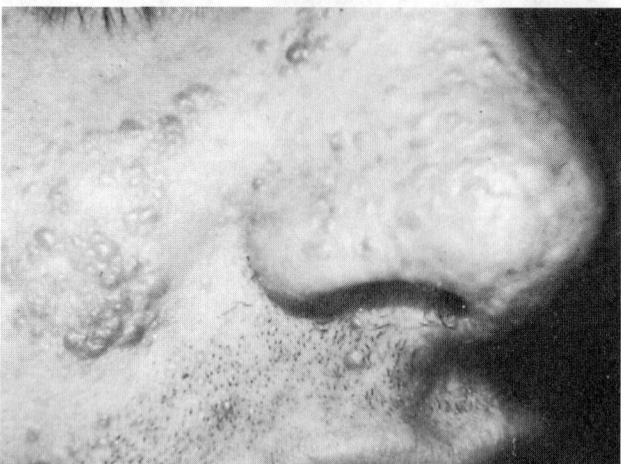

FIGURE 129.19. Angiofibromas were mistaken for acne in this adult with tuberous sclerosis.

lesions are mistaken for acne (Fig. 129.19), but the patient's age at the time of the lesions' appearance and the lack of comedones should exclude this diagnosis. Lesions may be treated by dermabrasion or laser therapy.

Papular Urticaria. Papular urticaria is a common, intensely pruritic disorder caused by hypersensitivity to insect bites. New lesions are papules with an erythematous flare that appear in crops (Fig. 129.20). Some lesions have a central punctum that represents the site of the insect's bite. Others, particularly those that appear in a linear arrangement or cluster, lack a punctum and are believed to be the result of allergens deposited at the time of a bite. Each crop of papules lasts several days but recurrences may be observed at intervals over many months. Most cases occur in the late spring and summer, but household exposure to fleas from animals can cause problems any time of year.

Fleas are the most common cause of papular urticaria, although mosquitos; lice; or grass, grain, or fowl mites also may be responsible. Secondary infections from excoriations are common and, in some children, the wheals may progress to bullae. Treatment success depends on eliminating the biting insects

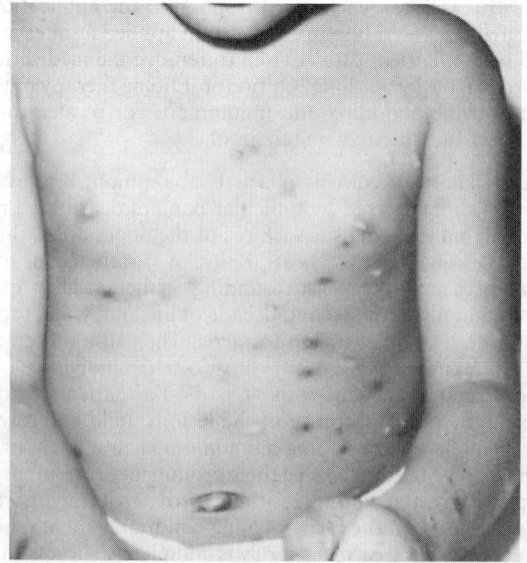

FIGURE 129.20. Papular urticaria. Resolving hyperpigmented papules and recent, erythematous papules with central puncta from flea bites.

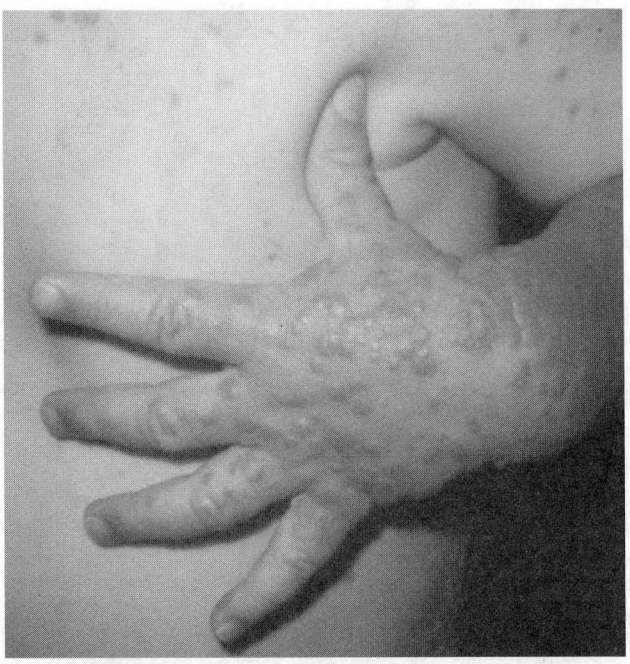

FIGURE 129.21. Numerous reddish papules are present over the arm, whereas the trunk is spared, in a patient with Gianotti-Crosti disease.

FIGURE 129.22. Pityriasis rosea. The diffuse papules may obscure the classic lesions, which are scattered, ovoid pink plaques.

from the child's environment and preventing insect bites. Animals should be examined; if infested, they should be treated appropriately and the household environment decontaminated. Established lesions may be treated with an appropriate topical corticosteroid or nonsensitizing anesthetic (e.g., pramoxine), or an oral antihistamine. If outdoor insects are implicated, patients may be advised to wear long sleeves and pants (that may be treated with permethrin to provide additional protection) and to apply an insect repellent to exposed skin. If present, secondary bacterial infection should be treated appropriately.

Gianotti-Crosti Syndrome. Gianotti-Crosti syndrome, also known as *papular acrodermatitis of childhood*, has a distinctive clinical picture because of the predominant location of the erythematous papules on the face, extremities, and buttocks with relative sparing of the trunk (Fig. 129.21). The papules generally measure from 1 to 5 mm in diameter and may appear to be vesicular; they tend to be of similar size, usually appear rapidly, and may be associated with pruritus.

Gianotti-Crosti syndrome is believed to be a cutaneous reaction to infection with any of a number of viruses, including hepatitis B, Epstein-Barr virus, parainfluenza virus, coxsackieviruses B and A16, cytomegalovirus, poliovirus, parvovirus B-19, rubella virus, human immunodeficiency virus, and respiratory syncytial virus. It also has occurred following immunizations.

There is no specific treatment for Gianotti-Crosti syndrome; however, the rash resolves within 3 to 8 weeks. If pruritus is severe, a topical corticosteroid or nonsensitizing anesthetic, or oral antihistamine may be prescribed.

Papulosquamous Disorders

Papulosquamous disorders are diseases characterized by elevated, scaling lesions.

Pityriasis Rosea

Pityriasis rosea typically produces oval thin plaques composed of tiny papules with a fine scale. At times, particularly in more deeply pigmented patients, papules may be prominent (Fig. 129.22). The cause of pityriasis rosea is unknown but is believed by many to be viral. The disorder occurs most commonly in teenagers and young adults but has been described in infants. Recurrent episodes are uncommon, and small epidemics have been reported among individuals in close contact.

In about one-half of patients, pityriasis rosea begins with the appearance of a herald patch, a solitary erythematous patch, or a minimally elevated plaque. At times, this lesion may be mistaken for tinea corporis. One to two weeks later, the typical generalized eruption begins. The ovoid lesions of pityriasis rosea are concentrated on the trunk and have their long axes parallel to lines of skin stress. Thus, their distribution on the patient's back gives the appearance of the boughs of a fir tree. Often viewing the rash from across the room facilitates seeing this characteristic pattern. Individual lesions are minimally elevated and erythematous or hyperpigmented. Most lesions are covered by a fine, wrinkled scale (Fig. 129.23). At times, particularly

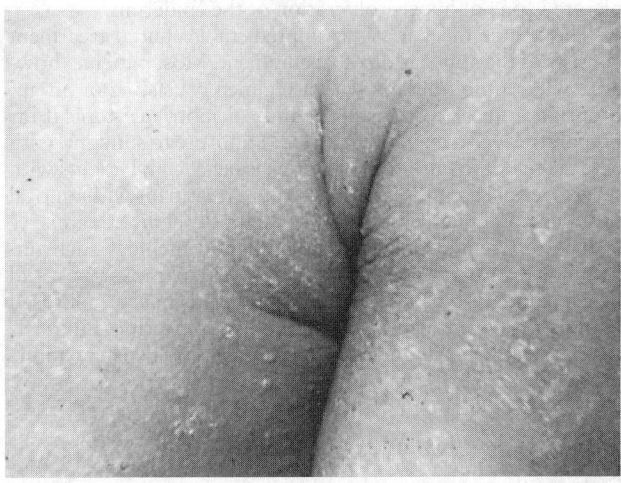

FIGURE 129.23. The fine scale on the ovoid plaques is characteristic of pityriasis rosea.

in more deeply pigmented individuals, lesions may be more papular in appearance or the eruption may involve the extremities and face, sparing the trunk (i.e., inverse pityriasis rosea). Occasionally, the lesions may be urticarial wheals or bullae, or may become purpuric.

The lengthy course of this disorder should be emphasized to the patient or the parents. The eruption itself develops over a 2-week period, persists for 2 weeks, and then fades over another 2 weeks. This pattern varies greatly, however, and rashes lasting 3 to 4 months are not unusual. Pruritus occurs in up to one-half of patients and may be managed with an emollient containing menthol and phenol, a topical nonsensitizing anesthetic (e.g., pramoxine), or an oral antihistamine. Judicious exposure to sunlight (avoiding burning) may hasten the resolution of the eruption. One report suggested that erythromycin was effective but its results have not been confirmed.

The differential diagnosis of pityriasis rosea includes dry nummular eczema and psoriasis. Secondary syphilis may produce an eruption similar to pityriasis rosea, although patients usually are ill, have lymphadenopathy, and exhibit lesions on the palms and soles. Nevertheless, a serologic test for syphilis should be considered if the patient is sexually active.

Psoriasis

Psoriasis is an inherited disorder whose onset occurs before 16 years of age in 25% to 45% of patients. Usually, the lesions are distinctive, with well-demarcated, erythematous papules or plaques covered with a silvery scale (see color Fig. 68.18 in color section). The scale tends to build up in layers, and its removal may cause a bleeding point (Auspitz sign). The papules enlarge to form plaques. Usually, the distribution is symmetric, with plaques commonly appearing over the knees and elbows because they are sites of repeated trauma. Other common sites of involvement are the eyebrows, ears, umbilicus, and gluteal cleft. Frequently, the scalp shows a thick, adherent scale; often, the nails demonstrate punctate stippling or pitting or become discolored and thickened, and the palms and soles may show scaling and fissuring. The Koebner phenomenon (i.e., the appearance of rash at sites of physical, thermal, or mechanical trauma) often is evident.

A variety of inciting factors in addition to trauma have been associated with the appearance of psoriatic lesions. An interesting factor in children is the development of guttate psoriasis, a condition characterized by multiple, small, teardrop-like lesions associated with pharyngeal or perianal *Streptococcus pyogenes* infection (Fig. 129.24). Other factors implicated are sunburn, drug eruptions, and viral infections. The histologic picture is one of hyperproliferation of the epidermis.

The course of psoriasis is unpredictable. Initial treatment consists of the application of an emollient. Most patients, however, will require therapy with a regimen consisting of an appropriate topical corticosteroid and calcipotriene; topical tar preparations also may be employed. Exposure to sunlight, with care taken not to burn the skin, often is beneficial. Patients with severe, recalcitrant disease may require treatment with an oral psoralen combined with ultraviolet light or methotrexate.

The differential diagnosis in childhood includes such uncommon disorders as pityriasis rubra pilaris, parapsoriasis, and lichen planus. Occasionally, atopic dermatitis may be confused with psoriasis, but psoriasis typically is not pruritic. Pityriasis rosea, tinea corporis, and seborrheic dermatitis also may mimic psoriasis.

Juvenile Dermatomyositis

Scaly, erythematous papules are characteristic of juvenile dermatomyositis. The lesions, called *Gottron papules*, classically are found over the knuckles, elbows, and knees. A violaceous

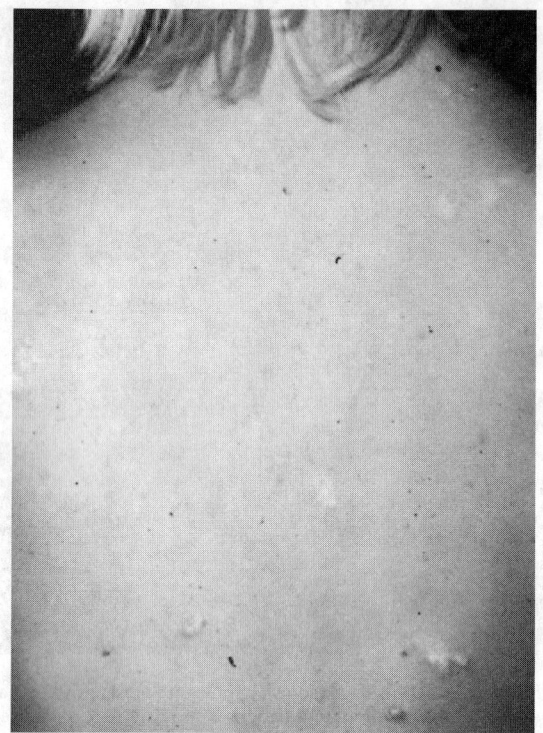

FIGURE 129.24. The sudden widespread appearance of small, scaly plaques is characteristic of guttate psoriasis.

discoloration of the upper and lower lids (i.e., heliotrope) and malar area and nailfold telangiectases frequently are present.

Juvenile dermatomyositis may be limited to the skin (i.e., amyopathic dermatomyositis, dermatomyositis sine myositis) or be associated with symmetrical muscle pain and proximal muscle weakness. Evaluation of patients suspected of having juvenile dermatomyositis should include measurement of muscle enzymes, including creatine kinase, aldolase, aspartate aminotransferase, and lactic dehydrogenase. Occasionally, muscle biopsy, electromyography, or magnetic resonance imaging is required. Systemic corticosteroids are the mainstay of therapy, although topical corticosteroids or hydroxychloroquine may be used to control skin disease.

Lupus Erythematosus

A wide variety of rashes have been associated with systemic lupus erythematosus (SLE). The so-called butterfly rash, a slightly raised, erythematous or violaceous thin plaque or patch with fine scale located over the malar areas and bridge of the nose, is most often associated with SLE. Patients may also exhibit discoid lesions, round, well-demarcated, erythematous to violaceous plaques with fine telangiectases, an adherent scale, and areas of atrophy. The lesions appear most commonly on the face and scalp and in the ears. Other cutaneous lesions include transient erythematous annular lesions in sun-exposed areas (subacute cutaneous lupus erythematosus), red or purple nodules, scaling patches on the dorsa of the fingers, and scarring and nonscarring alopecia.

Lichen Planus

The papules in lichen planus, a disorder found mostly in adults, characteristically are polygonal. When the lesions are examined closely, the flat-topped papules seem to form rectangles, squares, and other shapes (Fig. 129.25). The classic lesions are violaceous and occur most frequently on the wrists and

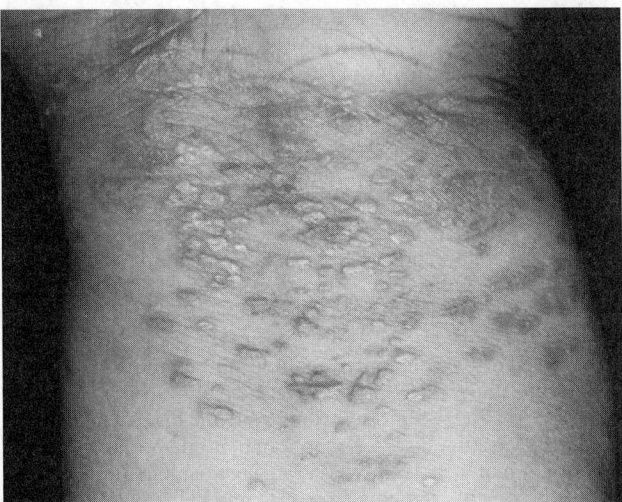

FIGURE 129.25. The classic papules of lichen planus are not only flat-topped but also purple and polygonal. (Courtesy of Alan B. Fleischer, Jr., MD.)

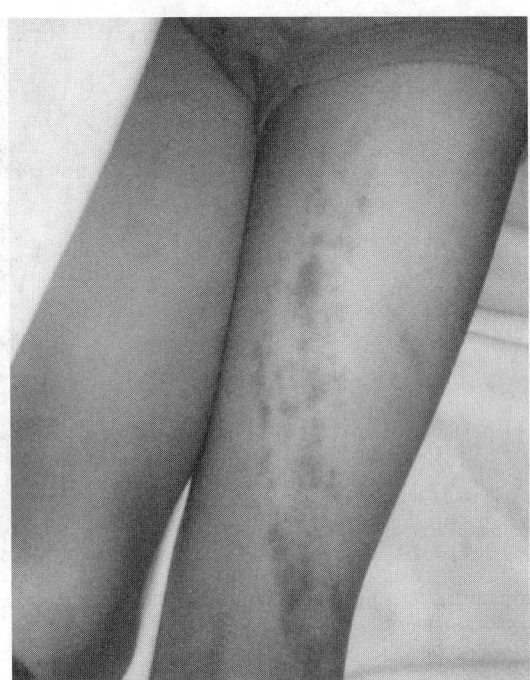

FIGURE 129.26. Linear arrangement of confluent papules in lichen striatus.

extensor surfaces of the forearms. They may coalesce to form plaques. Significant scaling of the lesions may occur on the lower extremities. Oral lesions, consisting of tiny white papules in lacy patterns, may occur on the buccal mucosa. Nail dystrophy, including roughening of the nail surface or longitudinal ridging, is not common in children with lichen planus.

Lichen planus is intensely pruritic. Excoriations can lead to secondary infection and to the occurrence of lesions at sites of trauma. The cause of the eruption is unknown, and the lesions persist for 8 to 18 months. Therapy consists of the application of a moderate- to super-potent corticosteroid and the administration of an antihistamine to control pruritus. In severe or unresponsive cases, oral corticosteroids or retinoids may be indicated.

Pityriasis Rubra Pilaris

Pityriasis rubra pilaris is an uncommon disorder of unknown cause characterized by erythematous, scaly papules that may coalesce to form plaques. The papules are centered about follicles and have tapered tips. A characteristic feature is the presence of islands of normal tissue between the joined plaques. Patients also develop thick, adherent scale on the scalp (similar to that seen in psoriasis) and thickening of the palms and soles, which may be marked. The degree of skin involvement varies widely. Pruritus is absent or minimal. Most cases of pityriasis rubra pilaris occur sporadically but familial clustering has been observed.

The course of pityriasis rubra pilaris usually is prolonged, interspersed by remissions and exacerbations. For patients with mild forms of the disease, topical agents, including emollients, keratolytics, tretinoin, or corticosteroids, may be beneficial. Oral retinoids and other systemic therapies are required for those with severe disease.

Pityriasis Lichenoides

Pityriasis lichenoides is an uncommon disorder with two variants: an acute form (known as *pityriasis lichenoides et varioliformis acuta* [PLEVA]) and a chronic type (known as *pityriasis lichenoides chronica*). Both produce a generalized erythematous papular and macular eruption, usually over the trunk and extremities. The lesions persist for months or recur in periodic eruptions. The acute form produces lesions that may

be hemorrhagic, vesicular, pustular, or even necrotic. Initially, the eruption may be mistaken for varicella. The chronic form is characterized by reddish brown papules that have an adherent scale and range from a few millimeters to 1 cm in diameter. The wafer-like plaques may be confused with pityriasis rosea. The cause of pityriasis lichenoides is unknown. Some cases resolve with exposure to ultraviolet light; others improve with prolonged erythromycin therapy.

Lichen Striatus

Lichen striatus, a self-limited eruption most common in children, is characterized by the rapid development of multiple small papules arranged in a linear, band-like pattern over an extremity (Fig. 129.26). The bands may be 1 to several centimeters in width, irregular or fairly uniform, and continuous or interrupted; they occur most commonly on the lower extremities. The papules may be scaly and generally are skin-colored or erythematous, although in deeply pigmented individuals they may be hypopigmented. The cause of this distinctive lesion is unknown. It has a duration of a few weeks to as long as 3 years. As resolution begins, papules disappear, leaving hypopigmentation that may persist for several months. Topical corticosteroids and keratolytics may hasten its resolution. Linear epidermal nevi, linear psoriasis, and linear lichen planus are included in the differential diagnosis.

Nodules

Erythematous

Pyogenic Granulomas. Pyogenic granulomas are benign vascular proliferations precipitated by trauma or infection, although the mechanism for growth stimulation is not known. The lesions grow rapidly, may be papular or nodular, and often are pedunculated. They usually are solitary and dark red to purple, with a surface that generally is moist, crusted, or eroded and that may bleed easily when traumatized (Fig. 129.27).

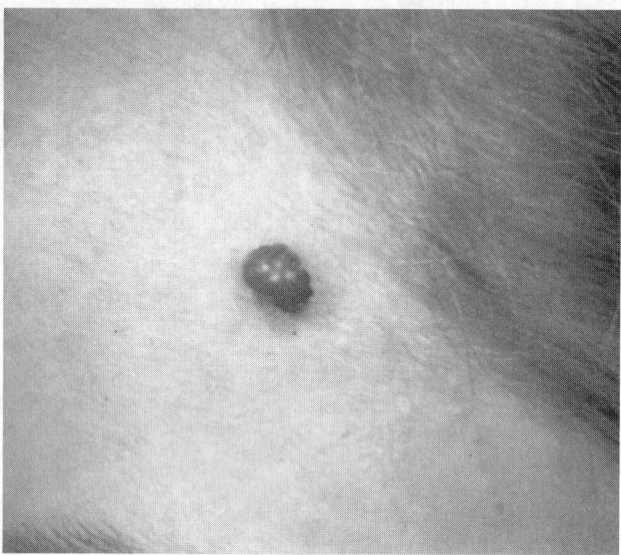

FIGURE 129.27. This pyogenic granuloma of the forehead is red, pedunculated, and moist.

The differential diagnosis of pyogenic granuloma includes warts, molluscum contagiosum, and superficial hemangiomas. The best treatment is excision and electrodesiccation of the base, although pulsed dye laser may be employed.

Erythema Nodosum. Erythema nodosum presents usually as painful, erythematous, warm nodules with indistinct borders most often located on the pretibial surfaces (Fig. 129.28). The number of nodules may vary from one to many. Their bright-

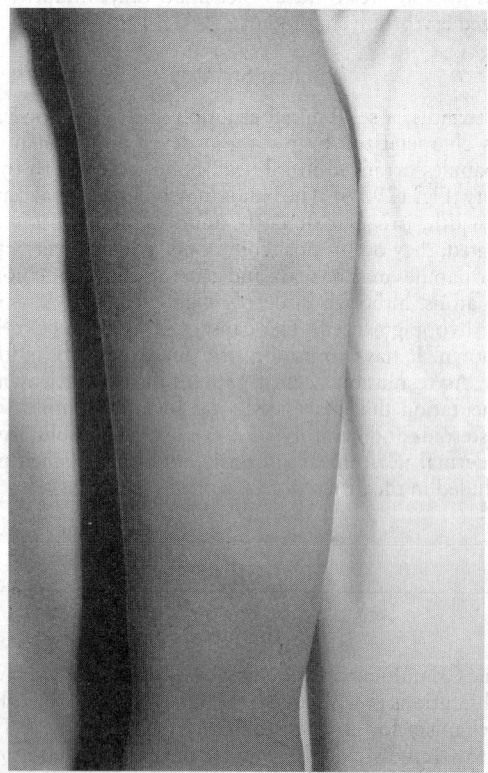

FIGURE 129.28. Erythema nodosum. Tender erythematous nodules over the pretibial surface. See Color Figure 129.28 in color section.

red color changes in a few days to brown-red or purple and later to yellow-green, as seen with a bruise. Lesions may occur on other body sites, including the arms and face. Erythema nodosum represents a hypersensitivity reaction to various infections, drugs, and other conditions. It is a form of panniculitis, an inflammation of the subcutaneous fat.

The most common precipitating agent in erythema nodosum in children in the United States is a preceding streptococcal infection. In the past, tuberculosis was the foremost cause. Other, less common precipitants include infection with Epstein-Barr virus or *Yersinia enterocolitica*, histoplasmosis, coccidioidomycosis, and leptospirosis. An association with inflammatory bowel disease and sarcoidosis has been noted. Drugs most frequently incriminated include sulfonamides, diphenylhydantoin, and oral contraceptive agents. Chronic or recurrent episodes suggest more serious systemic disorders, such as a collagen vascular disease, lymphoma, or inflammatory bowel disease. In many cases, however, a trigger is not found.

The lesions of erythema nodosum initially may be confused with areas of cellulitis, insect bites, or bruises. Arthralgias occur in some cases, and arthritis may be present, suggesting rheumatic disorders. Biopsy samples of lesions reveal intense inflammation in the subcutaneous fat, including around vessels. If a precipitating factor is identified, it should be managed appropriately. Most patients respond to relative rest and an oral nonsteroidal antiinflammatory agent. Typically, erythema nodosum resolves in 2 to 3 weeks.

Panniculitis. The term *panniculitis* denotes inflammation of the subcutaneous fat. The blood vessels usually are affected also, with resultant fat necrosis. The clinical appearance commonly is one of erythematous, enlarging nodules that frequently are painful to palpation. The lesion size may vary considerably, from less than 1 cm to many centimeters in diameter. As the lesions subside, the overlying skin becomes less erythematous, eventually leaving macular areas of hyperpigmentation. With resolution, a depression in the overlying skin is common.

The causes of panniculitis vary. Cold-exposure panniculitis is common on infants' cheeks. Some cases are associated with connective tissue diseases, particularly lupus erythematosus. Weber-Christian disease features recurring inflammatory subcutaneous nodules with systemic symptoms, particularly fever. The withdrawal of corticosteroids also may result in the appearance of panniculitis.

Skin-Colored

Epidermal Cysts. Most epidermal cysts occur after puberty. Clinically, they appear as discrete, enlarging, raised, somewhat compressible nodules of variable size. The overlying skin is normal, although a dilated follicular orifice that communicates with the underlying cyst may be appreciated. If the cyst ruptures, the lesion will become painful and erythematous. Epidermal cysts occur most frequently on the face, scalp, and back. Rarely, they may be associated with Gardner syndrome, other features of which include polyposis of the gastrointestinal tract, particularly the colon, multiple osteomas, and cutaneous fibromas. If treatment of an epidermal cyst is desired, excision is preferred.

Lipomas. The subcutaneous tumors typical of lipomas are spongy and often are lobulated. They occur most frequently in the subcutaneous tissue of the back and abdominal wall. The overlying skin is unaffected and not attached to these lesions, which are nontender and slow-growing and may be solitary or multiple. No therapy is required but lesions may be excised. Lesions in the midline lumbosacral area should be evaluated for underlying spinal dysraphism.

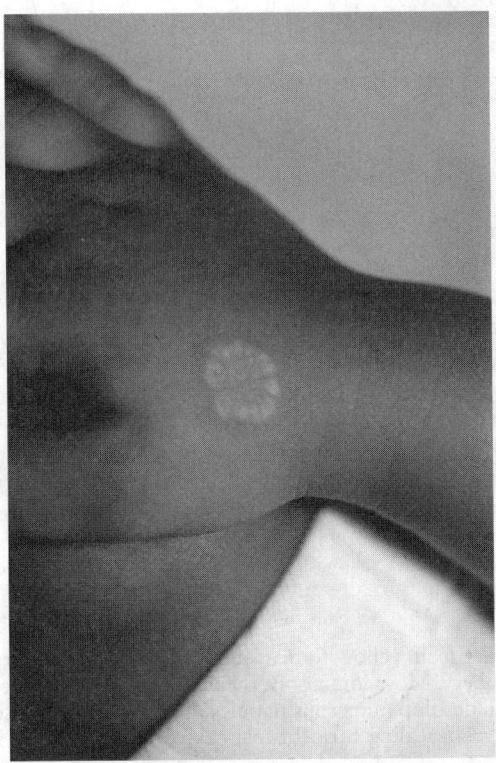

FIGURE 129.29. Ring-like lesion with papular border characteristic of granuloma annulare.

Granuloma Annulare. Granuloma annulare, a benign, self-limited disorder, produces small nodules within the dermis. Individual nodules enlarge to form ring-like lesions with a clearing center and an elevated, papular border (Fig. 129.29). Lesions are asymptomatic, skin-colored or violaceous, and usually are located on the hands, feet, or ankles. Occasionally, granuloma annulare produces papules located on the hands or fingers (papular granuloma annulare) or nodules overlying the pretibial surfaces (subcutaneous granuloma annulare). The cause of granuloma annulare is unknown. Biopsy reveals focal degeneration of collagen within the dermis with reactive inflammation.

The lesions of granuloma annulare resolve over months to years; approximately 75% of lesions disappear within 2 years. No therapy is required, but if it is desired options include the use of a topical or intralesional corticosteroid or cryotherapy. Because of its ring-like appearance, granuloma annulare often is mistaken for tinea corporis. However, the firm border and absence of scale should suggest the diagnosis.

Pilomatricomas. Pilomatricomas are firm to hard, multilobulated, slow-growing tumors. Most are skin-colored, but some may be reddish or bluish. They occur most commonly on the head and neck and almost always are solitary. Pilomatricomas are benign but often are removed for cosmetic reasons. They occur most commonly in the first two decades of life.

Connective Tissue Nevi. Connective tissue nevi are firm, skin-colored papules, nodules, or plaques. They often are grouped together, creating an orange peel appearance. Connective tissue nevi represent localized collections of dermal collagen and elastic tissue. Most often, lesions represent isolated cutaneous findings but they may be associated with tuberous sclerosis (i.e., the shagreen patch) or other syndromes.

Dermatofibromas. Dermatofibromas are solitary, hard, well-defined, dome-shaped nodules that occur occasionally in children. They are fixed firmly to the skin, and their color varies from skin-colored to red-brown to tan or black. Lesions rarely exceed 2 cm in diameter. Applying lateral pressure to the lesion causes dimpling of its surface. Dermatofibromas may arise spontaneously or following trauma such as an insect bite. No therapy is necessary and lesions will persist.

Neurofibromas. Neurofibromas are skin-colored or brown nodules that when depressed may be reduced temporarily as if through a button hole. They represent benign tumors of Schwann cells. Larger lesions that feel like a "bag of worms" on palpation are termed plexiform neurofibromas. Although they may occur as an isolated phenomenon, neurofibromas are one diagnostic feature of neurofibromatosis type 1. In those who have neurofibromatosis type 1, neurofibromas typically do not appear until after the first decade.

Hyperpigmented

Mastocytosis. Mastocytosis represents a spectrum of disorders characterized by excessive numbers of mast cells in the dermis and, occasionally, other organs (e.g., bone marrow, gastrointestinal tract) and the symptoms produced by the elaboration of mediators derived from these cells. In some cases, the disorder is caused by mutations in the *c-KIT* gene that result in an abnormal proliferation of mast cells.

Mastocytosis can be categorized into cutaneous and systemic forms. The most common type, particularly in children, is cutaneous mastocytosis, in which mast cell accumulation is limited to the skin. Four types of cutaneous disease are recognized: urticaria pigmentosa (UP), solitary mastocytomas, diffuse cutaneous mastocytosis, and telangiectasia macularis eruptiva perstans (TMEP). The most common form of cutaneous mastocytosis is UP, accounting for 70% to 90% of all cases. Lesions typically appear during the first year of life and increase in number, although they may be present at birth. They are small, red-brown, tan, or yellow macules or minimally elevated plaques that possess an orange peel appearance (Fig. 129.30). Approximately 10% to 20% of children with cutaneous mastocytosis have solitary mastocytomas, single or as many as five macules or thin plaques. They are larger than

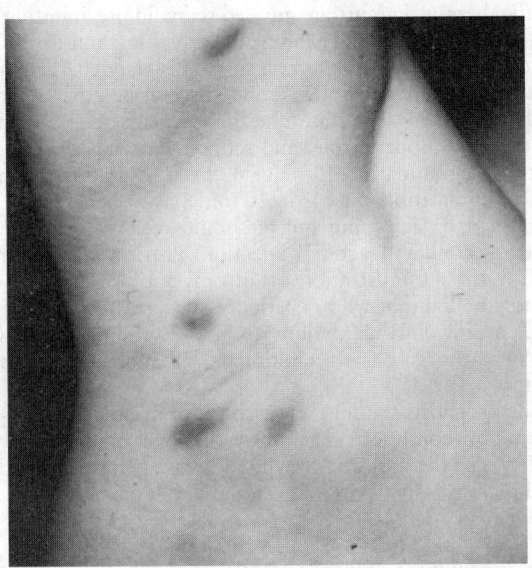

FIGURE 129.30. Multiple pigmented nodules of urticaria pigmentosa in the axilla. Rubbing causes an erythematous flare and swelling.

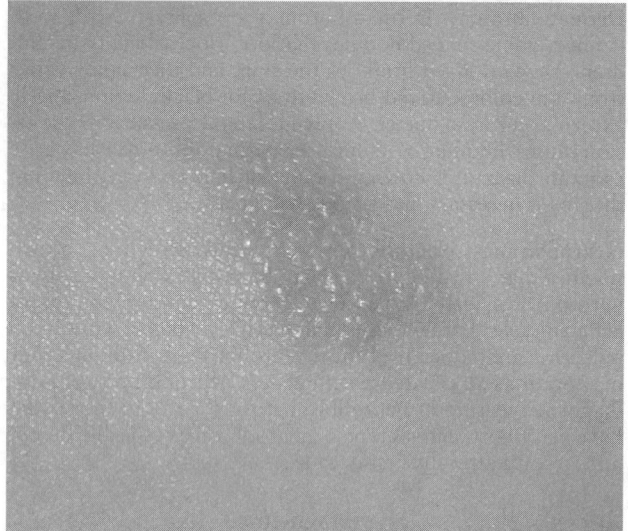

FIGURE 129.31. A solitary mastocytoma demonstrating an orange-peel appearance.

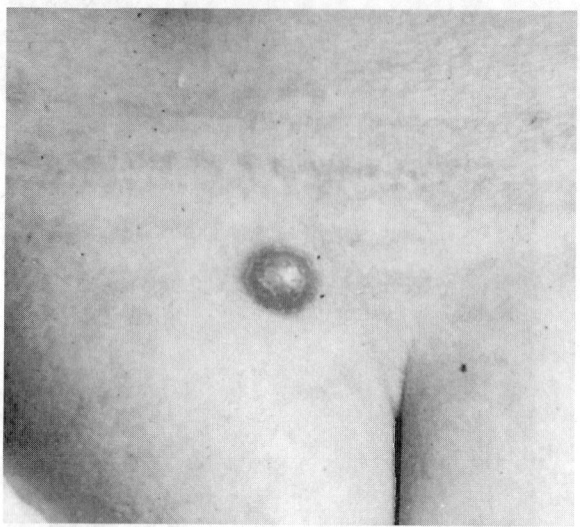

FIGURE 129.32. A yellowish nodule of juvenile xanthogranuloma in the sacral area.

the lesions of UP but have a similar time of onset, color, and appearance (Fig. 129.31). Diffuse cutaneous mastocytosis and TMEP occur rarely in children. The former variant appears in the neonatal period and is characterized by widespread infiltration of the skin with mast cells; discrete lesions are absent but the skin is thickened with numerous tiny papules. TMEP produces hyperpigmented macules and telangiectasias.

Children who have cutaneous mastocytosis may be well or experience symptoms resulting from mast cell–derived mediators, including histamine and various cytokines. Localized mast cell degranulation, as results from rubbing, causes lesions to become erythematous, edematous, and pruritic and, occasionally, to form vesicles or bullae (Darier sign). In rare cases, elevated levels of mediators produce systemic symptoms, including generalized pruritus, flushing, tachycardia, syncope, diarrhea, or respiratory distress. In addition to friction, mediator release may be precipitated by a number of drugs (e.g., acetylsalicylic acid, alcohol, codeine, dextromethorphan, meperidine, morphine, procaine, and reserpine).

Most children with mastocytosis are well and require no specific therapy. Parents are advised to avoid precipitating factors, including vigorous rubbing after bathing and drugs that cause mast cell degranulation. If surgery is planned, it is imperative that the anesthesiologist and surgeon be advised of the child's condition as certain anesthetic agents (e.g., atropine, halothane, d-tubocurarine, and scopolamine) also may cause mast cell degranulation. If frequent blister formation is a problem, the application of a corticosteroid may be beneficial. Once established, vesicles and bullae should receive local care to prevent secondary bacterial infection. Pruritus may be managed by the administration of an oral antihistamine or oral cromolyn. Children who experience syncope, respiratory distress, chronic diarrhea, failure to thrive, or bone pain or who have hepatomegaly merit additional evaluation and aggressive therapy.

The prognosis for children with UP or mastocytomas is excellent; both conditions generally resolve over time, typically by puberty. For the minority in whom disease persists into adulthood there is a small risk of eventual development of systemic involvement.

Xanthogranuloma. Juvenile xanthogranulomas start to appear in the first few months of life. They begin as small papules and enlarge into 0.5- to 1.0-cm nodules (Fig. 129.32). The le-

sions vary from yellow to brown to red and generally are firm and rubbery. Most commonly, there is a single lesion but some children develop numerous papules. The disorder represents a benign, self-healing form of histiocytosis whose cause is unknown.

Generally, no treatment is necessary, because approximately one-third disappear within 6 months, and another one-third are gone within 12 months. Rarely, cutaneous xanthogranulomas are associated with extracutaneous disease. Xanthogranulomas of the eye may lead to hyphema or glaucoma, or may be mistaken for an intraocular tumor. Children with neurofibromatosis and juvenile xanthogranuloma are at an increased risk for the development of juvenile chronic myeloid leukemia.

Vesicles

Disorders with Grouped Vesicles

Impetigo. Bacterial infections of the skin are among the most common dermatologic conditions for which children are brought to physicians. Superficial infections account for the great majority of these infections, and impetigo is the most common pyoderma. Impetigo may be divided into crusted (nonbullous) and bullous (discussed in Bullae, later) forms. *Staphylococcus aureus* is the agent primarily responsible for crusted impetigo, although *Streptococcus pyogenes* occasionally is implicated.

Crusted impetigo begins with tiny vesicles that rupture. Drying of serous fluid leads to the formation of a golden or "honey-colored" crust (Fig. 129.33). The lesions tend to spread locally. Family members often are infected as well. Any area of the body may be involved (although lesions often are located around the nares), and any break in the skin (e.g., abrasions, excoriations, lacerations, burns) may provide access.

When *S. pyogenes* was the most common bacterium responsible for impetigo, secondary nonsuppurative complications, such as poststreptococcal glomerulonephritis, were common in some areas of the United States and other countries. Acute rheumatic fever, however, has never been reported to follow impetigo.

When impetigo is widespread, antibiotic therapy with an oral agent active against *S. aureus* (e.g., cephalexin, dicloxacillin, etc.) is indicated. For localized diseases, mupirocin, applied topically, is effective.

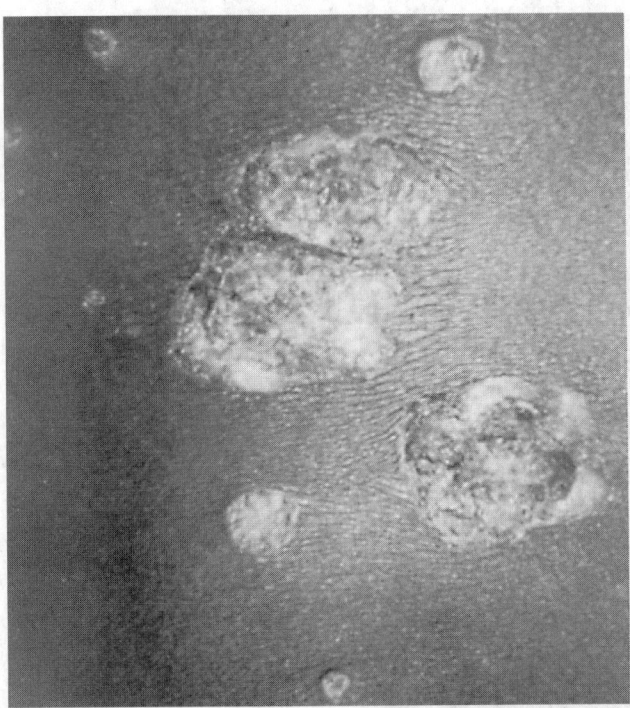

FIGURE 129.33. Crusted lesions of superficial pyoderma in a perioral distribution.

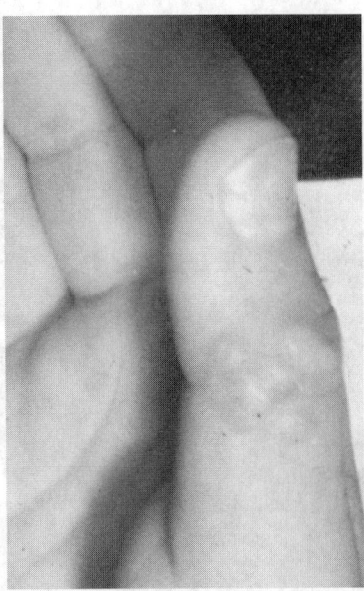

FIGURE 129.34. Herpes simplex infection always should be considered when grouped vesicles are present.

Herpes Simplex Virus Infection. Cutaneous herpes simplex virus (HSV) infections typically produce grouped vesicles on an erythematous base. The vesicles rapidly become pustular and then rupture, forming erosions that crust. Several forms of infection may occur. Neonatal HSV infection is discussed in the section Skin Lesions in the Neonatal Period. In older infants and toddlers, symptomatic primary infections most often involve the oral cavity (herpes gingivostomatitis), where multiple vesicles on the gums and buccal surfaces rapidly erode to form ulcers. The illness is accompanied by high fever, irritability, increased salivation, refusal to drink, and swollen, friable gingivae. When affected children suck their fingers, autoinoculation may lead to the appearance of vesicles there as well (Fig. 129.34).

Other common forms of cutaneous HSV infection include herpes labialis (the most common form of recurrent HSV infection), herpetic whitlow (infection of one or more digits that may be mistaken for bacterial infection), and herpes gladiatorum (cutaneous HSV infection seen in wrestlers and others who participate in sports that involve close physical contact). In these individuals, lesions are clustered vesicles on an erythematous base. Over several days, the lesions become pustular and then rupture, forming erosions that crust.

In children with atopic dermatitis, HSV infection may become widespread and potentially severe, a condition known as eczema herpeticum. Affected children exhibit vesicles, pustules, crusts, and "punched out" ulcers (Fig. 129.35). The lesions tend to be grouped and any area may be affected. Skin lesions are accompanied by fever, anorexia, vomiting, or diarrhea. Genital HSV infection usually is caused by HSV-2. In males, grouped vesicles on an erythematous base typically appear on the penis or other parts of the genitalia, while females often experience painful ulcers on the genital mucosae.

In children with localized cutaneous HSV infection, the treatment is supportive. In particular, oral and topical antiviral agents are of limited benefit in those with herpes labialis, reducing the duration of disease by 1 day or less. However, if infection is widespread or severe, or if a patient has eczema her-

peticum, antiviral therapy (e.g., with acyclovir or other agents) is indicated.

Herpes Zoster. Herpes zoster, or shingles, is an acute vesicular eruption that occurs in a dermatomal distribution and is caused by varicella-zoster virus, the same virus responsible for varicella. Development of herpes zoster requires previous varicella. The virus remains dormant in the dorsal root ganglia following primary infection until it is reactivated.

The lesions of herpes zoster often are preceded by painful stinging or burning sensations for a few days. Right lower quadrant involvement of the abdomen may be mistaken for appendicitis. Lesions begin as erythematous papules that form vesicles over the next week. The lesions appear in a band-like, dermatomal distribution and rarely cross the midline (Fig. 129.36). The vesicles may not be continuous in a band and, on occasion, more than one dermatome is involved. In a minority of patients, especially those who are immunocompromised, zoster may become generalized. The infection clears within 7 to 14 days, but 10% of such cases may last longer. Persistent

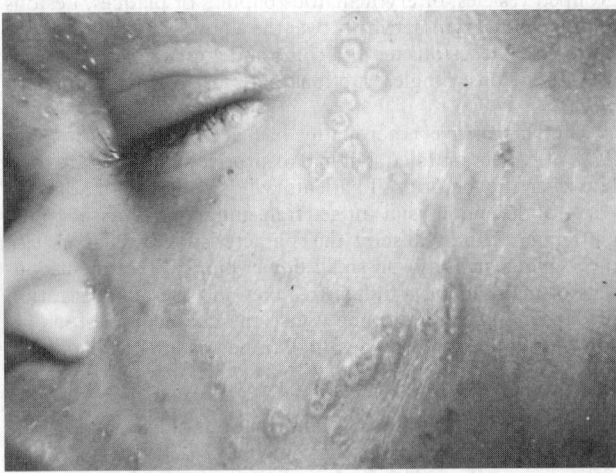

FIGURE 129.35. Eczema herpeticum. "Punched-out" ulcers caused by infection with herpes simplex virus in a patient with atopic dermatitis.

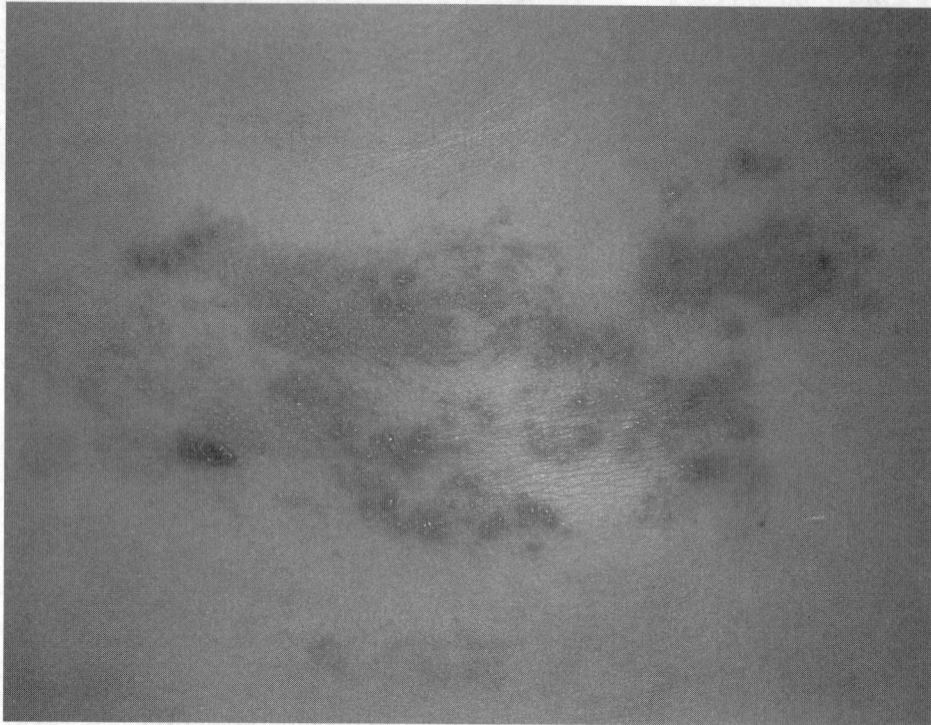

FIGURE 129.36. Clustered vesicles in a dermatomal distribution characteristic of herpes zoster.

pain in the area previously affected by herpes zoster is unusual in young children but may occur in adolescents and adults.

Lesions that appear at the tip of the nose or around the eye should be noted carefully; they may be associated with significant ophthalmic involvement (e.g., keratitis). Most infections can be managed by the use of compresses to dry the lesions, keep them clean, and relieve the itching or pain. The application of a topical antibiotic may help prevent secondary bacterial infection. In extensive cases or those occurring in immunocompromised individuals, parenteral antiviral therapy should be instituted. If eye involvement is suspected, consultation with an ophthalmologist is indicated. It should be recalled that the lesions of zoster are infectious. Although herpes zoster may be a presenting sign of malignancy in adults, it rarely is so in children.

Dermatitis Herpetiformis. Dermatitis herpetiformis is an uncommon autoimmune disorder characterized by pruritic, grouped vesicles, or erythematous papules or plaques. Lesions are distributed symmetrically over the elbows, knees, scalp, and buttocks. The lesions tend to come and go with exacerbations and remissions. Single eruptions may last for a few days to weeks.

Gluten-sensitive enteropathy has been found in 85% to 95% of patients studied, but malabsorptive symptoms are rare. However, the majority of patients will have IgA antibodies directed at the endomysial antigen transglutaminase (tissue transglutaminase) and will show the characteristics of celiac disease (i.e., villous atrophy) on small bowel biopsy. Treatment consists of maintaining a gluten-free diet and the administration of dapsone or sulfapyridine. Once the cutaneous lesions resolve, drug therapy may be discontinued as long as the diet is followed.

Lymphatic Malformations. Malformations of lymphatic tissue (also known as *lymphangiomas*) may be classified as microcystic or macrocystic. The microcystic forms are more common and may be present at birth or develop later. They produce deep-seated, tense vesicles. Most are small (1 to 3 mm in diameter) and clear to hemorrhagic (color Fig. 68.7 in color section). The surface of the lesions may be smooth or rough. Occasionally, a clear or hemorrhagic fluid may leak from traumatized lesions. In contrast, macrocystic malformations (e.g., cystic hygromas, cavernous lymphangiomas) are ill-defined, spongy masses that vary considerably in size. The overlying skin surface may appear normal or discolored. They are present at birth or develop within the first 2 years of life and often are located on the neck, axilla, or chest wall.

In contrast to hemangiomas, lymphatic malformations do not regress spontaneously and management must be individualized. Surgical excision is difficult and recurrences are common. The superficial, vesicular component of microcystic lesions may be treated with laser therapy.

Disorders with Generalized Vesicles

Varicella. Varicella (chickenpox) is a highly contagious childhood disease caused by the varicella-zoster virus. Infection usually follows contact with children infected with varicella, but zoster lesions also are infectious. The initial lesion is an erythematous macule or papule that becomes vesicular within a few hours. Occasionally, the vesicles may appear like a drop of water on an erythematous base (the so-called "dew drop on a rose petal"). The vesicles then become pustular and umbilicated, rupture, and are covered with a crust in 1 to 2 days. The characteristic lesions occur in crops, with varying types (e.g., vesicle, crust) present simultaneously. Mucous membrane involvement is common. Lesions initially are scattered on the trunk, face, and scalp, with the extremities becoming involved within a short time.

The incubation period of varicella is 10 to 21 days, with most cases appearing 14 days after exposure. Pruritus often is marked, and fever is common. Generally, the disease is fairly mild, except in adults, immunocompromised children, and neonates. Secondary infections are common. When large, glistening erosive lesions or bullae appear, secondary staphylococcal infection is likely. Complaints of pain in lesions usually indicate a secondary infection.

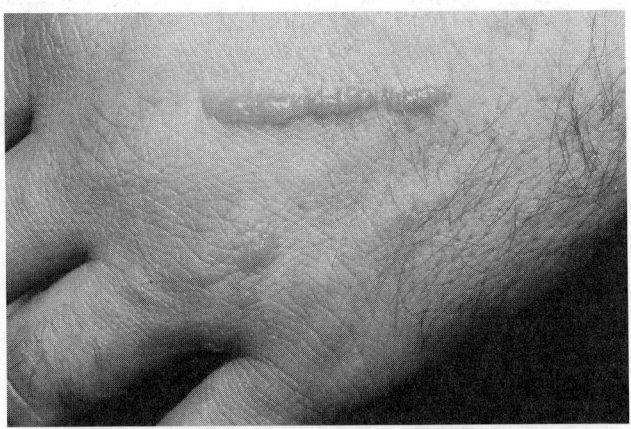

FIGURE 129.37. Linear vesicles in a patient with contact dermatitis due to poison ivy.

Treatment of uncomplicated varicella is symptomatic. Aspirin should be avoided because of its association with Reye syndrome. The application of a shake lotion (e.g., Calamine) and cool compresses may reduce the itching and can enhance drying of the lesions. Oral acyclovir should be considered for immunocompetent individuals at risk for severe disease, such as those older than 12 years of age, those with chronic cutaneous or pulmonary diseases, or those receiving chronic salicylate therapy or brief courses of systemic or inhaled corticosteroids. In immunocompromised patients, intravenous acyclovir is recommended. If the diagnosis is in question, a Tzanck smear, polymerase chain reaction test, or viral culture should be performed. The Tzanck smear can be performed rapidly and will demonstrate multinucleated giant cells suggestive of herpesvirus infection.

Disorders with Linear Vesicles

Contact Dermatitis Due to Plants. The appearance of vesicles, bullae, and erythematous papules in a linear arrangement on exposed areas suggests contact dermatitis due to plant allergens (i.e., urushiol present in poison ivy, poison oak, or poison sumac) (Fig. 129.37). Contact dermatitis occurs when an antigen penetrates the epidermis and sensitizes T lymphocytes, which then circulate through the skin and other organ systems. For potent antigens such as urushiol, sensitization takes only 7 to 10 days; weaker agents may require multiple exposures over many weeks. If sensitization occurs, reexposure to the antigen will cause contact dermatitis to develop within 12 to 24 hours.

Potent antigens such as urushiol typically cause an acute dermatitis that consists of vesicles, bullae, erythematous papules, and edema. New lesions may continue to appear over several days. If untreated, the dermatitis may persist for 3 to 4 weeks. In contrast, weaker antigens produce a subacute dermatitis that is characterized by erythema, scaling, and lichenification (i.e., thickening of the skin caused by scratching). Examples of antigens that produce this form of contact dermatitis include nickel (present in jewelry, belt buckles, or clothing snaps); potassium dichromate (present in some shoes); neomycin, thimerosal, or formaldehyde (used in topical medications); or Balsam of Peru or other fragrances (used in perfumes or soaps).

The key to recognizing contact dermatitis is the observation that the eruption is limited to certain skin areas. Linear vesicles or bullae on exposed surfaces suggest exposure to plant allergens. Nickel dermatitis occurs at sites of contact with jewelry (e.g., on the earlobes or other sites of piercing, neck, or wrists) or below the umbilicus where there is contact with a belt buckle

or clothing snap. An eruption on the dorsa of the feet should raise the suspicion of shoe dermatitis.

If the contact dermatitis is mild, a topical corticosteroid may be applied. However, when more than 10% to 15% of the body surface is involved, the disease is severe, or areas such as the face or perineum are significantly affected, oral prednisone is recommended with a tapering treatment course of 12 to 21 days. Oral antihistamines produce a sedative effect that offers relief from itching. Prevention of further episodes is an important part of the management of patients who have contact dermatitis. Individuals who have experienced plant dermatitis should learn to recognize and avoid poison ivy, sumac, and oak. When exposure may be unavoidable, wearing protective clothing or applying a barrier preparation may be useful.

Disorders with a Unique Distribution of Vesicles

Hand-Foot-and-Mouth Disease. The characteristic feature of hand-foot-and-mouth disease is the distribution of the lesions as suggested by the name. This viral exanthem occurs most often in the summer months, often in mini epidemics. The most frequent site of lesions is the mouth, where vesicles erode rapidly, leaving shallow, 1- to 5-mm ulcers with erythematous borders. Lesions on the hands and feet are small erythematous macules and oval vesicles with rims of surrounding erythema (Fig. 129.38). Occasionally, the buttocks and thighs may be involved. Coxsackievirus A16 is associated most frequently with this disease, but other coxsackieviruses, echoviruses, and enteroviruses occasionally are implicated. The primary disorder to differentiate from hand-foot-and-mouth disease is herpes gingivostomatitis. Treatment of hand-foot-and-mouth disease is symptomatic, and the disease usually resolves within 1 week.

Scabies. The characteristic feature of scabies is intense pruritus. Typically, lesions are erythematous papules, nodules, or linear burrows, although vesicles commonly are present. In infants, the rash is generalized involving the trunk, extremities, and head. Children and adolescents exhibit lesions concentrated in flexural areas, such as the interdigital spaces, wrists, axillae, on the areolae in women, and on the penis and scrotum in males. Scabies is discussed in detail in Pruritic Lesions, later.

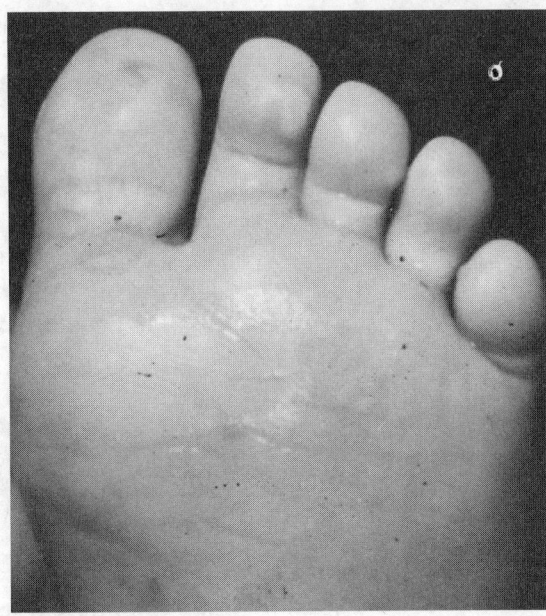

FIGURE 129.38. Erythematous papules and oval vesicles in hand-foot-and-mouth disease.

Tinea Pedis. Tinea pedis usually produces erythema, scaling, and fissuring in the interdigital webs of the toes, especially between the third and fourth and fourth and fifth toes. However, vesicles or bullae, often located on the instep, may be observed. An id reaction (a reaction to the fungal antigen) also may occur, resulting in papules or vesicles on the palms or fingers. Tinea pedis is discussed in detail in the section Scaling and Dry Lesions, later.

Dyshidrotic Eczema. Dyshidrotic eczema likely represents a variant of atopic dermatitis. The condition affects the hands and feet, particularly the palms and soles and lateral aspects of the digits, with deep-seated, intensely pruritic vesicles. If the vesicles rupture or are traumatized by scratching, affected areas become erythematous and crusted. Occasionally, bullae may be present. Despite the name of the condition, the eccrine apparatus is not affected.

Contact dermatitis and id reactions of tinea pedis, in addition to primary fungal infections, must be considered in the differential diagnosis. Treatment includes the application of a mid- to high potency corticosteroid and compresses to promote drying of erosions.

Bullae

Many of the vesicular lesions mentioned in the preceding section may also produce bullae. In addition, the following conditions are characterized by blisters.

Bullous Impetigo

The classic lesions of bullous impetigo, a staphylococcal toxin-mediated disorder, are bullae filled with cloudy fluid and surrounded by a thin margin of erythema. Characteristically, the bullae rupture rapidly, leaving round or oval erosions that become crusted (Fig. 129.39). The lesions most recently ruptured have an erythematous, shiny base, whereas older lesions are dry with a collarette or rim of scale, the remnant of the blister roof. In infants and toddlers, the diaper area is affected most frequently. *S. aureus* is the organism responsible for this infection, with the exfoliative toxin (exfoliative toxins A and

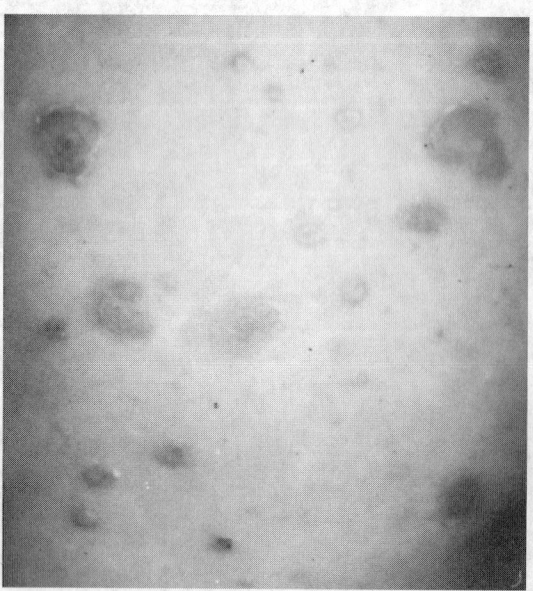

FIGURE 129.39. Bullae and round erosions of bullous impetigo complicating varicella.

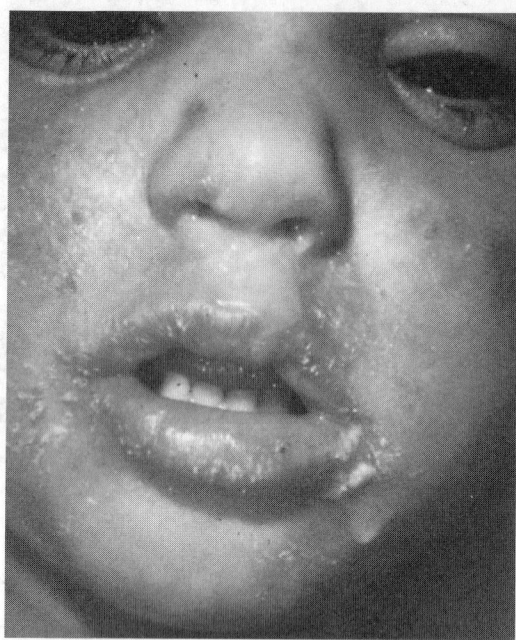

FIGURE 129.40. The purulent nasal discharge is the likely site of infection in this child with staphylococcal scalded skin syndrome. Note the early perioral scaling.

B) causing superficial intraepidermal cleavage and subsequent bulla formation. If diagnostic uncertainty exists, culture of blister fluid will reveal the causative organism. Treatment is with an oral antistaphylococcal antibiotic (e.g., cephalexin, dicloxacillin, etc.).

Staphylococcal Scalded-Skin Syndrome

Staphylococcal scalded skin syndrome (SSSS) is caused by certain strains of *S. aureus*, usually those belonging to phage group II, that produce exfoliative toxins (exfoliative toxins A and B). The toxins cause superficial intraepidermal cleavage resulting in blister formation and skin sloughing. Initially, there is generalized cutaneous erythema and pain. Within 24 hours, blisters and wrinkling of the skin are observed, followed by sloughing. Bullae may appear in areas of trauma or in areas that are rubbed or simply touched, the *Nikolsky sign*. A characteristic feature is crusting in a radial pattern (i.e., sunburst) around the mouth, nose, and eyes (color Fig. 68.13 in color section, Fig. 129.40).

The skin separation in SSSS is intraepidermal rather than deeper, at the epidermal basement membrane, as occurs in Stevens-Johnson syndrome and toxic epidermal necrolysis. As a result, SSSS is a milder disease with an excellent prognosis. Nevertheless, attention to potential fluid loss through the disrupted epidermis, temperature control, and skin care are essential. In mild forms of the disease, children may be treated with an oral antistaphylococcal antibiotic; those more severely affected should receive antibiotics parenterally. The differential diagnosis of SSSS includes thermal burns, Stevens-Johnson syndrome, and toxic epidermal necrolysis. In the latter two disorders, however, usually mucous membranes are severely affected, and no sunburst of crusting occurs around the mouth and eyes.

Stevens-Johnson Syndrome/Toxic Epidermal Necrolysis

Stevens-Johnson syndrome (SJS) (formerly called erythema multiforme major) and toxic epidermal necrolysis (TEN) represent severe and potentially life-threatening hypersensitivity reactions to drugs (e.g., antibiotics, anticonvulsants, or nonsteroidal antiinflammatory agents) or, less commonly, infectious agents (e.g., *Mycoplasma pneumoniae*). Both are characterized by large areas of epidermal necrosis. Although some controversy exists, many experts believe that SJS and TEN are the same disease, differing only in extent. In both disorders, patients experience prodromal symptoms, including fever, sore throat, rhinitis, cough, headache, vomiting, or diarrhea. Within 14 days, erythematous macules and patches appear on the trunk and extremities. Blisters form rapidly and leave large areas of denuded skin. In SJS there is epidermal loss of less than 10% of the body surface, while TEN is diagnosed when patients lose more than 30% of the epidermal surface (see color Fig. 68.14 in color section); those with 10% to 30% involvement are said to have SJS/TEN overlap. In SJS and TEN, target lesions (seen in erythema multiforme) are absent or few in number. Mucosal involvement is prominent with hemorrhagic crusting of the lips, oral ulcers, and purulent conjunctivitis. The mucosa of the trachea, bronchi, and gastrointestinal tract also may be involved.

Patients with SJS or TEN ideally should be managed in a burn unit or intensive care unit with careful attention to fluid and electrolyte status, nutrition, skin and eye care, and the potential for secondary bacterial infection. Intravenous immunoglobulin may be beneficial; the role of systemic corticosteroids is controversial. Long-term complications of SJS/TEN involve the eye, skin, and nails.

Blistering Distal Dactylitis

Blistering distal dactylitis usually is manifested by a single pus-filled bulla on the volar aspect of the distal phalanx of one finger. It nearly always is caused *Streptococcus pyogenes*, although *S. aureus* and group B streptococci have been implicated. Treatment includes incision and drainage of large bullae and the administration of an appropriate oral antibiotic.

Insect Bites

Although the characteristic lesions of insect bites are erythematous papules, often with a central punctum, bullae may develop in involved areas in individuals who are highly sensitive to insect bites (Fig. 129.41).

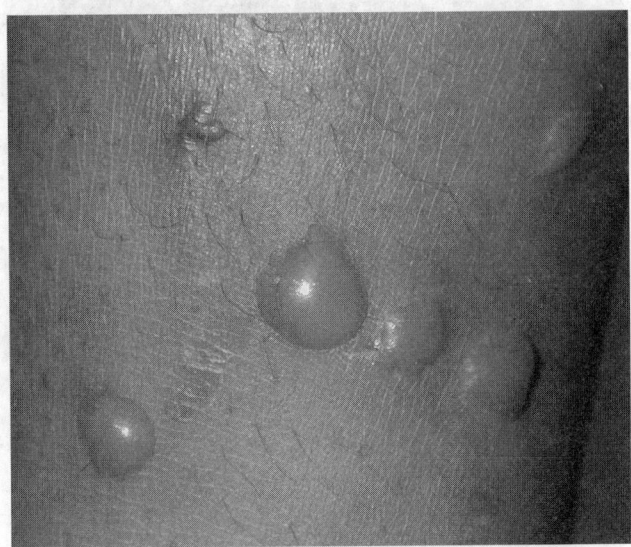

FIGURE 129.41. Bullae resulting from insect bites.

Chronic Bullous Disease of Childhood

Chronic bullous disease of childhood (also known as *linear IgA dermatosis*) is an acquired autoimmune disorder. It occurs sporadically, most commonly in the first decade of life (18 months to 8.5 years), is characterized by spontaneous remissions and exacerbations, and has a duration of 2 to 4 years. The clinical spectrum of the disease often renders accurate diagnosis difficult, bullous impetigo being the most frequent misdiagnosis. The bullae are tense (unlike the flaccid bullae of bullous impetigo) and clear or hemorrhagic, arising on normal or erythematous skin. Bullae may be round or sausage-shaped and often develop at the margins of prior lesions, creating the appearance of a "string of pearls," "rosette," or "cluster of jewels." The lesions occur most frequently on the buttocks, genitalia, thighs, and perioral areas. The mucous membranes may be involved, most commonly with oral erosions.

Pathologically, the blisters are subepidermal and can be separated from similar-appearing blisters by immunohistochemical studies, which demonstrate linear IgA deposits at the dermal–epidermal junction in uninvolved perilesional skin. Dapsone, prednisone, or sulfapyridine may be employed to control the disease. Spontaneous remission generally occurs within 5 years of the onset of disease.

Pemphigus Vulgaris and Pemphigus Foliaceus

Pemphigus encompasses a group of autoimmune disorders in which antibodies directed at desmosomal proteins prevent keratinocyte adhesion resulting in blister formation. Pemphigus occurs rarely in children; the two forms most likely to be encountered are pemphigus vulgaris and pemphigus foliaceus. The cutaneous lesions of pemphigus vulgaris often are preceded by oral ulcers. When blisters form on the skin, they progress rapidly to erosions. In pemphigus foliaceus, the blister roofs are so thin and fragile that fluid may not accumulate. As a result, the presentation often is one of crusted erosions, scaling, oozing, or blistering that may be confused with seborrheic dermatitis or impetigo. The eruption then progresses to the trunk and extremities, producing erythematous, crusting plaques. The mucous membranes are not involved. Diagnosis of both forms of pemphigus requires immunofluorescent stains performed on skin biopsies, and both forms are treated with systemic corticosteroids. Pemphigus foliaceus is a milder condition than pemphigus vulgaris and has a better prognosis.

Bullous Pemphigoid

Bullous pemphigoid is a disease of the elderly that only rarely occurs in children. It is an autoimmune disorder in which antibodies directed against desmosomal proteins result in the formation of subepidermal blisters. The disease is characterized by tense blisters and erythematous plaques with a predilection for flexural areas. Involvement of the vulvae may produce hemorrhagic blisters and erosions that may be mistaken for signs of sexual abuse. The mucous membranes of the mouth and eyes often are affected. Diagnosis requires the performance of immunofluorescent studies and treatment is with systemic corticosteroids. The prognosis of bullous pemphigoid is good and the condition often is self-limited.

Epidermolysis Bullosa

Epidermolysis bullosa (EB) represents a group of hereditary mechanobullous diseases. The disorders result from defects in proteins involved in anchoring the epidermis to underlying structures. As a result, in response to trauma, vesicles, bullae, or erosions occur. Three major forms of EB exist: EB simplex, junctional EB, and dystrophic EB (Table 129.2).

EB simplex encompasses a number of diseases that are inherited in an autosomal dominant fashion and may be localized or

TABLE 129.2

MAJOR TYPES OF EPIDERMOLYSIS BULLOSA

Type	Inheritance	Clinical Features
Epidermolysis bullosa simplex (generalized and localized [Weber-Cockayne syndrome] forms)	Autosomal dominant	Onset at birth; hands, feet, elbows, and knees involved (in Weber-Cockayne syndrome only hands and feet involved); no scarring; oral mucous membranes may be involved (but minimally); often improves over time.
Junctional epidermolysis bullosa (letalis)	Autosomal recessive	Onset at birth or shortly thereafter; life-threatening; involves perioral region, scalp, trunk, and extremities; lesions heal with scarring; perioral granulomatous ulcers are common; ulcers of gastrointestinal, respiratory, or genitourinary mucosa may occur; loss of nails; dysplastic teeth; complications: infection, growth failure, anemia.
Dominant dystropic epidermolysis bullosa	Autosomal dominant	Onset at birth; hyperkeratotic lesions develop at sites of blistering; variable severity; nail loss; milia; risk for squamous cell carcinoma.
Recessive dystrophic epidermolysis bullosa	Autosomal recessive	Onset at birth; progressive scarring and deformity; mitten-like deformities of hands and feet; contractures of joints; oral mucosal involvement; esophageal strictures; risk for squamous cell carcinoma.

generalized in their distribution. The most common type is the Weber-Cockayne syndrome that has its onset in late infancy or childhood and is characterized by superficial blisters that occur on the hands and feet following frictional stress. In contrast, some forms of EB simplex result in generalized blistering and may be present at birth or the immediate neonatal period (color Fig. 68.16 in color section). One such form, the Dowling-Meara type, causes extensive and potentially life-threatening blistering with involvement of the oral and laryngeal mucosae.

Junctional epidermolysis bullosa, a group of autosomal recessive disorders, may present at birth or shortly thereafter. One form, Herlitz, may seem benign at first with few blisters, but often it is progressive. Death is common, although it may occur after weeks or years later. Large granulomatous ulcers usually appear in the perioral area (Fig. 129.42). The nails are lost, and teeth are dysplastic. Mucous membranes frequently are involved early in the course of the disease, and strictures of the esophagus can develop. Scarring may be present. Complications include anemia from chronic blood loss and secondary infections.

The dystrophic forms of EB are characterized by scarring and may be inherited in an autosomal dominant or recessive mode. The most severe and devastating form of epidermolysis bullosa is the recessive dystrophic type. The bullae and erosions usually are present at birth, and the entire skin surface may be affected at different times by minor trauma. Scarring, milia formation, and nail loss are prominent features. Oral involvement leads to scarring with the tongue bound down, and swallowing is affected by esophageal strictures. The hands and feet become mitten-like, and contractures develop in the large joints. The prognosis is poor, even with the best of care. Secondary skin infections, anemia, growth retardation, amyloidosis, and skin cancer are complications.

Treatment of EB consists of careful attention to the skin to prevent friction, manage blisters and erosions that develop, treat secondary infection and anemia, and maintain adequate nutrition.

Vesiculopustules

Folliculitis and Furunculosis

Infections of the hair follicle unit are caused most frequently by *S. aureus*. Folliculitis is a superficial infection; a small rim of

erythema surrounds the hair follicle, which is topped by a small, white or yellow pustule. Furuncles are deeper infections with a larger rim of erythema, more swelling, and, often, a cavity of pus in the center.

Common sites for these infections include the scalp in children who have their hair pulled tightly, the buttocks in those wearing occlusive clothing, the beard area in some teenagers, and areas of the skin that are rubbed by padding in athletes. If localized, folliculitis can be treated successfully with the use of an antibacterial soap and application of a topical antibiotic

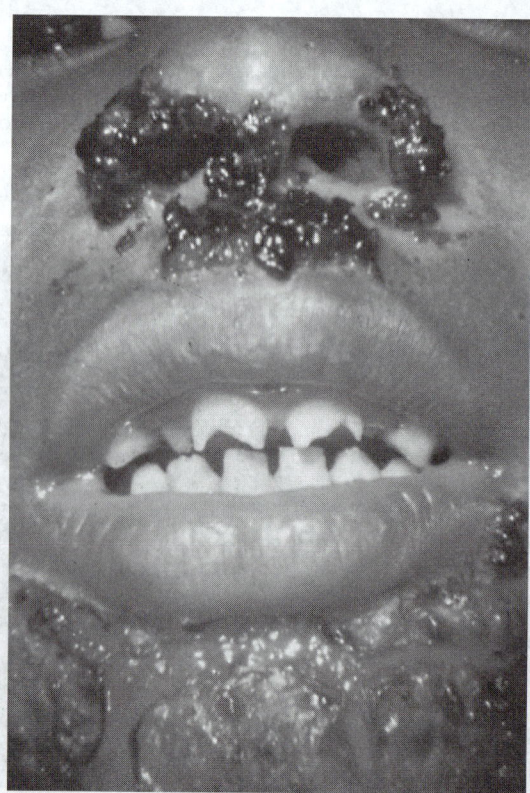

FIGURE 129.42. In junctional epidermolysis bullosa, erosions with hemorrhagic crusting are typical in the perioral area.

(e.g., clindamycin). More widespread disease or furunculosis usually requires treatment with a systemic antistaphylococcal antibiotic.

A gram-negative folliculitis may occur in teenagers who have acne and are treated with systemic antibiotics. The key to suspecting the diagnosis is a sudden flare of inflammatory papules and pustules in an individual receiving an oral antibiotic. Treatment generally requires withdrawal of antibiotic therapy and initiation of isotretinoin.

Hot tub or whirlpool folliculitis is characterized by the appearance of erythematous macules, papules, or pustules 8 to 48 hours after immersion in these tubs or after using a swimming pool or water slide. The lesions may occur on any part of the body immersed in the hot tub but often are located under swimsuits. The bacterial agent responsible is *Pseudomonas aeruginosa*; because the infection is superficial, normally no treatment is required. Hot tubs should be chlorinated and the pH maintained appropriately.

Miliaria Pustulosa

Obstruction of sweat ducts with an ensuing inflammatory response may produce a folliculitis-like eruption (Fig. 129.4). The lesions appear most commonly on areas subject to occlusion, particularly the neck, groin, and axilla, in warm weather or artificially produced warm environments. Treatment consists of the removal of excessive clothing and exposure to air.

Candidiasis

Yeast infections are caused most commonly by *Candida albicans*, a dimorphic fungus that occurs in both budding and mycelial phases. *Candida* thrives in warm, moist places; the diaper area of infants is an ideal site for proliferation (Fig. 129.43). The earliest lesions of *Candida* are small vesiculopustules on erythematous bases. The lesions enlarge and tend to become confluent. Their roofs then are lost rapidly, leaving the red bases. Characteristically, the inguinal creases are involved in candidal infections, which produce a confluent erythema, often with maceration and fissuring. Satellite lesions, erythematous papules or pustules, may be observed adjacent to areas of confluent erythema. Other common sites of candidal infection include the axillae, the neck in young infants, and the corners of the mouth.

Infants commonly have "thrush," which appears as adherent, white plaques of candidal infection in the mouth. Infection of the nails and paronychia also may develop in young children who suck their fingers or in individuals who immerse their hands in water for extended periods on a regular basis.

Unlike a bacterial paronychia, that due to *Candida* is chronic and characterized by a nontender, erythematous swelling at the base of the nail with loss of the cuticle. Often the nail becomes thickened and dystrophic. Outside the neonatal period, overt candidal infections are uncommon. Resistant, recurrent, or persistent *Candida* infection beyond infancy might suggest the presence of diabetes mellitus, hypoparathyroidism, Addison disease, an altered immunologic response to infection, acquired immunodeficiency syndrome, or malignancy.

Usually, cutaneous infection with *Candida* can be treated effectively with the application of an anticandidal agent, such as nystatin, or an imidazole antifungal agent (e.g., clotrimazole, miconazole).

Infantile Acropustulosis

Infantile acropustulosis is a highly pruritic skin disorder with a characteristic presentation. The lesions are vesicles and pustules located primarily on the palms and soles that occur in crops lasting 5 to 7 days (Fig. 129.44). Onset is between 2 to 10 months of age. The pustules are filled with polymorphonuclear neutrophils and, occasionally, eosinophils. Each crop may be followed by a remission of a few weeks before another bout occurs. Lesions occasionally appear on the extremities, trunk, and face.

The cause of infantile acropustulosis is unknown. Often, the condition is mistaken for scabies because of the associated intense pruritus and its appearance on the palms and soles. Treatment is symptomatic; an antihistamine may be administered to provide relief from pruritus and a mid- to high potency topical corticosteroids may be applied cautiously. In severe cases, dapsone has been used with success. Because of the intense scratching, secondary bacterial infection may occur. The disorder abates by 2 to 3 years of age.

Pustular Psoriasis

Psoriasis is a papulosquamous disorder characterized by elevated lesions that form scale (see Papulosquamous Disorders, earlier). Rarely, a pustular form may occur. Innumerable tiny pustules form on erythematous skin; lesions may be localized or widely distributed. The 2- to 3-mm pustules tend to coalesce, rupture, scale, and heal, often in waves. The mucous

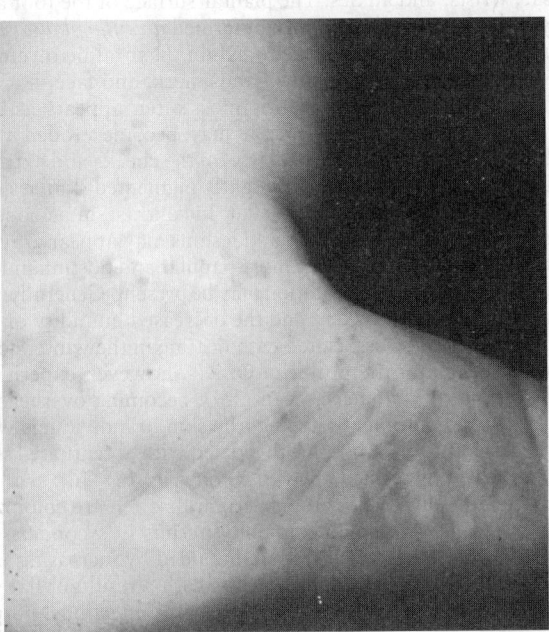

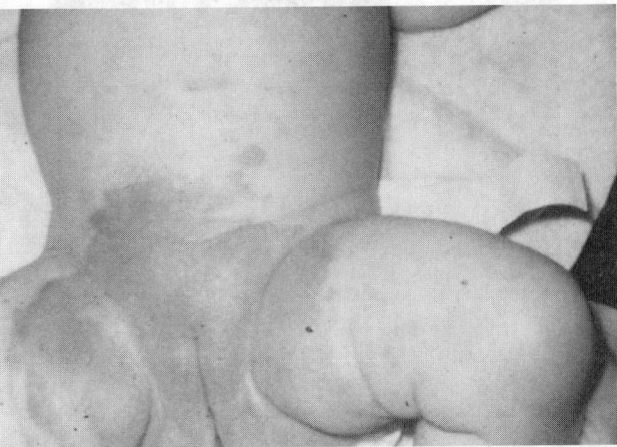

FIGURE 129.43. Candidal diaper dermatitis is characterized by involvement of the inguinal creases and satellite papules or pustules.

FIGURE 129.44. Intensely pruritic vesicles and pustules of the hands and feet are characteristic of infantile acropustulosis.

membranes of the mouth may be involved, and the tongue may appear to have a geographic pattern. The skin is tender, and systemic toxicity is common.

The cause of pustular psoriasis is unknown. A genetic predisposition is possible. Triggering factors include infection, sunburn, and abrupt cessation of oral corticosteroids. Treatment of localized forms includes topical corticosteroids, calcipotriene, or tar preparations. Widespread disease may require hospitalization and treatment with oral retinoids or methotrexate.

Eosinophilic Pustular Folliculitis

Eosinophilic pustular folliculitis is an uncommon disorder that usually occurs in neonates. However, a more widespread and persistent form has been described in children with human immunodeficiency virus infection. The disease is characterized by recurrent crops of pruritic, follicular, papulopustular lesions. The lesions tend to coalesce into plaques and occur most commonly on the scalp, face, chest, and back. Smears from the pustules show eosinophils, and peripheral eosinophilia is common. The lesions are sterile. The cause of the lesions is not known, and the course varies. Treatment with topical steroids of moderate potency has met with modest success.

Scaling and Dry Lesions

Atopic Dermatitis

Atopic dermatitis, also known as *eczema*, is the most common chronic skin condition of childhood. As many as 20% of children may develop the disease. Its cause is unknown but seems to be multifactorial; heredity plays a role, modified by environmental factors. The basic problem seems to be a sensitivity of the skin to numerous stimuli, all of which produce pruritus.

Atopic dermatitis has its onset before the age of 1 year in 60% to 80% of affected children and before the age of 5 years in 90%. The appearance varies with the patient's age and racial background. Infants and toddlers, for example, have a generalized distribution of lesions with involvement of the face, scalp, extremities, and trunk. In older children, the eruption is concentrated in flexural areas, such as the antecubital and popliteal fossae, wrists, and ankles. The plantar surface of the foot also may be involved, a clinical variant termed *juvenile plantar dermatosis*. Adolescents continue to exhibit flexural involvement but may develop lesions on the hands, neck, and face.

The rash of atopic dermatitis most often appears as dry, sometimes scaling patches, but it may become eroded with weeping of serous fluid, particularly on the cheeks and extremities (Fig. 129.45). In those with lightly pigmented skin, lesions are erythematous and tend to be flat. In contrast, in persons of color, erythema is less obvious and lesions may appear gray. In addition, the eruption often is more papular and postinflammatory hypo- or hyperpigmentation may be present. Generally, the skin of most patients is dry, and the decreased humidity of the environment that is associated with heating in the winter commonly accentuates the problem. Others, however, experience flares during the summer as a result of becoming overheated. In response to chronic scratching, the skin of individuals with atopic dermatitis may become thickened with accentuated skin creases, a finding termed *lichenification* (Fig. 129.46).

Since individuals with atopic dermatitis often are colonized with *S. aureus*, scratching commonly results in secondary infection. The presence of infection, heralded by increasing erythema and erosions, worsens pruritus with a resultant flare in the rash. Atopic skin also is prone to viral infections; herpes simplex may spread rapidly and extensively over the entire skin surface, resulting in severe disease and even death; this condi-

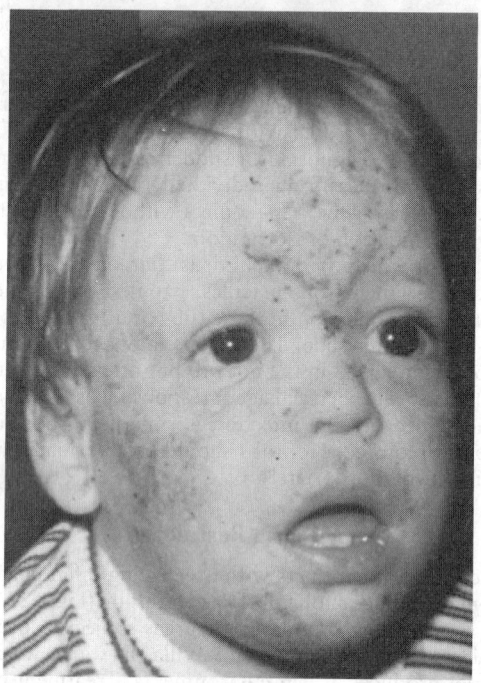

FIGURE 129.45. Typical morphology and facial distribution of infantile atopic dermatitis.

tion is called *eczema herpeticum* (see Fig. 129.35). Molluscum contagiosum also can be extensive on atopic skin.

The diagnosis of atopic dermatitis is made clinically; the major and minor criteria are listed in Box 129.1. Because this disorder is chronic and relapsing, treatment involves a great deal of teaching parents and children and of prescribing medications. Management rests upon daily skin care (designed to prevent disease flares) and treatment of exacerbations.

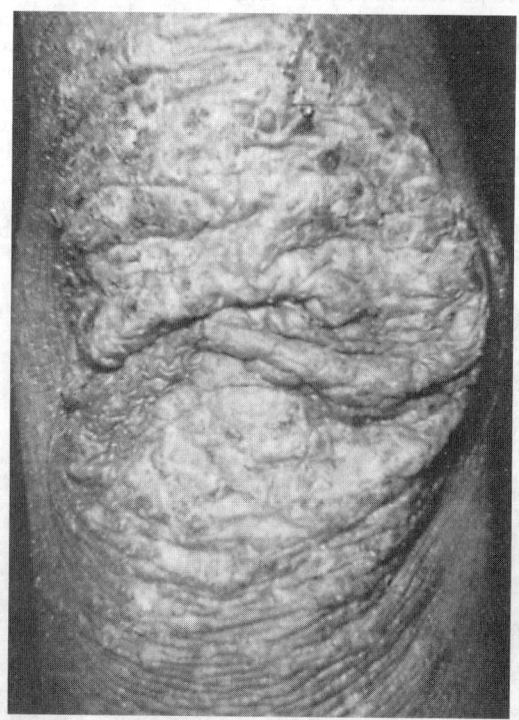

FIGURE 129.46. Dramatic lichenification from chronic scratching in atopic dermatitis.

ration of the skin condition. Allergic contact dermatitis also usually has a shorter course than does atopic dermatitis.

Pityriasis Alba

Pityriasis alba is a common condition characterized by hypopigmented macules or patches with minimal to no fine scale. The lesions, which generally are round to oval, occur most commonly on the face and less often on the neck, upper trunk, and proximal extremities. The borders of lesions are somewhat ill-defined with a gradual transition from normal to abnormal pigmentation. The lesions commonly occur in atopic individuals and likely represent an area of mild dermatitis with a resulting disturbance in the process of pigmentation. In less pigmented individuals, pityriasis alba often becomes apparent following sun exposure; the normal skin becomes darker but affected areas do not, accentuating contrast between the two. Treatment is with an appropriate topical corticosteroid for 2 to 3 weeks to reduce inflammation. The patient and family should be counseled that repigmentation may take as long as 1 year. The differential diagnosis includes tinea corporis, tinea versicolor, vitiligo, and psoriasis.

Xerosis

Xerosis, or dry skin, occurs most commonly during the winter months, when the indoor environment becomes dry from heating. Too frequent bathing and harsh soaps may contribute to the problem. Generally, the skin is dry and often has areas of erythematous, scaly patches, particularly on the extremities (sometimes called *winter eczema* or *eczema craquelé*). Pruritus is common. Treatment consists of the application of an emollient, decreasing the frequency of bathing to the extent possible, and the use of a humidifier or vaporizer to increase environmental humidity. For localized areas of winter eczema, an appropriate topical corticosteroid may be applied.

Seborrheic Dermatitis

Seborrheic dermatitis is a common skin condition with a predilection for two pediatric age groups, infants and adolescents. In infants between 2 and 10 weeks of age, seborrheic dermatitis generally begins on the scalp, producing a greasy, yellowish scale (cradle cap). The base may or may not be erythematous. Commonly, erythematous or salmon-pink patches also involve the eyebrows, nose, and retroauricular folds. In deeply pigmented individuals, significant hypopigmentation may accompany the rash (Fig. 129.47). The diaper area also may be involved with an erythematous, scaling eruption that involves the suprapubic area and inguinal folds. Infantile seborrheic dermatitis clears by 8 to 12 months of age. If scalp involvement is mild, shampooing, during which the scalp is scrubbed with a soft brush, may be sufficient. If scaling persists, an antiseborrheic shampoo may be used. Skin lesions may be treated with the application of a low-potency corticosteroid. Persistent scaling of the scalp should suggest other disorders, including tinea capitis, atopic dermatitis, and, rarely, Langerhans cell histiocytosis.

In adolescents, scaling occurs most commonly on the scalp, eyebrows, and eyelashes; erythematous scaling patches also occur in the nasolabial folds, postauricular creases, and presternal and interscapular regions. Scalp involvement is treated with an antiseborrheic shampoo (e.g., one containing zinc pyrithione, selenium sulfide, ketoconazole, or tar). If signs of inflammation are present, a midpotency corticosteroid solution may be applied as needed at bedtime. Skin lesions respond to the application of 2% ketoconazole cream or 1% hydrocortisone cream.

The cause of seborrheic dermatitis is not clear, although it may represent an inflammatory response to the yeast *Pityrosporum ovale*. The idea that the condition is related to sebaceous

---

BOX 129.1   Diagnostic Criteria for Atopic Dermatitis

Major criteria (three of four required)
Pruritus
Typical morphology and distribution
    Adults: flexural involvement (e.g., antecubital and popliteal fossae)
    Children and infants: face and extensor surfaces of the extremities involved
Chronic or relapsing course
Personal or family history of atopy

Minor criteria (three or more required)
Xerosis
Ichthyosis/keratosis pilaris/palmar hyperlinearity
Tendency to skin infection
Hand or foot dermatitis
Recurrent conjunctivitis
Dennie-Morgan infraorbital fold
Keratoconus
Orbital darkening
Facial pallor or erythema
Pityriasis alba
Involvement of anterior neck folds
Itch when sweating
Intolerance to wool and lipid solvents
Perifollicular accentuation
Food intolerance
Course influenced by environmental or emotional factors
White dermographism or delayed blanch

Modified from Hanifin JM, Rajka G. Diagnostic features of atopic dermatitis. *Acta Derm Venereol Suppl (Stockh)* 1980; 92:44.

Daily measures are intended to hydrate the skin (since most patients with atopic dermatitis have dry skin that contributes to itching and scratching) and control pruritus (primarily through the avoidance of precipitants). Factors that may precipitate pruritus include soaps; sweating and (conversely) exposure to cool air; certain materials, especially wool and synthetic fibers; and stress. Well-controlled studies have demonstrated food sensitivity in as many as 5% of affected children. The foods most frequently implicated are eggs, milk, wheat, peanuts, soybeans, and fish. The role of inhalants (pollen, mold, and dust mites) is not clear.

During disease flares, the keys to management are to reduce inflammation (through the application of a topical corticosteroid or noncorticosteroid immunomodulator), control pruritus (by using a sedating antihistamine at bedtime), and treat secondary infection, if present. As an exacerbation improves, topical corticosteroids may be withdrawn or tapered in strength and the antihistamine discontinued. For those with dry skin, emollients often must be continued, particularly after bathing.

The prognosis for atopic dermatitis usually is good; 80% to 90% of infants experience a spontaneous resolution or improvement in symptoms by adolescence. Atopic dermatitis may be confused with seborrheic dermatitis in young infants. Scabies, which also is characterized by pruritus, should be differentiated easily from atopic dermatitis by the presence and distribution of the papulovesicular lesions and the short du-

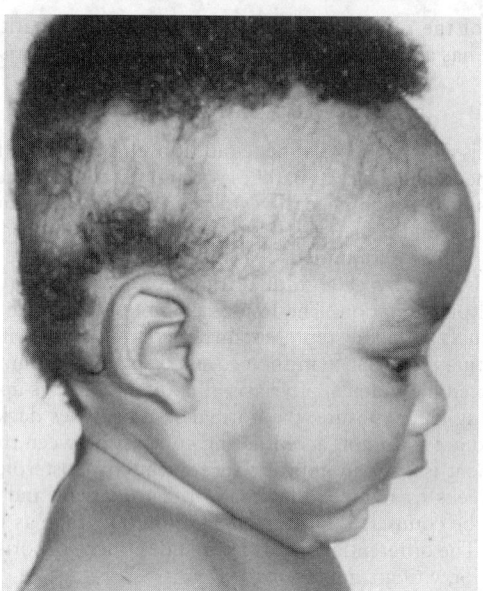

FIGURE 129.47. Note the facial hypopigmentation and scalp hair loss without prominent scaling in this child with seborrheic dermatitis.

FIGURE 129.48. Hyperpigmented scaling macules of tinea versicolor located on the chest.

gland function is supported by development of the dermatitis in areas with the highest density of these glands. The appearance of seborrheic dermatitis in infants probably reflects the effect of transiently elevated androgen levels; reappearance of the condition during puberty occurs with the resurgence of sex hormones.

Leiner Disease

Leiner disease is a rare disorder characterized by a generalized seborrheic dermatitis-like eruption combined with severe diarrhea, failure to thrive, and recurrent infections. The disease usually has its onset in the first few months of life. Generally, the skin is erythematous, with pronounced scaling. Dysfunction of the fifth component of complement has been demonstrated in some cases.

Tinea Versicolor

The characteristic clinical presentation of tinea versicolor is the gradual appearance and spread of hyper- or hypopigmented macules and patches on the neck, chest, and back (Fig. 129.48). The lesions have well-defined borders and may be erythematous, brown, or whitish. The macules may be ovoid or coin-shaped and have a fine adherent scale. Pruritus is uncommon. Most cases occur after puberty, but facial lesions in infants have been described, probably resulting from contact with affected parents.

The diagnosis may be confirmed by microscopical examination of the scale (to which potassium hydroxide has been added) for the presence of the budding cells and hyphae of *Pityrosporum orbiculare*, which give a spaghetti-and-meatballs appearance. A Wood light examination in a dark room should reveal a yellow to yellow-blue fluorescence, unless the patient has bathed recently.

Treatment of tinea versicolor consists of selenium sulfide 2.5% lotion applied to the affected area. Although various therapeutic routines exist, one common plan is to apply the lotion to all affected areas for 10 minutes daily for 7 days. Although this usually produces good results, relapses of the infection are common. To prevent recurrences, patients may be advised to apply the medication for 8 to 12 hours once every 1 to 2 months for a total of 4 to 6 months. Ketoconazole, itra-

conazole, or fluconazole orally may be used to treat those with resistant infections.

Tinea Cruris

Tinea cruris produces erythematous patches involving the proximal thighs and crural folds. Lesions are well-defined patches with erythematous, slightly raised, scaling borders. Tinea cruris may be unilateral or bilateral and typically spares the penis and scrotum. The condition is the result of infection from *Trichophyton mentagrophytes* or *Epidermophyton floccosum* and commonly occurs in adolescents and young adults. Application of an imidazole antifungal agent (e.g., miconazole, clotrimazole) usually is effective. The differential diagnosis includes candidiasis, intertrigo, and irritant and allergic contact dermatitis. Another condition that may mimic tinea cruris is *erythrasma*, a superficial corynebacterial infection. Patients with this disorder exhibit reddish-brown patches in flexural areas, such as the groin or axillae. Unlike tinea cruris, however, lesions do not have an elevated border and do not produce scale. The diagnosis of erythrasma may be confirmed by examining affected areas with a Wood lamp in a darkened room; in those affected a coral-red fluorescence will be observed. Erythromycin will eradicate the infection; localized forms may be treated topically, while more widespread infection should be managed with oral therapy.

Ichthyosis

Ichthyosis refers to a group of disorders characterized by the accumulation of visible scales and a general dryness of the skin surface. The four most common types of ichthyosis and some of their characteristic features are listed in Table 129.3.

Ichthyosis vulgaris, as the name suggests, is the most common form (Fig. 129.49). Most cases are mild and are overlooked easily on routine examination. Affected individuals have fine, plate-like scales with elevated edges that have the appearance of having been pasted on. Usually the extensor surfaces of the lower extremities are involved. Ichthyosis vulgaris commonly is associated with atopic dermatitis.

In the X-linked type of ichthyosis, the scales are larger and yellowish brown. The palms and soles are not involved, but the face, scalp, and neck characteristically are. Lamellar ichthyosis occurs in two forms, both of which present at birth, often with a collodion membrane (color Fig. 68.17 in color section). Later the classic form is characterized by large, greasy, brown

TABLE 129.3

PRIMARY FORMS OF ICHTHYOSIS

Type	Inheritance	Onset	Clinical Features
Ichthyosis vulgaris	Autosomal dominant	3 months–5 years	Thin scales with elevated edges that creates a "pasted on" appearance Extensor surfaces of lower extremities primarily affected Hyperlinearity of the palms Face, antecubital and popliteal fossae spared
X-linked ichthyosis	X-linked recessive	Infancy (may be present at birth)	Scales on the face, scalp, posterior neck, trunk and extensor surfaces of the extremities Scales become thicker and darker with time Spares palms, soles, antecubital and popliteal fossae
Lamellar ichthyosis	Autosomal recessive	Birth	Newborns have a collodion membrane, ectropion, and eclabium Once the collodion membrane is shed, the skin becomes erythematous and plate-like scales develop that affect all body surfaces, including the flexural creases, palms, and soles
Congenital nonbullous ichthyosiform erythroderma	Autosomal recessive	Birth	Newborns have a collodion membrane, ectropion, and eclabium Generalized erythema with fine white scale
Epidermolytic hyperkeratosis (congenital ichthyosiform erythroderma)	Autosomal dominant	Birth	Widespread scaling, erosions, bullae By childhood, patients exhibit thick, warty, yellow scales on the flexural surfaces of the elbows and knees, as well as on the trunk, palms, and soles

plate-like scales. The flexural creases, palms, soles, and scalp also are involved. Lamellar ichthyosis is relatively uncommon.

Bullous ichthyosis (congenital bullous ichthyosiform erythroderma, epidermolytic hyperkeratosis) is manifested at birth by widespread blistering and erythema (color Fig. 68.15 in color section). The lesions are especially prominent in the flexural creases. The scale is thick and gray to brown. Harlequin fetus is an extremely rare form of ichthyosis characterized by a dense, armor-like covering of the skin at birth, with severe deformity of the soft tissues and skeleton. There typically is severe ectropion and eclabium. Restrictions in movement

may lead to respiratory insufficiency and difficulty feeding. Infants often die within the first few days of life. Ichthyosis is seen also in numerous other syndromes, including Sjögren-Larsson, keratitis-ichthyosis-deafness, Refsum, and Conradi-Hünermann-Happle syndromes, among others.

Considerable research into the pathogenesis of the ichthyoses has led to a better understanding of these disorders. In all forms, genetic deletions or mutations appear to be responsible for alterations in epidermal differentiation. X-linked ichthyosis, for example, results from deletions or mutations that lead to a deficiency of steroid sulfatase.

The ichthyoses are chronic diseases that can be managed but not cured. Initially, treatment is with emollients that prevent evaporation of moisture from the skin. If the response is unsatisfactory, an emollient containing urea or an alpha-hydroxy acid (e.g., lactic acid or ammonium lactate) applied once or twice a day will improve the skin's ability to bind water. To control scale, preparations containing salicylic acid may be prescribed. Severe forms of ichthyosis, like epidermal hyperkeratosis, occasionally require treatment with an oral retinoid.

Nummular Eczema

As the name denotes, nummular eczema is characterized by the presence of coin-shaped plaques. The lesions may be "dry" (i.e., covered with scale) or "wet" (i.e., characterized by erythematous erosions and crusting). They are well-defined, often on an erythematous base, and may be hyperpigmented or may have undergone lichenification. Pruritus is variable. Lesions appear most commonly on the extensor surfaces of the arms and legs and on the dorsa of the fingers and hands.

An association seems to exist between a dry environment and appearance of the lesions. Frequent bathing with drying soaps may aggravate the rash. Treatment consists of the application of a topical corticosteroid. Decreasing the frequency of bathing (to the extent possible) and the application of an emollient may be beneficial. The differential diagnosis includes allergic contact dermatitis, atopic dermatitis, psoriasis, tinea corporis, and impetigo.

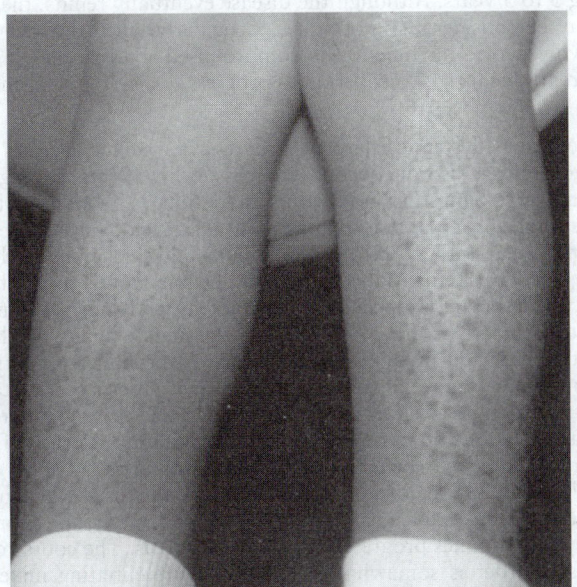

FIGURE 129.49. Large, plate-like scales of the lower legs in a patient with ichthyosis vulgaris.

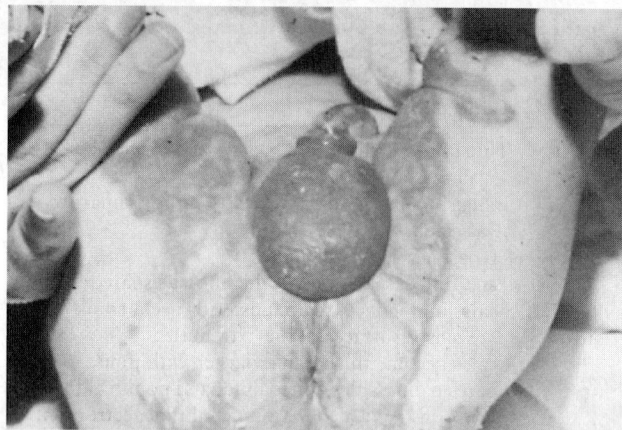

FIGURE 129.50. Erythematous, scaling, well-demarcated perianal dermatitis in an infant with acrodermatitis enteropathica.

Subacute or Chronic Contact Dermatitis

In acute contact dermatitis, the skin usually is erythematous and features vesicles and oozing (see Contact Dermatitis Due to Plants). In contrast, in subacute or chronic contact dermatitis, such as that resulting from nickel, the skin often is lichenified and scaling (see Pruritic Lesions, later).

Acrodermatitis Enteropathica

Acrodermatitis enteropathica is an autosomal recessive disorder in which a defective transport protein in the gastrointestinal tract results in impaired absorption of dietary zinc. Because human milk has a protein that facilitates zinc absorption, clinical manifestations often appear after an infant is weaned from human milk to formula or cow milk. Zinc deficiency also may occur in patients who have chronic malabsorption due to cystic fibrosis or celiac disease, or those who are maintained on parenteral nutrition without zinc supplementation.

Zinc deficiency leads to altered keratin synthesis and resultant skin lesions. The primary clinical appearance usually is one of crusted erosions with sharply marginated borders (Fig. 129.50). The lesions begin around the body orifices (i.e., mouth, eyes, or perianal areas). Lesions develop on the hands and feet as well, and with time, other areas of the body similarly may be involved. Crusting of the scalp and alopecia may occur, and the nails may be lost.

The diagnosis of acrodermatitis enteropathica is confirmed by the finding of a low zinc level. With supplementation, cutaneous lesions improve rapidly. While awaiting improvement, a topical corticosteroid may be applied to affected areas.

Disorders Involving Abnormal Skin Texture

Sclerosis

Scleroderma. Scleroderma is a rare connective tissue disorder that is believed to have an autoimmune cause. It may be separated into localized and systemic forms. Localized scleroderma, the most common form, begins as areas of indurated skin that have violaceous borders. Over time, the violaceous color is lost, and the skin takes on a waxy, ivory appearance. As the disease remits, previously affected areas become atrophic and hypo- or hyperpigmented (Fig. 129.51). Three clinical patterns of localized scleroderma have been described: linear scleroderma, morphea, and generalized morphea. In linear scleroderma, lesions appear in a band-like distribution, typically are unilateral, and usually involve the extremities, although the face and trunk

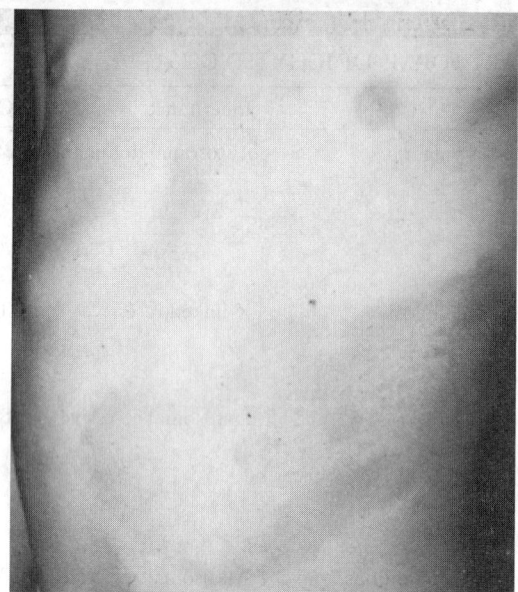

FIGURE 129.51. An irregularly pigmented patch of morphea on the abdomen. The skin has lost its elasticity and feels firm.

may be affected. The abnormal tissue may span joints, resulting in diminished range of motion or deformity, and may extend to soft tissue, muscle, or bone. In morphea, one or two discrete areas are affected, often on the trunk. Generalized morphea is characterized by the presence of widespread or coalescent lesions.

Treatment of active disease (i.e., areas that appear to be expanding and have violaceous borders) generally involves topical or intralesional corticosteroids or topical calcipotriene. Systemic therapies, such as methotrexate alone or combined with pulsed systemic corticosteroids, are reserved for those with recalcitrant disease. Other systemic therapies that have been advocated include penicillamine and ultraviolet A light. Physical therapy should be prescribed to maintain range of motion if lesions involve the skin overlying joints.

In most instances, localized scleroderma is self-limited, lasting 3 to 5 years. Although the disease eventually remits, there may be considerable morbidity, particularly when the face is involved or joint function is compromised. Fortunately, it is rare for localized scleroderma to progress to a systemic form.

Progressive Systemic Sclerosis. Progressive systemic sclerosis is a generalized disorder of connective tissue that affects the lungs, heart, gastrointestinal tract, joints, and kidneys, in addition to the skin. The initial lesions almost always develop on the distal extremities, with an insidious tightening and thickening of the involved areas. Invariably, Raynaud phenomenon is seen. The involved skin may appear shiny and blotchy, and finger swelling and contractures are common. The tightness extends up the extremities and involves the face. Pits of the finger pulp are common, as are telangiectases of the nail cuticles. The fatal course may be as short as 1 year, but it often lasts for many years. There is no cure for progressive systemic sclerosis. D-penicillamine may be effective in treating some patients.

The CREST syndrome (subcutaneous *c*alcinosis, *R*aynaud phenomenon, *e*sophageal dysfunction, *s*clerodactyly, and *t*elangiectasia) mimics progressive systemic sclerosis. The course of this disorder is somewhat less severe. Differentiating mixed connective-tissue disease from progressive systemic sclerosis may be difficult in the early stages. The causes of all these disorders are unknown.

Lichen Sclerosus et Atrophicus. The characteristic features of lichen sclerosus et atrophicus are patches of atrophy and hypopigmentation. The surface of the skin is white and thin, almost resembling cigarette paper and often is atrophic. The most common site of involvement in females is the perineum, where the lesions encircle the vulva and anus in an hourglass shape. Pain and pruritus lead to excoriation and secondary infection. Occasionally, patients develop erosions or purpura that may be mistaken for signs of sexual abuse. Some develop pain with defecation that may lead to stool withholding, or bleeding from anal fissures. In males, the foreskin may be involved, leading to phimosis.

The cause of lichen sclerosus et atrophicus is not known. Females are affected ten times as often as are males. Three-fourths of children have symptomatic improvement in 3 to 5 years. Although no curative therapy appears to be available, the application of a mid- to high potency topical corticosteroid often is effective. Although some success with testosterone cream has been reported in adults, this agent should not be used in children due to the potential for virilization.

Scleredema. Scleredema is a rare disorder of unknown cause characterized by the appearance of large areas of induration. Usually, the onset is sudden, often starting on the posterior neck and extending over the shoulders to the chest, face, upper extremities, and back. A strong association with a preceding streptococcal infection has been found in cases that have their onset within 6 weeks of a febrile illness.

The disease reaches its maximum extent in 2 to 6 weeks and most cases improve spontaneously in 6 months to 2 years. Perhaps one-fourth of affected children show only partial improvement. The induration and thickening of the skin may interfere with joint mobility and respiration. No effective therapy is known.

Loose Skin

Ehlers-Danlos Syndrome. Ehlers-Danlos syndrome (EDS) represents a group of ten inherited disorders in which abnormal collagen synthesis results in skin hyperelasticity and skin fragility (Fig. 129.52). The basic problem is a hereditary disorder of collagen. The skin feels velvety and when stretched, returns quickly to its previous position. Lacerations may produce thin scars resembling cigarette paper. Blood vessels also are fragile, with easy bruising being a common feature. The most severe form is EDS IV, characterized by translucent skin, marked bruising, and rupture of the arteries, bowel, or uterus. No effective therapy for EDS is available. Management is supportive. Recognition is important, particularly for those with EDS IV, or if surgery is contemplated, because care must be taken in wound closure.

Cutis Laxa. In cutis laxa, the skin hangs and sags, as a result of abnormal or absent elastic fibers, and gives the affected individual an aged or bloodhound-like facial appearance. Two forms have been recognized: an autosomal recessive type, which is severe, and a relatively benign autosomal dominant form. Systemic associations of this uncommon disorder include pulmonary emphysema, pneumothoraces, diverticula of the gastrointestinal and genitourinary tracts, rectal prolapse, and hernias. No treatment for this disorder is known.

Pseudoxanthoma Elasticum. Pseudoxanthoma elasticum is a rare genetic disorder with both dominant and recessive forms. The characteristic feature is the development of soft, yellowish papules and plaques on the neck, creating a cobblestone effect; the appearance resembles that of plucked chicken skin or orange peel. With age, the skin becomes inelastic and hangs in folds. The relatively benign skin changes belie the severity of ocular and cardiovascular problems. Angioid streaks—gray to brown linear bands—appear on the retina and, as fibrosis develops, central vision may be lost. In adults, significant vessel disease may occur, including coronary artery disease and gastrointestinal bleeding.

Depressed Lesions

Striae. As linear, shallow depressions of the skin commonly seen in adolescents, striae occur in areas where the skin has been subjected to stretching. Common sites include the shoulders, abdomen, hips, buttocks, thighs, and breasts. Initially, the lesions may appear red or red-blue, but they become skin-colored with time. The cause is not known but they are believed to result from breaks in connective tissue. There is a familial predisposition to striae and they are more likely to occur in individuals who are receiving systemic steroids, have Cushing disease, or receive potent topical corticosteroids for a prolonged period. Striae may appear after severe illness, such as infections, after oncologic therapy, or after excessive weight loss or gain. Patients may be counseled that the appearance of striae improves with time. No universally effective therapy exists. Topical tretinoin and pulsed dye laser have been reported to improve the appearance of lesions.

Corticosteroid Atrophy. Depressions in the skin may develop at sites of intramuscular injections of corticosteroids or after the prolonged application of a potent topical corticosteroid. The dermis and subcutaneous fat demonstrate local atrophy. In most cases, the tissues regenerate. The overlying skin appears normal.

Macular Atrophies. A number of types of anetoderma, or atrophy of the skin, may develop during childhood, although these conditions are uncommon. The characteristic feature is the appearance of white, pink, or bluish macules in which elastic tissue is lost. Most of these macules are round or ovoid. The skin may appear slightly depressed in the lesions, but outpouchings occur with time. Anetodermas may be primary or result from inflammatory conditions, such as varicella or acne.

Necrobiosis Lipoidica Diabeticorum. Necrobiosis lipoidica diabeticorum is a degenerative disorder of the skin that is characterized by the appearance of atrophic plaques on the

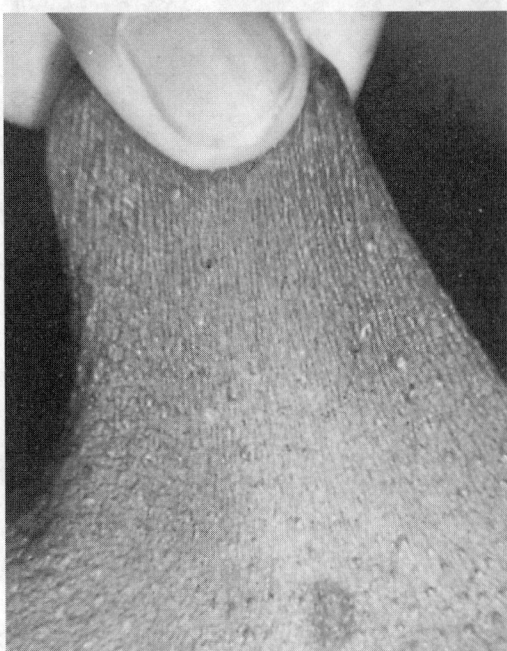

FIGURE 129.52. Striking hyperextensibility of the skin of the forearm in a patient with Ehlers-Danlos syndrome.

anterior surface of the lower legs. The lesions begin as reddish papules or nodules that enlarge gradually to form oval yellowish plaques with purplish borders. The surface may appear waxy and centrally depressed, with prominent telangiectases. Association with diabetes mellitus is strong; 90% of affected individuals have the disorder or a strong family history of it, or they will have diabetes eventually. The pathogenesis seems to involve microangiopathy, which alters dermal collagen. No satisfactory therapy is available.

Discoid Lupus Erythematosus. The classic lesions of discoid lupus erythematosus are well-demarcated, slightly raised, indurated, red to purple plaques. The lesions appear most commonly over the face and scalp. An adherent scale is typical, as are telangiectases, and central atrophy is common. Changes in pigmentation occur with time. In young children, therapy might include the judicious use of a midpotency topical corticosteroid along with sunscreens and avoidance of the sun. If this therapy fails, oral hydroxychloroquine may be used. Neonatal lesions of lupus frequently appear discoid. No therapy is necessary for these lesions; they resolve with time, although telangiectases may remain at the sites of involvement.

Macules and Patches

Hyperpigmented

Mongolian Spots. Importantly, mongolian spots, which are benign lesions, must not be confused with bruises, particularly bruises caused by child abuse. See Skin Lesions in the Neonatal Period, earlier.

Nevi. Lesions that represent collections of nevus cells, which are variants of normal melanocytes, are termed *nevi* or (by laypersons) *moles*. The disorders come in a number of varieties and often are cause for controversy and alarm.

Congenital Melanocytic Nevi. See discussion in Skin Lesions in the Neonatal Period.

Acquired Melanocytic Nevi. Acquired melanocytic nevi may appear at any time after birth, with peaks in appearance occurring between the ages of 2 and 3 years and again between 11 and 18 years. The average number of nevi in Caucasian adults is approximately 40, but the range is large. African American individuals have many fewer lesions. Acquired melanocytic nevi are divided into three clinical types, differentiation of which may not be easy. In the junctional nevus, which occurs predominantly in children, all the nevus cells are contained within the epidermis. The lesions are macular or only slightly raised and are smooth and hairless. Compound nevi have nevus cells both at the dermal–epidermal junction and within the dermis. The lesions are raised and smooth-bordered and often contain hair. Intradermal nevi have their nevus cells entirely in the dermis. They are raised, dome-shaped, smooth-bordered, and even in pigmentation.

The appearance of nevi varies considerably and ranges from deeply pigmented to colorless. Acquired nevi do not have to be removed routinely, unless they develop worrisome signs of change suggestive of melanoma. Although malignant change is uncommon in children, melanomas may develop at any age. Features that should suggest further evaluation include asymmetry, border irregularity, color variation within the lesion (particularly pink, red, blue, or white) or those with a diameter of greater than or equal to 6 mm. Evaluation also is indicated if a lesion is increasing in size, undergoes spontaneous bleeding or ulceration, develops satellite lesions, or becomes painful or pruritic.

Atypical (Dysplastic) Nevi. Attention has been drawn to the propensity of melanoma to develop in certain families. Members of these families seem to have an abnormally large number of acquired pigmented lesions, many of which are termed *atypical* or *dysplastic*. Atypical lesions are larger (5 to 12 mm) than are common nevi and are characterized by irregular and ill-defined borders. Often, their color is variegated, tan to dark brown, sometimes with a pink background. At times, lesions have a central elevated component, making their appearance simulate that of a sunny side up fried egg. Dysplastic nevi begin in adolescence and continue to appear into adulthood.

The risk for melanoma development among affected persons varies with the number of atypical nevi and the family history. For those who have a few atypical nevi but no family history of melanoma, the lifetime risk of developing melanoma is only minimally elevated. However, for the individual with atypical nevi in whom there is a family history of melanoma in two or more first-degree relatives, the risk approaches 100%.

Halo Nevi. Nevi occasionally develop a hypopigmented ring around them and, over time, disappear (Fig. 129.53). Such halo nevi represent an apparent immunologic attack by the body against its own melanocytic cells. Interestingly, some individuals with halo nevi also have areas of vitiligo. Halo nevi almost always are benign; further evaluation is warranted if the nevus or halo is irregular, particularly if the halo is incomplete.

Spitz Nevi. Spitz nevi are benign melanocytic tumors that occur most commonly in young children at approximately 3 years of age and in adolescents. Usually, they are solitary, occurring most commonly on the cheeks. The typical lesion is dome-shaped, has a smooth surface and distinct border, is hairless, and is pinkish (Fig. 129.54). Spitz nevi tend to grow rapidly over a 3- to 12-month period. Usually, they are removed because of concern about a true melanoma or for cosmetic reasons.

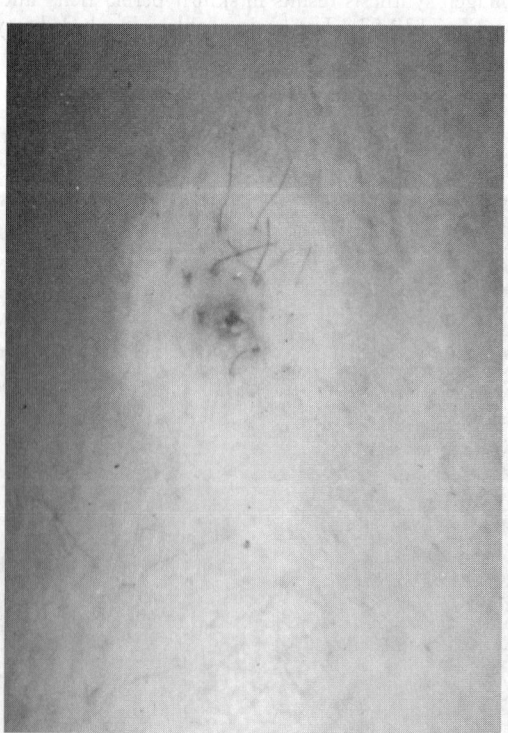

FIGURE 129.53. Depigmentation of the central nevus and surrounding skin in a halo nevus.

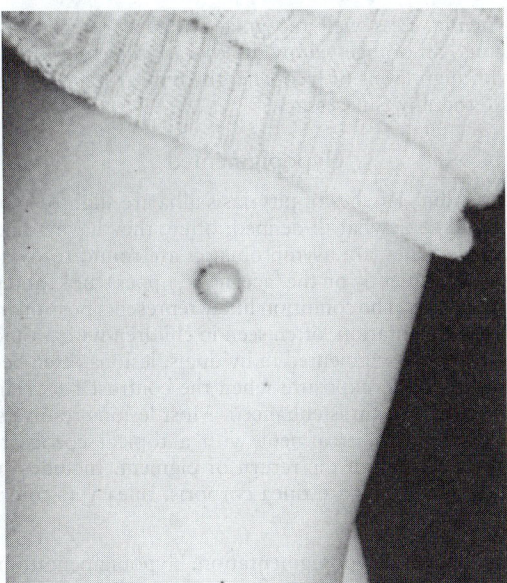

FIGURE 129.54. A well-circumscribed, pigmented spindle cell or Spitz nevus in a typical location, the upper arm.

Blue Nevi. The blue nevus is a benign lesion that also may be mistaken for a melanoma. Blue nevi usually are solitary, blue to blue-black, and generally less than 15 mm in diameter. They tend to occur most frequently on the hands, feet, buttocks, and face. No malignant changes have been reported.

Becker Nevi. Becker nevus, a relatively common condition that occurs most frequently around the time of puberty, is characterized by acquired areas of pigmentation of the skin. The typical site is the shoulder, but lesions, which seem to develop fairly rapidly, have been described on any cutaneous surface. Often, the borders are irregular, the pigmentation is spotty, and hair growth in the area almost always is increased (Fig. 129.55). The lesions occur more frequently in males than in females. The cause is unknown, although androgen stimulation is thought to play a role. On biopsy, differentiating this lesion from normal skin is difficult. Becker melanosis is a benign lesion for which no treatment is necessary.

Ephelides. Ephelides or freckles are tan to brown, small macules that develop early in childhood particularly in red-haired,

fair-skinned individuals. Inherited as an autosomal dominant trait, the lesions develop only on sun-exposed areas and become more prominent in the summer months. After adolescence, they are less noticeable.

Lentigines. Unlike freckles, lentigines develop not only on sun-exposed skin but on unexposed areas. They are small (0.2 to 1.0 cm), discrete, dark brown to black, round to oval macules. Lentigines may be present at birth but usually they develop in childhood and increase in number with age.

Although usually an isolated finding, lentigines may be associated with a number of different disorders. The Peutz-Jeghers syndrome features multiple lentigines, usually involving the lips, in association with intestinal polyposis. The LEOPARD syndrome is an acronym for the association of *l*entigines with *e*lectrocardiographic abnormalities, *o*cular hypertelorism, *p*ulmonic stenosis, *a*bnormalities of the genitalia, *r*etardation of growth, and *d*eafness. Finally, in Carney syndrome, individuals have two or more of the following abnormalities: hyperpigmented skin lesions (e.g., lentigines or ephelides), cardiac myxomas, cutaneous myxomas, myxoid mammary fibroadenomas, testicular tumors, adrenocortical disease, or pituitary adenomas with gigantism or acromegaly.

Café au Lait Macules. Café au lait macules (CALMs) are discrete light-brown macules that are present at birth or develop thereafter. Usually, they are seen as an isolated finding, especially among darkly pigmented individuals. The presence of multiple CALMs may provide an important cutaneous clue to neurofibromatosis type 1 (NF1). Six or more CALMs measuring 0.5 cm or more in diameter in prepubertal children or 1.5 cm or more in diameter in postpubertal individuals should prompt careful examination for other findings of this autosomal dominantly inherited disorder with protean features. Among children with six or more CALMs, 89% will meet diagnostic criteria for NF1 within 3 years. The diagnostic criteria for NF1 are presented in Box 129.2.

The presence of CALMs (rarely exceeding five or six) may be associated with other disorders as well, including Russell-Silver syndrome, multiple lentigines, ataxia-telangiectasia, tuberous sclerosis, McCune-Albright syndrome, Fanconi anemia, Proteus syndrome, and Turner syndrome.

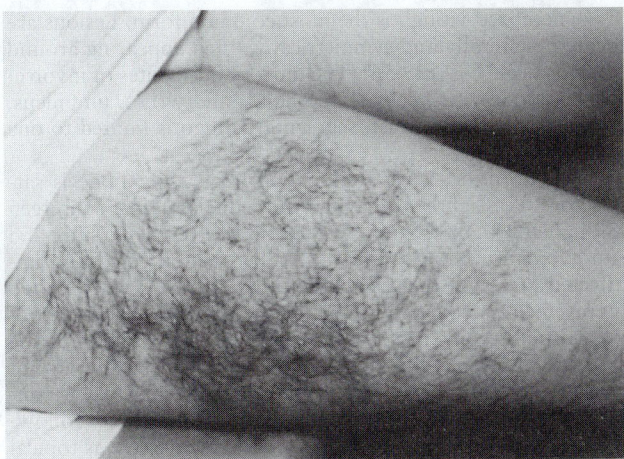

FIGURE 129.55. A large patch of irregular hyperpigmentation with hypertrichosis is characteristic of Becker melanosis.

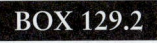

BOX 129.2   Diagnostic Criteria for Neurofibromatosis Type 1

Diagnosis Requires the Presence of Two or More of the Following

- Six or more café au lait macules measuring ≥0.5 cm in diameter in prepubertal individuals and ≥1.5 cm in those who are postpubertal.
- Two or more neurofibromas of any type or one or more plexiform neurofibroma(s) (neurofibromas are present in 20% of affected individuals by age 10 years and in more than 90% of adults).
- Freckling in the axillary or inguinal region (occurs in 85% of patients by age 10 years).
- Optic glioma
- Two or more Lisch nodules (iris hamartomas present in 25% of patients by age 5 years, 50% by age 10, and 95% by age 20).
- An osseous lesion (e.g., dysplasia of the sphenoid bone or dysplasia or thinning of long bone cortex).
- A first-degree relative with neurofibromatosis type 1.

Postinflammatory Hyperpigmentation. Darkening of the skin at sites of preceding inflammation or irritation is a common phenomenon, especially in deeply pigmented individuals. The pathophysiology of the deposition of melanin is unclear. Generally, the pigmentation fades with time.

Urticaria Pigmentosa. Collections of mast cells in the skin may create hyperpigmented macules, plaques, or nodules. See Mastocytosis in the section Nodules, earlier.

Phytophotodermatitis. A macular hyperpigmentation, phytophotodermatitis results from contact with photosensitizers present in certain plants. Crushing of these plants releases furocoumarins, the photobiologically active portion of which—psoralen—induces a dermatitis on exposure to ultraviolet light. Lime juice, particularly from lime skin, is a relatively common culprit. Other plants producing a similar effect include lemon, celery, parsnip, and fig. Initially, affected areas may be erythematous or form blisters. Hyperpigmentation follows with many unusual shapes, depending on the type of exposure (e.g., linear in areas where the juice has dripped, or in the form of a hand print). These lesions have been confused with bruises caused by child abuse.

Fixed Drug Eruption. A fixed drug eruption is a localized drug reaction characterized by the appearance of one or more purple to red plaques with clearly demarcated borders. Occasionally, they may appear urticarial or eczematous. Lesions heal over 10 to 14 days, leaving intense hyperpigmentation. Common drugs responsible for these lesions include salicylates, tetracyclines, barbiturates, sulfonamides, and phenolphthalein (present in many laxatives). The reason for such localized reactions from systemically administered drugs is unknown. Each time the drug is given, the eruption recurs in the same spot.

Acanthosis Nigricans. Acanthosis nigricans is manifested characteristically by the appearance of a hyperpigmented, somewhat velvety thickening of the skin. The most common sites of involvement are the nape and sides of the neck, the axillae, and the groin; the elbows and knuckles also may be affected. Although acanthosis nigricans may be associated with an internal malignancy in adults, this association is extremely rare in children. The problem most commonly associated with the disorder is obesity and insulin resistance. In some cases in which the disease onset is early in life, a familial association may be found. The presence of acanthosis nigricans should alert one to the possible coexistence of endocrinologic abnormalities, including insulin resistance and diabetes mellitus. No effective therapy is available for the lesions; however, lesions may regress with weight loss.

Maculae Ceruleae. Discrete, round, barely perceptible gray to bluish macules (also known as *taches bleuâtres*), maculae ceruleae occasionally are seen on the lower abdomen, thighs, and thorax of individuals who are infested with *Pediculosis pubis*. The discoloration seems to occur at the feeding sites of the lice and may be mistaken for a bruise.

Yellow

Carotenemia. Carotenemia is a common yellowish to orange skin discoloration caused by the ingestion of excessive amounts of carotene-containing foods. Occasionally, carotenemia is associated with hypothyroidism, diabetes mellitus, or nephrosis. Foods commonly connected with the disorder are carrots, squash, and other yellow vegetables. The areas most often involved are the face, palms, and soles. The disorder is asymptomatic and noninjurious; the main reason for concern is its possible confusion with jaundice. The sclerae are not yellow in carotenoderma.

Lycopenemia. Less well recognized than carotenemia is lycopenemia, an orange-yellow discoloration of the skin associated with high levels of lycopene, the red carotenoid of tomatoes. No therapy is necessary.

Hypopigmented

Pityriasis Alba. Patches of pityriasis alba are slightly hypopigmented and somewhat ill-defined; often, they have a fine, adherent scale. They are asymptomatic, are round to oval, and occur most frequently on the face, neck, upper trunk, and proximal extremities. The condition likely represents postinflammatory hypopigmentation, often seen in children with atopic dermatitis. In lightly pigmented individuals, lesions often become apparent after sun exposure when the contrast between normal and affected skin is enhanced. Most lesions resolve spontaneously, although treatment with a topical corticosteroid and emollients hasten the return of pigment. Included in the differential diagnosis are tinea corporis, tinea versicolor, and vitiligo.

Postinflammatory Hypopigmentation. Hypopigmentation may occur in areas of inflammation such as those affected by atopic dermatitis. These areas will regain their normal color, although as much as a year may be required.

Tinea Versicolor. Tinea versicolor is discussed in the section Scaling and Dry Lesions. This condition is most commonly seen in adolescents and young adults.

Seborrheic Dermatitis. Hypopigmented areas are common on the forehead, eyebrows, scalp, nasolabial folds, and other areas affected by seborrheic dermatitis. Usually, a greasy or fine scale is associated with the hypopigmentation. Although the hypopigmentation is seen most commonly in infants, it may occur in any age group affected. Topical ketoconazole is effective in clearing lesions. A low-potency topical corticosteroid will reduce the inflammation that causes the loss of pigmentation. Seborrheic dermatitis occurs during the first year of life and not again until the onset of puberty. See additional information under Scaling and Dry Lesions.

Vitiligo. The lesions of vitiligo are well-defined macules or patches that are depigmented and, therefore, are much lighter than those of the disorders listed earlier. This disorder destroys the pigment cells in the skin. The cause of vitiligo is unknown, but autoimmune, autocytotoxic, and neuronal dysfunction mechanisms have been suggested. It is more common than most people suspect; as many as 2% of the general population may have vitiligo, and 50% of those have the problem before age 20 years.

Generalized vitiligo is the most common form. Lesions are located bilaterally and symmetrically, often appearing around body orifices (Fig. 129.56). The most frequent sites of involvement are the face, backs of the hands and wrists, umbilicus, and genitalia. In contrast, segmental vitiligo is limited to one area of the skin.

Several options exist for treating vitiligo but none is satisfactory. For lightly pigmented individuals, use of sunscreen (SPF greater than or equal to 50) and protective clothing and sun avoidance reduce the contrast between affected and unaffected areas and may be sufficient. For others with limited involvement, a covering cosmetic may be applied. Potent topical corticosteroids result in the return of normal color to the skin in approximately 20% of treated patients, and 50% of those treated will have 75% or more repigmentation. A concern, however, is the potential for local skin atrophy following prolonged use. Topical tacrolimus is as effective as topical corticosteroids, but without the potential for inducing atrophy. Treatment with psoralens and ultraviolet A light, ultraviolet B light, or autologous grafting of unaffected epidermis or

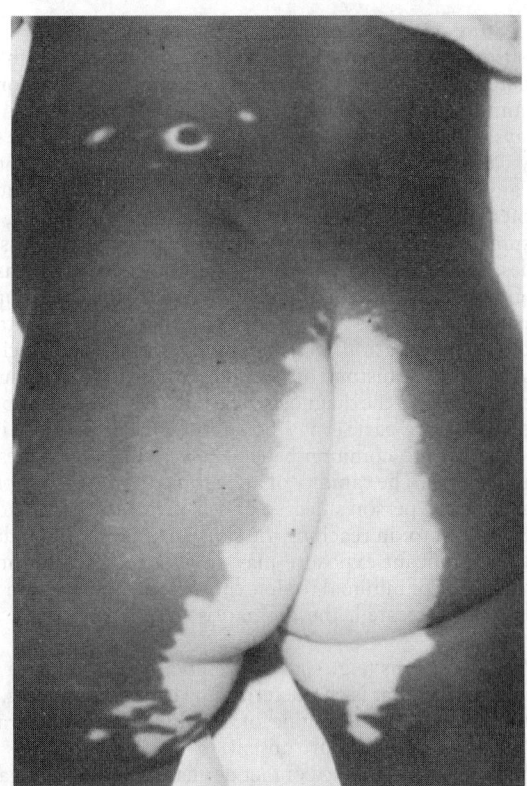

FIGURE 129.56. In vitiligo, depigmentation with distinct borders frequently involves the perineum.

cultured melanocytes should be reserved for older children with significant disease who fail other therapies. Care must be taken to protect the depigmented skin from sunburn.

Albinism. Albinism may affect the skin, hair, and eyes (oculocutaneous albinism [OCA]) or the eyes alone (ocular albinism). A number of types of OCA have been described. In all forms there is a defect in melanin synthesis that results in reduced or absent pigmentation. The severity and natural history of the disease depend on the type. Some individuals have a total absence of pigment with blue irides, pink pupils and skin, and white hair. Others develop evidence of pigmentation over time with the appearance of yellow hair and tan skin. Children with OCA may have severe reductions in visual acuity with photophobia and nystagmus. Most forms of OCA are inherited in an autosomal recessive fashion and result from one of several genetic mutations. No treatment is available for the hypopigmentation; patients and families should be advised about the need for sun protection and consultations with an ophthalmologist and geneticist arranged.

Piebaldism. Piebaldism also is known as *partial albinism*, because the area of skin involved is limited. The sites most commonly affected by the congenital absence of pigment are the hair, which has a white forelock, and the forehead, which has a triangular area of hypopigmentation. However, hypopigmented patches may be located on the anterior trunk or midportion of the extremities. A characteristic finding is the presence of normally pigmented small macules within patches of hypopigmentation. Piebaldism is an autosomal dominant disorder caused by mutations in the *KIT* protooncogene. It may be associated with deafness, and some affected individuals have Hirschsprung disease or cerebellar ataxia. No therapy exists for the depigmentation; a cosmetic cover-up may be used.

Waardenburg Syndrome. Waardenburg syndrome, a disorder inherited by the autosomal dominant route, is characterized by varying expressions of lateral displacement of the lacrimal puncta, a broad nasal root, partial or total heterochromia of the iris, piebaldism of the skin or hair, and congenital deafness. Patients with some forms of the disease may have associated Hirschsprung disease. Waardenburg syndrome accounts for as much as 1% of all deafness in children. Four types of the disease are recognized, all resulting from one of four genetic mutations.

Tuberous Sclerosis. Often, hypopigmented macules are the initial clue to tuberous sclerosis, a neurocutaneous disorder inherited in an autosomal dominant manner. The hypopigmented lesions are small, ovoid, and scattered, and their number varies. Larger lesions, known as *ash-leaf spots*, may have jagged edges resembling a leaf. Any child with unexplained seizures should be examined carefully for cutaneous clues, particularly hypopigmented macules. Shagreen spots—connective tissue nevi resembling raised, leather-like lesions—generally appear later, as does adenoma sebaceum, manifested by angiofibromas on the face. Many normal individuals have an isolated hypopigmented macule without underlying disorders.

Hypomelanosis of Ito. Hypomelanosis of Ito is characterized by unusual linear or swirled hypopigmented patches distributed along the lines of Blaschko (Fig. 129.57). The hypopigmentation usually is present at birth and may be limited or extensive (see discussion under Skin Lesions in the Neonatal Period). Hypomelanosis of Ito is the result of cutaneous mosaicism. Early reports suggested that this form of hypopigmentation was associated with abnormalities of the central nervous system (e.g., seizures and mental retardation), eye, bone, teeth, and hair (e.g., alopecia), but only a minority of children with hypomelanosis of Ito have extracutaneous problems. Therefore, if the history and examination otherwise are normal, investigation for occult abnormalities is not warranted. The mode of inheritance is not clear, and most cases seem to be sporadic. No treatment is available.

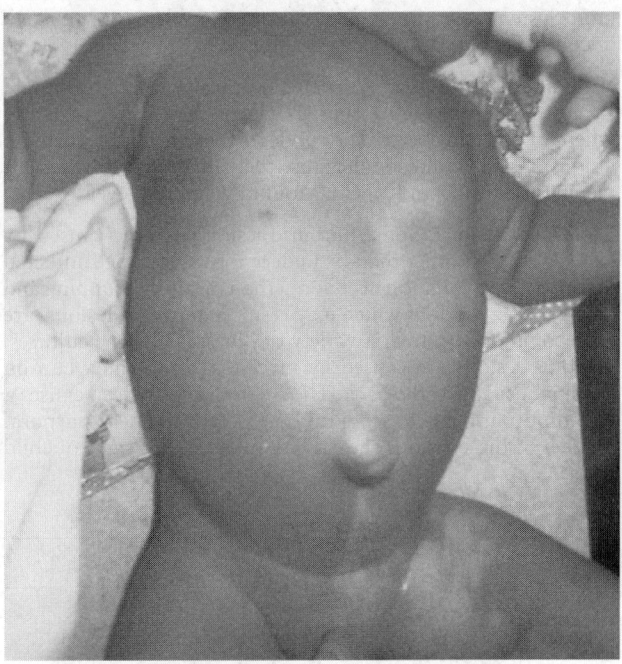

FIGURE 129.57. Swirling hypopigmentation in an infant with hypomelanosis of Ito.

Nevus Depigmentosus. Nevus depigmentosus is characterized by patches of hypopigmentation (not depigmentation) that have irregular borders. The lesions occur most frequently on the trunk and extremities and usually are present at birth (see discussion under Skin Lesions in the Neonatal Period). Rare associations with neurologic defects have been reported. No treatment is available. Affected areas require sun protection.

Purpura

Henoch-Schönlein Purpura. The rash of Henoch-Schönlein purpura (HSP) is classically purpuric but, early on, may appear urticarial, macular, or papular. The characteristic distribution of the rash helps to determine the diagnosis. The rash is located primarily in dependent areas, which for ambulatory patients includes the buttocks and lower extremities. The upper extremities are involved less frequently, the face even less commonly, and the trunk only rarely. The characteristic lesion is that of a leukocytoclastic vasculitis (i.e., palpable purpura), but the purpuric lesions may be macular, small or large and, in severe cases, may develop necrotic centers. Striking areas of edema involving the scalp, hands, feet, scrotum, or other areas may appear.

Generally, individuals with HSP have associated problems. Arthritis, typically involving the knees and ankles, occurs in more than two-thirds of the cases. Abdominal pain, gastrointestinal bleeding, and glomerulonephritis also are common. The purpuric lesions may appear in waves. One-third of the cases resolve within 2 weeks, another one-third in 2 weeks to 2 months, and the remaining one-third in 2 to 6 months. The cause of HSP is unknown but circulating immune complexes have been implicated. Skin biopsy specimens reveal IgA deposits around blood vessels. Infections due to *S. pyogenes*, Epstein-Barr virus, and hepatitis B, as well as exposures to food dyes and cold, have been implicated. Therapy is mainly supportive, although gastrointestinal symptoms and severe joint pain may respond to courses of systemic corticosteroids.

Acute Hemorrhagic Edema of Infancy. Acute hemorrhagic edema of infancy mimics HSP. Generally, it occurs in children younger than age 2 years. The purpuric lesions are annular in shape and are located acrally; involvement of the face is common. Systemic symptoms and associated problems are unusual, in contrast to HSP. The cause is unknown.

Vasculitis. The presence of palpable purpuric lesions should suggest an underlying vasculitis. (Its causes are discussed elsewhere in this textbook.) The sudden development of purpuric lesions in an ill child should cause the pediatrician to consider meningococcemia and Rocky Mountain spotted fever.

Factitious Lesions. Some purpuric lesions may be caused by external forces rather than by underlying disease. Self-inflicted lesions are less common in children than in adults. Cupping and coin rubbing, both of which may result in purpuric lesions, are used commonly to treat a variety of illnesses in some cultures. Cupping lesions are caused by inversion of a heated cup on the skin, usually of the back. The suction so produced causes a round purpuric patch. Coin rubbing results in linear purpura. Neither of these lesions should be confused with signs of child abuse.

Pruritic Lesions

Contact Dermatitis

Contact dermatitis has been discussed under several different sections in this chapter, depending on its cause (due to plants is discussed on p. 847; due to nickel and other weak antigens, on p. 856). In allergic contact dermatitis, pruritus is a promi-

nent feature. Contact dermatitis occurs when an antigen penetrates the epidermis and sensitizes T lymphocytes, which then circulate through the skin and other organ systems. For potent antigens such as urushiol, sensitization takes only 7 to 10 days; weaker agents may require multiple exposures over many weeks. If sensitization occurs, reexposure to the antigen will cause contact dermatitis to develop within 12 to 24 hours.

Potent antigens such as urushiol (present in poison ivy, oak, and sumac) typically cause an acute dermatitis that consists of vesicles, bullae, erythematous papules, and edema. The rash of poison ivy or *Rhus* dermatitis may be localized with groups of erythematous papules and vesicles, may have widely scattered lesions, or, on occasion, may be limited to the face, which appears swollen. A history of contact with eruption-producing plants is helpful to the diagnosis. The linear vesicles (or papules, if the lesions are early) may be subtle. Often, pruritus is severe. Contrary to common belief, the vesicular fluid does not spread the rash. The rapidity of appearance of the rash depends on the affected person's degree of sensitivity to the toxin and the amount of toxin reaching the skin. In sensitive individuals, areas of significant exposure may show a rash within hours, whereas areas of minimal toxin exposure may not show a rash for days. If untreated, the dermatitis may persist for 3 to 4 weeks.

Weaker antigens (e.g., nickel, preservatives) produce a subacute dermatitis that is characterized by erythema, scaling, and lichenification (i.e., thickening of the skin caused by scratching). Vesicles and bullae are absent.

The key to recognizing contact dermatitis is the observation that the eruption is limited to certain skin areas. Linear vesicles or bullae on exposed surfaces suggest exposure to plant allergens. Nickel dermatitis occurs at sites of contact with jewelry (e.g., on the earlobes or other sites of piercing, neck, or wrists) or below the umbilicus where there is contact with a belt buckle or clothing snap. An eruption on the dorsa of the feet should raise the suspicion of shoe dermatitis, usually caused by rubber additives or potassium dichromate. Involvement of the face and areas around the eyes suggests an allergy to agents in cosmetics, perfumes, or moisturizers.

If the contact dermatitis is mild, an appropriate topical corticosteroid may be applied. However, when more than 10% to 15% of the body surface is involved, the disease is severe, or areas such as the face or perineum are significantly affected, oral prednisone is recommended with a tapering treatment course of 12 to 21 days. Oral antihistamines produce a sedative effect that offers relief from itching. Topical anesthetics containing benzocaine and topical antihistamines (e.g., diphenhydramine) should be avoided because they may induce a contact dermatitis. Prevention of further episodes is an important part of the management of patients who have a contact dermatitis. Individuals who have experienced plant dermatitis should learn to recognize and avoid poison ivy, sumac, and oak. When exposure may be unavoidable, wearing protective clothing or applying a barrier preparation may be useful.

Contact dermatitis should not be confused with atopic dermatitis, which is a chronic disorder. Usually, atopic dermatitis begins in early childhood and has a unique morphology and distribution. If the foot is involved, contact dermatitis may be mistaken for tinea pedis; however, this infection typically involves the interdigital spaces. If the rash involves the dorsum of the foot, an allergic contact dermatitis is likely. In contrast, if the dermatitis appears on the weight-bearing surface, usually contact dermatitis can be ruled out.

Pediculosis

Infestation with head lice is an extremely common problem, and eradicating it is difficult, despite the best efforts of schools, health agencies, and physicians. The human head louse (*Pediculus humanus capitis*) is an obligate human parasite; it cannot survive away from its host for more than 26 hours in the adult form. The insect, which is 2 to 4 mm in length and ivory-colored, often is difficult to see. The egg cases of lice (nits) are the usual sign of infestation. Firmly cemented to the hair shaft they resemble dandruff but cannot be removed easily. The eggs hatch within 10 to 12 days.

Usually, *P. humanus capitis* results in pruritus of the scalp. Common accompaniments to the scratching are folliculitis and impetigo. The lice are spread easily through close contact, combs and brushes, and clothing, especially hats. Permethrin 1% is the standard form of therapy; alternate therapies include pyrethrins and malathion. Due to concerns about potential toxicity, lindane should be used with extreme caution and only if other treatments have failed. Treating symptomatic family members and close contacts is important as well. African American individuals rarely are infested with head lice, perhaps because head lice in the United States have claws that are not able to grasp hairs whose cross section is oval rather than round.

Infestation with the body louse (*Pediculus humanus humanus*) is a much less common problem in the United States. These lice live in the seams of clothing and feed on the skin, producing small, red papules and wheals. Although patients should be treated with permethrin 5% for 8 to 14 hours, the key to treatment is to rid clothing and bedding of lice and eggs. Clothing should be washed and dried at high temperature or dry-cleaned. Mattresses should be sprayed with a pediculicide.

Usually, pubic lice are acquired through contact during sexual intercourse; thus, sexual abuse must be considered in a finding of pubic lice in a child. Although the lice usually cling to pubic hair, in young children they may attach to body hair. Nits may be found in the eyelashes as well. The primary symptom is pruritus, and excoriations are common in heavy infestations. The nits on hair shafts are seen more commonly than is the louse itself, which is broader and shorter than are head and body lice. Sometimes, infestation is manifested by the appearance of bluish gray, faint purpuric lesions. Known as *maculae ceruleae*, these spots are sites of feeding by the louse. Treatment consists of an application of permethrin 1% to affected areas for 10 minutes. Alternate therapies include a pyrethrin or lindane, although the latter should be used with caution, particularly in children. Pediculicide treatment should be repeated in 7 to 10 days. Clothing and bedding should be laundered. If the eyelashes are involved, petrolatum, applied several times daily for 7 days, may prove effective.

Scabies

Scabies is an infestation with the mite, *Sarcoptes scabiei*. The 0.2- to 0.4-mm female mite burrows into the stratum corneum where it deposits eggs. The clinical picture, which usually develops 2 to 3 weeks after infestation, is thought to be the result of sensitization to the mite and its products. A person can have mites on the body and transmit them to others without having symptoms and signs of the disorder.

Usually, the pruritus of scabies is intense and unremitting. A characteristic feature is that it seems worse at night, perhaps as a result of a rise in skin surface temperature and increased activity of the scabies mites. The lesions of scabies are papules, tiny vesicles, and pustules. Most are excoriated and, in long-standing cases, lichenification may be extensive. Burrows (i.e., linear tracks) commonly are not seen in children. Usually, the distribution of lesions is located from the neck down, although young infants and children can have scalp and even facial involvement. Characteristically, the lesions are most numerous on the hands, particularly in the webs of the fingers in older children and adults and on the palms and soles in infants; on the wrists; in the axillae; at the belt line; on the areolae of women; and on the penis and scrotum in males. In infants, scabies can produce nodules or vesicles on the palms and soles

that can mimic pyoderma. Secondary bacterial infections occur frequently.

Although the clinical picture may be typical of scabies, an attempt to identify the mite in a scraping from one of the lesions always is prudent. A simple technique is to choose a nonexcoriated vesicle or papule, place a drop of immersion oil on it, scrape it with a scalpel blade to open it, collect the oil from the skin, place the oil on a glass slide with a coverslip on top, and look for the mite, eggs, or feces.

Usually, treatment of scabies can be accomplished effectively by the application of 5% permethrin cream to the entire body surface, including the head in infants. The permethrin cream should remain on for 8 to 14 hours and then should be washed off. Since permethrin is not always ovicidal, a second application 7 to 10 days later often is recommended. An alternative to permethrin 5% is lindane applied for 6 to 8 hours. Concerns about potential toxicity if it is used inappropriately or inadvertently ingested limit its use and, at present, it should be considered a second-line therapy. Lindane should not be used in the treatment of pregnant women and is best avoided in infants and young children. Regardless of the treatment used, the pruritus may take a week or more to resolve after treatment.

All asymptomatic family members and close contacts should receive a single treatment at the time the index case is initially treated. Failure to do so often results in cycles of reinfection. Many contacts may be infested despite a seeming absence of lesions. Clothing worn and bedding used by the family before treatment should be washed or stored for 72 hours before reuse to prevent reinfestation by mites.

Papular Urticaria

The red papules and wheals associated with papular urticaria, a reaction to insect bites, occur most commonly in the spring and summer. A more complete discussion of this topic is found in the section Erythematous Papules, earlier.

Varicella

The vesicles of chickenpox are pruritic, sometimes intensely so. Generally, the lesions are present in a variety of stages, including erythematous papules, vesicles, pustules, and crusts. A shake lotion (e.g., calamine) or topical nonsensitizing anesthetic (e.g., pramoxine), or oral antihistamine may help to relieve the pruritus. Varicella is discussed more fully in the section Vesicles, earlier.

Swimmer's Itch

A pruritic, allergic response to larval forms of schistosomes may occur in individuals who swim in freshwater lakes that are frequented by ducks, birds, and other carriers. Humans are accidental hosts of the schistosomes, which use snails as the intermediate host. The first exposure to the cercarial larvae produces no reaction; subsequent penetrations by this organism result in an allergic response. Tiny erythematous papules appear in the first hour after exposure and increase in size and pruritic effect over the next few days. The lesions appear most frequently on exposed body surfaces. Treatment is symptomatic with a topical corticosteroid or topical nonsensitizing anesthetic, or oral antihistamine.

Seabather's Eruption

Seabather's eruption occurs when larvae of *Linuche* sp. of jellyfish release nematocysts upon contacting the skin. In contrast to swimmer's itch, seabather's eruption occurs in areas covered by a swimsuit or wetsuit. The rash is composed of numerous pruritic papules or macules that appear within hours of exposure and persist for up to 2 weeks. A topical corticosteroid, topical nonsensitizing anesthetic (e.g., pramoxine), or oral antihistamine may be employed to control the symptoms of this self-limited condition.

Cutaneous Larva Migrans

Most cases of cutaneous larva migrans represent infection with the larva of the dog and cat hookworms (*Ancylostoma braziliense* and *A. caninum*). The larvae penetrate the skin and migrate through the superficial layers of the epidermis, creating characteristic serpentine patterns. A small, erythematous papule designates the entrance site of the hookworm larva. The tracks are a few millimeters in diameter, pink or skin-colored, and may advance 1 to 2 cm/day. Pruritus is prominent. Most frequently, the lesions appear on the feet, the body part that most commonly is exposed to the soil that contains the larvae. Infection is most frequent in warm, humid regions with sandy soil. Secondary bacterial infection may result from scratching. The condition is self-limited, resolving in weeks to months. Treatment is with topical thiabendazole or oral albendazole.

Grouped Lesions

Herpes Simplex Virus Infection

The appearance of erythematous papules that rapidly become vesicles and are clustered together on an erythematous base should suggest the diagnosis of herpes simplex. (See Vesicles, earlier.)

Insect Bites

The pruritic, erythematous papules of insect bites, particularly flea bites, commonly are grouped together. A central punctum on top of the papule or wheal is strong evidence that the papule is the result of a bite.

Contact Dermatitis

The erythematous papules and vesicles of contact dermatitis may be grouped according to cause. *Rhus* dermatitis (poison ivy) is characterized by linear papules and vesicles. (See Pruritic Lesions, earlier.)

Lymphangioma Circumscriptum

Grouped, tense, small vesicles may indicate the presence of an underlying localized abnormality of the lymphatic system. The vesicles most commonly are deep-seated, their surface may be rough, and the fluid may appear hemorrhagic rather than clear. The lesions are seen most frequently around the neck, the upper trunk, and the proximal extremities. Lymphatic malformations are discussed in detail in the section Vesicles, earlier.

Chronic Bullous Disease of Childhood

As the name implies, chronic bullous disease of childhood is a chronic disorder. The bullae or vesicles are grouped around the margins of an erythematous plaque, which represents an area of clearing. Multiple lesions usually are present. For more detail, see Bullae, earlier.

Diffuse Erythema

Scarlet Fever

Scarlet fever is a common condition resulting from pharyngeal infection with Group A beta-hemolytic streptococci that produce an erythrogenic toxin. The disease seems to have become milder over time and, as a result, it frequently is not diagnosed because typical features are lacking. The most constant finding is an eruption composed of fine erythematous papules that have a rough or "sandpaper" texture. The rash often first appears and is most concentrated in skin folds (e.g., the folds of the neck, axillae, and groin). Pastia lines (i.e., petechiae flexural creases like those of the antecubital fossae), circumoral pallor, and a "strawberry" tongue are seen frequently. Patients often are febrile and exhibit pharyngeal exudates. Parents should be advised that their child's hands and feet may exhibit significant sheets of desquamation in 7 to 14 days.

Staphylococcal Scalded Skin Syndrome

The diffuse erythema seen in staphylococcal scalded skin syndrome is, as implied by the name, strikingly suggestive of a scald or burn of the skin (see color Fig. 68.13 in color section). For a more detailed discussion of this syndrome, see Bullae, earlier.

Toxic Shock Syndrome

Toxic shock syndrome (TSS) is caused by infection with certain toxin-producing strains of *S. aureus*. In the absence of protective immunity, the toxins, TSS toxin-1 and staphylococcal enterotoxins, induce the formation of cytokines that produce characteristic symptoms and signs. The rash of TSS is a diffuse sunburn-like erythema. Additional signs include hyperemia of the conjunctivae and other mucous membranes, fever, shock, and multisystem failure. When first described, 90% of cases of TSS occurred in association with menses, often in women using super-absorbent tampons. With the institution of preventive measures, the incidence of TSS has declined and, at present, approximately 50% of cases are associated with menses. Nonmenstrual TSS may occur following staphylococcal infection of the respiratory tract (e.g., bacterial tracheitis or sinusitis), sites of trauma, burns, or surgical wounds. The diagnostic criteria for TSS are presented in Box 129.3. Treatment is supportive; patients should receive a parenteral antistaphylococcal antibiotic.

Arcanobacterium haemolyticum–Induced Rash

A rash similar to that of scarlet fever has been described in individuals infected with *Arcanobacterium haemolyticum*. The infection, which produces a sore throat with pharyngeal erythema and exudate, occurs most often in teenagers and young adults. The rash is diffuse, erythematous, and macular, and it blanches when pressed. A fine, papular component occurs, most frequently distally on the extensor surfaces of the extremities, and then spreads centrally to the trunk within a few days. A mild desquamation may follow in 1 or 2 weeks.

Acrodynia

Metallic mercury poisoning has become rare, although children's fascination with liquid-like metallic mercury still gives rise to occasional cases. Typical cases of acrodynia are unforgettable. Children are anorectic, irritable, and hypotonic. They sweat profusely and have a prominent rash similar to miliaria in addition to a background erythema of the skin. Their hands and feet are strikingly puffy, pink, perspiring, and painful, and they rub them together, causing desquamation. Hypertension is common.

Photosensitivity Disorders

Sunburn

The erythema resulting from damage to the skin by ultraviolet radiation is known as *sunburn*. Sunburn appears within 4 hours

BOX 129.3 — Diagnostic Criteria for Toxic Shock Syndrome

The diagnosis of toxic shock syndrome is considered probable if five criteria are present and confirmed if all six are present.

- Fever ≥38.9°C (≥102°F).
- Rash: a diffuse macular or scarlatiniform erythema that is accentuated in skin flexures.
- Desquamation that occurs 1 to 2 weeks after the onset of the illness and is particularly prominent on the palms and soles.
- Hypotension: systolic blood pressure ≤90 mm Hg for adults or <5th percentile for age for those <16 years of age; or orthostatic decline of ≥15 mm Hg supine to sitting, orthostatic syncope, orthostatic dizziness.
- Multisystem involvement (three or more of the following must be present).
  - Gastrointestinal: vomiting or diarrhea.
  - Muscular: severe myalgia or creatine kinase greater than two times the upper limit of normal.
  - Mucous membranes: vaginal, oropharyngeal, or conjunctival hyperemia.
  - Renal: blood urea nitrogen or creatinine greater than two times the upper limits of normal, or pyuria in the absence of a urinary tract infection.
  - Hepatic: total bilirubin, alanine aminotransferase, or aspartate aminotransferase concentration greater than two times the upper limit of normal.
  - Hematologic: platelets ≤100,000/mm^3.
  - Central nervous system: disorientation or alteration in consciousness without focal neurologic signs when fever and hypotension are absent.
- Laboratory criteria: negative results on the following tests if performed: throat, blood, or cerebrospinal fluid cultures (a blood culture may be positive for *Staphylococcus aureus*); no rise in titers for Rocky Mountain spotted fever, leptospirosis, or measles.

Adapted from American Academy of Pediatrics. Toxic shock syndrome. In: Pickering LK, ed. *Red Book 2003 Report of the Committee on Infectious Diseases,* 26th ed. Elk Grove Village, IL: American Academy of Pediatrics; 2003:625.

BOX 129.4 — Sun Protection Strategies

- To the extent possible, minimize prolonged outdoor activities during the hours of 10:00 AM and 4:00 PM.
- Wear protective clothing such as wide-brimmed hats, long-sleeved shirts, and long pants. Several manufacturers produce lightweight clothing that has an SPF of 50 or more, even when wet (see http://store.yahoo.com/coolibar/index.html, http://radicoolcanada.com/products.asp?IID=1, or http://tugasunwear.com). For clothing such as tee shirts, consider using a laundry additive that will increase the SPF value (e.g., Sungard).
- Use a sunscreen regularly. Choose a product with an SPF of 15 or greater that provides UVA and UVB protection.
  - Apply liberally 30 minutes before beginning outdoor activities, even on cloudy days.
  - Apply every 2 hours, particularly if swimming or sweating.
- Wear sunglasses labeled "maximum of 99% UV protection or blockage," "special purpose," "UV absorption up to 400 nm," or "meets ANSI UV requirements."

A key element of anticipatory guidance, therefore, is to counsel patients and their families about the risks of sun exposure and elements of sun protection. These are summarized in Box 129.4. The need for sun protection varies with skin type, specifically, the degree of skin pigmentation. Those with the greatest need for protection are fairly complexioned Caucasians who burn easily and do not tan; often these individuals have red hair and freckles. In contrast, deeply pigmented individuals who never burn are at little risk. Those with intermediate degrees of skin pigmentation may tan or burn and, therefore, require counseling about sun protection.

Drug Photosensitivity

Drug reactions to light have been divided into two types, toxic and allergic. *Phototoxic reactions* are due to nonimmunologic mechanisms (e.g., free radical damage to cells) and are manifested as erythema (that mimics a sunburn) or, occasionally, bullae on sun-exposed surfaces 2 to 6 hours after sun exposure. Doxycycline, tetracycline, sulfonamides, nonsteroidal antiinflammatory agents, phenothiazines, furocoumarins (responsible for phytophotodermatitis), and furosemide often are implicated.

Most *photoallergic reactions* result from delayed hypersensitivity. After sensitization, within 24 hours of reexposure to the drug and sun, a pruritic, eczematous eruption appears on sun-exposed and partially covered skin. Agents responsible for photoallergic reactions include tetracycline, griseofulvin, barbiturates, chlorothiazide diuretics, oral hypoglycemic agents, and phenothiazines. Treatment of drug photosensitivity reactions rests upon removal of the offending agent.

Phytophotodermatitis

Certain plants, particularly limes, contain natural furocoumarins, which may result in phototoxic drug reactions when present on the skin. (See Hyperpigmented Macules and Patches, earlier.)

of exposure and peaks between 6 and 24 hours. In addition to erythema and pain, individuals may develop vesicles or blisters. Once present, sunburn may be treated with cool compresses and an oral nonsteroidal antiinflammatory agent.

Beyond its acute effects (i.e., sunburn), sun exposure is linked to the development of skin cancer and skin aging. In 2002, it was estimated that 1.3 million Americans would develop skin cancer. The majority of these are nonmelanoma skin cancers (e.g., basal cell and squamous cell carcinomas) that are associated with cumulative sun exposure. However, in 2003, it was estimated that 54,200 persons would develop malignant melanoma and that 7,600 of these would die from their disease. Melanoma is linked to intermittent, intense sun exposure, such as that which produces blistering sunburns. Of note, the use of artificial tanning devices also is associated with an increased risk of skin cancer. Through its effects on dermal fibroblasts, arterioles, collagen, and elastin, ultraviolet radiation also is associated with photoaging, manifest as wrinkling and laxity of the skin, mottled pigmentation, and open comedones.

Lupus Erythematosus

A wide variety of rashes have been associated with systemic lupus erythematosus (SLE). Many patients with this disease are photosensitive and demonstrate a rash as their initial manifestation. The so-called butterfly rash, a slightly raised, erythematous or violaceous eruption with fine scale located over the malar areas and bridge of the nose, is most often associated with SLE. Patients may also exhibit discoid lesions, round, well-demarcated, erythematous to violaceous plaques with fine telangiectases, an adherent scale, and areas of atrophy. The lesions appear most commonly on the face and scalp and in the ears. Other cutaneous lesions include transient erythematous annular lesions in sun-exposed areas (subacute cutaneous lupus erythematosus), red or purple nodules, scaling patches on the dorsa of the fingers, and scarring and nonscarring alopecia.

Dermatomyositis

A butterfly distribution of erythema and swelling occurring after sun exposure or at least resembling a persistent sunburn may be the initial clue to or presentation of dermatomyositis (See Papulosquamous Lesions, earlier).

Polymorphous Light Eruption

As the name implies, the clinical presentation of polymorphous light eruption (PMLE) is variable. The lesions, which represent a reaction to ultraviolet light, range from small papules and vesicles to plaques. They may appear eczematous (with erythematous macules, papules, and vesicles) and often are pruritic, thus causing confusion with atopic dermatitis. PMLE often has its onset in childhood with the rash appearing in the spring and continuing through the summer. The eruption begins within several hours to days of exposure. Lesions last up to 1 week before resolving; recurrences following renewed sun exposure are common. Although the rash appears on sun-exposed areas (e.g., the face, ears, and upper chest), not all such areas are affected. Topical or systemic corticosteroids may provide relief from acute lesions, but sun protection is the ultimate therapy. In some cases, prolonged treatment with antimalarial agents may be necessary. PMLE often remits or becomes less severe over time.

Juvenile Spring Eruption (Hydroa Estivale)

Juvenile spring eruption (hydroa estivale) is a rare disorder that has its onset in childhood and shows some improvement in the late teenage years. The lesions, which are pruritic, consist of erythema, edematous papules, and vesicles. Crusted erosions on sun-exposed areas may be a clue to the diagnosis. The rash generally appears in the spring or summer months, occurs 1 to 2 days after sun exposure, lasts 1 week, and may return the following spring. Treatment consists of avoidance of sunlight.

Porphyrias

The porphyrias are an uncommon group of disorders caused by enzymatic defects in the metabolic pathway leading to the biosynthesis of porphyrins and heme. For patients with porphyria, sun avoidance and protection are mandatory; treatment with beta carotene may be beneficial.

Erythropoietic Protoporphyria. Erythropoietic protoporphyria generally is a mild disease characterized by burning, itching, and stinging of sun-exposed areas of skin. The skin may become erythematous, edematous, and thickened, but rarely does it become blistered or scarred. Liver disease occurs in some of the individuals affected by erythropoietic protoporphyria, which has an autosomal dominant pattern of inheritance. The disease results from a deficiency of ferrochelatase. Results of the free erythrocyte protoporphyrin test are unusually high in this disorder.

Congenital Erythropoietic Porphyria. Congenital erythropoietic porphyria is a destructive, severe disorder that is inherited in an autosomal recessive manner. It is caused by mutations in uroporphyrinogen III cosynthase. Symptoms occur early in life, often within the first month, with severe photosensitivity resulting in scarring and hypertrichosis. Teeth may appear red or brown. Hemolytic anemia and splenomegaly are common. The passage of red urine may be the first sign of the disease; progressive mutilation of the skin follows. Plasma, urine, and erythrocyte levels of uroporphyrins and coproporphyrins are increased. When examined with a Wood light, urine from affected individuals fluoresces a red color.

Hepatoerythropoietic Porphyria. Hepatoerythropoietic porphyria is a rare autosomal recessive disorder characterized by photosensitivity beginning in infancy. Severe erythema and blistering occur, and scarring of sun-exposed areas is prominent. Affected individuals have more facial hair than normal, and their urine may be red. Levels of red blood cell free erythrocyte protoporphyrin are increased.

Variegate Porphyria. Variegate porphyria rarely begins in childhood. The primary clinical manifestations are photosensitivity, neurologic symptoms, or abdominal pain. Skin changes include fragility and blistering of sun-exposed areas.

Porphyria Cutanea Tarda. Porphyria cutanea tarda, which is characterized by a photosensitive dermatosis, is extremely rare in children. The diagnosis is based on the finding of high levels of uroporphyrins and coproporphyrins in the plasma and urine.

Syndromes Involving Photosensitivity

A number of uncommon syndromes feature photosensitivity as a major presenting clue. Brief descriptions of a few of these disorders conclude this section.

Xeroderma Pigmentosum. Xeroderma pigmentosum is a rare, progressive, autosomal recessive, degenerative disease characterized by severe photosensitivity developing in the first few years of life. Erythema, bullae, pigmented macules, hypochromic spots, and telangiectases develop rapidly. The skin becomes atrophic, dry, and wrinkled. A variety of benign and malignant growths appear early in life. In affected individuals, the ability to repair DNA after exposure to ultraviolet radiation is defective.

Cockayne Syndrome. Individuals with Cockayne syndrome appear normal at birth but, by late childhood, clearly demonstrate short stature, microcephaly, and developmental delay. The eyes appear sunken, the ears large, and the limbs long. Progressive neurologic degeneration occurs, with deafness, loss of vision, dysarthria, gait disturbances, and ataxia. The skin is sensitive to light and develops erythema, blisters, and telangiectasia. The hands and feet are cool and often cyanotic. The mode of inheritance is autosomal recessive.

Bloom Syndrome. The first clue to the diagnosis of Bloom syndrome, an autosomal recessive disorder, usually is the development of plaques of telangiectatic erythema over the butterfly area and dorsa of the hands and forearms after exposure to sunlight. The prenatal onset of growth deficiency continues after birth. Malar hypoplasia, a small nose, and a high-pitched voice are typical. Bloom syndrome results from abnormalities in DNA repair and chromosome structure. Malignancy and recurrent infections account for the majority of deaths in individuals with this disorder.

Hartnup Disease. A rare autosomal recessive disorder, Hartnup disease is caused by defective transport of neutral amino acids by the intestinal mucosa and renal tubules. The skin changes resemble those of pellagra: an erythematous to vesicular eruption develops, with scaling, lichenification, and hyperpigmentation over the sun-exposed areas of the body, particularly the face, back of the neck, and hands. Neurologic signs resemble those of cerebellar ataxia, and psychiatric disturbances are common. The diagnosis can be confirmed by the finding of neutral amino acids in the urine. Treatment is with nicotinic acid or nicotinamide, and a high-protein diet.

Rothmund-Thomson Syndrome. The striking cutaneous picture of Rothmund-Thomson syndrome develops within a few years of birth. The first sign is erythema that becomes reticulated. Later, hyper- or hypopigmentation, small areas of atrophy, and telangiectases (collectively termed poikiloderma) appear. Photosensitivity occurs in one-third of patients. Short stature is common and one-half of children develop cataracts. The risk of malignancy, particularly of osteosarcoma, is increased.

Annular Lesions

Tinea Corporis

Superficial fungal infections probably are the most readily identified annular lesions of the skin. The ring-like lesions are recognized by most laypersons, although not all ringed lesions are tinea corporis. Because the infection of nonhairy areas of the skin by dermatophytes is limited to the epidermis, only the most superficial layers of the skin are involved. The rings generally are erythematous. As the inflammation spreads, the active infection in the center of the lesions resolves, and this area clears, resulting frequently in the picture of an advancing border with central clearing. The border generally is scaly and slightly elevated, and, on close inspection, may contain microvesicles and pustules (Fig. 129.58). The lesions, which may be single or multiple, are not always round. Bizarre shapes and, occasionally, a coalescence of lesions may be noted, and borders may not be

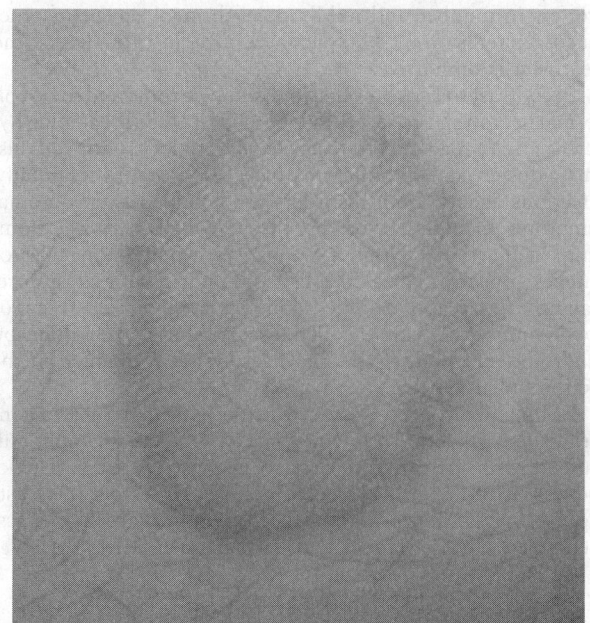

FIGURE 129.58. Annular lesion of tinea corporis with a raised border and scaling.

continuous. Tinea corporis usually is asymptomatic, although pruritus may be present.

The organism responsible for most cases of tinea corporis is *Trichophyton tonsurans*. *Microsporum canis*, *M. audouinii*, and *Trichophyton mentagrophytes* infections also are seen. The diagnosis may be confirmed by a potassium hydroxide preparation that reveals branching hyphae. The lesions do not fluoresce with a Wood lamp. The conditions most frequently confused with tinea corporis are granuloma annulare, the herald patches of pityriasis rosea, and nummular eczema. Treatment consists of application of one of the topical antifungal agents, such as an imidazole (e.g., miconazole). Application twice daily for 2 to 3 weeks or until the lesion clears is recommended. If lesions are multiple or involvement extensive, oral therapy may be indicated.

Pityriasis Rosea

The herald patches of pityriasis rosea may appear annular (See Papulosquamous Disorders, earlier).

Granuloma Annulare

Granuloma annulare is characterized by papules or nodules that form a ring (see Fig. 129.29). Lesions may be single or multiple and typically are violaceous, although they may be skin-colored. Most often lesions are located acrally, involving the ankles, dorsal surfaces of the feet or hands, or volar aspects of the wrists. Occasionally, granuloma annulare presents as one or more subcutaneous nodules overlying the tibiae. Although granuloma annulare often is confused with tinea corporis, the key to its differentiation from the latter disorder is a careful examination of the borders: in granuloma annulare, the surface of the lesion is devoid of vesicles, pustules, or scale, and skin markings are normal. In tinea corporis, the border of the lesion is scaly, often with microvesicles and pustules, and the color of the lesions varies from skin-colored to erythematous. The lesions of granuloma annulare are asymptomatic, being neither pruritic nor tender.

The cause of granuloma annulare is unknown. Most lesions resolve spontaneously within 2 years, but some may last for decades. In adults, an association with diabetes mellitus has been reported, but this has not been noted in children. On biopsy samples, these lesions resemble rheumatoid nodules, but no association is made with connective tissue diseases. Because the nodules regress, no treatment generally is required.

Psoriasis

Annular lesions also may be seen in psoriasis. These lesions usually can be differentiated from other conditions characterized by annuli by the presence of a thick, adherent, silvery scale; clear demarcation of the erythematous borders; and symmetry of distribution. See Papulosquamous Disorders, earlier, for a more complete discussion of psoriasis.

Nummular Eczema

Lesions of nummular eczema are coin-shaped, as the name implies. The lesion surface generally is thickened and dry, and the borders are fairly discrete. Central clearing is not typical. The cause is not known but seems to be related to dry skin. See Scaling and Dry Lesions, earlier, for further discussion.

Lichen Spinulosus

The lesions of lichen spinulosus often are grouped and, therefore, may appear as annuli. Lesions are tiny papules, each centered about a follicle and possessing a spiny projection of keratinaceous material emanating from the follicular orifice.

Lichen spinulosus is discussed in detail in Skin Colored Papules, earlier.

Urticaria

Urticaria is common in both children and adults. The lesions result from localized vasodilation and transudation of fluid from capillaries and small blood vessels. Individual wheals are transient, lasting a few hours and never longer than 24 hours. They are erythematous papules and plaques that may be round or oval, or form rings or arcs. Stasis of blood in the center of lesions frequently creates an appearance of purpura. Pruritus is a common feature. Approximately one-half of patients with urticaria have associated angioedema, a process analogous to urticaria that occurs in the submucosa, deep dermis, and subcutaneous tissue. Angioedema is characterized by poorly defined areas of swelling, often located around the eyes or lips.

Urticaria is a manifestation of the release of mediators, principally histamine, from cutaneous mast cells, which increase vascular permeability. It may be separated into acute (lasting less than 6 weeks) and chronic (lasting 6 weeks or more) forms. Acute urticaria has many causes but the agents most often responsible include drugs, foods, infections, and arthropod bites and stings (Box 129.5). Less common causes are contactants (e.g., latex), systemic diseases (e.g., collagen vascular diseases, inflammatory bowel disease), occult infections (e.g., sinusitis, dental abscesses), blood products, and physical agents (e.g., heat, cold, pressure, light, vibration, water). Cholinergic urticaria is a fairly distinctive form manifested by the appearance

---

BOX 129.5   Common Causes of Acute Urticaria in Children

Drugs
- Antibiotics (penicillins, cephalosporins, sulfonamides, and others)
- Nonsteroidal antiinflammatory agents
- Immunizations

Foods
- Nuts
- Shellfish
- Strawberries
- Peanuts
- Milk
- Wheat

Infections
- *Streptococcus pyogenes*
- Viral (adenovirus, enterovirus, Epstein-Barr virus, hepatitis B, others)
- Parasites

Insect stings and bites
- Bees
- Wasps

Inhalants
- Pollen
- Molds
- Animal dander

Collagen vascular diseases
- Systemic lupus erythematosus (and others)

---

of 2- to 3-mm papules surrounded by large erythematous flares. These flares are very pruritic and follow the onset of sweating. Given the wide variety of possible agents, pinpointing the cause of urticaria often is difficult, particularly for chronic urticaria. In most series, the cause of the problem has been uncovered in fewer than 20% of the cases. The presence of urticarial lesions that persist for more than 24 hours should raise the suspicion of urticarial vasculitis. A skin biopsy of one of the lesions will be diagnostic.

The disorders that may be confused with urticaria are erythema multiforme and urticarial vasculitis. Although the lesions of erythema multiforme are annular, unlike those of urticaria, they remain fixed in location for 7 days or more; are concentrated on the distal extremities and face; do not assume unusual shapes such as large plaques or arcs; and develop a central change, such as violaceous discoloration, vesicle, or crust. If urticarial-appearing wheals persist longer that 24 hours, it should raise suspicion of urticarial vasculitis. A skin biopsy of one of the lesions will be diagnostic.

The first step in treatment is to remove, treat, or avoid an identified cause. A first-generation (e.g., sedating) antihistamine will reduce pruritus and hive formation. If drowsiness occurs or control of symptoms is incomplete, a second-generation (e.g., nonsedating) agent may be substituted or added. Systemic steroids generally are not required.

Erythema Multiforme

Erythema multiforme (EM) is a cutaneous hypersensitivity reaction that traditionally has been separated into two types, minor and major, depending on the extent and severity of lesions. However, at present, the minor form is simply called erythema multiforme, while the major form is termed Stevens-Johnson syndrome. EM often is caused by herpes simplex virus infection; approximately 50% of affected children have a history of herpes labialis 3 to 14 days before the onset of the disease. Prodromal symptoms are absent. The rash is composed of erythematous macules or thin plaques that have a predilection for acral surfaces, including the palms, soles, and face, with relative sparing of the trunk. Lesions remain fixed in location for up to 3 weeks before resolving. Over several days, a central violaceous discoloration, a vesicle, or crust develops. Approximately one-half of children with EM have oral erosions that are few in number and mildly painful; involvement of other mucosal sites is rare. EM typically resolves in 1 to 2 weeks and treatment is supportive.

In contrast to EM, Stevens-Johnson syndrome and toxic epidermal necrolysis are severe and potentially life-threatening hypersensitivity reactions to drugs (e.g., antibiotics, anticonvulsants, nonsteroidal antiinflammatory agents) or, less commonly, infectious agents. Both disorders are heralded by prodromal symptoms, including fever, sore throat, cough, headache, vomiting, or diarrhea. Within 2 weeks, erythematous macules or patches appear on the skin. Blisters rapidly form and rupture, leaving large areas of denuded skin. Target lesions are absent or few in number. A more detailed discussion of Stevens-Johnson syndrome and toxic epidermal necrolysis is presented in the section Bullae, earlier.

EM may be confused with urticaria but often the two conditions may be differentiated clinically. Pruritus is common in patients with urticaria and less so in those with EM. Unlike the lesions of EM, those of urticaria are evanescent (i.e., lasting less than 24 hours) and of varied and unusual shapes (arcs, incomplete circles, plaques with serpiginous borders).

Erythema Marginatum

The clinical appearance of the skin lesions occasionally seen in acute rheumatic fever is not pathognomonic. Erythema marginatum begins as erythematous blotches or papules that spread centrifugally forming polycyclic or serpiginous lesions. The margins are sharp, and the lesions advance and change shape rapidly. Dull red, pink, or violaceous, the lesions may resemble urticaria, but they are not pruritic. Their rapid change distinguishes them from erythema multiforme.

Erythema marginatum occurs in approximately 10% of patients with acute rheumatic fever. The rash is not specific for acute rheumatic fever, however, having been reported also in patients with juvenile rheumatoid arthritis. It occurs most commonly on the trunk and inner aspects of the upper arms and thighs. A skin biopsy of the lesion may be helpful in establishing an early diagnosis of acute rheumatic fever.

Erythema Migrans

Erythema migrans is the earliest clinical manifestation of Lyme disease, being present in 80% to 90% of those with documented infection. Seven to 14 days following the bite of an infected tick, an erythematous papule or macule appears at the site of the bite. Without antibiotic treatment, the rash enlarges, forming an erythematous patch or ring, or concentric rings. The lesions usually are flat or slightly elevated and persist 1 to 2 weeks. The rash usually is asymptomatic, but burning, pruritus, or pain may be present. Days to weeks following the onset of erythema migrans, dissemination of the organism may result in small secondary cutaneous lesions at sites distant from the bite. The organism *Borrelia burgdorferi*, which is responsible for Lyme disease, is transmitted by the ticks, *Ixodes scapularis* and *Ixodes pacifica*. Treatment of erythema migrans is doxycycline (for those 8 years of age or older) or amoxicillin (for all ages).

Syphilis

Secondary syphilis may produce a rash composed of brownish to dull red macules that may appear annular and resemble pityriasis rosea. The lesions generally are discrete and follow lines of skin stress on the trunk, similar to those of pityriasis rosea. Reddish brown lesions on the palms and soles should be a clue to this diagnosis in sexually active patients. In addition, patients often have flu-like symptoms and generalized lymphadenopathy. The rash appears 6 to 8 weeks after the primary syphilitic lesion, and it may last from a few hours to months.

Lupus Erythematosus

A wide variety of cutaneous lesions may be seen in systemic lupus erythematosus. The butterfly rash is known best, but annular lesions may be early signs of the disorder. Lesions of discoid lupus erythematosus, which occur mainly on the face and sun-exposed areas, are indurated plaques that are violaceous and have an adherent scale. They occasionally appear annular in configuration. Lupus erythematosus is discussed in greater detail in Papulosquamous Disorders, earlier.

Sarcoidosis

Sarcoidosis is a multisystem disease that is believed to represent a granulomatous reaction to infectious agents or allergens. A rash develops in approximately 25% of affected children. The most common cutaneous eruptions are soft, red to yellowish-brown or violaceous, flat-topped papules, found most frequently on the face. Sometimes, these papules take on an annular configuration. Larger, violaceous, plaque-like lesions may be found on the trunk, extremities, and buttocks. Other cutaneous manifestations of sarcoidosis include nodules, ulcers, subcutaneous tumors, and erythema nodosum.

Linear Lesions

Contact Dermatitis

The most common linear eruption seen in children is caused by contact with the *Rhus* toxins produced by poison ivy, oak, or sumac (see Fig. 129.37). (See Disorders with Linear Vesicles, earlier.)

Lichen Striatus

Lichen striatus is characterized by the sudden onset of rapidly spreading, discrete, tiny papules in a linear band 1 to several centimeters wide. The lesions occur most commonly on the extremities. The papules are not always continuous but sometimes appear to skip over areas of normal skin. They usually are skin-colored or pink and sometimes are topped by a fine, adherent scale. In deeply pigmented individuals, the bands may appear hypopigmented (see Fig. 129.26). If a finger or toe is involved, the nail may become dystrophic. The cause of this unusual phenomenon is unknown. The papules regress spontaneously over 6 to 12 months, although hypopigmentation may last 1 to 2 years. Since the condition is self-limited, no therapy is necessary. Topical corticosteroids may hasten the disorder's resolution.

Linear Scleroderma

Morphea or localized scleroderma may take on a linear configuration. (See Disorders Involving Abnormal Skin Texture, earlier.)

Nevus Depigmentosus

Nevus depigmentosus usually presents as a patch of hypopigmentation, although some lesions are linear. The cause of these lesions, some of which appear after birth, is not known. Treatment of the cutaneous changes is not available. For additional discussion see Hypopigmented Macules and Patches under Skin Lesions in the Neonatal Period, earlier.

Incontinentia Pigmenti

Incontinentia pigmenti, an unusual genodermatosis, is manifested by four stages of cutaneous abnormalities. The first is vesicles, typically in a linear arrangement, that are present at or shortly after birth (see color Figure 68.11 in color section). The next stage is the appearance of verrucous (wart-like) lesions, not necessarily in the same areas as the inflammatory lesions. The verrucous stage peaks at 12 to 26 weeks and resolves gradually, usually within 1 or 2 years. The third stage is one of hyperpigmentation. These lesions are tan to slate-gray and may be arranged in irregular linear streaks or whorls. Sometimes, a pattern reminiscent of a marble cake may be seen. This stage also resolves gradually over the years. The final stage, which may or may not be present, consists of subtle, hypopigmented, atrophic patches of skin, especially on the legs. Incontinentia pigmenti is discussed in detail in the section Vesicles and Pustules under Skin Lesions in the Neonatal Period, earlier.

Linear Epidermal Nevi

Epidermal nevi may take on a linear configuration. Generally present at birth, they usually are unilateral and singular, are flesh-colored to yellowish brown, and become rougher and more wart-like with age (see Fig. 129.12). Most epidermal nevi are small and represent isolated cutaneous findings. However, extensive lesions may be associated with mental retardation, seizures, strabismus, hemihypertrophy, kyphoscoliosis, and eye and kidney lesions, and may be a feature of the Proteus and

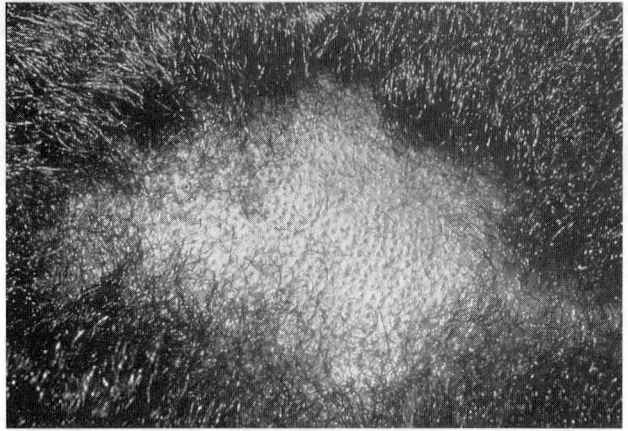

FIGURE 129.59. Hair loss and "black dot" hairs (infected hairs broken at the scalp line) in tinea capitis caused by *Trichophyton tonsurans*.

CHILD syndromes. The occurrence of epidermal nevi seems to be sporadic, although some may be associated with genetic mosaicism. These lesions represent hamartomas with thickening of the epidermis and overgrowth of sebaceous and apocrine glands. If desired, small lesions may be excised. Larger lesions, for which excision may not be practical, may be treated with a topical keratolytic to reduce thickness of the lesion and associated scale.

Disorders of the Scalp

Scaling

Tinea Capitis. Tinea capitis is a common problem in the United States, particularly for African American children. The organism responsible for 95% of infections is *Trichophyton tonsurans*. Infection with this organism produces a variety of lesions, most commonly one or more patches of hair loss within which are "black dot" hairs, the remnants of broken hairs within follicles (Fig. 129.59). However, children also may experience widespread scaling of the scalp with less obvious alopecia (the "seborrheic" form of tinea capitis). See Alopecia, later.

Seborrheic Dermatitis. Seborrheic dermatitis may produce scaling of the scalp in two groups of individuals: infants below the age of 1 year and those who have experienced adrenarche. In infants, scaling of the scalp begins between 2 and 10 weeks of age. The dermatitis can cause erythema and, occasionally, hair loss. The rash commonly affects the forehead, eyebrows, retroauricular areas, and other flexures, as well as the diaper area. In deeply pigmented infants, hypopigmentation of the involved areas may be prominent. In adolescents, scaling of the scalp is the most common symptom of seborrheic dermatitis, although they may develop erythematous, scaling patches of the eyebrows, nasolabial folds, and presternal area.

Although the cause of seborrheic dermatitis is unknown, it appears to be related to the presence of androgens and their effects on sebaceous glands, and may represent an inflammatory response to the yeast *Pityrosporum ovale*.

The scalp of an affected infant usually can be treated with mild shampoo and fine combing or brushing to remove the scale. In recalcitrant cases, an antiseborrheic shampoo (e.g., one containing zinc pyrithione or selenium sulfide) may be helpful. A low-potency corticosteroid applied topically will suppress areas of inflammation on the scalp. In adolescents, shampoos containing zinc pyrithione, selenium sulfide, keto-conazole, or tar are effective. Areas of scalp erythema may be treated with the application of a midpotency topical corticosteroid solution, gel, or lotion. For further discussion of seborrheic dermatitis, see Scaling and Dry Lesions, earlier.

Atopic Dermatitis. Scaling of the scalp in children who have atopic dermatitis is common and often is mistaken for seborrheic dermatitis. The scale generally is fine and white, and the scalp typically is pruritic. Excoriations of the scalp may be prominent, and secondary infections may occur. Excessive hair washing may exacerbate rather than help the problem, as it does in seborrheic dermatitis. Clues to the presence of atopic dermatitis usually are found on other areas of the skin. Treatment of the scalp in atopic dermatitis includes the use of a keratolytic shampoo and the application of an appropriate topical corticosteroid solution, gel, or lotion. Atopic dermatitis is discussed in detail in the section Scaling and Dry Lesions, earlier.

Psoriasis. In most children with psoriasis of the scalp, other areas of the skin also are involved, showing the typical erythematous plaques (see color Fig. 68.18 in color section). Occasionally, however, only the scalp may be affected. The base of the scalp lesion always is inflammatory; thus, erythema underlies the whitish scale. The scale sometimes forms large plaques, resulting in hair loss with combing. The hairline often is involved. Treatment involves the use of a keratolytic shampoo, such as one containing salicylic acid or tar. In addition, a mid- to upper potency corticosteroid and calcipotriene solution also may be employed. Thick, adherent scaling may require the use of a softening agent such as phenol and saline (P & S Liquid, Baker Cummins Dermatologicals, Inc., Miami, FL).

Pityriasis (Tinea) Amiantacea. The thick, adherent scaling of pityriasis (tinea) amiantacea usually is mistaken for tinea capitis. The scales are silvery and tend to overlap, often trapping hair and thereby causing thinning of the scalp hair. Despite its name, tinea amiantacea is not caused by a fungal infection. The cause is not clear, although many suspect a relationship to psoriasis, atopic dermatitis, or seborrheic dermatitis. Aggressive applications of scale-softening agents, similar to those used in psoriasis of the scalp, often are helpful.

Langerhans Cell Histiocytosis. Langerhans cell histiocytosis frequently is manifested by erythematous scaling patches that affect the scalp, retroauricular areas, flexures, and diaper area. Vesicopustules and brown or erythematous papules also may be present. Although the scaling areas may be mistaken for seborrheic dermatitis, a clue to the diagnosis is the presence of petechiae underlying the scale (Fig. 129.60). This diagnosis always should be considered in any recalcitrant scaling eruption of the scalp.

Pustules

Tinea Capitis. As noted previously, tinea capitis can take on many appearances on the scalp. In inflammatory forms, patients may exhibit scattered pustules or a kerion, a boggy, indurated, mass, the surface of which lacks hair and is studded with pustules (Fig. 129.61). On first glance, the kerion resembles a bacterial abscess. Inflammatory tinea capitis should be treated with griseofulvin. Although bacterial culture obtained from the surface of a kerion often reveals *S. aureus*, antibiotic therapy is not necessary. Children who have kerions generally experience complete regrowth of hair. (See Alopecia, later.)

Traction Folliculitis. Prolonged or excessive traction on hair from tight braiding may result not only in hair breakage and loss but also in the development of pustules at the borders of the areas of pulled hair. Resolution of the problem usually can be accomplished by removal of the traction. Occasionally, a

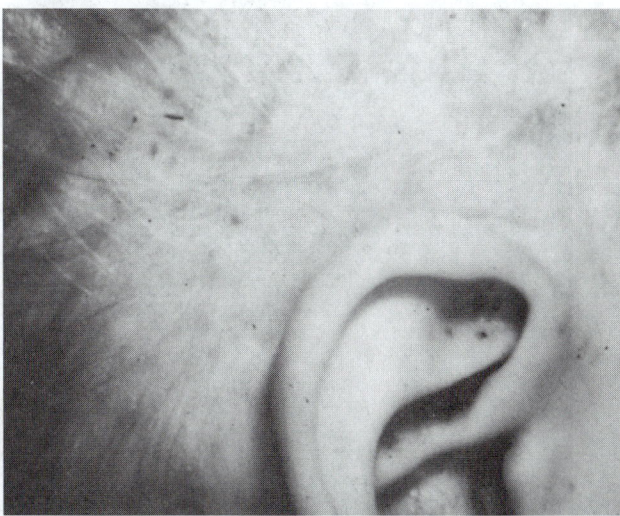

FIGURE 129.60. Seborrhea-like scaling of the scalp with underlying petechiae in a patient with Langerhans cell histiocytosis.

secondary bacterial infection, most commonly staphylococcal in origin, may become established in the hair follicles that were damaged by the pulling. In such cases, treatment with a topical or systemic antibiotic may be indicated.

Impetigo. Pustules and crusting of the scalp may be the result of secondary infection. A variety of stimuli may cause pruritus and subsequent excoriations of the scalp, preparing the way for bacterial infections. Precipitating causes include atopic dermatitis, occlusion from oils and greases, and head lice. The bacteria most frequently responsible are streptococci and staphylococci. Treatment with topical antibiotics may be effective but, with extensive lesions, systemic therapy may be required.

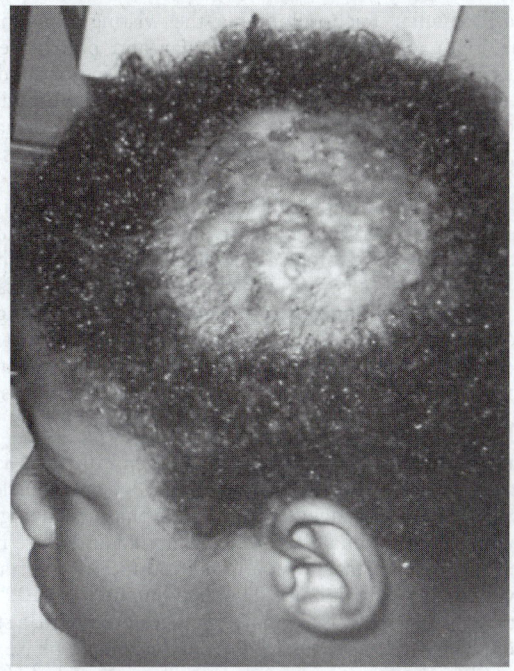

FIGURE 129.61. This boggy, oozing mass with pustules and hair loss is a kerion, one of the many varieties of tinea capitis.

BOX 129.6	Classification of Alopecia by Pattern and Time of Onset

Acquired localized alopecia
Nonscarring
  Alopecia areata
    Severe variants include alopecia totalis, alopecia universalis
  Tinea capitis
  Traumatic alopecia
    Trichotillomania
    Friction
    Traction
Scarring
  Kerion associated with tinea capitis
  Physical injury (e.g., burns)
  Lupus erythematosus
  Lichen planus

Acquired diffuse alopecia
Telogen effluvium
Endocrine (e.g., hypothyroidism, hypopituitarism, hypoparathyroidism, androgenetic alopecia)
Lamellar ichthyosis
Acrodermatitis enteropathica
Multiple rare syndromes and disorders

Congenital localized alopecia
Sebaceous, epidermal nevi
Melanocytic nevi
Hemangiomas
Aplasia cutis congenita
Incontinentia pigmenti
Focal dermal hypoplasia
Hallermann-Streiff syndrome (sutural alopecia)

Congenital diffuse alopecia
Genetic syndromes
  Ectodermal dysplasias
  Congenital hypothyroidism
  Marinesco-Sjögren syndrome
  Atrichia congenita
Cartilage hair hypoplasia
Hair shaft abnormalities
  Trichorrhexis nodosa
  Pili torti
  Monilethrix
  Trichorrhexis invaginata
  Trichothiodystrophy

Adapted from Datloff J, Esterly NB. A system for sorting out pediatric alopecia. *Contemp Pediatr* 1986;3:53.

Alopecia

See Box 129.6.

Tinea Capitis. Tinea capitis is the most common cause of localized hair loss in children. In the United States, 95% of infections are caused by *Trichophyton tonsurans*, an organism that is spread from person to person or by fomites, such as shared hats, combs, or brushes. For reasons unclear, nearly all of those infected with this organism are African American. *T. tonsurans* infection may produce a variety of clinical presentations, the most common of which is one or more patches of alopecia and scaling. Within the patches are "black dot" hairs, the remnants of infected hairs within follicles. Children may also experience widespread scaling of the scalp with less obvious hair loss (the "seborrheic" form). Finally, if an inflammatory response to the fungal agent develops, scattered pustules or a boggy, tender mass (i.e., a kerion) may be present.

Tinea capitis also may result from infection with *Microsporum canis*, an organism spread from dogs or cats to humans. Infected children exhibit one or more patches of scaling and alopecia. However, unlike infections caused by *T. tonsurans*, *M. canis* produces areas of alopecia in which hairs are broken not at the scalp (thus, "black dot" hairs are not present) but more distally. Kerions may also occur in *Microsporum* infections.

A potassium hydroxide preparation performed on hairs removed from the scalp by gentle scraping can be useful to confirm the presence of infection. In *Trichophyton* infections, spores will be seen within "black dot" hairs. In contrast, hairs infected by *M. canis* will be longer and spores and hyphae are seen on the surface of the hair. Alternately, a fungal culture may be performed by placing scale and hairs on the surface of an appropriate medium, such as dermatophyte test medium.

Tinea capitis should be treated with griseofulvin at a dose of 15 to 20 mg/kg/day of the microsize preparation for 8 weeks. It may be given as a single daily dose with a meal, preferably one high in fat content. For those who fail griseofulvin therapy, terbinafine, itraconazole, and fluconazole have been used successfully. Selenium sulfide 1% or 2.5% may be used as a shampoo twice weekly to reduce the shedding of organisms from the scalp. Care should be taken to examine other household members for signs of infection.

Alopecia Areata. The hallmark of alopecia areata is the appearance of well-circumscribed round or oval patches of complete or relatively complete hair loss. The scalp appears normal, without scale, erythema, or scarring. The lesions tend to appear rapidly and may be single or multiple. Short hairs that are broader distally than proximally (i.e., exclamation point hairs) often are seen at the periphery of lesions. If all scalp hair is lost, the term alopecia totalis is applied; alopecia universalis describes the loss of all body hair. Individuals with alopecia areata often exhibit pitting of the nails, tiny punctate depressions in the nail surface. The cause of alopecia areata is not known, although it likely represents an autoimmune phenomenon.

The course of alopecia areata is unpredictable. Even without therapy 90% or more of children regrow hair within 1 year, although nearly one-third of these will experience a recurrence. When hair regrows, it often is light or white. Individuals in whom alopecia areata appears in band-like distribution around the scalp (i.e., ophiasis) often eventually lose all scalp hair and have a poor prognosis.

The treatment of alopecia areata is disappointing. A wide variety of therapeutic techniques have been tried with variable effect. Hair regrown during a course of systemic corticosteroids is lost again when the corticosteroids are discontinued. Therefore, these agents should not be used. Other therapies include intralesional or potent topical corticosteroids, anthralin, and contact sensitization (e.g., with squaric acid dibutyl ester or other agents). Topical tacrolimus and imiquimod have been advocated, and topical minoxidil also has been employed. The key to treatment is careful, empathetic education of the patient and the parents. Consultation with a dermatologist and referral to support groups (e.g., the National Alopecia Areata Foundation) may be beneficial. Artificial hairpieces may help some patients to maintain a positive body image.

Traction Alopecia. The hair loss in traction alopecia is secondary to prolonged tension on the hair shaft, usually from

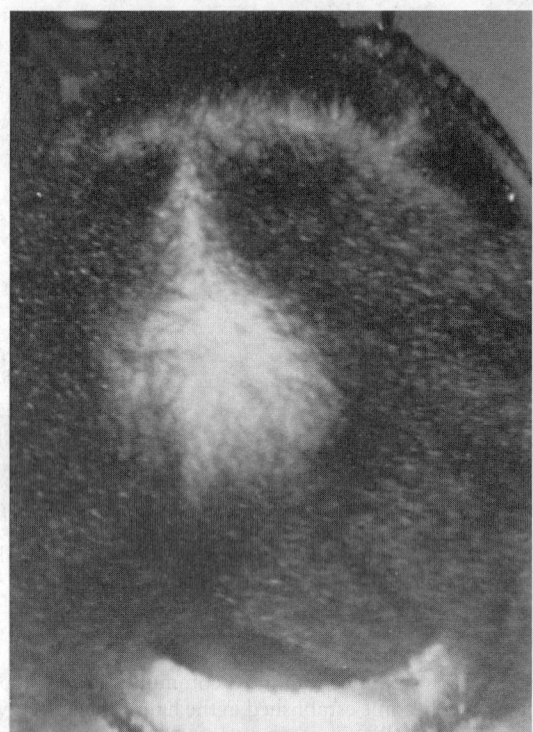

FIGURE 129.62. Traction alopecia over the midline of the occiput as a result of braiding.

braiding of the hair. Traction most commonly produces hair loss at the margins of the scalp or as oval or linear areas in part lines (Fig. 129.62). Permanent hair loss may result if pressure is maintained for a long time.

Friction Alopecia. Pressure alopecia is most common in young infants, who lie supine and rub their occiputs on the bedding. Persistent rubbing of the scalp by any means may result in hair breakage and loss.

Trichotillomania. Trichotillomania, the twisting or pulling out of one's hair, often results in irregular and poorly defined patches of alopecia (Fig. 129.63). The hair loss in this condition is never complete and within patches of relative alopecia are hairs of differing lengths. The scalp usually appears normal, although petechiae may be seen, particularly if the hair has been pulled out.

In most children and adolescents, trichotillomania represents a habit. In others, it may be a reaction to stress or evidence of a more severe psychological problem. Management should include an open discussion with the patient and parents. Patients should be encouraged to refrain from hair twisting and provided with positive reinforcement. Over time, most children discontinue the habit spontaneously. For those with severe trichotillomania, referral to a mental health professional for evaluation and therapy may be warranted.

Telogen Effluvium. The hair loss in telogen effluvium is diffuse, not localized. Normally, 90% to 95% of hair follicles on the scalp are in the anagen (or growing) phase, which generally lasts for approximately 3 years. The remainder are in the telogen (or resting) state, which lasts for 3 to 6 months and is followed by shedding of hairs. The shedding of 50 to 100 hairs from the scalp each day is normal. In telogen effluvium, a stressful event causes many of the follicles in the anagen phase to be converted to the telogen stage. Inciting factors include febrile illnesses, drug reactions, and delivery of a baby. Hair loss begins 4 to 16 weeks after the inciting event; the hair returns to

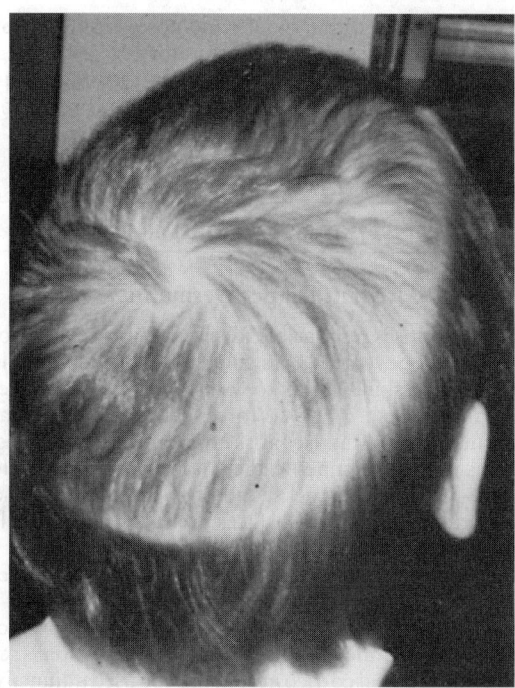

FIGURE 129.63. Alopecia with various hair lengths in an unusual configuration is characteristic of trichotillomania.

normal by 5 to 6 months. The diagnosis may be confirmed by pulling out a few hairs and examining the roots. Anagen hairs have a large pigmented bulb; telogen hairs have smaller bulbs that lack pigment. In telogen effluvium, the number of hairs in the telogen phase is unusually high. No treatment is necessary for telogen effluvium.

Loose Anagen Syndrome. In loose anagen syndrome, hairs in the anagen phase can be pulled easily from the scalp. Affected children have sparse, usually blond hair that rarely requires cutting. On hair pulling, the normal anagen sheath over the root is missing and the root bulb is misshapen. The length and density of the hair tend to increase with age.

Other Causes of Hair Disorders. Scalp hair may be absent, sparse, or abnormal for a wide variety of reasons, including reactions to drugs or chemicals, congenital defects in the hair shaft itself, and endocrine (e.g., hypothyroidism) or systemic disorders. Space limitations do not permit a review in this chapter of all the causes of alopecia. Box 129.6 presents a systematic classification of alopecia.

Disorders of the Nails

This section is limited to the description of only the most common nail disorders.

Dystrophic Nails

Psoriasis. As many as 50% of individuals with psoriasis exhibit nail abnormalities. When the skin eruption is not diagnostic of psoriasis, the presence of nail abnormalities may help to establish the diagnosis. A variety of lesions may occur, including pits, discoloration, and separation of the nail plate from its bed distally. Subungual thickening, crumbling, and grooving of the nails also may be found. Unfortunately, no universally effective therapy for nail involvement is available. Topical corticosteroids occasionally may be beneficial.

Alopecia Areata. Fine stippling of the nails and, occasionally, ridging may occur in association with alopecia areata. The pitting is much finer than that associated with psoriasis.

Nail-Patella Syndrome. The nail-patella syndrome is an inherited disease that is characterized by distorted or atrophic nails with triangular lunulae in association with absent or hypoplastic patellae. Some persons may have associated renal abnormalities, resulting in renal failure in adulthood. The condition is inherited as an autosomal dominant trait.

Beau Lines. Transverse grooves, the result of thinning of the nails, may be caused by trauma to the nail matrix or may follow a systemic disease.

Idiopathic Trachyonychia. Idiopathic trachyonychia (also known as *twenty-nail dystrophy*) begins in childhood and affects some or all of the nails. Typically, the nails have longitudinal ridges and are thickened. As the name suggests, the cause is unknown, although in some children it is inherited in an autosomal dominant fashion. No satisfactory treatment exists but the appearance of the nails may improve with time.

Nail Infections

Onychomycosis. Fungal infection of the nail, also known as *onychomycosis* or *tinea unguium*, is caused most often by *Trichophyton rubrum, T. mentagrophytes,* and *Epidermophyton floccosum.* These infections are not seen commonly in young children but may appear in adolescents. The infection usually presents with thickening of the nail and a yellow discoloration distally or laterally that indicates separation of the nail from the nail bed (distal and lateral subungual onychomycosis, respectively). Debris tends to accumulate beneath the nail plate. Occasionally, only the surface of the nail is involved with white discoloration and a fine, powdery scale (superficial white onychomycosis). Oral therapy with terbinafine or itraconazole generally is recommended. Griseofulvin requires prolonged therapy and has a low cure rate. Topical agents generally are ineffective but may have benefit in those with superficial white onychomycosis.

Candidal Infections. Infections with *Candida* are seen most often in young children who suck their fingers or in adults whose occupations require repeated immersion of the hands in water. The key to diagnosis is the observation of swelling and erythema of the skin at the base of the nail and lateral to it. The cuticle is absent and the nail itself is discolored, often greenish, and thickened, and separates from the nail plate distally. Treatment consists of removal of the source of continued wetness as well as application of a topical anticandidal agent to the infected nail and surrounding skin.

***Pseudomonas* Infections.** *Pseudomonas* infections of the nail often resemble *Candida* infections, with the nail bed taking on a greenish-blue discoloration. If present, paronychial involvement causes the skin surrounding the nail to be more tender in *Pseudomonas* than in *Candida* infections. Given that continuous immersion in water is an important contributing factor in this infection, keeping the nails dry is of utmost importance. Application of or soaking the nail in bleach three times daily may be effective in clearing the infection.

Vascular Disorders

Congenital vascular lesions or those that appear in the first month of life are discussed in the section Skin Lesions in the Neonatal Period. This section describes a few of the less common acquired cutaneous vascular lesions.

Spider Angioma

Spider angiomas present as tiny erythematous macules or papules that blanch with pressure. The lesions consist of a central arteriole from which other vessels radiate peripherally. Lesions often develop early in childhood and commonly are located on the face, hands, and arms. Most spider angiomas do not regress with age. If cosmetically indicated or desired, pulsed laser therapy will eradicate the lesion.

Pyogenic Granulomas

Pyogenic granulomas are benign vascular proliferations precipitated by trauma or infection, although the mechanism for growth stimulation is not known. The lesions grow rapidly, may be papular or nodular, and often are pedunculated. They usually are solitary and dark red to purple, with a surface that generally is moist, crusted, or eroded and that may bleed easily when traumatized (see Fig. 129.27). The differential diagnosis of pyogenic granuloma includes warts, molluscum contagiosum, and superficial hemangiomas. The best treatment is excision and electrodesiccation of the base, although pulsed dye laser may be employed.

Ataxia-Telangiectasia

The appearance of telangiectases, usually first on the bulbar conjunctivae, may be a clue to the cause of a child's ataxia, which usually has appeared by the age of 2 years. The telangiectases generally develop between 3 and 5 years of age and become increasingly extensive over time (Fig. 129.64). Typically, they involve the face and ears. Ataxia-telangiectasia is the result of mutations of the *ATM* gene and is inherited as an autosomal recessive manner. Affected children experience progressive ataxia and recurrent sinopulmonary infections. They also are at increased risk for the development of lymphoproliferative or central nervous system malignancies. Death usually occurs during the second decade of life as the result of infection or malignancy.

Hereditary Hemorrhagic Telangiectasia

Osler-Weber-Rendu syndrome is an autosomal dominant disorder that is characterized by the appearance of numerous small erythematous macules or papules that represent telangiectases. The lesions generally begin to appear late in the first decade of life and are located primarily around the mouth and on the

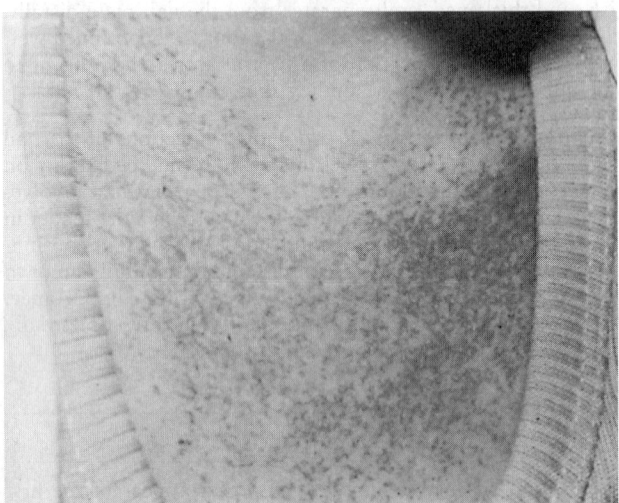

FIGURE 129.64. Diffuse telangiectasia on the upper chest of an adolescent with ataxia telangiectasia.

mucous membranes of the mouth and nose. Lesions also may be present on the mucosae of the respiratory or gastrointestinal tracts or in the brain. The most common presenting complaint is epistaxis, but gastrointestinal blood loss with chronic anemia is another frequent complication.

Diaper Dermatitis

Irritant Diaper Dermatitis

Irritant dermatitis is responsible for the majority of eruptions in the diaper area. Several factors contribute, including moisture (that reduces the skin's ability to withstand frictional forces applied by the diaper), frictional forces (applied by the diaper), and enzymes in stool that act as skin irritants. The result is erythematous patches or superficial erosions located on the lower abdomen, perineum, buttocks, and proximal thighs. Typically, the convexities of the skin surfaces are involved with relative sparing of the creases.

A key to managing irritant diaper dermatitis is to reduce moisture through frequent diaper changes. Application of a barrier preparation, such as zinc oxide paste, will protect the skin from moisture and allow healing. If inflammation is severe, a low-potency topical corticosteroid may be used adjunctively.

Candidal Diaper Dermatitis

Candidal diaper dermatitis, caused by infection with *C. albicans*, is characterized by the appearance of a rash that involves both the skin creases and convexities. Involved areas are bright red patches or erosions (see Fig. 129.43). Scaling may be present at the margin of affected areas and satellite papules or pustules often are observed. Treatment involves the application of an antiyeast preparation such as nystatin or an imidazole (e.g., clotrimazole, miconazole).

Seborrheic Dermatitis

Seborrheic dermatitis is a condition of unknown cause that begins during the first weeks or months of life and resolves by 1 year of age. In the diaper area, the disorder produces salmon-colored patches with greasy scale that involve the convexities and creases. Other sites of involvement include the scalp (termed *cradle cap*) and skin folds behind the ears, of the neck, and of the axillae. Treatment of seborrheic dermatitis in the diaper area is with a low-potency topical corticosteroid as needed.

Bullous Impetigo

Bullous impetigo, caused by infection with strains of *S. aureus* that produce an epidermolytic toxin, often has a predilection for the perineum. Since the blisters created by this condition are fragile and rupture easily, they may not be present at the time of examination. Rather, one commonly observes round or oval crusted erosions that possess a rim of scale, the remnant of the blister roofs. The disease nearly always is limited to the skin and systemic spread occurs only rarely. Bullous impetigo is treated with an oral antibiotic active against *S. aureus* (e.g., cephalexin, dicloxacillin).

Noduloulcerative Diaper Dermatitis

Noduloulcerative diaper dermatitis (also known as *Jacquet's diaper dermatitis*) is characterized by well-defined erosions or ulcers surmounting papules or nodules. It likely represents a severe variant of irritant diaper dermatitis and is treated in the same manner.

Psoriasis

Psoriasis is unusual during infancy but when present often involves the diaper area because of the trauma induced by chronic irritation (see color Fig. 68.18 in color section). Because the environment is moist, the scale characteristic of psoriasis elsewhere on the body is absent. Treatment includes the application of an emollient or a lowpotency topical corticosteroid.

Acrodermatitis Enteropathica

Acrodermatitis enteropathica is an autosomal recessive disorder in which a defective transport protein in the gastrointestinal tract results in impaired absorption of dietary zinc. Zinc deficiency leads to altered keratin synthesis and resultant skin lesions. The primary clinical appearance usually is one of crusted erosions with sharply marginated borders. The lesions often appear in the diaper area and around the mouth and eyes (see Fig. 129.50). The diagnosis of acrodermatitis enteropathica is confirmed by the finding of a low zinc level. With supplementation, cutaneous lesions improve rapidly. While awaiting improvement, a topical corticosteroid may be applied to affected areas twice daily.

Langerhans Cell Histiocytosis

The presence of a recalcitrant diaper eruption composed of purpuric papules, petechiae, and erosions or ulcers involving the creases should raise concern about Langerhans cell histiocytosis. Usually, however, cutaneous disease is present elsewhere (e.g., the scalp) and symptoms and signs of systemic involvement are evident (e.g., diarrhea, failure to gain weight, lymphadenopathy, hepatomegaly). Patients suspected of having Langerhans cell histiocytosis should be referred to a pediatric oncologist and dermatologist.

Acne

Acne Vulgaris

Acne vulgaris undoubtedly is the most common skin problem of adolescents. It is a chronic disorder that may last for years and cause emotional distress and permanent scarring. Although there is no cure for acne, medications can control the disease and prevent scarring.

Pathogenesis. Acne is a disorder of the pilosebaceous follicle, composed of a follicle, sebaceous gland, and rudimentary or vellus hair. The concentration of pilosebaceous follicles is highest on the face, chest, and back, thus explaining the appearance of acne lesions in these areas. Although the exact cause of acne is not known, several factors contribute.

Androgens play a key role in the causation of acne. At the time of adrenarche, the adrenal glands produce increasing amounts of the androgen dehydroepiandrosterone sulfate (DHEAS). Rising levels of DHEAS, perhaps after conversion to more potent androgens such as testosterone and dihydrotestosterone, cause sebaceous glands to enlarge and produce more sebum. Sebum from patients with acne is deficient in linoleic acid, a factor that also may contribute to altered keratinization.

Propionibacterium acnes is an anaerobic, gram-positive diphtheroid that colonizes pilosebaceous follicles following increases in sebum production. *P. acnes* produces chemoattractant factors that cause polymorphonuclear neutrophils (PMNs) to enter pilosebaceous follicles. As PMNs ingest *P. acnes,* hydrolytic enzymes are released that damage the follicle wall. Follicular contents can then enter the surrounding tissue, where they incite inflammatory reactions that are manifest clinically as erythematous papules, pustules, or nodules.

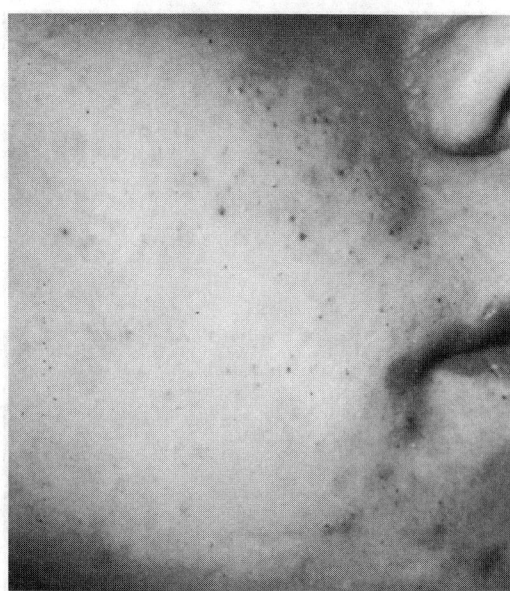

FIGURE 129.65. Open comedones predominate in this adolescent with acne.

In persons with acne, for reasons unclear, epithelial cells lining the follicle are not shed properly and become more cohesive. The result is a collection of cells and sebum that accumulate within the follicle. This process, called comedogenesis, is central to the development of acne lesions. Although familial trends are well recognized in patients with acne, an exact pattern of inheritance has not been defined. In addition, because the disease is common and modified by external factors, it is not possible to predict the severity of disease in an individual patient based on family history.

Clinical Manifestations. Initially, obstruction within the follicle is microscopic and cannot be perceived clinically; such lesions are termed microcomedones. As comedones enlarge, they become apparent as open comedones (blackheads) or closed comedones (whiteheads). Open comedones represent follicles with a widely dilated orifice (Fig. 129.65). Closed comedones are small white papules without surrounding erythema. They represent follicles that have become dilated with cellular and lipid debris but possess only a microscopic opening to the skin surface.

Patients with inflammatory acne manifest erythematous papules, pustules, or nodules. Papules and pustules are small, measuring less than 5 mm in diameter. Nodules measure greater than or equal to 5 mm in diameter and often involve more than one follicle (Fig. 129.66). After inflammatory lesions resolve, erythematous or hyperpigmented macules may remain for as long as 12 months and are often mistaken for true scars.

Some patients with acne develop scars as inflammatory lesions resolve. In general, scarring is most likely in those adolescents with large papules or nodules, but even small inflammatory lesions may produce scars. On the face, acne scars have the appearance of pits, while on the trunk they usually look like small hypopigmented spots. Rarely, patients develop hypertrophic or keloidal scars. True cysts, compressible nodules that lack overlying inflammation, also may be observed in patients with acne.

Adolescents and their families should be advised about the causes of acne and possible exacerbating factors. Myths about acne (e.g., the role of diet) should be dispelled. They should be advised that a realistic goal of treatment is to reduce the number and severity of lesions and to prevent scarring. It is also important to warn patients that 6 to 8 weeks may be required

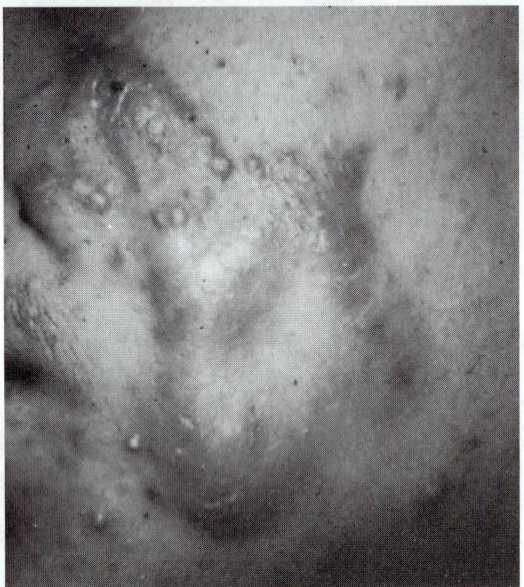

FIGURE 129.66. Large cysts and pustules are characteristic of acne conglobata, a severe form of acne.

for medications to work. Although there is no standardized treatment plan for acne, guidelines exist (Table 129.4). Medications used to treat acne may be separated into topical and systemic preparations.

Topical Therapies. *Benzoyl peroxide* (BP) primarily has an antibacterial effect and is useful in controlling inflammatory acne. It may also decrease the formation of free fatty acids, thereby improving obstructive (comedonal) disease. These two actions make it a useful first-line drug in the management of patients with mild inflammatory or mixed (i.e., inflammatory and comedonal) acne. BP also prevents the emergence of antibiotic resistance among *P. acnes*; therefore, it may be used adjunctively for patients receiving long-term antibiotic therapy. The application

of a product containing a 5% concentration once or twice daily is adequate for most patients. Common adverse effects include drying, erythema, and burning.

Topical antibiotics reduce concentrations of *P. acnes* and inflammatory mediators. As a result, these agents are most useful in treating mild to moderate inflammatory acne that is limited to the face. Topical clindamycin and erythromycin are available and are applied twice daily. Products that combine BP 5% and clindamycin or erythromycin are more effective than either drug alone.

For patients with numerous comedones, a *topical retinoid* will normalize the keratinization process within follicles, reducing obstruction and the risk for follicular rupture. Many experts recommend, however, the adjunctive use of a topical retinoid in those with moderate to severe inflammatory acne, even in the absence of clinical evidence of obstructive lesions. Options include tretinoin (Retin-A and others) or adapalene (Differin). Many adolescents who use tretinoin experience irritation, redness, or dryness, although this may be avoided by initiating therapy with a low-strength preparation (e.g., tretinoin cream 0.025% or adapalene). Other adverse effects include an apparent temporary worsening of acne 2 to 3 weeks after beginning treatment and increased sensitivity to sunlight caused by skin irritation.

Azelaic acid 20% (Azelex) is both antibacterial and anticomedonal. It is applied twice daily and appears to be well tolerated, although some patients experience pruritus, burning, stinging, tingling, or erythema. It is an alternative for patients with mild to moderate inflammatory and comedonal acne, or those with obstructive lesions who cannot tolerate tretinoin.

Systemic Therapies. *Oral antibiotics* possess greater efficacy than topical preparations and, for this reason, are prescribed for patients with severe or extensive inflammatory acne. They exert their antiinflammatory effect by decreasing bacterial colonization and inhibiting neutrophil chemotaxis; however, they also reduce the concentration of free fatty acids in sebum.

Although many antibiotics have been used to treat acne, tetracycline and erythromycin are most often prescribed initially, typically at a dose of 250 to 500 mg twice daily, although the higher dose usually is favored. The primary adverse

---

TABLE 129.4

OPTIONS FOR THE INITIAL MANAGEMENT OF FACIAL ACNE

Acne Severity	Lesion Type	Initial Treatment
Mild	Comedonal	Benzoyl peroxide once daily, or topical retinoid[1] once daily
	Inflammatory	Benzoyl peroxide once daily (or topical antibiotic[2] or combination preparation[2] bid)
	Mixed	Benzoyl peroxide once daily (or topical antibiotic[2] or combination product[2]) alone or combined with topical retinoid,[1] or azelaic acid twice daily
Moderate	Comedonal	Topical retinoid once daily[1]
	Inflammatory	Topical antibiotic[2] or combination product[2] bid, or oral antibiotic[3,4] if chest and back involved
		Many experts recommend the adjunctive use of a topical retinoid in those with moderate inflammatory acne
	Mixed	Topical antibiotic[2] or combination product[2] daily or bid (or oral antibiotic[3,4] if chest and back involved), and topical retinoid[1] once daily, or azelaic acid twice daily
Severe	Comedonal	Topical retinoid[1] once daily
	Inflammatory	Oral antibiotic[3,4]
		Many experts recommend the adjunctive use of a topical retinoid in those with severe inflammatory acne
	Mixed	Topical retinoid[1] once daily and oral antibiotic[3,4]

[1] For example, tretinoin cream 0.025% adapalene.
[2] For example, clindamycin, erythromycin, or benzoyl peroxide/clindamycin, benzoyl peroxide/erythromycin.
[3] For example, tetracycline or erythromycin 250 to 500 mg twice daily.
[4] For example, experts advise the use benzoyl peroxide in patients treated with oral antibiotics to prevent the emergence of antibiotic resistant *Propionibacterium acnes*.

effect of erythromycin is gastrointestinal upset that may be avoided by taking the medication with food. Tetracycline, like erythromycin, may cause gastrointestinal disturbances and should not be used during pregnancy or for patients less than 9 years of age due to potential discoloration of teeth. Tetracycline occasionally has caused esophageal ulceration, photosensitivity, vulvovaginal candidiasis, and, uncommonly, pseudotumor cerebri, hyperpigmentation, and onycholysis. For those who fail to respond to or cannot tolerate tetracycline or erythromycin, doxycycline or minocycline often are effective.

As with other acne therapies, 6 to 8 weeks often are required before oral antibiotics produce a significant clinical effect. Once the appearance of new lesions has ceased or been satisfactorily reduced, the dose may be tapered or eventually withdrawn in favor of topical agents.

Isotretinoin (13-cis retinoic acid, Accutane and others) is an oral analog of vitamin A that is highly effective for the treatment of severe, scarring acne. It typically is prescribed at a dose of 0.5 to 1.0 mg/kg/day for a course of 16 to 20 weeks. Despite its efficacy, oral isotretinoin therapy may be associated with important adverse reactions, the most serious of which is teratogenicity. For this reason, the drug should only be prescribed by those physicians with considerable experience in its use. Presently, all physicians wishing to prescribe isotratinoin must register with the Food and Drug Administration (FDA). Reports to the FDA have raised concern that isotretinoin use, through mechanisms unknown, may predispose patients to the development of depression or suicide. Although an association has not been clearly demonstrated, clinicians caring for patients who are receiving isotretinoin should remain alert to the presence or development of mental health disorders, including depression and suicidal ideation.

Combined *oral contraceptives* (OCs), those containing an estrogen and progestin, may improve acne by reducing free testosterone and ovarian androgen production. Despite this, these agents are not viewed as a primary therapy for acne but as an adjunct to standard medications.

Acne Variants

Acne Neonatorum. Acne neonatorum (neonatal acne) refers to the presence of inflammatory papules and pustules and, occasionally, comedones that typically appear within the first month of life. It occurs in 20% of neonates and males are affected more often than females. Generally, no treatment is required since lesions resolve spontaneously. If treatment is desired, a low-potency benzoyl peroxide preparation (e.g., 2.5%) or erythromycin may be applied.

Neonatal Cephalic Pustulosis. Neonatal cephalic pustulosis is a recently described entity that resembles neonatal acne. It appears during the first month of life and is characterized by erythematous papules and pustules that are located on the face, scalp, and neck. Comedones are not present. The condition may be the result of an inflammatory reaction to *Malassezia* sp. yeasts. The condition is self-limited but may be treated with a topical antiyeast preparation such as an imidazole.

Infantile Acne. Infantile acne begins at 3 to 6 months of age and may last until 12 to 18 months of age. Inflammatory papules and pustules, as well as comedones, are present, primarily on the face. For those with significant disease, the application of tretinoin or erythromycin often is beneficial.

Steroid Acne. Steroid acne is a result of the administration of oral or intravenous corticosteroids in large doses. The characteristic lesions—smooth, dome-shaped, erythematous papules of uniform size—appear suddenly in a crop (Fig. 129.67). Comedones are absent, and pustules are uncommon initially, although they may appear later.

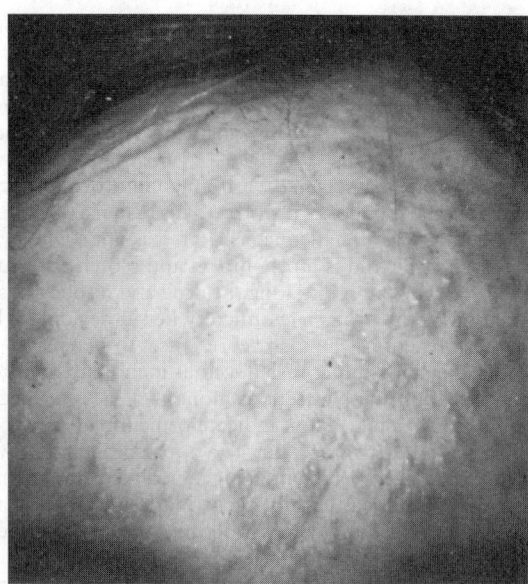

FIGURE 129.67. Monomorphous inflammatory papules appeared in this patient after steroid therapy.

Cosmetic Acne. Cosmetic acne refers to the appearance of typical acne lesions after prolonged application of comedogenic cosmetics. Cocoa butter, a favorite moisturizer, is a proved comedogenic agent.

Mechanical Acne. The typical lesions of mechanical acne occur in areas subject to repeated trauma; examples are lesions of the forehead caused by brushing or combing of the hair or lesions of the forehead and chin caused by a helmet or its straps. Rubbing may result in rupture of the sebaceous follicle unit below the skin surface.

Acne Conglobata. A severe variant of inflammatory acne is acne conglobata. It is characterized by cysts, abscesses, and multichanneled draining sinuses that involve the face, neck, and trunk. Extensive scarring may occur. Treatment is with an oral antibiotic or isotretinoin.

Acne Fulminans. Acne fulminans usually affects males, many of whom are receiving oral antibiotics for mild to moderate acne vulgaris. The onset is marked by the sudden onset of painful nodulocystic lesions that evolve into hemorrhagic nodules and plaques that ulcerate and drain. The back and chest usually are involved, although the face may be affected. Patients often experience fever, chills, weight loss, arthralgias, and myalgias. Osteolytic lesions mimicking osteomyelitis may affect the sternum, clavicles, or pelvis. Treatment usually is with a systemic corticosteroid and isotretinoin.

Drug Reactions

One of the main difficulties in dermatologic differential diagnosis is deciding whether a rash is drug-induced. Obviously, if the child is not taking a medication currently or has not received a drug recently, this is not a possibility. All too frequently, however, a febrile child is prescribed an antibiotic and later erupts in a rash. Is it an allergic reaction? Should the antibiotic be discontinued? Determining the answers to such questions is often difficult, because drug rashes can resemble almost any other kind of cutaneous eruption.

In studies of types of drug reactions, four cutaneous types have been found to make up almost 90% of the rashes. Nearly one-half of the rashes that are associated with drug reactions are *similar to exanthems*. These lesions may be maculopapular, morbilliform, macular, or scarlatiniform. They have no characteristic features that distinguish them readily from viral or bacterial exanthems. Penicillins, sulfonamides, trimethoprim-sulfamethoxazole, and erythromycin all are capable of producing this type of reaction.

The rash that is associated with ampicillin or amoxicillin presents a special diagnostic problem. This rash may be allergic or, more commonly, nonallergic. The latter is not a true hypersensitivity reaction and is morbilliform and blotchy. It usually begins 5 to 10 days after initiating the drug and resolves despite continuation of the drug. The difficulty lies in deciding which one of these reactions the rash represents. An extensive, erythematous, maculopapular rash develops in more than 80% of children and adults with infectious mononucleosis who receive ampicillin. This rash does not indicate penicillin allergy.

Urticarial eruptions account for approximately 25% of drug eruptions. These reactions are IgE-mediated, and their onset generally is sudden, usually occurring hours or days after drug exposure. The individual wheals are transient, but the entire process may last for 4 to 6 weeks. Penicillins, sulfonamides, barbiturates, and acetylsalicylic acid are drugs well known to cause this type of reaction.

Fixed drug reactions in children are less common than in adults; they are localized to a small area rather than being generalized, as usually is the case with drug reactions. The lesions are discrete, violaceous plaques that often are single or few in number and generally are asymptomatic. If the same drug is administered again, the rash will appear in the identical location. As many as 10% of drug reactions are of the fixed type.

Reactions resembling *erythema multiforme*, which feature concentric rings, or targets, occasionally with bullous or purpuric centers, account for 5% of drug reactions. Sulfonamides, penicillins, hydantoin, barbiturates, and griseofulvin have been implicated in this type of drug reaction. Infections and some systemic disorders can cause a similar eruption, however.

Other forms of drug reactions run the gamut of cutaneous lesions. Photosensitive dermatitis, vasculitic lesions with palpable purpura, vesicular or bullous eruptions, exfoliative lesions, erythema nodosum, and eczematous contact-type reactions all have been described. The child with a rash who is receiving a medication will continue to present diagnostic problems until sensitive and reliable tests for drug allergy are developed.

Acknowledgment

Gail Demmler, MD, contributed to the sections on warts and molluscum contagiosum.

Resources

Electronic Atlases

http://dermatlas.med.jhmi.edu/derm/
Johns Hopkins University DermAtlas. Contains over 7,000 images of pediatric dermatologic disorders. Each image is accompanied by a brief case history. One may search by diagnosis, disease category, or body site involved. There is a quiz to test your knowledge.
http://tray.dermatology.uiowa.edu/DermImag.htm
An atlas of general dermatology maintained by the Department of Dermatology at the University of Iowa. Images of conditions are listed alphabetically.
http://www.dermis.net/doia/mainmenu.asp?zugr=p&lang=e
Dermatologic Online Image Atlas maintained by the University of Erlangen, Germany. It contains over 4,500 images of adult and pediatric dermatologic disorders. Conditions may be searched alphabetically or by body area. There is a quiz to test your knowledge.

Suggested Readings

Acne

Krowchuk DP, Managing adolescent acne: A guide for pediatricians. *Pediatr Rev* 2005;26:244.
James WD. Acne. *N Engl J Med* 2005;352:1463.

Alopecia

Atton AV, Tunnessen WW Jr. Alopecia in children: the most common causes. *Pediatr Rev* 1990;12:25.

Atopic Dermatitis

Eichenfield LF, Friedlander SF. Coping with chronic dermatitis. *Contemp Pediatr* 1998;15:53.
Ellis C, Luger T. International consensus conference of atopic dermatitis II (ICCAD II): clinical update and current treatment strategies. *Br J Dermatol* 2003;148:3.
Williams HC. Clinical practice. Atopic dermatitis. *N Engl J Med* 2005;352:2314.

Birthmarks

Alper JC, Holmes LB. The incidence and significance of birthmarks in a cohort of 4,641 newborns. *Pediatr Dermatol* 1983;1:58.

Contact Dermatitis

Friedlander SF. Contact dermatitis. *Pediatr Rev* 1998;19:166.

Diaper Dermatitis

Arnsmeier SL, Paller AS. Getting to the bottom of diaper dermatitis. *Contemp Pediatr* 1997;14:115.
Singalavanija S, Frieden IJ. Diaper dermatitis. *Pediatr Rev* 1995;16:142.

Drug Reactions

Salkind AR, Cuddy PG, Foxworth JW. Is this patient allergic to penicillin? An evidence-based analysis of the likelihood of penicillin allergy. *JAMA* 2001;285:2498.
Shin HT, Chang MW. Drug eruptions in children. *Curr Probl Pediatr* 2001; 31:207.

Hypersensitivity Reactions

Prendiville J. Stevens-Johnson syndrome and toxic epidermal necrolysis. *Adv Dermatol* 2002;18:151.
Tamburro JE, Estely NB. Hypersensitivity syndromes. *Adolesc Med* 2001; 12:323.
Weston WL, Badgett JT. Urticaria. *Pediatr Rev* 1998;19:240.

Head Lice

Frankowski BL, Weiner LB. Head lice. *Pediatrics* 2002;110:638.
Roberts RJ. Head lice. *N Eng J Med* 2002;346:1645.

Ichthyosis

Shwayder T. Ichthyosis in a nutshell. *Pediatr Rev* 1999;20:5.

Neonatal Dermatology

Johr RH, Schachner LA. Neonatal dermatologic challenges. *Pediatr Rev* 1997; 18:86.
Nehal KS, Pebenito R, Orlow SJ. Analysis of 54 cases of hypopigmentation or hyperpigmentation along the lines of Blaschko. *Arch Dermatol* 1996;132:1167.
Vasiloudes R, Morelli JG, Weston WL. A guide to rashes in newborns. *Contemp Pediatr* 1997;14:156.

Nevi

DeDavid M, Orlow SJ, Provost N, et al. A study of large congenital melanocytic nevi and associated melanomas: review of cases in the New York University Registry and the world literature. *J Am Acad Dermatol* 1997;36:409.
Morelli JG, Weston WL. Sun, kids, moles, and melanoma. *Contemp Pediatr* 1999;16:61.

Vascular Lesions

Bruckner AL, Frieden IJ. Hemangiomas of infancy. *J Am Acad Dermatol* 2003; 48:477.
Drolet BA, Esterly NB, Frieden IJ. Hemangiomas in children. *N Eng J Med* 1999;341:173.
Tallman B, Tan OT, Morelli JG, et al. Location of port wine stains and the likelihood of ophthalmic and/or CNS complications. *Pediatrics* 1991;87:323.

CHAPTER 130 ■ SPORTS MEDICINE

GREGORY L. LANDRY

Pediatricians involved in primary care practice sports medicine on a daily basis. In most practices, at least one patient each day is involved in athletic pursuits and brings to the physician an agenda related to sports participation. Athletically inclined children and their parents ask difficult questions that are different from those of other patients seeking primary medical care. Advances in the diagnosis and treatment of medical problems in athletes have provided answers to many of those questions.

Sports medicine in the United States traditionally has been a subspecialty of orthopedic surgery. It developed from the evaluation and treatment of injuries occurring in professional and Olympic athletes. Techniques were discovered in the diagnosis and treatment of these conditions in athletes that minimized time lost from their sport as a result of injury. These techniques were applied quickly to college athletes, trickled down to high school athletes, and currently have many applications in youth sports. More and more families are demanding the same kind of treatment and care for younger patients that is provided for college and professional athletes. It no longer is acceptable simply to explain the diagnosis of and treatment for a particular injury or illness. Young athletes want to know how soon they can return to participation in their sport and what they can do to speed their recovery. When an illness or injury strikes, "When can I . . . ?" becomes the patient's chief concern in the disposition. To maximize safe return to activity, a physical therapist or an athletic trainer may assist with rehabilitation of the injury. In addition, if the child cannot perform a favorite athletic activity, an alternative activity should be suggested to enable the patient to maintain some degree of fitness during rehabilitation.

To care for young athletes, physicians need not be knowledgeable about sports (although it helps), but they must be sensitive to the importance of sports activities in the lives of athletic children. Similar in a sense to children with special educational needs, young athletes also have special needs. Athletes may be physically talented, and medical illness or injury may take on more significance than it would in children who are less physically talented. The principles of sports medicine have applications in pediatrics in a broader sense, however. For example, young musicians who are ill or injured and who are working toward a musical performance have needs similar to those of injured athletes who are working toward an athletic performance.

Once thought to be a passing fad, sports medicine has become an important area of health care. This chapter addresses some of the most common medical questions that may be encountered by a pediatrician who cares for children who participate in athletic activities.

PREPARTICIPATION HEALTH INVENTORY

Children should have a yearly health checkup with a primary care health provider that includes a preparticipation health inventory for those patients who participate in sports activities. Unfortunately, this is not always possible. Adolescents tend to seek health care infrequently and often only when they are required to do so by an employer or when it is a contingency for athletic participation. Most states require that athletes obtain a physician's statement of approval before they participate in sports activities, and this preparticipation visit provides an opportunity to address many health issues that may not come up at visits made for injuries.

The goals of a preparticipation health inventory vary somewhat from those of a routine health inventory in a nonathlete. In addition to assessing general health and diagnosing treatable conditions, conditions should be identified that may interfere with athletic participation or worsen as a result of it, especially any condition that may cause sudden death. Education related to the prevention of athletic injuries also should be included in the inventory process.

Group Examinations

Some physicians are faced with providing evaluations for a large number of athletes at one time. The most inefficient method practiced traditionally is for one or two physicians to perform a cursory examination of each athlete in a locker room. Instead, when large numbers of athletes require examination, the use of revolving stations provides the opportunity for more thorough and highly efficient evaluation. If additional health providers are recruited, the physical examination can be divided by organ systems into stations, and the tasks can be divided among the examiners. A list of possible stations appears in Table 130.1. Parents and coaches may help in administration of the process.

A few drawbacks to the station method deserve consideration. In a large group, the athletes face multiple examiners; with little time available in which to develop rapport, it is difficult to address sensitive topics such as sexual issues or drug use or to perform examinations of breasts and external genitalia in girls. For this reason, one-on-one evaluation by the primary care provider always is preferable.

Areas of Highest Yield

The history and orthopedic examination portions of the preparticipation inventory yield the most useful information. Most important in the history are questions pertaining to past injuries and to risk factors for sudden death. Athletes should be questioned regarding any family history of premature, nonaccidental death and about fainting or dizziness with exercise. Some of the cardiac causes of sudden death in the young athlete can be identified (Table 130.2). The low prevalence of these problems in the general population makes it difficult to justify the cost of an electrocardiogram and echocardiogram for every athlete. Some common causes of sudden death in athletes are familial, such as hypertrophic cardiomyopathy, prolonged

STATIONS FOR THE PREPARTICIPATION EVALUATION WITH SUGGESTIONS ABOUT PERSONNEL, EQUIPMENT, AND SPACE NEEDS

1. History: parent or coach—must be completed before the athlete proceeds to any station
2. Blood pressure: athletic trainer or nurse—must have thigh cuffs available for large athletes; should be right arm, sitting
3. Visual acuity: athletic trainer or nurse—Snellen chart best; need well-lit area
4. Head and neck: physician or nurse practitioner—disposable specula, extra batteries
5. Heart and lungs: physician or nurse practitioner—need quietest area available
6. Abdomen: physician or nurse practitioner—gloves for male genitalia and hernia examinations
7. Orthopedic: physician or athletic trainer—large examination table
8. Laboratory: medical or nursing assistant—gloves and specimen containers
9. Review and disposition: physician—best if it is the team physician

QT syndrome, and aortic rupture associated with Marfan syndrome. Because athletes with Marfan syndrome are at risk for sudden death caused by aortic rupture, examiners should scrutinize tall, thin athletes for findings consistent with the syndrome, such as scoliosis, pectus excavatum, hyperextensible joints, and a click and murmur consistent with mitral valve prolapse. Sudden, unexplained death in the family, fainting with exercise, or findings consistent with Marfan syndrome warrant further evaluation.

A good screening orthopedic examination can be performed in 90 seconds by primary care physicians as part of a general physical examination. The screening orthopedic examination is outlined in Table 130.3. If a history of any injury or a positive finding on the screening orthopedic examination exists, a more thorough evaluation is necessary.

Disposition

Most athletes fear that something will be discovered during the evaluation that will result in their disqualification from sports participation. Examiners should work toward allowing participation and should not disqualify any youngster who is physically and emotionally fit. In the group setting, the disposition should be made very clear. Ideally, the disposition should be written. If further medical evaluation is necessary, it should be

CARDIAC CAUSES OF SUDDEN DEATH IN YOUNG ATHLETES

Cardiomyopathy
Hypertrophic cardiomyopathy*
Congenital heart disease
Anomalous left coronary artery
Aortic rupture*
Hypoplastic coronary arteries
Prolonged QT syndrome*
Unknown

*Causes of death that are potentially preventable through detection of a family history of sudden, unexplained death or symptoms during exercise.

ORTHOPEDIC SCREENING EXAMINATION

Athletic Activity (Instructions)	Observation
Stand facing examiner	Acromioclavicular joints; general habitus
Look at ceiling, floor, over both shoulders; touch ears to shoulders	Cervical spine motion
Shrug shoulders (examiner resists)	Trapezius strength
Abduct shoulders 90 degrees (examiner resists at 90 degrees)	Deltoid strength
Rotate arms fully externally	Shoulder motion
Flex and extend elbows	Elbow motion
Arms at sides, elbows flexed 90 degrees, move wrists into pronation and supination	Elbow and wrist motion
Spread fingers; make fist	Hand or finger motion and deformities
Tighten (contract) quadriceps; relax quadriceps	Symmetry and knee effusion; ankle effusion
"Duck walk" four steps (away from examiner with buttocks on heels)	Hip, knee, and ankle motion
Back up to examiner	Shoulder symmetry; scoliosis
Knees straight, touch toes	Scoliosis, hip mition; hamstring tightness
Rise up on toes (raise heels)	Calf symmetry, leg strength

Reprinted with permission from Garrick JG. Sports medicine. *Pediatr Clin North Am* 1977;24:737.

made clear to the athlete that this either precludes participation or simply is a recommendation for further care.

ROLE OF THE TEAM PHYSICIAN

Immediate, and often ongoing, care of injuries in the estimated 20 million young athletes in the United States falls into the hands of coaches. Eighty percent of the sports injuries that occur in this country may be evaluated and treated first by coaches. This statistic points to a need to promote greater involvement by health professionals and to educate coaches regarding sports injuries. Pediatricians may feel unqualified to help with athletic teams because of the number of orthopedic injuries that occur. Actually, pediatricians make excellent team physicians because of their broad knowledge of primary care and their sensitivity to the young athlete psychologically. Most college and professional sports teams involve both a primary care physician and an orthopedic surgeon in team care. Few of the injuries that occur require extensive musculoskeletal evaluation on the field, but many do require a physician who is knowledgeable about sports injuries.

The basic requirements for a team physician are interest and a willingness to read about problems unique to the field of sports medicine. Team physician duties typically are voluntary, and most of us do the job because it is fun.

The specific duties of a team physician must be defined. Some medicolegal problems can be avoided if these responsibilities are delineated clearly in writing. Physicians' responsibilities vary greatly from team to team, and defining the responsibilities protects a physician to some extent from incurring an excessive time commitment. Most coaches and athletic directors welcome physician involvement, because they recognize their expertise in caring for medical problems and injuries. Occasionally, however, an overzealous coach cannot understand why an athlete with a particular injury cannot participate. To minimize this problem, the team physician's authority regarding the ability of the athletes to play in the event of any medical illness or injury should be clarified in writing.

Ideally, the school or team should enlist the services of a certified athletic trainer. The expertise of an experienced certified athletic trainer in assessing an injury and evaluating a player's ability to participate can be invaluable. In addition, a trainer can provide rehabilitation for the injury. If a school or team does not have one, hiring a trainer should be one of the first investments made toward improving the medical care of its athletes. The trainer will make the job of a team physician much easier.

The equipment available to a physician on the field is limited by cost considerations. The minimum requirements include a first aid kit, water jug, and ice chest containing plastic bags. These items are inexpensive, and the importance of having water available for hydration and ice available for injuries cannot be emphasized too strongly to both coaches and athletes.

The supplies included in the medical bag can be extensive, especially if those that usually are available in a trainer's bag are provided. A checklist for the medical bag appears in Table 130.4. Not all these items are required, but the team physician may want to consider them for adequate on-the-field coverage.

MANAGEMENT OF ATHLETIC INJURIES

Emergencies

When physicians provide medical coverage for any event, they must be prepared for any eventuality. They should have a plan in the event of a catastrophic injury, such as a spinal cord injury or cessation of pulse and breathing in an athlete. Team physicians also should be prepared to care for spectators in the event of a crisis. The ability to communicate with sources of emergency help can be critical. Do you have a cellular phone? Will it work in the remote area of the sports field? The location of the nearest telephone always should be known. If it is a pay telephone, loose change must be available to those individuals who are responsible for the care of the spectators and athletes; medical help can be delayed if coins for a pay telephone are not available. Determining in advance those individuals who will call for help if an ambulance is needed and those who should be called, including the location of the closest ambulance service, saves valuable time. This information probably should be written on the medical bag and the coach's first aid kit.

Management on the Field

Management of injuries on the field is applied first aid. When an athlete goes down on the playing surface, physicians should remain calm, because other people look to them for direction. Whenever possible, using the athlete's name has a calming effect. Once the athlete's attention is gained, the physician should ask the child to indicate where the pain is located. If the athlete is unresponsive, basic principles of life support (i.e., "A, B, C," for *a*irway, *b*reathing, and *c*irculation) should be followed.

An unconscious athlete who has been injured in a contact sport, such as football, should be treated as if a fracture of the cervical spine has been sustained. If any pain in the neck or back occurs, palpation of the cervical spine and back should be performed before the athlete is allowed to move. If any suggestion of a significant neck or back injury exists, the athlete

TABLE 130.4

SPORTS MEDICINE BAG: ITEMS THE TEAM PHYSICIAN MAY WANT TO INCLUDE IN THE ON-THE-FIELD MEDICAL BAG FOR SPORTS EVENT COVERAGE

Airway supplies
Oral airways
Nasal airways
Ambu bag with face mask and endotracheal tube adapter
Laryngoscope with light source and blades
Cricothyrotomy kit with tracheostomy tubes

Medications
Epinephrine 1:10,000 for resuscitation
Lidocaine hydrochloride, 100-mg vial, for arrhythmias
Lactated Ringer's solution with intravenous tubing and catheters
Epinephrine 1:1,000 for endotracheal tube instillation or subcutaneous use for anaphylaxis
Diazepam, 10-mg vial, for seizures
Methylpednisolone for spinal cord injury
Ophthalmologic saline for irrigation
Antibiotic ointment
Beta-agonist inhaler

Equipment
Stethoscope
Otoscope/ophthalmoscope
Thermometer
Penlight
Swiss Army knife
Sphygmomanometer
Tongue blades
Surgical towel clip, for SC dislocation

Dressings
White bandage tape
Sterile gauze pads
Cotton swabs
Elastic bandages
Sterile suture kits (gloves, suture material, syringes, and lidocaine)
Steri-Strips
Tincture of benzoin
Povidone-iodine solution or hexachlorophene
Bandage scissors
Finger splints
Plaster bandages and cotton web roll

should be transported by an emergency vehicle to the nearest emergency facility for radiography. Injuries to the extremities should be assessed by visual observation and palpation and by determination of range of motion and stability. Immediate swelling, bony tenderness, deformity, lack of range of motion, or instability indicates that the athlete may need assistance in leaving the field of play.

An examination should be repeated after the athlete has left the playing surface. In the absence of suspicion of fracture, ligamentous instability, or any neurovascular compromise, the question of the child's ability to play arises.

Determining an Athlete's Ability to Play

Determining an athlete's ability to play can be a challenge, even to a physician who has vast experience in sports injuries. Simple guidelines are helpful in dealing with medical problems that arise in the heat of the action.

Once the injury has been evaluated and determined to be relatively minor, the athlete's ability to play is assessed by functional evaluation. The athlete should be asked to perform a function that is similar to, or related to, actions that are required during the athletic event. If any pain, weakness, or instability is experienced during the functional examination, participation should be disallowed. For example, the athlete with a mildly sprained ankle can be asked to jump up and down on the toes of the injured foot while avoiding weight bearing on the uninjured foot. If this task can be performed without difficulty, return to play is reasonable. Other functional tests may be added, such as running in a figure-of-eight pattern or in zigzag sprints. Playing when an injury is present can increase the risk of further injury, and a functional examination shows the athlete that some degree of impairment exists. Functional testing takes some of the guesswork out of this sometimes difficult decision.

Stability should be assessed immediately after an injury occurs, because a ligament examination can be obtained best before swelling, hemorrhage, and inflammation have started to cause pain and protective muscle guarding. Any instability or increased joint laxity precludes athletic participation. Whereas the first examination is best for determining stability in regard to the athlete's ability to return to play, the extent of the injury may become clearer 15 to 20 minutes after the injury has occurred, when tissue damage has caused more inflammation. Protective taping or bracing will not, and should not, be used to permit an athlete with a significant injury to participate, but it may be used to protect a mild injury from exacerbation when the athlete returns to play.

HEAT ILLNESS

Heat illness is relevant to physicians in both cool and warm climates, because sporting events occur indoors as well as outdoors. Our understanding of the pathophysiology of heat illness has improved markedly, which is important, because life-threatening heat illness (heat stroke) probably is entirely preventable.

The terminology in this area can be confusing and often is misunderstood. Heat cramps, heat syncope, heat exhaustion, and heat stroke are part of a continuum.

Heat Cramps

Heat cramps are painful and forceful muscle contractions that usually occur in the gastrocnemius or hamstring muscles. They probably are related to heat, dehydration, and lack of training. Treatment includes rest, stretching, and the ingestion of copious amounts of water or a sports drink, if available. Occasionally, the cramps are the result of salt depletion in addition to the other factors, and the athlete needs more dietary sodium chloride.

Heat Syncope

Heat syncope is a term often used to describe a phenomenon that is common in runners in which they stop running at the end of a race and experience hypotensive syncope as a result of venous pooling. This is not life-threatening but is indicative of hypovolemia and the redistribution of blood volume that is caused by sweating and mild hyperthermia. Treatment consists of rest and the ingestion of generous amounts of water or a sports drink.

Heat Exhaustion

Heat exhaustion is manifested by pale skin color, vasoconstriction, dizziness, visual disturbances, syncope, and a moderately elevated rectal temperature (38° to 40°C, or 101° to 105°F). As with muscle cramps, treatment involves rest and rehydration. Ice packs and a fan may speed recovery. In some cases, intravenous fluid therapy may be required because of nausea and vomiting. Most authorities recommend normal saline, which approximates the composition of the sweat that has been lost.

Heat Stroke

The presence of central nervous system symptoms such as delirium, convulsions, and coma is indicative of heat stroke. A rectal temperature greater than 41°C (106°F) characteristically is seen in acute exercise-induced heat stroke. In the absence of exercise, heat stroke is associated with the absence of sweating and the presence of warm, flushed skin. The young, exercising athlete with heat stroke, however, usually still is sweating profusely and may have peripheral vasodilation. The central nervous system symptoms are more specific for heat stroke and indicate a medical emergency. Heat stroke can be fatal if it is not treated. Immediate immersion of the athlete in ice water is the most efficient means of cooling, but if this not available, the athlete should be packed in ice bags applied to the head, neck, and groin areas. Intravenous fluids (normal saline) should be administered as soon as possible, and immediate transport to a hospital is imperative. Because heat stroke may cause multisystem failure, the athlete may require admission to the hospital for observation.

Prevention of Heat Illness

The environmental conditions that cause the greatest heat stress must be considered. These include high environmental temperatures, high levels of relative humidity (as measured by a wet-bulb thermometer), and high levels of solar radiation (as occurs during the hottest part of the day). Evaporation is less effective when there is little wind. The greatest risk probably occurs on relatively warm days that follow cooler weather, especially in the early spring when athletes have not had time to adjust to the temperature change.

Susceptible Individuals

Certain types of individuals are at greater risk for sustaining heat injury, including those who are obese, poorly trained, dehydrated, or not used to heat. Age also is a risk factor, primarily for young children and the elderly. Anyone with a history of heat stroke is at risk for recurrence.

Football players are more susceptible to heat illness than are other athletes because their ability to lose heat through evaporation is abolished almost completely. Football uniforms cover most of the body, and practices start during some of the hottest days of the summer. Because coaches often are the only ones in contact with these athletes, they bear the main responsibility for preventing heat illness. Football players often have two practices a day, and they may not rehydrate their bodies before each practice. To address this problem, coaches should require that weight measurements be taken before and after each practice. The weights are recorded on a chart in the locker room next to the scales. At the beginning of a practice session, athletes who have lost 3% or more of their body weight are observed carefully and should not be allowed to participate, because they are at higher risk of the development of heat illness. Most coaches modify practices on hot days and allow the players to wear shirts and shorts for all or part of the practice session.

In addition to identifying risk factors, unlimited water or a sports drink should be provided to the athletes. Children drink more fluid if it tastes good, so a sports drink should be provided when possible.

COMMON MEDICAL ILLNESSES IN ATHLETES

Common Viral Infections

Exercise causes changes in the immune system, the significance of which is unknown. Exercise causes transient granulocytosis and lymphocytosis as well as an increase in circulating endogenous pyrogen. Despite these changes, athletes are just as susceptible as nonathletes to common viral illnesses. For individuals participating in team sports, the exposure rate probably is as high as it is for other children and adolescents attending school.

Few scientific data exist regarding common viral illnesses in relation to the ability of a child to participate in sports activities. The objective finding of fever is helpful. Excellent studies have shown increased cardiopulmonary effort and reduced exercise capacity in response to fever. Fever also is associated with poor tolerance of orthostatic stress, poor tolerance of submaximal exercise, and abnormal temperature regulation. For these reasons, fever should preclude participation in most instances.

Some physicians are extremely conservative because of the fear of precipitating myocarditis in an athlete who exercises in the presence of viral infections. The only suggestion of this occurred in an animal study, which showed that coxsackievirus B27 infection in mice produced a significant incidence of myocarditis when exercise was forced. No studies in humans have proven this connection. If exercise is a precipitating factor, it would seem that a much higher incidence of myocarditis would be seen in athletes. Most physicians use the presence of fever and the severity of symptoms to determine an athlete's ability to play.

Many of the common cold viruses are well known to cause significant impairment of small airways for several weeks after the infection. Exercise-induced chest tightness or cough should alert the physician that reactive airways may be impairing the athlete's performance, especially in any athlete who has known reactive airways. Exercise-induced asthma is as common in athletes as it is in nonathletes. Rather than automatically restricting the athlete from competition because of cough, wheezing, and shortness of breath, the bronchospasm should be treated aggressively with a beta$_2$-sympathomimetic aerosol, such as albuterol. This controls asthmatic symptoms in at least 80% of children who have exercise-induced symptoms.

Treatment with albuterol can safely provide marked improvement in symptoms. Additional agents such as cromolyn, nedrocromil, or a corticosteroid may be necessary for adequate treatment of the athlete with symptoms caused by bronchospasm.

Infectious Mononucleosis

Most practicing pediatricians care for athletes who have infectious mononucleosis. In almost all sports, this illness usually has a significant effect on the individual's ability to participate in sports activities. Infectious mononucleosis is of special concern in collision and contact sports because of the high incidence of splenomegaly and the risk of splenic rupture. A review of the literature regarding splenic rupture reveals that it is a rare event and that most ruptures occur during the first 3 weeks of the illness. Moreover, in more than 50% of the splenic ruptures reported, the spleen was not palpable during the initial examination.

The duration of illness and degree of splenomegaly vary greatly from person to person. Rather than setting an arbitrary interval during which an athlete must not participate in a sport, each individual should be observed on a weekly basis, with the ability to play determined by clinical symptoms and physical examinations. Most athletes with mononucleosis are too ill to consider resuming competition before 3 to 4 weeks after the onset of the illness. By the 3- to 4-week mark, they are past the period of high risk for splenic rupture and should be allowed to play sports if they feel able to do so.

Occasionally, athletes have a mild case of mononucleosis, and their symptoms abate as early as 2 weeks after the onset of the illness. Because palpation on physical examination is a poor method of assessing splenic size, radiologic evaluation should be considered, especially in an athlete who is participating in collision sports such as football or hockey. Plain radiographs of the abdomen are approximately 70% accurate in assessing splenic size. Ultrasound, if it is available, provides an accurate measurement of splenic volume. With documentation by radiography or sonography that the spleen is not enlarged, return to competition probably carries little risk. The athlete certainly should avoid physical stress early in the illness when fever and other symptoms are present. Light workouts probably can be resumed when the athlete feels able; however, the effects of exercise on the severity and duration of mononucleosis have not been studied. In a study of infectious hepatitis in army personnel, no difference was found in recovery time (4 weeks) or relapse rate between patients who performed regular exercise and light work and patients those who were kept at rest.

SPORTS NUTRITION

Nutrition is an increasingly important aspect of sports medicine. Unfortunately, many athletes do not ask for nutritional information from health professionals but seek advice from their coaches and teammates. Many experts in the field of sports medicine believe that the most significant advances made in sports medicine in the future will be in the area of nutrition. The pregame meal, fluid replacement, and weight gain and loss methods are common topics that pediatricians may be asked to address by athletes and coaches.

Pregame Meal

The meal that is eaten just before an athletic contest is important to athletes who want to be at their best at game time. Most athletes are not comfortable exercising on a full stomach. Ideally, the meal should be consumed 2 to 4 hours before exercise, and it should consist mostly of complex carbohydrates. High-fat meals tend to prolong the full feeling and take longer to digest.

A "quick-energy" candy bar or simple sugar snack consumed immediately before an event is more likely to be detrimental than helpful to an athlete. Rebound hypoglycemia may occur during athletic activity as a result of the relative hyperinsulinemia that occurs after the sugar load. This effect has been demonstrated in studies of patients who underwent aerobic exercise on a treadmill after sugar loading.

Fluid Replacement

During most athletic events that last less than 2 hours, the most practical fluid to use for rehydration is cold water. It certainly is the cheapest and most easily obtainable fluid. Most of the commercial sports drinks are pleasant tasting, replace sodium loss, and provide a source of carbohydrate. The carbohydrate and electrolyte composition of the replacement fluid probably is important only in endurance events that involve 30 minutes or more of continuous exercise. Hypertonic solutions once were thought to impede gastric emptying and intestinal absorption, but research has shown that oral solutions containing as much as 6% glucose are absorbed rapidly and provide an important source of carbohydrate for endurance athletes. Athletes should be reminded that thirst is not a sensitive indicator of hydration status and that they should replace fluid before they feel thirsty.

Weight Gain

An athlete who is interested in gaining weight to improve performance in a particular sport, such as football, should be trying to gain lean body mass. The athlete may be tempted to buy all kinds of nutritional products that are claimed to promote rapid weight gain. Numerous amino acid supplements are available, but studies have not shown them consistently to have any effect other than being an additional source of calories.

Free amino acid supplements cause both proven and theoretic harm to the athlete, and use is associated with a significant incidence of diarrhea and abdominal pain. Physiologically, polypeptides are absorbed more efficiently in the gut than are free amino acids. Animal studies on amino acid supplementation show a high incidence of nephropathy, but this never has been shown in humans. Creatine monophosphate is expensive and appears to produce few side effects. It has shown promise in studies on strength training and power sports and may have a detrimental effect on endurance athletes. The long-term effects of this popular supplement are unknown.

A careful dietary analysis often is helpful in assessing the daily caloric intake of an athlete, and it may reveal a level of caloric intake that is insufficient for adequate weight gain. If the athlete needs to increase the total daily caloric intake, ingesting more carbohydrates should be emphasized, because the diets of most U.S. residents already are rich in protein. While attempting to gain weight, the athlete should be involved in a strength training program so the gain is more likely to be in lean body mass.

Weight Loss

For some athletes, thinness is vital to their success. Ballet dancers, wrestlers, gymnasts, and distance runners often feel pressured to stay thin or to lose weight. These athletes are just as prone as are nonathletes to use unhealthy rapid weight loss methods, and they may be at risk for the development of eating disorders.

In general, athletes should use the same sensible weight loss methods as nonathletes, by decreasing their caloric intake while increasing their caloric expenditure. For most athletes, a reasonable maximum weight loss per week is 0.90 kg (2 lb). Faster weight loss probably will result in ketosis, loss of muscle mass, and dehydration. Use of saunas, rubber suits, or diuretics to lose weight should be discouraged strongly because of the associated risks of electrolyte disturbance and excessive dehydration. Fortunately, many of the unhealthy eating behaviors seen in athletes are transient, practiced only during participation in the particular sport, and do not become integrated permanently into their behavior patterns.

DERMATOLOGIC CONCERNS IN ATHLETES

Few skin problems disqualify athletes from playing sports, but contagious skin infections do rule out competition in sports that involve close contact, such as wrestling or rugby. Impetigo and herpesvirus infections are seen most commonly, although tinea corporis also is contagious enough to warrant disqualification. Impetigo and herpes infections can spread through a team quickly unless the athletes and coaches are cognizant of the importance of early diagnosis and treatment. With aggressive treatment, the amount of time lost from participation can be minimized.

Impetigo

The athlete with impetigo usually is infected by the same organism as is the nonathlete, predominantly *Staphylococcus aureus* or *Streptococcus pyogenes*. The diagnosis of impetigo may be more difficult in the wrestler because any bulla or crust may be rubbed off during a match or in the shower. Moreover, the lesions occur anywhere on the body, and they may not look much more impressive than do fresh abrasions. An athlete with recurrent impetigo may suspect infection early in the course of the infection and seek medical care. Skin cultures do not distinguish pathogens from normal flora and probably need not be performed unless recurrences are frequent or treatment response is poor.

Treatment involves good local care, including scrubbing with an antiseptic soap and applying an antibacterial ointment such as mupirocin. Systemic antibiotics should be used more liberally in most athletes, to speed recovery and decrease contagiousness to the other participants.

The ability of an athlete with impetigo to participate in a sport is subjective, but a waiting period of at least 24 to 48 hours after the initiation of a systemic antibiotic is necessary. Covering lesions with an occlusive dressing often is impractical because of perspiration and constant trauma to the dressing.

Impetigo can be prevented by frequent washing of the mats that serve as fomites. Athletes with impetigo should be disqualified promptly from competition. It may be reasonable for some athletes who are particularly susceptible to impetigo to take an antibiotic prophylactically during a designated period. This may be useful especially toward the end of the season, just before tournaments. The use of a prophylactic antibiotic increases the risk that resistant bacteria will develop, however, and this possibility should be weighed against the benefit of preventing an outbreak. Methicillin-resistant *S. aureus* (MRSA) has been reported in wrestlers.

Herpes Simplex

Herpetic infection in athletes who are involved in high-contact sports such as wrestling sometimes is called *herpes gladiatorum*. Lesions develop anywhere on the trunk or extremities and are more likely to occur in a break in the skin caused by an abrasion. The signs and symptoms are the same as for herpes simplex infections occurring elsewhere on the body, except the lesions often are more widespread.

Treatment includes disqualification until all vesicles are crusted over. As with impetigo, evaluation of a player's ability to participate is subjective. Some athletes have outbreaks that last for 5 to 7 days, which is a significant time away from competition. Systemic therapy with acyclovir or a similar agent should be instituted as soon as possible to speed recovery and reduce contagion.

As athletes become better educated about acyclovir, they are quicker to seek treatment because it speeds recovery. Some wrestling team physicians are using acyclovir prophylactically. Prophylactic acyclovir, 400 mg twice a day, or valacyclovir, 500 mg once a day, has been shown to be effective against recurrent herpetic lesions in other populations.

COMMON INJURIES INVOLVING THE HEAD AND NECK

Head and neck trauma can be anxiety provoking for the athlete, family, and physician covering an athletic event. Fortunately, in most sports, severe injuries are rare, but mild head and neck traumatic injuries are common occurrences in contact sports such as football and ice hockey.

Assessment on the Field

When physicians evaluate the extent of an athlete's injury while he or she still is on the field, they should ask the athlete whether any neck pain is present. Even when neck pain is denied, if the athlete has sustained a concussion, the neck should be palpated carefully along the cervical spine for any area of tenderness. It also is important, before the athlete is allowed to sit up or to stand, to ask him or her whether any neurologic symptoms are felt in the extremities, such as numbness, tingling, or weakness. If any neck pain exists, especially any cervical spine tenderness, the athlete must be considered to have sustained a neck fracture and must not be moved. After being immobilized properly, the athlete should be transported by trained personnel to an emergency facility. If the individual is unconscious, he or she must be assumed to have a neck fracture and should be treated accordingly. If an airway must be established, this potential injury must be assumed. In sports that involve the use of protective helmets, the team physician should be prepared to remove the face mask in case of a head or neck injury requiring access to the airway. Using a screwdriver or knife to remove the fasteners connecting the face mask to the helmet allows quick removal of the face mask and access to the airway without moving the athlete's neck.

Concussions

Concussions occur frequently in contact sports, and determining an athlete's ability to return to play afterward can be difficult. Some physicians unnecessarily disqualify athletes with even the mildest head trauma. The diagnosis of a concussion should be made in any athlete who sustains a transient loss of cognitive ability as a result of trauma to the head. The mildest form of concussion is commonly referred to as the *ding*, and it consists of a few seconds of confusion, loss of balance, and "seeing stars." This can be brief enough to go undetected by teammates and coaches.

Criteria for return to play after concussion are similar to those after other injuries; the athlete must pass a functional examination. Gait analysis and balance should be evaluated on the sideline. The most sensitive examination is a test for memory. In addition to asking simple information about the athlete's address or events that took place earlier in the day, it is helpful to have a teammate discuss the higher cognitive aspects of the game. If the athlete stumbles when being asked

questions about the game plan or the assignments, then return to competition is forbidden. These cognitive abilities may return during the event, and the athlete may return to competition at that time if no nausea, vomiting, or headache is noted and no other symptoms occur. If symptoms persist longer than 15 minutes, an athlete usually should not return to the same contest.

The longer the athlete experiences loss of higher cognition, the more severe is the concussion. The athlete should be questioned carefully about events that occurred earlier in the day. The presence of retrograde amnesia signals a more severe concussion, even without a history of loss of consciousness. The athlete with evidence of retrograde amnesia will be unlikely to regain full cognition during the game, will have a headache, and should not be allowed to compete.

Any athlete who loses consciousness for more than a brief time (a few seconds) during a competition should be disqualified from further participation in that competition. In sports that require headgear for participation, nonparticipation almost is guaranteed if the physician retains the athlete's headgear. In the heat of the moment, especially if he or she is not thinking clearly, the athlete may try to resume competition against medical advice. In contrast to other sports injuries, it usually is not a good idea to send to the showers an athlete who has sustained a head injury, because medical personnel may not be available to accompany the individual. The athlete must be observed closely after sustaining a concussion, and the team physician can usually best keep an eye on the athlete on the sidelines.

The headache that an athlete experiences after sustaining a concussion can last for days or weeks. Because headache indicates some cerebral dysfunction, an athlete should not be allowed to participate in sports in the presence of headache after a concussion. When the headache resolves, the athlete may be allowed to do some light jogging and, eventually, sprinting. If running produces headache, the athlete should not be allowed to proceed to competition. Occasionally, an athlete has postconcussion syndrome, with frequent headaches, poor concentration, irritability, and loss of certain cognitive abilities for days to weeks after the injury. An athlete with a persistent headache or a progressively worsening headache warrants a computed tomographic scan or a magnetic resonance imaging study, and a neurologic or neurosurgical evaluation should be considered.

Once an athlete has received a concussion, his or her risk of sustaining another concussion is increased. Traditionally, physicians have disqualified athletes from participating in a sport when they have sustained three concussions. The "three concussions and you are out" rule may be appropriate in some cases, but every patient must be approached individually. Both the severity of the concussions and the time between their occurrence should be considered. The possibility of delayed cerebral dysfunction, documented in professional athletes who have sustained recurrent concussions, should be kept in mind when counseling the athlete and the family.

Brachial Plexus Injuries

Many spectators of football, ice hockey, or wrestling are familiar with the athlete who comes off the field dangling or shaking an arm. Frequently, this athlete has sustained an injury commonly known as a *burner* or *stinger,* which is often a stretch or direct blow to the brachial plexus. The burning pain with associated shoulder and arm weakness usually abates in a few minutes; in a few instances, weakness may persist for a few days to a few months. This injury is thought to be caused by a blow that hyperextends the neck or causes lateral flexion of the neck away from the side of the injury, with or without a concomitant blow to the shoulder. Traction of the brachial plexus produces paresthesias in the shoulder, radiating down the arm and frequently into the hand. The athlete may complain of pain in the area of the trapezius muscle, but the injury seldom, if ever, should be associated with true cervical spine pain. Bilateral symptoms are strongly suggestive of spinal cord injury rather than plexus injury. The athlete should be removed from the game, and appropriate imaging studies should be taken to rule out the possibility of spinal stenosis in an individual with bilateral paresthesias or weakness.

Occasionally, symptoms of a burner are caused by pinching of a cervical root resulting from compression from a blow to the head. If cervical spine tenderness is present, this should not be considered a burner, and the athlete should be disqualified from participation until further evaluation of the neck can be performed. Cervical disc herniation also may present as a burner. Careful questioning of the athlete may reveal pain originating from the cervical spine. Manual axial compression of the head and neck often reproduces the symptoms. Suspicion of a cervical disc disorder warrants further evaluation such as a magnetic resonance imaging scan and consultation with a surgeon.

Brachial plexus injuries have been classified as first, second, or third degree, based on clinical and electromyographic study results. Most brachial plexus nerve injuries fall into the category of grade I and last for seconds to minutes. Theoretically, an interruption in function has occurred without anatomic damage. The decision regarding return to play is based on a careful strength assessment of the upper extremities. When the athlete feels completely recovered, his or her head and neck should be put through a range of motion against resistance. The shoulder girdle musculature and forearm muscles also should be tested against resistance. If no pain or weakness is reported by the athlete, return to competition may be allowed. Occasionally, an athlete may have persistent weakness that lasts for several weeks or several months. This indicates that a grade II injury with anatomic axonal damage has been sustained. A grade III brachial plexus nerve injury produces motor and sensory deficits of at least 1 year's duration. Fortunately, this injury is rare.

Any persistent weakness disqualifies an athlete with a brachial plexus injury from further sports activity. The trapezius pain frequently persists beyond the paresthesia and need not disqualify an athlete from competition. The cause of trapezius pain is not well understood. The athlete should be reexamined 24 to 48 hours after injury, because neuronal dysfunction resulting from edema may be delayed. Appropriate cervical spine films, including anteroposterior (AP), lateral, oblique, and flexion and extension lateral views, should be taken the first time any athlete sustains this injury, to ascertain whether congenital anomalies are present.

The athlete who sustains a burner in football or hockey should be fitted with a protective collar over the shoulder pads to limit neck movement. Other methods of limiting neck motion (e.g., straps) also exist and probably offer some protection against brachial plexus injury. Increasing overall neck strength is an important aspect of preventing these injuries.

INTRODUCTION TO ORTHOPEDIC INJURIES

In general, musculoskeletal problems are the most common reason for athletes to seek medical attention. Athletes are likely to delay seeking care until significant disability is present because they are taught to deny pain at an early age. In other words, most athletes tend to disregard minimal injuries and to obtain health care only when something is seriously wrong. Although most injuries are exacerbated and recovery is prolonged by continued participation in a sport, some injuries do not preclude participation, and in some the athlete may play safely in the presence of pain.

Definitions

The terms *strain* and *sprain* frequently are used incorrectly; often, the former is meant to suggest a minor injury and the latter to indicate a more significant injury. A sprain is defined accurately as any injury to a ligament or joint capsule. A strain is any injury to a muscle or tendon. Acute traumatic orthopedic injuries may warrant a visit to the pediatrician, but many of the visits are prompted by overuse injuries caused by cumulative microtrauma instead of one single impact, or macrotrauma. Strenuous athletic activity frequently produces microscopic tissue breakdown, but the body's capacity to heal usually repairs this breakdown before significant injury occurs. When the tissue trauma exceeds the body's healing capacity, tissue damage and edema result in pain, a signal that a clinical injury has occurred. Repetitive microtrauma to a tendon may produce tendinitis. Once thought to be a tenosynovitis, a painful tendon in an athlete usually is a result of tissue damage within the substance of the tendon, rather than inflammation of the synovial sheath. It may be more appropriately called tendonopathy. With repeated loading of bone, a stress fracture may be produced. In the skeletally immature athlete, especially during a period of rapid growth, muscle-tendon overload at the traction growth plate apophysis may produce a stress reaction. This injury is called an apophysitis. Tibial tubercle apophysitis (Osgood-Schlatter syndrome), calcaneal apophysitis (Sever syndrome), and iliac crest apophysitis are but a few examples of this phenomenon. Although the suffix *-itis* is used for many of these overuse injuries, most injuries involve a minimal inflammatory response. With most overuse injuries, simple rest helps, but a rehabilitation program speeds recovery and aids in preventing recurrences. Many overuse injuries develop when a change in the training regimen causes an increase in repetitive microtrauma. For example, a runner with an overuse injury should be questioned about any change in weekly mileage, terrain, or intensity of the workout. Identifying the cause of the overuse injury is important in providing treatment and preventing repetitive injury.

Grading of Injuries

Quantifying the severity of a sports injury is somewhat subjective, but grading systems do exist that make classification reasonably objective for most injuries. A sprain is graded as being either first, second, or third degree. A grade I sprain is one in which a few fibers within a ligament are torn. Clinically, little pain and swelling, a full range of motion, and no increased joint laxity occur. In a grade II sprain, significant numbers of fibers are torn and a detectable increase in joint laxity exists, but at least a few fibers are intact. Clinically, significant pain and swelling exist, with impairment of range of motion. In a grade III sprain, the entire ligament has been disrupted, and marked laxity is evident when the ligament is stressed.

Strains, or injuries to the muscle, are more difficult to evaluate than are sprains. Grading is based primarily on the clinical findings. In a grade I strain, only a few fibers are torn, and, clinically, only a little pain or contraction of the muscle against resistance is present. Strength testing reveals little, if any, loss of strength. In a grade II strain, significant numbers of muscle fibers have been injured, and, clinically, marked pain is noted on palpation and muscle contraction against resistance, as well as significant loss of strength (resulting more from a protective inhibition of recruitment than from actual muscle injury). A grade III strain involves a complete rupture of the muscle. This rupture actually occurs most commonly at the muscle-tendon junction, and it usually requires surgical repair.

Overuse injuries, such as tendinitis, are graded from I to III based on symptoms. A grade I injury produces pain only during athletic activity. A grade II injury produces pain for some time after the athletic activity. A grade III injury causes pain throughout the day and may disrupt sleep.

Treatment Modalities

Cryotherapy often is administered effectively by placing ice in a resealable plastic bag and applying the bag to the site of injury. The application of ice reduces edema and inflammation by causing vasoconstriction. Maximal vasoconstriction is produced in 15 to 20 minutes. Heat should not be applied to any acute injury for at least 72 hours, because the vasodilation it produces may increase bleeding and edema.

Antiinflammatory medications have been used liberally in sports medicine in an effort to reduce inflammation and edema in patients with acute and chronic injuries. They have not been studied well for use in soft tissue injuries in athletes, and, with newer evidence that they may impede healing, the use of these drugs has become more controversial. Their use for analgesia may be helpful during the rehabilitation period. Acetaminophen is the least expensive analgesic medication, and ibuprofen is more effective in some athletes. Athletes should be discouraged from using medication before practice and competition. Pain should be used as a guide in determining appropriate level of activity and for monitoring progress.

BACK INJURIES

Low back pain in athletes can be quite disabling, but the pain generally resolves within 2 weeks, often before medical care is sought. Athletes who seek medical care for back pain often have had pain for several weeks or intermittently for months and have tried to continue their sport until they are unable to compete. The differential diagnosis of back pain in the athletically active child or adolescent is very broad. In addition to mechanical causes, metabolic, neoplastic, and infectious origins should be kept in mind. In young athletes, however, the most common causes of back pain are mechanical.

Muscle Strain

Probably the most likely cause of low back pain in young athletes is acute or chronic muscle strain. This tends to occur in children who have a functional hyperlordosis of the lumbar spine in the standing position. The athlete usually has loss of flexibility and benefits from regular back exercises that increase flexibility. Significant hamstring muscle tightness also is a common finding and contributor. A flexibility program should include these muscles.

Spondylolysis

Spondylolysis is another significant cause of low back pain in the adolescent athlete. Young athletes who participate in sports that involve repetitive hyperextension of the low back, such as gymnastics, may sustain stress fractures of the pars interarticularis of the lower lumbar spine. While bending, these patients frequently can touch their toes or even put their palms on the floor with their knees extended, yet most have marked hamstring tightness. The spondylolysis may be unilateral or bilateral. When radiography is ordered, it always should include oblique views, because these may provide the only means of detecting this lesion (Fig. 130.1).

Lifters of heavy weights and football linemen who sustain loading of the spine in extension may experience pain from spondylolysis. When the pars defect is bilateral, there may be some slippage of the vertebrae on occasion, which is called spondylolisthesis. Increased slippage is uncommon, but it should be evaluated by an orthopedist.

Epiphyseal Injury

A less common condition in an athlete is Scheuermann epiphysitis, which typically occurs in the thoracic area. Irregularities of the epiphyses may be evident on radiography. Scheuermann disease is associated with a kyphotic deformity and wedging of the vertebrae. The athlete must limit athletic activities. Occasionally, a brace is necessary to halt progression of the deformity.

Herniated Disc

Disc protrusion should be considered in the evaluation of an adolescent with low back pain. Although it occurs less

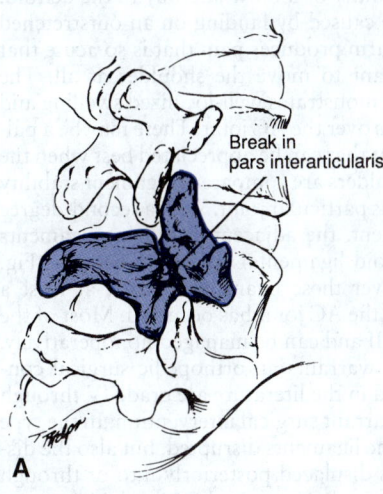
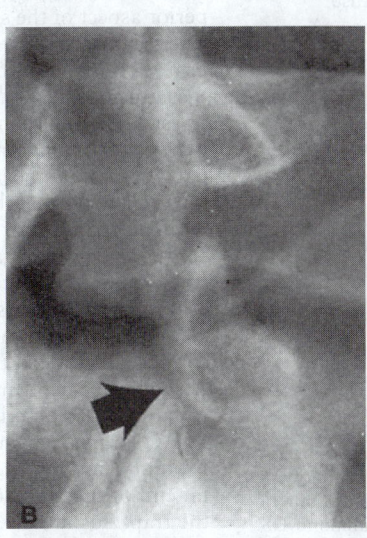

Break in pars interarticularis

A

B

FIGURE 130.1. Anatomy (**A**) and radiographic evidence (**B**) of spondylolysis. Spondylolysis is a break in the continuity of the pars interarticularis, which can be seen as a lucency on the oblique radiograph.

frequently in young athletes than in adults, disc protrusion tends to occur in athletes who are loading the spine repeatedly, predominantly during participation in football and basketball. The diagnosis can be difficult to make in adolescent athletes because they often do not have sciatica, which is the radiating pain down the sciatic nerve that is associated with disc disease in adults. Avoidance of heavy lifting, use of an antiinflammatory agent, and a regular back exercise program often allow the individual to resume athletic activities once the symptoms abate.

Evaluation of Back Pain

In evaluating the athlete who has low back pain, the history may not be as helpful as the physical examination. The athlete may not volunteer neurologic symptoms, and these must be inquired about specifically. In addition, the physician should ask about any changes in bladder or bowel control that the patient may have experienced. Pain that occurs only with athletic activity, especially in hyperextension, is suggestive of spondylolysis. A family history of back pain, especially that caused by disc pathology, may be indicative of a familial predisposition to the problem.

The examination of the athlete with low back pain should begin with careful observation of the individual standing as well as walking. Assessment of range of motion should be performed while the patient is standing. The presence of pain with flexion, extension, or lateral movement should be noted. The athlete also should be asked to twist in both directions to see whether this produces pain; pain produced with this maneuver is suggestive of spondylolysis or disc protrusion. Pain that occurs when the patient extends the back while standing on one leg (single leg hyperextension test) also is suggestive of spondylolysis.

The athlete should be asked to lie prone on the examining table for palpation of the entire spine and back. Deep palpation to localize the maximal area of tenderness may be diagnostic (Fig. 130.2). The neurologic status of the lower extremities should be examined. Straight leg raising tests should be per-

formed to determine whether stretching of the sciatic nerve reproduces pain. Care should be taken not to confuse the discomfort produced on stretching of the hamstrings with stretching of the sciatic nerve. Hamstring flexibility is more appropriately tested with the hip flexed to 90 degrees. Many athletes with low back pain of various origins have inflexible hamstrings that either contribute to or are a result of the pathologic process that is present.

Radiography of the spine should be performed in most cases. In a patient with acute low back pain and no history of trauma, it may be reasonable to wait for 2 weeks after the injury before obtaining radiographs, because the pain often resolves within that interval. Studies of back pain in children and adolescents, however, have shown that the yield of pathologic features on plain radiographs is much higher than that in adults with low back pain. If the history and physical examination are suggestive of spondylolysis, oblique views of the lumbosacral spine should be obtained to look for a pars interarticularis defect. A technetium bone scan may be necessary to confirm the clinical suspicion of acute spondylolysis.

Treatment

In general, even when the cause of low back pain is unclear, a trial of rest, antiinflammatory medication, and a back exercise program is helpful. Because of the poor flexibility of many of these athletes, consultation with a physical therapist often is beneficial for instruction in a back exercise program. As with adults, young athletes benefit from sleeping on their side in a fetal position on a very firm mattress. Occasionally, significant muscle spasm is associated with the low back pain. Heat usually relieves the spasm, but muscle relaxants may be warranted in a few cases. In terms of competition, as with many other injuries, athletes can use pain as their guide, avoiding maneuvers that produce pain. The athlete will need to understand that back pain usually does not resolve quickly and that the exercise program probably is the most important part of the treatment.

INJURIES TO THE UPPER EXTREMITY

Acromioclavicular Sprains

The most common acute shoulder injury is the acromioclavicular (AC) sprain, also known as a shoulder separation. The mechanism of injury of the AC sprain involves a blow to the superior aspect of the shoulder or a blow laterally to the deltoid. The sprain also may be caused by landing on an outstretched arm. Abduction of the arm produces pain that is so acute that the athlete may not want to move the shoulder at all. The physical examination demonstrates well-localized swelling and marked point tenderness over the AC joint. There may be a palpable step-off at the joint that can be appreciated best when the injured and normal shoulders are compared. Ligament stability is difficult to assess at this particular joint. With a second-degree sprain of the AC ligament, the adjacent stabilizing ligaments (the trapezoid and conoid ligaments) also must be torn (Fig. 130.3). If tenderness over these ligaments occurs, at least a second-degree sprain of the AC joint has occurred. Most of the sprains are graded I to III and can be managed nonoperatively. A significant deformity warrants an orthopedic surgical consultation. Also described in the literature are grade IV through VI AC sprains, which warrant surgical intervention. In the type IV injury, not only are the ligaments disrupted, but also the distal end of the clavicle is displaced posteriorly into or through the trapezius muscle. A grade V sprain disrupts the ligaments and the muscle attachments with a marked displacement of the

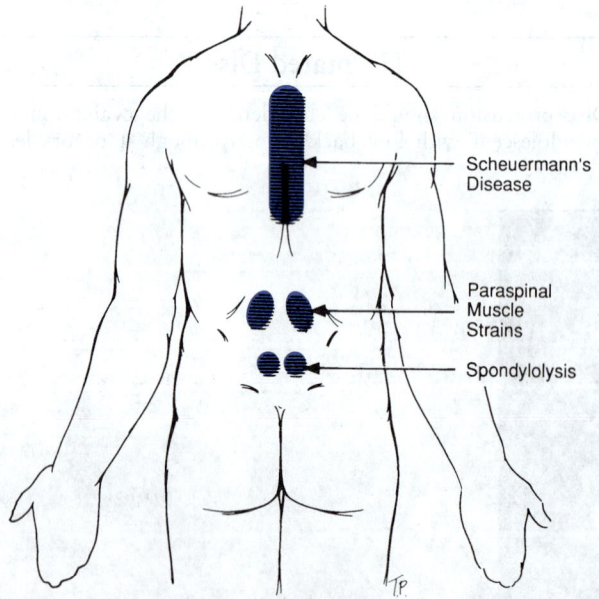

FIGURE 130.2. Palpation of the back and mechanical causes of low back pain. Pictured are the sites of pain and tenderness in the following causes of mechanical low back pain: Scheuermann epiphysitis, muscle strain, and spondylolysis. (Modified from Keene JS, Drummond DS. Mechanical low back pain in the athlete. *Compr Ther* 1985;11:7.)

Scheuermann's Disease

Paraspinal Muscle Strains

Spondylolysis

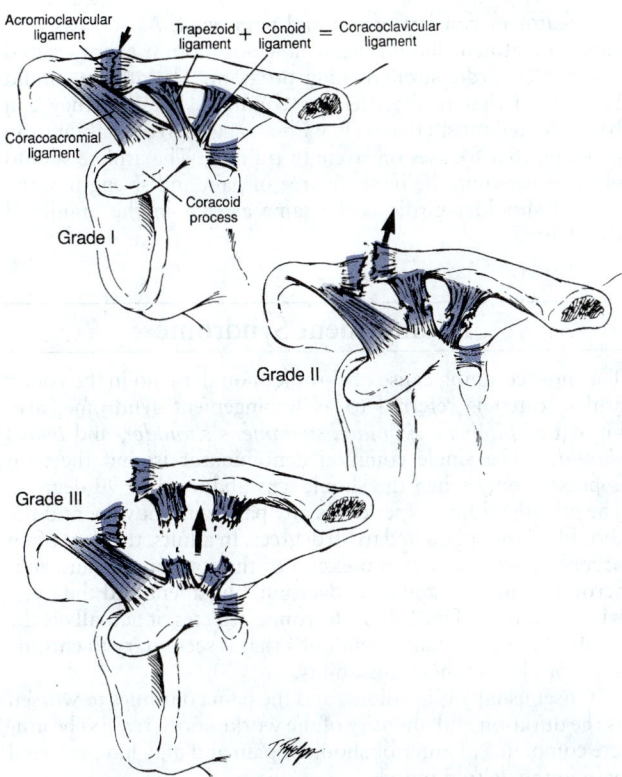

Acromioclavicular ligament   Trapezoid ligament + Conoid ligament = Coracoclavicular ligament

Coracoacromial ligament

Coracoid process

Grade I

Grade II

Grade III

FIGURE 130.3. Acromioclavicular (AC) sprains. A grade I sprain implies damage to the AC ligament without displacement of the clavicle. A grade II sprain means subluxation of the AC joint caused by disruption of the AC ligament and damage to the trapezoid and conoid ligaments. In the grade III sprain, all three of these ligaments are disrupted completely.

distal clavicle superiorly. The grade VI injury produces an inferior dislocation of the distal clavicle in which the distal clavicle is inferior to the coracoid process and posterior to the biceps and coracobracialis tendons.

Radiography may show an elevation of the distal clavicle. Distinguishing a second- from a third-degree injury by AP views with and without weights is not necessarily helpful. Both injuries are best treated functionally nonoperatively. An axillary view may help the clinician to determine the position of the distal clavicle as described in grade IV through VI injuries.

Treatment of the grade I through III AC sprain involves immobilization for pain relief. As soon as possible, as pain improves, range-of-motion and strengthening exercises should be started. The athlete should be warned that there may be some cosmetic defect after an AC sprain, and there may be a noticeable bump with callus formation.

Surgical management of third-degree sprains is controversial, but it usually is performed for cosmetic reasons only. Analgesic medication for pain relief and intermittent icing are helpful adjuncts to the exercise program. With collision sports such as hockey and football, additional padding such as a foam doughnut pad or a more rigid Orthoplast (a moldable plastic) splint under the shoulder pad helps the athlete feel more secure in competition and helps to prevent repeat injury. To return to competition, the athlete must have full range of motion of the shoulder with no pain and must have full strength of the shoulder girdle muscles.

Sternoclavicular Sprains

Although significantly less common than the AC sprain, the sternoclavicular (SC) sprain can be just as painful and dis-

abling, and in some cases it can be life-threatening. If complete disruption of the ligaments occurs, anteriorly or posteriorly, dislocation of the clavicle may occur. If the dislocation is posterior, it can be life-threatening as a result of compression of the trachea and great vessels in the neck. To treat this injury, outward traction on the arm and posterior shoulder traction may reduce the posterior dislocation. If that is unsuccessful, grasping the proximal clavicle with a surgical towel clip and pulling the clavicle anteriorly should reduce the dislocation. For this life-threatening injury, a towel clip should be kept in the medical bag on the field. In the skeletally immature individual, an SC injury usually is not a dislocation but a physis fracture of the proximal clavicle, with anterior or posterior displacement of the fracture.

The physical examination is remarkable for well-localized tenderness and swelling over the SC joint, and any movement of the shoulder, especially adduction, may produce pain. The SC joint and proximal physis of the clavicle are difficult to see on plain radiographs, but generally they are seen best on the serendipity view (an AP view of the SC joint, with 30 degrees of cephalad tilt of the x-ray beam). Tomograms or computed tomographic scanning may be required for differentiation of fracture and dislocation.

Treatment of a first-degree SC sprain is entirely symptomatic. A sling is used for the first few days, and then the patient is provided with range-of-motion exercises. A second- or third-degree sprain is treated with a figure-of-eight appliance for approximately 3 to 6 weeks, as is a reduced fracture.

Glenohumeral Dislocation

Anterior shoulder dislocations are far more common than posterior dislocations, and they have a high recurrence rate regardless of how they are treated. There still is a great deal of controversy regarding the best method of conservative management of these injuries. Some studies document that the recurrence rate is no different between patients treated with an early functional rehabilitation program that is begun as soon as the patient can tolerate it and those who are rigidly immobilized for 3 weeks. Return to competition is not allowed in either case until full range of motion and essentially equal strength in comparison with that of the uninjured shoulder returns.

Glenohumeral Subluxation

Glenohumeral subluxation probably is more common than frank dislocation in young athletes. Shoulder subluxation can be more difficult to diagnose, but it can cause just as much pain and disability as dislocation. Subluxations may occur anteriorly, posteriorly, and, occasionally, inferiorly.

Anterior subluxations occur as a result of a forceful abduction and external rotation, such as happens in making an arm tackle. The athlete is aware immediately that the shoulder slid. Treatment is the same as for the anterior dislocation, and the recurrence rate is similarly high.

Posterior subluxation usually occurs with the arm outstretched, such as when a baseball player slides headfirst. This produces posterior pain, but the athlete may not have noticed any pop or feeling of instability at the time of the injury. Subluxation of the shoulder posteriorly probably can be produced in more than 50% of physiologically normal individuals on clinical examination. With this in mind, the uninjured shoulder always should be evaluated as well.

Examination of the shoulder reveals guarding, with marked tenderness over the glenohumeral joint in the area of the subluxation. After an anterior subluxation, the athlete often has apprehension when the shoulder is taken into abduction and

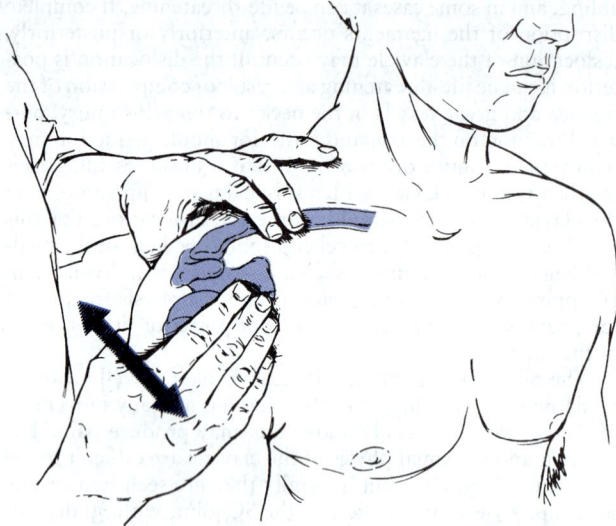

FIGURE 130.4. The shoulder drawer test (also called the *glide test*). To demonstrate anterior and posterior glenohumeral instability in the right shoulder, the left hand is placed on top of the shoulder so the clavicle and the scapula are stabilized. The right hand is free to create traction on the humeral head to push or pull it in and out of the glenoid fossa.

external rotation. Pain is produced when traction is placed on the humeral head in the direction of the subluxation. This can be demonstrated by performing a shoulder drawer test (Fig. 130.4).

Treatment consists of rest and pain relief. As soon as possible, the athlete should begin range-of-motion exercises and a shoulder girdle strengthening program. The athlete should be advised that recurrences are common, but that they can be prevented most effectively with an aggressive rehabilitation program that focuses on strength training. The athlete should not compete until he or she is free of pain and strength in the injured shoulder girdle is the same as that in the uninjured shoulder.

Impingement Syndrome

The most common cause of chronic shoulder pain in the young athlete often is referred to as impingement syndrome, also known as *pitcher's shoulder, swimmer's shoulder,* and *tennis shoulder.* The single common denominator is that the pain is present only when the shoulder is abducted to 90 degrees. The athlete seldom experiences any pain with movement if the shoulder is not abducted to 90 degrees. In adults, the pain often occurs as a result of compression of the rotator cuff and subacromial bursa by the coracoacromial ligament and the overlying acromion (Fig. 130.5). In young athletes, it actually is the result of a supraspinatus tendinitis that is secondary to chronic anterior glenohumeral instability.

Onset usually is insidious, and the pain continues to worsen as the duration and intensity of the workouts increase. The athlete complains of anterior shoulder pain and may have referred pain in the deltoid muscle.

On examination, the athlete usually experiences the greatest tenderness to palpation over the greater tuberosity, just anterior

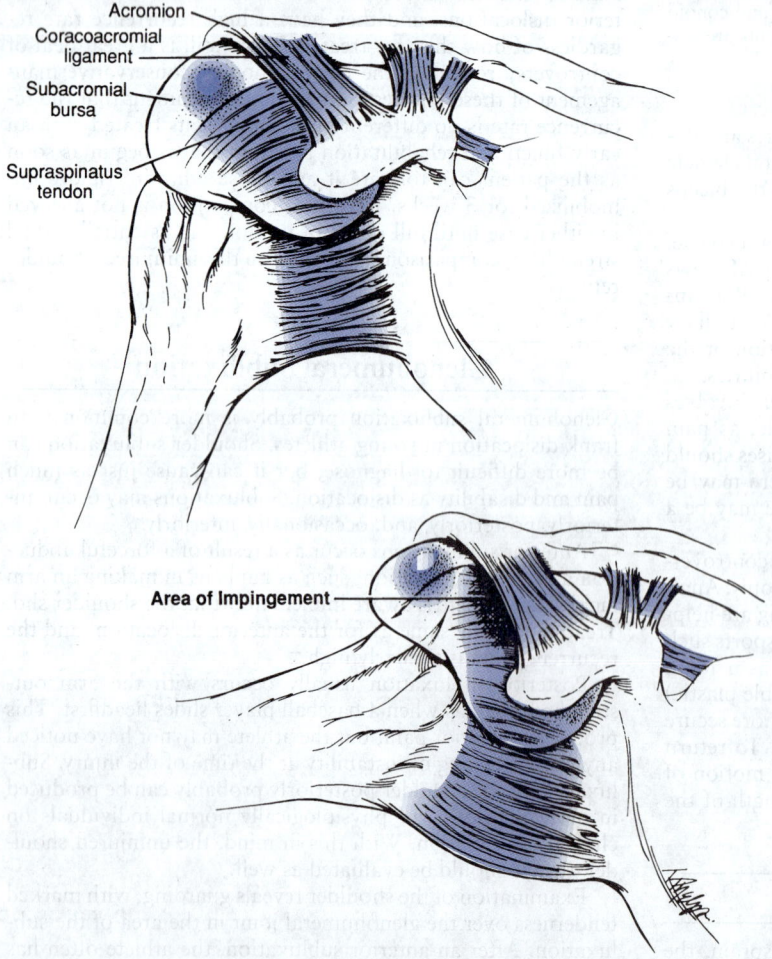

Acromion
Coracoacromial ligament
Subacromial bursa
Supraspinatus tendon

Area of Impingement

FIGURE 130.5. Anatomic basis for impingement syndrome. Impingement syndrome involves the compression and inflammation of the subacromial bursa and the supraspinatus tendon between the humerus and the coracoacromial ligament along the inferior edge of the acromion.

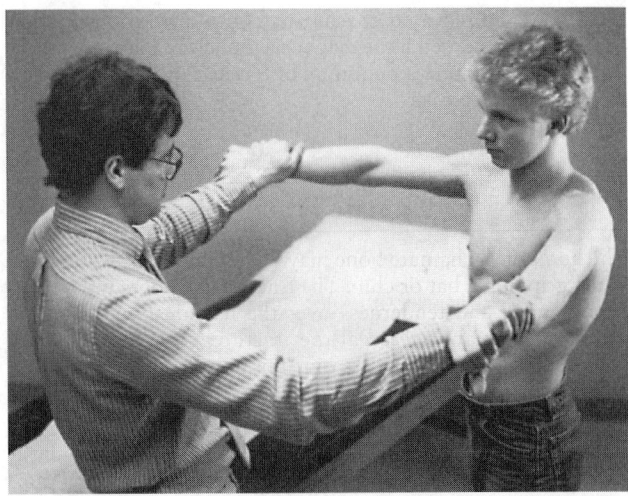

FIGURE 130.6. Strength assessment of the supraspinatus muscle. With the patient standing and facing the examiner, the patient's arms are abducted to 90 degrees, forward flexed 30 degrees to the parasagittal plane, and placed in internal rotation. Resistance to elevation of the arms (examiner pushes downward) selectively tests the supraspinatus muscles.

and lateral to the edge of the acromion. Typically, the athlete has pain with tests for impingement. One impingement test requires taking the shoulder up to 180 degrees of forward flexion actively or passively. This may produce pain, especially if the shoulder is adducted across the face. Another impingement test is performed by placing the shoulder at 90 degrees of abduction and 30 degrees of forward flexion with the arm held in internal rotation. Forced internal rotation may reproduce the pain. Palpation of the bicipital groove may reveal tenderness, because biceps tendinitis also may occur in those with chronic impingement syndrome. An athlete with impingement syndrome may have relatively weak muscles involved in external rotation and poor flexibility in internal rotation. Pain may be produced with strength testing of these muscles, especially the supraspinatus, which is the most superior muscle in the rotator cuff group. This is tested best by placing the arms in 90 degrees of abduction, forward flexed to 30 degrees and internally rotated. Resistance to further elevation of the arms selectively tests the supraspinatus (Fig. 130.6). Tests for glenohumeral instability also should be performed.

Treatment of impingement syndrome involves rest, or at least a decrease in activity. Ice applied to the subacromial area for 15 to 20 minutes after activity helps to reduce pain and inflammation. Analgesic medication also provides some relief. As in many overuse injuries, rehabilitation is the key to treatment of this injury. A strengthening and stretching program for the supraspinatus usually is different from any exercises the athlete previously has been taught. The strengthening program is especially important in the young athlete because the pain is usually secondary to glenohumeral instability. As in many overuse injuries, it may take 6 to 8 weeks to resolve this problem entirely. After 3 or 4 weeks of intense rehabilitation, however, the athlete usually notes significant improvement. In a small percentage of patients, conservative management fails, and a surgical procedure for stabilization or decompression is required.

Acute Elbow Injuries

Acute trauma to the elbow is important because fractures of the elbow tend to involve the physes. Radiography of the

elbow should be performed if any swelling or significant bony tenderness is present. In the absence of an obvious fracture, the radiograph should be examined carefully for an effusion, which usually is evident on the lateral view because of elevation of the fat pad in the coronoid fossa. The fat pad sign on the lateral view is diagnostic of hemarthrosis with an acute injury. This usually warrants orthopedic consultation for further studies to identify the cause of the effusion as well as to determine treatment.

Olecranon Bursitis

Swelling over the olecranon may be caused by olecranon bursitis. A blow over the end of the olecranon may cause bleeding into the bursa, with immediate swelling and tenderness. This injury is painful, but low risk exists for permanent disability. Occasionally, the bursa is tense enough to limit motion. In some cases, sterile preparation of the skin and needle aspiration are warranted for pain relief. After the bursa is drained, a tight pressure dressing should be applied, and the elbow should be rested for at least 24 hours. The elbow is a difficult area to pad, although an athlete can fashion a doughnut-type foam pad to relieve some of the pressure over the bursa.

Lateral Epicondylitis

Commonly known as *tennis elbow*, lateral epicondylitis is an overuse injury of the extensor muscles and tendon that attach over the lateral epicondyle of the distal humerus. It essentially is small tears in the tendinous insertion. This injury is associated with racket sports because of the persistent contraction of the wrist extensors that is required to maintain a strong grip on a racket. Lateral elbow pain in a tennis player often can be traced to a change in racket, a change in grip, a significant increase in playing time, or an attempt to learn to put topspin on the ball. However, lateral epicondylitis is unusual in an adolescent athlete. Subacute or chronic lateral elbow pain needs to be evaluated for Panner disease (osteochondrosis of the humeral capitellum), especially in a gymnast or pitcher who has lateral elbow pain.

Point tenderness over the lateral epicondyle at the insertion of the extensor mass in the elbow is indicative of lateral epicondylitis. Forced resistance to extension also produces pain. There should be no swelling about the elbow and no loss of range of motion. Radiography probably is not necessary early in this problem, unless a history of an injury exists.

The key to the treatment of lateral epicondylitis is a diligent rehabilitation program outlined by a physical therapist or trainer. This involves regular stretching and strengthening of the extensor muscle-tendon unit. Ice applied after exercise helps to reduce some of the pain and inflammation. An anti-inflammatory medication makes the athlete more comfortable. Rest speeds healing, although it is not always necessary for the athlete to refrain totally from activities. This problem takes at least 6 to 8 weeks to resolve, and the athlete often needs a lot of encouragement along the way. Most experts believe that local injections of corticosteroid or surgical procedures rarely are necessary.

Flexor-Pronator Tendinitis

Flexor-pronator tendinitis usually is seen in patients who are involved in throwing and racket sports. Athletes complain of pain over the medial aspect of the elbow. This condition is seen often in young pitchers when they are learning to throw breaking pitches. This throwing motion creates valgus stress, loading the medial aspect of the elbow, including the ulnar collateral ligament and the pronator teres muscle and tendon. Associated with stress and inflammation of the medial structures is inflammation of the ulnar nerve. Ulnar nerve symptoms in the adolescent usually are indicative of dislocation or subluxation of the ulnar nerve.

Examination of the elbow usually demonstrates the maximal area of tenderness to be the pronator mass and, to a lesser extent, the area at the medial epicondyle. Pain frequently is present, with resistance to pronation and flexion of the wrist. Occasionally, the medial collateral ligament (MCL) may be inflamed, and stress on the ligament with the elbow flexed at 30 to 40 degrees may produce pain. Pain may be produced with palpation of the ulnar nerve and the groove. Percussion of the nerve may reproduce paresthesia if any edema or inflammation of the nerve in the groove exists. If tenderness over the ulnar nerve is found, the nerve should be examined for dislocation or subluxation when the elbow is flexed past 90 degrees. A careful neurologic examination of the hand should be performed to check for evidence of ulnar nerve dysfunction.

Radiography should be performed in any young athlete who has acute medial pain to determine whether the medial physis has been disrupted. Stress of the physis may cause an avulsion fracture, which classically has been associated with excessive Little League pitching and has been called *Little League elbow*. Little League elbow is a misused term that has been applied to virtually any child with elbow pain, however, and is not a specific diagnosis.

As with lateral epicondylitis, flexor-pronator tendinitis is treated with rest, antiinflammatory medication, and rehabilitation. Ice applied to the elbow after any kind of activity helps to reduce some of the pain and swelling. Rehabilitation is the key to successful treatment in the long term. Stretching and strengthening of the pronator teres muscle help to resolve the problem and prevent recurrences. In sports that involve throwing, a change in the athlete's throwing mechanics often is helpful as well.

Wrist Sprains

The most common injury to the wrist involves the disruption of one or more of the numerous ligaments in the wrist. Many mechanisms of injury may cause ligament damage to the wrist, but there may not be much swelling or pain with this injury. Pain to palpation and pain with stress of the corresponding ligaments are consistent with the diagnosis of a sprain (e.g., tenderness dorsally and pain with hyperflexion of the wrist). Radiography should be performed because it may be difficult to distinguish a fracture from a sprain based on physical examination alone. Treatment involves immobilization in the form of a wrist splint, application of ice, and use of antiinflammatory medication. The time required for healing is variable.

Navicular Fractures

Falling on an outstretched hand may cause a fracture of the carpal navicular (scaphoid) bone. This fracture may not always produce noticeable swelling, but palpation of the anatomic "snuff box" produces pain. The navicular bone has a marginal blood supply, and this may lead to delayed healing or, on occasion, to avascular necrosis, especially when the diagnosis of fracture is delayed. Radiography should be performed with navicular views. When tenderness is present, even if the radiography results are negative, the patient should be cast in a thumb spica cast for 2 to 3 weeks. Physical and radiographic examina-

tion should be repeated at that time. Orthopedic consultation should be considered if the diagnosis is unclear. Navicular fractures usually require a minimum of 8 weeks of immobilization in a thumb spica cast.

Hamate Fractures

The hook of the hamate bone may be fractured during a fall or while gripping a bat or club. The fracture produces wrist pain, a poor grip, and tenderness over the hamate bone. Routine radiography may not reveal the fracture, so a carpal tunnel view should be obtained. Treatment is immobilization in a cast with incorporation of the little finger. An orthopedist should be consulted, because the rate of nonunion is high.

Finger Injuries

The most common injury involving the hand is the finger sprain. Sometimes called a *jammed finger*, it usually is the result of hyperextension of the proximal or distal interphalangeal joint. The sprain may produce moderate swelling and tenderness, with some limitation of motion. Careful palpation of the finger reveals tenderness about one or both of the collateral ligaments and frequently tenderness over the volar plate (palmar ligament). Flexion and extension should be examined carefully at each joint in the finger to rule out a disruption of the flexor or extensor mechanisms, such as mallet finger (disruption of the terminal extensor mechanism) or the boutonnière deformity (rupture of the insertion of the central extensor tendon). Stability of the joint should be assessed, by comparing ulnar and radial laxity with stress and AP laxity with stress with the contralateral joint in the other hand.

Radiographic evaluation should be considered in all patients with significant finger injuries. The degree of swelling or tenderness does not distinguish sprains from fractures. One should be quick to obtain films of the dominant hand in an athlete, especially of the thumb and index finger, which are so important functionally.

Finger sprains are treated in a position of function, with splints applied for comfort. As soon as it is comfortable, the finger should be taken out of the splint to allow for range-of-motion exercises. If the finger is left in the splint indefinitely, the fibrosis that occurs after hematoma can cause stiffness and loss of motion. Splints should be used to protect the finger from further injury as long as any tenderness remains over the joint. One of the easiest and most comfortable methods used to splint the sprained finger is by "buddy taping" (taping the injured finger to the adjacent finger).

The athlete's ability to return to play should be determined on an individual basis, because the severity of the sprain, the athlete's position on the team, and the type of sport are important considerations. Sometimes the injured finger is easy to protect. For example, a football lineman can have the entire hand bandaged in a fist, thus giving the injured finger a great deal of protection.

One particular sprain in the hand can be quite troublesome. The *skier's thumb* or *gamekeeper's thumb* is a sprain of the ulnar collateral ligament of the metacarpal-proximal phalangeal joint. This sprain is produced when an athlete lands on an outstretched hand and the thumb is deviated excessively radially. If a third-degree sprain occurs and is treated inadequately, the result may be long-term instability of the joint. The third-degree sprain warrants orthopedic consultation, because open repair or casting may be required.

INJURIES TO THE LOWER EXTREMITY

Iliac Crest Contusion

In contact sports, a blow to the iliac crest may produce a periosteal hematoma, which often is painful and disabling. Commonly known as a *hip pointer,* this injury can cause the athlete to miss several days or weeks of practice time and games. Usually, the contusion involves the anterior superior iliac crest. Treatment consists of ice and rest. When the athlete can sprint at full speed without a limp, return to competition is allowed. Reinjury is painful but is unlikely to result in any permanent disability. Padding of the area can be achieved with a large foam doughnut pad.

Iliac Apophysitis

Iliac apophysitis is seen almost exclusively in adolescent cross-country and distance runners. The aching pain over the iliac crest is insidious in onset. There usually is marked tenderness to palpation of the iliac crest, most often at the anterior superior iliac crest. AP and oblique radiography should be performed in any patient who has an acute onset of symptoms to rule out an avulsion fracture of the anterior superior iliac spine.

Treatment of this entity involves rest, ice application, and antiinflammatory medication. The athlete should discontinue running until no pain exists on palpation of the involved area. The pain usually resolves completely after 4 to 6 weeks of complete avoidance of running. Permanent sequelae from this injury have not been reported.

Quadriceps Contusion

A blow to the thigh may result in a large contusion within the quadriceps muscles. There may be massive bleeding to the point that shock may be induced. This injury can be painful and debilitating. On physical examination, a large, tender mass can be palpated within the muscle, and pain is produced with flexion of the knee. The severity of the damage cannot be assessed until 24 to 48 hours after the injury has occurred, but it correlates highly with the expected amount of time that will be lost from play and the risk that myositis ossificans will develop. If knee flexion is greater than 90 degrees, the injury is categorized as being grade I. If flexion is 45 to 90 degrees, it is grade II, and if less than 45 degrees of knee flexion exist, the injury is considered to be grade III. The incidence of myositis ossificans in grade III injuries is high, even if they are treated properly. Application of ice to the area and cessation of athletic activity are important to stop the acute bleeding. For at least 72 hours after the injury occurs, rest, ice, compression, and elevation should be used to minimize bleeding and edema. The use of heat may increase bleeding. Crutches should be used if the patient limps. The key to rehabilitation of this injury is the initiation of gentle, painless stretching of the quadriceps muscles as the hematoma resolves. Strengthening of the quadriceps also is important. Return to competition is based on full and painless range of motion, no pain to palpation, a minimum of 85% strength of the quadriceps compared with that in the uninjured leg, and completion of the running program (Table 130.5).

Femoral Stress Fracture

If a young running athlete has persistent vague thigh pain, a femoral stress fracture should be considered strongly. Usually

TABLE 130.5

RUNNING PROGRAM*

1. Jog 1/2 to 1 mile. Stop immediately if you are limping or if there is pain. Wait until tomorrow to start the program again. If there is no pain or limp during your jog, you may proceed to:
2. Six to eight 80-yard sprints at one-half speed. If no pain or limp, then do:
3. Six to eight 80-yard sprints at three-quarter speed. If no pain or limp, then do:
4. Six to eight 80-yard sprints at full speed, followed by four to six full-speed starts. If no pain or limp, then do:
5. Six to eight 80-yard cutting sprints (changing directions every 10 yards) at half speed. Then do:
6. Six to eight 80-yard cutting sprints at full speed.

After every workout, ice should be applied immediately to the injured area. (Do not stand around.)

Once you can perform all the previously listed tasks with no pain and minimal swelling, you may return to competition. If you take shortcuts on this program, you are only fooling yourself and are risking reinjury or possibly a more serious injury and a much longer time out of competition.

*This is a running program that can be given to the athlete so the criteria for return to competition are clear and the athlete can work toward a goal.

seen in high-mileage distance runners, the injury can be overlooked for weeks. The aching pain occurring with exercise has an insidious onset, and the physical examination often is non-localizing or the pain appears to be muscular in origin. If the pain has persisted for several weeks, the periosteal reaction may be seen only on oblique radiography. If the results of plain radiography are negative, a technetium bone scan is necessary to make the diagnosis.

Vague anterior groin pain may represent a femoral neck stress fracture. Prompt diagnosis with radiography or a technetium bone scan is important, because delay in diagnosis can lead to a displaced fracture, which is associated with a high risk of poor long-term outcome. Magnetic resonance imaging is also being used to diagnose stress fractures in the long bones.

Medial Collateral Ligament Sprains

In contrast to ankle injury, knowledge of the mechanism of injury can be helpful in determining the diagnosis of the acutely injured knee. The MCL sprain probably is the most common knee ligament injury to occur in contact sports. It occurs with valgus stress, such as happens with a blow to the lateral aspect of the knee. If the injury is mild, it may not produce much immediate disability, and the athlete may be able to continue to play for several more minutes. With significant bleeding and inflammation over the ligament, the athlete usually has a limp and must leave the game or practice.

In patients with an isolated MCL injury, examination of the knee reveals a trace to mild effusion. The presence of a large and tense knee effusion usually is indicative of an intraarticular injury or a patellar dislocation and is not consistent with an isolated MCL sprain. Point tenderness exists over the MCL, often at the middle portion of the ligament. Full extension may be limited because it stretches the MCL, and the ligament is more relaxed at 30 degrees of flexion. Pain is produced with stress of the MCL, which is examined best with the patient lying supine and the knee in 20 to 30 degrees of flexion. With the table supporting most of the weight of the leg, the femur is stabilized with one hand, and the ankle is grasped with the

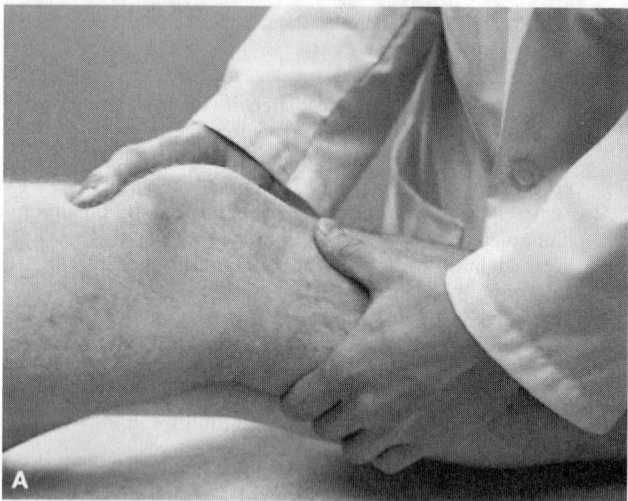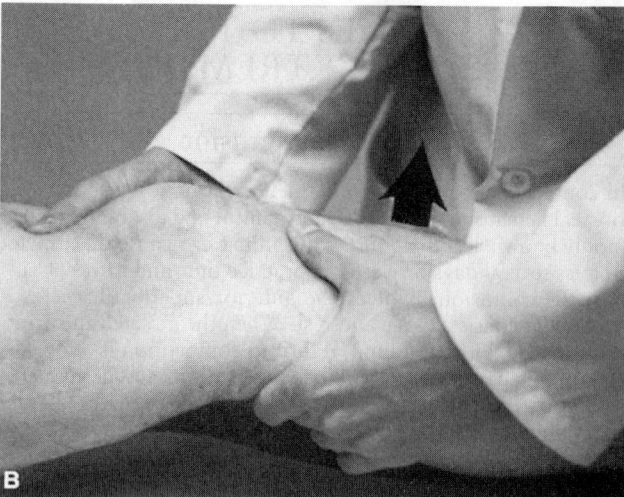

FIGURE 130.7. Lachman test. With the patient supine, the knee is flexed to 20 to 30 degrees. **A:** While the femur is stabilized with one hand, the tibia is grasped with the other hand. **B:** When pulled anteriorly in the absence of the anterior cruciate ligament, the tibia moves excessively anteriorly.

other hand. Outward stress is applied gently to the ankle to produce valgus stress to the knee, and the severity of the sprain is graded according to the degree of laxity noted. The knee should be examined for other ligament injury as well.

Radiography should be performed to rule out a fracture. If the physes are open, stress radiographs must be taken. The MCL sprain is treated in a fashion similar to the ankle sprain. Rest for 2 to 3 days and the use of crutches often provides pain relief, along with antiinflammatory medication, ice, compression, and elevation. As with the ankle sprain, rehabilitation is the key to ensuring a quick return to competition. Even with a third-degree sprain, rehabilitation is vital, and MCL injuries no longer are treated surgically unless another injury is involved. The criteria for an athlete's return to play are similar to those for ankle sprain. The athlete must have no pain, full range of motion, strength equal to at least 85% of that of the uninjured leg, and no swelling, and he or she must have completed the running program without pain or limp (see Table 130.5).

Anterior Cruciate Ligament Sprain

In contrast to the MCL sprain, an anterior cruciate ligament (ACL) sprain produces swelling of the knee in the first several hours after the injury occurs. Bleeding from the ligament usually produces a tense hemarthrosis. The ACL sprain almost always is a third-degree sprain, meaning that the ligament is disrupted completely.

The ACL tear usually is a noncontact injury caused by hyperextension of the knee or sudden deceleration of the leg with the foot flexed. Frequently, the athlete hears a loud pop. The injury is very painful, and the athlete seldom is capable of continuing to play.

If the athlete is evaluated on the field, stability testing for the ACL injury is extremely important. In the absence of bleeding or inflammation, the athlete will have less guarding, and the examination will be more accurate. Several hours after the injury, the knee is tender and swollen, and the athlete may object to any movement of the knee, which makes examination difficult. The large, tense effusion that is seen 24 hours after the injury is grossly bloody on aspiration. More than 85% of all acute tense hemarthroses are caused by ACL disruptions. (Patella dislocations are the second most common cause of acute hemarthroses.)

On physical examination, the most important test to perform is the Lachman test. The traditional anterior drawer test, performed with the knee at a 90-degree angle, is not as sensitive. The Lachman test is an anterior drawer test with the knee held in 20 to 30 degrees of flexion. One hand is placed on the femur to stabilize it, the other hand is used to grasp the proximal tibia, and anterior stress is applied to the tibia (Fig. 130.7). Loss of ACL integrity allows excessive anterior motion, compared with motion in the normal knee. Any hamstring spasm negates the results of this test. Occasionally, the athlete may injure the MCL in addition, and examination for this injury should be performed also.

Radiography should be performed, especially in an adolescent with open physes who may have a tibial plateau fracture instead of an ACL tear. (This is an avulsion fracture of the ACL, and it requires urgent attention from an orthopedic surgeon.) For an ACL tear, treatment with a knee immobilizer, crutches, and pain relief is reasonable; a surgical consultation should be obtained within the next 2 weeks. Arthroscopy or magnetic resonance imaging often is used to examine the menisci, because a meniscus tear also is demonstrated in 30% to 40% of patients with ACL tears.

Treatment of the acute ACL tear in most, but not all, cases requires surgery. A patient with an ACL-deficient knee is likely to have recurring instability. Surgical advances have led to excellent results in patients who have chosen surgical stabilization. Careful evaluation and discussion with the athlete about his or her preference are critical. Cast immobilization of an isolated ACL tear is to be condemned; it does not allow for healing and only adds to muscle atrophy and prolongs the rehabilitation process.

Posterior Cruciate Ligament Sprain

Far less common than the ACL sprain, injury to the posterior cruciate ligament (PCL) also is not as disabling. The injury is caused by a forceful blow to the tibia that drives it posteriorly, usually with the knee flexed (e.g., sustaining a fall on the knee with the foot in plantar flexion, striking the tibia, may disrupt the PCL). The athlete usually complains of posterior knee pain but does not have instability. On physical examination, an effusion is found, but it usually is small. The Lachman test results seldom are positive; a positive finding may indicate a more extensive injury. With the knee flexed to 90 degrees, on palpation of the medial and lateral femoral condyles and the anterior tibial plateau, an 8- to 10-mm plateau step-off is noted in the normal knee. If the step-off is completely lost, the tibia is displaced posteriorly, and the diagnosis of a complete PCL injury is made readily. Radiography should be performed in patients with suspected PCL injuries, because bony avulsion of the PCL may occur in the pediatric age group. Patients with bony avulsion of the PCL should be treated surgically; excellent static results can be achieved.

Treatment for a PCL injury is similar to that for an MCL sprain, including rest, ice, antiinflammatory medication, and a rehabilitation program. Isolated PCL deficiency rarely is a problem of functional instability once the athlete has completed a rehabilitation program, although some athletes have significant early traumatic arthritis. Surgical treatment of isolated PCL injury is controversial, because the prevalence of traumatic arthritis in athletes with a PCL-deficient knee is unknown. The results of surgical stabilization are not yet satisfactory.

Patellar Dislocation and Subluxation

Although not as common as the ACL tear, the combination of patellar dislocation subluxation is the second leading cause of acute hemarthrosis. The athlete occasionally says that the kneecap "went out of joint." With the knee flexed and some degree of valgus stress applied, the athlete feels the knee give way and may report an audible pop; he or she may indicate that the knee went back into the joint when it was straightened.

The diagnosis often can be made based on the physical examination alone. With careful palpation, marked tenderness is demonstrated over the medial aspect of the patella, the medial retinaculum, or the adductor tubercle. For subluxation or dislocation of the patella to result, there must be disruption of the medial retinaculum and the vastus medialis muscle, which is attached to the adductor tubercle and the intermuscular septum. The adductor tubercle is located just superior to the proximal attachment of the MCL (Fig. 130.8). The knee also should be examined for any ligament injury. Radiography should be per-

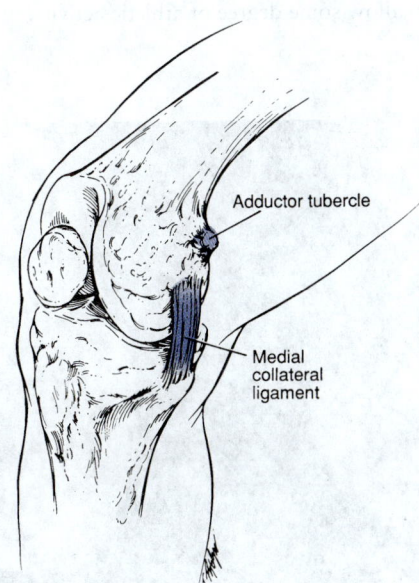

FIGURE 130.8. Adductor tubercle. When the patella is dislocated, the medial retinaculum often is torn at its attachment to the adductor tubercle. The adductor tubercle can be palpated easily just superior to the proximal attachment of the medial collateral ligament.

formed, because subluxation and dislocation can produce an avulsion fracture. If a fracture is present, surgical intervention may be required.

Treatment of the athlete for pain relief consists of the use of a knee immobilizer and crutches. Antiinflammatory medication or a narcotic agent may be necessary to achieve adequate pain relief during the first few days after injury. Although the risk of recurrence is high, few surgeons operate for a first episode unless a significant fracture occurs. Regaining range of motion and strengthening the upper leg muscles are imperative for an athlete to be able to resume play. Each patient must be assessed individually, but knee immobilization usually is maintained for only 3 to 5 days. The time required for full rehabilitation is variable. When the knee is rehabilitated completely, a patellar stabilizing device such as a Palumbo or a Bioskin knee sleeve helps to prevent recurrences (Fig. 130.9). These knee sleeves are designed to give the patella lateral pressure to prevent lateral excursion of the patella in the femoral groove.

Prepatellar Bursitis

A blow to the patella can cause contusion of the prepatellar bursa and bleeding within the bursa. Sometimes the injury is called *turf knee* or *wrestler's knee* because it usually results from a fall that strikes the patella on hard turf or a wrestling mat.

Physical examination reveals marked anterior swelling directly over the patella. Palpation of the center of the patella reveals ballotable fluid; in contrast, joint effusion demonstrates fluid around the patella but not directly anterior to it. Flexion of the knee is painful. Treatment includes ice, compression, and, rarely, aspiration of the bursa. Aspiration of the bursa invites infection, and the injury usually can be managed conservatively. Padding the area is difficult, and recurrences are common. The swelling does not preclude participation if the athlete has full range of motion and symmetric strength and can pass a functional examination.

Peripatellar Contusion

A blow to the soft tissues around the patella can cause a large hematoma to develop. A second mechanism of this injury is forced knee flexion while the quadriceps muscles are contracted. A tearing in the distal vastus medialis muscle causes bleeding into the subcutaneous tissue about the knee. The resolving hematoma in either case may develop into a large fluid collection around the patella. When the contusion is severe, the large amount of blood may take weeks to reabsorb, thus slowing efforts at rehabilitation. If the hematoma is aspirated, hemorrhage frequently recurs unless significant compression is applied, and the patient must refrain from activities involving knee flexion. Management is similar to that for the quadriceps contusion (see previous discussion).

Patellofemoral Stress Syndrome

The most common complaint heard in most sports medicine clinics is that of chronic patellar pain. Sometimes known as *chondromalacia*, this entity also is called runner's knee, peripatellar pain syndrome, patellalgia, and patellofemoral stress syndrome (PFSS). Chondromalacia is an inappropriate term for most of these chronic pain conditions because it is a specific pathologic diagnosis. When patients with this problem are examined surgically, no abnormality of the articular surface is found in more than 50% of them. The most appropriate term for the condition is PFSS. This syndrome is a common problem

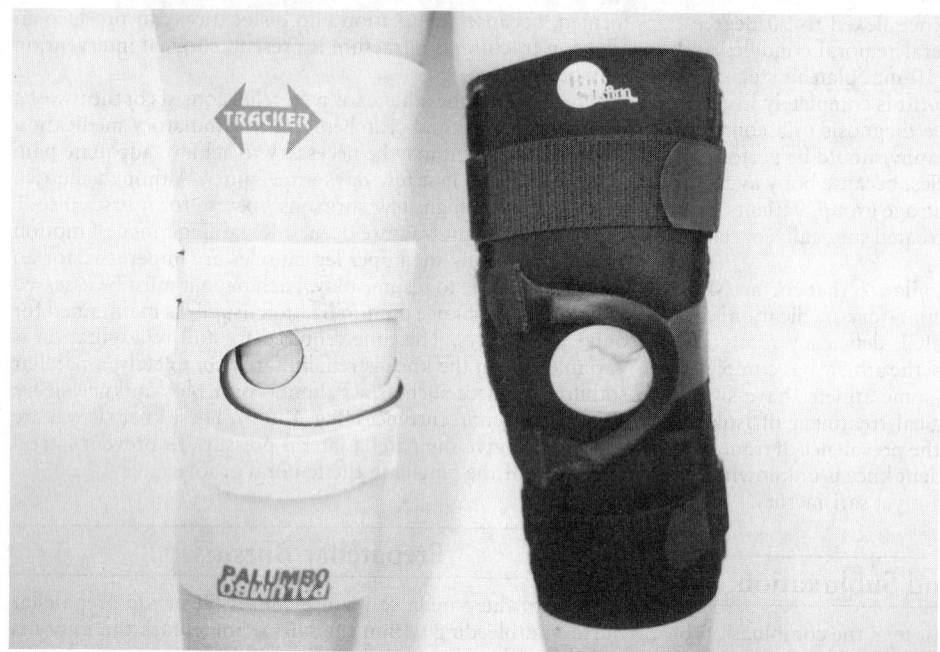

FIGURE 130.9. Patellar stabilizing devices. Shown are the Palumbo (on this athlete's right knee) and Bioskin (on the left knee) knee sleeves, which are designed to give the patella lateral pressure to prevent subluxation and dislocation.

in athletes who run; many chronic injuries to the lower extremity occur in distance runners or in athletes who participate in sports that involve running, such as soccer.

The origin of the pain in patients with PFSS is thought to be subchondral stress or synovial inflammation. Patients typically have a history of dull, aching knee pain that is difficult to localize. Movement of the knee may be associated with a clicking or popping sound. The pain is worse with activity, especially running and going up and down stairs. Exacerbations may occur with prolonged sitting, especially in the back seat of a car with the knees fully flexed. The pain also is brought on or aggravated by any trauma to the patella. There may be "giving way" of the knee, which commonly is associated with pain. There usually is no history of swelling. The history or presence of swelling should prompt consideration of another diagnosis.

On physical examination, firm palpation of the patella often reveals tenderness over the medial facet. This may require some medial displacement of the patella with palpation of its undersurface medially. There also may be tenderness over the lateral facet of the patella or at any point along the patellofemoral joint line. Compression of the patella in the femoral groove produces pain, which sometimes is called a positive compression test result. Patellofemoral pain is associated with hypermobile patellae as well as patella alta (high-riding patella). Often, the athlete has evidence of malalignment, such as femoral anteversion and external tibial torsion. Gait analysis often reveals ankle valgus and excessive pronation of the foot (Fig. 130.10). This also may be seen by examining the patient's worn shoes, which show breakdown of the heel counters medially and a worn sole medially.

Radiography should be performed in any athlete with more than 4 to 6 weeks of pain. Any history or evidence of swelling also warrants radiography. AP, lateral, tunnel, and patellar views should be obtained for complete evaluation of the knee. The sunrise view no longer is considered optimal for assessment of the patellofemoral joint. The Laurin and Merchant views are more helpful in diagnosing patellofemoral disorders, especially patellar subluxation. Performed with less knee flexion, each of these views is obtained using a different radiologic technique. The tunnel view is especially important for the growing adolescent, who is at risk for osteochondritis dissecans, usually of the medial femoral condyle.

The treatment of PFSS usually is not surgical. Modification of activities to avoid full flexion of the knee and stress of the patellofemoral joint is imperative. A strengthening program for the quadriceps mechanism and a stretching program, especially for the hamstring muscles, often improve the patient's symptoms. Some athletes also benefit from exercises that strengthen their hip muscles. In the athlete with excessive foot pronation, treatment should include the use of semi-rigid orthoses. Judicious use of ice and antiinflammatory medication usually is helpful. The athlete should be warned that patellar pain tends to be chronic, with exacerbations and remissions. The pain can be a lifelong problem, depending on the patient's activities. The goals are to educate the athlete about means of controlling the pain and to allow some degree of athletic activity.

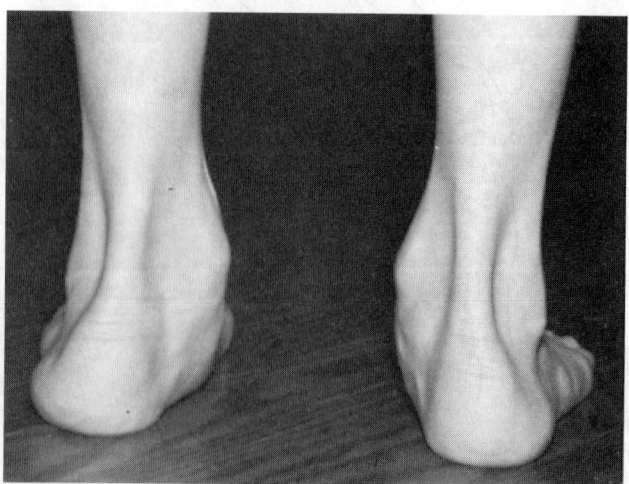

FIGURE 130.10. Ankle valgus and excessive foot pronation. This patient has marked ankle valgus bilaterally and excessive foot pronation standing.

Patellar Tendinitis

Another common cause of chronic anterior knee pain is patellar tendinitis. Also known as *jumper's knee,* it is seen most often in athletes who participate in sports that involve running and jumping, especially basketball and volleyball. The onset of pain is insidious, and it rarely is disabling. The injury consists of a microscopic fatigue tear at the insertion of the patellar tendon into the inferior pole of the patella.

The physical examination reveals point tenderness of the patellar tendon at the infrapatellar pole in 80% to 90% of patients. The remaining patients have tenderness of the quadriceps tendon at the superior attachment to the patella. Frequently associated with this problem is poor flexibility of the quadriceps and hamstring muscles.

Treatment includes rest, ice, antiinflammatory medication, and frequent stretching of the quadriceps and hamstring muscles. The athlete may continue to engage in the sport, but this may prolong the course of the tendinitis. With complete rest from running or jumping for 6 to 8 weeks, an athlete may be able to recover fully. Recurrences are common, and the pain can become more resistant to treatment as a result of scarring within the tendon.

Osgood-Schlatter Disease

In skeletally immature athletes with open tibial physes, swelling and point tenderness at the tibial tubercle are indicative of Osgood-Schlatter disease, which is associated with running and jumping in these individuals. This condition probably represents tiny stress fractures in the apophysis and is associated with a rapid growth spurt. Ice, antiinflammatory medication, and a decrease in activity help the young athlete to manage this problem. Treatment is similar to that of PFSS. The only permanent sequela is a prominence of the tibial tubercle, which rarely represents a cosmetic problem. Immobilization through the use of a knee immobilizer or crutches occasionally is necessary in patients who have severe pain. A few athletes continue to play until they are unable to walk without a limp. Regardless of the severity of the condition, the long-term prognosis is excellent, and chronic pain or disability is uncommon.

Iliotibial Band Friction Syndrome

The most common cause of lateral knee pain in a runner is known as iliotibial (IT) band friction syndrome. The IT band crosses the lateral femoral epicondyle before inserting into the tibia. Friction and pain can be produced when the IT band is taut, such as occurs in the downside leg when the athlete runs on banked roads consistently against traffic. No history of swelling or giving way occurs, but the runner describes dull, aching pain associated with the activity.

On occasion, demonstration of tenderness in this area on physical examination may be difficult, so it may be helpful to examine the runner after he or she has completed a workout. It should be possible to reproduce the patient's symptoms by applying firm pressure over the IT band at the lateral femoral epicondyle while flexing and extending the knee (Noble test).

Treatment for this problem consists of rest, a course of antiinflammatory medication, and the use of a flexible orthosis with a 1/8-in. medial heel wedge. Probably the most important aspect of treatment is instruction of the patient in IT band stretching, which must be done faithfully. This problem may not resolve without a minimum of 6 weeks of rest from running. The athlete should be cautioned about running consistently on only one side of the road, with its inherent drainage pitch. Running on alternating sides of the road or on level ground is encouraged. A tight IT band also may produce a friction syndrome over the greater trochanter at the hip (trochanteric bursitis). The pathophysiology of this condition is similar, and stretching of the IT band again is an important part of the treatment regimen. In both areas, the chronic bursitis may persist; if rest and stretching fail to provide relief, a local injection of soluble corticosteroid into the bursa should be considered.

Shin Splint Syndrome

Lower leg pain is a common reason for a young runner to seek medical attention. The most common cause of this pain is shin splint syndrome, which also is known as medial tibial stress syndrome. The athlete complains of aching pain that increases gradually in intensity throughout the exercise regimen. The pain improves greatly with rest. Shin splints often are related to overtraining, especially in the school-aged athlete who has not been doing much distance running before cross-country or track season begins. On physical examination, marked diffuse tenderness occurs over the posteromedial aspect of the tibia at the insertion of the soleus muscle. The tenderness with shin splint syndrome usually is present over the distal half of the tibia, as opposed to a tibial stress fracture, which tends to produce tenderness somewhere in the proximal half of the tibia. Ankle valgus and excessive pronation of the foot frequently are seen on gait analysis. Mechanically, the excessive pronation stresses the soleus muscle at its origin at the posterior medial aspect of the tibia. Treatment of the excessive pronation with better footwear or semi-rigid orthoses usually is key to producing resolution and preventing recurrences. Rest, ice, and antiinflammatory medication are helpful along with frequent calf stretches, which stretch all the ankle plantar flexor muscles. Some runners benefit from strengthening the ankle dorsiflexors. Athletes usually do not have to stop running completely, but they must decrease significantly the intensity and duration of their workouts.

Tibial and Fibular Stress Fractures

If the athlete with shin pain has a well-localized area of tenderness over the tibia or fibula, a stress fracture should be considered. An athlete with this condition often complains of pain at the start of the running activity that lasts for the duration of the workout. On physical examination, diffuse tenderness may be noted along the medial aspect of the tibia or lateral aspect of the fibula, but one area usually is significantly more tender than the rest. A stress fracture may be difficult to demonstrate radiographically, because the only abnormality seen may be a small area of periosteal reaction at the site of the fracture, without an actual cortical defect. Moreover, plain radiographs do not reveal evidence of a stress fracture until it has caused pain for at least 2 weeks. When a stress fracture is suspected, AP, lateral, and both oblique views should be obtained, because more of the periosteum is visualized tangentially. A technetium bone scan may be required to make the diagnosis. Most tibial stress fractures heal with rest from running and do not require cast immobilization. When point tenderness on palpation or pain with running has abated, the athlete may resume training. The fracture usually takes approximately 6 to 8 weeks to resolve, but some individual variability exists in the rest period required for healing. To maintain cardiovascular fitness while allowing the fracture to heal, the athlete should bike, swim, or run in water, as long as these activities do not produce pain.

Chronic Compartment Syndrome

Lower leg pain that is worse after running should raise the concern of a chronic compartment syndrome. Instead of pain that occurs during the entire workout, the athlete reports that the first 5 to 10 minutes of the run are essentially free of pain. Once the muscles are warmed up, however, aching, pounding leg pain may persist for several minutes to hours after the workout is completed. The athlete localizes the pain to a diffuse area of one of the muscle compartments, most commonly the anterior lateral. The pain is caused by elevated pressure within the muscle compartment resulting from a relative inadequacy of the musculofascial compartment size. The athlete may complain of numbness or weakness corresponding to nerve compression in that compartment. For example, the anterior lateral compartment may involve the peroneal nerve, with tingling over the dorsum of the foot and weakness to dorsiflexion of the great toe.

Physical examination may be normal or reveal tenderness to palpation of the medial tibia or anterior fibula, but careful palpation reveals that the maximum area of tenderness really is a diffuse area of one of the muscle compartments. To confirm the diagnosis, the athlete requires compartmental pressure measurements after exercise. If the pressure is elevated, fascial release is necessary to allow the patient eventually to train without pain. Rarely, an athlete may have an acute compartment syndrome and require an emergency fascial release.

Ankle Sprains

The most common acute injury to the lower extremity is the ankle sprain. The athlete usually reports twisting the ankle, but may not remember the details of the injury. There may be an audible pop at the time of the injury. Unlike in other sports injuries, knowledge of the mechanism of injury of an ankle sprain is not very helpful. A fair amount of swelling often is noted, with disruption of the ankle ligaments as a result of bleeding. Approximately 90% of ankle sprains are of the lateral ligaments, caused by inversion of the ankle or a combination of inversion and plantar flexion of the ankle. A small percentage are medial sprains involving eversion of the ankle.

Physical examination of the ankle involves the application of applied surface anatomy. Careful palpation of the structures reveals the maximal area of tenderness to be over the ligaments. If any bony tenderness is present, a fracture should be suspected, and radiography should be obtained. Stability testing may be difficult to perform if the athlete is seen a day or two after the injury, because of marked pain and muscle spasm. The most common ankle sprain involves one or both of the lateral ligaments, which are the anterior talofibular and the calcaneofibular ligaments. The anterior talofibular ligament is examined with the anterior ankle drawer test. With the tibia stabilized with one hand and the calcaneus grasped with the other hand, the examiner places traction on the talus anteriorly (Fig. 130.11). Increased laxity, as compared with laxity in the uninjured ankle, implies that at least a second-degree sprain has occurred. If a poor end-point exists (i.e., a marked diminution in resistance to stress of the ligament), a third-degree sprain of that ligament has occurred. Inversion testing with the ankle in slight plantar flexion tests the calcaneofibular ligament. Comparison with the patient's uninjured ankle is imperative, because ligament laxity varies a great deal from athlete to athlete. Eversion testing with the ankle in a neutral position reveals any instability of the deltoid ligament. In some ankle sprains, there may be a great deal of pain but no increased laxity. Careful palpation may reveal tenderness over the deltoid ligament, the lateral ligaments, and anteriorly over the inferior tibiofibu-

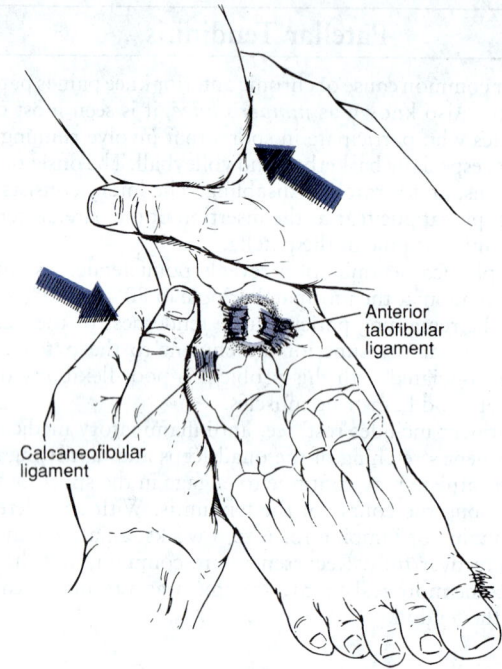

FIGURE 130.11. Anterior ankle drawer sign. To test the integrity of the anterior talofibular ligament, the tibia is stabilized with one hand, and the calcaneus and talus are grasped with the other. With the ankle in slight plantar flexion and internal rotation, the talus is given traction anteriorly. Excessive motion with this maneuver with a poor end-point is a positive drawer sign and implies a third-degree sprain of the anterior talofibular ligament.

lar ligament. This type of sprain at first may appear to be minor because no appreciable ankle laxity occurs, but the sprain also involves a tear of the interosseous membrane between the tibia and the fibula. Sometimes descriptively called the *ring-around-a-rosy* or *high sprain*, this injury usually takes longer to rehabilitate than do other, milder sprains.

Radiography should be performed in any ankle injury that produces more than minimal swelling or pain with weight bearing. AP, lateral, and mortise views should be included to enable adequate assessment of the ankle mortise. Careful examination of the talar dome radiographically is important because any small fracture seen on the radiograph is indicative of a larger chondral defect.

Treatment of the ankle sprain initially is designed to minimize the hematoma and swelling. The mnemonic RICE is a helpful way to remember *r*est, *i*ce, *c*ompression, and *e*levation as the important modalities with which to achieve this goal. Most athletes benefit from 48 to 72 hours of avoidance of weight bearing through the use of crutches. Compression bandages take many different forms, but a snug elastic wrap suffices. The elastic wrap is even more effective if a U-shaped felt pad is placed over the malleolus to add pressure beneath the wrap. Elevation of the extremity above the level of the heart increases venous return. The worst thing that an athlete with an ankle sprain can do is to continue playing despite the pain. Contrary to popular belief, the common ankle sprain is associated with a significant amount of pain and disability.

The second aspect of treating an ankle sprain concerns resolution of the hematoma. This involves range-of-motion exercises, along with protective weight bearing. An ankle sprain resolves much more quickly with the help of a physical therapist or an athletic trainer who can direct an exercise program. It also is helpful for athletes to have an exercise program provided in writing, to outline goals as well as to provide instruction regarding reasonable progression through the program. Athletes should not ignore pain but should use it as a guide regarding their ability to engage in weight-bearing activities. As soon as they can hop up and down on the affected ankle several times without pain, the athletes are ready to begin the running program (see Table 130.5). Athletes may progress through sprinting and changing directions on the ankle, and they must not be allowed to return to competition until they are able to change direction at full speed on the ankle without experiencing pain or instability.

Protective taping has been shown to be effective in preventing recurrent ankle sprain. Because tape can be expensive and many young athletes do not have access to a coach or trainer who is skilled in ankle taping, a lace-up ankle brace helps to prevent recurrences. High-top shoes probably are helpful in giving the ankle some stability. Surgical intervention rarely is indicated for third-degree ankle sprains. Surgery should be considered in an elite ballet dancer or gymnast, however, because an athlete engaging in this type of activity is less tolerant of ankle instability.

Achilles Tendinitis

Chronic aching pain over the Achilles tendon in a runner usually is caused by Achilles tendinitis, which once was thought to be a tenosynovitis. Most cases probably do involve inflammation of the synovial sheath, but, more importantly, they represent tiny tears in the substance of the tendon.

The examination reveals tenderness located a distance corresponding to the width of approximately two to three fingers above the calcaneal insertion of the tendon. Minimal swelling and crepitus to dorsal and plantar flexion of the ankle may be noted.

Appropriate treatment includes rest, ice, antiinflammatory medication, and gentle static stretching of the muscle-tendon unit. Quarter-inch heel lifts placed in the footwear provide relief and help to reduce stress to the tendon. The athlete with excessive pronation benefits more from using semi-rigid orthoses (arch supports). The athlete who is not a runner may continue to engage in sport but must lighten workouts, especially if they involve any running activity. An athlete who is a runner usually must rest from running for a minimum of 12 to 14 days. When the area no longer is tender to palpation, gradual return to training may be resumed. On occasion, it may take as long as 6 to 8 weeks before the athlete can resume running.

Calcaneal Apophysitis

A school-aged or adolescent athlete who has heel pain associated with a running sport usually has apophysitis of the calcaneus, also known as Sever disease. It frequently is bilateral and rarely produces swelling or discoloration. Examination reveals tenderness on medial and lateral heel compression. Radiography usually is not necessary initially, but should be considered to rule out other diagnoses if the pain does not respond to treatment. Ice, antiinflammatory medication, rest, and heel lifts usually provide relief. Flexible orthoses with a 1/8-in. medial heel wedge should be considered instead of heel lifts for pronated feet. Total rest from weight-bearing activities is not imperative, but it speeds relief.

Plantar Fasciitis

In the older adolescent or teenage runner, chronic heel pain located over the plantar surface of the heel often is caused by plantar fasciitis. This may not come to the attention of a physician until it has been going on for several weeks or months.

Typically, an athlete complains that the pain is most problematic on rising in the morning. After warming up, he or she may be able to run with minimal pain. Palpation reveals marked tenderness over the calcaneus at the insertion of the plantar fascia.

Treatment for this condition consists of rest, antiinflammatory medication, ice, and, most importantly, flexible orthoses with a 1/8-in. medial heel wedge to relieve the stress on the plantar fascia at its insertion on the calcaneus. Some runners do well with new running shoes, which provide a better arch support. Treatment of plantar fasciitis should provide some relief in 6 to 8 weeks, but it often takes 4 to 6 months to resolve totally, even with complete rest.

CONCLUSION

Sports medicine has become an important area of concern in ambulatory pediatrics because the young athletic patient expects the same care that is provided to college and professional athletes. The physician should recognize that the ability to return quickly to play and competition frequently is first on the agenda of the athlete who is seeking medical care. The most common injuries confronting the pediatrician often require the help of a physical therapist or athletic trainer to instruct the athlete in a proper rehabilitation program. Rehabilitation frequently shortens the time necessary for the athlete to spend away from competition and minimizes his or her risk of reinjury on returning to the sport.

Suggested Readings

General

American Academy of Pediatrics, American Academy of Orthopedic Surgeons, Sullivan JA, et al, eds. *Care of the young athlete.* Chicago: American Academy of Orthopedic Surgeons, 2000.
Landry GL, Bernhardt DB. *Essentials of primary care sports medicine.* Champaign, IL: Human Kinetics, 2003.
Mellion MB, Walsh WM, Madden C, et al., eds. *The team physician's handbook,* 3rd ed. Philadelphia: Hanley & Belfus, 2002.

Preparticipation Health Inventory

American Academy of Family Physicians, American Academy of Pediatrics, American Medical Society for Sports Medicine, American Orthopedic Society for Sports Medicine, American Osteopathic Academy of Sports Medicine. *The preparticipation physical evaluation,* 2nd ed. New York: McGraw-Hill, 1997.
American Academy of Pediatrics. Medical conditions affecting sports participation. *Pediatrics* 2001;107:1205.
Feinstein RA. Preparticipation physical examinations: critical controversies. *Adolesc Med State Art Rev* 1997;8:149.
Maron BJ, Mitchell JH. Revised eligibility recommendations for competitive athletes with cardiovascular abnormalities (the 26th Bethesda Conference). *J Am Coll Cardiol* 1994;24:845.

Role of the Team Physician

Committee on Sports Medicine and Fitness, American Academy of Pediatrics. The team physician. In: Dyment PG, ed. *Sports medicine: health care for young athletes.* Elk Grove Village, IL: American Academy of Pediatrics, 1991:48.
Lombardo JA. Sports medicine: a team effort. *Physician Sports Med* 1985;13:72.

Management of Athletic Injuries

McKeag DB. On-site care of injured youth. In: Kelley VC, ed. *Practice of pediatrics,* vol 10. Philadelphia: Harper & Row, 1984:1.

Heat Illness

Armstrong LE, Epstein Y, Grenleaf JE, et al. American College of Sports Medicine position stand: heat and cold illnesses during distance running. *Med Sci Sports Exer* 1996;28:1.
Squire DL. Heat illness: fluid and electrolyte issues for pediatric and adolescent athletes. *Pediatr Clin North Am* 1990;37:1085.

Common Medical Illnesses

Eichner ER. Infectious mononucleosis: recognizing the condition, "reactivating" the patient. *Physician Sports Med* 1996;24:49.
Halstead ME, Bernhardt DB. Common infections in the young athlete. *Pediatr Ann* 2002;31:42.

Sports Nutrition

Bar-Or O. Nutritional considerations for the child athlete. *Can J Appl Physiol* 2001;26(suppl):S186.

Clark N. *Sports nutrition guidebook,* 2nd ed. Champaign, IL: Human Kinetics, 1997.

Earnest C. Preventing nutritional disorders athletes: focus on the basics. *Curr Sports Med Rep* 2002;1:172.

Dermatologic Concerns

Adams BB. Sports dermatology. *Adolesc Med State Art Rev* 2001;12:vii, 305.

Dienst WL, Dightman L, Dworkin MS, et al. Pinning down skin infections. *Physician Sports Med* 1997;25:45.

Common Injuries to the Head and Neck

Ghiselli Cantu RC, Schaadt G, McAllister DR. On-the-field evaluation of an athlete with a head or neck injury. *Clin Sports Med* 2003;22:445.

Hershman EB. Injuries to the brachial plexus. In: Torg JS, ed. *Athletic injuries to the the head, neck, and face.* St. Louis: Mosby–Year Book, 1991:338.

Landry GL. Central nervous system trauma: management of concussions in athletes. *Pediatr Clin North Am* 2002;4:723.

Introduction to Orthopedic Injuries

Adirim TA, Cheng TL. Overview of injuries in the young athlete. *Sports Med* 2003;3375.

Bernhardt DT, Landry GL. Sports injuries in young athletes. *Adv Pediatr* 1995; 42:465.

Back Injuries

Gerbina PG, Micheli LJ. Back injuries in the young athlete. *Clin Sports Med* 1995;14:571.

Metcalf TS, Landry GL. Evaluation and treatment of back pain in the young athlete. *Clin Fam Med* 1999;1:125.

Injuries to the Upper Extremities

Ireland ML, Hutchinson MR. Upper extremity injuries in young athletes. *Clin Sports Med* 1995;14:533.

Lee SJ, Montomery K. Athletic hand injuries. *Orthop Clin North Am* 2002; 33:547.

Metcalf TS, Bernhardt DT. Evaluation and managing shoulder injury in young athletes. *Contemp Pediatr* 1996;13:94.

Pappas AM. Overuse syndromes of the shoulder and arm. *Adolesc Med State Art Rev* 1991;2:181.

Injuries to the Lower Extremities

Biedert RM, Sanchis-Alfonso V. Sources of anterior knee pain. *Clin Sports Med* 2002;3:335.

Chambers HG. Ankle and foot disorders in skeletally immature athletes. *Orthop Clin North Am* 2003;34:445.

Hergenroeder AC. Diagnosis and treatment of ankle sprains: a review. *Am J Dis Child* 1990;144:809.

Quinn K, Parker P, DeBie R, et al. Interventions for preventing ankle ligament injuries. *Cochrane Database Syst Rev* 2000;(2):CD000018.

Waters PM, Millis MB. Hip and pelvic injuries in the young athlete. *Clin Sports Med* 1988;7:513.

CHAPTER 131 ■ FAILURE TO THRIVE

REBECCA T. KIRKLAND

Failure to thrive (FTT) is a sign that describes a particular problem rather than a diagnosis. The term is used to describe instances of growth failure or, more specifically, failure to gain weight in childhood, although in more severe cases linear growth and head circumference may be affected. As stated by Perrin et al., the underlying cause is "insufficient usable nutrition." FTT differs from other causes of poor weight gain or growth failure because of its lack of obvious organic etiology. FTT is attributed to a child usually younger than 2 years whose weight is below the fifth percentile for age on more than one occasion or whose weight is less than 80% of the ideal weight for that age, using the standard growth charts of the National Center for Health Statistics (NCHS). An inadequate rate of weight gain that results in the crossing of two percentiles line over time indicates FTT. Updated growth charts are available from the Centers for Disease Control (CDC) web site at www.cdc.gov.

EPIDEMIOLOGY

FTT is a problem common in pediatric practice, and it accounts for 1% to 5% of all referrals to children's hospitals or tertiary centers. In a rural primary-care setting, 10% of children in the first year of life have had failure to thrive. FTT occurs more frequently among children living in poverty. Up to one-third of cases of FTT in some groups may be undiagnosed.

PATHOGENESIS

Organic versus Nonorganic Etiologies

The distinction between organic causes of FTT and nonorganic or psychosocial etiologies has limited usefulness. In the child with congenital heart disease or other chronic disease, the nonorganic or environmental factors also may contribute to the FTT and should not be overlooked. Likewise, the child within an emotionally disturbed family also may have an organic problem. One-third to more than one-half of cases of FTT investigated in tertiary-care settings and almost all the cases in primary-care settings have nonorganic etiologies. About one-fourth of all cases include a combination of organic and psychosocial factors. In addition, children with FTT of any etiology have significant diminishment of immunologic function and an increased susceptibility for acquiring infections. Studies show that stunted children have higher cortisol levels than nonstunted children, which may contribute to immune responses and to behavioral responses and mental health symptoms.

DIAGNOSIS

A careful, thorough history and physical examination (Table 131.1) of the child whose only sign may be a diminished weight allows a logical, rational approach to the ordering of

TABLE 131.1

CLINICAL APPROACH AND MANAGEMENT FOR FAILURE TO THRIVE

Approach	Immediate Support	Long-Term Support
Careful history Thorough physical examination (plot height and weight on curves) Observation of infant's behavior Psychosocial evaluation (family and environmental factors, home health visits) Judicious approach to laboratory testing, radiology, and imaging	Nutritional support (plot daily intake and weights) Team approach (pediatricians, nurses, social workers, nutritionists, developmental specialists, community service workers, health educators, mental health support, home health visits, child-life workers, volunteers) or temporary/permanent foster home Treatment of uncommon underlying organic illness	Frequent follow-up visits (well-child maintenance, plot heights and weights, developmental assessments) and/or home health visits Developmental intervention Parental guidance/support (substance abuse treatment, housing advocacy, or job training)

laboratory tests and other investigations. Observing the infant at times other than feeding, as well as during feeding, and of the interaction of the child with guardian or parent, and making an assessment of the nutritional, social, and environmental factors yields valuable information regarding the physical ability to feed and swallow as well as the psychosocial milieu. In the absence of evidence for an organic problem in the initial history and physical examination, subsequent laboratory investigation is unlikely to reveal an organic cause.

History

The pediatric history of the patient who fails to thrive should include an elicitation of symptoms suggesting organic diseases. A detailed environmental assessment is essential. Adverse psychosocial circumstances are known to have an association with diminished weight gain and growth in infancy.

A detailed nutritional and feeding history includes information related to duration of feeding time, quantity of food consumed, type of food, and to efficiency of breast-feeding in the breast-fed infant. A deficient caloric intake due to increased losses of nutrients in the stool (malnutrition or diarrhea), vomiting or regurgitation, or impaired utilization can be clarified. A history of food preferences may indicate an avoidance of foods with certain textures. This may suggest an underlying dysfunction that the child is unable to elucidate; for example, the elimination of specific foods from the diet without adequate explanation may present in a child with inflammatory bowel disease, who may avoid foods that cause abdominal discomfort without verbalizing that those foods cause pain. A history of excessive low-calorie liquid or fruit juice ingestion may indicate inappropriate nutrient intake with losses due to fructose and sorbitol malabsorption. A history may reveal an inadequate intake of protein and vitamins in some vegetarian diets. A report of food allergies may lead to the inappropriate restriction of a certain nutrient. An assessment of the parents' knowledge of appropriate nutrition for an infant or child may reveal significant gaps and errors. If a psychosocial problem is suspected, caution should be used when interpreting a dietary history, because parental guilt may result in inaccuracies.

The psychosocial history should include an assessment of the true caretakers and family composition (absent parents), employment status, financial state, degree of social isolation (absence of a telephone or of nearby neighbors), and family stress. Poverty indicators, including eligibility for the Supplemental Food Program for Women, Infants and Children (WIC), should be sought. The history should include whether adequate food is available in the home or whether the caregiver runs out of food on occasion. Maternal factors relating to the pregnancy, such as planned or unplanned pregnancy, young maternal age, use of medications for illness, substance abuse, physical or mental illness, postpartum depression, or inadequate breast milk, may be significant. A maternal history of being abused as a child or of eating disorders may be significant. Assessment should be made of levels of knowledge about parenting and about how to provide an adequate diet.

Predisposing factors in the infant are low birth weight, intrauterine growth retardation, perinatal stress, prematurity, one of a multiple birth cohort, chronic disease, and frequency of intercurrent illness such as diarrhea, vomiting, or otitis media. In the dynamic interaction between the parent and the child, factors in the child, such as being "difficult," chronically ill, or giving diminished feedback, may contribute to the overall problem. Questions regarding the child's sleep pattern, other behaviors, and the amount of time spent alone may be helpful. Mothers who are stressed may use breast-feeding for their comfort as well as for the infant's comfort. In these situations, the stress may diminish the breast-milk supply, leading to frequent breast-feeding and food refusal with poor weight gain in an infant who is referred to as the "vulnerable child."

Family members' heights and weights, their history of illness, and any developmental delay in family members that may contribute to slow growth or constitutional short stature should be included in the assessment. Shorter parental height and higher parity have been shown to be related to slower weight gain in the infant in the Avon Longitudinal Study of Parents and Children. Support systems available to the family and frequency home-address changes should be examined. Initially, parents may avoid mentioning psychosocial problems such as marital discord or spousal abuse; the discussion of such issues should take place during several visits. These conversations should be conducted in a nonthreatening manner, demonstrating concern and compassion.

Simple Observation

The infant's behavior can give valuable clues regarding his ability to interact appropriately for age. Behavioral features suggestive of psychosocial or environmental deprivation may include avoidance of eye contact, absence of smiling or vocalization, and a lack of interest in the environment (Fig. 131.1). The negative response of the child to cuddling and an inability to be comforted may indicate a problem. The child may exhibit repetitive motions such as head-banging, self-stimulatory activity such as anogenital manipulation, or he may be relatively

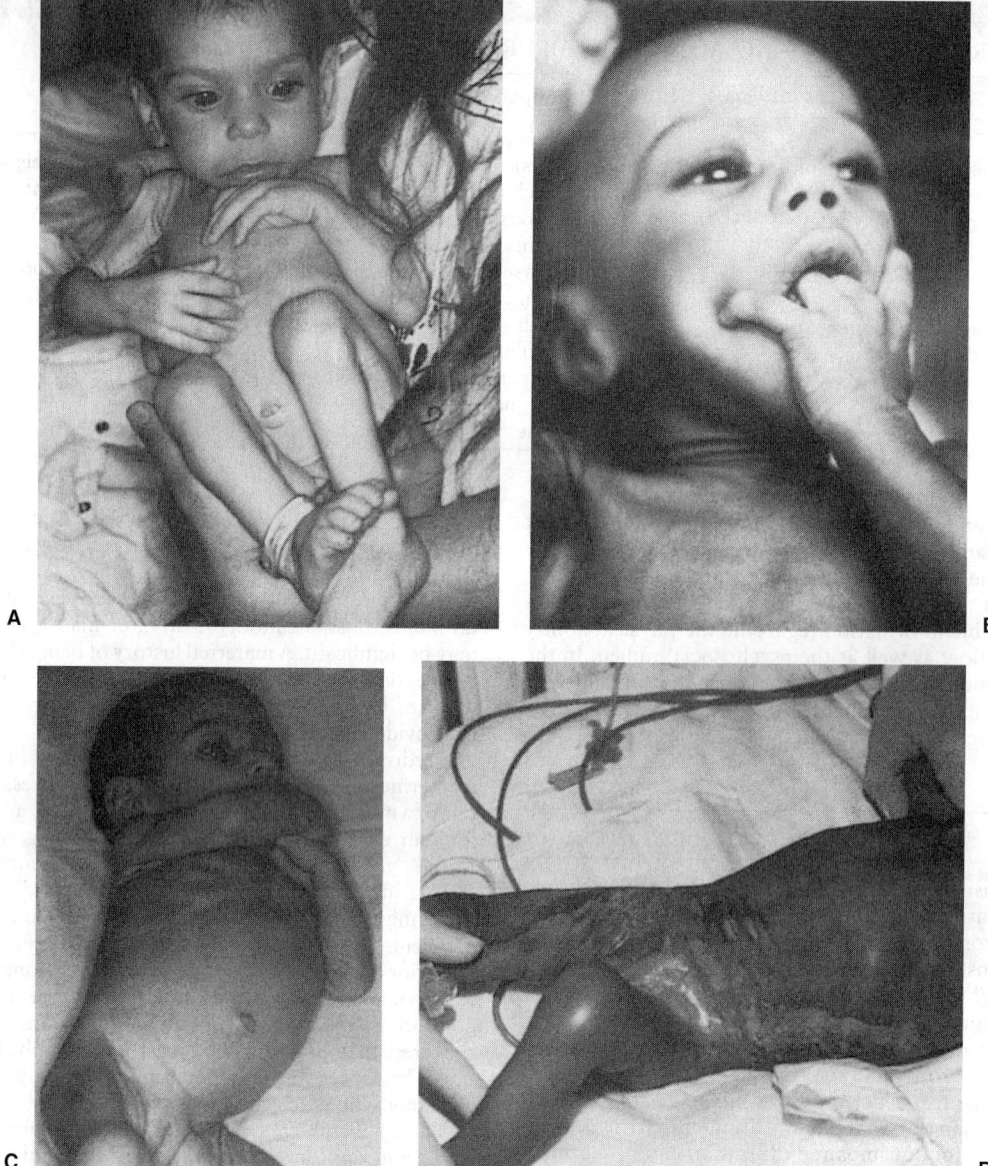

FIGURE 131.1. Physical signs of failure to thrive. **A:** Dull, apathetic eyes that avoid eye contact. **B:** Oral self-stimulatory behavior. **C:** Wasted extremities and protuberant abdomen. **D:** Severe diaper rash as a sign of overall neglect. (Reproduced with permission from Fleisher GR, Ludwig S, Baskin MN. *Atlas of pediatric emergency medicine.* Philadelphia: Lippincott Williams & Wilkins, 2004.)

immobile with infantile posturing. The infant may be withdrawn and socially unresponsive, even to the mother, and actually may look away from her. Some infants inappropriately seek affection from strangers. Historically, these behaviors have been described in institutionalized infants who suffer from lack of care and affection. Some infants are described as irritable secondary to malnutrition.

Observing the mother feeding the child may be helpful. Does she cuddle the infant or merely "prop" the bottle? Does she allow sufficient time for feeding? The parents' level of concern may be inappropriate if they are eager to relinquish the child to the health team quickly. Observing the parents' interactions with each other will indicate whether they are supportive of each other. Observing the child feeding can indicate oral motor or swallowing difficulties. Prolonged duration of feedings or an intolerance for foods of certain textures may suggest a mild neurologic dysfunction. The setting for eating may not be optimal for the child who is easily distracted. Feeding the child in front of the television set may distract the child from eating.

Physical Examination

An accurate assessment of the child's height, weight, and head circumference is essential. In the child younger than 2 years, the recumbent length rather than the standing height should be obtained carefully. This figure, along with weight and head circumference, should be plotted on the NCHS growth charts and related to previous measurements. The NCHS growth charts are gender-specific and appropriate for all races and nationalities. Attention to the percentile curves of length, weight, and head circumference may give valuable clues to the etiology of FTT. When all measurements are below the fifth percentile, the incidence of organic disease has been noted to be 70%, with a preponderance of neurologic or systemic diseases.

Gastrointestinal disorders are more common when only the weight is below the fifth percentile. When height and weight are affected, endocrine causes or a severe nutritional problem should be suspected (see Chapter 375, Growth, Growth Hormone and Pituitary Disorders, and 377, Neuroendocrine Disorders). The single assessment of height and weight may have limited usefulness without an indication of whether the child's pattern is deviating from the percentile or of how far below the curve the measurement may be. In intrauterine growth retardation, the child initially is small for height and weight; weight gain and growth velocity may be adequate, yet continue to be below the fifth percentile. Also, 5% of the normal population has had growth patterns at or below the fifth percentile (constitutional short stature). Therefore, determining the median age for the child's length (height or length age) and the median age for the child's weight (weight age) may be useful.

The complete developmental assessment is important. Careful evaluation should be made for dysmorphic features (clinical or genetic syndromes) and for signs of neurologic or central nervous system (hypotonia or spasticity), pulmonary, cardiac, or gastrointestinal (swallowing disorders, gastroesophageal reflux) disorders. Isolated defects in the soft or hard palate may indicate a feeding problem.

Signs of neglect may be indicated by a diaper rash, impetigo, flat occiput, poor hygiene, protuberant abdomen, lack of appropriate behavior, and inappropriate infantile postures (see Fig. 131.1) Child abuse may result in bruises and fresh lesions or healed, unexplained scars. Notation of drooling and bowel habits is essential.

Some of the many possible causes of FTT are listed in Table 131.2.

TABLE 131.2

CAUSES OF FAILURE TO THRIVE

Inadequate Caloric Intake		Inadequate Appetite or Inability to Eat Large Amounts	Inadequate Caloric Absorption: No Weight Gain during Refeeding; Increased Losses	Increased Caloric Requirements
Weight Gain during Refeeding	**No Weight Gain during Refeeding**			
Inappropriate feeding technique	Psychosocial problems*	Psychosocial problems (apathy)*	Psychosocial problems (refeeding diarrhea, intercurrent illnesses, hepatitis, rumination, regurgitation)*	Hyperthyroidism
Disturbed mother/child relationship*	Maternal/infant dysfunction, economic deprivation	Cardiopulmonary disease	Malabsorption—diarrhea (lactose intolerance, cystic fibrosis, cardiac disease, malrotation, inflammatory bowel disease, milk allergy, parasites, celiac disease)	Cerebral palsy
Inappropriate nutrient intake (excess fruit juice consumption, factitious food allergy, inadequate quantity of food, inappropriate food for age, neglect, inappropriate preparation of formula, food fads)	Mechanical problems (adenoidal hypertrophy, dental lesions, vascular slings)	Hypotonia (muscle weakness)		Malignancy
	Insufficient lactation in mother	Anorexia of chronic infection (chronic sinusitis) or immune deficiency diseases (HIV infection or AIDS)		Chronic systemic disease (juvenile rheumatoid arthritis)
	Cleft palate	Endocrine disorders (hypothyroidism, diabetes insipidus)	Vomiting or "spitting up" or diarrhea (gastroenteritis, congenital adrenal hyperplasia)	Chronic systemic infection (UTI, HIV, tuberculosis, toxoplasmosis)
Inappropriate parental knowledge of correct nutrition for infants and children	Nasal obstruction	CNS tumors	Intestinal tract obstruction (pyloric stenosis, hernia, malrotation, intussusception, chalasia)	Chronic respiratory insufficiency (bronchopulmonary dysplasia, cystic fibrosis)
	Sucking or swallowing dysfunction (CNS, neuromuscular, esophageal motility problems)	Genetic syndromes	Biliary atresia/cirrhosis	Congenital or acquired heart disease
	Regurgitation (gastroesophageal reflux)	Metabolic conditions (lead toxicity, iron deficiency, zinc deficiency)	CNS problems—increased intracranial pressure (subdural hematoma)	Anemia
	Malformation (posterior urethral valves)	Anemia	Chronic metabolic problems (hypercalcemia, storage diseases, and inborn errors of metabolism such as galactosemia, methylmalonic acidemia, renal tubular acidosis, diabetes mellitus, adrenal insufficiency)	Toxins (lead)
	Congenital syndromes (alcohol, phenytoin, drugs)	Chronic constipation		
	Genetic syndromes (Turner, trisomies 21, 18, 13)	Disturbance in appetite and satiety	Necrotizing enterocolitis or short bowel syndrome	

*Environmental causes are the most common source of problems.

DIAGNOSIS

A careful history and physical examination in the child with FTT may suggest clues to organic disease in the child who is found to have an organic diagnosis. The search for organic disease should be guided by the signs and symptoms found in the initial examination. If history suggests enrollment in a day-care center, recent travel, or living in a homeless shelter, enteric pathogens should be considered. Laboratory studies not suggested on the basis of the initial examination rarely are helpful. Simple routine testing, including hematocrit, urinalysis and culture of urine, blood urea nitrogen, calcium, electrolyte levels, human immunodeficiency virus enzyme-linked immunosorbent assay, and Mantoux tuberculin skin testing, is appropriate. Additional testing, radiographs, and imaging may be indicated specifically by the clinical examination (Box 131.1).

Hospitalization may not be helpful or necessary unless the child is seriously ill or is at risk of physical or sexual abuse, or parental concern and anxiety warrant it. Separation of the child from the family by hospitalization may promote anxiety and anorexia in the child, and cause a delay in feeding and supporting the child within her environment. Psychosocial factors also should be examined in children with organic problems.

In the past, hospitalization was considered essential to demonstrate rapid weight gain in the child with FTT, in order to distinguish between organic and nonorganic etiologies. Although immediate, rapid weight gain suggests evidence for a nonorganic cause of FTT, failure to gain weight does not rule out the nonorganic etiology. Children in whom the initial history and physical examination suggest an organic basis for FTT can either be admitted to an acute-care hospital or be evaluated as outpatients, if indicated. The child who has no evidence of organic disease, or who may have a combination of organic and psychosocial problems, can be evaluated and supported in either outpatient or inpatient settings.

Effective evaluation, whether inpatient or outpatient, requires the involvement of the parents from the beginning, with support provided by an interdisciplinary program. In addition to the pediatrician, the program may involve social workers, nurses, developmental specialists, nutritionists, child-life workers, psychiatrists, and workers from social and educational services in the community. The low self-esteem that many parents have suggests that the health-care providers should not focus blame, but should work with the strengths of the family to encourage the development of a nurturing environment.

THERAPY

Most experience in the evaluation and initial management of FTT has been in the inpatient setting in tertiary-care centers. Exhaustive investigations for organic causes and prolonged hospitalizations to evaluate family dynamics and poor infant weight gain have resulted in inefficiencies and often the lack of a diagnosis.

Nutrition and Growth Recovery

The goal is to enable catch-up weight gain at a rate that is greater than average for the age, so that the growth deficit is repaired and overcome (see Chapter 14, Feeding the Healthy Child). Nutritional requirements for the healthy infant at birth are 120 kcal/kg per day and at 1 year are an average of 100 kcal/kg of body weight per day. A child who fails to gain weight normally, and whose weight is below the fifth percentile, will not experience catch-up, and therefore requires a caloric intake that is higher than normal. In such cases, intake requirements may be 50% higher than normal, or 150 kcal/kg/day. A higher caloric intake may be needed when the infant's normal energy requirements in the state of good health are considered, as outlined in Table 131.3. A nutritionist can provide guidance in the modification of formula.

Malnourished infants require extra concern because of the anorexia that may accompany the malnutrition state. This anorexia occurs early in the process and may last for up to a week. Malnutrition can result in transient malabsorption during the refeeding process. The severely malnourished infant or child should be hospitalized. Environmental deprivation can result in the physiologic changes of hypopituitarism. The response of these secondary changes to treatment should be observed.

An aggressive approach to nutritional therapy is suggested. Supernormal caloric intake may be required to achieve catch-up, but frequently this increased intake is achieved by the child's own demands after entering the recovery phase. The following points may be a guide:

- Feeding and appropriate nutritional intake should be based on age and expected, not actual, weight.
- In the nutritionally deprived child, feeding should be allowed to proceed *ad libitum* as the child demands.
- After a child goes into the recovery phase, the *ad libitum* intake frequently will achieve 150% of the daily requirement or greater.
- During the catch-up growth phase, existing stores of vitamins may not be sufficient. A multivitamin preparation including iron and zinc is recommended.
- The child should be the guide as to when to increase the intake. This guideline applies to the child who is nutritionally deprived as a primary problem with no other abnormalities and who can take food by mouth.

| **BOX 131.1** | **Laboratory Testing and Diagnostic Imaging Studies** |

Initial laboratory screening to be considered:

- CBC, WBC, RBC, and erythrocyte sedimentation rate: occult infection, anemia, immune deficiency.
- UA and culture: check hydration status (specific gravity), acidosis (pH), and for evidence of infection.
- Serum electrolytes, blood urea nitrogen, creatinine, and calcium: check renal function, adrenal salt wasting, inappropriate formula preparation, hyper- or hypocalcemia.
- Liver function tests: signs of organomegaly or malnutrition and wasting.

Further tests that should be considered if physical examination suggests malnutrition exists:

- HIV testing if risk factors present.
- Tuberculosis skin testing.
- Genetic testing for syndromes.
- Sweat test for cystic fibrosis.
- Thyroid hormone levels.
- Other metabolic screening, growth hormone screening.
- Zinc levels in malnutrition.
- Diagnostic imaging studies not routinely helpful.
- Skeletal survey if abuse suspected.
- MRI/CT of head if congenital anomaly, microcephaly, macrocephaly, or trauma.
- Radiograph, particularly of knees, hand, and wrist, to evaluate for bone age, rickets.

TABLE 131.3

TREATMENT STRATEGIES FOR FAILURE TO THRIVE

Diet	Setting	Caretakers	Access to Resources	Follow
Increase calories to 1½–2 times daily recommended allowance of calories (i.e., 150 Kcal/day, limit fruit juices, low-calorie liquids, carbonated drinks, and grazing on low-nutrient snack foods). Content of meals: consider solids before liquids; consider protein and total calories before variety*; age-appropriate finger foods; consider meals for vitamins and zinc during catch up growth.	Consider frequency of feeding: every 2–3 hours with three meals and 2 or 3 snacks. Schedule feedings: same time each day (eat often but not constantly). Eliminate distractions such as feeding in front of television. Allow age-appropriate feeding and messiness: child should feed self if appropriate; ensure that the child can reach the food, e.g., chair is appropriate height—may need to add telephone book.	Understand who they are; meet all and reduce conflicts among them. Clarify who does the feeding; observe interactions with child, discuss appropriate feeding habits, e.g., no force feeding or bribing.	WIC . Food stamps. Food pantries. Community services: e.g., support for job training, substance abuse program, respite care, social services. Other resources: occupational therapy, physical therapy, behavioral psychology, psychiatry, speech nutrition.	Weekly to monthly: look for faster than normal-for-age weight gain**. Developmental intervention through early childhood programs or Head Start.

*The number of calories per ounce of formula can be increased by adding less water or by adding more carbohydrates. In infants, in addition to concentrating the formula, rice cereal can be added to applesauce or other pureed foods. In the infant who is receiving concentrated formula and high solid food, periodically assess electrolytes. In the older child, peanut butter and other fats provide sources of additional calories. The high-calorie milk drinks, 30 calories per ounce, are available through the Women, Infants, and Children (WIC) Program and can be used instead of whole milk, 19 calories per ounce.

The average caloric replacement recommendations are: 1 month, 120 Kcal/kg/day; 1–2 months. 115 Kcal/kg/day; 2–3 months, 105 Kcal/kg/day; 3–6 months, 95 Kcal/kg/day; 6 months—5 years, 90 Kcal/kg/day.

**If weight gain is not appropriate, or if the psychosocial conditions suggest that the child is at risk for neglect or abuse, then the child should be hospitalized.

The primary goal for improved nutrition must be accompanied by addressing any psychosocial difficulties. Hospital volunteers, when available, may provide valuable role modeling, support, and aid in feeding. Home visitation may be helpful. Eligibility for WIC, food stamps, and Temporary Assistance for Needy Families (formerly Aid for Families with Dependent Children) should be considered and facilitated.

If weight gain does not occur in 4 to 6 weeks , the oral feedings should be supplemented with feeding by nasogastric tube. Tube feedings also can take place at home, and half of the daily calories can be delivered at night by continuous drip through a soft, silicone nasogastric tube (see Chapter 359, Short Bowel Syndrome). An assessment of feeding and occupational therapy to improve sucking and swallowing may be needed. Return to oral feedings can be resumed after weight gain has been demonstrated in 4 to 6 months. If weight gain is inadequate, feeding gastrostomy tube placement may be appropriate for children with severe malnutrition and neurodevelopmental conditions causing severe delay.

During the nutritional recovery, some children may experience the symptoms of a nutritional recovery syndrome, including sweatiness, hepatomegaly (caused by increased glycogen deposition in the liver), widening of the sutures (the brain growth is greater than the growth of the skull in infants with open sutures), and fidgetiness or a mild hyperactivity. Considerations for treatment strategies are shown in Table 131.3.

PROGNOSIS

Close follow-up and frequent contact with the health care team are essential for reinforcing nutritional recommendations and psychosocial support. Involvement with the family by community social service workers, visiting nurses, and nutritionists is important. Although the prognosis with respect to weight gain and growth is good, 25% to 60% of infants with FTT remain small. Because of the possibility that caloric deprivation in infancy will produce severe, irreversible developmental deficits, treatment should begin expeditiously. Neurodevelopmental and cognitive disorders are areas of great impact for long-term disability in FTT. Cognitive function is below normal in one-half of the children with FTT, and a high frequency of behavior problems and learning difficulties is found on follow-up. Whether these findings are a direct result of the FTT or of the contribution of continued adverse social circumstances is not known. One study showed that FTT did not account for lack of development in cognitive functioning and that maternal IQ was the single significant predictor of performance in every test of child cognitive abilities. The families need education and community services to help them to cope and to provide a nurturing environment for the children.

Suggested Readings

Ashenburg CA. Failure to thrive: newer concepts in treatment. In: *Pediatric Nutritional Challenges From Undernutrition to Overnutrition; Twenty-Eighth Ross Roundtable Report*. Columbus, Ohio, 1997;14.

Batchelor JA. Has recognition of failure to thrive changed? *Child Care Health Dev* 1996;22:235.

Berwick DM. Nonorganic failure to thrive. *Pediatr Rev* 1980;1:265.

Berwick DM, Levy JC, Kleinerman R. Failure to thrive: diagnostic yield of hospitalization. *Arch Dis Child* 1982;57:347.

Bithoney WG, Dubowitz H, Egan H. Failure to thrive: growth deficiency. *Pediatr Rev* 1992;13:453.

Black MM, Dubowitz H, Hutcheson J, et al. A randomized clinical trial of home intervention for children with failure to thrive. *Pediatrics* 1995;95: 807.

Blair PS, Drewett RF, Emmett PM, et al. Family, socioeconomic and prenatal factors associated with failure to thrive in the Avon Longitudinal Study of Parents and Children (ALSPAC). *Int J Epidemiology* 2004;33:839.

Boddy J, Skuse D, Andrews B. The developmental sequelae of nonorganic failure to thrive. *J Psychol Psychiatry* 2000;41:1003.

Corbett SS, Drewett RF. To what extent is failure to thrive in infancy associated with poorer cognitive development? A review of meta-analysis. *J Child Psychol Psychiatry* 2004;45:641.

Dykman RA, Casey PH, Ackerman PT, McPherson WB. Behavioral and cognitive status in school-aged children with a history of failure to thrive during early childhood. *Clin Pediatr* 2001;40:63.

Frank D. Failure to thrive. In: Parker S, Zuckerman B, eds. *Behavioral and developmental pediatrics*. Boston: Little, Brown and Company, 1995: 134.

Goldbloom RB. Growth failure in infancy. *Pediatr Rev* 1987;9:57.

Hannaway PJ. Failure to thrive: a study of 100 infants and children. *Clin Pediatr,* 1970;9:96.

Homer C, Ludwig S. Categorization of etiology of failure to thrive. *Am J Dis Child* 1981;135:848.

Maggioni A, Lifshitz F. Nutritional management of failure to thrive. *Pediatr Clin North Am* 1995;42:791.

Mitchell WG, Gorrell RW, Greenberg RA. Failure to thrive: a study in a primary-care setting. Epidemiology and follow-up. *Pediatrics* 1980;65:971.

O'Connor ME, Szekely LJ. Frequent breastfeeding and food refusal associated with failure to thrive. A manifestation of the vulnerable child syndrome. *Clin Pediatr* 2001;40:27.

Perrin E, Frank D, Cole C, et al. Criteria for determining disability in infants and children: failure to thrive. Evidence Report/Technology Assessment No. 72 (prepared by Tufts–New England Medical Center Evidence-Based Practice Center Under Contract No. 290-97-0019). AHRQ Publication NO. 03-E026. Rockville, MD: Agency for Healthcare Research and Quality, March 2003.

Parkinson KN, Wright CM, Drewett RF. Mealtime energy intake and feeding behavior in children who failure to thrive: a population-based case-control study. *J Child Psychol Psychiatry* 2004;45:1030.

Pollitt E, Eichler A. Behavioral disturbances among failure-to-thrive children. *Am J Dis Child* 1976;130:24.

Sills RH. Failure to thrive: the role of clinical and laboratory evaluations. *Am J Dis Child* 1978;132:967.

Zenel JA. Failure to thrive: a general pediatrician's perspective. *Pediatr Rev* 1997;18:371.

a: INFECTIOUS DISEASES

CHAPTER 132 ■ FEVER WITHOUT SOURCE

MARK A. WARD, MARTIN I. LORIN, AND MARK W. KLINE

Fever is one of the most common pediatric complaints. In the first few years of a child's life, fever is second only to routine care as the reason for office or clinic visits. Between 5% and 20% of febrile children have no localizing signs on physical examination and nothing in the history to explain the fever. Fever without source (FWS), like febrile illness in general, is most commonly seen in children younger than age 5, with a peak prevalence between 6 and 24 months of age.

We define FWS as fever of relatively brief duration, arbitrarily 7 or fewer days, without an apparent source on history or physical examination. If the unexplained fever persists for longer than 7 days, it is commonly referred to as fever of undetermined origin (FUO). Although overlap exists between FWS and FUO, the differential diagnoses and the clinical approaches are different.

In most cases, FWS resolves spontaneously, without a specific diagnosis being established, and presumably is caused by a viral infection. In some cases, a relatively minor infectious process, either focal (e.g., otitis media, pharyngitis) or nonfocal (e.g., roseola), becomes apparent a few days into the febrile illness. Examples of infections with lengthy prodromal periods during which fever may be the only manifestation include roseola, cytomegalovirus infection, and typhoid fever. Because the duration of FWS, by definition, is brief and because so many children with self-limited viral infections present with FWS, the incidence of persistent infections or noninfectious chronic inflammatory conditions (e.g., juvenile rheumatoid arthritis) is much lower than that among children with FUO. Infrequently, FWS in an infant or child represents a drug reaction, an allergic or hypersensitivity disorder, or heat illness. A small number of young children presenting with FWS will manifest features of Kawasaki syndrome after a few days.

SERIOUS BACTERIAL INFECTIONS

Except in the very young infant, most serious bacterial infections (SBIs) can be recognized by a careful history and physical examination. However, a small percentage of children with bacteremia cannot be identified by clinical examination alone. These children have occult bacteremia, which we define as the presence of a positive blood culture in a child who looks well enough to be treated as an outpatient and in whom the positive blood culture is not anticipated. Specifically, the child does not have any local infection that ordinarily would be associated with bacteremia (e.g., pneumonia or epiglottitis), although the child may have a minor infection, such as otitis media. Whereas less than 5% of children with FWS have occult bacteremia, more than 50% of children with occult bacteremia come from the pool of children with FWS (Fig. 132.1).

Occult bacteremia occurs with essentially the same frequency in lower, middle, and upper socioeconomic populations, and the prevalence varies more with the selection criteria for study than with the geographic or socioeconomic base of the study population. The highest frequency of occult bacteremia is in children younger than 2 years of age. For additional information about bacteremia in children, see Box 132.1.

Other SBIs of concern in children with FWS include meningitis and urinary tract infection (UTI). The former can occur in the absence of neurologic findings and without demonstrable neck stiffness or pain on flexion. Infants and young children with UTI may not have, or may not be able to express, abdominal pain, back pain, or pain on urination. Whereas bacterial enteritis also is considered a potential SBI in children with FWS, it is unlikely in the absence of diarrhea, although fever may precede the first loose stool by several hours.

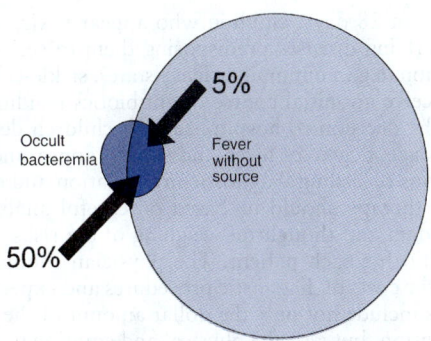

FIGURE 132.1. Relation of fever without source (FWS) and occult bacteremia. Many more cases of FWS than of occult bacteremia occur. Only 5% of cases of FWS are associated with occult bacteremia, but more than 50% of patients with occult bacteremia have FWS.

DIAGNOSTIC EVALUATION

Many of the diagnostic studies used to evaluate children with FWS are directed at excluding the presence of bacteremia or other SBIs. Failure to identify bacteremic children accurately subjects them to the potentially adverse sequelae of undiagnosed and untreated SBIs, including meningitis. Conversely, the indiscriminate use of diagnostic tests causes unnecessary expense and discomfort for the patient.

The advent of the *Haemophilus influenzae* type b vaccine, and more recently the conjugate pneumococcal vaccine, has markedly decreased the incidence of occult bacteremia and bacterial meningitis. The frequency of occult infection caused by *Neisseria meningitidis* and salmonellae has not changed. The decreased incidence of *H. influenzae* type b and pneumococcal infection in fully immunized children has led to a rethinking of the recommendations for the diagnostic and therapeutic management of children between 3 and 36 months of age with FWS. The current low risk of occult bacteremia or meningitis in these children no longer justifies *routine* blood culture, measurement of white blood cell (WBC) counts or other acute-phase reactants, or administration of antibiotics while awaiting

---

BOX 132.1	Studies of Bacteremia in Children with Fever Without Source

Children with fever without source (FWS) are more likely to be bacteremic than are children with minor outpatient infections. In one series, blood cultures were obtained from all febrile children younger than 2 years of age presenting to the emergency department. The prevalence of bacteremia in children with infections such as otitis media and pharyngitis was 1.5%; in those with FWS, the prevalence was 3.9%. In another series, 3% of febrile children with evidence of upper respiratory tract infections had occult bacteremia, in contrast to those with FWS, for whom the prevalence was 9%. These series were published prior to the advent routine immunization against *Haemophilus influenzae* type b and *Streptococcus pneumoniae*, and the total prevalence would now be much lower but the ratios might well be similar. Although most patients with FWS (even those with high fevers) do not have bacteremia, higher fever tends to be associated with a greater risk of bacteremia, a trend especially pronounced with *S. pneumoniae*.

---

results of blood culture in the nontoxic-appearing child who has received *H. influenzae* type b and pneumococcal vaccines. Because *S. pneumoniae* is associated more consistently with high fever and elevated WBC than are other organisms, these parameters will be less sensitive in children who have received the pneumococcal vaccine. The use of these vaccines will not impact the incidence of UTIs or bacterial enteritis.

Children between 3 and 36 months of age with FWS who appear toxic should be hospitalized for appropriate workup and initiation of intravenous antibiotics. Those who are at special risk for SBIs (e.g. sickle-cell disease or immunodeficiency) should have diagnostic studies, including a blood culture, and should be considered for empiric antibiotic therapy while awaiting the results of cultures. Those without special risk who look well and whose temperatures are less than 39.0°C require symptomatic therapy only.

For the child who has not received a complete course of pneumococcal immunizations and whose temperature is at or above 39°C, it is reasonable to obtain a WBC, differential count, and blood culture and to administer an antibiotic such as ceftriaxone if WBC counts are 15,000 per microliter or greater or absolute neutrophil counts (ANCs) are 10,000 per microliter or greater while awaiting the blood culture results. A chest roentgenogram generally is indicated only for those with clinical signs of lower respiratory infection but might also be considered for those with WBC counts of 20,000 per microliter or greater.

Use of clinical judgment is always required, and these recommendations are guidelines only. Several investigators have suggested that the use of clinical scoring systems for children with FWS may permit the selection of a subgroup of patients who appear well and have only a small or negligible risk of bacteremia or other serious bacterial illnesses. These clinical features include the child's appearance (e.g., normal hydration, lack of apparent toxicity, and lack of distress) and behavior (e.g., alert, playful, and eating, and drinking well). The studies on which this suggestion was based, however, included the full spectrum of febrile children presenting to the emergency department. A child with bacteremic pneumonia or bacteremic meningitis likely would look more ill than would a child with occult bacteremia. A study dealing only with children with "nonfocal, nontoxic-appearing illness (or uncomplicated otitis media)" treated as outpatients found that the Yale Observation Score was not clinically useful in detecting occult bacteremia. Thus, whereas clinical features can be helpful, they are not very accurate.

Two types of laboratory tests are used in evaluating children for occult bacteremia: *indirect tests*, such as the WBC count, erythrocyte sedimentation rate (ESR), and C-reactive protein (which reflect the body's response to infection), and *direct tests*, such as blood culture and rapid tests for the detection of bacterial antigens (which detect the organism itself). Indirect tests, such as the WBC count, serve only as screening tests to identify a subgroup of children at high risk of having bacteremia.

In a population with a low prevalence of a disease—as is the case with febrile children and bacteremia—even a sensitive and specific screening test has a low positive predictive value. In other words, the test does not discriminate well between the few patients with bacteremia and the many children with positive test results but without bacteremia. For children with FWS, a WBC count of 15,000 per microliter or greater has sensitivity and specificity of approximately 85% and 75%, respectively, for the detection of bacteremia. Even before immunizations against *H. influenzae* and *S. pneumoniae* were available, the positive predictive value was only approximately 10% to 15% at best. Nonetheless, the WBC count is the most widely used and probably the most practical screening test available. Other screening tests, such as the ESR and WBC morphology, also have a low positive predictive value.

Blood culture is an important diagnostic tool in the child with FWS. It is technically easy to perform and, unlike screening tests, is a direct and precise means of diagnosing bacteremia. Substantial cost savings result from reserving blood culture for children deemed by clinical criteria or a WBC count exceeding 15,000 per microliter to be at high risk for having bacteremia.

Bacterial pneumonia is infrequent in the absence of clinical signs (tachypnea, respiratory distress, rales, dullness to percussion, or decreased breath sounds) or hypoxemia by pulse oximetry. Most series of children with FWS have not included routine chest radiographs. Available data suggest that the incidence of occult bacterial pneumonia in children with FWS is probably 3% or less. However, some data suggest that the incidence is higher in children with temperatures at or above 39.0°C (102.2°F) and WBC counts of 20,000 per microliter or greater.

UTIs are common findings in infants and young children, and more than half of febrile UTIs in this age group are associated with upper tract involvement. In infants and toddlers, UTIs often are occult, presenting with fever and irritability only. Therefore, laboratory evaluation for UTIs should be considered for highly febrile children younger than 2 years of age. Urinalysis or dipstick for leukocyte esterase or nitrite is the usual screening test, but diagnosis can be established only by culture of an appropriately obtained urine specimen. For children with temperatures at or above 39.0°C, Baraff suggests a urine screening test for all males 1 year old or younger and all females 2 years old or younger. As these screens are less than 100% sensitive, he suggests culture regardless of the screen results in females younger than 1 year, males younger than 6 months, and uncircumcised males younger than 1 year.

MANAGEMENT

Antibiotic Treatment

Expectant antibiotic therapy can be justified for some children with FWS and high fever, WBC counts greater than 15,000 per microliter, absolute neutrophile counts greater than 10,000, or other risk factors for occult bacteremia (Table 132.1). Several retrospective studies and one prospective controlled study of occult bacteremia showed that children treated expectantly with antibiotics at the time of the initial visit fared better than did those who did not receive antibiotic therapy. Infants

TABLE 132.1

RISK OF OCCULT BACTEREMIA

	Low Risk	High Risk
Age	>3 years	<2 years
Temperature	<39.4°C (103°F)	>40°C (104°F)
WBC count (per microliter)	>5,000 and <15,000	<5,000 or >15,000
Observational variables	Normal	Abnormal
Other		History of contact with *Haemophilus influenzae* or *Neisseria meningitidis* History of bacteremic illness Immunologic impairment

WBC, white blood cell.

younger than 28 days, children who appear toxic, and those with underlying diseases predisposing them to serious bacterial infection (e.g., immunodeficiency states, sickle-cell disease) should receive an initial course of antibiotics pending culture results. The decision to hospitalize such children depends on the child's age, degree of fever, and clinical appearance.

Decisions regarding diagnostic investigation and expectant antibiotic therapy should be based on careful analysis of all available data and thoughtful weighing of the risks and cost–benefit ratio for each patient. The physician should be cognizant of the costs of diagnostic procedures and expectant therapy. Costs include not only the dollar amount of the tests and the medication, but also the physical and emotional trauma of blood drawing, the side effects of antibiotics, and the time and distress involved in clarifying false-positive results, lost specimens, and laboratory errors. The major potential benefit is the prevention of subsequent meningitis and other focal bacterial infections. Table 132.1 serves as a framework for assessing the risk of bacteremia in the individual patient.

Empiric antibiotic therapy should be directed against the three most common bacterial pathogens: *S. pneumoniae*, *N. meningitidis*, and *H. influenzae*. Amoxicillin (40 to 60 mg/kg/day) is a reasonable choice for most children. For children who have not been immunized against *H. influenzae* type b, coverage can be broadened to include ampicillin-resistant strains of that organism. Such therapy includes erythromycin-sulfisoxazole, trimethoprim-sulfamethoxazole, or amoxicillin-clavulanic acid, as well as several second- or third-generation cephalosporins. A single injection of ceftriaxone (50 to 75 mg/kg) provides 24 hours of coverage against *S. pneumoniae*, *H. influenzae*, and *N. meningitidis* without concern about compliance or vomiting.

Regardless of therapy, careful follow-up care is essential, and children should be reevaluated immediately if the clinical condition deteriorates, if signs or symptoms of serious focal infection develop, or if the blood culture yields a pathogen.

Infants Younger than 90 Days of Age

Infants younger than 90 days of age with FWS are of greater concern than are older children. The choice of 28, 60, or 90 days as dividing points is useful but arbitrary. Obviously, there is no biologic difference between a 59-day-old and a 61-day-old infant. Infants younger than 28 days of age are difficult to assess clinically, are at greater risk for acquiring SBIs than are older infants, and are vulnerable to infection by bacteria such as group B streptococci, *Escherichia coli*, and *Listeria monocytogenes*. They also are vulnerable to devastating and life-threatening infection by herpes simplex virus and enteroviruses. For these reasons, febrile infants 28 days of age or younger should have a blood culture and at least a complete blood count, urinalysis, and culture. A routine lumbar puncture is recommended by most (but not all) workers in this area and is mandatory if the infant is to receive antibiotics. If diarrhea is present, stools should be examined for the presence of leukocytes. Most authors recommend hospitalization of all febrile infants younger than 28 days of age, but this is not a universal recommendation and outpatient management can be considered if the infant looks well and is feeding well, provided careful follow-up can be assured.

Outpatient management of low-risk infants between 28 and 90 days of age, with or without empiric antibiotic therapy, may be considered if parents appear reliable and close follow-up is assured. Low-risk infants would be those who previously were normal and with normal complete blood counts and urinalysis (including dipstick for leukocyte esterase and nitrites), negative examination for fecal leukocytes if diarrhea is present, and normal spinal fluid if a lumbar puncture was done. Different authors have used different values for normal WBC and fecal leukocyte counts. In general, WBC counts between 5,000 and 15,000 per microliter would be considered normal, as would less than five fecal leukocytes per high power field.

Suggested Readings

Alpern ER, Alessandrini EA, Bell LM, et al. Occult bacteremia from a pediatric emergency department: current prevalence, time to detection, and outcome. *Pediatrics* 2000;106:505.

Baker MD, Bell LM, Avner JR. The efficacy of routine outpatient management without antibiotics of fever in selected infants. *Pediatrics* 1999;103:627.

Baraff LJ. Management of fever without source in infants and children. *Ann Emerg Med* 2000;36:602.

Baraff LJ, Bass JW, Fleisher GR, et al. Practice guidelines for the management of infants and children 0 to 36 months of age with fever without source. *Pediatrics* 1993;92:1.

Carroll WL, Farrell MK, Singer JI, et al. Treatment of occult bacteremia: a prospective randomized clinical trial. *Pediatrics* 1983;72:608.

Hoberman A, Wald ER, Hickey RW, et al. Oral versus initial intravenous therapy for urinary tract infections in young febrile children. *Pediatrics* 1999; 104:79.

Lee GM, Fleisher, GR, Harper, MB. Management of febrile children in the age of the conjugate pneumococcal vaccine: a cost-effectiveness analysis. *Pediatrics* 2001;108:835.

Roberts KB, Charney E, Sweren RJ, et al. Urinary tract infection in infants with unexplained fever: a collaborative study. *J Pediatr* 1983;103:864.

Stoll ML, Rubin LG. Incidence of occult bacteremia among highly febrile young children in the era of the pneumococcal conjugate vaccine: a study from a Children's Hospital Emergency Department and Urgent Care Center. *Arch Pediatr Adolesc Med* 2004;158:671.

Strait RT, Kelley KJ, Kurup VP. Tumor necrosis factor-alpha, interleukin-1 beta, and interleukin-6 levels in febrile, young children with and without occult bacteremia. *Pediatrics* 1999;104:1321.

Teach SJ, Fleisher GR. Efficacy of an observation scale in detecting bacteremia in febrile children three to thirty-six months of age, treated as outpatients. *J Pediatr* 1995;126:877.

CHAPTER 133 ■ FEVER OF UNKNOWN ORIGIN

MARTIN I. LORIN AND RALPH D. FEIGIN

The definition of fever of unknown origin (FUO) in children has evolved during the past few decades; a prolonged period of documentation of fever and in-hospital workup no longer are required for use of this term. These rigid criteria arose from studies of adults performed at a time when our understanding of this entity was relatively primitive and modern diagnostic techniques were unavailable. The length of time a child must be febrile before being labeled as having an FUO varies among different authors and investigators. Here, we use the term FUO to describe the condition of a child who is febrile for 8 or more days and in whom a careful history, physical examination, and preliminary laboratory evaluation (inpatient or outpatient) fail to reveal a probable cause for the fever. Youngsters who have been febrile without explanation for fewer than 8 days should be considered as having fever without source (FWS), which carries a different set of diagnostic probabilities and requires a different diagnostic approach (see Chapter 132). The causes of fever of unknown origin in children are shown in Table 133.1.

GENERAL PRINCIPLES

Most children with FUO do not have rare or exotic diseases, which has been shown to be true even in series from major pediatric referral centers. For example, in a series of 100 children evaluated at the Children's Hospital Medical Center in Boston, only three patients had diseases that would be considered rare (undefined vasculitis, Behçet syndrome, and ichthyosis).

Although the relative frequencies are somewhat different, the three causes of FUO most commonly identified in children are the same as those in adults: infectious diseases, rheumatologic disorders, and malignancies. The prognosis in children is somewhat better than that in adults, but FUO often represents a serious condition even in children. The mortality rate was 9% in the series of Pizzo and colleagues and 17% in that of Lohr and Hendley. McClung reported that 40% of the children in his study had "serious or lethal diseases." Infection, the leading cause of FUO at all ages, accounts for an even greater percent-

age of cases in children (more than 50% in some reports) than in adults. Rheumatologic diseases occur with approximately the same frequency in pediatric and adult series, whereas neoplasms are a less common cause of FUO in children than in adults.

The percentages of specific causes in different reports vary with factors such as criteria for inclusion in the study, availability of diagnostic expertise, and classification of patients with probable but uncertain diagnoses. In many cases of FUO in children, a specific diagnosis never is established and the condition eventually resolves spontaneously.

INITIAL APPROACH TO CLINICAL EVALUATION

The clinical approach to the child with FUO should be individualized for each patient. For most patients, diagnostic evaluation may be initiated in the office or the clinic. However, young infants, children who appear toxic or chronically ill, and children who have been febrile for a prolonged period of time with associated findings such as weight loss should be hospitalized for evaluation. Hospitalization is useful not only for expediting laboratory tests, but also for providing an opportunity to document fever, explore the history further, repeat the physical examination, and maintain constant observation.

The child's age affects both the probability of various disorders and the urgency with which the workup is undertaken. Young infants present a pressing problem; bacteremia and meningitis are more difficult to recognize than in the older child. Neonates and young infants also are susceptible to certain organisms such as group B streptococci and *Listeria monocytogenes*, which are rare findings in older patients. On the other hand, *Neisseria gonorrhoeae* as a cause of prolonged fever usually is seen in adolescents. Rheumatologic diseases occur more commonly in older children. Pizzo and colleagues reported an incidence of connective tissue disease approximately four times greater in children older than 6 years of age with

TABLE 133.1

CAUSES OF FEVER OF UNKNOWN ORIGIN IN CHILDREN

Infectious Diseases
Bacterial
  Bacterial endocarditis
  Brucellosis
  Cat-scratch disease
  Leptospirosis
  Liver abscess
  Mastoiditis (chronic)
  Osteomyelitis
  Pelvic abscess
  Perinephric abscess
  Pyelonephritis
  Salmonellosis
  Sinusitis
  Subdiaphragmatic abscess
  Tuberculosis
  Tularemia

Viral
  Cytomegalovirus
  Hepatitis viruses
  Epstein-Barr virus (infectious mononucleosis)

Chlamydial
  Lymphogranuloma venereum
  Psittacosis

Rickettsial
  Q fever
  Rocky Mountain spotted fever

Fungal
  Blastomycosis (nonpulmonary)
  Histoplasmosis (disseminated)

Parasitic
  Malaria
  Toxoplasmosis
  Visceral larva migrans

Unclassified
  Sarcoidosis
  Collagen vascular disease
  Juvenile rheumatoid arthritis
  Polyarteritis nodosa
  Systemic lupus erythematosus
  Malignancies
  Hodgkin disease
  Leukemia/lymphoma
  Neuroblastoma

Miscellaneous
  Central diabetes insipidus
  Drug fever
  Ectodermal dysplasia
  Factitious fever
  Familial dysautonomia
  Granulomatous colitis
  Infantile cortical hyperostosis
  Nephrogenic diabetes insipidus
  Pancreatitis
  Periodic fever
  Serum sickness
  Thyrotoxicosis
  Ulcerative colitis

FUO than in those younger than 6 years. The patient's gender also is relevant. Autoimmune disease occurs more commonly in girls, and certain immunologic deficiencies, such as Bruton agammaglobulinemia, Wiskott-Aldrich syndrome, and Chédiak-Higashi syndrome, are restricted to boys. Pelvic inflammatory disease, of course, occurs only in girls.

The patient's history should be searched carefully for any possible clues, however trivial or remote. A history of transfusion or the use of blood products would raise the possibility of a variety of transmittable viral and parasitic agents, including human immunodeficiency virus (HIV). Animal contact always is important. Dogs can harbor brucellosis or leptospirosis, and cats are vectors for cat-scratch disease and toxoplasmosis. Birds are a source of ornithosis and histoplasmosis. Rodents carry tularemia, leptospirosis, *Spirillum minus*, and *Streptobacillus moniliformis*. A history of travel, even in the distant past, is notable. Endemic diseases in Africa, India, and Asia include malaria, amebiasis, and schistosomiasis, which may manifest months to years after the person returns from an endemic area. Leprosy endemics even in parts of the United States and coccidioidomycosis endemics in the southwestern portion of the United States are examples of other diseases that may not become apparent clinically until months or years after initial exposure to the causative organism.

EVALUATION

After a careful and thorough history and physical examination have been completed, evaluation of the child with FUO should proceed along three lines: follow-up of all diagnostic clues, screening tests, and continued observation and reexamination.

Follow-Up of Diagnostic Clues

The most important aspect of the evaluation of a youngster with FUO is meticulous and complete follow-up of all potential clues, however insignificant they may appear to be. The results of the history and physical examination and all available laboratory data must be scrutinized closely for any abnormalities or positive features. Pizzo and colleagues found that in one-half of their cases, failure to use existing laboratory data correctly was a major reason for not establishing the proper diagnosis before the patient was hospitalized. A history of abdominal pain or diarrhea, even weeks before the onset of the fever, may be a clue to an enteric infection or an intraabdominal abscess. The slightest tenderness over the sinuses or mastoid area may be indicative of an underlying chronic infection. Even a mild peripheral eosinophilia may be a clue to a parasitic infection, immunodeficiency, or occult malignancy.

Screening Tests

When no clues exist to guide the workup or when follow-up of such clues fails to yield an answer, the physician must rely on an initial battery of screening tests. Even when clues are present, proceeding with some preliminary screening tests while following up on specific clues is not unreasonable. Basic screening tests include a complete blood count, erythrocyte sedimentation rate and C-reactive protein, chest roentgenography, urinalysis and culture, tuberculin skin test, blood culture, analysis of levels of hepatic enzymes and alkaline phosphatase, and analysis of blood urea nitrogen and creatinine. Further tests would include those for serum antibody titers against brucellosis, tularemia, rickettsial diseases, Epstein-Barr virus, HIV, and cytomegalovirus. Testing for antinuclear antibody titers may be useful, especially in the older child with prolonged fever. Serum rheumatoid factor results usually are negative in patients with the acute systemic form of juvenile rheumatoid arthritis (JRA). If these tests fail to yield a diagnosis, a gallium scan should be considered to look for a focus of inflammation. Other imaging studies such as bone scan, radiographic skeletal survey, roentgenography of the sinuses and mastoids, and abdominal ultrasound or computed tomographic (CT) examination generally should be performed only if specific clues or indications are present or if fever persists for an inordinate period of time. Bone marrow aspiration generally is most useful in diagnosing or ruling out hematologic disorders such as leukemia and hemophagocytic syndrome, but it may yield an unexpected organism on culture or may permit visualization of a viral or rickettsial agent by electron microscopy. Lumbar puncture usually is necessary only in young infants or in the child with meningeal or neurologic signs or symptoms, including mental status changes.

Hospitalization, Observation, and Reexamination

Hospitalization for the child who requires it for clinical indications or because of persistent fever with an unrevealing outpatient workup affords an opportunity not only to facilitate diagnostic testing, but also to obtain additional historical data from the patient, parents, and even other family members who may visit. Frequently, parents recall a pertinent event, such as travel or animal exposure, or a relevant family history only after the child has spent days in the hospital. The patient must have a complete physical examination on admission and a relatively complete follow-up examination daily. Daily repeating of items such as retinoscopic examination, detailed neurologic examination, or rectal examination is not necessary unless specifically indicated. Often, pulmonary rales, cardiac murmurs, skin rashes, areas of tenderness, pain on motion of a joint, and even abdominal masses appear while the child is hospitalized. All available data should be reviewed continually for clues that were not apparent initially. The pattern of fever should be observed. A high fever that spikes once or twice a day may be an indication of an occult abscess or the systemic form of JRA. The patient should be examined during an episode of fever; the rash of JRA may be present only at this time.

A youngster who looks well, has no tachycardia, and does not feel warm at the time of alleged fever may have factitious fever. In the age of the electronic thermometer, the attendant routinely remains at the bedside while measuring the temperature, rendering factitiously elevating the temperature reading difficult for the patient or parent. However, the oral reading can be influenced by ingesting hot liquids before the temperature measurement is taken. The ingenuity of some patients or parents in falsifying temperature readings and feigning illness is extraordinary, and, undoubtedly, such individuals will find ways to circumvent modern technology.

The response to antipyretic agents should be noted. Lack of response may indicate factitious fever or a neurologic basis for the fever. Temperature elevations secondary to neurologic dysfunction often are unresponsive to antipyretic drugs. Children with recurrent periodic fever frequently respond poorly or not at all to these agents.

ETIOLOGY

Infectious Causes

In the United States, the most common infectious agents to be considered in children with FUO include Epstein-Barr virus; cytomegalovirus; hepatitis virus; HIV; spirochetes such as leptospira, *Treponema pallidum*, and *Borrelia burgdorferi* (Lyme disease); rickettsia; mycobacteria; *Salmonella*; *Brucella*; *Francisella tularensis*; and *Bartonella henselae*.

The most common localized infections that may present as FUO include sinusitis, urinary tract infection, osteomyelitis, and occult abscesses, including those of the subdiaphragmatic, hepatic, pelvic, or perinephric regions.

Brucellosis

The presentation of brucellosis as FUO is explained by the nonspecificity of its symptomatology and by the chronicity of untreated infection. Physicians tend to ignore the possibility of this disease and often neglect to ask for a history of exposure to animals or animal products, such as cheese made from unpasteurized goat milk.

Leptospirosis

Leptospirosis is caused by a family of organisms with multiple serogroups and serotypes. Transmission of infection from animals to humans may occur during direct contact with the blood, urine, or organs of infected animals, or indirectly by exposure to an environment contaminated by leptospires. The organism may be acquired from soil or water. Reports suggest that leptospirosis is not a rare occurrence. Most infections no longer are associated with occupational exposure, and urban and suburban cases now occur more frequently than do cases reported from rural areas.

The clinical manifestations of leptospirosis, other than its appearance as Weil syndrome (icteric from of leptospirosis), are not specific. A variety of laboratory tests are available, but appropriate handling and collecting of specimens is imperative. In many cases, a definitive diagnosis cannot be established because of negative culture results and failure to demonstrate an increase in antibody titer to these organisms. These factors do not exclude the possibility that active infections are present because the organism may not be present in the specimens that have been cultured. Moreover, the antibody titer may have peaked before an acute-phase specimen was collected, and antibiotic therapy can suppress the development of positive titers or delay their appearance.

Salmonellosis

Salmonella sp. are found as contaminants in many food products. The nonspecificity of signs and symptoms that may be associated with salmonellosis accounts for its association with FUO in children. Repetitive blood and stool cultures are most helpful in establishing a diagnosis. Serologic tests generally are not useful. *Salmonella* should be considered in any child with FUO who recently returned from a trip abroad, especially from India or neighboring areas.

Tularemia

Francisella tularensis may be acquired from contact with a variety of animal species, as well as from mosquitoes, lice, fleas, ticks, flies, and contaminated water. The organism may penetrate mucous membranes and even unbroken skin. It also may be inhaled or swallowed. Questioning patients and their parents not only about ingestion of rabbit and squirrel meat but also about other animal contact and a history of tick bite is crucial.

Tuberculosis

Tuberculosis is an infrequent but important cause of FUO in children. Nonpulmonary tuberculosis (disseminated, peritoneal, pericardial, hepatic, or genitourinary) presents as FUO more frequently than does pulmonary tuberculosis. Active disseminated tuberculosis has been documented in children with normal chest radiographic results and negative tuberculin test results. The bone marrow and liver frequently are involved in children with miliary tuberculosis, and in select cases, liver specimens and bone marrow aspirates should be obtained and processed for morphologic evaluation and appropriate cultures. Gastric aspirates should be cultured in patients suspected of having miliary tuberculosis, even in the presence of a normal chest roentgenographic result. The demonstration of acid-fast organisms on smears of gastric secretions does not necessarily indicate *Mycobacterium tuberculosis* infection because nontuberculous *Mycobacterium* sp. may be present in the gastric contents of normal individuals.

Bacterial Endocarditis

Infective endocarditis is an infrequent cause of FUO in children. Endocarditis is a rare finding in infants, increasing in frequency with advancing age. The absence of a cardiac murmur does not exclude the possibility of endocarditis and is a particularly common finding when infection involves the right side of the heart. Endocarditis also may occur in the absence of a positive blood culture result, especially in association with the following factors: right-sided cardiac lesions; prior use of antibiotics; prolonged duration of disease; infection caused by organisms that do not grow well on routine culture media, such as *Brucella* sp. or *Coxiella burnetii*; and use of inadequate culture methods for the detection of anaerobic organisms. Associated laboratory findings include anemia, leukocytosis, and elevated erythrocyte sedimentation rate. Five or six blood cultures should be obtained both aerobically and anaerobically over a period of several days. Echocardiography may reveal vegetations, but a negative study result does not exclude endocarditis.

Bone and Joint Infections

Infections of the bones and joints usually can be diagnosed clinically but occasionally may present as FUO, a phenomenon more commonly associated with osteomyelitis than with septic arthritis. Infection of the pelvic bones is implicated most often in this regard. Radioisotopic bone scanning is more sensitive than is radiographic examination of the bones.

Liver Abscess and Other Hepatic Infections

Pyogenic liver abscesses are encountered most frequently in the immunocompromised child, but they also may be seen in the normal child. In some children, fever is the only finding. Blood culture results usually are sterile, and liver function test results and serum levels of hepatic enzymes often are within normal limits. Hepatomegaly and right upper quadrant abdominal tenderness may be present. Diagnosis can be established by examining the liver using ultrasound, CT scan, or radioisotopic scanning techniques. Bacterial hepatitis, as well as cholangitis, can occur in the absence of jaundice. Amebic liver abscesses generally are seen in children who have traveled to developing areas.

Granulomatous hepatitis is a syndrome characterized by granuloma formation within the liver, rather than a specific disease. In many cases, the specific cause never is determined. Most cases have been reported in adults, but examples in children also have been seen. In some cases, diagnosis can be established only by liver biopsy. Many of these cases have been found to be caused by cat-scratch disease (*B. henselae*). Usually, the diagnosis of cat-scratch disease can be made on the basis of the clinical history, physical examination, and imaging studies of the liver and spleen, without the necessity of biopsy. Serologic tests for *B. henselae* also are available.

Intraabdominal Abscesses

Subphrenic, perinephric, psoas, and pelvic abscesses all may present as FUO. A history of intraabdominal disease, recent abdominal surgery, abdominal pain, or vague abdominal complaints heightens suspicion for an intraabdominal collection of pus. Careful abdominal, pelvic, and rectal examinations are important in confirming suspicion of such an abscess. The organisms involved most commonly include *Escherichia coli*, anaerobic flora, *Staphylococcus aureus*, and streptococci. Routine laboratory tests usually are not helpful. Even with perinephric abscesses, the urinalysis generally is normal. The diagnosis is made by ultrasound examination or CT scanning.

Viral Infections

Infection by most viruses results in an illness that is brief and self-limited. However, hepatitis viruses, cytomegalovirus, Epstein-Barr virus, HIV, and certain arboviruses are exceptions to the rule. In all of these disorders, symptomatology may be variable and signs and symptoms nonspecific. Thus, these viral infections should be considered in the differential diagnosis of patients with FUO.

Upper Respiratory Tract Infection

Infections of the upper respiratory tract and related organs can present as FUO. Although obvious symptoms and signs would be expected, the complaints often are trivial and ignored. Physical findings may be absent, especially in cases of mastoiditis or sinusitis. Chronic or recurrent pharyngitis, tonsillitis, and otitis media should be considered in the differential diagnosis of patients with FUO.

Immunodeficiency

A variety of immunodeficiency states, both congenital and acquired, can present as FUO. Infection with HIV may present as FUO, often with nonspecific findings such as malaise, listlessness, and weight loss. Diagnosis can be established by serologic evaluation for HIV infection. Measurement of serum immunoglobulins and complement, a total leukocyte count with differential, and a nitroblue tetrazolium dye test will detect the most common immunodeficiency disorders.

Parasitic Infections

Malaria should be considered in children as a cause of FUO. In addition to fever, splenomegaly usually is present. A history of travel to endemic areas should be sought but is not found invariably. If an appropriate mosquito vector is present, infection may be transmitted from an individual who has visited an endemic area to one who has not. Malaria also may be acquired by blood transfusion or by the use of needles and syringes contaminated by the parasite. Demonstration of the organism on appropriately stained thin or thick smears of blood is diagnostic.

Connective Tissue Diseases

Connective tissue disorders and vasculitis are the second leading cause of FUO in children, and JRA accounts for most pediatric cases of rheumatologic diseases presenting as FUO. Although all three clinical forms of this disorder (acute systemic, pauciarticular, and polyarticular) may be associated with fever, the acute systemic form is most likely to present as FUO. The classic pattern of fever in this disorder is one or two fever spikes daily. Most serologic test results for rheumatoid factor are negative in children with the acute systemic form of JRA, rendering the disease difficult to diagnose. The diagnosis usually is made clinically by observation over a period of time and by ruling out other causes of the fever.

Malignancy

Malignancies are the third most frequent cause of FUO in children. Most cases are caused by leukemia or lymphoma. Rarely, neuroblastoma or other solid cancers such as hepatoma or rhabdomyosarcoma may present as unexplained fever.

Factitious Fever

Factitious fever always must be considered in the evaluation of a child with FUO. When the patient is an infant or young child, the parent or other caretaker is the one who is fabricating. In bizarre cases, the parent actually may induce fever by injecting the child with infectious or noxious materials. In the case of the older child or adolescent, the patient usually is the one falsifying information. In most cases, factitious fever can be excluded by having the nurse or physician stay in the room while the temperature is taken. Occasionally, the temperature must be taken rectally to ensure that the youngster has not drunk or rinsed the mouth with hot liquids before the temperature measurement is performed. In rare cases, measuring the temperature of a freshly voided urine specimen can be helpful.

Periodic Disorders

Familial Mediterranean fever (FMF) is an exceedingly rare autosomal recessive disorder seen mostly in Arabs, Armenians, and Sephardic Jews. FMF is characterized by acute episodes of fever and inflammation of serosal tissue such as the peritoneum, pleura, or joint synovia. Episodes occur at irregular intervals.

In contrast to FMF, most other periodic disorders are characterized by recurrent episodes of fever at fairly regular intervals. In many cases, the febrile attacks initially tend to occur 3 or 4 weeks apart, but as the illness persists, the interval between episodes often lengthens to 5 or 6 weeks. Between episodes, the patient is normal and asymptomatic. Some patients have neutropenia at the time of having fever, suggesting a variant of cyclic neutropenia. Others may have arthralgias, pharyngitis, aphthous stomatitis, or cervical lymphadenopathy with each episode of fever. The nature of most of these periodic disorders remains unknown, but many cases of periodic fever in children, with or without stomatitis and adenopathy, now are recognized as being associated with the hyperimmunoglobulinemia D syndrome.

Other Causes

Other causes of FUO include serum sickness, drug reactions, inflammatory bowel disease, thyrotoxicosis, Behçet syndrome, histiocytosis, sarcoidosis, ectodermal dysplasia, diabetes insipidus, chronic brain syndrome, subdural hematoma, infantile cortical hyperostosis, familial dysautonomia, and thyrotoxicosis. Several cases have been reported of infants receiving furosemide who have had otherwise unexplained fever lasting for many months. We have observed this phenomenon and noted that the fever remitted when the furosemide was discontinued and recurred when it was restarted. Whether the temperature elevation is caused by dehydration or another mechanism is unknown.

Familial dysautonomia is an inherited disease seen most frequently in individuals of Ashkenazi Jewish descent. Characteristic features include periods of hypo- and hyperthermia, hypertension or postural hypotension, hypo- and hyperhidrosis, flushing and blanching of the skin, crying without tears, diminished peripheral sensitivity to pain, diminished deep tendon reflexes, emotional lability, severe gastroesophageal reflux, and, in some patients, the development of scoliosis.

Mucocutaneous lymph node syndrome (Kawasaki syndrome) should be considered in the differential diagnosis of any young child with FUO, but usually it can be diagnosed or ruled out by the presence or absence of clinical features. Occasionally, however, fever and irritability may be the only findings for up to 10 days. The cause of this presumably infectious disease has not been determined.

Infrequently, an apparent FUO is only an exaggerated normal circadian temperature pattern, a misinterpretation of normal temperature that may be as high as 38°C (100.4°F) in infants or young children, or an unfortunate (but not remarkable) series of self-limited viral infections.

Finally, in as many as one-fourth of all cases of FUO in children, no definite diagnosis ever is established. Most of these cases resolve spontaneously.

Suggested Readings

D'Acremont V, Ambresin AE, Burnand B, Genton B. Practice guidelines for evaluation of fever in returning travelers and migrants. *J Travel Med* 2003;10:25.

Feigin RD, Shearer WT. Fever of unknown origin in children. *Curr Probl Pediatr* 1976;6:2.

Frenkel J, Houten SM, Waterham RJ, et al. Clinical and molecular variability in childhood periodic fever with hyperimmunoglobulinemia D. *Rheumatology* 2001;40:579.

Gartner JC Jr. Fever of unknown origin. *Adv Pediatr Infect Dis* 1992;7:1.

Jacobs RF. Bartonella henselae as a cause of prolonged fever of unknown origin. *Clin Infect Dis* 1998;26:80.

Lohr JA, Hendley JO. Prolonged fever of unknown origin: a record of experiences with 54 childhood patients. *Clin Pediatr* 1977;16:768.

Lorin MI. *The febrile child: clinical management of fever and other types of pyrexia.* New York: Wiley, 1982:94.

Marshall GS, Edwards KM, Butler J, Lawton AR. Syndrome of periodic fever, pharyngitis and aphthous stomatitis. *J Pediatr* 1987;110:43.

McClung HJ. Prolonged fever of unknown origin in children. *Am J Dis Child* 1972;124:544.

Miller LC, Sisson BA, Tucker LB, Schaller JG. Prolonged fevers of unknown origin in children: patterns of presentation and outcome. *J Pediatr* 1996;129:419.

Miller ML, Szer I, Yogev R, Bernstein B. Fever of unknown origin. *Pediatr Clin North Am* 1995;42:999.

Pizzo PA, Lovejoy FH, Smith DH. Prolonged fever in children: review of 100 cases. *Pediatrics* 1957;55:468.

Reimann HA, McCloskey RV. Periodic fever: diagnostic and therapeutic problems. *JAMA* 1974;228:1662.

Steele RW, Jones SM, Lowe B, Glasier CM. Usefulness of scanning procedures for diagnosis of fever of unknown origin in children. *J Pediatr* 1991;119:526.

CHAPTER 134 ■ PATHOGENESIS OF FEVER AND ITS TREATMENT

MARTIN I. LORIN

Fever often is defined simply as an elevation of body temperature above an arbitrary upper limit of normal. However, a more proper definition is an elevation of body temperature as part of a specific biologic response, mediated and controlled by the central nervous system (CNS). This definition distinguishes fever from other types of elevated body temperature, such as heat stress and heat illness.

PATHOPHYSIOLOGY

Fever is only one of a large array of responses elicited by chemical mediators of the inflammatory process. These mediators are termed endogenous pyrogenic cytokines, the best-known of which are interleukin-1 (IL-1) (which is composed of IL-1α and IL-1β), tumor necrosis factor-alpha (TNF-α), IL-6, and interferon gamma (IFN-γ). These mediators are synthesized by a variety of blood and tissue cells, including macrophages. In addition to inducing fever, these pyrogenic cytokines increase the synthesis of acute-phase proteins by the liver, decrease serum iron and zinc levels, provoke leukocytosis, and accelerate skeletal muscle proteolysis. IL-1 also induces slow-wave sleep, perhaps explaining the somnolence frequently associated with febrile illnesses.

Fever is the result of a highly coordinated series of events that begins peripherally with the synthesis and release of IL-1 and other mediators by cells in the blood or tissues. Molecules of IL-1 enter the blood and are carried to the CNS, where they induce an abrupt increase in the synthesis of prostaglandins, especially prostaglandin E_2, in the region of the anterior hypothalamus. This increase results in elevation of the set-point (or reference point) of the thermostat mechanism in this area of the brain. The temperature control region of the anterior hypothalamus then sees current body temperature as too low in comparison to the new set-point and initiates a series of events to elevate body temperature to a height equal to the new set-point. This adaptation involves the augmentation of heat production by increased metabolic rate and increased muscle tone and activity; in addition, it involves decreased loss of heat, primarily through diminished perfusion of the skin. Body temperature rises until a new equilibrium is achieved at the elevated set-point.

Fever: Friend or Foe?

How important is fever as a defense mechanism? The general assumption is that such a complex reaction must represent an integral and functional part of the inflammatory response and not simply an incidental or accidental biologic effect. However, answering the question of whether this response always is beneficial is more difficult. Defense mechanisms can go awry.

Fluid retention in congestive heart failure is one example of a situation in which a defense mechanism in excess may do more harm than good.

The question often posed is: Is fever a friend or a foe? A more appropriate question would be: Under what conditions is fever beneficial and under what conditions is it harmful? Even granting that fever does have a role in defending the host against infection, in some circumstances fever still may do more harm than good. Also, fever may be a less important defense mechanism in higher animals, such as mammals with well-developed immunologic systems, than in fish and reptiles with more primitive immunologic systems. Many animal experiments that demonstrated a survival benefit due to fever involved cold-blooded animals (poikilotherms), such as fish and lizards, which do develop fever in response to infection but do so strictly by behavioral mechanisms, by moving to the warmest external environment available. Despite the differences between the immunologic systems of these animals and primates, poikilothermic animals often have been selected as laboratory models for the study of fever because of the convenience with which fever can be prevented without confounding the study by introducing drugs such as aspirin.

Studies in lizards and goldfish infected with *Aeromonas hydrophila* have demonstrated a higher mortality rate when the febrile response is prevented by denying the animals access to a warmer environment. A study in young adult volunteers with the common cold found prolonged viral shedding in those given aspirin compared to those given a placebo. In view of the current knowledge of the immunosuppressive effects of aspirin, studies that used this drug to evaluate the effect of fever reduction on morbidity or mortality, either in animals or humans, must be considered suspect because they do not distinguish between whether the effect was caused by the suppression of fever or by the antipyretic drug itself. One study found increased time to total scabbing of lesions in children given acetaminophen (which has no antiinflammatory effect) versus those given placebo.

The growth or survival of some pathogenic bacteria or viruses is impaired at temperatures in the range of 40°C (104°F). Many pathogenic bacteria require iron for their growth, and fever has been shown to be associated with a decrease in serum iron and a simultaneous increase in serum ferritin, resulting in reduced levels of free iron in the blood. Because these bacteria have an enhanced need for iron at high temperatures, some researchers have suggested that this response is a coordinated host defense mechanism designed to deprive bacteria of free iron when they need it most. *In vitro* studies have demonstrated the enhancement of several human immunologic functions at moderately elevated ambient temperatures. These functions include increased lymphocyte transformation response to mitogen, increased bactericidal activity of polymorphonuclear leukocytes, and increased production of interferon. However, as temperatures approached 40°C

(104°F) in these experiments, most of the functions decreased to below baseline levels.

In one study of rabbits infected with *Pasteurella multocida*, survival rates increased with moderate fever, but with fevers greater than 2.25°C above baseline, survival rates were lower than in the euthermic state. Another study demonstrated increased mortality rates associated with fever in rats infected with *Salmonella enteritidis*. Thus, fever, especially fever of moderate degree, appears to enhance several aspects of the immunologic response. At high body temperatures, however, these effects may be diminished or even reversed.

Fever also can have undesirable effects other than the immunologic changes described earlier. Fever often makes patients uncomfortable. It is associated with an increased metabolic rate, increased consumption of oxygen and production of carbon dioxide, and increased demands on the cardiovascular and pulmonary systems. For the normal child, these stresses are of little or no consequence. However, for the child with an underlying disorder, especially of the heart or lungs, these increased demands may be significantly detrimental.

Fever can precipitate febrile convulsions in susceptible children between 6 months and 5 years of age. Although such seizures generally are benign, they are disturbing to the parent and child and may lead to the use of invasive procedures such as lumbar punctures, as well as to considerable expense.

An experiment in monkeys demonstrated the deleterious effect of fever on injured cerebral tissue. A standardized insult was introduced to one cerebral hemisphere in each experimental animal. One-half of the monkeys were maintained in the euthermic state and one-half were maintained at a core temperature of 40°C (104°F) for 2 hours after the injury. All animals then were sacrificed. A 40% increase in edema was found in the traumatized hemisphere of the hyperthermic animals as compared with the euthermic animals. Bleeding also was more profuse in the experimental group.

TREATMENT

Although our current state of knowledge does not permit rigid recommendations regarding the symptomatic treatment of fever, we can make some reasonable suggestions. Clearly, fever need not always be treated, and body temperature need not always be restored completely to normal. It is appropriate to treat high fever (40°C [104°F] or greater), as well as fever in children in the age group at risk for having febrile convulsions and in children with underlying neurologic or cardiopulmonary disease. Fever also should be treated in cases of septic shock and in any situation in which a component of heat illness is a consideration. Until more data are available, the treatment of fever to establish the patient's comfort should not be condemned.

Once a decision is made to treat a patient's fever symptomatically, the choice of a specific therapeutic modality should be based on several considerations. Because fever is the result of an elevation of the set-point in the hypothalamic thermoregulatory center, the most rational way to treat fever is to restore this set-point to normal; agents such as aspirin, acetaminophen, and ibuprofen all work on this basis. Aspirin and acetaminophen are equally effective at similar doses, whereas ibuprofen is effective at a somewhat lower dose and has a longer duration of action. Given the minimal differences in efficacy of these agents, selection should be based on potential toxicities and cost rather than efficacy. In a therapeutic dosage, aspirin is the most toxic of these agents. Gastritis, gastrointestinal bleeding, impaired platelet function, diminished urinary excretion of sodium, and blunted immune response occur frequently with aspirin, less often with ibuprofen, and hardly at all with acetaminophen. Correct therapeutic doses of acetaminophen are remarkably free of side effects. The association of aspirin with Reye syndrome has led to the virtual abandonment of this drug for antipyretic therapy in infants and children. The association with Reye syndrome is not shared by acetaminophen or ibuprofen.

Although the mechanisms are different, an overdose of any of these agents can be lethal. Fatal aspirin overdose has been associated primarily with a mixed metabolic acidosis and respiratory alkalosis; the major cause of death in cases of overdose of acetaminophen has been hepatic necrosis. Although an overdose of ibuprofen appears to be less severe and more easily managed than does an overdose of either aspirin or acetaminophen, deaths in children from CNS depression and apnea caused by overdoses of ibuprofen have been reported. With regard to toxicity associated with an ordinary therapeutic dosage, acetaminophen clearly is preferable for routine use. Whereas studies have shown a somewhat greater and more prolonged reduction in fever with the use of ibuprofen as compared to acetaminophen, this difference has not been proven to be clinically important. Furthermore, no published studies involve a rescue strategy to show whether patients who fail to respond to acetaminophen respond to ibuprofen. No data have been gathered to document either safety or increased efficacy of combined therapy with acetaminophen and ibuprofen, and several theoretic risks (especially renal injury) are associated with the concomitant administration of both drugs. Until further information is available, the practice of combining or alternating these agents should be discouraged.

Although acetaminophen often is prescribed on the basis of age, a weight-based dosage is more accurate. In general, the dose of acetaminophen is 10 to 15 mg/kg every 4 to 6 hours. Some sources suggest limiting the total dosage to no more than five times per day. Some reports have raised concern of acute liver injury secondary to an excessive therapeutic dosage of acetaminophen over the course of several days. The half-life of many drugs is prolonged significantly in the newborn and very young infant; therefore, antipyretics should be used with caution and at a reduced dosage in these age groups.

Under certain circumstances, the use of external cooling, generally by sponging, to reduce body temperature is necessary or advisable, either in addition to or instead of the administration of antipyretic drugs (Table 134.1). External cooling is the treatment of choice for heatstroke and other forms of heat

---

TABLE 134.1

USE OF EXTERNAL COOLING IN TREATING ELEVATED TEMPERATURE

Cooling Method	Indications
Tepid sponging *instead of* antipyretic drugs	Very young infants
	Severe liver disease
	History of hypersensitivity to antipyretic drugs
Tepid sponging *plus* antipyretic drugs	High fever [>40°C (104°F)]
	History of febrile seizures, neurologic disorders, or brain damage
	Infection plus suspicion of overheating or overwrapping
	Septic shock*
Cold sponging alone	Heat illness

*May require cold sponging.

illness. However, for fever, external cooling is indicated only in specific situations. External sponging is advisable in any situation in which suspicion exists that the cause of the elevated temperature may be a form of heat illness. Some patients with infections also may have a component of heat illness from over-wrapping, dehydration, or drugs.

For the previously well child with a non-life-threatening febrile illness, sponging adds little but increased discomfort for the patient. The antipyretic effect of oral acetaminophen plus sponging with tepid water is only slightly more rapid than is the effect of oral acetaminophen alone. Sponging with ice water is more rapid but more discomforting, and is necessary only for treating heat illness. Sponging often is useful in patients with neurologic disorders because many of these children have abnormal temperature control and respond poorly to antipyretic agents. Sponging also would be preferable to the use of antipyretic agents in children with hypersensitivity to these agents and in patients with severe liver disease. As mentioned earlier, in very young infants, the half-life of acetaminophen is prolonged, and so sponging may be preferable to the use of this agent.

Sponging should be done with tepid water [generally at approximately 30°C (85°F)]. Alcohol should not be used because it may be absorbed across the skin and because its fumes are absorbed across the alveolar membrane, resulting in CNS toxicity.

Suggested Readings

Banet M. Fever and survival in the rat. The effect of enhancing the cold defense mechanism. *Experientia* 1981;37:985.

Clasen RA, Pandolfi S, Laing I, Casey D. Experimental study of relation of fever to cerebral edema. *J Neurosurg* 1974;41:576.

Crocetti M, Moghbeli N, Serwint J. Fever phobia revisited: have parental misconceptions about fever changed in 20 years? *Pediatrics* 2001;107:1241.

Dinarello CA. Thermoregulation and the pathogenesis of fever. *Infect Dis Clin North Am* 1996;10:433.

Doran TF, DeAngelis C, Baumgardner RA, et al. Acetaminophen: more harm than good for chickenpox? *J Pediatr* 1989;114:1045.

Klastersky J, Kass EH. Is suppression of fever or hypothermia useful in experimental and clinical infectious diseases? *J Infect Dis* 1970;121:81.

Kluger MJ, Kozak W, Conn CA, et al. The adaptive value of fever. *Infect Dis Clin North Am* 1996;10:1.

Lorin MI. *The febrile child: clinical management of fever and other types of pyrexia.* New York: John Wiley & Sons, 1982:27.

Mackowiak PA. Fever: blessing or curse? A unifying concept. *Ann Intern Med* 1994;120:1037.

River-Penera T, Gugig R, Davis J, et al. Outcome of acetaminophen overdose in pediatric patients and factors contributing to hepatotoxicity. *J Pediatr* 1997;130:300.

Roberts NJ, Steigbigel RJ. Hyperthermia and human leukocyte function. *Infect Immun* 1977;18:673.

Rumack BH. Aspirin versus acetaminophen: a comparative view. *Pediatrics* 1978;62(Suppl):943.

Stanley ED, et al. Increased virus shedding with aspirin treatment of rhinovirus infection. *JAMA* 1975;231:1248.

Steele RW, Tanaka PT, Lara RP, Bass JW. Evaluation of sponging and of oral antipyretic therapy to reduce fever. *J Pediatr* 1970;77:824.

CHAPTER 135 ■ SEPSIS AND SEPTIC SHOCK

KENNETH M. BOYER AND PAUL N. SEVERIN

U.S. Supreme Court Justice Potter Stewart once wrote, "I can't define obscenity; but I know it when I see it." Most pediatricians would feel that statement could be applied equally well to sepsis, septic shock, and the related life-threatening systemic infections that can occur in children.

Since the late 1980s, intensive study has led to an improved understanding of the basic biochemistry and pathophysiology of serious infection. Fundamental to this new knowledge is the discovery that a great variety of illnesses—including such noninfectious conditions as immune-mediated organ injury, multiple trauma, and malignancy—have in common with infection the endogenous production of certain key inflammatory mediators that result in similar physiologic consequences.

TERMINOLOGY

Subspecialists in infectious diseases and critical-care medicine now generally agree regarding the terms that should be used to classify serious infections, despite less experience with their application in pediatrics (and neonatology). Currently accepted definitions include the following:

- *Systemic inflammatory response syndrome (SIRS)*: The systemic inflammatory response to a variety of clinical stresses. The response is manifested by two or more of the following conditions (one of which must be abnormal temperature or leukocyte count): temperature greater than 38.5°C or less than 36°C; heart rate greater than the 95th percentile or less than the 5th percentile for age; respiratory rate greater than the 95th percentile for age; and white blood cell count greater than 15,000 cells per microliter, less than 5,000 cells per microliter, or with greater than 10% immature (band) forms.

- *Infection*: Microbial phenomenon characterized by an inflammatory response to the presence of microorganisms or the invasion of normally sterile host tissue by those organisms.

- *Bacteremia*: The presence of viable bacteria in the blood. *Viremia, fungemia,* and *parasitemia* are the terms to be used when the corresponding organisms are isolated.

- *Sepsis*: The systemic response to documented infection (sepsis = SIRS + infection).

- *Severe sepsis*: Sepsis associated with organ dysfunction, hypoperfusion, or hypotension. Signs of hypoperfusion may include, but are not limited to, lactic acidosis, oliguria, or an acute alteration in mental status.

- *Septic shock*: Sepsis with hypotension that persists after adequate fluid resuscitation, along with the presence of perfusion abnormalities that may include, but are not limited to, lactic acidosis, oliguria, or an acute alteration in mental status. Patients with septic shock who are on

BOX 135.1	Bacterial Etiologies of Sepsis in Previously Normal Pediatric Patients, by Apparent Source

Occult
Streptococcus pneumoniae, Haemophilus influenzae type b, *Neisseria meningitidis, Staphylococcus aureus*

Focal Source
Skin and musculoskeletal: *S. aureus, Streptococcus pyogenes, H. influenzae* type b
Respiratory tract: *S. pneumoniae, H. influenzae* type b, *S. aureus,* oral anaerobes,* *S. pyogenes*
Gastrointestinal tract: *Salmonella* species, *Shigella* species, *Yersinia enterocolitica*
Peritoneum: enteric gram-negative rods,[†] enteric anaerobes,[‡] *Enterococcus faecalis*
Heart or pericardium: *S. aureus, H. influenzae* type b
Urinary tract: enteric gram-negative rods
Genital tract: *Neisseria gonorrhoeae,* enteric anaerobes
Meninges: *S. pneumoniae, N. meningitidis, H. influenzae* type b

Acquired Barrier Disruption
Abdominal surgery or penetrating trauma: enteric gram-negative rods, enteric anaerobes, *Enterococcus faecalis*
Cardiac surgery: staphylococci,[§] multiply resistant gram-negative rods**
Orthopedic surgery or compound fracture: staphylococci

Craniofacial surgery: staphylococci, *S. pyogenes, S. pneumoniae, H. influenzae* type b, oral anaerobes
Vascular access device-related: staphylococci, multiply resistant gram-negative rods, *Acinetobacter* species, *Candida albicans*
Burn wounds: *S. pyogenes, S. aureus, Pseudomonas aeruginosa*

Bite Wounds
Human: *Eikenella corrodens,* staphylococci, oral anaerobes
Dog: *Capnocytophaga canimorsus* (DF-2), *Pasteurella multocida,* staphylococci, oral anaerobes
Cat: *P. multocida,* oral anaerobes
Rat: *Streptobacillus moniliformis, Spirillum minus*
Flea: *Yersinia pestis*
Tick: *Francisella tularensis, Ehrlichia chaffeensis, Rickettsia rickettsii, Borrelia hermsi*

Peptostreptococcus, Fusobacterium species, *Prevotella melaninogenicus, Veillonella.*
[†]*Escherichia coli, Klebsiella* species, *Enterobacter* species.
[‡]*Bacteroides fragilis, Clostridium perfringens, Clostridium septicum, Fusobacterium* species.
[§]*S. aureus,* coagulase-negative staphylococci.
**Enterobacter* species, *P. aeruginosa, Klebsiella* species, *Stenotrophomonas maltophilia, Serratia marcescens.*

inotropic or vasopressor agents may have blood pressures in the normal range despite the presence of perfusion abnormalities.

■ *Multiple organ dysfunction syndrome (MODS)*: Presence of altered organ function in an acutely ill patient such that physiologic homeostasis cannot be maintained without multiple life support interventions, such as pressor infusions, mechanical ventilation, or transfusion of blood products.

Unlike the situation in adult medicine, SIRS and sepsis as defined here are common "problem statements" in pediatrics. Because pediatric patients compensate well for shock states with tachycardia and vasoconstriction, septic shock and MODS by these definitions become relatively uncommon (but ominous) clinical entities.

ETIOLOGY

Typically, sepsis and the various septic syndromes are caused by bacterial infections of an advanced or rapidly progressive nature. Contrary to popular belief, most patients with sepsis do *not* have documented bacteremia, which accounts for some of the recent changes in definitions. However, the probability of having positive blood cultures increases as one progresses down the classification list to septic shock and MODS. Even with negative blood cultures, bacterial etiology often can be established by positive Gram stains and cultures at focal sites of infection, characteristic alterations in hematologic parameters, tests for the presence of bacterial exotoxins, or clinical responses to empiric antimicrobial therapy.

The common (and some of the unusual) bacterial etiologies of sepsis in previously normal children are presented in

Box 135.1, according to the presence or absence of a focal source and according to the presence of accidental or surgical alterations in integumentary and mucosal barriers. A working knowledge of these organisms and the clinical settings in which they are most likely to present provides a rational basis for the selection of empiric antibiotic regimens. (The causes of neonatal infections are discussed comprehensively in Chapters 71 through 88. A complete description of the causes of community-acquired and nosocomial sepsis in compromised hosts can be found in Chapter 88.) Sepsis of a critical nature, even in a previously normal child, should prompt consideration of an important defect in host defense. For example, meningococcemia should suggest an abnormality in the terminal complement pathway.

The encapsulated organisms—*Streptococcus pneumoniae, Neisseria meningitidis,* and *Haemophilus influenzae* type b—have been the most common causes of sepsis (and bacteremia) of occult origin. These organisms occur most frequently in children aged 3 months to 5 years and commonly are preceded by viral upper respiratory illnesses. Peaks in incidence correspond to the nadir in transplacentally acquired maternal IgG antibodies. Use of infant vaccination has reduced dramatically the incidence of *H. influenzae* and *S. pneumoniae* sepsis in recent years in the United States.

A focus of infection always should be sought in patients with bacteremia. Often, the identity of a bloodstream isolate can be a clue to its origin. *Staphylococcus aureus* bacteremia, for example, always should suggest the possible presence of osteomyelitis, endocarditis, or pericarditis.

In sepsis of focal origin, likely bacterial etiologies are suggested by the site of the infection and often are determined by the normal flora of a contiguous surface. For example, urinary tract infections often are caused by enteric flora. Generally, first episodes are caused by antibiotic-susceptible *Escherichia coli.*

Recurrent episodes separated by periods of prophylactic antibiotics (to the extent that prophylaxis has altered enteric flora) will be caused by *Klebsiella* species, *Enterococcus* species, *Enterobacter* species, or *Pseudomonas aeruginosa* with multiple-drug resistance.

Generally, sepsis associated with bacterial enteritis is caused by *Salmonella*, *Shigella*, or *Yersinia enterocolitica*. Often, *Salmonella* enteric fever is associated with bacteremia. Shigellosis, on the other hand, rarely is bacteremic but may be associated with sepsis and septic shock, especially if *Shigella dysenteriae* is involved.

Disruption of skin or mucosal barriers may be accidental or surgical. Bite wounds can be associated with unusual oral pathogens, depending on the source. For example, dog bites generally are inoculated with *Staphylococcus* and oral anaerobes, but they may be contaminated also with *Pasteurella multocida* or *Capnocytophaga canimorsus*. Often, the latter two species are associated with bacteremia and sepsis. Generally, infections affecting surgical sites involve normal flora that contaminate surgically damaged tissue at the site of operation. For example, sepsis complicating craniofacial surgery is caused by the normal flora of the skin, scalp, and upper respiratory mucosal surfaces, including staphylococci, *Haemophilus* species, *S. pneumoniae*, and oral anaerobes.

In addition to severe bacterial infections sepsis has a broad differential diagnosis, as summarized in Box 135.2. Included are nonbacterial infections, such as viral, rickettsial, and spirochetal infections, and responses to bacterial products, such as the Jarisch-Herxheimer reaction that occurs after treatment of relapsing fever. Although it is not a final diagnosis, sepsis is an appropriate problem statement for such conditions. Shock states that may be confused with septic shock include supraventricular tachycardia with cardiogenic shock (often triggered by an acute febrile illness) and gastroenteritis with hypovolemic shock (also commonly associated with fever). Recognizing the former is particularly important because aggressive fluid resuscitation can lead to deterioration, rather than improvement, in cardiovascular status.

PATHOGENESIS

In the past, septic shock has been considered synonymous with endotoxin shock. Lipopolysaccharides purified from the cell membranes of a variety of such gram-negative organisms as *E. coli*, *Salmonella*, *Pseudomonas*, and *N. meningitidis* are capable of eliciting the characteristic picture of sepsis in experimental animals. The accidental infusion of contaminated intravenous fluids containing large amounts of endotoxin (but without viable organisms) has been found to trigger septic shock in humans. Experimental infusion of low doses of endotoxin in volunteers elicits characteristic physiologic and laboratory changes. Anti-endotoxin antibodies in pooled sera or in the form of specific monoclonal antibodies can block the response and have been studied intensively as adjunctive therapy in critically ill patients. Thus, endotoxin is unquestionably one of the trigger mechanisms of sepsis.

Other organisms can produce septic syndromes, either by virtue of their production of exotoxins or by sheer force of numbers. Both staphylococcal and group A streptococcal toxic

---

| BOX 135.2 | Differential Diagnosis of Sepsis |

Infection

Viral illness (influenza, enteroviruses, SARS coronavirus, dengue hemorrhagic fever, dis-seminated herpes)
Encephalitis (arbovirus, enterovirus, herpes)
Rickettsial infection (Rocky Mountain spotted fever, *Ehrlichia*, Q fever)
Spirochetal infection (syphilis, relapsing fever; Jarisch-Herxheimer reaction)
Vaccine reaction (pertussis, whole-virus influenza, typhoid)

Cardiopulmonary

Pneumonia (bacterial, viral, mycobacterial, fungal, *Pneumocystis*)
Pulmonary emboli (air, thrombus, fat)
Congestive heart failure
Arrhythmia (with cardiogenic shock)
Pericarditis (with pericardial tamponade)
Myocarditis

Metabolic-Endocrine

Adrenal insufficiency (adrenogenital syndrome, Addison disease, steroid withdrawal)
Diabetes insipidus
Diabetes mellitus
Inborn errors of metabolism (organic acidurias, urea cycle defects, carnitine deficiency)
Hypoglycemia
Reye syndrome
Neuroleptic malignant syndrome
Malignant hyperthermia

Gastrointestinal

Gastroenteritis with hypovolemic shock (viral, bacterial, parasitic)
Malrotation with midgut volvulus
Intussusception
Appendicitis or appendiceal abscess
Peritonitis (spontaneous, perforation, dialysis)
Hepatitis
Hemorrhage

Hematologic

Anemia (sickle cell, blood loss, nutritional)
Splenic sequestration crisis
Leukemia, lymphoma

Neurologic

Intoxication (drugs, carbon monoxide, intentional or accidental overdose)
Intracranial hemorrhage
Trauma (child abuse, accidents)
Guillain-Barré syndrome
Myasthenia gravis

Other

Collagen-vascular disease (systemic lupus erythematosus, juvenile rheumatoid arthritis)
Anaphylaxis (food, drug, insect sting)
Kawasaki syndrome
Erythema multiforme
Heatstroke
Opiate withdrawl (including iatrogenic)

shock syndromes are potentially lethal conditions, the clinical picture of which is caused by the circulation of well-characterized exotoxins from the site of infection. Bacteremia may accompany toxic shock but is not a necessary condition. Although the clinical features differ somewhat, toxemias arise in association with *S. dysenteriae* dysentery and with the acute hemorrhagic colitis caused by verotoxin-producing *E. coli* 0157:H7. Their exotoxins are biochemically similar; both can lead to the hemolytic uremic syndrome. As with staphylococcal and streptococcal toxic shock, blood cultures generally are negative. Finally, researchers have shown in experimental animals that the high-level intravenous infusion of even relatively nonvirulent gram-positive bacteria, such as coagulase-negative staphylococci, can induce the physiologic changes of sepsis and septic shock. For these reasons, gram-negative endotoxin no longer can be considered the sole microbiologic trigger of sepsis and septic shock.

Septic shock now is recognized to result from the sequential release of endogenous mediators. These substances, called *cytokines*, are products of monocytes, macrophages, T lymphocytes, endothelial cells, mast cells, polymorphonuclear leukocytes, and other cell types. Production of these cytokines is triggered by "toll-like receptors" (TLRs) in their cell membranes that interact with bacterial products such as endotoxin. The signals that comprise the inflammatory cascade presumably evolved as part of the mechanisms for controlling relatively localized infections or trauma. However, when a human host is confronted by a more massive challenge, various cytokines may be produced excessively, leading to a response so vigorous as to be potentially fatal. The cytokine that initiates the inflammatory cascade is tumor necrosis factor–alpha (TNF), a product of monocytes and macrophages. Injection of TNF in experimental animals completely mimics the clinical response (fever, hypotension, coagulopathy, multiple organ failure, and death) seen after injection with endotoxin, but the response has a shorter latency time. Circulating levels of TNF directly correlate with prognosis, as has been demonstrated in meningococcal disease.

Other mediators appear to be responsible for other specific clinical features. The interleukins (ILs), particularly IL-1, IL-2, and IL-6, mediate hypotension and fever. Hageman factor (factor XII) and platelet-activating factor (PAF) mediate coagulopathy. Interferon-gamma activates macrophages. Heparin binding protein triggers endothelial capillary leak. Granulocyte colony-stimulating factor and granulocyte-macrophage colony-stimulating factor (GCSF and GMCSF, respectively) stimulate production of phagocytic cells. The integrins on white cells (CD11 and CD18) and the intercellular and vascular adhesion molecules on endothelial cells (ICAMs and VCAMs) control leukocyte margination and diapedesis. The complement system produces substances (C3a and C5a) that are the major chemotactic attractants for leukocytes. Nitric oxide is a potent vasodilator of the microcirculation and is the final pathway of hypotension and septic shock. The list of mediators is ever-increasing, and a clear picture of the sequence is not yet complete.

The consequence of an excessive release of these mediators is the development of sepsis. Progression to septic shock and multiorgan system dysfunction or failure depends on the pathogens involved and the degree to which mediators and effector cells (as well as antimicrobial therapy) are capable of localizing and killing them. The most prominent physiologic features of septic shock are fever and cardiovascular compromise or collapse. The cardiac response to sepsis is characterized by an initial increase in cardiac output followed by a period of poor myocardial performance, probably caused by one or more myocardial depressant factors. The effect of sepsis on the vascular bed is complex but is characterized by direct injury to endothelial cells and their adhesion to one another, resulting in alterations

of vascular tone and in capillary leak. The alterations of tone result in decreased systemic vascular resistance and abnormal perfusion patterns to vital organ systems, which may lead to organ dysfunction or complete organ failure. Capillary leak allows the egress of fluid and proteins from the vascular system and results in hypovolemia and the severe edema often encountered during therapy of severe cases.

The effects of compromised perfusion and capillary leak are unique to each organ system. Mortality rates are directly proportional to the number of organs that fail. Capillary leak and intrapulmonary right-to-left shunting may lead to the acute respiratory distress syndrome (see Chapter 454). Initially, decreased renal perfusion leads to oliguria. In the presence of uncorrected hypotension, acute tubular necrosis may develop (see Chapter 454). Decreased cerebral circulation leads to confusion, disorientation, and obtundation. Compounding these changes is the frequent occurrence of disseminated intravascular coagulation (see Chapter 298), which can reduce perfusion of vital organs further or, through the depletion of clotting factors, can lead to major hemorrhage.

CLINICAL MANIFESTATIONS AND COMPLICATIONS

Recognition of the septic child may be difficult. The pediatrician's fundamental dilemma is differentiating the child with a potentially life-threatening infection from among the many children with self-limited or readily treated infections that are not life-threatening. An awareness of the presence of predisposing conditions to infection in individual children probably is the most helpful guide. However, not all seriously ill children have identified defects in their host defenses, particularly in infancy.

Most children with sepsis have obvious and significantly elevated temperatures. However, in the very young and those with advanced disease, temperatures actually may register in the hypothermic range. Rigors and hyperthermia (temperature greater than 41° C [105.8° F]) imply the presence of bacteremia.

Behavioral changes can be helpful indicators of serious illness. Four of the six items on the Yale Observational Scale—quality of cry, reaction to parent stimulation, state variation, and response to social overtures—are behavioral. Children with febrile illness, a weak cry, poor responsiveness, no smile, and lack of facial expression are likely to be septic. In some cases, these changes reflect compromised cerebral circulation; occasionally, they indicate complicating meningitis.

Although changes in respiratory pattern generally point to pulmonary disease, tachypnea and acrocyanosis also may reflect metabolic acidosis and poor peripheral perfusion—both characteristic of sepsis.

A careful evaluation of circulatory adequacy is important. Measuring blood pressure is basic, but one should recognize that children often compensate well for early shock states, so that blood pressure may be in the normal range. Difficulty in measuring a sick child's blood pressure is more likely to be a reflection of marginal circulation than of a technical problem with the blood pressure apparatus. Even if measured blood pressure registers in the normal range, circulatory inadequacy usually is manifested by cool extremities, acrocyanosis, absent or diminished peripheral pulses, and capillary refill times of more than 3 seconds. Although "warm shock" may be seen early in sepsis, it is a relatively unusual occurrence in children.

Cutaneous manifestations of sepsis may be extremely helpful as warning flags. Between 8% and 20% of patients with fever and petechiae have a serious bacterial infection, and 7% to 10% have meningococcemia or meningococcal meningitis. Purpuric lesions or ecchymoses of the distal extremities (purpura fulminans) raise these probabilities even higher. Diffuse erythroderma in the presence of fever and septic shock should suggest toxic shock syndrome.

DIAGNOSIS

Laboratory manifestations of sepsis include positive blood cultures and positive cultures from such other sites as urine, cerebrospinal fluid, stool, joint or bone aspirates, exudates, abscesses, and cutaneous lesions. Continuing efforts should be made to identify the site of origin of a septic process or sites of metastatic spread, using multiple cultures of multiple sites if necessary. Blood cultures that are persistently positive in spite of administration of appropriate empiric treatment imply the presence of resistant organisms or an endovascular origin of infection.

Hematologic parameters are useful in initial and continuing evaluations. Leukocytosis is the norm; leukopenia is more prognostically ominous. In some instances, leukopenia is the initial response, with remarkable leukocytosis the later response to successful therapy. Elevated band counts, toxic granulation, and Döhle bodies imply bacterial sepsis. Thrombocytopenia implies the presence of disseminated intravascular coagulation, which should be confirmed with documentation of prothrombin time, partial thromboplastin time, fibrinogen levels, and the presence of fibrin split products. Band counts (decreasing) and platelet counts (increasing) are useful serial studies implying successful treatment.

Metabolic acidosis, manifested by decreased serum bicarbonate, pH, and increased serum lactate, is a frequent biochemical manifestation of diminished end-organ perfusion. Compensatory respiratory alkalosis is a common early abnormality. Persisting metabolic acidosis during therapy is an ominous indicator of inadequate tissue oxygen delivery. Prerenal azotemia and uremia are the usual manifestations of diminished renal perfusion and acute tubular necrosis, respectively. Often, hypoalbuminemia develops during management of severe sepsis, the consequence of both a catabolic state and capillary leak of colloid into the interstitium.

THERAPY

The cornerstones of treatment for sepsis and septic shock are the maintenance of adequate oxygen and nutrient delivery to vital organs and eradication of the infecting organisms. After recognition of the situation, an orderly but rapid sequence of initial interventions to achieve these goals is mandatory.

Patients with severe sepsis should be monitored for all five vital signs: respiration, heart rate, blood pressure, temperature, and oxygen saturation (by pulse oximetry). Providing an adequate airway and ensuring peripheral oxygen saturation are top priorities. If abnormal, they should be supported immediately by administration of oxygen and, if necessary, by intubation and mechanical ventilation.

Circulation also should be assessed rapidly and, if it is marginal or inadequate, vascular access must be achieved by peripheral or central venous catheter or by the intraosseous route. Initial blood (or bone marrow) cultures should be obtained when access is achieved. If cardiogenic shock can be excluded reasonably, normal saline, in 20 mL/kg bolus infusions, should be administered. Large amounts of fluid resuscitation may be needed to re-establish tissue and organ perfusion (80 mL/kg total or more) in patients with septic shock. Aggressive volume resuscitation will assist in the early identification of patients with volume–refractory shock and, therefore, the need for inotropic or vasopressor support.

Concomitant with fluid resuscitation; initial empiric antibiotic therapy by the parenteral route should be initiated. An assessment of probable etiology should be made, with consideration of the likely infecting organisms (as presented in Box 135.1). The other key element in antibiotic choice is the likelihood of encountering resistance, the two major determinants of which are whether the infection was acquired in the hospital setting and whether the patient has received antimicrobial therapy recently. In the former instance, knowledge of previous bacterial isolates from a hospitalized child may be very helpful. In the latter, one can suspect an overgrowth phenomenon requiring an alternative drug or combination. The parenteral antibiotics used most frequently in the treatment of sepsis, their dosages, and their usual indications are summarized in Table 135.1. Occult, community-acquired sepsis is treated appropriately with ceftriaxone or cefotaxime. If staphylococcal infection is possible, empiric regimens should now include vancomycin because of the increasing prevalence of methicillin-resistance. Nosocomial sepsis is treated best empirically with multiple agents. The broad combination of vancomycin, a third-generation cephalosporin, and an aminoglycoside is used commonly in this setting. One should recall that an organism resistant to all the antimicrobial agents in an empiric regimen essentially is not being treated. No amount of supportive intervention can compensate for this inadequacy.

The goals of initial empiric antimicrobial therapy are clearing of the bloodstream, penetration to infected sites, and control of the progress of the infectious process. With more definitive microbiological data, regimens should be changed to the specific drugs of choice for the organisms isolated—as single agents or synergistic combinations, depending on identity. Often, gram-positive organisms are treated effectively with single agents; gram-negative rods are managed best with synergistic combinations. With the exception of children with bacterial meningitis (see Chapter 136), corticosteroid therapy is not beneficial. With clarification of the source of a problem, surgical drainage, or removal of hardware may be required as therapeutic adjuncts. When a source or infecting organism is not defined or results are delayed, modification of regimens may be needed if clinical response is suboptimal.

The elements of supportive care given after the patient has been admitted to an intensive care unit include continued monitoring of vital signs and oxygen saturation. In addition, invasive monitoring of central venous pressure and arterial pressure generally is indicated. Non-invasive echocardiography is useful in monitoring critically ill children with sepsis. Evaluation of contractility and afterload by this safe method will allow the physician to make appropriate adjustments of fluid and inotropic supports. Pulmonary artery (Swan-Ganz) catheters are invasive and can be technically difficult in the pediatric patient. Multiorgan system dysfunction, in which the pressure demands of mechanical ventilation may affect cardiovascular performance adversely, is the setting in which pulmonary artery catheters occasionally are considered. They permit more rigorous management of intravascular volume status, ventilator settings, and pressor infusions.

Management of pressor infusions, acute respiratory distress syndrome, acute tubular necrosis, and disseminated intravascular coagulation are discussed further in Chapters 453, 454, 456, and 298, respectively. Subspecialist consultation and a team management approach to septic shock are essential components of management. Conflicting priorities are common occurrences in managing these complex patients. One common situation is the need for the administration of multiple blood products, total parenteral nutrition, and numerous drugs and infusions, in the face of pulmonary edema, marginal myocardial performance, and renal failure. This situation may be handled by the use of slow continuous ultrafiltration or continuous arteriovenous hemofiltration, which can maintain euvolemia despite massive infusion volumes. Because they are continuous, these approaches are much more physiologic than is intermittent hemodialysis.

TABLE 135.1

RECOMMENDED DOSAGE SCHEDULE FOR THE ANTIMICROBIAL AGENTS USED MOST FREQUENTLY IN EMPIRIC TREATMENT OF PEDIATRIC PATIENTS WITH SEPSIS

Agent	Dosage (mg/kg/d) and Intervals of Administration	Maximum Daily Dosage	Most Commom Target Organisms
Amikacin	15–22.5 div q8h	1–2 g[a]	Hospital gram-negative rods
Ampicillin	100–300 div q4–6h	10–12 g	Community encapsulated organisms
Ampicillin-sulbactam[b]	150–300 div q4–6h	10–12 g	Community encapsulated organisms, anaerobes
Amphotericin B	0.5–1.0 g 1–2 d	—[a]	Invasive fungal infection
Aztreonam	120 div q6h	6–8 g	Hospital gram-negative rods
Cefepime	100–150 div q8–12h	6 g	Hospital gram-negative rods, staphylococci
Cefotaxime	100–200 div q6h	8–10 g	Community encapsulated organisms
Ceftazidime	100–150 div q8h	4–6 g	Hospital gram-negative rods
Ceftriaxone	50–100 div q12–24h	2 g	Community encapsulated organisms
Cefuroxime	100–150 div q6h	4–6 g	Community encapsulated organisms, staphylococci
Clindamycin	60–100 div q8h	2–4 g	Anaerobes, community staphylococci
Doxycycline	2–4 q24h	200 mg	Rickettsiae
Gentamicin	5.0–7.5 div q8h	500 mg[a]	Community gram-negative rods
Imipenem-cilastatin	60–100 imipenem div q8h	4–6 g	Hospital gram-negative rods, anaerobes
Levoflococin[b]	5–10 g 24h	500 mg	Hospital gram-negative rods, staphylococci
Linezolid	30 div q8h	1200 mg	Hospital enterococci, staphylococci
Meropenem	60 div q8h	4–6 g	Hospital gram-negative rods, anaerobes
Metronidazole	30 div q8h	2–4 g	Anaerobes
Oxacillin	150–200 div q4–6h	10–12 g	Community staphylococci
Nafcillin	150 div q6h	10–12 g	Community staphylococci
Piperacillin	200–300 div q4–6h	18–24 g	Community *Pseudomonas*
Piperacillin-tazobactam[b]	240 piperacillin div q8h	18 g	Community *Pseudomonas*, staphylococci
Tetracycline	25–50 div q8–12h	1–2 g	Rickettsiae
Ticarcillin	200–300 div q4–6h	18–24 g	Community *Pseudomonas*
Tobramycin	5.0–7.5 div q8h	500 mg[a]	Hospital gram-negative rods
Trimethoprim-sulfamethoxazole	8–20 trimethoprim div q12h	1–2 g[a]	*Salmonella, Shigella, Pneumocystis*
Vancomycin	40 div q6–12h	2–4 g[a]	Hospital staphylococci, enterococci, resistant pneumococci

[a]Serum concentration or toxicity monitoring desirable.
[b]Not licensed by U.S. Food and Drug Administration for pediatric use. Use should be limited to critical illness with high probability of resistant microorganisms.

Another major concern is the maintenance of adequate nutrition. Sepsis mediators create a hypermetabolic state that rapidly depletes body stores and exceeds the caloric content of conventional intravenous fluids. Early and aggressive parenteral administration of nutrition is necessary to keep up with these demands and to provide sufficient calories to promote tissue regeneration and healing.

Research in sepsis and septic shock therapy is ongoing. During the past two decades, clinical trials of monoclonal antibodies and receptor antagonists aimed at blocking critical steps in the cytokine cascade have been disappointing in sepsis but have led to a great advance in the treatment of rheumatologic conditions. Research attention has been directed recently to the close relationship of coagulation and inflammation. The abnormal interaction of cytokines and coagulation at the endothelial level has been implicated in septic shock, multiorgan dysfunction syndrome, and cell death. Activated protein C (APC) acts to alter this imbalance. It has antithrombotic, profibrinolytic, and antiinflammatory properties. Recombinant human APC (activated drotrecogin alpha) has been shown to reduce the relative risk of death by almost 20% and to improve survival rates in septic adult patients. However, clinical trials in pediatrics have recently been suspended because of marginal efficacy and hemorrhagic complications.

PREVENTION

Dramatic reductions in the incidence of invasive *H. influenzae* type b and, more recently, *S. pneumoniae* systemic infections are the welcome result of the widespread use of polysaccharide conjugate vaccines in infancy. Meningococcal and pneumococcal polysaccharide vaccines also have had an impact on the incidence of invasive infection in high-risk children older than age 2 years. Conjugate meningococcal vaccines have recently been introduced for routine vaccination of pre-adolescents, adolescents, and young adults. Attenuated typhoid vaccine (Ty21a) and Vi polysaccharide vaccine (alone or in combination) provide excellent protection for foreign travelers. Prevention of sepsis in compromised hosts is discussed in Chapter 134.

Suggested Readings

Bone RC, Balk RA, Cerra FB, et al. Definitions for sepsis and organ failure and guidelines for the use of innovative therapies in sepsis. *Crit Care Med* 1992; 20:864.

Carcillo JA. Pediatric septic shock and multiple organ failure. *Crit Care Clin* 2003;19:413.

Carcillo JA, Fields AI. Clinical practice parameters for hemodynamic support of pediatric and neonatal patients in septic chock. *Crit Care Med* 2002;30:1365.

Fekade D, Knox K, Hussein K, et al. Prevention of Jarisch-Herxheimer reactions by treatment with antibodies against tumor necrosis factor alpha. *N Engl J Med* 1996;335:311.

Goldstein B, Giroir B, Randolph A, et al. International pediatric sepsis consensus conference: Definitions for sepsis and organ dysfunction in pediatrics. *Pediatr Crit Care Med* 2005;6:2.

McCarthy PL, Sharpe MR, Spiesel SZ, et al. Observation scales to identify serious illness in febrile children. *Pediatrics* 1982;70:802.

Michelow IC, McCracken GH, Jr. Antibacterial therapeutic agents. In: Feigin RD, Cherry JD, Demmler GJ, et al. *Textbook of Pediatric Infectious Diseases* (5th ed.) 2004;2987.

Thomas L. *The lives of a cell.* New York: Viking, 1974:75.

Wheeler DS, Wong HR. The impact of molecular biology on the practice of pediatric critical care medicine. *Pediatr Crit Care Med* 2001;2:299.

CHAPTER 136 ■ BACTERIAL MENINGITIS BEYOND THE NEWBORN PERIOD

RALPH D. FEIGIN

Meningitis is an inflammation of the meninges. Between 1986 and 1995, the U.S. incidence of bacterial meningitis in children aged 1 month to 5 years decreased 87%, primarily because of the introduction of conjugate vaccine for *Haemophilus influenzae* type b (Hib) for children younger than 2 years of age. However, because death can occur in more than 5% of cases and morbidity may occur in 30% of survivors, it is still a feared childhood infection. Because of their different characteristics, neonatal and tuberculous meningitis are discussed in Chapters 72 (Meningitis) and 177, respectively.

EPIDEMIOLOGY

Common causes of bacterial meningitis in children older than 1 month of age are *Neisseria meningitidis*, *Streptococcus pneumoniae* and, until recently, Hib. Most cases occur in children between 1 month and 5 years of age, with the highest risk being in infants aged 6 to 12 months. Table 136.1 shows the incidence by age for the five most common organisms. Since the introduction of conjugate Hib vaccine, the average age of U.S. cases has increased to approximately 25 years, up from 15 months in 1986. Before the introduction of conjugate Hib vaccine, approximately 65% of U.S. bacterial meningitis was caused by Hib, with the remainder caused primarily by *N. meningitidis* and *S. pneumoniae*. Other countries had different rates. For example, in Spain, *N. meningitidis* caused approximately 68% of cases of childhood bacterial meningitis. Nonspecific risk factors for meningitis from these organisms include young age, close contact with carriers or those with invasive disease, and host factors such as asplenia or immunodeficiency.

N. *meningitidis* is a gram-negative diplococcus with 12 capsular polysaccharide serotypes. Approximately 90% of meningococcal disease is caused by groups A, B, and C. Serogroup prevalence differs throughout the world and changes with time. The most prevalent forms in the United States are groups B and C, with some serogroup Y outbreaks reported. Increases in rates of serogroup C have been reported in Canada, the United States, and the United Kingdom. U.S.

group A epidemics occurred as recently as the mid-twentieth century. Epidemics of group A *N. meningitidis* occur every 8 to 12 years in the "meningitis belt" of sub-Saharan Africa, where attack rates of 500 per 100,000 can occur.

The incidence of meningococcal meningitis in U.S. children aged 1 to 23 months is 4.5 per 100,000. The U.S. childhood mortality rate has been estimated at 8%. Meningococcal disease is more common in males and is increased in frequency in the later teens. The disease generally is acquired from carriers who can harbor the organism for months. The U.S. carriage rate is 15%, but it increases to more than 30% during outbreaks, and the carriage rate of unrelated subgroups increases as well. The incidence of disease peaks in winter, and the disease occurs in newly infected individuals rather than by breakthrough in chronic carriers. The risk of developing severe meningococcal disease is 1% in family contacts, approximately 1,000 times greater than the community risk. The risk for daycare contacts is 1 per 1,000. The incubation period is from 1 to 10 days.

Host factors, such as terminal complement deficiency (C5 to C9), complement-depleting diseases, or properdin deficiency, increase susceptibility to disease. Individuals with such deficiencies may develop disease late; in one study, patients developed disease at an average age of 17 years. Influenza or mycoplasma outbreaks in the preceding 2 to 3 weeks are associated with subsequent meningococcal outbreaks, possibly because of impaired pharyngeal defenses or lowered immunity.

S. *pneumoniae* is a gram-positive diplococcus with approximately 90 capsular polysaccharide serotypes. Sepsis and meningitis occur most frequently with serotypes 4, 6B, 9V, 14, 18C, 19F, and 23F. The meningitis rate in U.S. children aged 1 to 23 months is 6.6 per 100,000. The U.S. childhood mortality rate has been estimated at 15%. Meningitis is associated with viral upper respiratory infections and is most prevalent in winter. Carriage is transient, and it is a risk factor for development of infection.

Host factors are important with *S. pneumoniae* meningitis. The risk of developing meningitis in the U.S. black population is increased 5 to 36 times, and this risk is independent of income

TABLE 136.1

ESTIMATED AGE-SPECIFIC INCIDENCE OF BACTERIAL MENINGITIS (CASES PER 100,000 POPULATION), UNITED STATES, 1995

Age Group	*Haemococus influenzae*	*Streptococus pneumoniae*	*Neisseria meningitidis*	Group B Streptococcus	Listeria
<1 mo	0	15.7	0	125.0	39.2
1–23 mo	0.7	6.6	4.5	2.8	0
2–29 yr	0.1	0.5	1.1	0.1	0.04

Adapted from Schuchat A, Robinson K, Wenger JD, et al. Bacterial meningitis in the United States in 1995. *N Engl J Med* 1997;337:970.

or population density. In the absence of antibiotic prophylaxis, one in 24 children with sickle cell disease may develop *S. pneumoniae* meningitis by age 4 years, a rate 36 times that of black children without sickle cell disease.

The incidence of meningitis caused by penicillin-resistant *S. pneumoniae* has increased dramatically in recent years. In 1998, Centers for Disease Control and Prevention (CDC) surveillance from multiple areas around the United States found that 24% of invasive pneumococcal infections were nonsusceptible to penicillin and 14% of isolates were nonsusceptible to cefotaxime. Rates of resistance were highest in children younger than 5 years of age.

Hib is a gram-negative coccobacillus. Historically, it was the leading cause of bacterial meningitis in many developed countries. The incidence in children younger than 5 years of age ranged from 20 to 30 per 100,000 in certain countries to 409 per 100,000 in Alaskan Eskimos. In countries where Hib immunization is started when children are 2 months of age, a dramatic decrease in the incidence of disease has occurred. In Canada, a 98% reduction in the number of infections caused by Hib occurred from 1985 to 1995. The United States has experienced a similar decline, with a current incidence of 0.4 per 100,000 in children between 1 and 23 months. The U.S. mortality rate has been estimated at 2.3%. In countries where Hib vaccination is not yet widespread, the disease continues to be a common occurrence, with a peak incidence occurring in late autumn or early winter. The normal carriage rate of 2% to 5% is declining because the vaccine also protects against nasopharyngeal colonization. The risks of transmission of infection to a family contact are 6% and 2% for members younger than 1 year and 4 years of age, respectively. The risk of secondary infection developing in home contacts within 30 days of an index case is 585 times greater than the age-adjusted risk in the general population.

Host factors are important because meningitis occurs with increased frequency in children with diabetes mellitus, Cushing syndrome, and coma secondary to drug overdose. Genetic factors also may play a role. In one study, HLA-B12 was found in 52% of children with invasive *H. influenzae* disease versus 16% in a control group. HLA-Bw40 was present in 24% of children without invasive disease, but it was absent in those with systemic Hib infection. Additional studies have identified other genetic risk factors.

Other bacteria, such as group B streptococcus, *Listeria monocytogenes*, *Salmonella*, and *Fusobacterium necrophorum*, can cause meningitis in normal children. Host factors, both congenital and acquired, can be important in the development of meningitis caused by these bacteria. Skin flora should be suspected in children with a dermoid sinus, meningomyelocele, or hydrocephalus and a cerebrospinal fluid (CSF) shunt. Meningitis occurring after cochlear implantation has been reported. Cystic fibrosis or burn patients may develop *Staphylococcus aureus* or *Pseudomonas aeruginosa* meningitis after colonization. In a humidified atmosphere, *P. aeruginosa* or *Serratia marcescens* infection may occur. Children with sickle cell disease, congenital asplenia, or splenosis are especially susceptible to *Salmonella* infection, in addition to *H. influenzae* and *S. pneumoniae*. Children who have reticuloendothelial malignancies, are undergoing chemotherapy, or have indwelling catheters may develop meningitis from organisms of low virulence, such as *Streptococcus mitis*. In immunocompromised children, *Bacteroides fragilis* is a frequent anaerobic cause of meningitis. Congenital or acquired anatomic defects, such as a stapedial footplate defect or cribiform plate fracture, should be investigated in cases of recurrent meningitis.

Meningitis with two bacterial types in a CSF culture may occur in 1% of cases. Meningitis with a bacteria and a virus or fungus occurs rarely. The clinical course usually is that of bacterial meningitis.

PATHOGENESIS

Initially, upper respiratory tract infection occurs. Bacteremia follows, with opsonization and phagocytosis inhibited by bacterial capsules. Meningeal seeding occurs, most likely in the cerebral capillaries and choroid plexus. Invasion from a contiguous infection (e.g., mastoiditis) also can occur. Meningitis that develops after otitis media usually is from bacteremia rather than direct invasion. Meningitis also can develop subsequent to skull or vertebral column osteomyelitis.

Organisms initially are found in the lateral and dorsal longitudinal (sagittal) sinuses. Central nervous system (CNS) blood flows may be reduced by 25% to 50%. Dural inflammation slows the flow from the subarachnoid space to the sinuses, thereby permitting spread of infection. A meningeal exudate occurs over the brain. The spinal cord may be encased in pus. Purulent material may develop in the ventricles (ventriculitis) and the ventricular wall and around the veins and venous sinuses.

Cerebral cortex damage produces the neurologic sequelae of meningitis, such as impaired consciousness, seizures, retardation, and nerve deficits. These symptoms result from complications such as nerve inflammation, cerebral edema, increased intracranial pressure (ICP), cerebral vascular changes, hypoglycorrhachia (reduced CSF glucose), acidosis, and the host inflammatory response.

Nerve inflammation leads to meningeal symptoms and signs. Early pressure on peripheral nerves may lead to motor or sensory deficits. Subarachnoid cranial and spinal nerves often are involved in the inflammatory process. Deafness and vestibular disturbances occur most commonly, and optic nerve involvement also may occur. Hearing loss appears to result from inflammatory cells and mediators that reach the inner ear from the CSF via the cochlear aqueduct. Cochlear damage with loss of the organ of Corti may result. Inflammation and swelling of the facial nerve in the stylomastoid foramen and the auditory nerve in the internal acoustic meatus may compromise their blood supply. Transtentorial herniation also may cause nerve compression.

Cerebral edema results from vasogenic, interstitial, and cytotoxic processes. Vasogenic edema results from increased permeability of the blood brain barrier. Interstitial edema occurs with decreased CSF resorption as proteins, leukocytes, and debris interfere with the function of the arachnoid villi. Cytotoxic edema results from host and bacterial toxic factors, which increase intracellular water and sodium and loss of intracellular potassium.

Increased ICP often exceeds 300 mm H_2O. Hypoxemia and ischemia from decreased perfusion may result. Papilledema is a rare occurrence because of the brief duration of increased pressure. Hydrocephalus rarely occurs beyond the neonatal period. Communicating hydrocephalus may result from adhesive arachnoid thickening about the basal cisterns. Obstructive hydrocephalus may result from fibrosis and reactive gliosis obliterating the aqueduct of Sylvius or the foramina of Magendie and Luschka. In some cases, meningitis is associated with the syndrome of inappropriate antidiuretic hormone release (SIADH), causing water retention and a relative sodium loss by the kidney. SIADH increases the risk of developing electrolyte abnormalities, increased ICP, and seizures. Dehydration also can occur from increased insensible losses and decreased intake.

Cerebral vascular changes include vasculitis and major vascular events such as venous sinus occlusion or subarachnoid hemorrhage from necrotizing arteritis. Cerebral necrosis can result with or without vascular thrombosis. Combined with increased intraventricular pressure, it may lead to infarction or dissolution of the cerebrum. Autoregulation also may be destroyed, in which case, cerebral perfusion is a function of the systolic blood pressure.

Hypoglycorrhachia and acidosis result in part from increased glucose use and decreased glucose transport across the inflamed choroid plexus. Increased glucose use results in the excess production of lactate production and the depletion of the high-energy compounds adenosine triphosphate and phosphocreatine. The resultant acidosis may contribute to a loss of cerebral autoregulation and tissue damage. Increased concentrations of lactate also occur from anaerobic metabolism secondary to hypoxemia.

Increased CSF protein is caused partly by the flow of albumin-rich fluid into the subdural space secondary to inflammation and increased vascular permeability. With resolution of the inflammatory process, vascular permeability decreases, but continued transudation from newly formed subdural capillaries may persist. Subdural effusions may occur by these processes.

Host inflammatory responses in the CSF seem to rely on two mechanisms to clear bacteria. One requires a type-specific antibody, a functional classic complement system for opsonization, and competent neutrophils for phagocytosis. The second system is dependent on the interaction of nonspecific antibody and the alternative complement system for opsonization of the organism. Clearance by this system occurs without neutrophils.

Low concentrations of CSF antibody and complement initially permit bacterial proliferation. A low level of release occurs of cell wall fragments, consisting of endotoxin from gram-negative bacteria and teichoic acid from gram-positive bacteria. The interaction between these fragments and the blood brain barrier endothelium results in increased barrier permeability. Serum albumin, complement, and other proteins flow into the CSF. Early increased regional blood flow and ICP also may occur.

The host inflammatory response remains only partially understood and appears to be somewhat different for each type of organism. It includes a complex interaction of leukocytes, cytokines, complement, arachidonic acid products, platelet-activating factor (PAF), nitric oxide (NO), toxic oxygen products, and excitatory amino acids. Pathologic changes have been noted in the cerebral cortex, consisting of reactive microglia and astrocytes, without evidence of cortical bacterial invasion. Experimental studies show that neurologic outcome may be a function of subarachnoid inflammation and that neutrophils may do little to control the subarachnoid infection. Bacterial concentrations do not differ between normal and neutropenic animal models. In experimental models, leukocyte migration inhibition is associated with improved outcomes, including increased rates of survival and decreased brain edema, disruption of the blood brain barrier, and tissue damage.

Antibiotic therapy results in a large release of bacterial fragments, which promotes production of the cytokines IL-1β (IL-1β) and tumor necrosis factor–alpha (TNF-α). These cytokines trigger a cascade of mediators, including IL-6, IL-8, IL-10, IL-12, phospholipase A2, and interferon-gamma. IL-1β and TNF-α also stimulate endothelial cells to activate receptors that promote leukocyte attachment, leading to leukocyte migration into the CSF. In experimental studies, antibodies to IL-1β and TNF-α prevented the development of CSF leukocytosis. Although IL-1β and TNF-α are not directly toxic to neurons, CSF IL-1 levels are correlated with CSF inflammation, increased TNF-α concentration, and adverse outcome. CSF TNF-α causes increased vascular permeability by virtue of the toxic effects on endothelial cells and, in vitro, it causes myelin and oligodendrocyte necrosis. In one study, it was correlated with the number of febrile hospital days. Increased soluble TNF-α receptor, a regulatory protein for TNF-α, has been correlated with adverse neurologic sequelae.

Complement is involved early in the host response. In experimental studies, complement depletion delayed the appearance of leukocytes in the CSF. The complement cascade product C5a is a potent early chemoattractant for leukocytes.

The ILs (6, 8, 10, 12) and interferon-gamma have multiple roles, a few of which are described here. IL-6 works with IL-1 to promote B-cell growth and induces acute-phase reactants such as C-reactive protein (CRP). It also produces fever and activates the complement and clotting cascades. IL-8 is a chemoattractant that also stimulates the production of reactive oxygen metabolites and neutrophil degranulation. IL-10 regulates TNF-α levels and decreases NO and reactive oxygen metabolite synthesis. It also increases the release of soluble TNF-α receptors. IL-12 enhances cytolytic activity in T cells, natural killer cells, macrophages, and lymphokine-activated killer cells. IL-12 also stimulates release of interferon-gamma, which, among other actions, promotes phagocytosis and the secretion of reactive oxygen metabolites. CSF interferon-gamma levels and the ratio of TNF-a to IL-10 were found to be significantly different between patients with pneumococcal meningitis and those with Hib or meningococcal meningitis.

Phospholipase A$_2$ leads to the production of arachidonic acid from cell membranes; it then is converted to prostaglandins (PG), thromboxanes, and leukotrienes (LT). PGE$_2$ and prostacyclin reduce TNF-α mRNA production, providing a feedback system. In experimental studies, PGE$_2$ given with C5a resulted in decreased CSF leukocytosis. Arachidonic acid products provide a late stimulus for the recruitment of leukocytes that is independent of complement. Certain inhibitors of arachidonic acid (such as the cyclooxygenase inhibitor oxindanac) were associated with decreased leukocytosis and improved experimental survival. Indomethacin, a PGE$_2$ inhibitor, reduced cerebral edema but did not affect ICP. LTB$_4$ promotes the migration of neutrophils, among other actions, and can be produced by neutrophils. This process is inhibited by dexamethasone.

Phospholipase A$_2$ also leads to PAF production. Whereas the role of PAF in meningitis is not clear, *in vitro* it induces chemotaxis and platelet degranulation, triggers the coagulation cascade, and increases capillary permeability. In high concentrations, PAF is toxic to neurons and causes endothelial tissue damage.

IL-1β, TNF-α, PGE$_2$, PAF, NO, and LTB$_4$ are among the many mediators that increase ICP and cerebral edema by altering cerebral blood flow and blood brain barrier permeability. In experimental meningitis, an early increase in cerebral blood flow and blood pressure occurs within hours of initial development of infection. This increase may be mediated by NO, which is elevated in bacterial meningitis. When TNF-α was injected into the cisterna of experimental animals, NO mediated oxygen uptake and CSF–to–blood glucose ratios were reduced, whereas ICP and lactate concentrations were increased.

Other factors in the host response include neutrophil enzymes, oxygen radicals, and excitatory amino acids, all of which may cause neuronal death. Superoxide and hydrogen peroxide are secreted by brain microglial cells and leukocytes. The experimental infusion of superoxide dismutase prevents early increased regional blood flow, loss of autoregulation, ICP changes, and edema. These findings may point to an early role for peroxynitrite, a toxic metabolite formed from superoxide anions and NO. Increased concentrations of certain amino acids also have been found in bacterial meningitis. In one adult study, patients who had high CSF glutamate concentrations several days after starting antibiotics developed severe neurologic complications or died. Glutamate is an excitatory amino acid implicated in neuronal damage. It can be secreted by macrophages.

Significant additional discoveries may be made in the coming years. Pharmaceutical interventions designed to block inappropriate portions of the host response are being developed.

CLINICAL MANIFESTATIONS AND COMPLICATIONS

Meningitis can develop slowly over the course of several days, or it can be fulminant, with onset occurring within hours. The fulminant form is associated with severe brain edema, which can lead to cerebral herniation.

Fever and meningeal inflammation symptoms occur in 85% of patients. Symptoms of patients with meningitis are summarized in Table 136.2. They include headache, irritability, confusion, hyperesthesia, photophobia, nuchal rigidity, and seizures. Nuchal rigidity may appear late, especially in a young child. Seizures occur in 30% of cases at some time before or during the course of illness; in 20% of cases, seizures occur before admission. Infants may have a bulging fontanelle, but such appears late and in only approximately 30% of infants. In one study, bulging fontanelles occurred in 13% of children without meningitis. Older children frequently have headaches, and symptoms may proceed to altered mental status, hypertension, and bradycardia from increased ICP. In one series, approximately 15% of patients were semicomatose or comatose at admission, conditions more common with pneumococcal or meningococcal disease. Papilledema is a rare development; if present, a search for other processes (e.g., brain abscess, venous sinus occlusion, subdural empyema) should be performed.

TABLE 136.2

SELECTED SYMPTOMS AND SIGNS OF BACTERIAL MENINGITIS

Infants
Fever, hypothermia
Lethargy
Respiratory distress
Jaundice
Vomiting, diarrhea
Poor feeding
Restlessness, irritability
Decreased muscle tone
Full fontanelle
Seizures

Children
Fever, chills
Photophobia
Anorexia
Confusion, altered consciousness, coma
Cranial nerve palsies
Upper respiratory symptoms
Petechial or purpuric rash
Myalgia, arthralgia
Nuchal rigidity
Headache
Nausea, vomiting
Malaise, restlessness
Lethargy
Ataxia
Hyperesthesia
Back pain
Seizures
Kernig sign
Brudzinski sign

Transient or permanent cranial nerve damage may cause deafness, vestibular disturbance, ataxia, and extraocular or facial nerve paralysis. Optic-nerve arachnoiditis may lead to optic atrophy and blindness. Focal neurologic deficits may exist on admission in 15% of children and in 30% of children with pneumococcal meningitis. When focal signs are present without seizures, cortical necrosis, occlusive vasculitis, or thrombosis of cortical veins probably has occurred. Infants may have only restlessness, irritability, poor feeding, or unstable temperature. Adolescents may present with behavioral abnormalities that may be confused with drug abuse or psychiatric disorders.

Kernig sign (while supine with the leg flexed at the hip to 90 degrees and the knee flexed, pain occurs on leg extension beyond 135 degrees) and Brudzinski sign (while supine, leg flexion occurs when the neck is flexed) may be absent in 50% of cases, especially if antibiotics have been given. One study found that 1.5% of cases had no meningeal signs during hospitalization.

Other symptoms and signs may be present. Subdural effusions may occur in 50% of cases. Although usually asymptomatic, they may cause increasing head circumference, abnormal transillumination, vomiting, seizures, full fontanelle, focal neurologic signs, or persistent fever. They usually resolve spontaneously. Meningomyelitis or spinal cord infarction may lead to spastic paraparesis, with or without sensory loss. Early arthritis may be caused by invasions of the organism itself, whereas late arthritis more likely is immunologically induced. Transient arthritis occurs more commonly during meningococcal meningitis and rarely may be the only presenting sign. Arthralgia and myalgia also may occur. Pericardial effusions usually resolve with the administration of antibiotic therapy. However, pericardial effusion with persistent fever may require drainage. Facial cellulitis, pneumonia, epiglottitis, and endophthalmitis also can be presenting signs of meningitis. In one study of buccal cellulitis, 8% of patients had bacterial meningitis, most without meningeal signs.

In one-half or more cases of meningococcal disease, the patient may have purpura or petechiae (a nonblanching rash) during the course, but it may occur in any vasculitic process. Only a few petechiae may be present, so the physician should maintain a high degree of suspicion.

Shock with profound hypotension may occur in 5% of meningococcal and Hib meningitis cases, but it can be associated with any overwhelming bacteremia. Disseminated intravascular coagulation may occur. Both the classic and alternative complement paths are activated in meningococcal meningitis. Death can occur within hours, despite the administration of adequate therapy.

DIAGNOSIS

No single symptom or sign is pathognomonic for meningitis because any, none, or all of the clinical manifestations described may be present. Definitive diagnosis is established through a positive identification of the organism in the CSF, by culture or by other diagnostic techniques.

Lumbar Puncture

A lumbar puncture (LP) must be performed if meningitis is suspected. Increased numbers of neutrophils and increased protein and decreased glucose concentrations suggest the presence of bacterial infection. Usual initial CSF findings in CNS suppurative diseases are shown in Table 136.3.

In children with positive blood culture results but no meningeal signs, an LP should be performed if fever persists. Bacteremia can progress to meningitis within hours. Rarely,

TABLE 136.3

INITIAL USUAL CEREBROSPINAL FLUID FINDINGS IN SUPPURATIVE DISEASES OF THE CENTRAL NERVOUS SYSTEM AND MENINGES

Condition	Pressure (mm H$_2$O)	Leukocytes Per Microliter; Predominant Type	Protein (mg/dL)	Glucose (mg/dL)	Specific Findings
Acute bacterial meningitis	Elevated; average, 300	0–60,000; average, a few thousand; PMNs	100–500; occasionally >1,000	<40 in more than one-half of cases	Organism seen on smear or culture in 90% of cases
Subdural empyema	Elevated; average, 300	<100 to a few thousand; PMNs	100–500	Normal	No organisms seen
Brain abscess	Elevated	10–200; lymphocytes	75–400	Normal	Fluid is rarely acellular
Ventricular empyema (rupture of brain abscess)	Considerably elevated	Several thousand to 100,000; >90% PMNs	Several hundred	<40	Organism may be seen on smear of culture
Cerebral epidural abscess	Slightly elevated	Few to several hundred; lymphocytes	50–200	Normal	No organisms seen
Spinal epidural abscess	Reduced with spinal block	10–100; lymphocytes	Several hundred	Normal	No organisms seen
Thrombophlebitis (associated with subdoral empyema)	Often elevated	Few to several hundred; PMNs and lymphocytes	Slightly elevated	Normal	No organisms seen
Bacterial endocarditis (with embolism)	Normal to slightly elevated	Few to <100; PMNs and lymphocytes	Slightly elevated	Normal	No organisms seen
Acute hemorrhagic encephalitis	Elevated	Few to >1,000; PMNs	Moderately elevated	Normal	No organisms seen
Tuberculous infection	Elevated; may be low with dynamic block in advanced stages	25–100; rarely, >500; 80% PMNs in early stages, then lymphocytes	100–200; may be higher if dynamic block	Reduced; <50 in 75% of cases	Acid-fast organisms may be seen on smear of protein coagulum or culture
Cryptococcal infection	Elevated; average, 225	0–800; average, 50; lymphocytes	20–500; average, 100	Reduced in >50% cases; average, 30	Organisms seen in india ink preparation and Sabouraud culture medium
Syphilis (acute)	Elevated	Average, 500; lymphocytes with rare PMNs	Average, 100; gamma-globulin often high	Normal (rarely reduced)	Positive reagin test result; no organisms seen by usual techniques
Sarcoidosis	Normal to considerably elevated	0 to <100; monocytes	Slight-to-moderate elevation	Normal	No specific findings

PMNs, polymorphonuclear neutrophils.
Adapted with permission from Feigin RD, Cherry JD, eds. *Textbook of pediatric infectious diseases*, 5th ed. Philadelphia: Saunders, 2003.

meningitis can develop after an LP that presumably was performed during bacteremia. This development does not appear to be caused by seeding; it occurs more frequently in children younger than 1 year of age.

Contraindications to performing an LP are cardiopulmonary compromise, signs of possible increased ICP (e.g., papilledema, altered respiratory efforts, focal neurologic signs), and skin infection over the LP site. Herniation rarely may occur with increased ICP. Papilledema is a late sign of increased ICP, so a careful neurologic examination should be done. In children with suspected increased ICP or altered mental status, antibiotics should be given immediately after taking blood cultures

and an emergency computed tomographic (CT) scan should be done before the LP is performed. Some investigators contend that an LP should be withheld until altered mental status resolves. However, a delay can lead to an incorrect choice of antibiotics and a failure to treat contacts. A reliance on blood cultures and clinical signs is inadequate because both may be misleading, particularly if prehospital antibiotics have been given. If an LP cannot be performed, meningitic doses of antibiotics should be administered until the procedure can be performed.

When an LP is performed, CSF pressure should be measured. In one study, the mean pressure was 180 ± 70 mm H$_2$O, twice the upper normal limit. When ICP is elevated

TABLE 136.4

CEREBROSPINAL FLUID CELL COUNTS IN INFANTS WITHOUT MENINGITIS

Age (mo)	White Blood Cells (Cells per Microliter)
<1.5	3.7 ± 3.4
1.5–3.0	2.9 ± 2.9
3–6	1.9 ± 2.0
6–12	2.6 ± 2.5
>12	1.9 ± 2.7

Adapted with permission from Portnoy JM, Olson LC. Normal cerebrospinal fluid values in children; another look. *Pediatrics* 1985;75:484.

significantly, the minimum amount of fluid necessary for studies should be removed. CSF color should be recorded. Xanthochromia is associated with hemorrhage, bilirubin staining in icteric patients, or increased CSF protein.

Microscopy should include a total leukocyte count and differential. In children older than 12 months, a normal CSF leukocyte count is less than six cells per milliliter. Table 136.4 shows normal cell counts by age. Most (95%) healthy children older than 3 months of age have no CSF neutrophils, which are the initial leukocytes in the CSF. A later change to monocytes and lymphocytes occurs during recovery. If the LP is traumatic, a safe approach is to wait for culture results.

A Gram stain should be performed. Most results will be positive. The Gram-stain result may be positive in 90% of pneumococcal meningitis cases in young children and in more than 50% in older children. Prehospital administration of antibiotics may reduce Gram-stain yields to 40% to 60%. False-positive stain results may occur if an unoccluded LP needle is used because it may introduce skin organisms.

Normal CSF may be found in as many as 10% of cases of meningococcal meningitis; hence, a strong index of suspicion is necessary. Cultures should be performed regardless of fluid appearance or cell count. If an organism cannot be identified from an LP, alternative identification methods can be used, but this development should delay therapy. Blood cultures may be positive in as many as 90% of cases if antibiotics have not been given, but they frequently are of little value if pretreatment has occurred. Routine prehospital antibiotics generally do not have a significant effect on CSF cell counts, but they may reduce culture yields to less than 50% from a normal yield of 70% to 85%.

A Gram stain from purpuric or petechial skin lesions may reveal the organism. A urine culture should be obtained in a child younger than 1 year of age before giving antibiotics, if possible. Treatment should not be withheld in patients with suggested bacterial meningitis if a urine sample cannot be secured immediately by asking the child to void or by catheterization. Throat or nasopharyngeal cultures are not helpful because colonization by one organism can occur with infection by another.

CSF glucose values of less than two-thirds of the blood glucose level frequently are found. Several studies of meningococcal meningitis have reported normal glucose values in approximately 50% of patients. CSF protein usually is elevated. Normal protein levels in children older than 2 months are less than 40 mg/dL.

Rapid Diagnostic Tests

Because countercurrent immunoelectrophoresis and latex particle agglutination tests provide results rapidly, these tests are used most commonly, but both have limitations. Enzyme-linked immunosorbent assays (ELISA), polymerase chain reaction assay (PCR), and others are helpful in some cases.

Countercurrent immunoelectrophoresis in 1 hour identifies Hib, *S. pneumoniae*, *N. meningitidis* (types A, C, D, and W135), group B streptococcus, and other bacteria. A commercially available group B meningococcal antiserum generally is considered unreliable. Concurrent evaluation of CSF, urine, and serum increases the likelihood of establishing a diagnosis. A negative countercurrent immunoelectrophoresis result does not exclude bacteremia or meningitis caused by these organisms.

Latex particle agglutination tests of the CSF may be useful, but reported sensitivities and specificities vary widely. A negative latex particle agglutination result rarely affects the decision to give antibiotics. In one study, latex particle agglutination tests of CSF yielded positive results in 28% of specimens, but in only 3% of cases was it the only positive study.

A PCR analysis of CSF has been used to detect microbial DNA in patients with bacterial meningitis. Primers are available for detection of *S. pneumoniae*, *N. meningitidis*, and Hib simultaneously. Species-specific amplicons have been detected in 89% of patients with proven streptococcal, meningococcal, or Hib meningitis. No false-positive results were noted.

PCR is most useful in rapidly documenting viral antigens within the CSF, thus reducing the use of antibiotics in selected patients who are treated for presumptive bacterial disease but who may have viral meningitis. The great sensitivity of oligoprobes also has been demonstrated on amplified DNA for the diagnosis of *H. influenzae*, streptococcal, and *Mycobacterium tuberculosis* meningitis.

Rapid detection tests are not necessary for all patients. They may be helpful in situations such as a traumatic LP or in a patient who has been pretreated with antibiotics.

A diagnostic dilemma occurs when the LP cell count is less than 100 per microliter, the Gram-stain result is negative, and the CSF–to–blood glucose ratio is normal. Viral meningitis may be present, but these results also are consistent with bacterial meningitis. In such a case, empiric treatment should be considered. However, if the child is older than 1 year of age and has not been pretreated with antibiotics, withholding antibiotics for 6 to 12 hours and then repeating the LP may be a reasonable course of action.

If viral meningitis could be diagnosed with high accuracy, the administration of antibiotics and hospitalization might be avoided. Measurement of CSF beta-lactamase, TNF-α, beta-glucuronidase, lactate, pH, creatine phosphokinase, glutamic oxaloacetic transaminase, elastase-alpha proteinase inhibitor, staphylococcal coagulation, and leukocyte aggregation all show differing degrees of promise in distinguishing bacterial from viral meningitis, but they need further evaluation or development.

Differential Diagnosis

Many other processes produce signs and symptoms that mimic meningitis. High on the list should be infection with mycobacteria, fungi, viruses, or protozoa. Other noninfectious processes include a CNS abscess, bacterial endocarditis with embolism, subdural empyema, and brain tumor.

TREATMENT

Because of increasing penicillin resistance in *S. pneumoniae*, most centers use cefotaxime (225 to 300 mg/kg/day in three to four divided doses) or ceftriaxone (100 mg/kg/day in two divided doses) for children older than 3 months of age. In children aged 1 to 3 months, ampicillin (400 mg/kg/day in four divided doses) should be added because of the possible presence of *L. monocytogenes* or enterococcal infection. Because of the high frequency of *S. pneumoniae* resistant to penicillin and to third-generation cephalosporins, vancomycin (60 mg/kg/day in four divided doses) should be given with cefotaxime or ceftriaxone until an organism is identified and its sensitivities determined. If an organism other than *S. pneumoniae* is suspected, such as when a Gram stain shows gram-negative organisms in a meningococcal outbreak, alternative therapy can be considered.

In the United States, approximately 46% of *S. pneumoniae* strains now are relatively resistant to penicillin. In some U.S. locations, up to 25% resistance to third-generation cephalosporins has been found. Resistance to penicillin occurs more often in children who receive antibiotics within a month of developing meningitis. Although cefotaxime and ceftriaxone are effective against most penicillin-resistant pneumococci, caution is urged. Resistance is not beta-lactamase mediated, so beta-lactamase–resistant antibiotics are of no value. Pneumococci should be tested for susceptibility to penicillin, cephalosporins, vancomycin, meropenem, and rifampin. *S. pneumoniae* resistant to cephalosporins and vancomycin should be reported to the appropriate health department.

N. meningitidis penicillin resistance also is widely variable. In the United States, rates of less than 5% were reported in the late 1980s and early 1990s. However, rates of resistance to penicillin of 20% to 40% were reported in Spain during the same period.

Ceftriaxone and cefotaxime are third-generation cephalosporins with broad antimicrobial activity against gram-positive and gram-negative organisms. They penetrate the blood brain barrier well and have excellent CSF bactericidal activity. Because of its long serum half-life, ceftriaxone may be given every 12 to 24 hours. In meningitis, every 12 hours is recommended. Mild, self-limited diarrhea and biliary pseudolithiasis have been noted in some children who receive ceftriaxone. Ceftriaxone also can displace bilirubin from albumin and, therefore, should be given with caution when hyperbilirubinemia is present. Cephalosporins other than cefotaxime and ceftriaxone have higher minimum inhibitory concentrations than do these two drugs and, therefore, should not be used if *S. pneumoniae* is suspected.

Vancomycin combined with ceftriaxone or cefotaxime appears to be synergistic. It should not be used as monotherapy. Whereas initial experimental studies showed poor CSF penetration when vancomycin was used with dexamethasone, later studies have indicated that adequate penetration may occur when the proper dosing is used. As soon as CSF culture and tube dilution sensitivities document that an organism is sensitive to a drug other than vancomycin, it should be discontinued. When cephalosporin resistance is demonstrated or patients are allergic to cephalosporins, vancomycin can be combined with rifampin.

Meropenem, a carbapenem, either alone (120 mg/kg/day every 8 hours) or in combination with other drugs, may be effective for treating patients who cannot tolerate vancomycin.

The duration of antibiotic therapy depends on the causative agent and the clinical response. Minimal duration for Hib and *S. pneumoniae* is 10 days. A minimum of 7 days is required for meningococcal meningitis. The patient should be afebrile for 5 days before halting therapy. Although outpatient therapy is less costly than is hospitalization and it returns patients to their normal environment sooner, it currently is not recommended. Gram-negative meningitis should be treated for a minimum of 3 weeks.

If clinical improvement is slow, if dexamethasone is used, or if a resistant strain is identified on the initial culture, a repeat LP is indicated after 24 to 48 hours of therapy. Cell counts, protein, and glucose levels may be abnormal, but a repeat LP must have a negative Gram stain and sterile culture results. If *S. pneumoniae* is present in the repeat culture, rifampin (20 mg/kg/day in two divided doses) should be added. Another LP should be performed 24 to 48 hours after starting rifampin.

Adjunctive Therapy

Because the effect of bacterial meningitis is affected greatly by the host response, corticosteroids have been suggested as adjunctive therapy. In experimental meningitis, corticosteroids reduce meningeal inflammation, thereby reducing ICP and significantly increasing cerebral perfusion.

Sensorineural hearing loss is an important sequela of bacterial meningitis. In children with Hib meningitis, numerous studies have shown that dexamethasone (0.15 mg/kg per dose every 6 hours for 2 days) given rapidly just before or with administration of antibiotics significantly reduces hearing loss. Studies of corticosteroids in pneumococcal meningitis are more limited. Some have shown a benefit, but others have not. A 1997 meta-analysis found that dexamethasone given before the first dose of antibiotics in pneumococcal meningitis resulted in improved outcome for severe hearing loss. However, statistical significance was dependent on one particular study. In meningococcal meningitis, the use of corticosteroids has not been studied adequately.

The benefit of administering corticosteroids for other neurologic sequelae also is controversial. Some studies of patients treated with corticosteroids have shown a decreased rate of neurologic sequelae, but others have not. A meta-analysis of nine controlled trials of corticosteroid use in bacterial meningitis failed to document that corticosteroids reduced the risk of death or development of neurologic abnormality at hospital discharge or follow-up examination. A 1997 meta-analysis failed to demonstrate a benefit of corticosteroids for other neurologic deficits in pneumococcal meningitis.

Corticosteroid benefit in bacterial meningitis may vary by organism because of differences in the disease pathophysiology. Both Hib and *N. meningitidis* have endotoxin as the primary pathogenic material, but the hearing loss, shock, and other aspects of the diseases occur at significantly different rates. The primary pathogenic material in *S. pneumoniae* is lipoteichoic acid, which may trigger a different inflammatory response than does endotoxin. These differences, and others yet to be discovered, may explain why corticosteroids help with one organism and not another.

The use of corticosteroids is not benign. They may delay CSF sterilization, especially in pneumococcal meningitis. In the 1997 meta-analysis, patients who received corticosteroids had an increased incidence of secondary fevers. Corticosteroids should not be used for more than 2 days because studies have shown no improvement with a longer course. The risk of gastrointestinal bleeding occurring is not significantly increased in a 2-day course. Dexamethasone also can suppress clinical signs, leading to a false sense of clinical improvement.

The Committee on Infectious Diseases of the American Academy of Pediatrics recommends that dexamethasone therapy should be considered for suspected bacterial meningitis in children older than 6 weeks, after the risks and benefits of dexamethasone have been considered. Currently, dexamethasone is recommended for Hib meningitis and should be considered in pneumococcal and meningococcal meningitis. It should not be used in children with partially treated bacterial meningitis, nonbacterial meningitis, or CNS abnormalities.

Supportive Care

The first 3 or 4 days of treatment for bacterial meningitis are the most critical. Vital signs should be taken every 15 to 30 minutes until the patient is stable, then hourly for 48 hours, with rectal temperatures measured every 4 hours. The patient's body weight, urine specific gravity, serum electrolytes (sodium, potassium, chloride, and bicarbonate), and osmolality of serum and urine should be measured on admission and every 6 to 12 hours for the first 24 to 36 hours. A complete blood count with differential and platelets should be performed on admission and repeated as indicated. Coagulation factors should be checked if petechiae, purpura, or abnormal bleeding is present.

A complete neurologic evaluation should be performed on admission, followed by brief neurologic checks every 2 to 4 hours for the first several days. Complete neurologic evaluation should be performed daily. In children younger than 18 months, daily head circumference measurements and transillumination should be done. These procedures may permit the detection of subdural effusion or hydrocephalus.

To prevent vomiting and aspiration, and to allow better assessment of fluid intake, the patient should receive nothing by mouth initially. A careful intake and output record is required. All patients should be assessed carefully for hydration status and development of SIADH. The best indicators of SIADH are absence of signs of dehydration, increased body weight, decreased serum osmolality, and continued sodium excretion despite hyponatremia. If SIADH is demonstrated, fluids should be given at 1,000 mL/m^2/day. A solution with 40 mEq/L of sodium chloride, 35 mEq/L of potassium, and 20 mEq/L of acetate or lactate should be used. Fluids can be liberalized to maintenance requirements (1,600 mL/m^2/day) as the serum sodium level normalizes, usually within 1 day. Restriction of fluids should not occur in all patients. Antidiuretic hormone secretion in bacterial meningitis may be secondary to dehydration. In these circumstances, ADH secretion is a normal physiologic response and is not appropriately termed SIADH. If dehydration is present, maintenance fluids plus sodium and water deficit replacement over the course of 24 to 48 hours can be given. Loss of autoregulation may occur, and fluid restriction in dehydrated patients can decrease cerebral blood flow to ischemic levels.

In patients with septic shock, fluid must be provided to maintain circulation and blood pressure. Fluids should be given to maintain a systolic blood pressure of 80 to 90 mm Hg, a urine output greater than 500 mL/m^2/day, and adequate cerebral perfusion, as evidenced by mental status. Central venous pressure monitoring helps to avoid fluid overload. Plasma or albuminized saline and dopamine and dobutamine may improve blood pressure while minimizing fluid intake.

When signs of increased ICP such as a bulging anterior fontanelle or progressive lethargy occur, elevation of the head to 30 degrees may help. Increased ICP with deterioration of mental status or signs of cerebral herniation may be treated with intravenous mannitol (0.5 g/kg over 30 minutes, repeated as necessary) and, if necessary, placement of an ICP monitoring device. ICP should be kept at less than 20 mm Hg. Hyperventilation may compromise cerebral blood flow and increase the risk of infarction. The efficiency of high-dose pentobarbital and oral glycerol is still somewhat unproven.

In the absence of focal neurologic signs, a CT scan is not needed to identify effusions because they are part of the normal pathophysiology of the disease. A scan can identify cerebrovascular abnormalities and monitor the progression of hydrocephalus. Other indications for obtaining a CT scan include focal neurologic signs, prolonged obtundation, focal seizures, rapidly increasing head circumference, persistently increased CSF protein, persistent CSF granulocytosis, or chronically recurring meningitis. Radioisotope imaging may be helpful in some patients to show collections of purulent material.

Seizures must be controlled with emergency management and anticonvulsants as needed. If the seizures no longer are apparent by the third or fourth hospital day, anticonvulsants can be discontinued. An electroencephalogram may be indicated when (a) focal seizures are noted, (b) seizures persist beyond the third hospital day, or (c) prolonged alteration of consciousness occurs. The treatment of subdural effusions usually is not necessary unless the effusions are suspected as being the cause of focal seizures or increased ICP, or the source of prolonged fever. Subdural empyema should be drained and treated with antibiotics.

Intravenous heparin (1 mg/kg every 4 hours) may be beneficial in disseminated intravascular coagulation, although no controlled studies have documented the benefit of this course of action.

Fever lasts for 5 days in most children. If fever lasts longer than 8 days, a thorough search for brain abscess, subdural or pleural empyema, septic arthritis, thrombophlebitis, or pericarditis should be done. Nosocomial infections and drugs may prolong the duration of fever. Persistent fever also may arise from poor therapeutic response associated with the presence of organisms resistant to the antibiotics chosen for therapy.

Although serum CRP is not sensitive enough to distinguish bacterial from aseptic meningitis on admission, an admission CRP determination can be drawn and compared with subsequent CRP levels. A secondary increase in CRP or a slow decline may indicate complications not yet clinically evident.

CSF glucose and protein concentrations may be abnormal in more than 25% of cases at hospital discharge. They normalize slowly. Performing a predischarge LP normally is not necessary.

PROGNOSIS

Poor prognosis occurs with young age, untoward delays before appropriate antibiotics are started, and the presence of disorders that compromise the host response to infection. Patients whose CSF cultures grow more than 10^7 organisms frequently have more seizures, subdural effusions, bacteremia, speech disturbance, hearing loss, and prolonged fevers. Elevated CNS IL-1β and TNF have been associated with a higher risk of developing neurologic sequelae, as has very low CSF white blood cell count. Complications such as focal neurologic findings at admission, focal deficits, seizures during the infection, SIADH, purpura, shock, hypothermia, or a low white or red blood cell count at admission all have been associated with poor prognosis.

Death rates vary widely. Rates up to 55% have been reported in developing countries, with up to 15% in their major cities. In the United States, a meta-analysis found the death rate to be approximately 4% for Hib, 8% for *N. meningitidis*, and 15% for *S. pneumoniae*. Similar results from other developed countries have been reported.

Meningitis sequelae include hearing loss, mental retardation, seizures, spasticity and paresis, hydrocephalus, blindness, behavior disorders, and neuropsychological or auditory dysfunctions that adversely affect academic performance. Table 136.5 lists some of the major chronic complications of meningitis. Historically, as many as 50% of survivors had sequelae, but in one U.S. meta-analysis, sequelae were present in only 16% of cases. In a large prospective study, 33% of cases had detectable neurologic abnormalities, including paralysis, seizure, persistent tone, ataxia, hydrocephalus, and vision or

TABLE 136.5

CHRONIC COMPLICATIONS OF BACTERIAL MENINGITIS

Hearing loss
Behavior disorders
Mental retardation
Neuropsychiatric dysfunction
Seizures
Auditory dysfunction
Spasticity, paresis
Diabetes insipidus
Hydrocephalus
Transverse myelitis
Blindness
Polyarteritis

auditory problems at discharge. Five years later, only 11% of cases had a detectable neurologic deficit, although this rate increased to 14% at 15 years because of the occurrence of late seizures. Even major neurologic deficits may resolve with time. Therefore, cautious optimism must be maintained in discussing long-term complications with parents.

Some studies have found that survivors have IQs and middle-school grades comparable with those of siblings. Other studies noted small but significant deficits, particularly in verbal skills. The academic success of survivors may require additional school and family support.

The incidence of sequelae varies by organism. In one study, discharge morbidity was 21% for Hib, 9% for *N. meningitidis*, and 38% for *S. pneumoniae*.

Hearing loss is the most common neurologic sequela, with deafness present in approximately 10% of survivors. Evoked-response audiometry has revealed auditory nerve deficits in 6% of Hib meningitis cases, 10% of meningococcal meningitis cases, and 31% of pneumococcal meningitis cases. Generally, it is not related to the severity of illness. The time interval over which the relative risk of developing increasingly severe sensorineural hearing loss remains unclear. Some evidence indicates that hearing loss occurs early and may be associated with an early low CSF glucose level. Permanent or transient deafness often is noted early and occurs despite the rapid administration of appropriate therapy. In our own studies, a markedly depressed CSF–to–blood glucose ratio, seizures before admission, duration of fever after initiation of therapy, and treatment with oral antibiotics before establishment of diagnosis all were associated with increased risk of deafness occurring. Children presenting with ataxia are at high risk for having hearing loss, because vestibular and auditory branches of the eighth cranial nerve may be affected simultaneously. Hearing evaluations with evoked response audiometry, or pure-tone audiometry in older children, should be performed before or soon after hospital discharge in all children with bacterial meningitis. With the advent of cochlear implantation, determining the exact location of the damage, which can be conductive, sensorineural, or central, is important. In children with cochlear damage but intact auditory nerves, rapid evaluation for cochlear implantation should be performed before osteoneogenesis occurs.

Seizures that are difficult to control, persist beyond the fourth hospital day, or are focal in nature increase the risk of developing sequelae. Seizure frequency is similar for Hib and *S. pneumoniae* and is double that of meningococcal meningitis. Seizures do not necessarily result in epilepsy, but a high association between focal neurologic signs and afebrile seizures up to 15 years later has been noted. The risk of developing seizures

in the 20 years after illness is approximately 13% for those with early seizures and 3% for those without early seizures. Seizures are associated with CSF bacterial counts higher than 10^7 colony-forming units per milliliter, TNF-α concentrations higher than 103 pg/mL, and high lipopolysaccharide concentrations.

Cerebral infarction has been noted on CT scans within 1 day of onset of fever. Acute or delayed spinal cord infarction may result in quadriplegia or respiratory arrest. The speed with which the diagnosis is established and therapy is instituted has not been related to the risk of developing either cerebral or spinal cord infarction. Focal neurologic signs at admission are correlated with mental retardation and abnormal neurologic examinations at 1 year after discharge. Children with subdural effusions have no greater incidence of neurologic complications than do those without effusions.

Brain abscess as a complication is an extremely unusual event. If an abscess is found, it may have preceded the meningitis, and a search for infections at other locations (such as endocarditis) should be done. The response of the abscess to antimicrobials can be followed by serial CT scans. Relapse after administration of third-generation cephalosporin now occurs in fewer than 1% of cases.

PREVENTION

Prophylaxis can prevent the spread of *N. meningitidis* and *H. influenzae*. Pneumococcal prophylaxis is not recommended because contacts are not at significantly increased risk of developing infection. Anyone who develops fever after exposure to patients with any form of bacterial meningitis should get prompt medical attention. For the most current recommendations, refer to the reports of the Committee on Infectious Diseases of the American Academy of Pediatrics. In the United States, *N. meningitidis* and Hib cases must be reported to the appropriate health department.

N. meningitidis prophylaxis with rifampin (10 mg/kg, with a 600 mg maximum, every 12 hours for 2 days) should be given within 24 hours of case recognition. Household, day-care, and close contacts of the patient during the previous 7 days should receive rifampin, but casual school or work contacts should not. Often, deciding who had close contact is difficult because infections have occurred after exposure on school buses and school trips. Medical personnel exposed to the patient's secretions in the first 24 hours after the start of antibiotics should receive prophylaxis. Rifampin may turn urine, sweat, and tears orange. Contact lenses may stain permanently, and serum levels of oral contraceptives and other drugs may be reduced. *N. meningitidis* resistance to rifampin of up to 27% has been reported. Ciprofloxacin (500 mg orally in one dose) can be used for contacts older than 18 years of age. With those *N. meningitidis* sensitive to sulfonamides, sulfisoxazole may be given. The dose is 500 mg/day in infants younger than 1 year of age, 500 mg every 12 hours for children 1 to 12 years, and 1 g every 12 hours for patients older than 12 years. Sulfisoxazole should be given for 2 days. Ceftriaxone (125 mg intramuscularly in those younger than 12 years of age and 250 mg for those older than 12 years) is an effective alternative to rifampin and can be used. The index patient should receive prophylaxis on discharge unless treated with ceftriaxone or cefotaxime.

Hib prophylaxis with rifampin (20 mg/kg, with a 600 mg maximum, once daily for 4 days) eliminates most nasopharyngeal carriage of Hib. Rifampin is recommended for all nonpregnant household contacts, including adults, if a vaccinated child of any age or unvaccinated child younger than 48 months lives in the home. Rifampin should be given to day-care or nursery school contacts if two or more cases occur within 60 days.

Children who have received Hib vaccine should receive prophylaxis.

Vaccines

Hib conjugate vaccine (0.5 mL per dose) has two dosing schedules. The child should receive HbOC or PRP-T at 2, 4, and 6 months or PRP-OMP at 2 and 4 months. All three forms require a 12- to 15-month booster. If possible, the same vaccine should be used for all doses.

A few vaccine failures have been reported. Subnormal IgG2 or IgM levels have been noted in some failures, although probably no direct link exists between these immunoglobulin types and failure because the predominant antibody response is IgG1.

Hib conjugate vaccine is recommended routinely for children to prevent invasive Hib disease. *S. pneumoniae* vaccine (Pneumovax 23, 0.5 mL per dose) contains 25 μg each of the 23 polysaccharide antigens responsible for more than 90% of childhood pneumococcal bacteremia and meningitis. Although it is effective in children older than 17 months, it is recommended for use after 2 years of age for high-risk children, such as those with sickle cell disease, functional or anatomic asplenia, nephrotic syndrome, or immunocompromise, or when the effect of infection could be severe, as in children with certain congenital heart diseases. It is not recommended for the prevention of respiratory tract infection or otitis media in young children.

A seven-valent conjugate pneumococcal vaccine has been shown to be effective in preventing invasive pneumococcal disease caused by the serotypes contained in the vaccine. This vaccine is recommended for all children younger than 24 months of age and generally is given at 2, 4, 6, and 12 months of age (four doses).

N. meningitidis vaccine is recommended for individuals at high risk for the acquisition of disease. The American Academy of Pediatrics has recommended that congugate mcv4 vaccine should be given to adolecents 11–12 years of age, to adolescents at high school entry and to college freshman living in dormitories. This quadrivalent vaccine consists of capsular polysaccharides A, C, Y, and W135 in each 0.5-mL dose. Immunization with meningococcal polysaccharide quadrivalent vaccine (mpsv4) recommended for children 2 years of age and older in high-risk groups, including those with anatomic or functional asplenia, and those with terminal deficiencies of the complement system or with properdin deficiency. It also is recommended for individuals travelling to hyperendemic areas or in an epidemic due to a meningococcal type contained in the vaccine.

Research is under way to produce an effective serogroup B vaccine. The serogroup B polysaccharide is poorly immunogenic. New vaccines under development are derived from outer membrane proteins and the substitution of chemical groupings on the capsular polysaccharide, among other approaches.

Suggested Readings

Baraff LJ, Lee SI, Schriger DL, et al. Outcomes of bacterial meningitis in children: a meta-analysis. *Pediatr Infect Dis J* 1993;12:389.

Dicuonzo G, Lorino G, Lilli D, et al. Use of oligoprobes on amplified DNA in the diagnosis of bacterial meningitis. *Eur J Clin Microbiol Infect Dis* 1999;18:352.

Feigin RD, McCracken GH, Klein JO. Diagnosis and management of meningitis. *Pediatr Infect Dis J* 1992;11:785.

Feigin RD, Pearlman E. Bacterial meningitis beyond the neonatal period. In: Feigin RD, Cherry JD, Demmler GJ, Kaplan SL, eds. *Textbook of pediatric infectious diseases*, 5th ed. Philadelphia: Saunders, 2003;443.

McIntyre PB, Berkey CS, King SM, et al. Dexamethasone as adjunctive therapy in bacterial meningitis. *JAMA* 1997;278:925.

Pickering LK, ed. *2003 Red Book: Report of the Committee on Infectious Diseases*, 26th ed. Elk Grove Village, IL: American Academy of Pediatrics, 2003.

Van Vliet KE, Glimaker M, Lebon P, et al. Multicenter evaluation of the Amplicor Enterovirus PCR test with cerebrospinal fluid from patients with aseptic meningitis. *J Clin Microbiol* 1998;36:2652.

CHAPTER 137 ■ OPPORTUNISTIC INFECTIONS IN THE COMPROMISED HOST

CHRISTIAN C. PATRICK

Immunocompromised patients are at increased risk of developing an infection because of having one or more deficits in their host defense. This patient population is increasing in number because of the expanded use of immunosuppressive drugs and the ability to support patients with congenital or acquired immunodeficiencies (Table 137.1).

Microorganisms infecting immunocompromised patients can be well-recognized pathogens or organisms such as commensal organisms, once considered nonpathogenic. This latter point renders distinguishing an infection from a contaminated specimen difficult.

The type of immunodeficiency, based on the dysfunction of the immune system (phagocytic, cell-mediated immunity, humoral immunity, complement system), allows the physician some rationale to predict the cause of the opportunistic infection.

NEUTROPHIL DYSFUNCTION

The phagocytic system, along with the physical integument, represents the first line of defense against infecting microorganisms. The neutrophil or polymorphonuclear cell is the predominate cell of the phagocytic system.

Neutrophil dysfunction can manifest itself either by quantitative or qualitative defects. Quantitative defects are seen most commonly, and these are classified as hereditary or acquired.

TABLE 137.1

OPPORTUNISTIC INFECTIONS IN THE COMPROMISED HOST

Predisposing Causes (Selected Examples)	Opportunistic Organisms Isolated Most Frequently	Suggested Mechanism
Anatomic defect		
Central venous catheter	*Staphylococcus epidermidis, Staphylococcus aureus*, Enterobacteriaceae	Deficient skin barrier; presence of foreign body
Dermal sinus tracts	*S. epidermidis*, diphtheroids	Bypasses skin barrier
Respirators	*Pseudomonas* species Serratia	Serves as portal of entry; nidus of infection
Acquired immunodeficiencies		
Viral infections	Herpes viruses, bacterial infections (Epstein-Barr virus, human immunodeficiency virus, cytomegalovirus)	T-cell deficits, cytopenia
Immunosuppressive therapy	*Pneumocystis Jiroveci*, bacterial and fungal infections	Dependent on agent used
Inherited immunodeficiencies		
Phagocytic defects	*S. aureus*, Nocardia, Serratia, Candida	Defect in bacteriocidal killing
Humoral immune defects	*Streptococcus pneumoniae, Haemophilus influenzae, Neisseria meningitidis*	Low to absent antibody level
Complement deficits	Same as for humoral immune defects	Reduced chemotaxis, deficient opsonization
Cellular immunity defects	*P. carinii, Candida* species	Reduced T-cell numbers, diminished lymphoproliferative responses
Splenic deficiencies		
	S. pneumoniae, H. influenzae	Loss of opsonic activity decrease in phagocytosis
Collagen vascular diseases		
	Fungal infections, *S. aureus, Pseudomonas* species	Deficits in reticuloendothelial system
Other		
Malnutrition	Measles virus, herpes simplex virus, varicella-zoster virus, *Myobacterium* species (malnutrition), *S. aureus, Pseudomonas* species (cystic fibrosis)	Impaired T-cell function (malnutrition, uremia), impaired ciliary function (cystic fibrosis)
Renal disease		
Cystic fibrosis		
Diabetes mellitus		

Qualitative defects are divided into defects in microbicidal activity or those involving cell migration.

Quantitative neutropenia is stratified by the extent of neutropenia. An absolute neutrophil count (ANC) of 1,000 or fewer metamyelocytes, band forms, and neutrophils per microliter is considered significant neutropenia; an ANC of 100 or fewer per microliter is considered profound neutropenia.

The etiology of neutropenias commonly is classified as functional deficits or neutropenia secondary to an etiologic factor. Functional classifications of neutropenias include (a) disorders of proliferation of committed stem cells (e.g., cyclic neutropenia, reticular dysgenesis); (b) disorders of committed myeloid stem cells (e.g., infantile genetic agranulocytosis of Kostmann, acquired neutropenias); (c) disorders associated with immune dysfunctions or metabolic disturbances (e.g., cartilage hair hypoplasia, metabolic disorders); and (d) disorders associated with decreased neutrophil survival (e.g., immune neutropenias, viral infections).

The acquired neutropenias are associated most commonly with disorders of committed myeloid stem cells. Causes include infections (Box 137.1), drugs (e.g., antibiotics such as trimethoprim-sulfamethoxazole, penicillin; anticonvulsants such as phenytoin; barbiturates; and other miscellaneous drugs such as thiazides and propranolol), chemical and environmental toxins (e.g., benzene, DDT), anticancer chemotherapy (e.g., doxorubicin [Adriamycin], methotrexate, cytosine arabinoside), and infiltration of bone marrow (e.g., leukemia, lymphoma, neuroblastoma).

Because of the increasing and intensive use of chemotherapeutic agents in patients with cancer, this patient population

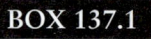

BOX 137.1   **Infectious Causes of Acquired Neutropenia**

Bacterial
Overwhelming sepsis
Typhoid
Tularemia
Brucellosis

Viral
Hepatitis A and B
Cytomegalovirus
Epstein-Barr virus
Varicella virus
Human immunodeficiency virus
Measles virus
Rubella virus
Respiratory syncytial virus

Protozoan
Malaria
Toxoplasmosis
Rickettsial
Rocky Mountain spotted fever
Scrub typhus
Epidemic typhus
Rickettsial pox

TABLE 137.2

ETIOLOGIC AGENTS IMPLICATED IN PATIENTS WITH NEUTROPHIL DEFICITS, HUMORAL DYSFUNCTIONS, AND CELLULAR IMMUNE DYSFUNCTION

Neutrophil Deficits	Humoral Dysfunction	Cellular Dysfunction
Bacteria	**Bacteria**	**Bacteria**
Gram-positive	*Haemophilus influenzae*	*Legionella pneumophila*
Coagulase-negative staphylococci	*Neisseria meningitidis*	*Listeria monocytogenes*
Viridans streptococci	*Streptococcus pneumoniae*	*Mycobacterium tuberculosis*
Staphylococcus aureus		*Mycobacterium avium* complex
Corynebacterium jeikeium		*Nocardia* species
Fungi		*Salmonella* species
Candida species		*Serratia marcescens*
Aspergillus species		**Fungi**
Histoplasma capsulatum		*Candida* species
		Cryptococcus neoformans
		Coccidioides immitis
		Histoplasma capsulatum
		Viruses
		Cytomegalovirus
		Epstein-Barr virus
		Herpes simplex virus
		Rotavirus
		Varicella-zoster virus
		Protozoa
		Cryptosporidium
		Pneumocystis jiroveci
		Toxoplasmosis gondii
		Helminth
		Strongyloides stercoralis

has become a paradigm for patients with neutropenia and presumed infection. The infecting organisms for this patient population are the gram-positive bacteria, primarily *Staphylococcus epidermidis*, *Staphylococcus aureus*, and viridans streptococci (Table 137.2). *Corynebacterium jeikeium* is associated with catheter-related infections. Of the gram-negative bacteria, *Enterobacter* species can be problematic because they easily induce beta-lactamase, rendering these organisms resistant to the cephalosporins and penicillin. Fungal infections occur most commonly in patients with prolonged neutropenia on broad-spectrum antibiotics. The predominate fungal organisms are *Candida* species, emanating from the patients' own gastrointestinal tract, and *Aspergillus* species, acquired from the respiratory route.

In 1966, Bodey et al. were the first to establish the relationship between the incidence of infection and the magnitude of neutropenia. At an ANC of 500 per microliter or less, the frequency of infection increased, and at an ANC of 100 per microliter or less, patients were at extreme risk, including a hazard for gram-negative bacteremia. The risk of developing infection is linked not only to the depth of neutropenia but to the rapidity of the decline in the ANC. Thus, patients with a slow decline, as seen in those with aplastic anemia, are at a lower risk than are patients who have been administered high-intensity chemotherapy.

The duration of neutropenia also is related to the risk of infections. Patients with neutropenia lasting 2 weeks or longer are at appreciable risk, including the risk of acquiring fungal infections.

Patients with leukemia or lymphoma have qualitative defects in neutrophil function. These qualitative defects also are evident during treatment using certain chemotherapeutic agents (e.g., methotrexate, anthracyclines, corticosteroids) or craniospinal irradiation.

A standardized plan is required to define patients with fever and neutropenia and to initiate therapy to provide appropriate

care, taking into account the hospital's epidemiology. Fever can be defined as a single oral temperature of at least 38.3°C or two oral temperatures of at least 38.0°C taken 1 hour apart. Fever is the most important indicator of infection, and pain also is a reliable symptom for the possible presence of infection.

In patients with fever and neutropenia, blood cultures should be obtained from a peripheral vein and the central venous catheter before antibiotics are administered. Specimens for culture should be obtained from any suspicious site. Chest radiographs are controversial, but they can be used for future comparisons.

Management of Fever and Neutropenia

The management of patients who are neutropenic with fever consists of providing appropriate antibiotics and supportive care. The ability to stratify patients according to risk for a serious infection has led to truncating intravenous therapy, either to oral therapy or no therapy in selected settings. The initial management of the febrile, neutropenic patient should include administration of broad-spectrum antibiotics that have bactericidal activity. The selection of the antibiotics should take into account the antibiotic susceptibility data of the hospital and those of the geographic area, the patient's colonizing isolates, the pharmacokinetic properties of the antibiotics, the possibilities for occurrences of drug interactions, and the presence of a focal site of infection (e.g., central venous catheter infection).

The Infectious Disease Society of America has attempted to standardize the use of antibiotics in the febrile, neutropenic patient. Three broad antibiotic regimens should be considered, depending on the patient's renal status, focal findings, type of chemotherapy given, and the epidemiology of possible infecting organisms. These regimens are (a) vancomycin plus an aminoglycoside plus a third-generation cephalosporin or vancomycin and a third-generation cephalosporin, (b) duotherapy with two beta-lactam antibiotics (e.g., a third-generation cephalosporin, such as ceftazidime) plus an antipseudomonal beta-lactam antibiotic or a beta-lactam antibiotic plus an aminoglycoside; or (c) monotherapy (e.g., cefepime, ceftazidime, or meropenem). The physician should first decide whether vancomycin is needed because of the presence of severe mucositis, colonization with methicillin-resistant S. aureus, or penicillin- or cephalosporin-resistant S. pneumoniae, catheter-related infection, previous quinolone prophylaxis, or hypotension.

Qualitative deficiencies elicit the specific risks of developing infection, depending on the underlying deficit. Chronic granulomatous disease is a microbicidal deficiency of neutrophils caused by a heterogenous group of biochemical and genetic disorders of the phagocytic nicotinamide-adenine dinucleotide phosphate oxidase complex. This defect results in the inability of phagocytes to generate superoxide anion and other oxygen species, thus allowing the development of infections by those bacteria and fungi that produce catalase. These organisms include staphylococci, gram-negative Enterobacteriaceae (e.g., Serratia marcescens, Salmonella species), Pseudomonas species, Nocardia, yeasts, and filamentous fungi such as Aspergillus fumigatus. Patients present early in life with infections of the skin, lungs, and bones of the hands and feet, as well as abscesses of the liver, appendix, and subphrenic or retroperitoneal spaces. Treatment must be aggressive, with abscess drainage and the administration of intravenous antibiotics. The etiology of pneumonia should be pursued aggressively using bronchoalveolar lavage or open lung biopsy. Other defects of the microbicidal mechanism include glutathione synthetase deficiency, myeloperoxidase deficiency, glucose-6-phosphate dehydrogenase deficiency, and glutathione peroxidase deficiency.

Cell migration defects include Chédiak-Higashi syndrome, leukocyte adhesion deficiency, special granule deficiency syndrome, actin dysfunction, Job syndrome, lazy leukocyte syndrome, glycogen storage disease (type 1B), hyperimmunoglobulin E syndrome, and impaired generation of serum-derived chemotaxis. Chédiak-Higashi syndrome is a rare autosomal recessive disorder characterized by recurrent pyogenic infections, neutropenia, peripheral neuropathy, and partial oculocutaneous albinism. The disease occurs with variable severity. Phagocytosis is normal; however, leukocyte dysfunction is evident in impaired chemotaxis, delayed intracellular killing, and defective natural killer cell activity. Infections are caused predominately by S. aureus, but other organisms such as group A streptococci, Haemophilus influenzae, gram-negative enterics, and fungal organisms can play a role.

CELLULAR IMMUNE DYSFUNCTION

Cell-mediated immunity involves thymus-derived lymphocytes, or T lymphocytes, which affect target cell cytolysis and the secretion of cytokines. T lymphocytes provide assistance to the B lymphocytes of the humoral immune system; thus, defects in cell-mediated immunity often result in a secondary defect in humoral immunity.

Assessing cell-mediated immunity should begin with a measurement of the total lymphocyte number. At any time, the lymphocyte count should be greater than 1,200 per microliter of blood. Lymphopenia may be indicative of congenital or acquired disorders. Flow cytometry can be used to measure the total number of T cells using anti-CD3 or T-lymphocyte subsets using anti-CD4 or anti-CD8.

To measure T-lymphocyte function, the activation of T cells can be achieved using global activators such as mitogens (e.g., phytohemagglutinin and concanavalin that predominately activate T cells or pokeweed mitogen that stimulates B

TABLE 137.3

INFECTIOUS AGENTS IMPLICATED IN PATIENTS WITH CELLULAR IMMUNE DYSFUNCTIONS

Bacteria
Legionella pneumophila
Listeria monocytogenes
Mycobacterium tuberclosis
Mycobacterium avium complex
Nocardia species
Salmonella species
Serratia marcescens

Fungi
Candida species
Cryptococcus neoformans
Coccidiodes immitis
Histoplasma capsulatum

Viruses
Cytomegalovirus
Epstein-Barr virus
Herpes simplex virus
Rotavirus
Varicella-zoster virus

Protozoa
Cryptosporidium
Pneumocystis carinii
Toxoplasma gondii

Helminth
Strongyloides stercoralis

cells) or antigens that stimulate cells specific to that particular antigen.

Skin tests using vaccine or microbial antigens to which the child has been exposed are used to assess delayed hypersensitivity. These tests often are absent in children younger than the age of 2 years and have a low specificity.

Chest radiographs are used in infants to assess the presence or absence of a thymic shadow.

Intracellular pathogens are evident in patients with cell-mediated immunity deficits because these organisms are particular targets of T-cell immunity (Tables 137.1 and 137.3). Viral infections are particularly problematic, with fungal and protozoan organisms seen. Because of the associated humoral immunodeficiency, recurrent bacterial infections, such as otitis media and pneumonia, often occur.

DiGeorge syndrome, or congenital thymic aplasia, has a profound T-lymphocyte abnormality caused by interference in the embryonic development of the thymus and parathyroid glands at approximately 12 weeks of gestation. The syndrome manifests with hypoparathyroidism, cellular immunodeficiency, congenital heart disease, and characteristic abnormal facies. Affected individuals have low total lymphocyte counts but normal concentrations of serum immunoglobulins. They are susceptible to intracellular organisms such as Mycobacterium tuberculosis, Listeria monocytogenes, and viruses (e.g., cytomegalovirus, varicella-zoster virus, measles, enterovirus, rotavirus). Fungi (e.g., Candida albicans, Cryptococcus neoformans, Histoplasma capsulatum) and certain bacteria (e.g., Streptococcus pneumoniae, H. influenzae) can be problematic because of a failure in B- and T-cell collaboration that results in an impairment in production of specific antibodies.

Chronic mucocutaneous candidiasis is considered a specific defect in T-lymphocyte immunity against Candida species. This entity represents a spectrum of diseases with no gender predilection but a familial occurrence. It often is associated with endocrine abnormalities such as hypothyroidism, hypoparathyroidism, pernicious anemia, and diabetes mellitus. *Candida* infections usually are localized, affecting the nails, skin, or mucous membranes, and are not systemic. These patients have a normal lymphocyte count and normal mitogen indices but an abnormal T-cell response to *Candida* antigens.

Wiskott-Aldrich syndrome is an X-linked recessive disorder that can present with recurrent infections, usually of the upper respiratory tract and skin; thrombocytopenia; and an eczematoid rash. T-lymphocyte and antibody defects are present. Leukemia or Hodgkin disease frequently complicates the syndrome. The cause of death primarily is infection, with bleeding being the next most common cause.

Ataxia-telangiectasia is an autosomal recessive primary immunodeficiency with clinical findings of cerebellar ataxia, developmental arrest, and oculocutaneous telangiectasias. Infections include sinopulmonary disease with encapsulated bacteria (e.g., *S. pneumoniae*, *H. influenzae*), leading to bronchiectasis.

Severe combined immunodeficiency disease occurs in X-linked, autosomal, or sporadic forms and is characterized by a severe deficiency in both T- and B-cell immunity. A deficiency of adenosine deaminase is found in approximately 50% of patients. Clinical features include failure to thrive, diaper dermatitis, chronic thrush, intractable diarrhea, and fulminant or prolonged pneumonia that usually is caused by *Pneumocystis carinii*. These patients are particularly prone to the development of infection with viruses (e.g., cytomegalovirus, Epstein-Barr virus, enteroviruses), fungi (e.g., *Candida* species), bacteria, and protozoa (e.g., *P. Jiroveci*). An antigen-compatible bone marrow transplant is the treatment of choice.

Secondary T-cell defects are seen far more commonly than are the primary immunodeficiencies. They include infection (e.g., human immunodeficiency virus, measles, tuberculosis), immunosuppressive therapy (e.g., cytotoxic drugs, corticosteroids, irradiation, cyclosporine), and malnutrition.

HUMORAL IMMUNE DYSFUNCTION

Humoral immunity involves the production of antibodies to soluble antigens. A dichotomy is made by antigens that require T-cell help (T-dependent), such as proteins, and those that do not (T-independent), such as polysaccharides that elicit predominately IgM antibodies.

Humoral immunodeficiencies usually are associated with pyogenic infections of the respiratory tract, including otitis media, sinusitis, and pneumonia. The infecting organisms usually are encapsulated bacteria and respiratory viruses (Table 137.4). Patients with humoral immunodeficiencies have difficulty eradicating infections caused by echoviruses, adenoviruses, and coxsackieviruses, and they can have chronic enteroviral meningoencephalitis.

The workup of a patient with a presumed humoral immunity deficit should include the serum immunoglobulin quantification, isohemagglutinin titers, T- and B-cell enumeration, and hemolytic complement determination. Antibody titers to diphtheria and tetanus toxoids, and IgG subclasses may be assessed in children with abnormalities in the functional production of antibodies.

X-linked agammaglobulinemia, or Bruton disease, is a B-cell deficiency. The concentrations of all serum immunoglobulins are decreased markedly after maternal antibody dissipates. Peripheral blood lymphocyte numbers are normal, but B cells and plasma cells are reduced or absent in lymphoid tissue. Infections begin in the first 6 months of life, as maternal antibody wanes. The most common infections are of the upper and lower respiratory tracts, with gastrointestinal infec-

TABLE 137.4

ETIOLOGIC AGENTS COMMONLY ASSOCIATED WITH HUMORAL IMMUNE DYSFUNCTION

Bacteria
Haemophilus influenzae
Neisseria meningitidis
Streptococcus pneumoniae

Virus
Echoviruses
Coxsackieviruses
Adenoviruses
Other respiratory viruses

tions being second. Infections with encapsulated bacteria (*S. pneumonias*, *H. influenzae*) along with *P. Jirocevi* are common occurrences. Diarrhea commonly is caused by *Giardia*, but *Salmonella*, *Shigella*, *Camplyobacter*, or rotavirus should be considered. Vaccine-associated polio and enterovirus arthritis or encephalitis can occur.

Selective IgA deficiency is the most common immunodeficiency, occurring in one of 500 to 800 normal white individuals. Most individuals with this deficiency are asymptomatic. The absence of secretory IgA can result in recurrent infections of the respiratory, gastrointestinal, and urogenital tracts. An association of selective IgA deficiency with atopy and autoimmune diseases has been noted.

Common variable immunodeficiency refers to a heterogeneous group of disorders that possess a variable degree of T- and B-cell activities. Specific pathogens are similar to those implicated in X-linked agammaglobulinemia.

COMPLEMENT DYSFUNCTIONS

The complement system is a series of proteins that solubilize and clear immune complexes that promote bacterial lysis and immunologic hemostasis. Deficiencies of the complement components are associated with recurrent infections, autoimmune disorders, and glomerulonephritis.

Defects in the classical complement pathway are identified with the total hemolytic complement (CH_{50}) assay.

C3 deficiency is a rare autosomal recessive trait in which patients present with recurrent pyogenic infections with encapsulated bacteria (*S. pneumonia*, *H. influenzae*, and *N. meningitidis*). Collagen vascular disease and membranoproliferative glomerulonephritis often are associated.

Deficiencies in the C5 to C9 components of the complement cascade are associated with recurrent and disseminated infection caused mainly *N. meningitidis*. Deficiencies in the early complement components such as C1–C4 cause increased susceptibilities to infections with encapsulated organisms (e.g., *S. pneumonia*, *H. influenzae*).

Suggested Readings

Babior BM, Woodman RC. Chronic granulomatous disease. *Semin Hematol* 1990;27:247.

Chinen J, Kline MW, Shearer WT. Primary immunodeficiencies. In: Feigin RD, Cherry JD, eds. *Textbook of pediatric infectious diseases*, 5th ed. Philadelphia: Saunders, 2004:967.

Hughes WT, Armstrong D, Bodey GP, et al. 2002 Guidelines for the use of antimicrobial agents in neutropenic patients with cancer. *Clin Infect Dis* 2002;34:730.

Mermel LA, Farr BM, Sherertz RJ et al. Guidelines for the management of intravascular catheter-related infections. *Clin Infect Dis* 2001;32:1249.

Patrick CC, ed. *Clinical management of infections in immunocompromised infants and children*. Philadelphia: Lippincott Williams & Wilkins, 2001.

Patrick CC, Shenep JL. Outpatient management of the febrile neutropenic child with cancer. *Adv Ped Infect Dis* 1999;14:29.

Patrick CC, Slobod KS. Opportunistic infections in the compromised host. In: Feigin RD, Cherry JD, eds. *Textbook of pediatric infectious diseases,* 4th ed. Philadelphia: Saunders, 1998:980.

Shackelford PG. Infectious complications of antibody deficiency. In: Long SS, Pickering LK, Prober CG, eds. *Principles and practice of pediatric infectious diseases.* New York: Churchill Livingstone, 1997:705.

Stiehm DR, Chin TW, Haas A, et al. Infectious complications of the primary immunodeficiencies. *Clin Immunol Immunopathol* 1986;40:69.

Viscoti C, Varnier O, Machetti M. Infections in patients with febrile neutropenia: epidemiology. Microbiology, and risk stratification. *Clin Infect Dis* 2005; 40:S240.

Weintrub PS. Infectious complications of complement deficiency. In: Long SS, Pickering LK, Prober CG, eds. *Principles and practice of pediatric infectious diseases.* New York: Churchill Livingstone, 1997:711.

CHAPTER 138 ■ BIOTERRORISM

ROBERT J. LEGGIADRO

The intentional delivery of *Bacillus anthracis* spores through mailed letters or packages established the clinical reality of bioterrorism in the United States in late 2001. An understanding of the epidemiology, clinical manifestations, and management of the more credible biologic agents is critical to limiting morbidity and mortality from a bioterrorism attack.

The implementation of an effective response to a deliberate release of biologic agents by terrorists requires the detection and reporting of cases as soon as possible. A prompt recognition of unusual clinical syndromes and increases above seasonal levels in the incidence of common syndromes or deaths caused by infectious agents is critical to launching an effective response.

EPIDEMIOLOGY

Potential biologic weapons share several characteristics. Ease of acquisition and production is a primary consideration. Other ideal properties include the potential to be aerosolized (particle sizes of 1 to 10 μm) and dispersed over a wide geographic area, as well as resistance to sunlight, dessication, and heat. The potential to cause lethal or debilitating disease and person-to-person transmission are important features, as is lack of effective therapy or prophylaxis.

Any small or large outbreak of disease merits evaluation as a potential biologic event. Unusually high rates of disease, as well as unusual clinical syndromes (e.g., a cluster of life-threatening pneumonia in otherwise healthy adults), should signal a warning. Once the case definition and attack rate have been determined, an epidemic curve can be calculated based on the number of cases over the course of time. The epidemic curve in a biologic event triggered by a point-source exposure most likely would be compressed, with a peak reached in a matter of hours or days. The occurrence of a second curve peak is possible with contagious agents, as a result of person-to-person transmission. The steep epidemic curve expected in a bioterrorism attack is similar to that seen with other point-source exposures, such as foodborne outbreaks.

Several epidemiologic clues may be helpful in determining whether further investigation into an outbreak as a potential biologic attack is warranted. A large epidemic, especially one occurring in a discrete population; more severe disease than expected for a given pathogen; and a disease unusual for a given geographic area (e.g., pulmonic tularemia in an urban setting) represent major indicators. Multiple simultaneous epidemics of different diseases, outbreaks with both human and zoonotic

consequences, and unusual strains or susceptibility profiles are additional helpful parameters. Variable attack rates as a function of an agent released relative to the interior or exterior of a building also are useful. Although most bioterrorism attacks will be covert, intelligence revealing plans for an attack, terrorist claims of a deliberate release, or direct physical evidence of an attack obviously point to such an event.

The emergence of mosquito-borne West Nile (WN) virus encephalitis in New York City in the summer of 1999 is an example of a naturally occurring outbreak that had elements of a potential bioterrorist attack. This outbreak represented a disease occurring in an unusual (previously nonendemic) area as well as one with zoonotic (birds) in addition to human consequences. It marked the first documented appearance of WN virus in the Western hemisphere and the first arboviral outbreak in New York City since the yellow fever epidemics of the nineteenth century. A large avian die-off, affecting primarily crows, preceded the outbreak in humans by at least several weeks.

CRITICAL BIOLOGIC AGENTS

In addition to anthrax, critical biologic agents include plague, tularemia, smallpox, viral hemorrhagic fever, and botulinum toxin (Table 138.1). These credible biologic agents are discussed further.

Anthrax

B. anthracis is a large, sporulatory gram-positive rod with three distinct life cycles featuring multiplication of spores in soil,

TABLE 138.1

CRITICAL BIOLOGIC AGENTS

Bacteria
Anthrax
Plague
Tularemia
Viruses
Smallpox
Viral hemorrhagic fevers
Toxins
Botulinum toxin

animal (herbivore) infection, and human infection. Anthrax continues to occur in developing countries where the organism is highly endemic and the use of animal anthrax vaccine is not comprehensive (e.g., Iran, Iraq, Turkey, Pakistan, and sub-Saharan Africa). Human cases may be classified as either agricultural or industrial. Herders, butchers, and slaughterhouse workers in direct contact with infected animals are susceptible to acquisition of agricultural infection, whereas workers in animal-hair processing mills and those handling bone meal may acquire industrial infection.

The three forms of human anthrax are cutaneous, inhalational, and gastrointestinal. The most common form is cutaneous, which is acquired through contact with an infected animal or animal products. The much less common inhalational form results from deposition of spores in the lungs, and gastrointestinal anthrax occurs after ingestion of infected meat. Because human-to-human transmission of anthrax has not been reported, standard precautions are recommended for hospitalized patients with all forms of anthrax infection. In the United States, 224 cases of cutaneous anthrax were reported between 1944 and 1994. Most cases in recent decades were a result of exposure to wool or animal hair.

The clinical presentation and course of the first ten confirmed cases of inhalational anthrax associated with bioterrorism in the United States were reported in late 2001. Epidemiologic investigation indicated that the outbreak was a result of the intentional delivery of B. anthracis spores through mailed letters or packages. The median incubation period was 4 days, ranging from 4 to 6 days. Several clinical features of these patients were not emphasized in earlier reports of inhalational anthrax, a previously rare disease. Drenching sweating, nausea, and vomiting were frequent symptoms of the initial phase of illness in this outbreak. Pleural effusions were a remarkably consistent clinical feature. No predominant underlying diseases or conditions were noted.

None of the ten patients had an initially normal chest radiograph. In addition to characteristic mediastinal widening, paratracheal or hilar fullness, pleural effusions, and parenchymal infiltrates were noted. Computed tomography (CT) of the chest was more sensitive than was chest radiography in revealing mediastinal lymphadenopathy, and an elevation in the proportion of neutrophils or band forms represented an early diagnostic clue.

Inhalational anthrax previously was reported to be a biphasic illness with influenza-like symptoms (i.e., fever, cough, malaise, fatigue, and chest discomfort) manifesting in the first phase, followed briefly by 1 to 2 days of improvement before development of the acute phase 2 to 5 days later. However, this brief period of improvement between initial and fulminant phases of illness was not observed in the first intentional outbreak associated with mail.

The 55% survival rate in these patients was higher than previously reported (less than 15%). Limited data on the treatment of survivors suggest that early treatment with a fluoroquinolone and at least one other active drug (e.g., rifampin, clindamycin, or vancomycin) may improve survival.

Nasal congestion, rhinorrhea, and sore throat, infrequently seen in this series, might help to distinguish influenza-like illness from inhalational anthrax. Newer diagnostic methods for B. anthracis include polymerase chain reaction (PCR), immunohistochemistry, and sensitive serologic tests. Optimal management, including combination antimicrobial regimens, as well as adjunctive therapies (e.g., immunoglobulin antitoxin and corticosteroids), remains to be defined.

Cutaneous anthrax is characterized by a skin lesion evolving from a papule, through a vesicular stage, to a depressed black eschar, often surrounded by significant edema and erythema (Fig. 138.1). The lesion, which may mimic a spider bite, usually is painless and located on exposed parts of the body such as

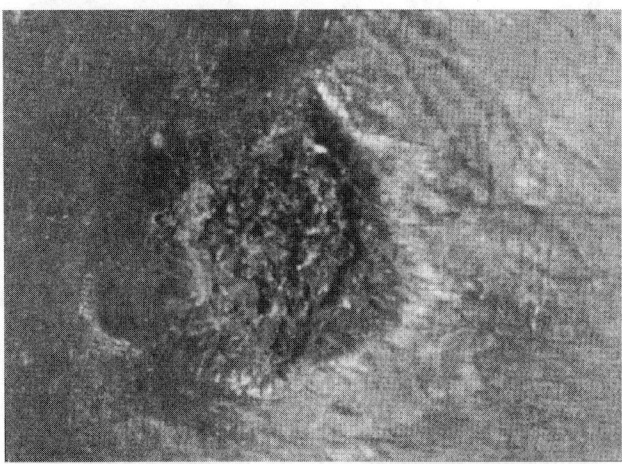

FIGURE 138.1. Cutaneous anthrax-eschar lesion. Public Health Image Library, CDC.

the face, neck, and arms. The incubation period ranges from 1 to 12 days but often is less than 7 days. Fatalities seldom occur (less than 1%) with the administration of effective antimicrobial therapy. Cutaneous anthrax occurred in a 7-month old infant who was exposed at his mother's workplace as a result of the 2001 attack. This infant displayed severe microangiopathic hemolytic anemia with renal involvement, coagulopathy, and hyponatremia, unusual findings with cutaneous anthrax.

The organism grows readily on sheep blood agar, forming rough, gray-white colonies of 4 to 5 mm, with characteristic comma-shaped or "comet-tail" protrusions. B. anthracis is differentiated from other Bacillus species by an absence of the following: hemolysis, motility, growth on phenylethyl alcohol blood agar, gelatin hydrolysis, and salicin fermentation. Biosafety level 2 conditions for safe specimen processing in the microbiology laboratory and prompt confirmation of suspected isolates at the Centers for Disease Control and Prevention (CDC) or the United States Army Medical Research Institute of Infectious Diseases (USAMRIID) in Fort Detrick, MD are warranted.

Postexposure vaccination with an inactivated, cell-free anthrax vaccine may be indicated, along with ciprofloxacin, doxycycline, or amoxicillin chemoprophylaxis, after a proven biologic event has occurred. Preexposure vaccination may be indicated for the military and other select populations or for groups for which a calculable risk can be assessed.

Smallpox

After a worldwide eradication program was initiated, the last known endemic case of smallpox occurred in Somalia in 1977, and the World Health Organization (WHO) declared smallpox eradicated in 1980. No animal reservoir exists. Current recognized stocks of variola virus are authorized to exist only at the CDC in Atlanta and a Russian state laboratory in Koltsovo. However, evidence indicates that additional variola isolates, either long-held unreported or acquired through security breaches, also may exist. Because vaccination against smallpox ceased in the United States in 1972, virtually the entire population now may be considered susceptible, as immunity wanes over the course of time. Release of an aerosol would be the most likely route of transmission during an act of bioterrorism. Any confirmed case of smallpox represents an international emergency and must be reported to national authorities through local and state health departments.

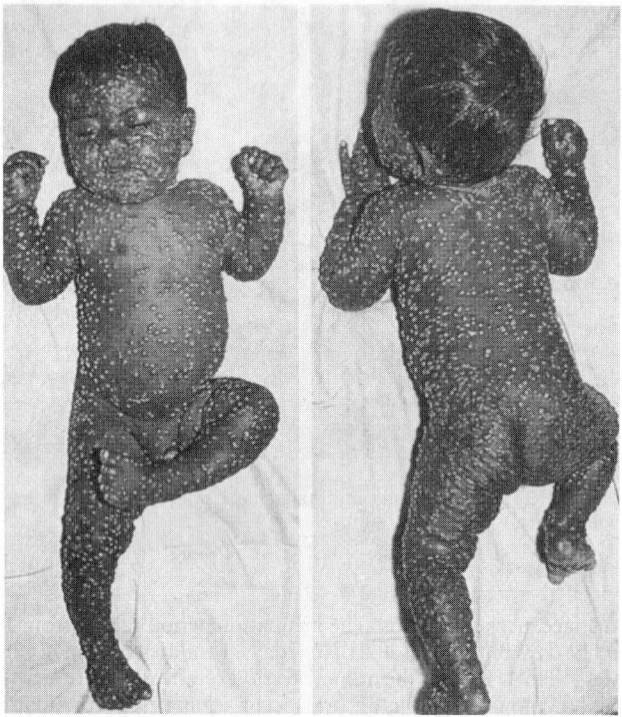

FIGURE 138.2. The lesions of smallpox are at the same stage of development on each area of the body, are deeply embedded in the skin, and are more densely concentrated on the face and extremities. (Reprinted with permission from Henderson DA. Smallpox: clinical and epidemiologic features. *Emerg Infect Dis* 1999;5:537.)

Smallpox is transmitted by respiratory secretions, requiring close person-to-person contact. The incubation period generally is 12 to 14 days, with a range of 7 to 17 days. Prodromal illness of classic variola major features acute onset of malaise, fever, rigors, vomiting, headache, and backache. Two to 3 days later, a discrete rash appears on the face, hands, forearms, and mucous membranes, spreading to the legs and then centrally to the trunk during the second week of illness (Fig. 138.2). Lesions progress from macules to papules to pustular vesicles over the course of 4 to 7 days. Umbilicate scabs form 8 to 14 days after onset, leaving depressions and depigmented scars.

In contrast to varicella (chickenpox), the rash of smallpox is centrifugal, with a concentration of lesions on the face and extremities, including palms and soles, compared to the trunk. Smallpox lesions also are synchronous in stage of development, whereas lesions of chickenpox appear in crops every few days, resulting in lesions at very different stages of maturation in different areas of skin.

Historically, the mortality rate for smallpox was 30% for unvaccinated contacts, and currently no antiviral therapy of proven efficacy exists. Supplies of vaccinia vaccine and vaccinia immune globulin are available only through the CDC. Mandatory smallpox vaccination was initiated in December 2002 for select members of the U.S. armed forces and personnel who serve in high-risk areas of the world. Smallpox vaccination was administered on a voluntary basis to U.S. Public Health response and health care teams beginning in January 2003. Postexposure vaccination and strict quarantine are indicated for all household and other face-to-face contacts of suspected smallpox cases.

In a limited outbreak with few cases, hospitalized patients should receive care in negative pressure rooms with high-efficiency particulate air filtration. Precautions using gloves, gowns, and masks also are indicated. Home isolation and care is appropriate for most patients in larger outbreaks.

Plague

Plague, a zoonotic illness caused by the gram-negative bacillus *Yersinia pestis*, primarily is a disease of rodents, with transmission occurring through infected fleas. Human disease is acquired through rodent flea vectors as well as respiratory droplets from animals to humans and humans to humans. Transmission of plague to humans in the United States occurs primarily via the bites of fleas from infected rodents. From 1970 to 1995, 341 cases of human plague were reported in the United States, most commonly from Arizona, California, Colorado, and New Mexico. Indications of a deliberate release of plague bacilli would include the occurrence of cases in locations not known to have enzootic infection, in persons without known risk factors, and in the absence of prior rodent deaths.

The three clinical forms of human plague are bubonic, primary septicemic, and pneumonic. Bubonic plague, characterized by the development of an acute regional lymphadenopathy, is the most frequent clinical form, accounting for 80% to 90% of U.S. cases. However, the pneumonic form would be the most likely presentation as a result of an aerosol release during a biologic attack. This clinical form is the least common, but it has the highest mortality rates; it is almost always fatal if antibiotics are not begun within 24 hours of onset of symptoms. Septicemic plague without obvious lymphadenopathy may be more difficult to diagnose than is bubonic plague because of its nonspecific manifestations (i.e., fever, chills, abdominal pain, nausea, vomiting, diarrhea, tachycardia, tachypnea, and hypotension). Delay in establishing diagnosis and initiating appropriate therapy may lead to death.

The incubation period for primary pneumonic plague is 1 to 3 days. Fever, chills, headache, and rapidly progressive weakness are characteristic of all clinical forms of plague. Cough, dyspnea, and hemoptysis are characteristic of primary pneumonic plague. The sudden appearance of a large number of previously healthy patients with fever, cough, shortness of breath, chest pain, and a fulminant course leading to death should suggest immediately the possibility of pneumonic plague or inhalational anthrax. The presence of hemoptysis would strongly suggest plague. *Y. pestis* may be identified in clinical specimens by Gram, Wright-Giemsa, Wayson, and immunofluorescent staining methods, in addition to standard bacterial cultures. Appropriate clinical specimens include lymph node aspirates and blood, as well as tracheal washes or sputum smears, if pneumonic plague is suspected. Tests used to confirm a suspected diagnosis, including antigen detection, IgM enzyme immunoassay, and PCR, are available only through state health departments, the CDC, and military laboratories.

Effective therapy is available in the form of streptomycin, gentamicin, chloramphenicol, doxycycline, and ciprofloxacin. Parenteral aminoglycoside therapy is recommended in a contained casualty (modest number of patients requiring treatment) setting; oral therapy is recommended in a mass casualty scenario. The potential benefits of administering doxycycline and ciprofloxacin in the treatment of pneumonic plague infection in children substantially outweigh the risks. An inactivated, whole-cell *Y. pestis* vaccine was discontinued by its manufacturers in 1999, and it no longer is available.

In addition to standard precautions, droplet precautions are indicated for all patients with suspected plague until pneumonia is excluded and appropriate therapy has been initiated. Droplet precautions should be continued in patients with confirmed pneumonic plague for 48 hours after the initiation of appropriate therapy. Only standard precautions are recommended for bubonic plague.

Tularemia

The etiologic agent of tularemia, a zoonotic illness, is *Francisella tularensis*, a gram-negative coccobacillus. The disease may be acquired from ticks and deer flies, contact with animals such as rabbits and rodents, ingestion of contaminated water, or inhalation of aerosols. In a bioterrorist event, inhalation of an aerosol would be the most likely route of infection. Human-to-human transmission of tularemia never has been reported. The annual incidence of tularemia in the United States is less than 200 cases; all suspected or confirmed cases must be reported to health authorities.

Clinical forms of the disease include ulceroglandular, glandular, oculoglandular, oropharyngeal, pneumonic, and typhoidal, reflecting the organism's portal of entry. Either pneumonic alone or typhoidal, with or without a pneumonic component, is the most likely clinical presentations of tularemia as a result of an aerosol release during a biologic attack. The incubation period for tularemia is 3 to 6 days, with a range 1 to 21 days. Typhoidal tularemia may present as fever of unknown origin. Standard precautions are indicated for hospitalized patients with all forms of tularemia.

Diagnosis usually is established by serological testing, and isolation of *F. tularensis* from clinical specimens requires cysteine-enriched media or inoculation of laboratory mice. In addition to requiring special media, the laboratory always should be informed when tularemia is suspected because of the potential hazard that exists to laboratory personnel. Suspected isolates should be confirmed by the CDC or USAMRIID through local or state health departments.

Effective therapy includes streptomycin, gentamicin, tetracycline, ciprofloxacin, or chloramphenicol; administration of postexposure prophylaxis with doxycycline or ciprofloxacin may be considered. The benefits of tetracycline or ciprofloxacin therapy may outweigh risks for children younger than 8 years of age in select clinical situations, including tularemia. A live-attenuated vaccine for preexposure use is available through USAMRIID.

Botulism

Seven distinct but related neurotoxins, A through G, are produced by different strains of *Clostridium botulinum*, an anaerobic gram-positive rod. The most common types in U.S. foodborne outbreaks are A, B, and E; outbreaks with unusual botulinum toxin types (i.e., C, D, F, and G, or E not acquired from an aquatic food) suggest a deliberate release. Classic neuroparalytic disease is acquired through the ingestion of preformed neurotoxin. Other forms include localized infection (wound botulism) and *C. botulinum* intestinal colonization in infants with *in vivo* toxin production (infant botulism). Botulism in the United States usually occurs in small clusters or single cases associated with home-canned foods. Although airborne transmission of botulinum neurotoxin does not occur naturally, aerosolization of preformed toxin would be the most likely route of transmission in a bioterrorism event. Sabotage of food supplies also could occur. Botulism is not transmitted from human to human; standard precautions are recommended for hospitalized patients.

The incubation period for foodborne botulism generally is 12 to 36 hours (range, 6 hours to 8 days). Clinical manifestations of disease acquired by inhalation are the same as those for foodborne botulism. Early manifestations include blurred vision, diplopia, and dry mouth. Patients are afebrile with a clear sensorium.

Later clinical features indicative of more severe disease include dysphonia, dysarthria, dysphagia, ptosis, and symmetrical, descending, progressive muscular weakness, with respiratory failure. Clinical suspicion is critical because a recognized source of exposure may be absent in a biologic attack. Botulism is a reportable disease.

A toxin-neutralization bioassay in mice is used to identify botulinum toxin in serum, stool, or food. *C. botulinum* also may be cultured from stool and food. Electromyography can be helpful diagnostically. Botulinum antitoxin of equine origin, available from CDC and state or municipal health departments, should be administered as soon as possible to patients who are symptomatic with botulism after testing for hypersensitivity to equine sera. A pentavalent toxoid of *C. botulinum* toxin types A, B, C, D, and E is available as a vaccine under investigational drug status through the CDC or Department of Defense.

Viral Hemorrhagic Fever

The term viral hemorrhagic fever (VHF) refers to a clinical illness associated with fever and a bleeding diathesis caused by a virus belonging to one of four distinct families: Filoviridae (e.g., Ebola and Marburg), Arenaviridae (e.g., Lassa fever), Bunyaviridae (e.g., Rift Valley fever), and Flaviviridae (e.g., yellow fever). VHF agents are RNA viruses normally transmitted to humans from animal reservoirs or arthropod vectors, although the natural reservoirs and vectors of the Ebola and Marburg agents are unknown. Most of these viruses are considered serious, potential biologic agents because of their potential to be aerosolized and their very high morbidity and/or mortality rates. Clinical features vary with the specific virus, but all are capable of causing fever, myalgia, prostration, petechiae, hemorrhage, and shock.

Treatment generally is supportive, although ribavirin has some *in vitro* and *in vivo* activity against arenaviruses and bunyaviruses but not against filoviruses or flaviviruses. VHF-specific barrier precautions, as well as airborne precautions, are recommended for any patient with suspected or documented VHF. Effective prophylaxis for post-exposure to a VHF agent is not available.

Suggested Readings

Arnon SS, Shechter R, Inglesby TV, et al. Botulinum toxin as a biologic weapon. Medical and public health management. *JAMA* 2001;285:1059.
Bartlett JG, Ingelsby TV, Borio L. Management of anthrax. *Clin Infect Dis* 2002;35:851.
Bartlett JG, Borio L, Radonovich L, et al. Smallpox vaccination in 2003: key information for clinicians. *Clin Infect Dis* 2003;36:883.
Borio L, Inglesby T, Peters CJ, et al. Hemorrhagic fever viruses as biologic weapons. Medical and public health management. *JAMA* 2002;287:2391.
Breman JG, Henderson DA. Diagnosis and management of smallpox. *N Engl J Med* 2002;346:1300.
Freedman A, Afonja O, Chang MW, et al. Cutaneous anthrax associated with microangiopathic hemolytic anemia and coagulopathy in a seven-month-old infant. *JAMA* 2002;287:869.
Dennis DT, Inglesby TV, Henderson DA, et al. Tularemia as a biologic weapon. Medical and public health management. *JAMA* 2001;285:2763.
Henderson DA, Ingelsby TV, Bartlett JG, et al. Smallpox as a biologic weapon. Medical and public health management. *JAMA* 1999;281:2127.
Inglesby TV, O'Toole T, Henderson DA, et al. Anthrax as a biologic weapon, 2002. Updated recommendations for management. *JAMA* 2002;287:2236.
Inglesby TV, Dennis DT, Henderson DA, et al. Plague as a biologic weapon. Medical and public health management. *JAMA* 2000;283:2281.
Jernigan JA, Stephens DS, Ashford DA, et al. Bioterrorism-related inhalational anthrax: The first 10 cases reported in the United States. *Emerg Infect Dis* 2001;7:933.
Patt HA, Feigin RD. Diagnosis and Management of suspected cases of bioterrorism: a pediatric perspective. *Pediatrics* 2002;109:685.

CHAPTER 139 ■ PEDIATRIC HUMAN IMMUNODEFICIENCY VIRUS INFECTION

EDINA H. MOYLETT AND WILLIAM T. SHEARER

As we journey into the twenty-first century, human immunodeficiency virus (HIV) remains a rapidly expanding modern-day plague. According to the World Health Organization (WHO), at least 42 million people are infected with HIV worldwide, 3.2 million of whom are children younger than 15 years old; 14,000 new infections occur daily, 2,000 of which are in children younger than 15 years of age. Best current projections suggest that an additional 45 million people will become infected with HIV by the year 2010, unless the world succeeds in mounting a drastically expanded global prevention effort.

For those living in most of the developed world, the future for HIV/AIDS (acquired immune deficiency syndrome) is not so bleak. The epidemic of HIV infection among children has changed substantially during recent years, with declining numbers of newly HIV-infected infants coincident with the widespread and effective implementation of recommended antiretroviral therapy to reduce perinatal transmission. In addition, the availability and implementation of highly active antiretroviral therapy (HAART) for use during pregnancy, as well as initial therapy in infected infants and children, have had the effect of further reducing the incidence of transmission and greatly improving the quality of life for HIV-infected individuals. Improved use of prophylaxis for opportunistic infections (OIs) has had an additive effect and further increased the numbers of HIV-infected children surviving into teenage years and beyond.

Despite these advances in the care of individuals with HIV, in excess of 10,000 children are living with HIV infection in the United States, with an estimated annual death rate of at least 100. Despite best efforts at preventing *in utero* transmission, newly infected infants continue to contribute to the numbers of children who require care for HIV. Adolescents are an emerging at-risk group: 20,000 new cases of HIV infection were reported among individuals 13 to 25 years old in the United States in 2003. With the significant immigrant population in U.S. cities, coupled with these statistics, anyone practicing pediatric medicine today must be familiar with key elements of pediatric HIV infection. Therefore, the purpose of this chapter is to review the fundamental aspects of this largely preventable infectious disease.

EPIDEMIOLOGY

The first cases of pediatric HIV infection were reported in November 1982, approximately 1 year after the first cases in adult patients were reported. In the early 1990s, at the peak of the AIDS epidemic, as many as 30% of pregnant women in the United States transmitted HIV to their newborn infants. This mode of acquisition of HIV accounted for close to 90% of the cases of pediatric HIV infection; the remaining cases were ascribed to the receipt of blood or blood products, sexual abuse, and rarely accidental exposure (e.g., contaminated-needle stick injury). Currently, in the United States and the rest of the developed world, the figures for maternal–fetal transmission have dropped significantly, to less than 2%, thanks primarily to the implementation of potent intrapartum chemoprophylaxis and advances in obstetric care. However, as of the end of 2001, the Centers for Disease Control and Prevention (CDC) National Center for HIV/STD and Tuberculosis Prevention, Division of HIV/AIDS Prevention, reported that almost 86,000 U.S. women of childbearing age (15 to 44 years) are living with HIV/AIDS.

In developing countries, principally sub-Saharan Africa, the story is in stark contrast. Seroprevalence rates of HIV infection among pregnant women are documented to be as high as 40%, and maternofetal transmission rates range from 25% to 40%. Breast-feeding increases the risk of transmission by approximately 15%. As of the end of 2002, figures from The Joint United Nations Programme on HIV/AIDS (UNAIDS) and WHO reported that an estimated .5 million children younger than 15 years of age died as a result of HIV infection, and approximately 2.8 million children were infected with the virus.

In other parts of the world, across all social divides, the HIV epidemic only now is beginning to have a significant impact on the social structure. At the end of 2002, in the Asia-Pacific region, which is home to 60% of the world's population, 7 million infections already have been recorded, with 1 million new infections reported in the year 2002. According to the United Nations, China can expect to have 10 million cases by 2010, and in India the number of carriers is expected to skyrocket from 4 million to between 20 and 25 million by 2010. Without significant education and assistance from international organizations, the numbers of children born with HIV infection, as well as orphaned by this modern-day plague, will continue on an upward trajectory.

After a plethora of reports in the early to mid-1980s of the development of acquired immunodeficiency syndrome (AIDS) in patients who had received blood products (including clotting factors, blood, and blood products), these blood products were recognized as being sources of the transmission of HIV infection. Since the implementation of universal screening of blood and blood products for antibodies against HIV in 1985, the incidence of acquired HIV infection after receiving blood products has been decreasing from accounting for as many as 20% of pediatric cases in the 1980s to less than 1% today. Additionally, the application of recombinant technology to the production of human blood factors (e.g., factor VIII) has eliminated transmissible disease risk.

PATHOGENESIS

HIV-1, a cytopathic RNA virus in the Retroviridae family, consists of a virion measuring 100 to 150 nm in diameter housing an electron-dense cylindrical core surrounded by a lipid envelope (Fig. 139.1). The envelope, acquired as the virus buds from the host cell, consists of a lipid bilayer containing the

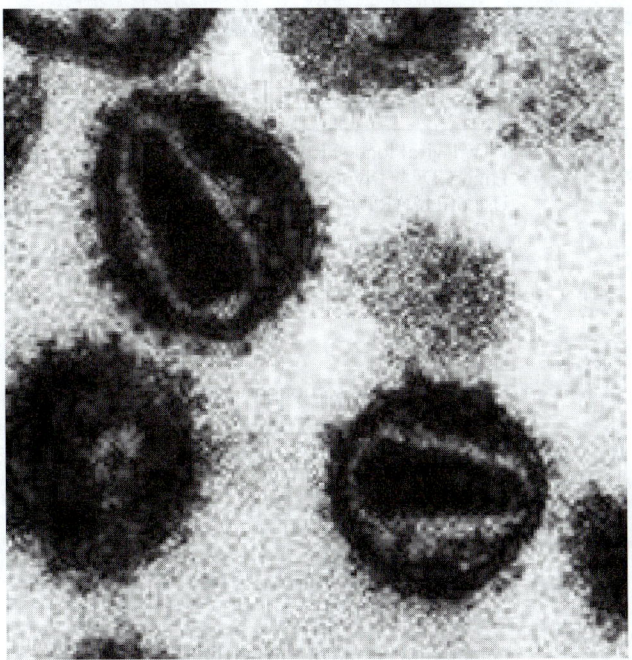

FIGURE 139.1. Human immunodeficiency virus. High-power electron microscopy view of human immunodeficiency virus particles. Note visible central core and envelope glycoproteins (gp120).

BOX 139.1	Pathogenesis of HIV

More than 90% of primary HIV infections involve M-tropic (R5, utilizes CCR5) strains, which readily infect macrophages and monocytes *in vitro*. M-tropic virus typically is non-syncytium inducing. An initial docking step with CD4+ triggers an HIV-envelope conformational change to enable gp120 to bind to CCR5 and initiate viral gp41-mediated virus-cell fusion. The virus replicates efficiently in CD4+/CCR5+-bearing cell types, macrophages, monocytes, and T-cells of lymph nodes, producing some billions of virions per day throughout the typical 10-year and longer course of infection. Most patients infected with subtype (or clade) B HIV strains (the predominant strains in the United States and Europe) experience a mutational transition in their HIV envelope gene, which alters the cell tropism to permit CXCR4 utilization (X4- or T-cell-tropic preference), so that the mutated virus can replicate in CXCR4-bearing cells, including immortalized T-cell lines *in vitro*. These isolates are encountered more frequently in late-stage disease and are syncytium-inducing. The switch in viral phenotype from R5 to X4 is associated with decline in the number of CD4+ T-cells and rapid progression of disease.

---

surface (gp120) and transmembrane (gp41) major envelope proteins, in addition to selected host cell-membrane proteins. The viral core, composed of capsid (p24), matrix (p17), and nucleocapsid (p7) structural proteins, contains two copies of single-stranded viral genomic RNA and several virally encoded enzymes (reverse transcriptase, protease, and integrase).

HIV-1 is characterized by its ability to replicate rapidly and mutate within its host. Although an individual may be infected with a predominant strain, as replication ensues, numerous viral variants, also known as *quasispecies*, are generated.

One of the major milestones in HIV research has been the discovery that chemokine receptors, primarily CCR5 and CXCR4, serve as co-receptors (along with the T-cell recognition molecule CD4+) and allow HIV infection to occur. Additional information about this process is presented in Box 139.1.

Consequent to the discovery of HIV-1 co-receptors was the discovery that polymorphisms of certain chemokines and chemokine receptors may modify the transmission of HIV-1 and progression of disease. The 32-bp deletion in the coding region of the CCR5 gene impedes cellular expression of the HIV-1 co-receptor and provides a strong, but not absolute, resistance to M-tropic viral infection in adults. However, unlike in adults, CCR5 delta-32 homozygosity in children has not been associated thus far with reduced infectivity (vertical transmission); additionally, the heterozygous genotype in children born to HIV-1-seropositive mothers does not confer resistance to infection, but it substantially slows the development of HIV-related disease. Unlike newly infected adult patients, newly infected pediatric patients experience a steep increase in HIV RNA within weeks after birth, followed by a very slow decline in RNA level for several years.

Distinct patterns of disease progression are encountered among perinatally infected infants, those with rapidly progressive disease or "rapid progressors," and conversely "nonprogressors" or "long-term survivors." Independent of HAART, some infants are noted to be rapid progressors, whereas others maintain immunologic control of their infection with years (more than 5) of slow decline before the development of AIDS. This phenomenon is not well explained; it is likely that multiple factors, including the aforementioned chemokine polymorphisms, genetically determined functional and structural defects in HIV-1 genes (e.g. *nef*), as well as a more robust production of HIV antibody and HIV-specific cytotoxic T-lymphocyte (CTL), are at play. Slow progressors constitute approximately 70% to 80% of all HIV-infected children, who have 5- and 6.5-year survival rates of 71% and 68%, respectively.

Transmission

The principal mode of transmission of HIV infection among children 15 years of age and younger is maternal-infant transmission, also known as *vertical transmission*. This mode may occur during pregnancy, immediately prior to birth, or during delivery.

Pregnancy

Current evidence suggests that most maternal-infant transmission of HIV occurs late in pregnancy or during labor and delivery. In a recent Thai study that examined the timing of vertical transmission of HIV among 218 HIV-positive mothers who gave birth to live infants, the overall transmission rate was 22.5%; 5.5% of infections were attributed to *in utero* transmission as defined by a positive HIV DNA polymerase chain reaction (PCR) at an age of less than 72 hours, and 75.5% of infections were acquired peripartum, as defined by a negative result at birth and a later sample that was HIV-1 positive.

Many risk factors have been identified that increase viral transmission from mother to infant (Table 139.1). Maternal plasma HIV viral load appears to be the best predictor of vertical transmission. Little or no transmission occurs with plasma viral loads of fewer than 1,000 copies/mL regardless of use of zidovudine (ZDV) (also known as azidothymidine [AZT]). Transmission rates between 20% and 60% have been reported

TABLE 139.1

FACTORS ASSOCIATED WITH RISK OF PERINATAL HIV TRANSMISSION

Maternal	Increased Risk	Decreased Risk
Ante-partum	HIV-1 viral load >1,000 copies/mL	HIV-1 viral load <1,000 copies/mL
	Low CD4$^+$ T-lymphocyte count	High CD4$^+$ T-lymphocyte count
	Vitamin A deficiency	Use of HAART
	Malnutrition	
	Illicit drug use	
	Cigarette smoking	
	Chorionic villus sampling	
	Amniocentesis	
Intra-partum	High maternal cervicovaginal HIV-1 levels	Use of HAART
	Ruptured membranes >4 hours	Elective cesarean section prior to ROM
	Premature delivery	
	Fetal scalp electrode use	
	Active genital ulcer disease	
	Vaginal laceration	
	Chorioamnionitis	
	Episiotomy	
Post-partum	Breast-feeding	
	Mastitis with breast-feeding	
Fetal/Neonatal		
	Birth weight <2,500 g	Enhanced β chemokine expression
	Presenting infant of multiple birth	CCR5 homozygous mutation*
		ART post-partum

HAART, highly active antiretroviral therapy; ROM, rupture of membranes.
*Modifies disease progression.

with plasma viral loads ranging from fewer than 100,000 to more than 100,000 copies/mL, respectively. Although the maternal viral load at delivery is very useful for determining the risk of transmission, no level exists above which transmission always occurs nor is there a level below which transmission is never encountered.

The levels of HIV in the maternal genital tract secretions may affect vertical transmission. Antiretroviral therapy (ART) has been shown to decrease HIV RNA levels in cervicovaginal lavage and reduce vertical transmission. Results from the Women–Infant Transmission Study (WITS) in relation to obstetric factors and vertical transmission identified that rupture of membranes 4 hours or more prior to delivery almost doubled the risk (odds ratio, 1.82) for transmission of infection to the infant. Additional factors independently associated with increased transmission were illicit drug use during pregnancy, low antenatal CD4$^+$ lymphocyte count, and a birth weight of less than 2,500 g. Low CD4$^+$ lymphocyte counts and low infant birth weight presumably reflect more advanced maternal disease status and an overall greater risk for transmission of the virus. Additionally, HIV-specific cytotoxic T-lymphocytes are thought to play an important role in the control of HIV replication, thereby slowing disease progression. Low infant birth weight also has been associated with a greater likelihood of *in utero* transmission occurring.

The role of the placenta in supporting or preventing the vertical transmission of HIV is unclear. *In vitro* studies indicate that placental trophoblasts actually are infected by HIV-1, mediated by a process that does not utilize those co-receptors normally facilitated for entry of virus (CD4/chemokine receptors). Infection appears to be mediated by the up-regulation of adhesion molecules. In addition, infected T-cell blasts transfer the infection more efficiently than does free virus. Infected placental cells possibly in turn pass the virus to fetal T-lymphocytes in a similar manner, employing integrins and adhesion molecules. These findings would support the increase in the incidence of transmission of HIV in the presence of chorioamnionitis as well as high maternal viral load.

Postpartum and Beyond

Mothers can transmit HIV infection to their offspring in the postnatal period via breast milk. Breast-feeding approximately doubles the risk of vertical transmission, which may occur at any time during the breast-feeding period. In a study from South Africa, which examined vertical transmission in association with breast-feeding, the highest overall rate of vertical transmission occurred in exclusively breast-fed children (39%), with the lowest rate being in infants who never had been breast-fed (24%). Mixed feeding has been shown to further increase the risk for breast milk-related transmission of HIV, possibly because mixed feedings allow both exposure to HIV and increased risk of gastrointestinal infections and the consequent disruption of mucosal integrity. In addition, the risk of HIV transmission from breast-feeding has been estimated to be almost twice as high among women who acquire HIV after birth. HIV viral loads in breast milk correlate with plasma viral loads and reach their peak during and just after seroconversion occurs. More advanced and symptomatic maternal disease, as well as mastitis, have been associated with an increased risk for HIV transmission.

However, the role of breast milk in the transmission of HIV remains somewhat controversial. In developed nations, HIV-infected mothers no longer administer breast milk to their infants, given the increased risk of postpartum transmission. This practice is not feasible in resource-poor countries. Given the unfavorable financial situations, in addition to suboptimal sanitation, in many parts of third-world nations, breast milk often is the sole form of nutrition for newborn infants, especially in their first 3 months of life.

Blood Products

Fortunately, the stringent testing of blood donors has decreased the risk of transfusion-acquired HIV infection significantly.

Blood donations in the United States have been screened for antibody to HIV-1 since March 1985, and for type 2 (HIV-2) since June 1992. Prior to screening for the presence of HIV-1 p24 antigen, an estimated one in 450,000 to 660,000 donations per year were deemed infectious for HIV. With current testing methodology, the risk of acquiring HIV infection through blood products is approximately 1 per 1,000,000 units transfused.

Sexual Contact

At present, sexually transmitted HIV infection remains a significant risk for adolescents and young adults who engage in high-risk behaviors. In day-to-day practice, pediatricians must be aware of *acute HIV syndrome* as a differential diagnosis for an unexplained febrile illness in adolescents and young adults.

DIAGNOSIS

The diagnosis of HIV infection differs in pediatric and adult populations. The transplacental transfer of maternal antibody of the IgG class necessitates performing viral-based confirmatory tests for making early pediatric diagnoses in neonates and infants up to 18 months of age. Thereafter, HIV enzyme-linked immunoabsorbent assay (ELISA) is the standard test, as in adult practice. An early establishment of the diagnosis of neonatal HIV infection is instrumental in the initiation of early and effective antiretroviral therapy that results in improved clinical outcomes.

Currently, of the diagnostic viral-based assays available, HIV DNA PCR is utilized most frequently for infant diagnostic purposes. Qualitative DNA PCR is used to detect cell-associated proviral DNA. Isolation of the virus by peripheral blood lymphocyte co-culture is the gold standard for HIV infection diagnosis; however, high cost and intensive labor requirements limit its use. Culture techniques may be falsely negative in the presence of HAART. Although quantitative plasma RNA PCR assays are available as an alternative for infant diagnostics, care should be exercised when results are in the low quantitative range, given the risk of false-positive results. In the absence of breast-feeding, utilizing viral-based assays, HIV-infected infants can be diagnosed accurately by the time they are 3 to 6 months of age and in some cases as young as 6 weeks old.

The diagnosis of HIV infection after 18 months of age is based primarily on serologic testing. The Western blot (WB) assay (HIV viral proteins of different molecular weights transferred to a polyacrylamide gel) has greater specificity and sensitivity than does the enzyme immunoassay, but it is more labor-intensive. The results of a WB assay are interpreted as follows: negative, absence of all bands; positive, presence of detectable antibodies to at least two of the following three proteins; the core protein (p24) and two envelope proteins (gp41, gp120/160) *or* three or more bands with one band from each *gag, pol,* and *env; or* bands for either p24 or p31 *and* gp41 or gp120/160; indeterminate, one of the three major bands. An indeterminate result should be repeated; if it persists, a viral-based test should be performed. Detection of a band to p24 antigen commonly is associated with an indeterminate result. Following HIV infection, antibody to p24 antigen typically is the first to develop; results should be positive within 2 to 3 months. Advanced HIV disease or agammaglobulinemia may result in false-negative serology; in such instances, viral-based assays should be used.

The recommended tests used to check for the presence of HIV infection in neonates and infants follow:

- Viral-based tests ideally should be performed at birth, between 1 and 2 months of age, and again between 3 and 6 months of age. Acceptable diagnostic viral-based tests include HIV DNA PCR/HIV RNA PCR/HIV lymphocyte co-culture; two of the same tests or any combination of the three tests is acceptable; HIV DNA PCR and HIV co-culture currently are preferred in neonates.
- HIV-specific antibody tests (EIA/WB) are performed at birth and again at 6, 12, and 18 months of age until loss of maternal antibodies is documented.

Recommended guidelines for the diagnosis of HIV infection in neonates and infants follow:

- HIV infection is confirmed if two consecutive viral-based tests are positive. A positive test should be confirmed with a repeat test on a new specimen as soon as possible.
- In the absence of breast-feeding, a perinatally exposed infant is deemed not HIV-infected if viral-based tests are negative up to and including 4 months of age.
- Beyond the neonatal period, in the absence of hypogammaglobulinemia or clinical evidence of HIV disease, HIV infection can be *reliably excluded* if two or more HIV-specific IgG antibody tests performed after the infant reaches 6 months of age, with an interval of at least 1 month between tests, are negative.
- After the infant reaches 18 months of age, HIV infection *is ruled out* with negative HIV IgG serology, absence of clinical disease, and hypogammaglobulinemia and previously negative viral-based tests.

CLINICAL MANIFESTATIONS AND COMPLICATIONS

For the most part, infected newborns are asymptomatic, without evidence of HIV acquisition. Infrequently, infection acquired *in utero* may manifest in a manner similar to that of other congenitally acquired viral infections, with resultant growth retardation, skin rash, lymphadenopathy, hepatosplenomegaly, and cytopenias. Pediatric HIV disease occurs primarily as a result of maternofetal transmission, and, therefore, the acute viral syndrome encountered in adult patients rarely is appreciated, with the exception of adolescent-age patients practicing high-risk behavior.

Advances in the management of pediatric HIV infection are reflected by the trend in incidence of opportunistic and other infectious complications. During the second decade of the pediatric HIV epidemic, a dramatic decrease has occurred in the frequency of OIs, as reported to the CDC. Advances accountable for this favorable change include the implementation of guidelines to prevent perinatal transmission, development of guidelines and initiation of therapy to prevent OIs, and, finally, an expansion in ART with the formulation of highly active medications suitable for pediatric administration.

Important differences exist between HIV-related clinical entities in adults and those in children:

- Prior to the advent of HAART, children had more rapid disease progression.
  Pneumocystis jiroveci injection (causing *pneumocystis* pneumonia PCP) and encephalopathy occur early in rapid progressors. Children have a higher prevalence of bacteremia and lymphocytic interstitial pneumonitis (LIP).
- However, Kaposi sarcoma, toxoplasmosis, cryptococcosis, and cytomegalovirus (CMV) infection seldom are encountered.

Additionally, age-related changes in CD4+ T-lymphocyte counts exist, as outlined in Table 139.2.

TABLE 139.2

IMMUNOLOGIC CATEGORIES BASED ON AGE-SPECIFIC CD4+ T-LYMPHOCYTE COUNTS AND PERCENTAGE OF TOTAL LYMPHOCYTES

Immunologic Category	<12 Months		1–5 Years		6–12 Years	
	μL	%	μL	%	μL	%
No suppression	≥1,500	(≥25)	≥1,000	(≥25)	≥500	(≥25)
Moderate suppression	750–1,499	(15–24)	500–999	(15–24)	200–499	(15–24)
Severe suppression	<750	(<15)	<500	(<15)	<200	(<15)

Adapted with permission from Centers for Disease Control and Prevention: 1994 Revised classification system for human immunodeficiency virus infection in children less than 13 years of age. *MMWR* 1994;43:6.

To discuss all the OIs and clinical manifestations associated with HIV disease is beyond the scope of this chapter; therefore, only those encountered more frequently are discussed in the subsequent sections. Box 139.2 outlines the revised classification system for HIV infection in children younger than 13 years of age, as established by the CDC.

Recurrent Bacterial Infections

HIV infection results in the progressive dysfunction of cellular and humoral immunity. The polyclonal activation of B-lymphocytes results in the increased spontaneous production of immunoglobulin and measurable hypergammaglobulinemia.

BOX 139.2 — Clinical Staging of HIV Infection in Children Younger than 13 Years of Age

Category N. *Not symptomatic*

Children who have no signs or symptoms considered to be the result of HIV infection or only one of the conditions listed in Category A.

Category A. *Mildly symptomatic*

Children with two or more of the conditions listed below but none of the conditions listed in Categories B and C.

Lymphadenopathy (greater than or equal to 0.5 cm at more than two sites; bilateral, equal one site)
Hepatomegaly
Splenomegaly
Dermatitis
Parotitis

Category B. *Moderately symptomatic*

Children who have symptomatic conditions other than those listed for Category A or C that are attributed to HIV infection.

Anemia (less than 8 gm/dL), neutropenia (less than 1,000/mm³), or thrombocytopenia (100,000/mm³) for 30 days or longer
Bacterial meningitis, pneumonia, or sepsis (single episode)
Oropharyngeal candidiasis, persisting longer than 2 months in children older than 6 months
Cardiomyopathy
Cytomegalovirus infection, with onset before 1 month of age
Diarrhea, recurrent or chronic
Hepatitis
HSV stomatitis, recurrent (more than two episodes within 1 year)
HSV bronchitis, pneumonitis, or esophagitis with onset before 1 month of age
Herpes zoster (shingles) involving at least two distinct episodes or more than one dermatome
Leiomyosarcoma
LIP or pulmonary lymphoid hyperplasia
Nephropathy
Nocardiosis
Persistent fever (longer than 1 month)
Toxoplasmosis (onset younger than 1 month of age)
Disseminated varicella

Category C: *Severely symptomatic*

Serious bacterial infections, multiple or recurrent of the following types: septicemia, pneumonia, meningitis, bone or joint infection, or abscess of an internal organ or body cavity.
Candidiasis, esophageal or pulmonary
Coccidioidomycosis, at site other than or in addition to lungs or cervical or hilar lymph nodes
Cryptococcosis, extrapulmonary
Cryptosporidiosis or isosporiasis with diarrhea persisting longer than 1 month
Cytomegalovirus disease with onset of symptoms at age greater than 1 month (at a site other than liver, spleen, or lymph nodes)
Encephalopathy
HSV causing a mucocutaneous ulcer for longer than 1 month; or bronchitis, pneumonitis, or esophagitis for any duration affecting a child older than 1 month of age
Histoplasmosis, at a site other than or in addition to lungs or cervical or hilar lymph nodes
Kaposi sarcoma
Lymphoma
Mycobacterium tuberculosis, disseminated or extrapulmonary
MAC or *Mycobacterium kansasii*, disseminated (at site other than or in addition to lungs, skin, cervical or hilar lymph nodes)
Pneumocystis carinii pneumonia
Progressive multifocal leukoencephalopathy
Salmonella (nontyphoidal) septicemia, recurrent
Toxoplasmosis of the brain with onset at older than 1 month of age
Wasting syndrome in the absence of a concurrent illness other than HIV

Adapted with permission from Centers for Disease Control and Prevention: 1994 Revised classification system for human immunodeficiency virus infection in children less than 13 years of age. *MMWR* 1994;43:6.

HSV, herpes simplex virus; LIP, lymphoid interstitial pneumonia; MAC, mycobacterium avium complex.

Despite having high levels of circulating IgG, most patients have increased levels of poorly functioning antibody. Impaired neutrophil function, leukopenia, abnormal production of cytokine, and splenic dysfunction also contribute to increased susceptibility to bacterial pathogens.

Recurrent bacterial infections (defined as two or more bacteriologically documented, systemic bacterial infections—including septicemia or bacteremia, meningitis, pneumonia, osteomyelitis, septic arthritis, or abscesses of body cavity or internal organ—occurring within a 2-year period) are second only to PCP as AIDS-defining infections. Pneumonia and sepsis are among the most common presentations; the rate of infection is more significant for those with low CD4$^+$ counts, but not exclusively so, and infection may occur across the entire spectrum of CD4$^+$ counts. Typical pathogens mirror those as seen in immunologically intact children; the range of isolates can be predicted from the site of infection or the clinical infection syndrome. Early in the HIV epidemic, the most common offending pathogens were *Streptococcus pneumoniae*, *Salmonella* species, and *Haemophilus influenzae* type B (Hib). In the current era, *S. pneumoniae* predominates, with *Salmonella* species and other gram-negative rods evident in developing countries. *Pseudomonas aeruginosa* is a significant cause of bacteremia in advanced HIV disease.

Prophylaxis against bacterial infections should include administering vaccination with Hib and heptavalent pneumococcal (PCV7) (9-valent conjugate vaccine currently under investigation) conjugate vaccines during infancy at 2, 4, and 6 months, with a booster dose given when the child is 12 to 15 months of age. HIV-infected children 24 to 59 months of age are considered to have a high risk of having pneumococcal infection, and two doses of PCV7 are recommended (2 months apart), followed in 2 months by administration of the 23-valent pneumococcal vaccine (PCV23). For children who already have received PCV23, PCV7 can be used to prime their immunologic response, with two doses of PCV7 given at 2 or more months following the receipt of PCV23. In the pre-HAART era, the monthly administration of intravenous immunoglobulin (IVIG) was proven to be efficacious in the prevention of recurrent bacterial infections, most notably for those patients with CD4$^+$ counts less than 200/μL. Trimethoprim-sulfamethoxazole has been shown to be as efficacious as IVIG. With the advent and success of HAART, many centers reserve the use of IVIG for patients with recurrent serious bacterial infections; however, its use is limited by the risks of transmitting of blood-borne pathogens, expense, inconvenience, and shortage.

Mycobacterium avium Complex

Mycobacterium avium complex (MAC) includes two closely related species, *Mycobacterium avium* and *Mycobacterium intracellulare*. As in adults, disseminated infection with MAC in pediatric patients is associated with a significant degree of immunosuppression (CD4$^+$ counts less than 50 cells/mm^3). However, the frequency of occurrence of disseminated MAC infection is less in children than in adults, possibly as a result of a lesser degree and duration of environmental exposure among pediatric patients. Both the gastrointestinal and respiratory tracts have been identified as portals for acquisition of the pathogen; the former is thought to be the most common site for colonization and subsequent dissemination.

Although the more characteristic manifestation of MAC infection among patients with AIDS is disseminated disease, localized manifestations may occur and include cervical adenitis, pneumonitis, skin lesions, and abscess formation. Presenting features typically are nonspecific and include fever, weight loss, fatigue, night sweats, diarrhea, and abdominal pain. Diagnosis is established by isolation of the organism from a sterile body site, most typically blood, bone marrow aspirate, or bone marrow core biopsy.

A major advance in the management of disseminated MAC has been the development of the newer macrolides, clarithromycin and azithromycin. Monotherapy for the treatment of disseminated disease, as with conventional mycobacterial tuberculosis therapy, results in the rapid development of resistance, inferring a need for combination therapy with two or more drugs. Recommended first-line agents include clarithromycin or azithromycin in combination with ethambutol and or rifabutin. Additional agents may be indicated depending on the severity of the disease and the results of drug-susceptibility testing. Prophylaxis (azithromycin or clarithromycin) for preventing initial MAC infection should be offered to HIV-infected children with the following CD4$^+$ cell counts:

- 6 years of age or older, fewer than 50 cells/mm^3
- 2 to 6 years of age, fewer than 75 cells/mm^3
- 1 to 2 years of age, fewer than 500 cells/mm^3
- Younger than 12 months of age, fewer than 750 cells/mm^3

Fungal Infections

Pneumocystis Jiroveci

PCP (pneumocystis pneumonia) historically has been the hallmark OI of the pediatric AIDS epidemic. Approximately 2,700 cases were reported to the CDC through 1997, representing 33% of AIDS-defining conditions in children younger than 13 years of age; only 15 cases were reported in 1997. PCP is an infection of early infancy; most infants are infected when they are between 4 and 6 months of age. The risk of acquiring PCP in the first year of life for perinatally HIV-infected children who are not receiving prophylaxis is estimated at approximately 12%. The dramatic reduction in the number of new cases of PCP in HIV-infected children is a result of the routine prescription of prophylactic therapy. The initial guidelines, as published in 1991, included CD4$^+$ T-lymphocyte number as a determining feature; however, it soon became apparent that many infants developed PCP at much higher CD4$^+$ counts than did adults, and even if they were not known to be HIV-infected at the onset of PCP. These findings led to revisions in the guidelines, which now recommend that prophylaxis be given to all HIV-exposed infants, independent of CD4$^+$ counts and HIV infection status, starting at 4 to 6 weeks of age until they are 4 months old, at which time a definitive diagnosis of HIV infection can be made.

The classic tetrad of clinical features of PCP are tachypnea, dyspnea, cough, and fever. Onset typically is insidious. Physical findings usually are limited to fine crepitations, low-grade fever, and universal hypoxemia. Fiberoptic bronchoscopy with bronchoalveolar lavage (BAL) has been shown to be a safe and sensitive method for establishing the diagnosis of PCP. Success with induced sputum or tracheal aspirates for intubated patients depends on the experience of the practitioner. Open lung biopsy typically is reserved for children with inconclusive results from less invasive methods and worsening clinical status.

Therapy for PCP should include treatment with trimethoprim-sulfamethoxazole or pentamidine, intravenous steroids, and intensive respiratory support. Medications may be switched to the oral route when clinical improvement is sustained. Although no controlled trials have been conducted in pediatric patients, many investigators have reported anecdotally improved clinical outcome with the administration of adjunctive steroid therapy. Steroids typically are administered for 4 to 5 days and subsequently weaned over the course of antimicrobial therapy.

Children who should receive PCP prophylaxis include the following:

- All HIV-infected and indeterminate children from 4 weeks to 12 months of age (prophylaxis may be discontinued if HIV is excluded after more than 4 months of age)
- HIV-infected children
  - 1 to 5 years of age; CD4$^+$ cell count less than 500/μL, CD4$^+$ % less than 15
  - 6 to 12 years of age; CD4$^+$ cell count less than 200/μL, CD4$^+$ % less than 15
  - All HIV-infected children treated for PCP

Candidiasis

Severe oral candidiasis may be the first clinical indication of the presence of HIV infection in exposed infants. Invasive disease rarely is encountered among pediatric patients, but mucosal disease occurs frequently. Mucocutaneous candidiasis in HIV-infected patients resembles that seen in immunocompetent patients but is more extensive and persistent. Recurrent mucocutaneous candidiasis is problematic in patients with poorly controlled retroviral disease. Patients presenting with oropharyngeal candidiasis and concurrent dysphagia, odynophagia, or retrosternal pain may have developed more serious invasive disease, such as esophageal or tracheobronchial candidiasis. Coexisting herpes simplex virus (HSV) or CMV infection may be present, necessitating endoscopy and diagnostic biopsy. However, many clinicians reserve endoscopy for cases unresponsive to therapy. Treatment for oropharyngeal disease usually is limited to topical nystatin; systemic therapy with either fluconazole or itraconazole is reserved for more persistent disease, and esophageal or tracheobronchial disease mandates systemic therapy, either oral or intravenous depending on disease severity.

Viral Infections

Cytomegalovirus

The incidence and prevalence of CMV infection in pediatric practice is significantly less than that encountered in adult practice. Manifestations of CMV disease include chorioretinitis, esophagitis, colitis, pneumonitis, and disseminated disease. As in adult practice, these disease entities occur in children with very low CD4$^+$ cell counts. CMV retinitis typically occurs when the CD4$^+$ T-cell count decreases to less than 100×10^6/L. CMV viremia clearly either precedes or is coincident with end-organ disease. As a result, it is possible to monitor for disease activity (PCR for detection of DNA in plasma, detection of CMV antigen in blood buffy coat) in the highest-risk patients (CMV-seropositive with low CD4$^+$ cell counts).

Patients usually report floaters or blurred vision, depending on the extent of retinal involvement. Large lesions in the periphery may be asymptomatic, whereas smaller areas of retinitis in the macula or near the disc can produce dramatic visual dysfunction. The classic lesion is a hemorrhagic necrotizing retinitis that follows the retinal vasculature. Clusters of small white dots representing retinal infiltration may precede the leading edge of the lesion as it advances.

Once CMV disease is diagnosed, treatment is warranted; ganciclovir, valganciclovir, foscarnet, and cidofovir are the current antiviral drugs of choice. Unilateral CMV retinitis is at risk for spreading to the contralateral eye, necessitating the need for initiating systemic therapy. Prior to the advent of potent ART, patients with CMV retinitis could expect life-long suppressive therapy; however, maintenance therapy has been safely withdrawn from patients with prolonged immune recovery resulting from HAART. Despite the advances in antiviral therapy, poor compliance, active retroviral disease, and drug resistance remain significant problems, with disease relapses and serious risk of blindness.

Varicella Zoster

Aside from the increased morbidity that occurs in association with varicella zoster virus infection, this virus rarely is associated with increased mortality rates in pediatric patients with AIDS. Severe herpes zoster or shingles (disease affecting more than one dermatome) may be the presenting illness in some HIV-infected children. Recurrent episodes occur more frequently in those children who acquired their primary varicella in the setting of low CD4$^+$ counts. However, unlike some of the OIs, episodes of herpes zoster typically are not associated with CD4$^+$ lymphocytopenia.

Acyclovir therapy has been the mainstay of treatment for patients with varicella zoster infections, oral therapy often being the initial choice and parenteral therapy for those with severe disease. The advantages of valacyclovir, the oral prodrug of acyclovir, with its ability to produce acyclovir levels nearing those associated with parenteral therapy, have not been extended to the pediatric population because of the lack of a suitable oral formulation for younger children. Similarly, famciclovir, an oral agent with good activity against varicella-zoster virus, has had limited use in pediatric-age patients and is not in a suitable oral preparation at this time.

Lymphocytic Interstitial Pneumonitis

LIP originally was an AIDS-defining diagnosis in the 1987 CDC classification of AIDS in children. The revised classification reflected the recognition that children with LIP as a first AIDS-indicator disease had improved survival, compared with other AIDS-indicator diseases, and LIP has been redefined as a stage B disease indicator. In a prospective birth cohort of HIV-infected children, the cumulative incidence of LIP (nodular changes persisting for more than 6 months) was 8%. The etiology of LIP remains uncertain. The principal hypotheses suggest that LIP represents an abnormal lymphoproliferative response, either to HIV alone or to superinfection with another virus, the most likely candidate being the Epstein-Barr virus. The pathology consists of a diffuse infiltration of lymphocytes (CD8$^+$ cells) in the interstitium and scattered nodules of mononuclear cells (lymphocytes, histiocytes, and plasma cells).

The onset of LIP is insidious. It may present with a chronic cough, generalized lymphadenopathy, hepatosplenomegaly, and clubbing; the median age of onset is 2.5 to 3 years. Persistent parotid gland enlargement is a useful marker for the presence of LIP in pediatric HIV infection. Physical findings on lung examination are few; radiologic findings include diffuse bilateral reticulonodular shadowing of between 1 and 5 mm, with frequently associated hilar enlargement. In the absence of an infectious agent isolated from BAL, it may be prudent to proceed with a lung biopsy to confirm the diagnosis, especially in the setting of increased endemic *M. tuberculosis* activity. However, a presumptive diagnosis of LIP can be made based on the clinical findings and typical radiologic changes lasting more than 2 months.

Children with LIP have an approximate threefold higher rate of hospital admission secondary to bacterial pneumonia than do their non-LIP counterparts. Treatment for LIP is supportive; response to steroids is controversial without controlled clinical trials.

TABLE 139.3

INDICATIONS FOR INITIATION OF ANTIRETROVIRAL THERAPY IN CHILDREN <12 MONTHS OF AGE INFECTED WITH HUMAN IMMUNODEFICIENCY VIRUS (HIV) INFECTION

Clinical Category		CD4+ Cell Percentage	Plasma HIV RNA Copy Number*	Recommendation
Symptomatic (Clinical category A, B, or C)	OR	<25% (Immune category 2 or 3)	Any value	Treat
Asymptomatic (Clinical category N)	AND	>25% (Immune category 1)	Any value	Consider Treatment†

*Plasma HIV RNA levels are higher in HIV-infected infants than older infected children and adults. This may be difficult to interpret in infants <12 months of age because overall HIV RNA levels are high and overlapping HIV RNA levels occur between infants who have and those who do not have rapid disease progression.
†Because HIV infection progresses more rapidly in infants than older children or adults, some experts would treat all HIV-infected infants <6 months or <12 months of age, regardless of clinical, immunologic, or virologic parameters.
Adapted with permission from Guidelines for the Use of Antiretroviral Agents in Pediatric HIV Infection–January 20, 2004, http://www.hivatis.org.

HIV-associated Encephalopathy

Encephalopathy is divided into three clinical types: rapidly progressive encephalopathy, progressive encephalopathy with plateau periods, and static encephalopathy. Rapidly progressive encephalopathy usually manifests with symptoms in the first or second year of life, profound developmental delay or loss of milestones, and spasticity or pyramidal tract signs. The less severe form has plateau periods in which the patient does not acquire new milestones but does retain already achieved skills. By contrast, children with static encephalopathy continue to gain new skills and abilities, but at a slower rate than that of their non-HIV infected counterparts.

According to the CDC classification system, establishing the diagnosis of encephalopathy in HIV-infected children requires one of the following findings to be present for at least 2 months in the absence of other identifiable causes:

- Failure to attain or loss of developmental milestones or loss of intellectual ability, verified by standard developmental scale or neuropsychological testing
- Impaired brain growth or acquired microcephaly demonstrated by head circumference measurements or brain atrophy demonstrated by neuroimaging with serial imaging in children younger than 2 years of age
- Acquired symmetric motor deficit manifested by two or more of the following: paresis, pathological reflexes, ataxia, or gait disturbance

Computed tomography (CT) imaging may show evidence of cortical atrophy, prominent sulci, enlarged ventricles, and decreased attenuation of white matter suggestive of progressive multifocal leukoencephalopathy. Seizures are notably an infrequent occurrence, probably reflective of the fact that HIV infection affects primarily the white matter.

Therapy for HIV-associated encephalopathy is focused on potent antiretroviral therapy, in particular using drugs with a demonstrable penetration of the blood–brain barrier. With advances in pediatric HIV treatment, a notable delay in the onset of encephalopathy has occurred, with improved survival outcome achieved for those children initiated on HAART prior to the onset of clinical disease.

HIV-associated Cardiac Manifestations

Cardiac disease in HIV-infected children becomes more evident with increasing age; usually, it is not encountered in infants or young children, but it may contribute significantly to mortality in children older than 10 years of age. In the multicenter Pulmonary and Cardiac Complications of HIV (P^2C^2HIV) study, cardiac dysfunction was documented in 18% to 39% of HIV-infected children and associated with an increased risk of death from the time of first diagnosis (cumulative mortality rate 1 year after diagnosis of congestive heart failure, 52.5%). In the latter ongoing prospective study, increased left ventricular mass with resultant dysfunction was documented in a large proportion of

TABLE 139.4

INDICATIONS FOR INITIATION OF ANTIRETROVIRAL THERAPY IN CHILDREN >1 YEAR OF AGE INFECTED WITH HUMAN IMMUNODEFICIENCY VIRUS (HIV)

Clinical Category		CD4+ Cell Percentage		Plasma HIV RNA Copy Number	Recommendation
AIDS (Clinical category C)	OR	<15% (Immune Category 3)		Any value	Treat
Mild–Moderate Symptoms (Clinical category A or B)	OR	15–25%* (Immune Category 2)	OR	>100,000 copies/mL†	Consider treatment
Asymptomatic (Clinical category N)	AND	>25% (Immune Category 1)	AND	<100,000 copies/mL†	Many experts would defer therapy and closely monitor clinical, immune and viral parameters

*Many experts would initiate therapy if CD4+ cell percentage is between 15% to 20%, and defer therapy with increased monitoring frequency in children with CD4+ cell percentage 21% to 25%.
†Controversy exists among pediatric HIV experts regarding the plasma HIV RNA threshold warranting consideration of therapy in children in the absence of clinical or immune abnormalities; some experts would consider initiation of therapy in asymptomatic children if plasma HIV RNA levels were between 50,000 to 100,000 copies/mL.
Adapted with permission from Guidelines for the Use of Antiretroviral Agents in Pediatric HIV Infection—January 20, 2004, http://www.hivatis.org.

TABLE 139.5

RECOMMENDED ANTIRETROVIRAL REGIMENS FOR INITIAL THERAPY FOR HUMAN IMMUNODEFICIENCY VIRUS (HIV) INFECTION IN CHILDREN

Protease Inhibitor-Based Regimens:	
Strongly recommended:	Two NRTIs* *plus* Lopinavir/Ritonavir or Nelfinavir or Ritonavir
Alternative recommendation:	Two NRTIs* *plus* Amprenavir (children >4 years old)[†] *or* Indinavir
Non-Nucleoside Reverse Transcriptase Inhibitor-Based Regimens:	
Strongly recommended: Children >3 years:	Two NRTIs* *plus* Efavirenz[‡] (with or without Nelfinavir)
Children <3 years or who can't swallow capsules:	Two NRTIs* *plus* Nevirapine[‡]
Alternative recommendation:	Two NRTIs* *plus* Nevirapine[†] (children >3 years)
Nucleoside Analogue-Based Regimens:	
Strongly recommended:	None
Alternative recommendation:	Zidovudine *plus* Lamivudine *plus* Abacavir
Use in special circumstances:	Two NRTIs*
Regimens that Are Not Recommended:	
	Monotherapy[§]
	Certain two NRTI combinations*
	Two NRTIs *plus* Saquinavir soft or hard gel capsule as a sole protease inhibitor**
Insufficient Data to Recommend:	
	Two NRTIs1 *plus* Delavirdine
	Dual PIs, including Saquinavir soft or hard gel capsule with low dose Ritonavir, with the exception of Lopinavir/Ritonavir[§]
	NRTI *plus* NNRTI *plus* PI[††]
	Tenofovir-containing regimens
	Enfuvirtide (T-20)-containing regimens
	Emtricitabine (FTC)-containing regimens
	Atazanavir-containing regimens
	Fosamprenavir-containing regimens

*Dual NRTI combination recommendations:
   Strongly recommended: zidovudine plus didanosine or lamivudine; or stavudine plus lamivudine
   Alternative: abacavir plus zidovudine or lamivudine; or didanosine plus lamivudine
   Use in special circumstances: stavudine plus didanosine; or zalcitabine plus zidovudine
   Insufficient data: tenofovir- or emtricitabine-containing regimens
   Not recommended: zalcitabine plus didanosine, stavudine, or lamivudine; or zidovudine plus stavudine.
[†]Amprenavir should not be administered to children under age 4 years due to the propylene glycol and vitamin E content of the oral liquid preparation and lack of pharmacokinetic data in this age group.
[‡]Efavirenz currently is available only in capsule form, although a liquid formulation currently is under study to determine appropriate dosage in HIV-infected children under age 3 years; nevirapine is the preferred NNRTI for children under age 3 years or those requiring a liquid formulation.
[§]Except for ZDV chemoprophylaxis administered to HIV-exposed infants during the first 6 weeks of life to prevent perinatal HIV transmission; if an infant is confirmed as HIV-infected while receiving ZDV prophylaxis, therapy should either be discontinued or changed to a combination antiretroviral drug regimen.
**With the exception of lopinavir/ritonavir, data on the pharmacokinetics and safety of dual PI combinations (e.g., low-dose ritonavir pharmacologic boosting of saquinavir, indinavir, or nelfinavir) are limited; use of dual PIs as a component of initial therapy is not recommended, although such regimens may have utility as secondary treatment regimens for children who have failed initial therapy. Saquinavir soft- and hard-gel capsules require low-dose ritonavir boosting to achieve adequate levels in children, but pharmacokinetic data on appropriate dosing are not yet available.
[††]With the exception of efavirenz plus nelfinavir plus 1 or 2 NRTIs, which has been studied in HIV-infected children and shown to have virologic and immunologic efficacy in a clinical trial.
NRTI: Nucleoside analogue reverse transcriptase inhibitor; NNRTI: Non-nucleoside analogue reverse transcriptase inhibitor.
Adapted with permission from Guidelines for the Use of Antiretroviral Agents in Pediatric HIV Infection–January 20, 2004, http://www.hivatis.org.

HIV-infected patients and served as a clinically important indicator of survival. Additionally, the rate of death was highest in the rapid-progressor group (12.9 per 100 child-years versus 6.1 per 100 child years).

Various potential causes have been postulated in HIV-related heart disease and include myocardial infection with HIV itself, OIs, viral infections, autoimmune response to viral infection, drug-related cardiotoxicity, nutritional deficiencies, and prolonged immunosuppression. To date, long-term exposure to ZDV has not been associated with direct cardiotoxicity; however, complications such as lipodystrophy, insulin resistance, high levels of low-density lipoprotein, and high triglyceride levels develop in as many as 60% of patients treated with HAART regimens and may complicate underlying cardiomyopathy. Encephalopathy, wasting, decreased CD4[+] count, and a prior history of a serious cardiac event all are predictors of cardiac complications associated with HIV infection in chil-

dren. Affected children may present with cardiomegaly, cardiac tamponade, and conduction disturbances. Given the prevalence of ventricular hypertrophy with subsequent functional impairment and risk of serious cardiac events, having HIV-infected children undergo routine echocardiographic surveillance for cardiac abnormalities is recommended.

HIV-associated Nephropathy

HIV-infected patients are at risk of developing a variety of acute and chronic renal diseases. The most common cause of chronic renal failure is HIV-associated nephropathy (HIVAN). This focal segmental glomerulosclerosis results in rapid deterioration in renal function. It is overwhelmingly a disease of blacks, with almost 90% of cases occurring in that ethnic group. Murine and human studies have shown clearly that HIVAN is caused

TABLE 139.6

PEDIATRIC AIDS CLINICAL TRIALS GROUP (PACTG) 076 ZIDOVUDINE (ZDV) REGIMEN

Time of ZDV Administration	Regimen
Antepartum	Oral administration of 100 mg ZDV five times daily*, initiated at 14–34 weeks gestation and continued throughout the pregnancy.
Intrapartum	During labor, intravenous administration of ZDV in a 1-hour initial dose of 2 mg/kg body weight, followed by a continuous infusion of 1 mg/kg body weight/hour until delivery.
Postpartum	Oral administration of ZDV to the newborn (ZDV syrup at 2 mg/kg body weight/dose every six hours) for the first 6 weeks of life, beginning at 8–12 hours after birth.[†]

*Oral ZDV administered as 200 mg three times daily or 300 mg twice daily is currently used in general clinical practice and is an acceptable alternative regimen to 100 mg orally five times daily.

[†]Intravenous dosage for full-term infants who cannot tolerate oral intake is 1.5 mg/kg body weight intravenously every 6 hours. ZDV dosing for infants <35 weeks gestation at birth is 1.5 mg/kg/dose intravenously, or 2.0 mg/kg/dose orally, every 12 hours, advancing to every 8 hours at 2 weeks of age if >30 weeks gestation at birth or at 4 weeks of age if <30 weeks gestation at birth.

by a direct effect of renal cell infection by HIV-1 and that the virus actively replicates within renal cells. Initially, HIVAN was thought to be a late manifestation of AIDS because it appeared in patients with low CD4+ counts and a history of OIs; however, evidence of HIVAN at the time of seroconversion now exists. HIVAN significantly alters the mortality rates of HIV-infected patients.

Clinically, patients present with heavy proteinuria and hypoalbuminemia. Typically, they are normotensive. Until the introduction of HAART, no effective therapy for HIVAN was available. Steroids and angiotensin-converting enzyme inhibitors have played a small role in controlling disease manifestations. However, a reduction in the incidence of HIVAN and improved survival rates depend on the effective control of viral replication using HAART.

TREATMENT

Multidrug Therapy

Current therapeutic interventions focus on the administration of aggressive combination antiretroviral regimens to suppress viral replication maximally, preserve immune function, and reduce the development of resistance. Unfortunately, the rapidity and magnitude of viral turnover occurring during all stages of HIV infection is greater than previously recognized; plasma virions are estimated to have a mean half-life of only 6 hours. ZDV (AZT) does interrupt the vertical transmission of HIV, and ZDV monotherapy has demonstrated significant benefit. Although combination nucleoside reverse transcriptase inhibitors are effective, the introduction of the non-nucleoside reverse transcriptase inhibitors (nevirapine and efavirenz) and the protease inhibitors (nelfinavir and ritonavir) has led to dramatic improvements in outcome. Fortunately, the antiretroviral armamentarium to treat pediatric HIV infection continues to expand.

Factors to be considered prior to initiation of therapy include the risk of disease progression as determined by CD4+ percentage and plasma HIV RNA copy number, the potential benefits and risks of therapy, and the ability of the caregiver to adhere to the administration of the therapeutic regimen. Issues associated with adherence should be assessed fully, discussed, and addressed with the child, if age appropriate, and caregiver before the decision to initiate therapy is made. Given the pathogenesis of HIV in infants, the consensus among experts caring for newly diagnosed infants is to initiate aggressive antiretroviral therapy. The Public Health Service supports the option of deferring administration of therapy for children older than 1

year of age who are in good health and whose CD4+ lymphocyte count is in the normal range for age.

Tables 139.3 and 139.4 outline current recommendations concerning when to initiate ART in HIV-infected infants and children, according to the Working Group on Antiretroviral Therapy and Medical Management of HIV-Infected Children. Table 139.5 outlines preferred antiretroviral combinations (Guidelines for the Use of Antiretroviral Agents in Pediatric HIV Infection—January 20, 2004, http://www.hivatis.org). Additional information regarding all aspects of pediatric antiretroviral therapy is reviewed under these guidelines.

PREVENTION

The report of the Pediatric Aids Clinical Trials Group (PACTG-076) in 1994 forever altered the future of pediatric AIDS, which demonstrated the effectiveness of ART in the prevention of perinatal HIV transmission. Subsequent to the results of that study, in which transmission rates were reduced by almost 70% in the face of administration of ZDV (Table 137.6), widespread recommendations concerning the management of HIV-infected pregnant women were generated. The additional benefit of elective cesarean section performed prior to rupture of the membrane varies greatly depending on the stage and control of maternal HIV infection. Up-to-date guidelines concerning the management of pregnant HIV-infected women at all stages of pregnancy, labor, and delivery, as well as administration of ART to exposed newborn infants, are reviewed in the latest guidelines from the U.S. Public Health Service Task Force.

CONCLUSIONS

Remarkable progress has been made in improving treatments for children infected with HIV. The availability of an extended armamentarium of antiretroviral agents, including those specifically formulated for pediatric consumption, has had a great impact on treatment outcome. Despite improvements that have been made in combination drug therapy, many obstacles exist in managing HIV-infected children and adolescents. Noncompliance with the vastly complicated drug regimens results in problems with drug resistance. Unfavorable adverse effects associated with the many different medication types only compounds this problem. HIV vaccines and alternative drug classes (e.g., receptor blockers) are areas of active research. The advances made in resource-rich countries for children with HIV must be extended to all children infected with HIV, regardless of the wealth of the nation in which they live.

Suggested Readings

American Academy of Pediatrics. Human Immunodeficiency Virus Infection. In: Pickering LK, ed. *Red Book: 2003 Report of the Committee on Infectious Diseases,* 26th ed. Elk Grove Village, IL: American Academy of Pediatrics; 2003:360.

Centers for Disease Control and Prevention. U.S. Public Health Service Task Force recommendations for use of antiretroviral drugs in pregnant HIV-1 infected women for maternal health and interventions to reduce perinatal HIV-1 transmission in the United States. *MMWR Morb Mortal Wkly Rep* 2002;51(Rr-18):1.

Deng H, Liu R, Ellmeier W, et al. Identification of a major co-receptor for primary isolates of HIV-1. *Nature* 1996;381:661.

Misrahi M, Teglas JP, N'Go N, et al. CCR5 chemokine receptor variant in HIV-1 mother-to-child transmission and disease progression in children. French Pediatric HIV Infection Study Group. *JAMA* 1998;279:277.

Connor EM, Sperling RS, Gelber R, et al. for The Pediatric AIDS Clinical Trials Group Protocol 076 Study Group. Reduction of maternal-infant transmission of human immunodeficiency virus type 1 with zidovudine treatment. *N Engl J Med* 1994;331:1173.

Landesman SH, Kalish LA, Burns DN, et al. Obstetrical factors and the transmission of human immunodeficiency virus type 1 from mother to child. The Women and Infants Transmission Study. *N Engl J Med* 1996;334:1617.

John-Stewart G, Mbori-Ngacha D, Ekpini R, et al. for the Ghent IAS Working Group on HIV in Women and Children. Breast-feeding and transmission of HIV-1. *J Acquir Immune Defic Syndr* 2004;35:196.

Recommendations of the U.S. Public Health Service and the Infectious Diseases Society of America. Guidelines for preventing opportunistic infections among HIV-infected persons. *MMWR Morb Mortal Wkly Rep* 2002;51(Rr-8):1.

Starc TJ, Lipshultz SE, Easley KA, et al. Incidence of cardiac abnormalities in children with human immunodeficiency virus infection: the prospective P2C2 HIV study. *J Pediatr* 2002;141:327.

Stringer JR, Beard CB, Miller RF, et al. A new name (Pneumocystis jiroveci) for pneumocystis from humans. *Emerg Infect Dis* 2002;8:891.

CHAPTER 140 ■ ANTIRETROVIRAL THERAPY IN PEDIATRIC ACQUIRED IMMUNODEFICIENCY SYNDROME

ROSS E. MCKINNEY, JR.

The ultimate goal of antiretroviral therapy for human immunodeficiency virus (HIV) is to cure the patient of infection. Because this objective is not yet achievable, the second target is to provide a simple, inexpensive, well-tolerated regimen that is able to control the infection for a long period, even indefinitely. Unfortunately, even this objective is elusive, and current treatment strategies generally are complex, rigid, and burdened by toxicities. Their efficacy is time-limited, and their effectiveness is marginal. Nonetheless, progress has been made, and newer, more potent antiretroviral agents have allowed HIV-infected people to live longer, healthier lives. Much of this progress has been attributable to a better understanding of HIV and its biologic behavior, thus rendering drug selection and use a more rational process. This chapter describes the antiretroviral drugs currently available and outlines some basic strategies for their use.

BIOLOGY OF HUMAN IMMUNODEFICIENCY VIRUS AND ANTIRETROVIRAL THERAPY

The antiretroviral drugs in current clinical use target critical steps in the life cycle of the virus. Fusion inhibitors block the movement of the virus from its attachment point on the cell surface to the cytoplasm. Reverse transcriptase inhibitors act on the genetic replication of the virus by inhibiting the virus protein that makes a cDNA copy of the viral genomic RNA. Protease inhibitors (PIs) act at a later stage in the virus life cycle by blocking the step when the viral protease cleaves the viral *gag-pol* polyprotein into the subunits required to make a fully mature, infectious virion. Additional viral targets such as the virus attachment protein (gp120) and the coreceptors (CXCR4 and CCR5) are the subject of drug development efforts, and

potentially useful antiviral drugs directed at these other targets currently are in clinical trials.

Two classes of reverse transcriptase inhibitors exist: nucleoside reverse transcriptase inhibitors (NRTIs) and nonnucleoside reverse transcriptase inhibitors (NNRTIs). NRTIs are modified nucleosides designed lacking a 3'OH group. They are phosphorylated by host cell kinases and then are incorporated into the elongating viral polynucleotide chain. Their incorporation produces a prematurely terminated cDNA molecule because another nucleotide cannot add to the chain given the absent 3'OH bonding site. Because the viral reverse transcriptase has a greater relative affinity for the modified nucleosides than does the human DNA polymerase (which generally rejects them), NRTIs have a tolerable therapeutic index. The NNRTIs act through a different mechanism than do the NRTIs. The NNRTIs interfere with nucleotide binding at the active site of the reverse transcriptase, blocking the inititiation of reverse transcription, and have no effect on cellular DNA polymerases because they are very enzyme specific. In fact, they are so specific that the NNRTIs have no effect on the reverse transcriptase of HIV-2. NNRTIs and NRTIs also have very different side effect profiles. NNRTIs can be used in combination with NRTIs, often with synergistic activity. Box 140.1 lists the different categories of drugs used in the treatment of HIV, including the NRTIs and NNRTIs.

HIV's *gag* virion structural proteins and the *pol* proteins are synthesized as a long polyprotein. The polyprotein must be cleaved into many smaller proteins by the viral protease to produce a fully mature and infectious virion. The HIV protease is an aspartyl protease with some similarities to cellular aspartyl proteases, but several relatively specific inhibitors of the HIV protease have been developed, with excellent antiviral activity.

Suboptimal antiretroviral dosing or noncompliance can permit continued viral replication in the presence of low concentrations of drug, thus promoting the development of resistance

BOX 140.1 Classification of Antiretroviral Drugs

Nucleoside Reverse Transcriptase Inhibitors
Abacavir
Didanosine
Emtricitabine
Lamivudine
Stavudine
Tenofovir
Zalcitabine
Zidovudine

Nonnucleoside Reverse Transcriptase Inhibitors
Delavirdine
Efavirenz
Nevirapine

Protease Inhibitors
Amprenavir
Fosamprenavir
Lopinavir
Indinavir
Nelfinavir
Ritonavir
Saquinavir

Fusion Inhibitor
Enfuviritide

to the agents. The development of resistant viruses can have important implications for the long-term efficacy of antiretroviral therapeutic regimens.

The recommended doses of antiretroviral agents are summarized in Table 140.1. The table includes doses both for drugs approved by the Food and Drug Administration (FDA) and, so readers may have some appreciation of drugs currently undergoing development, for antiretroviral drugs in advanced stages of clinical development. Dosing and indications may change, and new side effects and drug interactions may become known. The physician should consult a current version of the package insert when prescribing antiretroviral agents, particularly newer agents, or federal guidelines. Many antiretroviral drugs have serious side effects and potentially harmful interactions with other drugs. Patients must be monitored carefully for these potential problems. Antiretroviral therapy should be managed by or in close consultation with an expert in the care of pediatric HIV infection.

ANTIRETROVIRAL DRUGS

Nucleoside Reverse Transcriptase Inhibitors

The NRTIs were the first class of antiretroviral drugs to be used in HIV infection. They can be divided into two categories: thymidine derivatives and nonthymidine NRTIs. The thymidine derivatives are zidovudine (ZDV) and stavudine (d4T), and because of its resistance pattern, tenofovir (TDF). ZDV and d4T do not work well together, probably because ZDV inhibits the phosphorylation of d4T to d4T-triphosphate; the latter is the active form of d4T. In general, most combination regimens include at least two NRTIs.

The effective pharmacokinetic properties of the NRTIs are determined by the pharmacokinetic properties of the active, intracellular triphosphate form of the drug. The serum half-life of the unphosphorylated native drugs is relatively short, and most are excreted rapidly, some after hepatic glucuronidation. However, within the cell, the phosphorylated forms of the drugs may have a prolonged half-life, which allows for less frequent dosing intervals than the serum half-life would suggest.

The NRTIs as a class can produce mitochondrial toxicity. Although it can be tolerated in most patients for years of therapy, in some patients a syndrome of lactic acidosis and hepatic steatosis can develop. The usual symptoms are nausea, vomiting, abdominal pain, and weakness in a patient who has been receiving nucleosides for 6 months or longer. This syndrome occurs more commonly in adults, female patients, and overweight individuals, and it is a particular concern in pregnant women. The incidence is probably approximately 1% of people receiving long-term NRTI therapy. Information regarding clinical trials in NRTIs is presented in Box 140.2.

Abacavir

Abacavir (Ziagen) is a relatively potent carbocyclic guanosine analogue nucleoside that has excellent activity when used as first-line antiviral therapy. If used in first-line therapy, it appears to be one of, if not the most, potent NRTIs. Its use has been somewhat limited by the relatively severe hypersensitivity syndrome seen in roughly 5% of patients who use it. Both tablet and liquid preparations are available. Abacavir is also available in a fixed ratio combination tablet (Trizivir) with ZDV and 3TC.

Pharmacokinetics. Abacavir is administered on a schedule of one dose every 12 hours. The serum half-life is approximately 1 hour. Food has no effect on absorption. Abacavir crosses the blood brain barrier in a manner similar to that of ZDV, with a ratio of cerebrospinal fluid to plasma of approximately 0.2.

Antiviral Effects. Abacavir is an effective nucleoside, perhaps the most potent of current compounds as initial therapy, but resistance occurs frequently in patients who have been treated previously with other NRTIs. Most studies of abacavir have involved combinations with other antiretroviral agents. When used with PIs in therapy-naive adults, abacavir produced 2 log decreases in RNA copy number. Substantial cross-resistance exists between abacavir and other nucleosides. The key resistance sites appear to be at reverse transcriptase codons 65, 74, 115, 184, and the standard thymidine resistance mutations (41, 67, 70, 210, 215, 219).

Adverse Effects. The main concern with using abacavir is an idiosyncratic hypersensitivity reaction that occurs most often in the first weeks of therapy and is manifested by rash, fever, nausea, and vomiting. If it occurs, abacavir rechallenge should not be considered; patients have progressed to shock and even death as a result of rechallenge after an episode of hypersensitivity. This reaction can be difficult to distinguish from the rash syndrome of nevirapine (NVP) and even from some infectious conditions (adenovirus, scarlet fever).

Didanosine

Didanosine (ddI; Videx) is an NRTI metabolized from dideoxyinosine to its active form, dideoxyadenosine (ddA). It has a good side effect profile for children, but its use is limited by inconvenient dosage regimens in young children. These problems are caused principally by ddI's chemical instability in acid conditions such as those found in the stomach and the consequent requirement for oral coadministration of a buffering agent. ddI is available as a liquid mixed in antacid (usually Maalox), as a chewable and dissolvable tablet, or in its most convenient preparation, an enteric-coated, delayed-release capsule.

TABLE 140.1

DOSING OF ANTIRETROVIRAL DRUGS

Drug	Pediatric Dose	Adult Dose	Comments
Nucleoside Reverse Transcriptase Inhibitors			
Zidovudine (Retrovir)	Prematures: 1.5 mg/kg q12h to age 2 weeks, then 2 mg/kg q8h; infants: 2 mg/kg/dose q6h or 1.5 mg/kg q6h intravenously; pediatric: 180 mg/m^2/dose q8h or 240 mg/m^2/dose q12h	300 mg bid or 200 mg tid	Child perinatal prophylaxis: dose, 2 mg/kg q6h for 6 weeks. Maternal perinatal prophylaxis: dose, ACIG 076 trial established 100 mg five times per day, although 200 mg tid or 300 mg bid is probably acceptable.
Stavudine (Zerit)	Neonates: not known; pediatric: 1 mg/kg bid to 30 kg	>60 kg: 40 mg q12h; ≤60 kg: 30 mg q12h	
Lamivudine (Epivir)	Neonates (<30 days): 2 mg/kg bid; pediatric: 4 mg/kg bid	>50 kg: 150 mg bid; ≤50 kg: 2 mg/kg bid	
Didanosine (Videx)	Neonates (<90 days): 50 mg/m^2/dose q12h; pediatric: 90 mg/m^2/dose q12h	>60 kg: 200 mg bid; ≤60 kg: 125 mg bid	If tablets are used, at least two must be used with each dose to achieve adequate antacid dose. Available as a powder for pediatric oral solution, which is mixed with an antacid during reconstitution and is poorly stable.
Zalcitabine (HIVID)	Neonates: unknown; pediatric: 0.01 mg/kg q8h	0.75 mg tid	
Abacavir (Ziagen)	8 mg/kg dose bid	300 mg bid	Dosing information tentative.
Tenofovir disfumerate (Viread)	Unknown	300 mg qd	Pediatric dosing under evaluation.
Nonnucleoside Reverse Transcriptase Inhibitors			
Nevirapine (Viramune)	Neonates: 5 mg/kg qd for 14 days, then 120 mg/m^2 q12h for 14 days, then 200 mg/m^2 dose q12h; pediatric: 120–200 mg/m^2/dose q12h; for the first 14 days, dose is 120 mg/m^2 qd, then escalate as tolerated	200 mg q12h. For first 14 days, use one-half of dose, then increase	
Delavirdine (Rescriptor)	Unknown	400 mg tid	
Efavirenz (Sustiva)	10–15 kg: 200 mg qd; 16–20 kg: 250 mg qd; 21–25 kg: 300 mg qd; 26.0–32.5 kg: 350 mg qd; 32.6–40.0 kg: 400 mg qd; >40 kg: 600 mg qd	600 mg qd	Capsules only: 50, 100, and 200 mg. Efavirenz is probably not useful in patients in whom prior nonnucleoside reverse transcriptase inhibitor therapy failed because of cross-resistance.
Protease Inhibitors			
Nelfinavir (Viracept)	Neonate: 10 mg/kg tid; pediatric: 20–30 mg/kg tid	750 mg tid	Neonatal dose is an unproved estimate. Some people believe q8h is more appropriate than tid schedule.
Ritonavir (Norvir)	Neonate: unknown; pediatric: 400 mg/m^2 q12h; begin dosing at 250 mg/m^2 q12h, then increase over 5 days to full dose	600 mg bid. Initiate at 300 mg bid, then escalate as tolerated over 5 days	
Indinavir (Crixivan)	500 mg/m^2/dose q8h	800 mg q8h	Pediatric dose is still unproved.
Saquinavir (Invirase)	Unknown	1,000 mg bid	
Amprenavir (Agenerase)	Capsule: 20 mg/kg bid; liquid: 1.5 mL/kg bid (liquid is 15 mg/mL)	>50 kg: 1,200 mg bid; ≤50 kg: 20 mg/kg bid	Dosages tentative; clinical trials in progress. Capsules are 150 mg each.
Lopinavir (Kaletra)	Liquid: 7–14 kg: 12 mg/kg bid; 15–40 kg: 10 mg/kg bid; >40 kg: 400 mg Pobid	400 mg LPV bid	Combined with RTV at a 4:1 ratio in liquid and capsules.

BOX 140.2   Clinical Trials of Antiretroviral Drugs

Nucleoside Reverse Transcriptase Inhibitors
Abacavir
The first pediatric study to use abacavir, Pediatric AIDS Clinical Trials Group (PACTG) Protocol 330, evaluated abacavir monotherapy in a cohort of children who had extensive experience with therapy. Unfortunately, in that setting, the drug had little virologic effect. The study included a phase in which a second nucleoside reverse transcriptase inhibitor (NRTI) was added to the abacavir monotherapy, but again little benefit was seen, probably because of already established antiviral resistance. Studies of abacavir in adults have demonstrated good antiviral activity, comparable with protease inhibitors (PIs) and nonnucleoside reverse transcriptase inhibitors (NNRTIs). Monotherapy in adults with limited antiretroviral exposure (up to 12 weeks of zidovudine [ZDV]) led to average decreases of 1.5 to 2.1 logs. Abacavir is synergistic with other nucleosides, so it generally is used in combination. A pediatric trial in Europe (PENTA 5) found that abacavir/lamivudine (3TC) or abacavir/ZDV was superior to ZDV/3TC when used in an initial treatment regimen.

Didanosine (ddI)
PACTG Protocol 152 demonstrated that monotherapy with ddI was more effective than was ZDV alone and perhaps as effective as was combination ZDV/ddI. However, PACTG Protocol 300 then found that both ZDV/3TC and ZDV/ddI were more effective than ddI monotherapy, both clinically and with regard to surrogate markers.

Emtricitabine (FTC)
The first study of FTC in children is PACTG 1021, which at 60 weeks has shown good safety and efficacy for a regimen of FTC, ddI, and efavirenz (EFV), each administered once daily.

Lamivudine (3TC)
PACTG Trial 300 compared ZDV/3TC with monotherapy ddI. The combination was superior with regard to clinical outcomes and surrogate markers. Recently, studies have explored the combination of 3TC with ddI and EFV, and the combination appears to have good efficacy.

Stavudine (d4T)
Trials of d4T in children have demonstrated a good safety profile. It has been studied as monotherapy and in combination with ddI and 3TC (Adult ACTG Trial 306). The clinical effects of combination therapy with ddI or 3TC are similar to those seen with ZDV. d4T also can be combined with PIs or NNRTIs. It should not be coadministered with ZDV.

Tenofovir (TDF)
Clinical information on use of TDF in children is still relatively limited. Concerns about bone mineralization effects have contributed to slowed pediatric development.

Zalcitabine (ddC)
Two large trials of ddC in children, PACTG studies 138 and 190, have been completed. The first was a phase II/III trial of two dosage regimens of ddC monotherapy for children whose infection had progressed on ZDV or were intolerant of that drug. In that study, ddC generally was well tolerated. More than one-half of the children had stabilization of growth and a decline in p24 antigen concentrations. Thirty percent of the children had an increase in CD4 counts and gained weight. In PACTG 190, ddC (0.03 mg/kg/day) or placebo was added to ZDV in patients who were clinically stable. Relatively few differences in the two study groups were found, although children who received ZDV/ddC had a slower decline in CD4 cell counts.

Zidovudine (ZDV)
The first comparative, placebo-controlled trial of ZDV in adults demonstrated the effectiveness of ZDV when the study was halted early in 1986. Two hundred eighty-two patients with acquired immunodeficiency syndrome (AIDS) or advanced AIDS-related symptoms were treated with ZDV or placebo. Of the 145 ZDV-treated patients, only one died. In comparison, 16 of 137 patients in the placebo group died. The outcome was highly significant. Although this result unequivocally showed the short-term clinical benefit of ZDV, many questions were left unanswered.

The first pediatric trial of ZDV was performed from 1986 through 1987. It demonstrated that ZDV could be used in children in a manner similar to that for adults, although children may have had fewer adverse events. Benefits of ZDV treatment included weight gain faster than anticipated, decreased hepatosplenomegaly, and lowering of immunoglobulin G (IgG) and IgM concentrations toward more normal values. The first large phase II trial of ZDV in children had very similar results, confirming the positive effects of ZDV treatment on growth.

PACTG Trial 152 demonstrated that both ZDV/ddI and ddI alone were clinically superior to ZDV monotherapy. Similarly, PACTG Trial 300 demonstrated that both combination ZDV/ddI and ZDV/3TC were superior to ddI monotherapy. ACTG Trial 338 demonstrated that combination regimens containing ritonavir (RTV) and ZDV/3TC or d4T produced better short-term virus suppression than did ZDV/3TC alone. As a result of such studies, ZDV virtually is never used as a monotherapy but instead is used in combinations.

ACTG Protocol 076 established that ZDV monotherapy had a role in the prevention of vertical HIV transmission (mother to infant). In that study, ZDV (200 mg) was administered to the mother five times each day, intravenous ZDV was infused after the onset of labor (a 2-mg/kg bolus, then 1 mg/kg/hour), and the baby was given oral ZDV for 6 weeks (2 mg/kg/dose every 6 hours). This regimen decreased the transmission rate from 26% to 8%. Subsequently, through the use of combination therapy, rates for vertical transmission of HIV have decreased to less than 2% and to less than 1% in mothers whose virus is able to be fully suppressed. However, the therapies required for transmission rates this low are expensive and generally are not available in the developing world.

(Continued)

BOX 140.2   (Continued)

Case-control studies have suggested that ZDV is beneficial in the prevention of transmission of HIV in other contexts, particularly after needlestick accidents. As a result, the Centers for Disease Control and Prevention issued guidelines for preventing needlestick-related transmission of HIV that include ZDV in the treatment regimens. For individuals with high-risk needlestick accidents (hollow-bore needles, deep penetration, blood from a highly viremic patient), combination therapy with ZDV and 3TC, with or without a third drug, which should be chosen after consultation with an HIV care specialist, is suggested. A reasonable theoretic rationale exists for the prophylactic use of an NRTI because it blocks the initial steps in virus replication. If the virus RNA is not transcribed fairly quickly into DNA, it will biodegrade and become noninfectious.

Nonnucleoside Reverse Transcriptase Inhibitors
Efavirenz (EFV)

EFV appears to be approximately as effective as is a PI, provided the other agents in the combination regimen are active in the particular patient. A once-daily regimen of FTC, ddI, and EFV in children has been studied in PACTG Protocol 1021 and preliminarily appears to be active and well tolerated.

Nevirapine (NVP)

NVP has been used in a number of pediatric studies in combination with NRTIs. It shows consistent efficacy, although combination regimens including other active drugs for the specific patient are important. As perinatal prophylaxis, PACTG 316 evaluated the addition of NVP to the mother's standard regimen. No effect could be seen, but the transmission rate in the placebo group was lower than expected, so demonstrating a therapeutic benefit was difficult, while at the same time showing the potency of the prophylactic effect of the other components of the regimens. HIVNet 012 demonstrated a role for two-dose NVP prophylaxis in vertical transmission. Mothers were given a single dose of NVP (200 mg) during labor, and the infants received 2 mg/kg of NVP at 48 to 72 hours old. The transmission rate dropped by almost 50%, from 21% for infants whose mothers received short-course ZDV (the control group) to 12% in mother-infant pairs given NVP.

Protease Inhibitors
Amprenavir (APV)

Clinical experience with APV remains relatively limited, especially in children. It has good virologic effect when used in combination with NRTIs, producing undetectable viral loads in most treatment-naive patients.

Lopinavir (LPV; LPV/r)

In clinical trials, LPV/r has proved to be one of the most potent PIs. In its initial trials in children, 80% of therapy-naive HIV-infected children had viral suppression to fewer than 400 copies/mL at week 48, whereas 71% of therapy-experienced children were fully suppressed. Both results are excellent. The average therapy-naive child had an increase of 404 CD4+ lymphocytes/mm^3, whereas experienced children demonstrated a mean increase of 284 lymphocytes/mm^3. Only 2% of children dropped out of the study.

Indinavir (IDV)

Pediatric experience with IDV was primarily in studies at the National Cancer Institute and the Merck-PACTG collaborative Protocol 395. The latter phase I/II study showed good virologic effect but a significant rate of adverse events. In adults, when IDV and 3TC were added to patients who had been on long-term ZDV, the effects were striking. Twenty-eight of the 31 patients treated with three drugs reached fewer than 500 RNA copies/mL by week 24, compared with none of the patients who received only 3TC in addition to ZDV and 12 of 28 who added only IDV.

Nelfinavir (NLV)

The phase I/II trial of NLV in children demonstrated a potent antiviral effect when NLV was given in combination with NRTIs. The best effect was seen in children who received at least one new NRTI about the time NLV was started. In those children, eight of 11 followed to 34 weeks had undetectable virus loads. NLV may be somewhat less effective in children who have been treated already with multiple agents, although several centers have found that CD4+ lymphocyte counts improve even after the level of virus suppression becomes marginal. In adults, NLV combined with ZDV/3TC in treatment-naive patients was very effective. Eighty-one percent of adults treated with 750 mg of NLV were able to reach undetectable RNA levels, compared with 18% of subjects assigned ZDV/3TC alone.

Ritonavir (RTV)

The pediatric benefits of RTV have been demonstrated by PACTG Protocol 338. RTV-containing regimens (ZDV/3TC/RTV or d4T/RTV) had a larger suppression of viral load and a better CD4 cell response than did a ZDV/3TC-containing regimen when given to stable, therapy-experienced children. The study was not designed to answer clinical efficacy questions.

Saquinavir (SQV)

Little clinical information exists on SQV in children. The soft-gel capsules improved the clinical effects seen in adults. In antiretroviral-naive patients, SQV/ZDV/3TC was able to drop 61% of patients below the level of detection (20 copies/mL).

Fusion Inhibitor
Enfuviritide (T-20)

T-20 has been studied in relatively few children, although the numbers continue to increase. It appears to be well-tolerated, although discomfort occurs at the injection sites, sometimes associated with a small subcutaneous lump and localized erythema. Ninety-eight percent of patients have some form of reaction at the injection site, although it generally is not sufficient to terminate drug use.

Pharmacokinetics. Because ddI is acid labile, steps must be taken to neutralize stomach acid; ddI typically is given to young children as a premixed suspension in flavored antacid. The intracellular half-life of the active form of the drug (ddA triphosphate) is quite long (more than 24 hours); therefore, once-daily administration of ddI is possible, providing a considerable advantage given the complexity of many antiretroviral regimens. The enteric-coated capsules are more convenient than are the liquid suspensions or chewable tablets once the child is large enough to take them.

ddI should be given, when possible, on an empty stomach, ideally 1 hour before or 2 hours after a meal. However, with small children who eat often, implementing this regimen may not be possible, and the importance of the daily schedule for compliance should be weighed against the loss in absorption because of food.

ddI liquid is not stable. It must be stored under refrigerated conditions, and some clinics give patients ice chests to use in transporting ddI suspension home from the pharmacy. The shelf life, even refrigerated, is only 30 days. The chewable/dispersible tablets are somewhat more convenient, but the taste can be challenging for children. If tablets are used, the minimum dose is two tablets at a time because the tablets are mixed with antacid and two will supply an adequate buffering capacity.

Antiviral Effects. ddI monotherapy has antiviral effects similar to those of ZDV as measured by surrogate markers. It has somewhat better durability as monotherapy, but it is given now only in combinations. The resistance mutation most often associated with ddI is at codon 74, although demonstrating antiviral resistance to ddI *in vitro* is difficult. Because the drug's beneficial effects can be exhausted (as demonstrated by surrogate marker changes), failure to show resistance *in vitro* does not mean that resistance does not occur. Resistance also has been associated with codons 65, 151, and 184.

Adverse Effects. ddI generally is well tolerated in children. The most common adverse events are peripheral neuropathy and pancreatitis. The neuropathy usually presents as paresthesias, most often of the feet, and may appear as a gait disturbance in younger children. Pancreatitis typically presents as abdominal pain, nausea, and vomiting. In contrast to other causes of abdominal pain, pancreatitis usually is associated with an increase in amylase and lipase levels and may be confirmed in some instances with ultrasonography. However, it is not useful to monitor serum amylase levels routinely in patients taking ddI because most episodes of pancreatitis are relatively acute and are signaled first by pain. In addition, high amylase concentrations often are released by the salivary glands in children with HIV infection. To determine whether elevated serum amylase is attributable to pancreatitis or parotitis, a fractionated amylase determination can be performed. This assay can separate pancreatic from salivary isoenzymes. However, the isoenzymes may overlap, so a very high salivary amylase value can give a falsely elevated pancreatic fraction. To improve the predictive value of amylase measurements, a serum lipase determination can be obtained. In most instances in which both enzyme concentrations are high, pancreatitis should be suspected.

Additional effects may include abdominal symptoms such as diarrhea, pain, or nausea from ddI. Some of the effects may be from the antacid. Recently, the combination of d4T and ddI has been perceived as causing an undesirable rate of lactic acidosis and hepatic steatosis in pregnant women, and the combination is not recommended in that situation. Although the issue of the combination of ddI and d4T has been raised most frequently in pregnancy, many clinicians no longer use this pairing because of the concerns about mitochondrial toxicity.

Emtricitabine

Emtricitabine (FTC; Emtriva) is a relatively new drug with limited pediatric information. It has the same resistance pattern as lamivudine (3TC), although it has a longer half-life and somewhat greater activity on a gram-for-gram basis. It is available currently only as capsules or liquid.

Pharmacokinetics. FTC primarily is renally excreted. The plasma half-life is 10 hours, and the drug can be administered on a once-daily schedule.

Antiviral Effects. The effects of FTC are very similar to those of 3TC. Resistance is mediated primarily by M184V.

Adverse Events. FTC generally has been well tolerated. Hyperpigmentation of the palms and soles has been reported.

Lamivudine

3TC (Epivir) is derived from cytosine and is a relatively potent NRTI. The drug is well tolerated, has beneficial interactions with ZDV and d4T, and is a frequent component of combination regimens. Liquid and tablet preparations are available. 3TC also is available in fixed-ratio combinations with ZDV (Combivir) and ZDV and abacavir (Trizivir). These preparations are convenient for children large enough to take them.

Pharmacokinetics. 3TC has a relatively long half-life and is renally excreted. Dosage should be reduced in patients with renal impairment. It may be given every 12 to 24 hours. No food-related interactions occur.

Antiviral Effects. As monotherapy, 3TC can produce 1 log decreases in HIV RNA. However, resistance to 3TC monotherapy occurs quickly and requires only a single-point mutation at amino acid 184 in the reverse transcriptase gene. 3TC virtually always is used in combination with other NRTIs. The benefits of 3TC were confirmed in Pediatric AIDS Clinical Trials Group (PACTG) Protocol 300, in which ZDV/3TC was found to be clinically superior to monotherapy ddI.

Adverse Effects. 3TC is a well-tolerated compound. The only major side effect is pancreatitis, which occurred primarily in a very ill group of children treated with multiple antiretroviral agents at the National Cancer Institute. Subsequent studies have demonstrated that pancreatitis is a rare development. For example, no instances of 3TC-associated pancreatitis were found in PACTG 300 (patients followed a median of 11 months), whereas eight cases of pancreatitis occurred in patients treated with regimens containing ddI. 3TC occasionally causes headaches, gastrointestinal upset, fatigue, and elevated hepatic transaminases, none of which is a common reason to adjust dosage. It has been reported to cause mitochondrial toxicity and lactic acidosis, although at a low frequency.

Stavudine

d4T (Zerit) is a thymidine-derived nucleoside with clinical potency roughly equivalent to that of ZDV. The advantages to d4T are that it can be given on a twice-daily dosing schedule, side effects are relatively uncommon in children, and timing with food intake is not an issue. d4T is available in an FDA-approved liquid preparation and in capsule form. For adults, an extended-release capsule also is available.

Pharmacokinetics. Standard d4T has a relatively long intracellular half-life (3 to 4 hours) and can be given on a twice-daily schedule. No special arrangements for mealtime are required because d4T is absorbed well on either a full or empty stomach. Because d4T is renally excreted, dosage adjustment may be required in patients with renal problems. d4T is phosphorylated intracellularly to become active. Because ZDV may inhibit that phosphorylation, ZDV and d4T should not be used simultaneously. An extended-release d4T capsule has been approved for once-daily dosing in adults and may be suitable for some adolescents.

Antiviral Effects. d4T is similar to ZDV in effect, producing a 0.7 to 0.8 log decrease in virus titer when used as monotherapy. Resistance to d4T involves mutations at reverse transcriptase amino acid residue 75, as well as the standard thymidine analog mutations (41, 67, 70, 210, 215, and 219, with 215 being most significant).

Adverse Effects. Generally, d4T is well tolerated by children. In adults, d4T is associated with peripheral neuropathy in a high proportion of patients. However, neuropathy appears to occur less commonly in children. d4T also is associated rarely with anemia, pancreatitis, headache, and gastrointestinal disturbances. It is also the NRTI most often associated with lactic acidosis and hepatic steatosis, especially when used with ddI. Consequently, ddI and D4T generally are not used as a combination unless other options have been exhausted.

Tenofovir

(TDF, Tenofovir disfumerate Viread) is a nucleotide. A nucleotide is a phosphorylated nucleoside, which means the first step in the activation process has already been completed.

Pharmacokinetics. TDF is a prodrug that is converted to TDF in the gastrointestinal tract. The active form of the drug is TDF diphosphate. Oral bioavailability in adults is roughly 25%. The terminal plasma half-life is 5.5 hours. TDF is cleared renally, with no involvement of the cytochrome P-450 system.

Antiviral Effects. TDF is similar to ZDV in potency. As monotherapy, it produces a 0.5 to 0.7 log decrease in virus titer. Resistance is conferred by mutations at reverse transcriptase codons 65, 41, 210, and 215. TDF interacts with ddI, increasing ddI exposure, in many cases to a sufficient degree that the ddI dose should be adjusted downward. TDF exposure is not affected significantly.

Adverse Effects. TDF can decrease bone mineral density. The significance of this toxicity has not been defined completely in children, but bone mineral density should be monitored.

Zalcitabine

Zalcitabine (ddC; Hivid) has been used relatively sparingly in children. No liquid preparation has been developed, and the available capsular formulation is designed for adult dosing.

Pharmacokinetics. ddC is given every 8 hours. Some medications that affect ddC's renal clearance include cimetidine, amphotericin, foscarnet, and aminoglycosides. Antacids may decrease absorption.

Antiviral Effects. ddC is roughly comparable to ddI in activity and has a considerable degree of cross-resistance with the latter compound. In general, once a patient has had experience with ddI, little benefit is gained from a shift to ddC. The most important resistance mutations occur at reverse transcriptase amino acid residues 65, 69, 74, and 184.

Adverse Effects. ddC has been associated with peripheral neuropathy that most frequently affects the distal extremities, especially the feet. Although the symptoms of neuropathy usually begin with numbness or paresthesias, they can become quite painful and may persist for several weeks after discontinuation of ddC. ddC is associated rarely with pancreatitis or painful oral ulcerations. Headache and fatigue occur occasionally.

Zidovudine

ZDV (azidothymidine; Retrovir) was the first FDA-approved antiretroviral drug. ZDV is a chain-terminating, thymidine-derived NRTI. The drug has substantial, although tolerable, side effects and demonstrated clinical efficacy in children. However, although ZDV monotherapy has clinical benefits, resistance develops over time; hence, except for occasional use in the setting of regimens designed to interrupt vertical transmission, the drug is used only in combination regimens. ZDV is available in both liquid and capsule form.

Pharmacokinetics. ZDV has a short serum half-life (roughly 1 hour) in children beyond the first few months of life. The drug is first glucuronidated in the liver, then is renally excreted. In young infants, the half-life is prolonged because of both limited glucuronidation capability and immature renal function. The active form of ZDV is ZDV triphosphate. The drug is phosphorylated by cellular kinases. The intracellular half-life is approximately 3 hours, explaining why ZDV can be given as infrequently as twice per day.

Antiviral Effects. As monotherapy, ZDV typically produces a 0.5 to 0.7 log decline in RNA copy number. The effect lasts for several months to years. In children, ZDV monotherapy produces only mild improvements in CD4 numbers. It improves weight growth, at least in the short term, and can improve cognitive function in children with HIV encephalopathy. The primary resistance mutations to ZDV are at codons 41, 70, 215, and 219. The first to appear is at codon 70, whereas the most important site is 215. Mutations at codon 151 may produce multinucleoside resistance.

Adverse Effects. Alone or in combination, ZDV has a significant adverse event profile. The most common problems are hematologic: anemia and neutropenia. They may respond to dose adjustment, although care should be taken to remain in a therapeutic range. Some physicians use erythropoietin or granulocyte colony-stimulating factor to combat these side effects. Thrombocytopenia rarely is produced by ZDV, which reliably produces an increase in red cell volume and can lead to erythrocytic macrocytosis of more than 100 fL. Indeed, the absence of an increase in red cell volume in patients for whom ZDV has been prescribed can be a clinically useful indicator of poor compliance. ZDV also has been associated with myopathy and cardiomyopathy. ZDV frequently produces restlessness, mild headaches, nausea, and fatigue, particularly in older children. Some theoretic concerns exist regarding the potential long-term and transplacental carcinogenicity of ZDV and presumably other NRTIs, but no human data support these concerns.

Nonnucleoside Reverse Transcriptase Inhibitors

Three licensed NNRTIs exist: efavirenz (EFV), NVP, and delavirdine (DLV). They are similar in activity. EFV is used most widely, but pharmacokinetic data for dosing children younger than 3 years of age are not available. Information regarding clinical trials of NNRTIs is presented in Box 140.2. NVP is available in a well-studied liquid preparation as well as capsules, but it seems to have more side effects than does EFV. DLV rarely is used in children and lacks a pediatric preparation. These three NNRTIs have broad cross-resistance. New NNRTIs are being developed with distinct resistance profiles.

Delavirdine

DLV (Rescriptor) was the second FDA-approved NNRTI. It has no liquid formulation and almost no data exist about its use in children. It must be given three times per day, a high level of cross-resistance occurs with NVP, and the major side effect (rash) is less severe than that of NVP.

Efavirenz

EFV (Sustiva) was approved by the FDA in September 1998 for adults and children older than 3 years of age. A solid formulation is available, and a liquid version is in development. EFV has a long half-life, which allows once-daily administration.

Pharmacokinetics. EFV is hepatically excreted. The drug induces cytochrome P-450 isoform CYP3A4, which may decrease PI concentrations. The half-life is long, 40 to 55 hours, allowing once-daily dosing. Good penetration into the central nervous system (CNS) occurs.

Antiviral Effects. EFV resistance is similar to that of other NNRTIs because mutation K103N in the reverse transcriptase gene produces a nearly 20-fold decrease in susceptibility. Mutations at codon 181 produce a threefold reduction in EFV susceptibility, as opposed to a 30-fold decrease in NVP susceptibility. However, this differential has not provided clear advantage for EFV in clinical trials. Other EFV resistance substitutions have been seen at codons 106, 188, and 191.

Adverse Effects. The most common problems with EFV are rash, dizziness, and other minor CNS problems. Rash, most often a maculopapular eruption, occurs in 40% of children, with 7% reporting severe rash. Elevated liver function tests also have been seen in some children, although the rate of severe liver disease seems to be less than with NVP. The greatest toxicity concern relates to pregnant women. Although EFV has not been documented to cause birth defects in humans, three of 13 pregnant monkeys given EFV gave birth to infants with significant birth defects. The three had cleft palate, microphthalmia, and anencephaly with unilateral anophthalmia. Women are advised not to become pregnant while taking EFV.

Nevirapine

NVP (Viramune) is a benzodiazepine NNRTI that was developed simultaneously for children and adults, although the adult preparation was FDA-approved substantially earlier than was the pediatric preparation. The drug is quite potent, even as monotherapy, but rapidly selects for resistant virus.

Pharmacokinetics. The pharmacokinetics of NVP is complex. The drug is lipophilic and distributes into body tissues well. NVP administration autoinduces metabolism, so the same dose given over time leads to a decreasing serum concentration. The change in clearance is approximately 1.5- to twofold. Because a finite degree of induction occurs, NVP is given once daily for the first week, then twice-daily dosing is initiated. However, given its long half-life (approximately 25 hours in adults), in some cases NVP is administered on a once-daily schedule. In neonates, hepatic immaturity means that NVP metabolism is very slow, and a single oral dose can produce a therapeutic concentration for several days. This effect of NVP, combined with its potency and the fact NVP crosses the placenta well, is the reason that NVP is used to decrease mother-to-child HIV transmission in the developing world.

Antiviral Effects. A single point mutation at codon 103 of the reverse transcriptase leads to high-level NVP resistance. Codons 181, 188, and 106 also can decrease NVP sensitivity. When the drug is used as monotherapy, almost complete NVP resistance can be seen as soon as 4 to 6 weeks. When NVP is part of a combination, the drug has activity similar to that of PIs.

Adverse Effects. NVP is associated with two primary adverse effects. First, early after initiation of therapy, hepatitis, elevated hepatic transaminase levels, or both can develop. The other major side effect is rash, which occurs in approximately 8% of children. NVP rash begins as a macular-papular eruption, most often within 5 weeks of starting therapy. In most cases, the rash evolves to include fever and malaise. Administration of NVP should be stopped if rash occurs because the exanthem can evolve to severe Stevens-Johnson syndrome. In addition, patients demonstrating the rash should have liver function tests performed.

Protease Inhibitors

The PIs are effective because they can inhibit specifically the HIV protease while not affecting human proteases. The most closely related human proteases are in the renin-angiotensin-converting enzyme family. Most of the current PIs are peptidomimetic: they emulate the substrate of the enzyme but bind in the protease rather than being cleaved. Unfortunately, working with PIs pharmacologically is difficult because they are not readily made into suspensions or water-based solutions, they taste bad, and they interact with the hepatic cytochrome P-450 system in complex ways. Some PIs induce certain P-450 isoforms while inhibiting others. For example, RTV is a relatively broad inhibitor of the P-450 enzyme system that induces its own metabolism and also complicates the use of many other drugs. Information about clinical trials of PIs is presented in Box 140.2.

Amprenavir

Amprenavir (APV; Agenerase) has a unique resistance pattern, rendering it a candidate for use in combination with other PIs or as second-line PI therapy. The drug has been approved by the FDA for children older than 4 years of age.

Pharmacokinetics. AMP is cleared by the cytochrome P-450 system, which it also inhibits. However, APV does not appear to induce or inhibit its own metabolism. Specifically, APV inhibits the CYP3A4 isoform of the cytochrome P-450 system, the most common isoform. The plasma half-life is somewhat variable but averages approximately 7 hours, a length suitable for twice-daily dosing. However, the dosage forms are somewhat inconvenient, requiring a large numbers of bulky tablets.

Antiviral Effects. APV has a potent antiviral effect similar to those of other PIs. The major resistance mutations have been found at protease codons 50 and 84, with contributions from 46, 47, 54, 82, and 90. APV has been evaluated in combination with other PIs, and sufficient differences are apparent in its resistance pattern to render APV use with other PIs beneficial.

Adverse Effects. The most common adverse effects with APV are gastrointestinal. Some patients have headache, malaise, or fatigue, and cutaneous reactions can occur. Stevens-Johnson syndrome is a particular concern that should result in discontinuation of APV.

Fosamprenavir. Fosamprenavir (Lexiva) is a phosphate ester prodrug of APV. It has very similar biologic behaviors, but the esterification allows for greater absorption and more convenient dosing. Pediatric experience is quite limited.

Lopinavir

Lopinavir (LPV; in combination with ritonavir [RTV], Kaletra; LPV/r) is a potent PI with a unique resistance pattern and a short serum half-life. To compensate for the half-life, LPV is sold in a fixed-ratio (4:1) combination with RTV. Thus boosted, LPV can be administered on a 12-hour schedule.

Pharmacokinetics. LPV has a relatively short half-life on its own but can be given every 12 hours as LPV/r. The drug is hepatically cleared by the cytochrome P-450 enzyme system. LPV/r inhibits the clearance of many hepatically metabolized drugs, so caution is important concerning drug-drug interactions.

Antiviral Effects. LPV is among the most potent of the PIs. Resistance occurs at PI codon 82, the same site as for RTV and indinavir (IDV). However, other site mutations affecting RTV and IDV seem to have less effect on LPV. The fact that LPV has a distinct resistance pattern, as well as the combination with RTV, means that LPV/r often is combined with other PIs in late-stage regimens for advanced disease in previously treated patients.

Adverse Effects. Liquid Kaletra tastes better than liquid RTV, but both are bad-tasting medicines, containing roughly 42% ethanol (around 85 proof). The problems most commonly reported are the taste, vomiting, and loose stools. However, the drug generally is well tolerated if the child can be convinced to take it. The capsule formulation has considerable advantages in this regard.

Indinavir

IDV (Crixivan) generally has fallen out of favor, and pediatric experience is, in any case, very limited. IDV is potent and has a resistance pattern similar to that of RTV, but it has the potential to produce several distinct types of adverse effects. IDV also is difficult to administer because it should be administered every 8 hours in children and should be given on an empty stomach.

Pharmacokinetics. IDV is only soluble at a low pH; thus, it should be taken on an empty stomach. Once absorbed, IDV is carried on plasma proteins and is metabolized by glucuronidation and the cytochrome P-450 system. Some IDV is excreted through the kidneys. Because of urine's neutral pH, the IDV can precipitate and produce kidney stones. IDV has interactions with many drugs that are metabolized by the cytochrome P-450 system, most commonly to slow the metabolism of the other drug. IDV is an example of a therapeutic agent for which the pediatric pharmacokinetic profile is distinct from that of adults. It has rapid absorption, which leads to higher peak concentrations, followed by more rapid clearance than in adults. The result is a shorter dosing interval and, because of the high-peak concentrations, probably more side effects than in adults.

Antiviral Effects. IDV is a potent agent, comparable to RTV. The pattern of mutations seen is almost identical to that of RTV, and a high degree of cross-resistance occurs. In the initial IDV trials, researchers discovered that low doses of the agent allowed the evolution of PI-resistant quasispecies. When patients subsequently were switched to higher doses of IDV, no antiviral effect was seen because of the existence of mutations that had evolved at the lower dose. Thus, subtherapeutic dosing, either by misprescription or erratic compliance, allows permanent PI resistance to occur. This phenomenon also is true for other antiretroviral drugs.

Adverse Effects. Because of its solubility characteristics, IDV can form crystals in the kidney after filtration through the glomerulus. These crystals can agglomerate into small kidney stones. To minimize the formation of IDV stones, patients should drink lots of water or other fluids after taking the drug. The proportion of children who will have stones is not known, but some studies have suggested that the higher serum peak of IDV after oral dosing may lead to formation of more stones.

Other side effects of IDV include hyperbilirubinemia, which occurs in 5% to 10% of patients, nausea, abdominal pain,

headache, and, rarely, diabetes. A pattern of fat redistribution was seen in patients with chronic IDV use and has been described with the use of other PIs.

Nelfinavir

Nelfinavir (NLV; Viracept) is a less convenient drug to administer than RTV but has fewer adverse reactions. The medication is available in tablets and a granular powder. The powder is somewhat bulky, and bioavailability is not uniform. NLV is less potent than LPV/r, and some studies suggest it may not protect as well against the development of resistance mutations in the other drugs with which it is used in combination.

Pharmacokinetics. NLV is hepatically metabolized by multiple cytochrome P-450 isoforms, including CYP3A. The adult plasma half-life is 3.5 to 5.0 hours. The drug is highly protein bound, and relatively little is cleared through the kidneys. Most of the drug is excreted through the gastrointestinal tract and feces. The standard dosage is given every 8 to 12 hours. The 12-hour interval has not been demonstrated clearly to be clinically equal to every 8 hours but is better for patient compliance with the regimen.

Antiviral Effects. NLV is similar to other PIs in its antiviral effect. The most important resistance mutation is D30N, which was found by 12 to 16 weeks in 56% of patients who received NLV monotherapy. Marked cross-resistance occurs between NLV and the other PIs. Patients in whom NLV treatment fails and who still have low-level resistance may respond to other PIs or PI combinations. However, 65% to 80% of isolates with more than tenfold resistance to NLV also had more than a fourfold increase in resistance to other PIs, and NLV rarely works well if resistance to other PIs already has been documented.

Adverse Effects. NLV has a tolerable level of adverse drug effects. The most common side effect is diarrhea, which generally is manageable with symptomatic measures. However, diarrhea in some children may be such that they are unable to tolerate NLV. Less common problems include tiredness, abdominal pains, and rashes. Diabetes occurs rarely, as is the case with all PIs.

Ritonavir

RTV (Norvir) was the first PI approved by the FDA for children. RTV is available in both a liquid formulation and gel caps. Unfortunately, the liquid has an unpleasant taste and contains 43% ethanol. RTV is very potent, but because of significant side effects and drug interactions, it should be used with care. The most common use of RTV takes advantage of its potent effect on the metabolism of some other antiretroviral drugs. A low dose of RTV is given as an inhibitor of hepatic metabolism, which then extends the half-life of other drugs such as LPV or APV.

Pharmacokinetics. The pharmacokinetics of RTV is complicated by its effect on hepatic enzymes. RTV is hepatically metabolized by the cytochrome P-450 system. RTV generally inhibits P-450, but in contrast to the general rule, it induces its own metabolism. As a result, RTV is begun at one-half the standard dose, then increased after a period of induction. Although this strategy of beginning with a low dose and moving to a higher one seems counterintuitive to the general scheme of dose management in PIs (start or stop all medications at once), in this case the concentrations of drug remain fairly constant. Because RTV metabolism appears to be saturable, increasing doses may produce higher than expected levels. RTV is absorbed well orally, regardless of food. The half-life is 3 to 4 hours. Many interactions that occur with other medications can affect the metabolism of the RTV, as well as the other compounds. As noted earlier, RTV often is used as a pharmacologic booster for other drugs, to increase their half-life.

Antiviral Effects. RTV is very potent and has a relatively complex pattern of resistance mutations. The resistance mutations to RTV are almost identical to those of IDV, so a switch from one drug to the other for resistance reasons is unlikely to be beneficial. The main mutations associated with RTV resistance have been at HIV protease codons 82, 84, and 90. Some patients with high-level resistance to NLV also are refractory to RTV treatment, although it depends on which anti-NLV mutations are present.

Adverse Effects. RTV is associated with many problematic side effects: nausea and vomiting are produced by both the RTV itself and the ethanol solvent. In some children, the nausea becomes chronic and does not decrease with time. RTV also can produce diarrhea, anorexia, headaches, circumoral paresthesias, and elevated hepatic transaminases. In rare circumstances, it may produce diabetes. Hypercholesterolemia and hypertriglyceridemia both are common findings in laboratory tests when RTV is used at therapeutic dosing levels, although they are less problematic at the lower doses used for pharmacologic boosting. Care should be taken in coadministering any drug with RTV. A long list of absolute and relative contraindications includes many drugs commonly used in HIV disease. The common thread is clearance by the cytochrome P-450 enzyme system.

Saquinavir

Although it was the first PI approved for adult use, very little pediatric dosing information exists for saquinavir (SQV; Invirase or Fortovase [soft-gel capsule]). Because of its poor bioavailability, SQV usually is used in combination with RTV. This combination is rational both because SQV has a distinct resistance pattern and because RTV increases serum SQV levels. Some patients in whom other PI regimens have failed may respond to the combination of RTV and SQV, although they will do best if new NRTIs are introduced at the same time.

Although no pediatric dose for SQV has been established yet, the probable dosing interval will be every 8 hours. The drug interactions of SQV are very much like those of the other PIs, although they are less significant than those of RTV.

Pharmacokinetics. If given without an RTV boost, SQV is administered as a soft-gel capsule. The hard tablet formulation is not adequately bioavailable (less than 5% absorbed) to use without boosting. Although absorption of the soft-gel capsules in children is similar to that in adults, children appear to clear oral SQV somewhat more rapidly, and a higher milligram per kilogram dose is required. Food increases absorption of SQV in the soft-gel formulation. SQV is cleared almost entirely by cytochrome P-450 CYP3A4. Concomitant NLV, IDV, or RTV therapy increases levels of SQV by inhibiting hepatic metabolism (approximately fourfold, sixfold, and 20-fold, respectively). In fact, RTV can increase the serum half-life of SQV such that only twice-daily dosing is required. SQV does not penetrate the cerebrospinal fluid.

Antiviral Effects. SQV has a unique resistance pattern among the licensed PIs. The key mutations are G48V and L90M. In its soft-gel preparation, SQV probably is similar to other PIs in potency.

Adverse Effects. SQV generally is well tolerated. The most common adverse experiences are diarrhea, abdominal pain, headache, and nausea. Diabetes rarely may occur. Because photosensitivity can occur with SQV, use of sunscreen and protective clothing is suggested.

Fusion Inhibitor

Enfuvirtide

Enfuvirtide (T-20; Fuzeon) is the only available fusion inhibitor. The drug is a 36-amino acid peptide that binds to the gp41 subunit of the virus attachment protein. It prevents fusion of the virus' lipid bilayer with that of the cell, thereby blocking virus entry into the cell. This mechanism is unique to T-20, so cross-resistance is not a particular problem. The largest problem with T-20 is the need to inject the drug subcutaneously twice a day. This has limited its use to late-stage regimens. Additional information about clinical trials in T-20 is presented in Box 140.2.

Pharmacokinetics. T-20 needs to be injected subcutaneously. The metabolism of the drug is catabolic breakdown, with recycling of the amino acids. The half-life is 3.8 hours, and the drug is administered every 12 hours.

Antiviral Effects. T-20 binds to the gp41 of the virus attachment protein, preventing the virus from being able to fuse with its cellular target. Resistance does occur and is mediated by changes in the gp41 protein at codons 38, 43, 36, 40, 42, and 45. T-20, like other antiretroviral drugs, is best used in combination and in particular with combinations of agents that still retain activity against a patient's viral quasispecies.

TREATMENT WITH ANTIRETROVIRAL DRUGS

Several decisions affect management of antiretroviral drugs. The art of antiretroviral treatment is complicated: rules and principles evolve constantly. Given the high stakes of mismanagement (e.g., permanent loss of effective therapeutic options), in most cases the management of antiretroviral drugs should be left to physicians with specialized expertise and experience.

The first decision is whether to start therapy. Because surrogate markers are of limited value for predicting progression of disease in children younger than 2 to 3 years old, nearly all children younger than 2 years old are treated. Children at this age also have the greatest risk of developing CNS disease, and effective antiretroviral treatment can be very protective of CNS function. The worst risk in treatment of young children is actually the challenge of giving the medication itself. Infants and toddlers can be very oppositional, and many parents have difficulty giving bad tasting medications to well-appearing children. Add in an overlay of parental guilt and perhaps an element of denial and the situation becomes one with a high potential for partial adherence and its associated high risk of drug resistance. Thus, great care should be taken during teaching about the initiation of therapy, with a particular focus placed on why good adherence is so critical.

In older children, the decision regarding when to start treatment becomes more like the decision in adults. Any child with serious HIV-related symptoms should be treated, as should children older than 3 years with CD4$^+$ counts less than 350 cells/mm^3. Patients with a high viral load probably warrant treatment as well, although the viral load threshold for "mandatory" treatment has not been defined clearly. In all cases, the child and parent should "buy in" to treatment before they are sent home with prescriptions, because partial adherence is such a risk factor for the loss of valuable therapeutic options.

With the exceptions of some prophylaxis schemes, all antiretroviral treatment regimens now involve combinations of multiple agents. Clinical trials have demonstrated that drugs from different classes should be included in each regimen. Nearly all regimens begin with two or more NRTIs. In adolescents and adults, the NRTIs often are given as fixed-ratio combinations such as Combivir (ZDV and 3TC) or Trizivir (abacavir, ZDV, and 3TC). Recent trends have favored once-daily regimens, such as ddI and FTC, although they are not available as fixed-ratio combinations and still are relatively untested in children.

To the NRTI combination core, either an NNRTI or a PI, and sometimes a drug from each class, usually is added. Among the NNRTIs, NVP tends to be used in young children because of its liquid preparation and EFV in older children because of its established once-daily dosing and side effect profile. Among the PIs, NLV and LPV/r often are selected as first-line agents, although fashions in PI selection have shifted over the course of time.

Second- and third-line treatment regimens for patients who have disease progression during their initial therapy often involve combinations with more agents, including combinations of PIs. Drugs that are more difficult to administer, such as the injectable fusion inhibitor T-20, may be used, whereas they would not be acceptable as first-line therapy for convenience reasons. Unfortunately, second-line regimens tend to be less active than are first-line ones. Certain drugs, such as abacavir, also are unlikely to be beneficial in second-line regimens or for people who have been treated with other drugs in the same class (atazanavir, NLV, any NNRTI).

The key element to therapeutic success in antiretroviral treatment is adherence. Although initially many options may be available, low barriers to resistance in some drugs (NNRTIs, 3TC, NLV) and the potential for the development of cross-resistance (all classes) mean that great care must be taken to instruct the patient who is starting treatment. With good adherence, HIV disease in most patients can be controlled and good quality of life maintained, the primary objectives of antiretroviral therapy.

Suggested Readings

Butler KM, Husson RN, Balis FM, et al. Dideoxyinosine in children with symptomatic human immunodeficiency virus infection. *N Engl J Med* 1991;324:137.

Centers for Disease Control and Prevention. Case-control study of HIV seroconversion in health-care workers after percutaneous exposure to HIV-infected blood: France, United Kingdom, and United States, January 1988–August 1994. *MMWR Morb Mortal Wkly Rep* 1995;44:929.

Centers for Disease Control and Prevention. Update: provisional Public Health Service recommendations for chemoprophylaxis after occupational exposure to HIV. *MMWR Morb Mortal Wkly Rep* 1996;45:468.

Connor EM, Sperling RS, Gelber R, et al. Reduction of maternal-infant transmission of human immunodeficiency virus type 1 with zidovudine treatment. *N Engl J Med* 1994;331:1173.

Englund JA, Baker CJ, Raskino C, et al. A trial comparing zidovudine, ddI, and combination therapy for initial treatment of symptomatic HIV-infected children. *N Engl J Med* 1997;336:1704.

Fischl MA, Richman DD, Grieco MH, et al. The efficacy of azidothymidine (AZT) in the treatment of patients with AIDS and AIDS-related complex: a double-blind, placebo-controlled trial. *N Engl J Med* 1987;317:185.

HIV Paediatric Prognostic Markers Collaborative Study Group. Short-term risk of disease progression in HIV-1-infected children receiving no antiretroviral therapy or zidovudine monotherapy: a meta-analysis. *Lancet* 2003;362:1605.

Kline MW, Van Dyke RB, Lindsey JC, et al. A randomized comparative trial of stavudine (d4T) versus zidovudine (ZDV, AZT) in children with human immunodeficiency virus infection. *Pediatrics* 1998;110:214.

Luzuriaga K, Bryson Y, Krogstad P, et al. Combination treatment with zidovudine, didanosine, and nevirapine in infants with human immunodeficiency virus type 1 infection. *N Engl J Med* 1997;336:1343.

McKinney RE, Maha MA, Connor EM, et al. A multicenter trial of oral zidovudine in children with advanced human immunodeficiency virus disease. *N Engl J Med* 1991;324:1018.

McKinney RE, Johnson GM, Stanley K, et al. A randomized study of combined zidovudine-lamivudine versus didanosine monotherapy in children with symptomatic therapy-naive HIV-infection: the Pediatric AIDS Clinical Trials Group Protocol 300 Study. *J Pediatr* 1998;133:500.

Mueller BU, Butler KM, Stocker VL, et al. Clinical and pharmacokinetic evaluation of long-term therapy with didanosine in children with HIV infection. *Pediatrics* 1994;94:724.

Pediatric Network for Treatment of AIDS (PENTA). Comparison of dual nucleoside-analogue reverse-transcriptase inhibitor regimens with and without nelfinavir in children with HIV-1 who have not previously been treated: the Penta 5 randomised trial. *Lancet* 2002;359:733.

Van Dyke RB, Lee S, Johnson GM, et al. Reported adherence as a determinant of response to highly active antiretroviral therapy in children who have human immunodeficiency virus infection. *Pediatrics* 2002;109:e61.

Working Group on Antiretroviral Therapy and Medical Management of HIV-Infected Children. *Guidelines for the use of antiretroviral agents in pediatric HIV infection.* http://AIDSinfo.nih.gov; accessed 5/21/2004.

CHAPTER 141 ■ PROPHYLAXIS FOR EXPOSURE TO HUMAN IMMUNODEFICIENCY VIRUS

KENNETH L. DOMINGUEZ

Disclaimer: The use of trade names is for identification only and does not imply endorsement by the Public Health Service or the U.S. Department of Health and Human Services.

BACKGROUND

Postexposure prophylaxis (PEP) is the timely administration of antiretroviral (ARV) chemoprophylaxis to reduce the probability of becoming infected with HIV after an acute well-defined exposure and can be categorized as occupational (oPEP) or nonoccupational (nPEP). This chapter describes the epidemiology of various types of HIV exposures that may call into question use of PEP, recent animal and human studies supporting the use of PEP, current U.S. Public Health Service (USPHS)/Department of Health and Human Services (HHS) recommendations for oPEP and nPEP, and special considerations regarding pediatric nPEP. (See http://aidsinfo.nih.gov for most recent updates.) The USPHS oPEP recommendations continue to recommend a two-tiered system of three ARVs versus two ARVs, depending on the level of risk. The chapter highlights a change in the HHS nPEP recommendations, which now emphasize the importance of using three drug regimens, when feasible, to be consistent with the current standard of care regarding treatment of established HIV infection.

oPEP

Current Centers for Disease Control and Prevention (CDC) oPEP guidelines define health care personnel (HCP) as persons whose activities involve contact with patients or with patients' blood or other body fluids in a health care, laboratory, or public-safety setting. Occupational exposures that could place HCP at risk for HIV infection include (a) percutaneous injury (e.g., a needlestick or cut with a sharp object) or (b) contact of mucous membrane or nonintact skin (e.g., exposed skin that is chapped, abraded, or afflicted with dermatitis) with blood, tissue, or other body fluids that are potentially infectious. Nonintact skin exposures with potentially infectious body materials are not considered to be of risk except for direct contact (i.e., without barrier protection) with concentrated HIV in a research laboratory or production facility. Other body fluids include (a) semen, vaginal secretions, or other body fluids contaminated with visible blood that have been implicated in the transmission of HIV infection and (b) fluids with an undetermined risk of HIV transmission (i.e., cerebrospinal, synovial, pleural, peritoneal, pericardial, and amniotic fluids). In the absence of visible blood in the fluid or substance, exposure to saliva, tears, sweat, urine, or HIV feces is not considered to pose a risk for transmission of and does not require postexposure follow-up. Although mother-to-child transmission (MTCT) of HIV can occur through breast-feeding, exposure to breast milk has not been implicated in occupational transmission of HIV.

nPEP

Examples of nonoccupational exposures to HIV include exposure to HIV through unprotected sex or through sharing needles with HIV-infected persons. More common pediatric consultations for nPEP involve sexual abuse or exposure to discarded needles.

Studies of the Biologic Plausibility of PEP

In 1990, the USPHS published the first statement on oPEP at which time there was a lack of convincing data on the efficacy of PEP. Since then, additional data provide a stronger rationale for HIV PEP, including information regarding primary HIV pathogenesis, the biologic plausibility of the effectiveness of ARV drug administration for the PEP, and the effectiveness of ARV drugs for PEP in animal and human studies.

Primary HIV Pathogenesis and Biologic Plausibility of PEP Effectiveness

In primate models, simian immunodeficiency virus (SIV) travels within the inoculation site to dendritic-like cells during the first 24 hours, to regional lymph nodes in the next 24 to 48 hours, and to peripheral blood within 5 days of inoculation. Therefore, it seems biologically plausible that PEP, if started within hours after HIV exposure, could prevent spread of infection beyond the initially infected cells or lymph nodes.

Effectiveness of PEP in Animal and Human Studies

Animal and human data support the biologic plausibility of the effectiveness of HIV PEP. Animal models of the effectiveness of PEP vary by type of animal, type of virus, route and strength of inoculation, drug used for PEP, and the number, timing, and duration of doses of PEP. In primate models, macaques inoculated with SIV either intravenously or orally and treated with PEP at various time points using ZDV or (R)-9-(2-phosphonylmethoxypropyl) adenine (PMPA or tenofovir) exhibited a range of effectiveness in preventing infection or decreasing the severity of the initial infection, depending on the model. In general, early initiation of PEP, within a few hours of exposure, was associated with the highest effectiveness.

Human studies have been primarily observational. A case control study evaluated HIV seroconversion in HCP in the United States, France, and the United Kingdom with percutaneous exposure to HIV-infected blood. PEP (consisting of 1,000 mg/day of ZDV for 3 to 4 weeks) was received by 9 of 33 (27%) cases and 247 of 679 (36%) of controls. The likelihood of developing HIV infection among HCP who received PEP with ZDV was approximately 81% lower than among those who did not receive such PEP. Observational studies and registries designed to collect information about nPEP are being conducted and established, and thus far no seroconversions have been reported among registries in the United States, France, Switzerland, and Australia among individuals who received nPEP after exposure to HIV.

Studies of nPEP in Pediatric Practice

Few data exist regarding PEP in pediatric patients; however, nPEP surveys indicate that few hospitals or clinics have institutional policies for nPEP and patients often fail to complete a 4-week course of nPEP. Financial concerns, side effects, additional psychiatric and substance abuse issues, and the degree of parental involvement influenced whether PEP and HIV follow-up testing was completed. Many studies suggest that a successful PEP program should include psychosocial support, early follow-up with a physician knowledgeable about pediatric ARV therapy to assess compliance, and a written institutional protocol to provide a coordinated and standardized approach.

EPIDEMIOLOGY OF EXPOSURES TO HIV

Exposures in HCP

The average risk for HIV infection for HCP exposed to HIV-infected blood has been estimated at 0.3% for percutaneous exposures and 0.09% for mucous membrane exposures. The risk is unknown for skin exposures, but it is thought to be less than that for mucous membrane exposures. As of December 31, 2002, the CDC has received reports of 57 U.S. HCP with documented HIV seroconversion temporally associated with occupational HIV exposure and has been informed of an additional 139 HCP who report occupationally acquired HIV infection without such documentation. The risk of HIV transmission occurring from exposures that involve a larger volume of blood, especially when the source patient's viral load is probably high, is estimated to exceed the average risk of 0.3%.

There are very limited epidemiologic data on the most common exposures to blood for HCP in pediatric health care settings. Up to 6 sharp object injuries (SOIs) per 100 employees per year have been reported in pediatric health care settings

BOX 141.1   Preventing and Managing Bottle Switches in Day Care Centers*

1. Make sure that parents label each child's bottle of formula or breast milk with the child's name and the date.
   - Use only a bottle labeled for that child on that date
   - Never accept an unlabeled bottle from a parent
   - Do not use any unlabeled bottles that have been accepted accidentally
2. In the event that a child has mistakenly been given another child's bottle of expressed breast milk, do the following:
   - Inform the parents of the child who was given the wrong bottle that:
     - Their child was given another child's bottle of expressed breast milk
     - The risk of transmission of HIV is very small (see discussion below)
     - They should notify the child's physician of the exposure
     - The child should have a baseline test for HIV
   - Inform the mother who expressed the breast milk of the bottle switch and ask:
     - If she has ever had an HIV test and, if so, if she would be willing to share the results with the parents
     - If she does not know if she has ever had an HIV test, if she would be willing to contact her obstetrician

and find out and, if she has, share the results with the parents
   - If she has never had an HIV test, if she would be willing to have one and share the results with the parents and
   - When the breast milk was expressed and how it was handled prior to being brought to the facility
   - Provide the exposed child's physician information on when the milk was expressed and how the milk was handled prior to being brought to the facility.
3. Risk of HIV transmission from expressed breast milk drunk by another child is believed to be low because:
   - In the United States, women who are HIV-infected and aware of that fact are advised not to breast-feed their infants
   - Chemicals present in breast milk act, together with time and cold temperatures, to destroy the HIV present in expressed breast milk.

*Adapted from Hale CM et al. The ABCs of safe and healthy child care: A handbook for child care providers. Atlanta: Department of Health and Human Service, Centers for Disease Control and Prevention Publication, 1996.

---

involving mainly needles and most often among phlebotomists, nurses, and physicians. In addition, one-third of the approximately 12 human bite exposures per 10,000 occupied hospital beds that occur per year involved children and have failed to result in HIV seroconversion.

Prevention

Measures to prevent occupational HIV exposures include strict adherence to standard precautions and Office of Safety and Health Administration (OSHA) guidelines. Examples include the use of safer medical devices where appropriate, properly restraining patients when drawing lab samples, being well trained in doing procedures involving sharp objects, and using gloves when managing patients who might be combative or when manipulating the oral cavity. When handling breast milk, the use of gloves is not necessary except in situations where exposures to breast milk might be frequent, as in breast milk banking, or if the HCP has nonintact skin.

Exposures among Children in Health Care Settings

Children are present in hospitals either as patients or visitors and are subject to situations that could place them at risk for HIV infection. There have been case reports of children that were probably exposed inadvertently to blood from an HIV-infected person in the hospital or during in-home health care. Newborns have been inadvertently fed the expressed breast milk intended for another infant. Such exposures to breast milk would generally be considered to carry a low risk for HIV exposure unless the hospital is located in a geographic area with a high seroprevalence in women of child-bearing age.

Prevention

Measures to prevent pediatric exposures to HIV in health care settings include rapid disposal of used needles in sharps containers located out of the reach of children but readily accessible to HCP and use of standard procedures for labeling and dispensing bottles of expressed breast milk. Health care institutions may consider adapting existing recommendations related to bottles of expressed breast milk designed for day-care centers to hospital settings (Box 141.1). A bottle of expressed breast milk that has been properly labeled with the mother's and infant's hospital identifiers should always be checked against the infant's identification bracelet prior to providing bottle-feedings of expressed breast milk. In addition, health care institutions that allow feeding of infants with human donor milk should use donor milk banks that adhere to existing state laws or regulations or national guidelines that ensure proper screening of donors and sterilization of milk.

Exposures among Children Outside the Health Care Setting

Children can be exposed to HIV outside the hospital setting. Examples of such exposures include sexual abuse involving oral, anal, or vaginal penetration by an HIV-infected perpetrator, needle sticks in the home or public areas with recently discarded syringes containing HIV-infected blood, exposures to HIV-containing breast milk, and human bites that compromise the skin's integrity and involve an exchange of HIV-infected blood.

Sexual Abuse

There were 88,238 cases of various types of sexual abuse in children younger than 18 years of age reported in the United

States during 1999, including 26 cases of sexual abuse (17 confirmed, 9 suspected) among children with AIDS. These cases probably represent an underestimate due to the underreporting of such abuse.

Among adults, the probability of HIV transmission associated with a single act of unprotected receptive anal intercourse has been estimated to be between 0.008 and 0.032 and with vaginal intercourse to be between 0.0005 and 0.0015. The medical literature suggests that child sexual abuse may be a more efficient means of transmitting HIV than is adult sexual abuse because of anatomic differences and a higher frequency of repeated molestations and longer term abuse in children.

Any sexually assaulted child should be assessed within 72 hours of the assault. The clinician should (a) review the local HIV/AIDS epidemiology and assess risk for HIV infection in the assailant; (b) evaluate circumstances of the assault that may affect risk for HIV transmission; (c) consult with an HIV specialist if considering PEP; (d) discuss PEP, including its toxicity and unknown efficacy with the caregiver; (e) if indicated, provide enough medication to last until the return visit 3 to 7 days later, at which time the child can be reevaluated, including for his or her tolerance of the medication (if PEP is prescribed); and (f) perform HIV testing at baseline and then at 6 weeks, 3 months, and 6 months later.

The following situations are associated with a high risk of transmission of sexually transmitted infections (STIs), and HIV testing should be performed if (a) one or more children in a household has signs or symptoms of an STI; (b) the suspected assailant is known to have an STI or to be at high risk for STIs (e.g., the individual has multiple sexual partners or a history of STIs); (c) the patient or his or her parent(s) requests testing; (d) there is a high prevalence of STIs in the community; (e) there is evidence of genital, oral, or anal penetration or ejaculation; or (f) the assault involved traumatic mucosal injuries of the anus or vagina, associated with bleeding and contact with the semen of a known HIV-infected assailant. An example of a lower risk exposure is the sexual abuse of a child by a perpetrator with unknown HIV infection status in an area with low HIV seroprevalence.

Prevention. Examples of strategies to prevent the sexual abuse of children include (a) educating caretakers about teaching children to refuse to engage in abusive situations, to avoid keeping secrets related to abuse, and to disclose abusive situations to someone who is trusted; and (b) educating parents to select day-care centers with licensed day-care workers, open and visible play areas, and policies that allow parental visitation and do not allow for individual instruction in isolated settings.

Breast Milk Exposures

Globally, breast milk transmission of HIV represents an important mode of MTCT of HIV. In the United States, exposure to breast milk from an unknown or unscreened source is unlikely to result in HIV transmission, but each exposure must be considered on a case-by-case basis. Such exposures may occur through the switching or mislabeling of bottles containing expressed breast milk (e.g., in day-care settings), allowing an infant to breast-feed from a wet nurse with unknown HIV infection status, or using expressed, unpasteurized human milk that has not been screened for HIV or pasteurized. The likelihood that HIV is present in the breast milk of an unknown or unscreened source is low in the United States because the seroprevalence of HIV among pregnant women has been estimated at less than 2 per 1,000. The USPHS guidelines recommended that pregnant woman undergo HIV testing and that HIV-infected women should not breast-feed their infants. The

risk of such an exposure would increase if the source individual is determined to have a history of behaviors that put her at risk for HIV transmission or comes from a community with a high HIV seroprevalence.

Prevention. The CDC recommends that prenatal HIV testing should be offered to all pregnant women and routine rapid HIV testing should be offered to all pregnant women whose HIV status is still unknown at the time of delivery. HIV-infected mothers in resource-rich settings should be counseled to avoid breast-feeding, and clinicians should provide education to HIV-infected mothers regarding feeding options. Every effort should be made to avoid exposure to HIV-contaminated breast milk. Other prevention strategies are listed in the section on pediatric exposures in health care settings.

Discarded Needles or Syringes

The risk of HIV transmission occurring from discarded needles in public places is thought to be low. It is estimated that the probability of HIV transmission associated with a puncture wound involving a known HIV-contaminated needle in a health care setting is 0.0032. It is likely that discarded needles in outdoor public settings have a lower risk for transmission due to the effect of environmental factors and the length of time between injection drug use and a subsequent, accidental puncture wound. The stability of HIV under various environmental conditions has been shown to decrease over time and rarely has been detected in needles used for intramuscular or subcutaneous injections in HIV-infected persons. At room temperature, survival of HIV in syringes is halved for every tenfold decrease in blood volume and HIV is detected in less than 1% of syringes after more than a week. The following factors are likely to increase the risk or are required for HIV transmission in needle-stick injuries: presence of blood in a needle or syringe emptying into the wound, large needle bore size, deep puncture wounds, a needlestick injury directly into a vein or artery, a short lag time from time of discarding the needle or syringe to time of injury, positive HIV infection status of source individual, and a high seroprevalence among persons frequenting the geographic area where the needle was discarded (Table 141.1). For example, a child injured by picking up a freshly discarded syringe containing blood from a known HIV-infected injection drug user would be at higher risk of acquiring HIV infection. However, most pediatric needlestick injuries do not occur under such

---

TABLE 141.1

LOGISTIC REGRESSION ANALYSIS OF RISK FACTORS FOR HIV TRANSMISSION AFTER PERCUTANEOUS EXPOSURE TO HIV-INFECTED BLOOD*

Risk Factor	Adjusted Odds Ratio	(95% Confidence Interval)
Deep injury	15	(6.0–41)
Visible blood on device	6.2	(2.2–21)
Procedure involving needle in a vein or artery	4.3	(1.7–12)
Terminal illness in source patient	5.6	(2.0–16)
Postexposure use of zidovudine	0.19	(0.06–0.52)

*Table reprinted from Cardo DM, Culver DH, Ciesielski CA, et al. A case-control study of HIV seroconversion in health care workers after percutaneous exposure. Centers for Disease Control and Prevention Needlestick Surveillance Group. *New Engl J Med* 1997;337:1485.

circumstances and would be considered to have a very low risk for transmission.

Prevention. Children should be educated to avoid playing in areas known to be frequented by injecting drug users and to avoid playing with discarded needles and syringes. Needle exchange programs may play a role in decreasing the number of discarded needles in public places.

Human Bites

It has been estimated that 250,000 human bites occur annually in the United States. Fifty percent of children at one day-care center were bitten at least once in a year. There is currently no evidence that human bites without the presence of blood-tinged saliva in the wound pose an HIV infection risk to the victim. Although biting has been cited as a possible mode of transmission in several case reports, in all of the well-documented reports, the bites were by adults and involved severe biting with blood exchange. Seroconversion was documented in a man bitten by an HIV-infected commercial sex worker with blood-tinged saliva.

Management of bite wounds should include an evaluation for breaks or abrasions in the skin of the bite victim. Should such breaks or abrasions occur, the person who inflicted the bite should be evaluated for the presence of blood in the mouth or oral lesions, which may cause the wound to be contaminated with blood. Proper wound care includes irrigation, debridement, immobilization, and elevation of the affected body part and antimicrobial prophylaxis.

Prevention. Biting in day-care centers may be deterred by setting limits for a child's behavior, teaching and reinforcing coping skills, and providing other acceptable avenues or activities for children to release or redirect their anger.

Sports-Related and Day-Care–Related Bleeding Injuries

The risk of transmitting HIV or other bloodborne pathogens through sports-related injuries during athletic activities is considered to be low. To transmit a bloodborne pathogen during an athletic activity, blood from a bleeding wound or exudative skin lesion of an HIV-infected athlete would have to contaminate the skin lesion or exposed mucous membranes of another athlete. The likelihood of transmission of bloodborne pathogens in contact sports is estimated at 1 in 4 million/players/games for HIV. There have been no substantiated cases of HIV transmission and two cases of hepatitis B virus (HBV) transmission between athletes during an athletic event.

Similar to sports-related injuries, the incidence of injuries in day-care centers in the United States is low; the overall reported incidence of injuries in day-care settings has ranged from 0.25 to 2.50 per 100,000 child hours, with about one-third of such injuries requiring sutures in Washington state.

Prevention. Guidelines to prevent bloodborne pathogen transmission during athletic activities or at day-care facilities have been described. Once a child or athlete has suffered a bleeding injury, the physical activity associated with the injury should be stopped until the wound has been cleaned and dressed, the bleeding has stopped, blood-contaminated skin has been washed with soap and water, and blood-contaminated mucous membranes have been flushed with ample water. Gloves should be made available to staff in charge of cleaning wounds or surfaces contaminated with blood. Blood-contaminated surfaces should be cleaned with bleach solution (1 part bleach/100 parts water or 1 tablespoon bleach/1 quart water or 1/4 cup of bleach/1 gallon of water) and allowed to dry before reusing.

USPHS oPEP RECOMMENDATIONS

The USPHS oPEP recommendations underscore the need to balance the risk for infection against the potential toxicity or ARV agents. Because PEP is potentially toxic and side effects are common, its use is not justified for exposures that pose a negligible risk for transmission. For exposures that represent an increased risk for transmission, aggressive treatment using a highly active expanded regimen that includes three ARV drugs is recommended. However, most exposures do not represent an increased transmission risk and, for these exposures, the CDC recommends a basic two-drug regimen (Tables 141.2 and 141.3). In addition, the 2001 HIV oPEP recommendations also address oPEP for HBV and hepatitis C virus (HCV). (See http://aidsinfo.nih.gov for the most recent updates.)

First Steps in Management of Exposures, Considerations for Determining the Level of Risk in Occupational Exposures, and the Appropriateness of Offering PEP

Care of the Exposure Site

Wound and skin sites exposed to blood or body fluids should be washed with soap and water. Mucous membranes should be flushed with water. PEP may be instituted immediately and discontinued at a later time should the detailed evaluation determine that the exposure does not warrant continued PEP prophylaxis.

TABLE 141.2

BASIC AND EXPANDED PEP REGIMENS FOR OCCUPATIONAL EXPOSURES

Regimen Category/Application	Suggested 28-day PEP Drug Regimens*
Basic two-drug Occupational HIV exposures for which there is recognized transmission risk (see Table 141.1)	Select one of the following dual regimens: ZDV + 3TC 3TC + d4T d4T + ddI
Expanded three-drug Occupational HIV exposures that pose an increased risk for transmission (e.g., larger volume of blood and/or higher virus titer) (see Table 141.1)	Basic two-drug regimen + one of the following: **Recommended:** Indinavir (IDV) Nelfinavir (NFV) Efavirenz (EFV) Abacavir (ABC)
	Use as PEP with expert consultation: Ritonavir (RTV) Saquinavir (SQV) Amprenavir (AMP) Delavirdine (DLV) Lopinavir/Ritonavir
	Generally not recommended for use as PEP: Nevirapine (NVP)

*See doses in Table 141.3.

TABLE 141.3
DOSES OF ARVs USED FOR OCCUPATIONAL PEP

Drug Preparations	Neonatal Dose	Pediatric Dose	Adult Dose
Nucleoside Analogue Reverse Transcriptase Inhibitors (NRTIs)			
Zidovudine (AZT, ZDV) 10 mg/mL syrup; 100-mg capsules 300-mg capsules	2 mg/kg q6h	90–180 mg/m² q8h	200 mg tid; 300 mg bid
Lamivudine (3TC) 10 mg/mL solution; 150-mg tablets	2 mg/kg bid (<30 days of age) (Ref: ATIS 12/14/01)	4 mg/kg bid (3 months–16 years) (max. 150 mg bid)	150 mg bid
Stavudine (d4T) 1 mg/mL solution 15-, 20-, 30-, and 40-mg capsules	Birth–13 days of age: 0.5 mg/kg/dose q 12 hr ≥14 days of age and <30 kg: 1 mg/ kg/dose q12h	1 mg/kg q12h (up to weight of 30 kg.)	40 mg bid (weight ≥60 kg) 30 mg bid (weight <60 kg)
Didanosine (ddI) 10 mg/mL solution (reconstituted with antacid)	2 weeks–8 months 100 mg/m² bid (50 mg/m² bid <90 days)	>8 months of age 120 mg/m² bid	200 mg bid (weight ≥60 kg) on empty stomach 125 mg bid (weight <60 kg) on empty stomach
25-, 50-, 100-, 150-, and 200-mg chewable tablets with buffers	NONE	>8 months of age 120 mg/m² bid	200 mg bid (weight ≥60 kg) on empty stomach 125 mg bid (weight <60 kg) on empty stomach
100-, 167-, 250-mg buffered powder for oral solution	2 weeks–8 months 100 mg/m² bid	>8 months of age 120 mg/m² bid	250 mg bid (weight ≥60 kg) on empty stomach 167 mg bid (weight < 60 kg) on empty stomach
125-, 200-, 250-, 250-mg delayed release capsules (Videx EC)	NONE	NONE	400 mg qd (weight ≥60 kg) 250 mg qd (weight <60 kg)
Abacavir (ABC) 20 mg/mL solution; 300-mg tablets	<3 months of age NONE	(3 months–13 years of age) 8 mg/kg bid (max.: 300 mg bid)	300 mg bid
Nonnucleoside Reverse Transcriptase Inhibitors (NNRTIs)			
Efavirenz (EFV; DMP-266) 50-, 100-, and 200-mg capsules	NONE	(≤3 years of age; q day) 200 mg: 10 to <15 kg 250 mg: 15 to <20 kg 300 mg; 20 to <25 kg 350 mg; 25 to <32.5 kg 400 mg; 32.5 to <40 kg 600 mg; >40 kg	600 mg once daily
Protease Inhibitors (PIs)			
Amprenavir (APV)	NONE	(<50 kg; 4–12 years of age or 13–16 years of age <50 kg) See www.aidsinfo.nih.gov for dosing.	1,200 mg (eight 150-mg capsules) bid; see adult treatment guidelines for APV/RTV combination bid or QD treatment regimen
Indinavir (IDV) 200- and 400-mg capsules	NONE	500 mg/m² q8h* Smaller surface area: 300–400 mg/m² q8h*	800 mg q8h 200 mg, on empty stomach
Nelfinavir (NFV) 200 mg/tsp powder 250 mg tablet	40 mg/kg q12h*	20–30 mg/kg/dose tid >6 years of age: 50–55 mg/kg/dose bid*	1,250 mg bid, with meals or snack 750 mg tid, with meals or snack
Lopinavir/Ritonavir (ABT 378, LPV/RTV Kaletra)	NONE	See www.aidsinfo.nih.gov for dosing. Dosing scheme is complicated, and varies by weight and by concomitant NVP or efavirenz use	

*Dose is under study in clinical trials.

BOX 141.2   Recommendations for Contents of Occupational Exposure Report

- Date and time of exposure
- The procedure being performed
  - How and where exposure occurred and if a sharp device was involved, type of device
- The exposure
  - Type of exposure: Percutaneous injury (e.g., needlestick or other penetrating sharps, etc.), mucous membrane exposure (e.g., splash in eye, etc.), nonintact skin exposure (e.g., broken or abraded skin, etc.), bites resulting in blood exposure to either person involved
  - Type and amount of fluid/tissue: Blood, fluids containing blood, or potentially infectious fluid or tissue (semen; vaginal, cerebrospinal, synovial, pleural, peritoneal, pericardial, and amniotic fluids)
  - Severity of exposure, depth of wound, duration of contact, condition of skin
  - Likelihood of presence of HIV, HBV, or HCV in source material
- The source of exposure:
  - Infection status of person
    - HIV: presence of HIV antibody
    - HBV: presence of HbsAg
    - HCV: presence of HCV antibody
    - or other infectious disease
  - Stage of disease, history of antiretroviral therapy, antiretroviral resistance information, viral load, CD4+ T-cell count, liver enzymes (e.g., ALT)

- If infectious status unknown, determine risk for HIV, HBV, or HCV infection.
  - Known sources: Consider medical diagnoses, clinical symptoms (e.g., acute syndrome suggestive of primary HIV infection), history of risk behaviors
  - Unknown sources: Consider likelihood of bloodborne pathogen infection among patients in the exposure setting
- Susceptibility of exposed person
  - Hepatitis B vaccination and vaccine-response status
  - HIV, HBV, and HIV immune status
- Details about care of exposed site: Washing of wound, flushing of mucous membranes
- Details about counseling, postexposure management, and follow-up
- Current medication history of exposed person and ability to swallow pills

---

Abbreviations: HBV, hepatitis B virus; HCV, hepatitis C virus; HIV, human immunodeficiency virus.
Reprinted from Centers for Disease Control and Prevention. Updated U.S. Public Health Service Guidelines for the management of occupational exposures to HBV, HCV, and HIV and recommendations for post exposure prophylaxis. *MMWR Morb Mortal Wkly Rep* 2001;50:1.

The Occupational Exposure Report and Considerations for Determining Level of Risk

For the purposes of PEP, how does one determine whether the exposed person should be given PEP, and if so, whether the basic or expanded regimen should be given and how this should be documented? Box 141.2 contains a list of the details regarding the occupational exposure and the postexposure management, which should be noted in the exposed person's medical record, in addition to any other local, state, or federal requirements.

Tables 141.4A and 141.4B take into account both the details of the occupational exposure and the HIV status of the exposure source to determine the appropriate level of risk and recommendations for follow-up. In general, the following types of injuries or exposures require further evaluation: (a) percutaneous injuries, mucous membrane exposures, or skin exposures with compromised skin integrity (e.g., dermatitis, abrasion, or open wound) to blood, fluids that contain blood, or potentially infectious fluids; (b) exposures to blood-filled hollow needles or visibly bloody devices; (c) direct contact with concentrated virus in a research laboratory or production facility; and (d) bites with blood exposure to either person involved.

Evaluation of the Source and Exposed Individuals for Evidence of Bloodborne Infections, Including HIV, HBV, and HCV

The source individual should be informed of the exposure, and once informed consent is obtained, should be tested for HbsAg, anti-HCV, and HIV antibody. In addition, the source person's medical record information available at the time of exposure (e.g., previous medical history, laboratory test results, and diagnoses) may help confirm or exclude bloodborne virus

infection. A Food and Drug Administration (FDA)-approved rapid HIV-antibody test such as the Ora-quick test should be considered for use. The HHS nPEP guidelines recommend that such rapid testing should be conducted within an hour after exposure. Repeatedly reactive HIV enzyme immunosorbent assay (EIA) (non-p24 antigen type) or rapid HIV antibody tests are suggestive of infection and can be used to make initial decisions on PEP management. Additional information on HIV rapid tests can be found at www.cdc.gov/hiv/pubs/rt.htm. Confirmation by HIV Western blot of a reactive result should be conducted before notifying the source patient of the final results. A negative HIV EIA or rapid HIV antibody test is an excellent indicator of the absence of HIV antibody. Direct virus assays such as HIV RNA viral load tests or HIV p24 antigen EIA tests for routine screening of source patients are not recommended due to concerns about high false-positive rates in this setting. Because source testing can take some time to complete, and given that PEP may not be effective if not given soon after exposure, clinicians may have to make a decision about PEP based on incomplete information (e.g., prior to initiating HIV testing or obtaining HIV testing results). A baseline evaluation of HIV-exposed HCP should include testing for HIV within hours after exposure unless the source person is known to be HIV-seronegative, and information about current medication history and any medical conditions or circumstances that might influence drug selection (e.g., pregnancy, breast-feeding, hepatic or renal disease) should be obtained. The HIV-exposed HCP should be counseled about the signs and symptoms of acute retroviral syndrome and to return quickly for evaluation should an acute HIV infection be suspected. The exposed person should be reevaluated within 72 hours postexposure to determine whether additional information about the exposure or source person has become

TABLE 141.4A

RECOMMENDED HIV PEP FOR PERCUTANEOUS INJURIES

	Infection Status of Source				
Exposure Type	HIV-Infected Class 1*	HIV-Infected Class 2*	Source of Unknown HIV Status[†]	Unknown Source[‡]	HIV-Uninfected
Less severe[§]	Recommend basic two-drug PEP	Recommend expanded three-drug PEP	Generally, no PEP warranted; however, consider basic two-drug PEP[‖] for source with HIV risk factors[1]	Generally, no PEP warranted; however, consider two-drug PEP[‖] in settings where exposure to HIV-infected persons is likely	No PEP warranted
More severe[2]	Recommend expanded three-drug PEP	Recommend expanded three-drug PEP	Generally, no PEP warranted; however, consider basic two-drug PEP[‖] for source with HIV risk factors[1]	Generally, no PEP warranted; however, consider two-drug PEP[‖] in settings where exposure to HIV-infected persons is likely	No PEP warranted

*HIV-Infected, Class 1: Asymptomatic HIV infection or known low viral load. HIV-Infected, Class 2: Symptomatic infection, AIDS, acute seroconversion, or known high viral load. If drug resistance is a concern, obtain expert consultation. Initiation of PEP should not be delayed pending expert consultation, and because expert consultation alone cannot substitute for face-to-face counseling, resources should be available to provide immediate evaluation and follow-up care for all exposures.
[†]HIV infection status of source is unknown (e.g., deceased individual with no samples available for HIV testing).
[‡]Unknown source (e.g., a needle from a sharps disposal container).
[§]Less severe (e.g., solid needle and superficial injury).
[‖]The designation "consider PEP" indicates that PEP is optional and should be based on an individualized decision made between the exposed person and the treating clinician.
[1]If PEP is offered and taken and the source is later determined to be HIV-uninfected, PEP should be discontinued.
[2]More severe (e.g., large-bore hollow needle, deep puncture, visible blood on device, or needle used in patient's artery or vein).
Reprinted from Centers for Disease Control and Prevention. Updated U.S. Public Health Service Guidelines for the management of occupational exposures to HBV, HCV, and HIV and recommendations for post exposure prophylaxis. *MMWR Morb Mortal Wkly Rep* 2001;50:1.

TABLE 141.4B

RECOMMENDED HIV PEP FOR MUCOUS MEMBRANE EXPOSURES AND NONINTACT SKIN* EXPOSURES

	Infection Status of Source				
Exposure Type	HIV-Infected Class 1[†]	HIV-Infected Class 2[†]	Unknown HIV Infection Status of the Source Patient[‡]	Unknown Source[§]	HIV-Uninfected
Less severe[‖]	Consider basic two-drug PEP	Recommend expanded three-drug PEP[1]	Generally, no PEP warranted; however, consider basic two-drug PEP[1] for source with HIV risk factors[2]	Generally, no PEP warranted; however, consider two-drug PEP[1] in settings where exposure to HIV-infected persons is likely	No PEP warranted
Large volume[3]	Recommend basic two-drug PEP	Recommend expanded three-drug PEP	Generally, no PEP warranted; however, consider basic two-drug PEP[1] for source with HIV risk factors[‖]	Generally, no PEP warranted; however, consider two-drug PEP[1] in settings where exposure to HIV-infected persons is likely	No PEP warranted

*For skin exposures, follow-up is indicated only if there is evidence of compromised skin integrity (e.g., dermatitis, abrasion, or open wound).
[†]HIV-infected, Class 1: Asymptomatic HIV infection or known low viral load. HIV-infected, Class 2: Symptomatic infection, AIDS, acute seroconversion, or known high viral load. If drug resistance is a concern, obtain expert consultation. Initiation of PEP should not be delayed pending expert consultation, and because expert consultation alone cannot substitute for face-to-face counseling, resources should be available to provide immediate evaluation and follow-up care for all exposures.
[‡]HIV infection status of the source patient is unknown (e.g., deceased individual with no samples available for HIV testing).
[§]Unknown source (e.g., splash from inappropriately disposed blood).
[‖]Small volume (i.e., a few drops).
[1]The designation "consider PEP" indicates that PEP is optional and should be based on an individualized decision made between the exposed person and the treating clinician.
[2]If PEP is offered and taken and the source is later determined to be HIV-uninfected, PEP should be discontinued.
[3]Large volume (i.e., major blood splash).
Reprinted from Centers for Disease Control and Prevention. Updated U.S. Public Health Service Guidelines for the management of occupational exposures to HBV, HCV, and HIV and recommendations for post exposure prophylaxis. *MMWR Morb Mortal Wkly Rep* 2001;50:1.

available. If the source person is found to be definitively HIV-uninfected and has no symptoms of HIV infection or AIDS, the exposed person no longer needs to be followed up (e.g., no need for baseline HIV testing or PEP). If the source individual is found to be HIV-infected, the exposed HCP should be retested periodically for a minimum of 6 months after exposure (e.g., 6 weeks, 12 weeks, and 6 months after exposure). If the exposed individual is not on oPEP and is within the window period for initiating it, oPEP should be offered. A 12-month follow-up HIV test is indicated in exposed HCP if they become HCV-infected following exposure to an HIV–HCV coinfected source individual. Similarly, any exposed HCP who develops an illness compatible with an acute retroviral syndrome should undergo HIV testing regardless of the interval since exposure. Confidentiality of the source and exposed individuals should be maintained. If the HIV infection status of the source patient is unknown or cannot be determined, decisions about PEP should be made on a case-by-case basis, considering the risk of transmission from the exposure and the likelihood that the source patient is HIV-infected. Information about seroprevalence rates of HIV, HBV, or HCV in the community or institution from which the source material or source person originates may be helpful in evaluating the risk for exposure. The reliability and interpretation of tests of needles or other sharp instruments implicated in exposures is unknown and not recommended. The possible need for prophylaxis against HBV also should be considered. Additional guidelines on the management of occupational exposures to HBV and HBC can be accessed at the following Web site: www.cdc.gov/mmwr/PDF/rr/rr5011.pdf.

HIV Treatment Principles Used in Developing oPEP Recommendations

The selection of the regimens recommended for oPEP reflects the consideration of efficacy data, site of activity in the HIV replication cycle, and drug side effects. The USPHS emphasizes, however, that the determination of which agents to use, number of agents to use, and when to alter a PEP regimen is empiric. Selected drugs from three classes of ARV agents are recommended for use for oPEP: nucleoside analogue reverse transcriptase inhibitors (NRTIs), nonnucleoside reverse transcriptase inhibitors (NNRTIs), and protease inhibitors (PIs).

Combination regimens have been shown to be more effective than is monotherapy in reducing viral load and therefore, are recommended for oPEP. Highly active antiretroviral therapy (HAART) regimens containing, for example, NRTIs with a PI and/or an NNRTI have been shown to be superior to dual therapy alone in reducing HIV viral load. Although there are no studies to support the idea that using other ARV drugs in addition to ZDV will enhance the effectiveness of PEP, it is felt that the same factors that improve the efficacy of HIV treatment might similarly improve PEP efficacy. Because ARVs have associated adverse effects, the USPHS oPEP guidelines reserve the use of HAART regimens with three or more drugs for more severe exposures. These guidelines describe a two-tiered paradigm of "basic" or "expanded" prophylaxis for less severe and more severe exposures, respectively. Although some treatment regimens include HAART combinations of more than three drugs, current oPEP guidelines recommend the use of triple drug regimens for more severe exposures to maximize adherence and reduce the likelihood of side effects. In addition, the emergence of resistance to ARV drugs and development of new ARV drugs has prompted some changes in the list of drugs recommended for oPEP.

Basic and Expanded oPEP Regimens

The USPHS has developed guidelines for basic and expanded oPEP regimens, based on the level of HIV transmission risk (Table 141.5). A basic or dual-drug regimen, including ZDV/3TC as the basic combination of choice, should be considered

TABLE 141.5

BASIC AND EXPANDED PEDIATRIC PEP REGIMENS

A. Basic PEP regimens		
Strongly recommended		ZDV + [3TC* or ddI]
		d4T + 3TC
Alternative recommendation with expert consultation		ABC + [ZDV or 3TC]
		ddI + 3TC
Use in special circumstances		d4T + ddI or ZDV + ddC
Not recommended		ddC + [ddI or d4T or 3TC]
		ZDV + d4T
B. Expanded HAART Pediatric nPEP drug regimens		
Strongly recommended	Recommended basic regimen from above	+ Nelfinavir or Lopinavir/Ritonavir
	Recommended basic regimen from above	+ Efavirenz†
Alternative recommendation	Recommended basic regimen from above	+ Amprenavir‡ or IDV§
	ZDV + 3TC	+ ABC‖
Not recommended	Basic regimen from above	+ Nevirapine
	Basic regimen from above	+ Saquinavir

*ZDV + 3TC available as a combination formulation (Combivir). Such a combined formulation would decrease pill burden and improves likelihood of adherence.
†Efavirenz recommended for children >3 years of age. May not be used in pregnant women due to birth defects seen in animal studies.
‡Amprenavir recommended for children ≥3 years of age.
§IDV recommended for older children who can tolerate swallowing solid tablets or caplets.
‖ABC + ZDV + 3TC available as a combined formulation. Such a combined formulation would decrease pill burden and improves likelihood of adherence, but consider potential side effects.
Adapted from Centers for Disease Control and Prevention. Antiretroviral postexposure prophylaxis after sexual, injection-drug use, or other nonoccupational exposure to HIV in the United States: Recommendation from the U.S. Department of Health and Human Services. *MMWR Morb Mortal Wkly Rep* 2005;54:1.

TABLE 141.6

MAIN ADVERSE EVENTS ASSOCIATED WITH ARVs

Antiretroviral Class/Agent	Primary Side Effects and Toxicities
Nucleoside reverse transcriptase inhibitors (NRTIs)	**Mainly nausea or diarrhea**
Zidovudine (ZDV; AZT)	Anemia, neutropenia, nausea, headache, insomnia, muscle pain, and weakness
Lamivudine (3TC)	Abdominal pain, nausea, diarrhea, rash, and pancreatitis
Stavudine (d4T)	Peripheral neuropathy, headache, diarrhea, nausea, insomnia, anorexia, pancreatitis, increased liver function tests (LFTs), anemia, and neutropenia
Didanosine (ddI)	**Pancreatitis,**[*] lactic acidosis, neuropathy, diarrhea, abdominal pain, and nausea
Abacavir (ABC)	Nausea, diarrhea, anorexia, abdominal pain, fatigue, headache, insomnia, and hypersensitivity reactions
Nonnucleoside reverse transcriptase inhibitors (NNRTIs)	**Severe skin reactions (Stevens-Johnson syndrome, toxic epidermal necrolysis)**
Nevirapine (NVP)	Rash (including cases of Stevens-Johnson syndrome), fever, nausea, headache, hepatitis, increased LFTs, rarely fatal hepatic necrosis
Delavirdine (DLV)	Rash (including cases of Stevens-Johnson syndrome), nausea, diarrhea, headache, fatigue, and increased LFTs
Efavirenz (EFV)[†]	Rash (including cases of Stevens-Johnson syndrome), **insomnia, somnolence, dizziness,** trouble concentrating, and **abnormal dreaming**
Protease inhibitors (PIs)	**New-onset diabetes mellitus, hyperglycemia, diabetic ketoacidosis, exacerbation of preexisting diabetes mellitus, and dyslipidemia**
Indinavir (IDV)	Nausea, abdominal pain, **nephrolithiasis,**[‡] and indirect hyperbilirubinemia
Nelfinavir (NFV)	**Diarrhea,**[§] nausea, abdominal pain, weakness, and rash
Ritonavir (RTV)	Weakness, diarrhea, nausea, circumoral paresthesia, taste alteration, and increased cholesterol and triglycerides
Saquinavir (SQV)	Diarrhea, abdominal pain, nausea, hyperglycemia, and increased LFTs
Amprenavir (AMP)	Nausea, diarrhea, rash, circumoral paresthesia, taste alteration, and depression
Lopinavir/ritonavir	Diarrhea, fatigue, headache, nausea, and increased cholesterol and triglycerides

[*]Fatal and nonfatal pancreatitis in patients treated >4 weeks.
[†]See text regarding use of EFV, d4T + ddI, IDV, and ZDV + 3TC in pregnant women.
[‡]Nephrolithiasis less of a problem with good hydration (see text).
[§]Diarrhea may be controlled with antimotility agents.
Reprinted from Centers for Disease Control and Prevention. Updated U.S. Public Health Service Guidelines for the management of occupational exposures to HBV, HCV, and HIV and recommendations for post exposure propylaxis. *MMWR Morb Mortal Wkly Rep* 2001;50:1.

for lower risk exposures. ZDV/3TC is available as a combination formulation, which may improve adherence. However, recent data suggest that ZDV and 3TC resistance mutations may be common in certain locales. Therefore, clinicians may choose other NRTIs or ARV combinations based on local clinical experience and knowledge. Table 141.5 lists other dual regimens aside from ZDV/3TC to be considered for basic oPEP regimens.

The addition of a third drug, a PI or an NNRTI, to the basic dual drug regimen is recommended to create the expanded, triple-drug PEP regimen, thereby enhancing the ARV activity of the basic regimen in higher risk exposures. In addition, if the patient becomes HIV-infected, inclusion of a third drug should increase the effectiveness of treatment during this early phase of infection after seroconversion. Table 141.5 lists selected three-drug combinations in three categories: (1) recommended, (2) use as PEP with expert consultation, and (3) generally not recommended for use as PEP. The drugs recommended for use with expert consultation are those which might be used in cases of development of drug resistance to those drugs included in the recommended list and which may require special monitoring due to the potential for adverse events (e.g., hypersensitivity reactions with abacavir). Although nevirapine (NVP) is recognized as a highly potent ARV, it is not generally recommended for PEP due to case reports of serious adverse events related to multidose NVP taken for PEP, including hepatotoxicity and fulminant liver failure requiring liver transplantation, hypersensitivity syndrome, skin reactions, and rhabdomyolysis

(Table 141.6). It is important to distinguish this recommendation to avoid multidose NVP for PEP from separate recommendations concerning the use of the two-dose NVP regimen (one dose to the mother at labor, one dose to the infant shortly after birth) for prevention of MTCT of HIV.

In general, clinical experience or judgment may influence an individual practitioner to use alternate drug combinations for either the basic or expanded PEP regimens. When possible, persons with expertise in the management of HIV-infected patients should be consulted in the selection and implementation of PEP regimens.

Timing of Initiation and Duration of PEP after Exposure

PEP should be implemented as soon as possible after exposure, preferably within hours. Animal studies suggest that PEP is less effective when initiated after 24 to 36 hours, but the interval after which no benefit is gained from PEP for humans is not known. The HHS has updated its nPEP guidelines (formerly USPHS nPEP guidelines) to recommend initiating nPEP as soon as feasible within 72 hours after exposure, with the caveat that clinicians may consider administering nPEP for patients seeking care more than 72 hours after experiencing a significant exposure if they believe the benefits outweigh the risks. Although the appropriate duration of PEP is not known, based on the CDC case control study and results from an animal study, a 28-day regimen is recommended.

PEP Drug Toxicity Monitoring

Among HCP on PEP enrolled in a national surveillance system and registry, 50% experienced adverse symptoms and nearly 33% stopped taking PEP because of adverse signs and symptoms. Such side effects and discontinuation of PEP were more common among HCP taking three-drug versus two-drug combination regimens in two studies. The most common side effects associated with ARV agents and methods used to lessen certain of these side effects are well described (Table 141.6).

NVP toxicity deserves special mention as severe toxicity has been reported in 22 patients taking NVP-containing ARV regimens, including two cases of life-threatening liver failure, one of which required liver transplantation, and other cases of hepatotoxicity, skin reaction (including one documented and two possible cases of Stevens-Johnson syndrome), and rhabdomyolysis. Of the 22 cases, 16 adults received oPEP, 5 adults received nPEP, and 1 child who had suffered a needlestick exposure received PEP. Most regimens contained three drugs (range: one to five). Onset of symptoms occurred between 3 to 36 days, with the median occurring onset at 14 days. Because of severity and rapidity of onset of these severe toxicities, NVP is not recommended for use as PEP.

Toxicity monitoring should include a complete blood count and renal and hepatic chemical function tests at baseline and 2 weeks after starting PEP (Table 141.7). Potential toxicities and measures to minimize these effects, drug interactions, and methods for monitoring these side effects should be discussed with patients to maximize adherence to PEP regimens. The following side effects should be reported immediately to the clinician: rash, fever, back or abdominal pain, pain on urination or blood in the urine, and symptoms of hyperglycemia (e.g., increased thirst and/or frequent urination). The FDA (telephone: 800-332-1088 in the United States) and/or the manufacturer should be informed of unusual, serious, or unexpected toxicity associated with receipt of ARV drugs. In addition, pregnant HCP who are exposed to ARVs through PEP should be reported to the Antiretroviral Pregnancy Registry (telephone: 800-258-4263 in the United States, or write to the Antiretroviral Pregnancy Registry, 1011 Research Park, 1011 Ashes Drive, Wilmington, NC 28405). Finally, HCP receiving PEP who become HIV-infected should be encouraged to contact the CDC (telephone: 800-893-0485 or 404-639-1250) regarding enrollment into a clinical protocol to evaluate such events.

Considerations Involving Pregnant HCP

Certain ARV drugs or combinations of drugs either are not recommended or should be used with caution in pregnant women. Efavirenz (EFV) is associated with teratogenic effects in primate studies. Stavudine (d4T) in combination with didanosine (ddI) has been associated with fatal and nonfatal lactic acidosis in pregnant women. Indinavir (IDV) may lead to hyperbilirubinemia in newborns; therefore, it should not be administered to women shortly before delivery. Finally, the combination of ZDV and 3TC has been reported as possibly related to two cases of mitochondrial toxicity and death in HIV-uninfected infants exposed to the drugs perinatally in France. However, no similar deaths have been found in an exhaustive review of 20,000 infants in the major U.S. perinatal cohorts.

Resistance to ARV Agents

Despite the documentation of resistance mutations in source patients and the transmission of resistant HIV strains after occupational exposure, the relevance of such exposures to resistant virus is not fully understood. Although it is recommended that resistance testing information on the source be collected at the time of the initial exposure and taken into account in the selection of the PEP regimen, resistance testing of all source

patients is not recommended because it is unlikely that results would arrive in time to make adjustments in the 28-day PEP regimen, and no data support such an approach.

HIV Postexposure Counseling and Education

HIV-exposed HCP should be counseled regarding the prevention of secondary transmission, particularly during the initial 6 to 12 weeks after exposure when seroconversion might occur. Specifically, sexual abstinence and the use of condoms should be encouraged, while breast-feeding and the donation of blood, plasma, organs, tissue, or semen should be discouraged. Exposed persons also should be encouraged to seek medical advice should the following signs and symptoms of acute HIV infection or viremia appear: fever, rash, myalgia, fatigue, malaise, or lymphadenopathy. Early initiation of HAART relative to HIV seroconversion may improve the immune system's long-term ability to combat HIV infection. Information about adherence to the PEP regimen and management of side effects should emphasize the need to complete the full course of the regimen, the potential side effects and drug interactions, and ways in which these can be minimized and monitored. The following side effects should be reported immediately to the health care provider: rash, fever, back or abdominal pain, pain on urination or blood in the urine, and symptoms of hyperglycemia (e.g., increased thirst and/or frequent urination). Patients also should be told how to prevent and manage side effects including drinking at least 48 ounces of fluid per 24-hour period to limit the incidence of nephrolithiasis associated with IDV, and the use of prescription antimotility agents to limit the diarrhea associated with nelfinavir (NFV), saquinavir, and ritonavir. When recommending or offering PEP, physicians also should inform patients that knowledge about the efficacy and toxicity of PEP is limited. A summary of recent human and animal PEP efficacy data also may be provided.

HIV nPEP FOR EXPOSURES IN CHILDREN AND ADOLESCENTS

Since 1999, at least four states—California, Massachusetts, New York, and Rhode Island—have published either nPEP guidelines or clinical advisories. The American Academy of Pediatrics has recently released its own guidelines. The HHS guidelines for nPEP were updated in 2005. The recommendations for nPEP in children and adolescents in this chapter are based on oPEP and nPEP guidelines and adult and pediatric HIV treatment guidelines.

New Policy Recommendations Pertinent to Pediatric nPEP

The CDC's stance in 1998 as a result of its initial consultation with the USPHS on nPEP was that it was a clinical intervention of unproven efficacy but did not recommend or discourage its use and did not make specific ARV drug recommendations. Recent data from animal models, such as that of Otten et al., were presented earlier in this chapter that support the use of nPEP as late as 72 hours after an exposure to reduce the likelihood of HIV transmission. In the revised HHS nPEP guidelines, it is noted that data from animal models, perinatal clinical trials, studies of health care workers receiving oPEP, and observational nPEP studies suggest that nPEP may be effective in reducing the risk of HIV acquisition and recommend that specific ARV drug regimens be used based on the most current HHS adult ARV treatment guidelines. Individuals exposed to an HIV-infected person with a significant risk for HIV

TABLE 141.7

SUMMARY OF MANAGEMENT AND FOLLOW-UP OF PEP

	Time between HIV Exposure and Initiation of PEP	Time from Onset of PEP					
		2 Weeks	4 Weeks	6 Weeks	12 Weeks	6 Months	12 Months
PEP	1. Clean exposure site and determine if PEP is indicated. 2. Choose PEP regimen: consider exposed person's medication history and medical conditions or circumstances (i.e., pregnancy, breast-feeding, renal or hepatic disease). See Tables 141.2 to 141.6 and 141.8. 3. If indicated, start PEP within hours, but no more than 72 hours after HIV exposure. May consider initiating PEP before all workup completed if HIV results delayed >1 hour.		Stop PEP after 30 days or sooner if source determined to be HIV seronegative.				
HIV testing	Baseline HIV test of source: If source is HIV seronegative, do not start PEP or provide further PEP follow-up to exposed person. If source's HIV infection status is unknown, determine if PEP is indicated on a case-by-case basis. Re-evaluate within 72 hours if more information about source becomes available. If source is HIV seropositive, conduct baseline testing of exposed person.			Repeat	Repeat	Repeat	Repeat if exposed person becomes HCV-infected following exposure to source coinfected with HCV-HIV.
Monitor for ARV toxicity	Baseline tests: At a minimum: CBC; renal and hepatic function tests If PI given: Monitor for hyperglycemia. If IDV given: Monitor for crystalluria, hematuria, hemolytic anemia, and hepatitis. If toxicity noted, consider modifying regimen and other diagnostic procedures	Repeat					
Counsel exposed person	Counsel exposed person: 1. Instruct patient to use precautions to prevent secondary HIV transmission during follow-up. 2. If PEP is prescribed, inform patient about possible drug toxicities and the need for monitoring and possible drug interactions.	Period of time during which exposed person most most likely to transmit if recently HIV-infected and experiencing HIV viremia: person on PEP should use precautions to prevent secondary HIV transmission *especially* during this time period: • Exercise sexual abstinence or use condoms. • Refrain from donating blood, plasma, organs, tissue, or semen. • Refrain from breast-feeding.					

| BOX 141.3 | Comparison of Selected nPEP Policies | | |

Policy State/Date of release	Offer PEP within how many hours?	No. of PEP drugs	Pediatric recommendations
New York State Department of Health AIDS Institute March 2002	36 hours	"In general three drugs," but no consensus reached between two or three drugs. Notes common use of AZT/3TC/nelfinavir	Detailed recommendations
State of California 2001	72 hours	Two or three drugs depending on level of risk	Consult pediatric HIV specialist
Massachusetts Dept. Health Clinical Advisory October 20, 2000	72 hours	Not specified	Not specified
Rhode Island Department of Health August 1, 2002	72 hours, but may be given afterwards in special circumstances	Two or three drugs depending on level of risk	Special considerations listed in terms of dosing, support services, informed consent, necessity for caretaker involvement
American Academy of Pediatrics (AAP) 2003	72 hours	Physician choice: many physicians will choose three; some will prefer two	Detailed instructions
Health and Human Services 2005 (nPEP Guidelines)	72 hours	Three drugs from list of preferred and alternative regimens; consider two drugs if concerned about potential adherence or toxicity issues	Refers reader to AAP nPEP guidelines and The Working Group on Antiretroviral Therapy and Medical Management of HIV-Infected Children Guidelines

transmission and presenting for care within 72 hours of exposure would be eligible to receive an nPEP ARV regimen based on the most current ARV HIV treatment recommendations, with the caveat that those individuals presenting after 72 hours of exposure with a significant risk could be offered nPEP if the caregiver considers the benefits of nPEP to outweigh the risks.

Current UPSHS oPEP guidelines recommend three-drug regimens for more severe or increased risk exposures and two-drug regimens for less severe exposures because evidence is insufficient to support three-drug regimens for both levels of exposure. Based on the assumption that HAART's ability to maximally suppress viral replication translates into a higher likelihood preventing the establishment of HIV infection in an exposed person, HHS nPEP guidelines recommend a 28-day course of a three-drug HAART regimen for all persons presenting for care within 72 hours of nonoccupational exposures that represent a significant risk of HIV transmission with a *known* HIV-infected source. In addition, because no evidence suggests that a three-drug HAART regimen is more effective than is a two-drug regiment, nPEP guidelines suggest that a two-drug regimen could be considered when there is a concern about potential difficulties with adherence or adverse events requiring immediate medical attention.

A list of selected nPEP recommendations by selected states or national organizations is provided in Box 141.3. Most recommend offering PEP within 72 hours and using two-drug or three-drug regimens. The New York State Department of Health AIDS Institute generally recommends three drugs, but their Committee could not reach a consensus on the number of drugs to be used because of the issues of better adherence with two-drug regimens versus the superiority of three-drug

regimens for HIV treatment purposes. The American Academy of Pediatrics acknowledges that many clinicians would use three drugs but that two drugs may be considered in certain situations including issues related to toxicity and ease of adherence.

Principles for Pediatric PEP

The PEP recommendations for children in this chapter are based on both the oPEP recommendations for HCP with occupational exposures and for persons with nonoccupational exposures and the guidelines on HIV ARV therapy in children and adults. (See http://aidsinfo.nih.gov for most recent updates.) However, nPEP for exposed children always should be initiated in close consultation with a physician expert in the care of HIV-infected children. Based on a review of HHS nPEP guidelines and current data from oPEP and nPEP studies, the following are essential principles to be considered for administering pediatric HIV treatment and nPEP.

1. The effectiveness of combination therapy is greater than that of monotherapy to treat HIV infection. Similarly, the effectiveness of combination PEP is assumed to be greater than that of monoprophylaxis to prevent HIV infection.

Three-drug regimens are recommended for treatment of HIV-infected pediatric patients. Two-drug regimens are recommended only under special circumstances. Triple-drug combinations that include a PI are superior to the dual NRTI combination regimens alone in reducing viral load to undetectable levels and increasing CD4+ lymphocyte number.

2. Monotherapy for HIV infection should be avoided based on its poor efficacy relative to HAART and rapid emergence of resistance to a number of drugs. Similarly, it is assumed that monoprophylaxis to prevent transmission of HIV should be avoided, except for prevention of MTCT.

Prophylaxis with ZDV is recommended during the first 6 weeks for an HIV-exposed infant after birth to an HIV-infected mother.

3. Because the duration of PEP is only 28 days, drugs that do not require graded dosing schemes and are maximally effective throughout the entire course should be considered drugs of choice for PEP.

Ritonavir is an example of a drug that requires a graded dosing scheme of 5 days when initiating therapy. Although it is appropriate for treatment of HIV, it would not be a first choice nPEP medication because the patient would not be on the maximally inhibitory dose of the medication until 5 days after starting nPEP.

4. Two-drug NRTI combinations are not optimal for and are used under special circumstances for treatment of HIV and are considered the basic oPEP regimen for lower risk HIV exposures.

The revised nPEP recommendations are permissive of the use of two-drug regimens in significant exposures when adherence or drug toxicity is a consideration.

5. Triple-drug combinations are used as part of the expanded oPEP regimen for higher risk HIV exposures and are considered the first-choice regimen for HIV treatment and for nPEP based on the revised nPEP guidelines.

The triple-drug combination of choice is a highly active PI (NFV) in combination with two NRTIs (ZDV and 3TC). The dual NRTI combination of choice to be used with the PI is ZDV and 3TC. ZDV and ddC are a less preferred choice for use in combination with a PI. The PI of choice for PEP is NFV because it has fewer side effects and does not require stepwise dosing. Lopinavir/ritonavir is the only protease inhibitor approved by the U.S. FDA for use in children 6 months of age or older. Although no other protease inhibitor aside from lopinavir/ritonavir is FDA-approved for children younger than 2 years of age, the current treatment guidelines recommend the use of pediatric formulations of ritonavir and NFV in infants, with the understanding that optimal dosing of these agents in young infants has not been defined but is under study in clinical trials. NFV would be preferable to ritonavir, because of ritonavir's graded dosing schedule.

6. Pill burden, side effects, potency, and formulations of medications are important considerations in choosing a PEP regimen.

Because it has been shown that it is difficult for both adults and children to adhere to a full 28-day course of PEP, clinicians should take these factors into account in choosing a PEP regimen.

7. Approved ARV drugs for adults may be used in children despite lack of FDA approval for pediatric formulations (see Table 141.8).

Some recommended ARV drugs are not yet FDA-approved for use in children or for use in all age groups among children. However, current pediatric ARV treatment guidelines state that the absence of clinical trials addressing pediatric-specific manifestations of HIV infection does not preclude the use of any approved ARV drug in children and that all ARV drugs approved for treatment of HIV infection may be used for children when indicated—irrespective of labeling notations. However, because some physicians may wish to assign priority to particular ARV regimens for PEP purposes based on the FDA-approval status of the drugs, more detailed information about age-specific considerations is provided in the next section.

8. Clinicians faced with a decision regarding PEP should consult with a physician with expertise in pediatric HIV care.

TABLE 141.8

ARVs APPROVED BY THE U.S. FDA FOR TREATMENT OF HIV INFECTION IN CHILDREN BY AGE CATEGORY

Drug	0 to <3 Months	3 Months to <2 Years	≥2 Years
NRTIs			
Abacavir	No	Yes	Yes
ddC	No	No	Yes, ≥13 years of age
ddI	Yes, ≥2 weeks	Yes	Yes
d4T	Yes	Yes	Yes
ZDV	Yes	Yes	Yes
3TC	No*	Yes	Yes
NNRTIs			
Delavirdine	No	No	Yes, ≥16 years of age
Efavirenz	No	No	Yes, ≥3 years of age
Nevirapine	No	Yes (>2 months)	Yes
Protease Inhibitors			
Indinavir	No	No	Yes (adolescents/ adults)
Lopinavir/ Ritonavir (Kaletra)	No	Yes (≥6 months)	Yes
Nelfinavir	No	No	Yes
Ritonavir	No	No	Yes
Saquinavir	No	No	Yes, >16 years of age

*Use of 3TC recommended in children <3 months of age, despite absence of FDA approval.

Pediatric ARV therapy is a rapidly evolving field and physicians with expertise in pediatric HIV care should be consulted whenever possible when deciding on PEP regimens (Box 141.4).

Age-Specific Considerations for PEP in Children

The choice of drugs available for treatment of HIV is more limited for children than for adults. Some drugs available for treatment of adults are not FDA-approved, are not recommended for use in children, or lack formulations suitable for small children; however, current pediatric ARV guidelines state that FDA labeling practices should not necessarily limit use of ARVs in children. Pediatric ARV therapy is a rapidly evolving field. Clinicians faced with a decision regarding PEP should consult with a physician with expertise in pediatric HIV care and consider the most current local and national recommendations. However, a reasonable approach must take into account which pediatric formulations are available in a particular area, which are available through compassionate use programs, which are accessible in the appropriate time frame for PEP, and which have age-appropriate dosing schemes available for the child in question. Other alternate drugs for nPEP are listed in Table 141.5, as are drugs not recommended for nPEP. The dosing for the ARV drugs used in pediatric PEP is generally the same for that used to treat pediatric HIV infection, and the duration of treatment is usually 4 weeks. Physicians should consult http://aidsinfo.nih.gov for the most recent pediatric ARV treatment guidelines. In addition, although nevirapine (NVP) is approved for treatment of HIV infection in children older than 2 months of age, multiple-use NVP is not currently recommended for PEP in the United States due to its toxicity.

BOX 141.4	PEP Management Resources 52(1)

National Clinicians' Postexposure Prophylaxis Hotline (PEP line)
Run by University of California-San Francisco/San Francisco General Hospital staff; supported by the Health Resources and Services Administration Ryan White CARE Act, HIV/AIDS Bureau, AIDS Education and Training Centers, and the CDC.

Phone: (888) 448-4911

Internet: http://www.ucsf.edu/hivcntr

Needlestick!
A Web site to help clinicians manage and document occupational blood and body fluid exposures. Developed and maintained by the University of California, Los Angeles (UCLA), Emergency Medicine Center, UCLA School of Medicine, and funded in part by the CDC and the Agency for Healthcare Research and Quality

Internet: http://www.needlestick.mednet.ucla.edu

Hepatitis Hotline

Phone: (888) 443-7232
Internet: http://www.cdc.gov/hepatitis
Phone: (800) 893-0485

Reporting to CDC: Occupationally acquired HIV infections and failures of PEP
HIV Antiretroviral Pregnancy Registry

Phone: (800) 258-4263
Fax: (800) 800-1052
Internet: http://www.APRegistry.com

Reporting unusual or severe toxicities
Contact manufacturer directly or FDA

FDA: 1-800-332-1088

Selected NPEP guidelines
American Academy of Pediatrics

http://aappolicy.aappublications.org/cgi/content/full/pediatrics;111/6/1475
PEP in Children & Adolescents for Nonoccupational Exposure to HIV

New York State Dept. of Health AIDS Institute

www.hivguidelines.org
HIV PEP for children beyond the perinatal period
HIV PEP following sexual assault

State of California

http://www.dhs.ca.gov/ps/ooa/reports/PDF/HIVProphylaxisfollowingsexualassault.pdf
Offering HIV Prophylaxis Following Sexual Assault: Recommendations for the State of California

Commonwealth of Massachusetts

http://www.state.ma.us/dph/aids/guidelines/ca_exposure_nonwork.htm
Clinical Advisory: HIV Prophylaxis for Non-occupational Exposures

Rhode Island Dept. Health/Brown University AIDS Program

http://www.health.ri.gov/disease/NPEPFinalDraftJuly26.pdf
Nonoccupational Human Immunodeficiency Virus postexposure prophylaxis guidelines for Rhode Island health care practitioners

Adapted from Centers for Disease Control and Prevention. Updated U.S. Public Health Service Guidelines for the management of occupational exposures to HBV, HCV, and HIV and recommendations for post exposure prophylaxis. *MMWR Morb Mortal Wkly Rep* 2001;50:1.

Term Infants, Age Less than 3 Months

ZDV is an FDA-approved ARV drug for both HIV therapy and prophylaxis from the time of birth. ddI and d4T are approved for treatment of infants younger than 3 months of age. However, d4T is not recommended in combination with ZDV. In addition, experts feel that enough data exist regarding 3TC dosing for infants younger than 3 months of age to consider it safe to use for therapy of HIV-infected infants (see Table 141.3 for 3TC dose under study for infants younger than 3 months

of age). For infants exposed to HIV after birth, prophylaxis with ZDV and 3TC is considered the PEP two-drug regimen of choice in this and other age groups, unless there is a high level of resistant mutations to these drugs in the community. d4T is also FDA-approved in children 5 weeks of age or older, but it is not recommended in combination with ZDV. An expanded regimen for infants using a PI and two NRTIs (including ZDV) might be considered for higher risk exposures using investigational dosing schemes.

Children, Age at Least 3 Months but Less than 2 Years

ZDV, 3TC, ddI, d4T, abacavir, nevirapine, and lopinavir/ritonavir are the only FDA-approved ARVs for HIV therapy in this age group; however, liquid formulations of NFV and ritonavir are recommended for use in older infants and NVP is not recommended as a PEP agent. The nPEP regimens of choice in this age group include the two-drug nPEP regimen of ZDV/3TC and a three-drug regimen adding NFV or lopinavir/ritonavir. An investigational dose for NFV is noted in Table 141.3. Lopinavir/ritonavir is an approved PI combination in this age group for children 6 months of age and older.

Children, Age 2 to 13 years of age

ZDV, 3TC, ddI, d4T, abacavir, NVP, NFV, lopinavir/ritonavir, and ritonavir have been approved by the FDA for therapy of HIV infection for this entire age group. In addition, the following drugs have been approved for the following age groups: amprenavir (4 years or older), ddC (13 years or older), delavirdine (16 years or older), EFV (3 years or older), saquinavir (older than 16 years), and IDV (adolescent/adults). The nPEP regimens of choice in this age group include the two-drug nPEP regimen of ZDV/3TC and a three-drug regimen adding NPV or Kaletra or EFV as the third drug. Multidose NVP is not recommended as a PEP agent.

Adolescent Dosing

Adolescent dosages should be prescribed according to Tanner staging of puberty and not by age. Therefore, those in Tanner stages I and II should be dosed according to pediatric schedules and those in Tanner V should be dosed using adult schedules. Youths undergoing growth spurts (Tanner III females and Tanner IV males) should be closely monitored for medication efficacy and toxicity when using adult or pediatric dosing guidelines.

Considerations for Determining Level of Risk in Nonoccupational HIV Exposures and the Appropriateness of Administering PEP

In addition to the considerations for determining level of risk for occupational exposures (Tables 141.4A and 141.4B) and those described earlier in this chapter by type of exposure, the following generic considerations should be taken into account for nonoccupational HIV exposures: (a) the likelihood that the source is infected with HIV; (b) the likelihood of transmission, including the many cofactors that might increase or decrease transmission risk; (c) characteristics (e.g., viral load, stage of infection) of an HIV-infected source; (d) isolated versus recurrent HIV exposures; (e) time delay between possible exposure and presentation for medical care; and (f) ability to adhere to the ARV regimen. Factors to consider in determining level of risk in pediatric exposures are described earlier in this chapter. Each case must be evaluated individually, taking into account the specifics of each situation. In general, the HHS nPEP guidelines consider significant exposures to be exposures of the vagina, rectum, eye, mouth, or other mucous membrane, non-intact skin, or percutaneous contact with blood, semen, vaginal secretions, rectal secretions, or any body fluid that is visibly contaminated with blood to a source who is known or suspected to be HIV-infected. These guidelines recommend consideration of the use of nPEP in individuals with significant exposures presenting for care within 72 hours after exposure to a source patient known to be HIV-infected. In addition they suggest that similar exposures to a source patient with unknown HIV status be considered for nPEP on a case-by-case status.

Prophylaxis for Infectious Agents Other than HIV after Accidental Needlesticks with Discarded Needles and Sexual Assault

Recommendations for management of percutaneous exposures to infectious agents other than HIV have been described, and guidelines for HBV and HCV exposures have been incorporated recently into the HIV oPEP guidelines. Because HBV may survive on fomites for at least several days, one should check the HBV vaccination status of a child with a percutaneous exposure. For children who have completed their HBV immunization regimen, no further action is needed. Children who have not completed their regimen should receive an additional HBV vaccination and be scheduled to receive their remaining doses. Experts differ in their opinions on the need to administer hepatitis B immune globulin (HBIG) to children who have not completed the HBV immunization regimen. HCP with occupational bloodborne exposures should be screened for HCV in addition to HBV and HIV. Should the clinician elect to test for HCV in a pediatric nPEP exposure, it should be done at the time of injury and then 6 months later with a confirmatory test for positive tests. It is thought that the risk for transmission for hepatitis A virus (HAV) and HCV through discarded needles is very low, and therefore administration of immune globulin for HAV is not recommended. In addition, tetanus toxoid and tetanus immune globulin should be administered based on the vaccination history of the person who has been stuck.

Children or adolescents who are victims of sexual abuse should receive a baseline evaluation and then follow-up evaluations at 2 and 12 weeks afterward for detection of STIs. Sexual contacts of patients who have acute HBV should receive HBIG and begin the hepatitis B vaccine series within 14 days after the most recent sexual contact.

SUMMARY

In general, either a basic or expanded combination ARV regimen is recommended for oPEP, depending on the level of risk, and should be continued for 4 weeks. The combination of ZDV with 3TC is recommended as the two-drug or basic regimen of choice, and the combination of ZDV with 3TC and NFV is recommended as the three-drug or expanded regimen of choice. Alternate regimens also may be considered. Based on recent animal data and human studies, it appears that nPEP should be considered as a means of reducing HIV transmission after significant exposures to HIV-infected persons or those suspected of being HIV-infected among individuals presenting within 72 hours of exposure. The therapeutic principles established for oPEP and pediatric HIV therapy may be applied to nPEP for children and adolescents with some exceptions. Optimal therapy for most HIV-infected children and adults includes the use of triple combination ARV drug therapy. Recently updated HHS nPEP guidelines encourage the use of triple-drug ARV PEP regimens for all exposures that warrant nPEP, except for those where adherence or toxicity may be an issue. Although NVP is approved for use in treatment of HIV-infected children, multiple-use NVP is not recommended for use in HIV PEP due to its severe toxicity associated with both oPEP and nPEP. Determining the level of risk in these situations must be done on a case-by-case basis. Table 141.7 summarizes the important points to keep in mind for occupational PEP; however, most are applicable to nPEP as well. In addition to preventing infection in exposures that have already occurred, there needs to be continuing public health and clinical emphasis on preventing these exposures from occurring in the first place in both occupational and nonoccupational settings.

Acknowledgment

I would like to acknowledge Drs. Mary Glenn Fowler, Dawn Smith, Alan Greenberg, and Allyn Nakashima for their insightful comments, and the assistance of Ms. Hang Nguyen in the preparation of this manuscript.

Suggested Readings

Abdala N, Reyes R, Carney JM, Heimer R. Survival of HIV-1 in syringes: effects of temperature during storage. *Subst Use Misuse* 2000;35:1369.

American Academy of Pediatrics, American Public Health Association, National Resource Center for Health and Safety of Children. *Caring for our children: national health and safety performance standards: guidelines for out-of home child care programs,* 2nd ed. 2002.

American Academy of Pediatrics, Committee on Sports Medicine and Fitness. Human immunodeficiency virus [acquired immunodeficiency syndrome (AIDS) virus] in the athletic setting. *Pediatrics* 1991;88:640.

American Association of Blood Banks. *Standards for blood banks and transfusion services,* 21 ed. Bethesda, Md.: 2002.

Cardo DM, Culver DH, Ciesielski CA, et al. A case-control study of HIV seroconversion in health care workers after percutaneous exposure. Centers for Disease Control and Prevention Needlestick Surveillance Group. *New Engl J Med* 1997;337:1485.

Centers for Disease Control and Prevention. Antiretroviral postexposure prophylaxis after sexual, injection-drug use, or other nonoccupational exposure to HIV in the United States: recommendations from the U.S. Department of Health and Human Services. *MMWR Morb Mortal Wkly Rep* 2005; 54:1.

Centers for Disease Control and Prevention. Guidelines for preventing transmission of human immunodeficiency virus through transplantation of human tissue and organs. Centers for Disease Control and Prevention. *MMWR Morb Mortal Wkly Rep* 1994;43:1.

Centers for Disease Control and Prevention. Serious adverse events attributed to nevirapine regimens for postexposure prophylaxis after HIV exposures–worldwide, 1997–2000. *MMWR Morb Mortal Wkly Rep* 2001;49: 1153.

Centers for Disease Control and Prevention. Sexually transmitted diseases treatment guidelines 2002. *MMWR Morb Mortal Wkly Rep* 2002;51:1.

Centers for Disease Control and Prevention. Update: universal precautions for prevention of transmission of human immunodeficiency virus, hepatitis B virus, and other bloodborne pathogens in health-care settings. *MMWR Morb Mortal Wkly Rep* 1988;37:377.

Centers for Disease Control and Prevention. Updated U.S. Public Health Service Guidelines for the management of occupational exposures to HBV, HCV, and HIV and recommendations for post exposure prophylaxis. *MMWR Morb Mortal Wkly Rep* 2001;50:1.

Centers for Disease Control and Prevention. Updated U.S. Public Health Service Guidelines for the management of occupational exposures to HIV and recommendations for post exposure prophylaxis. *MMWR Morb Mortal Wkly Rep* 2005;54:1.

DeGruttola V, Seage GR III, Mayer KH, Horsburgh CR Jr. Infectiousness of HIV between male homosexual partners. *J Clin Epidemiol* 1989;42:849.

Downs AM, DeVincenzi I. Probability of heterosexual transmission of HIV: relationship to the number of unprotected sexual contacts. European Study Group in Heterosexual Transmission of HIV. *J Acquir Immune Defic Syndr* 1996;11:388.

Garner JS. Guideline for isolation precautions in hospitals. The Hospital Infection Control Practices Advisory Committee. *Infect Control Hosp Epidemiol* 1996;17:53.

Havens PL, and the Committee on Pediatric AIDS. Postexposure prophylaxis in children and adolescents for nonoccupational exposure to human immunodeficiency virus. *Pediatrics* 2003;111:1475.

Myles JE, Bamberger J. Offering HIV prophylaxis following sexual assault: recommendations for the state of California. 2001:1-33. Available at: http://www.aids-ed.org/pdf/guidelines/pepassault.pdf. Accessed July 15, 2005.

New York State Department of Health, Committee for the Care of Children and Adolescents with HIV Infection. HIV post-exposure prophylaxis for children beyond the perinatal period 2002:19-1. Available at: www.hivguidelines.org. Accessed on July 15, 2005.

Otten RA, Smith DK, Adams DR, et al. Efficacy of postexposure prophylaxis after intravaginal exposure of pig-tailed macaques to a human-derived retrovirus (human immunodeficiency virus type 2). *J Virol* 2000;74:9771.

Public Health Service Task Force. Public Health Service Task Force recommendations for use of antiretroviral drugs in pregnant HIV-1-infected women for maternal health and interventions to reduce perinatal HIV-1 transmission in the United States. *MMWR Morbid Mortal Wkly Rep* 2002. Available at: http://www.aidsinfo.nih.gov. Accessed July 15, 2005.

Resnick L, Veren K, Salahuddin SZ, et al. Stability and inactivation of HTLV-III/LAV under clinical and laboratory environments. *JAMA* 1986;255:1887.

Spira AI, Marx PA, Patterson BK, et al. Cellular targets of infection and route of viral dissemination after an intravaginal inoculation of simian immunodeficiency virus into rhesus macaques. *J Exp Med* 1996;183:215.

The Panel on Clinical Practices for Treatment of HIV Infection. Guidelines for the use of antiretroviral agents in HIV-1 infected adults and adolescents [HIV/AIDS Treatment Information Service, April 7, 2005]. Available at: http://www.aidsinfo.nih.gov. Accessed July 15, 2005.

The Perinatal Safety Review Working Group. Nucleoside exposure in the children of HIV-infected women receiving antiretroviral drugs: absence of clear evidence for mitochondrial disease in children who died before 5 years of age in five United States cohorts. *J Acquir Immune Defic Synd* 2000;25:261.

The Working Group on Antiretroviral Therapy and Medical Management of HIV-Infected Children. Guidelines for the use of antiretroviral agents in pediatric HIV infection [HIV/AIDS Treatment Information Service, March 24, 2005]. Available at: http://www.aidsinfo.nih.gov. Accessibility verified on July 15, 2005.

U.S. Department of Labor, Occupational Safety and Health Administration. *Occupational exposure to blood-borne pathogens; needlesticks and other sharps injuries.* Federal Register 56, 64004, 1991.

CHAPTER 142 ■ MYCOPLASMA AND UREAPLASMA INFECTIONS

W. PAUL GLEZEN

Mycoplasmas are classified as bacteria, but they are unique because they lack a rigid cell wall. For this reason, their morphology depends on the environment in which they grow, they are not detectable by the usual bacterial obtaining methods, and they are not susceptible to antibiotics that act on the cell wall, such as the penicillins.

Mycoplasmas are causes of economically important diseases in animals that may involve the respiratory tract, joints, or central nervous system. The first mycoplasma identified was the bovine pleuropneumonia organism (*Mycoplasma mycoides*), and the species discovered subsequently were called pleuropneumonia-like organisms (PPLOs). These tiniest of free-living organisms were recognized to be similar to bacteria denuded of their cell walls (spheroplasts or L-forms). Only three mycoplasmas have been associated with disease in humans. *Mycoplasma pneumoniae* causes primary atypical pneumonia and is the only pathogen of this group that is an important cause of disease in children. *Mycoplasma hominis* and *Ureaplasma urealyticum* are genital mycoplasmas and may cause illness in the neonatal period.

MYCOPLASMA PNEUMONIAE

Epidemiology

M. pneumoniae is the most common cause of pneumonia and tracheobronchitis in school-aged children and young adults treated in the outpatient setting. The average annual rate is approximately 5 in 1,000 school-aged children. *M. pneumoniae* is an uncommon cause of lower respiratory tract disease in infants and young children and usually does not result in hospitalization of children without chronic conditions. College students and military recruits may be confined to bed with *M. pneumoniae* pneumonia.

Epidemics of *M. pneumoniae* disease usually are long in duration and smoldering, and they may begin in the summer, with peak activity reached in autumn. Sporadic infections can occur throughout the year. In experimentally inoculated volunteers, the incubation period from the day of infection to the onset of pneumonia was approximately 14 days, but the average interval between the onset of an index case and the onset of a secondary case in the same household ranges from 3 weeks to as long as 3 months. The longer interval may be explained by the fact that pharyngeal carriage may persist, even in patients who have been treated with appropriate antibiotics.

Pathogenesis

When growing on human respiratory epithelium, the organism is a small, filamentous structure, approximately 0.1 to 2.0 μm. Infection of a susceptible person probably occurs through contact with *M. pneumoniae*-containing droplet nuclei that are coughed into the environment. Dissemination by aerosol has been demonstrated experimentally and deduced from descriptions of remarkable outbreaks occurring in closed populations. Human infection by aerosol may be accomplished by as little as one colony-forming unit (CFU), whereas approximately 100 CFUs are needed to infect volunteers by nose drops. The concentration of organisms in sputum specimens from patients with pneumonia has ranged from 10^2 to 10^6 CFU/mL.

The organism attaches to ciliated respiratory epithelial cells by a specialized tip. The attachment protein has been isolated, and specific antibodies have been demonstrated in serum and respiratory secretions of immune subjects. These antibodies apparently block attachment and thereby prevent acquisition of infection. Uninhibited attachment of *M. pneumoniae* to ciliated cells leads to ciliostasis, then loss of cilia, and, eventually, the desquamation of epithelial cells. Mononuclear cells infiltrate the submucosa of affected bronchi and bronchioles. An exudate consisting of debris from the desquamated cells, polymorphonuclear leukocytes, macrophages, and mucus develops as the disease progresses and may lead to a productive cough.

Clinical Features

The main clinical features of *M. pneumoniae* disease are fever, malaise, sore throat, and a dry, hacking cough. The onset usually is gradual, developing over the course of several days. The affected school-aged child may not appear particularly ill, and the examiner may be surprised when chest auscultation reveals rales and rhonchi. The chest roentgenogram may show peribronchial thickening and infiltration of one or both lower lobes, with some subsegmental atelectasis. Pleural effusion is not a prominent finding. The peripheral white blood cell count usually is in the normal range. The severity of the illness may be exaggerated in children with sickle cell disease. These children appear toxic, with prolonged high fever and peripheral white blood cell counts greater than 25,000 cells/μL, and they require hospitalization. Chest roentgenography may reveal dense infiltrates involving more than one lobe and prominent pleural effusion.

The progress of the infection may be aborted in some children who have fever and pharyngitis. A larger proportion of children will have a prominent cough and rhonchi in the larger airways on auscultation; in these children, a diagnosis of tracheobronchitis is warranted.

Some children not known to wheeze previously may have expiratory wheezing on examination. A nondescript rash may accompany the infection. A few children present with acute otitis media or bullous myringitis. The total course of the illness with or without treatment may encompass 2 weeks, with a bothersome night cough persisting even longer.

Complications

Many different extrapulmonary complications have been attributed to *M. pneumoniae* infection. The complication best documented in children is erythema multiforme bullosum, or Stevens-Johnson syndrome; the organism has been isolated from skin lesions on occasion. Hemolytic anemia with or without renal failure has been reported in adults. A plethora of neurologic syndromes, including meningoencephalitis, Guillain-Barré syndrome, transverse myelitis, and cerebral infarction, has been attributed to the infection; in most cases, however, the only evidence of infection is either an increase in the level of complement-fixing antibodies or a single high titer. Some cases have been reported in the absence of evidence of significant respiratory tract infection. The neurologic diseases that occur in the presence of cold agglutinin-positive pneumonia, at least, are more acceptable as putative neurologic complications. Isolation of the agent from respiratory secretions should be required to establish the association between *M. pneumoniae* infection and a neurologic condition.

Diagnosis

The diagnosis of *M. pneumoniae* infection can be suspected in a child who has the typical clinical picture described previously. The clinical impression can be reinforced by the presence of cold agglutinins in the serum at a titer of 1:64 or greater. Cold agglutinins are immunoglobulin M (IgM) antibodies that may appear early in the course of the infection, probably because the organism has an antigen similar to the I antigen on the red blood cell membrane. Cold agglutinins are not specific for *M. pneumoniae* infection and are present in only approximately 50% of affected persons, but this finding in a child with no chronic underlying condition is helpful because the likelihood of finding a titer of 1:64 or greater increases with the severity of the illness.

A specific diagnosis can be made by isolating the organism. *M. pneumoniae* is relatively easy to grow and to identify on enriched PPLO agar containing antibiotics to inhibit normal pharyngeal bacterial flora. Approximately 1 week is required for the growth of colonies on agar when they are incubated in a humidified incubator with 5% carbon dioxide. The colonies are small (visible with 10 times magnification), granular, and embedded in the agar without surface growth. When overlaid with a thin layer of sheep blood agar, they produce complete hemolysis in less than 24 hours, thus allowing presumptive identification to be established because

M. pneumoniae is the only respiratory tract mycoplasma that is hemolytic. Another test for presumptive identification is the application of sheep red blood cells in suspension that adsorb to the colonies. In broth culture, *M. pneumoniae* ferments glucose, so a decrease in the pH level is evidence that this bacterium may be present. Specific identification is accomplished by inhibition of growth on agar by a disk soaked with specific antiserum.

Rapid methods for antigen detection are now available to make the diagnosis within 24 hours. They include enzyme immunoassays and quantitative polymerase chain reaction. Although these tests are specific, they may lack sensitivity compared with either culture or antibody tests.

Serologic diagnosis has been accomplished by documenting a fourfold or greater increase in the level of complement-fixing antibodies between serum obtained when a patient is in the acute phase of the disease and that obtained when the patient is convalescent. More specific serologic tests, such as the growth inhibition test, generally are not available in the clinical laboratory. Because the infection usually is indolent and may have progressed for 14 or more days before clinical presentation, a clinically useful diagnosis can be established with a single serum specimen collected at first contact. Enzyme immunoassays measuring IgM and IgG antibodies usually are diagnostic.

Treatment

The treatment of choice for children with *M. pneumoniae* infection is erythromycin. Therapy should be started early for optimal response, which may not be dramatic under even the best of circumstances. Controlled clinical trials have shown that use of either erythromycin or tetracycline shortens the duration of the clinical course and hastens improvement of the chest roentgenographic findings. The usual dosage of erythromycin is 5 to 10 mg/kg given every 6 hours for 7 days. Other macrolides (e.g., clarithromycin or azithromycin) or tetracyclines may be used but are more expensive than erythromycin. Clarithromycin or azithromycin may be more convenient to use than erythromycin and should be as effective. Treatment may not eradicate the organism; *M. pneumoniae* often can be recovered from respiratory secretions after therapy is discontinued. Occasionally, the disease may recrudesce, and the patient may require treatment again. The prognosis generally is good, and few sequelae of infection have been reported.

M. pneumoniae has not gained high priority for vaccine development. Although morbidity rates related to infection are high, the consequences usually are not great. Consideration has been given to incorporating antigens from the attachment protein into an orally administered vector with the goal of stimulating both mucosal and humoral immunity to protect against infection. A safe, effective, and inexpensive vaccine given orally would help to reduce acute respiratory disease in children and young adults.

GENITAL MYCOPLASMAS

Mycoplasma hominis

M. hominis usually is found in the genital tract. This organism grows on routine bacterial media. The colonies are visible on agar without magnification but often are obscured by bacterial overgrowth. The colonies have a typical fried-egg appearance resulting from surface growth surrounding the central colony embedded into the agar. *M. hominis* has been isolated from the blood of women with postpartum fever and from the cerebrospinal fluid or blood of "septic" infants during the neonatal period. *M. hominis* is sensitive to tetracyclines and clindamycin.

Ureaplasma urealyticum

Organisms of the genus *Ureaplasma* are more fastidious in their growth requirements than are the mycoplasmas. The first strains discovered were called T (for tiny) strains. These bacteria have the ability to hydrolyze urea with the production of ammonia; this property is used for presumptive identification by including urea and an indicator in broth cultures. The first association between ureaplasmas and human disease came from studies of nongonococcal urethritis; however, subsequent studies revealed the contemporaneous presence of *Chlamydia*, which clouds the etiologic significance of ureaplasma for this condition. Other investigators have suggested that ureaplasma may be associated with chorioamnionitis and premature labor, but the etiologic significance of these observations remains to be established. This agent has been found along with other genital organisms in the respiratory tract of premature infants with pneumonia. Whether these organisms contribute to the pathology of this disease is uncertain. Ureaplasmas also occasionally are isolated from cerebrospinal fluid of premature infants, with or without accompanying pleocytosis. In some instances, clearing has occurred without administration of specific therapy. Most strains of *Ureaplasma* are inhibited by erythromycin, other macrolides, and tetracyclines, which can be given if treatment seems appropriate.

Suggested Readings

Cassell GH, Waites KB, Crouse DT. Mycoplasma infections. In: Remington JS, Klein JO, eds. *Infectious diseases of the fetus and newborn infant*, 5th ed. Philadelphia: WB Saunders, 2001:733.

Collier AM. Attachment by mycoplasmas and its role in disease. *Rev Infect Dis* 1983;5:S685.

Collier AM, Clyde WA Jr. Appearance of *Mycoplasma pneumoniae* in lungs of experimentally infected hamsters and sputum from patients with natural disease. *Am Rev Respir Dis* 1974;110:765.

Denny FW, Clyde WA Jr, Glezen WP. *Mycoplasma pneumoniae* disease: clinical spectrum, pathophysiology, epidemiology, and control. *J Infect Dis* 1971;123:74.

Fernald GW. Infections of the respiratory tract due to *Mycoplasma pneumoniae*. In: Chernick V, Boat TF, eds. *Kendig's disorders of the respiratory tract in children*, 6th ed. Philadelphia: WB Saunders, 1998:526.

Harris RJ, Williamson J, Hahn C, Marmion BP. Laboratory diagnosis of *Mycoplasma pneumoniae* infection. In: Tully JG, Razin S, eds. *Molecular and diagnostic procedures in mycoplasmology*, vol 2. San Diego: Academic Press, 1996:211.

Heggie AD, Jacobs MR, Butler VT, et al. Frequency and significance of isolation of *Ureaplasma urealyticum* and *Mycoplasma hominis* from cerebrospinal fluid and tracheal aspirate specimens from low birth weight infants. *J Pediatr* 1994;124:956.

Hu PC, Fernald GW. Prospects for the development of *Mycoplasma pneumoniae* vaccines. *Semin Pediatr Infect Dis* 1991;2:217.

Hu PC, Huang CH, Collier AM, et al. Demonstration of antibodies to *Mycoplasma pneumoniae* attachment protein in human sera and respiratory secretions. *Infect Immunol* 1983;41:437.

Pacifico L, Panero A, Roggini M, et al. *Ureaplasma urealyticum* and pulmonary outcome in a neonatal intensive care population. *Pediatr Infect Dis J* 1997;16:579.

CHAPTER 143 ■ CHLAMYDIAL INFECTIONS

MARGARET R. HAMMERSCHLAG

Chlamydiae are obligate intracellular bacteria that are ubiquitous in nature. Members of the genus possess both DNA and RNA, divide by binary fission, contain their own ribosomes, and are susceptible to antimicrobial agents. Although chlamydiae have a gram-negative envelope without detectable peptidoglycan, recent genomic analysis has revealed that both *Chlamydia trachomatis* and *C. pneumoniae* encode for proteins forming a nearly complete pathway for synthesis of peptidoglcan, including penicillin-binding proteins. All members of the genus share a common (group) lipopolysaccharide antigen. They also share a unique developmental cycle involving an infectious, metabolically inactive extracellular form, the elementary body (EB), and a noninfectious metabolically active intracellular form, the reticulate body (RB). The EBs, which are 200 to 400 μm in diameter, attach to the host cell by a process of electrostatic binding and are taken into the cell by endocytosis independent of the microtubule system. Once within the host cell, the EB remains within a membrane-lined phagosome. Fusion of the phagosome with the host cell lysosome fails to occur. The EBs differentiate into RBs, which undergo binary fission. After some 36 hours, the RBs differentiate back into EBs. At perhaps 48 hours, release may occur by cytolysis or by a process of exocytosis or extrusion of the whole inclusion, leaving the host cell intact. Thus, a biologic basis exists for prolonged subclinical infection.

Chlamydiae cause a variety of diseases in animal species at virtually all phylogenic levels. Until recently, the order contained one genus, *Chlamydia*, with four recognized species: *C. trachomatis*, *C. psittaci*, *C. pneumoniae*, and *C. pecorum*.

C. trachomatis and *C. pneumoniae* are the most significant human pathogens. *C. psittaci* is an important zoonosis. Recent taxonomic analysis using the 16S and 23S rRNA genes has suggested splitting the genus *Chlamydia* into two genera, *Chlamydia* and *Chlamydophila*. Two new species, *Chlamydia muridarum* (formerly the agent of mouse pneumonitis-MoPn) and *Chlamydia suis* (causes conjunctivitis, nasopharyngitis, and enteritis in pigs) would join *C. trachomatis*. *Chlamydophila* would contain *C. pecorum* (infections in sheep, cattle and koalas), *C. pneumoniae*, and *C. psittaci*, as well as three new species split off from *C. psittaci*: *Chlamydia abortus*, *Chlamydia caviae* (formerly *C. psittaci* Guinea pig conjunctivitis strain), and *Chlamydia felis* (causes feline keratoconjunctivitis). Controversy continues regarding this reclassification, but we will continue to refer to *Chlamydia* in this chapter. The routes of transmission, susceptible populations, and clinical presentations differ markedly for the three species that cause infection in humans (Table 143.1).

INFECTION CAUSED BY *CHLAMYDIA PSITTACI*

C. psittaci is widespread among many avian species, with psittacine birds, such as parrots and parakeets, and turkeys being the most common; it is a major cause of respiratory and gastrointestinal disease. Humans usually contract the disease from infected birds. The birds may be ill, but inapparent

TABLE 143.1

CHARACTERISTICS OF THREE CHLAMYDIAL SPECIES THAT CAUSE DISEASE IN HUMANS

Characteristic	C. trachomatis	C. psittaci	C. pneumoniae
Number of serovars	15	At least 4	1
Percent DNA homology to C. pneumoniae	<5	<10	94–100
Plasmid	Yes	Yes	No
Contains glycogen	Yes	No	No
Sensitive to sulfonamides	Yes	No	No
Morphology of elementary body	Round	Round	Round or pear shaped
Natural host	Humans	Birds	Humans, koalas, other mammals, amphibians
Population	Sexually active adults, infants	Poultry workers, veterinarians, bird fanciers	All ages
Mode of transmission	Sexual, mother to infant	Aerosol: bird to person	Aerosol: person to person
Diseases	Nongonococcal urethritis, cervicitis, salpingitis, neonatal conjunctivitis, infantile pneumonia, lymphogranuloma venereum	Pneumonia: "psittacosis"	Pneumonia, bronchitis

TABLE 143.2

LABORATORIES THAT TEST HUMAN SPECIMENS FOR *CHLAMYDIA PSITTACI*

Laboratory	Tests Performed	Telephone Number
Respiratory Diseases Laboratory Section, Centers for Disease Control and Prevention, Atlanta, GA	MIF CF PCR Culture	(404) 639–3563
Focus Technologies, Cypress, CA	IFA PCR Culture	(800) 445–4032
Laboratory Corp. of America Burlington, NC	Culture Polyclonal antibody	(800) 334–5161
Specialty Labs, Santa Monica, CA	MIF	(800) 421–4449

CF, complement fixation; IFA, immunofluorescent antibody; MIF, microimmunofluorescence; PCR, polymerase chain reaction.
Reprinted from Centers for Disease Control and Prevention. Compendium of measures to control *Chlamydia psittaci* infection among humans (psittacosis) and pet birds (avian chlamydiosis). *Morb Mortal Wkly Rep MMWR* 2000;49(RR-8):3.

infection also can occur. Psittacosis is likely to occur in poultry workers, veterinarians, and bird fanciers. Person-to-person spread is unusual. Psittacosis is a major problem for the poultry industry worldwide. Several serious outbreaks in turkey farms in the United States occurred during the late 1970s. In 1995, the Centers for Disease Control and Prevention (CDC) investigated an outbreak of avian chlamydiosis in a shipment of more than 700 pet birds sent from a Florida bird distributor to the Atlanta, Georgia area. Affected birds included parrots, parakeets, finches, lovebirds, cockatiels, conures, and canaries. Clinical psittacosis or serologic evidence of *C. psittaci* infection was found in 30.7% of households with birds from the infected flock. An average of 21 days (range, 1 to 47) elapsed between purchase of the bird and the onset of symptoms. Most infected individuals had mild or asymptomatic illnesses. Among persons in exposed households, illness occurred more frequently if the recently purchased bird had become ill or had died. Kissing or nuzzling, handling, and feeding the birds all were associated significantly with the development of clinical psittacosis, but in contrast to earlier studies, cleaning the birdcage was not. The risk of developing clinical psittacosis varied significantly by the type of bird to which the individual was exposed. The attack rate was highest for individuals exposed to parrots. Inhalation of infectious aerosols derived from feces, fecal dust, or secretions of *C. psittaci*-infected animals is thought to be the primary route of infection. The source birds can be infected asymptomatically or can show signs of infection such as anorexia, ruffled feathers, depression, and watery green droppings. Psittacosis frequently is a systemic infection in birds. The turkey strains can induce severe pericarditis. The gastrointestinal tract commonly is infected also.

The clinical course of psittacosis in humans varies, with incubation periods of 7 to 15 days or longer. Often, it starts suddenly with chills and high fever (38° to 40.5°C). Headache, often diffuse and severe, is a common chief complaint, as are malaise and nausea. The headache can be so severe that meningitis can be considered a possibility; 33% of the patients in one series underwent lumbar punctures. A persistent dry, hacking cough usually is present. The physical findings may belie the extent of the pulmonary involvement as seen on chest radiography. Rales may be heard, but changes indicative of consolidation usually are not seen. Chest radiography reveals soft, patchy infiltrates radiating from the hilum or, less frequently, a reticulonodular pattern. Most of the individuals in the Atlanta outbreak had very mild disease characterized by fever, headache, and cough.

The diagnosis of human infection caused by *C. psittaci* has not changed substantially for many years. The mainstay of diagnosis remains serology using the complement fixation (CF) test. According to the recommendations from the CDC for the year 2000, a confirmed case of psittacosis requires a compatible clinical illness, usually with a good history of avian exposure. Laboratory confirmation can be made by one of the three following methods: (a) culture of *C. psittaci* from respiratory secretions, (b) a fourfold or greater increase in CF or microimmunofluorescence (MIF) titer in sera collected at least 2 weeks apart, and (c) MIF immunoglobulin M titer of 16 or greater. A probable case should be epidemiologically linked to a confirmed case or have a single CF or MIF antibody titer of 32 or greater in a least one serum obtained after onset of symptoms. Early initiation of treatment may delay antibody response for several weeks. In its current recommendations for the control of *C. psittaci* infection among humans and pet birds, the CDC provides a list of laboratories that test human specimens (Table 143.2).

The treatment of choice in children 8 years of age and older is tetracycline, given for 21 days. Erythromycin may be an alternative but also may be less effective. *C. psittaci* is resistant to sulfonamides.

INFECTIONS CAUSED BY *CHLAMYDIA TRACHOMATIS*

Trachoma

Trachoma probably is the greatest single preventable cause of blindness in the world. It is endemic in the Middle East and Southeast Asia and (to a small extent) among the Navajo people in the southwestern United States. The disease is spread from eye to eye; flies are a frequent vector. Trachoma starts as follicular conjunctivitis, usually in early childhood. The follicles heal, leading to conjunctival scarring, which may result in turning of the eyelid so the lashes abrade the cornea (entropion and trichiasis). Eventually, corneal ulceration secondary to the constant trauma leads to scarring and blindness. Bacterial superinfection also may contribute to the scarring. The end result occurs years after the patient has had active disease.

Trachoma can be diagnosed clinically. The World Health Organization suggests that at least two of the following four criteria be met for diagnosis: lymphoid follicles on the upper tarsal conjunctivae, typical conjunctival scarring, vascular pannus, and limbal follicles. The diagnosis is confirmed by culture or staining methods performed during the active stage of the disease. Serologic tests are not helpful clinically because of the long duration of the disease and the high background prevalence of antibody in many populations in which trachoma is endemic.

Poverty and lack of sanitation are important factors in the spread of trachoma. As socioeconomic conditions improve, the incidence of the disease decreases substantially.

Lymphogranuloma Venereum

Lymphogranuloma venereum (LGV) is a systemic, sexually transmitted disease caused by the LGV biovar of *C. trachomatis*. LGV strains tend to be more aggressive *in vitro* and *in vivo* than are strains belonging to the trachoma biovar. Some 20 cases of LGV have been reported in children. Fewer than 1,000 cases are reported in adults in the United States each year. Unlike the trachoma biovar, LGV strains have a predilection for lymph node involvement.

The clinical course of LGV occurs in three stages. The first stage is characterized by the appearance of the primary lesion, a painless, usually transient papule on the genitals. The second stage is characterized by lymphadenitis or lymphadenopathy. Most patients are seen at this time with enlarging, painful buboes, usually in the groin. The nodes may break down and drain. Men are more likely to have this symptom. In women, the lymphatic drainage of the vulva is to the retroperitoneal nodes. Fever, myalgia, and headache also are common. In the tertiary stage, a full-blown genitoanorectal syndrome is seen, with rectovaginal fistulas, rectal strictures, and urethral destruction.

LGV can be diagnosed either through culture of *C. trachomatis* from a bubo aspirate or serologically. Most patients with LGV have CF antibody titers greater than 1:16. The recommended therapy is 2 to 3 weeks of tetracycline or sulfisoxazole. Tetracycline should not be given to children younger than 9 years of age.

Oculogenital Infections in Adults

The trachoma biovar of *C. trachomatis* also is responsible for a large spectrum of diseases that occur in sexually active adults. In men, it is the cause of 30% to 50% of all cases of nongonococcal urethritis. The CDC has estimated that probably one to three cases of chlamydial urethritis occur for every reported case of gonococcal urethritis. The symptoms are less acute than are those of gonorrhea, and the discharge usually is mucoid rather than purulent. As many as 50% of men with gonorrhea are coinfected with *C. trachomatis*.

C. trachomatis also is the major cause of epididymitis in men younger than 35 years. It also can cause proctitis. Proctocolitis may develop in individuals who have rectal infection with an LGV strain. Asymptomatic urethral infection frequently occurs in sexually active men. Autoinoculation from the genitals to the eyes can lead to inclusion conjunctivitis in both men and women.

In women, *C. trachomatis* infects the endocervix; women may have mucopurulent cervicitis but frequently are asymptomatic. The prevalence of cervical chlamydial infection among sexually active women has been reported to range from 2% to 35%, depending on the population studied. Some of the highest prevalence rates have been found in adolescent girls. *C. trachomatis* also can infect the urethra, leading to the urethral syndrome of dysuria with "sterile" pyuria. Complications of genital chlamydial infections in women include perihepatitis (Fitz-Hugh-Curtis syndrome) and salpingitis. The latter may cause significant morbidity, leading to infertility and ectopic pregnancy. *C. trachomatis* appears to be a frequent cause of salpingitis in adolescents.

The current standard for diagnosis remains isolation by culture of *C. trachomatis* from the endocervix and urethra in adults and adolescents and from conjunctiva, nasopharynx, vagina, or rectum of infants and children. *Chlamydia* culture has been defined further by the CDC as isolation of the organism in tissue culture and confirmation by microscopic identification of the characteristic inclusions by fluorescent antibody staining. Several nonculture methods have Food and Drug Administration (FDA) approval for diagnosis of chlamydial conjunctivitis. They include enzyme immunoassays (EIAs), direct fluorescent antibody tests (DFAs), DNA probes, and nucleic acid amplification tests (NAATs). EIAs and DFAs appear to perform well with conjunctival specimens, with sensitivities greater than or equal to 90% and specificities greater than or equal to 95% compared with culture. Unfortunately, the performance with nasopharyngeal specimens has not been as good, with sensitivities ranging from 33% to more than 90%. The DNA probe, Pace II (GenProbe, San Diego, CA), has FDA approval for only cervical and urethral sites in adults, in whom its performance has been similar to that of most of the approved EIAs available. It does not have FDA approval for any site in children.

A major advance in the diagnosis of *C. trachomatis* infection during the past decade has been the introduction of NAATs. These tests have high sensitivity, perhaps even 10% to 20% greater than culture, while retaining high specificity. Currently, three NAATs are FDA approved and are commercially available: polymerase chain reaction (PCR), Amplicor (Roche Molecular Diagnostics, Nutley, NJ); transcription-mediated amplification (TMA) (GenProbe, SanDiego, CA); and strand displacement amplification (SDA) (ProbeTec, Becton Dickson, Sparks, MD). PCR and SDA are DNA amplification tests; TMA is an RNA amplification assay. A fourth NAAT, ligase chain reaction (LCR)- LCx *Chlamydia trachomatis* Assay (Abbott Diagnostics, Abbott Park, IL), was withdrawn from the market in July 2002. The NAATs currently available have FDA approval for cervical swabs from women, urethral swabs from men, and urine from men and women. Data on use of NAATs in children are limited. Preliminary data suggest that PCR is equivalent to culture for detection of *C. trachomatis* in the conjunctiva and nasopharynx of infants with conjunctivitis. NAATs are not approved for testing those organisms in the rectogenital sites in children. The use of noninvasive specimens such as urine is especially useful in high-prevalence populations such as sexually active adolescents.

A single 1-g dose of azithromycin or a 7-day course of doxycycline (100 mg twice daily) now is recommended by the CDC as a first-line regimen for the treatment of uncomplicated genital infection in men and nonpregnant women. Amoxicillin now is recommended as the first-line regimen for treatment of pregnant women. It has microbiologic efficacy equivalent to those of the several erythromycin regimens and has significantly fewer side effects. Because *C. trachomatis* may be responsible for 25% to 50% of all cases of salpingitis, any therapeutic regimen also should contain doxycycline. Sexual partners should be treated as well.

Perinatally Transmitted Infections

Cervical chlamydial infection has been reported in 2% to 30% of pregnant women, depending on the population surveyed. An infant may acquire infection during passage through an infected birth canal. The overall risk of transmission is almost 50%. The organism can be inoculated into the conjunctivae, nasopharynx, rectum, and vagina. Clinically, the infant may have conjunctivitis or pneumonia.

Inclusion Conjunctivitis

Before the institution of universal prenatal screening and treatment of pregnant women, *C. trachomatis* was the most frequent identifiable infectious cause of neonatal conjunctivitis. The risk of acquisition by infants born to untreated mothers infected with the organism is perhaps 30% to 50%. The incubation period is 5 to 14 days after delivery. The presentation varies extremely, ranging from mild conjunctival infection with scant mucoid discharge to severe conjunctivitis with copious purulent discharge, chemosis, and pseudomembrane formation. The conjunctivitis must be differentiated from gonococcal ophthalmia because overlap can occur in both the incubation period and the clinical presentation of these disorders. At least 50% of infants with chlamydial conjunctivitis also have nasopharyngeal infection. The best diagnosis is made by culture of a conjunctival scraping or by one of the antigen detection methods, both of which perform very well in this setting. Oral erythromycin, 50 mg/kg/day for 14 days, is the therapy of choice. It permits better and faster resolution of the conjunctivitis and also treats any concurrent nasopharyngeal infection, which will prevent the development of pneumonia. Additional topical therapy is not needed.

Although an initial study suggested that neonatal ocular prophylaxis with erythromycin ointment could prevent the development of chlamydial ophthalmia, studies performed subsequently have not confirmed this finding. Ocular prophylaxis with silver nitrate, erythromycin, or tetracycline ointments or drops is not effective for the prevention of neonatal chlamydial conjunctivitis or pneumonia. Identification and treatment of pregnant women before delivery appear to be the best methods of preventing chlamydial infection in infants.

Pneumonia

Pneumonia develops in approximately 10% to 20% of all infants born to women with active chlamydial infection. *C. trachomatis* and respiratory syncytial virus probably are the two most common causes of pneumonia in infants younger than 6 months of age. The clinical presentation of chlamydial pneumonia is distinctive. The onset usually occurs in children between 1 and 3 months of age and is characterized by an insidious course, with a persistent cough, tachypnea, and lack of fever. Auscultation reveals rales; wheezing is an uncommon finding. The finding of peripheral eosinophilia (more than 400 cells/μL) is common. The most consistent finding on chest radiography is hyperinflation accompanied by interstitial or alveolar infiltrates. Erythromycin given for 2 to 3 weeks is the treatment of choice and results in clinical improvement and elimination of the organism from the respiratory tract.

Diagnosis of Chlamydial Conjunctivitis and Pneumonia

Culture of chlamydia from the conjunctiva or nasopharynx is diagnostic. Nasopharyngeal specimens can be obtained with a posterior nasopharyngeal swab or by aspiration. Dacron-tipped swabs with wire shafts are preferred. DFAs and EIAs also can be used for testing conjunctival and nasopharyngeal specimens. These tests appear to perform well at these sites, with sensitivities and specificities of not less than 90%. Preliminary data suggest that PCR is equivalent to culture for detection of *C. trachomatis* in the conjunctiva of infants with conjunctivitis and possibly is superior to culture for detection of the organism in nasopharyngeal specimens. The diagnosis

of chlamydial pneumonia also can be made serologically. An immunoglobulin M titer greater than 1:32 on the microimmunofluorescence test is very suggestive.

Infections in Older Children

C. trachomatis has not been associated with any specific clinical syndrome in older infants and children. Children who have been sexually abused may acquire anogenital infection. These infections usually are asymptomatic. Whether *C. trachomatis* causes vaginitis is not known. Accumulating evidence, however, suggests that perinatally acquired rectal and vaginal infections may persist for at least 3 years; thus, the presence of *C. trachomatis* in the vagina or rectum of a prepubertal child cannot be used as absolute evidence of sexual abuse. Cultures should be obtained from these sites only when a prepubertal child is being evaluated. DFAs and EIA tests both have been associated with many false-positive results when used on specimens from these anatomic sites in children and adults and are not approved by the FDA for this indication.

INFECTIONS CAUSED BY *CHLAMYDIA PNEUMONIAE*

The first isolates of *C. pneumoniae* were obtained serendipitously during studies of trachoma in the 1960s. Subsequent serologic studies demonstrated that the organism was responsible for a 1978 outbreak of mild pneumonia among Finnish schoolchildren. In 1986, Grayston and associates at the University of Washington isolated the organism from the respiratory tract of several college students with acute respiratory disease. DNA studies have found less than 5% relatedness between *C. pneumoniae* and *C. trachomatis* or *C. psittaci* (see Table 143.1). Ultrastructural studies demonstrated a unique EB morphology distinct from that of the other two species. *C. pneumoniae* shares the chlamydia lipopolysaccharide genus antigen.

Transmission is thought to occur from person to person through respiratory droplets. Spread of the infection has been documented among family members in the same household. Studies in the United States that have used culture in addition to serology suggest that *C. pneumoniae* may be responsible for 10% to 20% of community-acquired "atypical" cases of pneumonia (including acute chest syndrome in children with sickle cell disease), 10% of bronchitis cases, and 5% to 10% of pharyngitis cases. Clinically, infections caused by *C. pneumoniae* cannot be differentiated readily from those caused by other agents, especially *Mycoplasma pneumoniae*. Coinfections with both organisms and *Streptococcus pneumoniae* also are frequent findings. Asymptomatic respiratory infection occurs in 2% to 5% of adults and children. Serologic surveys have documented a rising prevalence of *C. pneumoniae* antibody beginning in school-aged children and reaching 30% to 45% by adolescence, a finding suggesting that clinically inapparent infection may be fairly common. However, infection as documented by culture occurs as frequently in young children as in adults; young children often lack antibody detectable by the MIF assay. Respiratory infection with *C. pneumoniae* has been associated with reactive airway disease, provoking bronchospasm in patients with no history of asthma and possibly causing acute exacerbations of the disease in individuals with asthma. One study also isolated *C. pneumoniae* from the middle-ear fluids of 8% of children with acute otitis media.

The specific diagnosis of *C. pneumoniae* infection is based on isolation of the organism in tissue culture. No FDA-approved NAATs for detection of *C. pneumoniae* are commercially available. Data suggest poor correlation between culture and serology, especially in young children. The optimum site for culture appears to be the posterior nasopharynx, and the specimen should be collected with wire-shafted swabs in a manner similar to that used for *C. trachomatis*. Few published data have described the response of *C. pneumoniae* infection to antibiotic therapy. Many of the patients first described by Grayston and colleagues were treated with erythromycin, 1 g/day for 10 days, with generally poor clinical response. *C. pneumoniae* is sensitive *in vitro* to tetracyclines; to macrolides including erythromycin, azithromycin, and clarithromycin; and to quinolones, but it is resistant to sulfonamides. Results of a multicenter study comparing erythromycin suspension with clarithromycin suspension for 10 days in children aged 3 to 12 years who had radiographically proved pneumonia found both drugs to be equally efficacious, eradicating the organism in 86% and 79% of the children, respectively. A second study examining a 5-day course of azithromycin in children and adults with pneumonia found a pathogen-eradication rate of 79%.

Suggested Readings

Alexander ER, Harrison HR. Role of *Chlamydia trachomatis* in perinatal infection. *Rev Infect Dis* 1983;5:713.

Bell TA, Stamm WE, Wang SP, et al. Chronic *Chlamydia trachomatis* infections in infants. *JAMA* 1992;267:400.

Block S, Hedrick J, Hammerschlag MR, et al. *Mycoplasma pneumoniae* and *Chlamydia pneumoniae* in community acquired pneumonia in children: comparative safety and efficacy of clarithromycin and erythromycin suspensions. *Pediatr Infect Dis J* 1995;14:471.

Centers for Disease Control and Prevention. Compendium of measures to control *Chlamydia psittaci* infection among humans (psittacosis) and pet birds (avian chlamydiosis). *Morb Mortal Wkly Rep MMWR* 2000;49(RR-8):3.

Centers for Disease Control and Prevention. Sexually transmitted diseases treatment guidelines 2002. *Morb Mortal Wkly Rep MMWR* 2002;51(RR-6):1.

Centers for Disease Control and Prevention. Screening tests to detect *Chlamydia trachomatis* and *Neisseria gonorrhoeae* infections-2002. *Morb Mortal Wkly Rep MMWR* 2002;51(RR-15):1.

Dowell SF, Peeling RW, Boman J, et al. Standardizing *Chlamydia pneumoniae* assays: recommendations from the Centers for Disease Control and Prevention (USA) and the Laboratory Centre for Disease Control (Canada). *Clin Infect Dis* 2001;33:492.

Grayston JT, Campbell LA, Kuo CC, et al. A new respiratory pathogen: *Chlamydia pneumoniae* strain TWAR. *J Infect Dis* 1990;161:618.

Hammerschlag MR. Diagnosis of chlamydial infection in the pediatric population. *Immun Invest* 1997;26:151.

Hammerschlag MR. Advances in the management of *Chlamydia pneumoniae* infections. *Exp Rev Antiinfect Ther* 2003;1:493.

Hammerschlag MR. Pneumonia due to *Chlamydia pneumoniae* in children: epidemiology, diagnosis and treatment. *Pediatr Pulmonol* 2003;36:384.

Hammerschlag MR, Roblin PM, Gelling M, et al. Use of polymerase chain reaction for the detection of *Chlamydia trachomatis* in ocular and nasopharyngeal specimens from infants with conjunctivitis. *Pediatr Infect Dis J* 1997;16:293.

Rockey DD, Lenart J, Stephens RS. Genome sequencing and our understanding of chlamydiae. *Infect Immun* 2000;68:5473.

Yung AP, Grayson ML. Psittacosis: a review of 135 cases. *Med J Aust* 1988;148:228.

CHAPTER 144 ■ RICKETTSIAL DISEASES

RALPH D. FEIGIN AND ANTHONY M. HLAVACEK

The rickettsial diseases are caused by microorganisms that have characteristics common to both bacteria and viruses. Rickettsiae depend on the intracellular milieu of animal cells for growth and reproduction and are considered to occupy a position between bacteria and viruses. They are, however, predominantly bacterial in character, as indicated by the following properties: They contain both DNA and RNA; they multiply by transverse binary fission; they possess enzymes of Krebs cycle, of protein synthesis, and of electron transport; at least one species contains muramic acid; they are retained by a filter; and their growth can be inhibited by a variety of antibacterial agents. They resemble viruses primarily because they grow only within living cells.

Rickettsiae also are agents that are similar in size and shape to one another, and they can be seen under light microscopy as coccobacillary forms. The characteristic pathologic lesion in all rickettsial diseases is a widespread vasculitis of small blood vessels. The exception is Q fever, in which pneumonitis assumes equal import. The rickettsial agents multiply within cells of susceptible hosts.

All rickettsial diseases are characterized clinically by fever, headache, and rash, with the exception of Q fever (which has no rash) and ehrlichiosis (which frequently has no rash). In the early stages of rickettsial diseases, all infections are susceptible to numerous broad-spectrum antibiotics. All rickettsiae assume a characteristic red when they are stained by the Gimenez method (Table 144.1).

All rickettsiae infections, with the exception of rickettsialpox, Q fever, and ehrlichiosis, induce agglutinins against strains of the bacillus *Proteus vulgaris*, such as OX19, OX2, or OXK (Weil-Felix reaction). Rickettsial organisms all exist under natural conditions in insects such as lice and fleas or arachnids such as ticks and mites. These arthropods serve as vectors for the transmission of all rickettsiae diseases, with the exception of Q fever, to humans.

All rickettsial organisms, with the exception of those that cause ehrlichiosis and the heterogeneic strains of scrub typhus, produce complement-fixing antibodies. The clinical and epidemiologic features of the disease in an individual case, supplemented by the measurement of complement fixation titers, constitute the principal means for establishing the diagnosis of rickettsial infection.

Immunity produced by any one of the rickettsial infections usually is of long duration against reinfection by the same agent. The single exception to this rule is scrub typhus.

Four major groups of rickettsial disease occur within the tribe Rickettsiae. Ehrlichiosis is caused by organisms within a separate rickettsial tribe, *Ehrlichieae*. With the exception of ehrlichiosis, infection caused by an organism belonging to one of these groups confers partial or complete immunity against infection caused by any of the other rickettsiae belonging to the same group. In contrast, little or no immunity is conferred by infections that are caused by rickettsiae belonging to different groups. However, a minor degree of serologic cross-reaction

TABLE 144.1
CLINICAL MANIFESTATION OF RICKETTSIAL DISEASES

Disease	Fever	Rash	Headache	Liver and Spleen Enlarged	Central Nervous System Involvement	Cardiac Involvement	Pulmonary Involvement
Rocky Mountain spotted fever (transmission by tick)	Yes 100–104°F	Maculopapular, petechial and/or purpuric. Extremities first, then trunk	Yes	Unusual	Yes (Common)	Yes (Frequent)	10–40% of cases
Mediterranean spotted fever (transmission by tick or mite)	Yes 100–104°F	Local skin lesion (*tache noire*) at site of bite, rash on extremities which spreads to trunk	Yes	Liver (33%) Spleen (20%)	Unusual	Bradycardia	Unusual
Rickettsialpox (transmission by mite)	Yes 100–101°F	Red papule at site of mite bite-evolves into vesicle then scab.	Yes	No	Very rare	No	No
		Then scattered nonpruritic macules noted on trunk, face and extremities	Yes	No	Yes (Common)	Myocarditis and pericarditis occur, but uncommon	Occasional
Epidemic typhus (louse borne)	Yes 100–104°F or higher	Maculopapular rash on trunk, spreading to extremities	Yes	Uncommon	Yes (Common)	May occur	May occur
Endemic typhus (transmission by fleas)	Yes 100–102°F	Maculopapular rash on trunk, spreading to extremities	Yes (mild)	No	Uncommon	Rare	Rare
Tsutsugamushi fever (transmission by chiggers)	Yes 100–102°F	Maculopapular rash on trunk, spreading to extremities	Yes	Yes (Common)	Deafness and tinnitus may occur	Occasional	Sometimes
Q Fever (airborne)	Yes 100–104°F	No	Yes	Yes (Frequent)	Unusual	Endocarditis, Pericarditis	Almost always is primary characteristic
Ehrlichiosis (human monocytic) (transmission by tick)	Yes 100–103°F	Macular, petechial	Yes	Yes (30–40%)	Uncommon but does occur	Uncommon	Uncommon
Ehrlichiosis (human granulcyte) (transmission by tick)	Yes 100–103°F	Yes (only 10%)	Yes	Uncommon	Uncommon	Uncommon	Uncommon

exists between some rickettsiae of the spotted fever groups and typhus. Generally, immunity that develops after natural infection is more prolonged than that which follows immunization.

Another general characteristic is that arthropods and mammals serve as natural hosts for rickettsiae. However, infection also can occur by an airborne route when infectious microorganisms acquire access to respiratory surfaces or the conjunctivae. The airborne route appears to be the most common method of spread when the infection occurs in laboratories. Humans are an accidental blind-end host for rickettsiae and do not contribute to the survival of the rickettsial species, except for louse-borne typhus.

Rickettsial diseases vary markedly in severity, from benign and self-limited to severe, fulminating diseases. The survival of the patient depends on a prompt establishment of diagnosis and the institution of appropriate therapy.

SPOTTED FEVERS

The spotted fevers are a group of infectious diseases caused predominantly by *Rickettsia rickettsii*. Because most are transmitted by ticks, they are called tick typhuses.

Rocky Mountain spotted fever is the most severe and important of the spotted fever group that appears in the temperate zones of North America. An illness almost identical to Rocky Mountain spotted fever occurs in South America, where it is called Sao Paulo disease. Other less severe forms of tick typhus occur in Asia, Africa, Australia, and Europe. They can be distinguished by geographic location as well as by differences in the spotted fever rickettsiae that cause them. Important epidemiologic characteristics of the spotted fever group and of other rickettsiae diseases are provided in Table 144.2.

Rocky Mountain Spotted Fever

Rocky Mountain spotted fever is a disease caused by *R. rickettsii*; it was recognized first in areas of Idaho and Montana, around the turn of the twentieth century. Its occurrence is not limited to the Rocky Mountain area, however; the disease actually is most prevalent in the southeastern United States. The incidence of Rocky Mountain spotted fever in the Rocky Mountain region began a steady decline before the introduction of antibiotic therapy in the 1950s and, by 1988, fewer than 20 cases of Rocky Mountain spotted fever were reported

TABLE 144.2

IMPORTANT EPIDEMIOLOGIC CHARACTERISTICS OF RICKETTSIAL DISEASES

Disease	Agent	Epidemiologic Features		
		Geographic Occurrence	Usual Mode of Human Transmission	Mammalian Host
Typhus Group				
Epidemic typhus	*R. prowazekii*	Worldwide	Infected louse feces rubbed into broken skin or as aerosol to mucous membranes	Humans, flying squirrels
Brill-Zinsser disease	*R. prowazekii*	Worldwide	Recrudescence months or years after primary attack of epidemic typhus	Humans
Murine typhus	*R. typhi*	Scattered pockets, worldwide	Flea bite	Rodents
Murine typhus-like	*R. felis*	United States	Flea bite	Opossums
Spotted Fever Group				
Rocky Mountain spotted fever	*R. rickettsii*	Western Hemisphere	Tick bite	Wild rodents, dogs
Tick typhuses (Mediterranean spotted fever)	*R. conorii**	Mediterranean, Caspian, and Black sea coastal regions; Africa; Southeast Asia	Tick bite	Wild rodents, dogs
Rickettsialpox	*R. akari*	Worldwide	Mite bite	Mice
Scrub Typhus	*Orientia tsutsugamushi*	Japan, Southeast Asia, west and southwest Pacific	Mite bite	Wild rodents
Q Fever	*Coxiella burnetii*	Worldwide	Inhalation of infected particles from environment of infected animals	Mammals
Ehrlichiosis Group[†]				
Human monocytic ehrlichiosis	*Ehrlichia chaffeensis*	Worldwide	Tick bite	Deer, dogs, humans
Human granulocytopenic ehrlichiosis	*Anaplasma phagocytophila*	United States, Europe	Tick bite	Deer, humans, other mammals

*In addition, *Rickettsia australis* (Queensland tick typhus) in Australia, *Rickettsia siberica* (Siberian tick typhus) in North Asia, and *Rickettsia japonica* (Oriental spotted fever) in Japan are antigenically and geographically distinct entities.
[†]*Ehrlichia ewingii*, which causes a variant of human granulocytic ehrlichiosis, and *Neorickettsia sennetsu*, the cause of Sennetsu fever, also are included in this group.
Adapted with permission from Edwards MS, Feigin RD. Rickettsial diseases. In: Feigin RD, Cherry JD, eds. *Textbook of pediatric infectious diseases*, 5th ed. Philadelphia: Saunders.

in the Rocky Mountain and Pacific coast areas. Most of the cases that have occurred in the past 20 years have been reported from the southeastern United States. Between 1993 and 1996, the Centers for Disease Control and Prevention collected and summarized 2,313 cases of Rocky Mountain spotted fever. During that time, the annual incidence per 1 million U.S. population rose from a low of 1.8 in 1993 to 3.3 in 1996. (The overall incidence has dropped, however, over the last 20 years from a high of 5.8 per million in 1981.) Fifty percent of confirmed cases were reported from only three states (Oklahoma, North Carolina, and Virginia). The incidence of confirmed cases was highest among children 5 to 9 years of age (3.7 per million).

Rocky Mountain spotted fever is the most common fatal tick-borne disease in the United States (more than 600 people died from Rocky Mountain spotted fever between 1983 and 1998). Rocky Mountain spotted fever also is the most prevalent rickettsial disease in the United States.

Despite the use of chloramphenicol or tetracyclines, Rocky Mountain spotted fever has an overall case fatality rate of 3.9%. A considerable number of the deaths can be attributed to failure to consider and establish the diagnosis early enough for appropriate therapy to be beneficial.

Etiology, Epidemiology, and Transmission

R. rickettsii is a small coccobacillary microorganism measuring 0.3 to 0.4 μm in length and 0.3 to 0.5 μm in diameter. The organisms usually occur singly or in strands. In stained specimens, a diplobacillus with pointed ends and a transparent band between the two bacilli are noted. Rickettsiae must penetrate cells to grow and multiply. They can be grown most readily in the yolk sacs of embryonated eggs. Rickettsiae may remain viable for several days in blood at 4°C; thus, a specimen of blood from a patient suspected to have rickettsial disease can be held for more days in a refrigerator before a definitive isolation procedure is performed. The Gimenez stain turns *Rickettsiae* red. *R. rickettsii* organisms have a soluble antigenic moiety shared with all the antigenic variants in the spotted fever group, as well as with rickettsialpox.

Because Rocky Mountain spotted fever rickettsiae primarily are parasites of ticks, human disease generally is associated with the biology of the ticks that transmit it. However, disease can be transmitted by the aerosol route in the laboratory or by blood transfusion.

The wood tick (*Dermacentor andersoni*) in the West, the Lone Star tick (*Amblyomma americanum*) in the Southwest, and the dog tick (*Dermacentor variabilis*) in the East all are carriers and vectors of this disease. Rocky Mountain spotted fever rickettsiae do not kill the arthropod host, but they can be passed from generation to generation of ticks transovarially. Congenitally acquired rickettsiae in tick eggs can persist through the various larval and nymph stages into the adult stage of a 2-year cycle of the tick. Infected adult ticks may survive for as long as 4 years.

The important epidemiologic features of Rocky Mountain spotted fever include seasonal characteristics because most cases occur during the period of greatest tick activity between April and September. Two-thirds of the cases in the United States occur in children younger than 15 years of age. The disease also is focal (i.e., relatively small areas within a state may account for a high percentage of that state's recorded cases of Rocky Mountain spotted fever).

Pathogenesis

The principal pathologic lesion of Rocky Mountain spotted fever is a vasculitis that develops after the bite of an infected tick. Rickettsiae multiply within the endothelial cells lining small blood vessels and are disseminated widely by the bloodstream. The rickettsiae can be demonstrated in both the cytoplasm and the nucleus of cells. Numerous mechanisms for cellular injury that have been suggested include injury to cell membranes resulting from penetration by multiple rickettsiae; depletion of adenosine triphosphate by intracellular rickettsiae, causing failure of the sodium pump and an influx of water; damage to the cell by toxic products of the rickettsial metabolism; and competition by *R. rickettsii* for crucial metabolic substrates.

Vascular lesions account for the more prominent clinical features noted, including rash, mental confusion, headache, heart failure, and shock. Pneumonia can be acquired by laboratory inhalation.

The vascular lesions are found everywhere, but they are appreciated most readily in the skin, adrenal glands, and gonads. Inflammation accompanies vasculitis of the heart and nervous system. Interstitial myocarditis is demonstrated readily in the location of the rickettsiae by immunofluorescence, which coincides with the distribution of the myocarditis. In neural tissue, both proliferative glial nodules (which usually are related topographically to inflamed blood vessels) and mononuclear infiltrations are seen. In the kidney, inflammation involves vessels of the interstitium, and acute tubular necrosis may occur in some patients. In the lung, rickettsial involvement of the pulmonary microcirculation results in interstitial pneumonia. Hepatic lesions include portal triaditis, portal vasculitis, and sinusoidal leukocytosis.

Changes in nitrogen balance are extreme. Early in this infection, large amounts of nitrogen may be excreted in the urine. Subsequently, nitrogen imbalances are related to an insufficient intake of protein. The serum albumin concentration is depressed as the result of losses of protein, hepatic dysfunction related to the disease process itself, and leakage of protein through the damaged endothelium of blood vessels.

Hyponatremia may be profound. Reported causes of the hyponatremia include a loss of sodium in the urine, a shift in water from the intracellular to the extracellular space, and an exchange of sodium for potassium at the cellular level. The intracellular sodium level increases slightly. The destruction of cells results in an increase in the serum concentration of potassium and in enormous losses of potassium in the urine. Plasma concentrations of antidiuretic hormone and aldosterone have been increased in some individuals with this disease.

Clinical Manifestations

Fever, headache, and rash are the hallmarks of Rocky Mountain spotted fever, as well as of other rickettsial diseases, although the complete triad may be present in only 45% to 62% of all cases. Mental confusion and myalgia also are common features of Rocky Mountain spotted fever. The onset of disease in children usually occurs 2 to 8 days after a bite is sustained from an infected tick. The onset of clinical manifestations may be gradual or abrupt. Body temperature increases rapidly to 40°C, with a pattern that is characterized by persistence, although many patients do have temperature oscillations of 1.8° to 2.8°C over several hours (Fig. 144.1).

The rash associated with Rocky Mountain spotted fever is one of the more pathognomonic features of this disease. It generally appears by the second or third day of illness, although it may be delayed for a week. Initially, the lesions are erythematous macules that can blanch on pressure. The lesions rapidly become petechial and, in untreated patients, even hemorrhagic (Fig. 144.2). Sometimes skin necrosis occurs. The rash appears peripherally on the wrists and ankles, spreading within hours up to the extremities and onto the trunk. The rash also appears frequently on the palms and soles. The absence of rash, however, does not exclude a diagnosis of Rocky Mountain spotted fever.

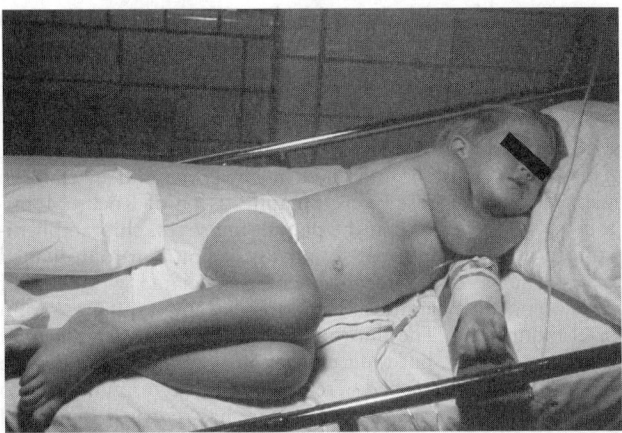

FIGURE 144.1. Patient with Rocky Mountain Spotted Fever. Rash is most extensive on extremities, with lesser intensity on trunk. Lesions are maculopapular, petechial, and purpuric. Facial edema and swelling of feet are evident. The protuberant abdomen is related to enlargement of the liver and spleen in this patient.

Headache in older children and adults is a characteristic finding. The headache is persistent night and day and is intractable. Young children, however, may not complain of this symptom. Signs of meningoencephalitis are common findings and may be appreciated because the patient is irritable, apprehensive, or restless or exhibits signs of mental confusion or delirium. Occasionally, children may become comatose. Meningismus may be present, but it is not accompanied always by abnormalities in the cerebrospinal fluid (CSF). In fact, the CSF generally is clear, with minor elevations seen in the lymphocyte count (less than 10 cells per microliter). Seizures (grand mal or focal) have been observed. Central deafness (persistent or transient) and cortical blindness have been described. Other reported neurologic involvement includes sixth-nerve paralysis, spastic paralysis, and ataxia. Rocky Mountain spotted fever also seems to exert a consistent effect on intellectual function, and several investigators have suggested that a higher probability of disability and difficulty in school performance exists in children who have had this disease.

Cardiac involvement is a frequent finding, and it requires an evaluation of each patient with clinically defined illness by electrocardiography, echocardiography, and other techniques, if necessary. Congestive heart failure and arrhythmias are common occurrences.

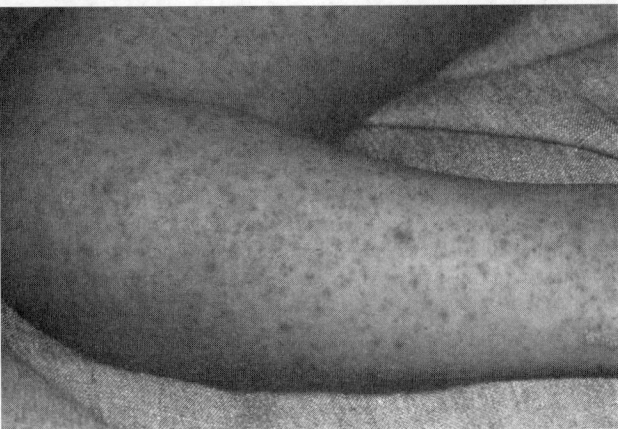

FIGURE 144.2. Close-up picture of extremity showing intense rash with many maculopapular, petechial, and purpuric lesions.

Muscle tenderness is a common feature of Rocky Mountain spotted fever. Characteristically, the patient complains when the calf or thigh muscles are squeezed.

Pulmonary involvement occurs in 10% to 40% of reported cases and may be associated with abnormal chest radiographic results and abnormal arterial blood gas measurements. Chest radiography may reveal cardiomegaly, focal infiltrates, or pulmonary edema.

Generalized edema of the face and extremities usually occurs and, in occasional cases, nuchal rigidity and conjunctival suffusion are seen. Acute tubular necrosis and glomerulonephritis can occur. Enlargement of the liver and spleen infrequently develops. Other gastrointestinal symptoms and signs, including nausea, vomiting, abdominal pain, and diarrhea, arise frequently during the early course of Rocky Mountain spotted fever. Icterus has been reported, but it is a relatively rare event, except in severe cases.

Diagnosis

Specific treatment should be initiated promptly because, in most cases, laboratory evaluations do not permit a specific cause to be identified before therapy must be instituted. *R. rickettsii*, however, can be identified by fluorescent or peroxidase-tagged antibody technique of a skin specimen obtained by biopsy on days 4 through 8 of the illness, and sometimes for a longer period. This technique is a practical means of confirming the diagnosis during the stages of the disease before positive serologic reactions can be obtained. One must recognize, however, that an experienced technologist usually is needed to interpret the immunofluorescent test result and that false-positive and false-negative results do occur. A negative immunofluorescent test result never excludes the diagnosis of Rocky Mountain spotted fever.

Specific serologic results usually are not positive before day 10 or 12 of the illness. Twenty percent of untreated patients with Rocky Mountain spotted fever die, most within the first 10 to 12 days of illness. For this reason, the provision of appropriate therapy never can await a definitive diagnosis.

Selected laboratory clues may be helpful. During the first 4 or 5 days after the onset of disease, the white blood cell (WBC) count is normal or may reveal a leukopenia. As the disease progresses, secondary bacterial infections may occur, and leukocyte counts may increase to as high as 30,000 cells per microliter. Thrombocytopenia of varying severity develops in most cases.

Historically, the Weil-Felix test was used in the diagnosis of Rocky Mountain spotted fever. This test, however, is insensitive and nonspecific, and it should not be used as a diagnostic tool in rickettsial diseases.

Tests available for establishing a specific diagnosis include an enzyme immunoassay, a complement fixation test, an indirect hemagglutination reaction test, microimmunofluorescence tests, and latex agglutination and microagglutination tests. Each of these tests has limitations with regard to sensitivity or specificity. The complement fixation and microagglutination tests are highly specific but lack sensitivity. Indirect hemagglutination and latex agglutination tests are highly sensitive and specific but are not suitable for seroepidemiologic diagnosis because the immunoglobulins detected by these tests (IgM) are short-lived. The microimmunofluorescence test is the most specific and sensitive test available, but it is subject to observer bias.

A microtiter enzyme-linked immunosorbent assay (ELISA) has been developed to characterize the IgG and IgM response in Rocky Mountain spotted fever. The ELISA is both sensitive and accurate. The value of this test is limited, however, because IgG and IgM seroconversions cannot be demonstrated until 6 days after the onset of illness. This test is useful in seroepidemiologic studies.

Investigators have shown that serum from patients with Rocky Mountain spotted fever has a unique profile when analyzed by frequency-pulsed electron capture-gas-liquid chromatography. Typical profiles can be noted as early as 1 day after the onset of disease and before any antibody test result becomes positive. A polymerase chain reaction (PCR) assay that enables the detection of specific sequences of DNA at the theoretic limit of one organism has been developed. The assay is a specific and useful screening test and diagnostic tool for the most common rickettsial illnesses in the United States. This test detects as few as 30 organisms per sample and can be completed in 48 hours, thus permitting therapeutic intervention during the acute illness.

The diagnosis of Rocky Mountain spotted fever can be confirmed by isolation of *R. rickettsii* in embryonated eggs of guinea pigs from blood drawn during the first week of illness before specific antibodies have developed. The isolation techniques are expensive, usually unavailable, and consequently rarely utilized.

Differential Diagnosis

Meningococcemia and measles are the disorders confused most frequently with Rocky Mountain spotted fever. A petechial rash involving the palms and soles that spreads in a centripetal manner suggests a diagnosis of Rocky Mountain spotted fever. The atypical measles syndrome can produce a similar rash. Therefore, a history of receiving previous measles immunization, particularly with a killed vaccine preparation, is important. One should note that killed measles virus vaccine has not been used in the United States for many years. Differentiating from meningococcemia can be difficult because WBC counts may be low or normal and signs of meningeal irritation and moderate pleocytosis may be seen in both diseases. The inability to differentiate meningococcemia from Rocky Mountain spotted fever does not justify delaying the administration of antimicrobial therapy because both diseases potentially are fatal. Treatment should be initiated promptly with one of the tetracyclines or chloramphenicol and penicillin G if the diagnosis of either disease is entertained and neither can be excluded immediately. When the appropriate diagnosis is certain, the inappropriate drug can be discontinued.

Other illnesses that should be considered in the differential diagnosis include typhoid fever, leptospirosis, rubella, scarlet fever, disseminated gonococcal disease, infectious mononucleosis, secondary syphilis, rheumatic fever, enterovirus infection, idiopathic thrombocytopenic purpura, thrombotic thrombocytopenic purpura, immune complex vasculitis, hypersensitivity reaction, and other rickettsial diseases.

Therapy

Doxycycline is the drug of choice for treating Rocky Mountain spotted fever. The 1997 Report of the Committee on Infectious Diseases of the American Academy of Pediatrics allows for the use of tetracyclines (doxycycline preferred) in this setting for children who are younger than 8 years of age. The reasons cited by the committee include: (a) tetracycline staining of teeth is dose-related and it is unlikely to occur in association with one or two short courses of therapy; (b) doxycycline is less likely to stain developing teeth than are other tetracyclines; and (c) tetracyclines also are the treatment of choice for ehrlichiosis, which can be confused clinically with Rocky Mountain spotted fever. For children weighing less than 45 kg, the dosage of doxycycline is 2 mg/kg orally or intravenously twice daily on the first day of treatment and once or twice daily thereafter. Older children should receive l00 mg twice daily on the first day and once or twice daily thereafter. If tetracyclines are provided, 30 to 40 mg/kg/24 hours may be given in four divided doses orally or 20 mg/kg/24 hours may be given intravenously (maximum dose, 2 g/24 hours).

Chloramphenicol also is highly effective when it is given early in the course of the disease and at an appropriate dosage. In children, we treat seriously ill patients with intravenous chloramphenicol at a dosage of 100 mg/kg/24 hours, in four divided doses up to a total dose of 2 to 4 g, with determination of optimal dosage by measurement of serum concentrations. This dosage must be modified in newborns and in children with serious liver disease as a manifestation of Rocky Mountain spotted fever. When the patient improves, chloramphenicol can be given orally at 50 mg/kg/24 hours in four divided doses. The use of chloramphenicol is associated with a risk of developing idiosyncratic aplastic anemia, and it requires serum level monitoring. The fluoroquinolones are another potential treatment option, but their efficacy in treating human disease has not been established. Treatment can be terminated 3 to 4 days after the patient's temperature has returned to normal for a full 24-hour period. The duration of therapy usually is 7 to 10 days.

Thrombocytopenia and disseminated intravascular coagulation may develop in the course of Rocky Mountain spotted fever. Providing adequate antimicrobial therapy is essential to prevent this complication.

Endothelial damage is widespread in Rocky Mountain spotted fever and other rickettsial infections. The need for providing supportive care cannot be overemphasized. Careful evaluation of serum and urine electrolyte concentrations, body weight, and renal function is important to guide fluid therapy. Hyponatremia is treated best by providing maintenance fluids (1,500 mL/m²/24 hours) or, in the case of severe hyponatremia, by instituting modest fluid restriction. The administration of sodium-rich fluids precipitates cardiac decompensation and pulmonary edema in critically ill patients with Rocky Mountain spotted fever without raising the serum sodium concentration substantially. Patients who have concomitant hypotension and hypoalbuminemia may be given albumin (1 g/kg immediately). When the clotting time is prolonged in patients without disseminated intravascular coagulation, the administration of vitamin K (2 mg intramuscularly immediately) has been helpful. Anemia of a severe degree may require blood transfusion. Several investigators have suggested that corticosteroid therapy has been helpful in shortening the febrile period. When corticosteroids are given in sufficient doses to any febrile patient, the febrile period should be diminished, but other specific therapeutic benefits related to this course of action in Rocky Mountain spotted fever have not been proved.

Prevention

Principal preventive measures that are effective include avoidance of contact with ticks and inoculation with killed vaccines. Individuals who are in a tick-infested area should examine themselves frequently and remove ticks from their bodies and clothing. Frequent removal of ticks is particularly valuable because infected ticks must be attached and feeding for 4 to 6 hours or more before they can transmit the disease. The application of substances such as dimethyl phthalate to clothes and other exposed parts of the body may provide additional protection against ticks.

Killed vaccines have been valuable in preventing death, but they do not protect reliably against the acquisition of disease. The vaccine most recently available is a chicken embryo vaccine that is superior to the more generally available yolk sac vaccine. Studies have demonstrated that the chicken embryo vaccine is safe and that two doses elicit low concentrations of antibodies to *R. rickettsii* in 50% of those vaccinated. Although vaccination provides only partial protection against Rocky Mountain spotted fever, it ameliorates the illness when it occurs. An attack of Rocky Mountain spotted fever is followed by solid immunity. No live rickettsial vaccine has been licensed.

Prognosis

The mortality rate from Rocky Mountain spotted fever was approximately 25% before appropriate antimicrobial therapy became available. If appropriate antibiotics are provided before the end of the first week of illness, recovery generally is the rule. The overall mortality rate remains 4% to 7%, however, principally because establishment of diagnosis and initiation of therapy are delayed in many patients until the second week of illness. Between 1993 and 1996, the average case fatality rate was 2.4% and varied between 4.7% in 1993 and 1.2% in 1996. When death occurs, it usually is the result of heart failure, vascular collapse, renal failure, or thrombocytopenia, either alone or in combination. Central nervous system involvement and disseminated intravascular coagulation are common occurrences.

Complications develop less commonly in patients who receive appropriate therapy early. Bronchopneumonia may develop in critically ill patients, and the infusion of sodium-rich parenteral fluid may precipitate both cardiac failure and pulmonary edema.

Mediterranean Spotted Fever

Mediterranean spotted fever was described first in 1910; it is a tick-borne infection caused by *R. conorii*. Other names given to this illness include boutonneuse fever, Kenya tick-bite fever, African tick typhus, India tick typhus, Israeli spotted fever, and Marseilles fever. A resurgence of this disease in Mediterranean countries such as Spain, Italy, and Israel has occurred.

Epidemiology

R. conorii is an obligate intracellular parasite of mites, which inoculate the microorganisms directly into the dermis during feeding. In the Mediterranean area, the vector is the brown dog tick, *Rhipicephalus sanguineus*. Various species of mites may act as vectors in other geographic areas.

The epidemiology of Mediterranean spotted fever is determined by the biology of the tick, which results in a consistent seasonal peak from late June to mid-October. Humans are accidental hosts and become a dead end in the transmission chain. Habitual contact with dogs appears to be the most common factor among people who acquire the infection. *Rickettsiae* also may be inoculated by scratching and via the conjunctival route. Laboratory infection by accidental inoculation has been described.

The exact prevalence of Mediterranean spotted fever is unknown, although seropositivity rates of antibodies to *R. conorii* have been reported to be as high as 70% in some regions of Spain.

Clinical Manifestations

The infecting bite passes unnoticed in most cases, and the incubation period varies from 6 to 10 days. Late in the incubation period, a small indurated lesion, called a tache noire (black spot), develops at the site of the tick bite. The lesion is not painful and rarely is pruritic. It becomes necrotic at its center, develops an eschar, and gives rise to enlargement of regional lymph nodes. The tache noire is pathognomonic but not always is present, with reported incidence rates varying from 30% to 90%. The tache noire is localized predominantly on the heads of children and on the legs of adults.

The onset of disease usually is abrupt, with severe headache, malaise, and a temperature that reaches 39°C to 40°C within the first 2 or 3 days. The fever continues for 6 to 12 days, and antibiotics can shorten the febrile period. Generalized myalgias, especially of the leg muscles, are a prominent feature. A rash usually appears on the third, fourth, or fifth febrile day.

The initial lesions are on the extremities; after 24 to 36 hours, the rash spreads to the trunk, neck, face, buttocks, palms, and soles. The first lesions are macular, pink, and irregularly defined; they become maculopapular after a few hours. Generally, they measure 1 to 4 mm in diameter. The rash persists for 10 to 20 days after the remission of clinical symptoms. The cutaneous manifestations result from the involvement of the vascular structures of the dermis by a vasculitis that is similar to the one seen with Rocky Mountain spotted fever.

Bradycardia is the most consistent cardiovascular finding in Mediterranean spotted fever, but other dysrhythmias have been reported. Phlebitis of the lower limbs is the main vascular complication. Venous thrombosis is a recognized complication, particularly in pregnant patients. More seriously ill patients may have pericarditis, heart failure, myocarditis, nephritis with acute renal failure, pneumonitis, pleuritis, the adult respiratory distress syndrome, or involvement of the central nervous system.

The liver is palpable in one-third of the patients, and the spleen may enlarge in 20% of children. Tests of hepatic function reveal an increase in levels of serum transaminases in more than one-half of the cases. Alkaline phosphatase concentrations are elevated in one-third of the patients. Needle biopsy of the liver reveals foci of hepatocellular necrosis and a predominantly mononuclear reaction to the necrosis at sites of infection caused by *R. conorii*.

Other systemic symptoms may occur. Photophobia and bilateral conjunctivitis have been reported. Severe unilateral conjunctivitis suggests transmission of the disease via the conjunctival route.

Occasionally, Mediterranean spotted fever may follow a rapidly fatal course. The rapid progression of the disease is characterized by a widespread vasculitis resulting in irreversible shock, disseminated intravascular coagulopathy, encephalopathy, and renal failure.

Diagnosis

If biopsy is performed early in the course of the disease, rickettsial organisms can be detected by immunofluorescence or by restriction fragment length polymorphism analysis of a PCR product from the tache noire. *R. conorii* cannot be isolated from blood cultures by means of routine laboratory procedures. The clinical presentation, geographic location, and epidemiologic considerations are helpful in establishing the diagnosis. Laboratory diagnosis is an important adjunct and involves the serologic identification of serum antibody.

Complement fixation, microagglutination, ELISA, and indirect immunofluorescence tests are available. The identification of specific IgM by immunofluorescence helps to differentiate acute infection from a carrier state. A latex agglutination test for the detection of antibodies to *R. conorii* is both sensitive and specific. The test is simpler and more rapid than is microagglutination.

Differential Diagnosis

Before the rash appears, differentiating Mediterranean spotted fever from other acute infections is difficult. Even after the appearance of the rash, the disease can be confused with measles, meningococcemia, toxicodermatosis, secondary syphilis, and leukocytoclastic angiitis. Other rickettsial diseases should be considered, especially in the absence of a tache noire. Cross-reactions among rickettsiae occur with immunofluorescence testing. Differentiation from typhoid fever can be established when agglutinins against antigens of typhoid or paratyphoid bacilli develop.

Treatment and Prevention

Mediterranean spotted fever generally runs a benign course and rarely is fatal. Doxycycline is the drug of choice, but tetracycline, chloramphenicol, or ciprofloxacin are acceptable alternatives. Recommended dosages are 100 to 200 mg/day for doxycycline and 2 g/day for tetracycline hydrochloride. The optimal duration of specific therapy has not been established definitively.

The major effective methods of control are concerned with the avoidance of tick bites. Natural immunity occurs after infection, and specific antibodies have been shown to persist for as long as 4 years after acute illness. Effective vaccines are not available.

OTHER TICK TYPHUS FEVERS

Three other antigenically distinct rickettsiae are *R. sibirica*, *R. australis*, and *R. japonica*, the causative agents of Siberian tick typhus, Queensland tick typhus, and Oriental spotted fevers, respectively. These agents share the same antigen as *R. rickettsii*, but they have distinguishing type-specific antigens demonstrated by complement fixation and neutralization tests. Siberian tick typhus has been diagnosed throughout central Asia, Queensland tick typhus is found in eastern Australia, and Oriental spotted fever is found in Japan.

Dogs constitute the principal mammalian reservoir, but ticks also act as reservoirs by virtue of transovarial transmission. All three diseases have similar clinical, pathologic, and epidemiologic patterns. They produce a mild disease, similar to that of Mediterranean spotted fever.

Treatment is similar to that for Rocky Mountain spotted fever.

Rickettsialpox

Rickettsialpox first was recognized in New York City, in 1946, as a benign rickettsial infection caused by *R. akari*. This organism is related antigenically to the spotted fever group. Certain features of the disease that distinguish rickettsialpox from other rickettsial infections include transmission by the body mite, an eschar at the site of the infectious mite bite, a vesiculopapular rather than maculopapular rash, and the absence of Weil-Felix agglutinins.

Organisms, Epidemiology, and Transmission

The causative agent, *R. akari*, grows in the nucleus as well as the cytoplasm of cells and is a soluble antigen that cross-reacts with Rocky Mountain spotted fever and three other tick typhus rickettsiae. Its clinical, epidemiologic, and serologic features distinguish it from other diseases of the spotted fever group.

Most cases of rickettsialpox in the United States have been reported from New York City, although some have been observed in other cities in the eastern portion of the country. A similar disease has been described in Ukrainian cities in the former Soviet Union. A disease that is clinically consistent with rickettsialpox has been reported in the Republic of South Africa.

House mice are the natural hosts of the mite that transmits rickettsialpox in the United States, but rats have been found to be infected in Russia, and wild rodents are suspected of carrying the disease in South Africa.

Clinical Manifestations

The incubation period of rickettsialpox is 9 to 14 days, but determining it precisely is difficult because most patients have continual exposure to the vector in their homes. Initially, a red papule develops at the site of the mite bite. The lesion slowly develops into a papulovesicular lesion, which soon becomes

a black scab or eschar at the time the fever begins. The lesion most often is solitary, although two eschars have been described in selected cases. Regional lymphadenopathy related to the primary eschar occurs almost invariably.

The temperature is irregular, fluctuating between 37.8°C and 39.5°C, and fever rarely lasts longer than 1 week. The disease characteristically is accompanied by headache, fever, cough, nausea, vomiting, and abdominal pain. The rash develops rapidly from scattered nonpruritic macules that become firm maculopapules in 1 or 2 days. In another day, the papules become vesicles. The lesions usually appear on the face, trunk, and extremities, but they also may be seen on the palms, soles, and mucous membranes. The number of lesions varies from five to more than 100. The characteristic papulovesicular lesions are distributed so haphazardly that this disorder is difficult to distinguish from varicella.

Diagnosis

The diagnosis can be made with complement fixation or immunofluorescence tests. Weil-Felix tests are useless because no *Proteus* agglutinins are produced. The major differential diagnosis is chickenpox.

Treatment

Deaths have not been reported. Doxycycline is the drug of choice for rickettsialpox, but chloramphenicol is an acceptable alternative. A treatment course of 3 to 5 days is sufficient. In infants and young children with mild illness, antibiotics can be withheld because the disease is self-limiting.

TYPHUS GROUP

The typhus group consists of three diseases: louse-borne typhus, Brill-Zinsser disease, and murine flea-borne typhus. These diseases are similar clinically but distinct epidemiologically.

Primary Louse-Borne Typhus

Primary louse-borne or epidemic typhus is an acute infectious disease transmitted by the body louse to humans. Louse-borne typhus has occurred predominantly in Europe, Asia, and Africa and is seen only intermittently in the United States. It has played a major role in the history of many nations since the fifteenth century. After World War I, more than 30 million people in Eastern Europe were infected with typhus and an estimated 3 million died.

Etiology, Epidemiology, and Transmission

The etiologic agent of louse-borne typhus fever is *R. prowazekii*. The morphology, metabolism, growth, toxin production, and staining characteristics of this organism are similar to those of rickettsiae of the spotted fever group.

Initially, the causative agent of epidemic typhus was thought to exist only in the human-louse-human cycle, and individuals who recovered from typhus were thought to constitute the principal reservoir of *R. prowazekii* during periods between epidemics. However, the findings of sporadic *R. prowazekii* infection, particularly in the United States, suggest that the agent of epidemic typhus may be perpetuated in an animal reservoir.

The louse becomes infected during a blood meal from a febrile patient. After a 5- to 10-day incubation period in the louse, a large number of rickettsiae can be found in louse feces. Transmission of rickettsiae from an infected louse to a new host can occur in several ways. A louse defecates as it feeds, and infected feces can be rubbed into the louse-bite wound. Dried louse feces can gain access to the mucous membrane of the eye or respiratory tract. The typhus spreads through a community as an epidemic, primarily because the louse prefers to feed on people with a normal body temperature. Hence, infected lice leave febrile patients as well as dead patients and prefer to feed on newer hosts who are healthy. Crowding, as occurs during wars or periods of famine, permits the ready transfer to new hosts.

Clinical Manifestations

One to 2 weeks after an infected louse bites a human host, the illness usually begins abruptly. The principal manifestations are fever, headache, and rash. The temperature increases to 40°C or higher. In an untreated patient, it may remain at this level, fluctuating only minimally until recovery or death ensues.

The rash usually appears on the trunk by days 4 to 7 of the illness, spreading peripherally to the extremities and generally sparing the face, palms, and soles. Initially, the rash is macular and the macules fade on pressure. The rash soon becomes maculopapular and, later, petechial-hemorrhagic. Severe, intractable headache is characteristic of this and other rickettsial diseases.

Typhus fever can present as encephalitis, meningitis, or meningoencephalitis. Severe, untreated cases can progress to prostration, stupor, or delirium with terminal myocardial and renal failure. Uncommon complications include gangrene, parotitis, otitis media, acute pericarditis, myocarditis, pericardial effusion, pleurisy, pleural effusion, and pneumonia.

Case fatality rates in untreated cases correlate with patient age. Mortality is an uncommon event in young children, but the rate may range from 10% in young adults to as high as 60% to 70% in individuals older than 50 years of age. Recovery from an attack gives rise to a lasting immunity. However, a relapse of louse-borne typhus occurs rarely (see section, Brill-Zinsser Disease).

Diagnosis

The rash of louse-borne typhus begins centrally and spreads peripherally, permitting this disorder to be distinguished clinically from Rocky Mountain spotted fever because the rash of Rocky Mountain spotted fever begins peripherally and spreads to the trunk. Moreover, the rash on the palms and soles, which occurs so frequently in Rocky Mountain spotted fever, rarely occurs in louse-borne typhus.

Complement fixation and immunofluorescence tests are diagnostic; however, with louse-borne typhus, the *R. prowazekii* strains are used as antigens. Antigenic crossing between any members of the typhus and spotted fever groups of organisms occurs frequently.

ELISA and latex agglutination tests were evaluated and found to be sensitive and reproducible. As a result of the antigenic crossover between the typhus group of rickettsiae, work is under way to isolate the species-specific protein for *R. prowazekii* so that it may be used for both immunodiagnosis and immunoprophylaxis. The PCR assay permits establishing confirmation of rickettsial infection within 48 hours, allowing therapeutic intervention to be made during the acute illness.

Therapy

Tetracyclines, chloramphenicol, or a fluoroquinolone are the antimicrobial agents of choice, using the dosages listed for Rocky Mountain spotted fever. Therapy is given until the child is afebrile for 48 to 72 hours. The usual duration of therapy is 7 to 10 days.

Prevention

Vaccination and louse control are the best means of controlling typhus epidemics. Killed vaccines produced from yolk sacs grown in chicken embryos have been highly effective in preventing death, but they do not prevent infection routinely.

Dichlorodiphenyltrichloroethane and other insecticides, such as malathion and lindane, have proved effective in reducing louse infestation during typhus epidemics. Insecticides should be dusted onto the clothes of louse-infected populations; when this is done, lice frequently are eliminated from the community.

Brill-Zinsser Disease

Brill-Zinsser is the name given to the relapse or recrudescence of louse-borne typhus that occurs many years after the primary attack. This relapsing form of typhus occurs because the rickettsiae remain dormant somewhere in the body, presumably within cells of the reticuloendothelial system. Many years later, during a course of stress or some other factor, the rickettsiae multiply and produce a second acute attack. As a result of partial immunity from the primary typhus attack, recrudescent infection almost always is a shorter, milder, and less debilitating illness. The causative agent is the same as for the primary disease (*R. prowazekii*), and the symptoms and signs are similar in type. Brill-Zinsser disease rarely occurs in the United States, with only one case reported to the Centers for Disease Control and Prevention in the 1980s.

Because recrudescent typhus usually does not occur in young children, tetracycline is the drug of choice. A single dose of doxycycline may lead to a prompt resolution of the clinical symptoms in selected cases.

Murine Typhus

Murine or epidemic typhus is a disease of rats that is passed from rat to rat by the rat flea and is transmitted only occasionally and accidentally to humans by the bite of an infected rat flea. This disease occurs worldwide and is particularly prevalent along coastal areas and around granaries. It was highly prevalent along the Atlantic seaboard and Gulf coastal areas of the United States during the first half of the twentieth century. Murine typhus also is known as urban fever because it is the only rickettsial infection that commonly is acquired in cities.

Etiology, Epidemiology, and Transmission

The causative agent of murine typhus is *R. typhi* (formerly *R. mooseri*), which is similar to *R. prowazekii* in its metabolism, growth, staining characteristics, and toxin production. *R. typhi* is slightly smaller and more uniform in size than is *R. prowazekii*. A new rickettsial agent tentatively designated as the ELB agent also has been identified as a cause of murine typhus.

Murine typhus usually is acquired by humans from the rat flea, *Xenopsylla cheopis*. This flea becomes infected when feeding on an acutely ill rat. The rickettsiae multiply in the flea without causing any ill effects, but the feces of the infected flea are infected for the remainder of the flea's life. Rat fleas prefer to feed on rats, but they feed on people when rats are unavailable. When an infected flea sucks blood, it ejects the rickettsiae into the open wound; alternatively, infected feces may be rubbed into the bite wound or transferred by a dried aerosol to the conjunctivae or respiratory tract. Laboratory-acquired infection also has been documented. In California, sporadic cases have been recorded as a result of the transmission by fleas of

R. typhi from opossums to humans. In the early 1940s, approximately 5,000 cases of murine typhus were reported annually in the United States. Currently, only approximately 60 to 80 cases are reported annually; approximately 80% of them come from Texas. Most cases occur from April through August.

Clinical Manifestations

The incubation period ranges from 6 to 14 days. Symptoms and signs include headache, fever, and rash, and the disease appears almost identical to that of louse-borne typhus. The principal difference is that murine typhus is milder and the duration of illness is shorter. The temperature generally does not increase much above 39°C, and the fever tends to be intermittent. The febrile period terminates after 9 to 13 days. Headache is less severe, and the maculopapular rash is less extensive than that in epidemic typhus. Complications are uncommon developments, and the mortality rate is 1% or less.

Diagnosis

Complement fixation and immunofluorescent tests performed with *R. typhi* antigens are used to diagnose the disease more explicitly. The isolation of *R. typhi* protein antigens has been attempted so that these antigens can be used ultimately to eliminate the problem of an antigenic crossover when complement fixation reactions are performed. The use of PCR assays permits establishing confirmation of rickettsial infection within 48 hours and allows administering therapeutic intervention during the acute illness.

Treatment

As with other rickettsial infections, doxycycline is the drug of choice. Chloramphenicol, tetracycline, or a fluoroquinolone also may be used.

Prevention

Eradication of rats is the principal means of preventing the spread of murine typhus to humans. Rat populations can be reduced by poisoning, trapping, and rat-proofing buildings.

Tsutsugamushi Fever (Scrub Typhus)

Tsutsugamushi fever is an acute infectious disease transmitted to humans by chiggers. The disease is restricted almost exclusively to a triangular area in Southeast Asia and the southwest Pacific. The points of the triangle are Japan, Pakistan, and the Solomon Islands. Individuals who are seen with scrub typhus infection elsewhere generally contracted the disease in this area.

Etiology, Epidemiology, and Transmission

The causative agent, *Orientia* (formerly *Rickettsia*) *tsutsugamushi*, is distinguished by antigenic heterogeneity, which is responsible for the differences seen in the severity of this disease in the same and different locations. It has thwarted all efforts to develop an effective vaccine or a widely specific and applicable serologic test. A modification of the Gimenez method is required to stain scrub typhus rickettsiae bright red.

Trombiculid mites are the reservoirs and vectors of this disease. They transmit rickettsiae to their own progeny via infected ova. They also transmit to the small rodents on which they feed.

Because of the prolonged persistence of *O. tsutsugamushi* in the human host, transplacentally acquired fetal infection can occur.

Pathology

The pathology of scrub typhus is a perivasculitis of small blood vessels similar to that of other rickettsial diseases. An eschar or necrotic inflammatory lesion develops at the site of the mite bite, followed by regional lymphadenopathy similar to that seen with rickettsialpox. Generalized lymphadenopathy is a common finding in scrub typhus, but it is rare to absent in all other rickettsial diseases.

Clinical Manifestations

An initial lesion develops into a necrotic eschar in more than 50% of cases. Mites are acquired when people walk through brush; therefore, the initial lesion generally is on the lower limbs. Regional lymphadenopathy accompanies the primary lesion in most cases. The incubation period is 7 to 14 days. At approximately the time that the initial mite bite, lesion, or eschar is noted, other features of the disease develop, namely, headache, fever, rash, and generalized lymphadenopathy. After regression of the eschar, a scar often remains and may persist for as long as 25 years.

A macular rash generally appears on the trunk for only a brief period, between the fifth and eighth days of illness. In selected cases, the rash persists and becomes maculopapular, extending onto the extremities. The generalized lymphadenopathy is prominent. Hepatosplenomegaly and conjunctival injection are seen commonly in patients with this disorder. Deafness and tinnitus may occur and are helpful diagnostic features when they appear. Atypical pneumonia, overwhelming pneumonia resembling the adult respiratory distress syndrome, myocarditis, and disseminated intravascular coagulation have been reported.

Diagnosis

The Weil-Felix OXK strain agglutination reaction may be the only serologic test result that is available in many less developed countries. It can aid in confirming a tentative diagnosis made during the acute phase of the disease, when administration of specific therapy can be life-saving. Only 50% of patients with scrub typhus ever have a positive OXK agglutination titer result, however.

Immunofluorescence tests are more diagnostic and reliable. Because of the multiplicity of scrub typhus strains, however, eight or more of the antigenic strains must be included in the immunofluorescence test for scrub typhus. These tests are available in few laboratories.

The antibody to *O. tsutsugamushi* that is measured by immunofluorescence is short-lived; as a result, the true incidence of scrub typhus in endemic areas likely is greater than described. An indirect immunoperoxidase test is available and provides specific, sensitive, and reproducible results. No cross-reactivity exists in testing against other diseases; this test is superior to the Weil-Felix reaction and comparable with the immunofluorescence test in the serodiagnosis of scrub typhus.

A dot immunoassay using nitrocellulose sheets that strongly absorb proteins and nucleic acids has been applied to the serodiagnosis of scrub typhus. The results are interpreted easily by untrained personnel because the differences in color intensity between positive and negative reactions can be distinguished readily by the naked eye.

Therapy

Chloramphenicol and tetracyclines are effective in treating scrub typhus, as described for the other rickettsial diseases. One study documented that a single 200-mg dose of doxycycline was as effective as a 7-day course of tetracycline in treating patients with this disease. In that particular study, therapy was not instituted until day 10 of the disease. Another study done in

Thailand with 39 patients (where resistance to doxycycline has been seen) documents that roxithromycin, a newer macrolide, may be equally effective. With antibiotic treatment, fatalities are rare occurrences.

Immunity begins to develop only in the second week of illness. Because both chloramphenicol and doxycycline are rickettsiostatic, patients with scrub typhus who are treated during the first week of illness may require intermittent courses of antibiotic therapy to prevent relapse. The wide heterogenicity of scrub typhus strains is thought to account for the frequent reinfections that occur after an initial infection. Reinfections rarely or never are seen in other rickettsial diseases.

Prevention

Exposed skin surfaces and clothing can be impregnated with dimethyl or dibutyl phthalate. The short-term control of vectors on camping grounds can be accomplished by cutting, burning, or bulldozing vegetation and spraying insecticides such as lindane or dieldrin.

The use of chemoprophylaxis also is possible for individuals who are in high-risk exposure areas for short periods. Doxycycline given at a dose of 200 mg once a week provides effective chemoprophylaxis for naturally transmitted scrub typhus if treatment is started before exposure to infection and is continued for 6 weeks afterward.

No satisfactory vaccine for this disease has been produced.

Q FEVER

Q fever is a rickettsial disease that occurs worldwide. Q fever is characterized by fever, headache, and pneumonia in more than 50% of cases. Q fever is unique among the human rickettsial infections in that it is primarily a disease of animals that is transmitted to humans by inhalation rather than by an arthropod bite, although it can be transmitted to humans by ticks.

Etiology, Epidemiology, and Transmission

The rickettsiae that cause Q fever is *Coxiella burnetii*. The organism is highly resistant to heat, a unique quality among rickettsial agents, as well as to desiccation and chemicals. It fails to produce cross-reacting *Proteus* strain agglutinins (Weil-Felix reaction).

Q fever primarily is a zoonosis infecting cattle, goats, sheep, and rodents on a worldwide basis and marsupials in Australia. Humans acquire the disease when they come in contact with infected animals and materials contaminated by these animals.

Epidemics of Q fever may occur in areas where animals are slaughtered, particularly when infected animals are pregnant, causing contamination of workers and creating aerosols that are carried by air-conditioning systems and that may infect personnel far removed from the slaughtering areas. Sheep or cattle used in research increase the possibility of occurrence of laboratory-acquired infections, and outbreaks of Q fever have been reported in many research laboratories. Q fever also occurs commonly in textile plants where wool is processed and in tanneries or shearing camps. In addition, Q fever is a common occurrence among children in rural areas who are exposed during the spring lambing season. Parturient cuts also have been implicated in outbreaks of fever.

The prevalence of Q fever probably is underestimated because more than 40% of individuals who have frequent contact with farm animals have been found to be seropositive for antibodies to *Coxiella*. The disease is being diagnosed in an increasing number of children younger than 3 years of age and

should be considered during a workup for fever of unknown origin.

Pathology

Mortality from Q fever is an extremely rare event. *C. burnetii* has been documented in lung macrophages at autopsy and in specimens obtained at transbronchoscopic lung biopsy or at the time of lobectomy. *C. burnetii* also may infect the liver, producing hepatosplenomegaly and abnormal liver function test results. Biopsy of the liver in an infected patient demonstrates granulomatous changes, with a dense fibrin ring surrounding a lipid vacuole. Rickettsial organisms are not found in these lesions. Similar granulomas have been noted in bone marrow. Vegetations on heart valves are seen when endocarditis complicates this disease. Rickettsiae have been isolated from affected valves.

Clinical Manifestations

After an incubation period of 9 to 20 days, the disease begins with chills, high fever, general malaise, myalgias, chest pain, and an intractable headache similar to that seen with other rickettsial diseases. This particular rickettsial disorder, however, is not accompanied by a rash.

Physical findings in the chest generally are minimal, and radiography may be necessary to appreciate the pulmonary pathology. In approximately 50% of patients, multiple round segmental opacities may be seen on chest radiography. Other, less common findings include linear atelectasis, lobar consolidation, or pleural effusion.

Although pneumonitis is a primary characteristic of Q fever, Q fever is a systemic disorder, as are the other rickettsioses. Hepatosplenomegaly occurs frequently, and gastroenteritis and hemolytic anemia have been reported.

The disease usually is mild and self-limited, lasting 1 to 2 weeks, with a mortality rate of 1% or less. Patients in whom Q fever and endocarditis or chronic Q fever develop, however, have a mortality rate between 30% and 60%. Other reported complications include myocarditis, pericarditis, meningoencephalitis, hepatitis, inappropriate secretion of antidiuretic hormone, and glomerulonephritis.

Diagnosis

Complement fixation or immunofluorescence tests that measure anti-phase I and anti-phase H antibody are effective in diagnosing Q fever. Specific IgM to *C. burnetii* can be measured by ELISA or by complement fixation or immunofluorescence tests. Anti-phase H antibody is present early in primary disease, and anti-phase I antibody is present in patients with chronic disease or those who have granulomatous hepatitis or endocarditis.

A PCR test that has the ability to detect as few as one to ten organisms is available. The assay can distinguish between strains of *C. burnetii* that cause acute disease and strains that are associated with endocarditis and chronic Q fever.

An immunoenzymatic test for the detection of anti-*C. burnetii* antibodies has proved more sensitive than has the indirect fluorescent antibody test for detecting low levels of antibody in individuals who have not developed disease. This test is particularly useful for seroepidemiologic surveys of Q fever.

Attempts to isolate the organism may be successful but are unrealistic because they predispose laboratory personnel to infection.

Therapy

Q fever responds promptly to tetracyclines or chloramphenicol, and relapses are rare. The most appropriate drug and the duration of therapy necessary for patients with endocarditis resulting from Q fever remain unclear. Combination therapy that includes quinolones has been shown to be effective. Tetracycline, chloramphenicol, rifampin, lincomycin, cotrimoxazole, and trimethoprim-sulfamethoxazole all have been used with differing degrees of success.

Prevention

Experimental Q fever vaccines have been developed and tested in human volunteers, but the development and production of a safe and effective vaccine have not been accomplished.

Controlling infection in domestic animals has proved difficult. Research laboratories that use sheep should be separated physically from other laboratories. Sheep never should be transported through any patient care area, and any transport should be accomplished in a cart that is designed to protect the environment from fomite and aerosol transmission.

Prognosis

The mortality rate from uncomplicated Q fever is 1% or less. Most patients recover completely within 30 to 60 days, with or without antimicrobial therapy. Antibiotics shorten the course of infection. When myocarditis, pericarditis, or endocarditis occurs, permanent disability and fatality are reported in 30% to 60% of patients.

EHRLICHIOSIS

Two human tick-borne diseases caused by organisms within the tribe *Ehrlichieae* have been recognized in the United States since 1986. The two diseases, human monocytic ehrlichiosis (HME) and human granulocytic ehrlichiosis (HGE), have similar presentations including fever, headache, myalgias, and anorexia, with associated leukopenia or pancytopenia. Sennetsu fever, which is limited geographically to Japan and the Far East, is a third human disease caused by organisms within the *Ehrlichieae* tribe. It is a mononucleosis-like illness.

Organism

Initially, the members of the genus *Ehrlichia* were classified into three genogroups based on morphologic findings and host cell tropism. Recent advances in genetic sequencing have led to a reclassification of these pathogens into three closely related genera instead of the single genus *Ehrlichia*. The genus *Ehrlichia* includes *Ehrlichia canis*, *E. ewingii*, and *E. chaffeensis*—the causative HME agent. The organism responsible for HGE, previously termed the HGE agent, is now known to be genetically indistinguishable from the organisms previously identified as *E. equis* and *E. phagocytophila* and now is termed *Anaplasma phagocytophila*. *Ehrlichia sennetsu*, which causes Sennetsu fever, and *E. risticii* now are members of the *Neorickettsia* genus.

Epidemiology and Transmission

Since the initial report of human illness, more than 700 cases of HME in adults have been described. Every state except North Carolina and South Dakota has reported infection. Illness occurs in the months when ticks are prevalent, from March to October. Approximately 80% of the patients diagnosed with infection recall having tick contact or a bite within the 4 weeks before the onset of symptoms.

Although most ehrlichia patients are adults, pediatric infections are well documented. Infection occurs commonly in children, yet the majority are subclinical. Seroprevalence studies done on 2,000 children at seven academic centers in the southeastern and south-central United States revealed that 13% of children studied have *E. chaffeensis* titers of 1:80 or greater, with 3% having titers greater than 1:160. Similar studies were done with children in North Carolina, where 22% had titers exceeding 1:80, and Missouri, where 9% had titers greater than 1:160.

The Lone Star tick (*A. americanum*) is the likely principal vector of HME. Alternative tick vectors, such as *D. variabilis*, probably exist in some geographic regions. The reservoir for HME has not been clarified. However, deer and livestock are the preferred hosts of *A. americanum*, and proximity to a wildlife reserve is a risk factor for acquisition of HME in some case clusters.

HGE infections have been reported most commonly in Wisconsin, Minnesota, and Connecticut, with evidence of infections existing in seven other states. More than 600 patients have been identified. The deer tick *Ixodes scapularis* and the dog tick *D. variabilis* are the proposed vectors of infection. Most HGE infections are diagnosed during months when the ticks are most active (April to September).

Pathogenesis and Pathology

The pathogenesis of ehrlichiosis has not been elucidated completely. Granulocytes are the primary target cells for HGE, and macrophages are the primary target cells for HME.

The organisms enter the cytoplasm of host cells and multiply in phagosomes into elementary bodies. These individual organisms multiply by binary fission into immature inclusions called elementary bodies. Mature groups of elementary bodies form morulae that are released by the rupture of the cell to reinitiate the infecting process.

Intraleukocytic inclusions have been observed in lymphocytes, monocytes, and neutrophils in some cases of human infection. This finding has not been a consistent or prominent feature of the disease, however, in part because most infections have been documented by retrospective serologic analysis.

Clinical Manifestations

The estimated incubation period for HME is 12 to 14 days. Similar to Rocky Mountain spotted fever, HME is an acute febrile illness that causes fever, headache, anorexia with or without vomiting, and myalgias (Table 144.3). Hepatosplenomegaly and a systolic murmur occur in 30% to 40% of patients. Rash, which may be macular, maculopapular, or petechial, rarely occurs in adults. Among pediatric infections, rash has occurred commonly, with a distribution that often includes both the trunk and the extremities.

Meningitis as a manifestation of HME has been reported in a small number of children, with symptoms ranging from irritability and meningismus to obtundation with response only to painful stimuli. Initial examination of the CSF fluid revealed pleocytosis ranging from approximately 50 to 1,400 WBCs/mm^3, with a predominance of either neutrophils or lymphocytes; between five and 40 red blood cells; mildly elevated protein levels (85 to 120 mg/dL); and a normal to slightly low glucose value. Each of the seven children recovered fully.

TABLE 144.3

CLINICAL AND LABORATORY FEATURES OF ADULT AND PEDIATRIC MONOCYTIC EHRLICHIOSIS

	Percentage of Cases	
Feature[a]	Audit (N = 46)	Pediatric (N = 20)
Fever	96	100
Anorexia	76	78
Headache	80	100
Myalgia	74	67
Rash	20	65
Leukopenia[b]	61	72
Thrombocytopenia[c]	52	78
Elevated aspartate aminotransferase levels[d]	76	83

[a]Some features were not specified for all patients.
[b]White blood cell count less than 4,000 per microliter.
[c]Platelets less than 150,000 per microliter.
[d]More than 55 U/L.
Reprinted with permission from Edwards MS, Feigin RD, Rickettsial disease. In: Feigin RD, Cherry JD, eds. *Textbook of pediatric infectious diseases*, 4th ed. Philadelphia: Saunders, 1998:22:39.

One-half to two-thirds of affected adults and children have mild leukopenia and thrombocytopenia. One child has had a documented decline in the WBC count from 13,000 to 1,600/mm³ over a period of several hours. Usually, thrombocytopenia is not associated with clinical bleeding; however, disseminated intravascular coagulopathy has been reported. Elevations of aspartate aminotransferase, which usually are modest, peak at approximately 1 week into the illness, with values ranging from twice normal to several thousand. Other uncommon manifestations of illness include elevation of renal function test results (occasionally of sufficient severity to require dialysis), hyponatremia, hypoalbuminemia, and toxic shock syndrome. These manifestations presumably are a consequence of the generalized vasculitis that accompanies the infection.

The mortality rate for HME is less than 2% in adults. Only one fatality caused by HME has been reported in a child. The child died of nosocomial pneumonia.

The clinical features of HGE are similar to those of HME in that fever, malaise, myalgia, and headache occur commonly. However, rash occurs in only 10% of cases, and hepatosplenomegaly and cardiac murmurs are uncommon findings. Thrombocytopenia occurs in most patients, mild leukopenia occurs in approximately 50%, and elevated serum aspartate aminotransferase levels occur in 90% of patients. The mortality rate for HGE ranges from 5% to 10%.

Diagnosis and Differential Diagnosis

The diagnosis of HME is established by documenting a fourfold increase in *E. chaffeensis* antibody titer or a single titer of at least 64 in a patient with a consistent history. Confirmation of HGE requires a single titer of greater than 80 or a fourfold increase in antibody titer to *A. phagocytophila* by the indirect fluorescent antibody test. Sera should be collected for serologic analysis at the time of establishing the diagnosis and then 2 to 4 weeks after the onset of the illness. A case also may be confirmed by PCR amplification of ehrlicheal DNA from a clinical sample or by detection of an intraleukocytic morula and a single IFA titer of 1:64 or greater.

Human ehrlichiosis must be distinguished from other tick-borne diseases, especially Rocky Mountain spotted fever. The illnesses are similar in that both have manifestations of diffuse vasculitis. Clinically, ehrlichiosis is less likely to be manifest by rash and more likely to have leukopenia or pancytopenia as a laboratory feature. The similarity of ehrlichiosis and Rocky Mountain spotted fever is emphasized by two retrospective serosurveys in which approximately 10% of the specimens, taken from patients lacking the serologic criteria for the diagnosis of Rocky Mountain spotted fever, fulfilled the criteria for the diagnosis of ehrlichiosis. Other tick-borne illnesses, such as Lyme disease, babesiosis, Colorado tick fever, relapsing fever, and tularemia, should be included in the differential diagnosis.

Simultaneous infection with *E. chaffeensis* and *Borrelia burgdorferi* has been described. Whether this case represents dual infection or is an instance of antigenic cross-reactivity is not known. In children, Kawasaki disease may present with features mimicking ehrlichiosis; paired sera from a group of children with Kawasaki disease have failed to react with a panel of *Ehrlichia* antigens.

Treatment

The treatment of choice for human ehrlichiosis is a tetracycline, preferably doxycycline. The dosage is the same as that for spotted fevers. Several children have received treatment with chloramphenicol with apparent improvement, but cases of treatment failure when chloramphenicol was used also have been reported. Rifampin has been used successfully in children with HGE, but further prospective therapeutic trials are needed before it can be recommended for critically ill children. Mild clinical illness is self-limited, and recovery without specific antimicrobial treatment has been described, although fever may be protracted. Because human ehrlichiosis may have a fatal outcome, doxycycline treatment should be initiated when the diagnosis is suspected, without regard for the age of the child.

Suggested Readings

Brettman CR, Lewin S, Holymein RS, et al. Rickettsialpox report of an outbreak and a contemporary review. *Medicine (Balt)* 1981;60:363.

Brown GW, Saunders JP, Singh S, et al. Single dose doxycycline therapy in scrub typhus. *Trans R Soc Trop Med Hyg* 1978;72:412.

Centers for Disease Control and Prevention. Current trends. Outbreak of murine typhus-Texas. *MMWR Morb Mortal Wkly Rep* 1983;32:131.

Edwards MS, Jones JE, Leass DI, et al. Childhood infection caused by *Ehrlichia canis* or a closely related organism. *Pediatr Infect Dis J* 1988;7:651.

Edwards MS, Feigin RD. Rickettsial diseases. In: Feigin RD, Cherry JD, eds. *Text book of pediatric infectious diseases*, 5th ed. Philadelphia: Saunders, 2003:2497.

Hunt JG, Field PR, Murphy AM. Immunoglobulin responses to *Coxiella burnetii* (Q fever): single serum diagnosis of acute infection using an immunofluorescence technique. *Infect Immunol* 1983;39:977.

Jacobs RF, Schutze GE. Ehrlichiosis in children. *J Pediatr* 1997;131:184.

Krause PJ, Corrow CL, Bakken JS. Successful treatment of human granulocytic ehrlichiosis in children using rifampin. *J Pediatr* 2003;112:e252.

Lantos P, Krause, PJ. Ehrlichiosis in children. *Semin Pediatr Infect Dis* 2002; 13:249.

Lee KY, Hyung SL, Ja, HH, et al. Roxithromycin treatment of scrub typhus (tsutsugamushi disease) in children. *Pediatr Infect Dis J* 2003;22:130.

Linneman CC: Skin biopsy in diagnosis of Rocky Mountain spotted fever. *J Pediatr* 1980;96:781.

Liu CT, Hilmas DE, Griffin MJ, et al. Alterations of body fluid compartments and distribution of tissue water and electrolytes in monkeys during Rocky Mountain spotted fever. *J Inject Dis* 1978;138:42.

McDade JE. Ehrlichiosis—a disease of animals and humans. *J Infect Dis* 1990; 161:609.

McDade JE, Shepard CC, Redus MA, et al. Evidence of *Rickettsia prowazekii* infections in the United States. *Am J Trop Med Hyg* 1980;29:277.

Paddock CD, Holman RC, Krebs JW, et al. Assessing the magnitude of fatal Rocky Mountain spotted fever in the United States: comparison of two national data sources. *Am J Trop Med Hyg* 2002;67:349.

Philip RN, Casper EA, MacCormack JN, et al. A comparison of serologic methods for diagnosis of Rocky Mountain spotted fever. *Am J Epidemiol* 1976;3:51.

Treadwell TA, Holman RC, Clarke MJ, et al. Rocky Mountain spotted fever in the United States, 1993–1996. *Am J Trop Med Hyg* 2000;63:21.

Zinsser H. *Rats, lice and history*. New York: Blue Ribbon Books, 1943.

CHAPTER 145 ■ CONTROL OF NOSOCOMIAL INFECTIONS

MARK W. KLINE

The goals and methods of infection control in hospitalized children are no different, in theory, from those in hospitalized adults. In practice, however, the higher percentage of children admitted to hospitals with overt, asymptomatic, or incubating infection, the increased morbidity of certain pathogens in some children, and the close contact required in the care of any young child necessitate modifying traditional methods of hospital infection control. General guidelines by which any hospital or patient care facility may establish a system of infection control are published regularly by the Centers for Disease Control and Prevention (CDC), the American Hospital Association, and the American Academy of Pediatrics. These guidelines, along with state and local requirements and those of the Joint Commission on the Accreditation of Hospitals, are the basis for an effective infection control program.

EPIDEMIOLOGY OF NOSOCOMIAL INFECTIONS IN CHILDREN

Infection that was neither present nor in incubation at the time of hospital admission but was acquired by a patient during a hospital stay is termed *nosocomial*. In general, nosocomial infection rates are lower for children than for adults hospitalized in comparable facilities. For children, attack rates are highest among infants, lowest among adolescents, and intermediate among toddlers and school-aged children. Nosocomial infection rates are highest in large teaching hospitals and lowest in nonteaching hospitals, a finding reflecting, in part, the severity of underlying illnesses and the extent to which invasive diagnostic or therapeutic procedures are performed in the various settings. Children hospitalized in neonatal or pediatric intensive care units are at particularly high risk for acquiring a nosocomial infection.

Virtually any microorganism can act as a nosocomial pathogen under circumstances conducive to its growth and transmission. *Staphylococcus aureus* and coagulase-negative staphylococci lead the list of bacterial isolates found in pediatric and newborn services, followed by *Escherichia coli*, *Pseudomonas aeruginosa*, and miscellaneous enteric gram-negative bacteria. *Candida* is the leading fungal isolate. Viruses are a major cause of nosocomial disease in children. Overall, rotavirus may be second only to *S. aureus* as a cause of nosocomial infection in children. Other viral agents, including respiratory syncytial virus, parainfluenza virus, adenovirus, and enteroviruses, contribute substantially to the rate of nosocomial respiratory and gastrointestinal illnesses. Outbreaks of infections in hospitals occasionally are caused by viruses associated with exanthematous diseases of childhood, including measles, varicella, and rubella.

Direct person-to-person transmission (contact or airborne) is the major mode of spread for most nosocomial pathogens. Prevention of direct transmission is complicated by the social nature of children in hospitals, fecal incontinence and lack of personal hygiene among young children, and mouthing behavior. Intimate contact with visiting parents and siblings provides a portal of entry for infectious agents from the community. Hospital personnel may be intermediaries in the chain of transmission within the hospital by hand carriage of nosocomial pathogens. For this reason the CDC recommends against health care workers' having acrylic nails or long nails (longer than 1/4"), especially in intensive care unit settings.

The inanimate environment is implicated less frequently than is person-to-person spread in nosocomial infections. Some respiratory and enteric pathogens in particular, however, may contaminate and survive on surfaces for long periods. Toys may act as vectors for the spread of infection. Building construction has been implicated in the dissemination of fungal spores and disease among immunocompromised patients in hospitals.

GOALS OF INFECTION CONTROL

Any hospital infection control program should attempt to achieve the following: prevent nosocomial infections and cross-infections (infections spread specifically between patients); provide isolation when required, without denying the patient appropriate care; prevent the spread of disease among patients, hospital employees, and visitors; and educate all potential contacts on means of preventing the spread of infections.

INFECTION CONTROL TEAM

The infection control team is charged most immediately with carrying out the infection control program. Local and state law and the size and character of an institution (e.g., acute versus chronic care patient mix) help to determine the size of the infection control team. The team consists of an infection control committee, which sets general policy, receives information, and gives direction to the other members of the team, the hospital epidemiologist, and the infection control practitioner.

An infection control committee generally has representation from all the hospital services involved in direct patient care (i.e., the various medical and surgical services and nursing staff), from hospital services involved in the hospital environment (e.g., housekeeping and laundry), and from other services relevant to patient care and health (e.g., dietary service). Many hospitals either employ a person specially trained in hospital epidemiology or designate a member of the infection control committee to work with both the committee and the infection control practitioner.

The infection control practitioner in most hospitals is a nurse with special training or experience in hospital infection control and epidemiology. This individual has a pivotal role in the daily functioning of the infection control and surveillance

TABLE 145.1

STANDARD PRECAUTIONS*

A. Hand washing

Wash hands after touching blood, body fluids, secretions, excretions, and contaminated items, whether or not gloves are worn.

Wash hands immediately after gloves are removed, between patient contacts, and when otherwise indicated to avoid transfer of microorganisms to other patients or environments.

It may be necessary to wash hands between tasks and procedures on the same patient to prevent cross-contamination of different body sites.

Use a plain (nonantimicrobial) soap for routine hand washing.

Use an antimicrobial agent or a waterless antiseptic agent for specific circumstances (e.g., control of outbreaks or hyperendemic infections), as defined by the infection control program.

B. Gloves

Wear gloves (clean, nonsterile gloves are adequate) when touching blood, body fluids, secretions, excretions, and contaminated items.

Put on clean gloves just before touching mucous membranes and nonintact skin.

Change gloves between tasks and procedures on the same patient after contact with material that may contain a high concentration of microorganisms.

Remove gloves promptly after use before touching noncontaminated items and environmental surfaces; before going to another patient, wash hands immediately to avoid transfer of microorganisms to other patients or environments.

C. Mask, eye protection, and face shield

Wear a mask and eye protection or a face shield to protect mucous membranes of the eyes, nose, and mouth during procedures and patient care activities that are likely to generate splashes or sprays of blood, body fluids, secretions, or excretions.

D. Gown

Wear a gown (a clean, nonsterile gown is adequate) to protect skin and prevent soiling of clothing during procedures and patient care activities that are likely to generate splashes or sprays of blood, body fluids, secretions, or excretions.

Select a gown that is appropriate for the activity and amount of fluid likely to be encountered.

Remove a soiled gown as promptly as possible, and wash hands to avoid transfer of microorganisms to other patients or environments.

E. Patient care equipment

Handle used patient care equipment soiled with blood, body fluids, secretions, and excretions in a manner that prevents skin and mucous membrane exposures, contamination of clothing, and transfer of microorganisms to other patients and environments.

Ensure that reusable equipment is not used for the care of another patient until it has been cleaned and reprocessed appropriately.

Ensure that single-use items are discarded properly.

F. Environmental control

Ensure that the hospital has adequate procedures for the routine care, cleaning, and disinfection of environmental surfaces, beds, bed rails, bedside equipment, and other frequently touched surfaces, and ensure that these procedures are followed.

G. Linen

Handle, transport, and process used linen soiled with blood, body fluids, secretions, or excretions in a manner that prevents skin and mucous membrane exposures and contamination of clothing and avoids transfer of microorganisms to other patients and environments.

H. Occupational health and blood-borne pathogens

Take care to prevent injuries when using needles, scalpels, and other sharp instruments or devices; when handling sharp instruments after procedures; when cleaning used instruments; and when disposing of used needles.

Never recap used needles or otherwise manipulate them using both hands or any other technique that involves directing the point of a needle toward any part of the body; rather, use either a one-handed scoop technique or a mechanical device designed for holding the needle sheath.

Do not remove used needles from disposable syringes by hand and do not bend, break, or otherwise manipulate used needles by hand.

Place used disposable needles and syringes, scalpel blades, and other sharp items in appropriate puncture-resistant containers, which are located as close as is practical to the area in which the items were used, and place reusable syringes and needles in a puncture-resistant container for transport to the reprocessing area.

Use mouthpieces, resuscitation bags, or other ventilation devices as an alternative to mouth-to-mouth resuscitation methods in areas where the need for resuscitation is predictable.

I. Patient placement

Place a patient who contaminates the environment or who does not (or cannot be expected to) assist in maintaining appropriate hygiene or environmental control in a private room.

If a private room is not available, consult with infection control professionals regarding patient placement or other alternatives.

*Standard precautions apply to all patients regardless of their diagnosis or presumed infection status. Standard precautions apply to any planned or potential contact with (a) blood, (b) all body fluid secretions and excretions except sweat, regardless of whether they contain visible blood; (c) nonintact skin; and (d) mucous membranes. Reprinted from Garner JS, Hospital Infection Control Practices Advisory Committee. Guidelines for isolation precautions in hospitals. *Infect Control Hosp Epidemiol* 1996;17:53.

programs. The duties and responsibilities of the infection control nurse are quite broad. He or she makes regular rounds through the hospital and seeks out suspected cases of nosocomial infection or cross-infection. The infection control nurse answers questions regarding isolation and other infection control practices during these rounds. He or she works closely with the microbiology laboratory so culture results from individual patients and environmental culture results are incorporated into the general infection control plan. The nurse acts as a liaison for any of the hospital services and personnel who have questions regarding infection control issues. The infection control nurse coordinates all activities relating to infection

TABLE 145.2

TRANSMISSION-BASED PRECAUTIONS*

Airborne precautions

A. Patient placement

Place the patient in a private room that has (a) monitored negative air pressure in relation to the surrounding areas, (b) six to 12 air changes per hour, and (c) appropriate discharge of air outdoors or monitored high-efficiency filtration of room air before the air is circulated to other areas in the hospital.

Keep the room door closed and the patient in the room.

When a private room is not available, place the patient in a room with a patient who has active infection with the same microorganism but with no other infection, unless otherwise recommended.

When a private room is not available and cohorting is not desirable, consultation with infection control professionals is advised before patient is placed.

B. Respiratory protection

Wear respiratory protection when entering the room of a patient with known or suspected infectious pulmonary tuberculosis.

Susceptible persons should not enter the room of patients known or suspected to have measles (rubella) or varicella (chickenpox) if other immune caregivers are available.

If susceptible persons must enter the room of a patient known or suspected to have measles or varicella, they should wear respiratory protection.

Persons immune to measles or varicella need not wear respiratory protection.

C. Patient transport

Limit the movement and transport of the patient from the room to essential purposes only.

If transport or movement is necessary, minimize the patient's dispersal of droplet nuclei by placing a surgical mask on the patient, if possible.

D. Additional precautions for preventing transmission of tuberculosis

Consult the Centers for Disease Control and Prevention. "Guidelines for Preventing the Transmission of Tuberculosis in Health Care Facilities" for additional prevention strategies.

Droplet precautions

A. Patient placement

Place the patient in a private room.

When a private room is not available, place the patient in a room with a patient or patients who have an active infection with the same microorganism but with no other infection.

When a private room is not available and cohorting is not achievable, maintain spatial separation of at least 3 feet between the infected patient and other patients and visitors.

Special air handling and ventilation are not necessary, and the door may remain open.

B. Mask

Wear a mask when working within 3 feet of the patient (logistically, some hospitals may want to implement the wearing of a mask to enter the room).

C. Patient transport

Limit the movement and transport of the patient from the room to essential purposes only.

If transport or movement is necessary, minimize patient dispersal of droplets by placing a surgical mask on the patient, if possible.

Contact precautions

A. Patient placement

Place the patient in a private room.

When a private room is not available, place the patient in a room with a patient or patients who have active infection with the same microorganism but with no other infection.

When a private room is not available and cohorting is not achievable, consider the epidemiology of the microorganism and the patient population when determining patient placement; consultation with infection control professionals is advised before patient is placed.

B. Gloves

Wear gloves (clean, nonsterile gloves are adequate) when entering the room.

During the course of providing care for a patient, change gloves after having contact with infective material that may contain high concentrations of microorganisms (fecal material and wound drainage).

Remove gloves before leaving the patient's environment and wash hands immediately with an antimicrobial agent or a waterless antiseptic agent.

After glove removal and hand washing, ensure that hands do not touch potentially contaminated environmental surfaces or items in the patient's room to avoid transfer of microorganisms to other patients or environments.

C. Gown

Wear a gown (a clean, nonsterile gown is adequate) when entering the room if you anticipate that your clothing will have substantial contact with the patient, environmental surfaces, or items in the patient's room or if the patient is incontinent or has diarrhea, an ileostomy, a colostomy, or wound drainage not contained by a dressing.

Remove the gown before leaving the patient's environment.

After gown removal, ensure that clothing does not contact potentially contaminated environmental surfaces to avoid transfer of microorganisms to other patients or environments.

D. Patient transport

Limit the movement and transport of the patient from the room to essential purposes only.

If the patient is transported out of the room, ensure that precautions are maintained to minimize the risk of transmission of microorganisms to other patients and contamination of environmental surfaces or equipment.

E. Patient care equipment

When possible, dedicate the use of noncritical patient care equipment to a single patient (or a cohort of patients infected or colorized with the pathogen requiring precautions) to avoid sharing between patients.

If the use of common equipment or items is unavoidable, then adequately clean and disinfect them before use for another patient.

F. Additional precautions for preventing the spread of vancomycin resistance.

Consult the Hospital Infection Control Practices Advisory Committee report on preventing the spread of vancomycin resistance for additional prevention strategies.

*Transmission-based precautions are followed, when indicated, in addition to standard precautions.
Reprinted from Gamer JS. Hospital Infection Control Practices Advisory Committee. Guidelines for isolation precautions in hospitals. *Infect Control Hosp Epidemiol* 1996;17–53.

TABLE 145.3

CLINICAL SYNDROMES OR CONDITIONS WARRANTING EMPIRIC USE OF TRANSMISSION-BASED PRECAUTIONS TO PREVENT TRANSMISSION OF EPIDEMIOLOGICALLY IMPORTANT PATHOGENS UNTIL INFECTION WITH THESE MICROORGANISMS IS EXCLUDED*

Clinical Syndrome or Condition[†]	Potential Pathogens[‡]	Empiric Precautions
Diarrhea		
Acute diarrhea with a likely infectious cause in an incontinent or diapered patient	Enteric pathogens[§]	Contact
Diarrhea with a history of recent antibiotic use	*Clostridium difficile*	Contact
Meningitis	*Neisseria meningitidis*	Droplet
Rash or exanthems, generalized, etiology unknown		
Petechial/ecchymotic with fever	*N. meningitidis*	Droplet
Vesicular	Varicella	Airborne and contact
Maculopapular with coryza and fever	Rubeola (measles)	Airborne
Respiratory infections		
Cough/fever/upper lobe pulmonary infiltrate in a patient with negative results for HIV or a patient at low risk for HIV infection	*Mycobacterium tuberculosis*	Airborne
Cough/fever/pulmonary infiltrate in any lung location in an HIV-infected patient or a patient at high risk for HIV infection	*M. tuberculosis*	Airborne
Paroxysmal or severe persistent cough during periods of pertussis activity	*Bordefella pertussis*	Droplet
Respiratory infections, particularly bronchiolitis and croup, in infants and young children	Respiratory syncytial or parainfluenza virus	Contact
Risk of multidrug-resistant microorganisms		
History of infection or colonization with multidrug-resistant organisms[‖]	Resistant bacteria	Contact
Skin, wound, or urinary tract infection in a patient with recent hospital or long-term care in a facility where multidrug-resistant organisms are prevalent	Resistant bacteria	Contact
Skin or wound infection		
Abscess or draining wound that cannot be covered	*Staphylococcus aureus*, group A streptococci	Contact

HIV, human immunodeficiency virus.

*Infection control professionals are encouraged to modify or adapt this table according to local conditions. To ensure that appropriate empiric precautions always are implemented, hospitals must have systems in place to evaluate patients routinely according to these criteria as a part of their preadmission and admission care.

†Patients with the syndromes or conditions listed may present with atypical signs or symptoms (e.g., pertussis in neonates and adults may not be associated with paroxysmal or severe cough). The clinician's index of suspicion should be guided by the prevalence of specific conditions in the community, as well as clinical judgment.

‡The microorganisms listed are not intended to represent the complete, or even the most likely, diagnosis, but rather possible etiologic agents that require precautions in addition to standard precautions until they can be ruled out.

§These pathogens include enterohemorrhagic *Escherichia coli* 0157:H7, *Shigella*, hepatitis A virus, and rotavirus.

‖Resistant bacteria judged by the infection control program, based on current state, regional, or national recommendations, to be of special clinical or epidemiologic significance.

Reprinted from Garner JS. Hospital Infection, Control Practices Advisory Committee. Guidelines for isolation precautions in hospitals. *Infect Control Hosp Epidemiol* 1996;17:53.

surveillance. Finally, he or she reports on these various activities to the infection control committee. The infection control nurse usually is a full voting and participating member of the infection control committee.

INFECTION SURVEILLANCE

Knowledge of the rates of infection within a hospital is key to effective infection control. Surveillance data on actual patient infections have proved useful in the design of effective infection control programs. Although environmental micro-

biologic sampling was practiced widely in the past, the data generated often were difficult to interpret and to use for infection control planning. Environmental cultures should be obtained only when other factors (e.g., *Legionella* outbreaks in patients receiving mechanical ventilation or in certain units) point to a possible common environmental source of infection. Cultures performed to evaluate colonization of patients by various microorganisms (especially around invasive appliances and devices) can be helpful not only for providing patient care, but also for allowing the infection control team to monitor the spread of hospital organisms before they cause disease. Records are kept on the types of organisms grown in the various cultures, and the antibiotic resistance and susceptibility patterns of these organisms are monitored so appropriate isolation and antibiotic therapy can be ordered.

In addition to concerns regarding infection that may be present in the hospital at any given time, infection control personnel also should monitor infections that may have been acquired in the hospital but do not manifest clinically until days or weeks after the patient's hospital discharge.

ISOLATION PRACTICE

The CDC recommends a two-tier approach to isolation precautions. *Standard precautions* apply to all patients receiving care in hospitals, regardless of diagnosis or presumed infection status. In the second tier are three categories of *transmission-based precautions* that apply only to patients with known or suspected infection by certain pathogens. Airborne precautions are used for patients known or suspected of having serious illnesses transmitted by airborne droplet nuclei (e.g., measles, varicella, and tuberculosis) that can be carried on air currents over substantial distances. Droplet precautions are used in situations of known or suspected serious illness that can be transmitted by large particle droplets that travel only short distances (less than 3 feet) before settling, including those of invasive *Haemophilus influenzae* type b or *Neisseria meningitidis* disease, certain bacterial respiratory infections (e.g., diphtheria or pertussis), and some viral infections (e.g., adenovirus, influenza, mumps, and rubella). Finally, contact precautions apply to patients known or suspected of having serious illnesses easily transmitted by direct patient contact or by contact with items in the patient's environment. Examples of such illnesses include the following: gastrointestinal, respiratory, skin, or wound infections or colonization with multidrug-resistant bacteria; certain enteric infections; respiratory syncytial virus, parainfluenza virus, or enteroviral infections in infants and young children; certain skin infections; and viral hemorrhagic conjunctivitis. The components of standard and transmission-based precautions are shown in Tables 145.1 and 145.2, respectively. Table 145.3 lists clinical syndromes and conditions warranting empiric use

of transmission-based precautions, in addition to standard precautions, to prevent transmission of epidemiologically important pathogens until infection with these microorganisms is excluded.

HAND HYGIENE

Hand hygiene is the best proven technique for infection control. Nonetheless, physicians have been shown to exhibit only 19% to 26% compliance with well-accepted hand-washing guidelines; nurses have better compliance rates of 40% to 63%. The fact that hand-washing compliance can increase to more than 90% during hand-washing campaigns is encouraging; however, compliance usually drops abruptly when the campaign is over. The CDC recommends hand hygiene as the cornerstone of its standard precautions, including the use of alcohol-based gels. In 2002, the CDC recommended use of alcohol-based gels as an alternative to hand washing to increase compliance among health professionals except when hands are visibly soiled. New formulations have reduced irritation or drying caused by these gels, and allergic contact dermatitis is uncommon. Gloves are a useful adjunct, but they do not replace hand sanitation by either washing or use of a gel.

Suggested Readings

American Academy of Pediatrics. Infection control for hospitalized children. In: *Report of the Committee on Infectious Diseases,* 26th ed. Elk Grove Village, IL: American Academy of Pediatrics, 2003:146.

Garner JS, Hospital Infection Control Practices Advisory Committee. Guidelines for isolation precautions in hospitals. *Infect Control Hosp Epidemiol* 1996;17:53.

Huskins WC, Goldmann DA. Nosocomial infections. In: Feigin RD, Cherry JD, Demmler GJ, Kaplan SL, eds. *Textbook of pediatric infectious diseases,* 5th ed. Philadelphia: WB Saunders, 2004:2874.

Huskins WC, Goldmann DA. Prevention and control of nosocomial infections in health care facilities that serve children. In: Feigin RD, Cherry JD, Demmler GJ, Kaplan SL, eds. *Textbook of pediatric infectious diseases,* 5th ed. Philadelphia: WB Saunders, 2004:2925.

CHAPTER 146 ■ DIAGNOSTIC MICROBIOLOGY FOR PEDIATRIC INFECTIONS

JAMES VERSALOVIC

Since the late nineteenth century, diagnostic microbiology has contributed to our understanding of infectious agents, their relevance to human pathology, and the practice of medicine. The development of staining techniques for the direct visualization of microbial pathogens by light microscopy made rapid assessment of infections possible. Microbial culture techniques permitted the isolation and complete identification of bacterial and fungal pathogens. Morphologic examination by microscopy in the laboratory has been effectively coupled to biochemical testing, immunoassays including agglutination tests,

and DNA probe testing for culture confirmation. Specific viral pathogens and obligate intracellular bacteria may require culture in specialized mammalian cell lines. Advances such as rapid shell-vial culture methods and direct detection by nucleic acid amplification have reduced the need for conventional viral culture techniques. Culture-independent approaches such as serologic testing, direct antigen detection, and molecular diagnostics complement culture-based strategies by facilitating the characterization of fastidious or unculturable pathogens. Finally, molecular methods have added the dimension of

TABLE 146.1

SUMMARY OF METHODS FOR DIAGNOSIS OF INFECTIONS

Methods	Details
Rapid	
Antigen detection	Immunochromatography; direct immunofluorescence (DFA); latex agglutination; rapid enzyme immunoassay
Microscopic smears	Fungal (potassium hydroxide or Calcofluor); Gram stain; routine or modified acid-fast bacillus (AFB)
Nucleic acid (DNA/RNA) amplification	Branched DNA (bDNA) detection; hybrid capture; nucleic acid sequence–based amplification (NASBA); polymerase chain reaction (PCR); reverse transcription-polymerase chain reaction (RT-PCR); strand-displacement amplification (SDA); transcription-mediated amplification (TMA)
Serology (antibody testing)	Immunochromatography (card-based assays); rapid enzyme immunoassays; immunofluorescence
Routine	
Culture	Antimicrobial susceptibility testing; biochemical testing; immunoassays (agglutination); DNA probe confirmation
Histology	Hematoxylin and eosin (H&E); immunohistochemistry; special stains (acid-fast bacillus [AFB], Brown-Brenn, Brown-Hopps, Gomori methenamine silver [fungal], Warthin-Starry silver)
Serology	Direct or indirect immunofluorescence (DFA or IFA); enzyme immunoassays (e.g., ELISAs)

quantitative or viral load testing and genotyping for mutation detection.

This chapter is divided into two sections. The first section describes various methodologic approaches and how different methods may be applied for the diagnosis of pediatric infections (Table 146.1). The second section describes classes of infections and how the laboratory may address specific diagnostic concerns relative to different types of infections (Tables 146.2 and 146.3).

DIAGNOSTIC METHODS

Direct Visualization

In the late nineteenth century, Christian Gram developed a stain (later known as the Gram stain) as a tool for the direct visualization of bacterial pathogens. The direct Gram stain remains a primary method for the rapid assessment of blood cultures

TABLE 146.2

DIAGNOSTIC STRATEGIES FOR PEDIATRIC INFECTIONS

Possible Infection	Primary Test(s)*	Secondary Test(s)†
Acute pharyngitis	Rapid *Streptococcus pyogenes* (GAS) antigen testing	Direct antigen testing for respiratory viruses (enzyme immunoassays or immunofluorescence)
Bronchitis or bronchiolitis	Direct antigen testing for respiratory viruses (enzyme immunoassays or immunofluorescence)	*Bordetella pertussis* PCR; *Chlamydia pneumoniae* or *Mycoplasma pneumoniae* serologies or PCR; respiratory Gram stain and culture; respiratory virus culture; RT-PCR for human metapneumovirus
Colitis or gastroenteritis	*Clostridium difficile* enterotoxin testing; O&P; rotavirus antigen immunoassays or stool electron microscopy; stool culture (including *Campylobacter*)	Antigen (*Cryptosporidium*, *Giardia*) immunoassays; EHEC stool Shiga toxin antigen testing or PCR; *Yersinia* stool culture; RT-PCR for noroviruses.
Encephalitis	Herpes simplex virus PCR of CSF	*M. pneumoniae* IgM serology; *M. pneumoniae* PCR of CSF; West Nile virus CSF/serum IgM or RT-PCR; PCR of CSF for EBV, CMV, VZV.
Meningitis	CSF Gram stain and culture; enterovirus RT-PCR	Blood culture; *Neisseria meningitidis* PCR of CSF
Neonatal sepsis	Blood culture; CSF Gram stain and culture	Enterovirus RT-PCR; *Streptococcus agalactiae* rapid antigen or PCR
Osteomyelitis	Blood culture	Bone biopsy culture
Pneumonia	Blood culture; sputum (respiratory) Gram stain and culture	*Legionella* culture; *L. pneumophila* urinary antigen; *Streptococcus pneumoniae* urinary antigen; M. pneumoniae IgM serology or PCR.
Septic arthritis	Blood culture; synovial fluid Gram stain and culture	
Urinary tract infection (cystitis or pyelonephritis)	Urinalysis; urine culture	Blood culture

CSF, cerebrospinal fluid; EHEC, enterohemorrhagic *Escherichia coli*; GAS, group A streptococcus; IgM, immunoglobulin M; O&P, ova and parasite examination; PCR, polymerase chain reaction; RT, reverse transcriptase.
*Primary: indicates testing recommended as routine laboratory or point-of-care evaluation.
†Secondary: indicates testing by special request or as adjunctive or confirmatory studies.

TABLE 146.3

SELECTED PATHOGENS AND CORRESPONDING DIAGNOSTIC TESTS

Organism	Primary	Secondary
Bordetella pertussis	PCR of nasopharyngeal aspirates or swabs	Culture; DFA
Coagulase-negative staphylococci	Culture	
Chlamydia pneumoniae	PCR or serology	
Escherichia coli (enteric bacteria)	Culture	EHEC Shiga toxin antigen or PCR testing
Enterovirus	RT-PCR	Viral culture
Herpes simplex virus	PCR or viral culture; DFA of skin lesions	Serology
Legionella pneumophila	Culture or urinary antigen testing	Antigen testing (DFA)
Moraxella catarrhalis	Culture	
Mycoplasma pneumoniae	PCR or serology	
Neisseria meningitidis	Culture or PCR	Antigen testing
Respiratory viruses (influenza A and B, parainfluenza 1 to 4, respiratory syncytial virus)	Direct antigen testing, enzyme immunoassays, or immunofluorescence	Viral culture
Rotavirus	Stool antigen testing	Electron microscopy
Streptococcus agalactiae	Culture	PCR or antigen testing
Staphylococcus aureus	Culture	
Streptococcus pneumoniae	Culture	Urinary antigen
Streptococcus pyogenes	Culture; rapid antigen testing	Serology; DNA probe hybridization or PCR

DFA, direct immunofluorescence; EHEC, enterohemorrhagic *Escherichia coli;* PCR, polymerase chain reaction; RT, reverse transcription.

and sterile body fluids. The lower limit of detection of the Gram stain is approximately 10^5 organisms/mL, requiring a relatively high organism load for direct visualization. Following primary assessment by Gram stain, routine cultures are monitored for growth, and positive cultures are evaluated by Gram stain in combination with biochemical, DNA probe, and immunologic tests for identification.

Alternative special stains have been developed for the visualization of mycobacterial, fungal, and parasitic pathogens. The acid-fast and modified acid-fast stains provide important tools for the assessment of infections with mycobacteria and filamentous bacteria. Fluorochroming methods using fluorescence microscopy (e.g., auramine-rhodamine staining) represent the standard approach for primary screening of mycobacteria in respiratory specimens owing to superior sensitivity, as compared with traditional acid-fast stains (e.g., Kinyoun). Modified acid-fast techniques rely on the application of dilute acids to detect partially acid-fast pathogens such as *Nocardia* directly in clinical specimens or cultures.

Fungi may be visualized directly by potassium hydroxide (KOH) or improved fluorochroming techniques with fungus-specific fluorophores such as calcofluor white. Calcofluor white staining techniques in the laboratory (similar to other fluorochroming methods) provide greater sensitivity for the primary detection of fungal pathogens and are recommended for laboratory-based evaluation. Diagnostic parasitology continues to rely heavily on the application of various staining techniques for the direct visualization of pathogens. The ova and parasite (O&P) examination of stool specimens by light microscopy is a routine approach for the evaluation of patients with gastrointestinal infections.

Antigen Detection

In the 1970s, key advances in immunology such as the development of monoclonal antibodies fueled rapid advances in the formulation of pathogen-specific immunoassays for diagnostic microbiology. Cerebrospinal fluid (CSF) bacterial antigen detection has been used for the detection of *Escherichia coli* K1, *Haemophilus influenzae* serotype b, *Neisseria meningitidis* (serogroups A, B, C, Y, W135), group B streptococcus,

and *Streptococcus pneumoniae.* Unfortunately, CSF bacterial antigen detection is not clinically useful in most circumstances, especially with the advent of vaccination for *H. influenzae* serotype b. In a comprehensive study by Perkins and associates that included 478 CSF specimens, all true-positive samples by latex agglutination were positive by Gram stain. Rapid bacterial antigen detection by latex agglutination yielded false-positive results in 54% of the antigen-positive samples. The additional false-positive results resulted in additional costs and prolonged hospitalizations.

Antigens may be effectively concentrated in the genitourinary tract, thus establishing urine as a specimen of choice for bacterial antigen detection. Urinary antigen detection is a reliable approach for the diagnosis of *Legionella pneumophila* serogroup 1 infection and should be performed in parallel with culture for the assessment of *Legionella* infections. The respiratory pathogen, *S. pneumoniae,* may be detected by urinary antigen testing as an adjunctive approach. Disseminated fungal infections such as blastomycosis or histoplasmosis may be reliably detected by commercially available serum or urinary antigen testing.

Stool antigen detection represents a convenient strategy for the diagnosis of gastrointestinal infections. Screening for protozoal pathogens in stool by O&P examination is tedious and time consuming. In a study from Alberta, reported by Kabani and colleagues, with 2,652 stool specimens from 1,532 children, the O&P examination rarely uncovered enteric parasites in hospitalized children (4%) as compared with children in the pediatric gastroenterology clinic (13%). Reliable commercial antigen detection assays are available for *Giardia lamblia* and *Cryptosporidium parvum* that may exceed O&P tests with respect to sensitivity. The gastric bacterial pathogen, *Helicobacter pylori,* may be diagnosed and monitored following treatment by enzyme immunoassay-based stool antigen detection with excellent specificity and sensitivity, exceeding 95% in children. Antibiotic-associated colitis may be diagnosed by stool-based detection of the common antigen or enterotoxins of *Clostridium difficile.* A study by Markowitz and associates highlighted the necessity to test for *C. difficile* enterotoxins A and B as a combination for the diagnosis of *C. difficile* infections in children. The enterotoxin A assay missed 41.5% of *C. difficile* infections, and the enterotoxin B assay failed to detect 34.9% of these infections. Rotaviruses may be detected by widespread immunoassay-based testing of stool specimens in the diagnostic evaluation of viral gastroenteritis.

Antibody Detection

Antibody detection is especially useful for the diagnosis of infections with unculturable or fastidious pathogens. Purified or recombinant antigen preparations are used in commercial assays for detection of pathogen-specific immunoglobulin M (IgM), IgG, or total antibodies in sera or CSF. The combination of nonspecific and specific serologic testing for two-step screening and confirmatory testing represents an established strategy for the diagnosis of spirochetal infections. For example, primary screening for syphilis by nonspecific rapid plasma reagin (RPR) testing is followed by confirmatory specific serologic findings if the screening test is positive. A screening test with greater sensitivity and reduced specificity is followed by a confirmatory test with greater specificity. A similar approach is used routinely for the diagnosis of Lyme disease (*Borrelia burgdorferi* infection) in which less specific enzyme-linked immunosorbent assay (ELISA)-based screening is employed before confirmatory immunoblot-based IgM or IgG (serum or CSF) testing.

Antibody detection is a prominent strategy in clinical virology because of the difficulty in culturing many viruses in established cell lines in the laboratory. The diagnosis of Epstein-Barr virus (EBV) infection by antibody detection is a two-step process akin to syphilis testing. Children suspected of infectious mononucleosis may be screened by heterophile testing (i.e., monospot) and confirmed with EBV-specific serologic testing. The diagnostic algorithms for hepatitis C virus (HCV) and human immunodeficiency virus type 1 (HIV-1) infection are similar in that primary ELISA-based screening is followed by more specific immunoblot assays. By contrast, hepatitis B virus (HBV) infections are evaluated with combination panels of antigen and antibody tests. Serologic testing for antibodies to *Toxoplasma gondii* is an important strategy for the diagnosis of toxoplasmosis. Serum IgM and IgG testing is performed routinely for the assessment of possible vertical transmission in newborns as well as disseminated infections in immunocompromised children.

Molecular Methods

Molecular methods have fostered the development of more rapid and accurate diagnostic tests for diverse microbial pathogens, as reported by Tang and colleagues and by Versalovic and Lupski. Beyond culture confirmation, nucleic acid amplification methods provide opportunities for the direct detection of pathogens in clinical specimens. Real-time polymerase chain reaction (PCR) methods are rapidly replacing older end-point PCR methods in applications for microbial detection and quantitation. Direct detection of *Mycobacterium tuberculosis* in respiratory specimens facilitates timely patient management and isolation, thus limiting potential spread of this infectious agent and reducing overall hospitalization costs, as noted by Kaul. Commercial kits approved by the Food and Drug Administration (FDA) are available for nucleic acid amplification of *M. tuberculosis* directly in smear-positive (PCR and transcription-mediated amplification [TMA]) or smear-negative specimens (TMA). In contrast to respiratory specimens, PCR was not useful for the detection of *M. tuberculosis* in gastric aspirates from pediatric patients, in a report by Neu and colleagues.

Viral load testing provides opportunities for monitoring of treatment responses in patients undergoing antiviral therapy for chronic viral infections. Whereas serologic testing establishes the diagnosis of HIV-1 infection, viral load testing at baseline and during antiviral therapy permits the monitoring of treatment responses and surveillance for drug-resistant HIV-1. During the acute phase of HIV-1 infection, viral load testing may indicate sharply elevated HIV-1 levels in the plasma before seroconversion. Viral load testing is also widely used for the management of patients infected with HBV or HCV. Viral load testing for CMV, EBV, and other human herpesviruses is a valuable approach for monitoring of immunocompromised children following solid organ transplantation, as noted by Bai and associates.

Genotyping or mutation detection strategies have an increasingly important role for the evaluation of infections with drug-resistant bacteria or viruses. Methicillin-resistant *S. aureus* (MRSA) may be identified by DNA amplification of the *mecA* gene. Real-time PCR approaches may combine species identification and MRSA detection. Drug-resistant HIV-1 may be characterized by sequencing (genotyping) of the HIV-1 reverse transcriptase (RT) and protease (P) genes. Because mutation profiles may be complex, interpretative algorithms have been developed that provide drug susceptibility patterns based on HIV-1 RT and P genotypes. DNA sequencing represents a supplemental approach for diagnostic bacteriology. According to Tang and colleagues, sequencing of bacterial 16S rRNA genes has facilitated the accurate identification of bacterial pathogens from clinical specimens.

Burke reported that infection control is recognized as an important patient safety issue, providing opportunities for molecular epidemiology to support hospital surveillance and outbreak detection efforts. Conventional microbiology including biochemical and antimicrobial susceptibility testing (AST) lacks the strain-level resolution necessary for effective pathogen tracking. Molecular methods such as pulsed-field gel electrophoresis (PFGE) and PCR-based typing are being used for DNA-based profiling of individual bacterial or yeast clones. Infection control efforts are supported by the rapid detection of point source outbreaks or patient-to-patient transmission. In addition to outbreak studies, multiple blood culture isolates of the same species from individual patients may be evaluated by DNA typing to distinguish central line infections from skin-borne contaminants and assess possible reinfection versus recrudescence.

Antimicrobial Susceptibility Testing

Antimicrobial susceptibility testing (AST) is performed routinely in diagnostic microbiology laboratories to facilitate the selection of optimal treatment regimens. Established criteria promulgated by the Clinical and Laboratory Standards Institute (CLSI) have been published for multiple AST approaches with different gram-negative or gram-positive bacterial pathogens. The simplest approach is disc diffusion or Kirby-Bauer testing, which does not yield a minimum inhibitory concentration (MIC). Each disc contains one antibiotic at a defined concentration, and relative growth inhibition zones are compared to determine whether a patient's isolate is resistant or susceptible to each of several antibiotics. Commercial systems (e.g., Vitek, bioMerieux, Durham, NC) perform alternative turbidity-based (non-MIC) testing for the determination of resistance or susceptibility to specific antimicrobial agents. Bradford noted that defined patterns of cephalosporin resistance with antibiotic panels may highlight the presence of extended-spectrum beta-lactamases, usually in gram-negative enteric bacteria such as *E. coli* and *Klebsiella pneumoniae*. Narrow-spectrum beta-lactamases may be detected rapidly by discs containing defined substrates (e.g., nitrocefin).

In addition to convenient non-MIC tests, laboratory strategies for the determination of specific MICs may be important for particular pathogen-antibiotic combinations. The antimicrobial gradient strip (e.g., E-test) test has become a popular method for MIC determinations on plated media. Each paper strip contains one antibiotic with a continuous antibiotic concentration gradient. By evaluating the elliptic zone of growth inhibition, MICs may be determined directly. Agar plate MIC determinations are used to determine penicillin MICs of clinically significant viridans streptococci or *S. pneumoniae* from blood cultures. MRSA and vancomycin-resistant enterococci (VRE) colonize children and may require MIC strategies following disc diffusion–based screening. Alternatively, molecular studies may indicate the presence of the drug resistance genes, *mecA* (in MRSA) or *vanA/B* (in VRE), and they may represent confirmatory studies for resistant organisms. Antibiotic combinations may be tested in synergy testing protocols. *Enterococcus* synergy testing is performed on plated media to determine resistance to cell wall–active agents (e.g., beta-lactams) or high-level resistance to aminoglycosides. Either pattern of resistance would negate potential synergies of antibiotic combination therapy.

CLINICAL UTILITY OF DIAGNOSTIC MICROBIOLOGY

Bloodstream Infections Including Sepsis

Causative agents of sepsis are identified routinely by blood culture techniques using continuously monitoring blood culture systems. In contrast to the general hospital setting, aerobic blood cultures are performed routinely without anaerobic blood cultures in pediatric settings. Modern blood culture systems have rich media formulations that enhance pathogen and contaminant detection and place a premium on sterile collection techniques. Pre-adolescent children generally have higher bacterial loads (10^2 to 10^3 colony-forming units [CFU]/mL) in peripheral blood than do adults (fewer than 10^1 CFU/mL) and generate positive signals in comparable time periods despite reduced blood collection volumes (1 to 5 mL).

The distinction of contaminants from pathogens in blood cultures is an issue of paramount importance. According to Weinstein and associates, species identification is a primary criterion for consideration of the clinical significance of positive blood cultures. Organisms such as *S. aureus, S. pneumoniae*, gram-negative enteric bacteria, and *Candida* species are considered true pathogens when isolated from peripheral blood. Typical contaminants include *Bacillus, Corynebacterium* (including diphtheroids), and *Propionibacterium* species. Organisms such as coagulase-negative staphylococci (CoNS), diphtheroids, and viridans streptococci may require further evaluation including the clinical status of the patient and the numbers of positive blood culture sets (if greater than one set is submitted). Notably, polymicrobial bacteremias with multiple pathogens may be apparent in patients with positive blood cultures. In a large-scale study in Finland reported by Saarinen and colleagues, 4.8% of invasive infections in children were polymicrobial.

The most common bacterial pathogens isolated from blood cultures include *S. aureus*, CoNS, *S. pneumoniae, S. agalactiae* (group B streptococcus), *E. coli, K. pneumoniae*, and *Pseudomonas aeruginosa*. Yeast pathogens from routine blood cultures include several *Candida* species, with *C. albicans* being the most common. In neonatal sepsis, pathogens commonly are identified in routine blood cultures. There has been a shift from gram-positive to gram-negative pathogens as causative agents of early-onset neonatal sepsis, as noted by Stoll and colleagues. Organisms such as group B streptococcus (*S. agalactiae*), *E. coli*, or *Listeria monocytogenes* are cultured in commercial blood culture systems and are considered pathogens whenever

isolated. Verboon-Maciolek and associates reported that enteroviruses also should be considered in infants younger than 2 months of age and may be detected by RT-PCR of serum specimens. Alternative blood culture approaches may be required for unusual or fastidious pathogens. The successful culture of mycobacteria or filamentous fungi (molds) from peripheral blood requires specialized culture media that may or may not be compatible with commercial blood culture systems. Lysis-centrifugation strategies with immediate plating on selective plated media may be required for successful isolation.

The diagnosis of catheter-related bloodstream infections represents an ongoing challenge for the microbiology laboratory. The standard approach is either quantitative or semiquantitative (most common method) culture of the catheter tip. The chief limitation with both methods is that the catheter must be removed for microbiologic studies to be performed. Microbiologists have attempted to develop strategies for assessment of catheter-related infections without the need for catheter removal. When paired blood cultures from the catheter in question and a peripheral site were compared by DesJardin and associates, only negative culture results from the catheters in question were helpful. Earlier time to positivity (more than 120 minutes) for catheter-derived blood cultures versus peripheral blood cultures represents another strategy that may facilitate the diagnosis of line-related sepsis, as reported by Blot and colleagues.

Central Nervous System Infections

The evaluation of acute bacterial meningitis and viral encephalitis places a premium value on rapid and accurate diagnosis for effective patient management. Immediate laboratory evaluation by CSF Gram stain is performed for the visualization of the most common agents of acute bacterial meningitis including *N. meningitidis* and *S. pneumoniae*. Gram stain results should be correlated with CSF glucose and protein levels in addition to the CSF cell counts. CSF cultures are routinely performed for the isolation and definitive identification of bacterial pathogens. The most important pathogens in children, *N. meningitidis* and *S. pneumoniae*, usually are cultured on blood or chocolate agar plates in 24 to 48 hours, followed by AST by disc diffusion (i.e., Kirby-Bauer testing).

Direct detection of bacterial DNA in CSF specimens may augment culture-based diagnostic studies. Efforts in the United Kingdom have demonstrated the utility of molecular methods for the rapid and accurate diagnosis of meningococcal meningitis. More than 4,000 CSF specimens were screened by real-time PCR in one study from the United Kingdom, reported by Corless and colleagues, and the improvement in the meningococcal detection rate was 2.9%; that is, 87 additional cases of meningococcal meningitis were identified by PCR alone. Bacterial antigen testing no longer is recommended for routine screening because the Gram stain is more comprehensive and matches the sensitivity of antigen testing. Rapid CSF antigen testing for *Cryptococcus neoformans* is clinically useful whenever cryptococcal meningitis is suspected in immunocompromised patients.

Important viral central nervous system (CNS) infections in children require rapid laboratory assessment and include aseptic meningitis and viral encephalitis. Molecular methods play an important role in distinguishing aseptic from acute bacterial meningitis. Aseptic meningitis may be diagnosed rapidly by RT-PCR-based detection of enterovirus RNA directly in CSF specimens. The rapid diagnosis of aseptic meningitis by enterovirus RT-PCR has reduced hospital stays for patients and decreased overall health care costs, as reported by Ramers and associates. Tang and colleagues noted that amplification of herpes simplex virus (HSV) DNA directly in CSF specimens is now considered the "gold standard" for the diagnosis of HSV meningitis or encephalitis. For West Nile virus meningoencephalitis, the detection of CSF IgM is considered the test of choice for establishing the diagnosis, although concurrent serum IgM testing is recommended. According to Bitnun and colleagues, the diagnosis of meningoencephalitis caused by *Mycoplasma pneumoniae* in children may be established by the direct amplification of *M. pneumoniae* DNA in CSF specimens. The causes of encephalitis usually are not found. Glaser and associates reported that despite extensive testing in a mixed-age population in California, 62% of cases were unexplained.

Gastrointestinal Infections

The clinical microbiology laboratory routinely performs stool cultures for the isolation of common enteric pathogens. In contrast to blood and CSF, stool is nonsterile and contains a plethora of bacterial organisms. Prominent enteric pathogens that are grown routinely from stool specimens include *Campylobacter*, *Salmonella*, and *Shigella* pathogens. Diagnostic laboratories routinely culture *Campylobacter* species by the application of selective media and elevated temperature (42°C) incubation in a microaerobic atmosphere. By contrast, *Yersinia* pathogens are not cultured routinely and should be specifically requested if *Yersinia* enterocolitis is suspected.

In addition to stool culture, rapid stool antigen detection methods facilitate the timely and cost-effective diagnoses of specific enteric bacterial infections. *C. difficile*, causative agent of antibiotic-associated colitis and diarrhea, is commonly detected by stool ELISA-based detection of glutamate dehydrogenase (GDH; common antigen) or enterotoxins A and B. Up to 50% of infants may acquire toxigenic *C. difficile* in the nursery, and very young children frequently test positive for *C. difficile* antigens without *C. difficile*-associated disease, according to Wilkins and Lyerly. For convenience and because of rapid turnaround times, many laboratories have adopted stool *C. difficile* enterotoxin (A/B combination testing) detection. Clinical evaluations of *C. difficile* enterotoxin ELISA studies have documented sensitivities exceeding 80%.

Enterohemorrhagic *E. coli* (EHEC) and Shiga toxin-producing *E. coli* (STEC) represent important causes of hemorrhagic colitis and the hemolytic uremic syndrome (HUS). Detection of Shiga toxin genes or antigens is an important strategy for the diagnosis because many non–serotype O157 isolates have been characterized in recent years, as reported by Kehl. Many laboratories utilize sorbitol-containing MacConkey agar to screen stool specimens for the presence of EHEC serotype O157:H7 by traditional culture methods. However, 25% to 50% of EHEC isolates are now considered to be non–serotype O157 organisms and may utilize sorbitol, meaning that culture-based screening methods are relatively insensitive. More recent approaches have targeted Shiga toxins I and II in stool specimens to detect the enterotoxins directly, regardless of the serotype.

Evaluation of parasitic infections of the gastrointestinal tract relies on tedious O&P examinations of stool specimens. Characteristic sizes and morphologies of cysts and trophozoites provide diagnostic information for establishing the causes of these infections. Few parasites can be cultivated in the laboratory, and thus culture-independent strategies are emphasized in diagnostic parasitology. Direct antigen detection methods have been developed for the more common pathogens including *C. parvum* and *G. lamblia*. Such pathogen-specific strategies must be used selectively to enhance the laboratory's abilities to diagnose important parasitic infections in a cost-effective manner. Stool antigen detection by enzyme immunoassay is an attractive approach for rotavirus detection because these viruses are difficult to culture, and electron microscopic studies are

not possible in most settings, as noted by Wilhelmi and colleagues. Astroviruses, enteric adenoviruses, noroviruses, and caliciviruses are important causes of gastroenteritis in children and are missed by immunoassays targeting rotaviruses. RT-PCR for neroviruses in stool may be a useful test.

Genitourinary Infections

Urine cultures frequently are requested in diagnostic microbiology laboratories for the evaluation of urinary tract infections (UTIs) and urosepsis. Urine specimens usually are obtained as nonsterile "clean-catch" specimens and require semiquantitative cultures to facilitate the evaluation of bacterial isolates. Alternative urine specimens include catheter-assisted collection, urine obtained by cystoscopy, and suprapubic aspiration. Cultured bacteria present in concentrations exceeding 10^3 CFU/mL are characterized in the laboratory to various extents, depending on the method of urine collection and complexity of different organisms isolated. The most common urinary tract pathogens, including gram-negative enteric bacteria (e.g., *E. coli*, *K. pneumoniae*, *Proteus*) and gram-positive pathogens (*Enterococcus*), are isolated by routine culture procedures. Direct Gram stains of urine specimens are not routinely obtained, and urinalyses should be performed for rapid urine screening. In addition to bacteria, yeast pathogens (e.g., *Candida* species) are important causes of UTIs in hospitalized patients and may be cultured by routine methods. According to Langley and associates, *Candida* species follow *E. coli* as the second most common group of pathogens isolated in children with nosocomial UTIs. Nosocomial UTIs are typically associated with urethral instrumentation in neonates and infants.

Respiratory Tract Infections

The assessment of acute pharyngitis is probably the most common indication for diagnostic testing of possible respiratory infections in children. *Streptococcus pyogenes* (group A streptococcus) is the most common cause of acute bacterial pharyngitis and represents the only definite indication for antibiotic treatment of pharyngitis, as reported by Bisno and colleagues. *S. pyogenes* is estimated to cause 15% to 30% of cases of acute pharyngitis in pediatric patients. Therefore, rapid antigen testing and selective culture of *S. pyogenes* from throat swabs are primary strategies for point-of-care and laboratory testing in this setting. Bourbeau noted that with sensitivities of 62% to 96%, rapid point-of-care antigen testing represents a useful primary strategy. In pediatrics, it is recommended that negative rapid antigen tests be supported by throat cultures. DNA probe tests for *S. pyogenes* are commercially available, and sensitivities have ranged from 88.6% to 94.8%.

According to Hall and Carroll, the role of the laboratory in the diagnosis of acute bronchitis and bronchiolitis in children is limited chiefly to the rapid detection of respiratory viruses. Respiratory viruses (adenovirus, influenza A and B, parainfluenza types 1 to 4, respiratory syncytial virus) account for most of these infections. Because conventional viral culture methods for respiratory viruses require several days or more for isolation, direct antigen detection by immunofluorescence and enzyme immunoassays represent attractive options with rapid turnaround times. Immunofluorescence-based viral antigen detection with nasopharyngeal specimens offers reduced time to detection and superior sensitivity (80% to 90%) when compared with enzyme immunoassays (approximately 70%). Kehl and colleagues noted that a commercially available multiplex RT-PCR assay (Hexaplex, Prodesse Inc., Madison, WI) provides a RNA detection strategy for the simultaneous evaluation of parainfluenza viruses types 1 to 3, respiratory syncytial virus, and influenza viruses A and B in diverse respiratory specimens. A newly recognized respiratory paramyxovirus, human metapneumovirus (hMPV), was described by Williams and Mullins and their colleagues as an important cause of pediatric bronchiolitis, pneumonia, and croup. In a study by Williams and associates, 20% of previously virus-negative lower respiratory tract illnesses in children were positive for hMPV, and 59% of hMPV-positive cases included a diagnosis of bronchiolitis. This virus is not isolated by routine respiratory viral cultures. Children lacking a cause for a lower respiratory tract illness after initial testing should be considered for nucleic acid amplification (e.g., RT-PCR)–based detection of hMPV in respiratory specimens.

Direct Gram stains are a basic part of the evaluation of respiratory specimens. Gram stain assessment of sputa and tracheal aspirates permits evaluation of specimen quality and possible significance of culture findings. The presence of abundant neutrophils and the finding of a single predominant organism in specimens of sufficient quality are consistent with a diagnosis of acute bacterial pneumonia. *S. pneumoniae* continues to be the most commonly isolated cause of community-acquired acute bacterial pneumonia. *S. pneumoniae* is readily visualized in sputum Gram stains and is isolated in respiratory cultures in 24 to 48 hours. Susceptibility testing of respiratory *S. pneumoniae* isolates is a more recent trend, reflecting the increased prevalence of antimicrobial resistance (including penicillin resistance) in pneumococci.

According to Miller and Gilligan, patients with cystic fibrosis (CF) have a distinct profile of prominent respiratory bacterial pathogens including *Burkholderia cepacia* complex, *P. aeruginosa*, and *S. aureus*. Both *P. aeruginosa* and *S. aureus* can be cultured using routine procedures for respiratory specimens, although mucoid *P. aeruginosa* isolates in patients with CF may not be identifiable by commercial systems. *B. cepacia* complex presents a formidable challenge for the laboratory because this species complex includes nine or more genomovars. The genomovars *B. multivorans* and *B. cenocepacia* comprise the majority (more than 85%) of clinical *Burkholderia* isolates from patients with CF. The data suggest that patients infected with *B. cenocepacia* should be evaluated carefully before lung transplantation is performed and are at risk for the cepacia syndrome. Because the characterization of *B. cepacia* complex organisms in patients with CF may have serious consequences for management, definitive identification of *B. cepacia* genomovars requires molecular studies including 16S rRNA gene sequencing.

Approximately 5% to 16% of patients with community-acquired pneumonia have concurrent bacteremia, and blood cultures are recommended for patients hospitalized with pneumonia, according to Skerrett. Serologic testing in this setting generally is reserved for atypical pathogens such as *M. pneumoniae* and *Chlamydia pneumoniae*. Serum IgM and acute-convalescent serum IgG titer comparisons may be helpful for supporting the diagnosis of atypical pneumonia. Urinary antigen testing for specific respiratory pathogens provides an attractive option for diagnosis, independent of organism isolation by culture. Urinary antigen testing is now available for the detection of *S. pneumoniae* as a possible adjunct to respiratory cultures. If legionellosis is suspected, culture on buffered charcoal yeast extract (BCYE) media may yield different *Legionella* species and should be coupled with urinary antigen testing for *L. pneumophila* serogroup 1.

Molecular methods have contributed to recent advances in accurate and rapid diagnosis of respiratory tract infections. PCR-based amplification of *Bordetella pertussis* or *B. parapertussis* DNA in nasopharyngeal aspirate or swab specimens is now considered the gold standard for the diagnosis of pertussis in children. Tilley and Sloan and their colleagues reported that DNA amplification is superior to culture or serologic testing by offering markedly improved sensitivity and higher predictive values. Agents of atypical pneumonia are notoriously difficult to culture and represent attractive targets for molecular diagnostics. PCR amplification of *M. pneumoniae* DNA in throat swabs or sputum specimens correlates with disease and establishes the diagnosis of atypical pneumonia. The sudden acute respiratory syndrome (SARS)-associated coronavirus is a newly identified and divergent coronavirus associated with epidemics of respiratory disease in Asia and North America. The entire SARS virus genome was sequenced within weeks of discovery, providing sequence data for the development of RT-PCR–based detection strategies.

Suggested Readings

Bai X, Rogers BB, Harkins PC, et al. Predictive value of quantitative PCR-based viral burden analysis for eight human herpes viruses in pediatric solid organ transplant patients. *J Mol Diagn* 2000;2:191.

Bisno AL, Gerber MA, Gwaltney JM Jr, et al. Practice guidelines for the diagnosis and management of group A streptococcal pharyngitis: Infectious Diseases Society of America. *Clin Infect Dis* 2002;35:113.

Bitnun A, Ford-Jones EL, Petric M, et al. Acute childhood encephalitis and *Mycoplasma pneumoniae*. *Clin Infect Dis* 2001;32:1674.

Blot F, Schmidt E, Nitenberg G, et al. Earlier positivity of central venous versus peripheral blood cultures is highly predictive of catheter-related sepsis. *J Clin Microbiol* 1998;36:105.

Bourbeau PP. Role of the microbiology laboratory in diagnosis and management of pharyngitis. *J Clin Microbiol* 2003;41:3467.

Bradford PA. Extended-spectrum beta-lactamases in the 21st century: characterization, epidemiology, and detection of this important resistance threat. *Clin Microbiol Rev* 2001;14:933.

Burke JP. Infection control: a problem for patient safety. *N Engl J Med* 2003;348:651.

Carroll KC. Laboratory diagnosis of lower respiratory tract infections: controversy and conundrums. *J Clin Microbiol* 2002;40:3115.

Corless CE, Guiver M, Borrow R, et al. Simultaneous detection of *Neisseria meningitidis*, *Haemophilus influenzae*, and *Streptococcus pneumoniae* in suspected cases of meningitis and septicemia using real-time PCR. *J Clin Microbiol* 2001;39:1553.

DesJardin JA, Falagas ME, Ruthazer R, et al. Clinical utility of blood cultures drawn from indwelling central venous catheters in hospitalized patients with cancer. *Ann Intern Med* 1999;131(9):641.

Glaser CA, Gilliam S, Schnurr D, et al. In search of encephalitis etiologies: diagnostic challenges in the California Encephalitis Project, 1998–2000. *Clin Infect Dis* 2003;36:731.

Hall CB. Respiratory syncytial virus and parainfluenza virus. *N Engl J Med* 2001;344:1917.

Kabani A, Cadrain G, Trevenen C, et al. Practice guidelines for ordering stool ova and parasite testing in a pediatric population: the Alberta Children's Hospital. *Am J Clin Pathol* 1995;104:272.

Kaul KL. Molecular detection of *Mycobacterium tuberculosis*: impact on patient care. *Clin Chem* 2001;47:1553.

Kehl SC. Role of the laboratory in the diagnosis of enterohemorrhagic *Escherichia coli* infections. *J Clin Microbiol* 2002;40:2711.

Kehl SC, Henrickson KJ, Hua W, et al. Evaluation of the Hexaplex assay for detection of respiratory viruses in children. *J Clin Microbiol* 2001;39:1696.

Langley JM, Hanakowski M, Leblanc JC. Unique epidemiology of nosocomial urinary tract infection in children. *Am J Infect Control* 2001;29:94.

Markowitz JE, Brown KA, Mamula P, et al. Failure of single-toxin assays to detect *Clostridium difficile* infection in pediatric inflammatory bowel disease. *Am J Gastroenterol* 2001;96:2688.

Miller MB, Gilligan PH. Laboratory aspects of management of chronic pulmonary infections in patients with cystic fibrosis. *J Clin Microbiol* 2003;41:4009.

Mullins JA, Erdman DD, Weinberg GA, et al. Human metapneumovirus infection among children hospitalized with acute respiratory illness. *Emerg Infect Dis* 2004;10:700.

Neu N, Saiman L, San Gabriel P, et al. Diagnosis of pediatric tuberculosis in the modern era. *Pediatr Infect Dis J* 1999;18:122.

Perkins MD, Mirrett S, Reller LB. Rapid bacterial antigen detection is not clinically useful. *J Clin Microbiol* 1995;33:1486.

Ramers C, Billman G, Hartin M, et al. Impact of a diagnostic cerebrospinal fluid enterovirus polymerase chain reaction test on patient management. *JAMA* 2000;283:2680.

Saarinen M, Takala AK, Koskenniemi E, et al. Spectrum of 2,836 cases of invasive bacterial or fungal infections in children: results of prospective nationwide five-year surveillance in Finland. Finnish Pediatric Invasive Infection Study Group. *Clin Infect Dis* 1995;21:1134.

Skerrett SJ. Diagnostic testing to establish a microbial cause is helpful in the management of community-acquired pneumonia. *Semin Respir Infect* 1997;12:308.

Sloan LM, Hopkins MK, Mitchell PS, et al. Multiplex LightCycler PCR assay for detection and differentiation of *Bordetella pertussis* and *Bordetella parapertussis* in nasopharyngeal specimens. *J Clin Microbiol* 2002;40:96.

Stoll BJ, Hansen N, Fanaroff AA, et al. Changes in pathogens causing early-onset sepsis in very-low-birth-weight infants. *N Engl J Med* 2002;347:240.

Tang YW, Ellis NM, Hopkins MK, et al. Comparison of phenotypic and genotypic techniques for identification of unusual aerobic pathogenic gram-negative bacilli. *J Clin Microbiol* 1998;36:3674.

Tang YW, Mitchell PS, Espy MJ, et al. Molecular diagnosis of herpes simplex virus infections in the central nervous system. *J Clin Microbiol* 1999;37:2127.

Tang YW, Procop GW, Persing DH. Molecular diagnostics of infectious diseases. *Clin Chem* 1997;43:2021.

Tilley PA, Kanchana MV, Knight I, et al. Detection of *Bordetella pertussis* in a clinical laboratory by culture, polymerase chain reaction, and direct fluorescent antibody staining; accuracy, and cost. *Diagn Microbiol Infect Dis* 2000;37:17.

Verboon-Maciolek MA, Nijhuis M, van Loon AM, et al. Diagnosis of enterovirus infection in the first 2 months of life by real-time polymerase chain reaction. *Clin Infect Dis* 2003;37:1.

Versalovic J, Lupski JR. Molecular detection and genotyping of pathogens: more accurate and rapid answers. *Trends Microbiol* 2002;10(suppl):S15.

Weinstein MP. Blood culture contamination: persisting problems and partial progress. *J Clin Microbiol* 2003;41:2275.

Weinstein MP, Towns ML, Quartey SM, et al. The clinical significance of positive blood cultures in the 1990s: a prospective comprehensive evaluation of the microbiology, epidemiology, and outcome of bacteremia and fungemia in adults. *Clin Infect Dis* 1997;24:584.

Wilhelmi I, Roman E, Sanchez-Fauquier A. Viruses causing gastroenteritis. *Clin Microbiol Infect* 2003;9:247.

Wilkins TD, Lyerly DM. *Clostridium difficile* testing: after 20 years, still challenging. *J Clin Microbiol* 2003;41:531.

Williams JV, Harris PA, Tollefson SJ, et al. Human metapneumovirus and lower respiratory tract disease in otherwise healthy infants and children. *N Engl J Med* 2004;350:443.

CHAPTER 147 ■ ASSAYS FOR THE DIAGNOSIS OF INFECTIOUS DISEASES

JAMES A. WILDE AND ROBERT H. YOLKEN

Establishing the accurate diagnosis of an infectious disease is a crucial initial step in the proper management of an infectious process. Obtaining a rapid laboratory diagnosis of an infection is particularly important to a pediatric practitioner because infections in the pediatric age group often present with few specific signs or symptoms. Pediatricians are often the first clinicians consulted to interpret the results of diagnostic assays. The goal of this chapter is not to review specific assays for the diagnosis of specific diseases, but rather to present the general principles involved in the performance and interpretation of assays used to diagnose pediatric infectious diseases.

TYPES OF DIAGNOSTIC ASSAYS

Assays for the diagnosis of infectious diseases can be divided into two general categories: those that directly identify microbial products in a body fluid site and those that measure immunoglobulins specifically directed at microbial antigens. The characteristics of these assays are presented in Table 147.1.

Direct Assays

Generally, the direct assays are most useful for the diagnosis of an active infection because they involve the direct measurement of microbial components. Furthermore, because direct assays can be quantitative, they also can be used to monitor the level of the infecting microorganism and to assess the course of the infection and the response to antimicrobial treatment.

Although assays that measure the immune response to an infecting organism are useful in many situations, several advantages are inherent in assays that directly assess the presence of microbial organisms in body fluids. Until recently, the direct detection of microbial pathogens was accomplished by immunoassays designed to detect antigenic components of the microorganism. These assays are similar in design to the immunoassays used for measuring antibodies in that they measure the interaction between antigens and antibodies. However, antigen detection assays differ because they involve the interaction of antigens in a sample with an antibody of known specificity. This interaction generally is accomplished by labeling the antibody with a suitable marker such as a radioactive isotope, enzyme, or latex particle (see Table 147.1). In general, the enzyme-based assays offer the highest levels of sensitivity and specificity; however, the particle-based assays can be useful in situations outside clinical laboratories in which rapid results are needed. For example, particle agglutination assays are used widely in clinical settings to detect antigens from group A streptococci rapidly.

Assays for the direct detection of microbial agents offer numerous advantages in establishing diagnoses of acute infections. Because they do not require the generation of an active immune response, they can be used to ascertain the presence of an infectious process before the patient has had sufficient time to generate detectable antibodies. Furthermore, these assays can be used for diagnosing infections in immunocompromised individuals, neonates, and other patients who would not be expected to generate a predictable immune response to infection. The principal drawback of antigen detection assays is that they are limited by the kinetics of the antigen-antibody reactions used to make the diagnostic measurement. Although this limitation can be overcome partially by selecting antigens that are present in multiple copies in microbial organisms (e.g., the capsular polysaccharide of *Haemophilus influenzae*), many important pathogens do not contain antigens that can be used for this purpose. In such cases, the presence of more than 1,000 organisms may be required before a detectable signal could be obtained, meaning that the assays would not be useful for the diagnosis of infection early in the course of disease, when the antigen load is low. In addition, the generation of an effective immune response to infection generally leads to the production of antibodies that bind to the microbial antigens that

TABLE 147.1

ASSAYS USED IN DIAGNOSIS OF INFECTIOUS DISEASES

Assay	Results
Antigen Detection	
Counterimmunoelectrophoresis	Line of precipitation produced when test specimen containing antigen migrates in gel toward anode and antigen-specific antibody migrates toward cathode
Latex particle agglutination	Antigen-specific antibody-coated latex beads agglutinate when test specimen containing specific antigen is added. In some cases, erythrocytes or other particles used in place of latex beads
Enzyme immunoassay	Antigen in specimen binds to antigen-specific antibody bonded to plastic plate. Antigen-specific antibody labeled with enzyme added, binds antigen in sandwich. Substrate for the enzyme added; rate of reaction as measured by color change reflects quantity of antigen in specimen
Fluorescent antibody	Fluoresceinated antigen-specific antibody binds antigen from specimen. Fluorescence after unbound antibodies washed away an indication of the presence of antigen
DNA probe	Enzyme or radiolabeled segment of target-specific DNA binds to homologous nucleic acid in sample. Signal remaining after unbound probe is washed away reflects quantity of target
Polymerase chain reaction	Uses thermostable DNA polymerase and specific primers to amplify target nucleic acid from undetectable to detectable levels. Variety of methods to detect products of reaction
Antibody Detection	
Complement fixation	Sample containing antibody is combined with target antigen and known amount of complement. Antigen-antibody complexes cause fixation (consumption) of complement. Sensitized red cells added, unfixed complement causes lysis. Degree of complement fixation reflects quantity of antibody
Radioimmunoassay	Iodine-125 used to label target Igs in a sample. Reaction with antigen and unlabeled Ig (competitively inhibits labeled Ig) as measured by radioactivity level reflects amount of labeled Ig
Enzyme immunoassay	Antibody in specimen binds to antigen bound to plastic microtiter plate or a similar surface. Antihuman Ig labeled with enzyme added; bound enzyme is reacted with substrate. The rate of reaction as measured by color change reflects the quantity of antibody in the clinical sample. Ig class or subclass measurable by the use of the specific enzyme-labeled antihuman Ig (e.g., antihuman IgM or antihuman IgG_1)
Neutralization reactions	Serial dilutions of sample containing antibody added to viral culture media along with target virus. Presence of antibody neutralizes virus, preventing growth in tissue culture
Hemagglutination inhibition	Antibody in sample reacted with specific antigen. Amount of unreacted antigen quantitated by binding of the antigen to erythrocytes. In some cases, antigen contains hemagglutinin and can bind directly to the erythrocytes (e.g., influenza virus). In other cases, binding of the erythrocytes to the unreacted antigen accomplished by coating the erythrocytes with specific antibody

Ig, immunoglobulin.

are the targets of the immunoassay reagents. Such antibodies can interfere with the sensitivity of the immunoassay, thus decreasing the utility of these assays late in the course of a chronic infectious process.

A principal limitation of direct assays is that the levels of the infecting microorganism in some disease states may be quite low, in which case only assays capable of detecting small quantities of microorganisms would be able to establish accurate diagnoses in all infected patients. Another limitation is that direct assays require the presence of the organism or its antigens in an accessible body site for a diagnosis to be made. Hence, diagnosing some infections, such as those caused by hepatitis A virus, *Mycoplasma pneumoniae*, and human immunodeficiency virus (HIV), in which symptoms generally occur after microbial replication has reached its peak, is difficult.

Antibody Detection Assays

Many different assays are available for the detection of antibodies to infectious agents. Although these assays are named for the method that is used for the measurement of the antigen-antibody reaction, all the assays make use of a similar basic reaction, namely, the binding of the patient's immunoglobulin to a defined microbial antigen.

Some of the problems of direct detection are overcome by the use of assays that measure the immune response to microbial infection. In such assays, serum (or, in some cases, urine or another body fluid) is tested for the presence of immunoglobulins directed at specific microbial organisms or at microbial components. The advantage of this procedure is that the organism need not be present in the sampled site when the measurement of an immune response is performed. Furthermore, because even a small quantity of infecting antigen can give rise to a large number of activated B cells, high degrees of sensitivity generally are not required for the detection of specific antibodies. Finally, because the immune response to an infecting microorganism persists for an extended period, antibody detection assays allow for the diagnosis of an infection after microbial replication has declined. These assays thus can be used for the diagnosis of infections that lead to chronic disease processes, such as infections with hepatitis C virus, dengue viruses, *Borrelia burgdorferi*, and *Treponema pallidum*.

In the case of lifelong infections such as those caused by HIV, the detection of antibody (in the absence of maternal antibody derived prenatally) is diagnostic for the disease process. In many other cases, this persistence of detectable antibody constitutes one of the principal limitations of antibody detection assays, in that the antibody can be present long after the infectious process is completed or the patient has undergone successful treatment. For this reason, the detection of antibody often cannot, by itself, be considered diagnostic of a current infection. For example, a child with antibodies to enteroviruses may have acute bacterial meningitis at the time of testing, a patient with antibodies to Epstein-Barr virus may have acute streptococcal pharyngitis, and a patient with a high antibody titer to histoplasmin antigen may have tuberculosis. This problem can be overcome partially by measuring antibody classes that are associated with an early immune response to infection, such as immunoglobulin M (IgM) and (IgA). Such measurements are useful particularly in the diagnosis of infections that occur during the prenatal period. Because IgM and IgA class antibodies do not cross the normal placenta in appreciable quantities, the detection of these antibodies in the infant can be used to distinguish maternal from fetal infections. This method has been used to detect perinatal infections with cytomegalovirus, rubella virus, *Toxoplasma* and, more recently, HIV. Of note is that in the case of infections that occur later in life, the persistence of these acute-phase antibodies varies, rendering their detection unreliable as specific indicators of recent infection, particularly when one uses more sensitive assays, which detect small concentrations of IgM antibody long after the initial infection occurs. The possibility of false-positive results caused by the presence of rheumatoid factors and other autoimmune reactants also limits the specificity of these reactions for the definitive diagnosis of the infectious process.

One approach to improving the specificity of antibody detection assays for the diagnosis of recent infectious diseases takes advantage of the finding that certain components of infecting microorganisms often are selected by the immune system as the initial targets of the immune response. The measurement of antibodies to such early antigens is thus a reflection of a recent infection, especially if it occurs in the absence of antibodies to other components of the organism that develop later in the course of infection (late antigens). Such assays are useful particularly for the diagnosis of infections caused by cytomegalovirus, Epstein-Barr virus, and other herpesviruses, in which the viral targets of an early and late immune response have been well characterized. The recent characterization of the timing of the immune response to *B. burgdorferi* also indicates that the measurement of antibodies to different microbial components can be used as a more accurate way to characterize the status of patients presumed to have Lyme disease. As the immune response to other microbial organisms becomes better characterized, the measurement of early antigens will play a more important role in the diagnosis of a recent infection in children.

Most antibody assays involve the measurement of immunoglobulins in blood or serum specimens. Recently, measuring antibodies in mucosal body sites has become possible. Studies have indicated that antibodies to infectious antigens can be measured accurately in mucosal sites such as saliva and urine. These antibodies can arise either from transudation from the systemic circulation or in response to antigenic stimulation at the mucosal surface. In either case, the measurement of antibodies at the mucosal site provides an assessment of the immune response to the infecting microorganism.

Being able to measure a range of antibodies in readily accessible body fluids would be extremely helpful in diagnosing infections in young infants and in monitoring immune responses in a clinical practice setting. Table 147.1 presents examples of the antibody detection assays that may be useful to the pediatric practitioner. Current assay methods vary considerably in their ability to detect specific antibodies and hence in their sensitivity and specificity. In general, the solid-phase immunoassays [exemplified by solid-phase enzyme immunoassays, also known as *enzyme-linked immunosorbent assays* (ELISA)] offer the highest degree of sensitivity while allowing for objective quantitation and the inclusion of controls for maintaining specificity. The explosion of knowledge of the antigenicity of microbial proteins and techniques for their cloning and production in recombinant forms should lead to development of more sensitive and specific solid-phase assays for detecting antibodies to a wide range of infecting microorganisms.

Older assays such as complement fixation and immunofluorescence remain useful in situations in which highly purified components of the infecting microorganism are not widely available, as is generally the case with bacteria and *Mycoplasma*. In infections with these microorganisms, the components against which antibodies are directed have not been well characterized and hence cannot be used as antigens for the solid-phase assays.

Another group of widely used assays are those that rely on agglutination. In most agglutination assays, particles made of latex or similar materials are coated with antigen. When they react with serum that contains antibody, cross-bridging causes the beads to bind to each other in a recognizable pattern of agglutination. Antibody-coated erythrocytes also can be used in place of synthetic particles, in which case a pattern of hemagglutination in reaction with antibody is observed. Although the particle agglutination assays are less sensitive than are solid-phase immunosorbent assays, they are rapid and simple to perform and can be used outside central laboratory settings. They are ideal for use in situations in which qualitative, rather than quantitative, results are needed. For example, such assays are useful to determine whether an individual is lacking antibody to rubella virus and thus is susceptible to infection with this virus.

One problem inherent in the use of assays for the detection of antibodies is the way in which the results are reported by the laboratory and interpreted by the clinician. Box 147.1 presents additional information about this problem.

Nucleic Acid Assays

A newer class of diagnostic assays that has sufficient sensitivity for establishing early diagnoses of a wide range of infectious diseases has been developed. These assays are based on the measurement of microbial nucleic acids in the body fluids of infected infants and children. Like the antigen assays, assays for the direct detection of nucleic acids measure components of the infecting microorganism. Instead of measuring antigens derived from the organism, however, they rely on the detection of genetic material specific for the pathogenic agent. In the case of viruses, the detection of virions requires the detection of the appropriate genomic nucleic acid, which is DNA in the case of DNA-containing viruses, such as herpesviruses, hepatitis B virus, and adenoviruses, and RNA in the case of viruses such as influenza, parainfluenza, measles, rotavirus, and hepatitis A and hepatitis C. Retroviruses such as HIV and human T-cell lymphotropic virus require RNA detection for the identification of intact virions, but because retroviruses undergo integration into the cellular genome in the form of a reverse transcribed copy of DNA, such agents also can be detected in infected cells in the form of DNA. Conversely, viruses with a DNA genome, such as the herpesviruses, usually generate messenger RNA when they are undergoing active replication and thus can be detected in their RNA form in infected cells. The ability to detect both DNA and RNA provides considerable information, not only in terms of the presence of the microbial agent, but also with regard to the stage of infection.

The detection of nucleic acids offers numerous striking advantages in terms of establishing rapid diagnoses of infectious diseases in the pediatric age group. First, because nucleic acids from all microorganisms are composed of combinations of the same four nucleotides (A, T, G, and C for DNA and A, U, G, and C for RNA), they allow for the detection of virtually any infectious pathogen in the same reaction format. For example,

How the Results of Assays Are Reported

Traditionally, results are reported in terms of a *titer*, in which the maximum dilution that results in a positive reaction is reported (i.e., a titer of 1:8 means that the sample gave a reaction when diluted eightfold but not when diluted 16-fold). The disadvantage of this system is that it does not take into account the inherent sensitivity of the assay that is used for the measurement of the antibody, which is particularly problematic when the more sensitive immunoassays are used for antibody measurement: a serum that has a titer of 1:8 as measured by an insensitive complement fixation assay may have a titer of more than 1:1,000 when measured by means of a solid-phase immunosorbent assay. This variation can cause problems in interpreting laboratory test results and can complicate the comparison of assays performed in different laboratories. Another problem with end-point titers is that, regardless of the assay, they are difficult to reproduce. If a laboratory reports a change in titer in samples obtained over the course of time, whether the change is caused by the generation of antibody in the patient, indicating an active infection, or by day-to-day variations in the sensitivity of the assay system used for the performance of the measurements is not always clear.

Fortunately, the solid-phase immunosorbent assays are quantitative in nature and lend themselves to standard curves and accurate reproducibility. In addition, they allow for reporting assay results in standard units, thus enabling the performance of control reactions and the standardization of results between different test runs and among different laboratories. Standard units also allow for higher degrees of accuracy because they do not require the traditional fourfold increase to achieve clinical significance; cutoff values and levels of significance can be established for each assay system. Although the units may be less familiar to the clinician than are titer measurements, assays reported in terms of standard units generally are more reproducible and allow for making more reliable comparisons with reference values. The universal reporting of antibody values in standard units therefore would represent a major step forward in the clinician's ability to interpret serologic data and to use the results in the management of the pediatric patient.

Until standard units become available universally, clinical laboratories should provide clinicians with data indicating the sensitivity of the assay and the expected assay-to-assay variation in the test results. Moreover, when a fourfold increase in titers over the course of time is used to make a diagnosis, acute and convalescent samples must be tested simultaneously to avoid the problems associated with day-to-day variability.

it should be possible to detect viral, bacterial, mycoplasmal, fungal, and chlamydial agents of pneumonia using the same set of reactions, varying only the order of the nucleotides and the size of the probes. Second, because nucleic acids can be extracted free from blocking immunoglobulins and other agents that could interfere with immunoassays, nucleic acid detection methods can be used to detect microorganisms in virtually any body fluid and at any stage in the disease process. Third, as discussed previously, the measurement of DNA or RNA can be used to determine whether an agent is undergoing active replication and thus whether it is latent or actually is contributing

to the acute disease process. Finally, the repetitive nature of nucleic acids allows for the performance of amplification reactions in which small quantities of nucleic acid are amplified by means of controlled chemical reactions to amounts that are easily detectable. Nucleic acid amplification assays, exemplified by the polymerase chain reaction, offer extreme degrees of sensitivity and theoretically allow for the millionfold amplification of nucleic acids and hence the detection of very small numbers of infectious microorganisms. Furthermore, the nucleic acid amplification reactions can be performed with small amounts of blood or other body fluids, so these tests are well suited for diagnosing infections in infants and small children.

The extreme sensitivity of nucleic acid amplification assays also results in numerous problems in interpreting the assays. Because small amounts of genetic material can be amplified to a great extent, contamination of samples by as little as one organism or a single copy of amplified DNA during the collection or processing steps can lead to false-positive results. For this reason, great care must be taken to prevent contamination, which is monitored by processing multiple negative controls in the extraction and amplification steps. In addition, numerous modifications to the nucleic acid amplification format are being included to minimize the chances of false-positive results caused by sample contamination. Until such modifications are shown to obviate contamination, clinicians who use these assays must demand that the laboratory include appropriate controls for contamination in each assay run and that data be reported from only assay runs certified to be free from contamination.

Additional limitations of current nucleic acid amplification assays are that they must be performed in specialized laboratories, require extended periods of time to complete, and cost significantly more than other assay systems. For these reasons, nucleic acid amplification assays are not warranted for detection of infectious agents in which sufficient quantities of antigen are present to allow for detection by means of antigenic assays. Hence, nucleic acid detection assays are not likely to replace antigenic assays for detecting antigens from group A streptococci, hepatitis B virus, or rotavirus. However, nucleic acid amplification assays do play an important role in the diagnosis of diseases in which the microbial load is too low to be detectable by immunoassay systems. Such assays play an important role in establishing the diagnosis of HIV infection in the child's first year of life, in detecting hepatitis C virus in the blood, and in detecting herpesviruses in the cerebrospinal fluid. In addition, nucleic acid amplification assays will play a crucial role in identifying new pathogens and in characterizing them as agents of disease in the pediatric population.

INTERPRETATION OF ASSAY RESULTS

The performance characteristics of individual assays generally are expressed in terms of sensitivity, specificity, and positive and negative predictive values. Understanding these concepts is crucial for properly interpretating laboratory tests for establishing the diagnosis of infectious diseases. *Sensitivity* is a measure of the assay's ability to identify a true-positive result accurately (i.e., to detect the microorganism or antibody in situations in which it actually is present) (Box 147.2). *Specificity* is a measure of the assay's ability to identify a true-negative result accurately (i.e., to yield a negative result in situations in which the microorganism or antibody is absent). In practice, no diagnostic assay achieves 100% sensitivity or specificity, so clinicians often must determine whether a positive result means that the infection actually is present or a negative result means that an infection truly is absent. This question is addressed

---

BOX 147.2 | **Definition of Assay Sensitivity and Specificity**

	Test result positive (+)	Test result negative (−)	Total
Disease present	a (true +)	b (false −)	a + b
Disease absent	c (false +)	d (true −)	c + d
Total	a + c	b + d	a + b + c + d

Sensitivity $= \dfrac{a}{a + b} =$ true-positive/total with disease

Specificity $= \dfrac{d}{c + d} =$ true-negative/total without disease

Positive predictive value $= \dfrac{a}{a + c} =$ true-positive/all test positive

Negative predictive value $= \dfrac{d}{b + d} =$ true-negative/all test negative

---

by the predictive value of the test: Given a positive result, what is the likelihood of a true positive (*positive predictive value*), or given a negative result, what is the likelihood of a true negative (*negative predictive value*)? Predictive values depend directly on the prevalence of the condition in the study population. As prevalence decreases, positive predictive value decreases, but negative predictive value increases. As prevalence increases, positive predictive value increases, but negative predictive value decreases.

An example will help to illustrate this important point (Box 147.3). Suppose in two populations of 1,000 people you wanted to test for disease X. In population A, the prevalence

of X is 20%, whereas in population B it is 1%. Now suppose you wanted to test for disease X using an assay with 90% sensitivity and 95% specificity. What are the predictive values of positive and negative results in these populations?

As can be seen in Box 147.3, the predictive value of a positive test is highly dependent on the prevalence of the disease in the population. In population A, most of the positive results occur in persons who actually have the disease (220 results are positive, of whom 180 have the disease; positive predictive value = 82%). The occurrence of a positive result therefore has a reasonable correlation with the presence of the disease state. Conversely, in low-prevalence population B, of 59 persons who have positive results, only nine (15%) actually have the disease. In this population, many false-positive results will occur for each true-positive result, despite the apparently high specificity of the test. In both cases, the negative predictive value is high; an individual whose test result is negative is unlikely to have the disease. However, the negative predictive value goes down as the prevalence in the population increases. Because no assay can be assumed to be 100% sensitive, the presence of an infectious disease cannot be ruled out completely by a negative assay result. Further diagnostic tests and treatment may be indicated if the clinical state of the patient does not match the test results.

What are the implications of these points about positive predictive value and negative predictive value? The most important is that the role of the physician is of paramount importance in deciding which tests to order. Many infectious diseases in the developed world have very low prevalence rates. If the test for disease X were used indiscriminately on all children in the United States to test for infection, the predictable result would be that most of the people identified as infected would, in fact, be in the false-positive category. If, however, the test were used only on people who had signs and symptoms known to be characteristic of infection with disease X, the prevalence rate in this group would be greater, and thus the predictive value of a positive reaction would be higher. Hence, assays for detecting antigens from group A streptococci are more useful when employed on samples from individuals with pharyngitis than when used on samples obtained from asymptomatic individuals, and assays for detecting HIV are more predictive when employed for the analysis of samples from high-risk populations. Of importance is that assays for infectious diseases should not be ordered on a routine basis or in the form of a large battery, but rather only after the likelihood of disease has received careful consideration in light of the patient's clinical condition and the epidemiology of the suspected infectious process.

Another concern in the interpretation of laboratory results involves the study population in which the assay's original sensitivity and specificity data are collected. The problem is this: data derived from the sampling of one population may not be applicable to the interpretation of assay results in another. For example, assays with high degrees of sensitivity for the detection of *Chlamydia* infections in symptomatic male subjects may not be appropriate for the detection of infection in asymptomatic female subjects. Similarly, assays for the diagnosis of Epstein-Barr virus infection based on the heterophile reaction are quite sensitive when applied to adolescents but lack sensitivity for the detection of this infection in infants.

For each assay, the manufacturer may claim a certain sensitivity and specificity, but these numbers may come from study populations quite different from the one of interest. The appropriateness of the study group always should be considered when interpreting the results of a laboratory test, especially when the patient has underlying immune activation or is from an age group or a geographic area in which the assay system has not been evaluated.

The concepts of sensitivity and specificity imply that a "gold standard" exists by which new assays can be assessed. In some

---

BOX 147.3 | **Predictive Values of an Assay in a High-Prevalence and Low-Prevalence Population**

High-Prevalence Population (n = 1,000)

Prevalence = 0.2
Sensitivity = 0.90
Specificity = 0.95
Test result

	+	−	Total
Disease present	180	20	200
Disease absent	40	760	800
Total	220	780	1,000

Positive predictive value = 180/220 = 82%
Negative predictive value = 760/780 = 97%

Low-Prevalence Population (n = 1,000)

Prevalence = 0.01
Sensitivity = 0.90
Specificity = 0.95
Test result

	+	−	Total
Disease present	9	1	10
Disease absent	50	940	990
Total	59	941	1,000

Positive predictive value = 9/59 = 15%
Negative predictive value = 940/941 = 99.9%

cases, such as the diagnosis of acute bacteremia and meningitis, currently available culturing techniques, although slower than direct detection assays, possess good levels of sensitivity and specificity and generally can be used to assess the performance characteristics of newer assay systems. However, for infections caused by viruses, mycobacteria, and other slower-growing microorganisms, current assays do not detect every case of infection, and, thus, a definitive standard does not exist yet. In such cases, a rapid test can produce truly positive results in situations in which the standard test does not detect the presence of the infecting agent, which is particularly likely with the nucleic acid amplification assays, in light of their high sensitivity. For example, a physician may have to decide what plan of action to follow in the case of a patient who has a positive result for a sexually transmitted disease by a nucleic acid amplification assay but a negative result by a less sensitive antigen detection assay. This question can be addressed only if the true sensitivity and specificity of both assays can be determined.

Documenting that a more sensitive assay can detect a microbial pathogen not detected by a less sensitive assay requires experiments using animal models, sequential analysis of infected individuals, and studies of disease transmission in defined outbreaks of infection. Although such studies can be difficult and expensive to design and perform, they are crucial to the development of a database on the performance characteristics of the newer, more sensitive assay systems. Such studies also are necessary to distinguish microbial carriage from disease because the more sensitive assays may detect microorganisms in clinical situations not previously recognized by less sensitive assays. Thus, performing carefully controlled clinical trials is essential for obtaining these data and represents a crucial step in making these assays useful for the pediatrician.

Numerous new diagnostic assays based on enzyme immunoassay and polymerase chain reaction techniques have been developed since the mid-1990s and have provided pediatricians with ever more powerful tools to diagnose infectious diseases. Table 147.1 shows how some of these diagnostic tests may be useful to the pediatric practitioner. These tests have enormous potential value to the practice of medicine, but they must be ordered selectively and interpreted carefully by physicians who are cognizant of the principles discussed in this chapter to derive the maximal benefit for their patients.

Acknowledgments

Work supported by Grant No. 5 U01 AI30420 from the National Institute of Allergy and Infectious Diseases of the National Institutes of Health.

Suggested Readings

Baseler MW, Stevens RA, Metcalf JA. Immunologic monitoring of patients with human immunodeficiency virus infection. In: Rose NR, deMacario EC, Fahey JL, et al., eds. *Manual of clinical laboratory immunology*, 4th ed. Washington, DC: American Society for Microbiology, 1992.

Benenson AS, Peddecord KM, Hofherr LK, et al. Reporting the results of human immunodeficiency virus testing. *JAMA* 1989;262:3435.

Bobo L, Coutlee F, Yolken RH, et al. Diagnosis of *Chlamydia trachomatis* cervical infection: an enzyme immunoassay for detection of DNA amplified by the polymerase chain reaction. *J Clin Microbiol* 1990;28:1968.

Dienstag JL, Feinstone SM, Kapikian AZ, Purcell RH. Faecal shedding of hepatitis A antigen. *Lancet* 1975;1:765.

Feldman WE. Diagnostic and prognostic values of bacterial antigen detection. In: Wicher K, ed. *Microbial antigenodiagnosis*, vol 2: *Practical applications*. Boca Raton, FL: CRC Press, 1987:143.

Fleisher G, Henle W, Henle G, et al. Primary infection with Epstein-Barr virus in infants in the United States: clinical and serologic observations. *J Infect Dis* 1979;139:553.

Fuccillo DA, Vacante DA, Sever JL. Rapid viral diagnosis. In: Rose NR, deMacario EC, Fahey JL, et al., eds. *Manual of clinical laboratory immunology*, 4th ed. Washington, DC: American Society for Microbiology, 1992:545.

Harcourt GC, Best JM, Banatvala JE. Rubella-specific serum and nasopharyngeal antibodies in volunteers with naturally acquired and vaccine-induced immunity after intranasal challenge. *J Infect Dis* 1980;142:145.

Henrickson KJ. Advances in the laboratory diagnosis of viral respiratory diseases. *Pediatr Infect Dis J* 2004;23:S6-10.

Hollinger FB, Dienstag JL. Hepatitis viruses. In: Lennett EH, Balonis A, Hausler WJ Jr, Shadomy HJ, eds. *Manual of clinical microbiology*, 4th ed. Washington, DC: American Society for Microbiology, 1985:813.

Juto P, Settergren B. Specific serum IgA, IgG, and IgM antibody determination by a modified indirect ELISA-technique in primary and recurrent herpes simplex virus infection. *J Virol Methods* 1988;20:45.

Kenny GE, Kaiser GG, Cooney MK, Foy HM. Diagnosis of Mycoplasma pneumoniae pneumonia: sensitivities and specificities of serology with lipid antigen and isolation on soy peptone medium for identification of infections. *J Clin Microbiol* 1990;28:2087.

Lieu TA, Fleisher GR, Schwartz JS. Cost-effectiveness of rapid latex agglutination testing and throat culture for streptococcal pharyngitis. *Pediatrics* 1990;85:246.

Nahmias A, Yolken R, Keyserling H. Rapid diagnosis of viral infections: a new challenge for the pediatrician. *Adv Pediatr* 1985;32:507.

Niesters, HG. Molecular and diagnostic virilogy in real time. *Clin Microbiol Infect* 2004;10:5.

Pang J, Modlin J, Yolken R. Use of modified nucleotides and uracil-DNA glycosylase (UNG) for the control of contamination in the PCR-based amplification of RNA. *Mol Cell Probes* 1992;6:251.

Pepple JM, Moxon ER, Yolken RH. Indirect enzyme-linked immunosorbent assay (ELISA) for the quantitation of the type specific antigen of *Haemophilus influenzae* B: a preliminary report. *J Pediatr* 1980;97:233.

Relmer CB, Black CM, Phillips DJ, et al. The specificity of fetal IgM: antibody or anti-antibody? *Ann NY Acad Sci* 1975;254:77.

Saiki RK, Gelfland DH, Stoffel S, et al. Primer-directed enzymatic amplification of DNA with a thermostable DNA polymerase. *Science* 1988;239:487.

Schacter J, Cles L, Ray R, Hines P. Failure of serology in diagnosing chlamydial infections of the female genital tract. *J Clin Microbiol* 1979;10:647.

Schwartz JS, Dans PE, Kinosian BP. Human immunodeficiency virus test evaluation, performance, and use: proposals to make good tests better. *JAMA* 1988;259:2574.

Sever JL, Tzan NR, Shekarchi IC, Madden DL. Rapid latex agglutination test for rubella. *J Clin Microbiol* 1983;17:52.

Tobin Jr, Berkowitz ID, Yolken R. The clinical laboratory and pediatric clinical care. *Crit Care Rep* 1991;2:406.

Viscidi RP, Yolken RH. Molecular diagnosis of infectious diseases by nucleic acid hybridization. *Mol Cell Probes* 1987;1:3.

Watts NB. Medical relevance of laboratory tests: a clinical perspective. *Arch Pathol Lab Med* 1988;112:379.

Weiner AJ, Kuo G, Bradley DW, et al. Detection of hepatitis C viral sequences in non-A, non-B hepatitis. *Lancet* 1990;335:1.

Wilde J, Yolken R, Willoughby R, Eiden J. Improved detection of rotavirus shedding by polymerase chain reaction. *Lancet* 1991;337:323.

Yolken RH. Solid phase immunoassays for the detection of viral diseases. In: van Regenmortel MHV, Neurath AR, eds. *Immunochemistry of viruses: the basis of serodiagnosis and vaccines*. Amsterdam: Elsevier, 1985.

Yolken RH. Nucleic acids or immunoglobulins that are the molecular probes of the future. *Mol Cell Probes* 1988;2:87.

Yolken RH. Laboratory diagnosis of viral infections. In: Galasso GJ, Whitley RJ, Merigan TC, eds. *Antiviral agents and viral diseases of man*, 3rd ed. New York: Raven, 1990:141.

Yolken RH. New methods for the quantitation of microbial nucleic acids. *Pure Appl Chem* 1991;63:1127.

Yolken RH. Gastroenteritis viruses. In: Lennett EH, ed. *Laboratory diagnosis of viral infections*, 2nd ed. New York: Marcel Dekker, 1992:381.

Yolken RH, Coutlee F, Viscidi RP. New prospects for the diagnosis of viral infections. *Yale J Biol Med* 1989;62:131.

Yolken RH, Hart W, Perman J. Viral infection and gastrointestinal dysfunction in children with HIV infection. In: Pizzo PA, Wilfert CM, eds. *Pediatric AIDS: the challenge of HIV infection in infants, children, and adolescents*. Baltimore: Williams & Wilkins, 1990:277.

Yolken RH, Stopa PJ. Analyses of non-specific reactions in enzyme-linked immunosorbent assay testing for human rotavirus. *J Clin Microbiol* 1979;10:703.

CHAPTER 148 ■ KAWASAKI DISEASE

RALPH D. FEIGIN, FRANK CECCHIN, AND SCOTT D. WISSMAN

Kawasaki disease is an acute, febrile, multisystem syndrome of unknown etiology that predominantly afflicts children younger than 5 years. The disease also is termed *mucocutaneous lymph node syndrome*. The diagnosis is based entirely on clinical features because no pathognomonic laboratory findings are extant.

The disease was recognized first by Tomisaku Kawasaki in 1967. Subsequently, numerous cases of the disease have been recognized throughout the world in all racial groups. Kawasaki disease is one of the most common causes of inflammatory arthritis and now is the leading cause of acquired heart disease in children in North America and Japan.

EPIDEMIOLOGY

Kawasaki disease affects children worldwide, primarily patients of Asian descent. Japan still has the highest incidence rate of Kawasaki disease of any country or population group at 108 to 111 cases per 100,000 children younger than 5 years of age, followed by persons of Japanese descent not living in Japan, who have a rate of 40 to 50 cases per 100,000 children younger than 5 years of age. The lastest published data from Japan show that the incidence rate in Japan has been increasing steadily during the last 11 years. The rate in 1998 was more than 1.5 times higher than in 1987.

Cases reported to the Centers for Disease Control and Prevention (CDC) indicate that the average yearly incidence among children 5 years old or younger in the United States is estimated to be approximately 12 to 15 cases per 100,000. Recent studies suggest that the incidence of Kawasaki disease has not changed markedly in the United States during the past decade. The incidence among Asian American children is three times higher than that in African American children and more than six times higher than that in white and Hispanic children. The incidence in the United States also varies by region, with the highest numbers of cases reported in the the Northeast and the West.

Kawasaki disease has been seen almost exclusively in children, and the male-to-female ratio is 1.5:1.0 in virtually all countries. Almost 80% of all cases occur in children younger than 5 years old, and 90% of all cases involve children younger than 8 years old. The median age of children diagnosed with Kawasaki disease in the United States is 2.3 years. Only 1.7% of cases occur in very young infants 90 days or younger, and fewer than 10 cases have been reported in the neonatal period, the youngest being less than 2 weeks old. This incidence pattern, which has been noted with other infectious diseases, suggests that transplacental antibody may offer some protection in young infants and that when maternal immunoglobulin G (IgG) concentrations begin to decline and infants no longer are

immune, a cohort of susceptible children is produced. Because individuals have either clinical disease or acquired immunity to an as yet unknown agent, the incidence may decline toward zero. The foregoing incidence pattern, however, cannot be accepted as proof of an infectious cause for Kawasaki disease.

Fewer than 10% of cases are in children 8 years old and older, but this age group has a higher prevalence of abnormal echocardiograms. The diagnosis generally is made much later in the course of the illness in these patients, and, hence, treatment is delayed; this may account for the increased frequency of cardiac abnormalities. Rarely are cases reported in the adult population. In several adult cases, the reported illness more likely was caused by toxic shock syndrome than by Kawasaki disease.

Kawasaki disease is seen at all seasons of the year. However, in the United States and Japan, a slight increase in the number of cases occurs in the winter and spring months. An association also has been noted between Kawasaki disease and residence within 180 m (200 yards) of a body of water as well as history of humidifiers in the home. Some studies have found a greater proportion of patients from families with higher socioeconomic backgrounds, and one study suggested that a greater number of cases occurred in children whose parents work in the health profession.

Clustering of cases of Kawasaki disease has been observed. Often, families of children with the disease have had contact with other children who had Kawasaki disease. Outbreaks have been reported in several cities in the United States, Australia, and Japan. One outbreak in Japan started in Tokyo and spread northward and southward to involve the entire country within 6 months. An increased incidence of second cases occurs among siblings of children with Kawasaki disease. During epidemics of the disease in Japan, the rate of second cases among siblings was 10 to 30 times greater than the incidence in the general population.

In several outbreaks, children with Kawasaki disease had a higher incidence of antecedent illness—primarily of respiratory origin—than did control patients. A report of two cases of Kawasaki disease strongly suggested person-to-person transmission between first cousins, with a latent period of 16 to 18 days. Secondary or coprimary cases are rare, and nosocomial infection has not been reported. The recurrence rate of the disease is about 4%.

ETIOLOGY

Arguments that Favor an Infectious Etiology

The cause of Kawasaki disease is still unknown. Most investigators have favored the possibility of an infectious agent or an immune response to an infectious agent or agents. This hypothesis has been supported by the epidemiologic patterns of the disease and the clinical appearance of oropharyngeal inflammation and cervical adenitis, which is consistent with the acquisition of a replicating agent by droplet transmission, of inflammation of the respiratory tract mucosa, of toxic appearance of children with fever, and of involvement of other organ systems. Laboratory features, which may include an elevated white blood cell count with a left shift, elevated levels of acute-phase reactants, and pyuria, also suggest an infectious origin.

Attempts to incriminate specific infectious agents have failed, and all attempts to culture bacteria or viruses have been unsuccessful. No culture or serologic evidence of infection with Lancefield group A streptococci or staphylococci exists with respect to the genesis of Kawasaki disease. Several investigators have proposed that a variant strain of *Propionibacterium acnes* may play a causative role in Kawasaki disease and that house dust mites may play a role as vectors. A causative link has not been established, however, despite multiple investigations. Single-case reports have documented recovery of various bacterial agents, among them *Yersinia pseudotuberculosis*, *Salmonella*, and *Pseudomonas aeruginosa*.

Several investigators have provided evidence of an agent similar to *Rickettsia*, but others have been unable to substantiate these findings. However, Kawasaki disease does not respond to treatment with antibiotics known to be effective against rickettsial agents, and most known rickettsial diseases are vector borne and seasonal. *Mycoplasma pneumoniae* also has been proposed as a causatice agent as has *Chlamydia pneumoniae*, but studies remain inconclusive.

The immunologic and clinical manifestations of Kawasaki disease bear remarkable similarity to diseases associated with superantigen production. The classic example is toxic shock syndrome, in which the staphylococcal enterotoxin functions as a superantigen that induces massive expansion of T cells expressing a specific Vbeta region on the T-cell receptor. This event, in turn, leads to excess cytokine production, causing clinical illness. Patients with acute Kawasaki disease have been shown to have selective expansion of T cells expressing T-cell–receptor variable regions Vbeta2 and Vbeta8, typically detected during the second week of illness. Further research to elucidate the source of the superantigen is ongoing.

Although many viruses have been implicated, an abnormal immune response to Epstein-Barr virus (EBV) is postulated. One study of patients with Kawasaki disease in Hawaii, however, showed no association between patients with EBV infection and control patients. In fact, none of the herpesviruses, including EBV, cytomegalovirus, human herpesvirus 6, varicella-zoster virus, and herpes simplex virus types 1 and 2, display a dominant role in the pathogenesis of Kawasaki disease in Hawaii. Patients studied during two outbreaks in Japan did have increased antibodies to adenovirus type 2, but no supportive data regarding a causative role exist. Some studies have suggested unusual immune responses to rubeola, rubella, and parainfluenza viruses.

Investigators have detected RNA-dependent DNA polymerase (reverse transcriptase) activity in cultured peripheral blood mononuclear cells from patients with Kawasaki disease. One study demonstrated that cultures taken between the third and ninth weeks after the onset of fever are the most likely to be associated with reverse transcriptase activity. In the early convalescent phase of Kawasaki disease, the cell can be detected most easily in older patients who mount a marked humoral immune response. However, all serologic tests for human immunodeficiency virus type 1 and human T-cell leukemia-lymphoma viruses types I and II have been negative. Other studies also rule out any retroviral cause.

Although frequently hypothesized, Kawasaki disease has not been associated consistently with exposure to environmental pesticides, chemicals, heavy metals, toxins, or pollutants. Usually, poisoning with environmental agents does not simulate an acute infectious disease, although similarities between acrodynia (mercury poisoning) and Kawasaki disease have been noted. Children with Kawasaki disease have had normal mercury levels, with the exception of six patients from the Great Lakes area whose urinary excretion of mercury was increased.

An outbreak of Kawasaki disease in Denver, Colorado was considered to be associated with the use of rug shampoo. Eleven of 23 patients with the syndrome had been exposed to rug shampoo in the 30 days before the onset of illness. Six case-control studies have been completed in an attempt to delineate the association between Kawasaki disease and rug shampooing. It was hypothesized that anionic detergents could trigger a hypersensitive response, or a causitive agent, either infectious or allergenic, was aerosolized during the cleaning process. Three of the studies demonstrated a significant association, whereas the other three did not.

Another suggestion is that Kawasaki disease may be an allergic phenomenon. Several studies suggest that the incidence of allergies in children with Kawasaki disease or in members of their families is higher than in control patients. The prevalence of atopic dermatitis in children with Kawasaki disease is nine times greater than in age-matched control children. In addition, numerous children with Kawasaki disease show a twofold to fourfold elevation in total serum IgE levels during the acute phase of the illness, followed by a decline to the normal range in the ensuing 1 to 2 months. Peak IgE levels do not correlate with the severity of disease or the incidence of arthritis and carditis. The relationship of IgE to the pathogenesis of Kawasaki disease remains unclear.

Relationship of Kawasaki Disease to Infantile Periarteritis Nodosa

A pathologic similarity between infantile periarteritis nodosa and fatal infantile Kawasaki disease appears to exist. Discussions of the similarities between these disorders have been published by numerous investigators. The two diseases cannot be shown to be identical because their causes are entirely unknown, and experience with gross and histologic investigation is relatively embryonic. Distinguishing infantile periarteritis nodosa with coronary artery involvement from fatal infantile Kawasaki disease pathologically is impossible. Clinically, most patients with infantile periarteritis nodosa associated with coronary artery involvement do not meet the other criteria established by the CDC for Kawasaki disease. However, when pathologic and clinical criteria are combined, the two diseases appear to be indistinguishable, thus raising a question about the novelty of Kawasaki disease. This issue is true particularly in the United States, where infantile periarteritis nodosa has been documented since the 1940s, whereas Kawasaki disease was not recognized as a clinical entity until 1974. A male-to-female ratio of 3:1 exists in patients with periarteritis nodosa. Whether any of the cases of periarteritis nodosa with coronary artery aneurysms were examples of Kawasaki disease is speculative because histories in the past often were scant, and deaths often were attributed, perhaps erroneously, to other disorders, such as scarlet fever.

PATHOLOGY

Grossly, cardiac hypertrophy is common. Multiple single bead-like or fusiform aneurysms of the coronary arteries and their branches usually are found in fatal cases. During the various clinical stages, specific pathologic findings are noted, and during days 0 to 9 of the illness, the coronary arteries have perivasculitis and endarteritis but medial sparing. Pericarditis, myocarditis, endocarditis, valvulitis, and conduction system inflammation are observed, with polymorphonuclear infiltrates. During days 12 to 25, coronary artery panvasculitis and aneurysm formation occur, with inflammation and necrosis of the media resulting in "true" aneurysms. By the second week, the inflammatory infiltrate has evolved into lymphocytic and plasma cell dominance.

Resolution of the coronary inflammation occurs near day 30, with subsequent granulation formation. Coronary artery scarring, stenosis, and endocardial fibroelastosis are described after day 40. Aneurysms of other arteries, such as the renal, iliac, and brachial arteries, may be found. Phlebitis is common, with vascular inflammation that most often and most severely affects larger musculoelastic arteries in their extraparenchymal portions. Sites of arteritis include the lung, pancreas, spleen, kidney, testis, mesentery, adrenal gland, and gastrointestinal tract.

CLINICAL MANIFESTATIONS

The classic clinical manifestations of Kawasaki disease in accordance with the CDC diagnostic criteria are given in Table 148.1. Atypical Kawasaki disease has been described with increased frequency in the literature and refers to the presentation of fever with fewer than four of the listed criteria and can be associated with coronary artery aneurysm. Atypical cases tend to occur in younger patients, especially in the infant cases reported, and these patients have a higher risk of developing cardiac sequelae.

Kawasaki disease occurs in four discrete phases, and usually children with this type of illness must be hospitalized. In the first—*acute*—phase, previously healthy children become febrile and irritable. Fever is relentless, and the temperature exceeds 40.6°C (105.8°F) in 40% of such patients. Nonsuppurative cervical lymphadenopathy, usually in the anterior triangle and frequently bilateral, may be present but may disappear rapidly. It is the least commonly observed of the diagnostic criteria. Within several days, rash and bilateral conjunctival injection appear. Usually, at the end of this phase, the physician first is consulted. This phase lasts between 1 and 2 weeks.

The second—*subacute*—phase begins 1 to 3 weeks into the course of the illness and is characterized by a continuing high, spiking fever that is unresponsive to standard antipyretic regimens or to antibiotics. The mean duration of fever is 12 days if the patient is not treated with aspirin or intravenous immunoglobulin (IVIG). The child is febrile and irritable and of-ten appears quite ill. Usually, cervical lymphadenitis is present. Bilateral injection of the conjunctivae, primarily bulbar, is impressive, and unilateral subconjunctival hemorrhage may occur. Anterior uveitis may be found by slit-lamp examination in 80% of all such patients. The anterior uveitis is self-limited, and the prognosis is good. Other ocular symptoms may include vitreous opacities, punctate keratitis, and papilledema. Chorioretinal and vitreous inflammation have been noted. Purulent conjunctivitis and blepharitis may occur, and photophobia may be apparent. The patients' lips are bright red, dry, and cracked. A strawberry tongue may be noted, and generally the oral mucosa is hyperemic. Meningeal findings are rare, although nuchal rigidity and lethargy have been reported.

A rash, particularly prominent over the trunk, consists of maculopapular, ill-defined erythematous plaques of variable size. At times, coalescent areas suggest the possibility of scarlet fever. Occasionally, vesicles and sterile pustules are seen. Petechiae, pinpoint rashes, and erythema multiforme have been described in selected cases. The rash has been noted also in the diaper area and on the face. Erythema and induration occur at the site of bacille Calmette-Guérin (BCG) immunizations in those patients who are from countries where BCG is given routinely. This condition is caused by cross-reactivity of T cells in patients between specific epitopes of mycobacterial and human heat shock proteins.

Occasionally, hepatomegaly and splenomegaly are detected, but they usually resolve quickly. Diarrhea may occur in the early subacute phase of the illness. Severe abdominal pain, paralytic ileus, and icterus are common occurrences. As the subacute phase progresses, erythema of the palms and soles may develop (Fig. 148.1). The hands and feet become edematous, and arthralgia and arthritis of large joints may be noted. In male patients, meatitis may be visible. In females, vulvitis has been described.

Desquamation is a constant feature of Kawasaki disease and signifies the the end of the subacute phase. Sometimes, desquamation can be seen several days before the fever abates, which occurs at a mean of 10 days after the onset of the illness. Usually, it is noted first in the periungual region, although other parts of the body may be involved. Desquamation may be particularly prominent in the diaper area. During the period of desquamation, arthralgias and arthritis may be noted, even though they were not present earlier. Most often, the large weight-bearing joints are involved. Disappearance of the rash and resolution of the adenopathy herald the end of the subacute phase of illness.

When all clinical signs resolve, the third—*convalescent phase*—begins, usually 6 to 8 weeks after the start of the acute phase of the illness. This third phase lasts until the normalization of the erythrocyte sedimentation rate. Beau lines

---

TABLE 148.1

DIAGNOSTIC CRITERIA FOR KAWASAKI DISEASE

Fever of 5 or more days' duration associated with at least four of the five following changes*:
  Bilateral conjunctival injection
  One or more changes of the mucous membranes of the upper respiratory tract, including pharyngeal injection, dry fissured lips, injected lips, and "strawberry tongue"
  One or more changes of the extremities, including peripheral erythema, peripheral edema, periungual desquamation, and generalized desquamation
  Rash, primarily truncal
  Cervical lymphadenopathy
Disease not explained by some other known disease process

*A diagnosis of Kawasaki disease can be made if fever and any of the changes listed are present in conjunction with coronary artery disease documented by two-dimensional echocardiography or coronary angiography.
Modified from previously published diagnostic criteria for Kawasaki disease from the Centers for Disease Control and Prevention and the American Heart Association Committee on Rheumatic Fever, Endocarditis, and Kawasaki Disease.

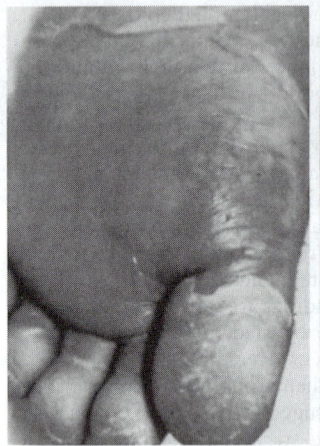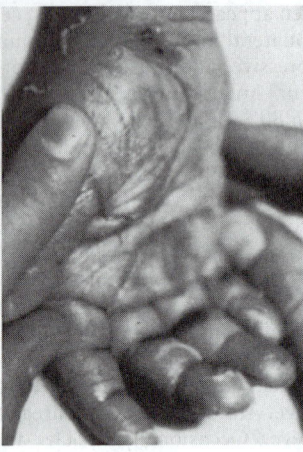

FIGURE 148.1. Erythema and edema of the feet and hands, characteristic of the second phase of Kawasaki disease.

(transverse depressions in the fingernails and toenails) and alopecia may be seen in the weeks and months after recovery.

Although rare, a fourth phase of illness is recognized in only a minority of cases. This phase is characterized by ongoing inflammation, subacute vasculitis, and an increased incidence of death from cardiac involvement.

LABORATORY DATA

The white blood cell count is elevated, with a left shift. Counts in excess of 30,000 cells/μL are noted in approximately 15% of patients, and counts in excess of 20,000 cells/μL are observed in approximately 50% of patients. A peripheral smear reveals an increased percentage of toxic neutrophils characterized by cytoplasmic swelling, vacuolation, and toxic granulation, especially with coronary lesions. Toxic granulation and Döhle bodies are seen. The erythrocyte sedimentation rate, C-reactive protein titer, alpha-2-globulin value, and alpha-1-antitrypsin level are elevated, but they normalize by 8 to 12 weeks. Usually, an elevated sedimentation rate and C-reactive protein level are not present with viral exanthems, hypersensitivity reactions, and measles. Mild anemia may be noted. Severe hemolytic anemia has been described but is unusual. Bone marrow examination has revealed normal number and morphology of megakaryocytes. Increased fibrinogen levels and prolongation of the partial thromboplastin time have been noted.

Often, an acute rise and convalescent fall in the levels of all classes of immunoglobulins occur. The elevation in the IgG level is seen predominantly in subclasses IgG1 and IgG3. The serum complement value is normal or high. Transaminase levels may be elevated, but usually they are not more than three times the upper limit of normal. Hypoalbuminemia, hyponatremia, and hypophosphatemia have been described. Urinalysis may reveal proteinuria and moderate sterile pyuria, usually reflecting urethritis. In patients in whom lumbar punctures have been performed, 10 to 50 white blood cells/μL, predominantly mononuclear, have been noted, but the cerebrospinal fluid protein and glucose levels generally are normal.

Thrombocytosis is another constant feature of this phase of illness, with platelet counts ranging from 500,000 to 3 million/mm^3. Thrombocytosis is seen rarely in the first week of illness. Usually, it appears in the second week, peaks in the third week, and returns gradually to normal approximately 1 month after onset in uncomplicated cases.

Electrocardiograms are abnormal in 77% of patients with Kawasaki disease and in all those who have pancarditis. The most common abnormalities, in order of frequency, are as follows: flattened T waves initially, followed by peaked T waves in convalescence; first-degree heart block; ST-segment elevation or depression; and QT-interval prolongation. Auscultation may reveal sinus tachycardia, a gallop rhythm, distant heart sounds, or a frictional rub. Chest radiography may reveal infiltrates and some cardiomegaly in selected patients.

COMPLICATIONS

Cardiovascular Complications

The most serious complications of Kawasaki disease are cardiovascular and include aneurysms of the coronary arteries and other large arteries, aneurysmal rupture, hemopericardium, myocarditis, coronary thrombosis, pericardial effusions, cardiac tamponade, mitral valve disease, and arrhythmias. Other complications that have been described are aneurysms of the aorta and the cerebral, vertebral, subclavian, axillary, internal, common and external iliac, hepatic, and renal arteries. In most cases, peripheral aneurysms have been associated with coronary artery aneurysms.

Other Complications

Acalculous cholecystitis has been noted repeatedly during the second phase of Kawasaki disease. Usually, children with hydrops of the gallbladder have abdominal pain, a soft palpable mass in the right upper quadrant, and abdominal distention. The diagnosis can be made by ultrasonography. Most cases resolve spontaneously.

Other complications include sterile purulent otitis media, mastoiditis, retropharyngeal mass, necrotic pharyngitis, pleural effusion, myositis, renal infarcts, nephritis and nephrosis, and gangrene of the fingers and toes. Further complications are encephalopathy, facial nerve paralysis, hemiparesis, ataxia, and evidence of cerebral aneurysms, cerebral embolus, subarachnoid hemorrhage, and sensorineural hearing loss. Several cases of hemophagocytic syndrome associated with Kawasaki disease also have been reported.

DIFFERENTIAL DIAGNOSIS

The diagnosis of Kawasaki disease is made clinically by exclusion. Children who meet the CDC criteria should be considered strongly to have Kawasaki disease. Infants are more likely to have an atypical Kawasaki presentation, and, in fact, children younger than 6 months may have coronary involvement, even though they do not fulfill the classic diagnostic criteria. The most common conditions that mimic Kawasaki disease are measles and group A beta-hemolytic streptococcal infection. Other disorders with which Kawasaki disease can be confused initially include roseola infantum, meningococcemia, Rocky Mountain spotted fever, leptospirosis, rubella, infectious mononucleosis, selected viral infections caused by the enteroviruses, rat-bite fever, toxoplasmosis, acrodynia, collagen vascular diseases—particularly infantile polyarteritis nodosa and juvenile rheumatoid arthritis, Reiter syndrome, and Behçet syndrome. Toxic shock syndrome may need to be excluded. Infantile papular acrodermatitis associated with hepatitis B surface antigen (Gianotti syndrome) can be confused with Kawasaki disease during the early stages of the disorder.

Drug reactions also have been confused with Kawasaki disease, including Stevens-Johnson syndrome.

TREATMENT

The goals of therapy for Kawasaki disease are to decrease the inflammatory response and to reduce the severity of the cardiovascular complications. The combination of IVIG and aspirin effectively remains the standard of care to meet these goals.

Controlled studies of the effect of giving IVIG plus aspirin within the first 10 days of the onset of fever versus that of administering aspirin alone have shown that high-dose IVIG significantly decreases the incidence of aneurysm development in such patients. A metaanalysis of treatment studies revealed that the prevalence of coronary artery abnormalities in Kawasaki disease depends highly on IVIG dose but is independent of salicylate dose. A large multicenter U.S. study supports the use of a single dose of IVIG at 2 g/kg given in a 10- to 12-hour infusion. Compared with the four-dose schedule of 400 mg/kg/day, the single-dose schedule of 2 g/kg is equally efficacious in reducing the risk of coronary disease and is superior in inducing rapid defervescence, thus shortening the duration of fever. Concentrations of phase reactants return to normal more rapidly. Although single-dose therapy is safe, the patient's pulse, heart rate, and blood pressure should be obtained at the beginning of the infusion, then at 30 minutes, 1 hour, and every 2 hours thereafter during the infusion. Despite the substantial fluid and protein load associated with this dosage, it has not been found to increase the risk of congestive heart failure, even in patients with decreased myocardial function. Additional information on the mechanism by which IVIG suppresses coronary artery lesions can be found in Chapter 149.

Aspirin appears to be a particularly important therapeutic modality. Although it does not have an immediate antipyretic effect, aspirin can help to reduce the height and duration of fever and serves as an important antithrombotic agent. The aspirin dose studied most thoroughly in the United States is 80 to 100 mg/kg/day divided into four doses until fever defervescence occurs or until day 14 of illness. The dosage then should be reduced to 3 to 5 mg/kg/24 hours to maintain an antiplatelet effect and continued at this level until 6 to 8 weeks after the initial onset of the illness.

The use of steroids for treating Kawasaki disease remains controversial, and the general consensus is that steroids should not be part of initial treatment. However, pulsed doses of methylprednisolone may be effective in reducing cardiac sequelae in children with persistent or recrudescent fever after a second treatment of 2 g/kg of IVIG.

Most children with Kawasaki disease are hospitalized in the initial period after diagnosis because of irritability and fever and because of the difficulties of administering fluids orally. Intravenous fluids may be required to prevent dehydration. Generally, bed rest is suggested until the second or third week after the onset of fever because of the myocarditis associated with this disease. Close follow-up after discharge from the hospital is essential to monitor for cardiac sequelae and persistent or recrudescent disease. The recrudescence of fever on low-dose salicylate therapy is a poor prognostic sign and usually heralds the onset of cardiovascular complications. Commonly, retreatment with IVIG is performed for persistent fever.

Generally during treatment, the peripheral white blood cell count, sedimentation rate, C-reactive protein, and platelet count should be monitored twice each week. High C-reactive protein levels have been shown to correlate with an increased risk of cardiac sequelae, especially in infants younger than 12 months. However, the negative predictive value is low if C-reactive protein levels are used for the diagnosis of Kawasaki disease. One study showed that 54% of patients with Kawasaki disease had normal C-reactive protein levels. In the age group 6 months to 1 year, this number increased to 64%. The peripheral pulses and capillary circulation should be monitored daily for evidence of vascular insufficiency. During the initial 2 weeks of illness, it is recommended to perform one to two echocardiograms, which may reveal early cardiac involvement, especially proximal coronary aneurysms. Another echocardiogram should be obtained 4 to 6 weeks after the disease onset, but follow-up and monitoring must be individualized for every patient. Angiography is indicated if significant coronary dilation or aneurysm formation occurs. If the coronary, renal, and other peripheral arteries appear normal at angiography, signs of vascular insufficiency are likely to appear during the next 10 years. Subtle coronary endothelial changes not visible on angiography may predispose to the development of coronary atherosclerosis during the second or third decade of life. Long-term evaluation of all patients with Kawasaki disease is recommended to detect the early onset of coronary artery disease or renovascular hypertension.

If coronary or peripheral artery aneurysms are found in the acute or convalescent stages of this illness, aspirin, at 3 mg/kg/24 hours, should be continued for at least 12 months. Dipyridamole, at 3 to 5mg/kg/day, also has been used for long-term cardiac sequelae as has warfarin therapy. At that time, the patient can be studied again by angiography. Regression of aneurysms seen previously occurs in more than 50% of patients; in the others, one may note persistent coronary artery abnormalities, such as stenosis, which develop in approximately 18% of patients with aneurysms, or thickening of the walls of these vessels.

The presence of coronary aneurysms predisposes an individual to platelet deposition, embolic phenomena, and progressive intimal fibrosis with luminal obstruction, which may lead to decreased coronary artery blood flow, with resultant angina and myocardial infarction. Fibrinolytic agents, such as streptokinase, urokinase, or tissue plasminogen activator, may be used to treat myocardial infarction. If coronary artery bypass grafting is indicated, internal mammary artery grafts are the best choice, as compared with saphenous vein grafts, because of their long-term patency and good growth potential.

Few guidelines are available for the treatment of patients with coronary artery aneurysms because long-term management has been studied less thoroughly. Some patients have recovered uneventfully from Kawasaki disease only to have angina and myocardial infarction occur between 1 month and 35 years after the acute illness. Children with persistent coronary artery abnormalities should undergo exercise myocardial perfusion studies with thallium or an exercise stress test on a treadmill or bicycle. Recent perfusion study trials have used dipyridamole vasodilator stress to detect regional areas cardiac hypoperfusion. In the hospitalized child in whom aneurysms form, a reasonable approach includes a period of 1 to 2 weeks of close observation and cardiac monitoring, with attempts made to assess whether the disease is progressing, has stabilized, or is regressing, as determined by observation of signs and symptoms, performance of serial echocardiography, and determinations of platelet count, body temperature, white blood cell and differential cell counts, and erythrocyte sedimentation rate. When the condition has stabilized, the decision may be made to discharge the patient, with plans for regular follow-up and follow-up angiography.

PROGNOSIS

Normally, Kawasaki disease is acute and self-limited, although cardiac damage may be progressive if it is sustained when the disease is active. Studies have shown that treatment within the first 10 days of illness is most beneficial in preventing such sequalae. Coronary artery aneurysms are detectable by angiography or by two-dimensional echocardiography in 20% of patients who are not treated with IVIG, as compared to 3% of those who receive IVIG within the first 10 days of illness. Usually, these abnormalities occur between days 7 and 28 of the illness; about 50% of these aneuryms resolve within 1 to 2 years of the initial illness. The risk of coronary abnormalities at 8 weeks remains 15% in infants younger than 1 year of age even when they are treated with IVIG.

Most deaths related to Kawasaki disease result from coronary artery thrombosis. Japanese surveys conducted between 1997 and 1998 on patients with Kawasaki disease suggest an average case-fatality rate of 0.16% in children younger than 1 year of age and 0.05% in children older than 12 years, with an overall rate of 0.08%. United States surveillance data suggest a 2.8% case-fatality rate in this country, but most investigators believe that this number is inflated artificially as a result of the selective reporting of deaths caused by this disease. However, a safe assumption is that deaths can be expected to occur in approximately 1% of affected children in the United States.

The mortality for Japanese boys with Kawasaki disease is twice that of healthy boys of the same age. No significant difference in mortality is found between girls with Kawasaki disease and healthy girls. The male-to-female ratio of deaths related to Kawasaki disease is much higher in infants, with nearly 90% of the infant fatalities occuring in male children. Overall, more severe outcomes are seen in patients who are younger than 1 year of age and who are male, have a longer fever duration, or have continuation of fever after an afebrile period.

Suggested Readings

Bell DM, Brink EW, Nitzkin J, et al. Kawasaki syndrome: description of two outbreaks in the United States. *N Engl J Med* 1981;304:1558.
Chung KJ, Brandt L, Fulton DR, et al. Cardiac and coronary arterial involvement in infants and children from New England with mucocutaneous lymph node syndrome (Kawasaki disease): angiocardiographic-echocardiographic correlations. *Am J Cardiol* 1982;50:136.
Fujiwara MT, Furukawa D. Kawasaki disease and parents in the medical profession. *Pediatr Infect Dis J* 2000;19:769.
Fukuda T, Ishibashi M, Yokoyama T, et al. Ischemia in Kawasaki disease: evaluation with dipyridamole stress technetium 99m tetrofosmin scintigraphy. *J Nucl Cardiol* 2002;9:632.
Fukushigi J, Nihill MR, McNamara DG. Spectrum of cardiovascular lesions in mucocutaneous lymph node syndrome: analysis of eight cases. *Am J Cardiol* 1980;45:98.
Furusho K, Nakano H, Shinomiya K, et al. High-dose intravenous gamma globulin for Kawasaki disease. *Lancet* 1984;2:1055.
Homan RC, Curns AT, Belay ED. Kawasaki syndrome hospitalizations in the United States, 1997 and 2000. *Pediatrics* 2003;112:495.
Kato H, Sugimurs T, Akagi T, et al. Long-term consequences of Kawasaki disease: a 10- to 21-year follow-up study of 594 patients. *Circulation* 1996;94:1379.
Laupland KB, Davies HD. Epidemiology, etiology, and management of Kawasaki disease: state of the art. *Pediatr Cardiol* 1999;20:177.
Leung DYM, Meissner HC, Schlievert PM. The etiology and pathogenesis of Kawasaki disease: how close are we to an answer? *Curr Opin Infect Dis* 1997;10:226.
Melish ME, Hicks RM, Dean AG. Kawasaki syndrome in Hawaii. *Pediatr Res* 1979;13:451.
Momena T, Sanatani S, Potts J, et al. Kawasaki disease in the older child. *Pediatrics* 1998;102:e7.
Morens DM, O'Brien RJ. Kawasaki disease in the United States. *J Infect Dis* 1978;137:91.
Palazzi DL, McClain KL, Kaplan SL, et al. Hemophagocytic syndrome after Kawasaki disease. *Pediatr Infect Dis J* 2003;22:663.
Rowley AH, Shulman ST. Kawasaki syndrome. *Pediatr Clin North Am* 1999;46:313.
Ruey-Kang R, Chang, MD. Hospitalizations for Kawasaki disease among children in the United States, 1988–1997. *Pediatrics* 2002;109:e87.
Sireci G, Dieli F, Salerno A. T cells recognize an immunodominant epitope of heat shock protein 65 in Kawasaki disease. *Mol Med* 2000;6:581.
Stanley TV, Grimwood K. Classical Kawasaki disease in a neonate. *Arch Dis Child* 2002;86:F135.
Witt MT, Minich LL, et al. Kawasaki disease: more patients are being diagnosed who do not meet American Heart Association Criteria. *Pediatrics* 1999;104:e10.
Yamada K, Fukumoto T, Shinkai A, et al. The platelet functions in acute febrile mucocutaneous lymph node syndrome and a trial of prevention for thrombosis by antiplatelet agent. *Acta Hematol Japon* 1978;41:791.
Yanagawa H, Nakamura Y, Yashiro M, et al. Incidence survey of Kawasaki disease in 1997 and 1998 in Japan. *Pediatrics* 2001;107:e33.

CHAPTER 149 ■ CARDIOVASCULAR ASPECTS OF KAWASAKI DISEASE

JUNICHIRO FUKUSHIGE

Kawasaki disease, Kawasaki syndrome, or infantile acute febrile mucocutaneous lymph node syndrome is the clinical entity of an acute febrile syndrome of unknown cause that is observed predominantly in children younger than 5 years of age. Cardiac involvement occurs in 20% to 25% of patients, and the disease is the leading cause of acquired heart disease in children.

EPIDEMIOLOGY

For epidemiology of Kawasaki disease, please see Chapter 148.

PATHOLOGY

The pathologic basis of this syndrome is an acute nonspecific and systemic vasculitis. Cardiovascular lesions of this syndrome are classified into four stages according to the duration of illness. Stage I (days 0 to 12) is characterized by acute vasculitis of the microvessels and small arteries and by acute perivasculitis and endarteritis of the major arteries, especially of the coronary system. Stage II (days 12 to 25) is characterized by panvasculitis and aneurysm formation of the coronary arteries, resulting in embolus formation and local obstruction. In stage III (days 26 to 40), granulation of the medium-sized arteries and the disappearance of inflammation in the microvessels and smaller arteries are evident. In stage IV (day 40 and beyond), scarring, thickening of the intima, calcification, embolus formation, and recanalization are seen. Arteritis is particularly severe and frequently affects the coronary and iliac arteries, but major arterial branches of the aorta, such as mesenteric, renal, celiac, subclavian, carotid, and hepatic arteries, also are sites of involvement. Interstitial myocarditis, pericarditis, inflammation of the sinoatrial and atrioventricular conduction system, endocarditis, and valvulitis also occur.

CLINICAL MANIFESTATIONS

The clinical manifestations include prolonged fever, conjunctival injection without exudate, reddening of the lips and oral mucosa, and reddening and indurative edema of the palms and soles in the initial stage, followed by membranous desquamation of the fingertips in the convalescent stage, polymorphous exanthem, and cervical nonpurulent lymphadenopathy.

The similarities of the clinical features and pathologic findings in Kawasaki disease to those in infantile polyarteritis nodosa have been confirmed by investigators.

CARDIOVASCULAR FINDINGS

The most serious complications of Kawasaki disease are cardiovascular, and they usually occur in the second week of illness. Auscultation of the heart reveals a gallop rhythm and distant heart sound in 80% of the patients, usually in the second week of illness. Rarely, a murmur of mitral regurgitation is heard. Cardiomegaly is revealed on chest roentgenography for more than 30% of the patients. Electrocardiographic (ECG) changes are common findings and include low-voltage and ST-segment depression in the first week of illness and PR prolongation, QTc prolongation, and ST-segment elevation during the second and third weeks. Arrhythmias are rare occurrences and are temporary. Development of paroxysmal supraventricular tachycardia, atrial fibrillation, ventricular tachycardia, or complete atrioventricular block is associated with serious coronary arterial lesions. ECG changes are common occurrences in patients with cardiomegaly, congestive heart failure, and heart murmur.

Dilatations or aneurysms of the coronary arteries caused by vasculitis are recognized in approximately 50% of the patients who have not received intravenous immunoglobulin (IVIG) therapy beginning on days 7 or 8 of the illness. The left coronary artery is involved more commonly than is the right, and the proximal parts of the left or right coronary arteries are involved frequently. More distal parts of the coronary arteries are involved occasionally. The dilatations or aneurysms remain even after the acute phase in 10% to 20% of these patients. With the widespread use of IVIG, however, coronary artery lesions now occur in 10% to 15% percent of patients, yet 1% develop giant aneurysms greater than 8 mm in diameter.

According to Kato and colleagues, of 128 patients who had documented coronary aneurysms during the acute phase, angiographic findings became normal in 73 (57%) within 1 to 2 years, a finding suggesting regression of the aneurysms in 1 to 2 years after the acute illness. A giant coronary aneurysm with a diameter of 8 mm or more and saccular, sausage-shaped, or multiple aneurysms are considered to be important risk factors in the progression to stenosis or occlusion. Ischemic heart disease may develop in fewer than 3% of the patients.

The patients with the following clinical symptoms and signs are more likely to develop coronary artery involvement:

- Male gender and age younger than 1 year
- A prolonged fever for more than 16 days or recrudescent fever

- Peripheral leukocyte count greater than 30,000/mm^3
- Erythrocyte sedimentation rate (ESR) greater than 101 mm/hour
- Elevated ESR or C-reactive protein titer for more than 30 days of illness
- Recrudescence of the ESR or C-reactive protein titer
- ECG abnormality (e.g., abnormal Q wave in leads II, III, aVF)
- Symptoms of myocardial infarction

For the early prediction of coronary involvement in the acute phase, elevated plasma thromboglobulin levels and hypoalbuminemia have been reported to be sensitive indicators for differentiating patients with coronary aneurysms from those with normal coronary arteries. No absolute criteria accurately predict which patient will develop coronary arterial lesions. Although an uncommon occurrence, an aneurysm or dilatation can develop in the more distal part of the coronary arteries, and the normal echocardiographic appearance of the proximal right or left coronary arteries may not exclude coronary lesions completely. Most patients with coronary artery lesions have normal ECGs, chest roentgenograms, and auscultatory findings.

Pericarditis, usually with a small amount of pericardial effusion, occurs in approximately 30% of the patients in the first to second week of illness. It rarely progresses to cardiac tamponade, and usually special treatment is not needed. Mitral regurgitation caused by valvulitis or ischemia of the papillary muscle is observed in approximately 1% of the patients in the acute phase. It usually is mild and improves, but in rare cases, congestive heart failure develops and requires digitalis, diuretics, and vasodilators. Aortic regurgitation and pulmonary regurgitation caused by valvulitis occur infrequently.

Myocardial infarction caused by thromboembolic occlusion of aneurysms or progression of the stenotic lesions accounts for most deaths caused by Kawasaki disease. An analysis of 104 deaths in Japan showed that 60 patients (57%) died of acute myocardial infarction and 7 patients (9%) died of congestive heart failure and myocardial infarction. Infarction developed within 1 year of the onset of the disease in 73% of the cases complicated by myocardial infarction and within 3 months in 40% of those cases. Asymptomatic myocardial infarction also is a common occurrence.

Peripheral aneurysms are found in 1% to 3% of the patients, usually with severe clinical symptoms of the acute phase and associated with coronary lesions. Ischemic necrosis of the distal extremities is a rare but potentially severe complication of Kawasaki disease.

DIAGNOSIS

The diagnosis of Kawasaki disease depends primarily on the clinical manifestations and the exclusion of other diseases. No definite diagnostic test exists. Diagnosis and evaluation of coronary artery lesions in Kawasaki disease by two-dimensional echocardiography are well established, and the diagnostic sensitivity is reported to be 80% to 90% (Fig. 149.1). Stenotic lesions may be detectable by two-dimensional echocardiography studies, but they are not demonstrable in most cases.

TREATMENT

According to the reports by the Japanese investigators in the early days, coronary lesions were recognized in 22% of the patients treated with aspirin alone, in 39% of those treated with flurbiprofen, and in 27% of those treated with prednisolone and dipyridamole after 1 month of illness. At 1 year after the

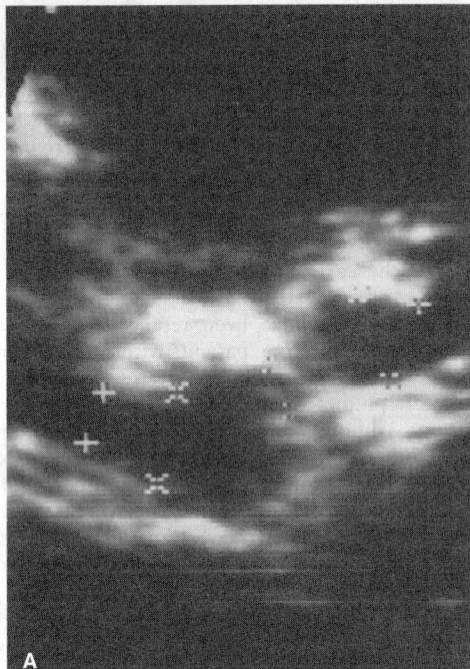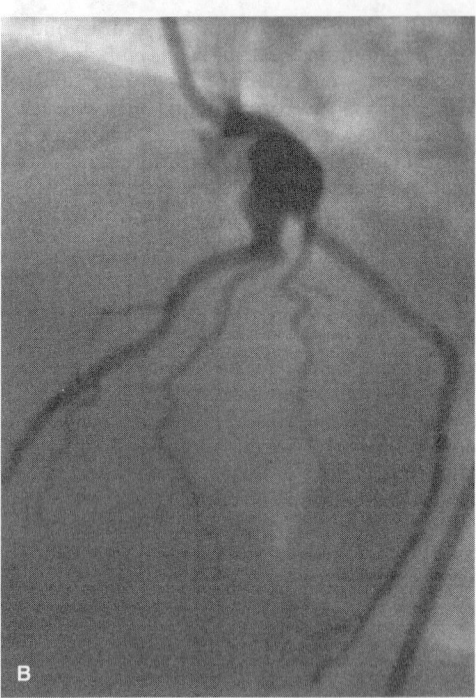

FIGURE 149.1. Two-dimensional echocardiography (**A**) and coronary angiogram (**B**) of a girl at 2 years 7 months of age, who had Kawasaki disease at 1 year 5 months, with a left coronary artery aneurysm.

acute illness began, coronary artery abnormalities were observed in only 1% of the patients treated with aspirin alone but in 12% of those treated with flurbiprofen and in 9% of those treated with prednisolone and dipyridamole.

High-dose IVIG therapy has been provided with increasing frequency in the United States and Japan. The nationwide survey conducted in Japan revealed that IVIG was administered to 86.4% of the patients in 2001 and 2002. In the United States, all children with Kawasaki disease are recommended to receive high-dose IVIG within 10 days of the onset of illness, preferably with 2 g/kg as a single infusion over the course of 10 to 12 hours. The controlled study by the U.S. Multi-center Kawasaki Syndrome Study Group indicated that a single-dose regimen (2 g/kg) of IVIG is as safe as and more effective than the conventional 4-day regimen given at a dosage of 400 mg/kg/day for 4 consecutive days. In addition, high-dose aspirin is administered with an initial dose of 100 mg/kg/day in four divided doses for 2 weeks or until defervescence of fever. Most Japanese physicians, however, have been using 30 to 50 mg/kg/day of aspirin administered in three divided doses. In any case, monitoring of the blood salicylate level is recommended to avoid development of toxicity (i.e., vomiting, hyperpnea, lethargy, liver dysfunction) and to maintain the level at 18 to 28 mg/dL because aspirin absorption is decreased and clearance is increased during the acute phase of illness.

To reduce the cost of treatment and the need for hospitalization, studies have been performed to construct risk scoring systems to give IVIG only to those children thought to be at highest risk of developing coronary artery lesions. Those scoring systems are not yet completely reliable in predicting which children will develop coronary abnormalities.

Not all patients respond to a single dose of IVIG. Approximately 10% of the patients who received IVIG therapy have persistent or recurrent fever, and some require a second dose of IVIG (1 to 2 g/kg), which may result in defervescence. Some patients who are resistant to IVIG may respond to intravenous pulse steroid therapy.

The mechanism by which high-dose IVIG reduces the development of coronary artery lesions is speculative. Possible

mechanisms are blockade or modulation of Fc receptor, neutralization of the etiologic agent or toxin by antiidiotypic antibodies or induction of suppressor T cells, and downregulation of cytokine production. The efficacy and safety of IVIG may differ according to the different preparation or various lots of the same brand.

Hospitalization and bed rest are the general recommendations during the acute phase of Kawasaki disease. The use of a single infusion of IVIG that was associated with rapid resolution of the fever and other inflammatory manifestations, especially a lower frequency and severity of coronary abnormalities, permits hospital discharge to occur much earlier than previously was possible. Patients with coronary artery involvement are at the highest risk for development of coronary embolism and myocardial infarction, and death, during the second and third weeks of illness. For symptoms of myocardial infarction, oxygen, vasodilators (e.g., nitroprusside, nitroglycerin), and catecholamines (e.g., dopamine, dobutamine) should be administered under close observation, and the patient should be monitored carefully. Anticoagulation with heparin and urokinase or tissue plasminogen activator by direct infusion into the coronary arteries, if possible, is advised. Defibrillation, cardiac pacing, or the administration of an antiarrhythmic drug such as lidocaine (Xylocaine) may be indicated.

A complete blood count, platelet count, C-reactive protein titer, ESR, serum transaminases, serum protein and protein electrophoresis, urinalysis, blood urea nitrogen level, creatinine, ECG, chest roentgenogram, and two-dimensional echocardiography study should be obtained at least once a week, preferably at twice-weekly intervals. If coronary or peripheral artery abnormalities are detected, dipyridamole (2 to 5 mg/kg/day) may be added to the usual dose of aspirin. Patients with coronary artery abnormalities may be discharged unless they have a considerable risk of developing an embolism or infarction.

For patients without coronary lesions as confirmed by two-dimensional echocardiography, continuing to take aspirin (3 to 5 mg/kg/day) for 8 weeks is recommended. No restriction of activities is necessary. Although these patients are extremely unlikely to develop any signs or symptoms of cardiovascular abnormalities, yearly follow-up is recommended. Any patient who had Kawasaki disease in infancy may be predisposed to the development of atherosclerosis of the coronary arteries early in adult life.

The American Heart Association has recommended guidelines for long-term follow-up. Patients with coronary lesions are provided with a daily dose of aspirin (3 to 5 mg/kg/day in single dose). A dose of 2 mg/kg/day of flurbiprofen may be provided in place of aspirin. Dipyridamole (2 to 5 mg/kg/day in three divided doses) often is used in addition because a single antithrombotic agent may be insufficient. The addition of warfarin to aspirin therapy also is recommended for those patients with giant aneurysms greater than 8 mm. Evaluations by ECG, chest roentgenogram, two-dimensional echocardiography study, and an exercise test on a treadmill or bicycle once every 2 to 3 months should be planned. Radionuclide scintigraphy may be added to evaluate and identify coronary artery obstructions. Regression of the coronary lesions is expected, especially in patients with fusiform dilatation of a mild degree with a diameter of less than 8 mm. Symptoms such as chest pain or severe arrhythmias are signs that suggest the need for immediate angiographic evaluation. For patients with coronary abnormalities but without obstructive lesions, no general restriction of daily activities is necessary, but strenuous exercises such as short dashes, marathon runs, and competitive sports should be discouraged, or advice should be provided on an individual basis.

Patients with obstructive lesions may be asymptomatic or may suffer from angina pectoris, myocardial infarction, or even sudden death. Antithrombotic therapy is indicated, but dipyridamole may not be recommended in cases with severe obstructive lesions. Patients with angina pectoris may be treated with calcium antagonists, beta-blocking agents, and nitrites, or they may require coronary bypass surgery. Patients should be followed closely with ECG, two-dimensional echocardiography studies, an exercise stress test, and thallium myocardial scintigraphy. The role of selective coronary angiography in evaluating and managing patients with Kawasaki disease is controversial. For patients with coronary abnormalities beyond the acute stage, especially for those with a large aneurysm, obstructive lesions, or both, angiographic evaluation is recommended 6 to 12 months after the onset of the disease to locate the coronary arteries precisely, so plans for long-term follow-up can be established. Repeated coronary angiography is recommended for patients with worsening clinical symptoms or if the results of noninvasive tests have worsened. The follow-up interval depends on the condition of the individual patient. Some patients require weekly evaluation, whereas others need only monthly or quarterly visits. Activities of the patients with obstructive lesions should be determined in light of the clinical symptoms and the results. Some patients with coronary artery stenoses and/or obstruction may require revascularization by catheter interventional treatment and/or bypass surgery. According to the guidelines established in 1987 by the Research Committee on Kawasaki disease, coronary artery bypass surgery is considered in patients with severe occlusion of the main trunk of the left coronary artery or of more than one vessel, severe occlusion in the proximal portion of the left anterior descending artery, or jeopardized collateral vessels.

The great saphenous vein and the internal thoracic artery have been used as autologous graft materials. In view of the long-term patency of the grafts, the internal thoracic artery has been used with increasing frequency. Bilateral use of the internal thoracic artery is recommended whenever indicated because it does not adversely affect the development of the chest wall in children. The gastroepiploic artery has been used

in combination with the internal thoracic artery with favorable early results.

Catheter interventions in patients with Kawasaki disease include percutaneous transluminal coronary angioplasty (PTCA), percutaneous transluminal coronary rotational ablation (PTCRA), directional coronary atherectomy (DCA), and stent implantation. According to a nationwide study in Japan, the immediate success rate was 74% for PTCA (n = 25), 100% for PTCRA (n = 13), 100% for DCA (n = 4), and 86% for stents (n = 7). Although restenosis after PTCA was observed in 24% and development of new coronary aneurysms associated with the use of high-pressure balloon inflation is an unfavorable complication, catheter intervention seems to be a promising therapeutic modality in the management of coronary stenosis as a sequela of Kawasaki disease.

For patients who have a history of Kawasaki disease but who have not been examined by a physician, we recommend obtaining a careful history and physical examination, chest roentgenogram, an exercise ECG, and two-dimensional echocardiography study. Some of these patients may require selective coronary angiography, but this technique may be replaced soon by digital subtraction angiography, magnetic resonance imaging, and x-ray computed tomography.

PROGNOSIS

The average mortality rate for Kawasaki disease is 0.1% to 2%. The short-term prognosis is excellent for 99% of the patients. The possible long-term effects of vasculitis and formation of aneurysms in the coronary arteries have not been assessed. Although regression of the coronary artery lesions of Kawasaki disease is well known, the coronary arteries most likely do not return completely to normal. All patients with a history of Kawasaki disease, including those who have no apparent cardiovascular abnormalities, should be examined at regular intervals. The persistently abnormal lipid levels in Kawasaki disease may increase the risk of development of premature coronary disease in young adults.

Suggested Readings

Akagi T, Ogawa S, Ino T, et al. Catheter interventional treatment in Kawasaki disease: a report from the Japanese Pediatric Interventional Cardiology Investigation group. *J Pediatr* 2000;137:181.

Dajani AS, Taubert KA, Takahashi M, et al. Guidelines for long-term management of patients with Kawasaki disease: report from the Committee on Rheumatic Fever, Endocarditis, and Kawasaki Disease, Council on Cardiovascular Disease in the Young, American Heart Association. *Circulation* 1994;89:916.

Fukushige J, Nihill MR, McNamara DG. Spectrum of cardiovascular lesions in mucocutaneous lymph node syndrome: analysis of eight cases. *Am J Cardiol* 1980;45:98.

Fujiwara H, Hamashima Y. Pathology of the heart in Kawasaki disease. *Pediatrics* 1978;61:100.

Furusho K, Kamiya T, Nakano H, et al. High-dose intravenous gamma globulin for Kawasaki disease. *Lancet* 1984;2:1055.

Guidelines for treatment and management of cardiovascular sequelae in Kawasaki disease. Subcommittee of Cardiovascular Sequelae, Subcommittee of Surgical Treatment, Kawasaki Disease Research Committee. *Heart Vessels* 1987;3:50.

Kato H, Sugimura T, Akagi T, et al. Long-term consequences of Kawasaki disease: a 10-to-21-year follow-up study of 594 patients. *Circulation* 1996;94:1379.

Kawasaki T, Kosai F, Okawa S, et al. A new infantile acute febrile mucocutaneous lymph node syndrome (MLNS) prevailing in Japan. *Pediatrics* 1977;59:651.

Newburger JW. Kawasaki disease: current treatment options. *Cardiovasc Med* 2000;2:227.

Newburger JW, Takahashi M, Beiser AS, et al. Single intravenous infusion of gamma globulin as compared with four infusions in the treatment of acute Kawasaki syndrome. *N Engl J Med* 1991;324:1664.

Taubert K. Epidemiology of Kawasaki disease in the United States and worldwide. *Prog Pediatr Cardiol* 1997;6:181.

CHAPTER 150 ■ *AEROMONAS*

RALPH D. FEIGIN

Aeromonas species cause opportunistic infections and are identified increasingly as pathogens in healthy persons. *Aeromonas* organisms are found as normal flora in nonfecal sewage and can be isolated from rivers, streams, canals, and tap water. These organisms cannot be recovered from water sources in which the saline content approaches that of sea water. *Aeromonas* can survive readily on work surfaces and can be recovered from moistened paper towels.

Aeromonas organisms are asporogenous, gram-negative, facultatively anaerobic, motile rods that have a single polar flagellum. These organisms are oxidase- and catalase-positive and produce acid or gas during carbohydrate fermentation. *Aeromonas* organisms grow well on blood agar, and most strains produce a large zone of beta-hemolysis on this medium. *Aeromonas* organisms also grow on *Salmonella-Shigella*, MacConkey, eosin-methylene blue, and triple sugar-iron media.

Aeromonas organisms are confused most often with *Enterobacteriaceae*. The oxidase tests aid in differentiation: *Aeromonas* species generally are oxidase-positive, whereas Enterobacteriaceae are oxidase-negative. *Aeromonas* species are susceptible to ceftriaxone, cefamandole, chloramphenicol, gentamicin, fluoroquinolones, and trimethoprim-sulfamethoxazole. *Aeromonas* species consistently are resistant to penicillin, ampicillin, streptomycin, cephalothin, and carbenicillin.

PATHOGENESIS

A. hydrophila produces alpha- and beta-hemolysins that are significant virulent factors in the pathogenesis of *A. hydrophila* infection. Alpha-hemolysin released from cells can produce dermonecrosis and may be cytotoxic to HeLa cells and human embryonic lung fibroblasts. Beta-hemolysin also may produce dermonecrosis and is cytotoxic to HeLa cells and to human diploid lung fibroblasts. Antibodies to either hemolysin neutralize both toxins.

Aeromonas species elaborate a cytotoxic enterotoxin that stimulates the cyclic adenosine monophosphate-mediated sequence of events in cells. This enterotoxin may cause diarrhea in humans. An association between enterotoxigenicity and multiple drug-resistant isolates has been established. Serum-resistant strains have been shown to cause more fluid accumulation in rabbit ileal loops than do drug-resistant isolates. *Aeromonas* species also produce endopeptidase, fibrinolysin, leukocidin, proteinase A and B, and staphylolytic enzyme.

Agglutinating, precipitating, and antihemolysin antibodies to *A. hydrophila* have been detected in patients with systemic *Aeromonas* infections but not in those with superficial infections. Antihemolysin titers as high as 1:1,280 and agglutinin titers up to 1:640 have been found. A specific opsonizing antibody in normal serum and the normal bactericidal activity of neutrophils are required to prevent invasive *A. hydrophila* infections.

CLINICAL MANIFESTATIONS

Septicemia caused by *Aeromonas* has been reported in more than 40 children, but because this infection is not a reportable disease, the total number of affected children is unknown. Although septicemia caused by *Aeromonas* has occurred in physiologically normal children, most patients have had a disorder known to impair the normal host response to infection. Clinical manifestations of septicemia are similar to those of other gram-negative enteric bloodstream infections. High fever and shock are common manifestations, and ecthyma gangrenosum, seen more commonly in *Aeromonas* infections, has been described. The reported fatality rate has been 50%, despite the introduction of antibiotic therapy. The high fatality rate may be related to the severity of the underlying disorder and does not reflect an unusual virulence of this microorganism.

Meningitis caused by *Aeromonas* has been reported in children. In almost all cases, the course has been fulminant, and the patients have died despite having received antibiotic therapy.

Gastroenteritis caused by *Aeromonas* has been described in a newborn nursery and in older children. Because *Aeromonas* is carried in the stool of healthy persons, its isolation from a patient with diarrhea does not necessarily imply an infection caused by *Aeromonas* organisms. In a prospective study of 1,156 children with diarrhea and an equal number of age- and gender-matched controls, enterotoxigenic *Aeromonas* was isolated from 10.2% of children with diarrhea compared with 0.6% of healthy children. The same study described three clinical syndromes of *Aeromonas* gastroenteritis: vomiting, low-grade fever, and watery diarrhea in 41% of patients; diarrhea with blood and mucus in the stool in 22%; and prolonged diarrhea of more than 2 weeks' duration in 37%.

A. hydrophila has been recovered from skin and wound infections in children, most of whom were normal hosts. Exposure to some water source was documented in 40% of these patients. I have recovered *Aeromonas* from skin lesions resulting from tick bites. In each case, an area of purple discoloration surrounded the bite, and nonpurulent drainage from the center of the lesion yielded the organism.

Uncommonly, *Aeromonas* has been described as a cause of osteomyelitis, peritonitis, endocarditis, myositis, urinary tract infections, pneumonia after near drowning, and ocular infections in physiologically normal and immunocompromised children. One case of epiglottitis caused by *Aeromonas* was reported in a patient with thalassemia. The extraintestinal manifestations associated with *Aeromonas* infection almost always are preceded by exposure to water or trauma.

Intussusception, internal hernia strangulations, hemolytic uremic syndrome, and failure to thrive have been reported as complications of *Aeromonas* infections.

A. caviae and *A. sobria* have been isolated from stool specimens of patients with gastroenteritis, the former found predominantly among breast-fed babies. *A. punctata* has been recovered from the stool of patients with gastroenteritis. Bacteremia caused by *A. sobria* and *A. punctata* has been described.

DIAGNOSIS

Aeromonas can be considered as a possible cause of infection in children who have any disorder in which the immune system has been compromised. It always should be considered as a possible cause of bacteremia, gastroenteritis, and skin infections in immunocompromised hosts.

A. hydrophila can be detected in food by an immunosorbent assay. These organisms also have been identified in environmental samples by use of 16S rDNA-targeted oligonucleotide primers.

TREATMENT AND PROGNOSIS

In vitro, *Aeromonas* species generally are susceptible to trimethoprim-sulfamethoxazole, fluoroquinolones, chloramphenicol, aminoglycosides except streptomycin, aztreonam, and the third-generation cephalosporins. Chloramphenicol and third-generation cephalosporins have proved efficacious. Ticarcillin-clavulanate generally is active against *Aeromonas*.

A drug to which the organism is sensitive should be provided intravenously in most cases. The duration of treatment depends on the site of infection and the clinical response to therapy.

Suggested Readings

Albert MJ, Ansaruzzaman M, Talukder KA, et al. Prevalence of enterotoxin genes in *Aeromonas* spp. isolated from children with diarrhea, health controls, and the environment. *J Clin Microbiol* 2000;38:3785.
Feigin RD. *Aeromonas*. In: Feigin RD, Cherry JD, Demmler GJ, Kaplan SL, eds. *Textbook of pediatric infectious diseases*, 5th ed. Philadelphia: WB Saunders, 2003.
Gracey M, Burke V, Robinson J. *Aeromonas*-associated gastroenteritis. *Lancet* 1982;2:1304.
Gracey M, Burke V, Rockhill RC, et al. *Aeromonas* species as enteric pathogens. *Lancet* 1982;1:223.
Hazen TE, Fliermans CB, Hirsch RP. Prevalence and distribution of *Aeromonas hydrophila* in the United States. *Appl Environ Microbiol* 1978;36:731.
Kampfer P, Christmann C, Swings J, et al. *In vitro* susceptibilities of *Aeromonas* genomic species to 69 antimicrobial agents. *Syst Appl Microbiol* 1999;22:662.
Kuijper EJ, Peeters MF, Steigenwalt AG, et al. Clinical and epidemiologic aspects of members of *Aeromonas* DNA hybridization groups isolated from human feces. *J Clin Microbiol* 1989;27:1531.
McCracken AW, Barkley R. Isolation of *Aeromonas* species from clinical sources. *J Clin Pathol* 1972;25:970.
Meeks MV. The genus *Aeromonas*: methods for identification. *Am J Med Technol* 1963;29:361.
Preuthipan A, Chantarojanasin T, Suwanjutha S, et al. *Aeromonas hydrophilia* epiglottitis: a case report. *J Med Assoc Thail* 1993;76:225.
Reina J, Hervas J, Serra A, et al. Estudio de las caractersticas clinicas y microbiológicas de 282 pacientes pediátricos con aislamiento de *Aeromonas* mesófilas en heces. *Enferm Infecc Microbiol Clin* 1993;11:366.
Shackelford PG, Ratzan SA, Shearer WT. Ecthyma gangrenosum produced by *Aeromonas hydrophila*. *J Pediatr* 1973;83:100.
Singh DV, Sayal SC. Relationship between enterotoxicity and multiple drug resistance in *Aeromonas* spp. *J Diarrhoeal Dis Res* 1995;13:172.

CHAPTER 151 ■ ACTINOMYCOSIS

JEFFREY R. STARKE

Actinomycosis, a rare infection in children, is marked by chronic granulomatous or suppurative inflammation and formation of external sinus tracts. Another hallmark of this infection is contiguous spread unimpeded by the usual anatomic tissue barriers. Metastatic spread to distant sites also occurs. Infection occurs when these endogenous oral commensal organisms invade tissues of the face and neck, thorax, or intestines. Actinomycosis occurs worldwide and usually is not an opportunistic infection. The organism can be isolated from the saliva, dental surfaces, gingiva, or tonsillar crypts of 30% to 50% of normal adults, if specimens are cultured properly, and may be part of the normal intestinal flora. Gender, race, season, and occupation are not important epidemiologic factors. The infection is reported in children less frequently than in adults, probably because the major predisposing factor for invasive infection is chronically poor oral hygiene. Children who are predisposed to aspiration may be at higher risk of developing thoracic actinomycosis.

Actinomycosis in humans was reported first in 1857. The organism *Actinomyces bovis* (literally, "ray fungus of the cow") was seen first in 1877 in granules from cattle with lumpy jaw syndrome. In 1878, similar granules were seen in human autopsy material; by 1885, actinomycosis in humans had been characterized. For decades, the etiologic agents of actinomycosis in cattle and humans were thought to be the same, but in 1940 *A. bovis* and *A. israelii* were shown to be distinct species.

Before the 1940s, the term actinomycosis designated infection from any actinomycete. In 1943, Waksman and Henrici separated the pathogenic Actinomycetaceae using oxygen requirements and mycelial fragmentation. Microaerophilic and anaerobic actinomycetes were placed in the genus *Actinomyces*, and aerobic pathogens were assigned to the genus *Nocardia*. Current classification places the aerobic actinomycetes in a separate family, Nocardiaceae.

ETIOLOGIC AGENTS

Actinomycosis may be caused by any of several agents that have been placed in the genera Actinomyces and Arachnia. These organisms are gram-positive, facultative or strict anaerobes,

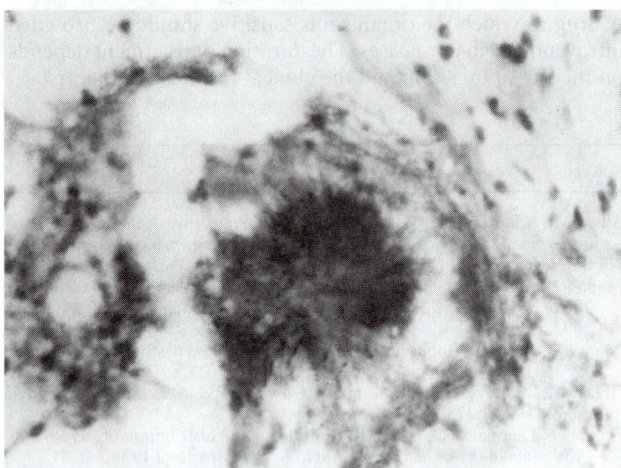

FIGURE 151.1. Sulfur granule found in a lung biopsy taken from a child with thoracic actinomycosis caused by *Actinomyces naeslundii*. The central core, made up of mycelian mass and calcium phosphate, is surrounded by a fringe of eosinophilic clubs. (Courtesy of Mr. David Hines, Texas Chidren's Hospital, Houston, TX.)

with a morphology that varies from diphtheroid to mycelial. Branching is a characteristic feature, but demonstrating it in clinical samples may be difficult. Members of both genera are oral commensals.

A characteristic of all organisms that cause actinomycosis is the propensity to form sulfur granules (Fig. 151.1). These granules are hard, gritty, and yellow or white, and average 2 mm in diameter. Usually, they are round basophilic masses with a fringe of eosinophilic clubs, and granules caused by other organisms (such as fungi, *Nocardia*, *Streptomyces*, and *Staphylococcus*) lack the characteristic clubbed fringe. Granules may be difficult to find, especially in chronic infections, and they may be in an abscess wall or sinus tract rather than in the pus or drainage. The granule represents a mycelian mass held together by calcium phosphate and, therefore, cannot form *in vitro*.

The most common agent of human actinomycosis is *A. israelii*. Grown on artificial media, the early colonies are branched filaments radiating from the center "spider" colony. Usually, the mature colonies are white, opaque, and rough. In enriched thioglycolate broth, discrete breadcrumb-like colonies form and, after 7 to 10 days of growth on solid media, they have a heaped and lobulated appearance, like the surface of a molar tooth.

Several other species of *Actinomyces* have been isolated from human cases of actinomycosis. *A. naeslundii* has been isolated from blood, thoracic abscess, cervicofacial infection, gallbladder, and pleural empyema. Granules are seen less commonly, and free mycelia are found more commonly than in infection caused by *A. israelii*. *A. naeslundii* and *A. israelii* have similar biochemical features, although growing *A. naeslundii* on artificial media may be slow or difficult.

Other species that have been implicated in human actinomycosis include *A. viscosus*, *A. odontolyticus*, and *A. meyeri*. The organism *Arachnia propionica* originally was called *A. propionicus* until it was discovered to be part of a serologically distinct genus. It is similar morphologically and biochemically to *A. israelii* and has been implicated in cervicofacial, intracranial, and pleuropulmonary infections, bite wounds, and renal abscess.

Usually, the pathologic lesions and sulfur granules of actinomycosis contain other bacteria. Some investigators have found these aerobic and anaerobic associates in all lesions, but others have found them in many but not all. The most common as-

sociates are other oral commensals, including *Actinobacillus actinomycetemcomitans*, *Haemophilus* species, *Eikenella corrodens*, streptococci, and oral anaerobes. Usually, antibiotic therapy directed at *Actinomyces* effects a cure, even if the associates are resistant to the drug used. The pathogenic role of these associates is unknown.

CLINICAL MANIFESTATIONS

Although actinomycosis may affect almost any organ in the body, three major areas of infection (in decreasing order of frequency) in adults and children are cervicofacial, abdominal, and thoracic. Cervicofacial actinomycosis is caused by the organisms entering the tissue through trauma to the mucous membranes of the mouth, carious teeth, or the tonsils. Poor dental hygiene usually is a predisposing factor. In children, tooth eruption of a molar or a dental procedure may provide a portal of entry. Two distinct patterns of cervicofacial actinomycosis occur. The first, commonly called lumpy jaw, is a slowly enlarging, painless, fluctuant swelling, usually located at the lower border of the mandible. The second form is painful and widespread and may simulate an acute pyogenic infection of the submandibular area. Both forms spread slowly, without regard to tissue planes, which differentiate cervicofacial actinomycosis from most other head and neck infections. Trismus can occur, and one or more sinus tracts may form (Fig. 151.2).

In the acute, rapidly progressive form, the degree of trismus and tissue edema may be disproportionate to the amount of inflammation. Lymphadenopathy usually does not develop, but a cold abscess or pseudotumor may form. No bone involvement occurs in the early stages of the disease, although, as infection progresses, radiographs of involved bone may reveal periosteal reaction, sclerosis, or lytic destruction.

Primary infection can occur in the scalp, palate, lacrimal gland, orbit, tongue, hypopharynx, larynx, trachea, salivary glands, paranasal sinus, mastoids, or maxilla. Infection may spread through the sinus tracts to the cranial bones, eventually causing meningitis.

Abdominal actinomycosis, which is an unusual occurrence in children, usually results from previous abdominal surgery, acute perforating gastrointestinal disease (especially appendicitis), or blunt or penetrating abdominal trauma. A hallmark of abdominal actinomycosis is delayed diagnosis, frequently

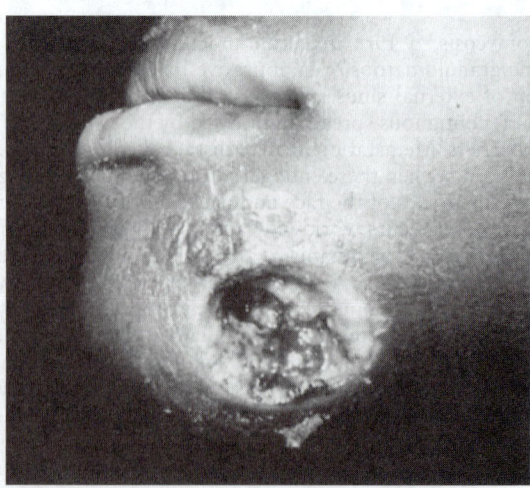

FIGURE 151.2. Large draining sinus tract caused by cervicofacial *Actinomyces israelii* infection. (Courtesy of Dr. Carol J. Baker, Baylor College of Medicine, Houston, TX.)

due to a latent period of many months between the precipitating event and the development of infection. The most common symptoms are indolent abdominal pain, fever, chills, and weight loss; the presentation is similar to that of tuberculous peritonitis.

Abdominal actinomycosis occurs most frequently in the ileocecal region and may cause chronic appendicitis. The infection may spread in any direction, involving other areas of the bowel or abdominal organs, the pelvis, the retroperitoneum, or the abdominal muscles. Bone involvement seldom occurs. Hepatic involvement complicates approximately 20% of cases of abdominal actinomycosis, often arising from direct extension of a subdiaphragmatic or subhepatic abscess. The first clue to the diagnosis of abdominal actinomycosis often is development of a sinus tract or mass involving the rectum, back, or abdominal wall. Primary pelvic actinomycosis can complicate induced abortions, the use of intrauterine devices, or retained surgical sutures, producing tuboovarian abscess, endometritis, or pelvic inflammatory disease.

Approximately 25% of the thoracic actinomycosis cases occur in children. Causative factors include the spread of an existing infection, such as cervicofacial actinomycosis, to the mediastinum and thorax; hematogenous seeding; inhalation of a foreign body; or, most commonly, inhalation or aspiration of organisms in the oral cavity. The infection spreads across tissue planes and frequently extends through the chest wall, causing one or more sinus tracts. Although the clinical manifestations and radiologic appearance are not specific for this infection, the most common presentation is that of an indolent, chronic pneumonitis that is resistant to antibiotic therapy. Cavitation of the lung and pleural effusion are common findings, but pericardial involvement rarely occurs. Presence of a mass or sinus tract should suggest this diagnosis. Symptoms include fever, productive cough, weight loss, chest pain, and retrosternal or back pain, which may accompany mediastinal lesions. Thoracic actinomycosis can resemble tuberculosis, lung abscess, and malignancy, but actinomycosis commonly involves the adjacent ribs or vertebral bodies, and bone involvement rarely occurs with other infections. Distant sites of metastatic infection occur in as many as 40% of thoracic actinomycosis cases. Diagnosis rarely is established before a sinus tract, soft tissue mass, bony lesion, or metastatic site of infection is detected.

Other forms of actinomycosis are rare occurrences in children. Actinomycosis of the central nervous system may result from direct extension from the paranasal sinuses but usually develops secondary to infection at distant sites. The most common forms are brain abscess (67%), meningitis or meningoencephalitis (13%), actinomycoma (7%), subdural empyema (6%), and epidural abscess (6%). However, the prognosis is poor, usually because establishment of diagnosis and initiation

of treatment are delayed. Primary actinomycosis of an extremity may develop secondary to penetrating trauma from a knife, toothpick, or other object, but most extremity infections are caused by hematogenous spread from another focus.

TREATMENT

The basic principles for treating actinomycosis have remained unchanged since the early 1960s, when Peabody and Seabury emphasized the use of intense and prolonged antibiotic therapy combined with surgical drainage of abscesses and excision of sinus tracts. Penicillin, in large doses given over the course of weeks or months, is the drug of choice. Usually, cervicofacial infection responds to antibiotics alone, as do some cases of thoracic and abdominal disease. The usual dosage schedule for intravenous penicillin G is 200,000 to 300,000 U/kg/day for 4 to 6 weeks, followed by oral penicillin for an additional 6 to 12 months. Specific considerations, such as dissemination, inoperability, or central nervous system disease, may alter this treatment schedule. Occasionally, penicillin alone is ineffective, usually because of an undrained abscess or the persistence of a resistant bacterial associate, such as *A. actinomycetemcomitans*. Tetracyclines, erythromycin, clindamycin, and third-generation cephalosporins are effective if penicillin cannot be used or is not effective. Although some cases of extensive abdominal or thoracic actinomycosis have been cured with antibiotics alone, most require extensive surgical resection of affected tissues, excision of sinus tracts, and drainage of suppuration.

Suggested Readings

Berardi RS. Abdominal actinomycosis. *Surg Gynecol Obstet* 1979;149:257.
Bramley P, Orton HS. Cervico-facial actinomycosis. A report of eleven cases. *Br Dent J* 1960;109:235.
Dobson SRM, Edwards MS. Extensive *Actinomyces naeslundii* infection in a child. *J Clin Microbiol* 1987;25:1327.
Golden N, Cohen H, Weissbrat J, et al. Thoracic actinomycosis in childhood. *Clin Pediatr* 1985;24:646.
Goussard P, Gie R, King S, et al. Thoracic actinomycosis mimicking primary tuberculosis. *Pediatr Infect Dis J* 1999;18:473.
Skoutelis A, Petrochilow J, Bassaris H. Successful treatment of thoracic actinomycosis with ceftriaxone. *Clin Infect Dis* 1994;19:161.
Smego RA Jr. Actinomycosis of the central nervous system. *Rev Infect Dis* 1987;9:855.
Snape PS. Thoracic actinomycosis: an unusual childhood infection. *South Med J* 1993;86:222.
Spinola SM, Bell RA, Henderson FW. Actinomycosis. *Am J Dis Child* 1981;135:336.
Weese WC, Smith IM. A study of 57 cases of actinomycosis over a 36-year period. *Arch Intern Med* 1975;135:1562.

CHAPTER 152 ■ NOCARDIOSIS

JEFFREY R. STARKE

Nocardiosis is a localized or disseminated infection caused by an aerobic actinomycete. It was described first in humans in 1890, 2 years after an aerobic actinomycete was observed in bovine farcy, an emaciating disease of cattle that causes pulmonary lesions and cutaneous abscesses. In humans, the soil-borne agent usually causes a pulmonary lesion that may be clinically silent or may provoke chronic bronchopulmonary disease. Hematogenous dissemination from the lungs may infect the central nervous system (CNS), bones, liver, spleen, or other soft tissues. Reports suggest an increasing incidence or recognition of primary lymphocutaneous forms of nocardiosis in children, usually involving the face or an extremity.

Most reported cases of nocardiosis have occurred in immunocompromised hosts, especially in patients with hematologic malignancy or in those being treated with immunosuppressive drugs, with human immunodeficiency virus (HIV) infection, with chronic granulomatous disease, or with chronic underlying pulmonary disease. Only the lymphocutaneous form of nocardiosis occurs commonly in immunocompetent patients.

EPIDEMIOLOGY

Nocardia are distributed widely in nature. Their natural habitat is soil and decaying vegetable matter. Infection in humans occurs by inhalation or by direct skin inoculation of soil or organic particles. Because these organisms rarely are part of the normal flora of humans and are not a common laboratory contaminant, their isolation from a clinical specimen suggests disease.

Some studies support the concept that *Nocardia* can be respiratory saprophytes. No definite evidence for animal-to-person or person-to-person transmission exists, although one cluster of cases has suggested the latter possibility. Tick bites and animal scratches have been proposed as the causes of several cases of cutaneous nocardiosis. Traumatic introduction of *Nocardia* into tissues has caused endophthalmitis, poststernotomy mediastinitis, and mycetoma lesions. Nosocomial cases have been described; they include an outbreak of nocardiosis in renal transplant patients that was related to organisms in the dust and air of the hospital unit.

Between 500 and 1,000 recognized cases of nocardiosis, of which 85% are serious pulmonary or systemic infections, occur in the United States each year. Cases occur in a random geographic distribution, with no seasonal or occupational predilection. Affected men outnumber women by three to one. Although persons of any age can develop nocardiosis, most patients are between 21 and 50 years of age.

ETIOLOGIC AGENTS

Before 1943, cases of nocardiosis were included under the term actinomycosis. Waksman and Henrici separated the pathogenic *Actinomycetaceae* into two groups: The microaerophilic and anaerobic actinomycetes were placed in the genus *Actinomyces*, and aerobic forms were assigned to *Nocardia*. Current classification places the aerobic actinomycetes in a separate family, Nocardiaceae.

Nocardia reproduce by fragmentation into bacillary and coccoid elements, but they are differentiated by their propensity for filamentous growth with true branching. The organisms grow over a wide range of temperatures on simple laboratory media, such as blood agar. Colonies on agar may be smooth and moist or rough. Their color varies from cream to brick red. *Nocardia* may grow poorly on antibiotic-containing media used for isolation of fungi. Colonies in pure culture often grow after 48 hours of incubation, but growth can take up to several weeks in mixed cultures from clinical material.

The usual microscopical appearance of *Nocardia* is a delicate, weakly gram-positive, beaded branching filament (Fig. 152.1). Most *Nocardia* are acid-fast but retain fuchsin less avidly than do mycobacteria. Acid and alcohol solutions (i.e., Ziehl-Neelsen stain) decolorize *Nocardia*, but more basic solutions do not. A modified Ziehl-Neelsen stain using 1% sulfuric acid is the best solution to demonstrate *Nocardia* in clinical specimens.

Nocardia asteroides is the predominant pathogen, involved in as many as 90% of human nocardiosis cases. *N. brasiliensis* now is recognized as a common cause of lymphocutaneous nocardiosis in immunocompetent patients and as the major cause of mycetoma in Central and South America. In experimental animals, *N. brasiliensis* is more virulent than are other *Nocardia* species. The association of skin trauma with lymphocutaneous nocardiosis suggests that, once beyond the skin barrier, *N. brasiliensis* can cause local disease despite normal host defenses. Other species, including *N. otitidiscaviarum* (*caviae*), *N. nova*, *N. farcinica*, and *N. transvalensis*, rarely are involved in human disease.

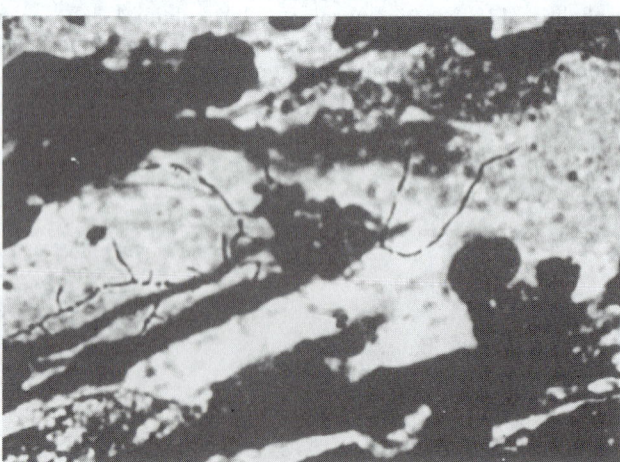

FIGURE 152.1. Microscopical appearance of *Nocardia brasiliensis.* Beaded, branching filaments are visible in pus from a cutaneous abscess.

PATHOGENESIS AND PATHOLOGY

N. asteroides usually infects humans through the respiratory tract, although the gastrointestinal tract may be the site of entry. Dissemination from the initial site is a common occurrence and can involve the liver, spleen, kidneys, CNS, or skin. Primary cutaneous nocardiosis is preceded by trauma and can take the form of mycetoma, cellulitis, pyoderma, or infection of a compound fracture.

Although most nocardiosis cases occurring before 1961 were primary infections, 85% of the current cases are associated with an array of debilitating diseases and conditions, especially lymphoreticular neoplasms, HIV infection, chronic granulomatous disease, long-term corticosteroid usage, organ transplantation with associated immunosuppressive treatment, dysgammaglobulinemias, and alcoholism. Many of the antecedent conditions involve dysfunction of cellular immunity, but immunoglobulin and leukocyte defects also predispose to this infection.

The host reaction to *Nocardia* infection is complex and poorly understood. Neutrophils are mobilized to the site of infection, but killing of organisms is limited. The major responses in animals include macrophage activation, development of cell-mediated immunity, inhibition of growth by polymorphonuclear leukocytes, and induction of a T-cell population capable of direct lymphocyte-mediated toxicity to *N. asteroides*.

Nocardiosis causes a suppurative lesion with abscess formation and necrosis. Pulmonary lesions usually consist of multiple abscesses, although a single abscess or nodule may occur. The suppuration resembles that seen with bacterial pyogenic infections. Little evidence of encapsulation exists, which may account for the ready dissemination of *Nocardia* from the pulmonary focus.

CLINICAL MANIFESTATIONS AND DIAGNOSIS

The most common form of nocardiosis in immunocompromised patients is pulmonary infection. Specific presentations include bronchopneumonia, lobar pneumonitis, and necrotizing pneumonia with single or multiple abscesses or empyema. Endobronchial nocardiosis rarely occurs. Pulmonary involvement often is chronic but can be acute, with rapid dissemination.

Clinical symptoms are nonspecific and include fever, anorexia, weight loss, productive cough, pleural pain, dyspnea, and hemoptysis. Chest radiography shows great variability, but the most common findings are alveolar or interstitial infiltrates, segmental bronchopneumonia (with or without thin-walled cavitation), subpleural plaques, and single or multiple nodules; rarely, miliary lesions or thick-walled cavities are seen. The radiographic pattern often is confused with tuberculosis, metastatic malignancy, bacterial pneumonia, actinomycosis, or pyogenic abscess.

Frequently, clinical manifestations occur in sites distant to the lung as a result of direct extension or hematogenous dissemination. Related problems seen most often include tracheitis, peritonsillar abscess, pericarditis, peritonitis, muscle abscess, perirectal abscess, endophthalmitis, sinusitis, mediastinitis with superior vena cava obstruction, septic arthritis, osteomyelitis, and a disseminated miliary form. *Nocardia* infection of virtually every organ has been reported, and it should be suspected when an infection does not respond to usual therapy, especially if trauma is a predisposing factor.

The skin, subcutaneous tissues, and lymph nodes are common sites for *Nocardia* infection in children. Lymphocutaneous infection can occur secondary to dissemination from a silent

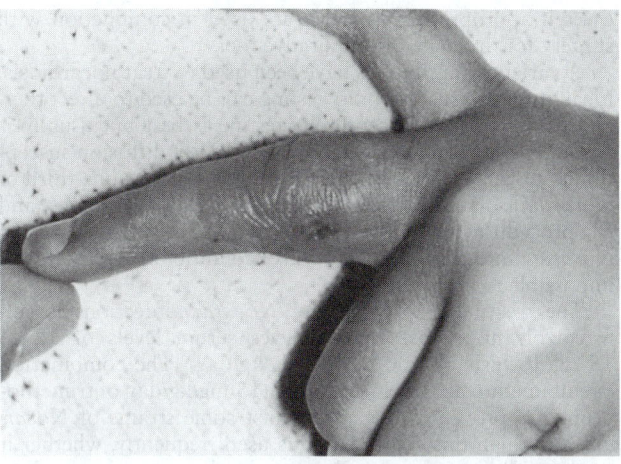

FIGURE 152.2. Cutaneous lesion caused by *Nocardia brasiliensis* in a 4-year-old girl. This lesion was accompanied by markedly tender epitrochlear adenitis. (Courtesy of Dr. Moise L. Levy, Department of Dermatology, Baylor College of Medicine, Houston, TX.)

pulmonary lesion or by direct inoculation through traumatized skin. *N. brasiliensis* is the most common species involving the skin. Subcutaneous abscesses related to disseminated disease can be single or multiple, usually are firm (but may be fluctuant), and usually lack induration, extensive erythema, or warmth. In children, a cervicofacial syndrome usually consists of a pustular facial lesion associated with submandibular or cervical adenitis. This presentation can be confused with tularemia, cat-scratch disease (*Bartonella*), actinomycosis, or cutaneous diphtheria. Nocardia occasionally form multiple subcutaneous nodules on an extremity, mimicking sporotrichosis. Primary cutaneous infection involves the inoculation site and the regional lymph nodes (Fig. 152.2), although dissemination from the skin to other organs occurs.

The CNS is involved in approximately one-third of immunocompromised patients with disseminated nocardiosis. The fatality rate of CNS nocardiosis is 40% to 70%, with most deaths resulting from delay in establishing the diagnosis and instituting specific therapy. Brain involvement may dominate the clinical presentation, although usually it is associated with other manifestations. Multiloculated brain abscesses are seen most commonly, but meningitis rarely occurs. Involvement of the CNS with *Nocardia* also can be caused by penetrating trauma of the skull or by placement of a ventriculoperitoneal shunt.

Diagnosing pulmonary nocardiosis may be difficult because the organism is seen in the sputum of only one-third of affected patients. Bronchoalveolar lavage or open lung biopsy often are required to establish the diagnosis and to differentiate nocardiosis from myriad other infections that have similar clinical and radiographic appearances in immunocompromised hosts. *Nocardia* are isolated readily from lymphocutaneous lesions and can be detected microscopically by using the appropriately modified weak acid-fast stain of pus. *N. asteroides* may be recovered from blood cultures in immunosuppressed patients. Tests for humoral antibodies or delayed cutaneous hypersensitivity are not useful clinically.

TREATMENT

Sulfonamides have been recognized as the drugs of choice in nocardiosis since their release in the 1940s. Previous therapy had been supportive, and spontaneous remissions rarely occurred. Cure of *Nocardia* infection can be expected in most cases if appropriate antibiotics are used in conjunction with surgery for drainage of suppurative foci.

A variety of antibiotics have been used to treat nocardiosis. Ideally, *in vitro* susceptibility testing can be used to direct therapy. Tube dilution susceptibility testing is best but usually is available only at reference laboratories. Disk diffusion susceptibility testing can be difficult because as many as one-third of *Nocardia* isolates do not grow adequately on agar plates, and test procedures are not well standardized. The relative rarity of *Nocardia* infections renders controlled antibiotic trials almost impossible to perform.

The treatment of choice for *Nocardia* infections is sulfisoxazole at a dose that achieves serum levels of 12 to 15 μg/dL (usually 100 to 150 mg/kg/day). The combination of sulfamethoxazole-trimethoprim (15 mg/kg/day of trimethoprim) has proven synergistic against some strains of *Nocardia*. Although this combination is used frequently, whether it has any advantage over sulfisoxazole alone remains unclear. A second antibiotic, such as tetracycline or ampicillin, may be necessary to effect a cure. For patients who cannot tolerate sulfa drugs, doxycycline, erythromycin, and amikacin may be used. Some of the other beta-lactam antibiotics (e.g., cefotaxime, cefuroxime, ceftriaxone) and amoxicillin-clavulanate are active *in vitro* against *Nocardia*, but clinical data are lacking. More recently, linezolid has been effective in treating some life-threatening infections that did not respond to other antimicrobial agents.

The optimal duration of therapy is uncertain. A minimum of 6 weeks is recommended, but usually sulfonamide therapy is continued for as long as 6 months because of the likelihood of relapse or appearance of metastatic abscesses with a shorter treatment duration. Some authors suggest that patients with HIV should be treated indefinitely. The appearance of a metastatic abscess during administration of appropriate therapy usually represents the evolution of a metastasis seeded previously, which may progress until adequate surgical drainage is achieved. Most lymphocutaneous sites of *Nocardia* infection require surgical drainage for cure, but pulmonary, brain, and other deep-seated infections often can be cured with antibiotics alone.

Suggested Readings

Beaman BL, Beaman L. Nocardia species: host-parasite relationships. *Clin Microbiol Rev* 1994;7:213.

Bross JE, Gordon G. Nocardial meningitis: case reports and review. *Rev Infect Dis* 1991;13:160.

Idriss ZH, Cunningham RJ, Wilfert CM. Nocardiosis in children: report of three cases and review of the literature. *Pediatrics* 1975;55:479.

Lampe RM, Baker CJ, Septimus EJ, et al. Cervicofacial nocardiosis in children. *J Pediatr* 1981;99:593.

Law BJ, Marks MI. Pediatric nocardiosis. *Pediatrics* 1982;70:560.

Moylett EH, Pacheco SE, Brown-Elliott BA, et al. Clinical experience with linezolid for treatment of nocardia infection. *Clin Infect Dis* 2003;36:313.

Smego RA Jr, Gallis HA. The clinical spectrum of *Nocardia brasiliensis* in the United States. *Rev Infect Dis* 1984;6:164.

Smego RA Jr, Moeller MB, Gallis HA. Trimethoprim-sulfamethoxazole therapy for *Nocardia infections*. *Arch Intern Med* 1983;143:711.

Stites DP, Glezen WP. Pulmonary nocardiosis in childhood. *Am J Dis Child* 1967;114:101.

Van Burik JA, Hackman RC, Nadeem SQ, et al. Nocardiosis after bone marrow transplantation: a retrospective study. *Clin Infect Dis* 1997;24:1154.

CHAPTER 153 ■ ANAEROBIC INFECTIONS

ITZHAK BROOK AND LISA M. DUNKLE

Diseases caused by anaerobic bacteria or intoxication have been known since the time of Hippocrates, when tetanus first was described. The existence of anaerobic organisms was recognized by Pasteur in his observations of bacterial fermentation. In 1896, Welch began the process of identifying specific etiologic agents with the description of what now is recognized as *Clostridium perfringens*. Disease is caused by relatively few representatives of the vast taxonomic spectrum of anaerobic organisms. The genus *Clostridium* includes several of the most prominent pathogens and causes the most characteristic disease patterns of all anaerobic infections, mainly by the production of potent toxins. Nonclostridial anaerobic bacteria cause less typical disease patterns, and their clinical importance has been recognized only within the last half of the twentieth century.

Clostridium organisms are characterized as anaerobic, gram-positive, spore-forming bacilli, although a few exceptions to each of these characteristics exist. Clostridial spores are found worldwide and are ubiquitous in soil, dust, dirt, and human and animal feces. Most species are considered nonpathogenic, although differentiating pathogens from nonpathogens in a polymicrobial infection may be difficult. The protein exotoxins produced by some of these organisms are among the most potent poisons known, and frequently the toxin-produced diseases occur without inflammation of tissues.

CLOSTRIDIUM TETANI

Etiology and Epidemiology

Clinical tetanus is caused by the exotoxin tetanospasmin, a 67-kd protein elaborated by the vegetative form of *C. tetani*. Tetanospasmin is a potent neurotoxin that is lethal to humans at a dose of less than 150 μg. Because the spores of *C. tetani* are ubiquitous and resist heat and disinfection, they can contaminate wounds readily. Most tetanus occurs without a history of apparent wound contamination, although puncture wounds and grossly contaminated lacerations commonly are tetanus-prone.

C. tetani is distributed worldwide and has been isolated from diverse sites including soil, feces, house dust, and contaminated heroin. Tetanus ranks high among the infectious diseases as a cause of death throughout the world, and in developing countries it is an important cause of neonatal death. The incidence of tetanus varies widely throughout the world; in the United States, a sharp decline in the rate of tetanus has occurred, although 50 to 100 cases are reported annually (average incidence, 0.03 cases per 100,000 persons). Neonatal tetanus is rare in the United States. This decline reflects the efficacy of the aggressive immunization program in the United States, especially as compared with developing countries, where mortality rates still are high. Unhygienic childbirth practices in most of the developing world and inadequate immunization of mothers explain most cases of neonatal tetanus. Often, nonmedical abortions and lack of attention to penetrating wounds are responsible for development of tetanus in adults. Climate and soil pH in the tropics probably contribute to the prevalence of *C. tetani* and its availability to contaminate wounds. In the absence of vigorous hygiene and immunization programs, tetanus remains a major killer.

Pathophysiology

After introduction into tissues, spores convert to vegetative forms, multiply, and elaborate tetanospasmin. This process occurs only if the oxidation-reduction potential of the inoculated tissue is sufficiently low to allow anaerobic growth to occur. Often, no associated inflammation or local infection is present.

Tetanospasmin enters the peripheral nerve at the site of injury and travels through the nerve to the central nervous system (CNS). The toxin's effect on the nervous system occurs centrally and peripherally. At the presynaptic nerve ending, the toxin binds to gangliosides in the neuronal membrane, prevents release of neurotransmitters, and affects polarization of postsynaptic membranes in complex polysynaptic reflexes. The resultant lack of inhibitory impulses is manifested in the characteristic spasms, seizures, and sympathetic overactivity of tetanus. The toxin has no apparent effect on mental status, and consciousness is not impaired directly by this disease.

The neuronal transport of the toxin is consistent with the observation that the time that transpires between the occurrence of the injury and the development of disease correlates with the distance between the wound and the CNS. Usually, the incubation period lasts between 3 days and 3 weeks; the most severe cases develop after the shortest incubation periods. In some instances, the toxin remains localized to the neurons associated with the wound, producing a localized form of tetanus. More commonly, the toxin affects the entire nervous system, causing generalized tetanus. In rare cases, the toxin affects only cranial nerves, a condition known as *cephalic tetanus*.

Tetanospasmin binds irreversibly to neurons and thereafter cannot be neutralized by antitoxin. The course and duration of established disease are determined by the location and "dose" of bound toxin. Usually, the complete course of tetanus lasts from 2 to 4 weeks, but it is influenced greatly by the patient's age and the development of complications.

The worldwide mortality is 45% to 55%; the mortality rate is approximately 1% in localized tetanus, but mortality rates of more than 60% are reported for tetanus neonatorum. Although survivors generally experience no neurologic sequelae, prolonged convalescence with residual muscle rigidity is observed for several months.

Clinical Manifestations

Usually, the clinical presentation of tetanus falls into one of three categories: localized, generalized, or cephalic. Neonatal tetanus, a generalized form of the disease, warrants discussion because of its occurrence worldwide.

Localized Tetanus

An unusual manifestation of tetanus, localized disease is thought to occur when circulating antitoxin prevents general spread of the toxin but is insufficient to prevent local uptake at a wound site. The condition results in prolonged, steady, and painful muscle contractions in the region of the wound; it lasts several weeks and eventually resolves completely. The condition has a low mortality rate (less than 1%). Localized tetanus may go unrecognized or may be mistaken for pain-induced muscle spasms. It may be unrecognized before generalized tetanus supersedes.

Generalized Tetanus

The most common form of clinical tetanus, generalized disease may occur after relatively minor injuries and commonly after non-tetanus-prone wounds. Although the onset may be insidious, the typical initial complaint of trismus caused by spasms of the parapharyngeal and masseter muscles occurs in 50% of cases. Common complaints include pain and difficulty with swallowing and unilateral or bilateral neck and other muscle group stiffness, such as abdominal or thoracic musculature. Persistent trismus is responsible for risus sardonicus, a classic finding of tetanus.

With disease progression, additional muscle groups become involved; the most striking is the paraspinal musculature. Their tonic spasms may result in severe opisthotonos; in young infants, the soles of the feet may touch the head. Vertebral fractures are common occurrences in this situation. Tetanic contractions progress over the course of several days; recruitment of additional muscle groups and significant worsening of symptoms are to be expected after the initial presentation.

In addition to the tonic contractions, painful spasms and contractions occur and further contort and distort the patient's posture. They affect all voluntary muscles and may involve the larynx, a complication that can be fatal. The force produces fractures of vertebrae or other bones and hemorrhage into muscles. These spasms are extraordinarily painful and are not true seizures, as they are not associated with the characteristic electroencephalographic changes of convulsions and are more appropriately called *tetanus spasms*. The spasms are stimulus-dependent, and the stimuli may be minor (e.g., light, drafts, noises or voices, and light touch). Because patients remain fully conscious throughout these spasms, anxiety and pain further complicate management and contribute to the severity of the untreated disease.

The effect of tetanospasmin on the autonomic nervous system results in characteristic cardiovascular instability. Labile hypertension, sometimes of a marked degree, is a common occurrence, as are episodes of tachycardia or other tachyarrhythmias. Fever can result also from sympathetic overactivity or from superinfections, such as pneumonia. In the intensive care setting, where ventilatory support and therapeutic paralysis are available, cardiovascular complications are the primary problem in management. As is the case with spasms, cardiovascular complications occur most commonly during the first week and resolve slowly during the ensuing 2 to 4 weeks.

Cephalic Tetanus

A rare manifestation of the disease, cephalic tetanus exclusively involves the cranial nerves after entry of *C. tetani* into wounds or chronic infections of the head and neck. Cranial nerve VII is involved most frequently, although any of the cranial nerves may be affected singly or in combination, causing weakness of the affected nerve. Cephalic tetanus may precede generalized disease, and isolated cephalic tetanus can occur and follows a chronology similar to that of generalized disease. Mortality rates are significant for these patients, but survivors demonstrate no sequelae.

Neonatal Tetanus

Tetanus in the newborn is a generalized form of the disease. Infants delivered vaginally to mothers who have not been immunized are at significant risk for development of neonatal tetanus. Birth practices in developing countries, such as applying mud or feces to the umbilical stump, greatly increase risk and are responsible for a large proportion of cases. Mortality rates are high, with infants dying of such complications as pneumonia and pulmonary hemorrhage, CNS hemorrhage, and laryngeal spasms.

The risk of neonatal tetanus in the United States should not be dismissed, particularly in unusually contaminated deliveries and if the maternal immunization status is uncertain. Passive immunization should be administered in these circumstances.

Differential Diagnosis

Tetanus is an uncommon occurrence in developed nations, where immunization and hygiene practices largely have eliminated the disease. The classic presenting complaint of trismus and of muscle spasms, stiffness, and pain with dysphagia and cranial nerve weakness can be seen in other conditions, although the classic picture is sufficiently characteristic to support the diagnosis of tetanus. Other conditions that can mimic some manifestations of tetanus include parapharyngeal and peritonsillar abscesses, poliomyelitis and other forms of viral encephalomyelitis, Bell palsy, meningoencephalitis (including rabies), hypocalcemic tetany, and dystonic reactions to phenothiazines. These other conditions are differentiated relatively easily from tetanus by specific laboratory or radiographic evaluations or by the clinical course. The absence of altered consciousness in tetanus is an important point in differentiating the disorder from CNS infections. A parapharyngeal inflammatory process can be suspected from clinical examination or radiographs of the airway. Usually, hypocalcemic tetany is confirmed by low serum levels of calcium; idiosyncratic dystonia caused by a phenothiazine resolves promptly after intravenous administration of diphenhydramine.

Confirming a specific diagnosis of tetanus by routine laboratory tests is difficult. Routine blood counts are normal or elevated slightly; cerebrospinal fluid (CSF) evaluations are normal; and electroencephalograms and electromyograms are normal and nonspecifically abnormal, respectively. Gram stains and anaerobic cultures of wounds reveal the characteristic gram-positive bacilli with terminal spores in as many as one-third of patients with tetanus. Although positive cultures from wounds may support the diagnosis in patients with clinical disease suggestive of tetanus, a positive culture from a contaminated wound in the absence of symptoms does not indicate that tetanus intoxication will develop.

Management and Prognosis

Without specific confirmatory laboratory tests, appropriate treatment based on the clinical diagnosis is warranted. The goals of therapy are to eradicate *C. tetani*, to neutralize its toxin, and to provide appropriate supportive care (Box 153.1).

Specific therapy includes intramuscular administration of tetanus immune globulin (TIG) to neutralize circulating toxin before it binds to neuronal cell membranes. The American Academy of Pediatrics Committee on Infectious Diseases (AAP CID) recommends a dose of 3,000 to 6,000 units for children and adults. The recommended dose for neonatal tetanus is 500

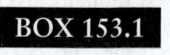

BOX 153.1 **Things to Consider in the Management of the Child with Tetanus**

The goals of therapy are to:

1. Eradicate *Clostridium tetani*: Metronidazole, 30 mg/kg/day given q6h for 10 to 14 days, or parenteral penicillin G, 100,000 U/kg/day given q4–6h.
2. Neutralize the toxin: IM administration of tetanus immune globulin (TIG to children and adults, 3,000–6,000 units; to neonates, 500 units).
3. Provide supportive care: Local wound care, including surgical débridement, meticulous nursing care, maintenance of adequate nutrition and hydration ventilatory support, and pharmacologic intervention to stabilize vital signs, institute sedation, and manage hypertension and muscle relaxation (including diazepam, phenothiazines, and curariform drugs).

units. The efficacy of additional intrathecal administration of TIG has not been proven. Equine tetanus antitoxin given early in the disease may prevent spread of the toxin within the CNS; however, this antitoxin is associated with serum sickness in 10% to 20% of patients, and it no longer is produced in the United States.

Additional specific therapy should include antimicrobial therapy for *C. tetani*. The AAP CID recommends oral or intravenous metronidazole, 30 mg/kg/day given every 6 hours for 10 to 14 days. Alternatively, parenteral penicillin G, 100,000 U/kg/day given every 4 to 6 hours, may be administered. Oral tetracycline and intravenous vancomycin are effective against *C. tetani*, but the cephalosporins are not reliably active.

Local wound care, including surgical débridement, is essential. Foreign bodies must be removed, and wounds must be irrigated well and left open. Local antibiotic or TIG instillation is not of proven benefit. Excision of necrotic tissue may be required, but excision of the umbilical stump no longer is recommended in cases of neonatal tetanus.

Supportive care of patients with tetanus always involves meticulous nursing care, ventilatory support, and intense pharmacologic intervention to stabilize vital signs (Box 153.2). If possible, patients should be managed in an intensive care setting of a tertiary-care center. Transfer to such a setting should be accomplished early in the course of the disease, before the severity of spasms precludes moving affected patients; the clinical condition deteriorates during the first week of the disease.

Equipment and facilities that should be available include a quiet darkened room, suction equipment and oxygen, cardiac and respiratory monitors, a ventilator, and tracheostomy equipment. In the initial days of the illness, minimizing external

BOX 153.2 **Equipment and Facilities That Are Needed to Manage Patients with Tetanus**

1. An intensive care unit setting in a quiet darkened room
2. Suction equipment and oxygen
3. Cardiac and respiratory monitors
4. A ventilator and tracheostomy equipment

stimuli and maintaining intravenous hydration may be sufficient supportive care. Sedation and muscle relaxation should be instituted, usually with diazepam. Diazepam in a dose of 0.1 to 0.2 mg/kg given intravenously every 4 to 6 hours provides smooth, safe muscle relaxation and may be adequate for relatively mild cases. Additional sedation with phenothiazines may be used, although these drugs alone are less effective than is diazepam. If spasms are not controlled adequately, therapeutic paralysis must be induced. These patients must be treated by experienced caregivers highly skilled in ventilatory support and maintenance of cardiovascular stability.

Neuromuscular blockade can be accomplished with the curariform drugs. The agents used most often are pancuronium and vecuronium. Vecuronium is an intermediate-acting neuromuscular blocking agent; in an initial dose of 0.08 to 0.10 mg/kg intravenously, with maintenance doses of 0.01 to 0.15 mg/kg every 30 to 60 minutes as needed, it appears to have fewer adverse effects on blood pressure and heart rate, a significant benefit in patients for whom hypertension and tachycardia are major complicating factors. Doxacurium, a long-acting agent of the same class with a similar safety profile for the cardiovascular system, may offer smoother patient management and more prolonged effect with each dose. The recommended initial dose is 0.03 to 0.05 mg/kg intravenously, followed by 0.01 mg/kg in 60 to 90 minutes, as needed. Subsequent intervals between maintenance doses may be lengthened or shortened by the administration of smaller or larger doses. Patients who undergo therapeutic paralysis must be sedated to avoid the anxiety that occurs in a conscious patient.

Therapy may be required also to manage the hypertension that results from sympathetic overactivity. Beta-blocking agents appear to be the agents of choice, with propranolol used most commonly (usual dose, 0.01 to 0.10 mg/kg every 6 to 8 hours). Propranolol may be useful for the management of tachyarrhythmias. For either indication, the dosage must be titrated to achieve optimal effect. The duration of these pharmacologic manipulations is dictated by the duration of effect of tetanospasmin but ranges from 2 to 3 weeks. Careful monitoring of all vital signs and activities and their correlation with drug effect will indicate when the toxin's effects have resolved.

Maintenance of adequate nutrition and hydration is mandatory. Because of the likely duration of the disease and the undesirability of oral or nasogastric feedings, usually parenteral nutrition is required for children with tetanus. Optimal nutritional support can minimize the severe weight loss that traditionally has been considered an expected outcome, and maintenance of adequate electrolyte balance can improve management of arrhythmias. Careful attention must be paid to skin care, especially in the paralyzed patient, and excretory functions must be monitored closely for urinary retention or serious constipation.

In the absence of optimal tertiary-care facilities and personnel for modern management, minimal stimulation, muscle relaxation, sedation short of respiratory depression, and adequate hydration may be the best that can be achieved. Tracheostomy may be needed (preferably on an elective rather than on an emergency basis) to avoid fatal laryngospasm, which greatly increases the mortality rate of the disease.

An important aspect of treatment is initiation of active immunization with tetanus toxoid. Patients must be immunized to prevent further disease because the amount of toxin required to produce disease is far less than that needed to stimulate immunity.

Although tetanus still is a very serious disease, the prognosis with modern techniques of intensive care is markedly better than that predicted by earlier statistics. With appropriate intensive care, the ultimate mortality rate of tetanus in the United States has been reduced greatly. The overall case-fatality rate in the United States has declined from 91% in 1947, to 24% during 1989 to 1991, to 11% during 1995 to 1997. Age plays an important part in outcome, with only 5% mortality rate for patients younger than 50 years of age, as compared with 42% for those older than 50. No mortality was observed in the United States between 1995 and 1997 in individuals younger than 25 years of age. Survivors are left largely without sequelae of tetanus, although the sequelae of modern intensive care may occur in time.

The primary predictors of prognosis remain the rapidity of symptom onset and the rate of progression from trismus to severe spasms. Poor outcome is predicted by an interval between injury and trismus shorter than 7 days or by progression from trismus to spasms in less than 3 days.

Prevention

Tetanus is an entirely preventable disease, and the fact that fewer than 5% of cases in the United States between 1995 and 1997 occurred in children younger than age 20 years attests to the efficacy of vigorous primary immunization. (A comprehensive immunization schedule is presented in Chapter 15.) The primary series of tetanus toxoid, administered as diphtheria and tetanus toxoids and pertussis vaccine to children at 2, 4, and 6 months and a booster between 12 and 18 months later, ensures protection in childhood. Boosters of tetanus toxoid should be administered each decade throughout life, with further tetanus prophylaxis given after acute wounds occur, as advocated by the AAP CID (Table 153.1).

Patients who have documentation of full primary immunization and appropriate boosters need no tetanus prophylaxis beyond appropriate local wound care for clean minor wounds, but they should receive a toxoid booster after sustaining a dirty, tetanus-prone injury if the most recent dose was received more than 5 years previously. Patients who are not known to have completed the primary series require a tetanus toxoid booster after incurring any penetrating wound and TIG after sustaining a tetanus-prone injury. The prophylactic dose of TIG is 250 to 500 units, given intramuscularly. A human gamma-globulin

---

TABLE 153.1

TETANUS PROPHYLAXIS IN WOUND MANAGEMENT

Immunization History	Type of Wound	
	Clean, Minor	All Others
Three or more doses of tetanus toxoid	No TIG; toxoid only if >10 year since last dose	No TIG; toxoid only if >5 year since last dose
Fewer than three doses or uncertain history	No TIG; toxoid, 0.5 mL	TIG*; 500 units; toxoid, 0.5 mL

*Equine tetanus antitoxin should be used when TIG is not available. TIG, tetanus immune globulin.
Adapted from the Report of the Committee on Infectious Diseases, 20th ed. Evanston, IL: American Academy of Pediatrics, 1997.

product, TIG does not carry the risk of serum sickness seen with equine antitoxin, and performing skin testing for hypersensitivity is unnecessary. U.S. statistics reveal that only 13% of patients who subsequently developed tetanus received appropriate tetanus toxoid boosters at the time of injury and that TIG was not given to any of the patients who should have received it. A continuing effort to educate the public about the need for tetanus immunoprophylaxis after childhood is necessary to prevent this disease. Prevention is much less costly than is treatment.

CLOSTRIDIUM BOTULINUM

Etiology and Epidemiology

Botulism represents acute neurologic disease caused by another potent clostridial toxin, elaborated by *C. botulinum*. Botulinal toxin is the most potent poison known, causing death in mice that receive as little as 10 pg. Disease is caused in humans by less than 100 ng. Seven antigenically distinct botulinal toxins are distinguished (i.e., types A through G) and are produced by four groups of *C. botulinum*, each distinguished by its characteristic biochemical activities. The production of each toxin appears to depend on the presence of a plasmid that encodes the toxin gene. Elimination of the plasmid renders the bacteria nontoxigenic. The molecular weights of the toxins, which now are thought to be cellular proteins released during lysis, vary within the range of 130 to 150 kd. The active moiety of the protein may be as small as 10 kd. The toxin is destroyed by heat and pressure (e.g., 100°C for 10 minutes or 80°C for 30 minutes), but it is resistant to chemical deactivation. The bacterial spores highly resist heat, but they may be killed by autoclaving at 120°C for 20 minutes.

Botulinal toxin acts at the neuromuscular junction, where it inhibits the release of acetylcholine, producing a flaccid paralysis. It has no effect on the CNS or on mentation, although the earliest effect is seen on the cranial nerves. Progression of paralysis occurs in a characteristic descending fashion, ultimately affecting the entire peripheral nervous system. Respiratory failure is the major cause of death as the paralytic effect of the toxin reaches the muscles of respiration.

Botulinum spores are common in soil, dust, lakes, and other environmental matter and can contaminate fruits, vegetables, meats, and fish. Honey has become recognized as a potential source of *C. botulinum* spores in one form of botulism.

In view of the widespread occurrence of *C. botulinum* spores and their remarkable resistance to destruction, the epidemiology of the disease correlates most closely with circumstances in which contaminated foods are heated inadequately and the preformed toxin is ingested. Often, the contaminated food correlates with geographic location and the type of botulinal toxin involved. Most cases of botulism in humans are caused by types A, B, and E; more than one-half of foodborne cases in the United States are type A, and 25% are type B. Type A causes two-thirds of cases in the western half of the United States, and type B exhibits similar prevalence east of the Mississippi. Usually, cases of type E botulism involve fish from the Pacific Northwest and Alaska; worldwide, most type E disease occurs in Japan, Scandinavia, and the former Soviet Union, presumably because of dietary habits.

Most outbreaks of botulism in the United States are associated with food products (e.g., home-canned vegetables) that are not heated adequately before consumption and in which spores generate and form toxins. Other food products that have been incriminated include smoked meats, raw and fermented fish products, and potato salad and commercial frozen pot pies prepared improperly at home.

Ingestion of *C. botulinum* spores may lead to generation of toxin in the intestine of susceptible hosts and to botulism. This mechanism is operative in infantile botulism, which has been linked to the addition of honey (a natural, unpasteurized product) to infant formula. This form of botulism, which represents two-thirds of reported cases in the United States, first was recognized and still predominates in the western United States among families favoring "natural" food products, although now it is recognized throughout the country. A similar mechanism of acquisition of botulinal toxin has been implicated in rare cases in older children and adults. Prolonged or recurrent paralysis in some patients with typical foodborne botulism may be caused by intestinal infection with *C. botulinum* and resultant continued elaboration and absorption of toxin. Rarely, contamination of wounds with *C. botulinum* results in parenteral absorption of botulinal toxin and in "wound botulism."

Pathophysiology

Botulism is caused by the binding of botulinal toxin to the neuromuscular junction. Whether from absorption of toxin from the gastrointestinal tract or from locally infected wounds, the toxin enters the lymphatics and bloodstream and circulates and gains access to neuromuscular junctions. The toxin does not cross the blood brain barrier, but it is bound to the cytoplasmic membrane of peripheral cholinergic nerve endings, where it inhibits the exocytosis of acetylcholine, resulting in flaccid paralysis. The toxin is bound irreversibly, like tetanus toxin, and recovery occurs only with regeneration of nerve endings. Unbound toxin may be neutralized with antitoxin early in the course of the disease, indicating the importance of early establishment of the diagnosis and institution of therapy.

The incubation period, duration, and severity of botulism are related directly to the quantity of toxin absorbed and bound to nerve endings. Speed of recovery depends entirely on the extent of involvement of nerve endings, which must be regenerated to replace those inactivated by botulinal toxin.

Clinical Manifestations

The clinical manifestations of botulism are related in some measure to age, with considerably less specific symptoms in infants than in older patients. At 18 to 48 hours after ingestion of tainted food, patients with botulism typically present with cranial nerve dysfunction manifested by diplopia, dysphagia, and difficulty speaking. Patients remain lucid, although anxiety and agitation may develop. Generally, fever is absent unless superinfection occurs. Additional signs may include pupillary dilation, vertigo, tinnitus, and dry mouth and mucous membranes. The descending progression of paralysis in botulism occurs at various rates, spreading and involving muscles of respiration and most voluntary musculature. The major manifestation is respiratory embarrassment, which may appear gradually or suddenly. If progression is slow, repeated measurements of tidal volume and other pulmonary function tests may be useful to predict the need for ventilatory support.

Involvement of the gastrointestinal tract varies and is related somewhat to the toxin serotype. Types A and B, the most common causes of botulism in the United States, cause abdominal complaints (e.g., abdominal pain, bloating, cramps, diarrhea) in approximately one-third of patients. These complaints are replaced quickly by constipation or obstipation. Type E produces more significant gastrointestinal complaints than do the other types. Gastrointestinal complaints do not accompany wound botulism. The incubation period spans 4 to 14 days, and the progression of paralysis otherwise is similar to that in foodborne disease.

Botulism in infants may present suddenly with respiratory failure, and infant botulism has been implicated in some cases of apparent sudden infant death syndrome. More commonly, weakness and flaccidity are insidious, with slow progression from poor feeding and constipation to weakness, hypotonia, and respiratory insufficiency. Most parents describe a weak cry and diminished movement. Ptosis, loss of the gag reflex, and poor head control are common findings.

The duration of flaccidity and respiratory embarrassment in all forms of botulism may be fairly prolonged. The typical duration of symptoms exceeds 1 month, and full recovery from weakness and fatigability may require as long as 1 year. Usually, recovery is complete. Although no additional specific complications of botulism intoxication are listed, the potential complications of prolonged paralysis, assisted ventilation, and nutritional support are significant. Patients who progress to significant respiratory compromise should be treated in tertiary-care centers where experienced ventilatory support teams are available. The susceptibility to hospital-acquired infections of skin, respiratory tree, urinary tract, and indwelling intravascular devices defines the additional clinical signs and symptoms that may be present in these patients.

Diagnosis and Differential Diagnosis

The clinical constellation of acute onset of symmetric descending flaccid paralysis, initially involving cranial nerves but sparing mentation and unassociated with fever, should be considered botulism, regardless of whether a history of consuming tainted food can be obtained. The entities confused most frequently with botulism are Guillain-Barré syndrome, myasthenia gravis, cerebrovascular accidents, other paralytic food poisonings, and some drug toxicities. Infectious encephalomyelitis may be confused with botulism in older children. Infant botulism is mistaken easily for septicemia, hypoglycemia, encephalitis, Werdnig-Hoffmann disease, or congenital myopathies.

Infectious conditions of the CNS can be differentiated from botulism by inflammatory changes in the CSF. Neither CSF pleocytosis nor chemical changes are characteristic of botulism. Similarly, Guillain-Barré syndrome is differentiated by its characteristic elevated CSF protein (i.e., albuminocytologic dissociation). The diagnosis of myasthenia gravis rests on a positive response to edrophonium (i.e., Tensilon test), and radiographic or nuclear imaging of the CNS usually demonstrates cerebrovascular accidents. Differentiating other forms of paralytic food poisonings (e.g., ciguatera) may be difficult without a positive ingestion history, but such forms probably are extraordinarily rare in the United States. Toxicity caused by aminoglycosides, phenothiazines, or atropine can be determined by affected patients' histories.

Electromyography may reveal suggestive changes in the form of diminished amplitude of muscle action potentials or brief, small, abundant motor-unit action potentials. However, absence of these changes does not rule out botulism. Electrophysiologic studies may help in identifying other possible diagnoses, such as primary myopathy. Routine hematologic and biochemical testing does not produce diagnostically useful findings, although changes suggesting acute infection may direct clinicians' attention toward some other condition.

Diagnosis is confirmed by demonstration of botulinus toxin or *C. botulinum* in suspected food, vomitus, and, occasionally, serum. The only reliable confirmatory test is the mouse inoculation toxin neutralization assay. Suggestive confirmatory evidence may be derived from the recovery of *C. botulinum* from vomitus, feces, intestinal contents, and, rarely, viscera.

Blood and stool samples should be obtained and refrigerated for transport to a laboratory (usually state health departments) equipped to determine botulinal toxin. These specimens must be handled with utmost care because exposure of percutaneous or mucous membranes to minute quantities of the toxin may cause fatal disease. Stools should be cultured for *C. botulinum* because this organism is not normal flora, and its identification in stool confirms the clinical diagnosis.

Management and Prognosis

Management involves providing optimal supportive care and administering specific therapy directed at neutralizing unbound toxin and eradicating any infection with *C. botulinum*. Speed is essential in establishing the diagnosis with reasonable certainty so that the circulating toxin can be neutralized before it binds to nerve endings. Because the only available licensed antitoxin is of equine origin and, therefore, carries a significant risk of serum sickness, every effort, including performing electromyography, Gram stain, culture of any infected wounds, and an exhaustive history of food intake in the previous 7 to 10 days, should be made to substantiate the diagnosis.

Suspected cases of botulism must be reported to local and state health authorities and to the Centers for Disease Control and Prevention (CDC) (telephone: 404-639-2206 [day]; 404-639-2888 [nights]), from which equine trivalent antitoxin for types A, B, and E is available. Patients with botulism should be treated with appropriate health care precautions, probably including blood and enteric isolation.

Human-derived immune globulin preparation currently is being investigated and has been approved by the FDA only as an investigational new drug treatment for use with infant botulism. It is available from the California Department of Health Services (telephone: 510-540-2646).

Oral or parenteral antimicrobial agents such as penicillin have limited value but may destroy some viable *C. botulinum* organisms. No data address the safety or efficacy of oral vancomycin for the eradication of enteric *C. botulinum*, despite its demonstrated efficacy in *C. difficile* enteric infections. Systemic antibiotic therapy is warranted only if superinfection occurs. Because aminoglycosides can affect the neuromuscular junction and potentiate the effect of botulinal toxin, they should be avoided.

Supportive care for patients with botulism involves the availability of equipment and experienced personnel for the meticulous and prolonged maximal ventilatory support of totally paralyzed patients. Because the ultimate extent of paralysis cannot be predicted early in such patients' courses, they should be transferred to tertiary intensive care facilities when the diagnosis is entertained. Monitoring with pulmonary function studies is a sensitive means of assessing the progression of paralysis and of determining the need for providing ventilatory support. Affected patients also need nutritional support, usually with total parenteral nutrition because of the prevalence of adynamic ileus. Every effort should be made to ensure optimal caloric intake because paralysis may be quite prolonged. Careful attention to skin care and to bowel and bladder function must be maintained to minimize complications.

The prognosis of botulism is related to the dose of toxin acquired and the duration and severity of paralysis. A patient's age is relevant. The overall mortality rate is 30% to 35%, but, for patients younger than 20 years of age, the mortality rate is 10%. The mortality rate for infant botulism is less than 5%. A correlation may be seen with the antigenic type; type B appears to have a lower mortality than that of type A. Most deaths from botulism occur in hospitals and can be attributed to failure to recognize the need for ventilatory support, failure of ventilatory equipment, and development of nosocomial pulmonary or

---

| BOX 153.3 | Complications Associated with Infant Botulism |

Secondary infections
  Acute otitis media
  Pneumonia
  Urinary tract infections
  Sepsis
  Clostridium difficile colitis
Muscular dysfunction
Seizures due to hypoxia or hyponatremia
Respiratory distress syndrome
Autonomic instability
Excessive production of antidiuretic hormone

---

systemic infections. The associated complications are listed in Box 153.3. Early recognition of the disease, provision of adequate supportive care, and meticulous attention to life-support systems markedly improve the outcome of botulism. Ordinarily, survivors recover without neurologic or neuromuscular sequelae, although full recovery may require many months. Weakness and easy fatigability are prolonged.

Prevention

Although botulinal toxoid is immunogenic and presumably protective, the rarity of this disease renders administration of active immunization impractical. The best preventive measure is to ensure adequate care of food products and infant feedings. After a case has been recognized, health authorities must be notified so that other potential cases can be identified and treated expediently.

Because the commercial food industry is attentive to appropriate temperatures and aseptic conditions, few cases of botulism are traced to such sources. In the home preparation of food, all hot foods should be brought to the appropriate temperature before consumption, with particular attention given to canning and preserving foods. The elimination of viable *C. botulinum* spores is ensured by the use of sterile containers and pressure cookers in which temperatures of 120°C can be reached and maintained for 30 minutes. Boiling home-preserved foods for 10 minutes before consuming them inactivates the toxin. Neither microwaves nor the temperatures commonly achieved in microwave ovens are adequate to kill *C. botulinum* spores or to inactivate the toxin. Home-preserved foods should be cooked in traditional equipment.

Prevention of infant botulism involves eliminating honey and other uncooked or inadequately preserved foods from the diets of infants younger than 12 months of age. *C. botulinum* spores have been recovered from corn syrup, although no cases have implicated this source. Breast-feeding apparently diminishes the severity of infant botulism, although cases have occurred in breast-fed infants who received honey in supplemental feedings. Adhering to standard recommendations for infant feeding practices can eliminate this risk.

CLOSTRIDIUM PERFRINGENS

C. perfringens is a ubiquitous bacterium associated with several exotoxin-mediated clinical diseases. Twelve recognized toxins are listed (i.e., alpha through nu), and the species is divided into types A through E on the basis of the spectrum of toxins produced. Disease syndromes caused by *C. perfringens* include food poisoning, necrotizing enteritis, and gas gangrene.

Clostridial Food Poisoning

Often, acute self-limiting gastroenteritis caused by contaminated food products is associated with *C. perfringens* and its toxins. In some years, *C. perfringens* has been documented as the third most common etiologic agent in outbreaks of foodborne disease (after *Salmonella* and *Staphylococcus aureus*). This variety of food poisoning occurs as a result of ingesting vegetative *C. perfringens* forms that have developed in foods (e.g., meats and gravies) that have been allowed to reach and stand at temperatures between 30°C and 50°C.

Primary contamination of meat with *C. perfringens* spores occurs commonly, and temperatures of cooked meat must exceed 120°C to ensure that spores are killed. At lower temperatures, spores may be converted to vegetative forms during cooling of the food, risking growth of *C. perfringens* in the gastrointestinal tract. The toxins produced by these organisms are responsible for subsequent development of symptoms.

Pathophysiology

Although the symptoms of *C. perfringens* food poisoning are attributable largely to the action of enterotoxins, usually they are formed in the gastrointestinal tract after ingestion of the entire organism. Ingestion of preformed toxin results in diarrhea only if gastric acidity has been neutralized. The enterotoxin formed *in vivo* is a 35-kd peptide that is heat- and acid-labile and is inactivated by some proteolytic enzymes. In animals, the toxin inhibits glucose absorption and secretion of water, sodium, and chloride, and it strips the epithelium of villous tips. The *in vitro* cytotoxic effect is similar to that of *Shigella* toxin, but it differs from that of cholera or *Escherichia coli* enterotoxins. Adenyl cyclase appears not to be involved in the mediation of *C. perfringens* toxin activity. The resultant gastroenteritis demonstrates components of secretory and inflammatory diarrhea.

Clinical Manifestations

C. perfringens food poisoning is an acute, self-limiting diarrheal illness with an onset 8 to 24 hours after ingestion of contaminated food. Commonly, crampy abdominal pain accompanies watery diarrhea, which does not contain blood or mucus. Fever, nausea, and vomiting rarely occur. The duration of disease commonly is less than 24 hours, and usually medical intervention is not warranted or sought, except in the case of outbreaks. Occasionally, fluid loss sufficient to require intravenous rehydration may occur, particularly in young infants.

Differential Diagnosis

Differentiating this acute diarrheal disease from the numerous other viral, bacterial, and toxic causes of diarrhea may be difficult on clinical grounds unless an outbreak has occurred. The absence of fever, nausea, vomiting, or blood or mucus in stools renders *Salmonella*, *Shigella*, *Campylobacter*, *Yersinia*, or rotavirus an unlikely cause. Usually, the duration of infection caused by these agents is more prolonged than that of *C. perfringens* food poisoning. Diagnosis can be substantiated reliably only by culture of large quantities of *C. perfringens* from the suspected food and the patient's fecal samples. Immunologic testing for enterotoxin may be used to detect contaminated food, but it is not useful in establishing a clinical diagnosis.

Management and Prognosis

By virtue of the self-limiting nature of this disease, medical intervention rarely is warranted. Generally, oral rehydration with hypotonic fluids suffices, although in unusual circumstances (particularly in infants), intravenous hydration may be required. Symptomatic antidiarrheal therapy is used infrequently because of the short duration of symptoms, but it probably is not contraindicated and may be useful in large outbreaks. Antibiotics serve no useful purpose in this disease and should not be used; no antitoxin is available.

Prevention

As is the case in most foodborne diseases, the best means of prevention is appropriate handling of cooked foods, especially meats. Meats should reach at least 120°C during cooking and, if not consumed while hot, should be stored at less than 5°C. Meat allowed to stand at room temperature is prime material for contamination with vegetative forms of *C. perfringens*. Preformed toxin is destroyed with reheating to serving temperature, although spores are not affected by this temperature. Inhomogeneous heating, as may occur in microwave ovens, can leave some toxins undestroyed and should be avoided.

Necrotizing Enteritis

Necrotizing enteritis caused by *C. perfringens* (i.e., pig-bel) is a rare, frequently fatal condition seen almost exclusively in highland natives of New Guinea. The disease is caused by *C. perfringens* type C; this organism elaborates the potent beta-toxin, which is responsible for extensive cytotoxicity and tissue necrosis. The beta-toxin is highly susceptible to proteolysis, and the disease is seen in hosts who lack intestinal proteolytic enzymes, presumably because of a largely vegetarian diet. Pig-bel is seen after ritual feasting on roast pig.

Although the equivalent of pig-bel has not been described in the developed world, the pathology and pathophysiology of the disease have led to speculation about the role of *C. perfringens* in other forms of necrotizing enteritis. In pig-bel, the beta-toxin causes extensive destruction and gangrene of the jejunum and ileum. Intramural gas (i.e., pneumatosis cystoides intestinalis) is common, an observation that long has interested pediatricians and neonatologists. The clinical manifestations of pig-bel include anorexia, severe abdominal pain, hematochezia, prostration, shock, and death. Diagnosis is clear-cut and specific in the appropriate epidemiologic setting. Proof that the same pathophysiology is operative in developed societies has not been obtained.

The management of pig-bel is largely supportive; no antitoxin or antibiotics are available or useful. Treatment of necrotizing enteritis of any type in the developed world requires supportive care, management of hypovolemia, and probably antimicrobial therapy directed at potential secondary invading organisms from the gastrointestinal tract. The prognosis is relatively poor; New Guinea natives rarely recover from pig-bel. Protective antibodies for the prevention of pig-bel can be induced by immunization with a beta-toxoid. The role of this observation in the larger context of *C. perfringens* foodborne diseases is unclear.

Gas Gangrene

Skin and soft tissue infections are caused infrequently by clostridial organisms; when this manifestation occurs, usually it takes place in the context of a polymicrobial infection involving other anaerobes, aerobes, and frequently both. Clostridial myonecrosis (i.e., gas gangrene) is a rare but extraordinarily serious condition caused largely by *C. perfringens*. More than 90% of cases of gas gangrene are caused by this species, although *C. novyi*, *C. septicum*, *C. histolyticum*, *C. sordellii*, and *C. fallax* rarely have been associated with the disease.

Gas gangrene affects muscle tissue that has been compromised by surgery, trauma, or vascular insufficiency and is contaminated with *C. perfringens* spores, usually from such foreign material as clothing, dirt, or hardware. The ubiquitous nature of *C. perfringens* spores in dirt, soil, and clothing and on skin, especially of the lower trunk, ensures availability of these organisms for inoculation into tissues with appropriate wounds. The metabolic requirements of *C. perfringens* for growth are the major factors in the establishment of clostridial myonecrosis. *C. perfringens* will not replicate in a redox potential (Eh) greater than −80 mV; the Eh of healthy muscle is +120 to +160 mV. With vascular embarrassment or tissue death caused by trauma, the Eh may fall to −150 to −250 mV and thus allow growth of clostridia. Prior bacterial infection lowers tissue pH and promotes clostridial growth because the tolerable Eh for *C. perfringens* at low pH (less than 7.0) is significantly higher than at physiologic pH. The occurrence of clostridial myonecrosis depends much more on appropriate physiologic conditions for growth than on the likely presence of *C. perfringens*. Approximately 70% of cases occur after trauma, 20% to 30% occur after controlled surgical procedures, and the remainder arise spontaneously in compromised hosts or after intramuscular injections. Wounds usually producing gas gangrene are those involving missiles, severe compound fractures, and crush injuries. Uterine myonecrosis can occur after septic abortion and may be encountered in pediatric and adolescent practices.

After infection with *C. perfringens* is established in the muscle, the severe, rapidly progressive myonecrosis results from the toxins elaborated by the organism, principally the alpha-toxin. The alpha-toxin is a lecithinase that rapidly lyses cell membranes and causes hemolysis, myofibrillar injury, and vascular permeability. The absence of detectable circulating alpha-toxin suggests that this toxin is not responsible for the overwhelming systemic toxicity, vascular collapse, shock, and changes in mental status that characterize gas gangrene. These symptoms appear to be caused by undefined toxins or by products released from the necrotic muscle. Although toxins elaborated by the other infrequent causative agents of gas gangrene are not all lecithinases, the pathophysiology of the disease appears similar.

Pathophysiology

After inoculation of *C. perfringens* into an appropriate wound and generation of replicative organisms from the spores, the toxins that are produced rapidly lyse myofibers and increase vascular permeability, and marked edema is an early concomitant of the ongoing tissue destruction. Gas produced within the disrupted myofibers is responsible for the more familiar name of the syndrome. Vascular congestion in the area of infection does not occur, and no inflammatory exudate is observed, but a thin, watery, foul-smelling interstitial fluid is produced. Pathologic examination of affected tissues reveals myofiber destruction, marked edema, gas formation, and extensive invasion with the characteristic large, blunt-ended, gram-positive bacilli of *C. perfringens*. No spores are present when the organism grows in tissue.

Massive tissue necrosis occurs at the site of local gas gangrene, but death from the disease usually is caused by resultant systemic symptoms. Tachycardia, hypotension, vascular collapse, and shock occur late in the course of the disease; massive hemolysis may occur, and renal failure may result from shock or hemoglobinuria. The latter symptoms have not been associated clearly with specific clostridial toxins, and only removal of necrotic muscle has been effective in ameliorating the symptoms. C. *perfringens* enterotoxin pathogenicity may be partially mediated by release of interleukins-1 and -6, tumor necrosis factor alpha, and interferon-gamma from human peripheral cells.

Clinical Manifestations

The clinical picture of gas gangrene is so characteristic that the diagnosis can be established with fair certainty on clinical grounds. The major problem is that the rarity of the disease may lower clinical suspicion and may hamper decisive action, thereby allowing massive destruction and systemic disease to occur. Characteristically, the disease begins 6 hours to 5 days after an injury has occurred. The initial symptom is pain in the affected area and an accompanying "heaviness" of the limb. The overlying skin appears normal at the onset but quickly becomes cool, pale, and waxy. Pain remains the most prominent symptom as the pallor and edema progress; serous fluid begins to exude from wounds and into spontaneously appearing blisters filled with clostridia. Frank necrosis of the skin is preceded by appearance of blotches of brown discoloration, both of which spread within hours to involve ever-larger areas of skin. Usually, underlying crepitus is obscured by the severe edema. Generally, uterine myonecrosis presents as an intraabdominal crisis, the diagnosis of which rests on the history of recent abortion.

Tachycardia, widespread myalgia, anxiety, and diaphoresis despite low-grade fever appear early and progress rapidly to hypotension, poor perfusion, and changes in mental status. Without administration of definitive therapy, the disease progresses inexorably to high fever (often with rigors), shock, renal failure, coma, and death. Clostridial septicemia may be a terminal event.

Surgical excision of affected tissues is the definitive therapy for gas gangrene and must be performed early to minimize the extent of muscle necrosis. At operation, the muscle initially appears pale and watery, with greatly diminished contraction after transection. Hours later, the tissue is dull red, lacks contractility, and does not bleed from cut surfaces. Necrosis of overlying skin and soft tissues occurs late and generally is an indication for amputation or, in areas for which amputation is not possible (e.g., the abdominal wall), wide excision.

Differential Diagnosis

The major conditions from which gas gangrene must be differentiated are other forms of severe, progressive necrotizing cellulitis (e.g., progressive synergistic gangrene, necrotizing fasciitis). The laboratory evaluation most likely to differentiate these entities is a Gram stain of tissue fluid revealing the sheets of gram-positive bacilli (without associated leukocytes) characteristic of gas gangrene. Progressive synergistic gangrene is a polymicrobial infection, usually involving gram-positive and gram-negative anaerobes, aerobic streptococci, and staphylococci, all of which are seen on Gram-stained smears of tissue aspirates. The exudate recovered from necrotizing fasciitis reveals the etiologic agents of *S. aureus* and *Streptococcus pyogenes*. Necrotizing fasciitis results in dissolution of the fascia; the overlying skin no longer is anchored and can be elevated easily. Both of these conditions may be associated with systemic toxicity, shock, and death, but the changes in mental status characteristic of gas gangrene are not seen. At operation, the typical picture of myonecrosis is absent. Additional laboratory evaluation is not particularly useful for confirming the diagnosis of gas gangrene or for eliminating the alternatives. Endometritis and septic shock caused by septic abortion may be clinically indistinguishable, although the characteristic distribution of gas in the myometrium may be apparent radiographically.

Management and Prognosis

The cornerstone of management is early and complete surgical débridement of the affected muscle. Delay in establishing the diagnosis or performing surgery allows progression and spread of the myonecrosis, leading to extensive loss of tissue and worsening systemic toxicity. The extent of débridement depends on the viability of muscle, which is determined at operation. Commonly, several surgical procedures must be performed before all nonviable tissue is removed because surgeons attempt to save as much tissue as possible, and subsequent operations are needed to remove tissue that proves to be nonviable. Aggressive surgical management must be encouraged early in the disease if a successful outcome is to be achieved.

Specific antimicrobial therapy directed at *Clostridium* should be administered to minimize the growth of the bacterium, recognizing that the anoxic and acidic environment of dead muscle is not conducive to antimicrobial efficacy. The drug of choice is penicillin G in a dose of 200,000 to 400,000 U/kg/day intravenously, divided for administration every 4 hours. Clindamycin has an advantage over penicillin because it suppresses synthesis of bacterial toxin and can be given with penicillin. Other antimicrobials include chloramphenicol, metronidazole, carbapenems, ampicillin, cephalosporins, and vancomycin. Treatment should be continued until bacteremia has cleared and symptoms have resolved.

Provision of supportive care is essential to the management of gas gangrene, and patients should be treated in centers capable of supporting vital signs, cardiovascular output, and renal function. Although no controlled data are available and pediatric studies are lacking, hyperbaric oxygen appears to be useful in treating gas gangrene in centers capable of managing its complications. The major advantage may be in minimizing tissue loss and in diminishing the extent of débridement required. Complications, including oxygen toxicity, changes in mental status, and perforation of tympanic membranes, are significant, and the prognosis for survival may not be improved with the aggressive surgical approach. The use of specific antitoxin has been advocated, but substantive supportive data are not available. The polyvalent antitoxin is of equine origin (carrying the risk of serum sickness) and has not been shown to improve outcome.

The prognosis for survival from gas gangrene depends on the location and extent of disease and speed with which appropriate débridement is performed. Mortality rates range from 5% with early establishment of diagnosis and aggressive débridement to virtually certain death if surgical treatment is delayed (e.g., in a wartime situation). With competent treatment, the overall survival rate appears to be 75% to 90%.

Prevention

The key to preventing clostridial myonecrosis is adequate cleaning and débridement of contaminated wounds. Antimicrobial treatment is considered therapeutic rather than prophylactic in this setting and should be administered to patients with heavily contaminated wounds, and care should be taken to avoid the anaerobic environments created by closing the wounds. Giving meticulous attention to the principles of surgical wound management prevents most cases of surgical wound gas gangrene.

CLOSTRIDIUM DIFFICILE

Antibiotic-associated colitis is a potentially serious diarrheal illness that initially was attributed to the direct toxic effects of some antibiotics, but it has been shown conclusively to be caused by toxigenic C. *difficile*. C. *difficile* produces two toxins—A and B—both of which cause disease. A toxin C has been described, but its role in production of disease is not yet clear. The prevalence of *C. difficile* in the gastrointestinal flora seems to vary widely depending on the age of the patient, underlying disease, and history of hospitalization or antibiotic usage. Carriage rates in asymptomatic neonates and infants may reach 50%, but the organism exists in fewer than 2% of older children and adults without diarrheal disease. Patients with cystic fibrosis demonstrate higher-than-average rates of asymptomatic carriage. Positive assays for *C. difficile* toxin without clinical symptoms suggest that factors providing protection against *C. difficile* colitis may be operative in infants and patients with cystic fibrosis. Infection frequently is acquired nosocomially, and hospitalized individuals constitute an important reservoir. Disease occurs epidemically and endemically in hospitals. Risk factors include increasing age, exposure to antibiotics or chemotherapy, colonization or acquisition of toxin-producing strains of *C. difficile,* and lack of circulating antibody to *C. difficile* toxin A.

Symptomatic *C. difficile* colitis is an unusual finding in pediatric patients. Whatever host factors play a role in protecting newborns and infants probably influence the incidence of symptomatic infection throughout childhood. Sporadic, community-acquired diarrhea unrelated to antibiotics rarely is associated with *C. difficile* cytotoxin. The incidence and pattern of *C. difficile* diarrhea in children younger than 2 years of age in day care is similar to that of *Giardia lamblia* and *Cryptosporidium.*

Virtually all antibiotics with antibacterial properties (except vancomycin) have been associated with the development of *C. difficile* colitis. The association of this disease with only clindamycin has been disproved. The drugs implicated most commonly are ampicillin, the cephalosporins, and clindamycin. Dose, route of administration, and duration of treatment are not related to the development of colitis.

Pathophysiology

C. difficile colitis is caused by the toxins produced by intestinal infection with *C. difficile*. Symptoms may occur during administration of an antibiotic or as long as 6 weeks after its discontinuation. Overgrowth with *C. difficile* is presumed to occur after suppression of the normal enteric flora with antibiotics and, with the production of toxin, colitis ensues. The predominant effect appears on the colon, with erythema and edema visible on sigmoidoscopy. The characteristic lesion (lending the condition one of its names) is that of pseudomembranous plaques that appear as gray-white exudates in a nodular configuration. The characteristic plaques are loosely adherent and are composed of fibrin, inflammatory cells, bacteria, mucus, and sloughed epithelial cells. If plaques are not visible to the naked eye, pathologic examination of biopsy material is diagnostic. Increased toxigenic strains of *C. difficile* have been recently noted in the U.S.

Clinical Manifestations

Some degree of watery diarrhea, infrequently with blood or mucus, develops in most patients. The extent of other abdominal complaints or systemic symptoms varies from mild to severe. The disease may be fatal. Abdominal pain, cramps, and lower quadrant tenderness are common symptoms, as are fever and leukocytosis. Severe dehydration and vascular collapse are rare occurrences at any age and are virtually unseen in children, but they should be considered. Generally, in individuals with mild disease not requiring specific therapy, the duration of symptoms ranges from 7 to 10 days after discontinuation of the instigating antibiotic. More prolonged symptoms or significant toxicity may indicate specific antimicrobial intervention. Addi-

tional complications include ileus, toxic megacolon, intestinal perforation, and arthritis.

Diagnosis and Differential Diagnosis

C. difficile pseudomembranous enterocolitis must be differentiated from all the other infectious causes of diarrheal disease, especially hospital-acquired infections. *Salmonella, Shigella, Campylobacter, Yersinia,* and rotavirus can be differentiated by culture or antigen assay of stool. A history of antibiotic therapy in the 4 to 6 weeks before onset, in conjunction with the detection of *C. difficile* toxin in fecal samples, strongly supports the diagnosis of *C. difficile* colitis. Detection of the toxin is relatively simple by assay of stools for *C. difficile* toxin— usually an enzyme immunoassay that will detect toxin A and B. Sigmoidoscopic examination revealing characteristic pseudomembranous plaques confirms the diagnosis. In extremely ill patients, necrotizing enterocolitis and toxic megacolon should raise the question of Hirschsprung disease, and the abdominal pain and tenderness of *C. difficile* colitis occasionally may mimic peritonitis. The potential complications are presented in Box 153.4.

Management and Prognosis

Supportive therapy, especially rehydration only, is generally adequate for patients with mild diarrhea and no systemic complications. Overall, the prognosis is excellent, with most patients recovering after discontinuation of the instigating antibiotic, with replacement of fluid and electrolytes as needed. Those with severe symptoms or persistent diarrhea require aggressive therapy. Vancomycin is effective but is expensive, tastes bad, and is associated with up to 20% relapse rate. Vancomycin, which is not absorbed from the gastrointestinal tract, is administered in doses of 10 to 40 mg/kg/day in four divided doses for 7 to 14 days; the lower dose is adequate in most patients.

Cholestyramine, an anion exchange resin that binds both *C. difficile* toxins, is an alternative to vancomycin. It is more likely to result in primary treatment failure than is vancomycin but is less likely to be followed by relapse. Metronidazole and bacitracin also can be used. Metronidazole orally has similar efficacy to vancomycin orally in mild and moderate cases, is less expensive, and does not select enterococcal resistance to vancomycin. Disadvantages of metronidazole are occasional resistance of *C. difficile*, rare induction of colitis, lack of approval by the Food and Drug Administration (FDA) for this

---

BOX 153.4	**Complications of *Clostridium difficile* Colitis in Children**

Dehydration
Electrolyte imbalance
Hypotension
Hypoalbuminemia with anasarca
Acquired malnutrition
Hypogammaglobulinemia
Lymphopenia
Ascites
Pleural effusions
Toxic megacolon
Transverse volvulus
Colon perforation
Secondary systemic infection (i.e., bacteremia)

indication in children, absence of convenient preparations for children, and its complete absorption at the upper gastrointestinal tract so that bactericidal levels are achieved erratically in the lower gastrointestinal tract. Antimotility agents, including loperamide, diphenoxylate hydrochloride with atropine, and opioids, should be avoided because they can adversely affect the ability to clear the toxins.

Fever, systemic manifestations, and severe diarrhea generally improve within 1 to 2 days of therapy, but diarrhea may last for 4 to 5 days. Relapses may be caused by reacquisition or persistence of spores in the colon. Most patients with a relapse respond to the retreatment, but they may experience multiple recurrences.

Options for management of multiple relapses include vancomycin or metronidazole plus the use of probiotics (with *Saccharomyces*, *Lactobacillus*, and *Bifidobacterium*) or Fleischmann's baker's yeast or followed by cholestyramine with or without lactobacilli; intravenous immunoglobulin; solution of fresh stool from healthy donor; and broth culture bacteria and donor stool.

Surgical intervention may be required in severe cases unresponsive to medical therapy or to manage complications such as toxic megacolon or colonic perforation. In fulminate colitis, careful vigilance is necessary to detect early signs of peritonitis and abdominal cellulitis that can indicate underlying intestinal perforation.

Prevention

C. difficile colitis is an endogenous infection induced to produce symptoms by antibiotic therapy. Few means exist to predict those in whom it may occur, and no active or passive immunity has been shown to be protective. Epidemiologic studies of *C. difficile* in hospitals have demonstrated that it is spread within health care institutions and that outbreaks can occur with relative ease. The organism is transmitted by hands of personnel caring for symptomatic or colonized patients and by fomites. Because patients in hospitals may be at significant risk because of prior antibiotic treatment and underlying disease, every effort should be made to prevent spread of *C. difficile* within the hospital setting. Patients who are known to be excreting *C. difficile* should be maintained in enteric isolation. Spores of *C. difficile* can survive on counter tops and other surfaces for weeks to months. Commonly used disinfectants are ineffective against spores of *C. difficile*. Sodium hypochlorite (500 ppm or greater of available chlorine) and 2% acid or alkaline glutaraldehyde are effective sporicidal agents.

NONCLOSTRIDIAL ANAEROBIC INFECTIONS

When sought, anaerobes have been found to cause 5% to 10% of all clinically significant bacteremic episodes in infants and children. Infections that are often caused by anaerobes include peritonitis, aspiration pneumonia, dental and chronic head and neck infections and their complications, abscesses, intraabdominal and pelvic infections, human and animal bite infections, and a variety of soft tissue infections. Although anaerobic infections in children occur less frequently than in adults, they should be considered in high-risk situations or cases of unexplained clinical sepsis.

Epidemiology and Pathophysiology

Usually, infection by nonclostridial anaerobic organisms involves endogenous flora. The species encountered most com-

TABLE 153.2

ANAEROBIC SPECIES COMMONLY ENCOUNTERED IN CLINICAL INFECTIONS

Site of Infection	Gram-Positive Species	Gram-Negative Species
Upper half of body	*Peptostreptococcus* *Eubacterium*	*Prevotella* *Porphyromonas* *Fusobacterium*
Lower half of body	*Clostridium* *Peptostreptococcus*	*Bacteroides fragilis* *Fusobacterium* *Veillonella*

monly (and their most likely locations) are listed in Table 153.2. Usually, anaerobic infection develops after some alteration in the physical barrier to endogenous microbes and further compromise in the viability of infected tissues have occurred. Devitalized tissue provides the necessary environment for the growth of anaerobic organisms. The anaerobic environment is enhanced by concomitant inoculation with several microbes, resulting in a synergistic infection. Deficiencies in host defense mechanisms caused by malignancy, prematurity, and drug- or disease-induced immunosuppression are associated with development of serious anaerobic infections. Compromise of tissues in the otherwise normal host by surgery, injury, or vascular embarrassment and the development of chronic infection (especially in the upper respiratory tract) predispose the patient to development of anaerobic infection.

Anaerobes are isolated most frequently from children with *peritonitis* caused by appendicitis or gastrointestinal perforation. The organisms recovered represent fecal flora, the *Bacteroides fragilis* group being the most common isolate. In most children with peritonitis, the infection is polymicrobial, and *E. coli* and other Enterobacteriaceae often are isolated concurrently. Virtually all cases of secondary peritonitis and associated wound infections yield anaerobes. Anaerobes also predominate in liver, spleen, and other intraabdominal and retroperitoneal abscesses.

Anaerobic bacteremia in children generally occurs after dissemination from a focus in the gastrointestinal tract, including the oral cavity. Alternately, it may occur in patients with chronic disease or compromised host defenses (e.g., leukemia). The organisms recovered from patients with septicemia are *Bacteroides*, *Prevotella*, *Porphyromonas*, *Fusobacterium*, *Clostridium*, and *Peptostreptococcus*. Occasionally, osteomyelitis and septic arthritis complicate anaerobic bacteremia, but they also can occur after trauma. The clinical manifestations do not differ from those of bone and joint infections caused by more common aerobic pathogens. Specimens for anaerobic culture should be obtained if drainage or biopsy procedures are performed, and anaerobic infections should be considered seriously in osteomyelitis of unknown cause.

Almost invariably, brain abscesses yield anaerobic organisms of oropharyngeal flora origin in children, as in adults. The predominant anaerobes in these abscesses include *Peptostreptococcus*, *Bacteroides fragilis* group, *Prevotella*, *Fusobacterium*, and microaerophilic streptococci. Usually, these uncommon infections occur in patients with chronic otitis, mastoiditis, or sinusitis that also is caused by these organisms. Other forms of anaerobic CNS infection are rare and usually have been reported as a complication of surgery or implantation of foreign body. The predominant anaerobe isolate in these infections is *Propionibacterium acnes*.

Often, cutaneous abscesses and wounds in sites proximal to the oropharynx and the gastrointestinal and genitourinary tracts yield anaerobes. The organisms generally are those that originate from the proximal endogenous bacterial flora: *Prevotella*, *Porphyromonas*, and *Fusobacterium* are recovered in infections of oral origin, and *B. fragilis* group and *Clostridium* in those of the lower gastrointestinal tract. Anaerobes of oral origin predominate in bite wounds, chronic mastoiditis, sinusitis, otitis and aspiration pneumonia, lung abscess, and empyema. Deep cellulitis and formation of an abscess around the oropharynx, including peritonsillar abscess, periodontal disease, dental abscess, and secondary facial cellulitis, most commonly involve *Prevotella*, *Fusobacterium*, *Peptostreptococcus*, and *Porphyromonas*; occasionally, *B. fragilis* or other *Bacteroides* species are involved. Often, aerobes are isolated concomitantly. Beta-lactamase-producing anaerobes exist in substantial numbers in tonsillar crypt abscesses, deep within chronically inflamed tonsils, and in parapharyngeal abscesses. These organisms may interfere with the action of the penicillins on other sensitive anaerobic or aerobic strains, and prudence warrants consideration of penicillin-resistant anaerobes as potential etiologic agents in serious parapharyngeal and respiratory infections.

In addition to those in sites associated prominently with anaerobic infection, virtually any local infection may yield anaerobes. Specific cultures for these organisms should be performed in cases of deep-seated infection, particularly in patients with underlying diseases that predispose them to opportunistic infection and in sites involving devitalized tissue.

The pathogenesis of anaerobic infections reflects the complex interaction of host defense mechanisms, including tissue blood supply and viability, and the virulence factors peculiar to each organism. The multiple proteolytic exotoxins and enzymes elaborated by many of the anaerobic organisms probably are responsible for the necrotizing nature of many anaerobic infections, such as necrotizing pneumonia and cellulitis. These toxins may contribute to the pathogenesis of the synergistic infections common to anaerobes, in which several relatively nonpathogenic organisms contribute to each other's virulence.

Some cell wall virulence factors have a direct role in the pathogenesis of clinical manifestations. The extensively studied animal model of peritoneal infection that develops after gastrointestinal perforation has shown that the capsular polysaccharide of *B. fragilis* group is solely responsible for the promotion of abscess formation. A T-cell–mediated immune reaction to the polysaccharide capsule of *B. fragilis* occurs, and lymphocytic cellular reaction is crucial in the development of intraabdominal abscess after fecal contamination of the peritoneum. Cellular immunity to the polysaccharide can be induced, and protection from formation of an abscess may result.

Interaction with host defenses contributes to pathogenesis, but it is understood incompletely. Certain strains of *Bacteroides* and *Fusobacterium* can activate complement by classic and alternate pathways, resulting in the generation of chemotactic factors and local accumulation of leukocytes. Most strains of *B. fragilis* are resistant to killing by serum mediated by complement.

Clinical Manifestations

The common clinical syndromes that may be caused in children by nonclostridial anaerobic organisms are listed in Table 153.3. In general, the clinical appearance of these infections is not different from that of similar infections caused by facultative organisms. Formation of gas may occur with facultative organisms, as with *Clostridium* and other anaerobes. The major clinical distinction is the foul odor associated with anaerobic infection. Anaerobes may cause infection in most of the

TABLE 153.3

INFECTIONS COMMONLY ASSOCIATED WITH ANAEROBIC BACTERIA

Associated with organisms of oral origin
Brain abscess
Chronic sinusitis
Chronic otitis and mastoiditis
Parapharyngeal and peritonsillar abscesses
Dental abscess and periodontitis
Ludwig angina
Branchial cleft cyst infection
Human bite wound infection and paronychia
Necrotizing and aspiration pleuropulmonary infection
Septicemia secondary to any of the foregoing

Associated with organisms of gastrointestinal or vaginal origin
Peritonitis and peritoneal abscess
Abdominal surgical wound infection
Pelvic inflammatory disease
Ascending cholangitis
Cellulitis, particularly perirectal
Blood infection after gastrointestinal disease or immunocompromise

same sites as in adults, although pleuropulmonary and pelvic anaerobic infections are unusual findings in children. Occasionally, anaerobic osteomyelitis, soft tissue cellulitis and abscesses, chronic head and neck infections, and perinephric and scrotal abscesses develop in children. Rarely, meningitis caused by anaerobic organisms is reported in children.

Because of the toxins produced, significant systemic disease may accompany local anaerobic infections. Endotoxin is elaborated by gram-negative anaerobes, and typical endotoxic shock can occur in serious anaerobic infections. Hemolysis, vascular collapse, jaundice, and severe toxigenic diarrhea also may occur.

The classic syndromes of gas gangrene, progressive synergistic gangrene, synergistic necrotizing cellulitis, nonclostridial crepitant cellulitis, chronic burrowing ulcer, and necrotizing fasciitis are manifestations of anaerobic or mixed soft tissue infections and are rare findings in children. This outcome probably reflects the generally healthy vascular supply to the tissues of children. If the blood supply is compromised, these characteristic infections can occur as they do in adults.

Commonly, abdominal infections and associated septicemia are caused by *B. fragilis* group, *Fusobacterium*, and *Clostridium*. Primary anaerobic septicemia in immunocompromised children is caused most frequently by these organisms, probably from invasion by gastrointestinal microbes. Ascending cholangitis in infants who have undergone surgical palliation for biliary atresia is a complication that may involve anaerobic and aerobic gastrointestinal organisms. Certain strains of *B. fragilis* may elaborate an enterotoxin that may cause diarrhea.

The syndrome of Ludwig angina has a characteristic clinical picture of rapidly progressive, submental, spreading cellulitis that elevates the tongue from the floor of the mouth and may encroach on the airway. Usually, systemic toxicity is severe, and the organisms involved are *Fusobacterium* and anaerobic cocci. Spirochetes may be seen in aspirated material.

Wounds contaminated with anaerobic organisms may result in polymicrobial soft tissue infections. Typically, wound infections of human or animal bites involve oral anaerobes among their polymicrobial flora.

The clinical manifestations of brain abscess caused by anaerobes are indistinguishable from those involving only aerobes.

Diagnosis

The diagnosis of anaerobic infection requires an alert physician and Gram stain and culture of appropriately collected material. Culture of the organisms is the only method of confirming clinical suspicion. Specimens should be sent in special transport media suitable for anaerobic bacteria. Aspirated fluid is preferred to swab specimens. Aspirated fluid can be sent to the laboratory in a plastic syringe if it is processed within 20 minutes of collection. Specimens should be obtained by aspiration that bypasses the mucosal and skin flora. Those appropriate for anaerobic culture include all normally sterile body fluids (e.g., blood, joint, pleural fluids), material obtained by puncture from a closed space (e.g., abscess, sinus), urine through suprapubic aspiration, sputum through transtracheal aspiration or protected specimen brush, and material obtained from culdocentesis after decontamination of the vagina. Gram-stained smears of all aspirated material should be examined for characteristic forms and should be used to complement culture results, which may be compromised by the fastidious nature of many anaerobic pathogens. Radiographs demonstrating gas in infected tissues may be helpful, but they are nonspecific.

Methods of processing cultures for anaerobic organisms are evolving and incorporating new techniques for the identification of organisms. Commercialized kits using DNA probes, monoclonal antibodies to specific sites of certain strains, and polymerase chain reaction are being developed. The field of anaerobic microbiology is undergoing rapid change, and considerable controversy surrounds the best procedures to be used in the clinical microbiology laboratory. Nonetheless, most hospital laboratories are equipped to identify organisms or groups of organisms.

Management and Prognosis

The treatment of anaerobic infection involves appropriate drainage, débridement, and antibiotic therapy. Deep abscesses in the abdominal cavity should be opened and drained, and the area should be irrigated with physiologic saline, if possible. Generalized peritonitis also may respond best to this therapy. Anaerobic lung abscess and empyema (rare in children) require drainage, but irrigation rarely is indicated. Small liver or other intraabdominal abscesses may respond to antimicrobial therapy, but larger abscesses may require percutaneous drainage. Oropharyngeal abscesses respond to incision and drainage without irrigation. Excision of malformations (e.g.,

branchial cleft cyst) should be performed. Large abscesses in the brain respond best to drainage, although computed tomography has documented the resolution of some large abscesses with medical therapy alone. The occurrence of multiple or loculated abscesses may render performance of surgical drainage impractical. Most authorities agree that abscesses larger than 2 cm in diameter have improved outcome if drainage is performed and that excision is the treatment of choice for well-encapsulated lesions. Commonly, smaller lesions and those documented before encapsulation respond to prolonged medical therapy alone.

Management of anaerobic cellulitis frequently requires prompt and extensive débridement and antibiotic therapy to prevent spread and to lessen tissue loss, especially for cases of clostridial gas gangrene, and also is necessary for cases of progressive synergistic gangrene, necrotizing fasciitis, and anaerobic myositis. Unlike aerobic soft tissue infections, severe anaerobic cellulitis frequently does not respond to antibiotics alone, probably because many antibiotics function poorly in the markedly reduced pH and oxygen tension of anaerobic infections.

Because susceptibility testing is time-consuming, costly, and often unreliable, the choice of antibiotics is based on recognizing the organisms likely to be involved in various anatomic sites and on known trends in antimicrobial susceptibilities. Specific antimicrobial susceptibility may be available in specialized laboratories. Susceptibility testing is important in closed-space infection (e.g., meningitis), bacteremia, and the immunocompromised host.

The antimicrobials of choice for anaerobic bacteria are listed in Table 153.4. Most gram-positive cocci and bacilli and about half of the gram-negative anaerobic bacilli are sensitive to penicillin. Semisynthetic penicillin derivatives (e.g., ampicillin, methicillin, oxacillin, and nafcillin) are less active than is the parent compound, but the very high levels of these drugs achieved with the parenteral administration of large doses may be adequate in some cases. Penicillin G should be used in dosages of 200,000 to 400,000 U/kg/day for infections caused by penicillin-sensitive anaerobes. Penicillin V is less effective. The comparable dosage of intravenous ampicillin, oxacillin, and methicillin is 200 mg/kg/day and of nafcillin is 100 mg/kg/day. B. fragilis group and a growing proportion of pigmented Prevotella and Porphyromonas, Fusobacterium, and some Clostridium species are penicillin-resistant through the production of beta-lactamase.

Antibiotics that exhibit high degrees of activity against penicillinase-producing anaerobes include chloramphenicol, the combinations of a penicillin (e.g., amoxicillin, ticarcillin) with a beta-lactamase inhibitor (e.g., clavulanic acid, tazobactam),

---

TABLE 153.4

ANTIMICROBIALS OF CHOICE FOR ANAEROBIC BACTERIA

Anaerobic Bacterial Species	First Choice	Alternate
Peptostreptococcus	Penicillin	Clindamycin, chloramphenicol, cephalosporins
Clostridium	Penicillin	Metronidazole, chloramphenicol, cefoxitin, clindamycin
Clostridium difficile	Vancomycin	Metronidazole
Gram-negative bacilli* (BL−)	Penicillin	Metronidazole, clindamycin, chloramphenicol
Gram-negative bacilli* (BL+)	Metronidazole, a carbapenem, a penicillin plus beta-lactamase inhibitor, clindamycin	Cefoxitin, chloramphenicol, piperacillin

BL− = non beta-lactamase producer
BL+ = beta-lactamase producer
*Bacteroides fragilis group, Prevotella species, Porphyromonas species, Fusobacterium species.

a carbapenem (e.g., imipenem, meropenem, ertapenem), metronidazole, and clindamycin. Cephalosporins exhibit various degrees of activity against anaerobic strains and should not be relied on for empiric therapy; however, two second-generation cephalosporins—cefoxitin and cefotetan—are the most effective ones. The amoxicillin or ticarcillin and clavulanic acid combinations are the drugs of choice for most anaerobic pediatric infections. Oral therapy with amoxicillin and clavulanic acid in a dosage of 45 mg/kg/day every 12 hours or clindamycin in a dosage of 20 to 30 mg/kg/day every 8 hours may be used for relatively uncomplicated infections. Serious infections above the diaphragm should be treated with intravenous ticarcillin with clavulanic acid in doses of 200 to 400 mg/kg/day every 8 hours. The doses of imipenem with cilastatin or meropenem (carbapenems), when chosen for broad coverage of aerobic and anaerobic organisms, is 40 mg/kg/day divided into four daily (for imipenem) and three daily (for meropenem) intravenous doses. Treatment of infections below the diaphragm should be directed at *B. fragilis* and Enterobacteriaceae, using a combination of penicillin plus a beta-lactamase inhibitor or a carbapenem.

The ureidopenicillins demonstrate broader activity than do the cephalosporins, but their inhibitory concentrations are significantly higher than those of the first-line drugs. First-generation cephalosporins and aminoglycosides have no activity against the *B. fragilis* group.

Before a CNS abscess has become encapsulated and localized, administration of antimicrobial therapy accompanied by measures to control the increase in the intracranial pressure is essential. Once an abscess has formed, surgical excision or drainage combined with a long course of antibiotics (4 to 8 weeks) remains the treatment of choice. Metronidazole, 7.5 mg/kg/day every 6 hours after a single loading dose of 15 mg/kg (plus penicillin), or chloramphenicol succinate in a dose of 100 mg/kg/day every 6 hours remains the proven drug of choice. Monitoring blood levels of chloramphenicol, modifying doses, and monitoring for potential toxicities are necessary. Penicillin should be added to metronidazole to cover microaerophilic streptococci and gram-positive anaerobes.

The duration of therapy for anaerobic infections generally is longer than that for comparable infections caused by aerobic organisms, ranging from 10 to 14 days for minor soft tissue infections, 10 to 21 days for septicemia, 6 weeks or more for bone infections, 4 to 6 weeks for chronic sinusitis, and 6 to 8 weeks for brain abscesses.

Hyperbaric oxygen has been recommended for the treatment of rapidly progressive anaerobic infections, but the value in children is uncertain. It should be administered only by experienced physicians in adequate facilities, without obviating standard therapy with surgery and antibiotics.

The outcome of severe anaerobic infections generally is related to the speed with which effective antibiotic or surgical treatment is administered and to the severity of underlying disease. Peritonitis, peritoneal abscess, and their associated secondary septicemia and abdominal wound infection in otherwise normal hosts carry good prognoses if their anaerobic causes are recognized, surgical drainage and débridement are performed, and an antibiotic therapy effective against *B. fragilis* group and Enterobacteriaceae is administered. If endotoxic shock, disseminated intravascular coagulopathy, or metastatic foci of infection supervene, the chances of a favorable outcome diminish. Anaerobic sepsis in patients with malignancy or other immunosuppressive conditions carries a poor prognosis, as does any generalized bacterial infection.

Data on the prognosis of anaerobic bacteremia in infants are conflicting and probably reflect the different circumstances under which cultures are obtained. Transient anaerobic bacteremia in newborns occurs approximately one-tenth as often as does aerobic bacteremia and appears to carry little or no morbidity or mortality, but anaerobic bacteremia associated with significant underlying clinical disease, such as necrotizing enterocolitis, carries a mortality rate as high as 30% to 40%.

Abscesses and cellulitis surrounding the oropharynx have an almost uniformly good prognosis with adequate drainage and antimicrobial therapy. The complications of airway compromise, spontaneous rupture into the pharynx or trachea, carotid artery invasion, jugular venous thrombosis, and dissection into the neck or mediastinum are rare findings. Cavernous sinus thrombosis is a potentially fatal complication of sinusitis.

Superficial anaerobic cellulitis and abscesses respond well to débridement and appropriate antibiotics. However, in progressive soft tissue infections caused by such toxin-producing anaerobes as *Clostridium*, the prognosis for saving the affected limb is poor, and as many as 15% of patients die despite administration of vigorous therapy.

The prognosis in patients with intracranial infection is related almost entirely to the location of the abscess, the ease with which it can be drained surgically, and the degree to which the mass effect of the abscess and surrounding edema compromise intracranial contents. Overall, the mortality rate approaches 15%; lesions in the cerebral hemispheres carry a prognosis significantly better than do those in the cerebellum or brainstem structures. Commonly, death occurs after rupture of the abscess into the ventricular system, brainstem herniation, or iatrogenic intracranial hemorrhage, which occurs in approximately 10% of patients undergoing needle aspiration. Patients with severely altered mental status have a very poor prognosis.

Prevention

Because most anaerobic infections are caused by endogenous flora, usually prevention through isolation techniques or immunization is not possible. Prophylactic use of antimicrobials is indicated in elective intraabdominal or oropharyngeal surgery. Cefoxitin has been used for such prophylaxis. Often, severe anaerobic infections caused by bowel flora after gastrointestinal compromise or perforation can be prevented by early, judicious surgery combined with appropriate antibiotic coverage for *B. fragilis* group and for Enterobacteriacae. This therapy constitutes early treatment for infection rather than prophylaxis. Similar management of other potentially contaminated sites may prevent the development of severe infection.

Superficial wounds thought to be contaminated by anaerobes should be irrigated copiously and allowed to heal by secondary intention, particularly if they are ragged lacerations caused by animal or human bites. Administration of appropriate antibiotics may help to prevent severe infection.

Suggested Readings

American Academy of Pediatrics. Tetanus (lockjaw). In: Peter G, ed. *2000 Red Book: report of the Committee on Infectious Diseases*, 25th ed. Elk Grove Village, IL: American Academy of Pediatrics, 2000:563.

Bartlett JG. *Clostridium difficile*-associated enteric disease. *Curr Infect Dis Rep* 2002;4:477.

Brook I. *Pediatric anaerobic infections: diagnosis and management*, 3rd ed. New York: Marcell Dekker Inc, 2002.

Brook I. *In vitro* susceptibility vs *in vivo* efficacy of various antimicrobial agents against the *Bacteroides fragilis* group. *Rev Infect Dis* 1990;13:1170.

Brook I. Anaerobic bacteria in upper respiratory tract and other head and neck infections. *Ann Otol Rhinol Laryngol* 2002;111:430.

Centers for Disease Control and Prevention. CDC surveillance summaries. Tetanus surveillance—United States, 1980–1994. *MMWR Mortal Morbid Wkly Rep* 1998;47:1.

Dunkle LM, Brotherton TJ, Feigin RD. Anaerobic infection in children: a prospective survey. *Pediatrics* 1976;57:311.

Ernst ME, Klepser ME, Fouts M, Marangos MN. Tetanus: pathophysiology and management. *Ann Pharmacother* 1997;31:1507.

Finegold SM. *Anaerobic bacteria in human disease.* New York: Academic Press, 1977.

Gorbach SL, Bartlett JG. Anaerobic infections. *N Engl J Med* 1974;290:1177.

Jousimies-Somer H, Summanen P. Recent taxonomic changes and terminology update of clinically significant anaerobic gram-positive and gram-negative bacteria (excluding spirochetes). *Clin Infect Dis* 2002;35(Suppl 1): s17.

Long SS. Infant botulism. *Pediatr Infect Dis J* 2001;20:707.

Nord CE. The role of anaerobic bacteria in recurrent episodes of sinusitis and tonsillitis. *Clin Infect Dis* 1995;20:1512.

Onderdonk AB, Cisneros RL, Finberg R, et al. Animal model system for studying virulence of and host response to *Bacteroides fragilis. Rev Infect Dis* 1990;12:S169.

Rasmussen BA, Bush K, Tally FP. Antimicrobial resistance in anaerobes. *Clin Infect Dis* 1997;24:S110.

Shapiro RL, Hatheway C, Swerdlow DL. Botulism in the United States: a clinical and epidemiologic review. *Ann Intern Med* 1998;129:221.

Sears CL, Myers LL, Lazenbjam A, Van Tussell RL. Enterotoxigenic *Bacteroides fragilis. Clin Infect Dis* 1995;20:S142.

Turton K, Chaddock JA, Acharya KR. Botulinum and tetanus neurotoxins: structure, function and therapeutic utility. *Trends Biochem Sci* 2002;27:552.

Warmy M, Pepin J, Fang A, et al. Toxin production by an emerging strain of *Clostridium difficile* associated with outbreaks of severe disease in North America and Europe. *Lancet* 2005;366:1079.

CHAPTER 154 ■ BARTONELLOSIS

BARBARA W. STECHENBERG

Bartonellosis is caused by *Bartonella bacilliformis*, which produces two illnesses that are distinctive clinically and temporally: Oroya fever, a disease characterized by severe, febrile, hemolytic anemia, and verruca peruana, an eruption of hemangioma-like lesions, and a subclinical asymptomatic infection. Carrión disease, an eponym that refers to both forms of the disease, is found only in an area of South America that includes parts of Peru, Ecuador, and Colombia.

ETIOLOGY AND PATHOGENESIS

B. bacilliformis is a small, gram-negative, motile organism with a brush of ten or more unipolar flagella. It is an obligate aerobe that grows best at 28°C in semisolid nutrient agar with 10% rabbit serum and 0.5% rabbit hemoglobin.

The vector of this disease is the sand fly, *Phlebotomus noguchi*. After inoculation, *Bartonella* enter the endothelial cells of the blood vessels, where they proliferate during the incubation period. These organisms, which can be found throughout the reticuloendothelial system and in many specific organs, then reenter the bloodstream and parasitize the erythrocytes. The resulting hemolytic anemia is caused by the destruction of these parasitized cells, which may constitute as many as 90% of the erythrocytes. Patients who survive the acute phase of Oroya fever may or may not develop the cutaneous manifestations of the disease, which appear as nodular hemangiomatous lesions or verrucae ranging in size from a few millimeters to several centimeters.

CLINICAL MANIFESTATIONS

The incubation period ranges from 2 to 14 weeks. In patients who are totally asymptomatic, diagnosis can be obtained only by blood culture. Other patients may develop such symptoms as headache, malaise, and occasional fever without anemia despite recovery of *B. bacilliformis* from blood cultures. Patients with severe anemia or Oroya fever are febrile, and *Bartonella* can be observed parasitizing the erythrocytes. The anemia develops rapidly, and patients present with a peculiar discoloration of the skin and sclera caused by the combination of slight icterus and severe anemia. Often, other symptoms referable to severe anemia are present. Delirium and clouding of the sensorium are rather common symptoms that usually are mild but may progress to overt psychosis. On physical examination, the signs of severe anemia and icterus may be accompanied by generalized lymphadenopathy.

The anemia is macrocytic and hypochromic, with anisocytosis and poikilocytosis. The erythrocyte count may drop to 500,000 cells per cubic millimeter in the first 2 to 4 weeks of the disease, and the reticulocyte count may increase to 50%. The pathognomonic sign of the disease is the identification of *B. bacilliformis* in Giemsa-stained erythrocytes, appearing as red-violet rods. The critical stage of the anemia is the period of transition in which the organisms suddenly disappear from the erythrocytes. During this time, the organisms change from rod-shaped to more coccoid forms. The anemia may decrease at this time, but in some cases, illness may become more severe, suggesting the development of intercurrent infection (usually with *Salmonella*).

In the preeruptive stage, patients may complain of pain in the joints, muscles, and bones, and cramps or paresthesias may occur. Such inflammatory reactions as phlebitis, parotitis, pleuritis, erythema nodosum, and encephalitis may occur. The anemia and lymphadenopathy of the invasive stage usually disappear. The appearance of verrucae is pathognomonic of the development of the disease in the eruptive stage. Usually, these verrucae are seen in the skin, but they may be found in mesenchymal tissue.

DIAGNOSIS

The diagnosis of bartonellosis is based on the clinical manifestations in conjunction with a blood smear showing typical organisms or blood cultures. In the preanemic stage and for patients without the typical anemia who reside in an endemic area, the diagnosis can be made on the basis of blood cultures alone. In the eruptive phase, the diagnosis may be made by the appearance of the typical verruca.

TREATMENT

B. bacilliformis is sensitive to many antibiotics, including penicillin, tetracycline, streptomycin, and chloramphenicol. Usually, treatment takes effect rapidly, lowering fever and eradicating the organisms from the blood. The choice of antibiotics should be guided by considerations other than simple eradication of the organism, including the risk of development of intercurrent infection. Chloramphenicol is considered the drug of choice because it is useful also in the treatment of salmonellosis. Blood transfusions may need to be given during the period of severe anemia. Treatment for verruca peruana is not necessary unless particularly large lesions interfere with function and, therefore, require surgery. Oral tetracycline may be used to aid in healing the lesions.

PREVENTION

In endemic areas, people can protect themselves by avoiding particular areas at night and by using insect repellents. Use of insecticides has been effective in controlling the disease by eliminating the vector.

Suggested Readings

Bass JW, Vincent JM, Person DA. The expanding spectrum of *Bartonella* infections: I. Bartonellosis and trench fever. *Pediatr Infect Dis J* 1997; 16:2.
Koehler JE. *Bartonella* infection. *Adv Pediatr Dis* 1996;11:1.

CHAPTER 155 ■ RELAPSING FEVER

BARBARA W. STECHENBERG

Relapsing fever is a vector-borne, spirochetal infection characterized by recurring febrile episodes of a remitting nature. It is caused by several species of *Borrelia*. *Borrelia* are loosely coiled spirochetes that easily stain with Wright or Giemsa stain, allowing diagnosis to be established by examination of the blood smear. They also can be grown on artificial media. The organism undergoes spontaneous antigenic variation *in vivo* and *in vitro*. Different antigenic variants result in repeated episodes of dense spirochetemia and account for the cyclic nature of the disease. With each remission, antibodies are produced to a specific strain, which then is immobilized and removed from the circulation.

EPIDEMIOLOGY

Louse-borne epidemic relapsing fever is caused by *Borrelia recurrentis*. Lice become infected by feeding on spirochetemic humans. Transmission to humans takes place when the bite wound is contaminated with the infectious hemolymph of the louse as it is crushed or wounded. This form of relapsing fever no longer is found in the United States, but it occurs in Africa and South America, particularly in areas of crowding, cold weather, and poor hygiene.

Endemic relapsing fever is transmitted by ticks of the genus *Ornithodoros*. *B. hermsii* and *B. turicatae* are the most common species in North America, but many species are implicated worldwide. After the tick becomes engorged on an infected host, *Borrelia* invade all tissues, and the tick remains capable of transmitting infection for years. These ticks occur in many areas of the world; in the United States, they are seen primarily in forested mountain areas of the western states, particularly in areas or dwellings with large rodent nests. The bite of these ticks is painless, and the ticks feed for short periods (10 to 30 minutes), often at night.

CLINICAL MANIFESTATIONS

After an incubation period of 5 to 11 days, the illness begins abruptly with high fever (39°C to 41°C), chills, prostration, headache, myalgia, and arthralgia. Diarrhea, chest pain, and cough may occur. Splenomegaly is a common finding; other physical findings may include conjunctival suffusion, hepatomegaly, and abdominal tenderness. Some patients experience a fleeting, truncal rash, especially at the end of the primary episode. Neurologic involvement is seen occasionally, particularly in louse-borne disease.

The primary febrile episode characteristically lasts from 3 to 6 days and is followed by a period of 7 to 10 days of decreased symptoms (i.e., patients are afebrile but weak). Relapses are associated with similar influenza-like symptoms, but they can be shorter than the primary episode. Louse-borne disease may relapse up to four times and tick-borne disease up to 10 to 12 times.

DIAGNOSIS

The most important aspect of diagnosis is clinical suspicion of the disease in patients who have traveled to or live in an endemic area. The diagnosis can be established by demonstrating the organism by Wright or Giemsa stain of a peripheral blood smear. Examination of dehemoglobinized thick smears or buffy coat smears may increase the yield. Intraperitoneal injection of infective blood into young mice, with demonstration of the organism in 1 to 14 days, may be used to confirm the diagnosis.

Serologic testing usually is not clinically helpful, although patients with relapsing fever may have elevated Proteus Ox-K agglutinins. Specific antibody testing is available from the Centers for Disease Control and Prevention. Other laboratory findings may include thrombocytopenia, hyperbilirubinemia, and elevated liver function test results.

TREATMENT

Relapsing fever has been treated successfully with tetracycline, which usually is considered the drug of choice, and with chloramphenicol, erythromycin, or penicillin. In louse-borne disease, single-dose regimens of tetracycline and erythromycin have proven to be effective. A single dose of tetracycline (500 mg or 10 mg/kg for children older than 8 years) or erythromycin (500 mg or 10 mg/kg for children younger than 8 years) may eradicate the organism.

Antibiotic therapy typically induces a Jarisch-Herxheimer reaction, with severe rigors, fever, and hypotension. When treating tick-borne disease in children in the United States, use of a more conservative regimen may be prudent. A single initial oral or parenteral dose of penicillin may attenuate this reaction because penicillin kills the organisms gradually. Because of the Jarisch-Herxheimer reaction, providing supportive measures is particularly important during the first few hours of treatment.

This reaction cannot be prevented by prior administration of hydrocortisone but can be treated with fluids and antipyretics. After defervescence, a 7- to 10-day course of penicillin V, erythromycin (40 to 50 mg/kg/day), or tetracycline (for patients older than 8 years) is given to prevent relapse.

Prevention of relapsing fever requires the avoidance or elimination of the arthropod vector. Cases should be reported immediately, particularly if they can be traced to public recreational settings.

Suggested Readings

Butler T, Jones PK, Wallace CK. *Borrelia recurrentis* infection: single dose antibiotic regimens and management of the Jarisch-Herxheimer reaction. *J Infect Dis* 1978;137:573.

Dworkin MS, Anderson DE, Schwan TG, et al. Tick-borne relapsing fever in the Northwestern United States and Southwestern Canada. *Clin Infect Dis* 1998;26:122.

Le CT. Tick-borne relapsing fever in children. *Pediatrics* 1980;66:963.

Shapiro ED. Tick-borne diseases. *Adv Pediatr Infect Dis* 1997;13:187.

Spach DH, Liles WC, Cambell GL, et al. Tick-borne diseases in the United States. *N Engl J Med* 1993;329:936.

CHAPTER 156 ■ LYME DISEASE

BARBARA W. STECHENBERG

Lyme disease, recognized in 1975, was first brought to medical attention by two women from Lyme, Connecticut, who were concerned about an illness spreading in their community. Their inquiries sparked an intensive investigation of this disorder and its protean manifestations.

Because of epidemiologic characteristics, such as geographic and seasonal case clustering, and reports of resolution of the early rash (i.e., erythema migrans [EM]) with empiric treatment, an infectious cause that was probably bacterial and associated with a vector was sought. In 1982, Burgdorfer and colleagues isolated a spirochete from the midgut of the tick *Ixodes scapularis*. This organism causes EM-like disease in laboratory animals, and its etiologic role was soon confirmed by isolation of the spirochete from blood, skin, and cerebrospinal fluid of patients with Lyme disease.

The spirochete has irregular coils and is 10 to 30 μm long and 0.18 to 0.25 μm in diameter. It grows on artificial media, particularly a modified Kelly medium. It was designated *Borrelia burgdorferi*, which has now been divided into three genomic groups.

associated with this disease is *I. pacificus*. In Europe, cases of EM, with or without neurologic findings, have occurred primarily in the geographic range of the *I. ricinus* tick. The taiga tick, *I. persulcatus*, is responsible for disease in Asia. The disease is more widespread than previously thought, implicating other potential vectors. A rash similar to EM has been described in humans residing in the southeastern and south-central United States. It is associated with the lone star tick *Amblyomma americanum*. This Lyme-like rash has been named Southern tick-associated rash illness (STARI).

The occurrence of Lyme disease peaks during summer and early fall. Cases cluster in sparsely settled and wooded areas. However, the conversion of farmland to woodland and finally to wooded suburbs has contributed to the spread of the increasing populations of deer and white-footed mice to more densely populated human areas and to the increasing prevalence of Lyme disease. As many as 67% of the patients in many studies do not report a history of tick bite, probably because of the small size (i.e., no larger than a pinhead) of the unengorged nymphal tick.

EPIDEMIOLOGY

The best documented vector is the deer tick, *I. scapularis*, whose geographic distribution correlates with the endemic foci in the eastern United States. The major areas where this organism is found are the eastern seaboard (e.g., Massachusetts, Rhode Island, Connecticut, New York, New Jersey, Maryland), the upper Midwest (e.g., Wisconsin, Minnesota), and the West (e.g., California, Nevada, Utah, Oregon). In the West, the tick

PATHOGENESIS

B. burgdorferi adapts to markedly different environments, the tick and its mammalian hosts, to complete its life cycle. The spirochete survives in the dormant state in the midgut of the nymphal tick during the fall, winter, and early spring. In the midgut, the organism primarily expresses OspA. With feeding in late spring or early summer, OspA is down-regulated, and OspC, required for infection of the mammalian host, is up-regulated. The spirochete also binds mammalian plasminogen and its activators, present in the blood meal, thus facilitating spread of the organism.

Immune cells first encounter the organism at the site of the bite. Complement-mediated lysis of the organism may be the first line of defense. As part of the innate immune response, macrophages opsonize and kill the organism. Inflammatory cells within the skin lesions produce primarily Th1 proinflammatory cytokines. Within days, most patients mount an IgM antibody response to OspC or the 41-kDa flagellar protein. Both innate and adaptive cellular elements are mobilized to control the infection.

Within days to weeks after onset, *B. burgdorferi* often disseminates by binding to certain host proteins and adhering to integrins, proteoglycans, or glycoproteins on host cells or tissue matrices. As in the tick, this may be facilitated by the binding of plasminogen and its activators. Despite an active immune response, *B. burgdorferi* may survive during this phase by changing or minimizing antigenic expression of surface proteins and by inhibiting certain critical host immune responses. Certain lipoproteins may also contribute. Ultimately, both innate and adaptive immune responses are required to control the dissemination of infection. Even without antibiotics, these immune mechanisms may control infection and symptoms resolve. However, the organism may still survive in localized niches such as joints for years. Months after onset, about 50% of untreated patients experience intermittent attacks of arthritis associated with neutrophil extravasation into joints to set up joint inflammation. These patients often have high antibody responses to many spirochetal proteins, suggestive of hyperimmunization. Eventually, even in untreated patients, most experience resolution of attacks of arthritis, as immune mechanisms seem to successfully eradicate the organism from the joints.

CLINICAL MANIFESTATIONS

The manifestations of Lyme disease can by divided into three stages (Box 156.1). These findings can be seen in isolation or concurrently. The incubation period usually is 3 to 32 days. The most common clinical finding is the skin rash (EM) (Fig. 156.1),

---

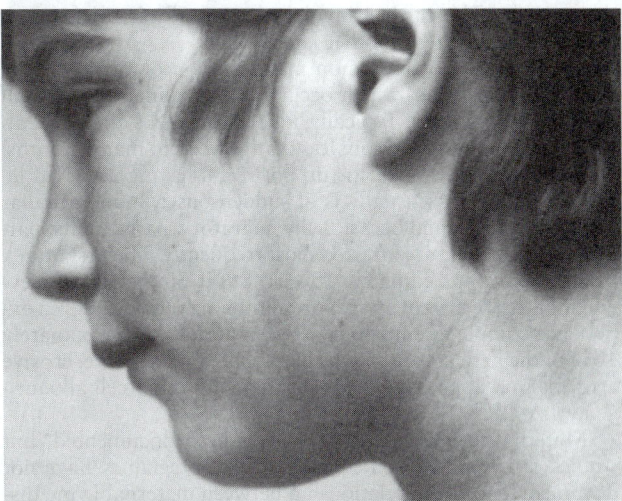

FIGURE 156.1. An enlarging lesion and multiple smaller annular lesions on the face of an 11-year-old boy diagnosed with Lyme disease who had been hiking in Westchester, NY.

---

which usually begins 4 to 20 days after the tick bite. An erythematous macule or papule forms at the site of the bite and gradually enlarges to form a large, plaque-like erythematous annular lesion with a median diameter of 16 cm. Early EM commonly has homogenous or central redness. The middle of the lesion often becomes clear, but it can be indurated or uniformly erythematous. It may have a vesicular or necrotic center. These lesions can occur anywhere on the body, but the usual sites are the thigh, buttocks, and axillae. Multiple secondary annular lesions are seen on approximately one-half of the patients (early dissemination—stage 2). The average duration of the untreated skin lesion is approximately 3 weeks. Often, EM is associated with systemic symptoms, most commonly malaise, fatigue, headache, stiff neck, and arthralgia. Fever usually is low grade, but it may be as high as 40°C. Lymphadenopathy, which is usually regional and associated with EM, and anicteric hepatitis, conjunctivitis, or pharyngitis also may occur. Infrequently, the flu-like symptoms may be seen without the characteristic rash. Respiratory and gastrointestinal symptoms are notably absent. These symptoms usually resolve over the course of several days, but they may occur intermittently for several weeks.

Neurologic involvement usually occurs within 4 weeks after the tick bite occurs. Meningitis, cranial nerve palsies, and peripheral radiculoneuropathy constitute the triad of neurologic Lyme disease. Lyme meningitis is characterized by excruciating headache and stiff neck, often associated with nausea and vomiting and emotional liability. Compared to viral meningitis, Lyme meningitis is more likely to have a longer duration of symptoms, lower temperature at presentation, and associated papilledema, EM rash, or cranial neuropathy. Cerebrospinal fluid in Lyme meningitis has a lower white blood cell count and a greater percentage of mononuclear cells than in viral meningitis. The seventh cranial nerve, either unilateral or bilateral, is involved most frequently in association with meningitis or as the sole neurologic manifestation. It usually lasts 2 to 8 weeks before complete resolution occurs. Less common neurologic abnormalities include meningoencephalitis, chorea, cerebellar ataxia, Guillain-Barré syndrome, pseudotumor cerebri, and myelitis. Eye involvement, which may be seen rarely, includes iritis, retinitis, and panophthalmitis.

Cardiac abnormalities occur in a small percentage of patients (primarily young men) within several weeks after the bite. These abnormalities range from fluctuating degrees of atrioventricular block to myocarditis and left ventricular

---

BOX 156.1   **Clinical Stages of Lyme Disease**

Stage 1: Early infection
Erythema migrans
Flu-like symptoms
Regional adenopathy

Stage 2: Disseminated infection
Multiple erythema migrans lesions
Hepatitis, musculoskeletal complaints
Acute neurologic disease
    Cranial nerve palsies, especially VII
    Meningitis
Cardiac involvement
    Atrioventricular Block

Stage 3: Late disease
Arthritis
Neurologic syndromes
    Encephalitis
    Radiculopathies
Late skin involvement

dysfunction. The cardiac involvement usually is brief, but it may be associated with other late findings.

The second most common manifestation of Lyme disease after EM is arthritis, which occurs in approximately one-half of untreated patients. Typically, it begins 4 weeks after EM, although the time varies from less than 1 week to many months. Some patients with arthritis do not recall having any skin lesions. The arthritis usually is of sudden onset, monoarticular or oligoarticular, and occasionally migratory. Large joints, particularly the knee, are affected most frequently. The first attack usually lasts approximately 1 week, but it can persist for several months; recurrent attacks are common events. Children experience complete remissions between attacks. Approximately 10% of the patients with Lyme disease develop a severe, erosive arthritis that appears to be associated with the B-cell alloantigen HLA-DR4.

Maternal-to-fetal transmission has been documented, but studies of Lyme disease occurring during pregnancy have not documented a causal relationship between maternal Lyme disease and any specific adverse outcome.

DIFFERENTIAL DIAGNOSIS

Differential diagnosis depends on the presentation of the illness. When the characteristic EM rash is recognized, the diagnosis should be fairly obvious. If the rash is not identified as EM, it may be confused with streptococcal cellulitis, erythema multiforme (if multiple lesions exist), or erythema marginatum. Lyme disease must be differentiated from acute rheumatic fever. Fortunately, the specific characteristics of rheumatologic and cardiac involvement differ and, in Lyme disease, no evidence exists of antecedent streptococcal infection.

Forms of arthritis that may be confused with Lyme disease are pauciarticular juvenile rheumatoid arthritis; reactive arthritis associated with *Salmonella*, *Shigella*, or *Yersinia*; Reiter syndrome; or postinfectious arthritis associated with several viral illnesses.

The major neurologic manifestation of aseptic meningitis may be confused with enteroviral, leptospiral, or early tuberculous meningitis. If neurologic signs and symptoms are chronic, the physician must consider sarcoidosis, Mollaret meningitis, Behçet syndrome, and multiple sclerosis.

DIAGNOSIS

The diagnosis of Lyme disease is made best on clinical and epidemiologic grounds; early in the illness, the gross appearance of the skin lesions is diagnostic. Routine laboratory test results usually are nonspecific and not useful. The yield from culture or direct visualization techniques is too low to be practical. Specific serologic tests can be used to confirm the diagnosis for patients with late complications or with no history of EM. The clinical picture is important in the interpretation of serologic results. Serologic testing should not be undertaken for nonspecific symptoms. Enzyme-linked immunosorbent assay (ELISA) is more sensitive than is indirect fluorescent antibody testing. Marked interlaboratory variability in results has been documented. A two-test approach is recommended because of the high rate of false-positive ELISA tests. A positive or equivocal ELISA result should be confirmed by Western blot assay and interpreted using criteria developed by the Centers for Disease Control and Prevention (CDC). A negative ELISA requires no further testing. IgM-specific antibody usually peaks between 3 and 6 weeks after onset; IgG antibody develops more slowly. Elevated antibody (i.e., IgG) response to *B. burgdorferi* persists for years. Polymerase chain reaction (PCR) or comparison of cerebrospinal fluid (CSF) and serum antibody may be helpful

in certain clinical settings, such as unusual presentation of joint or neurologic disease. However, false-positive results are common occurrences and accuracy is highly dependent on careful sample collection and laboratory techniques.

TREATMENT

Even before the causative agent was identified, antibiotic treatment with penicillin or tetracycline was shown to be associated with more rapid resolution of the rash and with prevention of late complications. The type and route of antimicrobial therapy is determined by the clinical features and stage of disease (Box 156.2). For children older than 8 years who are in the early stages of Lyme disease, the treatment is doxycycline, 100 mg twice a day for 10 to 21 days. In younger children, amoxicillin administered orally in a dosage of 30 to 50 mg/kg/day in two or three divided doses for 10 to 21 days is recommended, with cefuroxime axetil, 30 mg/kg/day in two divided doses, being an alternative. Recent studies have suggested that 10 to 14 days may be as effective as 3 weeks. For penicillin-allergic children who cannot take a cephalosporin or doxycycline, oral erythromycin or azithromycin may be used; however, they may

---

BOX 156.2	**Treatment for Lyme Disease**

Early localized disease

≥8 years	Doxycycline, 100 mg orally, twice a day for 10–21 days
All ages	Amoxicillin, 30–50 mg/kg/day orally, in two or three divided doses (max: 2 g/day) for 10–21 days
Alternative	Cefuroxime axetil, 30 mg/kg/day orally in two doses (max: 500 mg/dose) for 10–21 days

Early disseminated disease

Multiple EM rash
    Oral regimen as above for 21 days
Isolated cranial nerve palsy
    Oral regimen as above for 21–28 days
Meningitis or cranial nerve palsy with CNS involvement
    Ceftriaxone 75–100 mg/kg/day IV, in single dose (max: 2 g) for 14–28 days
            or
    Penicillin G 300,000 U/kg/day IV, in six divided doses for 14–28 days
Carditis
    Ceftriaxone or penicillin G IV as above for 14 days; mild involvement may be treated orally for 14–28 days

Late disease

Arthritis
    Same oral regimens as above for 28 days with nonsteroidal antiinflammatory agents
Persistent or recurrent arthritis
    Consider a second course of oral therapy or IV regimens as above for 14–28 days
CNS or peripheral nervous system disease
    IV therapy as above for 28 days

CNS, central nervous system; EM, erythema migrans.

not be as effective, and patients should be monitored carefully. Resolution of EM usually is rapid; nonspecific symptoms often resolve slowly.

Flu-like illness during summer is a difficult issue, since most cases are not caused by *B. burgdorferi*. In highly endemic areas, treatment may be indicated in a patient with fever, headache, and musculoskeletal complaints in the absence of respiratory or gastrointestinal complaints. Initial serologic testing may help. Although babesiosis and anaplasmosis (formerly human granulocytic ehrlichiosis) often are asymptomatic, coinfection with these agents does occur and should be considered in a patient with more severe flu-like symptoms, high fever, leukopenia, thrombocytopenia, and/or liver function abnormalities. Anaplasmosis also is treated with doxycycline.

For patients with isolated facial palsy or early arthritis, a similar oral regimen can be used for longer duration (28 days). Any child with facial nerve palsy and other neurologic symptoms such as headache should have a CSF examination; if abnormalities are found, treatment should be initiated with ceftriaxone. Children with other neurologic manifestations or established arthritis may be treated with ceftriaxone or high-dose parenteral penicillin. The sensitivity of *Borrelia* to ceftriaxone renders it an attractive choice. Parenteral therapy should be continued for a minimum of 14 days.

PROGNOSIS

The long-term prognosis for children with Lyme disease is excellent. Unfortunately, a widespread misconception that Lyme disease is difficult to diagnose and treat has led to much anxiety and overtreatment. A small subset of patients, primarily adults, have been diagnosed with refractory or chronic Lyme disease. This event probably does not represent active infection but may be caused by other clinical entities. Two controlled trials of adult patients with persistent symptoms showed no efficacy of prolonged antimicrobial therapy.

PREVENTION

The prompt recognition of this disease with its diverse manifestations should lead to early treatment and resolution. Avoiding contact with the tick vector prevents infection, and awareness of the brushy, wooded locations where the tick is found and prompt removal of the tick after a bite can contribute to prevention (Box 156.3). Detachment is particularly important, because at least 24 to 36 hours of attachment are required to allow transmission of the organism. Judicious use of insect repellents such as N,N-diethyl-meta-toluamide (DEET) for skin and permethrins for clothing may be helpful. Routine prophylactic antimicrobial therapy after a tick bite is not recommended, particularly because of the prolonged duration of attachment required for transmission. Although a single dose of 200 mg of doxycycline is effective for prevention of EM after prolonged deer tick attachment in adults in highly endemic areas, this reg-

---

BOX 156.3 **Prevention of Lyme Disease**

- Avoid heavily infested areas (woods, brush)
- Wear light-colored clothing with long sleeves, long pants tucked into socks
- Use insect repellent with N,N-diethyl-meta-toluamide (DEET)
- Use permethrin on clothing
- Inspect for ticks at least every 24 hours
- Remove ticks appropriately
  - Grasp with tweezers as close to skin as possible
  - Remove by pulling tick straight out
  - Do not use burning, chemicals, or other agents to "kill" tick
  - If mouthparts remain, leave alone—they will eventually be extruded
  - Swab area with antiseptic

imen may be associated with frequent adverse effects and is not recommended. Amoxicillin has not proven to be effective for prophylaxis.

Suggested Readings

Gerber MA, Shapiro ED, Burke GS, et al. Lyme disease in children in southeastern Connecticut. *N Engl J Med* 1996;335:1270.

Klempner MS, Hu LT, Evans J, et al. Two controlled trials of antibiotic treatment in patients with persistent symptoms and a history of Lyme disease. *N Eng J Med* 2001;345:385.

Krause PJ, McKay K, Thompson CH, et al. Disease-specific diagnosis of co-infecting tickborne zoonoses: babesiosis, human granulocytic ehrlichiosis and Lyme disease. *Clin Infect Dis* 2002;34:11844.

Nadelman RB, Nowakowski J, Fish D, et al. Prophylaxis with single-dose doxycycline for the prevention of Lyme disease after an *Ixodes scapularis* tick bite. *N Engl J Med* 2001;345:379.

Qureshi MZ, New D, Zulquarini NJ, et al. Overdiagnosis and overtreatment of Lyme disease in Children. *Pediatr Infect Dis J* 2002;21:12.

Salazar JC, Gerber MA, Goff CW. Long-term outcome of Lyme disease in children given early treatment. *J Pediatr* 1993;122:591.

Seltzer EG, Shapiro ED. Misdiagnosis of Lyme disease: when not to order serology tests. *Pediatr Infect Dis* 1996;15:762.

Shapiro ED. Doxycycline for tick bites—not for everyone. *N Eng J Med* 2001; 345:133.

Smith RP, Schoen RT, Rahn DW, et al. Clinical characteristics and treatment outcome of early Lyme disease in patients with microbiologically confirmed erythema migrans. *Ann Int Med* 2002;136:421.

Steere AC. Medical progress: Lyme disease. *N Engl J Med* 2001;345:115.

Steere AC, Coburn J, Glickstein L. The emergence of Lyme disease. *J Clin Invest* 2004;113:1093.

Steere AC, Grodzicki RL, Kernblatt AN, et al. The spirochetal etiology of Lyme disease. *N Engl J Med* 1983;308:733.

Szer IS, Taylor E, Steere AC. The long-term course of Lyme arthritis in children. *N Engl J Med* 1991;325:159.

Wormser GP, Nadelman RB, Dattwyler RJ, et al. Practice guidelines for the treatment of Lyme disease. *Clin Infect Dis* 2000;31:S1.

Wormser GP, Ramanathan R, Nowakowski J, et al. Duration of antibiotic therapy for early Lyme disease. A randomized, double-blind, placebo-controlled trial. *Ann Intern Med* 2003;138:697.

CHAPTER 157 ■ *CAMPYLOBACTER* AND *HELICOBACTER*

LARRY K. PICKERING, BENJAMIN D. GOLD, AND GUILLERMO M. RUIZ-PALACIOS

Campylobacter and *Helicobacter* are among the most common bacterial pathogens that infect humans. The genus *Helicobacter* was distinguished formally from *Campylobacter* and other gram-negative curved bacilli in 1989 after analysis of enzymatic activities, growth characteristics, fatty acid and nucleic acid hybridization profiles, 16S rRNA sequence analysis, and genome sequencing were accomplished.

CAMPYLOBACTER

Since 1909, *Campylobacter* has been recognized as an animal pathogen associated with abortion in cows and sheep. *Campylobacter* was discovered in 1957 to cause human infections when a pregnant woman was found to have bacteremia caused by *Campylobacter fetus*. *Campylobacter* originally was regarded as a rare, opportunistic pathogen, and the clinical spectrum resulting from infection with *Campylobacter* is broad and includes diarrhea and other localized infections, bacteremia, systemic illness, and immunoreactive complications. Data from the Centers for Disease Control and Prevention (CDC) Foodborne Diseases Active Surveillance Network (FoodNet) show that *C. jejuni* and *Salmonella* are the leading causes of bacterial diarrhea in the United States.

Etiology

The family Campylobacteraceae includes three closely related genera: *Campylobacter*, *Arcobacter*, and *Sulfurospirillum*. *Campylobacter* (from the Greek word meaning curved rod) are slender, S-shaped or spirally curved, mostly microaerobic, motile, gram-negative bacilli with a flagellum at one or both ends. More than 16 species have been identified in the *Campylobacter* genus, but not all of them are considered pathogenic in humans (Table 157.1). The diagnosis of *Campylobacter* infection relies on pathogen isolation, mainly from stools and occasionally from blood. *C. jejuni* is the species most commonly isolated from children. *C. fetus* is a rare cause of bloodstream and systemic infections, occurring primarily in immunocompromised and debilitated hosts. *C. fetus* also is associated with perinatal infections and abortion. With respect to disease manifestations associated with *Campylobacter* genus, *C. jejuni* is the prototype for enteric infections, and *C. fetus* is the prototype for extraintestinal infections. Other *Campylobacter* species are associated with symptoms and signs including diarrhea, abdominal pain, fever, and vomiting, and with lung, perianal, groin, and axillary abscesses.

Epidemiology

Campylobacter species are mainly zoonotic, with a variety of animals and birds implicated as reservoirs for infection. Both *C. jejuni* and *C. coli* have been isolated from the gastrointestinal tracts of cattle, sheep, pigs, and numerous wild and commercially raised birds. Contamination of meat during slaughter may be the route by which bacteria enter the human food chain. The main source of *C. jejuni* and *C. coli* infections in humans is poultry, although pet dogs, cats, and hamsters are potential sources. Transmission of *Campylobacter* species occurs via the fecal-oral route through contaminated food and

---

TABLE 157.1

RESERVOIR AND CLINICAL SYNDROMES OF *CAMPYLOBACTER* SPECIES

Organism	Reservoir	Disease Produced in Humans
Campylobacter jejuni subspecies jejuni	Poultry, cattle, dogs, cats, sheep, monkey	Diarrhea, bacteremia, meningitis
C. jejuni subspecies doylei	Pigs	Diarrhea, less commonly bacteremia
C. coli	Pigs, poultry, cattle, dogs	Diarrhea
C. lari	Seagulls, dogs, cats, poultry, monkeys, fur seals	Diarrhea, less commonly colitis, appendicitis, bacteremia
C. upsaliensis	Dogs, cats	Diarrhea, less commonly bacteremia, abscesses
C. fetus	Cattle, sheep, poultry, reptiles, swine	Bacteremia, meningitis, vascular infections, less commonly diarrhea
C. hyointestinalis	Pigs, cattle, hamsters, dogs, cats	Diarrhea, less commonly bacteremia, proctitis
C. concisus	Human oral cavity	Periodontal disease, diarrhea, less commonly bacteremia
C. sputorum	Human oral cavity	Abscesses
C. curvus	Human oral cavity	Periodontitis, alveolar abscess
C. rectus	Human oral cavity	Periodontitis
C. mucosalis	Human oral cavity, pig	Diarrhea
C. gracilis	Human oral cavity	Periodontitis, appendicitis, bacteremia, abscesses

water or by direct contact with fecal material from infected animals or people. Reservoirs for *Campylobacter* species are shown in Table 157.1. Humans appear to be the only reservoir for the periodontal pathogens.

Outbreaks of diarrhea caused by *C. jejuni* and *C. coli* have been associated with consumption of improperly handled or undercooked poultry and, less frequently, red meat, unpasteurized milk, and contaminated water. Person-to-person transmission of *Campylobacter* has been reported, specifically when the index cases were young children who were incontinent of stool, such as children in child-care facilities and neonates of infected mothers. Intrafamilial spread is an uncommon finding.

According to a FoodNet surveillance report, the incidence of infection with *C. jejuni* in 2003 decreased to 12.6 per 100,000 persons. This incidence rate is close to the 2010 national health objective of 12.3 cases per 100,000 persons and appears to be due in part to programs directed at providers and health care consumers and improvements in food safety programs. The incidence of *C. jejuni* infection follows a bimodal age distribution, with the highest isolation rates occurring in infants and young children, followed by a second peak in people 15 to 30 years of age. The rate of asymptomatic carriage is low in economically developed countries, but may be as high as 40% in economically developing nations, particularly in areas with poor hygiene, limited access to water, free-roaming poultry in houses, and areas that lack adequate excreta disposal. In developing countries, isolation rates of *Campylobacter* are 20% to 40% among young children with diarrhea, with an annual incidence of two infections per child. Asymptomatic infections are common occurrences, especially in older children. Male and female subjects have equal rates of infection. In temperate climates, infections occur more frequently in summer and early fall, but in tropical climates, the incidence appears to be greater during the rainy season.

C. fetus subspecies *venerealis* causes abortion in sheep and cattle and has been isolated from bile, blood, intestine, and placenta of these animals. *C. fetus* subspecies *fetus* is associated primarily with bacteremia and extraintestinal infections in humans, with isolation rates peaking in children younger than 1 year of age. In adults, infection occurs predominantly in patients with other comorbidities, including underlying illnesses that may be associated with immunoincompetence. Perinatal infections caused by *C. fetus* have been associated with maternal infections during pregnancy or at the time of delivery. Infection with *C. fetus* comprises less than 0.5% of all *Campylobacter* species reported. *C. fetus* is not a recognized cause of gastroenteritis, but because the organism does not grow well at 42°C, at which stool cultures for *Campylobacter* are held, and because of the uncommon occurrence of disease, the incidence of *C. fetus* infection is unknown.

Pathogenesis

After ingestion, *C. jejuni* are killed rapidly by gastric acid, which is an effective barrier against infection. Controlled studies have shown a wide variation in the number of *C. jejuni* organisms needed to produce an infection. Although some people have symptoms after ingesting 500 organisms, others ingest more than 10^6 organisms without effect. Thus, the critical inoculum size is not characterized completely. If organisms survive the gastric milieu, they must attach to the intestinal epithelial cells for infection to persist. This attachment apparently occurs because of the ability of *C. jejuni* to penetrate the mucous layer and to adhere to apical surfaces of host intestinal cells. *In vitro* adherence occurs through both specific and nonspecific adhesion-receptor interactions that involve numerous bacterial surface-associated proteins and glycolipids, namely, flagella, lipopolysaccharides, and surface structures of the outer membrane of bacteria. The attachment and subsequent uptake of *C. jejuni* into enterocytes is regulated at least by nonfimbriated bacterial surface proteins that bind to specific fucosylated oligosaccharide cell receptors.

After *C. jejuni* adhere to epithelial cells, the organisms are capable of causing illness by three postulated mechanisms. The first involves cell attachment and production of an enterotoxin, similar to cholera toxin, with subsequent development of secretory diarrhea. Second, like *Shigella*, bacteria can penetrate and proliferate within the intestinal epithelium and produce at least two cytotoxins, causing cell damage and death, that can be manifested as bloody diarrhea. The third mechanism, referred to as translocation, manifests by bacteria penetrating the epithelial lining without causing cellular damage and then proliferating in the lamina propria and mesenteric lymph nodes. These organisms then can reach the bloodstream to cause extraintestinal infection such as mesenteric adenitis, arthritis, meningitis, and cholecystitis. *C. jejuni* infection also has resulted in a variety of immune-mediate conditions.

Clinical Manifestations

Clinical manifestations of infection caused by *Campylobacter* depend on the species involved and characteristics of the host, such as age, immunosuppression, or underlying chronic and debilitating diseases. Acute diarrhea is the most common clinical presentation, and more than 90% of diarrheal cases caused by *Campylobacter* species are due to *C. jejuni* and *C. coli*. However, overall estimates may be inaccurate because culture techniques used in many laboratories may not detect other species or differentiate between these two species, which are clinically indistinguishable. Approximately 5% to 10% of cases of diarrhea caused by *C. jejuni* in the United States are caused by *C. coli*. After an incubation period of 1 to 7 days, patients typically experience prodromal symptoms of fever, headache, and myalgia. Diarrhea, accompanied by nausea, vomiting, and abdominal cramps, usually occurs within 24 hours, with stools that vary from loose and watery to grossly bloody. Substantial differences in the clinical presentation of diarrhea occur in children from economically developed compared with children residing in developing countries. The incidence of bloody diarrhea is greater than 50% in most studies conducted in developed countries, but in developing nations, watery diarrhea is the most frequent presentation; bloody diarrhea occurs in fewer than 20% of cases. In economically developing countries, however, *C. jejuni* is the pathogen most commonly isolated from children with dysentery, followed by *Shigella*, *Escherichia coli*, and *Entamoeba histolytica*. The frequency of stools varies, but many patients have at least 1 day with more than ten stools. Acute resolution is the rule, but diarrhea lasts longer than 2 weeks in 20% of cases, and chronic diarrhea accompanied by failure to thrive may occur in some children.

Abdominal pain affects more than 90% of patients older than 2 years of age and can be severe enough to mimic appendicitis. The complex of acute colitis with bloody stools, tenesmus, and low-grade fever has been reported and needs to be distinguished from inflammatory conditions such as ulcerative colitis or Crohn colitis. Thus, when this symptom complex occurs in an older child or adolescent, the illness can be confused easily with ulcerative colitis. Exclusion of *C. jejuni* infection is important if a diagnosis of inflammatory bowel disease is suspected. Immunoreactive complications as a result of *Campylobacter* infection have been described and include Guillain-Barré syndrome, a leading cause of acute flaccid paralysis; the Miller-Fisher syndrome, a variant characterized by ophthalmoplegia, areflexia, and ataxia; or a more dramatic presentation of an acute motor axonal neuropathy, a rapidly progressive tetraplegia associated with respiratory failure; reactive arthritis; Reiter syndrome (asymmetric arthritis, urethritis, and ophthalmitis in HLA B27-positive patients); erythema nodosum; and immunoproliferative states.

Bloodstream and extraintestinal infections are uncommon events, occurring more frequently in malnourished children or patients with chronic debilitating illnesses or immunosuppression. Bacteremia has been estimated to occur in one in 3,000 children with enteritis and in one in 170 in the elderly. Bacteremia almost always is transient and asymptomatic, although secondary bacteremia with a focal infection, such as meningitis, pneumonia, endocarditis, or thrombophlebitis, can occur. Additionally, infection can be severe or chronic with relapses that can persist for weeks, mostly in immunosuppressed patients. *C. jejuni* is the *Campylobacter* species most commonly isolated from immunosuppressed patients, followed by *C. fetus*. In developing countries, however, other species, including *C. jejuni* subspecies doylei, *C. upsaliensis*, and *C. hyointestinalis* have been isolated. *C. fetus* infections in children occur mainly during the perinatal period. This predilection may be caused by the ability of *C. fetus* to colonize the genital tract and colon and by tropism for fetal tissue. Perinatal *C. fetus* infections can induce abortion, stillbirth, premature labor, or neonatal sepsis and meningitis, with considerable morbidity and mortality rates that can be as high as 80%. Extraintestinal infections caused by *C. jejuni* are rare occurrences. Septicemia, meningitis, cholecystitis, hepatitis, pancreatitis, peritonitis, urinary tract infection, and septic arthritis have been reported. Other species of *Campylobacter* infect humans less commonly (Table 157.1).

Campylobacter are microaerophilic, requiring 5% oxygen, 10% carbon dioxide, and 85% nitrogen for optimal growth. Gas-generating envelopes that reproducibly provide the correct environment are available commercially. Although all *Campylobacter* species grow at 37°C, the optimal temperature for growth of a thermophilic group of *Campylobacter* composed of *C. jejuni*, *Campylobacter coli*, and *Campylobacter lari* is 42°C. The slow growth of *Campylobacter* requires selective media that allow isolation from more rapidly growing enteric flora. Because *C. jejuni* is the species that usually causes intestinal illness, many laboratories place stool specimens on one of the selective media and incubate stool cultures at 42°C to help optimally isolate this organism. With this method, several other species will be missed, especially those not thermotolerant and susceptible to cephalothin.

Agglutination, complement fixation, bactericidal selection, immunofluorescence, enzyme immunoassays, and DNA probes have been used for making a serologic diagnosis of *C. jejuni* infection, but they are of limited value in the clinical arena. Polymerase chain reaction (PCR) for detection of *Campylobacter* in feces has been developed; PCR has been shown to be more sensitive than is culture and can be used to differentiate species.

Isolation of *Campylobacter* from blood and other sterile body sites does not present the same problem as does isolation from feces, although sensitivities of systems vary. Growth occurs in standard blood culture media, but the organism grows slowly, requiring that culture bottles be kept for at least 7 days. *C. fetus* infection usually is diagnosed by blood culture; these organisms rarely are isolated from stool.

Diagnosis

Clinical diagnosis of *Campylobacter* diarrhea is difficult to establish because of variations in the clinical presentation, from watery to grossly bloody diarrhea, and a similarity in presentation to other causes of diarrhea. However, when inflammatory diarrhea with bloody stools, fever, and abdominal pain occurs, *Campylobacter* always should be considered in the differential diagnosis. A microbiologic diagnosis is needed to differentiate *C. jejuni* from other causes of colitis such as *Salmonella*, *Shigella*, Shigatoxin-producing *E. coli*, or *E. histolytica*. Direct examination of stool with Wright stain often shows the presence of fecal leukocytes. Rectal swabs can be cultured for *C. jejuni*, but rectal swabs are less effective than are stool samples for growing the organism. A stool transport media should be used, especially for rectal swabs. *Campylobacter* species have fastidious culture requirements, and these organisms can be slow growing. In addition, species other than *C. jejuni* and *C. coli* may be significantly underdiagnosed as causes of gastrointestinal tract disease because of (a) use of selective media and growth conditions that lack hydrogen that may inhibit their growth, (b) procedures used in many microbiology laboratories that do not identify *Campylobacter* isolates to the species level, and (c) lack of use of stool filtration techniques.

Ideally, for isolating *Campylobacter* from feces, two systems are used: selective enrichment media containing antimicrobial agents to specifically suppress the colonic microflora and a filtration method using cellulose membranes. The use of the filtration method allows for isolation of species such as *C. jejuni* subspecies doylei, *C. upsaliensis*, *C. fetus*, and *C. hyointestinalis* that are inhibited by antimicrobial agents contained in the selective enrichment medium. Studies using both the selective medium and the filtration method demonstrate that *Campylobacter* species other than *C. jejuni* may account for 30% to 60% of all *Campylobacter* isolates from patients with diarrhea. When both isolation methods were used, 73% of all *Campylobacter* isolates were *C. jejuni*, 13% were *C. upsaliensis*, and 12% were *C. coli* in one study.

Treatment

Due to the primarily self-limited behavior of most *Campylobacter* infections, supportive therapy is the preferred initial approach. Thus, rehydration and correction of electrolyte abnormalities are the mainstay of treatment for patients with break; *C. jejuni* enteritis. Most patients with *Campylobacter* gastroenteritis do not require antimicrobial therapy because infections generally are self-limited. Appropriate antimicrobial therapy should be considered if patients are acutely ill at the time bacteriologic diagnosis is established or if they have complications, systemic infection, or immunosuppression. Symptoms in patients who have been exposed to someone with known *Campylobacter* diarrhea may warrant giving empiric treatment pending culture results. Treating toddlers in child-care centers may be reasonable to prevent secondary spread of the organism. When antimicrobial therapy is indicated, azithromycin or erythromycin is recommended. Erythromycin resistance in the United States generally is stable at less than 5%, whereas higher resistance patterns to azithromycin and erythromycin have been reported from some countries. Several placebo-controlled studies have shown erythromycin therapy to be of no clinical benefit if given late in the course of disease, although erythromycin does decrease fecal shedding of the organism. Excretion of the organism can persist for 2 weeks to 3 months in immunocompetent hosts not treated with an appropriate antimicrobial agent. If antimicrobial therapy is initiated early in the illness, reduced excretion of the organism and rapid resolution of symptoms occur (Table 157.2).

Fluoroquinolone compounds (e.g., ciprofloxacin, ofloxacin) are useful agents in treating *C. jejuni* infections of the gastrointestinal tract in adults, although an alarming emergence of resistance has been documented worldwide. In the United States, resistance has been increasing over the course of time as reported in the CDC National Antimicrobial Resistance Monitoring System (NARMS) (http://www.cdc.gov/NARMS/). Ciprofloxacin is licensed in the United States as treatment for *C. jejuni* enteritis for people 18 years of age and older.

TABLE 157.2

RECOMMENDED ANTIMICROBIAL THERAPY FOR *CAMPYLOBACTER JEJUNI* AND *CAMPYLOBACTER FETUS* INFECTIONS

Organism	Recommended	Alternative
Campylobacter jejuni/coli	Azithromycin Erythromycin Fluoroquinolone*	Gentamicin
C. fetus	Gentamicin Meropenem Imipenem	Tetracycline[†]

*Not licensed for people younger than 18 years of age.
[†]Generally not recommended for pregnant women or children younger than 8 years of age.

Infections with *C. fetus* usually are systemic and require antimicrobial therapy. Although *C. fetus* often is susceptible to erythromycin, the preferred drugs are aminoglycosides, meropenem, or imipenem, depending on the susceptibility pattern. Ampicillin, chloramphenicol, and extended-spectrum cephalosporins also may be effective against serious *C. fetus* infections.

HELICOBACTER

Helicobacter pylori have been implicated as a cause of chronic, chronic-active, and atrophic gastritis and as the causative agent in the pathogenesis of duodenal and, to a lesser extent, gastric ulcers. In addition, *H. pylori* infection is an important cause of gastric adenocarcinoma and B-cell gastric mucosa–associated lymphoid tissue (MALT) lymphomas. *H. pylori* infection often is acquired during childhood, and often persists for decades or for a person's lifetime. In children and adults, the infection usually is asymptomatic. However, although no studies to date have demonstrated a definitive association, *H. pylori* infection may be associated with upper gastrointestinal tract symptoms (e.g., nausea, vomiting, anorexia) or chronic persistent epigastric abdominal pain. Moreover, *H. pylori* infection can cause failure to thrive and now has satisfied Koch's postulates as causing iron deficiency anemia. Gastric *Helicobacter* primarily inhabit the stomach either within or beneath the mucous layer adjacent to the epithelium but may adhere tightly to the gastric epithelia via specific (ligand-receptor) and nonspecific mechanisms. To date, no documented isolations of *H. pylori* from extra gastric sites or from the bloodstream have been reported. Evidence-based clinical practice guidelines for evaluating and treating children with *H. pylori* infection have been developed in Canada, Europe, and the United States.

Etiology

The Helicobacteriaceae family (Greek, *helicos*, spiral; *baktron*, rod) comprises spiral-shaped, gram-negative, microaerobic bacteria with multiple (four to six) flagella. The genus *Helicobacter* contains 20 species validated by international rules of nomenclature, with other species pending. Nine species, including *H. cinaedi*, *H. heilmannii*, and *H. fennelliae*, have been identified in stomachs or intestines of humans. The genus includes spiral or curved bacilli ranging from 0.3 to 1.0 μm in width and 1.5 to 10.0 μm in length. Most *Helicobacter* species grow poorly or not at all in routine aerobic atmospheres. Human *Helicobacter* have been observed and isolated from the gastrointestinal and hepatobiliary tracts of other mammals including dogs, cats, ferrets, sheep, and rodents and from chick-

ens. Sequencing of *C. jejuni* and *H. pylori* genomes has emphasized differences between *Campylobacter* and *Helicobacter* organisms.

Epidemiology

Helicobacter strains are species-specific. *H. pylori* predominantly causes human infection but occasionally occurs in domestic animals, such as kittens, puppies, and pigs, which are thought to become infected through human feces. *H. pylori* have been isolated from patients with gastrointestinal tract symptoms and asymptomatic persons from different parts of the world. *H. pylori* are ubiquitous pathogens, with prevalence rates that differ among populations and ethnic groups. Seroepidemiologic studies in different countries have shown an age-related increase in the prevalence of antibodies to *H. pylori*. *H. pylori*-specific antibodies seldom are found among asymptomatic children from industrialized countries, but children from developing regions acquire the infection early in life, as seen by a prevalence of more than 70% among children younger than 10 years of age in countries like Bolivia or Soweto. Although only 40% of adults from developed countries have antibodies, the prevalence among adults is greater than 90% in developing countries. The annual incidence of *H. pylori* infection in children is approximately 4% to 15% in economically developing countries and approximately 6% to 8% by the time the individual reaches age 10 years in economically developed countries. Serologic studies of Australian Aboriginals, who are known to be free of duodenal ulcers, have demonstrated a prevalence of *H. pylori* antibody of approximately 2%, but in regions of the world with a high prevalence of duodenal ulcers and gastric cancer, such as Japan, Hawaii, central Africa, southern China, and Mexico, antibody prevalence is high.

Transmission of *H. pylori* to humans may occur by one of three modes: iatrogenic, fecal-oral, and oral-oral. Iatrogenic transmission occurs through contaminated fiberoptic endoscopes and nasogastric tubes and may be an occupational hazard in health care providers. The fecal-oral route has been implicated as an important mode of transmission. *H. pylori* have been isolated from feces, mainly in children, and have been identified by PCR in stools. Contaminated drinking water and vegetables irrigated with contaminated water have been associated with a significantly higher prevalence of *H. pylori* infection. Evidence of oral-oral transmission exists from studies in Africa, where a greater risk of development of infection in children was shown when food was premasticated by mothers to feed their infants. The isolation and presence of *H. pylori* DNA in dental plaque, saliva, and vomitus suggest that oral-oral or gastro-oral transmission occurs.

H. pylori infection is transmitted primarily in the household by direct person-to-person spread. Several studies have demonstrated a clustering of *H. pylori* infection in families, with a significantly higher proportion of infected household members when a child, particularly if younger than 6 years of age, is found to be colonized with this organism. Specific hygiene practices and intimate contact may be associated with intrafamily spread of the organism. Evidence supports the notion that children serve as the primary source of infection in families.

The importance of crowding has been suggested by several studies, which consistently have shown that the chance of *H. pylori* infection occurring is greater in crowded conditions. In addition, a higher prevalence of *H. pylori* antibodies in orphans and institutionalized mentally delayed persons also suggests person-to-person spread. *H. pylori* also may be transmitted by animals, as suggested by the higher prevalence of infection among slaughterhouse workers, who have direct contact with freshly cut animal parts; among persons exposed to cattle; or among persons who consume internal organs. The finding of *H. pylori* in secretions and feces of cats and sheep indicates a possible zoonotic transmission. In summary, documented risk factors include low socioeconomic status, household crowding, poor sanitation or hygiene, and living in an economically developing country.

Pathogenesis

H. pylori overlays gastric epithelium and is associated with active inflammation of the mucosa. Gastritis associated with *H. pylori* affects primarily the mucus-secreting antral-type gastric epithelium and eventually involves the stomach fundus. These lesions are known as *chronic active* or *chronic gastritis*. *H. pylori* have not been associated with chemical (alcohol or nonsteroidal antiinflammatory drugs) or atrophic autoimmune fundal-type gastritis, which may be seen in association with pernicious anemia and which occurs when parietal cells are destroyed but mucus-secreting cells are not affected. *H. pylori*–associated gastritis has been reproduced experimentally in volunteers, and several animal models of gastritis have been developed. Animal models for ulcers (mice) and cancer (mongolian gerbils) also have been developed. The histologic changes of gastritis associated with detection and isolation of *H. pylori* revert with specific antimicrobial treatment, and if reinfection occurs, the gastroduodenal mucosal inflammation returns.

H. pylori have a unique biologic niche for which they are particularly adapted. The organism does not colonize any other epithelial cell type except gastric epithelia, it is not found systemically (i.e., in the bloodstream), and it is not found further down the intestinal tract. The presence of gastric metaplasia tissue in the duodenum provides a supportive milieu for *H. pylori* colonization just distal to the stomach. Active inflammation results in development of a duodenal ulcer. In patients with recurrent duodenal ulcers, *H. pylori* are found in the margins of the ulcer and in the inflamed antral mucosa. Several putative virulence factors of *H. pylori* have been implicated in the pathogenesis of gastritis and include flagella, which allow penetration and motility through the thick viscous gastric mucous layer; production of protease with mucolytic activity, thereby elaborating urea that is abundant in the gastric mucus and is a major substrate of *H. pylori* metabolism; adhesins, which confer the ability to attach to gastric epithelial cells; production of a potent urease enzyme that facilitates survival of organisms in the hostile gastric acid environment via urea metabolism and ammonia/CO_2 elaboration; the *vacA* protein; and cytotoxin. One of the dominant virulence factors associated with *H. pylori* pathogenesis is the *cag* (cytotoxicity associated gene) pathogenicity island present in most *H. pylori* strains. However, many recent studies demonstrated that disease outcomes in humans infected by *H. pylori* are not just the direct cause of a more virulent strain or strains. Conversely, it is the combination of a genetically programmed host immune/inflammatory response and infection with a specific *H. pylori* strain type, potentially modulated by environmental exposures (i.e., diet) that results in the varying severity of disease phenotypes.

H. pylori have been associated with gastric neoplasia. Sufficient epidemiologic evidence from a number of case-control and nested case-control cohort studies shows a high risk of development of gastric adenocarcinoma in adults infected with *H. pylori* and a stronger association when anti-*cagA* antibodies are found in serum. Original case-control studies demonstrated that a significant association exists among gastric cancer incidence, patient mortality, and *H. pylori* seropositivity. More recently, studies demonstrated a much higher prevalence of gastric adenocarcinoma and precursor lesions in families with a clustering of specific immune response determinant polymorphism (interleukin 1-beta). A low-grade primary gastric lymphoma, or more properly low-grade lymphoma, is another neoplastic lesion that occurs less frequently than does gastric adenocarcinoma. MALT lymphoma appears to have an even more definitive association with *H. pylori* infection, especially with *cagA*-expressing strains. Studies in adults and even children demonstrated that early stages of MALT lymphoma are cured by eradication of *H. pylori* with antimicrobial agents. In children with nodular gastritis, *cagA*-positive strains are identified more frequently than are *cagA*-negative strains, although whether this type of gastritis progresses to MALT lymphoma, atrophy, and gastric adenocarcinoma or persists as a chronic gastritis is unknown.

Clinical Manifestations

The spectrum of clinical manifestations of this chronic infection in children has not been defined well. The main clinical manifestations are present during adulthood, when the diagnosis is made, but little information exists on the natural history of *H. pylori* infection in its early stages during childhood, when the infection often is acquired. Although primary infection appears to be mainly asymptomatic, a similar spectrum of disease has been described in the pediatric population as in adults, ranging from gastritis, duodenal and (to a lesser extent) gastric ulcers, MALT lymphoma, and atrophic gastritis and intestinal metaplasia (i.e., precursor lesion for gastric cancer).

What appears to be clear is that the location of the gastric inflammatory infiltrate is one of the best predictors of disease sequelae, with antral predominant gastritis tending to be associated with higher levels of acid secretion, and is associated primarily with duodenal ulceration. Conversely, corpus or body-predominant, almost pan-gastritis is associated with the eventual development of gastric atrophy, decreased overall acid production, intestinal metaplasia, and eventually neoplasia and cancer. Studies are needed with large cohort sizes in disparate populations to determine which bacterial, host, and/or environmental factors dictate or influence disease outcomes.

Infection in young infants can present as an acute illness characterized by protracted vomiting that can be confused with upper gastrointestinal tract obstructive disorders. The youngest reported case of *H. pylori* infection, which presented with hematemesis, was a 5-month-old infant.

Symptoms of *H. pylori* Infection

Currently, the existence of a causal relationship between *H. pylori* infection and recurrent abdominal pain of childhood is not proven, in part because of poor study designs, lack of validated symptom-assessment instruments, and no placebo-controlled eradication trials with appropriate endpoints. In addition, although a relationship seems to exist between ulcer disease and abdominal symptoms, whether chronic gastritis causes symptoms in children remains unclear.

The relationship of social and familial factors with *H. pylori* infection and recurrent abdominal pain in children was analyzed in a population-based, cross-sectional study among preschool children aged 5 to 8 years. A clear association was found between recurrent abdominal pain with social and familial factors, but not with *H. pylori* infection.

The absence of symptoms may in itself not mean that no underlying gastroduodenal pathology is present, and a number of reports describe silent peptic ulcer disease. Thus, at present, more studies are needed to document clearly the association of symptoms with *H. pylori* infection and determine which individuals are more at risk for having long-term severe disease sequelae. Clinical entities associated with *H. pylori* infection are as follows: gastritis; acute active gastritis; and chronic gastritis, duodenitis, and duodenal ulcers.

Acute Active Gastritis. Although difficult at times to detect, anecdotal reports observed that after infection, symptoms may begin with epigastric pain, nausea, and vomiting that may last for a few days. Patients may improve rapidly and remain clinically asymptomatic, or mild symptoms that do not cause them to seek the care of a physician may persist. The pH of gastric juice usually is neutral or alkaline as a result of a decrease in gastric acid output, although this effect may be transient and hyperacidity can be found in some patients. This hypochlorhydria may persist for several weeks and may present with halitosis and mild gastrointestinal tract disturbances.

Chronic Gastritis, Duodenitis, and Duodenal Ulcer. The triad of antral gastritis, duodenitis, and duodenal or gastric ulcer visualized by endoscopy is associated with chronic and more severe gastrointestinal tract symptoms. Children may present with severe chronic and recurrent abdominal pain, anorexia, and failure to thrive or with persistent vomiting. Occasionally, hematemesis may be the first symptom. If *H. pylori* infection is associated with chronic gastritis alone, the only symptom may be recurrent abdominal pain or symptoms associated with nonulcerative dyspeptic syndrome or, occasionally, chronic diarrhea associated with nonulcerative dyspeptic syndrome. Frequent endoscopic findings are nodular antritis and pyloric hyperemia, although normal gastric mucosa with histologic evidence of active gastritis is not an unusual finding.

The histopathology of the gastric mucosa in infected children from a population at high risk for developing gastric cancer was compared to the findings with infected children from a lower-risk population. In both populations, the inflammatory lesions were seen predominantly in the antrum. Compared with children from the lower-risk populations, children from the higher-risk population exhibited more severe polymorphonuclear neutrophil infiltration, stromal and intraepithelial lymphocyte infiltration, mucus depletion, *H. pylori* colonization density, lower regenerative activity, and increased representation of T lymphocytes and macrophages, whereas more abundant B lymphocytes were found in the lower-risk population. The immune phenotype differences observed in high- versus low-risk populations were considered by the authors to contribute to the pathogenesis of gastric cancer.

Estragastrointestinal Diseases and *H. pylori*

The role of *H. pylori* in hematologic diseases—in particular, idiopathic thrombocytopenic purpura (ITP) in adults and iron-deficiency anemia in children—has been studied. Eradication of *H. pylori* has been associated with platelet recovery in adults with ITP, but results of studies in children with ITP and *H. pylori* infection have been mixed. Additional research into the involvement of *H. pylori* infection in ITP in children is needed.

Studies have demonstrated that iron-deficiency anemia may be due to clinically inapparent *H. pylori* gastritis. In addition, *H. pylori* eradication in children with long-standing iron deficiency anemia was associated with stable normalization of iron stores. *H. pylori* infection may be involved in select cases of iron deficiency anemia of unknown origin.

Diagnosis

Tests for diagnosis of *H. pylori* infection can be categorized as invasive or noninvasive. Invasive tests are based on endoscopy and direct assessment of gastric biopsies, and noninvasive tests are based on immunologic response (serum or salivary antibodies against *H. pylori*), detection of metabolic products of *H. pylori* (urease activity), or stool antigen detection. *H. pylori*

rarely are isolated from blood, but enterohepatic *Helicobacter* organisms may cause invasive infections in adults but have not been described in children. Unlike *Campylobacter*, *H. pylori* usually is diagnosed by nonculture methods such as histology, serology, PCR, or urease testing. However, in some patients, organisms may be needed for susceptibility testing.

Upper gastrointestinal endoscopy with biopsies remains the "gold standard" in diagnosing *H. pylori*. Routine duodenal biopsies yield additional pathologic findings that otherwise could have been missed, and thus offer an important observation to incorporate into clinical practice.

For isolation of *Helicobacter* species from clinical specimens, homogenized biopsies from the gastric antrum should be transported in appropriate media to the laboratory, where specimens are placed in a selective and enriched medium at 37°C under microaerobic conditions for 5 to 10 days. The organism has been isolated almost exclusively from gastric mucosa; isolates seldom are obtained from stool specimens. *H. pylori* also have been isolated from dental plaque. PCR for amplification of a conserved region of the 16S rRNA gene is a specific and sensitive method. PCR has been used to amplify *H. pylori* DNA in saliva, stools, gastric mucosa, and gastric juice. PCR assays also have been developed to amplify *H. pylori* virulence markers, such as the *cagA* and *vacA* genes and *vacA* gene regions, directly from gastric biopsies.

Organisms usually can be visualized easily on histologic sections using Gram, hematoxylin-eosin, silver, Giemsa, Genta, or acridine orange staining. For obtaining a presumptive diagnosis, several commercial tests are available for detection of urease production in biopsy specimens, although their sensitivity and specificity are lower than are those of silver stains of histologic preparations.

H. pylori produce a urease, which degrades host urea into ammonia and that neutralizes its microenvironment, and carbon dioxide, which can be detected by breath tests used to detect *H. pylori*. Noninvasive, commercially available tests include serum antibody detection by enzyme immunoassay and the 13C and 14C urea breath tests. The breath test is based on the finding that *H. pylori* hydrolyze urea, which is metabolized to ammonia and bicarbonate. The bicarbonate is absorbed and excreted as CO_2 by the lungs. If urea is labeled with 13C or 14C and the labeled urea is metabolized, it can be detected in the breath as labeled CO_2, which can be measured and used as a marker for *H. pylori* infection. A high rate of false-positive breath tests occur in children younger than 6 years of age. Detection of antibodies in saliva using a commercial device has had promising results and may simplify establishing the diagnosis.

The urea breath test using techniques such as a novel laser associated ratio analysis (LARA) 13C urea breath test and the stool antigen test, particularly new-generation monoclonal stool antigen tests, have been studied and demonstrate promise for use in the pediatric population. These investigations demonstrated the utility of these noninvasive diagnostic assays in the pediatric population both for diagnosis of *H. pylori* infection and as a test for cure in a wider range of age groups. However, further validation is required for these assays in children younger than 6 years of age. The polyclonal stool antigen tests demonstrate variable performance and have less favorable accuracy compared to the breath test and newer-generation monoclonal stool antigen tests. The noninvasive urea breath test and stool antigen test have been adopted as part of the standard of care for children with suspected *H. pylori* infection in Europe, but they have yet to be incorporated into clinical practice guidelines in North America.

The ^{13}C urea breath test is the method of choice to follow the response to treatment. *H. pylori* titers decrease after 3 to 6 months in subjects who have had their infections eradicated, but 50% do not become seronegative, even after prolonged follow-up. Therefore, the recommendation is that serology testing not be included in the clinical management, for both diagnosis and a test for cure, in children suspected to have *H. pylori* infection.

Treatment

H. pylori infection is curable with regimens of multiple antimicrobial agents. Antimicrobial resistance and noncompliance are leading causes of treatment failure. Multiple therapeutic regimens have been shown to be effective in curing patients infected with *H. pylori*. Use of single agents has been found to be ineffective for curing infection in most patients. Two or three drugs taken for 14 to 21 days are recommended for treatment. Treatment is indicated in symptomatic children only when *H. pylori* infection has been confirmed by culture, serology, or breath test. Treatment is not recommended in asymptomatic children or in children with nonspecific gastrointestinal tract symptoms, although close follow-up is recommended. Success in treatment of *H. pylori* infection depends on several factors including the susceptibility of the isolate or at least the susceptibility pattern in the specific geographic area where the patient lives.

Antibiotic resistance is still a significant factor affecting the outcome of *H. pylori* treatment and may be the sole reason for tertiary care center referrals for people infected with *H. pylori*. During recent years, multiple studies around the world have shown a high resistance of *H. pylori* to metronidazole and clarithromycin. Until now, resistance to amoxicillin has not been observed in Europe. However, cases of amoxicillin-resistant *H. pylori* strains from other parts of the world have been reported. Moreover, *H. pylori* resistance to clarithromycin appears to be higher in children than in adults for reasons that are yet to be determined. In addition, the *H. pylori* Antimicrobial Resistance Monitoring Program (HARP) is a multicenter network that provides ongoing prospective antimicrobial resistance and associated risk factor data for *H. pylori* in North America. HARP has shown that resistance to antimicrobial drugs used commonly to treat *H. pylori* infection is widespread and varies from year to year, particularly for clarithromycin and metronidazole.

The goal of treatment is eradication of *H. pylori*, which can be achieved only with a multidrug therapy consisting of a proton pump inhibitor and two or three of the following drugs in various combinations: clarithromycin, metronidazole, or amoxicillin or, in adults, tetracycline (Table 157.3). Bismuth-based salts have been replaced by proton pump inhibitors (lansoprazole, omeprazole, pantoprazole, esomeprazole, rabeprazole) or histamine$_2$ antagonists (cimetidine, famotidine, nizatidine, ranitidine), with a higher efficacy and fewer side effects. The current standard of practice is to treat with a triple-therapy regimen. Triple therapy should be given for 7 to 14 days, and the outcome should be followed with either the breath test or, if indicated, an endoscopy and gastric biopsies and culture. For patients in whom eradication therapy fails, the risk of developing antibiotic resistance is high. Referral to a gastroenterologist is, therefore, indicated for endoscopy and susceptibility testing of organisms obtained. Clearly, multicenter studies of *H. pylori* infection in the pediatric population, which include specific, randomized controlled eradication trials, are needed critically to extend current knowledge, develop better predictors of disease outcome, and determine which populations should be targeted for eradication therapy.

Suggested Readings

Campylobacter

Allos BM, Blaser MJ. *Campylobacter jejuni* and the expanding spectrum of related infections. *Clin Infect Dis* 1995;20:1092.

Bourke B, Chan VL, Sherman P. Investigation of an outbreak of *Campylobacter upsaliensis*: waiting in the wings. *Clin Microbiol Rev* 1998;11:440.

Centers for Disease Control and Prevention. National Antimicrobial Resistance Monitoring System (NARMS) for enteric bacteria Web site. Available at: www.cdc.gov/NARMS. Accessed.

Centers for Disease Control and Prevention. Preliminary FoodNet data on the incidence of foodborne illness—selected sites, United States, 2003. *MMWR Morb Mortal Wkly Rep* 2004;53:338.

Hadden RD, Gregson NA. Guillain-Barré syndrome and *Campylobacter jejuni* infection. *J Appl Microbiol* 2001;90:145s.

Pickering LK. Antimicrobial resistance among enteric pathogens. *Semin Pediatr Infect Dis* 2004;15:71.

Wassenaar TM. Toxin production by *Campylobacter* spp. *Clin Microb Rev* 1997; 10:466.

Helicobacter

Brown LM. *Helicobacter pylori*: epidemiology and routes of transmission. *Epidemiol Rev* 2000;22:283.

Drumm B, Koletzko S, Oderda G. *Helicobacter pylori* infection in children: a consensus statement. European Task Force on *Helicobacter pylori*. *J Pediatr Gastroenterol Nutr* 2000;31:207.

Duck WM, Sobel J, Pruckler JM, et al. Antimicrobial resistance incidence and risk factors among *Helicobacter pylori*—infected persons, United States. *Emerg Infect Dis* 2004;10:1088.

Gold BD, Abbott M, Colletti R, et al. Evidence based guidelines for an approach to the diagnosis and treatment of *Helicobacter pylori* infection in children: recommendations for diagnosis and treatment. *J Pediatr Gastroenterol Nutr* 2000;31:490.

Gottrand F, Kalach N, Spyckerelle C, et al. Omeprazole combined with amoxicillin and clarithromycin in the eradication of *Helicobacter pylori* in children with gastritis: a prospective randomized double-blind trial. *J Pediatr* 2001;139:664.

Höcker M, Hohenberger P. *Helicobacter pylori* virulence factors-one part of a big picture. *Lancet* 2003;362:1231.

Imrie C, Rowland M, Bourke B, Drumm B. Limitations to 13C-urea breath testing for *Helicobacter pylori* in infants. *J Pediatr* 2001;139:734.

McMahon BJ, Hennessy TW, Bensler JM, et al. The relationship among previous antimicrobial use, antimicrobial resistance, and treatment outcomes for *Helicobacter pylori* infections. *Ann Intern Med* 2003;139:463.

Passaro DJ, Chosy EJ, Personnet J. *Helicobacter pylori*: consensus and controversy. *Clin Infect Dis* 2002;35:298.

Pérez-Pérez GI, Sack RB, Reid R, et al. Transient and persistent *Helicobacter pylori* colonization in native American children. *J Clin Microbiol* 2003;41: 2401.

Sherman P, Hassall E, Hunt RH, et al. Canadian *Helicobacter pylori* Study Group Consensus Conference on the approach to *H. pylori* infection in children and adolescents. *Can J Gastroenterol* 1999;13:553.

Solnick JV, Schauer DB. Emergence of diverse *Helicobacter* species in the pathogenesis of gastric and enterohepatic diseases. *Clin Microbiol Rev* 2001;14:59.

Suerbaum, S, Michetti P. *Helicobacter pylori* infection. *N Engl J Med* 2002; 347: 1175.

TABLE 157.3

THERAPY FOR *HELICOBACTER PYLORI* INFECTIONS

Drug of Choice	Alternative Drugs
Proton pump inhibitor*	Bismuth subsalicylate plus
Plus clarithromycin	Metronidazole plus tetracycline†
Plus either amoxicillin or metronidazole	Plus either a proton pump inhibitor or H2-blocker*

*Proton pump inhibitors available in the United States are lansoprazole, omeprazole, pantoprazole, esomeprazole, and rabeprazole. Available H$_2$ blockers include cimetidine, famotidine, nizatidine, and ranitidine.
†Tetracycline generally is not recommended for pregnant women or children younger than 8 years of age.

CHAPTER 158 ■ CAT-SCRATCH DISEASE

KENNETH M. BOYER

Cat-scratch disease is a subacute, regional lymphadenitis syndrome that occurs after cutaneous inoculation. Contact with cats, in the form of a scratch by claws or teeth, is associated strongly with the illness, although cases without known cat contact have been reported. A fastidious proteobacterium, *Bartonella henselae*, is the cause. Complications of the disease occur, but generally it has an indolent chronic course for 2 to 3 months, followed by spontaneous resolution.

ETIOLOGY

Discovery of the cause and transmission mechanism of cat-scratch disease has been one of the fascinating recent stories in the field of infectious diseases. The initial breakthrough was the visualization of small, pleomorphic bacilli in biopsy materials obtained from nodes and primary granulomas and stained by the Warthin-Starry silver impregnation technique. In lymph nodes, the bacilli were seen intracellularly in capillaries and in macrophages lining sinuses in or near the germinal centers.

B. henselae was identified first in 1990 in patients with acquired immunodeficiency syndrome (AIDS) who had unique opportunistic infections, either bacillary angiomatosis or bacillary peliosis hepatitis. Lesions in both conditions had been noted to contain argyrophilic bacteria similar to those seen in children with cat-scratch disease. Polymerase chain reaction amplification of ribosomal RNA in biopsy specimens led to identification of bacterial genetic material most closely related to *B. quintana*, the rickettsia-like agent known to cause trench fever, and *B. bacilliformis*, the cause of bartonellosis. After successful cultivation, the new species has been named *B. henselae*. Frequently, children with cat-scratch disease develop specific antibodies against this organism, which now has been cultured from affected lymph nodes and also from the blood of epidemiologically related cats. In addition, *B. henselae*-specific DNA sequences have been amplified from cat-scratch skin test antigens.

EPIDEMIOLOGY AND TRANSMISSION

Cat-scratch disease is transmitted by cutaneous inoculation. In the great majority of cases, a history of a cat scratch, often by a kitten younger than 6 months, can be elicited. Play may be more frequent with kittens than with older cats, and kittens are less likely to have been declawed. Interestingly, bacillary angiomatosis in adult patients with AIDS frequently is associated with a history of cat scratch.

Cat-scratch disease occurs more commonly in children than in adults, with the peak in case numbers falling in patients between the ages of 5 and 14 years. Frequently, clustering of cases within families has been noted, generally in association with the acquisition of new pets. Veterinarians as an occupational group appear to have a greater likelihood of exposure to the disease. An increased prevalence of skin test reactivity among veterinarians and asymptomatic relatives within family case clusters indicates that some infections may be subclinical.

Cats are the zoonotic reservoir of *B. henselae*. In one study, 81% of cat sera were positive for antibodies. In another, 41% of apparently healthy cats were bacteremic. Cat fleas (*Ctenocephalides felis*) appear to be the major vector for transmission among cats. Their possible role in transmission to humans is unknown.

PATHOLOGY

The pathology of the primary inoculation site is similar to that of the affected regional lymph node. Both show a characteristic central avascular necrotic area surrounded by lymphocytes, with some giant cells and histiocytes. Three evolutionary stages are recognized within affected lymph nodes; all may coexist in the same node. Initially, generalized enlargement of the node with thickening of the cortex and hypertrophy of the germinal centers occurs. Lymphocytes are the predominant cell type, and epithelioid granulomas containing multinucleate giant cells may be scattered throughout the node. In the middle stage, granulomas become distributed more densely, fuse, and are infiltrated with polymorphonuclear leukocytes. Central necrosis of the epithelioid granulomas begins at this stage. Progression of the process leads to formation of large, pus-filled sinuses that are the chief late feature. The capsule of the node may rupture, allowing pus to drain into surrounding tissues, in turn resulting in a fibrotic inflammatory reaction and binding of the node to adjacent structures. The early stage of the lesion may resemble lymphoma or sarcoidosis; in later stages, the histopathology resembles tularemia, lymphogranuloma venereum, brucellosis, or infection with mycobacteria.

CLINICAL MANIFESTATIONS

After an incubation period ranging from 3 to 30 days (usually between 7 and 12 days), one or more red papules measuring 2 to 5 mm in diameter develop at the site of cutaneous inoculation, often within the line of a previous cat scratch. Although often overlooked, such primary lesions were uncovered in more than 90% of affected patients after a careful search in one series. They persist until the development of lymphadenopathy, which generally occurs in 1 to 4 weeks.

Chronic lymphadenitis is the hallmark of cat-scratch disease, most frequently affecting the first or second sets of nodes draining the site of inoculation. Intervening lymphangitis does not occur. The sites affected most frequently, in decreasing order of incidence, are the axillary, cervical, submandibular, preauricular, epitrochlear, femoral, and inguinal lymph node groups. Involvement of more than one lymph node group, either within the same regional drainage or at an unrelated site, is present in 10% to 20% of cases. At a given site, approximately one-half of all cases will involve a single node, and the other half will involve multiple nodes.

Usually, affected nodes are tender, and the overlying skin becomes warm, red, and indurated. Between 10% and 40% of the nodes eventually suppurate, occasionally with formation of a sinus tract to the skin surface. The duration of lymph node enlargement is 4 to 6 weeks, with persistence lasting as long as 12 months in exceptional cases. Frequently, nodes that have drained to the skin surface produce some residual scarring. Most patients lack constitutional symptoms. Elevated temperatures are documented in approximately 30% of patients and, when present, generally range between 38°C and 39°C. Other nonspecific symptoms may include malaise, anorexia, fatigue, and headache.

A distinctive manifestation of cat-scratch disease is Parinaud oculoglandular syndrome. The site of primary inoculation is the conjunctiva of one eye or the eyelid. Mild to moderate conjunctivitis accompanies the primary lesion. Preauricular lymph nodes are the corresponding unilateral site of adenopathy. The involved preauricular nodes may be within the substance of the parotid gland, but exocrine tissue typically is not involved. Although the oculoglandular syndrome may be induced by other agents, notably *Francisella tularensis*, the most common cause appears to be cat-scratch disease.

The most serious complication of cat-scratch disease is involvement of the central nervous system in the form of encephalopathy or encephalitis. High fever and convulsions develop within 6 weeks of the onset of lymphadenopathy, followed by alteration in the level of consciousness, headache, and muscle weakness. The cerebrospinal fluid is normal or shows minimal pleocytosis or elevated protein content. Electroencephalograms reveal diffuse slowing or focal abnormalities in most patients. Recovery has occurred without residua in nearly all the well-documented cases in the literature. A few patients have had a prolonged convalescence and required anticonvulsant therapy for persistent seizure foci. The incidence of encephalopathy is low, but it can be the presenting manifestation of cat-scratch disease.

Osteolytic bone lesions have been noted in several well-documented cases. In one affected patient, biopsy of a lesion in the ilium revealed a granulomatous reaction typical of cat-scratch disease. In all the reported cases, the involved bone site was anatomically remote from the site of primary inoculation, suggesting hematogenous spread.

Granulomatous hepatitis is another newly recognized systemic manifestation of cat-scratch disease. It typically presents as prolonged fever and abdominal pain, with or without lymphadenopathy. The reported cases have shown characteristic multiple hypodense lesions in the liver on computed tomographic scanning.

A distinctive clinical presentation of ocular involvement by *B. henselae* consists of acute visual loss, optic neuritis/neuroretinitis, and a striking pattern of stellate macular lipid exudates ("macular star"). Recovery of vision has occurred in most reported cases.

Other rare complications that have been ascribed to cat-scratch disease include erythema multiforme, thrombocytopenic purpura, mesenteric lymphadenitis, arthralgia, lymphedema, thyroiditis, and nontraumatic atlantoaxial dislocation (Grisel syndrome).

DIFFERENTIAL DIAGNOSIS

Several sets of criteria for the diagnosis of cat-scratch disease have been proposed. A current version assigns one point for subacute or chronic regional lymphadenopathy, two for cat contact, two for an inoculation site on physical examination, and two for a positive serologic test for antibodies against *B. henselae* by indirect immunofluorescence or enzyme immunoassay. A total of five points is strongly suggestive of the diagnosis; seven is definitive. *B. henselae* can be cultivated from affected nodes and detected by polymerase chain reaction amplification, but these techniques are available only in research settings. The cat-scratch skin test is considered obsolete.

The differential diagnosis of cat-scratch disease can include virtually all known causes of lymphadenopathy. As a general rule, the diagnosis is favored by chronicity, unilateral occurrence, tenderness, and characteristic sites of involvement, such as axillary, epitrochlear, and preauricular nodes. Cervical, femoral, inguinal, and generalized lymph node involvement is less specific for cat-scratch disease and necessitates more care in differential diagnosis.

The most common diagnoses in 85 patients with adenopathy and negative cat-scratch skin tests in one series were pyogenic lymphadenitis or abscess (29 patients), benign or malignant neoplasm (12 patients), and cervical adenitis caused by mycobacteria (10 patients). Malignant neoplasm can be ruled out definitively only by biopsy. Other conditions, such as tularemia, toxoplasmosis, plague, and Kawasaki disease, must be considered because of the need for specific therapy.

TREATMENT AND PROGNOSIS

Most often, the diagnosis of cat-scratch disease is considered when acute lymphadenitis fails to respond to empiric treatment with dicloxacillin or an oral cephalosporin. *In vitro* susceptibility of *B. henselae* has been demonstrated with penicillin G, amoxicillin, gentamicin, rifampin, erythromycin, clarithromycin, and azithromycin (which has the lowest minimal inhibitory concentration). In one uncontrolled retrospective study of hepatosplenic cat-scratch disease, rifampin treatment was associated with resolution of fever. Another small controlled trial demonstrated more rapid resolution of enlarged lymph nodes in children who had cat-scratch disease and were treated with azithromycin, 5 mg/kg/day (loading dose, 10 mg/kg) for 5 days. Suppurative nodes are treated best by needle aspiration, which should be repeated when necessary. Aspirated pus should be cultured, with an emphasis on the recovery of pyogenic organisms and mycobacteria. Generally, surgical excision of affected nodes is unnecessary, but it is indicated when uncertainty about the diagnosis or an atypical or prolonged course occurs. Incision and drainage should not be performed, as this procedure leads to prolonged drainage and formation of scars. In most patients, cat-scratch disease follows a benign course. Usually, systemic symptoms last less than 2 weeks. Affected nodes may be painful for several weeks and may remain enlarged for a number of months. Generally, in patients with such complications as encephalopathy, hepatic granulomas, neuroretinitis, or bone lesions, the disease runs a more prolonged course, but such patients also have a good long-term prognosis. More prolonged courses of azithromycin combined with rifampin have been used successfully in some cases. Reinfection appears to be an extremely rare occurrence.

PREVENTION

The only preventive approach to cat-scratch disease might be to avoid contact with cats, particularly aggressive play with young kittens. Control of flea infestation is a practical approach to preventing transmission between cats. There is no indication for destroying a family pet to which cases of cat-scratch disease have been attributed because the capacity for disease transmission appears to be transient. Declawing such a pet might be considered.

Suggested Readings

Adal KA, Cockerell CJ, Petri WA. Cat scratch disease, bacillary angiomatosis, and other infections due to *Rochalimaea* [*Bartonella henselae*]. *N Engl J Med* 1994;330:1509.

Arisee ES, Correa AG, Wagner ML, et al. Hepatosplenic cat-scratch disease and treatment. *Clin Infect Dis* 1999;28:778.

Bass JW, Freitas BC, Freitas AD, et al. Prospective, randomized, double-blind, placebo-controlled evaluation of azithromycin for treatment of cat scratch disease. *Pediatr Infect Dis J* 1998;17:447.

Carithers HA. Cat-scratch disease: notes on its history. *Am J Dis Child* 1970; 119:200.

Carithers HA. Oculoglandular syndrome of Parinaud: a manifestation of cat-scratch disease. *Am J Dis Child* 1978;132:1195.

Carithers HA, Margileth AM. Cat scratch disease. Acute encephalopathy and other neurologic manifestations. *Am J Dis Child* 1991;145:98.

Chomel BB, Kasten RW, Floyd-Hawkins K, et al. Experimental transmission of *Bartonella henselae* by the cat flea. *J Clin Microbiol* 1996;34:1952.

Corey B, Corey D. More on pet-associated illness. *N Engl J Med* 1986;315:461.

Giladi M, Kletter Y, Avidor B, et al. Enzyme immunoassay for the diagnosis of cat-scratch disease defined by polymerase chain reaction. *Clin Infect Dis* 2001;33:1852.

Herz AM, Lahey JM. Optic neuritis due to *Bartonella henselae*. *N Engl J Med* 2004;350:e1.

Wear DJ, Margileth AM, Hadfield TM, et al. Cat-scratch disease: a bacterial infection. *Science* 1983;221:1403.

Zangwill KM, Hamilton DH, Perkins BA, et al. Cat scratch disease in Connecticut. Epidemiology, risk factors, and evaluation of a new diagnostic test. *N Engl J Med* 1993;329:8.

CHAPTER 159 ■ DIPHTHERIA

JULIA A. MCMILLAN AND RALPH FEIGIN

Corynebacterium diphtheriae may infect the skin or the respiratory tract. Acute disease results when the infecting strain elaborates an extracellular protein toxin and the human host is not protected by antitoxin antibody.

ETIOLOGY

C. diphtheriae is a gram-positive, nonmotile, nonsporulating, pleomorphic bacillus. The organism was first described in 1826 by Brettoneau, who called it *la diphtherite* (Greek for *leather*) because of the leathery membrane formed in the throat of infected individuals. The clubbed shape of the organism led to the name *Corynebacterium*, from *coryne* (Greek for *club*). In 1884, Löffler grew *C. diphtheriae* in pure culture from patients with diphtheria and produced disease in animals. Subsequent investigation demonstrated that infection causes local invasion but that widespread complications, including neuropathy, carditis and arrhythmias, and adrenal hemorrhage are the result of a protein exotoxin. The toxin is produced only in *C. diphtheriae* that are lysogenic for a phage carrying the gene for toxin production. The quantity of toxin elaborated by lysogenic strains is increased by reduced concentration of inorganic iron in culture media and by exposure to ultraviolet light. The clinical significance of these *in vitro* findings is not known.

C. diphtheriae may be grown on a variety of selective media, including tellurite agar or specially enriched Löffler, Pai, or Tinsdale medium. Gram staining of typical colonies may provide presumptive identification after 24 to 48 hours. Toxin production is confirmed using the Elek immunoprecipitin technique, polymerase chain reaction, or an *in vivo* toxin neutralization test in guinea pigs. Toxigenic strains are not distinguishable by growth characteristics or morphology. Three biotypes of *C. diphtheriae*—*mitis*, *intermedius*, and *gravis*—are distinguishable by colony morphology, hemolysis, and fermentation reactions, but the toxin elaborated by all three is identical, and the severity of disease generally is not determined by the biotype isolated.

EPIDEMIOLOGY

Infection due to *C. diphtheriae* occurs throughout the world. Humans are the only known reservoir, although other "diphtheroids" are ubiquitous in nature. In the United States, approximately 125,000 cases were reported per year during the 1920s, with approximately 13,000 to 15,000 deaths annually. Frequency of disease fell sharply after widespread use of the diphtheria toxoid vaccine so that, during the 1980s and 1990s, five or fewer cases of respiratory disease were reported per year (51 total cases).

C. diphtheriae is acquired through contact with respiratory secretions or skin of an infected or colonized individual. Rarely, contaminated dust, fomites, or food has been thought to be the source of cutaneous infection. Asymptomatic carriage occurs but is infrequent in countries where vaccine use is prevalent. Immunization of 70% to 80% of a population is postulated to prevent endemic spread of disease.

Historically, diphtheria has occurred most often in children younger than 15 years, who usually are not immunized. In highly immunized populations, however, proportionally more older adolescents, adults, and elderly individuals are susceptible because of waning vaccine-related immunity. The U.S. goal of eradication of diphtheria among individuals up to 25 years old by the year 2000 was prompted by the success of widespread immunization. Less than five cases per year have been reported in the United States during the past 5 years.

The incubation period after exposure is approximately 2 to 5 days. Communicability among untreated infected persons continues for up to 2 weeks and is reduced to fewer than 4 days with treatment. Chronic carriage persists occasionally, even in treated individuals. Among nonimmunized populations, diphtheria occurs most often during fall and winter, although summer outbreaks have occurred. Disease spreads more quickly and is more prevalent in poor socioeconomic conditions where crowding occurs and immunization rates are low. The vulnerability of populations in which large numbers of children and adults remain unprotected by vaccine was demonstrated during the early 1990s in the newly independent states of the former Soviet Union. In the largest diphtheria outbreak reported since the 1960s, more 157,000 cases and 5,000 deaths were documented between 1990 and 1998, with a case fatality rate of 3% to 23%. Infant immunization rates in those countries had fallen as low as 60% in the early 1990s, partially due to public perception regarding the risks of immunization. School-age children were affected in some countries, but 60% to 80% of cases were older than 15 years of age.

Serologic surveys in countries in which childhood immunization rates are high, including the United States, have demonstrated that susceptibility persists among adults who have not received booster doses of vaccine.

PATHOGENESIS

Respiratory infection is initiated when C. *diphtheriae* enter the mucosal surfaces of the nose, mouth, eye, or genitalia. The skin may also serve as a point of entry, usually at a site of previous minor trauma. If the infecting organism is lysogenized by the βtox^+ bacteriophage, toxin will be elaborated and released after the incubation period of approximately 2 to 5 days. Diphtheria toxin is a protein made up of two fragments. The B fragment attaches to host cell receptors and brings about entry of the toxin into the cell. The A fragment interrupts cellular protein synthesis by preventing elongation of amino acid chains.

Toxin acts locally to produce necrosis and edema. In the mouth or throat, a patchy exudate appears, followed by deeper tissue involvement and the development of a gray-black, adherent membrane composed of epithelial cells, fibrin, inflammatory cells, erythrocytes, and organisms. The membrane may become so extensive that it causes upper airway obstruction and even suffocation. At the site of cutaneous infection, an ulcer with sharp borders develops and becomes covered with a gray membrane. Infection of the skin or throat often is complicated by coinfection with group A streptococcus.

As it is produced, toxin is disseminated by the hematogenous route and through the lymphatics to reach distant organs. Absorption of toxin varies depending on the site of initial infection; nasal diphtheria may result only in a mild serosanguineous discharge, without systemic illness, as absorption of toxin from the nose is limited.

Effects of toxin on cardiac and nervous tissue can be life-threatening. In the heart, cellular infiltrate develops with fatty accumulation, particularly involving the conducting system. Clinically apparent cardiac involvement may be present during the first few days of illness, although it often is delayed until the second week or later. Fatty degeneration of the myelin sheaths of nerves can cause paralysis both locally (in the muscles of the palate and hypopharynx) and at distant sites (including the muscles of respiration). Neurologic consequences of toxin generally are not seen until 2 to 3 weeks after onset of infection and may appear as late as 10 weeks. Necrosis of renal tubules and hepatic parenchyma, amegakaryocytic thrombocytopenia, and adrenal hemorrhage may also occur as a result of dissemination of toxin.

Antitoxin neutralizes circulating diphtheria toxin, but it has no effect once toxin has entered cells. To be effective in preventing serious consequences of disease, therefore, it should be given as early as possible.

CLINICAL MANIFESTATIONS

Severity of disease due to C. *diphtheriae* depends on the site of infection, the immunization status of the patient, and the dissemination of toxin, the last being influenced by adminis-

tration of antitoxin. Initial infection usually is localized and is categorized by the site of involvement. Tonsillar and pharyngeal diphtheria are most common; symptoms begin with a sore throat, usually in the absence of systemic complaints. Fever, if it occurs, is usually less than 102°F, and malaise, dysphagia, and headache are not prominent features. In nonimmune, infected individuals, membrane formation begins after the 2- to 5-day incubation period and grows to involve the pharyngeal walls, tonsils, uvula, and soft palate. It may even extend to the larynx and trachea, causing airway obstruction and eventual suffocation. Underlying tissue of the throat and neck becomes edematous, and lymphadenopathy develops. Marked edema of the neck may lead to a bull-neck appearance, with a distinct collar of swelling; the patient throws his or her head back to relieve pressure on the throat and larynx. "Erasure" edema associated with pharyngeal diphtheria obliterates the angle of the jaw, the borders of the sternocleidomastoid muscle, and the medial border of the clavicles. Swallowing may be made difficult by unilateral or bilateral paralysis of the muscles of the palate. If toxin production is unopposed by antitoxin and severe disease occurs, early localized signs and symptoms give way to circulatory collapse, respiratory failure, stupor, coma, and death. If antitoxin is given promptly, less severe disease resolves with the sloughing of the membrane within 7 to 10 days (or earlier). Disseminated effects of toxin, including myocarditis and nervous system complications, may occur late in the illness, even if the initial respiratory disease was mild.

In a minority of cases, the larynx is the initial site of infection, with initial presenting symptoms similar to laryngotracheobronchitis from other causes. Initial hoarseness may progress to loss of voice and severe respiratory tract obstruction in these patients.

Infection localized to the nares is less likely to result in serious systemic disease because toxin is not well absorbed from nasal tissues. Initially, nasal diphtheria may appear as a common viral upper respiratory tract infection, but the initially clear nasal discharge later becomes serosanguineous and then mucopurulent, with excoriation of the upper lip and nares. A membrane may develop on the nasal septum, either unilateral or bilateral. A foul odor may develop. This form of diphtheria is most common in infants. Unless diagnosed accurately and treated with antitoxin and antibiotics, these patients may develop prolonged infection and will be a continued source of infection to contacts.

Cutaneous diphtheria may occur at one or more sites, usually localized to areas of previous mild trauma or bruising. It is more common in tropical climates, but outbreaks have occurred in the United States. Pain, tenderness, and erythema at the site of infection progress to ulceration with sharply defined borders and formation of a brownish gray membrane. Local disease may persist for weeks to months. Antitoxin prevents systemic complications but has little effect on skin lesions.

Other sites of infection have included the external ear, the eye (usually the palpebral conjunctivae), and the genital mucosa. Rare, sporadic cases of endocarditis have been reported, usually due to nontoxigenic strains. Septicemia caused by C. *diphtheriae* is rare but universally fatal.

COMPLICATIONS

Airway obstruction by the diphtheritic membrane and peripharyngeal edema combine to pose a risk of death for patients with diphtheria. Toxin-related complications can occur despite the use of appropriate antibiotics, especially if antitoxin administration is delayed.

Cardiac complications may arise during the first 10 days of illness or may be delayed until 2 to 3 weeks after onset, when pharyngeal disease is subsiding. In a review of 312 patients during the 1940s, 48% had some manifestation of cardiac dysfunction. Cardiac involvement is thought to be responsible for 50% to 60% of the deaths associated with diphtheria. The first sign of toxin-induced myocardiopathy is tachycardia disproportionate to the degree of fever. A variety of dysrhythmias, including first-, second-, or third-degree heart block, atrioventricular dissociation, and ventricular tachycardia, can develop, and congestive heart failure may be a consequence of myocardial inflammation. An echocardiogram may demonstrate dilated or hypertrophic cardiomyopathy. In patients who survive, cardiac muscle regeneration and interstitial fibrosis lead to recovery of normal cardiac function, unless toxic damage has led to a permanent arrhythmia.

Demyelination of nervous tissue is seen in all fatal cases of diphtheria. Frank paralysis occurs in 10% to 20% of patients and most often involves the muscles of the palate and the hypopharynx, beginning as early as the first 10 days of illness. Difficulty swallowing and nasal speech often are the first indication of neurologic impairment. Involvement of other cranial nerves, which may be delayed until as late as 7 weeks after infection, results in oculomotor paralysis and blurred vision. Diffuse, usually bilateral, motor deficits resulting from involvement of the anterior horn cells of the spinal cord may be seen as late as 3 months after initial disease, with progression of weakness either from proximal to distal regions or, more commonly, from distal to proximal regions. Involvement of the phrenic nerve may cause diaphragmatic paralysis at any time between the first and seventh weeks of illness. Elevation of cerebrospinal fluid (CSF) protein can be seen and may lead to an erroneous diagnosis of Guillain-Barré syndrome. Recovery from neurologic damage usually is complete in patients who survive.

DIAGNOSIS

Early diagnosis of diphtheria is important so that appropriate antibiotics and antitoxin can be administered promptly. In patients whose clinical presentation suggests diphtheria, a portion of the membrane or a swab specimen of material beneath the membrane should be sent for culture. The laboratory should be notified in advance of the suspicion of diphtheria, so that the sample can be cultured on appropriate media. In addition to media selective for *C. diphtheriae*, a blood agar plate should be inoculated so that concomitant infection with group A streptococcus can be identified. Direct microscopical identification of *C. diphtheriae* using Gram stain or fluorescent antibody testing is unreliable. *C. diphtheriae* survives drying, so a silica gel pack or any sterile container may be used to send swab specimens to a reference laboratory.

If suspicious diphtheria organisms are isolated, a test should be performed to determine whether the isolate is a toxigenic strain. The gel diffusion test (Elek test) commonly is used, or toxin may be demonstrated by intradermal guinea pig inoculation. The Schick test, which involves intracutaneous injection of diphtheria toxin, has been used in the past to determine the immune status of the patient, but this test is not useful for early diagnosis. Coryneform bacteria are frequent contaminants, but any such bacteria isolated from sterile sites or from mucocutaneous samples from patients with suggestive disease should be identified to the species level, with appropriate tests for toxin production for any *C. diphtheriae* isolated.

Other laboratory tests in patients with diphtheria are nonspecific. The white blood cell count may be normal or slightly elevated. If neuropathy is present, the CSF protein may be slightly elevated and a mild CSF pleocytosis may exist. The electrocardiogram may demonstrate ST or T wave changes or dysrhythmia. Depending on dissemination of toxin, hepatic enzymes or blood urea nitrogen may be elevated.

Pharyngeal diphtheria may be distinguished from streptococcal pharyngitis, adenovirus, and mononucleosis by the presence of a firmly attached membrane and by the initial relative paucity of fever and other systemic complaints in patients with diphtheria. Clinical findings usually prevent confusion with other pharyngeal infections and their complications, including mucositis in patients treated with chemotherapy, oropharyngeal candidiasis, Vincent angina, retropharyngeal or peritonsillar abscess, and jugular vein thrombophlebitis. Conditions involving the trachea and larynx, including severe laryngotracheobronchitis, bacterial tracheitis due to staphylococci or streptococci, epiglottitis, foreign-body aspiration, and masses (e.g., laryngeal papillomas, hemangiomas, and lymphangiomas), are best distinguished from diphtheria by the presence or absence of an adherent membrane seen at laryngoscopy.

TREATMENT

Treatment should be undertaken as soon as the diagnosis is suspected, even if culture results are not yet available. Both neutralization of toxin using equine antitoxin and eradication of the organism with antibiotics are important in achieving effective therapy. The dose of antitoxin recommended depends on the location and size of the diphtheritic membrane, the degree of toxicity, and the duration of illness. For patients who have been ill for at least 48 hours, 20,000 to 40,000 units should be administered for pharyngeal or laryngeal diphtheria and 40,000 to 60,000 units for nasopharyngeal lesions. Patients with extensive involvement, including extensive swelling of the neck, or illness of at least 3 days' duration should receive 80,000 to 120,000 units. Some experts recommend that 20,000 to 40,000 units be used in patients with cutaneous diphtheria, as toxic sequelae have been reported, but antitoxin probably is of no value in isolated skin disease. Antitoxin should be administered intravenously. Intravenous immune globulin contains antibodies to diphtheria toxin, but its use has not been approved in the treatment of diphtheria, and optimal doses have not been established.

Only horse antidiphtheria antiserum is available in the United States. Approximately 10% of individuals have preexisting hypersensitivity to horse serum, and approximately 8% will develop serum sickness with its administration. Immediate hypersensitivity mediated by IgE should be assumed in patients with a previous history of asthma and allergy symptoms from exposure to horses, and therefore antitoxin should be administered only with great caution. Anyone who has previously received animal serum also is at increased risk for developing an allergic reaction or serum sickness if given antitoxin. Before antitoxin administration, even in the absence of these risk factors, a scratch test using a 1:1,000 dilution of antitoxin in saline should be performed. If negative, this can be followed by intradermal administration of 0.02 mL of a 1:1,000 dilution of antitoxin in saline. Sensitivity is indicated by a wheal surrounded by an area of erythema at least 3 mm larger than a negative physiologic saline control injection in either the scratch test or the intradermal test.

If the patient's history or the sensitivity tests suggest a risk for reaction, desensitization should be undertaken using injections of decreasing dilutions and increasing amounts of antiserum at 15-minute intervals in a protocol recommended in 2003 by the Committee on Infectious Diseases of the American Academy of Pediatrics. Consultation is also available at all times through the Centers for Disease Control and Prevention (telephone: 404-639-2889 or -2888). Despite these precautions, anaphylaxis can occur with administration of antitoxin.

Antibiotic therapy is no substitute for antitoxin but should be used concomitantly to eradicate the organism. Both erythromycin (40 to 50 mg/kg/day orally or parenterally, to a maximum of 2 g/day for 14 days) and penicillin (penicillin G, 100,000 to 150,000 U/kg/day intravenously in four divided doses, or procaine penicillin, 25,000 to 50,000 U/kg/day intramuscularly, to a maximum of 1.2 million units in two divided doses for 14 days) are acceptable therapies for respiratory or cutaneous diphtheria. Other antibiotics, including fluoroquinolones, rifampin, clarithromycin, and azithromycin have good *in vitro* activity against *C. diphtheriae*, but their use in treating or preventing disease has not been clinically evaluated. Because patients may not develop effective immunity after infection, diphtheria toxoid should be administered once patients have recovered, to complete the recommended series of immunizations.

Patients with respiratory diphtheria should be placed in isolation, and droplet precautions should be followed. Contact precautions are recommended for patients with cutaneous diphtheria. Isolation should continue until two cultures taken 24 hours after antimicrobial therapy has been completed are negative. These cultures should be taken from both the nose and throat of patients with respiratory diphtheria or from the skin of patients with cutaneous diphtheria.

Public health officials should be notified promptly when diphtheria is suspected. Nasal and pharyngeal swab cultures should be obtained from all close contacts, regardless of immunization status, to identify asymptomatic carriers. After cultures are obtained, all household contacts and others with habitual, close contact with the patient should be treated with oral erythromycin (40 to 50 mg/kg/day, to a maximum of 2 g/day) for 7 days or with a single intramuscular dose of benzathine penicillin G (600,000 units for those weighing less than 30 kg, and 1.2 million units for larger children and adults). Contacts identified as asymptomatic carriers should be isolated until at least two subsequent cultures taken a minimum of 24 hours after completion of antibiotic therapy are negative for *C. diphtheriae*. Repeat cultures at 2 weeks after cessation of therapy should be performed, and any patient whose culture is positive should be treated with an additional course of antibiotics. Antitoxin therapy is not necessary for asymptomatic carriers. Immunization should be undertaken or completed for all contacts who are not completely immunized against diphtheria.

In addition to administration of antitoxin and antibiotics, attention to details of patient management can avoid complications and enhance recovery. An artificial airway should be placed expectantly in patients with laryngeal and oropharyngeal diphtheria. Careful monitoring of cardiac status with frequent electrocardiography will provide early detection of cardiac complications. Strict bed rest along with administration of a high-calorie diet during the early phase of illness is important for maintaining nutrition and avoiding exertion that might exacerbate cardiac complications. Steroid therapy has not been shown to be helpful in reducing or alleviating complications or avoiding death.

PROGNOSIS

Death due to mechanical airway obstruction or cardiac involvement with circulatory collapse occurs in at least 10% of patients with respiratory tract diphtheria. Mortality has not improved; it approximated 20% in the outbreak in the new independent states of the Soviet Union during the early 1990s. Prognosis depends on the virulence of the organism (with the gravis strain usually accounting for the most severe disease), the age and immunization status of the patient, the site of involvement, and the speed with which antitoxin is administered. For patients in whom disease is recognized on day 1 and therapy is initiated promptly, the mortality is approximately 1%. If appropriate treatment is withheld until day 4, the mortality rises to 20%.

PREVENTION

Diphtheria toxoid is prepared by formaldehyde treatment of toxin followed by adsorption to aluminum salts to enhance potency. The toxoid dose used for immunization of children younger than 7 years contains 7 to 25 limit of flocculation (Lf) units and should be administered at 2, 4, and 6 months of age, with booster doses given at 18 months and again before school entry at 4 to 6 years of age. Because of a higher likelihood of adverse reactions, children older than 6 years and adults should receive only the reduced dose of 2 Lf. For those who have completed the initial immunization series, diphtheria toxoid (dT) should be administered every 10 years along with tetanus toxoid (TT). For nonimmunized older children and adults, two initial doses of dT should be given 1 to 2 months apart, followed by a third dose 6 to 12 months later. The only contraindication to use of diphtheria toxoid is a history of neurologic complication or anaphylactic reaction to a previous dose. Precautions and contraindications regarding pertussis and tetanus immunizations should be considered when administering those products concomitantly.

A serum concentration of 0.01 to 0.10 IU/mL of antibody against diphtheria toxin is considered protective. Multiple studies performed in countries in which universal childhood immunization is recommended or provided without cost to patients have demonstrated inadequate antitoxin antibody concentrations in adults, presumably because of waning immunity and inadequate adult immunization.

Vaccines that protect against diphtheria, tetanus, and pertussis have recently been licensed for use in adolescents and adults. Recommendations for their use are pending at the time of this writing. Current immunization recommendations can be found at www.aap.org.

Suggested Readings

Committee on Infectious Diseases, American Academy of Pediatrics. Diphtheria. In: Pickering L, ed. *Report of the Committee on Infectious Diseases*, 26th ed. Elk Grove Village, IL: American Academy of Pediatrics, 2003:263.

Dittmann S, Wharton M, Vitek C, et al. Successful control of epidemic diphtheria in the states of the former Soviet Socialist Republics: lessons learned. *J Infect Dis* 2000;181:S10.

Farizo KM, Strebel PM, Chen RT, et al. Fatal respiratory disease due to *Corynebacterium diphtheriae*: case report and review of guidelines for management, investigation, and control. *Clin Infect Dis* 1993;16:59.

Hodes HL. Diphtheria. *Pediatr Clin North Am* 1979;26:445.

Overturf G. *Corynebacterium diphtheriae*. In: Long SS, Pickering LK, Prober CG, eds. *Principles and practice of pediatric infectious diseases*. New York: Churchill Livingstone, 2003:771.

CHAPTER 160 ■ DIARRHEAGENIC *ESCHERICHIA COLI*

JAMES P. NATARO AND LARRY K. PICKERING

Escherichia coli is the predominant aerobic gram-negative organism of the human intestine. Whereas most *E. coli* isolates are harmless intestinal commensals, several highly adapted *E. coli* have developed the ability to cause a spectrum of human diseases. The diarrheagenic *E. coli* can be subdivided into six distinct categories, each having a characteristic mode of pathogenesis (Fig. 160.1), epidemiology, and clinical presentation (Table 160.1). These categories include several

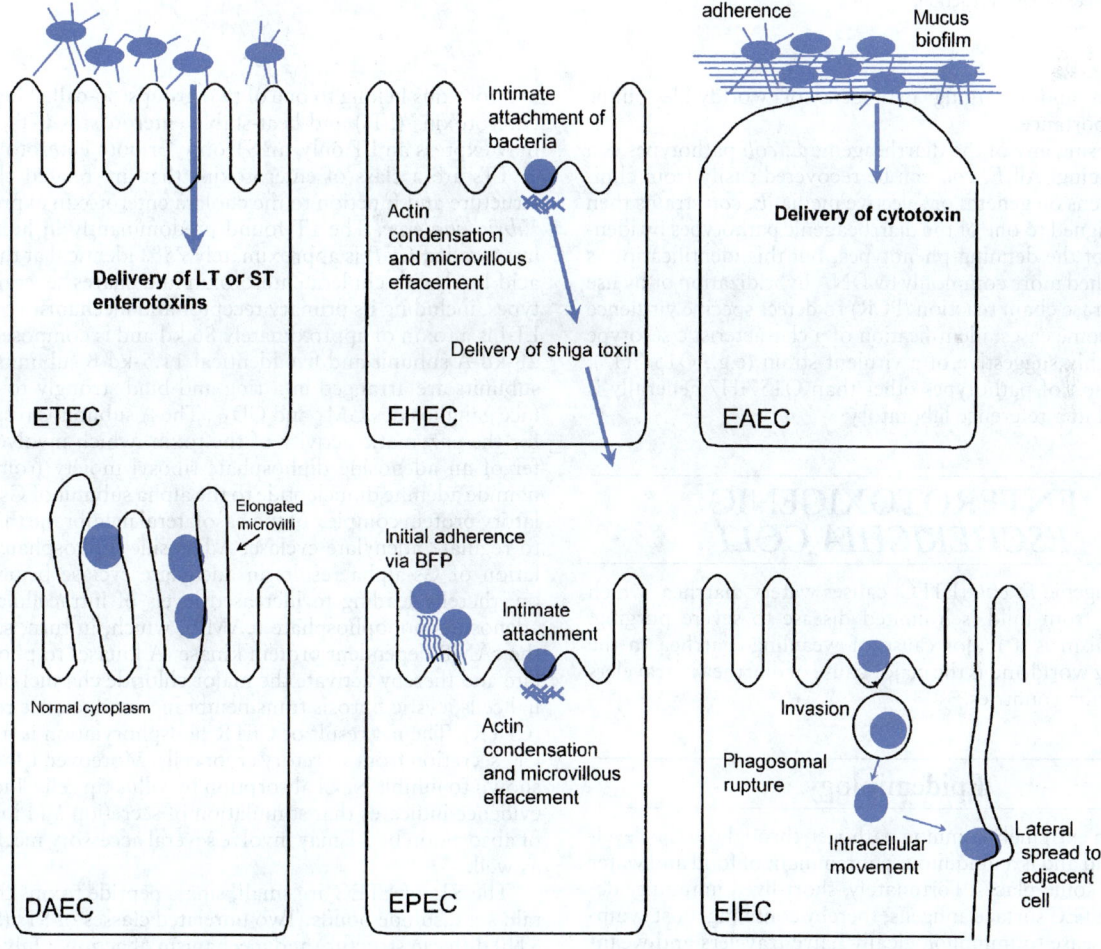

FIGURE 160.1. Pathogenic mechanisms of diarrheagenic *Escherichia coli*. The six pathotypes of diarrheagenic *E. coli* have distinct pathogenic strategies, illustrated here as their respective interactions with an intestinal epithelial cell. Enterotoxigenic *E. coli* (*ETEC*) adheres to the small bowel mucosa and delivers secretory enterotoxins. Enterohemorrhagic *E. coli* (*EHEC*) adheres intimately to the colonic mucosa ("attaching and effacing") and transduces a signal, resulting in secretory diarrhea. Concurrently, the organism releases shiga toxin, resulting in local and systemic effects. Enteroaggregative *E. coli* (*EAEC*) adheres in a thick mucous gel and causes intestinal secretion and damage. Diffusely adherent *E. coli* (*DAEC*) has been shown to elicit elongation of microvilli *in vitro*, although this effect has not been demonstrated *in vivo*. Enteropathogenic *E. coli* (*EPEC*) elicits the attaching and effacing lesion in the small bowel, resulting in intestinal secretion. Enteroinvasive *E. coli* (*EIEC*) invades the colonic mucosa, giving rise to an inflammatory enteritis. BFP, bundle-forming pilus. (Reprinted with permission from Nataro JP, Kaper JB. Diarrheagenic *Escherichia coli*. *Clin Microbiol Rev* 1998;11:1.)

TABLE 160.1

CATEGORIES OF DIARRHEAGENIC *ESCHERICHIA COLI*

Category	Clinical Syndrome	Epidemology	Diagnosis
Enterotoxigenic *E. coli*	Watery diarrhea	Weaning infants and travelers to developing countries	Detection of heat-stable or heat-labile toxins by enzyme immunoassay or genotype
Enteropathogenic *E. coli*	Watery diarrhea	Infants younger than 2 years, mostly in developing countries	Adherence to HEp-2 cells; gene probe, PCR
Enterohemorrhagic *E. coli*	Watery diarrhea, hemorrhagic colitis, hemolytic uremic syndrome	Epidemic and sporadic diarrhea, mostly in developed countries	Detection of characteristic serotypes (i.e., O157:H7, O111:H8, O26:H11); detection of shiga toxin; gene probe, PCR
Enteroaggregative *E. coli*	Watery, persistant diarrhea	All ages but predominantly infants	Adherence to HEp-2 cells; gene probe, PCR
Enteroinvasive *E. coli*	Watery diarrhea, dysentery	All ages; occurs in developing and developed countries	Invasion of cells in culture or guinea pig eye; gene probe, PCR
Diffusely adherent *E. coli*	Watery diarrhea	Older children	Adherence to HEp-2 cells; gene probe, PCR

PCR, polymerase chain reaction.

established and emerging pathogens of worldwide public health importance.

Diagnosing any of the diarrheagenic *E. coli* pathotypes can be challenging. All *E. coli* can be recovered easily from clinical specimens on general or selective media. *E. coli* strains then can be assigned to one of the diarrheagenic pathotypes by identification of the defining phenotypes, but this identification is accomplished more commonly by DNA hybridization or by use of polymerase chain reaction (PCR) to detect specific virulence genes. In some cases, identification of a characteristic serotype can be highly suggestive of a virulent strain (e.g., O157:H7). Identification of pathotypes other than O157:H7 generally is performed in a reference laboratory.

ENTEROTOXIGENIC ESCHERICHIA COLI

Enterotoxigenic *E. coli* (ETEC) causes watery diarrhea, which can range from mild, self-limited disease to severe purging. The organism is a major cause of weanling diarrhea in the developing world and is the major cause of diarrhea in travelers to developing countries.

Epidemiology

ETEC is an extremely common pathogen throughout the developing world and is a ubiquitous contaminant of food and water sources in some places. Fortunately, short-lived immunity develops to ETEC surface antigens, thereby confining most symptomatic disease to immunologically naive travelers and weaning infants; in developing countries, ETEC may cause as many as one-third of cases of sporadic infant diarrhea. In endemic areas, asymptomatic infection occurs frequently. ETEC infection occurs occasionally in the United States, and several large foodborne and waterborne outbreaks have been reported.

Pathogenesis

ETEC colonizes the surface of the small bowel mucosa and elaborates enterotoxins, giving rise to a net secretory state. The enterotoxins belong to one of two groups: so-called heat-labile enterotoxins (LTs) and heat-stable enterotoxins (STs). Strains may express an LT only, an ST only, or both enterotoxins.

LTs are a class of enterotoxins that are related closely in structure and function to the cholera enterotoxin expressed by *Vibrio cholerae*. The LT found predominantly in human isolates (called *LT-I*) is approximately 75% identical at the amino acid level with cholera enterotoxin and shares several phenotypes, including its primary receptor and mechanism of action. LT-I is a toxin of approximately 86 kd and is composed of one 28-kd A subunit and five identical 11.5-kd B subunits. The B subunits are arranged in a ring and bind strongly to cell surface gangliosides GM_1 and GD_{1b}. The A subunit is responsible for the enzymatic activity of the toxin, which involves transfer of an adenosine diphosphate-ribosyl moiety from nicotinamide adenine dinucleotide to the alpha subunit of Gs, a regulatory protein complex of the basolateral membrane that serves to regulate adenylate cyclase. Adenosine diphosphate ribosylation of Gs-alpha results in adenylate cyclase being locked on, thereby leading to increased levels of intracellular cyclic adenosine monophosphate (cAMP), which, in turn, stimulate the cAMP-dependent protein kinase (A kinase) to phosphorylate and thereby activate the major chloride channel of epithelial cells, cystic fibrosis transmembrane conductance regulator (CFTR). The net result of CFTR phosphorylation is increased Cl^- secretion from secretory crypt cells. Moreover, LT has been shown to inhibit NaCl absorption by villus tip cells. Increasing evidence indicates that stimulation of secretion and inhibition of absorption by LT may involve several accessory mechanisms as well.

The STs of ETEC are small, single peptide toxins that contain six disulfide bonds. Two unrelated classes of STs (STa and STb) differ in structure and mechanism of action. Only STa has been associated with human disease.

The mature STa toxin is an 18- or 19-amino-acid peptide with a molecular mass of approximately 2 kd. Two STa variants, designated STp (porcine) or STh (human), exist; both can be found among human ETEC isolates and are presumed to be equally pathogenic. STh and STp are nearly identical in the 13 residues that are necessary and sufficient for enterotoxic activity, and of these 13 residues, six are cysteines that form three intramolecular disulfide bridges.

The major receptor for STa is membrane-spanning guanylate cyclase C (GC-C), which belongs to a receptor cyclase family that includes the atrial natriuretic peptide receptors GC-A and GC-B. Binding of STa to GC-C stimulates guanylate cyclase activity, leading to increased intracellular cyclic guanosine monophosphate (GMP), which, in turn, activates cGMP-dependent, cAMP-dependent, or both types of kinases.

ETEC adheres to the intestinal mucosa via one or more proteinaceous fimbrial colonization factors, or CFAs. These organelles may have the appearance of rigid rods (of approximately 7 nm in diameter), thinner wiry structures, or wavy bundles of filaments. A large number of antigenically diverse CFAs have been characterized, yet epidemiologic studies suggest that approximately 75% of human ETEC worldwide express CFA-I, CFA-II, or CFA-IV.

Clinical Manifestations

The incubation period of ETEC diarrhea is 1 to 3 days in adult volunteers. Diarrhea usually begins abruptly and is watery in nature without blood, mucus, or fecal leukocytes. Patients may experience vomiting, but they generally do not have fever. ETEC infection usually is self-limited to less than 5 days.

Diagnosis

ETEC is best diagnosed by detection of the enterotoxins ST or LT. Several phenotypic and immunologic tests exist to identify the toxins. Enzyme immunoassays are available commercially. Genetic detection techniques are available in research and reference laboratories and include DNA probes and PCR.

Treatment

Maintaining adequate hydration is the cornerstone of management of ETEC diarrhea. Administration of antibiotics to which ETEC is susceptible will hasten resolution of symptoms. Trimethoprim-sulfamethoxazole has been recommended traditionally; however, increasing resistance to this agent has been documented, and alternative agents such as fluoroquinolones, ampicillin, and cefixime may be considered.

ENTEROPATHOGENIC *ESCHERICHIA COLI*

Enteropathogenic *E. coli* (EPEC) is a common cause of watery diarrhea among infants in the developing world and is defined as *E. coli* that causes a characteristic "attaching and effacing" (AE) lesion in the small bowel. EPEC does not secrete the enterotoxins LT, ST, or shiga toxin.

Epidemiology

EPEC primarily is an infection of infants younger than 2 years of age. Volunteer studies suggest that adults are susceptible but only after receiving high doses with gastric neutralization. In the 1940s and 1950s, EPEC caused outbreaks of severe, watery diarrhea in nurseries in industrialized countries, but since the 1970s, most EPEC disease has been shown to occur as sporadic endemic diarrhea in developing areas. The vehicle for EPEC transmission is not known with certainty.

Pathogenesis

The full mechanism of EPEC pathogenesis is not understood, but the AE histopathology is required for diarrheagenicity. This striking phenotype is characterized by effacement of the microvillous brush border and intimate adherence between the bacterium and the epithelial plasma membrane. Directly beneath the adherent bacterium are marked cytoskeletal changes, which include accumulation of polymerized actin, disorganization of the endoplasmic reticulum, and clearing of the apical cytoplasm. At times, the plasma membrane can be seen to wrap partially around the adherent bacterium, forming a distinctive cup or pedestal-like phenotype.

A three-stage model has been proposed to describe the interaction of EPEC with the epithelial cell and formation of the AE lesion: (a) distant adherence, (b) signal transduction, and (c) intimate adherence of the bacterium to the plasma membrane. These stages may occur concurrently. Distant adherence to, and presumably initial colonization of, the small bowel epithelium is mediated by the plasmid-borne bundle-forming pilus. Signal transduction refers to the ability of the bacterium to stimulate changes in cytoskeletal protein phosphorylation and ion fluxes, steps that are mediated by proteins that are injected from the bacterium into the affected epithelial cell. The secreted proteins and their dedicated secretion apparatus are clustered within a chromosomal locus of EPEC-specific genes termed a pathogenicity island. Also encoded on the pathogenicity island are intimin, a 94-kd outer membrane protein mediating intimate adherence, and the intimin receptor, a 78-kd protein called *Tir*.

Clinical Manifestations

EPEC causes watery diarrhea with an absence of fecal leukocytes. The diarrhea often is associated with vomiting and low-grade fever. The incubation period is 1 to 5 days. Diarrhea can be severe, leading to rapid dehydration of affected infants. Some studies suggest that EPEC may elicit a chronic diarrhea with malabsorption and sustained AE histopathology throughout the small intestine.

Diagnosis

EPEC can be identified using genotypic or phenotypic methods. Traditionally, EPEC was identified by detection of certain serotypic markers; however, identification of specific virulence determinants has rendered this method obsolete. Antisera to the EPEC serotypes no longer are widely available. The most common genetic assay is detection of the plasmid-borne adhesin genes with a DNA probe or PCR. Identification of a characteristic localized pattern of adherence to HEp-2 cells in culture also is a sensitive and specific method for detection of EPEC.

Treatment

EPEC nursery outbreaks in the 1940s and 1950s were accompanied by high mortality rates, but with proper attention to hydration and other supportive measures, infants usually can be managed successfully. Antibiotic therapy lessens the severity of symptoms and decreases the duration of shedding. Nonabsorbable aminoglycosides (especially colistin sulfate) have been the mainstay of therapy.

ENTEROHEMORRHAGIC *ESCHERICHIA COLI*

Enterohemorrhagic *E. coli* (EHEC, also known as *verotoxigenic* or *shiga toxin–producing E. coli*) are defined as organisms that form an AE lesion and elaborate shiga toxin. EHEC causes two distinctive syndromes: hemorrhagic colitis and hemolytic uremic syndrome (HUS), which may be preceded by hemorrhagic colitis or watery diarrhea. Like EPEC, EHEC elicits an AE lesion of the intestinal mucosa (but in the colon). All EHEC strains produce shiga toxin, which induces hemorrhagic colitis and is responsible for the systemic sequelae of this infection.

Epidemiology

EHEC is an emerging cause of foodborne illness in many parts of the world. Large outbreaks accompanied by deaths from HUS have focused public attention on issues of food safety. EHEC is a common isolate from the intestines of bovine species (and perhaps from other mammalian species as well) and, as such, the pathogen may contaminate beef products or other foods in contact with bovine-exposed soil. Beef products (particularly ground beef), other meats, vegetables, and apple cider have been implicated in outbreaks. EHEC outbreaks also have been linked to fecally contaminated drinking and recreational water. The infectious dose required to initiate EHEC infection is extremely low (less than 100 organisms), enabling large point-source outbreaks and person-to-person transmission to occur. EHEC infects patients of all ages, but HUS is seen most commonly in children and elderly adults.

EHEC infection has a geographic distribution with high rates occurring in Canada and the northern tier of the United States. In some developed areas, O157:H7 is reported as frequently as is *Campylobacter* or *Salmonella*, but EHEC appears to be an unusual occurrence in most developing countries. Most outbreaks of EHEC infection have been linked to O157:H7 strains, suggesting that this serotype is in some way more virulent or more transmissible than are other serotypes. Nonetheless, other serotypes have been implicated in both sporadic disease and outbreaks, and the occurrence of these other serotypes is considered to be on the rise.

Pathogenesis

The prominent features of EHEC pathogenesis include development of the AE lesion (see Enteropathogenic *Escherichia coli*, Pathogenesis) on the colonic mucosa, followed by elaboration of shiga toxin. The latter accounts at least in part for the severe mucosal damage that distinguishes EHEC enteritis from the less severe EPEC disease. EHEC also imparts epithelial cell signal transduction events that are similar to those elicited by EPEC. EHEC strains carry a chromosomal pathogenicity island and express intimin.

The shiga toxin family contains two related but immunologically non-cross-reactive groups called *Stx1* and *Stx2*. A single EHEC strain may express Stx1 only, Stx2 only, or both toxins. Stx1 from EHEC is identical to shiga toxin from *Shigella dysenteriae* 1.

The shiga holotoxin is composed of one A subunit, conferring the enzymatic activity, and five B subunits, conferring binding to the glycolipid receptor, Gb3. The A1 peptide is an N-glycosidase that removes a single adenine residue from the 28S rRNA of eukaryotic ribosomes, thereby inhibiting protein synthesis and causing cell death. The presence of the Gb3 receptor on enterocytes and renal endothelial cells is thought to account for the clinical manifestations of EHEC infection and its

sequelae. Shiga toxin is thought to damage the glomerular endothelial cells, leading to narrowing of capillary lumina and occlusion of the glomerular microvasculature with platelets and fibrin. Stx2 may be more potent in its ability to cause HUS than is Stx1.

Clinical Manifestations

EHEC enteritis comprises a clinical spectrum ranging from mild watery diarrhea to severe hemorrhagic colitis. EHEC infection typically begins with the development of watery diarrhea after an incubation period of 1 to 5 days. Vomiting and abdominal cramps are common occurrences. After 1 to 2 days, the diarrhea becomes bloody (defining hemorrhagic colitis) in most patients, and typically the illness lasts 4 to 10 days. The diarrhea usually is not associated with fever. Most patients do not have mucus or pus in the stool, and polymorphonuclear cells generally are not found. Intestinal hemorrhage may be profuse, and colonic necrosis and perforation may occur. Barium enema of patients with hemorrhagic colitis often reveals a characteristic thumbprinting pattern of the colon. The classic intestinal histopathology of hemorrhagic colitis caused by EHEC includes hemorrhage and edema of the lamina propria. Colonic biopsies may reveal focal necrosis and infiltration by neutrophils.

HUS consists of the triad of microangiopathic hemolytic anemia, thrombocytopenia, and renal failure, but partial forms have been described. Two to 13% of pediatric patients with O157:H7 infection develop HUS, typically in the second week of illness and after diarrhea has resolved. The typical human renal histopathology includes swollen glomerular endothelial cells and deposition of platelets and fibrin within the glomeruli. Of the patients who develop HUS, chronic renal failure persists in 4% to 10%; other forms of chronic renal disease or hypertension persist in 12% to 39%. HUS that is not caused by EHEC infection (atypical HUS) usually has a worse prognosis.

Other complications of EHEC infection include cholecystitis, pancreatitis, posthemolytic biliary lithiasis, rectal prolapse, appendicitis, hepatitis, hemorrhagic cystitis, pulmonary edema, myocardial dysfunction, and neurologic abnormalities, including stroke. Whereas most studies suggest that a more severe clinical course early in the disease predicts a higher risk of developing sequelae, the specific features associated with this risk are not well delineated.

Diagnosis

All licensed clinical laboratories in the United States should have the capability of detecting O157:H7. Because most O157:H7 isolates do not ferment sorbitol, cultivation of *E. coli* on sorbitol MacConkey medium is a convenient method for detection of this serotype, but confirmation of presumptive isolates with O157:H7 antiserum is required. Several other assays are available to detect O157 or its products in stool; these tests include enzyme immunoassays for O157 and shiga toxin, latex agglutination tests for the O157 antigen, and rapid strip-mounted monoclonal antibodies to detect the O157 antigen in stools. All of these tests have been shown to have good sensitivity and specificity in detection of EHEC, with the caveat that analysis of stool for the presence of the pathogen should be performed as early as possible in the diarrheal illness. Studies suggest that by 1 week after the onset of diarrhea caused by EHEC (and before most cases of HUS are manifest), most stools no longer yield the pathogen. Studies also suggest that all patients with bloody diarrhea should have their stools cultured for EHEC, but the clinician should communicate suspicion of this infection to laboratory personnel.

Molecular techniques for detection of the genes encoding intimin and shiga toxin have been used widely in research studies. These tests are sensitive and specific and offer the advantage of detecting EHEC of serotypes other than O157:H7.

Treatment

The approach to a patient with O157:H7 infection is controversial. As yet, antibiotics have not been shown to be effective in ameliorating diarrhea caused by EHEC or preventing the development of HUS. Some experts suggest that antibiotics may increase the risk of developing HUS. The administration of antimotility agents during the diarrhea phase has been associated with aggravated diarrhea and a higher risk of developing neurologic sequelae. Fluid and electrolyte balance should be maintained throughout the illness. When HUS supervenes, aggressive support can be lifesaving, and early dialysis is associated with improved outcome. A large number of complementary therapeutic interventions, all of which are designed to prevent absorption of the toxin or its systemic effects, have been proposed. As yet, no such interventions have been approved for clinical use. Patients with proven infection caused by EHEC and their contacts should be followed carefully for development of HUS-associated features.

ENTEROAGGREGATIVE *ESCHERICHIA COLI*

Enteroaggregative *E. coli* (EAEC) is an established cause of watery diarrhea in infants. EAEC are defined as *E. coli* that do not secrete enterotoxins LT or ST and that adhere to HEp-2 cells in an aggregative pattern. These organisms are being identified with increasing frequency in developed and developing areas.

Epidemiology

EAEC is associated with acute and, especially, persistent diarrhea (longer than 14 days) among children in the developing world. The vehicle for development of sporadic disease caused by EAEC is not known, but several foodborne outbreaks of diarrhea caused by EAEC have been described in developed countries. In addition to causing diarrhea, some evidence suggests that even asymptomatic EAEC infection may be associated with growth faltering in some children.

Pathogenesis

EAEC causes diarrhea by binding to the intestinal mucosa and releasing enterotoxins and cytotoxins. EAEC characteristically enhances mucus secretion from the mucosa, with trapping of the bacteria in a mucus-containing biofilm. Evidence indicates that both the small bowel and large bowel can be sites of human disease.

Some EAEC strains induce cytotoxic effects on the intestinal mucosa. The lesion is characterized by shortening of villi, hemorrhagic necrosis of the villous tips, and a mild inflammatory response with edema and mononuclear infiltration of the submucosa. The bacteria adhere to enterocytes without formation of the attaching and effacing lesion. A high-molecular-weight (greater than 100 kd) enterotoxin/cytotoxin has been described.

An ST-like toxin (EAST1) may be involved in intestinal secretion by EAEC, although this toxin can be found in other pathotypes of *E. coli* and in nonpathogenic flora.

Diagnosis

Establishing the diagnosis of EAEC infection can be difficult for several reasons. First, it is likely that not all organisms that exhibit the typical aggregative adherence pattern are, in fact, pathogenic. Identification of the critical virulence factors and redefinition of this group probably will occur. In addition, asymptomatic shedding of EAEC occurs commonly. Thus, an EAEC strain should not be presumed to be the cause of a patient's diarrhea unless the organism is isolated repeatedly in the absence of another pathogen. Molecular methods have been developed for diagnosing EAEC infection; these tests detect the presence of the virulence regulator AggR.

Clinical Considerations

Diarrhea caused by EAEC usually is watery and mucoid but may contain blood. Fever is present in a minority of patients. The diarrhea often persists for 2 weeks or more and may even continue for several days after the administration of appropriate antibiotic therapy.

Treatment

Patients with persistent diarrhea may require aggressive nutritional intervention to complement the management of fluids and electrolytes. No randomized prospective studies have evaluated the effectiveness of antibiotic therapy for EAEC infection. EAEC frequently is resistant to antimicrobial agents, but nonabsorbable aminoglycosides and fluoroquinolones are likely to be effective agents.

ENTEROINVASIVE *ESCHERICHIA COLI*

Enteroinvasive *E. coli* (EIEC) is biochemically, genetically, and pathogenetically closely related to *Shigella* species and is defined by its ability to invade epithelial cells. EIEC may cause an invasive inflammatory colitis and occasionally dysentery, but, in most cases, the organism elicits watery diarrhea indistinguishable from that caused by other *E. coli* pathogens.

Epidemiology

EIEC has been implicated in outbreaks of diarrhea, which usually are foodborne or waterborne. The infectious dose for EIEC in volunteers is higher than that for *Shigella* and, thus, the potential for person-to-person transmission is lessened. Endemic sporadic disease occurs in some areas, but epidemiologic features are not well characterized.

Pathogenesis

EIEC infection is thought to represent an inflammatory colitis, although many patients appear to manifest a secretory, small bowel syndrome. The current model of EIEC pathogenesis comprises (a) epithelial cell penetration, followed by (b) lysis of the endocytic vacuole, (c) intracellular multiplication, (d) directional movement through the cytoplasm, and (e) extension into adjacent epithelial cells. Movement within the cytoplasm is mediated by nucleation of cellular actin into a tail that extends from one pole of the bacterium. Genes required to effect this complex pathogenetic scheme are encoded on a 140-Md plasmid. Although EIEC is invasive, dissemination of the organism past the submucosa rarely occurs.

Clinical Manifestations

EIEC occasionally can cause dysentery syndrome, with fecal blood, mucus, and polymorphonuclear cells, but more commonly the infection manifests as secretory or mild inflammatory diarrhea. The infection usually is self-limiting. Antibiotic therapy is effective in ameliorating symptoms and decreasing the duration of shedding. Trimethoprim-sulfamethoxazole is the preferred agent when the strain is susceptible; ampicillin, cefixime, and quinolones are alternatives.

Diagnosis

EIEC can be detected by phenotypic or genotypic analyses of lactose-negative E. coli isolated from stool. Demonstration of invasiveness in cell culture or the guinea pig keratoconjunctivitis test is the classical phenotypic assay. However, gene probes and PCR assays may be both more readily available and more convenient.

DIFFUSELY ADHERENT ESCHERICHIA COLI

Diffusely adherent E. coli (DAEC) is defined by its characteristic diffuse pattern of adherence to HEp-2 cells in culture. Whether DAEC strains are true diarrheal pathogens is unclear because adult volunteers fed these strains have not developed diarrhea and no outbreaks have been documented. Characteristics of DAEC-induced diarrhea have not been well characterized, although some investigators have suggested that a mild watery diarrhea occurs. Limited epidemiologic data suggest that DAEC may be a cause of sporadic diarrhea in children outside infancy. A characteristic ultrahistopathologic lesion has been described. The management of possible DAEC-induced diarrhea has not been studied.

Suggested Readings

Clarke SC, Haigh RD, Freestone PP, Williams PH. Virulence of enteropathogenic *Escherichia coli*, a global pathogen. *Clin Microbiol Rev* 2003;16:365.

Huilan S, Zhen LG, Mathan MM, et al. Etiology of acute diarrhea among children in developing countries: a multicentre study in five countries. *Bull World Health Organ* 1991;69:549.

Nataro JP, Kaper JB. Diarrheagenic *Escherichia coli*. *Clin Microbiol Rev* 1998; 11:1.

Ochoa TJ, Cleary TG. Epidemiology and spectrum of disease of *Escherichia coli* O157. *Curr Opin Infect Dis* 2003;16:259.

Paton JC, Paton AW. Methods for detection of STEC in humans. An overview. *Methods Mol Med* 2003;73:9.

Ray PE, Liu XH. Pathogenesis of shiga toxin-induced hemolytic uremic syndrome. *Pediatr Nephrol* 2001;16:823.

Robins-Browne RM, Hartland EL. *Escherichia coli* as a cause of diarrhea. *J Gastroenterol Hepatol* 2002;17:467.

Safdar N, Said A, Gangnon RE, Maki DG. Risk of hemolytic uremic syndrome after antibiotic treatment of *Escherichia coli* O157:H7 enteritis: a meta-analysis. *JAMA* 2002;288:996.

Sears CL, Kaper JB. Enteric bacterial toxins: mechanisms of action and linkage to intestinal secretion. *Microbiol Rev* 1996;60:167.

Slutsker L, Ries AA, Greene KD, et al. *Escherichia coli* O157:H7 diarrhea in the United States: clinical and epidemiologic features. *Ann Intern Med* 1997;126:505.

CHAPTER 161 ■ *HAEMOPHILUS INFLUENZAE*

SHELDON L. KAPLAN

Haemophilus influenzae is a fastidious, gram-negative, pleomorphic coccobacillus that is responsible for serious systemic and local infections in children.

MICROBIOLOGY

H. influenzae is differentiated from other *Haemophilus* species by its requirement for factors X (i.e., heat-stable hematin) and V [i.e., heat-labile nicotinamide adenine dinucleotide (NAD)] for growth. Encapsulated strains of *H. influenzae* are classified by capsular polysaccharides types a through f. The polysaccharides are negatively charged, high-molecular-weight polymers that comprise repeating subunits of a disaccharide. In the prevaccine era, approximately 95% of invasive diseases were caused by the type b strain, for which the repeating subunit is polyribosyl ribitol phosphate (PRP). The partial deletion of IS1006-bexA, an insertion element, appears to be associated with increased capsule production and thus virulence for serotypes b and a. Unencapsulated strains (i.e., nontypable strains) primarily are etiologic agents in upper respiratory tract infections such as otitis media and sinusitis, but they also cause systemic disease, especially in the neonate or immunocompromised host.

H. influenzae organisms have several outer membrane proteins (OMP) that can be differentiated by sodium dodecylsulfate, polyacrylamide gel electrophoresis. Based on the OMP pattern, 21 subtypes of *H. influenzae* type b (Hib) can be described, although five subtypes account for more than 90% of the systemic isolates. OMP patterns have proved useful for epidemiologic investigations. Unlike type b strains, the OMP patterns of nontypable *H. influenzae* are highly variable. Hib strains also have been characterized by the electrophoretic mobility of 17 metabolic enzymes (i.e., multilocus enzyme electrophoresis). Most invasive disease in the United States is caused by clonal isolates of two related multilocus genotypes. *H. influenzae* isolates can be characterized into two primary phylogenetic divisions with serotypes c, e, and f capsules belonging to a single division and serotypes a and b occurring in divisions I and II.

H. influenzae contains a lipopolysaccharide that differs from lipopolysaccharides of Enterobacteriaceae in that it lacks repeating O side chains and is classified as a lipooligosaccharide. The lipid A component and core oligosaccharide of *H. influenzae* lipopolysaccharide are similar in structure to enteric lipopolysaccharide. Lipopolysaccharide has a role in the adherence and colonization of the respiratory tract by *H. influenzae* organisms.

H. influenzae produce an IgA1 protease that can cleave specifically the hinge region of the heavy chain of human IgA1. Both typeable and non-typeable *H. influenzae* have at least 5 major adhesins (high molecular weight proteins (HMW) 1 and 2, *Haemophilus* adherence and penetration protein (Hap), Hia/Hsf and hemagglutinating pili. These adhesins are involved in attachment and colonization as well as invasion of the respiratory tract.

H. influenzae type b was the first organism for which the entire bacterial genome was sequenced enabling scientists to more completely study virulence factors and host-pathogen interactions.

EPIDEMIOLOGY

In the United States, approximately 20,000 cases of systemic Hib infection occurred yearly before the introduction of the Hib protein conjugate vaccines. Most cases were bacterial meningitis. The estimated annual age-specific attack rate of Hib infection was 100 cases per 100,000 children younger than 5 years of age. The highest age-specific attack rate occurred in children between the ages of 6 and 11 months; the next highest rate was among those between the ages of 12 and 17 months. Overall, approximately one in 200 children developed a systemic infection due to Hib by the time they reached 5 years of age.

After the administration of the conjugate Hib vaccines to infants became routine, the incidence of invasive Hib infections in children fell dramatically. In Centers for Disease Control and Prevention (CDC) surveillance studies in the United States, conducted during 1998 to 2000, a total of 824 cases of invasive *H. influenzae* disease was reported among children younger than 5 years old; rates were 1.4 to 1.6 per 100,000 children. Of the isolates available for serotyping, only 22% were Hib in 2000, when the annual invasive disease rate for children younger than 5 years old was 0.3 per 100,000, a 99% decline in invasive Hib disease compared with the rate in 1990 (Fig. 161.1). The estimated incidence of invasive *H. influenzae* type b disease in US children in 2004 was 0.09 cases/100,000 for children <5 years old. As a result, nontypable strains and other non-b serotypes (especially type f) now cause a higher proportion of invasive *H. influenzae* infections. Serotypes a and f have been associated with meningitis and pneumonia in children younger than 5 years of age; 25% or more have an underlying illness.

Certain risk factors for systemic Hib infections have been identified. African American, Hispanic, and Native American children have higher rates of infection than do white, non-Hispanic children. The highest endemic incidence of disease in the prevaccine era occurred among native Alaskan Eskimos. Children younger than 4 years of age, who are household contacts of a patient with Hib disease, have a much higher risk for acquiring this disease than does the general population. Children with underlying immune deficiencies and anatomic or functional asplenia (e.g., hemoglobinopathies) are more likely to develop systemic *H. influenzae* infections. Other risk factors for the development of invasive Hib infections are attendance in day-care facilities, crowded households, frequent infections, and socioeconomic status. Additional risk factors for developing local infections caused by nontypable *H. influenzae* include viral respiratory infections, allergies, exposure to smoke, and anatomic abnormalities like cleft palate.

Breast-feeding for infants between 2 and 5 months of age appears to be a relatively protective factor.

PATHOGENESIS

Unencapsulated *H. influenzae* are common inhabitants of the upper respiratory tract under normal conditions in children and adults. Hib could be isolated from as many as 5% to 7% of young children at any time in the prevaccine era. Higher colonization rates occurred among children in day-care centers; much lower rates are observed in children after immunization with the *H. influenzae* protein conjugate vaccines.

Invasive disease caused by Hib frequently follows a viral upper respiratory infection, which may disrupt mucosal barriers and interrupt the normal activity of respiratory cilia. In infant rats, prior intranasal inoculation with influenza virus promotes bacteremia after the intranasal administration of Hib. In human nasopharyngeal organ cultures infected with Hib, organisms can be identified within the epithelium in an intercellular location by 24 hours. This invasion is preceded by disruption of the tight junctions between nonciliated cells. Presumably, after it passes the mucosal barrier, the organism can invade the bloodstream directly. In a susceptible host, bacteria multiply readily, and after a critical bacterial density is reached, dissemination occurs.

For local infections caused by unencapsulated strains, a preceding viral upper respiratory infection frequently disrupts the normal physiologic clearance mechanisms and permits

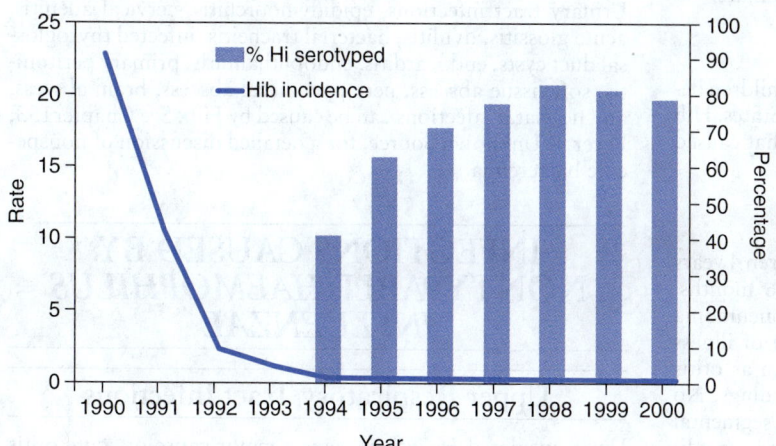

*Per 100,000 persons.

FIGURE 161.1. Incidence rate* of *Haemophilus influenzae* type b (Hib) invasive disease and percentage of *Haemophilus influenzae* (Hi) isolates serotype among children aged younger than 5 years, in the United States, 1990–2000. (Reprinted with permission from Centers for Disease Control and Prevention. Progress toward elimination of *Haemophilus influenzae* type b invasive disease among infants and children—United States, 1998–2000. *MMWR;*2002:51:234.)

invasion of the sinuses or middle ear by normal respiratory flora (e.g., *S. pneumoniae*, nontypable *H. influenzae*, and *Moraxella catarrhalis*). However, certain nontypable strains may possess one or more virulence factors that may mediate bloodstream invasion and the erosion of host defenses and help explain why invasive infections caused by nontypable *H. influenzae* may occur. Nontypable strains can colonize the female genital tract and thus be associated with neonatal infection. Often, acute chorioamnionitis and villitis are present in the placenta of mothers whose infants have early-onset sepsis.

HOST IMMUNITY

Antibody to the capsular polysaccharide is the major component of the host defense against Hib. The inverse relation between PRP antibody concentrations and susceptibility to systemic infection is well known. Children who develop serum anti-PRP antibody concentrations of at least 1 μg/mL 3 weeks after immunization with PRP are protected against invasive disease. Antibody to PRP is an important opsonin, is bactericidal in combination with complement, and promotes neutrophil chemotaxis. Functional differences exist for IgG and IgM and for the IgG subclasses (e.g., IgG1, IgG2), antibodies directed against PRP, but the relative contributions of the immunoglobulin classes to host defenses are unclear. Mucosal anti-PRP antibody (IgA) develops after natural diseases and parenteral immunization with PRP, but the clinical significance of IgA anti-PRP is unknown.

Antibodies to other noncapsular polysaccharide antigens, such as OMPs and lipooligosaccharides, may play some role in immunity against *H. influenzae*. Hib lipooligosaccharide is an important inducer of the inflammatory response, related to the production of cytokines, such as tumor necrosis factor (TNF) or interleukin-1 (IL-1). The macrophages of the reticuloendothelial system are key components for intravascular clearance of Hib.

Several surface antigens (ex. HMW1/HMW2) have been considered as vaccine candidates in studies of immunity to nontypable *H. influenzae*.

CLINICAL MANIFESTATION AND COMPLICATIONS

Infections Caused by *Haemophilus influenzae* Type B

After Hib bacteremia develops, invasion of most sites in the body can occur, but certain sites of infection predominate.

Meningitis

Hib was the leading cause of bacterial meningitis in children between the ages of 1 month and 4 years in the United States. Hib meningitis cannot be differentiated clinically from that caused by *N. meningitidis* or *S. pneumoniae*.

Pneumonia

Hib pneumonia occurs more commonly among children 4 years of age or younger. The mean age of patients is 26 months. The signs and symptoms are similar to those of pneumonia caused by other organisms, except that the course of illness may be more prolonged. Associated infections, such as otitis media, meningitis, and epiglottitis, are common findings. No characteristic pattern on chest radiography exists; segmental infiltrates, single or multiple lobe involvement, lobar consolidation, pleural effusion, and pneumatoceles may be observed.

Septic or Pyogenic Arthritis

Hib can cause septic arthritis in children younger than 2 years of age. Large joints, such as the knee, hip, ankle, and elbow, are affected most often. Single joints are infected more frequently than are multiple joints. Associated infections are common findings. An immune complex or noninfectious arthritis associated with systemic Hib infections, predominantly meningitis, may develop several days after appropriate antibiotic therapy has been initiated. Hib is an uncommon cause of osteomyelitis.

Cellulitis

A characteristic cellulitis caused by Hib can develop in children younger than 2 years of age. These children often have an upper respiratory infection that is followed by the acute onset of cellulitis. Usually, no history exists of trauma to the involved area. The cheek or buccal region and the periorbital area are the most common sites of infection. Why Hib so frequently is related to buccal cellulitis is unknown. The role of lymphatic seeding of the buccal soft tissues from otitis media is debatable. The area of cellulitis generally has indistinct margins and is tender and indurated. A violaceous or blue-purple color is a common finding but is not diagnostic. Concomitant infections, especially meningitis, may complicate the diagnosis. In young children with a buccal cellulitis thought to be caused by Hib, lumbar puncture is indicated if meningitis cannot be excluded clinically. Blood culture results are positive in as many as 80% of the patients, and Hib often can be recovered from an aspirate of the cellulitis.

Pericarditis

Hib can cause bacterial pericarditis. These patients usually are between 2 and 4 years of age and often have had an antecedent upper respiratory tract infection. Fever, respiratory distress, and tachycardia are consistent findings. Associated infections also are common findings. The etiologic diagnosis may be established by blood culture or by culture, Gram stain, or antigen detection of pericardial fluid. Optimal management includes pericardiectomy, which effectively drains purulent material from the pericardial sac and minimizes the chances of the development of pericardial tamponade and constrictive pericarditis.

Acute Epiglottitis

Acute epiglottitis is a dramatic, rapidly fulminating infection. It occurs predominantly in children 2 to 7 years of age.

Miscellaneous Infections

Urinary tract infections, epididymoorchitis, cervical adenitis, acute glossitis, uvulitis, bacterial tracheitis, infected thyroglossal duct cysts, endocarditis, endophthalmitis, primary peritonitis, soft tissue abscess, periappendiceal abscess, brain abscess, and neonatal infections can be caused by Hib. See Chapter 133, Fever of Unknown Source, for a detailed discussion of nonspecific bacteremia.

INFECTIONS CAUSED BY NONTYPABLE *HAEMOPHILUS INFLUENZAE*

Upper Respiratory Tract Infections

Unencapsulated *H. influenzae* is a major cause of acute otitis media and acute sinusitis in children. Since the introduction of the pneumococcal conjugate vaccine, NT *H. influenzae* may be the most common organism causing acute otitis media in children. In adults, nontypable *H. influenzae* is associated with bronchitis. Nontypable strains also are common causes of conjunctivitis in children.

A syndrome of concomitant purulent conjunctivitis and otitis media caused by nontypable *H. influenzae* occurs in young children. Spread among family members is a common occurrence.

Neonatal Infection

In the neonate, nontypable *H. influenzae* is a more common pathogen than are the type b strains. Septicemia, pneumonia, and respiratory distress syndrome with shock, meningitis, and conjunctivitis have been reported. In the Neonatal Research Network, *H. influenzae* was the third most common organism, accounting for early-onset sepsis (12%) in very low-birth-weight infants.

Miscellaneous Infections

Bacteremia, meningitis, lung cyst, thyroglossal duct cyst infection, rectal abscess, septic arthritis, and cerebrospinal fluid (CSF) shunt infections may be caused by nontypable *H. influenzae*. Systemic infections caused by unencapsulated *H. influenzae* occur predominantly in immunocompromised hosts, although pneumonia caused by nontypable strains is a common finding in children living in developing countries. Invasive infections caused by nontype-b *H. influenzae* should prompt an investigation for an underlying anatomic or immune defect.

DIAGNOSIS

Cultures of blood, CSF, and other body fluids and sites yield *H. influenzae* in most children with invasive infections. Gram stain of appropriate specimens frequently demonstrates the characteristic pleomorphic coccobacilli of *H. influenzae*, although other organisms can have similar morphology. Polysaccharide for Hib antigen is detected readily by latex agglutination in a variety of body fluids, especially CSF, urine, and serum. Polymerase chain reaction may detect evidence of *H. influenzae* type b in CSF when culture and latex agglutination are negative. Because antigen may be detected in urine for as long as 1 month after the receipt of some Hib vaccines, it is not a reliable predictor of systemic infection in this instance. *H. influenzae* isolated from middle-ear fluid or conjunctival scrapings also indicates an etiologic diagnosis.

THERAPY

Strains of *H. influenzae* may be resistant to commonly used antibiotics, and several different mechanisms may be involved in this resistance. In the United States over 25% of *H. influenzae* strains recovered from respiratory sources produce beta-lactamase enzymes (TEM-1 or ROB-1), the predominant mechanism of ampicillin resistance. The gene coding for the production of this enzyme usually is contained within a plasmid that can be transferred. In some strains, this gene is located on a chromosome. A small percentage of ampicillin-resistant strains has a mechanism of resistance related to altered penicillin-binding proteins. These strains test negative for beta-lactamase but are resistant to ampicillin.

Because beta-lactamase and cloramphenicol acetyltransferase enzymes are plasmid-mediated, strains of Hib can be resistant to ampicillin and chloramphenicol. Although this resistance is not a common occurrence in the United States, it is a major problem in some parts of the world.

Several other classes of antibiotics have excellent activity against *H. influenzae* isolates. Cefuroxime, cefotaxime, and ceftriaxone are parenteral cephalosporins with proven efficacy in the treatment of systemic *H. influenzae* infections. Ampicillin- and chloramphenicol-resistant strains remain susceptible to these cephalosporins. Trimethoprim-sulfamethoxazole, cefpodoxime, cefixime, cefuroxime axetil, cefdinir, and the combination of amoxicillin and clavulanic acid (a beta-lactamase inhibitor) are oral agents useful for treating infections caused by ampicillin-resistant *H. influenzae*. However, some beta-lactamase-producing strains of nontypable *H. influenzae* are not inhibited by amoxicillin-clavulanic acid. The activity of cefprozil *in vitro* against *H. influenzae* is inferior to those of cefixime, cefpodoxime, cefdinir, and cefuroxime. *In vitro* azithromycin has greater activity than does clarithromycin. Fluoroquinolones have excellent *in vitro* activity against *H. influenzae* isolates and may be a treatment consideration for selected patients.

Several treatment options are available for the initial management of the child with suspected invasive infection caused by Hib. Cefotaxime or ceftriaxone is the treatment most commonly recommended for bacterial meningitis, for which cefuroxime should be avoided.

After Hib is isolated and the antimicrobial susceptibility is determined, the most appropriate antibiotic can be continued. Ampicillin remains the treatment of choice for infections caused by susceptible strains. Cefuroxime (not meningitis), cefotaxime, or ceftriaxone should be used if ampicillin-resistant strains are identified. Cefotaxime or ceftriaxone should be used to treat infections caused by strains of Hib resistant to ampicillin and chloramphenicol. Ceftriaxone is particularly convenient for administration once daily if home parenteral therapy is considered. Chloramphenicol rarely is used to treat invasive Hib infections in the United States, but it is an important agent in resource-poor countries.

In some instances, after the signs and symptoms of the acute non-CNS infection have resolved, therapy can be completed with an oral agent. The duration of therapy is discussed in the chapters describing specific infections. Bacteremia, cellulitis, and pneumonia typically are treated for 10 days. Septic arthritis is treated for 14 days.

The initial treatment of acute otitis media or sinusitis possibly caused by *H. influenzae* usually is amoxicillin. If the physician suspects that ampicillin-resistant strains are involved, amoxicillin-clavulanate or one of the several oral agents previously mentioned can be administered. Oral therapy of bacterial conjunctivitis caused by nontypable *H. influenzae* appears to be effective in preventing acute otitis media, which occurs in a high percentage of these patients. The choice of a specific agent is based partly on *in vitro* activity against *S. pneumoniae* isolates as well as personal preference, cost, and ease of administration.

PREVENTION

The development of the Hib protein conjugate vaccines is one of the most important advances in preventive pediatrics. Children younger than 2 years of age do not develop protective antibodies after immunization with the purified polysaccharide capsule (PRP) of Hib. However, conjugating PRP to a protein enhances the immunogenicity of PRP in infants by converting a T-cell-independent antigen to a T-cell-dependent one. The three available Hib protein conjugate vaccines differ in composition (Table 161.1). The oligosaccharide conjugate Hib vaccine (HbOc) and PRP-OMP vaccines prevented

TABLE 161.1

HAEMOPHILUS INFLUENZAE TYPE b PROTEIN CONJUGATE VACCINES

Abbreviation	Commercial Name	Polysaccharide	Protein Conjugate	Recommended Ages	Source
HbOc	HibTITER	Oligosaccharide	CRM197 mutant	2, 4, 6, 15 mo	Wyeth-Lederle Vaccines
PRP-OMP	PedvaxHib	Native	Outer membrane protein of *N. meningitidis* group B	2, 4, 12, mo	Merck
PRP-OMP/Hep B	Comvax	As above	As above	As above	Merck
PRP-T*	ActHib OmniHIB	Native	Tetanus toxoid	2, 4, 6, 15 mo	Sanofi-pasteur

*PRP-T combined with acellular diphtheria, tetanus, and pertussis vaccine (Tripedia) is approved for booster dose only.

development of systemic Hib infection in large field trials. The American Academy of Pediatrics and the CDC recommend routine immunization with the HbOc, PRP-OMP, or PRP-T vaccine beginning at 2 months of age. The vaccine administration schedules are different because of differences in the kinetics of antibody response to HbOc or PRT-T versus PRP-OMP. Combining Hib conjugate vaccines and DTaP in the same syringe results in a decreased antibody level to PRP compared with the vaccines administered at separate sites. Thus, the combined PRP-T/DTaP vaccine is approved only for the booster dose at 15 to18 months. A combination vaccine containing PRP-T, diphtheria and tetanus toxoids, inactivated poliomyelitis vaccine and acellular pertussis vaccine is available in Canada and is under review by the US Food and Drug Administration for use in infants starting at 2 months of age. After one PRP conjugate is administered, the series should be completed with the same vaccine when possible, although the PRP conjugate vaccines are interchangeable. Children who develop invasive disease after receiving 2 or 3 or more doses of Hib conjugate vaccine should undergo an immune evaluation. Dosing schedules of the Hib conjugate vaccine in infants at 2, 3, and 4 months of age without a booster may not lead to reliable long-lasting immunity, based on the experience in the United Kingdom.

To prevent secondary infection, rifampin prophylaxis is indicated for all family contacts of persons with Hib disease, if another family member younger than 4 years of age who has not completed the Hib immunization series is residing in the same household. Rifampin is administered to children at a dose of 20 mg/kg (not to exceed 600 mg) once daily for 4 consecutive days. Parents are given 600 mg/day for 4 days. The index patient should receive rifampin because systemic antibiotics do not eradicate nasopharyngeal colonization of Hib reliably. Parents should be told that an increased risk of acquiring secondary infection exists in the household and that they should seek prompt medical attention for any suspicious signs or symptoms in their child. Parents of children exposed to a single case of systemic Hib infection in a child-care center or nursery school should be warned similarly. Rifampin should be administered to all infants and child-care personnel if two or more cases of invasive disease have occurred among the children or employees within 60 days and unvaccinated or incompletely vaccinated children attend the child-care facility. Although not perfect, rifampin prophylaxis is effective in preventing secondary infections.

Suggested Readings

Adderson EE, Byington CL, Spencer L, et al. Invasive serotype a *Haemophilus influenzae* infections with a virulence genotype resembling *Haemophilus influenzae* type b: emerging pathogen in the vaccine era? *Pediatrics* 2001;108. http://www.pediatrics.org/cgi/content/full/108/1/e18.

Black SB, Shinefield HR, Fireman B, et al. Efficacy in infancy of oligosaccharide conjugate *H. influenzae* type b (HbOc) vaccine in a United States population of 61,080 children. *Pediatr Infect Dis J* 1991;10:97.

Block SL, Hedrick J, Harrison CJ, et al. Community-wide vaccination with the heptavalent pneumococcal conjugate significantly alters the microbiology of acute otitis media. *Pediatr Infect Dis J* 2004;23:829.

Bodor FF, Marchant CD, Shurin PA, Barenkamp SJ. Bacterial etiology of conjunctivitis-otitis media syndrome. *Pediatrics* 1985;76:26.

Centers for Disease Control and Prevention. Progress toward elimination of *Haemophilus influenzae* type b invasive disease among infants and children– United States, 1998–2000. *MMWR* 2002;51:234.

Committee on Infectious Diseases, American Academy of Pediatrics. *H. influenzae* infections. In: Pickering LK, ed. *Red Book: 2003 Report of the Committee on Infectious Diseases*, 26th ed. Elk Grove Village, IL: American Academy of Pediatrics, 2003:293.

Dajani AS, Asmar BI, Thirumoorthi MC. Systemic *Haemophilus influenzae* disease: an overview. *J Pediatr* 1979;94:355.

Heilmann KP, Rice CL, Miller AL, et al. Decreasing prevalence of beta-lactamase production among respiratory tract isolates of *Haemophilus influenzae* in the United States. *Antimicrob Agents Chemother* 2005;49:2561.

Jorgensen JH. Update on mechanisms and prevalence of antimicrobial resistance in *Haemophilus influenzae*. *Clin Infect Dis* 1992;14:1119.

Meissner HC, Pickering LK. Control of disease attributable to *Haemophilus influenzae* type b and the National Immunization Program. *Pediatrics* 2002;110:820.

Murphy TF. Respiratory infections caused by non-typeable *Haemophilus influenzae*. *Curr Opin Infect Dis* 2003;16:129.

Musser JM, Kapur V. Molecular population genetics of *Haemophilus influenzae* in Ellis RW and Granoff DM (eds). *Development and Clinical Uses of Haemophilus b Conjugate Vaccines*. Marcel Dekker, Inc. New York, NY 1994.

O'Neill JM, St. Geme III JW, Cutter D, et al. Invasive disease due to nontypeable *Haemophilus influenzae* among children in Arkansas. *J Clin Microbiol* 2003;41:3064.

Rodriguez CA, Avadhanula V, Buscher A, et al. Prevalence and distribution of adhensins in invasive non-type b encapsulated *Haemophilus influenzae*. *Infect Immun* 2003;71:1635.

Rotbart HA, Glode MP. *Haemophilus influenzae* type b septic arthritis in children: report of 23 cases. *Pediatrics* 1985;75:254.

Schuchat A, Robinson K, Wenger JD, et al. Bacterial meningitis in the United States in 1995. *N Engl J Med* 1997;337:970.

Urwin G, Krohn JA, Deaver-Robinson K, et al. Invasive disease due to *Haemophilus influenzae* serotype f: clinical and epidemiologic characteristics in the *H. influenzae* serotype b vaccine era. *Clin Infect Dis* 1996;22:1069.

Wallace RJ, Baker CJ, Quinones FJ, et al. Nontypable *Haemophilus influenzae* (bio-type 4) as a neonate, maternal, and genital pathogen. *Rev Infect Dis* 1983;5:123.

CHAPTER 162 ■ *LEGIONELLA*

MORVEN S. EDWARDS

A constellation of illnesses caused by *Legionella* has been defined since the late 1970s. When epidemic pneumonia was diagnosed among delegates attending the 1976 American Legion convention in Philadelphia, the descriptive term *Legionnaires disease* was coined. An estimated 182 people developed pneumonia, and 29 died. A 3-year-old child was among those with documented seroconversion. Within months, a "new" bacterium was discovered: *Legionella pneumophila*. Serologic testing of various population groups revealed that the bacillus had existed for decades and accounted for numerous previously unexplained outbreaks of pneumonia.

Many of the members of the genus *Legionella* are recognized agents of human infection (Table 162.1). Legionnaires disease and Pontiac fever are caused by *L. pneumophila*. The former is a long-incubation, lower respiratory tract infection, and the latter is an influenza-like illness without pneumonia, named in 1968 for an outbreak in Pontiac, Michigan. In 1979, the Pittsburgh pneumonia agent, now designated *L. micdadei*, was isolated from the lung tissue of two renal transplant recipients. Most infections caused by *L. micdadei* are nosocomial and occur in immunocompromised patients.

MICROBIOLOGY

Legionella organisms are small, pleomorphic, gram-negative bacilli that are approximately 0.5 μm wide and 3 μm long. Their ultrastructural features are typical of gram-negative bacilli and include a cell wall with trilaminar cytoplasmic and outer membranes. *L. pneumophila* has a single polar flagellum; other species, except *L. oakridgenesis*, have polar or subpolar flagella.

The best medium for isolating *Legionella* is buffered charcoal-yeast extract agar supplemented with alpha-ketoglutarate. Cysteine and amino acids are required for growth. Growth occurs optimally at 35°C in 5% carbon dioxide. Colonies of *L. pneumophila* and other species are 1 to 2 mm in diameter, have a ground-glass appearance, are gray to gray-white in color, and exhibit a sticky consistency when lifted with a loop. The addition of dyes to the agar, fluorescence techniques, and modification of L-cysteine requirements may be used in the laboratory to differentiate species.

TABLE 162.1

CLINICAL FORMS OF INFECTION CAUSED BY *LEGIONELLA* SPECIES AND THEIR CAUSATIVE ORGANISMS

Clinical Form of Infection	Causative Organisms
Legionnaires disease	*L. pneumophila*
Pontiac fever	*L. pneumophila*
Pittsburgh pneumonia	*L. micdadei*
Bronchopneumonia	*L. pneumophila*, *L. micdadei*, *L. bozemanii*, *L. dumoffii*, *L. longbeachae*, and others

Of the 42 species of *Legionella*, fewer than one-half have been associated with human disease. *L. pneumophila* is the most pathogenic and accounts for 90% of legionellosis cases. *L. pneumophila* has 14 serogroups, each of which has been associated with human infection. Serogroup 1 accounts for 80% of reported infections.

Legionella from clinical specimens are not visible by Gram stain. Special stains, such as the Gimenez and Dieterle silver impregnation, are necessary for visualization. When obtained from tissue specimens, *L. micdadei* is acid-fast by a modified Ziehl-Neelsen stain or Kinyoun carbol-fuchsin technique. Other species are not acid-fast.

EPIDEMIOLOGY AND TRANSMISSION

Legionella spreads by the airborne route, and Legionnaires disease is transmitted by inhalation, particularly of water vapor-containing aerosolized bacteria. Outbreaks have been linked to the evaporative condensers of air cooling systems, which amplify spread of the bacteria, and to soil-associated sites of excavation, whirlpool spas, showers, respiratory therapy equipment, and the ultrasonic humidifier of a grocery store mist machine.

The incidence of Legionnaires disease peaks in the late summer and early fall and has a male gender dominance. Person-to-person spread has not been documented. The incidence peaks in the sixth decade of life, and infection is an uncommon occurrence in the first two decades. Risk factors for infection in adults include smoking and alcoholism. Major predisposing features for all ages include organ transplantation, immunosuppression, malignancy, and renal disease. Underlying respiratory disease may be a risk factor in childhood.

Seroconversion to *L. pneumophila* or a closely related or cross-reacting organism in association with mild or inapparent clinical infection appears to be a common occurrence among young children. In one longitudinal 5-year study, more than one-half of the participants younger than 4 years of age at enrollment developed a fourfold or greater rise in titer that was not associated with acute illness. In another investigation, the frequency of reciprocal antibody titers of at least 256 was 25% among children ages 2 to 9 years of age, some of whom were tested during episodes of respiratory tract infection. The infrequency with which *L. pneumophila* can be implicated as a cause of acute pneumonia in physiologically normal children was illustrated by a study of 110 children who ranged in age from 1 week to 17 years and were hospitalized with pneumonia. Only two cases of Legionnaires disease—one confirmed and one possible—were identified.

PATHOPHYSIOLOGY

Legionnaires disease is initiated by inhalation of *L. pneumophila*. The bacillus gains entry into the cytoplasm of macrophages through phagocytosis and has the capacity to resist monocytic microbicidal mechanisms and to replicate intracellularly. The resultant cellular infiltrate in the alveolar spaces consists of macrophages and neutrophils. Because the organisms are clustered in macrophages, pulmonary tissue is not damaged severely. The predominant sites of involvement are the terminal bronchioles and alveoli. In radiographs, this mode of invasion causes a patchy lobular consolidation, which may progress to severe multilobular involvement and bilateral consolidation. A nodular infiltrate occurs in some 20% of patients. Small abscesses may occur, but frank abscess formation rarely occurs.

Bacteremic spread is the proposed route for dissemination of infection in immunocompromised patients. The reticuloendothelial system often is involved in infections having a fatal outcome. Focal involvement of such organs as the heart (e.g., myocardium, pericardium, endocardium), kidneys, brain, and peritoneum has been observed. Cellular rather than humoral immunity has a major role in host defense.

CLINICAL MANIFESTATIONS

The incubation period for Legionnaires disease is 2 to 10 days. Prodromal symptoms include malaise, myalgias, and headache. The illness is characterized by sudden onset of high fever and shaking chills with systemic toxicity. Nonbloody, watery diarrhea occurs in one-third to one-half of patients and may begin with the onset of fever or at any time during the first week of illness. A dry, nonproductive cough usually is apparent by the second day of illness. The sputum is nonpurulent or minimally purulent. Without intervention, pulmonary signs become more prominent and progress to consolidation with or without pleuritis. Dyspnea is a prominent feature at the peak of illness. In the physiologically normal host, spontaneous resolution of symptoms begins on days 7 to 10 of the illness.

Most symptomatic pediatric infections have been diagnosed in children with identifiable risk factors for Legionnaires disease, but cavitary pneumonia can occur in immunocompetent hosts. Nosocomial Legionella pneumonia has been described in term and preterm neonates, with water distribution systems as the source of infection. In immunocompromised children, symptoms may progress to respiratory failure with fatal outcome, often accompanied by renal failure and neurologic manifestations. Among pediatric renal or bone marrow transplant recipients or those with leukemia in relapse, the initial features of legionellosis are similar to those enumerated for healthy hosts, but the disease is likely to progress rapidly, resulting in opacification of an entire hemithorax, or to have findings of extrapulmonary foci of infection. Five of eight adult heart transplant recipients had consolidation with eventual cavitation.

The usual laboratory features include leukocytosis (i.e., 15,000 to 20,000 leukocytes/mm^3) with a neutrophil predominance, hyponatremia from inappropriate secretion of antidiuretic hormone, hypophosphatemia, and abnormal liver function tests. Arterial blood gases document hypoxemia and hypocapnia. Abnormalities of renal function are unusual findings. Chest radiography reveals distal air space disease, usually in a segmental or lobar distribution. Initially, infiltrates usually are unilateral, but bilateral involvement may be a feature of progressive disease, even after the initiation of therapy. Small pleural effusions may be evident, particularly early in the course of infection.

Pontiac fever is a self-limited disease and has been diagnosed only in epidemic situations. The onset of influenza-like symptoms occurs so rapidly after exposure (i.e., 6 hours to 2 days) that symptoms may represent a toxic or allergic response to the bacillus rather than a response to replication of the bacteria in pulmonary macrophages.

DIAGNOSIS

Legionellosis can be diagnosed by isolation of the organism, direct staining techniques, detection of antigen, or demonstration of a rise in specific antibody titer in paired sera. For laboratories with experience in isolating the organism, blood, lower respiratory tract secretions, and lung tissue are the best sources; after 2 to 6 days, Legionella may be recovered in 50% to 70% of infections, thus providing definitive evidence of infection.

Direct immunofluorescence may be used to detect the organism in respiratory tract secretions, pleural fluid, or lung tissue. For patients able to produce sputum, the technique has a sensitivity ranging from 25% to 75% and a specificity exceeding 90%, and it may provide a diagnosis within hours.

Tests to detect Legionella antigens in urine also permit establishing a rapid diagnosis. Commercially manufactured Legionella urinary antigen tests are available as radioimmunoassay or enzyme immunoassay. These tests have high sensitivity (60% to 80%) and specificity (99%), especially for L. pneumophila serogroup 1. Antigen remains detectable in urine for days or weeks, even during the administration of antibiotics.

Assays based on the polymerase chain reaction (PCR) have been used to detect Legionella in such clinical samples as urine or bronchoalveolar lavage fluid. The PCR-based tests are highly specific, but they are not more sensitive than is culture.

Legionellosis may be diagnosed serologically by indirect immunofluorescence antibody assays. A fourfold rise between acute and convalescent antibody titers obtained 1 to 3 weeks after the onset of illness to a titer of 1:128 or greater is diagnostic. Among some patients, seroconversion may not occur until the twelfth week of illness. For L. pneumophila serogroup 1, the sensitivity and specificity of the indirect fluorescent antibody assay in adult patients are 70% and 95%, respectively. Because of the low prevalence of disease in children, the predictive value of seroconversion probably is lower, but it has not been investigated. The positive predictive value of single convalescent titer of 1:256 or greater is low and does not establish definitive evidence of recent infection.

Community-acquired legionellosis may resemble Mycoplasma infection, psittacosis, Q fever, influenza, or other viral lower respiratory tract infections. The differential diagnosis for sporadic infection in hospitalized immunocompromised children also includes the fungal, mycobacterial, and protozoan agents that cause atypical pneumonia.

TREATMENT

Because of its superior lung tissue penetration and its ease of administration, azithromycin has replaced erythromycin as the drug of choice for the treatment of Legionella infections. Initially and until a definite clinical response has occurred, it should be administered intravenously in a single daily dose of 10 mg/kg/day (maximum, 500 mg). Once improvement has been noted, a 5- to 10-day course of treatment may be completed using the same regimen orally.

Use of rifampin in addition to azithromycin is recommended as adjunctive therapy for patients with severe infection, but it should not be given as a single agent because resistant strains may emerge. Fluoroquinolones, such as ciprofloxacin, levofloxacin, and gatifloxacin, are bactericidal and effective but are not approved to use in patients younger than 18 years of age. Trimethoprim-sulfamethoxazole and doxycycline are active in vitro and are potential alternative treatment options, but doxycycline should not be used for children younger than 8 years of age. Penicillins, cephalosporins, and aminoglycoside antibiotics are ineffective.

Appropriate supportive care should be provided for lower respiratory tract infection, respiratory failure, or inappropriate secretion of antidiuretic hormone.

OUTCOME

Clinical response usually is evident within 2 to 5 days after initiation of therapy. Fever may persist for as long as 1 week. The resolution of pneumonia proceeds slowly and may require 1 month. Among immunocompetent adults, fatality rates are as low as 4% to 7% with appropriate treatment. The overall fatality rate for patients managed appropriately is 15% to 25%, but rates as high as 80% have been reported for immunocompromised patients. Apparent relapses have been encountered after an appropriate treatment course and are an indication for retreatment.

Suggested Readings

Andersen RD, Lauer BA, Fraser DW, et al. Infections with Legionella pneumophila in children. J Infect Dis 1981;143:386.

Benin AL, Benson RF, Besser RE. Trends in legionnaires disease, 1980–1998: declining mortality and new patterns of diagnosis. Clin Infect Dis 2002; 35:1039.

Carlson NC, Kuskie MR, Dobyns EL, et al. Legionellosis in children: an expanding spectrum. Pediatr Infect Dis J 1990;9:133.

Edelstein PH. Legionnaires' disease. Clin Infect Dis 1993;16:741.

Famiglietti RF, Bakerman PR, Saubolle MA, et al. Cavitary legionellosis in two immunocompetent infants. Pediatrics 1997;99:899.

Fields BS, Benson RF, Besser RE. Legionella and Legionnaires' disease: 25 years of investigation. Clin Microbiol Rev 2002;15:506.

Finegold SM. Legionnaires' disease: still with us. N Engl J Med 1988;318:571.

Kovatch AL, Jardine DS, Dowling JN, et al. Legionellosis in children with leukemia in relapse. Pediatrics 1984;73:811.

Mahoney FJ, Hoge CW, Farley TA, et al. Community wide outbreak of Legionnaires' disease associated with a grocery store mist machine. J Infect Dis 1992;165:736.

Muder RR, Yu VL. Infection due to Legionella species other than L. pneumophila. Clin Infect Dis 2002;35:990.

Muldoon RL, Jaecker DL, Kiefer HK. Legionnaires' disease in children. Pediatrics 1981;67:329.

Orenstein WA, Overturf GD, Leedom JM, et al. The frequency of Legionella infection prospectively determined in children hospitalized with pneumonia. J Pediatr 1981;99:403.

Schwebke JR, Hackman R, Bowden R. Pneumonia due to Legionella micdadei in bone marrow transplant recipients. Rev Infect Dis 1990;12:824.

Stout JE, Yu VL. Legionellosis. N Engl J Med 1997;337:682.

Winn WC Jr. Legionnaires' disease: historical perspective. Clin Microbiol Rev 1988;1:60.

CHAPTER 163 ■ LEPTOSPIROSIS

RALPH D. FEIGIN

Leptospirosis is a disease caused by a single family of organisms that contains multiple serogroups and serotypes. The disease is characterized by a broad spectrum of clinical findings.

EPIDEMIOLOGY

Virtually all mammals can be infected by leptospires (i.e., tightly coiled spirochetes) and can transmit disease caused by this genus of organisms. In various parts of the world, field mice, rats, moles, gerbils, hedgehogs, shrews, foxes, jackels, mongooses, civets, bandicoots, dogs, skunks, raccoons, opossums, and cattle have been implicated as sources of human infection. Leptospires also have been isolated from reptiles and birds. A host species may serve as a reservoir for one or more serotypes of leptospires, and a particular serotype may be hosted by many different animal species. Two or more animal hosts for the same serotype may exist in the same geographic area. Virtually any animal susceptible to infection by leptospires may become a temporary urinary shedder of the organisms.

Transmission of leptospires to humans occurs through contact with urine, blood, tissues, or organs of infected animals or exposure to an environment that has been contaminated by leptospires. Humans generally represent a dead end in the chain of infection, although person-to-person transmission can occur. Human-to-human transmission has been reported through human milk obtained by a breast-fed infant from a lactating mother who was infected with *Leptospira interrogans*. Leptospires may enter breaks in the skin or may penetrate the mucous membranes of the conjunctiva, nasopharynx, or vagina.

Leptospires may be transmitted from soil or water to humans. A warm climate (warmer than 25°C), moisture, and soil or surface water with pH values between 6.2 and 8.0 are optimal environments for survival of leptospires. These conditions are found commonly in many tropical regions throughout the year and in temperate zones during the late spring, summer, and autumn months.

The role of occupation as a major risk factor in leptospirosis was emphasized in the 1960s. Since then, however, increasing numbers of cases have been reported among children who live in urban areas and who participate in outdoor recreation. In rural areas, leptospires may be acquired from swimming in farm ponds or in contaminated rivers and streams.

Leptospirosis has become increasingly prevalent among children, students, and housewives. Cases from urban and suburban communities have been reported more frequently than have cases from rural areas. The dog has been incriminated increasingly as an important vector and reservoir of this disease.

PATHOPHYSIOLOGY

Leptospires penetrate the skin or mucous membranes and then invade the bloodstream and spread throughout the body to produce a wide variety of manifestations. The organism appears to bore through connective tissue and invade various tissues, including the anterior chamber of the eye and the subarachnoid space, without eliciting a significant inflammatory response.

Avirulent and virulent strains of leptospires are taken up by fixed phagocytes and reticuloendothelial tissue *in vivo*. The severity of the lesions produced correlates positively with the number of organisms. Specific resistance apparently is mediated by antibodies, which increase the efficacy of clearance of leptospires from the bloodstream by improving phagocytosis and thereby enhancing opsonization. Polymorphonuclear leukocytes are not an efficient defense factor against pathogenic leptospires in nonimmune hosts. The virulence of leptospires appears to be related to their ability to resist killing by neutrophils and serum components.

Selected clinical and histologic findings in human leptospirosis suggest that pathogenicity may result partially from enzymes, toxins, or other metabolites that are elaborated by or released by lysed leptospires. Endotoxin has been demonstrated in extracts of leptospires, but its precise role in the pathogenesis of leptospirosis remains unknown.

The development of jaundice and hemolytic anemia in patients with leptospirosis suggests that hemolysis may play a role in the pathogenesis of this disease. Hemolysis may persist during leptospirosis, a finding suggesting that circulating hemolysin is adsorbed by erythrocytes early during the course of leptospirosis and that the erythrocytes subsequently lyse despite the development of serum antibody.

In humans, a profound derangement in hepatic function has been associated with leptospirosis. Necrosis of liver cells is an infrequent occurrence, however, and the activity of serum glutamic oxaloacetic and pyruvic transaminases generally is elevated only slightly. The most prominent clinical manifestations of hepatic dysfunction include icterus and impaired production of the clotting factors dependent on vitamin K, decreased serum albumin, and increased serum globulins. These abnormalities have occurred in both icteric and anicteric patients with leptospirosis.

Renal failure is an important cause of death in patients with leptospirosis. In patients who die during the first week of disease, renal changes include cloudy swelling or isolated tubular epithelial cell necrosis. In those who die during the second week of illness, numerous foci of tubular epithelial necrosis are apparent. When patients die after the twelfth day of illness, an inflammatory infiltrate in the kidney is widespread, involving the medulla and the cortex. Impaired renal blood flow appears to constitute a fundamental alteration of the nephropathy associated with leptospirosis. Diminution in renal perfusion is suggested by hypotension, hypovolemia, and circulatory collapse. Reversible oliguria observed during the course of leptospirosis has been attributed to reduced renal blood flow resulting from hypotension, a deficit of extracellular fluid, or both. Rarely, adrenal insufficiency may occur after hemorrhagic infarction of the adrenal glands.

Cardiac dysfunction can lead to hypoperfusion in severe leptospirosis. Focal hemorrhagic myocarditis, pericarditis, and cardiac arrhythmias have been documented. Cardiac malfunction may occur secondary to hypotension, electrolyte imbalance, hypovolemia, or uremia. Other pathologic alterations of leptospirosis include acute hemorrhagic lobar pneumonia and massive hemoptysis, meningitis, meningoencephalitis and encephalitis, radiculitis, myelitis, and peripheral neuritis.

The intraocular fluid provides a protective environment for leptospires. Despite the development of high antibody titers in serum, leptospires may remain viable in the anterior chamber of the eyes for many months. This phenomenon appears to be responsible for the recurrent, chronic, or latent uveitis syndromes of patients with leptospirosis.

Myalgia is a common complaint in patients with all forms of leptospirosis. Myalgia appears to be the result of patho-logic changes, including vacuolation of the cytoplasm of the myofibrils.

CLINICAL MANIFESTATIONS

Common Leptospirosis

Leptospirosis is an acute systemic infection characterized by generalized vasculitis. Diminished awareness of this disorder, coupled with the diversity and nonspecificity of its presentation, accounts for the significant number of cases that go unrecognized.

The usual incubation period is 7 to 12 days, but a range of 2 to 20 days has been reported. The variation in incubation periods is not serotype-specific and has no prognostic significance.

The first (septicemic) stage of leptospirosis is characterized by the development of an acute systemic infection with an abrupt onset of symptoms. Fever, myalgia, arthralgia, and conjunctivitis may be noted. This phase terminates in approximately 4 to 7 days, with symptomatic improvement and defervescence. These changes coincide with the disappearance of leptospires from the blood, cerebrospinal fluid (CSF), and all other tissues except the aqueous humor of the eye and renal parenchyma. Antibody titers to leptospires develop rapidly, heralding the onset of the second (immune) stage of the illness. This stage, which lasts 4 to 30 days, may be associated with additional signs and symptoms of central nervous system involvement including stiff neck, photophobia, and irritability. Leptospiruria occurs commonly and continues for 1 week to 1 month. This immune phase of the disease generally is unaffected by antibiotic therapy. Meningitis and hepatic or renal involvement and meningitis reach peak intensity during this stage of disease.

Clinical leptospirosis can follow an icteric or an anicteric course. At least 90% of all the patients with leptospirosis are anicteric. Therefore, they escape definitive diagnosis, largely because icterus and azotemia are absent. The onset of the septicemic phase of anicteric leptospirosis is heralded by fever, malaise, myalgia, headache, chills, and abdominal pain. Fever abates by lysis, and other symptoms resolve. Death rarely occurs in patients with the first stage of anicteric leptospirosis. The second stage of anicteric disease is characterized by fever, uveitis, rash, headache, and meningitis. Usually, the fever is of brief duration and has a lower peak than during the septicemic phase.

Physical examination performed during the septicemic stage may reveal muscle tenderness, conjunctival suffusion, dehydration, generalized lymphadenopathy, hepatosplenomegaly, and skin rashes, which can be macular, maculopapular, urticarial, erythematous, petechial, purpuric, hemorrhagic, or desquamating. The skin lesions are most prominent over the trunk, but any area of the body can be affected. Pharyngitis, rales, arthritis, nonpitting edema, and tachycardia may occur. Hypotension is a rare finding in anicteric disease. Muscle pain and tenderness may be generalized, but the muscles of the calf, lower spine, and abdomen are affected most frequently. Conjunctival suffusion, photophobia, ocular pain, and conjunctival hemorrhage are more helpful diagnostic signs. Suffusion is more marked on the bulbar than on the palpebral conjunctiva. Nonobstructive, toxic dilatation of the gallbladder that may require cholecystotomy often occurs in children with leptospirosis. Pain associated with this problem must be differentiated from myositis, subperitoneal or subserosal hemorrhages, pancreatitis, or abdominal wall causalgia, all of which may occur in patients with either anicteric or icteric leptospirosis. Other signs and symptoms of the septicemic phase of anicteric leptospirosis include parotitis, orchitis, epididymitis, prostatitis, arthralgia, arthritis, and otitis media.

The immune phase of anicteric disease is reflected by CSF pleocytosis, with or without meningeal signs or symptoms. As an antibody titer develops, leptospires are cleared rapidly from the CSF. If examination of the CSF is performed during the second week of illness, a meningeal reaction can be demonstrated in more than 80% of the patients with anicteric disease, but only 50% of patients have clinical signs and symptoms of meningitis.

Lumbar punctures may reveal various CSF pressures, with mean values less than 200 mm H$_2$O. Cell counts within the CSF vary from normal to 500 cells/mm^3. Polymorphonuclear leukocytes predominate early during the immune phase, but mononuclear cells predominate subsequently. Protein concentrations within the CSF range from normal to 300 mg/dL. Glucose concentrations generally are normal.

Encephalitis, spasticity, paralysis, cranial nerve paralysis, peripheral neuritis, nystagmus, radiculitis, seizures, visual disturbances, myelitis, or Guillain-Barré syndrome may appear during or after the immune stage of anicteric disease. Leptospiruria is the rule during the immune stage of anicteric leptospirosis, and it is not associated with impaired renal function. Anicteric or icteric leptospirosis developing during the first two trimesters of pregnancy seems to increase the risk of spontaneous abortion.

Icteric Leptospirosis

The icteric form of leptospirosis also is known as *Weil syndrome*. This nomenclature is a distinctive clinical expression for severe leptospirosis, but it does not refer to a specific serotype. The mortality rate increases with age and, despite optimal supportive care, is between 5% and 10%. Weil syndrome is dominated by symptoms of renal, hepatic, or vascular dysfunction. Icterus and azotemia may be so severe that the biphasic course of illness is not observed.

Icterus remains the hallmark of Weil syndrome, with the patient's bilirubin concentrations rising as high as 60 to 80 mg/dL, although concentrations usually are less than 20 mg/dL. Direct- and indirect-reacting bilirubin increase, and modest elevations in serum alkaline phosphatase and depressed activity of plasma prothrombin occur. The hypoprothrombinemia responds to the parenteral administration of vitamin K. Serum albumin generally is depressed.

Hepatomegaly develops in approximately one-fourth of these patients, a frequency no greater than that in anicteric cases. Transient intrahepatic biliary obstruction may occur, but acholic stools generally are not observed. Acalculous cholecystitis occurs in some 55% of children with icteric leptospirosis.

Renal dysfunction may be seen in all forms of leptospirosis, regardless of the severity of the disease or the serotype causing infection. Proteinuria is the most frequent abnormality, but usually it is mild. Hyaline or granular casts and cellular elements may be found in the urinary sediment. Gross or microscopic hematuria probably reflects a hemorrhagic diathesis rather than a glomerular injury. Oliguria or anuria may develop early and may persist. Renal failure generally is reversible, but it also is the principal cause of death in patients with leptospirosis.

Cardiac involvement occurs relatively infrequently. Congestive heart failure and cardiovascular collapse occur, and cerebrovascular accidents are observed in patients with leptospirosis.

Hyponatremia is a consistent finding in patients with severe icteric leptospirosis. The hyponatremia appears to result from the failure of the sodium pump that causes sodium to move intracellularly in exchange for potassium and from a redistribution of fluid such that the extracellular fluid space is expanded at the expense of the intracellular space. Hyponatremia in these patients may be unresponsive to sodium replacement and fluid restriction. It is treated best by fluid restriction, which can be continued unless hypotension ensues. Clinical improvement generally follows a spontaneous increase in serum sodium, which may be seen before any other evidence of clinical improvement.

LABORATORY DIAGNOSIS

A confirmed case of leptospirosis, as defined by the Centers for Disease Control and Prevention (CDC), must fulfill the following criteria: clinical specimens that are culture positive for leptospires or clinical symptoms compatible with leptospirosis and either seroconversion or a fourfold or greater rise in the microscopic agglutination titer between acute and convalescent serum specimens obtained 2 or more weeks apart and studied at the same laboratory.

Presumptive leptospirosis is defined as showing clinical symptoms compatible with leptospirosis and a microscopic agglutination titer of at least 1:100, a positive macroscopic agglutination slide test reaction on a single serum specimen obtained after the onset of symptoms, or a stable microscopic agglutination titer of at least 1:100 in two or more serum specimens obtained after the onset of symptoms.

Leptospires can be recovered from blood or CSF during the septicemic stage of the illness and from urine during the immune phase. Media for the inoculation of leptospires usually contain a buffered solution, with or without peptone, and with or without 0.1% or 0.2% agar to which rabbit serum has been added to provide a final concentration in the medium of 5% to 10%. A pH between 7.2 and 7.8 is essential. For routine use, Fletcher semisolid medium or Ellinghausen-McCullough-Johnson-Harris semisolid medium is recommended. Stuart medium has been used to prepare and maintain antigens for serologic tests. Tween 80-albumin medium (OAC) is available commercially and appears to be superior for primary isolation of leptospires.

Multiple cultures should be obtained because the concentration of organisms at any given time may be very low. Urine is the main source from which leptospires can be isolated during the immune and convalescent phases of leptospirosis. A clean-voided urine specimen can be inoculated directly into an appropriate semisolid medium. Diluting urine specimens with sterile buffered saline solution is imperative to ensure growth. The best results are obtained by adding 0.1 mL of urine to 0.9 mL of buffered saline before inoculation into 5 mL of semisolid medium.

Leptospires may be observed by darkfield examination, but a concentration of 10,000 to 20,000 leptospires/1 mL of fluid is needed to observe these organisms. Leptospires can be stained by several silver impregnation techniques.

Fluorescent antibody techniques have been applied successfully to the detection of leptospires in urine or tissues. A positive and negative control specimen should be obtained at the time the unknown specimen is being tested. Positive results are considered presumptive evidence of infection. DNA hybridization techniques or nucleic acid amplification procedures, including polymerase chain reaction protocols using leptospiral-specific cDNA probes or oligonucleotide primers, can be used to detect the presence of leptospires in body fluids or culture supernatants.

Serologic tests are available for the diagnosis of leptospirosis. The microscopic agglutination test performed with live organisms at the CDC is one of the methods of choice. The enzyme-linked immunosorbent assay (ELISA) has been compared with the microscopical agglutination test for the serologic diagnosis of leptospirosis. The results suggest that this test is a sound alternative to the microscopic agglutination test because of its sensitivity, standardization, and simplicity. Rapid serodiagnosis of leptospirosis with the use of an immunoglobulin M (IgM)-specific dot ELISA has proved to be as sensitive and specific as microscopic agglutination tests. The dot ELISA uses minute volumes of leptospiral antigens.

The IgM-PK ELISA is an assay for IgM that employs a proteinase K-treated antigen. This test was compared with the Leptoteste-S macroagglutination test and with the standard microscopic agglutination test for the diagnosis of leptospirosis. Thirty-eight percent of patients with leptospirosis were identified earlier with either test than with the standard microscopic agglutination test. The IgM-PK ELISA had a sensitivity of 89.9% and a specificity of 97.4% and has been suggested as the test of choice in laboratories equipped to perform ELISA.

A slide agglutination ELISA also is available; it is inexpensive and can be performed more quickly and easily than ELISA. This test is extremely useful in laboratories that are not as well equipped as those in which IgM ELISA is performed.

Lepto Dipstick, a dipstick assay for detection of *Leptospira*-specific IgM antibodies in sera, also is available, and results using this test correlate well with results obtained by the IgM ELISA leptospiral antigen detection method (93.2% observed agreement). The dipstick is a useful rapid screening test for leptospirosis.

A passive microcapsule agglutination test also has been developed. Compared with the standard microscopic agglutination test, the passive microcapsule agglutination test showed a relatively greater degree of genus specificity and four- to 32-fold higher titers. This test is simple to perform and is reproducible; it can be employed routinely in the laboratory.

A fourfold increase in titers between acute and convalescent sera is indisputable evidence of active leptospirosis when this result is obtained using any of the specific serologic tests. Other tests that may be used for the serologic diagnosis of leptospirosis include a complement fixation assay, a hemolytic test, an indirect immunofluorescent test, an erythrocyte-sensitizing substance test, and countercurrent immunoelectrophoresis.

TREATMENT

Treatment is most beneficial when administered early. Treatment with penicillin or tetracycline (except in children younger than 8 years of age) should be initiated if the diagnosis of leptospirosis is suspected. Parenteral aqueous penicillin G administered as 6 to 8 million U/m^2 of body surface/day in six divided doses is optimal. For patients sensitive to penicillin, tetracycline administered as 10 to 20 mg/kg/day should be provided intravenously, or 25 to 50 mg/kg/day can be given orally in four divided oral doses for 1 week.

Management of leptospirosis requires attention to supportive care. Fluid and electrolyte balance must be maintained meticulously. Dehydration, acute renal failure, and cardiovascular collapse require prompt and specific treatment.

PREVENTION

Hygienic conditions should be encouraged in farmyard buildings, swimming pools, and slaughterhouses. Immunization of workers at high risk for development of leptospirosis has been used successfully in other parts of the world. Leptospire bacterins are available commercially and have been evaluated for safety and efficacy in laboratory animals and in domestic livestock. The degree of protection attained in these animals depends largely on the antigenic potential of the immunizing agent.

Suggested Readings

Brandão AP, Camargo ED, da Silva ED, et al. Macroscopic agglutination test for rapid diagnosis of human leptospirosis. *J Clin Microbiol* 1998;36:3138.

Everard CO, Edwards CN, Everard JD, et al. A twelve-year study of leptospirosis on Barbados. *Eur J Epidemiol* 1995;11:311.

Feigin RD. Leptospirosis. In: Feigin RD, Cherry JD, Demmler GJ, Kaplan SL, eds. *Textbook of pediatric infectious diseases*, 5th ed. Philadelphia: WB Saunders, 2003:1708.

Feigin RD, Lobes LA, Anderson DC, et al. Human leptospirosis from immunized dogs. *Ann Intern Med* 1973;79:777.

Heath CW Jr, Alexander AD, Galton MM. Leptospirosis in the United States. *N Engl J Med* 1965;273:857.

Peter G. Leptospirosis: a zoonosis of protean manifestations. *Pediatr Infect Dis* 1982;1:282.

Shahed Y, Shpilberg O, Samara D, et al. Leptospirosis in pregnancy and its effect on the fetus: case report and review. *Clin Infect Dis* 1993;17:241.

Smits HL, Ananyina YV, Chereshsky A, et al. International multicenter evaluation of the clinical utility of a dipstick assay for detection of *Leptospira*-specific immunoglobulin M antibodies in human serum specimens. *J Clin Microbiol* 1999;37:2904.

Sulzer CR, Glosser JW, Rogers F, et al. Evaluation of an indirect hemagglutination test for the diagnosis of human leptospirosis. *J Clin Microbiol* 1975;2:218.

Watt G, Alquize LM, Padre LP, et al. The rapid diagnosis of leptospirosis: a prospective comparison of the dot enzyme-linked immunosorbent assay and the genus-specific microscopic agglutination test at different stages of illness. *J Infect Dis* 1988;157:840.

CHAPTER 164 ■ LISTERIOSIS

MORVEN S. EDWARDS

Listeria monocytogenes was described in 1911 as a bacillus that produced minute nodular lesions in the liver of a rabbit. It was shown to have infective capacity in laboratory animals in 1926 and was isolated from the blood of a patient with a mononucleosis syndrome in 1929. The first perinatal infection caused by *L. monocytogenes* was described in 1936. The organism was called *Listerella* at that time; the current designation was adopted in 1939 in honor of Lord Lister.

MICROBIOLOGY

L. monocytogenes is a short, non-spore-forming, gram-positive bacillus. In log phase of growth and in cerebrospinal fluid (CSF), organisms may appear predominantly coccoid and may form short chains that may be mistaken on Gram stain for pneumococci or group B streptococci. Older cultures may stain Gram variable, and they can be confused morphologically with *Haemophilus influenzae*. *L. monocytogenes* grows well on most laboratory media. On sheep-blood agar, the colonies are 1 to 2 mm in diameter, gray-white, and translucent, with a narrow zone of alpha-hemolysis that may be most evident on lifting a colony from the plate. Almost all strains of *L. monocytogenes* are motile, a feature most pronounced at room temperature in a semisolid motility medium. The organism is catalase-positive and oxidase-negative, and it hydrolyzes esculin. Optimal temperatures for growth range from 20° to 37°C, and although growth is faster at 30° to 37°C, the organism's capacity to replicate at low temperatures is a helpful differentiating feature. *L. monocytogenes* may be confused in the laboratory with corynebacteria, group B streptococci, enterococci, and diphtheroids.

Somatic and flagellar antigens have been used to classify *L. monocytogenes* into serotypes, designated numerically. Currently, at least 17 have been identified, with types 1/2a, 1/2b, and 4b accounting for 90% of cases of listeriosis.

EPIDEMIOLOGY AND TRANSMISSION

L. monocytogenes is widespread in nature. The organism is found in dust, soil, water, sewage, and vegetation. It has caused naturally acquired infection in more than 50 species of animals, including mammals, birds, rodents, crustaceans, and fish. It has been isolated from insects, but they are not considered an important vector of infection. The organism's capacity to withstand dry, alkaline conditions may account for its persistence in soil and its widespread distribution in nature. Between 1% and 5% of asymptomatic adults harbor this organism in the gastrointestinal tract.

The incidence of human infection is highest in the spring and summer months, but infection in animals occurs more frequently during the winter. Infection in humans is a sporadic occurrence and usually cannot be traced to animal contacts. Most cases probably result from soilborne infection. The acquisition of *L. monocytogenes* beyond the neonatal period likely results in asymptomatic colonization or infection of the mucous membranes of the throat or gastrointestinal tract, with transient or persistent fecal shedding. Infection may be acquired transplacentally or perinatally after delivery through the birth canal of a colonized parturient. *Listeria* may be transmitted genitally from person to person, but transmission by the respiratory route has not been documented. Epidemic neonatal listeriosis may be transmitted among infants by contact with the hands of hospital personnel. A nosocomial outbreak was associated with contaminated mineral oil used for infant bathing. Clusters of infections with no evident source also have been described in newborn nurseries and among hospitalized immunocompromised hosts.

Numerous foodborne outbreaks have been documented. In one of them, cabbage used in coleslaw was contaminated, presumably from the manure of a flock of sheep, one of which had died of listeriosis. Pasteurized milk was the source in another outbreak. The milk came from dairy cows that had suffered from *Listeria* encephalitis. Mexican-style cheese contaminated with *L. monocytogenes* serotype 4b was implicated in an outbreak in which 58 of 86 cases occurred in mother and infant pairs.

PATHOPHYSIOLOGY

Fecal carriage rates and serologic assessment indicate that many people are exposed to *L. monocytogenes*, although few develop invasive infection. Most infections are observed in neonates and older persons, a finding suggesting a host-associated immune defect. Also predisposed are persons with reticuloendothelial dysfunction caused by diabetes or cirrhosis, those requiring immunosuppressive or corticosteroid therapy, and patients with malignancy, particularly lymphoma or Hodgkin disease, solid organ transplantation, pregnancy, or human immunodeficiency virus infection. The propensity for listeriosis in persons with T-cell dysfunction demonstrates the important role of thymus-derived lymphocytes and mononuclear phagocytes in host response to this intracellular pathogen. *Listeria* replicates within the cytoplasm of host cells and usurps their actin-based contractile mechanism to form filopods that are ingested by adjacent cells. This cell-to-cell spread avoids direct contact with the extracellular environment. Thus, cell-mediated immunity is highly important in listeriosis. Immune globulins and complement also function in host defense, but only limited protection is conferred by these T-cell-independent mechanisms.

L. monocytogenes can invade the eyes and skin of humans by direct exposure or inoculation, but invasion of the bloodstream from a gastrointestinal tract source is the most likely route. The organism has tropism for the central nervous system (CNS), particularly the meninges. Hematogenous maternal infection is presumed to seed the placenta and to cause fetal infection through the umbilical vein, with dissemination to multiple organs. Human listeriosis is characterized by the formation of nodular granulomas that vary in site and number according to the mode of infection, the dose of organisms, and the age and resistance of the host. In neonates, the liver usually is involved diffusely, and granulomas also are observed in the lungs, spleen, adrenal glands, and lymph nodes. The organisms cause necrosis followed by proliferative activity of cells of the reticuloendothelial system. The granulomas undergo central necrosis. At the periphery of the necrotic focus, chronic inflammatory cells and organisms may be seen.

CLINICAL MANIFESTATIONS

Listeria infections affecting children can be divided into three broad categories: maternal infections, neonatal infections, and infections beyond the neonatal period in children with or without predisposing conditions.

Maternal Infections

Maternal infection is manifested as an influenza-like illness with chills, fever, vomiting, myalgia, and headache that occurs in the days or weeks before abortion or delivery. Patients may have abdominal or urinary symptoms, cough or upper respiratory tract congestion, or fever alone. Intrauterine infection can cause amnionitis, premature labor, spontaneous abortion, stillbirth, or early-onset neonatal infection. Green or brown staining of the amniotic fluid often is observed.

Neonatal Infections

Three syndromes of listeriosis occur in neonates: granulomatosis infantisepticum, early-onset sepsis with or without pneumonia, and late-onset meningitis.

Granulomatosis infantisepticum is the designation for classic disseminated listeriosis, with generalized septicemia, extensive pustular or petechial rash, and marked hepatomegaly. This overwhelming form of listeriosis frequently results in death *in utero*. Liveborn infants often are depressed at birth and usually die in the first hours of life as a result of respiratory distress, meningitis with seizures, or shock. In one report, 15 of 21 infants born alive had fatal outcomes.

Early-onset listeriosis is defined by the onset of symptoms within the first 7 days of life. Most infants are symptomatic at or within hours after delivery. Also referred to as the *septicemic* form of the illness, early-onset listeriosis is associated with obstetric complications and premature onset of labor. Respiratory distress and shock with cardiac dysfunction are the predominant symptoms. In one report, ten of 14 liveborn infants with listeriosis had respiratory symptoms at delivery; three infants developed illness at 12 hours, 3 days, and 4 days of age, respectively. One infant was asymptomatic. Meningitis occurred in four patients, each of whom was symptomatic at birth. Nonspecific findings of neonatal sepsis, such as hypothermia, fever, cyanosis, poor feeding, and vomiting, may accompany early-onset infection. Types 1/2a and 1/2b predominate in early-onset disease, although outbreaks caused by type 4b also have been described. The case fatality rate is 20% to 30%.

Late-onset listeriosis occurs 2 to 4 weeks after delivery. Infection can result from acquisition of the organism during passage through the birth canal or from environmental sources. Also called the *meningitic* form of disease, late-onset listeriosis generally occurs in full-term infants whose mothers have had a benign obstetric course. It is almost always manifested as meningitis or meningoencephalitis, with symptoms typical of purulent meningitis, including fever, irritability, and poor feeding. Presenting features include a bulging fontanelle, seizures,

respiratory distress, and vomiting or diarrhea. Examination of the CSF reveals pleocytosis, usually ranging from 100 to several thousand cells per cubic millimeter, an elevated protein, and a depressed glucose level. Neutrophils or mononuclear cells may predominate, and the predominant cell type may shift to neutrophils or mononuclear cells during the course of illness. Type 4b predominates in late-onset disease. With proper treatment, the fatality rate is less than 10%, but some infants sustain neurologic damage from meningitis.

Infection after the Neonatal Period

Listeriosis in childhood or adolescence is an uncommon event. Among 87 patients between the ages of 2 months and 20 years for whom sufficient data are available, 54% had no underlying diseases known to predispose to *Listeria* infections. Approximately one-fourth had hematologic malignancies, were organ transplant recipients, or were receiving medications that caused immunosuppression. Miscellaneous predisposing conditions, including cirrhosis, portal hypertension, diabetes mellitus, tuberculosis, renal disease, systemic lupus erythematosus, and pregnancy, may have enhanced susceptibility in the remainder of patients. Infection may present as the following: bacteremia with no focus; focal infection, such as endocarditis, osteomyelitis, peritonitis, or ocular infection; or CNS infection. The manifestations of meningitis for this older group of children are similar to those with other etiologic agents.

Several CNS manifestations of listeriosis have been described. With its propensity to affect the brain or brainstem, *Listeria* may cause diffuse encephalitis or rhombencephalitis, characterized by dizziness, vomiting, and cranial nerve palsies. Primary involvement of the brainstem follows a biphasic pattern in which a nonspecific prodrome of headache, vomiting, and fever is followed by cranial nerve palsies most commonly involving the sixth, seventh, ninth, and tenth nerves. Among 14 cases of *L. monocytogenes* brain abscess, seven occurred in patients with leukemia or renal allografts, and four occurred in patients without predisposing features. With the exception of an unusually high frequency of associated bacteremia and meningitis, the features of *Listeria* brain abscess were not distinctive.

Foodborne transmission now is recognized as a major source of human listeriosis manifesting as gastroenteritis. Outbreaks have been associated with unwashed raw vegetables, with ready-to-eat foods including soft cheese, deli foods, and pâté, and with unpasteurized milk. After an incubation period of approximately 24 hours, the common symptoms are fever, chills, nonbloody diarrhea, and abdominal cramps. Symptoms subside after several days, but they can be severe enough to warrant hospitalization.

DIAGNOSIS

The only means by which *L. monocytogenes* infection can be diagnosed reliably is by isolating the organism from clinical specimens. Cultures should be obtained from appropriate sources that may include blood, CSF, purulent collections, and bone marrow. For suspected early-onset neonatal infection, the placenta, amniotic fluid, and maternal vagina and lochia may provide evidence of infection. Neonatal surface cultures from the throat, conjunctivae, or feces are indicative only of colonization and are not clinically useful. A Gram stain of CSF or purulent collections that reveals short, gram-positive coccobacillary organisms supports the diagnosis. Cultures usually yield the organism within 24 to 48 hours of incubation, but a longer interval may be required. Serologic tests have not been useful for establishing a diagnosis of *Listeria* infection in individual patients. The presence of peripheral blood monocytosis or a mononuclear cell predominance in CSF should enhance the suspicion that *L. monocytogenes* infection is present. However, the absence of these findings does not exclude the diagnosis.

Although other *in utero* infections, such as disseminated cytomegalovirus infection, should be considered in the differential diagnosis, the features of granuloma infantisepticum usually are so distinctive as to be pathognomonic. The septicemic form of early-onset listeriosis, with or without respiratory distress, cannot be differentiated clinically from septicemia associated with other bacteria that cause early-onset infection, particularly group B streptococci and the Enterobacteriaceae. Similarly, *Listeria* meningitis cannot be differentiated from other bacterial infections of the meninges. CSF Gram-stained smears may be confused with group B streptococci, *Streptococcus pneumoniae*, *Corynebacterium*, and *H. influenzae*. *Listeria* meningitis, particularly rhombencephalitis, has been misdiagnosed as tuberculous meningitis. Among immunocompromised patients, *Listeria* meningitis may present in a manner similar to that of cryptococcal or pneumococcal meningitis. If T-cell function is abnormal, *Nocardia asteroides* should be considered in the differential diagnosis of brain abscess.

TREATMENT

Successful treatment of *L. monocytogenes* infection with ampicillin or penicillin alone has been reported. However, because of reported *in vitro* tolerance or resistance to penicillin alone and studies showing *in vitro* synergy and increased clinical efficacy, combination therapy with ampicillin and gentamicin is the initial regimen of choice. In neonates, an ampicillin dose of 150 to 200 mg/kg/day for nonmeningeal infections or 300 to 400 mg/kg/day for *Listeria* meningitis is indicated. The higher dose is appropriate for treating infection in immunocompromised hosts. After clinical response occurs or for less severe infections in immunologically normal hosts, ampicillin or penicillin alone can be given. Treatment should be continued for 10 days for bacteremia without a focus, for 14 to 21 days for meningitis or meningoencephalitis, and for 4 to 6 weeks for such serious focal infections as brain abscess or endocarditis.

Alternative antibiotics to which *Listeria* is susceptible *in vitro* include tetracycline, chloramphenicol, trimethoprim-sulfamethoxazole, and erythromycin. Data on which to base a recommendation for vancomycin as alternative therapy are insufficient. Cephalosporins are ineffective and have no role in treatment. Trimethoprim-sulfamethoxazole is active against *L. monocytogenes*, achieves good penetration of the CNS, and is the best alternative single agent for penicillin-allergic patients. Newer antibiotics that appear to be effective include mezlocillin, imipenem, and ciprofloxacin.

COMPLICATIONS

Untreated, listeriosis usually is fatal within 4 days. Even with treatment, the fatality rates are 60% to 70% among patients with underlying immunosuppression and those with granuloma infantisepticum. Proportionately lower rates are found among neonates and otherwise healthy older children. The bacteremic and meningitic forms of listeriosis can be cured, but complications may develop despite prompt antimicrobial treatment. Sequelae such as hydrocephalus, strabismus, and retardation may occur after CNS infections.

PREVENTION

General recommendations for the prevention of listeriosis are same as for the prevention of other foodborne infections. They include cooking thoroughly raw food from animal sources, washing raw vegetables thoroughly before cooking, keeping uncooked meats separate from vegetables and from cooked and ready-to-eat foods, avoiding unpasteurized milk or foods made from unpasteurized milk, and washing hands, knives, and cutting boards after handling uncooked foods. Persons at high risk for developing listeriosis, including pregnant women and those with a weakened immune systems, should follow these general recommendations. In addition, those at increased risk should refrain from eating soft cheeses, refrigerated pates and meat spreads, refrigerated smoked seafood (unless it is contained in a cooked dish), hot dogs, luncheon meats, and deli meats unless they are cooked until steaming hot. Cross-contamination of other foods, utensils, and food preparation surfaces with fluids from hot dog packages should be avoided. Washing one's hands after handling hot dogs, luncheon meats, or deli meats is recommended.

Suggested Readings

Bortolussi R, Schlech WF III. Listeriosis. In: Remington JS, Klein JO, eds. *Infectious diseases of the fetus and newborn infant,* 5th ed. Philadelphia: Saunders, 2000:1157.

Boucher M, Yonekura ML. Perinatal listeriosis (early-onset): correlation of antenatal manifestations and neonatal outcome. *Obstet Gynecol* 1986;68:593.

Braden CR. Listeriosis. *Pediatr Infect Dis J* 2003;22:745.

Dalton CB, Austin CC, Sobel J, et al. An outbreak of gastroenteritis and fever due to *Listeria monocytogenes* in milk. *N Engl J Med* 1997;336:100.

Dee RR, Lorber B. Brain abscess due to *Listeria monocytogenes*: case report and literature review. *Rev Infect Dis* 1986;8:968.

Evans JR, Allen AC, Stinson DA, et al. Perinatal listeriosis: report of an outbreak. *Pediatr Infect Dis* 1985;4:237.

Larsson S, Cornberg S, Winblad S. Listeriosis during pregnancy and neonatal period in Sweden 1958–1974. *Acta Paediatr Scand* 1979;68:485.

Lennon D, Lewis B, Mantell C, et al. Epidemic perinatal listeriosis. *Pediatr Infect Dis* 1984;3:30.

Linnan MJ, Mascola L, Lou XD, et al. Epidemic listeriosis associated with Mexican-style cheese. *N Engl J Med* 1988;319:823.

Lorber B. Listeriosis. *Clin Infect Dis* 1997;24:1.

Mylonakis E, Paliou M, Hohmann EL, et al. Listeriosis during pregnancy. *Medicine (Baltimore)* 2002;81:260.

Safdar A, Armstrong D. Antimicrobial activities against 84 *Listeria monocytogenes* isolates from patients with systemic listeriosis at a comprehensive cancer center (1955–1997). *J Clin Microbiol* 2003;41:483.

Schlech WF III. Foodborne listeriosis. *Clin Infect Dis* 2000;31:770.

Schuchat A, Lizano C, Broome CV, et al. Outbreak of neonatal listeriosis associated with mineral oil. *Pediatr Infect Dis J* 1991;10:183.

Schuchat A, Swaminathan B, Broome CV. Epidemiology of human listeriosis. *Clin Microbiol Rev* 1991;4:169.

Southwick FS, Purich DL. Intracellular pathogenesis of listeriosis. *N Engl J Med* 1996;334:770.

Tim MW, Jackson MA, Shannon K, et al. Non-neonatal infection due to *Listeria monocytogenes*. *Pediatr Infect Dis* 1984;3:213.

CHAPTER 165 ■ MENINGOCOCCAL INFECTIONS

C. MARY HEALY, MORVEN S. EDWARDS, AND CAROL J. BAKER

Great strides have been made in our understanding of the meningococcus since the initial descriptions of "epidemic cerebrospinal meningitis" by Vieusseux in 1805, and of "petechial or spotted fever" the following year by Elisha North. More than a century ago, the causative organism, then called *Diplococcus intracellularis meningitidis*, was described by Weichselbaum, who observed that it was found almost exclusively within neutrophils, and that it could be differentiated morphologically from the pneumococcus.

The introduction of serum therapy in 1907, the later addition of sulfonamides and penicillin in the 1940s, and the current availability of intensive care support have dramatically improved the outcome of these infections. However, *Neisseria meningitidis* causes fulminant infections that are fatal within hours after the onset of symptoms, and Herrick's statement, in 1919, that "no other infection so quickly slays" still holds true. Many problems must be resolved before meningococcal disease is successfully eradicated.

MICROBIOLOGY

Neisseria is a member of the family Neisseriaceae, which also contains the genera *Kingella, Eikenella, Simonsiella,* and *Alysiella*. *N. meningitidis* is differentiated from *N. gonorrhoeae* and less pathogenic *Neisseria* species on the basis of carbohydrate fermentation reactions. *N. gonorrhoeae* ferments only glucose, but most strains of *N. meningitidis* ferment glucose and maltose. Laboratory identification of the few strains that fail to produce acid from either carbohydrate may be particularly difficult.

Meningococci are fastidious. For optimal growth, they require enriched media, such as chocolate, blood, or Mueller-Hinton agar, and a 3% to 10% CO_2 atmosphere. Colonies are 1 to 5 mm in diameter, translucent, and nonhemolytic. *N. meningitidis* is a gram-negative, biscuit-shaped or coffee bean-shaped diplococcus with rounded outer and flattened inner margins; it has a polysaccharide capsule to protect it from phagocytosis. Specific capsular polysaccharide antigens allow the classification of meningococci into at least 13 serogroups. Serogroups A, B, C, Y, and W135 are responsible for human disease. The other groups are designated D, X, Z, 29-E, H, I, K, and L. The principal noncapsular cell-wall antigens include lipooligosaccharide, which is analogous to the lipopolysaccharide of enteric gram-negative bacilli, and the outer membrane protein (OMP). At least 12 different lipooligosaccharide serotypes exist. Groups B and C can be subdivided into at least 15 protein types on the basis of antigenically distinct OMPs. The OMPs allow the organism acquire iron (required for growth) by binding to host heme, transferrin, and lactoferrin, and are part of a lipoprotein-lipopolysaccharide complex that is responsible for the endotoxinlike effect observed in invasive infection.

Meningococci also contain pili or fimbriae that enhance attachment to nasopharyngeal epithelial cells, thus allowing colonization and invasion.

EPIDEMIOLOGY

Meningococcal infection is primarily a disease of childhood. In general, an inverse relation exists between age and attack rate, with the exception of an increased incidence among 15- to 24-year-olds who account for up to 20% of meningococcal-related deaths. More than 50% of the patients are younger than 4 years, and the highest age-specific attack rate is found among infants less than 12 months of age. Infection has been described during the first month of life. Among children, the genders are affected equally. Outside of infancy, persons aged 16 to 18 years and college freshmen living in dormitories also are at increased risk of acquiring infection.

Meningococcal disease has a worldwide distribution. The incidence of disease varies from year to year because of the superimposition of 3- to 5-year epidemic cycles on the base of endemic disease activity. Since *N. meningitidis* was classified into serogroups in 1950, epidemic and endemic serogroups have been identified. Historically, group A strains were associated with worldwide epidemics until 1963, when a serogroup shift occurred, and epidemic group B disease was observed. These shifts have continued, to group C in 1967, and to groups A and B in 1976. Clusters of group C disease have been reported in schoolchildren after epidemic influenza. In sub-Saharan Africa, in an area called the "meningitis belt," meningococcal infection is caused almost exclusively by group A; groups B and C cause the bulk of disease in other countries, although groups Y and W135 also occur.

The reasons for shifts in serogroup prevalence are unclear. One group of investigators described the clonal population structure of more than 400 strains of *N. meningitidis* group A that were isolated from 23 outbreaks. Most epidemics or outbreaks were characterized by a single or predominant clone. Similar clonal analyses have been carried out for serogroups B and C. A limited number of clones have been responsible for the epidemics since 1915. Hypothetically, epidemic outbreaks may begin only when changes in herd immunity coincide with the appropriate seasonal and climatic conditions that promote the carriage and transmission of one or more strains.

Sporadic cases usually are caused by serogroup B or C. Until recently, these infections were likely to be caused by group B strains in the 6- to 24-month age group and by group C strains in older children. In the United States, group Y disease, which often is associated with pneumonia and other focal manifestations of disease, has been observed with increasing frequency throughout the 1990s, and in one study, it accounted for 26% of cases observed from 1992 through 1996. Currently in the United States, group B predominates in children younger than 5 years of age, but more than two-third of cases in other age groups are attributable to groups C and Y.

Meningococcal disease occurs in a typical seasonal pattern worldwide. In the "meningitis belt," disease recurs annually, in waves, with attack rates rising at the end of the dry season and declining after the rainy season begins. In the rest of the world, the attack rate peaks in winter and early spring months, a typical disease season in the Northern hemisphere running from November through March. This seasonal pattern coincides with a concomitant rise in the incidence of viral upper respiratory tract infections, lending weight to the theory that viruses may act as cofactors in the development of invasive disease.

Infections that develop within 24 hours of onset in the index case are designated as coprimary, whereas onset at least 24 hours after exposure to the index case is referred to as a secondary case. Sporadic cases are to be distinguished from a cluster of cases, in which two or more cases of the same serogroup occur more closely than expected in a population, and from an outbreak, in which increased transmission of infection in a population occurs.

PATHOGENESIS AND PATHOLOGY

Humans are the only natural host for meningococcal infection, and the oropharynx is its reservoir. Acquisition of nasopharyngeal infection by inhalation or direct contact results in transient, intermittent, or chronic carriage. The prevalence of asymptomatic carriage during nonepidemic periods ranges from 2% to 38%, and the median duration of carriage is 10 months. It is estimated that only 1% of carriers in Norway during the 1970s developed invasive disease. The carriage rate is increased in situations of overcrowding, in lower socioeconomic groups, and by passive and active smoking. In most hosts, infection of the upper respiratory tract elicits the formation of serum bactericidal antibody 7 to 10 days later. This immune response does not eliminate carriage, but it does protect the host from symptomatic infection. Susceptibility to invasive disease exists in the interval between acquisition of the organism in the nasopharynx and development of bactericidal antibody in the serum. Pili mediate the attachment of meningococci, and parasite-directed endocytosis promotes their entry into nonciliated cells of the nasopharyngeal mucosa. Dissemination occurs when the organism penetrates the nasopharyngeal mucosa of the nonimmune host and enters the bloodstream, where it replicates. From there, it may disseminate to the meninges, joints, myocardium, or elsewhere. Injury to the nasopharyngeal mucosa by preceding respiratory viral infection or smoking may promote invasiveness, but this hypothesis is contested.

The prevalence of passively or naturally acquired bactericidal antibody is inversely related to the incidence of invasive infection. Maternally derived antibodies probably provide some protection for most infants during the first few months of life. Passively acquired antibody concentrations reach a nadir between the ages of 6 and 24 months. Nasopharyngeal carriage of meningococci from serogroups with low pathogenicity may elicit cross-reactive antibodies that protect against invasiveness of pathogenic serogroups A, B, and C. Similarly, gastrointestinal colonization with bacteria containing antigens that cross-react with meningococci may contribute to the development of naturally acquired immunity.

Specific antibody and complement are important for immunity. Specific bactericidal IgG antibodies bind to meningococci and may activate the classic or alternative complement pathways. Bacterial killing can be mediated by serum, which requires the membrane attack complex, or by phagocytes. Patients who are deficient in specific antibody must rely more heavily on the integrity of complement-dependent bactericidal activity. Fatal or recurrent meningococcemia has been associated with congenital deficiencies of the alternative (properdin deficiency) or terminal complement pathways (components C5 through C9). These hosts must kill the organism by phagocytic rather than complement-mediated mechanisms. Defects

in alternative and terminal complement pathways are easily assessed by the AP50 and CH50 assays, respectively. Partial compensation for this opsonic deficiency can be provided by eliciting specific antibodies through immunization. Acquired complement deficiency, as occurs with systemic lupus erythematosus (SLE), chronic liver disease, and nephrotic syndrome, also predispose to meningococcal infection. Some people develop serum IgA antibody (i.e., blocking antibody) that renders the bactericidal IgG or IgM antibody ineffective and results in disease susceptibility.

The predominant pathologic feature of fulminant meningococcemia is diffuse vascular damage and disseminated intravascular coagulation (DIC). In DIC, thrombin is persistently and recurrently elaborated, and fibrinogen, platelets, and coagulation factors such as anti-thrombin III and protein C (which may also have antiinflammatory effects) are consumed, with resulting haphazard activation and inhibition of fibrinolysis. Bleeding into any organ may occur. Histopathologically, the vascular changes consist of endothelial damage, vessel wall inflammation, necrosis, and thrombosis. These changes presumably are mediated by the effects of endotoxin, because the degree of septic shock correlates closely with endotoxin levels, and the effects are reproducible in animal models. A correlation between C3 activation products and the level of endotoxin supports the concept that complement activation contributes to multiple organ failure in overwhelming disease. Increased vascular permeability with leakage of plasma proteins, changes in vasomotor tone with maldistribution of intravascular volume, impaired myocardial function, and disordered cellular metabolism all interact to cause the circulatory collapse and myocardial dysfunction that is the major cause of death.

CLINICAL MANIFESTATIONS AND COMPLICATIONS

The clinical expression of meningococcal disease in children may be categorized as meningococcal bacteremia without sepsis, meningococcal sepsis without meningitis, meningitis, and other manifestations. The initial replication of meningococci in the bloodstream usually causes the nonspecific symptoms of fever, malaise, myalgia, and headache. Bacteremia without a focus may be considered as a possible diagnosis and, depending on the degree of toxicity, these patients may inadvertently be sent home, with or without antimicrobial therapy. When one group of 13 children in whom occult bacteremia had been diagnosed were reassessed, the bloodstream cleared without antimicrobial therapy in three patients, four developed meningitis, and the remainder were clinically improved with amoxicillin therapy. In another series of 37 children with unsuspected meningococcal infection when they first presented for medical attention, 17 subsequently developed meningitis, one hypotension, one respiratory failure, two pericardial effusion, and one died. Therefore, although some children with meningococcal bacteremia clear their bloodstream without antimicrobial therapy, the risks of developing meningitis (and/or other focal disease) or recurrent bacteremia with or without sepsis, warrant a full diagnostic evaluation including lumbar puncture and treatment with appropriate antimicrobials once meningococcal bacteremia is detected. Chemoprophylaxis also should be given to the contacts of these children.

Acute meningococcal bacteremia without meningitis begins with influenzalike symptoms (fever, upper respiratory signs, lethargy) that may last hours to days and are very nonspecific. Eventually, most affected children are septic. The majority of these children have cutaneous manifestations, which initially may take the form of a nonspecific maculopapular, morbilliform, or urticarial rash. Evolution to a petechial or purpuric

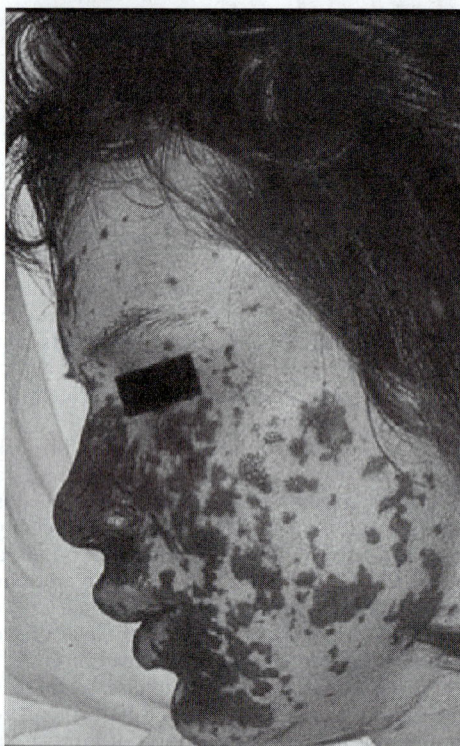

FIGURE 165.1. Purpura fulminans in a child with fulminant meningococcal sepsis. Purpura may evolve rapidly even in an initially non-toxic appearing child.

rash within hours or days is the rule. Purpura, usually most extensive on the buttocks and lower extremities, is a feature of fulminant disease (Fig. 165.1). In fulminant disease, the patient is toxic and ill-appearing and clinical deterioration is rapid, sometimes occurring within minutes. Hypotension, oliguria, DIC, myocardial dysfunction, and vascular collapse (often irreversible) lead to death in approximately 10% to 20% of the patients. When the course is less fulminant, and shock is responsive to therapy, the occasional fatal infection usually is due to the consequences of direct invasion of the myocardium, manifested by congestive failure, poor contractility, and pulmonary edema.

Only one-third to one-half of the children with meningococcal meningitis have petechiae or purpura at the time of initial evaluation. Among the remainder, the clinical presentation often is that of bacterial meningitis, characterized (except in very young infants) by nuchal rigidity, altered level of consciousness, and signs or symptoms of increased intracranial pressure. Most children (95%) with meningococcal meningitis survive and have a better outcome than those with meningitis caused by *Streptococcus pneumoniae*. The most common cause of death is cerebral edema with herniation.

Children with meningitis or suspected meningococcal bacteremia have higher bacterial counts in their bloodstream than do those with unsuspected meningococcal bacteremia or other manifestations of infection. However, at the time of hematogenous dissemination, other sites may be seeded. The primary presentation reflects the particular focus in which a nidus for infection was established. Primary meningococcal pneumonia, periorbital cellulitis, pericarditis, peritonitis, cervical adenitis, endocarditis, purulent conjunctivitis, and endophthalmitis are rare, but they have been reported in children. Primary meningococcal infection of bone and joint (not be confused with immune complex–mediated disease) also has been described and is associated with benign outcome in most cases. Occasion-

ally, manifestations of disease usually attributed to *N. gonorrhoeae*, such as vulvovaginitis or pelvic inflammatory disease, prove to be caused by *N. meningitidis*. The syndrome of chronic meningococcemia, in which persistent meningococcal bacteremia is associated with fever, skin lesions resembling gonococcemia, and arthritis, also is extremely rare in childhood.

DIAGNOSIS

The diagnosis of a confirmed case of infection with *N. meningitidis* is established by the growth of the organism from blood, cerebrospinal fluid (CSF), synovial fluid, petechial or purpuric lesion, or other usually sterile sites. The yield is lower if pretreatment with antimicrobials has occurred. The presence or absence of meningitis cannot be diagnosed by clinical signs alone, and lumbar puncture always should be performed during the course of the illness, even if it is deferred initially in an unstable patient. A low white cell count in the CSF does not exclude the diagnosis of meningococcal meningitis, because it may indicate either early disease or even severe infection, in which overwhelming sepsis does not allow an appropriate inflammatory response. Serogroup-specific polymerase chain reaction (PCR), a method of amplifying deoxyribonucleic acid (DNA) in the bacterial genome, increasingly is used for meningococcal diagnosis in some countries where the disease is common, but PCR is not as yet widely available in the United States. The presence of gram-negative diplococci in stained smears of CSF, petechiae, buffy coat of blood, and other usually sterile fluid defines a presumptive case. The procedure of pressing a clean glass slide against a lanced petechial or purpuric lesion is simple and yields the organism in as many as 83% of the attempts when performed before or promptly after initiation of antimicrobial therapy. Bacterial antigen detection in the CSF by latex agglutination supports the diagnosis of a probable case in the setting of a compatible clinical illness, but a negative test does not exclude infection. Latex agglutination tests are less sensitive and less specific than culture, and they are not recommended for serum or urine. They may be helpful in detecting highly immunogenic meningococcal serogroups (A, C, W135, Y), but they are less successful in detecting group B meningococcal polysaccharide and may cross react with other bacterial species.

The predictive value of fever and petechiae in the diagnosis of meningococcal infection is variable. For example, of 411 children with fever and petechiae attending an emergency center, less than 2% had invasive bacterial disease (0.5% meningococcal disease); however, in another review of 129 children with these symptoms, 20% had invasive bacterial disease and 11% had meningococcal infection. Although most children with fever and a petechial rash do not have meningococcal disease, the diagnosis should be considered in any child presenting with these symptoms. Low-grade bacteremia and/or pretreatment with antimicrobials may lessen the chances of isolating meningococcus in cultures. The presence of purpura rather than petechiae renders the diagnosis of meningococcal infection far more likely. Rocky Mountain spotted fever, epidemic typhus, ehrlichiosis, atypical measles, staphylococcal sepsis, and viral infections (particularly echovirus and adenovirus) are other differential considerations. The noninfectious or unclassified disorders that should be considered include Kawasaki disease, idiopathic thrombocytopenic purpura, Henoch-Schönlein purpura, vasculitis, drug reactions, and leukemia.

Early in the course of infection, meningococcal symptoms and signs are very nonspecific. Skin lesions may be absent, macular, or maculopapular. Meningococcal bacteremia should, therefore, be considered in any child with signs of toxicity, particularly during the winter and early spring, even if the rash appears benign. Urticarial rash occurring soon after the initiation of penicillin therapy is likely to be a manifestation of meningococcal bacteremia, rather than of penicillin allergy. In the absence of rash, the features of meningococcal meningitis are not distinctive, and the presenting findings are similar to those of other types of bacterial meningitis.

THERAPY

Aqueous penicillin G, administered intravenously at a dose of 250,000 U/kg/day (maximum 12 million U/day), is the treatment of choice for meningococcal infections. Cefotaxime (200 mg/kg/day), ceftriaxone (80 to 100 mg/kg/day), or ampicillin (300 mg/kg/day) also is effective. For the rare child with penicillin allergy characterized by anaphylaxis, in whom a cephalosporin may pose some risk for cross-allergenicity, chloramphenicol (75 to 100 mg/kg/day) is recommended. Strains of *N. meningitidis* with reduced sensitivity or resistance to penicillin (minimal inhibitory concentration, 0.1 to 1.0 μg/mL) have been recovered with increasing frequency since 1986 in Spain, Italy, parts of Africa, and sporadically in the United States. Penicillin-resistant strains remain susceptible to chloramphenicol, cefotaxime, and ceftriaxone. Given the low prevalence of isolates in North America that exhibit increased resistance to penicillin, routine penicillin susceptibility testing of invasive isolates currently is not recommended.

Meningococcal bacteremia constitutes a medical emergency, because patients may deteriorate extremely rapidly. The initial dose of antimicrobial therapy should be administered before the transport of an acutely ill patient with a petechial or purpuric rash. Adequate resuscitation and supportive care is critical for favorable outcome. Many patients develop shock shortly after the initiation of antimicrobial therapy, and so this endotoxin-mediated course should be anticipated and treated aggressively. It is mandatory to continuously monitor vital signs, including blood pressure, clinical status (e.g., urine output, peripheral perfusion), and blood electrolytes and chemistries in an intensive care setting. Anticipatory therapy with volume resuscitation or pressor agents should be provided as indicated. Unlike meningitis due to *Haemophilus influenzae* type b, no proven benefit exists in administering steroids in meningococcal meningitis in children. The advisability of administering steroids to patients with possible adrenal hemorrhage (i.e., Waterhouse-Friedrichsen syndrome) is debated, but data are lacking that this approach favorably affects the outcome in critically ill patients. Treatment should be provided as indicated for control of increased intracranial pressure, seizures, and correction of anemia and electrolyte abnormalities. For meningococcal bacteremia or meningitis, 5 to 7 days of parenteral antimicrobial therapy are required.

Clinical trials of many initially promising adjuvant therapies have shown variable results. One of the more promising therapies is activated protein C, levels of which are severely reduced in fulminant meningococcemia. One large multicenter trial in adults demonstrated significantly reduced mortality from both gram-negative and gram-positive sepsis in patients treated with activated protein C who were at low risk for treatment-associated side effects (e.g., hemorrhage). More recently, the pharmacokinetics, pharmacodynamic effects, and safety profile of activated protein C in children were found to be similar to those reported in adults. However, the results of efficacy trials in children are disappointing. The mainstay of treatment for meningococcal infections remains a high index of clinical suspicion, early antibiotics, and adequate resuscitation and supportive care.

TABLE 165.1

CLINICAL AND LABORATORY PARAMETERS ASSOCIATED WITH POOR PROGNOSIS IN MENINGOCOCCAL INFECTION

Clinical	Laboratory
Extremes of age	Leukopenia
Purpura (especially if rapidly evolving)	Thrombocytopenia
Hypothermia or skin-rectal temperature difference >3°C	Abnormal coagulation
Shock	Metabolic acidosis
Seizures	Meningococcemia without meningitis
Focal neurologic signs	Low CSF white blood cell count
Coma	

PROGNOSIS

Approximately 20% of children with meningococcal bacteremia with sepsis die, although mortality rates as low as 5% to 10% have been reported in specialized centers. The usual cause of death is irreversible shock, and most deaths occur within 48 hours of hospital admission. Fatality rates for children with meningococcal bacteremia plus meningitis are lower (approximately 5%), presumably because these patients constitute a subset who have survived meningococcal bacteremia long enough to develop meningeal seeding. Several prognostic signs recognized at the time of hospital admission predict poor survival (Table 165.1).

The complications of meningococcal infections may be classified as early and late (Table 165.2). Early complications are the direct result of disseminated infection and include myocarditis, pericarditis, pneumonia, hemorrhage, and arthritis. Meningococcal meningitis may be complicated acutely by seizures, cranial nerve palsies (particularly of the third, fourth, and sixth cranial nerves), ataxia, or cerebral herniation. Subdural effusion, almost universally sterile, may be seen during convalescence. The most common neurologic residual of meningococcal meningitis is deafness, which usually is bilateral, sensorineural, and permanent. Reported for 5% to 10% of the survivors, hearing loss occurs significantly more often among children with leukocytosis (20,000 cells or more per cubic millimeter), leukopenia (5,000 cells or less per cubic millimeter), or CSF cells (10,000 or more per cubic millimeter) at the time of admission than in patients with an uncomplicated course. Neurologic sequelae generally are limited to deafness, but residual cranial nerve palsy or retardation occur occasionally.

Late, allergic, hypersensitivity, immune complex-mediated, and *reactive* all are terms that have been used to describe the complications of meningococcal disease that occur during recovery from infection. Late complications, manifested as cutaneous vasculitis, arthritis, pericarditis, or rarely, episcleritis, occur in 10% of the survivors. Although these complications present with inflammatory features, the clue to the noninfectious cause of the complications is the timing of onset—usually 5 to 10 days into infection. Pericardial or joint fluid may contain leukocytes in excess of 50,000 per cubic millimeter, with a neutrophil predominance, but the fluid invariably is sterile. Patients with the admission findings of shock, extensive rash, leukocytosis, or leukopenia, and those with fever persisting more than 5 days into therapy, are at risk for these complications.

TABLE 165.2

RELATIVE FREQUENCY OF COMPLICATIONS OF MENINGOCOCCAL INFECTION

Complication	Frequency
Early	
Cardiovascular	
Pericarditis	+
Myocarditis	+++
Pulmonary	
Pneumonia	++
Pleural effusion or empyema	+
Neurologic	
Seizures*	++++
Cranial nerve palsy	+
Ataxia	++
Cerebral herniation	+
Subdural effusion	+++
Hearing loss	+++
Miscellaneous	
Arthritis	++
Hemorrhage	+++
Late	
Arthritis	+++
Vasculitis	++
Pericarditis	++
Episcleritis	+

+, rare; ++, 1–5%; +++, 5–10%; ++++, more than 10%.
*At hospital admission.

TABLE 165.3

CHEMOPROPHYLAXIS REGIMENS FOR HIGH-RISK CONTACTS AND INDEX CASES

Age of Patient	Dose	Duration
Rifampin		
≤1 mo	5 mg/kg orally every 12 hr	2 d
>1 mo	10 mg/kg (maximum, 600 mg) orally every 12 hr	2 d
Ceftriaxone		
≤15 yr	125 mg intramuscularly	Single dose
>15 yr	250 mg intramuscularly	Single dose
Ciprofloxacin*		
≥18 yr	500 mg orally	Single dose

*Not recommended for use in pregnant women.

The treatment consists of drainage (only if needed for symptomatic relief) and administration of nonsteroidal anti-inflammatory agents. Occasionally, prednisone (60 mg/m^2/day initially) may be required to reduce inflammation in patients with pericarditis. Antimicrobial therapy should not be prolonged beyond the duration required for uncomplicated infection. Arthritis and vasculitis usually resolve fully within 2 to 3 weeks, but full recovery from pericarditis may require several months.

PREVENTION

Antimicrobial Prophylaxis

Chemoprophylaxis to eradicate the nasopharyngeal carriage interrupts the spread of meningococcal infections. Among household contacts, the secondary attack rate varies from 3 per 1,000 for sporadic disease to 3 per 100 exposed persons during epidemic situations. High-risk contacts of index cases of invasive meningococcal disease, for whom chemoprophylaxis is recommended, include household contacts (especially young children and those who have slept or eaten in the same dwelling as the index patient or had secretion contact with the patient), child-care or nursery-school contacts (within the 7 days before the index patient's admission), and those who have had unprotected contact during mouth-to-mouth or nasotracheal intubation resuscitation efforts. Chemoprophylaxis is not recommended for school contacts, indirect contacts, or medical personnel who have not been directly exposed to secretions. However, a few outbreaks among school classmates have been reported and, in this setting, chemoprophylaxis should be undertaken only after consultation with local public health

authorities. Because high-dose penicillin suppresses the colonization of the nasopharynx only transiently, the index patient should receive treatment for nasopharyngeal carriage eradication at the conclusion of parenteral therapy, unless the patient received a full course of ceftriaxone or cefotaxime.

Rifampin is the antimicrobial most often used for chemoprophylaxis in children (Table 165.3). Rifampin eradicates the carrier state rapidly, but resistant strains have emerged. The drug usually is well tolerated, but recipients should be alerted that it stains urine and tears red-orange and may interfere with the efficacy of oral contraceptives, seizure-prevention, and anticoagulant medications. Ceftriaxone administered as a single 125 mg (to patients 15 years of age or younger) or 250 mg (to patients older than 15 years) dose intramuscularly is an alternative to rifampin that also is highly effective in eradicating carriage. It is not recommended for routine use, because efficacy has been documented only for serogroup A, but it has the advantage of being easy to administer (hence increasing compliance) and, unlike rifampin, is recommended during pregnancy. A single 500-mg dose of ciprofloxacin orally is effective in eliminating carriage, but although past and ongoing studies have demonstrated that it and other fluoroquinolones are relatively safe in children, currently it is approved for use only in nonpregnant patients who are 18 years of age or older and in children with complicated urinary tract infections caused by multiply resistant organisms.

Monthly injections of benzathine penicillin G have prevented the recurrence of invasive disease in patients with a terminal complement protein deficiency.

Immunoprophylaxis

Immunization is recommended for persons older than 2 years who have anatomic or functional asplenia and deficiencies of properdin or terminal complement components. It also is recommended for those traveling to areas with hyperendemic or epidemic meningococcal disease and during outbreaks of meningococcal disease caused by a vaccine-preventable strain. Two cohorts of adolescents should be immunized routinely: (1) young adolescents at the 11–12 years visit; and (2) adolescents at high school entry or 15 years of age, whichever comes first. Entering college students who plan to live in dormitories should also be immunized. Physicians also should immunize students if requested by them or their parents, or if required by the educational institution or state law. Because the duration of eradication of pharyngeal colonization may be as short as 6 weeks after chemoprophylaxis, and the time required to elicit an immune response after immunization is approximately 10 to 14 days, secondary cases can occur several weeks or more after the diagnosis of disease in an index patient. The administration of vaccine should be considered as an adjunct to chemoprophylaxis among household and intimate contacts. Vaccine has been used successfully to halt the spread of epidemic disease.

Until recently, the only vaccine available in the United States for immunoprophylaxis against invasive meningococcal infection was a quadrivalent preparation containing polysaccharides of groups A, C, Y, and W135 (Menomune, sanofi pasteur, Swiftwater, PA). This vaccine consists of 50 μg of each purified polysaccharide, and it is safe and well tolerated. The group A polysaccharide is immunogenic for infants as young as 3 months, although an optimal response is not elicited until the age of 4 or 5 years. For the control of an epidemic caused by group A meningococci, two doses of the vaccine administered 3 months apart have been given to children younger than 18 months. Groups C, Y, and W135 are immunogenic for children 2 years of age and older. However, group C polysaccharide in particular is poorly immunogenic in children younger than 2 years, in whom group C causes 25% of disease. Serum antibody concentrations decline rapidly over 2 to 3 years and, therefore, revaccination should be considered if indications still exist within 3 to 5 years after immunization. Children who were vaccinated first when younger than 4 years should be considered for revaccination after 2 to 3 years if they remain at risk. The rapid waning of antibody levels, and concerns that repeated vaccine doses may cause immune tolerance and a reduced antibody response have, therefore, precluded the routine use of this polysaccharide vaccine except in populations at high risk of contracting meningococcal infection or for control of outbreaks.

A group C vaccine, in which the polysaccharide is conjugated to a carrier protein, has been developed. This serogroup C polysaccharide-conjugate vaccine is safe, has an acceptable reactogenicity profile, demonstrates immunogenicity for all age groups (including young infants less than 2 years of age), and induces immunologic memory. It is licensed in Europe and Canada for routine use in infants and children, where it has been extremely efficacious in reducing group C disease.

In the United States, where more than two-thirds of meningococcal infection in persons over 5 years of age is caused by groups C, Y, and W135, a quadrivalent A, C, Y, W-135 polysaccharide-conjugate vaccine was licensed in 2005 for use in persons aged 11 to 55 years. This vaccine contains 4 μg each of A, C, Y, and W135 polysaccharide conjugated to diphtheria toxoid (Menactra-sanofi pasteur). It has demonstrated acceptable safety, reactogenicity, and immunogenicity in adults and, when compared to the polysaccharide vaccine, has comparable or superior seroconversion rates and serum bactericidal responses to each serogroup. It is recommended for use in children aged 11 to12 years, concomitant with other adolescent immunizations (e.g., tetanus-diphtheria toxoid); at high school entry or age 15 years, whichever comes first; and college freshman living in dormitories, and high-risk populations. It is the preferred vaccine for outbreak control or for travelers to epidemic areas for those aged 11 years and older. Although a welcome development, issues remain regarding meningococcal immunization. The conjugate vaccine is costly, and development of a suitable infrastructure to implement the approved adolescent immunization program will be required. The optimal timing of booster vaccination with the conjugate vaccine is unknown. While research is ongoing, currently no similar vaccine is available for younger age groups.

The group B polysaccharide is poorly immunogenic in humans. The possibility of using group B surface proteins, such as OMPs, is being investigated. However, to date, this approach has had limited success because multiple group B serotypes are circulating in most countries, and OMPs do not induce cross-reactivity between different serotypes.

Suggested Readings

American Academy of Pediatrics. Committee on Infectious Diseases. Prevention and control of meningococcal disease: Recommendations for use of meningococcal vaccines in pediatric patients. *Pediatrics* 2005;116:496.

Barton P, Kalil AC, Nadel S, et al. Safety, pharmacokinetics, and pharmacodynamics of drotrecogin alpha (activated) in children with severe sepsis. *Pediatrics* 2004;113:7.

Bernard GR, Vincent JL, Laterre PF, et al., Efficacy and safety of recombinant human activated protein C for severe sepsis. *N Engl J Med* 2001;344:699.

Blondeau JM, Yaschuk Y. *In vitro* activities of ciprofloxacin, cefotaxime, ceftriaxone, chloramphenicol, and rifampin against fully susceptible and moderately penicillin-resistant *Neisseria meningitidis*. *Antimicrob Agents Chemother* 1995;39:2577.

Edwards MS, Baker CJ. Complications and sequelae of meningococcal infections in children. *J Pediatr* 1981;90:540.

Feigin RD, Baker CJ, Herwaldt LA, et al. Epidemic meningococcal disease in an elementary-school classroom. *N Engl J Med* 1982;302:1255.

Harrison LH, Armstrong CW, Jenkins SR, et al. A cluster of meningococcal disease on a school bus following epidemic influenza. *Arch Intern Med* 1991;151:1005.

Healy CM, Butler KM, Smith EO, et al. Influence of serogroup on the presentation, course, and outcome of invasive meningococcal disease in children in the Republic of Ireland, 1995–2000. *Clin Infect Dis* 2002;34(10):1323.

Kirsch EA, Barton RP, Kitchen L, Giroir BP. Pathophysiology, treatment and outcome of meningococcemia: a review and recent experience. *Pediatr Infect Dis J* 1996;15(11):967.

Mandl KD, Stack AM, Fleisher GR. Incidence of bacteremia in infants and children with fever and petechiae. *J Pediatr* 1997;131:398.

Morley SL, Pollard AJ. Vaccine prevention of meningococcal disease, coming soon? *Vaccine* 2001;20(5–6):666.

Peltola H. Meningococcal disease: still with us. *Rev Infect Dis* 1983;5:71.

Pollard AJ, Britto J, Nadel S, et al. Emergency management of meningococcal disease. *Arch Dis Child* 1999;80(3):290.

Potter PC, Frasch CE, van der Sande WJM, et al. Prophylaxis against *Neisseria meningitidis* infections and antibody responses in patients with deficiency of the sixth component of complement. *J Infect Dis* 1990;161:932.

Raymond NJ, Reeves M, Ajello G, et al. Molecular epidemiology of sporadic (endemic) serogroup C meningococcal disease. *J Infect Dis* 1997;176:1277.

Rosenstein NE, Perkins BA, Stephens DS, et al. The changing epidemiology of meningococcal disease in the United States, 1992–1996. *J Infect Dis* 1999; 180(6):1894.

Rosenstein NE, Perkins BA, Stephens DS, et al. Meningococcal disease. *N Engl J Med* 2001;344(18):1378.

Ross SC, Rosenthal PJ, Berberich HM, et al. Killing of *Neisseria meningitidis* by human neutrophils: implications for normal and complement-deficient individuals. *J Infect Dis* 1987;155:1266.

Stephens DS, Farley MM. Pathogenic events during infection of the human nasopharynx with *Neisseria meningitidis* and *Haemophilus influenzae*. *Rev Infect Dis* 1991;13:22.

Sullivan TD, LaScolea LJ, Jr. *Neisseria meningitidis* bacteremia in children: quantitation of bacteremia and spontaneous clinical recovery without antibiotic therapy. *Pediatrics* 1987;80:63.

Van Esso D, Fontanals D, Uriz S, et al. *Neisseria meningitidis* strains with decreased susceptibility to penicillin. *Pediatr Infect Dis J* 1987;6:438.

Van Nguyen Q, Nguyen EA, Weiner LB. Incidence of invasive bacterial disease in children with fever and petechiae. *Pediatrics* 1984;74:77.

Wang VJ, Kuppermann N, Malley R, et al. Meningococcal disease among children who live in a large metropolitan area, 1981–1996. *Clin Infect Dis* 2001; 32(7):1004.

Wong VK, Hitchcock W, Mason WH. Meningococcal infections in children: a review of 100 cases. *Pediatr Infect Dis J* 1989;8:224.

Woods CR, Smith AL, Wasilauskas BL, et al. Invasive disease caused by *Neisseria meningitidis* relatively resistant to penicillin in North Carolina. *J Infect Dis* 1994;170:453.

CHAPTER 166 ■ GONOCOCCAL INFECTIONS

LORI E. R. PATTERSON

Although gonorrhea is most familiar as a urogenital infection in sexually active adults, disease caused by *Neisseria gonorrhoeae* occurs at a variety of anatomic sites in all age groups. Improved diagnostic methods and aggressive treatment have contributed to an overall decline in incidence, but changing patterns of antibiotic susceptibility pose treatment challenges. In children beyond the neonatal period, the infection usually is a marker for sexual abuse or contact.

MICROBIOLOGY

N. gonorrhoeae is a small, gram-negative, aerobic, nonmotile, oxidase-positive diplococcus with flattened adjacent surfaces. Its ultrastructure is typical of the gram-negative organisms. The outer lipid membrane contains pili, lipooligosaccharide, and several distinct proteins. The most prevalent of these, porin, acts as an anion channel through the hydrophobic cell membrane. Other outer membrane proteins facilitate adherence and block host humoral immunity to the gonococcus. Pili also contribute to adherence; nonpiliated strains are avirulent.

Differentiating gonococcal strains aids in epidemiologic study. In addition to being serotyped by its porin antigen pattern, a strain may be classified by its ability to grow on various nutrient-deficient media, a system known as *auxotyping*. Combined auxotype and serotype data have defined more than 100 distinct strains of *N. gonorrhoeae*. Antibiotic resistance patterns also can distinguish strains, although this property may not remain fixed. Resistance may be conferred either by chromosomal alterations (producing intrinsic resistance to a variety of antimicrobials) or by plasmid-mediated mechanisms (important for penicillin and tetracycline).

EPIDEMIOLOGY

The number of new gonorrhea infections reported in the United States has declined from a peak in the mid 1970s, but the incidence has remained steady at about 130 cases per 100,000 population in recent years. This far exceeds the Centers for Disease Control and Prevention's (CDC's) Healthy People 2010 goal of 19 cases per 100,000, and it renders gonorrhea second only to chlamydia in cases reported. Authorities estimate that approximately 600,000 infections actually occur each year. Young adults account for most cases, followed closely by older adolescents. Young women aged 15 to 19 years have the highest incidence of any group. In young adults, more episodes are reported in men, possibly because of underrecognition of infection in asymptomatic women. Demographic risk factors for gonorrhea include young age, unmarried status, nonwhite race, urban residence, low socioeconomic status, and men having sex with men. Asymptomatic men and prostitutes are important reservoirs of infection and contribute to the difficulty in eradicating the disease.

Gonorrhea is found in humans only and is transmitted through direct physical contact with infected mucosa or secretions. In adolescents and young adults, this spread occurs via sexual contact. Neonates and young children usually are infected intrapartum or by sexual abuse, respectively. Conjunctivitis in older children occurs by autoinoculation. Rectal gonorrhea may be acquired by receptive anal intercourse or by perineal contamination by genitourinary secretions. Pharyngeal infection presumably occurs after orogenital contact. Transmission by fomites has been implicated in nursery outbreaks but is rare. The incubation period generally is 2 to 7 days.

Since the late 1970s, the prevalence of antibiotic-resistant strains of *N. gonorrhoeae* has risen markedly. The U.S. Gonococcal Isolate Surveillance Project monitors trends in antimicrobial susceptibility, and data are used to formulate treatment strategies. Although the proportion of gonococci exhibiting plasmid-mediated or chromosomally mediated resistance to penicillin and/or tetracycline has declined since the mid-1990s, these strains still account for approximately 16% of isolates. Resistance to quinolones is endemic in Hawaii and California and is becoming an increasingly common occurrence in other areas; azithromycin resistance has been identified recently in a small number of isolates. Cephalosporin resistance has not been clinically significant.

PATHOGENESIS

Once introduced to a mucosal surface, the gonococcus adheres to the host cell, aided by its outer membrane pili. The bacteria penetrate tissue by endocytosis through or between epithelial cells, disrupting the mucosal integrity. Lipooligosaccharide exerts a toxic effect on the ciliated epithelial cells. An intense inflammatory response with influx of neutrophils and other phagocytes produces the characteristic profuse exudate; gonococcal peptidoglycan contributes to inflammation by activating complement. As gonococci invade the subepithelial space, deeper tissue destruction occurs through the action of extracellular enzymes and the cytotoxic and endotoxin-like effects of lipooligosaccharide. Invasion of local blood vessels and lymphatics may lead to dissemination. Eventually, scarring and fibrosis develop in the untreated patient.

The host's mucus production, pH, hormonal milieu, and normal flora probably influence progress of infection in the early stages. Prepubertal girls, whose vaginal secretions are alkaline and whose epithelium lacks the effects of estrogen, are more likely to develop vulvovaginitis than are adolescents, in whom cervicitis occurs more commonly. Disseminated or complicated gonorrhea occurs more commonly during menses and with the use of intrauterine devices and less commonly during pregnancy or with the use of oral contraceptives.

Although specific host defenses against gonococcal infection are not understood fully, clinical and laboratory observations give important clues. Humoral and secretory immunoglobulins against *N. gonorrhoeae* appear in response to infection, but they are not totally protective against subsequent episodes. One possible explanation is that gonococci readily alter the antigenic structure of pili (i.e., phase variation) and certain outer membrane proteins, thus evading recognition by the host. Pili themselves appear to interfere with host cell phagocytosis. All gonococci produce a protease that cleaves immunoglobulin A1, thwarting the protective action of this mucosal surface antibody. Complement activation may play a role in protecting against disseminated disease, because complement-deficient patients are at increased risk for developing gonococcemia. The role of cellular immunity in defense against the gonococcus is unknown.

Most strains of *N. gonorrhoeae* are susceptible to the bactericidal action of normal serum. Strains that cause invasive disease lack this serum sensitivity, have different growth characteristics and nutritional requirements, and are more likely to be highly sensitive to penicillin than are serum-sensitive strains.

CLINICAL MANIFESTATIONS AND COMPLICATIONS

Gonococcal infection may be localized to a mucosal surface or disseminated hematogenously. Many infected adults are asymptomatic, but how this fact translates to pediatric infection is uncertain.

Ophthalmia Neonatorum and Other Neonatal Disease

Gonococcal ophthalmia neonatorum (GON), the most common form of neonatal gonorrhea, usually occurs after intrapartum contact with the mother's infected genital secretions, but cesarean delivery does not preclude its development. Risk factors include prematurity, prolonged rupture of amniotic membranes, lack of prenatal care, lack of postpartum antimicrobial prophylaxis, and a maternal history of drug abuse or sexually transmitted disease. Onset of the conjunctivitis usually occurs when the infant is 2 to 5 days old. The ocular discharge is classically bilateral, mucopurulent, and profuse; marked eyelid edema and chemosis are present. Unilateral and milder cases also are seen. Without prompt treatment, corneal ulceration, invasion of deeper ocular structures, and globe perforation occur, with subsequent loss of vision.

Other localized disease in the neonate includes rhinitis, funisitis, vaginitis, anorectal infection, and scalp abscess after fetal monitoring. Invasive infection (sepsis, meningitis) rarely occurs. A form of neonatal septic arthritis usually appears 1 to 4 weeks after delivery and after several days of prodromal symptoms, involves one to four distal joints, and is not associated with skin lesions.

Vaginitis and Cervicitis

Uncomplicated gonococcal infection of the female genital tract presents with mild to profuse vaginal discharge, local pruritus, and dysuria. In young girls, urinary symptoms may predominate, and edema, erythema, and tenderness of the vulva are common findings. Once a girl undergoes puberty, her infection is more likely to be endocervical and often is silent. In addition to having vaginal discharge and dysuria, she may have localized labial swelling and tenderness that reflect infection of the Bartholin and Skene glands. Systemic symptoms and signs are rare findings.

The most serious complication of genital gonorrhea, seen in 10% to 20% of infected female patients, is pelvic inflammatory disease (PID). Children and adolescents are more likely to develop this syndrome than are adults. Risk factors include multiple sexual partners, use of an intrauterine device, and vaginal douching. Ascent of the gonococcus from the vagina or cervix leads to endometritis, salpingitis, and, occasionally, pelvic or abdominal abscesses. Frequently, other genital microbes (particularly chlamydia and anaerobes) are found in the diseased structures, with or without gonococci; the relative role of each of these organisms in the pathogenesis of PID is undefined. The resultant fallopian tube fibrosis leads to obstruction and sterility in 12% of first-time infections, increasing to 50% to 75% after three episodes. Other women later have an increased incidence of ectopic pregnancy or chronic pelvic pain. PID is suggested clinically by lower abdominal pain, discomfort on motion of the cervix, and tenderness of the adnexal structures, which may show a masslike enlargement. Fever and genital bleeding or discharge also may be present. Alternatively, symptoms may be minimal or absent. More extensive spread of the gonococcus, with or without other organisms, leads to perihepatitis (i.e., Fitz-Hugh–Curtis syndrome), with fever and right upper quadrant pain or tenderness.

Urethritis

Purulent urethral discharge and dysuria are hallmarks of gonococcal infection of the urethra in either gender, although the infection rarely is confined to this structure in female patients. Urinary frequency and urgency are not seen. Asymptomatic men constitute a small percentage of cases. Epididymitis and prostatitis are rare complications, but scarring may result in urethral strictures.

Other Localized Disease

Gonococcal conjunctivitis in older children and adolescents resembles that in neonates. Pharyngeal and anorectal gonorrhea most often are asymptomatic, although the latter may present with tenesmus, rectal bleeding, and pruritus. Cervical adenitis may accompany gonococcal pharyngitis. Mucopurulent exudate may be seen with pharyngitis or proctitis.

Disseminated Gonococcal Infection

Hematogenous spread of gonococci to joints and other sites occurs more frequently in children and adolescents than in adults. Disseminated gonococcal infection (DGI) usually develops after asymptomatic mucosal infection. Unlike the arthritis in neonates, joint symptoms in older children mimic the adult presentation and take one of two forms. The first, "arthritis-dermatitis syndrome," consists of migratory polyarthralgia, tenosynovitis, skin lesions, and systemic symptoms. Knees, ankles, and wrists are involved most commonly. Skin lesions are distributed sparsely on the dorsal extremities and appear as painful papules or petechiae that rapidly become hemorrhagic, pustular, necrotic, or ulcerated. Blood and skin biopsy cultures usually show gonococci, but no growth is obtained from synovial fluid. The second syndrome is characterized by a monoarticular purulent arthritis with minimal systemic signs. A joint aspirate is likely to show the organism on smear or culture, but bacteremia is not demonstrable. This is the most common form of septic arthritis in young adults.

Other forms of DGI are extremely rare findings in children. Meningitis and endocarditis with valvular involvement have been reported.

DIAGNOSIS

Because pediatric gonorrhea occurs in a variety of forms and may mimic other conditions, a high index of suspicion is necessary for establishing its diagnosis. In children past the neonatal period and in adolescents without a history of consensual sexual activity, isolation of *N. gonorrhoeae* indicates sexual abuse until proven otherwise. In addition, a search for gonorrhea must be undertaken in any sexually active adolescent who presents with consistent symptoms.

The patient history should make note of risk factors for acquisition of gonorrhea and details of alleged abuse. In adolescents, information must be obtained about sexual activity and symptoms in partners. *N. gonorrhoeae* infection in other household members should be recorded. The patient should be examined gently but thoroughly for urogenital discharge and signs of trauma, such as perineal bruising or lacerations. Samples for culture should be collected from the urethra in male patients (alternatively, culture of urethral discharge alone is sufficient, if present), the vagina in prepubertal female patients, the endocervix in older female patients, and other sources (e.g., rectum, pharynx, joint fluid, blood, skin biopsy) as appropriate. A self-obtained swab from the adolescent vagina may be more acceptable to the patient and does not sacrifice sensitivity. Use of gel lubricants or cotton swabs may interfere with isolation of the gonococcus and should be avoided; warm water and synthetic swabs are suitable alternatives. A first-void urine may be centrifuged; then the sediment can be cultured. Isolation of *N. gonorrhoeae* confirms the diagnosis.

Gonococci are fastidious in their growth requirements and do not tolerate drying. Success in isolation requires immediate plating of specimens onto room temperature media. Specialized transport systems may be useful if performing this technique is not feasible. Generally, modified Thayer-Martin medium (i.e., chocolate agar plus vancomycin, colistin, trimethoprim, and nystatin) is used for isolation. The added antibiotics suppress growth of accompanying normal flora, but they also may impair isolation of vancomycin-sensitive strains of *N. gonorrhoeae*. If the specimen is taken from a normally sterile site (e.g., synovial fluid), chocolate agar alone is sufficient. Optimal growth occurs at 35°C to 37°C in an atmosphere enriched with 5% carbon dioxide, which may be obtained with use of an incubator and a candle jar. If DGI is suspected clinically but blood cultures are negative, isolation of gonococci from mucosal surfaces supports the diagnosis.

A Gram stain of purulent secretions that shows gram-negative diplococci *within* neutrophils helps to diagnose gonococcal urethritis and conjunctivitis but not other clinical conditions because of morphologically similar normal flora. *N. gonorrhoeae* cannot be distinguished from nonpathogenic *Neisseria* by appearance alone. Speciation of oxidase-positive, gram-negative diplococcal isolates should be determined by the pattern of acid production from carbohydrates (i.e., gonococci metabolize glucose but not maltose, lactose, or sucrose). Chromogenic enzyme substrate systems, rapid coagglutination techniques using monoclonal antibodies against the gonococcus, and fluorescence-tagged monoclonal antibodies also may be used to identify *N. gonorrhoeae*. Because of the medicolegal implications of a pediatric diagnosis of gonorrhea, at least two of these culture-based identification methods should be performed.

Nonculture tests represent an important advance for detecting gonorrheal infection in high-prevalence populations. The most recent of these tests, the nucleic acid amplification tests (NAATs), also are the most sensitive and can be performed on swabs of discharge or on urine; specimens also can be tested for coincident chlamydial infection. Unfortunately, their usefulness in children is unknown. Because the legal ramifications of a positive test are so great, use of NAATs is not recommended in preadolescents at this time. Enzyme immunoassay or nucleic acid probes may detect the gonococcus directly in clinical specimens, but their utility is limited to making a presumptive diagnosis in populations with a high prevalence of gonorrhea.

DIFFERENTIAL DIAGNOSIS

Time of onset and Gram stain of drainage may distinguish GON from infection by chlamydia, herpes simplex, or other bacteria and from chemical conjunctivitis caused by silver nitrate. Nongonococcal urethritis, with discharge that typically is less purulent than that from *N. gonorrhoeae*, may be caused by chlamydiae or trichomonads and perhaps by *Ureaplasma* species; these agents also can cause vaginitis, as does *Candida albicans*.

The arthritis of DGI may resemble other septic arthritides or that seen in some collagen-vascular diseases. Associated tenosynovitis or the typical rash suggests gonorrhea. PID may be difficult to distinguish from other intraabdominal conditions such as appendicitis, mesenteric adenitis, ectopic pregnancy, ovarian cyst, and urinary tract infection. Leukocytosis and elevated sedimentation rate or C-reactive protein are common findings, but normal values do not exclude the diagnosis of PID. Ultrasonography of pelvic structures, endometrial biopsy, or laparoscopy may be helpful. Failure to identify a cause for abdominal pain or arthritis in a sexually active or abused woman or a child of either gender, respectively, should prompt a workup for gonorrhea.

THERAPY

Antibiotic resistance has forced the abandonment of such historically useful drugs as penicillin and tetracycline for most cases of gonorrhea. Treatment strategies now focus on drugs that have an efficacy approaching 100% for all strains after one dose, are well tolerated, and preferably are inexpensive. Pediatric gonorrhea treatment has not been studied extensively; recommendations often are based on small series or extrapolated from adult data. Treatment options are listed in Table 166.1; other regimens may be effective. "Test of cure" culture is unnecessary after standard therapy has been implemented, but it is recommended if treatment other than ceftriaxone (or in older teens, a quinolone) is used. Performing follow-up cultures several weeks after initiation of treatment also is advisable in teens who remain sexually active, because reinfection occurs commonly. If symptoms persist, affected patients should undergo reculture, and antibiotic sensitivity should be performed on any isolate.

Regardless of the form of disease, medical and legal imperatives are finding and treating the source of pediatric gonorrhea. The possibility of sexual abuse always must be investigated, and all household members should be evaluated for gonorrheal infection. Children and adolescents who have had sexual exposure to an individual with gonorrhea should themselves be cultured and treated. The partners of sexually active adolescents must be notified and treated, often with the help of public health officials. Because other sexually transmitted infections (e.g., chlamydia, syphilis, human immunodeficiency virus, hepatitis B) frequently coexist with gonorrhea, they should be sought in all patients. Detecting chlamydial infection can be difficult, so concurrent empiric therapy for this condition is recommended for all children past the neonatal period.

TABLE 166.1

TREATMENT OF GONOCOCCAL INFECTION IN CHILDREN

Patient Age and Infection	Treatment of Choice and Alternatives
Neonates	
Ophthalmia neonatorum*	Ceftriaxone 25–50 mg/kg (maximum 125 mg) IV or IM once
Sepsis, arthritis, meningitis, scalp abscess[†]	Ceftriaxone 25–50 mg/kg IV or IM daily for 7 days (meningitis, 10–14 days) Or Cefotaxime 25 mg/kg IV or IM q12h for 7 days (meningitis, 10–14 days)
Older Children[‡]	
Vaginitis, cervicitis, urethritis, proctitis, pharyngitis	Ceftriaxone 125 mg IV or IM once Or Cefixime 400 mg PO once[§] Or Spectinomycin 40 mg/kg (maximum 2 g) IM once[‖] Or Ciprofloxacin 500 mg PO once[#] Or Ofloxacin 400 mg PO once[#] Or Levofloxacin 250 mg PO once[#]
Conjunctivitis*	Ceftriaxone 50 mg/kg (maximum 1 g) IV or IM once
Sepsis, arthritis	Ceftriaxone 50 mg/kg (maximum 1 g) IV or IM daily for 7 days
Meningitis, endocarditis	Ceftriaxone 25 mg/kg (maximum 2 g/day) q12h IV for 10–14 days (meningitis) or for at least 28 days (endocarditis)
Pelvic inflammatory disease	Therapy individualized; generally use cefoxitin + doxycycline, or clindamycin + gentamicin, until 24 hours after improvement, then doxycycline or clindamycin alone to complete 14-day course

IM, intramuscularly; IV, intravenously; PO, per os (by mouth).

*Accompany with frequent saline eye washes; a formal eye examination for complications is recommended.

[†]Cefotaxime is preferred for neonates with hyperbilirubinemia or who are premature.

[‡]Evaluate for sexual abuse. All children past the neonatal period should receive concomitant treatment for possible chlamydia infection: erythromycin (40–50 mg/kg/day in four divided doses PO for 14 days), or azithromycin (20 mg/kg, maximum 1 g, PO once) for children younger than age 8, or doxycycline (100 mg twice/day PO for 7 days) or azithromycin (1 g PO once) for older children.

[§]For older adolescents. It may be effective in younger children but has not been evaluated in this group.

[‖]Spectinomycin is not effective for gonococcal pharyngitis.

[#]Generally, quinolones are not recommended for children younger than 18 years. Because of high prevalence of resistant strains, quinolones should not be used for infections acquired in Asia, Hawaii, or California.

Neonates

Infants born to mothers with untreated gonorrhea should receive a single parenteral dose of ceftriaxone, 25 to 50 mg/kg (maximum, 125 mg), after gastric and rectal cultures are obtained. If signs of infection develop, affected patients should be hospitalized, and the appropriate regimen should be instituted (see Table 166.1).

Older Children

A single dose of ceftriaxone is the treatment of choice for uncomplicated genitourinary, pharyngeal, or rectal gonorrhea. Cefixime is a possible oral alternative, but its use has not been studied in children. Spectinomycin is another choice, as are quinolones for older adolescents.

DGI requires parenteral therapy; generally, hospitalization is necessary for serious disease or when noncompliance is an issue. Intraarticular antibiotics and surgical drainage of an infected joint (except perhaps the hip) are not necessary, although serial joint space aspirations may be needed.

Because PID usually results from polymicrobial infection, therapy must be individualized. Culture results and clinical response should be considered. Therapy in an inpatient setting is recommended if other intraabdominal disease cannot be ruled out, if noncompliance or medication nontolerance is an issue, or if the patient is quite ill. Suggested antibiotic regimens include cefoxitin and doxycycline, or clindamycin and gentamicin, for at least 24 hours after improvement is seen. Doxycycline or clindamycin should be continued at least 10 to 14 days.

PROGNOSIS

When treated promptly with appropriate antibiotics, most gonococcal infections can be cured. Usually, permanent sequelae (e.g., blindness from GON, sterility from PID) result from delay in seeking medical attention.

PREVENTION

Interrupting the spread of gonorrhea from mother to neonate may be accomplished best by identifying infected women at the first prenatal visit. Every culture-positive woman and any sexual partner must be treated at that time. Women at high risk of reexposure should be cultured again in the third trimester and retreated if reinfection has occurred.

Extensive experience has proved the efficacy of the Credé procedure (instillation of 1% silver nitrate solution into the conjunctival sac within 60 minutes of birth) in preventing GON. The use of topical 1% tetracycline ophthalmic ointment or 0.5% erythromycin ophthalmic ointment has been advocated as alternative prophylaxis because these agents do not cause chemical conjunctivitis and appear to be as effective. In areas with chromosomally mediated resistance to tetracycline, use of that antibiotic may be inadvisable. None of these topical preparations reliably protects against nonocular infection or chlamydial conjunctivitis.

Educating children and adolescents about sexually transmitted diseases may help them make informed choices that can help interrupt disease spread. Among sexually active adolescents, use of condoms and spermicide should be encouraged as a means of preventing gonorrhea and other sexually transmitted diseases. Every effort should be made to identify and treat the sexual contacts of known patients with gonorrhea.

Suggested Readings

American Academy of Pediatrics. Gonococcal infections. In: Pickering LK, ed. *Red Book: 2003 Report of the Committee on Infectious Diseases*, 26th ed. Elk Grove Village, IL: American Academy of Pediatrics, 2003:285.

Britigan BE, Cohen MS, Sparling PF. Gonococcal infection: a model of molecular pathogenesis. *N Engl J Med* 1985;312:1683.
Centers for Disease Control and Prevention. Screening tests to detect *Chlamydia trachomatis* and *Neisseria gonorrhoeae* infections: 2002. *Morb Mortal Wkly Rep MMWR* 2002;51:1.
Centers for Disease Control and Prevention. Sexually transmitted disease surveillance 2003 supplement. Gonococcal isolate surveillance project (GISP) annual report: 2003. Atlanta, GA: U.S. Department of Health and Human Services, 2004.
Centers for Disease Control and Prevention. Sexually transmitted diseases treatment guidelines 2002. *Morb Mortal Wkly Rep MMWR* 2002;51:1.
Hammerschlag MR. Appropriate use of nonculture tests for the detection of sexually transmitted diseases in children and adolescents. *Semin Pediatr Infect Dis* 2003;14:54.
Hammerschlag MR, Cummings C, Roblin PM, et al. Efficacy of neonatal ocular prophylaxis for the prevention of chlamydial and gonococcal conjunctivitis. *N Engl J Med* 1989;320:769.
Handsfield HH, McCormick WM, Hook EW, et al. A comparison of single-dose cefixime with ceftriaxone as treatment for uncomplicated gonorrhea. *N Engl J Med* 1991;325:1337.
Knapp JS, Rice RJ. *Neisseria* and *Branhamella*. In: Murray PR, Baron EJ, Pfaller MA, et al, eds. *Manual of clinical microbiology*, 6th ed. Washington, DC: American Society for Microbiology, 1995:324.
Rawstron SA, Hammerschlag MR, Gullans C, et al. Ceftriaxone treatment of penicillinase-producing Neisseria gonorrhoeae infections in children. *Pediatr Infect Dis J* 1989;8:445.
Woods, CR. Gonococcal infections. In: Feigin RD, Cherry JD, Demmler GJ, Kaplan SL, eds. *Textbook of pediatric infectious diseases*, 5th ed, vol 1. Philadelphia: WB Saunders, 2004:1280.

CHAPTER 167 ■ *PASTEURELLA MULTOCIDA*

MORVEN S. EDWARDS

The organism now designated *Pasteurella multocida* was isolated first by Kitt in 1878 and subsequently by Pasteur, who identified it as the causative agent of fowl cholera. Originally, *Pasteurella* species causing "hemorrhagic septicemia" were classified according to the animal source from which they were isolated. Recognition of interspecies transmission of infection and common biochemical features led to the grouping of isolates from all sources as *P. multocida* in 1939. These organisms are common commensals in the respiratory tract of animals, and human infection usually can be linked to contact with animals.

MICROBIOLOGY

P. multocida is one of 11 *Pasteurella* species, most of which are associated more commonly with animal disease than with human disease. *P. multocida* includes three subspecies: *multocida*, *septica*, and *gallicida*. *P. multocida* is the most virulent species in animals. Most human *Pasteurella* infections are caused by organisms identified as *P. multocida* subspecies *multocida* and subspecies *septica*, followed by *P. canis*, *P. stomatis*, and *P. dagmatis*. *P. multocida* is indole and urease positive and is characterized by absence of hemolysis when grown on blood agar. It grows well on a variety of routine media that do not contain bile, including blood, chocolate, and Mueller-Hinton agars; it

does not grow on the bile-containing MacConkey agar. On blood agar, its colonies resemble enterococci. Optimal growth occurs at 37°C under aerobic or facultatively anaerobic conditions.

P. multocida is a small, nonmotile, gram-negative rod that occurs singly, in pairs, or in short chains and may exhibit bipolar staining. These organisms may be confused microscopically with *Haemophilus influenzae*, *Neisseria* species, and *Acinetobacter* species.

EPIDEMIOLOGY AND TRANSMISSION

The incidence of asymptomatic respiratory tract or oral cavity colonization with *P. multocida* approximates 70% to 90% in cats, 50% to 70% in dogs, 50% in pigs, and 15% in wild rats. Carriage has been documented in larger felines (e.g., lions, tigers, leopards, panthers, lynx) and in a variety of other animals, including horses, cattle, sheep, rabbits, and water buffalo.

Most *P. multocida* infections in humans are the result of direct inoculation by animal bites or scratches, and this pathogen has been implicated in 80% of infected cat bites and in 50% of infected dog bites. No seasonal or gender predilection for infection exists. *P. multocida* infections for which specific exposure to a bite cannot be elicited usually are the result of contact with animal secretions. Occasionally, asymptomatic upper respiratory tract colonization may precede dissemination of infection in humans, and *P. multocida* has been isolated from asymptomatic persons who have frequent contact with animals. Close contact with the family cat during breast-feeding was the source for transmission through oropharyngeal colonization to an infant who developed meningitis and bacteremia caused by *P. multocida*. In some cases, no animal contact can be established. Although exquisitely susceptible to direct sunlight, the organism can survive in water or soil for approximately 3 weeks. Human-to-human transmission has not been documented, but an animal-soil-human route could account for some cases that cannot be linked directly to animals.

PATHOGENESIS AND PATHOLOGY

The pathogenesis of *P. multocida* infections may be understood by examining the several potential routes of inoculation. The most common way in which infection is established is direct implantation of organisms beneath the skin from an animal bite or scratch. Inoculation is likely to be deeper and to penetrate the periosteum or a joint space if the source is a cat bite (i.e., puncture wound injury) rather than a dog bite (i.e., laceration wound). The rapidly established and intensely painful local cellulitis that results may be attributed in part to the production by *P. multocida* of neuraminidase and endotoxin. The discharge from wounds is gray and serosanguineous. Localized infections are characterized by an infiltration of neutrophils that may manifest as abscess formation, osteomyelitis, septic arthritis, or tenosynovitis.

Nasopharyngeal colonization with *P. multocida* may occur before respiratory tract infection develops. Invasive infection occurs almost exclusively in the setting of underlying respiratory tract disease, such as chronic bronchitis or bronchiectasis.

In experimental models of infection, intraperitoneal or parenteral inoculation promotes rapid replication in extracellular tissues, with subsequent hematogenous dissemination and invasion of reticuloendothelial organs. Bacteremic infection in humans is a particular risk in the setting of hepatic dysfunction. Patients with bacteremia may have foci of infection, the most common of which are intraabdominal abscess formation and meningitis.

CLINICAL MANIFESTATIONS

The three major clinical manifestations of *P. multocida* infections are soft tissue, respiratory tract, and disseminated infections. Cellulitis caused by *P. multocida* characteristically has a rapid onset, often within a few hours after an animal bite or scratch occurs. The average time of onset is 12 to 24 hours, with a range of 3 hours to 3 days. Erythema, pain, edema, and discharge described as watery and gray, odorous, or serosanguineous are the predominant local features, and 20% to 30% of patients have regional adenopathy. Depending on the location and extent of the wound, infection may be complicated by formation of an abscess, tenosynovitis, arthritis, or osteomyelitis. Direct inoculation presumably is required to establish infection in the tendon sheath, joint, or bone. The extremities usually are affected, but osteomyelitis and brain abscess have complicated a bite wound to the head in children. Joint stiffness with cellulitis of the hand is a sign of involvement of the tendon sheath, and surgical exploration should be undertaken. Even with appropriate drainage, wound infections caused by *P. multocida* heal slowly, particularly if poorly vascularized tissues such as the tendon are involved.

Respiratory tract infections occur in the setting of chronic pulmonary disease, such as bronchitis or bronchiectasis, and are rare in children. Organisms colonizing the nasopharynx are of low virulence and have minimal invasive potential except in the presence of preexisting injury.

Disseminated infection in children most commonly presents as bacteremia with or without meningitis. Most of the reported cases have occurred in infants younger than 1 year of age. A history of nontraumatic animal contact, such as facial licking by household pets, commonly is elicited. Presenting symptoms for infants with *Pasteurella* meningitis are those of purulent meningitis and include lethargy, vomiting, irritability, and fever.

P. multocida has been isolated from the female genital tract, and neonatal sepsis associated with maternal chorioamnionitis has been described. Bacteremia is a rare complication of wound infection. A few patients have had appendicitis caused by *P. multocida*. The isolates were recovered from peritoneal fluid, appendiceal abscesses, or incisional wound abscesses. The source and pathogenesis of infection in these patients are uncertain; at the time appendicitis was evident, bacteremia did not coexist in the patients who underwent blood culture.

DIAGNOSIS

The diagnosis of *P. multocida* infection is established by culture of the organism from blood, wound, abscess, or, in the case of meningitis, cerebrospinal fluid. When cultures are obtained from wound infections, laboratory personnel should be alerted to the possible presence of *Pasteurella*. The Gram stain may produce confusion with the following organisms: *Haemophilus influenzae*, which, unlike *P. multocida*, requires factors X and V for growth; *Neisseria*, which is differentiated by indole production; and *Acinetobacter* species, which grow on bile-containing media. Clinically, the features of rapid onset and grayish drainage aid in differentiating between cellulitis caused by *P. multocida* and staphylococcal or streptococcal wound infections. In the context of exposure to cats, tularemia, plague, and cat-scratch disease are differential considerations, but each of these diseases has a longer incubation period than *Pasteurella* infections.

TREATMENT

Penicillin is the drug of choice for *P. multocida* infections. For uncomplicated wounds managed on an outpatient basis, penicillin V at a dosage of 50,000 U/kg/day administered four times daily is recommended. If the severity of the wound warrants hospitalization, aqueous penicillin G should be administered at a dosage of 200,000 U/kg/day, given every 6 hours. Parenteral therapy always is indicated under the following circumstances: if bite wounds are associated with signs of systemic toxicity; if involvement of tendon, bone, or joint is a consideration; if wound cellulitis has progressed despite administration of oral therapy; and in children with impaired immune function, particularly reticuloendothelial system dysfunction.

P. multocida strains are almost universally susceptible to penicillin, having a median minimal inhibitory concentration of approximately 0.1 μg/mL. However, penicillin susceptibility testing should be confirmed in serious infections or in those patients who fail to show the expected response to therapy because rare isolates may be penicillin resistant. Other anti-microbials to which isolates of *P. multocida* are susceptible include the following: the penicillin derivatives ampicillin, ticarcillin, piperacillin, and mezlocillin; the second- and third-generation parenteral cephalosporins; quinolones; and trimethoprim-sulfamethoxazole. Antibiotics that are inadequate for treating *P. multocida* infections include dicloxacillin, erythromycin, clindamycin, vancomycin, the aminoglycosides, and first-generation cephalosporins. Broad-spectrum oral cephalosporins, such as cefixime, cefpodoxime, or ceftibuten, may prove effective. If *P. multocida* may be one of several pathogens in an infected animal or human bite wound, the following antimicrobials are appropriate for empiric treatment: ampicillin-sulbactam sodium or ticarcillin with clavulanate, administered parenterally, or amoxicillin with clavulanate, given orally. In patients allergic to penicillin, trimethoprim-sulfamethoxazole plus clindamycin is an alternative regimen that can be administered orally or intravenously, depending on the severity of the infection.

The usual duration of treatment for cellulitis or a localized wound abscess caused by *P. multocida* is 7 to 10 days. With adequate drainage, 2 to 3 weeks of treatment usually suffice for treatment of arthritis or tenosynovitis, and 3 to 4 weeks for osteomyelitis. Recovery among infants and children with meningitis caused by *P. multocida* has been reported with regimens including ampicillin (200 to 300 mg/kg/day) or penicillin G (300,000 to 400,000 U/kg/day) for a 14-day (mean) course of therapy.

OUTCOME

Recovery is the rule, but bone and joint infections caused by *P. multocida* may have residua consisting of decreased joint mobility or ankylosis and chronic osteomyelitis, depending on the extent of the initial injury. Most survivors of meningitis have had a normal outcome, but hemiparesis has been reported.

Suggested Readings

Arons MS, Fernando L, Polayes IM, et al. *Pasteurella multocida:* the major cause of hand infections following domestic animal bites. *J Hand Surg* 1982;7: 47.

Boerlin P, Siegrist HH, Burnens AP, et al. Molecular identification and epidemiological tracing of *Pasteurella multocida* meningitis in a baby. *J Clin Microbiol* 2000;38:1235.

Clapp DW, Kleiman MB, Reynolds JK, et al. *Pasteurella multocida* meningitis in infancy: an avoidable infection. *Am J Dis Child* 1986;140:444.

Green BT, Ramsey KM, Nolan PE. *Pasteurella multocida* meningitis: case report and review of the last 11 years. *Scand J Infect Dis* 2002;34:213.

Kumar A, Devlin HR, Vellend H. *Pasteurella multocida* meningitis in an adult: case report and review. *Rev Infect Dis* 1990;12:440.

Raffi F, David F, Mouzard A, et al. *Pasteurella multocida* appendiceal peritonitis: report of three cases and review of the literature. *Pediatr Infect Dis* 1986;5:695.

Schuur PMH, Haring AJP, van Belkum A, et al. Use of random amplification of polymorphic DNA in a case of *Pasteurella multocida* meningitis that occurred following a cat scratch on the head. *Clin Infect Dis* 1997;24:1004.

Thompson CM, Pappu L, Levkoff AH, et al. Neonatal septicemia and meningitis due to *Pasteurella multocida. Pediatr Infect Dis* 1984;3:559.

Weber DJ, Wolfson JS, Swartz MN, et al. *Pasteurella multocida* infections: report of 34 cases and review of the literature. *Medicine (Baltimore)* 1984;63: 133.

Zaramella P, Zamorani E, Freato F, et al. Neonatal meningitis due to a vertical transmission of *Pasteurella multocida. Pediatr Int* 1999;41:307.

CHAPTER 168 ■ PERTUSSIS

JAMES D. CHERRY

Pertussis (i.e., whooping cough) is an acute, communicable, respiratory illness that affects susceptible persons of all ages but is particularly serious in infants. The illness can be controlled relatively effectively by universal immunization of infants and children.

ETIOLOGY AND EPIDEMIOLOGY

Pertussis is caused by *Bordetella pertussis* and, less frequently, by *Bordetella parapertussis*. Both are fastidious gram-negative aerobic bacilli that require special media for growth.

EPIDEMIOLOGY

The epidemiology of reported clinical pertussis is very different from the epidimiology of *B. pertussis* infection, resulting in much confusion relating to the epidemiology of pertussis. The epidemiology of reported pertussis is affected extensively by the degree of vaccine use. Pertussis occurs in all parts of the world, and humans are the only known hosts of *B. pertussis*. Transmission occurs from person to person by respiratory secretion droplets, and contagion is extremely high in nonimmunized populations. Spread occurs from children, adolescents, and adults with disease to susceptible contacts; asymptomatic carriers are not important in transmission. Adults with protracted cough illnesses (i.e., unrecognized pertussis) are an important source of *B. pertussis* infection among nonimmunized or partially immunized children.

In nonvaccinated populations, approximately 10% of reported cases occur in children younger than 1 year of age, 40% in children 1 to 4 years old, 45% in children 5 to 9 years old, and 5% in persons older than 9 years of age. In highly immunized populations today, such as in the United States, 30% of the reported cases occur in the first year of life, another 11% occur in children younger than age 5 years, 10% occur in children between 5 and 9 years of age, 29% occur in children and adolescents, and the remaining 20% are reported in adults.

Reported pertussis occurs in epidemic cycles with intervals of 2 to 5 years. In the prevaccine era in the United States, the average yearly reported attack rate was 157 per 100,000 persons. Immunization reduced this rate of reported pertussis to fewer than 1 per 100,000 in the 1970s. Since 1984, a modest increase in reported pertussis, from less than 1 to 8 cases per 100,000, has occurred. The major incidence of mortality from pertussis occurs among infants. Of reported cases of pertussis in the United States, 0.6% of the patients younger than 1 year of age die. The clinical attack and mortality rates of pertussis are higher for female than for male patients.

In contrast with the cyclic nature of reported pertussis, the epidemiology of *B. pertussis* infection is not cyclic but endemic in adolescents and adults. *B. pertussis* infection is the cause of 13% to 20% of prolonged cough illnesses in adults. Serologic survey data suggest that infection rates in adolescents and adults are between 1% and 8%. The rate in adolescents and adults of cough illness caused by *B. pertussis* infection is in the range of 0.4% to 1.5%.

PATHOPHYSIOLOGY

Pertussis is predominantly a disease of the ciliated epithelium of the respiratory tract. The *B. pertussis* organism has many unique, biologically active antigens, and studies have suggested roles for these antigens in the pathogenesis of disease. In the pathogenesis of pertussis, four steps are important: attachment, evasion of host defenses, local damage, and systemic manifestations.

After the airborne transmission of respiratory secretions containing *B. pertussis* occurs, the organisms attach to the cilia of the respiratory epithelial cells of the new host. Filamentous hemaggluttinin (FHA), pertussis toxin (PT), pertactin, and fimbriae (types 2 and 3) are *B. pertussis* antigens that are most important in the attachment process. Of these four proteins, pertactin is the most important adhesion. After attachment, the infection proceeds because of the profound adverse effect on host immune effector cell function by adenylate cyclase toxin and PT.

Tracheal cytotoxin is likely to be the main cause of local tissue damage of the ciliated respiratory epithelium, and this damage may be, at least in part, the cause of the paroxysmal cough. Pertussis is a unique disease in that systemic manifestations are rare. The characteristic lymphocytosis is caused by PT.

CLINICAL MANIFESTATIONS

Classic pertussis is a lengthy illness, commonly lasting 6 to 12 weeks and characterized by three stages: catarrhal, paroxysmal, and convalescent. The catarrhal stage has its onset after an incubation period of 7 to 10 days. The onset of illness is subtle and resembles a mild upper respiratory tract infection with coryza, mild conjunctival injection, and mild cough. The upper respiratory symptoms continue, and, during the next 7 to 10 days, coughing becomes more persistent and frequent. Mild fever may occur during the catarrhal stage.

The paroxysmal stage is manifested by increasingly forceful coughing in the form of episodic paroxysms, which occur particularly frequently at night. In classic pertussis, episodes of repetitive severe coughing are followed by a single sudden massive inspiration. The characteristic *whoop* sound results from the forceful inhalation and a narrowed glottis. Each coughing paroxysm consists of 10 to 30 forceful coughs in a series. The patient's face becomes increasingly cyanotic; the tongue protrudes to the maximum; and mucus, saliva, and tears stream from the nose, mouth, and eyes, respectively. Episodes of paroxysmal cough may be singular, or several may occur in rapid succession. Twenty to 200 or more sessions of paroxysmal cough may occur each day. The paroxysmal episodes are exhausting, and young children appear apathetic and dazed after attacks. Paroxysms are precipitated by eating, drinking, and any physical activity. Between attacks, patients usually show few signs of illness, and fever is not characteristic of uncomplicated cases. In young infants, apnea and bradycardia may

accompany coughing fits, and a whoop is less likely to occur after a paroxysm.

After the paroxysmal stage, which lasts from 1 to 4 weeks or more, the convalescent stage is heralded by a lessening in the severity and frequency of paroxysms. The duration of the convalescent stage varies. Paroxysmal-type coughing often reoccurs for 6 months or more after a child has recovered from pertussis in association with other respiratory infections. Weight loss or failure to gain weight is a conspicuous feature of severe pertussis, especially in infants. Studies indicate that only 60% of pertussis cases in children have the classic picture; 40% of children have milder disease, with a total duration of cough of less than 4 weeks and generally less frequent and less severe paroxysms. Children in whom vaccine has failed also tend to have less severe disease.

COMPLICATIONS

Complications of pertussis occur commonly and can be grouped into three categories: respiratory, central nervous system, and secondary pressure effects. The rate of complications is inversely related to age. Bronchopneumonia, the most common complication, is caused by secondary infection with common respiratory pathogens (i.e., *Haemophilus influenzae, Streptococcus pneumoniae, S. pyogenes,* and *Staphylococcus aureus*), or it can be caused by a more extensive *B. pertussis* infection. If pneumonia is the result of secondary infection, significant fever and tachypnea are the usual findings. Other respiratory complications include atelectasis, bronchiectasis, interstitial or subcutaneous emphysema, and pneumothorax. Although atelectasis may persist for months after illness, carefully performed follow-up studies have not demonstrated permanent pulmonary sequelae. Young infants with *B. pertussis* pneumonia often have pulmonary hypertension, which often leads to death in spite of aggressive respiratory management. Otitis media is a frequent complication, especially in infants.

Central nervous system complications occur relatively commonly during the paroxysmal stage of pertussis. Data from the Centers for Disease Control and Prevention indicate that 1.4% of infants younger than 6 months of age experience seizures with pertussis, and approximately 0.2% suffer encephalopathy. Severe disease usually is manifested by convulsions and then semicoma or coma. Hemiplegia, paraplegia, ataxia, aphasia, blindness, deafness, and decerebrate rigidity may occur. After an encephalitis-like illness, permanent sequelae are common findings. Approximately one-third of patients die, one-third survive with residua, and one-third survive and appear normal. Sequelae include mental retardation, seizure disorders, and changes in personality and behavior.

Secondary pressure effects that occur during the paroxysmal stage of severe pertussis may cause epistaxis, melena, petechiae, subdural hematoma, umbilical or inguinal hernias, and rectal prolapse.

DIAGNOSIS

Typical pertussis can be reliably diagnosed clinically on the basis of characteristic history and physical findings. However, in infants, children with only mild cases, adults, and individuals with cases modified by immunization, establishing the diagnosis may be more difficult. A careful history usually reveals contact with a person or persons having a prolonged illness with cough. These contact cases are likely to be adolescents or adults.

The absence or presence of only minimal fever is strong evidence for the diagnosis of pertussis rather than a similar type of illness caused by a respiratory virus. In classic pertussis, the leukocyte count is elevated because of lymphocytosis. Leukocytosis develops at the end of the catarrhal stage and during the paroxysmal stage of the disease. Absolute lymphocyte counts usually are greater than 10,000 and often are more than 30,000 cells/dL. Young infants and patients with mild or modified disease may not exhibit the typical lymphocytosis.

Establishing the specific diagnosis of pertussis depends on isolation of the organism or its demonstration by a rapid identification method. *B. pertussis* can be isolated from nasopharyngeal secretions during the catarrhal and early paroxysmal stages of disease. With optimal specimen collection, fresh culture medium, and experienced technicians, 80% of the suspected cases can be confirmed by culture in outbreak situations. Specimens for culture should be obtained from the nasopharynx with the use of Dacron or calcium alginate swabs or by nasopharyngeal aspiration. These specimens should be inoculated directly onto or into selective media (e.g., Regan-Lowe charcoal agar, modified Stainer-Scholte broth, or fresh Bordet-Gengou agar). Alternatively, Regan-Lowe transport medium should be inoculated and the specimen transported to a diagnostic laboratory. Prior antibiotic treatment may markedly reduce the isolation rate.

Direct fluorescence antibody (DFA) identification of *B. pertussis* in nasopharyngeal specimens is a reasonably accurate procedure when performed with good reagents by experienced personnel. This technique is particularly useful if antimicrobial therapy has been given, thus decreasing the likelihood of obtaining a positive culture. In many laboratories, rapid diagnosis now is performed by the use of the polymerase chain reaction (PCR). In general, PCR has greater sensitivity and specificity than does DFA, and it frequently is more sensitive than is culture. Extreme care is necessary in the PCR laboratory because contamination can lead to false-positive results.

Pertussis also can be diagnosed serologically, but because all standard tests usually depend on the demonstration of an increase in antibody titer, these techniques usually are not useful for early diagnosis. The demonstration of a fourfold rise in agglutinin titer is firm evidence that the illness was pertussis. Enzyme-linked immunosorbent assay (ELISA) techniques that use several different pertussis antigens (e.g., PT, FHA, whole cell) and measure antibody in different immunoglobulin fractions (e.g., IgA, IgG) have been used successfully in research and investigational settings. ELISA is available in many routine laboratories.

B. pertussis infection in adolescents, adults, and children who have not been vaccinated recently can be diagnosed by single serum ELISA. Most useful in this regard is a high IgA or IgG value against PT. Antibody to FHA is less specific because it could result from an infection with *B. parapertussis* or a cross-reaction caused by other infectious agents.

TREATMENT

B. pertussis is susceptible to erythromycin and other macrolides, and the administration of these antibiotics to children during the incubation period or the catarrhal stage will prevent or modify clinical disease. Erythromycin therapy also can alter the clinical course of pertussis if treatment is initiated early in the paroxysmal stage. Treatment initiated later in the paroxysmal stage does not lessen the duration or severity of clinical illness, although patients should be treated to reduce the risk of spread to other susceptible contacts. The dosage of erythromycin is 40 to 50 mg/kg/day, orally (adults, 2 g/day), given in four doses for a total of 14 days. The findings of a relatively large study suggested that a 7-day course of treatment with erythromycin was as effective as a 14-day course. Azithromycin, 10 mg/kg on day 1 and 5 mg/kg on days 2 to 5 as a single dose for 5 days (maximum 600 mg/day) for chil-

dren, and 500 mg on day 1 and 250 mg on days 2 to 5 for adults, or clarithromycin 15 to 20 mg/kg/day, given orally in two divided doses (maximum 1 g/day) for 7 days for children or 1 g/day for adults, is also effective but less well studied. Because both azithromycin and clarithromycin have fewer severe side effects in older patients, they generally are better choices for treatment and prophylaxis in adolescents and adults.

In a small but significant number of neonates, erythromycin treatment given during the first 2 weeks of life has been associated with hypertrophic pyloric stenosis. Therefore, infants in this age group should be observed carefully for signs of this illness while undergoing treatment. The macrolide doses listed earlier should be used for both treatment and prophylaxis. In rare instances, *B. pertussis* has been resistant to erythromycin and other macrolides. Trimethoprim-sulfamethoxazole is an alternative to erythromycin, but its efficacy is less well documented.

Because pertussis is a highly contagious infectious disease, patients should be placed in respiratory isolation for 5 days after the initiation of erythromycin or other macrolide therapy. If therapy has not been given, the patient should remain in isolation until 3 weeks after the onset of paroxysms. The younger the child, the more likely is the need for hospitalization. In severe cases, ventilatory therapy may be lifesaving.

Most infants should receive oxygen, and gentle suction should be used to remove secretions. Supportive care includes avoidance of situations that provoke attacks of coughing and maintenance of hydration and nutrition. Although corticosteroids and salbutamol (albuterol) have been used as adjuncts to therapy, no controlled data have indicated the usefulness of either type of medication.

PREVENTION

Universal immunization with pertussis vaccines in children has been extraordinarily successful in controlling epidemic pertussis in the United States. Until relatively recently, the only available vaccines in the United States and in all areas of the world except Japan were suspensions of inactivated *B. pertussis* cells (i.e., whole-cell vaccines). In the mid-1990s, eight efficacy trials with eight candidate acellular pertussis-component diphtheria-tetanus-pertussis vaccines (DTaP) were completed, and, after favorable results occurred with these trials, DTaP vaccines were licensed for the primary immunization of infants in the United States and many other countries throughout the world. Acellular pertussis vaccines are available in the United States only in combination with diphtheria and tetanus toxoids (DTaP vaccines); the combination products are adsorbed with aluminum salts. A successful immunization program for children consists of five doses of DTaP. The primary immunization series consists of an initial three doses given at approximately 2, 4, and 6 months of age, with a fourth dose given at 15 to 18 months. The fifth dose (i.e., booster) is given at the time of school entry, at 4 to 6 years of age.

If pertussis is prevalent in a community, the immunization schedule can be adjusted so the first dose is given during the third week of life and the next two doses at monthly intervals.

DTaP vaccines contain one or more of the following *B. pertussis* antigens: PT toxoid, FHA, pertactin, and fimbriae 2 and 3. All DTaP vaccines contain toxoid PT, and lipooligosaccharide (endotoxin) has been removed from all of them. All DTaP vaccines are immunogenic and stimulate antibody responses to their respective components after the patient has received two or three doses. All DTaP vaccines also are less reactogenic than DTP vaccines.

When the results of the eight efficacy trials are reviewed carefully and allowances are made for bias and study weaknesses, multicomponent vaccines that contain pertactin are found to be more efficacious than two-component (PT toxoid/FHA) or single-component (PT toxoid) vaccines. In addition, a five-component vaccine (PT/FHA/pertactin/fimbriae 2/fimbriae 3) was more efficacious than was a three-component vaccine (PT/FHA/pertactin). In general, whole-cell pertussis vaccines have greater short-term efficacy than do acellular pertussis vaccines. However, the two DTaP vaccines that contain pertactin and are available in the United States have good efficacy against both mild and typical pertussis. The duration of vaccine-produced immunity is relatively short (5 to 10 years), although illness usually is less severe in previously vaccinated persons than in nonvaccinated individuals. DTaP vaccines are given intramuscularly in a volume of 0.5 mL per dose.

In the past, pertussis immunization was not performed routinely in persons 7 years of age or older because severe pertussis was a disease of young children, and reactions to DTP immunization were thought to increase with age. However, the successful control of pertussis and *B. pertussis* circulation in the future will necessitate giving booster immunizations to adolescents and adults, as recommended for diphtheria and tetanus toxoids. These adolescent- and adult-formulated vaccines (Tdap) already have been developed and are licensed in Canada, Australia, and some European countries. In June and October of 2005, the ACIP recommended using Tdap instead of Td for preadolescents, adolescents, and adults 10 through 64 years of age.

Reactions associated with DTP immunization occurred commonly and occasionally were alarming. In general, reactions that occur after immunization with DTaP vaccines are markedly less frequent and less severe than those that occur after administration of DTP and occur at a rate and magnitude similar to those that occur after administration of DT immunization. With the primary DTaP series (first three doses), the following reactogenicity rates can be expected: injection site—redness, 17%; swelling, 12%; and pain, 2%; systemic—fever, 11%; fussiness, 7%; drowsiness, 18%; anorexia, 9%; and vomiting, 5%. Persistent crying of 3 hours duration or longer that occurred in 1% of DTP recipients is a rare occurrence after administration of DTaP immunization (approximately 1 per 2,000). Hypotonic-hyporesponsive episodes and seizures are rare events after administration of DTaP immunization (less than 1 per 10,000).

Of some concern are the recent observations of increased frequency and severity of local reactions (erythema and induration) occurring after administration of the fourth and fifth doses of DTaP vaccines. These events likely are Arthus reactions caused by the higher concentrations of diphtheria toxoid and toxoided PT in the DTaP vaccines compared with the concentrations in the DTP vaccines that were used previously in the United States. Also of concern has been the occasional observation of extensive swelling of the thigh after administration of booster doses of DTaP vaccines.

Pertussis vaccines do not cause sudden infant death syndrome or encephalopathy. DTP vaccines did on occasion induce the first seizures in children who were destined to develop infantile epilepsy, and these instances often incorrectly were called pertussis vaccine encephalopathy. Because fever is an uncommon occurrence after administration of DTaP immunizations, this association now is much less likely.

Contraindications for immunization have evolved since the late 1960s because of the presumed complications of the pertussis component of DTP vaccine. Although no evidence of the validity of these contraindications exists, the prudent practitioner will observe them to avoid misunderstandings about the cause of temporally associated events. Children who have had an immediate anaphylactic reaction after receiving DTaP immunization should not receive any further immunization with the vaccine until an immunologic evaluation has been carried out and possible desensitization has occurred; then further immunization with tetanus toxoid may be implemented. Children who develop unexplained encephalopathy within 7 days after receiving DTaP vaccine generally should not receive additional doses of pertussis vaccines. Physicians should seek up-to-date immunization advice from the Report of the Committee on Infectious Diseases of the American Academy of Pediatrics or Reports of the Advisory Committee on Immunization Practices because recommendations change frequently.

Immunization programs can be successful only if virtually all infants are immunized. When contraindications are overinterpreted and many children remain nonimmunized, a significant risk of contracting disease exists for those who most need protection. The benefits of pertussis immunization substantially outweigh any possible risks of immunization.

Certain control measures are necessary in situations of exposure. In day-care centers and in families, individuals who are exposed should be given erythromycin for 14 days, azithromycin for 5 days, or clarithromycin for 7 days. Booster doses of vaccine should be given when indicated.

Suggested Readings

American Academy of Pediatrics. Pertussis. In: Pickering LK, ed. *Red book: 2003 report of the Committee on Infectious Diseases,* 26th ed. Elk Grove Village, IL: American Academy of Pediatrics, 2003:472.

Cherry JD, Heininger U. Pertussis and other *Bordetella* infections. In: Feigin RD, Cherry JD, Demmler GJ, Kaplan S, eds. *Textbook of pediatric infectious diseases,* 5th ed. Philadelphia: WB Saunders, 2003:1588.

Cherry JD, Gornbein J, Heininger U, Stehr K. A search for serologic correlates of immunity to *Bordetella pertussis* cough illnesses. *Vaccine* 1998;16:1901.

Cherry JD, Karzon DT, Brunell PA, Golden GS. Report of the task force on pertussis and pertussis immunization: 1988. *Pediatrics* 1988;81(suppl):939.

Cherry JD, Olin P. The science and fiction of pertussis vaccines. *Pediatrics* 1999; 104:1381.

Olin P, Rasmussen F, Gustafsson L, et al. Randomised controlled trial of two-component, three-component, and five-component acellular pertussis vaccines compared with whole-cell pertussis vaccine. *Lancet* 1997;350:1569.

CHAPTER 169 ■ PLAGUE

RALPH D. FEIGIN AND LORI P. ZINK

Plague, which is caused by *Yersinia pestis*, has caused the most devastating epidemics in human history. The epidemic spread of this disease through most of Europe in the 1300s became known as the *Black Death*. One-third of the population of Europe died as a result of this epidemic.

The bacillus responsible for plague was identified first in 1894, and, at nearly the same time, the role of fleas and rats in transmitting the disease was recognized. In 1900, plague was introduced into San Francisco by rats aboard ships. The disease rapidly spread to rodents of the American Southwest, and plague is now enzootic throughout the western United States, Central and South America, and other parts of the world.

In 1943, antibiotics effective against *Y. pestis* became available. As a result of these advances, plague is a rare occurrence in the United States today. However, plague continues to be endemic in many parts of the world, leading to recent outbreaks in Madagascar, Peru, and India. Although antibiotics have been effective in the treatment and prophylaxis of plague, antibiotic resistance is an increasing concern. Furthermore, the potential use of aerosolized *Y. pestis* as a biologic weapon is being investigated, leading to renewed interest in the understanding and study of *Y. pestis*.

MICROBIOLOGY

Y. pestis is a pleomorphic, nonmotile, gram-negative bacillus of the family Enterobacteriaceae. When the bacillus is stained with Gram, Giemsa, or Wayson stain, it reveals a bipolar morphology. *Y. pestis* grows best on brain-heart infusion and Mac-Conkey agar. Positive cultures show pinpoint colonies within 24 to 48 hours after inoculation. However, laboratories that are fully automated or semiautomated may not detect *Y. pestis*.

Y. pestis grows optimally at 28°C. Organisms can be isolated from blood, sputum, cerebrospinal fluid, feces, urine, or aspirates of enlarged lymph nodes. These body fluids can be examined for the typical bacilli. Isolated bacteria can be identified by their nonmotile activity at 37° and 22°C. Usually, the organism is negative for urea hydrolysis, but it may be positive in freshly isolated specimens. The response is positive for catalase, nitrate, methyl red, esculin, and beta-galactosidase. The indole, oxidase, and Voges-Proskauer reactions are negative. *Y. pestis* ferments maltose, xylose, glucose, arabinose, salicin, dextrin, mannitol, and trehalose. It does not produce acid from lactose, sucrose, rhamnose, melibiose, adonitol, cellobiose, sorbose, or dulcitol. *Y. pestis* does not use citrate or grow in potassium cyanide, nor does it respond to lysine, ornithine decarboxylase, or arginine dihydrolase.

The organism can be identified by lysis of the isolate by known strains of bacteriophage, agglutination with specific *Y. pestis* antiserum, animal inoculation, and detection of fraction 1 antigen by fluorescent antibody staining. The genome of *Y. pestis* has been sequenced. Polymerase chain reaction (PCR) is available for detection of the plasminogen activator gene of *Y. pestis*. A rapid PCR has been developed that can detect 10^2 colony-forming units (CFUs) of *Y. pestis* in sputum 5 hours after the sample is collected.

The virulence of *Y. pestis* strains varies, depending on the development of the envelope of fraction I antigen, absorption of hemin from medium, production of V and W antigens, synthesis of purines, and generation of toxins. The presence of a fraction I envelope or V and W antigens renders the strain resistant to phagocytosis and permits the organism to multiply. A plasmid of 9-kb pairs contains the determinant of secretory protein that kills other bacterial strains. A plasmid of 72-kb pairs, which all pathogenic *Y. pestis* strains contain, confers the requirement for environmental calcium, which is necessary for the organism to grow at 37°C. When grown under this condition, *Y. pestis* produces the V and W antigens necessary for virulence. Toxins have been produced by all fully virulent strains. Endotoxin and exotoxin appear to contribute to the morbid effects of plague. Transferable plasmid-mediated resistance, including multidrug transport systems, has been isolated.

TRANSMISSION

Historically, plague typically was transmitted by fleas that had fed on infected rats. This form of transmission is more likely to occur in urban, rat-infested, and crowded dwellings and may result in epidemics. In the United States, this form of spread rarely occurs where plague is transmitted to humans after contact with an enzootic focus. Wild rodents perpetuate the plague bacillus by virtue of their ability to withstand an inoculum of *Y. pestis* many times greater than that which causes disease in domestic animals or humans. After being inoculated, the wild rodent becomes bacteremic and can infect the fleas that feed on it. The fleas then can transmit the plague bacillus to another rodent. Hibernating animals are particularly resistant to clinical infection and, if inoculated before going into hibernation, may survive the winter and succumb to the infection only after they emerge from their burrows, thus carrying the bacillus into a new season. Carnivores are relatively resistant to infection but contribute to the spread of the organism by transporting infected fleas from one area to another.

Plague is transmitted to humans by the bite of an infected flea, the inhalation of infected droplets from a patient with pneumonic plague, or the skinning and evisceration of infected animals. Rarely, *Y. pestis* can enter through the conjunctiva and the pharynx. Assymptomatic transient pharyngeal carriage has been described in contacts of bubonic plague cases; the incidence of this carriage is unknown.

Domestic animals play a significant role in bridging the gap between sylvatic plague and human infection. Cats and dogs are susceptible to both natural and experimental plague. Between 1977 and 1998, 23 cases of feline-associated human plague infection were reported. Epizootics in cats have been observed in conjunction with plague epidemics in humans. Domestic animals' fleas are more likely than are rodent's fleas to bite humans. The Oriental rat flea is the most efficient transmitter of the plague bacillus because of the frequency with which it bites humans and its propensity for regurgitating large numbers of *Y. pestis* in the process of biting. Because cats and dogs are susceptible to natural and experimental plague and because of their extensive contact with humans, domestic animals may be responsible for some cases of human plague.

Sylvatic plague depends on the rodent flea as a vector. This flea is not as efficient as a rat flea in transmitting *Y. pestis*, but it may become a reservoir of the organism by surviving for a year or more after the original host dies. Between epizootics, *Y. pestis* can survive in soil, which may serve as a means for transmission of plague.

In urban areas, the organism usually is introduced from an enzootic population into a susceptible rat population. In areas where humans and rats live in proximity, an epizootic in rats may be followed by an epidemic in people. In the United States, children become infected by direct contact with a sylvatic reservoir of this infection. Adult cases are the result of working or hunting in plague-infected areas.

PATHOGENESIS AND PATHOLOGY

The portal of entry of the *Y. pestis* organism determines the form the disease takes. The most common site of entry is the skin, after the bite of an infected flea has occurred. Broken skin provides an easy route for direct inoculation while handling infected animals. After the organism has bypassed the skin barrier to cause infection, it moves by lymphatics to regional lymph nodes. The infection may be localized at this site, with subsequent formation of antibodies and ultimate recovery of the patient. This form of the disease has been called *pestis minor*.

Frequently, *Y. pestis* is disseminated through the bloodstream. Involvement of the liver, spleen, lungs, kidneys, and meninges may occur. Disseminated intravascular coagulation, a common finding in fatal cases, includes an elevation of split-fibrin products, thrombocytopenia, and fibrin deposition in the glomeruli.

The major determinant of the severity of the disease appears to be the presence of high levels of circulating endotoxin. Virulent *Y. pestis* organisms are phagocytized but are not killed. They replicate unimpeded in macrophages, permitting the accumulation of endotoxin.

If the primary portal of entry is the lung, the resulting disease usually is fulminant. Plague bacilli can replicate freely in the alveolar spaces, resulting in severe and overwhelming pneumonitis, septicemia, and endotoxemia. In fatal cases, lymph nodes in the thoracic region have shown infarction, liquefaction necrosis, and formation of pus. The mucosa of the trachea and bronchi may be covered by a frothy, bloody exudate. Submucosal hemorrhages and necrotic areas surround the trachea. Pleural surfaces contain hemorrhagic lesions and fibrinous adhesions. The lung may show signs of acute edema or consolidation. The most prominent histologic feature is an alveolar exudate consisting of polymorphonuclear leukocytes and histiocytes. The kidneys may appear grossly hemorrhagic, and areas of necrosis may be evident. Glomeruli with fibrin thrombi are found frequently in patients who have disseminated intravascular coagulation.

CLINICAL MANIFESTATIONS

The incubation period of *Y. pestis* is approximately 3 or 4 days, but it can be as short as 1 to 2 hours or as long as 2 weeks. The onset of illness usually is abrupt, beginning with malaise, headache, fever, and weakness. Often, fever is accompanied by shaking chills. Development of a visible or palpable mass of nodes, known as a *bubo*, may be preceded by tenderness or pain at the site.

On physical examination, the patient appears to be apprehensive, toxic, and tachycardic. The site of inoculation at the skin may or may not be evident. In some cases, the inoculation site is covered by a carbuncle. In bubonic plague, large, fixed, tender, and edematous lymph nodes are evident at one anatomic site. The areas of nodal involvement are the groin, axilla, and neck, in decreasing order of frequency. Any involved lymph node, including the intraabdominal nodes, can suppurate, which may produce the picture of an acute abdominal emergency.

Neurologic manifestations resulting from the effects of toxin on the brain are common findings. Patients with plague may report insomnia or may suffer from weakness, delirium, stupor, gait disturbances, disorders of speech, loss of memory, or vertigo. Meningitis may occur. Children younger than 15 years of age seem to be more susceptible, and septicemic patients are four times more likely to develop meningitis than are patients with bubonic plague. Meningitis often manifests itself while the patient is well into a course of antibiotic therapy for bubonic or septicemic plague. Intravascular coagulation may herald the onset of renal involvement, which can present clinically as an acute cortical or tubular necrosis. Involvement of the liver is evidenced by mildly elevated liver enzymes.

Pneumonic plague has identical constitutional symptoms, but the course is more fulminant, and the pulmonary component is more pronounced. Within 20 to 24 hours after the onset of illness, dyspnea, tachypnea, and a bloody, mucopurulent, productive cough are evident. If effective treatment is not instituted immediately, most patients die.

DIAGNOSIS

Bubonic plague can be confused with any other disorder of the skin or lymph nodes. The diagnosis of staphylococcal or streptococcal lymphadenitis is established by appropriate culture. A more indolent disorder known as *lymphogranuloma venereum* usually presents with mild localized or systemic disease and commonly is associated with anogenital ulcers. Adenitis caused by *Treponema pallidum* (i.e., syphilis) usually is not tender. Adenopathy that develops as a result of *Pasteurella multocida* infections or cat-scratch fever usually is associated with few constitutional symptoms and a history of exposure to animals. The onset of adenopathy associated with *Francisella tularensis* infection (i.e., tularemia) occurs more gradually. The ulcerated skin lesions of anthrax may resemble those of plague in the later stages.

The buboes of plague are very tender. Bacterial staining of lymph node tissue by Wright, Gram, or Wayson stains should show bipolar plague organisms. Fluorescent antibody staining of direct smears and tissues can provide a rapid presumptive diagnosis of plague. Newer rapid diagnostic tests for plague—F1 antigen detection, immunoglobulin M enzyme immunoassay, immunostaining, and PCR—are available at some health departments, the Centers for Disease Control and Prevention (CDC), and military laboratories. The passive hemagglutination antibody detection assay is mostly of retrospective value as days to weeks pass between onset of disease and development of antibody. The laboratory should be notified that plague is suspected. The laboratory should split the culture, incubating one at 28°C and one at 37°C for identification of the F1 antigen. Antimicrobial suceptibility testing should be performed at a reference laboratory.

TREATMENT

Definitive diagnosis can be made only by culture of *Y. pestis* from infected tissue or body fluid. Therapeutic decisions must be made before culture results are available.

The CDC recommends treatment of all suspected cases of plague. Patients who do not require hospitalization can be treated with tetracycline or chloramphenicol. Tetracycline can be given to patients 8 years old and older at a dosage of 25 to 50 mg/kg/day every 4 to 6 hours up to a total daily dose of 1 g in children and 2 g in adults. If outpatient treatment is provided, the patient should be followed for the first 3 days to ensure resolution of the disease. Sulfonamides may be used for prophylaxis in pediatric patients as an alternative to the tetracyclines. For acutely ill patients, streptomycin remains the drug of choice. Streptomycin should be administered intramuscularly at a dosage of 20 to 30 mg/kg/day in two divided doses. If plague meningitis is considered, chloramphenicol, administered at 50 to 100 mg/kg/day intravenously in four divided doses, after an initial dose of 25 mg/kg, is the treatment of choice. Other intravenous antibiotics that can be useful, particularly in the presence of hypotension, are kanamycin, administered at 15 mg/kg/day in three divided doses up to a maximum dose of 1.5 g/day, and gentamicin, administered at 7.5 mg/kg/day for children or 3 to 5 mg/kg/day for adults in three divided doses. The duration of therapy must be determined by the severity and length of the disease. Treatment should be continued for at least 7 days for patients with uncomplicated disease.

Antibiotic resistance has become an increasing concern with regard to Y. pestis. The nonsterile flea midgut is an excellent environment for conjugative transfer of antibiotic resistance genes. Transferrable plasmid-mediated, high-level resistance to streptomycin has been insolated in Madagascar from at least two individual cases. Multidrug resistance transport systems have been isolated as well. Isolates with resistance to streptomycin, rifampin, kanamycin, spectinomycin, trimethoprim-sulfamethoxazole, ampicillin, tetracycline, minocycline, and doxycycline have been reported; one isolate from a 16-year-old boy in Madagascar contained a plasmid that conferred resistance to ampicillin, chloramphenicol, kanamycin, streptomycin, spectinomycin, sulfonamides, tetracycline, and minocycline. To date, outbreaks of multidrug-resistant plague have not been reported. However, continued survey of resistance patterns is important; modification of empiric therapy may be necessary to conform with local susceptibility patterns.

Patients suspected of having any form of plague should be placed on strict respiratory isolation until at least 48 hours of antimicrobial therapy has been given, pneumonia has been ruled out, and sputum cultures are negative. All criteria must be met.

BIOTERRORISM

The epidemiology of plague after its use as a biologic weapon would differ substantially from that of naturally occurring infection. Intentional dissemination of plague most likely would occur via an aerosol of Y. pestis, resulting in an outbreak of pneumonic plague. The size of the outbreak would depend on the quantity of the biologic agent used, characteristics of the strain, environmental conditions, and methods of aerosolization. In 1970, the World Health Organization (WHO) reported that, in a worst-case scenario, if 50 kg of Y. pestis were released over a city of 5 million, pneumonic plague could occur in as many as 150,000 persons, with 36,000 expected to die. Indications that plague has been disseminated artificially would be the occurrence of cases in locations not known to have enzootic infection, among individuals with no known risk ractors (e.g., animal contact), and the absence of prior deaths of rodents.

After a deliberate attack, aerosolized inhaled Y. pestis would cause primary pneumonic plague, with the time from exposure to the development of first symptoms usually being 2 to 4 days with a range of 1 to 6 days. The sudden appearance of large numbers of previously healthy persons with fever, cough, shortness of breath, chest pain, rapidly progressive pneumo-

nia or bronchopneumonia, and a fulminant course leading to death immediately should cause concern regarding pneumonic plague or inhalational anthrax. Hemoptysis in this setting would strongly suggest plague. Buboes would be absent, except for rare cervical buboes.

In a contained casualty setting, in which a modest number of people would require treatment, parenteral antibiotic therapy with streptomycin (15 mg/kg intramuscularly twice daily, maximum daily dose 2 g) or gentamicin (2.5 mg/kg intramuscularly or intravenously three times daily in children or 5 mg/kg intramuscularly or intravenously once daily for adults) would be the treatment of choice (Table 169.1). Alternative choices are ciprofloxacin, doxycycline, or chloramphenicol. In a mass casualty setting, administering intravenous or intramuscular therapy may not be practical or possible, so oral therapy, preferably with doxycycline (if 45 kg of heavier, 100 mg orally twice daily or if less than 45 kg, 2.2 mg/kg orally twice daily) or tetracycline or ciprofloxacin (20 mg/kg orally twice daily; maximum 500 mg orally twice daily), should be administered for 10 days. Patients with pneumonic plague require substantial advanced medical support, and complications of gram-negative sepsis including acute respiratory distress syndrome, disseminated intravascular coagulation, shock, and multiorgan failure would be expected.

PROGNOSIS

Mortality rates for untreated cases of plague range between 40% and 70%. Almost invariably, pneumonic plague is fatal without treatment. If antimicrobial therapy is provided promptly, the overall mortality rate for plague should be as low as 5%. Complications of plague during convalescence may include lung abscess, suppuration of buboes (which may be delayed), and polyarthritis. Secondary infection with *Pseudomonas* species and *Staphylococcus aureus* may occur, particularly within lymph node tissue.

PREVENTION

Eradication of rats and their removal from areas inhabited by humans are the best means for limiting urban epidemics of plague. Vector control is achieved by the use of insecticides in fields and housing areas. Control of rodents can be achieved by trapping and poisoning the animals and by fumigating their burrows. Control of fleas should precede the destruction of the rodents. Educating the public is important. Children should be taught not to handle sick or dead rodents, and care must be exercised in removing fleas from household pets. Trash should not be permitted to accumulate near living areas.

Victims of plague should be isolated until they are bacteriologically sterile. Because plague is a reportable disease, the WHO should be notified within 24 hours of the diagnosis of a case. Contacts of patients with pneumonic plague should receive chemoprophylaxis with tetracycline (25 to 50 mg/kg/day every 4 to 6 hours up to a total daily dose of 1 g in children and 2 g in adults for 5 days) if they are older than 8 years of age or with streptomycin (20 mg/kg/day in two divided doses) if they are younger than 8 years of age. Trimethoprim-sulfamethoxazole, at 40 mg/kg/day in two divided doses, also has been used. Duration of treatment is 7 days. A 6-day quarantine period is observed for contacts of patients with regard to international travel.

No plague vaccine currently is available commercially in the United States. A formaldahyde inactivated whole-cell vaccine was developed and is partially efficacious against bubonic plague. An effective vaccine against pneumonic plague has yet to be developed.

TABLE 169.1

RECOMMENDED THERAPY

Contained Casualty Setting
Children[||]
Preferred choices:
Streptomycin, 15 mg/kg IM twice daily (maximum daily dose 2 g)
Gentamicin, 2.5 mg/kg IM or IV three times daily[†]
Alternative choices:
Doxycycline,
If ≥45 kg, give 100 mg IV twice daily or 200 mg IV once daily
If <45 kg, give 2.2 mg/kg IV twice daily (maximum 200 mg/day)
Ciprofloxacin, 15 mg/kg IV twice daily (maximum 800 mg/day)[‡]
Chloramphenicol, 25 mg/kg IV four times daily (maximum 4g/day)[§]

Pregnant Women[¶]
Preferred choice:
Gentamicin, 5 mg/kg IM or IV once daily or 2 mg/kg loading dose followed by 1.7 mg/kg IM or IV three times daily[†]
Alternative choices:
Doxycycline, 100 mg IV twice daily or 200 mg IV once daily
Ciprofloxacin, 400 mg IV twice daily[‡]

Mass Casualty Setting and Postexposure Prophylaxis[#]
Children[||]
Preferred choices:
Doxycycline,[**]
   If ≥45 kg give 100 mg orally twice daily
   If <45 kg then give 2.2 mg/kg orally twice daily
Ciprofloxacin, 20 mg/kg orally twice daily (maximum 1 g per day)
Alternative choice:
Chloramphenicol, 25 mg/kg orally four times daily[§,††]

Pregnant Women[¶]
Preferred choices:
Doxycycline, 100 mg orally twice daily and
Ciprofloxacin, 500 mg orally twice daily
Alternative choice:
Chloramphenicol, 25 mg/kg orally four times daily[§,††]

IM, intramuscular; IV, intravenous.

*These are consensus recommendations of the Working Group on Civilian Biodefense and are not necessarily approved by the U.S. Food and Drug Administration. See "Therapy" section for explanations. One antimicrobial agent should be selected. Therapy should continue for 10 days. Oral therapy should be substituted when the patient's condition improves.
[†]Aminoglycosides must be adjusted according to renal function. Evidence suggests that gentamicin, 5 mg/kg IM or IV once daily, would be efficacious in children, although this is not yet widely accepted clinical practice. Neonates up to 1 week of age and premature infants should receive gentamicin, 2.5 mg/kg IV twice a day.
[‡]Other fluoroquinolones can be substituted at doses appropriate for age. Ciprofloxacin dosage should not exceed 1 g/day in children.
[§]Concentration should be maintained between 5 and 20 μg/mL. Concentrations greater than 25 μl/mL can cause reversible bone marrow suppression.
[||]Refer to "Management of Special Groups" for details and discussion of breast-feeding women; in neonates, a gentamicin loading dose of 4 mg/kg should be given initially.
[¶]Refer to "Management of Special Groups" for details. In children, ciprofloxacin dose should not exceed 1g/d, and chloramphenicol should not exceed 4 g/d. Children younger then 2 years should not receive chloramphenicol.
[#]Duration of treatment of plague in the mass casualty setting is 10 days. Duration of postexposure prophylaxis to prevent plague infection is 7 days.
[**]Tetracycline could be substituted for doxycycline.
[††]Children younger than 2 years should not receive chloramphenicol. Oral formulation is available only outside the United States.
Adapted from Inglesby TV, Dennis DT, Henderson DA, et al. *JAMA* 2000;283:2281.

Suggested Readings

Cantey JR. Plague in Vietnam. *Arch Intern Med* 1974;133:280.
Centers for Disease Control and Prevention. Plague vaccine. *MMWR Morb Mortal Wkly Rep* 1982;31:301.
Centers for Disease Control and Prevention. Plague in the United States, 1982. *MMWR Morb Mortal Wkly Rep* 1983;32:SS19.
Finegold MJ. Pathogenesis of plague. *Am J Med* 1968;45:549.
Guiyoule A, Gerbaud G, Buchrieser C, et al. Transferable plasmid-mediated resistance to streptomycin in a clinical isolate of *Yersinia pestis*. *Emerg Infect Dis* 2001;7:43.
Goldstein MD. Plague. In: Feigin RD, Cherry JD, Kaplan S, Demmler, eds. *Textbook of pediatric infectious diseases*, 5th ed. Philadelphia: WB Saunders, 2003:1487.
Inglesby TV, Dennis DT, Henderson DA, et al. Plague as a biological weapon: medical and public health management. Working Group on Civilian Biodefense. *JAMA* 2000;283:2281.
Kant S, Nath LM. Control and prevention of human plague. *Indian J Pediatr* 1994;61:629.
Kaufmann AF, Boyce JM, Martone WJ. Trends in human plague in the United States. *J Infect Dis* 1980;141:522.
Loiez C, Herwegh S, Wallet F, et al. Detection of *Yersinia pestis* in sputum by real-time PCR. *J Clin Microbiol* 2003;41:4873.
Mann JM, Schaudler L, Cushing A. Pediatric plague. *Pediatrics* 1982;69:762.
Rattan A, Kumar R. Laboratory diagnosis of plague. *Indian J Pediatr* 1994;61:625.

CHAPTER 170 ■ PNEUMOCOCCAL INFECTIONS

RALPH D. FEIGIN AND SHELDON L. KAPLAN

Disease caused by *Streptococcus pneumoniae* remains one of the leading causes of morbidity and mortality in children. Almost all children experience some manifestations of pneumococcal infection. *S. pneumoniae* is the leading cause of acute otitis media and acute sinusitis and a frequent cause of pneumonia, bacteremia, and meningitis in children. The emergence of pneumococcal strains resistant to multiple antibiotics has complicated the therapy of suspected and proved *S. pneumoniae* infections.

MICROBIOLOGY

S. pneumoniae is a gram-positive, lancet-shaped diplococcus that usually occurs in pairs. Under certain conditions, pneumococci may form chains, the length of which depends on the type of media in which the organism has been grown. *S. pneumoniae* is encapsulated, and capsular size varies considerably. With Gram stain, pneumococci may resemble other organisms, particularly alpha-hemolytic streptococci.

On solid media, encapsulated pneumococci produce shiny, round colonies approximately 1 mm in diameter. Serotypes 3, 8, and 37 form larger, mucoid colonies. As the cultures age, the center of the colony regresses, creating a central dimple. When grown on media containing blood, all pneumococci cause alpha-hemolysis of the surrounding erythrocytes. Pneumococci are facultative anaerobes and may be grown aerobically or anaerobically. Rarely, strains of *S. pneumoniae* are obligate anaerobes.

Optochin is helpful in identifying pneumococci because usually these organisms are sensitive to this agent and beta-hemolytic streptococci are resistant. Discs impregnated with Optochin are laid on pneumococcal cultures, and the plate is incubated overnight. Sensitivity is manifested by a zone of inhibition around the disc.

Pneumococci also may be identified by a bile solubility assay. When bile is added to a culture of pneumococci, prompt dissolution of the cocci occurs. The Quellung reaction permits rapid identification of pneumococci. This reaction is carried out by mixing equal volumes of the suspension of bacteria, antiserum, and methylene blue on a slide and examining the bacteria by light microscopy. Capsular swelling identifies genus, species, and serotype. The use of the Quellung reaction permits immediate identification of pneumococci from cultures or body fluids.

A rapid test to identify pneumococci growing in liquid culture uses latex particles coated with antibodies to all currently identified serotypes. This test is extremely useful, although selected strains of alpha-streptococci may cross-react with pneumococci.

EPIDEMIOLOGY

Pneumococci typically are found in the pharynx of healthy people. *S. pneumoniae* organisms are spread from person to person in droplets from respiratory secretions. Infection of the upper respiratory tract aids the spread. In temperate climates, colonization and disease caused by pneumococci are seen more commonly in the winter and spring. Outbreaks of pneumococcal infection can occur in physically crowded settings, such as military barracks, prisons, and day-care centers.

Rates of colonization vary widely and depend on numerous variables, including age, race, population studied, and degree of exposure to children. The prevalence of colonization typically has been found to be between 25% and 50%, with some studies finding rates as high as 97%. Most children develop colonization at some point during their first few years of life. Rates of colonization gradually increase with age over the first 1 or 2 years of life, and the highest rates are associated with children receiving institutional care.

With the increase throughout the world in the prevalence of penicillin- and multiantibiotic-resistant pneumococci, numerous studies have attempted to define risk factors for colonization with resistant organisms. Factors that have been implicated include recent therapy with antimicrobial agents, age younger than 2 years, attendance in a child-care facility, residence in a chronic care facility, and recent hospitalization.

Ninety serotypes of *S. pneumoniae* have been identified worldwide, with the distribution of serotypes that account for infections varying according to region. A difference also has been noted between serotypes causing infections in adults and those infecting children. In North America, serotypes 4, 6B, 9V, 14, 18C, 19F, and 23F are associated most commonly with infections in the pediatric age group. These same serotypes also have been found to account for most organisms with antibiotic resistance. Serotypes 1, 3 and 5 are found more commonly in older children and adults.

Immunity to *S. pneumoniae* depends on the presence of type-specific antibody to the capsular antigen of the organism. Immunity during the first few months of life apparently is derived from maternal antibody transferred passively to the fetus. Children younger than 2 years old respond poorly to the capsular polysaccharide antigen. This finding may explain the frequency of pneumococcal bacteremia in children between the ages of 3 months and 2 years.

Pneumococcal infection occurs more frequently in blacks than in whites, a finding that is not explained fully by the frequency of sickle cell disease in the black population, as well as in some Native American populations.

PATHOGENESIS

Pneumococci may invade from a site of colonization by hematogenous spread or by direct extension. Pneumococcal meningitis usually occurs after pneumococcal bacteremia, but it can also result from direct spread to the meninges as a sequela of a cerebrospinal fluid (CSF) leak that occurs after a temporal or basilar skull fracture. Pneumococcal otitis media usually results from the spread of pneumococci colonizing the nasopharynx via the eustachian tube into the middle ear.

Pneumococcal pneumonia is caused by aspiration of pneumococci that reside in the pharynx. Several studies document that a viral infection, including influenza, may compromise pulmonary defense mechanisms and predispose the individual to invasion by pneumococci. Although pneumococci most commonly produce otitis media, sinusitis, pneumonia, bacteremia, and meningitis, any organ system can be affected.

Identification of the specific factors responsible for pneumococcal infection and subsequent injury to the host continues to be an area of active research. The capsule of *S. pneumoniae* is known to aid the pneumococci by resisting phagocytosis, but the capsule itself is nontoxic. Specific serotypes associated with large capsules appear to be more virulent and to cause greater morbidity and mortality than do serotypes characterized by smaller capsules. Rough strains of pneumococci lacking a capsule are avirulent. Serotypes 1 and 3 more commonly cause pneumonia complicated by empyema than do other serotypes.

Some serotypes are associated more commonly with specific sites of infections than are others. For example, serotype 1 is found primarily in children with pneumonia, serogroup 19 with mastoiditis, and serotype 14 with pneumonia and cellulitis. Most researchers concur that elements of the cell wall are responsible for the initiation of the inflammatory response seen in pneumococcal infection. Specifically, peptidoglycan and teichoic acid have been found to be the two most potent inflammatory components of the cell wall and appear to initiate an inflammatory response by activating complement factor C3 via the alternative pathway.

Numerous pneumococcal proteins that may serve as virulence factors have been identified. Pneumolysin, an intracellular protein, is the best characterized of these proteins. Although it is not secreted by pneumococci, it is released on cell lysis as the infection progresses or on initiation of antimicrobial therapy. Pneumolysin has been shown to have numerous effects *in vitro*. At high concentrations, it forms transmembrane pores and results in lysis of most of the cell types found in the lung. It also has been shown to inhibit ciliary motion, to disrupt epithelial membranes, to interfere with neutrophil and lymphocyte function, and to stimulate the production of inflammatory cytokines. Other possible virulence factors include an immunoglobulin A protease, a neuraminidase, and an autolysin enzyme.

Deficiency of the terminal components of complement has been associated with recurrent pyogenic infection, including that caused by *S. pneumoniae*. Deficiency of complement factor C2 also appears to be associated with *S. pneumoniae* infection. Invasive pneumococcal disease is much more prevalent among persons with anatomic or functional asplenia and is particularly prevalent in patients with sickle cell disease and other hemoglobinopathies. These patients appear to be unable to activate C3 by the alternative pathway or to fix opsonin to the pneumococcal cell wall. Ineffective clearance of bloodborne bacteria in the absence of type-specific antibodies and abnormal activation of the alternate pathway for complement metabolism place the asplenic patient at risk for development of overwhelming infection. The efficacy of phagocytosis for *S. pneumoniae* is diminished in patients with B-cell and T-cell deficiency syndromes that lack opsonic anticapsular antibody and fail to produce agglutination and lysis of bacteria. These observations suggest that opsonization of the pneumococcus depends on the classic and alternate complement pathways and that recovery from pneumococcal disease depends on the development of anticapsular antibodies that act as opsonins and enhance phagocytosis and intracellular killing of pneumococcus.

Low levels of factor B or impairment of the properdin pathway and defective opsonization occur in physiologically normal persons during acute pneumococcal disease, findings suggesting that pneumococcal infection may develop in some people because of a transient preexisting depression of factor B or that acute pneumococcal infection may be accompanied by consumption of this component of the complement system. Complement factors C3 through C9 produce chemotactic and opsonic properties in serum, and each plays an important role in protection against pneumococcal infection.

Within body tissues, particularly the lung, the spread of infection is enhanced by the antiphagocytic properties of the capsular-specific soluble substance. Edema-promoting factors also play important roles in the pathogenesis of infection within the lung. After infection is established, the alveoli fill with serous fluid. Subsequently, polymorphonuclear leukocytes accumulate in the infected alveoli, causing consolidation. Ultimately, macrophages replace the leukocytes, and the exudate resolves. This sequence of events evolves over the course of 7 to 10 days, but it can be modified by the use of appropriate antimicrobial therapy.

CLINICAL MANIFESTATIONS

The clinical manifestations are related to the site of infection. *S. pneumoniae* can cause otitis media, mastoiditis, sinusitis, bacteremia including purpura fulminans, meningitis, pneumonia with or without empyema, cellulitis, abscesses, pericarditis, peritonitis, septic arthritis, osteomyelitis, endocarditis, and epidural or brain abscess. Bacteremia may be followed by an infection at virtually any site. Lobar consolidation on chest radiograph, along with a white blood count exceeding 15,000/mm^3, is suggestive of pneumococcal pneumonia. Epiglottitis caused by *S. pneumoniae* has been observed in immunocompromised children.

Pneumococcal bacteremia without a focus may occur in children, who are most commonly between ages 3 months and 3 years and have unexplained fever and no localizing signs or symptoms. Subcutaneous abscesses have been reported after occult pneumococcal bacteremia, and endocarditis has been documented. Renal glomerular and cortical arterial thromboses have been associated with pneumococcal bacteremia. Gangrenous lesions of the skin on the face or extremities, localized gingival lesions, and disseminated intravascular coagulation also are reported manifestations of pneumococcal disease. Pneumococcal infection is an uncommon but well-described etiologic agent in hemolytic uremic syndrome.

DIAGNOSIS

The isolation of pneumococci from the nasopharynx does not permit establishing a diagnosis of pneumococcal disease because pneumococcal carriage is so prevalent. Blood cultures should be obtained from all children with meningitis, pneumonia requiring hospitalization, septic arthritis, or other serious infections. Blood cultures may be positive in in children ages 3 to 36 months who have unexplained fever and leukocytosis without localized signs of infection. Urinary excretion of *S. pneumoniae* presumably represents seeding of the urine from a remote site of pneumococcal infection. Pneumococci should be sought in CSF, pleural fluid, joint fluid, or other appropriate sites.

Pneumococci can be identified in selected body fluids such as CSF or joint fluid by Gram stain as gram-positive, lancet-shaped diplococci. Latex particle agglutination test can establish a diagnosis rapidly and is useful mainly in detecting polysaccharide capsular antigen in CSF. Early in the course of pneumococcal meningitis, numerous *S. pneumoniae* organisms may be revealed by Gram stain in relatively acellular CSF. New diagnostic tests are being developed using polymerase chain reaction technology. A commercial urinary antigen test (Binax

NOW) to detect urinary pneumococcal is not useful for distinguishing pneumococcal from other forms of pneumonia because nasopharyngeal colonization alone may lead to a postive result.

TREATMENT AND PROGNOSIS

Penicillin remains the drug of choice for patients with pneumococcal disease caused by penicillin-susceptible isolates. Since the early 1990s, a rapid increase in the prevalence of both penicillin-nonsusceptible [minimal inhibitory concentration (MIC), 0.1 to 1.0 μg/mL] and penicillin-resistant (MIC, 2 μg/mL or greater) strains has occurred throughout the world. Decreased susceptibility to beta-lactam antibiotics for pneumococci is based on alteration in penicillin-binding proteins and not the production of beta-lactamase enzymes. In addition, many of these isolates also have displayed resistance to other classes of antibiotics such as macrolides (erythromycin), trimethoprim-sulfamethoxazole, tetracycline, chloramphenicol, and rifampin. The prevalence of antibiotic-resistant strains continues to increase, with more than 50% of isolates found to be either nonsusceptible or resistant to penicillin in some countries. Some of the highest rates of resistance have been reported in Korea, Spain, and Hungary. In the United States, the prevalence of penicillin-resistant pneumococci varies widely, with approximately 40% to 50% of all isolates being nonsusceptible to penicillin. Isolates recovered from children younger than 2 years old and from upper respiratory sites (middle ear fluid) tend to have the highest rates of resistance. In some areas, more than half of the penicillin-resistant isolates are resistant to one or more other classes of antibiotics. However, the rates of resistance appear to be declining in the United States following the widespread use of the 7-valent pneumococcal conjugate vaccine (PCV7).

All pneumococci isolated from normally sterile body fluids should have antibiotic susceptibility patterns evaluated to help determine the most appropriate therapy. *S. pneumoniae* is the only organism and the extended-spectrum cephalosporins, cefotaxime or ceftriaxone, are the only antibiotics for which the National Committee for Clinical Laboratory Standards has established different interpretive breakpoints depending on the site of infection. For pneumococcal isolates recovered from patients with bacterial meningitis, the interpretive breakpoints for cefotaxime/ceftriaxone are as follows: susceptible, 0.5 μg/mL or less; intermediate, 1.0 μg/mL; resistant,

2.0 μg/mL or greater. For isolates associated with noncentral nervous system (CNS) infections, the breakpoints are as follows: susceptible, 1.0 μg/mL or less; intermediate, 2.0 μg/mL; resistant, 4.0 μg/mL or greater. These different breakpoint interpretations have major implications with respect to using cefotaxime or ceftriaxone in the treatment of invasive pneumococcal infections.

In a normal host, pneumococcal infection, other than that of CNS, caused by either penicillin-susceptible or penicillin-nonsusceptible isolates with MICs for penicillin up to 2 μg/mL generally can be treated successfully with penicillin. For more serious infections other than meningitis, the recommended dosages of penicillin G for pneumococcal infections in childhood (e.g., septicemia) in children are 200,000 to 300,000 U/kg/day; for meningitis dosage see Table 170.1. For invasive non-CNS pneumococcal infections caused by isolates having penicillin MICs greater than 2 μg/mL, cefotaxime, ceftriaxone, or cefuroxime is the preferred agent when the organism is susceptible or intermediate for these agents. Clindamycin is an important option for treatment of non-CNS invasive pneumococcal infections caused by clindamycin-susceptible isolates that are resistant to beta-lactam antibiotics or for patients allergic to beta-lactam antibiotics.

Penicillin V is available for oral use only and should be used for only such infections as pneumonia caused by penicillin-susceptible isolates. The recommended dosage of penicillin V is 25 to 50 mg/kg/day. Other penicillins, such as ampicillin and other related compounds, show excellent activity against penicillin-susceptible pneumococci. Amoxicillin is the oral penicillin most often administered because of its preferred taste. Amoxicillin or amoxicillin-clavulanate is the agent of first choice for the treatment of acute otitis media. The dose of amoxicillin for treatment of pneumococcal infections is 90 mg/kg/day. Oral cephalosporins such as cefuroxime axetil, cefdinir, or cefpodoxime also are important options for completing treatment of local upper respiratory or invasive pneumococcal infections. Macrolide antibiotics may be used for mild pneumococcal disease in children who are allergic to penicillin, although few data are available documenting the efficacy of macrolides in the treatment of pneumococcal pneumonia specifically in children as opposed to community-acquired pneumonia in general.

For children with presumed bacterial meningitis or with positive CSF Gram stains for gram-positive cocci, empiric antibiotic coverage should be directed at the treatment of a possible penicillin- or cephalosporin-resistant organism. Initial

TABLE 170.1

TREATMENT OF PNEUMOCOCCAL MENINGITIS IN CHILDREN: MODIFICATIONS BASED ON ANTIBIOTIC SUSCEPTIBILITIES OF THE *STREPTOCOCCUS PNEUMONIAE* ISOLATE

Penicillin MIC (μg/mL)	Cefotaxime/Ceftriaxone MIC (μg/mL)	Therapy	Dosage*	Maximum Dose
<0.1	≤0.5	Penicillin	300,000–400,000 units in three to four doses	24×10^6 units/day
≥0.1	≤0.5	Cefotaxime or	200–225 mg in three or four doses	4 g q8h or 3 g q6h
		Ceftriaxone	100 mg in one or two doses	2 g q12h or 4 g q24h
	1.0–2.0	Cefotaxime or	300 mg in three or four doses	4 g q8h or 3 g q6h
		Ceftriaxone plus	100 mg in one or two doses	2 g q12h or 4 g q24h
		Vancomycin	60 mg in four doses	0.5 g q6h
	>2.0	Same as for 2.0 μg/mL plus rifampin	20 mg in two doses	300 mg q12h

MIC, minimum inhibitory concentration; qxh, every x hours.
*Doses are given as amounts per kilogram per day.
Reprinted from Kaplan SL. Management of pneumococcal meningitis. *Pediatr Infect Dis J* 2002;21:589.

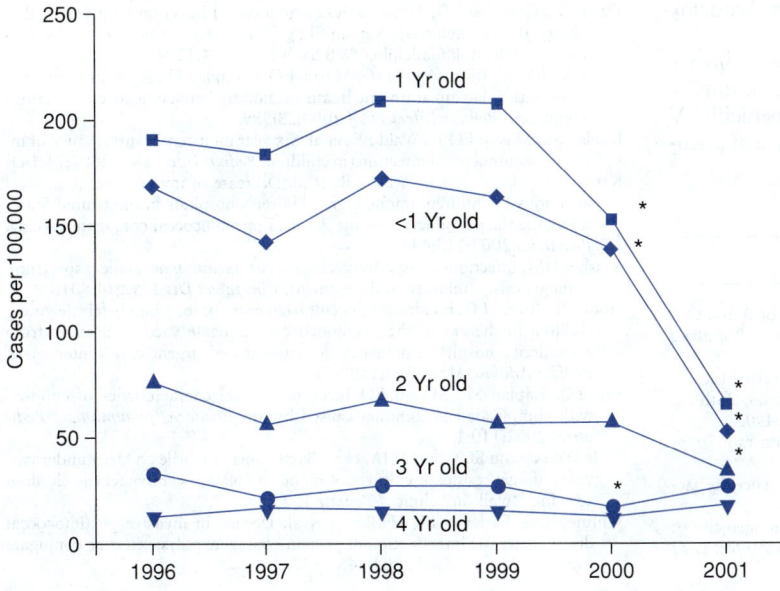

FIGURE 170.1. Rates of invasive pneumococcal disease among children younger than 5 years old, according to age and year. Data are from the Active Bacterial Core Surveillance from 1996 through 2001. The 1996 and 1997 rates do not include data from New York State. Asterisks indicate $P <.05$ for comparisons of the rate in 2000 or 2001 with combined rate for 1998 and 1999.

antibiotics should include a third-generation cephalosporin (e.g., cefotaxime or ceftriaxone) and vancomycin. Administration of this combination can be continued until antibiotic susceptibilities are available. Recommended dosages for intravenous administration may be found in Table 170.1. Treatment is modified once antibiotic susceptibilities are available. Penicillin-susceptible organisms can be treated with penicillin alone. Penicillin-nonsusceptible (MIC, 0.1 μg/mL or greater) organisms fully susceptible to cefotaxime/ceftriaxone (MIC, up to 0.5 μg/mL) should be treated with cefotaxime or ceftriaxone alone. Vancomycin should be discontinued when susceptibility to extended-spectrum cephalosporins is established. Meningitis caused by *S. pneumoniae* isolates resistant to extended-spectrum cephalosporins (MIC, 1.0 μg/mL or greater) should be treated with the combination of vancomycin and cefotaxime or ceftriaxone. Vancomycin should not be used alone for therapy of meningitis. Addition of rifampin (20 mg/kg/day in two divided doses) to this combination may be beneficial in patients with isolates that have cefotaxime/ceftriaxone MICs greater than 2.0 μg/mL.

Repeat lumbar puncture to document sterility of the CSF after 36 to 48 hours of therapy is recommended for any patient who is not improving as expected or who has a pneumococcal isolate for which the cefotaxime/ceftriaxone MIC is 2.0 μg/mL or greater. Dexamethasone remains controversial for pneumococcal meningitis, and each physician must weigh the potential risks and benefits of this adjunctive therapy.

The prognosis of pneumococcal disease depends on the age of the host, integrity of the immune system, virulence of the infecting organism, site of infection, and adequacy of therapy.

PREVENTION

A pneumococcal conjugate vaccine (PCV7) composed of the polysaccharides of the seven most common serotypes (4, 6B, 9V, 14, 18C, 19F, and 23F) causing invasive pneumococcal infections in children conjugated to a mutant of diphtheria toxin (CRM$_{197}$) is available. The conjugate vaccine leads to development of protective antibody concentrations in young children after at least three doses. In addition, the PCV7 is associated with a reduction in nasopharyngeal colonization by pneumococcal isolates of the serotypes contained in the vaccine. The PCV7 was shown to be approximately 90% efficacious in pre-

venting invasive pneumococcal disease in a large randomized controlled trial. The PCV7 is recommended for routine administration to infants at 2, 4, 6, and 12 to 15 months of age. The schedule for infants who did not receive the PCV7 at these ages is outlined in the American Academy of Pediatrics recommendations.

The incidence of invasive pneumococcal infections has declined approximately 70% since the PCV7 was licensed for routine administration in 2000 (Fig. 170.1). If the incidence of pneumococcal bacteremia continues to decline, the approach to the immunized infant and child with high fever without a source will likely require modification; that is, the value of a screening peripheral white blood cell count and/or blood culture will be greatly diminished. In addition, in one study, the proportion of pneumococcal isolates recovered from children with invasive disease that were resistant to penicillin declined significantly 2 years after the introduction of the PCV7. Studies are ongoing to determine whether pneumococcal isolates with serotypes not in the PCV7 will begin to emerge as more common causes of invasive disease, so-called serotype replacement. For otherwise healthy children with invasive pneumococcal infections who have had three or more doses of PCV7 or who have received the age-appropriate number of doses if older than 12 months of age when first immunized, the pneumococcal isolates should be preserved for serotyping, if at all possible. Thus far, most such children have infection caused by nonvaccine serotype isolates. If the isolate has a serotype of the 7-valent vaccine, an immunologic evaluation should be considered.

A 23-valent pneumococcal polysaccharide vaccine is available. Current recommendations are to provide pneumococcal vaccine to children age 2 years and older with functional or anatomic asplenia, including patients with sickle cell disease and other hemoglobinopathies, and to children with nephrotic syndrome or chronic renal failure, conditions associated with immunosuppression, human immunodeficiency virus infection, CSF leaks, or cochlear implants. Other patients for whom pneumococcal vaccine should be considered are children with chronic cardiovascular, pulmonary, or hepatic disease. The 23-valent pneumococcal vaccine also should be administered to those children considered at high risk for development of invasive pneumococcal infection who already have received the recommended doses of the PCV7. The reader interested in further details of the indications for use of the PCV7 or the 23-valent pneumococcal vaccine is encouraged to review the recommendations established by the American Academy of Pediatrics.

Penicillin or ampicillin should be given to children who are age 5 years or younger and are anatomically or functionally asplenic. Controlled studies suggest that the use of penicillin V administered on a daily basis may reduce the incidence of pneumococcal bacteremia in these patients.

Suggested Readings

American Academy of Pediatrics Subcommittee on Management of Acute Otitis Media. Diagnosis and management of acute otitis media. *Pediatrics* 2004;113:1451.

American Academy of Pediatrics. Pneumococcal infections. In: Pickering LK, ed. *Red book: 2003 report of the Committee on Infectious Diseases,* 26th ed. Elk Grove Village, IL: American Academy of Pediatrics, 2003:490.

Appelbaum PC. Epidemiology and *in vitro* susceptibility of drug-resistant *Streptococcus pneumoniae. Pediatr Infect Dis J* 1996;15:932.

Austrian R, Gold J. Pneumococcal bacteremia with especial reference to bacteremic pneumococcal pneumonia. *Ann Intern Med* 1964;60:759.

Black S, Shinefield H, Fireman B, et al. Efficacy, safety and immunogenicity of heptavalent pneumococcal conjugate vaccine in children. *Pediatr Infect Dis J* 2000;19:187.

Dagan R, Greenberg D, Jacobs MR. Pneumococcal infections. In: Feigin RD, Cherry JD, Demmler GJ, Kaplan SL, eds. *Textbook of pediatric infectious diseases,* 5th ed. Philadelphia: WB Saunders, 2004:1204.

Gonzalez BE, Martinez-Aguilar G, Mason EO Jr, Kaplan SL. Azithromycin compared with β-lactam antibiotic treatment failures in pneumococcal infections in children. *Pediatr Infect Dis J* 2004;23:399.

Kaplan SL, Mason EO Jr, Wald ER, et al. Six year multicenter surveillance of invasive pneumococcal infections in children. *Pediatr Infect Dis J* 2002;21:141.

Kaplan SL, Mason EO Jr, Wald ER, et al. Decrease of invasive pneumococcal infections in children among eight children's hospitals in the United States following the introduction of the 7-valent pneumococcal conjugate vaccine. *Pediatrics* 2004;113:443.

Musher DM. Infections caused by *Streptococcus pneumoniae*: clinical spectrum, pathogenesis, immunity, and treatment. *Clin Infect Dis* 1992;14:801.

Stool ML, Rubin LG. Incidence of occult bacteremia among highly febrile young children in the era of the pneumococcal conjugate vaccine: a study from a children's hospital emergency department and urgent care center. *Arch Pediatr Adolesc Med* 2004;158:671.

Tan TQ, Kaplan SL, Mason EO Jr, et al. Clinical characteristics of children with complicated pneumonia caused by *Streptococcus pneumoniae. Pediatrics* 2002;110:1.

Teele DW, Pelton SI, Grant MJA, et al. Bacteremia in febrile children under two years of age: results of cultures of blood in 600 consecutive febrile children seen in a "walk-in" clinic. *J Pediatr* 1975;87:227.

Whitney CG, Farley MM, Hadler J, et al. Decline in invasive pneumococcal disease after the introduction of protein-conjugate polysaccharide conjugate vaccine. *N Engl J Med* 2003;348:1737.

CHAPTER 171 ■ *PSEUDOMONAS* AND RELATED GENERA

RALPH D. FEIGIN

Pseudomonas species usually are strict aerobes; however, they can grow anaerobically in the presence of nitrates. Aerobic pseudomonads can use any carbon source, and they multiply readily in almost any moist environment containing minimal concentrations of organic compounds. Most *P. aeruginosa* strains are motile by a single, polar flagellum and possess fine projections called *pili*. These organisms grow readily on standard laboratory media. When strains are obtained from a clinical specimen, beta-hemolysis may be observed on blood agar. A blue-green phenazine pigment and fluorescein are produced by more than 90% of *P. aeruginosa* organisms. *Pseudomonas* strains can be differentiated from one another by phage typing, serologic typing, ribotyping, and pyocin typing.

The genus *Pseudomonas* has undergone reclassification, and four of the five homology groups I to V have been reclassified into separate genera: *Burkholderia cepacia* (formerly *P. cepacia*), *Stenotrophomonas maltophilia* (previously *Xanthomonas maltophilia*), *Burkholderia pseudomallei* (previously *P. pseudomallei*), and *Burkholderia mallei* (formerly *P. mallei*).

EPIDEMIOLOGY

Pseudomonas organisms are ubiquitous and may be found in water, in soil, and on vegetation. Between 5% and 30% of physiologically normal persons carry *Pseudomonas* in their gastrointestinal tracts. These organisms frequently are found in hospitals, and the dissemination of these organisms may occur by aerosol, as well as by direct physical contact with patients or contaminated environmental sites. Potential environmental sites in which these organisms can be found growing include distilled water, antiseptic solutions, whirlpools, eyedrops, irrigation fluids, dialysis fluids, and, often, equipment used for inhalation therapy or respiratory care. *Pseudomonas* also can be found growing in swimming pools, hot tubs, water parks, cosmetics, illicit injectable drugs, and the inner soles of sneakers.

B. cepacia has been recognized increasingly as a cause of sporadic nosocomial outbreaks of infection in intensive care units. Those outbreaks have been traced to contaminated automated peritoneal dialysis machines, blood gas analyzers, povidone-iodine solution, and chlorhexidine. It also is a common cause of colonization and endobronchial infection in patients with cystic fibrosis.

S. maltophilia has caused pneumonia, urinary tract infections, endocarditis, meningitis, and peritonitis in hospitalized patients and in patients with cystic fibrosis. *B. pseudomallei* is the cause of melioidosis, a disease described in Box 171.1. *B. mallei* is the cause of glanders, a disease described in Box 171.2.

PATHOGENESIS

Pseudomonas organisms usually are noninvasive, even after colonization and infection of the skin. Pseudomonads produce a variety of virulence factors, including an endotoxin,

---

BOX 171.1   Melioidosis

Melioidosis is a rare disease that is most prevalent in Southeast Asia and northern Australia. It increased in frequency in the United States with the return of U.S. residents from Vietnam and is seen rarely in immigrants from Southeast Asia. The causative agent is *Burkholderia pseudomallei*. Infection with this organism develops after direct contamination of abrasions or wounds with contaminated soil or water or inhalation of contaminated dust. Transmission from animals to humans has not been reported.

Melioidosis may remain latent for months or years before the clinical manifestations appear. The disease may present as a single primary skin lesion (e.g., vesicle, bulla, pustule, urticaria) in a patient who has no other underlying disease. Occasionally, septicemia occurs, and multiple abscesses develop in every organ of the body. Meningitis, encephalitis, and endophthalmitis have been observed in normal and immunocompromised hosts during or after an episode of septicemia. Myocarditis, endocarditis, pericarditis, intestinal abscesses, acute gastroenteritis, cholecystitis, septic arthritis, osteomyelitis, paraspinal abscess, urinary tract infections, and generalized lymphadenopathy may be caused by *B. pseudomallei*.

Chronic melioidosis occurs more commonly in white than in Asian individuals. Chronic melioidosis may involve every organ in the body except the brain. Melioidosis may remain dormant, with exacerbations occurring years after primary infection when host defenses are impaired as a result of burns, corticosteroid use, or other processes. Diagnosis is established by culture of blood, skin lesions, or other purulent material. The organism grows in media commonly used for isolation of gram-negative bacteria.

Serologic tests are more useful in establishing the diagnosis of melioidosis in latent or asymptomatic forms of the disease. Hemagglutination, indirect hemagglutination, complement fixation tests, and an enzyme-linked immunosorbent assay (ELISA) are available. Diagnostic titers are 1:40 or greater for the hemagglutination test and 1:10 or greater for the complement fixation test. Both tests should be performed because the sensitivity of serologic tests varies. Hemagglutination antibodies usually are evident within 7 to 14 days after the onset of illness, but the complement fixation test does not become positive until 4 to 6 weeks into the disease process. Peak titers for both tests are observed at 4 to 6 months. An ELISA that detects specific immunoglobulin G (IgG) and IgM antibody to *B. pseudomallei* is available as a screening test for melioidosis; it is more sensitive than are the IgG indirect fluorescent antibody and the indirect hemagglutination tests for melioidosis.

BOX 171.2   Glanders

Glanders, a zoonotic disease that infects primarily horses and other equine animals, is caused by *Burkholderia mallei*. Glanders is spread from diseased to healthy animals directly or indirectly. Human infection is seen primarily in persons with direct or indirect contact with diseased animals or their tissues. Infection is particularly prevalent among veterinarians or laboratory workers. Infection in children is unusual but has been reported.

The incubation period usually is 1 to 14 days, but extended incubation periods have been described. The prodrome may consist of fever, anorexia, nausea, vomiting, myalgia, and icterus. An erysipelas-like swelling of the face or limbs and painful nodules may be observed. The nodular eruption spreads rapidly and is followed by a generalized pustular skin eruption. Nasal involvement may include a thick, purulent discharge and erosion of the nasal structures. Lymphadenopathy and pneumonia are common findings. Severe septicemia with metastatic abscesses, pneumonitis, and death in 2 to 4 weeks may occur with the acute forms of glanders. A chronic form of this disorder with acute exacerbations also has been described.

The most important feature in the history is animal contact. The clinical manifestations are not specific and may resemble typhoid fever, melioidosis, erysipelas, tuberculosis, or syphilis.

Diagnosis is made by direct smear of discharges and exudates and identification by staining or use of fluorescent antibody techniques, bacteriologic isolation from purulent material or biopsy, intraperitoneal inoculation of guinea pigs or hamsters with exudates, or skin testing. Agglutination and complement fixation tests are available. The agglutination test is more sensitive, but complement fixation is more specific.

Before the antibiotic era, human glanders was fatal. Most strains of *B. mallei* are sensitive to sulfonamides and tetracyclines. The efficacy of these agents in children with glanders is difficult to establish because of the paucity of cases.

---

an enterotoxin, and multiple extracellular enzymes. The *Pseudomonas* endotoxin is weak compared with the endotoxins produced by other gram-negative organisms, and it may produce a diarrheal syndrome. The *Pseudomonas* enterotoxin has an unclear role in causing diarrhea in humans.

Pseudomonas produces many extracellular products, including caseinase, collagenase, elastase, exotoxin A, fibrinolysin, gelatinase, hemolysin, lecithinase, lipase, and phospholipase C.

The elaboration of these proteolytic enzymes may result in localized necrosis of skin or lung and corneal ulceration. These proteases can degrade numerous plasma proteins, including complement and coagulation factors. Destruction of lecithin and solubilization of this material (i.e., surfactant) may play an important role in the atelectasis seen in pulmonary infections caused by *Pseudomonas*. A leukocidin that in part may be capsular material has been described, and exotoxin S has been identified as still another virulence factor.

Attachment of *Pseudomonas* to mucosal surfaces is mediated by a battery of adhesins, which are produced in large quantities in these organisms. *P. aeruginosa* binds preferentially to normal respiratory mucin, in contrast to other Enterobacteriaceae. Competitive binding inhibition assays suggest that asialo GM_1, an apical membrane receptor expressed by regenerating respiratory epithelial cells, is a receptor for *P. aeruginosa* and that epithelial repair represents a major event for *P. aeruginosa* adherence. The glycocalyx (extracellular slime layer) is important in allowing *P. aeruginosa* organisms to adhere to each other and to form microcolonies that impair phagocytosis and antibiotic activity. Elevated serum concentrations of immunoglobulin

G4 (IgG4) antibodies to opsonic determinants may inhibit normal pulmonary clearance of *P. aeruginosa* by pulmonary macrophages *in vivo*. The pathogenicity of *P. aeruginosa* depends on its ability to resist phagocytosis. The persistence of these organisms in the lungs of patients with cystic fibrosis may be related to factors in the sputum that interfere with the bactericidal activity of fresh, normal serum against this organism.

CLINICAL MANIFESTATIONS

Pseudomonas can produce disease in healthy children after the organism has been introduced into a minor wound and a localized abscess that exudes blue or green pus has developed. The skin lesions, which may be caused by direct inoculation or secondary to septicemia, begin as pink macules, progress to small hemorrhagic nodules, and eventually become necrotic lesions, with associated eschar formation. The central area may be surrounded by an intense red areola (i.e., ecthyma gangrenosum). Rarely, *P. aeruginosa* causes septicemia, meningitis, endocarditis, otitis externa, mastoiditis, pneumonia, peritonitis, corneal infections, or urinary tract infections in normal children. Osteomyelitis caused by *P. aeruginosa* or other *Pseudomonas* strains may develop after puncture wounds of the foot or other bones have occurred.

Outbreaks of urinary tract infections, dermatitis (folliculitis), otitis externa, and mastitis caused by *P. aeruginosa* have been reported in healthy children after the use of community swimming pools, family-owned hot tubs, or other recreational whirlpool baths. Skin lesions may develop several hours to 5 days or longer after contact with these contaminated water sources. The pruritic or painful skin lesions may be macular, pustular, or erythematous, measuring between 5 and 30 mm. In selected cases, nodules develop. Illness may vary from extensive truncal involvement in some patients to only a few scattered lesions in others. Occasionally, malaise, vomiting, sore throat, conjunctivitis, rhinitis, fever, and breast swelling may be associated with the skin lesions. Multiple serotypes of *P. aeruginosa* have been associated with these outbreaks.

Otitis externa caused by *P. aeruginosa* has been reported in healthy persons who frequently swim in pools contaminated with this organism. A malignant form of otitis externa has been associated with *Pseudomonas* infection in which a necrotizing infection of the external ear canal and surrounding soft tissue and bone occurs. This infection may spread to include the mastoid and the petrous parts of the temporal bone, leading to skull base osteomyelitis, as well as paralysis of the facial nerve. Most children with malignant forms of otitis externa have an immunodeficiency secondary to leukopenia, disordered leukocyte function with normal numbers of leukocytes, acquired immunodeficiency syndrome (AIDS), malnutrition, or diabetes mellitus. An increasing number of patients with AIDS and persistent ear pain or otorrhea who do not respond to conventional treatment for external otitis are seen in outpatient clinics.

P. aeruginosa produces infection somewhat more often during the neonatal period than later in life. Septicemia that occurs early, in the first few hours of life, is associated with a high rate of morbidity and mortality, with a clinical course similar to those of other forms of gram-negative septicemia. Late-onset septicemia in the neonate is associated with indwelling foreign bodies (i.e., endotracheal tubes, vascular catheters, and urinary catheters).

Disorders reported with other *Pseudomonas* species in healthy children include pneumonia and abscesses caused by *B. cepacia*, abscesses caused by *P. fluorescens*, otitis media caused by *P. putrefaciens* or *P. stutzeri*, and cellulitis and septicemia caused by *S. maltophilia*. Septicemia and endocarditis associated with *S. maltophilia* primarily have been seen in in-travenous drug abusers. Septicemia and peritonitis caused by *B. cepacia* have been associated with contamination of equipment used for peritoneal dialysis.

Cystic Fibrosis

Death in patients with cystic fibrosis usually results from obstructive, chronic pulmonary disease (see Chapter 236). *P. aeruginosa* can be recovered from cultures of the respiratory tract of most children with cystic fibrosis. Recovery of *P. aeruginosa* from the sputum of these patients does not imply the presence of infection or pneumonitis. Colonization of sputum may reflect the extensive use of mist tents, inhalation therapy, and continuous broad-spectrum antibiotic therapy. However, some observations suggest a more specific correlation between cystic fibrosis and *Pseudomonas*.

P. aeruginosa organisms isolated from patients with cystic fibrosis are almost all mucoid and produce excessive amounts of capsular slime. Eradicating the organism by administering continuous antibiotic therapy is almost impossible. The lung in the patient with cystic fibrosis is thought to trigger a switch to a cluster of genes that encode for the abundant production of the mucoid polysaccharide (alginate), giving rise to the mucoid phenotype. Mucoid *P. aeruginosa* seldom is recovered from patients who do not have cystic fibrosis (0.5% to 1.7%).

Bacterial infection in patients with cystic fibrosis is limited almost entirely to the lung, and septicemia is rare. The pulmonary infection is chronic, and bronchitis, bronchiectasis, and bronchiolitis are common findings. Some patients develop necrotizing pneumonitis.

B. cepacia is an increasingly frequent cause of asymptomatic colonization, pneumonia, and septicemia. The incidence of colonization increases with the severity of the disease and increasing age. The frequent colonization of the respiratory tract with *B. cepacia* in patients with cystic fibrosis has been associated with increased morbidity and mortality rates in some cystic fibrosis centers since the mid-1980s.

Colonization of patients with cystic fibrosis by *S. maltophilia* has been increasing. Prolonged colonization may be associated with progressive deterioration in pulmonary function.

Burns and Wound Infection

The surfaces of burns and wounds often are colonized by *P. aeruginosa*. Colonization does not imply infection, but it is a prerequisite to development of invasive disease. Septicemia caused by this organism is a major problem in burned patients. The administration of antibiotics may diminish the susceptible microbial flora, but it permits selective strains of *Pseudomonas* to grow and become more numerous. In burned patients, abnormalities of neutrophil function precede the onset of septicemia. Thermal injury also is associated with abnormalities in the killing of *Pseudomonas* by neutrophils, delayed rejection of homografts, abnormal responses to antigens, abnormal vascular responses, impaired delayed hypersensitivity responses, diminished uptake of particles by the reticuloendothelial system, and altered antimicrobial pharmacokinetics.

Malignancy and Immunosuppression

Patients with neutropenia, particularly children with leukemia who are receiving immunosuppressive therapy, are susceptible to *Pseudomonas* septicemia and pneumonia. Infection usually is a result of invasion of the bloodstream by *Pseudomonas*, with which the patient already is colonized (e.g., in the gastrointestinal tract). Generalized vasculitis may develop, and hemorrhagic necrotic lesions may be found on the skin as purple nodules or ecchymotic areas that become gangrenous. Gangrenous perirectal cellulitis or abscesses may occur. Anorexia, nausea, vomiting, diarrhea, fever, ileus, and profound hypotension may develop. The single most important factor predisposing children with cancer to the development of infection is granulocytopenia. Mortality rates associated with *P. aeruginosa* bacteremia were higher for patients with solid tumors, an absolute neutrophil count of less than $100/\mu L$, perineal skin lesions, and bacteremia during remission or induction therapy rather than relapse. Heat-stable opsonins specific for *P. aeruginosa* may be depleted in children with acute leukemia who are receiving combination chemotherapy; fatal infections with this organism may be related to deficiencies of a specific opsonin. Infection by *P. aeruginosa*, particularly pneumonia, is an increasing problem for children or adults with advanced human immunodeficiency (HIV) disease. The diagnosis should be considered in patients with advanced HIV disease who present with new respiratory symptoms. The associated immunosuppression, use of systemic *Pneumocystis* prophylaxis or broad-spectrum antibiotics, and sinus disease are important risk factors for patients with advanced HIV disease.

Other Predisposing Conditions

Pseudomonas septicemia occurs with increased frequency in children who have indwelling intravenous or urinary catheters. Pneumonia and septicemia caused by *Pseudomonas* also are increased in frequency in children receiving respiratory support or inhalation therapy. Children with dermoid sinus tracts or dermoids that extend down to or communicate with the meninges or neural tissue are prone to develop abscesses and meningitis caused by *Pseudomonas*. *Pseudomonas* septicemia may occur in children with congenital or acquired neutropenia and in any person with deficient leukocyte function.

Bacteremia with *S. maltophilia* usually results from the presence of an intravascular device or an infection of the respiratory, gastrointestinal, or urinary tract. Other infections of children with *S. maltophilia* occur primarily after these patients experience trauma or undergo instrumentation. Rare disorders caused by *Burkholderia* species include melioidosis (see Box 171.1) and glanders (see Box 171.2).

DIAGNOSIS

The diagnosis of *Pseudomonas* infection depends on recovery of the organism from a localized site of infection or from the blood or cerebrospinal fluid. Recovery of the organism from the surface of the skin, throat, or bronchial secretions may reflect colonization and is not diagnostic of infection. Although the bluish, nodular skin lesions and ulcers with ecchymotic and gangrenous centers (i.e., ecthyma gangrenosum) once were considered pathognomonic of *Pseudomonas* infection, similar lesions have been seen after septicemia caused by Enterobacteriaceae, *Aeromonas*, *Serratia*, and other gram-negative organisms, in addition to *Aspergillus* and *Fusarium* in immunocompromised patients. Immunoglobulin antibodies to *P. aeruginosa* surface antigens in serum have been detected reliably by enzyme-linked immunosorbent assay. Antibody titer increases are associated with active disease caused by *P. aeruginosa* in patients with cystic fibrosis. Antibody titers normalize after *Pseudomonas* infections are brought under control by effective antimicrobial therapy. This assay is helpful in differentiating early infections from colonization. Antibodies to *P. aeruginosa* also may be detected by immunoblotting (e.g., Western blot).

TREATMENT AND PROGNOSIS

Pseudomonas infections should be treated promptly with an antibiotic to which the organism is sensitive *in vitro*. Septicemia should be treated with an aminoglycoside (gentamicin, tobramycin, netilmicin, or amikacin) combined with a beta-lactam antibiotic (antipseudomonal penicillin, third- or fourth-generation cephalosporin, or carbapenem). The combination of an aminoglycoside and a beta-lactam antibiotic may be synergistic against the organism. Rifampin may be added to the combination therapy if the clinical response is not adequate. Use of either the beta-lactam antibiotics or the fluoroquinolones alone for treating *Pseudomonas* septicemia is not advisable because strains of this organism rapidly become resistant to these agents. The dosages of some of the aminoglycosides more commonly used are gentamicin and tobramycin, 3.0 to 7.5 mg/kg/day, or amikacin, 15.0 to 22.5 mg/kg/day, in three divided doses given intramuscularly or intravenously over the course of 1 hour. Ceftazidime has proved useful in selected patients with this disease and can be provided in a dosage of 75 to 200 mg/kg/day in three divided doses. Azlocillin and piperacillin have proved effective against *P. aeruginosa* when combined with an aminoglycoside. These antibiotics can be given intramuscularly in dosages of 200 to 300 mg/kg/day in three divided doses. Abscesses caused by *Pseudomonas* should be incised and drained.

Ciprofloxacin has been evaluated for the treatment of acute and chronic *P. aeruginosa* infection in adolescents and adults with cystic fibrosis. This antibiotic can be given orally or intravenously. Ciprofloxacin should not be used until after the patient has reached puberty because it may bind to cartilage and arrest growth. If it is used, it may be given in a dose of 10 to 15 mg/kg/day in two divided doses administered intravenously. Oral administration may be given in a dose of 20 to 30 mg/kg/day in two divided doses, which should not exceed 1,000 mg/day for patients who weigh less than 40 kg or 1,500 mg/day for patients who weigh more than 40 kg.

Pseudomonas meningitis can be treated with ceftazidime, 200 mg/kg/day in four divided doses, and an aminoglycoside given intravenously. Concomitant intraventricular or intrathecal treatment with gentamicin may be required to sterilize the cerebrospinal fluid. Gentamicin can be placed into the ventricular or lumbar cerebrospinal fluid in a total dosage of 1 or 2 mg once daily. Fluoroquinolones are possible alternatives in the treatment of *P. aeruginosa* infections of the central nervous system if conventional therapy has failed.

Meropenem penetrates cerebrospinal fluid and can be used when *P. aeruginosa* is resistant to ceftazidime. Meropenem is the preferred carbapenem because the high doses of imipenem required to treat central nervous system infections may be associated with toxicity. Ciprofloxacin, pefloxacin, and aztreonam are possible alternatives.

Acute systemic melioidosis is treated with the combination of ceftazidime, 120 mg/kg/day, or chloramphenicol, 50 to 75 mg/kg/day, plus an aminoglycoside (kanamycin, 20 to 30 mg/kg/day, or amikacin, 15 to 20 mg/kg/day) and sulfisoxazole, 120 to 150 mg/kg/day, for 4 weeks. Patients with chronic melioidosis can be treated with chloramphenicol or tetracycline over a period of many months. Trimethoprim-sulfamethoxazole no longer is recommended because most *B. pseudomallei* organisms are resistant.

Recent studies showed that ceftazidime in a dosage of 120 mg/kg/day intravenously in three divided doses was associated with a 50% lower overall mortality rate when compared with other forms of therapy. These data suggest that ceftazidime combined with an aminoglycoside and sulfisoxazole now should be considered the treatment of choice for severe melioidosis.

Soft tissue infections caused by *B. pseudomallei* should be treated for 4 to 6 months with tetracycline (in children older than 8 years) in a dosage of 50 mg/kg/day in four divided doses. In younger children, trimethoprim-sulfamethoxazole (8 mg/kg/day of trimethoprim and 40 mg/kg/day of sulfamethoxazole) in two divided doses can be used. Therapy may be supplemented with sulfonamides. The duration of therapy must be guided by clinical findings. Therapy for many months may be required for patients with *Pseudomonas* osteomyelitis.

Prognosis depends on the nature of the underlying disease process. Septicemia is a leading cause of death in children with leukemia, and *Pseudomonas* is responsible for one-half of these deaths.

PREVENTION

The prevention of *Pseudomonas* infection depends on continuous surveillance of the hospital environment and eradication of the source of *Pseudomonas* as quickly as possible. The prevention of follicular dermatitis is possible by maintaining pool water at a pH of 7.2 to 7.8 and free available chlorine concentrations at 70.5 mg/L.

Pseudomonas infection in newborn nurseries usually is transmitted by the hands of hospital personnel. Strict attention to hand washing, preferably with a liquid iodophor, before and between contacts with newborn infants can prevent transmission. The growth of *Pseudomonas* on suction catheters can be prevented by rinsing the catheter in an acetic acid solution.

Solutions used for total parenteral alimentation should be prepared meticulously, and similar care should be exercised in the insertion and maintenance of other catheters. Daily replacement of all apparatus used for intravenous administration reduces the hazard of extrinsic contamination by *Pseudomonas* and other gram-negative organisms.

The efficacy of active immunization of burned patients with specific strains of *Pseudomonas* or the administration of hyperimmune globulin to prevent development of *Pseudomonas* septicemia has been demonstrated. *Pseudomonas* infection in burned patients has been minimized by the use of topical applications of 10% mafenide acetate cream or topical silver nitrate (0.5% solution). *Pseudomonas* vaccine has been suggested as a possible method for preventing septicemia in patients with acute leukemia or cystic fibrosis.

Suggested Readings

Brady MT. *Pseudomonas* and related species. In: Feigin RD, Cherry JD, Demmler GJ, Kaplan SL, eds. *Textbook of pediatric infectious diseases,* 5th ed. Philadelphia: WB Saunders, 2003:1557.

Campell WN, Hendrix E, Cryz S, et al. Immunogenicity of a 24-valent *Klebsiella* capsular polysaccharide vaccine and an eight-valent *Pseudomonas* O-polysaccharide conjugate vaccine administered to victims of acute trauma. *Clin Infect Dis* 1996;23:219.

Feder HM Jr, Grant-Kels JM, Tilton RC. *Pseudomonas* whirlpool dermatitis. *Clin Pediatr* 1983;22:638.

Gilligan PH, Whittier S. *Burkholderia, Stenotrophomonas, Ralstonia, Brevundimonas, Comamonas,* and *Acidovorax.* In: Murray PR, Baron, EJ, Pfaller MA, et al, eds. *Manual of clinical microbiology,* 7th ed. Washington, DC: ASM Press, 1999:526.

Horn KL, Gherini S. Malignant external otitis of childhood. *Ann J Otol* 1981; 2:402.

Nelson JD, Bradley JS. *Pocketbook of pediatric antimicrobial therapy,* 12th ed. Baltimore: Williams & Wilkins, 2000–2001:68.

Neu HC. The role of *Pseudomonas aeruginosa* in infections. *J Antimicrob Chemother* 1983;11(suppl):B1.

Patamasucon P, Pitchyangkura C, Fischer GW. Melioidosis in childhood. *J Pediatr* 1975;87:133.

Pennington JE, Reynolds HY, Wood RE, et al. Use of *Pseudomonas aeruginosa* vaccine in patients with acute leukemia and cystic fibrosis. *Am J Med* 1975;58:629.

Stechenberg BW, Feigin RD. Glanders. In: Feigin RD, Cherry JD, eds. *Textbook of pediatric infectious diseases,* 2nd ed. Philadelphia: WB Saunders, 1987:1140.

Tsai MJ, Teng CJ, Teng RJ, et al. Necrotizing bowel lesions complicated by *Pseudomonas septicaemia* in previously healthy infants. *Eur J Pediatr* 1996; 115:2168.

Vishwanath S, Ramphal R. Adherence of *Pseudomonas aeruginosa* to human tracheobronchial mucin. *Infect Immunol* 1984;45:197.

White NJ, Chaowagul W, Wuthiekanum V, et al. Solving of mortality of severe melioidosis by ceftazidime. *Lancet* 1989;2:697.

Wider AF, Wenzel RP, Trilla A, et al. Outbreak of *Pseudomonas aeruginosa* infections in a surgical intensive care unit: probable transmission via hands of health care worker. *Clin Infect Dis* 1993;16:372.

Zuravleff JJ, Yu VL. Infections caused by *Pseudomonas maltophilia* with emphasis on bacteremia: case reports and review of the literature. *Rev Infect Dis* 1982;4:1236.

CHAPTER 172 ■ RAT-BITE FEVER

RALPH D. FEIGIN AND MARK E. HELM

Rat-bite fever describes either one of two distinct clinical syndromes. Streptobacillary rat-bite fever is reported more commonly in North America, whereas spirillary rat-bite fever, also called soduku, appears more often in Asia. Either form is transmitted by the bite of a rat or other rodent or by contact of the skin or mucous membrane with an infected animal. Transmission of the streptobacillary form to humans from mice, squirrels, weasels, gerbils, and domestic animals that prey on rodents also has been reported. The causative agent of streptobacillary rat-bite fever also can be transmitted by ingestion of contaminated water or unpasteurized milk products. The illness that occurs after such ingestion is called *Haverhill fever,* and it may appear as epidemic outbreaks. Rat-bite fever is considered a rare disease, with incidence dependent on contact with rats or other carriers. The true incidence is unknown, and the condition likely is underdiagnosed.

CAUSATIVE AGENTS

Streptobacillus moniliformis causes streptobacillary rat-bite fever and Haverhill fever in humans. This nonencapsulated, nonmotile, gram-negative rod is pleomorphic and fastidious, but it can be grown on current culture media supplemented

TABLE 172.1

CLINICAL FEATURES OF RAT BITE FEVER

Streptobacillus Moniliformis Streptobacillary Form	*Streptobacillus Moniliformis* Haverhill Fever Form	*Spirillum Minus*
Incubation period of 1–10 days (usually <7)	Incubation period of 1–3 days	Incubation period of 14–18 days
Fever	Fever	Induration at site of inoculation
Chills	Chills	Lesion may progress to ulcer and
Headache	Rash	eschar
Vomiting	Arthritis	Fever
Maculopapular rash (2-4 days after disease onset;	Upper respiratory illness	Chills
rash may become petechial or purpuric and	Gastrointestinal complaints	Regional lymphadenopathy
desquamate)		(common)
Septic arthritis		Relapses (common)
Lymphangitis, lymphadenitis (rare)		Rash: purple to red brown with
Endocarditis		occasional indurated erythematous
Pneumonia		plaques
Relapses (rare)		Severe diarrhea (common)
		Weight loss (common)
		Anemia (common)
		Meningitis
		Endocarditis
		Myocarditis
		Nephritis
		Hepatitis

with serum, ascitic fluid, or blood. *In vitro* growth may be inhibited by sodium polyanethol sulfate found in most aerobic, but not anaerobic, blood culture bottles. *S. moniliformis* may produce variants without cell walls in the presence of penicillin or suboptimal growth conditions, but these forms usually revert under appropriate conditions to parent forms. These L-phase variants are resistant to penicillin, may deposit in tissues, and may prolong duration of symptoms of infection.

Spirillum minus, responsible for the spirillary form of rat-bite fever, is a 2- to 5-μm aerobic gram-negative spirochete with a terminal flagellum. Researchers generally agree that this organism, like other spirochetes, cannot be grown on artificial media.

CLINICAL MANIFESTATIONS

The clinical manifestations of the two forms of rat bite fever caused by *S. moniliformis* and that caused by *S. minus* are shown in Table 172.1.

Streptobacillary rat-bite fever may occur 1 to 10 days (typically less than 7 days) after inoculation of *S. moniliformis*. Although the incubation period may be as long as 22 days, shorter incubation times are reported more commonly among younger patients. The site of inoculation characteristically heals without complication. Streptobacillary disease typically begins with the acute onset of fever with chills, headache, nausea, and vomiting. A macular-papular rash potentially involving the palms and soles may be seen 2 to 4 days after the onset of the illness in roughly three-fourths of patients. The rash may persist for as long as 3 weeks and can become generalized or may develop petechial, purpuric, or pustular characteristics. One in five patients with rash may experience desquamation. Within the first week, approximately half of sufferers will develop arthralgia or extremely painful arthritis, potentially with joint effusion. The arthritis tends to be asymmetric, involving large joints, and over time may become migratory. Lymphangitis and lymphadenitis are uncommon manifestations. Other reported rare complications of streptobacillary rat-bite fever includeendocarditis (universally fatal before antibiotics), pneumonia, ab-

scess formation in or below the skin or within organs (including the brain), meningitis, mastoiditis, pericardial effusion, septic arthritis, chorioamnionitis, and periarteritis nodosa. In untreated streptobacillary rat-bite fever, the fever and arthritis may persist or follow an irregularly relapsing course. Most untreated disease will resolve spontaneously within 2 weeks, but untreated infection is associated with a 10% to 13% mortality rate. In patients younger than 3 months of age, the risk of mortality is increased even in patients who receive adequate treatment. With treatment, the mortality rate is thought to be less than 1%.

Disease caused by ingestion of *S. moniliformis*, or Haverhill fever, occurs after 1 to 3 days of incubation. This illness is characterized by abrupt onset of fever, chills, rash and arthritis, with upper respiratory and gastrointestinal complaints common. The rash of Haverhill fever tends to be small and uniform, and recurrence of fever is rare. The only reported complication of Haverhill fever is iron deficiency anemia, and no fatalities have been reported.

Soduku, or spirillary rat-bite fever, has a longer incubation period compared with the other form, averaging 14 to 18 days and ranging from 1 to 36 days. In contrast to the other form, spirillary rat-bite fever begins with induration at the superficially healed site of inoculation, coinciding with fever and chills. The lesion may progress to formation of a chancre or ulceration and formation of an eschar. Regional lymphadenopathy is a common development in spirillary rat-bite fever. The patient's temperature may rise over the course of 2 to 4 days to 41°C in increments and then abruptly fall. Six to eight relapses of fever may occur, separated regularly by afebrile periods of 3 to 7 days. Myalgia, headache, and vomiting are seen often during febrile episodes. Roughly half of patients infected with *S. minus* develop a macular purple to red-brown rash with occasional indurated erythematous plaques or urticarial lesions. In children, severe diarrhea, weight loss, and anemia are common complications. More severe complications reported in protracted, untreated disease include meningitis, endocarditis, nephritis, myocarditis, and hepatitis. Duration of untreated diseases usually is 3 to 8 weeks, but relapses may continue for months or years. Fatality rates in untreated spirillary rat-bite fever reportedly are 6% to 7%.

DIAGNOSIS

Diagnosis of rat-bite or Haverhill fever depends primarily on clinical history and suspicion of exposure to rodents. When bites are involved, differentiation between the two forms is suggested by the incubation period, the presence of lymphadenopathy or arthritis, and the development of swelling and/or ulceration at the site of inoculation.

Isolation and identification of *S. moniliformis* or *S. minus* from an affected patient provide definitive diagnosis, but both organisms present challenges in this regard. *S. moniliformis* can be grown from blood or joint fluid on artificial media, with careful attention given to growth requirements, but identification requires biochemical testing typically available only in a reference laboratory. Evidence of *S. moniliformis* infection has been demonstrated using enzyme-linked immunosorbent assay and polymerase chain reaction techniques. If the bacterium can be isolated, identification can be accomplished by analysis of fatty acid profiles using gas-liquid chromatography. Protein electrophoresis has been used to identify the strain causing Haverhill fever. Serologic testing for *S. moniliformis* has proven unreliable. *S. minus* has been identified on peripheral blood smear or by darkfield examination of ulcer exudates. Isolation of *S. minus* usually requires animal inoculation.

TREATMENT

Penicillin is the treatment of choice for both *S. moniliformis* and *S. minus* infection. Although *S. minus* is more sensitive to penicillin, thus potentially permitting a lower dose, therapy should begin before definitive identification of the causative agent has been made and should be adequate to treat either infection. Most strains of *S. moniliformis* are susceptible to intramuscular procaine penicillin G at doses of 600,000 units every 12 hours for 7 to 10 days, or 5 days of procaine penicillin

G, followed by oral penicillin for an additional 7 days. Patients with allergies to penicillin or with strains resistant to penicillin may be treated with oral tetracycline (2 g/day for older patients) or intramuscular streptomycin (15 mg/kg/day divided in two doses). Ampicillin, cefotaxime, or cefuroxime may be useful alternatives to penicillin. Erythromycin, chloramphenicol, and clindamycin have been used with some success. None of these agents has been studied rigorously. Prophylactic antibiotic treatment administered after a bite has been incurred is of unknown efficacy in preventing rat-bite fever.

Suggested Readings

American Academy of Pediatrics. Rat-bite fever. In: Pickering LK, ed. *Red book: 2003 report of the Committee on Infectious Diseases,* 26th ed. Elk Grove Village, IL: American Academy of Pediatrics; 2003:521.

Berger C, Altwegg M, Meyer A, et al. Broad range polymerase chain reaction for diagnosis of rat-bite fever caused by *Streptobacillus moniliformis. Pediatr Infect Dis J* 2001;20:1181.

Boot R, Oosterhuis A, Thuis HC. PCR for the detection of *Streptobacillus moniliformis. Lab Anim* 2002;36:200.

Byington CL, Basow RD. *Spirilum minus.* In: Feigin RD, Cherry JD, Demmler GJ, Kaplan SL, eds. *Textbook of pediatric infectious diseases,* 5th ed. Philadelphia: WB Saunders, 2004:1687.

Byington CL, Basow RD. *Streptobacillus moniliformis.* In: Feigin RD, Cherry JD, Demmler GJ, Kaplan SL, eds. *Textbook of pediatric infectious diseases,* 5th ed. Philadelphia: WB Saunders, 2004:1722.

Centers for Disease Control and Prevention. Rat-bite fever: New Mexico, 1996. *JAMA* 1998;279:740.

Costas M, Owen RJ. Numerical analysis of electrophoretic protein patterns of *Streptobacillus moniliformis* strains from human, murine and avianinfections. *J Med Microbiol* 1987;23:303.

Edwards R, Finch RG. Characterisation and antibiotic susceptibilities of *Streptobacillus moniliformis. J Med Microbiol* 1986;21:39.

Hockman DE, Pence CD, Whittler RR, et al. Septic arthritis of the hip secondary to rat bite fever. *Clin Orthop* 2000;380:173.

Shanson DC, Gazzard BG, Midgley J, et al. *Streptobacillus moniliformis* isolated from blood in four cases of Haverhill fever. *Lancet* 1983;322:92.

Tattersall RS, Bourne JT. Systemic vasculitis following an unreported rat bite. *Ann Rheum Dis* 2003;62:605.

Wallet F, Savage C, Loiez C, et al. Molecular diagnosis of arthritis due to *Streptobacillus moniliformis. Diagn Microbiol Infect Dis* 2003;47:623.

CHAPTER 173 ■ *SALMONELLA* INFECTIONS

LARRY K. PICKERING

Salmonellosis is a term that refers to infections caused by the genus *Salmonella,* which contains approximately 2,500 serotypes. Two broad clinical syndromes are produced by organisms in the genus *Salmonella.* The first includes nontyphoidal *Salmonella* organisms that infect a range of hosts, cause disease of the gastrointestinal tract in many animals including humans, are especially problematic in immunosuppressed hosts, are distributed widely in nature in the gastrointestinal tracts of wild and domestic mammals, birds, reptiles, and insects, and are important foodborne pathogens. The nontyphoidal, animal-adapted *Salmonella* organisms are important public health problems in industrialized countries, where ingestion of contaminated foods often results in large outbreaks of disease. The second group includes a few *Salmonella* serotypes, especially *Salmonella* serotypes Typhi and Paratyphi, which are adapted to humans, have no other known natural hosts, and

cause the protracted bacteremic illness of typhoid and paratyphoid enteric fever. *Salmonella* serotypes Typhi and Paratyphi are endemic in many economically disadvantaged countries that lack safe drinking water and food. Increasing resistance of many *Salmonella* serotypes has complicated antimicrobial therapy in infected individuals.

ETIOLOGY

Salmonellae are gram-negative, non-spore-forming, facultatively anaerobic bacilli that belong to the Enterobacteriaceae family. Classification and nomenclature of *Salmonella* species are confusing. On the basis of DNA hybridization studies, *Salmonella* isolates are classified in a single species, *S. enterica.* The species *S. enterica* contains approximately 2,500 different serotypes. *Salmonella* serotypes and isolates (previously known as species) were classified on the basis of host range, surface antigen structure, and biochemical characteristics, and the terms they were given appeared to designate them as separate species (e.g., *S. typhimurium*). The current correct taxonomic name would be *S. enterica* serotype Typhimurium. Commonly (although taxonomically incorrect), serotypes are designated as species (e.g., *S. typhimurium*).

Salmonella can be subdivided into serotypes on the basis of three types of surface antigens: cell-wall somatic or O antigens, flagellar or H antigens, and polysaccharide or Vi antigens. Generally, *Salmonella* serotypes were named for the city in which they were defined. Many hospital laboratories perform agglutination reactions that define specific O antigens into serogroups designated *Salmonella* A, B, C_1, C_2, D, and E. This grouping confirms identification of the genus and may be useful epidemiologically, but final serotyping generally requires a reference laboratory. *S. typhi* may be identified rapidly (serogroup D, Vi-antigen positive) by using commercially available agglutination tests, but identifying serotypes in other serogroups requires additional testing. For example both *S. typhimurium*, a cause of diarrhea, and *S. paratyphi*, a cause of enteric fever, are in serogroup B. *S. typhimurium* and *S. enteritidis* (serogroup D) are the two most common causes of human *Salmonella* infections in the United States. Other serotypes commonly associated with human disease include *S. newport* (serogroup C_2), *S. heidelberg* (serogroup B), *S. infantis* (serogroup C_1), *S. hadar* (serogroup C_2), and *S. agona* (serogroup B). The complete genome sequence has been determined for a multidrug-resistant strain of *Salmonella* serotype Typhi.

EPIDEMIOLOGY

Animals, including poultry, livestock, and pets, including reptiles, are the major reservoirs for nontyphoidal *Salmonella*. Reptiles maintain fecal carriage rates of *Salmonella* of more than 90%, rendering salmonellosis associated with reptiles a continuing public health concern. Other sources include contaminated animal products, meat-processing plants, contaminated water, and infected humans; fruits and vegetables, including sprouts, are less common sources. *Salmonella* serotype Typhi infects only humans, and *Salmonella* serotype Paratyphi has a reservoir primarily in humans. Methods of transmission include the following: ingestion of contaminated food, milk, water, medications, or dyes; contact with infected animals; fecal-oral transmission resulting in person-to-person spread; and, rarely, contact with contaminated medical instruments or even blood or blood product transfusions such as platelets. Most cases of salmonellosis are foodborne, with outbreaks caused by ingestion of contaminated eggs, cheese, ice cream premix, juice, sprouts, dry cereal, raw almonds, and fresh fruits and vegetables. Volunteer studies using adults have shown that between 10^5 and 10^6 viable organisms must be ingested for clinical disease to occur, although data from foodborne outbreaks of salmonellosis indicate that the infective dose for various *Salmonella* serotypes and for people with immune deficiencies may be lower.

Infections with nontyphoidal strains of *Salmonella* are common. Approximately 40,300 cases were reported in 2004 to the Centers for Disease Control and Prevention (CDC). *Salmonella* is one of the most frequently reported causes of foodborne outbreaks, cases, and deaths in the United States. Before 1996, most data regarding salmonellosis in the United States were derived from a passive surveillance system. These data estimated that 800,000 to 3.7 million infections actually occurred per year in the United States. In 1996, an active surveillance system for foodborne illness, referred to as the Foodborne Diseases

TABLE 173.1

CONDITIONS THAT PREDISPOSE TO INVASIVE SALMONELLOSIS

Acquired immunodeficiency syndrome
Bartonellosis
Collagen-vascular disease
Diabetes mellitus
Extremes of age
Focal lesions (kidney stones or gallstones, endovascular lesions, prosthetic devices)
Hemolytic anemia, including sickle cell disease
Inflammatory bowel disease
Malaria
Malignancy
Malnutrition
Organ transplantation
Recipients of immunosuppressive therapy
Rheumatologic disorders
Schistosomiasis

Active Surveillance Network (FoodNet), was established by the CDC (www.cdc.gov/foodnet). Since 1997, *Salmonella* and *Campylobacter* have been the two most frequent laboratory-confirmed enteric pathogens.

Age-specific attack rates peak in the first year of life and are higher for children younger than 5 years of age and for persons 25 to 64 years of age. Most reported cases of *Salmonella* infection are sporadic, but transmission by contaminated food and water frequently results in outbreaks of disease. Many outbreaks of *Salmonella* serotype Enteritidis have been associated with ingestion of contaminated eggs. *Salmonella* serotype Enteritidis infects the upper oviduct and contaminates the contents of eggs that appear to have intact shells. Morbidity and mortality after infection occurs more commonly in certain groups of people (Table 173.1).

Salmonella serotype Typhi colonizes only humans, and *Salmonella* serotype Paratyphi colonizes humans and some primates; therefore, disease can be acquired only through close contact with a person with typhoid fever or with a carrier of one of these organisms or by ingestion of food or water contaminated with human feces from a carrier. Since the early part of the twentieth century, the incidence of typhoid fever in the United States has changed dramatically. *Salmonella* serotype Typhi infection has become an uncommon occurrence as compared with nontyphoidal salmonellosis. Approximately 400 cases of typhoid fever are reported annually in the United States. Most cases of typhoid fever in the United States are associated with foreign travel; most domestically acquired cases result from contact with food contaminated by a chronic carrier. Worldwide, typhoid fever is a major health problem, generally in economically developing countries, with an estimated 16 million new cases and 600,000 deaths/year.

The incubation period for *Salmonella* gastroenteritis is 6 to 72 hours. The incubation period for enteric fever is 3 to 60 days (usually 7 to 14 days).

PATHOGENESIS

Exposure to gastric acid (pH less than 3.5) is lethal to *Salmonella*. If the number of bacteria swallowed is large enough, if gastric acid is neutralized by ingested food, or if conditions of reduced gastric acidity (achlorhydria as occurs in infants and in people with pernicious anemia, gastric surgery, or treatment with antacids, H_2-receptor antagonists, or proton-pump inhibitors) are present, sufficient bacteria may survive passage to enter the small intestine. To become established in the intestine and to colonize the ileum and colon, *Salmonella* also must elude removal by intestinal motility. The use of antiperistaltic drugs can render the condition worse or can lead to systemic invasion. Alteration of the normal intestinal flora by antimicrobial agents renders the host more susceptible to salmonellosis. Lower inocula may cause disease in persons with deficiencies of host defense mechanisms, including persons with radiation-induced intestinal damage.

Symptoms of *Salmonella* infection are associated with mucosal invasion with inflammation or production of toxins. Some *Salmonella* strains elaborate a heat-labile toxin that may function as an enterotoxin or cytotoxins that inhibit protein synthesis. After attachment, organisms must resist both nonspecific and specific host defense mechanisms long enough to multiply to sufficient numbers to damage underlying cells and tissues. Once attached to mucosal cells, *Salmonella* organisms then can invade the mucosa. The M cells, which are specialized epithelial cells overlying Peyer patches, probably are the site of internalization of *Salmonella* serotype Typhi and less commonly other serotypes. Organisms then interact with macrophages and lymphocytes in Peyer patches and other lymphoid tissue in the mucosa of the small intestine. After several weeks of infection, Peyer patches enlarge and become necrotic and most likely are responsible for the abdominal pain that occurs during the course of typhoid fever. As *Salmonella* organisms invade through Peyer patches, they are transported in phagocytic cells to mesenteric lymph nodes and through the thoracic duct to the bloodstream; circulating bacteria are removed by reticuloendothelial cells in liver, spleen, and bone marrow. Some organisms can reach distant target organs or tissues, such as the gallbladder, where they can multiply and secondarily seed the intestine. Symptoms of typhoid fever occur when a critical number of organisms has replicated. Serotypes vary in their potential to invade the bloodstream. Infection with *Salmonella* serotype Typhi induces systemic and humoral immunity and cellular responses that often confer incomplete protection against relapse and reinfection. *Salmonella* serotypes contain a wide variety of plasmids and genes that encode virulence factors and antimicrobial resistance.

CLINICAL MANIFESTATIONS

Several clinical syndromes are associated with *Salmonella* infections caused by various *Salmonella* serotypes: the chronic carrier state; acute gastroenteritis; bacteremia; enteric fever, including typhoid and paratyphoid fevers; and dissemination with localized suppuration, which manifests as intravascular infection, abscesses, osteomyelitis, arthritis, or meningitis. These clinical syndromes may overlap.

Every serotype can produce any of the clinical patterns, but certain *Salmonella* serotypes are associated consistently with specific clinical syndromes. The transient asymptomatic carrier may occur more commonly than does gastroenteritis. By the third month after infection with nontyphoidal *Salmonella*, more than 90% of infected persons have stopped excreting the organism. Higher proportions of neonates have prolonged carriage. Persons who excrete the organism for longer than 1 year are considered chronic carriers. Asymptomatic fecal excretion of *Salmonella* serotype Typhi for longer than 1 year occurs in approximately 3% of adults after they have an episode of acute typhoid fever and in 0.3% of patients with nontyphoidal salmonellosis. Gallbladder disease predisposes to chronic carriage.

The most frequent manifestation of disease caused by nontyphoidal *Salmonella* is gastroenteritis, which occurs most commonly in infants during their first year of life, decreases abruptly in early childhood, and remains relatively constant throughout adulthood. Manifestations include diarrhea, abdominal cramps and tenderness, and fever. The most prominent symptom is diarrhea, ranging from a few stools to profuse, bloody diarrhea to a cholera-like syndrome. Usually, diarrhea is self-limited and lasts 3 to 7 days. Fever generally resolves within 72 hours. In uncomplicated gastroenteritis, bacteremia occurs in 5% to 10% of cases, with higher rates occurring in groups at high risk (see Table 173.1).

Enteric fever most often is produced by *S. typhi*, *S. paratyphi* A, *S. paratyphi* B, and *S. paratyphi* C, but fever may be caused by any serotype. The term *typhoid fever* refers to illness caused by *Salmonella* serotype Typhi. Clinical manifestations usually are more severe when the causative organism is *Salmonella* serotype Typhi. Typically, the onset of enteric fever occurs 7 to 14 days after ingestion of the organism and is gradual, with elevated fever, headache, malaise, anorexia, lethargy, and abdominal signs and symptoms, including constipation and (less frequently) diarrhea. Physical findings vary, but an erythematous pharynx, hepatosplenomegaly, and lymphadenopathy with or without the presence of rose spots (faint salmon-colored maculopapular 2- to 3-mm lesions on the trunk) are common signs. Relative bradycardia has been described but is not uniform. Complications of untreated typhoid fever include intestinal hemorrhage and perforation and focal infections, which usually occur in the third or fourth week after onset of symptoms. Without antimicrobial therapy, most infections resolve after 4 weeks of infection, without development of complications. However, complications occur in 10% to 15% of patients and include intestinal bleeding and perforation and typhoid encephalopathy. Relapse occurs in 5% to 10% of patients, usually 2 to 3 weeks after resolution of fever.

The major significance of nontyphoid or nonparatyphoid *Salmonella* bacteremia is the risk of developing disseminated focal infections. *S. choleraesuis* and *S. dublin* are nontyphoid serotypes that produce a syndrome of sustained bacteremia. *Salmonella* organisms have a propensity for infection of vascular sites and high-grade bacteremia. Chronic *Salmonella* bacteremia has been associated with concomitant *Schistosoma mansoni* infection.

Focal infections occur in approximately 10% of patients with *Salmonella* bacteremia. Osteomyelitis and meningitis are the most common focal infections, followed in descending order by pyelonephritis, endocarditis, vascular infections, pneumonia, septic and reactive arthritis, and abscesses in other organs. *Salmonella* osteomyelitis is a problem in children and adolescents with sickle cell disease. *Salmonella* infection occurs more frequently in persons with human immunodeficiency virus (HIV) infection than in the general population, and recurrent *Salmonella* bacteremia is an acquired immunodeficiency syndrome (AIDS)—defining illnesss.

DIAGNOSIS

Gastroenteritis caused by *Salmonella* can be established by stool culture. The diagnosis of *Salmonella* bacteremia is made by obtaining cultures of blood and bone marrow aspirate, and in enteric fever, cultures from any foci of infection, including rose spots, urine, and stools, also are useful. Approximately 60% to 80% of patients with typhoid or paratyphoid fever have positive blood or bone marrow cultures during the first week of illness. The sensitivity of blood culture is reduced by prior use of antimicrobial agents and is increased by culturing a large volume of blood. The sensitivity of stool cultures increases over time and depends on the amount of feces cultured. Bone marrow culture is the most sensitive procedure for recovery of *Salmonella* serotype Typhi. Communication with microbiology laboratory personnel about appropriate specimen collection and transport will optimize organism isolation.

TABLE 173.2

ANTIMICROBIAL THERAPY FOR *SALMONELLA* INFECTIONS

Clinical Manifestation	Agents	
	Children	Adults
Chronic carrier state with *Salmonella* serotype Typhi	Amoxicillin plus probenecid	Fluoroquinolone
Acute gastroenteritis*	None	None
Bacteremia or dissemination with localized suppuration	Cefotaxime, ceftriaxone, ampicillin, trimethoprim-sulfamethoxazole, or chloramphenicol	Ceftriaxone, cefotaxime, or a fluoroquinolone
Typhoid fever	Ceftriaxone, cefotaxime, ampicillin, chloramphenicol, trimethoprim-sulfamethoxazole or azithromycin	Fluoroquinolone or ceftriaxone

*Most cases resolve spontaneously without antimicrobial therapy. Patients who may benefit from therapy include those who are infants (especially ≤3 months of age), elderly, or immunosuppressed and those with systemic signs or symptoms.

Often, serologic tests for *Salmonella* agglutinins are part of the febrile agglutinin panel, which includes the Widal test. This procedure, which measures the antibody response to somatic and flagellar antigens of *Salmonella* serotype Typhi, is unreliable because of frequent false-positive and false-negative results. Many typhoid carriers may have antibody titers against the Vi capsular polysaccharide of *Salmonella* serotype Typhi. The test may be useful for identifying chronic carriers associated with outbreaks of typhoid fever. DNA probes and polymerase chain reaction assays to detect protein antigens of *Salmonella* serotype Typhi may become of value in diagnostic testing for *Salmonella* serotype Typhi in samples of body fluid from patients suspected of having typhoid fever.

TREATMENT

Table 173.2 shows recommended antimicrobial therapy for various clinical manifestations of *Salmonella*. Both the specific syndrome and characteristics of the host associated with *Salmonella* infection influence selection and duration of antimicrobial therapy. Antimicrobial agents are not recommended in persons who are nontyphoidal *Salmonella* carriers or in most patients with gastroenteritis because antimicrobial agents have been shown to prolong the duration fecal excretion, increase the risk of developing complications, produce a relapse, and enhance development or selection of resistant strains. The use of antimicrobial agents should be considered in patients with gastroenteritis if the disease appears to be evolving into enterocolitis or into one of the systemic syndromes. Antimicrobial agents also should be considered in severely malnourished children, in infants up to 3 months of age, in the elderly, in patients with hemoglobinopathies, and in immunosuppressed patients, including persons with AIDS and patients receiving immunosuppressive therapy who have uncomplicated gastroenteritis, in whom the risk of developing bacteremia or metastatic infection is high. Treatment of *Salmonella* infection includes the following: patients with typhoid fever, bacteremia caused by nontyphoid strains, or dissemination with localized suppuration; selected patients with acute gastroenteritis; and persons who are chronic carriers of *Salmonella* serotype Typhi isolates.

Antimicrobial agents used to treat patients with various *Salmonella* syndromes include chloramphenicol, ampicillin, amoxicillin, trimethoprim-sulfamethoxazole, cefotaxime, ceftriaxone, and fluoroquinolones. Despite *in vitro* activity, first- and second-generation cephalosporins and aminoglycosides have been ineffective in treating patients with *Salmonella* infection and should not be used. The selection of antimicrobial agents for therapy is complicated by the emergence of *Salmonella* strains that are resistant to multiple antimicrobial agents.

In patients with disseminated infections, ampicillin, chloramphenicol, ceftriaxone, or cefotaxime can be used if organisms are susceptible. For enteric fever, ceftriaxone is the drug of choice for children, and ceftriaxone or a fluoroquinolone is the drug of choice for adults. Quinolones are not approved for use in people younger than 18 years of age for this indication.

For intravascular infections, such as endocarditis or infection of an aneurysm, ampicillin, ceftriaxone, or cefotaxime are preferred over chloramphenicol because of their bactericidal activity. For *Salmonella* meningitis, cefotaxime or ceftriaxone is recommended. Ciprofloxacin is the drug of choice for adult chronic carriers of *Salmonella* serotype Typhi, whereas in children with normally functioning gallbladders without cholelithiasis, ampicillin or amoxicillin combined with probenecid is the treatment of choice for chronic carriers of *Salmonella* serotype Typhi. Patients who have gallstones and who fail to respond to 6 weeks of antimicrobial therapy may require cholecystectomy if eradication of the organism is necessary.

Broad selective pressure appears to affect rates of resistance for *Salmonella* serotypes in various reservoirs. This pressure includes antibiotic use in poultry (a reservoir for *Salmonella* serotype Heidelberg) and in cows (a reservoir for *Salmonella* serotype Typhimurium). Nontyphoid *Salmonella* species have become progressively more resistant to chloramphenicol, ampicillin, and trimethoprim-sulfamethoxazole. Resistance to five or more antimicrobial agents is highest for Typhimurium and Newport isolates. Studies of Typhi isolates in the United States in 2001 and reported by the National Antimicrobial Resistance Monitoring Systems showed that 23% were resistant to two or more antimicrobial agents. All *Salmonella* isolates from persons who require antimicrobial therapy should have susceptibility testing performed.

Aspirin has been associated with precipitous declines in temperature and shock and should be avoided in patients with enteric fever syndromes; this decline has not been observed with acetaminophen or ibuprofen in children. Corticosteroids may be administered to patients with severe typhoid fever and for whom prompt therapy for toxemia may be lifesaving, although some reports correlate the use of steroids with intestinal perforation. The duration of steroid therapy is 48 hours; courses of longer duration may increase the rate of relapse. Dexamethasone (3 mg/kg intravenously, followed by eight doses of 1 mg/kg every 6 hours) is the usual regimen.

PREVENTION

The most important aspects of prevention of *Salmonella* infection are education and avoidance. Proper food handling, storage, and preparation techniques should be used. Fresh eggs

TABLE 173.3

TYPHOID VACCINES

Vaccine	Type	Route	Age at Receipt	Number of Doses	Interval between Doses	Boosting Interval
Ty21a*	Live-attenuated	Oral	≥6 years	Four	2 days	Every 5 years
ViCPS	Polysaccharide	Intramuscular	≥2 years	One	—	Every 2 years

CPS, capsular polysaccharide.
*Contraindicated in immunocompromised people and in patients taking antimicrobial agents.

should be stored at temperatures up to 7°C (up to 45°F), and eggs should be cooked until both the yolk and the white are firm. Pasteurized egg products should be substituted for raw eggs in dishes served without further cooking. All dairy products should be pasteurized before being ingested. *Salmonella* organisms usually grow at 35° to 37°C, but they can grow at lower temperatures. To minimize problems, foods should be held at or lower than 2° to 5°C at all times. Travelers should be advised to follow appropriate practices when eating abroad. Surveillance is an important mechanism to characterize trends in occurrence of *Salmonella* infection and to identify outbreaks of disease. Information about safe ownership of reptiles is available at www.cdc.gov/healthypets/animals/reptiles/.

Two typhoid vaccines are available for use in the United States: (a) an oral live-attenuated vaccine (Vivotif, Berna Products, Coral Gables, FL), manufactured from the Ty21a strain of *Salmonella* serotype Typhi by the Swiss Serum and Vaccine Institute; and (b) a capsular polysaccharide vaccine for intramuscular use (TYPHIM Vi vaccine, manufactured by Sanofi Pasteur, Lyon, France and distributed by Sanofi Pasteur, Swiftwater, PA). Another vaccine, an acetone-inactivated parenteral vaccine, currently is available only to the armed forces. Typhoid fever vaccination is indicated for administration to travelers who go to typhoid-endemic regions and may be exposed to contaminated food and drink, household contacts of known *Salmonella* serotype Typhi carriers, and microbiology laboratory technicians who work with *Salmonella* serotype Typhi.

Although no prospective, randomized trials comparing typhoid vaccines licensed in the United States have been conducted, several field trials have demonstrated the efficacy of each vaccine. Table 173.3 shows a comparison of the main characteristics of live oral Ty21a vaccine and parenteral Vi polysaccharide vaccine. The oral vaccine has not been tested adequately in children younger than 6 years of age and is not licensed for use in this age group. It is also contraindicated in immunosuppressed patients, including people infected with HIV.

Suggested Readings

Baumler AJ, Tsolis RM, Ficht TA, Adams LG. Evolution of host adaptation in *Salmonella enterica. Infect Immun* 1998;66:4579.

Centers for Disease Control and Prevention. Preliminary FoodNet data on the incidence of infection with pathogens transmitted commonly through food: selected sites, United States, 2003. *MMWR Morb Mortal Wkly Rep* 2004;53:338. Information available at www.cdc.gov/foodnet/.

Centers for Disease Control and Prevention. Reptile-associated salmonellosis: selected states, 1998–2002. *MMWR Morb Mortal Wkly Rep* 2003;52:1206.

Glynn MK, Bopp C, Dewitt W, et al. Emergence of multidrug-resistant *Salmonella enterica* serotype Newport infections resistant to expanded spectrum cephalosporins in the United States. *J Infect Dis* 2003;188:1707.

Hohmann EL. Nontyphoidal salmonellosis. *Clin Infect Dis* 2001;32:263.

Hornick RB, Greisman SE, Woodward TE, et al. Typhoid fever: pathogenesis and immunologic control. *N Engl J Med* 1970;283:686.

Misra S, Diaz PS, Rowley AH. Characteristics of typhoid fever in children and adolescents in a major metropolitan area in the United States. *Clin Infect Dis* 1997;24:998.

National Center for Infectious Diseases. Centers for Disease Control and Prevention. National Antimicrobial Resistance Monitoring Systems (NARMS) for Enteric Bacteria Web site. Available at www.cdc.gov/NARMS.

Noyola DE, Fernandez M, Kaplan SL. Reevaluation of antipyretic in children with enteric fever. *Pediatr Infect Dis J* 1998;17:691.

Parry CM, Hien TT, Dougan G, et al. Typhoid fever. *N Engl J Med* 2002;347:1770.

Patrick ME, Adcock PM, Gomez, TM, et al. *Salmonella enteritidis* infections, United States, 1985–1999. *Emerg Infect Dis* 2004;10:1.

Pickering LK. Antimicrobial resistance among enteric pathogens. *Semin Pediatr Infect Dis* 2004;15:71.

Schutze GE, Schutze SE, Kirby RS. Extraintestinal salmonellosis in a children's hospital. *Pediatr Infect Dis J* 1997;16:482.

Telzak EE, Budnick LD, Greenberg MSZ, et al. A nosocomial outbreak of *Salmonella enteritidis* infection due to the consumption of raw eggs. *N Engl J Med* 1990;323:394.

CHAPTER 174 ■ SHIGELLOSIS

THERESA J. OCHOA AND THOMAS G. CLEARY

Shigellosis is the most common cause of dysentery and a leading cause of death in developing countries. It is characterized by acute febrile diarrhea with abdominal pain, often with mucus or blood in the feces. Complications and extraintestinal manifestations of infections are not rare developments.

MICROBIOLOGY

Shigella species are members of the Enterobacteriaceae family. The shigellae are gram-negative, aerobic, nonmotile bacteria that do not use lactose or use it only during prolonged periods of incubation. The *Shigella* genus consists of four species (with more than 40 serotypes) that are biochemically differentiated. Group A, *S. dysenteriae*, has 13 serotypes. Group B, *S. flexneri*, has 6 serotypes and 13 subserotypes (1a, 1b, 2a, 2b, 3a, 3b, 4a, 4b, 5a, 5b, 6, X variant, and Y variant). Group C, *S. boydii*, has 18 serotypes; and group D, *S. sonnei*, has a single serotype. Although important differences in virulence genes and clinical features among *Shigella* serotypes exist, these organisms traditionally are discussed together because of their microbiologic and clinical similarities.

EPIDEMIOLOGY

Shigellae are spread by the fecal-oral route. They are hardy organisms that can survive in water for as long as 6 months. Unlike most other agents that cause diarrhea, the inoculum size required to cause illness is very low. Some adult volunteers have become ill after ingesting only ten shigellae. Although shigellae are like other enteric pathogens in that they can be spread through contaminated food or water, they are atypical in that they are passed easily from person to person.

The peak incidence of symptomatic *Shigella* infection occurs during the first 4 years of life. Despite the small inoculum required to produce disease, infants in the first few months of life rarely are symptomatically infected. The reason is unclear. The exact incidence of *Shigella* infection is unknown because many infections are asymptomatic, and infections associated with illness not always are diagnosed or reported. The annual number of *Shigella* episodes worldwide was estimated to be 164.7 million, of which 163.2 million were in developing countries (with 1.1 million deaths) and 1.5 million in industrialized countries. More than one-half of the episodes and deaths occur in children younger than 5 years of age. Approximately 18,000 cases of *Shigella* are diagnosed each year in the United States.

Shigellosis often is seen in outbreaks involving day-care centers, nursing homes, prisons, troops, and cruise ships. Outbreaks of infection are difficult to control because of the low infectious dose and ease of person-to-person transmission. Some settings in the United States, such as custodial care institutions and Indian reservations, have unusually high isolation rates. Native Americans have a risk of acquiring shigellosis that is approximately four times that of the remainder of the population. Sexually transmitted shigellosis occurs among those having unprotected anal intercourse. Day-care centers are an important focus for outbreaks of shigellosis in the United States. The small inoculum required for production of disease, the pooling of susceptible children, and the frequent lack of adherence to basic hygienic procedures contribute to this situation.

In the developing world, where carriers are common, the frequency of infection is even greater, with infants routinely exposed to *Shigella* early in life. Studies by Leonardo Mata of 45 Guatemalan infants whose stools were cultured weekly during their first 3 years of life documented 1,032 positive cultures for *Shigella* species. Although these studies were done many years ago, the risk for children in the developing world probably has not decreased.

The peak occurrence in the United States is between July and October. In tropical regions, the peak period is during the rainy season.

Important geographic variations in the prevalent serotypes of *Shigella* exist. In the United States and other industrialized countries, most shigellosis is caused by *S. sonnei*, followed by *S. flexneri*. In most of the developing world, *S. flexneri* is seen more commonly than is *S. sonnei*. In some areas, *S. dysenteriae* serotype 1 causes epidemic disease.

PATHOGENESIS

The virulence of *Shigella* results from its ability to invade, multiply, spread to adjacent epithelial cells, and induce inflammation within the intestine. *Shigella* species infect the large intestine primarily. When the pathogen reaches the colon, bacteria are taken up by the M cells. After translocation, *Shigella* organisms are phagocytosed by dendritic cells and resident macrophages in Peyers patches. *Shigella* causes apoptosis of the macrophages, thus allowing access to the basal side of the epithelial cells, where bacteria can enter efficiently. The infected macrophages release large amounts of inflammatory cytokines. This early inflammatory process leads to disruption of the epithelial barrier, thereby facilitating further invasion of *Shigella*.

The most fundamental virulence property shared by all shigellae and by the enteroinvasive *Escherichia coli* is the ability to invade mammalian cells. Most of the genes responsible for invasion are located on the *Shigella* virulence plasmid. *Shigella* that lack this plasmid are avirulent. This plasmid carries two types of genes: the *ipa* and *ipg* genes encoding the entry-mediating proteins and the *mxi* and *spa* genes encoding the type III secretion system. This secretion system is found in many other pathogenic gram-negative bacteria; its function is to transport proteins from the bacterial cytoplasm into the host cell plasma membrane and cytoplasm on contact with host cells. In addition to the key plasmid-encoded invasion proteins, shigellae have chromosomally encoded traits that enhance their pathogenicity. The *Shigella* species also produce several toxins. Shiga toxin, a protein synthesis inhibitor produced in high amounts by *S. dysenteriae* serotype 1, may account for the severity of infection caused by this serotype compared with other shigellae. This toxin is involved in the pathogenesis of the hemolytic uremic syndrome (HUS), a major complication of infection with *S. dysenteriae* serotype 1. Enterotoxins also have been described that may contribute to the watery diarrhea.

The pathogenesis of the neurologic manifestations in shigellosis is as yet unclear. Data from animal models and epidemiologic studies previously linked Shiga toxin to the development of neurologic disturbances. However, Shiga toxin is not a neurotoxin. Children who have neurologic symptoms during shigellosis usually are infected with *Shigella* that do not produce Shiga toxin.

Immune responses to shigellae are both humoral and cellular. Volunteer studies show that tumor necrosis factor-alpha and interferon-gamma increase in stool within 24 to 48 hours of infection. Antibody-secreting cells are present in blood by 4 to 7 days after infection, and humoral antibody develops by 7 to 14 days. Antibodies to lipopolysaccharides and the invasion plasmid antigens are produced during natural infection. Some epidemiologic, serologic, and clinical data suggest that the concentration of serum immunoglobulin G (IgG) antibodies to the O-specific polysaccharide component of lipopolysaccharide is related to immunity to shigellosis.

Children with shigellosis have a persistent activation of the innate immune response in the convalescent phase. Children have delayed accumulation of mast cells and eosinophils and reduced neutrophil counts in the rectum, compared with adults. These factors may affect the clinical course in children.

PATHOLOGY

The most obvious pathologic changes in shigellosis are those found in the colon. The rectosigmoid and distal segments of the colon typically are more involved than are proximal areas. Erythema, mucosal edema, friability, focal hemorrhages, and adherent mucopurulent pseudomembranes all may be found. The microscopic findings include edema, capillary congestion, capillary thromboses, focal hemorrhages, crypt hyperplasia, crypt abscesses, goblet cell depletion, mononuclear and polymorphonuclear infiltrates, shedding of epithelial cells, and ulcerations. The cellular infiltrate persists for a month or more.

CLINICAL MANIFESTATIONS

Shigella enteric infection has several typical clinical presentations. Some children have a biphasic illness, presenting with severe abdominal cramps associated with fever and watery diarrhea, followed in 24 to 48 hours by colitis with small-volume, bloody stools, whose passage is associated with tenesmus (an ineffectual urge to defecate) and pain. Other children present with a picture of colitis. In still others, watery diarrhea never progresses to the colitic phase. Approximately 40% of children with *Shigella* infection have blood in their stools, and 50% have emesis. Clinical presentation vary with *Shigella* species. Patients with *S. sonnei* infection usually have watery diarrhea, whereas those with *S. flexneri, S. boydii,* and *S. dysenteriae* infection typically have bloody diarrhea and more severe systemic symptoms. *S. dysenteriae* serotype 1 typically produces more severe colitis. The incubation period varies from 1 to 7 days but typically is 2 to 4 days.

Physical findings include fever (e.g., more than two-thirds have rectal temperatures higher than 38.9°C), evidence of toxicity, dehydration, and lower quadrant abdominal tenderness. Because the disease involves distal segments of colon more than proximal areas, rectal examination may demonstrate an unusual degree of tenderness. Without therapy, fever and diarrhea may persist for a week or more. Chronic diarrhea can occur not only in children with acquired immunodeficiency syndrome (AIDS), but also in immunologically normal children. Mild dehydration and electrolyte disturbances are common findings. Despite frequent bowel movements, less than 30 mL/kg/day of fluid is lost during the dysenteric phase. Hyponatremia and hypoglycemia are major metabolic abnormalities that are associated with adverse outcomes. Hyponatremia occurs most commonly with *S. dysenteriae* infection. Because stool sodium losses do not appear to account for the degree of hyponatremia, researchers have postulated that the abnormality is produced by inappropriate antidiuretic hormone secretion. The prevalence of hypoglycemia is higher among patients with shigellosis than among patients with diarrhea from other causes. The low concentrations of insulin and elevated concentrations of glucose regulatory hormones (e.g., growth hormone, glucagon, epinephrine, norepinephrine, cortisol) suggest failure of gluconeogenesis as the cause of hypoglycemia. Shigellosis causes protein-losing enteropathy, which can aggravate or provoke malnutrition and lead to death. Shigellosis probably is the most frequent enteric infection resulting in the progression of marginal malnutrition to overt protein-calorie malnutrition. Postshigellosis persistent diarrhea is not uncommon. A community-based study of Bangladeshi children found that, despite the use of nalidixic acid in dysenteric episodes, persistent diarrhea occurred in 23% of children with shigellosis.

Complications and extraintestinal manifestations of shigellosis include seizures and other neurologic symptoms, bacteremia, HUS, Reiter syndrome, toxic megacolon and perforation, and toxic encephalopathy (Ekiri syndrome). In various series, 10% to 35% of affected children have seizures or other neurologic symptoms. Seizures have been considered the most frequent extraintestinal manifestation of shigellosis. Lethargy and seizures may occur before diarrhea develops. Their frequency is disproportionate to the expected incidence of febrile convulsions, a finding suggesting that shigellae directly or indirectly trigger seizures. In patients whose course is complicated by convulsions, the outcome usually is good. Although

a few patients have died, most children recover and have no neurologic residua, even with prolonged or focal seizures. Encephalopathy can occur during an enteroinvasive *E. coli* infection or a *Shigella* infection. Severe encephalopathy is a more ominous complication than is convulsion; patients can present with obtundation or coma or with abnormal neurologic signs, such as decorticate or decerebrate posturing. Cerebral edema, necrosis, and hemorrhage have been described. This toxic encephalopathy in children is characterized by extreme hyperpyrexia (sometimes higher than 41.7°C), hypotension, and a rapidly fatal course, without sepsis or severe dehydration. The pathogenesis of this syndrome, called *Ekiri* in the Japanese literature, is not well understood, although some data suggest that hypocalcemia may be important. Ekiri, predominantly associated with *S. sonnei* infection, was responsible for many deaths in Japan before and immediately after World War II.

The development of HUS is associated with *S. dysenteriae* serotype 1. Hemolysis and thrombocytopenia are triggered by vascular damage caused by Shiga toxin-mediated inhibition of protein synthesis. Some *E. coli* (e.g., *E. coli* O157:H7, *E. coli* O26:H11) organisms are like *S. dysenteriae* serotype 1 in that they produce massive amounts of Shiga toxin or a closely related protein (Shiga toxin 2). These *E. coli* organisms are associated with afebrile hemorrhagic colitis and HUS.

Bacteremia is an uncommon finding in watery diarrhea caused by *Shigella* species. However, sepsis with disseminated intravascular coagulation may complicate severe dysentery. Bacteremia that occurs during shigellosis may be caused by either the *Shigella* or other enteric organisms. Children infected with *S. dysenteriae* serotype 1 are at least twice as likely to develop bacteremia as are those infected with other serotypes. Overall, the bacteremia-associated mortality rate is almost 50%, although for *S. dysenteriae,* the mortality rate is 85%. Individuals at highest risk of dying include infants in the first year of life and children who are not breast-fed, are malnourished, or are afebrile. Patients with AIDS who develop *Shigella* infection may become bacteremic. Extraintestinal localization of infection during bacteremia is rare. The bacteriology of the bronchopneumonia that is common among very ill children has not been well defined. Evidence obtained at autopsy suggests that the pneumonia often is caused by pathogens other than *Shigella.*

Focal nonbacteremic extraintestinal shigellosis occurs rarely. Vaginitis with a bloody discharge with or without associated diarrhea is associated more commonly with *S. flexneri* than with other serogroups. In some girls, symptoms last for months if no therapy or inadequate therapy is given. Keratitis, conjunctivitis, iritis, and iridocyclitis are other rare complications of shigellosis in young children. Eye involvement may occur without diarrhea. Patients positive for HLA-B27 are at risk of developing reactive arthritis, or Reiter syndrome (i.e., arthritis, urethritis, conjunctivitis), after a bout of shigellosis.

The mortality rate of isolated enteric infection is well below 1% in industrialized societies. In preindustrial societies, however, 10% to 30% of children with severe dysentery die. Although complications have been reported most commonly in patients infected with *S. dysenteriae* type 1, infection with any species of *Shigella* may be fatal.

DIAGNOSIS

Although stool culture is the usual basis for diagnosis, many *Shigella* infections are not detected with current methods. Adult volunteer studies have shown that even daily stool cultures fail to yield the organism in approximately 20% of ill patients who have ingested shigellae. Optimal recovery of shigellae from stool or rectal swab specimens is achieved by promptly inoculating selective and nonselective media. Serotype-related differences in yield with common media exist. *S. dysenteriae* serotype 1, unlike other shigellae, is isolated more consistently on MacConkey media than on *Salmonella-Shigella* agar. Complete identification of shigellae depends on biochemical and serologic criteria. Because almost all *Shigella* species have O antigens related to common *E. coli* O antigens, serology alone is inadequate to define *Shigella*.

Ancillary laboratory studies sometimes are helpful in making a presumptive diagnosis before culture results are available. The fecal leukocyte examination commonly is positive in children with bacillary dysentery. Blood counts often show leukocytosis with a left shift; approximately one-third of the children have more than 25% band forms. Leukemoid reactions with leukocyte counts greater than 50,000 occurred in as many as 10% of the patients in some series. *S. dysenteriae* serotype 1 characteristically is associated with higher leukocyte counts than are other serotypes of *Shigella*. Cerebrospinal fluid of children who have seizures usually is normal, although a few children have mild lymphocytic pleocytosis.

More recently developed molecular methods may help to improve the speed, sensitivity, and specificity of diagnosis. These methods include pulsed-field gel electrophoresis, plasmid analysis by polymerase chain reaction, and enzyme-linked immunosorbent assay.

The clinical picture of colitis can be caused by shigellae and by enteroinvasive *E. coli*, Shiga toxin-producing *E. coli* (STEC) (e.g., *E. coli* O157:H7), *Salmonella*, *Campylobacter jejuni*, *Yersinia enterocolitica*, *Clostridium difficile*, *Entamoeba histolytica*, and inflammatory bowel disease. Establishing definitive diagnosis of these illnesses on presentation is difficult, although differential points may be present in some cases. Epidemiologic evidence of person-to-person spread suggests shigellosis or STEC. Convulsions occur commonly with *Shigella* but are uncommon occurrences with the other forms of colitis. Bloody diarrhea in the first few months of life is more likely to be caused by *Salmonella* than by *Shigella*. A history of antibiotic use (particularly clindamycin or ampicillin) suggests the presence of *C. difficile*. A negative fecal leukocyte examination may suggest the presence of *E. histolytica*, particularly if the patient is afebrile and has a history of foreign travel; the fecal leukocyte examination often is positive with the other illnesses included in the differential diagnosis. Afebrile hemorrhagic colitis suggest STEC infection. Negative study results may suggest enteroinvasive *E. coli*, particularly if nonmotile, lysine decarboxylase-negative *E. coli* organisms are isolated. The differentiation of *Shigella* from other causes of watery diarrhea may not be possible on presentation if the patient is afebrile and has negative study results for fecal blood and fecal leukocytes.

TREATMENT

Antibiotics have a major role in the management of bacillary dysentery. Shigellosis should be treated routinely with antibiotics. Treatment of shigellosis by appropriate agents has proven efficacious in shortening the duration of fever, diarrhea, and toxemia and may reduce the risk of development of lethal complications. Whether treatment prevents hemolysis or HUS is not known. The excretion of the pathogen in stools is shortened significantly, thus reducing the spread of the infection. The major disadvantages associated with treatment are cost, drug toxicity, and selection of resistant organisms. Plasmids commonly carry the genes for resistance to multiple antibiotics. Thus, selective pressure of a single antibiotic may allow a strain to emerge that is resistant to many drugs. Recently, plasmid-encoded extended-spectrum beta-lactamase in *Shigella* species has been reported.

The choice of drugs for eradicating shigellosis is problematic. The emergence of resistant shigellae has been a recurring theme since the late 1950s. High levels of resistance to ampicillin, trimethoprim-sulfamethoxazole (TMP-SMX), chloramphenicol, and tetracycline have been reported worldwide. Local resistance patterns dictate the choice of empiric therapy. Susceptibility data may differ dramatically in cities separated by a short distance. Furthermore, *in vitro* susceptibility does not always predict clinical efficacy: for example, oral gentamicin is poor therapy despite having good *in vitro* susceptibility. Because of year-to-year fluctuations, continuous surveillance is necessary. If the pathogen is sensitive to TMP-SMX and the child is treated with this agent, improvement is expected to occur within 1 or 2 days, although normal stools may not be seen for as long as 9 days. This response appears to be better than that seen in patients infected with an ampicillin-sensitive *Shigella* infection treated with ampicillin, who typically remain ill for several days despite receiving therapy. Patients with *S. dysenteriae* serotype 1 infection respond more slowly to antibiotic therapy than do others with bacillary dysentery.

A third-generation cephalosporin currently may be the best empiric choice for treating suspected shigellosis of unknown susceptibility. Both oral cefixime, where available, and parenteral ceftriaxone are efficacious. One study suggests that azithromycin is at least equivalent (and probably superior) to cefixime for treating severe dysenteric illness. Pivmecillinam, where available, also is an acceptable alternate drug. Nalidixic acid usually is effective in treating infections caused by *Shigella* strains that are resistant to ampicillin and TMP-SMX. However, resistance to nalidixic acid usually becomes prevalent within a few years of the drug's introduction into a community for treatment of shigellosis. The rate of clinical cure associated with the use of nalidixic acid is equivalent to that achieved with ampicillin, although eradication of *Shigella* from the stool may take longer. The newer quinolones have been used successfully in the treatment of shigellosis in adults and children. Although resistance to fluoroquinolones rarely has been reported, these drugs often are recommended as empiric therapy in areas with high resistance to *Shigella*. A randomized trial comparing ciprofloxacin and pivmecillinam for childhood shigellosis showed that a 5-day course of ciprofloxacin is effective and safe for multiresistant childhood shigellosis.

The timing of therapy is important. If a strong clinical suspicion of shigellosis exists, the patient should be started empirically on antibiotics before culture results become available. The patient who has high fever, severe abdominal pain, small and frequent stools with blood and mucus, and a positive fecal leukocyte examination should be treated without delay. If an outbreak of one of the other organisms known to cause these symptoms is in progress, it may be reasonable to aim therapy at that pathogen. In areas where *Campylobacter* infection is a particularly common occurrence, starting therapy directed at both *Shigella* and *Campylobacter* may be advisable for dysenteric illness. If *Shigella* was not suspected initially because the patient had a watery diarrhea syndrome without colitis, therapy should be started after cultures suggest that *Shigella* is the likely cause.

The duration of therapy required for shigellosis is shorter than that for many other common infections. Although single-dose regimens are almost as effective as are multiple-dose regimens in relieving symptoms in older children, single doses are less effective in clearing the feces of the organism. Because one of the goals of therapy is the prevention of intrafamilial spread, multiple doses typically are used. This strategy is debatable in developing nations, where asymptomatic excretion is a common finding, and eradication of a single focus of infection may have less effect on secondary cases. Whether the choice of antibiotics is ampicillin, TMP-SMX, a third-generation cephalosporin, nalidixic acid, ciprofloxacin, or azithromycin, a 5-day course of therapy is recommended.

Antimotility agents, such as diphenoxylate hydrochloride with atropine (Lomotil), should be avoided in children with shigellosis. These agents appear to prolong the duration of fever and excretion of the organism. Although data on adults suggest that loperamide combined with an appropriate antimicrobial treatment is useful, no studies in children have been reported.

PREVENTION

After many years of study and numerous clinical studies, there are no licensed vaccines for shigellosis. A recent small study showed that two experimental *Shigella* conjugate vaccines (for *S. flexneri* and *S. sonnei*) were safe and immunogenic in 1- to 4-year-old children. Because day-care centers represent a major source of *Shigella* infection in young children in the United States, attention given to basic infection control measures should be encouraged. These measures typically include emphasis on hand washing, exclusion of sick children, and exclusion of food preparers from diaper-changing duty. Parents also should be instructed about the importance of hand washing. In developing nations, the best means of preventing infection of the young child appears to be prolonged breast-feeding. Whether breast-feeding decreases shigellosis by preventing the consumption of contaminated food, by providing secretory IgA and lactoferrin and thus impairing bacterial virulence, by loading the gut with receptor glycolipids that bind Shiga toxin, or by nonspecific gut flora-modifying factors remains uncertain.

Suggested Readings

Ahmed F, Ansaruzzaman M, Haque E, et al. Epidemiology of post-shigellosis persistent diarrhea in young children. *Pediatr Infect Dis J* 2001;20:525.

Ashkenazi S, Dinari G, Zevulunov A, et al. Convulsions in childhood shigellosis: clinical and laboratory features in 153 children. *Am J Dis Child* 1987;141:208.

Basualdo W, Arbo A. Randomized comparison of azithromycin versus cefixime for treatment of shigellosis in children. *Pediatr Infect Dis J* 2003;22:374.

Bennish ML. Potentially lethal complications of shigellosis. *Rev Infect Dis* 1991;13:319.

Blocker A, Jouihri N, Larquet E, et al. Structure and composition of the *Shigella flexneri* "needle complex," a part of its type III secretion. *Mol Microbiol* 2001;39:652.

Gruenheid S, Finlay BB. Microbial pathogenesis and cytoskeletal function. *Nature* 2003;422:775.

Kotloff KL, Winickoff JP, Ivanoff B, et al. Global burden of *Shigella* infections: implications for vaccine development and implementation of control strategies. *Bull World Health Organ* 1999;77:651.

Munoz C, Baqar S, Van de Verg L, et al. Characteristics of *Shigella sonnei* infection of volunteers: signs, symptoms, immune responses, changes in selected cytokines and acute-phase substances. *Am J Trop Med Hyg* 1995;53:47.

Passwell JH, Ashkenazi S, Harlev E, et al. Israel *Shigella* Study Group: safety and immunogenicity of *Shigella sonnei*-CRM9 and *Shigella flexneri* type 2a-rEPAsucc conjugate vaccines in one- to four-year-old children. *Pediatr Infect Dis J* 2003;22:701.

Prado V, Lagos R, Nataro JP, et al. Population-based study of the incidence of *Shigella* diarrhea and causative serotypes in Santiago, Chile. *Pediatr Infect Dis J* 1999;18:500.

Salam MA, Bennish ML. Antimicrobial therapy for shigellosis. *Rev Infect Dis* 1991;13:332.

Sansonetti P. Host-pathogen interactions: the seduction of molecular cross talk. *Gut* 2002;50:112.

Speelman P, Kabir I, Islam M. Distribution and spread of colonic lesions in shigellosis: a colonoscopic study. *J Infect* 1984;150:899.

Struelens MJ, Patte D, Kabir I, et al. *Shigella* septicemia: prevalence, presentation, risk factors and outcome. *J Infect Dis* 1985;152:784.

Zimbabwe, Bangladesh, South Africa (Zimbasa) Dysentery Study Group. Multicenter, randomized, double blind clinical trial of short course versus standard course oral ciprofloxacin for *Shigella dysenteriae* type 1 dysentery in children. *Pediatr Infect Dis J* 2002;21:1136.

CHAPTER 175 ■ STAPHYLOCOCCAL INFECTIONS

CHRISTIAN C. PATRICK, UMBEREEN S. NEHAL, AND RALPH D. FEIGIN

Staphylococci are ubiquitous bacteria that colonize and are pathogenic for humans and animals. *Staphylococcus aureus* is the predominant pathogen causing a variety of infections. Coagulase-negative staphylococci (CoNS) are pathogens in neonates, compromised hosts, and patients with foreign bodies, and they may cause urinary tract infection in physiologically normal hosts.

MICROBIOLOGY

Staphylococci are gram-positive, nonmotile, aerobic, or facultative anaerobic bacteria. They are not fastidious and grow well on ordinary media. All members are catalase-positive. Staphylococci are categorized by their ability to produce coagulase; *S. aureus* is coagulase-positive. Currently, 29 species are CoNS. *S. aureus* and some CoNS produce a capsule for which the clinical importance is unclear, but it is the basis of a vaccine strategy currently being tested. *S. aureus* produces a unique cell wall

protein, protein A, that possesses antiphagocytic properties and has a high affinity for the Fc portion of certain immunoglobulin subclasses.

Coagulase-positive staphylococci elaborate numerous extracellular toxins that generally are thought to be responsible for the virulence of these organisms. The clinically important staphylococcal extracellular products include the following: alpha-, beta-, and delta-hemolysins; coagulases; leukocidin; hyaluronidase; staphylokinase; the epidermolytic toxins; erythrogenic toxins; toxic shock syndrome (TSS) toxin 1 (TSS-1); and enterotoxins.

EPIDEMIOLOGY

Staphylococci are widely distributed in nature and are common inhabitants of the normal human flora. *S. aureus* is found in the nares, fingernails, and, occasionally, skin. Nasal colonization is a risk factor for development of infection in hospitalized patients. Neonates become colonized early in life. *S. aureus* is carried by 20% to 40% of adults; 30% are long-term carriers.

Staphylococci usually are tolerated by the human body; they cause localized disease (e.g., in patients with open wounds or those with an intravenous catheter) or systemic infections in immunocompromised individuals (e.g., patients who are immunosuppressed or have diabetes mellitus). Viral respiratory infection may alter the natural host defense and allow the development of staphylococcal pneumonia. Recurrent staphylococcal infections can be caused by autoinfection from an asymptomatic carrier state.

Staphylococcal infections can occur as an epidemic or as a sporadic event. Person-to-person spread (particularly via the hands) appears to be the most common form of transmission, although airborne transmission can occur. Contact with contaminated objects also may spread infection.

PATHOGENESIS

The pathologic effects on *S. aureus* can be attributed to direct tissue invasion or toxin production and liberation. Colonization factors allow *S. aureus* to adhere to host fibrinogen, fibronectin, laminin, collagen, and other surface-binding proteins. Binding to fibrinogen also allows *S. aureus* to bind to indwelling foreign bodies. Evasion of host defenses can be caused by staphylococcal protein A, teichoic acid, and, rarely, a capsule.

Some enzymes and toxins produced by *S. aureus* are known virulence factors. Enzymes involved in the pathogenesis include catalase, hyaluronidase, beta-lactamase, lipase, and fatty acid–modifying enzyme. Hyaluronidase or spreading factor facilitates spread of infection in the early stages. beta-Lactamase inactivates a class of antibiotics. Catalase converts hydrogen peroxide (H_2O_2) to water and oxygen, reducing H_2O_2 as a host defense mediator in phagocytosis. Lipase facilitates invasion.

S. aureus produces a variety of toxins, five of which are membrane-damaging toxins (alpha, beta, delta, and the leukocidins). Other toxins include the enterotoxins A through E, epidermolytic toxins A and B, and TSS–1. Leukocidins have several biologic effects, but their foremost action is the lysis of macrophages. The enterotoxins cause foodborne diseases; however, enterotoxins B and C are associated with TSS. The epidermolytic toxins cause scalded skin syndrome and divide the epidermis at the stratum granulosum layer. Most cases of TSS are associated with TSS-1.

The polymorphonuclear leukocyte appears to be the most important line of defense after the skin barrier has been breached. Inherited or acquired defects in chemotaxis, opsonization, or intracellular killing predispose to development of staphylococcal infection, and the incidence of such infections is highest in patients with defects in this area of host defense. Granulocytopenia of any origin predisposes to development of infection with endogenous bacteria, including staphylococci.

PATHOLOGY

The formation of an abscess is characteristic of staphylococcal infections in humans, and the skin is the usual portal of entry. Tissue necrosis of the lesion occurs. Invasion and spread of the organism are promoted by increased connective tissue permeability secondary to local multiplication and the production of enzymes. Liquefaction necrosis occurs rapidly, with a fibrin wall surrounding a center of organisms and leukocytes. Thrombosis of blood vessels with formation of fibrin clots can occur. Trauma that breaks the fibroelastic barrier may spread the infection, often initiating bacteremia with spread to bones, joints, heart valves, and so forth.

CLINICAL MANIFESTATIONS

The clinical manifestations vary with the portal of entry of the organism and the immune status and general health of the patients. *S. aureus* infections of the skin are among the most common bacterial infections. Lesions include impetigo, bullous impetigo, folliculitis, furuncles (i.e., boils), carbuncles, paronychia, cellulitis, ecthyma, staphylococcal scalded skin syndrome, staphylococcal scarlatiniform eruption, and TSS. These last three are toxin-mediated.

Musculoskeletal infections commonly are caused by *S. aureus*, the most frequent cause of acute osteomyelitis and discitis. In most cases, the bacteria reach the bone by hematogenous spread from a skin lesion, but they also can do so from a contiguous focus of infection. The organism usually localizes in the metaphyseal end of a long bone. The clinical syndrome may be preceded by trauma, pyoderma, or other antecedent infection. Osteomyelitis is associated with irritability, fever, anorexia, vomiting, local warmth, and point tenderness.

Staphylococcal bacteremia usually occurs with a focus of infection. Sources of bacteremia vary and often are obscure, but the skin, respiratory tract, or intravenous access should be considered. Bacteremia may have an acute onset or may be slowly progressive, with shaking chills, fever, and metastatic abscess in organs such as the lung, bone, joints, kidneys, heart, brain, or deep tissues.

Pyarthrosis also is caused frequently by *S. aureus* and most commonly involves the hip, knee, ankle, and elbow. Muscle abscesses usually present with a subacute onset of moderate muscle pain, followed by fever. An associated increase in serum muscle enzymes without evidence of septicemia occurs. These muscle abscesses are seen more often in tropical areas (i.e., tropical pyomyositis) but have been described in the United States with increased frequency in recent years.

Peritonsillar abscess, purulent conjunctivitis, otitis media, retropharyngeal abscess, sinusitis, acute mastoiditis, bacterial tracheitis, and parotitis can be caused by *S. aureus* either alone or with other bacteria. Staphylococcal pneumonia must occur as a primary infection or secondary to a viral infection. This illness begins as an upper respiratory tract infection with fever, nasal discharge, cough, and anorexia, with progression to symptoms and signs of increasing cough, tachypnea, dyspnea, and retractions. Radiographic findings associated with staphylococcal pneumonia include pneumatocele, empyema, pneumothorax, abscesses, and consolidation. Other head and neck infections caused by *S. aureus* include thyroiditis, cervical adenitis, orbital cellulitis, blepharitis, and hordeolum.

Visceral findings of staphylococcal infections can include hepatic, renal, perinephric, spleen, or pancreas abscesses. These abscesses can be difficult to diagnose if symptoms are nonspecific. Diffuse proliferative glomerulonephritis is a renal manifestation of staphylococcal bacteremia that is not thought to be associated with actual bacterial seeding of the kidney.

Staphylococcal enterocolitis is food poisoning caused by ingestion of contaminated food. When left at room temperature, certain foods (e.g., dairy products, bakery products, meats) are fertile soil for the production of enterotoxins. The illness has a sudden onset, occurring 1 to 6 hours after ingestion of preformed toxin in contaminated food. The illness is manifested by profuse diarrhea, abdominal cramps, and nausea. Symptoms improve within 8 to 24 hours. Staphylococcal enterocolitis also can be caused by bacterial overgrowth in the bowel after undergoing antibiotic therapy. The symptoms are the same as those of food poisoning, with the addition of fever.

Central nervous system (CNS) infections that may be caused by *S. aureus* include meningitis, brain subdural-epidural abscesses, and cerebral venous thrombosis. Meningitis caused by *S. aureus* is a rare occurrence and generally results from hematogenous spread after surgery in patients with a foreign body, but it can occur by contiguous extension of otitis media, sinusitis, mastoiditis, or osteomyelitis of the skull and vertebrae.

Cardiovascular infections include endocarditis, pericarditis, and septic thromboses. Endocarditis is manifested by high fever, progressive anemia, and metastatic abscesses and has a high mortality rate.

S. aureus is the second most frequent cause of infections in foreign body infections after *Staphylococcus epidermidis,* attributable to such items as central venous catheters, CNS shunts, and peritoneal dialysis catheters. These infections often require removal of the foreign body. Infection by *S. aureus* in neonates includes omphalitis, breast abscess, parotitis, and cervical adenitis.

COMMUNITY-ACQUIRED METHICILLIN-RESISTANT *STAPHYLOCOCCUS AUREUS*

Methicillin-resistant *S. aureus* (MRSA) first was identified as a nosocomial pathogen. However, in recent years, strains of MRSA have emerged as distinct community-acquired organisms (CA-MRSA) with increasing prevalence. MRSA is considered community acquired if a positive culture is isolated from an outpatient or within 72 hours of hospitalization, and if risk factors for nosocomial MRSA are absent. These risk factors include a history of (a) frequent or recent hospitalization or surgery, (b) dialysis, (c) indwelling device or catheter, or (d) residence in a long-term facility. Accurate identification of CA-MRSA is hindered by inconsistent awareness of among health care providers, varying definitions, and availability of historical data.

CA-MRSA initially was described in the 1980s but has been increasingly identified, especially in the United States. At a Chicago hospital, CA-MRSA increased about 25-fold in a 5-year period, whereas other, more recent studies estimate a more modest increase. Polymerase chain reaction analysis of CA-MRSA reveals a unique gene, *SCCmec IV,* which codes for its methicillin resistance. It differs from the *SCCmec* types I–III found in nosocomial MRSA and suggests development of a novel clone rather than extension of nosocomial MRSA to the community. Although nosocomial MRSA often is multidrug resistant, most non-beta-lactam antibiotics remain effective against CA-MRSA. Studies have shown that most CA-MRSA is susceptible to clindamycin, trimethoprim-sulfamethoxazole, gentamicin, and vancomycin. Both nosocomial MRSA and CA-MRSA have a high resistance to erythromycin. However, when the D-test is performed on erythromycin-resistant, clindamycin-sensitive CA-MRSA, inducible clindamycin resistance is rare.

The demographics and clinical manifestations of CA-MRSA resemble those of community-acquired methicillin-sensitive *S. aureus* (CA-MSSA). No risk factors predisposing to CA-MRSA have been identified in children, and asymptomatic carriage of CA-MRSA occurs among healthy children. Transmission of CA-MRSA has been reported in day-care centers, among military recruits, and via contact sports. Skin and soft tissue are predominant sites of infection for both community-acquired types. Although one study found that CA-MRSA was associated with longer hospital stays than was CA-MSSA, it demonstrated no differences in presence or length of bacteremia, days in an intensive care unit, complication rates, or surgical intervention between the two.

Several case series, however, have described serious consequences from CA-MRSA and CA-MSSA. In 1999, the Centers for Disease Control and Prevention reported the deaths from CA-MRSA of four children who had been treated with cephalosporins at presentation. Most recently, a case series from Houston described severe CA-MRSA and CA-MSSA sepsis in 14 previously healthy adolescents that resulted in three deaths. These children presented with joint involvement and pulmonary disease. Surprisingly, the *S. aureus* clones isolated were genetically similar to those prevalent in that community. Further research is needed to elucidate risk factors for and indicators of serious disease from community-acquired *S. aureus*.

CA-MRSA presents a new challenge to community pediatricians who must treat presumed staphylococcal infections empirically. Maintaining a suspicion for CA-MRSA renders clindamycin, instead of cephalosporins, the preferred empiric therapy. In light of the high resistance to erythromycin among CA-MRSA, however, it is important for clinicians to obtain a culture, request a D-test, and adjust antimicrobial therapy accordingly. Vigilant monitoring for signs of multiorgan disease and sepsis is vital to prevent serious complications from community-acquired *S. aureus* strains.

DIAGNOSIS

A presumptive diagnosis of staphylococcal infection can be obtained by identifying gram-positive cocci in clusters on a Gram stain of clinical material (e.g., aspirate of pus, sputum, and blood). Joint fluid or bone aspirates may be obtained in an effort to discern the cause of septic arthritis or osteomyelitis. A definitive diagnosis depends on isolation of the organism on liquid or solid medium from an otherwise sterile site or aspiration from a wound or lesion. At least two blood cultures should be obtained. When routine culture and sensitivity results show erythromycin-resistant and clindamycin-susceptible isolates, a D-test should be performed to evaluate inducible clindamycin resistance.

Serologic assays used to evaluate the host antibody response to multiple staphylococcal antigens have promise but are not widely available. The antigens used are teichoic acid, collagen-binding protein, and alpha-toxin. The sensitivity of each assay depends on the type of disease. Enzyme-linked immunosorbent assay, gel diffusion, and counterimmunoelectrophoresis methods for the detection of antibodies to teichoic acid have been shown to be highly specific for detection of staphylococcal infection. More than 50% of patients with bacteremia, 70% with staphylococcal osteomyelitis, and 90% with staphylococcal endocarditis have detectable antibodies. These antibodies are not detected in persons without staphylococcal disease or in those with superficial staphylococcal infections. Antibodies may be detected in some patients who do not have bacteremia but who do have staphylococcal osteomyelitis, septic arthritis, and pneumonia.

The diagnosis of staphylococcal food poisoning usually is made on a clinical basis. Suspicion of the presence of disease can be substantiated by Gram stain and culture of the presumed food source and by demonstration of toxin-producing staphylococci.

TREATMENT

The therapy for staphylococcal infections depends on the general health and immune status of the patient, the site of infection, and the results of antimicrobial susceptibility testing. Focal infections with collections of purulent material require adequate drainage. Serious staphylococcal infections require systemic bactericidal antibiotics. Because staphylococcal infections can persist and recur, prolonged antibiotic therapy may be required.

Penicillin G (100,000 to 250,000 U/kg/day intravenously every 4 hours) is active against penicillin-susceptible, non–penicillinase-producing staphylococci and is the treatment of choice. However, approximately 90% of community- and hospital-acquired staphylococci are resistant to penicillin.

For organisms resistant to penicillin, the semisynthetic penicillins, such as methicillin, nafcillin, or oxacillin, and for oral use, cloxacillin or dicloxacillin, are administered.

MRSA is widespread, necessitating the use of vancomycin. Vancomycin (40 to 60 mg/kg/day intravenously every 6 hours) is the drug of choice for treating organisms resistant to penicillin or to penicillin derivations and is recommended for treating severe infections empirically in areas with high levels of MRSA before antimicrobial susceptibility test results are known.

Patients who are allergic to penicillin should be treated with alternative antibiotics to which *S. aureus* may be susceptible. They may include clindamycin, trimethoprim-sulfamethoxazole, and meropenem. Sensitivity testing of isolates is imperative because of the resistance that both community- and hospital-acquired *S. aureus* may have to penicillin and semisynthetic penicillin derivatives.

The antimicrobial armamentarium for the treatment of MRSA has been expanded. Linezolid has demonstrated significant activity against MRSA. It is available in both an oral and an intravenous formulation. Quinupristin-dalfopristin is a newer injectable streptogramin antibiotic combination that has been found effective in the treatment of MRSA. Both these agents should be restricted to specific situations for which other alternatives are not feasible. Both these newer agents also have high costs.

In July 2002, the first documented case of infection caused by vancomycin-resistant *S. aureus* in the United States was reported. This organism was susceptible to chloramphenicol, minocycline, linezolid, trimethoprim-sulfamethoxazole, and quinupristin-dalfopristin.

Alternative therapy for skin, soft tissue, bone, and joint infection is clindamycin. In treating endocarditis, brain abscess, or meningitis caused by *S. aureus*, vancomycin can be used, but serum antibiotic levels should be monitored.

COMPLICATIONS

Staphylococcal bacteremia may be complicated by disseminated intravascular coagulation and thrombocytopenia. Staphylococcal osteomyelitis can lead to pyogenic arthritis, sterile arthritis, subperiosteal abscesses, or subcutaneous abscesses. Untreated staphylococcal osteomyelitis may be complicated by the formation of a Brodie abscess. This low-grade infection, which produces a necrotic core surrounded by granulation tissue, can persist for years. Staphylococcal endocarditis can lead to septic pulmonary emboli if the infection is right-sided. Infection in the nasolabial areas of the face may be associated with cavernous sinus thrombosis and infection. Staphylococcal pneumonia can be complicated by congestive heart failure, fibrothorax secondary to inadequate drainage of an empyema, bronchopleural fistulas with subsequent pneumothorax, abscess formation, or empyema. Staphylococcal enterocolitis can result in shock and dehydration caused by excessive fluid loss.

PREVENTION

The possibility of developing a vaccine against *S. aureus* appears realistic. Capsular polysaccharide conjugate vaccines promote antibody production in humans, thus facilitating opsonophagocytosis.

Preventing staphylococcal infections is difficult because of the organism's ubiquitous nature. However, because most infections are caused by direct contact from a hospital staff member to a patient or from one patient to another, good personal hygiene and hand washing with an effective detergent containing hexachlorophene, chlorhexidine, or an iodophor are effective preventive measures. Mupirocin antibiotic ointment has been used to eradicate the nasal carriage state.

Food poisoning can be prevented by excluding persons with staphylococcal infections from the preparation and handling of food. Optimal cooking and refrigeration of meat, dairy products, and bakery goods help to prevent the disease.

INFECTIONS CAUSED BY COAGULASE-NEGATIVE STAPHYLOCOCCI

Historically, CoNS have been regarded as harmless, commensal saprophytes, but certain species now are considered pathogens and are implicated in a wide range of infections, particularly among immunocompromised patients and those with a foreign body. *S. epidermidis* is the prominent species in infections. New epidemiologic and molecular techniques can be useful to identify strain characteristics in nosocomial outbreaks of disease.

CoNS have been implicated in a variety of clinical infections. They are a primary cause of nosocomial bacteremia in neonates and immunocompromised patients who have cancer or have undergone a bone marrow transplant. CoNS also are the major pathogens in patients with infected central venous catheters, CNS shunts, or peritoneal dialysis catheters. Two nonnosocomial infections caused by CoNS are recognized: *S. epidermidis* can cause native valve endocarditis, and *S. saprophyticus* causes urinary tract infections in young, sexually active women.

CoNS have few virulence factors. Certain species can adhere to catheters and secrete a slime substance or glycocalyx that coats the staphylococci, thus allowing them to evade their host's defenses. Numerous exotoxins are produced by CoNS. Extracellular metalloprotease has elastase activity. A cysteine protease degrades human secretory immunoglobulin A, immunoglobulin M, serum albumin, fibrinogen, and fibronectin. An extracellular serine protease is involved in epidermin processing. Lipases have been postulated to cause skin colonization. Delta-toxin, an enteropathogenic toxin, has been associated with necrotizing enterocolitis in infants. Peptidoglycan and teichoic acid of *S. epidermidis* stimulates human monocytes to release tumor necrosis factor-alpha, and interleukins-1 and 6.

A basic difficulty in interpreting clinical studies of CoNS exists because of the different criteria used to define a clinically significant culture. The Committee on Infectious Diseases of the American Academy of Pediatrics has suggested the following considerations to distinguish pathogenic, rather than contaminant, CoNS: (a) growth within 24 hours, (b) multiple positive blood cultures, (c) symptoms of infection in the patient, (d) presence of an intravascular catheter for 3 days or more, and (e) multidrug resistance of the CoNS strain.

Clinical presentation of infections caused by CoNS generally are more indolent and may present with a subacute or chronic course. CoNS now are the single most frequent cause of late-onset septicemia among premature infants, especially low-birth-weight infants. These organisms also are a cause of neonatal meningitis and have been implicated as a cause of necrotizing enterocolitis.

CoNS are a common cause of infection in patients with leukemia and lymphoma and have become the primary pathogen causing bacteremia in hematopoietic stem cell transplant recipients (usually during periods of agranulocytosis before marrow engraftment). Infections associated with central venous catheters are caused primarily by CoNS, and these organisms also cause infections in patients with peripheral catheters composed of steel and polyethylene.

CoNS account for 60% to 75% of all bacterial courses of shunt infections. These shunts previously were infected by organisms from the skin of the patients at the time the catheters were inserted. Seventy percent of ventriculoperitoneal shunt infections occur within 2 months of placement of the shunt. CoNS also are common causes of infection of peritoneal dialysis catheters and of prosthetic heart valves and other indwelling prosthetic devices. *S. saprophyticus* is the most common CoNS cause of urinary tract infections, which occur predominantly in young, healthy, sexually active women.

Antibiotic therapy against CoNS should be directed by susceptibility testing because these organisms often are resistant. Cross-resistance occurs between the semisynthetic penicillinase-resistant penicillins and the cephalosporins; as a rule, methicillin resistance can be interpreted as resistance to all beta-lactam antibiotics. Vancomycin is the drug of choice for organisms resistant to penicillinase-resistant penicillin and also is recommended for empiric treatment of severe infections. Gentamicin and rifampin have been shown to be synergistic with vancomycin against methicillin-resistant CoNS.

Vancomycin and rifampin comprise the mainstay of therapy for persistent foreign body infections. Clindamycin and rifampin also may be useful in some cases. Quinupristin-dalfopristin and linezolid may be therapeutic options for vancomycin-intermediate susceptible isolates.

Removal of indwelling catheters that are infected or of prosthetic devices may be required to eradicate the source of infection. Standard therapy for ventriculoperitoneal shunt infections had included removal of the shunt system coupled with systemic administration of antibiotics. More recent studies suggest that these infections may be treated successfully by externalization of the peritoneal shunt and administration of both intraventricular and systemic antibiotics.

TOXIC SHOCK SYNDROME

TSS is an uncommon but potentially devastating illness. TSS is an acute febrile illness with an erythroderma rash and multisystem involvement with a high complication rate.

Etiology

TSS-1, produced by *S. aureus*, is a significant mediator of the pathogenicity of TSS. Other mediators include enterotoxins B and C. These toxins are thought to act as superantigens that stimulate the host response. Although TSS is caused mainly by *S. aureus*, group A, beta-hemolytic streptococci can produce a similar syndrome.

Epidemiology

TSS was described first in 1978. In 1980, it was recognized with increasing frequency in young, menstruating women using a particular brand of tampons. TSS can occur at any age but has been recognized more frequently in teenage and young women. Individuals with focal infection caused by *S. aureus*, which can be occult, are at risk.

Pathology

The most striking finding is the lack of inflammation. Skin biopsies reveal mild lymphocytic dermal perivasculitis and a subepidermal cleavage plane. Evidence of a shock state in the kidneys, liver, and lungs has been noted.

Clinical Manifestations

Patients with TSS usually describe a prodrome of nausea and vomiting, sore throat, profuse watery diarrhea, and myalgia. Patients typically have a prominent fever (38.8°C or greater), hypertension, and a diffuse, sunburn-like rash. The erythroderma is most prominent on the trunk and usually is not pruritic. Conjunctival hyperemia without purulent exudate and pharyngeal hyperemia with a strawberry tongue are common findings. Hypotension leads to multiple organ system dysfunction. Petechiae, vesicles, or bullae are uncommon findings. The Nikolsky sign usually is negative. Desquamation of the palms, soles, fingers, and toes occurs 2 to 4 weeks after the onset of the illness.

Diagnosis

The diagnosis of TSS should be considered when a patient meets the definition of TSS, which includes all the major criteria: (a) fever of 38.8°C or higher, (b) rash or erythroderma with subsequent desquamation, and (c) hypertension. Minor criteria require any three of the following: (a) mucous membrane inflammation (vaginal, oropharyngeal, or conjunctival hyperemia), (b) gastrointestinal abnormalities (vomiting or diarrhea), (c) muscle abnormalities (elevated creatine kinase, severe myalgia), (d) CNS abnormalities (obtundation, coma, no focal findings), (e) hepatic abnormalities (elevated bilirubin or transaminases twice the upper limit for age), (f) renal abnormalities (urinalysis with five or more white blood cells per high-power field or blood urea nitrogen or serum creatinine greater than twice the upper limit for age), and (g) hematologic abnormalities (platelet count of less than 100,000/μL). Additionally, culture results must be negative for other causes except for *S. aureus* and negative serologic test results for Rocky Mountain spotted fever, leptospirosis, and measles, as indicated. A focus of *S. aureus* infection should be sought aggressively.

The differential diagnosis of TSS is lengthy but includes sepsis, septic shock (e.g., meningococcemia), leptospirosis, Rocky Mountain spotted fever, scarlatiniform eruptions, ehrlichiosis, staphylococcal scalded skin syndrome, severe streptococcal infections, Kawasaki disease, urinary tract infections, viral syndromes, toxin-induced diarrhea, and drug reactions.

Treatment

Prompt intervention is mandatory for shock and multiorgan involvement. Drainage of the infected sites or removal of a potentially infectious medical device is imperative. Appropriate antibiotics, usually a penicillinase-resistant penicillin such as nafcillin, should be administered. Clindamycin also may be given to inhibit staphylococcal protein synthesis and thus toxin production. In severe cases, intravenous immunoglobulin may be administered to provide antitoxin antibodies, methylprednisolone may be given to suppress cytokine production, or both intravenous immunoglobulin and methylprednisolone may be administered.

Acknowledgments

This work is supported by National Cancer Institute Center Support Grant P30 CA 21765 and by the American Lebanese Syrian Associated Charities.

Suggested Readings

Ayliffe GA. The progressive intercontinental spread of methicillin-resistant *Staphylococcus aureus. Clin Infect Dis* 1997;24(suppl 1):S74.

Centers for Disease Control and Prevention. Four pediatric deaths from community-acquired methicillin-resistant *Staphylococcus aureus:* Minnesota and North Dakota, 1997–1999. *JAMA* 1999;282:1123.

Chesney PJ, Davis JP. Toxic shock syndrome. In: Feigin RD, Cherry JD, Demmler, GJ, Kaplan, SL, eds. *Textbook of pediatric infectious diseases,* 5th ed. Philadelphia: WB Saunders, 2003:836.

Daum RS, Ito T, Hiramatsu K, et al. A novel methicillin-resistance cassette in community-acquired methicillin-resistant *Staphylococcus aureus* isolates of diverse genetic backgrounds. *J Infect Dis* 2002;186:1344.

Dietrich DW, Auld DB, Mermel LA. Community-acquired methicillin-resistant *Staphylococcus aureus* in southern New England children. *Pediatrics* 2004; 113:e347.

Fattom AI, Naso R. Staphylococcal vaccines: a realistic dream. *Ann Med* 1996; 28:43.

Gonzalez BE, Martinez-Aguilar G, Hulten KG, et al. Severe *Staphylococcus* sepsis in adolescents in the era of community-acquired methicillin resistant *Staphylococcus aureus. Pediatrics* 2005;115:642.

Herold BC, Immergluck LC, Maranan MC, et al. Community-acquired methicillin-resistant *Staphylococcus aureus* in children with no identified predisposing risk. *JAMA* 1998;279:593.

Hussain FM, Boyle-Vavra S, Daum RS. Community-acquired methicillin-resistant *Staphylococcus aureus* colonization in healthy children attending an outpatient pediatric clinic. *Pediatr Infect Dis J* 2001;20:763.

Kluytmans J, Van Belkum A, Verbrugh H. Nasal carriage of *Staphylococcus aureus:* epidemiology, underlying mechanisms, and associated risks. *Clin Microbiol Rev* 1997;10:505.

Martinez-Aguilar G, Hammerman WA, Mason EO Jr, Kaplan SL. Clindamycin treatment of invasive infections caused by community-acquired, methicillin-resistant and methicillin-susceptible *Staphylococcus aureus* in children. *Pediatr Infect Dis J* 2003;22:593.

Nakamura MM, Rohling KL, Shashaty M, et al. Prevalence of methicillin-resistant *Staphylococcus aureus* nasal carriage in the community pediatric population. *Pediatr Infect Dis J* 2000;21:917.

Rodriguez, C, Patrick CC. Coagulase-negative staphylococcal infections. In: Feigin RD, Cherry JD, Demmler, GJ, Kaplan, SL, eds. *Textbook of pediatric infectious diseases,* 5th ed. Philadelphia: WB Saunders, 2003:1129.

Rupp ME. Coagulase-negative staphylococcal infections: an update regarding recognition and management. *Curr Clin Top Infect Dis* 1997;17:51.

St. Geme JW III. *Staphylococcus epidermidis* and other coagulase-negative staphylococci. In: Long SS, Pickering LK, Prober CG, eds. *Principles and practice of pediatric infections diseases.* New York: Churchill Livingstone, 1997:793.

Sattler CA, Correa A. Coagulase-positive staphylococcal infections (*Staphylococcus aureus*) In: Feigin, RD, Cherry, JD, Demmler, GJ, Kaplan, SL. *Textbook of pediatric infectious diseases,* 5th ed. Philadelphia: WB Saunders, 2003:1099.

Sattler CA, Mason EO Jr, Kaplan SL. Prospective comparison of risk factors and demographic and clinical characteristics of community-acquired, methicillin-resistant versus methicillin-susceptible *Staphylococcus aureus* infection in children. *Pediatr Infect Dis J* 2003;22:593.

CHAPTER 176 ■ GROUP A STREPTOCOCCAL INFECTIONS

JULIA A. MCMILLAN AND RALPH D. FEIGIN

MICROBIOLOGY

Streptococcus pyogenes (group A streptococcus) is a gram-positive coccus that produces clear (beta) hemolysis on blood agar. This bacteriologic feature aids in the recognition and differentiation of *S. pyogenes* from viridans (alpha) streptococci and from nonhemolytic (gamma) streptococci. Selected strains of group A streptococci hemolyze slowly and produce a greenish hemolysis on the surface of blood agar plates, similar to that produced by viridans streptococci. These strains can be identified by their ability to produce clear hemolysis under anaerobic conditions.

Group A hemolytic streptococci can be differentiated from other hemolytic streptococci by laboratory identification of their group-specific cell wall carbohydrate. A commonly used office laboratory identification technique takes advantage of the finding that 95% of group A streptococci are unable to grow in the presence of bacitracin. Definitive identification of group A streptococci is established by the use of techniques that use group-specific antisera.

More than 60 types of group A streptococci have been identified on the basis of their serologically distinct surface proteins (i.e., M proteins). The M protein plays a role in the pathogenesis of infection caused by the group A streptococcus because it renders this organism resistant to phagocytosis.

Protruding from the surface of the group A streptococcal cell and into a hyaluronic capsule layer are hairlike fimbriae that are responsible for adhering group A streptococci to epithelial cells. These fimbriae contain lipoteichoic acid. The M protein also is associated with these fimbriae. Other surface proteins that have been identified are the T and R proteins, which bind nonspecifically to the Fc fragment of gamma globulins, and serum opacity reaction proteins. The specific function and precise location of each of these proteins on the surface of the organism have not been identified. However, evaluation of these characteristics has proven useful in the course of epidemiologic studies of streptococcal infections.

The carbohydrate substance that is responsible for group specificity is found in the cell wall. The group A carbohydrate is a polymer of rhamnose units with side chains of *N*-acetylglucosamine, which is responsible for its group specificity. The cell membrane lies within the cell wall and is composed primarily of lipoprotein complexes or lipid and protein. This membrane is the outer surface of the protoplasts or L-forms of streptococci, which lack cell walls and are resistant to penicillin and other cell wall–inhibiting antibiotics.

The group A streptococci release many biologically active extracellular products into surrounding media (Box 176.1). Streptolysin O (i.e., oxygen-labile hemolysin) and streptolysin S (i.e., oxygen-stable hemolysin) can injure cell membranes.

Streptolysin O is antigenic, but streptolysin S is not. Three erythrogenic or pyrogenic toxins may be elaborated. These substances, identified as A, B, or C, are similar to endotoxin in their ability to exhibit primary toxicity or a secondary toxicity that results from the acquisition of host hypersensitivity. Individual reports and local outbreaks beginning in the late 1980s of a toxic shock–like syndrome caused by streptococci are thought to be associated with the reappearance of strains making pyrogenic exotoxin A. Strains with the M protein types M_1 and M_3 also appear to be associated disproportionately with the streptococcal toxic shock syndrome, and both the M protein type and the presence of pyrogenic exotoxin A may play some role in the virulence of the strains involved.

Other extracellular products of group A streptococci include DNAases (i.e., A, B, C, D), the streptokinases, a hyaluronidase, an amylase, a proteinase, an nicotinamide adenine dinucleotidase (NADase), and an esterase. Several of these are antigenic (e.g., streptokinase, DNAase B, hyaluronidase, NADase), and measuring antibodies to these antigens has proven useful in documenting clinical infection.

The production of streptococcal skin infections (i.e., pyoderma, impetigo) appears to require disruption of the cutaneous epithelium by trauma, preexisting skin disease, or insects. Group A streptococci often are found on normal skin, but they do not produce disease unless some means of access exists.

TRANSMISSION

Studies of patients with streptococcal pharyngitis suggest that airborne routes of spread and environmental contamination play little or no role in the spread of this form of streptococcal infection. Close contact is required for the spread of streptococcal pharyngitis; direct projection of large droplets or physical transfer of respiratory secretions containing the bacteria is necessary. The spread of group A streptococcal pharyngitis within families or in classrooms is common.

The period of greatest contagion for streptococcal pharyngitis or scarlet fever occurs during the acute stage of illness. Penicillin therapy rapidly suppresses the growth of group A streptococci and, if continued, usually eradicates the group A streptococcus from the upper respiratory tract. The patient can be considered much less contagious after 24 to 48 hours of antimicrobial therapy. If they are afebrile, children can return to school by that time with little risk of spread of the organism to close contacts.

Prolonged carriage (weeks to months) of group A streptococci may occur in the throat and has been reported in approximately 10% to 20% of school-aged children. Anal carriers of group A streptococci have been identified and have been proven to be the source of epidemic spread of the disease in hospitals. Rectal or anal carriage occurs more often than was suspected previously. Contaminated milk or food may result in outbreaks of streptococcal infection of the throat; more often, these outbreaks are caused by group C or group G streptococcus.

EPIDEMIOLOGY

Group A streptococci are pathogenic for humans but are found infrequently in other species (Box 176.2). Streptococcal impetigo occurs with the greatest frequency in preschool children, but streptococcal pharyngitis is predominantly a disorder of school-aged children. Outbreaks of streptococcal respiratory tract infections have been observed in day-care centers. Streptococcal impetigo seems to be a recurrent disease in preschool and school-aged children.

Tonsillitis and pharyngitis caused by streptococci are particularly common in cold and temperate climates. Streptococcal impetigo and pyoderma occur with greater frequency in tropical climates. Streptococcal pharyngitis is more frequent during the winter and spring, and streptococcal impetigo generally is a disease of the summer months in temperate climates and appears with relatively equal frequency throughout the year in tropical countries.

PATHOGENESIS

The development of pharyngitis appears to depend on the attachment of group A streptococci to epithelial cells, which is accomplished by their fimbriae. The streptococci must compete with the other pharyngeal flora, which have the ability to interfere with colonization of group A streptococci in the throat.

Skin lipids are lethal for group A streptococci *in vitro* and may provide a barrier against the establishment of streptococcal infection of the skin under normal conditions. Invasion of tissues by group A streptococci is facilitated by various toxins and enzymes that attack hyaluronic acid and fibrin. The M protein is antiphagocytic and contains a substance that is cytotoxic in the presence of non–type-specific antibody. Type-specific antibody against M protein enhances phagocytosis, but usually this is not detectable until 6 to 8 weeks after the onset of infection. The primary role of type-specific antibody against M protein may be its prevention of reinfection by the same serologic type. Surface phagocytosis by monocytes and, subsequently, by polymorphonuclear leukocytes appears to be the primary mechanism for defense in the early stages of streptococcal infection.

The spread of streptococci to regional lymph nodes is common, particularly when infection occurs in the pharynx or tonsils. Bacteremia is uncommon in older children and adults, but it occurs more frequently in infants with streptococcal disease.

The rash of scarlet fever has been attributed to the elaboration of erythrogenic toxin. Streptococcal toxic shock syndrome may result from a direct influence of the pyrogenic exotoxins or the M protein acting as a "superantigen" to cause polyclonal stimulation of T cells that mediate the production of a variety of lymphokines (e.g., tumor necrosis factor-beta, interleukin-2, and interferon-gamma).

CLINICAL MANIFESTATIONS

Streptococcal pharyngitis and tonsillitis are relatively brief illnesses, with incubation periods of several hours to 3 or 4 days. The infection varies in severity, from subclinical (i.e., no symptoms) to relatively extreme toxicity characterized by nausea, vomiting, high fever, and hypotension. The onset is acute and may be characterized by pharyngitis, headache, fever, and abdominal pain, particularly in children. The tonsils and pharynx may appear inflamed and are covered by an exudate in 50% to 80% of patients. The exudate usually appears by the second day of the disease, is characteristically whitish to yellow, and may become confluent. Swollen and tender anterior cervical lymphadenopathy affects 30% to 60% of the patients. Clinical manifestations of the disease subside in 3 to 5 days unless complications such as sinusitis or parapharyngeal, peritonsillar, or retropharyngeal abscess develop. Nonsuppurative complications such as acute nephritis (see Chapter 325) may be seen 10 days and rheumatic fever (see Chapter 285) an average of 18 days after the onset of group A streptococcal pharyngitis.

A form of streptococcal infection known as *streptococcal fever* or *streptococcosis* may occur in infants. This illness is characterized by a chronic low-grade fever, generalized lymphadenopathy, persistent mucoserous nasal discharge, and little evidence of localized pharyngeal inflammation.

Scarlet fever is unusual in infancy, possibly because of the transplacental transfer of maternal antibody to erythrogenic toxins. Apparently, hypersensitivity to these exotoxins must occur before a person can develop scarlet fever as a manifestation of streptococcal disease. The frequency of scarlet fever after infancy has increased since the late 1980s. It usually presents with fever, nausea, vomiting, and the appearance of the typical rash. Abdominal pain and vomiting may precede the development of the rash by 12 to 48 hours. Although sore throat usually is present, it may not be as troublesome as in patients with pharyngitis alone. The erythematous maculopapular rash usually begins on the trunk and spreads to cover the entire body within hours to days. The rash has the texture of sandpaper. The forehead and cheeks are flushed, and the area around the mouth is pallid (i.e., circumoral pallor). The rash generally fades on pressure and ultimately desquamates. Deep red,

nonblanching, or petechial lesions may be seen in the folds of the joints (i.e., Pastia lines) or in other parts of the extremities. Early in the course of illness, the dorsum of the tongue has a white coat, through which edematous and red papillae project (i.e., white strawberry tongue). Several days later, the white covering desquamates, and the tongue becomes swollen, red, and mottled (i.e., red strawberry tongue).

A scarlatiniform rash may appear in patients with streptococcal wound infections or impetigo. An enanthema is characterized by bright red or hemorrhagic spots that appear on the interior pillars of the tonsil fossae and the soft palate. The cervical nodes are enlarged and tender, but the pharyngeal signs usually are minimal. The rash may desquamate over 7 to 21 days. Eosinophilia is common during the recovery phases from scarlet fever; the number of eosinophils may reach 30% of the differential leukocyte count in this disorder.

Streptococcal impetigo may develop up to several weeks after a strain of group A streptococci is detected on normal skin. The patient usually is afebrile, and the lesion is painless. The lesion appears initially as a superficial vesicle with little surrounding erythema and progresses to a pustule that becomes thick and yellow. The pustule may last for days to a week. A secondary staphylococcal infection occurs commonly in the pustular and subsequently crusted forms of this disease. Removal of the crust, which is a part of local therapy, reveals a moist or purulent undersurface early during the course of the disease. On healing, depigmentation may occur, but permanent scarring is uncommon because the infection does not involve the dermis.

Acute poststreptococcal nephritis (see Chapter 325) can follow impetigo or other forms of streptococcal skin infection or streptococcal pharyngitis. This disorder is produced by specific nephritogenic strains of streptococci. Rheumatic fever (see Chapter 285) has not been associated with streptococcal skin infections. The latent period for acute nephritis is longer after skin infection (average, 3 weeks) than after throat infection (average, 10 days). The serologic streptococcal types associated with nephritis after skin infection usually are different from those that produce nephritis after throat infection.

Streptococcal pyoderma may be superimposed on eczema, burns, wounds, scabies, or other diseases that provide access through the barrier of the skin. Ecthyma is a deeper and more chronic form of streptococcal pyoderma found predominantly in tropical areas.

Erysipelas is a form of streptococcal infection involving the skin and the adjacent mucous membranes. Erysipelas is characterized by an elevated red lesion often associated with bullae filled with yellowish fluid that may crust over after rupture. A well-demarcated advancing border, which appears redder and more edematous at the edge than centrally, is seen. The central red area may fade and may even appear normal as the lesion progresses. Erysipelas usually involves the face; the extremities and the rest of the body are affected less often. The acute onset of erysipelas often is accompanied by systemic toxicity. The lesion may persist for several days to several weeks, and relapses are common; recurrences usually develop at the same body site.

Other infections that may be caused by the group A streptococcus include otitis media, sinusitis, mastoiditis, pneumonia, empyema, necrotizing fasciitis, septicemia without localized infection, meningitis, and toxic shock syndrome. The number of cases of toxic shock syndrome caused by group A, beta-hemolytic streptococci has increased significantly. This syndrome is characterized by high fever (higher than 38.9°C), diffuse macular erythroderma, hypotension, and involvement of at least three of the following organ systems: gastrointestinal, muscular, renal, mucous membranes, hepatic, hematologic, and central nervous system. The currently accepted case definition of streptococcal toxic shock syndrome appears in Table 176.1.

TABLE 176.1

CASE DEFINITION FOR THE STREPTOCOCCAL TOXIC SHOCK SYNDROME*

I. **Isolation of group A streptococci (*Streptococcus pyogenes*)**
   A. From a normally sterile site (e.g., blood, cerebrospinal, pleural, or peritoneal fluid, tissue biopsy, surgical wound)
   B. From a nonsterile site (eg., throat, sputum, vagina, superficial skin lesion)

II. **Clinical signs of severity**
   A. Hypotension: systolic blood pressure ≤90 mm Hg in adults or <fifth percentile for age in children
   and
   B. Two or more of the following signs:
      Renal impairment
      Coagulopathy
      Liver involvement
      Adult respiratory distress syndrome
      Generalized erythematous macular rash that may desquamate
      Soft tissue necrosis, including necrotizing fasciitis or myositis, or gangrene

*An illness fulfilling criteria IA and II (A and B) can be defined as a *definite* case. An illness fulfilling criteria IB and II (A and B) can be defined as a *probable* case if no other etiology for the illness is identified.

Group A beta-hemolytic streptococci may be found in 50% of patients with peritonsillar or retropharyngeal abscesses and may act synergistically with anaerobic bacteria to produce the characteristic clinical picture. Although puerperal sepsis is now rare, nursery outbreaks of bacteremia, omphalitis, and meningitis still occur. Disseminated intravascular coagulation, purpura fulminans, gangrene, perianal cellulitis, and vaginitis have been reported in children as a result of group A streptococcal infection. Streptococcal infections of the thumb have preceded the development of subpectoral abscesses and pleural effusion; this presumably is the result of a spread of streptococci along lymphatic channels that drain the area of the thumb. Streptococci also have been implicated in bacteremia and in secondary skin, muscle, or bone infection in patients with varicella.

An association between group A streptococcal infection and two additional nonsuppurative conditions has been proposed. Flares of guttate psoriasis in genetically susceptible individuals are thought to be caused by activation of CD4$^+$ T cells by streptococcal superantigen. Antibiotic therapy has not consistently ameliorated the condition or prevented future flares. In recent years, an association between obsessive-compulsive and tic disorders in children has been linked to streptococcal infection in a syndrome referred to as pediatric autoimmune neuropsychiatric disorder associated with group A streptococcal infection (PANDAS). Some investigators have described improvement in neuropsychiatric symptoms with antibiotic therapy.

STREPTOCOCCAL RESPIRATORY CARRIER STATE

Many normal persons harbor group A streptococci in the upper respiratory tract for prolonged periods without evidence of disease or an immunologic response. Approximately 10% of school-aged children are carriers, and that rate may increase to as high as 30% during periods of peak streptococcal activity in the community. Carriers only rarely spread the organism to close contacts. The risk of a carrier's developing rheumatic fever appears to be significantly less than that of a person with active streptococcal pharyngeal infection. Streptococcal pharyngitis often is diagnosed mistakenly in patients who are colonized by group A streptococci but whose symptoms are caused by a viral infection. The carrier state may be recognized by throat culture or by antigen detection testing after symptoms have resolved.

DIAGNOSIS

For patients with acute pharyngitis or tonsillitis, the physician must rely on the clinical appearance of the patient, culture results, and epidemiologic findings to confirm the probability of streptococcal infection. The physician's problem in identifying group A streptococcal pharyngitis is difficult because these organisms are found in the throats of physiologically normal children (i.e., carriers) and those whose clinical findings are caused by many other agents, including gonococci, Epstein-Barr virus, and *Mycoplasma pneumoniae*. Pharyngitis caused by *Corynebacterium diphtheriae* was sometimes mistaken for that caused by group A streptococcus in the past, but this infection is now extremely rare in the United States. There is some evidence that in adolescents and young adults pharyngitis mimicking streptococcal pharyngitis may be caused by *Arcanobacterium haemolyticum*. The rash often associated with this infection may be indistinguishable from scarlet fever. *A. haemolyticum* is more reliably eradicated by erythromycin than by penicillin. Many viruses produce pharyngitis that closely mimics streptococcal pharyngitis and can be excluded only by the absence of a positive culture result for group A streptococci.

Most streptococcal infections are short-term illnesses. Antibody responses appear relatively late, and streptococcal antibody titers are useful only retrospectively in the diagnosis of acute streptococcal infection. However, titers play an important role in supporting the diagnosis of nonsuppurative complications of group A streptococcal disease, such as acute nephritis and rheumatic fever. The measurement of antibody titers may be useful if obtaining a culture of the primary site of infection (e.g., osteomyelitis) is difficult or if the patient has been treated with antibiotics to which the group A streptococcus is susceptible.

Clinical manifestations that suggest streptococcal disease include high fever, exudative pharyngitis, tender anterior cervical nodes, a history of contact with a documented case of streptococcal infection, and a scarlatiniform rash. The concurrent findings of hoarseness, cough, rhinorrhea, or conjunctivitis render the diagnosis of streptococcal pharyngitis less likely.

The diagnosis of streptococcal pharyngitis can be confirmed by culture, but recovery of group A streptococcus from the pharynx does not in itself differentiate the streptococcal carrier state from streptococcal disease. Rapid techniques (i.e., 5 to 60 minutes) for identifying group A streptococci in the upper respiratory tract are available commercially. These techniques involve extraction of the group-specific carbohydrate from the cell wall of the organism and subsequent identification of the organism by agglutination or immunologic reaction detected by a color change. Currently available data suggest that the specificity for these tests exceeds 90% and that the sensitivity ranges from 85% to 95%. These tests have the advantage of rapid identification of group A streptococci and are particularly appealing because faster treatment clearly is associated with an earlier clinical response. Because the sensitivity of these rapid tests is not 100%, however, a negative result in a patient whose symptoms suggest group A streptococcal pharyngitis should be followed by a confirmatory throat culture. Rapid antigen detection tests also can be useful in the detection of group A streptococci from streptococcal pyodermalike lesions. Neither throat culture nor antigen detection generally is recommended in children less than 3 years old or whose symptoms are suggestive of viral infection (cough, hoarseness, coryza, conjunctivities, anterior stomatitis, diarrhea). A positive result in such patients is likely to represent carriage.

Clinically, the pharyngeal exudate of infectious mononucleosis tends to be thicker, whiter, and more extensive than that of streptococcal pharyngitis; the clinical impression of Epstein-Barr virus infection can be confirmed by the heterophile spot test or specific Epstein-Barr virus antibody determinations. Diphtheritic pharyngitis can be differentiated by the usually more adherent membrane and the extension of the membrane onto the uvula. The diphtheritic membrane is characterized by a sweet to fetid odor. Simultaneous infection with streptococci and *C. diphtheriae* may produce the clinical picture of bull-neck diphtheria.

In many patients with impetigo, group A beta-hemolytic streptococci and *Staphylococcus aureus* can be isolated concurrently, but usually *S. aureus* is the primary pathogen. Group A streptococcus is the only pathogen isolated in 5% of cases of impetigo, whereas *S. aureus* is the sole isolate in 50% to 60% of cases. Occasionally, the vesicles of chickenpox resemble those of a bullous impetigo, but the former usually are less transient and tend to involve the trunk more than the extremities. The lesions of chickenpox tend to itch, and the crusts are not as thick as those of streptococcal impetigo. However, the lesions of varicella can be infected secondarily with streptococci.

Humoral immune responses to numerous somatic components of the streptococcal cell have been demonstrated. Antibody to the M protein is particularly important because it is the basis of immunity to or protection against reinfection from the same serologic type. Type-specific antibody also may be transferred from the mother to the fetus. The development of type-specific antibody can be inhibited by prompt treatment with penicillin.

Antibody determinations are particularly useful in providing a strict method for defining streptococcal infection in certain clinical and epidemiologic situations and in supporting the possibility of a preceding streptococcal infection in patients with rheumatic fever or glomerulonephritis.

The antistreptolysin O titer is the streptococcal antibody test used most frequently. Because streptolysin O also is produced by groups C and G streptococci, the test is not specific for group A infection. The antistreptolysin O response is weak in patients with streptococcal impetigo and pyoderma, but anti-DNAase B and antihyaluronidase responses are measurable after both skin and throat infections.

The Streptozyme (Carter-Wallace, Cranbury, NJ) agglutination test is based on the antibody agglutination of erythrocytes coated with a mixture of streptococcal extracellular antigens. This test has the appeal of speed, simplicity, and reaction with a variety of streptococcal antigens. Antibody responses measurable by this assay have been demonstrated within the first 7 to 10 days after the onset of infection. This contrasts with the development of neutralizing antibody titers to streptolysin O, which appear after 3 to 6 weeks, and to anti-DNAase B, which appear after 6 to 8 weeks. Because of problems with standardization of this reagent, producing variable results with different lots, this test should be interpreted with caution.

TREATMENT

Penicillin remains the drug of choice for the treatment of group A beta-hemolytic streptococcal infections unless the patient is allergic to this antibiotic. No strains of group A streptococcus resistant to penicillin have been isolated. Although penicillin tolerance has been described, its clinical significance has not been defined. Eradication of group A streptococci from the nasopharynx or the upper respiratory tract may be difficult because of noncompliance with prescribed antibiotics, reinfection from family or classroom contacts, or persistence of colonizing group A streptococcus. Moreover, beta-lactamase–producing organisms in the nasopharynx or the production of inhibitory substances by other organisms may allow the persistence of the group A streptococcus. Antibiotics other than penicillin, particularly the cephalosporins, more consistently eradicate group A streptococcus from the pharynx in patients with pharyngitis. It is likely, however, that these other antibiotics merely appear more effective, because they more reliably eradicate streptococci in individuals with a positive culture for group A streptococcus whose symptoms were mistakenly attributed to that organism.

Erythromycin is the drug of choice in patients who are allergic to penicillin. Group A beta-hemolytic streptococci resistant to erythromycin have been reported, and in countries where the use of erythromycin is higher than that in the United States (Japan, Spain, Finland), resistance rates as high as 20% have been found. In the United States, erythromycin resistance generally is seen in less than 5% of group A streptococcal strains; however, one study suggests that increased use of azithromycin for treatment of respiratory tract infections has led to increasing erythromycin resistance at least in some locales. Sulfonamides suppress but do not eradicate group A streptococci, and many group A streptococci are resistant to tetracycline.

The rationale for the use of penicillin in the treatment of streptococcal pharyngitis is to relieve symptoms and to prevent the development of acute rheumatic fever, which can be accomplished with low-dose therapy maintained over a rather long period. Administration of a single intramuscular injection of benzathine penicillin G (600,000 U for children weighing less than 27 kg, or 1.2 million U for children weighing more than 27 kg or for adults) is another method of accomplishing this objective. Alternatively, penicillin V (250 mg for children weighing less than 27 kg and 500 mg for heavier children) in two or three divided doses over 10 days is the treatment of choice. In patients who are allergic to penicillin, erythromycin (20 to 40 mg/kg/day of erythromycin estolate or 40 mg/kg/day of erythromycin ethyl succinate) in two to four divided doses should be used. Clarithromycin and azithromycin are equally effective. Clindamycin (30 mg/kg/day for 10 days) also can be used for the treatment of streptococcal pharyngitis in patients who are allergic to penicillin. Other antibiotics that have been used successfully in the therapy of group A beta-hemolytic streptococcal pharyngitis or tonsillitis include amoxicillin, amoxicillin with clavulanic acid, and several cephalosporins. Treatment with these broader-spectrum antibiotics is not associated with a reduced rate of clinical or bacteriologic relapse compared with treatment with penicillin alone.

Patients with streptococcal bacteremia, deep soft tissue infections, erysipelas, pneumonia, or meningitis should be treated with penicillin parenterally, preferably intravenously. The dosage and duration of therapy must be based on the nature of the disease process, and daily dosages as high as 400,000 U/kg/day may be required in the most severe infections. Intravenous clindamycin in addition to intravenous penicillin has been recommended by some experts to treat streptococcal toxic shock syndrome and necrotizing fasciitis.

In patients with streptococcal impetigo, local skin care, such as removal of crusts and use of special bacteriostatic soaps, coupled with the use of local antibiotic ointments, may be sufficient for the management of patients with a few skin lesions, but these measures are not adequate for those with more widespread impetigo. A topical antibiotic ointment such as mupirocin (Bactroban) is effective therapy for some patients with localized impetigo, even when parenteral therapy has not been initiated. Oral or parenteral penicillin or oral macrolide in the doses prescribed for the treatment of streptococcal pharyngitis should be used in patients with multiple impetiginous lesions or if multiple family members, child care contacts, or athletic team members are affected. If culture of the lesion is not available or if staphylococcal superinfection is suspected, a first-generation cephalosporin often provides appropriate treatment for both pathogens.

Penicillin treatment has not been proved to reduce the frequency of nephritis after treatment of skin infections, and substantial clinical experience suggests that patients with skin infection caused by a nephritogenic streptococcal strain may develop this complication despite penicillin therapy. One study suggests that penicillin therapy may lower the risk of this complication in patients with streptococcal pharyngitis caused by a nephritogenic strain.

PREVENTION

No satisfactory method has been developed yet to prevent streptococcal disease by immunization. The spread of group A beta-hemolytic streptococci is decreased by limiting the density of persons living within the home environment, isolating the contagious patient, and, especially, treating with antibiotics patients known to have this infection. For populations with streptococcal infection occurring at an epidemic level over an extended period (e.g., selected military populations), institution of mass prophylaxis, usually with injections of benzathine penicillin, may be necessary.

INFECTIONS CAUSED BY STREPTOCOCCI OTHER THAN GROUPS A AND B

The classification of streptococci can be confusing because of their separation on the basis of hemolysis and their separate identification by Lancefield typing. These two methods of identification are not mutually exclusive; Table 176.2 shows

TABLE 176.2

CORRELATION OF STREPTOCOCCI IDENTIFIED BY LANCEFIELD GROUPING AND HEMOLYTIC REACTIONS WITH SITES OF HUMAN COLONIZATION AND DISEASE

Lancefield Group	Species	Usual Reaction on Sheep Blood Agar	Usual Human Habitat	Most Common Human Disease
A	S. pyogenes	Beta-hemolysis	Pharynx, skin, rectum	Pharyngitis, erysipelas, impetigo, septicemia, wound infections, rheumatic fever, acute glomerulonephritis, necrotizing fasciitis, cellulitis, otitis media, meningitis, pneumonia, conjunctivitis, acute endocarditis
B	S. agalactiae	Beta-hemolysis	Pharynx, vagina	Puerperal sepsis, endocarditis, neonatal sepsis, meningitis, otitis media, osteomyelitis, pneumonia
C	S. equi, S. equisimilis, S. dysgalactiae, S. zooepidemicus	Beta-hemolysis	Pharynx, vagina, skin	Wound infection, puerperal sepsis, cellulitis, endocarditis
D	Enterococcus faecalis, E. faecium; S. bovis	Gamma-hemolysis	Colon contents	Endocarditis, urinary tract infection, biliary tract infection, intestinal infection, peritonitis
E	S. infrequens	?	?	?
F	S. minutus anginosus	Beta-hemolysis	Mouth, pharynx	Sinusitis, meningitis, brain abscess, pneumonia
G	S. canis	Beta-hemolysis	pharynx, vagina, skin	Puerperal infection, skin or wound infection, endocarditis
H	S. sanguis*	Alpha-hemolysis	Mouth	Endocarditis, brain abscess
K	S. salivarius*	Alpha-hemolysis	Mouth	Endocarditis, sinusitis, meningitis, brain abscess
L		Beta- or alpha-hemolysis	Mouth	Endocarditis, abscess, parotitis, neonatal sepsis
M		Beta- or alpha-hemolysis	Mouth, pharynx, vagina	Endocarditis, septicemia
N	S. lactis-cremoris	Alpha- or gamma-hemolysis	Pharynx	Meningitis, septicemia?
O		Alpha- or beta-hemolysis	Pharynx, conjuctiva, vagina	Pneumonia, endocarditis, septicemia
Nontypable	S. viridans	Alpha-hemolysis	Pharynx	Endocarditis, intravascular catheter-related infections
Nontypable	S. mutans	Alpha-hemolysis	Pharynx	Endocarditis, intravascular catheter-related infections
Nontypable	S. pneumoniae	Alpha-hemolysis	Nasopharynx	Sepsis, meningitis, otitis media, pneumonia, sinusitis

*These organisms are isolated frequently from the bloodstream as alpha-hemolytic streptococci. Along with many nongroupable alpha-streptococci, they are often called S. viridans, a term that incorrectly implies a specific species. Nevertheless, as a group, they cause most episodes of endocarditis and are usually exquisitely sensitive to penicillin.

Adapted from Keusch GT, Weinstein L. *Streptococcal disease.* Kalamazoo, MI: Upjohn Company, 1973.

the classification of streptococci by Lancefield type and by the hemolytic reactions on blood agar, as well as their correlation with human colonization and disease.

As early as 1938, hemolytic streptococci belonging to Lancefield group B were related causally to severe human disease. Group B streptococcal infection is discussed in Chapter 75.

Human infections with streptococci groups C to H and K to O and with nontypable strains have been reported in normal infants and children. The classification of these organisms and infections with which they have been associated are shown in Table 176.2. With the exception of group D streptococci and several alpha-hemolytic strains, penicillin G provides effective therapy for non–group A streptococci. Increasing frequency of penicillin and cephalosporin resistance in *S. pneumoniae* has become a worldwide problem (see Chapter 170). Enterococci generally are susceptible to ampicillin or vancomycin; however, increasing resistance has been seen, usually in hospital-associated infections.

Bacterial endocarditis in children may be caused by *S. viridans*. Some *S. viridans* organisms require vitamin B_6 or thiol compounds for optimal growth in the laboratory, and supplemental media are necessary for their isolation and sensitivity testing. Some of these organisms are tolerant or relatively tolerant to penicillin, and therapy with penicillin and aminoglycosides is recommended until the results of sensitivity studies are available. If endocarditis is caused by enterococci, therapy with ampicillin plus an aminoglycoside is recommended.

Suggested Readings

Bisno AL, Gerber MA, Gwaltney JM, et al. Practice guidelines for the diagnosis and management of group A streptococcal pharyngitis. *Clin Infect Dis* 2002;35:113.

Bratcher DF. *Arcanobacterium haemolyticum*. In: Long SS, Pickering L, Prober CG, eds. *Principles and practice of pediatric infectious diseases,* 2nd ed. Philadelphia: Churchill Livingstone, 2003:766.

Committee on Infectious Diseases, American Academy of Pediatrics. Severe invasive group A streptococcal infections: a subject review. *Pediatrics* 1998;101:136.

Darmstadt GL. A guide to superficial strep and staph skin infections. *Contemp Pediatr* 1997;14:95.

Gerber MA, Tanz RR. New approaches to the treatment of group A streptococcal pharyngitis. *Curr Opin Pediatr* 2001;13:51.

Gerber MA, Tanz RR, Kabat W, et al. Potential mechanisms for failure to eradicate group A streptococci from the pharynx. *Pediatrics* 1999;104:911.

Kaplan EL, Gerber MA. Group A, group C, and group G beta-hemolytic streptococcal infections. In: Feigin RD, Cherry JD, Demmler, GJ, Kaplan, SL, eds. *Textbook of infectious diseases,* 5th ed. Philadelphia: WB Saunders, 2003:1142.

Martin JM, Green M, Barbadora KA, Wald ER. Erythromycin-resistant group A streptococci in schoolchildren in Pittsburgh. *N Engl J Med* 2002;346:1200.

Perrin EM, Murphy ML, Casey JR, et al. Does group A beta hemolytic streptococcal infection increase risk for behavioral and neuropsychiatric symptoms in children? *Arch Pediatr Adolesc Med* 2004;158:848.

Rasmussen JE. The relationship between infection with group A beta hemolytic streptococci and the development of psoriasis. *Pediatr Infect Dis J* 2000;19:153.

Siegel AC, Johnson EE, Stollerman GH. Controlled studies of streptococcal pharyngitis in the pediatric population. I. Factors related to the attack rate of rheumatic fever. *N Engl J Med* 1961;265:559.

Stetson CA, Rammelkamp CH Jr, Krause RM, et al. Epidemic acute nephritis: studies on etiology, natural history and prevention. *Medicine (Baltimore)* 1955;34:431.

Stevens DL, Tanner MH, Winship J, et al. Severe group A streptococcal infections associated with a toxic shock–like syndrome and scarlet fever toxin A. *N Engl J Med* 1989;321:1.

Wannamaker LW. Differences between streptococcal infections of the throat and of the skin. *N Engl J Med* 1970;282:23.

Wilson GJ, Talkington DF, Gruber W, et al. Group A streptococcal necrotizing fasciitis following varicella in children: case reports and review. *Clin Infect Dis* 1995;20:1333.

Working Group on Severe Streptococcal Infections. Defining the group A streptococcal toxic shock syndrome: rationale and consensus definition. *JAMA* 1993;269:390.

CHAPTER 177 ■ TULAREMIA

RICHARD F. JACOBS

Tularemia is an acute, febrile, zoonotic illness caused by the grain-negative bacterium *Francisella tularensis*. Tularemiais distributed widely in the northern hemisphere, with numerous infections occurring in humans over relativelylarge areas of the United States, Europe, and Asia. Tularemia is a disease of small animals, but humans are highly susceptible hosts.

MICROBIOLOGY

F. tularensis is a small, nonmotile, gram-negative coccobacillary organism that requires cysteine for growth. In 1959, *F. tularensis* was divided into two types: *F. tularensis* subspecies *tularensis* (type A) and *F. tularensis* subspecies *palaearctica* (type B) are the official nomenclatures.

F. tularensis tularensis, found predominantly in North America, is highly virulent, causing severe disease in mammals and mild to severe disease in humans. *F. tularensis palaearctica* has been identified in Asia, Europe, and North America.

The species frequently is linked to environmental sources and waterborne diseases of rodents and appears to be less virulent in mammals. Descriptions of strains of the organism in Central Asia and Japan added further complexity to the subspecies differentiation. Apparently, the biochemical characteristics and virulence of *F. tularensis* strains do not reflect their genetic character, as judged by molecular techniques using 16S rRNA. Strains isolated from the Central Asian area of the former Soviet Union and Japan belong to genotype A, although the virulence and some of the biochemical characteristics conform to those of the genotype B strains, which means that strains of *F. tularensis tularensis* are not restricted to the North American continent. However, the highly virulent strains of the organism possibly are restricted to North America.

The organism can be cultured on media using glucose-cysteine agar, a temperature of $37°C$, and a pH of 6.9, but selected media may be necessary for optimal growth. Clinicians should be aware that the organism does grow on routine blood and wound cultures (e.g., lymph node aspirate), which may present a health hazard in the microbiology laboratory because of aerosolization among laboratory workers. Because as few as ten organisms have been shown to induce experimental infection in humans, biosafety level 2 is recommended for clinical laboratory work. Clinicians should notify the laboratory if tularemia is included in the differential diagnosis. All strains of *F. tularensis* appear to be serologically identical. Despite this serologic homogeneity, future epidemiologic studies will implement molecular identification using 16S rRNA to divide the isolates into genotypes A and B.

EPIDEMIOLOGY

F. tularensis is a ubiquitous organism found in the Northern Hemisphere between 30 and 71 degrees northern latitude. It has been reported throughout the United States, but it occurs most commonly in the western and south central states, with the highest incidence in regions of Oklahoma, Missouri, Arkansas, Louisiana, Tennessee, Texas, Illinois, and Virginia. Although the incidence peaks during the late spring through the summer months, the year-round distribution of cases probably reflects the multiple vectors of transmission of this organism (Fig. 177.1). The major vector of *F. tularensis* is the tick, and the disease is seen primarily in children and young adults during the major tick seasons of spring, summer, and early fall. The disease is transmitted to humans by vector (e.g., ticks, lice, fleas, deer flies, mosquitoes), animal bites, or ingestion of infected, inadequately cooked animal tissues or contaminated water. *Amblyomma americanum* (Lone Star tick), *Dermacentor andersoni* (wood tick), and *Dermacentor variabilis* (dog tick) are the main reservoirs for *F. tularensis*. Inhalation of the organisms, which occurs primarily while working or being exposed to contaminated land or water or both (Scandinavia), skinning animal carcasses, and working with the organism in the microbiology laboratory, has been identified as a common cause of tularemia pneumonia. It may be transferred mechanically by claws or teeth of domestic pets that have preyed on infected animals. Rabbits, hares, muskrats, voles, rats, mice, and more than 100 other animal species harbor *F. tularensis*. Cases of infection in older children and adults in the winter months typically are associated with rabbit or deer hunting or contamination through contact with infected animal tissues.

Contrary to earlier reports of tularemia as "rabbit fever," tick exposure is the vector for 71% of pediatric and adults cases. The reported incidence of rabbit exposure is similar for adults (11%) and children (7%). Tularemia in children has been documented after a cat bite, a squirrel bite, and exposure to other domestic animals.

PATHOGENESIS

F. tularensis gains access to the human body through the skin, conjunctiva, oropharynx, respiratory tract, or gastrointestinal tract. It spreads by lymphatics or hematogenously, and bacteremia usually develops during the first week of infection. Skin, regional lymph nodes, liver, spleen, and lungs can be involved, and the lesions can occur in the gastrointestinal tract and the central nervous system.

The classic lesion is one of focal necrosis and granuloma formation. After a tick bite, a hallmark presentation for *F. tularensis* infection is the resultant eschar, ulcer, or papule with regional lymphadenitis (Fig. 177.2). The organism elicits humoral and cell-mediated immune responses, but seroconversion may take 1 or 2 weeks after infection. Despite reports of recurrent disease, the initial infection with *F. tularensis* usually confers lasting immunity.

CLINICAL MANIFESTATIONS

The average incubation period for tularemia is 3 to 4 days (range, 1 to 21 days). The onset of symptoms usually is abrupt, with a temperature usually greater than 39.4°C (103°F), chills, pharyngitis, myalgias, arthralgias, nausea and vomiting, and, occasionally, headache, cough, and photophobia. The predominant signs of tularemia include the following: regional lymphadenopathy or lymphadenitis; an ulcer, eschar, or papule at the site of tick embedment; and hepatosplenomegaly. Some patients develop conjunctivitis (Table 177.1). In untreated cases of tularemia, fever may persist for 2 to 3 weeks or longer. No characteristic peripheral blood profile has been established for

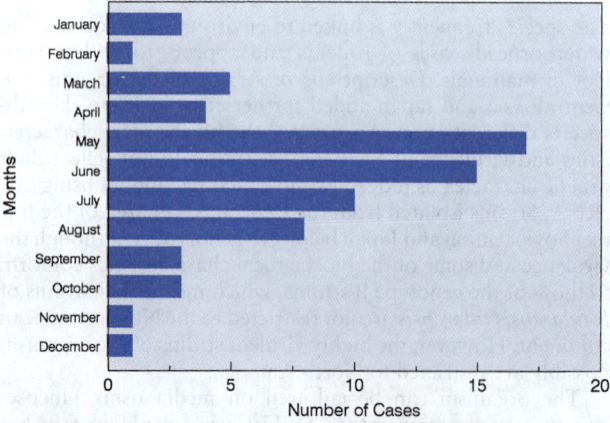

FIGURE 177.1. Distribution of tularemia cases in children. (Adapted from Jacobs RF, Condrey YM, Yamauchi T. Tularemia in adults and children: a changing presentation. *Pediatrics* 1985;76:818.)

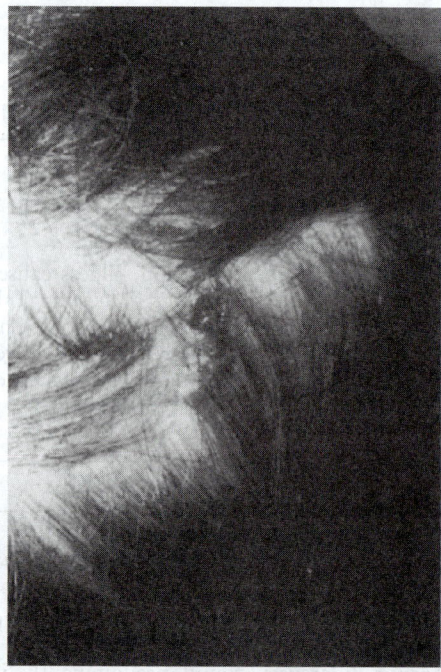

FIGURE 177.2. A papule with an ulcerative base on the scalp of a child with ulceroglandular tularemia presenting with fever and unilateral cervical lymphadenitis.

TABLE 177.1

CLINICAL TYPES AND PRESENTATION OF TULAREMIA IN CHILDREN

Clinical Type	Percentage	Signs and Symptoms*	Percentage
Ulceroglandular	45	Lymphadenopathy	96
Glandular	25	Fever (≥38.3°C)	87
Oculoglandular	2	Pharyngitis	43
Pneumonic	14	Ulcer, eschar, papule	45
Oropharyngeal	4	Myalgias, arthralgias	39
Typhoidal	2	Nausea, vomiting	35
Unclassified	6	Hepatosplenomegaly	35

*Additional signs and symptoms: headache (9%), cough (9%), diarrhea (4%), conjunctivitis (4%).
Adapted from Jacobs RF, Condrey YM, Yamauchi T. Tularemia in adults and children: a changing presentation. *Pediatrics* 1985;76:818.

tularemia. Various skin rashes (macular, morbilliform, pustular, and erythema nodosum) have been described, but the predominant feature is regional lymphadenopathy or lymphadenitis. Subcutaneous nodules have been reported.

In one study, fever developed in 87% of children, with 48% having temperatures greater than 39.4°C. The mean temperature peak for these patients was 39.2°C (range, 38.3° to 41.7°C), and the mean duration of fever was 19.4 days (range, 3 to 60 days).

The classification of six forms of tularemia depends on the portal of entry. The distribution of the clinical manifestations of tularemia in children in one large series was as follows: (a) 45% ulceroglandular; (b) 25% glandular; (c) 14% pneumonic; (d) 4% oropharyngeal; and (e) 2% oculoglandular and typhoidal, with 6% of the cases remaining unclassified. The most common forms of tularemia are ulceroglandular and glandular, in which organisms gain access through the skin, usually after a tick bite. Approximately 2 days after the onset of symptoms, the regional lymph nodes become tender and swollen. Within 24 hours, a painful, swollen papule develops distal to the regional nodes. This papule ruptures and progresses to ulceration and eschar (see Fig. 177.2). In untreated cases, the ulcer may become indolent, and the lymph nodes may suppurate and spontaneously drain. In children, regional lymphadenopathy typically is seen in the cervical area, and in adults it occurs in the inguinal area, probably reflecting the most frequent sites of tick bites. Generalized lymphadenopathy, although uncommon, has been described in cases of tularemia. Glandular tularemia is identical to the ulceroglandular form, except the portal of entry cannot be identified. The other four forms of tularemia are relatively uncommon compared with the ulceroglandular and glandular types (see Table 177.1). In oculoglandular tularemia, the portal of entry typically is the conjunctival sac. Numerous sharply defined nodules or ulcers are apparent on the palpebral conjunctivae, and regional nodes in the preauricular area are involved, developing as a Parinaud complex. Before the development of preauricular lymphadenopathy, pain is a major symptom. The adenopathy typically is painful, thus differentiating it from a similar clinical presentation of cat-scratch disease.

After *F. tularensis* invades the oropharyngeal route (i.e., oropharyngeal tularemia), local involvement consists of pharyngitis, acute tonsillitis, and cervical adenitis. Complaints of sore throat frequently are out of proportion to the visible pathologic features, and exudate is an uncommon finding, although a pseudomembrane resembling that caused by *Corynebacterium diphtheriae* can be present.

The pneumonic form of tularemia previously was thought to be relatively rare in children and to be a severe and lethal form of the disease, but studies on the changing epidemiology and clinical manifestations of this disease have shown that pneumonic tularemia is not an uncommon event. In one study, 14% of children younger than 19 years with confirmed tularemia had abnormal chest roentgenography results and were diagnosed with pneumonia. Although most of these children had other clinical forms of tularemia, approximately one-third presented with isolated pneumonia unresponsive to traditional antibiotic therapy.

The typhoidal (gastrointestinal) form of tularemia seldom occurs in children. This form of the disease may present with fever of long duration and should be considered in the evaluation of patients who present with fever of unknown origin. In typhoidal tularemia, invasion is secondary to ingestion of the causative agent, and necrotic lesions occur throughout the gastrointestinal tract. This form of the disease may present as a fever of unknown origin, or it may present with acute septicemia. Frequently, hepatosplenomegaly and, occasionally, diarrhea occur. Rhabdomyolysis may be the predominant clinical feature in the sepsis presentation.

DIAGNOSIS

The diagnosis of tularemia is suggested by the history and aided by the physician's awareness in endemic areas. In nonendemic areas, the diagnosis of tularemia may be difficult to establish. History of contact, although often unavailable, should take into account the season of the year, the clinical manifestations of the disease, the unresponsiveness to antibiotics not effective against tularemia, and the endemic rate of disease in that area.

The diagnosis is confirmed by serologic tests. The commercially available standard agglutination test is reliable. Microagglutination and an enzyme immunoassay using outer membrane proteins have become the standard tests because of their enhanced sensitivity compared with the standard agglutination test. Unfortunately, they do not provide a diagnosis early in the course of disease. Agglutinating antibody titers often are not detectable until the second week of illness (days 10 to 14). In some cases, seroconversion has not been described until the illness has persisted 4 to 6 weeks. In rare cases, patients may never exhibit agglutinating antibodies. A fourfold increase in the specific agglutination titer confirms the diagnosis, but a presumptive diagnosis should be considered with acute titers of greater than or equal to 1:160. This titer may indicate current or past infection, but in a clinically compatible case, it should be considered an indication for administering presumptive therapy. Patients with active disease often develop titers equal to or greater than 1:1,280 as the initial manifestation of seroconversion. Other laboratory studies, including a complete blood cell count, erythrocyte sedimentation rate, urinalysis, and *Proteus* OX2/OX19 titers, are not useful in establishing the diagnosis or in managing the patient. The agglutination test is specific, but cross-reactions do occur with *Brucella* species and have been seen in recent recipients of cholera vaccine. Other serologic tests (e.g., lymphocyte stimulation, antigen detection in urine, and polymerase chain reaction) have been reliable and confirm the diagnosis early in disease. Generally, these tests are not available outside research and reference laboratories.

Gram-stained smears of material from exudates, lymph node aspirates, or sputum do not reveal the organism reliably, but they are useful because positive smear results may rule out other bacterial pathogens. Lymph node aspirates from patients with cervical lymphadenitis may be undergo Gram staining safely in the laboratory. If gram-positive cocci in chains or clusters are identified, the most likely diagnosis of pyogenic cervical lymphadenitis caused by *Staphylococcus aureus* or group A beta-hemolytic *Streptococcus* can be confirmed. Cultures of *F. tularensis* should not be perfomed routinely in the diagnostic microbiology laboratory because of the danger of aerosolization to laboratory personnel. If confirmation by culture is indicated, appropriate laboratory precautions, including notifying the laboratory of the potential for the specimen to contain *F. tularensis*, is the duty of the clinician. Appropriate laboratory precautions with biosafety level 2 then can be maintained, and state health department laboratories can perform direct fluorescence antibody testing to confirm the identification of the organisms as *F. tularensis*.

DIFFERENTIAL DIAGNOSIS

The differential diagnosis of tularemia depends on the clinical form of the infection. Ulceroglandular and glandular tularemia must be differentiated from disease caused by *S. aureus, Streptococcus pyogenes, Mycobacterium tuberculosis*, nontuberculous *Mycobacterium*, and *Bartonella henselae*. In cases of inguinal lymphadenopathy, the diagnosis of lymphogranuloma venereum, granuloma inguinale, and other ulcer adenopathy sexually transmitted diseases should be considered in older patients. Occasionally, sporotrichosis and infectious mononucleosis are diagnosed in these patients. Oculoglandular tularemia is more distinctive, but disease caused by common pathogens must be excluded. Oropharyngeal tularemia must be differentiated from streptococcal tonsillopharyngitis and corynebacterial disease. Typhoidal tularemia resembles bacteremia and must be differentiated from other more traditional bacterial and enteric diseases and from classic typhoid fever. Tularemia pneumonia may present a significant clinical challenge to the physician. Tularemia pneumonia must be differentiated from other bacterial forms of pneumonia and other forms of lower respiratory tract infection unresponsive to traditional antibiotic therapy. Pathogens and disorders include *M. tuberculosis, Mycoplasma pneumoniae, Chlamydia pneumoniae, Legionella*, psittacosis, Q fever, fungal infections, viral pneumonia, and rickettsial infections.

TREATMENT

Streptomycin has been considered the drug of choice. The recommendation for 30 to 40 mg/kg/day divided into two daily intramuscular injections for a 7-day course is effective. An alternative regimen is streptomycin at a dosage of 30 to 40 mg/kg/day administered intramuscularly for the first 3 days, with subsequent reduction to 15 to 20 mg/kg/day given intramuscularly for the final 4 days. A Jarisch-Herxheimer reaction has been observed in the beginning of therapy with aminoglycosides. In severe cases or if a child does not establish an afebrile, asymptomatic course within a few days, extension of treatment beyond 7 days is indicated and should be based on clinical assessment. Streptomycin-resistant strains have been reported, but they are rare. Defervescence and symptomatic response are prompt, usually within several days. The response may be somewhat delayed if the lymph nodes have progressed to suppuration.

Gentamicin has become a more popular choice for treatment. In hospitalized children, intravenous gentamicin at standard dosages of 2.5 mg/kg/dose given every 8 hours (or 5.0 mg/kg/dose every 12 hours) for 7 days has been used. If clinical defervescence does occur, outpatient management with intramuscular gentamicin can be pursued. Consideration for once- to twice-daily dosing of gentamicin (5.0 mg/kg/dose) currently is recommended by some experts based on their clinical experience. Standard intramuscular or intravenous therapy with gentamicin should use 5.0 mg/kg/dose every 12 hours. The streptomycin guidelines for length of therapy with time to defervescence and symptom relief should be used in gentamicin therapy.

Although no randomized trial data exist to compare aminoglycoside with quinolone treatment of tularemia, ciprofloxacin has been used successfully in Scandanavia. Fluoroquinolones, specifically ciprofloxacin, now are recommended for the treatment of tularemia in older adolescents and adults due to *F. tularensis*, subspecies *palearctica*.

Although tetracycline and chloramphenicol have activity against *F. tularensis*, they are considered to be poor alternatives for children. Anecdotal reports of unacceptable rates of relapse of clinical symptoms after discontinuation of tetracycline or chloramphenicol indicate that these agents should not be used as standard therapy in children. Reconsideration of the use of tetracycline in children younger than 8 years of age has been accepted, and tetracycline (25 to 50 mg/kg/day in four divided doses), doxycycline (2 to 4 mg/kg/day in two divided doses), and chloramphenicol (50 mg/kg/day in four divided doses intravenously) have been used successfully as alternative regimens. An oral formulation of chloramphenicol no longer is available in the United States. Children treated successfully with tetracycline for a differential diagnosis that included tickborne infections (e.g., *Rickettsia, Ehrlichia*) should not be given gentamicin or streptomycin routinely after confirmation of serologic tests for tularemia. The parents should be counseled that a relapse can occur, and if it does with symptomatic disease, gentamicin or streptomycin should be initiated at that point. Other antibiotics with acceptable *in vitro* minimal inhibitory concentrations (Table 177.2) have not been proven effective.

The major adverse reaction to streptomycin in children is ototoxicity. Children should be monitored for development of tinnitus, which indicates the need for a reduction of the daily dose. Hearing screening before initiation of streptomycin or gentamicin therapy should be considered. If hearing loss has occurred, the alternative streptomycin regimen or gentamicin therapy with monitoring of serum levels in severe cases can be considered. Audiologic evaluation is indicated after therapy in these cases.

In one study, no deaths occurred in a series of pediatric patients, but suppurative adenitis occurred in 16% of the overall population, with late suppuration after antibiotic therapy occurring in 33% of children with the ulceroglandular or glandular forms. Surgical intervention, which was required for 19 of these patients, involved repeated needle aspiration in seven, incision and drainage in eight, and excisional biopsy in four patients. Cultures of late suppurative nodes did not yield *F. tularensis*. In asymptomatic patients, specimens from the lymph nodes should not be cultured or evaluated.

TABLE 177.2

ANTIBIOTIC SUSCEPTIBILITY TO *FRANCISELLA TULARENSIS*

Antibiotic	MIC_{50}* (μg/mL)
Penicillin	>8.0
Ampicillin	>8.0
Tetracycline	2.0
Chloramphenicol	1.0
Streptomycin	2.0
Gentamicin	1.0
Cefotaxime	2.0
Ceftriaxone	2.0

*MIC_{50} is the concentration (μg/mL) at which 50% of the isolates are inhibited.
Adapted from Baker CN, Hollis DG, Thornsberry C. Antimicrobial susceptibility testing of *Francisella tularensis* using a modified Mueller-Hinton broth. *J Clin Microbiol* 1985;22:212.

Supportive therapy is indicated for severely ill patients. Although uncommon, patients with typhoidal or pneumonic tularemia with bacteremia have presented with sepsis or the sepsis syndrome. Appropriate monitoring and intensive care therapy are indicated for these patients. The prognoses for patients treated appropriately are excellent. The clinical course of the illness usually is less than 1 month. The mortality rate is less than 1%, except in the subgroups of fulminant pneumonia or typhoidal tularemia.

PREVENTION

Prevention of acquisition of human tularemia depends on the prevention of contact with vectors and provision of protection during the handling of contaminated animal tissues. Children should be cautioned against handling sick or dead rabbits or rodents. Rabbit or rodent carcasses should be disposed of by burial or incineration. Rubber gloves should be worn when preparing game animals. Children who live in tick-infested areas should have their skin and hair checked frequently for the presence of ticks, which should be removed carefully and appropriately. Children in an area of tick endemicity should wear clothing with tightly fitting cuffs at the ankles and wrists. Common tick repellents can be used cautiously to prevent the attachment and feeding of ticks on children.

The only tularemia vaccine available in the United States is an attenuated live vaccine that is unlicensed and classified as an investigational product. The vaccine is reserved for persons in constant contact with *F. tularensis* organisms. Physicians who have patients at risk can obtain information about the vaccine from the Centers for Disease Control and Prevention.

Suggested Readings

Baker CN, Hollis DG, Thomsberry C. Antimicrobial susceptibility testing of *Francisella tularensis* using a modified Mueller-Hinton broth. *J Clin Microbiol* 1985;22:212.

Centers for Disease Control and Prevention. Tularemia: Oklahoma 2000. *MMWR Morb Mortal Wkly Rep* 2001;50:704.

Ikaheimo I, Syrjala H, Karhukorpi J, et al. *In vitro* antibiotic susceptibility of *Francisella tularensis* isolated from humans and animals. *J Antimicrob Chemother* 2000;46:287.

Jacobs RF, Condrey YM, Yamauchi T. Tularemia in adults and children: a changing presentation. *Pediatrics* 1985;76:818.

Jacobs RF, Narain JP. Tularemia in children. *Pediatr Infect Dis* 1983;1:487.

Johansson A, Berglund L, Gothefors L, et al. Ciprofloxacin for treatment of tularemia in children. *Pediatr Infect Dis J* 2000;19:449.

Mason WL, Figelsbach HT, Little SF, et al. Treatment of tularemia, including pulmonary tularemia with gentamicin. *Am Rev Respir Dis* 1980;121:39.

Pullen RL, Stuart BM. Tularemia analysis of 225 cases. *JAMA* 1945;129:495.

Sandstrom G, Sjostedt A, Forsman M, et al. Characterization and classification of strains of *Francisella tularensis* isolated in the Central Asian focus of the Soviet Union and in Japan. *J Clin Microbiol* 1992;30:172.

CHAPTER 178 ■ SYPHILIS

CHARLES R. WOODS

Worldwide, syphilis, a venereal disease of adolescence and adulthood, remains important in pediatrics as an acquired and a congenital infection. Syphilis was recognized as a disease in Europe during the fifteenth century and initially was called the "great pox," in distinction from smallpox. *Treponema pallidum*, the etiologic agent of syphilis, was described in 1905, but symptoms specific to syphilis were not determined until 1938 because of frequent dual infection with gonorrhea. Humans are the sole natural host of *T. pallidum*.

MICROBIOLOGY

T. pallidum is a member of the genus *Treponema* (order Spirochaetales), which contains three other pathogens [*T. pertenue* (yaws), *T. carateum* (pinta), and *T. endemicum* (endemic syphilis, or bejel)], and at least six nonpathogens that can be normal flora in the oral cavity and in the genitourinary and intestinal tracts. Treponemes are microaerophilic gram-negative bacteria that are 6 to 20 μm long and 0.1 to 0.5 μm in diameter. Morphologically, they are rod-shaped, with 8 to 14 flat waves that give a helical appearance. They possess six axial fibrils that are intracellular, flagellumlike organelles that extend pole to pole, vary in length, and determine the shape and characteristic motility of the microbe. Treponema reproduce by transverse fission.

Survival outside an infected host is very limited. Difficulties in cultivating *T. pallidum* have hampered efforts to understand the pathogenesis of disease caused by these organisms. Virulent strains have been propagated by intratesticular inoculation in rabbits, and limited *in vitro* culture on monolayers of several cell types has been achieved, but *in vitro* culture for diagnostic purposes remains unavailable.

EPIDEMIOLOGY

Syphilis occurs most often in adolescents or in adults via sexual contact. The risk of acquiring infection per sexual contact with an infected partner is approximately 30%. The microbe can invade intact mucous membranes or areas of abraded skin. Acquisition by direct contact with an infected lesion rarely occurs, but health care providers can become infected by contact if appropriate barrier precautions are not used. Congenital syphilis occurs through the transplacental passage of *T. pallidum* from an infected mother to a fetus or by contact with an infectious lesion in the birth canal. Transplacental transmission can occur throughout pregnancy. The risk of vertical transmission is greater among pregnant women with primary or secondary syphilis than with latent disease, and this risk diminishes after the fourth year of untreated infection. In children with acquired syphilis manifesting in childhood, sexual transmission should

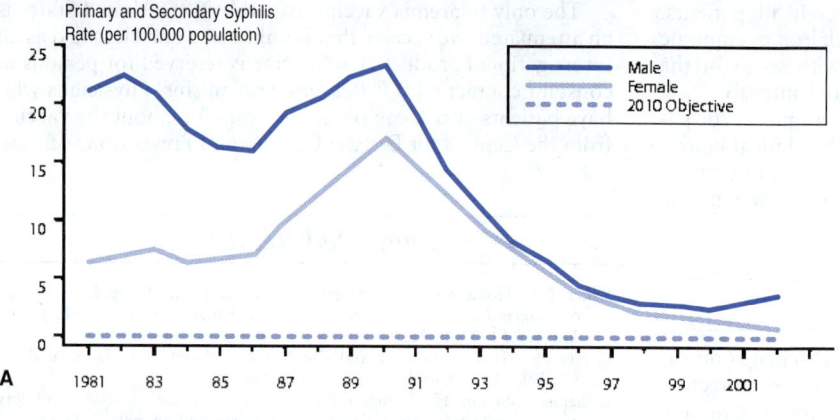

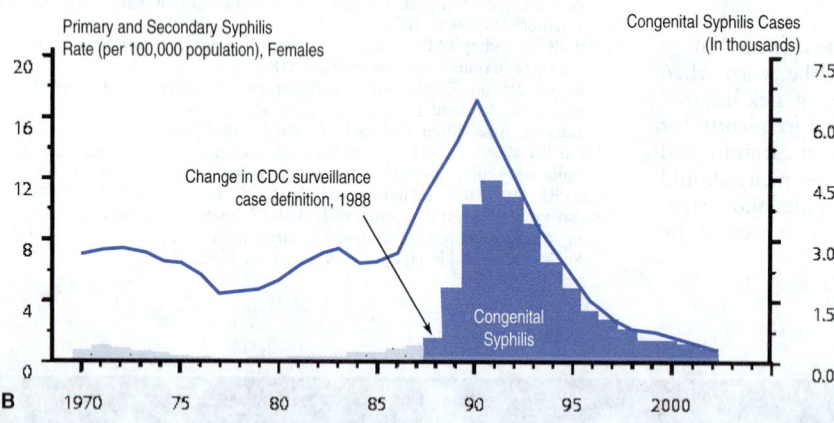

FIGURE 178.1. A: Incidence of primary and secondary syphilis in men and women in the United States, 1981 to 2002, with comparison to the *Healthy People* year 2010 national objective. **B:** Reported cases of congenital syphilis in the United States, 1970 to 2002, illustrating the correspondence of the number of cases with rates of syphilis among women. (Modified with permission from Centers for Disease Control and Prevention. *Sexually transmitted disease surveillance 2002 supplement, syphilis surveillance report.* Atlanta, GA: U.S. Department of Health and Human Services, Centers for Disease Control and Prevention, January 2004.)

be assumed unless another mechanism is identified. Syphilis seldom is found in children who have been sexually abused.

An upsurge in the number of syphilis cases in the United States during the late 1980s subsequently diminished during the 1990s (Fig. 178.1A). Risk factors associated with this increase, and with many current cases, include poverty, crack cocaine use, trading sex for drugs and money, and infection with human immunodeficiency virus (HIV). Dual infection with gonorrhea is present in 8% of cases. Syphilis is more prevalent in men than in women, and the gender gap in primary and secondary syphilis cases that had been closing in the United States during the 1990s began to widen again in 2001 (Fig. 178.1A). In 2002, the national rate among men was 3.8 cases/100,000 compared with 1.1 among women. The increase in male cases occurred primarily among men who have sex with men.

African Americans have had rates higher than those of other groups in the United States, but this disparity narrowed from more than 50-fold compared with non-Hispanic whites in 1991 to eightfold in 2002. The peak age range of syphilis is 15 to 55 years, coinciding with increased sexual activity. Female case rates are higher than those of males from ages 15 to 19 years, reflecting sexual activity with older males who have higher infection rates. The rates of syphilis vary widely across the United States (Fig. 178.2). In 2002, the South continued to have higher rates (3.1 per 100,000) than those of the West (2.3 per 100,000), Midwest (2.1 per 100,000), and Northeast (1.7 per 100,000), although rates increased in the latter three regions in 2002.

The rates of congenital syphilis in the United States have declined since 1991 and correspond closely with those of acquired syphilis in women of childbearing age (Fig. 178.1B). Inadequacy or lack of prenatal care is a risk factor for vertical transmission to the fetus or newborn (the mother goes untreated). Syphilis remains a considerable public health issue in developing countries and Eastern Europe. Congenital syphilis increased 26-fold in the Russian Federation from 1991 to 1999.

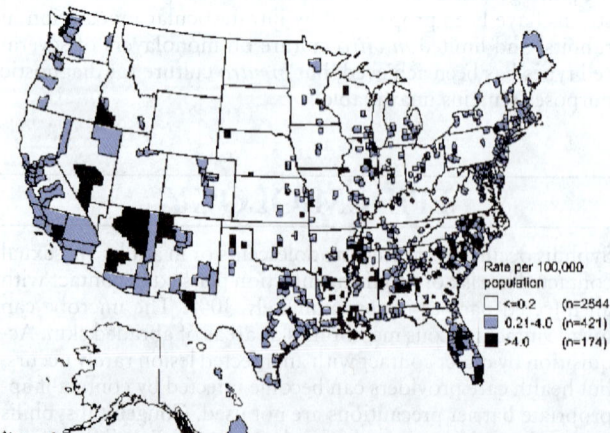

FIGURE 178.2. Primary and secondary syphilis in the United States, 2002—Counties with rates above and below the *Healthy People* year 2010 objective of 0.2 cases per 100,000 population. (Reproduced with permission from Centers for Disease Control and Prevention. *Sexually transmitted disease surveillance 2002 supplement, syphilis surveillance report.* Atlanta, GA: U.S. Department of Health and Human Services, Centers for Disease Control and Prevention, January 2004.)

PATHOGENESIS

Four stages of syphilitic disease are defined: primary, secondary, latent, and tertiary (Fig. 178.3). Syphilis begins when *T. pallidum* penetrates the skin or mucous membrane at a site of

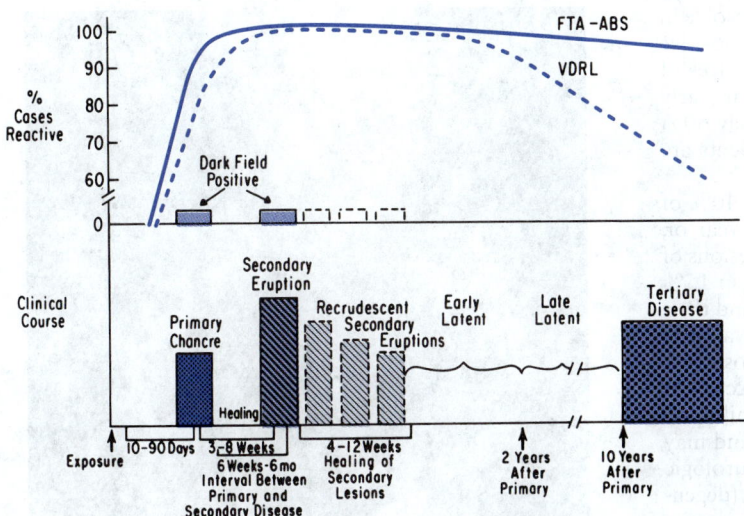

FIGURE 178.3. The course of untreated syphilis. (Reproduced with permission from Sánchez PJ, Gutman LT. Syphilis. In: Feigin RD, Cherry JD, Demmler GJ, Kaplan SL, eds. *Textbook of pediatric infectious diseases*, 5th ed. Philadelphia: W.B. Saunders, Co., 2004.)

exposure. An outer membrane protein of the microbe appears to attach to a receptor(s) on the host cell surface, initiating invasion. The organism multiplies locally and spreads through the perivascular lymphatic system to the systemic circulation, which disseminates the infection widely even before a primary lesion is evident. Capillary cells are a prime target of parasitism. During the typical 3-week incubation period, a local, intense inflammatory response by plasma cells, macrophages, and lymphocytes ensues, with obliterative endarteritis in the area of inflammation. This response produces the red, indurated, ulcerative, spirochete-filled lesion of primary syphilis: the chancre. A concomitant cellular proliferation in the regional lymph nodes produces adenopathy.

The secondary lesions of syphilis, a consequence of dissemination, are caused by an inflammatory response in ectodermal tissue of skin, mucous membranes, and the central nervous system (CNS). The host response to these lesions is similar to that which occurs to primary lesions. The condylomata lata (venereal warts) of secondary syphilis are characterized by epithelial hyperplasia, hyperkeratosis, plasma cell infiltrate, and presence of spirochetes.

Tertiary syphilis can involve any organ and is caused by slowly developing immune-mediated host responses to the infection. This stage is characterized by a diffuse, chronic inflammation in affected tissues, generally skin, CNS, and cardiovascular tissues. Gummata are late-appearing focal areas of nonsuppurative inflammatory necrosis surrounded by fibrotic scarring. Viable organisms are rare findings or absent in these lesions, which appear to result from a granulomatous hypersensitivity reaction.

Congenital syphilis from the transplacental passage of treponemes during maternal spirochetemia can occur as early as 9 to 10 weeks of gestation. Pathologic changes have been observed as early as 15 weeks. Transmission *in utero* causes the wide dissemination of the organism in the fetus. The organs affected most severely include brain, liver, lung, and the skeletal system. Early infection can lead to spontaneous abortion of syphilitic fetuses, generally after 18 weeks of gestation. Infected fetuses and newborns may have extramedullary hematopoiesis. The placenta typically is large and thickened, having hypercellular villi with acute and chronic inflammation, as well as proliferative fetal vascular changes. The umbilical cord often contains abscesslike necrotic foci around the vessels within the Wharton jelly. Spirochetes are present in the umbilical vessel walls.

IgM and IgG antibodies are detectable by the time the chancre appears, but humoral immunity is insufficient to control the infection. Cell-mediated immunity is suppressed during the primary and secondary stages of infection. After effective treatment, IgM antibody declines over the course of 1 to 2 years, but IgG antibodies usually persist throughout the life of the infected person. The host immune response is not protective, such that reinfection after treatment commonly occurs.

CLINICAL MANIFESTATIONS AND COMPLICATIONS

Most cases of syphilis encountered in pediatric practice are seen in infants (congenital) or in sexually active adolescents. The stages of acquired syphilis are based on the different clinical manifestations and underlying pathophysiology. The hallmark of primary syphilis is the chancre, a skin lesion that appears at an inoculation site after a mean incubation period of 21 days (range, 3 to 90 days). The chancre, usually single and nontender, occurs most often on the genitalia and is associated with nontender lymphadenopathy. Regional lymphadenopathy may be the only readily apparent sign of primary syphilis in women when chancres occur on the cervix or vaginal wall. Primary syphilis heals spontaneously in 3 to 12 weeks.

Symptoms of secondary syphilis appear 2 to 12 weeks after the onset of primary syphilis and result from the dissemination of treponemes. Symptoms include low-grade fever, sore throat, headache, malaise, and diffuse lymphadenopathy. The most notable manifestation is a rash that consists of macular, maculopapular, papular, or pustular lesions that inevitably harbor organisms. The classic rash begins on the trunk and, at this stage, is generalized and maculopapular, eventually involving most of the body, including the palms and soles. Secondary syphilis may cause condylomata lata, which are hypertrophic papular skin lesions found in such moist areas as the anus or vulva. All skin and mucous membrane lesions of secondary syphilis are highly contagious. Neurosyphilis occurs in approximately 30% of patients during the course of secondary syphilis. Pleocytosis and proteinosis are present in the cerebral spinal fluid (CSF) and may be clinically silent or become manifest as meningeal and cranial or spinal nerve involvement that are reversible with proper therapy. Immune complexes comprised of treponemal antigen, fibronectin, antibody, and complement are implicated in the pathogenesis of iritis, anterior uveitis, arthritis, and nephrotic syndrome that can occur during secondary syphilis.

The rash and other findings of secondary syphilis resolve in 1 to 2 months, giving way to a latent period, defined by positive syphilis serology with no evidence of disease. Recurrences of secondary manifestations can occur during the first year (early latency) but not thereafter (late latency). Approximately 60% of untreated patients will have persisting latency. Patients are relatively immune to reinfection during latency.

Tertiary, or late, infection occurs in approximately 40% of untreated patients after a latent period of at least 1 year or, more frequently, 3 to 10 years. Gummata, the classic lesions of tertiary syphilis, develop in skin, soft tissue, and bone in 15% of cases. These lesions have minimal clinical impact, and their presence has been called benign late syphilis. Cardiovascular syphilis, including syphilitic aortitis with medial necrosis, occurs in 10% of patients with late syphilis, with onset occurring usually 10 to 40 years after primary disease. Neurosyphilis persists in approximately one-half of untreated patients and may remain asymptomatic or mimic almost any other neurologic disease. Common presentations include tabes dorsalis (degeneration of dorsal columns of the spinal cord), paresis, dementia, meningitis, and amyotrophic lateral sclerosis (ALS). The interval between primary syphilis and the onset of late neurosyphilis usually is more than 5 years, but disease may progress more rapidly in children than in adults.

Congenital Syphilis

Untreated syphilis that occurs during pregnancy is transmitted to the fetus in nearly all cases and can lead to spontaneous abortion (usually after the first trimester), stillbirth, premature delivery, and nonimmune hydrops fetalis. Live-born infected infants may be asymptomatic (as many as two-thirds) or manifest early signs (those appearing in the first 2 years of life) and/or late signs (those appearing later, over the first two decades of life). Any organ system can be affected because of the widespread dissemination that occurs after transplacental infection. In the newborn, congenital syphilis can have presentations similar to those of congenital infections caused by cytomegalovirus, toxoplasmosis, herpes simplex virus, rubella, bacterial sepsis, blood group incompatibility, and numerous other neonatal conditions.

Early signs vary, and their presence at birth versus later onset may depend on the timing of infection *in utero*. Hepatomegaly occurs in more than 90% of affected infants. Liver function may be normal, but jaundice due to syphilitic hepatitis is associated with elevated serum transaminase and alkaline phosphatase concentrations. Direct hyperbilirubinemia occurs commonly, due to cholestasis, and prothrombin time may be prolonged. Liver disease, when present, may resolve slowly and even transiently worsen after treatment. Splenomegaly is present in one-half of cases and usually is associated with extramedullary hematopoiesis. Generalized nonsuppurative lymphadenopathy, including epitrochlear adenopathy, is evident in as many as 50% of infants.

Skin involvement commonly occurs and usually appears during the first 2 weeks of life. The classic eruption consists of small copper-red maculopapular lesions. When widespread and bullous, it is called syphilitic pemphigus. Hands and feet are affected most severely, and these areas undergo desquamation and crusting over the course of 1 to 3 weeks. Bullous fluid teems with spirochetes. Nasal mucous membrane involvement takes the forms of snuffles (syphilitic rhinitis), which appears after the first week of life; the blood-tinged discharge is filled with spirochetes. Purulence may indicate bacterial superinfection. Condylomata appear on other mucous membranes or other areas of skin affected by moisture or friction. Mucous patches may been seen in the mouth and genitalia. Fissures may occur around the lips, nares, or anus.

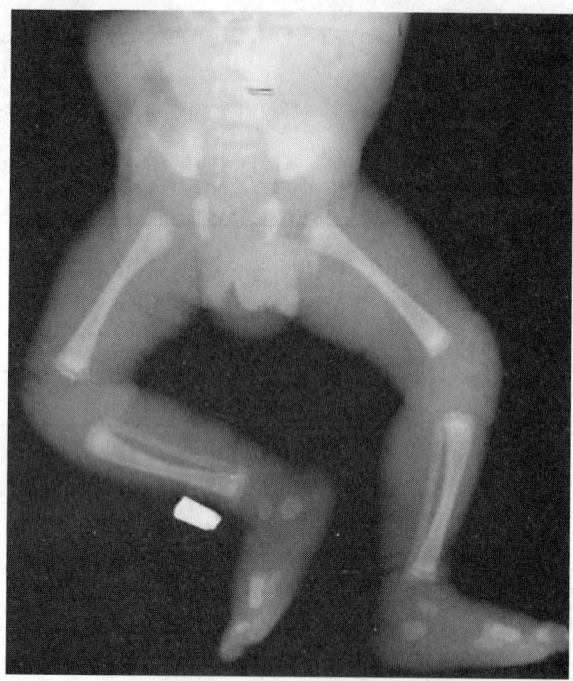

FIGURE 178.4. Skeletal radiograph of legs, showing diffuse metaphysitis in a child with congenital syphilis. (Courtesy of Dr. Milton Wagner, Baylor College of Medicine, Houston, TX.)

Bone involvement occurs in 60% to 80% of cases and usually is multiple and symmetric. Periostitis occurs in the metaphyses and diaphyses of long bones, whereas osteochondritis affects the joints, primarily knees, ankles, wrists, and elbows (Fig. 178.4). Pain associated with bony involvement can be striking and can lead to refusal to move the involved extremity, termed pseudoparalysis of Parrot. Demineralization or destruction of the upper medial tibial metaphysis, when evident radiographically, is called Wimberger sign. Bone changes usually resolve spontaneously during the first 6 months of life.

The involvement of the CNS often is asymptomatic and may arise after the neonatal period, if the disease goes untreated. It may present as acute syphilitic leptomeningitis or chronic meningovascular neurosyphilis. Cranial nerve palsies, seizures, or hydrocephalous can occur. CSF findings are considered suggestive of neurosyphilis in infants with more than 25 white blood cells (WBC)/mm^3 and protein greater than 150 mg/dL (greater than 170 mg/dL in premature infants). Reactive CSF VRDL generally indicates the presence of neurosyphilis, although false-positive results may occur. CNS infection can be present even in the face of normal CSF studies. Ocular involvement presents most commonly as chorioretinitis, but congenital glaucoma and uveitis also occur.

Anemia, thrombocytopenia, leukopenia, and leukocytosis are common developments in congenital syphilis. Hemolytic anemia that is Coombs test-negative can occur and persist for weeks after effective treatment has been given. *Pneumonia alba*, a fibrotic pneumonia, may be seen in congenital syphilis (Fig. 178.5). A slowly resolving, diffuse pulmonic infiltrate also may be documented on chest radiography. Other findings include failure to thrive, pancreatitis, nephritis, nephrotic syndrome, myocarditis, ileitis, malabsorptive gastrointestinal fibrosis, testicular masses, alopecia, nail exfoliation, and pituitary gumma.

Late congenital syphilis occurs in 40% of untreated survivors and has multiple manifestations, many of which are residual to early lesions. The identification and treatment of neonates with congenital syphilis has nearly eliminated these consequences in developed countries. Many of these lesions

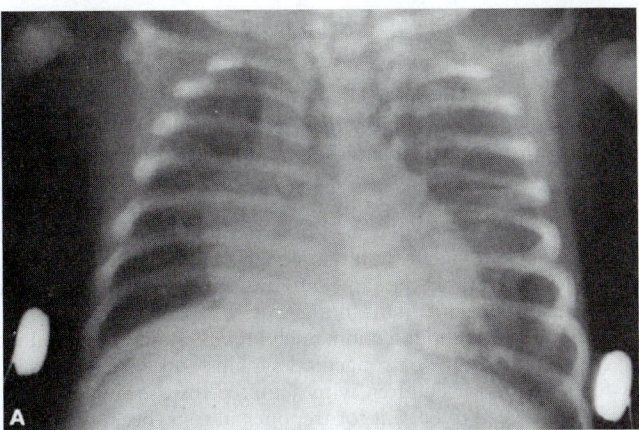
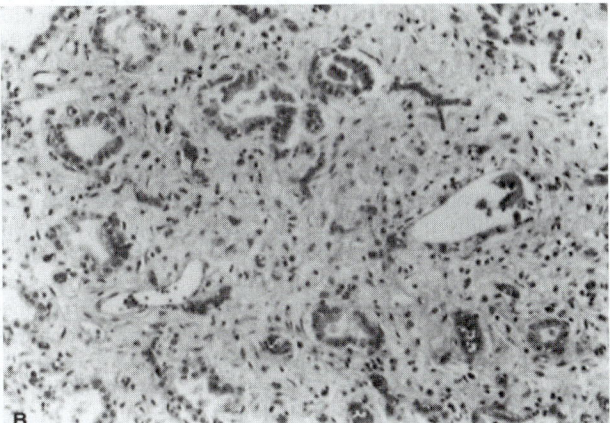

FIGURE 178.5. A: Chest radiograph of an infant with congenital syphilis pneumonia. No distinguishing characteristics differentiate bacterial or certain viral pneumonias of infancy. (Courtesy of Dr. Milton Wagner, Baylor College of Medicine, Houston, TX.) **B:** Histologic section from a more extensive pneumonia than is evident in A. Note extensive fibrosis with loss of normal pulmonary architecture. (Courtesy of Dr. Claire Langston, Baylor College of Medicine, Houston, TX.)

are destructive in nature, such that damage that occurs prior to the administration of treatment often is irreversible. Nasal cartilage destruction that occurs during snuffles can lead to a saddle-nose deformity. Prolonged periostitis can lead to frontal bossing (olympian brow), thickening of the sternoclavicular portion of the clavicle (Higoumenakis sign), anterior bowing of the mid-tibia (saber shins), and scaphoid scapula. Clutton joints are symmetric, painless, sterile, synovial effusions, usually localized to the knees. Perforation of the hard palate is a classic finding.

Dental anomalies include Hutchinson teeth (peg-shaped, notched central incisors), mulberry molars (multicuspid first molars), and enamel anomalies predisposing to caries. Eye involvement leads to interstitial keratitis in patients between ages 4 and 30 years, secondary glaucoma, or corneal scarring. Once present, keratitis is not affected by penicillin. Eighth-nerve deafness can develop, usually in children between ages 8 and 10 years, and often starts with high-frequency hearing loss. Together, Hutchinson teeth, interstitial keratitis, and eighth-nerve deafness comprise the Hutchinson triad. Rhagades are spoke-like scars around the mouth, anus, and genitalia that began as fissures. Involvement of the CNS can include meningovascular involvement and paresis. Cranial nerve palsies and optic atrophy can develop. Other findings that occur during early congenital syphilis can persist and progress.

DIAGNOSIS

Syphilis is diagnosed through clinical findings and through the direct identification of treponemes in clinical specimens or through y positive findings on treponemal-specific or nonspecific serology (Box 178.1). The rabbit-infectivity test remains the reference standard for confirmation of syphilis, but it is not available outside research laboratories. Clinically, the definitive laboratory diagnosis is made either by direct visualization of treponemes by dark-field microscopy of exudate from a primary chancre or an active secondary lesion or by direct fluorescent antibody (DFA) testing of clinical specimens.

Probable cases of syphilis can be established by means of serologic findings in association with compatible clinical findings. Specific tests for antibody to *T. pallidum* include the fluorescent treponemal antibody absorption (FTA-ABS) test and the treponemal-specific microhemagglutination test (MHA-TP). The MHA-TP largely has been replaced by the *T. pallidum*

particle agglutination test (TP-PA). The TP-PA is used more widely than is the FTA-ABS. These tests are positive in 75% (TP-PA) to 85% (FTA-ABS) of patients with primary syphilis and in 100% of patients with secondary syphilis. False-positive results are rare but may occur in patients with other spirochetal diseases, including Lyme disease, leptospirosis, relapsing fever, or those caused by other pathogenic *Treponema* species. Specific treponemal tests usually become positive earlier in the course of disease than do nonspecific tests and usually remain positive for life. Disadvantages of the treponemal-specific tests include greater expense, longer assay times, and lack of correlation of titers with disease activity. Efforts to develop immunoblotting tests for anti-treponemal IgM or IgA, which may be useful in establishing the diagnosis of congenital syphilis in cases in which the IgG could be of maternal origin, are ongoing. Polymerase chain reaction (PCR)-based tests have been evaluated in research settings.

The nontreponemal tests for syphilis involve detection of antibodies to cardiolipin, a component of membranes and mammalian tissue (purified cardiolipin in lecithin-cholesterol liposomes is used in current tests). The two nontreponemal tests currently in use are the rapid plasma reagin (RPR) test and the Venereal Disease Research Laboratory (VDRL) test. The RPR

BOX 178.1	Diagnostic Tests for Syphilis

Diagnostic identification of *Treponema pallidum*
Dark-field examination of exudate
Direct fluorescent antibody to *T. pallidum* (exudate)

Specific treponemal serologic tests
Fluorescent treponemal antibody absorption test (FTA-ABS)
Microhemagglutination test for *T. pallidum* (MHA-TP)
T. pallidum particle agglutination test (TP-PA)

Nontreponemal serologic tests
VDRL test
Rapid plasma reagin card test (RPR)

is positive in approximately 85% of cases of primary syphilis and in 98% of cases of secondary syphilis, whereas the VDRL test is positive in approximately 80% of primary cases and in 95% of secondary cases. Nontreponemal titers reflect disease activity: fourfold decreases suggest adequate therapy, whereas fourfold increases indicate active disease (treatment failure or reinfection). Patients usually become seronegative to nontreponemal tests within 1 year of receiving adequate treatment of primary syphilis and within 2 years for secondary syphilis. In rare cases, a serofast state occurs, in which a positive (but usually low) titer persists despite adequate therapy. These tests are inexpensive but are less sensitive than are the specific treponemal tests. These are used primarily for screening and monitoring therapy, whereas the treponemal tests are used to establish presumptive diagnosis. The VDRL test is the only one approved for testing the reactivity of spinal fluid.

False-positive reactions with nontreponemal tests occur in approximately 1% of normal adults. The reaginic antibody cross-reacts with more than 200 non-*T. pallidum* antigens (although not with the agents of Lyme disease). False-positive reactions can occur during some viral infections (e.g., infectious mononucleosis, varicella, measles, and perhaps HIV infection), systemic lupus erythematosus, lymphoma, malaria, tuberculosis, hepatitis, and endocarditis, and among injection-drug users. False-negative results can occur when a high concentration of antibody inhibits agglutination (the prozone phenomenon), which can be avoided with serial dilutions of the serum. Over the course of time, some untreated patients may become seronegative. In the absence of definitive laboratory confirmation, specific treponemal tests should be used to confirm diagnoses suspected on the basis of clinical findings or positive nontreponemal tests.

Laboratory Evaluation

In addition to serologic testing, children with suspected or confirmed syphilis, after thorough physical examination, should have complete blood counts (including platelet count and differential) and CSF analysis (cell count, protein, and VDRL testing). Routine CSF analysis in adolescents is not needed unless they have neurologic or ophthalmologic signs or symptoms, evidence of tertiary syphilis, or coinfection with HIV. Decisions to obtain radiographs of the chest or long bones, liver function tests, ophthalmologic exams, or hearing tests can be based on clinical findings.

Congenital Syphilis

The diagnosis of congenital syphilis is suggested by a maternal history of syphilis during pregnancy or clinical findings in the neonate. The maternal serologic status for syphilis should be determined for all newborn infants prior to hospital discharge. Testing of maternal serum is preferred, because infant serum can be nonreactive if maternal titers are low or the mother was infected late in pregnancy. Cord blood should not be used for testing because of unacceptable false-positive and false-negative rates. As in acquired disease, confirmation of the diagnosis of congenital syphilis in mothers or symptomatic infants is achieved best (but infrequently) through direct identification of *T. pallidum* from a lesion, by either dark-field microscopy or DFA. A mother whose only evidence of active syphilis is a newly positive nontreponemal test should have her diagnosis confirmed with a treponemal test before the evaluation and treatment of an asymptomatic infant is initiated for congenital syphilis, unless the wait for such results would unduly delay providing appropriate care for the infant. Establishing sero-

logic diagnoses can be difficult in infants because of transplacentally acquired maternal IgG.

Infants are considered to have proved or highly probable congenital syphilis if they have one or more of (a) physical, laboratory, or radiographic evidence of active disease (in conjunction with evidence of maternal syphilis if the following criteria are absent); (b) the presence of treponemes in the placenta or umbilical cord, detected by dark-field or DFA examinations; (c) reactive CSF VDRL; or (d) serum nontreponemal titer at least fourfold higher than that of their mother, using the same test and preferably the same laboratory. The last circumstance is uncommon, and infant:mother ratios of less than four do not exclude congenital infection. Such infants should be examined carefully for signs of congenital syphilis and evaluated as set forth above for children with acquired disease. Infant serum does not need to be sent for treponemal tests, because positive tests do not distinguish between infant or maternal origin of the antibody, and negative tests do not rule out infection.

Infants with possible congenital syphilis include those who have (a) a normal physical examination *and* (b) serum nontreponemal titers the same or less than fourfold higher than maternal titers *and* any of the following maternal histories: (a) mother received inadequate or no treatment or has no documentation of treatment; (b) mother was treated with a nonpenicillin regimen; (c) mother was treated with an appropriate penicillin regimen but did not have the expected fourfold decline in nontreponemal titer; (d) mother was treated 30 days or less before delivery (efficacy of treatment cannot be assumed); or (e) mother was treated before pregnancy but has no documentation of serologic follow-up to assess response to therapy or reinfection. In addition to the evaluation recommended for infants with highly probable congenital syphilis, these infants should have long-bone radiographs, which are one of the most sensitive clinical studies in detecting congenital syphilis in otherwise asymptomatic infants. When possible, the placenta or umbilical cord of these infants also should be examined. Findings consistent with congenital syphilis would reclassify these infants as having proved or highly probable disease for treatment purposes.

Asymptomatic infants with nontreponemal titers the same or less than fourfold of their maternal titers can be considered in two groups: those born to (a) mothers who were treated during pregnancy more than 4 weeks prior to delivery with a penicillin regimen appropriate to the stage of disease and who had a fourfold decrease in nontreponemal titer if early syphilis or stable low titer if late syphilis (with no evidence of reinfection or relapse), and (b) mothers who were treated before pregnancy and had stable, low nontreponemal titers (VDRL of 1:2 or less, or RPR of 1:4 or less) before and during pregnancy and at delivery. This distinction is made for treatment considerations. Neither infant group requires laboratory investigation for evidence of congenital syphilis.

THERAPY

Parenteral penicillin G is the preferred drug for all stages of syphilis. Penicillin resistance has not developed in *T. pallidum*. Dosage and duration depend on the stage and clinical manifestations. Penicillin G is the only agent documented to be effective for patients with neurosyphilis, congenital syphilis, or syphilis during pregnancy. In these scenarios, penicillin-allergic patients generally should be desensitized and then treated with penicillin. If they cannot be treated, expert consultation should be obtained. The Jarisch-Herxheimer reaction, which consists of fever, headache, myalgia, and malaise, occurs in some patients 2 to 12 hours after receiving therapy for active syphilis (especially early stages). The reaction is thought to be produced by the release of treponemal endotoxin through the action of penicillin. It is a rare finding in newborns but may occur in later infancy.

Acquired Syphilis

Early acquired syphilis (primary, secondary, or early latent syphilis) can be treated with 50,000 U/kg of benzathine penicillin G intramuscularly in a single dose (not to exceed the adult dose of 2.4 million units). In nonpregnant patients 8 years old or older who are allergic to penicillin, 14-day courses of doxycycline or tetracycline may be given. These agents may be considered for younger children if the benefits of therapy are considered greater than the risks of dental staining. Limited data suggest that ceftriaxone should be effective for early syphilis. The optimal regimen is undefined, but some experts recommend 1 g daily intramuscularly or intravenously for 8 to 10 days in adolescents and adults. A single dose is not effective. A single oral dose of azithromycin, 2 g, may be effective in some patients. Close follow-up is essential when any of the nonpenicillin regimens is used. In children younger than 8 years old, especially those for whom close follow-up is not assured, consideration should be given to hospitalization and desensitization, followed by treatment with penicillin G.

Latent or tertiary syphilis existing for more than 1 year with no evidence of neurosyphilis can be treated with benzathine penicillin G at a dosage of 50,000 U/kg/dose (not to exceed 2.4 million units), administered intramuscularly for 3 successive weeks. In patients who are allergic to penicillin, either tetracycline or doxycycline can be given for 4 weeks, but only in cases in which neurosyphilis has been excluded by lumbar puncture.

Children with neurosyphilis should be given aqueous crystalline penicillin G intravenously, 200,000 to 300,000 U/kg/day divided every 4 to 6 hours, for 10 to 14 days. The recommended regimen in adolescents and adults is aqueous crystalline penicillin G, 12 to 24 million U/day (2 to 4 million units every 4 hours), given intravenously for 10 to 14 days. If compliance can be assured, adolescents or adults may be treated with an alternative regimen of 2.4 million units of procaine penicillin intramuscularly as a single daily dose combined with probenecid, 500 mg/dose orally four times per day, both for 10 to 14 days. Some experts add the treatment course for tertiary syphilis above after the neurosyphilis regimen is completed.

Incubating syphilis may be eliminated with penicillin, ampicillin, amoxicillin, ceftriaxone, or azithromycin (but not spectinomycin) treatments given for gonorrhea or chlamydia infection.

Follow-up

Patients who acquired syphilis less than 1 year before receiving treatment (early) should have quantitative nontreponemal tests at 3, 6, and 12 months after finishing treatment. Those with syphilis for more than 1 year (late) should have repeat testing at 12 and 24 months. If nontreponemal titers rise or do not fall fourfold within 6 months for early disease or 12 to 24 months for late disease, patients should be evaluated for neurosyphilis and HIV infection and retreated using the late-disease regimen. Twofold changes in titers may represent interassay variability rather than true change. Patients with neurosyphilis should undergo repeat CSF examinations every 6 months. If CSF cell counts do not decrease within the first 6 months or normalize in 2 years, retreatment should be considered.

Evaluation for Sexual Abuse

Syphilis is an uncommon complication of sexual abuse in children. However, the diagnosis of syphilis in children beyond their early infancy raises questions of and the need for investigation for possible sexual abuse. Distinguishing late (and previously undiagnosed) congenital syphilis from acquired syphilis can be difficult. Antibiotics administered for common childhood infections inadvertently may provide partial treatment for congenital syphilis and alter its presentation. The child should be thoroughly examined for the presence of late manifestations of congenital syphilis and should be referred to clinicians skilled in the evaluation of children who potentially have been sexually abused.

Congenital Syphilis

Infants identified as having proved or highly probable disease, before or after clinical and laboratory evaluation, are treated with either (a) intravenous aqueous crystalline penicillin G, 50,000 U/kg per dose every 12 hours (100,000 U/kg/day) during the first 7 days of life and every 8 hours (150,000 U/kg/day) thereafter for a total of 10 days or (b) intramuscular procaine penicillin G, 50,000 U/kg/day as a single dose for 10 days. Intravenous aqueous penicillin provides higher CSF concentrations of penicillin G than does intramuscular procaine penicillin, but both are considered adequate therapy for congenital syphilis. If more than 1 day of therapy is missed, the entire course should be restarted. A full 10-day course of penicillin is preferred, even if the infant received ampicillin initially for possible sepsis.

Infants initially identified as having possible congenital syphilis may be treated with a single intramuscular dose of benzathine penicillin G, 50,000 U/kg, if the full evaluation (including CBC, CSF studies, and long-bone radiographs) is normal and follow-up is certain. Otherwise, the full 10-day course of aqueous or procaine penicillin G should be administered. Some specialists recommend the single-dose treatment without evaluation if the infant's nontreponemal test is nonreactive, risk of infection is low, and close serologic follow-up is assured. If any part of the infant's evaluation is abnormal or uninterpretable (e.g., CSF contaminated by blood), the full 10-day course is recommended. Some experts prefer the 10-day course for all infants in this category. Others prefer it if the mother had untreated early syphilis at delivery.

For asymptomatic infants born to mothers with appropriate treatment and response to treatment during pregnancy, the single-dose benzathine penicillin (as noted earlier) is recommended. Some experts would not treat these infants but would provide close serologic follow-up. For asymptomatic infants born to mothers who have had appropriate therapy and response prior to pregnancy, treatment is not mandatory, but some experts would treat with a single dose of benzathine penicillin, especially if follow-up is uncertain.

When congenital syphilis of any stage is identified beyond the neonatal period, the treatment regimen for acquired neurosyphilis generally should be used.

Follow-up

Infants treated for congenital syphilis should be evaluated at 1, 2, 3, 6, and 12 months of age. Nontreponemal tests should be repeated every 2 to 3 months after treatment until they are nonreactive or diminished fourfold. Nontreponemal antibodies of maternal origin usually become negative within 3 months and should be negative by the time the child is 6 months of age, if the infant was not infected. If nontreponemal titers remain stable or increase after the infant reaches ages 6 to 12 months, he or she should be re-evaluated (including CSF analysis) and treated with a 10-day parenteral course of penicillin G. Maternally derived treponemal-specific antibodies may persist for as long as 15 months, such that treponemal tests are of little help during infancy. Reactivity at 18 months can be used to confirm that congenital infection had occurred.

Infants with congenital neurosyphilis (abnormal or unin-terpretable CSF WBC count or protein or positive CSF VDRL) should have repeat clinical and CSF evaluations every 6 months until their CSF examinations are normal. A reactive CSF VDRL test at any 6-month evaluation is an indication for retreatment. If CSF WBC counts still are not decreasing at each examination or remain abnormal at 2 years, retreatment also is indicated.

Syphilis and Human Immunodeficiency Virus Infection

Because the risk factors for acquisition of syphilis and HIV in-fection are similar, coinfection is not an unusual occurrence. Patients diagnosed with either infection should be assessed for the presence of the other, as well as other sexually transmit-ted diseases. HIV-infected patients may have increased risks of developing neurologic complications during early syphilis and higher rates of treatment failure with recommended regimens. Serologic tests for syphilis in patients with HIV generally can be interpreted as for HIV-negative persons, but false-negative results have been reported. Treatment generally is the same as for HIV-negative persons, although some experts recommend using the late-syphilis regimen, even for patients with early syphilis. Some physicians also recommend that all coinfected patients have CSF examination prior to beginning therapy, with follow-up studies performed in those with initial abnormalities. Treatment of neurosyphilis is the same as for HIV-negative patients.

PREVENTION

All persons diagnosed with syphilis should be reported to local public health authorities for contact investigation and should undergo testing for other sexually transmitted diseases. Sex-ual contacts within the past 3 months of persons with pri-mary and within the past 6 months of persons with secondary syphilis should be treated because of the high risk of the pres-ence of early syphilis that still may be seronegative. All pregnant women should undergo serologic screening early in pregnancy and again at delivery. Women at high risk for syphilis should un-dergo testing again at 28 weeks' gestation. Moist, open lesions and blood from persons with acquired primary or secondary syphilis, as well as infants with congenital syphilis, should be considered contagious until 24 hours of treatment has been completed. Gloves should be worn for all patient contact dur-ing this period.

Suggested Readings

Centers for Disease Control and Prevention. Sexually transmitted diseases treat-ment guidelines 2002. *MMWR Morb Mortal Wkly Rep* 2002;51(RR-6):18.

Christian CW, Lavelle J, Bell LM. Preschoolers with syphilis. *Pediatrics* 1999;103:e4. URL: http://www.pediatrics.org/cgi/content/full/103/1/e4.

Committee on Infectious Diseases, American Academy of Pediatrics. Syphilis. In: *2003 Red Book*. Elk Grove Village, IL: American Academy of Pediatrics, 2003;595.

Michelow IC, Wendel GD, Norgard MV, et al. Central nervous system infection in congenital syphilis. *N Engl J Med* 2002;346:1792.

Moyer VA, Schneider V, Yetman R, et al. Contribution of long-bone radiographs to the management of congenital syphilis in the newborn infant. *Arch Pediatr Adolesc Med* 1998;152:353.

Sánchez PJ, Gutman LT. Syphilis. In: Feigin RD, Cherry JD, Demmler GJ, Kaplan SL, eds. *Textbook of pediatric infectious diseases*, 5th ed. Philadelphia: W.B. Saunders Co, 2004;1724.

Sheffield JS, Sánchez PJ, Morris G, et al. Congenital syphilis after maternal treat-ment for syphilis during pregnancy. *Am J Obstet Gynecol* 2002;186:569.

Sison CG, Ostrea EM, Reyes MP, et al. The resurgence of congenital syphilis: a cocaine-related problem. *J Pediatr* 1997;130:289.

Stoll BJ, Lee FK, Larsen S, et al. Clinical and serologic evaluation of neonates for congenital syphilis: a continuing diagnostic dilemma. *J Infect Dis* 1993;167:1093.

Tikhonova L, Salakhov E, Southwick K, et al. Congenital syphilis in the Russian Federation: magnitude, determinants, and consequences. *Sex Transm Infect* 2003;79:106.

CHAPTER 179 ■ TUBERCULOSIS

JEFFREY R. STARKE

Tuberculosis remains the most important chronic infectious disease in the world in terms of morbidity, mortality, and cost. An estimated 2 billion people worldwide are infected with the tubercle bacillus, and 1 to 3 million deaths from tuberculosis occur annually. Children in developing countries account for 1.3 million cases and 450,000 deaths annually from tuberculo-sis. In the United States, an estimated 10 to 20 million people have latent tuberculosis infection, 16,000 people develop tu-berculosis each year, and 2,000 die with complications of the disease.

After *Mycobacterium tuberculosis* enters the lung and be-gins to multiply, the person has tuberculosis infection. The hall-mark of tuberculosis infection is a positive tuberculin skin test result, but chest radiography is normal or reveals only a healed granuloma, and the child is free of signs and symptoms. Tu-berculosis disease occurs when clinical manifestations of pul-monary or extrapulmonary tuberculosis become apparent by chest radiography or clinical findings. The word *tuberculosis* usually refers to disease. Most untreated infected adults never develop disease. The time between the onset of tuberculosis infection and the beginning of disease may be several weeks or many years. In adults, usually a clear distinction between in-fection and disease exists. However, among children in whom disease usually develops as an immediate complication of the primary infection, the two stages are less distinct. An infected child with radiographic or clinical manifestations consistent with tuberculosis is considered to have disease, even if no symp-toms are present.

ETIOLOGY

The genus *Mycobacterium* is classified in the order Actinomy-cetales and the family Mycobacteriaceae. The major agents of human tuberculosis are *M. tuberculosis* and *M. bovis*. Infections caused by *M. bovis* are rare in most areas the United States because of the slaughter of infected cattle and the almost universal pasteurization of milk. However, in San Diego, California, one-third of culture-proven cases of tuberculosis in children are caused by *M. bovis*, the initial infection likely occurring in another country before immigration to the United States.

Tubercle bacilli are nonmotile, non-spore-forming, pleomorphic, weakly gram-positive, curved rods approximately 2 to 4 μm long. They may appear beaded or clumped. They are obligate aerobes and grow in simple synthetic media with glycerol or other compounds as the carbon source and ammonium salts as the nitrogen source. The bacilli grow best at 37°C to 41°C, have a characteristic colony morphology, and lack pigmentation. They often grow as intertwining, serpentine cords.

A hallmark of mycobacteria is acid fastness (i.e., the capacity to form stable mycolate complexes with arylmethane dyes such as carbol-fuchsin, crystal violet, auramine, and rhodamine). The dyes are not removed readily by rinsing with ethanol plus hydrochloric acid. The bacilli appear red when stained with fuchsin (i.e., Ziehl-Neelsen or Kinyoun stains) and purple when stained with crystal violet; they exhibit yellow-green fluorescence under ultraviolet light when stained with auramine and rhodamine (Truant stain).

The cell wall of mycobacteria contains 20% to 60% lipids bound to proteins and carbohydrates. This lipid-rich cell wall accounts for hydrophobic properties, acid fastness, and resistance to the bactericidal actions of antibody and complement. True waxes, mycolic acid, and glycolipids are unique to the cell wall of mycobacteria.

Identification of mycobacteria is based on their growth characteristics, staining properties, and biochemical or metabolic characteristics. Speciation depends on the following: the temperature of optimal growth; catalase production, which is present in virulent, isoniazid-susceptible *M. tuberculosis* but absent in some isoniazid-resistant strains; the secretion of niacin, which is characteristic of *M. tuberculosis;* sensitivity to sodium chloride; the reduction of tellurite; and the capacity to produce carotenoid pigments on exposure to light (i.e., photochromogen), equally in light and dark (i.e., scotochromogen), or not at all (i.e., nonphotochromogen). In most modern mycobacteriology laboratories, the identification of *M. tuberculosis* is established by a DNA probe of colonies on a plate, organisms in broth, or high pressure liquid chromatography analysis of the mycolic acids, which are unique to each strain of mycobacteria.

EPIDEMIOLOGY

The incidence of tuberculosis in the United States declined 5% to 6% each year for several decades until 1985, when it leveled. From 1986 to 1992, the reported number of cases increased to 26,000 per year. From 1992 to 2003, case numbers again declined to approximately 15,000 in 2004. From 1985 through 2003, more than 90,000 additional cases of tuberculosis were reported in the United States than would have been expected if the previous decline had continued. Four major factors often are cited to explain the increase from 1986 to 1992. One cause was the human immunodeficiency virus (HIV) epidemic because coinfection with HIV infection is the greatest risk factor known for the development of tuberculosis disease in an adult infected with the tubercle bacillus. An increasingly important factor was the increase in the number of immigrants to the United States from countries with a high prevalence of tuberculosis. In 2003, more than 50% of U.S. tuberculosis cases occurred among foreign-born patients, compared with 22%

TABLE 179.1

HIGH-RISK GROUPS FOR TUBERCULOSIS IN THE UNITED STATES

Increased risk of exposure to an infectious adult
Foreign-born persons from high-prevalence countries
Residents of correctional institutions
Residents of nursing homes
Homeless persons
Users of intravenous and other street drugs
Some health care workers
Children living with adults in the categories listed previously
Increased likelihood that disease will develop after infection occurs
Human immunodeficiency virus coinfection
Medical risk factors (e.g., diabetes mellitus)
Immunosuppressive diseases or therapies
Malnutrition
Infancy

in 1985. A third factor, verified by new methods of DNA typing of organisms, was the discovery of transmission of *M. tuberculosis* in a variety of settings, including hospitals, nursing homes, schools, churches, and bars. Finally, the general decline in public health services and access to medical care in parts of the United States hindered identification of high-risk individuals, rapid diagnosis, treatment, and completion of contact investigations.

In the early twentieth century, the risk of being exposed to an adult with infectious tuberculosis was higher and more uniform across the entire population than it is currently. Tuberculosis has retreated into fairly well-defined groups of high-risk persons (Table 179.1). Cities with populations of more than 250,000 account for 18% of the nation's population but more than 42% of its tuberculosis cases. Case rates also are high in the Appalachian Mountain region and along the southern border of the United States.

Although tuberculosis case rates in the United States generally have increased with patient age, a trend toward an increased case rate has occurred in young adults, especially among urban minority populations. Case rates are always lowest among children 5 to 14 years of age; most childhood tuberculosis occurs among children younger than 5 years.

Certain environments in our society contain sizable numbers of adults at high risk for developing tuberculosis, which promotes its transmission. Tuberculosis rates in jails, prisons, nursing homes, homeless shelters, and migrant camps often are 10 to 50 times higher than in the general community. Many of these environments house persons at increased risk for acquiring HIV infection. HIV-seronegative adults with untreated tuberculosis infection have a 5% to 10% lifetime risk of developing tuberculosis disease. HIV-seropositive adults also infected with the bacillus develop tuberculosis at a rate of 5% to 10% per year. Although fewer cases of children with coexisting HIV infection and tuberculosis have been reported, the increased rate of childhood tuberculosis from 1986 to 1992 could be linked partially to the spread of tuberculosis infection from HIV-infected adults with tuberculosis.

Children with tuberculosis represent 5% to 6% of the total annual number of cases. Since 1976, the decline in incidence of childhood tuberculosis had been slower than that for older populations. Between 1987 and 1991, the number of pediatric tuberculosis cases in the United States increased by 39%, to 1,656 per year. This increase undoubtedly was linked to the increased case rates among young adults. From 1992 to 2003, the number of tuberculosis cases in U.S. children again declined slightly. The pediatric tuberculosis case rate reflects the effect of the disease on childhood health and serves as a public health marker of ongoing tuberculosis transmission within a community. As long as the disease persists in adults, susceptible children will become infected.

Although the number of cases of childhood tuberculosis has increased, the epidemiology in the United States has remained fairly constant. Approximately 60% of childhood cases occur in children younger than 5 years old. The disease affects both genders equally. Although most children acquire infection with *M. tuberculosis* in their home or neighborhood from relatives or adult family friends, epidemics of childhood tuberculosis, almost always caused by contact with an infectious adult, continue to occur within schools, churches, day-care centers, and nursery schools.

M. tuberculosis is transmitted from person to person, usually by droplets of mucus that become airborne when an infected person coughs, sneezes, laughs, or sings. The duration of exposure required to transmit *M. tuberculosis* depends on the infectiousness of the source case. Adults with cavitary disease harbor the greatest number of tubercle bacilli for the longest time. The best predictor of contagiousness is a positive acid-fast stain of sputum from an adolescent or adult with pulmonary disease. Most adults are no longer infectious after several days to 2 weeks of therapy, but this period may increase for patients with advanced cavitary disease who continue to cough. Children with pulmonary tuberculosis rarely infect other children. Tubercle bacilli are sparse in the endobronchial secretions of children, who usually do not cough with sufficient force to transmit infection. However, those rare children who develop adult-type tuberculosis, with upper lobe infiltrate or cavity, severe cough, and sputum production, may be infectious to others.

PATHOGENESIS

The primary (Ghon) complex of tuberculosis consists of disease at the portal of entry and the regional lymph nodes that drain the area of the primary focus. The infection may occur anywhere in the body, but the primary site is the lung in more than 95% of cases. Tubercle bacilli on particles larger than 10 μm usually are caught in the mucociliary mechanisms of the bronchi and are expelled. Smaller particles are inhaled beyond the clearance mechanisms. In the alveoli or alveolar ducts, bacilli multiply, and an inflammatory exudate is present. Some of the bacilli are carried by macrophages through the lymphatic channels to the regional lymph nodes. While the primary complex is developing, tubercle bacilli spread by the bloodstream and lymphatics to many parts of the body. This dissemination can involve large numbers of bacilli, leading to miliary tuberculosis or, more commonly, small numbers of bacilli that leave tuberculous foci scattered in various tissues. These foci may or may not develop into significant extrapulmonary tuberculosis later in life. After 4 to 8 weeks, cell-mediated immunity develops. At this time, the primary complex usually heals to the extent that it is not visible on chest radiography, and further dissemination is arrested. These events usually produce no signs or symptoms.

The parenchymal portion of the primary complex often heals completely after undergoing caseating necrosis and encapsulation. Further healing occurs by fibrosis or calcification. The nodal component has a decreased tendency to heal completely. Even after calcification occurs, viable tubercle bacilli may persist for many years in the node or in distant sites. Although children usually develop tuberculosis disease during the primary infection, most cases in adults are caused by endogenous regrowth of latent bacilli resident in the body from the time of the primary infection (i.e., adult or postprimary tuberculosis). The most common form of postprimary tuberculosis

affects the apical region of the lung. The apex of the lung has the highest oxygen tension, and the many organisms deposited there during hematogenous dissemination are those most likely to reactivate.

Without specific therapy, tuberculosis disease develops in 5% to 10% of immunologically normal adults with tuberculosis infection at some time during their lives. The risk for children is greater; as many as 40% of children younger than 1 year of age with untreated tuberculosis infection develop radiographic evidence of disease, compared with 24% of children between the ages of 1 and 5 years and 15% of those between the ages of 11 and 15 years. Although infants and young children are more likely to develop immediate complications of the initial infection, children who are older when infected are more likely to develop postprimary disease as adults.

A predictable timetable of tuberculosis infection and its possible complications exists. Massive lymphohematogenous spread leading to miliary or acute meningeal tuberculosis occurs approximately 2 to 6 months after the initial infection develops. Endobronchial tuberculosis, with segmental pulmonary changes, occurs within 9 months. Clinically important lesions of bones or joints do not appear until at least 1 year after infection develops, and renal lesions develop 5 to 25 years after initial infection develops. In general, complications in children occur within the first 5 years (especially the first year) after they develop the initial infection. Complications later in life are caused by reactivation of previously dormant latent bacilli at a site of dissemination.

DIAGNOSIS

The diagnosis of tuberculosis disease in adults is mainly bacteriologic, but in children, it usually is epidemiologic and indirect. In the absence of a positive culture result, the strongest evidence for tuberculosis in a child is history of exposure to an adult with contagious disease. The importance of an adequate history and exposure tracings cannot be overemphasized. Less direct methods, such as the tuberculin skin test and other laboratory tests, offer supportive information.

Tuberculin Skin Test

A positive tuberculin skin test result is the hallmark of tuberculosis infection. Within 8 years of his discovery of the tubercle bacilli, Robert Koch found that subcutaneous injection of a broth culture filtrate of tubercle bacilli, which he called *tuberculin*, produced fever, chills, vomiting, and induration at the injection site in a person with tuberculosis. The diagnostic usefulness of this test was described in the early twentieth century. In 1934, Florence Seibert developed a purified protein derivative (PPD) from broth cultures, which became the standard known as *PPD-S*.

The gold standard tuberculin test is the Mantoux, an intradermal injection of 5 tuberculin units (TU) of PPD in 0.1 mL of diluent containing the stabilizing agent polysorbate 80. This test is standardized and quantitative; results are interpreted as the transverse diameter of induration at 48 to 72 hours. The Mantoux test is subject to a variety of influences related to the test procedure (Table 179.2). The testing technique must be precise and consistent. Although experienced health care providers demonstrate good intraobserver agreement in interpretation, inexperienced observers, especially parents, often report results inaccurately.

A variety of host-related factors, such as age, nutrition, immunosuppression, viral infections or immunization with live viral vaccines, administration of corticosteroids, and the presence of overwhelming tuberculosis, can depress tuberculin

TABLE 179.2

FACTORS THAT CAN INFLUENCE MANTOUX TEST RESULTS

Factors related to the host
Presence of other infections (viral, bacterial, fungal)
Recent inoculation with live virus vaccine
Metabolic derangements
Malnutrition
Immunosuppression by disease or drug treatment
Age (very old or young)
Overwhelming tuberculosis disease
History of bacille Calmette-Guérin vaccination

Factors related to the environment
Prevalence of nontuberculous mycobacteria

Factors related to the testing procedure
Improper administration or interpretation
Antigen overload with simultaneous tests
Boosting exerted by previous skin tests
Loss of strength of purified protein derivative because of improper storage
Variations in commercial products

reactivity. Approximately 10% of adults and children with culture-documented tuberculosis do not react initially to PPD; delayed hypersensitivity often appears after appropriate treatment is started. In adults, initial anergy to tuberculin is related to a poor prognosis, but it does not appear to be true for children. A negative skin test result never rules out tuberculosis.

Recent exposure to environmental nontuberculous mycobacteria (NTM) can result in cross-sensitization and a false-positive reaction to PPD. This problem is especially common in the southeastern United States, where NTM occur in the environment, especially the soil. Cross-sensitization with NTM usually causes a reaction of less than 10 mm to a 5-TU Mantoux test, although reactions up to 15 mm can occur. This cross-sensitization tends to wane over a period of months. Prior immunization with bacille Calmette-Guérin (BCG) also may cause a significant Mantoux reaction, which often is smaller than 10 to 12 mm and usually wanes within 3 to 5 years. Because the effect of BCG on the skin test is variable and a reaction of 10 mm or more in a previously BCG-vaccinated child usually indicates infection with *M. tuberculosis,* the interpretation of the skin test result should be the same for a BCG-vaccinated child as it would be for a comparable, nonvaccinated child. Prior receipt of BCG vaccine is not a contraindication to receiving a tuberculin skin test.

The important issue for interpreting the Mantoux test result is the amount of induration that should be considered as likely to indicate tuberculosis infection. This amount varies with the population tested and depends on epidemiologic factors. Some overlap in reaction to the Mantoux test between groups of people with and without tuberculosis infection always occurs. False-positive and false-negative results always will occur, no matter what amount of induration is selected. Because of the critical contribution of epidemiology to the interpretation of the skin test, the size of induration considered positive should vary for groups according to their risk for acquiring tuberculosis infection. For adults and children at the highest risk of having tuberculosis infection progress to disease—those who are recent contacts of adults with infectious tuberculosis, who have abnormalities on chest radiography or clinical evidence of tuberculosis, or who are infected with HIV or have other causes of immune compromise—induration of 5 mm or more is classified as positive, indicating likely infection with *M. tuberculosis.* For other high-risk groups (see Table 179.1), including all infants, and for children living with adults in high-risk groups,

induration of 10 mm or more is a positive result. Although raising the amount of induration considered positive to 15 mm for children at low risk for acquiring tuberculosis may be a scientifically sound practice in some locales, this strategy presents some practical problems, the most important of which is the difficulty of establishing that a child truly has no risk factors for acquiring tuberculosis infection. The American Academy of Pediatrics and Centers for Disease Control and Prevention recommend that children from low-prevalence populations with no specific risk factors should not be tested routinely, but if they are tested, 15-mm or larger indurations should be considered positive.

Laboratory Tests

Routine laboratory tests, such as a complete blood count and differential, erythrocyte sedimentation rate, and urinalysis, rarely aid in establishing the diagnosis of tuberculosis. Abnormalities of serum liver enzyme tests may be helpful in diagnosing miliary tuberculosis. Analyses of infected body fluids (e.g., pleural, joint, cerebrospinal) demonstrating lymphocytes, elevated protein, and decreased glucose suggest tuberculosis. These fluids and sputum should be examined microscopically with acid-fast stain to detect mycobacteria.

The most important laboratory test for establishing the diagnosis and managing tuberculosis is the mycobacteria culture. In adults, isolation of the organism confirms the diagnosis, and susceptibility test results direct therapy. Isolation of *M. tuberculosis* is not essential to the diagnosis of tuberculosis in children if epidemiologic, skin test, clinical, and radiographic findings are compatible with the disease. If culture and susceptibility tests are available from the adult source case, cultures from the child add little to management. However, when the source case is unknown, especially in areas with high rates of drug resistance, attempts should be made to isolate the organism from the child. Cultures should be obtained in any child with suspected extrapulmonary tuberculosis to confirm the diagnosis. Sputum produced by an older child or adolescent with pulmonary tuberculosis often yields *M. tuberculosis.* Younger children rarely produce sputum spontaneously, but it may be induced by use of hypertonic saline aerosol treatment. Gastric aspirates yield the organism in 30% to 40% of children; the yield is even greater in infants. When obtained correctly, gastric aspirates have a greater yield than do samples from bronchoalveolar lavage. Aspiration should be done early in the morning, as the child awakens, before the overnight accumulation of secretions swallowed from the respiratory tract is emptied from the stomach. The aspirates should be collected using saline-free fluid, and the pH should be neutralized if processing will be delayed for more than several hours.

Traditional culture methods using classic media such as Löwenstein-Jensen or simple synthetic media such as Middlebrook 7H10 require 4 to 6 weeks for isolation of the organism and another 2 to 4 weeks for susceptibility testing. The radiometric system uses liquid media containing fatty acid substrates labeled with carbon-14. As the mycobacteria metabolize the fatty acids, carbon dioxide-14 is released and measured as a marker of bacterial growth. A second substrate is used to differentiate NTM from *M. tuberculosis.* This system yields culture and susceptibility results within 7 to 10 days and is more sensitive than are traditional media for sputum cultures.

Many laboratories now use DNA probes to identify and speciate mycobacteria after they have been isolated in media. These probes use DNA sequences that are complementary to specific RNA or DNA sequences of *M. tuberculosis.* The sensitivity and specificity of these probes when used on isolated organisms approach 100%. Unfortunately, the sensitivity decreases precipitously when these probes are used directly on patient samples.

The technique of nucleic acid amplification (NAA) markedly increases the sensitivity of DNA testing directly on patient samples. The target DNA is isolated, replicated thousands of times using DNA polymerase and thermal cycling, and then detected using a nucleic acid probe or specially stained electrophoresis gels. The sensitivity and specificity of NAA for *M. tuberculosis* on sputum samples from adults with pulmonary tuberculosis that test positive with acid-fast stain have been greater than 95%, and the results can be available in less than 48 hours. Unfortunately, the various NAA techniques are approved for use only on samples that have positive results from the acid-fast stain because the specificity of the test is too low for routine testing of stain-negative samples. Several studies of the use of NAA on gastric aspirate samples from children with pulmonary tuberculosis have demonstrated a sensitivity slightly greater than culture (approximately 50%), but false-positive results also occur. The NAA for *M. tuberculosis* may be especially valuable to evaluate children with HIV infection who may have pulmonary tuberculosis. The various techniques are being adapted for use on other samples and tissues to aid in the diagnosis of extrapulmonary tuberculosis.

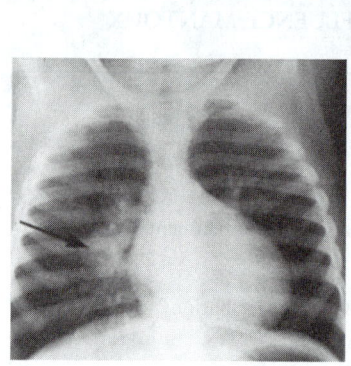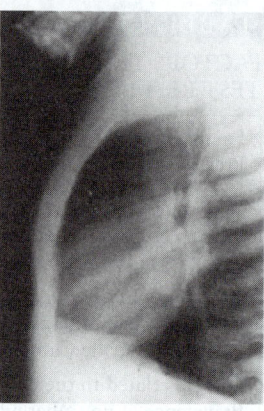

FIGURE 179.1. Chest radiographs of hilar adenopathy (*arrow*) caused by a primary tuberculosis infection in an infant. Notice the mass lesion at the hilum, seen best in the lateral view. (Courtesy of Dr. Katharine H. K. Hsu.)

Diagnostic Criteria

The diagnosis of tuberculosis disease in children often is based on epidemiologic, clinical, radiographic, and skin test information, rather than mycobacteriologic data. The diagnosis of tuberculosis disease is confirmed if *M. tuberculosis* is isolated from any body site or if the clinical, radiographic, or histologic findings are consistent with tuberculosis and at least two of the following criteria are met: (a) a 5-TU Mantoux test yields more than 5 mm of induration, (b) other disease entities are ruled out and the subsequent clinical course and response to therapy are consistent with tuberculosis, and (c) an adult source case with contagious tuberculosis is discovered. Various clinical scoring systems, which assign points to various signs and symptoms, have been developed, but none has been subjected to clinical trials and most are considered to have limited usefulness.

CLINICAL MANIFESTATIONS

Endothoracic Disease

Asymptomatic Primary Tuberculosis

Asymptomatic, primary tuberculosis is an infection associated with tuberculin skin reactivity in the absence of clinical or significant radiographic findings. This type of infection is seen more commonly in school-aged children than in young infants; 80% to 95% of infected older children have clinically silent tuberculosis infections, but only 50% to 60% of infected infants remain asymptomatic. These children usually are treated with a single antituberculosis drug. Contact tracing to determine the origin of the infection is important, especially for infants and young children who were infected recently.

Primary Pulmonary Tuberculosis

The initial pulmonary complex includes the parenchymal focus and regional lymphadenitis. Approximately 70% of primary foci are subpleural, and localized pleurisy is a common component of the primary complex. The primary infection begins with the deposition of infected droplets into lung alveoli. The initial parenchymal inflammation usually is not visible on chest radiography, but a localized, nonspecific infiltrate may be seen. All segments of the lung are at equal risk of being seeded. In 25%

of cases, multiple primary foci are present in the lungs. The infection spreads early to regional (usually hilar or mediastinal) lymph nodes. If tuberculin hypersensitivity develops within 3 to 10 weeks after infection occurs, the inflammatory reaction in the lung parenchyma and lymph nodes intensifies. The hallmark of primary tuberculosis in the lung is the relatively large size and importance of the adenitis compared with the relatively small size of the initial parenchymal focus. Because of the patterns of lymphatic drainage, a left-sided parenchymal focus often leads to bilateral hilar adenopathy, but a right-sided focus is associated with right-sided adenitis only.

In most cases, the parenchymal infiltrate and adenitis resolve early. In some children, especially infants, the hilar lymph nodes continue to enlarge (Fig. 179.1). Bronchial obstruction begins as the nodes compress the associated regional bronchus. Inflammation intensifies, and the nodes may erode through the bronchial wall, leading to formation of thick caseum in the bronchial lumen and eventual occlusion of the bronchus. The common sequence for the development of endobronchial disease is hilar adenopathy, localized emphysema (caused by partial obstruction), and then atelectasis. The resulting radiographic shadows have been called *collapse-consolidation* or *segmental* tuberculosis (Fig. 179.2). The radiographic findings are similar to those seen with foreign body aspiration. Segmental lesions are seen most commonly in infants because of the small diameters of their bronchi. These lesions tend to occur within 6 months of the development of initial infection.

Physical signs and symptoms of hilar adenopathy and segmental lesions are surprisingly uncommon and usually are found in young infants. Occasionally, the beginning of infection is marked by low-grade fever and mild cough. As the primary complex progresses, nonspecific symptoms such as fever, cough, and weight loss may occur. Pulmonary signs usually are absent. Some children have localized wheezing or diminished breath sounds, which may be accompanied by tachypnea or rarely by frank respiratory distress. Nonspecific symptoms and pulmonary signs sometimes are alleviated by antibiotics, a finding suggesting that bacterial superinfection distal to the obstruction may play a role.

Most cases of tuberculous bronchial obstruction in children resolve. Occasionally, residual calcifications of the primary focus or regional lymph nodes are present. Calcification implies that the lesion has been present for at least 6 months. Healing of the segment rarely is complicated by scarring or contraction associated with cylindric bronchiectasis, which occurs primarily in the lower lobes and is an extremely rare

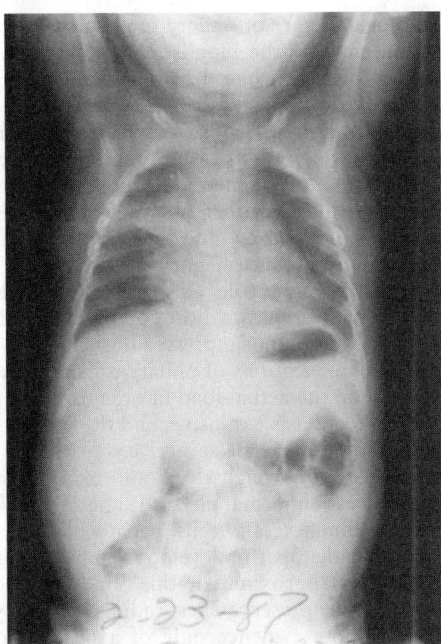

FIGURE 179.2. Chest radiograph shows a segmental lesion during a primary tuberculosis infection in an infant. Volume loss on the right is manifested by atelectasis and a displaced horizontal fissure.

occurrence in children who have undergone timely and appropriate chemotherapy.

Progressive Primary Pulmonary Tuberculosis

A rare but serious complication of childhood tuberculosis occurs when the primary focus enlarges steadily and develops a large caseous center. The radiograph shows bronchopneumonia or lobar pneumonia. Liquefaction may result in the formation of a thin-walled primary cavity associated with large numbers of tubercle bacilli. A tension cavity may develop as a result of a valve-like mechanism, allowing air to enter but not escape the cavity. The enlarging focus may slough necrotic debris into an adjacent bronchus, leading to further intrapulmonary dissemination. Rupture into the pleural cavity leads to bronchopleural fistula or pyopneumothorax; rupture into the pericardium or mediastinum also can occur.

Significant signs and symptoms frequently are seen in locally progressive disease. High fever, severe cough with sputum production, weight loss, and night sweats are common symptoms. If sputum production occurs, these children may be contagious to others. Physical signs include diminished breath sounds, rales, and dullness and egophony over the cavity. Before antituberculosis chemotherapy was developed, the prognosis was poor, with a fatality rate of 30% to 50%. The current prognosis for full recovery is excellent. Superinfection of a simple primary tuberculous focus with a bacterial pneumonia may have a clinical and radiographic presentation similar to that of progressive primary tuberculosis. Antimicrobial agents effective against *Staphylococcus*, *Klebsiella*, and anaerobes may be indicated along with antituberculosis drugs.

Pleural Effusion

Localized pleural effusion occurs so frequently in primary tuberculosis that it is almost a component of the primary complex. Clinically significant pleurisy with effusion occurs in 5% to 30% of young adults with tuberculosis but infrequently in children younger than 6 years old and very rarely in those younger than 2 years. Pleurisy occurs within 6 to 12 months of the development of initial infection and is caused by extension of a subpleural focus. It almost never is associated with a segmental lesion or miliary tuberculosis. The effusion usually is unilateral and may be small or extensive.

Chronic Pulmonary Disease

Chronic pulmonary tuberculosis (i.e., adult or reactivation tuberculosis) represents endogenous reinfection from a site of tuberculosis infection established previously in the body. This form of tuberculosis always has been rare in childhood, but it may occur in adolescence. Children with a healed tuberculosis infection acquired before they are 2 years of age rarely develop chronic pulmonary disease, which is seen more commonly in those who acquire their initial infection after reaching 7 years of age. The most common pulmonary sites are the original parenchymal focus, the regional lymph nodes, or the apical seedings (i.e., Simon foci) established during the early bacillemia from the primary focus. This form of disease usually remains localized to the lungs because the presensitization of the tissues to tuberculin evokes an excellent immune response that prevents further lymphohematogenous spread.

The initial lesion usually is a small area of pneumonia that may progress to caseation, liquefaction, and cavitation (Fig. 179.3). The most common clinical features are cough, fever, chest pain, weight loss, and, eventually, hemoptysis. This form of tuberculosis is highly contagious if significant sputum production and cough are present. The prognosis is excellent for patients given appropriate antituberculosis therapy.

Cardiac and Pericardial Tuberculosis

Involvement of the myocardium may occur in miliary disease. Direct extension of tuberculosis to the myocardium from mediastinal nodes or lung parenchyma is an exceedingly rare event. Tuberculous endocarditis has been described in only several case reports.

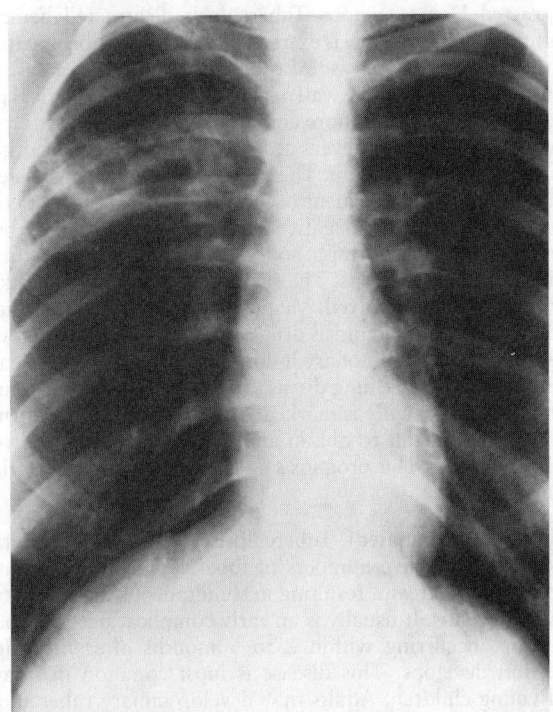

FIGURE 179.3. Chest radiograph shows two tuberculous cavities in an adolescent girl.

The most common form of cardiac tuberculosis is pericarditis, but it is rare, occurring in between 0.4% and 4.0% of children with tuberculosis. Pericarditis usually arises by direct invasion or lymphatic drainage from subcarinal lymph nodes. Early in the course, the pericardial fluid is serofibrinous or occasionally hemorrhagic. Fibrosis may obliterate the pericardial sac, with the development of constrictive pericarditis over a period of years. The presenting symptoms are nonspecific and include low-grade fever, malaise, and weight loss; chest pain seldom occurs. A pericardial friction rub or distant heart sounds with pulsus paradoxus may be present. An acid-fast stain of the pericardial fluid rarely reveals the organism, but cultures are positive in 30% to 70% of cases. Pericardial biopsy with histology and culture may be necessary to confirm the diagnosis. Results of therapy with antituberculosis drugs and corticosteroids are excellent. Partial or complete pericardiectomy may be required when constrictive pericarditis is present.

Lymphohematogenous Spread

Tubercle bacilli are disseminated to distant sites from the lymphadenitis or primary focus of the primary complex in all cases of tuberculosis infection. Experimental animals given local injections of bovine tuberculosis develop dissemination within hours. Autopsy studies of people who died within days or weeks after acquiring initial infection with *M. tuberculosis* have demonstrated organisms in many organs, most commonly the liver, spleen, skin, and apices of the lungs. The clinical picture produced by the lymphohematogenous dissemination depends on the host immune response and the quantity of organisms released. Three basic clinical forms occur: occult lymphohematogenous spread, protracted hematogenous tuberculosis, and miliary tuberculosis.

Occult Lymphohematogenous Spread. Occult lymphohematogenous spread is the most common form, and it occurs in all cases of asymptomatic tuberculosis infection. This event may lead to the development of extrapulmonary tuberculosis months or years after the initial infection.

Protracted Hematogenous Tuberculosis. Protracted hematogenous tuberculosis now is extremely rare. It probably is caused by the intermittent release of tubercle bacilli when a caseous focus erodes through the wall of a blood vessel. The clinical picture may be acute, but more commonly, it is indolent and prolonged. High, spiking fevers accompany the release of organisms into the bloodstream. The fever occasionally is persistent. Multiple organ involvement occurs frequently; the most common signs are hepatomegaly, splenomegaly, adenitis of both deep and superficial lymph nodes, and papulonecrotic tuberculids occurring in crops. The skeletal system, joints, and kidneys may become involved. Meningitis occurs late in the course and, before antituberculosis drugs became available, often was a terminal event. Pulmonary lesions are rare occurrences early in the course; diffuse lung disease appears later. The tuberculin skin test result usually is markedly positive. Culture confirmation can be difficult to obtain and may require bone marrow or liver biopsy. The prognosis is excellent with appropriate therapy.

Miliary (Disseminated) Tuberculosis. Miliary tuberculosis arises when massive numbers of tubercle bacilli are released into the bloodstream, resulting in simultaneous disease in two or more organs. It usually is an early complication of primary infection, occurring within 2 to 6 months after the initial infection develops. This disease is most common in infants and young children. Adults may develop miliary tuberculosis as a result of the breakdown of a previously healed or calcified lesion that formed years earlier.

The pathologic picture of miliary tuberculosis is caused by tubercle bacilli entering the bloodstream from a caseous focus that erodes through a blood vessel. The organisms lodge in small capillaries in various sites and form tubercles of relatively uniform size, ranging from 2 mm to several centimeters. Different tissues have different susceptibilities to infection. Lesions are larger and more numerous in the lungs, spleen, liver, and bone marrow than in other tissues. This difference may be explained by blood supply and by the numbers of reticuloendothelial cells and tissue phagocytes. The patient's general immune status may play a role, as suggested by findings that this form of tuberculosis occurs more commonly in infants and in malnourished or immunosuppressed hosts.

The clinical manifestations of miliary tuberculosis are protean and depend on the actual load of organisms that disseminates. Rarely, the onset is explosive, and the patient becomes gravely ill over the course of several days. Most often, the onset is insidious, with weight loss, anorexia, malaise, and low-grade fever. Few abnormal physical signs are present early in the course. Within several weeks, hepatosplenomegaly and generalized lymphadenopathy develop in approximately one-half of patients. At approximately this time, fever as high as 39°C to 40°C may be present. Chest radiography may be normal initially or show evidence only of a primary complex; few respiratory signs or symptoms are observed. Within 3 to 4 weeks after onset of symptoms, the lung fields usually become filled with tubercles (Fig. 179.4). The child may develop respiratory distress and diffuse rales or wheezing. Pneumothorax, pneumomediastinum, and pleural effusion also can complicate miliary tuberculosis. Signs or symptoms of meningitis or peritonitis are found in 20% to 30% of these patients. In a patient with miliary tuberculosis, headache almost always indicates the presence of meningitis, and the presence of abdominal pain or

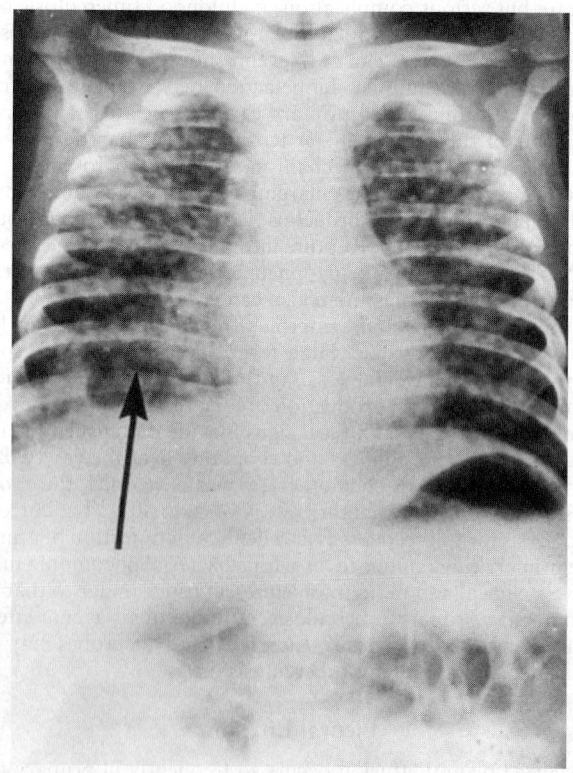

FIGURE 179.4. Chest radiograph of a child with miliary tuberculosis shows typical tubercles and an air-filled cavity (*arrow*). (Courtesy of Dr. Katharine H. K. Hsu.)

tenderness usually signals tuberculous peritonitis. Cutaneous lesions, including papulonecrotic tuberculids, nodules, or purpuric lesions, may occur in crops. Choroid tubercles appear several weeks after the onset of disease in 13% to 87% of the patients. Diagnosis can be difficult to establish, and a high index of suspicion on the part of the examiner is required. The patient often presents with a fever of unknown origin. As many as 50% of these patients have a negative tuberculin skin test result, especially late in the course of the disease. Chest radiography may be characteristic. Early sputum cultures have a low sensitivity; the yield from gastric aspirates or bronchial washings is greater. Biopsy of the liver or bone marrow, with appropriate bacteriologic and histologic examinations, may facilitate a more rapid diagnosis. The most important clue may be a history of a recent exposure to an adult with contagious tuberculosis.

Even with proper treatment, the resolution of miliary tuberculosis may be slow. Fever usually declines within 2 to 3 weeks, but the chest radiographic abnormalities may not resolve for several months, and weight gain in small children often is delayed. Corticosteroids occasionally hasten symptomatic relief, especially when air block, peritonitis, or meningitis occur. Most patients recover fully with adequate chemotherapy.

Extrathoracic Disease

Central Nervous System Tuberculosis

Involvement of the central nervous system (CNS) is the most serious complication of tuberculosis in children. Before the development of effective therapy, CNS tuberculosis was uniformly fatal. Several different forms of CNS tuberculosis exist, including meningitis, tuberculoma, and brain abscess.

The pathogenesis of CNS tuberculosis results from formation of a metastatic caseous lesion in the cerebral cortex or meninges during occult lymphohematogenous dissemination of the initial infection. This lesion (Rich focus) may increase in size and discharge tubercle bacilli into the subarachnoid space. A thick, gelatinous exudate infiltrates the cortical or meningeal blood vessels, producing inflammation, obstruction, or infarction. The brainstem usually is the site of greatest involvement, which accounts for the frequent involvement of cranial nerves III, VI, and VII. The basal cisterns usually become obstructed, leading to hydrocephalus. This is a communicating hydrocephalus because all four ventricles are open to the flow of cerebrospinal fluid (CSF), but the flow to the spinal column is obstructed.

Tuberculous meningitis complicates one in 300 untreated tuberculosis infections in children. This disease is almost unheard of in infants younger than 4 months because it takes at least that long for the inciting pathologic events to develop. It occurs most commonly in children younger than 4 years and usually occurs within 2 to 6 months of the development of the initial infection.

The clinical onset of tuberculous meningitis may be abrupt or insidious. The more rapid progression of disease tends to occur in young infants, who may experience symptoms for only several days before the onset of acute hydrocephalus, brain infarction, or seizures. More commonly, the onset is gradual, occurring over the course of several weeks. The usual course can be divided into three stages. The first stage, which may last 1 to 2 weeks, is characterized by nonspecific symptoms such as fever, headache, irritability, drowsiness, and malaise. No focal neurologic signs are present, but infants and young children may experience a loss or stagnation of developmental milestones. The second stage usually begins abruptly,

with lethargy, convulsions, nuchal rigidity, positive Kernig or Brudzinski signs, increased deep tendon reflexes, hypertonia, vomiting, and cranial nerve palsies. The appearance of this clinical picture correlates with the development of hydrocephalus and increased intracranial pressure, combined with meningeal irritation and, in some cases, vasculitis with infarction. Some patients have relatively few signs of meningeal irritation but show signs of encephalitis, such as disorientation, abnormal movements, and speech abnormalities. The third stage is marked by coma, irregular pulse or respirations, hypertension, hemiplegia or paraplegia, decerebrate posturing, and eventually death.

The most important aid to establishing the correct diagnosis is a history of recent contact with an adult who has pulmonary tuberculosis. The tuberculin skin test result is negative in as many as 50% of patients, especially infants and young children. The most important test is examination and culture of the lumbar CSF. The CSF leukocyte count usually ranges from 10 to 500 cells/μL. Early evaluation may reveal a predominance of polymorphonuclear leukocytes, but in most cases, lymphocytes predominate. The glucose level typically is less than 40 mg/dL, but it rarely drops to less than 20 mg/dL, as it does in bacterial meningitis. The protein level is elevated and may be markedly high (more than 400 mg/dL) because of hydrocephalus and spinal block. The lumbar CSF protein is not indicative of the ventricular CSF protein, which often is normal or only slightly elevated. The success of microscopic examination of stained CSF and mycobacterial culture is related directly to the amount of CSF sampled. If 5 to 10 mL of CSF is obtained, acid-fast stain of spun CSF may be positive in as many as 30% of cases, and the culture result is positive in 70%. Examination of small (1 mL or less) amounts of CSF is unlikely to demonstrate the organism. Culture of other sites, such as gastric aspirates or urine, may help confirm the diagnosis. Computed tomography may help establish a diagnosis of tuberculous meningitis and aids in evaluating the success of therapy. Evidence of brainstem meningitis, hydrocephalus, or focal infarcts may be present. One or several tuberculomas may be present at diagnosis, or they may appear while ultimately successful chemotherapy is given.

Skeletal Tuberculosis

Skeletal tuberculosis usually results from lymphohematogenous dissemination of tubercle bacilli early in the course of the initial infection. Bone infection occasionally is initiated by direct extension from a contiguous lymph node or by extension from a neighboring infected bone. Involvement of bone complicates 1% to 2% of untreated infections in childhood, usually occurring within 12 to 24 months of formation of the primary complex. The pathologic process begins in the metaphysis because of its rich blood supply. Granulation tissue and caseation develop, destroying bone by direct infection and pressure necrosis. Cold soft tissue abscesses and extension of the infection through the epiphysis into the joint often accompany the primary bone lesion.

The most commonly affected bones are the vertebrae, causing tuberculosis of the spine (i.e., Pott disease). Although any vertebral body can be infected, a predilection exists for the thoracic vertebrae, especially T12. Involvement of two or more vertebrae is fairly common, and skip areas between lesions may occur. The body of the vertebra usually is affected, causing destruction and collapse (Fig. 179.5). The progression to tuberculous spondylitis viewed on radiographs is from narrowing of a disc space to collapse and wedging of the vertebral body, with subsequent angulation of the spine (i.e., gibbus) or severe kyphosis. Paraspinal abscess, psoas abscess, or retropharyngeal abscess may develop from the bone lesion. The most frequent

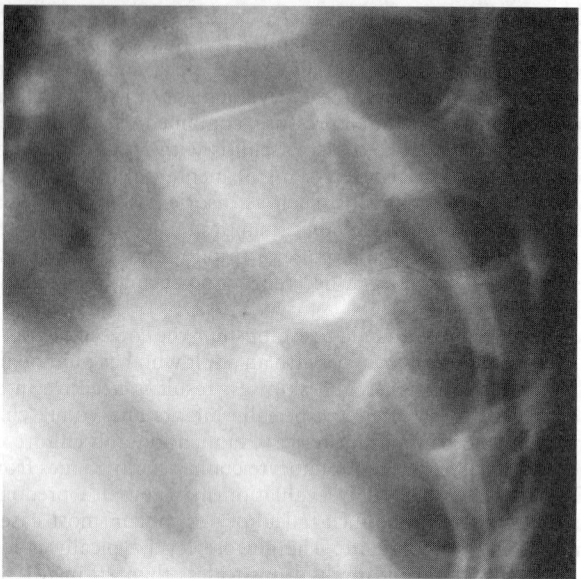

FIGURE 179.5. Radiograph shows destruction and collapse of the twelfth vertebra caused by tuberculous spondylitis. (Courtesy of Dr. Gail J. Demmler.)

clinical signs and symptoms of tuberculous spondylitis include low-grade fever, restlessness, pain, and abnormal positioning or gait. Rigidity of the spine is caused by muscle spasm, often initiated by the patient's effort to minimize pain by immobilization. Intermittent referred pain caused by associated radiculitis may occur.

Abdominal and Gastrointestinal Tuberculosis

Tuberculosis of the oral cavity and pharynx is quite unusual today; most cases in the past were associated with bovine tuberculosis acquired from infected milk. The usual lesion is a painless ulcer on the mucosa, palate, or tonsil, accompanied by swelling of a regional lymph node. Tuberculosis of the larynx may cause hoarseness. Tuberculosis of the esophagus is an exceedingly rare finding in children.

Tuberculous enteritis is caused by ingestion of infected milk, superinfection of the mucosa caused by swallowed tubercle bacilli discharged from a patient's own lungs, or hematogenous spread. The regions most commonly affected are the jejunum and ileum, especially near the Peyer patches or appendix. Shallow ulcers are the most common lesions that cause pain, diarrhea or constipation, and weight loss. Mesenteric adenitis accompanying the enteritis may cause intestinal obstruction or may erode through the omentum and cause peritonitis. The clinical presentation of tuberculous enteritis mimics many other conditions; the diagnosis is confirmed by the presence of pulmonary sites of tuberculosis, a positive tuberculin skin test result, and biopsy and culture of the ulcerative lesion.

Tuberculous peritonitis occurs mainly in young men and is a rare finding in children. Generalized peritonitis may occur as a result of hematogenous dissemination. Localized peritonitis is caused by direct extension from a lymph node, intestinal focus, or tuberculous salpingitis. The lymph nodes, omentum, and peritoneum often are matted together and are palpated as a doughy irregular mass that is relatively nontender. Ascites may occur, usually accompanied by fever. The tuberculin skin test result virtually always is positive. Paracentesis may confirm the diagnosis, but the procedure must be done carefully to avoid entering matted, immobilized intestine.

Renal Tuberculosis

Renal tuberculosis is a fairly rare finding in children because it does not develop for several years after the initial infection. Tubercle bacilli reach the kidney during lymphohematogenous dissemination. Organisms can be recovered from the urine in many cases of miliary tuberculosis and in some cases of pulmonary tuberculosis before renal parenchymal disease develops. Small caseous tubercles develop in the renal parenchyma and discharge tubercle bacilli into the tubules. A large mass may develop near the cortex and discharge large numbers of organisms through a fistulous tract into the renal pelvis. Infection can spread locally to involve the ureter, gallbladder, prostate, or epididymis.

Usually no symptoms are present early in the course of renal tuberculosis. The development of "sterile" pyuria, hematuria, dysuria, or vague flank pain first suggests the presence of infection. Superinfection with other bacteria may cause delay in diagnosing the underlying tuberculosis. Intravenous pyelography or ultrasound may reveal a mass lesion or hydronephrosis if ureteral stricture is present. The urine culture result almost always is positive for *M. tuberculosis*, although cultures may be positive intermittently. Microscopic examination of sediment from an adequately large early morning urine specimen frequently reveals acid-fast bacilli. The tuberculin skin test result usually is positive. Surgical intervention rarely is required for establishment of diagnosis or treatment if adequate chemotherapy is given.

Superficial Lymph Node Tuberculosis

Tuberculosis of the superficial lymph nodes (i.e., scrofula) is the most common form of extrathoracic disease, complicating 3% to 6% of infections. In most cases, it is an early manifestation of lymphohematogenous dissemination, occurring within 6 to 9 months of the primary infection. Some cases arise years after the initial infection and may herald a reactivation of infection.

Regional lymphadenitis is part of the primary complex of tuberculosis. The nodes most commonly involved are in the tonsillar and submandibular regions because of extension of a primary lesion in the upper lung fields or the abdomen. Enlarged nodes in the inguinal, epitrochlear, or axillary regions result from skin or skeletal infections in the extremities.

In the early stage of infection, the lymph nodes are firm, discrete, and nontender. Multiple nodes in one region often are involved. Scrofula in the neck usually is unilateral, but because of the drainage patterns of lymphatics from the chest, it may be bilateral. Other than low-grade fever, systemic signs and symptoms usually are absent. The lymph nodes may enlarge gradually. Occasionally, rapid enlargement occurs, associated with high fever, tenderness, and fluctuation. This picture can be caused by tuberculosis or a bacterial superinfection. The initial presentation rarely is a fluctuant mass with overlying cellulitis or discoloration of the skin.

Many other conditions, including infection caused by NTM, cat-scratch disease, tularemia, brucellosis, malignant tumor, bronchial cleft cyst, cystic hygroma, and pyogenic infection, can be confused with tuberculous adenitis. The most frequent problem in diagnosis is differentiating infection caused by *M. tuberculosis* from NTM adenitis in geographic areas where NTM commonly occurs. Evidence of thoracic lymph node or pulmonary involvement on chest radiography is seen more commonly in tuberculosis but can occur with NTM disease. The induration caused by a 5-TU PPD Mantoux test usually is greater than 15 mm with *M. tuberculosis* infection and less than 10 mm with NTM disease; reactions of 10 to 15 mm can be caused by either infection. The most important part of an evaluation is determining whether exposure to a tuberculous adult has occurred. In many cases, the correct diagnosis can be established only by biopsy and culture of tissue from the involved lymph node.

If left untreated, tuberculous adenitis causes caseation and necrosis of the lymph node. The capsule breaks down, leading to the spread of infection to adjacent lymph nodes. The skin overlying this mass of lymph nodes becomes thin, shiny, and erythematous. Rupture through the skin may result in formation of a sinus tract. Lymphadenitis caused by *M. tuberculosis* responds well to antituberculosis chemotherapy, although the lymph nodes may not return to normal size for months or years. Surgical removal is not adequate therapy because the lymph node disease is but one part of a systemic infection, and involved nodes frequently extend into the mediastinum, where they are difficult to remove. However, a surgical biopsy and culture frequently must be performed to differentiate tuberculous adenitis from other entities, especially NTM infection. Excisional biopsy is preferred over incisional biopsy because of an increased risk of subsequent development of sinus tract formation or severe scarring with the latter procedure.

Perinatal Tuberculosis

True congenital tuberculosis caused by the spread of infection through the placenta or amniotic fluid has been reported in only 400 infants. Transplacental transmission occurs through the umbilical vein from a mother with primary hematogenous or genital tuberculosis. This hematogenous "inoculation" of the fetus leads to miliary tuberculosis. The major site of disease is the liver, which is enlarged. Pulmonary disease usually has a miliary pattern but may be more localized. Generalized lymphadenopathy and meningitis occur in approximately 50% of these patients. The exact clinical manifestations depend on the infecting "dose" of bacilli and the time of transmission. Stillbirth has been associated with tuberculosis in the fetus. Although the onset of symptoms may be delayed for several weeks, symptoms most commonly begin around the second week of life and include lethargy, decreased feeding, nasal discharge, jaundice, respiratory distress, and abdominal distention from hepatosplenomegaly.

Several cases of congenital tuberculosis have been caused by aspiration of amniotic fluid infected with *M. tuberculosis* from a mother with tuberculous endometritis. Pulmonary symptoms and signs dominate the clinical picture, but hepatomegaly usually is present.

Diagnosis of true congenital tuberculosis is likely to be delayed, especially if the diagnosis of tuberculosis has not been established in the mother. Signs and symptoms in the neonate are similar to those caused by other congenital bacterial or viral infections. The tuberculin skin test is not helpful in diagnosing infants. Demonstration of acid-fast bacilli in a gastric, endotracheal, or bone marrow aspirate or biopsy tissue is required to establish the diagnosis. The mortality rate remains high because of delayed establishment of diagnosis and the overwhelming nature of the infection.

Perinatal tuberculosis caused by inhalation of tubercle bacilli expelled by an adult who handles the infant occurs much more commonly than does true congenital tuberculosis. More than 50% of untreated infants infected with *M. tuberculosis* at or near birth can be expected to develop clinically significant disease, usually in the lungs or cervical lymph nodes. The newborn infant should be separated from any adult known or thought to have pulmonary tuberculosis until the disease no longer is contagious. If significant exposure has occurred or is likely to occur at home, the infant should undergo baseline chest radiography and then be started on isoniazid (10 to 15 mg/kg/day). Isoniazid is continued for 3 months after the last possible exposure, and a Mantoux tuberculin test then is

performed. If the test result is positive, isoniazid is continued as in standard therapy of tuberculosis infection; if the test result is negative, the drug is discontinued. Babies who are breast-fed must receive pyridoxine in conjunction with isoniazid. If isoniazid cannot be given or if the adult source case has multiply resistant tuberculosis, BCG vaccination of the infant should be considered. If the mother or other family members have old cases of treated tuberculosis or untreated inactive infection, no risk to the infant exists, and treatment is not recommended. However, performing tuberculin skin tests at 6-month intervals for the first year of life may be prudent.

THERAPY

Approaches to the treatment of tuberculosis have undergone radical changes since the early 1980s. Most cases of tuberculosis should be cured, but the limiting factor often is human behavior: poor adherence to treatment, leading to relapse and the emergence of drug resistance.

Chemotherapeutic Agents

Various chemotherapeutic agents are available for treating patients with tuberculosis (Table 179.3). The first-line drugs, which include isoniazid, rifampin, pyrazinamide, ethambutol, and streptomycin, usually are used for initial treatment. The second-line drugs, including *para*-aminosalicylic acid, ethionamide, capreomycin, kanamycin, fluoroquinolones (levofloxacin, gatifloxacin and moxifloxacin), and cycloserine, are used when drug resistance or intolerance is encountered.

Isoniazid

Since its release in 1952, isoniazid has been the mainstay of antituberculosis therapy. At the usual dose of 10 mg/kg, the peak plasma concentration exceeds the minimal inhibitory concentration (MIC) for *M. tuberculosis* (0.02 to 0.05 μg/mL) by a factor of 30 to 80. These high concentrations persist in the plasma and sputum for many hours. Concentrations in the CSF, even in the absence of inflammation, are 50% to 100% of plasma concentrations. Low concentrations are present in breast milk. Tablets frequently are given with food, although poor absorption in some children has been reported when the drug is given this way. Isoniazid is metabolized in the liver by acetylation. The rate and degree of acetylation are determined genetically, but they usually are of little significance for treatment or drug toxicity in children.

Most children tolerate isoniazid so well that only clinical monitoring is necessary. Transient elevation of hepatic enzymes has been documented in 10% of adult patients, with overt clinical hepatitis occurring in only 1%. Both problems are rare occurrences in children, but they occur slightly more commonly in adolescents. Routine serum liver enzyme testing is unnecessary for children taking isoniazid unless they have a history of liver disease, are taking other hepatotoxic drugs (especially anticonvulsants), or develop clinical signs and symptoms of toxicity. Significant hepatic toxicity is more likely to occur if the dose exceeds 10 mg/kg/day and rifampin also is being given and if the patient has severe disseminated tuberculosis (e.g., miliary or meningeal disease).

Peripheral neuritis, caused by the competitive inhibition of pyridoxine metabolism, can occur when isoniazid is given to patients with poor nutrition. Although this problem is fairly common in adults, children's pyridoxine levels are depressed, but clinical manifestations rarely occur. Children with reasonably balanced diets do not need pyridoxine supplementation. However, breast-fed infants receiving isoniazid always should

TABLE 179.3

ANTITUBERCULOSIS DRUGS USED IN CHILDREN

Drug	Dose (kg/day)	Route of Administration	Drug Toxicity	Available Preparations
Isoniazid	5–15 mg	Oral, intravenous, intramuscular	Hepatotoxicity; peripheral neuritis; rash	100- and 300-mg scored tablets; 10 mg/mL suspension
Rifampin	10–15 mg	Oral, intravenous	Hepatotoxicity; staining of contact lenses; flulike syndrome	150- and 300-mg capsules
Pyrazinamide	20–40 mg	Oral	Hepatotoxicity; arthritis or arthralgias; gout	500-mg scored tablets
Streptomycin	20 mg up to 1 g total	Intramuscular	Eighth nerve damage (vestibular loss more common than hearing loss)	1-g vials
Ethambutol	15–25 mg	Oral	Optic neuritis; red-green color blindness	100- and 400-mg scored tablets
Ethionamide	10–20 mg	Oral	Gastric irritation; teratogenic	250-mg tablets
Capreomycin	10–15 mg	Intramuscular	Nephrotoxicity; eighth nerve damage (hearing loss more common than vestibular loss)	1-mg vials
Kanamycin	15–30 mg	Intramuscular, intravenous	Nephrotoxicity; eighth nerve damage (hearing loss more common than vestibular loss)	100-mg, 500-mg, and 1-g vials
Cycloserine	10–20 mg up to 1 g total	Oral	Neurologic and psychiatric	250-mg capsules
Paraamino Parasalicylic acid	250–300 mg	Oral	Severe gastric irritation	Packets (three per day is the adult dose)

receive supplementation because of the low pyridoxine concentrations present in breast milk.

Infrequent adverse effects of isoniazid include convulsions (with overdose), psychosis, severe headache, allergic manifestation, and a lupus-like syndrome. Isoniazid can increase levels of phenytoin and carbamazepine and cause significant toxicity by blocking their metabolism in the liver.

Rifampin

A key drug in the modern management of tuberculosis, rifampin is absorbed readily from the gastrointestinal tract. Oral doses of 10 to 15 mg/kg result in peak plasma concentrations of 6 to 32 μg/mL, far exceeding the MIC for *M. tuberculosis* (0.5 μg/mL). Rifampin diffuses readily into all body tissues and fluids, achieving CSF concentrations of 60% to 90% of plasma levels. Its metabolism and excretion occur in the liver and kidneys, respectively.

Rifampin usually is well tolerated. However, the preparation is an orange-red dye that stains all body fluids, including urine, tears, sweat, and feces. It may permanently stain contact lenses. Hepatic toxicity is a rare (less than 1%) occurrence unless rifampin is used in conjunction with isoniazid doses that exceed 10 mg/kg/day. Gastrointestinal irritation, leukopenia, thrombocytopenia, and a peculiar influenza-like syndrome that is immunologically mediated may occur. Rifampin can render oral contraceptives inactive and may interact adversely with several other drugs, including quinidine, sodium warfarin, and corticosteroids.

Although the usual dose of rifampin is 10 to 15 mg/kg/day, proprietary formulations include only 150- and 300-mg capsules. A suspension can be made by most pharmacies for the desired dose and concentration. Rifampin should not be given with food because its absorption becomes erratic. Rifamate, a capsule with a fixed combination of isoniazid (150 mg) and rifampin (300 mg), may be useful for adults and some children or adolescents.

Pyrazinamide

First developed in 1949, pyrazinamide has been rediscovered as an important antituberculosis drug. In adults, an oral dose of 30 mg/kg produces plasma levels of approximately 20 μg/mL. The pharmacokinetics of pyrazinamide are not described adequately for children. Daily doses of 30 mg/kg are tolerated well by children, and the CSF levels are similar to those obtained in adults, 50% to 75% of plasma levels. Pyrazinamide is an unusual drug that is not bactericidal *in vitro* but does contribute to killing *M. tuberculosis in vivo*. It is active only at a pH of approximately 5.5, which is the pH inside macrophages. It is metabolized by the liver, and hepatotoxicity may occur, especially if the dose exceeds 40 mg/kg/day. Pyrazinamide and its metabolites inhibit urinary excretion of uric acid. Approximately 10% of adults develop arthralgias, arthritis, or gout, but these complications are extremely rare in children.

Streptomycin

Although it is used less frequently than in the past, streptomycin is important for drug-resistant tuberculosis. It must be given intramuscularly. Streptomycin penetrates inflamed meninges well, but CSF levels are low in the absence of inflammation. The principal adverse effect is eighth nerve toxicity. The most common complication is damage to the vestibular branch, resulting in vertigo or ataxia. Hearing loss occurs less frequently, but auditory acuity should be monitored if streptomycin is used for more than a few weeks.

Ethambutol

At the usual dose of 15 to 25 mg/kg/day, ethambutol reaches a peak plasma concentration of 3 to 5 μg/mL, a level that is bacteriostatic for *M. tuberculosis*. At higher doses, however, the drug may be bactericidal. It is absorbed rapidly from the gastrointestinal tract and is excreted in the urine, mainly as the parent compound. Although ethambutol can cause optic neuritis or red-green color blindness, these toxicities are extremely rare in children. At the usual doses, ethambutol rarely causes optic toxicity in adults, and it has not been reported in children. Ethambutol is not used routinely in small children because their visual activity and color perception are difficult to monitor, but it should be used in cases of drug-resistant tuberculosis or when the risk of resistance is high.

Second-Line Drugs

If drug resistance to first-line drugs or toxicity becomes a problem, second-line drugs are used. *Para*-aminosalicylic acid previously was an important agent for the treatment of tuberculosis. However, it is only bacteriostatic and is associated with severe gastric irritation at usual doses. A newer granular formulation is better tolerated with fewer gastrointestinal side effects. Certain aminoglycosides, such as capreomycin, kanamycin, and amikacin, are active against most strains of *M. tuberculosis*, including those resistant to streptomycin. Cycloserine rarely is used in children because of its propensity to cause a variety of neurologic and psychiatric disturbances. Ethionamide is effective and well tolerated by children. It is bacteriostatic but achieves excellent CSF concentrations. It should not be used in pregnant women because of its teratogenic effects in animals. Several fluoroquinolones have excellent activity against *M. tuberculosis*. Fear of damage to growing cartilage, a theoretic risk suggested by animal data, precludes their routine use in children, but these drugs may be used in cases of multidrug-resistant tuberculosis.

Rationale for Multidrug Therapy

The traditional approach to antituberculosis chemotherapy is combined use of a potent bactericidal drug, usually isoniazid, with a second drug given to prevent the emergence of resistance to isoniazid. Some drugs, such as pyrazinamide and streptomycin, can kill *M. tuberculosis* but are not as effective in preventing emergence of resistance to other drugs. Rifampin, isoniazid, ethambutol, and *para*-aminosalicylic acid effectively prevent the development of resistance to other agents. This approach requires 12 to 24 months of treatment to produce a bacteriologic cure. Modern methods of combination drug treatment are designed for rapid killing of *M. tuberculosis* to sterilize the lesions as quickly as possible.

Short-Course Therapy

Treating patients for the shortest possible period is important for several reasons. Expense is decreased markedly compared with longer, traditional therapy, which is an important consideration in developing countries with limited resources. More time and program resources can be allocated to ensuring adherence with medications and clinic or physician visits, and the patient is exposed to potentially toxic drugs for a shorter period of time. In addition, if a patient quits treatment early, a greater likelihood exists that bacteriologic cure will have been achieved.

Numerous short-course therapy trials have been conducted on adults with drug-susceptible pulmonary tuberculosis. A 9-month course of treatment with isoniazid and rifampin cures 98% of cases. Both drugs usually are given daily for the first 2 to 8 weeks; thereafter, they can be given daily or twice weekly, with equivalent results. When given twice weekly, the rifampin dose is the same as the daily dose, but the isoniazid dose is increased to two to three times the daily dose. Twice-weekly therapy is effective because after 2 months, the replication of

the organisms is slow and the drugs have a long elimination half-life. Twice-weekly medications always should be administered under the direct observation of a health care professional (directly observed therapy) because of the adherence problems associated with virtually every tuberculosis control program.

Therapy with isoniazid and rifampin lasting less than 9 months has led to unacceptably high relapse rates (10% or greater) in adults. Shorter durations can be successful if more than two drugs are used initially. Because pyrazinamide and streptomycin have their greatest effect early in therapy, a dualistic approach of intensive three- or four-drug therapy (e.g., isoniazid, rifampin, pyrazinamide, ethambutol) for 2 months, followed by isoniazid and rifampin for 4 months, is effective in 98% of cases. Unfortunately, regimens of shorter duration than 6 months are not as effective. The current American Thoracic Society recommendation for pulmonary tuberculosis in adults is a 6-month regimen using isoniazid, rifampin, pyrazinamide, and ethambutol for 2 months, followed by 4 months of isoniazid and rifampin.

Intensive, short-course antituberculosis therapy has proven to be highly effective for children with drug-susceptible pulmonary tuberculosis. The best-studied regimen consists of isoniazid and rifampin given for 6 months, supplemented with pyrazinamide during the first 2 months. This regimen yields cure rates approaching 100%, relapse rates approaching 0%, and an incidence of mild adverse drug reactions of approximately 1%. It is desirable to have medications administered daily for the first 2 to 4 weeks of therapy; thereafter, they can be given daily or twice weekly. All treatment for tuberculosis disease should be observed directly by a health care worker. For patients for whom social issues or other constraints prevent them from receiving reliable daily administration of drugs even in the initial phase of treatment, drugs can be given two to three times per week from the beginning. If initial isoniazid or rifampin resistance is deemed more likely because of epidemiologic factors, a fourth drug should be added until the drug susceptibility pattern is established.

Most forms of extrapulmonary tuberculosis respond well to the 6-month, 3-drug regimen used for pulmonary tuberculosis. One exception may be bone and joint tuberculosis, which often requires 9 to 12 months of treatment to effect a cure, especially if surgical intervention is not undertaken. Although tuberculous meningitis probably can be cured with 6 months of therapy if isoniazid, rifampin, and pyrazinamide are given initially, the lack of data leads many experts to recommend extending therapy to 9 to 12 months. Most experts add a fourth drug initially, usually ethionamide, ethambutol, or an aminoglycoside, to protect against unsuspected drug resistance.

Drug Resistance

The incidence of drug-resistant tuberculosis is increasing throughout the world, with rates as high as 35% in some locales (e.g., Southeast Asia, parts of Central America, South America, Africa). Rates in the United States from 1988 to 1994 varied from less than 1% to 15% along the Mexican border and more than 30% in New York City. Primary resistance occurs when a person is infected with an organism that is already resistant to a drug. Secondary resistance occurs when drug-resistant organisms emerge as a dominant population during therapy. Poor patient adherence or improper administration of medications by the physician lead to secondary resistance.

Patterns of drug resistance among children mirror those found in adults in a given population. Certain epidemiologic factors, such as immigration from a country with a high resistance rate or a history of prior treatment for tuberculosis, correlate with drug resistance in adult patients and their contacts. When drug resistance is suspected, initial therapy must include at least three or four drugs. Subsequent therapy must be tailored to the resistance pattern.

For isoniazid resistance, a regimen of rifampin, pyrazinamide, and ethambutol given for 9 to 12 months usually is effective. For rifampin-resistant tuberculosis, the combination of isoniazid, pyrazinamide, and ethambutol plus one additional drug is effective. For isoniazid and rifampin resistance, a regimen using at least two bactericidal drugs must be designed based on the exact susceptibility pattern of the isolate. In this situation, cure rates in adults are often less than 80%, even under the best conditions.

Corticosteroids

Although data on their efficacy are relatively sparse, corticosteroids have found a place in the treatment of some forms of tuberculosis. However, they never should be used unless effective antituberculosis drugs are given simultaneously. Corticosteroids may be of benefit if the host inflammatory reaction is contributing to tissue damage or impairment of function. Convincing evidence suggests that corticosteroids aid patients with tuberculous meningitis and increased intracranial pressure caused by brainstem inflammation and resultant hydrocephalus. Children with endobronchial disease (e.g., localized air trapping, collapse-consolidation lesion) frequently benefit from corticosteroids. Other forms of tuberculosis that may benefit from corticosteroids are miliary disease with alveolocapillary block, pericarditis, peritonitis, and pleural effusion. Prednisone is the drug used most commonly, 1 to 2 mg/kg/day for 4 to 6 weeks, with gradual withdrawal over several weeks.

PREVENTION

Primary prevention, such as vaccination, is designed to prevent the establishment of tuberculosis infection. Secondary prevention, such as isoniazid therapy, aims at preventing the development of active disease after infection has occurred.

Bacille Calmette-Guérin Vaccination

BCG was derived from a strain of *M. bovis* that was attenuated through years of serial passage in culture. The many BCG vaccines derived from the original strain vary greatly in antigenicity and efficacy. The BCG vaccine activates host cell-mediated immunity to mycobacterial antigens in an attempt to prevent infection or progression to disease if a subsequent infection with *M. tuberculosis* occurs.

Variations in strains and lack of experimental standardization have hampered evaluation of many BCG trials. Intradermal injection of BCG is the most precise and effective technique, but multiple-puncture techniques are popular because of the ease of administration. The usual local reaction to an intradermal BCG vaccination is a papule that develops a permanent scar (Fig. 179.6). Painless enlargement of the regional lymph nodes frequently occurs but usually resolves within several weeks.

The efficacy of the BCG vaccines in preventing subsequent tuberculosis disease in children has ranged from 0% to 80% in various studies. BCG is given to newborns in some countries, to 1-year-old children in others, and to adolescents in still others. Little is known about the effectiveness of revaccination. The most important and consistent effect of the BCG vaccines is to limit significantly the development of serious disseminated tuberculosis (e.g., miliary disease, meningitis) in young children. Vaccinated children who subsequently develop tuberculosis tend to have localized thoracic disease.

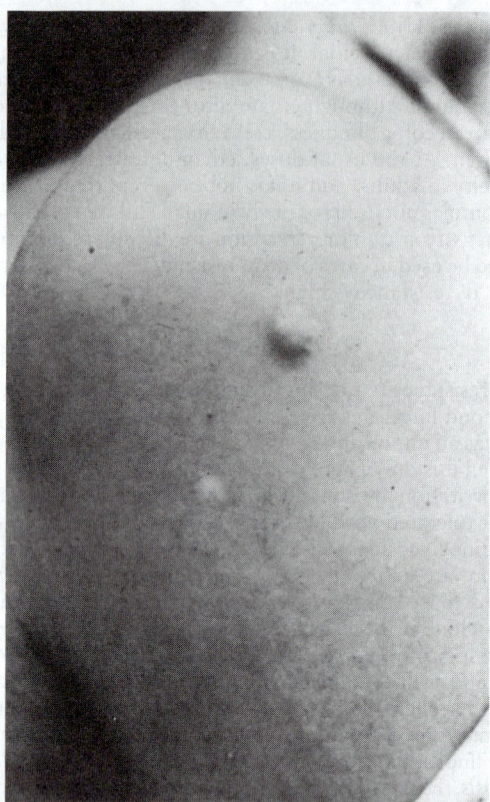

FIGURE 179.6. Bacille Calmette-Guérin vaccination scar on a young child.

Adverse reactions to BCG are uncommon in immunocompetent children. Localized ulceration, adenitis, and osteomyelitis have been reported. Disseminated infection and death have been reported only in children with severe immunodeficiencies.

The BCG vaccine is used rarely in the United States. A disadvantage of the vaccine is that BCG can produce, in approximately one-half of vaccinated newborns, a transient hypersensitivity to tuberculin and a positive Mantoux reaction (usually less than 12 mm) that may persist for as long as 5 years. Because a skin test reaction caused by BCG cannot be differentiated from one caused by infection with *M. tuberculosis*, the safest course is to attribute any significant reaction to tuberculosis infection, regardless of the BCG status of the patient. In the United States, BCG may be useful in protecting persons likely to have unavoidable exposure to tuberculosis, such as an infant whose mother has active tuberculosis or a child who may become exposed to multidrug-resistant tuberculosis.

TREATMENT OF TUBERCULOSIS INFECTION

The treatment of asymptomatic, tuberculin-positive patients to prevent development of tuberculosis disease is an established practice in the United States. The widespread use of the term *chemoprophylaxis* is unfortunate because it actually is treatment of a subclinical infection. Therapy with isoniazid does not alter the tuberculin reaction in most children infected with *M. tuberculosis*, but extensive clinical trials have demonstrated that 1 year of daily isoniazid therapy (10 mg/kg/day) prevents the development of active tuberculosis for at least 30 years.

Isoniazid is indicated for children with a positive tuberculin test result but no clinical or radiographic evidence of disease, children with a negative tuberculin test result who have had known recent exposure to an adult with contagious tuberculosis, and persons of any age who show recent conversion (from negative to positive) of the tuberculin skin test after exposure to a contagious case. (Children with a negative tuberculin test result after known exposure may be an example of primary prophylaxis. Infection may have occurred already, but the skin test result has not yet become positive.) For established infection in children and adolescents, isoniazid is given for 9 months. Daily therapy is preferred, but twice-weekly directly observed therapy is acceptable if self-supervision is unreliable. Therapy with rifampin for 6 months is used for persons known to be infected with isoniazid-resistant strains of *M. tuberculosis*. However, data are scarce, and treatment failures have been reported.

Suggested Readings

American Thoracic Society, Centers for Disease Control and Prevention, Infectious Disease Society of America. Treatment of tuberculosis. *Am J Respir Crit Care Med* 2003;167:603.

American Thoracic Society, Centers for Disease Control and Prevention. Targeted tuberculin testing and treatment of latent tuberculosis infection. *Am J Respir Crit Care Med* 2000;161:S221.

Khan K, Muenning P, Behta M, et al. Global drug resistance patterns and the management of latent tuberculosis infection in immigrants to the United States. *N Engl J Med* 2002;347:1850.

Lincoln EM, Sewell EM. *Tuberculosis in children*. New York: McGraw-Hill, 1963.

Marias BJ, Gie RP, Hesseling AC, et al. The clinical epidemiology of childhood pulmonary tuberculosis: a critical review of literature from the prechemotherapy era. *Int J Tuberc Lung Dis* 2004;8:278.

Miller FJW. *Tuberculosis in children*. New York: Churchill Livingstone, 1981.

Schaaf HS, Beyers N, Gie RP, et al. Respiratory tuberculosis in childhood: the diagnostic value of clinical features and special investigations. *Pediatr Infect Dis J* 1995;14:189.

Starke JR, Correa AG. Management of mycobacterial infection and disease in children. *Pediatr Infect Dis J* 1995;14:553.

Starke JR. Transmission of *Mycobacterium tuberculosis* to and from children and adolescents. *Semin Pediatr Infect Dis* 2001;12:115.

Swanson DS, Starke JR. Drug-resistant tuberculosis in children. *Pediatr Clin North Am* 1995;42:455.

Ussery XT, Valway SE, McKenna M, et al. Epidemiology of tuberculosis among children in the United States. *Pediatr Infect Dis J* 1996;15:697.

CHAPTER 180 ■ NONTUBERCULOUS MYCOBACTERIA

JEFFREY R. STARKE

Mycobacteria other than *Mycobacterium tuberculosis* and *M. leprae* are known by several names, including *nontuberculous*, *atypical*, *unclassified*, *environmental*, and *opportunistic* mycobacteria. *Nontuberculous mycobacteria* (NTM) is probably the preferred and most accurate nomenclature. These organisms were discovered almost a century ago, but their role in causing pulmonary and lymph node disease was not described until 1948.

EPIDEMIOLOGY

In the early 1950s, 1% to 2% of the patients in tuberculosis sanatoria in Georgia and Florida had disease that was epidemiologically distinct from tuberculosis. Those with NTM disease were more likely to be older and white, and they usually had underlying chronic pulmonary disease, such as bronchiectasis or silicosis. Reaction to a tuberculin skin test occurred less commonly than among patients with tuberculosis, and close contacts tended to have negative test results for tuberculin. As more reports of NTM disease were published, marked geographic variability in the incidence of NTM disease and in the specific NTM species causing illness became apparent.

Between 1958 and 1970, large numbers of Navy recruits were skin-tested with purified protein derivative (PPD) from *M. tuberculosis* (PPD-S), *M. intracellulare* (PPD-B), and *M. scrofulaceum* (PPD-G). As many as 70% of the recruits from the southeastern states reacted to NTM skin test antigens, compared with 10% to 40% of recruits from the northern, midwestern, or western states. None of these sensitized recruits had ever experienced disease, thus demonstrating that most NTM infections are asymptomatic.

Although it has never been proved, NTM organisms probably are inhaled or introduced into the mouth, nose, or throat. NTM can be found in the environment in soil, water, or vegetation. The organisms may be present in some animals, but animal-to-human or person-to-person transmission has not been demonstrated. Certain mycobacteria that cause cutaneous granulomas may be present in water, including oceans, ponds, swimming pools, aquariums, and hot tubs. Children are more likely to have NTM cutaneous granulomas or superficial lymph node disease, and adults are more prone to pulmonary infections.

Changes in the epidemiology of NTM infections have occurred because of infections in adults and children with human immunodeficiency virus (HIV) and nosocomial infections. NTM disease occurs commonly in patients with advanced HIV infection (CD4+ count of less than 100) from all areas of the United States, even those where background infection rates (based on historic skin test results) are low. Their disease tends to be disseminated and difficult to control with current medications. The number of reports of instances or clusters of nosocomially acquired NTM infections in immunocompromised and immunocompetent hosts has grown, most associated with surgery or an indwelling catheter.

ETIOLOGY

At least 30 *Mycobacterium* species are associated with human disease, and several more may be encountered in clinical specimens. In 1959, Runyon proposed a grouping of mycobacteria exclusive of *M. tuberculosis*, *M. bovis*, and *M. leprae* based on pigmentation, growth rate, and colony morphology. Although this grouping is one way of organizing the species, more sophisticated methods of species identification, based on DNA typing or high performance liquid chromatography (HPLC) analysis of the mycolic acids in the cell wall, now commonly are used. By conventional methods, using solid media, the growth of most of the NTMs is slow; exact speciation and susceptibility testing may take as long as 6 to 10 weeks. Only the so-called rapid-grower NTM (M. fortuitum, M. chelonae, and M. abscessus) can be isolated on solid media in less than 10 days. The radiometric culture system has reduced the time required for the isolation of most NTM to 2 weeks or less. A special substrate permits immediate differentiation of NTM from M. tuberculosis: NTMs grow freely in this substrate, but the growth of M. tuberculosis is inhibited.

Although isolation of an NTM is the best method to confirm disease, many NTMs are plentiful in the environment and can be encountered as colonizers. Five characteristics can help distinguish true infection from colonization: (a) quantity of growth, which increases with true disease; (b) repeated isolation of the same organism; (c) isolation from a deep-seated anatomic site, which is more meaningful; (d) whether the species of NTM isolated is known to cause disease at the site; and (e) whether the host has risk factors for NTM disease, such as immunocompromised state or cystic fibrosis.

PATHOGENESIS

Most people who encounter NTM have asymptomatic infection. Inhaled or ingested mycobacteria deposit on the mucous membranes of the nose, mouth, and throat. Local manifestations of infection are rare occurrences. When disease develops, the histopathologic findings are similar to those caused by M. tuberculosis infection. Lymph nodes affected by NTM develop necrosis within areas of caseation early in the course. Nonspecific acute and chronic inflammatory changes occur more often than do true granulomas. Acid-fast stains of tissue are positive in 30% to 60% of the cases. Even the most experienced pathologist cannot reliably differentiate NTM adenitis from tuberculous adenitis by microscopical or histologic examination.

Pulmonary disease is a rare occurrence in children, and the clinical picture includes hilar adenopathy, patchy infiltrates of multiple lobes, and lobar pneumonia. The pathologic and clinical findings are similar to those of tuberculosis in children.

Patients with coexistent NTM and HIV infections tend to have more severe and disseminated disease. NTM infection occurs primarily in the lungs, bone marrow, liver and spleen, gastrointestinal tract, and kidneys. Blood and stool culture results usually are positive. HIV-infected patients tend not to form granulomas; their inflammatory reaction is a less specific mix of chronic and acute changes. However, infected tissues may have an enormous number of organisms that are seen readily on acid-fast stain preparations.

CLINICAL MANIFESTATIONS AND COMPLICATIONS

Superficial Lymph Nodes

In children, the most common sites of clinically significant NTM infection are the superficial lymph nodes of the head and neck. When this clinical picture first was described, M. scrofulaceum was the most common infecting agent. More recent cases have been caused by M. avium and M. intracellulare (which together make up the M. avium complex), but M. kansasii and M. fortuitum occasionally cause this form of disease (Table 180.1). An increasing number of cases of NTM

TABLE 180.1	
MOST COMMON SITES OF INFECTION FOR NONTUBERCULOUS MYCOBACTERIA	
Site	**Most Common Organisms**
Lymph node	M. avium complex, M. kansasii, M. fortuitum, M. genavense, M. haemophilum, M. abscessus, poorly characterized mycobacteria
Pulmonary	M. kansasii, M. avium complex, M. xenopi, M. chelonae, M. fortuitum, M. haemophilum, M. szulgai, M. gordonae, M. malmoense
Disseminated	M. avium complex, M. kansasii, M. fortuitum, M. chelonae, M. xenopi, M. haemophilum, M. gordonae

lymph node disease are caused by poorly characterized mycobacteria that cannot be isolated on usual media but can be demonstrated by polymerase chain reaction (PCR) testing of the tissue. Scrofula caused by NTM occurs most commonly in young children because of their tendency to put objects contaminated with soil, dust, or standing water into their mouths. The younger the child, the more likely that scrofula is caused by NTM.

Children living in rural or suburban settings are more likely to develop NTM cervical adenitis. Adenitis caused by NTM usually involves a group of nodes, most often located in the anterior superior cervical chain or submandibular area. Preauricular, postauricular, and submental lymph nodes also may be infected. In rare cases, infection of an axillary, epitrochlear, or inguinal node occurs secondary to cutaneous inoculation. The disease usually is unilateral. The nodal swelling may be explosive over the course of several days, but more often it develops insidiously, occasionally after an upper respiratory tract infection. The nodes usually are painless, nontender, and firm initially. As the infection progresses, the nodes soften and often develop fluctuance. The skin becomes shiny and thin, with an erythematous or violaceous hue. Untreated nodes frequently rupture through the skin, causing drainage and eventual formation of a sinus tract that can persist for months or years. Healing is marked by fibrosis and scarring of the skin. Low-grade fever may be present initially, but other systemic signs or symptoms are rare findings. A high fever or a toxic appearance of the child may indicate superinfection with pyogenic bacteria.

The differential diagnosis of NTM adenitis includes tuberculosis, cat-scratch disease, tularemia, brucellosis, actinomycosis, nocardiosis, toxoplasmosis, mononucleosis, malignancies, cystic hygroma, and rarer conditions. The greatest difficulty usually is differentiating NTM adenitis from adenitis caused by M. tuberculosis. The chest radiograph of a patient with tuberculous adenitis often is abnormal, but some children with NTM adenitis have significant mediastinal or hilar adenopathy; rarely, segmental pulmonary lesions are present. Lack of contact with an adult who has tuberculosis, a normal chest radiograph, small reaction to a standard tuberculin skin test, and poor response to antituberculosis therapy suggest the likelihood of an NTM scrofula.

Pulmonary Infection

Pulmonary disease caused by NTM in adults frequently resembles chronic pulmonary tuberculosis, causing upper lobe infiltrates and cavitary lesions. Most of these patients have preexisting chronic lung diseases, such as silicosis, malignancy, cystic fibrosis, or healed tuberculosis. The most frequent etiologic agents are *M. kansasii*, *M. avium* complex, and *M. fortuitum*. Because NTM may be isolated from the sputum of adults with no lung disease, a single positive sputum culture result is not sufficient to establish the diagnosis. More invasive procedures, such as bronchial lavage or biopsy, may be necessary, especially because more than one pathogenic organism may be present.

Primary childhood pulmonary disease caused by NTM is a rare event. Some affected children have enlarged hilar lymph nodes with endobronchial breakthrough and segmental lesions, similar to those seen in tuberculosis. Disease caused by *M. kansasii* is most likely to resemble tuberculosis in a child. Other patients have more diffuse lung disease, involving all of one or more lobes. Most children do not have underlying chronic pulmonary disease. The onset of illness can be insidious or acute, with fever, cough, and listlessness. Diagnosis is difficult to establish because the clinical, radiographic, and skin test data can mimic tuberculosis; NTM, especially *M. gordonae*, *M. kansasii*, and *M. avium* complex, can be isolated from the gastric aspirates of healthy children. NTM pulmonary disease should be suspected in a young child with the clinical picture of tuberculosis who has no known source case or risk factors for tuberculosis, a mildly or nonreactive tuberculin skin test result, and no evidence of tuberculosis infection in the family and who does not respond well to antituberculosis medications.

An increasing number of cases have been reported of NTM isolated from the respiratory secretions of patients with cystic fibrosis. Because these patients tend to be older and have more extensive underlying pulmonary disease, assessing the role of an NTM infection in an individual patient's clinical course may be difficult. The incidence of isolation of an NTM in adult patients with cystic fibrosis has ranged from 3% to 20%. *M. avium* complex, *M. kansasii*, and the rapidly growing NTMs are isolated most often. Occurrence or worsening of cough, sputum production, fever, weight loss, or other systemic symptoms, in association with initial isolation of an NTM from sputum, suggest NTM-related disease.

Cutaneous Infection

The most common form of cutaneous NTM infection is the skin granuloma, usually caused by *M. marinum* or *M. balnei*. The organisms are introduced by contaminated water that enters a skin abrasion or cut. Direct trauma from contact with shrimp, barnacles, coral, or fishhooks may lead to infection. The granulomatous lesions evolve slowly. They usually are painless and progress from small wartlike nodules to ulcers, with or without drainage, over the course of several weeks. A sporotrichotic form has been described. Regional adenopathy is not routinely part of the primary lesion. The clinical diagnosis is substantiated by biopsy or culture of the ulcer discharge. Although some lesions heal spontaneously, chemotherapy usually is given. Extensive ulcers may require débridement and skin grafting.

The rapidly growing *M. fortuitum*, *M. chelonae*, and *M. abscessus* can cause skin disease resulting from the contamination of a wound or needle puncture site. These organisms can be found on the skin, or they may be present in the hospital environment, especially in the operating room. Surgical wound infections, abscess formation after childhood immunizations, and infection complicating puncture wounds to the foot have been described. Central venous catheter infections have been described and usually involve the skin and subcutaneous tissues at the catheter entrance site. Removal of the catheter is an essential part of treatment. Seropurulent drainage, poor wound healing, and development of sinus tracts frequently complicate these infections. Diagnosis is established readily by culture of the infected site.

Disseminated Infection

Disseminated NTM disease was a rare occurrence before the HIV epidemic. A literature review in 1972 revealed that only 12 cases involving children had been reported. All 12 children had died; nine had steadily progressive disease, and three had periods of remission and reactivation. Lesions of the lungs, long bones, liver, gastrointestinal tract, and bone marrow were common findings. The histopathology and clinical picture of several children bore a striking resemblance to acute nonlipoid reticuloendotheliosis. In recent years, researchers have demonstrated that several patients and family cohorts with disseminated NTM infections have defects in the interferon-gamma receptor or with production of specific cytokines.

Patients with untreated, advanced HIV infection may develop disseminated NTM infection, usually caused by *M. avium* complex or *M. kansasii*. Typical involvement exhibits massive numbers of organisms in the gastrointestinal tract, lungs, bone marrow, liver, kidneys, and rarely the central nervous system. Blood and stool culture results usually are positive. The most common signs and symptoms are nonspecific and include weight loss, malaise, fever, dyspnea, and diarrhea. Almost all patients have coexisting infections, and determining which infectious agent is causing a specific problem or symptom is difficult. Although even massive NTM infection rarely is the cause of death in patients with HIV infection, it contributes to their wasting and the deterioration of immunologic function. Patients with acquired immune deficiency syndrome (AIDS) and disseminated NTM have shorter lifespans than do patients with AIDS and similar CD4+ counts who do not have NTM infection. Treatment of the NTM infection leads to clinical improvement in most of these patients.

Other Sites of Infection

Skeletal NTM infection in the absence of disseminated disease is a rare event and usually occurs as a complication of surgery or trauma. The rapidly growing mycobacteria most often are the etiologic agents. In children, central nervous system disease caused by NTM is a rare occurrence, with only nine cases reported in the pre-HIV era. Meningitis occurs more commonly than does brain parenchymal disease. Several episodes of infection of indwelling vascular catheters caused by *M. fortuitum* or *M. chelonae* have been described, and porcine heart valves have become infected by these rapid growers. Several reports and series have shown that *M. abscessus* is a fairly frequent cause of middle-ear infections in children who have had ear drainage tubes for a prolonged time. Most of these patients had received several courses of antibiotics and eardrops containing corticosteroids. These infections can extend, causing mastoiditis and temporal bone involvement. The organism is isolated easily from middle-ear fluid. Response to chemotherapy is slow and often incomplete; surgical excision usually is an important part of therapy.

DIAGNOSIS

Nonspecific laboratory tests, such as blood counts, urinalysis, and serum chemistry tests, are of no value in diagnosing NTM infection. The most direct diagnostic method is appropriate mycobacterial culture of involved tissue, including lymph nodes, sinus tract drainage, skin granuloma, or bronchial secretions. Unfortunately, the culture result is positive for only one-half of the cases of probable mycobacterial cervical adenitis. Differentiating NTM isolates from *M. tuberculosis* is based on growth characteristics, serum chemistry tests, and DNA or

HPLC typing. Drug susceptibility tests should be performed on all mycobacterial isolates except *M. avium* complex: for this one complex of organisms, drug susceptibility testing does not accurately predict clinical response. Histopathologic examination of tissues can differentiate mycobacterial infection from other lesions but does not help determine whether the infecting agent is an NTM or *M. tuberculosis*.

Skin testing can be a valuable aid in establishing a diagnosis. An immunocompetent person with NTM infection often has a 5- to 12-mm reaction to a 5-TU Mantoux tuberculin (PPD-S) test. Larger reactions are seen, but rarely exceed 18 mm. A similar reaction to PPD-S may be caused by infection with *M. tuberculosis*, but most patients with tuberculosis have reactions larger than 15 mm. The skin test result is most useful when combined with other information. For example, a 2-year-old child with cervical adenitis who has had no known exposure to tuberculosis but has a normal chest radiograph, has an 11-mm reaction to PPD-S, and lives in the southeastern United States probably has NTM adenitis. Lymph node biopsy and culture may need to be obtained to confirm the diagnosis. Skin testing with PPD-S is of no value in differentiating the various NTM species. The reaction to PPD-S in persons with NTM infection wanes after resolution of the disease, but patients with tuberculous adenitis retain their delayed hypersensitivity indefinitely. Skin testing rarely is helpful for patients with skin granulomas or infections or in immunosuppressed patients, who usually are anergic.

THERAPY

Specific therapy depends on the location and extent of the infected tissue and the species of NTM involved. Surgery usually plays a more important role in the management of NTM disease than it does for tuberculosis. Most NTM infections are localized in the body and are amenable to surgical removal.

Some cases of NTM cervical adenitis resolve spontaneously, but severe scarring and recurrence commonly occur. Removal of the nodes usually is required for diagnosis and treatment. In the neck, multiple infected nodes located near vital structures, such as the facial nerves and carotid artery, may preclude removing all involved tissue. Removal of most of the diseased tissue usually leads to resolution, although approximately 10% to 15% of the infections recur locally, requiring a second surgical procedure. The procedure of choice is excisional biopsy. Incisional biopsy may lead to a chronic sinus tract, poor healing, and increased scarring, although an incision and curettage procedure has been used successfully by some experienced surgeons. The usual agents of NTM adenitis, *M. avium* complex, are relatively resistant to most antimycobacterial drugs. Several published reports relate successful treatment of NTM adenitis using clarithromycin or azithromycin combined with rifampin, ethambutol, or both for 3 to 6 months, without surgery. This approach often fails, however, and excisional biopsy remains the treatment of choice. Small local recurrences after an incomplete excision may respond to chemotherapy. Some cases of NTM adenitis caused by *M. kansasii* may respond to rifampin and ethambutol, without surgery.

Many skin granulomas caused by NTM heal spontaneously, but some persist and require treatment. Surgical excision has been used frequently, but subsequent skin grafting may be necessary. Lesions caused by *M. marinum* or *M. kansasii* may respond to rifampin and ethambutol given for 8 to 12 weeks.

Doxycycline and trimethoprim-sulfamethoxazole have been effective in a few patients.

Skin and deep tissue infections caused by *M. fortuitum*, *M. chelonae*, or *M. abscessus* require a different approach. Few lesions heal spontaneously, and systemic therapy usually is required. These three species are not susceptible to the typical antimycobacterial drugs. Combinations of drugs, using amikacin, cefoxitin, erythromycin, doxycycline, and trimethoprim-sulfamethoxazole, may be effective. The new antibiotic linezolid has a high level of activity against most NTMs, including the rapid-grower species. Disk susceptibility testing performed in a reference laboratory can help determine the optimal drug combination. Infected catheters and other implanted devices must be removed to effect a cure.

Treating pulmonary or disseminated NTM infections often is difficult. *M. avium* complex organisms usually are resistant to isoniazid and pyrazinamide and have variable susceptibility to rifampin and streptomycin. Ethambutol, rifabutin, and clofazimine may have some activity against these species. The newer macrolides, clarithromycin and azithromycin, are important drugs for the treatment of most NTM infections, regardless of anatomic site. They are particularly useful for disease caused by *M. avium* complex or rapid-grower NTM. They have vastly improved the treatment of disseminated infections. The effective treatment of pulmonary disease usually requires medical therapy administered for 1 to 2 years; surgery also may be necessary in some cases. Disseminated infection caused by NTM in HIV-infected patients is difficult to eradicate unless the immune system can be reconstituted with anti-HIV drugs. Most patients improve shortly after specific therapy is administered.

Suggested Readings

Albright JT, Pransky SM. Nontuberculous mycobacteria infections of the head and neck. *Pediatr Clin North Am* 2003;50:503.

Chesney PJ. Nontuberculous mycobacteria. *Pediatr Rev* 2002;23:300.

Contreras MA, Cheung OT, Sanders DE, et al. Pulmonary infection with nontuberculous mycobacteria. *Am Rev Respir Dis* 1988;137:149.

Gupta SK, Katz BZ. Intrathoracic disease associated with *Mycobacterium avium-intracellulare* complex in otherwise healthy children: diagnostic and therapeutic considerations. *Pediatrics* 1994;94:741.

Hale YM, Pfyfler GE, Salfinger M. Laboratory diagnosis of mycobacterial infections; new tools and lessons learned. *Clin Infect Dis* 2001;33:834.

Horsburgh CR Jr. *Mycobacterium avium* complex infection in patients with acquired immunodeficiency syndrome. *N Engl J Med* 1991;324:1332.

Lincoln EM, Gilbert LA. Disease in children due to mycobacteria other than *Mycobacterium tuberculosis*. *Am Rev Respir Dis* 1972;105:683.

Nolt D, Michaels MG, Wald ER. Intrathoracic disease from nontuberculous mycobacteria in children: two cases and a review of the literature. *Pediatrics* 2003;112:e 434.

Oliver KN, Weber DJ, Wallace, Jr. RJ, et al. Nontuberculous mycobacteria. I. Multicenter prevalence study in cystic fibrosis. II. Nested cohort study of impact on cystic fibrosis lung disease. *Am J Respir Crit Care Med* 2003;167:828, 835.

Phillips MS, von Reyn CF. Nosocomial infections due to nontuberculous mycobacteria. *Clin Infect Dis* 2001;33:1363.

Remus N, Reichenbach J, Picard C, et al. Impaired interferon-gamma–mediated immunity and susceptibility to mycobacterial infection in childhood. *Pediatr Res* 2001;50:8.

Starke JR. Nontuberculous mycobacterial infections in children. *Adv Pediatr Infect Dis* 1992;7:123.

Starke JR, Correa AG. Management of mycobacterial infection and disease in children. *Pediatr Infect Dis J* 1995;14:455.

Wallace RJ Jr., Brown BA, Griffith DE, et al. Clarithromycin regimens for pulmonary *Mycobacterium avium* complex infection in children with acquired immunodeficiency syndrome. *J Pediatr* 1994;124:807.

Woods GL, Washington JA II. Mycobacteria other than *Mycobacterium tuberculosis*: review of microbiologic and clinical aspects. *Rev Infect Dis* 1987;9:275.

CHAPTER 181 ■ *YERSINIA ENTEROCOLITICA*

THERESA J. OCHOA AND THOMAS G. CLEARY

Yersinia enterocolitica produces acute gastroenteritis in younger children and mesenteric adenitis in older children. It also has been associated with a variety of extraintestinal manifestations. Although initially reported in the cooler regions of Europe and North America, the organism has been recognized worldwide as a cause of human infection.

ETIOLOGY AND EPIDEMIOLOGY

The genus *Yersinia* belongs to the family Enterobacteriaceae. Three of the eleven species are pathogenic to humans: *Y. pestis*, *Y. enterocolitica*, and *Y. pseudotuberculosis*.

Y. enterocolitica is an oxidase-negative, nonlactose-fermenting, aerobic, gram-negative coccobacillus. It ferments glucose, galactose, and mannose; reduces nitrates; and does not produce hydrogen peroxide. The organism is motile at $22°C$ to $25°C$ but not at $37°C$. These properties help to differentiate it from *Y. pestis* and other Enterobacteriaceae. *Y. enterocolitica* grows well on ordinary media, such as blood, MacConkey medium, heart infusion, and *Salmonella-Shigella* agars, although a selective agar medium has been developed specifically for its isolation. *Y. enterocolitica* strains have been differentiated into approximately 70 serogroups (based on somatic O antigens) and six biotypes. Eleven of the serogroups of *Y. enterocolitica* commonly cause human disease. Most animal and environmental isolates are avirulent for humans. Biogroups 1B, 2, 3, 4, and 5 are associated with human infection. Biogroup 1A includes nonpathogenic environmental isolates. Serologically, the most frequent serogroups associated with human infection are 0:3, 0:5, 27, 0:8, and 0:9.

Y. enterocolitica is widespread in nature. It is present in the gastrointestinal tract of wild and domestic mammals, in the environment (surface water, sewage), and in certain foods (meats, dairy products, seafood, and vegetables). Most of the known pathogenic biogroups are associated with definitive animal hosts, especially the pig. In case-control studies, a correlation has been demonstrated between infection and the consumption or handling of raw or undercooked pork products such as chitterlings.

Gastrointestinal infection with *Y. enterocolitica* appears to be most common in developed countries within the temperate zones. Most cases occur during the winter. The organism is cold-adapted and capable of multiplication at low temperatures. Water- and food-borne infections have been documented, as has person-to-person transmission in family and community outbreaks. The significance of food-product contamination during processing is underscored by the organism's ability to grow in properly refrigerated food, including raw and cooked meat and milk. *Y. enterocolitica* has emerged as a significant cause of transfusion-associated sepsis. Factors contributing to this are the ability of the bacterium to multiply at $4°C$ and to utilize iron liberated from aging erythrocytes.

The incubation period for intestinal infection is typically 4 to 6 days, varying from 1 to 14 days. The excretion of the bacteria in stools continues for a few weeks after cessation of the symptoms.

PATHOGENESIS

Y. enterocolitica usually causes diffuse inflammation of the ileum and colon, with infiltrates in the lamina propria and superficial ulcerations in the terminal ileum and colon. Mesenteric lymphadenitis, with reactive germinal centers and sometimes microabscess formation, often is associated. In most cases, the appendix is grossly and histologically normal or shows only mild inflammation.

The usual route of acquisition of *Y. enterocolitica* is through the ingestion of food or water contaminated with the bacteria. Prior to the initiation of an infectious process, this microorganism undergoes a temperature adaptation in the human host, making use of both chromosomal and plasmid-associated virulence determinants that are temperature regulated. Once attached to M cells (overlaying Peyer patches), the bacteria penetrate these cells to gain access to and multiply in adjacent tissue. The pathogenic strains carry a plasmid for *Yersinia* virulence (pYV) coding for virulence proteins such as the *Yersinia* outer proteins (Yops) and the *Yersinia* adhesion A (YadA). These strains also express chromosomally encoded virulence factors including enterotoxins and those proteins related to invasion and serum resistance. Pathogenic *Yersinia* species share the Yop virulon, which is the core of the *Yersinia* pathogenicity machinery. The Yop virulon is an archetype of the Type III Secretion System, which enables bacteria to secrete and inject bacterial proteins into the cytosol of eukaryotic host cells. The Yops perturb the cytoskeleton, disrupting phagocytosis and blocking the production of proinflammatory cytokines, thus favoring the survival of the invading *Yersinia*. In addition, pathogenic *Yersinia* species produce antiinflammatory proteins.

Susceptibility to systemic infection is enhanced by iron overload and the administration of deferoxamine, an iron-chelating agent. Although *Y. enterocolitica* produces no detectable iron-binding compounds, it can multiply in the intestine by using siderophores produced by other bacteria. To multiply in tissue, the organism must compete with host iron-binding proteins for the available iron. Extraintestinal infection of *Yersinia* is facilitated by iron overload. Iron bound to deferoxamine can also be utilized.

CLINICAL MANIFESTATIONS AND COMPLICATIONS

Y. enterocolitica is primarily a gastrointestinal tract pathogen, with a propensity for extraintestinal spread under appropriate host conditions (immunosuppression, iron overload). Gastrointestinal infection may present as an enterocolitis in young children or as an acute mesenteric lymphadenitis and terminal ileitis mimicking appendicitis in older children. Acute gastroenteritis is the most common presentation in young children (under 3 years of age). Symptoms include diarrhea, usually accompanied by fever, vomiting, and abdominal pain. Stools usually are mucoid or bloody. The severity of diarrhea varies. The abdominal pain usually is colicky, diffuse, or localized to the right lower abdomen. The disease is self-limited, usually lasting from 2 to 3 weeks, although prolonged diarrhea has been described with severe ileitis. In children older than 5 years and adults, severe abdominal pain and fever may predominate with minimal diarrhea, suggesting acute appendicitis. The diagnosis of these patients frequently is made only after surgery. Intra-abdominal complications of enteric infection include perforation, peritonitis, intussusception, toxic megacolon, mesenteric vein thrombosis, chronic ileitis, and gangrene of the bowel wall. The infection also may be associated with exudative pharyngitis and headache. In some cases, infection is entirely asymptomatic, as documented by serologic studies or the recovery of the organism from stool specimens of asymptomatic family contacts.

Extraintestinal manifestation and complications are relatively rare in children. Sepsis occurs in the first year of life and in children with iron overload (as well as deferoxamine therapy of iron overload) or with underlying diseases, such as diabetes mellitus, malignancy, cirrhosis, thalassemia, or sickle cell disease. Septicemia complicates enteritis, particularly in children in the first year of life. Rare complications included hepatic abscess (especially associated with hemochromatosis, diabetes, cirrhosis); kidney, spleen, and lung abscess; osteomyelitis; septic arthritis; pneumonia; meningitis; carditis; panophthalmitis; thyroiditis; and primary cutaneous infection. *Y. enterocolitica* triggers secondary immunologically induced sequelae such as reactive arthritis, erythema nodosum, Reiter syndrome, glomerulonephritis, and myocarditis. Eighty percent of individuals experiencing post-*Yersinia* reactive arthritis are HLA-B27 positive.

DIAGNOSIS

Y. enterocolitica can be recovered from stools, mesenteric lymph nodes, throat swabs, peritoneal fluid, or blood. Isolation from otherwise uncontaminated material, such as blood or lymph nodes, is not difficult because *Y. enterocolitica* grows on ordinary media. Isolation from stools is more difficult. Although it can be recovered from stools using conventional media, the organism can be overlooked because the colonies are very small at 24 hours of incubation. Cold enrichment of stool samples has proved to be of marginal value for the recovery of pathogenic serogroups. In most instances, isolates recovered after cold enrichment have been predominantly nonpathogenic environmental isolates (biogroup 1A). Recovery can be improved by the use of selective media, such as cefsulodin-Irgasan-novobiocin medium. When recovered from a stool specimen, biotyping and serotyping should be attempted. Fecal leukocytes and blood commonly are found in patients with enteritis. Cerebrospinal fluid may have pleocytosis despite negative cultures.

Serology can aid diagnosis, especially during outbreaks. Infection can be confirmed by demonstrating increases in serum antibody titer after infection. Antibodies usually are detected from 8 to 10 days after the onset of clinical symptoms and persist for several months. Serologic response often is absent in infants. *Y. enterocolitica* can cross-react with *Y. pseudotuberculosis* and with other organisms, including *Escherichia coli* 0157 and *Brucella*, *Vibrio*, *Salmonella*, and rickettsia species.

The differential diagnosis in young children includes *Shigella*, enteroinvasive *E. coli*, *Salmonella*, and *Campylobacter*. In older children, preoperative differentiation from acute appendicitis may be impossible. *Y. pseudotuberculosis* can cause an identical clinical picture. These two species can be differentiated only by antigenic structure, biochemical activities, and sensitivity to various *Yersinia* phages.

THERAPY

Y. enterocolitica usually is susceptible to trimethoprim-sulfamethoxazole, aminoglycosides, tetracycline, chloramphenicol, fluoroquinolones, and third-generation cephalosporins. It is resistant to penicillin, ampicillin, carbenicillin, erythromycin, clindamycin, and cephalothin. The role of antibiotic therapy in the management of children with *Y. enterocolitica* enteritis is controversial. Controlled studies have found that antibiotics (ampicillin, trimethoprim-sulfamethoxazole) did not alter the clinical or bacteriologic course of the disease or reduce intrafamilial spread, despite *in vitro* susceptibility of the organism. Antibiotic therapy is not indicated in uncomplicated gastroenteritis, which usually is self-limited. It should be initiated for complicated infections and compromised hosts, especially children with systemic iron overload (e.g., those with hemolytic states). The mortality for patients with septicemia may be as high as 50%, despite antibiotic therapy. Bacteremic children generally respond well to cefotaxime.

PREVENTION

The prevention of human infections depends on using uncontaminated food and water, minimizing contact with potentially infected animals, and appropriate cooking practices in the handling of pig products.

Suggested Readings

Abdel-Haq N, Asmar BL, Abuhammour WM, Brown WJ. *Yersinia enterocolitica* infection in children. *Pediatr Infect Dis J* 2000;19:954.

Bottone EJ. *Yersinia enterocolitica*: overview and epidemiologic correlates. *Microbes Infect* 1999;1:323.

Cornelis GR. *Yersinia* type III secretion: send in the effectors. *J Cell Biol* 2002; 158:401.

Fredriksson-Ahomaa M and Korkeala H. Low occurrence of pathogenic *Yersinia enterocolitica* in clinical, food and environmental samples: a methodological problem. *Clin Micro Rev* 2003;16:220.

Gayraud M, Scavizzi MR, Mollaret HH, Guillevin L, Hornstein MJ. Antibiotic treatment of *Yersinia enterocolitica* septicemia: a retrospective review of 43 cases. *Clin Infect Dis* 1993;17:405.

Hoogkamp-Korstanje JA, Stolk-Engelaer VM. *Yersinia enterocolitica* infection in children. *Pediatr Infect Dis J* 1995;14:771.

Lee LA, Taylor J, Carter GP, et al. *Yersinia enterocolitica* O:3—an emerging cause of pediatric gastroenteritis. *J Infect Dis* 1991;163:660.

Marks MI, Pai CH, Lafleur L, et al. *Yersinia enterocolitica* gastroenteritis: a prospective study of clinical, bacteriologic and epidemiologic features. *J Pediatr* 1980;96:26.

Naqvi SH, Swierkosz EM, Gerard J, Mills JR. Presentation of *Yersinia enterocolitica* enteritis in children. *Pediatr Infect Dis J* 1993;12:386.

Robins-Browne RM, Prpic JK. Effects of iron and desferrioxamine on infections with *Yersinia enterocolitica*. *Infect Immun* 1985;47:774.

CHAPTER 182 ■ *YERSINIA PSEUDOTUBERCULOSIS*

THERESA J. OCHOA AND THOMAS G. CLEARY

Yersinia pseudotuberculosis causes gastroenteritis and mesenteric lymphadenitis. It also mimics Kawasaki disease and rarely causes septicemia.

ETIOLOGY

Y. pseudotuberculosis belongs to the genus *Yersinia* and family Enterobacteriaceae with two other human pathogens: *Yersinia enterocolitica* and *Yersinia pestis*. *Y. pseudotuberculosis* is closely related to *Y. pestis* (97% to 100% DNA homology) and more distantly related to *Y. enterocolitica*. Although genetically it is closely related to *Y. pestis*, clinically it behaves like *Y. enterocolitica*.

Y. pseudotuberculosis is a non-lactose-fermenting, aerobic, gram-negative coccobacillus. This oxidase-negative and urease-positive organism reduces nitrates and ferments glucose, galactose, maltose, mannose, and xylose. It often is motile when grown at 22°C to 25°C, but nonmotile at 37°C. It grows better at 4°C in buffered saline than most other common bacteria.

Six serogroups (I through VI) have been defined antigenically on the basis of somatic O antigens. Four flagellar (H) antigens (A through D) are recognized. Serotypes are defined by both O and H antigens. Most human infections (approximately 80%) are related to serogroup 1.

PATHOGENESIS

The oral infection of guinea pigs with *Y. pseudotuberculosis* causes necrotic Peyer patches in the terminal ileum and cecum, with caseous necrosis in the mesenteric lymph nodes. The infected lymph nodes are enlarged and inflamed, with hemorrhages on their surface, microabscess formation, and the occasional development of a granulomatous reaction with giant cells. The intestinal tract, particularly the terminal ileum, may have edema, leukocyte infiltration, and superficial ulcerations. The appendix usually is grossly and microscopically normal or is mildly inflamed, but some cases of acute phlegmonous appendicitis associated with this organism have been described.

Human infection occurs via the ingestion of contaminated food or water. After reaching the gastrointestinal tract, the organism is taken up by M cells overlying Peyer patches, and it spreads from there to mesenteric nodes. Infection usually is contained at this point, but systemic spread occurs occasionally.

Pathogenic strains of *Y. enterocolitica*, *Y. pestis*, and *Y. pseudotuberculosis* carry a plasmid for *Yersinia* virulence (pYV), which codes for several virulence proteins, including the type-III secretion system, the surface-exposed adhesion (YadA), and the effector proteins (Yops, for *Yersinia* outer proteins). The type-III secretion system enables the bacteria to secrete and inject bacterial proteins into host cells. This system is composed of a needle-like structure, a translocation machinery, and at least six effector proteins. Pathogenic strains also carry chromosomal genes for attachment and invasion.

EPIDEMIOLOGY

Y. pseudotuberculosis is found in animals worldwide. The bacteria have been recovered from a wide range of domestic and wild animals and birds. Rodents and fowl, especially turkeys, pigeons, ducks, and canaries, frequently are infected and represent important reservoirs. The organism is excreted in feces and animal-to-animal transmission has been documented.

Human infections by these bacteria are infrequent occurrences and are reported mainly in northern Europe, generally as sporadic cases for which the source of the infection is not found. Direct or indirect contact with infected animals probably represents the major mechanism of infection. Household pets often are the source of infection for children. The organism also has been recovered from foods, milk, water, soil, and other environmental sources. A history of drinking well water or mountain stream water is common. Most infected patients are children older than 5 years or adolescents. Human infections occur more frequently during fall and winter months. The incubation period typically is 4 to 6 days, varying from 1 to 14 days.

Epidemics of *Y. pseudotuberculosis* are rare events. One outbreak of undetermined source was caused by serogroup III in Finland. The infected cases were scattered over a large geographic area, without clustering in families, thus leading to the conclusion that the level of infectivity was low, at least for this strain. The disease was more severe in children than in adults.

CLINICAL MANIFESTATIONS AND COMPLICATIONS

The most common manifestation of *Y. pseudotuberculosis* is mesenteric lymphadenitis, with abdominal pain and fever. Because tenderness in the right lower quadrant is a frequent finding, the clinical picture may be indistinguishable from that of acute appendicitis. The diagnosis often is considered only after laparotomy reveals a normal appendix and enlarged mesenteric lymph nodes. The infection usually is self-limited, with complete recovery beginning around the fifth day of the disease, although symptoms may persist for 1 week to 6 months. Enterocolitis, the usual manifestation of *Y. enterocolitica*, is relatively unusual with infection caused by *Y. pseudotuberculosis*.

Less commonly, an illness mimicking Kawasaki disease has been described. This syndrome involves fever lasting 5 days to 2 weeks, rash (scarlatiniform, maculopapular, erythema multiforme-like, or urticarial), periungual desquamation, strawberry tongue, cracked lips, conjunctivitis, sterile pyuria, and thrombocytosis. Coronary artery aneurysms also have been documented to follow *Y. pseudotuberculosis* infection.

Typical Kawasaki disease-like findings developed in approximately 9% of patients with *Y. pseudotuberculosis* infection.

Renal involvement of *Y. pseudotuberculosis* is unique and not well explained. Approximately 10% to 14% of patients develop azotemia with or without oliguria, sterile pyuria, and glycosuria. Renal biopsies demonstrate tubulointerstitial nephritis. Onset is 2 to 14 days (mean 6) after onset of fever, and the course is almost always benign, with complete recovery in 4 weeks. Renal ultrasound typically shows large kidneys with hyperechogenicity in the cortex.

The most lethal complication of the disease is septicemia. It usually occurs in patients with underlying diseases, such as malnutrition, diabetes mellitus, cirrhosis, immunosuppressive therapy, hemodialysis, or iron overload caused by hemochromatosis, hemolytic disease, polycythemia, and chronic venous congestion. This organism, like *Y. enterocolitica*, is unable to produce iron-binding compounds. Its multiplication in tissues and the subsequent development of septicemia depends on the availability of host iron. The administration of deferoxamine, an iron-chelating substance that is sometimes used in these patients, allows virulent *Y. pseudotuberculosis* to thrive, because the organism can use the bound iron.

Post-infectious complications have been identified following infection with some, but not all, serotypes. The rate of complications (14% to 53%) varies depending in part on the serotype of the outbreak. The most common post-infectious complications are erythema nodosum, reactive arthritis, iritis, and nephritis. Other reported complications are intra-abdominal abscesses, pleural effusion, myocarditis, uveitis, intussusception, and hemolytic uremic syndrome. Some infected persons identified during the investigation of family contacts are completely asymptomatic.

DIAGNOSIS

Y. pseudotuberculosis can be recovered from inflamed mesenteric lymph nodes during surgery. Histologic examination of lymph nodes removed during an operation may aid in the diagnosis. The recovery rate of this organism from stools is low. Although it grows on ordinary media, colonies often are small after incubation for 24 hours but are apparent after 48 hours; it may, therefore, be overgrown by other flora in stool specimens. Selective media, such as cefsulodin-Irgasan-novobiocin (CIN) medium, are useful, especially for mixed cultures. Cold enrichment increases the yield of positive cultures, but may take up to 3 weeks.

Serologic examinations, although less definitive than culture, are sometimes helpful. *Y. pseudotuberculosis* serogroups II and IV cross-react with *Salmonella* strains and, in some instances, with *Y. enterocolitica*, *Escherichia coli*, and *Brucella*. Antibody titers during the acute phase may be low; a second serum titer is needed to demonstrate a fourfold increase. Hemagglutination titers of 1:160 or higher are considered significant.

A polymerase chain reaction (PCR)–based assay can be used for the detection of chromosome- and plasmid-borne virulence genes of *Y. pseudotuberculosis* and can provide a rapid and reliable genotypic characterization of field isolates.

The main differential diagnosis for the most common clinical presentation is acute appendicitis; other diseases that may cause enlarged ileocecal lymph nodes or ileitis include tuberculosis, salmonellosis, actinomycosis, *Y. enterocolitica*, regional ileitis, and ulcerative colitis. The differential diagnosis for children who present with a Kawasaki-like illness includes staphylococcal or streptococcal infection, leptospirosis, Stevens-Johnson syndrome, and collagen vascular disease.

THERAPY

Because mesenteric lymphadenitis usually is self-limited, with complete spontaneous recovery, antibiotic therapy may not be indicated. Antibiotics should be used when children with underlying disorders are infected or when septicemia or other complications are suspected. The mortality associated with septicemia is high, reaching 70% despite antibiotic therapy. Unlike *Y. enterocolitica*, *Y. pseudotuberculosis* usually is susceptible *in vitro* to ampicillin, chloramphenicol, aminoglycosides, cephalosporins, and tetracycline. Which of these agents represents optimal therapy remains uncertain. Ampicillin therapy of the Kawasaki-like variant of *Y. pseudotuberculosis* infection shortens duration of positive cultures but does not appear to change the clinical course.

Suggested Readings

Abe J, Onimaru M, Matsumato S, Noma S, et al. Clinical role for a superantigen in *Y. pseudotuberculosis* infection. *J Clin Invest* 1997;99:1823.

Attwood SEA, Mealy K, Cafferkey MT, et al. *Yersinia* infection and acute abdominal pain. *Lancet* 1987;2:529.

Cornelis GR. *Yersinia* type III secretion: send in the effectors. *J Cell Biol* 2002;158:401.

Koo JW, Park SN, Choi SM, et al. Acute renal failure associated with *Yersinia pseudotuberculosis* infection in children. *Pediatr Nephrol* 1996;10:582.

Lee VT, Schneewind O. Type III secretion machines and the pathogenesis of enteric infections caused by *Yersinia* and *Salmonella* spp. *Immunol Rev* 1999;168:241.

Ljungberg P, Valtonen M, Harjola VP, et al. Report of four cases of *Yersinia pseudotuberculosis* septicemia and a literature review. *Eur J Clin Microbiol Infect Dis* 1995;14:804.

Press N, Fyfe M, Bowie W, Kelly M. Clinical and microbiological follow-up of an outbreak of *Yersinia pseudotuberculosis* serotype Ib. *Scand J Infect Dis* 2001;33:523.

Sato K, Ouchi K, Taki M. Ampicillin versus placebo for *Yersinia pseudotuberculosis* infection in children. *Pediatr Infect Dis* 1988;7:686.

Tertti R, Vuento R, Mikkola P, et al. Clinical manifestations of *Yersinia pseudotuberculosis* infection in children. *Eur J Clin Microbiol Infect Dis* 1989;8:587.

Viboud GI, So SS, Ryndak MB, Bliska JB. Proinflammatory signalling stimulated by the type III translocation factor YopB is counteracted by multiple effectors in epithelial cells infected with *Yersinia pseudotuberculosis*. *Mol Microbiol* 2003;24:1305.

CHAPTER 183 ■ MISCELLANEOUS BACTERIAL INFECTIONS

RANDALL G. FISHER

MISCELLANEOUS GRAM-POSITIVE COCCI

Aerococcus

The genus *Aerococcus* contains four species: *A. viridans, A. urinae, A. christensenii* sp. nov., and *A. sanguicola* sp. nov. The latter two are newly described species, the former of which was isolated from a vaginal specimen and the latter from a blood culture. Aerococci are catalase-negative, nonmotile, gram-positive cocci that appear preferentially in tetrads. These relatively slow-growing organisms produce translucent alpha-hemolytic colonies on blood agar. Like enterococci, most aerococci grow in 6.5% salt.

Epidemiology and Pathophysiology

Aerococci are distributed worldwide as contaminants of air and dust. They have been found also on meats, in raw vegetables, and on human skin in small numbers. In most circumstances, aerococci are saprophytic. Aerococci have been cultured from all areas of hospitals, including operating suites and delivery rooms. Disease in humans is distinctly uncommon. *A. viridans* can be isolated from 0.9% of patients with pneumonia. Most affected patients are elderly, but pediatric infections have been reported. Immunocompromised patients, particularly those with neutropenia, are at risk of developing infection. Adhesion factors may play a role. Additional information about the clinical manifestations, diagnosis, and treatment of infections caused by aerococci is presented in Box 183.1.

Leuconostoc

Leuconostoc species are facultatively anaerobic gram-positive cocci that usually appear in pairs or chains. They are catalase-negative and often alpha-hemolytic on blood agar and may react with group D streptococcal antiserum. These properties are shared by viridans streptococci, with which *Leuconostoc* species often are confused. Differences include the production of gas from glucose and high-level vancomycin resistance.

Epidemiology and Pathophysiology

Commonly, *Leuconostoc* species are found on plants, especially sugar cane and leafy vegetables. They also are found in dairy products and wine. They are used in industry as starter cultures in food production. Although not a part of the normal human flora, occasionally they are recovered from vaginal swabs in healthy individuals. *Leuconostoc* rarely is pathogenic. Studies also have shown colonization of mucosal surfaces in some hospitalized individuals. Case reports of human infection began to appear in 1985. Risk factors are thought to include underlying disease states or immune compromise, gastrointestinal tract disease, prior or current antibiotic therapy (especially vancomycin), venous or gastrointestinal tract access devices, recent invasive procedures, and infancy. Of the first 21 cases reported in the English-language literature, 12 were in children, and 10 of those were in patients younger than 1 year of age. Documented portals of entry include central lines and gastrostomy tubes.

Clinical Manifestations and Complications

Bacteremia is by far the most common clinical manifestation of *Leuconostoc* infection, heralded by fever and usually

---

| BOX 183.1 | Clinical Manifestations, Diagnosis, and Treatment of *Aerococcus* Infection |

Clinical Manifestations and Complications
Most cases of *A. viridans* bacteremia have been found in association with signs and symptoms of subacute infective endocarditis. *A. urinae* causes a febrile urinary tract infection. Lymphadenitis has been reported recently. Bacteremia and meningitis also have been described. Meningitis may present as a prolonged illness associated with seizures or abnormal neurologic examination in an otherwise normal host. Bone and joint infections and wound or other localized infections are exceedingly rare.

Diagnosis and Treatment
Appearance on Gram stain and growth in culture are keys to the diagnosis of aerococcal infection. Aerococci may resem-

ble staphylococci on Gram stain and viridans group streptococci on blood agar. In their bile esculin hydrolysis and growth in 6.5% salt, they resemble enterococci. Aerococci, however, are pyrrolidone carboxylyl peptidase-negative and do not form chains. Most aerococci are sensitive to penicillin, ampicillin, the cephalosporins, and the macrolides, and all are susceptible to vancomycin. Despite good minimal inhibitory concentrations (MICs), however, time-kill studies show that neither penicillin nor vancomycin produces rapid bactericidal effect against aerococci; therefore, in treating endocarditis, the combination of penicillin or vancomycin with an aminoglycoside is required. Usually, they are intermediately susceptible or resistant to sulfonamides and aminoglycosides.

leukocytosis. Gastrointestinal disturbances, especially diarrhea, are common occurrences. Infants are prone to emesis. Pneumonia, dental infections, peritonitis, ventriculoperitoneal shunt infection, and meningitis also have been described.

Diagnosis and Treatment

Usually, cultures are positive within 24 to 48 hours. *Leuconostoc* species are somewhat fastidious. All are intrinsically vancomycin resistant. The identification of vancomycin-resistant streptococci should raise suspicion of *Leuconostoc* infection and prompt further biochemical studies. Usually, *Leuconostoc* is sensitive to the primitive beta-lactam antibiotics, especially penicillin and ampicillin. Tolerance to penicillin is fairly common; treatment with relatively high doses frequently is successful. Combination of penicillin and gentamicin probably is synergistic. Resistance increases with later generations of cephalosporins.

Pediococcus

Like *Leuconostoc* species, pediococci are intrinsically vancomycin-resistant, facultatively anaerobic, gram-positive cocci. They appear most characteristically in tetrads on Gram stain, although they may appear in pairs or clusters. They are catalase- and oxidase-negative. Most isolates react with Lancefield group D streptococcal antibodies. They are leucine aminopeptidase-positive, which distinguishes them from *Leuconostoc* species. They produce white, opaque, nonhemolytic colonies on sheep's blood agar.

Epidemiology and Pathophysiology

Like *Leuconostoc* species and other lactic-acid bacteria, pediococci are found on plants, in dairy products, and in alcohol-containing beverages. They also are used in the formation of silage and as starter cultures for some meat products. They are not thought to be part of normal human flora. Although formerly thought to be nonpathogenic, they now are considered rare opportunistic pathogens of minimal virulence.

Many cases of blood isolates are seen in patients without symptoms of infection or in polymicrobial cultures in which the significance of the isolate cannot be assessed adequately. Clear-cut cases of sepsis have occurred. Risk factors for bacteremia, with or without symptoms, appear to be extremes of age, recent abdominal surgery or tube feedings, broad-spectrum antimicrobial therapy, and the presence of severe underlying disease states.

Clinical Manifestations and Complications

Most patients are either asymptomatic or exhibit fever as the only symptom. Most reported cases of *Pediococcus* bacteremia have had concomitant pneumonia. Reported pediatric cases are in patients with underlying gastrointestinal tract anomalies. Isolation of *Pediococcus* as part of a polymicrobial process in localized infections is a common finding, especially from abdominal sites. Assessing the relative importance of *Pediococcus* in these sites is difficult. Bacteremic pneumonia in a previously healthy pregnant woman has been reported.

Diagnosis and Treatment

Diagnosis of infection with *Pediococcus* is made by identifying vancomycin-resistant, gram-positive cocci in its characteristic tetrads. Many pediococci initially are misidentified as *Streptococcus equinus*, *Streptococcus constellatus*, or group D streptococci, not enterococci, although they do not form chains. Hence, reported cases of pediococcal infection may represent only a fraction of the total number of infections. Generally, pediococci are susceptible to penicillin, ampicillin, imipenem, and

first- and second-generation cephalosporins. Pediococci, like *Leuconostoc*, are intrinsically resistant to vancomycin. Generally, sensitivity to ticarcillin and cefotaxime is poor, despite large zones of inhibition by disc susceptibility testing. Aminoglycoside sensitivity is variable.

MISCELLANEOUS GRAM-POSITIVE BACILLI

Arcanobacterium

The genus *Arcanobacterium* has one clinically relevant species, *A. haemolyticum* (formerly *C. haemolyticum*), now recognized as a cause of exudative pharyngitis and maculopapular rash in adolescents and young adults. *A. haemolyticum* is an asporogenous, facultatively anaerobic, catalase-negative, gram-positive rod.

Epidemiology and Pathophysiology

A. haemolyticum is recovered from 0.5% to 10.0% of children and adolescents presenting with pharyngitis. Selectivity for older children is unexplained. Organisms survive intracellularly, which may contribute to the difficulty encountered in eradicating penicillin-susceptible organisms.

Clinical Manifestations and Complications

A. haemolyticum causes a pharyngitis that resembles that seen in group A streptococcal infection except that palatal petechiae and strawberry tongue usually are absent. Circumoral pallor also is a rare finding. Approximately one-half of infections are associated with a maculopapular rash that typically is confined to extensor surfaces, sparing the trunk, palms, and soles. It often is scarlatiniform. Peritonsillar abscesses sometimes are seen. Infections other than pharyngotonsillitis are distinctly less common findings. However, reports of sinusitis and orbital cellulitis, including subperiosteal abscess requiring surgical debridement, have appeared. Soft-tissue abscesses and cellulitis are reported. Visceral infection or bacteremia is a rare occurrence; endocarditis in an intravenous drug abuser has been reported. Skin infection resembling ecthyma gangrenosum has been noted in tropical areas.

Diagnosis and Treatment

A. haemolyticum grows poorly on tellurite medium, which helps distinguish it from *Corynebacterium diphtheriae*. Tolerance for penicillin sometimes is noted, which may explain treatment failures with penicillin. Erythromycin is the treatment of choice for pharyngitis. Peritonsillar abscesses require prompt surgical therapy as well as appropriate antimicrobials.

Bacillus

Bacillus species are large, straight, endospore-forming, gram-positive rods. Organisms are aerobic or facultatively anaerobic. Endospores are very resistant to adverse conditions. *B. anthracis* and *B. cereus* are significant causes of disease. Less frequent pathogens are *B. brevis*, *B. licheniformis*, *B. subtilis*, *B. sphaericus*, and *B. thuringiensis*.

Epidemiology and Pathophysiology

B. anthracis can infect both domestic herbivores and many different types of wild animals. In the past, almost all cases of anthrax in the United States were cutaneous, caused by the contact of broken or abraded skin with spores or live bacilli. In late 2001, respiratory cases related to domestic terrorism were reported. The current global environment continues to favor the possibility of bioterrorism events, and *B. anthracis* is a potential weapon. The extreme stability of anthrax spores allows this potential misuse. Considering the scarcity of naturally occurring inhalational anthrax, all cases should be presumed to be secondary to bioterrorism. *B. anthracis* contains three virulence factors: (a) edema toxin, (b) lethal toxin, and (c) a thick capsule. Edema toxin causes extravasation of fluid, leading to the edema characteristic of cutaneous disease. Lethal toxin increases proinflammatory cytokines, including tumor necrosis factor-alpha (TNF-α) and interleukin 1-beta (IL-1β). The capsule makes it difficult for the immune system to kill phagocytosed organisms.

B. cereus produces virulence factors, including a necrotizing enterotoxin, an emetic toxin, phospholipases, proteases, and hemolysins. *B. cereus* colonization of intravenous catheters may be aided by localization in adherent biofilms. Food-borne outbreaks of gastrointestinal illness are the most common manifestation of significant *B. cereus* infections; diarrhea caused by enterotoxin or vomiting from the emetic toxin are common complications after consumption of contaminated food. Improperly cooked fried rice may pose the greatest risk of *B. cereus* spore germination and toxin elaboration.

Clinical Manifestations and Complications

B. anthracis causes three distinct forms of disease: cutaneous, inhalational, and gastrointestinal.

- Cutaneous disease usually begins as a pruritic, painless papule. Over the course of time, the papules go on to vesiculate. The vesicles rupture, leaving a dry eschar. Significant local edema may develop. Antibiotic treatment does not alter the progression of the lesions. Regional adenopathy sometimes is found. Children may be highly febrile and have an associated leukocytosis. A perimeter of smaller satellite vesicles, called "pearly wreath," is highly suggestive of cutaneous anthrax, but it is seen only occasionally.
- Inhalational anthrax generally presents as a nonspecific syndrome of low-grade fever, dry cough, fatigue, myalgias, malaise, and drenching sweats. Other symptoms may include chest pain or discomfort. Nausea and vomiting are not uncommon occurrences. The radiologic hallmarks of inhalational anthrax, widened mediastinum and pleural effusion, may be subtle or absent early in the disease process. After a 2- to 3-day period of seeming improvement, the patient with undiagnosed inhalational anthrax undergoes rapid decompensation, with stridor, dyspnea, air hunger, and respiratory failure developing over the course of hours.
- Gastrointestinal anthrax is an uncommon occurrence. It occurs 1 to 7 days after consuming contaminated meat. Initial symptoms are diffuse abdominal pain, nausea, and vomiting. Emesis may be blood-tinged. Bloody diarrhea develops in almost all patients. Severe abdominal pain with rebound tenderness consistent with acute abdomen has been reported. As the pain subsides, massive ascites ensues. Computed tomographic (CT) scan displays mesenteric lymphadenopathy. The disease progresses to shock and death within days. The prognosis is much better for those with oropharyngeal anthrax, which can cause massive edema of the soft tissues of the neck in conjunction with pseudomembranous pharyngitis. This form of disease is rare.

Nonanthracis species of *Bacillus* can cause local and disseminated infection after traumatic injury, burns, or surgery. Local infection may be indolent, marked only by increased drainage at wound sites. *B. cereus* now is thought to be second only to *Staphylococcus epidermidis* as a cause of serious ophthalmic infection that develops after traumatic injury. A corneal ring abscess is the classic manifestation of eye infection. Findings include pain, chemosis, proptosis, and retinal hemorrhage. Eye infections are very aggressive, in part because of the elaboration of extracellular toxins and enzymes in the closed space of the globe.

B. cereus causes two food-poisoning syndromes, characterized by either diarrhea or vomiting. The diarrheal syndrome begins approximately 8 to 16 hours after consumption of contaminated food (usually meat) and resolves within 12 hours. The emetic toxin elaborated by growth of *B. cereus* in rice or pasta produces an illness similar to that of food poisoning caused by *Staphylococcus aureus*. After ingestion of toxin and a short incubation period of 1 to 5 hours, nausea, vomiting and, occasionally, diarrhea develop. Typically, affected individuals recover within 24 hours with minimal or supportive care.

Diagnosis and Treatment

A definitive diagnosis of cutaneous anthrax requires obtaining culture specimens prior to the institution of antibiotic therapy. Punch biopsy of the edge of the cutaneous lesion should be obtained for immunohistochemical testing and silver staining. Establishing the diagnosis of inhalational anthrax is difficult in the absence of an exposure history. Mediastinal widening is a helpful sign but may resemble that seen with mediastinal histoplasmosis. The diagnosis is established firmly if smears and cultures of pleural fluid and/or blood are positive for *B. anthracis*. Public health department reference laboratories have available specialized testing, such as polymerase chain reaction (PCR) or direct fluorescent antibody testing. Serologic testing has good sensitivity and specificity, but it is not positive until approximately 10 days into the disease.

Most *B. anthracis* isolates are sensitive to fluoroquinolones, rifampin, vancomycin, the carbapenems, tetracycline, the aminoglycosides, and clindamycin. They generally are resistant to cephalosporins and trimethoprim-sulfamethoxazole. Although most isolates are sensitive to penicillins, some contain penicillinases that may be inducible, which would render the organisms resistant to penicillin at some point during the course of treatment. Treatment recommendations largely are speculative and based largely on animal models of infection because of the paucity of human cases. Patients with bacteremia or other invasive disease generally are treated with more than one antibiotic; the combination of ciprofloxacin or tetracycline and an aminoglycoside or clindamycin often is used. Because tetracycline does not cross the blood brain barrier well, it should not be used for those patients with meningitis. In theory, clindamycin may be beneficial in decreasing the production of toxin, although this reduction has not been demonstrated specifically with regard to *B. anthracis*. Duration of therapy has not been established clearly; for cutaneous anthrax, 10 days usually is sufficient, but 60 days is the current standard for inhalational disease. Adjunctive measures such as chest tube drainage of pleural effusions and careful management of fluids and electrolytes are of paramount importance. Systemic steroids probably are beneficial for patients with massive edema and for patients with meningitis.

Bacillus species are common contaminants of blood cultures. Physicians must be alert to possible recovery of *Bacillus* as a pathogen. *Bacillus* species often are true pathogens in association with central venous lines in patients with neutropenia. Differentiating among individual species can be difficult. Usually, *B. cereus* can be distinguished from *B. anthracis* by phenotypic features of motility, beta-hemolysis, and penicillin resistance. Vancomycin and clindamycin are recommended for the treatment of serious *Bacillus* species infections; organisms commonly are resistant to penicillins and cephalosporins. Removal of the line is the most important aspect of treatment in neutropenic patients with line infections. Effective débridement of local infection may be required for cure. Consultation with an ophthalmologist should be sought early for the management of eye infection.

Corynebacterium (Non-diphtheriae species)

Corynebacterium species derive their name from their clublike shape. Organisms are facultatively anaerobic or aerobic and do not produce spores. They are nonmotile and catalase-positive and contain mycolic acid in their cell walls. Clinically relevant species include *C. diphtheriae* (see Chapter 159, Diphtheria), *C. amycolatum*, and *C. jeikeium* (formerly *Corynebacterium* group JK). The last one can be a major nosocomial agent of bacteremia and endocarditis.

Epidemiology and Pathophysiology

Commonly, *Corynebacterium* species are recovered as normal flora in hospitalized patients. Nosocomial acquisition of *C. jeikeium* has been characterized most completely. Not surprisingly, patient-to-patient transmission in the hospital environment can occur, and selective antibiotic pressure augments colonization with *Corynebacterium* species. In some series, *C. amycolatum* is the most common isolate; in the past, many isolates were misidentified as *C. striatum*, *C. ulcerans*, or *C. xerosis*. *Corynebacterium* species, particularly *C. jeikeium*, possess lipophilic properties, which may account for their ability to proliferate on skin that has a higher lipid content. Infections have been described in neonates and immunocompromised older children. Intravascular access devices and breach of skin integrity are important risk factors for the development of local infection and bacteremia. Other risk factors include male gender, neutropenia, broad-spectrum antibiotic exposure, and prolonged hospital stay. Catalase production may be responsible for the rare infection with non-JK *Corynebacterium* species in children with chronic granulomatous disease.

Clinical Manifestations and Complications

Immunocompromised patients infected with *C. jeikeium* may demonstrate a local inflammatory lesion at the site of infection or may demonstrate a disseminated, hemorrhagic, or necrotic papular exanthem. *C. jeikeium* also is recognized to be one of the most common causes of prosthetic valve endocarditis in adults.

Although primarily a pathogen in sheep and goats, *C. pseudotuberculosis* can cause a localized granulomatous lymphadenitis in humans; almost all cases are associated with animal contact. *C. amycolatum* is a rare cause of endocarditis, catheter infections, and surgical wound infections. It has been reported as a cause of secondary septic arthritis and of fatal sepsis in a premature neonate. *C. xerosis*, *C. pseudodiphtheriticum*, and *C. striatum* are rare causes of pulmonary infection and endocarditis. *C. ulcerans* is a zoonotic pathogen that produces an ulcerative pharyngitis after contact with an infected animal or consumption of contaminated raw milk. Some strains of *C. ulcerans* produce diphtheria toxin and can cause serious illnesses that precisely mimic cutaneous or respiratory diphtheria. *C. urealyticum* (formerly *Corynebacterium* group D2) is a rare cause of alkaline-encrusted cystitis and sometimes pyelitis.

Diagnosis and Treatment

A diagnosis of *Corynebacterium* infection is based on isolation of the organism from clinical material. Vancomycin is recommended for empiric therapy of suspected *Corynebacterium* infection until susceptibilities are known. Almost all isolates also are susceptible to teicoplanin, which has been used successfully in some reported cases. Two-drug therapy that includes an aminoglycoside commonly is used for treatment of *Corynebacterium* endocarditis. Scrupulous attention to skin hygiene may reduce colonization of hospital personnel and the incidence of patient-to-patient transmission of pathogenic strains.

Erysipelothrix rhusiopathiae

Erysipelothrix rhusiopathiae, also called *E. insidiosa*, was identified by Rosenbach, in 1884, as a cause of the cutaneous disease erysipeloid. The organism is a slender, pleomorphic, nonmotile, gram-positive, unencapsulated rod that produces 0.1-mm bluish colonies on blood agar. Some strains produce alpha-hemolysis in 48 to 72 hours. Inoculated gelatin stab culture inconsistently forms a test-tube brush appearance that is diagnostic for this organism.

Epidemiology and Pathophysiology

Erysipelothrix is a common commensal of wild and domestic animals and may be a saprophyte of soil. The organism is an important cause of epidemic disease in swine. Accordingly, those at risk for exposure to *Erysipelothrix* include fish handlers, meat processors, poultry workers, veterinarians, abattoir workers, and food handlers.

Usually, human infection results from contamination of skin abrasions exposed in handling colonized material. Males are infected more commonly than are females, perhaps because of increased exposure. The disease usually is self-limiting and most often involves the hands. Biopsy of the skin lesions reveals a marked inflammatory response. Childhood *Erysipelothrix* infection is unusual. Additional information about the clinical manifestations, diagnosis, and treatment of infections caused by *Erysipelothrix* is presented in Box 183.2.

Rhodococcus equi

Rhodococcus equi is a catalase-positive, urease-positive, oxidase-negative, gram-positive rod that has assumed an increasingly visible role as a pathogen in immunocompromised patients. The organism assumes a more coccoid morphology in solid media and a more bacillary form in liquid media. Its cell wall contains mycolic acid, rendering it acid-fast when grown on Löwenstein-Jensen media and stained with Kinyoun stain.

Epidemiology and Pathophysiology

Despite the common occurrence of this pathogen as a cause of veterinary infections, most reported human cases have not had farm or animal exposure. The organism lives in soil. Person-to-person transmission has not been documented. The appearance of pyogranulomatous lesions in the lung is consistent with the role of *R. equi* as a respiratory pathogen containing mycolic acid, a possible virulence factor in the cell wall. CD4$^+$ lymphocytes may be essential for pulmonary clearance, which explains why persons infected with human immunodeficiency virus (HIV) comprise two-thirds of patients with proven *R. equi* infection. The appearance of an unusual appearing granulomatous inflammation, termed *malakoplakia*, in lung biopsy should raise suspicion of the presence of *R. equi* infection.

Clinical Manifestations and Complications

Symptoms of a slowly progressive pneumonia are common occurrences. Although most infections occur in patients with the acquired immunodeficiency syndrome (AIDS), malignancy and transplantation also pose risks. Often, pulmonary infection is pleura-based and associated with cavitation. Extrapulmonary

ized patients with altered host defenses. When the microbiology laboratory reports the isolation of an oxidase-negative, lactose-nonfermenting, gram-negative rod, *Acinetobacter* is by far the most likely organism. The taxonomy can be confusing, but the most common isolates of the genus are *A. baumannii*, *A. lwoffi*, *A. haemolyticus*, and *A. johnsonii*. These aerobic, oxidase-negative, catalase-positive organisms grow on standard agar between 33°C and 35°C.

Epidemiology and Pathophysiology

A. calcoaceticus is distributed widely as a water-dwelling saprophyte and commensal in animals and humans. In hospitals, *Acinetobacter* has been isolated from personnel and from environmental sources. Most cases of *Acinetobacter* infections occur in patients who require endotracheal intubation or intravenous access. Risk factors include recent surgery, antibiotic therapy, and immunosuppression. Patients with serious underlying illnesses can become colonized rapidly with *Acinetobacter* from a highly contaminated environment. Often, a seasonal incidence of infection is observed, with a peak occurring during the late summer. Outbreaks have been reported from neonatal intensive care units (ICUs). Strict infection control is critical in halting such outbreaks.

Clinical Manifestations and Complications

Acinetobacter infection shares several features with other forms of gram-negative infection. Bacteremic patients present with fever and hypotension; patients rarely are asymptomatic. The lung is the most common site of primary infection, but infection associated with intravenous catheters occurs frequently. Often, other microbes are isolated from blood cultures that yield *Acinetobacter*, a finding that is associated with a poor prognosis.

Diagnosis and Treatment

Diagnosis is based on isolation of *Acinetobacter* from clinical material. Because of its coccobacillary shape, this organism may appear similar to *Haemophilus* or *Neisseria* on Gram stain. Its inability to grow anaerobically in any medium readily differentiates *Acinetobacter* from enteric bacteria. Prompt initiation of appropriate antimicrobial therapy and management of local infection caused by *Acinetobacter* usually results in a good outcome. However, selection of an antimicrobial agent may be complicated by the emergence of multiply resistant strains that display high-level resistance to aminoglycosides. Combination antibiotic therapy and third-generation cephalosporins have shown some efficacy in some cases. The carbapenems (imipenem/cilastatin and meropenem) were thought to be safe choices, but carbapenem resistance is emerging, and clonal spread of resistant organisms within communities has been well described. In some case series of multidrug-resistant *Acinetobacter* infections, ampicillin/sulbactam has led to decreased mortality rates. Final antibiotic choice should be based on detailed evaluation of the organism's susceptibility.

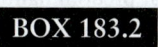

BOX 183.2

Clinical Manifestations, Diagnosis, and Treatment of *Erysipelothrix* Infection

Clinical Manifestations and Complications
Localized cutaneous infection, the erysipeloid of Rosenbach, is the most common manifestation of *Erysipelothrix* disease. After a 1- to 4-day incubation period, an acute, localized, purple-red lesion appears at the side of an abrasion contaminated with *Erysipelothrix*. Absence of suppuration and involution without desquamation help to differentiate this lesion from streptococcal or staphylococcal infections. Fever and other constitutional symptoms are uncommon findings, occurring in fewer than 10% of cases unless bacteremia supervenes. Usually, untreated infection is self-limiting, with an average duration of 3 weeks. Pediatric bacteremia, joint, and pulmonary infections have been reported, although they are unusual. Endocarditis is an uncommon but important complication of *Erysipelothrix* infection. Although patients with rheumatic or congenital heart disease are at increased risk for development of endocarditis, previously normal heart valves can be infected.

Diagnosis and Treatment
For localized disease, establishing the diagnosis depends largely on the clinical appearance of the lesion and an appropriate history of exposure. Attempts to culture the organism from material collected by swab or aspirate from a local lesion usually are unsuccessful. However, biopsies of affected skin cultured in broth usually yield the offending bacteria. Commonly, *Erysipelothrix* is isolated from the blood of patients with septicemia or endocarditis. Occasionally, these organisms are misidentified as enterococci or lactobacilli. The organism is exquisitely sensitive to penicillin. Localized disease can be treated with oral medication, but high parenteral doses are necessary for treatment of endocarditis or disseminated disease.

---

disease occurs in 7% of patients with *R. equi* pneumonia. Pericarditis and brain abscess have been reported.

Diagnosis and Treatment

Although sputum specimens may be positive for the organism, bronchoalveolar lavage or lung biopsy may be required. *R. equi* may coexist with other pathogens. Positive findings on Gram stain and Kinyoun stain should be interpreted in the context of clinical information. Commonly, clinical isolates are resistant to penicillins and cephalosporins. Erythromycin, clindamycin, rifampin, aminoglycosides, vancomycin, fluoroquinolones, and imipenem are active against *R. equi*. Combination antibiotic therapy and surgical resection often are required for cure.

MISCELLANEOUS GRAM-NEGATIVE BACTERIA

Acinetobacter

Acinetobacter, a genus of coccobacillary bacteria in the family Neisseriaceae, is a distinctly uncommon pathogen in healthy persons, but it is seen with increasing frequency in hospital-

Achromobacter (Alcaligenes)

Organisms of the genus *Achromobacter* (formerly called *Alcaligenes*) are nonfermenting, motile, aerobic gram-negative bacilli that live in aqueous environments and moist soil. They grow well on both blood and MacConkey agar. They alkalinize organic salts and amides. They may be confused with other nonfermenting gram-negative rods, especially *Pseudomonas* species.

Epidemiology and Pathophysiology

Like *Pseudomonas* species, *Achromobacter* live in aqueous environments. In some people, they also may be part of the normal flora of the gastrointestinal and respiratory tracts. These organisms establish a niche within the hospital environment and have been recovered from ventilators, humidifiers, "sterile" saline, intravenous fluids, and even disinfectant solutions. Infection can be life-threatening in neonates and in immunocompromised hosts.

Achromobacter species are weakly virulent bacteria. Medical care provides the conduit through which organisms are introduced into their host. Preterm or small-for-gestational-age term infants are at particular risk of acquiring disseminated *Achromobacter* infections. Vertical transmission is rare. An increased incidence of infection has been reported for patients with neoplasms and for those with immunodeficiency states. Patients with cystic fibrosis may acquire *Achromobacter* infection. Infection with *Achromobacter* species may develop after a penetrating trauma has occurred in an otherwise normal host.

Clinical Manifestations and Complications

A. xylosoxidans sepsis or meningitis in newborns tends to present later and more insidiously than do infections with the usual vertically acquired pathogens. Newborns with *A. xylosoxidans* sepsis or meningitis may develop a distinctive rash, in which 1- to 2-cm, sharply demarcated red patches appear, especially in the head and neck region. Cerebrospinal fluid (CSF) profiles may resemble those usually associated with viral meningitis. Neonatal disease has an extremely poor prognosis, with high rates of death, neurologic morbidity, and intracranial hemorrhage.

A. xylosoxidans usually is not suspected clinically in older patients, except in the circumstance of a common source outbreak. Infections do occur in patients with AIDS, but whether having HIV disease is an independent risk factor is unclear. A case in which a persistently infected lymph node became a nidus for 14 separate incidents of bacteremia in a child with hyper-IgM syndrome has been reported.

Diagnosis and Treatment

The diagnosis of *Achromobacter* infections rests on recovery of the organism from clinical samples. The clinician should suspect *A. xylosoxidans* when the laboratory reports a *Pseudomonas*-like species that is resistant to all aminoglycosides. Key differentiation features include the antibiogram and the morphology of the organism, with its distinctive peritrichous flagella.

Typically, *Achromobacter* species are resistant to a large number of antibiotics. The combination of piperacillin or imipenem with trimethoprim-sulfamethoxazole (TMP-SMX) is reasonable empiric therapy for suspected *Achromobacter* infection, until susceptibilities are known. Removal of infected catheters may speed recovery.

Chromobacterium violaceum

Chromobacterium violaceum is a long, motile, facultatively anaerobic, gram-negative rod that is a saprophyte of soil and water, especially in tropical and subtropical climates. Most isolates produce an intense insoluble pigment (violacein) that causes colonies on solid media to appear dark purple to black. Infection with *C. violaceum*, when it does occur, is a serious disease with a high mortality rate.

Epidemiology and Pathophysiology

Commonly, *C. violaceum* is found in soil and water of areas with tropical or subtropical weather patterns, but in the United States, it has been recovered from soil as far north as New Jersey. Almost all infections in humans have occurred in the southeastern part of the United States. Cases occur predominantly in summer, and most patients are younger than 14 years of age. Human infection is a relatively rare occurrence. Differences in virulence between soil strains and those recovered from patients may exist. Usually, infection is acquired through cuts or abrasions that come in contact with contaminated soil or water. A disproportionately high number of *C. violaceum* infections have occurred in patients with chronic granulomatous disease or other killing defects of the white blood cells. Local infection can be followed by dissemination of infection to distant sites.

Clinical Manifestations and Complications

The sequence of illness in all reported patients is similar, beginning with a contaminated inoculation site and localized disease consisting of nodular or pustular skin lesions. In some cases, the original site is the eye, and purulent conjunctivitis is the presenting symptom. Regional lymphadenopathy follows, and hematogenous spread to visceral organs may occur. One of the hallmarks of infection with *C. violaceum* is the formation of numerous microabscesses in multiple organs, especially the liver, lung, and kidneys. Severe disease is heralded by high fever (39°C to 41°C), confusion or lethargy, abdominal pain, headaches, nausea and vomiting, and (sometimes) myalgias. Hepatosplenomegaly and jaundice may be present. Progression to septic shock with disseminated intravascular coagulation and multisystem organ failure is precipitous.

Diagnosis and Treatment

Diagnosis is made by recovery of the organism from blood, lymph nodes, skin lesions, or abscesses. Sometimes, gram-negative bacilli can be seen in smears of material from skin lesions. Laboratory values can include leukocytosis or leukopenia with left shifts, anemia, elevated liver enzymes, and rising serum creatinine. Identifying the organism is easy if it produces the characteristic violet pigment, but infection with nonpigmented strains can occur. A compatible clinical history should arouse suspicion of *C. violaceum* infection, especially in patients with chronic granulomatous disease.

C. violaceum is sensitive *in vitro* to chloramphenicol, gentamicin, fluoroquinolones, tetracyclines, imipenem, and TMP-SMX. All isolates are resistant to vancomycin and rifampin, and often the organism is resistant to penicillins and cephalosporins. Most survivors have been treated with chloramphenicol, gentamicin, or both. A case of a 4-month-old infant who was treated with ciprofloxacin and TMP-SMX and survived *C. violaceum* sepsis has been published. Prolonged therapy with several different antibiotics may be required for cure.

Citrobacter

Citrobacter, a genus of enteric, gram-negative rods closely related to *Salmonella*, has been associated increasingly with human disease. The organisms of this genus most commonly isolated are *C. freundii*, *C. koseri* (formerly *C. diversus*), and *C. amalonaticus*.

Epidemiology and Pathophysiology

From 1970 to 1979, 4% of neonatal meningitis cases were caused by *Citrobacter*, and *C. koseri* was the species isolated most often. Generally, these cases occur sporadically, but occasional clusters of *C. diversus* meningeal infection have been reported. The prevalence of neonatal colonization in outbreaks has been as high as 79%. *Citrobacter* is an unusual cause of infection after the first several months of life and primarily is an opportunistic pathogen in the older child.

The newborn can become colonized in the birth canal of a colonized mother or in the hospital nursery. Broad use of antimicrobial agents can produce selective pressure leading to increased colonization with *Citrobacter*. Increased bacterial density combined with a blunted immune response may produce invasive disease.

Clinical Manifestations and Complications

Most neonatal *Citrobacter* infections occur within 7 days of birth, although "late-onset" sepsis (after 3 weeks of age) also has been reported. Preterm infants are at particular risk. Common signs and symptoms are fever, lethargy, poor feeding, vomiting, irritability, bulging fontanelles, seizures, and jaundice. Occasionally, umbilical infection and surgical manipulation of colonized umbilical stumps have preceded development of bacteremia and meningitis. Neonatal meningitis caused by *C. koseri* is particularly severe and is complicated by multiple brain abscesses in as many as 75% of these patients.

Although *Citrobacter* can be isolated from stools of asymptomatic patients, the organism has been implicated in gastrointestinal disease. In a retrospective pediatric emergency department study, *C. freundii* accounted for 1.2% of urinary tract isolates. Bone and soft tissue infections occur but extremely rarely in children.

Diagnosis and Treatment

Citrobacter organisms are isolated readily on standard media as gray, opaque, round colonies that produce a strong fetid odor. Treating *Citrobacter* meningitis is rendered difficult by the frequent formation of abscesses and the variable penetration of aminoglycosides into the central nervous system. The combination of a third-generation cephalosporin and an aminoglycoside often is used; however, resistance of *Citrobacter* to aminoglycosides has been a common occurrence in some institutions, and careful attention should be paid to antibiotic susceptibility in planning therapy. Cephalosporin resistance of these isolates also is on the rise. Most isolates are susceptible to carbapenems, cefepime, and the newer fluoroquinolones.

Follow-up lumbar puncture 72 hours into therapy should be performed to see if sterility of the CSF has been achieved. Total duration of therapy should be at least 21 days after sterility and 4 to 6 weeks if abscesses or encephalomalacia develop. Neurosurgery should be involved anticipatorily in the care. Organisms may persist at intracranial sites long after apparent clinical recovery has occurred. Cranial CT scans are helpful for evaluating such complications as hydrocephalus and multicystic encephalomalacia. Ventriculostomy and craniectomy for open drainage of abscesses have been required to effect bacteriologic cure in some children. Therapy for *Citrobacter* infection beyond the neonatal period requires appropriate antibiotic treatment, drainage of abscesses, and débridement of wounds. Outbreaks of neonatal *Citrobacter* infections have been aborted by isolating patients and caregivers, but multiple sources of infection may limit the effectiveness of this approach.

Edwardsiella tarda

Edwardsiella tarda is a non-lactose-fermenting, gram-negative bacillus that is indole-positive and produces H_2S. It ferments only glucose and maltose, hence the species name *tarda*. Resistance to colistin distinguishes it from *Salmonella*.

Epidemiology and Pathophysiology

E. tarda is an organism associated with fresh water and marine life. Case reports of human disease have implicated ornamental fish, pet turtles, snakes, and catfish as sources of infection. Such host factors as chronic liver disease, chronic alcohol abuse, steroid therapy, hemoglobinopathy, or iron overload predispose to development of infection with *E. tarda*. Infection with *E. tarda* occurs more commonly in tropical and subtropical climates. The elderly and the very young are at increased risk of severe illness.

Clinical Manifestations and Complications

Infections with *E. tarda* can be divided into two types: intestinal and extraintestinal. Gastrointestinal infection usually causes a secretory self-limited enteritis, with intermittent watery diarrhea and low-grade fever. Wound infection is the most common extraintestinal infection. Most infected wounds are caused by fish fins or snakes; cellulitis or abscesses may develop. A case in which *E. tarda* soft tissue infection progressed to myonecrosis in a normal host has been reported. Septicemia with *E. tarda* is a rare but serious complication typically seen in patients with liver disease, iron overload, or immune suppression. It presents with high fever, shock, and disseminated intravascular coagulation and carries a mortality rate of approximately 45%. In one case, a neonate developed sepsis with a strain of *E. tarda* presumably acquired by the mother from freshwater swimming at 6-months' gestation. Meningitis also has been reported. Patients with hemoglobin disorders, especially SC hemoglobinopathy, may be predisposed to bony infection with *E. tarda*, as they are with salmonellae.

Diagnosis and Treatment

Diagnosis rests on identification of *E. tarda* in culture. The major pitfall is mistaking it for *Salmonella* species. *E. tarda* is sensitive *in vitro* to most antibiotics routinely used in the treatment of gram-negative infections, including beta-lactams, cephalosporins, aminoglycosides, and fluoroquinolones. Gastrointestinal disease does not require treatment. Severe disease probably should be treated with the combination of a beta-lactam and an aminoglycoside, although synergy has not been demonstrated.

Eikenella corrodens

Eikenella corrodens is a facultatively anaerobic, straight, nonmotile, oxidase-positive, gram-negative rod or coccobacillus. It grows slowly on blood or chocolate agar but poorly or not at all on MacConkey agar. The species name *corrodens* reflects the fact that approximately 50% of isolates pit the agar. It is a pathogen of periodontitis in both adults and children and is a common isolate from wounds that have been contaminated by oral secretions.

Epidemiology and Pathophysiology

E. corrodens is a normal inhabitant of the mouth and of the gastrointestinal and genitourinary tracts of humans. Infection occurs when mucosal or skin barriers are disrupted. Classically, high-risk groups have been intravenous drug abusers, the elderly, and those with advanced carcinomas; however, children now also are recognized as being at high risk for acquisition of *E. corrodens* infections. Reported thyroid abscesses and purulent thyroiditis all have occurred in children. In one review, more than 20% of *E. corrodens* pleuropulmonary infections occurred in children younger than 14 years of age, and more than 50% of abdominal infections were seen in patients younger than 25 years. *E. corrodens* orbital cellulitis, empyema, peritonsillar abscess, paronychia, and osteomyelitis also have been observed in children. Cases of discitis have been reported. Approximately 40% of childhood infections with *E. corrodens* involve the head and neck.

Often, *E. corrodens* infections are polymicrobial and may include other anaerobes or gram-negative rods. However, *E. corrodens* is accompanied most frequently by alpha-hemolytic streptococci. Abscesses are the hallmark of CNS infection and most intraabdominal infections. Skin abscesses tend to recur even after presumed adequate drainage has been achieved.

Clinical Manifestations and Complications

Infections with *E. corrodens* are indolent; the time from inoculation to onset of symptoms generally is 1 week or longer. Many cases show initial improvement with therapy, only to relapse days later, even with appropriate therapy. Infection of periodontal sites may be associated with rapid progression and bone resorption. Craniofacial and neck infections may require repeated drainage procedures and long courses of antimicrobials. Often, CNS infections are preceded by sinus infections, but they have been seen also in children with congenital heart disease.

Pleuropulmonary infections are marked by fever, cough, and chest pain. Effusions or empyema are noted in 30% of these patients, and cavitation is seen in 8%. Children with a predisposition toward aspiration may be at higher risk. Endocarditis is associated with large, friable vegetations and frequent emboli and often requires valve replacement.

Most commonly, abdominal *E. corrodens* infections occur as complications of ruptured appendicitis, but they have been associated also with abdominal trauma and surgery. Soft tissue infections may require wide débridement and skin grafting. Infection of underlying joints, tendons, or bones is not an infrequent occurrence and can be necrotizing and even lead to amputation.

Diagnosis and Treatment

A definitive diagnosis rests on recovery of *E. corrodens* in culture. This task can be difficult to perform, however, because of the organism's slow growth. *Eikenella* tends to be overgrown by hardier species when it is part of a polymicrobial process, and it may be missed, especially if it does not pit the agar. In addition, it is misidentified frequently.

E. corrodens has an unusual antimicrobial susceptibility pattern. Most isolates are sensitive to penicillin, ampicillin, and third-generation cephalosporins but resistant to semisynthetic penicillins such as methicillin and nafcillin. Additionally, they uniformly resist clindamycin and metronidazole, drugs commonly used to treat anaerobic infections. Penicillin usually is the drug of choice, although some strains produce beta-lactamases.

Incision and drainage of abscesses and débridement of necrotic tissue are essential to recovery from these infections. Therapy should be prolonged after patients apparently have recovered, because early cessation of antibiotic therapy is associated with relapse.

Enterobacter

Enterobacter species are gram-negative enteric bacteria commonly found in soil, water, and sewage. They are facultatively anaerobic, motile bacteria. *E. cloacae*, *E. aerogenes*, and *E. sakazakii* are the species recovered most frequently from clinical material. A neonatal outbreak of *E. gergoviae* bacteremia has been reported.

Epidemiology and Pathophysiology

Enterobacter most commonly is encountered as a hospital-acquired pathogen in patients with chronic illness. *Enterobacter* is one of the pathogens most commonly encountered in pediatric and neonatal ICUs. The vertical spread of *Enterobacter* from mother to infant may occur at the time of birth. Both environmental and endogenous sources have been cited in colonization and disease. Spread from contaminated intravenous fluids and colonized hospital personnel is particularly well-documented.

Often, newborn infants are colonized by *Enterobacter* species in the first month of life. Generally, colonization rates are lower in breast-fed infants and in older children. Antibiotic therapy increases the risk of acquiring resistant organisms in infants, children, and adults, owing to the presence of an inducible beta-lactamase. Neutropenia, central venous catheters, intubation, and urinary tract catheterization increase the risk of acquiring infection. Some *Enterobacter* species are more virulent than are others, and organisms may acquire virulence factors from other species.

Clinical Manifestations and Complications

Infection caused by *Enterobacter* frequently is indistinguishable from illness caused by other enteric pathogens, with some exceptions. *E. sakazakii* causes a particularly devastating neonatal meningitis. Mortality rates reach 50%. Almost all survivors suffer severe neurologic complications consistent with the development of multiple infarctions of the brain. Commonly, necrotizing enterocolitis complicated by peritonitis yields *Enterobacter* species.

In older immunocompromised children, bacteremia with septic shock is a significant risk. Some *Enterobacter* species recovered from children with diarrhea have been reported to produce enterotoxin.

Diagnosis and Treatment

A diagnosis of infection caused by *Enterobacter* relies primarily on isolation of the organism in culture from clinical material. Molecular diagnostic techniques offer promise in identification of pathogens and characterization of outbreaks. Therapy of *Enterobacter* infection is rendered problematic by frequent resistance to cephalosporins, penicillins, and aminoglycosides. Resistance to cephalosporins is mediated by a chromosomal cephalosporinase gene that expresses the enzyme on exposure to cephalosporin therapy. It follows that some strains will acquire resistance to cephalosporins during the course of therapy, despite initially favorable susceptibility studies. Administration of third-generation cephalosporins or prolonged hospitalization increases the risk of multidrug-resistant clinical isolates. Administration of empiric combination therapy that includes an aminoglycoside is appropriate until susceptibilities are known. Extended-spectrum penicillins are less likely to induce the production of broad-spectrum beta-lactamases. Carbapenems or cefepime are important alternatives in severely ill patients in whom multidrug-resistant organisms are suspected. Rarely, resistance to carbapenems and cefepime occurs.

In cases of neonatal *E. sakazakii* meningitis, physicians should anticipate the potential development of abscesses, infarctions, and cysts. Neurosurgery should be involved early, and prolonged antibiotic therapy is required.

Chryseobacterium (Flavobacterium)

Members of the genus *Chryseobacterium* (formerly *Flavobacterium*) seldom are associated with human infection; most cases occur after exposure to a contaminated environmental source. These organisms are long, thin, catalase-positive, gram-negative rods with slightly swollen ends. They grow on solid agar as 1-mm, yellow, convex, glistening colonies of buttery consistency. The clinically relevant species include *C. meningosepticum*, *C. balustinum*, and *C. odoratum*.

Epidemiology and Pathophysiology

Chryseobacterium species are distributed widely as saprophytes in fresh and salt water. In hospitals, these organisms have been found to be ubiquitous colonizers of the environment, including such places as flower vases, ice machines, vials of intravenous drugs, eyewashes, nebulizers, and sink traps. In some instances, these reservoirs have been implicated in nosocomial outbreaks of disease. Ribotyping has proved useful in epidemiologic studies of hospital outbreaks.

C. meningosepticum is an uncommon cause of neonatal infection but can be responsible for nursery epidemics. More than 50% of infected infants weigh less than 2,500 g, and more than 50% of the patients manifest illness before reaching age 7 days.

Most cases of invasive human disease caused by *Chryseobacterium* are thought to result from heavy environmental contamination with *C. meningosepticum*, which then spreads to compromised newborns or debilitated older patients. Some neonatal infections may be caused by colonization of affected infants during passage through the birth canal. Neonatal flavobacterial infection in underdeveloped countries could be related to the use of contaminated ground water for bathing of newborn infants and to poor feminine genital hygiene.

Clinical Manifestations and Complications

Neonatal sepsis and meningitis caused by *C. meningosepticum* share signs and symptoms with other forms of neonatal bacterial infection. However, the development of meningitis may be insidious, and several days of infection may pass before the symptoms become apparent. The prognosis is extremely poor, with mortality rates exceeding 60%. One-half of survivors develop significant neurologic complications, including hydrocephalus. Childhood chryseobacterial infection occurring beyond the newborn period is a rare event, although this organism has been implicated in meningitis, sepsis, endocarditis, and pneumonia.

Diagnosis and Treatment

Rapid identification of *Chryseobacterium* infection is urgent to ensure administration of proper therapy, to hasten initiation of appropriate infection control, and to forestall epidemic outbreaks. Identification of *C. meningosepticum* is hindered by the characteristically long periods required for oxidation of carbohydrates and by weak or delayed indole production. Clinical isolation of an unidentified gram-negative rod that is catalase- and oxidase-positive and that shows multiple antibiotic resistance should raise the suspicion of presence of *C. meningosepticum* infection.

The treatment of *C. meningosepticum* meningitis is a true challenge. Characteristically, *Chryseobacterium* species are resistant to ampicillin and aminoglycosides, and a delay in identifying the organism may lead to prolonged periods of suboptimal therapy and consequent persistence of organisms in the CSF. Drugs that have been used with some success alone or in combination include erythromycin, vancomycin, TMP-SMX, cefotaxime, and rifampin. Because of the complication of hydrocephalus and the possible need for intraventricular therapy, neurosurgeons are essential to the management teams.

Hafnia alvei

Hafnia alvei (previously *E. hafnia*) is a facultatively anaerobic, catalase-positive, oxidase-negative, gram-negative bacil-

lus. It grows well on blood or MacConkey agar as a nonlactose fermenter, producing gray-white, slightly elevated, glistening colonies.

Epidemiology and Pathophysiology

H. alvei has been found in soil, dairy products, sewage, and the feces of humans and animals. The incidence of carriage of the organism probably ranges between 2% and 10%. Long regarded as a nonpathogen, *H. alvei* now has been associated clearly with enteritis and rarely has been isolated in pure culture from other sites, including blood, CSF, peritoneal fluid, and urine. Infection appears to be opportunistic.

The pathophysiology of *H. alvei* has been investigated most thoroughly as a cause of gastroenteritis. Although it is not invasive and does not produce enterotoxins, *H. alvei* does cause diarrhea in experimental animals, probably by attachment-effacement, as does enteropathogenic *Escherichia coli*.

Clinical Manifestations and Complications

Most patients with gastroenteritis secondary to *H. alvei* report 6 to 12 episodes of watery diarrhea per day, low-grade or no fever, and nausea, with or without vomiting. Sometimes, mucus (but not blood) is found in stools. Illness is self-limited. Approximately 9 cases of septicemia caused by *H. alvei* occur per year in the United States. *H. alvei* may be a cause of necrotizing enterocolitis, especially in older children after they have undergone bone marrow transplantation. Adult cases of cholecystitis, liver abscesses, and appendicitis have been reported.

Diagnosis and Treatment

Diagnosis is made by isolating the organism from stools or from normally sterile body fluids. No comprehensive antibiotic susceptibility studies are available for *H. alvei*. Case reports show that most isolates are resistant to ampicillin but are sensitive to aminoglycosides, second- and third-generation cephalosporins, aztreonam, imipenem, chloramphenicol, and TMP-SMX. Treatment is not necessary for most cases of gastroenteritis. Empiric therapy for systemic infection with a third-generation cephalosporin and an aminoglycoside is reasonable pending results of susceptibility testing.

Klebsiella

Klebsiellae are gram-negative enteric rods that lack motility and grow as large mucoid colonies on solid media. Organisms are defined serologically by their capsular polysaccharide (K antigens) and lipopolysaccharide (O antigens). *K. pneumoniae* represents the most common human pathogen in this genus, followed by *K. oxytoca*; other species are recovered uncommonly as clinical isolates.

Epidemiology and Pathophysiology

Klebsiella species are common opportunistic nosocomial pathogens of the urinary tract, respiratory tract, and biliary tract. They are second only to *E. coli* as causes of bacterial sepsis. They are the most common gram-negative organism causing invasive infection in transfusion-dependent patients with thalassemia major. Sources of infection include colonized hospital staff and environmental sources. Plasmid-mediated beta-lactamase resistance can be responsible for the rapid spread of resistant organisms to susceptible patients.

By 1985, nearly 50% of reported *Klebsiella* outbreaks occurred in neonatal ICUs, and newborn outbreaks of *K. pneumoniae* and *K. oxytoca* continue to be frequent occurrences worldwide. Local and distant spreads of resistant organisms have been observed in intensive care populations.

Pneumonias caused by *Klebsiella* usually arise from colonization of the upper respiratory tract followed by aspiration of organisms to the lower respiratory tract. Typically, colonization of newborns occurs by the time they reach age 1 month (or earlier in breast-fed infants); it occurs also in older children and adults. However, illness and antibiotic use have been observed to promote overgrowth of *Klebsiella*; host and bacterial factors contribute to adherence of organisms to oral epithelium. Capsular polysaccharide (K antigens), lipopolysaccharide antigens, and (perhaps) fimbriae act as virulence factors. Generally, *K. pneumoniae* lags behind group B streptococcus and *E. coli* as a cause of "early-onset" or "late-onset" newborn infection. *Klebsiella* is an unusual cause of pulmonary or urinary tract infection in otherwise healthy older children.

Clinical Manifestations and Complications

Pulmonary infection should suggest the possibility of underlying immunodeficiency or significant malnutrition, if not suspected previously. Lung abscesses or massive lung ischemia leading to necrosis may occur as a complication. Mortality rates have ranged from 5% to 20%, with higher death rates occurring in children infected with aminoglycoside-resistant strains.

Diagnosis and Treatment

Isolation of *Klebsiella* from clinical material is the mainstay of diagnosis. Citrate-containing media can be used to facilitate isolation of *Klebsiella* strains because these organisms can use citrate as a sole carbon source. Serotyping with specific antisera can be accomplished, but molecular diagnostic techniques offer some advantages over conventional serology in characterization of outbreaks.

Antimicrobial therapy should be guided by an understanding of contemporary local antimicrobial susceptibilities of *Klebsiella*. *Klebsiella* species not uncommonly harbors extended-spectrum beta-lactamases, which leads to resistance to many beta-lactam agents. Generally, combination therapy with an aminoglycoside and cephalosporin or penicillin is recommended for critically ill or immunocompromised patients with bacteremia; imipenem or meropenem may be effective for multidrug-resistant strains. Final antibiotic choice should be based on results of susceptibility testing. Strict adherence to infection control policies may help to prevent spread of resistant *Klebsiella* strains.

Morganella morganii

Morganella morganii (formerly *Proteus morganii*) is a motile gram-negative rod commonly found in feces of humans, other mammals, and reptiles. Most strains do not ferment lactose and are indole-positive and ornithine decarboxylase–positive. *M. morganii* produces urease but does not demonstrate swarming activity on 1.5% agar.

Epidemiology and Pathophysiology

Like *Proteus mirabilis*, *M. morganii* commonly invades the catheterized urinary tract of the elderly and of patients requiring intensive care. In contrast to well-described nursery epidemics of *P. mirabilis* infection, no *M. morganii* neonatal outbreaks have been described, and CNS infections are rare findings in newborns. *E. coli* and *P. mirabilis* account for the vast majority of urinary tract infections in children, but *M. morganii* has been implicated in some cases of cystitis and pyelonephritis. In adults, in contrast to *Proteus* infections, which almost always start in the urinary tract, serious *Morganella* infection is more likely to originate from the biliary tree. *Morganella* splits urea but appears to be less efficient than is *P. mirabilis*, which may account in part for its lower frequency as a cause of urinary tract infections.

Clinical Manifestations and Complications

Often, urinary tract infection with *M. morganii* is associated with an elevated urinary pH. Urolithiasis can occur, although perhaps less frequently than during *P. mirabilis* infection. *M. morganii* has been recovered from fewer than 10% of adult bacteremic episodes, but mortality rates have exceeded 20%. Other reported complications identified in immunocompromised or instrumented patients include meningitis, arthritis, empyema, peritonitis, and skin infection. *M. morganii* has been recovered alone or in combination with other organisms from surgical wounds and soft tissue abscesses in children.

Diagnosis and Treatment

M. morganii produces a reddish-brown pigment when cultured on nutrient media supplemented with 5% tryptophan. Generally, it ferments only glucose and mannose and does not produce a red coloration on lysine iron agar. Effective treatment of local infections or septicemia relies on appropriate antibiotic choice, often including an aminoglycoside. Most urinary tract infections respond to ampicillin or third-generation cephalosporins; failure to clear bacteriuria should alert physicians to the possibility of the presence of urolithiasis or a structural abnormality.

Pantoea agglomerans (Erwinia)

The genus *Erwinia* has an extended domain as an infectious microbe. The clinically relevant species, *Pantoea agglomerans* (*E. agglomerans*, *E. herbicola*), is a facultatively anaerobic, fermentative, H_2S-negative, gram-negative rod that grows well at 37°C on standard agar.

Epidemiology and Pathophysiology

Erwinia species are common plant and insect pathogens. In humans, *P. agglomerans* first was isolated in the 1920s from stool specimens of patients with typhoid fever. Additional saprophytic human strains subsequently were identified, and the first reports of *P. agglomerans* as a human pathogen appeared in the 1960s. Subsequently, a nationwide outbreak of *P. agglomerans* was traced to contaminated liners from caps of parenteral solution bottles.

Commonly, *P. agglomerans* is associated with other organisms from clinical specimens, but isolation of this organism in pure culture from infected sites leaves little doubt that this microbe can be a human pathogen. Most strains appear to act as saprophytes, but the organism has been isolated from purulent wounds of the extremities acquired by laceration or thorn pricks. Insidious cases of septic arthritis and osteomyelitis caused by *P. agglomerans* have developed after plant thorn injuries and wood splinter injuries. Most serious infections have occurred in persons with diminished host defenses.

Clinical Manifestations and Complications

Often, *P. agglomerans* bacteremia is associated with fever, shaking chills, and systemic toxicity characteristic of gram-negative sepsis. Frequently, these symptoms have been misinterpreted in hospitalized patients who unknowingly were given contaminated intravenous fluids. Eye and skin infections caused by *P. agglomerans* are particularly prominent, and the organism has been associated with osteomyelitis and neonatal meningitis in rare cases.

Diagnosis and Treatment

Incorrect identification of *P. agglomerans* occurs commonly, and even when identified in isolates from human sources, often it is considered a contaminant or saprophyte. The growth of yellow colonies on standard media and the characteristic microscopic spindle-shaped bodies aid in making the identification.

Most localized infections respond to treatment that includes an aminoglycoside. Failure to clear localized infection should prompt a careful search for a retained organic foreign body. In view of the rarity of bacteremia caused by *Pantoea* species, single sporadic cases should be investigated, and clusters of two or more cases should prompt making an immediate inquiry into a possible common source of infection. Formal surveillance programs have been key to the early termination of epidemics.

Pasteurella Species other than *P. multocida*

The genus *Pasteurella* consists of a group of pleomorphic gram-negative coccobacilli that are part of the normal flora of many animals. These organisms are frequent animal pathogens. (*Pasteurella multocida* is discussed in Chapter 167.) The other species of the genus *Pasteurella* are rare but occasionally serious causes of infection in humans. These organisms grow readily on most common laboratory media except MacConkey. These small, coccoid or rod-shaped bacilli may show prominent bipolar staining on Gram stain. Colonies are nonhemolytic and have a distinctive musty or "mushroom" odor. Some species have been reclassified as *Actinobacillus* or *Mannheimia*. Clinically recovered species other than *P. multocida* include *Actinobacillus ureae*, *Mannheimia haemolytica*, *Actinobacillus pneumotropica*, *P. dagmatis*, *P. canis*, *P. aerogenes*, *P. bettyae*, and *P. stomatis*. *P. caballi* has caused wound infections to develop after horse bites.

Epidemiology and Pathophysiology

Infection occurs when the organisms are inoculated into subcutaneous tissues either from animal teeth that break the skin or from animal saliva that comes in contact with nonintact skin. Animal bite wounds produce cellulitis, abscesses, tenosynovitis, or bone or joint infection, but infection can become generalized, especially in patients with immune compromise. CNS infection with these organisms has developed after head trauma or neurosurgery. Pulmonary infections also can occur. Most cases of serious infection occur in patients with underlying disease states, such as diabetes mellitus, chronic alcoholism, or liver disease. Such risk factors as household pet exposure, animal contact, or animal bites should heighten suspicion of the possible presence of *Pasteurella* infection.

Clinical Manifestations and Complications

Pasteurella infections produce pain, swelling, pus, and (sometimes) formation of an abscess at the site of inoculation within 24 to 36 hours. Clinically, these infections are not distinguishable from wound infections with staphylococci. Gram stain may show the characteristic pleomorphic bacilli with bipolar staining. Growth on standard agar is rapid. Patients with peritonitis, meningitis, osteomyelitis, or infectious endocarditis have symptoms typical of these diagnoses.

Diagnosis and Treatment

Establishing a diagnosis of *Pasteurella* infection can be difficult, because often it is misidentified. Other organisms of the same family, such as *Actinobacillus* species and *Haemophilus* species, have similar biochemical profiles. Notifying the bacteriology laboratory of suspicion of *Pasteurella* infection is helpful. Penicillin has been considered the drug of choice for *Pasteurella* infection in the past and, despite some reports of penicillin resistance, still is effective against most strains. Most *Pasteurella* species also are susceptible to ampicillin, beta-lactamase inhibitor combination drugs, tetracycline, ertapenem, and linezolid. Dicloxacillin and cephalexin, two drugs commonly prescribed for wound infections, have poor activity against *Pasteurella* species and should not be used as monotherapy for animal bite wounds.

Plesiomonas shigelloides

The genus *Plesiomonas* has only one species, *Plesiomonas shigelloides*. These organisms are facultatively anaerobic, motile gram-negative rods that are common inhabitants of surface water and fish. They have been implicated in gastrointestinal infections and (rarely) recovered from extraintestinal sites. They can be distinguished from Enterobacteriaceae by oxidase positivity. They grow well on MacConkey agar. A few isolates of *P. shigelloides* share common O antigen with *Shigella sonnei*.

Epidemiology and Pathophysiology

The organism is a ubiquitous fresh-water inhabitant at temperatures greater than 8°C. Sometimes, it is found also in estuaries in temperate or tropical climates, and it can exist in seawater during the summer months. It has been cultured from finfish, shellfish, pigs, birds, and dogs. Infection with *P. shigelloides* has been associated with ingestion of raw or improperly cooked fish (especially oysters). Asymptomatic carriage of *P. shigelloides* is a rare finding in developed countries.

Most often, infection is associated with gastroenteritis. Acquisition of disease has been linked specifically to consumption of raw seafood or untreated water and to foreign travel, especially to Mexico. The mechanism by which the organism produces disease is elusive. It is not invasive and does not produce a toxin. Inoculation of volunteers does not produce symptoms. Attachment to cultured intestinal cells and entry via endocytosis has been demonstrated in an *in vitro* model. Potential virulence factors are being evaluated. *P. shigelloides* rarely is a pathogen in extraintestinal sites. Osteomyelitis, endophthalmitis, cholecystitis, pseudoappendicitis, meningitis, and septicemia have been reported sporadically.

Clinical Manifestations and Complications

Patients with *P. shigelloides* gastroenteritis complain of diarrhea, crampy abdominal pain, nausea and vomiting, headache, and fever. Usually, symptoms begin 24 hours to 4 days after contact with the organism. Most cases occur during the summer. Diarrhea tends to be secretory. Blood or mucus may be present in the stools. Patients with *P. shigelloides* gastroenteritis tend to experience a more acute disease associated with more severe abdominal pain and of longer duration (one-third being sick for more than a month) than do patients with other enteropathogens. Septicemia or meningitis, or both, occur almost exclusively in immunocompromised hosts. Newborns make up most of the reported cases of *P. shigelloides* meningitis, for whom the mortality rate is 80%.

Diagnosis and Treatment

A clinical history of foreign travel or of ingestion of raw seafood or untreated water should raise suspicion of the possible presence of *P. shigelloides* infection. Oxidase tests should be performed on any predominant or solitary organisms to distinguish them from Enterobacteriaceae. Selective medium can be used if the index of suspicion is high.

Most strains of *P. shigelloides* produce a beta-lactamase, which seems to be specific for the penicillins. *P. shigelloides* is universally susceptible to TMP-SMX, the fluoroquinolones, the aminoglycosides, most cephalosporins (usually resistant to cefepime and ceftazidime), and chloramphenicol. Gastroenteritis may be prolonged, even with therapy. Extraintestinal infections carry a poor prognosis and should be treated aggressively. For meningitis, the cephalosporins are effective therapy against most isolates.

Proteus and *Providencia*

Proteus and *Providencia* (formerly classified as part of the *Proteus* genus) are associated increasingly with pediatric illness. These organisms are motile, gram-negative bacilli that do not ferment lactose and are differentiated from other Enterobacteriaceae by their ability to deaminate phenylalanine and lysine. Rapid and abundant urease production differentiates *Proteus* from *Providencia*.

Epidemiology and Pathophysiology

Proteus and *Providencia* are found in soil. Although they are normal inhabitants of the colon and perineum, they can be found in greater numbers in patients receiving antibiotic therapy. Approximately 4% of all neonatal meningitis cases are caused by *P. mirabilis*. After the first few months of life, *Proteus* infection most commonly involves the urinary tract. Although *E. coli* causes most urinary tract infections in children, *Proteus* and *Providencia* species often are implicated in reported series of cystitis and pyelonephritis. *P. mirabilis* is particularly common as a cause of male initial urinary tract infections and supplants *E. coli* as the major urinary tract pathogen in children prone to formation of renal stones.

Most cases of CNS infection caused by *Proteus* occur in the neonate. A propensity for the formation of brain abscesses remains unexplained. Several factors may predispose the urinary tract to invasion by *Proteus* and *Providencia*. *Proteus* splits urea, which increases local pH, resulting in toxicity to renal cells and potentiation of urolithiasis. Urinary tract stones provide a refuge for *Proteus* organisms and form a barrier to effective antimicrobial therapy. Factors conferring motility and allowing *Proteus* to "swarm" on agar assist invasion of urinary tract epithelial cells. *Providencia stuartii* manifests an extraordinary ability to persist within the catheterized urinary tract; bacteriuria may take weeks or even months to clear.

Clinical Manifestations and Complications

P. mirabilis infection of the newborn often presents with typical symptoms of neonatal sepsis; manifestations of sepsis may include encephalitis, septic arthritis, and osteomyelitis. The onset of infection after the first week of life occurs in a few patients, and meningitis may accompany early- or late-onset disease. Rarely, brain abscesses may develop for weeks or months before presentation. *Proteus* brain abscesses are associated with a high rate of mortality, frequent complications, and neurologic deficits in survivors. Hydrocephalus is a frequent complication and should be anticipated.

Urinary tract infections with these bacteria are associated with elevated urinary pH; clinical findings and urine abnormalities in these cases often are less striking than in cases of *E. coli* urinary tract infections. As many as 30% of these patients have recurrent infections more than 12 months after receiving the initial treatment. Prolonged urinary tract catheterization is an important risk factor for development of urinary tract infection and sepsis. In rare cases, infection with either of these genera can produce purplish discoloration of the urine bag in patients with long-term placement of catheters.

Proteus or *Providencia* bacteremia occurs infrequently in the pediatric age group. The genitourinary tract is the source identified most commonly. Mortality rates average less than 40% and depend on the severity of underlying disease in the host. Osteomyelitis, pneumonia, mastoiditis, and wound infections also occur in affected children.

Diagnosis and Treatment

Proteus is suspected easily because of its ability to swarm on the surface of moist agar. Species are distinguished by biochemical tests. Usually, *P. mirabilis* is sensitive to ampicillin; often, this drug, alone or in combination with an aminoglycoside, is suitable therapy for neonatal meningitis after the identity and susceptibility of the infecting organism are known. A third-generation cephalosporin is an alternative. Intraventricular antibiotics have not reduced mortality rates or morbidity significantly but have been used to clear ventricular colonization. Neurosurgical intervention may be required for complications of hydrocephalus or intracranial abscess.

The effective treatment of local infections or septicemia relies on appropriate choice of an antibiotic, often including an aminoglycoside, combined with surgical débridement and drainage of abscesses. Most *P. mirabilis* urinary tract infections respond to ampicillin, but failure to clear bacteria should alert physicians to the possibility of the presence of urolithiasis or a structural abnormality. Often, removal of a stone or surgical correction of anatomic defects is required for cure.

Serratia

The genus *Serratia* contains species increasingly associated with infection, particularly in the compromised host. *S. marcescens* is the chief species associated with disease. *Serratia* organisms are straight, motile, catalase-positive, gram-negative rods. Colonies are opaque, iridescent, and appear white, pink, or red on solid agar. Clinically relevant strains include *S. marcescens*, *S. liquefaciens*, *S. odorifera*, *S. ficaria*, and *S. plymuthica*. Chromogenic species can produce a blood-red color on contaminated foodstuffs.

Epidemiology and Pathophysiology

S. marcescens once was considered to be nonpathogenic and was used as a biologic marker of transmission. However, beginning in the 1950s, nosocomial infections were reported, heralding the importance of the organism as a hospital pathogen. Early outbreaks on a pediatric ward and neonatal nursery were attributed to contaminated intravenous solution and caps of bottles containing saline used to moisten umbilical cords. *S. marcescens* now is recognized as a major pathogen of compromised newborns. Environmental sources have been implicated in many hospital outbreaks, but hand-to-hand transmission appears to be the primary mechanism of nosocomial spread. Patient colonization can be nearly universal, persistent, and associated with increased rates of invasive disease. Molecular biology techniques can help define spread in the hospital environment.

The respiratory tract is a common location for disease. Often, *S. marcescens* produces a focal necrotizing pneumonia. The organism possesses proteases, hemolysins, and adherence properties that may contribute to virulence. Antibiotic resistance may be plasmid-mediated or chromosomal. Extended-spectrum beta-lactamases and multidrug efflux pumps have been described. Transposable plasmid elements may contribute to the rapid spread of multidrug resistance.

Clinical Manifestations and Complications

Commonly, disease in newborn ICUs is associated with high rates of underlying respiratory illness, necrotizing enterocolitis, intravenous catheters, and cardiac disease. Ventriculitis, brain abscesses, or porencephalic cysts are common complications of neonatal *Serratia* meningitis.

In older children and adults, *Serratia* species are isolated most frequently from the urinary tract, but respiratory infections, bacteremia, and endocarditis also occur. Instrumentation, catheterization, and clustering of susceptible patients are important risk factors. Compared to infection with other enteric pathogens, infection of the respiratory or genitourinary tract with *S. marcescens* is more likely to be complicated by bacteremia. However, bacteremia with *S. marcescens* is less likely to induce shock, pneumonia, or hemorrhage. At least two cases of sepsis and/or chorioamnionitis in pregnant women with loss of the fetus have been described. *S. marcescens* also is a rare post-operative pathogen.

Diagnosis and Treatment

The diagnosis of *Serratia* infection relies primarily on isolation of organisms from clinical material. Chromogenic species can impart a red color to bronchial secretions or urine; most strains are nonpigmented. Hydrolysis of gelatin distinguishes *S. marcescens* from *Klebsiella* and *Enterobacter* in the clinical microbiology laboratory.

An empiric antibiotic choice should be made in the context of susceptibilities of hospital flora. Therapy should be tailored once susceptibilities are known. In seriously ill newborns or immunocompromised older children, combination antibiotic therapy that includes a cephalosporin or penicillin and an aminoglycoside often is preferred. Meningitis and its complications should be anticipated in neonates with *Serratia* bacteremia. However, physicians need to be wary of potential resistance to cephalosporins and penicillins caused by the production of extended-spectrum beta-lactamases. Resistance to all aminoglycosides also can occur. In such circumstances, use of a carbapenem antibiotic may be valuable. In outbreaks, cohorting and removal of environmental sources may require several months of effort to be successful. Occasionally, neonatal ICUs have been closed to admissions to abort epidemics.

Stenotrophomonas maltophilia

Stenotrophomonas is a new genus with only one species, *S. maltophilia*. Until 1993, this aerobic, straight to slightly curved, gram-negative bacillus was known as *Xanthomonas maltophilia* and, before that, as *Pseudomonas maltophilia*. *S. maltophilia* is oxidase-negative and motile by means of polar multitrichous flagella. Growth on standard laboratory media produces large, glistening colonies that are lavender-green to gunmetal gray and give off the odor of ammonia. Increasingly, *S. maltophilia* is recognized as a nosocomial pathogen, mostly in debilitated patients and in those with long-term indwelling central venous catheters.

Epidemiology and Pathophysiology

S. maltophilia is a ubiquitous organism with natural habitat in water and soil. It has been cultured also from milk, sewage, frozen fish, and hospital disinfectants. These organisms have developed an ecologic niche in the hospital environment; 97% of *S. maltophilia* infections are hospital-acquired. Infections with *S. maltophilia* occur most commonly in patients with cancer, leukemia, debilitating disease, neutropenia, central venous catheters, or a combination of these risk factors. Prior treatment with broad-spectrum antibiotics also is a significant predisposing feature.

Like many pseudomonads, *S. maltophilia* is an organism of low virulence and limited invasiveness. An intact host immune system is an important deterrent to severe or life-threatening infection. Colonization with *S. maltophilia* is not an uncommon finding, especially in the respiratory tract. Infection occurs when colonizing organisms overgrow or when they gain access to sterile body sites. Usually, *S. maltophilia* infections are seen in patients with central venous catheters. Infection with *S. maltophilia* also has occurred after surgical procedures, clean intermittent catheterization, and intravenous drug use. Risk factors for infection in oncology patients are severe and/or prolonged mucositis, diarrhea, a large number of previous antibiotic courses, prolonged hospital length of stay, and receipt of metronidazole; in patients with AIDS, identified risk factors include advanced disease, neutropenia, central venous catheterization, steroids, and receipt of broad-spectrum antimicrobial agents. Community-acquired infection is a rare occurrence.

Clinical Manifestations and Complications

Infections with *S. maltophilia* separate broadly into two categories. First and most common is catheter-related bacteremia or septicemia, usually in patients with neutropenia. Patients have hectic or intermittent fevers for several days before blood cultures become positive. Catheter-related infection, in general, has a good prognosis. The second form of infection is septicemia complicated by pneumonia or shock. Pneumonia is an ominous clinical sign. In one series, only 36% of patients with pneumonia survived their *S. maltophilia* infection. The presence of clinical signs of shock at the onset of fever also is a poor prognostic sign. Precipitous decline in clinical status and death can occur before the organism has been identified by the laboratory.

Skin and soft tissue infections can present with lesions that appear like ecthyma gangrenosum or resemble the nodular skin lesions of disseminated fungal infections. Meningitis is a rare occurrence, and laboratory findings may be subtle; in a review of all reported meningitis cases, the highest CSF white blood cell count noted was 650 cells per cubic millimeter.

Patients with advanced cystic fibrosis can become colonized with *S. maltophilia*. The importance of this colonization is unknown; colonization does not alter short-term (3-year) survival, and the organism does not appear to be spread horizontally among patients with cystic fibrosis.

Diagnosis and Treatment

Diagnosis is made by isolating the organism from blood, pus, or other body fluids. Because nosocomial outbreaks have been reported, isolation of *S. maltophilia* from hospitalized patients should prompt notification of infection control. Occasionally, *Pseudomonas cepacia* is misidentified as *S. maltophilia*, especially in patients with cystic fibrosis. *S. maltophilia* is oxidase-negative and DNase-positive.

S. maltophilia is multidrug resistant. Virtually all isolates of *S. maltophilia* are resistant to penicillins, cephalosporins, and aminoglycosides, and all are highly resistant to imipenem. Imipenem therapy has been shown to be a predisposing factor for both *de novo* infection and conversion to infection in patients colonized with *S. maltophilia*. From 98% to 100% of isolates of *S. maltophilia* are sensitive to TMP-SMX, which usually is the drug of choice. Addition of ticarcillin-clavulanate may be warranted because TMP-SMX is not bactericidal. In cases of catheter-related infection, the catheter should be removed. Mortality rates are higher in patients whose catheters are not removed promptly. In some cases, removal of the catheter alone is curative. Late recurrence of infection is a common finding in patients whose lines are not removed.

Vibrio vulnificus

Vibrio vulnificus is a small, curvilinear, gram-negative rod of the family Vibrionaceae. Biochemical test results are similar to those of other members of the family except that *V. vulnificus* ferments lactose. This halophilic (salt-loving) organism grows in concentrations of sodium chloride of from 1% to 8%.

Epidemiology and Pathophysiology

V. vulnificus, like *V. parahaemolyticus*, is a marine organism that is a common inhabitant of offshore waters. It has been isolated from sediment, plankton, water, finfish, crabs, and oysters, with peak recovery occurring in the summer and early fall. Oysters from the Gulf of Mexico and the mid-Atlantic states have higher colony counts than do those from the North Atlantic, Pacific, and Canadian coast. No known method can ensure that commercial shellfish do not contain viable *V. vulnificus* because of the ubiquity of the organism and its ability to thrive under even the most careful conditions of sanitation, storage, and transport. Disease in humans is initiated by contact with the organism either through marine contamination of a wound or through the gastrointestinal tract after ingestion of the organism in raw shellfish, most commonly oysters. Ninety percent of reported patients are age 40 or older. Most childhood cases of septicemia have been associated with thalassemia major. Wound infections in previously healthy children and adolescents have been reported.

Local infection occurs after wound exposure to contaminated seawater. *V. vulnificus* elaborates a cytolysin, a collagenase, and a protease, which enhance its rapid spread in tissues. Histamine and bradykinin contribute to the intense inflammatory nature of these lesions.

Patients with hepatic disease have 40 to 80 times greater risk of developing septicemia and have a fatality rate 2.5 times higher than that of otherwise healthy individuals. *V. vulnificus* grows better in an excess of iron. Liver damage, excess iron, and deferoxamine therapy have been shown to decrease the lethal dose of *V. vulnificus* in experimental animals. Iron overload almost certainly underlies *V. vulnificus* septicemia in patients who require repeated transfusions and deferoxamine therapy for anemia. Sometimes, fatal septicemia is seen in patients with other chronic diseases.

Clinical Manifestations and Complications

Affected, otherwise healthy individuals have exhibited a mild, self-limited gastrointestinal illness similar to that caused by *V.*

parahaemolyticus. However, the most serious infection produced by *V. vulnificus* is primary septicemia, which occurs most commonly in patients who have liver disease and have ingested the organism in raw shellfish. Recalcitrant shock in patients with septicemia is secondary to toxins, loss of vascular tone, capillary leak, and (possibly) negative inotropy as in other forms of gram-negative sepsis.

Generally, patients with primary septicemia have a history of recent (6- to 72-hour) consumption of raw seafood. Illness is marked by the rapid onset of fever, hypotension, and septic shock. Prodromal symptoms such as malaise, chills, and fever are common findings. Vomiting and diarrhea are seen in approximately 20% of these patients. Shock progresses quickly, and reversal is difficult to achieve. Secondary skin lesions develop in approximately one-half of affected patients and may be bullous, petechial, or maculopapular. Mortality rates from primary septicemia have been reported to range from 46% to 79%. *V. vulnificus* rarely is isolated from such other sites as eyes, bones, and CSF. A single case report describes involvement of the deep brain nuclei demonstrated by magnetic resonance imaging (MRI) in a man with *V. vulnificus* meningitis.

Wound infections are marked by rapid progression; the formation of bullae, edema, vascular thromboses; and necrosis of involved tissues. Primary wound infection may progress to systemic infection and carries a mortality rate ranging from 7% to 24%.

Diagnosis and Treatment

The diagnosis of *V. vulnificus* infection is made by isolating the organism from blood, tissues, or stool. *V. vulnificus* grows best in cellobiose-colistin agar but may be recovered also from ordinary blood agar or MacConkey plates. The diagnosis of *V. vulnificus* wound infection or septicemia can be suspected on clinical grounds, and appropriate therapy can be initiated while awaiting culture results. The clinical history of shellfish ingestion or seawater contamination of a wound heightens suspicion. *V. vulnificus* infection should be given high consideration in patients with hemosiderosis, anemia with transfusion therapy, liver disease, or other chronic disease states.

In severe wound infections, rapid surgical therapy is of paramount importance. In primary septicemia, life support with adjunctive therapies for severe septic shock is of primary concern. Secondarily, appropriate antibiotic treatment for *V. vulnificus* should be started as early as possible. For additional information, see Box 183.3.

| **BOX 183.3** | Antibiotic Therapy in *Vibrio vulnificus* Infection |

In vitro, *V. vulnificus* is susceptible to many antibiotics. However, in animal models, the MICs obtained in the laboratory did not seem to correspond with response to therapy. This disparity was particularly large with regard to cefotaxime and gentamicin. Case reports showed favorable outcomes with tetracycline, doxycycline, chloramphenicol, or ciprofloxacin therapy. Animal models favor tetracycline. More recently, the combination of minocycline and cefotaxime has been shown to be synergistic *in vitro*, with the combination reducing the growth of the organism by six orders of magnitude when compared with either drug alone. This combination also was successful in a mouse model

of infection. No data compare the efficacy of tetracycline with that of minocycline. The available evidence, however, suggests that either tetracycline or minocycline in combination with cefotaxime should be considered the treatment of choice for known or suspected *V. vulnificus* infection. The possible role of newer fluoroquinolones has yet to be defined clinically, but some possess good *in vitro* activity. Patients with severe anemia, liver disease, hemosiderosis, or other debilitating chronic diseases or those receiving deferoxamine therapy should be advised against eating raw seafood of any kind. Patients with open wounds probably should avoid contact with seawater or brackish inland waters.

Suggested Readings

Berkowitz FE. The gram-positive bacilli: a review of the microbiology, clinical aspects, and antimicrobial susceptibilities of a heterogeneous group of bacteria. *Pediatr Infect Dis J* 1994;13:1126.

Blake PA, Merson MH, Weaver RE, et al. Disease caused by a marine *Vibrio*: clinical characteristics and epidemiology. *N Engl J Med* 1979; 300:1.

Bonadio WA. *Klebsiella* pneumoniae bacteremia in children. Fifty-seven cases in 10 years. *Am J Dis Child* 1989;143:1061.

Campbell JR, Diacovo T, Baker CJ. *Serratia marcescens* meningitis in neonates [review]. *Pediatr Infect Dis J* 1992;11:881.

Chow JW, Fine MJ, Shlaes DM, et al. *Enterobacter* bacteremia: clinical features and emergence of antibiotic resistance during therapy. *Ann Intern Med* 1991;115:585.

Dooley JR, Nims LJ, Lipp VH, et al. Meningitis of infants caused by *Flavobacterium meningosepticum*. *J Trop Pediatr* 1980;26:24.

Friedland I, Stinson L, Ikaiddi M, Harm S, Woods GL. Resistance in Enterobacteriaceae: results of a multicenter surveillance study, 1995–2000. *Infect Control Hosp Epidemiol* 2003;24:607.

Graham DR, Band JD. *Citrobacter diversus* brain abscess and meningitis in neonates. *JAMA* 1981;245:1923.

Grieco MD, Sheldon C. *Erysipelothrix rhusiopathiae*. *Ann N Y Acad Sci* 1970; 174:523.

Holst E, Rollof J, Larsson L, et al. Characterization and distribution of *Pasteurella* species recovered from infected humans. *J Clin Microbiol* 1992;30:2984.

Jones BD, Mobley HL. Genetic and biochemical diversity of ureases of *Proteus*, *Providencia*, and *Morganella* species isolated from urinary tract infection. *Infect Immun* 1987;55:2198.

Kim BN, Woo JH, Ryu J, Kim YS. Resistance to extended-spectrum cephalosporins and mortality in patients with Citrobacter freundii bacteremia. *Infection* 2003;31:202.

Macher AM, Casale TB, Fauci AS. Chronic granulomatous disease of childhood and *Chromobacterium violaceum* infections in the southeastern United States. *Ann Intern Med* 1982;97:51.

Marshall WF, Keating MR, Anhalt JP, et al. *Xanthomonas maltophilia*: an emerging nosocomial pathogen. *Mayo Clin Proc* 1989;64:1097.

Raffensperger JG. *Eikenella corrodens* infections in children. *J Pediatr Surg* 1986;21:644.

Raveh D, Rudensky B, Schlesinger Y, Benenson S, Yinnon AM. Susceptibility trends in bacteriemias: analyses of 7544 patient-unique bacteraemic episodes spanning 11 years (1990–2000). *J Hosp Infect* 2003;55:196.

Sanders WE Jr, Sanders CC. *Enterobacter* species: pathogens poised to flourish at the turn of the century. *Clin Micro Rev* 1997;10:220.

Talan DA, Abrahamian FM, Moran GJ, et al. Clinical presentation and bacteriologic analysis of infected human bites in patients presenting to emergency departments. *Clin Infect Dis* 2003;37:1481.

Yu VL. *Serratia marcescens*: historical perspective and clinical review. *N Engl J Med* 1979;300:887.

d: VIRAL INFECTIONS

CHAPTER 184 ■ ARBOVIRUSES AND RELATED ZOONOTIC VIRUSES

THEODORE F. TSAI AND MICHAEL BELL

The arboviruses (arthropod-borne viruses) are a heterogenous group of more than 500 viruses classified into 13 taxonomic families (Table 184.1). Despite their taxonomic diversity, the vector-borne and certain related zoonotic viruses are studied together because of their common natural reservoirs and overlapping modes of transmission. Table 184.2 lists these diseases, arranged by the principal clinical manifestation of infection, mode of transmission, and the frequency with which the disease

TABLE 184.1

CHARACTERISTIC OF ARBOVIRUSES AND CERTAIN ZOONOTIC VIRUSES

Virus (Family)	Representative Virus	Genome (Segments)	Vectors
Alphaviruses (Togaviridae)	EEE	Positive, single-stranded RNA (1)	Mosquitoes, ticks
Flaviviruses (Flaviviridae)	Yellow fever, dengue	Positive, single-stranded RNA (1)	Mosquitoes, ticks, vertebrates
Bunyaviruses, phleboviruses, nairoviruses, hantaviruses (Bunyaviridae)	La Crosse, sandfly fever, CCHF, Hantaan (respectively)	Negative and ambisense single-stranded RNA (3)	Mosquitoes, ticks, sandflies, vertebrates
Orbiviruses, coltiviruses (Reoviridae)	Colorado tick fever	Double-stranded RNA (10/12)	Mosquitoes, ticks
Lyssaviruses, vesiculoviruses, and others (Rhabdoviridae)	Rabies	Negative, single-stranded RNA (1)	Vertebrates, sandflies
Arenaviruses (Arenaviridae)	Lassa	Ambisense, single-stranded RNA (2)	Rodents
Filoviruses (Filoviridae)	Ebola	Negative, single-stranded RNA (1)	Unknown
Thogoto-like viruses (Orthomyxoviridae)	Thogoto	Negative, single-stranded RNA (6-7)	Ticks
Orthopoxviruses, yatapoxviruses, unassigned (Poxviridae)	Monkeypox	Double-stranded DNA	Vertebrates
Paramyxoviridae	Nipah	Negative, single-stranded RNA (1)	Vertebrates

EEE, eastern equine encephalitis; CCHF, Congo-Crimean hemorrhagic fever.

TABLE 184.2

ARBOVIRAL AND SELECTED ZOONOTIC VIRAL INFECTIONS BY GEOGRAPHIC AREA

Virus	Nondescript Febrile Illness	Febrile Illness with Rash	Febrile Illness with Arthritis	Meningo-encephalitis	Hemorrhagic Fever	Other
North America						
Mosquito-borne viruses						
Cache Valley	○			○		
California encephalitis				○		
Dengue 1–4		●		○		Hepatitis
Eastern equine encephalitis				○		
Everglades (VEE type II)				○		
Jamestown Canyon				○		Respiratory symptoms
Keystone				○		
La Crosse				●		
St. Louis encephalitis				●		
Snowshoe hare				○		
Tensaw				○		
Trivittatus				○		
Venezuelan equine encephalitis (sylvatic subtypes ID, IE)				○		Pneumonitis
West Nile§	●	●	●	●		Hepatitis, pancreatitis, myocarditis; Perinatal illness after congenital third-trimester infection
Western equine encephalitis				●		Perinatal illness after congenital third-trimester infection
Tickborne viruses						
Colorado tick fever	●			○	○	
Powassan				○		
Salmon river	○					
Zoonoses						
Bayou, Black Creek Canal						Noncardiogenic pulmonary edema, nephrosis, myositis
Monongahela New York, Sin Nombre						Noncardiogenic pulmonary edema
Lymphocytic choriomeningitis	○			○	○	Pneumonia, Parotitis, orchitis, arthritis, congenital CNS malformation
Modoc				○		
Rio Bravo	○			○		Pneumonia, orchitis
Seoul					○	Interstital nephritis
Sandfly-borne viruses						
Vesicular stomatitis (New Jersey and Indiana)	○			○		Respiratory illness
Central and South America						
Mosquito-borne Viruses						
Bussuquara	○					
Cache valley	○					
Catu	○					
Cotia	○					
Dengue 1–4		●		○	●	Hepatitis; perinatal illness after congenital third-trimester infection
Eastern equine encephalitis				○		
Fort Sherman	○					

(Continued)

TABLE 184.2

CONTINUED

Virus	Nondescript Febrile Illness	Febrile Illness with Rash	Febrile Illness with Arthritis	Meningo-encephalitis	Hemorrhagic Fever	Other
Group C viruses (Apeú, Carparu, Itaqui, Madrid, Marituba, Murutucu, Nepuyo, Oriboca, Ossa, Restan)	○					
Guama	○					
Guaroa	○			?		Hepatitis?
Ilheus	○			○		
Mayaro		●	●			
Mucambo (VEE type III)	○			○		
Piry	○					
Rocio				●		
St. Louis encephalitis	○			○		
Tacaiuma	○					Two cases with concurrent malaria fatal
Tonate (VEE Sylvatic subtype IIIB)	○			○		
Tucunduba				○		
Venezuelan equine encephalitis (epizootic IABC)	●			●		Abortion, CNS malformation after first-trimester infection
VEE (sylvatic subtypes ID, IE, IF)	○			○		Pneumonitis
West Nile		○		○		Perinatal illness after congenital third-trimester infection
Western equine encephalitis				●		
Wyeomyia	○					
Xingu	○					Hepatitis?
Yellow fever	●				●	Hepatitis
Sandfly-borne viruses						
Alenquer	○					
Candiru	○					
Chargres	○					
Changuinola	○					
Morumbi	○					
Oropouche	●	○		○		
Punta Toro	○					
Serra Norte	○					
Vesicular stomatitis (New Jersey and Indiana)	○			○		
Vesicular stomatitis (Alagoas)				○		
Zoonoses						
Juquitiba Andes, Bermejo Choclo, Laguna Negra, Lechiguanas, Oran, H39694						Noncardiogenic pulmonary edema, nephrosis
Guanarito					●	
Junin					●	Fatal congenital infection
Machupo					●	Fatal congenital infection
Rio Bravo	○			○		Pneumonia, orchitis
Sabia*					○	
Europe						
Mosquito-borne viruses						
Batai	○			○		
Inkoo	○			○		Respiratory illness
Sindbis	●	●	●			
Snowshoe hare				○		
Tahyna	●				○	Respiratory illness
West Nile§	●	○	○	●		Hepatitis, pancreatitis

(Continued)

TABLE 184.2

CONTINUED

Virus	Nondescript Febrile Illness	Febrile Illness with Rash	Febrile Illness with Arthritis	Meningo-encephalitis	Hemorrhagic Fever	Other
Sandfly-borne viruses						
Sandfly fever (Naples)	●					
Sandfly fever (Sicilian)	●					
Toscana	●			●		Hepatosplenomegaly, DIC
Tickborne viruses						
Bhanja	○			○		
Central European encephalitis[†,‡]	●			●		Hepatitis, thrombocytopenia
Congo-Crimean hemorrhagic[‡] fever					●	
Dhori	○			○		
Kemerovo				○		
Lipovnik				○		
Louping ill[‡]				○		
Thogoto	○			○		Hepatitis, optic neuritis
Tribec				○		
Zoonoses						
Erve				○		Thunderclap headache
Lymphocytic choriomeningitis	●			●	○	Pneumonia, arthritis, orchitis, parotitis; congenital CNS malformation
Belgrade-Dobrava	○				○	Interstitial nephritis, pantropic
Puumula	●			○	○	Interstitial nephritis, myocarditis
Seoul	○				○	Interstitial nephritis, pantropic
Asia						
Mosquito-borne viruses						
Batai	○			○		
Banna	○			○		
Beijing				●		
Chandipura	○			●		
Chikungunya		●	●	○	○	
Dengue 1–4	●	●		○	●	Hepatitis common; perinatal illness after third-trimester infection
Gansu				●		
Japanese encephailitis				●		Abortion after congenital first- and second-trimester infection
Kunjin		○	○	○		
Semliki Forest (Metri)				○		
Sindbis	●	●	●		○	
Snowshoe hare				○		
Tahyna	●			○		Respiratory illness
West Nile[§]	●	●	●	○		Hepatitis, pancreatitis, myocarditis
Yunnan	○					
Zika		●				
Sandfly-borne viruses						
Chandipura	○			○		
Sandfly fever (Naples)	●					
Sandfly fever (Sicilian)	●					

(Continued)

TABLE 184.2

CONTINUED

Virus	Nondescript Febrile Illness	Febrile Illness with Rash	Febrile Illness with Arthritis	Meningo-encephalitis	Hemorrhagic Fever	Other
Tickborne viruses						
Alkhumra‡				○	●	Hepatitis
Alma-Arasan	○					
Banna				●		
Congo-Crimean hemorrhagic‡ fever					●	
Dhori	○			○		
Ganjam	○					
Issyk-kul	○					
Karshi	○					
Kemerovo				○		
Kyasanur Forest				●	●	Pneumonitis, retinitis
Negishi				○		
Omsk hemorrhagic fever				●	●	
Powassan				○		
Russian spring-summer encephalitis				●		
Syr-Darya valley		○				
Tamdy	○					
Wanowrie				○	○	
Zoonoses						
Bangladesh				●		Pneumonia
Hantaan					●	Pantropic; interstial nephritis
Nipah				●		
Lymphocytic choriomeningitis	●			○		Pneumonia, arthritis, orchitis, parotitis; congenital CNS malformation
Seoul					●	Pantropic; interstitial nephritis
Africa						
Mosquito-borne viruses						
Babanki	●	●	●			
Bangui		○				
Banzi	○					
Bhanja	○			○		
Bunyamwera		●		○		
Bwamba		●		○		
Chikungunya		●	●	○	○	
Dengue 1–4	●	●		○	●	Hepatitis; perinatal illness after congenital third-trimester infection
Garissa		○		○	○	
Germiston		○		○		
IgboOra			○			
Ilesha		●		○	○	Hemorrhagic fever
Koutango		○				
Lebombo	○					
Ngari					●	
Nyando	○					
O'nyong-nyong		●	●			
Orungo	●					
Pongola			○			
Rift Valley fever	●			●	●	Hepatitis, retinitis
Semliki Forest	○			●		
Shokwe	○					
Shuni	○					
Sindbis		●	●		○	
Spondweni		○				
Tahyna	●			○		Respiratory illness
Tataguine		●				

(Continued)

TABLE 184.2

CONTINUED

Virus	Nondescript Febrile Illness	Febrile Illness with Rash	Febrile Illness with Arthritis	Meningo-encephalitis	Hemorrhagic Fever	Other
Usutu		○				
Wesselsbron	○					Hepatitis
West Nile§	●	●	●	●		Hepatitis, pancreatitis, myocarditis
Yellow fever	●				●	Hepatitis
Zika		○				
Sandfly-borne viruses						
Chandipura	○					
Sandfly fever (Naples)	●					
Sandfly fever (Sicilian)	●					
Tickborne viruses						
Abadina	○					
Bhanja	○			○		
Congo-Crimean hemorrhagic fever					●	
Dugbe	○			○		
Nairobi sheep disease	○					
Quaranfil	○					
Thogoto	○			○		Hepatitis, optic neuritis
Zoonoses						
Dakar bat	○					
Duvenhage				○		
Lassa					●	Pantropic; fatal congenital infection
Lymphocytic choriomeningitis	○			○	○	Pneumonia, arthritis, orchitis, parotitis; congenital CNS malformation
Mokola				○		
Monkeypox		●				
Tanapox		○				
Transmission cycle unknown						
Ebola (Zaire, Sudan, Ivory Coast)		●			●	Pantropic
Kasokero	○					
LeDantec				○		
Marburg		○			○	Pantropic
Australia						
Mosquito-borne viruses						
Barmah Forest			●	○		Glomerulonephritis
Dengue 1–4	●	●				Hepatitis; perinatal illness after congenital infection
Edge Hill			○			
Gangan			○			
Japanese encephalitis				○		
Kokobera			○			
Kunjin			○	○		
Murray Valley				●		
Ross River		●	●	○		Glomerulonephritis
Sepik	○					
Sindbis	○	○	○			
Trubanaman	○					
Zoonoses						
Ballina					○	
Hendra					○	Fatal pneumonia
Menangle	○					

○, rare, sporadic; ●, frequent, epidemic; CNS, central nervous system; VEE, Venezuelan equine encephalitis.
*Illness reported only after laboratory-acquired infection.
†Also transmitted by ingestion of infected milk products.
‡Also transmitted by contact with fresh meat of infected animals.
§Transmission via breast milk.

has been recognized. Several of these diseases are relatively uncommon, with only one or two cases of human infection reported, although antibody prevalence studies may suggest the possibility of more widespread infection.

The number of these agents may appear daunting, but a careful evaluation of the clinical syndrome, combined with the appropriate use of a reference diagnostic laboratory, can help to identify the etiology of infection in most cases. In addition to the syndromic and laboratory features of the illness, epidemiologic factors in the patient's history should be sought to identify contact with or potential exposure to an infectious source or vectors (e.g., appropriate season and place of exposure within the relevant incubation period preceding onset of illness). Many of the known arthropod-borne and related zoonotic viruses are orphan viruses with unknown disease potential; additionally, novel viruses and viral-disease associations continue to be identified as human incursions increase into rodent and other vector habitats.

Although the recognized arboviruses are distributed principally in developing countries, "tropical" infections are encountered increasingly in returned travelers and no longer can be considered exotic. Dengue fever, probably the arboviral infection most frequently acquired during travel, is diagnosed in approximately 50 travelers returning to the United States each year. Yet these cases undoubtedly represent only a small fraction of the true number of cases because of the illness's nonspecific presentation and because adequate diagnostic specimens are not obtained routinely. Examples of other arboviral infections imported by travelers include Mayaro fever acquired in Central and South America; Toscana and Central European tickborne encephalitis (CEE) from Europe; West Nile–associated viral myelitis from the Middle East; viral retinitis associated with Rift Valley fever (RVF), Lassa fever, Thogoto viral encephalitis, and Ilesha viral infections from Africa; Ross River viral arthropathy from Australia; and chikungunya infection and Japanese encephalitis (JE) from Asia. Cases of fatal yellow fever occurring in nonimmunized travelers underscore the importance of providing pretravel counseling and appropriate immunizations.

Several arboviral infections indigenous to the United States remain important to the public health, most notably West Nile encephalitis (WNE), which has spread at a remarkable pace in epidemics across the North American continent since its introduction in 1999. LaCrosse encephalitis is an important pediatric disease in areas of the Midwest, where its incidence exceeds that of herpes encephalitis and, in some locations, equals that of *Haemophilus influenzae* meningitis in the preimmunization era. The expansion of residential development into wooded locations and the increasing popularity of outdoor recreation in remote areas have been associated with the increased occurrence of numerous bacterial, rickettsial, or protozoal vector-borne diseases such as Lyme disease, ehrlichiosis, and babesiosis. These same trends also have led to increased transmission of viral infections, such as hantavirus pulmonary syndrome—now with confirmed cases in 31 states; Eastern equine encephalitis (EEE), which occurs in eastern marshlands; and Colorado tick fever, which is distributed chiefly in the Rocky Mountain states.

EPIDEMIOLOGY

Most arboviruses are maintained in natural cycles of infection between vector insects or ticks and vertebrate hosts, with seasonal variations in cycle amplitudes related to extremes of humidity, temperature, and other environmental factors. The viruses may be carried through the winter or dry months by vertical transovarial transmission in vector mosquitoes, by transtadial transmission in ticks (across tick developmental

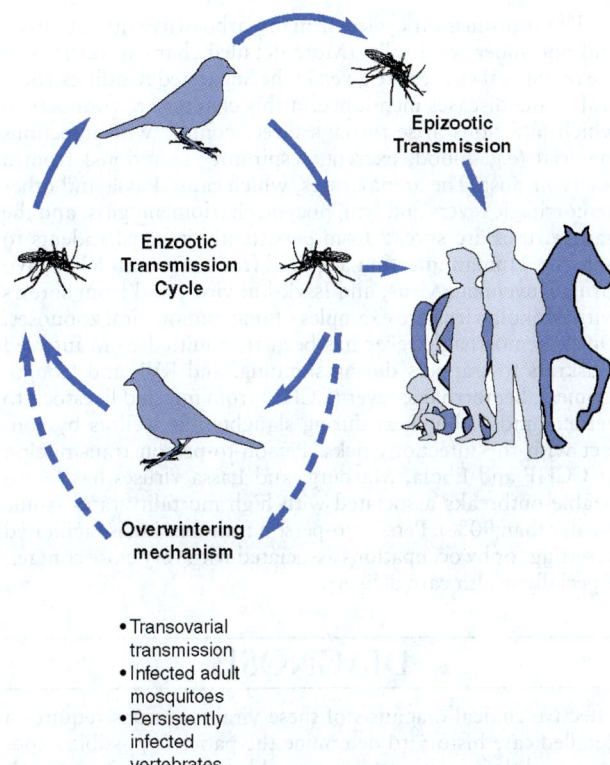

FIGURE 184.1. Typical arbovirus transmission cycle. The virus is amplified by an enzootic vector among birds [e.g., West Nile (WN), St. Louis, eastern equine (EEE), western equine encephalitis (WEE) viruses], and under conditions of increased transmission, spills over to cause tangential (epizootic) infections in humans and other dead-end hosts (e.g., horses can develop encephalitis from WN, EEE, WEE, and JE viruses). In cycles that involve an enzootic vector with a restricted feeding preference for birds, ancillary bridging vectors that feed upon birds and humans transmit are involved in epizootic transmission (e.g., for EEE and West Nile viruses). Transovarial transmission of the virus in mosquito eggs, larvae, or overwintering adult mosquitoes (*dashed arrows*), or persistently infected vertebrates, maintain the virus during winter.

stages, such as larval to nymphal to adult stage), or in persistently infected vertebrates; in tropical locations, transmission may occur continuously. A common pattern of enzootic transmission in a bird–mosquito cycle is illustrated in Figure 184.1. Human infections are most likely to occur in circumstances of intense viral transmission, when the virus "spills over" from the enzootic cycle. The enzootic foci of certain "place-specific" diseases, such as sylvatic yellow fever and Venezuelan equine encephalitis, may be maintained in relatively remote or inaccessible locations, so that humans are infected when they impinge on these otherwise isolated locations. Epizootic or bridging vectors are required to transmit infection to humans or other dead-end hosts in such diseases as EEE, for which the enzootic vector exhibits a narrow "biting preference" limited to the amplifying host. A different vector, therefore, is needed to deliver the virus to humans. Vertebrate-amplifying hosts must sustain viremias of sufficient titers (e.g., 10^4 pfu/mL or higher) and for sufficient periods (e.g., 3 to 5 days) to provide sufficient opportunity for enzootic vectors to become infected. Certain arboviruses, notably yellow fever, dengue, chikungunya, and Oropouche viruses, produce sufficient viremias in humans that anthroponotic (vector-borne interhuman) transmission is possible, with the possibility of pure human-driven epidemics occurring. In Africa, yellow fever epidemics arise when viremic persons traveling from areas of enzootic virus transmission introduce the virus into urban areas, where peridomestic breeding *Aedes aegypti* mediate a human–mosquito–human cycle.

The transmission cycles of many arboviruses are complex and not understood fully. (More detailed characterizations of the individual viruses are given in the Suggested Readings.) Several of the diseases mentioned in this chapter are zoonoses in which infections arise through direct contact with infectious material (e.g. blood, excreta, respiratory secretions) from a reservoir host. The arenaviruses, which cause Lassa and other hemorrhagic fevers and lymphocytic choriomeningitis, and the hantaviruses are spread from persistently infected rodents to humans. Human infection acquired from bats with Rio Bravo virus, Duvenhage virus, and Issyk-kul virus, and from shrews with Mokola virus are examples of uncommon viral zoonoses. Omsk hemorrhagic fever has been transmitted from infected muskrats to trappers during skinning, and RVF and Congo-Crimean hemorrhagic fever (CCHF) from infected livestock to herders and to butchers during slaughter, as well as by contact with the infectious ticks. Person-to-person transmission of CCHF and Ebola, Marburg, and Lassa viruses has led to sizable outbreaks associated with high mortality rates (some greater than 90%). Person-to-person transmission is facilitated in settings or by occupations associated with very close contact, especially health care delivery.

DIAGNOSIS

Effective clinical diagnosis of these viral infections requires a detailed case history to determine the patient's possible exposures and their relationships to established incubation periods for these infections. In general, arboviral infections are acute and preceded by an incubation period ranging from several days to no more than several weeks. A longer interval suggests an alternate diagnosis. A detailed list should be made of the dates and places of travel, the kinds of habitats encountered, dwellings occupied, and the activities in which the patient was engaged, in addition to any history of military service and residence in tropical areas (where previous asymptomatic infections may have been acquired). The evaluation should include a careful assessment of immunization history, including yellow fever, JE, or other arboviral vaccines.

Most arboviral infections produce a nonspecific febrile illness, and specific laboratory tests are needed to confirm their diagnosis. Often, patients are seen after the acute phase of illness, and serology is the only means by which the diagnosis can be made; however, several arboviruses, including those of dengue, chikungunya, yellow fever, Venezuelan equine encephalitis, and Colorado tick fever, can circulate in the blood for several days, whence they can be recovered in the acute febrile phase of the illness. Suckling mice, primary duck embryo cells, and continuous mosquito cell lines (e.g., C636) are especially sensitive systems for recovering most arboviruses, but Vero cells, which are more widely available, are an adequate system for viral culture in most cases. The intrathoracic inoculation of *Toxorhynchites* mosquitoes is a sensitive system for the isolation of dengue and yellow fever viruses. Neurotropic arboviruses should be sought by real-time polymerase chain reaction (PCR) of cerebrospinal fluid (CSF). Viral culture, immunohistochemical studies, or electron microscopy should be undertaken when a brain biopsy is obtained from patients with suspected viral encephalitis.

In most instances, the detection of viral-specific IgM in serum is the most rapid approach to making a presumptive laboratory diagnosis. Its detection in the CSF, reflecting an intrathecal antibody response, is diagnostic of acute central nervous system (CNS) infection, whereas IgM in a single serum specimen provides only a presumptive diagnosis, because specific IgM may persist beyond a single transmission season in some individuals. Infection is confirmed serologically by demonstrating seroconversion (i.e., fourfold or greater change

in titer) in appropriately timed serum specimens. The diagnosis is considered presumptive if a high titer is present in a serum pair or in a single serum specimen. Indirect immunofluorescence (IF) is used widely to measure IgM and IgG antibodies. Although IgG assays are sensitive, serologic cross-reactions to viruses within a taxonomic group frequently are encountered. The hemagglutination inhibition (HI) test, using goose erythrocytes, is a sensitive but broadly reactive assay for those arboviruses that exhibit the property of hemagglutination. Heterologous reactions may be encountered in patients previously infected by related viruses. The complement fixation (CF) test is more specific but is not entirely sensitive, because the antibody response is slow and unpredictable, and it can result in false-negative results. Although, in general, neutralization tests provide the highest specificity, they are inconvenient to perform.

The direct detection of viral genomic material or antigens in blood or other fluids is an important alternative to serology in diagnosing Ebola and other hemorrhagic fevers. Circulating antibodies against theses viruses may not be detectable for several weeks, and infection may cause death before the patient has had time to develop detectable antibodies. Establishing the diagnosis rapidly in the acute phase of illness is important for timely decisions to be made regarding both therapeutic management of the individual patient and public health and infection-control requirements to prevent additional cases. PCR analysis of acute serum samples is a sensitive and specific approach to laboratory diagnosis of dengue fever, Venezuelan equine encephalitis, O'nyong nyong, Ebola, and other infections producing relatively high viremia levels. In addition, viral particles can be visualized by electron microscopy on tissue culture supernatant after successful viral culture, offering useful information for several pathogens with distinctive morphologies. Viral antigens also can be visualized directly by immunohistochemistry in fixed or frozen tissues.

Serologic diagnostic testing is available through several private diagnostic laboratories, state health department laboratories, some university laboratories, and the U.S. Army Medical Research Institute of Infectious Diseases. Assays for all these agents, including viral isolation and viral antigen or genomic detection, are available after consultation from the Centers for Disease Control and Prevention (CDC). Until the specific etiology of a viral hemorrhagic fever is determined, all testing is performed best in a biosafety level 4 facility, because most of these agents are aerosol-infectious in a laboratory setting.

Cases of arboviral encephalitis should be reported to state health departments. Available public health control measures can reduce their transmission and epidemic threat. Because of the possibility of nosocomial transmission occurring and the availability of diagnostic assays, all suspect cases of viral hemorrhagic fever should be reported to the Special Pathogens Branch, CDC. Until the specific etiology of a viral hemorrhagic fever is determined, all testing should be performed in a biosafety level 4 (BSL-4) because of the high risk of occupational laboratory transmission occurring and the possibility of person-to-person spread of some of these viruses. High-risk laboratory procedures, such as centrifugation, which can generate infectious aerosols, require special precautions. All wastes and exhaust from BSL-4 facilities are sterilized before leaving the facility. Inactivated aliquots of a specimen can be removed from the BSL-4 facility for further assessment. Because of the transmissibility and potential severity of illnesses caused by many of these pathogens, appropriate reporting of cases is an important aspect of diagnosing. The laboratory diagnoses of arboviral encephalitis should be reported to the state health department so that public health measure (e.g., vector control) can be applied to reduce the risk of further transmission and a possible epidemic. Any suspected case of viral hemorrhagic fever poses a high risk of health care–associated transmission (e.g., to other patients, health care personnel, and laboratory personnel) and should be reported immediately to the viral Special Pathogens Branch, CDC, for appropriate diagnostic assessment.

Differential Diagnosis

Most arboviral infections lead to nonspecific illnesses consisting of fever, headache, musculoskeletal aches, and malaise, which cannot be differentiated clinically from the prodrome of viral hemorrhagic fevers or from a wide variety of viral bacterial and parasitic infections. The presence of rash can be somewhat helpful in guiding clinical diagnosing, although a lack of specificity limits its utility. Dengue and West Nile fever, certain other arboviral infections, Lassa fever, and filoviral hemorrhagic fevers can cause a morbilliform exanthem. Frequently, dengue has been misdiagnosed as measles or rubella, because these diseases also appear in outbreaks. The rash can be evanescent and difficult to detect in dark-skinned persons. A maculopapular rash can be seen in infections caused by enteroviruses, human parvovirus, rhinoviruses, reoviruses, parainfluenza viruses, rotavirus, hepatitis B virus, Epstein-Barr virus (EBV), cytomegalovirus (CMV), human herpesvirus 6, various rickettsia, and *Mycoplasma pneumoniae* infections. Scarlet fever, leptospirosis, relapsing fever, and medication-associated eruptions also can cause maculopapular rashes. Petechial eruptions can be seen in dengue, Colorado tick fever, alphavirus infections, and the hemorrhagic fevers, and these eruptions may appear similar to those seen in tickborne typhus, epidemic or murine typhus, meningococcemia, Brazilian purpuric fever, bacteremia from *H. influenzae*, certain enteroviral infections, and Henoch-Schönlein purpura. Sindbis and related alphaviral infections can produce a rash and polyarthritis resembling rubella. Their differential diagnosis also includes fifth disease, hepatitis A and B, EBV and certain enteroviral infections, *M. pneumoniae* infection, serum sickness, rat-bite fever, acute rheumatic fever, enteroarthritis, rheumatoid arthritis, and other infections producing acute symmetric polyarthritis.

Dengue, yellow fever, RVF, and CCHF viruses frequently produce a mild to moderate hepatitis, and in endemic areas, they should be considered in the differential diagnosis of ordinary viral hepatitis.

Arboviral CNS infections are not clinically distinctive, although a focal neurologic presentation is atypical. Focal signs suggestive of herpes encephalitis have been reported in isolated cases of western and snowshoe hare viral encephalitis, and they are a feature in approximately 25% of children with Powassan and La Crosse encephalitis. In addition, other treatable CNS conditions that should be ruled out are a partially treated bacterial meningitis, *M. pneumoniae* infection, Rocky Mountain spotted fever, leptospirosis, tuberculosis, Lyme disease, listeriosis, typhoid fever, cat-scratch encephalopathy, fungal meningitis, cerebral malaria, toxoplasmosis, cysticercosis, lead or other toxic encephalopathies, and heat stroke. An important consideration in the differential diagnosis, because a history of exposure to mosquitoes may be given, is encephalopathy from N,N-diethyltoluamide (DEET), which presents with encephalopathic signs and CSF pleocytosis. Rabies should be retained in the differential diagnosis even if no history of animal bite is given, because such exposures often are overlooked (especially in the case of bat exposure), the incubation period is variable, and hydrophobia may not be prominent.

The seasonal distribution of arboviral encephalitis cases in late summer and early autumn may be an important clue to the diagnosis, although this seasonality overlaps that of enteroviral infections, which are the leading cause of meningoencephalitis in this interval. Other viral causes of meningoencephalitis include infections from mumps virus and its vaccine, EBV, CMV, adenoviruses, influenza virus, and postinfectious encephalitis from the viruses associated with childhood exanthems. Polio may be encountered in unvaccinated persons and in immunocompromised persons exposed to vaccine strains. Infection with human immunodeficiency virus (HIV) type 1 may present with CNS signs before symptoms of systemic illness are noticed.

Other disorders of the CNS that should be considered in the differential diagnosis of meningoencephalitis include sarcoidosis, reactions to trimethoprim-sulfamethoxazole and other medications, vascular disorders of the CNS, space-occupying lesions, trichinosis, and CNS infections from free-living amoebae and *Baylisascaris procyonis*. Hemorrhagic shock–encephalopathy syndrome should be considered in the differential diagnosis for infants.

THERAPY

Research on therapeutic modalities has focused on the treatment of the hemorrhagic fevers because of their high case-fatality rates. In controlled trials of adults, ribavirin reduced mortality and morbidity rates in Lassa fever and hemorrhagic fever with renal syndrome (HFRS), and anecdotal experience suggests possible efficacy in Argentine hemorrhagic fever and CCHF. Immune plasma is an effective therapy for Argentine hemorrhagic fever, and passive immunization has been used empirically in the therapy or prophylaxis of other hemorrhagic fevers and after laboratory exposure to certain arboviruses. Immune globulins are available for CCHF and for tickborne encephalitis (TBE), but use of the latter in post-exposure prophylaxis and treatment of TBE has been associated with exacerbated illness in some cases. Although similar adverse experiences have not been reported in a limited number of JE and WNE cases treated with passive immunization, caution should be exercised. In one controlled trial, interferon alpha-2a therapy failed to improve the outcome of JE cases.

Supportive therapy for patients with encephalitis necessitates close attention to monitoring intracranial pressure (ICP), cardiorespiratory function, and fluid and electrolyte balance. Inappropriate secretion of antidiuretic hormone and hyponatremia is a frequent complication of arboviral encephalitis. Although patients with EEE, JE, and other arboviral infections of the CNS frequently exhibit clinical signs of elevated ICP, one controlled study of JE demonstrated that dexamethasone therapy did not improve outcome. Convulsions may be the initial presentation in some arboviral CNS infections, and status epilepticus is a complication in some cases; appropriate cardiorespiratory support, correction of metabolic disorders, and anticonvulsant therapy with lorazepam should be instituted promptly.

PREVENTION

Vaccines licensed in the United States or Europe are available for three arboviral infections: yellow fever, JE, and TBE. Attenuated yellow fever vaccine and inactivated JE vaccine (produced in Japan) are licensed and commercially available in the United States for use by travelers. Inactivated vaccines for TBE are produced in Europe and are used widely in some countries. Because the risk of acquiring TBE is low for most travelers, vaccination is not recommended routinely, and the vaccine is not available in the United States. Vaccines to prevent hemorrhagic fever with renal syndrome and Kyasanur Forest disease are licensed in Asia. Vaccine development is under way for WNE, dengue, and Ebola hemorrhagic fever, although not necessarily for travelers' use. Inactivated, canarypox-vectored and noted DNA equine vaccines for WNE are available commercially.

Vector-borne infections can be prevented by avoiding at-risk locations during transmission seasons or at high-risk times of the day (e.g., avoiding outdoor activity during the period when mosquito vectors are active). Use of protective clothing and repellents can reduce arthropod exposure and bites. Repellents containing picaridin (also known as icaridin or Autan® internationally) and DEET are the most effective formulations; oil of lemon eucalyptus may be as effective as low concentrations of DEET but it should not be used in children <3 years. N,N-diethyltoluamide (DEET)-containing repellents have been used widely since the 1960s, but picaridin, a designer molecule based on DEET, has equal or better repellent activity. In high concentrations, DEET can irritate the skin and produce deep ulcerations. Cases of encephalopathy, including fatal cases, have been reported in children from ages 17 months to 8 years after exposures to formulations containing as little as 10% DEET. Although percutaneous exposure was prolonged in most cases, small quantities and limited exposure have been associated with encephalopathy.

Permethrin [0.5%, Permanone (Louiston International Corp., Easton, PA)] sprayed on clothing and bed nets effectively repels and kills mosquitoes and ticks, and impregnated material remains effective even after several washings. Permethrin shampoo [1%, Nix (Warner Lambert, Morris Plains, NJ)] and permethrin cream [5%, Elimite (Allergen, Inc., Research Triangle Park, NC)] are approved for use on children older than 2 years of age to treat head lice and scabies, and permethrin has been used topically in powders and soaps to repel or kill body lice and other insects. Presumably, these preparations could be used on skin as protection against mosquitoes and ticks. Citronyl, derived from citronella oil, may be more effective than DEET in repelling certain sandflies.

TABLE 184.3

PRECAUTIONS WHEN USING INSECT REPELLENTS

- Apply repellents to clothing and, where ticks are a problem, to shoes and camping gear.
  Permethrin-containing repellents are best because they kill as well as repel insects and ticks and they are relatively waterfast; treated clothing will remain effective after laundering. Permethrin repellents are not approved for use on skin.
- Use repellents sparingly and apply only to skin not covered by treated clothing. Wear long sleeves, long pants, and a hat when possible.
- Use aerosols in an open area, as toxicity has occurred after inhalation or ingestion of DEET; safeguard containers to prevent accidental ingestion.
- Avoid applying repellent to hands of young children who may rub them into their eyes or mouth.
- Never use repellents on wounds, irritated skn, or mucous membranes.
- Use repellents sparingly; application will depend on product concentrations, ambient temperature, perspiration, water exposure, and other factors. Formulations of microencapsulated DEET may lengthen effectiveness and reduce potential for absorption and systemic toxicity.
- Wash repellent-treated skin after returning indoors.
- Wash treated skin and seek medical attention if a suspected reaction to insect repellent occurs; bring the repellent to the attending physician.

Other simple measures that reduce exposure to vector mosquitoes include covering exposed areas with clothing, avoiding outdoor activities at dusk and dawn when certain vectors are most active, and using mosquito bed nets and insecticidal room sprays. Ordinary insect nets and screens do not have a mesh sufficiently fine to exclude sandflies, which require finer meshes or permethrin-impregnated nets or clothing. When traveling in tick-infested areas, frequent inspection to remove adherent ticks from clothing, gear, and the body (including the scalp) is recommended.

From a public health perspective, arboviral diseases can be prevented or controlled by combining several approaches, including the elimination or reduction of vector mosquito–breeding sources, periodic application of larvicides or adulticides to reduce mosquito populations, and the emergency application of adulticides to lower vector populations in the face of an epidemic. Specific strategies are tailored to the breeding habitat and habits of individual vectors (Table 184.4).

Several arboviruses (e.g., WNE and St. Louis encephalitis) are transmitted to human populations only after an extensive period of amplification in natural reservoirs (e.g., birds). Surveying transmission in mosquitoes and birds helps to anticipate the likelihood of epidemic transmission occurring, allowing emergency vector control measures to be instituted at an early stage.

Certain arboviral and related zoonotic diseases of public health significance have been grouped below according to the major syndromes with which these agents generally are associated, although overlapping syndromes are common findings.

VIRAL HEMORRHAGIC FEVERS

Viral hemorrhagic fever (VHF) is a loosely defined category that includes infections from a number of viruses causing similar clinical syndromes and sharing a similar severity of disease. However, these viruses are dissimilar in many ways, including their taxonomy, reservoir hosts, and, thus, geographic distributions. Risk factors for exposure also vary among the infections, and specific control methods are required. Although the signs and symptoms of individual VHFs may overlap, their pathogenesis may not; thus, therapeutic approaches may differ as well.

Yellow Fever

Historically, yellow fever has been feared as one of the great plagues because of its potential to produce thousands of epidemic deaths and the ease of its spread through the movement of viremic humans and infected mosquitoes. In the United States, as recently as 1905, an outbreak in New Orleans produced 5,000 cases and 1,000 fatalities. Now, the transmission of yellow fever is confined to an endemic zone in tropical Africa between 15 degrees north and 10 degrees south and in parts of Central and South America between 10 degrees north and 40 degrees south (Fig. 184.2). The flavivirus is transmitted in a sylvatic or jungle cycle between forest mosquitoes and monkeys, leading to sporadic cases in tangentially infected humans. However, when the virus is introduced to urban locations infested by peridomestic Ae. aegypti, epidemic mosquito-borne human-to-human transmission can result.

In South America, the virus is transmitted in wandering epizootics among monkeys in basins of the Amazon, Orinoco, Catatumbo, Atrato, Magdalena, and other river systems. Tree-hole Haemagogus and Sabethes mosquitoes are the primary vectors. Approximately 100 to 200 human infections are

TABLE 184.4

EXAMPLES OF CONTROL STRATEGIES TO REDUCE TRANSMISSION OF ARBOVIRAL AND ZOONOTIC DISEASES

Disease	Permanent or Long-term Solutions to Reduce Breeding Sites	Annual or Periodic Maintenance Practices to Reduce Vectors	Emergency Measures to Reduce Vectors	Personal Protective Behaviors
Western equine encephalitis, St. Louis encephalitis, West Nile encephalitis in Western United States	Eliminate natural depressions that hold water; engineer ditches and water impoundments to reduce breeding sites; teach good irrigation water management	Apply larvicides to breeding sites; control irrigation run-off; distribute Gambusia (larvae-eating fish)	Aerial or ground ultra-low-volume application of adulticides	Avoid outdoor activity at dusk and dawn; use repellents when outdoors
Dengue	Create public awareness to eliminate peridomestic containers	Inspect premises for containers that hold water; destroy, empty, or treat with larvicides	Intensify destruction of breeding sites; application of adulticides is controversial	Air condition or screen houses; use indoor insecticides
Rodent-borne hemorrhagic fevers	Build rodent-proof houses and grain storage facilities; separate human habitation from grain and food stores	Clean up sources of rodent harborage; remove or make garbage and other rodent food sources inaccessible; use rodenticides, traps	Rodenticides, traps	Sleep off the ground

reported annually, from January to May, chiefly among pioneers, soldiers, and forestry and agricultural workers whose occupational activities take them into the jungle. Consequently, most cases occur in males between the ages of 15 and 40. Recent cases at the fringe of or introduced into major cities in Brazil and Bolivia have created a threat of epidemic urban yellow fever, prompting the establishment of mass immunization campaigns.

In the moist savanna of West and Central Africa, sylvatic mosquito vectors actively transmit the virus among monkeys and humans during the wet season, resulting in an endemic pattern of transmission, with cases frequently occurring in susceptible (unvaccinated) children. Where water storage is practiced and in urban locations, vector *Ae. aegypti* mosquitoes may be prevalent, holding a potential for epidemic transmission when the virus is introduced. The risk of epidemic transmission is associated with the presence of vectors in 5% or more of households.

Classically, the disease has been divided into three stages of infection, remission, and intoxication. After an incubation period of 3 to 10 days, fever, headache, malaise, and musculoskeletal pain occur suddenly, often accompanied by nausea

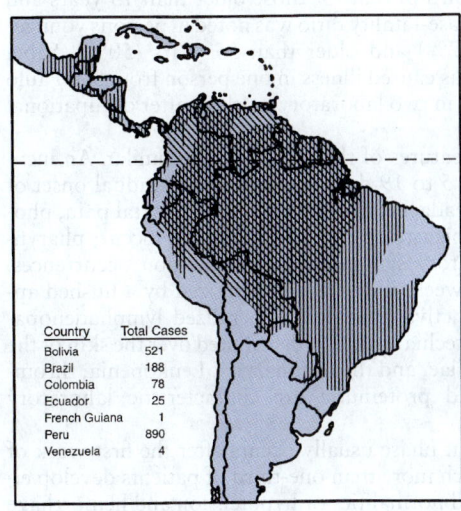

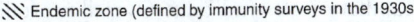

Country	Total Cases
Bolivia	521
Brazil	188
Colombia	78
Ecuador	25
French Guiana	1
Peru	890
Venezuela	4

\\\\ Endemic zone (defined by immunity surveys in the 1930s)

|||| Areas susceptible to periodic outbreaks

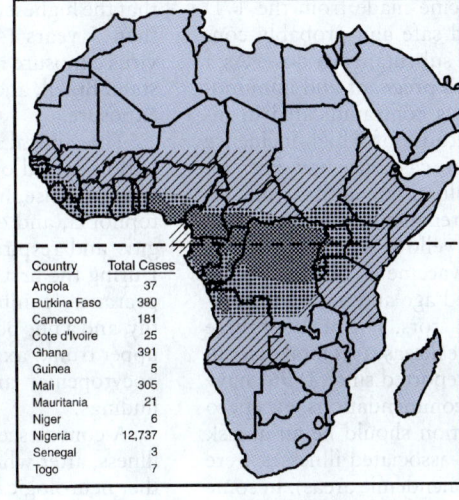

Country	Total Cases
Angola	37
Burkina Faso	380
Cameroon	181
Cote d'Ivoire	25
Ghana	391
Guinea	5
Mali	305
Mauritania	21
Niger	6
Nigeria	12,737
Senegal	3
Togo	7

▓ Enzootic zone (lower Guinea forest block)

▦ Endemic zone (forest/savanna mosaic, humid and semi-humid savannas)

/// Epidemic zone (dry savanna)

FIGURE 184.2. Areas at risk for yellow fever, by zone.

and vomiting. Few physical signs are present except conjunctivitis, flushing of the skin, and Faget sign, a relative bradycardia. In most cases, the fever resolves after a few days. However, in approximately 10% of cases, the remission is temporary, lasting only hours to a few days, whereupon illness resumes with the reappearance of toxicity, fever, vomiting, abdominal pain, jaundice, hematemesis, and other hemorrhagic manifestations. Typically, patients are jaundiced, dehydrated, hypotensive, and often oliguric; proteinuria is a characteristic feature and may serve as a helpful differential feature. Myocarditis may complicate the illness. Azotemia, encephalopathy, progressive liver damage, and bleeding lead to death in 30% to 50% of cases.

Clinical laboratory examination discloses leukopenia, elevated liver enzymes, and abnormalities of coagulation, including abnormal prothrombin, partial thromboplastin, and clotting times, with significant reductions of liver-dependent clotting factors. Evidence of disseminated intravascular coagulation (DIC) has been reported in some patients.

Numerous mucosal, serosal, and subcutaneous hemorrhages are seen at autopsy. The liver shows a pattern of widespread parenchymal necrosis in a characteristic midzonal distribution and microvesicular fatty accumulation, with a minimal mononuclear inflammatory infiltrate. Hepatocytes undergo hyaline degeneration to an apoptotic death, represented by their evolution to eosinophlic-staining Councilman bodies, often found in the canaliculi. The renal medullae are congested and swollen, and the convoluted tubules are damaged. Evidence of myocarditis also may be present.

A diagnosis cannot be made reliably on clinical features alone, because other viral hemorrhagic fevers, viral hepatitis, leptospirosis, malaria, typhus, typhoid fever, and some intoxicants produce a similar clinical presentation. A specific laboratory diagnosis can be made rapidly by identifying viral antigen or genomic sequences in blood or liver biopsy tissue. Serologic diagnosis by detecting specific IgM through enzyme-linked immunosorbent assay (ELISA) in serum is more readily available and also can provide a rapid diagnosis; however, cross reactions from other flaviviral antibodies can limit specificity. The virus can be isolated from blood or tissues in mosquito cell cultures or in suckling mice.

No specific therapy is available, but supportive therapy for hepatic, renal, and circulatory failure may be life-saving. Attention should be given to the prevention and treatment of secondary bacterial infection.

The attenuated yellow fever vaccine made from the 17D virus strain is highly efficacious and safe and probably confers lifelong immunity after a single subcutaneous dose. As a live vaccine, it should not be given to pregnant and immunocompromised persons. The vaccine is contraindicated in infants younger than age 4 months because of a high incidence of vaccine-associated encephalitis. Rare cases also have been reported in adult vaccinees. A potentially fatal multisystemic illness of hepatitis, vascular instability, renal failure, and bleeding diathesis compatible with wild-type yellow fever recently has been recognized as being potentially vaccine-associated, with a rate of 1 per million doses. Advanced age and a genetic component have been suggested as risk factors. The rarity of these events and the potential hazards of the disease (six fatal cases in nonimmunized travelers have been reported since 1996) have not prompted a change in vaccine recommendations, except to reconfirm that the traveler's destination should be an at-risk location (two of the serious vaccine-associated illnesses were in persons vaccinated for travel to nonendemic areas). In some instances, proof of immunization may be required under international travel regulations. Routine childhood vaccination in endemic areas has been recommended under the World Health Organization (WHO) Expanded Program for Immunization programs, but implementation has been fragmentary. The elimination of mosquito breeding sites of *Ae. aegypti* is a prerequisite for reducing the risk of epidemic transmission in areas of high human population densities.

New World Arenaviral Infections

Junin, Machupo, Guanarito, and Sabiá viruses, the etiologic agents, respectively, of Argentine (AHF), Bolivian (BHF), Venezuelan (VHF), and Sabiá-associated hemorrhagic fevers, are the only agents among 13 New World arenaviruses that cause human disease in nature, although Flexal and Pichinde viruses have been reported to cause a simple febrile illness after occupational laboratory exposures. These viruses are maintained in specific sigmodontine rodent reservoir hosts. The reservoirs for Junin, Machupo, and Guanarito viruses are *Calomys musculinus*, *Calomys callosus*, and *Zygodontomys brevicauda*, respectively; the reservoir of Sabiá virus has not yet been determined. The pattern of diseases caused by these viruses is enzootic, with intermittent periods of hyperendemic–epidemic transmission. Humans are infected directly from the rodent reservoir through infectious droplets of rodent excreta or by ingestion or direct contact with such infectious material.

AHF and BHF occur in relatively localized geographic foci—AHF chiefly in the agricultural pampas of Buenos Aires and Santa Fe provinces and BHF in the tropical savanna of northeastern Bolivia. VHF has been recognized only in the tropical grassy plains of Portuguesa and adjacent Barinas states in northwestern Venezuela, but the extent of its geographic distribution has not been studied systematically. AHF is almost exclusively an occupational disease of agricultural workers, who become infected during the harvest season from February to May. The adult population has been vaccinated progressively, and infections now are reported increasingly among children. Fetal infection and death have occurred commonly in pregnant women infected with Junin virus, with an associated increase in maternal mortality rates. Junin virus has been isolated from breast milk. BHF and VHF are acquired in a peridomestic setting, with cases occurring in both genders and all age groups. A review of all BHF cases from 1959 through 1962 established that the attack rate for children younger than 10 years of age (4%) was one-third of that for those older than 15 years and that the highest case-fatality ratio was noted in persons younger than 5 years (47%) and older than 55 years (50%). Sabiá virus exposure has caused illness in one person from São Paulo state, Brazil, and in two laboratory workers after occupational exposure.

The clinical features of these diseases are similar. An incubation period of 5 to 19 days is followed by gradual onset of fever, malaise, headache, and myalgia. Retroorbital pain, photophobia, and epigastric abdominal pain may occur; pharyngitis and respiratory symptoms are uncommon occurrences. During the first week, illness is characterized by a flushed appearance, conjunctival injection, generalized lymphadenopathy, and a fine petechial eruption distributed over the skin of the upper trunk, axillae, and the oropharynx. Leukopenia, thrombocytopenia, and proteinuria are characteristic laboratory findings.

A convalescent phase usually occurs after the first week of illness, after which more than one-third of patients develop either neurologic abnormalities or hypotension and hemorrhage associated with a capillary leak syndrome. Overall mortality rates range between 15% to 30%. Progression to neurologic or hemorrhagic syndromes is a strain-specific manifestation of tropic properties of the infecting virus.

The hypotensive-hemorrhagic phase is manifested by gastrointestinal and mucosal bleeding, petechiae, and hemoconcentration with an increasing hematocrit. Mental status changes, ataxia, and tremor are common symptoms but, even when severe, can be accompanied by a normal CSF. Acute renal failure and secondary bacterial infection are additional complications.

Early illness due to the New World arenaviruses cannot be differentiated clinically from other acute infections. Hemorrhagic manifestations may be confused with meningococcemia, leptospirosis, yellow fever, dengue hemorrhagic fever, and idiopathic thrombocytopenia, all of which can occur in the same geographic areas where AHF, BHF, and VHF are found. Establishing a definitive diagnosis requires identification of the virus, viral antigen, or RNA from blood or tissue or demonstration of a specific antibody response by IF, ELISA, or neutralization assays on appropriately timed serum specimens.

Specific therapy for AHF using specific immune plasma reduced mortality rates to less than 1% when 2 units were administered within 8 days of onset of illness. A complication of immune serum therapy is a late-onset neurologic syndrome with fever, ataxia, and tremor occurring 4 to 6 weeks later in 10% of treated patients. Most patients with this late neurologic syndrome recovered fully. Intravenous ribavirin should be considered if specific immune plasma is unavailable or if a patient with AHF presents later than 8 days after onset of disease. Patients must be monitored and treated promptly for shock, hemorrhage, and secondary infection.

Patient care and specimen handling should be performed using standard precautions. The special isolation of patients is not required. Human-to-human transmission has been reported but rarely occurs. An experimental vaccine for AHF (i.e., Candid-1) was more than 95% effective in a large-scale human trial and may be effective for BHF. This vaccine is undergoing phase II trials in children between ages 1 and 14 years. Although control of rodents has reduced outbreaks of BHF in towns, the rural distribution and wider geographic areas where AHF occurs limit the usefulness of rodent control for the latter disease.

Lassa Fever

Initially described in a series of nosocomial epidemics as a lethal hemorrhagic fever associated with a 50% mortality rate, Lassa fever now is known to be a relatively common, usually self-limited, febrile illness in West Africa. Nonetheless, Lassa fever causes as many as 300,000 cases and 5,000 deaths there each year and is a leading cause of fetal and maternal deaths. Lassa fever in children is a well-described syndrome and may account for as many as 10% of febrile illnesses in children admitted to hospitals in endemic areas.

Lassa virus is the only African arenavirus, of which there are five, that produces human disease. The virus is carried persistently by *Mastomys huberti* and *Mastomys erythroleucus*, the rodent reservoirs whose infectious excretions are the source of human infections in peridomestic and bush settings.

In adults and children, early illness includes fever, malaise, headache, and musculoskeletal pain. The nonspecific syndrome progresses over the course of 4 to 5 days to include painful pharyngitis, cough, chest pain, and abdominal complaints, including cramping pain, diarrhea, and vomiting. Patients appear ill, are weak, and can be hypotensive. In endemic areas, a purulent pharyngitis, with conjunctivitis, head and neck edema, and mucosal bleeding are highly specific signs of Lassa fever. Chest examination may reveal crepitant rales and evidence of pleural or pericardial effusions. Permanent sensorineural hearing loss can be a late sequela.

Pregnant women are at high risk for having spontaneous abortions and maternal deaths.

Near-term *in utero* infection appears to be invariably fatal for the newborn infant, and infected mothers have transmitted Lassa virus to nursing infants. Infants with Lassa fever can be severely ill with diarrhea, abdominal distention, and bleeding. The illness can be complicated by pneumonia or seizures and, in children older than 2 years, the mortality rate is 14%. One study in Liberia found a 27% mortality rate among children; of four reported deaths, three were infants with swollen-baby syndrome. This is a highly characteristic syndrome of Lassa fever among children younger than 2 years and is comprised of anasarca, abdominal distention, and bleeding.

Lassa fever typically resolves gradually over the course of 8 to 10 days. In severe cases, the illness may be complicated by hypovolemic shock, encephalopathy, and respiratory distress caused by laryngeal edema, pleural effusions, or pneumonitis. Gingival, gastrointestinal, and vaginal bleeding seem to be caused by circulating inhibitors of hemostasis, as well as platelet and endothelial dysfunction; the bleeding does not reflect DIC.

Patients can have an elevated hematocrit due to hemoconcentration. Leukopenia and proteinuria may be present. A poor prognosis is associated with elevated aspartate aminotransferase levels (150 U/mL) and high levels of circulating virus ($\geq 10^{3.6}/\mu L$).

Hepatocellular necrosis, indistinguishable from lesions associated with Marburg, Ebola, and yellow fever viral infections, is the most conspicuous pathologic finding. Splenic and adrenocortical necrosis, interstitial nephritis and pneumonia, and myocarditis also can be found on postmortem examination. High concentrations of virus are found in the absence of distinct pathologic lesions in some organs, including the placenta.

Death from Lassa fever is caused by circulatory collapse related to intravascular volume depletion caused by the dysfunction of capillary endothelium. Shock generally is not attributable to hemorrhage alone.

Rapid recognition of the disease is essential to allow prompt therapy to be initiated. Specific therapy for Lassa fever using intravenous ribavirin is more effective if administered within 6 days of onset of disease and is indicated for adults with markers of poor prognosis. Although the relevance of these prognostic markers in children is undefined, and ribavirin given over prolonged periods in high doses to rats has produced growth retardation, administering intravenous ribavirin to seriously ill children is reasonable, provided the risks and benefits have been explained to the parents.

Lassa virus infection can be diagnosed through viral isolation or the identification of viral antigen or genomic sequences amplified by PCR from blood. Specific IgM antibody against Lassa virus can be detected by ELISA or IF late in acute infections. Neutralizing antibodies may not be demonstrable immediately in recovered patients, and the immunologic mechanisms associated with recovery are undefined.

Supportive care should include the maintenance of fluid and electrolyte balance and respiratory support.

Lassa virus has been transmitted from person to person during hospitalization. All health care should be performed using standard precautions, with the addition of contact and droplet precautions when caring for patients with suspected or confirmed Lassa fever.

Eliminating peridomestic rodents, utilizing rodent-proof storage containers to prevent food contamination, minimizing the handling of trapped rodents, and ensuring thorough cooking of rodents consumed as food are the mainstays of prevention of Lassa fever.

Congo-Crimean Hemorrhagic Fever

CCHF, caused by a nairovirus in the family Bunyaviridae, is a potentially fatal illness transmitted by ticks and by contact with infectious body fluids. The virus reservoirs are *Hyalomma* ticks, widely distributed in Africa, the Mediterranean, eastern Russia, the Middle East, and western Asia. A broad range of animal species, including domestic livestock, are hosts for the ticks and can serve as both viral amplifiers and vectors. Human infections occur from bites by infectious ticks, from contact with blood of infected animals (e.g., during slaughter), and, in the health care setting, from contact with the body fluids of infected patients. Asymptomatic or mild infections occur, as evidenced by an antibody prevalence of 2% to 30% in farmers and shepherds in endemic areas. The incidence of CCHF is seasonal and follows the rise in tick density during spring and summer.

The incubation period for CCHF is from 2 to 9 days. Illness onset is abrupt and nonspecific, with fever, chills, rigors, intense headache, and generalized muscle aches. Early in the course of illness, the patient can experience chest pain, nausea, vomiting, or diarrhea, with hypotension, conjunctivitis, and tender hepatomegaly noted on examination. Onset of hemorrhagic symptoms occurs after 3 to 6 days of illness, with epistaxis, petechial and often dramatic ecchymotic bleeding into the skin, and upper and lower gastrointestinal tract bleeding. Endothelial dysfunction and capillary leakage are responsible for pulmonary edema and circulatory failure, leading to death in as many as 30% of cases.

Laboratory findings include lymphopenia, thrombocytopenia, and elevated bilirubin and transaminase levels. DIC occurs at the end-stage of illness, whereas early hemorrhagic symptoms are attributed to thrombocytopenia and endothelial and platelet dysfunction, among other factors yet to be described.

Virus RNA and viral antigens can be detected in blood, liver tissue, or autopsy materials obtained during acute infection. Later in the course of infection, specific IgM or IgG can be detected in serum specimens by IF assay, reverse passive hemagglutination inhibition assay, ELISA, or neutralization assays.

A pathologic examination typically reveals disseminated hemorrhages and widespread edema. The liver is involved extensively, with parenchymal necrosis.

Survival is correlated with an effective humoral immune response. Passive immunotherapy with immune plasma can be lifesaving if given early enough. Intravenous ribavirin shows therapeutic promise and might be useful for postexposure prophylaxis. Early suspicion of CCHF based on a clinical presentation and an appropriate epidemiologic history is important to allow consideration of these therapeutic interventions. Secondary bacterial infections are common findings, and they should be anticipated and treated appropriately. The administration of fluids (with careful attention to volume status and pulmonary function) and inotropic agents is indicated to treat circulatory failure.

Travelers to endemic areas should be aware of regional, seasonal, and occupational risk factors. Appropriate measures should be used to prevent tick bites; contact with livestock or freshly slaughtered carcasses should be avoided.

All health care should be provided using standard precautions. Patients with suspected or confirmed CCHF should be cared for by personnel using added droplet and contact precautions. Occupational transmission to health care personnel and secondary transmission to their family members has been documented. A mouse brain-derived vaccine has been developed, but data regarding its efficacy and side-effect profile are very limited. It is not available in the United States.

Filoviral Hemorrhagic Fevers

The hemorrhagic fevers associated with Marburg and Ebola viruses command attention because of their fulminant nature and lethality. Case-fatality during outbreaks are high, with 26% mortality rates among the 37 reported cases of Marburg disease and 53% (Sudan strain) to 88% (Zaire strain) among patients with Ebola hemorrhagic fever (EHF). Based on the size of the virion, its tubular morphology, and distinctive physicochemical properties, these viruses have been grouped in a family of RNA viruses, the Filoviridae. Four subtypes of Ebola virus (Reston, Sudan, Zaire, and Côte d'Ivoire) can be differentiated by genotype and by antigenic variation. The Sudan subtype of Ebola virus is less virulent in animals and is associated with a somewhat lower case-fatality rate in humans than is the Zaire subtype. A single human infection with the Côte d'Ivoire subtype has been confirmed by isolation of the virus. Reston virus was discovered in 1989, as the cause of a highly fatal epizootic hemorrhagic disease of monkeys imported from the Philippines. Despite explosive transmission, with possible airborne spread among colonies, only four humans had serologic evidence of infection; none was symptomatic, suggesting that the Reston subtype may have limited pathogenicity for humans.

The geographic and ecologic distribution of Marburg or Ebola viruses is poorly understood, beyond general descriptions of regions where outbreaks are thought to have originated. Certain features of outbreak amplification and transmission have been consistent from outbreak to outbreak. Unlike other hemorrhagic fevers, which are transmitted mainly from natural reservoirs, Ebola and Marburg virus outbreaks have relied on high-efficiency transmission from person-to-person, especially in the health care setting, where occupational infection caused by exposure to infectious body fluids and excreta is well-documented. In addition to contact with infectious material from human patients causing infection, contact with infected monkey tissues or blood also has been responsible for infection, creating new chains of transmission during an ongoing outbreak. Person-to-person transmission is by contact with broken skin, percutaneous inoculation (e.g., needlestick injuries), and splashes of infectious droplets that land on exposed mucous membranes. Transmission patterns during human outbreaks are consistent with these modes and have not been suggestive of true airborne transmission. However, the extraordinary virulence of these pathogens, combined with experience with Reston virus outbreaks in monkey colonies and limited experimental monkey data, warrants a conservative approach, using respiratory protection, especially when undertaking procedures that might result in the generation of fine aerosols.

All cases of human illness have occurred in Africa or, as in the European outbreak of Marburg disease, have had their source in that continent through the importation of infected vervet monkeys. The discovery of Reston-viral infections in macaque monkeys from Asia suggests a possibly much wider distribution of Ebola-related viruses. The natural reservoirs of the filoviruses have not been defined, although bats have been shown to support viral replication without disease and to shed virus in excreta.

Ebola and Marburg infections begin with an abrupt onset of similar symptoms, including fever, headache, and myalgia. Patients may appear restless and anxious, later becoming disoriented and delirious. A rash may be seen after 3 to 8 days, usually morbilliform, confluent, and nonpruritic, beginning on the upper trunk and spreading centrifugally to involve the entire body except the face and neck. Desquamation occurs 2 weeks later, in survivors. Profuse vomiting and watery, melenic diarrhea occur, accompanied by abdominal pain that can be intense, even suggestive of a surgical abdomen. Hemorrhagic complications occur in approximately half of patients and are not, on their own, life-threatening. Bleeding most commonly is from the gastrointestinal tract in the form of melena and coffee-ground emesis; gingival and vaginal bleeding occurs as well. Multisystem failure from pneumonitis, hepatitis, pancreatitis, and tubulointerstitial nephritis, combined with intractable hypotension, usually leads to death.

Laboratory studies demonstrate a white blood cell count with an absolute lymphopenia and a left-shifted differential, and Pelger-Huët anomalies may be seen in some polymorphonuclear cells. Transaminase levels are moderately elevated. Proteinuria and chemical evidence of prerenal or renal failure are seen.

The pathophysiology of bleeding and events leading to death are not understood fully. DIC may be a terminal or secondary event, and platelet and endothelial cell dysfunction may be the primary causes of hemorrhage and shock.

The liver shows eosinophilic degeneration, with prominent vacuolar changes. Interstitial pneumonia, interstitial nephritis, and follicular necrosis of the spleen are found, often with pathologic evidence of pantropic infection.

Filoviruses have been isolated from the semen 2 to 3 months after onset of disease, and they have been implicated in one case of sexually transmitted infection. Marburg virus has been isolated also from the anterior chamber of the eye from a convalescent patient with uveitis 80 days after the acute phase of illness, indicating the potential for viral persistence in some patients.

Diagnostic techniques that provide rapid confirmation of the diagnosis are important because isolating the patient and initiating appropriate infection-control practices are critical to preventing spread. In early disease, viral antigen can be identified in skin biopsy or autopsy tissues using immunohistochemistry, and in blood or serum by ELISA. High concentrations of virus are found in blood, various organs, and occasionally in urine. The direct visualization of characteristic viral particles can be achieved using electron microscopy. Reverse transcriptase–PCR (RT-PCR) has proven useful in rapidly confirming the virus subtype. The most reliable serologic test in use is ELISA; IF assay and CF are not specific.

Immune whole blood therapy has been used successfully, but experience is limited to a very small number of patients, and the attempts did not control for other predictors of survival. An S-adenosyl-homocysteine hydrolase inhibitor active against respiratory syncytial virus shows promise as a future therapeutic agent. Anticipation and prophylactic treatment of DIC with heparin were credited in the recoveries of two patients, but consensus regarding the safety and efficacy of this approach is lacking; such treatment should be attempted only in settings where appropriate supportive care can be provided, including accurate monitoring of coagulation profiles.

Appropriate infection-control practices remain the mainstay of outbreak interventions for these diseases. These practices include preventing the occupational exposure of health care personnel (e.g., personal protective equipment, and cohorting or isolation), correctly managing and disposing of sharps, and decontaminating or incinerating medical and other potentially infectious waste. These practices should be combined with community education to prevent unnecessary exposure to sick individuals outside the health care system and to prevent contact with potential sources of reintroduction of the virus (e.g., dead or sick primates).

Hemorrhagic Fever with Renal Syndrome

Hemorrhagic Fever with Renal Syndrome (HFRS) includes a group of diseases caused by Old World hantaviruses in the family Bunyaviridae. Hantaviruses persistently infect small murid rodents (e.g., field mice, voles, rats) that can shed virus in urine,

feces, or respiratory secretions. Humans are infected percutaneously or by direct exposure to infectious aerosols. Secondary person-to-person transmission does not occur. Infections occur in agricultural and peridomestic locations, with a fall and spring seasonality, representing major public health threats in such countries as China, where 40,000 to 100,000 cases are reported each year. Laboratory outbreaks have occurred, often associated with rodent colonies. Men, particularly agricultural and forestry workers, are at greatest risk for acquisition of infection in nondomestic settings. Cases among children are infrequent occurrences; symptomatic disease may be milder in this age group.

Epidemic hemorrhagic fever, the most severe form of HFRS, occurs principally in Asia and Eastern Europe. The disease is caused by Hantaan, Seoul, or Dobrava viruses, each of which has a specific murine rodent host. Seoul virus is distributed worldwide in persistently infected rats, but it has been implicated in only three reported cases of human illness in the United States and few cases in other developed countries. Illness begins abruptly, with fever, intense backache, gastrointestinal symptoms, headache, and myalgia during the initial stage of the illness. As the fever subsides, circulatory instability ensues, with periods of abrupt hypotension and hypertension. Generalized bleeding from mucous membranes, from the gastrointestinal tract, and rarely from petechial hemorrhages in the skin occurs, as does renal failure from acute interstitial nephritis. Recovery follows a diuretic phase. The principal therapeutic challenges are treatment of renal failure and shock, but pulmonary edema, stroke, primary encephalopathy, myocarditis, hepatitis, and pancreatitis may complicate the illness. The case-fatality rate is less than 5% when good supportive care is available. A residual inability to concentrate the urine may persist after recovery, and studies in the United States have suggested an association exists with hypertensive renal disease.

Nephropathia epidemica, a milder form of HFRS caused by the arvicoline rodent–associated Puumala virus, occurs in Scandinavia and Western Europe. Most cases are associated with a milder degree of renal insufficiency and without significant hemorrhagic phenomena. Epistaxis, macroscopic hematuria, and mild gastrointestinal bleeding occurs in 5% of affected patients, but most patients experience only a flu-like syndrome with proteinuria. Fatal cases are rare. Common findings are photophobia and blurred vision, caused by myopic shift with narrowing of the anterior chamber and thickening of the crystalline lens. Puumala infection has been associated with Guillain-Barré syndrome.

Two hantaviruses, Prospect Hill virus, a meadow vole-associated hantavirus enzootic in the United States, and Thailand virus from *Bandicota indicus* in Thailand, have not been associated with human illness.

Epidemic hemorrhagic fever may be confused with Waterhouse-Friderichsen syndrome, acute glomerulonephritis, pyelonephritis, leptospirosis, scrub typhus, dengue fever, thrombocytopenic purpura, or acute renal vein thrombosis. Nephropathia epidemica cannot be differentiated clinically from other nonspecific viral syndromes.

The pathologic examination of patients with epidemic hemorrhagic fever discloses widespread macroscopic and microscopic hemorrhages, capillary endothelial damage, and associated fluid transudation. The most striking abnormalities occur in the kidneys, which show a pale, swollen cortex with a sharp demarcation from a varyingly hemorrhagic medulla. Characteristic histopathologic changes include acute tubulointerstitial nephritis with interstitial edema, extravasation of red blood cells, and inflammatory infiltrates.

Laboratory diagnosis is made serologically, using an IgM capture ELISA or IF assays. HI or neutralization tests are needed to differentiate infections caused by different hantaviruses, which cross-react serologically. RT-PCR amplification has been used to establish the diagnosis and to differentiate hantaviral strains. Immunohistochemistry is useful for postmortem diagnosis. Virus can be recovered rarely from blood and various fluids and tissues, but routine viral isolation attempts have no diagnostic utility.

When given early in the illness, intravenous ribavirin ameliorates circulatory instability and renal insufficiency, thus improving rates of survival. Steroid therapy has been shown to ameliorate disease, but does not improve rates of survival. Public health measures have focused on the control of rodents and on building rodent-proof homes and grain storage facilities. Inactivated Hantaan virus vaccines are available commercially in Korea and China, but their effectiveness is unknown. A recombinant vaccinia-Hantaan virus and naked DNA vaccine are undergoing evaluation.

Hantavirus Pulmonary Syndrome

Hantavirus pulmonary syndrome (HPS) was recognized first in 1993, after a cluster of unexplained respiratory deaths occurred in the southwestern United States. It is now known to be a pan-American zoonosis caused by a number of New World hantaviruses. In contrast to their Old World cousins, these viruses persistently infect small sigmodontine rodents, indigenous only to the Americas, and cause a disease characterized by profound combined cardiopulmonary compromise. Humans are infected percutaneously or by direct exposure to infectious aerosols from infected rodents. Reports have cited secondary person-to-person transmission and nosocomial transmission of Andes virus in South America, but no similar reports exist for Sin Nombre virus infection in the United States and Canada. Infections occur in agricultural and peridomestic locations, depending on the habits of the specific rodent reservoir.

As in HFRS, recognized cases among children are rare findings. Fewer than a dozen of the cases reported from the United States have been among adolescents aged 12 to 16. A single case of mild illness in a 4-year-old child was discovered serendipitously in the United States. However, a case in a 9-year-old child was reported from Argentina, and other pediatric cases of HPS have been reported from South America. One-fifth of cases during a 1997 outbreak in Chile were in young children; three had petechia, and one died of frank hemorrhage.

Usually, patients present after a brief 3- to 5-day febrile prodrome, including myalgias, headache, nausea or vomiting, and diarrhea, that progresses to include cough and shortness of breath. Within 12 to 24 hours of presentation, most patients develop some degree of hypotension and evidence of pulmonary edema and hypoxia, usually requiring mechanical ventilation. Patients who do not survive have severe hypotension, frequently terminating with sinus bradycardia, electromechanical dissociation, or ventricular tachycardia or fibrillation. This terminal hemodynamic compromise can be independent of oxygenation status and occurs a median of 5 days after the onset of severe illness. Multiorgan dysfunction syndrome is seen rarely. Usually, survivors diurese before convalescence, if they were in positive fluid balance, and improve almost as rapidly as they decompensated. Initially, clinically differentiating from other severe pneumonias, leptospirosis, and rickettsial illnesses may be difficult.

Patients are febrile with tachypnea and tachycardia on presentation. Patients do not present with rash, hemorrhagic signs, pharyngitis, conjunctivitis, or peripheral or periorbital edema. In contrast to HFRS, overt hemorrhage is seen rarely in later stages of illness and only in severe cases in association with DIC. However, petechiae and flushing of the head and neck indicative of vascular fragility have been noted with some frequency among South American cases. Chest radiographs consistently are abnormal, with signs of interstitial edema

and occasional pleural effusions. Notable hematologic findings include leukocytosis with increased myeloid precursors, circulating immunoblasts, thrombocytopenia, and hemoconcentration, which is most pronounced in patients with florid pulmonary edema. Hypoalbuminemia, mild to moderate elevations of transaminases, creatine phosphokinase, and amylase also have been reported. Other abnormalities include the development of metabolic acidosis, rising serum lactate levels, and prolongation of prothrombin and partial thromboplastin times. As many as three-fourths of patients have proteinuria, and one-fifth have creatinine elevated above 2.0 mg/dL. Virus strain-specific clinical variants, such as marked renal insufficiency among cases infected with Black Creek Canal and Bayou viruses, have been noted.

Pathologic examination demonstrates generalized capillary dilation and edema, with major histopathologic lesions in the lung and spleen, which also are the sites where antigen is detectable. The lungs, in most cases, reveal a mild-to-moderate interstitial pneumonitis with variable degrees of congestion, edema, and mononuclear cell infiltration. The cellular infiltrate is a mixture of small and enlarged mononuclear cells with the appearance of immunoblasts, which also are prominent within the red pulp and periarteriolar sheaths of the spleen and paracortex and within sinuses of lymph nodes. Functional impairment of vascular endothelium appears to be central to the pathogenesis of HPS, but details of the origin and mechanism of this disturbance remain undefined.

Laboratory diagnosis is made by IgM capture ELISA or by a Western blot assay. Numerous native and recombinant antigens are used, but generally they are cross-reactive, and Sin Nombre virus antigens have shown excellent accuracy even for the more distant South American viruses. Because many of these viruses have not been isolated, neutralization tests are not available readily, and isolation of virus has no role in routine laboratory confirmation. RT-PCR assays of serum and subsequent sequencing have been used in establishing clinical diagnosis, and sequence comparison can differentiate hantavirus strains. Postmortem tissues can be examined by immunohistochemical staining.

Unlike its use in HFRS, intravenous ribavirin has been shown not to improve survival in HPS. The cornerstone of therapy remains early recognition and judicious hemodynamic support, providing fluid resuscitation coupled with the early use of inotropes, such as dobutamine. Public health measures have focused on reducing the numbers of peridomestic rodents and human exposures to them.

Rift Valley Fever

Rift Valley fever (RVF) is a disease of chiefly sub-Saharan African livestock, with intermittent epizootics associated with prolonged heavy rainfall and causing serious losses of sheep and cattle and abortions among domestic livestock. Although sporadic human infections and limited epidemics were recognized in East and South Africa as early as the 1930s, an unprecedented outbreak in Egypt in 1977 and 1978 produced an estimated 200,000 cases of human illness and 600 fatalities, demonstrating that the virus can spread rapidly under the right circumstances. In 1987, a subsequent outbreak involving hundreds of persons in West Africa was associated with a dam project. These outbreaks highlighted the epidemic potential of RVF infection, but they were dwarfed by the 1997 to 1998 outbreak in East Africa, where nearly 10% of the population in a widespread area was affected.

RVF virus is a phlebovirus in the family Bunyaviridae and is transmitted by a variety of mosquitoes, some of which serve as the natural reservoir. Other biting insects can spread RVF during epizootic conditions, although they do not amplify the virus. Ingestion, direct inoculation, and inhalation of infected aerosols from slaughtered or aborted animals have been the principal modes of transmission to humans. Occupational infections among laboratory personnel have been common occurrences during outbreaks. Person-to-person transmission has not been reported.

The usual incubation period is 3 to 6 days, but it may be as brief as 24 hours. In most cases, RVF is a self-limited dengue-like illness; fever, chills, headache, and severe muscle and back aches resolve over the course of a 3- to 6-day period. Upper respiratory tract symptoms, conjunctival injection, and hepatitis may occur. The most frequent complication of RVF infection is ocular disease, which begins approximately 1 to 3 weeks after onset of illness and has occurred in as many as 20% of infected patients. Retinal exudates, usually in a perimacular or macular location; retinal hemorrhages; and edema are the most common ocular findings. These lesions arise from a primary retinitis, with vasculitis causing thrombotic sequelae. Loss of visual acuity persists in one-half of affected patients.

Severe cases, with encephalitis or hemorrhagic fever, occur in approximately 1% of infections and can lead to death. Meningoencephalitis can develop 3 to 10 days after resolution of the acute febrile illness. Signs of meningeal irritation, confusion, and other alterations of mentation and extrapyramidal signs may develop. The outcome of meningoencephalitis in children usually is favorable, but fatalities have been reported. The potential for the delayed onset of ocular and CNS disease is of particular importance to clinicians caring for travelers returning from endemic areas, who might present with acute symptoms well after their return. Hemorrhagic fever is associated with generalized bleeding, especially from the gastrointestinal tract and into the skin; vomiting; hepatitis; and shock. An estimated 50% of patients with hemorrhagic fever die.

A pathologic examination discloses widespread areas of macroscopic and microscopic hemorrhages. Focal hepatocellular necrosis is a prominent and consistent finding. Fetal death is a common occurrence in infected livestock, but it has not been reported after human infections.

The diagnosis is made serologically through ELISA or IF by detection of antibody or antigen. The virus can be isolated readily from blood, tissues, and other body fluids. Immunohistochemistry and PCR also can be used for indirect viral detection.

An investigational inactivated vaccine exists but is not available for general use. No specific therapy is available. Although intravenous ribavirin had shown promise, based on *in vitro* studies and infection with related viruses, early data from a limited clinical trial have suggested that a possibly greater risk of development of encephalitic complications exists among recipients. The use of repellents against mosquitoes and other biting insects and avoidance of raw meat and ill animals are important precautions to prevent exposure.

CENTRAL NERVOUS SYSTEM INFECTIONS

West Nile Encephalitis

WN virus, a flavivirus antigenically related to the viruses of JE, St. Louis encephalitis, and Murray Valley encephalitis, is transmitted over a broad geographic range that includes Africa, parts of Europe and Russia, the Middle East, South Asia, and Australia and the western hemisphere; Kunjin virus represents an antigenic subtype distributed in Australia, New Guinea, and Asia. The virus is transmitted principally in a *Culex* mosquito–avian cycle, and migratory viremic birds or their infected parasitic ticks are suspected to contribute to the virus' dispersal.

In some locations, epizootic or "bridging" vectors that feed on both birds and mammals play an important role in transmitting the virus from its enzootic avian cycle to humans (Fig. 184.1). Although *Culex pipiens* complex mosquitoes (northern and southern house mosquitoes) are the principal enzootic vectors in the United States, a hybrid of this species with *Culex molestus* appears to be the principal epizootic vector responsible for human infections. Numerous alternative species transmit the virus in specific ecologic zones. Unlike St. Louis encephalitis, which shares a similar enzootic transmission cycle, WN virus is lethal to some avian species, whose deaths have provided a sensitive surveillance indicator. The virus also causes fatal encephalitis in horses.

The infection is a leading cause of nonspecific summer fevers in some areas of the Old World, resulting in antibody prevalence rates of 50% to 100% among children by the time they reach age 5 years. Major epidemics, with attack rates as high as 50%, have been reported with the introduction of the virus into immunologically susceptible populations (e.g., to Eastern Europe). After the virus was introduced into the United States in 1999, it quickly became established on the eastern seaboard and has spread across the continent to produce more than 16,000 cases in an ongoing nationwide epidemic (Fig. 184.3). The scale of the outbreak in 2003 was such that 0.02% of blood donations were virally infected during the transmission season and 14 transfusion-associated cases and other transplant-associated cases occurred. Although the height and duration of viremia in infected persons is too limited to permit anthroponotic (human-to-human, vector-mediated) transmission, direct introduction via blood or organs, particularly to immunosuppressed persons, can lead to infection and illness. Transmission via breast milk and perinatal congenitally acquired infections after third trimester maternal infection have been reported in anecdotal cases.

Most infections, particularly in children, are asymptomatic. In the 0.2% of persons in whom infection is symptomatic, the incubation period is 3 to 14 days. Generally, clinical manifestations are mild, with fever, malaise, anorexia, headache, myalgia, nausea, and vomiting constituting WN fever. Physical findings are nonspecific and include conjunctivitis, pharyngitis, polyarthropathy, and generalized, mildly tender lymphadenopathy, which has been reported in more than 75% of patients. The skin may be marked by indistinct mottling and macules and by a diffuse roseolar eruption affecting chiefly the trunk and upper extremities. The severity of illness correlates strongly with age, and children typically have asymptomatic or mild infections lasting 3 to 6 days. Illness in the elderly is more likely to be complicated by CNS infection, although meningoencephalitis has been reported in adolescents and children. The encephalitis syndrome may include—in addition to changes of consciousness—seizures, weakness and paralysis, ataxia, cranial nerve palsies and polyradiculitis, and myelitis. The syndrome of inappropriate antidiuretic hormone secretion (SIADH) may lead to hyponatremia. Fulminant hepatitis, pancreatitis, myocarditis, and poliomyelitis with residual flaccid paresis have been reported in anecdotal cases.

In tropical locations where dengue, Sindbis, and other arboviruses causing a nonspecific febrile illness cocirculate, WN fever cannot easily be differentiated. In the United States, summertime enteroviral infections enter into the differential diagnosis because of their seasonality and appearance in outbreaks that include aseptic meningitis (e.g., Echovirus 13). The differential diagnosis of WNE is broad, and it includes infectious and noninfectious causes of aseptic meningitis, acute encephalitis or encephalopathy, and myelitis.

A diagnosis can be made serologically by detecting viral-specific IgM in CSF or serum by ELISA or IFA, although the potential for cross reactions with St. Louis encephalitis virus may necessitate confirmation with neutralization tests or

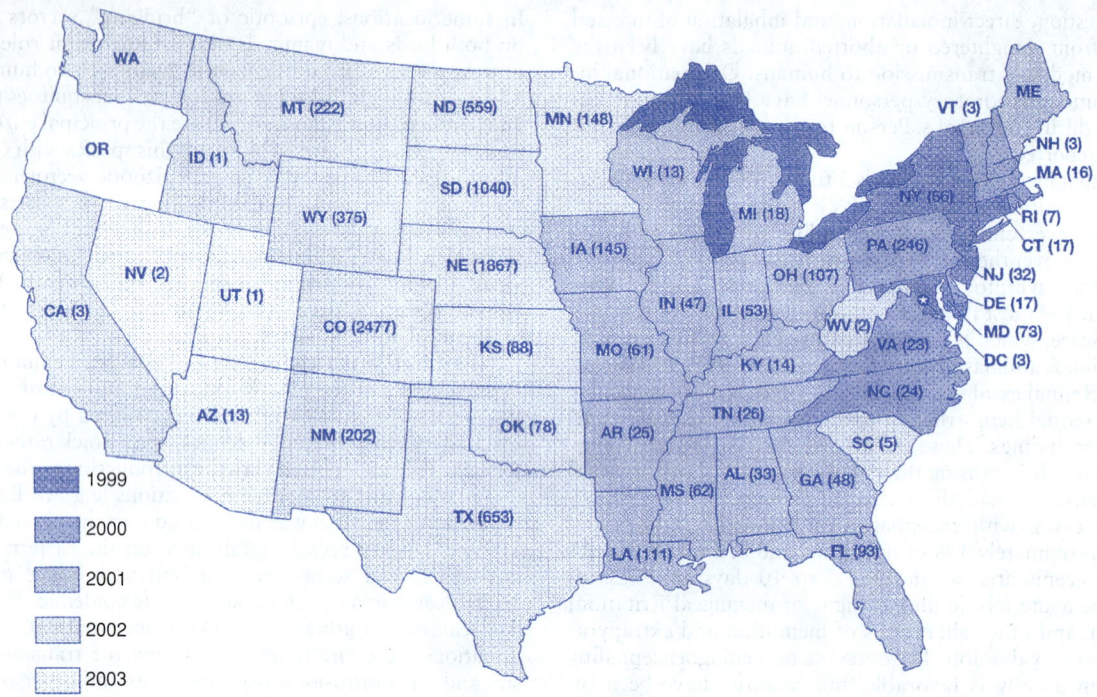

FIGURE 184.3. Human West Nile viral infections, United States, 1999 to 2003, by state and year first affected.

specific ELISAs. CSF specimens may be positive in real-time PCR assays.

The treatment is supportive. A trial of passive immunization with hyperimmune antibody is in progress. Public health interventions to reduce mosquito populations are the principal means of prevention, but individuals also should observe personal protective measures against mosquito exposure and bites. An inactivated vaccine and canarypox-vectored vaccine are licensed for horses and a live-attenuated vaccine for humans is undergoing development.

St. Louis Encephalitis

St. Louis encephalitis remains an important cause of epidemic viral encephalitis in the United States, periodically producing hundreds of cases in local or regional outbreaks. Sporadic cases and smaller outbreaks have been reported also in southern Canada, Mexico, and parts of Central and South America (Fig. 184.3; see Table 184.2). In the western United States, where the flavivirus is transmitted among *Culex tarsalis* mosquitoes and passerine birds in an enzootic cycle similar to that of western equine encephalitis, rare sporadic infections occur from July to October in rural areas (Fig. 184.4). In the eastern United States, *C. pipiens*– and *C. quinquefasciatus*–borne epidemics—analogous to recent outbreaks of WNE—emerge at unpredictable intervals, with the potential for producing hundreds of cases in the late summer and fall, principally in urban locations. In Florida, the *C. nigripalpus* mosquito transmits the virus in urban and suburban epidemics, with transmission extending through December in some instances.

Remarkably, only 1 in 300 infections progresses to clinical illness; however, except for advanced age, the host factors predisposing to neuroinvasive disease are undefined. Severity of illness and mortality are associated also with age, and in most outbreaks, the majority of cases occur in the elderly. The spectrum of illness ranges from a simple febrile illness with headache to aseptic meningitis or encephalitis. Although

St. Louis encephalitis generally causes a milder illness in children than that in adults, more than 85% of cases in patients younger than 20 years old manifest as meningitis or encephalitis. The overall case-fatality rate is 6%, but it is less than 1% in children younger than 5 years of age.

The onset often is insidious, with a prodrome of fever, headache, nausea, vomiting, myalgia, mental confusion, and clumsiness. Physical examination discloses fever, meningism, and an altered state of consciousness. Tremulousness, generalized weakness, hyporeflexia or hyperreflexia, and cranial nerve palsies are the most common neurologic abnormalities, whereas focal weakness and other localizing signs are observed less frequently.

A moderate CSF pleocytosis (i.e., 100 to 200 leukocytes per cubic millimeter) is a typical finding, but the initial examination may fail to reveal any evidence of inflammation. Limited experience with imaging studies has disclosed no abnormalities in most cases, but specific changes in the substantia nigra have been observed in a few cases. Hyponatremia caused by inappropriate antidiuretic hormone secretion occurs in approximately one-third of cases.

Pathologic examination of the CNS shows widespread focal neuronal degeneration in the midbrain, thalamus, brainstem, cerebral cortex, cerebellum, and spinal cord, accompanied by focal and perivascular inflammatory infiltrates.

The consequences of infection acquired during pregnancy are unknown, although in a single case in which encephalitis occurred in the second trimester, a normal full-term infant was delivered without viral-specific IgM in cord blood. Psychomotor sequelae have been reported in 25% of infants who recovered. In older children and adults, tremulousness, nervousness, headache, and memory impairment are frequent but temporary sequelae.

The diagnosis is made serologically through ELISA, IFA, HI, or CF, but heterologous reactions with dengue, WN virus, and other flaviviruses may obscure interpretations. The presence of specific IgM antibody in the CSF is diagnostic; in the serum, it is presumptive evidence of recent infection. CSF should be assayed by PCR, and brain tissue from biopsy or autopsy

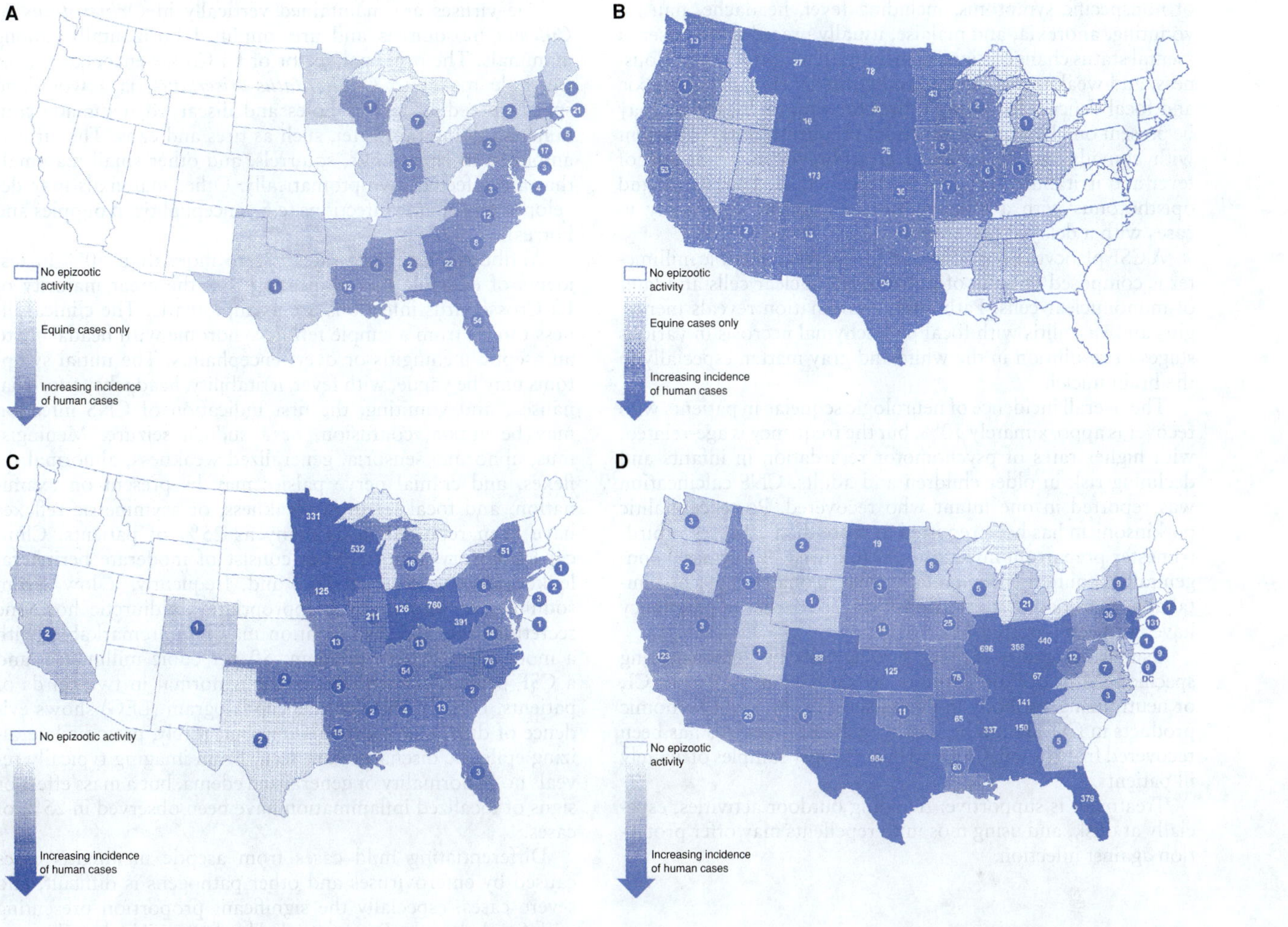

A

B

C

D

No epizootic activity

Equine cases only

Increasing incidence of human cases

FIGURE 184.4. Reported cases of arboviral encephalitis and relative incidence by state, United States, 1964 to 1997.

specimens should be examined by immunohistochemistry or IF for evidence of viral antigen.

No specific therapy is available. Heeding public health advisories to use mosquito repellents, to avoid outdoor activity in the evening, and to remain in air-conditioned or well-screened residences has been shown to be protective.

Western Equine Encephalitis

Western equine encephalitis is endemic to the western United States, Canada, Mexico, and areas of Argentina, and Uruguay (see Figs. 184.3, 184.4, 184.5 and Table 184.2) and periodically has produced outbreaks numbering in scores or hundreds of cases. In North America, the alphavirus is transmitted among birds and *C. tarsalis* mosquitoes in rural locations. Consequently, farmers, ranchers, and other persons who spend long hours outdoors (particularly in the evening) are at highest risk of acquiring infection. Incidence is almost two times higher in men than in women. A declining rural population, the increased prevalence of air-conditioned residences, and other lifestyle changes associated with suburban and urban life have led to a decline in the numbers of cases and infections, such that antibody prevalence in endemic areas now is in the range of 1% and fewer than 5 cases are reported annually. Age-specific incidence shows that risk is highest among the elderly.

Infections chiefly are asymptomatic. Clinical manifestations range from a mild illness with headache and fever to meningoencephalitis. The case-fatality rate is 3%. A brief prodrome

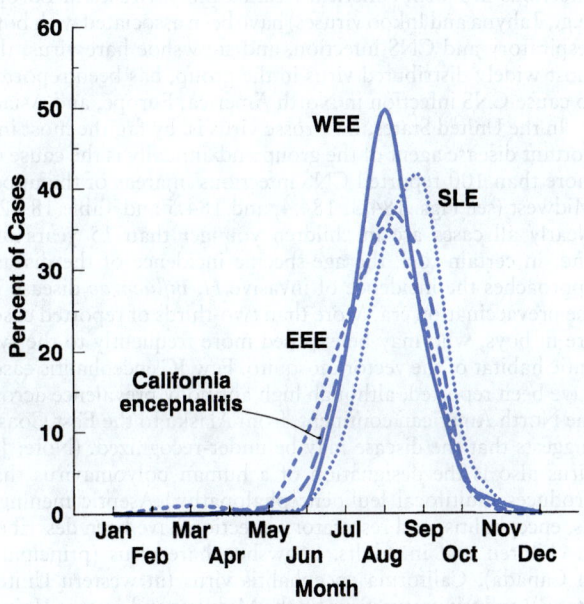

FIGURE 184.5. Month of onset for reported cases of arboviral encephalitis, United States, 1971 to 1983. EEE, eastern equine encephalitis; WEE, western equine encephalitis; SLE, St. Louis encephalitis.

of nonspecific symptoms, including fever, headache, nausea, vomiting, anorexia, and malaise, usually precedes the onset of mental status changes, signs of meningeal irritation, tremulousness, and weakness. Generalized hyporeflexia or hyperreflexia and focal deficits, localizing to frontotemporal locations, may be present on physical examination. Frequently, infants present with convulsions after having an abbreviated prodrome of fever and irritability. Progression to generalized spasticity and opisthotonus with a bulging fontanelle occur commonly in cases with a delayed presentation.

A CSF pleocytosis of 10 to 300 leukocytes per cubic millimeter is composed initially of polymorphonuclear cells and later of mononuclear cells. Pathologic examination reveals meningitis and vasculitis with focal parenchymal necrosis in various stages of resolution in the white and gray matter, especially in the brain nuclei.

The overall incidence of neurologic sequelae in patients who recover is approximately 10%, but the frequency is age-related, with higher rates of psychomotor retardation in infants and declining risk in older children and adults. CNS calcification was reported in one infant who recovered. Postencephalitic parkinsonism has been reported in more than 20 cases. Third-trimester prepartum infection was followed by perinatal congenitally acquired encephalitis in two neonates, but congenital abnormalities after infections acquired earlier in pregnancy have not been reported.

Usually, diagnosis is made serologically by demonstrating specific IgM in CSF or serum or by showing a rise in HI, CF, or neutralizing antibody in paired serum specimens. Genomic products in CSF should be sought by PCR. The virus has been recovered from blood, CSF, and brain biopsy samples of acutely ill patients.

Treatment is supportive. Avoiding outdoor activities, especially at dusk, and using mosquito repellents may offer protection against infection.

California Encephalitis

Several viruses in the California serogroup of bunyaviruses [e.g., La Crosse, Jamestown Canyon (JC), California encephalitis, and trivittatus viruses] are responsible for sporadic CNS infections in North America. Related bunyaviruses in Europe (e.g., Tahyna and Inkoo viruses) have been associated with both respiratory and CNS infection, and snowshoe hare virus, the most widely distributed virus in the group, has been reported to cause CNS infection in North America, Europe, and Asia.

In the United States, La Crosse virus is, by far, the most important disease agent of the group and annually is the cause of more than 100 reported CNS infections in areas of the upper Midwest (see Figs. 184.3, 184.4, and 184.5 and Table 184.2). Nearly all cases are in children younger than 15 years old and, in certain foci, the age-specific incidence of the disease approaches the incidence of invasive *H. influenzae* disease in the prevaccination era. More than two-thirds of reported cases are in boys, who may be exposed more frequently to the sylvatic habitat of the vector mosquito. Few JC encephalitis cases have been reported, although high antibody prevalence across the North American continent, from Alaska to the East Coast, suggests that the disease may be under-recognized. (Note: JC virus also is the designation of a human polyomavirus that produces multifocal leukoencephalopathy.) Aseptic meningitis, encephalitis, and respiratory infection have been described in children and in adults. Snowshoe hare virus (principally in Canada), California encephalitis virus (in western United States), and trivittatus virus (in the Midwest and eastern United States) have been associated with isolated cases of meningoencephalitis.

The viruses are maintained vertically in *Ochlerotatus* or *Culiseta* mosquitoes and are amplified horizontally among mammals. The principal vector of La Crosse encephalitis, the tree-hole mosquito *Ochlerotatus triseriatus*, is a woodland species breeding in tree holes and discarded manmade containers holding rainwater, such as tires and cans. The virus is amplified in chipmunks, squirrels, and other small mammals that are infected asymptomatically. Other mammals may develop symptomatic infections (e.g., encephalitis in puppies and horses).

Antibody prevalence rates rise to more than 50% in residents of endemic foci, indicating that the great majority of La Crosse virus infections are asymptomatic. The clinical illness ranges from a simple febrile syndrome with headache, to an aseptic meningitis or overt encephalitis. The initial symptoms may be vague, with fever, irritability, headache, anorexia, nausea, and vomiting; the first indication of CNS infection may be ataxia, confusion, or a sudden seizure. Meningismus, abnormal sensoria, generalized weakness, abnormal reflexes, and cranial nerve palsies may be present on examination, and focal seizures, weakness, or asymmetric reflexes have been reported in as many as 25% of patients. Clinical laboratory abnormalities consist of moderate peripheral leukocytosis with a left-shift and, frequently, a low serum sodium level caused by inappropriate antidiuretic hormone secretion. The CSF examination may be unremarkable, with a modest pleocytosis (median, 50 per cubic millimeter) and a CSF protein concentration that is normal in two-thirds of patients. Usually, the electroencephalogram (EEG) shows evidence of diffuse or focal slowing, but, rarely, periodic lateralizing epileptic discharges are seen. Brain imaging typically reveals no abnormality or generalized edema, but a mass effect or signs of localized inflammation have been observed in 25% of cases.

Differentiating mild cases from aseptic meningitis cases caused by enteroviruses and other pathogens is difficult, and severe cases, especially the significant proportion presenting with focal abnormalities, may not be distinguished easily from herpes simplex encephalitis. The diagnosis is confirmed serologically by identifying specific IgM in CSF or blood through ELISA or IF, or by showing a rise in IF, HI, or neutralizing antibody titers. Heterologous reactions in some serologic systems may interfere with the differentiation of La Crosse virus from snowshoe hare virus or other related agents. Viral genomic sequences have been detected in CSF samples, but the diagnostic value of PCR has not been evaluated adequately. Virus rarely has been recovered from CSF or from brain tissue.

Signs of elevated ICP and, rarely, deaths caused by brain herniation have been reported, but the overall case-fatality ratio is less than 0.5%, and generally, the outcome of patients who recover is good. Convulsions, as a single fit or status epilepticus, occur in 50% of cases. Behavioral abnormalities and poor psychometric test performance have been described in some recovered patients, but the significance of these observations is unclear, and the incidence of neurologic and psychologic sequelae has not been characterized well.

Supportive treatment consists of intensive monitoring and treatment of cardiorespiratory function, maintaining fluid and electrolyte balance, and the timely administration of anticonvulsants. Invasive monitoring of ICP may be indicated in some cases. Ribavirin has a viral inhibitory effect *in vitro*, and it is undergoing evaluation in a controlled trial. Where the disease is endemic, control measures that have been promoted include removing containers that serve as mosquito breeding sites, filling tree holes, and applying adulticides to vegetation around residential areas. Risk can be reduced further by urging children to play in open sunlit areas, to wear protective clothing, and to use mosquito repellents.

Eastern Equine Encephalitis

EEE is an exceptionally fulminant nervous system infection rivaling rabies in the gravity of its outcome. EEE occurs in relatively focal locations on the eastern and Gulf coasts of the United States, in some inland locations, and in the Caribbean (see Fig. 184.3). An antigenically distinct viral subtype of the alphavirus is transmitted in areas of Central and South America.

EEE virus is transmitted among birds by *Culiseta melanura*, an ornithophyllic mosquito found in a specific swampy habitat with mucky peat soils supporting a cedar, red maple, or loblolly bay flora. Other vector species (notably salt-marsh *O. sollicitans*, woodland *O. canadensis*, and freshwater *Aedes vexans* and *Coquillettidia perturbans*) that feed both on birds and mammals are required to bridge the enzootic cycle and transmit the infection to humans, horses, and, rarely, other dead-end hosts. A median of only three cases per year is reported in the United States. Most cases occur between July and September, but, in the deep South, the virus may be transmitted year-round (see Fig. 184.4).

After an incubation period of 4 to 10 days, a prodromal illness of variable duration precedes the onset of neurologic symptoms. The prodrome consists of intense headache, fever, malaise, nausea, vomiting, and myalgia. Although usually brief, nonspecific symptoms may last as long as several weeks in individual cases. Infants are more likely to present with generalized convulsions after having brief intervals of unexplained irritability, anorexia, and fever. Neurologic symptoms consist of confusion, delirium, and other changes in mentation followed by a rapid progression to coma. Various neurologic signs, including meningismus, focal weakness or paralysis, cranial nerve palsies, and abnormal reflexes, may be present. Signs of elevated ICP may develop.

One-third of cases are fatal, with a higher incidence of fatalities occurring in infants and in the elderly. Serious neurologic sequelae occur most frequently in young children and infants; more than 50% of surviving patients younger than 5 years old have been reported to have serious sequelae. The effects of EEE acquired during pregnancy are unknown; one woman with EEE in the third trimester delivered a healthy baby with no evidence of congenital infection.

A peripheral leukocytosis with a left-shift differential count and a massive CSF pleocytosis are common findings. The early predominance of neutrophils in the CSF may suggest a bacterial meningitis. An initial CSF white blood cell count of greater than 500 per cubic millimeter or a serum sodium of less than 130 mEq/mL has been associated with a poor prognosis.

The pathologic findings in the CNS include edema and disseminated foci of neuronal degeneration with neutrophilic or mononuclear inflammatory responses, reflecting the stage of illness when death occurred. An acute pyogenic meningitis may be present. Vasculitis and infarction are seen in some cases.

Because EEE seroprevalence is well below 1%, even in endemic areas, the presence of any level of EEE virus antibody (demonstrated by IFA, HI, CF, ELISA, or neutralization tests) in an acute specimen is strong evidence of the diagnosis. Brain tissue obtained by biopsy or at autopsy should be cultured and examined immunohistologically for evidence of virus or viral antigen. Viral genomic sequences in CSF have been detected by PCR; however, the procedure has been evaluated in few cases.

No specific therapy is available. Intensive supportive care, control of ICP, and respiratory support have reduced the case-fatality ratio among cases reported in the last 20 years. Avoiding known enzootic foci and using mosquito repellents are recommended to reduce the risk of infection. Large-scale applications of larvicides and adulticides have been used to reduce vector mosquito populations.

Lymphocytic Choriomeningitis

Lymphocytic choriomeningitis (LCM) is a worldwide zoonosis that is associated with the common house mouse, *Mus musculus*. LCM virus, an arenavirus, is shed in the urine and other excreta of persistently infected mice and Syrian hamsters, which can act as alternative reservoir hosts. Peridomestic infections have occurred among persons living in proximity with wild infected mice, from infected pet rodents, and among scientific workers whose laboratory rodents or cell lines were infected silently. One estimate from a large city suggests that as many as 5% of individuals had serologic evidence of previous infection, although an etiologic diagnosis of the acute illness rarely is made.

The virus was named after the lymphocytic meningitis that it produces in experimentally infected monkeys and mice; in humans, 90% or more of patients develop an influenza-like illness without signs of CNS infection. Usually, the systemic illness is characterized by fever, anorexia, and severe muscle aches, and (frequently) by nausea, vomiting, pharyngitis, lymphadenopathy, and upper respiratory symptoms. A biphasic fever occurs in one-fourth of cases.

A variety of complications, including aseptic meningitis (characterized by headache) and encephalitis, may follow the influenza-like prodrome. Other less common complications include arthritis, parotitis, orchitis, pneumonia, myocarditis, rash, pancreatitis, and mucosal bleeding. Patients with CNS infection can have meningism, an altered mental state, papilledema, cranial nerve palsies, generalized weakness, abnormal reflexes, and focal seizures. Polyneuritis, permanent flaccid paralysis, headaches, and a chronic meningoencephalitis have been reported as sequelae. Damage to the CNS may result in increased CSF pressure and may necessitate the implementation of a shunt. In rare cases, death has resulted from acute meningoencephalitis and after severe systemic illnesses complicated by pneumonia and generalized hemorrhages. The differential diagnosis of the meningitic disease manifestation includes other viral meningitides, in addition to tuberculous meningitis.

Patients may have a peripheral leukopenia. Examination of the CSF discloses a pleocytosis with as many as 5,000 leukocytes per cubic millimeter. Lymphocytes predominate, but as many as 25% of the cells may be polymorphonuclear. Hypoglycorrhachia is found in 25% of patients.

Infections that occur during the first trimester of pregnancy may cause spontaneous abortion, and infections that develop between the third and fifth months of pregnancy can result in a congenital LCM syndrome. Congenitally infected infants have presented with nonobstructive hydrocephalus with periventricular calcifications, chorioretinitis, and psychomotor retardation. More than one-half of cases are associated with severe neurologic sequelae, consisting of spastic paresis, visual loss, and developmental delay, and as many as one-third of affected infants die during the first 2 years of life. A pathologic examination of the brain has demonstrated ependymal proliferation, with a predominantly perivascular mononuclear infiltration, and signs of sclerosis. Cases have been reported in Russia and in Arizona, Iowa, Illinois, New Mexico, and Texas in the United States.

The laboratory diagnosis is made through IF or ELISA on serum or CSF, but LCM virus can be recovered from the CSF, blood, or throat washings in as many as 50% of patients. If mice are used in virus-isolation attempts, the colony must be certified to be free of LCM virus. In cases of suspected congenital infection, maternal serum, CSF, and blood of the affected infants should be examined serologically. Prevention hinges on eliminating house mice and avoiding contact with pet mice and hamsters, especially during pregnancy.

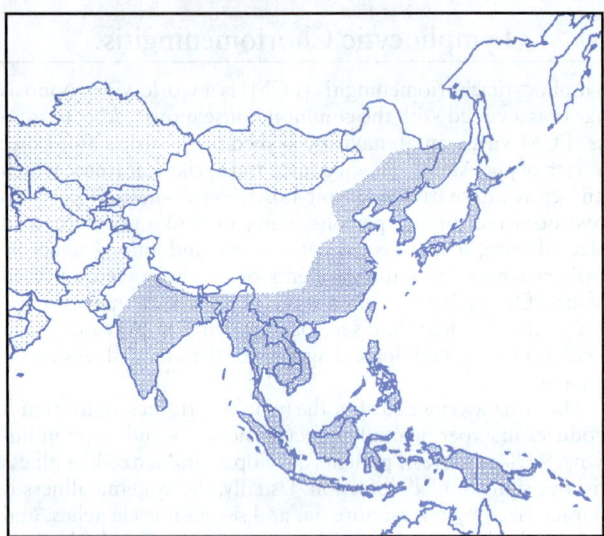

FIGURE 184.6. Areas of known or suspected Japanese encephalitis viral transmission.

Japanese Encephalitis

JE, the leading cause of viral encephalitis in Asia (where more than 45,000 cases are reported annually), also has been transmitted sporadically in the western Pacific and in far northern Queensland (Fig. 184.6). The mosquito-borne flavivirus is transmitted during the summer and early fall in temperate locations, during the wet season in subtropical locations, and throughout the year in tropical areas. Where rice cultivation depends on irrigation, JE vector populations and transmission of disease follow these human-dictated agricultural schedules.

This flavivirus, antigenically related to St. Louis encephalitis, WNE, and Murray Valley encephalitis viruses, is transmitted among domestic pigs or birds and *Culex mosquitoes*, chief among them, *C. tritaeniorhynchus*. The various vector species breed in ground pools, so risk of acquiring disease is greatest in rural areas where flooded rice paddies provide abundant vector habitats and domestic pigs coexist with humans.

In areas where transmission is endemic, infections occur at an early age, so that antibody prevalence and immunity in rural areas approach 100% by adulthood. Age-specific attack rates are highest in children younger than 10 years old, but immunologically susceptible travelers of all ages are at risk of acquiring the illness. The overall case-to-infection ratio is in the range of 1 in 300.

The incubation period ranges from 5 to 14 days. The onset of clinical illness may be gradual, with fever, headache, vomiting, and other nonspecific symptoms appearing over the course of several days and resolving over the course of 5 to 7 days in patients without neurologic infection. In other patients, the initial symptoms intensify with chills, continued fever and headache, stiff neck, and a rapid decline in consciousness. Frequently, the onset is abrupt, necessitating hospitalization for acute delirium, stupor, seizures, or paresis on the initial day of symptoms. A depressed level of consciousness is the essential clinical feature, but motor abnormalities are common, including random purposeless movements, facial and oculomotor palsies, generalized or focal spastic or flaccid paresis, tremor, and abnormal deep-tendon and plantar reflexes occur with variable frequency. Convulsions occur frequently in children. Rigidity, masked facies, and extrapyramidal signs may appear later in the illness. Clinical presentations with urinary incontinence or lower motor weakness caused by myelitis, Guillain-Barré syndrome, or acute psychosis have been reported. Infec-

tion during the first and second trimesters of pregnancy can produce lethal fetal infection and miscarriage.

The most frequent complications are pneumonia and other nosocomial infections and, with prolonged coma, stasis ulcers. Children younger than 10 years old have poorer outcomes, with higher rates of death and sequelae. Where intensive supportive care is available, the overall case-fatality rate ranges from 2% to 10%, although, in some locations, case-fatality rates remain as high as 35%, with neurologic sequelae occurring in an equal proportion of survivors. In some studies, preexisting neurocysticercosis was an important risk factor for development of illness and adverse outcome. Other clinical and laboratory parameters associated with poor outcomes include presence of virus and interferon in the CSF, low serum and CSF levels of specific IgG and IgM, and a depressed sensorium on hospital admission. The proportion of surviving patients with sequelae stands in inverse relation to the case-fatality ratio, reflecting the availability and quality of supportive care. Significant sequelae of psychomotor retardation, paralysis or paresis, convulsions, and extrapyramidal signs are reported in 10% to 30% of recovered patients, and residual EEG abnormalities are common sequelae in children. As many as 75% of recovered children may exhibit psychomotor retardation or behavioral disturbances.

An early peripheral polymorphonuclear leukocytosis frequently is seen. Examination of the CSF discloses several hundred leukocytes per cubic millimeter and an elevated protein concentration. Hyponatremia caused by secretion of inappropriate antidiuretic hormone is a frequent complication. Imaging of the head often shows abnormal signals in the midbrain and thalamus, with evidence of hemorrhages in the latter location.

Neuropathologic examination discloses a panencephalomyelitis, with scattered foci of infected neurons in the cerebrum, basal ganglia, brainstem, cerebellum, and spinal cord and perivascular and parenchymal inflammatory infiltrates.

The diagnosis is confirmed by demonstrating viral-specific IgM or by detecting viral nucleic acid by real-time PCR in the CSF. Acute serum may provide greater sensitivity as a PCR analyte.

No specific therapy has been proved. Interferon-alpha 2a was studied in a controlled trial, but it showed no benefit. Monoclonal antibody immunotherapy has been reported. Although clinical signs suggest elevated ICP in some patients, in a controlled trial, dexamethasone therapy did not improve outcome.

A formalin-inactivated vaccine purified from infected mouse brain (JEVax) is recommended for travelers who plan visits of 30 or more days during the transmission season to rural areas where the disease is endemic. Three doses, given on days 0, 7, and 30, are recommended and provide a protective efficacy of more than 90%. Only travelers at high risk of exposure should be immunized, because allergic reactions, consisting of generalized urticaria and angioedema, occur in 0.1% to 1.0% of vaccinees. Moreover, reactions are delayed until 1 to 3 days after vaccination. Rare, temporally related neurologic side effects have been reported, but a causal association with vaccination is unproved. Avoiding outdoor activity in the evening, wearing mosquito repellents, and sleeping under permethrin-impregnated bed nets are recommended to reduce risk of exposure.

Tickborne Encephalitis

The term *tickborne encephalitis* is applied to infections caused by three closely related flaviviruses in the tickborne-virus serocomplex. Throughout Europe, including Scandinavia and parts of western Russia, the virus of Central European encephalitis (CEE), transmitted chiefly by *Ixodes ricinus*, causes a biphasic febrile illness in which CNS symptoms are prominent during recrudescence. In the Far East and Russia, Russian spring-summer encephalitis virus, transmitted by *Ixodes persulcatus*, produces a more severe encephalitis, sometimes complicated by residual neurologic deficits. A Siberian viral subtype is transmitted in an overlapping geographic range centrally in the Eurasian continent. Other tickborne viruses of the complex that cause human disease include louping ill and related ovine viruses (transmitted in the British Isles and Europe), Omsk and Kyasanur Forest hemorrhagic fever viruses, and Langat and Powassan viruses.

TBE is chiefly an occupational disease of forestry workers and also is an avocational risk to persons frequenting forests and brushy areas that are the vector ticks' habitat (e.g., hiking). Many cases occur in children who play in these locations. Infections occur in the spring and summer (accounting for the disease name), with a peak incidence occurring in July. The disease also can be acquired by consuming raw milk products from infected cows, sheep, or goats or by contact with infected slaughtered animals.

After an incubation period of 7 to 14 days, a severe but rapidly resolving febrile illness develops, consisting of headache, myalgia, and upper respiratory symptoms. In the remaining 10% to 25% of patients, recovery is followed within a day to more than a week by aseptic meningitis, meningoencephalitis, or myelitis, and the recrudescence of fever, headache, and CNS signs such as neck stiffness, tremor, somnolence, disturbed mentation, cranial nerve palsies, generalized weakness, and cerebellar signs. In approximately 3% of patients with CNS involvement, a progressive course of paresis or paralysis affecting the proximal musculature and pharyngeal and respiratory muscles may ensue. A fatal outcome, frequently from bulbar paralysis, is reported in fewer than 1% of cases. Minor neuropsychiatric sequelae and residual EEG changes persist in some patients. CNS infection occurs more frequently and is more severe in the elderly.

The clinical course of Russian spring-summer encephalitis is more severe, resulting in a case-fatality ratio as high as 20% and in significant neurologic sequelae in one-half of the survivors. Residual chronic seizures and a characteristic, sometimes progressive, flaccid paralysis of the shoulder girdle have been described. Unlike the previously described biphasic course, the initial symptoms of fever, intense headache, nausea, vomiting, and photophobia progress directly into a neurologic syndrome of convulsions, mental status changes, meningism, and bulbar and extremity weakness.

Seijures should be controlled with anticonvulsants and ventilatory support in the event of bulbar paralysis may be needed. No specific therapy is available. Laboratory diagnosis rests on serologic confirmation of infection through ELISA, HI, or CF assays. PCR analysis of serum and CSF has been positive in rare cases when samples were obtained early in the infection. The differential diagnosis includes Borrelia infection and other viral causes of meningoencephalitis. In Western Europe, *Ixodes ricinus* is the vector of Lyme disease, anaplasmosis, and various rickettsial infections and can transmit Bartonella, Babesia, and CEE virus. Dual Borrelia-CEE infections have been reported to be unusually severe and have led to fatal illness.

Thrombocytopenia and elevated transaminases are seen. Imaging studies have shown distinctive changes in the thalamus and basal ganglia, corresponding to areas typically exhibiting pathologic changes. Histopathologic abnormalities are found chiefly in the gray matter of the cerebrum, brainstem, and anterior horn cells of the upper spinal cord. Nodular foci of neuronal necrosis with inflammatory cellular infiltrates, perivascular cuffs, and spongiform rarefaction typify the pathologic changes.

The detection of viral-specific IgM in CSF is diagnostic. Because of the biphasic course of illness, viral nucleic acid no longer is present in CSF at clinical presentation, and PCR has little diagnostic use. Effective inactivated vaccines for CEE are available to expatriates in Europe and Russia, but for travelers, vaccination is recommended only for those whose intineraries include high risk activities. TBE–specific immune globulin, available in Europe, may be given as preexposure prophylaxis for short-term, high-risk exposure. Specific immune globulin may be given to adults as postexposure prophylaxis; however, to be effective and to provide protection from immunopathologic complications, passive immunization must begin within 4 days of the tick-bite occurrence. Even with the prompt administration of immune globulin, illness may be exacerbated by postexposure prophylaxis. Because of the occurrence of adverse events and frequent breakthrough cases, in many countries, postexposure administration to children younger than 14 years of age is not approved.

Venezuelan Equine Encephalitis

Venezuelan equine encephalitis (VEE) periodically causes extensive epidemics and equine epizootics in Central and South America, leading to few human deaths but significant social and economic disruption. VEE outbreaks have produced as many as 30,000 human cases in a single year, with an equal number of fatal cases among horses in contemporaneous epizootics. Previously, epidemics occurred at intervals of approximately 10 years, principally in rural coastal locations of Colombia and Venezuela; in 1971, the most extensive recorded outbreak spread from Central America into Texas, where it caused 110 human and more than 1,500 equine cases. Although small, isolated outbreaks followed sporadically, 25 years passed before the next major outbreak occurred in 1995 to 1996, in Venezuela and Colombia, causing an estimated 75,000 human cases, 300 of them fatal.

During outbreaks, epizootic subtypes of VEE virus (i.e., IAB or IC) are spread directly among horses and burros by mosquito vectors, with tangential transmission to humans but no human-to-human spread. In contrast, the sylvatic VEE viral subtypes are transmitted continuously in cycles among forest-dwelling rodents and mosquitoes, occasionally causing sporadic cases or small outbreaks in equines and humans intruding on the sylvatic cycle. For example, subtype II, also known as Everglades virus, has been responsible for three isolated encephalitis cases in Florida. Although the reservoir and origin of epizootic viruses still are uncertain, genetic sequencing suggests that they arise by mutation from sylvatic strains.

Contrary to its name, VEE in humans usually produces a self-limited but prostrating grippe and results in encephalitis in fewer than 5% of cases. After an incubation period of 1 to 7 days, illness begins with an acute onset of intense headache, fever, and myalgia, so sudden that it often can be documented to an exact hour. Shaking chills, arthralgia, photophobia, ocular pain, nausea, vomiting, and other signs of toxicity force affected patients to bed or to seek medical attention. Recovery follows rapidly, the entire course of the illness lasting less than a week, but a recrudescence of symptoms and biphasic fever occur in some patients. Few physical findings are evident: the patient appears flushed and lethargic, has tender muscles, and may exhibit an injected pharynx and conjunctiva. Lymphadenopathy, splenomegaly, and signs of pneumonia are seen in some patients.

Neurologic symptoms occur infrequently in adults, but even in children, in whom the risk of development of CNS infection is greatest, fewer than 5% of the illnesses lead to meningoencephalitis. Various neurologic abnormalities, including a depressed sensorium, meningismus, generalized weakness, focal and generalized seizures, and pathologic reflexes, are reported. Among all patients with CNS involvement, the case-fatality ratio is 20%, but fatality rates are higher among children younger than 5 years old. Infections that occur during pregnancy have resulted in spontaneous abortion and congenital fetal infection, manifested by CNS and other malformations, and late fetal death.

The clinical laboratory evaluation discloses panleukopenia with an initial depression of lymphocytes followed by neutropenia. Elevated alanine amino transferase levels have been described in some patients.

Pathologic examination shows lymphoid depletion, follicular necrosis in the spleen and lymph nodes, and an interstitial pneumonia. The brain is congested, with evidence of a vasculitis. A specific diagnosis can be made serologically through HI, CF, IF, ELISA, or neutralization tests. Attempts to isolate virus from pharyngeal secretions or blood during the first 3 days of illness are fruitful in 50% of patients. Identification of the viral subtype with specific monoclonal antibodies provides important epidemiologic information about the likelihood of epidemic spread. Viral genomic products in blood can be detected by PCR in most acute phase samples.

The treatment is supportive. Live attenuated and killed vaccines are available for laboratory workers. Inactivated equine vaccines are administered routinely in some areas; however, inadequate inactivation resulting in residual infectious virus is suspected to have caused livestock deaths and epizootics. Travelers to enzootic areas should take precautions against mosquito bites.

Murray Valley Encephalitis

Four major outbreaks of encephalitis in the basin areas drained by the Murray and Darling rivers of southeastern Australia had been reported as an unknown disease before the causative flavivirus was isolated during an outbreak in 1951. The mosquito-borne flavivirus, named Murray Valley encephalitis virus, is the most important cause of arboviral encephalitis in Australia, but sporadic human and equine CNS infections also are caused by the closely related Kunjin virus, a subtype of WN virus.

In northern Australia, the viruses are transmitted in an avian enzootic cycle and are spread to humans by *Culex annulirostris* in an endemic pattern. *Aedes tremulus* mosquitoes may have a role in sustaining the virus during the dry season. Epidemics occur in heavily populated southeast Australia at infrequent intervals, usually in years following heavy spring rainfall in the north. This pattern has been associated with the Southern Oscillation–El Niño effect. Cases occur in the austral summer and fall, between January and June. With the exception of the last major outbreak in 1974, when 58 cases were reported over a broad area of Australia and New Guinea, most recent cases have been reported from the north, often in Aborigines and principally in children. The incidence of disease and severity of illness are greater in males. Overall, the case-fatality ratio is approximately 20%.

Nonspecific prodromal symptoms, including fever, headache, nausea, vomiting, and dizziness, precede the onset of neurologic signs and symptoms. A stiff neck, ataxia, tremor, slurred speech, confusion, and generalized convulsions are early manifestations of meningoencephalitis. Motor abnormalities can include spasticity and hyperreflexia or, conversely, a flaccid paralysis or hypotonia. Extrapyramidal signs occur in some patients. Bulbar paralysis may lead to respiratory failure. Signs of elevated ICP are evident in most patients. Permanent brain damage, leading to residual weakness or paralysis, psychomotor retardation, postencephalitic parkinsonism, or lesser disabilities, occur in one-third of patients who recover.

The CSF exhibits a moderate pleocytosis, with ten to several hundred leukocytes and a shift occurring from a predominance of polymorphonuclear cells in the first week of illness to a mononuclear pleocytosis. Destructive changes are prevalent in the cerebellum, particularly in the Purkinje cells and in the brainstem and spinal cord. Scattered foci of neuronal destruction and inflammation are found in the cortex. Perivascular and meningeal inflammation are pronounced.

The specific serologic diagnosis of Murray Valley encephalitis is hindered by heterologous reactions with Kunjin virus and other Australian flaviviruses. Fractionation of CSF or serum to obtain IgM for HI assay provides a more specific result than conventional IgM-capture ELISA.

Supportive therapy, particularly measures to lower elevated ICP and respiratory support, may be needed in severe cases. Public health surveillance of vectors and sentinel chickens is maintained to monitor epidemic threats.

Rocio Encephalitis

Rocio encephalitis first was recognized in a series of outbreaks between 1975 and 1977, in the Ribeira Valley and Santista Lowlands on the southern coast of Brazil, near São Paulo, when more than 1,000 acute encephalitis cases occurred, principally among men with outdoor occupations. Attack rates were high—approximately 35 in 1,000 inhabitants—and risk was even higher among poor families. Cases occurred in the fall, late in the wet season, between March and June. The case-fatality ratio was 5% among hospitalized patients. Sporadic cases continue to be reported from the region, but in 1996, eight cases were recognized outside the original epidemic area for the first time, in Bahia state.

The eponymous flavivirus is related antigenically to St. Louis encephalitis virus and is transmitted also among birds by mosquitoes, including *Aedes scapularis* and *Psorophora ferox*.

Clinical features are similar to those of other acute viral CNS infections. After an incubation period of 1 to 2 weeks, an initial phase of fever, malaise, nausea, vomiting, and severe headache lasting several days is followed by resolution of the illness or by progression to meningoencephalitis, manifested by neck stiffness, confusion, altered consciousness, and various neurologic findings, including weakness, pathologic reflexes, ataxia, and cranial nerve (particularly bulbar) palsy. Major neurologic sequelae were reported in one-fourth of survivors.

Neuropathologic lesions are distributed widely in the CNS but are most prominent in the brain nuclei and brainstem. Lesions in the cerebellum and of the anterior horn cells have been described.

Diagnosis is made serologically by identifying specific IgM in CSF or serum or by demonstrating seroconversion by HI, CF, or neutralization tests.

Intensive care, particularly of patients with bulbar palsy, may be lifesaving. An experimental inactivated vaccine had poor immunogenicity and was not investigated further. Mosquito repellents and other measures against mosquito bites are recommended.

Henipaviral Encephalitis

Hendra virus (formerly called equine morbillivirus) and Nipah virus are related, bat-associated members of the newly formed genus of *Henipavirus* in the family Paramyxoviridae. Both viruses have exhibited a potential for causing neurologic and respiratory infection and, of note, recurrent neurologic illness. Hendra virus was recognized first in association with clusters of respiratory and neurologic illnesses in horses and humans that occurred in 1994 and 1995, near Brisbane, Australia. Nipah virus was identified as the cause of a geographically extended outbreak of encephalitis that spread from Malaysia to Singapore between 1998 and 1999, principally among farmers and abattoir workers who were in close contact with infected pigs. A third, related virus may have been responsible for a series of outbreaks that occurred in western Bangladesh between 2001 and 2004.

Although human Hendra and Nipah infections were acquired, respectively, from acutely infected horses and pigs, those animals, in turn, had been infected from the principal viral reservoir of frugivorous *Pteropus* bats (fruit bats). The three recognized human Hendra virus infections presumably were acquired from respiratory secretions of infected horses that had acute pneumonia. Human Nipah viral infections occurred in an epidemic of nearly 300 cases that accompanied a widespread epizootic of respiratory infections among pigs. Pig-to-pig spread probably occurred by multiple routes of direct contact with infected urine, saliva, and pharyngeal and lung secretions and by veterinary procedures. The great majority of the human cases were occupationally acquired and involved close contact with pigs during assorted husbandry activities, in abattoirs, and during culling. The mass destruction of more than a million animals was the means by which the outbreak ultimately was contained. Isolated cases of infection acquired from dogs and human-to-human transmission were reported. In contrast to the principally zoonotic source of infection in these outbreaks, a relatively larger proportion of cases in Bangladesh have had no clear animal contact, and person-to-person spread could not be eliminated in some cases.

Of the three recognized cases of human Hendra virus disease, two patients had a respiratory illness with severe flu-like signs and symptoms; one of them died with pneumonia. Another patient recovered from acute meningitis only to relapse a year later with a progressive, ultimately fatal, encephalitis.

Infection with Nipah virus is asymptomatic in 10% of cases, but usually it is followed within 2 weeks (range 2 days to 2 months) by a prodrome of fever, vomiting, dizziness, and headache progressing to encephalitis. Drowsiness, mental status changes, hypotonia, areflexia, and myoclonus are common features of the neurologic infection. In addition, hypertension, tachycardia, and respiratory depression associated with brainstem infection and motor abnormalities localizing to the upper cervical cord have been noted. Some patients have had a respiratory illness, accompanied by radiographic changes of interstitial pneumonia. The illness is fatal in approximately 40% of cases. Thrombocytopenia, lymphopenia, mildly elevated transaminases, and hyponatremia, and pleocytosis and elevated protein in the CSF are the laboratory abnormalities most commonly reported. Disseminated focal hyperintense magnetic resonance imaging (MRI) lesions are found mainly in the white matter and occasionally in the cortex. This pattern may be helpful in distinguishing cases from JE, in which abnormalities and hemorrhage frequently localize to the thalamus.

A relapse of Nipah encephalitis within a mean interval of 7.6 months after initial recovery was reported in 12 patients (7.5% of those surveyed), and a delayed onset of encephalitis 8.4 months later in patients whose initial infection was asymptomatic or accompanied by a mild illness was reported in another 10 patients (3.7%). Late neurologic illnesses were acute in progression and manifested by fever, headache, seizures, and focal neurologic signs; four cases were fatal. The subacute or relapsing course of Hendra and Nipah cases has suggested that the viruses persist in the CNS.

The pathologic changes predominate in the brain, but also are found in the lungs, heart, and kidneys. Histologic examination discloses vasculitis with giant cell syncytia of the vascular endothelia and perivascular zones of microinfarction and ischaemia. Neuronal degeneration is followed by the formation of neuronophagia and microglial nodules.

Serologic testing can provide a clue to the diagnosis, but cross-reactions among the agents may limit specificity. Virus has been isolated from CSF, saliva, tracheal secretions, nasal secretions, and urine samples during the acute phase of illness. Viral antigen can be detected by immunohistochemistry.

No specific therapy has been studied in controlled trials, although ribavirin has been administered in a series of patients. Avoiding contact with wild or domestic animals and careful, frequent handwashing are recommended for travelers who cannot bypass areas with potential transmission.

UNDIFFERENTIATED FEBRILE ILLNESSES

Colorado Tick Fever

Colorado tick fever is a coltivirus infection transmitted in the western United States, in Canada, and in Mexico by the wood tick *Dermacentor andersoni*. Infections from antigenically related viruses in Asia tentatively have been reclassified as Seadnoviruses. The wood tick's distribution in high plains and woodland habitats at elevations between 4,000 and 10,000 feet defines the virus's distribution in the West; with rare exception, most patients give a history of travel to these locations (Fig. 184.7). More than 90% of cases give a history of tick bite or tick exposure, but occasional infections have occurred after exposure to fomites carrying ticks or after transfusion of infected blood. The virus is maintained transstadially in the tick vector and is amplified among small mammals. Either female or male adult ticks can transmit the infection to humans.

The illness is a prostrating grippe and is biphasic in approximately 50% of patients. An initial phase, occurring 3 to 4 days after a tick bite occurs, consists of fever, intense headache, retroorbital pain, acute myalgia with hyperesthetic,

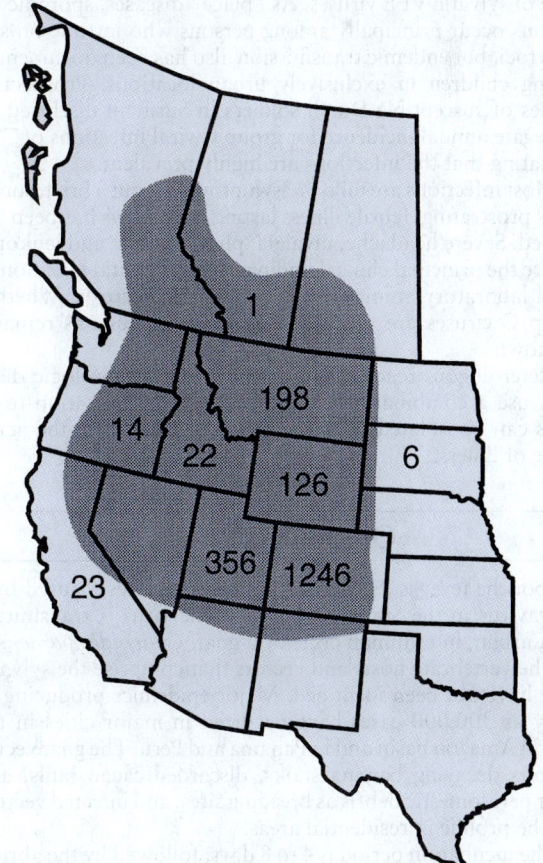

FIGURE 184.7. Distribution of *Dermacentor andersoni* ticks and reported Colorado tick fever cases by state, United States, 1980 to 1996.

painful skin, and lumbar back pain. After defervescence, a 2- to 3-day period of remission may be followed by one or (rarely) more recurrences. Hemorrhage, encephalitis, and death have been reported in children, but an uncomplicated recovery is the rule. Convalescent patients may complain of asthenia for weeks or months.

Lymphopenia occurs in two-thirds of patients with Colorado tick fever and is considered a hallmark of the disease. A moderate thrombocytopenia is a usual occurrence.

The virus infects erythrocyte precursors and circulates peripherally in infected mature erythrocytes. The diagnosis can be made by recovering virus from acute and (occasionally) from convalescent blood, by direct IF examination of the peripheral smear, by PCR analysis of blood, or serologically through ELISA or neutralization assays.

Colorado tick fever cannot be diagnosed reliably from clinical features alone, but a history of tick exposure in enzootic locations in the spring or early summer months should suggest the diagnosis. The absence of respiratory symptoms aids in differentiating Colorado tick fever from other summertime viral fevers. Treatment is supportive. Infected persons should not donate blood until viremia is proved to have cleared. Protective measures include impregnating clothing with permethrin and wearing trousers and long-sleeved, light-colored clothing, which should be inspected frequently to remove adherent ticks.

Group C Bunyavirus Infections

The group C bunyaviruses are comprised of 13 antigenically related viruses occurring chiefly in Central and South America. They are maintained in forested locations among small mammals and mosquitoes, in a pattern similar to the transmission cycle of sylvatic VEE viruses. As "place" diseases, sporadic infections occur principally among persons who intrude on sylvatic foci, but endemic transmission also has been documented among children in exclusively urban locations. Prospective studies of susceptible Dutch soldiers in Surinam disclosed an aggregate annual incidence for group C viral infections of 7%, indicating that the infections are highly prevalent.

Most infections are mild or asymptomatic, but a brief, sometimes prostrating, febrile illness lasting 2 to 7 days has been described. Severe headache, myalgia, photophobia, and leukopenia are the principal clinical findings. Experimental infection of small laboratory animals produces hepatic necrosis. Whether group C viruses are a cause of hepatitis in humans remains unknown.

Heterologous reactions necessitate that the serologic diagnosis use a combination of HI, CF, and neutralization tests. Virus can be isolated from the blood of patients in the acute phase of illness.

Oropouche Fever

Oropouche fever is a generally mild febrile illness caused by a bunyavirus in the Simbu serogroup. The virus is transmitted in an urban, interhuman cycle by a gnat, *Culicoides paraensis*, but the vertebrate hosts and vectors that comprise the sylvatic cycle have not been identified. Major epidemics producing as many as 300,000 cases have occurred in major cities in the central Amazon basin and in Panama and Peru. The gnat vector exploits decaying banana stalks, discarded cacao hulls, and other peridomestic debris as breeding sites, and infected vectors may be prolific in residential areas.

The incubation period is 4 to 8 days, followed by the abrupt onset of fever, muscle aches, chills, headache, photophobia, and (sometimes) nausea, vomiting, and diarrhea. An uncomplicated

aseptic meningitis has been reported in some cases. Leukopenia may be present in the acute phase of illness. An uncomplicated recovery that occurs after 5 to 7 days is the rule, but in some instances, residual asthenia and a recurrence of symptoms after stressful activity have been reported.

A specific diagnosis is made by recovery of virus from acute-phase blood. Serologic diagnosis is obtained through ELISA, HI, CF, or neutralization tests.

Phlebotomus or Sandfly Fever

Among the 35 phleboviruses in the family Bunyaviridae, three are important agents of human disease in the Mediterranean littoral and Central Asia. Sandfly fever Sicilian (SFS) and Naples (SFN) viruses caused large epidemics in World War II and remain prevalent agents of endemic infections from June to November in some areas of the Mediterranean, northern Africa, and as far east as India and Pakistan. In Europe, economic development and large-scale malaria control programs led to marked declines in the transmission of SFS and SFN viruses, whereas cases of aseptic meningitis caused by Toscana virus infections recently have been recognized to be prevalent throughout the Mediterranean littoral, leading to numerous cases of illness in residents and travelers to Spain, Cyprus, and Italy. Several sandfly-borne viruses of Central and South America produce nonspecific febrile illnesses. Although cases of clinical illness have been reported infrequently, high seroprevalence rates indicate that infections may be widespread.

SFS and SFN viruses are transmitted and maintained vertically, chiefly by *Phlebotomus papatasii* sandflies, and Toscana virus by *P. perniciosus*; horizontal transmission among vertebrates contributes to viral amplification. The short flight range of the vectors restricts the foci where risk of infection is encountered.

Sandfly fever is a remarkably brief, self-limited illness (i.e., lasting 2 to 4 days) that is typified by headache, myalgia, back pain, photophobia, and (sometimes) nausea and vomiting. Conjunctivitis and leukopenia are hallmarks of the disease. Even milder illnesses and subclinical infections are usual in children. Although Toscana virus usually produces an asymptomatic infection or mild febrile illness in children, it frequently leads to self-limited aseptic meningitis or, less frequently, encephalitis. The virus is the leading cause of pediatric CNS infection in areas of Italy. One atypical encephalitis case was accompanied by diffuse rash, lymphadenopathy, hepatomegaly, and epidymo-orchitis and was further complicated by DIC and only partial recovery with hydrocephalus.

Infections are diagnosed by viral isolation from acute blood or serologically through ELISA or by neutralization tests. Toscana CNS infections are diagnosed readily by PCR examination of CSF. A citronella extract is the most effective repellent against sandflies, although formulations containing DEET also are effective. Sandflies feed at night, but their small size renders ordinary screens and bed nets ineffective. Finer mesh screens or permethrin-impregnated netting or clothing is required.

ARTHROPATHIES

Chikungunya

Chikungunya (its descriptive name derived from an Acholi verb meaning "to bend up") is an acute mosquito-borne viral arthropathy transmitted in Asia, the Middle East, and Africa. The etiologic agent is an alphavirus related antigenically to the virus causing O'nyong nyong fever. In Africa, the virus is transmitted among forest monkeys and mosquitoes in a cycle analogous to that of yellow fever, resulting in an endemic pattern of human infections and occasional epidemics. The viral transmission cycle in Asia is characterized poorly, and the disease is noted in periodic, often dramatic, epidemics caused by person-to-person spread by *Ae. aegypti* mosquitoes. The intermittent epidemics, frequently occurring in cities, have resulted in attack rates as high as 20% to 50%, with a sharp age-related risk reflecting the interval since the last outbreak. The viral reservoir between these long cycles of epidemic transmission is unknown. Similar *Ae. aegypti*–borne epidemic transmission also occurs in Africa. A clinically similar illness caused by O'nyong nyong virus is transmitted in sub-Saharan Africa and was seen last in widespread outbreaks in Kenya and Uganda.

After a sudden onset of fever, malaise, and generalized musculoskeletal pain, the illness evolves with a disabling symmetric polyarthritis, affecting chiefly the metacarpophalangeal joints, wrists, elbows, shoulders, knees, ankles, and metatarsal joints. Redness and swelling of the pinnae occur in some patients. Joint pain may be so severe that patients cannot work or are forced to hobble or even to lie stiff and motionless, guarding against any movement of their joints. Conjunctivitis, generalized adenopathy, and a maculopapular, often pruritic, rash may be detected. Polyarthropathy with joint pain, stiffness, and swelling may persist in a fluctuating course for 6 to 18 months, although resolution without deformity is the rule. Infrequently, the acute illness is complicated by hemorrhagic fever with severe gastrointestinal, mucosal, and petechial bleeding and, in some cases, shock. In one series, convulsions occurred in a large proportion of affected infants, and encephalitis was suspected. Other cases with extraocular muscle palsy and polyneuropathy also suggest the possibility of neurologic involvement.

Clinically, chikungunya resembles O'nyong nyong, dengue, and Sindbis and WN fevers, which are transmitted in the same geographic distribution and cause similar syndromes of fever with musculoskeletal pain. Lymphadenopathy and frank joint involvement in chikungunya differentiates it from dengue, which produces principally myalgia. The onset of chikungunya may be more sudden, the period of fever somewhat shorter (2 to 4 days versus 3 to 7 days in dengue), and recovery (except for persistent arthritic complaints) more rapid than in dengue.

A slight leukocytosis and thrombocytopenia may be present, and C-reactive protein may be elevated. A specific diagnosis is made by isolating virus from an acute blood sample or by detecting specific IgM or a rise in HI or CF antibody titers. Virus may be recovered more easily from infants who are younger than 6 months and who sustain significantly higher viremia levels (although their illnesses are not more severe).

The treatment is symptomatic, emphasizing rest and nonsteroidal antiinflammatory compounds. Long-term prognosis is good. An experimental attenuated vaccine has been evaluated in early-phase clinical trials.

Ross River Arthropathy

Recurrent epidemics of polyarthritis in Australia had been described since 1926, but their etiology was not resolved until 1963, with the isolation of an alphavirus, named Ross River virus, from *Aedes vigilax* mosquitoes. The disease is endemic in Australia, Tasmania, New Guinea, and New Caledonia; in 1979 and 1980, it was introduced and became epidemic on Fiji, Samoa, Tonga, and the Cook Islands. More than 2,000 cases are reported annually in Australia, mainly along the coast and in the north of the country, with frequent outbreaks occurring along the inland rivers. Although cases are recognized throughout the year in eastern Australia, transmission occurs principally in the austral summer and autumn (January to May) after the seasonal densities of *Cx. annulirostris* and *O. vigilax*, the principal mosquito vectors, respectively, in inland and coastal

locations. The virus is transmitted in a cycle among mammals and marsupials, but interhuman transmission may contribute to epidemic spread in heavily populated areas in Australia, as occurred in the South Pacific, where *Aedes polynesiensis* was the epidemic vector. Frequently, cases are reported in returning travelers. A clinically indistinguishable disease caused by Barmah Forest virus, also a mosquito-borne alphavirus, occurs in an overlapping geographic and temporal distribution, but at a lower frequency, indicating as yet undissected differences in its transmission cycle.

Approximately 90% of infections are inapparent, resulting in a high accrual of immunity in persons living in endemic areas and a corresponding declining susceptibility of clinical illness in persons older than 40 years of age. Cases are recognized more often in women, and children are more likely to have a mild or asymptomatic infection. Increased frequencies of HLA-DR7 and Gma+X+b+ phenotypes have been reported among patients with Ross River polyarthritis.

The incubation period typically is 7 to 9 days (range, 2 to 21 days). The illness consists of constitutional symptoms; symmetric polyarthritis, especially of the wrists, knees, ankles, and small joints of the hands and fingers; and a morbilliform rash. Malaise, fatigue, and myalgia are the predominant initial symptoms, accompanied by diarrhea, headache, neck stiffness, pharyngitis, and tender lymphadenopathy in some cases, but by fever in only one-half of patients. Similarly, rash may be absent in one-third of cases, and its appearance with respect to symptoms is highly variable, occurring weeks before or afterward and sometimes with recurrences. Typically, the exanthem consists of small 1- to 5-mm papules, distributed on the trunk and limbs, that occasionally become vesicular or purpuric. An enanthem may be present. Joint pain, stiffness, and immobility are the principal symptoms prompting clinical attention. The affected joints, in decreasing order of frequency, are wrists, knees, ankles, small joints of the hands and fingers, elbows, toes and tarsal joints, shoulders, hips, and spine. Pathology varies, ranging from slight stiffness and warmth to significant impairments of function with redness and swelling, mimicking gout. Occasionally, periarticular and tendon swelling lead to nerve entrapment and paresthesias. Pain, limitation of movement, and swelling are self-limited (mean, 6 weeks) but may persist for more than 6 months in one-half of cases, with greater and lengthier periods of incapacity in older patients. Permanent deformity has not been reported.

Anecdotal cases of CNS infection or glomerulonephritis have been described as complications of both Ross River and Barmah Forest virus infection. The possibility of congenital infection without deformity has been reported.

The differential diagnosis includes infections from Barmah forest, Kunjin, Gan Gan, Stratford, and Edge Hill viruses (Australian arboviruses); chikungunya, dengue, *Mycoplasma pneumoniae*; rubella, parvovirus, EBV, hepatitis A and B, and other viruses causing symmetric polyarthritis; and rat-bite fever, Henoch-Schönlein purpura, serum sickness, rheumatoid arthritis, and enteroarthritis.

A peripheral leukopenia with atypical lymphocytes may be present, and usually the sedimentation rate is elevated. The joint fluid is clear, with a mononuclear cytosis of 1,500 to 15,000 per milliliter. Although viral antigen has been found in mononuclear cells, virus never has been recovered from joint fluid. No signs of immune complex formation or complement activation have been detected, and T-cell proliferative responses have not been correlated with disease activity.

A specific diagnosis can be made serologically by detecting specific IgM in an acute serum by demonstrating a fourfold rise in HI titer or by amplifying genomic products in acute blood by PCR. Symptomatic treatment with nonsteroidal antiinflammatory drugs is recommended. Personal protective measures are advised to reduce risk of infection (e.g., avoidance, applications of repellents, and protective clothing); an inactivated vaccine is undergoing evaluation.

Sindbis Virus Infection

Sindbis virus, a mosquito-borne alphavirus, is distributed widely in Africa, Asia, parts of Europe, and Australia, where it causes sporadic self-limited cases of febrile illness with headache, polyarthropathy, and a papulovesicular rash. Cases in Nordic regions (i.e., Ockelbo fever in Sweden, Pogosta disease in Finland, Karelian fever in Russia) and west and central Africa (i.e., Babanki viral infection) have been attributed to variants of the virus.

The virus is transmitted in an enzootic cycle among birds and *Culex* mosquitoes, *C. univittatus* and *C. neavei* in Africa, *C. tritaeniorhynchus* in Asia, and *C. annulirostris* in Australia. In northern Europe, *C. torrentium* and *Culiseta morsitans* are the principal enzootic vectors, but sylvatic *Aedes* species that feed both on birds and humans function as bridging vectors. Cases in Scandinavia occur on a 7 year cycle mainly from July to October among persons entering mosquito-infested woodlands to pick berries and mushrooms. Serological surveys in Finland have disclosed evidence of infection in 11% of the population. In South Africa, cases occur during the austral summer from December to April.

Often, the presenting features are joint pains or rash, with a mild fever appearing later or not at all. Headache, muscle aches, and lassitude are other early symptoms. The exanthem is variable with discrete macules, papules, and (less often) painful or pruritic vesicles appearing in crops over the course of several days and resolving in 5 to 10 days. The rash appears chiefly over the trunk and limbs, including the palms and soles; less often, the face and oral mucosa also are involved.

The second characteristic feature of the infection is polyarthritis, which appears concurrently or within a few days of the occurrence of the exanthem. Pain in large joints, especially in ankles and knees, may be disabling, and the hips, wrists, shoulders, fingers, and neck also may be affected. Redness, swelling, and a serous effusion may develop. Usually, joint symptoms resolve within weeks, although arthralgia persists in one-third of cases for 3 to 4 years. Hemorrhagic manifestations were reported in one case.

The diagnosis is made serologically by demonstrating specific IgM in acute serum or a rise in specific HI or CF antibody while being cognizant of cross-reactions. Virus rarely has been recovered from vesicular fluid.

Nonsteroidal antiinflammatory drugs provide symptomatic relief from joint symptoms. Mosquito repellents are recommended for persons entering northern European woodlands during the summer and other areas with enzootic transmission.

FEBRILE EXANTHEMS

Dengue Fever

Worldwide, dengue fever ranks as the most common arboviral infection and, in the form of dengue hemorrhagic fever (DHF), it causes tens of thousands of life-threatening infections annually in the tropics, principally in children. Four dengue virus serotypes (types 1 to 4) circulate in tropical America, Africa, Asia, Australia, and the Pacific. Infections are transmitted from person to person through the agency of *Ae. aegypti* (the principal mosquito vector worldwide) and (rarely) *Ae. albopictus* (an accessory vector in Asia). Epidemics arise in susceptible populations living in areas with competent vectors after the

virus is introduced by viremic persons. In areas where transmission is endemic, dengue is principally a disease of children, and infections occur in almost 100% of children before they reach age 12 years of age. In the absence of previous immunity, when new virus strains are introduced, or among travelers from nonendemic areas, infections occur in all age groups.

Cross-immunity among the serotypes is limited, and sequential infection predisposes to the risk for developing DHF, which is manifested by hemorrhagic phenomena and shock. Thus, the cocirculation of multiple dengue serotypes in a population establishes risk for endemic DHF, an epidemiologic pattern that is extant in Southeast Asia and that has emerged in Central and South America. Low avidity, heterotypic cross-reactive antibodies increase Fc receptor-mediated viral entry into mononuclear cells and augment viral replication (immune enhancement). The resulting exaggerated immune and cytokine response, with elaboration of vasoactive mediators, leads to capillary endothelial dysfunction, hemorrhages, and plasma leakage, producing shock. A polymorphism in the CD 209 promotor for dendritic cell-specific ICAM-3 grabbing nonintegrin, a receptor for dengue virus, white race, good nutrition, asthma, and other chronic diseases have been associated with increased risk for acquiring DHF, emphasizing the underlying role of host factors in DHF pathogenesis. DHF also can occur in primary dengue viral infections, particularly with types 1 and 3, indicating that factors other than immune enhancement contribute to the pathogenesis of DHF. DHF also occurs in infants in whom increased viral replication is enhanced by circulating, poorly neutralizing maternal antibodies.

The incubation period is 3 to 7 days. Classic dengue is a grippe-like, often biphasic illness that cannot be differentiated easily from influenza, measles, and other acute infections. Fever, muscle and joint pains, chills, headache, and lumbar back pain are the most common early symptoms, but, in comparison to other childhood febrile illnesses, dengue is accompanied more frequently by anorexia, nausea, and vomiting. Facial flushing is characteristic; in fair-skinned persons, a centrifugally spreading morbilliform rash may be detected late in the illness. Usually, illness resolves in 3 to 7 days and sometimes is complicated by minor hemorrhagic phenomena such as epistaxis and minor gingival, gastrointestinal, and vaginal mucosal bleeding. A positive tourniquet test and lower platelet, total leukocyte, and absolute monocyte and neutrophil counts—reflecting marrow suppression arising from dengue viral infection of bone marrow dendritic and adventitial reticular cells—are found more frequently in dengue than in other febrile illnesses; however, their discriminatory power is low. Anicteric hepatitis is a common occurrence, with transaminase levels exceeding 400 U/L in 10% of cases.

The foregoing self-limited hemorrhagic phenomena should be differentiated from the hemorrhagic-shock syndrome, which is characterized by severe generalized bleeding and sudden plasma leakage, pleural and peritoneal effusions, and, in advanced cases, hypovolemic shock with a case-fatality ratio of 1% to 5%. The onset of hypotension may be precipitous and typically occurs with defervescence. Poor perfusion results in pallor, cool extremities, and a thready pulse. Frequently, the liver is tender and enlarged, petechiae and purpuric bruising may appear, and bleeding internally and from venipuncture sites may occur. The interval of vascular instability may be as brief as 24 to 48 hours, and it reverses spontaneously. Onset is preceded clinically by thrombocytopenia, often to a level of <100,000 cells/mm^3 and by elevations of interferon-gamma, tumor necrosis factor–alpha, and soluble CD8 and interleukin-2 receptors above those seen in patients with dengue fever, consistent with an exaggerated TH1 cell response. Whereas a slightly higher hematocrit (reflecting hemoconcentration), lower platelet count and higher aspartate aminotransferase occur in patients who eventually develop DHF, these laboratory markers are not sufficiently specific or sensitive to be useful discriminants predicting DHF.

Occasionally, dengue can present with signs of CNS infection or encephalopathy, acute upper gastrointestinal bleeding, splenic rupture, or hemoptysis. The hemorrhagic manifestations of dengue can complicate late stages of pregnancy, and, in several cases, congenital infection has resulted in severe neonatal dengue with vascular instability, respiratory distress, and hemorrhages. Consideration should be given to cesarean delivery to minimize the risk of CNS hemorrhages occurring in infected infants.

Classic dengue is self-limited and is treated symptomatically with acetaminophen and bed rest. Where multiple dengue serotypes cocirculate with an attendant risk for DHF, aggressive clinical and laboratory monitoring, including early radiographic monitoring for pleural effusion, is indicated to identify DHF in its early stages. Sensitive clinical monitoring and supportive fluid and cardiovascular support have been shown to reduce DHF mortality from 25% to less than 0.5%. Ringer's lactate is indicated for initial fluid resuscitation in moderate shock cases and if a colloidal solution is needed, starch is preferred. Recombinant activated factor VII has been beneficial in controlling active bleeding in DHF.

Simple dengue cannot be differentiated clinically from WN fever, chikungunya, and commonplace viral illnesses. Laboratory diagnosis is essential and can be achieved readily by PCR analysis or by detecting specific IgM in acute serum specimens. Viral isolation to identify the specific viral type is accomplished easily in mosquito cell culture and is useful epidemiologically. Serologic testing of paired sera through HI, CF, and indirect measurements of IgG through ELISA or FA can be informative, but in areas where dengue and other flaviviral infections are endemic, cross-reactions among dengue serotypes and with other flaviviruses can interfere with interpretation.

The reduction of *Ae. aegypti* breeding sites in residential areas has been advocated as the key to community-wide dengue control. Common items that can hold water, such as flower pots, pet water dishes, barrels, and discarded tires and other debris are exploited by the vector. Public health campaigns aim to reduce the number of potential breeding containers and, in areas where drinking water is stored, to encourage the simple expedient of covering storage containers. Larvicides provide supplementary control. In the event of an epidemic, emergency ultra-low-volume applications of adulticides have been used, although the efficacy of this intervention is not proved. Experimental vaccines are being evaluated in human trials. Individuals can protect themselves by wearing repellents, staying in screened or air-conditioned locations, and using indoor insecticidal sprays.

Monkeypox

Human monkeypox is a severe systemic exanthem, clinically resembling smallpox and occurring as a sporadic zoonosis in rural rain forest villages of western and central Africa. The disease is caused by monkeypox virus, an orthopoxvirus transmitted to humans by inhalation of or mucocutaneous contact with infectious secretions of infected rodents. Serosurveys have implicated squirrels and other small mammals (e.g., *Funisciurus* and *Heliosciurus* species) as animal reservoirs, but details of the transmission cycle are poorly defined. Secondary person-to-person transmission occurs by contact and droplets and possibly small-particle aerosols, with an incubation period of approximately 12 days, similar to smallpox (range, 7 to 19 days). In early reports, secondary human-to-human spread accounted for approximately 28% of cases, and tertiary and quaternary chains of transmission were rare occurrences. With waning smallpox vaccine-induced immunity following cessation of vaccinia vaccination programs, secondary transmission has accounted for 75% of cases—occurring in as many as eight generations, although no evidence indicated that the virus could sustain itself in the human population without continued reintroductions from the wild. In contrast to this experience, however, in a U.S. outbreak that occurred after an introduction of infected African animals in 2003, none of the 81 cases was attributed to secondary transmission (i.e., all could be linked to direct animal contact).

In areas with endemic transmission, human monkeypox is predominantly a disease of children. The median age of patients is approximately 10 years, although one-fourth of patients are older than 15 years. A prodrome of fever accompanied by severe headache, backache, general malaise, vomiting, and prostration is followed a few days later by a centrifugally spreading rash that appears first on the face and may involve the palms and soles. As in smallpox, the lesions develop more or less simultaneously and evolve at the same rate, passing through stages of macules, papules, vesicles, and pustules before umbilication, drying, and desquamation, 3 weeks later. Usually, lesions are 0.5 cm in diameter and vary from a very few to several thousand; although lesions are more superficial than those from smallpox, residual pocks may mark the face. Oral lesions and retropharyngeal swelling can interfere with swallowing and breathing; some cases have been complicated by encephalitis. Pronounced lymphadenopathy is a principal differentiating feature from smallpox. The disease is most likely to be confused with chickenpox, however, despite the latter's centripetal pleomorphic rash. The proportion of fatal cases has ranged from 3.5% to 10%, but no cases were fatal in the U.S. outbreak.

Isolation of virus and viral PCR detection from lesions remain the gold standards for diagnosis of acute cases. Serologic diagnosis is problematic, but antibodies can be detected with varying accuracy by neutralization assays, HI, or new-generation Western blots and peptide ELISAs. Vaccination with vaccinia virus (i.e., smallpox vaccination) is protective and also is recommended in postexposure prophylaxis, preferably within 4 days. The therapeutic efficacy of cidofovir is unknown. Contact and droplet-based precautions should be used to prevent transmission in hospital settings. Preventive measures include restricting contact with and raw ingestion of wild-caught game (especially contact that may lead to scratching or biting) and washing hands after contact with such animals.

Suggested Readings

Anonymous. Notice to readers update: management of patients with suspected viral hemorrhagic fever-United States. *MMWR* 1995;44:474.

Feigin RD, Cherry JD, Demmler GJ, Kaplan SL, eds. *Textbook of pediatric infectious diseases*, 5th ed. Philadelphia: Saunders, 2004.

Fields BN, Howley PM, Griffin DE, et al., eds. *Field's virology*, 4th ed. New York: 2001.

Keystone JS, Kozarsky PE, Freedman DO, et al., eds. *Travel medicine*. St. Louis: Mosby, 2004.

Richman DD, Whitley RJ, Hayden FG. *Clinical virology*, 2nd ed. New York: Saunders, 2003.

CHAPTER 185 ■ CORONAVIRUSES

ROBERT L. ATMAR

Coronaviruses (CVs) account for 5% to 35% of all upper respiratory tract infections worldwide and are second to the rhinoviruses as a cause of the common cold in children and adults. CVs also have been implicated in lower respiratory tract disease of children and adults, in gastroenteritis, and, possibly, in central nervous system (CNS) disorders. A newly recognized illness, severe acute respiratory syndrome (SARS), is caused by a CV that appears to have originated in animals (a zoonotic illness). The CDC provides the latest information on SARS on the SARS website, www.cdc.gov/ncidod/sars/.

CAUSATIVE AGENT

Human coronaviruses (HCVs) were isolated first in human embryonic trachea organ culture. These agents and other CVs isolated from animals were characterized by electron microscopy as large, pleomorphic, spherical or elliptical, enveloped RNA viruses with a diameter of 80 to 200 nm. The envelope displays distinctive 20-nm long, petal-shaped projections that produce a solar corona appearance. The RNA genome is surrounded by a nucleoprotein that forms a helical nucleocapsid just beneath the envelope. Major antigens are the nucleocapsid and two or three envelope proteins. Based on antigenic relatedness, human isolates now are grouped into at least three serotypes: HCV-229E, HCV-OC43, and the SARS coronavirus. Two additional human strains, NL63 and HKU1, have recently been identified. The cell receptor for HCV-229E is human aminopeptidase N (CD13). Angiotensin-converting enzyme 2 is a functional receptor for the SARS coronavirus. The cellular receptor for HCV-OC43 has not been identified.

EPIDEMIOLOGY

HCVs are worldwide in distribution. Estimates of prevalence in any population vary with the sensitivity of serologic tests. Using HCV-229E and HCV-OC43 as antigens, regardless of the test used, 50% to 60% of adults older than 30 years of age have antibody to both serotypes. The most sensitive tests show prevalence rates approaching 90% to 100%. On the other hand, the SARS CV was recognized first to infect humans in southern China in late 2002; infection spread from China to other parts of southeast Asia and the rest of the world in 2003. Seroprevalence studies show no evidence of past infection in humans, suggesting that this virus has been introduced only recently into the human population.

Most HCV infections occur from midwinter to early spring. One serotype may predominate for 1 year, then may exhibit low activity for 1 year or more. Exceptions to these generalizations exist (e.g., studies in Germany and England showed the viruses to be present all during year, and a Seattle study found that both serotypes sometimes circulate in a population simultaneously).

HCVs demonstrate some age specificity. Geometric mean antibody titers tend to increase directly with age. In a Seattle study, children averaged one HCV infection per year, approximately three times as many as their parents. Many individuals experienced reinfection with the same virus, but in all cases, serial infections by the same virus were separated by at least 8 months. Thus, short-term immunity against homologous virus reinfection, but not against reinfection by the other serotypes, appears to exist. Whether infection with the SARS CV leads to short- or long-term immunity is not known.

Subclinical infection with HCVs is a common finding in healthy children and adults. In the Seattle study, the antibody titer in 40% of children and 36% of adults increased significantly without evidence of illness. Similarly, in an 8.5-year surveillance of healthy older children in Atlanta, only 38% (63 of 168) of children with HCV-229E seroconversion and 47% (44 of 93) of those with HCV-OC43 seroconversion reported any illness. Subclinical infection with the SARS CV appears to be an uncommon occurrence, although the frequency of asymptomatic infection is being evaluated.

PATHOGENESIS

HCVs appear to be transmitted via the respiratory route. Volunteers have been infected readily through an intranasal inoculation of virus. A natural transmission experiment in human volunteers using HCV-229E showed aerosol transmission may be the most common means, but hand-to-face transmission has not been excluded. The SARS CV is transmitted primarily by contact, although aerosol transmission probably also occurs. Other routes of CV transmission have not been documented in humans, but animal CVs can be spread by the fecal-oral route, and the SARS CV is excreted in stool.

In human volunteers, the incubation period of HCV colds ranges from 1 to 5 days, and for the SARS CV, the incubation period is as long as 10 days. HCVs replicate in the upper respiratory tract, are shed in nasal washings, and reach detectable levels at onset of symptoms. Illness generally lasts 6 to 7 days, but it can persist for 18 days. The SARS CV replicates in the lower respiratory tract, and peak titers are not detected until 7 to 10 days after the onset of symptoms.

Reinfection with HCVs is a common occurrence. Studies of children in Tecumseh, Michigan, and in Atlanta, Georgia, show a high rate of reinfection in individuals with prior antibodies. In addition, antibody did not appear to modify the severity of clinical illness. As many as 50% of individuals with symptomatic HCV infections do not have diagnostic increases in antibody titer.

The quantity of antibody seems related to protection. A study from England shows that individuals with high concentrations of serum-neutralizing antibodies and specific nasal IgA antibodies before challenge had fewer infections, reduced symptoms, and shortened durations of virus shedding. Studies also show that antigenic variability of HCV-OC43–related and HCV-229E-related strains affects the level of protection; immunity to a homotypic challenge seems to last at least a year, but immunity to heterotypic strains is slight. Thus, strain-specific antibody, high levels of serum-neutralizing antibodies, and specific secretory IgA antibodies all probably play protective roles but still may provide only transient immunity.

CLINICAL MANIFESTATIONS AND COMPLICATIONS

Upper Respiratory Disease

HCVs cause typical colds similar to those caused by rhinoviruses, but with less cough and more malaise and nasal discharge. Sore throat, cough, malaise, and headache are present in approximately 50% of adults, 20% of whom have fevers. Cervical adenitis, muscle aches, and rash are less common findings. Clinical findings in children also are typical of colds; however, manifestations frequently are more severe. In a study of Atlanta children, 40% had fevers higher than 37.6°C, and one-third reported having cervical adenitis.

Lower Respiratory Disease

In children, HCV infections are associated with asthma attacks, pneumonia, and bronchiolitis. When HCVs have been sought, they have been the second most common respiratory virus (after rhinovirus) to be associated with wheezing episodes in children older than age 2 years. A few cases of pneumonia in adults and immunocompromised patients have been reported. The clearest association of HCV infection with lower respiratory tract disease in adults is with chronic obstructive pulmonary disease.

The SARS coronavirus causes a lower respiratory tract illness that is associated with fever, cough, pulmonary infiltrates, and respiratory failure. Disease in the initial epidemic was recognized most commonly in adults. Disease in children seems to be milder than that in adults, although severe illness (respiratory failure) in children can occur.

Gastroenteritis

CVs are associated with diarrheal diseases in mammals, especially newborns. In 1975, coronavirus-like particles (CVLPs) were found by electron microscopy (EM) in stools from children and adults with nonbacterial gastroenteritis. However, in subsequent studies, CVLPs were found with equal frequency in asymptomatic individuals. CVLPs are difficult to propagate *in vitro*, and whether some EM reports of CVLPs represent true virus particles is debatable. Controversy on the etiologic role of HCVs as enteric pathogens is ongoing. The SARS coronavirus is present in the stool of infected persons and can cause watery diarrhea later in the course of the respiratory illness.

The most convincing association of CVLPs with human enteric disease is with necrotizing enterocolitis in neonates and diarrheal disease in children. In Arizona, CVLPs were found by EM in 49 of 126 children with diarrhea. Of these patients, 88% were younger than 2 years old and 71% were younger than 1 year old. Ages ranged from 1 month to 12 years. Peak months for occurrence of illness were September through January, and median duration of illness was 7 days. Population characteristics, symptoms, and duration of illness were similar to those seen with rotaviruses. Diarrhea occurred in 94%, vomiting in 51%, fever in 63%, and occult blood in stools in 18%, and 18% had at least one other enteric pathogen present. No grossly bloody stools were noted. Treatment should center around maintaining fluid and electrolyte balance, as for rotaviruses and other viral-caused gastroenteritis.

Central Nervous System Disease

Murine CVs JHM and A59 can produce acute encephalomyelitis, subacute demyelinating encephalomyelitis, or chronic asymptomatic demyelinating disease in mice. In humans, viruses are considered possible etiologic agents of multiple sclerosis (MS). In 1976, CVLPs were identified by EM in tissues from patients with MS. Correlations of MS with upper respiratory infections and HCV-229E infections further stimulate hypotheses of an etiologic role of HCV in this disease; however, the significance of these findings is controversial. Some studies have used *in situ* hybridization and reverse transcription-polymerase chain reaction (RT-PCR) to detect CV RNA in significantly higher proportions of patients with MS than in controls. Thus, the possible causative role of CVs in human CNS disease continues to be an intriguing, but unresolved, conjecture.

DIAGNOSIS

Four approaches are used in establishing the diagnosis of HCV infections. First, isolating and identifying HCVs in cell and organ culture is difficult and limited to a few research laboratories. Virus often must be detected by EM. Second, serodiagnosis relies on serum neutralization, hemagglutination inhibition (HCV-OC43 only), complement fixation, indirect fluorescent antibody, and enzyme-linked immunosorbent assay (ELISA); ELISA tests provide the most sensitive results. Third, viral antigens in clinical specimens are detected using immunofluorescence and ELISA. The ELISA test is sensitive and may require only a single clinical sample. Fourth, the most recent approach is the detection of viral nucleic acids using either labeled, virus-specific probes in hybridization assays or nucleic acid amplification through RT-PCR. All these approaches also work for the SARS CV, although isolation should be attempted only under biosafety level 3 conditions. None of these methods is sensitive for SARS CV during the first week of illness.

PREVENTION AND THERAPY

Successful prevention of HCV infection is not imminent. High reinfection rates, limited protective value of circulating antibody, unidentified viral types, and difficulty in propagating the organism in the laboratory render providing prevention by vaccination unlikely. Some success has been found with recombinant interferon-alpha nasal sprays.

No effective treatment for HCV infections is known. The role of vitamin C is controversial, and the use of aspirin should be avoided to prevent possible development of Reye syndrome.

Suggested Readings

Arbour N, Day R, Newcombe J, et al. Neuroinvasion by human coronaviruses. *J Virol* 2000;74:8913.

Bitnun A, Allen U, Heurter H, et al. Children hospitalized with severe acute respiratory syndrome-related illness in Toronto. *Pediatrics* 2003;112:e261.

Callow KA, Parry HF, Sergeant M, et al. The time course of the immune response to experimental coronavirus infection of man. *Epidemiol Infect* 1990;105:435.

Johnston SL, Patterson PK, Sanderson G, et al. Community study of role of viral infections in exacerbations of asthma in 9–11 year old children. *Br Med J* 1995;310:1225.

Kaye HS, Dowdle WR. Seroepidemiologic survey of coronavirus (strain 229E) infections in a population of children. *Am J Epidemiol* 1975;101:238.

McIntosh K. Coronaviruses and toroviruses. In: Feigin RD, Cherry JD, Demmler GJ, et al., eds. *Textbook of pediatric infectious diseases*, 5th ed. Philadelphia: Saunders, 2004:2379.

Mertsola J, Ziegler T, Ruuskanen O, et al. Recurrent wheezy bronchitis and viral respiratory infections. *Arch Dis Child* 1991;66:124.

Mortensen ML, Ray CG, Payne CM, et al. Coronaviruslike particles in human gastrointestinal disease. *Am J Dis Child* 1985;139:928.

Peiris JSM, Yuen KY, Osterhaus ADME, et al. The severe acute respiratory syndrome. *N Engl J Med* 2003;349:2431.

SARS website. CDC. www.cdc.gov/ncidod/sars/. Last accessed 5/18/05.

Schmidt OW, Allan ID, Cooney MK, et al. Rises in titers of antibody to human coronaviruses OC43 and 229E in Seattle families during 1975–1979. *Am J Epidemiol* 1986;123:862.

Turner RB, Felton A, Kosak K, et al. Prevention of experimental coronavirus colds with intranasal alpha-2b interferon. *J Infect Dis* 1986;154:443.

CHAPTER 186 ■ RHINOVIRUSES

ROBERT L. ATMAR

Rhinoviruses (RVs) cause approximately 30% to 50% of all acute respiratory illness. RVs are associated primarily with the common cold, but they also may be involved in bronchitis, sinusitis, pneumonia, and acute exacerbations of asthma.

The first recognized RV was isolated in 1954; now, at least 102 serotypes have been identified. The genus name was coined in 1963 to reflect the usual prominent nasal involvement. The RVs are one of four genera of human pathogens in the picornavirus family; the other genera include various enteroviruses (polioviruses, coxsackieviruses, echoviruses), parechoviruses, and hepatitis A (hepatovirus). Like the other picornaviruses, RVs are small (30 nm), nonenveloped (therefore, resistant to lipid solvents), and icosahedral (20-sided); they possess a single-stranded RNA genome. Several RVs have been sequenced completely, and they demonstrate much cross-homology among themselves and with the genomes of other picornaviruses. RVs differ from other picornaviruses in that they become noninfectious at a pH of less than 5. For all 102 RV serotypes, three binding sites exist where the virus attaches itself to the receptor on the cell: for 91 serotypes (the major receptor group), the binding site is intercellular adhesion molecule-1 (ICAM-1); for 10 serotypes (the minor receptor group), the binding site is a low-density lipoprotein receptor; and for serotype 87, the binding site is a third, as yet unidentified, molecule. After attaching to a cell, the RV probably is endocytosed within a vesicle, then the RNA is released into the cytoplasm. Viral replication occurs in the cytoplasm, and viruses are released by cell lysis.

RVs have been isolated from natural infections of cattle, chimpanzees, and humans. Human RVs infect only humans and chimpanzees; chimpanzee infections are subclinical.

EPIDEMIOLOGY

RV infections are found in varying degrees year round, but they show the greatest incidence in spring and early autumn. This seasonal pattern occurs worldwide. Several RV serotypes usually circulate simultaneously, frequently coincident with other respiratory viruses. However, all types generally are not equal in prevalence and do not spread to the same degree. In a University of Wisconsin student family study (Eagle Heights, Madison, WI) conducted between 1963 to 1965, 19 RV types were isolated, but only three types (43, 51, and 55) spread beyond the index family, and they spread widely. These dominant RV serotypes occur locally over relatively short periods but they do not extend over large geographic areas or for several years.

Unlike some major respiratory viruses [e.g., parainfluenza types 1 and 3 and respiratory syncytial virus (RSV)], individual RV serotypes seldom recur within a population from year to year. At Eagle Heights, ten RV types were found from 1963 to 1964 and nine types from 1964 to 1965, but only one type (RV15) occurred in both years. Also, RV43 and RV55 were predominant from 1963 to 1964, whereas RV51 prevailed from 1964 to 1965. Similar observations have been made in other epidemiologic studies.

The incidence of RV infections is highest in infants and lowest in older individuals. In Seattle, RV infection rates of 0.59 per person-year were found in family members with and without symptoms. Rates ranged from 0.8 to 1.2 for children aged 0 to 5 years to 0.2 to 0.3 for adults older than 20 years. Women of childbearing age, however, showed rates 1.2 to 1.5 times higher than those of men. The true incidence of RV infections probably is higher than reported, because RV diagnostic tests often are not very sensitive.

Prevalence studies show RV antibodies begin to appear early, increase throughout childhood and adolescence, peak in early adulthood, and then stabilize for years. In Charlottesville, Virginia, fewer than 10% of young children had serum antibodies to any of 56 RV types tested, whereas adults had antibodies to approximately 50%.

Transmission

Schoolchildren are the most important reservoir of RVs; home and school are locations of the highest rate of transmission. Dissemination within susceptible family members averages approximately 50% and, within a schoolroom, ranges from 0% to 50%. Long-term association with individuals with RV infections may be required for transmission to occur. Even then, transmission rates approach only 50%. Thus, short-term contacts such as occur when shopping, attending movies, visiting friends, and visiting a physician's waiting room are reasonably risk-free. However, transmission rates may be higher among young children in day-care facilities, where all respiratory viruses may spread readily.

Because RVs often seem to disseminate slowly, the route of transmission is important. RVs can be transmitted either by large droplet aerosol or by direct contact; the relative importance of these two routes remains an open question. Blocking transmission in various habitats such as the schoolroom and home may be possible. Using an experimental epidemiologic model featuring natural RV16 transmission among human volunteers, researchers were able to stop RV16 transmission with virucidal facial tissues. More practically, careful handwashing, especially around young children, should be utilized as a means to interrupt transmission.

PATHOGENESIS

Most infection is presumed to be through the respiratory route, although infection through the conjunctival route has been demonstrated. The incubation period normally is 2 to 3 days. Ciliary dysfunction can predispose to respiratory infection. RVs replicate well in the upper respiratory tract and generally cause rhinorrhea and nasal obstruction. Cough usually is present even in mild RV colds. RVs have been found in the lower bronchi, but no compelling evidence exists of viral replication in the lower respiratory tract.

RVs may be shed in large amounts (1,000 to 1 million infectious particles per milliliter of nasal washing) during the first 2 to 3 days of a cold and may continue to be produced for nearly a month. RVs seem to cause only mild pathologic changes in cells of the respiratory tract, even when producing a marked local response. Local secretion of kinins or other cytokines and chemokines can cause varied symptoms of inflammation. Approximately 24 hours after infection, a sharp increase in nasal IgA secretion occurs. After approximately 1 week, virus-specific antibody, predominantly IgA, appears in the nasal passages, tears, and parotid saliva. Serum antibody, usually IgG, appears at approximately 1 week and peaks at 1 month; however, specific serum antibody may not form in as many as 50% of cases.

The presence of serum antibody correlates positively with immunity, and resistance to infection is related to amount. Few individuals are infected who have homologous serum antibody levels of approximately 1 to 16. The relative importance and specific roles of serum and nasal-secretion antibody, as well as cell-mediated immunity, in protection against RV infection are unsettled. Serum antibody simply may be the indicator of immunity; nasal secretory antibody or cell-mediated immunity may be the active immune component.

Increased psychosocial stress, as measured by a variety of stress indices, is associated with increased suseptibility to infection and clinical disease. On the other hand, the physical-stress exposure to cold is not associated with more frequent rhinovirus infection or illness.

CLINICAL MANIFESTATIONS AND COMPLICATIONS

RV infections in any age group usually cause only mild respiratory tract illnesses (i.e., common colds with simple coryza). Complete recovery usually occurs in 1 or 2 weeks. However, since the discovery of the first RV serotypes, these viruses have been shown to cause serious lower respiratory illness, especially in young children.

Asthma

RVs are important precipitants of wheezy bronchitis or infectious asthma. This relationship was described first in 1973, in England. Since then, many clinical studies have shown RV infection to be associated with asthmatic exacerbations in both children and adults. No specific RV serotypes have been found to be particularly asthmagenic. RVs may be the most important cause of asthma attacks in children older than 1 to 2 years. In some series, more than 50% of wheezing illnesses are associated with a rhinovirus illness.

Other Respiratory Illnesses

RVs are implicated in cases of bronchiolitis, pneumonia, chronic bronchitis, sinusitis, and acute otitis media. Physicians disagree on the role of RVs in severe lower respiratory tract illnesses other than asthma. Nonetheless, in hospitalized infants in Bristol, England, RVs were second in importance to RSV, even in patients with bronchiolitis and pneumonia. In Rochester, New York, and Vienna, Austria, RVs were associated with serious lower respiratory disease in hospitalized infants; RV-caused illnesses could not be differentiated clinically from severe lower tract illnesses attributable to RSV.

Acute otitis media (AOM) primarily is a bacterial disease, but often it is preceded or accompanied by a viral upper respiratory illness. Clear, comprehensive evidence for viral extension from the nasopharynx to the middle ear has been established only recently. Antigen detection techniques identified viruses in 44% of 131 Finnish children with AOM. Twenty-four of these children had viruses in the middle-ear fluid, and only one of the 24 did not have the same viral antigen in both the middle-ear fluid and the nasopharyngeal secretions. From 1987 through 1988, pediatricians in Finland used traditional cell culture methodology to study the role of RVs in children with AOM. Viruses were detected in 42%; RV predominated over RSV by 24% to 13%, respectively. Subsequent studies found that patients in whom AOM was refractory to treatment harbored significantly more viral pathogens than did the controls, suggesting that the presence of viruses in the middle-ear fluids of children with AOM can delay response to antibacterial therapy.

RVs also have been identified in aspirates obtained by direct puncture of maxillary sinuses. When computed tomographic scans of the sinuses were performed in adults with natural colds, radiographic abnormalities (e.g., secretions, air–fluid level) of one or more sinuses were common findings. However, such diagnostic studies are not needed for routine patient care.

DIAGNOSIS

RV infections cause such a wide spectrum of respiratory illness that diagnosing them clinically is not possible. RV infections can be isolated year round, but a seasonal pattern of infection is recognized internationally; many mild to moderate respiratory infections of the spring, summer, and autumn months are caused by RVs. RVs have been found in the absence of symptoms, but only infrequently, at least in industrialized nations. Subclinical shedding from well children in the United States has ranged from 0.8% to 11.0%, whereas rates up to 50% have been measured in some Third-World populations. Nasal specimens are superior to throat swabs for RV isolation. The virus can be isolated relatively easily if details of specimen collection and culture procedures are followed; however, because more than 100 serotypes exist and none is predictably predominant, clinical diagnosis by serologic methods is impractical because it is costly. Use of the polymerase chain reaction (PCR) has increased the identification of RV infections 50- to 200-fold compared with culture alone. No methods currently exist for rapid diagnosis of RV infection.

PREVENTION AND THERAPY

Because of the number of serotypes, the development of a conventional vaccine seems unlikely. Numerous antiviral drugs (interferon-alpha, pleconaril, tremacamra [a soluble ICAM-1], viral protease inhibitors) have been evaluated in clinical trials, but none is available for clinical use. Thus, treatment is directed primarily toward the control of symptoms using sympathomimetic agents (e.g., phenylpropanolamine), first generation antihistamines, and mild nonsteroidal antiinflammatory drugs.

Alternative and complementary medications also have been evaluated in the treatment of RV colds. Vitamin C, echinacea, and zinc compounds have been proposed as preventives or treatments for colds. Overall, no clear indication has been established that treatment or prevention of the common cold is affected by these agents, although some trials have suggested a benefit from large doses of vitamin C or the administration of zinc lozenges. However, no data support the use of these agents in children.

Environmental controls under study include virucidal tissues and proper air handling and filtration.

Suggested Readings

Arola M, Ziegler T, Ruuskanen O. Respiratory virus infection as a cause of prolonged symptoms in acute otitis media. *J Pediatr* 1989;116:697.

Atmar RL. Rhinoviruses. In: Feigin RD, Cherry JD, Demmler GJ, et al., eds. *Textbook of pediatric infectious diseases,* 5th ed. Philadelphia: Saunders, 2004:2042.

Dick EC, Jennings LC, Mink KA, et al. Aerosol transmission of rhinovirus colds. *J Infect Dis* 1987;156:442.

Fendrick AM. Viral respiratory infections due to rhinoviruses: current knowledge, new developments. *Am J Ther* 2003;10:193.

Fox JP, Cooney MK, Hall CE, et al. Rhinoviruses in Seattle families, 1975–1979. *Am J Epidemiol* 1985;122:830.

Gwaltney JM Jr, Heinz BA. Rhinovirus. In: Richman DD, Whitley RJ, Hayden FG, eds. *Clinical Virology,* 2nd ed. Washington, DC: ASM Press, 2002:995.

Johnston SL, Patterson PK, Sanderson G, et al. Community study of role of viral infections in exacerbations of asthma in 9–11 year old children. *Br Med J* 1995;310:1225.

Kellner G, Popow-Kraupp T, Kundi M, et al. Clinical manifestations of respiratory tract infections due to respiratory syncytial virus and rhinoviruses in hospitalized children. *Acta Paediatr Scand* 1989;78:390.

Pitkaranta A, Virolainen A, Jero J, et al. Detection of rhinovirus, respiratory syncytial virus, and coronavirus infecitons in acute otitis media by reverse transcriptase polymerase chain reaction. *Pediatrics* 1998;102:291.

Schmidt HJ, Fink RJ. Rhinovirus as a lower respiratory tract pathogen in infants. *Pediatr Infect Dis J* 1991;10:700.

CHAPTER 187 ■ ADENOVIRUSES

JAMES D. CHERRY

Adenoviruses cause a diverse array of diseases in children, most commonly respiratory and gastrointestinal illnesses. Certain clinical manifestations of adenovirus infections are distinctive, although most illnesses are difficult to differentiate from those caused by other viral and bacterial pathogens.

ETIOLOGY

Adenoviruses are DNA viruses; 49 types are known to infect humans. Six subgroups are defined based on biochemical and biophysical criteria. Adenoviruses can be grown in tissue culture cell preparations of human epithelial origin. Exceptions are enteric adenovirus types 40 and 41, which were identified by electron microscopy and grow in Graham 293 cells and the PLC/PRF/5 cell line. Infected tissue cultures have a characteristic cytopathic effect in 1 day to 4 weeks.

EPIDEMIOLOGY

Adenoviral infections occur throughout the world. In temperate climates, sporadic disease occurs year round; epidemic disease commonly occurs in winter, spring, and early summer. Seasonal variation with adenoviral gastroenteritis has not been described.

Transplacental antibody appears to be protective in early infancy. However, when adenoviral infection occurs in the neonate, severe and rarely fatal pulmonary or multiorgan system diseases may occur. Adenoviral infections in children commonly are caused by types 1, 2, 3, and 5. Types 6 and 7 occur slightly less frequently. The incidence of adenoviral infection peaks in children between ages 6 months and 5 years. An increased susceptibility to adenoviruses is reported in neonates and small infants, in immunocompromised patients, and occasionally in male subjects.

The transmission of adenoviruses occurs through small droplets or the fecal-oral route and is facilitated by closed environments. Contaminated swimming pool water has been implicated in the spread of pharyngoconjunctival fever. The incubation period of adenoviruses is between 3 and 7 days. Viruses may be shed from the respiratory tract up to 2 days before and 5 days after clinical symptoms develop. Viruses may be found in the stool for several months. Adenoviruses commonly are isolated from the throat, conjunctiva, and stool.

PATHOGENESIS

The characteristics of adenoviral infections vary with the infecting serotype and the immune status of the host. Infection usually involves the upper respiratory tract and the conjunctivae. Spread to the lower respiratory tract may occur by progression or viremia. Rashes and multiorgan infections also may result from viremia. Swallowed virus is thought to cause gastrointestinal infection. Pathologic changes that occur in self-limited respiratory infections are not well studied. Autopsy material from lethal infections has revealed necrotizing bronchitis, bronchiolitis and pneumonia, focal hepatic necrosis, and cerebral edema with perivascular lymphocytic infiltrates. Characteristic small eosinophilic and larger basophilic intranuclear inclusions are seen in all infected tissues. Severe illnesses with manifestations of septic shock are associated with elevated serum levels of tumor necrosis factor–alpha, interleukin-6, and interleukin-8.

In humans, adenoviruses can cause lytic and latent infections. Oncogenic cell transformation is reported in animals but not in humans.

TABLE 187.1

CLINICAL MANIFESTATIONS OF ADENOVIRAL INFECTIONS BY SEROTYPE AND FREQUENCY

System/Organ	Illness Category	Frequency	Adenoviral Types
Respiratory	Common cold	Rare	1, 2, 3, 5, 7
	Nasopharyngitis, pharyngitis, and tonsillitis*	Common	1[†], 2[†], 3[†], 4, 5[†], 7[†], 7a, 14, 15 (21/H21 + 35)[‡]
	Acute respiratory disease*	Very common	2, 3, 4[†], 5, 7[†], 8, 11, 14, 21
	Acute laryngotracheitis	Occasional	1, 2, 3, 5, 6, 7
	Acute bronchiolitis	Occasional	3, 7, 21
	Pneumonia (civilian population)*	Common	1, 2, 3[†], 4, 5, 7[†], 7a[†], 8, 11, 21[†], (21/H21 + 35)[‡], 35
	Atypical pneumonia in military recruits*	Common	4[†], 7[†], 21
	Pertussis-like syndrome	Rare	1, 2, 3, 5, 12, 19
	Bronchiolitis obliterans	Rare	7, 21
	Unilateral hyperlucent lung	Rare	7, 21
Eye	Acute follicular conjunctivitis*	Common	1, 2, 3, 4, 6, 7, 9, 10, 11, 15, 16, 17, 19, 20, 22, 34, 37
	Pharyngoconjunctival fever*	Common	1, 2[†], 3[†], 4[†], 5, 6, 7[†], 7a[†], 8, 14[†], 37
	Epidemic keratoconjunctivitis*	Occasional	2, 3, 4, 5, 7, 8[†], 10, 11, 13, 14, 15, 16, 17, 19, 23, 29, 37
Skin	Morbilliform and rubelliform exanthem	Occasional	3, 4, 7, 7a
	Roseola-like	Occasional	1, 2
	Stevens-Johnson syndrome	Rare	7
	Petechial exanthem	Rare	7
Genitourinary	Acute hemorrhagic cystitis	Rare	7, 11, 21
	Nephritis	Rare	3, 4, 7a
	Orchitis	Rare	Unknown
	Oculogenital syndrome*	Rare	19, 37
Gastrointestinal	Gastroenteritis*	Common	1, 2, 3[†], 5, 7[†], 11, 12, 15, 17, 31[†], 32, 33, 40[†], 41[†]
	Mesenteric lymphadenitis	Rare	1, 2, 3, 5, 7
	Intussusception	Rare	1, 2, 3, 5, 6, 7
	Appendicitis	Rare	1, 2, 7
	Hepatitis	Rare	1, 2, 3, 5[†], 7 (11 + 35/H11 + 35)[‡]
Heart	Myocarditis	Rare	7, 7a, 21
	Pericarditis	Rare	7
Neurologic	Encephalitis and meningitis	Rare	1, 2, 3, 5, 6, 7, 11, 12, 32
Joint	Arthritis	Rare	7
Auditory	Deafness	Rare	3
Endocrine	Thyroiditis	Rare	Unknown

*Occurs in outbreaks.
[†]Most common.
[‡]Intermediate strain.

CLINICAL MANIFESTATIONS AND COMPLICATIONS

Respiratory Infections

Serologic surveys indicate that 10% of respiratory infections in children are caused by adenoviruses (Table 187.1). Rarely, adenoviruses cause common colds. Usually, respiratory infections with adenoviruses are characterized by fever and pharyngitis. Symptoms that occur with acute adenoviral pharyngitis include malaise, headache, sore throat, cough, cervical adenopathy, abdominal pain, and coryza, especially in the young. Pharyngeal exudates may be thin and spotty or thick and membranous. Laryngotracheitis, bronchitis, pneumonia, and rarely, bronchiolitis may occur concomitantly with pharyngeal disease. Illness of 5 to 7 days' duration occurs commonly, although symptoms may persist for 2 weeks.

Pulmonary infection with adenoviruses can be severe, especially in infants, toddlers, and immunocompromised patients. High fever, dyspnea, wheezes, and rhonchi are present in these cases, and radiography may reveal diffuse infiltrates, hyperin-

flation, lobar atelectasis, and rarely, pleural effusions. Associated symptoms may include seizures, lethargy, vomiting, diarrhea, and conjunctivitis. Manifestations of extrapulmonary involvement, including meningitis, encephalitis, hepatitis, myocarditis, nephritis, and exanthems, may be present. Severe infections result in bronchiectasis, bronchiolitis obliterans, and hyperlucent lung.

Epidemics of adenoviral respiratory disease have been recognized in military populations living in close quarters. The disease, termed *acute respiratory disease* (ARD), is characterized by an acute, febrile, respiratory infection lasting 1 to 4 weeks, with pulmonary involvement occurring in most cases. These epidemics usually are caused by adenovirus types 4 and 7 and, occasionally, by types 3, 11, 14, and 21.

Pertussis-like Syndrome

Adenoviral infections occasionally are associated with illness characterized by paroxysmal cough with associated post-tussive whoop, vomiting, apnea or hypoxemia, and lymphocytosis. The illness often begins with mild coryza without fever.

Convalescence occurs usually in 1 to 3 months. Studies suggest that most and probably all of these pertussis-like illnesses are *Bordetella* infections in which the adenovirus is a coinfecting agent.

Pharyngoconjunctival Fever

The constellation of acute fever, conjunctivitis, coryza, pharyngitis, and cervical adenitis occurring historically in summer epidemics, usually associated with inadequately chlorinated swimming pools, can be ascribed with some certainty to adenoviral infection. Both the bulbar and palpebral conjunctivae are involved. The palpebral conjunctiva may have a granular appearance. Initially, disease may be monocular, although the unaffected eye usually becomes involved. Bacterial superinfection of the conjunctiva is rare, and resolution is complete.

Epidemic Keratoconjunctivitis

Numerous adenoviruses have been found to cause epidemics of keratoconjunctivitis. The most common cause is type 37, and the most severe disease is associated with types 5, 8, and 19. Adenoviral keratoconjunctivitis is nonseasonal; primarily affects adults; and is transmitted by fomites, ophthalmic instruments and solutions, and bodies of fresh water. After 4 days to 2 weeks of incubation, a follicular conjunctivitis develops with symptoms of lacrimation, photophobia, and foreign-body sensation. Hyperemia and edema of the conjunctiva are present, and preauricular adenopathy is a common finding. Approximately one-half of affected persons have rhinitis and pharyngitis. Keratitis with punctate epithelial and sometimes subepithelial lesions develops as the conjunctivitis resolves. Visual disturbances may occur and persist for several years. Similar epidemics of keratoconjunctivitis associated with respiratory and constitutional symptoms have been described in infants and young children.

Skin Manifestations

Several types of adenoviruses cause exanthematous disease, usually an erythematous maculopapular rash. Exanthems of confluent morbilliform, petechial, and Stevens-Johnson syndrome have been reported. Other findings of adenoviral respiratory infection commonly are present.

Genitourinary Manifestations

Hemorrhagic cystitis caused by adenovirus begins acutely with dysuria and frequency; hematuria develops within 24 hours. Occasionally, concomitant suprapubic pain, fever, and upper respiratory tract symptoms are present. Resolution occurs in several days to 2 weeks and appears to be complete. This illness is not seasonal. Boys are affected more frequently than are girls.

Nephritis has been reported in cases of disseminated adenoviral infections and in rare instances with respiratory infections.

Adenoviruses reportedly have been isolated from genital lesions that clinically resemble herpes genitalis and from cervicitis occurring with pharyngoconjunctival fever. Hemolytic-uremic syndrome has been associated with adenoviral infection.

Gastrointestinal Manifestations

The adenoviral types commonly associated with respiratory illnesses also may cause vomiting and diarrhea. Adenovirus types 40 and 41, along with rotavirus, are thought to cause most gastroenteritis in infants and young children. The enteric adenoviruses are identified most easily by electron microscopy or enzyme-linked immunosorbent assay (ELISA) because they do not grow in commonly used tissue cultures. Watery diarrhea usually lasts 1 to 2 weeks and, in the initial days, may be associated with vomiting. Mild fever and, uncommonly, respiratory symptoms may occur with enteric adenoviral infections.

Mesenteric lymphadenitis with abdominal pain, fever, and other symptoms suggestive of appendicitis may be associated with adenoviral infections. Adenoviruses have been isolated from intraoperative specimens of mesenteric lymph nodes and the appendix. Acute and chronic adenoviral appendicitis occurs. Enlarged mesenteric lymph nodes often are thought to serve as lead points for intestinal intussusception. Observation of adenoviral intranuclear inclusions and seroconversion has associated a number of adenoviruses with intussusception.

Hepatitis has been reported with adenoviral infection in infants, young children, and immunocompromised patients.

Neurologic Manifestations

Central nervous system disease in adenoviral infection seldom occurs, but a variety of clinical manifestations have been noted. Both meningitis and encephalitis may be the major manifestations of adenoviral infections. Alternatively, neurologic illness may be associated with marked disease at other body sites.

Heart

Both myocarditis and pericarditis are rare findings in adenoviral respiratory infections.

Immunocompromised Host

Severe disseminated disease occurs and includes fulminant disease with multiorgan involvement, notably severe necrotizing pneumonia, and hepatitis with disseminated intravascular coagulation. Several different adenoviral types have been recovered from children with immunodeficiency diseases or malignancies; those who are receiving corticosteroid therapy, immunosuppressive therapy, or radiation therapy; and those who have undergone transplantation procedures.

Congenital and Neonatal Infections

Congenital and neonatal adenoviral infections may be severe, with multiple organ involvement. Illnesses suggest early-onset sepsis with hepatomegaly, progressive pneumonia, hepatitis, and thrombocytopenia.

DIAGNOSIS

The differential diagnosis for adenoviral illnesses differs with various clinical manifestations. Pharyngoconjunctival fever and keratoconjunctivitis often are recognized as adenoviral infections based on clinical findings because of their characteristic symptom complex and epidemic nature. Adenoviral pharyngitis must be differentiated from streptococcal, Epstein-Barr virus, influenza, parainfluenza, and enteroviral infections. Adenoviral pneumonia may be difficult to distinguish clinically from illness caused by other viral and bacterial pathogens. Eye disease must be distinguished from herpes simplex virus keratitis and, in the neonate, from conjunctivitis caused by *Neisseria gonorrhoeae* and *Chlamydia* species. Bacterial and parasitic intestinal infections sometimes produce symptoms like those of adenoviral infections.

Because of the occurrence of fever, lymphadenopathy, and exanthem and enanthem, adenoviral infections frequently are confused with Kawasaki disease.

Specific diagnosis commonly is achieved by tissue culture methods, specific antigen detection, or seroconversion. Respiratory adenoviruses can be isolated in most clinical laboratories. Specimens for culture should be obtained from the affected conjunctiva or throat by swabbing with cotton or Dacron swabs; or respiratory secretions, urine, or tissue may be submitted. Preferably, specimens are placed into viral transport media for transport to the virology laboratory. Rapid diagnostic tests [indirect fluorescent antibody test, ELISA, polymerase chain reaction (PCR), radioimmunoassay] are available. In general, except for PCR, their sensitivity is relatively low compared with culture, but specificity is high.

The serologic diagnosis of adenoviral infection is achieved by demonstrating an increase in complement-fixing antibody to the adenovirus-type–common hexon antigen or by demonstrating specific IgM serum antibody in a single serum by enzyme-linked immunosorbent assay.

THERAPY

No specific treatment exists for adenoviral infections. The patient should be discouraged from engaging in strenuous activity, and supportive care should be given. Corticosteroid treatment is to be avoided, and immunosuppressive regimens should be reduced or suspended. Corticosteroid preparations should be administered carefully to patients with pneumonia and wheezing. Corticosteroids may contribute to the development of severe disease and may complicate recovery. Experimental treatment of severe adenoviral infections has included the administration of immunoglobulins with high titers against the specific adenovirus types and intravenously administered ribavirin or cidofovir.

PREVENTION

Live attenuated viruses in enteric-coated capsules were effective and were used to immunize military recruits against adenovirus types 4 and 7. Subsequent asymptomatic intestinal infection protected against ARD. Trials of these vaccines in children showed similar efficacy. Unfortunately, adenoviral vaccines no longer are available, and the incidence of ARD in military recruits is again a significant problem.

Suggested Readings

Brandt CD, Kim HW, Vargosko AJ, et al. Infections in 18,000 infants and children in a controlled study of respiratory tract disease: I. adenovirus pathogenicity in relation to serologic type and illness syndrome. *Am J Epidemiol* 1969;90:484.

Cherry JD. Adenoviruses. In: Feigin RD, Cherry JD, Demmler GJ, Kaplan S, eds. *Textbook of pediatric infectious diseases,* 5th ed. Philadelphia: WB Saunders Co. 2004:1843.

Horwitz MS. Adenoviruses. In: Knipe DM, Howley PM, eds. *Virology,* 4th ed. Philadelphia: WB Saunders Co. 2001:2301.

Krajden M, Brown M, Petrasek A, Middleton P. Clinical features of adenovirus enteritis: a review of 127 cases. *Pediatr Infect Dis J* 1990;9:646.

Mitchell LS, Taylor B, Reimels W, et al. Adenovirus 7a: a community-acquired outbreak in a children's hospital. *Pediatr Infect Dis J* 2000;19:996.

Munoz FM, Piedra PA, Demmler GJ. Disseminated adenovirus disease in immunocompromised and immunocompetent children. *Clin Infect Dis J* 1998;27:1194.

CHAPTER 188 ■ INFLUENZA VIRUSES

JAMES D. CHERRY

Influenza viruses cause acute respiratory infections that usually occur in outbreaks or epidemics. In contrast to all other respiratory viral infections [except severe acute respiratory syndrome (SARS)] that occur in outbreaks, acute febrile illnesses occur in both adults and children. Influenza viral infections in children are associated with considerable morbidity and mortality, and the spectrum of clinical illness is broad. Influenza outbreaks and epidemics occur in birds, horses, pigs, and aquatic mammals, in addition to humans.

Influenza viruses are orthomyxoviruses. Three major antigenic types (A, B, and C) and multiple antigenic subtypes have been identified.

Influenza viruses are irregular, spherical particles 80 to 120 nm in diameter. The surface is composed of numerous hemagglutinin and neuraminidase "spikes." Inside the virus is a lipid bilayer, a matrix protein, and an RNA nucleocapsid.

Four important antigenic components have been described. The nuclear protein and matrix protein are antigenically type-specific and stable. The nuclear protein is the antigenic basis for typing strains as A, B, or C. Hemagglutinin and neuraminidase antigens are subtype-specific and variable. Fifteen different hemagglutinin subtypes (H1 to H15) and nine neuroaminidase subtypes (N1 to N9) occur in nature. Each of these subtypes has the potential to combine through genetic reassortment to yield a different viral strain. However, since 1874, only three separate hemagglutinins, H1, H2, and H3, and two separate neuraminidases, N1 and N2, have been recognized in influenza A viruses causing epidemics in humans. Variation in these two antigens (hemagglutinin and neuraminidase) is the basis for antigenic drift and shift in the prevalent viruses. *Drift* implies a minor change in the hemagglutinin or the neuraminidase without a change in subtype; *shift* implies a major change in either hemagglutinin or neuraminidase or both antigens, resulting in a change in subtype. Antigenic drift occurs in influenza A and B viruses, but shift occurs only in influenza A.

In the laboratory, influenza viruses can be cultivated in embryonated chicken eggs, in the MDCK cell line, and in primary monkey kidney tissue cultures.

Nomenclature for the classification of influenza virus strains specifies type, host (for strains of animal origin), geographic source, strain number, and year of isolation. To this, the code designations of hemagglutinin and neuraminidase subtypes are appended.

For example, recent strains that are included in the 2005–2006 vaccines are A/California/7/2004 (H3N2)-like, A/New Caledonia/20/99 (H1N1)-like, and B/Shanghai/361/2002-like.

EPIDEMIOLOGY

Pandemics of influenza caused by different influenza A subtypes occurred in 1874, 1889, 1900, 1918, 1933, 1946, 1957, 1968, and 1977. The 1918 pandemic resulted in 20 million deaths worldwide. Pandemics of influenza A result from antigenic shift. Wild aquatic birds are thought to be the influenza A virus reservoir in nature from which transmission to poultry, pigs, and other mammals occurs. Subsequently, influenza A viruses can be transmitted from pigs and poultry to humans. The pandemics of 1957 and 1968, associated with genetic shifts, were caused by reassortant influenza viruses that likely were generated in pigs. In more recent years, extensive outbreaks of influenza A infections have occurred in domestic poultry in many countries. The types of virus involved have been H7N7, H5N1, H9N2, H7N3, and H7N2. Transmission in these outbreaks has, on occasion, occurred directly from birds to humans. Fortunately, as yet, these viruses have not spread in the human populations. However, it is soon expected that human infection will result in genetic reassortment between a circulating avian strain and a circulating human strain, which will lead to a worldwide pandemic in humans with a virus having the hemagglutinin and neuroaminidase of an avian strain.

After pandemic influenza of a new subtype, epidemics of generally lesser intensity occur approximately every 2 to 3 years in association with antigenic drift. Outbreaks of influenza B are more variable and occur at roughly 4- to 7-year intervals, and these epidemics are the result of antigenic drift. Infection with influenza C virus is common in children, but the epidemiologic pattern of this virus is not determined.

Populated areas generally experience some influenza viral activity each year. Epidemics and outbreaks usually occur at times of cooler weather; in the tropics, epidemic disease usually occurs during the rainy season. The highest attack rate of influenza usually occurs in children, followed by secondary peaks of illness in adult populations. Case-fatality rates are greatest in infants and the elderly. Influenza is more likely to be fatal in persons with preexisting heart disease, chronic pulmonary disorders, diabetes mellitus, chronic renal disease, neuromuscular disorders, and neoplasms.

Influenza is spread from person to person via the respiratory route. The most common mechanism is inhalation of large airborne particles produced by coughing and sneezing. Spread also may occur by direct or indirect contact with fine-particle aerosols.

PATHOGENESIS

The major site of infection is the ciliated epithelium of the respiratory tract. Extensive necrosis of nasal and tracheal ciliated cells occurs as early as the first day after the onset of symptoms. It is followed by edema and infiltration with lymphocytes, his-

tiocytes, plasma cells, and polymorphonuclear cells. Repair of affected mucous membranes, indicated by mitoses in the surviving basal cells, begins by the third to fifth day of illness. A pseudometaplastic response of undifferentiated epithelium that reaches a maximum at 9 to 15 days after onset of infection occurs; thereafter, ciliary function and mucus production reappear.

Secondary bacterial infection is a common occurrence. More extensive inflammatory cell infiltration and destruction of the basal cell layer and basement membrane are seen, and delayed regeneration of the ciliated epithelium results.

Pneumonia may occur as a result of primary influenza viral infection, bacterial superinfection, or combined bacterial-viral infection. Although influenza is predominantly an infection of the respiratory tract, the heart, brain, and lymphoid tissues sometimes are involved in fatal cases. Specifically, focal and diffuse myocarditis, mediastinal lymph node disorganization and necrosis, and diffuse cerebral edema have been observed. In addition, Reye syndrome (diffuse encephalopathy and fatty degeneration of the liver) is a complication of influenza, particularly that caused by type B virus in children.

Influenza viral infection evokes a vigorous and complex immunologic response. Humoral, secretory, and cell-mediated mechanisms all are involved. Hemagglutination-inhibiting antibodies are important for virus neutralization, and antibodies against neuraminidase are associated with diminished severity of illness and reduced rates of person-to-person transmission. Local (IgA) antibodies probably are important as a first line of defense, if they are present.

After infection occurs, the duration of immunity and degree of protection against challenge by heterologous viral strains vary. In general, natural immunity against influenza A strains lasts approximately 4 years. As increasing antigenic drift occurs, previously infected persons are likely to have symptomatic reinfections; when antigenic shift occurs, antibody from the previous infection offers no protection.

CLINICAL MANIFESTATIONS AND COMPLICATIONS

Clinical manifestations of influenza follow a short, 2- to 3-day incubation period. Although the predominant manifestations of influenza viral infections are respiratory, systemic complaints are an integral part of the illness. In general, the manifestations of influenza in children fall into two categories based on age. The first category is school-aged children and adolescents, and the second category is younger children and infants. In school-aged children and adolescents, the illness is similar to that which occurs in adults (classic influenza). Illness onset is abrupt with fever, facial flush, chills, headache, myalgia, and malaise. Temperature varies between 39°C and 41°C and generally is lower in older patients. Systemic complaints, on the other hand, generally are more severe in the older patient. Initially, dry cough and coryza occur, but these symptoms are of lesser concern to the patient than are the severe systemic manifestations. Approximately one-half of patients complain of sore throat, which is associated with a nonexudative pharyngitis. Ocular symptoms are common findings and include tearing, photophobia, burning, and pain with eye movement. In uncomplicated illness, the fever lasts from 2 to 5 days. Occasionally, the temperature shows a biphasic pattern that may or may not be caused by secondary bacterial complications.

The course of illness changes by day 2 to 4 of illness, when the respiratory symptoms become more prominent and the systemic complaints begin to subside. Major coughing—dry and hacking—usually persists for up to a week. Occasionally, coughing persists well after other symptoms have subsided.

Influenza A and B infections generally are similar, although B viral infections may have more prominent nasal and eye complaints and fewer systemic findings, such as dizziness and prostration, than do comparable influenza A illnesses. Although influenza C outbreaks rarely are discerned, illness caused by this virus is indistinguishable from that caused by A and B viral types.

The leukocyte count in uncomplicated influenza usually is normal, but frequently leukopenia (less than 4,500 cells per microliter) occurs. Approximately one-third of patients have a relative lymphopenia, and one-third have a relative neutropenia. In general, approximately 10% of older children have clinical signs and radiographic evidence of pulmonary involvement.

In younger children and infants, the manifestations of influenza viral infections frequently are similar to those of other common respiratory viral infections. Laryngotracheitis, bronchitis, bronchiolitis, and pneumonia all occur. Frequently, primary infection is an undifferentiated febrile upper respiratory illness. Temperature usually exceeds 39.5°C. Affected children appear mildly toxic and have cough, coryza, and irritability. On examination, pharyngitis usually is noted and pulmonary involvement is common. Other findings include vomiting, diarrhea, otitis media, and fleeting erythematous or erythematous maculopapular discrete rashes.

Acute laryngotracheitis caused by influenza A virus occasionally is more severe than is infection caused by parainfluenza viruses. In neonates, influenza infection cannot be distinguished clinically from bacterial sepsis. Lethargy, poor feeding, petechiae, poor peripheral circulation with mottling of skin, and apneic spells all occur.

The most common complications of influenza are bacterial infections of the respiratory tract (pneumonia, otitis media, and sinusitis). Acute myositis is a particular complication of influenza B viral infections in children. Acute myositis is characterized by severe pain and tenderness in the calves of both legs. Onset is sudden, and usually the affected child refuses to walk. Serum creatinine phosphokinase and aspartate immunotransferase levels may be increased.

Reye syndrome is a complication of both influenza A and B infections in association with the administration of aspirin. In the past, outbreaks of Reye syndrome were related to epidemic activity of influenza.

Other rare complications of influenza viral infections include neurologic manifestations (encephalitis, acute necrotizing encephalopathy, Guillain-Barré syndrome, and transverse myelitis), pericarditis and myocarditis, and sudden death.

DIAGNOSIS

During outbreaks and epidemics, the clinical diagnosis of influenza can be made with some reliability. Important in the clinical diagnosis of influenza is the occurrence in the community of a similar illness with fever in both adults and children. The definitive diagnosis of influenza depends on either isolation of virus from respiratory secretions or a significant increase in serum antibody titer during convalescence. Rapid detection techniques (fluorescent antibody and enzyme immunoassay) for influenza antigens in nasopharyngeal epithelial cells are both sensitive and specific and available in most laboratories.

The serologic diagnosis of influenza classically used either complement fixation or hemagglutination-inhibition techniques. Complement fixation detects antibody against soluble nuclear protein antigens common to all strains of influenza A or B. Hemagglutination-inhibiting antibodies, which are subtype-specific, provide more definitive evidence of infection. The enzyme-linked immunosorbent assay often is used for the serologic diagnosis of influenza. Using this technique, specific IgM antibodies can be determined so that diagnosis can be made based on a single specimen obtained shortly after the onset of illness.

TREATMENT

Symptomatic treatment is the cornerstone of management and consists of rest, adequate hydration with oral fluids, control of fever and myalgia with acetaminophen, and maintenance of comfortable breathing by means of humidified air and, occasionally, nasal decongestants. Persistent irritating cough during convalescence often can be relieved with dextromethorphan or codeine.

The physician should be alert to the possibility of secondary bacterial infection. These infections are suggested by a prolonged febrile course or recrudescence of fever during early convalescence. Before antibiotic therapy is begun, the site of infection should be identified and appropriate cultures obtained. Most infections are caused by *Streptococcus pneumoniae, Haemophilus influenzae, Streptococcus pyogenes,* or less commonly, *Staphylococcus aureus.*

The antiviral agent amantadine hydrochloride is active *in vitro* against influenza A viruses and has prophylactic and therapeutic benefits. It seems reasonable to administer amantadine therapeutically to severely ill, hospitalized children if the illness is likely to have been caused by influenza A virus. Treatment with amantadine should be instituted within 48 hours of onset of illness. The prophylactic dose of amantadine for children is as follows: children 1 to 9 years old, 5 mg/kg per 24 hours, administered twice a day; children older than 9 years, 200 mg per 24 hours, administered twice a day. Influenza B viruses are not susceptible to amantadine.

Two neuraminidase inhibitors (Zanamivir and Oseltamivir) are approved for the treatment of both uncomplicated influenze A and B. Zanamivir is administered using a special breath-activated plastic inhaler. It is approved for children 7 years of age or older and it should be given within 2 days of onset of symptoms. It is administered twice a day for 5 days.

Oseltamivir is approved for children 1 year of age or older. The dose is 30 mg twice daily for children weighing 15 kg or less, 45 mg twice daily for those weighing between 16 and 23 kgs, 60 mg twice daily for those weighing between 24 and 40 kg, and 75 mg twice daily for those weighing more than 40 kg. Oseltamivir also is approved for prophylaxis in adolescents (13 years of age and older) with a dose of 75 mg daily.

Side effects of amantadine include nervousness, anxiety, insomnia, difficulty concentrating, lightheadedness, behavioral changes, delirium, hallucinations, agitation, and seizures. Patients with asthma have experienced respiratory function deterioration in association with zanamivir administration, and nausea and vomiting are side effects of oseltamivir.

PREVENTION

Influenza immunization is now recommended annually for all children aged 6 to 23 months. Influenza viral vaccines are safe and effective in preventing influenza, if the antigens in the vaccine correlate with circulating influenza viruses. Both inactivated influenza vaccines and a live-attenuated vaccine are available, and both can be used in children.

Inactivated influenza vaccines can be administered to all children who are 6 months of age or older. Children younger than 9 years of age, who have not previously received influenza vaccine, should receive two doses 1 month apart, and older children and those previously immunized need only receive one dose. The vaccine should be given intramuscularly.

The live-attenuated influenza vaccine is approved for use in healthy children and adolescents, 5 to 17 years of age and healthy adults, 18 to 49 years of age. The vaccine is administered intranasally; children younger than 9 years of age who are being immunized for the first time should receive two doses 6 to 10 weeks apart. Older children and those who have been previously immunized need only one dose. The vaccine should not be given to immunocompromised persons, to children receiving aspirin, or to individuals who have had Guillain-Barré syndrome.

Persons who have experienced anaphylaxis to chicken or egg protein may experience anaphylaxis following influenza immunization; in most instances, these children should not receive influenza vaccines. Influenza vaccines should be administered in the autumn season each year. Because vaccine recommendations frequently change, physicians should consult the latest recommendations of the Committee on Infectious Diseases of the American Adademy of Pediatrics or the Advisory Committee on Immunization Practices (ACIP) as well as manufacturers recommendations each fall.

Suggested Readings

American Academy of Pediatrics. Influenza. In: Pickering LK, ed. *Red Book: 2003 Report of the Committee on Infectious Diseases*, 26th ed. Elk Grove Village, IL: American Academy of Pediatrics, 2003:382.

Centers for Disease Control and Prevention. Prevention and control of influenza: recommendations of the Advisory Committee on Immunization Practices (ACIP). *MMWR* 2005;54(No. RR-8):1.

Glezen WP. Influenza viruses. In: R. D. Feigin, J. D.Cherry, Demmler, G. J., Kaplan, S., eds. *Textbook of pediatric infectious diseases*, 5th ed. WB Saunders Co, Philadelphia, PA. 2004;2252.

Peltola V, Ziegler T, Ruuskanen O. Influenza A and B infections in children. *Clin Infect Dis* 2003;36:299.

Terebuh P, Uyeki T, Fukuda K. Impact of influenza on young children and the shaping of United States influenza vaccine policy. *Pediatr Infect Dis J* 2003; 22:S231.

Thompson WW, Shay DK, Weintraub E, et al. Mortality associated with influenza and respiratory syncytial virus in the United States. *JAMA* 2003;289:179.

Webster RG, Shortridge KF, Kawaoka Y. Influenza: interspecies transmission and emergence of new pandemics. *FEMS Immunol Med Microbiol* 1997;18: 275.

CHAPTER 189 ■ PARAINFLUENZA VIRUSES

CAROLINE BREESE HALL

Major actors of the yearly show that fills
Each fall with varied forms of respiratory ills
and striking melodies that mimic far too well
The barking seal, the crowing cock, the brassy bell.
—*CBH*

The parainfluenza viruses (PIVs) cause ubiquitous infections with varied manifestations in childhood. Their spectrum of illness ranges from mild and asymptomatic upper respiratory tract illness to disease involving the lower respiratory tract in young children. Recognition of the PIVs as important worldwide human pathogens comes not only from their causing symptomatic illness early in life, but also from their ability to reinfect throughout life. The PIVs, especially types 1 and 2, have earned a distinctive notoriety from their being the most frequent causes of croup. In 1991, PIV-1 and PIV-2 infections were estimated to account for 250,000 visits to emergency rooms, 70,000 hospitalizations, and $190 million in medical care costs annually.

The first PIV was isolated from mice in Sendai, Japan a half century ago and received the name *Sendai virus*, or the hemagglutinating virus of Japan (HVJ). The PIVs subsequently were recognized to be widespread in animals. The first human PIV was isolated from infants with croup and was descriptively named *croup-associated (CA) virus*. With the subsequent recognition of PIV-1, PIV-3, and PIV-4, CA virus was renamed PIV-2.

VIRUS CHARACTERIZATION

The PIVs, along with respiratory syncytial virus (RSV), belong to the family of enveloped RNA viruses, *Paramyxoviridae*, which have nonsegmented, single-stranded, negative-sense genomes. The genomes of all four types of human PIVs code for at least one nonstructural and six structural proteins. The lipid envelope, derived from the host cell, is studded with the surface glycoproteins, hemagglutinin-neuraminidase (HN) and fusion (F) proteins. These two surface glycoproteins are integral to the immunity and pathogenesis of the PIVs. The HN facilitates the attachment of the virus to the host cell, and the F protein, along with HN, allows the virus to enter the host cell, by fusing the host and viral cellular membranes. Cell-to-cell spread of infection subsequently occurs.

The human PIVs possess common antigens, as demonstrated by their serologic responses to heterotypic parainfluenza strains and to mumps virus. The human PIVs may be divided into two major antigenic groups (PIV-1 and PIV-3 in one group, and PIV-2 and PIV-4, along with mumps virus, in the other). Minor antigenic variation occurs with all four PIV types.

EPIDEMIOLOGY

The PIVs have been found across the globe, and, although their seasonal pattern may vary according to the climate and geography, their clinical manifestations are similar. In the United States, the seasonal pattern of the PIVs in different parts of the country may have some variation, but PIV-1, -2, and -3 each has a character that is distinctive and yet interactive with the other serotypes (Table 189.1). The PIVs did not demonstrate their epidemic nature until the mid-1960s, when PIV-1 showed a notable pattern of outbreaks occurring every other year in the fall of odd-numbered years (Fig. 189.1). PIV-2 has a more unpredictable behavior than does PIV-1 or PIV-3 (Fig. 189.1). PIV-2 most often appears toward the end of the PIV-1 fall outbreak, but sporadically and with less intensity than does PIV-1. PIV-3 is present in the community for more months than are the other PIVs. It usually is most prominent in the spring to fall of each year. Relatively few isolations and outbreaks of PIV-4 have been reported, and disease associated with PIV-4 usually is mild. Thus, relatively little is known about the epidemiologic and clinical manifestations of PIV-4.

Most children have been infected with PIV-1, -2, and -3 by the time they reach 5 years of age, and many have been

TABLE 189.1

PARAINFLUENZA VIRUSES

	Type 1	Type 2	Type 3	Type 4
Seasonal Incidence	Fall of odd numbered years	Unpredictable Fall, Winter	Spring ⟶ Fall	Few isolated; seasonal variation uncertain
Site of Infection	Upper airway; may involve lower airway	Upper airway; may involve lower airway	Upper spreading to lower airway	Mostly upper airway
Viral Shedding	Average 4–7 days, range 12 days	Average 4–7 days, longer shedding may occur	2–3 weeks commonly, occasionally longer	
Major Clinical Manifestations	Croup, URI	Croup, URI	Bronchiolitis, Pneumonia, URI	URI

reinfected by this age. PIV-3 usually is the child's earliest infection, with one-half to two-thirds of infants acquiring infection within the first year of life. Infection with PIV-1 and PIV-2 usually occurs subsequently and more gradually, with approximately three-fourths of school-age children having antibody. Seroprevalence to PIV-2 is variable, ranging anywhere from 50% to 90%. Almost all adults have detectable antibody to PIV-1 and -3.

Repeated infections with the PIVs may occur at any age, but many (50% or more) are asymptomatic. Boys tend to be hospitalized more frequently, but infection rates in outpatients and in populations with repeated infections suggest that gender does not play a permanent role.

The importance of PIV-1, -2, and -3 in causing acute respiratory infections in children has been supported recently by data from the National Respiratory and Enteric Virus Surveillance System from the Centers for Disease Control and Prevention (CDC). Although the rate of hospitalization with PIV infection was widely variable in different years and locations, researchers estimated that rates of PIV-1, -2, and -3–associated hospitalizations ranged from 1.9 to 12 per 1,000 children younger than 1 year of age and between 0.5 and 2.0 per 1,000 children ages 1 to 4 years. These findings resulted in an estimated 7,600 to

48,000 hospitalizations for infants younger than 12 months of age, and 8,100 to 42,600 admissions for those 1 to 4 years of age. PIV-3 and PIV-1 were the most frequent causes of hospitalization, ranging from 8,700 to 52,000 annual hospitalizations for PIV-3 and 5,800 to 28,900 for PIV-1. PIV-2 generally was a less common cause, but with wide variation, causing 1,800 to 15,600 hospitalizations each year.

PATHOGENESIS

Transmission

The PIVs are highly contagious, as evidenced by the alacrity of spread among children in day-care centers and other groups of young children in close contact. Almost all children initially exposed to PIV-3 in these settings will acquire infection. Approximately 60% to 80% will acquire PIV-1 and PIV-2 under similar circumstances.

The mode of spread of the PIVs appears similar to that of RSV, thus requiring close person-to-person contact and direct exposure to the contaminated secretions of infected

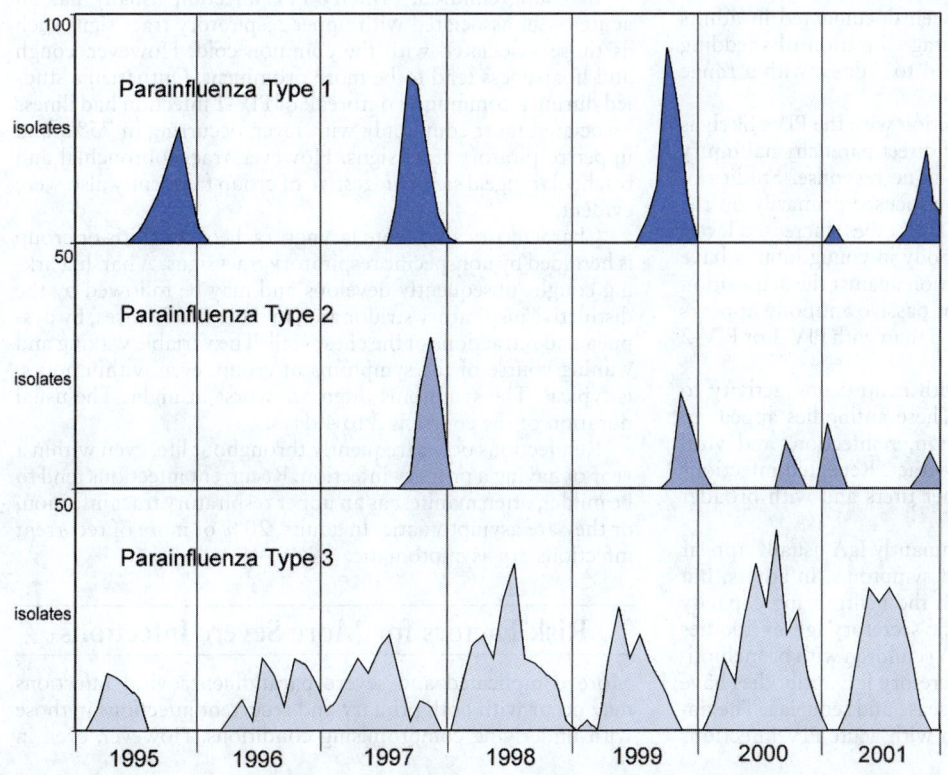

FIGURE 189.1. Patterns of seasonal activity of parainfluenza viruses types 1, 2, and 3 in Monroe County, New York from 1995–2001, are illustrated by the number of isolates obtained from ambulatory children as part of an ongoing community surveillance program for infectious diseases.

individuals. This exposure most likely occurs primarily via the large-droplet aerosols of respiratory secretions from infected contacts or by contact with contaminated fomites followed by self-inoculation. The large quantities of virus contained in the nasal secretions of young children, the frequency of both symptomatic and asymptomatic infections, and PIVs' ability to survive in the environment support the likelihood that these modes of transmission predominate. Experimentally, PIV-3 has been shown to be viable in a small-particle aerosol for 1 hour, but secretions most likely are disseminated via the coughs and sneezes that are so prominent in PIV infections. PIV-3 primarily is contained in large-particle aerosols for which close person-to-person contact is required.

Immunopathology

The inoculation of these viruses into the upper respiratory tract usually results in infection after an incubation period of 2 to 4 days. Attachment of the virus occurs via specific receptors on the cell membrane of the host's respiratory epithelium, with subsequent penetration occurring by fusion. Infections may be limited to the upper respiratory tract or subsequently spread to the lower respiratory tract, which most frequently occurs with PIV-3. Infections with PIV-1 and -2 tend to involve primarily the larynx and upper trachea, resulting in croup.

Few pathologic studies of children with PIV infection exist. The spread of the viral infection along the respiratory tract results in inflammation of the epithelium, with the accumulation of necrotic tissue and inspissated mucus. This inflammatory material may cause obstruction in both the upper and lower respiratory tracts. In the former, this obstruction may result in the characteristic nasal congestion and otitis media. Spread to the lower respiratory tract results in obstruction of the flow of air, with atelectasis, pneumonia, and bronchiolitis developing in the young child. Involvement of the subglottic tissues may be the prominent manifestation, resulting in stridor and croup.

In young children, viral shedding is most abundant and prolonged. With PIV-3 infection, shedding may be detected for as long as 2 to 3 weeks. Intermittent and an even longer duration of shedding with PIV-3 has been documented in adults with chronic lung disease. The average duration of shedding for children with PIV-1 infection is 4 to 7 days, with a range of up to 12 days.

The pathogenesis of clinical infection with the PIVs likely is engendered by a combined effect of direct parenchymal injury from the virus and the evoked immune response. Studies of adaptive immunity to the PIVs have focused primarily on the role of specific secretory and serum antibodies. Increased levels of maternal, passively derived antibody in young infants have been correlated with relative protection against the acquisition of infection. The protective effect of passive antibody appears to be less against infection with PIV-3 than with PIV-1 or PIV-2 infections.

PIVs evoke specific antibody with neutralizing activity to HN and F surface glycoproteins. These antibodies appear to correlate with resistance to infection, reinfection, and viral replication in the lower respiratory tract. Repeated infections result in specific antibodies in higher titers and with broader antigenic site–specific responses.

Secretory IgG, IgM, and predominantly IgA usually appear within 7 to 10 days of the onset of symptoms. In adults, but not in children, they correlate with the neutralizing capacity of the respiratory secretions. Specific secretory IgE antibodies also are produced, especially in young children with bronchiolitis. Higher titers of these specific secretory IgE antibodies have been correlated with more severe disease and sequelae. The nasopharyngeal secretions of children with acute PIV infections

also have been shown to contain chemokines, macrophage inflammatory protein-1alpha, and RANTES (regulated upon activation, normal T-cell expressed and secreted), which may be important in the pathogenesis and expression of PIV infection.

The impact of cell-mediated immune responses to PIV infections in humans has not been well studied but is likely to be pivotal in the control of the viral infection and in recovery. The increased duration and severity of PIV infections in immunocompromised hosts support this hypothesis.

CLINICAL MANIFESTATIONS AND COMPLICATIONS

The clinical presentation of infection with the PIVs depends on the age of the child, whether the infection is primary or recurrent, the infecting serotype, and the presence of an underlying compromising condition (Fig. 189.2). In general, the PIVs contribute proportionately more of the respiratory illnesses seen in outpatients than those seen in hospitalized patients. Second, the three major PIVs, types 1 through 3, can cause the same spectrum of respiratory illnesses, ranging from upper respiratory tract infections, which are most common, to those involving the lower respiratory tract, which occur most frequently in infants with primary infection. Approximately two-thirds of the lower respiratory tract infections requiring hospitalization occur in infants younger than 1 year of age.

In children with primary infection, each serotype of PIV has a characteristic, predominant association with a particular respiratory syndrome. Croup is associated most frequently with PIV-1 and PIV-2, although PIV-2 infections are less common than are PIV-1 infections. Bronchiolitis and pneumonia usually are caused by PIV-3. PIV-4, although infrequently isolated, appears to cause mostly afebrile upper respiratory tract infections. In a pediatric practice, overall PIVs type 1, 2, and 3 caused approximately two-thirds of the croup cases, one-fourth of those with tracheobronchitis, and approximately half of the upper respiratory tract illnesses, including the common cold, laryngitis, pharyngitis, and otitis media (Fig. 189.2).

In young children, primary PIV infection usually has an acute onset associated with upper respiratory tract signs such as those associated with the common cold. However, cough and hoarseness tend to be more prominent. Outpatients studied during a community outbreak of PIV-1 infection had illness associated most commonly with fever, occurring in 75%, and upper respiratory tract signs. However, tracheobronchial and tracheolaryngeal signs suggestive of croup frequently also were evident.

Characteristically, acute laryngotracheobronchitis or croup is heralded by nonspecific respiratory tract signs. A harsh, barking cough subsequently develops and may be followed by the distinctive inspiratory stridor and, in more severe cases, by dyspnea and retractions of the chest wall. The variable waxing and waning course of the symptoms of croup, even within hours, is typical. The symptoms often are worse at night. The usual duration of the course is 3 to 4 days.

Reinfections occur frequently throughout life, even within a year of having a primary infection. Recurrent infections tend to be milder, often manifest as an upper respiratory tract infection, or they are asymptomatic. In adults, 20% or more of recurrent infections are asymptomatic.

Risk Factors for More Severe Infections

More complicated and severe parainfluenza viral infections may occur with both primary and recurrent infections in those with underlying compromising conditions. However, even in

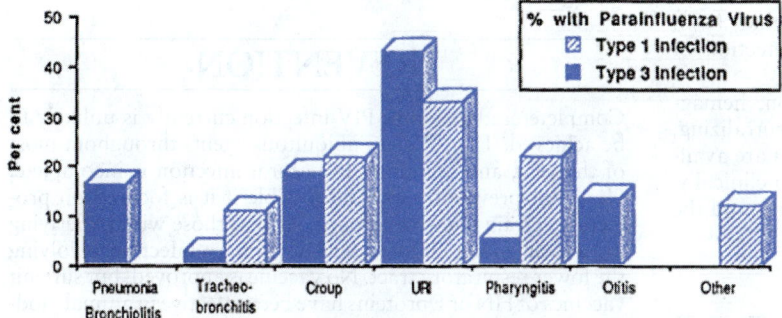

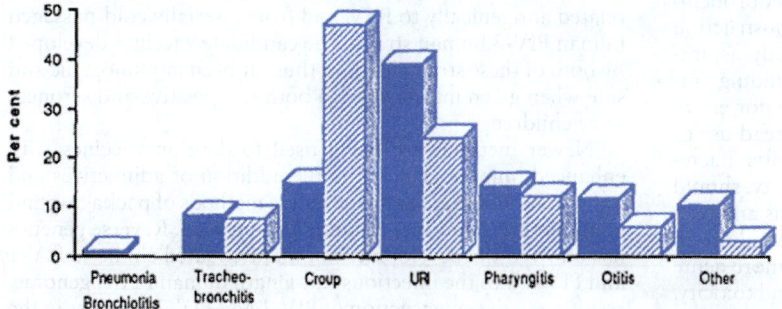

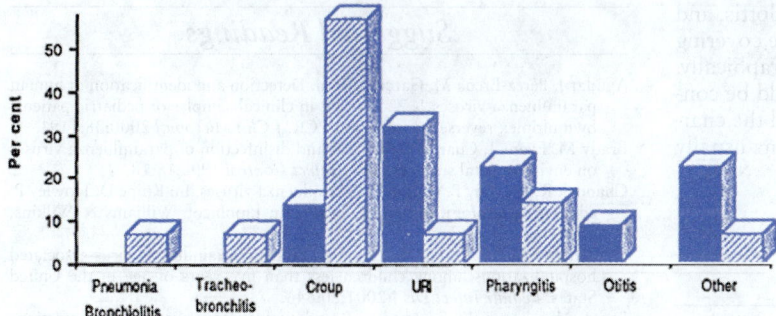

FIGURE 189.2. Type of illness with PIV-1 compared to PIV-3, according to age in outpatients from private pediatric practices presenting with acute respiratory and/or febrile illnesses. URI, upper respiratory tract infection. Data obtained 1984 through 1988 from the Community Infectious Disease Surveillance Program of the University of Rochester School of Medicine, Rochester, NY. (Reproduced with permission from Parainfluenza viruses. In: Feigin R, Cherry J., eds. *Textbook of pediatric infectious diseases* (5th ed). Philadelphia: WB Saunders, 2004;2:2277.)

normal children, complications occasionally may occur. In young infants, and in those with premature gestation, the course of primary PIV infection may be associated with apnea. Otitis media frequently complicates PIV infections in children, particularly in those younger than 1 year of age with PIV-3 infection. PIV-1 and PIV-3 are major contributors to the otitis media observed in children 1 to 5 years of age (Fig. 189.2). The otitis media accompanying PIV infection may be primarily viral, bacterial, or both. Rarely, a more severe bacterial infection, such as bacterial tracheitis, may complicate PIV infections. Upper respiratory tract PIV infections may cause recurrent episodes of wheezing, particularly in those patients with underlying hyperreactive airways.

Severe complications and fatal disease, however, rarely occur with PIV infections unless the patient has a chronic underlying condition, most commonly those involving the cardiopulmonary system. In such patients, the usually mild PIV infection may trigger an exacerbation of their serious, underlying chronic disease. Immunocompromised patients, especially those with compromised cellular immunity, have an augmented chance of having prolonged viral shedding and developing severe and fatal disease. Transplant recipients are at particular risk for developing lower respiratory tract disease, which may lead to respiratory failure and death in 20% of cases.

DIAGNOSIS

The diagnosis of parainfluenza viral infection in children may be suspected with a compatible clinical syndrome, especially croup, occurring during an outbreak of PIV infection in the community. However, in general, most respiratory infections from PIV in children cannot be differentiated from other such respiratory pathogens on clinical grounds alone but require specific diagnosis.

The laboratory confirmation of PIV infection may be made by viral isolation, rapid antigen detection assays, and newer detection methods, such as reverse transcriptase-polymerase chain reaction (RT-PCR), as well as by serologic assays. For viral isolation, nasopharyngeal or lower respiratory tract specimens should be obtained in viral transport media and maintained at approximately 4°C, because sitting at room temperature diminishes the viral infectivity. Although viral isolation traditionally has been considered the gold standard for diagnosing parainfluenza viral infections, its sensitivity is dependent on the expertise of the individual laboratory. Furthermore, it is labor-intensive and expensive.

Isolates of PIV usually may be detected after 3 to 7 days on sensitive cell lines by the hemadsorption of red blood cells or specific identification in cultures by more rapid antigen detection methods, such as immunofluorescence and enzyme immunoassay (EIA). PCR assays recently have been developed with a reported sensitivity and specificity of greater than 95%. Multiplex PCR assays allow the simultaneous detection of other respiratory viruses.

Serologic assays, including complement fixation, hemagglutination inhibition, hemadsorption inhibition, neutralizing, and EIAs may be used if acute and convalescent sera are available. Serologic diagnosis, however, rarely is of help clinically, and cross-reacting heterologous antibodies may confound the diagnosis.

Differential Diagnosis

PIV infections that manifest as acute laryngotracheobronchitis should be differentiated from other causes of obstruction of the airway producing stridor, such as foreign body aspiration and congenital anatomical abnormalities, including tracheomalacia and acute angioneurotic edema. The major entity that was differentiated before the advent of widespread use of *Haemophilus influenzae* type B vaccine was epiglottitis. Bacterial tracheitis, although an infrequently detected entity, should be considered within the differential. Both epiglottitis and bacterial tracheitis usually can be differentiated from viral croup by their clinical presentations. In both, the onset is more acute and the course rapidly progressive, with high fever and toxicity. The "seal's bark" and preceding upper respiratory tract infection of viral croup, along with its fluctuating course, usually are absent in epiglottitis and bacterial tracheitis. Roentgenograms of the neck in epiglottitis may reveal the swollen epiglottis, and in bacterial tracheitis, a shaggy exudative membrane covering the trachea may be visualized directly or roentgenographically. In a nonimmunized child, laryngeal diphtheria should be considered. This entity tends to be gradual in onset, and the characteristic exudative membrane in the posterior pharynx usually is visible.

THERAPY

In normal children, PIV infections usually are mild and self-limited. Thus, therapy primarily is supportive. No specific antiviral therapy is available for PIV infections. Ribavirin, with or without the concomitant administration of intravenous immunoglobulin, has been tried in a few uncontrolled studies of immunocompromised patients.

Children with croup caused by PIV require supportive care to ensure comfort, adequate hydration, and control of fever. The armamentarium of home therapies has been varied, colorful, and anecdotal, ranging from salves of plant extracts to cold night air. The purported successes of such remedies likely arise from the usual variable and fluctuating course of croup. Administration of cold air mist often is used, but a beneficial effect has not been proven.

Children with more severe croup may require hospitalization and treatment to alleviate their airway obstruction. The administration of aerosolized bronchodilators, such as racemic epinephrine, have resulted in some benefit. However, the effect is transient, requires close monitoring, and does not affect the hypoxemia if present. Currently, most of the more severely distressed children with croup are treated with corticosteroids. The past conflicting data on their benefit appears to have been related to the variation in the dose used. Corticosteroids currently recommended are parenteral dexamethasone, given IM or IV at a dose of 0.6 mg/kg to a maximum total dose of 10 mg, or dexamethasone given orally at a dose of 0.15 mg/kg or 0.6 mg/kg to a maximum total oral dose of 10 mg.

PREVENTION

Complete eradication of PIV infection currently is unlikely to be achieved. The PIVs are ubiquitous agents throughout most of the year, and immunity to natural infection is incomplete. However, prevention may be feasible if it is focused on protecting certain high-risk groups, such as those with underlying disease or young children with a primary infection involving the lower respiratory tract. No vaccine is approved, but subunit vaccines of HN or F proteins have been effective in animal models, and several live-attenuated vaccines appear to be promising candidates for children. PIV-3 live-attenuated candidate vaccines have been developed from bovine PIV-3, which is closely related antigenically to RSV, and from a serially cold-passaged human PIV-3 human strain. The candidate vaccines developed by both of these strategies have thus far been immunogenic and safe when given intranasally to both seropositive and seronegative children.

Newer methods are being used to develop vaccines with enhanced immunogenicity by the addition of adjunctives and immunomodulators, and alternative methods of packaging and administrating vaccines also are being trialed. Reverse genetics has allowed the development of an attenuated chimeric PIV-1 and PIV-2 into the infectious full-length human PIV-3 genome, resulting in the construction of PIV-1 and PIV-2 vaccines in the backbone of the attenuated PIV-3 genome.

Suggested Readings

Aguilar J, Pérez-Breña M, Garcí M, et al. Detection and identification of human parainfluenza viruses 1, 2, 3, and 4 in clinical samples of pediatric patients by multiplex reverse transcription-PCR. *J Clin Microbiol* 2000;38:1191.

Brady M, Evans J, Cuartas J. Survival and disinfection of parainfluenza viruses on environmental surfaces. *Am J Infect Control* 1990;18:18.

Chanock R, Murphy B, Collins P. Parainfluenza viruses. In: Knipe D, Howley P, eds. *Fields virology*, 4th ed. Philadelphia: Lippincott Williams & Wilkins, 2001:1341.

Couniham M, Shay D, Holman R, et al. Human parainfluenza virus-associated hospitalizations among children less than five years of age in the United States. *Pediatr Infect Dis J* 2001;20:646.

Fan J, Henrickson K, Savatski L. Rapid simultaneous diagnosis of infections with respiratory syncytial virus A and B, influenza viruses A and B, and human parainfluenza virus types 1, 2, and 3 by multiplex quantitative reverse transcription—polymerase chain reaction—enzyme hybridization assay (Hexaplex). *Clin Infect Dis* 1998;26:1397.

Glezen W. Incidence of respiratory syncytial and parainfluenza type 3 viruses in an urban setting. *Pediatr Virol* 1987;2:1.

Glezen W, Denny F. Epidemiology of acute lower respiratory disease in children. *N Engl J Med* 1973;288:498.

Glezen W, Frank A, Taber L, et al. Parainfluenza virus type 3: seasonality and risk of infection and reinfection in young children. *J Infect Dis* 1984;150:851.

Glezen W, Greenberg S, Atmar R, et al. Impact of respiratory virus infections on persons with chronic underlying conditions. *JAMA* 2000;283:499.

Hall C, Geiman J, Breese B, et al. Parainfluenza viral infections in children: correlation of shedding with clinical manifestations. *J Pediatr* 1977;91:194.

Hall C. Respiratory syncytial virus and parainfluenza virus. *N Engl J Med* 2001;344:1917.

Heikkinen T. Role of viruses in the pathogenesis of acute otitis media. *Pediatr Infect Dis J* 2000;19:S17.

Heikkinen T, Thint M, Chonmaitree T. Prevalence of various respiratory viruses in the middle ear during acute otitis media. *N Engl J Med* 1999;340:260.

Henrickson K, Kuhn S, Savatski L. Epidemiology and cost of infection with human parainfluenza virus types 1 and 2 in young children. *Clin Infect Dis* 1994;18:770.

Knott A, Long C, Hall C. Parainfluenza viral infections in pediatric outpatients: seasonal patterns and clinical characteristics. *Pediatr Infect Dis J* 1994; 13:269.

Laurichesse H, Dedman D, Watson J, et al. Epidemiological features of parainfluenza virus infections: laboratory surveillance in England and Wales, 1975–1997. *Eur J Epidemiol* 1999;15:475.

McIntosh K, Ellis E, Hoffman L, et al. The association of viral and bacterial respiratory infections with exacerbations of wheezing in young asthmatic children. *J Pediatr* 1973;82:578.

McIntosh K, Halonen P, Ruuskanen O. Report of a workshop on respiratory viral infections: epidemiology, diagnosis, treatment, and prevention. *Clin Infect Dis* 1993;16:151.

Murphy B, Collins P. Live-attenuated virus vaccines for respiratory syncytial and parainfluenza viruses: applications of reverse genetics. *J Clin Invest* 2002; 110:21.

Ng W, Rajadurai V, Pradeepkumar V, et al. Parainfluenza type 3 viral outbreak in a neonatal nursery. *Ann Acad Med Singapore* 1999;28:471.

Nichols W, Corey L, Gooley T, et al. Parainfluenza virus infections after hematopoietic stem cell transplantation: risk factors, response to antiviral therapy, and effect on transplant outcome. *Blood* 2001;98: 573.

Reed G, Jewett P, Thompson J, et al. Epidemiology and clinical impact of parainfluenza virus infections in otherwise healthy infants and young children <5 years old. *J Infect Dis* 1997;175:807.

Welliver R, Wong D, Sun M, et al. Parainfluenza virus bronchiolitis: epidemiology and pathogenesis. *Am J Dis Child* 1986;140:34.

Yanagihara R, McIntosh K. Secretory immunological response in infants and children to parainfluenza virus types 1 and 2. *Infect Immunol* 1980;30: 23.

CHAPTER 190 ■ HUMAN METAPNEUMOVIRUS

CAROLINE BREESE HALL

> *A player in the Mardi Gras of ills of years long past,*
> *Though only recently it's been unrobed*
> *and now unmasked.*
> *But just what role this respiratory reveler has to show*
> *in its occult genomic soul we've yet to know.*
>   —CBH

Human metapneumovirus (hMPV) recently has appeared on the stage of human respiratory pathogens. Currently, its role may be described best as an understudy to respiratory syncytial virus (RSV). Thus far, it has been associated with primarily upper and lower respiratory tract illnesses, and sometimes with asymptomatic infections. Human metapneumovirus infections occur across the age span, with increased severity at each end: the young child and the older, compromised adult. Although hMPV was discovered only recently, serologic data indicate that it probably has been an occult contributor to the burden of respiratory ills for some time.

Van den Hoogen et al. initially discovered this new member of the *Metapneumovirus* genus, which previously had consisted of only avian pneumovirus. The virus was identified in a retrospective survey of specimens collected over the course of 20 years from patients with respiratory illness from whom 28 specimens were identified as containing hMPV. Within the next 2 years, reports of this same metapneumovirus in respiratory specimens came rapidly from Australia, North America, Europe, and Asian countries.

VIRUS CHARACTERIZATION AND LABORATORY CHARACTERISTICS

hMPV is the mammalian metapneumovirus first associated with disease and, like RSV and the parainfluenza viruses, belongs to the Paramyxoviridae family. Within this family are two subfamilies. The first is the Paramyxovirinae subfamily, which contains the parainfluenza viruses and the Hendra virus, among others. The second is the Pneumovirinae subfamily, which contains two genera: the pneumoviruses, to which RSV belongs, and the metapneumoviruses, to which this new hMPV has been assigned. Initial phylogenetic analysis indicated hMPV was related most closely to the turkey avian metapneumovirus, subtype C. Subsequent morphologic, antigenic, and genomic data have confirmed this relationship.

Similar to RSV and other paramyxoviruses, hMPV is an enveloped RNA virus with a nonsegmented, single-stranded, negative-sense genome. The envelope consists of a lipid bilayer that is derived from the plasma membrane of the host cells. Electron micrographs show pleomorphic, spherical, and filamentous particles of various sizes. The spherical particles have a mean diameter of approximately 200 nm, with a range of 150 to 600 nm. The filamentous particles have an average size of 282 × 62 nm (Fig. 190.1). Small, 13 to 17 mm spikes project from the envelope.

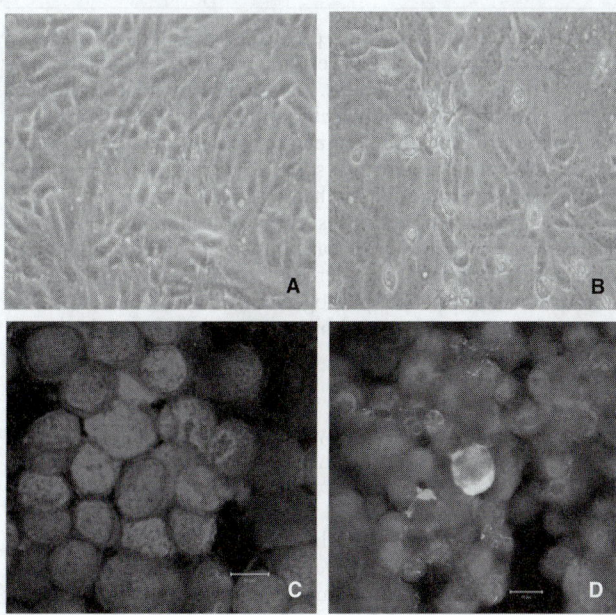

FIGURE 190.1. A: Vero 76 (African Green Monkey) uninfected and unstained monolayer. Magnification 1,000×. **B:** Cytopathic effect (CPE) of hMPV in Vero 76 cells, unstained preparation, 7 days after inoculation. CPE is characterized by foci of rounded and refractile cells. Magnification 1,000×. **C:** LLCMK-2, uninfected cells with indirect immunofluorescence using rabbit hyperimmune serum anti-hMPV and Alexa Fluor® 488 goat anti-rabbit IgG. Confocal microscope image. 1:1,000 Evans Blue counterstaining. Bar marker represents 10 μm. **D:** LLCMK-2 cells infected with hMPV, with indirect immunofluorescence (as in figure C). Pattern is granular in the cytoplasm, resembling that characteristic of human respiratory syncytial virus. (Courtesy of T. Peret, MD; Respiratory and Enteric Virus Branch, Division of Viral and Rickettsial Diseases, Centers for Disease Control and Prevention.)

A sequencing of the genome has been accomplished and shows it to have a length of about 13.4 kB and eight open reading frames (ORFs) that are transcribed into eight distinct structural proteins. These proteins include the surface transmembrane glycoproteins, the fusion (F), attachment (G), and the small nonglycosolated hydrophobic (SH) proteins; two matrix proteins (M, M2); and three proteins that are associated with the nucleocapsid, the nucleocapsid protein (N), the phosphoprotein (P), and polymerase (L). The surface transmembrane glycoproteins have an arrangement within the virion similar to that of RSV.

hMPV Strains

Considerable strain variation exists for hMPV. Analyses of isolates from multiple countries suggest that at least two major distinct lineages (groups A and B). These two lineages have a nucleotide homology of 80% to 88%, whereas the homology is 93% to 100% within each of these two clusters. The amino acid homology is higher both between (93% to 97%) and within (97% to 100%) the two lineages. Two sublineages or subgroups also appear to exist in each of these two genetic lineages. Although the epidemiologic behavior of these strain groups is still incompletely understood, both appear to circulate simultaneously, with A strains generally predominating, but in those over 3 years of age as many B as A strains occur. However, the immunologic and clinical importance of strain variation remains to be determined.

EPIDEMIOLOGY

The emerging epidemiologic picture of hMPV is based on a collage of mostly retrospective studies of relatively small numbers of patients. Nonetheless, the data accumulated thus far clearly show that hMPV is a ubiquitous agent with worldwide distribution that peaks in temperate climates during the colder autumn to spring months. In some countries, its seasonal pattern appears to be similar to that of RSV, although it generally is more variable; in countries with cooler climates, often its the peak of activity is less pronounced. The overall burden of respiratory illness engendered by hMPV compared to RSV and to other respiratory pathogens is still evolving, and direct comparisons are obfuscated by variations in the methods and populations analyzed.

The ubiquitous and early acquisition of hMPV has been shown by multiple serologic studies of various age groups. In Australia, specific antibody to hMPV was present in 90% of individuals by the time they reached the age of 5 years, and in 98% by 10 years of age. In the Netherlands, seroprevalence was similar, with 25% of subjects positive at 6 to 12 months of age, and almost all by age 5 years. Clinical disease, however, is detected in a much smaller proportion of children, suggesting that many infections are very mild or asymptomatic.

The proportion of acute respiratory illnesses caused by hMPV generally has been estimated in most recent reports as 1% to 3% in the general population of all ages, 5% to 9% in young children, and 2% to 7% in adults. The rates have been highly variable in different populations, but usually highest in those younger than 2 years, over 65 years, with underlying conditions, and those hospitalized or in long-term care facilities. Of banked specimens from individuals with respiratory disease submitted to diagnostic laboratories, hMPV has been identified in approximately 4% to 16%. hMPV has been detected in 1% to 4% of specimens from asymptomatic individuals. As with those infections caused by other respiratory pathogens of young children, those from hMPV resulting

in hospitalization occur 1.2 to 2.3 times more frequently in boys.

In a recent study (Williams et al.), specimens that had been collected over 25 years from healthy children younger than 5 years of age attending a vaccine clinic were analyzed by reverse transcription-polymerase chain reaction (RT-PCR) for the presence of hMPV. Nasal wash samples were examined from 687 visits for lower respiratory illnesses among 463 children, 57% of whom were 24 months of age or younger. Viruses other than hMPV were identified in 279 (41%), with RSV accounting for 103 of the 279 (37%) virus positive samples. In 248 of the virus-negative samples, hMPV was identified in 49 (20%), which, if extrapolated to the total cohort of children with lower respiratory tract disease would indicate that 12% of lower respiratory tract illnesses were caused by hMPV, similar to the 15% from RSV in this defined group of young children.

Two prospective population-based studies have examined the burden of lower respiratory disease caused by hMPV in hospitalized children, one in the United States (Mullins et al.) and one in Hong Kong (Peiris et al.). HMPV was identified by RT-PCR in 3.9% of the 668 samples obtained from children younger than 5 years of age hospitalized for acute respiratory illness in Rochester, New York and Nashville, Tennessee. In comparison, RSV was identified in 18.7%, parainfluenza viruses 1 to 3 in 6.7%, and influenza in 3.4%. The estimated hospitalization rates per 100,000 persons for hMPV were 114 cases for children younger than 12 months of age, 131 cases for 1- to 2-year-olds, and 10 cases for children 2 to 5 years of age.

In a similar population of 587 children 3 to 72 months of age hospitalized with acute respiratory illness in Hong Kong, the rate of hMPV-associated admissions was similar at 5.5%, and the annual rate of hMPV hospitalizations was estimated as 442 hospital admissions per 1,000 children younger than 6 years of age.

Although firm estimates of hMPV's role in causing respiratory illness are difficult to obtain from recent studies of varying populations and laboratory methods, clearly hMPV appears to be a major actor in the burden of acute respiratory illness borne by the young child and an epidemiologic mime of RSV.

PATHOGENESIS

The pathogenesis of hMPV has yet to be delineated. Some characteristics of infection that hMPV shares with RSV and the parainfluenza viruses have engendered the hypothesis that its pathogenesis also may involve both the viral cytopathic effect and immunologic mechanisms.

The acquisition of infection in the young child likely occurs from close contact with older caretakers because infection occurs in individuals of all ages when the virus is active in the community. Inoculation into the respiratory tract of the young child from direct contact with infected secretions or large-droplet aerosols from these close contacts is the putative scenario. The virus may be isolated in specimens from the upper and lower respiratory tract and blood, and it may be shed in respiratory secretions for a variable period, ranging from a few to 20 days in hospitalized infants. Of 17 infants who had both nasopharyngeal secretions and plasma tested for the presence of hMPV, seven had the virus identified in both the nasopharyngeal and plasma specimens. More prospective studies including suitable controls are required to delineate the average duration of shedding in various age groups and also to determine the clinical significance of detecting the virus in respiratory secretions for prolonged periods by highly sensitive techniques, such as real-time polymerase chain reaction (PCR).

A specific humoral-antibody response appears to be consistent and durable. Seroprevalence studies have identified specific IgG and neutralizing antibodies in individuals from birth to 99 years of age. The low rate of infection in infants in the first months of life and the high prevalence of passive maternal antibody at birth indicate that serum antibody is protective. With the decline of passive antibody that occurs during the infant's first few months of life, the rates of infection begin to climb. The greatest increase in seroprevalence occurs during the next 2 years, indicating that early childhood is the prime period for the acquisition of hMPV infection.

Repeated infections occur throughout life, as documented by the identification of hMPV in respiratory secretions of individuals at all ages. Furthermore, the mean titer of specific antibody has been higher in those older than 2 years of age, suggesting that anamnestic responses develop from repeated encounters with hMPV. Specific antibody, therefore, is neutralizing, durable, and uniformly produced, but it does not afford complete protection against infection. Whether this event results partly from less cross-protection against heterogeneous group strains is unknown. It is suggested by the observation that one immunocompromised child developed hMPV infection with a different subgroup strain in 2 subsequent years.

Both local and systemic cell-mediated immunity are likely to be important in controlling hMPV infection, but more information in deciphering their roles is needed.

CLINICAL MANIFESTATIONS AND COMPLICATIONS

Infection with hMPV may be manifest in both children and adults as respiratory infections with a range of severity from mild or asymptomatic disease to severe lower respiratory tract illness. Most reports thus far have involved patients who have been hospitalized with acute respiratory illness. In these patients, the overall clinical picture is similar to that produced by RSV.

In hospitalized children in whom hMPV infection is identified, the most frequent diagnoses are lower respiratory tract infection, primarily bronchiolitis and bronchitis, which account for one-fourth to two-thirds of the diagnoses. Pneumonia and exacerbation of reactive airway disease are reported as causing 2% to 30% of the illnesses. Acute laryngotracheobronchitis has been diagnosed in approximately 3% to 20% of children infected with hMPV, suggesting that this manifestation occurs less commonly than with the parainfluenza viruses but more frequently than with RSV infection. In the study of healthy children younger than 5 years of age enrolled in a vaccine clinic, croup was associated with 18% of hMPV infections, 11% of RSV infections, and 64% of parainfluenza infections. Pneumonia was associated less often with hMPV (8%) than with RSV (21%), but exacerbations of asthma were more frequent in children with hMPV (14%) than with RSV (3%). hMPV infection frequently is associated with upper respiratory tract infections at all ages, but less so in young children and the elderly. Otitis media has accompanied hMPV infection in about 10% to 40% of young children.

The most frequent signs and symptoms in children in the first 2 years of life are fever (usually low grade), cough, nasal congestion or rhinorrhea, and lower respiratory tract signs of crackles with or without wheezing. In children who are hospitalized, 50% to 90% have this constellation of signs. Sore throat and conjunctivitis also may occur but generally are reported less frequently.

In comparison to infections caused by RSV in young children, those from hMPV appear to cause clinical illness requiring medical attention less frequently and to occur in patients having an older mean age. In hospitalized children in Hong Kong, the mean age was 32 months, and in the United States, it was 11.5 months compared with 3 months for RSV infection. The overall course of hMPV infection usually is shorter than that for RSV, and the presentation more commonly is that of an upper respiratory tract infection or pneumonia. However, lower respiratory tract disease in young children may be as severe as that accompanying RSV infection. Of those children hospitalized with lower respiratory tract disease, one-third to one-half required oxygen, and 5% to 8% have been mechanically ventilated.

The chest roentgenogram of children hospitalized with lower respiratory tract disease commonly shows focal, bilateral infiltrates, peribronchial cuffing, and hyperinflation (Fig. 190.2). These findings usually are not distinctive from those observed with other lower respiratory tract infections from such agents as RSV and the parainfluenza viruses.

Complications may occur during the acute course of hMPV infection in hospitalized children, although most are not life-threatening. Apnea has been reported occasionally in conjunction with lower respiratory tract disease. Otitis media, as noted above, commonly is associated with hMPV infection, but whether it is caused by hMPV alone, by concurrent bacterial or viral infections, or by both, is unclear. Concurrent infections with other pathogens have been documented frequently. In infants, 30% or more of the hMPV infections are accompanied by another agent, which is most often RSV. The role that these co-infections play in the clinical presentation is unclear but confounds the etiologic diagnosis. In one study of 30 infants with severe RSV bronchiolitis, 70% had coinfection with hMPV, which the authors hypothesized as augmenting the severity of the RSV infection.

Hyperreactivity of the airway may occur after infection with hMPV, but it appears to be a less common sequela than that following RSV infection. The frequency of subsequent wheezing episodes or exacerbations of asthma after hMPV infection has been reported variably as occurring in 2% to 20% of children. Rawlinson et al. found hMPV infection commonly was present in children with exacerbations of asthma but infrequently in those whose asthma was currently asymptomatic. In contrast to RSV infection, hMPV infection may be a poor inducer of the chemokine RANTES, the chemotactic factor for eosinophils, but a good inducer of IL-8, which attracts neutrophils.

Repeated Infections

Recurrent infections may be asymptomatic or symptomatic and manifest as upper or lower respiratory tract infections. In a retrospective analysis by Boivin et al. of specimens from patients with respiratory illness in Canada, 38 hMPV isolates were obtained from 37 patients who were 2 months to 99 years of age (median age, 49 years). Seventy percent were hospitalized, and 19% were in chronic-care facilities. The majority had underlying conditions, including immunocompromised states and chronic pulmonary conditions. Thirty-five percent were younger than 5 years of age, and 46% were older than 65 years of age. In this group of patients, lower respiratory tract illness predominated, and some patients required intensive care. In those younger than 5 years of age, the median duration of hospitalization was 4 days, whereas in those older than 65 years of age, the median number of days of hospitalization was 10.5. An additional viral agent also was detected in 24% of the 38 samples containing hMPV.

Information is limited, especially with regard to previously healthy individuals, on the proportion of repeated infections that are asymptomatic, as well as on the clinical features most frequently noted in those repeated infections that are symptomatic. Information from the majority of studies has been

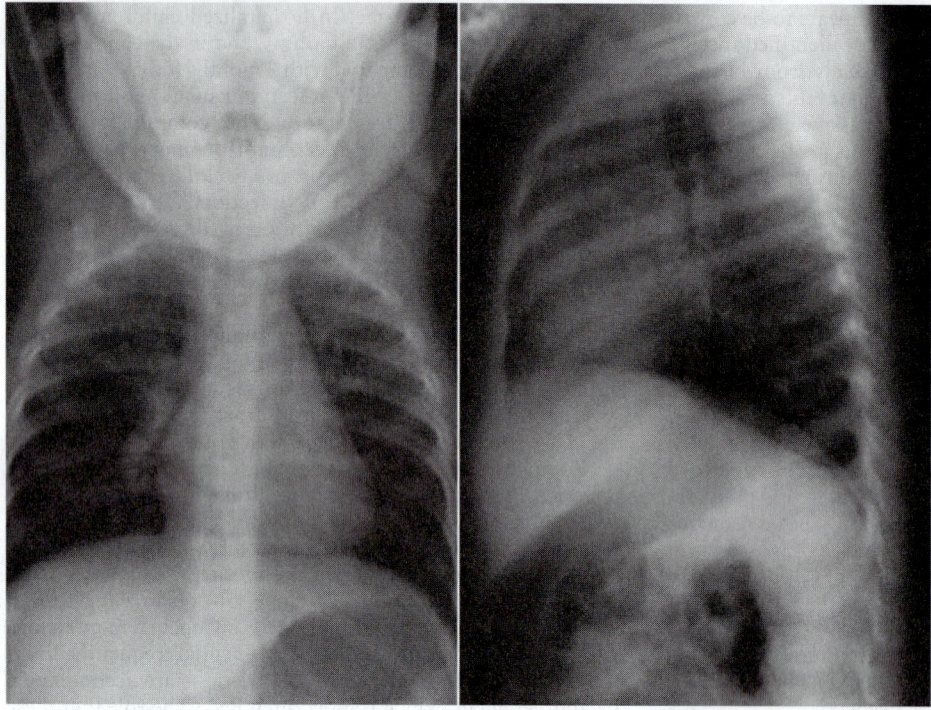

FIGURE 190.2. Chest radiographs of 6-month-old infant with hMPV bronchiolitis, showing hyperinflation and diffuse perihilar infiltrates. (Courtesy of John V. Williams, M.D.; Division of Infectious Diseases, Departments of Pediatrics.)

derived retrospectively from patients with underlying conditions, thus confounding the correlation of the onset and duration of hMPV shedding with the acquisition of hMPV infection, the onset of symptoms, and the role of any coinfecting agents.

One prospective study in Rochester, New York, included both healthy adults and high-risk adults with underlying cardiopulmonary diseases. In this study, hMPV infection was associated with 44 (4.5%) of 984 illnesses. However, hMPV also was detected in 9 (4.1%) of 217 asymptomatic infections. The rates of hMPV infection that were symptomatic and asymptomatic in the healthy elderly were 1.7% and 1.4%, respectively. In young, healthy adults, asymptomatic infection was found more commonly (9.5%) than was symptomatic infection (6.6%). In high-risk adults, symptomatic infection occurred twice as frequently as did asymptomatic infection (3% versus 1.5%). These data suggest that asymptomatic infection with hMPV may be a frequent occurrence at all ages, but it is more likely to be symptomatic in those individuals who have comorbid conditions.

Conditions Increasing Risk of More Severe Infection

Although a determination of all the risk factors for symptomatic and more complicated infection with hMPV still are incomplete, the information thus far suggests that, for both children and adults, those factors that increase the risk for acquiring severe disease are similar to those for RSV. In previously healthy individuals, exposure to smoke, day-care attendance, and young or older age have been associated with an elevated chance of having clinical severity.

Underlying conditions likely to augment the severity of disease include premature gestation, chronic lung disease, and immunocompromised states. The complication most frequently reported is involvement of the lower respiratory tract, predominately pneumonia. The marked severity reported in some of these cases appears related primarily to exacerbations of the underlying condition triggered by the hMPV infection.

DIAGNOSIS

The clinical and laboratory findings associated with hMPV infection in children generally are not distinctive from those associated with other viral respiratory infections. The complete blood cell count and C-reactive protein have been reported as being usually within the normal range. Identification of hMPV infection, therefore, requires both a high degree of suspicion that hMPV may be the cause of the infection and specific laboratory diagnosis.

Van den Hoogen et al. initially discovered hMPV by using a random PCR amplification strategy. It involved fingerprinting the RNA genome with a PCR employing arbitrary primers, followed by refining the primers to identify hMPV specifically. Currently, RT-PCR is the diagnostic method most frequently used, with primers that have varied according to the research laboratory.

RT-PCR appears to be the most sensitive of generally available methods. The RT-PCR assays currently employ primers directed at the conserved genomic areas of the F, M, N, and L ORFs. The relative sensitivity and reproducibility of the individual assays using these different primers for the most part have not been determined. One recent report developed a real-time RT-PCR using a LightCycler™ platform that the authors found to be specific, more sensitive, and less time consuming than a conventional RT-PCR.

hMPV also may be isolated from upper and lower respiratory tract specimens in tissue culture, usually in rhesus monkey kidney (LLC-MK2) or tMK cells. The sensitivity and feasibility of isolation is diminished by the long period required for a cytopathic effect to occur and by the variability of its presence and appearance in different cell lines. The expense also is augmented by the use and maintenance of noncontinuous cell cultures over a long period.

Several serologic assays have been used for diagnosis, primarily in research laboratories, because serologic diagnosis is not helpful in the management of the acute infection. Those assays currently utilized have included immunofluorescence assays on infected tissue culture, IgG EIA, and neutralization assays. More standard and rapid serologic assays are under development.

THERAPY

Currently, the management and therapy of hMPV infections are supportive. No clinically effective antiviral agent has been identified thus far. *In vitro* ribavirin and polyclonal intravenous immunoglobulin have been shown to have equivalent antiviral activity against hMPV and RSV, suggesting that this may be an option for hMPV infections, similar to that for RSV, in severely immunocompromised patients.

PREVENTION

Methods are needed for preventing hMPV infection. The number of cases of hMPV infection that are acquired nosocomially may be diminished by the use of appropriate infection control procedures.

The mode of transmission of hMPV is unknown, but it may be similar to that of RSV, which requires close contact with infectious respiratory secretions. With RSV infection, this contact may occur via large-droplet aerosols from an infected individual or via fomites with subsequent self-inoculation occurring from contaminated hands. Integral to the efficacy of infection control procedures for RSV is compliance by all medical personnel with methods of good hand cleansing. This need requires repetitive emphasis. Additional procedures include cohorting and screening of both visitors and health care workers for acute respiratory signs to diminish the introduction of hMPV onto the wards.

No vaccine for hMPV is available. However, for the closely related avian metapneumovirus, inactivated vaccines directed at the F protein and live vaccines have been developed.

Suggested Readings

Boivin G, Abed Y, Pelletier G, et al. Virological features and clinical manifestations associated with human metapneumovirus: a new paramyxovirus responsible for acute respiratory-tract infections in all age groups. *J Infect Dis* 2002;186:1330.

Boivin G, De Serres G, Cote S, et al. Human metapneumovirus infections in hospitalized children. *Emerg Infect Dis* 2003;9:634640.

Biovin G, MacKay I, Sloots, TP et al. Global genetic diversity of human metapneumovirus fusion gene. *Emerg Infect Dis* 2004;10:1154.

Esper F, Boucher D, Weibel C, et al. Human metapneumovirus infection in the United States: clinical manifestations associated with a newly emerging respiratory infection in children. *Pediatrics* 2003;111:1407.

Falsey A, Erdman D, Anderson L, et al. Human metapneumovirus infections in young and elderly adults. *J Infect Dis* 2003;187:785.

Mejias A, Chávez-Bueno S, Ramilo O. Human metapneumovirus: a not so new virus. *Pediatr Infect Dis J* 2004;23:1.

Mullins JA, Erdman DD, Weinberg GA, et al. Human metapneumovirus infection among children hospitalized with acute respiratory illness. *Emerg Infect Dis* 2004;10:700.

Nissen M, Siebert D, Mackay I, et al. Evidence of human metapneumovirus in Australian children. *Med J Aust* 2002;176:188.

Peiris J, Tang W, Chan K, et al. Children with respiratory disease associated with metapneumovirus in Hong Kong. *Emerg Infect Dis* 2003;9:628.

Peret T, Boivin G, Li Y, et al. Characterization of human metapneumoviruses isolated from patients in North America. *J Infect Dis* 2002;185:1660.

Rawlinson WD, Waliuzzaman Z, Carter IW, et al. Asthma exacerbations in children associated with rhinovirus but not human metapneumovirus infection. *J Infect Dis* 2003;187:1314.

Stockton J, Stephenson I, Fleming D, et al. Human metapneumovirus as a cause of community-acquired respiratory illness. *Emerg Infect Dis* 2002;8:897.

Van den Hoogen BG, Fouchier R. Clinical impact and diagnosis of Human metapneumovirus infection. *Pediatr Infect Dis J* 2004;23:S25.

Vicente D, Cilla G, Montes M, et al. Human metapneumovirus and community-acquired respiratory illness in children. *Emerg Infect Dis* 2003;9:602.

Williams JV, Harris PA, Tollefson SJ, et al. Human metapneumovirus and lower respiratory tract disease in otherwise healthy infants and children. *N Engl J Med* 2004;350:443.

Wyde PR, Chetty SN, Jewell AM et al. Comparison of the inhibition of human metapneumovirus and respiratory syncytial virus by ribavirin and immune serum globulin *in vitro*. *Antiviral Res* 2003;60:51.

CHAPTER 191 ■ RESPIRATORY SYNCYTIAL VIRUS

CAROLINE BREESE HALL

Chameleon of decades past and new
Can we yet find the way to conquer you?
For underneath your coat of guise there lies
A soul of genes programmed to yet surprise.
—CBH

Respiratory syncytial virus (RSV) is the major cause of lower respiratory tract illness in young children. Worldwide, acute respiratory illness is the leading cause of morbidity and mortality in young children, with an estimated 4 million deaths occurring annually in those within the first 5 years of life. Viruses have been shown to be the most frequent cause, and RSV is the leading agent identified. In the United States, the estimated cost associated with hospitalization for RSV in infants is $300 to $600 million each year. The additional burden engendered from illness in outpatients is unknown, but is considerable.

RSV was discovered in 1956, and it was christened the *chimpanzee coryza agent* (CCA) because it was isolated from a source colony of chimpanzees suffering from the common cold. Its subsequent isolation from infants with lower respiratory tract disease and its characteristic appearance in tissue culture resulted in its current appellation of *respiratory syncytial virus*.

VIRUS CHARACTERIZATION

RSV belongs to the *Paramyxoviridae* family within the genus *Pneumovirus*. This genus contains the morphologically and biologically similar pneumonia virus of mice, bovine RSV, ovine RSV, caprine RSV, turkey rhinotracheitis virus, and the recently discovered human metapneumovirus. RSV is an enveloped, medium-sized RNA virus with a nonsegmented, single-stranded, negative-sense genome. Three of the proteins (N, P, and L) are associated with the nucleocapsid, and five (F, G, SH, M, and M2) are associated with the envelope. Two proteins, NS1 and NS2, are nonstructural proteins of the virion. The two major surface glycosylated proteins, F and G, project from the surface, giving the envelope a thistle-like appearance. These glycoproteins appear to be of prime importance in the infectivity and pathogenesis of the virus.

RSV is a notably liable virus, poorly withstanding changes in temperature and pH. RSV in the secretions of patients may survive at room temperature on nonporous surfaces, such as countertops and furniture, for 3 to 30 hours depending on the humidity. On hands, RSV remains infectious for approximately 0.5 to 1 hour.

Two major strain groups, A and B, with subtypes within each group, have been identified through monoclonal antibody and genomic analyses. The major antigenic variations between these strain groups have been associated primarily with the G protein. Both group A and B strains usually circulate concurrently in a given community. The epidemiologic and clinical importance of infection caused by strains from group A versus group B remains unclear.

EPIDEMIOLOGY

RSV infection occurs globally, being identified in every geographic area studied. In most communities, RSV's seasonal pattern is singular, predictably producing a sizable outbreak of infections each year, especially in temperate climates. In the United States, RSV activity usually lasts for approximately 20 weeks, from November to May, with the peak period of circulation usually occurring during January through March.

The concurrent rise in bronchiolitis and lower respiratory tract illnesses in young children signals an RSV outbreak, even without laboratory confirmation. RSV spreads so effectively among the young that virtually all children have been infected within their first 2 to 3 years of life. During the first year of exposure to RSV, 50% or more of infants acquire infection, and 40% of these infections have been estimated to result in lower respiratory tract illness. Prospective studies of families in Houston showed that 69% of infants acquired RSV infection, and one-third of them had lower respiratory tract disease. In their second year, 83% of children became infected, and 16% had lower respiratory tract disease. Repetitive infections occurred frequently; one-third to one-half of these patients became reinfected in their third and fourth year. The risk of developing an infection is even greater for children in day-care centers, with 65% to 98% acquiring infection during each of their first 3 years.

Infection severe enough to cause hospitalization occurs primarily in infants younger than 12 months of age, especially in those younger than 6 months of age. Recent data from the Centers for Disease Control and Prevention (CDC) have indicated that the annual rates of hospitalization for bronchiolitis increased 2.4 times between 1980 and 1996. RSV was estimated to cause 51,000 to 82,000 bronchiolitis admissions yearly.

The risk factors associated with more severe disease include not only young age but also underlying cardiac or pulmonary disease and host factors of genetic susceptibility associated with specific gene polymorphisms. Other factors that have been associated with augmenting the chance of young children acquiring RSV disease include crowding, lower socioeconomic income, multiple siblings, older school-age siblings, and exposure to passive smoke.

PATHOGENESIS

RSV is acquired through the inoculation of respiratory secretions of infected individuals into the nose or eyes of another individual. Close contact with such individuals may result in inoculation from large-particle aerosols generated by sneezing or coughing or by contacting infectious secretions on fomites, with subsequent self-inoculation. After an incubation period of 3 to 6 days, the virus spreads during primary infection along the epithelium of the respiratory tract, producing bronchiolitis and/or pneumonia.

Early in the course of bronchiolitis, a lymphocytic peribronchiolar infiltration associated with edema of the walls and surrounding tissue is evident. Progression of the infection causes the characteristic necrosis and sloughing of the bronchiolar epithelium, resulting in the plugging of the infant's airways, which are particularly prone because of their small diameter. Impedance to the flow of air occurs during both inspiration and expiration, but it is augmented during expiration when the lumen is narrowed further by the positive expiratory pressure. Air trapped peripheral to the sites of partial occlusion results in the clinical manifestation of hyperinflation of the lung. When complete obstruction occurs, the trapped air may become absorbed, resulting in multiple areas of atelectasis. Lower respiratory tract involvement from RSV commonly exhibits pathologic findings of both bronchiolitis and pneumonia, with interstitial infiltration of mononuclear cells and alveolar filling. Recovery is marked by evidence of regeneration at the bronchiolar epithelium, usually within the first week, but the presence of ciliated cells and complete recovery may require weeks.

Immunity

An immunologic process has been hypothesized as integral to the pathogenesis of infant lower respiratory tract disease and its potential severity. This hypothesis has been based primarily on the observations that repeated infections occur throughout life, indicating the lack of a durable protective response and, second, by the experience with the initial RSV vaccine. This formalin-inactivated vaccine, given during trials in the 1960s, resulted in enhanced, even fatal, disease in some infants when they subsequently acquired natural RSV infection.

The potential role of the innate and adaptive immune response in RSV disease and protection remains undefined, but the research it has engendered has resulted in much information potentially applicable to the therapy and prevention of this ubiquitous infection.

The normal humoral immune response to initial RSV infection is marked by a transitory rise in specific IgM antibody in the serum. Subsequently, usually within 2 weeks, IgG antibody appears. The IgG antibody produced is durable, but the titer tends to decline over the course of the next 1 to 2 months. The neutralizing antibody responses to the F and G proteins have been correlated with subsequent protection against reinfection. However, the neutralizing antibody response to the glycosylated proteins, F and G, tends to be relatively poor in young infants. Passively derived maternal antibody also may inhibit the antibody response.

The local production of antibody may be important in controlling the infection as the virus spreads from cell to cell. Neutralizing activity has been identified in the nasal secretions of infected children and correlated with diminished viral shedding, but not with protection against illness or its severity. A specific secretory antibody response also has been identified in infants and includes IgM, IgA, IgG, and IgE antibodies bound to epithelial cells and free in nasal secretions. Their effect on the course of infection is not entirely clear.

Systemic and local cell-mediated immune responses are likely to be integral in effecting the clearance of virus and in recovery. However, their roles in protecting against reinfection and illness have not been demonstrated clearly. Nonetheless, the importance of the cellular immune response is supported by the observation that adults and children with compromised cellular immunity tend to have prolonged, severe, and sometimes fatal infection with RSV. Although laboratory measures of cell-mediated immunity, including lymphocyte transformation activity and cytotoxic T-lymphocyte responses, have been identified in both adults and infants after having RSV infection, they have not been associated clearly with affecting the course of the disease. Most of the information elucidating the function and importance of the multiple components of the immune response has come from animal models, and the results have been variable and sometimes conflicting.

Immunity to RSV may be summarized as being complex, with an effective response requiring a fine balance of the innate and adaptive components of immunity. First, these components appear to be affected by a variety of viral, environmental, and host factors, including genetic susceptibility. Second, the immunity evoked is not complete or durable, but some protection is afforded by natural infection, as supported by the observation that severe lower respiratory tract disease rarely occurs after the patient's first encounter with the virus.

CLINICAL MANIFESTATIONS AND COMPLICATIONS

Infection in Infants and Young Children

The initial encounter with RSV infection almost always is symptomatic, but it may have a range of severity from a mild upper respiratory tract infection to a life-threatening lower respiratory tract infection. The risk of lower respiratory tract disease developing during primary infection is high. Lower respiratory tract infections with the first RSV infection commonly are manifest as pneumonia or bronchiolitis and have been estimated to occur in approximately 30% to 70% of initial RSV infections. In crowded and closed populations of infants, such as those in day-care centers, the proportion of infants developing bronchiolitis or pneumonia may be even higher. Tracheobronchitis also may occur with primary infection, especially in infants who are outpatients. Croup is a relatively unusual manifestation of RSV. Of all croup cases, approximately 10% are attributed to RSV, in comparison to 5% to 40% of cases of pneumonia and bronchitis and 50% to 90% of bronchiolitis cases.

The initial manifestations of RSV infection in young children usually are those of an upper respiratory tract infection. Fever, usually low-grade, is a common occurrence during the first few days of illness, as are cough and nasal congestion. Hoarseness and laryngitis, however, usually are not prominent. Spread to the lower respiratory tract often is heralded by a worsening cough. Fever may no longer be present when lower-tract involvement becomes evident. As the disease progresses, dyspnea, tachypnea, and retractions of the intercostal muscles, along with diffuse crackles and the hallmarks of bronchiolitis, wheezing and hyperinflation, may be observed. In cases of pneumonia, localized or diffuse crackles and sometimes hyperinflation are present. In cases of both bronchiolitis and pneumonia, expiratory and inspiratory wheezing and crackles may be evident and characteristically are variable within short periods of time. Bronchiolitis and pneumonia thus often are difficult to differentiate clinically and may be a continuum of the course of the infection. Hypoxemia usually is present in infants requiring hospitalization. The diffuse spread of the virus results in significant areas of lung parenchyma in which the ratio of ventilation to perfusion is low, thus producing arterial hypoxemia. If an infant no longer is able to compensate for the disordered gas exchange by increasing ventilation, hypercarbia may ensue.

A roentgenogram of the chest can show a variety of findings, ranging from minimal findings of peribronchial thickening to multiple areas of interstitial infiltration and hyperinflation. Hyperaeration, evident in more than half of hospitalized children, is particularly characteristic of RSV infection. Approximately 20% to 25% of infants will have on their chest roentgenograms a consolidated area, most frequently subsegmental in the right upper or middle lobe, which may be from atelectasis. Characteristically, the roentgenographic findings do not correlate with the severity of illness.

One of the most frequent complications during the acute phase of the illness is otitis media. Through polymerase chain reaction (PCR), the virus has been detected in 75% of middle-ear effusions. RSV may be the only pathogen identified in the middle-ear fluid, but commonly it is present in conjunction with a bacterial pathogen, usually *Streptococcus pneumoniae*. Studies have suggested that otitis media caused by a co-infection of RSV and a bacterial pathogen result in a worse outcome and greater chance of failure with antibiotic therapy.

Apnea is a life-threatening complication of acute RSV, occurring in approximately 20% of hospitalized cases. Apnea is most likely to develop in premature infants and in those who have not yet reached a postconceptional age of 44 weeks. Apnea may be the initial sign of RSV infection, thus preceding any overt respiratory signs. A follow-up of infants presenting with apnea indicates that most of them do not have increased risk of apneic episodes occurring with subsequent respiratory infections.

Infants with RSV bronchiolitis may be at high risk for aspiration, which also may be manifest as wheezing. Recent studies have suggested that, in infants who received preventive therapy with thickened feedings and early ribavirin therapy, subsequent episodes of reactive airway disease were reduced significantly compared with infants who received no such therapy.

Secondary bacterial infection in developed countries is an unusual complication of RSV infection, occurring in fewer than 1% of cases. Although antibiotics frequently are administered to young infants with RSV infection, their use has not resulted in an improved rate of recovery.

Infections in Older Children and Adults

Recurrent RSV infections occur throughout life, sometimes with intervals of only months between infections. In healthy individuals, these recurrent infections generally are mild, most commonly manifesting as an upper respiratory tract infection or sometimes tracheobronchitis. The infection may be asymptomatic in approximately 15% of patients. The upper respiratory tract infections associated with RSV tend to be more severe and prolonged than those associated with other viral agents. The involvement of the sinuses and ear occurs more commonly, and the cough may be sufficiently prolonged to evoke the diagnosis of bronchitis. Wheezing may accompany the upper respiratory tract signs, and evidence of hyperreactivity of the airway may last as long as 8 weeks, even in previously healthy individuals. Although these repeated infections generally are less severe than is the initial infection, a significant portion still involve the lower respiratory tract and require medical attention.

Infections in Patients with Underlying Conditions

In contrast to infection in healthy individuals, repeated infection with RSV in individuals with compromised and chronic conditions, as well as in the elderly, may result in severe and sometimes fatal disease. Children most at risk for requiring hospitalization include those with premature birth, underlying chronic lung disease, congenital heart disease, immunosuppressive conditions, and other chronic diseases such as nephrotic syndrome. One-quarter to two-thirds of hospitalized young children with RSV infection have an underlying condition (Fig. 191.1). Infants younger than 32 weeks' gestation are seven times more likely to require hospitalization than are full-term infants. The presence of chronic lung disease further increases this risk. An estimated 17% of such infants will require hospitalization for RSV during the first 2 years of life, and an

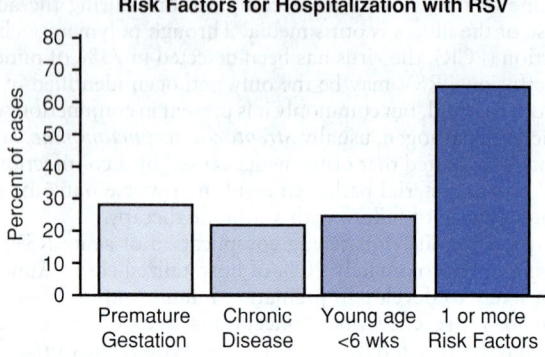

FIGURE 191.1. Risk factors occurring in 1,708 infants who were hospitalized with proven respiratory syncytial viral infections in Rochester, NY.

appreciable proportion will require intensive care and mechanical ventilation.

RSV recently has been recognized in immunosuppressed patients as an opportunistic agent associated with nosocomial outbreaks. In transplantation units, remarkably severe illness has resulted, with reported mortality rates of 30% to 100%. The control of RSV in immunosuppressed patients is confounded by its clinical manifestations being similar to those of other opportunistic agents that are more commonly considered and diagnosed in this group.

DIAGNOSIS

A reasonably accurate diagnosis of RSV infection in young children may be made on the basis of the distinctive epidemiology and clinical manifestations of RSV infection. In older children and adults, the findings are less distinctive and accurate. Specific laboratory diagnosis may be made by viral isolation, a rapid antigen detection assay RT-PCR, or serology. Viral isolation traditionally has been the standard method, but the expense and quality of cell lines and laboratory expertise, as well as the time involved, are disadvantages. The optimal specimen is a nasal wash or tracheal secretions. Because RSV is a liable virus, the specimen requires prompt transport to the laboratory without subjecting it to major temperature changes.

Commercially available rapid assays for detecting RSV antigen have become widely used because of their simplicity and value in making decisions concerning infection control and specific therapy. Most of them involve an enzyme immunoassay that may be performed in less than 1 hour. Their disadvantage is their variable sensitivity, ranging from 50% to 90%, usually 60% to 70%. These tests, therefore, should be used only during the RSV season, when the incidence of the virus in the community is high, and, if they are negative, the patient should be tested further by another method. Direct and indirect immunofluorescent assays generally are highly specific, but they require more time and technical expertise. Reverse transcriptase-polymerase chain reaction (RT-PCR) appears to have higher rates of specificity and sensitivity than do other currently available diagnostic methods, and with the inclusion of appropriate additional primers, it allows the simultaneous detection of multiple pathogens.

Serologic diagnosis rarely is of help in the management of the patient because of the requirement of acute and convalescent sera. Furthermore, maternally derived specific antibodies are present in all young infants, and all individuals subsequent to primary infection possess specific antibody. Neutralization and enzyme immunoassay (EIA) are the serologic assays used most frequently, and they offer the possibility of detecting specific antibody classes. Assays for IgM antibodies to RSV are of limited use because they commonly are not evoked in patients with proven infection and, if present, may not be detectable until 6 to 40 days after the onset of illness.

THERAPY

Most young children with RSV infection require no more than care given to provide comfort and to ensure the adequate intake of fluids. Supportive care is of even greater importance in the hospitalized infant. It should be based first on the recognition that the course and physical findings during RSV infection may fluctuate rapidly. Thus, in the more severely infected infant, obtaining documentation of blood gases is essential. Additional therapies have included mainly ribavirin, bronchodilating agents, corticosteroids, and antibiotics. In general, most of these agents have limited benefit, and their use should be highly selective and individualized. Nonetheless, these agents have been used in most infants hospitalized with RSV infection.

Ribavirin, a synthetic nucleoside analog, is the only specific treatment currently approved for RSV lower respiratory tract disease in hospitalized infants. Ribavirin has a broad spectrum of antiviral activity, and resistance to the drug has not been shown. It is administered by aerosol, usually for 8 to 24 hours per day, until clinical improvement occurs. It may be administered for shorter and intermittent periods. Although the drug generally has been well tolerated and shown clinical benefit in some studies, in others the short-term outcome has not been shown to be affected. The degree of benefit from ribavirin therapy relative to its cost must be considered on an individual basis.

Bronchodilators, including oral and inhaled beta$_2$ agonists, combined alpha and beta agonists, and anticholinergics, frequently are used in the management of bronchiolitis. Studies of these agents have given variable results, possibly partly because the hallmark manifestation of bronchiolitis, wheezing, can be engendered by several different mechanisms other than bronchial hyperreactivity. In the young infant, the small diameter of the airways renders them particularly vulnerable to obstruction from the inflammatory cellular material and mucus produced during RSV infection. A meta-analysis of bronchodilator therapies could not document their benefit because of the heterogenicity of the populations and methods used. Thus, use of bronchodilator therapy for the routine management of first-time wheezers younger than 1 year of age generally is not recommended.

Studies evaluating both inhaled and systemic corticosteroid therapy for bronchiolitis, as well as for proven RSV bronchiolitis, have yielded similarly conflicting results. One meta-analysis found that patients receiving systemic corticosteroid therapy had 0.43 days less of hospitalization and symptoms than did controls. However, these studies included infants with previous episodes of wheezing. In trials that excluded infants with a history of previous wheezing, no significant benefit was evident. Corticosteroid therapy, therefore, also is not recommended for the routine management of infants who are first-time wheezers.

Antibiotics also are administered commonly to young infants with bronchiolitis. The rarity of bacterial infection complicating RSV bronchiolitis supports the recommendation that antibiotics should not be used in cases without valid evidence of concurrent bacterial infection.

PROGNOSIS

Most infants do well and recover from the acute illness within 2 to 7 days. The cough, however, may persist for several weeks. The major sequela recognized is recurrent episodes of wheezing. After hospitalization for RSV lower respiratory tract disease, approximately 50% of patients experience subsequent reactive airway disease, primarily during the first couple of years. In most of these children, these manifestations diminish with age. Whether RSV has a direct role in producing the predisposition to having subsequent episodes of wheezing is not clear. The potential link between reactive airway disease and RSV infection, nonetheless, has engendered much research that has suggested that similar immune and neuronal pathways exist with RSV infection and reactive airway disease, which may be the mechanism linking the two.

PREVENTION

The prevention of RSV infection is the preferred method for control, but this goal remains unattained. Complete prevention of RSV infections currently is likely to be no more than a mirage. However, prevention in populations most at risk is an achievable goal and one toward which much already has been accomplished.

Infection Control

Avoiding RSV infection within the home is difficult and unlikely to be possible. General procedures aimed at diminishing the spread of infectious secretions on hands and fomites, nonetheless, may limit the spread of infection. These procedures include good hand washing, including the use of hand rub antiseptic products, and the cleansing of objects likely to be contaminated with secretions. In the hospital, however, recommended procedures for infection control for RSV can be clinically- and cost-effective.

RSV is spread by close contact with contagious secretions from infected individuals via large-droplet aerosols or fomites, with subsequent self-inoculation. Thus, careful hand washing is of prime importance in preventing nosocomial spread. Eye-nose goggles and gloves also have been used. Their use mainly discourages self-inoculation by personnel and may be particularly beneficial when compliance with hand washing is inadequate. Gowns utilized when in close contact with infected patients and isolation or cohorting of infected patients also may help. During the RSV season, visitors should be screened for signs of illness. Staff adherence to the recommended infection-control procedures is of prime importance and may be augmented by a review each year of the procedures prior to the advent of the RSV season.

Prophylaxis with Respiratory Syncytial Antibody Products

The passive administration of intravenous immunoglobulin containing high levels of RSV neutralizing antibody (RSV-IVIG) and, more recently, a monoclonal antibody (palivizumab) for intramuscular administration, has been given monthly during the RSV season to high-risk children to prevent the acquisition of severe RSV infection. RSV-IVIG when administered monthly has been shown to reduce the rate of hospitalization by 41% in children with premature gestation with or without chronic lung disease. The product subsequently developed, palivizumab, is a humanized mouse IgG monoclonal antibody that binds to the F protein of RSV. When administered monthly to high-risk infants, palivizumab gave similar results, reducing hospitalizations for RSV infection by 55%.

Palivizumab currently is the preferred product because of its ease of administration. The American Academy of Pediatrics recommends that prophylaxis with palivizumab be considered for children with chronic lung disease who are younger than 24 months of age and for infants of premature gestation, primarily those with gestational ages of less than 28 weeks. Children with congenital heart disease, who were not included originally in those recommended for prophylaxis because of concern for adverse effects, now are included based on more recent studies showing palivizumab prophylaxis to be safe. A more precise definition of the groups of infants who would most benefit from prophylaxis relative to its considerable cost remains unclear and controversial. Thus, decisions for its use must be individualized.

Immunization

Appreciable barriers exist to the development of an effective and safe vaccine against RSV, especially in infants. Ideally, the vaccine should be effective during the newborn period, when the immune response is not fully developed. The optimal vaccine also should provide better protection than does natural disease, which does not afford durable immunity.

Technologic advances have produced promising subunit, live-attenuated, and polypeptide candidate vaccines. The primary targets for subunit vaccines have been the two major surface glycoproteins, F and G. In trials, these vaccines have been shown to be safe and generally immunogenic in normal children, in those with underlying conditions, in healthy and elderly adults, and in women who are postpartum or in their third trimester of pregnancy.

Live viral candidate vaccines initially were developed using cold-adapted strains from temperature-sensitive mutants. These vaccines were unsuitable for young children because they produced unacceptable degrees of illness, were overattenuated, and were not immunogenic, or some strains were genetically unstable, with reversion to the wild-type virus. Current, more promising candidates have been developed by repetitive rounds of chemical mutagenesis to elicit mutations that provide the desirable attenuation, stability, and immunogenicity. New recombinant genetic engineering technology has allowed the precise manipulation of the genomic soul of RSV and the development of vaccines that once were no more than mirages may yet be possible.

Suggested Readings

Agency for Healthcare Research and Quality (AHRQ). Management of bronchiolitis in infants and children. *Agency for Healthcare Research and Quality: Evidence Report/Technology Assessment* 2003;03-E009:1.

Champlin R, Whimbey E. Community respiratory virus infections in bone marrow transplant recipients: the M.D. Anderson Cancer Center experience. *Biol Blood Marrow Transplant* 2001;7:8S.

Collins P, Chanock R, Murphy B. Respiratory syncytial virus. In: Knipe D, Howley P, eds. *Fields' virology*. Philadelphia: Lippincott Williams & Wilkins, 2001;1341.

Crowe J. Respiratory syncytial virus vaccine development. *Vaccine* 2002;20:S32.

Glezen W, Taber L, Frank A, et al. Risk of primary infection and reinfection with respiratory syncytial virus. *Am J Dis Child* 1986;140:543.

Hall C, Walsh E, Long C, et al. Immunity to and frequency of reinfection with respiratory syncytial virus. *J Infect Dis* 1991;163:693.

Hall C. Nosocomial respiratory syncytial virus infections: the "cold war" has not ended. *Clin Infect Dis* 2000;31:590.

Henderson F, Collier A, Clyde W, et al. Respiratory syncytial virus infections, reinfections and immunity. *N Engl J Med* 1979;300:530.

Meissner H. Selected populations at increased risk from respiratory syncytial virus infection. *Pediatr Infect Dis J* 2003;22:S40.

American Academy of Pediatrics. Revised indications for the use of palivizumab and respiratory syncytial virus immune globulin intravenous for the prevention of respiratory syncytial virus infections—Policy Statement, American Academy of Pediatrics. *Pediatrics* 2003;112:1447.

Shay D, Holman R, Roosevelt G, et al. Bronchiolitis-associated mortality and estimates of respiratory syncytial virus-associated deaths among U.S. children, 1979–1997. *J Infect Dis* 2001;183:16.

CHAPTER 192 ■ PARVOVIRUSES

JAMES D. CHERRY

Parvoviruses infect and cause disease in a great variety of insects and animals. The human parvovirus B19 was discovered serendipitously in 1974, and it was found to be associated with human disease in the early 1980s. B19 virus is the cause of erythema infectiosum (fifth disease) and transient red blood cell aplasia (aplastic crisis), as well as other less common clinical manifestations.

Parvovirus B19 belongs to the family Parvoviridae and the subfamily Parvovirinae, of which three genera have been identified: *Parvovirus*, *Dependovirus*, and *Erythrovirus*. Although B19 virus now is classified as the only member of the genus *Erythrovirus* and not a *Parvovirus*, contemporary literature still refers to it as human parvovirus B19.

Parvovirus B19 is a small (23 nm), single-stranded DNA, nonenveloped virus. It has been propagated in suspension cultures of human erythroid bone marrow and in primary fetal liver cells.

EPIDEMIOLOGY

Most epidemiologic information comes from studies of erythema infectiosum outbreaks. These outbreaks are most prevalent in the winter and spring and last for 3 to 6 months. The disease has a cyclic pattern similar to that of rubella. Peak periods of disease occur approximately every 6 years, with increased activity lasting an average of 3 years.

The case-to-case interval of erythema infectiosum usually is between 4 and 14 days, and the attack rate is high. In school-related outbreaks, attack rates of 25% are common. The highest attack rates are in children 5 to 14 years old; secondary cases occur in preschool children, teachers, and parents. In the home, secondary cases occur more commonly in mothers than in fathers.

Antibody studies indicate the following prevalence data: in children younger than 5 years old, 2% to 9%; in children and adolescents 5 to 18 years old, 15% to 35%; and in adults older than 18 years, 40% to 60%. The prevalence of antibody suggests that many infections are either asymptomatic or symptomatic but are unrecognized as typical B19 viral infections.

The mode of spread is by droplet via the respiratory tract.

PATHOGENESIS

After infection has occurred via the respiratory tract, viremia occurs in which 10^{10} or 10^{11} viral particles per milliliter of blood may be found. Associated with viremia (approximately 7 to 10 days after infection), a profound reticulocytopenia occurs. *In vitro* studies indicate that early erythrocyte precursor cells are susceptible to B19 virus infection. The blood group P antigen is the cellular receptor for B19 virus, and persons who lack this antigen are resistant to infection. Neutropenia, lymphopenia, and a decrease in the platelet count occur in conjunction with the reticulocytopenia. During the second week of infection, hemoglobin values decrease slightly.

In erythema infectiosum, the exanthem occurs approximately 17 to 18 days after infection develops, when virus no longer can be detected in throat swabs or blood specimens. At the time of rash, virus-specific IgM antibody is present, suggesting that the exanthem may be immune-mediated. However, the virus also has been identified in the rash by skin biopsy. In immunocompromised patients who fail to produce effective neutralizing antibodies, persistent infections occur.

CLINICAL MANIFESTATIONS AND COMPLICATIONS

Human parvovirus B19 can cause various manifestations that may depend on the immune status of the host (Table 192.1).

Erythema Infectiosum

Although erythema infectiosum is recognized classically by its distinct rash, studies in volunteers suggest a biphasic illness. Approximately 1 week after infection occurs, a nonspecific febrile illness with headache, chills, malaise, and myalgia develops. These symptoms last 2 to 3 days, followed by an asymptomatic interlude of approximately 7 days, and then the exanthematous phase of the illness begins.

The exanthem occurs in three stages. The first stage is the appearance of a fiery red rash on the cheeks ("slapped-cheek" appearance) and a relative circumoral pallor. The facial appearance is suggestive of scarlet fever, an allergic reaction, or collagen vascular disease. The facial exanthem may be accentuated when the affected person moves from outdoors to a warm room. The second stage follows the onset of facial involvement by 1 to 4 days, as an erythematous maculopapular rash on the trunk and extremities. Initially, this rash is discrete, but soon it takes on a characteristic lacy or reticular pattern. The third stage of the exanthem is characterized by changes in the intensity of the rash, with periodic evanescence and recrudescence. The duration of the third stage is highly variable;

TABLE 192.1

MANIFESTATIONS OF HUMAN PARVOVIRUS B19 INFECTION

Disease or Syndrome Host	Characteristics
Erythema infectiosum (fifth disease)	Normal Children
Polyarthritis	Generally immunocompetent adults (women > men)
Aplastic crisis (usually transient)	Individuals with hemolytic anemia
Chronic anemia	Immunocompromised hosts
Congenital infection (anemia or hydrops fetalis)	Fetus (generally first 20 weeks of pregnancy)

fluctuations are related to environmental factors such as exposure to sunlight and temperature. The rash often is pruritic, especially in adults, and generally is more prominent on the extensor surfaces. Occasionally, slight desquamation is noted in some patients.

Other symptoms and signs are uncommon findings in erythema infectiosum. Headache occurs in approximately one-fifth of affected children and one-half of affected adults. Enanthem is a rare finding, although children occasionally have pharyngitis. Joint pain and swelling and myalgia are particularly troublesome in adults.

In addition to typical erythema infectiosum, other cutaneous manifestations, such as a papular-purpuric glove and sock syndrome, erythema multiforme bullosum, and urticarial and morbilliform eruptions, have been noted.

Arthritis

The most common complication of erythema infectiosum is arthritis. It occurs in 80% or more of adults but in fewer than 10% of children with erythema infectiosum. The illness ranges in severity from mild arthralgia to frank arthritis. Involvement of the joints usually is transient, lasting only a few days, but in some adults these symptoms may persist for weeks or, rarely, months. Arthritis occurs more commonly in women than in men and most often involves the knees, ankles, and proximal interphalangeal joints; involvement usually is bilateral. The onset of arthritis usually occurs 1 to 6 days after the onset of the rash, but occasionally it has been noted before the exanthem. Many adults have arthritis without skin manifestations of infection.

Aplastic Crisis

In individuals with hemolytic anemias, the profound reticulocytopenia associated with acute B19 virus infection may result in critical depression of hemoglobin concentrations. This transitory arrest of production of erythrocytes is termed *aplastic crisis* and can occur in any individual whose erythrocytes have a short lifespan. Individuals at risk for developing aplastic crisis with acute B19 virus infections include those with sickle cell disease, hereditary spherocytosis, thalassemia, pyruvate kinase deficiency, and acquired hemolytic anemias.

In association with aplastic crisis, most patients have fever, malaise, and gastrointestinal symptoms; some also have respiratory symptoms. Typical erythema infectiosum is a rare occurrence.

Laboratory studies in afflicted patients reveal reticulocyte counts between 0% and 1% and hemoglobin values 10% to 30% less than baseline values. Approximately one-fourth of infected patients also have leukopenia and neutropenia, and more than one-third have thrombocytopenia.

Infection in Immunocompromised Patients

Chronic B19 virus infection occurs in some children with immunodeficiencies. Persistent anemia occurs because of a continuous lysis of red blood cell precursors. It has been noted most often in children with acute lymphocytic leukemia, but it also occurs in other acquired and congenital immunodeficiency states. Fatigue and pallor are the only clinical findings. Patients with chronic anemia have high, persistent concentrations of B19 virus in their serum (10^8 particles per ml), and viremia and anemia may, if untreated, persist for years.

Intrauterine Infection

Infection in pregnancy results in fetal hydrops, fetal death, and miscarriage. Studies indicate that maternal B19 virus infections result in a transplacental transmission rate of 33% and a fetal death rate of 9%.

Other Clinical Manifestations

Rarely, erythema infectiosum is complicated by transient hemolytic anemia and encephalitis, with and without residual damage. B19 viral infections associated with thrombocytopenic purpura, Henoch-Schönlein purpura, myocarditis, acute hepatitis, aseptic meningitis, chronic fatigue syndrome, parotitis, pneumonia, hemophagocytic syndrome, vasculitis, glomerulonephritis, and pseudoappendicitis also have been reported.

DIAGNOSIS

The exanthem of erythema infectiosum is characteristic, so the diagnosis is easy to establish during epidemics. Sporadic cases can be a problem because rubella, scarlet fever, and enteroviral infections can be confused with erythema infectiosum. Other differential diagnostic considerations are collagen vascular diseases, drug reactions, and allergic responses to environmental substances.

In patients with chronic hemolytic anemia, the occurrence of an aplastic crisis generally can be assumed to be caused by B19 virus infection. Other causes of moderate degrees of reticulocytopenia and general bone marrow suppression include systemic bacterial infections and marrow-suppressive drugs, such as chloramphenicol.

The specific diagnosis of a B19 viral infection can be made by demonstrating B19-specific IgM antibody in the serum of ill or convalescing individuals by using enzyme-linked immunosorbent assay (ELISA), radioimmunoassay, or immunofluorescence. In immunocompromised patients, antigen can be detected in the serum by DNA hybridization, polymerase chain reaction (PCR), or electron microscopy. Past infection and immunity is determined by the demonstration of specific B19 serum IgG antibody.

THERAPY AND PREVENTION

No specific treatment is available for B19 viral infections. Patients with aplastic crisis may require transfusion; otherwise, B19 viral infections rarely require therapy. Arthritis or arthralgia may be painful and can be treated with nonsteroidal anti-inflammatory agents.

In erythema infectiosum outbreaks, pregnant women should, when possible, avoid having contact with susceptible school-aged children. If B19 virus infection occurs during pregnancy, the pregnancy should be monitored carefully. At delivery, examination of cord blood or blood from the neonate for virus and IgM antibody reveals whether *in utero* infection occurred. Babies infected *in utero* should be examined periodically for delayed sequelae. Because congenital malformation has not been found to be causally related to B19 virus infection, therapeutic abortion is not indicated for infection during pregnancy.

During erythema infectiosum outbreaks, isolation of exanthematous patients is not useful because the patient no longer is contagious by the time the exanthem occurs. On the other hand, patients with aplastic crisis or immunodeficiency may still be excreting virus and should be isolated from other patients when hospitalized.

Immunocompromised patients with chronic B19 virus infections can be treated successfully with intravenous immunoglobin (IVIG), as can other patients without demonstrated immune deficiencies who have chronic infections. A suggested dose is 400 mg/kg/day for 4 days. Some patients have required repeated treatment courses.

Suggested Readings

American Academy of Pediatrics. Parvovirus B19 (Erythema Infectiosum, fifth disease). In: Pickering LK, ed. *Red Book: 2003 Report of the Committee on Infectious Diseases,* 26th ed. American Academy of Pediatrics, 2003:459.

Anderson MJ, Higgins PG, Davis LR, et al. Experimental parvoviral infection in humans. *J Infect Dis* 1985;152:257.

Bloom ME, Young NS. Parvoviruses. In: Knipe DM, Howley PM, eds. *Virology,* 4th ed. Philadelphia: WB Saunders Co. 2001:2361.

Cherry JD. Human parvovirus B19. In: Feigin RD, Cherry JD, Demmler GJ, Kaplan S, eds. *Textbook of pediatric infectious diseases,* 5th ed. Philadelphia: WB Saunders Co. 2004:1796.

Cherry JD. Parvovirus infections in children and adults. *Advances in Pediatrics,* vol. 46. St. Louis: Mosby, Inc., 1999;245.

Kerr JR. Pathogenesis of human parvovirus B19 in rheumatic disease. *Ann Rheum Dis* 2000;59:672.

Miller E, Fairley CK, Cohen BJ, Seng C. Immediate and long term outcome of human parvovirus B19 infection in pregnancy. *Brit J Obstet Gynaecol* 1998;105:174.

Nocton JJ, Miller LC, Tucker LB, Schaller JG. Human parvovirus B19-associated arthritis in children. *J Pediatr* 1993;122:186.

CHAPTER 193 ■ POLIOVIRUSES

JAMES D. CHERRY

Polioviruses are a subgroup of the enteroviruses. When a susceptible person is infected with a poliovirus, one of the following responses may occur: inapparent infection, minor illness (abortive poliomyelitis), nonparalytic poliomyelitis (aseptic meningitis), or paralytic poliomyelitis. Infection with and disease caused by polioviruses can be controlled completely by universal immunization with poliovirus vaccines.

Polioviruses are single-stranded RNA viruses. They are 30 nm in size and consist of a naked protein capsid and a dense central core of RNA. They grow readily in monkey kidney tissue culture and several different human tissue cultures, and they cause illness and pathology in infected monkeys.

The three distinct antigenic types of polioviruses are types 1, 2, and 3. Infection with a poliovirus results in lifelong immunity to the homologous virus type, but it confers no immunity to the other two viral types.

EPIDEMIOLOGY

The general epidemiology of polioviruses is similar to that of other enteroviruses and is discussed more fully in Chapter 194, Nonpolio Enteroviruses and Parechoviruses. The spread of polioviruses and the clinical manifestations of infection are affected markedly by the degree of vaccine use and the socioeconomic conditions of the population. The epidemiology of poliomyelitis was a mystery until researchers discovered that unrecognized infections were the main source of the spread of the virus. Historically, in populations with poor sanitation and hygiene, epidemics of poliomyelitis did not occur, but widespread dissemination of polioviruses occurred continually. In such populations, immunizing infections with all three poliovirus types occurred in infants who usually were protected from significant clinical disease by transplacentally acquired antibodies. In populations with improved standards of hygiene, immunizing infections in infants no longer occur regularly, so pools of susceptible children form in the population. When poliovirus is introduced into such a population, infection occurs in these older children, and poliomyelitis not infrequently occurs. The age spread of cases of poliomyelitis in a population depends on the overall hygienic standards of the population, as well as such factors as family size and crowding.

The evolution of poliomyelitis from an endemic to epidemic situation followed a characteristic pattern. Initially, only isolated cases occurred. Over the course of years, the endemic rate gradually increased, followed by periodic, then yearly, severe epidemics with high attack rates. Once a community reached a socioeconomic situation in which epidemic poliomyelitis occurred regularly, a gradual shift occurred in the incidence according to age. Relatively few cases occurred in infants, the peak occurred in the 5- to 14-year-old age group, and an increasing proportion of cases occurred in young adults.

The universal use of oral polio vaccines, beginning in the early 1960s, resulted in the elimination of infection with wild polioviruses in the Western Hemisphere and much of the developed world. In 1988, the World Health Assembly established the objective of global polio eradication. By the close of the year 2001, the area of endemic poliomyelitis had been reduced to 10 countries and a reporting of fewer than 1,000 cases.

PATHOGENESIS

The general pathophysiology of enteroviral infections is presented in Chapter 194, Nonpolio Enteroviruses and Parechoviruses.

The virus can be recovered from the blood, throat, and feces of the infected person 3 to 5 days after exposure. At this time, minor illness may occur, or the infection may be unrecognized. Major illness, with involvement of the central nervous system (CNS), has its onset approximately 10 days after infection. Most likely, the blood is the main pathway for viral invasion of the CNS in natural disease. Experimental infections in monkeys, however, have demonstrated that the virus can reach the CNS by traveling along axons of peripheral nerves.

The neuropathology of poliomyelitis usually is pathopneumonic. Neuronal damage is caused directly by multiplication of the virus in the cells; little evidence exists of infection in surrounding tissues except for slight histologic evidence of meningitis and perivascular cuffing. Neuronal lesions are found most commonly in the anterior horn cells of the spinal cord.

CLINICAL MANIFESTATIONS AND COMPLICATIONS

In susceptible persons, 90% to 95% of infections are inapparent and approximately 4% to 8% are classified as minor illness (abortive poliomyelitis); rarely does nonparalytic poliomyelitis (aseptic meningitis) or paralytic poliomyelitis develop. In general, older persons are more likely to have severe paralytic disease and higher mortality rates. Bulbar poliomyelitis may be precipitated by tonsillectomy at the time of inapparent infection; a history of tonsillectomy also is related to a higher rate of bulbar disease.

Abortive poliomyelitis (minor illness) is similar to many other enteroviral infections and frequently is unrecognized as a significant infection. The illness is mild and nonspecific, with low-grade fever, malaise, anorexia, and sore throat. On physical examination, no significant abnormalities are noted.

Nonparalytic Poliomyelitis (Aseptic Meningitis)

Nonparalytic poliomyelitis is similar to aseptic meningitis caused by many other enteroviruses. Initially, illness is characterized by nonspecific fever, malaise, and headache. Other complaints are anorexia, nausea, vomiting, constipation, and diarrhea. Fever usually is moderate (37.8°C to 39.5°C), and muscles usually ache. Soon thereafter, the neck, back, and hamstrings become stiff, and sometimes hyperesthesia and paresthesia occur. Occasionally, the illness is biphasic, with an initial phase (minor illness) consisting of fever and nonspecific complaints and a second phase (CNS or major illness) having symptoms that indicate CNS involvement.

On physical examination, nuchal-spinal signs can be observed. For example, when sitting, the patient uses the hands in a tripod supporting position, indicative of spinal rigidity. Nuchal rigidity can be noted by asking the patient to flex the chin to the chest. Kernig and Brudzinski signs usually are positive. In nonparalytic poliomyelitis, the reflexes usually are normal. Observing the reflexes over the course of time is important, however, because changes may indicate impending paralysis. The white blood cell count usually is normal or slightly elevated. Examination of cerebrospinal fluid (CSF) discloses changes similar to those seen in other enteroviral aseptic meningitides. The cell count range usually varies from 20 to 300 cells per microliter. Although the differential cell count usually has a predominance of lymphocytes, greater than 50% polymorphonuclear leukocytes may be seen early in an illness. The CSF glucose level usually is normal, and the protein concentration is normal or slightly elevated. In the usual case, recovery occurs in 3 to 10 days.

Paralytic Poliomyelitis

The initial findings in paralytic poliomyelitis are similar to those in nonparalytic poliomyelitis except that, occasionally, findings are more pronounced. Fever is likely to be higher, and muscle pain is more conspicuous. Before the onset of actual muscle weakness, superficial and deep tendon reflexes diminish or disappear. Patients destined to develop paralytic poliomyelitis often appear acutely ill, are restless and flushed, and have an anxious expression. Biphasic illness with a symptom-free interlude of several days between the initial illness phase and the development of paralysis commonly occurs in paralytic poliomyelitis.

The onset of paralysis may be sudden, with complete loss of function within a few hours, or it may progress gradually over the course of 3 to 5 days. Asymmetric involvement is typical, particularly in milder cases. Approximately 20% of affected patients have bladder paralysis, which is temporary; paralytic ileus caused by bowel atony is a common occurrence in severe cases. In general, lower limbs are affected more commonly than are upper limbs. In severe cases, quadriplegia occurs, as may functional loss of intercostal, abdominal, and trunk muscles. In affected areas, superficial and deep tendon reflexes are lost, and twitching and diffuse fasciculations of affected muscles may be noted transiently. Sensory abnormalities usually do not occur.

In bulbar disease, the tenth cranial nerve nuclei are involved most commonly, resulting in paralysis of the pharynx, soft palate, and vocal cord. Facial paralysis is seen less commonly, and ocular palsies are unusual findings. An encephalitic form of the disease is characterized by irritability, disorientation, drowsiness, and coarse tremors. Hypoxia and hypercapnia resulting from respiratory insufficiency caused by inadequate ventilation can produce disorientation without true encephalitis.

The most important complication of paralytic poliomyelitis is respiratory insufficiency caused by inadequate ventilation. Myocardial failure sometimes occurs, either secondary to pulmonary complications or as a direct result of acute myocarditis. Not infrequently, patients who have had paralytic poliomyelitis develop what appear to be new neuromuscular symptoms later in life. The late-onset weakness and muscle atrophy result from routine attrition of remaining anterior horn cells associated with aging rather than persistent neural infection with polioviruses.

DIAGNOSIS

Poliovirus infection should be considered in all unimmunized patients with aseptic meningitis with or without paralysis. If poliovirus infection is suspected, specimens for viral diagnostic studies should be obtained from the throat, stool, and CSF. All diagnostic virologic laboratories have the facilities to isolate polioviruses, and hospitals unequipped for virus isolation should refer specimens to regional laboratories. Poliovirus grows readily in appropriate tissue culture systems, and the presence of an enterovirus usually is noted in 3 to 4 days. Polioviruses can be separated from other enteroviruses and poliovirus vaccine strains can be identified by polymerase chain reaction (PCR).

Patients infected with polioviruses regularly develop neutralizing antibody to the type-specific virus. Therefore, the cause of the illness can be confirmed by examining acute and convalescent serum antibody titers to the three polioviral types. A fourfold increase in neutralizing antibody titer is indicative of infection. In acute illness, specific IgM neutralizing antibody for a specific poliovirus type also is diagnostic.

The differential diagnosis of nonparalytic poliomyelitis must include other enteroviral infections, as well as the numerous other causes of aseptic meningitis. The diagnosis of paralytic poliomyelitis during outbreaks should be no problem. Rarely, however, other enteroviruses (particularly enterovirus 71) cause paralytic syndromes similar to those caused by polioviruses. In sporadic instances of paralytic illness, several other diseases must be considered in the differential diagnosis. These illnesses include Guillain-Barré syndrome, peripheral neuritis (postinjection, toxic, herpes zoster), arboviral infections, rabies, tetanus, botulism, and tick paralysis.

In countries where live oral poliovirus vaccines (OPVs) are used, the consideration that a paralytic illness may be induced by polio vaccine also should be entertained.

THERAPY

The treatment of nonparalytic poliomyelitis is nonspecific. In mild cases, analgesics may be given for headache and muscle pain.

All patients with paralytic disease should be hospitalized. Impaired ventilation must be looked for and treated early. Increasing anxiety, restlessness, and fatigue are early indications that the patient needs mechanical ventilation. To handle secretions, tracheostomy frequently is indicated in patients with pure bulbar poliomyelitis, spinal respiratory muscle paralysis, and bulbar spinal paralysis. Patients with poliomyelitis usually are fully conscious and aware. All procedures relating to their care should be explained to them to reduce anxiety.

In bed, the patient with poliomyelitis should be in a neutral position with the feet at right angles, knees slightly flexed, and hips and spine straight. This position can be achieved by using boards, sandbags, and, occasionally, light splint shells. Active and passive motions are indicated as soon as muscle pain disappears. Consultation with other services (orthopedics and physiotherapy) should be obtained early in an illness so development of fixed deformities can be prevented.

PREVENTION

Poliomyelitis is a vaccine-preventable disease. Its control, as well as the control of the circulation of wild polioviruses, has been achieved in many areas of the world. Two effective poliovirus vaccines, trivalent live OPV and trivalent formalin-inactivated parenterally administered poliovirus vaccine (IPV), are available. OPV induces intestinal immunity, is simple to administer, is well accepted by patients, and results in immunization of some contacts of vaccinated persons; its use has eliminated endogenous disease caused by wild polioviruses in the United States. In rare instances (approximately 1 case per 800,000 first doses of vaccine), administration of OPV has been associated with paralysis in healthy recipients or their contacts. In contrast with OPV, IPV is less likely to result in herd immunity in diffuse and varied populations. IPV costs more than does OPV, is more difficult to administer, and produces a lesser degree of intestinal immunity; it lacks the ability to immunize contacts of some immunized persons and necessitates booster doses in older children and adults. The present global polio eradication program utilizes OPV and is based on four components: (a) maintenance of high vaccine coverage, (b) development of effective disease surveillance, (c) supplementary vaccine doses to all children during national immunization days, and (d) "mopping-up" vaccination campaigns in high-risk areas.

Because of concern about vaccine-associated paralytic poliomyelitis, both the Advisory Committee on Immunization Practices (ACIP) and the Committee on Infectious Diseases of the American Academy of Pediatrics have recommended since the year 1999 that only IPV be used in the United States, and OPV is no longer available. The primary series for IPV consists of three doses. The interval between the first two doses should be at least 4 weeks (preferably 8 weeks). The third dose should be given 6 to 12 months after the second dose. A booster dose is given to children 4 to 6 years of age before they enter school. The need for routinely administered additional booster doses is unknown, but adult booster doses may be necessary for continued community protection.

Full information regarding polio vaccine immunization practices is in the Report of the Committee on Infectious Diseases of the American Academy of Pediatrics (*Red Book*) and in the recommendations of the ACIP of the U.S. Department of Health and Human Services.

Known or suspected cases of poliomyelitis should be reported promptly to county or state health departments so that immediate epidemiologic investigations can be undertaken. Specimens should be obtained for viral studies. If a workup suggests wild poliovirus infection, a community immunization plan should be considered to prevent further cases.

Suggested Readings

American Academy of Pediatrics. Poliovirus infections. In: Pickering LK, ed. *Red Book: 2003 Report of the Committee on Infectious Diseases,* 26th ed. Elk Grove Village, IL: American Academy of Pediatrics, 2003:505.

Centers for Disease Control and prevention. Poliomyelitis prevention in the United States: updated recommendations of the Advisory Committee on Immunization Practices (ACIP). *MMWR* 2000;49(RR-5):1.

Cherry JD. Enteroviruses and Parechoviruses. In: Feigin RD, Cherry JD, Demmler GJ, Kaplan S, eds. *Textbook of pediatric infectious diseases,* 5th ed. WB Saunders Co, Philadelphia, PA. 2003;1984.

Nathanson N, Fine P. Poliomyelitis eradication—a dangerous endgame. *Science* 2002;296:269.

Technical Consultative Group to the World Health Organization on the Global Eradication of Poliomyelitis. "Endgame" issues for the global polio eradication initiative. *Clin Inf Dis* 2002;34:72.

de Quadros CA, Hersh BS, Olive JM, et al. Eradication of wild poliovirus from the Americas: acute flaccid paralysis surveillance, 1988–1995. *J Infect Dis* 1997;175(Suppl 1):S37.

CHAPTER 194 ■ NONPOLIO ENTEROVIRUSES AND PARECHOVIRUSES

JAMES D. CHERRY

The nonpolio enteroviruses and parechoviruses (coxsackieviruses, echoviruses, enteroviruses, and parechoviruses) are responsible for significant and frequent human illness with protean clinical manifestations. These viruses and the polioviruses were categorized together and named in 1957 by a committee sponsored by the National Foundation for Infantile Paralysis. They are grouped together because of the following: their natural habitat is the alimentary tract; they share common features in their epidemiology, clinical spectrum, and pathogenesis; and they have physical and biochemical similarities.

The enteroviruses and parechoviruses are two genera of the Picornaviridae (*pico*, small; *RNA*, ribonucleic acid) family; they are single-stranded RNA viruses. They are 30 nm in size and consist of a naked protein capsid and a dense central core of RNA. Most enteroviruses and parechoviruses grow in selected primate tissue cultures; some grow only when inoculated into suckling mice less than 24 hours old. A complete system for the primary recovery of enteroviruses and parechoviruses from patients includes the following: primary rhesus, cynomolgus, or African green monkey kidney; diploid human embryonic lung fibroblast cell strain; and RD (rhabdomyosarcoma) cell line tissue cultures and the intraperitoneal and intracerebral inoculation of suckling mice less than 24 hours old.

Twenty-three coxsackieviruses comprise group A, and 6 coxsackieviruses comprise group B; 30 echoviruses and 4 enteroviruses (designated enteroviruses 68 to 71) also exist. Former echoviruses 22 and 23 have been reclassified as parechoviruses 1 and 2, respectively.

Although some minor serologic cross-reactions occur among several enterovirus types, no common group antigens of diagnostic importance exist. Individual enteroviral types are identified by neutralization with type-specific antisera.

EPIDEMIOLOGY

Humans are the only natural host of nonpolio enteroviruses that infect people. Spread is from person to person and by the fecal-oral and, possibly, oral-oral (respiratory spread) routes. Transmission of infection by fomites and the contaminated hands of health care personnel has been documented in the hospital setting. Contaminated swimming and wading pools may serve as a means of spreading of enteroviruses during summer. Children are the main susceptible cohort; therefore, primary spread is from child to child. Secondary spread occurs to susceptible contacts in family groups. The incidence of infection and disease is related inversely to age, and the prevalence of specific antibodies is related directly to age. Epidemics and outbreaks depend on new susceptible individuals in the population; reinfection with clinical disease with a particular serotype is not thought to occur routinely. In temperate climates, enteroviral infections occur primarily in the summer and fall; in the tropics, infections regularly occur throughout the year.

Although 65 nonpolio enteroviral and parechoviral types exist, usually only a few viral types circulate in a community during any one season. From the early 1960s to 1990, echovirus type 9 was the most prevalent of the nonpolio enteroviruses. Other common types in widespread circulation were as follows: echoviruses 4, 6, 11, and 30; all coxsackie B viruses except B6; and coxsackieviruses A9 and A16. Since 1990, echoviruses 30 and 11 have been the most common circulating types. Recently, major epidemic disease caused by enterovirus 71 has occurred in Taiwan, Malaysia, Australia, and Japan.

PATHOPHYSIOLOGY

After an individual is exposed, an enterovirus becomes implanted in the pharynx and the lower alimentary tract. The infection quickly spreads to the regional lymph nodes, the virus multiplies, and minor viremia occurs on approximately the third day. This viremia results in involvement in many secondary infection sites, and viral multiplication in these sites coincides with the onset of clinical symptoms 4 to 6 days after exposure. As the virus multiplies at the secondary infection sites, major viremia begins during days 3 to 7 of infection. Involvement of the central nervous system may occur as a result of the initial minor viremia, or it may be delayed and be the result of major viremia. Major viremia usually lasts for 3 to

7 days. Cessation of viremia correlates with the appearance of antibody and the beginning of clinical recovery. Infection may continue, however, in the lower intestinal tract for prolonged periods.

Enteroviral illnesses vary from clinically unrecognized to severe fatal illnesses. Pathologic findings are described only in the more severe illnesses. The most striking findings in severe cases are in the heart (myocarditis), brain and spinal cord (meningitis and encephalitis), lungs (pneumonitis), adrenals (cortical necrosis), and liver (hepatic necrosis).

CLINICAL FINDINGS

Nonpolio enteroviral infections are exceedingly common findings in the United States. Virtually all children have one or more infections each summer and fall. Although few specific enteroviral diseases exist, a variety of interrelated syndromes and anatomically associated illnesses can occur. Table 194.1 presents the protean clinical spectrum of disease. Many illnesses and syndromes can be caused by different coxsackieviral, echoviral, and enteroviral types, and most types can produce a variety of clinical syndromes. In a few instances, clinical characteristics indicate one or two specific enteroviral types.

Asymptomatic Infection

Historically, the finding of enteroviruses in the stool of healthy children led to the assumption that most enteroviral infections were asymptomatic. This reasoning was in error because enteroviruses may be excreted in stool for months after acute infection occurs, and the finding of an enterovirus on a particular day is no indication of what happened when the infection first occurred. Although most enterovirus infections appear to go unrecognized, probably most affected persons have some symptoms, but usually the illnesses are trivial. The available data suggest that, on average, 50% or fewer of all infections are asymptomatic.

Nonspecific Febrile Illness

Nonspecific febrile illness is the most common manifestation of nonpolio enteroviral infections. This illness usually has an abrupt onset without prodrome. In young children, frequently only fever and malaise are observed. In older children, headache may be noted. Fever usually lasts 2 to 4 days and varies between 38.3° and 40.0°C. Occasionally, the fever is biphasic. Headache, malaise, and anorexia generally are related to the degree of fever. Additional findings in nonspecific febrile illness include mild nausea, vomiting, diarrhea, and abdominal discomfort. Enteroviruses are a significant cause of febrile convulsions in young children. Older patients may complain of sore throat.

In general, the findings on physical examination are benign. The usual duration of illness is 3 to 4 days, with extremes at 1 and 6 days.

Respiratory Manifestations

Respiratory manifestations are common findings with enteroviral infections. The most common manifestation is pharyngitis; in summer, nonpolio enteroviruses are the most common cause of this illness in children. Usually, enteroviral pharyngitis is abrupt in onset. Although physical examination reveals pharyngitis early in infection, the symptoms in younger

TABLE 194.1

CLINICAL MANIFESTATIONS OF NONPOLIO ENTEROVIRUSES AND PARECHOVIRUSES

Clinical Categories	Virus Types				
	Coxsackieviruses A	Coxsackieviruses B	Echoviruses	Enteroviruses	Parechoviruses
Nonspecific febrile illness	All types	All types	All types	All types	All types
Respiratory manifestations					
Common cold	Mainly 21, 24; rarely other types	Mainly 1–5; rarely 6	Mainly 2, 20; rarely other types	—	—
Pharyngitis	Probably all types; mainly 9	Probably all types; mainly 1–5	Probably all types; mainly 9, 11, 16, 19, 25, 30	71	—
Herpangina	1–10, 16, 22	1–5	6, 9, 16, 17, 25	—	1
Lymphonodular pharyngitis	10	—	—	—	—
Stomatitis and other lesions in the anterior mouth	5, 9, 10, 16	2, 5	9, 11, 20	71	—
Parotitis	not typed	3, 4	—	70	—
Croup	9	4, 5	4, 11, 21	—	—
Bronchitis	—	1, 4	8, 12–14	—	—
Bronchiolitis and asthmatic bronchitis	Many types	Many types	Many types	—	—
Pneumonia	9, 16	1–6	6, 7, 9, 11, 12, 19, 20, 30	71	—
Pleurodynia	1, 2, 4, 6, 9, 16	1–6	1–3, 6–9, 11, 12, 14, 16–19, 24, 25, 30	—	2
Gastrointestinal manifestations					
Nausea and vomiting	9, 16	2–5	2, 4, 6, 9, 11, 16, 18–20, 30	—	1
Diarrhea	1, 9, 16	2–5	3, 4, 6, 7, 9, 11–14, 16–21, 25, 30	—	1
Constipation	9	3–5	4, 6, 9, 11	—	—
Abdominal pain	9, 16	2–5	4, 6, 9, 11, 18, 19, 30	—	—
Pseudoappendicitis	—	—	1, 8, 14	—	—
Peritonitis	—	1	—	—	—
Mesenteric adenitis	—	5	7, 9, 11	—	—
Appendicitis	—	2, 5	—	—	—
Intussusception	—	3	7, 9	—	—
Hepatitis	4, 9, 10, 20, 24	1–5	1, 3, 4, 6, 7, 9, 11, 14, 20, 21, 30	—	—
Reye syndrome	2	4	14	—	1
Pancreatitis	9	3–5	—	—	—
Diabetes mellitus	—	1–5	—	—	—
Acute hemorrhagic conjunctivitis	24	—	—	70	—
Pericarditis and myocarditis	1, 2, 4, 5, 7–10, 16	1–5	1, 4, 6–9, 11, 14, 17, 19, 25, 30	—	1
Genitourinary manifestations					
Orchitis and epididymitis	—	1–5	6, 9, 11	—	—
Nephritis	—	4	6, 9	—	—
Hemolytic-uremic syndrome	4, 9	2–5	—	—	1
Pyuria, hematuria, or proteinuria	—	5	1, 6, 9	—	—
Myositis and arthritis	2, 9	4	9, 18, 24	—	—
Exanthem	2–5, 7, 9, 10, 16	1–5	1–7, 9, 11, 13, 14, 16–19, 21, 24, 25, 30, 32, 33	71	1
Neurologic manifestations					
Aseptic meningitis	1–14, 16–18, 21, 22, 24	1–6	1–9, 11–21, 24–27, 29–33	71	1, 2
Encephalitis	2, 4–7, 9, 10, 16	1–5	1–9, 11–21, 24, 25, 27, 30, 33	71	1, 2

(Continued)

TABLE 194.1

(CONTINUED)

Clinical Categories	Virus Types				
	Coxsackieviruses A	Coxsackieviruses B	Echoviruses	Enteroviruses	Parechoviruses
Paralysis (lower motor neuron involvement)	2, 4–7, 9–11, 14, 21	1–6	1–4, 6–9, 11, 12, 14, 16–19, 25, 27, 30, 31	70, 71	—
Guillain-Barré syndrome and transverse myelitis	2, 4–6, 9, 16	1–4	6, 7, 18, 19	70	1
Cerebellar ataxia	4, 7, 9	3, 4	6, 9, 16	—	—
Peripheral neuritis	—	—	9	—	—

children often are not particularly referable to the throat. The usual initial complaint is fever, and young children may exhibit malaise and anorexia. Older children may complain of sore throat, headache, and myalgia. Mild vomiting or diarrhea also may occur.

Herpangina is a particular specific enteroviral pharyngitis. In addition to having fever, children with herpangina have a characteristic exanthem. Vesicles and ulcers 1 to 2 mm in diameter appear on the anterior tonsillar pillars, soft palate, uvula, tonsils, pharyngeal wall, and, occasionally, the posterior buccal surfaces. The lesions usually are discrete and average approximately five per patient. Some patients have only one or two lesions, whereas others have 14 or more. The lesions are particularly characteristic when they occur on the soft palate. Early virologic studies indicated several coxsackieviruses A as the causative agents. Subsequent studies indicated that, in addition to group A coxsackieviruses, most group B coxsackieviruses and many echoviruses also cause herpangina.

The common respiratory viral illnesses of children that involve areas below the pharynx (croup, bronchitis, bronchiolitis, infectious asthma, pneumonia) may in sporadic instances be caused by enteroviral infections. Except for pneumonia, these illnesses, when caused by enteroviruses, generally are milder than are their counterparts caused by typical respiratory viral agents.

A specific enteroviral illness of the respiratory tract is pleurodynia (Bornholm disease). Historically, pleurodynia was an epidemic disease, with most cases occurring in older children and young adults. Today in the United States, most cases occur sporadically and outbreaks are rare occurrences. Most cases in adults probably are diagnosed incorrectly. The onset of illness is characterized by sudden occurrence of pain, typically located in the chest or upper abdomen. Pain is muscular in origin and of variable intensity. Often, the pain is excruciatingly severe and sudden and is associated with profuse sweating. The patient may appear pale, as though in shock. The pain occurs in spasms that last from a few minutes to several hours. During spasms, patients usually have rapid, shallow, grunting respirations that suggest pneumonia or pleural inflammation. In older children and adults, the pain often is described as stabbing or knifelike; in adults, the illness can be confused with a heart attack. The symptoms usually last only 1 to 2 days, but frequently the illness is biphasic, so a patient apparently recovers only to have a recurrence several days later.

Gastrointestinal Manifestations

Gastrointestinal manifestations are almost universal in nonpolio enteroviral infections. Some manifestations, such as nausea, vomiting, and diarrhea, are very common but usually are not severe and are only part of a more general overall illness. Conversely, abdominal pain may be a striking specific finding of enteroviral infections in young children.

Eye Findings

Mild conjunctivitis occurs frequently in many enteroviral illnesses, but usually it is not troublesome. A specific acute hemorrhagic conjunctivitis, however, occurs in major epidemics. This illness is caused mainly by enterovirus 70, but it has also been caused by coxsackievirus A24. Most epidemics have occurred in tropical and semitropical countries, but epidemics also have occurred in the continental United States. During epidemics, the highest attack rate is in school-aged children. The illness has a sudden onset, with severe eye pain, photophobia, blurred vision, lacrimation, erythema and congestion of the eye, and edematous and chemotic lids. Subconjunctival hemorrhages occur, and transient punctate epithelial keratitis, conjunctival follicles, and preauricular lymphadenopathy are noted frequently. Systemic symptoms, including fever, are rare. The illness lasts 7 to 12 days. In a few cases, a paralytic illness that is like poliomyelitis or Guillain-Barré syndrome develops after enterovirus 70 acute hemorrhagic conjunctivitis.

Cardiovascular Manifestations

Pericarditis and myocarditis are infrequent but important severe manifestations of nonpolio enteroviruses. The group B coxsackieviruses have been implicated most frequently. Group B coxsackieviruses also are etiologic factors in some cases of acute myocardial infarction in young adults.

Genitourinary Manifestations

Group B coxsackieviruses are second only to mumps as causative agents of orchitis. Orchitis frequently occurs as a second phase in a biphasic illness; the initial phase usually is nonspecific febrile illness, aseptic meningitis, or pleurodynia. Other rare genitourinary findings associated with nonpolio enterovirus infections are listed in Table 194.1.

Muscle and Joint Manifestations

After intraperitoneal inoculation into suckling mice, group A coxsackieviruses routinely cause myositis; these viruses, therefore, have been candidates for muscle infection in humans.

Although myalgia is a common complaint of illness caused by nonpolio enteroviruses, myositis associated with human enteroviral infections has been documented only in persons with immunologic disorders. In particular, dermatomyositis-like syndromes caused by echoviral infections have been noted in children with agammaglobulinemia. Occasionally, arthritis has been reported in association with enteroviral infections.

Skin Manifestations

The nonpolio enteroviruses cause a variety of skin manifestations. Specific exanthematous manifestations by frequency of viral type are listed in Table 194.2. In summer and fall, enteroviruses are the leading cause of exanthem in children.

Echovirus 9 is the agent most commonly associated with exanthem in children. This exanthem is erythematous, maculopapular, and usually discrete. Often, the exanthem is petechial and is noted in association with aseptic meningitis. The illness mimics meningococcemia. Other enteroviruses cause petechial and purpuric rashes (see Table 194.2), and they can be confused with septicemic illnesses.

The hand, foot, and mouth syndrome, which was caused most commonly by coxsackievirus A16 (Fig. 194.1), has been noted in outbreaks of enterovirus 71 and is a clearly recognizable enteroviral illness. The exanthem is predominantly vesicular and is located on the hands, feet, and buttocks. The enanthem usually involves the anterior mouth and consists of large, ulcerative lesions.

Neurologic Manifestations

Neurologic illness is a common finding in nonpolio enteroviral infections; aseptic meningitis occurs most often (see Table 194.1). The most common causes of aseptic meningitis are as follows: coxsackieviruses A9, B2, B4, and B5; echoviruses 4, 6, 9, 30, and 33; and enterovirus 71.

Paralytic illness similar to that caused by the polioviruses also is an occasional manifestation of the nonpolio enteroviruses. Paralysis caused by the nonpolio enteroviruses usually is less severe and causes less residual damage. Outbreaks of illness caused by enterovirus 71 have occurred.

Neonatal Infections

Nonpolio enteroviral infections in neonates result in a wide variety of clinical manifestations. Although these neonatal infections may be mild, significant numbers are particularly severe, and deaths are not uncommon. In particular, the infections may be generalized, with both myocarditis and meningoencephalitis. Outbreaks have occurred in newborn nurseries.

Of particular importance is a sepsis-like illness that can be the manifestation of several different nonpolio enteroviruses. This illness is characterized by fever, poor feeding, abdominal distention, irritability, rash, lethargy, and hypotonia. Patients also may have diarrhea, vomiting, seizures, and apnea. Severe fatal illness most often is caused by echovirus 11. In fatal cases, jaundice, hepatitis, disseminated intravascular coagulation, thrombocytopenia, and hypotension occur.

Chronic Enteroviral Infections in Immunocompromised Patients

Chronic unusual infections in children with agammaglobulinemia caused by a variety of enteroviruses have been reported.

The most common illness is meningoencephalitis; arthritis and polymyositis also frequently occur. Echovirus 11 has been the most common cause of chronic infection, but 19 other types also have been causative.

DIAGNOSIS

The clinical differentiation of enteroviral disease frequently is considered impossible. When all the circumstances of a particular illness are evaluated, however, enteroviral diseases often can be suspected on clinical grounds. The most important factors in the clinical diagnosis are the season of the year, the geographic location, exposure, the incubation period, and clinical symptoms.

Because some enteroviral infections mimic severe but treatable bacterial illnesses (meningitis and septicemia), frequently situations occur for which treatment with antimicrobial therapy should be administered until a bacterial origin is excluded.

All hospital viral diagnostic laboratories should have facilities for the recovery of the majority of enteroviruses that cause illness. Laboratories that are not thus equipped should send specimens to a reference laboratory. In general, in suspected enteroviral illness, specimens should be collected from multiple sites. In all cases, material from the throat and a stool specimen should be collected. If possible, the site of the major clinical manifestation (cerebrospinal fluid, pericardial fluid) also should be cultured.

Contrary to popular belief, many common enteroviruses grow rapidly in tissue culture, so isolation of an enterovirus as a cause of a specific illness frequently takes less than 1 week. The identification of an isolated enterovirus is more difficult and can take much longer. During the 1990s, many reports indicated the usefulness of the polymerase chain reaction for the rapid diagnosis of enteroviral infections. The polymerase chain reaction has been most useful in identifying enteroviruses in the cerebrospinal fluid of patients with meningitis and in the blood from infants with sepsis-like illnesses.

Except in special circumstances, the use of serologic techniques in the primary diagnosis of suspected enteroviral infections is impractical; therefore, every effort should be made to obtain culture for virus as early as possible in an illness. Many commercial laboratories offer serologic diagnostic panels for enteroviruses. These panels are expensive and lack sensitivity and specificity, leading to erroneous diagnoses. In certain circumstances, when specific etiologies are suspected, antibody titer increases may be useful in confirming a clinical diagnosis.

THERAPY

No specific antiviral agent is approved for the treatment of enteriviral infections. Commercially available immune globulins contain antibodies to most enteroviruses. In severe catastrophic enteroviral infections, such as those that occur in neonates, a reasonable approach is to administer intravenous immune globulin to the child, but this therapy has not been demonstrated to be beneficial. Intravenous immune globulin has a beneficial effect in the treatment of subacute and chronic enteroviral infections in patients with immune deficiencies.

PREVENTION

Passive protection with human immune globulin should be considered in nursery outbreaks of severe enteroviral disease. Some evidence indicates that immune serum was useful in the management of two nursery enteroviral outbreaks.

TABLE 194.2

CLINICAL EXANTHEMATOUS MANIFESTATIONS OF ENTEROVIRUSES

Clinical Feature	Virus Subgroup	Associated Viral Agents and Prevalence of Manifestation		
		Common	Occasional	Rare
Macular rash	Coxsackievirus A			
	B		1, 2, 5	
	Echovirus and enterovirus		2, 4, 5, 13, 14, 17, 19, 30	18, 71
Maculopapular rash	Coxsackievirus A	9	2, 4, 5, 10, 16	6, 7
	B		1–5	
	Echovirus and enterovirus	4, 9	2, 5–7, 11, 16–19, 25, 30, 71	1, 3, 13, 14, 27, 33
Vesicular rash	Coxsackievirus A	5, 16	8–10	4, 7
	B			1–3, 5
	Echovirus and enterovirus		11	6, 9, 17, 71
Petechial or purpuric rash	Coxsackievirus A	9	4	
	B		2–5	
	Echovirus	9	4, 7	
Urticarial rash	Coxsackievirus A	9	16	
	B		4, 5	
	Echovirus		11	
Erythema multiforme or Stevens-Johnson syndrome	Coxsackievirus A		9	10, 16
	B			4, 5
	Echovirus			6, 11
Exanthem and meningitis	Coxsackievirus A		2, 9	7
	B	1, 2, 4, 5		
	Echovirus and enterovirus	4, 9	6, 11, 17, 18, 25, 30	3, 14, 33, 71
Exanthem and pneumonia	Coxsackievirus A		9	7
	B		6	1
	Echovirus			9, 11
Hand-foot-and-mouth disease	Coxsackievirus A	16	5, 10	7, 9
	B			1, 3, 5
	Echovirus and enterovirus	71		
Hemangioma-like lesions	Coxsackievirus A			
	B			
	Echovirus			25, 32
Herpangina and exanthem	Coxsackievirus A		4	9
	B			2
	Echovirus		16, 17	
Roseola-like illness	Coxsackievirus A			6, 9
	B	5		1, 2, 4
	Echovirus		16, 25	9, 11, 27, 30
Anaphylactoid purpura	Coxsackievirus A			4
	B			
	Echovirus			9, 18
Zoster-like rash	Coxsackievirus A			
	B			
	Echovirus			5, 6
Pityriasis-like rash	Coxsackievirus A			
	B			
	Echovirus			6
Chronic or recurrent rash	Coxsackievirus A	16		
	B			
	Echovirus			11

Reprinted with permission from Cherry JD. Enteroviruses and parechoviruses. In: Feigin RD, Cherry JD, Demmler GJ, Kaplan S, eds. *Textbook of pediatric infectious diseases,* 5th ed. Philadelphia: WB Saunders, 2004:1984.

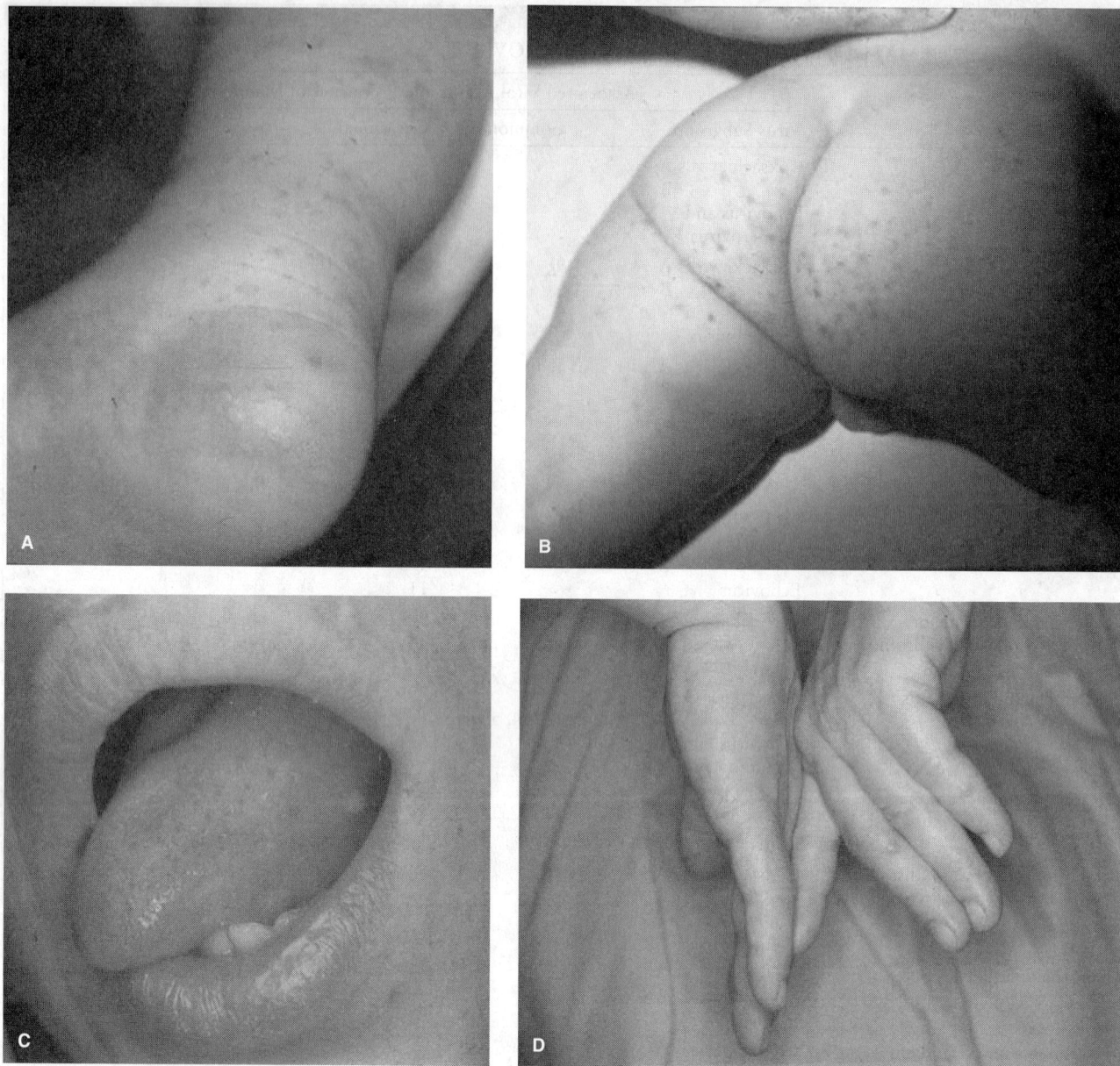

FIGURE 194.1. Hand, foot, and mouth syndrome due to coxsackievirus A16 in three family members. **A** and **B**: Lesions on the foot and buttocks of a 1½-year-old boy. **C**: Lesion on the tongue of a 21-year-old woman exposed to the child in **A** and **B**. **D**: Lesions on the hand of a 46-year-old woman exposed to the child in **A** and **B**. (Reprinted from Cherry JD, Jahn CL. Hand, foot, and mouth syndrome: report of six cases due to coxsackie virus, group A, type 16. *Pediatrics* 1966;37:639. Used by permission.)

Suggested Readings

Abzug MJ. Prognosis for neonates with enterovirus hepatitis and coagulopathy. *Pediatr Infect Dis J* 2001;20:758.

Byington CL, Taggart EW, Carroll KC, Hillyard DR. A polymerase chain reaction-based epidemiologic investigation of the incidence of nonpolio enteroviral infections in febrile and afebrile infants 90 days and younger. *Pediatrics* 1999;103:27.

Cherry JD. Enteroviruses. In: Remington JS, Klein JO, eds. *Infectious diseases of the fetus and newborn infant,* 5th ed. Philadelphia: WB Saunders, 2001:477.

Cherry JD. Enteroviruses and parechoviruses. In: Feigin RD, Cherry JD, Demmler GJ, Kaplan S, eds. *Textbook of pediatric infectious diseases,* 5th ed. Philadelphia: WB Saunders, 2004:1984.

Dagan R. Nonpolio enteroviruses and the febrile young infant: epidemiologic, clinical and diagnostic aspects. *Pediatr Dis J* 1996;15:67.

Dietz V, Andrus J, Olive JM, et al. Epidemiology and clinical characteristics of acute flaccid paralysis associated with nonpolio enterovirus isolation: the experience in the Americas. *Bull World Health Organ* 1995;73:597.

Wang S-M, Liu C-C, Tseng HW, et al. Clinical spectrum of enterovirus 71 infection in children in southern Taiwan, with an emphasis on neurological complications. *Clin Infect Dis* 1999;29:184.

CHAPTER 195 ■ EPSTEIN-BARR VIRUS INFECTION IN CHILDREN

KATHERINE LUZURIAGA AND JOHN L. SULLIVAN

In 1964, Anthony Epstein and Yvonne Barr isolated a new herpesvirus from Burkitt lymphoma tumor cells. This herpesvirus (the fifth to be described) was named *Epstein-Barr virus* (EBV) and, in 1968, Werner and Henle demonstrated that seroconversion to EBV occurred during the course of infectious mononucleosis (IM). Subsequent to the finding that EBV is the causative agent of IM, several additional clinical syndromes and malignant disorders have been linked to EBV infection.

EPIDEMIOLOGY

Since the 1970s, EBV has been recognized to transmit primarily through contact with oropharyngeal secretions. EBV also has been recovered from the genital tract, suggesting a sexual mode of transmission. EBV infection may be transmitted through blood transfusions in which latently infected B lymphocytes serve as the source of infecting virus.

Seroepidemiologic studies have demonstrated a wide variation in the age at which EBV infection is established. In many areas of the developing world, EBV infection occurs in early infancy, and by 2 years of age, more than 80% of children have experienced primary EBV infection. The majority of these infections are asymptomatic. Passively acquired maternal antibody apparently is protective, with the majority of primary infections occurring after 4 to 6 months of age. In some areas of the developed world, primary infection does not occur until adolescence. In the United States, approximately 10% to 15% of susceptible college students become infected each year, and the majority of these infections are associated with a mononucleosis syndrome.

PATHOGENESIS

Epstein-Barr virus (EBV), a member of the Herpesviridae family, is an enveloped virus with 172 kb linear double-stranded DNA genome that codes for approximately 100 proteins. EBV infects over 90% of the world's population and is spread by contact with oropharyngeal secretions from a virus carrier. The tonsils appear to be the initial site of viral entry and replication, but the virus persists throughout life in infected B lymphocytes. Whereas primary EBV infections usually are asymptomatic or only mildly symptomatic in young children, primary EBV infection in older children or adults may result in an infectious mononucleosis syndrome. EBV genome also has been detected in a variety of neoplasms, including Hodgkin disease, Burkitt lymphoma, and nasopharyngeal carcinoma, although EBV's role in their pathogenesis is not well understood. EBV-associated lymphoproliferative disease also is a common cause of morbidity in individuals undergoing transplantation.

Persistent EBV infection likely results from a dynamic interplay between viral evasion strategies and host immune responses. Potent T-cell activation occurs and high levels of

EBV-specific CD4+ and CD8+ responses are generated during acute EBV infection. How and why EBV persists despite these broad and vigorous immune responses is unclear, but recent studies have provided insight into potential EBV immune evasion strategies. An EBV IL-10 homologue (BCRF1) has been identified that has potent immunosuppressive activity. In addition, it appears that EBV exploits normal pathways of B cell differentiation to allow it to persist in a transcriptionally quiescent state in memory B cells and thus minimize immune recognition. EBV infection of resting naïve B cells occurs in the tonsillar mantle zone (Fig. 195.1) and results in generation of activated, proliferating B cell blasts through the expression of the viral growth program under the regulation of the transcription factor, EBV nuclear antigen 2 (EBNA 2). These EBV infected B cell blasts express many EBV proteins and are thus potentially subject to immune effector mechanisms, including lysis by EBV-specific CD8+ T-cells. However, some EBV-infected B cell blasts appear to escape immune surveillance and traffic to lymphoid follicles where they form germinal centers, turn off EBNA 2, and express a more restricted set of viral proteins (EBNA 1; latent membrane protein-1 or LMP-1; and latent membrane protein-2 or LMP-2). Survival of germinal center B cells normally requires signals from antigen on antigen presenting cells through the B cell receptor and on signals from CD40L on T helper cells through CD40. The expression of the EBV LMP-1

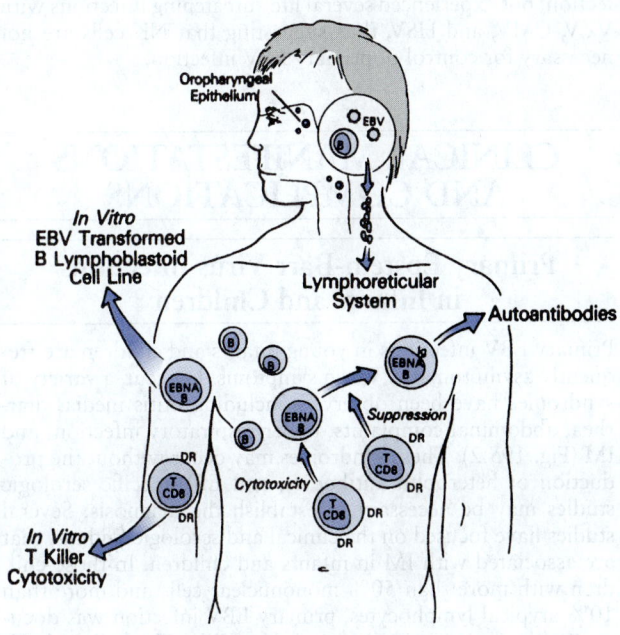

FIGURE 195.1. Immunopathogenesis of acute Epstein-Barr virus–induced infectious mononucleosis. DR, HLA-DR antigen; EBNA, Epstein-Barr nuclear antigens.

protein, a CD40 functional homologue and EBV LMP-2 protein, a B cell receptor functional homologue, may mimic these signals, allowing survival of the EBV-infected B cells and the acquisition of a memory B cell phenotype in which only limited EBV protein expression occurs. EBV-infected B cells leave the tonsil and circulate throughout the body as memory B cells with little transcriptional activity, thus likely escaping immune surveillance.

During acute Epstein-Barr virus (EBV) infection in humans, up to 44% of peripheral blood CD8+ T cells stain with EBV viral epitope-specific tetramers; virtually all tetramer-staining cells express CD45RO, HLA DR, and CD38 suggesting high-level activation and turnover of these cells in vivo (Fig. 195.1). Interestingly, responses to EBV lytic proteins appear to predominate during acute infection. In healthy, chronically EBV-infected individuals, up to 5% of peripheral blood CD8+ T-cells stain with tetramers; responses to lytic and latent proteins have been detected. During acute infection, the majority of tetramer-staining cells co-stain with markers of cellular activation (HLA-DR, CD38) and turnover (Ki67); the co-expression of these markers decreases during convalescence. Although the majority of tetramer-staining CD8+ T-cells during acute infection are of the RO phenotype, tetramer-staining cells that co-express CD45RA (naive T-cell) or CD45RO (memory T-cell) are identified in convalescent individuals.

Activated natural killer (NK) cells also are observed in the peripheral blood of acute IM patients as also seen with other viral infections. NK cells are considered to play a primary role in the immune surveillance against virally or neoplastically modified cells, because they require no *in vitro* stimulation or previous antigen exposure. Interestingly, NK cells alone are not sufficient to counteract the establishment of EBV-transformed B cell lines *in vitro*; however, they do contribute to improved B lymphoblastoid cell line regression in the presence of EBV-specific cytotoxic lymphocytes (CTL). This effect by NK cells may be due to either direct cytotoxicity or IFN production, because EBV and EBV-infected cells induce gamma-IFN production by NK cells, and alpha-IFN is known to inhibit EBV-induced B-cell proliferation *in vitro*.

Biron et al. described a patient with complete absence of natural killer cells who experienced an unremarkable EBV infection, but experienced several life-threatening infections with VZV, CMV, and HSV, thus suggesting that NK cells are not necessary for control of primary EBV infection.

CLINICAL MANIFESTATIONS AND COMPLICATIONS

Primary Epstein-Barr Virus Infections in Infants and Children

Primary EBV infections in young infants and children are frequently asymptomatic. When symptoms do occur, a variety of syndromes have been observed, including otitis media, diarrhea, abdominal complaints, upper respiratory infection, and IM (Fig. 195.2). These syndromes may occur without the production of heterophil antibodies, and EBV-specific serologic studies may be necessary to establish the diagnosis. Several studies have focused on the clinical and serologic findings that are associated with IM in infants and children. In those children with more than 50% mononuclear cells and more than 10% atypical lymphocytes, primary EBV infection was documented in the majority. Most of the children had clinical evidence compatible with IM (significant cervical adenopathy and tonsillar pharyngitis). Respiratory symptoms were frequently prominent, especially in young infants. Complications of EBV

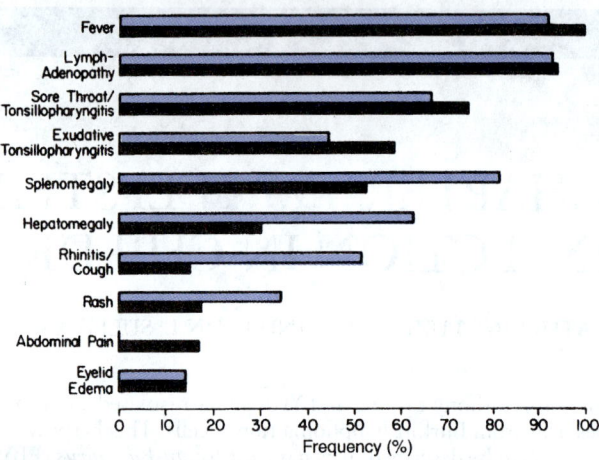

FIGURE 195.2. Frequency of clinical findings in two age groups: less than 4 years old (*open bars*) and 4 to 6 years old (*solid bars*). (Reprinted with permission from Sumaya CV, Ench Y. Epstein-Barr virus infections mononucleosis in children: I. clinical and general laboratory findings. *Pediatrics* 1985;75:1003.)

IM occur in approximately 20% of children, usually during or shortly after the peak of clinical illness. Table 195.1 lists the frequency of significant complications noted in one series of patients. Only 25% of infants 10 to 24 months of age demonstrated heterophil antibody responses, whereas 75% of children aged 24 to 28 months tested positive for heterophil antibody and only 60% of infants demonstrated VCA-IgM antibodies, compared with 100% of older children and young adults.

The IM syndrome is not uncommon among young children. The presence of atypical lymphocytes and lymphadenopathy in

TABLE 195.1

COMPLICATIONS PRESENT IN CHILDHOOD EPSTEIN-BARR VIRUS INFECTIOUS MONONUCLEOSIS

Complication	Number of Children (%)
Respiratory tract	
Pneumonia	6 (5.3)
Severe airway obstruction*	4 (3.5)
Neurologic	
Seizures	4 (3.5)
Meningitis/encephalitis	2 (1.8)
Peripheral facial nerve paralysis	1 (0.9)
Guillain-Barré syndrome	1 (0.9)
Hematologic	
Thrombocytopenia with hemorrhages	4 (3.5)
Hemolytic anemia	1 (0.9)
Infectious	
Bacteremia	1 (0.9)
Recurrent tonsillopharyngitis	3 (2.7)
Liver: jaundice	2 (1.8)
Renal: glomerulonephritis	1 (0.9)
Genital: orchitis	1 (0.9)
Total	31†

*Criteria consisted of nasal alar flaring, suprasternal retractions, or stridor.
†Four children had more than one of these complications; this total is composed of 24 different children, or 21.2% of the study group.
(Reprinted with permission from Sumaya CV, Ench Y. Epstein-Barr virus infectious mononucleosis in children: I. Clinical and general laboratory findings. *Pediatrics* 1985;75:1003.)

the absence of heterophil antibodies further documents the age-related differences in host responses to EBV. We have demonstrated that young infants can mount an EBV-specific cytotoxic T-lymphocyte response during acute EBV infection. These cytotoxic T-lymphocyte responses in young infants appear to be directed against the same epitopes recognized by young adults.

Infectious Mononucleosis in the Adolescent

The IM syndrome appearing in adolescents is characterized by fever, anterior and posterior cervical lymphadenopathy, exudative pharyngitis, and fatigue. The syndrome is self-limited, lasting an average of 2 to 3 weeks. An estimated 30% to 50% of students entering college in the United States are susceptible (seronegative) to EBV. Approximately 10% to 15% of seronegative persons become infected each year, and the majority of those infected show signs and symptoms of classic IM. Studies of West Point cadets have demonstrated an association of clinically apparent IM with the likelihood of being under stress.

Individuals experiencing acute IM may develop morbilliform rashes when treated with ampicillin or penicillin during the acute phase of the disease. Hepatosplenomegaly is commonly present and severe, but only rarely results in splenic rupture, after trauma, and fulminant hepatitis secondary to periportal necrosis. One of the most common causes of hospitalization during acute IM is severe pharyngitis with concern for airway obstruction. This complication, which usually resolves in 24 to 72 hours, may be severe enough to warrant empiric treatment with intravenous corticosteroids, although the efficacy of such treatment is not proved.

Secondary Hemophagocytic Lymphohistiocytoses (HLH)

A secondary HLH syndrome may occur in association with infections caused by viruses (including HIV-1), bacteria, fungi, or parasites; in patients with congenital or acquired immunodeficiency, especially the X-linked lymphoproliferative (XLP) syndrome associated with a predisposition to fatal EBV infection; and in association with malignant neoplasia (Box 195.1).

This syndrome is characterized by fever and generalized constitutional symptoms with myalgias and malaise. Physical examination reveals an enlarged liver and spleen, with generalized lymphadenopathy. Laboratory studies commonly demonstrate abnormal liver function test results, with a coagulopathy that is more severe than that expected on the basis of the abnormal liver function results. The patient is usually pancytopenic and may appear toxic. HLH has been observed most frequently in individuals with underlying immunosuppression, including allograft recipients, leukemia patients, and patients with severe collagen vascular disease receiving high-dose corticosteroids. The mortality in patients experiencing infection-associated HLH has been high; however, it is likely that the use of immunosuppressive agents in patients experiencing infection-associated HLH has contributed to the high mortality.

Some controversy surrounds the pathologic differentiation between secondary HLH and malignant histiocytosis. The pathologic features of secondary HLH vary with the time that biopsies are performed. Early in the disease, the bone marrow may be hypercellular with few infiltrating histiocytes. Erythrophagocytosis usually is demonstrated best in aspirate smears. Early in the disease, lymph nodes may exhibit an intense immunoblastic proliferative response with partial effacement of the lymph node architecture. Liver biopsy reveals large portal infiltrates of lymphocytes, immunoblasts, and histio-

---

BOX 195.1   Diagnostic Guidelines for HLH

The diagnosis of HLH can be established if one of either 1 or 2 below is fulfilled.

1. A molecular diagnosis consistent with HLH.
2. Diagnostic criteria for HLH fulfilled (five out of the eight criteria below).
   A. **Initial diagnostic criteria (to be evaluated in all patients with HLH).**

Clinical Criteria
- Fever
- Splenomegaly

Laboratory Criteria
- Cytopenias (affecting ≥ 2 of 3 lineages in the peripheral blood):
  - Hemoglobin (<90 g/L) (In infants <4 weeks: Hgb <100 g/L)
  - Platelets ($<100 \times 10^9$/L)
  - Neutrophils ($<1.0 \times 10^9$/L)
- Hypertriglyceridemia and/or hypofibrinogenemia (fasting triglycerides ≥ 3.0 mmol/L (i.e., ≥ 265 mg/dL, fibrinogen ≤ 1.5 g/L)

Histopathologic Criteria
- Hemophagocytosis in bone marrow, spleen, or lymph nodes. No evidence of malignancy.

   B. **New Diagnostic Criteria**
- Low or absent NK-cell activity (according to local laboratory reference).
- Ferritin ≥ 500 microgram/L.
- Soluble CD25 (i.e., soluble IL-2 receptor) $\geq 2,400$ U/ml.

Comments:

1. If hemophagocytic activity is not proven at the time of presentation, further search for hemophagocytic activity is encouraged. If the bone marrow specimen is not conclusive, material may be obtained from other organs. Serial marrow aspirates over time also may be helpful.
2. The following findings may provide supportive evidence for the diagnosis:
   a. Spinal fluid pleocytosis (mononuclear cells) and/or elevated spinal fluid protein,
   b. Histologic picture of the liver resembling chronic, persistent hepatitis (biopsy).
3. Other abnormal clinical laboratory findings consistent with the diagnosis are: cerebromeningeal symptoms, lymph node enlargement, jaundice, edema, skin rash, hepatic enzyme abnormalities, hypoproteinemia, hyponatremia, VLDL elevated, and HDL decreased.

The diagnosis of FHL is justified by a positive family history as well as disease-causing mutations in the perforin and Munc 13-4 genes, and parental consanguinity is suggestive. (Revised with permission from Henter et al. *Semin Oncol* 1991;18:2933.)

---

cytes. Immunologic studies have been reported in only a few patients. In the majority of patients studied, EBV was the associated infectious agent. Atypical lymphocytes, which are the hallmark of acute EBV infection, are absent or diminished, reflecting a decrease in activated CD8 T-cells normally seen in response to EBV. Underlying immunoregulatory disturbances may allow an inappropriate antiviral response. As this response progresses, cytokines secreted by activated T lymphocytes may elicit the proliferation and activation of histiocytes.

At present, no specific treatment exists for infection-associated HLH; patients presenting with symptoms compatible with infection-associated HLH should be thoroughly studied for evidence of acute EBV, cytomegalovirus, adenovirus, or other viral infections. Individuals with evidence of acute viral infection may not benefit from immunosuppressive therapy. A treatment protocol is available through the Histiocyte Society. Those individuals who survive their acute infection without any underlying immunodeficiency have an excellent prognosis. Individuals with XLP can present with infection-associated HLH in the face of acute EBV infection. In this instance (XLP with underlying SH2D1A mutation), treatment with B-cell–directed chemotherapy has resulted in some remissions and survival.

X-Linked Lymphoproliferative Syndrome

The X-linked lymphoproliferative (XLP) syndrome is characterized by a selective immunodeficiency to EBV manifested by severe or fatal IM and acquired immunodeficiency. Prospective studies in male subjects before EBV infection have demonstrated normal cellular and humoral immunity. During acute EBV infection, male subjects with XLP syndrome demonstrate vigorous cytotoxic cellular responses, which predominantly involve activated cytotoxic CD8 T-cells. Fatal EBV infections in male subjects with XLP syndrome usually result from extensive liver necrosis, and those who survive acute EBV infection demonstrate global cellular immune defects with deficient T-cell, B-cell, and NK cell responses. The germline mutations responsible for XLP have been localized to the SH2DIA gene on the X chromosome. The protein encoded by the XLP gene has been identified in T lymphocytes and has been named *signaling lymphocyte activation molecule-associated protein* (SAP). This adaptor protein appears to play an important role in T-lymphocyte signal transduction events. The relationship of SAP to EBV infection and T-cell signal transduction is under study. In patients with XLP syndrome, treatment of fulminant IM with B cell directed chemotherapy regimens have resulted in some remissions and survival. At present, the only curative therapy is bone marrow or cord blood stem-cell transplantation.

Burkitt Lymphoma

Burkitt lymphoma is the most common childhood malignancy in equatorial Africa and was first described in 1958, by the British surgeon Denis Burkitt. This unmistakable tumor typically presents in the jaws of young patients, and the majority of endemic cases occur in discrete geographic climates located along the malaria belt in Africa. Malaria is hypothesized to provide a chronic stimulator for proliferation of B lymphocytes, some of which carry latent EBV. In the rare instance during B-cell division that a specific reciprocal chromosomal translocation involving the c-*myc* locus on the long arm of chromosome 8 and one of the immunoglobulin loci on chromosome 14, 2, or 22 occurs, a Burkitt lymphoma may result. The ability of EBV to "growth transform" human B cells, along with the potential to induce malignant lymphomas in New World monkeys makes EBV a strong candidate for contributing the remaining transforming factors in the multistep process of Burkitt lymphoma development.

More than 95% of endemic Burkitt lymphoma tumor cells contain copies of the EBV genome, whereas only 15% to 20% of sporadic (outside high-incidence areas) cases of Burkitt lymphoma contain EBV genomes. Analysis of the EBV genome

terminal repeat frequency in endemic Burkitt lymphomas has demonstrated that the tumors originate in the lineage of a single EBV-infected B cell.

Although EBV-transformed B lymphocytes propagated *in vitro* typically express six EBNA proteins and two latent membrane proteins, new Burkitt lymphoma cells typically express only EBNA-1. It has been hypothesized that the translocation in the c-*myc* gene occurs in a EBV infected germinal-center cell that is on its way to becoming a memory cell, and the cell becomes stuck in the proliferating mode and only expresses EBNA-1. This process, along with reduced expression of MHC class I antigens and lack of adhesion molecules, likely contributes to the ability of these cells to escape T-lymphocyte surveillance.

Post-Transplant Lymphoproliferative Disorders

EBV is associated with lymphoproliferative disorders in individuals receiving organ allografts and immunosuppressive therapy. These lymphoproliferative disorders range from the benign polyclonal B-cell proliferations to malignant B-cell lymphomas. The frequency of post-transplant lymphoproliferative disorders after receipt of allografts is related to the degree and type of immunosuppression.

The most common form of lymphoproliferative disorder is the benign polyclonal B-cell proliferation frequently observed in individuals experiencing a primary EBV infection after transplant of the allograft. Systemic symptoms of fever and sore throat may be present. Prolonged symptoms and lymphadenopathy usually respond to a reduction in immunosuppressive therapy. The development of a monoclonal B-cell lymphoma may be preceded by benign polyclonal B-cell proliferation or by sudden development of a solid tumor mass in the organ allograft or any other tissue. These lymphomas are polymorphic with monoclonal B-cell proliferations and are resistant to treatment. The clinical course is usually one of an aggressive lymphoma, with survival of less than 1 year. In severe cases of polyclonal lymphoproliferative disorders, and in some cases of monoclonal B-cell lymphoma, infusion of donor leukocytes or EBV-specific T-cell lines has been successful in treating the lymphoproliferative disorders.

Malignancies and Human Immunodeficiency Virus Infection

In the setting of immunodeficiency associated with human immunodeficiency virus (HIV-1) infections, non-Hodgkin lymphomas have been shown to occur approximately 60- to 100-fold more frequently than expected. A study conducted in Los Angeles County, from 1984 to 1992, showed that EBV was associated with 39 of 59 (66%) HIV-related systemic lymphomas.

Given the profound immune defects in HIV-infected patients, along with the known role of cytotoxic T lymphocytes in controlling EBV-induced proliferation, it is not surprising that the number of EBV-infected B cells in the peripheral blood of those with HIV infection is higher than in the general population. HIV-associated non-Hodgkin lymphoma, usually of B-cell origin, is a relatively late manifestation of HIV infection. For unknown reasons, the majority of EBV-associated non-Hodgkin lymphomas in HIV-infected patients have presented as primary central nervous system lymphomas.

Another EBV-induced disease in HIV-infected individuals is oral hairy leukoplakia, an unusual wartlike disease of the lingual squamous epithelium. Virus replication is evident only in the upper layers of the epithelium and is effectively inhibited by acyclovir. Interestingly, the lesions of oral hairy leukoplakia appear to be relatively specific to HIV-related immunodeficiency; the disease is only rarely observed in patients with other immunodeficiencies.

Epstein-Barr Virus and Smooth-Muscle Tumors

Children infected with HIV experience an unusually high incidence of smooth-muscle tumors (leiomyomas and leiomyosarcomas). Ordinarily, the incidence of leiomyomas in children is extremely low. The demonstration that EBV can infect smooth-muscle cells in HIV-infected individuals may help explain the role of EBV in the pathogenesis of leiomyomas. Additional evidence for an etiologic role of EBV in the development of these neoplastic lesions is provided by the description of smooth-muscle tumors containing clonal EBV developing in three children after liver transplantation.

Hodgkin's Disease

EBV genomic DNA was first reported in Hodgkin disease in 1987. More recent evidence supports a role for EBV in the pathogenesis of Hodgkin disease, in which the malignant cells, including Reed-Sternberg cells, contain the EBV genome in up to 50% of Western cases. As with Burkitt lymphoma, the association of EBV with Hodgkin disease appears to vary geographically, because 94% of cases of classic Hodgkin disease occurring in Peru contain EBV transcripts within Reed-Sternberg cells. Healthy Western populations are infected with predominantly type 1 EBV and, not surprisingly, the majority of EBV detected in Hodgkin disease is type 1. A reasonable hypothesis suggests that a germinal-center B lymphocyte acquires a differentiation blocking mutation during acute EBV infection, and the presence of EBV genome with expression of LMP-1 and LMP-2 confers growth and survival signals that enhance tumor growth.

T-Cell Lymphoma

Until the mid-1990s, little evidence suggested that normal T-cell lymphocytes were susceptible to EBV infection. Studies have demonstrated EBV-infected tonsillar T lymphocytes in individuals with acute IM. This observation is consistent with the description of T-cell lymphomas in individuals with chronic EBV infection.

DIAGNOSIS

In the majority of young adults with IM, atypical lymphocytosis and heterophil antibodies are present. However, in young infants and children with primary EBV infection (whether or not associated with IM), heterophil antibody responses frequently are absent. Primary infection in childhood frequently requires EBV-specific serologic tests. A common approach to a patient suspected of having a primary EBV infection is to first perform a rapid slide test for heterophil antibodies; if the test result is positive (differential absorption with guinea pig kidney and beef red blood cell antigens should be performed), EBV-specific serology is unnecessary, but if the rapid slide test result is negative, the serum sample should be tested for EBV-specific antibodies.

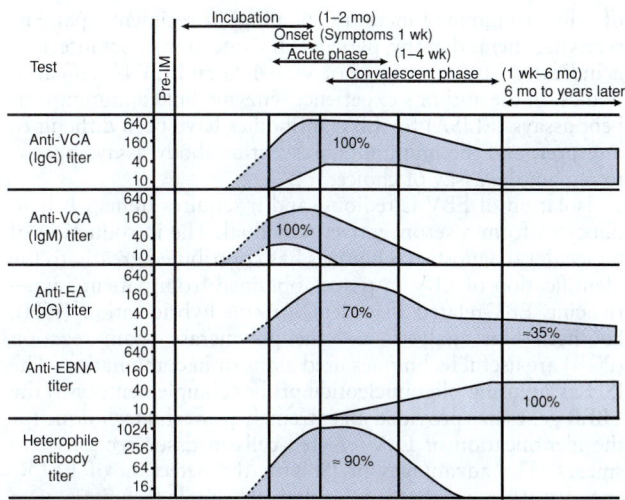

FIGURE 195.3. Characteristic Epstein-Barr virus–specific antibody responses observed in young adults with acute infectious mononucleosis (IM). EA, early antigens; EBNA, Epstein-Barr nuclear antigens; VCA, viral capsid antigen. (Adapted with permission from Henle G, Henle L, Horowitz CA. Epstein-Barr virus specific diagnostic tests in infectious mononucleosis. *Hum Pathol* 1974;5:551.)

Antibodies to three specific EBV antigens have been thoroughly studied and found to be of diagnostic importance: (a) viral capsid antigen (VCA), (b) early antigens (EAs), and (c) EBNAs. These antigens are detected by an indirect immunofluorescence assay. Individuals experiencing acute EBV-induced IM and the EBV-associated malignancies (Burkitt lymphoma and nasopharyngeal carcinoma) have been thoroughly studied, as well as normal controls, and certain characteristic antibody patterns have been described.

Figure 195.3 shows the characteristic antibody patterns observed in young adults experiencing EBV-induced IM. Before EBV infection, all three antibodies are absent, but during the acute phase of infection, high titers of IgM and IgG antibodies to VCA are seen. IgM antibodies are transient, and disappear after a few months. The majority of persons develop transient IgG antibodies against EAs, and many normal persons maintain moderate (1:20 to 1:40) antibody titers to EAs for years after primary infection. Antibodies directed against the EBNA proteins are produced early in infection; however, detectable titers by indirect immunofluorescence usually are not found until 1 to 2 months after acute infection. This pattern of late appearance is probably a reflection of the insensitivity of the complement-dependent indirect immunofluorescent antibody test. Healthy persons who have had past infection with EBV show VCA-IgG antibodies. VCA-IgM responses may be seen in only 60%, and EA responses in approximately 50%, of young infants during acute EBV infection.

In general, acute or recent primary infection is indicated by the following: (a) the presence of VCA-specific IgM antibodies; (b) high titers of VCA-specific IgG antibodies (1:320 or greater); (c) detection of anti-EA antibodies (1:10 or greater); and (d) the absence of anti-EBNA. Convalescent serum samples should be obtained to demonstrate the disappearance of VCA-IgM and the appearance of EBNA antibodies. EBV antibody titers should not be used to make a diagnosis of chronic IM or other EBV-associated syndromes on the basis of a mild to moderate elevation of VCA (1:160 to 1:320) or EA (1:20 to 1:40) antibodies because normal persons may show such titers years after uncomplicated infection. Elevated EBV titers are seen also in patients with EBV-associated malignancies and those with virtually any condition associated with suppression of cellular immune function (i.e., allograft recipients, patients receiving chemotherapy, patients HIV infection). Past infection is indicated by the presence of VCA-IgG and EBNA-IgG antibodies. In the author's experience, enzyme-linked immunosorbent assays (ELISA) for EBV antibodies have been difficult to interpret, and the immunofluorescent antibody assays appear to remain the assay of choice.

Isolation of EBV is tedious, and it requires human B lymphocytes from a seronegative individual. The introduction of molecular diagnostic techniques has contributed greatly to the identification of EBV in tissues obtained from patients experiencing EBV-related disorders. *In situ* hybridization (ISH), Southern blot analysis, and the polymerase chain reaction (PCR) are useful techniques used alone or in combination. The ISH assay using oligonucleotide probes complementary to the EBER genes has provided an extremely powerful technique for the identification of EBV-infected cells in tissue sections and smears. The advantages of ISH for the detection of EBER-encoded RNA are that it is a relatively simple technique, uses cheap stable probes, can be used on archival material, does not require radioactivity, and provides a permanent morphologic end point. Because latently infected cells may express millions of copies of EBER-RNA, ISH provides an extremely sensitive technique for the identification of even a few infected cells within a tissue. This technique now is applied widely, and it has been extremely useful in identifying EBV in entities such as Hodgkin disease, T-cell lymphoma, and hemophagocytic lymphohistiocytosis (HLH) and nasopharyngeal carcinoma. EBV DNA copy numbers in B lymphocytes can be quantitatively estimated using real-time PCR methods. Copy numbers range from 10^4 to 10^6 copies/10^6 B lymphocytes during acute EBV infection.

THERAPY

Symptomatic and Antiinflammatory

The mainstay of treatment for individuals with IM and other manifestations of primary EBV disease is supportive care. Acetaminophen or nonsteroidal antiinflammatory agents are recommended for the treatment of fever, throat discomfort, and malaise. The provision of adequate fluids and nutrition also is appropriate. Although getting adequate rest is prudent, bed rest *per se* is unnecessary.

The use of corticosteroids in the treatment of EBV-induced IM has been controversial. Studies reviewing the use of corticosteroids have been imperfect but do suggest that these agents induce a modest improvement, with diminution of lymphoid and mucosal swelling. A trial of corticosteroids in individuals with impending airway obstruction (manifested clinically by difficulty breathing or dyspnea in the recumbent position) may be warranted.

Some experienced clinicians recommend that corticosteroids should be administered in routine cases of IM, but these recommendations are based on anecdotal experience. The clinical illness of IM reflects the immune response to EBV, an agent that establishes lifelong latency and that has oncogenic potential. For this reason, the administration of immunomodulating agents, such as corticosteroids, during primary infection is theoretically contraindicated because of the possibility of altering the immune response and predisposing the patient to a long-term lymphoproliferative complication. Indeed, studies in individuals with IM who received corticosteroids many weeks earlier have demonstrated diminished numbers of B cells and T cells, including diminished numbers of CD4 helper T and CD8 cytotoxic/suppressor T cells. Because no long-term data obtained on individuals who receive corticosteroids dur-

ing primary EBV infection are available, it would seem prudent, despite the potential of short-term improvement, to withhold such treatment from most individuals, given the self-limited nature of this infection in the vast majority of cases.

Antiviral Treatment

Acyclovir is a nucleoside analogue that inhibits permissive EBV infection through the inhibition of EBV DNA polymerase but has no effect on latent infection.

The specific therapy of acute EBV infections using intravenous and oral formulations of acyclovir has been studied. Although short-term suppression of viral shedding can be demonstrated, significant clinical benefit has been lacking. These results are not surprising in view of the fact that little evidence exists for ongoing viral replication in the symptomatic phase of EBV-induced mononucleosis. The symptomatic phase of IM is likely secondary to the immunopathology generated in response to EBV-transformed B lymphocytes during the acute phase of the disease.

In the majority of the EBV-associated malignancies in which the stage of the virus life cycle has been characterized, little evidence exists for permissive (lytic) infection. Because acyclovir is effective only in inhibiting replication of linear EBV DNA, little is to be gained by its use in diseases associated with latent infection.

Anecdotal support exists for the use of acyclovir in EBV-induced HLH where evidence of replicating EBV was demonstrated. Anecdotal use of other agents such as interleukin-2, interferon-alpha, and intravenous immunoglobulins in EBV-associated diseases have been reported. No clear-cut benefits of such modalities have been demonstrated at this time.

PREVENTION

The wealth of evidence implicating EBV in the etiology of a variety of human neoplasms has made the prospect of developing a viral-based vaccine effective against human cancers very appealing. In endemic regions of the world, the vaccination of infants against EBV would potentially reduce the incidence of Burkitt lymphoma, whereas vaccine administration in developed countries would prevent the development of acute IM in young adults. With the annual incidence of acute IM estimated at 100,000 cases, EBV causes significantly more illnesses than mumps, for which a successful vaccination strategy exists. The recent epidemiologic descriptions linking prior EBV infection with the development of multiple sclerosis and systemic lupus erythematosus provides additional rationale for the development of a vaccine to prevent EBV infection.

Suggested Readings

Beaulieu BL, Sullivan JL. Epstein-Barr virus. In: Richman DD, Whitely RJ, Hayden F, eds. *Clinical virology.* New York: Churchill Livingstone, 2002: 479.

Biron CA, Byron KS and Sullivan JL. Severe herpesvirus infections in an adolescent without natural killer cells. *New Engl J Med,* 1989;320:1731.

Ebell MH. Epstein-Barr virus infectious mononucleosis. *Am Fam Phys* 2004; 70(7):1279.

Henle G, Henle L, Horowitz CA. Epstein-Barr virus specific diagnostic tests in infectious mononucleosis. *Hum Pathol* 1974;5:551.

Hjalgrim H, Askling J, Rostgaard K, et al. Characteristics of Hodgkin's lymphoma after infectious mononucleosis. *N Engl J Med* 2003;349(14):1324.

James JA, Kaufman KM, Farris AD, et al. An increased prevalence of Epstein-Barr virus infection in young patients suggests a possible etiology for systemic lupus erythematosus. *J Clin Invest* 1997;100:3019.

Kieff E, Rickinson AB. Epstein-Barr virus and its replication. In: Fields BN, Knipe DM, Howley PM, eds. *Field's virology,* vol. 2. Philadelphia: Lippincott-Raven, 2001:2511.

Levin LI, Munger KL, Rubertone MV, et al. Multiple sclerosis and Epstein-Barr virus. *JAMA* 2003;289:1533.

Macsween KF, Crawford DH. Epstein-Barr virus-recent advances. *Lancet Infect Dis* 2003;3(3):131.

Milone M, Tsai DE, Hodinka RL, et al. Treatment of primary Epstein-Barr virus infection in patients with X-linked lymphoproliferative disease using B-cell directed therapy. *Blood* 2005;105(3):994.

Precopio ML, Sullivan JL, Willard C, et al. Differential kinetics and specificity of EBV-specific CD4+ and CD8+ T cells during primary infection. *J Immunol* 2003;170(5):2590.

Sumaya CV, Ench Y. Epstein-Barr virus infection mononucleosis in children: I. Clinical and general laboratory findings. *Pediatrics* 1985;75:1603.

Thorley-Lawson, DA. Epstein-Barr virus: exploiting the immune system. *Nat Rev Immunol* 2001;1(1):75.

Thorley-Lawson DA, Gross A. Persistence of the Epstein-Barr virus and the origins of associated lymphomas. *N Engl J Med* 2004;350(13):1328.

Williams H, Macsween K, McAulay K, et al. Analysis of immune activation and clinical events in acute infectious mononucleosis. *J Infect Dis* 2004;190(1):63.

CHAPTER 196 ■ POSTNATAL HERPES SIMPLEX VIRUS

STEVE KOHL

Herpes simplex virus (HSV) is a moderately large virus consisting of an icosahedral capsid enclosing a core of double-stranded DNA and protein, surrounded by a lipid-containing envelope (Box 196.1). Two subtypes are distinguishable—types 1 and 2—with approximately 50% DNA homology. Although type 1 is regarded as the oral type and type 2 as the genital type, changing sexual habits and possibly other factors blur this distinction. Thus, the virus type is not a reliable indicator of the anatomic site of isolation.

EPIDEMIOLOGY

Although highly infectious, HSV is not transmitted casually from person to person. The enveloped virions are relatively unstable at atmospheric conditions, and close interpersonal contact usually is required for transmission. HSV can be transmitted via such body fluids as saliva and certainly can be acquired by direct apposition of infected with uninfected integument or mucous membranes. For example, virus has been transferred directly between wrestlers (herpes gladiatorum) and rugby players (herpes rugbeiorum, or "scrum pox"). Nurses and respiratory therapists may acquire HSV infections of the paronychial region (herpetic whitlow), presumably from ungloved hand contact with oropharyngeal secretions. Health care workers effectively may transfer HSV to their patients and actually can cause outbreaks of gingivostomatitis. Children with gingivostomatitis may acquire HSV whitlow by biting their nails or sucking their thumbs. Newborns may acquire HSV infection during passage through a virus-infected birth canal. Genital and anal HSV infections are acquired and transmitted through direct contact with infected genitalia or in connection with oral-genital, anal-genital, or oral-anal contacts. In all such cases, transmission may occur when the infected parties are asymptomatic and unaware of their own HSV infections. The presence of active lesions is associated with high titers of virus, which probably increases the likelihood that transmission will occur. Although HSV has been isolated from the hands of patients having an oral lesion and been shown to persist for several hours on inanimate objects or in distilled water, few data implicate inanimate sources as important reservoirs of persistence and spread of virus.

If the uninfected exposed skin or mucous membranes are abraded, damaged, or otherwise altered, the risk of transmission and spread is enhanced. For example, burned or abraded skin is more susceptible to HSV infection than is intact skin. Infants may acquire HSV infections in the area of a diaper rash; infants and children with eczema are at risk for development

---

BOX 196.1	**Herpes Simplex Virus (HSV) Genome**

The large HSV genome (approximately 100×10^6 kd) encodes for more than 90 polypeptides. Replication occurs after viral penetration and uncoating by an orderly cascade of gene products have occurred. Several important virus-encoded enzymes (products of beta genes), such as thymidine kinase and DNA polymerase, are necessary for viral DNA replication to occur and have served as important targets for antiviral compounds. Several major viral surface structural glycoproteins are enumerated. Some of them (e.g., gG) are type-specific, and some (gB, gD, gH) are critical for viral-cell interaction. Most of these glycoproteins are immunogenic and may be used in type-specific serologic assays (e.g., gG) or for vaccine candidates (e.g., gB or gD). The virus is assembled in the nucleus and buds through the nuclear membrane, acquiring its envelope, and is released at the cell surface.

HSV assumes a state of persistent latency in neural tissue (ganglion) after primary infection of the host has occurred. A limited number of RNA transcripts occurs during latency and appear to be necessary for efficient recurrences. Human HSV can be replicated in tissue cultures derived from a variety of species. The ready growth of HSV in the laboratory and the lack of species specificity distinguish this virus from other human herpesviruses. The rapidly progressive and relatively characteristic focal cytopathology induced by HSV in susceptible tissue cultures, coupled with reliable antigen detection techniques, permits simple, inexpensive recovery of this virus and its relatively easy identification and typing as 1 or 2.

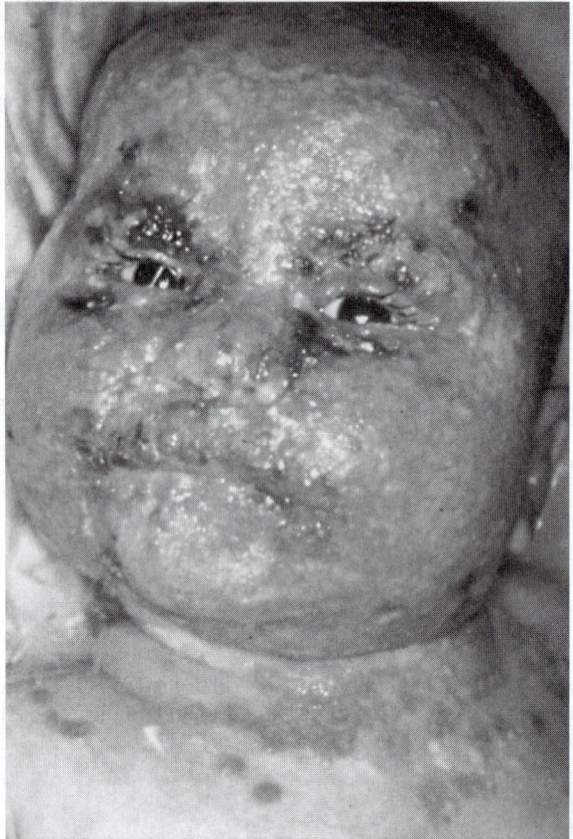

FIGURE 196.1. Extensive herpes simplex virus infection in an infant with atopic eczema (Kaposi varicelliform eruption). (Reproduced with permission from Kohl S. Postnatal herpes simplex virus infection. In: Feigin RD, Cherry JD, eds. *Textbook of pediatric infectious diseases*, 4th ed. Philadelphia: Saunders, 1998:1709.)

of serious disseminated HSV infections (Kaposi varicelliform eruption) (Fig. 196.1).

The epidemiology of HSV is dominated by symptomatic and asymptomatic infection in a huge pool of latently infected individuals. Symptomatic recurrences and asymptomatic shedding ensure the continued spread of HSV. Approximately 1% of individuals shed HSV orally, and 0.2% to 0.5% of women shed HSV genitally at any time. HSV-2 seropositive men and women shed HSV in the genital tract approximately 1% to 5% of the time. The numbers are higher for individuals who are high-risk or immunocompromised. Seroepidemiologic studies reveal that HSV infections are found in all populations. No definite seasonal pattern in HSV infections exists.

Most neonatal HSV infections are acquired from maternal genital strains and, thus, usually are caused by HSV-2. After the neonatal period, HSV-1 infections predominate and, depending on social and economic factors, 40% to 60% of young children of lower socioeconomic status are seropositive by age 5 years. Most such individuals exhibit HSV-1 antibodies by the time they reach adulthood. In one study of adolescents, 62% were seropositive for HSV-1 and 12% for HSV-2.

Studies have documented the acquisition of HSV-1 in child-care nursery or school settings, with clusters of infection and, in some cases, outbreaks of symptomatic illness occurring in as many as 13 children per outbreak. Typically, illness occurs in children 1 to 2 years old, with herpetic gingivostomatitis being the major manifestation. Studies of higher socioeconomic populations reveal seroepidemiologic evidence for HSV-1 infection in only 30% of university students. Reflecting its association with sexual activity, the prevalence of HSV-2 increases at approximately the time of puberty and early adolescence. The

percentage of HSV-2-seropositive adults ranges from 20% to 35%, with a 30% increase occurring in the last decade in the United States and a fourfold increase among adolescents.

The incidence of HSV genital infection has increased markedly since the late 1970s. Approximately 1 million new cases occur annually in the United States. In studies of sexually active university students, 4 to 16 per 1,000 acquire genital HSV infection annually. In family health clinics, the rate can be as high as 55 per 1,000.

Risk factors for the acquisition of HSV-2 in North America include gender (female greater than male), race (higher in blacks), lower socioeconomic status, multiple sex partners, failure to use condoms, and bacterial vaginosis. Transmission of HSV-2 from an infected individual to an HSV-2-seronegative individual occurs annually in approximately 10% of stable heterosexual couples. Higher rates occur in transmission from men to women (19%) and to HSV-1- and HSV-2-seronegative women (32%).

The reactivation of latent HSV infection is associated with a variety of influences, including exposure to sunlight (ultraviolet), certain febrile illnesses, local trauma, menstruation, and immunosuppression. These influences, therefore, define additional epidemiologic factors pertinent to HSV infections.

PATHOGENESIS

HSV tends to infect cells of ectodermal origin and, in most cases, initial viral replication occurs at the portal of entry, usually in skin or mucous membranes. The nuclei of infected cells manifest eosinophilic intranuclear inclusions. Because HSV has a predilection for cells that originate in embryonic ectoderm, these viruses may involve the central nervous system (CNS).

The incubation period for primary HSV infection varies from 2 to 20 days in most cases. After primary infection has occurred, the virus remains latent in sensory neural ganglia that innervate portions of the skin or mucous membranes originally involved. Thus, an individual with recurrent HSV almost always experiences reactivation of the HSV lesions in the identical region. In immunologically intact individuals, the recurrence generally is less severe than is the primary infection. In individuals previously infected with one type of virus (e.g., HSV-1, orally), infection with a second type (e.g., HSV-2, genitally) is not prevented but is less severe than in a host who has never been infected with either. Less commonly, an individual can acquire a reinfection with the same type (e.g., a second infection with a new strain of HSV-2 genitally in a patient with preexisting genital HSV-2 infection). Generally, the reinfection is mild and often is dismissed as an endogenous recurrence. These strains can be differentiated by DNA endonuclease restriction analysis of viral isolates. The pathophysiology of recurrent HSV is described in Box 196.2.

CLINICAL MANIFESTATIONS AND COMPLICATIONS

Most infections do not cause significant or specific symptoms. Although they harbor latent HSV, most seropositive persons are unaware of having ever encountered these viruses. The spectrum of symptomatic HSV infections ranges from minor localized recurrences, usually at mucocutaneous junctions, to severe and even fatal illnesses.

Gingivostomatitis

Gingivostomatitis is the most common form of HSV-induced primary illness seen in children. Symptomatic illness may occur

BOX 196.2

Pathophysiology of Recurrent Herpes Simplex Virus (HSV) Infection

After developing primary HSV infection, immuno-competent individuals have an early nonspecific response followed by a specific immunologic response. The former consists of mobilization of polymorphonuclear and mononuclear leukocytes to the site of infection, release of interferons and other cytokines, and activation of macrophages and natural killer cells. After several days, many types of specific antiviral antibodies are produced. In the second to third weeks of infection, specific cellular immunity manifested by blastogenesis of lymphocytes, production of immune lymphokines (as interferon-gamma, interleukin-2, migration inhibitory factor), a positive delayed hypersensitivity skin test, and T-cell cytotoxicity can be detected. In individuals with cellular immunologic defects (neonates, severely malnourished infants, patients with Wiskott-Aldrich syndrome and other primary immunodeficiencies, and patients receiving transplants or immunosuppressive chemotherapy), primary HSV infection can be a disseminated, life-threatening syndrome, probably because of a defect in cell-mediated immunity of the nonspecific or specific variety.

The immune response to recurrent infection is not well-characterized. It does not appear to be associated with marked alterations in the production of antibody, although fourfold elevations in titer and reemergence of IgA and IgM antiviral antibody may occur. The activity of natural killer cells and production of lymphokines increase, and relative defects in these and the blastogenesis of lymphocytes may be associated with frequent or severe recurrent infection. In the host with cellular defects, recurrences are common events and result in long duration and increased severity but usually do not cause widespread dissemination.

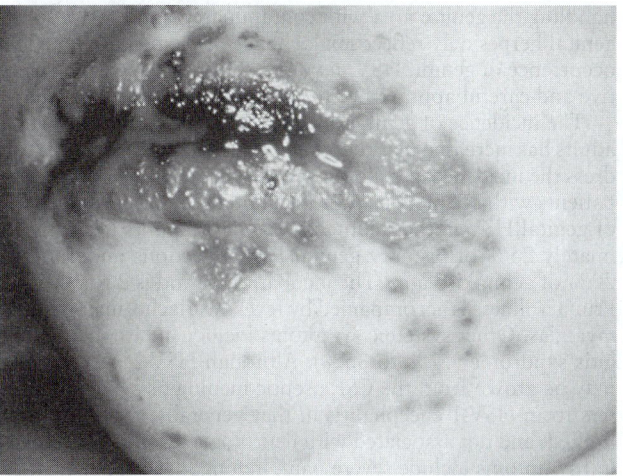

FIGURE 196.2. Primary herpes gingivostomatitis at the ulcerative vesicular stage in a normal toddler. (Reproduced with permission from Kohl S. Postnatal herpes simplex virus infection. In: Feigin RD, Cherry JD, eds. *Textbook of pediatric infectious diseases*, 4th ed. Philadelphia: Saunders, 1998:1706.)

in 30% or more of seropositive infants. Usually, it is seen in young children between ages 6 months and 3 years. In children younger than 6 months old, the presence of residual maternal antibody probably modifies or prevents the appearance of recognizable symptoms in association with HSV infection. Primary gingivostomatitis in children often is acquired from a family member with active primary or recurrent oral HSV infection. Although acute gingivostomatitis caused by HSV occurs relatively infrequently, it still is common enough that most pediatricians should become familiar with the condition and learn to distinguish this infection from herpangina.

The incubation period covers a few days, and the illness is ushered in by fretful behavior and fever. Usually, affected infants refuse to eat and may even refuse fluids. Vesicular lesions appear on and around the lips, along the gingiva, on the anterior tongue, and on the anterior (hard) palate (Fig. 196.2). Vesicles break down rapidly, and usually lesions appear as 1- to 3-mm shallow gray ulcers on an erythematous base. Generally, the gums are mildly hypertrophic, ulcerated, and erythematous. They may appear friable and frequently bleed on contact. Not uncommonly, vesicles extend about the lips and chin or down the neck in immunologically normal children. Often, the breath emits a foul odor (fetor oris). Affected children experience extreme discomfort and cannot or will not eat; if fluids are refused as well, such children may require hospitalization to maintain adequate hydration. The risk of dehydration occurring is compounded by the fever that usually accompanies this syndrome. The lesions bleed easily and may become covered with a black

crust. Often, cervical and submental nodes are swollen and tender. The process evolves for 4 to 5 days, and resolution requires at least an additional week. Autoinoculation may cause lesions on the hands (whitlow) and, less commonly, on the trunk or genital area.

HSV gingivostomatitis is differentiated from herpangina, a manifestation of enteroviral infection, by the predominance of ulcers in the anterior and posterior portions of the oropharynx; usually, herpangina is a posterior pharyngeal ulcerative condition. In addition, unlike HSV infection, herpangina often has a more acute onset, shorter duration, and seasonal occurrence. Although enterovirus-mediated hand-foot-and-mouth disease can present with oral ulcers and a vesicular eruption on the distal portion of extremities, its bilaterally symmetric distribution should differentiate it from HSV gingivostomatitis and concurrent HSV autoinoculation of a digit. Severe Stevens-Johnson syndrome (erythema multiforme) may mimic HSV, but the generalized macular rash with bull's-eye lesions is characteristic of erythema multiforme. HSV can be associated with erythema multiforme (see section, Erythema Multiforme and Herpes Simplex Virus Infection).

In adolescents and especially in college-aged patients, primary HSV infection often manifests as a posterior, occasionally exudative pharyngitis. The characteristic findings are shallow tonsillar ulcers with a gray exudate. In this setting, it must be differentiated from streptococcal infection, Epstein-Barr virus, adenovirus, *Arcanobacterium* and, rarely, diphtheria- or tularemia-induced pharyngitis. In one study of college students of high socioeconomic status, HSV was diagnosed most often (24%) as the etiology of acute pharyngitis. This manifestation usually is caused by HSV-1, but with the increased frequency of oral-genital sexual practices among both heterosexual and homosexual individuals, HSV-2 pharyngitis is encountered more commonly.

Considering the widespread publicity of HSV as a sexually transmitted disease, health care workers are advised to anticipate patient anxieties when making the diagnosis of HSV oral infection. Unless sexual contact or abuse is suspected, physicians should explain the normal mode of acquisition of oral HSV in young children.

Genital Infections

Primary herpetic vulvovaginitis may occur rarely in very young infants and children if HSV is introduced inadvertently in handling the genital area with contaminated hands. Moreover, genital herpes may reflect sexual abuse of young children. The occurrence of genital HSV in young children warrants a sensitive and careful appraisal of the family dynamics.

The incidence of genital infection in adolescents and young adults has increased markedly since the late 1970s; few data address the incidence in children. Approximately 35% to 50% of patients with the first episode of genital herpes report a history of genital HSV in their contacts. HSV-1 accounts for approximately 25% of primary genital HSV infections and 15% to 20% of genital isolates. The incubation period is 2 to 14 days. Primary illness is accompanied by fever, headache, malaise, and myalgias. Other systemic symptoms include an aseptic meningitis syndrome (11% to 35%). Although HSV-2 occasionally may be grown from the CSF, aseptic meningitis syndrome differs from HSV-1 encephalitis in that generally it is mild, self-limited, and not associated with neurologic residua. Local genital symptoms include severe pain, itching, dysuria, vaginal or urethral discharge, and tender inguinal adenopathy. In primary illness, lesions begin as painful vesicles or pustules and progress to wet ulcers and then to healing ulcers with or without crusts. Usually, crusts occur only on squamous epithelium. Lesions tend to last for 2 to 3 weeks before complete healing occurs. Virus shedding occurs for a mean of 11.5 days.

In addition to aseptic meningitis syndrome, the complications of primary HSV genital infection include sacral autonomic nervous dysfunction (manifested as poor rectal sphincter tone, constipation, sacral anesthesia, urinary retention, impotence), extragenital lesions, secondary yeast infections in women, and pharyngitis.

Beyond discomfort and embarrassment, the importance of HSV in the female genital tract relates to the potential impact of the virus on offspring, especially when a child is born to a mother with active viral shedding, particularly in connection with a symptomatic or asymptomatic primary or first episode of maternal infection (see Chapter 78, Herpes Simplex Virus). The presence of genital ulcer lesions, including those caused by HSV infection, increases the risk for the acquisition of human immunodeficiency virus (HIV) infection. An additional consideration is the effect of HSV on the self-image of the young, sexually active patient. Although some individuals cope easily with the illness and the likelihood of having recurrent disease, a sizable number exhibit profound depression, poor self-esteem, complete abstention from sexual activity, and general withdrawal. Self-help groups of individuals who have genital HSV are useful and are located in many cities of the United States.

Other Primary Herpes Simplex Virus Skin Infections

Virtually any part of the skin and mucous membranes may be involved in HSV infections. Often, altered skin provides a portal of entry for HSV. Vesicular lesions spread throughout the affected skin, usually crusting and resolving in approximately 1 week. In normal wrestlers, herpes gladiatorum usually involves the head (73%), extremities (42%), and trunk (28%). The illness accompanying eczema herpeticum can be severe and even fatal, although in most cases, the infection resolves without the administration of specific therapy and leaves no sequelae (see Fig. 196.1). Similar widespread herpetic lesions may occur in skin altered by abrasions or by thermal or chemical burns. In this situation, a secondary fever may occur, usually 1 week to several weeks after the initial insult. Careful inspection of the site or adjacent normal tissue may reveal vesicles or nonspecific ulcerative lesions. Several affected patients who did not receive therapy have died of disseminated HSV infection.

Herpetic whitlow is a painful, erythematous, swollen lesion occurring at a site of broken skin on the terminal phalanx of

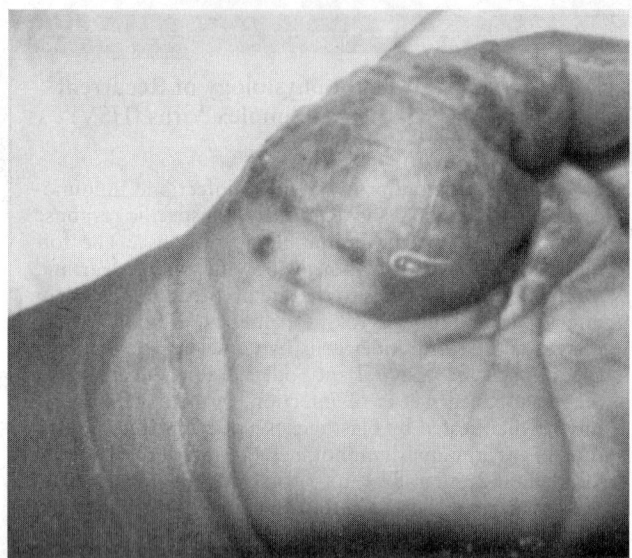

FIGURE 196.3. Herpetic whitlow in a toddler with oral herpes simplex virus infection. (Reproduced with permission from Kohl S. Postnatal herpes simplex virus infection. In: Feigin RD, Cherry JD, eds. *Textbook of pediatric infectious diseases*, 4th ed. Philadelphia: Saunders, 1998:1710.)

fingers (69%) and thumb (21%). Less commonly, toes are involved. The painful white swellings appear to be filled with pus, but, when opened for drainage, they are found to contain little fluid and no purulent material. Occasionally, the whitlow, which may persist for 7 to 10 days, initially is accompanied by a few vesicles that may give a clue to the etiology of the infection. Whitlows are seen in four typical situations. First, infants with herpetic gingivostomatitis may autoinoculate their fingers (Fig. 196.3). Second, whitlows are encountered in infants without obvious oral disease, sometimes caused by infected adults kissing their children's fingers. Third, in sexually active patients, more often the whitlow is a manifestation of concurrent genital disease, which should be investigated through appropriate history and physical examination. Fourth, dentists, respiratory therapists, nurses, and pediatricians who sometimes examine oral cavities or handle secretion-contaminated material without wearing gloves are at risk for developing herpetic whitlows. Because of the epidemiology of HSV, usually whitlows in children are caused by HSV-1. Importantly, the herpetic condition should be diagnosed because usually it is confused with a bacterial felon or paronychia and is incised and drained. This outcome is not indicated in the therapy of HSV whitlow. Only a needle aspiration and culture are necessary for diagnosis of herpetic whitlow. Appropriate infection-control measures will reduce the spread of virus due to whitlows.

Herpes Simplex Virus of the Eye

Primary HSV infection of the eye may manifest as a blepharitis or a follicular conjunctivitis, often accompanied by preauricular lymphadenopathy. If restricted to the conjunctiva, the infection, which can be accompanied by vesicular herpetic lesions elsewhere on the face or in the nose or mouth, usually resolves without sequelae. Herpetic infection of the eye may, however, progress to involve the cornea, with more serious potential consequences. For this reason, ophthalmologists always should examine and evaluate such cases.

Corneal involvement by HSV may manifest initially with minute vesicles at the corneal margin. The progress of corneal infection (best seen with the use of topical fluorescein dye) is marked by the appearance of branching lesions (a dendritic pattern) or the less diagnostic irregular (ameboid or geographic) ulcer. The affected child complains of severe photophobia, blurred vision, chemosis, and lacrimation. Primary eye infection may include stromal involvement, uveitis, and (rarely) retinitis. Spontaneous healing, which generally requires 2 to 3 weeks, can be expedited by the use of antiviral therapy (see section, Therapy, page 1256). Corticosteroids are contraindicated. The risk of developing visual impairment is enhanced with recurrences. With each bout of infection, the dendritic ulcers are more extensive and more liable to result in scarring and loss of sight. Rarely, in the immunocompromised host, HSV has been associated with retinal necrosis.

Herpes Simplex Virus Infections of the Central Nervous System

HSV is the most common identifiable cause of sporadic encephalitis, which usually is very serious. It accounts for 2% to 5% of all cases of encephalitis in the United States and for as many as 20% of all etiologic diagnoses (60% to 70% of cases of encephalitis remaining without a diagnosis). The case-fatality rate associated with untreated HSV encephalitis is approximately 70%, and survivors generally exhibit considerable permanent neurologic disability. The spread of HSV-1 to the CNS seems to proceed via neurogenic pathways. Although HSV encephalitis may involve virtually any area of the brain, it shows a striking tendency to involve the frontal and temporal lobes after the neonatal period.

An important step is to differentiate the HSV-induced aseptic meningitis syndrome—usually caused by HSV-2 and usually a complication of primary genital infection—from HSV encephalitis. In the former, signs of meningitis, including headache, photophobia, and stiff neck, appear shortly after genital lesions are noted. Usually, seizures and focal CNS findings are absent. An examination of the cerebrospinal fluid (CSF) reveals a lymphocytosis, with 300 to 2,600 white blood cells (WBCs) per cubic millimeter and sometimes a low glucose level. This syndrome may recur with genital recurrences. Usually, complete recovery occurs without the administration of specific therapy. HSV occasionally may be grown from the CSF.

In contrast to meningitis, HSV encephalitis is a highly lethal disease. In 96% of cases, it is caused by HSV-1. It may be a result of primary (30%) or recurrent (70%) infection. A larger percentage of cases of HSV encephalitis in younger individuals probably is due to primary infection. One-third of cases occur in the pediatric age range. As in most manifestations of HSV infection, but unlike most other common forms of viral encephalitis (enterovirus, arbovirus), HSV encephalitis has no seasonality. It is an acute illness with fever, malaise, irritability, and nonspecific symptoms lasting 1 to 7 days, progressing to signs and symptoms of focal CNS involvement in 3 to 7 days, and finally to coma and death (Table 196.1). The advent of sensitive HSV DNA polymerase chain reaction (PCR) diagnosis has confirmed that most cases are focal, although mild and atypical presentations occur more commonly than was thought. Fever and altered behavior in any child should evoke suspicion of encephalitis. Meningeal signs are uncommon findings. No correlation exists between the isolation of HSV from sites extrinsic to the CNS (e.g., the oropharynx or genital tract) and the diagnosis of HSV encephalitis. Thus, the presence of oral or genital lesions is not helpful in the diagnosis or exclusion of HSV encephalitis. Both identical and discordant viruses have been isolated simultaneously from the brain and oral secretions.

The CSF generally reveals a pleocytosis with as many as 2,000 WBCs per cubic millimeter, usually (80% of cases) more than 50 WBCs per cubic millimeter. In 90% of cases, more

TABLE 196.1
HISTORICAL AND CLINICAL FINDINGS IN HERPES SIMPLEX VIRUS ENCEPHALITIS

Findings	Incidence (%)
Historical findings	
Alteration of consciousness	97
Fever	90
Personality changes	71
Seizures	67
Vomiting	46
Hemiparesis	33
Memory loss	24
Findings at presentation	
Fever	92
Personality changes	85
Dysphasia	76
Autonomic dysfunction	60
Ataxia	40
Seizures	38
Focal	28
Generalized	10
Cranial nerve defects	32
Visual field loss	14
Papilledema	14

Reproduced with permission from Kohl S. Postnatal herpes simplex virus infection. In: Feigin RD, Cherry JD, eds. *Textbook of pediatric infectious diseases,* 4th ed. Philadelphia: Saunders, 1998:1706.

than 60% of cells are lymphocytes. Early in the infection, neutrophils may predominate. In 75% to 85% of cases, red blood cells, reflecting the hemorrhagic necrosis, are seen in the CSF. Between 5% and 25% of patients have hypoglycorrhachia, and 80% have elevated CSF protein levels (median, 80 mg/dL), which rise to striking levels with progression of the disease. The CSF is normal in 2% to 3% of patients with early HSV encephalitis. HSV almost never is grown from lumbar CSF and rarely from ventricular fluid. Thus, whereas the CSF examination is helpful, it is not diagnostic of HSV encephalitis unless PCR is used to detect HSV DNA.

The usefulness of neurodiagnostic tests is limited. The electroencephalography (EEG) probably is one of the more useful tests. A "typical" pattern of unilateral or bilateral (poor prognosis) periodic focal spikes against a background of slow (flattened) activity (paroxysmal lateral epileptiform discharges) is associated with HSV encephalitis. Other findings include large-amplitude irregular slow activity, sharp waves, and variable spikes. In 80% to 90% of patients, the EEG finding is not only abnormal but localizing. This test is one of the earliest localizing laboratory studies. The brain scan or computed tomography (CT) is less helpful early in the illness. Late in the illness, the CT appearance may be characteristic [i.e., low-density, contrast-enhanced lesions in the temporal area, mass effect, edema, and hemorrhage (Fig. 196.4)], but early in the illness, when diagnosis is critical, often the CT appearance is unremarkable. An abnormal CT scan is a poor prognostic factor. Magnetic resonance imaging (MRI), an early sensitive test for localizing HSV encephalitis (Fig. 196.5), is the radiologic technique of choice for making an early diagnosis of HSV encephalitis. The finding of focal abnormality on EEG, MRI, CT, or radionuclide brain scan is significantly more likely to occur in HSV encephalitis than in those other illnesses with which it is confused.

The clinical and laboratory data acquired by noninvasive methods are valuable only for increasing the index of suspicion for HSV encephalitis; they do not confirm the diagnosis. The differential diagnosis of this condition is relatively large and

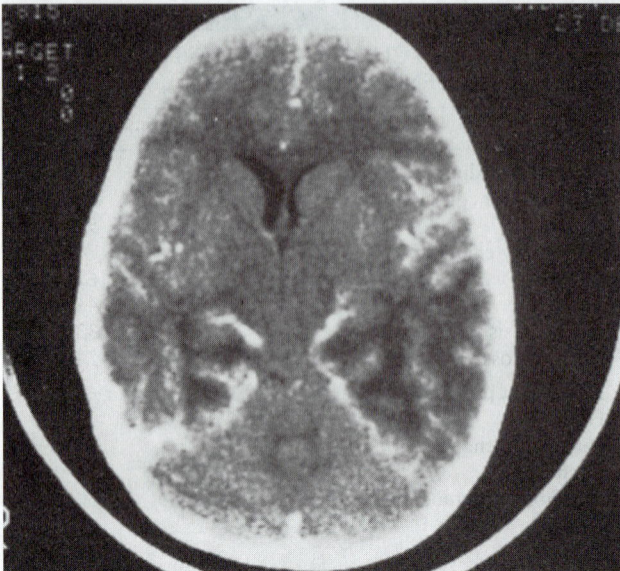

FIGURE 196.4. Computed tomographic scan obtained 1 week after onset of herpes simplex virus encephalitis in a 6-year-old child. Note the bilateral temporal low-density areas with dye enhancement and the mass effect. (Reproduced with permission from Kohl S. Postnatal herpes simplex virus infection. In: Feigin RD, Cherry JD, eds. *Textbook of pediatric infectious diseases*, 4th ed. Philadelphia: Saunders, 1998:1712.)

includes many treatable conditions (Box 196.3). HSV DNA PCR diagnosis of spinal fluid samples, performed in specialized laboratories, initially was shown to be more than 98% sensitive and 94% specific, when compared to brain biopsy. Indeed, the 94% specificity probably is higher because PCR is even more sensitive than is culture. One week of acyclovir therapy did not alter the PCR sensitivity. More recently, lower levels of sensitivity have been reported in samples obtained in the early phases of illness. False-positive results may be reported from less specialized laboratories as well. A repeat CSF PCR may be helpful. Unless reliable HSV DNA detection by PCR is positive, a brain biopsy test is essential in patients with suspected HSV

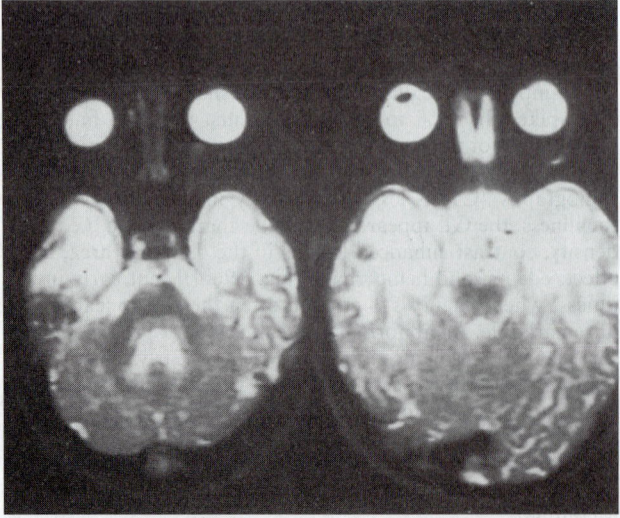

FIGURE 196.5. Magnetic resonance image of patient with early herpes simplex virus encephalitis. Note the bilateral temporal lobe enhancement. (Reproduced with permission from Kohl S. Herpes simplex encephalitis. *Pediatr Clin North Am* 1988;35:465.)

BOX 196.3	**Differential Diagnosis of Herpes Simplex Virus Encephalitis**

Infections
Fungal
    Especially *Cryptococcus*
Bacterial
    Abscess, cerebritis
    Listeria monocytogenes meningitis
    Subdural, epidural empyema
    Tuberculosis
    Bacterial endocarditis
    Lyme disease
    Syphilis
Mycoplasmal
Rickettsial
Protozoal
    Toxoplasmosis
    Amoebic
Viral
    Human herpesvirus 6
    Mumps virus
    Coxsackievirus, echovirus
    Arbovirus (especially St. Louis encephalitis)
    Postinfluenza encephalitis
    Reye syndrome
    Lymphocytic choriomeningitis virus
    Rabies virus
    Epstein-Barr virus
    Rubella virus
    Cytomegalovirus
    Adenovirus
    Tickborne encephalitis virus
    Human immunodeficiency virus type 1
    Progressive multifocal leukoencephalopathy
    Subacute sclerosing panencephalitis
    West Nile virus

Noninfectious Disorders
Tumor
Vascular disease
Arteriovenous malformations
Toxins
Alcoholic encephalopathy
Hematoma
Adrenal leukodystrophy

encephalitis, both to provide optimal aggressive therapy for that condition and to achieve a diagnosis for the 50% to 60% of patients without HSV infections, roughly one-half of whom would benefit from other specific therapies.

The risk of performing brain biopsy test is low. A national collaborative study of 182 biopsy tests revealed only three complications: hemorrhage in two patients and herniation of brain tissue in a third. Roughly 3% of brain biopsies were false-negatives, usually due to the biopsy being performed on the wrong site or to improper specimen handling.

Increasingly frequent reports cite a postherpetic encephalomyelitis with a probable autoimmune or demyelinating etiology and cite virus-positive recurrences of HSV encephalitis months after apparently successful therapy. These conditions can be differentiated and documented by PCR or biopsy using appropriate tissue histology and culture.

HSV-1 DNA is detected by PCR analysis accompanied by a transient anti-HSV antibody response in the CSF in patients with the classic syndrome of Mollaret meningitis.

Herpes Simplex Virus Infection of the Gastrointestinal Tract in Normal Hosts

Several publications have documented HSV esophagitis in normal patients. The presenting symptoms include severe odynophagia, retrosternal and subxiphoid pain, and the inability to eat. Generally, skin lesions are absent. Usually, double-contrast esophagrams reveal abnormalities. Esophagoscopy reveals ulcerations and fibrinous and, at times, hemorrhagic exudate. Usually, symptoms remit in 5 to 7 days with nonspecific therapy.

Delineating involvement of the other end of the gastrointestinal tract with HSV is important, especially when it manifests as an anorectal infection in homosexual males. HSV also is a rare cause of severe hepatitis, especially in pregnant women, usually associated with high fever, leukopenia, thrombocytopenia, and a high mortality rate.

Recurrent Herpes Simplex Virus Infections

All the sites discussed in connection with primary HSV disease may be involved also in recurrent infections. HSV infection may occur without manifestation of specific lesions. With the aid of co-cultivation techniques, HSV has been recovered from dorsal root ganglia subserving the areas of skin in which individuals have experienced recurrent herpes lesions. HSV-1 has been found in trigeminal ganglia, and HSV-2 has been recovered from sacral ganglia. By in situ hybridization and PCR, HSV DNA has been detected also in ganglia. Concomitant infection of oral and genital sites by HSV is most likely to result in recurrences in oral sites if it is type 1 virus and in genital sites if it is type 2 virus.

The most common manifestation of recurrent HSV infection is herpes labialis ("cold sores," "fever blisters"), which is estimated to occur in 25% to 50% of the general population. Most individuals experience a prodrome (pain, burning, tingling, or itching) at the site lasting 6 hours to several days. Then follows a progression from papules (lasting 12 to 36 hours) to vesicles (usually gone by 48 hours) to ulcers and crust (lasting 2 to 4 days). Most outbreaks are healed by 5 to 10 days. Most pain occurs during the vesicular stage. Virus is isolated readily from vesicles and less commonly from ulcers and crusts. Maximum virus titers in lesions (up to 10^7 to 10^8 viruses) are measured in the vesicles. Recurrences tend to occur at the same location or at closely related areas. In general, they occur on the lips, mucocutaneous junction, or other parts of the face. Recurrent lesions inside the mouth rarely are caused by HSV and more likely are aphthous lesions. Intraoral HSV recurrences tend to occur on tissue adjacent to bone, such as the gums or palate, and not on the lips or buccal mucosa. A differential diagnosis of the condition also includes pemphigus, lichen planus, ulcers caused by cyclic neutropenia, and ulcers associated with celiac disease, ulcerative colitis, Crohn disease, pernicious anemia, and Behçet syndrome.

Recurrent genital HSV probably is the second most common manifestation of HSV and one of the most bothersome. Recurrences occur much more commonly after primary HSV-2 (90%) than after HSV-1 (55%) infection. The mean rate of recurrence is 0.1 episode per month after primary genital HSV-1 infection and 0.3 episode per month after primary HSV-2 genital infection. Subclinical recurrences are very common events, accounting for one-third of total days of viral reactivation.

Only 5% to 12% of individuals with recurrent genital HSV have constitutional symptoms. Local symptoms include pain (averaging 4 to 6 days), itching, dysuria, adenopathy, and lesions lasting 4 to 5 days and progressing to crusting and healing by 9 to 11 days. Virus is shed for an average of 3 to 4 days. In dry areas, vesicles are seen, but the vesicles in wet areas rapidly break down into ulcers. Generally, symptoms are milder and their duration is shorter than in primary genital disease.

Other cutaneous recurrences may manifest at each anatomic site in which primary infection occurs. HSV may recur on the face or trunk in a typical dermatome distribution like that associated with varicella-zoster virus. Frequent repeated attacks of zosteriform-like lesions on any part of the body in a normal host suggest the presence of HSV and not varicella-zoster infection.

Erythema Multiforme and Herpes Simplex Virus Infection

Erythema multiforme may be an allergic response to recurrent HSV infection. In several series, approximately 15% of patients with erythema multiforme reported having recurrent HSV before skin eruption, which may be macular or urticarial, occurred. In one series, 5 of 80 patients who had recurrent oral HSV experienced a rash (presumably erythema multiforme) 8 to 14 days after the onset of a cold sore. Several studies document HSV antigen-antibody immune complexes present in the serum and skin of patients who had erythema multiforme after HSV infection.

HSV DNA has been detected in the biopsy samples of skin lesions of patients with erythema multiforme. In one study, HSV DNA was detected by PCR analysis of skin biopsy samples from 8 of 10 children with a history of HSV-associated erythema multiforme and from 8 of 10 children with idiopathic erythema multiforme minor (but not in unaffected skin or in biopsy samples from control patients). The skin manifestations may last for 14 to 21 days. Generally, therapy is directed toward the allergic and not the viral component of the illness or toward prevention of herpetic recurrences.

Herpes Simplex Virus Infection in the Immunocompromised Host

Box 196.4 lists the conditions associated with unusually severe HSV infections. (HSV infection in the neonatal period is discussed in Chapter 78, Herpes Simplex Virus.) Other than the several cases of HSV encephalitis in patients with agammaglobulinemia (and concomitant infections with enterovirus), the common links in these varied groups are either skin abnormalities (eczema, burns) or immunologic defects, primarily in the cell-mediated aspects of the immune system.

The incidence of severe HSV infection in these pediatric groups is defined poorly. The following statistics derive from patients not receiving prophylactic antiviral therapy. In series of adult and pediatric patients with renal, marrow, stem-cell or cardiac transplants, 70% to 90% of seropositive individuals excreted HSV, usually from the oropharynx and usually at the time of peak immunosuppression, in the first month after transplantation. HSV was isolated from 43% of the pediatric renal transplant recipients in one series. HSV in cardiac transplant recipients caused symptomatic illness in 45% to 85% of seropositive patients, depending on the intensity of immunosuppression. In bone-marrow transplant recipients, HSV (often in the absence of cutaneous or mucous membrane lesions) is one of the causes of interstitial pneumonitis, a disorder that accounts for approximately 5% to 10% of deaths. It has been

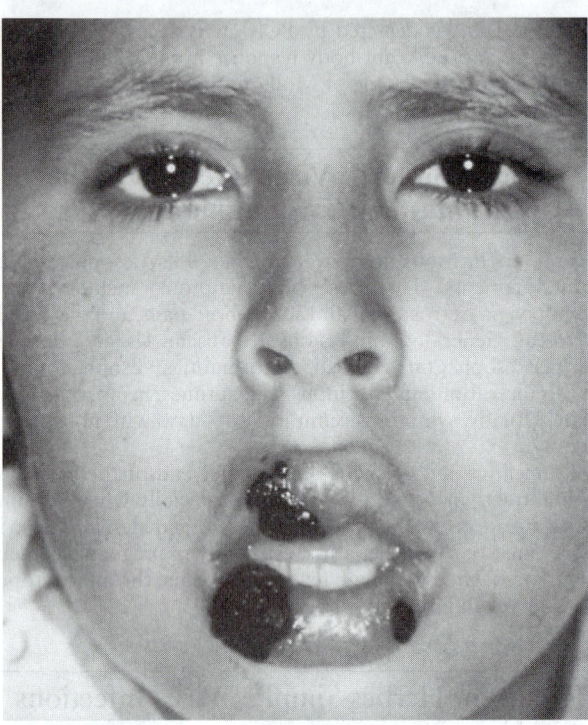

FIGURE 196.6. Chronic hemorrhagic herpes simplex virus infection in a girl with leukemia and a bone marrow transplant. (Reproduced with permission from Kohl S. Postnatal herpes simplex virus infection. In: Feigin RD, Cherry JD, eds. *Textbook of pediatric infectious diseases*, 4th ed. Philadelphia: Saunders, 1998:1717.)

chronic, bloody, coalescing, ulcerated, oozing lesions, eroding into the subcutaneous tissue, occasionally destroying underlying structures. The tissue is odorous, and the lesions are painful (Fig. 196.6). A similar syndrome may be seen in the perianal or genital area, usually caused by HSV-2 infection, and this is one of the characteristic syndromes in adolescent and adult patients with AIDS. Untreated lesions may lead to death caused by local destruction and hemorrhage or may regress as the immune status of the host improves or as antiviral chemotherapy is used. Poor response to antiviral therapy should prompt the performance of viral susceptibility testing to detect acyclovir-resistant virus. This problem most typically occurs in patients receiving chronic or frequent courses of therapy and accounts for approximately 5% of HSV isolates from immunocompromised patients.

In patients with burns, eczema, pemphigus, or abrasions, a similar syndrome may occur, often with conversion of second-degree tissue damage to third-degree damage. Possibly as a result of the more severe immunodeficiency occurring with several of these conditions, the local infection may progress to dissemination into visceral organs. The widespread necrotizing lesions commonly are known as *Kaposi varicelliform eruption* or *eczema herpeticum* (see Fig. 196.1).

These lesions must be differentiated from the bacterial infections caused by gram-positive or gram-negative organisms, chronic fungal infections (as seen with *Mucor* species, aspergillosis, blastomycosis), other viral infections (vaccinia, varicella), mycobacterial infections, and various noninfectious lesions, such as pyoderma gangrenosum or Sweet syndrome. Chemotherapy-induced mucositis may mimic and also be complicated by HSV infection.

Uncommonly, esophagitis caused by HSV has been reported in normal children, but it is a relatively common occurrence in immunocompromised patients. Pathologic studies suggest that approximately 25% of cases of autopsy-proven esophagitis are secondary to HSV infection. Underlying conditions include

reported as a cause of pneumonia in children with acquired immunodeficiency syndrome (AIDS). In children, HSV is a common cause of acute infection in the leukopenic leukemic patient in relapse, and it accounts for a significant number of deaths that occur during remission. HSV, typically oral infection, occurs in 5% to 15% of children with AIDS. In developing countries, disseminated HSV infection is not an unusual finding in severely malnourished children.

Several major syndromes are attributable to HSV in immunocompromised patients, with some overlap and occasional progression from one to another. The first is a local, chronic, often extensive cutaneous or mucocutaneous infection. The second is infection of one organ, usually contiguous to an orifice (e.g., esophagitis or pneumonitis). The most serious is widespread dissemination involving distant areas of skin or visceral organs (lungs, liver, adrenals) and the CNS. Except in the most immunosuppressed patients, disseminated disease probably most often represents primary infection, whereas the local syndromes may represent primary or (more often) recurrent illness.

The typical local syndrome begins in the mouth or about the lips, often appearing innocuously as an ordinary recurrence of herpes labialis. Over the course of several days, if untreated, the papules and vesicles progress to bullae, often with hemorrhagic fluid. The bullae or vesicles progress to huge,

burns, aplastic anemia, malignancies, organ transplantation, a variety of other serious medical problems, and nasogastric tube–induced trauma in postoperative patients. Approximately 20% to 50% of these patients have HSV involvement elsewhere (lungs, trachea and, less commonly, skin). The esophagitis may be asymptomatic or associated with dysphagia, odynophagia, epigastric discomfort, and retrosternal pain. The characteristic findings in the esophagus are ulcers with raised granular margins. Often, the ulcers are covered with fibrinous exudate and, in advanced cases, are confluent with progression to complete mucosal loss in large segments of the esophagus. Typically, visceral herpes infection is not suspected before death. Uncommonly, involvement of adjacent gastric tissue can be documented. Diagnostic evaluation should include barium swallow, which may demonstrate edema, nodules, and ulceration of the esophagus. Esophagoscopy with biopsy and viral culture is diagnostic and helps to exclude other common causes of this syndrome, including *Candida*, cytomegalovirus, and possibly other fungal and bacterial infection or chemotherapy-induced changes.

The organ second most commonly involved in immunocompromised hosts probably is the lungs. HSV pneumonia is a rare premortum diagnosis and occurs almost exclusively in immunosuppressed patients. In one series of 1,000 consecutive autopsies, HSV pneumonia was identified in 10 cases. In most cases in adults, the process is a result of endogenous viral mucocutaneous reactivation and involvement of lung tissue by contiguous spread, causing focal pneumonia (60% of cases). Hematogenous spread from an oral or genital site may result in diffuse pneumonitis. Patients had cough, dyspnea, fever, and hypoxia, and 50% had rales. Most had other concomitant pulmonary infections with bacteria, *Candida*, *Aspergillus*, and cytomegalovirus. HSV pneumonia cannot be diagnosed from the association of upper airway cultures with the radiographic picture. The diagnosis must be pursued aggressively using culture and histopathology from involved lung tissue.

Meningoencephalitis caused by HSV is not a common finding in immunocompromised patients. It may occur as part of widely disseminated disease or may be a localized condition. In immunocompromised patients, it may occur after a slowly evolving subacute form. The most severe form of HSV infection in the immunocompromised host is widely disseminated disease involving the liver, adrenals, lungs, spleen, kidney, marrow, and (often) the brain. In the absence of prophylactic antiviral therapy, this type of infection occurs in 10% to 25% of children with transplants and HSV infection. Usually, the clinical presentation is one of initial fever and mucocutaneous involvement that, instead of healing as expected, disseminates. The cutaneous dissemination may involve a widespread vesicular eruption that appears much like varicella or may involve more local, large, hemorrhagic vesicles and bullae. In approximately 20% of cases of disseminated disease, skin lesions are absent. The major target organs involved give rise to syndromes of hepatitis, pneumonia, shock, bleeding, disseminated intravascular coagulopathy, seizures, coma, renal failure, hypothermia, and death in days to weeks. Laboratory tests may reveal leukopenia, thrombocytopenia, elevated values on liver function tests, hyponatremia, azotemia, pneumonitis, hypoglycemia, CSF pleocytosis, abnormal EEG, and electrocardiographic abnormalities. Death is very common in this syndrome, even after the institution of antiviral chemotherapy. Less commonly, isolated organs, particularly the liver, may be involved, resulting in herpetic hepatitis.

DIAGNOSIS

Because HSV may be shed in response to fever, stress, or immunosuppression, the finding of HSV in certain secretions does not mean that the clinical condition is caused by HSV. In general, the virus must be isolated from the tissue in question to confirm the diagnosis, especially in immunosuppressed hosts.

Rapid, Nonspecific Methods

Electron microscopy and cytologic examination are rapid and very suggestive diagnostic modalities, but they are not entirely specific. Electron microscopy of vesicular fluid or tissue preparations may reveal the characteristic virus of the herpes family, but it cannot differentiate HSV from other herpesviruses.

Cytology can reveal the typical multinucleated giant cells and, less commonly, the Cowdry type A intranuclear inclusions characteristic of HSV, but these findings may be seen also with cytomegalovirus and varicella-zoster virus. In most series, 40% to 60% of culture-positive specimens are cytologically positive if examined by an experienced observer. False-positive examination results are unusual but do occur.

Rapid, Specific Methods

Several rapid, specific tests depend on immunologic reagents for antigen detection. Fluorescent antibody methods, enzyme-linked immunosorbent assays (ELISAs), immunoperoxidase-tagged antibody in ELISA or tissue sections, radiometric tests, and *Staphylococcus* protein A absorption tests are available or being investigated. Generally, these tests use relatively specific hyperimmune serum to HSV or monoclonal antibodies to specific HSV glycoproteins. Most studies reported a 50% to 90% sensitivity and more than 95% specificity. These tests are of widespread clinical utility, but they are not yet as sensitive as is culture.

PCR allows for a spectacularly sensitive detection of viral DNA. In most situations, it is not necessary for HSV diagnosis. In unusual settings, such as erythema multiforme, PCR of involved skin lesion biopsy material may establish HSV as the etiology and can influence decisions about future suppressive therapy. The most useful role for PCR is the detection of HSV DNA in the spinal fluid of patients with suspected HSV encephalitis. If a reliable laboratory reports positive results, the need for a brain biopsy test is obviated. The major problems with PCR are false-positive responses, primarily caused by poor laboratory technique, and false-negative results reported more recently. Test reliability depends highly on the competence of the performing laboratory.

Less Rapid, Specific Methods

The reference standard for HSV diagnosis outside the CNS remains tissue culture. HSV grows rapidly (mean, 2 to 3 days) in human and nonhuman cells, producing a typical cytopathic effect. Often, the use of shell-vial techniques allows for establishing definitive diagnosis in 18 to 24 hours. Occasionally, confusion is caused by high-titer specimens of varicella-zoster virus or cytomegalovirus. Definitive viral characterization is accomplished by antisera reaction causing neutralization, fluorescent antibody reaction, or several of the antigen detection tests mentioned. Typing can be accomplished using specific monoclonal antibodies, DNA analysis, or endonuclease restriction patterns (see section, Endonuclease Restriction Analysis).

A variety of antibody tests can be used to document primary HSV infection. Classic tests include viral neutralization, complement fixation, indirect hemagglutination, and fluorescent antibody assays. Newer tests include ELISAs to detect antibodies, radiometric assays, and Western blot analysis to detect antibody to specific viral polypeptides. Several precautions must be observed in analyzing the serologic response. Patients with documented prior HSV infections may have fourfold titer elevations with recurrences, and they may have IgM or IgA responses with recurrences. Rarely, severely immunosuppressed patients do not produce antibody. Thus, only when a patient's serum converts from negative to positive can a primary infection be diagnosed with confidence. Generally, patients with prior HSV infection (symptomatic or asymptomatic) remain seropositive for life (probably reflecting existing latency) with minor fluctuations. However, in some of the most important conditions—HSV encephalitis or early disseminated HSV in immunosuppressed hosts—serology is relatively useless because of a slow titer rise or late conversion. In addition, a significant percentage of these conditions represent recurrent and not primary disease. Although CSF-to-serum antibody ratios may be diagnostic in HSV encephalitis, often they are not so until several days or weeks into the illness and, thus, their clinical usefulness is limited. Reliable type-specific serologies with sensitivity of 80% to 95% and specificity greater than 96% have become available recently.

Endonuclease Restriction Analysis

Each HSV DNA has a specific cleavage pattern or "fingerprint" when digested by endonuclease restriction enzymes and subjected to electrophoresis in a gel. These cleavage patterns can be used to type the virus and to demonstrate relatedness or differences (strains) among isolates from different persons for epidemiologic purposes ("outbreaks," nosocomial transmission), among isolates obtained from different sites in the same individual during one illness, or among isolates obtained from the same site over the course of time. This analysis has added markedly to the understanding of the epidemiology of HSV, the examination of the possibility of exogenous reinfection versus recurrence, and the recognition of the ability to harbor more than one latent virus at the same site.

Drug Susceptibility Testing

Although not in uniform use, viral culture and sensitivity testing increasingly are available and important, especially in the care of immunosuppressed hosts. Inhibiting levels of 3 μg/mL or greater for acyclovir and 150 μg/mL or greater for foscarnet indicate viral resistance.

Experimental Methods of Viral Detection

The development of genetic engineering has permitted the production of complementary nucleic acid, enabling genetic probing of tissue. Nucleic acid hybridization or *in situ* PCR may detect virus or viral DNA or RNA in latent conditions, possibly virus-transformed cells or sites of very low levels of productive infection.

PROGNOSIS

HSV infections occurring after the fetal and neonatal periods are annoying, but usually they are not immediately life-threatening. The outcome of HSV encephalitis can be serious, ranging from extensive and permanent neurologic disability to death. HSV is one of the most common causes of infectious blindness in people living in industrialized countries. In immunocompromised patients, it is a major cause of morbidity and mortality. Genital HSV may not have life-threatening potential, but it is a significant cause of physical and psychological morbidity.

THERAPY

Oral Herpes Simplex Virus

A placebo-controlled trial in children with herpes gingivostomatitis treated with oral acyclovir (15 mg/kg five times daily for 7 days) demonstrated a decrease in oral lesions (4 days, versus 10 days in placebo) and more rapid disappearance of fever, extraoral lesions, and eating and drinking problems. A marked reduction in days that virus was shed (1 versus 5) also occurred. Intravenous acyclovir has been used in patients with severe primary gingivostomatitis when hospital admission was required to maintain hydration (Box 196.5). In these uncommon cases, the illness responded in several days, with defervescence and cessation of new lesion development. No data are available to determine whether this therapy would change the risk of recurrences occurring in later life.

Symptomatic therapy includes antipyretics and oral hydration with bland liquids and ice slurries. The use of oral anesthetics probably is not indicated and has resulted in self-injury when children chewed on anesthetized oral mucosa or lips. Topical acyclovir ointment therapy is not indicated in recurrent oral HSV infection except in immunocompromised patients with mild illness. Topical penciclovir and oral acyclovir have been shown to decrease minimally the number of days that normal adults with recurrent oral HSV experience symptoms and viral shedding, and these agents generally are not indicated.

Herpes Simplex Virus Keratitis

The pyrimidine nucleoside trifluridine in a 1% ophthalmic solution inhibits HSV DNA synthesis. It is the drug of choice for the local treatment of primary and recurrent HSV, such as keratitis, keratoconjunctivitis, and eyelid lesions, and for use after operations on eyes previously infected with HSV or for use in steroid therapy in similar eyes. Keratitis appears to respond more rapidly to trifluridine than to either idoxuridine or vidarabine ointment. Ulcers failing to respond to the latter two agents have responded to trifluridine. None of the local therapies affects the rate of recurrence. Continuous suppressive oral acyclovir (400 mg twice daily) results in 40% fewer recurrences in adults. Trifluridine is used as one drop per eye every 2 hours while awake (maximum, nine drops daily) until reepithelialization of corneal ulcers occurs, then as one drop every 5 hours while awake (maximum, 5 drops daily) for 7 additional days. The maximum duration of therapy is 21 days. Side effects consist of local stinging, burning, and edema (3% to 5% of cases).

The indications for and side effects of vidarabine ophthalmic ointment are similar to those of trifluridine, although the ointment preparation may be more useful in children (see Box 196.4). Dosage is 0.5 in. five times per day (at 3-hour intervals). If no improvement occurs in 7 days or reepithelialization is not complete in 21 days, trifluridine is indicated. In serious ocular infection, therapy often is initiated with intravenous acyclovir as well as topical preparations.

Individuals caring for children with HSV keratitis are advised strongly to undertake treatment in conjunction with an ophthalmologist familiar with this illness. The use of cycloplegic and antiinflammatory agents in this illness requires practical experience.

BOX 196.5   Therapy of Herpes Simplex Virus Infection in Children

Genital Disease
Primary
Oral acyclovir, 200 mg five times daily for 7 to 10 days (1 capsule = 200 mg)* or 400 mg three times daily for 10 days, pediatric dose 40 to 80 mg/kg per day divided in three or four doses for 5 to 10 days
Valacyclovir, 1 g twice daily for 10 days*
Famciclovir, 250 mg three times daily for 7 to 10 days*
Intravenous acyclovir, 15 mg/kg/day in three divided doses for 5 to 7 days

Recurrent
Oral acyclovir, 200 mg five times daily for 5 days or 400 mg three times daily for 5 days* or 800 mg twice daily for 5 days*
Oral valacyclovir, 500 mg twice daily for 3 to 5 days* or 1,000 mg once daily for 5 days*
Oral famciclovir, 125 mg twice daily for 5 days*

Suppressive
Oral acyclovir, 200 mg three to five times daily or 400 mg two to three times daily for up to 5 years*
Oral valacyclovir, 500 mg/day* or 1,000 mg/day*
Oral famciclovir, 250 mg twice daily*

Oral Disease
Primary: same as for primary genital infection. Oral dose for children should not exceed 80 mg/kg/day of acyclovir (15 mg/kg five times daily). (No pediatric dosing guidelines are available for valacyclovir or famciclovir.)
Recurrent: penciclovir, topical, every 2 hours while awake for 4 days

Encephalitis
Intravenous acyclovir, 30 mg/kg/day in three divided doses for 21 days†

Neonatal Disease
Intravenous acyclovir, 60 mg/kg/day in three divided doses for 14 to 21 days†

Immunocompromised Patients
Intravenous acyclovir, 15 to 30 mg/kg/day in three divided doses; duration as warranted clinically
Oral acyclovir, 200 mg three to five times daily, not to exceed 80 mg/kg/day; duration as warranted clinically

Acyclovir-resistant Isolates
Intravenous foscarnet, 120 mg/kg/day in three divided doses until infection resolution

Ocular Infection
Trifluorothymidine (Viroptic), 1% to 2% ophthalmic solution, one drop every 2 hours to a maximum of nine drops, then one drop every 4 hours (five drops daily), not to exceed 21 days
Vidarabine (Vira-A), 3% ophthalmic ointment, five times daily; change to different agent if no healing occurs in 7 to 9 days
Iododeoxyuridine (Stoxil), 0.1% ophthalmic solution or 0.5% ophthalmic ointment. Solution: one drop each hour during the day and every 2 hours during the night. Ointment: five times daily, every 4 hours and before bedtime; change to different agent if no occurs healing in 7 to 9 days
Acyclovir 400 mg orally twice daily for long-term suppression, pediatric dose 80 mg/kg/day in three divided doses, maximum 1,000 mg/day*

---

*These are adult doses. No licensed guidelines exist for pediatric doses in this condition. Oral acyclovir dose for children should not exceed 80 mg/kg/day. No pediatric dosing guidelines are available for valacyclovir or famciclovir.
†The large dose has been found effective and nontoxic in these particular clinical conditions and patients.
(Adapted with permission from Kohl S. Postnatal herpes simplex virus infection. In: Feigin RD, Cherry JD, eds. *Textbook of pediatric infectious diseases*, 2nd ed. Philadelphia: Saunders, 1987:1577.)

Herpes Simplex Virus Encephalitis

Intravenous acyclovir (10 mg/kg per dose three times daily for 21 days) is the drug of choice in the treatment of children with HSV encephalitis (see Box 196.5). As noted in earlier vidarabine studies, patients' mental status at initiation of therapy and speed of initiation of therapy markedly influence the outcome of patients with HSV encephalitis treated with acyclovir. Lethargic patients have a 15% mortality rate, whereas comatose patients have a 40% rate of mortality. Relapses, reported to occur from 5% to 25% of the time in children and associated with lower doses and shorter duration of therapy, often are associated with positive CSF PCR. Retreatment with acyclovir usually is successful. The use of longer-term oral suppressive therapy using oral valacyclovir is being investigated.

In addition to antiviral therapy, meticulous intensive care optimizes the outcome of these patients. Fluid management to prevent overhydration is critical. Often, direct intracranial pressure measurement is necessary to monitor and treat increased intracranial pressure effectively. The use of steroids is common but remains controversial and unstudied. Usually, an-

ticonvulsant therapy to manage severe and prolonged seizures and ventilatory support are necessary. The care of children with HSV encephalitis requires a team of pediatric intensivists, neurologists, neurosurgeons, and infectious-disease experts in a tertiary-care setting.

Genital Herpes Simplex Virus Infection

Acyclovir (Zovirax), an inactive drug, is the drug of choice for HSV genital infection in children (see Box 196.5). The inhibition of DNA synthesis requires its phosphorylation. In this regard, HSV thymidine kinase is much more active than is its mammalian counterpart. Thus, acyclovir becomes a specific antiviral agent in the presence of thymidine kinase-positive viruses. Thymidine kinase appears to be an important enzyme for viral virulence (Box 196.6).

Intravenous acyclovir has an impressive effect on primary genital HSV infection. Used in a dose of 5 mg/kg each 8 hours for 5 days, intravenous acyclovir shortened the duration of viral shedding and decreased local and systemic symptoms by 20% to 50%. Complications such as extragenital lesions and urinary

---

Acyclovir and Thymidine Kinase in HSV

Mutant, thymidine kinase-negative acyclovir-resistant isolates of HSV have been recovered from otherwise healthy patients in the course of acyclovir therapy for genital HSV infections. The patients (unlike immunocompromised patients; see section, Herpes Simplex Virus Infection in Immunocompromised Hosts) generally responded to acyclovir therapy. These viral mutants seem less virulent in animal models, and patients who were culture-positive for such mutants often have thymidine kinase-positive HSV isolates in their next recurrence. Thus, the clinical significance and epidemiologic importance of these mutants in normal hosts remain to be established.

---

retention were reduced significantly. Although intravenous acyclovir may shorten the duration of viral shedding and duration of symptoms in recurrences, it is not recommended for the treatment of recurrent genital disease.

Oral acyclovir has therapeutic effects on both primary and recurrent HSV infection in adults. In a dosage of 200 mg five times per day for 5 to 10 days, oral acyclovir significantly reduced viral shedding and the formation of lesions, duration of lesions, and duration and severity of symptoms in primary infection. In similar studies of adult patients with recurrent genital HSV infection, oral acyclovir (200 mg five times per day for 5 days) decreased the duration of viral shedding, time to healing, and development of new lesions, especially when administered early in the recurrence.

In these studies, in which patients were cautioned regarding hydration, no significant side effects were noted. Neither oral nor intravenous acyclovir reduces the rate of recurrence when used to treat either primary or recurrent genital infection (see section, Chemoprophylaxis). Oral acyclovir, in various doses, appears to be the drug of choice for treating genital HSV infection (see Box 196.5).

Two second-generation oral agents are effective in treating genital HSV. Famciclovir is converted to penciclovir after absorption and is 70% to 80% bioavailable, with a longer intracellular half-life than that of acyclovir. Valacyclovir is converted to acyclovir after adsorption, with a 55% to 60% bioavailability. These bioavailabilities are compared to those of 15% to 20% for oral acyclovir. In clinical trials, less frequent doses of these two agents have been found effective and comparable to acyclovir in the therapy and suppression of genital herpes and herpes zoster infections in adults. Currently, they are licensed for therapy in herpetic recurrences and initial infection, and as suppressive therapy (see Box 196.5). Pharmacokinetic studies are being performed in children, but licensed guidelines currently are approved for adults only. Toxicity is minimal, as with acyclovir, although famciclovir has been carcinogenic in some animal studies. Because both agents must be converted to the phosphorylated compound (as is the case with acyclovir), HSV that resists acyclovir because of absent or altered thymidine kinase also will resist valacyclovir and, generally, famciclovir. The main convenience of these two new agents is the less frequent dosing needed, but therapy will be more expensive than with generic acyclovir.

Symptomatic therapy of HSV lesions should be directed toward reducing local discomfort, promoting healing, and preventing autoinoculation and superinfection. Nonspecific creams and ointments probably delay healing and increase the risk of developing maceration and infection. Keeping lesions clean and dry is an important local measure. Urination can be made less painful by urinating in a bathtub or sitz bath. Some experts advise sitz baths with Burow solution or short compress treatment. Prolonged soaking delays healing.

Herpes Simplex Virus Infection in Immunocompromised Hosts

Clinicians must make the difficult determination of how serious the manifestation in immunocompromised hosts must be before initiating therapy, a course that may require hospitalization.

Acyclovir ointment appears to decrease pain, viral shedding, and the time to complete healing of lesions in immunocompromised individuals with mild, non-life-threatening mucocutaneous HSV infection. However, for mild illness, it essentially has been rendered obsolete by oral acyclovir in children (see Box 196.5). Patients with more severe illness should be treated with the intravenous preparation in a hospital setting.

Intravenous acyclovir has been analyzed extensively in immunocompromised patients with mucocutaneous HSV infection. When used early, acyclovir arrests the progression of infection. It decreases the time to cessation of new lesions, the time to crusting of lesions, and the time to healing, and it induces a more rapid cessation of pain and termination of viral shedding. Intravenous acyclovir is the drug of choice for treating moderate or severe HSV in immunocompromised hosts. The dose is 250 mg/m^2 or 5 mg/kg/day every 8 hours infused over the course 1 hour. In more serious disease (e.g., dissemination to visceral organs or the CNS), this dose should be doubled, although no controlled studies exist to demonstrate improved efficacy using higher doses of acyclovir in immunocompromised hosts. The major toxicity has been renal, with a reversible obstructive nephropathy and transient rises in serum creatinine levels (5% to 10% of patients). Usually, adequate hydration prevents this problem. Table 196.2 lists guidelines for dosages in patients with impaired renal function. Less commonly (1%), reversible neurologic symptoms (lethargy, agitation, tremor, disorientation, coma, and transient hemiparesthesia) and laboratory abnormalities (abnormal EEG results, increased CSF myelin basic protein) have developed in patients with marrow transplants. Usually, these patients have received interferon and CNS chemoprophylaxis for leukemia. Other less serious problems include phlebitis (14%) and hives (5%).

Oral acyclovir in dosages of 200 mg five times per day effectively promotes lesion healing and inhibits viral shedding. It is useful in treating mild illness in immunocompromised children. Few guidelines are available for treating children with oral acyclovir, and currently it is not licensed for use in children. All studies to date using acyclovir in immunosuppressed patients have noted the marked propensity of these individuals to continue to have recurrences when therapy is withdrawn.

TABLE 196.2

DOSAGE OF INTRAVENOUS ACYCLOVIR FOR PATIENTS WITH RENAL INSUFFICIENCY

Creatine Clearance (mL/min/1.73 m^2)	Dose (mg/kg)	Dosing Interval (hr)
50	5.0	8
25–50	5.0	12
10–25	5.0	24
0–10	2.5	24

Reproduced with permission from Kohl S. Herpes simplex virus infection. In: Kaplan SL, ed. *Current therapy in pediatric infectious diseases*. Toronto: BC Decker, 1993:209.

Both valacyclovir and famciclovir are effective in the oral therapy of HSV disease in the immunocompromised patient, and at higher doses, both agents can achieve serum levels similar to that seen with intravenous acyclovir therapy. Valacyclovir has been used at doses as high as 2,000 mg four times a day in the therapy of cytomegalovirus infection. In one such study in adult patients with AIDS, the unexpected adverse effect of a hemolytic uremic syndrome was observed, but this effect has not been seen in all such clinical trials. Valacyclovir thus should be used with caution in the immunocompromised patient.

Three HSV mutations give rise to acyclovir resistance. They include altered viral DNA polymerase, altered thymidine kinase, and absent thymidine kinase. The overwhelming majority of significant clinical isolates of acyclovir-resistant viruses is due to absence of thymidine kinase. These isolates have occurred and resulted in acyclovir-unresponsive illness in immunocompromised children, who usually have been treated with chronic or recurrent courses of acyclovir. Usually, this outcome manifests as lesions that fail to heal and will worsen during the course of adequate acyclovir therapy. Although documentation of viral resistance is optimal, in the immunocompromised patient with documented HSV infection who fails to respond after 4 to 7 days of intravenous acyclovir therapy, resistance should be assumed, and alternate therapy must be considered. Foscarnet (120 mg/kg/day in three divided doses administered intravenously by slow infusion) was efficacious in a controlled trial in a small number of HIV-infected adult patients with acyclovir-resistant HSV infection. It is a relatively toxic drug causing nephrotoxicity, electrolyte imbalance, and bone marrow toxicity, and it must be used with caution. Currently, foscarnet is the agent of choice for treating acyclovir-resistant HSV infection in immunocompromised hosts. Intravenous and topical cidofovir have been shown to be useful in the treatment of thymidine kinase-negative HSV infection. Mutations in the viral polymerase renders the virus resistant to foscarnet and cidofovir.

PREVENTION

Environmental Control or Barrier Prevention

Because HSV is sensitive to heat, light, and lipid solvents, the use of antiseptics, soap and hot water, or chlorine decreases the risk of transferring the virus in such settings as the home, spas, pools, and hospitals. Wrestlers with skin lesions should be excluded from participation in practice or competition until herpes infection is ruled out. Medical and dental personnel who handle respiratory or oral secretions and administer oropharyngeal and tracheostomy care should wear gloves and wash carefully before and after working with patients and their secretions. Parents and caretakers of infants with eczema or severe diaper rash should be especially careful to avoid directly or indirectly contacting this altered skin with an active HSV lesion. Burn patients should be protected against exposure to or direct contact with personnel or visitors who have active HSV lesions. Immunosuppressed patients who develop evidence of HSV infection usually are manifesting evidence of reactivation of latent virus. Primary HSV infections in immunosuppressed individuals, as in neonates, may be especially severe, and protecting these susceptible patients against exposure to HSV lesions is important. Hospital personnel with uncovered active cold sores or herpetic whitlow should not care for immunosuppressed patients. Although no human data are available, *in vitro* experiments have shown that condoms retard the passage of viable HSV. (The use of cesarean section to prevent neonatal HSV is discussed in Chapter 78, Herpes Simplex Virus.)

Immunoprophylaxis

Agents such as bacille Calmette-Guérin, smallpox vaccine, and many other compounds have been used in attempts to affect herpetic recurrences. They have proved to be ineffective and, at times, dangerous. In early clinical trials, a subunit glycoprotein-D vaccine was shown to decrease significantly the rate of symptomatic genital infection (by 73%) in HSV-1 and HSV-2 seronegative women. Phase three trials are ongoing.

Chemoprophylaxis

Oral acyclovir administered long term markedly suppresses recurrences in immunodeficient patients. Oral or intravenous acyclovir used at times of maximum immunosuppression, such as in the first months after a patient has undergone organ transplantation or during periods of neutropenia in individuals receiving antineoplastic chemotherapy, nearly completely prevents the predictable rate of HSV recurrence in seropositive individuals. Oral acyclovir (400 mg given two times per day) administered long-term decreases recurrence of genital HSV by 50% to 70% in immunocompetent patients with frequent recurrences and reduces the frequency of HSV DNA detection by 80%. Breakthrough recurrences are mild. Similar effects are seen with the suppressive therapy of frequently recurrent oral disease in adults. When oral acyclovir is discontinued, HSV recurrences revert to pretreatment frequency. Thus, oral acyclovir suppresses recurrences without curing the latent infection. Side effects are limited to mild gastrointestinal irritation. Similar results are seen using less frequent dosing with oral famciclovir (250 mg twice a day and valacyclovir (500 to 1,000 mg once a day).

Suggested Readings

Belongia EA, Goodman JL, Holland EJ, et al. An outbreak of herpes gladiatorum at a high school wrestling camp. *N Engl J Med* 1991;325:906.

Cherpes TL, Meyn LA, Krohn MA, et al. Association between acquisition of herpes simplex virus type 2 in women and bacterial vaginosis. *Clin Infect Dis* 2003;37:319.

Domingues RB, Tsanaclis AM, Pannuti CS, et al. Evaluation of the range of clinical presentation of herpes simplex encephalitis by using polymerase chain reaction assay of cerebrospinal fluid samples. *Clin Infect Dis* 1997;25:86.

Fleming DT, McQuillan GM, Johnson RE, et al. Herpes simplex virus type 2 in the United States, 1976 to 1994. *N Engl J Med* 1997;337:1105.

Frenck RW, Kohl S. Herpes simplex virus in the immunocompromised child. In: Patrick CC, ed. *Infections in immunocompromised infants and children*. New York: Churchill Livingstone, 1992:603.

Ito Y, Kimura H, Yabuta Y, et al. Exacerbation of herpes simplex encephalitis after successful treatment with acyclovir. *Clin Infect Dis* 2000;30:185.

Kohl S. Herpes simplex encephalitis. *Pediatr Clin North Am* 1988;35:465.

Kohl S. Postnatal herpes simplex virus infection. In: Feigin RD, Cherry JD, eds. *Textbook of pediatric infectious diseases*, 4th ed. Philadelphia: Saunders, 1998:1703.

Lakeman FD, Whitley RJ. Diagnosis of herpes simplex encephalitis: application of polymerase chain reaction to cerebrospinal fluid from brain-biopsied patients and correlation with disease. *J Infect Dis* 1995;171:857.

Mertz G, Loveless MO, Levin MJ, et al. Oral famciclovir for suppression of recurrent genital herpes simplex virus infection in women. A multicenter, double-blind, placebo-controlled trial. *Arch Intern Med* 1997;157:343.

Patel R, Bodsworth NJ, Wooley P, et al. Valacyclovir for the suppression of recurrent genital HSV infection: a placebo controlled study of once-daily therapy. International Valacyclovir HSV Study Group. *Genitourin Med* 1997;72:105.

Safrin S, Crumpacker C, Chatis P, et al. A controlled trial comparing foscarnet with vidarabine for acyclovir-resistant mucocutaneous herpes simplex in the acquired immunodeficiency syndrome. *N Engl J Med* 1991;325:551.

Stanberry LR, Spruance SL, Cunninghan AL, et al. Glycoprotein-D-ajuvant vaccine to prevent genital herpes. *N Engl J Med* 2002;347:1652.

Tyring SK, Baker D, Snowden W. Valacyclovir for herpes simplex virus infection: long-term safety and sustained efficacy after 20 years' experience with acyclovir. *J Infect Dis* 2002;186:S40.

Weston WL, Brice SL, Jester JD, et al. Herpes simplex virus in childhood erythema multiforme. *Pediatrics* 1992;89:32.

Whitley RJ, Cobbs CG, Alford CA, et al. Diseases that mimic herpes simplex encephalitis diagnosis, presentation and outcome. *JAMA* 1989;262:234.

CHAPTER 197 ■ HUMAN HERPESVIRUS TYPE 6

JULIA A. MCMILLAN AND CHARLES F. GROSE

Human herpesvirus type 6 (HHV-6) was first isolated in 1986 from the white blood cells of adult patients with lymphoproliferative disorders and human immunodeficiency virus (HIV) infection. Its morphologic similarity to other known members of the family of human herpesviruses (herpes simplex viruses types 1 and 2, varicella-zoster virus, cytomegalovirus, and Epstein-Barr virus), include its lipid envelope, icosahedral symmetry, and large nucleocapsid (162 capsomeres). The double-stranded DNA of HHV-6 is most similar to that of human herpesvirus-7 but it shares significant homology and genome organization with cytomegalovirus (CMV) as well. Two variants of HHV-6 have been designated (variant A and variant B). HHV-6 primarily infects T lymphocytes (CD4$^+$/CD8$^-$). The A and B variants of HHV-6 can be distinguished by monoclonal antibody and by growth characteristics *in vitro*.

EPIDEMIOLOGY

HHV-6 is transmitted through saliva and is acquired early in life, most frequently from close household contacts. Maternal antibody protects most infants from infection during their first few months of life, but 95% of children throughout the world become infected by 18 months. Virtually all infection in infants is due to the B variant. Latent virus persists throughout life in lymphocytes and monocytes and at low levels in various tissues. The virus is reactivated and intermittently shed in saliva, unaccompanied by symptoms, in healthy children and adults.

The A variant has been identified during reactivation in older individuals (including children) whose cellular immunity is compromised following bone marrow and organ transplantation.

PATHOGENESIS

Primary infection with HHV-6 is associated with antibody production and the presence of virus in peripheral blood mononuclear cells. The virus primarily infects CD4$^+$ T lymphocytes, resulting in apoptosis and cytokine release. Protection from infection during the first few months of life is presumably due to passively transmitted maternal antibody. Susceptibility to dissemination during suppression of cellular immunity (as occurs following bone marrow and organ transplantation) suggests that control of reactivation is largely a function of cell-mediated immune function.

In vitro studies of HHV-6 infection of T-lymphocytes indicate that the virus has an immunosuppressive effect, reducing cytokine production and lymphoproliferation.

CLINICAL MANIFESTATIONS AND COMPLICATIONS

Primary HHV-6 infection usually is unrecognized or results in mild symptoms. Isolation of HHV-6 from peripheral blood mononuclear cells concomitant with a rise in antibody against HHV-6 was reported in 10% to 15% of children younger than 2 years presenting with fever to a pediatric emergency center. Rash was observed in only a minority of these children, but many of them had otitis media. HHV-6 infection has been documented also during illness associated with rash but no fever. Other findings described in infants with primary HHV-6 infection include pharyngitis, otitis media, diarrhea, pneumonia, hepatomegaly, hepatocellular dysfunction, intussusception, and febrile seizures. Complete recovery from infection in these patients has been the rule.

Roseola

Japanese investigators discovered the link between HHV-6 and roseola in 1988. The percentage of children whose primary HHV-6 infection manifests as roseola is not known, but studies in the United States and elsewhere indicate that the clinical syndrome recognized as roseola affects only a minority. It is now recognized that both HHV-6 and HHV-7 can cause the clinical constellation that results in a clinical diagnosis of roseola.

As early as 1870, the mild illness now called *roseola infantum* or *exanthema subitum* was recognized and described as being distinct from other exanthematous diseases of childhood. Typically, roseola affects infants and young children between the ages of 6 months and 3 years, with 80% of the cases occurring before age 18 months. Initial fever may reach 40.0°C to 40.5°C (104°F to 105°F), has an abrupt onset, and typically persists, either continuously or intermittently, for 3 to 4 days. During this febrile period, affected infants or children usually maintain near-normal appetite and behavior, although they may exhibit periods of irritability during times of increased fever.

Physical examination during this preeruptive phase yields few findings to distinguish roseola from other, more worrisome illnesses. Sometimes, palpebral edema is described, and careful examination usually reveals suboccipital lymphadenopathy. Mild erythema of the pharynx may be seen in approximately one-third of affected patients. Sometimes, a bulging or tense fontanelle is noted in young infants with roseola. The beginning of febrile illness may trigger a brief, slight elevation in the white blood cell count, with a predominance of neutrophils. During the bulk of the febrile period, however, the white blood cell count typically falls to 3,000 to 5,000 cells per millimeter, with a relative lymphocytosis.

Usually, the rash of roseola coincides with abrupt termination of the febrile period. Typically, the rash is pale pink (rose) with discrete macules or, less commonly, maculopapules, predominantly on the neck and trunk. Most often, the rash persists for 1 to 2 days, but it may last only a few hours (Fig. 197.1). Pruritus and desquamation are not seen.

The rapidity of the initial temperature elevation is cited as the reason for the frequent association between febrile seizures and roseola. Encephalitis and transient hemiparesis have been reported in young infants with a febrile illness, followed by a

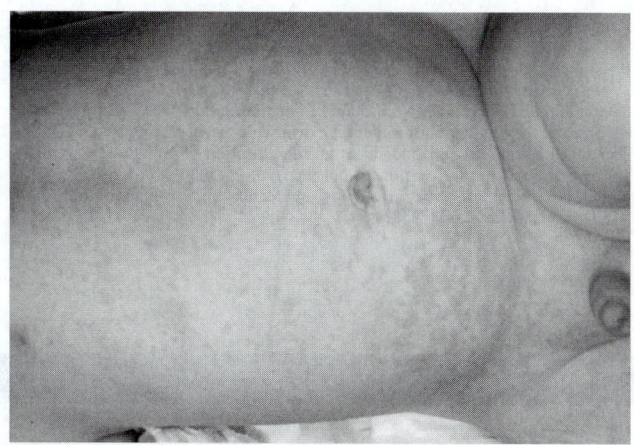

FIGURE 197.1. Roseola (Courtesy of Bernard A. Cohen, http://dermatlas.org.) (Reprinted with permission from Goodheart HP. *Goodheart's photoguide of common skin disorders: diagnosis and management.* Philadelphia: Lippincott Williams & Wilkins, 2003: 187.) See Color Figure 197.1 in color section.

rash characteristic of roseola. The young age of patients with roseola, combined with their high fever and occasional bulging fontanelle, often suggests the possibility of bacterial infection, including meningitis. Laboratory investigation and hospitalization for treatment with intravenous antibiotics may be undertaken while serious infection is being investigated.

Other Disorders

HHV-6 can be detected in saliva and in peripheral blood mononuclear cells in about 90% of the world's population. Asymptomatic shedding of virus from salivary glands of parents and other close contacts is likely the source of infection in infants and young children. Viral reactivation and shedding are almost always asymptomatic. Anecdotal reports of disease associated with reactivation of HHV-6 in immunocompetent individuals, however, include mononucleosis-like syndrome, fulminant hepatitides, lymphadenopathy, and encephalitis. Efforts to implicate HHV-6 as a cause or co-factor in multiple sclerosis and chronic fatigue syndrome have been inconclusive.

Infection in Immunocompromised Individuals

It has been difficult to determine the importance of reactivation of, or reinfection with, HHV-6 among immunocompromised patients. Aggressive immunosuppressive regimens, particularly following hematopoietic and solid organ transplantation, are known to result in reactivation of latent herpesvirus infections, including HHV-6, in some individuals. The frequency of reactivation detected depends upon the type of graft, the type of immunosuppression used, and the laboratory studies employed to detect reactivation. Reactivation appears to be more frequent among recipients of hematopoietic cell transplants (about 50%) than following solid organ transplantation (approximately 20% to 30%). Some studies suggest that reactivation of HHV-6 following transplantation may be less frequent among pediatric transplant recipients, compared to adults. In addition to reactivation, donor tissue may harbor latent virus as well, permitting reinfection of the recipient. It has been impossible to distinguish reliably the clinical consequences of reactivation and reinfection from those due to transplant rejection, intercurrent infection due to a variety of

other agents, and reactivation and infection due to other herpesviruses. Some evidence suggests that CMV and HHV-6 act synergistically to produce a variety of clinical manifestations. Clinical features that have been associated with HHV-6 following bone marrow and solid organ transplantation include fever, encephalitis/encephalopathy, bone marrow suppression, rash, hepatitis, thrombotic microangiopathy, interstitial pneumonitis, engraftment failure, and graft rejection.

HHV-6 appears to promote the replication of HIV *in vitro*, an observation that has led to investigation of a possible role for HHV-6 infection or reactivation in AIDS progression. To date, no substantiation of these suspicions has been observed in clinical studies. HHV-6 infection and reactivation has, however, been implicated as a cause of end-organ complications among patients with AIDS, including CNS infections, pneumonitis, and retinitis.

DIAGNOSIS

During the symptomatic phase of primary HHV-6 infection the white blood cell (WBC) count, particularly the lymphocyte count, is usually below normal for age. Cerebrospinal fluid (CSF) findings usually are normal in infants and children who undergo lumbar puncture because of seizures, encephalopathy, or as part of an evaluation for suspected bacterial infection.

Primary HHV-6 infection is confirmed when conversion occurs from seronegativity to seropositivity in association with detection of HHV-6 by culture or polymerase chain reaction (PCR) from peripheral blood mononuclear cells. Detection of a fourfold increase in IgG antibody titer alone does not indicate new infection, because periods of increased IgG antibody concentrations occur with asymptomatic reactivation of latent infection. In addition, the indirect immunofluorescence assay commonly used to measure HHV-6 antibody does not consistently distinguish between HHV-6 and HHV-7 antibodies. HHV-6 can be detected in peripheral blood cells and tissues in healthy, latently infected individuals, limiting the accuracy of this technique in linking clinical illness to HHV-6 infection. Studies in transplant recipients have indicated that the detection of HHV-6 genome in cell-free plasma using PCR, and quantitative assessment of HHV-6 DNA using the Taq-Man system, may be useful in detecting increased activity of HHV-6 and linking symptoms to the effects of the virus. These techniques are not widely available, however.

THERAPY

Most cases of HHV-6 infection are either unrecognized or only moderately symptomatic (clinical roseola) and, therefore, need no specific antiviral treatment. Antipyretic medication (acetaminophen) may be indicated for the amelioration of high fever. In a few instances, such as severe HHV-6 hepatitis, antiviral treatment is a consideration. HHV-6 replication is inhibited *in vitro* by both ganciclovir and foscarnet, but is not affected significantly by acyclovir. However, it should be noted that ganciclovir and foscarnet are not approved by the U.S. Food and Drug Administration to treat HHV-6 infection in humans.

Suggested Readings

Caserta MT, Mock DJ, and Dewhurst S. Human herpesvirus 6. *Clin Infect Dis* 2001;33:829.

Feldstein AE, Razonable RR, Boyce TG, et al. Prevalence and clinical significance of human herpesviruses 6 and 7 active infection in pediatric liver transplant patients. *Pediatr Transplantation* 2003;7:125.

Grose C. Childhood infections with human herpesviruses types 6, 7, and 8. *Adv Pediatr Infect Dis* 1997;12:181.

Hall CB, Caserta MT, Schnabel KC. Persistence of human herpesvirus 6 according to site and variant: possible greater neurotropism of variant A. *Clin Infect Dis* 1998;26:132.

Hall CB, Long CE, Schnabel KC, et al. Human herpesvirus-6 infection in children: a prospective study of complications and reactivation. *N Engl J Med* 1994;331:432.

Huang LM, Lee CY, Lin KH, et al. Human herpesvirus-6 associated with fatal haemophagocytic syndrome. *Lancet* 1990;336:60.

Kempe CH, Shaw EB, Jackson JR, et al. Studies on the etiology of exanthema subitum (roseola infantum). *J Pediatr* 1950;37:561.

Pruksananonda P, Hall CB, Insel RA, et al. Primary human herpesvirus 6 infection in young children. *N Engl J Med* 1992;326:1445.

Salahuddin SZ, Ablashi DV, Markham PD, et al. Isolation of a new virus, HBLV, in patients with lymphoproliferative disorders. *Science* 1986;234:596.

Yamanishi K, Shiraki K, Konda T, et al. Identification of human herpesvirus 6 as a causal agent for exanthem subitum. *Lancet* 1988;1:1065.

Yoshikawa T. Human herpesvirus-6 and -7 infections in transplantation. *Pediatr Transplantation* 2003;7:11.

CHAPTER 198 ■ HUMAN HERPESVIRUS TYPES 7 AND 8

CHARLES F. GROSE

HUMAN HERPESVIRUS TYPE 7

In 1990, the discovery of a new herpesvirus was reported. Human herpesvirus (HHV) type 7 was isolated from the peripheral blood lymphocytes of a healthy individual. The DNA of HHV-7 has been characterized extensively and was found to be distinct from previously known herpesviruses. Despite some DNA sequence homology with human herpesvirus type 6—the agent that causes roseola—HHV-7 now is considered to be sufficiently different to merit classification as a separate herpesvirus.

Epidemiology

In a series of seroepidemiologic studies, seroconversion to HHV-7 was observed in children who were already HHV-6-seropositive. Therefore, prior infection with HHV-6 did not protect against subsequent infection with HHV-7. In an analysis of a large number of serum samples, most children older than 2 years were immune to HHV-6 (as expected), but a majority of 2-year-old children had no HHV-7 antibody. These children seroconverted to HHV-7 over the next 3 to 5 years. Currently, HHV-7 diagnostic testing is performed mainly in individual herpesvirus research laboratories.

Clinical Manifestations and Complications

Usually, the disease caused by HHV-7 infection is not apparent, although HHV-7 seroconversion sometimes leads to a syndrome similar to roseola. HHV-7 frequently can be isolated from the saliva of healthy adults around the world. Transmission of HHV-7 has been documented clearly in multigenerational families living in the same household.

Transmission does not occur at parturition. However, nearly 100% of older children exhibit evidence of prior HHV-7 infection, as demonstrated by virus isolation from saliva. The percentage of children who acquire HHV-7 from their mothers is approximately 50%; those who acquire the disorder from their fathers, approximately 25%; and those who acquire the disease from other individuals, approximately 25% (Fig. 198.1).

HUMAN HERPESVIRUS TYPE 8 (KAPOSI SARCOMA HERPESVIRUS)

Yet another human herpesvirus was discovered in 1994. Scientists first detected the viral genome in samples of Kaposi

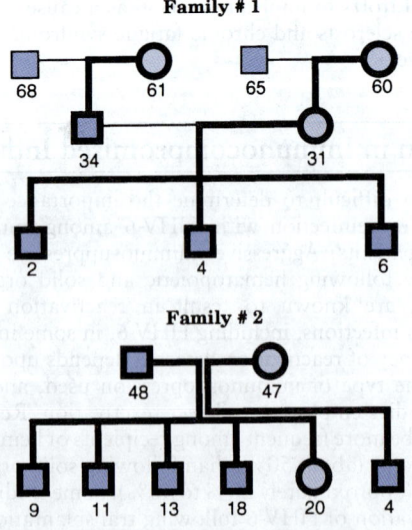

FIGURE 198.1. Transmission of human herpesvirus type 7 (HHV-7) through large multigenerational families. HHV-7 is transmitted from either father (grandfather) or mother (grandmother) to children by inadvertent exchange of saliva. Dark lines indicate route of transmission of the same HHV-7 strain between family members.

sarcoma tissues, using a technique called *representational difference analysis* to identify and characterize unique DNA sequences that are absent in nondiseased tissue obtained from the same patients. The viral DNA sequences are most similar to a simian herpesvirus called *herpesvirus saimiri* but also resemble portions of the Epstein-Barr virus genome. The viral genome sequence is designated *KSHV* or *HHV-8*.

Epidemiology

HHV-8 DNA sequences have been found in nearly all biopsies obtained from adults with Kaposi sarcoma, regardless of whether such patients also are infected with the human immunodeficiency virus (HIV). In Africa, where concomitant infection with HIV and KSHV is more common, Kaposi sarcoma occurs in children during their first 2 years of life. However, HHV-8 sequences have not been detected in a large number of other malignancies, including diffuse large cell lymphoma, non-Burkitt lymphoma, chronic lymphocytic leukemia, acute lymphocytic leukemia, acute nonlymphocytic leukemia, and Hodgkin disease.

Important questions about when children or adults contract their primary HHV-8 infection and about the modes of transmission are under active investigation. Enormous geographic differences exist in incidence rates. In studies of healthy adult blood donors in the United States, from 3% to 4% are positive for KSHV antibody. Almost no children in the United States or Europe are antibody positive. In contrast, in countries in central Africa, as well as Egypt, HHV-8 seroprevalence is 10% or more in late childhood and over 40% by adulthood. No differences are seen between males and females. These facts suggest an acquisition in childhood by nonsexual means. The most likely explanation is virus in saliva. This possibility is strengthened by

a report that KSHV can replicate in oral epithelial cells. Thus, sloughed cells containing the KSHV genome, in the mouth of a seropositive person, can carry the virus to a seronegative person after exchange of saliva.

Clinical Manifestations and Complications

Immunocompetent children may manifest a febrile maculopapular rash during primary infection, but then have no apparent sequelae until decades later. A recently discovered but rare complication is hemophagocytic lymphohistiocytosis in infants. Further studies are required to determine the conditions favoring the transmission of KSHV infectivity in different geographic areas, the complete disease syndrome in healthy children, as well as the long-term consequences of KSHV infection (other than Kaposi sarcoma).

Suggested Readings

Andreoni M, Sarmati L, Nicastri E, et al. Primary human herpes 8 infection in immunocompetent children. *JAMA* 2002;287:1295.

Chang Y, Cesarman E, Pessin MS, et al. Identification of herpesvirus-like DNA sequences in AIDS-associated Kaposi's sarcoma. *Science* 1994;266:1865.

Duus KM, Wagenaar T, Grose C, et al. Tropism of wild type KSHV isolated from the oropharynx of immune competent individuals for cultured oral epithelial cells. *J Virol* 2004;78:4074.

Grossman WJ, Radhi M, Schauer D. et al. Development of hemophagocytic lymphohistiocytosis in triplets infected with HHV-8. *Blood* 2005;106:1203.

Serrano D, Toma L, Andreoni M, et al. A seroprevalence study of human herpesvirus type 8 in eastern and central Africa and in the Mediterranean area. *Eur J Epidemiol* 2001;17:871.

Takahashi Y, Yamada M, Nakamura J, et al. Transmission of HHV-7 through multigenerational families in the same household. *Pediatr Infect Dis J* 1997;16:975.

CHAPTER 199 ■ VARICELLA-ZOSTER VIRUS INFECTIONS

CHARLES F. GROSE

Chickenpox is the common childhood exanthem caused by the human herpesvirus varicella-zoster virus (VZV). Before varicella vaccine was recommended for all susceptible children in 1995, most children acquired chickenpox during early school years, thereby developing lifelong immunity. However, approximately 10% of young adults are susceptible to primary VZV infection because they did not contract chickenpox as children and have not received varicella vaccine. After a person recovers from chickenpox, the virus remains in a latent state in the dorsal root ganglion cells for decades. As immunity wanes in late adulthood, occasionally the virus reactivates and causes the dermatomal exanthem known as *shingles* or *zoster*. Zoster also occurs in some children who have had chickenpox, often in association with treatment with immunosuppressive chemotherapy and irradiation for acquired disease (e.g., leukemia and lymphoma).

THE VIRUS AND ITS PATHOGENESIS

VZV is one of the eight known human herpesviruses. The other seven are herpes simplex type 1 (oral) and type 2 (genital), cytomegalovirus, Epstein-Barr virus, and the newly discovered human herpesviruses types 6, 7, and 8. The route by which primary VZV infection causes disease is illustrated in the schema for pathogenesis (Fig. 199.1). The interval between infection

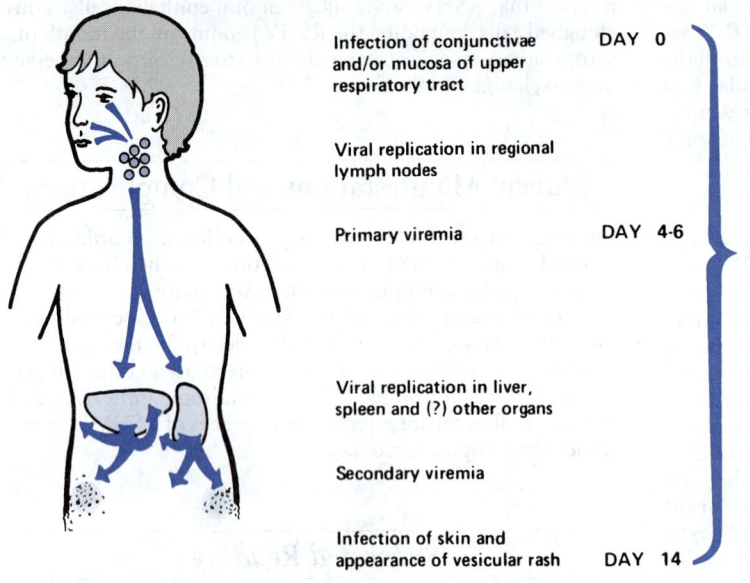

Infection of conjunctivae and/or mucosa of upper respiratory tract — **DAY 0**

Viral replication in regional lymph nodes

Primary viremia — **DAY 4-6**

Viral replication in liver, spleen and (?) other organs

Secondary viremia

Infection of skin and appearance of vesicular rash — **DAY 14**

INCUBATION PERIOD

FIGURE 199.1. The pathogenesis of chickenpox. Primary infection with varicella-zoster virus occurs when virus-laden water droplets contact the respiratory mucosa or conjunctivae of a susceptible host. The pathogenesis most likely includes a biphasic course with primary and secondary viremia followed by the typical vesicular exanthem of chickenpox. Based on this schema, varicella-zoster immune globulin must be given before primary viremia to prevent chickenpox in the exposed host. (Reprinted from Grose C. Varicella-zoster virus infections: chickenpox [varicella], shingles [zoster], and varicella vaccine. In: Glaser R, ed. *Human herpesvirus infections*. New York: Marcel Dekker, 1994:117.)

and appearance of the vesicular rash (incubation period) usually is 14 to 15 days, with a range of 10 to 20 days. The initial site of infection is the conjunctivae or upper respiratory tract. Then the virus replicates at a local site in the head or neck for approximately 4 to 6 days. Thereafter, the virus is transmitted throughout the body during the primary viremia. After a second cycle of replication, the virus is released in larger amounts 1 week later (secondary viremia) and quickly invades the cutaneous tissues. As the virus exits the capillaries and enters the epidermis, characteristic vesicles of chickenpox appear on the skin.

The entire VZV genome was sequenced in 1986. For some time, VZV was thought to be an identical virus around the world. However, in 1998 and 2002, two mutant viruses were discovered, one in Minneapolis, Minnesota, and the second in Vancouver, Canada. Whether these viruses will spread more widely is unknown.

EPIDEMIOLOGY

Chickenpox is transmitted by virus in water droplets carried by air currents from infected children to susceptible individuals. Epidemiologic observation studies document that children in the late incubation period may be infectious 1 or 2 days before the appearance of the exanthem. They remain infectious through the first few days of the rash but probably no longer than the sixth day. Affected children can return to school when lesions have become encrusted. Susceptible children can also contract chickenpox from elderly persons with zoster, although the period of contagion appears to be much shorter.

In most communities in North America, Japan, and Europe, outbreaks of chickenpox occur annually from January to May. The fewest cases occur in August and September. The periodicity of chickenpox derives from bringing susceptible children together in school every autumn. The epidemiology pattern in the United States is changing because of the introduction of varicella vaccination programs in 1995. However, chickenpox will continue to be seen in North America in the foreseeable future because neither Canada nor Mexico has a national varicella immunization program. Moreover, varicella immunization will not be given in most countries of South America, Africa, or Asia (except Japan).

CLINICAL FEATURES OF CHICKENPOX

The characteristic feature of chickenpox is the vesicle. In healthy children, the exanthem develops over 3 to 6 days, usually beginning along the hairline on the face. Each lesion begins as a macule that progresses to papule and vesicle, then to a crusted vesicle. Subsequently, the rash emerges in successive crops over the trunk, then the extremities. Lesions in different stages of development are present throughout the first week. The rash is more confluent wherever the skin has been abraded previously, such as the diaper area.

The typical course of chickenpox is documented meticulously in U.S. children. Usually, the prodrome is mild, with malaise and low-grade fever. Once the pox lesions appear, the temperature rises, but rarely to more than 102°F. The average number of skin lesions ranges between 200 and 300 in the index case within a family. Secondary cases may have a more severe course, with up to 500 or more pox lesions, presumably because such patients receive a larger inoculum of virus from infected siblings. By the end of the first week, infected children again are afebrile, and the cutaneous lesions continue to form crusts that dry and fall off. Infants younger than 1 year may have more severe disease; likewise, older teenagers and adults are at greater risk when they develop chickenpox. The mortality for chickenpox in otherwise healthy children (ages 1 through 14 years) is approximately 1 in 50,000, whereas that for infants younger than 1 year is 1 in 13,000. One subgroup at highest risk for fulminant chickenpox is children receiving high-dose corticosteroid therapy for such diseases as asthma.

The most frequent complication of chickenpox in a healthy child is bacterial infection of a vesicular lesion (Box 199.1). The most common infecting organism is group A *Streptococcus*, although staphylococcal infections also occur. Secondary diseases range from cellulitis and erysipelas to cutaneous abscesses, impetigo, and suppurative lymphadenitis. More serious, but less common, bacterial sequelae include septic arthritis and osteomyelitis, streptococcal necrotizing fasciitis, and staphylococcal pyomyositis.

The viral sequelae of chickenpox can involve virtually all organ systems and can include pneumonitis, hepatitis, arthritis, pericarditis, glomerulonephritis, orchitis, and involvement of

Complications of Chickenpox

Bacterial
Cellulitis
Erysipelas
Cutaneous abscess
Impetigo
Suppurative lymphadenitis
Septic arthritis
Osteomyelitis
Necrotizing fasciitis
Pyomyositis

Viral
Pneumonitis
Hepatitis
Arthritis
Cerebellar syndrome
Pericarditis
Glomerulonephritis
Orchitis
Meningoencephalitis
Myelitis
Polyneuritis

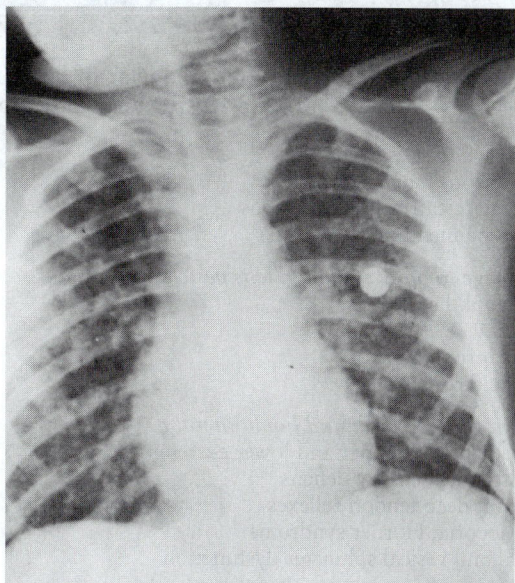

FIGURE 199.2. Varicella pneumonitis in a boy with leukemia and chickenpox. Symptoms include cough, dyspnea, tachypnea, and chest pain. Initial roentgenographic findings include peribronchial nodular infiltrates that may extend throughout the lung. Because varicella pneumonitis is a medical emergency, the patient should be admitted for intensive respiratory care as well as administration of antiviral chemotherapy.

the nervous system. Neurologic manifestations include meningoencephalitis, myelitis, and polyneuritis. In particular, the acute cerebellar syndrome is the most common VZV-induced neurologic disease in children. Usually, ataxia begins during the second week of the illness, but it can precede the exanthem. Often, cerebellar signs and symptoms persist for several weeks but resolve with no permanent neurologic deficits. The preferred method for diagnosis of viral cerebellitis is magnetic resonance imaging, which can detect abnormal signals within the cerebellum better than can computed tomography. Eye findings include unequal pupil size (anisocoria). Chickenpox also is associated temporally with Reye syndrome.

CHICKENPOX ASSOCIATED WITH CANCER AND IMMUNODEFICIENCY SYNDROME

Although chickenpox is a relatively benign condition in otherwise healthy children, VZV infection often is life-threatening when it occurs in children who are immunocompromised or immunosuppressed. The most relevant data about VZV-related morbidity and mortality were gathered before the development of effective antiviral agents. In children who had leukemia or lymphoma and who were receiving anticancer chemotherapy, chickenpox was a more prolonged disease. New lesion formation lasted an average of 9 days (range, 5 to 14 days) rather than 3 to 7 days. Visceral dissemination was apparent in one-third of the children, and approximately 8% of the children died. Often, this severe form of VZV infection is called *progressive chickenpox*. Almost every child who died had varicella pneumonitis (Fig. 199.2), which sometimes was associated with hepatitis and encephalitis. The only identifiable risk factor for VZV dissemination was a total lymphocyte count of less than 500 cells/mm^3 on the first day of exanthem. Children in such a risk group should be treated immediately with acyclovir (see

the later discussion of treatment). Progressive chickenpox has also occurred in children who have received gene replacement therapy for inherited immunodeficiencies.

The variable outcome of chickenpox in children infected with human immunodeficiency virus (HIV) depends on the immunologic status of the patient. In HIV-seropositive children without symptoms of acquired immunodeficiency syndrome (AIDS), chickenpox usually follows its typical course. In children with very low CD4 lymphocyte counts and AIDS, chickenpox may become a progressive disease, as described in children with leukemia. Most HIV-seropositive children should be considered in the higher risk category, and prevention with immune globulin or treatment with acyclovir should be undertaken (see later).

CONGENITAL VARICELLA INFECTION

Chickenpox in pregnant women can lead to intrauterine infection with embryopathy, especially during the first 20 weeks of gestation. The sequelae of VZV infection of the fetus involve mainly ectodermal derivatives and appear to be the consequence of viral destruction within the cervical and lumbosacral plexus and the brain. The most common deformities are hypoplasia and paresis of one of the extremities, together with cicatricial scarring over the skin on the involved limb. A more detailed enumeration of fetal embryopathy is included in Box 199.2. Documenting the diagnosis of congenital varicella syndrome other than by clinical examination is difficult because usually infants do not excrete virus, and the VZV-specific immunoglobulin M response is short-lived postnatally. The risk of fetopathy in pregnant women with chickenpox is less than 3% by most surveys. Infants born to women with gestational chickenpox, who have a normal newborn examination, do not develop virus-related sequelae later in childhood.

BOX 199.2	Neurologic Sequelae of Fetal Varicella-Zoster Virus Infection

Damage to sensory nerves
Cutaneous manifestations
Zigzag (cicatricial) skin lesions
Hypopigmentation

Damage to optic stalk and lens vesicle
Microphthalmia
Cataracts
Chorioretinitis
Optic atrophy

Damage to cervical and lumbosacral cord
Hypoplasia of upper and lower extremities
Motor and sensory deficits
Absent deep tendon reflexes
Anisocoria, Horner syndrome
Anal and vesical sphincter dysfunction

Damage to brain, encephalitis
Microcephaly
Hydrocephaly
Calcifications
Aplasia of brain

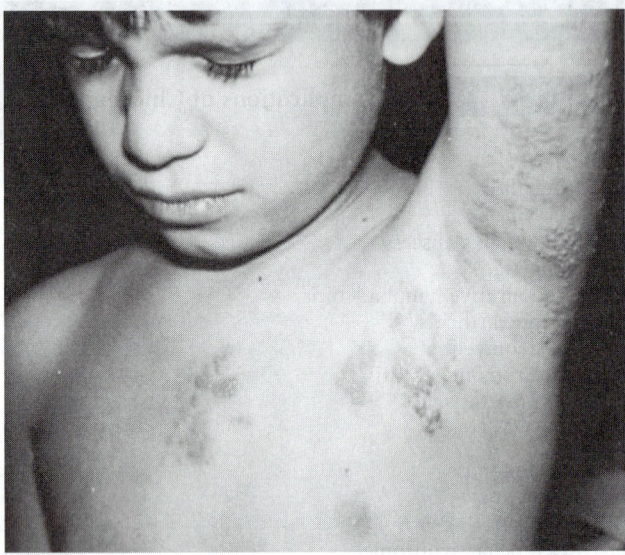

FIGURE 199.3. Zoster (shingles) in a child. The patient was receiving chemotherapy for treatment of leukemia when zoster was observed in the left first/second thoracic dermatome. The child had a history of chickenpox 3 years before the onset of cancer. (Reprinted from Grose C. Varicella-zoster virus infections: chickenpox [varicella], shingles [zoster], and varicella vaccine. In: Glaser R, ed. *Human herpesvirus infections*. New York: Marcel Dekker, 1994:117.)

ZOSTER (SHINGLES)

Zoster is the dermatomal exanthem that occurs when VZV reactivates from its site of latency and travels down a sensory nerve to the skin. Zoster is unusual in children. The estimated annual rate is approximately 1 case per 1,000 children between ages 1 and 19 years. The younger the child at the time of chickenpox (especially when younger than 2 years), the more likely it is that the child will develop zoster later in childhood. Zoster in younger children often occurs in dermatomes supplying the arms and legs.

As discussed, zoster occurs more often in immunocompromised children (Fig. 199.3). The incidence in children with leukemia and lymphoma (who have had chickenpox before diagnosis of malignancy) is approximately 20 cases per 1,000 per year, which is higher even than the rate in the elderly (6 to 8 cases per 1,000 per year). Zoster rarely is a life-threatening illness in such children. However, the morbidity is appreciable and includes extensive keloid formation, which is both unsightly and deforming when it affects an extremity. Therefore, all immunocompromised children with shingles should be treated promptly with acyclovir (see later).

DIAGNOSIS

Because of the characteristic vesicular rash, diagnosis of chickenpox usually can be made on physical examination. In certain cases, the rash can be confused with herpes simplex virus infection or other skin conditions, particularly when few vesicles are evident. Likewise, when zoster occurs in unusual locations, the diagnosis is not always apparent. In the past, the virus was identified by obtaining samples of the vesicle fluid for inoculation in cell culture, in which cytopathic effect usually is observable 3 to 7 days later. Currently, VZV infection is usually diagnosed within 2 to 3 hours by a rapid antigen detection technique. For this test, cells from the base of a vesicle are dried on a glass slide before being probed with a fluorescein-conjugated, VZV-

specific monoclonal antibody. The Tzanck smear is less specific and rarely is required. Past infection can be documented by persistence of anti-VZV antibody. However, children who are immunized with varicella vaccine may develop only low levels of antibody not detectable by commercial antibody kits available in most clinical virology diagnostic laboratories. Under these circumstances, a negative antibody titer does not indicate vaccine failure.

PREVENTION USING IMMUNE GLOBULIN

Chickenpox in healthy children rarely is a serious disease. Low-grade fever can be treated with acetaminophen. Aspirin should be avoided in children with chickenpox because of its link with Reye syndrome. For relief of itching, calamine lotion can be applied liberally to the skin. More severe pruritus, especially at night, may be ameliorated by giving diphenhydramine (Benadryl) elixir. Most children with chickenpox do not need to be seen by a physician unless they develop symptoms and signs of bacterial skin infection or one of the aforementioned viral complications.

The approach to exposed children receiving corticosteroids or chemotherapy for cancer or AIDS is much more emergent. If such children are known to be susceptible to VZV infection, varicella-zoster immune globulin (VZIG) should be administered in attempt to prevent or ameliorate infection. Other exposed patients for whom prevention of varicella using VZIG is recommended include the newborn whose mother developed chickenpox within 5 days before delivery or 48 hours after delivery, hospitalized premature infants 28 weeks' gestation or more whose mother lacks a reliable history of chickenpox, and hospitalized premature infants less than 28 weeks' gestation or up to 1,000 grams birth weight, regardless of maternal history. VZIG must be administered by intramuscular injection within 3 to 4 days after exposure to chickenpox (i.e., during the early incubation period before the virus has spread throughout the body; see Fig. 199.1). The dose of VZIG is one vial (approximately 1.25 mL) for each 20 pounds of body weight; the maximum dose is five vials of VZIG. It is anticipated that VZIG may no longer be available in the near future. Recommendation for use of intravenous immune globulin (IGIV) instead of VZIG have been made, but the efficacy of IGIV in preventing or ameliorating varicella has not been studied.

TREATMENT

If VZV-susceptible patients are beyond the fourth day after exposure, no beneficial effect derives from passive immunization with gamma globulin. Therefore, attending physicians must wait until chickenpox manifests itself and then should treat affected patients with acyclovir (Zovirax). Acyclovir is approved as both an intravenous and an oral formulation for the treatment of chickenpox. Intravenous acyclovir is administered to high-risk children at a dose of 500 mg/m^2 every 8 hours (total daily dose, 1,500 mg/m^2), usually for 7 days. The only serious side effect of acyclovir therapy is renal insufficiency. Therefore, serum creatinine levels should be monitored every 2 to 3 days.

An oral formulation of acyclovir is approved by the U.S. Food and Drug Administration for treatment of chickenpox in immunologically normal children. This recommendation was based on U.S. studies in which acyclovir suspension was administered orally in a dose of 80 mg/kg/day (20 mg/kg four times a day), beginning on the first day of the chickenpox rash. Three groups of children should be considered for acyclovir: children during the first year of life, adolescents who are known to be at a higher risk, and siblings of any age who sequentially contract chickenpox within the same household and often develop more severe disease. A fourth group includes all children who have chronic conditions (e.g., eczema, asthma, rheumatoid arthritis, diabetes) and who may benefit from a shortened course of chickenpox. The recommended dosage of acyclovir in older children weighing more than 40 kg and demonstrating normal renal function is 800 mg four times daily. Acyclovir is supplied in 200- and 800-mg capsules or as a suspension containing 200 mg/5 mL. Older adolescents of near adult size can be treated with a highly efficacious second-generation acyclovir derivative, for example, famciclovir at a dosage of 500 mg orally three times daily for 5 to 7 days. The more widespread use of varicella vaccine may diminish the need for antiviral treatment (see later).

VARICELLA VACCINATION

A live attenuated VZV vaccine called *Varivax* (Merck, West Point, PA) was approved in March 1995 for distribution in the United States. The current recommendation of the American Academy of Pediatrics is that all healthy children between the ages of 12 and 18 months receive one dose of the live attenuated varicella vaccine (Varivax) by subcutaneous injection. Recommendation for a second (booster) dose of varicella vaccine prior to school entry is anticipated (see www.aap.org for the most current recommendations). Children who are older than 18 months and have not had chickenpox also can be given varicella vaccine. Children at age 13 or older require two doses of vaccine given 4 to 8 weeks apart. In most cases, varicella vaccine should not be administered to children receiving corticosteroids or other immunosuppressive therapies, because of the small risk of disseminated infection. However, varicella vaccine should not be withheld from healthy children living in the same household with an immunosuppressed VZV-susceptible sibling, because the risk of acquiring wild-type varicella from an unimmunized sibling is greater than the risk of vaccine-related infection. Similarly, children cared for by a VZV-susceptible pregnant woman should be immunized despite the potential risk that the woman will acquire mild, vaccine-related infection.

Because varicella vaccine is a live attenuated vaccine, an effective immune response is dependent on virus replication in the inoculated child. A frequent side effect of replication is a skin rash 2 to 4 weeks after immunization. The rashes usually consist of 2 to 10 papules, although a few children develop a more widespread exanthem. Children with rashes can transmit the vaccine virus to persons who are not immune, although the risk is extremely small (3 documented cases after administering 30 million doses in the United States). Vaccinees without a rash do not appear to be contagious. Even in children without a rash, low-grade fever may occur 1 to 2 weeks after vaccination.

The 2003 *Redbook* lists the following rare but serious complications temporally associated with varicella vaccination: anaphylaxis, thrombocytopenia, erythema multiforme, Stevens-Johnson syndrome, nervous system (ataxia, encephalitis, seizures, neuropathy, Guillain-Barré-syndrome) manifestations, and secondary bacterial infection. The early concern that varicella vaccine could lead to an increased rate of zoster in vaccinees has not been substantiated; in fact, zoster may be dimished in vaccinees, but longer follow-up is required.

Varicella vaccination is 95% effective in preventing moderate to severe chickenpox. In this regard, severe varicella caused about 100 deaths/year in the United States in the past. Since 1995, however, it has become increasingly apparent that a subgroup of vaccinees will develop what is called breakthrough varicella (modified varicella), when exposed to wild-type chickenpox in the community. Breakthrough varicella generally is a much milder disease than typical wild-type chickenpox, with low-grade fever and short-lived rash (10 to 30 papulovesicles) lasting 2 to 3 days, because of the preexistent vaccine-induced immunity. Breakthrough varicella can be as contagious as wild-type chickenpox. In one report, an outbreak of modified varicella occurred in a day-care center in which all the children had been immunized. A total of 25 of 88 children developed chickenpox. At the present time, there is no explanation for this apparent vaccine failure, although again it was observed that none of the children developed severe varicella. Because of breakthrough chickenpox, the 2003 *Redbook* estimates the overall effectiveness of varicella vaccine to prevent chickenpox of any severity to range from 70% to 85%. Future investigations will certainly determine the reasons for breakthrough disease.

Suggested Readings

Grose C, Varicella vaccination of children in the United States: assessment after the first decade 1995–2005. *J Clin Virol* 2005;33: 89.
Pickering LK, ed. *Redbook 2003: report of the Committee on Infectious Disease.* Elk Grove Village, IL: American Academy of Pediatrics, 2003:672.

CHAPTER 200 ■ ACQUIRED CYTOMEGALOVIRAL INFECTIONS

STUART P. ADLER

Of all the viruses that infect humans, cytomegalovirus (CMV), a member of the herpes family of viruses, has the largest size genome, with approximately 230 kilobases of DNA. CMV is ubiquitous in the human population, and biologically CMV's interaction with its human host is extremely complex. CMV usually causes little or no disease, but it may induce illness, either after a first or primary infection or among immunocompromised patients after reactivated infection or secondary infection caused by reinfection with a second viral strain. CMV has adapted to the human immune system such that it adequately propagates itself with prolonged viral excretion in nearly all body fluids including urine, saliva, and semen, without a significant impact on the human immune system and inducing little if any disease. Disease associated with CMV infection occurs most often when the immune system is compromised because of immaturity, as occurs in the fetus, because of disease, as occurs in human immunodeficiency virus (HIV) infection, or for iatrogenic causes, as occurs in transplant recipients.

Within a 65-nm inner core of the CMV viral particle resides the large, double-stranded DNA. Included within the CMV genome are more than 200 open-reading frames. The inner core itself is contained within an icosahedral protein capsid composed of 162 capsomeres. This, in turn, is surrounded by a tegument layer and an outer enveloped membrane composed of glycoprotein. The CMV viral particles are structurally similar to those of other human herpesviruses. The CMV DNA encodes for at least 100 proteins, most of which are structural. The envelope glycoproteins are antigenic and are responsible for generating an immune response. Most of the neutralizing antibodies induced by CMV antigens are directed against the major CMV glycoprotein called gB, although a second envelope glycoprotein called gH also contains neutralizing epitopes. Cellular responses such as those generated by cytotoxic T cells are directed primarily against the major tegument protein, pp65.

CMV has only a single serotype; that is, antibodies directed against one viral isolate cross-react with almost all other isolates. Genetically, however, there are probably thousands of different strains. Each unrelated isolate of CMV differs genotypically from all other epidemiologically unrelated isolates. These genotypic differences have been important epidemiologic tools in tracking the virus as it is transmitted from one individual to another.

EPIDEMIOLOGY AND TRANSMISSION

In the United States, approximately 1% to 2% of the population acquires a CMV infection each year, and thus by age 70 years, nearly all individuals become infected with CMV. In many areas of the world, nearly 100% of a population is infected with CMV by age 2 years. Table 200.1 lists some of the modes by which CMV is transmitted among humans. Congenital infection accounts for a minority of acquired CMV infections. Between 1% and 2% of all newborns worldwide are infected with CMV at birth. Newborns are infected *in utero* either as the result of a primary maternal CMV infection during pregnancy or as a result of recurrent maternal infection that occurs when a mother has had a CMV infection before pregnancy. Recurrent maternal infections occur either following reactivation of latent maternal virus or by reinfection of the mother with a second CMV strain. If a woman's first CMV infection occurs during pregnancy, the CMV transmission rate from mother to the fetus is about 50%, but for women initially infected with CMV before pregnancy, the transmission rate to the fetus is only 1% to 3%. Congenital CMV disease occurs primarily following a primary maternal infection during pregnancy. This aspect of CMV infection is covered in Chapter 77.

Newborns who are not infected *in utero* may acquire CMV postnatally from two major sources. Approximately 10% to 13% of seropositive women excrete CMV in cervical or vaginal secretions, and infants delivered of a mother who is excreting CMV will often acquire CMV from this source. Perinatal acquisition of CMV via this mode by full-term healthy newborns causes no apparent disease. CMV transmission from mother to infant also occurs via breast milk. Between 25% and 50% of

TABLE 200.1

MODES AND FREQUENCY OF CYTOMEGALOVIRUS TRANSMISSION

Mode	Approximate Transmission Rate
Transplacental	
Primary maternal	50%
Recurrent maternal	0.5%–1%
Perinatal	
Breast milk	25%–50%
Cervical secretion	10%
Postnatal	
Day care	10%–70%
Intrafamilial	50%
Sexual	
Oral	Unknown
Genital	Unknown
Nosocomial	
Transfusion	2%–10% (with unscreened or filtered blood)
Hospital personnel	0%

seropositive women who breast-feed their infants will transmit CMV to these infants. Infants acquiring CMV via breast milk also have no apparent disease associated with CMV acquisition via this source.

Infants and children may also acquire CMV either via child-to-child transmission or via intrafamilial transmission. Child-to-child transmission has been studied intensely, particularly in the day-care setting. Of preschool children who attend large day-care centers, an average of 25% (range, 10% to 70%) will acquire a CMV infection from other children in the same day-care center. These children, especially those less than 2 years old, will, in turn, transmit the virus to their caretakers, including both parents and day-care workers. Infection rates for previously uninfected day-care workers are between 10% and 20%/year, compared with an annual infection rate of approximately 2% for the general population. The annual rate of CMV infections among parents who have not had a previous infection (seronegative) and who have a child who is less than 2 years old and is shedding CMV is approximately 50%, or 25-fold higher than for the general population.

Thus, the natural history of CMV transmission in day care is that a child who acquired CMV either congenitally or perinatally enters day care and then transmits the virus to other children, with subsequent transmission from children to seronegative day-care employees and seronegative parents. CMV transmission by young children is facilitated by the prolonged duration of viral excretion in both saliva and urine. For children less than 2 years of age who acquire CMV infection postnatally, CMV is excreted for an average of 18 months with a range of 6 to 40 months. In contrast, for older children and adults who acquire primary CMV infection, viral excretion in urine and saliva usually occurs for only a few days to several weeks, although some individuals may excrete the virus for longer periods.

CMV is excreted not only in urine and saliva but also in other secretions except tears. CMV is in highest concentrations in semen and is highly prevalent in cervical or vaginal secretions. Hence, it is assumed that CMV transmission occurs via sexual activity. CMV infections are associated with increased sexual activity among adolescents and those attending clinics for sexually transmitted diseases. Homosexual men also have very high rates of CMV infection, with nearly 100% having acquired CMV infection presumably via sexual activity.

Nosocomial transmission of CMV within the hospital occurs very infrequently. In numerous studies, CMV transmission from infected patients to hospital personnel has not been observed. Patient-to-patient transmission is rare and occurs only when patients are hospitalized side-by-side for prolonged periods. Thus, CMV seronegative women caring for young children or for other patients who may be excreting CMV can be reassured that there is little or no risk of acquiring CMV from patients. CMV may be transmitted by transfusion of whole blood. CMV is located in the white cell fraction. For immunocompromised patients requiring transfusion, the risk of CMV acquisition from a blood donor is eliminated either by selecting donors who are CMV seronegative or by using blood products with white cells removed.

In summary, the person-to-person transmission of CMV is facilitated by prolonged viral excretion (especially among young children) in nearly all body fluids. Transmission, however, is slow and requires frequent and prolonged "intimate contact" as occurs among family members, among those engaged in sexual activities, or among children cared for together for prolonged periods in day care. Casual transmission of CMV as could occur in a supermarket, movie theater, or other crowded place is very unlikely.

CYTOMEGALOVIRAL INFECTIONS IN THE IMMUNOCOMPETENT HOST

Most CMV infections are totally inapparent and asymptomatic. Disease manifestations, when present, may be associated with a syndrome resembling infectious mononucleosis. This syndrome, like that caused by Epstein-Barr virus, includes either mild, flu-like symptoms with low-grade fever and malaise, or a more full-blown syndrome resembling infectious mononucleosis and associated with hepatosplenomegaly, lymphadenopathy, atypical lymphocytosis, pharyngitis, and occasionally a rubelliform rash. Other less frequent symptoms include migratory polyarthritis, particularly in the fingers, knees, and toes, and rarely but occasionally pneumonia, particularly in young infants. In previously healthy individuals with an infectious mononucleosis–like syndrome caused by CMV, diagnosis may be difficult because signs and symptoms may mimic those of more serious diseases such as leukemia, systemic lupus erythematosus, and autoimmune hemolytic anemia. Primary CMV infection may also be associated with prolonged fever but no other signs or symptoms.

Symptomatic adults or children with postnatally acquired CMV infections will experience resolution of symptoms over several weeks or days without sequelae. Adults with acquired CMV infections are more likely to have disease manifestations and especially infectious mononucleosis–like syndrome. Both this syndrome and a variety of unusual manifestations associated with CMV infections are relatively rare, occurring in less than 1% of infected individuals. Thus, in older children and adults, the possibility of CMV should be considered in patients with nonspecific flu-like illnesses or infectious mononucleosis–like illnesses.

DISEASE IN THE IMMUNOCOMPROMISED HOST

In immunocompromised patients, CMV infections are a serious and frequent cause of morbidity and mortality. CMV replicates in almost every organ and tissue system, but infection is thought to occur primarily in endothelial cells. Hence, a compromised immune system may produce CMV disease in any organ or tissue system.

The primary types of immunocompromised patients for whom CMV infections are a potential problem include patients who have had organ transplantations, who are being treated for malignant disease, or who are immunocompromised as a result of HIV infection. The disease manifestations associated with CMV in these infections are protean but generally include fever, lymphadenopathy, hepatitis, pneumonia, or gastrointestinal infections with either gastritis or colitis. There may also be arthritis and, if immune suppression is severe enough, as occurs with HIV infection, encephalopathy and retinitis. Leukopenia, associated with disseminated CMV infection in immunocompromised patients, is common.

The pathogenesis of CMV infections among immunocompromised patients is complex. In these patients, CMV immunosuppression leads to the reactivation of latent virus, and the frequency and severity of CMV disease are related to the extent of immunosuppression. Among solid organ transplant recipients, latent CMV reactivates from the seropositive donor organ more than 90% of the time. CMV-seronegative patients who have received an organ from a CMV-seropositive donor are at highest risk for CMV disease. Depending on the immunosuppressive therapy used to prevent graft rejection, seropositive recipients of seronegative organs may also reactivate latent CMV after transplantation and may develop CMV disease. Among bone marrow transplant recipients, CMV always reactivates after transplantation if either the donor or the recipient was seropositive, and reactivation is often accompanied by severe CMV disease, especially pneumonitis.

HIV-infected patients have particular difficulties with CMV pneumonia, retinitis, gastrointestinal disease, and occasionally neuropathy and encephalitis. CMV disease among patients being treated for malignancy is less common than among recipients of solid organs or hematopoietic cells or those with HIV infection. The frequency of CMV disease among those receiving chemotherapy for malignancy is related to the intensity and duration of immunosuppression induced by the chemotherapy.

Among immunocompromised patients, CMV itself may induce further immunosuppression by a variety of mechanisms. Patients with CMV mononucleosis have depressed cell-mediated immune responses to a variety of mitogens and antigens. The virus also depresses natural killer cell activity and T-cell proliferation *in vitro*. CMV infection may enhance immunosuppression in patients with acquired immunodeficiency syndrome (AIDS), but this is controversial. Previously, there was circumstantial evidence that CMV infections increased the risk for bacterial infections in childhood; this is currently unsubstantiated.

Among transplant recipients, CMV infections may enhance organ rejection and graft-versus-host disease. CMV enhances both cytoplasmic and surface expression of HLA class 1 antigens *in vitro* and also induces many classes of autoantibodies. It is unknown, however, whether CMV infection is central in triggering rejection or simply is activated following immune suppression or treatment for rejection. Similarly, in HIV-infected patients, it is unclear whether progressive immunodeficiency allows the emergence of CMV disease or whether CMV disease allows HIV infections to progress more rapidly.

DIAGNOSIS

Diagnosis of primary CMV infections among immunocompetent patients is usually not difficult and relies on traditional serologic and virologic techniques. Following a primary CMV infection, individuals make immunoglobulin G (IgG) antibodies to CMV. These antibodies are detected by a variety of serologic methods such as complement fixation, enzyme immunoassay, or latex agglutination. These antibodies are usually detected 2 to 4 weeks after a primary CMV infection and rise to high levels, where they are generally sustained for life. Primary infection can also be identified among immunocompetent individuals by detecting CMV-specific IgM in the serum or low-avidity IgG antibodies to CMV using readily available commercial assays. The presence of IgM antibodies themselves does not necessarily indicate a primary infection because these antibodies may also occur following reactivation of CMV. IgM antibodies to CMV have been detected in 90% of homosexual men as well as in immunocompetent patients. Thus, IgM may not always be a specific indicator for primary acquired CMV infection. Low-avidity IgG antibodies against CMV persists up to 20 weeks after primary CMV infection. These low-avidity antibodies are then replaced by high-avidity antibodies (greater than 60% binding in presence of 5 M urea). Avidity is a sensitive and specific test for recent primary CMV infection.

Among immunocompetent patients, when reactivation occurs it is rarely associated with disease. For a symptomatic immunocompetent patient, a CMV diagnosis also requires exclusion of all other causes of infectious mononucleosis such as Epstein-Barr virus or toxoplasmosis. These disorders are usually excluded based on the absence of either Epstein-Barr

virus–specific or heterophile antibodies and for toxoplasmosis a lack of either IgG or IgM antibodies to toxoplasma antigens.

The diagnosis of CMV can be supported but not confirmed by detecting the virus in secretions, particularly in urine or saliva. Viral culture in human fibroblasts in tissue culture is the traditional method, and it is easy to perform but often time consuming, requiring 2 to 4 weeks to detect traditional cytopathic effects in tissue culture. A faster culture method, called the shell vial assay, is based on the detection of a protein made in the early stages of CMV infection. This test allows the detection of CMV in body fluids as rapidly as 48 hours after obtaining specimens. Hence, in an immunocompetent patient with a suspected CMV infection, one should use serologic techniques for detecting both IgG and IgM antibodies as well as virologic techniques for detecting CMV in urine, saliva, or other fluids. IgG should be absent or at low levels early in the course of illness resulting from primary infection and should rise during the ensuing 2 to 4 weeks.

Among immunocompromised patients, the diagnosis of CMV disease as opposed to CMV infection is much more difficult to establish. Seropositive immunocompromised patients often reactivate CMV following immunosuppression. Thus, the detection of antibodies of CMV in serum or the detection of virus in urine, saliva, or even in blood is sufficient to diagnose a CMV infection but not to diagnose disease caused by CMV. The detection of CMV antigenemia and a high viral load, as detected by polymerase chain reaction in the plasma of patients, particularly those who have received organ transplants, both have a good association with CMV disease.

Among immunocompromised patients, the diagnosis of CMV disease requires two factors. First, all other possible causes of inflammation or disease such as *Pneumocystis carinii* infection, toxoplasmosis, and other viral, fungal, or bacterial infections must be eliminated. Second, CMV must be detected in a biopsy specimen, for example, from lung tissue or alveolar lavage. The presence of CMV in inflamed tissues can be detected histologically using traditional staining. CMV induces a morphologic change in some cells characterized by a classic intranuclear inclusion. These cells are called "owl eye" cells and indicate high levels of virus in the infected tissue. CMV can also be detected by *in situ* nucleic acid hybridization or by the polymerase chain reaction both targeted to CMV DNA. These nucleic acid techniques are very sensitive and detect low levels of virus, which may not always establish disease, although it clearly establishes tissue infection. Thus, the presence of "owl eye" cells in a diseased tissue such as lung, liver, or brain, without the presence of another microorganism that may be producing the patient's symptoms, is usually sufficient for a diagnosis of CMV disease.

In summary, although the diagnosis of CMV infection is often possible in immunocompetent patients, the diagnosis of CMV disease in immunocompromised patients is usually more difficult. In general, CMV antigenemia or high viral load in blood associated with evidence of tissue inflammation and viral infection, or excretion of virus in body fluids, is necessary to diagnose CMV infection. When all these factors are present, as well as a consistent constellation of symptoms likely to be caused by CMV, a presumptive diagnosis of CMV is reasonable.

PROGNOSIS AND THERAPY

The prognosis for immunocompetent patients is always good, and no specific therapy is required. For immunocompromised patients, the outcome is uncertain and depends on the level and duration of immune suppression. Hence, for immunocompromised patients, antiviral therapy against CMV is important. Two forms of therapy are available. One is chemotherapy using drugs that inhibit CMV DNA replication. Ganciclovir is the most commonly used drug and is structurally similar to acyclovir but with greater inhibitory activity against CMV. Ganciclovir has been used successfully to treat CMV infections in immunocompromised patients and is licensed in the United States for the treatment of severe CMV infections. Although many of the studies with ganciclovir have been uncontrolled, controlled trials have shown benefit for patients with CMV retinitis and for bone marrow recipients. These and other patients with CMV disease generally respond to ganciclovir. The effect of ganciclovir alone in patients with CMV pneumonia has been more difficult to ascertain.

Ganciclovir inhibits viral replication via a mechanism similar to that of acyclovir. Cellular enzymes phosphorylate ganciclovir to a triphosphate, and the triphosphate acts as a competitive and reversible inhibiter of viral DNA synthesis, with little if any effect on cellular DNA replication. Ganciclovir reduces or eliminates the amount of virus excreted in urine and saliva and generally clears CMV from the blood. This antiviral effect occurs only while the patient is receiving the drug. After ganciclovir therapy is stopped, viral excretion and viremia rapidly reappear. In patients with AIDS, CMV relapses are common after ganciclovir therapy, and long-term administration of ganciclovir is often required.

The recommended therapeutic dose of ganciclovir is 5 mg/kg/dose twice daily intravenously for 2 to 3 weeks followed by 5 mg/kg daily intravenously for maintenance therapy. Ganciclovir is also available for oral administration in CMV-infected patients with AIDS but is poorly absorbed from gastrointestinal tract. Oral ganciclovir is used primarily to treat CMV retinitis. The oral dose is 1 g three times/day. Valganciclovir, a valine ester of ganciclovir, is well absorbed from the gastrointestinal tract and is effective at inhibiting CMV replication. Valganciclovir has been successfully used to treat CMV disease in adults, and the dose is 900 mg per day. For oral ganciclovir and valganciclovir, there are no specific dosages for children. The adverse effects associated with ganciclovir include mild leukopenia and neutropenia, which occur commonly. Because of drug toxicity, zidovudine and ganciclovir should not be administered simultaneously. Another drug for treating CMV retinitis in HIV-infected patients is foscarnet (90 to 180 mg/kg/day), which also inhibits CMV DNA synthesis, although by a different mechanism.

Another treatment for CMV infections among immunocompromised patients is immunoglobulin with high levels of IgG antibodies to CMV. Immunoglobulin is usually administered concurrently with ganciclovir and is especially important for patients who have had bone marrow or solid organ transplants. Among seropositive patients, it reduces the incidence and severity of posttransplant disease resulting from CMV. Ganciclovir is also effective for preventing progressive hearing deficit associated with symptomatic congenital CMV disease for newborns with evidence of central nervous system involvement.

PREVENTION

A live attenuated CMV vaccine, called the Towne Strain, is effective prophylactically in preventing or significantly reducing the incidence of CMV disease among seronegative patients who have received a kidney from a seropositive donor. Unfortunately, this vaccine is not commercially available. Thus, many transplant centers use a combination of passive immunization with immunoglobulin and prophylactic administration of ganciclovir to prevent CMV preemptively following organ transplantation.

Work is in progress to develop other vaccines against CMV. These experimental vaccines include other live attenuated strains of CMV and recombinant vaccines that use the major gB glycoprotein of CMV. Work in this area has been slow but steadily ongoing.

Suggested Readings

Adler SP. CMV and daycare. *Adv Pediatr Infect Dis* 1991;7:109.

Adler SP. Cytomegalovirus. In: Mayhall CG, ed. *Hospital epidemiology and infection control*, 2nd ed. Baltimore: Williams & Wilkins, 1999:559.

Bodeus M, Beulne P, Goubau P. Ability of three IgG-avidity assays to exclude recent cytomegalovirus infection. *Eur J Clin Microbiol Infect Dis* 2001;20: 248.

Bowden RA, Syers M, Fluornoy N, et al. Cytomegalovirus immune globulin and seronegative blood products to prevent primary cytomegalovirus infections after bone marrow transplantation. *N Engl J Med* 1986;314:1006.

Bueno J, Ramil C, Green M. Current management strategies for the prevention and treatment of cytomegalovirus infection in pediatric transplant recipients. *Paediatr Drugs* 2002;4:279.

Chou S. Acquisition of donor strains of cytomegalovirus by renal transplant recipients. *N Engl J Med* 1986;314:1418.

Collaborative DHPG Treatment Study Group. Treatment of serious cytomegalovirus infections with 9-(1,3 dihydroxy-20propoxymethyl) guanine in patients with AIDS and other immunodeficiencies. *N Engl J Med* 1986;314: 801.

Demmler GJ. Cytomegalovirus. In: Katz SL, Gerson AA, Hotez PJ, eds. *Krugman's infectious diseases of children*. St. Louis: Mosby-Year Book, 2004: 47.

Kimberlin DW, Lin CY, Sanchez PJ, et al. Effect of ganciclovir therapy on hearing in symptomatic congenital cytomegalovirus disease involving the central nervous system: a randomized, controlled trial. *J Pediatr* 2003;143: 16.

Lalezari J, Lindley J, Walmsley S, et al. A safety study of oral valganciclovir maintenance treatment of cytomegalovirus reinitis. *J Acquir Immune Defic Syndr Hum Retrovirol* 2002;30:392.

Merigan T, Renlund D, Keay S, et al. A controlled trial of ganciclovir to prevent CMV disease after transplantation. *N Engl J Med* 1992;326:1182.

Pescovitz MD, Rabkin J, Merion RM, et al. Valganciclovir results in improved oral absorption of ganciclovir in liver transplant recipients. *Antimicrob Agents Chemother* 2000;44:2811.

Snydman DR, Werner BG, Heize-Lacey B, et al. Use of cytomegalovirus immune globulin to prevent cytomegalovirus disease in renal transplant recipients. *N Engl J Med* 1987;317:1049.

Zanghellini F, Boppana SB, Emery VC, et al. Asymptomatic primary cytomegalovirus infection: virologic and immunologic features. *J Infect Dis* 1999; 180:702.

CHAPTER 201 ■ RUBELLA (GERMAN MEASLES)

ANDREEA C. CAZACU AND GAIL J. DEMMLER

Rubella is an acute infectious disease characterized by low-grade fever, erythematous maculopapular rash, and adenopathy. Rubella infection in early pregnancy may result in fetal infection with severe congenital anomalies. Rubella was described in the 1700s by German physicians, and in 1866, Veale, a Royal Artillery surgeon, described an outbreak of illness that he named "rubella." In 1941, Gregg, an Australian physician, described congenital defects in infants of mothers who had rubella during pregnancy. Rubella virus was isolated in tissue culture in 1962. Rubella and congenital rubella syndrome (CRS) became reportable in 1966 and 1969, respectively. Development of the hemagglutination inhibition (HAI) test in 1967 rendered possible the performance of large-scale surveillance studies and diagnostic testing. Attenuated rubella virus vaccine was developed in the late 1960s and was licensed in the United States in 1969. Vaccine use in children and in women of childbearing age dramatically reduced the number of cases of postnatally acquired rubella and congenital rubella.

ETIOLOGY

Rubella virus is a non-arthropod-borne, RNA-containing, heat-labile togavirus of the genus *Rubivirus*. It has no antigenic relationship with other togaviruses. Only a single type of rubella virus has been described. Several antigens have been defined, including an envelope antigen, a hemagglutinin, the inhibition of which by rubella specific antisera is the basis for the HAI test for rubella. Isolation of rubella virus in tissue culture from clinical specimens is achieved by viral interference. When African green monkey kidney cells are infected with rubella virus, they show no cytopathic effect, and when the same rubella-infected cells then are challenged with an appropriate enterovirus, they resist infection with the enterovirus and again demonstrate no cytopathic effect, or interference.

POSTNATALLY ACQUIRED RUBELLA

Pathogenesis and Epidemiology

Natural infection with rubella virus occurs only in humans, although several different animals have been infected experimentally with the virus. Transmission occurs by oral droplet in acquired rubella, compared with transplacentally in congenital rubella. In human volunteers, infection occurs easily after droplet presentation to the nasopharyngeal mucosa. The sequence of events includes replication of the virus in the nasopharyngeal mucosa, involvement of regional lymphatics, and subsequent viremia. The maximum titer of the virus in the nasopharynx is present several days before the rash appears, and an infected person is most contagious during this period. Periods of maximum communicability include the week before and the week after the appearance of the rash, and patients with known cases of acquired rubella should be isolated dur-

ing this period. Viremia clears quickly after appearance of the rash, but the virus may be shed from the nasopharynx after the resolution of the rash.

Rubella virus has been isolated from the nasopharynx, blood, skin, synovial fluid, cerebrospinal fluid (CSF), placenta, and other specimens. Infected hosts develop both humoral and cell-mediated immunity. After infection, antibodies in both immunoglobulin M (IgM) and G (IgG) classes develop rapidly after appearance of the rash. Rubella-specific IgM antibody usually persists approximately 12 weeks and may aid in diagnosis of an acute infection. Antibodies of IgG class persist for life and are markers for immunity.

In the prevaccine era, major rubella outbreaks occurred every 6 to 9 years, with the highest attack rates in school-aged children (5 to 10 years) and lesser attack rates in preschool-aged children. Rubella occurs worldwide, and outbreaks are seen in the winter and spring months in temperate climates. After widespread immunization with rubella vaccine was achieved, incidence rates or reported rubella decreased steadily and reached an all-time low in 1988. Since 1989, however, the number of reported cases has increased steadily each year, marking a moderate resurgence of postnatal rubella and subsequent concern for an increase in CRS.

Whereas increases in incidence of acquired rubella have occurred in all age groups, the most dramatic increase has occurred in persons older than 15 years of age. In 1990, 26 rubella outbreaks were reported, and they appeared to fall into two categories. One type of outbreak was associated with settings in which unvaccinated adolescents and adults congregated, such as prisons, colleges, workplaces (especially hospitals), and recreational settings. Another form of outbreak occurred among children and adults in religious communities with low levels of rubella vaccination. Information from both these types of outbreaks suggests that failure to vaccinate, not primary or secondary vaccine failure, was responsible for this increase incidence of rubella. In 1996, 196 provisional cases of indigenous rubella were reported; most cases occurred in adults 20 years of age or older. In 1998, more than 90% of infants with CRS were born to foreign-born mothers, 81% of whom were of Hispanic ethnicity.

Clinical Manifestations

Incubation periods for postnatal rubella range from 14 to 21 days, usually 15 to 18 days. Inapparent infection may occur in 25% or more of infected individuals. Prodromal symptoms, usually appearing 1 to 5 days before the rash, are seen more commonly among older children and adults; they consist of low-grade fever, coryza, conjunctivitis, cough, and lymphadenopathy (Table 201.1). An enanthem of rubella, Forchheimer spots, consists of discrete, erythematous pinpoint or larger lesions found on the soft palate in the prodromal phase or on the first day of the rash. These lesions are not pathognomonic for rubella, however. The lymphadenopathy associated with rubella may appear as early as 7 days before appearance of the rash. The suboccipital, posterior auricular, and cervical lymph nodes are involved most commonly, but

TABLE 201.1

COMPARISON OF COMMON CLINICAL MANIFESTATIONS OF CONGENITAL AND POSTNATAL RUBELLA

Congenital Rubella	Postnatal Rubella
Intrauterine growth retardation	Fever
Skin lesions	Maculopapular rash
Petechiae	Lymphadenopathy
Purpura	Polyarthralgia
Hepatosplenomegaly	Polyarthritis
Jaundice	Encephalitis
Ophthalmologic abnormalities	Thrombocytopenia
Cataracts	
Retinopathy	
Glaucoma	
Cardiac abnormalities	
Patent ductus arteriosus	
Pulmonary artery stenosis	
Meningoencephalitis	
Thrombocytopenia	
Hemolytic anemia	
Sequelae long-term	
Sensory neural hearing loss	
Neurodevelopmental disabilities	
Endocrinopathies	
Hypogammaglobulinemia	

generalized lymphadenopathy may occur. Maximum swelling of the lymph nodes and tenderness usually coincide with the first day of the appearance of the rash.

The exanthem of rubella may be the first indication of this infection in young children. It begins on the face and moves rapidly downward to the trunk and lower extremities. The exanthem lasts approximately 3 days; it may persist for 5 days or disappear within the first day. The rash of rubella is erythematous, discrete, and maculopapular, and it generally does not coalesce or darken as in rubeola. Fever in rubella is more often of low grade (less than 38.8°C) and does not persist for the length of the exanthem.

Arthritis is seen more commonly in adults and adolescents and more frequently in the female than the male population. Joint involvement usually is multiple (large and small joints) and appears as the rash nears resolution. It may be accompanied by recurrence of fever. Elevation of the sedimentation rate may occur in rubella arthritis. Symptoms usually abate within 15 days of appearance. Some studies suggest a relationship between rubella arthritis and subsequent development of rheumatoid arthritis.

Serious complications of postnatal rubella are rare. Encephalitis occurs in approximately 1 in 6,000 children, with the usual onset occurring after the appearance of the rash. The encephalitis usually is not fatal, and complete recovery can be expected in most cases. Mononuclear pleocytosis may occur in the CSF, along with a normal or slightly elevated protein level. Persistent abnormalities in the electroencephalogram have been described. Neuritis may occur during rubella infection, with paresthesia the chief complaint.

Thrombocytopenic purpura has occurred in rubella. In the majority of patients, the purpura resolves and the platelet counts return to normal within 15 days.

Differential Diagnosis

No pathognomonic findings occur in rubella, and with the reduced incidence of rubella, physicians must have a high index of suspicion to make the diagnosis. Helpful epidemiologic fac-

tors include age of the patient, history of contact cases with the period of incubation, documented status of immunization, and season of the year.

Included in the differential diagnosis of acquired rubella syndrome are illnesses associated with enteroviruses, mild rubeola, mild scarlet fever, mononucleosis, cytomegalovirus, toxoplasmosis, *Mycoplasma pneumoniae* infection, and human parvovirus B19 infection.

Diagnosis

Rubella virus may be isolated from nasal, blood, throat, urine, or CSF specimens obtained from individuals with postnatal rubella, and the isolation of the virus confirms the diagnosis. Isolating rubella virus is technically difficult, and the virology laboratory must be alerted that rubella virus is suspected so the specimen can be handled and processed appropriately. Because of limitations associated with culture of the rubella virus, the diagnosis of postnatal rubella usually is determined by serologic testing of acute and convalescent sera obtained 10 to 14 days apart. The traditional HAI test for rubella has been replaced by commercially available tests that are more sensitive and easier to perform. Serologic tests now performed include enzyme immunoassay (EIA), latex agglutination, and indirect immunofluorescence. One of the most widely used tests is the EIA with the capture technique. Results of this test may be reported as nonimmune or immune, or negative, low-positive, midpositive, or high-positive. Tests to detect rubella-specific IgM antibody are also commercially available; however, these tests may produce both false-negative and false-positive results.

A test result on paired sera that is reported as changing from nonimmune to immune, a fourfold rise in titer, or the determination of the presence of rubella-specific IgM antibody indicates a recent infection with rubella virus. Tests should be performed on the same sera, simultaneously in the same laboratory.

References laboratories also may detect the virus in clinical samples by reverse transcriptase–polymerase chain reaction (RT-PCR) methods.

Treatment

Treatment is largely supportive and includes use of acetaminophen for fever. Hospitalization rarely is required but may be necessary when complications occur. Rubella arthritis usually responds to antiinflammatory agents, such as aspirin, and rest of the involved joints.

CONGENITAL RUBELLA

The initial report of Gregg in 1941 described CRS as a triad of congenital cataracts, heart defects, and low birth weight in infants born after maternal rubella during early pregnancy. With the pandemic of rubella in 1964, the complexity of this syndrome was recognized, and the term "expanded rubella syndrome" became standard to describe the more extensive organ involvement observed in infants with congenital rubella.

Pathogenesis and Epidemiology

The timing of maternal rubella during pregnancy is important because it relates to the pathogenesis of congenital rubella. Maternal rubella infection, either apparent or inapparent, in the first month of pregnancy predictably results in maternal viremia with subsequent placental and fetal infection, widespread organ involvement, and persistent infection of the fetus. Early fetal infection results in hypoplastic organs and a subnormal number of cells. The risk of fetal infection after maternal rubella is greatest during the first month of pregnancy, and subsequent congenital anomalies are seen in 30% to 60% of these children. The risk of fetal infection appears to decline thereafter, but hearing loss, ocular abnormalities, and developmental disabilities have been described in children born to women who experienced rubella during the second trimester of pregnancy.

Rubella virus has been isolated from placental and fetal tissue from aborted fetuses and from nasopharynx, urine, CSF, cataracts, and almost every organ in infants with congenital rubella. Excretion of virus from the nasopharynx and in the urine may persist until the child is 1 year of age or older. Infants with congenital rubella develop both humoral and cell-mediated immunity. Differences exist in the immune response in congenital rubella and birth-acquired rubella, in that the rubella-specific IgM antibody persists in the sera of infants with congenital rubella until they are 6 months of age or older, and HAI antibodies may not persist for life and may disappear in later life (after 5 years of age).

The number of cases of CRS reported to the Centers for Disease Control and Prevention had declined each year since vaccine licensure in 1969 and reached an all-time low in 1988. Since 1989, however, an increase in the number of reported cases of CRS has occurred. This observed increase in incidence of CRS parallels the reported increase in that of postnatal rubella seen since 1989. Because CRS is the most severe and preventable consequence of rubella infection, CRS cases should be identified and investigated to estimate the incidence and identify opportunities to prevent rubella infection in pregnant women. For example, it is estimated that up to 25% of postpubertal girls and women lack antibody to rubella virus, and continued reports of outbreaks of rubella in populations of childbearing age indicate potential resurgence of CRS.

Clinical Manifestations

Clinical manifestations of CRS include intrauterine growth retardation (the most common manifestation and hardly ever an isolated finding), hepatosplenomegaly, generalized adenopathy, thrombocytopenia, hemolytic anemia, hepatitis, jaundice, meningoencephalitis (which may persist beyond the first year of life), bone lesions, large anterior fontanelle, pneumonitis, myocarditis, and nephritis (see Table 201.1).

Eye involvement may be manifested by cataracts (usually noted at birth), glaucoma, retinopathy that does not interfere with visual acuity, and micro-ophthalmia, usually associated with cataracts.

Sensorineural deafness is a common finding and may not be apparent until later in childhood. Heart defects are frequent findings; patent ductus arteriosus is the most common finding, followed by stenosis of the pulmonary artery. More than one heart defect may coexist in the same patient.

Numerous delayed manifestations with long-term implications have been described and include deafness, ocular damage, endocrinopathies (diabetes mellitus and thyroid dysfunction), progressive rubella panencephalitis, immunologic defects (particularly low levels of IgG), developmental and motor disabilities, behavioral problems, and learning disabilities.

Differential Diagnosis

Differential diagnosis includes congenital cytomegalovirus infection, syphilis, toxoplasmosis, neonatal herpes, and enteroviral infection of the newborn. Infants with congenital rubella are much more likely to be symptomatic at birth than are infants with the aforementioned infections.

Diagnosis

The diagnosis of CRS can be made with isolation in cell culture of the virus, demonstration of rubella-specific IgM antibody that may be present until the child is 6 to 12 months of age, or persistence of rubella IgG antibody beyond 6 months of age. Rubella virus may be isolated from throat, urine, cataracts, or CSF until the child is 1 year of age and in a small number of children beyond that age. Rubella panencephalitis can be diagnosed by demonstration of rubella-specific IgG and IgM antibody in the CSF. Detection of virus by RT-PCR methods also can be used in reference laboratories.

Treatment

No specific antiviral treatment for CRS exists. Treatment consists of the skillful identification of the child's cardiac, sensory, and neurodevelopmental problems and appropriate referrals for management. Emphasis should be placed on longitudinal assessment of these children, with the goal being early detection and intervention for hearing loss and developmental disabilities. Children with low levels of IgG may be referred to an immunologist and considered for gamma-globulin replacement therapy.

Management of the Pregnant Woman

Exposure of a pregnant woman to rubella virus requires immediate assessment of her immune status. If the exposed woman is known to be immune, she can be reassured of no risk. If her immune status is unknown and she presents for serologic testing as soon as the exposure occurred, the presence of antibody indicates immunity and no risk. If there is no detectable antibody at the time of exposure, further testing should be performed in 3 weeks; if antibody is present in the second specimen, infection is documented. If there is no antibody in the second specimen, a third specimen obtained 6 weeks after exposure should be evaluated for the presence of rubella antibody to see whether infection occurred. If this third specimen is negative, infection did not occur, no further testing is required, and the patient may be reassured. All testing should be performed on all sera simultaneously and in the same laboratory.

Postexposure prophylaxis of the pregnant woman with immune globulin (IG) is not recommended routinely and should be considered only if termination of pregnancy is not an option. The administration of IG, 0.55 mL/kg, may prevent or modify infection, but CRS has been documented in infants born to mothers who received IG after rubella exposure.

If clinical illness is present (i.e., rash), virus isolation should be attempted, and serologic testing should be performed. Seroconversion, a fourfold rise in titer, the presence of rubella-specific IgM antibody, or isolation of virus indicates a primary infection.

RUBELLA PREVENTION

Control Measures

Emphasis should be placed on immunization of children at an appropriate time. Some authorities recommend screening for rubella antibody in all personnel, including health care workers, who may have exposure to rubella-susceptible contacts. If these workers are not immune, they should be immunized.

Patients with acquired rubella should be considered contagious for 7 days after appearance of the rash and should be isolated during this period. Infants with CRS should be considered contagious for the first year of life and isolated from susceptible contacts at high risk, such as women of childbearing age, unless virus cultures of the nasopharynx and urine prove negative. Rubella is a reportable disease, and every effort should be made to diagnose all suspected cases of acquired and congenital rubella and to report them to the appropriate public health agency.

Vaccine Recommendations

The live rubella virus vaccine distributed in United States contains the RA 27/3 strain of rubella virus. Serum antibody is induced in more than 98% of recipients of the vaccine and appears to be lifelong. Rubella vaccine usually is administered in combination with measles and mumps vaccine (MMR) or the newly licensed measles, mumps, rubella, and varicella combination vaccine. The recommended routine childhood vaccination schedule includes a two-dose schedule of a rubella-containing vaccine, administered first at 12 to 15 months of age, followed by a second dose at age 4 to 6 years or at age 11 to 12 years.

Susceptible children who reside in households with pregnant women may be immunized, as may children with minor illness. Adverse reactions to rubella vaccine include rash, fever, and adenopathy 7 to 10 days after receiving the vaccine. Transient arthralgias, most commonly in postpubertal girls and women, also may occur 2 to 3 weeks after vaccination.

Contraindications to Vaccination

Contraindications to rubella vaccine exist in patients with immunodeficiency or immunocompromise. Persons with human immunodeficiency virus infection, however, may be vaccinated. Rubella vaccine should not be given to pregnant women, but it may be given post partum. If vaccine is given inadvertently to a pregnant woman, or if pregnancy occurs within 3 months of immunization, the patient should be reassured and counseled that CRS has not been documented in women who have received rubella vaccine during pregnancy. However, asymptomatic infection has occurred, and, therefore, it presents a theoretic risks to the fetus. Current, detailed recommendations and contraindications regarding rubella immunization and rubella epidemiology may be obtained from the following Web sites: www.aap.org (American Academy of Pediatric) and www.cdc.org (Centers for Disease Control and Prevention).

Suggested Readings

American Academy of Pediatrics. Rubella. In: Pickering L, ed. *Redbook: 2003 report of the Committee on Infectious Diseases,* 26th ed. Elk Grove Village, IL: American Academy of Pediatrics, 2003:536.

Best JM, O'Shea S. Togaviridae: rubella virus. In: Lennette EH, Halonen P, Murphy FA, eds. *Laboratory diagnosis of infectious diseases: principles and practice,* vol 2: *Viral, rickettsial and chlamydial diseases.* New York: Springer-Verlag, 1988:435.

Centers for Disease Control and Prevention. Control and prevention of rubella: evaluation and management of suspected outbreaks, rubella in pregnant women and surveillance for congenital rubella syndrome. *MMWR Morb Mortal Wkly Rep* 2001;50:1.

Centers for Disease Control and Prevention. Measles, mumps and rubella vaccine use and strategies for elimination of measles, rubella and congenital rubella syndrome and control of mumps: recommendations of the Advisory Committee on Immunization Practices (ACIP). *MMWR Morb Mortal Wkly Rep* 1998;47:1.

Cherry JD. Rubella. In Feigin RD, Cherry JD, Demmler GJ, Kaplan SK, eds. *Textbook of pediatric infectious diseases,* 5th ed, vol 2. Philadelphia: WB Saunders, 2004:2134.

Gregg NM. Congenital cataract following German measles in the mother. *Trans Ophthalmol Soc Aust* 1941;3:35.

Wesselhoeft C. Rubella (German measles). *N Engl J Med* 1947;236:943, 978.

CHAPTER 202 ■ MEASLES (RUBEOLA)

ANDREEA C. CAZACU AND GAIL J. DEMMLER

Infection with measles virus produces an illness characterized by a prodrome of fever, coryza, cough, conjunctivitis, an enanthem (Koplik spots), and development of a confluent, erythematous maculopapular rash. The mortality rate associated with measles is approximately 1 in 3,000 cases in the United States. A higher mortality and increased morbidity is seen in young infants, immunocompromised children, and pregnant women. In developing countries, such as Africa, mortality rates of 10% or higher occur in malnourished children who contract measles.

Measles epidemics were described in both the Roman Empire and ancient China. By the seventeenth century, differentiation between measles and smallpox was made, and reports of measles in London and colonial America were described. In the late 1800s, the pathognomonic enanthem of measles was reported in detail by Koplik.

In 1954, Enders and Peebles isolated measles virus in human and simian tissue culture lines. Cultivation of measles virus in chicken embryo tissue enabled vaccine development to proceed. Vaccine trials occurred in the late 1950s and early 1960s, with vaccine licensure in 1963.

ETIOLOGY

Measles virus, which has an internal core of RNA and an outer envelope of glycoproteins and lipids, is a member of the family of Paramyxoviridae, genus Morbillivirus. Two glycoproteins, hemagglutinin (H) and fusion (F), are important in immune protection responses. Immune responses to these two glycoproteins include hemagglutination antibody response in infected individuals (H) and fusion of nucleated cells with formation of multinucleated giant cells (F). Measles virus is monotypic, sensitive to both heat and cold, and inactivated by ultraviolet light.

EPIDEMIOLOGY

Measles is a highly contagious disease and occurs throughout the world as a winter–spring disease in temperate climates. Person-to-person transmission of the measles virus occurs by droplet spread of respiratory secretions with acquisition of infection by the nasopharyngeal route and possibly the conjunctivae. The highest period of infectivity is the catarrhal period before appearance of the exanthem. Person-to-person spread of measles occurs in the home among family members, in medical settings between patients and health care workers, and among students and teachers in day-care centers, schools, colleges, and universities.

In the prevaccine era, highest attack rates were seen in children 5 to 10 years of age, although in urban populations, a higher incidence was observed in preschool-aged children. In developing countries, the highest attack rates occur in children 2 years of age or younger. When the widespread use of measles vaccine began in 1965, the incidence of measles fell remarkably and in 1983 reached an all-time low. In 1986, however, the incidence of measles increased and in 1989 and 1990 reached epidemic proportions in many areas of North America. This increase in incidence of measles was most striking among unvaccinated preschool-aged children, adolescents, and young adults, especially those individuals who were foreign-born. However, vaccine failure, occurring in as many as 5% of individuals who received one dose of measles vaccine, also may have contributed to the observed increase in incidence of measles, and led to current recommendations that children receive two doses of measles vaccine prior to adolescence.

PATHOGENESIS AND PATHOLOGY

Measles virus infection of the nasopharynx respiratory epithelium spreads to regional lymphatics, resulting in viremia. This viremia is enhanced by replication of the virus in the reticuloendothelial system. The respiratory tract, skin, and conjunctivae are major sites of infection, but other organs may be involved. Viral replication peaks in all organs and the blood at approximately the same time that the rash appears, followed by development of immune responses and subsequent curtailment of the illness.

Formation of multinucleate giant cells—the result of cell fusion—characterizes the pathologic response to measles virus infection. These cells are found in the skin, respiratory tract, reticuloendothelial system, and other organs. They contain both intracytoplasmic and intranuclear eosinophilic inclusions.

Immune responses to infection with measles include hemagglutination inhibition (HAI) and production of neutralizing and complement fixing (CF) antibody. In natural infection, antibody responses appear at approximately 14 days and peak several weeks later, with a range of 4 to 6 weeks. The CF antibody appears later than HAI and does not usually persist. The IgM antibody response appears early in the illness, but rarely persists beyond 90 days.

Infected hosts develop cell-mediated immunity and interferon response in the serum. Delayed hypersensitivity responses are suppressed by infection with natural measles virus as well as by vaccine strains. Immunocompromised hosts, especially individuals with T-cell lymphocyte dysfunction, may have a prolonged course with measles, a prolonged duration of excretion of virus, and a high incidence of morbidity and mortality.

CLINICAL MANIFESTATIONS

Persons with measles virus infections fall into four distinct clinical groups: typical measles in the normal host; modified measles in a host with preexisting antibody; atypical measles in the host who received killed vaccine; and measles in immunocompromised, malnourished, or special hosts.

Typical Measles

The incubation period in typical measles is approximately 10 days, starting with a 3- to 5-day prodrome of malaise, fever, cough, coryza, and conjunctivitis. These symptoms increase over the 3- to 5-day prodrome period. Fever ranges from 39.4°C to 40.6°C, reaching its highest at the nadir of exanthem. About 2 days before the rash, Koplik spots (white, pinpoint lesions on a bright red buccal mucosa) appear first opposite the lower molars and quickly spread to involve the entire buccal and lower labial mucosa. Koplik spots resolve by the third day of exanthem. The exanthem of measles starts about the fourteenth day after exposure and appears first behind the ears and the hairline of the forehead. The rash progresses downward to the face, neck, upper extremities, and trunk and reaches the lower extremities by the third day. Initially, the rash is discrete, erythematous, and maculopapular, but it becomes confluent in the same progression as its spread (Fig. 202.1). Eventually the rash undergoes a brownish discoloration that does not blanch with pressure and may desquamate. The exanthem lasts 6 to 7 days, and resolution of the rash proceeds in the same order as that of its appearance. In uncomplicated measles, fever resolves in the first week; increased temperature beyond the third or fourth day of the exanthem suggests a complication.

Pharyngitis as well as generalized adenopathy may be seen during the period of exanthem. Splenomegaly is a common occurance. Diarrhea, vomiting, and abdominal pain may be prominent symptoms of measles, especially in young children. Leukopenia is a predictable finding.

Modified Measles

Modified measles occurs in children who have received immune serum globulin or intravenous immune globulin

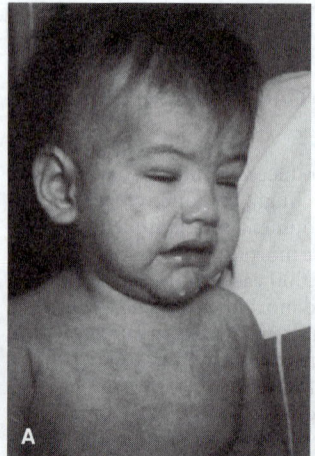
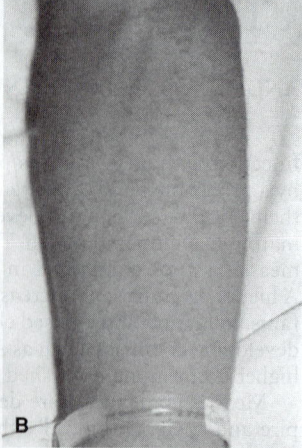

FIGURE 202.1. Maculopapular rash. **A:** Typical measles. (Courtesy of Dr. Gail J. Demmler.) **B:** Atypical measles. See Color Figure 207.1 in color section.

preparations, or in very young infants who still have transplacentally acquired maternal measles antibody. In addition, vaccine-modified mild measles, a form of secondary vaccine failure, can occur in individuals who were appropriately vaccinated with the live measles virus vaccine. In mild or modified measles, the prodrome period is shortened, symptoms are not as severe, and Koplik spots usually do not occur, and if present, they fade rapidly. The exanthem follows the progression of regular measles but appears faint and does not become confluent.

Atypical Measles

Atypical measles is rarely seen today. It occurred in persons immunized with killed measles virus vaccine who were exposed to natural measles. This illness may be observed today in older adults who received killed measles vaccine from 1963 to 1967 and were not reimmunized with live virus vaccine.

The incubation period for atypical measles is the same as for typical measles. The illness is characterized by sudden onset of fever (39.4°C to 40.6°C). Headache, myalgias, extreme weakness, and abdominal pain all may be present. Almost all patients have a dry, nonproductive cough.

The rash of atypical measles appears first on the distal extremities and is pronounced on the wrists and ankles (see Fig. 202.1). The rash may remain localized or spread to involve the upper and lower extremities as well as the trunk. The palms and soles are also involved. The rash of atypical measles typically is erythematous and maculopapular; however, it also may be vesicular, petechial, or purpuric in nature, and urticaria, edema of the hands and feet, and severe hyperesthesia also have been described. Koplik spots are rarely seen.

Pulmonary involvement occurs in almost all patients with atypical measles. Respiratory distress with tachypnea, dyspnea, and cough are prominent symptoms, and pneumonia, hilar adenopathy, and pleural effusions may be seen on chest radiograph. Pulmonary involvement also may occur in the absence of rash in atypical measles.

Measles in the Immunocompromised or Malnourished or Special Host

Measles may be severe or fatal in individuals whose immune system is compromised by chemotherapy, transplantation, human immunodeficiency virus (HIV) or acquired immunodeficiency syndrome (AIDS), or severe malnutrition. Giant cell pneumonia is a common complication of measles in the immunocompromised host. It may occur in the absence of an exanthem and may have an insidious onset or fulminant course. Encephalitis also may occur in these patients and progress with a more insidious, protracted course than in the normal host. Hemorrhagic measles also occurs in hosts with impaired immunity, often with a fatal outcome.

Measles occurring in the pregnant female may lead to pneumonia and increased mortality of the pregnant woman and a fetal effect of prematurity, spontaneous abortion early in pregnancy, or increased incidence of stillbirth. Perinatal measles, which has its onset in the first 10 days of life, is considered to be transplacentally acquired and has a high incidence of pneumonia with resulting mortality.

COMPLICATIONS OF MEASLES

Complications of measles include viral pneumonia, laryngitis, laryngotracheobronchitis, bronchiolitis, and otitis media (Table 202.1). Since differentiating between the patient who

TABLE 202.1

COMPLICATIONS OF MEASLES

Complication	Percent Frequency
Diarrhea	25%
Laryngotracheobronchitis	21%
Otitis media	10%
Pneumonia	5%
Encephalitis	0.1%
Subacute sclerosing panencephalitis	0.0001%

has viral pneumonia associated with measles and the patient who has a superimposed bacterial pneumonia often is difficult, antimicrobial treatment against the bacteria most commonly involved, such as *Streptococcus pneumoniae*, *Staphylococcus aureus*, *Haemophilus influenzae*, and *Streptococcus pyogenes*, should be considered. Other complications of measles include myocarditis, pericarditis, appendicitis, corneal ulcerations, and thrombocytopenic purpura. Hemorrhagic measles, seen frequently in former years, occurs rarely and probably was a result of disseminated intravascular coagulopathy.

Neurologic complications of measles include encephalitis, a rare but serious complication that occurs in approximately 1 of every 1,000 to 2,000 cases of measles. A mortality rate of 15% and morbidity of 25% among survivors has been reported. Encephalitis has its usual onset during the period of the exanthem, but onset during the prodromal period also may occur. Patients present with seizures, cerebral edema, and other neurologic deficits, and the cerebrospinal fluid (CSF) shows usually a mononuclear cell pleocytosis and a slightly elevated protein. The electroencephalogram is abnormal in measles encephalitis but also may be abnormal in the absence of clinically diagnosed encephalitis.

Subacute sclerosing panencephalitis (SSPE) is an uncommon degenerative central nervous system (CNS) disease associated with persistent measles virus infection of the CNS. The risk of development of SSPE is approximately 1 per 100,000 infections with natural measles and 1 per 1 million immunizations in vaccine-associated SSPE. The incubation period is shorter in vaccine-associated SSPE than it is with natural virus. SSPE has an insidious onset with intellectual deterioration, myoclonic jerks, progression to dementia, and finally decorticate rigidity and death. The clinical picture, the typical electroencephalogram, and exceptionally high titers of measles HAI antibody in the serum and CSF are the basis for the diagnosis. Brain tissue for detection of measles virus RNA by polymerase chain reaction (PCR)–based methods should be submitted to the Centers for Disease Control and Prevention (CDC) to determine if SSPE is caused by natural or vaccine-associated measles virus strain.

DIFFERENTIAL DIAGNOSIS

The differential diagnosis includes infections with those viruses that may cause erythematous maculopapular rashes: enteroviruses, adenoviruses, rubella, erythema infectiosum, rickettsial diseases such as Rocky Mountain spotted fever, Kawasaki syndrome, and infectious mononucleosis. Also considered in the diagnosis should be infections with *Mycoplasma pneumoniae* and drug eruptions associated with fever. It is more likely that these illnesses would be confused with the clinical presentation of modified or atypical measles rather than typical measles. In atypical measles, the age of the patient and a history of repeated measles immunizations (killed vaccine may have been administered several times) may help establish the diagnosis.

DIAGNOSIS

Isolation of measles virus may be attempted because commercially available reagents now allow many viral diagnostic laboratories to isolate and identify the measles virus in cell culture. The best specimens for isolation of measles are nasopharyngeal washes or swabs and urine sediment. The virus also may be isolated from peripheral blood lymphocytes and conjunctivae early in the course of illness and from tissue obtained from biopsy procedures. Clinicians should alert the laboratory and health department that measles is suspected and ensure that the specimens are transported promptly to the virology laboratory for maximum isolation rates.

The serologic diagnosis of measles also may be made. The HAI test has been widely performed, and many laboratories currently use the enzyme-linked immunosorbent assay (ELISA) technique. Antibodies usually are present in the patient's serum by day 1 to 3 of the exanthem and peak 2 to 6 weeks later. A patient with suspected measles, either in the prodromal period or with rash, should have a serum obtained immediately, followed by collection of a convalescent, paired serum specimen in 2 to 3 weeks. Both sera should be evaluated simultaneously in the same laboratory to determine the presence of antibody. A seroconversion or fourfold or greater rise in the antibody titer or the presence of IgM antibody in either serum as determined by ELISA confirms a serologic diagnosis of measles. In atypical measles, a patient's sera may have extremely high titers of HAI antibody. This also occurs in patients with SSPE, in whom HAI antibody also is found in the CSF.

Immunofluorescent studies have been performed on exfoliated cells and tissue from different organs to detect measles virus antigen. A paramyxovirus viral particle may be observed by using electron microscopy in lung tissue of patients with giant cell pneumonia. Molecular methods that employ reverse transcription PCR techniques are available also for detection of measles virus RNA in clinical samples.

THERAPY

No specific approved antiviral therapy for measles virus infection is available. Fever should be controlled with acetaminophen or ibuprofen, and room air should be humidified. Older children may complain of photophobia and prefer darkened rooms. Careful attention should be given to fluid intake, particularly in young infants who are commonly dehydrated. Antibiotics should be given for bacterial complications. Children with very serious complications of measles (e.g., pneumonia, encephalitis, croup) should be hospitalized and treated with fluids and respiratory support. Aerosolized or intravenous ribavirin has been used on a compassionate basis to treat measles pneumonia, although its effectiveness has not been rigorously evaluated in clinical trials. Treatment with vitamin A appears to decrease morbidity and mortality rates in children who contract measles in developing countries. Most experts also recommend supplementation and treatment with vitamin A in children 6 to 24 months of age who are hospitalized with measles or its complications, or in those younger infants who have underlying intestinal malabsorption, malnutrition, or recent immigration from areas of high measles mortality. Recommended doses include a single dose of 200,000 IU for children older than 1 year of age and 100,000 IU for younger infants. The dose may be repeated in 1 day, and in 1 month in patients with severe vitamin A deficiency.

Airborne precautions are recommended to prevent exposure to susceptible individuals. Children with measles are still considered contagious for 5 days after appearance of the rash, and immunocompromised persons with measles may be contagious longer and should be isolated for the duration of their illness.

MEASLES PREVENTION

General Considerations

Prevention of measles in the general population is possible by maintaining a high level of immunization among children aged 15 months or older. Many physicians have not seen a patient with measles and, therefore, must have a high index of suspicion when confronted with a patient with fever and a maculopapular exanthem. A suspected case of measles should be reported immediately to public health authorities, then confirmed serologically and virologically. Health care workers or students entering colleges or universities should furnish proof of immunization or be screened to determine their immunity to measles, and, unless contraindicated, nonimmune persons should be immunized.

Despite the availability of a safe and effective vaccine, measles-susceptible persons of all age groups are found in the United States, for many different reasons. Many parents delay immunization of children until they enter school, at which time immunization is required by law. Therefore, a number of children 15 months to 5 years of age are not immune. Children younger than 15 months of age may have no maternal antibody and, consequently, are susceptible to measles infection. Adults born after 1956 may never have been immunized or have had natural measles, and thus, are susceptible to infection. Persons immunized before 1977 may have been immunized at 12 months of age or younger and may no longer be immune. Persons who were immunized with killed virus vaccine (1963 to 1967) may not have been reimmunized with attenuated vaccine. Other reasons for nonimmune persons include vaccine failure (less than 5% of all persons who receive the measles vaccine) and immunization with unknown vaccine between 1963 and 1967. Persons who were immunized with attenuated live virus vaccine (other than Edmonston B) and who received immune globulin along with the vaccine may not be immune. Improperly stored measles vaccine also may fail to provide adequate protection. Therefore, since 1980, a stabilizer has been added to the vaccine preparation, making it more resistant to inactivation by heat, and education efforts have emphasized proper handling and storage of the vaccine. Persons immunized before 1980 may have received improperly handled vaccine, which could be ineffective in producing an immune response.

Vaccine Recommendations

All persons born after 1956 and who have no documentation of having received adequate measles immunization or of having had natural measles infection documented by physician diagnosis or serologic testing and who do not have a contraindication for measles vaccine should be immunized. Currently, a two-dose schedule, using a combined measles-mumps-rubella (MMR) vaccine, or the newly licensed quadrivalent measles-mumps-rubella-varicella (MMRV) vaccine is recommended for children. The first dose of measles-containing vaccine should be administered between 12 and 15 months of age. However, during epidemics, a first dose of monovalent measles vaccine should be given at age 6 months to provide early protection, followed by a routine MMR vaccine at 15 months of age. The second dose of measles vaccine or MMR may be administered at age 4 to 6 years or at age 11 to 12 years. Only constant vigilance controls measles. Physicians caring for children and adolescents should monitor measles epidemiology continuously in their area and comply with the recommendations of local public health officials. Updated information may be obtained from www.aap.org and www.cdc.org.

Vaccine Contraindications

Contraindications to measles vaccine include pregnancy, anaphylaxis to egg or neomycin, severely compromised immunity, or receipt of immune globulin within 3 months. MMR vaccine is recommended for all asymptomatic HIV-infected persons who are not severely immunosuppressed and who lack evidence of measles immunity. MMR vaccination of symptomatic HIV-infected persons should be considered if they (a) do not have evidence of severe immunosuppression and (b) lack evidence of measles immunity. A personal and family history of seizures should be evaluated on a case-by-case basis. Tuberculosis is not a contraindication for administration of measles vaccine.

Adverse Vaccine Reactions

As many as 15% of vaccines may have fever 5 to 12 days after vaccination, and may be accompanied by febrile seizures. Fever usually lasts 1 to 5 days. A small number of vaccinees develop a transient rash or thrombocytopenia. The frequency of neurologic disease and encephalopathy associated with administration of measles vaccine occurs with an estimated frequency of 1 per 3 million doses of vaccine. Epidemiologic studies do not support the concept that measles vaccine causes autism or inflammatory bowel disease.

PREVENTION FOR EXPOSED INDIVIDUALS

If given in the first 72 hours after exposure, live measles virus vaccine may prevent infection. Immune globulin may be given to prevent or modify illness in exposed individuals if given within 6 days of exposure. The recommended dose is 0.25 mL/kg (maximum dose is 15 mL). Immunocompromised children should receive 0.5 mL/kg with a maximum of 15 mL. Children with symptomatic HIV infection should receive immune globulin at the time of exposure regardless of vaccination status. Intravenous immune globulin preparations also contain antibody to measles virus. Immune globulin administra-

tion precludes vaccination for 3 months in children in whom there is otherwise no contraindication.

For detailed recommendations or contraindications for vaccine administration and passive immunoprophylaxis, the reader is referred to the *Report of the Committee on Infectious Diseases* (*Red Book*), 2003, 26th edition.

Suggested Readings

American Academy of Pediatrics. Measles. In: Pickering L. ed. *Report of the Committee on Infectious Diseases,* 26th ed. Elk Grove Village, IL: American Academy of Pediatrics, 2004:419.

Centers for Disease Control and Prevention. Status report on the childhood immunization initiative: United States, 1996. *MMWR Morb Mortal Wkly Rep* 1997;40:665.

Cherry JD. Measles. In: Feigin RD, Cherry JD, Demmler GJ, Kaplan SL, eds. *Textbook of pediatric infectious diseases,* 5th ed, vol 2. Philadelphia: Saunders, 2004:2283.

Dales L, Hammer SJ, Smith NJ. Time trends in autism and in MMR immunization coverage in California. *JAMA* 2001;285:1183.

Davis RL, Kramarz P, Bohlke K, et al. Measles-mumps-rubella and other measles-containing vaccines do not increase the risk for inflammatory bowel disease: a case-controlled study from the Vaccine Safety Datalink Project. *Arch Pediatr Adolesc Med* 2001;155:354.

Edmonson MB, Addiss DG, McPherson JT, et al. Mild measles and secondary vaccine failure during a sustained outbreak in a highly vaccinated population. *JAMA* 1990;263:2467.

Fulginiti VA, Eller JJ, Downie AW, et al. Altered reactivity to measles virus: atypical measles in children previously immunized with inactivated measles virus vaccine. *JAMA* 1967;202:1075.

Gindler JS, Atkinson WL, Markowitz LE, et al. Epidemiology of measles in the United States in 1989 and 1990. *Pediatr Infect Dis J* 1992;11:841.

Hussey GD, Klein M. A randomized, controlled trial of vitamin A in children with severe measles. *N Engl J Med* 1990;323:160.

Immunization Practices Advisory Committee. Measles prevention. *MMWR Morb Mortal Wkly Rep* 1989;38:11.

Katz SL. Measles (rubeola). In: Gershon AA, Hotez PJ, Katz SL, eds. *Krugman's infectious diseases of children,* 11th ed. St. Louis: Mosby, 2004:353.

Katz S, Krugman S, Quinn T, eds. Proceedings of the international symposium on measles immunization. Pan American Health Association, Washington, D.C., March 16–19, 1982. *Rev Infect Dis* 1983;5:389.

Koplik H. The diagnosis of the invasion of measles from a study of the exanthema as it appears on the buccal mucous membrane. *Arch Pediatr* 1986;13:918.

Littauer J, Sorensen K. The measles epidemic at Umanak in Greenland in 1962. *Dan Med Bull* 1965;12:43.

Measles—Los Angeles County, California, 1988. *MMWR Morb Mortal Wkly Rep* 1989;38:49.

Minnich LL, Goodenough F, Ray G. Use of immunofluorescence to identify measles virus infections. *J Clin Microbiol* 1991;29:1148.

Moench TR, Griffin DE, Obriecht CR, et al. Acute measles in patients with and without neurological involvement: distribution of measles virus antigen and RNA. *J Infect Dis* 1988;158:433.

Norrby E. Paramyxoviridae: measles virus. In: Lennette EH, Halonen P, Murphy FA, eds. *Laboratory diagnosis of infectious diseases: principles and practice. Vol 2: Viral, rickettsial, and chlamydial diseases.* New York: Springer-Verlag, 1988:525.

CHAPTER 203 ■ MUMPS

ANDREEA C. CAZACU AND GAIL J. DEMMLER

Mumps is a contagious disease characterized by swelling of the salivary glands, particularly the parotid glands. Inapparent infections may occur in 40% of infected individuals. In 1934, experiments by Johnson and Goodpasture demonstrated a mumps-like illness in rhesus monkeys receiving parotid secretions from patients with mumps. Filtered parotid secretions

from infected monkeys could be passed to other monkeys with resulting parotitis from a filterable agent, a virus.

Mumps virus subsequently was propagated in eggs, which allowed production of mumps antigen for a complement fixation test. Attenuation of the virus *in vitro* was accomplished by Enders in the 1940s; this accomplishment proved useful for vaccine development, and a vaccine was prepared and licensed in 1968.

ETIOLOGY

Mumps is a single-stranded RNA virus and a member of the family *Paramyxoviridae*, genus *Paramyxovirus*. It has two major surface glycoproteins: the hemagglutinin-neuraminidase and the fusion protein. Mumps virus is sensitive to heat and ultraviolet light.

EPIDEMIOLOGY

Mumps is transmitted by direct contact or infected droplets from the oropharynx. Communicability is present before parotid swelling occurs (1 to 7 days, but usually 1 to 2 days) and 7 to 9 days after onset of parotid swelling. The incubation period of mumps is approximately 18 days, but may be longer. Mumps occurs in winter and spring seasons and had its highest attack rates in 5- to 9-year-old children in the prevaccine era. Ascertaining the epidemiologic features of mumps is difficult because of the high incidence of inapparent infections and a common incidence of parotitis caused by other pathogens.

PATHOGENESIS AND PATHOLOGY

Mumps virus produces a generalized infection. After entry into the oropharynx, viral replication takes place, causing subsequent viremia and involvement of the glands or nervous tissue. The virus may be isolated from saliva, blood, urine, and cerebrospinal fluid (CSF). Affected glands show edema and lymphocyte infiltration.

CLINICAL MANIFESTATIONS

Parotitis

The classic illness of mumps is swelling of the parotid gland (i.e., parotitis). Systemic symptoms include low-grade fever, headaches, malaise, anorexia, and abdominal pain. Acid-containing foods may aggravate discomfort of the parotid gland. Ordinarily, the parotid gland is not palpable, but in mumps cases, it rapidly progresses to maximum swelling over several days. Unilateral swelling usually occurs first, followed by bilateral parotid involvement. Occasionally, simultaneous involvement of both parotid glands occurs. Unilateral parotid disease occurs in fewer than 25% of patients. Fever subsides within 1 week and disappears before swelling of the parotid glands resolves, which may require as long as 10 days. Other salivary glands may be involved, including both submaxillary and sublingual, and orifices of the ducts may be erythematous and edematous (Table 203.1).

Orchitis and Oophoritis

About one-third of postpubertal males develop unilateral orchitis. It usually follows parotitis within 1 week but may precede it or occur in the absence of it. Bilateral orchitis occurs much less frequently, and although gonadal atrophy may follow orchitis, sterility is rare, even with bilateral involvement. Prepubertal boys also may develop orchitis, but it is uncommon in those younger than 10 years. Orchitis is accompanied by high fever, severe pain, and swelling. Nausea, vomiting, and

TABLE 203.1

COMMON CLINICAL MANIFESTATIONS AND COMPLICATIONS ASSOCIATED WITH MUMPS

Clinical Manifestations	Complications
Salivary gland swelling	Gonadal involvement
Parotid	Orchitis
Others	Oophoritic
Fever	Gonadal atrophy
Malaise	Sterility
Abdominal pain	Meningoencephalitis
Inapparent infection (40%)	Peripheral neuritis
	Auditory nerve (deafness)
	Facial nerve (facial paralysis)
	Myocarditis
	Arthritis
	Hematologic abnormalities

abdominal pain are also common findings. Fever and gonadal swelling usually resolve in 1 week, but tenderness may persist.

Oophoritis in females is an uncommon finding and occurs in approximately 7% of infected females. It can be suspected if abdominal or pelvic pain occurs in a girl or woman with mumps.

Meningoencephalitis

Central nervous system (CNS) involvement with mumps may occur and more often is an aseptic meningitis than a true encephalitis. It may precede development of parotitis or appear in the absence of parotitis, but usually it occurs in the first week after parotitis develops. Headache, fever, nausea, vomiting, and meningismus are common. Marked changes in sensorium and seizures also may occur.

Pleocytosis of the CSF occurs commonly in mumps, even in the absence of clinical meningitis. The CSF may have a mononuclear pleocytosis, with a normal or low level of glucose, and usually a normal level of protein. Mumps virus may be isolated from CSF early in the illness. Mumps meningoencephalitis carries a good prognosis and usually is associated with an uneventful recovery.

Other clinical manifestations of mumps include pancreatitis accompanied by severe abdominal pain, chills, fever, and persistent vomiting. Thyroiditis, oophoritis, and mastitis occasionally occur.

COMPLICATIONS OF MUMPS

Neuritis of the auditory nerve may result in deafness. There is sudden onset of tinnitus, ataxia, and vomiting followed by permanent deafness. Other neurologic complications include facial nerve neuritis and myelitis. Less common complications include arthritis, myocarditis, and hematologic complications. Sterility has been rarely reported if bilateral postinfectious gonadal atrophy occurs.

DIFFERENTIAL DIAGNOSIS

Parotitis caused by other viruses—enteroviruses such as coxsackievirus, influenza, and parainfluenza viruses, cytomegalovirus, human immunodeficiency virus, and lymphocytic choriomeningitis virus—cannot be differentiated clinically from mumps parotitis. Suppurative parotitis and preauricular adenitis may mimic mumps, and these infections are commonly caused by *Staphylococcus aureus* or atypical mycobacteria or other bacteria. However, clinically the parotid gland is very tender and the overlaying skin is erythematous. Spontaneous drainage through sinus tract formation also may occur in suppurative adenitis and parotitis.

Adenitis, recurrent parotitis, calculus of Stensen duct, tumors of the parotid gland, and Mikulicz syndrome may be considered in the differential diagnosis of mumps.

Mumps meningoencephalitis is similar clinically to aseptic meningitis caused by common viruses such as the enteroviruses. However, it may be differentiated by CSF viral culture or detection of the virus by polymerase chain reaction–based methods.

DIAGNOSIS

The diagnosis of mumps usually is made clinically; however, laboratory confirmation can be helpful, especially in patients with unusual manifestations. The serum amylase level is often elevated when there is salivary gland or pancreatic involvement, and isoenzyme analysis can be performed to distinguish between these two sites of infection. The serologic diagnosis of mumps may be made by testing paired sera for mumps IgG antibody obtained early in illness and 2 to 4 weeks after illness. The diagnosis of mumps also can be made from a single serum specimen if the presence of mumps IgM antibody is detected. Most clinical virology laboratories perform mumps serology using enzyme immunoassay (EIA). In addition, the presence of complement fixing antibody (CF) to the soluble (S) component of the mumps virus suggests a recent infection, within the last 6 months. Mumps virus can be grown from saliva or swabs of material expressed directly from Stensen duct, as well as from urine and CSF. Obtaining viral cultures is encouraged because isolation of the virus confirms the diagnosis. Clinicians collecting specimens for isolation of mumps virus should alert the virology laboratory that mumps virus is suspected and transport the specimens promptly on wet ice.

TREATMENT

There is no specific antiviral agent available to treat mumps infection or its complications. However supportive treatment for fever or pain is indicated if severe symptoms are present. Testicular swelling and pain may be relieved with gentle support of the testicle and ice packs. Management of mumps aseptic meningoencephalitis is similar to that for other forms of aseptic meningitis associated with common viruses.

PREVENTION OF MUMPS

All children should receive two doses of mumps-containing vaccine; their first dose of mumps vaccine may be part of the combination measles-mumps-rubella (MMR) vaccine administered at 12 to 15 months of age, and the second dose may be administered at 4 to 6 years of age or between 11 and 12 years of age. Mumps vaccine also is a component of the new quadrivalent measles, mumps, rubella, and varicella (MMRV) combination vaccine. Individuals born before 1957 are likely immune to mumps as a result of natural infection. Adverse reactions attributed to mumps vaccination are exceedingly uncommon. For detailed, current recommendations and contraindications for administration of mumps vaccine, refer to www.aap.org and www.cdc.org.

Suggested Readings

American Academy of Pediatrics. Rubella. In: Pickering L, ed. *Report of the Committee on Infectious Diseases*, 26th ed., Elk Grove Village, IL: American Academy of Pediatrics, 2003:439.

Centers for Disease Control. Measles, mumps and rubella—vaccine use and strategies for elimination of measles, rubella and congenital rubella syndrome and control of mumps: recommendations of the Advisory Committee on Immunization Practices (ACIP). *MMWR Morb Mortal Wkly Rep* 1998;47:1.

Cherry JD. Mumps. In: Feigin RD, Cherry JD, Demmler G, Kaplan S, eds. *Textbook of pediatric infectious diseases*, 5th ed., Vol. 2. Philadelphia: WB Saunders, 2004:2305.

Gershon AA. Mumps (epidemic parotitis). In: Gershon AA, Hotez PJ, Katz SL, eds. *Krugman's infectious diseases of children*, 11th ed. St. Louis: Mosby, 2004;391.

Orvell C. Paramyxoviridae: mumps virus. In: Lennette EH, Halonen P, Murphy FA, eds. *Laboratory diagnosis of infectious diseases: principles and practice. Vol 2. Viral rickettsial and chlamydial diseases.* New York: Springer-Verlag, 1988:507.

Wharton M, Cochi SL, Hutcheson RH, et al. A large outbreak of mumps in the postvaccine era. *J Infect Dis* 1988;158:1253.

CHAPTER 204 ■ POLYOMAVIRUSES

JOHN A. VANCHIERE AND GAIL J. DEMMLER

Polyomaviruses are small DNA viruses that infect most humans, persist for life, and rarely cause disease. In patients who are severely immunosuppressed, however, polyomaviruses can produce serious illness of the central nervous system (CNS) or urinary tract. The polyomaviruses that infect humans include JC virus (JCV), BK virus (BKV), and simian virus 40 (SV40). Polyomaviruses, especially SV40, are named for their ability to cause tumors in laboratory animals, and they have been increasingly identified in human tumors, including tumors of the CNS, mesotheliomas, osteosarcomas, and lymphomas. In humans, these viruses are neurotropic, nephrotropic, and lymphotropic, with each virus having different affinities for each of these target organs.

JC VIRUS

Progressive multifocal leukoencephalopathy (PML) is a rare, demyelinating disease of the CNS seen in hosts who are immunosuppressed, most commonly in patients with acquired immunodeficiency syndrome (AIDS). The causative agent—JCV—first was isolated in fetal glial cell culture in 1971 from the brain homogenate of a patient (initials, JC) with fatal PML. Although PML is a rare, opportunistic disease, infection with JCV is a common occurance in childhood, especially in school-aged children; 65% of 14-year-old children have antibody to the virus. JCV usually causes few or no symptoms, although it has been associated with mild respiratory illness. The virus can reactivate and be detected in the urine of normal pregnant women, renal and bone marrow transplant recipients, and children and adults with malignancies.

Pathology

The histopathologic changes seen in the brains of patients with PML consist of multiple areas of gross demyelination, enlarged hyperchromatic nuclei of the oligodendrocytes, and proliferation of bizarre-appearing astrocytes. Neurons are typically unaffected. Electron microscopy reveals large numbers of polyomavirus particles in the nuclei of oligodendrocytes, and viral antigen can be identified by immunofluorescence. While viral DNA can be detected easily by DNA hybridization assays and polymerase chain reaction (PCR), a striking lack of inflammatory response is evident in the brains of patients with PML. This disparate finding is not surprising given the profound T-cell immune suppression that predisposes patients to PML.

Clinical Manifestations

The diagnosis of PML should be considered in any immuno-compromised host who develops a progressive, multifocal neurologic illness. Among adult patients with AIDS, PML has an incidence of nearly 5%, but it is much less common in children. PML often begins with personality and behavioral changes, altered mental status, hemiparesis, ataxia, aphasia, or cortical blindness and progresses to coma over a period of weeks to months. Death usually results in 2 to 4 months, although some patients have lived for 1 to 2 years. Paradoxically, the cerebrospinal fluid is often normal. The electroencephalogram shows diffuse and nonspecific slowing. Computed tomography (CT) of the brain reveals areas of demyelination.

Diagnosis

The diagnosis of PML may be suggested clinically in any immunocompromised patient who develops multifocal brain disease. Other neurodegenerative diseases of known or presumed viral etiology include multiple sclerosis, subacute sclerosing panencephalitis, herpesvirus infections of the CNS, and AIDS. A tentative diagnosis of PML can be made if CT or magnetic resonance imaging (MRI) shows areas of decreased density in the white matter areas of the brain.

Definitive diagnosis of PML is made by brain biopsy or by examination at autopsy. The unique histopathology usually establishes the diagnosis. Polyomavirus particles are demonstrated frequently in oligodendrocytes by electron microscopy, and JCV antigens may be detected in the brain by immunofluorescence. Given its high sensitivity and specificity, the detection of JCV DNA in spinal fluid by PCR has become the noninvasive assay of choice for diagnosis of PML in the appropriate clinical setting.

Therapy

Prompt restoration of T-cell immune function is required to slow the progression of PML. The disease usually is fatal within 6 months of diagnosis, although spontaneous remissions have been reported. For some patients with AIDS, highly active antiretroviral therapy (HAART) has been beneficial in halting the progression of PML. In patients receiving iatrogenic immunosuppression, immunosuppressive regimens should be reduced or discontinued, if possible. At present, there are no antiviral agents approved for the treatment of PML; however, anecdotal reports describing low-dose cidofovir have recently been reported, and other antiviral agents may available on an experimental basis in the near future.

BK VIRUS

BK virus first was isolated from the urine of a 39-year-old man (initials, BK) with allograft failure 4 months after undergoing renal transplantation. Infection with BKV occurs commonly in early childhood and may be asymptomatic or associated with a viral respiratory illness. Most children (90% to 100%) have antibody to BKV by age 10 years. BKV has been implicated also as a cause of viral cystitis in normal children and interstitial nephritis in an immunocompromised child. Normal pregnant women also may excrete BKV (and JCV) in their urine, but no conclusive evidence corroborates vertical transmission from mother to infant. The BKV rarely causes PML-like disease and, like JCV and SV40, BKV has been associated with some human CNS tumors.

Clinical Manifestations

Disease due to BKV is seen most commonly in renal transplant recipients, either due to reactivation of persistent BKV in the recipient or infection from the donor organ. Up to 40% of renal transplant recipients excrete BKV in their urine, and BKV-associated nephropathy (BKVN) has emerged as an important cause of graft dysfunction or loss. Ureteral stenosis in renal transplant recipients also has been associated with BKV, and hemorrhagic cystitis is a common, late manifestation of BKV in bone marrow transplant recipients.

Diagnosis

BKV replication in the urinary tract can be suspected by the presence of cytologically atypical cells called "decoy cells" in the urinary sediment. Virions can be detected by electron microscopy, and viral antigen in infected cell nuclei can be detected by immunofluorescence. PCR-based assays can detect and quantitate BKV DNA sequences in urine and blood plasma. Because BKV may be shed asymptomatically in the urine, a biopsy of the kidney, ureter, bladder, or other organ suspected to be involved showing documentation of BKV DNA by *in situ* hybridization may be necessary to support a pathogenic role.

Therapy

Recognized BKV infection is associated most commonly with T-cell immune deficiency or iatrogenic immunosuppression. Therefore, therapeutic efforts should focus on careful reduction or withdrawal of immunosuppression, if feasible. At present, no antiviral agents are approved for treatment of diseases associated with BKV infection, but controlled clinical trials are in progress because anecdotal reports suggest cidofovir, leflunomide, and ciprofloxacin may inhibit BKV replication and benefit selected patients.

SIMIAN VIRUS 40

SV40 is a polyomavirus virus of rhesus macaque origin that was introduced accidentally into the human population as a contaminant of poliovirus and adenovirus vaccines used between 1955 and 1963. Recent molecular and serologic studies suggest that SV40 may now be circulating in humans. Its mode of transmission is unknown, although it is excreted in the urine of some healthy and immune-compromised children and adults who could not have received contaminated vaccines. SV40 has been found in numerous human tumors, including ependymomas, choroid plexus carcinomas, lymphomas, mesotheliomas, and osteosarcomas. SV40 also has been found in the brain tissue of a patient with PML and in the urine of some patients with nephropathy after organ transplantation. Its spectrum of disease has not been fully elucidated, and little is known of the long-term sequelae of SV40 infection.

Suggested Readings

Erard V, Kim HW, Corey L, et al. BK DNA viral load in plasma: evidence for and association with hemorrhagic cystitis in allogeneic hematopoietic cell transplant recipients. *Blood* 2005;106:1130.

Farasati NA, Vats A, Shapiro R. Monitoring for polyomavirus BK and JC in urine: comparison of qualitative polymerase chain reaction with urine cytology. *Transplantation* 2005;79:984.

Hirsch HH, Steiger J. Polyomavirus BK. *Lancet Infect Dis* 2003;3:611.

Imperiale MJ. The human polyomaviruses, BKV and JCV: molecular pathogenesis of acute disease and potential role in cancer. *Virology* 2000;267:1.

Leung AY, Chan MT, Yuen KY, et al. Ciprofloxacin decreased polyoma BK virus load in patients who underwent allogeneic hematopoietic stem cell transplantation. *Clin Infect Dis* 2005;40:528.

Randhawa P, Vats A, Shapiro R. Monitoring for polyomavirus BK and JC in urine: comparison of quantitative polymerase chain reaction with urine cytology. *Transplantation* 2005;79:984.

Safak M, Khalili K. An overview: human polyomavirus JC virus and its associated disorders. *J Neurovirol* 2003;9:3.

Seth P, Diaz F, Major EO. Advances in the biology of JC virus and induction of progressive multifocal leukoencephalopathy. *J Neurovirol* 2003;9:236.

Smith JM, McDonald RA, Finn LS, et al. Polyomavirus nephropathy in pediatric kidney transplant recipients. *Am J Transplant* 2004;4:2109.

Vanchiere JA, Demmler GJ. Human polyomaviruses and papillomaviruses. In: Feigin R.Cherry J, Demmler G, Kaplan S, eds. *Textbook of pediatric infectious diseases*. Philadelphia: WB Saunders, 2004:1809.

Vilchez RA, Kozinetz CA, Arrington AS, et al. Simian virus 40 in human cancers. *Am J Med* 2003;114:675.

CHAPTER 205 ■ RETROVIRUSES

MARK W. KLINE AND RALPH D. FEIGIN

The known human retroviruses include human T-cell lymphotropic virus (HTLV) types I and II and human immunodeficiency virus (HIV) types 1 (formerly HTLV-III) and 2. Retroviruses possess a single-stranded RNA genome. A virus-encoded enzyme known as *reverse transcriptase* catalyzes the transcription of viral RNA into proviral DNA, which then integrates into the host cell genome. This characteristic is linked etiologically to several lymphoproliferative, immunosuppressive, and degenerative disorders. Although these disorders have been studied best in adult populations, clinically important pediatric diseases can result from retroviral infection.

ETIOLOGIC AGENTS AND PATHOGENESIS

All the human retroviruses belong to a single viral family, the *Retroviridae*. HTLV-I and HTLV-II belong to a subfamily known as the *oncornaviruses*, and HIV-1 and HIV-2 belong to the lentivirus subfamily. One other subfamily, the spumaviruses, includes human foamy virus, an agent with no known pathogenicity for humans.

The various retrovirus subfamilies have distinct *in vitro* and *in vivo* characteristics. Oncornaviruses transform cells in culture and can produce tumors in animals. Lentiviruses produce syncytia and cytopathic effects in cell culture and cause slowly progressive infections in the host. The spumaviruses induce vacuolization of cells in culture and do not cause apparent adverse effects in the host.

Human retroviruses have a peculiar tropism for lymphocytes. In the case of HIV, this tropism results from the high affinity of the viral envelope protein for the CD4 molecule on the surface of helper-inducer T lymphocytes. In addition to T lymphocytes, a variety of cells, including monocytes, macrophages, and microglial cells of the central nervous system (CNS), express the CD4 molecule. The hallmark of HIV infection is progressive loss of $CD4^+$ T lymphocytes with inexorable diminution of immune function. The frequent occurrence of nervous system disease in individuals infected with HIV may be attributable in part to the introduction of virus into the CNS via infected monocytes and macrophages.

HTLV-I induces expression of interleukin-2 receptors on $CD4^+$ T lymphocytes. The presence of excessive receptors for interleukin-2, a recognized T-cell growth factor, may help to explain the lymphoproliferation observed in some individuals infected with HTLV-I. Both HTLV-I and HTLV-II can cause *in vitro* proliferation of normal lymphocytes in the absence of exogenous antigens.

This chapter focuses on the epidemiology and clinical features of infection caused by HTLV-I and HTLV-II. For a thorough discussion of pediatric HIV infection and acquired immune deficiency syndrome, the reader is referred to Chapter 139.

EPIDEMIOLOGY

Seroepidemiologic studies of HTLV-I and HTLV-II have been hampered by the inability of screening antibody tests to differentiate between infections with the two viruses. HTLV-I infection appears to be most prevalent in southern Japan and the Caribbean basin. Other foci of infection include parts of Africa and Central and South America. The geographic distribution of HTLV-II is unknown. The prevalence of HTLV infection (types I and II) among U.S. blood donors is approximately 2 per 10,000.

Both HTLV-I and HTLV-II are highly cell associated, and transmission of either virus is thought to require passage of infected lymphocytes rather than of cell-free body fluids. Consequently, the efficiency of transmission of these viruses is thought to be less than that of HIV. The modes of transmission of HTLV-I are identical to those of HIV-1, including sexual activity, transfusion of infected cellular blood products, and breast-feeding. Perinatal transmission has been documented by detection of HTLV-I in cord blood. HTLV-II has been found predominantly among injecting-drug users and their sexual partners; infection has been documented also in some non-drug-using Native American populations. Preliminary data suggest that mother-to-infant transmission of the virus occurs infrequently.

CLINICAL MANIFESTATIONS

Individuals infected with HTLV-I have a lifetime risk of approximately 5% to 10% for development of adult T-cell leukemia-lymphoma (ATLL) or myelopathy/tropical spastic paraparesis (TSP). ATLL may result from HTLV-I infection acquired during the first few years of life—with a long period of latency averaging several decades—and the ultimate development of clinically evident disease, usually in middle age. Cases of ATLL attributable to blood transfusion have not been reported.

Clinical features of ATLL result from a malignant proliferation of mature T cells infected with HTLV-I. The disease course may be either indolent or fulminant. The most common findings at presentation include lymphadenopathy, hepatosplenomegaly, and polymorphous skin lesions. Leukocytosis may be present. The diagnosis of ATLL is suggested by the presence in the peripheral blood of abnormal lymphocytes with indented nuclei, but they are not identified in every case. Hypercalcemia and lytic bone lesions are found in most individuals with fulminant disease. Opportunistic infections occur commonly in individuals with ATLL. The spectrum of infectious agents observed is similar to that seen in the acquired immune deficiency syndrome caused by HIV-1.

Like that in ATLL, the clinical onset of HTLV-I–associated myelopathy/TSP typically occurs during middle age. The disease has been reported (rarely) in children as young as 5 to 10 years. The onset of myelopathy after receipt of a blood transfusion has been reported, with a mean latent period of approximately 2 years. The typical presentation of HTLV-I–associated myelopathy/TSP includes slowly progressive spastic weakness of the lower extremities, sometimes associated with numbness or dysesthesia. Physical examination reveals hyperreflexia. Abnormal lymphocytes similar to those seen in ATLL may be found in the peripheral blood or cerebrospinal fluid.

One other condition—the infective dermatitis syndrome—has been linked to HTLV-I infection. Typically, affected individuals have been young children with severe exudative eczema, chronic rhinitis, and recurrent infections. Mothers of several of these patients have been found to be HTLV-I-positive, and several of the children have developed ATLL during adolescence.

Initially, HTLV-II was isolated from a patient with a T-cell variant of hairy cell leukemia, but the association of the virus with that or any other disease is unclear. Adults with HTLV-II infection appear to be at increased risk for development of a variety of minor or more serious infections, including pneumonia, urinary tract infection, and tuberculosis.

DIAGNOSIS AND TREATMENT

The diagnosis of ATLL or HTLV-I–associated myelopathy/TSP is suggested by compatible clinical findings in a patient from a population with endemic HTLV-I infection. Serologic tests for HTLV-I, including enzyme immunoassay and Western blot assay, also detect cross-reacting anti–HTLV-II antibodies. Therefore, seropositive individuals are called *HTLV-positive* and not *HTLV-I-positive*. Further discrimination between HTLV-I and HTLV-II infections requires additional testing with newer assays, such as polymerase chain reaction or HTLV type-specific peptide serologic assays. Serologic tests for HTLV do not cross-react with those for HIV. The efficacy of antiretroviral agents for treatment of HTLV-I–associated disease remains to be defined.

Suggested Readings

Maloney EM, Wiktor SZ, Palmer P, et al. A cohort study of health effects of human T-cell lymphotropic virus type-I infection in Jamaican children. *Pediatrics* 2003;112:e136.
Poiesz BJ, Poiesz MJ, Choi D. The human T-cell lymphoma/leukemia viruses. *Cancer Invest* 2003;21:253.

CHAPTER 206 ■ SMALLPOX

JULIA A. McMILLAN

Smallpox is the human disease caused by variola virus, a member of the genus *Orthopoxvirus* in the Poxviridae family. Other members of the genus include monkeypox, cowpox, rabbitpox, and vaccinia, the virus used for immunization against smallpox. Humans are the only natural hosts for variola, a fact that made possible the eradication of smallpox through a worldwide vaccination effort during the latter half of the twentieth century. The last endemic case of smallpox occurred in Somalia in 1977. In 1980, the World Health Organization (WHO) declared that smallpox had been eradicated from the globe. In the United States, immunization of the general public ended in 1972, and routine immunization of health care workers was discontinued in 1976. Two WHO reference laboratories were established to maintain variola virus stocks, one in the United

States and one in Russia. All other countries agreed to destroy existing variola virus isolates. In recent years, concern has been raised that virus stored in the former Soviet Union may have been sold to individuals planning to use it as a weapon of bioterrorism. The possibility of its hostile release has led to renewed interest in smallpox, its treatment, and its prevention. Large segments of the world's population have never been vaccinated against smallpox, and immunity is unlikely to persist in individuals vaccinated as children more than 3 decades ago.

PATHOGENESIS

During natural infection, variola entered the lymph nodes, leading to an asymptomatic viremia about 3 to 4 days following infection. The virus replicated in the reticuloendothelial system before a second episode of viremia resulted in fever, headache, backache, and generalized malaise. This febrile prodrome was followed, after 2 to 3 days, by development of an enanthem and generalized rash. The disease was associated with an overall mortality rate of approximately 30%, with the highest rates noted among infected infants, elderly persons, and pregnant women. Death occurred most often during the second week of illness without apparent involvement of organ systems other than the skin and reticuloendothelial system. Electrolyte abnormalities, dehydration, and secondary bacterial infection were noted, but death was most often attributed to "toxemia."

Neutralizing, hemagglutinin-inhibiting, and complement-fixing antibodies developed during the disease, beginning at the end of the first week. Neutralizing antibodies may persist for many years, but the relationship between persistence of these antibodies and protection from smallpox is not understood.

EPIDEMIOLOGY

Historically, smallpox entered the body via the respiratory route via the oropharynx or nasopharynx in aerosolized or droplet secretions from an infected individual. Other means of spread, through direct contact with respiratory secretions or with contaminated bedding or clothing, also occurred. Infected individuals were not generally considered contagious until the onset of the rash, which occurred after an incubation period of 7 to 17 days (mean, 12 days). Infectivity persisted until all lesions scabbed over and the scabs separated from underlying skin. Scabs themselves contained infective virus, but they were not believed to be a frequent source of infection. Variola survives best in aerosolized form during periods of low temperature and humidity. Historically, therefore, outbreaks were more common during cold, winter months. Smallpox was not as easily spread from person to person as is measles, varicella, or influenza. Prolonged, close contact (face-to-face contact within 6 to 7 feet), usually in a household or hospital, was usually required for secondary spread. Immunity can be induced by vaccination or natural disease.

CLINICAL MANIFESTATIONS AND COMPLICATIONS

There are two known forms of variola virus, variola major and variola minor, or alastrim. The two types can now be distinguished virologically, but when smallpox was endemic only clinical distinction was possible. Variola major is historically more important because of its greater overall case fatality rate (ranging from 15% to 45%). Variola major was classified into five types based on the type of lesions produced and the progression of the disease. The disease type in an in-

dividual is thought to have been determined by host factors and virus virulence. Ordinary smallpox was the most common and was subdivided into three types according to the appearance of the skin lesions: ordinary-discrete (case fatality less than 10%), ordinary-semiconfluent (case fatality 25% to 50%), and ordinary-confluent (case fatality 50% to 75%). Flat smallpox, in which lesions evolved more slowly and finally coalesced, made up about 7% of cases and resulted in death in over 90%. Hemorrhagic smallpox accounted for approximately 3% of cases and resulted in near-100% mortality. This type was difficult to diagnose because of the absence of discrete vesiculopustular lesions. It was seen in all age groups but disproportionately affected pregnant women. Modified smallpox was a milder disease that evolved more rapidly than ordinary smallpox and was accompanied by fewer, smaller, and more superficial lesions. Mortality was rare; most affected individuals had been previously vaccinated. Variola sine eruptions occurred in infants who were young enough to retain maternal antibody against variola or in previously vaccinated contacts. As the name suggests, individuals with this type had no rash. They were asymptomatic or had brief periods of fever with associated flu-like symptoms, and they were not thought to be able to transmit infection to others.

Variola minor is a less severe form of smallpox. The mortality rate associated with this virus was about 1%. It was first recognized in the early twentieth century in South Africa and later appears to have spread to the Americas and to Europe.

High fever, malaise, headache, backache, and prostration were the symptoms of the preeruptive phase of typical smallpox. Vomiting, diarrhea, abdominal pain, and seizures sometimes occurred. After 2 to 3 days, the infected individual developed painful lesions in the mouth and throat, followed closely (within 24 hours) by a maculopapular rash predominantly on the face and extremities but gradually spreading to the entire body. The orpharyngeal lesions became ulcerated, releasing large numbers of virions into the saliva. It was at this stage that the individual was most contagious. The papules developed into vesicles 4 to 5 days after the rash appeared. The initially clear vesicular fluid became turbid and gave the lesions the appearance and texture of firm, tense pustules (Fig. 206.1). The lesions developed an umbilicated center and began to crust approximately 10 days to 2 weeks after the rash appeared. By the second week, the lesions had scabbed, and the crusts began to separate from the underlying skin. Scarring was seen in the majority of those who survived.

Widespread skin lesions led to fluid and electrolyte losses in individuals with severe smallpox. Intravascular volume depletion resulted in hypotension and renal failure as well. During

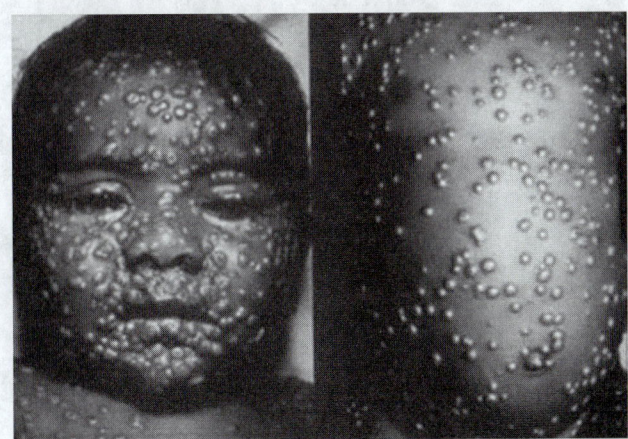

FIGURE 206.1. Photograph of a child with variola major. (Courtesy of the World Health Organization, Geneva.)

much of the long history of this disease, and even during the final decades before it was eradicated, intravascular fluid and electrolyte repletion was not available. The historical mortality rates are undoubtedly affected by limited medical resources. Complications also included secondary bacterial infection and, in about 1%, encephalitis. Disseminated intravascular coagulation was seen in patients with hemorrhagic smallpox. Among survivors, approximately 1% developed panophthalmitis and blindness because of viral keratitis or secondary bacterial infection of the eye. Approximately 2% of children developed arthritis. The cause of death among individuals who died of smallpox was attributed to "toxemia," circulating immune complexes, and shock.

DIAGNOSIS

Today, clinical suspicion of smallpox would constitute an international public health emergency, because it would imply the use of variola as a weapon of bioterrorism. During the preeruptive febrile prodrome, smallpox is indistinguishable from many other causes of acute febrile illness. Recognition of the distinct features of the rash, once it begins to erupt, would help to distinguish this infection from other rash-associated illnesses. The appearance of the lesions should be distinguishable from other viral eruptions such as rubella, measles, meningococcemia, rickettsial diseases, rat-bite fever, and enteroviral infections. The widespread distribution of the lesions of variola major should differentiate it from localized papulovesicular rashes such as impetigo, shingles, and insect bites. The viral infection most likely to be confused with smallpox is varicella. Differentiating these infections is particularly problematic now that widespread childhood immunization against varicella has left many physicians without clinical experience to recognize chickenpox easily. Several characteristics are helpful in differentiating one from the other (Fig. 206.2).

In the past, smallpox was mistaken for drug eruptions and erythema multiforme. Hemorrhagic smallpox was misdiagnosed as meningococcemia, severe acute leukemia, and hemorrhagic varicella.

Because of the potential biologic threat implicit in making a diagnosis of smallpox, it is critical that laboratory confirmation be sought. Samples should be collected only by individuals who have been vaccinated against smallpox. Even vaccinated health care providers, however, should wear protective gowns, masks, and gloves when collecting samples and caring

for a patient suspected of having smallpox. Vesicular or pustular fluid and/or scabs should be collected using a cotton swab. Blood and throat swab specimens should also be obtained. The swabs and blood samples should be placed in a container sealed with adhesive tape and then placed into a second, watertight, container. State health authorities should be contacted immediately. They should, in turn, contact the Centers for Disease Control and Prevention. All samples should be sent directly to a Biological Safety Level 4 laboratory where they can be processed safely.

Variola virus can be detected in the laboratory using electron microscopy, nucleic acid identification, immunohistochemical studies, and tissue culture using cell culture or chorioallantoic egg membrane.

TREATMENT

Any patient suspected of having smallpox should be cared for using contact and airborne isolation precautions, in addition to universal precautions. If possible, the patient should be cared for in a negative-pressure room. State and local public health officials should be notified immediately, so surveillance for additional cases can be initiated and smallpox vaccine can be made available. Anyone who has been in contact with the patient during the period of contagion, including family and community contacts, emergency medical personnel, and all hospital workers, should be immunized as quickly as possible. Immunization within 4 days of exposure attenuates illness caused by smallpox and often prevents disease entirely.

Patient management should include provision of fluid and electrolytes to prevent hypotension, electrolyte abnormalities, and renal failure. Nutritional support should be provided in recognition of the significant protein loss that can occur in patients with extensive lesions. If secondary bacterial infection of the skin or eyes is suspected, antibiotic therapy should be provided and should include an agent expected to be effective against *Staphylococcus aureus*. It has been suggested that corneal lesions be treated with topical idoxuridine, though there is no evidence of efficacy of this agent in treating smallpox. Studies in animals have indicated that cidofovir, a nucleoside analogue that inhibits DNA polymerase, has activity against variola *in vitro* and is effective in treating related infections in animals, including monkeypox, vaccinia, and cowpox, if it is administered early in the disease. This agent, which is licensed for treatment of cytomegalovirus infection, would likely

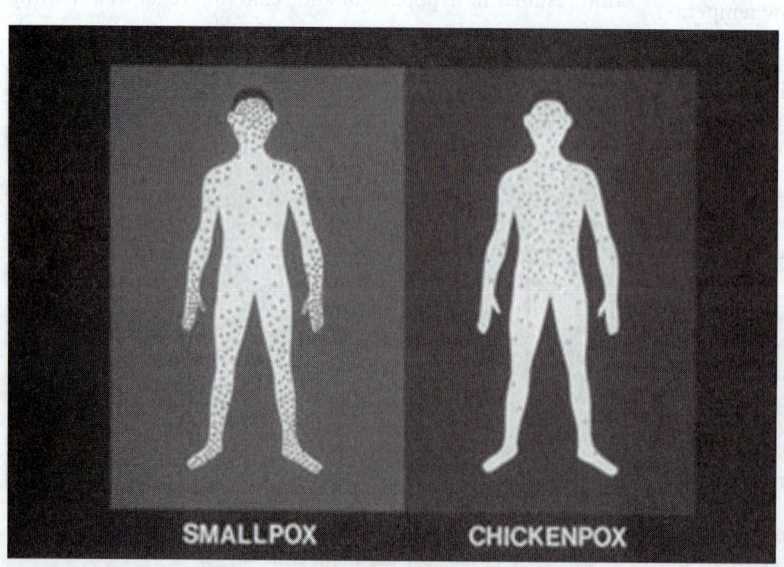

FIGURE 206.2. Typical distribution of the rash of smallpox compared with the distribution of the rash of varicella. (Courtesy of the World Health Organization, Geneva.)

be used under investigational protocol if smallpox were confirmed as the cause of illness. Vaccinia immune globulin (VIG), used to ameliorate adverse reactions to smallpox vaccination, does not improve the outcome for patients with smallpox.

PREVENTION

Since Jenner reported in 1798 that inoculation with cowpox provided protection against smallpox, vaccination has been the primary means of prevention. Widespread childhood vaccination was the primary method for prevention in developed countries throughout the nineteenth and twentieth centuries until worldwide eradication of the disease was declared in 1980. In developing countries in which smallpox had persisted during the second half of the twentieth century, eradication was finally brought about through surveillance and vaccination of contacts. This method was successful because vaccination within 3 to 4 days following exposure prevents or significantly ameliorates disease, thus interrupting the chain of transmission.

Vaccinia is the *Orthopoxvirus* used in vaccines available today to protect against smallpox. These vaccines also protect against related *Orthopoxvirus* species, such as monkeypox. Serologic reactivity can be demonstrated in more than 95% of vaccinated individuals, and protection is thought to persist for at least 5 years. Immunity following revaccination is thought to persist for at least 30 years. During the twentieth century, the vaccinia vaccine used was a live, lyophilized, preparation obtained from "lymph" collected from the skin of vaccinated calves. The vaccine (brand name Dryvax) is diluted and administered using multiple punctures with a bifurcated needle to inoculate vaccinia under the skin. There the virus multiplies and, if vaccination is successful, produces a characteristic "jennerian" pustule after 8 to 9 days, with crusting and scabbing after 2 weeks. Vaccinia virus vaccine is currently available for civilian use only through the Centers for Disease Control and Prevention. Recently, a tissue culture vaccine has been developed, but it is not yet available for use in humans.

Complications following vaccinia vaccination can affect both the vaccinated individual and contacts of the vaccinee (Box 206.1). Fever occurs in as many as 70% of primary vaccinees and in 35% after revaccination. Myalgia, malaise, soreness at the vaccination site, local lymphadenopathy, and erythema surrounding the inoculation site are also common events. The live vaccine virus can be inadvertently inoculated from the site of vaccination to the face, eyes, or other sites

---

BOX 206.2	Contraindications to Smallpox Vaccination

In the absence of a smallpox exposure or outbreak, smallpox vaccination is contraindicated for individuals who have or are in close contact with others who have the following conditions:

Compromised immune system
Eczema (past or present) or other types of extensive skin disease
Inflammatory eye disease
Pregnancy or intent to become pregnant within 28 days following vaccination
Women who are breast-feeding
Allergy to any component of the vaccine (polymyxin B sulfate, streptomycin sulfate, chlortetracycline hydrochloride, neomycin sulfate)
Anyone using ocular steroid medication
Moderate to severe illness

---

or to contacts of the vaccinee. Less frequent adverse events include erythema multiforme, postvaccinal encephalitis and encephalopathy, progressive vaccinia (vaccinia gangrenosa), eczema vaccinatum, generalized vaccinia, myocarditis, and fetal vaccinia. In the absence of smallpox exposure or recognition of a smallpox outbreak, vaccination is contraindicated for individuals who have or are in close contact with anyone who has any of the following: compromised immune system, eczema (past or present), other types of extensive skin disease, or inflammatory eye disease, as well as those who are pregnant or intend to become pregnant in the 28 days following vaccination (Box 206.2). In addition, women who are breast-feeding, individuals with allergy to any component of the vaccine (polymyxin B sulfate, streptomycin sulfate, chlortetracycline hydrochloride, neomycin sulfate), anyone who is using ocular steroid medication, and anyone with moderate to severe illness should not be vaccinated. Vaccinees should be prohibited from blood donation for 21 days, and tuberculin skin testing should be deferred for 1 month following vaccination.

Plasma from recently vaccinated individuals can be used to prepare VIG, which has been used to treat complications of smallpox vaccination. VIG is not effective in the treatment of postvaccinal encephalitis.

In the absence of recognized smallpox disease, smallpox vaccine is not recommended for individuals less than 18 years of age. The vaccine is contraindicated for infants less than 1 year old.

BOX 206.1	Adverse Events following Vaccinia Virus Vaccination

Fever
Erythema surrounding the injection site
Myalgia, malaise
Regional lymphadenitis
Inadvertent self-inoculation or inoculation of contacts
Erythema multiforme
Postvaccinal encephalitis or encephalopathy
Generalized vaccinia
Progressive vaccinia (vaccinia gangrenosa)
Eczema vaccinatum
Vaccinial myocarditis
Fetal vaccinia

Suggested Readings

American Academy of Pediatrics. Smallpox (variola). In Pickering LK, ed. *Redbook: 2003 Report of the Committee on Infectious Diseases*, 26th ed. Elk Grove Village, IL: American Academy of Pediatrics, 2003:554.

Breman JG, Henderson DA. Diagnosis and management of smallpox. *N Engl J Med* 2002;346:1300.

Henderson DA, Inglesby TV, Bartlett JG, et al. Smallpox as a biological weapon: medical and public health management. *JAMA* 1999;281:2127.

Lane JM, Ruben FL, Neff JM, et al. Complications of smallpox vaccination, 1968: results of ten statewide surveys. *J Infect Dis* 1970;122:303.

Mack T. A different view of smallpox and vaccination. *N Engl J Med* 2003;348:5.

Recommendations for using smallpox vaccine in a pre-event vaccination program: supplemental recommendations of the Advisory Committee on Immunization Practices (ACIP) the Healthcare Infection Control Practices Advisory Committee (HICPAC). *Morb Mortal Wkly Rep MMWR* 2003;52:1.

CHAPTER 207 ■ VIRAL GASTROENTERITIS

ANGELA J. PECK AND JOSEPH S. BRESEE

Viral gastroenteritis is a major cause of pediatric morbidity worldwide, and in developing countries, it is a leading cause of mortality. The medically important human gastroenteritis viruses include rotaviruses, caliciviruses, adenoviruses, and Astroviruses (Table 207.1). A variety of other viruses, such as coronaviruses, toroviruses, and picobirnaviruses, have been associated with gastroenteritis, but their clinical and public health importance remain unclear.

ROTAVIRUS

Rotaviruses are the most common cause of severe, dehydrating diarrhea among infants and young children worldwide. Rotaviruses cause an estimated 440,000 deaths each year among children younger than 5 years of age, and they cause 25% to 50% of all hospitalizations for gastroenteritis. Because of the high prevalence of rotavirus disease, several rotavirus vaccine candidates have been developed as a key strategy to prevent childhood mortality in developing countries and hospitalizations in developed countries.

Virology and Pathogenesis

Rotaviruses were discovered in 1973 by Bishop and colleagues in Australia, who found the viruses by using electron microscopy on duodenal biopsies from children with acute diarrhea. Soon after the initial discovery, virus also was detected in stool specimens of patients with gastroenteritis. By electron microscopy, rotaviruses are approximately 70 nm in diameter and have a wheel-shaped morphology (Latin, *rota* = "wheel"). Rotaviruses are nonenveloped viruses that belong to the family *Reoviridae*. They have three layers, including an inner and outer capsid surrounding an inner core, which contains a genome of 11 segments of double-stranded RNA. Rotaviruses

TABLE 207.1

THE RELATIVE CONTRIBUTIONS OF VIRAL PATHOGENS AS CAUSES OF CHILDHOOD GASTROENTERITIS AMONG CHILDREN IN COMMUNITIES AND THOSE REQUIRING HOSPITALIZATION

	Percent of Cases	
	Community-Based	Hospital-Based
Rotaviruses	5–20	25–50
Caliciviruses	10–25	20–30
Astroviruses	10–25	5–10
Adenoviruses 40/41	10–15	5–12
Coronaviruses	1–3	1–2
Toroviruses	Unknown	0–3.5
Picobirnaviruses	Unknown	<1

are classified primarily by group (A to G) and serotype. Group designation is determined by antigenic type of the major capsid protein, VP6, which forms the inner capsid of rotavirus. Although seven distinct antigenic groups have been described, group A viruses are the major cause of most human rotavirus infections. Group B rotaviruses have been reported in large diarrheal outbreaks in China and sporadic cases in India and Bangladesh, and group C has been associated with occasional outbreaks of gastroenteritis and possibly with biliary atresia, but neither appears to be a common cause of illness. None of the other groups has been found to cause human disease.

Group A rotaviruses are classified further on the basis of a dual classification scheme, based on two outer capsid proteins, that combines serotypic designation of VP7 (G serotype) and the genotypic designation of VP4 (P genotype). VP7 and VP4 are viral proteins that make up the outer capsid of the virus and are responsible primarily for eliciting an immune response to the virus in humans. Five (G1 to G4 and G9) of the 14 identified G types currently account for 80% to 90% of human infections. Of the 20 known P types, three (P[4], P[6], and P[8]) account for more than 90% of strains detected.

Although the genes that code for the VP7 and VP4 of rotaviruses segregate independently, only a few combinations of G and P types are responsible for the majority of infections. P[8],G1 strains are the predominant viruses worldwide, particularly in North America, with four other strains (P[4],G2; P[8],G3; P[8],G4; and P[6],G9) accounting for the majority of the other infections. Even so, rotavirus strains can be quite diverse, with a variety of strains prevalent in a community at any time, and serotype prevalence may change from season to season. Strain diversity is an especially common presence in developing countries. Thus, one challenge of developing vaccines has been to ensure that a vaccine can protect against a variety of naturally occurring strains.

Rotaviruses infect the mature upper villous enterocytes of the small intestine, which have both digestive and absorptive functions. The infectious dose is low (10^2 to 10^3 virus particles), but large amounts of rotavirus (10^{12} virus particles per gram) are shed in stool during acute infection, rendering transmission quite easy to occur. Diarrhea that occurs as a result of rotavirus infection is likely caused by a combination of osmotic diarrhea, resulting from loss of absorptive function due to loss of mature enterocytes, and secretory diarrhea, due to the opening of calcium channels, which results in an influx of calcium and efflux of sodium and water (associated with a nonstructural viral protein, NSP4). The intraenterocyte calcium concentration also leads to cell death. In a normal host, infection resolves as the number of susceptible mature enterocytes decreases due to cell death and as the host generates an immune response. Rotavirus is present in stool 1 to 2 days before onset of symptoms and generally is excreted for 2 to 3 weeks after cessation of diarrhea; however, by using sensitive molecular detection methods, researchers have detected virus in stool for up to 2 months after severe disease in young children. Recent studies have detected rotavirus antigen and nucleic acid in the blood of ill children and animals, indicating that rotavirus infection

TABLE 207.2

CHARACTERISTICS OF VIRAL AGENTS OF GASTROENTERITIS

Characteristic	Rotavirus	Calicivirus	Astrovirus	Adenovirus
Predominant age of illness	<5 years	All ages	<2 years	<2 years
Incubation period	1–3 days	12–48 hours	1–4 days	3–10 days
Symptoms				
Diarrhea	Explosive, watery (5–10 episodes/day)	Watery with acute onset	Watery; milder than rotavirus	Watery; milder than rotavirus; can be prolonged
Vomiting	80%–90%	>50%	Less common than rotavirus	Less common than rotavirus
Fever	Frequent	Less common, usually mild	Less common, usually mild	Less common, usually mild
Illness duration	2–8 days	Norovirus: 1–5 days Sapovirus: 1–4 days	1–5 days	3–10 days
Mode of transmission	Person to person via fecal–oral route, fomites	Person to person via fecal–oral route, fomites, food/water	Person to person via fecal–oral route	Person to person via fecal–oral route
Principal methods of clinical diagnosis	Stool EIA or LPA	None available	Stool EIA (not available in the United States)	Stool EIA
Other diagnostic assays	RT-PCR, EM, IEM, PAGE, serum EIA, virus isolation	RT-PCR, EM, IEM, stool or serum EIA	RT-PCR, EM, IEM, serum EIA, virus isolation	RT-PCR, EM, IEM, virus isolation

EIA, enzyme immunoassay; EM, electron microscopy; IEM, immune electron microscopy; LPA, latex particle agglutination; PAGE, polyacrylamide gel electrophoresis; RT-PCR, reverse transcriptase-polymerase chain reaction.

may be associated with viremia in some cases. The implications for diagnostics from these findings and the rate of this manifestation are unclear.

Epidemiology

Rotavirus gastroenteritis may occur in any age group but is most common in the first 5 years of life (Table 207.2). Most cases of severe, dehydrating gastroenteritis occur among children between 4 and 24 months of age, corresponding to the period in which the first infection with rotavirus occurs after immunity wanes from maternally acquired antibodies. Rotavirus illness generally occurs less frequently and less severely with age as a child develops immunity after having recurrent infections. Infections generally are sporadic, but outbreaks also are common occurrences among children in child-care settings. Adults, particularly those caring for rotavirus-infected children, can be infected, and outbreaks can occur when new antigenic strains of rotavirus emerge. By the time they reach age 5, more than 80% of children have serologic evidence of infection.

Worldwide, rotavirus causes approximately 2 million hospitalizations and a median of 440,000 deaths per year in children younger than 5 years of age, with deaths among children in the poorest countries accounting for more than 90% of the total. In hospital-based studies, rotavirus has been found to be responsible for 25% to 50% of the cases of acute gastroenteritis, and rotavirus has been found to cause 5% to 40% of cases in community-based studies. A higher prevalence in hospital-based studies reflects the more severe disease caused by rotavirus compared with other agents causing gastroenteritis. Children living in developing countries are more likely to have rotavirus gastroenteritis at a younger age and to be infected with uncommon serotypes. Estimates of disease burden indicate that in developed countries, hospitalization rates for rotavirus are between 2.5 and 5 per 1,000 in children aged younger than 5 years, whereas in developing countries it may

be as high as 30 per 1,000. In an assessment of the annual impact of rotavirus on the 1997 U.S. birth cohort, the Centers for Disease Control and Prevention (CDC) estimated that 70% (2,730,000) of the cohort was infected and 1 in 80 U.S. children were hospitalized for rotavirus infection. Deaths from rotavirus among children in the United States and other developed countries are rare occurrences (approximately 20 to 40 deaths occur annually in the United States) due to the availability of rehydration therapy and early access to health care. The total annual economic burden in the United States of rotavirus disease was $1 billion in 1997.

Rotavirus is transmitted person-to-person most likely by the fecal-oral routes, but researchers have hypothesized that respiratory transmission through large-droplet spread may play a role. Occasional outbreaks have occurred with evidence of foodborne and waterborne transmission, but these appear to occur rarely in developed countries. Rotavirus can be found on toys and hard surfaces in child-care centers, indicating that fomites also may play a role in transmission. Although rotavirus can infect many animal species and molecular analysis of some rotavirus strains has suggested the presence of animal and human genes, transmission from animals to humans is likely to be quite rare.

In general, the first episode of rotavirus diarrhea is the most likely to be severe and confers protection against subsequent symptomatic infection. Each subsequent infection generally leads to milder illness. Asymptomatic rotavirus infection does occur and may account for most of infections in older children, but stools from asymptomatic controls rarely are rotavirus-positive. Hence, detection of rotavirus in stool samples of children with gastroenteritis should be considered as confirmation of the cause of the illness and not as an incidental finding.

Rotavirus gastroenteritis occurs predominantly during winter months in countries with temperate climates. In North America, the annual season starts in autumn in Mexico and the southwestern United States and moves sequentially from the Southwest to the Northeast, ending in spring in maritime

Canada. In the United States, summertime rotavirus infections are rare occurrences and often are associated with immuno-compromised children or with errors in laboratory tests. Seasonality is less evident within tropical climates, where year-round disease commonly occurs, although disease often peaks in cool, dry months even in tropical areas.

Clinical Characteristics

Rotavirus has a mean incubation period of 1 to 3 days. Neonates are more likely to have asymptomatic infection because they have protection by transplacentally acquired maternal antibody and by antibodies and other factors in breast milk. Infants and young children typically have fever and abrupt onset of vomiting, followed by frequent, foul-smelling, watery stools. Vomiting and fever often precede diarrhea and resolve by the second or third day of illness, whereas diarrhea persists for several more days. In hospitalized patients, diarrhea lasts a median of 6 days (range 2 to 23 days). Stools generally do not contain blood or fecal leukocytes. Symptoms and asymptomatic viral shedding can be prolonged substantially in immunocompromised patients.

Other common clinical features include isotonic dehydration, compensated metabolic acidosis, and malabsorption. Simultaneous respiratory symptoms may occur but likely are due to concurrent wintertime respiratory viral infections. Recent case reports have indicated that rotavirus may be an uncommon cause of encephalitis. In addition, other extraintestinal rotavirus manifestations, including acute myositis, hemophagocytic lymphohistiocytosis, and polio-like paralysis, have been described, but their relationship to rotavirus infection remains unclear.

Diagnosis

Sensitive and specific assays to detect rotavirus antigen in stools are available and offer an easy and inexpensive method to diagnose the disease in children. Both enzyme immunoassays (EIAs) and latex particle agglutination tests for group A rotavirus detection are available commercially. These tests generally have a high (90% to 95%) sensitivity and specificity. Stool samples collected during the acute phase of illness are likely to contain sufficient virus for detection, and these assays sometimes can detect virus in stool samples obtained the week after symptoms have resolved.

Other methods for rotavirus detection include electron microscopy, viral isolation, polyacrylamide gel electrophoresis (PAGE) of RNA extracted directly from stool, and reverse transcriptase-polymerase chain reaction (RT-PCR), but these methods are used primarily in research or public health settings rather than for clinical diagnosis. PAGE has an advantage of being relatively simple and having good specificity (100%) and sensitivity (80% to 90%), and it can be performed relatively inexpensively in tropical countries without specific rotavirus reagents. PAGE also can be used for typing strains because the electrophoretic pattern of the 11 double-stranded RNA segments varies among human rotavirus strains. RT-PCR is more sensitive than are other methods and allows for detection of rotavirus in settings in which the virus titer might be quite low, such as late in the course of illness or in extraintestinal sites. However, the expense and expertise required to perform RT-PCR render its use impractical in most clinical settings. Serologic testing for rotavirus infection is possible but impractical, so it is not widely available in clinical care settings. Immune histochemical stains have been developed that allow for the identification of rotavirus antigen in pathologic tissues, and they are available in some research and public health settings.

In some cases, rotavirus can be detected using simple EIA for antigen detection on serum from ill children.

CALICIVIRUSES

Human caliciviruses were the first viral agents to be associated with gastroenteritis, when in 1972, Norwalk virus was identified by Kapikian and colleagues from the U.S. National Institutes of Health. The virus was detected using immune electron microscopy on stool specimens from human volunteers infected with stool filtrates collected during an outbreak of gastroenteritis in Norwalk, Ohio. Caliciviruses may be the most common causes of gastroenteritis outbreaks and are appreciated increasingly as common causes of sporadic childhood vomiting and diarrhea.

Virology

Caliciviruses are nonenveloped, positive-sense, single-stranded RNA viruses in the family *Caliciviridae* and measure 27 to 40 nm in diameter by electron microscopy. Human caliciviruses are divided into two genera, Norovirus and Sapovirus. Noroviruses include a number of genetically related viruses of which Norwalk virus is the prototype. These viruses have been referred to previously as small round-structured viruses and "Norwalk-like viruses," but *Norovirus* was determined in 2002 to be the official genus name. Sapoviruses, which also were designated officially in 2002, were described first in 1976 when detected in stools of patients with gastroenteritis. This group of viruses was referred to initially as classical caliciviruses and later as "Sapporo-like viruses" in reference to the location of the first detection of Sapporo virus, the prototype strain. By electron microscopy, viruses in the Norovirus genus have less distinct, rough outer edges, and viruses with the typical calicivirus morphology have characteristic cup-shaped depressions over the surface of the virion (Greek, *calyx* = "cup").

Noroviruses are divided further into five genogroups (I, II, III, IV, V), of which only three (I, II, and IV) cause human disease; these three genogroups are subdivided further into at least 20 genetic clusters or subgroups. The number of viruses in each genogroup continues to increase as additional viruses are identified as a result of more widespread application of molecular techniques.

Epidemiology

Caliciviruses cause infection in all ages and, like rotavirus, have a worldwide distribution. Calicivirus-associated gastroenteritis can occur sporadically or in outbreaks. Noroviruses are the most common cause of foodborne illness in the United States, estimated to account for 23 million illnesses a year in the United States and 93% of all nonbacterial outbreaks reported by the CDC between 1997 and 2000. Common sources of foodborne transmission include uncooked foods that become contaminated by ill food handlers who are shedding virus and shellfish harvested from contaminated water. However, at least half of norovirus-associated outbreaks occur through person-to-person spread in closed populations, such as nursing homes, child-care centers, hospitals, and cruise ships, where such transmission is facilitated. The impact of noroviruses on institutions can be dramatic: attack rates can require closing of hospital wards or suspension of cruises.

Noroviruses increasingly are appreciated for causing sporadic community-acquired gastroenteritis among children. In a recent community-based study of gastroenteritis among Finnish children between 2 months and 2 years of age, noroviruses were detected in 20% of stool specimens from gastroenteritis episodes, a percentage second only to that of rotaviruses, which were detected in 31% of stools. Among children in the study who were hospitalized, noroviruses were associated with 13% of the stools in which virus was detected. All age groups are infected by noroviruses, but serosurveys document that antibody is acquired at an early age, indicating that first exposure to these viruses occurs early in life.

Sapoviruses are associated most commonly with sporadic, non-outbreak-associated gastroenteritis, and most commonly among young children (similar to rotavirus). In the community-based Finnish study among children younger than 2 years of age, sapoviruses were detected in stools from 9% of all gastroenteritis episodes and in 4% of hospitalized case-patients. Although outbreaks due to sapoviruses have been reported, they occur less commonly and more often among elderly populations.

The infectious dose of caliciviruses is low (10 to 100 virus particles), and transmission occurs by the fecal-oral route, directly from a person to another person, or indirectly by fecally contaminated food or water or by fomites. Transmission also has been associated with exposure to vomitus, presumably by more widespread contamination of surfaces, with resulting fomite spread, or by large droplet spread. Infections occur throughout the year but appear to peak in the winter months in temperate climates.

Clinical Characteristics

The incubation period for norovirus-associated gastroenteritis is 24 to 48 hours, but it can be as short as 6 hours, and duration of illness generally lasts 12 to 72 hours. Profuse vomiting often is the initial symptom of norovirus infection, and it is a more predominant symptom in children than in adults. Watery, nonbloody diarrhea and abdominal cramps also generally are present. Low-grade fever occurs in one-third to one-half of patients. Studies with volunteers given stool filtrates have shown that asymptomatic infections may occur in as many as 30% of infections. For sapoviruses, the incubation period has been reported to be 2 to 3 days, and illness generally lasts for 1 to 4 days. Sapovirus infection often causes a milder disease than does norovirus infection and is characterized by predominant diarrhea, with vomiting in some cases, often without fever. For either virus, stools generally do not contain blood, mucus, or fecal leukocytes. Excretion of virus begins with onset of symptoms and may continue for 2 weeks after recovery. Duration of excretion can be longer in those patients who had more severe disease, and prolonged duration of excretion can occur in immunocompromised hosts. Some evidence suggests that noroviruses may be associated with chronic diarrhea in transplant patients. No long-term complications have been reported from calicivirus infection.

In the early 1980s, Kaplan and colleagues found that outbreaks that met simple criteria were likely to have been caused by noroviruses. The criteria included (a) failure to detect a bacterial or parasitic pathogen in stool specimens, (b) the occurrence of vomiting in at least 50% of patients, (c) mean duration of illness of 12 to 60 hours, and (d) mean incubation period of 24 to 48 hours. The Kaplan criteria were particularly useful as a diagnostic tool in the absence of specific laboratory methods, and they remain widely used by local health departments for the diagnosis of outbreaks.

Diagnosis

Commercial assays are not available currently outside of research and reference laboratories. Commercial EIA tests used in Europe and Japan have relatively poor sensitivity but may be useful in investigations of outbreaks. Although in the past, direct and immune electron microscopy of stool specimens and serum antibody detection were the most widely available tools for diagnosing calicivirus infections, since 1992, the increasing use of RT-PCR has improved the ability to diagnose norovirus infections. Even so, use of RT-PCR in clinical settings is limited by availability and expense. However, sequencing of the PCR product from clinical samples is a useful epidemiologic tool in investigations of outbreaks in linking cases to each other and to a common source, and RT-PCR now is the primary method for determining the cause of outbreaks of gastroenteritis. Caliciviruses have not been reproducibly propagated in cell cultures.

ASTROVIRUSES

Astroviruses were described first in 1975 when detected by electron microscopy in stool specimens of infants with gastroenteritis. Since 1990, with the development of sensitive and specific diagnostic methods, Astroviruses have been recognized as being common causes of community-acquired and nosocomial illness. Astroviruses may be the next most common viral cause of gastroenteritis among children after rotaviruses and possibly noroviruses.

Virology

Astroviruses are nonenveloped, positive-sense, single-stranded RNA viruses in the family Astroviridae. By electron microscopy, Astroviruses are 28 to 30 nm in diameter, and they have a smooth edge and sometimes a characteristic star-like appearance in the center (Greek, *astron* = "star"). At least eight distinct serotypes (HastV 1 to 8) of human Astroviruses exist. Serotype 1 is detected most commonly, but more than one serotype commonly circulates in communities during each season. Nonserotype 1 viruses can predominate in a season, and greater serotype diversity may be found in developing countries.

Epidemiology

Like rotaviruses and caliciviruses, Astroviruses have a worldwide distribution and have been detected, as a cause of both sporadic disease and outbreaks, in all countries in which sufficiently sensitive detection methods have been used. In developing countries, Astroviruses generally have been detected in fewer than 10% of young children treated for gastroenteritis in outpatient clinics or in hospitals, and the lower proportions reported from some studies (fewer than 1% to 3%) may reflect insensitive detection methods rather than true prevalence. Even so, one study in rural Mexico found Astrovirus to be the most common cause of diarrhea in the first 3 years of life: 26% of diarrheal episodes in a prospectively followed cohort were attributed to Astrovirus. Outbreaks of Astrovirus gastroenteritis have been reported in schools, day-care centers, hospitals, nursing homes, and households.

Outbreaks may cause very high attack rates, particularly in closed populations, such as child-care settings. Astroviruses have been reported to be responsible for 5% to 16% of nosocomial gastroenteritis in children's hospitals. Although Astroviruses have been detected in all age groups, most infections are in children younger than 2 years old. Serosurveys in the United States have shown that more than 90% of children will have antibody to human Astroviruses by 6 to 9 years of age. Disease in adults is an uncommon occurrence. In volunteer studies, most adults challenged with virus neither became infected nor developed diarrhea. However, in a large outbreak among schoolchildren, teachers also became ill, perhaps as a result of a large dose of virus in this type of setting or a different mechanism of transmission. Outbreaks have been reported among the elderly, probably due to waning immunity with increasing age.

Transmission occurs by the fecal-oral route, generally directly by person-to-person contact but also may occur via contaminated food and water. The infectious dose has not been established. In temperate climates, Astrovirus shows a seasonal distribution similar to that of Rotavirus, with a peak in the winter, but seasonality is less clear in tropical settings.

Clinical Characteristics

The incubation period for astrovirus infection is 1 to 4 days. Symptomatic illness occurs more commonly and with increased symptoms in infants and young children, although asymptomatic infections can occur in all ages. Clinical symptoms are similar to those caused by rotavirus, but generally milder, with 2 to 5 days of watery diarrhea, often accompanied by vomiting and less often by high fever and abdominal pain. Illness generally is mild and self-limited, but malabsorption and lactose intolerance have been reported after infection. Stools do not contain blood or mucus. Children may shed virus 1 to 2 days prior to illness, and the duration of excretion lasts a median of 5 days after the onset of symptoms. Prolonged duration of diarrhea has been reported among children with malnutrition and among immunocompromised patients. Asymptomatic excretion among healthy children has been reported to occur for 3 weeks when more sensitive detection methods have been used, and persistent excretion occurs in immunocompromised patients. Because most illness caused by astroviruses occurs in young children and elderly persons, protection from illness is assumed to be conferred by infection and to be relatively durable.

Diagnosis

Since 1990, great improvements have been achieved in the methods used to diagnose astrovirus gastroenteritis, including the adaptation to grow the virus in continuous cell lines, sequencing and elucidation of the structure of the genome, and development of improved methods of detection, including EIAs and RT-PCR. Commercial EIAs for detection of viral antigen in stools are available in Europe but not yet in the United States. RT-PCR, serologic assays, and electron microscopy are used primarily in research settings.

ENTERIC ADENOVIRUSES

Enteric adenoviruses are relatively common causes of gastroenteritis in infants and children. Early studies of enteric adenoviruses were hindered by the failure to propagate these viruses in conventional cell culture and the inability to demonstrate that conventional adenoviruses produce gastroenteritis. Similar to the case with Astroviruses, the development of rapid and sensitive diagnostic assays for the detection of enteric adenoviruses has increased our appreciation of their role as causes of diarrhea in children.

Virology

Adenoviruses are nonenveloped, double-stranded DNA viruses in the family Adenoviridae. The icosahedral capsid is 70 to 80 nm in diameter by electron microscopy. Six subgroups of adenoviruses, which contain at least 51 different serotypes, cause human infection. Serotypes 40 and 41 (subgroup F) are the two most clearly associated with gastroenteritis; however, serotype 31 has been associated with gastroenteritis in some studies and serotypes 42 to 29 have been reported as causes of diarrhea in HIV-infected patients. Unlike other adenoviruses, adenoviruses 40 and 41 require special transformed cell lines for growth.

Epidemiology

Like other viral agents of gastroenteritis, enteric adenoviruses have a worldwide distribution. They generally are considered to account for 5% to 10% of hospitalizations for acute gastroenteritis in children, and they may be a common cause of nosocomial diarrhea. Enteric adenoviruses generally have been detected in 1% to 4% of children with community-acquired diarrhea. In developing countries, enteric adenoviruses, compared with other viral agents, appear to account for a smaller proportion of diarrheal disease than in developed countries, although they are detected occasionally in rates similar to those of rotavirus. Most infections occur in children younger than 2 years old, and in the few studies that have examined the role of enteric adenoviruses in an adult population, they appear to be less important causes of gastroenteritis than they are in children.

Enteric adenoviruses are transmitted via the fecal-oral route from person to person. Foodborne and waterborne spread have not been described. No seasonality of enteric adenovirus infection has been recognized, but few studies have reviewed multiple seasons.

Clinical Characteristics

The incubation period for gastroenteritis associated with enteric adenoviruses is 3 to 10 days. Infections with enteric adenoviruses can range from being mild or asymptomatic to producing profuse, nonbloody, watery diarrhea and vomiting, but they generally are milder than are those associated with rotavirus. Watery diarrhea is the most prominent symptom, and children often have six to ten stools per day. The illness lasts 5 to 9 days, but diarrhea has been reported to have a long duration in some studies and can become chronic in immunocompromised children. Abdominal pain and 2 to 3 days of low-grade fever (less than 38.5°C) frequently also are present, whereas temperatures of 39°C or higher occur in 10% to 25% of children. Respiratory symptoms, including pneumonia, have been associated with enteric adenovirus infections but are present less commonly than with other adenoviruses. Immunity associated with enteric adenoviruses is poorly understood. Children can become ill when reinfected; however, illness among adults is an uncommon occurrence, even in settings of outbreaks where they have a high likelihood of exposure.

Diagnosis

Enzyme-linked immunosorbent assay (ELISA) and latex particle agglutination kits are available commercially and provide highly sensitive and specific antigen detection of enteric adenoviruses. Other possible diagnostic methods include immune electron microscopy, RT-PCR, and isolation of virus on specific transformed cell lines, but these methods are available and performed only in research laboratories.

TABLE 207.3

COMPOSITION OF COMMERCIAL ORAL REHYDRATION SOLUTIONS AND COMMONLY CONSUMED BEVERAGES

Solution	CHO (gm/L)	Na (mmol/L)	K (mmol/L)	Cl (mmol/L)	Base* (mmol/L)	Osmolarity (mosm/L)
Oral Rehydration Solutions						
WHO-ORS (2002)	13.5	75	20	65	10	245
WHO-ORS (1975)	20	90	20	80	10	311
ESPGHAN ORS	16	60	20	60	10	240
Infalyte†	30	50	25	45	34	200
Pedialyte‡	25	45	20	35	30	250
Rehydralyte‡	25	75	20	65	30	305
CeraLyte§	40	50–90	20	40–80	30	220
Commonly Used Beverages (Not appropriate for transfer treatment)						
Apple juice‖	120	0.4	44	45	—	730
Coca Cola¹	112	1.6	—	—	13.4	650
Gatorade²	46	23.5	2.5	17	3	330
Chicken broth‖	8	260	0.5	260	—	450
Tea‖	—	6	—	—	6	

*Actual or potential bicarbonate, such as lactate, citrate, or acetate.
†Mead-Johnson Laboratories, Princeton, NJ.
‡Ross Laboratories, Columbus, OH (data for flavored and freezer pop Pedialyte are identical).
§http://www.ceralyte.com/index.htm. Accessed April 25, 2003.
‖USDA.
¹Coca-Cola Corporation, Atlanta, GA (figures do not include electrolytes, which may be present in local water used for bottling; base = phosphate).
²The Gatorade Company, Chicago, IL.
Reprinted from Centers for Disease Control and Prevention. Managing acute gastroenteritis among children: oral rehydration, maintenance, and nutritional therapy. *MMWR Morb Mortal Wkly Reports* and Recommendations 2003;52:1.

OTHER GASTROENTERITIS VIRUSES

Other viruses, including human coronaviruses and toroviruses within the virus family *Coronaviridae*, and picobirnavirus, also are associated with gastroenteritis. Human coronaviruses have been detected in studies in several countries, but their association with gastroenteritis remains unclear. Misdiagnosis is problematic because no confirmatory test is available, and enteric coronaviruses must be identified by electron microscopy. Recent reports of the clinical characteristics of patients infected with the severe acute respiratory syndrome (SARS)-coronavirus have described diarrhea in approximately one-fourth of cases. Likewise, with toroviruses, the epidemiologic link of detection of virus in stool to illness remains unclear, although the viruses sometimes can be found in high proportions of stools from patients with diarrhea. Picobirnaviruses have been associated with disease in studies of HIV-infected adults. Other viruses, such as pestiviruses, some picornaviruses, parvoviruses and parvo-like viruses, reoviruses, enteroviruses, and other unclassified small round viruses, have been found in fecal specimens and implicated in gastroenteritis. However, many of these viruses have been reported only sporadically or have been associated with single outbreaks of illness, and the data are inconclusive regarding the relative importance and features for many of these viruses.

TREATMENT OF VIRAL GASTROENTERITIS

No specific therapies exist for any of the viruses that cause acute gastroenteritis. The mainstay of management is assessment, correction of fluid loss and electrolyte disturbances, and maintenance of adequate hydration. Oral rehydration therapy with appropriate glucose-electrolyte solutions is sufficient for most patients (Table 207.3). Intravenous rehydration is required for the patient with severe dehydration with shock or intractable vomiting. Children should maintain caloric intake as best as possible, with maintenance dietary therapy dependent on the age and diet history of the patient. Breast-fed infants should continue to nurse on demand, and formula-fed infants should continue their usual formula immediately upon rehydration. Children receiving semisolid or solid foods should continue to receive their usual diet during episodes of diarrhea, although substantial amounts of foods high in simple sugars (carbonated soft drinks, juice, gelatin desserts) should be avoided because the osmotic load might worsen diarrhea. Because most infectious gastroenteritis in children is caused by viruses, appropriate use of antibiotics in patients with acute gastroenteritis should be stressed.

Evidence suggests that administration of oral probiotics, such as *Lactobacillus* species, provide clinically significant benefits, such as reduction of diarrhea duration in acute gastroenteritis caused by rotavirus. Human or bovine colostrums and human serum immunoglobulin contain antibodies to rotavirus, and studies suggest that they may be beneficial in decreasing or preventing rotavirus diarrhea, but they are not used in routine practice.

PREVENTION OF VIRAL GASTROENTERITIS

Rotavirus Vaccines

Rotavirus vaccines offer the best prospect for prevention of rotavirus morbidity and mortality worldwide. Although no vaccines are used currently in immunization programs, several vaccines are in late-stage development or have been licensed. All rotavirus vaccines in clinical development are live, orally administered vaccines given in multiple doses. They are designed to mimic natural infection but replace a child's first exposure to wild-type rotavirus with attenuated strains that will generate an adequate immune response to confer protection.

A quadrivalent, reassortant rhesus rotavirus vaccine (Rotashield, Wyeth Laboratories) that contained viruses with serotype specificity for G1 to G4 proved highly effective in trials in developed and developing countries. The vaccine was approved for use in U.S. infants in a three-dose schedule given at 2, 4, and 6 months in 1998. However, the vaccine was withdrawn from use less than a year later after cases of intussusception occurring among vaccine recipients were reported. An estimated 1 case of intussusception occurred for every 10,000 infants immunized, although recent data indicate that the risk may be lower. The vaccine is not available for purchase and is not being manufactured. Two vaccines, including a pentavalent bovine-human reassortant vaccines and a monovalent attenuated human strain, have demonstrated excellent efficacy and safety in trials thus far and are likely to be licensed soon. Other vaccines are in clinical trials, including neonatal strains and other human-animal reassortants.

Although experimental vaccines against noroviruses are in early stages of development, proof that these vaccines could be protective remains to be established. No vaccines against other caliciviruses, Astroviruses, or enteric adenoviruses are yet in human trials.

Nonvaccine Approaches

Until effective vaccines are available, prevention strategies are limited. Breast-feeding confers some protection against rotavirus infection in young infants that likely is mediated through rotavirus antibodies in the milk and other nonimmunologic factors. Good hygiene and handwashing practices are effective prevention strategies and should be encouraged, particularly in institutional settings such as child-care centers and hospitals. Even so, reducing transmission of viral gastroenteritis is difficult because the disease generally requires a low infectious dose, high quantity of viruses are excreted in stool (and often vomitus) from infected persons, and the agents are quite stable in the environment. Therefore, virtually all children in both developed and developing countries become infected early in life.

Noroviruses are relatively resistant to environmental disinfection, but cleaning contaminated surfaces and food preparation areas with household chlorine bleach-based cleaners can decrease the spread of infection with these viral agents and likely is effective in settings where rotavirus and astrovirus outbreaks occur. Proper hand hygiene among child-care providers and food handlers also is likely to be an effective tool for preventing viral transmission.

Suggested Readings

Bishop RF, Davidson GP, Holmes IH, Ruck BJ. Virus particles in epithelial cells of duodenal mucosa from children with viral gastroenteritis. *Lancet* 1973;2:1281.

Bresee, JS, Glass RI, Gentsch JR, Ivanoff B. Current status and future priorities for rotavirus vaccine development, evaluation, and implementation in developing countries. *Vaccine* 1999;17:2207.

Blutt SE, Kirkwood CD, Parreno V, et al. Rotavirus antigenaemia and viraemia: a common event? *Lancet* 2003;362:1445.

Centers for Disease Control and Prevention. Managing acute gastroenteritis among children: oral rehydration, maintenance, and nutritional therapy. *MMWR* 2003;52:1.

Centers for Disease Control and Prevention. Norwalk-like viruses: public health consequences and outbreak management. *MMWR* 2001;50:1.

Centers for Disease Control and Prevention. Rotavirus vaccine for the prevention of rotavirus gastroenteritis among children. *MMWR* 1999;48:1.

Fankhauser RL, Monroe SS, Noel JS, et al. Epidemiologic and molecular trends of "Norwalk-like viruses" associated with outbreaks of gastroenteritis in the United States. *J Infect Dis* 2002;186:1.

Gentsch JR, Woods PA, Ramachandran M, et al. Review of G and P typing results from a global collection of rotavirus strains: implications for vaccine development. *J Infect Dis* 1996;174:S30.

Glass RI, Noel J, Mitchell DK, et al. The changing epidemiology of astrovirus-associated gastroenteritis: a review. *Arch Virol Suppl* 1996;12:287.

Hermann JE, Taylor DN, Echeverria P, et al. Astroviruses as a cause of gastroenteritis in children. *N Engl J Med* 1991;324:1757.

Kaplan JE, Feldman R, Campbell DS, et al. The frequency of a Norwalk-like pattern of illness in outbreaks of acute gastroenteritis. *Am J Public Health* 1982;72:1329.

Krajden M, Brown M, Petrasek A, et al. Clinical features of adenovirus enteritis: a review of 127 cases. *Pediatric Infect Dis J* 1990;9:636.

Matson DO, Estes MK. Impact of rotavirus infection at a large pediatric hospital. *J Infect Dis* 1990;162:598.

Mitchel DK, Pickering LK. Enteric infections. In: Patrick CC, ed. *Clinical management of infections in immunocompromised infants and children.* Philadelphia: Lippincott, 2001:413.

Murphy TV, Garguillo PM, Massoudi MS, et al. Intussusception among infants given an oral rotavirus vaccine. *N Eng J Med* 2001;334:564.

Parashar UD, Hummelman EG, Bresee JS, et al. Global illness and death caused by rotavirus disease in children. *Emerg Infect Dis* 2003;9:565.

O'Ryan M, Matson DO. Viral gastroenteritis pathogens in the day care center setting. *Semin Pediatr Infect Dis* 1990;1:252.

Velazquez FR, Matson DO, Calva JJ, et al. Rotavirus infection in infants as protection against subsequent infections. *N Engl J Med* 1996;355:1022.

e: FUNGAL DISEASES

CHAPTER 208 ■ CANDIDIASIS

WALTER T. HUGHES

Candidiasis is the opportunistic fungal infection encountered most frequently in infants and children. The spectrum of the disease extends from benign thrush to life-threatening disseminated (systemic) candidiasis. Debilitated and immunocompromised individuals and very low-birth-weight infants are at highest risk for acquiring serious infections.

ETIOLOGY

Several species of the genus *Candida* may cause infections in humans, but *Candida albicans* is the usual causative agent. Other species have come to prominence as causes of disease, especially in immunocompromised patients. These include *C. tropicalis*, *C. pseudotropicalis*, *C. paratropicalis*, *C. krusei*, *C. guilliermondii*, *C. parapsilosis*, *C. glabrata*, *C. dubliniensis*, *C. inconspicua*, *C. lusitaniae*, *C. rugosa*, and *C. stellatoidea*. These yeasts are round to oval vegetative cells that, under conditioned circumstances, produce pseudohyphae. Characteristically, *C. albicans* develops chlamydospore formation under stressful, controlled conditions, whereas other species of *Candida* do not exhibit such structures.

EPIDEMIOLOGY

Candida species are highly prevalent in nature and are found predominantly in association with humans and other warm-blooded animals. *C. albicans* may be isolated from soil, but usually only at sites where human or animal contamination has occurred. One species, *C. stellatoidea*, has been isolated only from humans. Within the animal kingdom, *C. albicans* has been isolated from a variety of wild and domestic animals.

Likely, transmission of *Candida* involves direct contact with a colonized site. Oral thrush in neonates results from organisms that are acquired during passage through the birth canal or from colonized nipples of the mother or a nursing bottle. Although *C. albicans* has been isolated from the air around patients with cutaneous candidiasis, the extent of airborne transmission has not been established. Colonization with *C. albicans* occurs in most infants and children and is not associated with discernible illness. Receptor sites on epithelial cells of the mucosa permit adherence of the yeast form and the establishment of colonization.

Several functions of the immune system actively defend against this organism in healthy hosts. Secretory and humoral IgA antibodies are generated, as are specific anticandidal IgE, IgG, and IgM antibodies. The organism can activate an alternate complement pathway. Neutrophils, monocytes, and eosinophils can ingest and kill the yeast. The organism can induce the formation of suppressor and mitogen-stimulated lymphocytes and thereby produce a lymphokine that will kill it. Lactoferrin has anticandidal activity. Although mucosal surfaces are colonized easily, the normal skin is relatively resistant to colonization and infection with *Candida* species.

At high risk for acquiring infections from *Candida* species are patients with acquired and congenital immune deficiency disorders, cancer, certain endocrinopathic conditions, diabetes mellitus, burns, trauma, and malnutrition; organ transplant recipients; individuals receiving immunosuppressive drugs such as corticosteroids; and very low birth-weight infants. Healthy individuals may be at increased risk for candidiasis of the mucous membranes during infancy, pregnancy, and old age. Invasive disseminated candidiasis has been encountered in 7% of children infected with the human immunodeficiency virus and in 11% of recipients of bone marrow transplants. Surveillance studies show the annual incidence of 8 per 100,000 population in the United States. The highest incidence (75 per 100,000) occurs among infants 1 year of age and younger. A significant shift has occurred in the epidemiology of hematogenous candidiasis caused by different *Candida* species. A relative decrease in *C. albicans* and *C. tropicalis* is associated with an increase in *C. krusei* and *C. glabrata*. This shift has been attributed in part to the use of fluconazole. The invasive form of candidiasis may be found in one-third of children with malignant tumors and febrile-neutropenic episodes that are not responsive to antibiotics. Approximately 10% of preterm infants with birth weights of less than 1,000 grams have infections caused by *Candida* species acquired in the neonatal intensive care unit and one-third of these infections are fatal.

PATHOLOGY

The initial step in infection is adherence of the yeast form of *Candida* to an epithelial cell surface. The adherent blastospore then develops a filamentous or pseudohyphal form, and the organism becomes invasive. In the case of mucous membranes, infection such as thrush develops as an adherent pseudomembrane composed of epithelial cells, leukocytes, keratin, food debris, and both yeast and pseudohyphal forms of *Candida*. Mucosal lesions may progress to well-demarcated ulcers, especially in the intestinal tract, with a base of granulation tissue covered by a fibrinous exudate and granulocytes. Organisms may invade blood vessels, may become bloodborne, and may disseminate to any organ in the body in immunosuppressed patients. From the mucosal portal of entry, a systemic disease evolves, with the kidneys, lungs, liver, brain, and spleen affected most frequently. The gut is the major site for entry of organisms in candidemia. In systemic disease, a pyogenic response occurs, with microabscess formation. Granulomatous reactions occur infrequently.

CLINICAL MANIFESTATIONS

The clinical features of candidiasis may be considered in three categories: those associated with mucous membranes, those associated with the skin, and those in which systemic invasion has occurred.

Mucous Membrane Candidiasis

Oropharyngeal candidiasis usually is recognizable on the mucosal surface as patches of pearly white pseudomembranes that resemble curds of milk. Removal of the pseudomembrane leaves a denuded erythematous lesion. The buccal mucosa, dorsal and lateral areas of the tongue, gingiva, and pharynx are involved most frequently. *C. albicans* is the species that usually causes thrush. With esophageal candidiasis, dysphagia and retrosternal pain may be presenting symptoms, but some lesions remain silent, especially in immunocompromised hosts. The inferior third of the esophagus is involved most commonly. Esophagoscopy or esophagography reveals ulcerations of the mucosa, producing a cobblestone pattern.

The clinical manifestations of gastrointestinal candidiasis are not defined well. Any portion of the gastrointestinal tract may be affected in severely immunosuppressed patients. Such lesions may provide a portal of entry for systemic disease.

Vaginal candidiasis causes pruritus and a whitish, watery vaginal discharge. Typical thrush lesions may be visualized on the vaginal mucosa. The mucosal surface of the respiratory tract may be colonized with *Candida* at any site. Candidiasis limited to the larynx and bronchi is rare and more often is associated with pulmonary and systemic disease.

Cutaneous Candidiasis

The most common form of cutaneous candidiasis is dermatitis in the diaper areas of infants. Usually, the groin, perineum, and lower abdominal areas are involved. Often, the rash is a confluent papulovesicular reaction with well-demarcated borders.

Other sites frequently involved include the intertriginous areas of the axilla and sites around the umbilicus.

Chronic mucocutaneous candidiasis is an uncommon syndrome that reflects an underlying immunodeficiency or, in some cases, an endocrinopathy. Skin, mucous membranes, and skin appendages are involved. Few patients recover from this infection unless the underlying abnormality is corrected.

Congenital cutaneous candidiasis is a rare infection acquired *in utero* and often associated with maternal candidal vulvovaginitis and intrauterine devices. Skin lesions appear in the first 6 days of life.

Systemic Candidiasis

Systemic or disseminated candidiasis implies hematogenous dissemination to deep organs of the body from a portal of entry at a mucous membrane or skin site. Any organ may be involved, but the lungs, liver, spleen, kidney, and brain are affected most frequently. This form of candidiasis occurs almost exclusively in severely immunosuppressed patients and debilitated, premature infants. Therefore, the clinical manifestations depend on the organs and tissues involved. Suspicion should be aroused in any immunosuppressed patient who has fever of unknown origin and neutropenia.

Certain low-birth-weight infants without fever may exhibit nonspecific signs and symptoms, such as respiratory abnormalities, apnea, bradycardia, hypotensive episodes, endophthalmitis, meningitis, and an erythematous and nodular rash. Neonates with candidemia for 5 or more days are likely to have renal, cardiac, or ophthalmic involvement.

A chronic disseminated form of candidiasis, with prominent lesions in the liver and spleen, has been reported more frequently in recent years in children with malignant tumors.

DIAGNOSIS

The lesions of oral thrush are unique, and the diagnosis can be made from visual examination in most instances. Infection in mucous membranes and skin, however, can be confirmed by direct examination of materials swabbed or scraped from the surface lesions and by culture of the specimens on the appropriate media. Specimens from surface lesions can be applied to 10% potassium hydroxide or to a drop of lactophenol cotton blue solution on a microscope slide with a coverslip and examined for budding yeast forms and pseudohyphae. The diagnosis of systemic candidiasis is difficult to establish and requires at least the isolation of *Candida* species from otherwise sterile body fluids, such as bone marrow, cerebrospinal fluid, or blood; the

demonstration of invasive yeasts or pseudohyphae in biopsy specimens; or both. Most commercially available automated continuous-monitoring blood culture systems in common use are satisfactory for the isolation of *Candida* sp. Computed tomography is useful in demonstrating lesions in the liver, spleen, kidneys, and brain. Often, such lesions are sufficiently characteristic to permit a presumptive diagnosis to be made. The usefulness of methods to detect *Candida* antigenemia, cell wall mannan and mannoproteins, and D-arabinitol-to-L-arabinitol ratios in urine has been limited. Although molecular probes using polymerase chain reaction methods offer promise, no generally accepted serologic method has evolved for the diagnosis of invasive disease.

The evaluation of a neonate in the intensive care unit with candidemia should include cultures of cerebrospinal fluid and urine; repeated blood cultures; ophthalmologic examination; ultrasonography of the kidneys, liver, spleen, and heart; computed tomography of the brain; and an echocardiogram.

TREATMENT

The type of organism and location of candidiasis are important in determining the appropriate approach to treatment. Amphotericin B resistance is uncommon with *C. albicans, C. tropicalis,* and *C. parapsilosis, but C. krusei, C. glabrata,* and *C. lusitaniae* may be resistant to the drug (Table 208.1). The following recommendations are in agreement with the Infectious Diseases Society of America Guidelines for Treatment of Candidiasis.

Mucous Membrane Candidiasis

Oropharyngeal candidiasis is treated with clotrimazole troches 10 mg five times a day or oral nystatin, 200,000 to 500,000 units every 4 to 6 hours, for 1 week or longer. Vaginal candidiasis is treated with clotrimazole or nystatin suppositories. Esophageal, gastric, and intestinal candidiasis can be treated in the same manner as that used for treating oropharyngeal candidiasis, provided that the nystatin suspension is swallowed.

Fluconazole, given orally or intravenously, has been effective in oral and esophageal candidiasis and should be considered for use in severe cases and in patients who are not responsive to the nonabsorbable drugs. The efficacy of itraconazole has been found equal to that of fluconazole in the treatment of esophageal candidiasis. Newer drugs, such as voriconazole 4 mg/kg twice daily by mouth or intravenously, or caspofungin are indicated for severe and/or refractory esophageal candidiasis.

TABLE 208.1

SUSCEPTIBILITY PATTERNS OF *CANDIDA* SPECIES (MODIFIED FROM PAPPAS, ET AL., 2004)

Drug	C. albicans C. tropicalis C. parapsilosis	C. lusitaniae	C. glabrata	C. krusei
Amphotericin B	+	+/−	+/−	+/−
Echinocandin	+	+	+	+
Fluconazole	+	+	+/−*	−
Flucytosine	+	+	+	+
Itraconazole	+	+	+/−*	+/−*
Voriconazole	+	+	+/−*	+/−

+, susceptible; −, resistant; +/−, susceptible or resistant; *, maximization of dosage and bioavailability necessary.

Cutaneous Candidiasis

Cutaneous candidiasis can be treated with topical nystatin, miconazole, or clotrimazole preparations. Chronic mucocutaneous candidiasis in some cases may be treated effectively with oral ketoconazole, fluconazole, or itraconazole.

Systemic Candidiasis

Candidiasis with deep organ involvement or hematogenous spread is treated systemically with amphotericin B. No drug has been shown to be more effective. The dosage of amphotericin B is 0.5 to 1.0 mg/kg/day as a daily infusion, given over 4 to 6 hours. Before this dose is initiated, a test infusion of 0.25 mg/kg/day is given over a period of 6 hours to assess the extent of possible adverse reactions to the preparation. Amphotericin B should be administered over a period of 4 to 6 weeks, or even longer in some cases. Especially important is the monitoring of patients who are receiving amphotericin B for adverse effects of the drug, which will be reflected in electrolyte imbalance and nephrotoxicity.

In randomized studies, fluconazole and amphotericin B were associated with similar clinical response rates and survival in the treatment of candidemia among nonneutropenic and neutropenic patients. However, drug-related adverse effects occurred more frequently with amphotericin B. Fluconazole 6 mg/kg every 12 hours, orally or intravenously, may be used as an alternative to amphotericin B for systemic cases of candidiasis in patients other than those with *C. krusei* infections. The echinocandin, caspofungin, may be considered as an alternative to amphotericin B and fluconazole.

Lipid formulations of amphotericin B (lipid complex or colloidal dispersion) now are available commercially for patients with treatment-limiting toxicity and certain treatment failures from the standard amphotericin B preparation. Therapeutic superiority of these preparations over amphotericin B deoxycholate has not been demonstrated for candidiasis.

Neonatal candidiasis can be treated effectively with amphotericin B deoxycholate 0.6 mg/kg/day or intravenous fluconazole 5 to 12 mg/kg/day. Treatment should be continued for 14 to 21 days after resolution of signs and symptoms and negative repeat cultures.

Prophylaxis

Certain severely immunocompromised individuals who are a high risk for developing invasive candidiasis may benefit from prophylaxis with antifungal drugs such as amphotericin B, fluconazole, and itraconazole. Recent studies suggest selected patients with prolonged neutropenia due to cancer chemotherapy or bone marrow or solid-organ transplant recipients may warrant antifungal prophylaxis. Kaufman et al. showed that the administration of intravenous fluconazole to preterm infants weighing less than 1,000 grams during the first 6 weeks of life significantly reduces both colonization and invasive fungal disease.

Suggested Readings

Darnstadt GL, Dinulos JG, Miller Z. Congenital cutaneous candidiasis: clinical presentation, pathogenesis and management guidelines. *Pediatrics* 2000;105:438.

Kao AS, Bradt MD, Pruitt WR, et al. The epidemiology of candidemia in two United States cities: results of a population-based active surveillance. *Clin Infect Dis.* 1999;29:1164.

Kaufman D, Boyle R, Hazen KC, et al. Fluconazole prophylaxis against fungal colonization and infection in preterm infants. *N Eng J Med* 2001;345:1660.

Marr KA, Seidel K, Slavin MA, et al. Prolonged fluconazole prophylaxis is associated with persistent protection against candidiasis-related death in allogenic marrow transplant recipients; long-term followup of a randomized, placebo-controlled trail. *Blood* 2000;96:2055.

Murray PR, Baron EJ, Jorgensen JH, et al. *Manual of clinical microbiology*, 8th ed. Washington D.C.: American Society for Microbiology Press, 2003:2113.

Nucci M, Anaissie E. Revisiting the source of candidemia: skin or gut? *Clin Infect Dis* 2001;33:1959.

Pappas PG, Rex JH, Sobel JD, et al. Infectious Diseases Society of America guidelines for the treatment of candidiasis. *Clin Infect Dis* 2004;38:161.

Powers JH, Dixon CA, Golberger MJ. Voriconazole versus liposomal amphotericin B in patients with neutropenia and persistent fever. *N Engl J Med* 2002;346:289.

CHAPTER 209 ■ THE DERMATOPHYTOSES

BERNHARD L. WIEDERMANN

Dermatophytosis refers to colonization of the skin with members of the dermatophytic fungi of the genera *Trichophyton*, *Microsporum*, and *Epidermophyton*. Clinical disease may appear as a consequence of the host's response to this colonization. The condition has been recognized since antiquity and was termed *herpes* by the Greeks, in reference to the tendency of lesions to creep in a circular fashion. Later, the Romans used the term *tinea*, meaning "worm" or "moth," to indicate a presumed association of the disease with insects. The modern term *ringworm* is a combination of these two historical names.

The affected body site is incorporated into commonly used clinical nomenclature. Thus, *tinea capitis* refers to dermatophytosis of the scalp, lesions of the trunk and extremities are termed *tinea corporis*, foot involvement is named *tinea pedis*, perineal disease is known as *tinea cruris*, and dermatophytosis of the nails is called *tinea unguium*.

ETIOLOGY

The three genera of dermatophytes refer to asexual (imperfect or anamorph) stages of the fungi. A completely different nomenclature is used to speak of the sexual (perfect or teleomorph) forms, which will not be discussed here. Confusion may arise from this distinct nomenclature and from the classification of dermatophytes according to natural habitat as *geophilic* (soil saprophyte), *zoophilic* (animals as primary hosts), or *anthropophilic* (humans as primary hosts). Nonetheless, this latter classification is useful in the evaluation of outbreaks or persistence of infection in individuals.

To date, approximately 40 different dermatophytes have been identified, but only 11 commonly cause disease in humans. The most common organisms causing disease in the United States are *Trichophyton tonsurans, T. rubrum, T. mentagrophytes, Microsporum canis,* and *Epidermophyton floccosum.*

EPIDEMIOLOGY

Age is a determinant for some dermatophyte infections. For example, tinea pedis is found commonly in adults but rarely in children. In contrast, tinea capitis occurs commonly in children but rarely after puberty. However, previous data suggesting that tinea capitis clears at puberty probably are incorrect; most cases resolve within a year regardless of therapy or age of the patient.

Gender also may play a role in some dermatophyte infections. Tinea capitis caused by *Trichophyton* in adults appears to occur more commonly in women. Tinea cruris occurs more commonly in men, which may be related in part to anatomic differences rather than genetic causes.

Similarly, associations of infections with specific populations, such as tinea capitis with African American children, may relate more to physical (coiling of hair shafts) than to genetic factors. Other environmental issues, such as geographic site, animal exposure, presence of trauma, or immunocompromising conditions (particularly those involving cell-mediated immunity) may predispose to development of dermatophytosis.

PATHOGENESIS AND PATHOLOGY

Infecting organisms are acquired from soil, animal, or human sources and colonize keratin-containing tissues. Direct contact may not be necessary for transmission. The dermatophytes possess the relatively unique ability to use keratin as a substrate for growth, which allows them to invade keratin-rich tissues. During the initial incubation period, the organism grows in the stratum corneum of the skin and then progresses in accord with the growth rate of the particular organism and the rate of squamous cell turnover in the host. The site of disease enlarges and spreads locally. Histopathologic features vary with the body site involved, but they generally consist of a mixed infiltrate of lymphocytes, histiocytes, eosinophils, and plasma cells in the stratum corneum. Fungal elements may be visualized using periodic acid-Schiff or methenamine silver staining. In circular lesions of the skin, active fungal invasion and growth occur at the rim of the lesion; the center of the lesion contains relatively few organisms. Formation of kerions in tinea capitis is marked by an intense polymorphonuclear cell infiltrate.

CLINICAL MANIFESTATIONS AND COMPLICATIONS

The clinical features of dermatophytoses vary with the site of the infection.

Tinea Capitis (Fig. 209.1)

Ringworm of the scalp in the United States usually is caused by *T. tonsurans; M. canis* and *Microsporum audouinii* are less

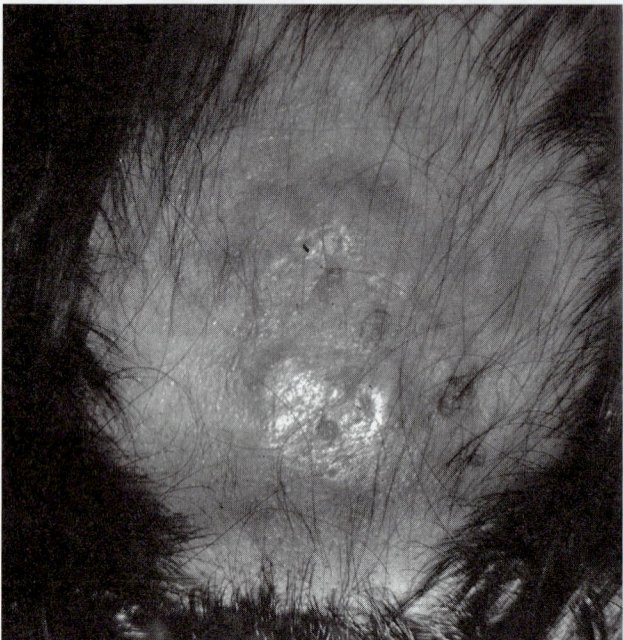

FIGURE 209.1. Tinea capitis. (Courtesy of George Cohen, M.D.)

common etiologic agents. In the noninflammatory variety, the lesion begins at the base of the hair shaft as an erythematous papule that then spreads peripherally as hairs break just above the level of the scalp, leaving areas of alopecia. Pruritus is a common finding. Patches, sometimes grayish, may appear at separate areas and may become confluent. The inflammatory type, more commonly associated with *M. canis,* may result in a pustular folliculitis and regional lymphadenopathy. Kerions are inflammatory, tender, purulent boggy masses that form as a result of the host's immune response and generally do not represent secondary bacterial infection.

Black-dot tinea capitis is the most common presentation of tinea capitis in the United States and usually is associated with *T. tonsurans.* It is characterized by numerous small, round patches where hair shafts have broken off at the level of the follicle and appear as dots on the skin surface.

Tinea Corporis (Fig. 209.2)

Tinea corporis refers to dermatophytosis involving the glabrous skin in all parts of the body, with the exception of the palms, soles, and groin. The most frequent causes are *T. mentagrophytes, T. rubrum,* and *M. canis.* The typical ringworm lesion is pruritic and appears as an erythematous, annular lesion with an elevated, scaly, papular, and sometimes vesicular border spreading in a centrifugal manner while clearing centrally. Formation of kerions rarely is seen. Occasionally, tinea corporis may be confused with secondary syphilis, psoriasis, or seborrheic dermatitis.

Tinea Cruris

Tinea cruris (jock itch) is similar to tinea corporis, except that tinea cruris appears almost exclusively in adolescent boys and adult men. The lesions are localized to the groin and often are associated with tight-fitting underclothing. *E. floccosum, T. rubrum,* and *T. mentagrophytes* account for most cases. The erythematous, slightly indurated patch spreads, forming

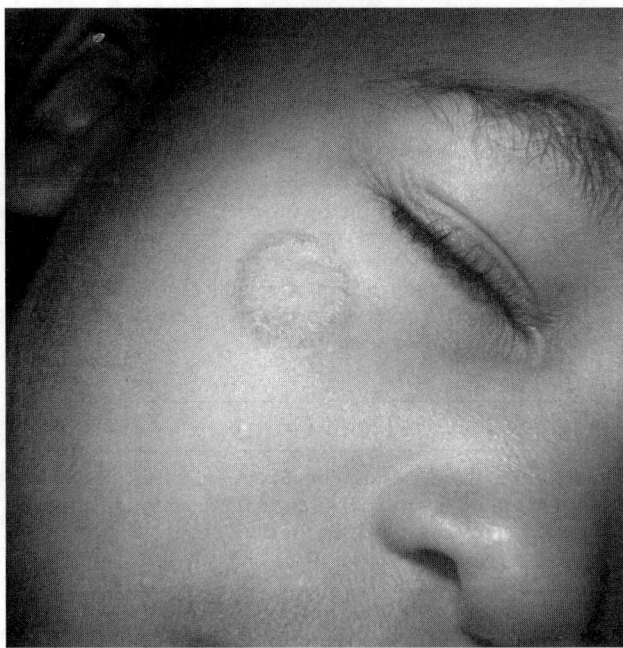

FIGURE 209.2. Tinea corporis. (Courtesy of George Cohen, M.D.)

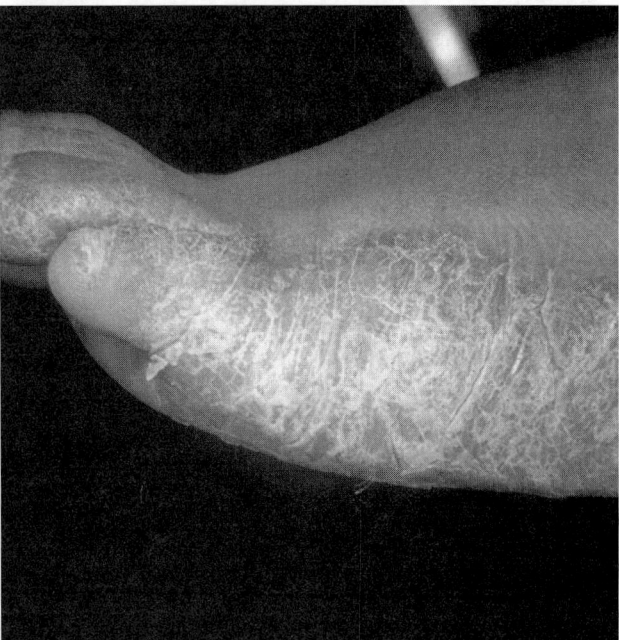

FIGURE 209.3. Tinea pedis. Note "moccasin" distribution. (Courtesy of George Cohen, M.D.)

tiny vesicles at the peripheral border. The lesions are intensely pruritic and may be painful, particularly if maceration or secondary bacterial infection occurs. The medial thighs may be involved. Tinea cruris may be confused with monilial skin infection or with erythrasma. Scrotal involvement is less common than with monilial infections in the groin area. Also, satellite lesions are more typical of monilial infection and can aid in making this clinical distinction. The pink coral fluorescence under Wood light characteristic of erythrasma may aid in differentiating it from tinea cruris.

Tinea Pedis (Fig. 209.3)

Tinea pedis (athlete's foot) is a relatively uncommon occurrence in young children and occurs most frequently in adolescent boys. Infection occurs more commonly in the summer months, particularly if occlusive shoes are worn. Use of communal baths, pools, and similar areas is a risk factor. *T. rubrum* and *T. tonsurans* are the most common etiologic agents. Typically, individuals present with fissuring, maceration, and scaling of the interdigital space webbing of the lateral (third and fourth) toes. The patient usually experiences pain and pruritus. In younger children, *T. mentagrophytes* may cause a vesicular-type reaction involving multiple areas of the foot. *T. rubrum* can cause a chronic hyperkeratotic rash of the sole of the foot in a so-called moccasin distribution, sometimes involving both feet and one hand. Secondary bacterial infection (erythrasma) may complicate tinea pedis, and the condition may be confused with contact dermatitis or eczema.

Tinea Unguium (Fig. 209.4)

Tinea unguium is a relatively uncommon occurrence in children, perhaps because of rapid nail growth in this age group, but youngsters can be infected during household epidemics. The most common etiologic agent is *T. rubrum*, but many species of dermatophytes have been implicated. Usually, a yellow or brown discoloration of the nail is seen, with thickening

and friability beginning at the distal and lateral borders of the nail. Tinea unguium may be confused with a large variety of nail disorders, including candidal infection, psoriasis, Reiter syndrome, and lichen planus.

Miscellaneous Dermatophytoses

Less common manifestations of dermatophyte infection include involvement of the hands (tinea manuum) and beard (tinea barbae). Id (dermatophytid) reactions may be seen, most

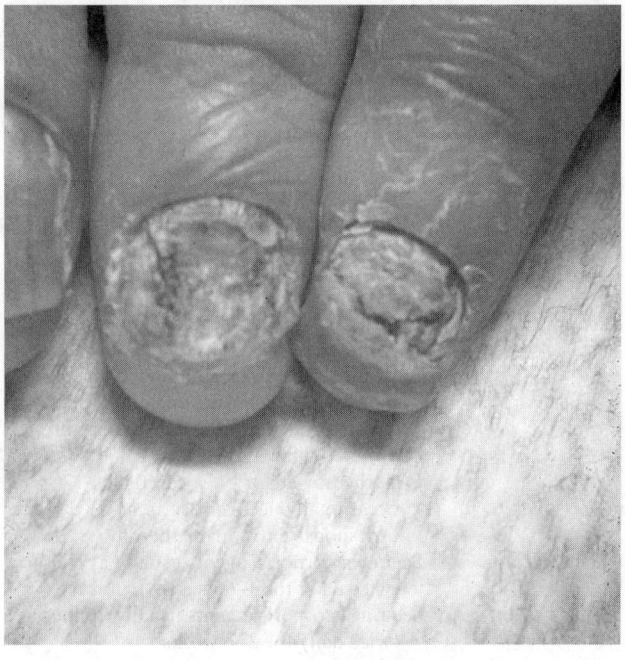

FIGURE 209.4. Tinea unguium. (Courtesy of George Cohen, M.D.)

commonly in association with tinea pedis. *Tinea incognito* refers to infections with atypical features, usually due to application of topical corticosteroids.

DIAGNOSIS

Dermatophytosis usually can be diagnosed solely on the basis of clinical features. Atypical features may require further study, however. Many authorities recommend routine culturing of suspected tinea capitis because prolonged therapy is needed and clinical response is slow, potentially causing delayed appreciation of misdiagnosis. For tinea capitis, Wood light examination no longer is particularly useful because the major pathogen, *T. tonsurans*, does not fluoresce. (*M. canis* and *M. audouinii*, among others, fluoresce bright green but, since the late 1950s, they have been much less common causes of tinea capitis.) If necessary, specimens of hair or skin can be collected by gently scraping with a scalpel or by gently brushing or swabbing a lesion. Nail clippings also may be examined. KOH examination of material might be useful if fungal hyphae are demonstrated, but a negative examination does not exclude the diagnosis. Dermatophyte test medium, a phytone dextrose agar containing cycloheximide, gentamicin, chlortetracycline, and phenol red dye, changes color from yellow to red within approximately 14 days of inoculation of clinical material containing dermatophytes.

THERAPY

Dermatophytosis treatment guidelines are listed in Table 209.1. With the exception of tinea capitis and most cases of tinea unguium, dermatophyte infections are treated topically.

Tinea Capitis

Although it can resolve spontaneously, tinea capitis should be treated. Microsize or ultramicrosize griseofulvin is the drug of choice, given orally for 4 to 12 weeks. Other oral drugs, such as itraconazole and terbinafine, may prove to be more effective than is griseofulvin, but oral terbinafine is not licensed yet for use in pediatric patients. Topical therapy with agents such as selenium sulfide shampoo can help to decrease shedding of spores, and corticosteroid therapy occasionally is a useful adjunct if formation of kerions is severe.

Tinea Corporis

Tinea corporis can be treated with any of several topical antifungal preparations, including terbinafine, miconazole, and clotrimazole. Severe cases of tinea corporis may require griseofulvin taken orally for several weeks.

Tinea Cruris

The patient with tinea cruris should wear loose-fitting clothing that allows good aeration. The topical preparations listed for tinea corporis can also be used for tinea cruris.

Tinea Pedis

Tinea pedis usually can be treated with topical powders such as tolnaftate or undecylenic acid. Additionally, the affected child should wear clean, absorbent socks and should keep the feet as dry as possible. Severe or unresponsive cases may require treatment with griseofulvin. Patients with secondary bacterial infection may benefit from oral antibiotics.

Tinea Unguium

Oral therapy is required for tinea unguium, and many cases are recalcitrant to oral griseofulvin. Oral itraconazole and terbinafine have been used successfully in adults, but these agents are not approved for treatment of tinea unguium in children.

PROGNOSIS

Most cases of superficial dermatophytosis respond to standard therapy. Tinea capitis may evolve to kerion formation as mentioned above, and children then may demonstrate systemic signs and symptoms. However, bacterial superinfection is rare. Spontaneous resolution is uncommon.

PREVENTION

Dermatophytoses are spread by direct contact, so prompt treatment of suspected cases is advisable to prevent spread to others in close contact with the index case. For children with tinea capitis, sharing of combs, brushes, and hair ornaments should be avoided. Children with tinea capitis who attend day care or school probably should receive topical treatment with selenium sulfide shampoo to reduce the chance of spread.

TABLE 209.1

DERMATOPHYTOSIS TREATMENT GUIDELINES

Condition	Standard Treatment
Tinea capitis	Microsize griseofulvin 15–20 mg/kg/day once daily, maximum 1 g, × 4–6 weeks. **or** Ultramicrosize griseofulvin 5–10 mg/kg/day once daily, maximum 750 mg, × 4–6 weeks Both should be given after a fatty meal
Tinea corporis	Topical therapy with miconazole nitrate, clotrimazole, terbinafine, or tolnaftate, once daily for 4 weeks Oral therapy as for tinea capitis occasionally needed for cases unresponsive to topical therapy
Tinea cruris	See tinea corporis; agents usually applied twice daily for 4–6 weeks
Tinea pedis	See tinea corporis; agents usually applied twice daily for 2–3 weeks
Tinea unguium	Oral griseofulvin as listed for tinea capitis above, administered for 6–18 months

Suggested Readings

Alston SJ, Cohen BA, Braun M. Persistent and recurrent tinea corporis in children treated with combination antifungal/corticosteroid agents. *Pediatrics* 2003;111:201.

Bakos L, Brito AC, Castro LCM, et al. Open clinical study of the efficacy and safety of terbinafine cream 1% in children with tinea corporis and tinea cruris. *Pediatr Infect Dis J* 1997;16:545.

Friedlander SF, Aly R, Krafchik B, et al. Terbinafine in the treatment of *Trichophyton* tinea capitis: a randomized, double-blind, parallel-group, duration-finding study. *Pediatrics* 2002;109:602.

Friedlander SF, Pickering B, Cunningham BB, et al. Use of the cotton swab method in diagnosing tinea capitis. *Pediatrics* 1999;104:276.

Fuller LC, Child FJ, Midgley G, et al. Diagnosis and management of scalp ringworm. *Brit Med J* 2003;326:539.

Gupta AK, Skinner AR. Onychomycosis in children: a brief overview with treatment strategies. *Pediatr Dermatol* 2004;21:74.

Lobato MN, Vugia DJ, Frieden IJ. Tinea capitis in California children: a population-based study of a growing epidemic. *Pediatrics* 1997;99:551.

Pomeranz AJ, Fairley JA. Management errors leading to unnecessary hospitalization for kerion. *Pediatrics* 1994;93:986.

Schwartz RA. Superficial fungal infections. *Lancet* 2004;364:1173.

CHAPTER 210 ■ ASPERGILLOSIS

WALTER T. HUGHES

Aspergillosis is caused by a monomorphic mold and may occur in several diverse disease forms. The clinical features depend on whether the infection results in colonization only, in hypersensitivity to the organism (allergic aspergillosis), or in invasive mycotic disease, which is found predominantly in the immunosuppressed host.

ETIOLOGY

Of the some 300 *Aspergillus* species, the most common ones affecting humans are *A. fumigatus* and *A. flavus*. Other species involved in infections include *A. niger, A. oryzae, A. glaucus, A. nidulans, A. restrictus, A. sydowi, A. terreus, A. versicolor, A. candidus, A. ustus,* and *A. amstelodami.*

EPIDEMIOLOGY

Aspergillus is ubiquitous in the environment in most parts of the world and may be found in soil, hay, compost piles, decaying vegetation, water, flour, house dust, bedding, food, chemical solutions, medications, surgical dressings, fireproofing material, shower stalls, and potted plants.

Allergic bronchopulmonary aspergillosis has been reported as a complication of asthma and cystic fibrosis. Invasive aspergillosis is found predominantly in the immunocompromised host.

Human-to-human and animal-to-human transmission are not known to occur. Host factors for susceptibility are of prime importance in the acquisition of the infection. At high risk are individuals with malignancy; organ transplant recipients; and patients with acquired immunodeficiency syndrome (AIDS), chronic granulomatous disease, and other immune deficiency disorders.

Nosocomial aspergillosis has been associated with airborne and waterborne organisms in the hospital environment of immunosuppressed patients. The high density of organisms associated with building construction and in fireproofing materials has been related to outbreaks of pulmonary aspergillosis in hospitalized patients. Furthermore, primary cutaneous aspergillosis may occur under surgical dressings and at Hickman catheter sites. Infrequently, invasive aspergillosis of the lung, sinuses, brain, and bone occurs in otherwise normal individuals.

PATHOLOGY

Allergic Aspergillosis

Allergic bronchopulmonary aspergillosis begins with the inhalation of *Aspergillus* conidia (spores). In a genetically susceptible (HLA-DR restriction) asthmatic patient or one with cystic fibrosis, the spores develop into hyphal forms as the bronchi become colonized. A local inflammatory reaction develops. Antigens of the hyphae react with IgE, IgG, and IgA antibodies as the response escalates to damage of the bronchial wall and infiltration with eosinophils. Antigen-specific CD4 Th2-like T lymphocytes produce increased levels of interleukin (IL)-4 and IL-5. The bronchial wall is infiltrated with mononuclear cells and eosinophils. Mucus and exudate, along with segments of the fungus, may fill the bronchi. The lung parenchyma may become involved with granulomatous reactions. Vasculitis is an uncommon finding with this type of pulmonary aspergillosis, and the lack of an acute neutrophil response is compatible with a delayed hypersensitivity response.

Invasive Aspergillosis

The pathogenesis of invasive aspergillosis differs considerably from that of allergic aspergillosis. Although pulmonary aspergillosis is found occasionally in presumably otherwise normal individuals, the usual host for any invasive form of the disease is one whose immune system has been compromised. Normally, inhaled *Aspergillus* conidia that reach the paranasal sinuses and lung are ingested and digested by polymorphonuclear leukocytes or alveolar macrophages. If this arm of the defense mechanism is impaired, as it is in patients with chronic granulomatous disease (in whom oxidative intracellular killing is impaired) and in patients with other phagocytic defects or quantitative deficits, the organism may colonize and develop hyphal and invasive forms. With this type of host-parasite relationship, the outcome often is hemorrhagic infarction and necrosis.

The pathologic pattern appears to be related, to some extent, to the severity of immunocompromise. A fibrosing granulomatous reaction or chronic, nonspecific inflammatory response may be found in an otherwise healthy patient. A severely compromised host exhibits massive hyphal invasion of blood vessels and no granulation tissue. In some patients, the infection may localize with formation of a cavity—the aspergilloma. The cavity is occupied partially by a ball of *Aspergillus* hyphae. Rarely, a chronic, necrotizing, granulomatous pneumonia is seen around a central zone of infarct-like necrosis of parenchyma resulting from angioinvasive aspergilli. These lesions tend to be found in the upper lobes. Paranasal sinuses infected with this fungus may exhibit a spectrum of tissue responses similar to the pattern described for the lung, or the site may be colonized only, with hypertrophy of the sinus mucosa.

CLINICAL MANIFESTATIONS

The clinical features of aspergillosis depend on the host response or, in most instances, on deficits in the host response. The lung and paranasal sinuses are the sites involved most frequently, but disseminated infection may affect several body organs. Another determinant of clinical manifestations is whether the disease is based on hypersensitivity to the organism or on invasion of tissues by the fungus. The clinical types of aspergillosis are described next.

Allergic Bronchopulmonary Aspergillosis

An asthmatic patient will experience wheezing and dyspnea. Acute attacks may be associated with fever. Cough may produce sputum with plugs of mucus and fungus. Eosinophilia may suggest aspergillosis as a cause of the illness.

Invasive Aspergillosis

Aspergillosis of the lung is characterized clinically by cough, hemoptysis, obstructive airway signs, and abnormalities associated with the underlying disease, such as neutropenia. Erosion of a major blood vessel may result in fatal hemorrhage. Pulmonary aspergillosis may progress to a disseminated invasive mycosis involving one or more other deep organs.

Sinusitis may be asymptomatic or associated with symptoms of fever, pain, and swelling. The maxillary sinus is the site involved most frequently.

The growth of *Aspergillus* species in the external otic canal usually is benign, and symptoms should not be attributed to its presence unless other causes are excluded.

Endophthalmitis may occur after trauma or surgery to the eye, or it may result from systemic infection. Ocular pain, ciliary injection, and uveitis may occur. Black corneal ulcers also may occur.

Cutaneous lesions have been described as primary infections at sites where Hickman catheters have been inserted and under surgical dressings. The signs are erythema, induration, and cutaneous or subcutaneous necrosis. Cutaneous lesions might also develop after systemic dissemination of infection from other sites (Fig. 210.1).

Hematogenous dissemination is a common occurrence in severely compromised hosts. It usually is seen in association with invasive pulmonary aspergillosis and neutropenia. One-half the patients with disseminated aspergillosis have extrapulmonary organ involvement. The brain, gastrointestinal tract, esophagus, heart, liver, and kidneys are the sites involved most frequently, but any organ, including bone, can be infected.

The signs and symptoms of aspergillosis are related to impaired function of the organ involved. Although all patients usually have fever, specific signs and symptoms can be absent, despite considerable infection of a deep organ.

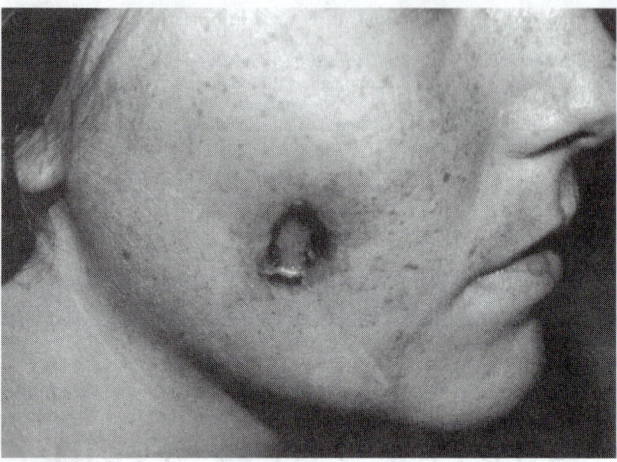

FIGURE 210.1. A necrotic, ulcerative, and indolent cutaneous lesion due to *Aspergillus fumigatus* in a child with malignancy and disseminated aspergillosis.

DIAGNOSIS

A definitive diagnosis requires the demonstration of typical septate, branching hyphae in tissues, and isolation of the organism in culture. *Aspergillus* species are cultured readily on all standard mycologic media, and growth is apparent within a few days.

Although *Aspergillus* is highly prevalent in the environment and may contaminate laboratory media if care is not taken, this organism is not found frequently as a part of the normal flora of the respiratory tract. The isolation of *Aspergillus* species from the sputum or nasal swab in an immunocompromised patient with pneumonia suggests the diagnosis of aspergillosis. Even in disseminated disease, the organism rarely is isolated from the blood. Aspirates and biopsies from infected sites should be cultured and studied histologically.

Serologic tests for antibody are helpful in cases of allergic bronchopulmonary aspergillosis and may yield detectable titers in some types of invasive disease. Used alone, however, such tests are not diagnostic.

Methods to detect the galactomannan of *Aspergillus* in serum, cerebrospinal fluid, bronchoalveolar fluid, and urine may aid in the diagnosis of invasive aspergillosis. The FDA-approved Platelia *Aspergillus* antigen immunoassay (MiraVista Diagnostics, Indianapolis) has approximately 81% sensitivity and 89% specificity for invasive aspergillosis. This test also is useful in monitoring antigenemia for response to treatment. Molecular tests using the polymerase chain reaction to identify *Aspergillus* DNA offer promise for diagnostic and epidemiologic uses.

TREATMENT

Allergic Aspergillosis

Treatment of allergic bronchopulmonary disease is drastically different from that of the invasive infection. In allergic bronchopulmonary aspergillosis, clinical improvement and regression of the infiltrate have occurred after the administration of corticosteroids. Remission of disease has been achieved with prednisone given every other day in a dosage of 0.5 mg/kg. Larger doses of 60 mg/day (total dose) have been associated with limited tissue invasion by the fungus. The appropriate duration of this therapy is not established, and caution should be practiced in its use. Current medical knowledge indicates that antifungal drugs are not beneficial for patients with this form of aspergillosis.

Invasive Aspergillosis

Until recently, amphotericin B, although far from ideal, has been the only drug available for the treatment of invasive aspergillosis. Newer drugs now approved by the FDA for this purpose include voriconazole, itraconazole, and caspofungin. Amphotericin B and voriconazole are considered first-line drugs, whereas itraconazole and caspofungin are secondary drugs for patients failing or intolerant to the primary drugs. Combinations of drugs have not been studied adequately for recommendations to be made at this time. The standard amphotericin B deoxycholate is administered intravenously, starting with a test dose for toxicity of 0.25 mg/kg and then increasing the daily dose by 0.25 mg/kg increments until a maintenance dose of 1.0 mg/kg/day is reached. Doses as high as 1.5 mg/kg/day may be warranted in some cases. Infusions are given over a period of 2 to 6 hours as tolerated. A course of 4 to 6 weeks is needed for all cases, and some patients may require a longer therapeutic period. The lipid-based formulations of amphotericin B (lipid complex, colloidal or liposomal) are associated with less toxicity than is the deoxycholate preparation, but no advantage in efficacy has been demonstrated. They are recommended for patients who cannot tolerate or who are not responding to conventional amphotericin B. The dose is 3 to 5 mg/kg/day, intravenously.

Voriconazole, a second-generation triazole, recently was compared with amphotericin B deoxycholate in a randomized trial of 277 patients with invasive aspergillosis. Herbrecht et al. found that initial therapy with voriconazole led to better responses, higher survival rates, and fewer severe adverse effects than when compared with amphotericin B. In individuals older than 12 years of age, the drug is administered intravenously in doses of 6.0 mg/kg every 12 hours for the first 24 hours, then 4.0 mg/kg every 12 hours for 7 days. Therapy then can be switched to 100 to 200 mg taken every 12 hours by mouth. Transient visual distortions may occur. Doses for infants and young children have not been established firmly.

Caspofungin, a new class of echinocandin agents, is indicated for treatment of invasive aspergillosis in patients refractory or intolerant to other therapies. Safety and effectiveness in pediatric patients have not been established.

Itraconazole has been effective in several patients with invasive aspergillosis nonresponsive to amphotericin B. A recent study by Gallin et al. strongly supports the use of itraconazole prophylactically in the management of chronic granulomatous disease. The use of antifungal agents in other immunocompromised hosts for the prevention of aspergillosis has not been established.

Surgical resection of well-localized pulmonary lesions probably is advisable when possible, but firm guidelines regarding surgical intervention are not available.

The results of treatment of invasive aspergillosis in immunosuppressed patients are poor and depend to a great extent on the reconstitution of immune responses, especially in patients with functional neutrophils in adequate number. The roles of recombinant colony-stimulating factors, such as granulocyte colony-stimulating factor, and granulocyte transfusions have not been established.

Suggested Readings

Abassi S, Shenep JL, Hughes WT, Flynn PM. Aspergillosis in children: a 34-year experience. *Clin Infect Dis* 1999;29:1210.

Denning WD. Invasive aspergillosis. *Clin Infect Dis* 1998;26:781.

Gallin JI, Alling DW, Malech HL, et al. Itraconazole to prevent fungal infections in chronic granulomatous disease. *N Engl J Med* 2003;348:2416.

Hebrecht R, Denning DW, Patterson TF, et al. Voriconazole versus amphotericin B for primary therapy of invasive aspergillosis. *N Engl J Med* 2002;347:408.

Hori A, Kami M, Kishi Y, et al. Clinical significance of extra-pulmonary involvement of invasive aspergillosis: a retrospective autopsy-based study of 107 patients. *J Hosp Infect* 2002;50:175.

Maertens J, Van Eldere J, Verhaegen J, et al. Use of circulating galactomannan screening for early diagnosis of invasive aspergillosis in allogenic stem cell transplant recipients. *J Infect Dis* 2002;186:1297.

CHAPTER 211 ■ COCCIDIOIDOMYCOSIS

ZIAD M. SHEHAB

EPIDEMIOLOGY

Coccidioidomycosis is an infection caused by the dimorphic fungus *Coccidioides immitis*. Usually, the primary pulmonary infection is self-limited, but disseminated and even fatal disease can occur. The infection is endemic in the Western Hemisphere in an area contained between 40 degrees of latitude north and south. In the United States, this area includes the deserts of the southwestern states: California, Arizona, New Mexico, and western Texas. This area corresponds to the Lower Sonoran life zone, which is characterized by arid to semiarid climate, hot summers and short winters, and limited rainfall with few freezes. The organism grows in the superficial layers of the soil to a depth of 20 cm. Arthroconidia are aerosolized during wind storms or when soil is disturbed, as by construction work, archaeologic digs, earthquakes, or farming. Prolonged droughts followed by rains increase the rate of primary infections, which are more likely to occur in the winter following germination of the organism in the soil after a rainy season. In endemic areas, infections occur in individuals without any predisposing condition at a rate estimated to be around 2% to 4% per year. On occasion, the infection has been transmitted through fomites, such as soil from potted plants.

In the Southwest, *C. immitis* results in 100,000 infections per year. It is seen also in other parts of the country in individuals who have lived or traveled to the endemic areas of the

Southwest. Although the infection rate in endemic areas has continued to drop, the rapid population growth in these areas continues to make coccidioidomycosis a significant health problem. While health care workers in endemic areas learn to suspect and identify the disease using the proper diagnostic tools, a high index of suspicion remains necessary, especially with increased exposure of larger numbers of travelers from nonendemic areas to the Southwest.

PATHOGENESIS AND PATHOLOGY

The organism's life cycle exhibits two distinctive phases: a saprophytic or vegetative phase and a parasitic phase. On culture media and in nature, the organism grows as a mycelium with branching, septate hyphae. After 5 to 7 days, the mycelia develop rectangular spores (arthroconidia, arthrospores), which are easily airborne. The arthrospores measure 2 to 8 μm, allowing them to reach the alveolar spaces when aerosolized. In the host tissues, the arthroconidia begin the parasitic phase of the life cycle. They enlarge and develop into spherules, which are double-walled structures of 20 to 100 μm diameter. The spherules undergo internal segmentation, leading to the formation of endospores that measure 2 to 5 μm. When the spherules rupture in the surrounding tissues, they release the endospores, leading to the formation of more spherules. The spherule is noninfectious. As a result, person-to-person transmission of coccidioidomycosis does not occur except in rare situations wherein the organism is allowed to revert to its mycelial form, such as growth on a plaster cast from a draining wound. Alternately, when the spherules rupture into the environment, the released endospores can lead to formation of hyphae, thus repeating the cycle in nature.

The organism grows readily on standard laboratory media, producing visible mycelial colonies in 3 to 4 days. During the second week, the colonies develop cobweb-like aerial hyphae that can be aerosolized and are infectious. Identification of the colonies is achieved by animal inoculation, demonstration of the spherule stage, demonstration of specific exoantigens, or identification of the organism using specific genetic probes.

Acquisition of *C. immitis* infection usually occurs via the respiratory route, which may result from infection with as little as a single spore. In most patients, the infection remains localized to the lungs and the hilar nodes. In a few (0.5%), dissemination to extrapulmonary sites occurs via the lymphatics or the bloodstream. Rarely, infection can be acquired by skin puncture with a contaminated object.

The pulmonary disease is manifested by a bronchopneumonia that may involve any lobe. As the disease progresses, cell-mediated immune responses, which are essential for control of the disease process, become defective, resulting in an ineffective type 2 helper T-cell response.

C. immitis can spread beyond the lung, a process that usually occurs within weeks or months after initial infection. Endogenous reactivation of primary disease also may occur, especially in immunosuppressed children. Extrapulmonary dissemination may occur after primary infection in normal hosts and after primary infection or reactivation in immunocompromised hosts. Once dissemination occurs, cell-mediated immune responses often are impaired, especially in severe infections. Dissemination may occur to any part of the body and usually involves the meninges, bones, joints, skin or soft tissues, or lymph nodes. The tissue reaction in disseminated disease is primarily granulomatous, with the lesions containing abundant giant cells and histiocytes. Usually, spherules are seen readily within the macrophages.

The rates of dissemination beyond the lungs vary considerably and are higher in Filipinos, Hispanics, blacks, pregnant women, and infants. Immunosuppressed hosts, especially those with human immunodeficiency virus (HIV) infection, are prone to severe pulmonary disease and dissemination.

CLINICAL MANIFESTATIONS

Primary Infection

Clinical manifestations of primary infection in children are thought to be similar to those described in adults. Infection typically is subclinical or may resemble a mild upper respiratory tract illness in approximately 60% of infected immunocompetent individuals. In the remainder, symptoms range from a mild febrile respiratory or influenza-like illness 1 to 3 weeks after exposure to severe lower respiratory tract illness with lobar pneumonia, pleural effusions, and, sometimes, pericarditis. Typically, the presentation is subacute and self-limited, but some patients will have a more complicated pulmonary illness and, rarely, may develop extrapulmonary disease.

Cough and fever are the most common presenting symptoms and often are associated with chest pain, dyspnea, fatigue, and chills. Fever occurs in about half the patients. Arthralgias, myalgias, and headaches also are reported (Table 211.1). Rarely, airway obstruction in infants may result in stridor. These symptoms are not readily distinguishable from those of other pulmonary infections. The presence of such associated findings as eosinophilia, pleuritic chest pain out of proportion to the other symptoms, and such cutaneous manifestations as erythema nodosum or erythema multiforme are helpful clinical clues. Early in the course of the infection, erythematous maculopapular rashes also may be seen. The appearance of erythema nodosum correlates with the development of cell-mediated immune responses and is associated with a low risk of dissemination. Rarely, patients may present with a picture of septic shock.

Radiologically, single or multifocal bronchopulmonary infiltrates are the most common presentation of primary coccidioidomycosis (Table 211.1). Segmental or lobar consolidation and nodular or patchy pulmonary infiltrates also may be seen. Hilar adenopathy with or without pulmonary infiltrates

---

TABLE 211.1

FEATURES OF PRIMARY COCCIDIOIDOMYCOSIS

- Clinical
  - Asymptomatic in 60%
  - Common
    - Cough
    - Fever
  - Less common
    - Chest pain, dyspnea
    - Fatigue, chills
    - Erythema nodosum
- Radiologic: Nonspecific
  - Most commonly bronchopulmonary infiltrates, often with hilar adenopathy
  - Segmental or lobar consolidation
  - Nodular or patchy infiltrates
  - Small pleural effusions
  - Nodules (rare)
  - Thin-walled cavities (rare)
  - Miliary pattern (especially in patients with human immunodeficiency virus infection or other severe immunosuppression)
  - In neonates: Focal consolidation with diffuse nodular densities

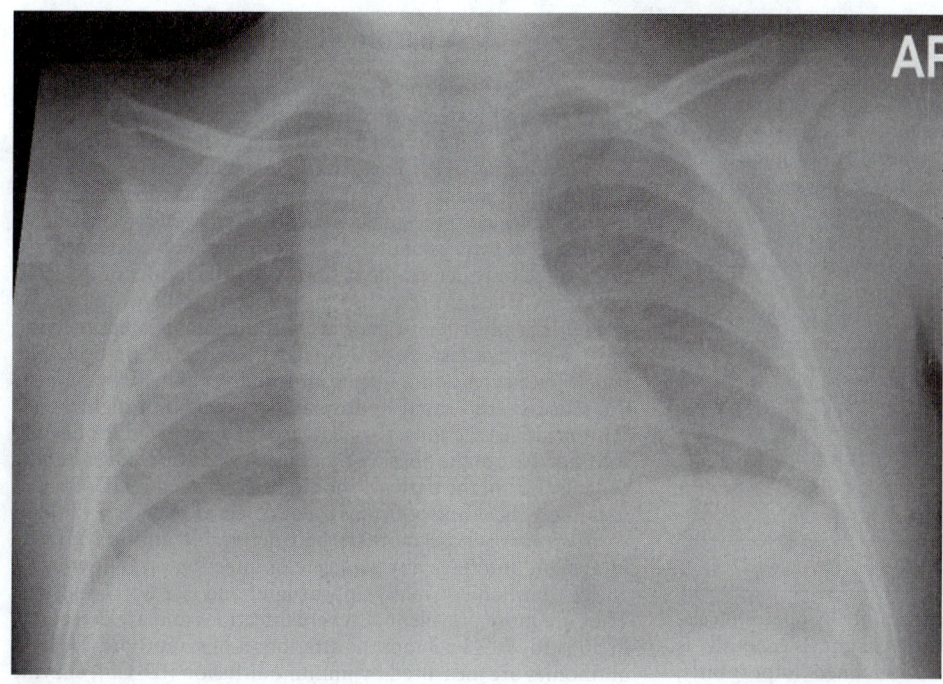

FIGURE 211.1. Right upper lobe infiltrate with hilar and paratracheal adenopathy due to coccidioidomycosis.

(Fig. 211.1) is seen in about 20% of the patients. Small pleural effusions are frequent and usually are sterile. In most cases these changes do not require any specific therapy and resolve spontaneously in 90% to 95% of patients. Cavitation, nodule formation, bronchiectasis, or calcification may develop later. Typically, the cavities are thin-walled and asymptomatic and only rarely require therapy; many regress spontaneously. Cavities rarely can lead to the development of abscesses or bronchopleural fistulas with pyopneumothorax, complications that occur more commonly in the immunosuppressed or diabetic patient. Nodules and thin-walled cavities develop in 5% of patients with coccidioidal pneumonia. Typically, these lesions are single and asymptomatic. Up to 10% of single nodules will calcify, but multiple calcifications are unusual. A miliary pattern is seen sometimes in immunosuppressed individuals and is unusual in normal hosts.

In neonates, the disease presents with a focal area of consolidation followed by diffuse nodular infiltrates and, commonly, evidence of hyperinflation. Pleural effusions and mediastinal adenopathy are uncommon. These findings may be associated with nonspecific respiratory symptoms and minimal clinical findings on auscultation of the chest. Untreated, this disease may be severe and occasionally fatal.

Primary cutaneous coccidioidal infection is rare. The lesion resembles a chancre and is associated with regional lymphadenitis. Although in adults the process tends to resolve spontaneously over 2 to 3 months, progressive and prolonged infection may be more common in children and may require antifungal therapy.

Disseminated Coccidioidomycosis

Dissemination is unusual in infected children (0.5%), except in young infants. Disseminated disease presents with persistent fever, toxicity, and the insidious development of lesions outside the chest; the spread manifests within a few weeks to a few months after primary infection. Rarely, dissemination can occur after an asymptomatic primary infection. Dissemination can occur to any site (Table 211.2). The areas most commonly affected are the central nervous system, bones and joints, skin and soft tissues, and genitourinary systems.

Meningitis can occur as part of widespread dissemination and often is the only site of extrapulmonary disease. The disorder may present acutely with the primary infection but more commonly presents up to 6 months later. The typical symptoms are headache, ataxia, sluggishness, and vomiting. Concomitant hydrocephalus frequently is seen at presentation but may also develop in the course of the disease. Focal neurologic findings may be present, and evidence of meningeal irritation often is lacking. Chorioretinitis may provide evidence for dissemination.

Bony involvement occurs most commonly in the vertebrae, tibia, metatarsals, skull, and metacarpals. Usually, it results in a chronic osteomyelitis, which may drain in soft tissues and form fistulas with the overlying skin. A single bone is involved in 60% of the cases. Contiguous spread resulting in meningitis is a concern in vertebral osteomyelitis. Dissemination to the skin most commonly presents with a verrucous granuloma at the nasolabial fold. The subcutaneous tissue may be involved, resulting in cold abscesses and chronic sinus tracts and ulcers. Coccidioidomycosis may involve the pelvic organs. Coccidioiduria may be a silent manifestation of renal involvement disseminated disease. Coccidioidomycosis occurs infrequently during pregnancy but is associated with serious complications when the disease develops in the third trimester or soon after delivery. Neonates born to mothers with pelvic disease can acquire the infection perinatally, presumably from inhalation or aspiration of infected decidua. Disease in such neonates and young infants is associated with high mortality. Most cases of coccidioidomycosis in newborns and infants are the result of

---

TABLE 211.2

MANIFESTATIONS OF DISSEMINATED COCCIDIOIDOMYCOSIS

- Pulmonary: Diffuse reticulonodular infiltrates on chest x-ray
- Central nervous system: Meningitis, often with hydrocephalus
- Musculoskeletal: Osteomyelitis, arthritis, abscesses
- Cutaneous: Ulcers, verrucous lesions, abscesses

environmental exposure. Congenital infection has been demonstrated in one case.

Patients with conditions that result in T-cell dysfunction, such as leukemia, lymphoma, and solid-organ or bone marrow transplantation, are predisposed to more severe forms of the disease, including dissemination, especially during primary infections. In addition, such children may experience disease as a result of reactivation of old infection. In patients with acquired immunodeficiency syndrome (AIDS), severity of the disease is enhanced in those with a CD4 level of less than 250 cells/μL. Mortality is high even with the use of antifungal therapy for those patients who develop diffuse severe pulmonary disease. Disseminated coccidioidomycosis constitutes an AIDS-defining illness. HIV-positive individuals who have a positive coccidioidal serology in the absence of disease often go on to develop active disease. The introduction of highly active antiretroviral therapy has been associated with a decline in the severity of disease in HIV-infected persons.

DIAGNOSIS

In endemic areas, the diagnosis is made readily by obtaining appropriate tests. In nonendemic areas, the diagnosis generally is not considered unless a travel history is obtained. Importantly, exposure in endemic areas may be very brief. The primary infection resembles many other lower respiratory tract illnesses, including those caused by viruses, bacteria, *Mycobacterium tuberculosis*, mycoplasma, and such fungi as *Histoplasma*. The hematologic findings are not specific and consist of elevated erythrocyte sedimentation rate and leukocytosis. The presence of severe eosinophilia (more than 20%) suggests dissemination. The diagnosis is established by the use of cultures, serologic studies, examination of respiratory secretions, and tissue examination.

Culture and Identification of the Fungus

Demonstration of the organism by culture or visualization of spherules in tissues or respiratory secretions establishes the diagnosis. Culture is more sensitive than stains for examination of respiratory secretions. The Papanicolaou smear is the most sensitive cytologic test for identification of the fungus in respiratory secretions and is more sensitive than KOH smears. Bronchoscopy may be indicated in patients with severe disease or in those in whom sputum examination and serology was nondiagnostic. The yield from other sources, such as pleural fluid, blood, or joint fluid, is lower. Only one-third of cerebrospinal fluid (CSF) specimens are culture-positive in the presence of meningitis, and direct examination of the CSF almost always yields negative results. With the exception of the rare primary cutaneous disease, demonstration of spherules outside the chest provides evidence of dissemination. Usually, the organism grows within 5 days on most routine laboratory media as a nonpigmented mold. These cultures represent a biohazard to laboratory workers, and plates growing suspicious colonies should be taped immediately and handled only in a biosafety cabinet. Final identification is usually performed using specific genetic probes.

Skin Test

Lysates of either the mycelial (coccidioidin, 1:100 dilution) or spherule phase (spherulin) are used to elicit delayed cutaneous hypersensitivity. The intradermal skin tests are primarily useful in epidemiologic studies and are not commercially available.

Serologic Studies

The initial serologic response to *C. immitis* infection is of the IgM type and is demonstrated by the precipitin reaction seen with primary infection. These responses are assessed by the tube precipitins (TPs), latex particle agglutination (LPA), enzyme immunoassay (EIA-IgM), or immunodiffusion (ID-TP) methods. Ninety percent of patients yield a positive result by the first 2 to 3 weeks of illness. Not uncommonly, the IgM antibody is the only detectable antibody in primary uncomplicated infections. The IgM response subsequently resolves so that, by 6 months, only 10% of patients with uncomplicated infection have a positive test. A positive IgM test by TP or by ID-TP usually indicates acute infection. The LPA and EIA-IgM tests are sensitive and rapid but are associated with a high rate of false-positive reactions; thus, any isolated positive LPA or EIA-IgM test (i.e., in the absence of a positive IgG or recovery of the organism from the patient) should be confirmed by ID-TP. Occasionally, IgM antibody has been detected in the cord blood of newborns whose mothers had detectable antibody. These infants did not have any evidence of infection on follow-up.

IgG antibodies usually appear later and last 6 to 8 months. They are more prevalent in severe infections and are detectable in 50% to 90% by 3 months after onset of symptoms. The IgG antibodies are measured by immunodiffusion (ID-CF), enzyme immunoassay (EIA-IgG), or complement fixation (CF). Usually, they are undetectable during the first week of infection and may appear as long as 3 months after onset of symptoms. The magnitude of the CF antibody response correlates closely with severity of disease and risk of dissemination. In most laboratories, a CF titer of 1:32 or higher correlates with disseminated infection. Rarely, the serologic test will remain negative in an immunocompromised host with coccidioidomycosis. At least 90% of people with a symptomatic primary infection will demonstrate an IgM or IgG response of modest magnitude.

The CSF of patients with meningeal coccidioidomycosis is usually characterized by mononuclear cell pleocytosis, high protein, and low glucose. Early on, however, a polymorphonuclear response may be seen. At the time of diagnosis, 70% of patients with meningitis have detectable serum or CSF CF antibody. Eventually, it becomes positive in almost all patients. Occasionally, patients with contiguous infections (vertebral osteomyelitis or epidural abscess) may have low levels of CF antibody in the CSF without other evidence of meningeal involvement.

THERAPY

Primary Infection

Primary coccidioidomycosis is self-limited in more than 90% of children, requiring only analgesia and rest. Antifungal therapy is not indicated for individuals without risk of dissemination who present with a primary pulmonary infection or with an asymptomatic pulmonary nodule or cavity. Antifungal therapy is recommended for those with continuous fever for 1 month or those with extensive, progressive or miliary pulmonary disease. In addition, pregnant women, most children from such high-risk populations as Filipinos, neonates, and most young infants should be treated, as should immunosuppressed children. Amphotericin B often is used for the initial therapy in severely ill patients, followed by therapy with the triazoles. End-points of therapy in children without dissemination are not well defined. Typically, initiation of therapy dictates continued therapy for a period of 6 to 12 months. Surgical treatment seldom is indicated in primary disease but may be necessary if pericardial involvement is complicated by tamponade or if cavities last more than a year, especially in symptomatic patients.

Disseminated Disease

All patients with extrapulmonary dissemination should be treated. General clinical improvement, lowering of CF titers, and conversion to culture negativity are favorable signs. Seropositive individuals with HIV also should be treated, even in the absence of detectable disease, as they are at high risk for dissemination.

The agent of choice in fulminant infections is amphotericin B. The therapy consists of 1.0 mg/kg/day once daily initially, then tapered to three times weekly. Most patients respond to a total dose of 15 to 45 mg/kg, whereas those with severe, protracted illness may need as much as 100 mg/kg. Amphotericin does not cross the blood–brain barrier, and its administration by the lumbar, cisternal, or intrathecal route is necessary when amphotericin B is used to treat meningitis. It is associated with a high rate of arachnoiditis. Over the last decade, the azoles have transformed the therapy of most forms of disseminated coccidioidal disease, especially meningitis. The agents used most commonly are itraconazole and fluconazole. The use of fluconazole in pregnancy should be assessed carefully as it has been associated with an embryopathy. Relapses are common after discontinuation of therapy.

Meningitis is treated best with fluconazole (12 mg/kg/day) or itraconazole, typically without concurrent use of amphotericin B. Generally, patients respond within 1 to 2 months, although abnormalities of the CSF may persist for prolonged periods. The therapy is associated with suppression of the infection but not eradication, and discontinuation of therapy is associated with a high relapse rate, thus requiring lifelong therapy.

In adults with musculoskeletal dissemination, itraconazole is more effective than fluconazole. In young children, this increased efficacy has to be weighed against the erratic absorption of the liquid preparation of itraconazole and the need for twice-daily administration.

Clinical progress coupled with decreases in CF titers gauge the response to therapy for coccidioidomycosis. Rises in CF titers may herald relapses of infection. Within endemic areas, a useful approach may be to screen serologically those immunosuppressed individuals or those infected with HIV and to offer them antifungal prophylaxis with one of the azoles.

PREVENTION

Currently, no effective mode of active immunization is available to prevent human coccidioidomycosis. Efforts have been aimed at dust control and eradication of the fungus from the soil. The efficacy of these methods is unproved. In endemic areas, immunocompromised children should be advised against activities with high exposure risk, such as digging soil, mountain biking, or participating in archaeologic expeditions.

Suggested Readings

Charlton V, Ramsdell K, Sehring S. Intrauterine transmission of coccidioidomycosis. *Pediatr Infect Dis J* 1999;18:561.

Dewsnup DH, Galgiani JN, Graybill JR, et al. Is it ever safe to stop azole therapy for *Coccidioides immitis* meningitis? *Ann Intern Med* 1996;124:305.

Feldman BS, Snyder LS. Primary pulmonary coccidioidomycosis. *Semin Resp Infect* 2001;16:231.

Galgiani JN, Ampel NM, Catanzaro A, et al. Practice guidelines for the treatment of coccidioidomycosis. *Clin Infect Dis* 2000;30:658.

Galgiani JN, Catanzaro A, Cloud GA, et al. Comparison of oral fluconazole and itraconazole for progressive nonmeningeal coccidioidomycosis. *Ann Intern Med* 2000;133:676.

Linsangan L, Ross L. *Coccidioides immitis* infection or the neonate: two routes of infection. *Pediatr Infect Dis J* 1999;18:171.

Panackal AA, Hajjeh RA, Cetron MS, et al. Fungal infections among returning travelers. *Clin Infect Dis* 2002;35:1088.

Pappagianis D. Serologic studies in coccidioidomycosis. *Semin Resp Infect* 2001;16:242.

Stevens DA. Coccidioidomycosis. *N Engl J Med* 1995;332:1077.

CHAPTER 212 ■ CRYPTOCOCCOSIS

STEPHANIE H. STOVALL AND STEVEN C. BUCKINGHAM

Cryptococcosis is a mycosis that predominantly affects the lung, central nervous system (CNS), skin, and bone. Nineteen species of the genus *Cryptococcus* have been identified, but only *C. neoformans* is pathogenic in humans. This organism was identified in 1894, and its pathogenic role in human CNS disease was discovered shortly thereafter. The majority of infections caused by *C. neoformans* occur in immunocompromised individuals.

MICROBIOLOGY

Cryptococci are nonfermenting, round to oval, aerobic yeasts of irregular sizes, averaging 4 to 8 μm in diameter. Reproduction occurs by budding with a narrow neck between parent and daughter cells. *C. neoformans* is surrounded by an antiphagocytic polysaccharide capsule (Fig. 212.1). The five capsular serotypes of this organism are grouped into two varieties: *C. neoformans* variant *neoformans* (serotypes A, D, and AD) and *C. neoformans* variant *gatii* (serotypes B and C).

EPIDEMIOLOGY

The two varieties of *C. neoformans* have distinct epidemiologic and pathogenic characteristics. *C. neoformans* variant *neoformans* causes disseminated infections, especially in individuals with impaired cellular immunity, and has a particular tropism

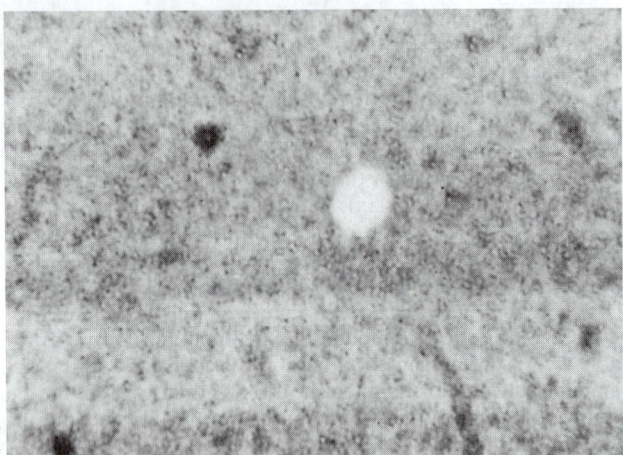

FIGURE 212.1. India ink preparation of cerebrospinal fluid showing budding yeast with prominent capsule.

for meninges. It is found in soil throughout the world, often in association with weathered bird droppings. *C. neoformans* variant *gatii* is associated with focal infections, particularly of the brain, in immunocompetent persons. It is endemic to regions of the world in which the red river gum tree, *Eucalyptus camaldulensis*, is found, including Australia, South America, Southeast Asia, and southern California. The remainder of this chapter will concern itself with *C. neoformans* variant *neoformans* unless otherwise stipulated.

Cryptococcosis is most often found in patients with acquired immunodeficiency syndrome (AIDS). One study reported that 89% of cryptococcosis cases occur in persons infected with human immunodeficiency virus (HIV). Infection with *C. neoformans* occurred in 5% to 15% of adults with AIDS prior to the widespread use of highly active antiretroviral therapy (HAART). Since the advent of HAART, the incidence of cryptococcosis has decreased by more than 50% in the adult population. Cryptococcosis was unusual in HIV-infected children even prior to the routine use of HAART. Among 473 HIV-infected children followed from 1987 to 1995, only four developed cryptococcosis (average annual incidence, 0.10%). Cryptococcal infection occurs rarely in children who are immunocompromised for reasons other than HIV infection (e.g., cancer chemotherapy or systemic lupus erythematosus).

PATHOGENESIS

Cryptococci are inhaled and gain access to the body via the lower respiratory tract, where the initial host response relies on phagocytosis of the organisms. The principal virulence factor of *C. neoformans* is the polysaccharide capsule, which prevents phagocytosis and down-regulates the host immune response by stimulating suppressor T cells. Opsonization by anticapsular antibodies or complement facilitates ingestion of cryptococci by phagocytic cells. Neutrophils kill the ingested organisms effectively, but macrophages are ineffective unless they are activated by interferon-gamma from helper T cells. Natural killer cells also appear to play a role in the host response. If the initial host response fails to contain the infection, the pulmonary fungal burden will increase and hematogenous dissemination to other organs may occur subsequently.

Individuals with deficient cellular immunity can rapidly develop disseminated disease after infection with *C. neoformans*. The CNS is the organ system most frequently affected in disseminated disease. There is frequently minimal inflammatory response, especially in the immunocompromised individual; in fact, the cerebrospinal fluid (CSF) leukocyte count is often only minimally elevated. Cryptococci may also spread to extrapulmonary sites in presumably immunocompetent hosts; in these individuals, the immunologic response is characterized by formation of granulomas, termed cryptococcomas, which are composed of multinucleate giant cells.

CLINICAL MANIFESTATIONS

Initial pulmonary infection is typically asymptomatic in immunocompetent hosts, though immunocompromised patients may experience cough, hemoptysis, chest pain, and significant constitutional symptoms. Radiographic findings in symptomatic patients range from solitary or multiple pulmonary nodules to diffuse infiltrates.

The most common manifestation of cryptococcal disease is meningitis, especially in the immunocompromised host. Symptoms of cryptococcal meningitis include fever, headache, vomiting, and altered mentation. The onset of symptoms usually is insidious but can sometimes be acute, especially in immunocompromised patients. Classic meningeal signs, such as Kernig and Brudzinski signs, are seen in 50% of patients. Approximately one-third of patients will experience cranial nerve palsies, visual disturbances, or papilledema, and about 15% have seizures. About 10% of patients with meningitis have no neurologic symptoms whatsoever. Lumbar puncture typically reveals an elevated opening pressure and findings on CSF analysis of lymphocytic pleocytosis, elevated protein, and low glucose.

Cryptococcomas of the CNS present with symptoms typical for elevated intracranial pressure, including headache, seizures, and focal neurologic deficits; hydrocephalus and uncinate herniation may occur. On computed tomographic scans or magnetic resonance imaging, the appearance of these lesions is similar to that of purulent abscesses or malignant metastases.

Extraneural cryptococcosis can involve virtually any organ of the body. Disseminated disease, including bloodstream and urinary tract infections, are seen more commonly in immunosuppressed individuals. Bone lesions, which are usually asymptomatic, are apparent radiographically in approximately 10% of patients with disseminated disease. Skin lesions also are seen in 10% of such patients and can be ulcerative, papular, or pustular. Eye involvement presents as retinitis. Other occasionally involved sites include the liver, spleen, heart, kidneys, and prostate.

DIAGNOSIS

Definitive diagnosis of cryptococcosis rests on isolation of the organism in culture. Cryptococcus grows readily on solid agar (without cycloheximide) or fungal culture media incubated at 37°C; recovery may be improved by the lysis-centrifugation technique. *C. neoformans* can be isolated from the CSF of 75% to 90% of patients with cryptococcal meningitis; however, large quantities of CSF should be cultured to enhance detection. Histologic demonstration of the organism in tissue using Gomori methenamine silver, Gridley, mucicarmine, or periodic acid-Schiff stains also supports the diagnosis.

Cryptococcal antigen detection by latex agglutination is more sensitive than the previously used India ink stain for the diagnosis of cryptococcal meningitis. In more than 90% of patients with cryptococcal meningitis, antigen will be detected in CSF, and in 50%, antigen will be detected in serum. During therapy the cryptococcal antigen titer can be followed as evidence of response to therapy; however, culture is the gold standard for ensuring sterility. The presence of rheumatoid factor in the serum may lead to false-positive latex agglutination results. India ink stains demonstrate encapsulated yeasts in the CSF of nearly 60% of patients with cryptococcal meningitis. Skin testing is of no diagnostic value.

THERAPY

Several antifungal agents are available for the treatment of cryptococcosis; however, uncertainty surrounds their optimal use in children. Given the decreasing incidence of AIDS in children, it is unlikely that randomized controlled trials will be done to determine the optimal therapy of cryptococcosis in children. Guidelines for the treatment of cryptococcosis in adults have been established, and to some extent these may be extrapolated to the pediatric population. This section will discuss the treatment of cryptococcosis in general, with specific comments on therapy in children as existing evidence allows.

Immunocompetent patients with asymptomatic pulmonary disease do not require antifungal therapy. Antifungal therapy is indicated for symptomatic immunocompetent patients and for all immunocompromised patients, though there are differences in therapeutic regimens and duration based upon immunologic status. Efforts should be made to normalize immune function in immunocompromised individuals if possible (e.g., HAART, weaning doses of steroids or other immunosuppressive drugs). Regardless of presenting symptoms or immunologic condition, all patients with cryptococcosis should be evaluated carefully for occult CNS infection.

When indicated, treatment of cryptococcal disease *that does not involve the central nervous system* in immunocompetent adults with mild to moderate symptoms may be accomplished with fluconazole (200 to 400 mg/day), administered for 6 to 12 months. Alternative regimens include itraconazole (200 to 400 mg/day) for 6 to 12 months or amphotericin B (0.4 to 0.7 mg/kg/day) for a total dose of 1 to 2 g. The optimal treatment of similar disease in immunocompetent children has not been rigorously evaluated. A conservative approach is to treat such children with amphotericin B at least until there is evidence of a therapeutic response, then to complete therapy with fluconazole (12 mg/kg/day) to complete 6 to 12 months of therapy. Therapy for similar disease in immunocompromised children and adults should continue at least until normal immune function is restored. It is presently recommended that HIV-infected children receive lifelong suppressive therapy with fluconazole after an episode of cryptococcosis.

Therapy for cryptococcosis *involving the central nervous system* is divided into primary therapy, the goal of which is to sterilize the CSF, and maintenance therapy, the goal of which is to prevent relapsing disease. Primary therapy for all patients should include amphotericin B (0.7 to 1 mg/kg/day) plus flucytosine (100 mg/kg/day). Traditionally, this therapy was continued for a minimum of 6 weeks and at least until repeat CSF examinations documented declining cryptococcal antigen titers. An alternative approach that has been studied in adult patients consists of induction therapy with amphotericin and flucytosine for a minimum of 2 weeks, followed by (provided CSF culture is sterile at this time) consolidation therapy with fluconazole (400 mg/day) for an additional 8 to 10 weeks. The induction/consolidation approach limits the need for intravenous access, reduces exposure to toxic side effects of amphotericin B and flucytosine, and eliminates need for monitoring of flucytosine serum levels. Unfortunately, the safety and efficacy of this approach in children have not been established. Primary therapy regimens that do not include amphotericin B (e.g.,

fluconazole or itraconazole alone or fluconazole plus flucytosine) are not recommended.

After primary therapy of CNS cryptococcosis has resulted in sterilization of CSF and declining CSF cryptococcal antigen titer, maintenance therapy is administered to prevent relapse. Fluconazole (6 mg/kg/day in children; 200 to 400 mg/day in adults), administered orally, is the most efficacious antifungal agent for this purpose. In adults with AIDS-associated cryptococcal meningitis, neither amphotericin B (1 mg/kg intravenously, one to three times per week) nor itraconazole (200 mg/day orally) prevents relapses as effectively as does fluconazole. All patients should receive a minimum of 6 to 12 months of maintenance therapy. In immunocompromised patients, this duration should be extended at least until normal immune function is restored (e.g., when cancer chemotherapy is terminated); in patients with AIDS-associated cryptococcal meningitis, maintenance therapy is generally continued for life. While consideration can be given to discontinuing maintenance therapy in patients with AIDS after HAART has restored cellular immune function (i.e., CD4 count greater than 200/μL in adults), insufficient evidence currently exists to routinely endorse this approach.

Ketoconazole has no role in the treatment of cryptococcosis. Although voriconazole is active against *C. neoformans in vitro*, its clinical efficacy for cryptococcosis has not been established. Caspofungin, the first commercially available echinocandin, is inactive against *Cryptococcus* species.

Intracerebral cryptococcomas should be removed if they are large (greater than 3 cm) or symptomatic, provided this is surgically feasible, as medical therapy alone is rarely adequate for such lesions. In addition, antifungal therapy as described above for CNS disease is indicated and can be guided by serial CSF evaluations.

PROGNOSIS

Several studies have identified patients who are at risk for poor outcomes from cryptococcal meningitis. Baseline findings associated with an increased risk of relapse or death include a pretreatment CSF or serum cryptococcal antigen titer of 1:32 or higher, CSF leukocytes numbering fewer than 20/μL, high CSF opening pressure, low CSF glucose, positive CSF India ink stain, and absent serum anticryptococcal antibody. Additional factors predictive of relapse after 4 weeks of therapy include cryptococcal antigen in CSF or serum of 1:8 or higher, lack of decline in CSF or serum antigen, and persistently low CSF glucose. In patients with AIDS-associated cryptococcal meningitis, poor outcomes have been associated with decreased mental status at diagnosis, elevated CSF cryptococcal antigen, CSF leukocytes numbering fewer than 20/μL, extraneural cultures positive for *C. neoformans*, hyponatremia, and age younger than 35 years.

Approximately 70% of patients with cryptococcal meningitis are cured with antifungal therapy. After therapy, neurologic evaluations are normal in 50% to 60% of these patients. The remaining patients have visual disturbances, cranial nerve palsies, motor dysfunction, or impaired mentation.

PREVENTION

No isolation measures beyond standard precautions are necessary for hospitalized patients with cryptococcosis. A prospective, randomized controlled trial demonstrated that prophylaxis with fluconazole reduces the frequency of cryptococcal disease in adults with AIDS, particularly those with CD4 cell counts of fewer than 50/μL. Because of the infrequency of cryptococcal infection and the frequency of adverse effects associated with daily fluconazole use, it is not recommended that all patients with AIDS or severe cell-mediated immunosuppression be treated prophylactically. Patients with a history of cryptococcosis, however, should receive maintenance antifungal therapy to prevent relapse.

No vaccine exists for the prevention of human cryptococcosis. A conjugate vaccine linking the capsular polysaccharide glucuronoxylomannan to tetanus toxoid protected against lethal cryptococcosis in mice, but elicited nonprotective and possibly deleterious, as well as protective, antibodies. Research continues on alternative approaches to vaccine design.

Suggested Readings

Abadi J, Nachman S, Kressel AB, Pirofski LA. Cryptococcosis in children with AIDS. *Clin Infect Dis* 1999;28:309.

American Academy of Pediatrics. *Red Book: 2003 Report of the Committee on Infectious Diseases*, 26th ed. Elk Grove Village, IL: American Academy of Pediatrics, 2003.

Fleuridor R, Lees A, Pirofski L. A cryptococcal capsular polysaccharide mimotope prolongs the survival of mice with *Cryptococcus neoformans* infection. *J Immunol* 2001;166:1087.

Gonzales CE, Shetty D, Lewis LL, et al. Cryptococcosis in human immunodeficiency virus-infected children. *Pediatr Infect Dis J* 1996;15:796.

Leggiadro RJ, Barrett FF, Hughes WT. Extrapulmonary cryptococcosis in immunocompromised infants and children. *Pediatr Infect Dis J* 1992;11:43.

Masur H, Kaplan JE, Holmes KK, et al. Guidelines for preventing opportunistic infections among HIV-infected persons—2002. Recommendations of the U.S. Public Health Service and the Infectious Diseases Society of America. *Ann Intern Med* 2002;137:435.

Mirza SA, Phelan M, Rimland D, et al. The changing epidemiology of cryptococcosis: an update from population-based active surveillance in 2 large metropolitan areas, 1992–2000. *Clin Infect Dis* 2003;36:789.

Muller FM, Groll AH, Walsh TJ. Current approaches to diagnosis and treatment of fungal infections in children infected with human immunodeficiency virus. *Eur J Pediatr* 1999;158:187.

Saag MS, Graybill RJ, Larsen RA, et al. Practice guidelines for the management of cryptococcal disease. Infectious Diseases Society of America. *Clin Infect Dis* 2000;30:710.

Speed B, Dunt D. Clinical and host differences between infections with the two varieties of *Cryptococcus neoformans*. *Clin Infect Dis* 1995;21:28.

Zhong Z, Pirofski LA. Opsonization of *Cryptococcus neoformans* by human anticryptococcal glucuronoxylomannan antibodies. *Infect Immun* 1996;64:3446.

CHAPTER 213 ■ HISTOPLASMOSIS

ROBERT J. LEGGIADRO

INTRODUCTION

Histoplasmosis, caused by the dimorphic soil fungus *Histoplasma capsulatum*, is the most common pulmonary and systemic mycosis in humans. Normal as well as immunocompromised hosts may be affected, and reactivation disease is believed to occur during immunocompromised states.

EPIDEMIOLOGY

Although it is distributed throughout temperate zones of the world, histoplasmosis is recognized to be most highly endemic in the central United States. Factors known to favor fungal growth in soil are relatively high humidity, temperatures ranging between 20°C and 30°C, and strict aerobic conditions and acidity, which are characteristics of the highly endemic river basins of the central United States.

Outbreaks of symptomatic histoplasmosis are associated with point sources, or microfoci, of infection. Such microfoci are almost always characterized by contamination with bird or bat manure and include bird roosts, bat caves, old buildings, urban parks, decayed trees or wood piles, and chicken coops. Activities associated with *H. capsulatum* exposure and acquisition through the respiratory route include clearing or cleaning bird roosts and chicken coops, spelunking, construction or excavation, wood gathering or cutting, camping, and gardening. Dusty conditions greatly increase the number of infective airborne spores.

PATHOGENESIS

Human infection with *H. capsulatum* generally results from inhalation of airborne spores. These spores germinate into yeast forms within alveoli and bronchioles in 3 to 5 days. After an initial neutrophilic response, macrophages parasitize the yeast forms that proliferate within these cells in nonimmune individuals, eventually resulting in cellular death. Infected macrophages may also effect subclinical dissemination through the lymphatic system to regional lymph nodes, the liver, or the spleen. After a period of 1 to 2 weeks, specific cell-mediated immunity develops, which contains the infection and leads to resolution. Healing occurs slowly. Necrotic and caseous pulmonary and lymphatic lesions become encapsulated and calcified over months (children) and years (adults). Although they may persist in the central areas of caseous or calcified lesions, yeast forms are unlikely to cause further active infection. However, such endogenous foci may explain the occurrence of active histoplasmosis in immunocompromised individuals during residence in a nonendemic area. Presumably, these patients acquired histoplasmosis while residing in an endemic area before their immunosuppression. A possible alternative explanation to endogenous reactivation in such situations is exogenous reinfection from *H. capsulatum* microfoci in the environment of a nonendemic area.

CLINICAL MANIFESTATIONS

Most infections are asymptomatic or self-limited and do not require antifungal therapy. However, treatment is indicated in

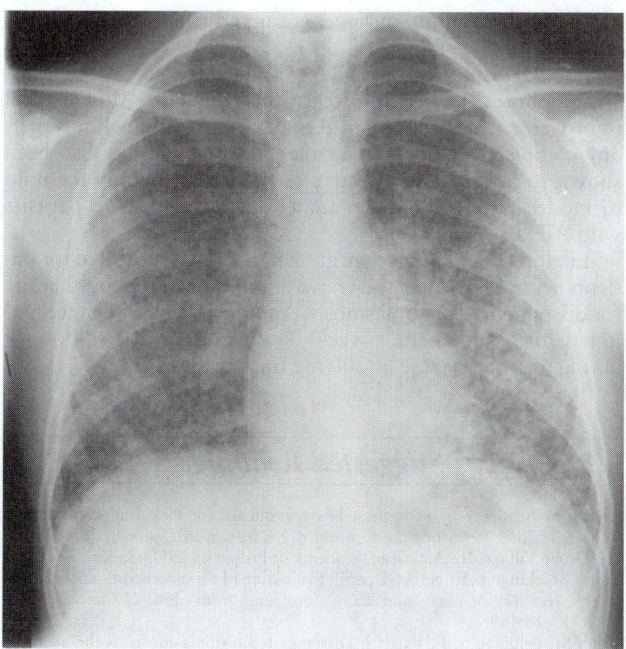

FIGURE 213.1. Miliary pulmonary histoplasmosis in an immunologically normal 10-year-old boy from Arkansas. There is a bilateral, diffuse, miliary, pulmonary parenchymal pattern of densities with greater involvement of the lower lobes. No hilar adenopathy or pleural effusion is present. (Reprinted from Robertson KR, James DH, Chesney PJ, et al. Miliary pulmonary histoplasmosis in a normal child. *Arch Pediatr Adolesc Med* 1994,148:833.)

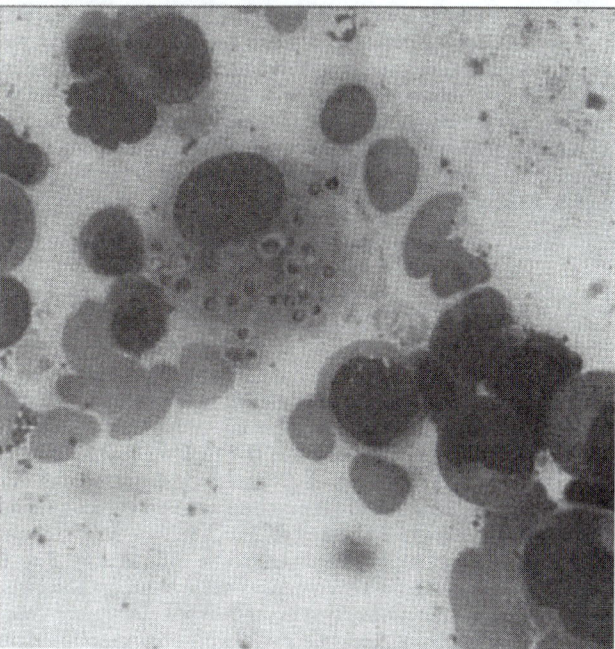

FIGURE 213.2. A digitally processed hematoxylin-eosin stain of bone marrow aspirate reveals several histiocytes containing intracellular yeast-like forms (original magnification ×1000). (Reprinted from Kane JM, Schmidt K, Conway JH. Fever, hepatosplenomegaly, and pancytopenia. *Arch Pediatr Adolesc Med* 2003;157:201.)

disseminated and some other forms of *H. capsulatum* infection. Clinical features of acute pulmonary histoplasmosis, the most common form of self-limited infection, include fever, cough, chest pain, and fatigue. Chest radiographic findings range from focal infiltrates to hilar or mediastinal adenopathy and, rarely, a miliary pattern after intense exposure (Fig. 213.1). In the absence of treatment, symptoms improve gradually after several weeks. Nearly 10% of these patients develop either pericarditis or arthritis with erythema nodosum. Antiinflammatory, not antifungal, therapy is indicated for these individuals.

Antifungal therapy is indicated for patients with chronic pulmonary histoplasmosis, which is manifested by productive cough, sweats, weight loss, fatigue, and fibrotic apical pulmonary infiltrates with cavitation.

Fibrosing mediastinitis is a progressive and often fatal form of histoplasmosis that does not respond to either antifungal or antiinflammatory therapy. This excessive fibrotic reaction to past infection may improve after surgical resection of fibrotic mediastinal masses that are impinging on vital structures, although operative mortality is high.

Disseminated histoplasmosis may be seen in otherwise normal, healthy infants living in endemic areas or in immunocompromised individuals, most commonly those infected with the human immunodeficiency virus who are residing in, or have a history of residing in, an endemic area. These patients most frequently present with fever, hepatosplenomegaly, and pancytopenia. Chest radiographic features range from normal to focal or diffuse miliary infiltrates and adenopathy.

DIAGNOSIS

Cultures for *H. capsulatum* are most helpful in patients with disseminated or chronic pulmonary histoplasmosis. In dissem-

inated disease, the highest yield is from bone marrow specimens. For an early diagnosis, examination of bone marrow material with silver stains may identify organisms compatible with *H. capsulatum* (Fig. 213.2). Wright-stain smear of buffy-coat preparation of peripheral blood may also provide an early diagnosis of disseminated histoplasmosis.

Blood cultures are also important in the diagnosis of disseminated histoplasmosis, and the lysis–centrifugation blood culture system is more sensitive and rapid than the conventional brain–heart infusion biphasic blood culture method of *H. capsulatum* isolation. In the study of Bille et al., the mean time for recovery of *H. capsulatum* from blood was 8 days by lysis–centrifugation, as compared with 24 days by biphasic brain–heart infusion. A significantly greater number of *H. capsulatum* isolates also were recovered by lysis–centrifugation in the same study. Histopathology and culture of liver biopsy material and oropharyngeal ulcers and culture of urine are additional useful diagnostic modalities in disseminated disease.

In addition to being a valuable rapid diagnostic test for disseminated histoplasmosis, the sensitive and specific radioimmunoassay for *H. capsulatum* antigen in urine has proved to be useful in assessing the efficacy of antifungal treatment and detecting relapses in children and adults with disseminated histoplasmosis. Antigen levels fall with successful induction therapy and increase with relapse.

Commercially available serologic tests for antibodies to *H. capsulatum* include complement fixation (CF) to mycelial and yeast antigens and immunodiffusion (ID) for precipitin bands to H and M antigens. In most symptomatic infections in normal hosts, antibodies develop 4 to 6 weeks after exposure. Antibody titers peak over several months. Development of ID antibodies lags behind the appearance of CF antibodies by 2 to 4 weeks, but ID precipitins persist longer than CF antibodies.

CF yeast-phase titers of 1:32 or greater should be regarded as highly suggestive of histoplasmosis and titers of 1:8 and 1:16 as presumptive evidence of infection. Mycelial titers of at least 1:8 and M or H bands by ID should also be regarded as highly suggestive of histoplasmosis. CF is more sensitive but also gives more false-positive results than does the more specific ID. Cross-reactions may be seen with the fungal infections blastomycosis, coccidioidomycosis, and paracoccidioidomycosis.

Although a useful epidemiologic tool, the histoplasmin skin test generally is not helpful in the diagnosis of acute histoplasmosis, especially in disseminated histoplasmosis of infancy and severe forms of infection.

TREATMENT

Treatment with amphotericin B remains the gold standard for patients with disseminated histoplasmosis and for those with severe manifestations of acute or chronic pulmonary histoplasmosis. Amphotericin B is dosed at 0.7 to 1 mg/kg/day with a total dosage of 30 to 35 mg/kg given during 4 to 6 weeks. Although data for children are limited, some experts recommend limiting amphotericin B therapy to 2 to 3 weeks, if substantial clinical improvement has occurred, to be followed by 3 to 6 months of itraconazole. Fever, nausea and vomiting, phlebitis, abnormal renal function, anemia, and hypokalemia are common adverse reactions. Treatment with liposomal amphotericin B improved survival among adults with AIDS compared to treatment with amphotericin B deoxycholate.

For most patients without human immunodeficiency virus infection or acquired immunodeficiency syndrome (AIDS) who have chronic pulmonary histoplasmosis or acute pulmonary histoplasmosis that necessitates antifungal therapy, the oral azole drug itraconazole is effective. Corticosteroids may be indicated in severe, acute pulmonary histoplasmosis as well. The pediatric dosage for itraconazole is 5 to 10 mg/kg/day orally once or twice a day (adult dose, 200 mg orally once or twice daily). Treatment with itraconazole for acute pulmonary histoplasmosis should continue for 2 to 3 months. Prolonged therapy with one of these agents for chronic pulmonary histoplasmosis is indicated because of the high relapse rate in this condition. The duration of treatment should be at least 12 months, and treatment should not be discontinued until the chest radiograph stabilizes (over 3 to 6 months of observation) and the sedimentation rate becomes normal.

Itraconazole requires an acidic environment for optimal solubilization and absorption and should be taken with food. Adverse effects include headache, nausea, vomiting, abdominal pain, anorexia, pruritus, rash, asymptomatic elevations of plasma aminotransferases, hepatitis, and impotence. Hypokalemia, hypertension, edema, and dizziness may also be seen with itraconazole use.

Drug interactions involving oral azole drugs are noteworthy. Antacids and H_2 receptor antagonists decrease itraconazole absorption, and phenytoin and rifampin increase its metabolism.

For AIDS patients with severe disseminated histoplasmosis, amphotericin B is the treatment of choice. After clinical improvement, amphotericin B may be discontinued and therapy completed with itraconazole. Itraconazole has also been shown to be safe and effective as induction therapy for mild to moderately severe disseminated histoplasmosis in patients with AIDS.

Lifelong maintenance antifungal therapy is indicated for patients with AIDS after they have completed induction therapy for disseminated histoplasmosis. Appropriate maintenance regimens for adults include weekly amphotericin B in a dose of 50 mg or itraconazole at 200 mg once or twice daily.

Suggested Readings

American Academy of Pediatrics. Histoplasmosis. In: Pickering LK, ed. *Red Book: 2003 Report of the Committee on Infectious Diseases*, 26th ed. Elk Grove Village, IL: American Academy of Pediatrics; 2003:353.

Bille J, Stockman L, Roberts GD, et al. Evaluation of a lysis-centrifugation system for recovery of yeasts and filamentous fungi from blood. *J Clin Microbiol* 1983;18:469.

Byers M, Feldman S, Edwards J. Disseminated histoplasmosis as the acquired immunodeficiency syndrome—defining illness in an infant. *J Pediatr Infect Dis* 1992;11:127.

Como JA, Dismukes WE. Oral azole drugs as systemic antifungal therapy. *N Engl J Med* 1994;330:263.

Fojtasek MF, Kleiman MB, Connolly-Stringfield PA, et al. The *Histoplasma capsulatum* antigen assay in disseminated histoplasmosis in children. *Pediatr Infect Dis J* 1994;13:801.

Goodwin RA, Loyd JE, DesPrez RM. Histoplasmosis in normal hosts. *Medicine* 1981;60:231.

Goodwin RA, Shapiro RL, Thurman GH, et al. Disseminated histoplasmosis: clinical and pathologic correlations. *Medicine* 1980;59:1.

Hughes WT. Hematogenous histoplasmosis in the immunocompromised child. *J Pediatr* 1984;105:569.

Kane JM, Schmidt K, Conway JH. Fever, hepatosplenomegaly and pancytopenia in a 5-month-old infant. *Arch Pediatr Adolesc Med* 2003;157:201.

Johnson PC, Wheat LJ, Cloud GA, et al. Safety and efficacy of liposomal amphotericin B compared with conventional amphotericin B for induction therapy of histoplasmosis on patients with AIDS. *Ann Intern Med* 2002;137:105.

Leggiadro RJ, Barrett FF, Hughes WT. Disseminated histoplasmosis of infancy. *Pediatr Infect Dis J* 1988;7:799.

Odio CM, Navarette M, Carillo JM, et al. Disseminated histoplasmosis in infants. *Pediatr Infect Dis J* 1999;18:1065.

Paya CV, Roberts GD, Cockerill FR. Laboratory methods for the diagnosis of disseminated histoplasmosis: clinical importance of the lysis-centrifugation blood culture technique. *Mayo Clin Proc* 1987;62:480.

Wheat LJ. Practice guidelines for the management of patients with histoplasmosis. *Clin Infect Dis* 2000;30:688.

Wheat LJ. Diagnosis and management of histoplasmosis. *Eur J Clin Microbiol Infect Dis* 1989;8:480.

Wheat LJ. Histoplasmosis: recognition and treatment. *Clin Infect Dis* 1994; 19:S19.

Wheat LJ, Connoly-Stringfield PA, Baker RL, et al. Disseminated histoplasmosis in the acquired immune deficiency syndrome: clinical findings, diagnosis and treatment, and review of the literature. *Medicine* 1990;69:361.

CHAPTER 214 ■ SPOROTRICHOSIS

MICHAEL R. MCGINNIS AND MICHAEL B. SMITH

Sporotrichosis is a chronic fungal infection typically limited to cutaneous and subcutaneous tissues. Dissemination of the infection is unusual. The causative agent is the dimorphic fungus *Sporothrix schenckii*. Sporotrichosis occurs worldwide but is found primarily in warm, temperate, and tropical regions. With few exceptions, the fungus gains entry into the body through trauma to the skin. In children, the infection often occurs as a solitary lesion on the face (Fig. 214.1A) or neck. Subsequent discrete nodular lesions tend to develop and spread along the lymphangitic system (Fig. 214.1B). Most cases of sporotrichosis occur in adults after intradermal inoculation of the fungus on contaminated thorns or splinters, reeds, or grasses. In many instances there is no memory of localized trauma. Floral nursery workers, gardeners, tree farmers, and others are at highest risk, although epidemic forms have been recorded in adults and children. In some endemic regions of Latin America approximately 60% of those infected are children under 15 years of age. Risk factors include playing in fields of crops and owning a cat. Cats have been associated as a risk factor by several investigators. Rare cases of disseminated sporotrichosis have been reported in patients with human immunodeficiency virus (HIV) infection. The pulmonary and extracutaneous forms are caused by inhalation of the fungus, which initially causes primary pneumonia. Secondary spread to joints, bone, muscle, and other organs is rare but may occur in the immunosuppressed host.

ETIOLOGY

S. schenckii is a dimorphic fungus that exists in a mycelial form in culture at 25°C. The invasive, yeast-like form is grown easily on enriched media, such as brain–heart infusion agar, at 37°C. The yeast is nearly round to oval and may form one or more daughter blastoconidia. Cigar-shaped blastoconidia are produced also from the parent yeast cells, most frequently in disseminated infections. The histologic picture in sporotrichosis is that of a mixed suppurative and granulomatous tissue reaction, with fibrosis and microabscess formation (Fig. 214.2). This tissue reaction is seen in both localized and disseminated infections. Typically, demonstration of fungi in tissue is very difficult. Culture of pus and biopsy material should be performed because the fungus is isolated easily in culture.

CLINICAL MANIFESTATIONS

The principal clinical forms of sporotrichosis are cutaneous and systemic. Lymphocutaneous infections are characterized by a linear series of painless nodules following the lymphatic drainage system from the primary nodular-ulcerative lesion occurring at the site of trauma. The first sign of infection may appear as soon as 5 days or as late as 6 months after traumatic inoculation; the average incubation time is 3 weeks. The first sign of disease is the appearance of a small, painless, movable subcutaneous nodule. The nodule enlarges to become a fluctuant mass with progression to ulceration. Similar painless subcutaneous nodules appear along the lymphatic channels. The clinical picture of an ulcer on the finger or wrist, with an associated chain of nodules present along draining lymphatics, is clinically pathognomonic of sporotrichosis. These lesions may persist for years if they are not treated. Infection of joints or bone may occur, probably by dissemination via the bloodstream from a cutaneous focus or, less commonly, from

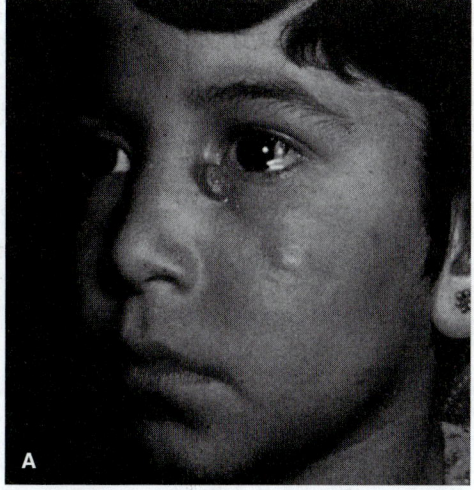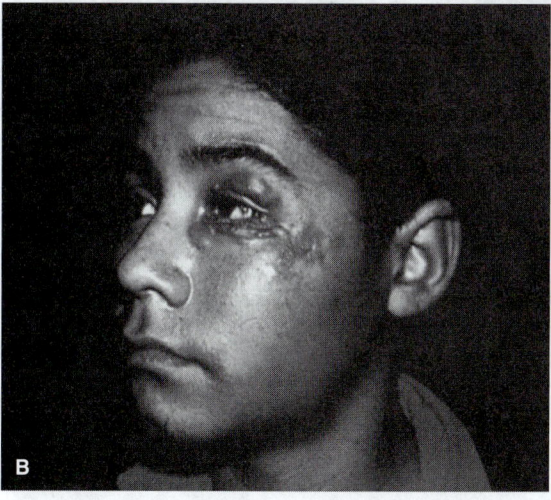

FIGURE 214.1. A: Sporotrichosis in its classic appearance as a solitary lesion on the face of a child. **B:** Sporotrichosis spread.

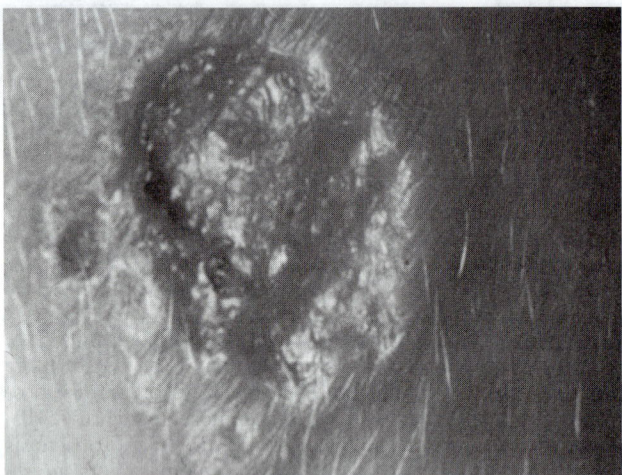

FIGURE 214.2. Magnified view of a sporotrichosis lesion.

a pulmonary source. In sporotrichosis of the joint, thickened synovium with cartilage degeneration is seen (Fig. 214.3). The knee is affected most commonly, with joint swelling, inflammation, and occasional sinus tracts. Extracutaneous sporotrichosis is rare in children, but involvement of the liver, spleen, pancreas, thyroid, myocardium, and central nervous system has been reported. Primary pulmonary sporotrichosis results from inhalation of the fungus, primarily in middle-aged alcoholic men or in patients with chronic obstructive pulmonary disease.

DIAGNOSIS

Definitive diagnosis of sporotrichosis requires the use of direct immunofluorescence or isolation of *S. schenckii* from in-

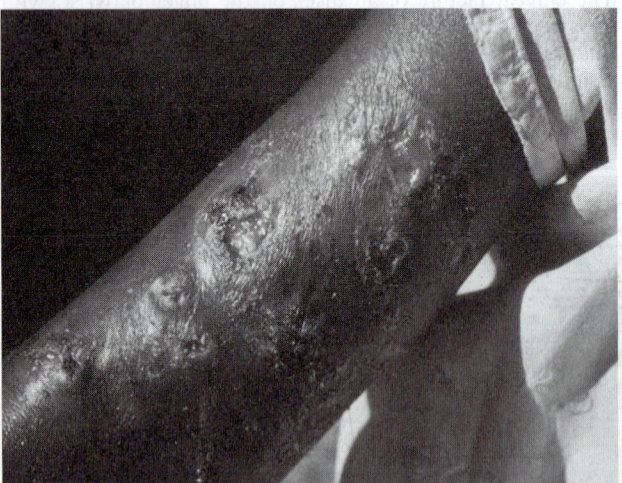

FIGURE 214.3. Sporotrichosis presenting on an arm.

fected tissue. The fungus is cultivated readily from tissue. Blood culture is unlikely to be positive except in immunocompromised patients with disseminated disease. The tube agglutination, latex agglutination, and indirect enzyme immunoassay tests are the most specific and reliable aids to diagnosis by serology. Though not commercially available, polymerase chain reaction–based assays to detect the fungus in clinical specimens have been developed that are specific.

TREATMENT

For many years, oral potassium iodide has been the treatment of choice for cutaneous sporotrichosis. Treatment schedules vary, but all involve rapidly increasing doses until 30 to 40 drops are given three times per day, usually until 4 weeks after symptoms have resolved. Recently, because of its effectiveness, dosing convenience, and lack of side effects, itraconazole (5 to 10 mg/kg/day as a single dose or divided into two doses; maximum 200 mg/day once or twice daily for 3 to 6 months) has replaced oral potassium iodide as the drug of choice for cutaneous infection. Amphotericin B is the drug most effective for pulmonary and disseminated sporotrichosis. With septic arthritis, itraconazole is the recommended drug, followed by amphotericin B and fluconazole, and surgical débridement may be necessary. For children with HIV lifelong maintenance therapy with itraconazole may be required.

PREVENTION

Risk of infection can be minimized by use of protective gloves and clothing during high-risk activities such as gardening or other activities that expose the skin to inoculation by thorns or other herbaceous materials.

Suggested Readings

American Academy of Pediatrics. Sporotrichosis. In: Pickering LK, ed. *Red Book: 2003 Report of the Committee on Infectious Diseases,* 26th ed. Elk Grove Village, IL: American Academy of Pediatrics, 2003:558.

Chandler FW, Watts JC. Sporotrichosis. In: Connor HD, Chandler FW, Schwartz DA, et al., eds. *Pathology of infectious diseases,* vol 2. Stamford, CT: Appleton & Lange, 1997:1089.

Dahl BA, Silberfarb PM, Sarosi GA, et al. Sporotrichosis in children. *JAMA* 1971;215:1980.

Hu S, Chung W-H, Hung S-I, et al. Detection of *Sporothrix schenckii* in clinical specimens by a nested PCR assay. *J Clin Microbiol* 2003;41:1414.

Karakayali G, Lenk N, Alli N, et al. Itraconazole therapy in lymphocutaneous sporotrichosis: a case report and review of the literature. *Cutis* 1998;61:106.

Kauffman CA, Hajjeh R, Chapman SW. Practice guidelines for the management of patients with sporotrichosis. *Clin Infect Dis* 2000;30:684.

Kwon KS, Yim CS, Jang HS, et al. Verrucous sporotrichosis in an infant treated with itraconazole. *J Am Acad Dermatol* 1998;38:112.

Lyon GM, Zurita S, Casquero J, et al. Population-based surveillance and a case-control study of risk factors for endemic lymphocutaneous sporotrichosis in Peru. *Clin Infect Dis* 2003;36:34.

Morris-Jones R. Sporotrichosis. *Clin Exp Dermatol* 2002;27:427.

Orr ER, Riley HD. Sporotrichosis in childhood: report of ten cases. *J Pediatr* 1971;78:951.

CHAPTER 215 ■ MISCELLANEOUS FUNGAL INFECTIONS

MICHAEL B. SMITH AND MICHAEL R. MCGINNIS

Numerous reports have implicated soil-borne fungi as causative agents of fungal diseases in a variety of clinical settings. Because most soil- and airborne fungi are rapid growers on culture media and may overgrow cultures from lesions resulting from nonfungal causes, the vast majority of reports published in the literature relating these fungi to disease are questionable. Rarely, however, a fungus not normally considered a pathogen may cause disease in particular circumstances. What should be remembered is that strain variation in fungi is great, as are types and degrees of compromised states, and some genetic changes may enhance pathogenic potential of otherwise harmless organisms in some patient populations. Distinguishing among infection, colonization, and contamination becomes critical in deciding on patient management.

Infection occurs when the fungus invades and grows within viable tissue and sterile body fluids. The body's response takes the form of signs and symptoms, which is disease. Disease results from either functional harm, damage, or a combination of these factors. Colonization pertains to the presence of a fungus growing in nonviable tissue. A contaminant is simply a fungus that is present, usually as conidia or hyphal fragments. Depending on the situation, infection, colonization, and contamination represent reference points on a continuum of potential host–fungus interactions.

Saprophytic fungi may be involved in disease in at least three manners. The first and most important is the ever-increasing list of opportunistic infections. They occur in the setting of immunologic compromise, either due to human immunodeficiency virus (HIV) infection or associated with the use of cytotoxins and steroids to treat neoplasia (particularly hematologic neoplasia), to prevent organ transplant rejection, and to treat certain collagen vascular and arthritic diseases. Often, the degree of immunosuppression dictates which fungal opportunists will be involved. The most common agents are *Candida albicans* and *C. tropicalis*, which come from mucosal reservoirs in the patient. The lungs are the entry portal for the common extrinsic opportunists *Aspergillus* species, Zygomycetes, and *Cryptococcus neoformans*. In addition to these commonly encountered opportunistic fungi, infections caused by many other fungi have been documented. *Fusarium* species in some cancer patient populations and *Pseudallescheria boydii* are prominent entries in the list of fungal opportunists; reports of their involvement in infection appear almost monthly. The list of opportunistic fungal pathogens is so long that two new disease entities have been defined: phaeohyphomycosis and hyalohyphomycosis.

The various types of phaeohyphomycosis are caused by phaeoid or dematiaceous fungi (the latter having constitutive melanin pigment in their cell walls) associated with soil and plants. Nearly 110 such agents have been documented, the majority since 1975. The microscopic and histologic appearance of one such agent, *Cladophialophora bantiana*, is shown in Fig. 215.1; the clinical disease is shown in Fig. 215.2. The forms of hyalohyphomycosis are caused by fungi that lack melanin pigment in their cell walls. More than 70 species have been confirmed as capable of causing infection. Phaeohyphomycosis tends to be more necrotic and erosive, and generally the causative agents do not respond to treatment with amphotericin B. In contrast, in hyalohyphomycosis, thrombotic phenomena with local invasion are common, and most organisms

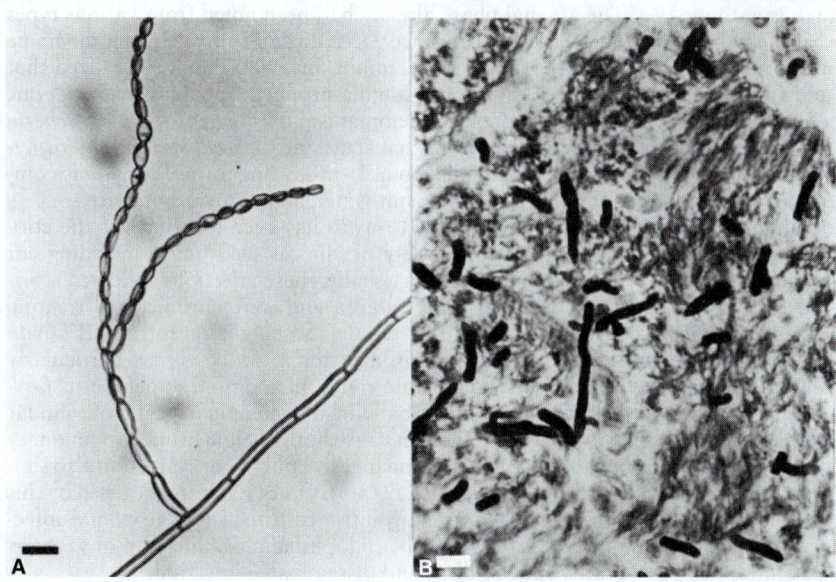

FIGURE 215.1. Phaeohyphomycosis. **A:** Microscopic section showing conidiation of the agent *Cladophialophora bantiana*. **B:** Typical histologic appearance of phaeoid septate hyphae in tissue *C. bantiana* (original magnification ×450).

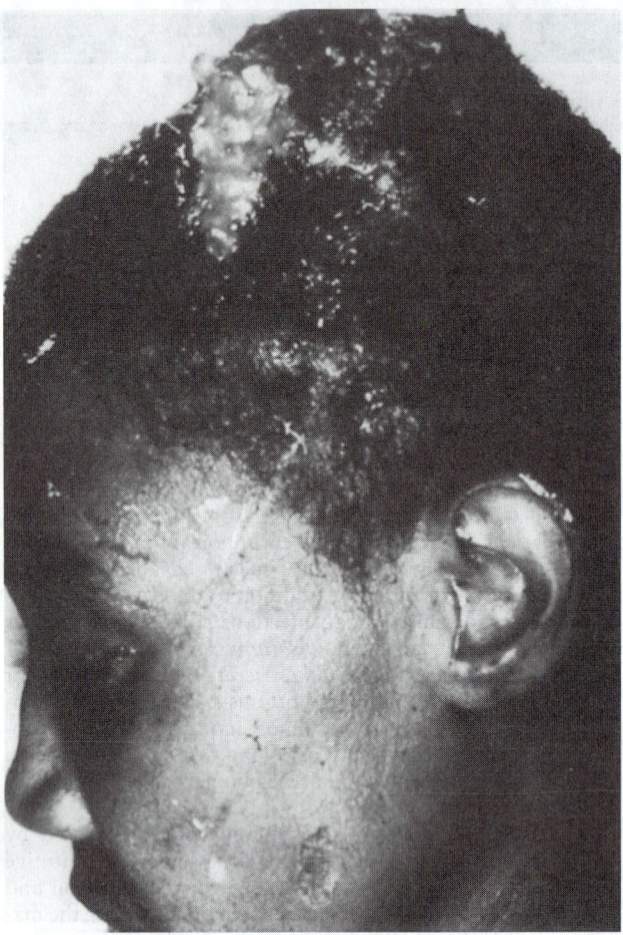

FIGURE 215.2. Cerebral phaeohyphomycosis. The organism *Clado-phialophora bantiana* was acquired by inhalation and disseminated to the brain, producing a massive tumor that eroded through the scalp.

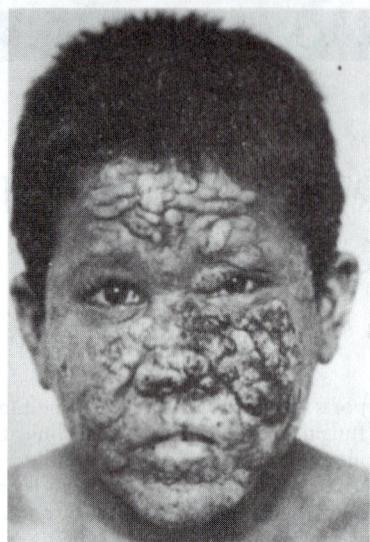

FIGURE 215.3. Phaeohyphomycosis caused by *Mycocentrospora acerina*, a pathogen of celery and other plants, in an Indonesian boy. No underlying condition could be detected.

otherwise healthy. Reported cases include *Mycocentrospora acerina* (a plant pathogen) infection of the face (Fig. 215.3), *Aureobasidium pullulans* (a soil saprophyte) involvement of the skin, progressive ulceration of the dermis by the water mold *Saksenaea vasiformis*, and granuloma of the lung containing the insect pathogen *Beauveria bassiana*.

HYALOHYPHOMYCOSIS

Approximately 70 agents have been recovered from the clinical entity known as *hyalohyphomycosis*. Most affected patients have been immunosuppressed. The agents gain entrance through the lungs, sinuses, indwelling catheters, dialysis tubing, and gastrointestinal tract. In tissue, all produce branching, septate, hyaline mycelia that are morphologically identical to that seen in invasive aspergillosis.

Allescheria boydii was described by Shear in 1922 as the causative agent of a mycetoma of the foot of a patient who lived in western Texas. The fungus was a homothallic (self-fertile) organism that produced sexual spores in a fruiting body. In addition, it produced at least two types of asexual conidia. The asexual phase already had been noted from various types of fungal diseases since 1899; in 1911, it was given the name *Monosporium apiospermum*. In 1944, Emmons realized that the sexual phase and conidia-producing phase were in fact one species. At present, the organism is known as *Pseudallescheria boydii* during the sexual stage and as *Scedosporium apiospermum* as the asexual conidia-producing form. *P. boydii* is common in sewage, stagnant water, and barnyard manure.

Since the 1890s, *P. boydii* has been identified as the etiologic agent of a variety of clinical syndromes, including ear infections in children. Usually, these infections followed a primary bacterial otitis externa and were chronic, and treating them was difficult. By far, the most common form of *P. boydii* infection is white-grain mycetoma, which is seen particularly in the world's temperate zones. In addition, sometimes *P. boydii* produces fungus balls in old pulmonary cavities, similar to *Aspergillus*, and can cause both allergic bronchopulmonary hyalohyphomycosis and invasive pulmonary infection also similar to *Aspergillus* (Fig. 215.4). Other syndromes caused by this species include osteomyelitis, arthritis, surgical wound infection, sinusitis, keratitis, endophthalmitis, infection of vascular grafts, endocarditis, and disseminated infection.

have some sensitivity to amphotericin B. Both these entities can be subdivided into superficial, cutaneous, subcutaneous, systemic, and allergic, depending on tissue involvement and mechanism of disease development.

A barrier break is the second circumstance by which soil organisms may gain entrance to protected organ systems. This factor is a predisposition much less common than is immunosuppression, but such cases do occur. Barrier breaks may be introduced by surgery, indwelling catheters, the use of nonsterile material in drug abuse, intrathecal injections, and ambulatory hemodialysis, among others. Reports have cited a mushroom growing on a mitral valve after open-heart surgery, of *Scopulariopsis* granulomas in the lung after the injection of crude opium, and of *Aspergillus* meningitis following the intrathecal use of contaminated steroids. Often, the same fungi involved in these diseases are found in the opportunistic categories.

Colonization of injured or debilitated tissue is the third category. Commonly, this predisposing situation is cited in reports of *Alternaria* invading the nose after a submucous resection, *Fusarium* colonizing burned skin, Zygomycetes infecting the injured foot of a diabetic, and *Pseudallescheria* infecting the knee after a soccer injury or auto accident. Many patients are not immunosuppressed. If viable tissue is invaded, the colonization becomes infection.

These three categories—opportunism, barrier break, and colonization of debilitated tissue—account for the vast majority of miscellaneous mycoses. Occasionally, a case occurs in which no predisposing factor is detected. The patient appears

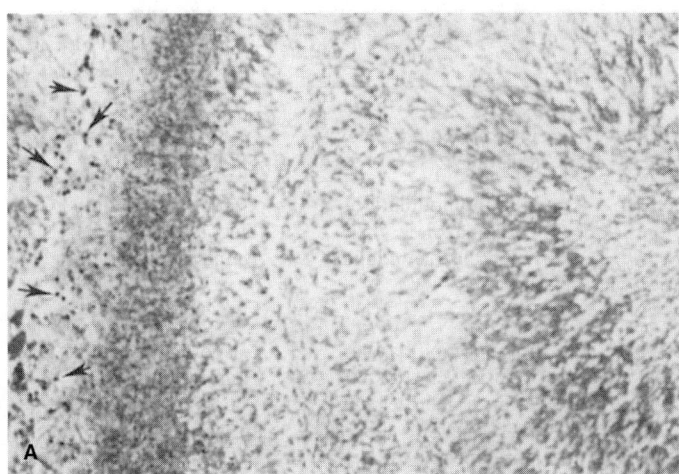 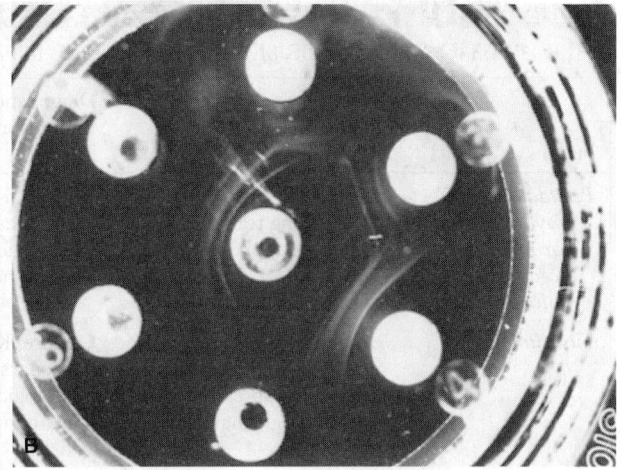

FIGURE 215.4. Pseudallescheriasis. **A:** Fungus ball in a preformed pulmonary cavity. *Aspergillus* is the most common agent of this disease but, in this section, concentric rings of growth can be seen, topped by single conidia (*arrows*), characteristic of *Pseudallescheria boydii*. **B:** Serology of a patient with fungus ball due to *P. boydii*. The patient's serum is in the center well. Five of the six surrounding wells contain various preparations of *P. boydii* antigen. Positive reactions have occurred. Well 5 (*bottom*) contains antigen to *Aspergillus* and is negative.

The rarity of *P. boydii* infections began to change in the 1960s and 1970s, when the generalized use of high-dose steroids, cytotoxins, and other immunosuppressive agents created a large susceptible patient population. Opportunistic infections of all types became common, and among these were fungus infections. *Candida*, *Aspergillus*, *Cryptococcus*, and Zygomycetes were encountered (in that order). Most affected patients had hematologic neoplasia and, if treatment resulted in neutropenia, fungus infections often quickly developed. In the 1980s, an additional population of organ transplant recipients increased the pool of susceptible individuals. The once rare infections caused by *P. boydii* have increased to the point that this organism now ranks just below the Zygomycetes in number of cases produced.

In the setting of immunosuppression, *P. boydii* infections usually begin in the lungs, with almost any organ becoming involved after hematogenous dissemination. A variety of changes in the lungs are visible on roentgenography, ranging from nonspecific infiltrates to cavitating lesions. Infections progress rapidly, producing necrotizing pneumonitis, pulmonary abscesses, and nodular infarcts. Dissemination occurs to the brain and other organs. Histologically, the branched, regularly septate mycelium seen in tissue sections is identical to those seen in disseminated aspergillosis.

Another form of *P. boydii* infection results from the aspiration of contaminated water or sludge or from the introduction of material into immunocompetent patients by injury or accident. In the first form, more than a dozen cases have been reported in children who aspirated stagnant water, sewer pond sludge, pig manure, or sheep dip, or who nearly drowned in swimming pools. An aspiration pneumonia results, and the organism disseminates. Often, the course is protracted. Football injuries, bruises from soccer playing, and motorcycle and automobile accidents have caused lacerations that later were followed by chronic osteomyelitis caused by *P. boydii*. Osteomyelitis in this setting usually does not respond to antifungal therapy, and amputation may be necessary in some cases.

Generally, *P. boydii* resists treatment with amphotericin B and many imidazole drugs. Ketoconazole and miconazole have been successful in a few cases, although the parenteral form of miconazole is not available in the United States (Table 215.1). Voriconazole, a new imidazole, and terbinafine, an allylamine

derivative, have shown promise as therapeutic agents for this fungus.

Approximately 15 species of *Fusarium* are known to cause infections, most frequently in immunocompromised patients. Of these, *F. oxysporum* and *F. solani* are the two species encountered most commonly. Members of this genus are soil saprobes and plant pathogens that occur throughout the world. The separation of *Fusarium* species is moving from morphology to genomic sequencing.

These fungi are known to cause onychomycosis, keratitis, osteomyelitis, cutaneous-subcutaneous and disseminated infections, mycetoma, and colonized cutaneous wounds. Disseminated infections occur in patients with malignancy and in organ transplant patients. Patients with granulocytopenia, such as resulting from chemotherapy, are at significant risk for developing this infection. Local tissue invasion in these patients, in onychomycosis for example, can result in angioinvasion and subsequent disseminated disease.

As with all opportunistic fungal infections, prompt diagnosis and management are essential. Cutaneous lesions resulting from hematogenous dissemination of the fungus are not uncommon. These lesions can present as skin nodules with central necrosis or target lesions or can resemble ecthyma gangrenosum. The lesions are easily accessible to biopsy and histologic evaluation; however, the hyphae present are indistinguishable from other hyaline molds such as *Aspergillus*, and culture is necessary for definitive identification. Disseminated infection has a poor prognosis and is often fatal unless granulocytopenia can be reversed. Those patients with immunosuppression, but without granulocytopenia (i.e., solid organ transplant patients), fare better, and cure is feasible. Frequently, *Fusarium* associated with burn wounds results in colonization of the burn eschar. A mat of hyphae bearing conidia can be seen on the surface of the wound. Sometimes sporodochia (cushion-like hyphal structures that bear conidia on their surface), like those formed on plant tissue, occur at the surface of the burn wound. A continuum exists between colonization and infection; histology becomes extremely important in determining how management should be approached. *Fusarium* is resistant to fluconazole and itraconazole. Amphotericin B is used, despite the fact that the minimum inhibitory concentration values often are greater than 1 g/mL. Voriconazole has limited activity (Table 215.1).

TABLE 215.1

THERAPEUTIC AGENTS FOR SELECTED FUNGAL INFECTIONS

Fungus	Underlying Host Conditions	Diagnostic Laboratory Tests	Therapy Fungus May Respond to	Agents Fungus is Often Resistant to
Pseudallescheria boydii (asexual form Scedosporium apiospermum)	Immunocompetent: Penetrating trauma Immunosuppression	Culture, KOH preparation Histologic examination of tissue	Immunomodulation Voriconazole Posaconazole (adults)	Caspofungin (adults) Fluconazole Amphotericin B
Fusarium spp.	Immunocompetent: Cutaneous burns Immunosuppression: Hematologic malignance	Culture, KOH preparation Histologic examination of tissue	Immunomodulation (GCSF or GMCSF) Surgical débridement Voriconazole Posaconazole (adults)	Caspofungin (adults) Amphotericin B Fluconazole Itraconazole
Trichosporon spp.	Immunosuppression	Culture, KOH preparation Histologic examination of tissue Cross-reactivity in some cases Cryptococcal latex agglutination test	Immunomodulation Fluconazole Posaconazole (adults)	Caspofungin (adults)
Scedosporium prolificans	Immunocompetent: Penetrating trauma Immunosuppression	Culture, KOH preparation Histologic examination of tissue	Immunocompetent: Surgical resection Immunosuppressed: Antifungals ineffective	Amphotericin B 5-Fluorocytosine Imidazoles and triazoles
Cladophialophora bantiana	Immunocompetent	Culture, KOH preparation Histologic examination of tissue	Posaconazole (adults) Liposomal amphotericin B Itraconazole Voriconazole	
Emmonsia spp.	Immunocompetent	Culture, KOH preparation Histologic examination of tissue	Amphotericin B 5-Flurocytosine Ketoconazole Itraconazole	
Rhinosporidium seeberi	Immunocompetent	Histologic examination of tissue	Surgical resection	Amphotericin B 5-Fluorocytosine Imidazoles and triazoles
Geotrichum spp.	Immunosuppression	Culture, KOH preparation Histologic examination of tissue	Amphotericin B Itraconazole (?) Voriconazole (?)	
Malassezia spp.	Immunocompetent Immunosuppression	Culture, KOH preparation	Azoles Remove central venous catheter Discontinue lipid parenteral nutrition	
Zygomycetes	Immunocompetent: Penetrating trauma; thermal burns Immunosuppression: Hematologic malignancy; diabetes mellitus (ketoacidosis)	Culture, KOH preparation Histologic examination of tissue	Liposomal amphotericin B (high doses) with or without recombinant cytokines Immunomodulation Surgical débridement Posaconazole (adults) Correct underlying medical condition	Caspofungin (adults) 5-Fluorocytosine Azoles

Note: These represent generalizations. Few controlled studies on antifungal therapy exist. Response may vary with the immune status of the patient, the individual fungal isolate, and other factors. Consultation with an infectious disease physician is recommended for individual cases.

Species of *Trichosporon* are associated with soil. They have also been isolated from water, human feces, and numerous other materials. Molecular studies have resulted in the proposal of several new species of *Trichosporon*. These fungi are agents of hair colonization (white piedra), summer-type hypersensitivity pneumonitis in Japanese patients, and colonization of the throat, lower gastrointestinal tract, and skin.

T. beigelii may cause infections in patients experiencing immunodeficiency due to treatment for neoplastic disease, immunosuppression for organ transplantation, or nonneoplastic cytopenia. *Trichosporon* are seen most commonly in patients with neoplastic disease, including acute leukemia, chronic leukemia, multiple myeloma, solid tumors, non-Hodgkin lymphoma, and Hodgkin lymphoma. Additional predisposing factors include cytotoxin-induced granulocytopenia, corticosteroids, prosthetic valve surgery, and hemochromatosis. For convenience, we are using the name *T. beigelii* rather than one of the proposed species names such as *T. asahii*.

In lung tissue, nodular infarcts are caused by angioinvasion and blood vessel occlusion by fungi. By hematogenous dissemination, bone marrow and such organs as the kidneys, heart, brain, liver, and spleen can be invaded. In tissue, the fungus may form a combination of varying amounts of septate hyphae (similar to *Aspergillus)* and pseudohyphae with some budding cells (such as *Candida*). The presence of arthroconidia produced by *Trichosporon* distinguishes this fungus from *Aspergillus* and *Candida*. Direct immunofluorescent staining of fungal elements in tissue sections can be used to differentiate and identify these three pathogens.

As with many other opportunistic pathogens, *Trichosporon* species tend to resist many antifungal agents. Amphotericin B and the azoles have been used with varying degrees of success. The combination of amphotericin B and 5-fluorocytosine has been said to have synergistic activity. As with many of these opportunistic fungal infections, recovery from granulocytopenia is extremely important for a positive outcome from a *Trichosporon* infection. Fluconazole is considered the optimal first-line antifungal. Echinocandins are not recommended (Table 215.1).

PHAEOHYPHOMYCOSIS

Phaeohyphomycosis is a newly described disease entity. The fungi that cause this type of infection appear as septate branching mycelium in tissue, with a discernible constitutive brown pigment (melanin) in their cell walls. More than 110 species, most of which are common soil inhabitants, have been described as agents of phaeohyphomycosis. Most have been recorded in only a few cases, almost all of which occurred in immunosuppressed hosts. However, two agents are fairly common in an entity called *subcutaneous phaeohyphomycosis*, which results from the traumatic introduction of the fungus on a splinter or other foreign body. *Exophiala jeanselmei* and *Wangiella dermatitidis* have been noted in more than 100 reports, many of which cite the disorder in immunocompromised hosts. A few patients have been treated with either amphotericin B or itraconazole or both antifungal agents. In others, a diagnostic surgical excisional biopsy has resolved the infection without the use of antifungal agents. In initial culture, both species occur as black yeasts, only later developing hyphae. In a number of instances, infections caused by *E. jeanselmei* have occurred in patients with undiagnosed diabetes mellitus, facilitating the detection of the diabetes.

Like hyalohyphomycosis, phaeohyphomycosis is a dynamic concept and can be subdivided in a similar manner. It can occur as cutaneous, subcutaneous, locally invasive, or disseminated disease. Although any site can be involved, the sinuses, the lungs, and the brain are most frequent. Some agents isolated as opportunists in phaeohyphomycosis also cause other types of infections. Most of the agents are phylogenetically related and normally occur in soil, on wood, and in decaying plant material. The list includes species of *Alternaria, Curvularia, Bipolaris, Exserohilum, Exophiala,* and *Wangiella*. The common agents of chromoblastomycosis, *Fonsecaea pedrosoi* and *Phialophora verrucosa,* have come from thousands of cases of that disease. In chromoblastomycosis, they occur as brown, planate-dividing, nonbudding cells without hyphae in tissue. These same species have been recovered from approximately a dozen patients with opportunistic phaeohyphomycosis, appearing in these patients as septate, branching, brown hyphae in tissue. A few rare reports of mycetoma caused by some of these fungi are known (e.g., *E. jeanselmei*).

In 1984, a second member of the genus *Scedosporium*, *S. prolificans* (syn. *S. inflatum*) was identified. Initially, all infections with this organism occurred in children who had suffered trauma. Wound contamination led to a chronic osteomyelitis that was unresponsive to antimycotic drugs. The organism *S. prolificans* appears to be worldwide in distribution, having been found in the United States, Australia, Venezuela, and Europe. Approximately 30 cases of disseminated disease due to this species are present in the literature, all of which occurred in immunocompromised patients, the vast majority of which were neutropenic. With the exception of two of the reported cases, all were fatal. *S. prolificans* is resistant to antifungals, and recovery from neutropenia appears to play a crucial role in control of the infection (Table 215.1). Restoration of immune competence is essential for survival.

A particularly interesting form of the disease is cerebral phaeohyphomycosis (see Figs. 215.2 and 215.3). More than 100 cases have been reported. This syndrome can occur in either immunosuppressed or immunocompetent individuals. The most common agent is *Cladophialophora bantiana* and is seen most frequently in patients without any underlying immunosuppressive illness. The clinical course often results in death, and at autopsy, masses of black-brown hyphae are seen in brain tissue. Early diagnosis and aggressive management are important. Surgical management appears to be critical along with treatment with voriconazole or itraconazole. Tissue débridement has been associated with improved outcome in a few cases. Long-term antifungal therapy and repeat surgical management may be required (Table 215.1).

ADIASPIROMYCOSIS

Adiaspiromycosis denotes the *in vivo* development without replication of adioconidia from the inhaled conidia of species of the fungal genus *Emmonsia*. The disease was described first in 1942 in desert rodents captured in Arizona. Examination of museum specimens of rodents and of newly captured animals has revealed that the disease is distributed worldwide. It has been found in animals that were captured in the early 1800s. The first human case was described during 1964 in France.

Approximately 50 human infections have been reported. Cases in children have been noted, particularly in Eastern Europe. As a result of these infections, one 11-year-old boy had functional impairment of the lung, and a 10-year-old boy required treatment with nystatin and amphotericin B by aerosol.

In tissue, the adioconidia are 10 to 13 μm in diameter when the causative agent is *E. parva*. Adioconidia as large as 40 μm in diameter can be produced in culture at 37°C. Because of the size and shape of these structures, coccidioidomycosis must be included in the differential diagnosis. Because they do not contain endospores and they have extremely thickened cell walls, their separation from *Coccidioides* is relatively easy.

The far more widely distributed *E. parva* variant *crescens* produces adioconidia as large as 220 μm in diameter in natural

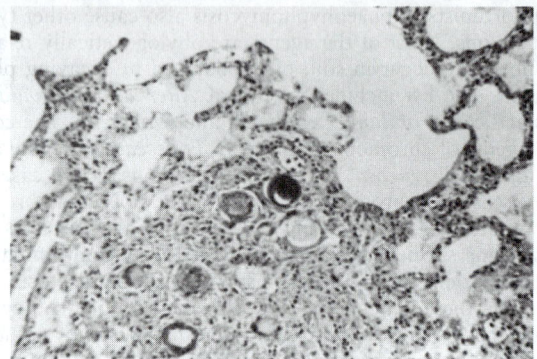

FIGURE 215.5. Adiaspiromycosis. Adioconidia in lung. The cells are 150 to 200 μm in diameter in this infection by *Emmonsia parva* variant *crescens*.

infections and as large as 400 μm in culture at 37°C (Fig. 215.5). These cells could be confused with *Rhinosporidium seeberi*. Their thick cell walls and the absence of spores allow for an accurate differentiation. This particular species has been the only *Emmonsia* species reported infecting humans to date, and all infections have been pulmonary.

Infection is limited to the lungs, and since reproduction of the fungus does not appear to occur *in vivo*, the amount of pulmonary impairment depends on the amount of initially inhaled conidia. Treatment depends on symptomatology, as in mild cases the infection could be self-limited. Amphotericin B, 5-flurocytosine, ketoconazole, and itraconazole singly or in various combinations have been used for treatment (Table 215.1).

RHINOSPORIDIOSIS

Rhinosporidiosis is an infection of the mucocutaneous tissue caused by the parasite *R. seeberi*. The organism has not been grown in culture, has been difficult to classify, and has been until very recently thought to be a fungus. Sequencing of 18S rRNA indicates that the organism is in fact an aquatic protist (class Mesomycetozoea, order Dermocystida) and not a fungus. The disease results in the production of polyps, tumors, papillomas, or wart-like vegetative growths that are hyperplastic, highly vascularized, friable, and sessile or pedunculated (Fig. 215.6). Most commonly, the nose and conjunctivae are involved. Nasal infection is common in damp tropical climates, whereas conjunctivitis is more common in dry, dusty areas. Infection of the anus, penis, vagina, ears, pharynx, and larynx may occur. The disease first was described independently in Tennessee, India, and Argentina. More than 4,000 cases have been reported in India, where the disease is so common that

tabulations are not kept. It is common also in Sri Lanka. Several hundred cases (in horses and humans) have been reported in Argentina and 50 or so have been reported in South Africa and the United States. In both South Africa and the United States, conjunctival disease is more common than is nasal infestation. The nasal form also is not unusual in dogs in the southeastern United States.

In tissue, the organism grows as a sporangium as large as 250 to 350 μm in diameter. The sporangia contain sporangiospores that are released at maturity through a pore. Then the sporangiospores enlarge to produce new sporangia. Surgical removal is the most common method of treatment, and recurrence is seen in about 10%. There is no antimicrobial therapy available.

GEOTRICHOSIS

Geotrichosis is a rare opportunistic infection caused by the yeast-like hyphomycete *Geotrichum candidum*. The organism is ubiquitous in the soil and air and is part of the normal flora of the skin and gastrointestinal tract. It has been found also in cottage cheese and other dairy products.

Hundreds of reports have linked *G. candidum* to a variety of disease types. In most cases, however, the pathogenic role of the fungus was not substantiated, and often its delineation from *C. albicans* is unclear. Probably no more than three dozen authentic cases are reported in the literature. One report described a female patient with leukemia in blast crisis after vincristine and prednisone therapy. She developed disseminated fungal disease. Only *G. candidum* was isolated from blood, urine, skin biopsy, and autopsy specimens. In tissue, septate hyphae and yeast-like cells that probably were arthroconidia were seen. *Geotrichum* produces arthroconidia, which resemble nonbudding yeasts. Possibly, two agents were present: a *Trichosporon* or a *Candida* in addition to *Geotrichum*. This finding emphasizes the difficulty of assessing fungi in histopathologic sections. Amphotericin B is the drug of choice in treating *G. candidum*. The azoles itraconazole or voriconazole also may be useful (Table 215.1).

MALASSEZIA

Malassezia consists of at least 11 species of lipophilic yeast that are part of the resident skin flora of humans and other warm-blooded animals. Members of the genus *Malassezia* may cause pityriasis versicolor, seborrheic dermatitis, folliculitis, nonfollicular pustulosis of the newborn, and nosocomial catheter-related sepsis in neonates receiving intravenous lipid emulsion in pediatric care units. Transmission is most likely from person to person, probably via the hands of medical

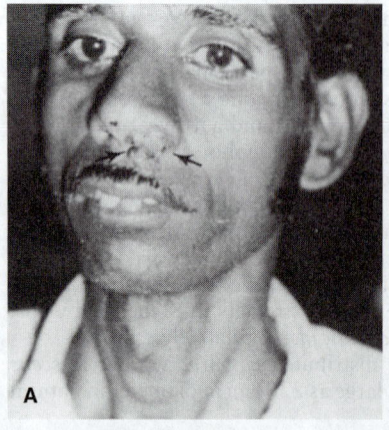

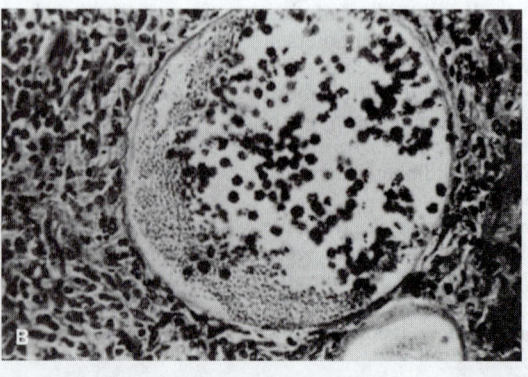

FIGURE 215.6. Rhinosporidiosis. **A:** Pedunculated lesions have formed on the nasal mucosa (*arrows*). **B:** Histologic section shows sporangium 350 μm in diameter (×450).

personnel. The yeast has also been associated with atopic dermatitis. Systemic *Malassezia* infections are only seen in neonates and immunocompromised patients. These patients develop intermittent low-grade fever that is of unclear etiology. Catheter removal and discontinuation of intravenous lipids are important for a successful outcome in fungemic cases.

The differentiation of the 11 species relies upon rRNA sequence data and other molecular information. The species in the genus include: *M. furfur, M. globosa, M. restricta, M. pachydermatis, M. sympodialis, M. obtuse, M. slooffiae, M. dermatis, M. nana, M. japonica,* and *M. yamatoensis. M. globosa* is recovered more frequently in younger subjects than in older individuals (15 years or older). Other species of interest are *M. obtuse, M. restricta, M. furfur,* and *M. slooffiae.* The largest concentrations of organisms are found on the skin of the face, scalp, neck, upper chest, and back, where there is the presence of high amounts of sebaceous skin lipids. *Malassezia* increases after puberty, which is presumably related to the increase in skin surface lipids that results from higher sebaceous gland activity during this period. Pityriasis versicolor in children under 1 year of age is not unusual in humid and hot climates. The hypochromic lesions are the main clinical manifestation, and the most affected site is the face.

The yeast is easily seen in the direct examination of skin scrapings. When fungemia is present, polymerase chain reaction may be a useful adjunct to blood cultures. The yeast can be recovered in the laboratory when the medium is supplemented with a small quantity of olive oil. There are specialized media available for the isolation of this yeast; however, these media are typically not available in clinical laboratories. Topical azoles can be used to manage skin infections.

ZYGOMYCOSIS

Zygomycosis can be a rapidly progressive infection that can result in death in a short period of time. Rapid diagnosis and aggressive management are critical for survival. In the pediatric population, critically ill premature newborns, and older children with underlying hematopoietic malignancies (Burkitt lymphoma, acute lymphoblastic leukemia), neutropenia, and bone marrow transplantation are at the greatest risk. Zygomycosis in children with solid organ transplants is rare. The most common form of the disease occurs as rhinocerebral infection in those who have diabetes mellitus ketoacidosis. Particular Zygomycetes species tend to be associated with specific types of infection: *Apophysomyces elegans* and cutaneous wounds following trauma, *Mucor* and *Rhizopus arrhizus* in thermal burns, and *Rhizopus arrhizus* and *Absidia corymbifera* in rhinocerebral and disseminated infection.

The diagnosis of zygomycosis relies heavily upon the observation of hyaline, sparsely septate, irregularly branching hyphae that are variable in diameter. The hyphae are readily seen in clinical specimens as well as tissue sections. Zygomycetes tend to invade blood vessels. In our experience, Zygomycetes are rarely isolated in the laboratory as a laboratory contaminant. Their isolation should be considered potentially significant until proven otherwise. The isolation of these fungi can be difficult if media containing large quantities of sugar (malt extract agar) are not used and if the tissue is homogenized prior to inoculation on the isolation media. Management is approached by surgical débridement, antifungal agents such as liposomal amphotericin B, and correction of the underlying problem. Azoles have not been effective in managing this infection. Preliminary information regarding posaconazole suggests that this triazole may have application for the treatment of zygomycosis.

Suggested Readings

Antachopoulos C, Walsh TJ. New agents for invasive mycoses in children. *Curr Opin Pediatr* 2005;17:78.

Abzug MJ, Walsh TJ. Interferon-gamma and colony-stimulating factors as adjuvant therapy for refractory fungal infections in children. *Pediatr Infect Dis J* 2004;23:769.

Greenberg RN, Scott LJ, Vaughn HH, Ribes JA. Zygomycosis (mucormycosis): emerging clinical importance and new treatments. *Curr Opin Infect Dis* 2004;17:517.

Mirhendi H, Makimura K, Zomorodian K, et al. A simple PCR-RFLP method for identification and differentiation of 11 *Malassezia* species. *J Microbiol Methods* 2005;61:281.

Walsh TJ, Groll A, Hiemenz J, et al. Infections due to emerging and uncommon medically important fungal pathogens. *Clin Microbiol Infect* 2004;10:48.

---

f: PARASITIC DISEASES

CHAPTER 216 ■ *ENTAMOEBA HISTOLYTICA*

BRADLEY HOWARD KESSLER

Amebiasis is defined as infection with *Entamoeba histolytica*, with or without overt clinical symptoms. Distribution of the disease is worldwide, affecting as much as 10% of the population. The highest prevalence is seen in developing areas and tropical regions. It has been estimated that approximately 1% to 5% of U.S. residents who have never traveled outside the United States have amebiasis; most of these are asymptomatic carriers. Severe disease, such as ulcerative amebic colitis or liver abscess, is relatively rare.

ETIOLOGY

Two forms of the protozoan parasite *E. histolytica*, cysts and trophozoites, are found in stool specimens. Trophozoites are motile, variably shaped organisms that are 7 to 30 μm in diameter and have a single nucleus and a granular, vacuolated cytoplasm. Trophozoites characteristically produce pseudopodia, which are finger-like projections from the main body that

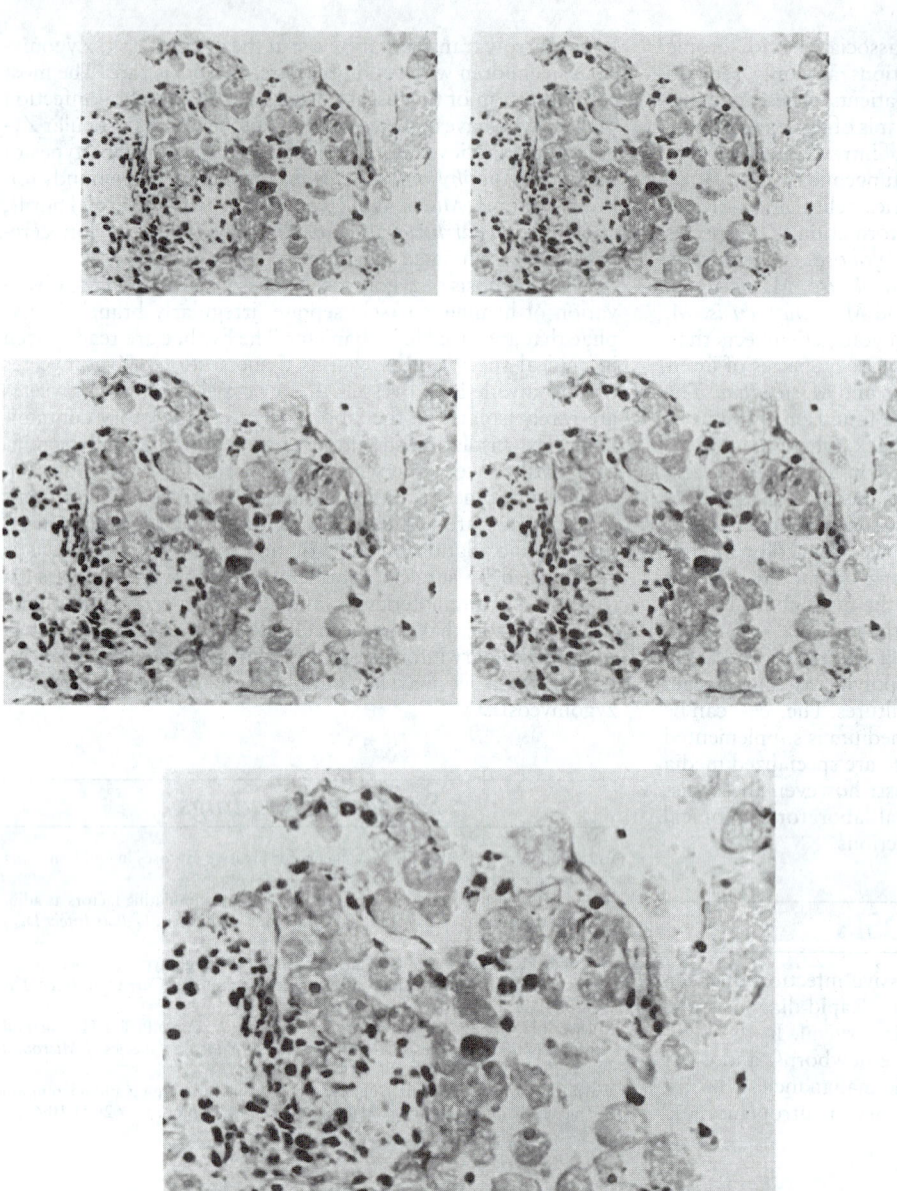

FIGURE 216.1. Trophozoite with hemophagocytosis. (Courtesy of Pathology Department of Good Samaritan Hospital Medical Center.)

participate in both motility and phagocytosis. This form of the parasite may be found in patients with symptomatic or asymptomatic amebiasis. In individuals with symptomatic amebiasis, the pathogenic trophozoites may contain ingested red blood cells in endoplasmic vacuoles and can be as large as 60 μm in diameter (Fig. 216.1). Phagocytosis may be an important virulence factor. Specific isoenzyme migration patterns or zymodemes obtained from starch gel electrophoresis are indirect markers of virulence. Certain strains of nonpathogenic *E. histolytica*, now classified as *E. dispar*, are associated only with asymptomatic carriage.

The nonmotile cyst form is similar in size to the trophozoite but may contain as many as four nuclei. Infection occurs only with ingestion of cysts. On ingestion, after excystation in the small bowel, each single cyst results in eight trophozoites. Encystation of the trophozoite completes the life cycle. Unlike the trophozoite, which is destroyed rapidly by external environmental conditions and gastric acid, the cysts are resistant to gastric acid and to the chlorine concentrations commonly used in domestic water purification, as well as to extreme temperature and drying. Cysts may survive outside the host for several weeks in a moist environment. Cysts excreted in the stool of infected individuals perpetuate the life cycle through fecal-oral spread.

EPIDEMIOLOGY

Fifty million cases of amebiasis are recorded annually. *E. histolytica* is the third leading parasitic cause of death in the world. Prevalence is highest in areas with poor sanitation and inadequate water treatment. Effective forms of water treatment include boiling and filtration. Infection with pathogenic tropho-zoites is not a major clinical problem in the United States, despite prevalence rates ranging from 0.1% to 50.0% in regional and institutional surveys. Overall, in the United States prevalence rates approach 2% to 4%. Amebic infection generally is confined to certain high-risk groups, including recent long-term travelers, immigrants, and immunocompromised hosts. The invasive trophozoites cause diarrhea and dysentery in 2% to 8% of infected patients. Trophozoites that enter the bloodstream may pass to the liver or other organs and cause abscesses. Such abscesses are found as a complication of intestinal disease in all endemic areas. Reports from endemic areas worldwide also indicate that of those children who develop amebic liver abscess, most are younger than 3 years, although amebic hepatic abscess is believed to be less common in children than in adults. Amebic abscess of the liver has been reported in 1% to 9% of patients with invasive amebiasis. Abscesses are seen more frequently in men, with the highest incidence in individuals 20 to 50 years of age.

Humans are the natural host and reservoir for *E. histolytica*. Fecal-oral transmission of cysts occurs frequently through contaminated water or foods such as vegetables. Major outbreaks occur in the United States, where disease transmission predominantly occurs by person-to-person spread. Infected food handlers play a major role in transmitting the infection. Outbreaks have been associated with pollution of the water supply by sewage. Amebic infection is common in homosexuals and infects as many as 30%, with *E. dispar* the predominant infecting species. Patients with the acquired immunodeficiency syndrome often harbor multiple enteric pathogens, and amebae frequently are detected in the stool of such patients. Most of these patients probably are infected with *E. dispar* and therefore are usually asymptomatic. The virulence of *E. histolytica* in specific areas, such as South Africa, Mexico, and India, may be explained by the strain of the parasite and by the nutritional status and bacterial flora in the intestine of the host.

PATHOGENESIS AND PATHOLOGY

Invasive amebiasis occurs through a number of steps: colonization in the colonic mucous blanket, penetration or depletion of the mucous layer with disruption of the epithelial barrier, and parasite lysis of responding host inflammatory cells, followed by deeper tissue penetration. Cytopathic effects of *E. histolytica* on monolayers of mammalian cells in tissue culture have been well described.

The factors that determine whether ingestion of *E. histolytica* will produce no infection, a commensal state, symptomatic colitis, or hepatic abscess are not well defined. Some factors implicated include the strain of the organism, the ability of the organism to produce cysteine proteases and pore-forming proteins (amoebapores), the adhesiveness of the organism to epithelial cells through a galactose/N-acetyl-D-galactosamine lectin-binding protein, the ability of the organism to engulf tissue elements through phagocytosis, and the interaction of the organism with the bacterial flora that is indigenous to the gastrointestinal tract. The identity of a high-affinity intestinal epithelial cell receptor is unknown. Adherence is necessary for cytolytic activity.

The mechanism of tissue invasion is not understood clearly. Some postulate that a toxin or lytic compound from the parasite provokes a generalized inflammatory response, possibly through an epithelial cell–induced cytokine, including interleukin-8, lymphokines, and activation of nuclear factor-kappa B. Activation of human caspase 3, a molecule important for apoptosis or cell death, occurs after amebic contact. In addition to tissue destruction, trophozoites may cause diarrhea by stimulating intestinal secretion by prostaglandin production. As the process continues, classic flask-shaped ulcers with undermined edges are formed. When amebae move into the bowel wall, some may be picked up in the portal circulation and become disseminated, first to the liver and then throughout the body.

The pathologic lesions described most frequently are ulcers that are scattered throughout the colon but affect predominantly the cecum and ascending colon. The sigmoid colon and rectum usually are less involved; the terminal ileum rarely is involved. As the disease progresses, the ulcer enlarges and extends into the submucosa and muscular coat. On rare occasions, this extension can lead to perforation. Histologic examination reveals a diffuse, nonspecific inflammation that is indistinguishable from other forms of idiopathic colitis, such as ulcerative colitis. Amebae frequently can be seen at the leading edge of the ulcer and in the overlying inflammatory exudate.

An amebic liver abscess usually is solitary, but multiple abscesses can occur. The right lobe of the liver is involved most often. The material within an abscess has been described as resembling anchovy paste or chocolate syrup. The parasite rarely is found in aspirated abscess fluid. Whether amebic hepatitis always precedes amebic abscess is not known.

CLINICAL FEATURES

Most infections are asymptomatic (luminal colonization), and elimination of the parasite from the gastrointestinal tract occurs within 12 months (Box 216.1). The incubation period for the illness varies but usually is 2 to 4 weeks. The severity of illness may vary from very mild symptoms to severe fulminating disease with mucosal inflammation, ulceration, and even perforation. Most patients with invasive amebiasis describe a gradual onset of cramping, abdominal pain, malaise, tenesmus (with rectal involvement), and frequent stools. Stools usually are blood stained and mucoid. Diarrhea may persist for weeks but can wax and wane, with alternating periods of constipation. In some patients, the onset of symptoms may be acute, with the following signs: fever; profuse, bloody, mucoid diarrhea; dehydration; and electrolyte abnormalities. This fulminant picture may mimic that seen in toxic megacolon, acute inflammatory bowel disease, and bacillary dysentery. More serious disease is associated with youth, pregnancy, malnutrition, corticosteroid therapy, and underlying systemic disease. Possible complications include intestinal perforation, hemorrhage, stricture, inflammation, peritonitis, and a local inflammatory mass or ameboma. On physical examination, tenderness usually is present throughout the lower abdomen.

Hepatic amebiasis and abscess are characterized by fever, abdominal pain, pleuritic pain, respiratory distress, and hepatomegaly. The pain usually is localized to the right upper quadrant, with radiation to the right shoulder and laterally to the chest. Patients frequently give no history of significant

---

BOX 216.1 **Clinical Disease Resulting from *Entamoeba histolytica***

Asymptomatic

Invasive amebiasis
Cramping
Abdominal pain
Malaise
Tenesmus
Frequent stools (may be blood stained and mucoid)
Fever

Complications
Intestinal perforation
Hemorrhage
Stricture
Inflammation
Peritonitis
Ameboma
Hepatic abscess

gastrointestinal symptoms. Amebic abscess develops in fewer than 1% of patients with intestinal amebiasis. Chest radiographs may show elevation of the right hemidiaphragm. Laboratory evaluation may reveal anemia, with an elevated leukocyte count and a left shift. The most common finding on physical examination is a large, tender liver. Icterus occurs infrequently, and its presence is an ominous sign. Examination of the chest may reveal rales, decreased breath sounds, and a friction rub. Complications involve the pleural cavity or intraabdominal extension of the abscess.

DIAGNOSIS

Because medical therapy is highly effective in all forms of amebiasis, the diagnosis should be made as early as possible. Distinguishing between amebiasis and inflammatory bowel disease is critical. The symptoms, findings on colonoscopy, and histologic findings on examination of biopsy material can mimic the findings in ulcerative colitis. Steroids, which are prescribed frequently for ulcerative colitis, may complicate the course of amebiasis and increase mortality.

Microscopic examination of repeated stool specimens is the definitive diagnostic test. When the test is performed correctly, the results of more than 90% of stool examinations are positive in infected patients. Stool samples should be examined immediately after defecation or should be preserved in a fixative such as polyvinyl alcohol or formalin ethyl acetate for later examination. Staining with thimerosal-iodine-formalin (merthiolate-iodine-formalin) increases the sensitivity. In addition to direct examination, concentration of the specimen treated with formalin ethyl acetate increases the sensitivity of the test. An experienced examiner competent in the diagnosis of parasitic infections should be consulted to distinguish the nuclear characteristics of the trophozoites and differentiate *E. histolytica* from other amebae that rarely are pathogenic. These include *Entamoeba hartmanni*, *Entamoeba coli*, and *Endolimax nana*. The stools *must* be collected before barium studies are performed, because barium decreases the yield of positive examination results. Rectal mucosal scrapings collected during proctosigmoidoscopy also can be examined and will increase the positive yield. Trophozoites can be seen on colonic biopsies in approximately 50% of cases. If stool examination results are negative and a high level of suspicion exists for intestinal amebiasis, serologic testing such as an indirect hemagglutination (IHA) test should be done. Serum antiamebic antibodies are present in 70% to 90% of the patients at the time of presentation. IHA test results are strongly positive (titer greater than 1:256) in 85% to 90% of patients with invasive colonic disease or liver abscess. A limitation of the IHA test is that the results can remain positive for more than 20 years and therefore may represent earlier illness. The gel diffusion precipitin test has a high predictive value for disease in symptomatic patients. Other common serologic tests include counterimmunoelectrophoresis, indirect immunofluorescent antibody, complement fixation, and enzyme-linked immunosorbent assay. Colonization with nonpathogenic strains rarely provides a serologic response. A newer assay using the polymerase chain reaction can detect *E. histolytica*–specific DNA. This assay can differentiate between pathogenic and nonpathogenic strains.

The key to recognizing an amebic liver abscess is suspecting the diagnosis in patients with fever and an enlarged, tender liver. Patients with a liver abscess usually do not have concurrent diarrhea. Laboratory test results generally are nonspecific. The serum alkaline phosphatase levels may be elevated. Bilirubin and liver transaminase levels may be normal or mildly elevated. In addition to serology, liver scanning (including ultrasonography, computed tomography, and technetium-99m sulfur colloid scanning) can help to detect a liver defect that

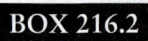

| **BOX 216.2** | **Treatment of Disease Resulting from *Entamoeba histolytica**** |

Asymptomatic carrier
Paromomycin, 25 to 35 mg/kg/day divided into three doses/day for 7 days OR Iodoquinol (formerly diiodohydroxyquin), 30 to 40 mg/kg/day (maximum, 2 g/day) divided into three doses/day for 20 days

Invasive amebiasis
Metronidazole (Flagyl), 35 to 50 mg/kg/day divided into three doses/day for 10 days followed by iodoquinol (as above) for 20 days

---

*For treatment of complicated infection, see text.

is consistent with an abscess. Needle aspiration may help to establish a diagnosis, although this is not undertaken commonly.

THERAPY

The specific therapy recommended for infection with *E. histolytica* depends on the site of involvement (luminal, intramural, or systemic) (Box 216.2). An *asymptomatic carrier* should be treated with paromomycin, 25 to 35 mg/kg/day in divided doses given every 8 hours for 7 days or iodoquinol (formerly diiodohydroxyquin), 30 to 40 mg/kg/day (maximum, 2 g/day) in divided doses given every 8 hours for 20 days. Iodoquinol has been reported to cause optic atrophy in rare cases. An alternative regimen is diloxanide furoate (Furamide), which is not available in the United States, 7 mg/kg three times daily for 10 days.

Invasive amebiasis of the intestine, liver, or other organs requires the additional use of a tissue amebicide such as metronidazole (Flagyl). This is administered at a dose of 35 to 50 mg/kg/day in divided doses given every 8 hours for 10 days. Because metronidazole is a less effective luminal amebicide, treatment should be followed by iodoquinol (as outlined earlier) for 20 days to eliminate parasites in the intestine.

If iodoquinol or metronidazole cannot be given or the course of illness is severe, dehydroemetine, 1.0 to 1.5 mg/kg/day (maximum, 90 mg/day) in divided doses given every 12 hours by the intramuscular route for 5 days, is an alternative. Dehydroemetine should be used with caution, because it can cause severe side effects, among which are cardiotoxicity, which can lead to fatal myocardiopathy, arrhythmias with T-wave changes, muscle weakness, and renal complications. Dehydroemetine therapy should be followed by paromomycin for 7 days or iodoquinol for 20 days (as outlined earlier).

An uncomplicated, deep, unruptured liver abscess may be treated medically. Liver abscess or other forms of extraintestinal disease should be treated with metronidazole followed by iodoquinol (as outlined earlier) or, alternatively, with dehydroemetine followed by chloroquine, 10 mg/kg/day for 14 to 21 days, plus iodoquinol (as outlined earlier). The patient's clinical condition usually will improve within 72 hours of the initiation of medical therapy. Clinical signs and radioisotope scanning or ultrasonography of the liver are useful guides to the effectiveness of the therapy. For the refractory case or the patient with impending rupture of the abscess, percutaneous needle aspiration or open drainage may be necessary. A high index of suspicion, early institution of medical therapy, and aspiration of abscesses having the potential for rupture are believed to have contributed to the better outcome in children.

Prophylaxis for travelers to endemic areas is not recommended. The best prophylaxis is exercising caution in unsanitary conditions and endemic environments.

Acquired cellular immunity to invasive amebiasis seems to occur. Work is under way to develop a subunit amebiasis vaccine via a number of strategies. This includes using recombinant antigens such as the Gal/GalNac-specific lectin. Vaccination would be the most cost-effective approach to prevention.

Suggested Readings

Guerrent RL. Amebiasis: introduction, current status, and research questions. *Rev Infect Dis* 1986;8:218.

Haque R, Huston CD, Hughes M, et al. Current concepts: amebiasis. *N Engl J Med* 2003;348:1565.

Houpe E, Barroso L, Lockhart L, et al. Prevention of intestinal amebiasis by vaccination with the *Entamoeba histolyica* Gal/GalNac lectin. *Vaccine* 2004; 22:611.

Katz DE, Taylor DN. Parasitic infections of the gastrointestinal tract. *Gastroenterol Clin North Am* 2001;30:797.

LaVia W. Parasitic gastroenteritis. *Pediatr Ann* 1994;23:556.

Li E. Protozoa: amebiasis. *Gastroenterol Clin North Am* 1996;25:471.

Merritt RJ, Coughlin E, Thomas DW, et al. Spectrum of amebiasis in children. *Am J Dis Child* 1982;136:785.

Nazir Z, Moazam F. Amebic liver abscess in children. *Pediatr Infect Dis J* 1993; 12:929.

Pickering LK. Therapy for acute infectious diarrhea in children. *J Pediatr* 1991; 118:S118.

Stauffer W, Ravdin JI. *Entamoeba histolytics*: an update. *Curr Opin Infect Dis* 2003;16:479.

CHAPTER 217 ■ BABESIOSIS

CHRISTIAN C. PATRICK

Babesiosis is an emerging tick-borne disease that is caused by an intraerythrocytic protozoan manifesting in hemolysis in susceptible animals. The disease has been noted since biblical times, largely owing to its significant economic impact on livestock. The first human case of babesiosis was reported in 1957. Humans are a rare host, but serologic studies demonstrate infection in children and adults in endemic areas.

MICROBIOLOGY

The genus *Babesia* belongs to the subphylum Apicomplexa, which includes *Toxoplasma* and the malaria parasite *Plasmodium*. Ninety-nine species of *Babesia* have been identified. *B. microti* (reservoir in mice), *B. divergens* (reservoir in cattle), and the recently identified species WA-1 and MO-1 (reservoir unknown) are implicated in human disease in the United States. *B. divergens* is the major pathogen in Europe.

Microscopically, *Babesia* organisms are small (1 to 5 mm long), round, oval, or pear shaped. Because *Babesia* produces an illness similar to that produced by *Plasmodium*, the distinguishing laboratory features used to differentiate the two include *Babesia*'s inability to produce pigments in red blood cells (RBCs) in the latter stages of its life cycle, the presence of extracellular merozoites, and the rare formation of tetrads of merozoites resembling a Maltese cross.

EPIDEMIOLOGY

In the United States, the Ixodidae family of small, hard-bodied ticks is the primary vector for *B. microti*. This tick infects the northeastern United States from Wisconsin and Minnesota to Maryland. Infections due to variants of *B. microti* have also been reported in Missouri and on the coast of the United States in Washington and California. *Ixodes scapularis* is the species predominantly incriminated and is the same species of the tick implicated in Lyme disease and human granulocytic ehrlichiosis. Transmission through blood transfusion and from transplanted organs as well as perinatal transplacental transmission have also occurred.

The tick's life cycle spans approximately 2 years and comprises three stages: larval, nymphal, and adult. The most common host for the larval form is the white-footed mouse, *Peromyscus leucopus*. The transformation of the larval form to the nymphal form occurs transtadial. The white-tailed deer is the major reservoir for the adult tick, allowing mating to occur. The deer reservoir has allowed an expansion of the scope of babesiosis due to an increase deer population allowing an associated rise in the tick population. *Babesia* is transmitted to humans predominantly by the nymphal form of the tick.

Babesiosis occurs most often in the United States during late summer and fall, which is the nymph's major feeding period. Most cases have been confined to the northeastern states, coinciding with the tick vector epidemiology.

PATHOGENESIS

Although the exact mechanisms that allow *Babesia* to enter the red cell are unknown, the complement C3b receptor has been shown to be involved in the parasite's entry into the RBC in mice infected with *B. rodhani*. Once inside the RBC, the organism reproduces asexually by budding into two to four merozoites, which are released from the RBCs at varying times, in contrast to malaria-causing plasmodia, which are released synchronously from RBCs. Thus, *Babesia* generally is marked by milder symptoms of RBC lysis. The actual mechanisms that lead to hemolysis are unknown. Acute renal failure can occur with massive hemolysis.

The spleen is intimately involved in the disease process. Splenic dysfunction generally causes a more severe case of babesiosis. Owing to the spleen's reticuloendothelial cell capacity to remove deformed (parasitized) RBCs, removal of the spleen can lead to a relapse of disease in treated patients.

Cell-mediated immunity appears critical to control infections, although a humoral immune response is manifested.

CLINICAL MANIFESTATIONS

In immunocompetent individuals, babesiosis generally is a mild or subclinical infection. Asymptomatic infection is frequent in children. Manifestations occur more often and are more severe in immunocompromised patients, including those with acquired immunodeficiency syndrome, those with asplenia, the elderly, and neonates. After an incubation period of 1 to 4 weeks after the bite of an infecting tick, the susceptible host experiences a gradual onset of fatigue, malaise, anorexia, and fever with temperature spikes to 40°C (104°F). Other symptoms may include shaking chills, myalgias, sore throat, nonproductive cough, arthralgias, headaches, nausea and vomiting, and dark urine. Rash may be present but is not a constant feature.

Physical examination may reveal pallor, mild splenomegaly, hepatomegaly, jaundice, and pharyngeal erythema. Laboratory findings include moderately severe hemolytic anemia with a positive direct Coombs test, decreased haptoglobin, and an increased reticulocyte count. The erythrocyte sedimentation rate may be elevated. The leukocyte count is normal or decreased. Elevated liver function tests are identified in approximately one-half of infected patients.

The natural history can be prolonged, lasting weeks to months. A fulminant course with high fever, hemolytic anemia, hemoglobinuria, jaundice, congestive heart failure, renal failure, and adult respiratory distress syndrome is seen rarely.

Because the same tick vector is able to transmit babesiosis, Lyme disease, and ehrlichiosis, coinfection can occur. This has been documented by serology.

DIAGNOSIS

Babesiosis is diagnosed by a combination of clinical findings including history of tick bite, residency in or travel to an endemic region, plus laboratory findings. The latter includes intraerythrocytic parasites visualized on Giemsa or Wright stains of thick and thin blood smears (Fig. 217.1), including a formation known as a Maltese cross, consisting of a tetrad of merozoites in the shape of a cross (Fig. 217.2). Similar to *Plasmodium*, *Babesia* produces a variety of intraerythrocytic forms. *Plasmodium* can be distinguished by pigment production, synchronous stages of development, and no extracellular merozoites. In babesiosis, parasitemia can be detected as long as 10 months after the onset of illness. Serologic assays for babesial antibody include enzyme-linked immunosorbent as-

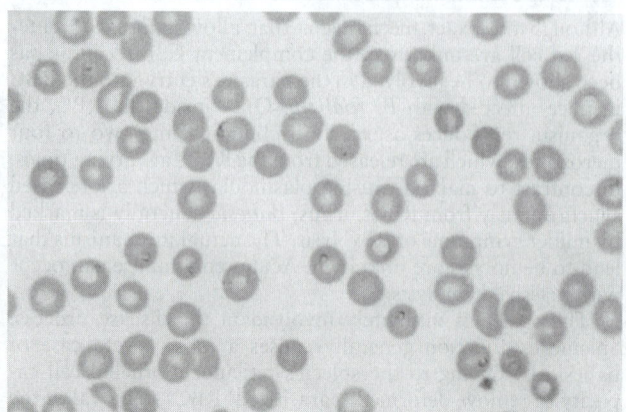

FIGURE 217.1. Peripheral blood smear showing intraerythrocytic ring forms.

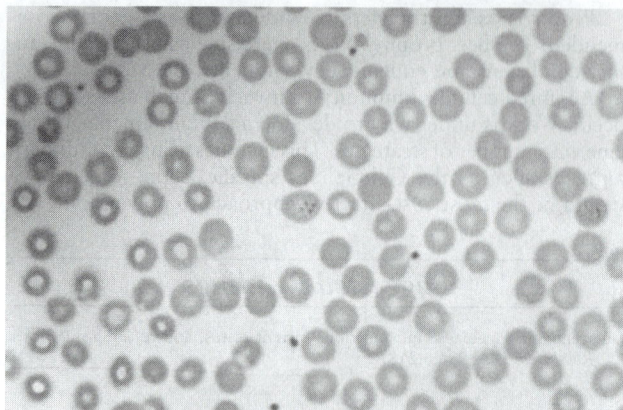

FIGURE 217.2. Peripheral blood smear revealing a tetrad form of merozoite (Maltese Cross form) in the middle of the micrograph.

say, immunoblot, and complement fixation tests. Polymerase chain reaction (PCR) analysis for *Babesia* is sensitive and comparable to blood smears, but requires a specialized laboratory.

TREATMENT

Babesiosis is largely self-limited, although therapy is required for those most at risk (splenectomized patients, immunosuppressed patients, and the elderly) and those with significant symptoms. A 7- to 10-day course of oral clindamycin (20 to 40 mg/kg/day divided into three doses, maximum 600 mg three times per day) and oral quinine (25 mg/kg/day divided into three doses, maximum of 650 mg three times per day) is the recommended treatment of choice, although treatment failure has been described. Recently, a combination of atovaquone (20 mg/kg twice a day, maximum 750 mg twice a day) and azithromycin (12 mg/kg daily, maximum 600 mg daily) for 7 to 10 days has shown equal efficacy in adult patients with fewer adverse effects. Exchange transfusions in combination with clindamycin and quinine have been successfully used but are reserved for life-threatening cases.

PREVENTION

Prevention consists of the avoidance of tick-infested areas, prevention of tick bites by use of insecticides, and the timely removal of ticks. This latter point is significant because a tick attachment of at least 24 hours is required for *Babesia* transmission to occur.

Suggested Readings

Aguilar-Delfin I, Wettstein PJ, Persing DH. Resistance to acute babesiosis is associated with interleukin-12 and gamma interferon-mediated responses and requires macrophages and natural killer cells. *Infect Immun* 2003;71:2002.

Boustani MR, Gelfand JA. Babesiosis. *Clin Infect Dis* 1996;22:611.

Clawson ML, Paciorkowski N, Rajan TV, et al. Cellular immunity, but not gamma interferon, is essential for resolution of *Babesia microti* in BALB/c Mice. *Infect Immun* 2002;70:5304.

Grunwaldt E, Barbour AG, Benach JL. Simultaneous occurrence of babesiosis and Lyme disease. *N Engl J Med* 1983;308:1166.

Herwaldt BL, Kjemtrup AM, Conrad PA, et al. Transfusion-transmitted babesiosis in Washington state: first reported case caused by a WA1-type parasite. *J Infect Dis* 1997;175:1259.

Homer MJ, Aguilar-Delfin I, Telford SR III. Babesiosis. *Clin Microbiol Rev* 2000; 13:451.

Jack RM, Ward PA. *Babesia rodhaini* interactions with complement: relationship to parasitic entry into red cells. *J Immunol* 1980;124:1566.

Jacoby GA, Hunt JV, Kosinski KS, et al. Treatment of transfusion-transmitted babesiosis by exchange transfusion. *N Engl J Med* 1980;303:1098.

Krause PJ. Babesiosis. *Med Clin N Am* 2002;86:361.

Krause PJ, Lepore T, Sikand VK, et al. Atovaquone and azithromycin for the treatment of babesiosis. *N Engl J Med* 2000;343:1454.

Krause PJ, Telford SR III, Pollack RJ, et al. Babesiosis: an underdiagnosed disease of children. *Pediatrics* 1992;89:1045.

Lantos PM, Krause PJ. Babesiosis: similar to malaria but different. *Pediatr Ann* 2002;31:192.

Pantanowitz L, Telford SR III, Cannon ME. The impact of babesiosis on transfusion medicine. *Trans Med Rev* 2002;16:131.

Rosner F, Zarrabi MH, Benach JL, Habicht GS. Babesiosis in splenectomized adults: review of 22 reported cases. *Am J Med* 1984;76:696.

Smith RP, Evans AT, Popovsky M, et al. Transfusion-acquired babesiosis and failure of antibiotic treatment. *JAMA* 1986;256:2726.

CHAPTER 218 ■ CRYPTOSPORIDIOSIS

WALTER T. HUGHES

Cryptosporidiosis is a common enteric infection of humans and animals that is caused by the coccidian protozoan *Cryptosporidium*. The first human case was described in 1976. The infection came to prominence in the early 1980s because of its association with the acquired immunodeficiency syndrome (AIDS) and other immunocompromised states. Furthermore, by the mid-1980s, it had become recognized as a frequent cause of diarrhea in otherwise physiologically normal children, especially those attending day-care centers.

ETIOLOGY

Cryptosporidium species are small, intracellular and extracytoplasmic protozoan parasites belonging to the protist phylum Apicomplexa, class Coccidia, family Cryptosporidiidae. The oocyst form of *Cryptosporidium* resides in the feces and is the infective stage. Each parasite completes its life cycle on intestinal surface epithelial cells. Sporozoites within the oocyst mature, undergo sporulation, and are released into the intestine, where they attach to the microvillar surface of epithelial cells. The organism is enveloped by the membrane of the host cell, thus forming a vacuole. Merogony, gametogony, and sporogony occur. Macrogametes and microgametes develop and on fertilization form an oocyst with four sporozoites. The oocyst is passed into the feces. At least ten species of *Cryptosporidium* have been identified. *Cryptosporidium parvum* causes most of the infections in humans, although *C. felis, C. muris,* and *C. meleagridis* have been found in a few cases.

EPIDEMIOLOGY

Human-to-human, animal-to-human, and human-to-animal transmission of *Cryptosporidium* has been reported. Outbreaks have been traced to contaminated water and food supplies.

Cryptosporidium is a common cause of enteric infection worldwide. Immunocompromised hosts with impaired cell-mediated immunity are at increased risk for acquiring cryptosporidiosis and expression of severe disease. Surveys of selected populations reveal carrier prevalence rates ranging from 0.6% to 4.0% in North America and from 4% to 20% in developing countries. Approximately 3% to 4% of patients with AIDS in the United States and 50% of those in Haiti and Africa are infected. *Cryptosporidium* has been isolated from the stools of 4.1% of hospitalized, immunocompetent patients with diarrhea in Australia, from 1.4% of a similar population in the United Kingdom, from 4.3% of Costa Rican children, and from 6.1% of immunocompetent patients with diarrhea in developing countries. Estimates are that diarrhea caused by *Cryptosporidium* occurs in 20 to 30 million children annually in Latin America. Because the oocyst is highly stable in the environment, contaminated drinking water, apple cider, spas, waterparks, fountains, hot tubs, and swimming pools are sources of outbreaks of infection. A contaminated public water supply resulted in an epidemic of more than 400,000 cases of cryptosporidiosis in Milwaukee, Wisconsin. Some studies indicate that *Cryptosporidium* oocysts are present in 65% to 95% of surface water (i.e., rivers, lakes, and streams) tested throughout the United States. Between 1989 and 2000, more than 170 outbreaks were associated with recreational water venues, with almost half resulting in episodes of gastrointestinal illness.

In the United States, 13% of children younger than 5 years, 38% of those 5 to 13 years of age, and 58% of adolescents and young adults 14 to 21 years of age are seropositive for antibodies to *C. parvum*. Several outbreaks of diarrhea attributable to *Cryptosporidium* have occurred in day-care centers in the United States, which currently are the setting of highest risk for otherwise normal children. In these outbreaks, other organisms, such as *Giardia lamblia*, also may be found in stool samples. When this occurs, however, *Cryptosporidium* usually is the causative agent of the diarrhea. Almost one-third of household members of children infected in a child-care center outbreak reported diarrhea, as compared with only 3% of household members of uninfected control children.

Person-to-person transmission has been reported in the hospital environment, a finding suggesting the need for enteric isolation precautions to protect susceptible immunocompromised patients. Animal-to-human transmission may occur, especially from calves. *C. parvum* oocysts have been found in the feces of 3% to 5% of cats. Flies can carry oocysts from unsanitary sites to other surfaces.

PATHOLOGY

The jejunum is the usual site of *C. parvum* infection, although in the severely immunocompromised host with AIDS, the entire intestinal tract from mouth to rectum, including the gallbladder and biliary duct, may be affected. The histologic pattern is one of organisms adherent to the surface of the enterocytes between the microvilli and the parasitiferous vacuole. Varying degrees of villous atrophy, crypt hyperplasia, and infiltration of the lamina propria with neutrophils and monocytes may occur. With mucosal infection, intraepithelial CD4 lymphocytes participate in host responses to control the infection, in part through production of interferon-gamma, which inhibits development of the organism in enterocytes. Moreover, infection is associated with increases in local cytokines, such as interleukin-12 and tumor necrosis factor-alpha in addition to interferon-gamma. Patients with peripheral blood CD4 lymphocyte counts less than 200 cells/mm³ are at increased risk of cryptosporidiosis. Responses of specific immunoglobulins G, A, M, E, and secretory A have been demonstrated, but infection and diarrhea may persist in patients with high levels of both serum and secretory antibodies. Diarrhea is associated with impaired intestinal absorption and enhanced excretion.

CLINICAL MANIFESTATIONS

Infection with *Cryptosporidium* may be asymptomatic or symptomatic. When the infection becomes clinically evident, the extent of the signs and symptoms generally is related to the degree of patient immunocompetence (Table 218.1). Immunologically normal children and adults have either asymptomatic infection or a self-limited illness.

Patients with AIDS or other severe immunodeficiency states usually have chronic diarrhea, often with cholera-like features. Diarrhea commonly is profuse, watery, and without blood. Fluid losses may be extensive, as great as several liters per day in adults. The pathophysiology of this extensive fluid loss has not been elucidated. These patients also may have abdominal pain, anorexia, weight loss, nausea, and vomiting, but they rarely are febrile. Symptoms, severe wasting, and oocyst shedding may persist for months and often until death in patients with AIDS.

In immunocompetent hosts, the illness resembles that of giardiasis, with watery diarrhea, abdominal pain, malaise, myalgias, weight loss, and anorexia. In careful studies of Finnish patients, the incubation period was 1 week, and the duration of the illness was approximately 12 days. Hospitalized children with cryptosporidiosis have experienced illnesses of similar duration, and, of those with diarrhea, more than 50% experience vomiting, nearly 50% exhibit fever, and approximately 85% have abdominal pain.

TABLE 218.1

CLINICAL FINDINGS IN PATIENTS WITH GASTROINTESTINAL INFECTION RESULTING FROM *CRYPTOSPORIDIUM*

Normal Host	Patient with AIDS or Other Severe Immunodeficiency
Asymptomatic	Gastroenteritis: four syndromes
Gastroenteritis	Chronic diarrhea: 36%
Watery diarrhea: 95%	Cholera-like diarrhea: 33%
Abdominal pain: 85%	Transient diarrhea: 15%
Vomiting: 50%	Relapsing diarrhea: 15%
Fever: 50%	Rarely: cholecystitis
Malaise	Duration: months
Weight loss	
Duration: about 12 days	

C. parvum infection of the respiratory tract has been associated with symptoms of laryngotracheobronchitis. Cryptosporidial cholecystitis with upper right quadrant pain, fever, and jaundice has been observed in severely compromised patients with AIDS and CD4 counts less than 50 cells/mm³.

DIAGNOSIS

The differential diagnosis for cryptosporidiosis includes all causes of diarrhea. Attention should be directed to this protozoan when the patient has AIDS or some other form of immunodeficiency or when he or she has attended a day-care center. Sporadic cases also may occur in otherwise healthy children.

The diagnosis of cryptosporidiosis is established by the identification of *Cryptosporidium* oocysts from fecal specimens in the absence of other enteric pathogens. More definitive is the demonstration of intracellular forms of the parasite in biopsy specimens of intestinal mucosa obtainable by endoscopy. The clinician must bear in mind that *Cryptosporidium* can be found in asymptomatic individuals. Fecal samples can be examined by several staining methods, including acid-fast stains, fluorescent auramine and rhodamine stains, periodic acid–Schiff stains, and carbolfuchsin-negative stains. These special stains must be specifically requested, because routine examination of stool for ova and parasites does not allow detection of *Cryptosporidium*.

Initially, an iodine-stained wet mount and an acid-fast–stained (modified Kinyoun or Ziehl-Neelsen) smear should be prepared. The 4- to 6-μg oocysts stain intensely red by the acid-fast techniques. Fecal specimens can be processed by centrifugation at 500 × G for 10 minutes and smear preparations made from the sediment.

Newer diagnostic tests are commercially available and in use in some clinical laboratories. For example, the direct and indirect fluorescent-antibody assays (Meridian Diagnostics, Inc., Cincinnati, OH) have close to 100% sensitivity and specificity. Similarly, enzyme immunoassays such as the ProSpecT enzyme immunoassay (EIA; Alexon, Inc., Ramsey, MN) appear to be promising.

Polymerase chain reaction amplification of *C. parum* DNA has provided highly sensitive methods for detection, but such techniques are not adequately developed and standardized for routine diagnostic use. Serologic tests for antibody to *Cryptosporidium* have been developed but are not in general use at this time and are not of diagnostic value.

TREATMENT

Specific therapy for cryptosporidiosis is limited. In most immunocompetent children, the course is self-limiting, but immunosuppressed patients may require intensive and prolonged supportive management. Studies have yielded equivocal results from the use of drugs such as azithromycin and paromomycin. The Food and Drug Administration approved a new drug, nitrazoxanide (Alinia, Romark Pharmaceuticals, Tampa, FL) for the treatment of cryptosporidiosis in children from 1 to 11 years of age, based on two studies. In one trial, 88% of children receiving nitrazoxanide compared with 38% of those given a placebo responded favorably. Another trial showed that 56% of malnourished children with the infection responded to nitrazoxanide compared with 23% given the placebo. The recommended dose of the oral suspension for patients 12 through 47 months of age is 100 mg (5 mL) every 12 hours for 3 days. Patients 4 to 11 years of age should receive 200 mg (10 mL) every 12 hours for 3 days. No significant adverse events have been encountered.

Experimental preparations of hyperimmune bovine colostrum and bovine transfer factor have undergone preliminary trials, with some evidence of efficacy. Effective antiretroviral treatment of AIDS is associated with resolution of symptoms of cryptosporidiosis.

PREVENTION

Because oocyst excretion may persist for as long as 2 weeks after clinical recovery occurs, enteric isolation precautions should be instituted for hospitalized patients, with special efforts to avoid exposure of immunosuppressed patients. Severely immunocompromised patients should avoid swimming in and drinking from lakes and rivers. Because chlorination does not kill the organism, the use of boiled tap water (1 minute) or the filtration of drinking water with submicron (less than 1 μg) personal-use filters is suggested. Commercially available bottled water is not standardized for microbial purity.

Suggested Readings

American Academy of Pediatrics. Cryptosporidiosis. In: Pickering LK, ed. *Redbook: 2003 report of the Committee on Infectious Diseases*, 26th ed. Elk Grove Village, IL: American Academy of Pediatrics, 2003:255.

Chen X-M, Keithly JS, Paya CV, LaRusso NF. Cryptosporidiosis. *N Engl J Med* 2002;346:1723.

Jokipii L, Kokipii MM. Timing of symptoms and oocyst excretion in human cryptosporidiosis. *N Engl J Med* 1986;315:1643.

Kelly P. Effect of nitrazoxanide on morbidity and mortality in Zambian children with cryptosporidiosis: a randomized controlled trial. *Lancet* 2002;360: 1375.

Leav BA, Mackay M, Ward HD. Cryptosporidiosis: new insights and old challenges. *Clin Infect Dis* 2003;36:903.

MacKenzie WR, Hoxie NJ, Proctor ME, et al. A massive outbreak in Milwaukee of *Cryptosporidium* infection transmitted through the public water supply. *N Engl J Med* 1994;331:161.

Maggi P, Larocca AM, Quarto M, et al. Effect of antiretroviral therapy on cryptosporidiosis and microsporidiosis in patients infected with human immunodeficiency virus type 1. *Eur J Clin Microbial Infect Dis* 2000;19:213.

Ortega YR, Arrowwood M. Cryptosporidium, cyclospora and isospora. In: Murray PR, Baron EJ, Jorgensen JH, et al., eds. *Manual of clinical microbiology*, 8th ed. Washington, DC: ASM Press, 2003:2008.

Rossignol JF, Ayoub A, Ayers MS. Treatment of diarrhea caused by *Cryptosporidium parvum*: a prospective, randomized, double blind, placebo-controlled study of nitrazoxanide. *J Infect Dis* 2001;184:103.

CHAPTER 219 ■ *GIARDIA LAMBLIA*

WILLIAM J. KLISH

Giardia lamblia holds the distinction of being the first protozoan parasite to be recognized. It was described in a letter by van Leeuwenhoek of Delft, the Netherlands, to the Royal Society of Medicine in 1681 after he observed this parasite in his stool while trying to evaluate his own intermittent chronic diarrhea. He made the important clinical observation that these "animalcules" could be found only in liquid stool, not in normal, formed stool.

EPIDEMIOLOGY

G. lamblia is a cosmopolitan parasite of worldwide distribution and is an important cause of traveler's diarrhea. *Giardia* is the most common intestinal parasite found in the United States. Its prevalence may be increasing. In 1979, *Giardia* was found in an average of 4% of stool specimens submitted to state diagnostic laboratories. This prevalence increased to 6% to 7% in the late 1980s and 1990s. The states in which it appears most frequently are located in the Midwest and the Northwest. *Giardia* also is prevalent in the mountainous western United States, where infection can be contracted by drinking water from mountain streams that have been contaminated by feces from humans, dogs, and other species susceptible to *G. lamblia*. The beaver acts as a reservoir for the organism during the summer months by becoming infected (presumably from humans) and then defecating directly into streams. Water can be disinfected by adding 13 mL of a saturated solution of iodine to 1 L of clear water, or 26 mL to 1 L of cloudy water. All organisms are killed after 15 minutes of incubation at 20°C;

at 3°C, however, this method is not totally effective. Boiling water for 10 minutes kills all organisms.

Giardia also can be spread by close person-to-person contact in which fecal contamination may occur, such as in daycare centers and residential institutions. In addition, contaminated food may act as a vector for this parasite. Human milk may contain secretory anti-*Giardia* antibodies that can prevent symptoms of diarrhea but not *Giardia* infection in breast-fed infants.

THE ORGANISM

Three species of *Giardia* have been described. *G. lamblia* is the species that is specific to humans, but it can be crosstransmitted to other animals, such as dogs, cats, rats, gerbils, guinea pigs, beavers, raccoons, bighorn sheep, and pronghorn antelope. *G. muris* infects rodents and birds; *G. agilis* is specific to amphibians. *G. lamblia* is the name used for the species infecting humans in North America. This same organism is called *G. intestinalis* in Europe and *Lamblia intestinalis* in Russia and Eastern Europe. It has also been called *G. duodenalis* and *G. enterica*.

G. lamblia is a flagellate protozoan belonging to the family Hexamitidae. The trophozoite or motile form is characterized by its symmetry: two oval, dorsally situated nuclei and four pairs of flagella. In addition, it has two median bodies and a ventral adhesive disc by which the parasite adheres to the intestinal mucosa and other surfaces. Attachment seems to be mediated through the cytoskeleton by contractile filaments and microtubules to lectin-binding sites on the mucosa. Interference in such binding can occur through the ingestion of lectins such as wheat-germ agglutinin normally consumed in the diet. The organism also exists in a cyst form, which results when the trophozoite rounds up and elaborates a cyst wall. These cysts allow the organism to survive passage out of the host. *Giardia* cysts are resistant to destruction in hypotonic solutions such as water and can survive for more than 2 months in water at 8°C but for only 4 days in water at 37°C. When cysts are ingested, the excystation process is induced by gastric acid and is completed in the duodenum with the emergence of trophozoites. Infection is established if the trophozoite can survive, attach to the intestinal mucosa, and multiply. This process may require nutrients within the intestinal fluid.

PATHOGENESIS

The pathogenesis of diarrhea and steatorrhea in giardiasis is not understood completely. Initially, the organisms were believed to damage the intestinal mucosa either through direct invasion or the elaboration of some toxin. Careful histologic studies with light and electron microscopy have shown some reduction in villous height and mild crypt hyperplasia, but this effect appears to be related to specific *Giardia* strains.

Mechanical blockage of nutrient absorption resulting from the mass of *Giardia* organisms adhering to the intestinal mucosa also has been postulated. Histologic examination of the intestinal mucosa of diseased individuals, however, usually does not reveal enough organisms to support this hypothesis. *Giardia* appears to have the capability to alter intestinal motility, which may play a role in the development of symptoms.

Finally, careful electron microscopy has revealed that *Giardia* seems to stimulate excessive mucus production by the intestinal mucosa. This excessive mucus causes thickening of the unstirred layer or glycocalyx adherent to the intestinal brush border and may result in a diffusion barrier for nutrients, ultimately causing diarrhea and malabsorption.

CLINICAL MANIFESTATIONS OF GIARDIASIS

Acute symptoms of giardiasis include watery diarrhea, nausea, bloating, belching (described as sulfurous), cramping, abdominal pain, and weight loss; these symptoms usually occur 1 to 2 weeks after the ingestion of cysts (Box 219.1). The illness usually is self-limited, lasting 2 to 6 weeks, but it may recur intermittently or become chronic. Chronic symptoms can include fatigue, nervousness, weight loss, growth retardation, steatorrhea, lactose intolerance, and, rarely, protein-losing enteropathy. Chronic giardiasis frequently is associated with immunodeficiency syndromes such as immunoglobulin A (IgA) and IgM deficiencies and the acquired immunodeficiency syndrome. Individuals who are carrying the disease chronically may be asymptomatic.

DIAGNOSIS

Routine laboratory values such as blood cell counts and electrolyte levels are normal in most patients. Nonspecific radiographic abnormalities that may be seen on barium contrast studies of the upper intestinal tract include thickening of the mucosal folds, hypersecretion with dilution of the barium column, and hypermotility.

Direct examination of feces for the presence of *G. lamblia* cysts or trophozoites remains the hallmark for diagnosis. Direct

---

> | **BOX 219.1** | Symptoms Associated with *Giardia lamblia* Infection |
>
> Asymptomatic
> Acute
>   Watery diarrhea
>   Nausea
>   Bloating
>   Belching
>   Cramping
>   Abdominal pain
>   Weight loss
> Chronic
>   Fatigue
>   Nervousness
>   Weight loss
>   Growth retardation
>   Steatorrhea
>   Lactose intolerance
>   Protein-losing enteropathy (rare)

fecal smears in physiologic saline are the easiest way to examine the stool microscopically. Recovery of the organism can be enhanced by a concentrating technique using either formal-ether or zinc sulfate flotation. Permanent slides then can be made using stains such as trichrome. Because *Giardia* cysts and trophozoites are not excreted continuously, however, even the best laboratories report as negative a significant number of stool specimens in patients with disease. If the diagnosis is suspected strongly, at least three stools should be collected on different days. If both a direct smear and a concentration test are performed on each stool, the chance of diagnosis is approximately 75% from one stool, 90% from two stools, and 97% from three stools.

The diagnosis is made readily by direct examination of the upper small intestine, either by mucosal biopsy or through the collection of jejunal contents. *Giardia* trophozoites can be seen in histologic sections of the small bowel, particularly if they are stained with trichrome. Their recovery can be enhanced via a "touch preparation" of the biopsy material. In this technique, the mucosal surface of the small intestinal biopsy sample is touched to a glass slide before it is immersed in fixative. The slide then is air dried, fixed in methanol, stained, and examined microscopically. Jejunal aspirates obtained by intubation also can be examined microscopically for the presence of *Giardia* trophozoites.

Several immunologic assays for *Giardia* antigen in stool specimens are now available. These tests appear more sensitive than the earlier tests used for the diagnosis of giardiasis with their sensitivity and specificity ranging as high as 90% and 100%, respectively, on a single stool specimen.

TREATMENT

Treatment is indicated whenever *Giardia* is found to cause acute diarrhea, chronic intermittent disease, subclinical symptoms, or infection in others (Table 219.1). Generally, treatment of asymptomatic carriers is not recommended. Children with nondiarrheal giardiasis, however, who exhibit other gastrointestinal symptoms or who have evidence of malabsorption should be considered for therapy. Public health considerations also may require that asymptomatic carriers be treated.

TABLE 219.1

AVAILABLE TREATMENT OPTIONS FOR *GIARDIA LAMBLIA* INFECTION

Agent	Dosage
Nitazoxanide (Alinia)	100 mg every 12 hours for 3 days (children 1 to 4 years) 200 mg every 12 hours for 4 days (children 4 to 11)
Metronidazole (Flagyl)	250 mg three times daily for 1 week (adults) 15 to 20 mg/kg/day divided into three doses (children)
Furazolidone (Furoxone)	100 mg four times daily for 7 to 10 days (adults) 6 mg/kg/day divided into four doses for 7 to 10 days (children)
Tinidazole	2 g in a single dose (adults) 50 mg/kg in a single dose (children)

The newest drug available in the United States for giardiasis is nitazoxanide (Alinia), and it is available as an oral suspension. The recommended dose for children 1 to 4 years of age is 100 mg every 12 hours for 3 days, and for children 4 to 11 years old, the dose recommended is 200 mg every 12 hours for 4 days. The traditional treatment for patients with both asymptomatic and symptomatic giardiasis is metronidazole (Flagyl). This is administered in dosages of 250 mg three times daily for 1 week in adults or 15 to 20 mg/kg/day divided into three doses for children. Another drug that can be used is furazolidone (Furoxone), 100 mg four times daily for 7 to 10 days in adults or 6 mg/kg/day divided into four doses for children. Tinidazole has been evaluated extensively since the early 1970s and is highly effective in adults when given as a single 2-g dose or in children given in a single dose of 50 mg/kg. It also is effective in children when given by suppository for 1 to 3 days, thereby avoiding upper gastrointestinal side effects. Bacitracin zinc, 120,000 units (USP) orally twice daily for 10 days, or neomycin, 120,000 units (USP), orally twice daily for 10 days, has been used successfully in adults.

Suggested Readings

Addiss DG, Juranik DD, Spencer HC. Treatment of children with asymptomatic and non-diarrheal *Giardia* infection. *Pediatr Infect Dis J* 1991;10:843.

Cody MM, Sottnek HM, O'Leary VS. Recovery of *Giardia lamblia* cysts from chairs and tables in child day-care centers. *Pediatrics* 1994;94:1006.

Davidson RA. Issues in clinical parasitology: the treatment of giardiasis. *Am J Gastroenterol* 1984;79:256.

Dvorak AM. *Giardia lamblia. N Engl J Med* 1993;338:1010.

Forthing MJG, Mata L, Uriutia JJ, Kronmal RA. Natural history of *Giardia* infection of infants and children in rural Guatemala and its impact on physical growth. *Am J Clin Nutr* 1986;43:395.

Garcia LS, Shimizu RY, Novak S, Chan F. Commercial assay for detection of *Giardia lamblia* and *Cryptosporidium parvum* antigens in human fecal specimens by rapid solid phase-phase qualitative immunochromatography. *J Clin Microbiol* 2003;41:209.

Katelaris PH, Naeem A, Farthing MJ. Attachment of *Giardia lamblia* trophozoites to a cultured human intestinal cell line. *Gut* 1995;37:512.

McIntyre P, Boreham PFL, Phillips RE, Shepperd RW. Chemotherapy in giardiasis: clinical responses and *in vitro* drug sensitivity of human isolates in axemic culture. *J Pediatr* 1986;108:1005.

Tee GH, Moody AH, Cooke AH, Chiodini PL. Comparison of techniques for detecting antigens of *Giardia lamblia* and *Cryptosporidium parvum* in faeces. *J Clin Pathol* 1993;46:555.

Wolfe MS. Giardiasis. *Pediatr Clin North Am* 1979;26:295.

Wright JM, Dunn LA, Upcroft P, Upton JA. Efficacy of antigiardial drugs. *Expert Opin Drug Saf* 2003;2:529.

CHAPTER 220 ■ LEISHMANIASIS

MURRAY WITTNER AND HERBERT B. TANOWITZ

The leishmaniases are vector-borne diseases caused by obligate intracellular protozoans or hemoflagellates of the genus *Leishmania*. The diseases affect the viscera, skin, and/or mucous membranes. They are transmitted by several genera and species of phlebotomine sandflies. Three major clinical syndromes are recognized: visceral (VL), cutaneous (CL), and mucocutaneous (MCL) leishmaniasis (Table 220.1). In each type of disease, macrophages are parasitized exclusively.

The clinical manifestations of leishmaniasis appear to depend upon a complex set of factors, including tropism and virulence of the parasite strain, as well as the susceptibility of the host that may be determined genetically. The host's cell-mediated immune responses appear to be a major factor moderating these syndromes. Each species of *Leishmania* has clinical variants that may cause similar patterns of disease in the same host species. Thus, in the case of VL (kala-azar), *L. donovani, L. chagasi, L. infantum,* and *L. amazonensis* invade cells of the reticuloendothelial system of the viscera, usually causing splenomegaly, hypergammaglobulinemia, occasionally hepatomegaly, and pancytopenia; untreated, the disease is progressive and usually fatal. In CL, *L. tropica* (with some notable exceptions), *L. major, L. aethiopica,* and *L. mexicana* usually are limited to reticuloendothelial cells of the skin; the infections generally are self-limited, healing spontaneously. Similarly, *L. braziliensis* invades the reticuloendothelial cells of the skin, although it has the propensity to metastasize to the mucous membranes of the nose, mouth, and pharynx, causing facial disfigurement and, occasionally, death. Strains of *L. tropica* have been found to cause viscerotropic disease. In individuals with human immunodeficiency virus (HIV) or acquired immunodeficiency syndrome (AIDS), leishmania infections have been recognized as opportunistic infections and may serve as a cofactor in the pathogenesis of HIV infection.

CAUSAL ORGANISM AND LIFE CYCLE (FIG. 220.1)

In vertebrates, leishmania are obligate intracellular organisms that exist only in the amastigote stage. The species that

TABLE 220.1

CLINICAL SYNDROMES CAUSED BY *LEISHMANIA* SPECIES AND THEIR GEOGRAPHIC DISTRIBUTION*

Clinical Syndromes	*Leishmania* Species	Location
Visceral leishmaniasis		
Kala-azar: generalized involvement of the reticuloendothelial system (spleen, bone marrow, liver)	L. (L.) donovani	Indian subcontinent, northern and eastern China, Pakistan, Nepal
	L. (L.) infantum	Middle East, Mediterranean littoral, Balkans, central and southwestern Asia, northern and northwestern China, northern and sub-Saharan Africa
	L. (L.) donovani (archibaldi)	Sudan, Kenya, Ethiopia
	L. (L.) spp.	Kenya, Ethiopia, Somalia
	L. (L.) chagasi	Latin America
	L. (L.) amazonensis	Brazil (Bahia State)
	L. (L.) tropica	Israel, India, and viscerotropic disease in Saudi Arabia (U.S. troops)
Post-kala-azar dermal leishmaniasis	L. (L.) donovani	Indian subcontinent, East Africa
	L. (L.) spp.	Kenya, Ethiopia, Somalia
Old World cutaneous leishmaniasis		
Single or limited number of skin lesions	L. (L.) major	Middle East, northwestern China, northwestern India, Pakistan, Africa
	L. (L.) tropica	Mediterranean littoral, Middle East, western Asiatic area, Indian subcontinent
	L. (L.) aethiopica	Ethiopian highlands, Kenya, Yemen
	L. (L.) infantum	Mediterranean basin
	L. (L.) donovani (archibaldi)	Sudan and East Africa
	L. (L.) spp.	Kenya, Ethiopia, Somalia
Diffuse cutaneous leishmaniasis	L. (L.) aethiopica	Ethiopian highlands, Kenya, Yemen
New World cutaneous leishmaniasis		
Single or limited number of skin lesions	L. (L.) mexicana (chiclero ulcer)	Central America, Mexico, Texas
	L. (L.) amazonensis	Amazon basin and neighboring areas, Bahia and other states in Brazil
	L. (V.) braziliensis	Multiple areas of Central and South America
	L. (V.) guyanensis (forest vaws)	Guyana, Suriname, northern Amazon basin
	L. (V.) peruviana (uta)	Peru (western Andes) and Argentinean highlands
	L. (V.) panamensis	Panama, Costa Rica, Colombia
	L. (V.) pifanoi	Venezuela
	L. (V.) garnhami	Venezuela
	L. (V.) venezuelensis	Venezuela
	L. (V.) colombiensis	Colombia and Panama
	L. (L.) chagasi	Central and South America
Diffuse cutaneous leishmaniasis	L. (L.) amazonensis	Amazon basin and neighboring areas, Bahia and other states in Brazil
	L. (V.) pifanoi	Venezuela
	L. (L.) mexicana	Mexico and Central America
	L. (L.) spp.	Dominican Republic
Mucosal leishmaniasis	L. (V.) braziliensis (espundia)	Multiple areas in Latin America

(L.), subgenus *Leishmania*; (V.), subgenus *Viannia*.
Modified from Pearson RD, Sousa AQ. Clinical spectrum of leishmaniasis. *Clin Infect Dis* 1996;22:1. Data from Lainson R, Shaw JJ. Evolution, classification and geographic distribution. In: Peters W, Killick-Kendrick R, eds., *The Leishmaniases in Biology and Medicine*. London: Academic Press, 1987:1.
*Reprinted by permission of Pearson RD. Leishmaniasis. In: Guerrant RL, Walker DH, Weller PF, eds., *Tropical Infectious Diseases:Principles, Pathogens and Practice*. Philadelphia: Churchill Lvingstone, 1999.

infect humans usually are morphologically indistinguishable from one another by both light and transmission electron microscopy. The amastigotes are round to oval bodies approximately 2 to 4 μm in diameter; they possess a single nucleus and a specialized mitochondrial structure that has extranuclear DNA, termed a *kinetoplast*, and they lack a free flagellum. Amastigotes are phagocytized by macrophages and reside within a parasitophorous vacuole of the macrophage. In this environment, they multiply by binary fission, eventually destroying the host cell. The life cycle of the organism is described in Box 220.1. They subsequently are phagocytized, and the process occurs repeatedly. No evidence shows that amastigotes actively penetrate host cells.

Promastigotes have surface molecules that bind to several macrophage receptors. Within the parasitophorous vacuole, phagocytized promastigotes transform to amastigotes, and multiplication occurs. Many of the invading promastigotes do not survive because mammalian tissue fluids contain cytolytic substances. Those organisms that are phagocytized transform to amastigotes and initiate replication. The organisms can be seen readily in tissues or smears by light microscopy, especially with Giemsa or Wright stain, with which the nucleus

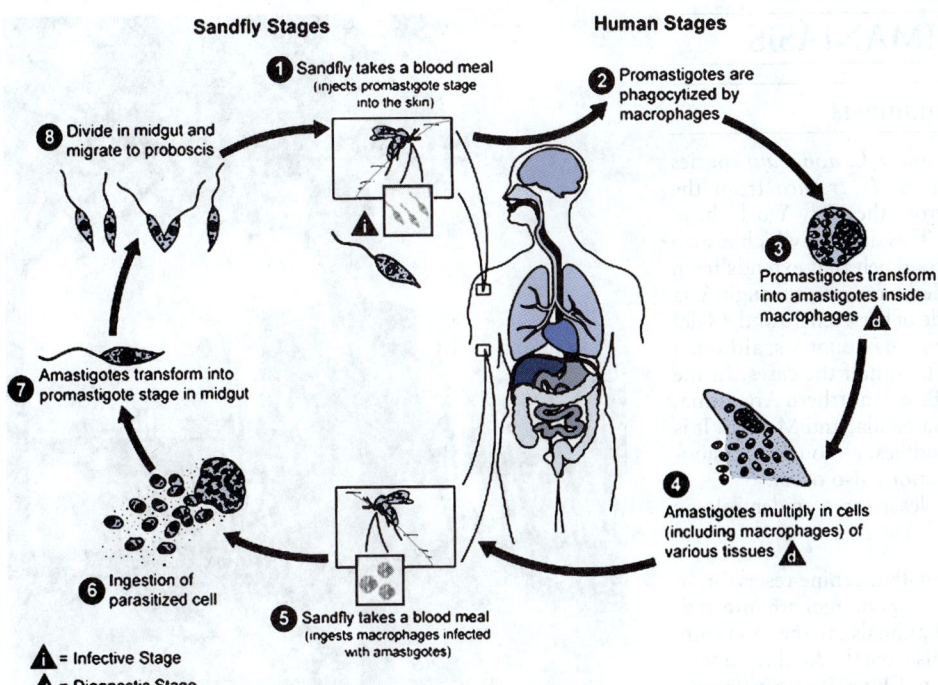

Sandfly Stages

❶ Sandfly takes a blood meal
(injects promastigote stage
into the skin)

❽ Divide in midgut and
migrate to proboscis

❼ Amastigotes transform into
promastigote stage in midgut

❻ Ingestion of
parasitized cell

❺ Sandfly takes a blood meal
(ingests macrophages infected
with amastigotes)

Human Stages

❷ Promastigotes are
phagocytized by
macrophages

❸ Promastigotes transform
into amastigotes inside
macrophages ⓓ

❹ Amastigotes multiply in cells
(including macrophages) of
various tissues ⓓ

ⓘ = Infective Stage

ⓓ = Diagnostic Stage

FIGURE 220.1. Life cycle of *Leish-maniasis donovani*, the causative agent of visceral leishmaniasis. (Courtesy of the Centers for Disease Control and Prevention.)

and kinetoplast stain bright red and the cytoplasm stains pale blue. In Novey, McNeal, Nicolle (NNN) culture medium at 24°C, the organisms grow readily, assuming the promastigote or insect form.

Clinical isolates are morphologically indistinguishable, and molecular biologic techniques have been utilized to characterize the strains and species of clinical isolates. These techniques include endonuclease restriction studies of the kinetoplast DNA (K-DNA), buoyant density of the K-DNA and mitochondrial DNA (M-DNA) on cesium chloride, leishmanial isozyme patterns, monoclonal antibody specificity, polymerase chain reaction (PCR) (employing species-specific oligonucleotide primers), and exoantigen secretory 4-factor serotyping.

| BOX 220.1 | Life Cycle of *Leishmania* |

When a female sandfly feeds on an infected individual, it may ingest an infected cell from blood or tissue. The amastigotes are liberated in the fly's midgut and, within a few hours, transform to the promastigote stage. These organisms are elongated flagellates, 15 to 25 μm long by 1.5 to 3.5 μm wide, with an anterior, free flagellum that is approximately 15 to 28 μm long and may vary morphologically from short and stumpy to elongated forms. Binary fission occurs within the fly's midgut, and the large numbers of promastigotes that are produced gradually move forward to the pharynx, buccal cavity, and mouth parts. At 8 to 20 days, depending on temperature and the species of sandfly, the mouth parts of the fly may be blocked partially or completely by large numbers of promastigotes and dislodged into the bite wound when the female sandfly (*Phlebotomus* spp., *Lutzomyia* spp.) feeds. In some instances, promastigotes may be inoculated mechanically into the bite wound (Fig. 220.2).

EPIDEMIOLOGY

The precise incidence of leishmaniasis is not known. However, the World Health Organization (WHO) has estimated that 350 million individuals are at risk and that the disease is endemic in more than 88 countries. It occurs in northern Argentine to southern Texas (except Uruguay and Chile) and in southern Europe, Asia (not Southeast Asia), the Middle East, and Africa. The estimated incidence of VL is 500,000 cases annually, and for CL and MCL, it is 1.5 million cases per year. Although the parasite usually is transmitted via the bite of the sandfly, it also may be transmitted as a result of a laboratory accident, direct person-to-person transmission, and blood transfusion. In addition, evidence exists that suggests it may be transmitted either *in utero* or during the peripartum period.

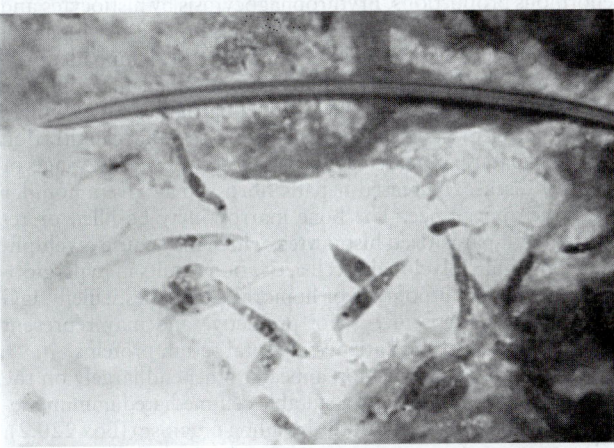

FIGURE 220.2. Promastigote forms from proboscis of crushed sandfly (*Phlebotomus*). (Courtesy of Dr. Herman Zaiman.)

TYPES OF LEISHMANIASIS

Visceral Leishmaniasis

VL is caused by various organisms in the *L. donovani* species complex, although recently, strains of *L. tropica* from the Middle East and *L. amazonensis* from the New World have been found to cause this syndrome. This disease, which is also known as kala-azar, is found in a broad belt that extends from the Straits of Gibraltar across the Mediterranean through Asia to the east coast of China, at a latitude of between 30 and 48 degrees north. VL has been reported from 47 countries, although Sudan and India account for more than half the cases. In the Western Hemisphere, it is found in Brazil, northern Argentina, Paraguay, Venezuela, Colombia, Guatemala, and Mexico. It is transmitted by various species of sandflies, although occasionally congenital and bloodborne infections also occur.

Kala-azar appears to exist in at least three epidemiologic forms:

1. A Mediterranean type of VL, with a canine reservoir, in which young children (1 to 4 years of age) are infected, and dogs, foxes, or other feral animals are the reservoirs (*L. infantum*). This type extends from the Mediterranean littoral through central Asia into China; it also is present in parts of South America (*L. chagasi*), where foxes and dogs are reservoir hosts. In Brazil, young males most often are infected.
2. An Indian type (*L. donovani*) of VL, with a human reservoir, in which the disease predominates in Indian children between 5 and 15 years of age; humans are the only known reservoir. Although sought, evidence of natural infection in dogs has not been found. No evidence of rodent reservoirs exists.
3. An African type of VL in which rodents are the reservoir hosts. The Nile rat in Sudan and probably the gerbil in Kenya are the reservoirs. In Kenya, kala-azar often is related to old or eroded termite mounds where young males often congregate (Fig. 220.3).

Pathology and Pathobiology

The principal pathologic lesions of VL are caused by reticuloendothelial hyperplasia. A pea-sized granuloma (i.e., leishmaniana) forms at the inoculation site. Subsequently, infected macrophages disseminate to local lymph nodes and then to the viscera, especially the spleen, liver, bone marrow, and intestines. The spleen gradually enlarges, sometimes assuming enormous proportions. Erythrophagocytosis by histiocytes and the anemia so typical of kala-azar may be the result in part of such sequestration of red cells. In early disease, lymphadenopathy caused by large numbers of parasite-filled macrophages is found. Kupffer cells, filled with amastigotes, are swollen and hyperplastic, and centrilobular necrosis or fatty infiltration of the hepatic parenchyma often is observed. In late-stage or chronic disease, increased hepatic fibrosis may give a nodular cirrhotic appearance. The bone marrow may be filled or replaced with parasitized histiocytes, which may cause myelophthisic anemia. Polyclonal B-cell activation results in hyperglobulinemia. This outpouring of humoral antibodies, chiefly IgG and largely nonspecific, is not protective and may represent more than half of the patient's the total serum proteins.

The outcome of infection appears to depend largely on the host's capacity to generate a suitable cell-mediated immune response and the virulence of the invading organism (Box 220.2). The genetics of human resistance and susceptibility remains unclear. The role of the sandfly in influencing disease has been appreciated recently. Sandfly saliva contains maxadilan, a potent vasodilatory salivary polypeptide. In Brazil, *L. chagasi*

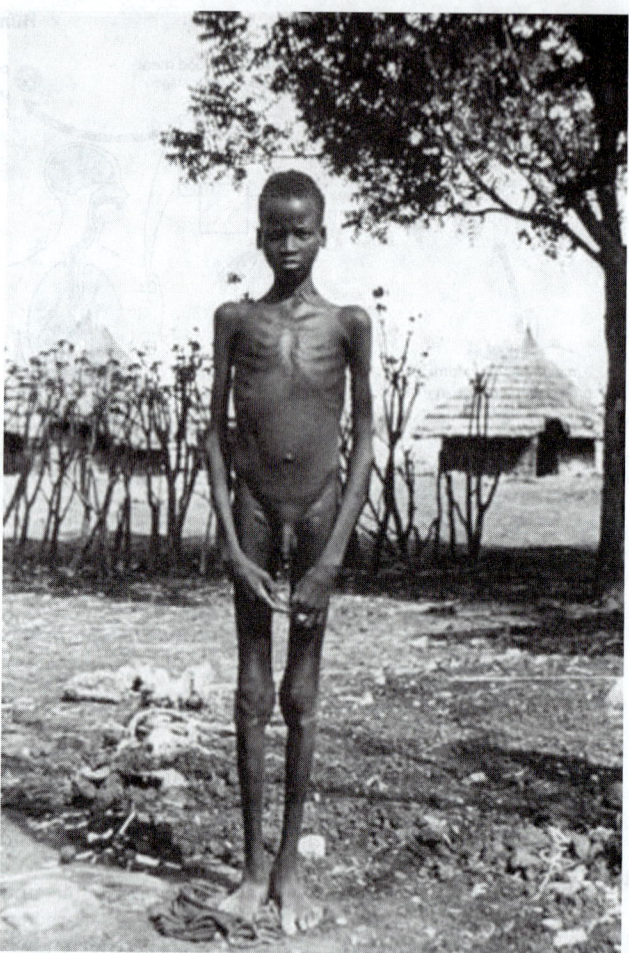

FIGURE 220.3. Emaciated young African male with visceral leishmaniasis. (Courtesy of Dr. Herman Zaiman.)

causes VL, and the sandfly (*Lutzomyia longipalpis*) that transmits VL has high levels of maxadilan in its saliva, promoting erythema and vasodilation. However, in Costa Rica, *L. chagasi* causes CL, and the sandfly (*L. longipalpis*) that transmits *L. chagasi* has very little maxadilan in its saliva, causing minimal vasodilation and erythema; the organisms multiply in the skin.

Clinical Manifestations

The clinical prepatent period varies widely from 6 weeks to 6 months but has been reported to be as early as 10 to 14 days and as long as 10 years. The primary skin nodule often is not noticed, although it is a more regular feature in African leishmaniasis.

Infantile VL may begin either suddenly with high fevers and vomiting or insidiously with irregular daily fever, anorexia, weight loss, lassitude, and pallor. Double daily fever spikes are a characteristic sign, the fever reaching more than 40°C. Splenomegaly gradually becomes evident by the end of the first month (Fig. 220.4). If the symptoms continue unabated, the spleen may extend to the umbilicus or even into the pelvis. Diarrhea or frank dysentery is not an unusual occurrence, and blood sometimes is observed. A general bleeding diathesis often becomes evident shortly before death occurs. After several months, if the disease goes untreated, patients usually die. Acute fulminant disease is seen more often in infants and young children.

In addition, infantile VL has been associated with alterations in lipoprotein metabolism. A handful of cases of presumed congenital VL have been reported. These infants were

BOX 220.2 — Pathobiology in Visceral Leishmaniasis

Experimentally, resistance in mice appears to be determined by a single autosomal gene. In experimental infections, the disease has been shown to be regulated by the Th$_1$ subset of CD4$^+$ and CD8$^+$ T cells. Cytokines such as interferon-alpha (IFN-α), interleukin-2 (IL-2), and tumor necrosis factor-alpha (TNF-α) have major roles. Cytokines activate macrophages to kill intracellular amastigotes by both oxidative and nonoxidative mechanisms. Murine and *in vitro* studies suggest that nitric oxide (NO) is an important factor in killing of amastigotes. The infection becomes clinically evident if the parasites are not eliminated or controlled by the host's cellular immune response. However, after chemotherapeutic cure has been achieved, acquired immunity emerges; delayed hypersensitivity, as demonstrated by the Montenegro (leishmanin) skin test, also becomes positive. Usually, immunity to visceral leishmaniasis (VL) is complete and long-lasting after chemotherapeutic cure has occurred. However, relapse, as seen in post-kala-azar dermal leishmaniasis, is characterized by delayed hypersensitivity, dermal localization of parasites, and moderate hypergammaglobulinemia. Although activation of macrophages with enhanced phagocytosis of parasites may occur, sterile cure may not occur. The appearance of dermal delayed hypersensitivity at the time acquired immunity appears suggests that cell-mediated immunity plays an important role in protection. Further work on this aspect of VL is needed.

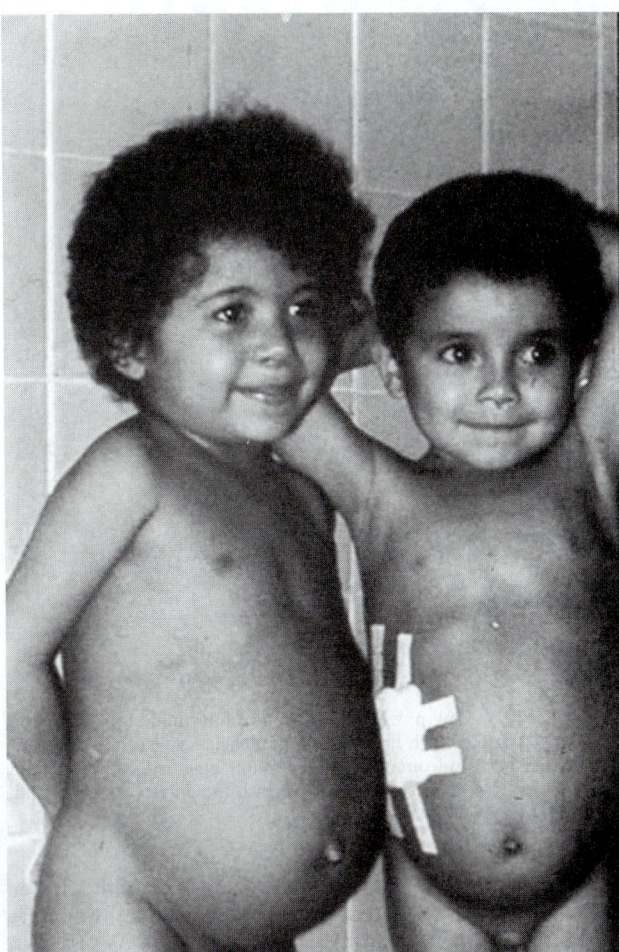

FIGURE 220.4. Two young boys suffering from visceral leishmaniasis (*Leishmania chagasi*) from Brazil. Both have abdominal distension due to hepatosplenomegaly. (Courtesy of WHO. Photograph by Dr. P. Marsden. WHO/TDR/Marsden.)

born of infected mothers, and some had evidence of parasitism of the placenta. However, whether these cases represent congenital or peripartum infection is not clear because sophisticated serologic techniques were not available.

In older patients, VL generally has a more chronic course, with marked emaciation, brittle hair, massive splenomegaly, lymphadenopathy, and a dusky slate-gray complexion (see Fig. 220.3). Hyperglobulinemia (i.e., IgG), leukopenia, and anemia typically are found. As a result of general debility, death often results from such intercurrent infections as pneumonia, amebic or bacillary dysentery, malaria, or cancrum oris in more than 90% of cases.

In India, the dark-gray appearance of the skin is known as kala-azar (black sickness). In some cases of VL, post–kala-azar dermal leishmaniasis (PKDL) occurs at variable times after resolution of VL and can be associated with relapse of visceral disease. In Sudan PKDL appears early, often within several months and in more than 50% of cases. High levels of interleukin (IL)-10 have been found at this time. The lesions are characterized by the appearance of hypopigmented, erythematous, or nodular lesions of the skin of the face, chest, neck, and buttocks. At times, the nodular lesions may resemble lepromatous leprosy.

Pancytopenia usually is seen. Characteristically, anemia always is evident, with hemoglobin levels below 8 g/dL. Survival of red cells is shortened as a result of several possible factors, including a Coombs-positive hemolytic anemia and hypersplenism. Leukopenia of 2,000 to 3,000 cells/mm^3 typically is found with neutropenia, relative lymphocytosis, an almost total absence of eosinophils, and thrombocytopenia. Serum albumin usually is less than 3 g/dL, and globulin levels (mostly IgG) often are greater than 5 g/dL (5 to 10 g/dL).

VL has been reported as an important opportunistic infection in patients infected with HIV/AIDS and who previously were not known to have had leishmaniasis. However, the leishmania infection (VL or CL) may have been acquired recently by a sandfly bite, or a latent infection may have been reactivated as the CD4 count fell below 150 to 200/μL. In this regard, latent leishmania infection also may reactivate after immunosuppression develops for other reasons, such as chemotherapy for malignant disease. Patients with AIDS often have typical VL. However, the diagnosis may be particularly difficult to establish in cases for which the presentation is atypical, with low-grade fever, fatigue, cough, and gastrointestinal complaints (Fig. 220.5). Similarly, atypical visceral disease caused by *L. tropica* was seen in individuals who participated in Operation Desert Storm in the Persian Gulf. Undoubtedly, while VL caused by *L. donovani* has been reported in U.S. troops who served in Iraq and Afghanistan, VL caused by *L. tropica* has not been confirmed as of yet.

Cutaneous Leishmaniasis: Old World Cutaneous Leishmaniasis

Old World cutaneous leishmaniasis is caused by *L. major* (rural), *L. tropica* (urban), *L. aethiopica*, *L. infantum*, and *L. donovani*. These organisms are found throughout the Middle East; along the Mediterranean basin and islands; and in East and West Africa, India, and southwestern Asia. In humans, infection by *L. tropica* usually produces self-limited skin ulcers in which intracellular (amastigote) parasites can be found situated in macrophages in and about the lesions. Recent reports

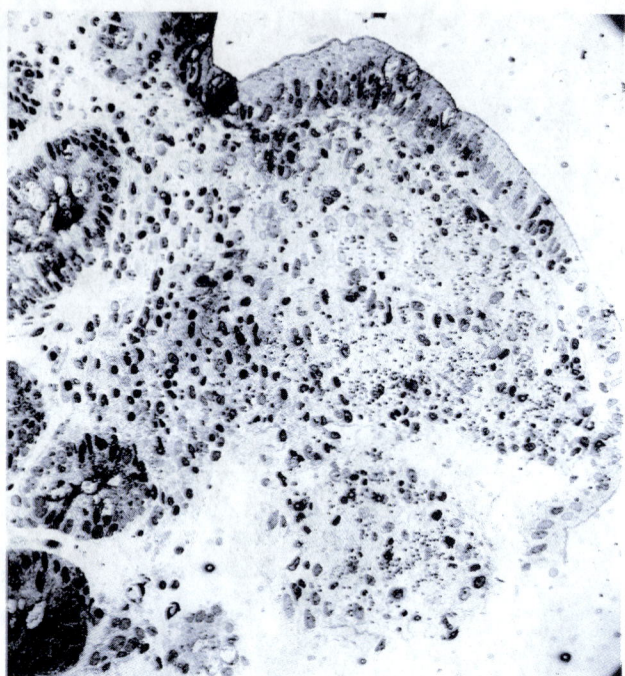

FIGURE 220.5. Low power thin section of intestinal biopsy from an 18-year-old patient with human immunodeficiency virus/acquired immunodeficiency syndrome with large volume diarrhea. Many nests of amastigotes present in the mucosa beneath the enterocytes. Original magnification ×660.

have described *L. tropica* isolates from patients with VL (see VL). Dogs, jackals, and rodents are infected naturally and are thought to be the natural reservoirs of infection. As with VL, various species of *Phlebotomus* (sandflies) transmit the infection, although person-to-person contact transmission can occur and is the basis of the long-time practice in middle and central Asia of immunizing with organisms of low virulence to prevent possible disfigurement by a natural infection.

CL, or Oriental sore (Delhi boil, Aleppo button), often is classified into "wet" and "dry" types. The wet or rural form is caused by *L. major* and is found chiefly in various rodents on the edge of deserts. The dry or urban type is anthroponotic preponderantly, caused by *L. tropica*, and transmitted by phlebotomine species that frequently feed on humans and dogs. The dry or urban form of CL is characterized by a long incubation period, long duration of active infection, and large numbers of parasites in the dermis (Fig. 220.6). By contrast, the moist or rural type has a relatively short incubation period, with rapid healing and few parasites in the skin. *L. aethiopica* is restricted to the mountain valleys of the Rift Valley of Ethiopia, Tanzania, and Kenya, where the rock and tree hyraxes are infected regularly (Fig. 220.7). Humans become infected when they intrude into these areas. This form of CL usually is self-limiting, although in a small number of individuals (1:100,000), non-healing diffuse cutaneous leishmaniasis (DCL) disease has been reported.

Pathology and Pathobiology

In CL caused by *L. tropica*, the development of the lesion may take weeks to months, and there are relatively few lymphocytes and plasma cells with large numbers of parasites in nests of macrophages. In CL caused by *L. major*, the onset occurs rapidly, with an outpouring of lymphocytes and plasma cells; parasites sometimes are difficult to find. In some cases, extensive formation of satellite lesions occurs in the proximity of the primary lesion so that local spread often is seen. The

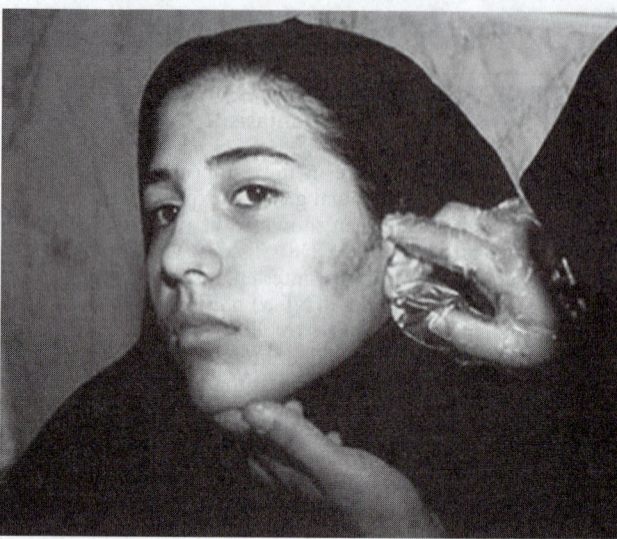

FIGURE 220.6. Iranian female from Isfahan with healed scar from cutaneous leishmaniasis, together with new lesions. (Courtesy of the WHO. Photograph by Andy Crump. WHO/TDR/Crump.)

pathologic reaction may be florid, with marked pseudoepitheliomatous hyperplasia that can be mistaken for carcinoma. Secondary bacterial infection may complicate the lesion and delay healing. However, once the ulcer heals, usually by fibrosis, the patient has long-lasting immunity.

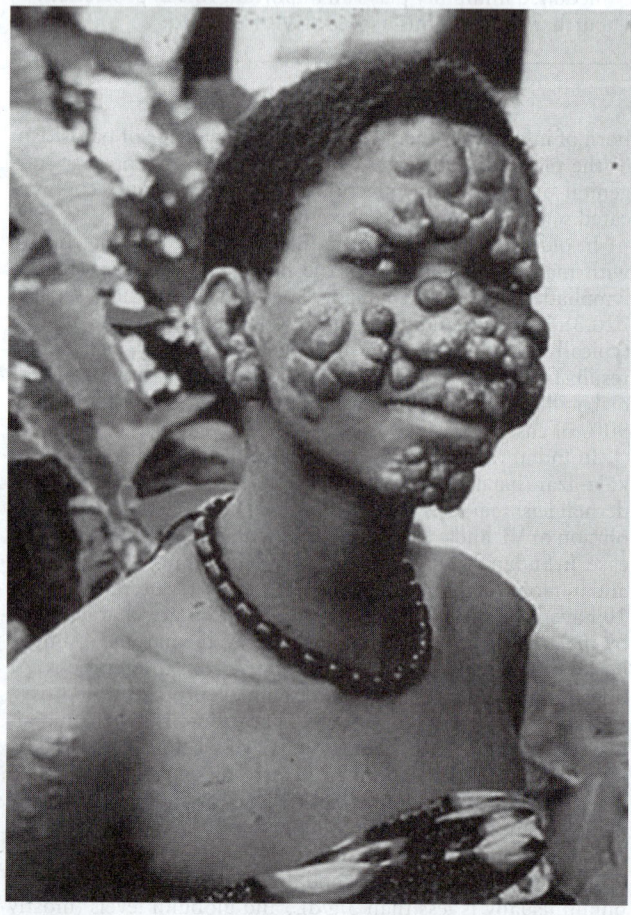

FIGURE 220.7. Tanzanian woman with *Leishmania aethiopica* infection. (Courtesy of the WHO. Photograph by Dr. I. Laufner. WHO/TDR/Laufner.)

BOX 220.3	Pathobiology of Cutaneous Leishmaniasis

In a small number of patients with cutaneous leishmaniasis (CL), evidently the inability to mount a suitable cell-mediated immune reaction is associated with specific anergy to leishmanin and an indolent nonhealing lesion (Fig. 220.8). This condition is known as *diffuse cutaneous leishmaniasis* (DCL), or leishmaniasis tegumentaria diffusa. Characteristically, lesions in DCL are filled with large, parasite-containing histiocytes, and lymphocytes are absent. Recent studies of DCL from the Dominican Republic suggest that immune suppression plays an important role in this form of the disease.

At the other extreme, a small group of patients whose cell-mediated immune response to infection with leishmanial organisms is exaggerated markedly, and these lesions heal by scarring. At the edge of the scar, however, new lesions appear, and the disease extends from the margins. Eventually, tissue damage may be rather extensive. On histologic examination, many lymphocytes, plasma cells, epithelioid cells, and large multinucleated giant cells can be seen. Organisms are difficult to locate but sometimes can be cultured from the lesions. This form of CL is called *leishmaniasis recidivans* (LR). Patients exhibit marked delayed hypersensitivity to leishmanin. The studies of Turk and Bryceson have provided the concept that CL may be a spectrum of diseases with DCL at one end of the spectrum (anergy) and LR at the other (marked delayed hypersensitivity).

In contrast to studies in mice, in which the outcome of *Leishmania tropica* infection is largely determined by Th_1/Th_2 responses, in humans the responses are more complex and not as evident. However, as in mice, interferon-gamma appears to be important in controlling human infection.

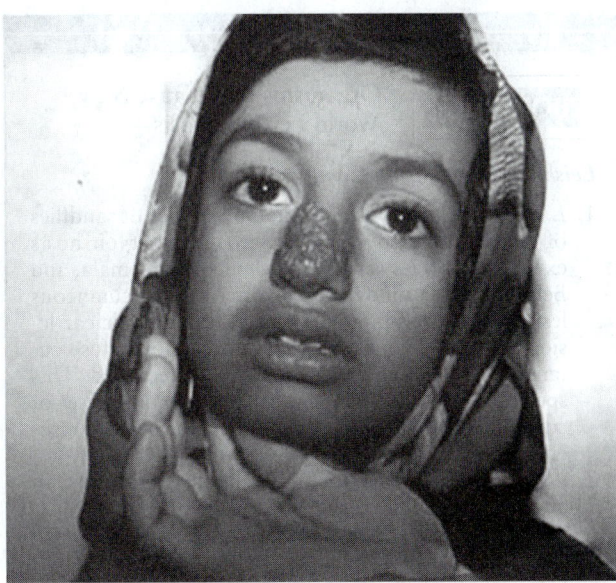

FIGURE 220.8. Nonhealing cutaneous leishmaniasis on the nose of a young Iranian girl. (Courtesy of the WHO. Photograph by Andy Crump. WHO/TDR/Crump.)

clinical picture. Whether indicating each of the clinical types of American CL by a separate species of *Leishmania* is justified is not clear. With regard to the American cutaneous forms, several main groups of organisms often are distinguished: the *L. mexicana* species complex, which includes *L. mexicana*, *L. amazonensis*, and *Leishmania venezuelensis*; the *Viannia* subgenus, which includes *L. (V.) braziliensis*, *L. (V.) panamensis*, and *L. (V.) guyanensis*; and *L. amazonensis*. Box 220.4 describes the *L. mexicana* complex and the *L. braziliensis* complex.

In MCL, as represented by espundia, nasal involvement may occur in as many as 80% of infections, 30% of which eventually may mutilate the mucous membranes of the mouth, nose, palate, larynx, and trachea. These cases often are fatal because of the intervening sepsis. Lesions of the mucous membranes often arise several years to decades after a cutaneous ulcer has healed. Once involvement of the mucous membrane occurs, the infection may be difficult to eradicate by chemotherapy.

Several forms of CL have been described and seem to be associated with the ability of the patient to develop cell-mediated immune mechanisms. Whether these mechanisms are directly responsible for protection in humans still is not certain (Box 220.3).

Clinical Manifestations

CL usually begins with the appearance of a pruritic, red, vesicular papule that appears weeks to months after the bite of a sandfly has occurred. The papule gradually enlarges, often measuring 1 to 2 cm in diameter. When the surface of the papule dries, it encrusts and drops off, revealing a shallow ulcer. The ulcer may or may not enlarge progressively and characteristically has raised, sharp, indurated margins. Healing usually takes place in 3 to 18 months, often leaving an obvious hypo- or hyperpigmented depressed scar. Frequently, however, single or multiple papules heal directly without extensive ulceration. If the lesions do not become infected secondarily, usually no complications develop.

American Cutaneous Leishmaniasis

In contrast to Old World CL, American cutaneous disease is tied closely to the forests of South, Central, and North America. Each variety has its own distinct epidemiologic, pathologic, and

DIAGNOSIS

In VL, diagnosis involves finding the organism in stained smears of spleen aspirate, peripheral blood, or bone marrow. In Indian kala-azar, the parasites may be found regularly in peripheral blood monocytes (i.e., buffy coat), but in African and Mediterranean forms, they may be difficult to find by this technique. Splenic puncture, liver biopsy, and bone marrow aspiration are the most rewarding procedures, although they are not without serious hazard in individuals with a bleeding diathesis. Contraindications include a soft or diffluent, acutely enlarging spleen. Patients with low platelets and/or prolonged prothrombin time should not have a needle biopsy. In children younger than 5 years of age, splenic aspiration should be performed only by a fully experienced physician.

Spleen and bone marrow aspirates should be placed in NNN or Schneider insect culture medium and smeared on slides, and saline-diluted aspirates should be inoculated into the peritoneal cavity of hamsters. Nonspecific tests reflecting the markedly elevated serum globulins, such as the formol gel and Sia water tests, are helpful in acute disease and are performed readily in the field, but the results can be positive in many conditions. Lack of specificity as well as sensitivity renders them unreliable.

BOX 220.4   Organisms that Cause New World Leishmaniasis

Leishmania mexicana Complex

1. *L. (M.) mexicana* is transmitted by species of sandflies of the genus *Lutzomyia*. Many rodent reservoir hosts exist. This species is found in Mexico, Guatemala, and Belize. It causes mild infection, often a single cutaneous lesion that is self-limited, or persistent chronic ear lesions. It causes Chiclero ulcer. One case of diffuse cutaneous leishmaniasis (DCL) has been recorded. This species probably is the cause of the occasional cases of cutaneous leishmaniasis (CL) that occur in the southern United States.
2. *L. (M.) amazonensis* is found along the Amazon basin and in Trinidad. It rarely infects humans but is transmitted by various species of *Lutzomyia* in rodents. In humans, it causes a mild and self-limited skin lesion. Occasionally, patients reportedly develop DCL.

Leishmania braziliensis Complex

1. *L. (V.) braziliensis* is transmitted by various species of *Lutzomyia* in Brazil and in the forest areas east of the Andes. This is the "prototype" of American or mucocutaneous leishmaniasis (MCL), or espundia. It may cause destructive ulcerative lesions of the nasooropharynx as a result of early or late metastases from a more superficial site (Fig. 220.9).
2. *L. (V.) guyanensis* is transmitted by species of *Lutzomyia* in Guyana, Surinam, Brazil, and Venezuela. It causes single or multiple spreading cutaneous ulcers over many parts of the body. It is thought to metastasize along lymphatics but does not visceralize (Fig. 220.10). It sometimes spreads to the nasooropharynx, causing mucosal disease. It sometimes is referred to as *pian bois*, or forest yaws.
3. *L. (V.) panamensis* is transmitted by species of *Lutzomyia* in Panama and possibly farther north and south. It may cause single to several superficial ulcers and may metastasize along the lymphatics or to the nasooropharynx.
4. *L. (V.) peruviana* is seen in Peru on the western slopes of the Andes to an altitude of 3,000 meters. It causes a single or a few self-healing ulcers. No oronasopharyngeal spread occurs. Often, it is referred to as *uta*. Dogs are regarded as the reservoir hosts.

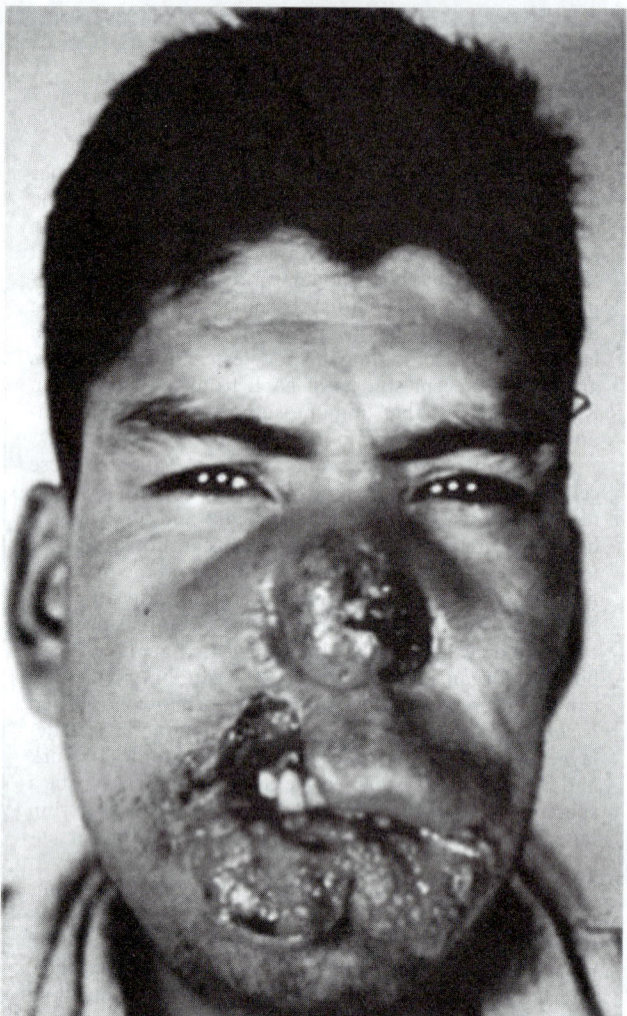

FIGURE 220.9. Mucocutaneous leishmaniasis in a Brazilian male caused by *Leishmania (V.) braziliensis*.

Other diagnostic tests that may be used in VL are described in Box 220.5.

In CL, microscopic examination of Giemsa or Wright stain smears of tissue obtained from nonnecrotic areas of the ulcer or from the base should be performed. Needle aspiration and culture of tissue fluid taken from the ulcer margin can be rewarding. Biopsy material taken from the edge of the ulcer should be examined histologically, as should small fragments macerated in saline and inoculated into NNN medium or Schneider insect medium. Examination of tissue impression smears can be rewarding. Clinically, the lesions often are characteristic, so that the diagnosis should be suspected in a patient who has visited an endemic area.

Although the leishmanin test usually is positive in patients with ulcerated lesions, the material is not readily available in the United States. However, a positive leishmanin skin test may help distinguish among a variety of skin lesions, such as syphilis, tropical phagedenic ulcer, yaws, tuberculosis, and various fungal diseases. The indirect fluorescent antibody or direct agglutination tests may be positive in this infection, although often at low titers and, therefore, are of little value.

In MCL, the fluorescent antibody test using amastigote antigen is most useful, being positive in 75% to 85% of cases, with declining titers after therapeutic cure. A direct agglutination test (DAT) employing promastigotes also is used frequently, as is enzyme-linked immunosorbent assay (ELISA). Recently, a DNA-DNA hybridization or dot-blot test has been used that is highly sensitive and species specific in tissue or biopsy specimens. Isozyme analysis of isolated organisms currently is being used to help identify the species causing the infection. This procedure is available at the Centers for Disease Control and Prevention (CDC).

THERAPY

For many years, VL and CL have been treated successfully with the pentavalent antimonial agents. Stibogluconate sodium (Pentostam; Wellcome Foundation, UK Triostam) is available through the CDC Drug Service and generally in English speaking-countries. Meglumine antimonate (Glucantime; Rhone Poulenc, France) is available in French-speaking

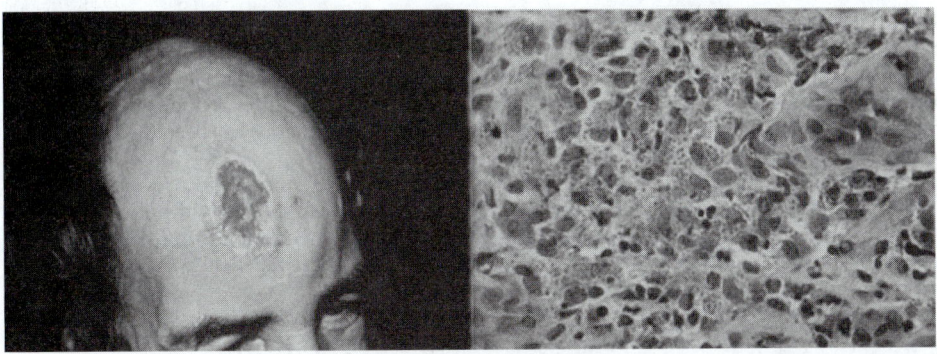

FIGURE 220.10. Skin ulcer caused by *Leishmania* (*V.*) *venezuelensis* from Venezuela treated successfully with sodium antimony gluconate. Tissue section from ulcer margin revealing numbers of amastigotes. Hematoxylin and eosin ×900.

countries and Latin America. The recommended pediatric and adult dose is 20 mg/kg daily, administered intramuscularly or intravenously for 28 days for VL and MCL and for 20 days for CL. Pediatric dosing can be determined according to body surface area when treating children weighing less than 20 kg.

Adverse reactions are common. Myalgias and arthralgias are especially common occurrences during the latter part of therapy. Nausea, vomiting, headache, anorexia, and abdominal pain also occur. Elevated levels of serum amylase and lipase, indicating pancreatitis, are encountered occasionally and can be severe. Electrocardiographic changes, including decreased T-wave amplitude, T-wave inversion, prolongation of the QTc, and nonspecific ST-T–wave changes are seen. These resolve shortly after therapy is concluded (treatment should be discontinued if the QTc interval exceeds 0.5 seconds). Deaths, presumably due to arrhythmias, have been reported in patients who were receiving more than 20 mg/kg/day. In HIV-infected patients, almost 25% fail to respond to antimony therapy and almost 40% of responders subsequently relapse.

In addition, liposomal amphotericin B (AmBisone; Fujisawa, Deerfield, IL) has been approved by the U.S. Food and Drug Administration (FDA) for the treatment of VL. Other lipid formulations including amphotericin B lipid complex (Ambelcet; Liposome Company, Princeton, NJ) and amphotericin B cholesterol sulfate (Amphtec; Sequus, Menlo Park, CA) are effective. The approved recommended regimen for immunocompetent patients (adults and children) with VL is 3 mg/kg/day on days 1 through 5 and 14 and 21.

However, the recommendation is that liposomal amphotericin B be administered on days 1 through 5 and 10 with the following daily doses: 3 to 4 mg/kg/day if the disease was acquired in Europe or Brazil; 3 mg/kg/day if the disease was acquired in Africa; and 2 to 3 mg/kg/day if the disease was acquired in India. Tolerance to these new lipid amphotericin formulations has been excellent, with few adverse reactions occurring. Treatment with amphotericin B lipid complex of VL in patients who are immunosuppressed or have HIV has given an almost 100% cure rate. However, most of these patients relapse. The recommended treatment is 4 mg/kg/day on days

---

BOX 220.5   Nonroutine Diagnostic Tests for Visceral Leishmaniasis

DNA-DNA hybridization tests, so-called dot-blot techniques, have exquisite specificity and sensitivity, detecting as few as 50 to 100 organisms. However, their potential use in routine diagnosis is hampered by the complex procedure of the hybridization. Polymerase chain reaction (PCR) may been used for the diagnosis of leishmaniasis. Unfortunately, PCR-based diagnostic methods have had a wide range of sensitivities and specificities. In a study from Sudan, PCR was reported to be more sensitive than was microscopy for the detection in lymph node and bone marrow aspirations, whereas sensitivity in blood of proven visceral leishmaniasis (VL) cases was only 70%.

A positive serologic test can occur as a result of past or subclinical inapparent infection. An enzyme-linked immunosorbent assay (ELISA) that detects antibodies to a cloned recombinant polypeptide antigen, K39, of *Leishmania chagasi* has been shown to be specific in active VL and could detect antibodies in patients with acquired immunodeficiency syndrome (AIDS). A recent study has demonstrated that this test could be applied to field situations.

The usual diagnostic tests may be negative in patients with human immunodeficiency virus (HIV) or *L. tropica* infection or in otherwise profoundly immunocompromised patients. Recently, however, two genomic fragments encoding portions of a single 210-kDa *L. tropica* protein have proved

useful for establishing the diagnosis of viscerotropic *L. tropica* infection in Desert Storm patients.

The leishmanin or Montenegro skin test is a measure of delayed hypersensitivity to leishmanial antigen. In VL, the test remains negative throughout the period of active disease. Once chemotherapeutic cure occurs, the test turns positive. Thus, recovery from VL is characterized by the development of cell-mediated immunity. The change from a negative to a positive leishmanin test in VL is regarded as an important prognostic sign that the patient is developing or has developed protective immunity. Because numerous reports have appeared recently noting positive leishmanin tests in individuals who have had no history of VL, researchers have postulated that many individuals in endemic areas may become immune by prior inapparent infection.

Antileishmanial antibodies usually are present in VL and can aid in establishing the diagnosis. The fluorescent antibody test is highly specific, as are the indirect hemagglutination and gel diffusion tests. However, the complement fixation test is positive in only 65% to 70% of cases. Sera from patients with VL are known to give false-positive results when patients who may have antibodies to *Trypanosoma cruzi* are present; in the Western Hemisphere, it may be necessary to absorb out these antibodies.

1 through 5 and days 10, 17, 24, 31, and 38. Without maintenance therapy, almost all of these patients relapse. Because of resistance to pentavalent antimonials in Bihar (India), amphotericin B is used and is highly efficacious. Liposomal amphotericin B has been effective for the treatment of VL presumably caused by *L. infantum* in immunocompetent children.

Parenteral pentamidine isethionate, intramuscularly 4 mg/kg three times weekly for up to 15 doses, has been used with limited success in antimony-resistant cases of VL. However, it is no longer necessary since the advent of liposomal amphotericin. An oral agent, miltefosine, has been shown to be highly effective for the treatment of VL in India. Originally it was developed as an antineoplastic agent. It is a phosphorylcholine ester of hexadecanol (hexadecyphosphocholine) that inhibits phospholipid and sterol biosynthesis. The treatment dose was 2.5 mg/kg/day for 4 weeks. It has also been used successfully for cutaneous disease.

Several reports suggest that recombinant interferon-gamma along with pentavalent antimonial drugs is helpful for successful therapy of VL. Because assessing whether a cure has been achieved is difficult, patients must be followed at 6-month intervals for up to 2 years. If PKDL occurs, treatment should be reinstituted.

PROGNOSIS

If untreated, VL is fatal in 75% to 85% of infantile and 90% of adult cases. Properly treated at an early stage, it can be cured in 85% to 95% of cases. The prognosis for patients who develop pancytopenia or bleeding diatheses or who fail to develop a delayed hypersensitivity skin reaction usually is poor.

CL resolves with antimony treatment. Lesions usually heal approximately 4 to 6 weeks after initiation of therapy, although large lesions may require additional time. Mucosal lesions caused by *L. braziliensis* do not heal unless therapy is instituted.

PREVENTION

Presently, many studies are being devoted to development of a leishmaniasis vaccine. These efforts include testing of killed or live-attenuated parasites, as well as many *Leishmania* antigens including recombinant protein. Recent studies indicate that DNA vaccines appear to induce, in animal models, preferentially a Th$_1$ immune response, which is necessary for the elimination of intracellular parasites. This approach holds out the possibility for the development of a protective vaccine in humans.

There are many aspects to the control of VL. Sandflies (*Phlebotomus* and *Lutzomyia*) can be eliminated readily by residual spraying. Because sandflies ordinarily do not fly very high, sleeping quarters should be above ground level. Permethrin-impregnated bed nets can be highly effective in preventing sandfly bites. Animal reservoirs, such as infected dogs and rodents, should be destroyed. Early therapy prevents transmission in families and neighborhoods.

Residual spraying for sandflies and vaccination for Old World CL have reduced and limited this disease in many areas of the Middle East and central Asia. However, because of the indolent nature of the healing with vaccination and the possibility of visceralization, this practice has been discontinued in Israel.

New World CL is extremely difficult to prevent because it is largely a forest disease. It can be avoided only by sleeping in tents under impregnated fine-mesh netting, wearing long-sleeved clothing, and using insect repellents.

Suggested Readings

Aguilar-Be I, da Silva Zardo R, Paraguai de Souza, et al. Cross-protective efficacy of a protective *Leishmania donovani* DNA vaccine against visceral and cutaneous murine leishmaniasis. *Infect Immun* 2005;73:812.

Belli A, Garcia D, Palacios X, et al. Widespread atypical cutaneous leishmaniasis caused by *Leishmania* (L.) *chagasi* in Nicaragua. *Am J Trop Med Hyg* 1999; 6:380.

Berman J. Recent developments in Leishmaniasis: epidemiology, diagnosis, and treatment. *Curr Infect Dis Rep* 2005;7:33.

Berman JD. Chemotherapy for leishmaniasis: biochemical mechanisms, clinical efficacy, and future strategies. *Rev Infect Dis* 1988;10:560.

Berman J. Current treatment approaches to leishmaniasis. *Curr Opin Infect Dis* 2003;16:397.

Bhattacharya SK, Jha TK, Sundar S, et al. Efficacy and tolerability of miltefosine for childhood visceral leishmaniasis in India. *Clin Infect Dis* 2004;38: 217.

Centers for Disease Control and Prevention. Cutaneous Leishmaniasis in U.S. military personnel Southwest/Central Asia, 2002–2003. *MMWR Morb Mortal Wkly Rep* 2003;52:1009–1012.

Dillon DC, Day CH, Whittle JA, et al. Characterization of a *Leishmania tropica* antigen that detects immune responses in Desert Storm viscerotropic leishmaniasis patients. *Proc Natl Acad Sci USA* 1995;92:7981.

Eltoum IA, Zijlstra EE, Ali MS, et al. Congenital kala-azar and leishmaniasis in the placenta. *Am J Trop Med Hyg* 1992;46:57.

Handman E. Cell biology of Leishmania. *Adv Parasitol* 1999;44:1.

Herwaldt BL. Leishmaniasis. *Lancet* 1999;354:1191.

Jha MD, Sundar S, Thakur CP, et al. Miltefosine, an oral, agent for the treatment of Indian VL. *N Engl J Med* 1999;341:1795.

Locksley RM, Pingel S, Lacy D, et al. Susceptibility to infectious diseases: leishmania as a paradigm. *J Inf Dis* 1999;179:S305.

Mary C, Auriault V, Faugere B, Dessein AJ. Control of *Leishmania infantum* infection is associated with CD8+ and gamma interferon- and interleukin-5 producing CD4+ antigen-specific T cells. *Infect Immunity* 1999;67:5559.

Martino L, Davidson RN, Giacchino R, et al. Treatment of Visceral leishmaniasis in children with liposomal amphotericin *B J Ped* 1997;131:1.

Medrano FJ, Hernandez-Quero J, Jimenez E, et al. VL in HIV-1-infected individuals: a common opportunistic infection in Spain? *AIDS* 1992;6: 1499.

Morales MA, Cruz I, Rubio JM, et al. Relapses versus reinfection in patients coinfected with *Leishmania infantum* and human immunodeficiency virus type 1. *J Infect Dis* 2002;185:1533.

Murray HW. Treatment of visceral leishmaniasis in 2004. *Am J Trop Med Hyg* 2004;71:787.

Singh S, Sivakumar S. Recent understanding in the treatment of visceral leishmaniasis. *J Postgrad Med* 2003;49:61.

Sundar S, Rai M. Laboratory diagnosis of visceral leishmaniasis. *Clin Diag Lab Immun* 2002;9:951.

Sundar S, Jha TK, Thakur CP, et al. Oral miltefosine for Indian visceral leishmaniasis. *N Eng J Med* 2002;347:1739.

Sundar S, Mehta H, Suresh AV, et al. Amphotericin B treatment for Indian visceral leishmaniasis: conventional versus lipid formulations. *CID* 2004;38:377.

Vega-Lopez F. Diagnosis of cutaneous leishmaniasis. *Curr Opin Infect Dis* 2003;16:97.

Yadav TP, Gupta H, Satteya U, et al. Congenital kala-azar. *Ann Trop Med Parasitol* 1989;83:535.

CHAPTER 221 ■ MALARIA

LAWRENCE M. BARAT AND SNEHAL N. SHAH

Each year in the United States, more than 7 million people travel to countries where malaria is endemic, approximately 1,400 persons receive diagnoses of malaria, and five to ten persons die from the infection. When malaria is diagnosed rapidly and treated correctly, severe morbidity and mortality from the disease can be prevented. The use of appropriate prevention strategies, including personal protection measures and chemoprophylaxis, can markedly reduce a traveler's risk of acquiring malaria.

BIOLOGY AND LIFE CYCLE

Four species of malaria cause clinical disease in humans: *Plasmodium falciparum* (Fig. 221.1), *P. vivax* (Fig. 221.2), *P. ovale*, and *P. malariae*. Transmitted by the bite of an infected female *Anopheles* mosquito during a blood meal, the parasite stage known as the *sporozoite* enters the blood of the human host and passes rapidly to the liver, infecting hepatocytes (Fig. 221.3). The infecting parasites, now called *tissue trophozoites*, undergo nuclear division to form schizonts, which yield multiple merozoites. This asexual cycle of the infection is called the *exo-erythrocytic cycle* and usually lasts from 5.5 to 16.0 days. During this period, the host is asymptomatic. Subsequently, merozoites are released into the blood and rapidly infect erythrocytes.

In the erythrocyte, the parasites undergo a second asexual cycle (erythrocytic cycle); trophozoites develop into schizonts, which produce merozoites. The erythrocytes rupture, releasing merozoites, which then infect other red blood cells. Persons are symptomatic during the erythrocytic cycle; in particular, spiking fevers generally occur with the release of merozoites. After a number of days, the release of merozoites may become synchronized, resulting in classic cyclic fevers. Typically, in *P. vivax* and *P. ovale*, merozoites are released in 48-hour cycles (tertian malaria) and, in *P. malariae*, in 72-hour cycles (quartan malaria).

Some merozoites, after infecting erythrocytes, mature into sexual forms known as *gametocytes*. Both male and female gametocytes must be ingested during a blood meal by a female *Anopheles* mosquito for the sexual life cycle to occur in the mosquito's gut. Sporozoites are produced in the wall of the mosquito's gut and pass to the salivary glands; they are transmitted when the mosquito takes its next blood meal, thus completing the life cycle.

With *P. vivax* and *P. ovale* infections, some liver trophozoites, known as *hypnozoites*, may remain dormant. Weeks to months, and rarely years, later (the pattern varying by the region in which the infection was acquired), hypnozoites can become active and develop into merozoites. The release of merozoites from the liver results in recurrent parasitemia and clinical illness, termed a *relapse*. Persons with *P. vivax* or *P. ovale* can have multiple relapses for up to 4 years (and occasionally longer) after the primary infection.

Recurrent parasitemia also can occur when parasites persist at low levels in the blood (below the limit of detection)

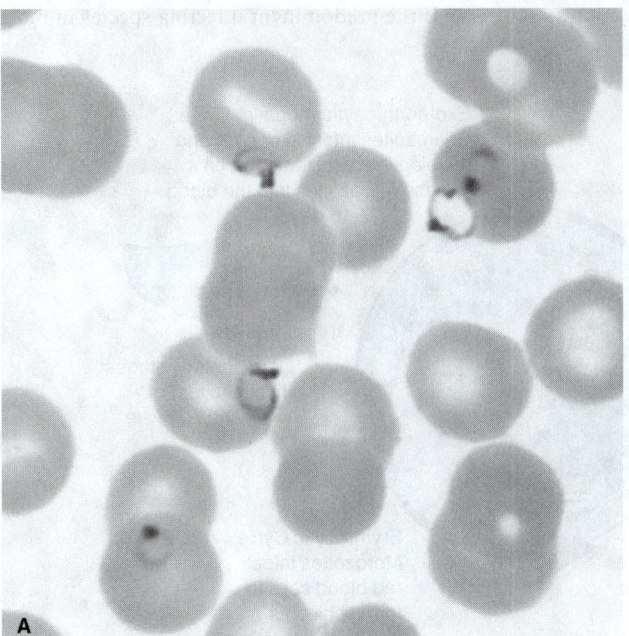
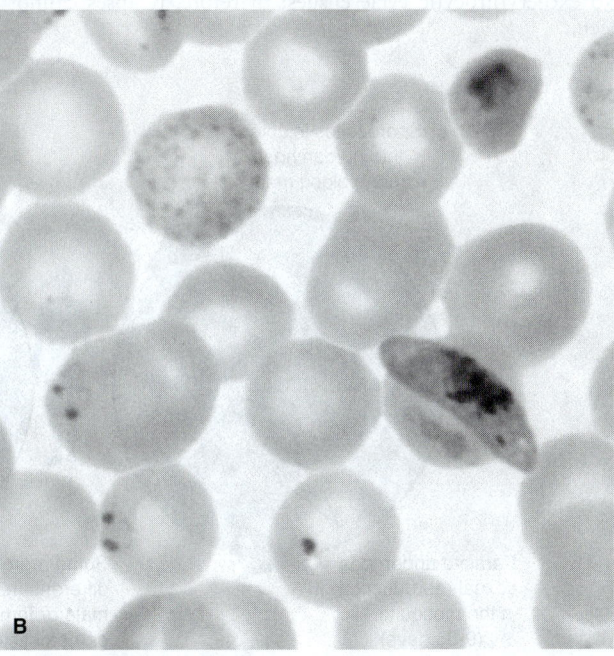

FIGURE 221.1. Microscopic image of *Plasmodium falciparum*. **A:** ring stage and **B:** gametocyte.

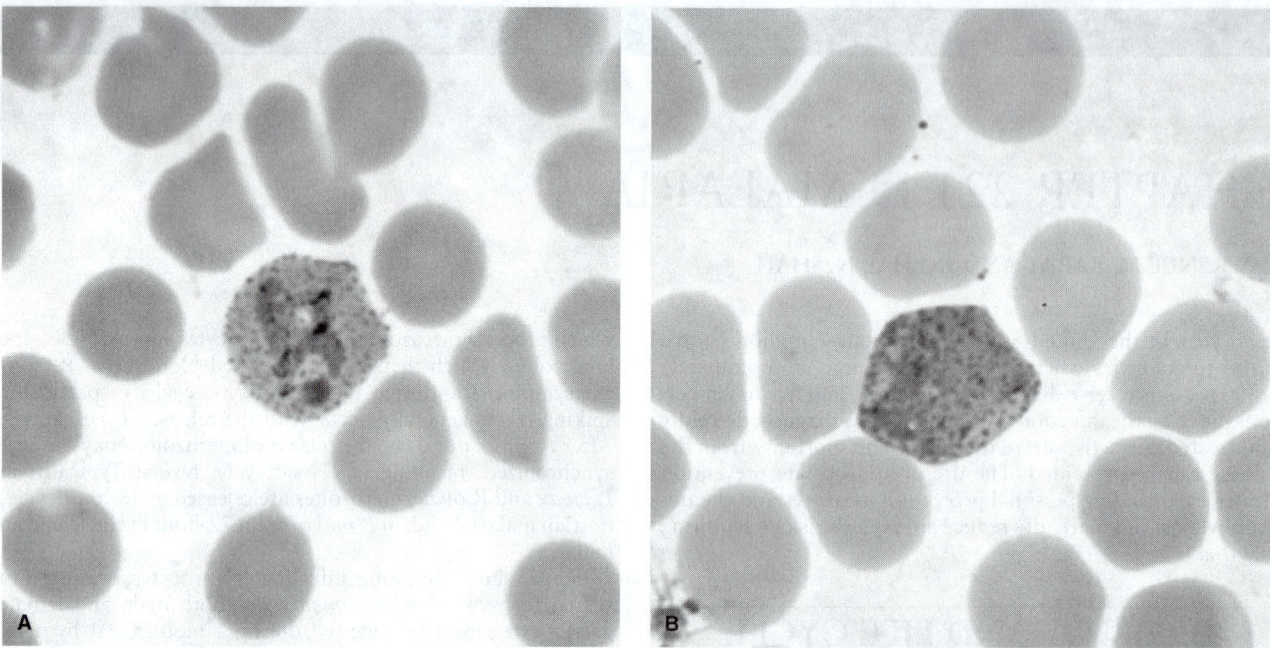

FIGURE 221.2. Microscopic image of *Plasmodium vivax*. **A:** trophozoite and **B:** gametocyte.

after the primary attack. The level of parasitemia may increase days to weeks later, causing another clinical attack. These repeat bouts, termed *recrudescences*, usually occur when patients receive drug treatment that does not eliminate all the blood-stage parasites. Recrudescences can occur with all four species.

Although the primary mode of transmission is from the bite of an infected *Anopheles* mosquito, malaria can be acquired from the transfusion of blood or blood products or the transplantation of organs from infected persons. Infection can be acquired congenitally from infected mothers. In the United States, fewer than ten transfusion-associated and congenital infections are diagnosed each year. In both these modes of transmission, persons are infected only with blood-stage parasites. No exo-erythrocytic cycle ensues; therefore, relapses cannot occur.

EPIDEMIOLOGY

The World Health Organization (WHO) estimates that 300 to 500 million clinical cases of malaria are diagnosed worldwide each year, resulting in 1 to 2 million deaths. More than 90% of deaths occur in children younger than age 5 years in sub-Saharan Africa, and malaria is one of Africa's leading causes of mortality in children under five years of age. *P. falciparum* is the species responsible for almost all malaria-associated severe morbidity and mortality.

Malaria is transmitted in approximately 100 countries in the tropical and subtropical regions of four continents (Fig. 221.4). The species distribution varies in different regions. In Africa, more than 90% of infections are caused by *P. falciparum*. In contrast, *P. vivax* is the predominant infecting species in most

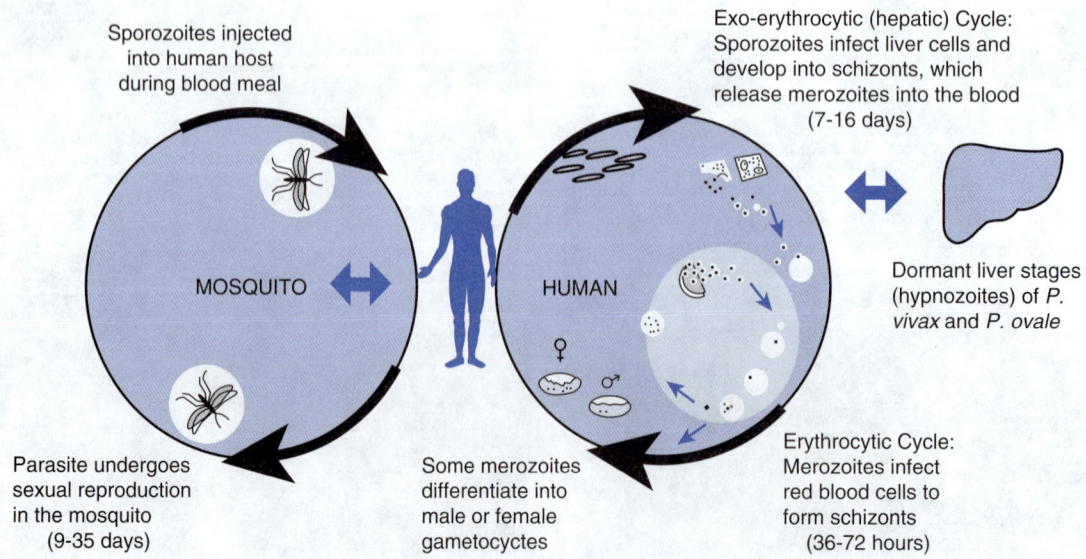

FIGURE 221.3. Malaria transmission cycle.

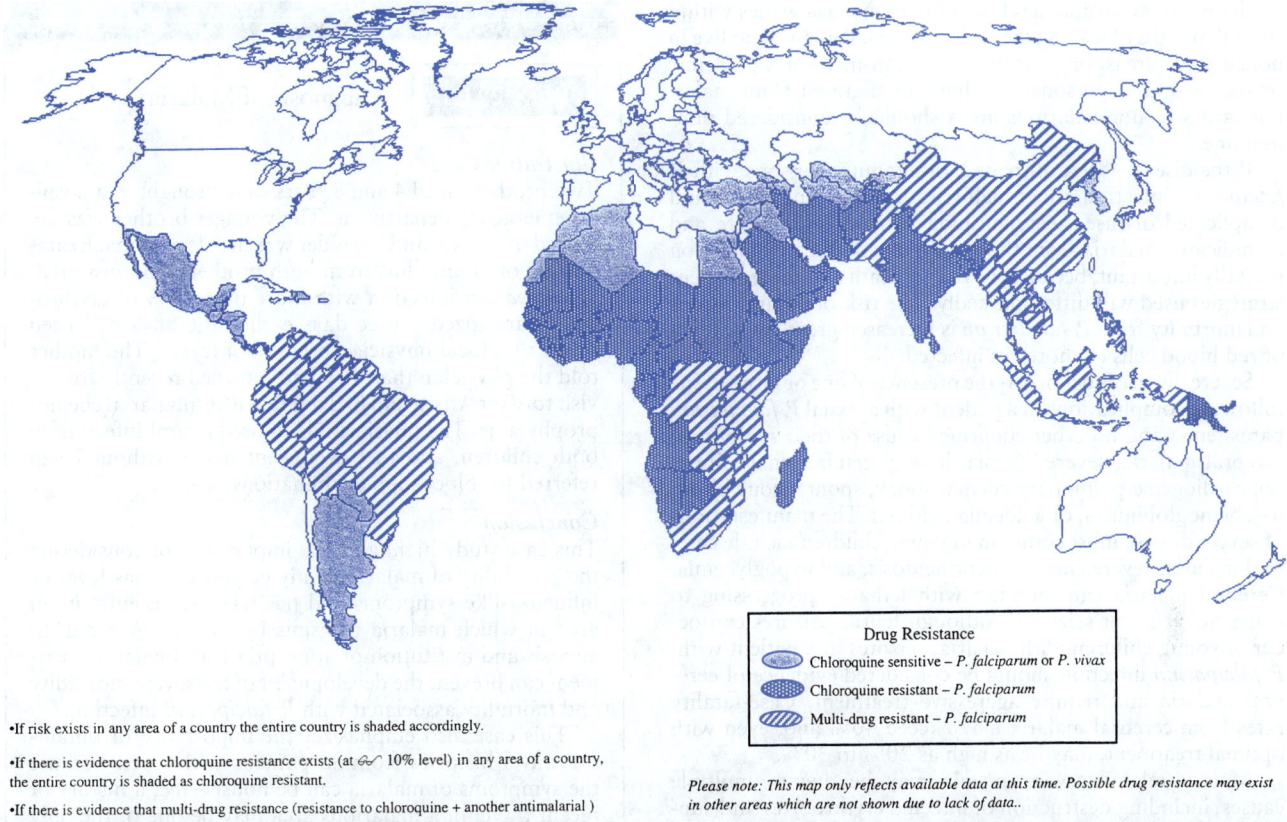

•If risk exists in any area of a country the entire country is shaded accordingly.

•If there is evidence that chloroquine resistance exists (at ⟨∼⟩ 10% level) in any area of a country, the entire country is shaded as chloroquine resistant.

•If there is evidence that multi-drug resistance (resistance to chloroquine + another antimalarial) exists (at ⟨∼⟩ 10% level) in any area of a country, the entire country is shaded as multi-drug resistant.

Drug Resistance
Chloroquine sensitive – *P. falciparum* or *P. vivax*
Chloroquine resistant – *P. falciparum*
Multi-drug resistant – *P. falciparum*

Please note: This map only reflects available data at this time. Possible drug resistance may exist in other areas which are not shown due to lack of data..

Drug resistance varies within countries; please refer to specific country for detailed risk and prophylactic information

FIGURE 221.4. Worldwide distribution of malaria, including distribution of drug-resistant *Plasmodium falciparum*, 1998.

malarious areas in the Americas, Asia, and Oceania. Together, *P. falciparum* and *P. vivax* account for more than 90% of all clinical infections worldwide.

Nearly all of the approximately 1,500 cases of malaria diagnosed yearly in the United States were acquired through international travel and could have been prevented using appropriate chemoprophylaxis. Rarely, malaria is transmitted via blood transfusion, contaminated needles or syringes, or through congenital infection.

CLINICAL MANIFESTATIONS AND COMPLICATIONS

The symptoms and signs of malaria are nonspecific, therefore the clinician must maintain a high index of suspicion and routinely elicit a travel history from patients. Almost all nonimmune persons with malaria will present with fever, either by history or confirmed on physical examination. Malaria should be considered in any patient with fever who has traveled into an area of endemic transmission. Fevers are generally high and spiking, with associated rigors and sweats. Febrile episodes have been described classically as having a predictable periodicity of 48 or 72 hours, with periods of symptomatic improvement between the paroxysms. However, patients with malaria, particularly those with *P. falciparum*, may not develop cyclic fevers. Therefore, lack of a cyclic fever pattern does not rule out the diagnosis of malaria. Hypotension and tachycardia may accompany the febrile paroxysms, particularly in patients with associated dehydration. Patients with malaria often will de-

scribe influenza-like symptoms, including myalgias, malaise, and headache. Diarrhea, vomiting, abdominal pain, and other gastrointestinal symptoms may be present. Cough, shortness of breath, and other respiratory symptoms occur less frequently and may indicate the onset of pulmonary complications or severe anemia. The presence of gastrointestinal or pulmonary symptoms or both should not lead the physician to rule out malaria.

Mild to moderate anemia, resulting in part from destruction of red blood cells or from suppression of erythropoiesis or both, is common and often is accompanied by an elevated reticulocyte count, hyperbilirubinemia, and hemoglobinuria. Inadequate reticulocyte response or microcytic anemia may indicate intercurrent iron deficiency. Mild thrombocytopenia often is present, resulting from peripheral destruction or splenic sequestration, but bleeding diatheses are rare. The leukocyte count can be normal or low. Hepatomegaly and splenomegaly also are common, and liver transaminases may be mildly elevated.

The risk of developing severe and complicated malaria is influenced greatly by whether an infected person has acquired immunity to infection. Persons living in areas that have year-round endemic malaria transmission often develop partial, nonsterilizing immunity after repeated infections. For lifelong residents of these areas, protective immunity typically develops during early childhood or after repeated infections, depending on the intensity of transmission. Persons with acquired immunity still can be infected with malaria parasites, but they generally have a milder febrile illness or may be asymptomatic. As immunity increases, the risk of major complications progressively decreases, although immune persons still may develop moderate to severe anemia. Immunity to malaria wanes within several months of leaving the endemic area. Persons who live in nonendemic areas, or in areas where transmission is epidemic or seasonal, and persons who have immigrated from malarious areas to nonmalarious areas should be considered nonimmune.

If the disease is left untreated, nonimmune persons with *P. falciparum* infection are at high risk of developing severe and complicated disease. Distinguishing patients with severe and complicated malaria from those with uncomplicated infection is vitally important, because the risk of death and the treatment strategies used will differ markedly. The risk of complications and mortality from *P. falciparum* is increased greatly when 5% of red blood cells or more are infected.

Severe disease is defined as the presence of one or more of the following complications in a patient with asexual *P. falciparum* parasitemia and no other confirmed cause of their symptoms: cerebral malaria, severe anemia, hypoglycemia, renal failure, noncardiogenic pulmonary edema, shock, spontaneous bleeding, hemoglobinuria, or acidemia-acidosis. The manifestations of severe disease most common in young children include cerebral malaria, severe anemia, lactic acidosis, and hypoglycemia. Cerebral malaria can manifest with lethargy progressing to coma or recurrent seizures. Although febrile seizures can occur in young children with malaria, seizures in a patient with *P. falciparum* infection should be considered evidence of cerebral malaria and require aggressive treatment. Case-fatality rates from cerebral malaria may exceed 40% and, even with optimal treatment, may be as high as 20% to 30%.

Malaria-related severe anemia may be due to multiple causes, including destruction of infected erythrocytes and suppression of erythropoiesis. Moderate to severe hypoglycemia may result from the consumption of glucose by the parasites, hyperinsulinemia, impaired gluconeogenesis, or a combination of these factors. Hypoglycemia usually is responsive to parenteral glucose supplementation. Patients with *P. falciparum* infection should undergo hemoglobin and blood glucose measurements every 8 to 12 hours during the initial treatment period to monitor for these complications.

Metabolic acidosis is associated with an increased risk of death in severe malaria. The acidosis frequently is attributable to lactic acidosis in children with malaria and severe malarial anemia. Poor tissue perfusion, inadequate oxygen delivery, and dehydration can lead to lactic acidosis, and treatment must be aimed at correcting any reversible cause of acidosis. Noncardiogenic pulmonary edema is an uncommon complication of malaria in children, usually associated with high-density infection. It can manifest as respiratory distress, tachypnea, and nonproductive cough. Chest radiography may demonstrate progressive bilateral interstitial and airspace disease. Respiratory failure can develop rapidly and may progress to death. Acute tubular necrosis is another rare complication of malaria in children, although elevation of blood urea nitrogen and creatinine due to dehydration is common.

Complications with other species are rare. Splenic rupture has been described in patients who have long-standing, untreated *P. vivax* infection and have developed massive splenomegaly. With effective chemotherapy, this complication is unusual. Nephritis is a rare complication of persistent *P. malariae* infection, but occurs more commonly in children.

Tropical splenomegaly syndrome, another rare complication in long-term residents of endemic areas, manifests as massive splenomegaly resulting from a hyperimmune response to infection. The diagnosis is supported by the detection of high levels of malaria-specific antibodies in a patient's serum. Tropical splenomegaly syndrome can be controlled with treatment of the acute infection and continual use of antimalarial chemoprophylaxis while the person remains in the endemic area. Symp-

---

BOX 221.1   Diagnosis of Malaria

Illustrative Case

Two brothers aged 4 and 8 years were brought to a hospital emergency department. The younger brother was deceased on arrival and the older was in a deep coma. Examination of blood films from both brothers demonstrated *P. falciparum* infection with more than 10% of erythrocytes parasitized. Three days earlier, the boys had been taken to a local physician because of fevers. The mother told the physician that they had returned recently from a visit to West Africa and had not taken antimalarial chemoprophylaxis. The physician diagnosed a viral infection in both children, and they were sent home without being referred for blood-film examinations.

Conclusion

This case study highlights the importance of considering the possibility of malaria in any person who has fever or influenza-like symptoms and has traveled recently in an area in which malaria transmission occurs. A rapid diagnosis and institution of appropriate antimalarial treatment can prevent the development of the severe morbidity and mortality associated with *P. falciparum* infection.

This case also emphasizes the importance of obtaining travel histories from all patients with fever. Because the symptoms of malaria can be nonspecific, a history of recent travel in a malarious area may be one of the only clues leading a clinician to consider malaria in the differential diagnosis. Malaria should be considered in any person with fever who has traveled recently in an area in which malaria is endemic.

---

toms should resolve, and chemoprophylaxis can be stopped once a person leaves the endemic area.

DIAGNOSIS

For an overview of diagnostic procedures, see Box 221.1.

The definitive diagnosis of malaria is based on the identification of parasites infecting erythrocytes on Giemsa- or Wright-Giemsa-stained peripheral blood films. Thick- and thin-blood films should be obtained without delay, because parasites will be present both during and between febrile paroxysms (Fig. 221.5). Thick films allow for the examination of a larger volume of blood, facilitating the detection of low-density infections. Thin films permit easier identification of the infecting species. If parasites are not seen on the initial blood films, repeat samples should be examined 8 hours later. To rule out malaria completely, repeat blood films should be taken every 8 to 24 hours (depending on the severity of a patient's illness) during the next 72 hours.

If parasites are detected, the examiner must distinguish between *P. falciparum* and the other species, because falciparum malaria causes almost all malaria-associated severe morbidity and mortality, and the approach to treatment will be different from that of the other three species. Usually, blood films containing *P. falciparum* will have a predominance of early trophozoites, known as *ring forms*, with few other developmental stages present. Ring forms derive their name from their signet-ring appearance, with a discrete dot of reddish purple

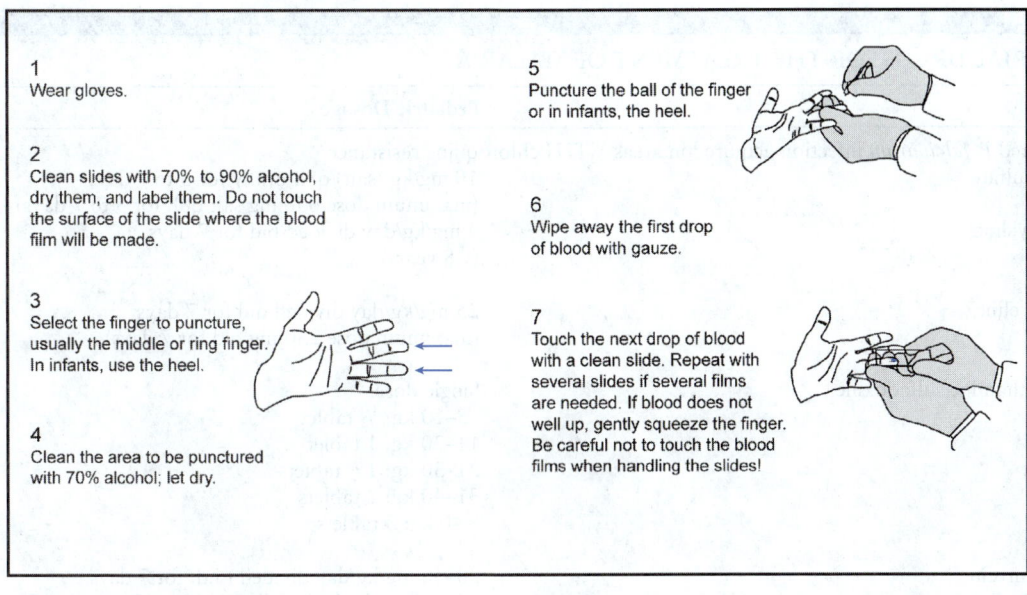

1 Wear gloves.

2 Clean slides with 70% to 90% alcohol, dry them, and label them. Do not touch the surface of the slide where the blood film will be made.

3 Select the finger to puncture, usually the middle or ring finger. In infants, use the heel.

4 Clean the area to be punctured with 70% alcohol; let dry.

5 Puncture the ball of the finger or in infants, the heel.

6 Wipe away the first drop of blood with gauze.

7 Touch the next drop of blood with a clean slide. Repeat with several slides if several films are needed. If blood does not well up, gently squeeze the finger. Be careful not to touch the blood films when handling the slides!

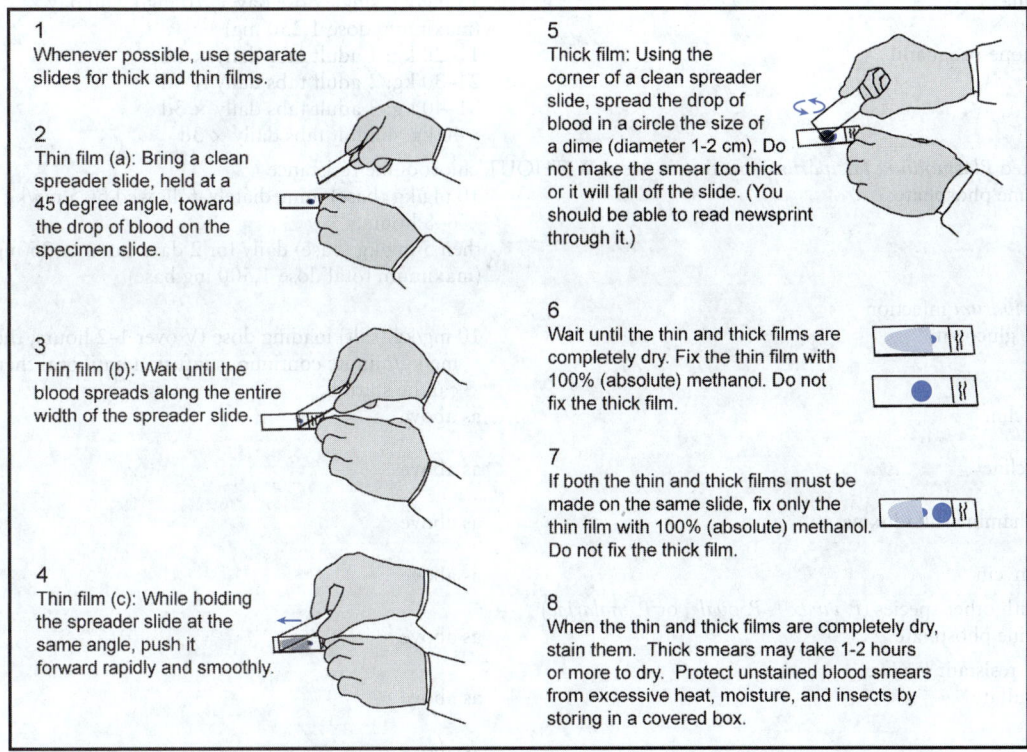

1 Whenever possible, use separate slides for thick and thin films.

2 Thin film (a): Bring a clean spreader slide, held at a 45 degree angle, toward the drop of blood on the specimen slide.

3 Thin film (b): Wait until the blood spreads along the entire width of the spreader slide.

4 Thin film (c): While holding the spreader slide at the same angle, push it forward rapidly and smoothly.

5 Thick film: Using the corner of a clean spreader slide, spread the drop of blood in a circle the size of a dime (diameter 1-2 cm). Do not make the smear too thick or it will fall off the slide. (You should be able to read newsprint through it.)

6 Wait until the thin and thick films are completely dry. Fix the thin film with 100% (absolute) methanol. Do not fix the thick film.

7 If both the thin and thick films must be made on the same slide, fix only the thin film with 100% (absolute) methanol. Do not fix the thick film.

8 When the thin and thick films are completely dry, stain them. Thick smears may take 1-2 hours or more to dry. Protect unstained blood smears from excessive heat, moisture, and insects by storing in a covered box.

FIGURE 221.5. Instructions for collection and preparation of thin and thick blood films.

chromatin and a gray-blue ring of cytoplasm. Later in the course of disease, banana-shaped gametocytes also may be present. Parasite densities greater than 2%, multiple infected erythrocytes, and double-chromatin dot rings are characteristic of *P. falciparum*, but occasionally can be seen with other species. The presence of mature trophozoites and schizonts suggests infection with other species, although these also can be seen with severe *P. falciparum* infection. Infected erythrocytes larger than uninfected cells and having a granular cell surface (Schüffner's granules) would suggest *P. vivax* or *P. ovale*. If the infecting species cannot be determined, the patient should be treated presumptively for *P. falciparum*, because this treatment will be effective against all four species of malaria. Treatment can be changed, if necessary, once the species is confirmed.

A determination of parasite density should be carried out by counting the number of infected red blood cells and the total number of erythrocytes in ten or more oil-immersion fields in an area in which the erythrocytes form a monolayer on a thin-blood film. Parasite density is calculated by dividing the number of parasitized cells by the total number of erythrocytes. Patients

TABLE 221.1

ANTIMALARIAL DRUGS FOR THE TREATMENT OF MALARIA

Drug	Pediatric Dosage
Uncomplicated *P. falciparum* infection acquired in areas WITH chloroquine resistance	
(i) Quinine sulfate	10 mg/kg (salt) q8h orally for 3 to 7 days*
PLUS	(maximum dose 650 mg salt q8h for 3 to 7 days)
a) Doxycycline[†]	4 mg/kg/day divided bid for 7 days
	(>8 years)
OR	
b) Tetracycline[†]	25 mg/kg/day divided qid for 7 days
	(maximum dose 250 mg qid for 7 days)
OR	
c) Pyrimethamine/sulfadoxine	Single dose:
	5–10 kg: ½ tablet
	11–20 kg: 1 tablet
	21–30 kg: 1½ tablets
	31–40 kg: 2 tablets
	>40 kg: 3 tablets
OR	
d) Clindamycin	20–40 mg/kg/day divided t.i.d. for 7 days
(ii) Mefloquine	15 mg/kg, single dose day 1, 10 mg/kg on day 2[‡]
	(maximum dose 1,250 mg)
(iii) Atovaquone-proguanil	11–20 kg: 1 adult tabs daily × 3d
	21–30 kg: 2 adult tabs daily × 3d
	31–40 kg: 3 adult tabs daily × 3d
	>40 kg: 4 adult tabs daily × 3d
Uncomplicated *Plasmodium falciparum* infection in areas WITHOUT chloroquine resistance	
(i) Chloroquine phosphate	10 mg/kg (base) immediately, followed by 5 mg/kg (base) in 6–8 hours,
	then 5 mg/kg (base) daily for 2 days (total of 25 mg/kg base)[§]
	(maximum total dose 1,500 mg base)
Severe *P. falciparum* infection	
(i) Quinidine gluconate**	10 mg/kg (salt) loading dose IV over 1–2 hours, then 0.02
PLUS	mg/kg/minute continuous infusion until oral therapy can be started.
a) Doxycycline[†]	as above
OR	
b) Tetracycline[†]	as above
OR	
c) Pyrimethamine/sulfadoxine	as above
OR	
d) Clindamycin	as above
Infections with other species (*P. vivax*[††], *P. ovale,* or *P. malariae*)	
(i) Chloroquine phosphate	as above
Chloroquine-resistant *P. vivax*	
(i) Quinine sulfate	as above
PLUS	
Doxycycline[†]	as above
OR	
Tetracycline[†]	as above
(ii) Mefloquine	as above
Prevention of relapses in *P. vivax* or *P. ovale* infection	
(i) Primaquine phosphate[‡‡]	0.6 mg/kg (base) daily for 14 days
	(maximum dose 30 mg base daily for 14 days)

*Quinine sulfate given for 3 days should be combined with a second drug such as doxycycline or tetracycline for 7 days, or a single dose of pyrimethamine-sulfadoxine (only if infection was acquired in an area free of sulfadoxine-pyrimethamine resistance). *P. falciparum* infections from some areas of Southeast Asia, most notably Thai–Cambodian and Thai-Burmese border areas, should be treated with 7 days of quinine sulfate and 7 days of doxycycline or tetracycline.

[†]Preferred regimen for nonimmune patients older than 8 years of age. The benefits of using doxycycline or tetracycline must be weighed against the known risks of adverse effects in children younger than 8 years. Alternatives include quinine plus pyrimethamine-sulfadoxine, quinine plus clindamycin, atovaquone-proguanil, or mefloquine alone. Sulfa-containing regimens may fail in infections from areas with sulfa resistance, such as parts of Southeast Asia, East and Southern Africa, and the Amazon basin.

(Continued)

TABLE 221.1

(CONTINUED)

‡Mefloquine at treatment doses has been associated with a greater risk of serious neuropsychiatric side effects (1/2,000 to 1/1,200). Incidence was higher among patients treated with 25 mg/kg and much higher (1/173) among patients receiving 25 mg/kg after failing 15 mg/kg. Splitting the dose (15 mg/kg on the first day followed by 10 mg/kg 24 hours later) may reduce side effects of high dose mefloquine. Mefloquine resistance is seen in South-East Asia and has been reported in South America. Quinine plus doxycycline is the most effective therapy available in the United States for the treatment of *P. falciparum* acquired in mefloquine-resistant areas.

§A standard dosing option: chloroquine phosphate 10 mg/kg (base) once daily for 2 days, followed by 5 mg/kg once on the third day.

**Quinine dihydrochloride can also be used, if available (not available in the United States.). Dosage: 25 mg/kg divided into three doses per day, infused over 1 to 2 hours every 8 hours until the patient is able to tolerate oral quinine sulfate.

††Some *P. vivax* parasites from Papua New Guinea, Indonesia, Burma, India, and South America (Guyana) have been shown to be resistant to chloroquine. Persons who acquire *P. vivax* in these areas should be treated with regimen used for chloroquine-resistant *P. falciparum*.

‡‡Primaquine is used to eradicate hypnozoites from the liver of infected persons. Patients who require primaquine should be screened for G6PD deficiency before therapy. Patients with mild G6PD deficiency (A variant, greater than 10% residual enzyme activity) can be treated with 0.9 mg/kg base (maximum dose 45 mg) once per week for 8 weeks. Severely deficient patients (B variant, less than 10% residual enzyme activity) cannot receive primaquine because of risk of potentially fatal hemolysis. Primaquine should not be used during pregnancy.

with *P. falciparum* infection and a parasite density of 5% or greater are at high risk of complications and death.

Alternative methods for diagnosis are available. Rapid diagnostic tests (RDTs) to detect the presence of parasite antigens by measuring either histidine-rich protein-2 (HRP-2) or parasite lactate dehydrogenase (pLDH) from a drop of capillary blood also are available. RDTs based on pLDH can differentiate *P. falciparum* from non-falciparum infections. None of these assays has been shown to be more sensitive than a thick-blood film examined by a competent microscopist. These assays are not approved by the U.S. Food and Drug Administration (FDA) and are not available in the United States. HRP-2 detection tests may remain positive for some time after clinical infection has resolved. A determination of parasite density is not possible using these methods. The polymerase chain reaction (PCR) method amplifies parasite DNA and may be more sensitive for detecting parasites than is microscopy. PCR is particularly valuable for identifying parasite species that cannot be determined by microscopy. Currently, PCR is used mostly as a research tool and is available only in reference laboratories. It should not be used for primary diagnosis. If any of these diagnostic tests are used, the diagnosis, species identification, and parasite density should be confirmed by blood-slide examination. Malaria serology detects antibodies to all four species but cannot be used to diagnose current infections. However, it may be useful for identifying an infective donor in transfusion-related malaria, investigating congenital malaria, confirming malaria diagnosis in empirically treated nonimmune persons, and diagnosing tropical splenomegaly syndrome.

THERAPY

Rapid diagnosis and institution of treatment are essential to prevent severe morbidity and mortality. The optimal treatment regimen depends on the patient's medical status, the infecting species, the region from which the infection was acquired, the presence of complications, and the density of infection (for *P. falciparum*). Most important is distinguishing between infections with *P. falciparum* and other species, because the initial approach to treatment differs. When the species cannot be determined, patients should be treated presumptively for falciparum malaria until a definitive species determination can be made.

Plasmodium falciparum Infection

In nonmalarious areas, patients with falciparum malaria should be hospitalized, because their clinical condition may deteriorate rapidly in the first 24 to 48 hours despite the insti-

tution of appropriate antimalarial therapy. Fluid replacement, with close monitoring of fluid intake and output, antipyretic agents, and management of anemia are important adjuncts to antimalarial treatment. Blood films should be repeated at least every 24 hours in uncomplicated infection and every 8 to 12 hours in severe and complicated disease to monitor the parasite density. Although parasite density may increase during the first 24 hours, a steady decrease should be seen thereafter. Blood film examinations should be repeated until asexual forms no longer are detectable. Monitoring of blood glucose and hemoglobin is essential, because hypoglycemia and severe anemia may develop rapidly. If a patient has an altered mental status, a lumbar puncture should be performed to rule out concurrent bacterial meningitis, although caution must be taken, because some patients with cerebral malaria may have increased intracranial pressure.

If no complications can be identified, fewer than 5% of erythrocytes are infected, and the patient can tolerate oral medications, he can be treated for uncomplicated infection. The clinician then must determine the geographic region from which the infection was acquired. Chloroquine-resistant *P. falciparum* has been identified in most areas of the world where malaria is endemic (see Fig. 221.4). Sulfadoxine-pyrimethamine (SP) resistance occurs in South-East Asia and South America and is becoming more prevalent in Africa. Mefloquine resistance is seen in South-East Asia and has been reported in South America.

For areas with chloroquine resistance, the mainstay of antimalarial treatment is combination therapy with quinine sulfate given for 3 days and doxycycline or tetracycline given for 7 days (Table 221.1). For children younger than 8 years, doxycycline or tetracycline can be replaced with a single-dose treatment of SP. SP should only be used in travellers from areas known to be free of SP resistance. Alternatively, combination therapy with quinine sulfate and clindamycin is safe and effective against chloroquine resistant malaria. For falciparum malaria acquired in areas with multidrug resistance, which includes the borders of Thailand with Cambodia and Myanmar, the western provinces of Cambodia, and the eastern areas of Myanmar, treatment with quinine should be extended to 7 days. In addition, the use of doxycycline or tetracycline should be considered for children younger than 8 years with malaria acquired in these areas, because of the high level of resistance to multiple drugs. In particular, the use of doxycycline or tetracycline in combination with quinine or quinidine could be considered for those with severe or complicated disease, because the risks associated with using this drug in young children (dental staining and deposition of drug in the bone epiphysis) are small when compared with the risks of complications and death from falciparum infection. Atovaquone-proguanil (Malarone™), approved by the FDA in June 2001, is effective against uncomplicated, multidrug resistant malaria. It is associated with fewer side effects than mefloquine, and a pediatric formulation is available. Newer drugs, including several drugs from the class of artemisinins (artesunate, dihydroartemisinin, artemether, and others) also are effective treatments for multidrug-resistant *P. falciparum* infection but currently are not available in the United States. Mefloquine is an alternative treatment for uncomplicated falciparum malaria, but is it associated with a high frequency of adverse reactions when used at treatment doses. Mefloquine alone should not be used for infections acquired in areas with multidrug resistance.

For persons with uncomplicated malaria acquired in areas in which chloroquine-resistant *P. falciparum* has not been identified (i.e., Mexico, Central America northwest of the Panama Canal, Haiti, the Dominican Republic, Argentina, and parts of the Middle East, primarily Syria, Jordan, and Iraq), chloroquine phosphate can be used (see Table 221.1).

If 5% of erythrocytes or greater are infected; complications are present, including cerebral malaria, noncardiogenic pulmonary edema, or renal failure; or the patient cannot tolerate oral medications, she should be given intravenous treatment regardless of where the infection was acquired (see Table 221.1). In the United States, where intravenous quinine is not available, quinidine gluconate is the drug of choice. It should be administered by continuous infusion until the parasite density has fallen to less than 1% and complications have resolved, at which point treatment can be completed using oral quinine sulfate. Because quinidine gluconate can cause prolongation of the QT interval and widening of the QRS complex (a rare complication in children) that may lead to fatal torsades de pointes, patients receiving this drug should be maintained on continuous cardiac monitoring. If the QT interval prolongs to more than 0.6 seconds or the QRS complex increases by more than 50% of baseline, the quinidine infusion should be discontinued temporarily and can be resumed once these abnormalities have resolved.

For patients in whom 10% of erythrocytes or greater are infected, and in those with complications, including cerebral malaria, quinidine gluconate supplemented with exchange transfusion can reduce the parasite density rapidly, resulting in the prevention or resolution of complications. The goals for exchange transfusion are the same as those for intravenous quinidine. Repeat blood films from patients receiving intravenous quinidine with or without exchange transfusion should be examined every 8 hours until the parasite density is less than 1%. Intravenous quinidine should be continued throughout the exchange transfusion.

Non-*falciparum* Malaria

Chloroquine phosphate remains the drug of choice for the treatment of blood-stage infection with *P. vivax*, *P. ovale*, and *P. malariae* (see Table 221.1). *P. vivax* infections resistant to chloroquine have been described in Papua New Guinea, Indonesia, and parts of Asia and South America, although chloroquine-resistant *P. vivax* is a significant problem only on the island of New Guinea (Papua New Guinea and Papua Indonesia). Failure of *P. vivax* to respond to chloroquine or recurrence of parasitemia within a month after treatment suggests that the infection may be chloroquine-resistant. In those cases, treatment with a 3-day course of quinine sulfate and 7 days of tetracycline or doxycycline is recommended. Mefloquine (15 mg/kg) also can be used also for the treatment of chloroquine-resistant *P. vivax*, particularly for children younger than 8 years. Limited data are available on the efficacy of atovaquone-proguanil for the treatment of chloroquine resistant *P. vivax*.

To eradicate the persistent liver-stage parasites and to prevent relapses in *P. vivax* and *P. ovale* infections, a 14-day course

of primaquine (0.6 mg/kg base daily) should be administered after completing chloroquine (see Table 221.1). Before starting primaquine, a patient's glucose-6-phosphate dehydrogenase (G6PD) level should be measured. Persons with severe G6PD deficiency (i.e., less than 10% residual enzyme activity) should not receive primaquine. Persons with greater residual enzyme activity may receive primaquine in a weekly dose of 0.9 mg/kg base for 8 weeks, with hemoglobin measurements after each dose. Patients receiving this regimen should be observed closely after the first dose, because some degree of hemolysis can be expected.

Consultation for the treatment of malaria can be obtained from state and local health departments or 24 hours per day from the Malaria Treatment Hotline at the Centers for Disease Control and Prevention [tel. (770) 488-7788].

PREVENTION

For persons traveling in malaria-risk areas, an optimal prevention strategy involves the use of personal protection measures to minimize contact with mosquitoes and correct use of antimalarial chemoprophylaxis. The provision of appropriate prevention advice requires knowledge of travelers' specific itinerary, timing of the trip, and accommodations. In many endemic areas outside sub-Saharan Africa, transmission occurs only in rural areas; persons visiting urban centers may not be at risk for malaria. Persons taking only day trips into endemic areas also are at reduced risk, because *Anopheles* mosquitoes generally take blood meals from dusk through dawn. Detailed information regarding malaria-risk areas, personal protection measures, and antimalarial chemoprophylaxis is available from the Centers for Disease Control and Prevention through the Health Information Hotline [tel. (800) 311-3435], the Web site (http://www.cdc.gov/travel), and the annual publication *Health Information for International Travel*.

Personal Protection Measures

Using a variety of personal protection measures reduces the risk of contact with *Anopheles* mosquitoes. These measures include the use of insect repellents, wearing of clothes covering most of the body, minimizing outdoor activities between dusk and dawn, using a room fan to prevent mosquitoes from flying, sleeping in screened or air-conditioned rooms. Insect repellents containing *N,N*,diethylmetatoluamide (DEET) in concentrations of less than 35% are effective when used as directed. When screened or air-conditioned rooms are not available, sleeping under mosquito netting treated with the synthetic pyrethroid insecticides (e.g., permethrin or deltamethrin) is recommended.

Chemoprophylaxis

Decisions regarding the use of chemoprophylaxis must weigh the risk of acquiring malaria, particularly *P. falciparum*, against the potential adverse reactions of the various chemoprophylactic agents. The choice of chemoprophylactic agent depends on the destination of travel and the duration of the travel. In most areas of the world in which malaria is transmitted, chloroquine-resistant *P. falciparum* has been identified (see Fig. 221.4), the options for prophylaxis include mefloquine, doxycycline and atovaquone-proguanil.

Mefloquine should be taken weekly starting 1 to 2 weeks before travel, weekly throughout the stay, and for 4 weeks after leaving the risk area. Randomized, controlled, double-blind studies have not demonstrated an increased risk of adverse reactions with mefloquine as compared with other chemoprophylactic agents. Children were excluded from these prophylaxis trials, but several studies of mefloquine for treatment of malaria have included children, and adverse reactions were rare, except for nausea and vomiting. Serious neuropsychiatric reactions, including seizures and acute psychosis (reported at the higher doses used for treatment), are rare at the dosage given for chemoprophylaxis and occur most often in persons predisposed to these conditions. Therefore, mefloquine should not be given to persons with a history of or medical conditions that predispose to seizures, nor to persons with major psychiatric conditions. It also is contraindicated in persons with cardiac conduction abnormalities. Studies of long-term mefloquine use in Peace Corps volunteers demonstrated that the risk of adverse reactions to mefloquine decreased with duration of usage.

Because mefloquine is available only in tablet form, dosing in young children, particularly those weighing less than 15 kg, can be difficult. Before travel, pharmacists should prepare the doses for young children by grinding the tablets, weighing out the correct amount based on the child's weight, and placing each dose in an empty gelatin capsule. Doses can be administered by mixing with food or formula. If the child vomits within a few minutes of the dose, it should be readministered after waiting for 30 minutes.

For children older than 8 years, doxycycline is an effective prophylactic drug when taken correctly (Table 221.2). Doxycycline should be started 1 to 2 days before entering a risk area, and it should be taken daily throughout the stay and for 4 weeks after leaving the area. Doxycycline should be taken with food and should not be taken at bedtime, because it can cause gastritis or esophagitis. Some persons taking this drug may become photosensitive; travelers taking doxycycline should take precautions to reduce sun exposure. Doxycycline should not be used for prophylaxis by pregnant women and by children younger than 8 years.

Atovaquone-proguanil (Malarone™) should be started 1 to 2 days before travel, taken daily during travel, and continuing daily for 7 days after leaving the malarious area. It should not be used in children weighing less than 11 kg or in patients with severe renal impairment. Doxycycline or atovaquone-proguanil are the drugs of choice for persons traveling into areas with multidrug resistance, which include parts of Thailand, Cambodia, Myanmar, and Vietnam.

For persons who will be traveling in areas in which medical services are not available within 24 hours, a treatment dose of atovaquone-proguanil may be brought along for presumptive self-management of febrile illness (see Table 221.2). Presumptive self-treatment with atovaquone-proguanil should not be used by persons already on atovaquone-proguanil prophylaxis. Such self-treatment should be considered only as a stop-gap measure, and medical attention should be sought as soon as possible. Families traveling with children should be advised to identify appropriate sources of medical care either before travel or shortly after arrival, in the event that their children develop fever or other symptoms suggesting malaria.

Chloroquine remains the chemoprophylactic agent of choice for persons traveling into areas in which chloroquine resistance has not been documented (see Fig. 221.4). Chloroquine phosphate should be taken weekly beginning 1 to 2 weeks before travel, throughout the stay, and for 4 weeks after leaving the risk area (see Table 221.2). Chloroquine is safe for all age groups. It is available only in tablet form in the United States, although syrup forms are available in other countries. If tablets

TABLE 221.2

CHEMOPROPHYLAXIS FOR THE PREVENTION OF MALARIA

Drug	Pediatric Dose
Areas WITH chloroquine-resistant *P. falciparum** (in no specific order)	
i) Mefloquine	<15kg: 5 mg/kg /week[†,‡]
	15–19 kg: ¼ tablet/week
	20–30 kg: ½ tablet/week
	31–45 kg: ¾ tablet/week
	>45 kg: 1 tablet/week
ii) Doxycycline alone	>8 years: 2 mg/kg daily[§]
	(maximum dose 100 mg/day)
iii) Atovaquone-proguanil**	11–20 kg: 1 pediatric tab daily
	21–30 kg: 2 pediatric tabs daily
	31–40 kg: 3 pediatric tabs daily
	>40 kg: 1 adult tab daily
Areas WITHOUT chloroquine-resistant *P. falciparum*	
i) Chloroquine phosphate	5 mg/kg base once weekly
	maximum adult dose of 300 mg base
Stand-by Treatment[††]	
(ii) Atovaquone-proguanil (Malarone™)	11–20 kg: 1 adult tabs daily × 3 d
	21–30 kg: 2 adult tabs daily × 3 d
	31–40 kg: 3 adult tabs daily × 3 d
	>40 kg: 4 adult tabs daily × 3 d

*In one study of European tourists traveling to East Africa, prophylactic effectiveness was 91% for mefloquine, and 42% for chloroquine alone. Atovaquone-proguanil and doxycycline effectiveness were not studied, but are believed to be comparable to mefloquine.
[†]Once weekly, starting 1 to 2 weeks before, during, and for 4 weeks after travel.
[‡]One tablet contains 250 mg salt. An exact dose for children less than 15 kg body weight has not been established; however, limited data suggest that mefloquine given at 5 mg/kg is as safe and effective in very young children as in adults.
[§]Once daily, starting 1 to 2 days before, during, and for 4 weeks after travel.
**Atovaquone-proguanil and doxycycline are regimens of choice for areas of known mefloquine-resistant *P. falciparum* in Southeast Asia. Few tourists, however, are actually exposed to mefloquine-resistant *P. falciparum*.
[††]Persons traveling in areas where medical services are not readily available should be given a treatment dose of atovaquone-proguanil for presumptive self-treatment to use in the event of febrile disease.

---

are used, doses for young children should be prepared as with mefloquine. If syrup is to be used, the amount of syrup required should be determined by calculating the correct dosage and administering the volume that contains that dosage, based on the syrup concentration of chloroquine. With the exception of mild gastrointestinal upset and vomiting of the dose, particularly in infants and young children, adverse reactions to chloroquine are rare.

Some persons will develop malaria even though they adhered to their recommended chemoprophylactic regimen and personal protection measures. With *P. falciparum*, symptoms develop most often within a few weeks after the last dose of the prophylactic drug and generally occur when the blood concentration of the prophylactic agent is less than the level that provides complete protection. Usually, infection occurs when doses of the drug were missed, but it can occur also when absorption is inadequate or metabolism of the drug is too rapid. Prophylaxis failures resulting from a drug-resistant infection are less common. In the cases of *P. vivax* or *P. ovale* infections, development of parasitemia, despite adherence with recommended preventive measures, usually occurs months after the last dose of the prophylactic agent and represents relapse infections. These cases are not considered prophylaxis failures, because none of the currently recommended chemoprophylactic agents are active against hypnozoites (the persistent liver stage of these species), which are responsible for the relapse. For this reason, a 14-day course of primaquine for terminal prophylaxis may be indicated to prevent these relapse infections in long-term visitors (e.g., missionaries and Peace Corps

volunteers) to high-transmission areas for *P. vivax* (e.g., Papua New Guinea and Papua Indonesia).

Any person who develops fever weeks to months after returning from an area endemic for malaria should be referred for a blood-film examination for malaria. If parasites are present, patient management should follow the recommendations outlined (see Table 221.1).

Case Reporting

Malaria is a nationally notifiable disease in the United States. All confirmed cases of malaria should be reported to the local health department, and a malaria case surveillance form must be completed. Further resources in the treatment and management of malaria are given in Box 221.2.

Disclaimer

The use of trade names in this chapter is for identification only and does not imply endorsement by the Public Health Service or the U.S. Department of Health and Human Services.

Suggested Readings

Barat LM, Bloland PB. Drug resistance among malaria and other parasites. *Infect Dis Clin North Am* 1997;11:969.
Bloland PB. *Drug resistance in malaria.* Geneva: World Health Organization, 2001. WHO/CDS/CSR/DRS/2001.4.
World Health Organization. Severe falciparum malaria. *Trans R Soc Trop Med Hyg* 2000;94(Suppl 1):S1.
English M, Sauerwein R, Waruiru C, et al. Acidosis in severe childhood malaria. *Q J Med* 1997;90:263.
Centers for Disease Control and Prevention. *Health information for international travel 2003–2004.* Atlanta: Department of Health and Human Services, 2003.
Lobel HO, Kozarsky PE. Update on the prevention of malaria for travelers. *JAMA* 1997;278:1767.
Lobel HO, Miani M, Eng T, et al. Long-term malaria prophylaxis with weekly mefloquine. *Lancet* 1993;341:848.
Miller KD, Greenberg AE, Campbell CC. Treatment of severe malaria in the United States with a continuous infusion of quinidine gluconate and exchange transfusion. *N Engl J Med* 1989;321:65.
Miller LH, Warrell DA. Malaria. In: Warren KS, Mahmoud AA, eds. *Tropical and geographic medicine,* 2nd ed. New York: McGraw-Hill, 1990:245.
Re VL, Gluckman SJ. Prevention of malaria in travelers. *Am Fam Phys* 2003; 68:509.
Steffen R, Fuchs E, Schildknecht J, et al. Mefloquine compared with other malaria chemoprophylactic regimens in tourists visiting East Africa. *Lancet* 1993;341:1299.
White NJ. The treatment of malaria. *N Engl J Med* 1996;335:800.
Zucker JR, Campbell CC. Malaria: principles of prevention and treatment. *Infect Dis Clin North Am* 993;7:547.

CHAPTER 222 ■ TOXOPLASMOSIS

RUTH LYNFIELD, FOLASHADE OGUNMODEDE, AND NICHOLAS G. GUERINA

Toxoplasma gondii is an obligate intracellular protozoan parasite found in many animal species throughout the world. Nicolle and Manceaux observed the parasites in the blood, liver, and spleen of a North African desert rodent, *Ctenodactylus gondii*. In 1909, the parasite was named *Toxoplasma* ("arclike form") *gondii* (after the rodent). In 1923, Janku reported cysts in the retina of an infant who had unilateral microphthalmia, hydrocephalus, and seizures. Subsequently, *Toxoplasma* was recognized as causing a variety of clinical syndromes in humans. Although infection usually is asymptomatic in normal hosts, serious disease may occur in the setting of congenital infection or in an immunodeficient host. Infection with *Toxoplasma* is lifelong. The acute stage of infection is characterized by parasitemia. The chronic stage occurs when the parasite becomes encysted in host tissues. *Toxoplasma* may break out of host cells, causing a local reactivation. In the setting of an inadequate immune response, reactivated disease may lead to systemic spread of the parasites.

LIFE CYCLE

Toxoplasma has a sexual cycle that occurs exclusively in felines and an asexual cycle that occurs in most warm-blooded animals (Fig. 222.1). Cats acquire the infection by ingesting oocysts in contaminated soil or tissue cysts in birds and rodents they hunt and kill. The sexual cycle takes place in the cat intestine, where gametocytes are formed and fertilized to form zygotes. Zygotes become encapsulated within a wall and are shed as oocysts. During a primary infection, a cat can shed millions of oocysts daily for a period of 1 to 3 weeks. The oocysts sporulate and become infectious 24 hours or more after excretion. Sporulated oocysts may remain infectious in soil for more than 1 year, especially in warm, humid environments. Although cats typically develop immunity to *T. gondii* after a primary infection, the duration of immunity to intestinal shedding is not known; however, reinfection with oocyst shedding has been observed.

An animal or human may ingest material contaminated by cat feces containing *Toxoplasma* oocysts. The oocyst ruptures in the intestine and releases sporozoites. The sporozoites divide in the intestinal cells and associated lymph nodes. Tachyzoites, the rapidly dividing form characteristic of the acute stage of infection, are formed and are dispersed via blood and lymph. When an effective immune response is established, the parasites become localized in tissue cysts composed of components from both the parasites and infected host cells. Within the tissue cysts are slowly dividing forms of *T. gondii* called *bradyzoites*; tissue cysts are the form characteristic of the chronic stage of infection. Bradyzoites within intact tissue cysts can survive for the life of the host. Tissue cysts can be found in any organ, but most typically are found in the brain, eye, heart, and skeletal muscles. Occasionally, tissue cysts may rupture, releasing bradyzoites. In the presence of an intact immune response, infection usually is controlled. In immunodeficient hosts, reactivation of chronic *Toxoplasma* infection may occur, with bradyzoites transformed

into tachyzoites, which may proliferate rapidly and induce tissue damage.

The infectious cycle may be perpetuated by tissue cysts when an infected animal is ingested by a carnivore; the bradyzoites are released, infect the intestinal epithelial cells, and are transformed into tachyzoites that disperse systemically. When an immune response is established, bradyzoites again are formed. Studies of cats indicate that the prepatent period (the time between infection and shedding of the oocysts) and the quantity of oocysts shed following a primary infection vary depending on the form of *T. gondii* ingested. Primary infection following ingestion of tissue cysts is associated with greater oocyst shedding and a shorter (3 to 10 days versus more than 18 days)

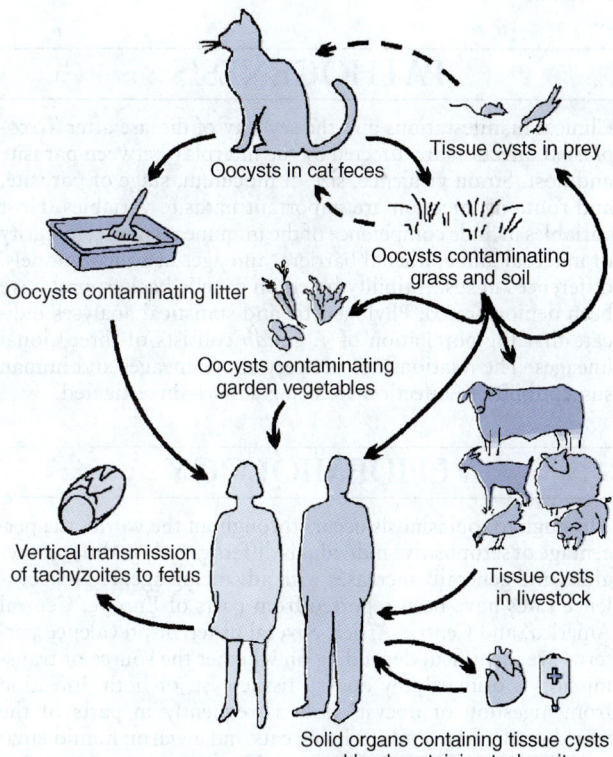

FIGURE 222.1. The *Toxoplasma gondii* life cycle and pathways for infection. The only source for the production of *T. gondii* oocysts is the feline intestinal tract. Acquired disease in humans occurs by direct ingestion of oocysts from contaminated sources (soil, cat litter, garden vegetables) or by ingestion of tissue cysts present in undercooked tissues from infected animals. Fetal infection most commonly occurs after acute maternal infection in pregnancy, but it can also occur after reactivation of latent infection in immunocompromised women. Pathways leading to human disease are indicated by *solid arrows*, and pathways leading to feline infection are indicated by *broken arrows*. (Reprinted from Lynfield R, Guerina G. Toxoplasmosis. *Pediatr Rev* 1997;18:75.)

prepatent period compared with primary infection after ingestion of oocysts.

TRANSMISSION OF INFECTION

Toxoplasma oocysts, bradyzoites, and tachyzoites can all cause infection in humans. Typically, isolated cases are identified, but outbreaks of toxoplasmosis have been linked to the ingestion of contaminated water, soil, and undercooked hamburger.

Ingestion or inhalation of oocysts may occur after the handling of contaminated soil or cat litter or after ingestion of contaminated water or food (e.g., unwashed garden produce). Oocysts are very hardy and can resist drying or treating with disinfectants, alcohols (95% ethanol, 100% methanol), or 10% formalin. They may be inactivated by heating (66°C).

Transmission can occur by ingestion of tissue cysts present in undercooked meat (especially pork and mutton). The bradyzoites in tissue cysts can be destroyed by heating (66°C) or gamma irradiation. Generally, freezing meat at −20°C also will kill tissue cysts. In addition to ingestion, bradyzoites can be transmitted via transplant of an organ containing tissue cysts. Rarely, tachyzoites may be transmitted through a blood transfusion, by a laboratory accident, or by ingestion of unpasteurized (goat's) milk. Tachyzoites are the most fragile infectious form and cannot withstand freezing and thawing, drying, or exposure to digestive enzymes. Fetuses may become infected through the placenta by tachyzoites after a primary maternal infection.

PATHOGENESIS

Clinical manifestations and the severity of disease after *Toxoplasma* infection are affected by the interplay between parasite and host. Strain virulence, size of inoculum, stage of parasite, and route of infection are important parasite variables. Host variables include competence of the immune response, integrity of mucosal and epithelial barriers, and age. In animal models, differences in susceptibility based on genetic background have been demonstrated. Phylogenetic and statistical analyses indicate that the population of *T. gondii* consists of three clonal lineages. The relationships between these lineages and human susceptibility to infection are being actively investigated.

EPIDEMIOLOGY

Although toxoplasmosis occurs throughout the world, the percentage of seropositive individuals differs greatly in different regions and generally increases with advancing age. High prevalence rates have been reported from parts of Europe, Central America, and Central Africa. Several different prevalence patterns are identified, depending on whether the source of transmission is primarily by oocyst, tissue cyst, or both. Infection from ingestion of oocysts occurs frequently in parts of the world with many outdoor-living cats and a warm, humid environment. In such areas as Central America, seropositivity begins at approximately 1 year of age, when children begin playing in oocyst-contaminated sand and soil, and it reaches 50% to 75% by adolescence. In other regions of the world, transmission occurs primarily through the ingestion of undercooked meat. In these areas, depending on eating customs, seropositivity may begin in adolescence (or sooner) and can continue throughout adulthood. In many parts of the world, the pattern is mixed. Studies in certain regions actually have found a decreasing seroprevalence. U.S. military recruits were found to have an overall seroprevalence of 9.5% in 1986 as compared with 14.4% in 1962, and studies of French pregnant women in

Paris noted a drop from approximately 87% during the period from 1960 to 1970 to approximately 70% in 1985. Seroprevalence rates among women of childbearing age in Europe vary from 50% in Brussels, Belgium, to 11% in Norway. In the United States, based on information from the National Health and Nutritional Examination Survey (NHANES), seroprevalence rates have remained stable over the last 10 years. The most recent NHANES, conducted in 1999 to 2000, estimated the overall *Toxoplasma* immunoglobulin G (IgG) seroprevalence rate at 15.8% and the seroprevalence among girls and women 12 to 49 years old at 15%.

With few exceptions, congenital infection occurs in the setting of primary maternal infection during pregnancy. The risk of congenital infection depends on the risk of acute acquired infection during pregnancy. This risk, in turn, depends on the yearly seroconversion rate for the particular population and on the age of the pregnant woman. Fetal infection may occur after reactivation of disease in immunocompromised pregnant women, and there are rare reports in the literature of fetal infection following chronic toxoplasmosis in pregnant women with no known immune dysfunction. The incidence of congenital *Toxoplasma* infection in some European countries with very high seroprevalence rates has declined in recent years, possibly owing to aggressive screening recommendations and national prevention programs. Brazil has the highest reported incidence of congenital infection in the Americas; 1 per 3,000 live births. In Massachusetts, where screening for congenital *Toxoplasma* infection has been part of the newborn screening program since 1986, the estimated incidence is 1 per 10,000 live births.

CLINICAL MANIFESTATIONS

Acquired Infection in Immunocompetent Hosts (Including Pregnant Women)

Most cases of *Toxoplasma* infection are subclinical in individuals with normal immune systems, and usually disease is self-limiting. Lymphadenopathy is the manifestation recognized most frequently, and the location most often is cervical, followed by axillary and then inguinal sites, although any group of lymph nodes may be involved. Adenopathy may occur more commonly at single sites in adults, but is more likely to occur at multiple sites in children. Usually, the lymph nodes are firm and movable and initially may be tender. They do not suppurate, and typically the lymph nodes are 1 to 2 cm in size, but they may be as large as 6 cm. Most cases of lymphadenopathy resolve over the course of 1 to 2 months.

Occasionally, disease may persist beyond 6 months. Adenopathy may be recurrent. The differential diagnosis of toxoplasmic lymphadenopathy includes lymphoma, leukemia, and other malignancies, infectious mononucleosis (Epstein-Barr virus), cytomegalovirus (CMV) infection, human immunodeficiency virus (HIV) infection, cat-scratch disease, bacterial lymphadenitis, atypical mycobacterial infection, tuberculosis, tularemia, and sarcoidosis. Other clinical presentations include an infectious mononucleosis–like illness with fever, malaise, and myalgia, although sore throat and hepatosplenomegaly are not typical with *Toxoplasma* infection.

Ocular disease may be associated with acute acquired infection in normal hosts but is associated more typically with congenital disease and reactivated disease. Although it is rare, severe systemic disease, including encephalitis, has been reported in apparently normal children (see further discussion later in this section). Other reported manifestations have included maculopapular rash, hepatitis, pneumonitis, myositis, myocarditis, pericarditis, and meningitis. Infection in immunologically normal hosts usually is self-limited. Severe disease more typically occurs in patients with a deficient immune system.

Infection in Immunocompromised Hosts

Toxoplasmosis in immunocompromised hosts may result from acute or reactivated infection. Disseminated infection may occur with fever and involvement of any and all organs, including brain, heart, and lung. It may result from primary infection in patients who are receiving immunosuppressive therapy (e.g., organ or bone marrow transplant recipients), in patients who have malignant disease (especially reticuloendothelial) and are undergoing chemotherapy, or in patients with acquired or congenital immunodeficiencies. Primary infection can occur also in transplant recipients via an infected organ or bone marrow or through blood transfusion. Diagnosing disseminated toxoplasmosis in such patients may be difficult because signs and symptoms are not specific to toxoplasmosis. However, the condition should be considered as a diagnostic possibility because the infection is rapidly fulminant. Early treatment can improve the outcome. Reactivation of latent infection may occur in the setting of altered immunity, such as immunosuppressive therapy after a transplant or decreasing immune function in a patient with acquired immunodeficiency syndrome (AIDS). Clinical findings include any of the following: retinal disease, encephalitis, pneumonitis, myocarditis, or multiorgan disease.

Toxoplasma encephalitis (TE) is a common opportunistic infection in adult patients with AIDS (10% to 50% of those seropositive for *Toxoplasma* with CD4 counts of fewer than 100 cells/μL), and typically it results from reactivation of infection in the setting of poor cellular immunity. In contrast to its incidence in adults, TE is uncommon in children with AIDS, most likely because of the low incidence of *T. gondii* infection. TE may present with fever, headache, and focal neurologic signs. Disturbances of consciousness, confusion, motor impairment, seizures, impaired coordination, and focal weakness can occur. Usually, the course is subacute, but it may be fulminant and rapidly fatal. Generally, focal hypodense mass lesions with contrast enhancement are seen. Magnetic resonance imaging with enhancement is thought to be more sensitive in detecting lesions than is computed tomography. Often, lesions are found in the basal ganglia and corticomedullary junction of the cerebral hemispheres. Usually, multiple lesions are found, but a solitary lesion can occur. Marked edema often is present. In patients with disseminated toxoplasmosis in the brain, contrast enhancement may be absent. An image finding that is highly suggestive but only present in approximately 25% of cases is the asymmetric (eccentric) target sign. This lesion is characterized by a ring of contrast enhancement with a small eccentric nodule along the wall, giving it a target-like shape. In developing countries, where neuroimaging and other sophisticated techniques may not be readily available, HIV-positive individuals with suspected intracranial masses should be empirically treated for TE. The main differential diagnosis of TE is primary central nervous system (CNS) lymphoma, especially in the presence of a single lesion. Other possibilities include progressive multifocal leukoencephalopathy, bacterial abscess, cryptococcosis, cytomegalovirus infection, tuberculosis, and focal viral encephalitis. Patients with TE may have coexisting intracranial diseases. Another CNS manifestation of toxoplasmosis is myelopathy, which has been reported in patients with AIDS.

Although TE is rare in individuals with intact immune systems, a report reviewing TE in children found that 9 of 32 reported cases occurred in children who had no known immunodeficiencies. In eight of these immunocompetent children, TE occurred with primary infection (one unknown).

Pulmonary toxoplasmosis may be seen in patients with AIDS with decreasing CD4 cell counts (typically, fewer than 100 cells/μL) or other immunosuppressed patients (primarily reported in adults). The clinical picture of pulmonary toxoplasmosis is similar to that of pneumocystis, although usually the course is more rapid. Patients present with fever, cough, and dyspnea. Often, diffuse bilateral interstitial pneumonitis is seen on chest radiography (although variously a miliary pattern, multiple nodules, lobar infiltrates, and pleural effusions have been described). Often, patients have a high lactate dehydrogenase level. The organism may be found in a bronchoalveolar lavage aspirate and in biopsy specimen, or in both, using appropriate histologic staining techniques. Thorascopic or open lung biopsy may be required to make a diagnosis in some cases.

Congenital Infection

The risk of fetal infection with *T. gondii* increases, but the severity of disease decreases, with the gestational age at which acute maternal infection occurs. The onset of fetal infection by *T. gondii* also is delayed after an acute maternal infection. The rate of maternal-fetal transmission may be as low as 1% or less with maternal infection in the periconceptional period and can approach 90% or greater with maternal infection in late gestation. Average transmission rates are approximately 15% or less overall for the first trimester (rate rapidly increases after 10 weeks of gestation), 30% for the second trimester, and 60% for the third trimester and are a function of the increasing efficiency of the placenta. Studies of twins have shown that monozygotic twins have nearly identical infection rates but dizygotic twins do not, further underscoring the importance of the placenta in fetal infection.

Although rare, there have been case reports of congenital *T. gondii* infection when maternal infection was documented before conception. There has also been a case report of congenital infection that was thought to result from maternal reinfection during pregnancy. Congenital infection following chronic maternal infection is a more frequent occurrence in the setting of maternal immunosuppression, such as women receiving cytotoxic or corticosteroid therapy or women with HIV infection. In these women, symptoms of reactivated maternal toxoplasmosis may be absent, and the fetal transmission risk as a function of the degree of maternal immunosuppression is not known.

In the absence of treatment of the fetus with combination anti-*Toxoplasma* drugs, most fetuses infected early in pregnancy die *in utero* or in the neonatal period or have severe neurologic and ophthalmologic disease. Those infected in the second and third trimesters typically have mild or subclinical disease. The delay in maternal-fetal transmission appears to diminish with increasing gestational age. Although most fetal infections are likely to occur within several weeks, a delay of more than 3 months has been described.

Most newborn infants with congenital *Toxoplasma* infection have subclinical infection with no overt disease at birth, but indirect ophthalmoscopy may reveal ocular disease, and examination of the cerebrospinal fluid (CSF) and intracranial radiographic imaging may reveal abnormalities of the CNS. The New England Newborn Screening Program measures *Toxoplasma*-specific IgM on all newborn infants in Massachusetts and New Hampshire. Over a 6.5-year period beginning in 1986, 52 infants with congenital *Toxoplasma* infection were identified from 635,000 infants screened. Fifty of the 52 infants had normal routine newborn examinations, but their *T. gondii* infection was identified through serologic screening, 48 had further testing that revealed abnormalities of either the CNS or the retina in 19 (40%). Most often, ocular lesions consisted of unilateral macular retinal scars, and CNS lesions were characterized by small, focal cerebral calcifications and mild to moderate elevations of CSF protein.

The principal clinical findings for infants and children with *symptomatic* congenital toxoplasmosis were described by Eichenwald in 1960. Such children were classified as having disease limited to the CNS and eyes (108 of 152) or more generalized (systemic) disease (44 of 152). The latter group evinced a lower incidence of CNS and ocular disease and a higher incidence of hepatosplenomegaly, lymphadenopathy, jaundice, and anemia. For all 152 infants, the incidences of neurologic and ocular abnormalities were as follows: intracranial calcifications, 37%; abnormal CSF profiles, 63%; chorioretinitis, 86%; convulsions, 41%; and hydrocephalus, 20%. Examples of brain and retinal lesions are shown in Figure 222.2.

Complications of Congenital *Toxoplasma* Infection in the Absence of Extended Treatment

Prospective studies have shown that although most infants with congenital *Toxoplasma* infection have mild or subclinical disease at birth, they remain at significant risk for long-term sequelae. Most studies have focused on the occurrence of ocular disease and show that the incidence of new-onset retinal lesions may approach 90% and that the risk for new lesions extends into adulthood. Severe visual impairment and blindness can occur. A few studies also have reported a significant incidence of neurologic problems, even when subclinical infection was present at birth. Specific complications include motor and cerebellar dysfunction, microcephaly, seizures, decreased intelligence quotient, mental retardation, and sensorineural hearing loss. Congenital toxoplasmosis has also been associated with precocious puberty secondary to hypothalamopituitary dysfunction.

Efficacy of Prophylaxis and Treatment of Congenital *Toxoplasma* Infection

Spiramycin has been shown to decrease *in utero* vertical transmission of *Toxoplasma*. In a prospective controlled study in France, the overall incidence of congenital infection was decreased from 58% to 23% when mothers were started promptly on spiramycin after seroconversion was identified. The severity of disease in those fetuses who became infected did not appear to be altered. The failure of spiramycin to prevent all cases of maternal-fetal transmission may result from the initiation of treatment after fetal infection has already occurred or from a demonstrated high variability of maternal serum and amniotic fluid spiramycin concentrations. In addition, some studies failed to demonstrate any difference in the rate of maternal-fetal transmission when groups receiving no antenatal treatment, antenatal spiramycin treatment, or antenatal pyrimethamine and sulfonamide-sulfadiazine were compared. Nonetheless, it is generally accepted that antenatal treatment is beneficial; initiating anti-*Toxoplasma* chemotherapy as soon as possible following maternal seroconversion (typically with spiramycin) and changing maternal therapy to a combination of pyrimethamine and sulfadiazine (plus folinic acid rescue) when infection is documented appear to decrease the risk for severe fetal disease significantly.

Experience with extended postnatal treatment regimens for congenital *Toxoplasma* infection is increasing. Although the optimal duration of therapy has not been determined, combination therapy for a 1-year period—most often with pyrimethamine (plus folinic acid) and sulfadiazine—appears to decrease the incidence of long-term complications significantly. The incidence of new-onset ocular disease may be decreased to as low as 10% after a 1-year treatment regimen, although longer-term follow-up (through adolescence) is needed for most studies. Significant neurologic complications are limited to children with compromising CNS disease at birth, although some of such children may do better than expected as compared with untreated children. The Chicago Collaborative Treatment Trial reported 37 congenitally infected infants who received extended treatment initiated within the first months of life. Thirty-four of these infants had signs of generalized or neurologic disease. Although some of these children had visual handicap, most did well in follow-up (mean period of follow-up, 3.5 years; longest, 10 years). Nineteen children (who did not have hydrocephalus) had normal or nearly normal neurologic function. Severe disabilities occurred in eight of ten children who had symptomatic hydrocephalus at birth and in two of eight who had symptomatic hydrocephalus identified in the first months of life. Risk factors associated with a poor outcome included delay in the diagnosis and initiation of treatment, prolonged uncorrected hydrocephalus, extensive visual impairment, and prolonged concomitant neonatal hypoxemia and hypoglycemia.

Ocular Disease

Toxoplasma is the most common cause of infectious chorioretinitis in immunocompetent children. In the past, ocular toxoplasmosis was thought to be primarily a sequela of congenital infection; however, more recent data suggest it may more frequently follow postnatally acquired infection. For example, Southern Brazil has a very high seroprevalence rate, and most *Toxoplasma* infections are thought to be acquired postnatally, yet 18% of the population has chorioretinal scars. Similarly, 20 of 97 (21%) individuals infected during a 1995 waterborne outbreak of toxoplasmosis in British Columbia went on to develop *Toxoplasmic* chorioretinitis. Strain or host differences or inoculum size may account for the high rate of acquired chorioretinitis in some settings. Usually, chorioretinal disease associated with acquired toxoplasmosis involves one eye. Disease associated with reactivation from congenital infection may be bilateral, although many cases are unilateral.

Mechanisms for new-onset retinal disease may include the new onset of an inflammatory reaction to old retinal tissue cysts, a hypersensitivity reaction to *Toxoplasma* antigens localized in the retina, and invasion of the eye after recurrent parasitemia. The peak incidence of recurrent chorioretinitis after congenital infection is thought to occur during the second to third decades of life. Recurrence can also follow acquired chorioretinitis. The frequency of recurrences may be reduced by long-term intermittent therapy with trimethoprim-sulfamethoxazole.

Ocular symptoms include blurred vision, photophobia, epiphora, and vision loss (including loss of central vision with macular involvement). Usually, the lesion of ocular toxoplasmosis is a focal necrotizing retinitis. Panuveitis is possible. The typical lesion starts as a yellow-white elevated patch with indistinct margins, often on the posterior pole and often near an old pigmented scar. The vitreous may fill with inflammatory cells, and focal retinal vasculitis is possible. Clusters of lesions may occur. With healing, lesions will atrophy, become pale, and develop black pigment. The differential diagnosis in infants includes other congenital infections associated with retinal lesions, such as CMV infection, herpes simplex, rubella, varicella, syphilis, congenital anomalies, and congenital hypertrophy of retinal pigmented epithelium. There can be associated microphthalmia, strabismus, cataract, nystagmus, and other ocular findings. In older children, the differential also includes fungal retinitis, tuberculosis, sarcoid, and *Toxocara* infection. Diffuse unilateral subacute neuroretinitis caused by *Baylisascaris procyonis* (raccoon roundworm) can be confused with *Toxoplasma* chorioretinitis. Complications of *Toxoplasma* chorioretinitis can include vision loss, retinal detachment, and neovascularization of the retina and optic nerve.

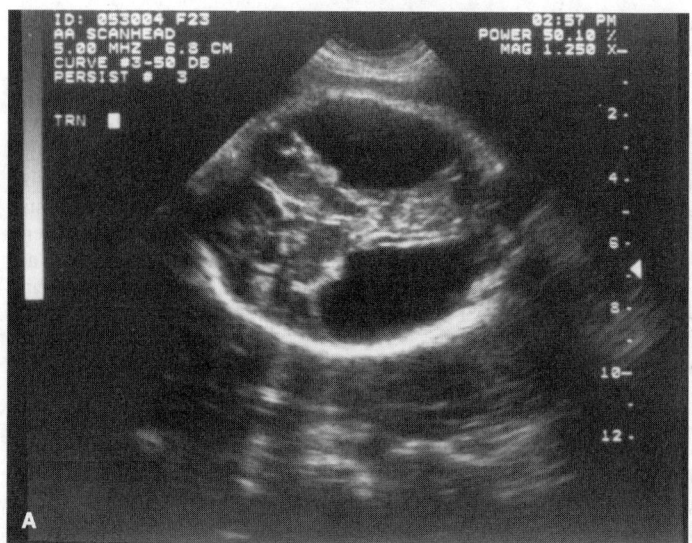

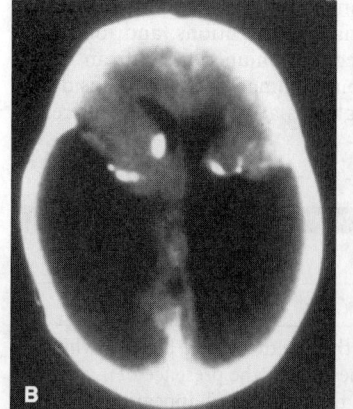

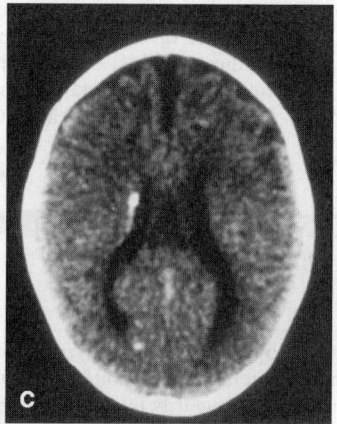

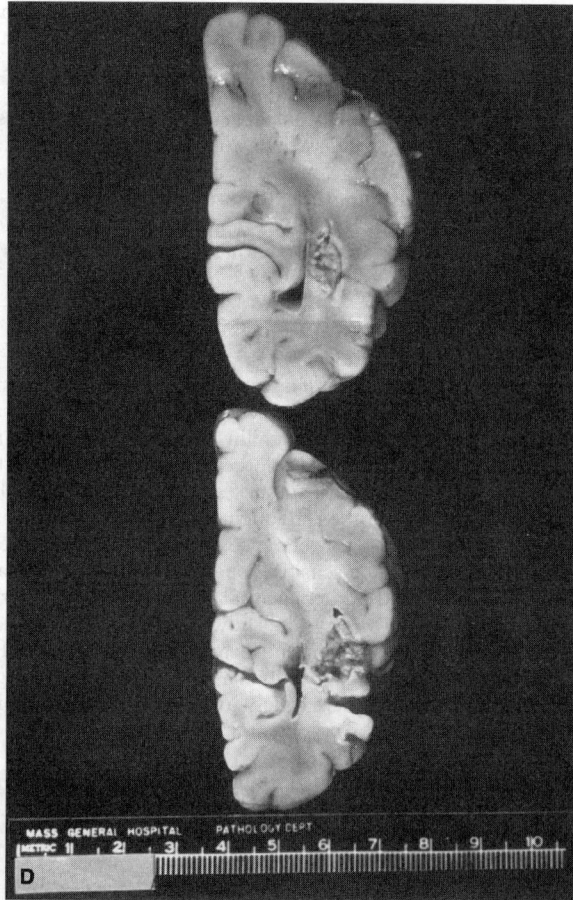

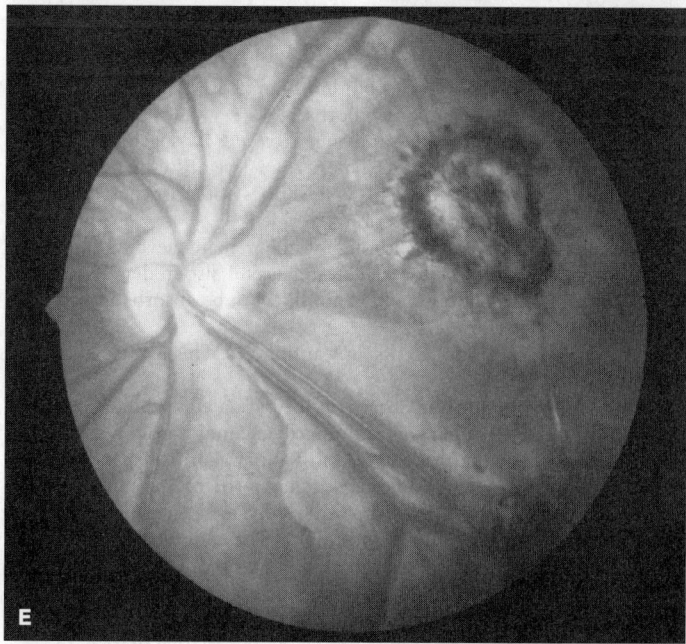

FIGURE 222.2. Brain and retinal lesions in congenital *Toxoplasma* infection. A, B: Hydrocephalus after first-trimester fetal infection. A: Dilated lateral ventricles were found during a fetal ultrasonography survey conducted owing to small fetal size for the estimated gestational age of 26 weeks. A 13-week-gestation maternal serum sample was retrieved, and *Toxoplasma* serology was consistent with acute maternal *Toxoplasma* infection acquired in the first trimester. The only intervention acceptable to the mother was treatment with pyrimethamine, sulfadiazine, and folinic acid. Fetal disease was already advanced, and the hydrocephalus progressed. B: At birth, the infant had monocular microphthalmia, chorioretinitis, and blindness, in addition to massive hydrocephalus. C–E: Focal parenchymal brain and chorioretinal lesions in newborn infants with a congenital infection. C: Brain computed tomographic scan showing small, calcified lesions. D: Necrotic lesion adjacent to the lateral ventricle in an infant who died of causes unrelated to *Toxoplasma* infection. *Toxoplasma* tissue cysts were identified in microscopic sections through the lesion. E: Chorioretinal scar with macular involvement. (Courtesy of Dr. Robert Peterson, Children's Hospital, Boston, MA.) (A to D, Reprinted from Lynfield R, Guerina G. Toxoplasmosis. *Pediatr Rev* 1997;18:75. B and D also published in Lynfield R, Eaton R. Teratogen update: congenital toxoplasmosis. *Teratology*. Copyright © 1995 Wiley-Liss, Inc.)

Other sequelae include cataracts, glaucoma, and changes in the iris. Many patients have episodic recurrences of chorioretinitis.

Immunocompromised patients may experience multiple active lesions in one or both eyes, often without evidence of old lesions. Frequently, the lesions are adjacent to blood vessels, suggesting hematologic dissemination. Histopathologic examination may reveal large numbers of tachyzoites in necrotic retinal tissue. A distinguishing feature of CMV retinitis is that typically it has minimal vitreous inflammation. Some patients with AIDS have dual infection with *Toxoplasma* and CMV.

DIAGNOSIS

Diagnostic tests for *T. gondii* infection include the measurement of *Toxoplasma*-specific antibodies, detection of *Toxoplasma*-specific DNA by polymerase chain reaction (PCR), isolation or histologic demonstration of the organism, and detection of *Toxoplasma* antigens in tissues and body fluids. Serology is the technique used most frequently to make a diagnosis of *Toxoplasma* infection. In reference laboratories, serologic assays have proven to be sensitive, specific, and often critical in diagnosing acquired and congenital infections. Some particularly useful serologic assays are shown in Table 222.1.

The enzyme-linked immunosorbent assays for IgG (IgG-ELISA) and IgM (double-sandwich IgM-ELISA, or DS-IgM-ELISA) have become increasingly available in many hospital-based and regional laboratories, but many of these laboratories use commercially available kits with limited sensitivity, specificity, or reproducibility. This finding is particularly true of the commercially available DS-IgM-ELISA, and consideration should be given to the confirmation of serologic results by a reference laboratory. The results of a single *Toxoplasma*-specific IgM test should be interpreted with caution and should not be used alone to diagnose acutely acquired infection or to institute further medical action, particularly in pregnant women. In 1997, the U.S. Food and Drug Administration published an advisory alerting providers to the limitations of commercial IgM test kits. All positive IgM tests should be confirmed by a reference laboratory.

In addition to the assays listed in Table 222.1, the indirect immunofluorescent antibody (IFA) test has proven to be a useful assay for many years, and it still is used by many laboratories. However, it is less sensitive than the ELISA, and it may yield a false-positive result in some clinical circumstances (e.g., patients with circulating antinuclear antibodies). Depending on the assay used, different ranges of antibody titers may be reported. Interpretation of titers requires consultation with the laboratory performing the assays. In addition, the significance of results, appropriate interventions, and follow-up studies should be determined in conjunction with an infectious disease expert. The Sabin-Feldman dye test is considered the "gold standard," although it is available only at reference laboratories.

TABLE 222.1

SEROLOGIC TESTS FOR THE DIAGNOSIS OF *TOXOPLASMA* INFECTION

Serologic Test	Comments
Sabin-Feldman dye test	This test makes use of the uptake by *Toxoplasma* tachyzoites of the dye methylene blue (in which organisms appear swollen and blue). The tachyzoite membranes lyse in the presence of complement and specific antibody (primarily IgG) resulting in thin, unstained-appearing organisms. This test has been used extensively as a screening test for *Toxoplasma* infection; it has been recommended as the test of choice for antenatal maternal screening, but it is available only in reference laboratories.
ELISA	This test has been adapted for the detection of *Toxoplasma*-specific IgG, IgM, IgA, and IgE.
IgG-ELISA	This test is readily available in most commercial laboratories but has limited utility in the determination of acute infection in adults, children, and newborns.
IgM-ELISA	The currently recommended form of this test is the double-sandwich *Toxoplasma*-specific IgM-ELISA. IgM titers may remain elevated from months to more than 1 year, so the test may not be reliable for determining the exact timing of infection. As IgM does not cross the placenta, the test may be very useful in determining congenital infection.
IgA-ELISA	*Toxoplasma*-specific IgA rises very early in infection and, although it may remain elevated for at least 26 weeks, high titers correlate with recent infection. The test is useful also in diagnosing congenital infection, as IgA does not cross the placenta and is not likely to be absorbed from breast milk.
IgE-ELISA	The duration of specific IgE appears to be briefer than IgM or IgA antibodies. This assay can be useful in the serologic diagnosis of acute infection.
IgG avidity	Avidity is determined from the ratio of antibody titration curves of serum treated to dissociate antibody-antigen complexes versus untreated serum. This is primarily a confirmatory test. High avidity levels are consistent with remote infection (more than 3 to 5 months prior depending on assay used) although the presence of low avidity antibodies is not diagnostic of acute infection.
ISAGA	This test measures *Toxoplasma*-specific antibody captured from sera by the agglutination of a particulate antigen preparation. Assays for detecting IgM and IgE have been developed and both tests may be complementary to ELISA procedures.
Differential agglutination test	This test compares agglutination titers for sera against formalin-fixed tachyzoites (HS antigen) with those against acetone- or methanol-fixed tachyzoites (AC antigen). The different test preparations display antigens present at different times in infection, so the relative titers with each preparation are indicative of acute versus remote infection.
PCR	Amplification and detection of *T. gondii* DNA. Usually 100% specificity, although sensitivity varies. PCR can be performed on blood, csf, amniotic fluid, and vitreous fluid. Particularly useful in diagnosis of congenital toxoplasmosis and toxoplasma encephalitis in AIDS patients. Generally not required to diagnose acute toxoplasmosis in immunocompetent persons.

ELISA, enzyme-linked immunosorbent assay; Ig, immunoglobulin; ISAGA, immunosorbent agglutination assay; PCR, polymerase chain reaction.
Adapted from Lynfield R, Guerina G. Toxoplasmosis. *Pediatr Rev* 1997;118:75.

Toxoplasma-specific IgG may be detected within 1 week of a primary infection, and peak titers are found 3 to 8 weeks later. In children and adults with normal antibody responses, IgG antibody typically lasts for life. The Sabin-Feldman dye test, IgG-ELISA, IgG-immunosorbent agglutination assay (IgG-ISAGA), or IgG-IFA may be used to detect specific IgG levels. *Toxoplasma*-specific IgM also can be detected within 1 week of infection, and peak titers occur 3 to 4 weeks later. Depending on the assay used, specific IgM titers may persist for months to more than 1 year after a primary infection. Because of the greater sensitivity and specificity, titers should be obtained using the DS-IgM-ELISA and IgM-ISAGA procedures. Furthermore, because IgG and IgM titers may be positive for an extended duration, the determination of acute infection often requires repeat testing at 3- to 4-week intervals. Accurate demonstration of a change in titer requires that the initial and follow-up serum samples be evaluated simultaneously. Other assays that may aid in the diagnosis of acute infection include the IgA-ELISA, IgE-ELISA, and the differential agglutination (AC/HS) test.

PCR for *Toxoplasma* DNA has been used to detect *T. gondii* in body fluids and tissue, including amniotic fluid, CSF, blood, urine, ocular fluid, and bronchoalveolar lavage specimens. Although studies regarding the utility of PCR in some of these sources have been limited, the test has been established as an important tool in the diagnosis of *Toxoplasma* infection when performed by reference laboratories. PCR is particularly useful in diagnosing intrauterine infections, because it can be used as soon as amniocentesis can be safely performed (after the fifteenth week of gestation), and it eliminates the need for more invasive procedures on the fetus. Amniocentesis is not recommended for HIV-positive women because of the risk of transmitting the HIV virus to the fetus during the procedure. Caution should be applied in interpreting PCR results, including taking into account the type of sample and the clinical setting. Often, special handling procedures are required for optimal results, and these should be reviewed with the laboratory performing the assay before the specimen is obtained.

Tachyzoites and tissue cysts can be visualized directly in histologic sections or cytologic preparations, although special staining techniques (e.g., peroxidase-antiperoxidase procedure) may be required. Typically, *Toxoplasma* lymphadenitis has characteristic findings on routine histology to allow a presumptive diagnosis, even though organisms are not usually found in tissue sections. Histologic findings are described as a triad of reactive follicular hyperplasia, focal distention of sinuses with monocytoid cells, and irregular clusters of epithelioid histiocytes located around the margins of the germinal centers. Usually, TE in patients with AIDS produces brain abscesses that have a central avascular area surrounded by a hyperemic area that contains an inflammatory infiltrate and perivascular cuffing. Areas of necrosis contain tachyzoites. A surrounding outer zone contains *Toxoplasma* cysts. Diffuse TE is characterized by numerous microglial nodules without abscesses located in the gray matter.

Isolation techniques for *T. gondii* involve inoculation into mouse peritoneum or tissue culture. These techniques are cumbersome and expensive, require 2 to 6 weeks for completion, and are available only in a few reference laboratories. Often, antigen detection assays are insensitive, and they are not as readily available as are serologic assays.

Acute Acquired *Toxoplasma* Infection in Immunocompromised Patients

Antibody production may be impaired in certain immunodeficient states, so diagnosing acute infection may be more difficult. Because disease progression may be fulminant in im-

munodeficient patients and because multiple pathologic conditions may coexist, aggressive testing, including biopsy of focal lesions, may be needed. PCR may be useful to diagnose acute systemic and focal infections. PCR on CSF may be particularly useful in the diagnosis of TE in adult patients with AIDS, although the sensitivity may be decreased in patients already receiving treatment. A presumptive diagnosis of TE also may be made in patients with AIDS who are *Toxoplasma* seropositive and have the classic radiographic and clinical findings of TE. In these patients, biopsies of brain lesions still may be required when the response to empiric therapy is inadequate.

Acute Maternal and Fetal *Toxoplasma* Infection in Pregnancy

Because pregnant women usually do not have symptomatic disease, the diagnosis of acute maternal infection in pregnancy relies on serologic screening. However, the United States does not have a systematic prenatal screening program, and if screening is done during pregnancy, usually only one serum sample is submitted, making diagnosis of acute maternal infection very challenging. Studies from Europe and from the Toxoplasmosis Serology Laboratory at the Palo Alto Medical Foundation Research Institute in Palo Alto, California, have demonstrated the usefulness of high-avidity IgG antibodies in excluding recent (within the past 3 to 5 months) *Toxoplasma* infections in pregnant women. This may be particularly useful when only one serum sample is available. If screening occurs early in pregnancy (especially up to 2 months' gestation), a positive Sabin-Feldman dye titer, IgG-IFA, or IgG-ELISA result and a negative DS-IgM-ELISA or IgM-ISAGA result will indicate that infection occurred most likely before conception, with very little risk to the fetus. Even if IgM titers are positive early in gestation, a high IgG titer that is stable or falling on follow-up testing 3 weeks later indicates infection before pregnancy. Interpreting first-time serologic testing later in pregnancy may be more difficult, and follow-up studies may be needed. If the IgG titer is positive and stable on retesting 3 weeks apart and the DS-IgM-ELISA and IgM-ISAGA results are negative, infection is likely to have occurred before conception. A positive IgM titer or rising IgG titer may reflect acute infection in pregnancy, and additional testing by IgA-ELISA, AC/HS, and IgG avidity may help to elucidate further the likely timing of infection. The interpretation of positive or equivocal test results should be performed in consultation with a reference laboratory and an infectious disease specialist.

Pregnant women who are seronegative on initial testing remain at risk for acute *Toxoplasma* infection for the remainder of their pregnancy. For this reason, some countries have established *Toxoplasma* screening programs that use repeated serologic testing at regular intervals throughout pregnancy. Once acute maternal infection has been identified, tests for fetal infection should be undertaken. Combination evaluation with ultrasonographic surveys for fetal anomalies plus amniocentesis for *Toxoplasma*-specific PCR on amniotic fluid have been used successfully to test for fetal infection by experienced maternal-fetal medicine personnel in collaboration with a *Toxoplasma* reference laboratory. In one study in France, 37 of 38 fetal infections (from among 339 fetuses tested) were identified by amniotic fluid PCR, including three missed by fetal blood testing and ultrasonographic screening. One was false-negative, and no false-positive test results occurred. The earliest time at which sufficient amniotic fluid for PCR testing can be obtained safely is approximately 15 weeks' gestation; however, some investigators have found the highest sensitivity of tested amniotic fluid to be at 20 weeks' gestation or later. In a recent multicenter study in Europe involving 271 women with proven primary *Toxoplasma* infection during pregnancy, amniotic fluid PCR was positive in 48 of 75 infected fetuses. The overall sensitivity was 64%, with a negative predictive value of 87.8%; specificity and positive predictive value were 100% each.

Congenital *Toxoplasma* Infection

The serologic diagnosis of congenital *Toxoplasma* infection in newborns and young infants is complicated by the presence in their serum of transplacentally derived maternal IgG. In addition, antibody responses may be delayed for months in some infants, and IgM antibody may be lost by the time of delivery for others. In some cases, interpretation of serology in the neonatal period may be complicated further by placental leakage of maternal IgM and IgA. For these reasons, infants born to mothers known to have had acute *Toxoplasma* infection in pregnancy should undergo further evaluation for signs of infection. Most such infants will appear normal at birth, but they should have a complete evaluation by a pediatric ophthalmologist and by cranial imaging to rule out focal brain lesions or hydrocephalus. A cranial computed tomography scan may be best, because usually it can be done without sedation in newborns, and it may be more sensitive than cranial ultrasonography in detecting small calcified lesions. Examination of the CSF for elevated protein, pleocytosis, and the presence of *T. gondii* by PCR (performed in a reference laboratory) may aid in the diagnosis. PCR testing on blood and urine specimens may also be useful, although studies have been limited thus far.

The serologic diagnosis of congenital *Toxoplasma* infection requires testing of blood samples from both the infant and the mother. Typically, immunologically normal women with acute *Toxoplasma* infection in pregnancy will have positive serology by IgG-ELISA and DS-IgM-ELISA or IgM-ISAGA. Diagnosis in the infant relies on the presence of IgM, but when titers by the DS-IgM-ELISA and IgM-ISAGA procedures are negative or equivocal, additional testing for IgA and IgE by ELISA should be performed. Studies from France have demonstrated the usefulness of Western blot assays for earlier detection of neonatal toxoplasmosis. Western blot compares the immunologic profiles of mothers and babies and differentiates between passively acquired antibodies and newly synthesized antibodies in the neonate. In one study, the combination of Western blot and established serologic tests was able to detect 94% of the cases of congenital *Toxoplasma* infection.

If all laboratory tests are negative for infection and no clinical abnormalities consistent with infection are found, follow-up serology is needed to confirm the absence of infection. Transplacentally derived maternal IgG titers may take months to fall to undetectable levels. Usually, this outcome occurs between 6 and 12 months, and infants with congenital infection typically have elevated IgG levels beyond 1 year. Prospective studies have shown that antibody levels may fall while infants are undergoing treatment with combination anti-*Toxoplasma* drugs. IgG levels may decrease significantly, and IgM levels may become negative. Serologic rebound of both IgG and IgM may occur when treatment is discontinued. The clinical significance of rebound is uncertain. In France, no difference in the incidence of new-onset retinal lesions in 133 children was demonstrated among (a) children with serologic rebound treated an additional 3 months with anti-*Toxoplasma* chemotherapy, (b) children with serologic rebound who did not receive additional therapy, and (c) children without serologic rebound. When no clinical abnormalities are detected but laboratory results are equivocal, consideration should be given to empiric therapy until follow-up studies further support the absence of infection.

Acute Ocular Toxoplasmosis

Most cases of acute, postnatal *Toxoplasma* chorioretinitis are thought to result from late sequelae of congenital infection, but some studies have suggested that chorioretinitis after acute acquired *Toxoplasma* infection may be more common than previously recognized. The detection of *Toxoplasma*-specific IgA or IgE antibodies or an acute pattern on the differential agglutination (AC/HS) test (see Table 222.1) indicates acute acquired *Toxoplasma* chorioretinitis. In cases of reactivated infection, *Toxoplasma* IgG may be at low levels, and *Toxoplasma* IgM typically is negative. Often, the diagnosis is made when characteristic retinal lesions are seen in a *Toxoplasma*-seropositive patient, but if the lesions appear atypical to an experienced ophthalmologist, other diagnoses should be considered. In addition to serologic assays, PCR on ocular fluid may be useful for differentiating between ocular toxoplasmosis and other causes of retinitis.

TREATMENT

Pyrimethamine and sulfadiazine (or trisulfapyrimidines) provide synergistic activity against *Toxoplasma* when these drugs are used in combination. Activity is against the tachyzoite form of *T. gondii*. Pyrimethamine is a folic acid antagonist and can cause bone marrow suppression. Usually, this suppression can be prevented by folinic acid (leucovorin), which should always be administered prophylactically. *T. gondii* cannot use exogenous folinic acid efficiently, so its use does not reduce the efficacy of treatment. Monitoring for drug toxicity includes frequent complete blood counts and platelet counts (weekly or biweekly) with extended therapy; periodic monitoring of liver function tests and renal function also may be beneficial. If treatment-associated neutropenia or anemia develops, the doses of folinic acid should be increased. Pyrimethamine (and in some cases sulfadiazine) dosing may have to be modified if severe bone marrow suppression occurs. Caution should be applied in using pyrimethamine in patients receiving zidovudine, because bone marrow toxicities may be additive, and zidovudine may interfere with the activity of pyrimethamine (although the clinical significance of this effect is unclear). Concurrent use of phenobarbital may decrease the half-life of pyrimethamine, and sulfadiazine may prolong the half-life of phenytoin by interfering with its metabolism via hepatic microsomal enzymes. Allergy to sulfa drugs may require a change from sulfadiazine to clindamycin, which is effective in combination with pyrimethamine. Suggested drug doses are listed in Table 222.2. The selection of a treatment regimen including dosing should be made in consultation with an infectious disease expert.

Other drugs being investigated in the treatment of *Toxoplasma* infection include the macrolides clarithromycin, azithromycin, and roxithromycin, as well as atovaquone. Atovaquone is attractive because it is active against both the tachyzoite and the cystic forms of *T. gondii*. The suspension form of atovaquone has better bioavailability than the tablet form. One study of 17 immunocompetent patients found it to be well tolerated and effective (together with a course of prednisone) for the treatment of ocular toxoplasmosis. Some investigators have cautioned against the use of atovaquone as a single agent in treatment or secondary prophylaxis of TE in immunosuppressed patients. It has been tried in combination therapy with either pyrimethamine or sulfadiazine in patients not able to tolerate standard regimens. Additional studies are needed on the efficacy and role of atovaquone-containing regimens.

Spiramycin is a macrolide antibiotic used in the prophylaxis against fetal transmission and sometimes is added to treatment

TABLE 222.2

DRUG DOSES FOR THE TREATMENT AND PROPHYLAXIS OF *TOXOPLASMA GONDII* INFECTION

Drugs	Doses
Treatment	
Adults	
Pyrimethamine plus	50–100 mg twice daily for the first day, then 25–75 mg* once daily
Sulfadiazine (preferred regimen) or	1.0–1.5 g per dose given four times daily
Clindamycin	300–600 mg per dose given four times daily[†]
Folinic acid (leucovorin)	10–20 mg once daily[‡]
Children	
Pyrimethamine plus	2 mg/kg once daily for 2 days (maximum, 50 mg), then 1 mg/kg once daily (maximum, 25 mg)[§]
Sulfadiazine (preferred regimen) or	100 mg/kg/day divided into two doses
Clindamycin	20–30 mg/kg/day divided into four doses
Folinic acid (leucovorin)	5–10 mg three times weekly**,[†]
Prophylaxis in HIV-Infected Patients ***	
Prophylaxis against Primary Acquired Infection[‖]	
TMP-SMX	
Adults	1 double-strength TMP-SMX tablet once daily
Children	150 mg TMP/750 mg SMX/m^2/day divided into two doses daily
Prophylaxis against Recurrent Disease (prior *Toxoplasma* Encephalitis)[‖]	
Adults	
Pyrimethamine	25–50 mg once daily
Sulfadiazine	500–1,000 mg/dose given four times daily
Folinic acid (leucovorin)	10–25 mg once daily[‡]
Children	
Pyrimethamine	1 mg/kg or 15 mg/m^2 (maximum, 25 mg) once daily
Sulfadiazine	85–120 mg/kg/day in two to four divided doses
Folinic acid (leucovorin)	5 mg every 3 days[†]

HIV, human immunodeficiency virus; TMP-SMX, trimethoprim-sulfamethoxazole.

For a particular clinical syndrome, review of a regimen, including dosing, with an infectious disease specialist is advised.

*For toxoplasmic encephalitis in a patient with acquired immunodeficiency syndrome (AIDS), pyrimethamine, 200 mg on the first day followed by 50 to 75 mg once daily, is recommended.

**For HIV-infected children use 10–25 mg of folinic acid once daily.

[†]For toxoplasmic encephalitis in a patient with AIDS, clindamycin, 600 mg per dose given four times daily, is recommended.

[‡]Folinic acid dose may be increased for pyrimethamine-associated bone marrow toxicity. Folinic acid should be continued one week after pyrimethamine is discontinued.

[§]For treatment of congenital toxoplasmosis in newborns, regimens have included 1 mg/kg/day of pyrimethamine for 2 or 6 months, followed by 1 mg/kg of pyrimethamine every other day (or Monday, Wednesday, and Friday) to complete a year.

[‖]In HIV-positive adults, primary toxoplasmosis prophylaxis may be discontinued when the CD4$^+$ T lymphocyte count has increased to more than 200 cells/μL for 3 months or longer, and secondary prophylaxis can be discontinued among patients with a sustained increase in CD4$^+$ counts (e.g., 6 months or longer) to more than 200 cells/μL on antiretroviral therapy.

***Adapted from Centers for Disease Control and Prevention. Treating opportunistic infections among HIV-exposed and infected children: recommendations from CDC, the National Institutes of Health and the Infectious Disease Society of America. *MMWR Morb Mortal Wkly Rep* 2004;53:RR-14; Centers for Disease Control and Prevention. Treating opportunistic infections among HIV-infected adults and adolescents: recommendations from CDC, the National Institutes of Health and the HIV Medicine Association/Infectious Disease Society of America. *MMWR Morb Mortal Wkly Rep* 2004;53:RR-15; and Guidelines for preventing opportunistic infections among HIV-infected persons—2002: recommendations of the U.S. Public Health Service and the Infectious Diseases Society of America. *MMWR Morb Mortal Wkly Rep* 2002;51:RR-8. (Alternative regimens also are described.)

regimens for congenital infection. The drug accumulates in the placenta, and it has been used in the first trimester without reported fetal complications. Spiramycin is licensed for use in Europe and Canada, and it is available in the United States from Rhône-Poulenc (Montreal, Canada) as an investigational drug regulated by the U.S. Food and Drug Administration.

Acquired Toxoplasmosis

Most cases of acquired toxoplasmosis in immunologically normal children and in nonpregnant adults are self-limiting, and specific drug therapy is reserved for the rare occurrence of severe or persistent clinical symptoms or for compromise of vital organs. Combination therapy is usually given, with pyrimethamine and sulfadiazine with folinic acid rescue. Therapy is continued until 1–2 weeks after symptoms resolve (approximately 3 to 6 weeks).

Infection in Immunocompromised Patients

In immunocompromised patients, acute or active infection should be treated regardless of symptoms, because such patients are at high risk of severe disease from *Toxoplasma*. Combination drug therapy with pyrimethamine and sulfadiazine (or clindamycin for sulfa drug–intolerant patients) plus folinic acid is given (see Table 222.2). In patients with AIDS, treatment for TE should be given for at least 6 weeks, provided there is clinical and radiologic improvement. Longer courses may be required. Adjunctive corticosteroids should be administered if indicated for treatment of mass effect or edema caused by focal lesions and should be discontinued as soon as feasible. Relapses of active disease are frequent, and an initial course of therapy should be followed by lifelong suppressive therapy against *Toxoplasma*. In adults and adolescents, if immune reconstitution as a consequence of highly active antiretroviral therapy (HAART) occurs, with a sustained increase in CD4 cells (more than 200 cells/μL for 6 or more months), suppressive therapy may be altered if the patient has completed initial therapy and is asymptomatic (see U.S. Public Health Service/Infectious Disease Society of America [USPHS/IDSA] guidelines for details). Table 222.2 outlines an adaptation of the USPHS/IDSA guidelines regarding secondary prophylaxis of TE in patients with AIDS who have had a prior episode of TE. Prevention of disease, particularly TE, is attempted by the administration of anti-*Toxoplasma* drugs to *Toxoplasma*-seropositive HIV-infected patients (see Table 222.2). USPHS/IDSA guidelines state that *Toxoplasma*-seropositive adolescents and adults whose CD4 lymphocyte counts are lower than 100 cells/μL should receive prophylaxis (although some clinicians start prophylaxis at CD4 counts of fewer than 200 cells/μL). Again, if immune reconstitution as a consequence of HAART occurs in adults and adolescents, with a sustained increase in CD4 cells (more than 200 cells/μL for 3 or more months), prophylaxis may be discontinued (see USPHS/IDSA guidelines). Primary prophylaxis with trimethoprim-sulfamethoxazole is recommended for *Toxoplasma*-seropositive HIV-infected children who have severe immunosuppression. Severe immunosuppression in children is defined using CD4 cells as a function of age, with fewer than 750 CD4 cells/μL (or less than 15%) for children younger than 12 months of age, fewer than 500 CD4 cells/μL (less than 15%) for children 1 to 5 years of age, and fewer than 200 CD4 cells/μL (less than 15%) for children 6 to 12 years of age. A benefit of trimethoprim-sulfamethoxazole is its availability in the developing world. If patients cannot tolerate this regimen, the alternative is dapsone and pyrimethamine plus folinic acid. Atovoquone can also be considered if other regimens are not tolerated. Please see the USPHS/IDSA guidelines for complete details. Secondary prophylaxis of TE in children with HIV infection should be pyrimethamine plus sulfadiazine together with folinic acid. Children with a history of toxoplasmosis should continue to receive lifelong secondary prophylaxis. The safety of discontinuing primary or secondary prophylaxis in children has not been determined.

Congenital Infection

Prophylaxis against Fetal Infection after Maternal Infection in Pregnancy

Spiramycin (1 g three times daily) prophylaxis against fetal transmission should be given to pregnant women with acute *Toxoplasma* infection. Therapy should be changed to pyrimethamine, sulfadiazine, and folinic acid if fetal infection is diagnosed subsequently; this regimen is not used in the first trimester of pregnancy, and it has generally been reserved for cases of proven fetal infection, because of potential toxicities to the mother and fetus. If fetal testing cannot be performed or maternal infection is not diagnosed until late in the second trimester or in the third trimester, the empiric use of pyrimethamine and sulfadiazine (plus folinic acid) may be appropriate. The empiric use of pyrimethamine and sulfadiazine (plus folinic acid) after the first trimester may be considered even when antenatal studies do not demonstrate fetal infection, because currently available testing cannot rule out fetal infection with certainty. Despite antenatal treatment, prevention of severe newborn disease cannot be guaranteed, and frequent fetal ultrasound surveys should be performed because parenchymal brain damage and hydrocephalus may develop rapidly. Good outcomes, however, have been reported for newborn infants with congenital *Toxoplasma* infection when maternal serologic screening was coupled with prompt antenatal treatment, even when fetal infection occurred in the first

trimester. Monitoring for drug toxicity should include frequent maternal complete blood counts.

Fetal transmission is very unlikely to occur in the setting of remote maternal infection unless maternal immunodeficiency is present. Consideration must be given to prophylaxis in HIV-positive pregnant women with prior *Toxoplasma* infection, but the selection of a prophylaxis regimen must consider the teratogenic potential of administering drugs in the first trimester and the potential for bone marrow toxicity to the mother and fetus (see the USPHS/IDSA guidelines). Infants born to dually infected mothers should be evaluated soon after birth, and, even if the initial assessment is negative for congenital *Toxoplasma* infection, close follow-up (including repeated serologic tests) should be performed.

Treatment and Follow-up of Infected Newborns

The optimal duration of treatment for congenital *Toxoplasma* infection is not known, but often a 1-year regimen with combination drug therapy is recommended. The drugs used most commonly are pyrimethamine and sulfadiazine with folinic acid rescue. Some treatment programs also have used spiramycin on an alternating schedule with pyrimethamine and sulfadiazine (plus folinic acid). The safety and efficacy of sulfadoxine-pyrimethamine-lactose (Fansidar) are being studied as a possible alternative treatment approach. Adjunctive carticosteroids are used to treat acute vision-threatening lesions or cerebrospinal fluid protein $\geq$ 1g/dL. Because of the risk for late sequelae with congenital *Toxoplasma* infection, clinical follow-up is recommended throughout early childhood. Routine ophthalmologic evaluations are especially important, because infants and young children cannot report vision changes.

Pharmacokinetic studies regarding pyrimethamine in infants have shown a serum half-life of 33 hours, with steady-state levels being nearly twice as high at daily dose of 1 mg/kg as compared with a dose of 1 mg/kg every other day. CSF drug levels that were achieved are active against *T. gondii in vitro*, but these levels were only 10% to 25% of serum levels. Based on this information, the daily dosing schedule of 1 mg/kg may be reasonable, especially for the initial portion of the treatment course (2 to 6 months; see Table 222.2, footnote). The principal side effect of therapy is drug-induced neutropenia, which usually is caused by pyrimethamine and resolves in response to increased folinic acid dosing. In some cases, modification of the pyrimethamine dose is required. Less commonly, neutropenia can result from sulfadiazine.

Ocular Toxoplasmosis

Active chorioretinitis should be treated in both children and adults. Combination therapy with pyrimethamine and sulfadiazine (plus folinic acid) generally is preferred, especially in children. Some experts use a regimen that includes clindamycin. One report found subconjunctival clindamycin efficacious. The duration of treatment is approximately 2 weeks after acute inflammation has resolved. Most experts also treat vision-threatening lesions with prednisone until acute inflammation resolves.

PREVENTION

Avoiding exposure to sources of *Toxoplasma* is an important way to prevent infection. This caution is particularly important for seronegative pregnant women and for immunocompromised patients. Individuals should be advised not to eat undercooked or raw meat. It is useful to store meat frozen at $-20°$F to inactivate tissue cysts. Meat should be cooked to an internal temperature of 66°C (150°F). Hands should be washed thoroughly after handling raw meat and vegetables and fruits, and raw vegetables and fruits should be washed thoroughly before they are eaten. Kitchen surfaces, cutting boards, and utensils should be cleaned after each use. Gloves should be worn, and hands should be washed thoroughly after handling such potentially contaminated materials as soil, cat litter, or sandboxes or after gardening. Cats should be kept indoors and should be fed only dry, canned, or cooked food. Cat litter should be changed daily (because oocysts do not sporulate in the first 24 hours after passage), preferably by someone not pregnant or immunocompromised. The possibility of transmission of infection via oocysts can be reduced further by soaking a cat's litter pan in near-boiling water for 5 minutes.

Suggested Readings

American Academy of Pediatrics. *Toxoplasma gondii* infections (toxoplasmosis). In: Pickering LK, ed. *Redbook: 2003 report of the Committee on Infectious Diseases,* 26th ed. Elk Grove Village, IL: American Academy of Pediatrics, 2003:631.

Centers for Disease Control and Prevention. Treating opportunistic infections among HIV-exposed and infected children: recommendations from CDC, the National Institutes of Health and the Infectious Disease Society of America. *MMWR Morb Mortal Wkly Rep* 2004;53:RR-14.

Centers for Disease Control and Prevention. Treating opportunistic infections among HIV-infected adults and adolescents: recommendations from CDC, the National Institutes of Health and the HIV Medicine Association/Infectious Disease Society of America. *MMWR Morb Mortal Wkly Rep* 2004;53:1.

Gilbert R, Gras L. European Multicentre Study on Congenital Toxoplasmosis: effect of timing and type of treatment on the risk of mother to child transmission of *Toxoplasma gondii. Br J Obstet Gynaecol* 2003;110: 112.

Guerina NG, Hsu HW, Meissner HC, et al. Neonatal serological screening and early treatment of congenital *Toxoplasma gondii* infection. *N Engl J Med* 1994;330:1858.

Hohlfeld P, Daffos F, Costa JM, et al. Prenatal diagnosis of congenital toxoplasmosis with a polymerase chain reaction test on amniotic fluid. *N Engl J Med* 1994;331:695.

McAuley J, Boyer K, Patel D, et al. Early and longitudinal evaluations of treated infants and children and untreated historical patients with congenital toxoplasmosis: the Chicago collaborative treatment trial. *Clin Infect Dis* 1994;18:38.

Mets MB, Holfels E, Boyer KM, et al. Eye manifestations of congenital toxoplasmosis. *Am J Ophthalmol* 1997;123:1.

Montoya JG. Laboratory diagnosis of *Toxoplasma gondii* infection and toxoplasmosis. *J Infect Dis* 2002;185(suppl 1):S73.

Pearson PA, Piracha AR, Sen HA, Jaffe GJ. Atovaquone for the treatment of *Toxoplasma* chorioretinitis in immunocompetent patients. *Ophthalmology* 1999;106:148.

Romand S, Wallon M, Franck J, et al. Prenatal diagnosis using polymerase chain reaction on amniotic fluid for congenital toxoplasmosis. *Obstet Gynecol* 2001;97:296.

CHAPTER 223 ■ THE NEMATODES

THOMAS CHERIAN

The phylum Nematoda constitutes one of the six classes included in the phylum Aschelminthes. It is the second largest phylum in the animal kingdom, comprising an estimated 500,000 species, most of which are free-living. A few species are parasitic, including some that are parasitic to humans. Nematodes are cylindrical organisms, tapering at the head and tail ends. Their bodies are encased in a thick, impervious cuticle. They have a body cavity that contains the organs. With rare exceptions, parasitic nematodes have separate genders.

The life cycle of parasitic nematodes varies considerably among species. These differences have clinical significance because some infections may be transmitted directly from infected to uninfected humans, whereas in others, the eggs must undergo an obligatory period of maturation outside the human host before they become infectious to other humans. Nematodes do not multiply within humans, the exception being strongyloidiasis in the immunocompromised host.

GLOBAL IMPACT AND EPIDEMIOLOGY

Nematode infections are among the most common infections in humans. The World Health Organization (WHO) estimates that over 2 billion individuals are infected by soil-transmitted helminths, namely *Ascaris,* hookworm, and *Trichuris,* worldwide, many being multiply infected with two or more nematodes. More than 300 million of these individuals suffer from associated severe morbidity and 155,000 deaths are reported annually. The numbers of people infected with *Ascaris,* hookworm, and *Trichuris* worldwide are estimated to be 1.4 billion, 1.2 billion, and 1 billion, respectively. More than three-fourths of those infected live in developing countries.

Nematodes are found most commonly in regions with warm, humid climates where malnutrition, poor living standards, and poor sanitation are common. Indiscriminate defecation and use of human feces as fertilizer are important risk factors. Nematode infections may be acquired through the ingestion of eggs (*Ascaris, Enterobius,* whipworm), by penetration of infective larvae (hookworm, *Strongyloides*), by insect bite (filarial worm), or by ingestion of infected meat (trichinella) or fish (*Capillaria, Anisakis*) (Table 223.1).

In areas where infection is endemic, maximum intensity occurs in school-aged children, adolescents, and young adults. This outcome is explained by age-related changes in exposure and the acquisition of immunity. Even among the high-risk section of the population, infection tends to be highly aggregated, so that a few persons harbor heavy worm burdens, although most harbor few parasites. Heavily infected individuals within a community are predisposed to this state by such as yet unidentified processes as behavioral and social factors, nutritional status, and genetic background. Heavy worm burdens in schoolchildren in developing countries directly or indirectly cause undernutrition, growth retardation, anemia, and impaired cognitive function. Many of these effects may be reversed by chemotherapy. It has been suggested that the immunologic responses to chronic helminthic infection may predispose to human immunodeficiency virus (HIV)/acquired immunodeficiency syndrome and tuberculosis and impair the

TABLE 223.1

SUMMARY OF THE COMMON INTESTINAL AND TISSUE NEMATODE INFECTIONS IN HUMANS

Organism	Geographical Distribution	Clinical Manifestations of Infestation	Diagnosis	Treatment
Intestinal Nematodes				
Ascaris lumbricoides	Worldwide, but more common in tropical regions with poor sanitation	Nonspecific colicky abdominal pain and distension; intestinal obstruction; obstruction of biliary on pancreatic ducts; Löffler syndrome	Demonstration of embryonate and nonembryonate eggs in feces	Pyrantel pamoate 11 mg/kg (maximum 1 g) as single dose; or mebendazole 100 mg twice daily for 3 days
Hookworms	Worldwide distribution but more common in areas with warm, humid climate	Ground itch; Löffler syndrome; epigastric pain, tenderness, and diarrhea; anemia and hypoproteinemia	Demonstration of characteristic ovoid eggs in feces	Mebendazole 100 mg twice daily for 3 days; pyrantel pamoate 11 mg/kg (maximum 1 g) for 3 days; supplemental iron
Trichuris trichuria	Worldwide, but more common in tropical regions with poor sanitation	Severe colitis and proctitis presenting with abdominal pain, bloody diarrhea, and rectal prolapse	Demonstration of characteristic lemon-shaped eggs in feces	Mebendazole 100 mg twice daily for 3 days
Enterobiasis vermicularis	Worldwide	Nocturnal perianal pruritus; vaginal discharge and vulval pruritus; rarely appendicitis and salpingitis	Demonstration of characteristic eggs	Single dose of pyrantel pamoate 11 mg/kg (maximum 1 g); or single dose of mebendazole 100 mg
Strongyloides stercoralis	Worldwide	Pruritic skin rash (larva currens); Löffler syndrome; epigastric pain, vomiting and diarrhea; hyperinfection in patients with HIV/AIDS	Demonstration of larvae in feces or in the duodenal fluid	Ivermectin 200 μg/kg/day for 1–2 days
Aberrant infection with intestinal nematodes				
Cutaneous larval migrans *Ancylostoma braziliense* or *A. caninum*	Worldwide, but more common in areas with warm, humid climate	Itching and typical serpiginous tracks	Generally made clinically	Thiabendazole (10%–15%) topically four times daily; or ivermectin 200 μg/kg daily for 1–2 days
Anisakiasis *Anisakis simplex* or *Pseudoterranova decipiens*	Worldwide with higher incidence where raw fish is eaten	Abdominal pain, nausea, and vomiting	Demonstration of parasite in stomach by endoscopy and biopsy	Self-limiting in most cases; endoscopic removal of parasite
Angiostrongylus cantonensis	Southeast Asia and Pacific	Eosinophilic meningitis	Serologic tests to detect antibody to organism	Supportive; repeated lumbar puncture to reduce headache
Tissue Cestodes				
Filariasis *Wuchereria bancrofti* or *Brugia malayi*	Africa, Asia, South and Central America, and Pacific islands	Lymphangitis; elephantiasis; hydrocele; chylous ascites; chyluria	Detection of microfilaria in blood, urine (in chyluria), and hydrocele fluid; antigen detection	Diethylcarbamazine 6 mg/kg/day in two to three divided doses for 12–14 days (for *W. bancrofti*) and 3–6 mg/kg/day for 6–12 days (for *B. malayi*)

(Continued)

TABLE 223.1

(CONTINUED)

Organism	Geographical Distribution	Clinical Manifestations of Infestation	Diagnosis	Treatment
Onchocerca volvulus	West and Central Africa, isolated foci in Latin America, and Yemen	Erythematous papular rash; lymphedema and depigmentation (leopard skin); chronic lymphadenopathy (hanging groin); iridocyclitis, optic atrophy, corneal fibrosis, and blindness	Demonstration of microfilaria in skin snips or in eye by slit lamp examination	Ivermectin 150 μg/kg repeated every 3 months; surgical excision of nodules on the head; doxycycline 100 mg daily for 6 weeks
Trichinella spiralis	Worldwide	Intestinal phase: abdominal pain, nausea, vomiting, and malaise Muscle invasion phase: eyelid edema, myalgia, weakness, fever, and eosinophilia	Demonstration of parasite on muscle biopsy; serologic tests and antigen detection assays	Mebendazole 200–400 mg three time daily for 3 days, then 400–500 mg three times daily for 10 days; or albendazole 400 mg twice daily for 8–14 days
Dracunculus medinensis (Guinea worm)	Sub-Saharan Africa	Painful papule followed by painful ulcer with protrusion of worm; fever, nausea, vomiting, diarrhea, dyspnea, urticaria, and eosinophilia	Characteristic clinical picture	Metronidazole 25 mg/kg/day (maximum 750 mg) in three divided doses for 10 days; removal of the worm

AIDS, acquired immunodeficiency syndrome; HIV, human immunodeficiency virus.

efficacy of vaccines against these or other diseases. However, this effect has yet to be conclusively demonstrated. At least one recent cohort study in Uganda did not show any evidence that helminthic infection contributed to a more rapid progression of HIV infection or that antihelminthic treatment had any of effect on the CD4 counts or viral load.

In developed countries (including the United States), nematode infections are encountered most commonly in travelers to developing countries and among immigrants and adoptees from endemic regions. With increasing air travel and immigration, the prevalence of nematode infections in the United States is bound to increase. Infection in travelers is common, although often asymptomatic, because of the low worm burden.

INTESTINAL NEMATODES

Ascaris lumbricoides

Ascaris lumbricoides is one of the largest and most common parasites in humans. In the United States, estimates posit that 4 million people are infected, mainly in the Southeast. The adult worm is 15 to 30 cm long and resides in the lumen of the jejunum and the ileum.

Life Cycle

Infection occurs by ingestion of embryonate eggs via contaminated fingers or food or by geophagia. The adult female worm produces on average 200,000 eggs per day, which are passed in the feces. The eggs develop in the soil in perhaps 2 to 3 weeks. On being swallowed, the eggs develop into second-stage larvae that penetrate the intestinal wall, enter the venous circulation, and travel to the lungs. A local hypersensitivity reaction

(Splendore-Hoeppli phenomenon) may occur at the site of entry of the larvae into the lung tissue. After further development in the lungs, the third-stage larvae ascend to the trachea, are expectorated, and then are swallowed. The resultant introduction of the fourth-stage larvae into the gastrointestinal tract allows them to develop into mature adults that establish residence in the jejunum and ileum, completing the cycle.

Clinical Features

The most common clinical manifestations are nonspecific colicky abdominal pain and distension. These symptoms are caused by metabolic products of the worms, which irritate the sensory receptors in the intestine and result in interference with normal peristalsis, spasmodic contraction, and ischemia of the bowel wall.

Chronic ascariasis is known to precipitate malnutrition in undernourished children, probably as a result of malabsorption. *Ascaris* infection causes fat and lactose intolerance and malabsorption of vitamin A. Protein absorption is improved in children after treatment of ascariasis.

Heavy infestation with *Ascaris* can result in small-bowel obstruction. Migration of worms can cause obstruction of biliary and pancreatic ducts. In regions where it is endemic, *Ascaris* is a common cause of acute abdominal emergencies and biliary and pancreatic disease.

Migration of larvae through the lungs may result in Löffler syndrome presenting as fever, productive cough, eosinophilia, and pulmonary infiltrates.

Diagnosis

Diagnosis is made by the demonstration of the distinctive golden-coated embryonate and nonembryonate eggs (Fig. 223.1); concentration techniques rarely are needed. Sometimes,

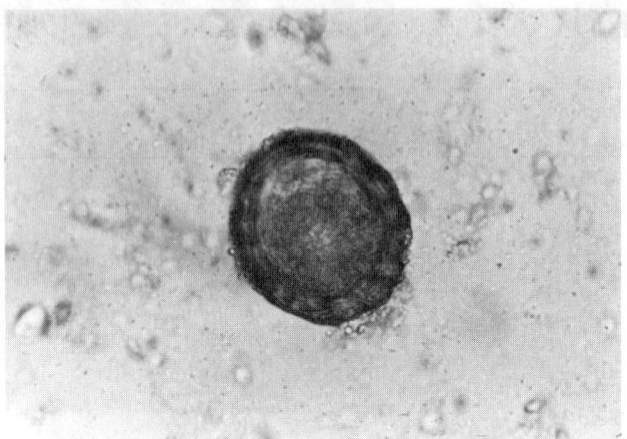

FIGURE 223.1. Eggs of *Ascaris lumbricoides* (×396) in freshly passed stool.

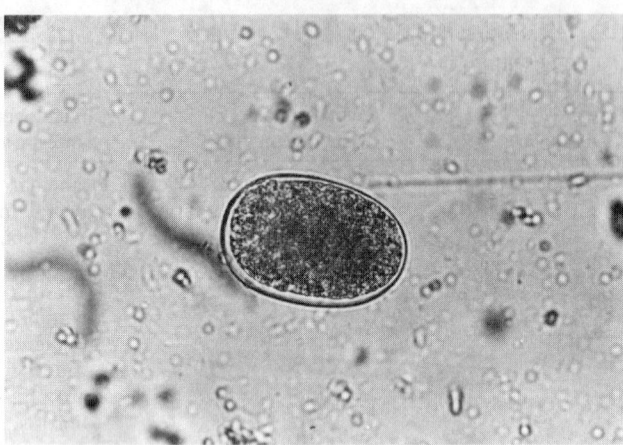

FIGURE 223.2. Hookworm ova (×396) in stool.

adult worms may be passed per rectum or, less commonly, coughed up through the mouth or nose. Eosinophilia is seen during the pulmonary migration phase of the larvae but might not be seen in uncomplicated intestinal infection.

Treatment

The recommended treatment for symptomatic or asymptomatic infection is pyrantel pamoate, 11 mg/kg, not to exceed 1 g, as a single dose; mebendazole in a fixed dose of 100 mg twice daily for 3 days or as a single dose of 500 mg; or albendazole in a single dose of 400 mg. Pyrantel pamoate and albendazole are approved drugs but considered investigational for this condition by the U.S. Food and Drug Administration (FDA). Experience with these drugs is limited in children younger than 2 years; nevertheless, these drugs do not seem to act differently in this age group as compared to older age groups.

In cases in which intestinal or biliary obstruction is suspected, piperazine citrate solution, 75 mg/kg/day, not to exceed 3.5 g, may be given through a gastrointestinal tube. Piperazine paralyzes the worms, allowing them to be passed by peristalsis without migrating into other sites. Piperazine is antagonistic to pyrantel pamoate, and the two should not be used together.

Hookworms

Infection with two species of hookworm, *Ancylostoma duodenale* and *Necator americanus*, affects approximately 1.2 billion people worldwide. Infection was prevalent in the southeastern United States until the 1930s, but transmission has since been reduced greatly, owing to eradication programs and improved sanitation; currently, most cases are imported. In developing countries, hookworm infection is a common cause of iron deficiency anemia and hypoproteinemia. More recently *A. caninum* has been reported as a cause of eosinophilic enteritis in northeastern Australia.

Life Cycle

Adult hookworms are cylindrical, grayish white, and approximately 1 cm long. They reside in the upper small intestine. The adult female worm may produce 9,000 to 30,000 eggs daily, which are passed in the feces. Under suitable soil conditions of temperature and humidity, the eggs hatch into larvae, molt, and become infective. Infective larvae penetrate exposed skin that comes into contact with contaminated soil, enter the venous circulation, and are carried to the lungs. In the lungs,

the larvae penetrate the alveoli, travel up the trachea, and are coughed up and swallowed. In the gastrointestinal tract, the larvae mature into adult worms that attach themselves to the jejunal mucosa, sucking minute quantities of blood. The worms change location every 4 to 8 hours, producing minute mucosal ulceration.

Clinical Features

An intense pruritus, erythema, and vesicular rash (ground itch) may develop at the site of the entry of the infective larvae. Passage through the lungs may cause Löffler syndrome–like effects, with cough, pulmonary infiltrates, and eosinophilia.

The intestinal phase of the infection results in epigastric pain, tenderness, and diarrhea. The major clinical manifestations of infection in children are anemia and hypoproteinemia as a result of chronic blood loss. The daily blood loss from a single adult worm is 0.16 to 0.34 mL for *A. duodenale* and 0.03 to 0.05 mL for *N. americanus*. Thus, moderate infection (100 to 500 worms) and severe infection (500 to 1,000 worms) can cause significant blood loss daily. Iron deficiency may lead to geophagia in young children, which in endemic areas may result in other nematode infection.

Diagnosis

The diagnosis is made by finding the characteristic ovoid eggs in the feces (Fig. 223.2). Direct examination of the feces is sufficient with egg counts of more than 1,200 per milliliter of feces; concentration techniques may be required for light infection.

Treatment

Mebendazole (100 mg twice daily for 3 days or 500 mg once) is the drug of choice. Albendazole (400 mg as a single dose) or pyrantel pamoate (11 mg/kg, not to exceed 1 g, for 3 days) also are effective; these drugs are approved but considered investigational for this indication by the U.S. FDA. Supplemental iron should be given for at least 3 months after the hemoglobin concentration reaches the threshold of 12 g/dL.

Trichuris trichiura (Whipworm)

Trichuriasis is among the common helminthic infections in humans, with an estimated 1 billion cases worldwide. Infection is most frequent in warm, humid regions. In the United States, trichuriasis is prevalent in the southeastern states. The normal habitat of *Trichuris trichiura* is the cecum and the ascending colon. The adult worms have a cylindrical body (mean length, 40 mm), with a thin whip-like anterior end that is anchored to the intestinal mucosa and a coiled thicker posterior end exposed to the lumen.

Life Cycle

The adult female worm daily produces approximately 13,000 eggs that are passed in the feces. The eggs mature in warm, moist soil in shady areas over a period of 3 weeks. Infection is acquired by the ingestion of the embryonate eggs. The larvae are released in the upper small intestine. Unlike other nematodes, *Trichuris* does not have the tissue migratory phase, and the complete development of the larvae to mature adult worms takes place during passage through the intestine.

Clinical Features

Most infections are asymptomatic. However, heavy infection (more than 1,000 worms) may cause severe colitis and proctitis presenting with abdominal pain, bloody diarrhea, and rectal prolapse. The clinical presentation may mimic Crohn disease. The worms also are known to suck minute quantities of blood (0.005 mL per worm per day), and heavy infections also may result in mild anemia.

Diagnosis

Demonstration of the characteristic lemon-shaped eggs in the stool establishes the diagnosis. Because eggs may be difficult to find in light infections, a concentration procedure is recommended.

Treatment

The drug of choice for the treatment of trichuriasis is mebendazole (100 mg twice daily for 3 days or 500 mg once, irrespective of age). A single dose of albendazole (400 mg) may be used for light and moderate infections, although a 3-day course is recommended for heavy infection.

Enterobius vermicularis

Enterobiasis, or pinworm, is the most common nematode infection in North America (an estimated 40 million persons infected) and Europe. Pinworm infections are most common in children and occur in all socioeconomic groups. Infection is more common in institutionalized children and within families. The adult worms are small (1 cm long) and thread-like and inhabit the cecum and adjacent gastrointestinal tract.

Life Cycle

The gravid adult female worms migrate at night to the perianal and perineal regions, where the eggs are deposited. The eggs embryonate within 6 hours and may be transferred to the clothes, bed linen, dust, and air. Infection occurs by ingestion of eggs, usually via the fingers contaminated from scratching or handling the contaminated clothes and bed linen. The larvae are released in the duodenum, molt twice, and mature into adult worms within 4 to 6 weeks.

Clinical Manifestations

Enterobiasis is asymptomatic in a large proportion of infected individuals. The most common presentation of infection is nocturnal perianal pruritus due to hypersensitivity to worm antigens. Migration of worms to the vulva and vagina may result in vaginal discharge and vulval pruritus. Rarely, migration of

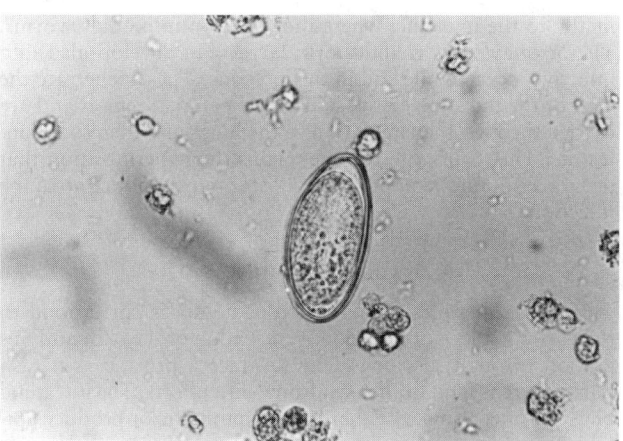

FIGURE 223.3. *Enterobius vermicularis* ova (×396) collected from the perianal skin.

the parasite may produce ectopic disease, such as appendicitis or salpingitis. Some anecdotal reports cite other symptoms, such as insomnia, irritability, weight loss, and bruxism, but no evidence substantiates a causal relationship of these symptoms to *Enterobius* infection.

Diagnosis

The characteristic ovoid eggs may be demonstrated by microscopical examination of cellophane tape applied to the perianal region in the early morning (Fig. 223.3); eggs usually are not seen in the feces on direct examination because of the low egg count.

Treatment

A single dose of pyrantel pamoate (11 mg/kg, not to exceed 1 g), mebendazole (100 mg), or albendazole (400 mg) is equally effective in eradicating the infection. Albendazole is approved but considered as investigational for this indication by the U.S. FDA. Treating all the members of the household is advisable, as several are likely to be infected, often without symptoms. Retreatment after 2 to 3 weeks may be administered to destroy adult worms that may have hatched from eggs swallowed around the time of the first treatment; none of the drugs destroys the eggs.

Strongyloides stercoralis

Although less common than other sources of nematode infection, *Strongyloides stercoralis* has the potential to cause overwhelming infection, particularly in immunosuppressed individuals. It is distributed widely throughout the world, particularly in the tropics, including the southeastern United States. The adult female worm is colorless and perhaps 2.2 mm long; the male worm is shorter (0.7 mm). The adult worms inhabit the upper small intestine.

Life Cycle

The life cycle of *S. stercoralis* is more complex than that of other nematodes. Mature female worms lay eggs that embryonate within the intestine and develop into rhabditiform larvae, which are deposited on the soil along with feces. In the soil, the larvae may develop either into free-living adult male or female larvae, which continue their existence in the soil, or into infective filariform larvae. The infective larvae penetrate the skin and enter the venous circulation and pass to the lungs and finally to the intestine, where they develop into adult worms. The *Strongyloides* rhabditiform larvae can develop also into infective larvae while still in the intestine. These penetrate the wall of the intestine or the skin of the perianal region and are carried through the circulation to the lungs and then to the intestine. This "autoinfection" explains the hyperinfection that occurs in immunocompromised hosts who cannot control the infection.

Clinical Features

The clinical manifestations of strongyloidiasis correspond to the various stages of infection. Penetration of the skin and migration through the lungs may produce a pruritic skin rash (larva currens) and Löffler syndrome–like effects. The intestinal phase of infection may either be asymptomatic or produce epigastric pain, vomiting, and diarrhea. In heavy infection, chronic malabsorption and weight loss may be seen. In immunocompromised individuals, including those infected with HIV, hyperinfection strongyloidiasis may be seen. Invasion of all tissues, including the central nervous system, may occur. In addition, penetration of the intestinal wall by filariform larvae may result in translocation of intestinal flora into the bloodstream, leading to sepsis.

Diagnosis

Diagnosis of strongyloidiasis depends on the demonstration of larvae in the feces or in the duodenal fluid. Sampling of duodenal contents is achieved by the use of the string test (Enterotest). Diagnosis of uncomplicated infection may be difficult, and repeated examination may be necessary. Eosinophilia (more than $500/\mu L$) is common. Larvae may be detected in the sputum of patients with disseminated infection.

Treatment

Ivermectin, 200 μg/kg/day for 1 to 2 days, is the drug of choice. An alternative is thiabendazole administered in a dose of 50 mg/kg/day (maximum 3 g per day) on 2 consecutive days.

CONTROL OF INTESTINAL NEMATODE INFECTIONS

Although intestinal nematode infections do not often cause acute illness or death, chronic infection causes considerable morbidity and economic hardship. Malnutrition in children and parasitic diseases have a strikingly similar geographic distribution. Animal experiments have established unequivocally that nutrition in all its forms is affected adversely by parasitic nematodes. Iron deficiency anemia is associated regularly with hookworm disease. Children with heavy *T. trichiura* infection have been shown to have impaired cognitive function. Many of these effects can be reversed with anthelminthic chemotherapy. Single oral doses of albendazole (400 mg) or mebendazole (500 mg) administered every 6 months have been shown to be effective in alleviating this morbidity. As schoolchildren have the most intense infection, which adversely affects their growth and school performance, they should be the targets for disease control. In areas where more than 25% of children are mildly to moderately underweight and parasites are known to be widespread, the children may be targeted for regular deworming programs. In highly endemic areas where more than 50% of the population is infected, mass treatment of the entire community is justified. The direct benefit of chemotherapy is that the worm burden is reduced, which immediately alleviates morbidity and may reduce transmission. Repeated doses keep the worm burden below the level at which it causes morbidity.

The epidemiology of intestinal nematode infections strongly suggests that infection produces natural protective immunity. This theory is supported by data from animal models showing that host responses can abbreviate infection, minimize reinfection, and stunt parasite growth and fecundity. Therefore, vaccines against intestinal nematode infections may provide an effective means for disease control. Although a few candidate vaccines have shown efficacy in animal models, none of them has reached the stage of human trials.

ABERRANT INFECTION WITH INTESTINAL NEMATODES

For a complete discussion of infection with *Toxocara canis*, see Chapter 224.

Cutaneous Larval Migrans (Creeping Eruptions)

Cutaneous larval migrans is caused most often by A. *braziliense* and less commonly by A. *caninum*, the dog and cat hookworms. The adult worms reside in the intestine and shed eggs that develop into larvae in the soil. Humans are infected by the larvae when they come in contact with contaminated soil (usually sandy beaches). Infection of humans with the larvae causes itching and typical serpiginous tracks that mark the route of migration of the parasite. Diagnosis is made clinically, and the parasite seldom is demonstrated in the lesions on biopsy. Treatment of choice is thiabendazole topically (10% to 15% aqueous suspension four times daily), ivermectin (200 μg/kg daily orally for 1 to 2 days), or albendazole (400 mg daily for 3 days); the latter two drugs are approved but considered investigational for this indication by the U.S. FDA.

Anisakiasis

Anisakiasis is caused by the accidental infections of humans with the larval stage of the *Anisakis* nematodes of saltwater fish and squid. Infection is acquired by the ingestion of raw or poorly cooked fish or squid. Two species associated most often with human infection are A. *simplex* and *Pseudoterranova decipiens*. Infection occurs worldwide but is more common in areas where fish is eaten raw (e.g., Japan, the Pacific coast of South America, and the Netherlands).

Clinical manifestations are caused by the penetration of the larvae into the stomach or small intestine, resulting in abdominal pain, nausea, and vomiting. Involvement of the lower small intestine may cause lower abdominal pain, mimicking appendicitis.

Diagnosis can be established by endoscopy and demonstration of the parasite in the stomach or by pathologic examination of the tissues. The symptoms are self-limited in most patients, but recovery is hastened by endoscopic removal of the parasite. Chemotherapy with mebendazole and albendazole has not been evaluated adequately.

Angiostrongylus cantonensis

Human infection with *Angiostrongylus cantonensis*, the rat lungworm, may result in invasion of the meninges by the larvae, causing meningitis with eosinophilic pleocytosis of the cerebrospinal fluid. The adult worms inhabit the lungs of rats, where eggs hatch and the larvae are swallowed and expelled in the feces. Further development takes place in mollusks, including snails, freshwater prawns, and crabs. Human infection occurs with ingestion of undercooked prawns, snails, or crabs. Signs and symptoms include headache, fever, and meningismus. Cranial nerve palsies may occur in a few patients. Severe infection can result in coma and death. Cerebrospinal fluid pleocytosis with eosinophilia that exceeds 10% is present in more than 95% of cases. Serologic tests based on enzyme-linked immunosorbent assay (ELISA) or Western blot have been used to detect antibodies to *A. cantonensis*. Most patients recover spontaneously. Treatment consists primarily of supportive measures aimed at reducing headache. Repeated lumbar punctures have been reported to produce symptomatic relief for patients with persistent headache. No drug is proven to be effective and some patients given thiabendazole, mebendazole, albendazole, or ivermectin have worsened as a result of severe host reaction to dying larvae.

TISSUE NEMATODES

Bancroftian and Brugian Filariasis

Bancroftian and brugian filariasis are clinically similar conditions caused by *Wuchereria bancrofti* and *Brugia malayi*, respectively. The total number of cases (infection and chronic disease) due to *W. bancrofti* worldwide is estimated to be 120 million. Ninety percent of cases are caused by *W. bancrofti*. The remainder of cases are caused by *B. malayi*, which is seen mainly in South and East Asia, especially India, Malaysia, Indonesia, the Philippines, and China. The largest number of cases occur in the age group of 15 to 44 years. However, 16.5 million cases of *W. bancrofti* infection and 2 million cases of *B. malayi* infection occur in children younger than age 15 years.

Life Cycle

Infection is acquired through the bite of an infected anopheline mosquito. The infective larvae pass into the lymphatic system, where they mature into thread-like adult worms; the male and female worms are 40 mm long and 100 mm long, respectively. The fertilized female larvae liberate microfilariae into the lymphatics. The microfilariae enter the bloodstream, usually in a surge during the nighttime, and are ingested by mosquitoes. The microfilaria mature into infective larvae in the mosquito, completing the cycle.

Clinical Manifestations

In endemic areas, a sizable proportion of the population may have microfilaremia without having any symptoms. The adult parasite worm induces dilation and proliferation of the lymphatic endothelium, which is associated with lymphatic dysfunction. In addition, inflammation, either due to a host immune response to the dying parasite or due to secondary bacterial or fungal infection, may occur. Usually, symptoms are caused by acute inflammation resulting in lymphangitis (presenting as painful cord-like swellings with reddish streaks on the overlying skin), lymphadenitis, acute epididymitis, orchitis or funiculitis, or lymphatic obstruction with lymphedema or hydrocele. In elephantiasis, the skin overlying the area of lymphedema becomes thick and warty (Fig. 223.4). Rupture of distended lymphatics into the peritoneal cavity or into the urinary tract results in chylous ascites and chyluria, respectively. Another filarial syndrome described in expatriate visitors to endemic regions consists of lymphangitis, lymphadenitis, and genital pain. Though the syndromes described above are mainly seen in adolescents and adults, lymphatic filariasis is often acquired in childhood. Initial damage to the lymphatic system remains subclinical or gives rise only to nonspecific presentations of adenitis/adenopathy and presents after puberty with the characteristic features of adult disease syndromes.

Diagnosis

Diagnosis is established by the demonstration of microfilaria in stained smears of blood, urine (in chyluria), or hydrocele fluid. Concentration techniques may be necessary when low microfilarial densities are suspected. Assays to detect circulating filarial antigen are now available and are regarded as the gold standard for diagnosing *W. bancrofti* infection. These assays are very specific and more sensitive than microscopy, but they do not detect *B. malayi*. Many lymphatic filariasis patients are amicrofilaremic and diagnosis may have to be made clinically.

Treatment

Diethylcarbamazine is the drug of choice for the treatment of filariasis in children. It is administered in a dose of 6 mg/kg/day in two to three divided doses for 12 to 14 days (for *W. bancrofti*) or 3 to 6 mg/kg/day in divided doses for 6 to 12 days (for *B. malayi*). For the chronic manifestations of lymphatic filariasis, such as hydrocele and elephantiasis, surgical treatment may be required. Intensive efforts to improve local hygiene and the use of antibiotic ointments decrease the frequency of recurrent

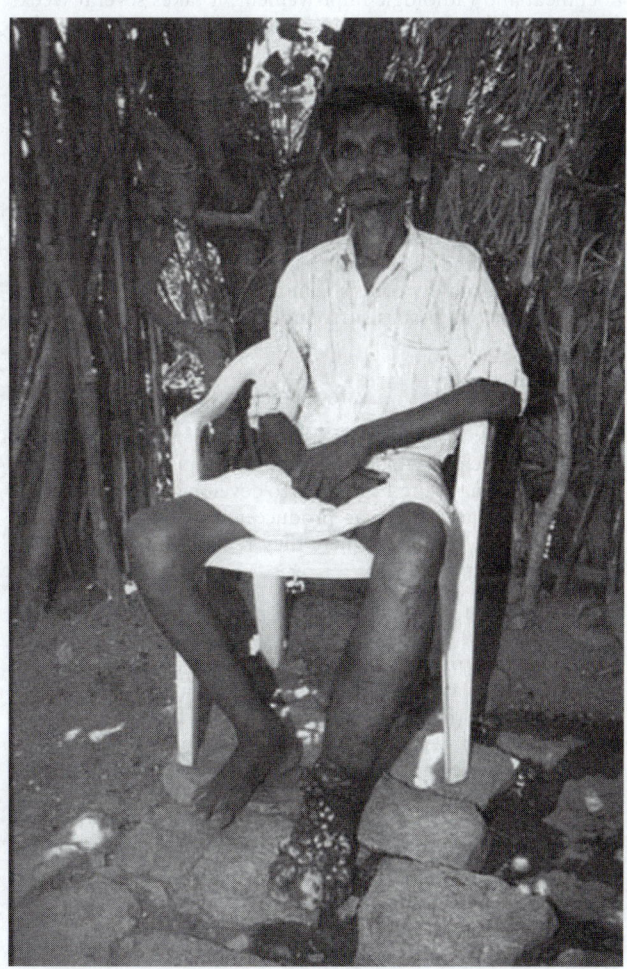

FIGURE 223.4. An elderly man with lymphatic filariasis. Available at: http://www9.who.int/tropical_diseases/databases/imagelib.pl?imageid=01021881.

infection episodes in patients with elephantiasis. Patients with chyluria require nutritional support.

Control

The two methods used for filariasis control include vector control and systematic individual or community chemotherapy. Vector control may be achieved by indoor spraying of houses with insecticides, use of mosquito net impregnated with pyrethroids, and larval control of mosquito breeding sites. Achieving such control is difficult in most endemic areas. The other option is to use yearly mass treatment to at-risk populations with a single-dose, two-drug regimen, selecting among albendazole and either ivermectin or diethylcarbamazine.

Tropical Pulmonary Eosinophilia

Tropical pulmonary eosinophilia is a syndrome caused by an immunologic hyperresponsiveness to *W. bancrofti* or *B. malayi*, especially in the lungs. The disease presents with dry nocturnal cough and wheezing. In some patients, low-grade fever, hepatomegaly, and lymphadenopathy also may occur. Striking eosinophilia is seen in the peripheral blood, and absolute eosinophil counts generally are in excess of 4,000 cells per cubic millimeter. Chest roentgenograms show diffuse reticulonodular opacities or a ground-glass appearance of the lungs; typically, the lung apices are spared. Treatment with diethylcarbamazine, 10 mg/kg/day in three divided doses for 2 to 3 weeks, results in clinical and radiologic improvement; it takes several weeks for eosinophil counts to return to normal levels.

Onchocerciasis (River Blindness)

Onchocerca volvulus is endemic mainly to West and Central Africa where 99% of infected people live, with isolated foci in Latin America and Yemen. It is estimated that 18 million people, 99% of whom are in Africa, are infected worldwide; 270,000 are blind. The adult female worm is 400 mm long, and the adult male worm is 3 mm. The worms are found in the subcutaneous tissues surrounded by characteristic fibrous nodules.

Life Cycle

Infection is transmitted by the bite of female blackflies (*Simulium* species), which breed along rivers and streams. Infective larvae may take 12 months to develop into adult worms. The fertilized female larvae produce unsheathed microfilaria that migrate to the skin, where they remain until they are ingested by biting blackflies.

Clinical Manifestations

Early infection produces an erythematous, papular rash. Severe infection is associated with lymphedema and depigmentation of the skin (leopard skin) (Fig. 223.5). The skin may lose its elasticity and, with chronic lymphadenopathy, gives rise to pedunculus sacs, particularly in the inguinal region (hanging groin). Adult worms in the subcutaneous tissue produce firm, mobile, nontender nodules located mainly over bony prominences. Microfilaria in the eyes may give rise to iridocyclitis, chorioretinitis, optic atrophy, and, ultimately, corneal fibrosis and blindness.

Diagnosis

Diagnosis is established by demonstration of microfilariae in skin snips or in the eye by slit lamp examination. Adult worms can be identified in excised nodules.

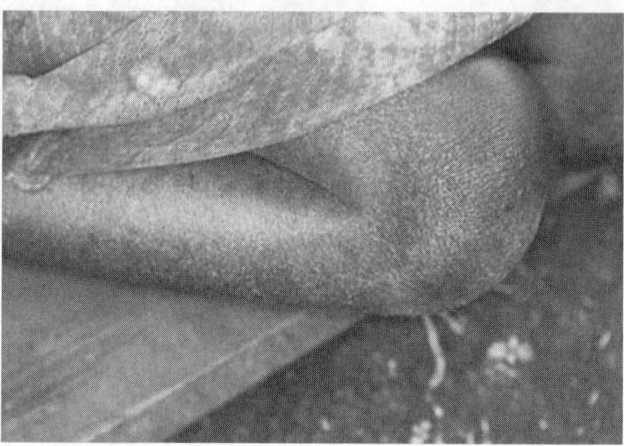

FIGURE 223.5. An 18-year-old girl with onchocercal dermatitis with leopard skin. Available at: http://www9.who.int/tropical_diseases/databases/imagelib.pl?imageid=01032071.

Treatment

Diethylcarbamazine no longer is the drug of choice for onchocerciasis because of the frequency with which it causes severe host (Mazzotti) reaction. The current drug of choice is ivermectin. This drug kills microfilariae but not the adult worm. However, a dose of 150 μg/kg repeated every 3 months will suppress the disease to a degree that will avoid complications. Surgical excision of nodules on the head, especially in children, may reduce the risk of blindness. *Wolbachia* are bacterial symbionts of filaria, including *Onchocercus volvulus*, and are essential for the fertility of their nematode hosts. Antibiotics targeted at *Wolbachia* have been shown to disrupt the embryogenesis of the female worm and result in prolonged absence of microfilaremia. In addition, recent studies have shown that *Wolbachia* are major contributors to the immunopathology of onchocerciasis. Doxycycline 100 mg daily for 6 weeks or 200 mg daily for 4 weeks results in depletion of *Wolbachia* and may be an important addition to the treatment and control of onchocerciasis.

Control

Control is achieved mainly from reduction of the vector population at the breeding sites. Such control is achieved by spraying insecticides and by teaching communities at risk how to avoid contact with blackflies.

Trichinosis

Of the five recognized species of *Trichinella*, *T. spiralis* is responsible for most human infection. *T. spiralis* is ubiquitous in its distribution and infects a wide variety of domestic and wild animals worldwide. Adult worms are small, with the females measuring 2 to 4 mm and the males 1.0 to 1.5 mm.

Life Cycles

Trichinosis is acquired by ingestion of animal muscle containing the encysted larvae. In the intestine, larvae are liberated from the cysts and enter the columnar epithelium of the intestine, where they mature into adults. The fertilized female adult worm produces larvae that enter the bloodstream and are disseminated throughout the body. On reaching the striated muscle, the larvae enter individual muscle cells, which transform into nurse cells. In a few weeks, the larvae become infective, and the nurse cells become thick-walled capsules (cysts).

Clinical Manifestations

Symptoms may be related to the intestinal, muscle invasion, and convalescent stages of infection. The intestinal phase of the infection starts 1 to 7 days after ingestion of infected meat and consists of abdominal pain, nausea, vomiting, and malaise. The muscle invasion phase occurs in the second week and may last 1 to 5 weeks or longer. It is characterized by eyelid edema, myalgia, weakness, fever, and eosinophilia. Less commonly encountered symptoms include headache, facial flushing, urticaria, profuse sweating, conjunctivitis, hoarseness, dyspnea, and dysphagia.

Diagnosis

Diagnosis is based on the clinical manifestations, history of ingestion of potentially infected meat, and demonstration of the parasite on muscle biopsy. Serologic tests are available but are not positive until the third week of infection. Antigen detection assays are available, and molecular diagnostic methods are under development.

Treatment

All cases of confirmed or suspected trichinosis should be treated to prevent the continued production of larvae. Mebendazole (200 to 400 mg three time daily for 3 days, then 400 to 500 mg three time daily for 10 days) or albendazole (400 mg twice daily for 8 to 14 days) is effective. Concomitant administration of prednisolone may be required to reduce the allergic and inflammatory symptoms.

Control

Control is achieved by inspection of carcasses and thorough cooking of pork and game. Freezing at $-30°C$ for 24 hours also kills the larvae.

Dracunculiasis (Guinea Worm Infection)

Dracunculiasis (or guinea worm infection) is caused by *Dracunculus medinensis*, the largest known nematode parasite in humans (60 to 100 cm). The areas currently endemic for dracunculiasis are all located in sub-Saharan Africa. About 75,000 cases were reported in 2000, of which 73% were in Sudan.

Life Cycle

Infection is acquired by drinking water containing infective larvae developing within the bodies of the crustacean intermediate host (*Cyclops* species). The larvae are released in the stomach, from whence they pass into the intestine, penetrate the mucosa, and migrate to the retroperitoneal space; here, they mature into adult worms. The fertilized female worm migrates to the subcutaneous tissues, usually of the legs. The overlying skin ulcerates, and a portion of the worm protrudes. On contact with water, large numbers of larvae are released and are ingested by crustaceans, wherein further maturation to infective larvae takes place, completing the cycle.

Clinical Manifestations

Infection is asymptomatic until the female worm reaches the subcutaneous tissues. A painful papule develops over the site. Fever, nausea, vomiting, diarrhea, dyspnea, urticaria, and eosinophilia may precede or accompany blistering of the skin. A painful ulcer develops, through which the worm protrudes. Larvae are discharged intermittently over the next few weeks, after which the worm gradually is extruded or absorbed and the ulcer heals. Multiple ulcers are common. Secondary bacterial infection of the ulcers or tetanus may occur.

Diagnosis

The clinical picture is characteristic. Larvae may be demonstrated in the discharge from the ulcer.

Treatment

Metronidazole (25 mg/kg/day; maximum 750 mg in three divided doses for 10 days) provides symptomatic relief and weakens the anchorage of the worms in the subcutaneous tissues, facilitating removal.

Suggested Readings

Intestinal Nematodes

Anonymous. Drugs for parasitic infections [Online]. *Med Lett Drugs Ther* 2002; April. Available at: http://www.medletter.com/freedocs/parasitic.pdf.

Crompton DW. How much human helminthiasis is there in the world? *J Parasitol* 1999;85:397.

Crompton DW. Ascaris and ascariasis [Review] [160 refs]. *Adv Parasitol* 2001; 48:285.

Crompton DW, Nesheim MC. Nutritional impact of intestinal helminthiasis during the human life cycle [Review] [129 refs]. *Annu Rev Nutr* 2002;22:35.

Centers for Disease Control and Prevention, Division of Parasitic Diseases. *Parasite image library.* Available at: http://www.dpd.cdc.gov/dpdx/HTML/Image_Library.htm.

de Silva NR. Impact of mass chemotherapy on the morbidity due to soil-transmitted nematodes. *Acta Tropica* 2003;86:197.

Fincham JE, Markus MB, Adams VJ. Could control of soil-transmitted helminthic infection influence the HIV/AIDS epidemic. *Acta Tropica* 2003; 86:315.

Koontz F, Weinstock JV. The approach to stool examination for parasites. *Gastroenterol Clin North Am* 1996;25:435.

Mahmoud AAF. Strongyloidiasis. *Clin Infect Dis* 1996;23:949.

Montressor A, Crompton DW, Gyorkos TW, Savioli L. *Helminth control in school age children.* Geneva: World Health Organization, 2002.

Ottensen EA, Nutman TB. Tropical pulmonary eosinophilia. *Annu Rev Med* 1992;43:417.

Ottesen EA, Ismail MM, Horton J. The role of albendazole in programmes to eliminate lymphatic filariasis. *Parasitol Today* 1999;15:382.

CHAPTER 224 ■ *TOXOCARA* INFECTIONS

B. KEITH ENGLISH

Human infection with the larval stage of the common dog roundworm, *Toxocara canis*, is the principal cause of two distinct clinical syndromes: visceral larva migrans (VLM) and ocular toxocariasis or ocular larva migrans (OLM). Most *Toxocara* infections occur in young children, and although infections most result in mild or inapparent disease, serious complications may occur. Humans do not act as a definitive host for these nematodes, but the larvae may migrate throughout the tissues and may provoke an eosinophilic inflammatory response that can result in striking symptoms and laboratory findings.

EPIDEMIOLOGY AND TRANSMISSION

T. canis, a nematode roundworm of the family Ascaridia, is a cosmopolitan parasite, infecting dogs (and other canids) in all tropical and temperate regions of the world. Toxocariasis in domestic dogs is prevalent almost uniformly in North America south of latitude 60 degrees north and has been reported in all 50 states. The adult worms reside in the proximal small intestine of dogs (the definitive hosts) and live for an average of 4 months. Adult female worms may produce 200,000 eggs/day; eggs passed in feces are not embryonate and thus are not infective. Depending on soil composition, temperature, and humidity, the eggs become infective in 2 to 5 weeks.

In adult dogs, embryonate eggs containing second-stage larvae hatch in the stomach and small intestine, penetrate the intestinal mucosa, travel via the portal circulation to the liver, then enter the systemic circulation, reaching the heart and lungs 3 to 5 days after infection (Box 224.1). Some larvae penetrate the bronchioles, travel to the trachea and pharynx, are swal-

lowed, and develop into adult worms in the small intestine. Other larvae invade the pulmonary vein, travel back to the heart, and spread via the systemic circulation throughout the body. In puppies, the tracheal route predominates, accounting for their importance in the transmission of disease to other hosts.

In humans and paratenic hosts (including mice, rats, lambs, and pigs), the tracheal route of migration leading to the development of adult worms does not occur. Larvae do travel to the liver via the portal circulation and to the systemic circulation via the lungs, however, and they lodge in small blood vessels in somatic organs. The larvae then bore through the walls of the blood vessels and migrate through the tissues. As in dogs, most of these larvae become dormant but may remain viable for many years.

Nearly all human toxocaral infections occur by ingestion of infective eggs from soil that is contaminated with excreta from puppies or from contaminated hands or fomites. Ingestion of uncooked organ and muscle meat from paratenic hosts (pigs, lambs, rabbits, snails, and, perhaps, chickens) is a documented (but uncommon) source of human infection. Pica for dirt (geophagia) is the principal risk factor for VLM in children and adults. Because embryonization requires more than 2 weeks, direct transmission from infected dogs presumably is uncommon. Therefore, frequent exposure to dogs (e.g., by veterinarians) alone is insufficient to predict an increased likelihood of *T. canis* infection. Although puppy ownership is associated with a higher incidence of *T. canis* infection, ample exposure may occur in children without a household dog: 10% to 30% of soil samples from public parks, sandboxes, and backyards are contaminated with *T. canis* eggs, which may survive for years.

Seroprevalence studies using an enzyme-linked immunosorbent assay (ELISA) for antibodies to *T. canis* have revealed that 4.6% to 7.3% of kindergarten children from different regions of the United States have been infected. Seroprevalence rates are higher in African Americans than in whites. For both African Americans and whites, seroprevalence rates increase with rural residence, crowding, and lower socioeconomic status. In some rural populations in the southeastern United States, seroprevalence rates exceeding 20% have been reported. A positive ELISA for *T. canis* also is associated with epilepsy, yet children with epilepsy of undefined origin do not have seroprevalence rates higher than those in children with epilepsy of known cause. This finding suggests that epilepsy is a risk factor for the acquisition of *T. canis* (e.g., through pica) rather than vice versa.

The epidemiologic features of VLM and OLM are strikingly different. Although both are associated with exposure to puppies, only VLM is associated clearly with pica. Patients with VLM usually are 1 to 4 years old, whereas patients with OLM have a mean age of 7 to 8 years. Most patients with OLM have no history of a syndrome similar to VLM, although ocular involvement may occur concomitantly with VLM, especially in very young children with severe disease or many years after VLM.

BOX 224.1   **Acquisition of *Toxocara canis* in Dogs**

Dogs may acquire *Toxocara canis* infection in five ways:

- Transplacental migration of larvae (the most important method of transmission, resulting in prenatal infection of almost 100% of puppies born to infected mothers)
- Transmammary passage of larvae to nursing pups in milk
- Ingestion of infective eggs
- Ingestion of larvae in tissues of paratenic hosts (see later)
- Ingestion of late-stage larvae or immature adult worms in vomitus or feces of infected pups

PATHOGENESIS

The clinical and pathologic features of *T. canis* infection in patients with VLM and OLM reflect primarily the brisk inflammatory response of the host, although the migrating larvae may cause direct tissue damage. Dead or dying larvae provoke a particularly intense inflammatory response. As described in the initial report linking *T. canis* larvae with VLM, the characteristic pathologic lesions are eosinophilic granulomas that surround larvae in various stages of disintegration; in advanced lesions, no evidence of the larvae remains. Most often in humans, the liver is the site of greatest involvement, but involvement of the lungs also is frequent. Eye involvement is an important complication of *T. canis* infection and occurs in many different forms. Although they are less common, larval infections of the myocardium, brain, pancreas, skin, kidney, intestine, and regional lymph nodes have been reported.

The contrasting epidemiology of VLM and OLM led Glickman to hypothesize that the dose of the organism ingested could determine whether VLM, ocular involvement, both, or neither developed in the patient. In this model, the ingestion of a few larvae would result in initially asymptomatic infection but could result in ocular disease in some cases. The ingestion of a moderate number of larvae could result in VLM because of a more dramatic inflammatory response; these patients would have a low risk of subsequent ocular involvement if the inflammatory response could prevent migration of larvae to the eye. Finally, ingestion of very many larvae could overwhelm the immune response, resulting in concomitant VLM and ocular disease; these patients would be at higher risk for larval infection of other sites (e.g., brain, myocardium) as well. Although there is some experimental support for features of this model, it remains largely speculative. Three human research subjects given a single dose of 100 to 200 larvae had no clinical evidence of disease but did develop moderate eosinophilia. It is also possible that certain *T. canis* strains exhibit tropism for ocular or visceral migration.

Experimental infection of paratenic hosts (including mice, rabbits, and the Japanese quail) with embryonate eggs of *T. canis* has provided important information regarding the pathogenesis of *Toxocara* infections. These studies have confirmed the importance of the host immune response in the development of tissue injury in this disease. Studies in mice (and *in vitro* studies of human T lymphocytes) indicate that the T-cell response to *Toxocara* infection is mediated primarily by cells of the helper-2 T-cell phenotype. Production of the cytokine interleukin-5 (IL-5) by helper-2 T cells appears to be the critical step in the development of eosinophilia during experimental *Toxocara* infection, and mice genetically deficient in IL-5 fail to develop eosinophilia after challenge with *T. canis*. Compared with control animals, IL-5–deficient mice exhibit no difference in tissue parasite burden after infection with the embryonate eggs of *T. canis*, yet they develop less extensive pulmonary damage.

CLINICAL FEATURES

Visceral Larva Migrans

The classic manifestations of VLM reflected the fact that only clinical diagnosis of *T. canis* infection was possible; fever, hepatomegaly, eosinophilic leukocytosis, and hypergammaglobulinemia defined the syndrome. Many affected patients also had pulmonary involvement (rales or wheezes) and rashes (often pruritic). Seizures were reported in more than 25% of patients in one early series. Most *T. canis* infections in children now are understood to be asymptomatic, and only a few symptomatic infections result in the full-blown VLM syndrome. The use of improved serologic tests should better define the clinical characteristics of less severe cases of VLM.

Hepatomegaly remains a common sign in VLM, and toxocariasis is one of the causes of granulomatous hepatitis. However, the most common symptoms of VLM are pulmonary and often mimic those of asthma or pneumonia. Chest radiographs demonstrate infiltrates in one-half of the patients with pulmonary symptoms and may reveal a nodular pattern. Severe lung disease is uncommon, but life-threatening pneumonitis with or without pleural effusions has been reported. *Toxocara* infection must be considered in the differential diagnosis of any patient with pneumonia and marked eosinophilia. Fever, generalized adenopathy, rash (often urticarial), and weight loss may occur. Ocular disease is unusual in association with VLM but may occur in severe cases. Unusual presentations of VLM that have been described include eosinophilic ascites and gastroenteritis, generalized lymphadenopathy, lymphedema, encephalitis, and myelitis. Long-term exposure to migrating *Toxocara* larvae also may result in more subtle clinical manifestations ("covert toxocariasis"), but high rates of *T. canis* seroprevalence (see earlier) make it difficult to determine whether nonspecific symptoms associated with a positive serologic test are related to *Toxocara* infection.

Leukocyte counts of 30,000 to 100,000/mm³ with pronounced eosinophilia are common in patients with VLM. The percentage of eosinophils usually is greater than 20% in acute cases and may reach 90%; eosinophilia often persists for months or years after symptoms resolve. Hypergammaglobulinemia often is present, with elevations of immunoglobulin E (IgE), IgM, and IgG. Isohemagglutinin titers (anti-A, anti-B) often are elevated because the *T. canis* larva expresses surface antigens that cross-react with epitopes of the blood group antigens.

The prognosis in most cases of VLM is excellent, complete recovery being the rule. Severe and even fatal cases have been reported, however. Myocardial involvement is rare but has been reported in several fatal cases and as an incidental finding at the time of open heart surgery in two patients. *T. canis* may cause eosinophilic meningitis; larvae have been found in the brain at autopsy in children with fatal infection and incidentally in children with unrelated causes of death. Although seizures may occur in VLM, this complication appears to be much less frequent than early reports suggested. The effects of asymptomatic and mild infection are largely unknown. Both a large cohort study and a large case-control study found small deficits in performance on neuropsychiatric tests in seropositive children as compared with seronegative controls. In the cohort study, confounding variables appeared to explain these differences; in the case-control study, small differences between seropositive and seronegative children remained after careful adjustment for potential confounding factors. Considering the frequency of *T. canis* infection in children, more careful study of the neurologic consequences of *Toxocara* infections is merited.

Ocular Toxocariasis

Extensive reviews of OLM have been published. Ocular involvement by nematode larvae first was reported in 1950 and in 1956 was shown to be caused by *T. canis*. Various clinical patterns have emerged, none of which is pathognomonic. OLM usually occurs in young school-aged children (mean age, 7 to 8 years), but it may occur in adults and infants. A history of pica frequently is not present, and eosinophilia is uncommon.

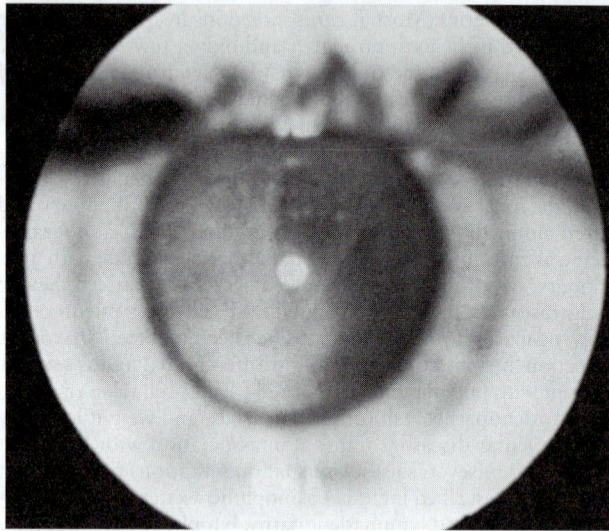

FIGURE 224.1. Pupillary view of retinal detachment in a patient with presumed toxocariasis and endophthalmitis. (Reprinted from Giles CL, Capone Jr A, Joshi MM. Uveitis in Children. In: Nelson LB, Olitsky SE, eds. *Harley's pediatric ophthalmology*, 5th ed. Philadelphia: Lippincott Williams & Wilkins, 2005:319.)

Usually, only one eye is involved, but bilateral disease has been reported. Patients commonly complain of decreased visual acuity.

Three clinical patterns are recognized most frequently. The best-known and perhaps most frequent pattern is *Toxocara* endophthalmitis, which is characterized by a yellow-white mass, retinal detachment, and cells in the vitreous; these features are shared by retinoblastoma, and clinically differentiating between the two disorders is often difficult (Fig. 224.1). A feared complication of this condition is the formation of a cyclitic membrane, which may lead to complete vision loss. The other two syndromes often recognized as consequences of *T. canis* ocular disease are posterior retinochoroiditis, which usually occurs in older children or adults, and peripheral retinochoroiditis, which may mimic pars planitis and may cause traction on the retina, resulting in retinal folds, which once were thought to be a congenital malformation. Other clinical patterns include optic papillitis, diffuse unilateral subacute neuroretinitis, the motile chorioretinal nematode syndrome (so-called OLM), keratitis, conjunctivitis, and lens involvement.

DIFFERENTIAL DIAGNOSIS

T. canis is the cause of most human cases of VLM and OLM, but other animal roundworms, including *T. cati* (cats), *Toxascaris leonina* (dogs and cats), and *Baylisascaris procyonis* (raccoons) occasionally may cause both VLM and OLM. Infection with other nematodes whose life cycle includes a tissue migratory phase (e.g., *Strongyloides stercoralis*, *Ascaris lumbricoides*, *Trichinella*, hookworms, and schistosomes) may cause marked eosinophilia and may mimic toxocaral VLM. Eosinophilic leukemia may be considered in some patients with severe eosinophilia. The eosinophilia associated with *T. canis* infection may persist for months or years, and it occurs in asymptomatic infected patients. Thus, silent or preceding *T. canis* infection should be considered in the differential diagnosis of unexplained persistent eosinophilia.

The differential diagnosis of OLM is broad and depends on the clinical pattern. The most difficult and important problem for the ophthalmologist is the distinction between *T. canis*

endophthalmitis and retinoblastoma. Although retinoblastoma more frequently is bilateral (30% versus a few case reports) and calcified (commonly versus rarely) than OLM, enough overlap exists to render these features unreliable. *Toxocara* endophthalmitis usually is not associated with much pain or photophobia. *T. canis* is one of several causes of pseudoretinoblastoma; others include Coats disease (retinal telangiectasia with exudation), persistent hyperplastic primary vitreous, retinopathy of prematurity, and ocular toxoplasmosis.

Although a presumptive diagnosis of VLM can be supported by abnormalities on a variety of laboratory tests (eosinophilia, hypergammaglobulinemia, elevated isohemagglutinin levels), such tests are nonspecific and usually are normal in cases of ocular disease. Various immunologic tests have been developed over the years but historically were largely unsuccessful, presumably because they used antigen prepared from adult worms.

The development of ELISA tests using antigen purified from larval forms of *T. canis* has greatly improved the diagnosis of *T. canis* infections. The *Toxocara* excretory-secretory (TES) ELISA uses an excretory or secretory antigen from the supernatants of *T. canis* larvae maintained *in vitro*. The TES ELISA has proved to be a sensitive and specific test in the diagnosis of VLM, and it appears to be useful in the diagnosis of OLM as well. *T. canis* can be distinguished from *T. cati* and other animal toxocarids by serologic methods and by use of the polymerase chain reaction.

For the diagnosis of VLM, the TES ELISA is superior to older methods. The reported sensitivity and specificity of the ELISA (for which a titer of 1:32 or greater is considered indicative of infection) are 78% and 92%, respectively. These figures compare with sensitivities of only 18% to 26% for the previously used indirect hemagglutination and bentonite flocculation tests; the former tests also were more than 90% specific. Laboratories performing the TES ELISA should provide, along with the results, guidelines for interpreting a specific titer.

The serologic diagnosis of OLM remains problematic. In ocular disease, TES ELISA titers usually are lower than are those in VLM. If a titer greater than 1:8 is considered indicative of infection, the ELISA has been reported to be 90% sensitive and 91% specific. Several false-negative results have been reported, however. Elevated titers in the absence of disease or false-positive results (representing asymptomatic *T. canis* infection in association with ocular disease of another origin) also would be expected to occur, especially in patients from groups with a high seroprevalence. Aspiration of aqueous humor or vitreous humor in affected patients may confirm the diagnosis by allowing the demonstration of antibody to *T. canis* in these fluids by ELISA, and positive results have been reported in the presence of a negative serum ELISA result. Although the procedure is invasive, aspiration of the aqueous humor may be considered in a patient in whom enucleation of the eye for possible retinoblastoma is planned. Use of the polymerase chain reaction technique to detect toxocaral nucleic acids in tissue specimens may prove useful in the future. Imaging techniques (e.g., ultrasonography and computed tomography) have been used to characterize *T. canis* ocular lesions but do not appear to distinguish these lesions clearly from other diagnoses, including retinoblastoma.

TREATMENT

Discussion of potential therapy of VLM or OLM must begin with consideration of the prognosis of untreated disease. The overall prognosis for VLM is excellent. Even in more severe cases, removal of the patient from the source of exposure usually is adequate to effect satisfactory recovery. Pharmacologic treatment of VLM should be considered when severe symptoms occur (e.g., severe respiratory distress) or when involvement of critical organs (myocardium, brain) is noted. In these situations, the use of corticosteroids may be indicated and has been reported to result in dramatic improvement of symptoms. The efficacy of antihelmintic drugs in the treatment of VLM remains uncertain, but many authorities recommend the use of these agents. The Committee on Infectious Diseases of the American Academy of Pediatrics recommends treatment with either albendazole or mebendazole.

The prognosis of OLM is more guarded and depends on the clinical pattern. Any child with known or suspected OLM should be referred promptly to an ophthalmologist experienced in the diagnosis and treatment of this condition. Steroids have proved beneficial in severe vision-threatening forms of this disease, and early surgery may prevent some of the complications. Laser photocoagulation may be used to eradicate meandering larvae if other attempts to remove the larvae fail. Anthelmintic agents have not been demonstrated to be effective and should be used cautiously, if at all, in the treatment of *T. canis* ocular infection.

PREVENTION

Newborn puppies are the principal source of infection in young children. All newborn puppies should be wormed before they reach 2 to 3 weeks of age, and worming should be repeated every 2 weeks until the puppy is 4 months old. Thereafter, fecal examinations should be performed twice yearly, with treatment as indicated. Scoop laws are of some benefit, because eggs that are not embryonate require 2 weeks or more to become infective. Pica should be discouraged, and good hygiene should be practiced. For young children with persistent pica, close supervision is recommended when they play outdoors in parks, backyards, or sandboxes.

Once soil is contaminated with *T. canis* eggs, it cannot be decontaminated. Efforts to prevent transplacental and trans-

mammary transmission of *T. canis* to puppies have been largely unsuccessful. Thus, efforts to prevent human toxocariasis must focus on a reduction in the environmental load of *T. canis* eggs by ensuring the early and regular treatment of puppies.

Suggested Readings

American Academy of Pediatrics. Toxocariasis. In: Pickering LK, ed. *Redbook: 2003 report of the Committee on Infectious Diseases,* 26th ed. Elk Grove Village, IL: American Academy of Pediatrics; 2003:630.

Beaver PC, Snyder CH, Carrera GM, et al. Chronic eosinophilia due to visceral larva migrans. *Pediatrics* 1952;9:7.

Del Prete GF, De Carli M, Mastromauro C, et al. Purified protein derivative of mycobacterium tuberculosis and excretory-secretory antigen(s) of *Toxocara canis* expand in vitro human T cells with stable and opposite (type 1 T helper or type 2 T helper) profile of cytokine production. *J Clin Invest* 1991;88: 346.

Despommier D. Toxocariasis: clinical aspects, epidemiology, medical ecology, and molecular aspects. *Clin Microbiol Rev* 2003;16:265.

Glickman LT, Magnaval JF. Zoonotic roundworm infections. *Infect Dis Clin North Am* 1993;7:717.

Glickman LT, Schantz PM. Epidemiology and pathogenesis of zoonotic toxocariasis. *Epidemiol Rev* 1981;3:230.

Jacobs DE, Zhu X, Gasser RB, et al. PCR-based methods for identification of potentially zoonotic ascaridoid parasites of the dog, fox and cat. *Acta Trop* 1997;68:191.

Marmor M, Glickman L, Shofer F, et al. *Toxocara canis* infection of children: epidemiologic and neuropsychologic findings. *Am J Public Health* 1987;77:554.

Schantz PM, Glickman LT. Current concepts in parasitology: toxocaral visceral larva migrans. *N Engl J Med* 1978;298:436.

Shields JA. Ocular toxocariasis: a review. *Surv Ophthalmol* 1984;28:361.

Takamoto M, Ovington KS, Behm CA, et al. Eosinophilia, parasite burden and lung damage in *Toxocara canis* infection in C57Bl/6 mice genetically deficient in IL-5. *Immunology* 1997;90:511.

Worley G, Green JA, Frothingham TE, et al. *Toxocara canis* infection: clinical and epidemiological associations with seropositivity in kindergarten children. *J Infect Dis* 1984;149:591.

Yamaguchi Y, Matsui T, Kasahara T, et al. *In vivo* changes of hemopoietic progenitors and the expression of the interleukin 5 gene in eosinophilic mice infected with *Toxocara canis. Exp Hematol* 1990;18:1152.

CHAPTER 225 ■ THE CESTODES

THOMAS CHERIAN

Human cestode infections may be caused either by the adult tapeworms residing in the intestinal lumen or by the larval forms that infect the tissues. Intestinal forms are acquired by ingestion of the larval forms in infected meat or fish. In this case, humans are the definitive hosts. In tissue infection with the larval forms, humans are accidental intermediate hosts.

INTESTINAL CESTODES

Adult cestodes (tapeworms) inhabit the intestinal lumen. Their bodies consist of three parts: the head, the neck, and the body. The head, or scolex, has two or more suckers or a knob of small hooks (rostellum) by which the parasite attaches itself to the intestinal wall. The scolex is attached to the body by a short neck. The ribbon-like body (the strobila) consists of segments, or proglottids. Each proglottid contains male and female re-

productive systems and is responsible for the production of the parasite eggs. Proglottids begin to develop in the neck region of the parasite. As they mature, they move downward in the strobila as newer segments are formed in the neck region. The fully mature proglottids break away from the strobila and degenerate, releasing the ova in the intestine, whence they are expelled in the feces. Alternatively, the mature proglottids may migrate to the anus and pass out in the feces. The eggs are ingested by the intermediate hosts and hatch in the intestine; there they release the oncosphere that penetrates the intestinal wall to reach the circulation. The oncosphere may lodge in one of many organs, where it matures into the parasite cyst variously called *cysticercus, cysticercoid, alveolar cyst,* or *hydatid cyst.*

The adult worms produce minimal disease in the intestine. They cause nonspecific intestinal symptoms and may be associated with decreased nutrient absorption. Immune response to the adult tapeworm may produce eosinophilia and

TABLE 225.1

SUMMARY OF THE COMMON INTESTINAL AND TISSUE CESTODE INFECTIONS IN HUMANS

Organism	Geographic Distribution	Clinical Manifestations of Infestation	Diagnosis	Treatment
Intestinal Cestodes				
Taenia saginata	Cattle breeding areas, especially central Asia, Near East, central and eastern Africa	Abdominal discomfort, hunger pains, and weight loss; intestinal obstruction may occur with multiple worms	Demonstration of ova or proglottids is feces or coproantigen by enzyme-linked immunosorbent assay	Praziquantel, 5–10 mg/kg as single dose Or Niclosamide, 50 mg/kg (2 g in adults) as single dose (not recommended for those <2 years of age)
Taenia solium	Mexico, Central and South America, Southeast Asia, India, Africa and southern Europe	Abdominal discomfort, hunger pains, and diarrhea	Same as above	Same as above
Diphyllobothrium latum	Siberia, Scandanavia, Baltic region, northern United States, Canada, South America	Abdominal discomfort, occasionally intestinal obtruction, and megaloblastic anemia	Recovery of ova or proglottids in stool	Same as above
Hymenolepsis nana	Worldwide	In those with heavy worm load anorexia, abdominal pain, nausea, vomiting, diarrhea, irritability, and dizziness	Demonstration of ova in feces	Praziquantel, 25 mg/kg as single dose
Tissue Cestodes				
Cysticercosis (*Taenia solium*)	Mexico, central and South America, India, sub-Saharan Africa	Neurocysticercosis: seizures, headache, altered mental status, visual problems, focal deficits, and hydrocephalus Extraneural: subcutaneous nodules, and myopathy and pseudohypertrophy with heavy muscular infection	Neuroimaging; immunodiagnostics	Praziquantel, 50–60 mg/kg/day in three divided doses for 15 days Or Albendazole, 15 mg/kg/day in two to three divided doses for 8–30 days May also require antiepileptic drugs and corticosteroids (see text)
Echinococcus granulosus (hydatid cyst)	China, India, Africa, Iraq, Mediterranean basin, Uruguay, Argentina, Chile	Often asymptomatic, clinical signs when present depend on location of cysts and the pressure effects on surrounding structures	Radiographic studies, serologic tests	Surgery; albendazole, 10–15 mg/kg/day in two to three divided doses in 28 day cycles with 14 days in between for at least three cycles as an adjunct to surgery or when surgery is not possible
Echinococcus multilocularis (alveolar cyst)	Sub-Arctic regions of Alaska, Canada, northern Europe, and northern United States	Same as above	Same as above	Same as above

immunoglobulin E (IgE) elevation, but the immune response does not alter the course of intraluminal infection.

Taenia saginata (Beef Tapeworm)

Taenia saginata, or beef tapeworm, is found commonly in the cattle-breeding areas of the world, especially in Central Asia, the Near East, and central and eastern Africa. The parasite measures 4 to 10 m, with 1,000 to 2,000 proglottids. The scolex, which measures 1 to 2 mm, has four suckers (but no hooks) by which the parasite attaches itself to the intestinal mucosa.

Life Cycle

Infection is acquired by the ingestion of raw or undercooked beef. In the intestine, the scolex evaginates from the cysticercus, attaches itself to the intestinal mucosa, and develops into the adult worm. Gravid proglottids appear 90 to 120 days after infection. Eggs may be liberated in the intestinal lumen by detached proglottids. Alternately, single proglottids may migrate actively through the anus or from the fecal mass after it has been passed. The eggs remain viable in the soil for days to weeks. After ingestion by cattle, the eggs hatch to release oncospheres that penetrate the intestinal mucosa and reach the bloodstream, where they are filtered out in the striated muscle. They develop into mature cysticerci within approximately 70 days. Reindeer and certain herbivorous wild animals are also known to harbor cysticerci of *T. saginata*.

Clinical Manifestations

Commonly, adult worms in the intestine are asymptomatic, although nonspecific abdominal discomfort, hunger pains, and weight loss have been reported. Infection with multiple worms may cause intestinal obstruction. The most common complaint is the discomfort and embarrassment caused by mature proglottids migrating out through the anus. Significant eosinophilia may occur in a small proportion of patients.

Diagnosis

Specific diagnosis is established by the recovery of the parasite proglottid. The proglottids of *T. saginata* may be distinguished from those of *T. solium* by the number of main lateral uterine branches. The eggs of *T. saginata* may be indistinguishable from those of *T. solium*.

Immunodiagnostic tests for *Taenia*-specific faecal antigen based on polyclonal rabbit antisera against *T. saginata* or *T. solium* proglottid extracts in capture-type enzyme-linked immunosorbent assay (ELISA) have been developed. These tests are more sensitive than microscopy and are highly specific.

Treatment

The treatment of choice is praziquantel. The drug is administered in a single dose of 5 to 10 mg/kg. It is not recommended in pregnancy, and its safety in children younger than 4 years of age has not been established.

The alternative drug is niclosamide. This drug is available as chewable 500-mg tablets. It is administered as a single dose that either should be chewed thoroughly or crushed and made into a paste before administration. The dose is 2 g for adults and 50 mg/kg in children. It is not recommended in pregnancy or in children younger than 2 years because of lack of safety data.

Taenia solium (Pork Tapeworm)

T. solium infection is endemic in Mexico, Central and South America, Southeast Asia, India, Africa, and southern Europe.

The adult worm has a scolex with four large suckers and a rostellum with a double row of hooks by which it anchors itself to the intestinal mucosa. A narrow neck connects the scolex to a strobila consisting of some 1,000 proglottids. Humans can be either the definitive host or the intermediate host for *T. solium*. Ingestion of eggs by humans results in cysticercosis (discussed later under tissue cestodes).

Life Cycle

The *T. solium* life cycle is similar to that of *T. saginata*. Infection is acquired by ingestion of infected pork that is raw or undercooked. The scolex evaginates and develops into the adult worm in the intestine. The eggs or proglottids are passed out in the feces. Unlike the proglottids of *T. saginata*, those of *T. solium* do not migrate actively. On ingestion by hogs or humans, the eggs hatch in the duodenum or jejunum. The released oncospheres penetrate the intestinal wall and are carried throughout the body via the bloodstream. They are filtered out in the subcutaneous tissues, muscle, eye, brain, and other body sites, where they develop into cysticerci, completing the cycle.

Clinical Manifestations

Usually, the adult worms do not cause any symptoms; however, they may cause occasional vague abdominal discomfort, hunger pains, and diarrhea. Cysticerci in human beings may cause symptoms, depending on the site of infection (see the later discussion of tissue cestodes).

Diagnosis

Diagnosis is established by demonstration of ova in the stool or by coproantigen detection by ELISA. However, differentiation from *T. saginata* may be difficult. DNA-based assays have been developed and used to differentiate between the two parasites.

Treatment

Treatment of *T. solium* is the same as for *T. saginata*. Because praziquantel is absorbed systemically, there is a small risk that patients who may have concomitant asymptomatic neurocysticercosis may develop neurologic complications (headache, seizures) as a result of the action of the drug on the cysts.

Diphyllobothrium latum (Fish Tapeworm)

Diphyllobothrium latum, or "fish tapeworm," belongs to the pseudophyllidean cestode group. This group has a scolex with two bothria (sucking organs) rather than the typical four seen in the *Taenia* group. The worms are large, measuring up to 25 m long, and consist of 3,000 to 4,000 proglottids that have a characteristic rosette-shaped uterus. An individual may be infected with more than one worm at a time. Areas of high endemicity include the lake and delta areas in Siberia, Scandinavia, the Baltic regions, and adjacent areas of the former Soviet Union, northern United States, Canada, and South America. Infection can be maintained in the absence of humans by fish-eating mammals.

Life Cycle

Infection is acquired by ingestion of raw, poorly cooked, or pickled freshwater fish. The worm matures 3 to 6 weeks after ingestion of eggs. After maturation, both eggs and proglottids are passed in the stool; often a partial chain of proglottids a few inches to several feet long may be passed. The eggs develop in fresh water, after which they hatch and release ciliated coracidium larvae that are ingested by the first intermediate hosts, the copepod. The copepods containing the second-stage larvae (procercoid) are ingested by fish and develop into more advanced stages in the muscles of the fish. If smaller fish are ingested by larger fish, the muscles of the larger fish are parasitized. The cycle is completed when infected fish are ingested by humans or fish-eating mammals.

Clinical Manifestations

Often, infection is asymptomatic, although patients may notice the passage of proglottids in the stool. Infection with multiple worms may lead to abdominal discomfort and, occasionally, intestinal obstruction. Chronic infection may be associated with megaloblastic anemia from vitamin B_{12} deficiency, a result of parasite-mediated vitamin B_{12} intrinsic factor dissociation, leading to decreased absorption and by uptake of the vitamin by the parasite itself. Megaloblastic anemia is seen much more commonly in Finland and adjacent areas than in North America. Increased uptake of vitamin B_{12} by strains of the parasite in Finland or a genetic predisposition to megaloblastic anemia may account for this phenomenon.

Diagnosis

Diagnosis is made by recovery of the characteristic eggs or proglottids in the feces.

Treatment

Both niclosamide and praziquantel are effective in the treatment of *D. latum*. The dose used is similar to that for *Taenia*. Severe vitamin B_{12} deficiency should be treated with parenteral vitamin injections.

Hymenolepis nana (Dwarf Tapeworm)

Hymenolepis nana infection is distributed worldwide and may be transmitted from person to person by fecal-oral transmission. The adult worm measures only 5 to 45 mm and has a scolex with four suckers and a short rostellum with 20 to 30 hooks.

Life Cycle

Generally, infection is acquired by ingestion of *H. nana* eggs from feces of infected individuals. The eggs hatch in the stomach or small intestine. The liberated oncospheres penetrate the villi of the upper small intestine. The larvae mature into the cysticercoid stage in the villi and then migrate back into the lumen, where the scolex evaginates and attaches itself to the mucosa. The adult worm matures within a few weeks.

Clinical Manifestations

Most patients infected with *H. nana* are asymptomatic. However, varied symptoms have been described, especially in patients with heavy worm burdens. These include anorexia or increased appetite, abdominal pain, nausea, vomiting, diarrhea, irritability, dizziness, and headache. Seizures have been described in patients in the former Soviet Union. Autoinfection, in which the eggs hatch in the intestine and complete the life cycle within the same host, may result in heavy infection in immunocompromised patients.

Diagnosis

Diagnosis is established by the demonstration of eggs in the feces; proglottids rarely are expelled in the feces. Egg morphology is seen better in fresh specimens or in those preserved in formalin-based fixatives. A single examination is not always enough to rule out infection.

Treatment

Niclosamide, praziquantel, and paromomycin are effective against *H. nana*. Because niclosamide and paromomycin are not active against the larval stage in the intestinal villi, a 7-day course of the drug is required. Praziquantel is effective in a single dose of 25 mg/kg and is considered to be the treatment of choice. Retreatment may be necessary for persistant infections.

TISSUE CESTODES

Cysticercosis

Cysticercosis occurs when humans are infected by the ingestion of *T. solium* eggs. The eggs are sticky and can be found attached to the perianal skin and under the fingernails of tapeworm carriers. They may be transmitted by direct contact or through food handled by a carrier. Internal autoinfection by regurgitation of proglottids into the stomach has been suggested but not proven. After ingestion, the oncospheres penetrate the intestinal mucosa and migrate throughout the body. Although the larvae are carried to almost every tissue in the body, they do not develop into mature cysts in most tissues. Most cysticerci are found in the central nervous system tissue, skeletal muscle, subcutaneous tissue, and eyes.

Epidemiology

The increasing availability of neuroimaging studies and serosurveys using the enzyme-linked immunotransfer blot assay has demonstrated clearly that cysticercosis is more widely prevalent than was estimated previously. Some estimate that approximately 50 million people are infected with the cyst stage worldwide, making it the most common parasitic disease of the central nervous system and a major public health problem in developing countries. The areas with highest prevalence are Mexico, Central and South America, India, and sub-Saharan Africa. Autopsy studies in Mexico showed the presence of at least one central nervous system cysticercus in 0.4% to 3.5% of unselected autopsies. In a large epidemiologic study from Togo, West Africa, evidence of cysticercosis was found in 2.4% of the population, including 39% of those with epilepsy. Studies in India have shown that up to one-half of all patients with afebrile seizures have serologic evidence of cysticercosis. With the influx of immigrants from Latin America and Asia, cysticercosis is being recognized increasingly in the United States.

Clinical Manifestations

Neurocysticercosis. The brain is the most common site for cysticercosis and also is the site that most often results in symptomatic disease. Seizures are the most common clinical manifestations and occur in 70% to 90% of cases. Less common manifestations include headache, visual problems, altered mental status (including psychosis), ataxia, focal deficits, and hydrocephalus.

Parenchymal neurocysticercosis usually presents with seizures, headache, and altered mental status. Seizures are most often generalized or focal with secondary generalization; one-third of patients have simple partial seizures. Focal neurologic deficits, when present, are generally transient over days, weeks, or months, with periods of remission and relapse. In children and adolescents, an encephalitic form, as a result of massive infection, has been described. Studies of cerebrospinal fluid (CSF) may reveal elevation of protein or pleocytosis. Most patients do well even without antiparasitic therapy. Generally, seizures are well controlled with a single anticonvulsant, and cysts generally resolve within 2 years.

Extraparenchymal neurocysticercosis takes one of two forms: *ventricular neurocysticercosis* and *subarachnoid cysticercosis*. Approximately 10% to 20% of patients with neurocysticercosis present with extraparenchymal cysts that primarily are found in the ventricles. Most patients with ventricular neurocysticercosis develop mechanical obstruction of CSF flow, which results in obstructive hydrocephalus. Patients with subarachnoid cysticercosis develop basal arachnoiditis and present with signs of meningeal inflammation and CSF findings of meningitis. Some patients develop communicating hydrocephalus, and others may develop stroke as a result of vasculitis.

Extraneural Cysticercosis. Cutaneous cysticercosis presenting as subcutaneous nodules is common in areas of high endemicity. Cysticerci in muscle are usually asymptomatic, but heavy infestation may cause myopathy, sometimes associated with muscular pseudohypertrophy. Cardiac cysticerscosis is known to occur but is generally asymptomatic.

The other site of infection is the eye. Cysts most often are found in the vitreous humor. They are found less commonly in the subretinal space, subconjunctiva, or anterior chambers.

Diagnosis

Neuroimaging and serologic tests are the main methods for the diagnosis of neurocysticercosis. The imaging techniques used most commonly are computed tomographic (CT) and magnetic resonance imaging (MRI) scans. The CT or MRI appearance depends on the phase of development of the onchospere, i.e. the vesicular, colloidal, granulonodular, or calcified phases (Fig. 225.1). In the viable vesicular phase, the CT scan depicts circumscribed, round hypodense areas without contrast enhancement, whereas the MRI shows CSF-like intensity signal with no surrounding high intensity signal on T_2-weighted images; a high-intensity 2- to 3-mm nodule, depicting the scolex may be seen within the cyst. As the cyst degenerates, an annular (colloidal phase) or nodular (nodular phase) enhancement with irregular perilesional edema is seen. Finally, when the cyst dies, it can disappear or become an inactive calcified nodule of homogenous high intensity on CT or low-intensity proton-weighted MRI. Most ventricular and cisternal cysts are not visualized directly on CT scan, although their presence may be suspected in the presence of obstructive hydrocephalus. Injection of metrizamide into the ventricular or lumbar CSF may help in delineating the cyst in such cases. MRI is more sensitive than CT scan in identifying extraparenchymal cysts, including ventricular and cisternal cysts.

The enzyme-linked immunotransfer blot assay is highly specific for *T. solium* infections. The assay is 100% sensitive in patients with multiple active parenchymal cysts or extraparenchymal neurocysticercosis. However, it has a low sensitivity in those with solitary or calcified cysts.

Because neuroimaging is rarely pathognomic and serologic assays do not have optimal sensitivity and specificity, a set of absolute, major, minor, and epidemiologic criteria was defined at a consensus meeting in 2000 on the basis of which a definite or probable diagnosis of neurocysticercosis may be made, as reported by Del Brutto and associates.

Treatment

Treatment, which depends on the number and location of the cysts, their viability, and the degree of inflammatory response, must be individualized. Numerous studies have reported on the use of antiparasitic drugs in the treatment of active neurocysticercosis. Praziquantel was the drug to be used first. The usual dose is 50 to 60 mg/kg/day in three daily doses for 15 days. Albendazole, at a dose of 15 mg/kg/day in two or three daily doses for 8 to 30 days, is equally effective. Both these drugs hasten the resolution of the cysts. However, some patients may develop worsening inflammation with resultant headache, vomiting, and seizures. Therefore, routine use of corticosteroids is recommended to prevent this complication. The most frequent recommendation for corticosteroid use is dexamethasone, between 1 and 1.5 mg/kg/day (maximum 10 mg/day) divided into four to six doses/day for 4 days. Prednisolone, 1 mg/kg/day, may replace dexamethasone when long-term steroid therapy is required. Although antiparasitic drugs do cause resolution of cysts and seizures, the results are not obviously different from the natural history of the disease, thus leading to a debate on the use of these drugs in neurocysticercosis.

Consensus guidelines have also been developed for the treatment of neurocysticercosis, as reported by Garcia and colleagues. There is consensus that growth of a parenchymal cyst deserves specific treatment either with antiparasitic drugs, surgery, or both. There is also consensus on the use of antiparasitic drugs with steroids for the treatment of patients with more than five viable cysts and subarachnoid cysts. In cases of calcified cysticerci or cysticercus encephaitis, the consensus is that antiparasitic therapy is not indicated; in the latter, initial therapy should be directed at reducing intracranial hypertension. There is no consensus on the use of antiparasitic therapy for other forms of parenchymal neurocysticercosis or in the treatment of cysticercus encephalitis after control of intracranial hypertesion.

Antiepileptic drugs are recommended for the control of seizures, and antiparasitic drugs should not be regarded as an alternative. Antiepileptic drugs can generally be safely withdrawn after resolution of the parasitic infection and normalization of the imaging studies.

Surgical therapy is recommended for the treatment of ventricular cysts, hydrocephalus, and spinal and ophthalmic cysticercosis.

Control

The main method of control of this disease consists of eradication of porcine cysticercosis through improved animal husbandry and meat inspection. Porcine infection can also be addressed by mass anthelmintic treatment and possibly in the future through immunization.

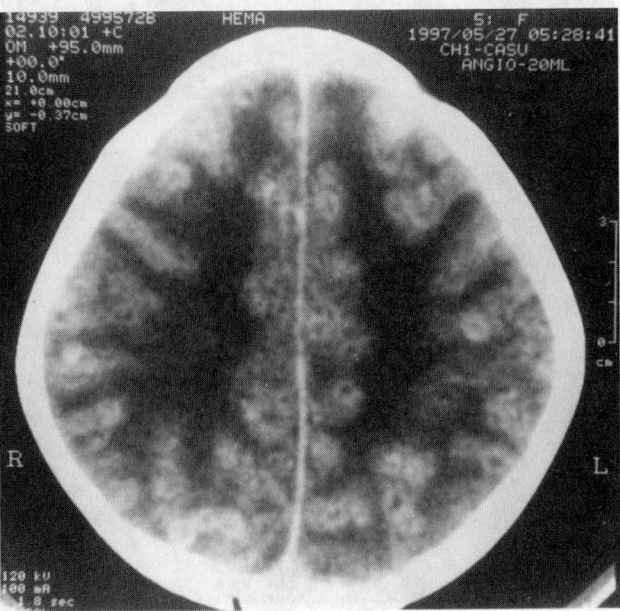

FIGURE 225.1. Computed tomographic scan of the brain showing multiple parenchymal neurocysticerci.

Echinococcosis (Hydatid Disease)

Echinococcosis is caused by the larval (metacestode) stage of various cestode species, two of which are important for reasons of medical and public health. *Echinococcus granulosus* is the cause of cystic echinococcosis and is the form most common in humans. *E. multilocularis*, the etiologic agent of alveolar echinococcosis, is less common, whereas *E. vogeli*, the cause of polycystic echinococcosis, is very rare. *E. oligarthrus* infection is limited to sylvatic animals in Central and South America, and no human cases have been reported.

Geographic Distribution

E. granulosus infection occurs worldwide. Areas of high endemicity are China, India, Africa, Iraq, the Mediterranean basin, Uruguay, Argentina, and Chile. Disease occasionally occurs in Great Britain, the United States, southern and eastern Europe, Australia, and New Zealand. The highest incidence probably occurs in the Turkana region of Kenya, a site of close association between humans and dogs.

E. multilocularis infection is limited to the Northern Hemisphere, mainly in the sub-Arctic regions of Alaska and Canada and northern Europe. The parasite has been discovered also in the northern United States (Montana, Wyoming, and South Dakota) and in South Carolina.

Life Cycle

Echinococcous **granulosus.** The definitive hosts of *E. granulosus* are dogs. The adult tapeworm, which is approximately 7 mm long, inhabits the intestine of dogs. Eggs or gravid proglottids passed in the feces are ingested by grazing animals, such as sheep, cattle, goats, horses, and camels or accidentally by humans. The oncospheres penetrate the intestinal wall and most frequently are carried to the liver but also to the lungs, brain, bone, peritoneum, kidneys, heart, and orbit. At these sites, the oncospheres develop into fluid-filled hydatid cysts having an inner germinal layer and an outer laminated wall, surrounded by fibrous reaction of the invaded tissue. The germinal layer proliferates inward and forms daughter cysts and brood capsules that produce the larval stage, the protoscolex. Often, the protoscoleces become detached and collect together in the cyst as "hydatid sand." The unilocular hydatid cysts grow within the invaded tissues and develop over several years. They measure perhaps 1 cm in diameter after 5 years and eventually may grow to 20 cm in diameter. The primary canine hosts become infected when they feed on the offal or carcasses of infected intermediate hosts. The protoscoleces attach themselves to the intestinal wall and develop into adult worms, thus completing the cycle.

Echinococcus multilocularis. The life cycle of *E. multilocularis* is similar to that of *E. granulosu*s. The definitive hosts are foxes, wolves, and dogs. The cysts (alveolar cysts) are sponge-like masses filled with a jelly-like matrix and differ from hydatid cysts in that they invade the host tissue by proliferating outward like a malignant growth that frequently metastasizes to other organs. The diffuse borders are not well delineated from the adjacent liver tissue. In humans, the cysts do not form protoscoleces or brood capsules.

Clinical Manifestations

Echinococcosis can mimic a variety of conditions, and symptoms depend on the location of the cysts. The course of the disease varies. Infection may occur in childhood, but because of the slow growth of the cysts, it may not produce symptoms until middle age.

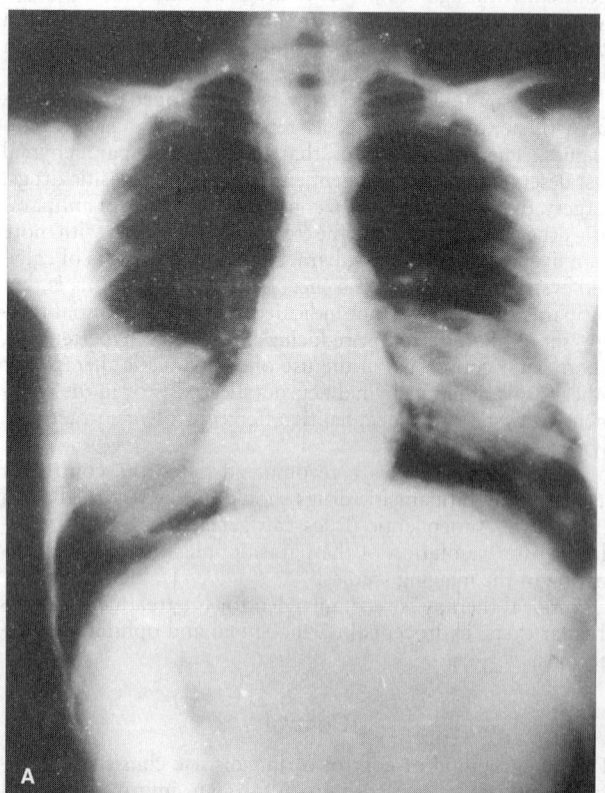
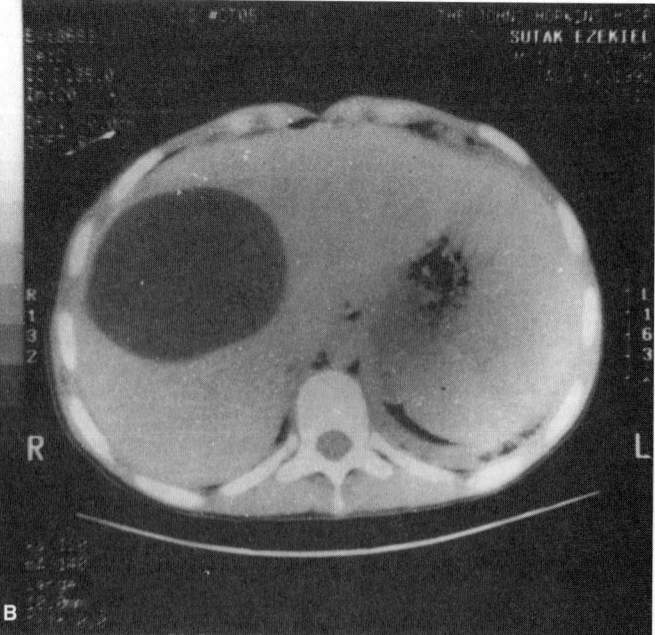

FIGURE 225.2. **A:** Chest roentgenogram showing bilateral pulmonary echinococcal cysts. **B:** Computed tomographic scan of the abdomen showing a solitary cyst in the liver of an 11-year-old boy.

E. granulosus cysts are found most often in the liver (65%) and lungs (25%). Conversely, *E. multilocularis* cysts occur almost exclusively in the liver (98%), but metastatic lesions can form in the lungs, brain, and other organs.

Not uncommonly, hydatid cysts can be asymptomatic and can be discovered accidentally on routine chest roentgenography or abdominal ultrasonography. When they do cause symptoms, usually they are related to compression of the surrounding structures. Hydatid cysts in the liver give rise to right upper quadrant and epigastric pain, hepatomegaly, jaundice, and portal hypertension. Lung cysts may present with hemoptysis, pleural effusion, and atelectasis. Cysts in the brain produce signs and symptoms of a cerebral tumor, whereas those in the kidney produce hematuria and may resemble a hypernephroma. Cysts in the bone may present as spontaneous fracture of the long bones or compression fracture of the vertebrae. Cysts may rupture spontaneously, resulting in fever, urticaria, and signs of anaphylaxis. Seeding of protoscoleces may result in secondary cysts at other sites. Fatalities are rare but may occur as a result of cyst rupture, compression of vital structures, or septicemia from infected cysts.

Alveolar cysts tend to grow rapidly and metastasize and therefore result in symptoms early in the course of disease. They are associated with high mortality if they are not diagnosed and treated early.

Diagnosis

A hydatid cyst must be suspected in any patient who comes from an endemic area and presents with signs and symptoms of a space-occupying lesion. Radiographic studies, such as chest roentgenography, ultrasonography, CT scan, and MRI, will reveal the presence of the typical fluid-filled cysts, sometimes with enclosed daughter cysts and brood capsules (Fig. 225.2). Older cysts may be partially calcified.

Numerous serologic tests using hydatid cyst fluid or antigen 5 are available. Serology is 80% to 100% sensitive and 88% to 96% specific for liver cysts; sensitivity is lower for pulmonary cysts (50% to 56%) and for cysts at other sites (25% to 56%). False-positive test results may occur with other cestode infection and also with malignancies and liver cirrhosis. Newer serologic tests using recombinant *Echinococcus* antigens or tests that detect IgG_1 subclass antibodies provide better specificity. At present, imaging remains more sensitive than serodiagnosis, and a positive scan suggests echinococcosis even when serology is negative.

Treatment

Surgery is the recommended treatment for single unilocular cysts of *E. granulosus*. Because of the risk of spreading infection if the cyst ruptures, the recommended procedure is to inject the cyst with a scolecidal agent, such as hypertonic (30%) saline, 95% ethanol, or iodophor, before attempting excision of the cyst. An ultrasound-guided percutaneous treatment using a technique called PAIR (puncture, aspiration, injection, reaspiration), with 95% ethanol as a scolecide agent, has also been used very successfully in the treatment of hydatid abdominal cysts (mainly hepatic).

Mebendazole and albendazole have been shown to be effective against echinococcal cysts and may be used as an adjunct to surgery, when surgery is not possible or is associated with significant morbidity (as with cysts in the brain or bone), or in the presence of multiple cysts. Albendazole is more effective than mebendazole and results in improvement in approximately 75% of cysts in the liver, lung, or peritoneum and cure in about 30%. Bone cyst cure rates are lower (25%), with improvement in perhaps one-half the patients. The recommended treatment schedule with albendazole is 10 to 15 mg/kg/day in two to three divided doses given as three 28-day cycles with 14 days between cycles. A minimum of three cycles is recommended; improvement rate is lower with shorter courses, and the chances of recurrences are higher, although very little further improvement is seen if treatment is continued beyond 6 months.

Preoperative use of albendazole before surgery renders the cysts nonviable and reduces the risk of recurrence after surgery. Albendazole, usually two 28-day cycles, may also be used postoperatively to reduce the risk of recurrences.

For alveolar cysts, wide surgical resection is recommended to ensure total removal of the cyst. Albendazole may be used as an adjuvant to surgery, either to reduce the size of the cyst preoperatively or to prevent intraoperative spread.

Control

Control measures include meat inspection, burning or burying of offal, control of the dog population, and reduction of tapeworm by testing and mass treatment of dogs.

Suggested Readings

Botero D, Tapowitz HR, Weiss LM, Wittner M. Taeniasis and cysticercosis. *Infect Dis Clin North Am* 1993;7:683.

Del Brutto OH, Rajshekhar V, White AC Jr, et al. Proposed diagnostic criteria for neurocysticercosis. *Neurology* 2001;57:177.

Garcia HH, Gonzalez AE, Evans CA, Gilman RH, for the Cysticercosis Working Group in Peru. Taenia solium cysticercosis. *Lancet* 2003;362:547.

Garcia HH, Evans CA, Nash TE, et al. Current consensus guidelines for treatment of neurocysticercosis. *Clin Microbiol Rev* 2002;15:747.

Horton RJ. Albendazole in treatment of human cystic echinococcosis: 12 years of experience. *Acta Trop* 1997;64:79.

Kammerer WS, Schantz PM. Echinococcal disease. *Infect Dis Clin North Am* 1993;7:605.

Morris DL. Pre-operative albendazole therapy for hydatid cyst. *Br J Surg* 1987; 74:805.

Morris DL, Taylor DH. Optimal timing of post-operative albendazole prophylaxis in *E. granulosus*. *Ann Trop Med Parasitol* 1988;82:65.

Perdomo R, Alvarez C, Monti J, et al. Principles of surgical approach in human cystic echinococcosis. *Acta Trop* 1997;64:109.

CHAPTER 226 ■ SCHISTOSOMIASIS

MARK W. KLINE

Schistosomiasis is a disease of the circulatory system caused principally by three species of trematodes: *Schistosoma mansoni*, *S. haematobium*, and *S. japonicum*. Some 200 to 300 million people worldwide are infected with one of these organisms. Travel to and from endemic areas of Africa, South America, and Asia has spread the disease well beyond its historical geographic boundaries to North America and Europe. In the United States, more than 400,000 people may be infected with one of the human schistosomes. Although transmission of the infection in the United States is not possible because of the absence of snail intermediate hosts, recognition of the clinical features of the disease is key to establishing the diagnosis and providing treatment for the prevention of long-term adverse sequelae.

LIFE CYCLE

Humans are the definitive hosts for the three principal schistosome species; certain snails serve as intermediate hosts (Fig. 226.1). Deposition of eggs (oviposition) occurs in the venules of the large intestine (*S. mansoni*), small intestine (*S. japonicum*), or urinary bladder (*S. haematobium*) of humans. Many eggs remain in the tissues or are carried via the bloodstream to the liver or other distant body sites. A few reach the lumina of the intestine or urinary bladder and are excreted.

Free-living miracidia are released when eggs contact warm fresh water. Miracidia swim until they find an appropriate snail intermediate host; then they penetrate its tissues and begin asexual reproduction. In a few weeks, infective larvae, or *cercariae*, are shed from the snail and may penetrate intact human skin. After penetration occurs, the parasite develops into a worm-like schistosomulum and passes through the skin and to the lungs via lymphatics or the bloodstream. After a total period of 1 to 3 weeks, schistosomula reach the liver, where maturation and sexual reproduction occur. Adult schistosomes descend through the venous system to their preferred sites in the intestine or urinary bladder. Oviposition occurs 4 to 12 weeks after cercarial penetration of the skin has occurred.

EPIDEMIOLOGY

The geographic distribution and prevalence of schistosomiasis change continuously. The transmission of schistosomes depends absolutely on the distribution of susceptible snails. Population shifts and the introduction of irrigation have led to an increased prevalence of infection in many endemic areas. Conversely, population treatment and snail eradication programs have affected the prevalence of infection favorably in certain areas. Inhabitants of endemic areas usually encounter schistosomes during childhood and may be infected repeatedly throughout their lives. The prevalence of infection may reach adult levels during the first decade of life. The incidence of initial infections, therefore, is low in comparison with the overall prevalence and is restricted largely to children. Most infected

persons have a low worm burden and pass only a few eggs in the stool or urine. Relatively small numbers of individuals are infected heavily, but they contribute disproportionately to environmental contamination and the transmission of infection. Control efforts often have been directed against these heavily infected individuals.

S. japonicum is endemic only in the Far East, with foci in China, Japan, the Philippines, Indonesia, Thailand, Laos, and Cambodia. A similar human schistosome of lesser importance, *S. mekongi*, first was reported from the Mekong River delta and probably is endemic throughout Southeast Asia.

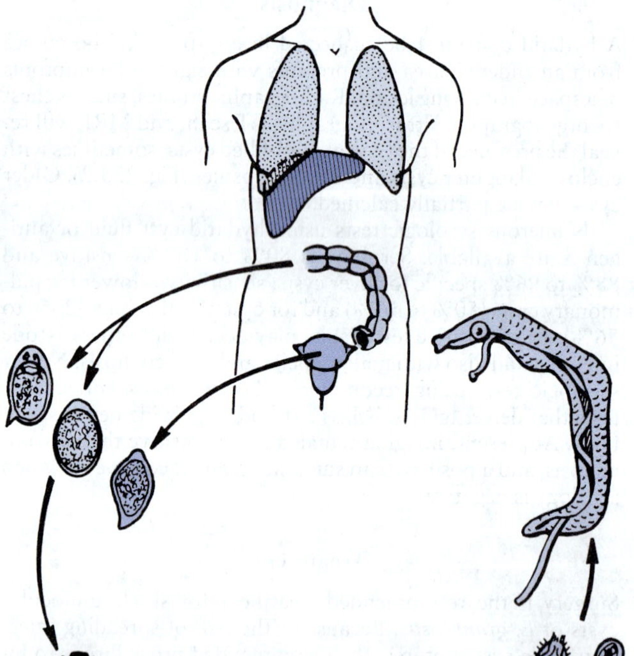

FIGURE 226.1. The life cycle of schistosomes (counterclockwise): parasite eggs passed into freshwater in human excreta hatch into miracidia that infect the intermediate host, an aquatic snail. Several weeks later, the snail releases free-swimming cercarial forms that seek and penetrate human skin, transforming into immature male or female larvae. Six to 8 weeks later, mature worms complete the cycle by mating in portal or urinary tract veins and releasing eggs into nearby viscera. (Reprinted from King CH, Mahmoud AAF. *Schistosoma* and other trematodes. In: Gorbach SL, Bartlett JG, Blacklow NR, eds. *Infectious diseases*, 3rd ed. Philadelphia: Lippincott Williams & Wilkins, 2004:2379.)

S. haematobium is endemic throughout Africa and in parts of Southwest Asia and the Middle East. *S. mansoni* is widespread in Africa and is the only human schistosome present in the Western Hemisphere, with endemic foci in Brazil, Suriname, Venezuela, and the Caribbean. Schistosomiasis in the United States occurs mainly among immigrants from endemic areas.

PATHOGENESIS AND CLINICAL MANIFESTATIONS

Adult schistosomes mask themselves by adsorption of host antigens onto their surfaces. Consequently, the adult parasites elicit minimal local inflammatory responses. Conversely, intense local inflammation may accompany cercarial penetration of the skin, and granulomatous inflammation often surrounds schistosome eggs in tissues. The clinical and pathologic features of schistosomiasis are determined in large part by host immune responses to the worms and eggs. Box 226.1 describes the three distinct clinical patterns of disease.

Cercarial penetration of the skin in a nonsensitized individual usually is an inconspicuous event clinically. Mild erythema and pruritus may develop locally within minutes of penetration of the skin. This initial reaction is transient. One to 2 weeks later, small (1- to 2-mm) pruritic papules may be noted at the same sites. Individuals previously sensitized to schistosomal antigens may have intense reactions on reexposure. Localized urticaria and pruritus occur initially, and pruritic papular lesions are noted within 24 hours. Lesions may persist for 7 to 10 days.

Differentiating schistosomal dermatitis from other skin diseases can be difficult. The diagnosis is suggested by a history of swimming, wading, or bathing in untreated water from areas endemic for schistosomiasis and by the occurrence of lesions only on water-exposed body surfaces. Biopsy specimens from early skin lesions may demonstrate the organisms.

Individuals heavily infected with *S. japonicum* and, to a lesser extent, with *S. mansoni* may experience the abrupt onset of an illness similar to serum sickness as oviposition commences. This condition is known as *Katayama fever*, and its clinical manifestations include high spiking fevers, abdominal pain, vomiting, anorexia, myalgias, and headache. Generalized lymphadenopathy and hepatosplenomegaly may be noted, and peripheral blood eosinophilia virtually always is present. Sigmoidoscopy and liver biopsy may be helpful in establishing the diagnosis of Katayama fever. Histopathologically, the liver is infiltrated by eosinophils, and schistosome eggs are seen occasionally. Katayama fever usually is self-limited, but it may persist for weeks to several months.

Much of the long-term morbidity and mortality associated with schistosomiasis reflect chronic effects of host immunologic responses to eggs in the tissues. In the wall of the human intestine, eggs of *S. mansoni* and *S. japonicum* incite granulomatous inflammation, which disrupts tissue architecture and function and ultimately leads to fibrosis. The clinical manifestations of intestinal schistosomiasis vary. Many individuals are asymptomatic, whereas others complain of abdominal pain, anorexia, vomiting, diarrhea, or blood in the stool. Children may experience growth failure. Occasionally, symptoms mimic those of cholecystitis or peptic ulcer disease. Colonic polyposis is an uncommon finding seen only in individuals infected with *S. mansoni*. Hepatosplenic schistosomiasis occurs when schistosome eggs cause embolization in the liver. A characteristic pattern of scarring, known as *pipestem* or *Symmers fibrosis*, is found around portal veins and eventually leads to portal hypertension. Often, hepatomegaly is the initial clinical manifestation of hepatosplenic schistosomiasis. In advanced cases, congestive splenomegaly and variceal bleeding are noted. Signs and symptoms of hepatocellular disease (e.g., icterus, ascites, elevated serum transaminase levels) usually are absent.

Deposition of *S. haematobium* eggs in the bladder and ureters produces granulomatous reactions and scarring, with nodular or ulcerative changes of the bladder and fibrosis of the ureters. Early manifestations of urinary tract schistosomiasis include urinary frequency, dysuria, and terminal hematuria. Intravenous pyelography or ultrasonography may demonstrate hydroureter and hydronephrosis in advanced cases. Carcinoma of the bladder occurs with increased frequency in individuals with *S. haematobium* infection.

Schistosome eggs may reach distant body sites via lymphatic or vascular channels. The deposition of eggs in the pulmonary vasculature leads to granuloma formation, obstruction of pulmonary blood flow, and schistosomal cor pulmonale. *S. mansoni* and *S. haematobium* may produce transverse myelitis by the deposition of eggs in the spinal cord. Mass lesions of the brain caused by *S. japonicum* are an important cause of focal seizures in the Far East.

DIAGNOSIS

Historical and clinical findings suggestive of schistosomiasis already have been described. Definitive diagnosis is based on the presence of viable eggs in stool, urine, or biopsy specimens. Quantification of eggs in the excreta is desirable because the severity of disease correlates with egg counts. Ordinary fecal smears are an insensitive means of diagnosing schistosomiasis. The thick smear method of Kato is simple and accurate and permits counting of schistosome eggs. Urine samples are collected best around noon to take advantage of the diurnal pattern of *S. haematobium* egg excretion. The urinary sediment is examined by routine methods. If present, eggs then can be enumerated by the Bell technique. If the results of stool and urine studies are negative, rectal biopsy may assist in establishing a diagnosis, particularly in individuals infected with *S. mansoni* or *S. japonicum*. Determining the viability of the eggs is important because nonviable or calcified eggs may persist for long periods after successful therapy or the death of adult schistosomes. Serodiagnostic and antigen detection methods for diagnosing schistosomiasis have not been developed to the level of routine clinical application.

TREATMENT

Praziquantel is the drug of choice for treatment of all forms of schistosomiasis. A single oral dose of 40 mg/kg is recommended for *S. mansoni* and *S. haematobium* infections. *S. japonicum* and *S. mekongi* infections require a larger total dose: 60 mg/kg, given in two or three divided doses in 1 day. Generally, praziquantel is well tolerated. Abdominal pain, nausea, headache, and rashes have been reported, but most adverse reactions are mild.

Treatment of schistosomiasis should not be undertaken unless viable eggs have been demonstrated in excreta or biopsy specimens. Generally, egg counts are reduced markedly by therapy, but complete eradication of eggs and schistosomes is not mandatory.

The prognosis of schistosomiasis is excellent when treatment is initiated early. Late effects of chronic schistosomiasis are not entirely reversible with therapy.

PREVENTION

Contaminated bodies of water in areas endemic for schistosomiasis should be avoided. Waterproof boots offer protection if wading is necessary. Exposed skin should be dried promptly and completely. Personal water supplies can be boiled or stored for several days to eliminate viable cercariae.

Suggested Readings

American Academy of Pediatrics. Schistosomiasis. In: Pickering LK, ed. *Redbook: 2003 report of the Committee on Infectious Diseases*, 26th ed. Elk Grove Village, IL: American Academy of Pediatrics, 2003:549.

Cioli D, Pica-Mattoccia L. Praziquantel. *Parasitol Res* 2003;90(suppl 1):3.

Elliott DE. Schistosomiasis: pathophysiology, diagnosis, and treatment. *Gastroenterol Clin North Am* 1996;25:599.

Ferrari ML, Coelho PM, Antunes CM, et al. Efficacy of oxaminiquine and praziquantel in the treatment of *Schistosoma mansoni* infection: a controlled trial. *Bull World Health Organ* 2003;81:190.

Grobusch MP, Muhlberger N, Jelinek T, et al. Imported schistosomiasis in Europe: sentinel surveillance data from TropNetEurop. *J Travel Med* 2003; 10:164.

Magnussen P. Treatment and re-treatment strategies for schistosomiasis control in different epidemiological settings: a review of 10 years' experiences. *Acta Trop* 2003;86:243.

Richter J. The impact of chemotherapy on morbidity due to schistosomiasis. *Acta Trop* 2003;86:161.

CHAPTER 227 ■ ARTHROPODA

TARA D. MILLER AND MOISE L. LEVY

Arthropods are a large and varied group of invertebrate animals with chitinous exoskeletons, jointed appendages, and segmented bodies. They are classified further as follows: arachnids, which have eight legs and include mites, ticks, spiders, and scorpions; insects, or hexapods, which have six legs and include lice, mosquitoes, flies, fleas, bees, wasps, and ants; and caterpillars and moths. This chapter focuses on those arthropods that commonly cause disease in the pediatric population.

ARACHNIDS

Mites

Epidemiology and Transmission

Mites are ubiquitous parasites that infest humans and domestic animals such as dogs and cats, as well as wild birds, chickens, bats, rodents, and even snakes. Humans encounter mites on pets or in their natural habitat while engaging in outdoor activities such as hiking and camping. The human itch mite, *Sarcoptes scabiei*, is transmitted by close personal contact and thus easily spread among children.

Clinical Manifestations

Although some mites are vectors for viral and rickettsial diseases, the most common clinical manifestation is local skin inflammation. The reaction, which typically occurs within minutes to hours of a bite occurring, may be the result of hypersensitivity to agents secreted during feeding. For example, chiggers, also known as harvest mites or red bugs, attach to the skin, inject proteolytic enzymes, and then feed on the degraded tissue. The chigger may remain attached for as long as 4 days, and then it drops off into the soil to mature into its adult form. The bite itself is painless, so hosts often do not know they have been bitten until pruritic macules appear 3 to 24 hours later. *Sarcoptes scabie* also is the cause of scabies. The female adult mite becomes pregnant and then burrows through the skin, leaving behind a trail of eggs, feces, and debris. Clinically, an intensely pruritic hypersensitivity reaction occurs in the form of erythematous papules, nodules, vesicles, or pustules. The clinical distribution varies depending on the age of the child. The feet, palms, axillae, and scalp are the usual sites of infestation in infants, whereas older children have burrows and lesions on the wrist, the genitalia, the waist or umbilicus, or in the finger webs. The diagnosis is confirmed by scraping the representative skin lesions and viewing the mites, eggs, and/or feces under the microscope.

Treatment and Prevention

Whereas most mite bites are treated symptomatically to reduce itching and to prevent secondary infections, the scabies mite completes its entire life cycle on the human host, and thus infestation may persist until an effective scabicide is used. Lindane was the recommended treatment of scabies; however, growing resistance and safety concerns over potential neurologic side effects in children have rendered other agents first-line therapy. Permethrin 5% cream is the treatment of choice for children older than 2 months of age and adults; precipitated sulfur (5% to 15%) in petrolatum is safe for infants (Table 227.1). A single dose of oral ivermectin [200 μg/kg (not for children < 15 kg)] also has been shown to be effective in treating scabies. Topical ivermectin and aqueous malathion (0.5%) are additional scabicides currently being investigated. To avoid reinfestation, all close contacts must be treated at the same time, and all

TABLE 227.1

TREATMENT FOR SCABIES AND HEAD LICE

	First-Line Agents	Second-Line Agents	New Agents
Scabies	>2 mo of age: permethrin 5% cream (Elimite) <2 mo of age: precipitated sulfur (5%–15%) in petroleum	Malathion 0.5% (Ovide)	Oral or topical ivermectin
Lice	Over-the-counter Permethrin 1% (Nix) Pyrethrin (0.18%–0.33%) with piperonyl butoxide (multiple shampoos, liquids, gels such as Rid or A-200)	Malathion 0.5% (Ovide) Permethrin 5% (Elimite)	Oral ivermectin

TABLE 227.2

TICK-TRANSMITTED INFECTIOUS DISEASES OF HUMANS

Agent	Disease
Arbovirus	Encephalitis
Babesia microti	Babesiosis
Borrelia burgdorferi	Lyme disease
Borrelia duttonii	Relapsing fever
Coxiella burnetii	Q fever
Ehrlichia chaffeensis	Human monocytic ehrlichiosis
Human granulocytic ehrlichiosis agent	Human granulocytic ehrlichiosis
Francisella tularensis	Tularemia
Orbivirus	Colorado tick fever
Rickettsia conorii	Fièvre boutonneuse
Rickettsia rickettsii	Rocky Mountain spotted fever
Other rickettsiae	Tick typhus

clothing, bedding, and other items in close contact with the patient must be washed and dried thoroughly.

Ticks

Epidemiology and Transmission

Ticks are macroscopic arthropods that may cause a local reaction after a bite but, more importantly, also can transmit several potentially serious infectious diseases to their human hosts (Table 227.2). Tick bites most commonly occur in the spring and summer when their hosts (e.g., dogs and children) can be found playing outside, especially in wooded areas. Most ticks that feed on humans attach themselves using barbed mouth parts called *chelicerae*. They then secrete a strong, cement-like substance that secures the attachment for as long as 7 days. After engorging themselves with blood, they drop off their hosts. Because the bite is painless, ticks often are noted only when the child bathes or is undressed.

Clinical Manifestations

The local reaction, thought to be mediated by complement, may result from hypersensitivity, injected toxins, or irritation to the tick's secretions. A pruritic red papule with or without swelling, blistering, and bruising usually occurs within days to weeks of being bitten. Most tick bites heal in 2 to 3 weeks, but the reaction may persist for months to years as a nodular tick-bite granuloma.

Some pregnant female ticks secrete a neurotoxin that causes tick paralysis, an acute neurologic syndrome characterized by an ascending lower motor neuron paralysis. The patient develops ataxia and areflexia 1 to 2 days after the tick attaches, and if the tick is not removed, the syndrome can progress to involve the trunk, upper extremities, pharynx, and tongue. Death may result from respiratory compromise. Tick paralysis can be diagnosed by clinical course only; the patient's neurologic symptoms improve once the tick is removed. Therapy otherwise is supportive.

Treatment and Prevention

The best treatment is prompt removal of the tick (usually within 48 hours) to prevent transmission of infection. The recommended method for removal of a tick is to grasp it with curved forceps or protected fingers as close to the skin as possible and then exert a steady pulling force until the tick is withdrawn from the skin. Remaining mouth parts (chelicerae) also should be removed.

Prevention of tick bites includes practical avoidance measures as well as the use of chemical repellants. The American Academy of Pediatrics recommends removing potential tick habitats by clearing brush and leaf litter, removing woodpiles, and keeping grass lawns mowed in endemic residential areas. Endemic wooded areas should be avoided entirely, but if this is not possible, the Academy recommends using (and not straying from) wide trails and not sitting on the ground. Selection of clothing is also important. Hats, long-sleeved shirts tight at the wrists, and long pants tight at the waist and tucked into socks are preferred. All items should be light in color to help identify the ticks. Repellants with N,N-diethyl-3-methylbenzamide (DEET) should be applied and reapplied every 1 to 2 hours for additional protection (for further discussion of DEET, please see mosquito treatment and prevention section). Another protective agent against ticks is permethrin, an insecticide that kills ticks on contact and is applied to clothing and outdoor equipment rather than the skin. Permethrin also is effective against mosquitoes, biting flies, chiggers, and scabies mites.

Spiders

In the United States, the two spiders that cause severe cutaneous and systemic reactions to envenomation are *Loxosceles reclusa*, the brown recluse spider, and *Latrodectus mactans*, the black widow spider.

Brown Recluse Spider

Epidemiology. Brown recluse spiders are dull yellow to dark brown and generally have a fiddle-shaped mark on the dorsal cephalothorax. This spider lives mainly in the south-central United States, especially the Midwest but can be found in many other areas. It prefers dark, secluded places and often is found in closets, storage boxes, barns, garages, and other little-used areas of the home.

Clinical Manifestations. Brown recluse venom contains proteolytic enzymes in addition to sphingomyelinase D, a protein that causes platelet aggregation and activates the complement cascade, attracting neutrophils into the wound. Shortly after sustaining a brown recluse spider bite, the patient may experience itching and tingling; the local area becomes swollen, red, and tender. The characteristic lesion may be described as a "target sign" with a central hemorrhagic vesicle surrounded by a ring of white ischemia and an outer ring of erythema. Within a few days, the bite may develop central necrosis and/or blebs in addition to regional lymphadenopathy and lymphadenitis. Systemic symptoms such as fever, chills, nausea, vomiting, and myalgias are seen more commonly in children and generally occur 12 to 24 hours after the bite. More severe envenomation may be complicated by thrombocytopenia, disseminated intravascular coagulation, hematuria, hemoglobinuria, renal failure, and shock. A complete blood cell count, platelet count, and urinalysis should be monitored carefully, particularly in young children.

Treatment. Treatment of uncomplicated cutaneous lesions from a brown recluse spider bite is best approached conservatively. Immobilization, ice, compression, and local wound care are suggested. Prescribing an antipruritic drug, such as diphenhydramine, and covering the wound help to prevent further trauma and thus the development of a secondary infection. If indicated, administration of prophylactic antibiotics and/or a tetanus booster also is recommended. Early surgical excision and intralesional corticosteroids have not proved beneficial for severe bites; however, systemic steroid therapy should be considered in severe systemic reactions. Dapsone, a leukocyte inhibitor, was shown in uncontrolled studies to reduce surgical complications as well as the time necessary for the wound to heal. Its use is controversial, and further studies with this agent are necessary before its general use can be considered in children.

Black Widow Spider

Epidemiology. The black widow spider can be indentified by a scarlet red "hourglass" on its abdomen.

Clinical Manifestations. Its venom, which can be fatal, especially in young children, contains a neurotoxin known as alpha-latrotoxin. Although the bite itself usually is painless, within minutes severe pain, burning, swelling, and inflammation of the bite site occur. Systemic symptoms, including weakness, leg pain, dizziness, hypertension, tremors, and abdominal muscle cramps and pain, then may develop. Cardiac arryhthmias, hemoglobinuria, and nephritis also have occurred in severe cases.

Treatment. Recommended treatment consists of icing, elevating, and immobilizing the involved extremity. Calcium gluconate can be helpful for abdominal and muscle spasms. Benzodiazepines and pain medications also are used as necessary. Antivenin (Merck, Sharp & Dohme, West Point, PA), of equine origin, can be administered in severe cases, provided the patient does not exhibit hypersensitivity to skin testing of this material.

INSECTS

Lice

Epidemiology and Transmission

Three types of lice attack humans: *Pthirus pubis* (the crab louse), *Pediculus humanus corporis* (the body louse), and

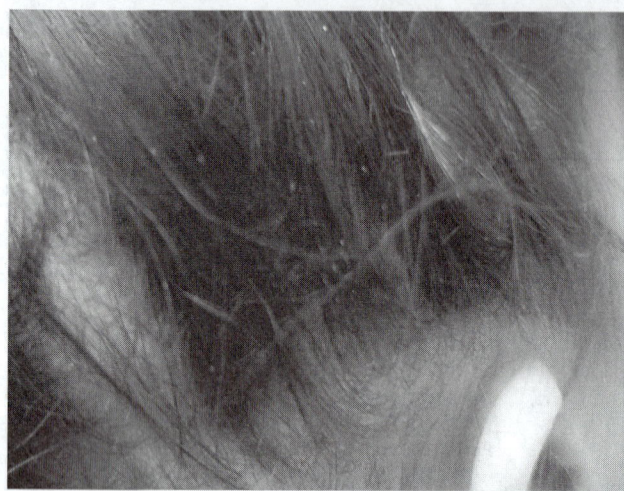

FIGURE 227.1. Extensive infestation with head lice. Note shiny, white nits on the hair shafts. (Courtesy of Christy Salvaggio, MD.) (Reprinted from Collazo E. Head lice. In: Greenberg MI, ed. Greenberg's text-atlas of emergency medicine. Philadelphia: Lippincott Williams & Wilkins, 2005:409.)

Pediculus humanus capitis (the head louse). Children of all socioeconomic levels are affected most commonly by the head louse, a 3- to 4-mm (about the size of a sesame seed) red, black, or gray-white parasite (Fig. 227.1). Because lice cannot jump or fly, transmission occurs by direct contact or contact with infested hair items such as combs, brushes, or hats. Lice feed exclusively on human blood, and whereas they can live as long as 2 months on the scalp, they can survive only 1 to 2 days away from their host.

Clinical Manifestations

Female head lice lay eggs, or nits, on the proximal hair shaft, approximately 1 cm from the scalp surface (although in warmer climates, the eggs may be further away from the scalp). The nits are silver-white "beads" that are less than 1 mm in length, and once the nymphs emerge from them, the casings remain behind, cemented to the hair shaft by chitin. The most common clinical manifestation is pruritus, especially of the occipital scalp.

Body and crab lice usually present with intense itching of the infested area. Unlike other types, body lice can also transmit systemic diseases such as typhus and relapsing fever, a recurring 3- to 6-day course of high fevers and chills, myalgias, arthralgias, and headache.

Treatment

The treatment of choice for head lice is permethrin 1% (Nix), a more potent and longer-lasting synthetic derivation of pyrethrin, a natural chrysanthemum extract found in other over-the-counter agents (see Table 227.1). Permethrin paralyzes the breathing muscles of the lice and thereby causes death through suffocation. Lice can shut down their respiratory systems for as long as 30 minutes when immersed in water; therefore, treatments should be applied to dry hair (wet hair also is suspected to dilute the products). In the past, lindane was the preferred treatment, but it no longer is recommended because of high resistance, questionable efficacy, and adverse effects including the potential for neurotoxicity and bone marrow suppression.

Growing resistance to first lindane and now permethrin can be attributed in part to the inappropriate use of the pediculicides: not following the product directions, using the product as a prophylatic agent, or misusing the product on conditions not related to lice, such as seborrheic dermatitis, or on nonviable nits and dead lice. Thus, not only is proper diagnosis imperative, but also parents must be instructed to follow the application directions precisely and to apply a second treatment 8 to 10 days later. If live lice are detected 8 to 10 days after the second treatment, a prescription second-line therapy such as permethrin 5% (Elimite), worn overnight under a shower cap, or malathion 0.5% lotion should be sought. Although malathion is not considered to be a first-line agent, an *in vitro* study in reported in 2001 in the *Archives of Dermatology* showed it to be the fastest-killing pediculicide and the most effective ovicide.

Oral ivermectin, a broad-spectrum antiparasitic drug, is an emerging therapy currently being investigated. As in scabies infestation, all family members should be treated at the same time, and the patient's personal hair items as well as recently used clothes, towels, and bedding should be washed in hot (130°F) water or dried at high heat. A preliminary study in *Pediatrics* in 2004 suggested that a new dry-on, suffocation-based pediculicide may be a future option.

Mosquitoes

Epidemiology and Clinical Presentation

Mosquitoes transmit diseases such as encephalitis, malaria, and yellow fever to more than 700 million persons annually (see also Chapter 221). They are attracted to bright clothing, heat, humidity, and human odors, particulary breath carbon dioxide levels. The characteristic pruitic erythematous papule is a reaction to the anticoagulant salivary secretions of the mosquito.

Treatment and Prevention

Although topical corticosteroids and antihistamines provide relief from the bites themselves, prevention of the bites is the key to preventing disease. Protection is achieved best by avoiding their habitats, staying indoors at dawn and dusk (peak mosquito-biting hours), wearing protective clothing, and using insect repellants.

Repellants interfere with the insect's sensory devices, causing it to become confused and thus unable to land on its host. One study compared the efficacy of different insect repellants against mosquito bites. The investigators tested both plant-derived essential oils (citronella, cedar, eucalyptus, peppermint, lemongrass, geranium, and soybean) and synthetic chemicals. The most effective plant-derived repellants were based on soybean oil and provided an average of 1.5 hours of protection. The other plant-derived products were effective for only 3 to 20 minutes. The most effective chemical repellants contained DEET. DEET is effective not only against mosquitoes, but also against biting flies, chiggers, fleas, and ticks. In general, the more DEET a product contains, the longer the repellant protects against bites; a 10% concentration affords approximately 2 hours of protection, whereas a 24% concentration provides an average of 5 hours. However, the effectiveness of DEET concentrations then plateaus, and strengths greater than 30% to 50% percent do not afford greater protection. Because it generally is recommended that DEET not be applied more than once a day, the choice of concentration should coincide with the expected length of time outdoors. Because of concerns of neurologic and cardiovascular toxicity, the American Academy of Pediatrics recommends that repellants used on infants and children should not contain more than 30% DEET. The Academy also recommends that DEET not be used on infants younger than 2 months of age.

Flies and Myiasis

Epidemiology and Transmission

Myiasis is the invasion of body tissues or cavities by the larval stage (maggots) of flies. Typically, eggs are deposited by a vector, such as a mosquito, in or around a body site, which ultimately is infested. Incubated by body heat, the eggs hatch, and larvae emerge to burrow into the body tissue or cavity. Although an uncommon finding in children of developed nations, myiasis may occur in malnourished, neglected children, in travelers to tropical climates, or after accidental exposure. Human myiasis has been linked to warm, humid climates, which provide a favorable environment for the breeding of flies. Epizootics in livestock and inadequate sanitation also are risk factors associated with myiasis.

Clinical Manifestations

By far the most common form of myiasis in otherwise normal children is cutaneous myiasis, or invasion of the skin by larvae. The most common fly associated with the cutaneous form is the human botfly or warble fly (*Dermatobia hominis*); although in North America, cutaneous myiasis generally is caused by *Cuterebra* species. After the larvae burrow into the skin, a painful, elevated, pruritic papule develops. The lesions, predominately located on the exposed areas of the body, enlarge and become more painful as the larvae increase in size. Serosanguineous material or the larvae themselves may be seen exuding from the lesion. The papules often are excoriated, and secondary bacterial infection with *Staphylococcus aureus*, *Streptococcus pyogenes*, or gram-negative bacilli may develop. With the appropriate host and history, cutaneous myiasis should be entertained as the cause of a discrete pruritic nodule that does not resolve with standard therapy.

The intestinal tract, lower genitourinary tract, external auditory canal, and oral and nasal cavities, as well as the orbits (ophthalmomyiasis), are other sites of human myiasis. The most serious forms of myiasis involve invasion of the nose and orbit. Nasal myiasis can extend into the sinuses, penetrate the cribriform plate, and reach the meninges and brain. Ophthalmomyiasis may cause massive destruction of orbital tissue, requiring exenteration of the orbital contents. Gonococcal conjunctivitis in children is thought to attract flies and predispose to larval infestation.

Treatment and Prevention

The treatment of myiasis basically entails the physical removal of larvae from the invaded tissue or cavity. Cutaneous myiasis may necessitate either simply applying gentle pressure to extrude the larvae or performing more extensive surgical intervention. Occlusive dressings (e.g., petroleum jelly, bacon fat) to deprive the larvae of oxygen encourage the larvae to migrate externally. In any case, the larva should be removed completely and examined under a microscope to ensure that it is intact. Once the larva is removed, the primary papule gradually resolves. More aggressive surgical approaches may be required for treating nasal or orbital myiasis. Administration of topical or systemic antibiotics is necessary if secondary bacterial infections have developed. Human myaisis can be prevented by controlling the source of the larvae, the female fly.

Fleas

Epidemiology and Transmission

Fleas are ubiquitous in our environment and thus their bites are common. Children are especially prone to bites because they tend to spend more time on and closer to the floor (a flea can jump to a maximum height of 18 cm). The fleas that most commonly attack humans are the human (*Pulex irritans*), cat (*Ctenocephalides felis*), and dog (*Ctenocephalides canis*) fleas, which rarely carry disease. However, rat fleas are the historical, although now rare, transmitters of the plague and murine typhus. New evidence now suggests that cat fleas may be the vectors of *Bartonella henselae*.

Clinical Manifestations

Clinically, a local reaction occurs as linear groups of inflammatory papules, most commonly found on the lower legs, hands, and forearms. Wheals and bullae may occur in sensitized individuals, especially young children. Children are more prone to these types of reactions because tolerance to the bites develops with age.

Treatment and Prevention

Treatment is symptomatic, and prevention entails treating the environment, both suspected animals and infested areas of the house and yard, with insecticide.

Bees, Wasps, and Ants

Bees, wasps, and ants all are stinging insects that belong to the order Hymenoptera.

Wasps and Bees

Epidemiology and Clinical Manifestations. Wasps and bees tend not to harm humans unless provoked. Their sting produces immediate local pain followed by hours of swelling and erythema. Systemic reactions such as edema, urticaria, serum sickness (fever, urticaria, angioedema, arthralgias), or even anaphylaxis may develop in some individuals.

Treatment and Prevention. Treatment depends on the individual's reaction. If the stinger remains in the skin, it should be scraped off promptly. Care should be taken not to grab the protruding end of the stinger because it contains the venom pouch, which, if squeezed, will inject more venom into the patient. Application of ice and an injection of lidocaine are suggested for local pain relief, and oral steroids and antihistamines are recommended for mild systemic reactions. Anaphylaxis is a medical emergency and usually develops within 20 minutes of the sting. It requires immediate administration of subcutaneous epinephrine. Children known to suffer such systemic reactions should wear a medical alert tag, and parents should carry an insect sting emergency kit. Desensitization, or immunotherapy, also is available.

Fire Ants

Epidemiology. Fire ants are the wingless stinging counterparts of bees and wasps. They are imported from South America and inhabit the southern United States.

Clinical Manifestations. The ant grips the skin with its mandibles, punctures its victim, then rotates around its jaws, inserting the stinger multiple times. The painful reaction initially is a cluster of erythematous papules that develop into pustules within 24 hours. The pustules eventually rupture and may leave small scars. Systemic reactions such as fever, edema, urticaria, gastrointestinal distress, or even fatal allergic reactions (especially in infants) can occur.

Treatment and Prevention. Treatment is symptomatic; immunotherapy also may be indicated. Whether the insects are flying or grounded, no insect repellant currently is available for stinging insects. The best prevention is avoidance.

Suggested Readings

American Academy of Pediatrics. Follow safety precautions when using DEET on children. http://www.aap.org/family/wnv-jun03.htm. Accessed December 31, 2004.

Angel TA, Nigro J, Levy ML. Infestations in the pediatric patient. *Pediatr Clin North Am* 2000;47:921.

Anderson PC. Spider bites in the United States. *Dermatol Clin* 1997;15:307.

Brown S, Becher J, Brady W. Treatment of ectoparasitic infections: review of the English-language literature, 1982–1992. *Clin Infect Dis* 1995;20: S104.

Burkhart CG, Burkhart NB, Burkhart KM. An assessment of topical and oral prescription and over-the-counter treatments for head lice. *J Am Acad Dermatol* 1998;38:979.

Committee on Infectious Diseases. Prevention on Lyme disease. *Pediatrics* 2000; 105:142.

Eichenfield LF, Colon-Fontanez F. Treatment of head lice. *Pediatr Infect Dis* 1998;17:419.

Foil L, Andress E, Freeland RL, et al. Experimental infection of domestic cats with *Bartonella henselae* by innoculation of *Ctenocephalides felis* (Siphonaptera: Pulicidae) feces. *J Med Entomol* 1998;35:625.

Fradin MS, Dav JF. Comparative efficacy of insect repellants against mosquito bites. *N Engl J Med* 2002;347:13.

Hansen RC, et al. Guidelines for the treatment of resistant pediculosis. *Contemp Pediatr* 2000;(suppl):4.

Jelinek T, Nothdurft HD, Rieder N, Loscher T. Cutaneous myiasis: review of 13 cases in travelers returning from tropical countries. *Int J Dermatol* 1995; 34:624.

Meinking TL, Entzel P, Villar ME, et al. Comparative efficacy of treatments for *Pediculus capitis* infestations. *Arch Dermatol* 2001;137:287.

Metry DW, Hebert AA. Insect and arachnid stings, bites, infestations, and repellants. *Pediatr Ann* 2000;29:39.

Paller AS. Scabies in infants and small children. *Semin Dermatol* 1993;12:3.

Pearlman DL. A simple treatment for head lice: dry-on, suffocation-based pediculicide. *Pediatrics* 2004;114:275.

Rao R, Nosanchuk JS, Mackenzie R. Cutaneous myiasis acquired in New York State. *Pediatrics* 1997;99:601.

Rolain JM, Frac M, Davoust B, Raoult D. Molecular detection of *Bartonella quintana, B. koehlerae, B. henselae, B. clarridgeiae, Rickettsia felis*, and *Wolbachia pipientis* in cat fleas, France. *Emerg Infect Dis* 2003;9: 338.

Sams HH, Dunnick CA, Smith ML, King LE. Necrotic arachnidism. *J Am Acad Dermatol* 2001;44:561.

Victoria J, Trujillo R. Topical ivermectin: a new successful treatment for scabies. *Pediatr Dermatol* 2001;18:63.

Walker GJ, Johnstone PW. Interventions for treating scabies. *Cochrane Database Syst Rev* 2000;CD000320.

SECTION II ■ DISEASES OF THE RESPIRATORY TRACT

CHAPTER 228 ■ CHRONIC COUGH IN CHILDREN

I. CELINE HANSON AND WILLIAM T. SHEARER

Chronic cough is a vexing and common problem for children, their caregivers, and health care providers. Effective treatment may be difficult, especially if the underlying cause of the cough cannot be determined. Etiologies are varied and include common infectious agents that cause both upper and lower respiratory tract disease, asthma, gastrointestinal reflux disease (GERD), foreign body aspiration, and chronic primary pulmonary disease (Box 228.1). Cough also may be associated with other chronic diseases including immune deficiency, cardiac disease, neurologic disease, and allergy. The approach to diagnostic evaluation of chronic cough can be frustrating and daunting to parents and the affected child if not approached systematically. This chapter will review the causes of chronic cough and provide an approach for diagnostic evaluation in children. Readers are referred to more extensive and specific discussions of specific chronic cough-associated disorders (e.g., asthma, GERD, cystic fibrosis), provided in this textbook.

EPIDEMIOLOGY

Chronic cough defined as daily cough for 3 to 4 weeks likely has been experienced by more than 50% of the pediatric pop-ulation at some time during the first 18 years of life. This can be explained by the variable prevalence of disorders associated with chronic cough. For example, in the United States, as many as 8.9 million children younger than 17 years of age were purported to have had a diagnosis of asthma in 2001 (NCHS data, Centers for Disease Control and Prevention). Asthma varies in prevalence by age, race, and exposure (infectious, environmental) in the United States. In children, using physician diagnosed asthma alone as an indicator of cough largely under-predicts its prevalence. In a study of Alaskan Native children, physician diagnosis of asthma missed more than 30% of children with self-reported symptoms of chronic cough.

The U.S. National Health Interview Survey of 1996 estimated that 16 of every 100 children younger than 18 years of age experienced an episode of acute bronchitis. Of these episodes, more than 90% were medically attended and their illness was accompanied by restricted activity days (average of 13 to 29 days dependent upon age at presentation). Most clinicians describe acute bronchitis as a febrile illness with cough, rhonchi, and referred breath sounds. Hence, simple lower respiratory tract infections (LRTIs) are common findings and likely to be associated with chronic cough as defined previously.

In a study of children with recurrent LRTIs, as many as 42% of those younger than 18 months of age had silent GERD by scintigraphy. Evaluation of children older than 18 months of age, when physiologic reflux can be excluded, still reported silent GERD in 27%. Hence, the risk for GERD being associated with chronic cough symptoms is a common occurrence in older toddlers and children.

Parental smoking has been reported to cause chronic cough in children; children with two parents who smoke are reported to have a chronic cough prevalence of over 50%. Since lung function does not fully mature until school age, the impact of acute and long-term pollution exposure has been carefully studied in children. U.S. investigators identified higher death rates in infants from 1 to 12 months of age when inhaled particulate matter of less than 10 mm was sustained at high levels. Studies have documented diminished lung function and bronchitic symptoms including chronic cough following long-term exposure in Polish, Austrian, and U.S. children.

Some of the chronic disorders associated with chronic cough have a defined genetic link and fewer individuals are impacted than as with LRTIs or asthma. Examples include cystic fibrosis estimated to occur in 1 in 2,500 North Americans of European ancestry. Primary immune deficiency disorders may vary from 1 in 300 with selective IgA deficiency to 1 in 200,000 with severe combined immune deficiency. Disorders with lesser prevalence, such as foreign body aspiration, may have significant morbidity that can be prevented with early detection and sensitive diagnostic tools. The use of such epidemiologic data is important as it can allow the clinician to develop a logical pattern for evaluation of chronic cough based on family history, individual clinical symptoms/examination, and disease likelihood.

BOX 228.1 | **Conditions Associated with Chronic Cough (3 Weeks or Longer)**

Asthma
Recurrent episodes of bronchitis infections (*Chlamydia*, pertussis, *Mycobacterium*)
Cystic fibrosis
Primary ciliary dyskinesia
    Kartagener syndrome
    Immotile cilia syndrome
Immunodeficiency
    Selective IgA deficiency
    Hypogammaglobulinemia (primary and secondary)
Anatomic lesions
    Foreign body
    Previous esophageal atresia repair
    Mediastinal tumors
    Congenital heart disease
Irritants
    Milk aspiration (gastroesophageal reflux, tracheoesophageal fistula)
    Tobacco smoke
    Pollution
    Occupational exposure
Psychogenic cough

PATHOGENESIS

Cough is intended to clear the airway of mucus and external debris and is a normal host response. The cough reflex involves forceful exhalation caused by the contraction of expiratory muscles against a closed glottis. Gas is expelled at high velocity, and matter is moved toward the oral cavity. Neural pathways, the cortex, and the brainstem control the cough reflex. This reflex may become exaggerated in cough-associated disorders as a result of increased particulate matter in the airway.

CLINICAL MANIFESTATIONS

Chronic cough is usually more worrisome to caregivers than to health care providers. Data suggest that parental and teacher reports of childhood cough may not always correlate with severity or even frequency of disease. Clinical presentation varies according to the associated disorder. For infectious agents, timing of cough, history of affected family members, and concurrent systemic symptoms may serve as important differentiators in the evaluation. In acute bronchitis, fever and cough almost invariably occur in connection with upper respiratory congestion (predominantly nasal). The patients' temperatures can range from 37° to 39°C (100° to 103°F). Usually, cough is dry, harsh, and without sputum production in young infants. Coughing can be accompanied by gagging and vomiting, leading to poor oral intake and dehydration. Occasionally, older children with persistent cough will produce sputum and may complain of chest-wall pain. Usually, the clinical illness is preceded by 24 to 48 hours of lassitude or malaise. Subsequently, fever and cough develop; these symptoms may persist for as long as 1 week. A relatively slow recovery phase, spanning 1 to 2 weeks, with persistent cough is characteristic. Secondary bacterial infection can complicate the recovery period, causing exacerbation of fever and other clinical findings.

Chronic bronchitis is an uncommon occurrence in children but when present is characterized by excessive production of mucus and by cough that is present on most days for a minimum of 3 months per year. Fever can accompany the cough, and the temperature can range from 37°C to 39°C (100F° to 103°F). Establishing a distinction between this typically infectious disorder and asthma may be difficult. Asthma, or reversible obstructive airway disease, can be distinguished by the patients' clinical response to the administration of traditional bronchodilators. Clinical symptoms of asthma may include persistent cough or audible spontaneous wheezing, which may be precipitated by upper respiratory infection/occult or symptomatic sinusitis, environmental exposures including airborne pollens, indoor allergens (animal dander, mites), weather changes, or irritants (strong odors, smoking). Exercise, stress, and undetected/untreated reflux are also well known to exacerbate childhood asthma. Night-time cough may be a common clinical presentation for the child with asthma and associated reflux.

Persistent LRTIs (e.g., pertussis) and *Chlamydia* and *Mycobacterium* infections can present with a complex of symptoms similar to chronic bronchitis or asthma. Their clinical presentation may not differ from an acute bronchitis syndrome. Pertussis has a unique clinical presentation with a typical catarrhal phase followed by a whoop/paroxysmal and then convalescent phase, which in total may span over 6 to 8 weeks.

Cystic fibrosis is typically accompanied by steatorrhea, nasal polyps, failure to thrive, and recurrent lower respiratory tract symptoms in association with cough. Primary ciliary dyskinesia encompasses the immotile cilia disorders and Kartagener syndrome (rhinosinusitis, bronchitis, or bronchiectasis

and situs inversus). Patients affected with these disorders exhibit a defect in mucociliary transport and present with chronic cough and recurrent lower respiratory disease.

Immune disorders associated most frequently with recurrent sinopulmonary infection and chronic cough include selective IgA deficiency (serum IgA level, 10 mg/dL or less), hypogammaglobulinemia (primary and secondary), IgG subclass deficiencies, and ataxia-telangiectasia. The clinical presentation is similar to those already described but may also include complications from normally low virulent organisms.

Environmental exposures increasingly have been implicated in the development of chronic cough complex. In these patients, clinical presentation may be indolent in nature. Symptoms may be difficult to associate with an exposure because caregivers are slow to identify them or are not forthcoming with exposure histories. Chronic cough may be associated with feeding, as in patients with overt reflux or tracheoesophageal fistulas. As previously noted, for many children the clinical symptoms of GERD may be only chronic cough without associated gastrointestinal symptoms commonly seen in older children and adults.

DIAGNOSIS/EVALUATION OF CHRONIC COUGH

The evaluation of chronic cough requires obtaining a good medical history and clinical examination. Box 228.2 identifies relevant history that can facilitate evaluation of cough. A history of other ill family members may assist the physician in searching for causative infectious agents. Associated systemic symptoms (fever, malaise, rash) in affected household members or known associates and description of their clinical course can help the physician in determining the likelihood for simple symptom resolution versus anticipated complications (tuberculosis, pertussis). Presence or absence of productive sputum can help to assess chronicity of disease and to distinguish an infectious etiology from allergic diatheses. Family history may identify chronic disorders such as primary immune deficiency or cystic fibrosis because these genetically inherited disorders may be present or have been reported in family members.

| BOX 228.2 | Relevant History for Evaluating Chronic Cough of Childhood |

History of affected household members or companions
Association with other symptoms
Failure to thrive, lymphadenopathy
Fever, night sweats
Sneezing, nasal or ocular pruritus, headaches
Chronic diarrhea, malabsorption
Audible wheezing, dyspnea, exercise intolerance
Timing/onset of cough
Daytime versus nighttime
Association with food intake
Association with environmental exposures (smoking, pollution, work/school)
Association with seasonal or weather changes
Association with position or exertion (e.g., recumbent position, exercise)
History for obstruction
Apnea
Sleep disruption or daytime somnolence
Snoring

Environmental history can be very helpful in identifying chronic smoke exposure, allergen exposures (animal dander, airborne pollens) chemicals/toxic substances exposures, and family/child dynamics that might render foreign body aspiration likely. Evaluation of activities of daily living (e.g., food ingestion patterns, bowel patterns, school performance, and play and sleep patterns) can provide insight for both systemic disorders such as cystic fibrosis or obstructive disorders including sleep apnea or asthma.

For most children with chronic cough, postinfectious cough is the most likely diagnosis, pulmonary function is normal, and no complications will occur. However, a full clinical examination should occur for all affected children as specific clinical findings can predict those children who require more than reassurance and supportive therapeutic intervention. Box 228.3 outlines clinical findings that provide clues for diagnostic evaluation. These criteria include evidence of systemic disease such as growth failure, lymphadenopathy, organomegaly, developmental delay, or neurologic abnormality. Chest-wall deformities, abnormal pulmonary auscultation, clubbing or edema, or abnormal cardiac auscultation might suggest the potential for primary or secondary pulmonary disease and referral as necessary for subspecialty evaluation.

Diagnostic evaluation for chronic cough is warranted when history and clinical examination findings as outlined in Boxes

---

BOX 228.3	Clinical Findings that Predict Diagnostic Evaluation

Failure to thrive or abnormal anthropometric measures
Clubbing of digits or peripheral edema
Cyanosis, central or peripheral
Chest deformities
Audible stridor, wheeze, labored breathing
Abnormal cardiac auscultation, evidence of cor pulmonale
Organomegaly, generalized lymphadenopathy, ascites
Developmental delay or neurologic findings (muscle weakness, tics)
Allergic findings (allergic salute, ocular tearing, sneezing)

228.2 and 228.3 are detected. Figure 228.1 outlines a diagnostic algorithm for the child with chronic cough. The approach is divided into (a) lack of clinical signs or history that suggest an associated disorder or (b) presence of suspect clues. Without clues to pathogenesis, simple chest radiograph, allergy testing

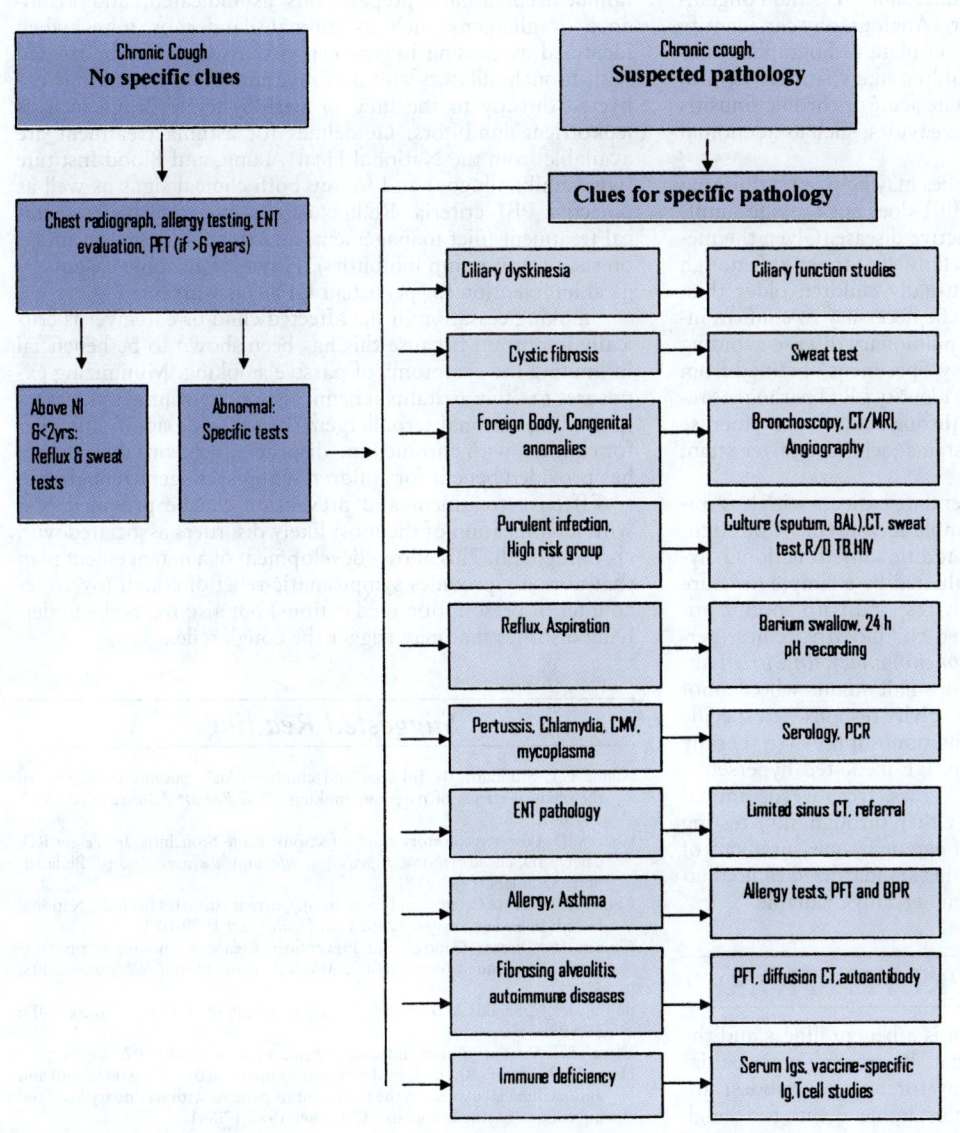

FIGURE 228.1. Algorithm for diagnostic evaluation of children with chronic cough. BAL, bronchoalveolar lavage; BPR, broncho provocation responses; CMV, cytomegalovirus; CT, computed tomography; ENT, ear/nose/throat; HIV, human immunodeficiency virus; MRI, magnetic resonance imaging; NI, normal study; PCR, polymerase chain reaction; PFT, pulmonary function test; R/O TB, rule out tuberculosis. (Modified with permission from Morice AJ, and Committee Members. Diagnosis and management of chronic cough. *Eur Respir J* 2004; 24:487.)

for children older than 3 years of age, evaluation of the oral airway passages (ear/nose/throat [ENT] referral), and, as appropriate, age pulmonary function tests (PFTs) can, as applicable, be considered. If these tests are normal and cough persists, then a sweat test and evaluation for GERD both radiographically and by pH probe is warranted. With negative results, the caregiver should be assured that no pathology exists.

For children with chronic cough and suspect clues linking the cough to an associated disorder, Figure 228.1 provides recommendations for diagnostic tools to assist in evaluation. Determination of elevated chloride (greater than 60 mEq/L) by sweat iontophoresis is diagnostic for cystic fibrosis in most patients. Gene testing using DNA analysis for mutations of the cystic fibrosis transmembrane conductance (CFTR) gene can assist when sweat test results are inconclusive. Of note, gene testing may require evaluation of multiple CFTR alleles to diagnose cystic fibrosis optimally, particularly when genetic counseling for at-risk parents is being considered. Immotile cilia disorders have a defect in mucociliary transport, as evidenced by a decrease in frequency of ciliary beat. Electron microscopy of bronchial cilia classically reveals structural defects, with absent dynein arms. This diagnosis is made by bronchial or occasionally nasal turbinate biopsy.

Imaging studies beyond chest radiographs can be most helpful in evaluating bronchiectasis (high resolution computerized tomography [CT]), specific primary pulmonary diseases such as those associated with fibrosis (diffusion CT), and congenital anomalies or mediastinal tumors. Angiography can identify cardiac anomalies not easily seen on plain radiographs. Limited CT of the sinuses in small children likely is more helpful than are plain radiographs to evaluate acute or chronic sinusitis and obstructive disease of the sinus cavities, such as adenoidal hypertrophy or polyps.

Bronchoprovocation (BPR) studies may help in establishing the diagnosis of asthma when the PFT does not provide significant evidence of reversible obstructive disease. Given the mechanics of this procedure, its use is limited to those old enough to adequately perform the PFT, usually children older than 6 years of age. Bronchoscopy may be necessary to confirm infection or to evaluate for primary pulmonary disease avoiding invasive procedures like lung biopsy. Specimens obtained from bronchoalveolar lavage (BAL) may identify LRTI pathogens responsible for chronic cough either through culture, polymerase chain reaction studies, or special stains (acid fast, silver stain, fungal stain) of lung fluid.

Immunologic studies can differentiate patients with low immunoglobulin levels through a simple measurement of circulating serum IgG, IgA, or IgM. Additionally, functional hypogammaglobulinemia can be evaluated by a simple measure of a child's ability to appropriately respond with specific antibody production to recommended childhood vaccines (pertussis, diphtheria, *Streptococcus pneumoniae*). *In vitro* lymphocyte studies may be necessary in small infants who cannot mount cutaneous delayed hypersensitivity responses to specific antigens or in patients requiring immunosuppressive therapy to control underlying lung disease. IgE-mediated hypersensitivity or allergy to aeroallergens (grass, tree, weed, animal dander, dust mite) can be tested either through skin testing in children as young as 2 years of age or by measurement of antigen-specific serum IgE levels using standardized radioallergoabsorbent technology that is commercially available.

THERAPY AND PREVENTION

Usually, acute respiratory infection is a benign illness and the associated postinfectious cough can be treated with palliative therapy (i.e., analgesic therapy for febrile episodes; antitussives, decongestants, and antihistamine agents for cough

and rhinitis). The efficacy of such approaches has not been proven for over-the-counter medications. It should be noted that in a recent review of randomized controlled pediatric trials of antitussives, expectorants, mucolytics, and antihistamine–decongestant combinations, efficacy could not be determined. The authors cautioned that the number of trials was small with very few participants, which may have impacted the inability to determine efficacy for each outlined drug group.

Persistent coughing with gagging and vomiting can precipitate dehydration and serum metabolic changes. Monitoring of these parameters in severely affected hosts and reconstitution of deficits by oral or parenteral rehydration are indicated.

When secondary bacterial infection is suggested by exacerbation of fever or by evidence of pneumonia on a chest radiograph, broad-spectrum antibiotic therapy may be indicated. Specific antimicrobial therapy should provide coverage for known or likely LRTI pathogens (e.g., *Haemophilus influenzae* or *S. pneumoniae*). When an associated disorder can be identified, the treatment of chronic cough should target that disorder. Such interventions would include appropriate antimicrobials for established infections. Delivery of childhood vaccines (pertussis-containing vaccines, measles-containing vaccines, and the conjugate polysaccharide vaccines against *H. influenzae* or *S. pneumoniae*) can prevent significant morbidity following exposure. Management of allergic diatheses includes nasal antiinflammatory preparations, oral antihistamine/decongestant preparations as indicated, and avoidance of allergens such as animal dander or mites when identified as causing hypersensitivity. Asthma can be treated with bronchodilators and antiinflammatory preparations delivered directly to the lung or with systemic drugs such as leukotriene inhibitors. Guidelines for asthma treatment are available from the National Heart, Lung, and Blood Institute (www.nhlbi.nih.gov) and follow both clinical signs as well as objective PFT criteria. Reflux usually is responsive to medical treatment (diet management, antacids, H_2 receptor antagonists, proton pump inhibitors). However, in some cases, surgical intervention for persistent GERD is warranted.

Smoking cessation in the affected child or caregiver is critically important because this has been shown to be beneficial in limiting the symptoms of passive smoking. Minimizing exposures to other irritants (chemicals) or environmental factors (pollution, seasonal aeroallergens) can provide significant relief for children with chronic lung disorders. Behavioral treatment has provided benefit for children with psychogenic cough.

Effective treatment and prevention can be provided best with identification of the most likely disorders associated with chronic cough. This allows development of a management plan that not only provides symptomatic relief of cough (over-the-counter or prescription medications) but also treats the underlying disorder that may trigger the cough reflex.

Suggested Readings

Aligne CA, Stoddard JJ. Tobacco and children. An economic evaluation of the medical effects of parental smoking. *Arch Pediatr Adolesc Med* 1997; 151:648.

Cherry JD. Lower respiratory tract infections: acute bronchitis. In: Feigin RD, Cherry JD, eds. *Textbook of pediatric infectious diseases,* 2nd ed. Philadelphia: Saunders, 1987:278.

Centers for Disease Control and Prevention. Current estimates from the National Health Interview Survey, 1996. *Vital Health Stat* 1999;10:1.

Centers for Disease Control and Prevention. Cigarette smoking-attributable morbidity—United States, 2000. *MMWR Morb Mortal Wkly Rep* 2003; 52:842.

deJongste JC, Sheilds MD. Cough 2: chronic cough in children. *Thorax* 2003; 58:998.

Glezen WP. Viral respiratory infections. *Pediatr Ann* 1991;20:407.

Henry D, Ruoff GE, Rhudy J, et al. Clinical comparison of cefuroxime axetil and amoxicillin/clavulanate in the treatment of patients with secondary bacterial infections of acute bronchitis. *Clin Ther* 1995;17:861.

Kubo AS, Funabashi S, Uehara S, et al. Clinical aspects of "asthmatic bronchitis" and chronic bronchitis in infants and children. *J Asthma Res* 1978;15:99.

Lewis TC, Stout JW, Martinez P, et al. Prevalence of asthma and chronic respiratory symptoms among Alaska Native children. *Chest* 2004;125:1665.

Morice AJ, and Committee Members. The diagnosis and management of chronic cough. *Eur Respir J* 2004;24:481.

Richards CS, Grody WW. Prenatal screening for cystic fibrosis: past, present and future. *Expert Rev Mol Diagn* 2004;4:49.

Schroeder K, Fahey T. Over-the-counter medications for acute cough in children and adults in ambulatory settings. *Cochrane Database Syst Rev* 2004;18:CD001831.

Schwartz J. Air pollution and children's health. *Pediatrics* 2004;113:1037.

Thomas EJ, Kumar R, Dasan JB, et al. Prevalence of silent gastroesophageal reflux in association with recurrent lower respiratory tract infections. *Clin Nucl Med* 2003;28:476.

Velissauriou IM, Dafetzis DA. Chronic cough in children: recent advances. *Expert Rev Anti-infect Ther* 2004;2:111.

CHAPTER 229 ■ BRONCHIOLITIS

I. CELINE HANSON AND WILLIAM T. SHEARER

Lower respiratory tract infection (LRTI) in children younger than 24 months of age is a common clinical occurrence and, during the past decade, has been associated with increasing hospitalization rates in children in the United States during winter months. The spectrum of pathologic involvement includes large and small airways (tracheobronchitis, bronchitis, bronchiolitis) and alveolar or interstitial lung involvement (pneumonia).

The term *bronchiolitis* was coined in the early 1900s. Criteria for the diagnosis of bronchiolitis include first episode of acute wheezing at age 24 months or younger, accompanying physical findings of viral infection (i.e., coryza, cough, fever), and exclusion of pneumonia or atopy as the cause of wheezing.

EPIDEMIOLOGY

Table 229.1 lists the infectious agents that have been associated with the clinical entity of bronchiolitis. Viruses, particularly respiratory syncytial virus (RSV), account for most of the pathogens isolated during clinical disease. In reviews of bronchiolitis-associated outpatient and hospital morbidity in Native American and Alaskan Native children, RSV was associated with between 50% and 80% of all cases of bronchiolitis. RSV infection is estimated to be a very common childhood event in all pediatric populations, affecting almost 60% of infants during the first year of life, and it is responsible for over 100,000 hospitalizations annually. The onset of illness

varies across the United States, but typically begins in October through December and ends in March to May.

Human metapneumovirus, a paramyxovirus first identified in 2001, has been identified increasingly as being responsible for acute lower tract respiratory infections, including bronchiolitis in all age groups, and severe clinical outcome in very young and/or immunocompromised children. In a retrospective study of over 2,000 healthy U.S. infants followed from 1976 through 2001, human metapneumovirus was identified in 12% of all lower respiratory illnesses and 59% of patients diagnosed with bronchiolitis. In this study, peak viral isolation occurred from December through April. A more recent evaluation of 1,500 Italian infants, children, and their families identified co-isolation of RSV or influenza virus in more than 16% of acute respiratory infections caused by human metapneumovirus.

Influenza viruses cause significant respiratory disease during the winter months, with an attributed 50,000 deaths each year in the United States (1990–1999). Death from influenza is not common in infants. Modeling data estimate about 92 deaths in U.S. children younger than 5 years of age occurred during the 1990s. Estimates for influenza-related hospitalizations were 114,000 per year in the United States during the 1990s. In a Canadian cohort of 182 infants hospitalized for influenza from 1999 through 2002, 27% were admitted with a diagnosis of LRTIs (not bronchiolitis) and 15% with asthma/bronchiolitis diagnoses.

Other viral agents (adenovirus, parainfluenza, mumps) have been reported in the literature in association with bronchiolitis. Seasonal patterns of isolation overlap for many of the listed viral agents (Table 229.1). Adenovirus isolation is unique, when compared with the other listed viral agents, in its more marked nasopharyngeal isolation during non-winter months. Like metapnuemovirus, adenovirus isolation may occur year round. Although *Mycoplasma pneumoniae* has been associated with lower respiratory tract disease and episodes of wheezing occasionally in infants and more commonly in older children, no bacterial agents have been implicated as inciting the wheezing.

TABLE 229.1

BRONCHIOLITIS: ETIOLOGIC AGENTS

Viral*	Months of Peak Illness
Respiratory syncytial virus	December–May
Metapneumovirus	October–May
Influenza viruses	October–May
Adenovirus (types 3, 7, 21)	October–June
Parainfluenza virus (type 3)	June–December (sporadic)
Mumps	Sporadic
Miscellaneous	
Mycoplasma pneumoniae	

*Viral agents are listed in order of decreasing presumed incidence based on reported isolation patterns.

PATHOGENESIS

The sites of inflammation in bronchiolitis are the small bronchi and bronchioles; the alveolar spaces are spared. Pathologic changes include necrosis and sloughing of respiratory epithelium, with destruction of ciliated cells, lymphocytic infiltration of epithelium, and intrabronchiolar plugs of fibrin and mucus and edema causing either complete or partial obstruction. Usually, 1 to 2 weeks are required before the respiratory epithelium is restored completely.

Airway obstruction from fibrinous debris and mucus plugs, combined with the abnormal mechanics of respiration in bronchiolitis, increases substantially the work of breathing for affected infants and also leads to mismatching of pulmonary ventilation and perfusion. Not surprising, arterial hypoxemia can be documented frequently during clinical disease. A retention of carbon dioxide is not a common problem, but, when it is present, it can result in acute respiratory acidosis and the need for prompt ventilatory assistance. Blood pH level abnormalities can be documented and may reflect contraction alkalosis related to the dehydration associated with poor oral intake and the contraction of extracellular spaces.

An investigation of immunologic responses at the site of injury after viral infection and bronchiolitis have occurred has led to speculation regarding the long-term complications and sequelae of bouts of bronchiolitis, including subsequent reactive airway disease. For most children, no such clinical correlation can be documented. However, in subpopulations of infants with elevated serum IgE levels and likely genetic predisposition to atopic disease, early onset of wheezing with bronchiolitis has been associated with documented pulmonary function changes consistent with asthma in their early school years.

Traditionally, inflammatory responses after viral infection are thought to be cell-mediated, with lymphocytic infiltration followed by the recruitment of macrophages to clear debris. In children with RSV-associated bronchiolitis, an evaluation of nasal and bronchial washings shows that the normal immune cytokine response is aberrant, with a shift towards a T helper cell type 2 (Th2) inflammatory response and poor or absent Th1 cytotoxic response. This shift in cytokine response likely is responsible for ineffective viral clearance and the production of proinflammatory cytokines that result in a continued inflammatory response. Therapeutic and/or preventive intervention for bronchiolitis will be defined better as more information on the immune response of bronchiolitis-associated pathogens and host response is determined.

CLINICAL MANIFESTATIONS AND COMPLICATIONS

Most often, bronchiolitis affects children between ages 2 and 12 months. The clinical presentation of bronchiolitis is that of a lower respiratory tract viral illness: fever [usually 38.3°C (101°F) or less], cough, dyspnea, and rhinitis. Hypoxia with cyanosis and increased work of breathing precipitates most hospitalizations for infants with bronchiolitis, but hypoxia frequently can be documented even without clinical evidence of desaturation (i.e., cyanosis or poor peripheral perfusion). On physical examination, tachypnea with chest retractions and wheezing with rhonchi are common findings, and mild conjunctivitis and otitis are not uncommon. Often, increased respiratory effort, fever, and cough lead to poor feeding and vomiting. Lethargy and dehydration often are observed.

Usually, radiographic abnormalities are nonspecific and may include air trapping, atelectasis, and peribronchial thickening and consolidation (Fig. 229.1). A diffuse interstitial infiltration pattern also has been reported, adding to the spectrum of chest radiographic abnormalities in this disease.

Children with significant cardiopulmonary disease or immunodeficiency are at much greater risk of having serious sequelae from bronchiolitis. Atelectasis, apnea, and respiratory failure are the most important acute complications of bronchiolitis. Immature ventilatory control and respiratory muscle fatigue lead to apnea and respiratory failure in the youngest patients with bronchiolitis. Once they are intubated and mechan-

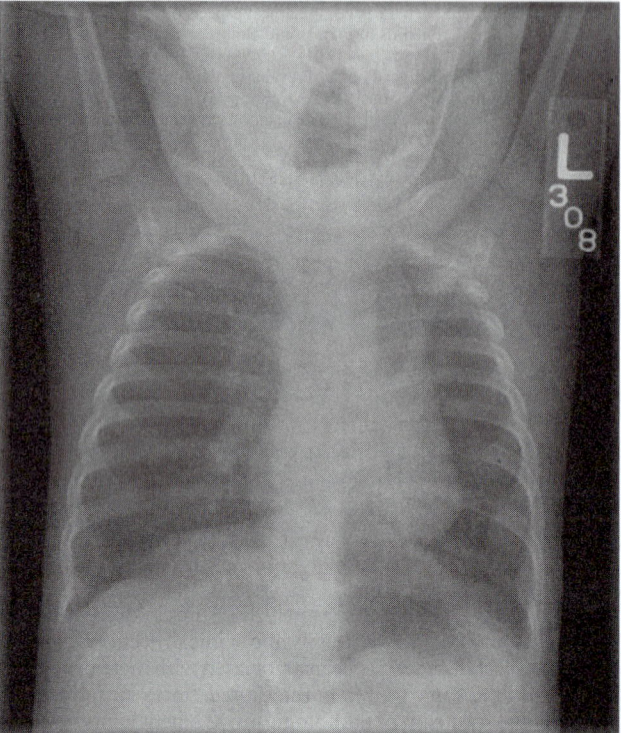

FIGURE 229.1. Chest radiograph of infant bronchiolitis showing typical findings of hyperinflation, air trapping and hilar prominence with peribronchial thickening. (Provided with the kind permission of MM Sockrider, M.D., Baylor College of Medicine, Texas Children's Hospital Pulmonary Medicine Clinic.)

ically ventilated, infants with bronchiolitis are at risk for developing pneumothorax and pneumomediastinum. Intubated patients should be monitored for changes in the amount of tracheal secretions and for secondary fever, which may indicate superinfection and the need for antibiotic therapy. Infants with chronic lung disease and who have been weaned from oxygen therapy may require supplemental oxygen at the time of discharge from the hospital after a bout of bronchiolitis.

Bronchiolitis obliterans is a complication of bronchiolitis caused by adenovirus types 3, 7, and 21; influenza viruses; *M. pneumoniae*; and *Pneumocystis carinii*. This disorder is characterized pathologically by diffuse destruction of distal small airways and physiologically by hypoxia and fixed air-flow obstruction. Bronchiolitis obliterans has not been described in association with RSV infection.

Concurrent genetic and environmental factors (including hyperactive airways that are prone to episodic obstruction) and parental smoking have been implicated in the development of recurrent wheezing after bronchiolitis. In a study of emergency visits for pediatric asthma and bronchiolitis, the prevalence of self-reported parental smoking was 41% despite good knowledge of the impact of environmental tobacco smoke on their child's disease. Significant pulmonary dysfunction noted in affected children in adult life may be coupled to subsequent environmental exposures, including adult smoking practices and exposure to pollution. Infants with predisposing conditions, specifically low- and very low-birth-weight infants, may be at increased risk of developing RSV bronchiolitis with severe sequela.

Differential Diagnosis

The differential diagnosis of bronchiolitis includes triggering of underlying reactive airway disease or asthma, other infectious lower respiratory tract diseases (e.g., pneumonia and chemical irritation, as with reflux or aspiration pneumonia), anatomic abnormalities (vascular ring, lung cysts), and extrapulmonary causes of wheezing (cardiac asthma, acidosis, poisoning). In severe disease, chest radiography may be helpful in excluding pneumonia. A barium swallow or pH probe determination can document reflux as a cause of recurrent lower respiratory tract diseases that are accompanied by wheezing. Evidence of cardiac disease may be identified by barium swallow; evidence of extrinsic bronchial constriction may be noted by echocardiography and electrocardiography.

The diagnostic distinction most difficult to make in infants is between intrinsic reactive airway disease and bronchiolitis. Reactive airway disease, or asthma, is a reversible obstructive airway disease; a 20% reduction in pulmonary function—forced expiratory volume in 1 minute—may be noted after cold or methacholine challenge and is reversible with inhaled bronchodilators. Use of this diagnostic technique is limited to children who are old enough to perform pulmonary function testing (older than age 6 years). In small children, establishing the diagnosis of asthma is more difficult; a clinical history or family predisposition, atopy, and recurrent bouts of wheezing that are responsive to bronchodilators assist in making a diagnosis. Recurrent episodes of bronchiolitis have been implicated in the occurrence of reactive airway disease in older children. Because most children with bronchiolitis have a viral illness, the diagnosis of bronchiolitis can be made on the basis of clinical and historical findings.

Children with cystic fibrosis can have bouts of bronchiolitis that manifest clinically as prolonged or unusually complicated or severe lower respiratory tract illnesses. The diagnosis of cystic fibrosis can be made by documenting elevated chloride levels (greater than 60 mEq/L) by sweat iontophoresis testing.

IgE-mediated hypersensitivity to foods, airborne allergens, or insect stings can precipitate systemic allergic reactions, including urticaria, wheezing, and hypotension. The history and physical examination can be very helpful in identifying allergies in children. Evidence that the administration of food is followed quickly by diarrhea, vomiting, angioedema, or hives and wheezing clearly suggests food allergy. Radioallergosorbent testing of serum for specific IgE response to food is helpful in confirming this clinical diagnosis. Often, wheezing with airborne allergen exposure is accompanied by symptoms of allergic rhinitis characterized by watery, clear rhinorrhea, nasal and ocular pruritus, and sneezing. Physical examination may reveal the classic stigmata of atopy (e.g., an upturned nose with a nasal crease, allergic shiners, follicular conjunctivitis, bluish boggy nasal mucosa, or a cobblestone appearance of the posterior pharynx). Allergic reactions to insect bites are common occurrences and should be suspected when physical examination reveals either typical lesions, such as vesicular skin lesions after fire ant bites, or an intact stinger still embedded in the skin after bee or wasp stings.

THERAPY

The treatment of bronchiolitis continues to rely primarily on supportive care, specifically, the provision of oxygen and appropriate fluid management. Secondary bacterial infection is rare, and antibiotics are rarely needed. Past therapeutic interventions for clinical management included bronchodilators, cholinergics, corticosteroids, and antivirals, but their efficacy has been disputed in more recent clinical trial reviews. Data on bronchodilator effectiveness in the treatment of bronchiolitis have yielded conflicting outcomes. In one series, 30% of infants with RSV bronchiolitis responded to nebulized albuterol with improvement in their pulmonary function. This improvement was, however, short-term and did not appear to reduce admission rates or decrease the duration of hospitalization. In

another series, the use of oral albuterol was no more beneficial than was placebo in infants with mild to moderate viral bronchiolitis. In a review of eight trials (394 children) evaluating bronchodilators in infants/children with bronchiolitis, drug response was only modest and short-lived.

Neither epinephrine nor anticholinergics have been shown to have significant proven benefit in the treatment of bronchiolitis. Data from multicenter controlled trials suggest that the use of nebulized adrenaline in emergency department treatment of acute bronchiolitis does not have a significant advantage over nebulized saline in reducing the number of hospital admissions or the duration of hospital stays. Similarly, in a review of six clinical trials using ipratropium bromide for wheezing precipitated by respiratory infection in children younger than 2 years of age, no significant difference in length of hospital stay or improvement in emergency room respiratory rate of oxygen saturation could be identified.

Clinicians have reported anecdotally the successful use of corticosteroids administered by varying methods (oral, inhaled, intramuscular) in RSV-related LRTI. In a review of systemic glucocorticoids use in acute viral bronchiolitis (13 trials), no benefit was found in either length of stay or clinical score for hospitalized infants/children with bronchiolitis. Three of these reviewed studies specifically evaluated readmission rates for wheezing and found no improvement in rehospitalization with glucocorticoid use.

Children with suspected bronchiolitis should be admitted to the hospital if they are tachypneic, have marked retractions, seem listless, or have a history of poor intake of fluids. Immunocompromised infants and those with underlying cardiopulmonary disease should be hospitalized if bronchiolitis develops. Increasing use of pulse oximetry has been suggested as being associated with an increased number of admissions of previously healthy infants with bronchiolitis during the past 2 decades. Such admission trends have led to the development of practice guidelines for the treatment of childhood bronchiolitis. The guidelines rely on careful clinical assessment and monitoring, with medical intervention offered only in selected settings. Physician adherence to developed guidelines varies according to severity of disease and the location of the child's care (routine hospital admission, emergency department, intensive care unit); children with severe disease or admitted to intensive care units are more likely to be treated with bronchodilators, epinephrine, corticosteroids, and antivirals.

The inpatient evaluation should include a chest film, arterial blood gas measurements, and oxygen saturation (S_aO_2) monitoring. Nasopharyngeal washings should be obtained for viral cultures and, more important, for RSV enzyme immunoassay or immunofluorescence (sensitivity of such assays as compared to culture averages 80% to 90%) or influenza rapid screening tests (sensitivity 45% to 90%, specificity 60% to 95%, as compared to viral culture) because results can be available immediately to clinicians (within 12 to 24 hours) and may have a great impact on the management of disease. The infant should receive intravenous fluids at maintenance rates, with additional fluids given to restore normal hydration. Care to avoid overhydration should be observed. Humidified oxygen should be started at 28% and adjusted to maintain the P_aO_2 at more than 60 mm Hg and the S_aO_2 at more than 90%. Nebulized epinephrine or beta$_2$ agonists may be given as needed but should be discontinued if significant improvement is not observed.

Intubation and mechanical ventilation are indicated for apnea, for a rising P_aCO_2 value, and for listlessness and retractions suggesting impending respiratory failure. Corticosteroids, bronchodilators, and furosemide all have been used in ventilated patients with bronchiolitis. Most patients ventilated for bronchiolitis require 7 to 14 days of mechanical support before they can be weaned from the ventilator.

Ribavirin is an antiviral agent that is effective against RSV and influenza viruses A and B. It is indicated for the early treatment of RSV in infants with congenital heart disease, bronchopulmonary dysplasia (now called chronic lung disease), lung and chest-wall anomalies, and immunodeficiency. Infants younger than age 6 weeks and severely ill patients (P_aO_2 less than 65 mm Hg, rising P_aCO_2) with bronchiolitis also are candidates for ribavirin therapy. Data do not support efficacy for the use of ribavirin in healthy infants with RSV bronchiolitis; that is, no shortening in length of stay or improvement of clinical scores was observed. In three trials of ribavirin use in previously healthy children with hospitalization due to LRTI caused by RSV, the mortality rate was modestly only improved over placebo (5% versus 9%, respectively; OR 0.58), respiratory deterioration was somewhat improved over placebo (7.1% versus 18.3%, respectively; OR 0.37), and the difference in days of hospitalization was 1.9 fewer days with ribavirin over placebo. Given the cost and delivery limitations for ribavirin use, its utility in the routine care of hospitalized RSV bronchiolitis is not well established.

The role of antibiotic therapy in bronchiolitis is minimal because few bacterial agents have been described as causative. The routine submission of nasopharyngeal specimens for bacterial culture is not warranted in RSV bronchiolitis. Antimicrobial therapy may be administered because of concomitant radiographic evidence of pneumonia. Traditional causative agents (*Haemophilus influenzae*, *Streptococcus pneumoniae*) should be considered and appropriate therapy initiated according to local sensitivity profiles. If secondary bacterial infection is a consideration, nosocomial infectious agents (*Staphylococcus aureus*) should be considered.

PREVENTION

The prevention of infection by etiologic agents that cause childhood bronchiolitis is the cornerstone for reducing disease morbidity. Vaccines are under development for RSV and parainfluenza and, although not yet approved for use, hold promise for the future. Two influenza vaccine types are available for use in the United States, an inactivated vaccine and a live viral cold-adapted intranasal vaccine (LAIV). In addition to a recommendation (ACIP; AAP and AAFP) for delivery to at-risk populations, inactivated influenza vaccine has been added to the general childhood immunization schedule for annual delivery (typically October through early March) to healthy infants 6 to 23 months of age. Viral antigen inclusion in both the inactivated and LAIV vaccines changes annually and is predicted using sophisticated modeling technology and principles of antigenic drift. LAIV or cold-adapted intranasal influenza vaccine is approved for use in healthy individuals older than 60 months of age and younger than 50 years.

The early identification of infected household members during influenza season and epidemics offers opportunities for disease prevention in high-risk children. Vaccine is the preventive measure of choice. Chemoprophylaxis for influenza has limited utility in children because only two drugs (amantidine and rimantidine) are approved by the U.S. Food and Drug Administration (FDA) for use in children older than 1 year of age and only against influenza A. Chemoprophylaxis often is offered during the 2 weeks following immunization and prior to the development of an immune response. Prophylaxis dosing for both drugs (amantidine and rimantidine) is 5 mg/kg/day, as two divided doses, not to exceed 150 mg/day for children 1 to 9 years of age.

Passive immunization against RSV has been approved by the FDA through the use of palivizumab (humanized mouse monoclonal antibody directed against an epitope of the A antigenic site of the F protein of RSV) and RSV intravenous immune globulin (RSV-IVIG, pooled human globulin from donors with high serum titers of RSV–neutralizing antibody) for children who are younger than 24 months of age with chronic lung disease and for certain preterm infants (less than 36 weeks' gestation). The administration of palivizumab or RSV-IVIG is monthly (every 30 days) at the onset of RSV season (October through December; regional differences are acknowledged). Five monthly doses (first delivered prior to the onset of RSV season, typically November) are recommended of each product (palivizumab 15 mg/kg/dose intramuscularly or RSV-IVIG 750 mg/kg per dose or 15 mL/kg per dose intravenously). Neither drug is approved for use in the treatment of RSV disease. Palivizumab can be used in selected infants (the decision should be made based on the degree of physiologic compromise) with hemodynamically significant congenital heart disease. RSV-IVIG is contraindicated for use in children with cyanotic congenital heart disease. Palivizumab does not interfere with the delivery of childhood immunizations. In contrast, the delivery of childhood immunization with varicella and measles-mumps-rubella vaccination should be deferred for 9 months after the last dose of RSV-IVIG has been given.

The routine childhood vaccination schedule provides opportunities for children to acquire protection from the bacterial antigens (*H. influenzae*, *S. pneumoniae*) that might be associated with superinfection of bronchiolitis. The full and timely immunization of infants is an important adjunct for controlling comorbidity of all lower respiratory infectious disease processes, including bronchiolitis.

Suggested Readings

Adcock PM, Stout GG, Hauck MA, et al. Effect of rapid viral diagnosis on the management of children hospitalized with lower respiratory tract infection. *Pediatr Infect J Dis* 1997;16:842.

Boeck KD. Respiratory syncytial virus bronchiolitis: clinical aspects and epidemiology. *Monaldi Arch Chest Dis* 1996;51:210.

Bolvin G, Abed Y, Pelletier G, et al. Virological features and clinical manifestations associated with human metapneumovirus: a new paramyxovirus responsible for acute respiratory-tract infection in all age groups. *J Infect Dis* 2002;186:1330.

Centers for Disease Control and Prevention. Bronchiolitis-associated outpatient visits and hospitalizations among American Indian and Alaska Native children—United States, 1990–2000. *Morb Mortal Wkly Rep* 2003;52:707.

Committee on Infectious Diseases: American Academy of Pediatrics. Revised indications for the use of palivizumab and respiratory syncytial virus immune globulin intravenous for the prevention of respiratory syncytial virus infections. *Pediatrics* 2003;112:1442.

Fitzgerald DA, Kilham HA. Bronchiolitis: assessment and evidence-based management. *Med J Aust* 2004;180:399.

Hartling L, Wiebe N, Russell K, et al. Epinephrine for bronchiolitis. *Cochrane Database Syst Rev* 2004;CD003123.

Kotagal UR, Robbins JM, Kini NM, et al. Impact of a bronchiolitis guideline: a multisite demonstration project. *Chest* 2002;121:1789.

Legg JP, Hussain IR, Warner JA, et al. Type and type 2 cytokine imbalance in acute respiratory syncytial virus bronchiolitis. *Am J Respir Crit Care Med* 2003;168:633.

Mallory MD, Shay DK, Garrett J, Bordley WC. Bronchiolitis management preference and the influence of pulse oximetry and respiratory rate on the decision to admit. *Pediatrics* 2003;111:e45.

Martinez FD, Wright AL, Taussig LM, et al. Asthma and wheezing in the first six years of life. The Group Health Medical Associates. *N Engl J Med* 1995;332:133.

Martinez FD. Respiratory syncytial virus bronchiolitis and the pathogenesis of childhood asthma. *Pediatr Infect Dis J* 2003;22:S76.

McConnochie KM. Bronchiolitis: what's in the name? *Am J Dis Child* 1983;137:11.

Patel H, Platt R, Lozano JM and Wang EE. Glucocorticoids for acute viral bronchiolitis in infants and young children. *Cochrane Database Syst Rev* 2004;CD004878.

Romero JR. Palivizumab prophylaxis of respiratory syncytial virus disease from 1998 to 2002; results from four years of palivizumab usage. *Pediatr Infect Dis J* 2003;22:S46.

Weisman LE. Populations at risk for developing respiratory syncytial virus and risk factors for respiratory syncytial virus severity: infants with predisposing conditions. *Pediatr Infect Dis J* 2003;22:S33.

Williams JV, Harris PA, Tollefson SJ, et al. Human metapneumovirus and lower respiratory tract disease in otherwise healthy infants and children. *N Engl J Med* 2004;350:443.

CHAPTER 230 ■ VIRAL AND ATYPICAL PNEUMONIA

KENNETH M. BOYER AND PHILLIP A. JACOBSON

Viral and atypical (nonbacterial) pneumonias are the pulmonary infections encountered most commonly in pediatrics. The varied causes of these illnesses, excluding bacteria and fungi, cover a broad taxonomic spectrum. With improvement in microbiologic techniques, the number of known causative agents continues to increase. Although most nonbacterial pneumonias have a good prognosis, occasionally they are life-threatening. Defining the etiology of these conditions in the past has been the province of epidemiologists and virologists, but a sufficient body of knowledge has accumulated to permit the practicing pediatrician to make informed clinical judgments and rapid specific diagnoses. Moreover, in selected instances, specific therapies and preventive measures now are available.

Viral pneumonia is defined as pulmonary infection in which a viral pathogen invades and elicits an inflammatory response in pulmonary parenchyma. Most viral pneumonia is acute in onset and produces diffuse, scattered, or interstitial infiltrates in radiographs. Atypical pneumonia is defined as pulmonary infection elicited by one of a group of fastidious pathogens, including mycoplasmas and chlamydiae. Most atypical pneumonia is subacute in onset but, like viral pneumonia, it is usually not associated with true radiographic consolidation. Other unusual pathogens, such as rickettsiae and protozoan parasites, occasionally may elicit pneumonia syndromes that resemble these two clinical patterns.

ETIOLOGY

At least 15 different virus groups, three *Mycoplasma* species, one rickettsia, three *Chlamydia* species, and one protozoan parasite have been associated with pneumonia syndromes in children. The overall importance of these agents is not measured simply by their incidence. Some agents, although they are fairly common, generally give rise to relatively mild illness; others encountered less frequently characteristically cause serious disease. In Table 230.1, the major agents causing disease in various age groups are presented according to their overall frequency, their typical degree of severity, and their usual mode of access to the lung.

Respiratory syncytial virus (RSV) is the most common cause of pediatric pneumonia, particularly if it is associated with bronchiolitis. Although infection with this virus is fairly common in all age groups, lower respiratory tract involvement is especially prominent in infancy.

The three parainfluenza viruses (types 1, 2, and 3) are second only to RSV as causes of lower respiratory tract disease in infants and younger children. Of these agents, parainfluenza virus 3 occurs most frequently in pneumonia; infection by parainfluenza viruses 1 and 2 generally produces laryngotracheitis.

Human metapneumovirus (hMPV) is a recently discovered respiratory virus that appears to be a significant cause of lower respiratory tract infection in infants and children. It is classified in the same family (*Paramyxoviridae*) and subfamily (Pneumovirus) as RSV. Its symptoms appear to be similar to those of RSV and influenza. It is estimated to be the cause of 12% of lower respiratory tract infections in children younger than the age of 5 years.

Influenza viruses A and B are not as prevalent overall as RSV, the parainfluenza viruses, and hMPV, but during periods of epidemic spread, they may become predominant isolates in ambulatory and hospitalized children with lower respiratory tract diseases.

Sometimes adenoviruses are isolated in children with pneumonia and with pertussis syndrome. Although the overall frequency of these viruses is somewhat less than that of the other common respiratory viruses, numerous fatal illnesses have been reported. Of the 31 known adenoviruses, types 1, 2, 3, 4, 5, 7, 8, 11, 21, and 35 have been associated clearly with pneumonia. Some degree of lower respiratory tract involvement by rhinoviruses is indicated by their documented role in exacerbations of asthma and bronchitis. Among the enteroviruses, primary virus pneumonia has been documented best with coxsackieviruses A9 and B1, although coxsackieviruses A16, B4, and B5 and echoviruses 9, 11, 19, 20, and 22 also have been reported.

The human coronaviruses HCoV-O43 and HCoV-229E have been implicated as causes of pneumonia in a few seroepidemiologic studies, but recovery of these agents in tissue culture has been rare. Two other newly described coronaviruses, HCoV-NL63 and HCoV-NH (possibly the same species), have been shown to be relatively common causes of acute respiratory illnesses in children in the Netherlands and in Connecticut. Their role in viral pneumonia is not yet defined.

Another newly discovered coronavirus is responsible for an important entity called severe acute respiratory syndrome, otherwise known as SARS. This disease first appeared in southern China in November of 2002 and rapidly spread to 29 countries. More than 8,000 cases were reported worldwide, resulting in more than 900 deaths. The epidemic now appears to have been controlled through an extraordinary global public health effort. Lower respiratory infection by the SARS coronavirus (SARS-CoV) frequently leads to acute respiratory distress syndrome with respiratory failure. Younger children appear to be affected much less severely than are teenagers and adults.

Pneumonia is the most common serious complication of measles. On careful radiographic study, at least one-half of all patients with routine cases of measles have pulmonary infiltrates early in the illness, a finding suggesting a viral rather than a bacterial cause. Secondary pneumonia in measles results from the common bacterial pathogens, particularly *Streptococcus pneumoniae* and *Staphylococcus aureus*. Progressive, fatal, primary measles pneumonia (Hecht giant cell pneumonia) can occur in patients with cell-mediated immunodeficiency, hematologic malignancy, or acquired immunodeficiency resulting from human immunodeficiency virus (HIV) infection. The characteristic measles rash often is absent.

TABLE 230.1

ETIOLOGIC AGENTS IN VIRAL AND ATYPICAL PNEUMONIA

Etiologic Agents	Frequency*			Usual Degree of Severity†			Mode of Access to Lung
	0–3 mo	4 mo–5 yr	6–16 yr	0–3 mo	4 mo–5 yr	6–16 yr	
Virus							
Respiratory syncytial virus	++++	++++	+	++	++	+	Respiratory
Parainfluenza viruses							
Type 1	+	++	+	++	++	+	Respiratory
Type 2	+	+	+	++	++	+	Respiratory
Type 3	++	+++	++	++	++	+	Respiratory
Human metapneumovirus	+	++	?	++	++	?	Respiratory
Influenza viruses							
Type A	++	+++	+++	++	++	++	Respiratory
Type B	++	++	+	++	++	++	Respiratory
Adenoviruses‡	+	++	++	+++	++	+	Respiratory
Rhinoviruses§	+	+	+	−	+	+	Respiratory
Enteroviruses‖	+	+	+	++	++	+	Respiratory (hematogenous)
Coronaviruses¶	+	++	+	+	++	+++	Respiratory
Measles virus	+	++	++	+++	++	++	Respiratory (hematogenous)
Rubella virus	+	−	−	++	−	−	Hematogenous
Human immunodeficiency virus	+	++	+	++	++	++	Hematogenous
Varicella-zoster virus	+	+	+	+++	+++	+++	Hematogenous (respiratory)
Cytomegalovirus	+++	+	+	++	+++	+++	Hematogenous (respiratory)
Epstein-Barr virus	−	+	++	−	++	+	Hematogenous (respiratory)
Herpes simplex virus	++	+	+	++++	+++	+++	Hematogenous (respiratory)
Mycoplasmas							
Mycoplasma pneumoniae	−	+	++++	−	++	+	Respiratory
Mycoplasma hominis	++	−	−	++	−	−	Respiratory
Ureaplasma urealyticum	++	−	−	++	−	−	Respiratory
Chlamydiae							
Chlamydia pneumoniae	−	+	+++	−	+	+	Respiratory
Chlamydia psittaci	+	+	+	−	++	++	Respiratory
Chlamydia trachomatis	+++	−	−	++	−	−	Respiratory
Rickettsiae							
Coxiella burnetii	−	+	+	−	++	++	Respiratory (hematogenous)
Protozoa							
Pneumocystis jerovici	+	++	+	+++	+++	+++	Respiratory

*++++, most frequent; +++, frequent; ++, infrequent; +, rare; −, no reported cases; ?, uncertain.

†++++, often fatal; +++, severe; ++, usually hospitalized; +, home management; −, no reported cases; ?, uncertain.

‡ Types 1, 2, 3, 4, 5, 7, 14, and 21.

§Ninety or more types known.

‖ Coxsackieviruses A9, A16, B1, B4, and B5; echoviruses 9, 11, 19, 20, and 22.

¶Human coronaviruses HCoV-OC43, -229E, -NL63, -NH, and SARS- CoV.

Viruses that may attack the lungs by hematogenous spread include varicella-zoster virus (VZV), Epstein-Barr virus (EBV), rubella, cytomegalovirus (CMV), herpes simplex viruses (HSV), and HIV. Rubella, CMV, and HSV may cause interstitial pneumonia in the infant infected congenitally or perinatally. CMV and VZV are causes of life-threatening pneumonia in immunocompromised hosts. Pneumonia has been noted in adolescents with infectious mononucleosis. Pulmonary infiltration is also a component of the fatal X-linked lymphoproliferative syndrome that is caused by EBV. Pulmonary lymphoid hyperplasia (lymphoid interstitial pneumonitis) is the most frequent cause of pneumonia in pediatric acquired immunodeficiency syndrome (AIDS). Whether this subacute to chronic condition is the direct result of pulmonary infection by HIV or is triggered by concomitant viral infection (e.g., by EBV) remains unclear.

Of the 15 known *Mycoplasma* species that can infect humans, only *M. pneumoniae* is a well-established cause of atypical pneumonia. In children younger than 2 years old, infection is common, but pneumonia is an unusual development. In children older than 5 years, *M. pneumoniae* is the most common cause of pneumonia. Genital mycoplasmas—*Ureaplasma urealyticum* and *M. hominis* in particular—have been associated with infant pneumonia acquired congenitally and perinatally.

Three *Chlamydia* species have been associated with pneumonia. *C. psittaci* is the well-recognized cause of psittacosis (ornithosis). *C. pneumoniae* is a recently described agent that is second only to *M. pneumoniae* as a cause of pneumonia in adolescents and young adults. *C. trachomatis,* the cause of inclusion conjunctivitis in neonates, causes a characteristic afebrile pneumonitis syndrome in infants ages 3 to 19 weeks. Its incidence has decreased in recent years with the widespread obstetric practice of screening and treating for *C. trachomatis* during pregnancy.

Of the rickettsiae, only *Coxiella burnetii* is associated with pneumonia, in the form of Q fever. This infection may be severe, but, because of its restricted ecologic niche, it rarely occurs in children. *Pneumocystis jerovici* (previously known as *P. carinii*), a protozoan parasite, is an important cause of pneumonia in children who are receiving chemotherapy and is the second major cause of pneumonia in children with HIV infection.

EPIDEMIOLOGY

The major contributors to the overall epidemiology of viral and atypical pneumonia in children are RSV, parainfluenza viruses, hMPV, *M. pneumoniae,* and influenza viruses A and B. Because of their brief incubation periods and high degree of communicability, these agents tend to spread through communities in well-defined waves. RSV, hMPV, and the influenza viruses occur predominantly in the winter months; parainfluenza viruses 1 and 2 usually are seen in the spring and fall. During intervals between epidemics, parainfluenza virus 3 and *M. pneumoniae* persist endemically.

New human viruses, such as avian influenza and SARS-CoV, may emerge as the result of recombination events with animal viruses. Such viruses, as seen recently with SARS, have the potential for pandemic spread.

Annual rates of childhood pneumonia show a rough inverse correlation with age, ranging from 40 per 1,000 children younger than 5 years to 7 per 1,000 adolescents ages 12 to 15 years. RSV is the most common causative agent in children younger than 5 years of age; *M. pneumoniae* is the most common one in older children.

In children, congenital heart disease and bronchopulmonary dysplasia are associated with viral pneumonia of greater severity, particularly that caused by RSV. Pulmonary deterioration in patients with cystic fibrosis has been shown to be associated with respiratory viral infection. Surprisingly, the common respiratory viruses have an impact in patients with hematologic malignancy and immunosuppressed states that is only moderately greater than that in physiologically normal hosts.

Most often, transmission of the more common agents of lower respiratory tract disease occurs by means of droplet spread resulting from relatively close contact with a source case. Direct inoculation at the alveolar level probably does not occur in most cases because of the extremely small size of aerosolized particles necessary to accomplish it. Studies of RSV infections transmitted nosocomially have shown the importance of adults with mild RSV upper respiratory tract infection as intermediates in transmission to susceptible young infants. The same nosocomial transmission mechanism probably applies to other viruses. Often, school-aged children introduce respiratory viral agents into households, with resulting secondary infections in parents and siblings. The increasing use of group day care by working parents has been associated with enhanced transmission of a number of respiratory pathogens and certainly has extended "school age" to include a population of younger children.

PATHOGENESIS AND PATHOLOGY

After inoculating the upper respiratory tract, the agents that cause viral pneumonia proliferate and spread by contiguity to involve more distal portions of the lower respiratory tract. Infected epithelium loses its ciliary appendages, rounds up, and sloughs into the air passages, resulting in stasis of mucus and accumulation of cellular debris. Relative expiratory obstruction causes hyperinflation and air trapping, with increased deadspace ventilation.

When infection extends to the terminal airways, alveolar lining cells lose their structural integrity, resulting in the loss of surfactant production, hyaline membrane formation, and pulmonary edema. These changes, combined with narrowing of the airway, lead to atelectasis and increased intrapulmonary shunting. Inflammatory responses at the site of tissue damage and in contiguous submucosal and interstitial structures impair gas exchange further. Four major pathologic expressions have been described in fatal viral infections, any or all of which may be present in a given case: acute bronchiolitis, necrotizing bronchiolitis, interstitial pneumonia, and alveolar pneumonia. Atypical pneumonia associated with *M. pneumoniae* or *C. pneumoniae* rarely has a fatal outcome.

Two important factors that influence the pathologic expression of viral and atypical pneumonia in children are anatomy and immunity. In young infants, the small caliber of the terminal airways, their limited cartilage support, and the absence of interconnections between alveolar spaces (pores of Kohn) contribute to wheezing and lobular atelectasis. Immunopathologic mechanisms have been invoked to explain the disparities between clinical expressions of infection by RSV and *M. pneumoniae* in infants and in older children. Interaction between RSV-infected epithelial cells and specific immunoglobulin E (IgE), leading to release of histamine, has been postulated as an immune mechanism for bronchospasm in RSV disease. Cumulative immunity after repeated natural infections by *M. pneumoniae* may account for the more impressive clinical expression of illness seen in older children and adults. *Mycoplasma*-specific, cell-mediated immunity, detectable at low levels in young children but increased in adults, probably contributes to the pathogenesis.

CLINICAL MANIFESTATIONS

Generally, acute viral pneumonia in infants or young children develops after 1 or 2 days of coryza, decreased appetite, and low-grade fever. The onset usually is gradual, with increasing fretfulness, respiratory congestion, vomiting, cough, and fever. In very young infants, fever may be minimal, and apneic spells ("near-miss" sudden infant death syndrome or "apparent life-threatening events") are the most prominent (and frightening) presenting complaints. The most reliable physical findings of pneumonia are those of respiratory distress—tachypnea, tachycardia, nasal flaring, and retractions. Patients with diminished functional residual capacity may exhibit grunting. Generally, cyanosis accompanies apneic spells or coughing attacks, but it may be present at rest if significant ventilation-perfusion mismatch has developed.

Other physical findings are fairly variable and may be normal. Wheezing is present in infants with bronchiolitis, stridor in children with laryngotracheobronchitis. Hyperresonance to percussion may be noted if significant air trapping is present. Diminished local percussion or breath sounds may indicate lobar consolidation or atelectasis. In patients with interstitial pneumonia, fine crackling rales may be present diffusely or locally. Also important in the initial assessment is an evaluation of a child's state of hydration because increased insensible losses from fever and hyperventilation, coupled with anorexia, can result in significant fluid deficits.

Chlamydia pneumonia in young infants, in contrast to the usual acute viral pneumonias affecting this age group, is subacute to chronic in its development and is nonseasonal. Characteristic features include the absence of fever, a "staccato" cough pattern (paroxysmal coughs separated by short inspirations), and diffuse rales on auscultation. Usually, radiographic findings consist of interstitial infiltrates with subsegmental atelectasis. Hypergammaglobulinemia and mild eosinophilia are common laboratory abnormalities.

Viral pneumonia and atypical pneumonia in older children and adolescents resemble the usual patterns seen in adults. Generally, premonitory complaints include such systemic symptoms as malaise, myalgia, and anorexia in addition to upper respiratory tract symptoms. "Chilliness" may occur, but generally rigors are absent. Usually, cough is irritative and nonproductive. A temperature higher than 39°C is an unusual finding. Although tachypnea, flaring, and retractions generally are present, they may be less apparent than those in infants or young children. Findings on chest examination are more reliable than are those of infants and may include local percussion dullness or diminished breath sounds and local or diffuse fine rales. Because apnea is a rare finding in older patients, cyanosis is an ominous sign of impairment of gas exchange. Although mild dehydration often is present, generally it is not evident on examination.

Radiologic findings vary according to the patient's age and the infecting agent. In infants and young children, bilateral air trapping and perihilar infiltrates are the most frequent findings of viral pneumonia. Patchy areas of consolidation may represent lobular atelectasis or alveolar pneumonia. In older children and adolescents, lobar involvement can be defined more often, but typically the affected areas are not consolidated completely. Although true lobar consolidation may occur in patients with viral or atypical pneumonia, this finding should be distinguished from atelectasis and is more consistent with a bacterial cause of disease. Similarly, although small pleural effusions may be detected in decubitus films in patients with viral or atypical pneumonia, effusions are much more suggestive of bacterial infection.

Peripheral leukocyte counts vary but generally are less than 15,000/mm³ in patients with viral or atypical pneumonia. A striking lymphopenia is characteristic of SARS in children. Gram stains of sputum or tracheal secretions show sloughed ciliated epithelial cells along with neutrophils, with a mixed bacterial population representing normal pharyngeal flora. Predominance of neutrophils and a uniform bacterial population are more consistent with bacterial infection.

DIFFERENTIAL DIAGNOSIS

In the differential diagnosis of viral and atypical pneumonia, the following factors must be considered: status of the host (normal or compromised), environment (family or school exposure), age of the patient, and season of the year. In certain epidemiologic settings, the specific cause of nonbacterial pneumonia may be guessed with relative certainty. Often, however, this category of pulmonary infection is a diagnosis of exclusion. The major conditions to be differentiated include noninfectious pulmonary diseases, bacterial pneumonias amenable to conventional antibiotics, and the more unusual bacterial, fungal, or parasitic infections that may require specialized forms of therapy.

Noninfectious conditions that may simulate nonbacterial pneumonia are summarized in Table 230.2. The demarcation between infectious and noninfectious conditions is not always sharp. In children with sickle cell anemia, for example, pulmonary vasoocclusive crisis presents with fever, leukocytosis, and patchy pulmonary infiltrates (the acute chest syndrome). Differentiating this condition from pneumococcal or *Mycoplasma* pneumonia, to which the child with sickle cell anemia has increased susceptibility, may be difficult or impossible. Early recognition of noninfectious conditions either mimicking or underlying pneumonia may prevent recurrence or may improve the prognosis. Recognition of the "snowman in a snowstorm" chest radiograph of total anomalous pulmonary venous return may lead to a curative open heart procedure. Recognition and treatment of cystic fibrosis may prevent early irreversible pulmonary damage.

Classically, pneumonias caused by pyogenic bacteria are lobar in distribution and exhibit consolidation on roentgenography. Atelectasis, conversely, is a common finding in viral pneumonia and must be distinguished from true consolidation. Pleural effusions, circular infiltrates, consolidations with convex margins, and pneumatoceles favor bacterial infection, as do high fever and significant leukocytosis. Acute-phase reactants, such as erythrocyte sedimentation rate and C-reactive protein level, are increased in patients with bacterial respiratory

---

TABLE 230.2

NONINFECTIOUS CONDITIONS THAT MAY SIMULATE OR UNDERLIE VIRAL AND ATYPICAL PNEUMONIA IN CHILDREN

Technical	Damage by physical agents	Collagen disease (SLE, JRA)
Poor inspiratory film	Lipoid pneumonia	Sarcoidosis
Underpenetrated film	Kerosene pneumonia	Neoplasm (primary, metastatic)
Physiologic	Near drowning	Histiocytosis X
Prominent thymus	Smoke inhalation	Bronchogenic cyst
Breast shadows	Iatrogenic pulmonary damage	Vascular ring
Chronic pulmonary disease	Drugs (bleomycin, nitrofurantoin)	Pulmonary sequestration
Asthma	Radiation pneumonitis	Cystic odenomatoid malformation
Bronchiectasis	Graft-versus-host disease	Congenital lobar emphysema
Bronchopulmonary dysplasia	Atelectasis	Alpha$_1$-antitrypsin deficiency
Pulmonary fibrosis	Mucus plug	Allergic alveolitis
Cystic fibrosis	Foreign body	Dust (farmer's lung)
Recurrent aspiration	Congestive heart failure	Mold (allergic aspergillosis)
Gastroesophageal reflux	Pulmonary infarction	Excreta (pigeon breeder's lung)
Tracheoesophageal fistula	Sickle vasoocclusive crisis	Pulmonary hemosiderosis
Cleft palate	Fat embolism	Desquamative interstitial pneumonitis
Neuromuscular disorders	Pleural effusion	Adult respiratory distress syndrome
Familial dysautonomia	Pleural reaction	

JRA, juvenile rheumatoid arthritis; SLE, systemic lupus erythematosus.

infection. However, these tests add little to a careful initial clinical examination, roentgenographic findings, differential white blood cell count, and (if accessible) Gram stain and culture of tracheal secretions in excluding a bacterial cause. Only positive results of cultures of blood, pleural fluid, or lung aspirates definitively prove the cause of bacterial pneumonia.

Among the less common causes of pneumonia, tuberculosis never should be forgotten. Tuberculin testing should be considered in the initial evaluation and is especially important for children who live in urban areas, for recent immigrants, and for Native Americans. Fungal pneumonia, particularly coccidioidomycosis, blastomycosis, and histoplasmosis, should be considered in children who live in or visit endemic areas and who fail to respond to conventional antibiotics. Often, a suggestive history, such as exposure to excavations (e.g., backyard swimming pools, geologic or archeologic digs), cleanup chores in old sheds and barns, and dust storms, can be elicited. Erythema nodosum and eosinophilia are common clinical clues to these entities. Other fungal pneumonias, such as aspergillosis and cryptococcosis, occur in the setting of immunosuppression. These conditions, coupled with the possibilities of infection with *Pneumocystis*, resistant bacteria, and CMV, may warrant the use of bronchoalveolar lavage or open lung biopsy as definitive approaches to diagnosis in the compromised host.

SPECIFIC DIAGNOSIS

The methods used for virologic and chlamydial isolation are available in most major medical centers and public health laboratories. With the possible exceptions of HSV and adenoviruses, respiratory viruses rarely are carried asymptomatically. Thus, identification of an agent in upper respiratory tract secretions is strong evidence for its causative role in pneumonia. Conventional virologic techniques provide the most specific means of identification. Rapid diagnosis of influenza A virus, parainfluenza viruses, RSV, and *Chlamydia* infections by means of fluorescent antibody techniques, enzyme-linked immunosorbent assays, direct DNA probes, or polymerase chain reaction has proved useful in numerous centers. Some of these techniques may actually be more sensitive than are conventional cultures. In individual cases, serologic diagnosis of respiratory viral infection generally is less satisfactory than is virologic diagnosis. The difficulties associated with serology relate to the timing when the specimen was collected, the choice of antigens to test, and variations in the quality and specificity of available reagents. In contrast, serologic diagnosis of chlamydial pneumonitis can be very helpful. Even at the onset of illness, affected infants have high titers of specific IgG and IgM antibodies. Similarly, a positive antibody test result for HIV infection constitutes strong evidence for either pulmonary lymphoid hyperplasia or opportunistic *Pneumocystis* pneumonia in a child with pulmonary infiltrates and a compatible maternal or social history.

Laboratory capability for the isolation of mycoplasmas is increasingly available in university medical centers, although cultures are used most often for genital mycoplasmas. DNA probes are available for the diagnosis of *M. pneumoniae*. However, serologic techniques are a more practical means of making a specific diagnosis. Acute-phase reactants (e.g., cold agglutinins) are helpful when the patient has an acute illness. Definitive diagnosis requires testing of paired sera for specific antibodies. Usually, *Pneumocystis* infection is diagnosed by visualizing organisms in specimens obtained by bronchoscopy or biopsy, using silver impregnation stains or fluorescein-labeled monoclonal antibodies.

Because of the epidemiologic behavior of viral respiratory infections, often a reasonable guess as to a specific cause can be made on the basis of such factors as the patient's age, the season of the year, and associated clinical features. If the presence of a particular viral agent in a community has been established by isolation or serologic means, the probability that other patients with similar manifestations have illness caused by that agent is increased greatly.

THERAPY

Therapy for viral pneumonia is primarily expectant and supportive. The course of uncomplicated viral pneumonia is not influenced by the administration of antibiotics. In most cases in which pulmonary involvement is uncovered, however, antibiotic therapy is used because bacterial disease cannot be ruled out with certainty. In the absence of a specific viral diagnosis, this approach is both reasonable and practical. Nonetheless, antibiotic therapy in routine cases must be appropriate for the most common treatable pathogens (penicillin-sensitive and penicillin-resistant *S. pneumoniae, Haemophilus influenzae,* and *M. pneumoniae*). In the immunocompromised host or one in whom nosocomial infection is a possibility, methicillin-sensitive and methicillin-resistant *S. aureus* and other hospital-associated and opportunistic pathogens must be considered. If aspiration is a possibility, coverage for penicillin-sensitive and penicillin-resistant oral anaerobes should be provided.

In certain fulminant viral pneumonias, such as varicella in a child with leukemia, antiviral chemotherapy with acyclovir may be lifesaving, but one should recall that as many as one-half of all patients with this condition have complicating bacterial sepsis amenable to antibiotic therapy. The treatment of pneumonia caused by CMV in immunocompromised hosts now consists of the combination of ganciclovir and intravenous hyperimmune globulin. Treatment with amantadine, rimantadine, oseltamivir, or zanamivir should be considered in children with viral pneumonia in the context of a community epidemic of influenza. Amantadine and rimantadine have therapeutic benefit for influenza A; oseltamivir and zanamivir are active against both influenza A and B.

The inhalational antiviral ribavirin inhibits replication of RSV but has very limited effect on clinical symptoms and length of hospital stay. Crystallization of drug in ventilator valves is a technical difficulty with its use that necessitates protective filters in the circuitry that require frequent changes. The drug also may be mutagenic, rendering it potentially hazardous to pregnant caretakers. Ribavirin may be considered for use in patients with the most severe underlying cardiopulmonary disease and/or those who are immunocompromised. When used, the drug should be administered as early as possible during an RSV illness for maximum benefit. It does appear to reduce morbidity and mortality rates in patients with bone marrow transplants who have been infected with RSV.

Specific antimicrobial therapy for mycoplasmal, chlamydial, and rickettsial pneumonias with macrolides or tetracycline shortens the course of the illness but generally has a less dramatic therapeutic effect than does specific antibiotic therapy for bacterial infections. The drug of choice for *Pneumocystis* pneumonia is oral or parenteral trimethoprim-sulfamethoxazole.

The elements of supportive therapy include adequate hydration, high humidity, maintenance of oxygenation, and mobilization of lower respiratory tract secretions. Because of increased insensible fluid losses as a result of fever, hyperventilation, and anorexia, mild dehydration often is observed initially, and continuing losses may occur during the acute phase of illness. Thus, restoration of deficits and adequate maintenance of intake of fluids are desirable. With regard to the latter, one should remember that fluid requirements increase by approximately 12% per degree Centigrade of fever and that hyperventilation increases fluid requirements by an additional 15%.

Mist tents have fallen into disuse because they hinder observation and because mist has little direct therapeutic benefit. However, a high level of humidity is required to prevent the drying effects of supplemental oxygen therapy. By slowing evaporation, it probably also serves to reduce the viscosity of mucus secretions and the magnitude of insensible fluid losses. Mobilization of respiratory secretions by means of vibration and postural drainage is indicated in patients with nonbacterial pneumonia complicated by atelectasis, but it is not helpful in the absence of excessive secretions or mucus plugging.

Because of ventilation-perfusion abnormalities and alveolocapillary block, most children with nonbacterial pneumonia have some degree of hypoxemia. In children with respiratory distress, provision of supplemental oxygen reduces anxiety and ventilation rates. Increases in inspired oxygen to approximately 30% are provided easily with nasal prongs or "face tents," which are the most convenient means of administering oxygen. More severe respiratory distress or cyanosis requires documentation of a patient's respiratory status by means of arterial blood gas determinations and more exact regulation of inspired oxygen administered by "high-flow" nasal prongs, hood, or face mask. Oximetry, capnography, or transcutaneous monitoring can reduce the need for frequent blood gas sampling and insertion of arterial lines. In patients with respiratory failure, mechanical ventilation is required to maintain oxygenation and to control carbon dioxide retention.

Apnea and bradycardia occur commonly in young infants with viral pneumonia, and these disorders are particularly frequent complications in patients with a history of premature birth. Although the mechanism for these episodes is unclear, continuous monitoring for apnea is prudent in young infants with viral pneumonia.

Acetaminophen or ibuprofen should be used to control fever. Although expectorants and cough suppressants are prescribed widely for upper respiratory tract infections in children and adults, these agents are not helpful in the initial treatment of nonbacterial pneumonia. Bronchodilators are used commonly in patients with viral pneumonia complicated by wheezing. Some studies show improved clinical scores when inhaled adrenergics are employed. Racemic epinephrine is more effective than is albuterol, presumably because it alleviates airway inflammation as well as bronchospasm. However, not all patients respond to bronchodilators, and they do not affect the duration of hospital stay. Careful assessment of the clinical response to these agents is warranted. They should be discontinued in patients with no clinical response as indicated by persistent wheezing and tachycardia. During convalescence, a persistent irritative cough that interferes with sleep may be alleviated by the judicious use of antihistamines, dextromethorphan, or codeine.

PROGNOSIS

Children who have recovered from pneumonia should be reevaluated clinically 2 to 3 weeks after the condition is diagnosed. If affected children are asymptomatic, have returned to normal activities, and have benign results on physical examination, follow-up radiography is not required. Repeated chest radiography is indicated in children with complicated clinical courses, underlying cardiopulmonary disease, or prior episodes of pneumonia or if signs or symptoms of respiratory difficulty persist at the time of follow-up. Approximately 20% of patients with uncomplicated cases of pneumonia have persistent radiographic abnormalities 3 to 4 weeks after diagnosis is established, but a selective approach to follow-up chest films permits the early recognition of atelectasis or chronic disease.

The incidence of long-term complications of nonbacterial pneumonias is unknown. However, these conditions likely play a role in the development of some cases of bronchiectasis, chronic pulmonary fibrosis, desquamative interstitial pneumonitis, and unilateral hyperlucent lung (Swyer-James syndrome). These complications are well-documented sequelae of measles and of adenovirus and influenza viral pneumonia, but they are rare occurrences now.

PREVENTION

Nosocomial spread of the common respiratory viruses occurs readily in pediatric wards and involves intermediate carriage by medical personnel who have acquired mild upper respiratory tract infections. A reasonable approach to interdicting nosocomial transmission is to group patients with pneumonia and to exclude personnel with symptomatic respiratory illness from ward duties. With the exceptions of measles, varicella, and SARS, mask or gown isolation has no effect on transmission. Avoiding close contact, washing hands, and wearing glasses or goggles will minimize the incidence of respiratory infections among personnel. Blood and secretion precautions (universal precautions) are recommended for all hospitalized patients.

Of the common viral causes of pneumonia, vaccines are available only for influenza viruses. Annual influenza vaccination using "split-product" vaccines is recommended strongly for children with chronic respiratory disease and other conditions that predispose them to the development of pneumonia. Routine immunization of infants 3 to 24 months of age has been recommended. Vaccination of adult health care personnel reduces the number of work days missed because of illness and can prevent nosocomial transmission. Vaccines against RSV, parainfluenza virus type 3, M. pneumoniae, and recently the SARS-CoV have received considerable investigative effort but have not proved yet to be of value. They present problems in vaccine development because of the possibility of triggering immunopathologic phenomena that could potentiate rather than prevent illness.

RSV bronchiolitis and pneumonia can be prevented in high-risk infants by passive immunization. Monthly palivizumab (a "humanized" monoclonal anti-RSV antibody) now is recommended for high-risk infants and has resulted in a marked decrease in the number of hospitalizations during the winter respiratory viral season. Breast-feeding, avoidance of secondhand smoke, and limiting attendance at day-care facilities and social functions also can be effective in preventing or attenuating RSV infections.

P. jerovici pneumonia can be prevented in pediatric patients with hematologic malignancy or AIDS by the prophylactic administration of trimethoprim-sulfamethoxazole. This medication has become part of the routine management of these conditions and has reduced the incidence of P. jerovici infection dramatically. Opportunistic pneumonia caused by CMV, which is a major hazard in seronegative, high-risk, premature infants and in recipients of allogeneic bone marrow transplants, can be prevented effectively by the exclusive use of CMV-seronegative blood products. In transplant recipients who are at risk for having primary or reactivated CMV disease, ganciclovir, valganciclovir, and intravenous immunoglobulin preparations have been shown to reduce rates of infection and interstitial pneumonia.

Suggested Readings

American Academy of Pediatrics, Committee on Infectious Disease. Reassessment of indications for ribavirin therapy. *Pediatrics* 1996;97:137.

Beem M, Saxon E. Respiratory-tract colonization and a distinctive pneumonia syndrome in infants infected with *Chlamydia trachomatis. N Engl J Med* 1977;296:306.

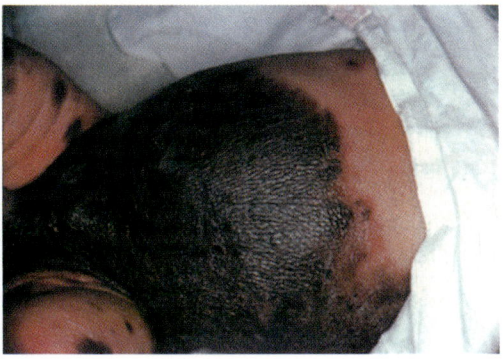

FIGURE 68.1. Giant congenital melanocytic nevus with atypical features, including a scalloped border, irregular pigmentation, and variable thickness.

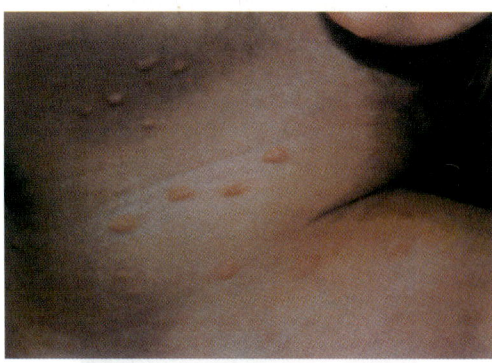

FIGURE 68.2. Multiple pinkish brown papules and nodules of generalized cutaneous mastocytosis.

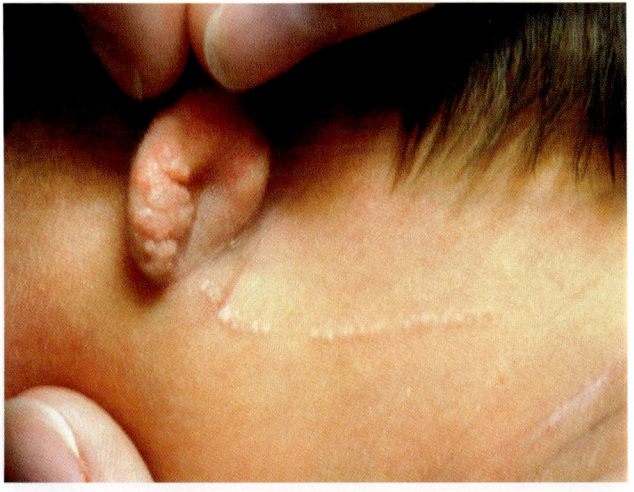

FIGURE 68.3. Linear nevus sebaceous on the neck and posterior ear with typical sharply demarcated, waxy, yellow-orange, pebbly appearance.

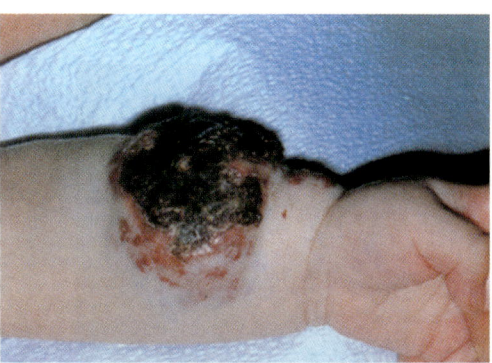

FIGURE 68.4. Mixed superficial and deep infantile hemangioma on the left forearm with ulceration and crusting. The superficial component is bright red; the deep component is blue.

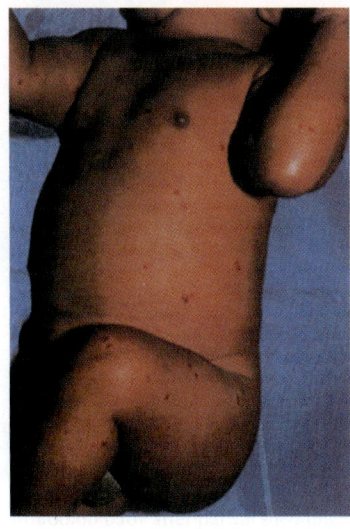

FIGURE 68.5. Newborn with multiple 1- to 4-mm, firm, red, papular cutaneous hemangiomas of the diffuse neonatal hemangiomatosis syndrome.

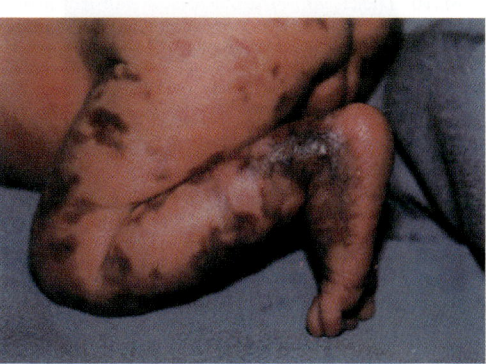

FIGURE 68.6. Reticulated mottling of cutis marmorata telangiectatica congenita with atrophy and telangiectasia of the skin.

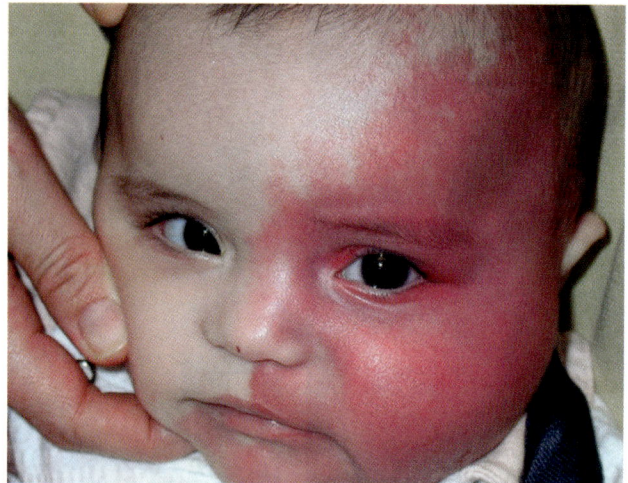

FIGURE 315.1. Capillary malformation (port-wine stain).

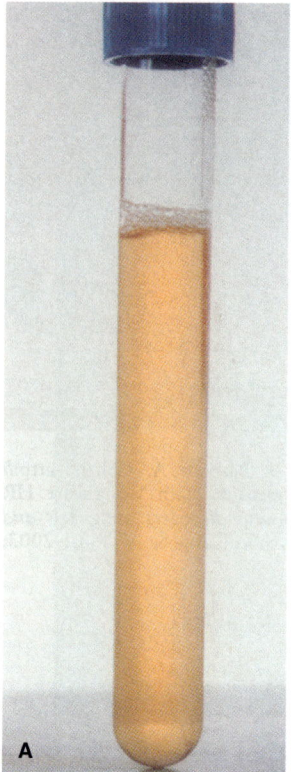
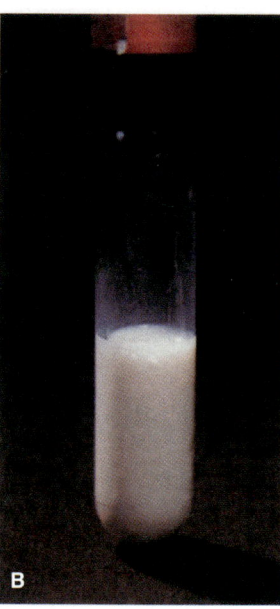

FIGURE 365.3. A: Ascitic fluid from a patient with cirrhosis, with its typical yellowish appearance. **B:** Ascitic fluid from a patient with chylous ascites, with its characteristic milky appearance.

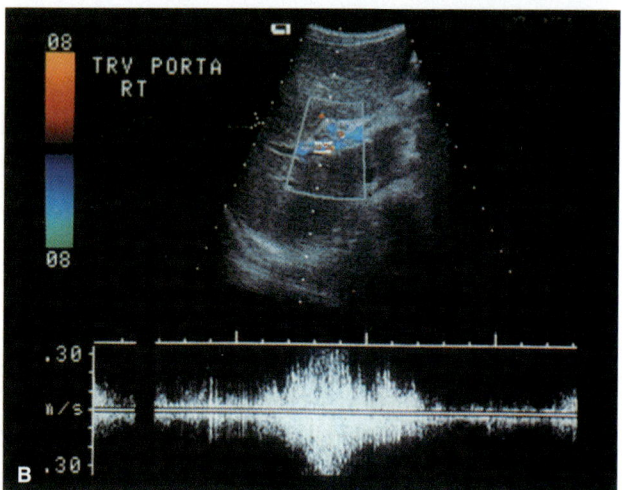

FIGURE 371.3. B: Doppler ultrasonographic study of the same patient; the collateral veins are enclosed in the rectangle. The collateral veins appear blue in that image.

Cherry JD, Krogstad P. SARS: the first pandemic of the 21st century. *Pediatr Res* 2004;56:1.

Denny FW, Clyde WA Jr. Acute lower respiratory tract infections in nonhospitalized children. *J Pediatr* 1986;108:635.

Fran J, Henrickson KJ, Savotski LL. Rapid simultaneous diagnosis of infections with respiratory syncytial viruses A and B, and human parainfluenza virus types 1, 2, and 3 by multiplex quantitative reverse transcription-polymerase chain reaction-enzyme hybridization assay (Hexaplex). *Clin Infect Dis* 1998;26:1397.

Hughes WT, Rivera GK, Schell MJ, et al. Successful intermittent chemoprophylaxis for *Pneumocystis carinii [jerovici]* pneumonitis. *N Engl J Med* 1987; 316:1627.

Juven T, Mertsola J, Waris M, et al. Etiology of community-acquired pneumonia in 254 hospitalized children. *Pediatr Infect Dis J* 2000;19:293.

McIntosh K. Community-acquired pneumonia in children. *N Engl J Med* 2002; 346:429.

McIntosh K. Coronaviruses in the limelight. *J Infect Dis* 2005;191:489.

Meissner HC, Long SS, Committee on Infectious Diseases, Committee on Fetus and Newborn. Revised indications for the use of palivizumab and respiratory syncytial virus immune globulin intravenous for the prevention of respiratory syncytial virus infections. *Pediatrics* 2003;112:1442.

Williams JV, Harris PA, Tollefson SJ, et al. Human metapneumovirus and lower respiratory tract disease in otherwise healthy infants and children. *N Engl J Med* 2004;350:443.

CHAPTER 231 ■ HYPERSENSITIVITY PNEUMONITIS

I. CELINE HANSON AND WILLIAM T. SHEARER

The term *hypersensitivity pneumonitis* defines a spectrum of pulmonary disorders that includes granulomatous, interstitial, and alveolar filling diseases. These respiratory disorders are associated causally with intense and frequently prolonged exposure to inhaled organic antigens. The range of implicated vegetable and animal antigens is broad.

EPIDEMIOLOGY

In the United States, bird-breeder's lung, farmer's lung, and ventilator hypersensitivity pneumonitis occur most often. Many diseases are related to specific adult occupations (e.g., pigeon-breeder's lung, farmer's lung disease, disease associated with oil mist exposure in metalworkers and popcorn factories), but children living in environments rich with these antigens occasionally also can be afflicted with these respiratory illnesses. Table 231.1 lists some of the most common offenders in children including avian proteins, molds, bacteria, and medica-

tions. For children, most of the exposures occur in the home setting and include exposure to family businesses (chicken or turkey farms), family pets, moldy homes or home settings such as basement showers, or outdoor exposures (riding schools and associated barn chores). As outlined, many fungi have been associated with hypersensitivity pneumonitis, especially thermophilic actinomycetes.

PATHOGENESIS

The name *hypersensitivity pneumonitis* and the association of the condition with the inhalation of a foreign antigen suggest that this disease entity is mediated by immunologic phenomena. Gell and Coombs divided immune tissue injury into four types of hypersensitivity reactions. Immunoglobulin E (IgE)–mediated, or type I, hypersensitivity may seem a likely cause of the lung disease observed clinically, yet no evidence exists to support this hypothesis. Serum IgE levels are normal in affected

TABLE 231.1

CAUSATIVE AGENTS OF HYPERSENSITIVITY PNEUMONITIS REPORTED IN THE LITERATURE IN CHILDREN (0 TO 18 YEARS)

Antigen	Antigen Source	Specific Exposures
Animal proteins	Bird species	Home exposure to doves, parakeets, pigeons, parrots, etc. (bird fancier's disease)
	Cat hair	Home environment
Molds	*Alternaria alternata*, *Aspergillus* species, *Micropolyspora faeni*, *Thermoactinomyces vulgaris*	Home environment; riding school (farmer's lung disease)
	Epicoccum nigrum	Basement shower
	Trichosporon species, *Cyrptococcus* species, *Fusarium napiforme*	Home environment only (summer-type hypersensitivity)
Other infectious diseases	*Mycobaterium-avium* complex	Hot tub/sauna exposure
	Dirofilariasis	Heartworm infestation
Medications	Methotrexate	

individuals; in fact, antigen-specific IgE levels rarely are elevated. Patients affected with hypersensitivity pneumonitis usually are not atopic. After antigen inhalation, rales, not wheezing, are the typical auscultatory findings, and evidence of bronchospasm is exceedingly rare. Pulmonary symptoms of dyspnea and cough rarely respond to the administration of traditional histamine blockers or mast cell stabilizers such as cromolyn sodium. All the information suggests that type I, IgE-mediated hypersensitivity plays little or no role in the pathogenesis of hypersensitivity pneumonitis.

No data conclusively support a role for type II hypersensitivity, or cytotoxic reactions, in hypersensitivity pneumonitis. Other data using rabbits as experimental models for hypersensitivity pneumonitis, however, suggest that types III (Arthus reaction or immune-complex) and IV (cell-mediated or delayed) hypersensitivity play roles in the pathogenesis of this disease entity. The role of immune complex-mediated reactions in the pathogenesis of hypersensitivity pneumonitis is supported most significantly by the Arthus-type reactions that are documented histologically after intradermal skin testing with the suspected offending antigen. Circulating serum immune complexes (i.e., serum precipitins) suggest that type III hypersensitivity reactions play a significant role in the early clinical response to antigen. The absence of immune complexes at sites of inflammation (i.e., lung biopsy) suggests that type III responses do not mediate this disease.

Evidence of type IV or cell-mediated hypersensitivity has been derived primarily from work with hypersensitivity pneumonitis induced in guinea pigs and rabbits. In these models, evidence of local T-lymphocyte activation has included enhanced local lymphokine production and increased numbers of local activated T cells recovered in bronchoalveolar lavage (BAL) fluid. Affected patients have evidence of granuloma formation at lung biopsy (as high as 70% in one review of patients with farmer's lung). The mechanisms for formation of granulomas include pulmonary macrophage and a T-helper-1–cell response that increases interleukin-1beta, tumor necrosis factor-alpha, and interferon-gamma production locally.

In summary, most immunologic investigations suggest that hypersensitivity pneumonitis probably is mediated by a combination of immunologic events, including immune complex formation and cell-mediated hypersensitivity.

CLINICAL PRESENTATION

The clinical presentation of hypersensitivity pneumonitis is variable and traditionally is separated into three somewhat distinct clinical entities: acute, subacute, and chronic. The acute form of hypersensitivity pneumonitis frequently is related to intermittent, intense inhalation of the offending antigen, with symptoms precipitated 4 to 6 hours after contact with antigen. Typical clinical symptoms include elevated temperature in the range of 38.3° to 40.0°C (101° to 104°F), dry cough, dyspnea, and malaise. Constitutional symptoms can persist for weeks after exposure, but they usually resolve within 24 hours. The patient appears ill on physical examination, and lung auscultation typically documents bilateral bibasilar rales. Wheezing or evidence of reversible reactive airway disease is an uncommon finding and provides evidence against the diagnosis of hypersensitivity pneumonitis.

The subacute presentation of hypersensitivity pneumonitis lacks the characteristic findings of fever, malaise, and dyspnea that are noted in the acute form of the disorder. Clinically, the patient may complain of persistent anorexia or weight loss and malaise. Pulmonary symptoms such as progressive shortness of breath or insidious onset of dyspnea on exertion may be late manifestations. The chronic form of hypersensitivity pneumonitis usually is related to long-term, low-dose antigen exposure. Clinical findings include a normal physical examination, with the exception of pulmonary rales detected on auscultation of the chest. Wheezing rarely accompanies chronic hypersensitivity pneumonitis. Lung disease related to the chronic form of the disorder usually is poorly responsive to traditional therapeutic intervention. Initial pulmonary findings include severe restrictive impairment (coupled with a diffusion defect), pulmonary fibrosis (determined radiographically and histologically, with noncaseating granulomas noted), and progressive nonreversible obstructive disease that is characterized by hyperinflation and sometimes is associated histologically with evidence of obliterative bronchiolitis and emphysema.

DIAGNOSIS

Characteristic laboratory findings in patients with an acute episode of hypersensitivity pneumonitis (which can be reproduced by antigen inhalation challenge also) include the following: leukocytosis, with white blood cell counts as high as 25,000/μL; eosinophilia (in approximately 10% of patients); polyclonal elevation of serum immunoglobulin levels; and nonspecific reactive rheumatoid factor results (Table 231.2). Because positive evidence of antigen-specific serum precipitins is documented well in both symptomatic and asymptomatic exposed individuals, using this measure solely to diagnose hypersensitivity pneumonitis is not always valid.

The best diagnostic test for this clinical entity is antigen inhalation challenge, although it does have some inherent problems. First, the patient must be able to perform pulmonary function testing adequately, so the procedure is best suited for the evaluation of older children and adults. Second, the patient can exhibit marked decreases in vital capacity and pulmonary function; testing is uncomfortable and, if it is not performed in a controlled setting, it can be catastrophic. Third, because the delivery of antigen to each individual cannot be measured precisely, establishing the exact dose of antigen that causes a positive response even in asymptomatic exposed individuals is difficult. Nonetheless, characteristic pulmonary findings include a restrictive lung pattern, with a decrease in the forced expiratory volume and forced vital capacity 4 to 6 hours after inhalation, and a gradual return to baseline capacities over the course of the subsequent 8 to 12 hours.

In adults, BAL has proved beneficial diagnostically in that patients with hypersensitivity pnuemonitis have prominent lymphocytosis and a depressed ratio of T-helper cells (CD4+ T lymphocytes) to T-suppressor cells (CD8+ T lymphocytes). In a study of pediatric patients with hypersensitivity pneumonitis, BAL findings of prominent lymphocytosis as identified in adults could be reproduced. A depressed CD4/CD8 ratio was not a consistent finding in the pediatric population studied. However, cellular activation was noted to be present as manifest by elevated human leukocyte antigen-DR expression on BAL lymphocytes and an increased number of natural killer cells.

Chest radiography of patients with acute hypersensitivity pneumonitis may reveal bibasilar interstitial infiltrates or multibasilar nodular densities (Fig. 231.1). In chronic disease forms, pulmonary fibrosis can be seen, with evidence of contracted lung tissue. When progressive obstructive lung disease complicates hypersensitivity pneumonitis, hyperinflation may be noted radiographically. Computed tomographic findings include decreased attenuation with mosaic perfusion, ground-glass opacification, and nodules and reticular pattern, in order of their prevalence.

A serum marker, high-molecular-weight, mucin-like antigen (KL-6 or MUC1) has been associated with interstitial pneumonitis. Levels are elevated in more than 60% of individuals

TABLE 231.2

LABORATORY AND RADIOGRAPHIC FINDINGS IN PEDIATRIC HYPERSENSITIVITY PNEUMONITIS

Peripheral Blood	Leukocytosis	Peripheral Eosinophilia (10% of Patients)	Polyclonal Gammopathy	Plus Rheumatoid Factor (50% of Patients)	Plus Antigen-Specific Precipitins
Pulmonary testing	Depressed total lung capacity/forced vital capacity	Depressed forced expiratory volume in 1 second without significant reversibility	Diminished functional residual capacity	Depressed residual capacity	Abnormal diffusion capacity
Radiographic findings					
Chest radiograph	Normal	Patchy alveolar infiltrates (lower lung fields >apices)	Military nodules		
Computed tomography scan	Acute HP: nonspecific airspace opacification	Subacute HP: small rounded opacities	Chronic HP: Linear fibrosis; Centrilobular nodules; ground-glass opacifications		

HP, hypersensitivity pneumonitis.

with pulmonary fibrosis, hypersensitivity pneumonitis, sarcoidosis, and radiation pneumonitis. KL-6/MUC1 appears to correlate better with disease activity than with specific disease differentation.

DIFFERENTIAL DIAGNOSIS

The differential diagnosis includes all disease states that cause interstitial infiltrates on radiography, such as lymphoid interstitial pneumonitis, which is seen characteristically in human immunodeficiency virus infection and in connective tissue diseases. Infectious causes of granulomatous disease (i.e., mycobacteria) should be excluded before a diagnosis of hypersensitivity pneumonitis is made. In the acute form, pyogenic or viral pneumonia often is misdiagnosed because of accompanying fever and leukocytosis. The recurrence of symptoms in characteristic exposure patterns, however, should alert the physician to the possible presence of hypersensitivity pneumonitis.

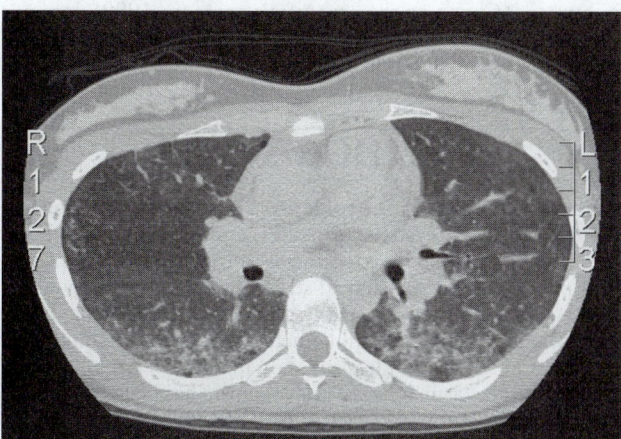

FIGURE 231.1. Computed tomography scan of the midthorax in a 19-year-old patient with hypersensitivity pneumonitis resulting from avian proteins. The radiographic image shows ground-glass opacifications of interstitial disease and nodularity in the midlung fields. (Courtesy of LL Fan, M.D., Baylor College of Medicine, Texas Children's Hospital Pulmonary Medicine, Houston, TX.)

This diagnosis can be made more definitively by obtaining a detailed history of environmental exposure and by observing typical laboratory findings of leukocytosis, a normal serum IgE level, a restrictive pulmonary function pattern, and evidence of offending antigen serum precipitins.

Because organic antigens are related causally to hypersensitivity lung disease, physicians frequently consider clinical patterns of other similar lung diseases to be equivalent. The most common misconception is the equation of acute bronchopulmonary aspergillosis with hypersensitivity pneumonitis. The two disease entities differ by the lack of wheezing noted on auscultation, the negative results of immediate hypersensitivity skin testing for a suspected offending antigen, and the normal serum IgE levels in hypersensitivity pneumonitis.

TREATMENT AND PREVENTION

The therapy of choice for patients with hypersensitivity pneumonitis is avoidance of the offending agent or agents, if it or they can be identified. Serum precipitins can be helpful in determining putative causative agents. For example, serum-specific IgG antibodies to *Penicillum frequentans* have been demonstrated in patients with suberosis, hypersensitivity pneumonitis caused by inhalation of cork dust. Recent clinical studies have identified additional etiologic agents in suberosis, *Aspergillus fumigatus*, and cork dust itself. DNA-based methodologies also have been used successfully to identify and causally link respiratory antigens to disease (e.g., mycobacteria and pseudomonads in modern metalworking fluids causing respiratory disease in exposed machine workers). Because causative agents often are related to a person's occupation, however, patients frequently are reluctant to limit their exposure to the offending antigen. For children, this option usually is not a difficult problem.

For acute and subacute forms of the disease, avoidance alone often is not sufficient to cause clinical improvement. In these instances, corticosteroid therapy has proven useful in controlling pulmonary exacerbations and in reversing some restrictive lung components. Methylprednisolone pulse therapy has been reported to be as effective as continuous therapy in improving pulmonary function testing and clinical symptoms. Monitoring serum KL-6/MUC1 levels has been offered as a predictive marker for determining response to high-dose corticosteroid therapy in idiopathic pulmonary fibrosis. Its efficacy in predicting clinical progression in hypersensitivity pneumonitis is not yet defined. Antihistamines and bronchodilators are ineffective therapeutic modalities in patients with acute and subacute hypersensitivity pneumonitis.

In patients with chronic lung disease (interstitial fibrosis, obliterative bronchiolitis), corticosteroid therapy usually is not effective in reversing pulmonary function deficits or improving clinical symptoms. Patients with chronic lung disease occasionally have evidence of obstructive lung disease and sometimes benefit from bronchodilator therapy. With appropriate clinical suspicion and astute and pertinent collection of historic data, these affected individuals should be identified before irreversible lung disease ensues. This identification is particularly critical for children in whom early establishment of a diagnosis of acute hypersensitivity pneumonitis or alveolitis can obviate long-term sequelae through administration of short-term treatment and simple avoidance of implicated agents.

Suggested Readings

Chen C, Kleinau I, Niggemann B, et al. Treatment of allergic alveolitis with methylprednisolone pulse therapy. *Pediatr Allergy Immunol* 2003;14:66.

Fan LL. Hypersensitivity pneumonitis in children. *Curr Opin Pediatr* 2002;14: 323.

Gell PGH, Coombs RRA. *Clinical aspects of immunology,* 2nd ed. Philadelphia: FA Davis, 1968.

Gudmundsson G, Hunninghake GW. Interferon-gamma is necessary for the expression of hypersensitivity pneumonitis. *J Clin Invest* 1997;99:2386.

Hansell DM, Wells AU, Padley SP, Muller NL. Hypersensitivity pneumonitis: correlation of individual CT patterns with functional abnormalities. *Radiology* 1996;199:123.

Kohno N. Serum marker KL-6/MUC1 for the diagnosis and management of interstitial pneumonitis. *J Med Invest* 1999;46:151.

Morell F, Roger A, Cruz MJ, et al. Suberosis: clinical study and new etiologic agents in a series of eight patients. *Chest* 2003;124:1145.

Patterson R, Greenberger PA, Castile RG, et al. Diagnostic problems in hypersensitivity pneumonitis. *Allergy Proc* 1989;10:141.

Ratjen F, Costabel U, Griese M, Paul K. Bronchoalveolar lavage fluid findings in children with hypersensitivity pneumonitis. *Eur Respir J* 2003;21:144.

Trout DB, Seltzer JM, Page EH, et al. Clinical use of immunoassays in assessing exposure to fungi and potential health efects related to fungal exposure. *Ann Allergy Asthma Immunol* 2004;92:483.

Yadav JS, Khan IV, Fakhari F, Soellner MB. DNA-based methodologies for rapid detection, quantification, and species-or strain-level identification of respiratory pathogens (Mycobacteria and Pseumomonads) in metalworking fluids. *Appl Occup Environ Hyg* 2003;18:966.

Yi ES. Hypersensitivity pneumonitis. *Crit Rev Clin Lab Sci* 2002;39:581.

Zacharisen MC, Schlueter DP, Kurup VP, Fink JN. The long-term outcome in acute, subacute, and chronic forms of pigeon breeder's disease hypersensitivity pneumonitis. *Ann Allergy Asthma Immunol* 2002;88:150.

CHAPTER 232 ■ *PNEUMOCYSTIS JIROVECI* PNEUMONIA

DONALD C. ANDERSON

The disease generally known as *Pneumocystis carinii* pneumonia (or PCP) is an opportunistic infection of increasing importance to pediatricians. A marked increase in the prevalence of this disorder in the United States since the 1970s has paralleled therapeutic advances in the management of immunologic and neoplastic diseases that have resulted in longer survival of children with these underlying disorders. Most important, this infection is occurring now in epidemic proportions in association with the acquired immunodeficiency syndrome (AIDS). PCP is especially common in human immunodeficiency virus (HIV)—infected infants in central, western, and southern Africa, where it is the cause of death in 30% to 50% of HIV-infected infants younger than 6 month old.

EPIDEMIOLOGY

Pneumocystis organisms were described first by Chagas in 1909 as possible morphologic variants of *Trypanosoma cruzi*. From the time of its discovery until late in the 1980s, *Pneumocystis* was widely thought to be a protozoan to be classified with *Toxoplasma*, but some microbiologists argued that *Pneumocystis* organisms exhibit morphologic similarities to those of fungi. It behaves as a protozoan in response to antiprotozoal drugs and as a fungus with respect to its periodic acid–Schiff and silver staining characteristics. In 1988, definitive classification using DNA analysis confirmed that *P. carinii* is a fungus, albeit an unusual example, lacking in ergosterol and very difficult

to propagate in culture. Subsequent genotypic studies of diverse *Pneumocystis* species in different mammals showed that the organism that causes human PCP is distinct. It is now termed *P. jiroveci* in recognition of the Czech parasitologist, Otto Jirovec, who is credited with the seminal descriptions of the microbe in humans. Changing the organism's name (in 1999) does not preclude the use of the acronym PCP because it can be read "*Pneumocystis* pneumonia."

PATHOGENESIS

Three developmental forms of *P. jiroveci* have been identified by light microscopy: cysts, sporozoites, and trophozoites. When they are identified in lung tissue or respiratory secretions, cysts are spheric or crescent-shaped structures approximately 5 μm in diameter, containing as many as eight oval bodies or sporozoites that are 1 to 2 μm in diameter. The natural habitat of *P. jiroveci* and its mode of transmission in humans remain largely unknown. The occurrence of this organism has been recognized in many wild and laboratory animal species over a wide geographic distribution, but an association between animal reservoirs and human infection has not been established. Before and during World War II, epidemics of interstitial plasma cell pneumonitis secondary to *P. jiroveci* were recognized in debilitated and premature infants throughout European institutions and nursing homes. The interruption of outbreaks by the introduction of strict isolation of affected patients suggested the probable importance of person-to-person spread of the disease within that setting. In the United States, PCP was not reported until 1956. In contrast to the early European patterns, U.S. cases primarily have been sporadic and have occurred almost exclusively in children with impaired host defenses. Necropsy studies have demonstrated that apparent (asymptomatic) infection occurs frequently in patients with cancer or other conditions that cause immunocompromise, but the epidemiologic importance of these asymptomatic carriers in the transmission of pneumocystic disease is unknown. *Pneumocystis* organisms are detected frequently in the sputum, pharyngeal secretions, or tracheal aspirates of symptomatic patients, and cysts have been shown to survive for several months in dried lung specimens maintained at room temperature. These observations suggest that infection probably occurs as a result of inhalation of the organism, which justifies respiratory isolation of symptomatic patients who are exposed to other highly susceptible patients.

The dramatic nature of PCP tends to obscure the fact that its severity is the result of the susceptibility of the host rather than the virulence of the parasite. That *P. jiroveci* is an organism of low pathogenicity is emphasized clearly by the rare occurrence of infections in intact hosts. Since the middle to late 1960s, PCP has occurred almost exclusively in patients with primary or acquired immunologic disorders or in those receiving immunosuppressive treatment of oncologic disease or organ transplantation. Of 194 cases reported to the Centers for Disease Control and Prevention (CDC) from 1967 through 1970, 29 occurred in infants younger than 1 year, 83% of whom had primary immunodeficiency disorders. In contrast, acute lymphocytic leukemia was the most common underlying disease in children older than 1 year. Of 1,251 children with malignant diseases at the Saint Jude Children's Research Hospital in Memphis, Tennessee, from 1962 to 1971, PCP occurred in 51 (4.1%). Within populations of patients with cancer, PCP occurs more commonly in individuals with generalized lymphoproliferative malignancy than in those with solid tumors. The risk of the development of *Pneumocystis* infections increases with the extent of malignant disease and the intensity of chemotherapy or radiotherapy provided. The precise mechanisms accounting for enhanced susceptibility in individual patients are not understood completely. PCP has been reported in association with congenital and acquired hypogammaglobulinemia, severe combined immunodeficiency disease, selective T-cell deficiency (DiGeorge syndrome), AIDS, and other secondary immunodeficiency states. The development of specific antibodies to *Pneumocystis* organisms in infected patients has been inconsistent. During the course of "epidemic" disease in malnourished infants, immunoglobulin M (IgM) values frequently increase markedly, with variable changes in IgG and IgA values. IgG antibody concentrations increase in the serum 4 to 6 weeks after infection and are thought to provide permanent immunity in those infants. Experimental evidence suggests that specific antibody fixes complement C3 fragments on the surface of *Pneumocystis* organisms and thereby enables their subsequent phagocytosis by alveolar macrophages. The importance of impaired cellular immunity in the pathogenesis of PCP is demonstrated by the ability of corticosteroids or cyclosporine to induce *Pneumocystis* infection in laboratory animals, the remarkable susceptibility of patients with AIDS to development of PCP (it occurs in at least 50% of these individuals), and the occurrence of PCP in malnourished hosts with significantly impaired cellular immune responses. In infants and children with AIDS, the quantity of peripheral blood CD4 T-helper lymphocytes serves as a useful predictor of PCP; as the level of CD4 lymphocytes decreases, the risk of developing this infectious complication increases.

P. jirovecii infections are unique in that the pathologic findings, with rare exceptions, are limited to the lungs, even in fatal cases. In the infantile epidemic form of the disease, essentially all alveoli contain large numbers of organisms. Extensive interstitial plasma cell infiltrates distend alveolar walls to five to 20 times their normal thickness, and almost no intraalveolar fibrinous exudate is noted.

CLINICAL MANIFESTATIONS AND COMPLICATIONS

In the childhood and adult forms of PCP, the histogenesis has been described in three stages. An initial stage is characterized by the presence of cysts and trophozoites attached to alveolar walls. No septal inflammatory or cellular responses are evident, and no clinical disease is associated with this stage. A second stage, which may or may not be associated with clinical signs and symptoms, is characterized by the desquamation of alveolar cells and an increase in the number of cysts within alveolar macrophages. A final stage that definitely is associated with clinical manifestations is typified by extensive reactive and desquamative alveolitis, manifested by marked cytoplasmic vacuolation of macrophages, mononuclear, and plasma cell infiltrates within alveolar septa, and clusters of organisms located predominantly within macrophages in the lumina of alveoli.

The natural course of *Pneumocystis* infections in children is highly variable and depends primarily on the status of host defenses in individual patients. Infantile epidemic pneumocystosis is typified in premature, debilitated, or marasmic infants between the ages of 2 and 6 months. These patients often have chronic diarrhea and weight loss before respiratory symptoms develop. Characteristically, the onset is insidious, with progression of cough, tachypnea, and respiratory distress occurring over a 1- to 4-week interval. Fever is either absent or low-grade in most cases. Symptoms in immunosuppressed children or adults may be more abrupt in onset and more rapidly progressive than in infantile epidemic cases; in these older patients, the severity and duration of disease before diagnosis is established are highly variable, but the mortality rate is approximately 100% if treatment is not provided. Unlike in infantile cases, fever generally is present and is high-grade, and it often precedes the onset of a nonproductive cough, tachypnea, and severe dyspnea or the appearance of pulmonary infiltrates on radiography.

Infants and children with AIDS usually are acutely ill at the time of onset with fever (79%), cough (86%), dyspnea (86%), tachypnea (88%), and an alveolar oxygen gradient greater than 30 mm Hg (95%). The median length of survival after a diagnosis of PCP is established in subjects with AIDS is approximately 2 months. The onset of clinical disease in high-risk patients is unpredictable, but it often has been observed to occur after the discontinuation of corticosteroid therapy or reduction in drug dosage. Observations suggest that the development of clinical disease depends in part on whether inflammatory responses are normal or are impaired somewhat as a result of the patient's underlying disease, therapeutic regimen, or both.

DIAGNOSIS

Physical examination at the time of initial presentation may reveal tachypnea, nasal flaring, and intercostal, subcostal, or supracostal retractions. An ashen color or cyanosis may be present or may develop rapidly. Auscultation of the chest frequently is characterized by a conspicuous absence of adventitious sounds despite rapid (80 to 100/minute), shallow respirations. Scattered rales, rhonchi, or wheezes usually are detected later in the clinical course as resolution occurs. Aside from variable temperature elevations, few physical abnormalities are noted except those attributable to pulmonary disease or secondary to the patient's underlying disease or treatment.

Various radiographic abnormalities have been observed in documented cases of isolated PCP. These variations in part are a result of observations being made at different stages in the course of the disease. Bilateral diffuse parenchymal infiltrates are seen most commonly, but no pattern is specific enough either to exclude or to confirm a consideration of a *Pneumocystis* infection. Although it initially is a reticulogranular interstitial process, PCP progresses to a predominantly alveolar process, with coalescence and air bronchogram formation. Late in the course of the disease, complete opacification of the lung fields may occur. Hilar adenopathy and pleural effusion are not characteristic unless they are a result of an underlying disorder.

Characteristic clinical features are not specific enough to differentiate PCP from other opportunistic pulmonary infections in highly susceptible pediatric patients. Furthermore, mixed infections involving viral, bacterial, fungal, or parasitic opportunists along with *Pneumocystis* organisms have been documented. These observations underscore the importance of establishing a definitive diagnosis before the institution of specific therapy. Because clinical features alone are of little value in making a differential diagnosis, a causative diagnosis can be ascertained only by the demonstration of *Pneumocystis* organisms in lung tissue or respiratory secretions.

Various techniques have been used to obtain suitable materials for diagnostic purposes. Although specimens obtained by noninvasive methods from sputum or pharyngeal, tracheal, or gastric secretions occasionally reveal *Pneumocystis* organisms in infected patients, these sources are not sufficiently reliable to exclude the diagnosis if organisms are not identified. Bronchoalveolar lavage, endobronchial brush biopsy, and transbronchial lung biopsy have been used successfully to establish a diagnosis of PCP in adult patients. Bronchoalveolar lavage has been shown to be safe and effective, especially in patients with AIDS. These techniques have been used successfully in infants as young as 2 months. Their routine use in children is not justified, however, given the limited experience and significant morbidity associated with these procedures in pediatric patients. Invasive techniques, including open lung biopsy, closed needle biopsy, and percutaneous needle aspiration, are the most reliable methods of confirming a diagnosis. Open lung biopsy provides the most reliable specimen for identification of both the organism and the extent of the infection; its chief disadvantage is that it requires general anesthesia. A closed needle biopsy procedure is less reliable for providing adequate tissue and is associated with significantly greater morbidity than is open thoracotomy. Percutaneous needle aspiration has proved to be a reliable and safe procedure in some centers. The methenamine silver nitrate method of Gomori and the less widely used but more rapid toluidine blue O stain are most useful for demonstrating cyst forms in tissue sections, aspirates, or imprints. For more detailed morphologic study of intracystic sporozoites and trophozoites, polychrome stains, including Giemsa, Wright, Gram, and methylene blue stains, are more suitable. In tissue sections, Gomori stain in combination with the hematoxylin-eosin stain enables the study of both the organism and the host tissue. Several studies have shown that *P. jiroveci* DNA can be detected by polymerase chain reaction techniques in lung tissues of infected children. This approach has been applied in epidemiologic studies to understand the prevalence of PCP in children dying of respiratory tract illnesses in the developing world. However, the low specificity of this approach currently precludes its use in clinical practice.

Serologic methods, including complement fixation, immunofluorescent testing, enzyme-linked immunosorbent assay, and latex agglutination testing, have been developed, but because of a lack of specificity or sensitivity, these techniques generally are not useful for diagnostic purposes. Moreover, the likelihood that impaired immune responses exist in affected patients precludes the interpretation of serologic results in most cases. A method developed for the detection of *Pneumocystis* antigenemia by countercurrent immunoelectrophoresis has proved unreliable as a means by which to confirm or exclude a diagnosis.

Before the availability of specific therapeutic agents, the overall prognosis of patients with PCP was poor. Despite supportive care, almost all infected patients with underlying neoplastic or immunodeficiency disorders died, and as many as 50% of affected infants in the European epidemics died as a result of this pulmonary infection. To control the European epidemics, Ivády and Páldy first suggested the use of pentamidine isethionate, a diamidine with previously demonstrated antifungal and antiprotozoal activities. Use of this therapeutic agent in infants during the next several years resulted in a dramatic reduction in mortality rates, from 50% to 3.5%. Pentamidine became available to investigators in the United States in 1967, through the CDC. During the next 3 years, of 163 children and adults with documented PCP who were treated with pentamidine, 43% recovered. Of 404 patients to whom the drug was administered for suspected or documented PCP, however, 189 (47%) experienced significant toxic manifestations. Toxicity ranged from localized reaction at injection sites (18%) to systemic effects, including impaired renal function (24%), liver toxicity (10%), hypotension (10%), and hypocalcemia (1%). Although pentamidine was effective treatment of this disorder, the high incidence of toxicity emphasized the need for an alternative therapeutic agent. With the advent of the AIDS epidemic, the intravenous administration of pentamidine was initiated, allowing a marked reduction in the number of injection site reactions that had been associated with intramuscular administration, but no decrease in the incidence of the other adverse effects.

THERAPY

Early animal studies and limited investigations in human patients suggested that a combination of pyrimethamine and sulfadiazine could be effective in the treatment of PCP. When a somewhat similar combination of trimethoprim and sulfamethoxazole (also known as cotrimoxazole) became available, prospective studies demonstrated the efficacy of this agent to be comparable with that of pentamidine in the treatment of PCP complicating childhood leukemia. Of great import, no significant toxicity secondary to trimethoprim-sulfamethoxazole therapy was observed in these investigations. In additional studies in pediatric patients with cancer, trimethoprim-sulfamethoxazole also was shown to be effective in the prevention of PCP. During one 2-year study period representing 30,000 patient-days, 17 of 80 placebo-treated patients (21%) contracted PCP, whereas no cases were recognized in 80 patients who were given trimethoprim-sulfamethoxazole prophylaxis. At present, trimethoprim-sulfamethoxazole appears to be the drug of choice for the treatment and prevention of PCP. The therapeutic doses are 20 mg of trimethoprim and 100 mg of sulfamethoxazole/kg/day orally in four equal doses. The intravenous doses are 15 mg of trimethoprim and 75 mg of sulfamethoxazole/kg/day in four doses.

Patients with AIDS demonstrate a high rate of adverse reactions to trimethoprim-sulfamethoxazole, as well as to pentamidine. Those who cannot tolerate the former should be treated with intravenous pentamidine at a single daily dose of 4 mg/kg. Some potential therapies for treating PCP have not been evaluated sufficiently in pediatric patients. Drugs with evidence of efficacy include trimethoprim-dapsone, pyrimethamine and sulfadoxine, trimetrexate, clindamycin and primaquine, and atovaquone. Animal studies suggest that a combination of erythromycin and sulfisoxazole has strong anti-*Pneumocystis* activity. In addition to antimicrobial agents, corticosteroids administered early in the course of moderately severe pneumonitis reduce the occurrence of respiratory failure and improve oxygenation among adult patients with AIDS.

PREVENTION

PCP can be prevented effectively by providing chemoprophylaxis with trimethoprim-sulfamethoxazole in pediatric patients at risk for this opportunisitic infection. For children 4 weeks of age or older, the American Academy of Pediatrics Committee on Infectious Diseases generally recommends trimethoprim-sulfamethoxazole (trimethoprim, 150 mg/m^2/day with sulfamethoxazole, 750 mg/m^2/day), orally in divided doses twice a day, three times per week on consecutive days. Use of this regimen or alternative regimens of this agent can prevent PCP in as many as 95% of high-risk patients, including those with cancer and primary immunodeficiency disorders and recipients of organ transplants. Revised guidelines for PCP prophylaxis in infants and children with AIDS have been developed by an expert committee at the CDC. Because all infants born of HIV-infected women theoretically are at high risk for development of PCP, it is recommended that PCP prophylaxis be started at or near the completion of HIV-1 prophylaxis (e.g., with zidovudine) at 4 to 6 weeks of age in all exposed infants but discontinued when HIV-1 infection is reasonably excluded. HIV-1-exposed infants who do become infected should remain on PCP prophylaxis regimens until they are 12 months of age. Use of chemoprophylaxis in this age group has been highly effective in HIV-infected infant populations. When these infants reach 1 year of age (or older), the use of chemoprophylaxis with recommended regimens of trimethoprim-sulfamethoxazole should be based on the level of the CD4 lymphocyte count and other AIDS-defining features. For patients who cannot tolerate trimethoprim-sulfamethoxazole, aerosolized pentamadine (300 mg administered once monthly via a Respigard II nebulizer) is an alternative for individuals 5 years of age or older. Daily oral dapsone (2 mg/kg or maximum of 100 mg) is another recommended alternative for children younger than 5 years of age. Although no clinical studies have been performed to evaluate these recommended regimens rigorously, these guidelines provide the most reasonable approach at this time. Although

chemoprophylaxis substantially reduces the risk of PCP in at-risk populations, pulmonary and extrapulmonary *P. jiroveci* infections have occurred in some HIV-1–infected children receiving these regimens. Such observations indicate that such agents do not eradicate *P. jiroveci* organisms, and patients at high risk are protected only while they are receiving chemoprophylaxis and remain susceptible to acquisition of infection when the drugs are discontinued.

Suggested Readings

American Academy of Pediatrics. In: Pickering LK, ed. *Redbook: 2003 report of the Committee on Infectious Diseases,* 26th ed. Elk Grove Village, IL: American Academy of Pediatrics, 2003.

Bommer W. Die interstitielle plasmacellulare Pneumoniae und *Pneumocystis carinii. Ergeb Mikrobiol* 1964;39:116.

Burke BA, Good RA. *Pneumocystis carinii* infection. Medicine (Baltimore) 1973; 52:23.

Chintu C, Mudenda V, Lucas S, et al. Lung diseases at necropsy in African children dying from respiratory illnesses: descriptive necropsy findings. *Lancet* 2002;369:985.

Doppman IL, Geelhoed GW, DeVita VT. Atypical radiographic features in *Pneumocystis carinii* pneumonia. *Radiology* 1975;114:39.

Graham SM. Prophylaxis against *Pneumocystis carinii* pneumonia for HIV-exposed infants in Africa. *Lancet* 2002;360:1966.

Hughes WT. Trimethoprim-sulfamethoxazole therapy for *Pneumocystis carinii* pneumonitis in children. *Rev Infect Dis* 1982;4:602.

Hughes WT, Feldman S, Chaudhary S, et al. Comparison of pentamidine isethionate and trimethoprim-sulfamethoxazole in the treatment of *Pneumocystis carinii* pneumonitis. *J Pediatr* 1973;92:285.

Hughes WT, Kuhn S, Chaudhary S, et al. Successful chemoprophylaxis for *Pneumocystis carinii* pneumonitis. *N Engl J Med* 1977;297:1419.

Hughes WT, Price R, Kim H, et al. *Pneumocystis carinii* pneumonitis in children with malignancies. *J Pediatr* 1973;82:404.

Ivády G, Páldy L. A new form of treatment for interstitial plasma-cell pneumonia in premature infants with pentavalent antimony and aromatic diamides. *Monatsschr Kinderheilkd* 1958;106:10.

Kasolo F, Lishimpi K, Chintu C, et al. Identification of *Pneumocystis carinii* DNA by polymerase chain reaction in necropsy lung samples from children dying of respiratory tract illnesses. *J Pediatr* 2002;140:367.

King S, Committee on Pediatric AIDS and Infectious Diseases and Immunization Committee. Evaluation and treatment of the human immunodeficiency virus 1–exposed infant. *Pediatrics* 2004;114:497.

Perera D, Western KA, Johnson HD, et al. *Pneumocystis carinii* pneumonia in a hospital for children: epidemiologic aspects. *JAMA* 1970;214:1074.

Stringer JR, Beard CB, Miller RF, et al. A new name (*Pneumocystis jiroveci*) for *Pneumocystis* from humans. *Emerg Infect Dis* 2002;9:891.

Walzer PD, Schultz MG, Western KA, et al. *Pneumocystis carinii* pneumonia and primary immune deficiency diseases of infancy and childhood. *J Pediatr* 1973;82:416.

CHAPTER 233 ■ BACTERIAL PNEUMONIA

JOHN F. MODLIN

In the United States, infection of the lower respiratory tract is recognized annually in 15 to 20 of 1,000 infants younger than 1 year of age and in 30 to 40 of 1,000 children 1 to 5 years old. Whereas respiratory viruses and *Mycoplasma pneumoniae* are the most common agents of lower respiratory tract disease in children and young adults, the weight of evidence suggests that pyogenic bacteria are responsible for 20% to 40% of cases. Bacterial pneumonia is observed most commonly in the winter

and early spring and occurs almost twice as frequently in boys as in girls.

Diseases involving the airways, such as bronchopulmonary dysplasia, cystic fibrosis, and bronchiectasis, and such anatomic defects as cleft palate or tracheoesophageal fistula predispose affected individuals to the development of bacterial pneumonia. Pneumonia and lung abscesses are common infections in children with severe cognitive neurologic disorders or diminished levels of consciousness. Children with hemoglobinopathies, especially sickle cell disease, demonstrate higher rates of bacterial pneumonia. Children who are immunodeficient on the basis of inherited or acquired disease or immunosuppressive therapy are at increased risk of developing pneumonia from a wide spectrum of bacteria and at additional risk from viruses, fungi, protozoa, and parasites. The diagnosis and management of opportunistic pulmonary infections that occur in immunocompromised children are covered in Chapter 232.

In practice, distinguishing bacterial pneumonia from other forms of pneumonia usually is difficult because infants and young children do not produce adequate sputum for Gram stain and culture and because routine chest radiographs do not commonly demonstrate abnormalities specific for bacterial infection. Furthermore, invasive procedures are warranted only in severely ill patients or in patients with underlying immunodeficiency.

ETIOLOGY

Age and the presence of underlying disease are the two most important patient characteristics determining the cause of bacterial pneumonia. Bacterial pneumonia presenting in the patient's first 5 days of life, which generally is considered to be acquired *in utero* or intrapartum, is caused by the same organisms responsible for generalized neonatal sepsis (i.e., group B streptococci, *Listeria monocytogenes*, *Haemophilus influenzae*, and gram-negative enteric bacilli). Most cases of perinatally acquired pneumonia occur among low-birth-weight infants and infants who have peripartum complications. These infants may be at increased risk of developing nosocomial pneumonia caused by *Pseudomonas aeruginosa*, *Escherichia coli*, or other gram-negative bacilli if they require endotracheal intubation and mechanical ventilation. *Chlamydia trachomatis*, a pathogen acquired from the maternal genital tract at delivery, may not cause respiratory symptoms until the child's second month of life.

After the neonatal period, *Streptococcus pneumoniae*, *Moraxella catarrhalis*, and group A streptococci are responsible for most cases of bacterial pneumonia in otherwise healthy children. *Neisseria meningitidis* seldom is reported. *Staphylococcus aureus* pneumonia now is seen rarely in infants and toddlers, and pneumonia caused by *Bordetella pertussis* and *H. influenzae* type b (Hib) has been controlled effectively in the United States and other developed countries by universal immunization. *M. pneumoniae* and *Chlamydia pneumoniae* infections are uncommon findings in children younger than age 3 years.

For school-aged children and adolescents, the etiologic spectrum for bacterial pneumonia narrows to *M. pneumoniae*, *C. pneumoniae*, and *S. pneumonia*. Many sources cite *M. pneumoniae* as the most common cause of bacterial pneumonia between 5 and 30 years of age.

PATHOGENESIS

The respiratory tract below the vocal cords normally is sterile; microorganisms are excluded from the tracheobronchial tree by nonspecific host defenses, including the blanket of mucus covering the mucosal epithelium, the ciliary transport activity, and the cough reflex. Secretory immunoglobulin A antibody present in mucosal secretions helps to protect against reinfection with specific organisms. Within the lung parenchyma, bacteria are cleared by lymphatic channels that drain to regional lymph nodes and by macrophages that line the terminal bronchioles and alveoli. The lung is protected also by systemic humoral and cell-mediated immune mechanisms, including passively acquired maternal antibody, which protects against pneumococcal and Hib infections in the child's first 4 to 6 months of life. Alteration of any of these protective mechanisms is likely to predispose the child to the development of bacterial pneumonia.

Bacterial pathogens that cause pneumonia in children are transmitted from person to person by close personal contact or airborne spread. Colonization of young children's upper respiratory tract with pathogenic bacteria is a common finding; the prevalence of carriage of pneumococci is 25% to 40% during the winter months and somewhat lower during other seasons. Pneumonia results from aspiration of pathogenic bacteria into the lower respiratory tract; often, the process is aided by concurrent viral infection, particularly with the influenza viruses and measles virus. Careful studies have documented the coexistence of a respiratory virus in 30% to 50% of children with bacterial pneumonia. Acute viral infection serves to disrupt the normal anatomic and physiologic barriers of the respiratory tract mucosa and briefly may suppress the activity of phagocytic leukocytes in the airways and lung.

Less commonly, bacteria spread to the lung hematogenously from a distant focus (e.g., bacterial endocarditis or septic jugular venous thrombosis). In such instances, pneumonia may occur in the setting of widespread pyogenic infection or other sites, including the meninges, bones, and joints.

CLINICAL MANIFESTATIONS

The signs and symptoms of bacterial pneumonia vary with affected children's ages, with the organism, and with the presence or absence of underlying disease. Characteristically, older children and adolescents present with fever, chills, headache, dyspnea, productive cough, chest pain, abdominal pain, and nausea or vomiting. However, infants are likely to have mostly nonspecific symptoms of fever, lethargy, poor feeding, vomiting, or diarrhea. Apnea may be a prominent sign among infants younger than 2 months. Tachypnea may be overlooked by the parents, and cough, if present, often is not a prominent finding in very young infants. Similarly, the physical examination findings in young infants with pneumonia are less definitive; usually, percussion and auscultation do not elicit the characteristic dullness to percussion and decreased breath sounds found in older children and adults with pneumonia, and distinguishing rales from the sounds produced by a congested upper respiratory tract may be difficult.

DIAGNOSIS

In practice, the diagnosis of pneumonia is made with the demonstration of infiltrates on anteroposterior and lateral chest radiography. False-negative results sometimes are attributed to dehydration. Conversely, many noninfectious diseases of the lung, including malignancy, collagen-vascular disease, congestive heart failure, pulmonary embolus, allergic alveolitis, pulmonary hemorrhage, hemosiderosis and drug toxicity, may mimic the radiographic appearance of pneumonia. A pattern of peribronchial or "patchy" infiltrates (bronchopneumonia) does not distinguish viral or *M. pneumoniae* pneumonia from bacterial pneumonia, but demonstration of hyperinflation is most consistent with viral infection. The presence of lobar consolidation or pleural effusion suggests bacterial infection, whereas pneumatoceles and abscess cavities are virtually diagnostic (Fig. 233.1). Lobar consolidation, which is present in approximately one-half of children with bacterial pneumonia, correlates with the presence of bacteremia. Roentgenograms demonstrate bilateral disease in 20% to 25%

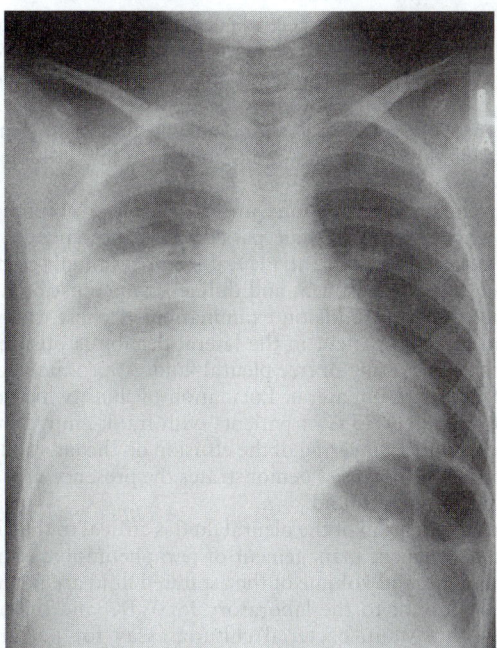

FIGURE 233.1. A child with bacterial pneumonia. This radiograph of the chest shows lobar consolidation and a pleural effusion on the right. Note the meniscus indicating the presence of fluid in the pleural cavity. (Reprinted from Fleisher GR, Ludwig S, Baskin MN, eds. *Atlas of pediatric emergency medicine*. Philadelphia: Lippincott Williams & Wilkins, 2004:196.)

of pediatric patients. Spheric infiltrates, which seldom are seen early in the course of pneumococcal pneumonia, initially may be confused with a focal fungal, mycobacterial, or parasitic infection or with a metastatic neoplasm. The resolution of the pulmonary infiltrates lags behind clinical improvement of the patient. Routine follow-up radiographs contribute little to the management of the child with an uncomplicated course of pneumonia.

Computed tomography (CT) of the chest provides better resolution and thus is more sensitive than is radiography for the detection of pulmonary infiltrates. However, the expense of CT scanning justifies its use only when such complications as adenopathy, empyema, cavitation, or pericarditis are suspected.

A complete blood count and either an erythrocyte sedimentation rate or C-reactive protein determination should be performed for all pediatric patients with suspected pneumonia to help distinguish bacterial from viral pneumonia; one should keep in mind that the predictive value of all nonmicrobiologic assays is less than absolute. Gram staining of expectorated sputum may be valuable in establishing the diagnosis of pneumonia in school-aged children or adolescents, especially when a single organism is seen in association with polymorphonuclear leukocytes; usually, culture of an adequate sputum specimen yields the pathogenic organism. The use of antigen detection tests performed on expectorated sputum is discouraged because these assays lack sensitivity. Infants and young children are incapable of producing a spontaneous sputum specimen, and efforts to induce sputum usually are not successful.

Cultures of blood and pleural fluid (if present) should be obtained from children requiring hospitalization. Cultures of the nasopharynx and throat are not useful and should not be attempted because of the risk of producing misleading information. Such invasive procedures as bronchoalveolar lavage or open lung biopsy are justified in cases of pneumonia that are severe or complicated by underlying disease. Direct transthoracic needle aspiration of the lung is a very useful procedure in cases in which recovery of an organism is critical for management.

ANTIBIOTIC MANAGEMENT

Children with mild to moderate bacterial pneumonia often are managed as outpatients, with an oral antibiotic chosen to cover the most likely bacterial pathogens based on the child's age and the epidemiologic setting. High-dose amoxicillin (80 mg/kg/day) is recommended for outpatient management of pneumonia for infants and children between 3 months and 5 years of age. Although as many as 40% of isolated *S. pneumoniae* organisms are not fully susceptible to penicillin or ampicillin by *in vitro* criteria, the ampicillin serum concentration achieved with this regimen is sufficient to treat most infections other than those of the central nervous system. Alternatively, a second-generation cephalosporin with good activity against *S. pneumoniae* (i.e., cefuroxime or cefpodoxime) should be used, keeping in mind that not all cephalosporins possess optimal activity against penicillin-nonsusceptible *S. pneumoniae*.

An oral macrolide (e.g., erythromycin, clarithromycin, or azithromycin) is the first-line treatment for ambulatory school-aged children and adolescents because of the activity of these agents against *M. pneumoniae* and *C. pneumoniae*. Erythromycin may be given in a dose of 30 to 50 mg/kg/24 hours in two to four divided doses with a maximum dose of 1 to 2 g/day. Azithromycin is given in a dose of 5 to 12 mg/day only once each day with a maximum dose of 600 mg. Clarithromycin may be given in a dose of 15 mg/kg/day in two divided doses with a maximum of 1 g/day. Because some *S. pneumoniae* organisms and a few group A streptococci may be macrolide-resistant, amoxicillin or a second-generation cephalosporin should be added to the regimen of patients with lobar pneumonia and/or a pleural effusion, or when there is no response to macrolides. Studies in adults with community-acquired pneumonia have shown nearly equal efficacy of erythromycin and beta-lactam antibiotics for outpatient management.

Children hospitalized with more serious disease require maintenance of adequate oxygenation and antibiotics; chest physical therapy and intermittent positive-pressure treatments usually provide little additional benefit. Initial antibiotic therapy should be guided by the results of a sputum Gram stain and should be modified, if necessary, once the results of cultures of blood, sputum, or pleural fluid are reported. A second- or third-generation cephalosporin frequently is given parenterally for empiric treatment, and an intravenous or oral macrolide should be added for children older than age 5 years until a diagnosis of *M. pneumoniae* pneumonia is excluded.

PNEUMONIA CAUSED BY SPECIFIC BACTERIAL PATHOGENS

S. pneumoniae is a common cause of pneumonia at all ages. Serotypes 1, 3, 6, 7, 14, 18, 19, and 23 are the most common of the 84 serotypes found in children, differing slightly from the distribution of serotypes that cause bacteremic pneumonia in adults. Pleural effusion occurs in a minority of cases, but frank empyema is an unusual finding, and pneumatocele formation is rare. Approximately 30% of children with pneumococcal pneumonia have positive blood cultures on presentation, a finding associated with more severe disease. Rapid resolution of fever and dyspnea with appropriate antibiotic therapy is the rule, but prolonged courses occur, especially with extensive lung involvement and with empyema. The mortality of pneumococcal pneumonia in children is approximately 10%. With recovery, residual impairment of lung function is minimal. Rare complications include pericarditis, meningitis, endocarditis, arthritis, and bursitis. The introduction of heptavalent pneumococcal conjugate vaccine in 2000 has reduced the incidence of bacteremic pneumococcal pneumonia by 90% and the incidence of all chest radiographically confirmed pneumonia in young children by approximately 20%.

Respiratory disease caused by *M. pneumoniae* also is covered in Chapter 230. *M. pneumoniae* causes an "atypical" pneumonia that is distinguishable from disease caused by pyogenic bacteria by a 2- to 3-week incubation period and by a longer duration of a prodrome of fever, malaise, headache, sore throat, and cough. The usual pediatric patient appears less ill than do patients with pyogenic bacterial pneumonia and usually has a relative absence of chest physical examination abnormalities. Chest radiographic findings are indistinguishable from those found with viral pneumonia, including a low incidence of pleural effusion. Fever, cough, and nonrespiratory symptoms may persist for 2 to 3 weeks before slowly resolving. *M. pneumoniae* pneumonia generally is self-limited, but patients with sickle cell disease and primary B-cell immunodeficiencies may have more severe and prolonged disease. Antibiotic treatment reduces the duration of symptoms, but not dramatically. Macrolide antibiotics are most appropriate for pediatric patients, although fluoroquinolones and tetracyclines also possess excellent activity against *M. pneumonia*. No effective vaccine exists.

Hib pneumonia is clinically and radiographically indistinguishable from pneumococcal pneumonia. In the early 1990s, *H. influenzae* equaled *S. pneumoniae* as a cause of pneumonia in children younger than 2 years before the introduction of Hib immunization of infants, but now it is quite rare. As many as 90% of children with Hib pneumonia have positive blood cultures, and 40% to 75% have accompanying pleural effusions. Of children with Hib, 10% to 30% also have meningitis, epiglottitis, or other serious pyogenic infection. The mortality is 5% to 10%.

S. aureus pneumonia appears to be less common than it was in the 1950s and 1960s, but it remains an important cause of serious pneumonia in infants younger than 6 months of age and in all pediatric patients with influenza. Staphylococcal pneumonia initially presents like pneumonia caused by other bacteria but characteristically progresses to pneumatocele formation and empyema, even in the presence of appropriate antibiotic therapy. Although staphylococci can be recovered from the blood in only 10% of infants, usually organisms are present in large numbers in a gram-stained tracheal aspirate. Mortality from staphylococcal pneumonia is 20% to 30%, and recovery in survivors may take weeks. The emergence of methicillin-resistant *S. aureus* infections now requires the empiric use of vancomycin when *S. aureus* is suspected as the cause of community-acquired pneumonia.

COMPLICATIONS

A parapneumonic effusion (the presence of fluid in the pleural space) may be caused by congestive heart failure, malignancy, collagen-vascular disease, and infection within the parenchyma of the lung. The composition of the parapneumonic effusion secondary to infection can vary from a thin, serous transudate with few white blood cells (WBCs), low protein content, and a pH of more than 7.2 to a thick, purulent exudate (or empyema) in which the WBC count is greater than 15,000 cells/mm³, the protein content is more than 3.0 g/dL, and the pH is less than 7.2. A serous exudate and empyema may represent the extremes in the natural history of pleural space involvement from underlying bacterial infection of the lung, which progresses from an exudative phase to a fibropurulent phase with accumulation of polymorphonuclear leukocytes and fibrin, and then to an orga-

nizing, fibrous layer or "peel" that adheres to pleural surfaces and ultimately may restrict expansion of the lung. *S. pneumoniae*, *S. aureus*, and group A streptococci are the major causes of empyema. Parapneumonic effusions secondary to viruses, *M. pneumoniae*, and *C. pneumoniae* are uncommon findings and usually are composed of an exudate of low volume when they occur.

Parapneumonic effusions are found more commonly in young children and in male patients. The presence of an inflammatory exudate in the pleural space results in continued fever, chest pain, dyspnea, and dullness to percussion and diminished breath sounds on examination. A chest radiograph with an affected patient in the lateral decubitus position will demonstrate layering of free pleural fluid. Approximately one-half of cases are unilateral. Loculation of fluid, which occurs in approximately 75% of patients with frank empyema, may inhibit dependent layering of the effusion on the lateral decubitus film. CT of the chest demonstrates the presence and extent of loculated pleural fluid.

Characterization of the pleural fluid is critical to the diagnosis and subsequent management of parapneumonic effusions. The character and volume of the aspirated fluid are noted, and samples are sent to the laboratory for WBC and differential count, Gram stain, bacterial culture, assay for pneumococcal and Hib polysaccharide antigens, pH measurement, and determination of glucose, protein, and lactate dehydrogenase content. Studies in adults have shown that concentrations of glucose of less than 40 mg/dL, a lactate dehydrogenase level greater than 1,000 IU/dL, and a pH of less than 7.2 are better predictors of a positive bacterial culture and need for thoracotomy tube drainage than are WBC and protein content.

Management of parapneumonic effusions associated with bacterial pneumonia consists of administration of an antibiotic and drainage of the pleural fluid. Frequently, drainage can be accomplished by needle aspiration during the exudative stage, although more than one aspiration procedure may be required. Empyema requires the insertion of one or more thoracotomy tubes, which sometimes must be repositioned to drain loculated areas of purulent fluid. CT-guided chest catheter placement and video-assisted thoracoscopy represent methods recently introduced for drainage of pleural fluid and débridement of loculations. Chest tubes are withdrawn when drainage ceases, usually after a period of 2 to 5 days. The clinical response to management of empyema characteristically is slow; fever, chest pain, and irritability may persist for 1 to 2 weeks, although stabilization of vital signs and improvement of systemic oxygenation occur more rapidly. Clearing of abnormalities on chest radiography may take weeks to months. In most children, gradual improvement of pulmonary function occurs, with little or no long-term restrictive lung abnormality. Surgical decortication of the organized peel no longer is performed in children, except in unusual circumstances. The overall mortality rate for empyema in children is 6% to 12%, but it may be higher in infants and in patients with staphylococcal empyema.

Pneumatoceles are thin-walled cavities that develop in the lung in the course of bacterial pneumonia. Pneumatoceles complicate approximately 40% of cases of *S. aureus* pneumonia and are unusual complications of pneumonia caused by *S. pneumoniae*, *H. influenzae*, and group A streptococci. Pneumatoceles are asymptomatic except when they rupture into the pleural space and cause pneumothorax or pyopneumothorax. Most persist for 2 to 3 months and resolve spontaneously.

Lung abscesses arise at the site of necrotizing pneumonia that occurs after aspiration of oropharyngeal secretions. Children with severe mental-motor retardation, seizure disorders, poor oral hygiene, and periodontal disease are particularly susceptible to the development of lung abscesses. Dependent segments of the lung (i.e., the posterior segment of the right upper lobe and the superior segments of the right and the left lower lobes) are the usual locations of formation of abscesses. Anaerobic bacteria play a prominent role in formation of abscesses. Usually, one or more species of anaerobes, with or without other oral bacteria, will be recovered from abscess cavities.

Fever, cough, tachypnea, and a fetid breath odor are the major presenting manifestations of lung abscess. Chest radiography reveals a focal infiltrate surrounding a cavity that may contain an air-fluid level; approximately 10% of patients have more than one cavity. Fiberoptic bronchoscopy may be used to obtain a specimen directly from the abscess cavity for diagnostic purposes. A 3- to 4-week course of metronidazole or ampicillin combined with a beta-lactamase inhibitor (e.g., amoxicillin-clavulanate [Augmentin], ampicillinsulbactam [Unasyn]) is appropriate therapy for lung abscess. Clarithromycin and azithromycin are effective antibiotic options.

Suggested Readings

Bartlett JG, Mundy LM. Community-acquired pneumonia. *N Engl J Med* 1995; 333:1618.

Black SB, Shinefield HR, Ling S, et al. Effectiveness of heptavalent pneumococcal conjugate vaccine in children younger than five years of age for prevention of pneumonia. *Pediatr Infect Dis J* 2002;21:810.

Buckingham SC, King MD, Miller ML. Incidence and etiologies of complicated parapneumonic effusions in children, 1996 to 2001. *Pediatr Infect Dis J* 2003;23:499.

Freij BJ, Kusmiesz H, Nelson JD, et al. Parapneumonic effusions and empyema in hospitalized children: a retrospective review of 227 cases. *Pediatr Infect Dis* 1984;3:578.

Glezen WP, Loda FA, Clyde WA, et al. Epidemiologic patterns of acute lower respiratory disease of children in a pediatric practice. *J Pediatr* 1971;78:397.

Hughes JR, Sinha DP, Cooper MR, et al. Lung tap in childhood: bacteria, viruses, and mycoplasmas in acute lower respiratory tract infections. *Pediatrics* 1969;44:477.

Jadavji T, Law B, Lebel MH, et al. A practical guide for the diagnosis and treatment of pediatric pneumonia. *Can Med Assoc J* 1997;156:S703.

Juvén T, Mertsola J, Waris M, et al. Etiology of community-acquired pneumonia in 254 hospitalized children. *Pediatr Infect Dis J* 2000;19:293.

Klein JO. Diagnostic lung puncture in the pneumonias of infants and children. *Pediatrics* 1969;44:486.

McIntosh K. Community acquired pneumonia in children. *N Engl J Med* 2002; 346:429.

Peter G. The child with pneumonia: diagnostic and therapeutic considerations. *Pediatr Infect Dis J* 1988;7:453.

Schutze GE, Jacobs RF. Management of community-acquired bacterial pneumonia in hospitalized children. *Pediatr Infect Dis J* 1992;11:160.

Vuori-Holopainen E, Salo E, Saxén H, et al. Etiological diagnosis of childhood pneumonia by use of transthoracic needle aspiration and modern microbiological methods. *Clin Infect Dis* 2002;34:583.

CHAPTER 234 ■ LARYNGEAL DISORDERS

RICHARD J. H. SMITH AND BENJAMIN B. CABLE

ANATOMY

Anatomic considerations are discussed in Box 234.1.

LARYNGOMALACIA

Stridor is a high-pitched, musical sound that is produced by airflow turbulence resulting from partial obstruction of the airway. It must be differentiated from other airway sounds, such as stertor, wheezes, rhonchi, and rales. Although the etiology of stridor is multifactorial, often the location of the airway obstruction can be determined by careful listening. For example, inspiratory high-pitched stridor with a relatively normal voice usually denotes supraglottic obstruction; biphasic (inspiratory and expiratory) stridor of intermediate pitch is heard with glottic or subglottic obstruction; and expiratory stridor associated with a "barking" cough indicates intrathoracic tracheal obstruction.

Congenital laryngeal stridor or laryngomalacia is the most common form of stridor in infants and accounts for approximately 80% of all cases of pediatric stridor. It is characterized by an inspiratory, harsh, high-pitched stridor that arises from medial prolapse of the epiglottis, aryepiglottic folds, or arytenoid cartilages (Fig. 234.6). Usually, the tissues obstructing the laryngeal inlet are the aryepiglottic folds and the arytenoids (67% of cases), although combined posterior and anterior obstruction caused by the arytenoids and epiglottis, respectively, is not an infrequent finding (30% of cases). However isolated, anterior (epiglottic) obstruction is rare (fewer than 3%). The pathophysiology of laryngomalacia includes poor neurologic control or hypotonia, redundant laryngeal soft tissue, and inadequate cartilaginous support (hence the name *laryngomalacia* or *soft larynx*). The differential diagnosis includes subglottic stenosis, vocal cord paralysis, and tracheomalacia, a relatively rare disorder presenting either as idiopathic tracheomalacia or as secondary to extrinsic compression, often from a vascular malformation.

Nearly always, laryngomalacia is noticed within the first few weeks or months of life, and an initial diagnosis of laryngomalacia made after the age of 2 years should be questioned. The stridor is intermittent and mild and occasionally becomes exacerbated by crying, supine positioning, and upper respiratory infections. Cyanosis, hoarseness, feeding difficulties, atypical stridor, failure to thrive, and apneic spells indicate the need for a complete diagnostic evaluation and possible operative intervention. However, most cases resolve spontaneously by the time this child reaches age 12 to 18 months.

The diagnosis of laryngomalacia can be made with a high degree of certainty on the basis of an office examination complemented by flexible fiberoptic laryngoscopy. Although some investigators recommend that all children with laryngomalacia undergo direct laryngoscopy and bronchoscopy, or flexible fiberoptic bronchoscopy, to rule out concomitant airway disease, a review by Mancuso and colleagues reported a significant second airway lesion in only 4% of 233 children with laryngomalacia. More importantly, the nine children with other airway lesions had atypical histories and unusual stridor. Although prudence would prompt evaluation of the entire airway in infants with laryngomalacia, unless the pattern of

BOX 234.1   Anatomic Considerations in Laryngeal Disorders

A neonatal larynx differs from an adult larynx not only in size but also in relative dimensions and location. A neonate's larynx is approximately one-third the size of its adult counterpart. The average cross-sectional area of an infant's glottis is approximately 15 mm², which is relatively small when compared with an adult glottis. The epiglottis is proportionately larger (1.38:1.00), and this relative difference in size and the position of the larynx high in the neck are instrumental in allowing infants to suckle and breathe simultaneously. During swallowing, the epiglottis abuts the soft palate to create lateral digestive channels that funnel food into the piriform fossae and esophagus while the midline airway remains patent and effectively separated. Olfaction also may be enhanced by the neonate's ability to breathe while swallowing.

Descent of the larynx to a lower position in the neck begins at age 2 years. During infancy, the inferior border of the cricoid cartilage is located at the fourth cervical vertebra, but by puberty, its location is at the level of the seventh cervical vertebra. This change in position creates a confluence of the digestive and respiratory tracts and results in a longer vocal tract, which is ideal for complex speech and articulation. However, this lengthening abolishes the ability to suckle and breathe simultaneously. Growth of the larynx continues until puberty, by which time full laryngeal development has occurred.

The membranoskeletal framework of the larynx is composed of several cartilages to which are attached muscles and folds of tissue that render respiration, phonation, and deglutition possible. The intricacies and subtleties of these structures are complicated, but their basic anatomy is relatively simple. The major cartilages of the larynx are the cricoid, thyroid, epiglottis, and arytenoids.

Only the cricoid, with a broad arch posteriorly and a narrow arch anteriorly, forms a complete ring. Attached superiorly is the sharply flexed, shieldlike thyroid cartilage; its more important features include paired superior and inferior horns, lateral plates or laminae, and the thyroid notch. In lateral profile, the notch forms an anteriorly projecting angle known as the *laryngeal prominence* or *Adam's apple*. Facets on the inferior horns articulate with the posterior arch of the cricoid, establishing a hinge motion between the two cartilages (Fig. 1).

The leaflike epiglottis is tucked within the thyroid cartilage. It is made of fibroelastic cartilage and is attached inferiorly to the thyroid cartilage just above the level of the true vocal cords. From its midportion, the epiglottis is attached to the tongue by the median and lateral glossoepiglottic folds. From both lateral borders of the epiglottis, quadrangular membranes arise and arch posteriorly to the arytenoids. So named because of their shape, the quadrangular membranes are as tall as the epiglottis anteriorly and are only as high as the ipsilateral arytenoid posteriorly. Both the superior and the inferior borders of each quadrangular membrane are free (Figs. 2 and 3).

The arytenoid cartilages are paired paramedian structures. Each has an apex, a concave base that rests on the underlying cricoid cartilage, a lateral process to which attach many of the intrinsic muscles of the larynx, and an anteriorly projecting vocal process. A second laryngeal membrane—the triangular membrane or conus elasticus—originates from this anteriorly projecting vocal process and continues

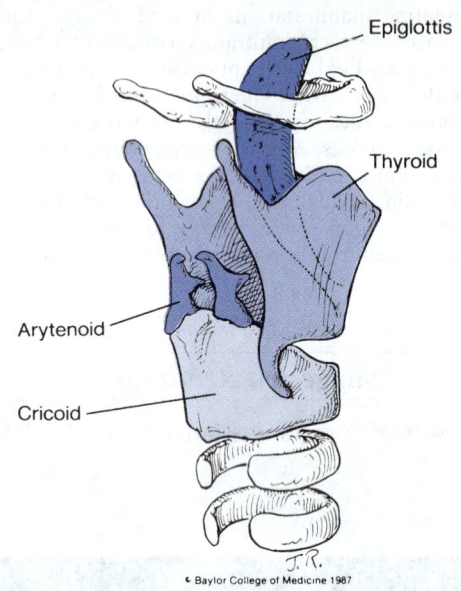

BOX 234.1. FIGURE 1. Posterior oblique view of laryngeal cartilaginous framework.

anteriorly to the thyroid cartilage. Its superior edge is thickened and forms the vocal ligament. Inferiorly, the triangular membrane attaches to the cricoid cartilage (see Fig. 3). Two minor paired cartilages also are present. The corniculate cartilage lies on the superior portion of the arytenoids and contributes to the height of the posterior glottis. The small and sometimes rudimentary cuneiform cartilages are located in the aryepiglottic folds and may act like a batten to stiffen the folds.

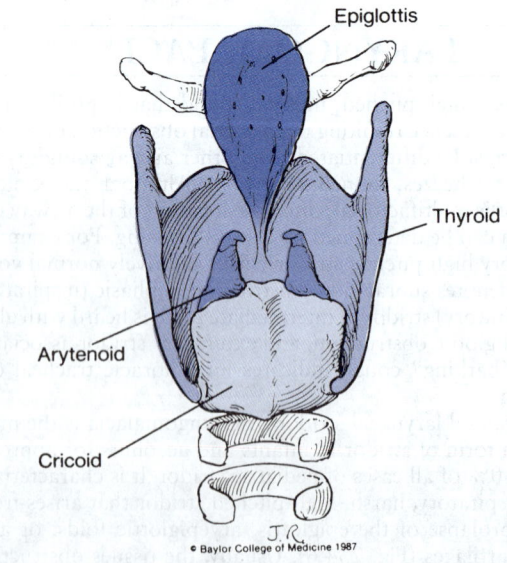

BOX 234.1. FIGURE 2. Posterior view of the laryngeal cartilages.

(Continued)

BOX 234.1   (Continued)

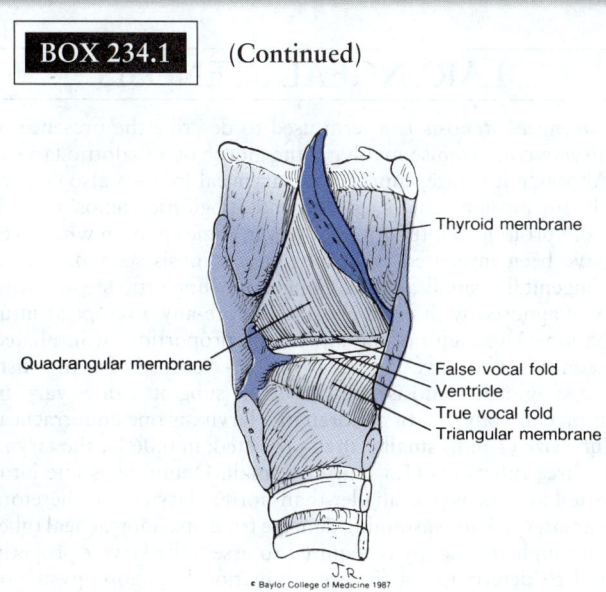

BOX 234.1. FIGURE 3. Quadrangular and triangular membranes as they attach to the laryngeal cartilages.

Overlying these structures are the laryngeal muscles and mucosa. To aid in our understanding of the anatomic associations, we divide the intrinsic muscles of the larynx into two groups. One group, comprising the thyroarytenoid, the thyroepiglottic, and the aryepiglottic muscles, is associated with the quadrangular membrane. The second group, comprising the posterior cricoarytenoid, the lateral cricoarytenoid, and the interarytenoid muscles, acts on the arytenoid cartilages.

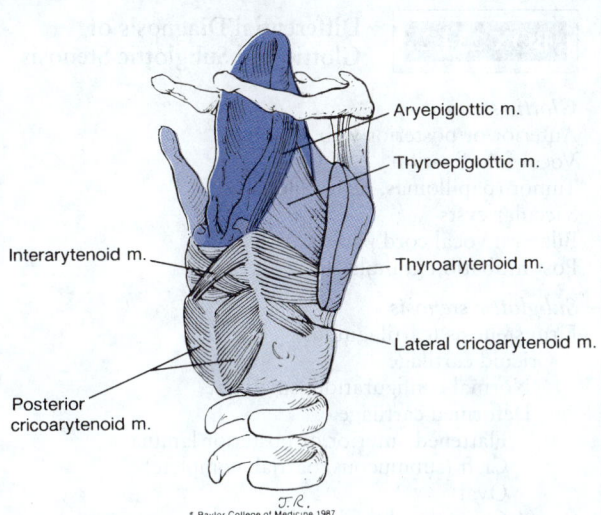

BOX 234.1. FIGURE 4. Laryngeal muscles associated with the laryngeal membranes.

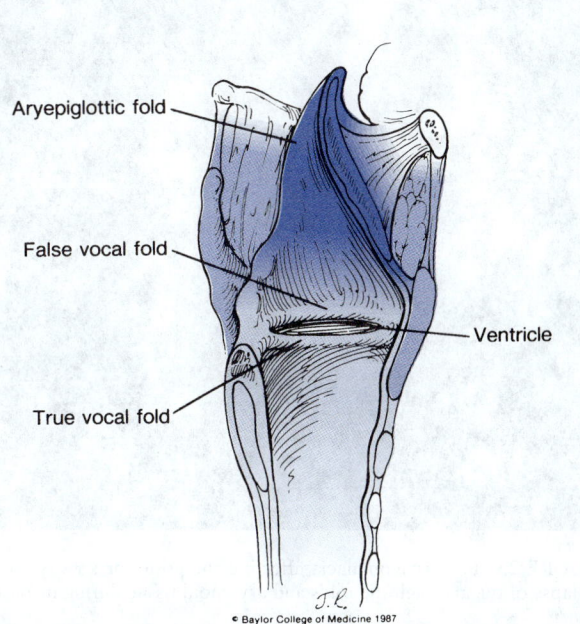

BOX 234.1. FIGURE 5. Overlying mucosa that creates three important folds: the aryepiglottic folds, the false vocal cords, and the true vocal cords.

A seventh muscle, the vocalis muscle, parallels the vocal fold and is part of the thyroarytenoid muscle (Fig. 4).

The overlying mucosa forms three important folds: the aryepiglottic folds, the false vocal cords (representing the inferior borders of both quadrangular membranes), and the true vocal folds. With the exception of the true vocal folds, which are covered by stratified squamous epithelium, the mucosa from the trachea to the aryepiglottic folds is pseudostratified ciliated columnar epithelium (Fig. 5).

The major functions of the larynx—respiration, phonation, and deglutition—require certain positions of the vocal cords for optimal operation. On maximal respiration, the vocal cords become flattened. During phonation, they are lightly juxtaposed. During swallowing, maximal closure of the airway occurs by the coordinated apposition of the vocal cords, the sphincteric action of the aryepiglottic folds, and elevation of the larynx to the tongue base.

Trauma or pathologic changes involving the larynx may affect the dynamics of the vocal cord. If function becomes compromised, such symptoms as stridor, hoarseness, and aspiration can develop. They are the harbingers of potentially serious laryngeal problems and dictate that an adequate laryngeal evaluation be performed. Examination may require simple flexible fiberoptic visualization or a more detailed study using rigid laryngoscopes and bronchoscopes with the patient under general anesthesia.

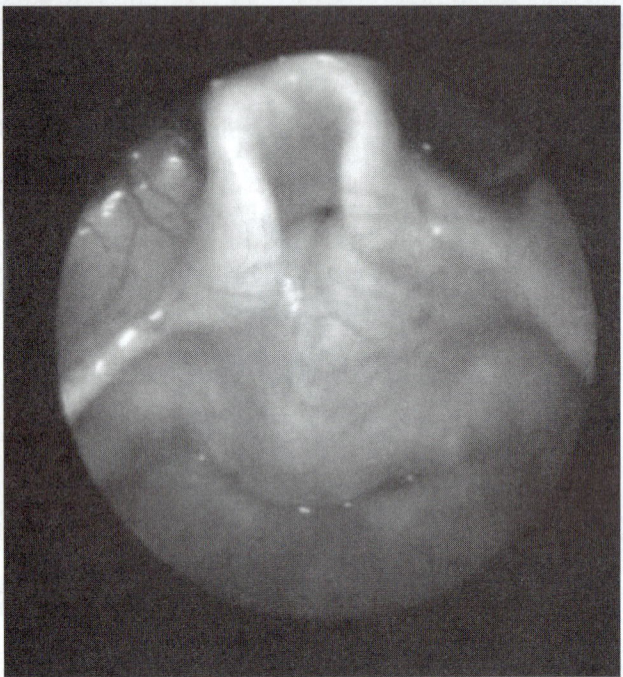

FIGURE 234.6. Laryngomalacia affecting the posterior airway with collapse of the aryepiglottic folds and arytenoid tissue during inspiration.

obstruction of the airway suggests that the laryngomalacia is unusually severe or otherwise atypical, routine direct laryngoscopy and bronchoscopy or flexible fiberoptic bronchoscopy are not cost effective.

Gastroesophageal reflux disease (GERD) also may play a role in stridor and laryngomalacia. Little and associates reported on the high incidence of GERD in children with laryngeal anomalies, in particular laryngomalacia, as compared with children without laryngeal disorders. Possible explanations for this association include GERD-induced triggering of neurologic laryngeal reflex pathways, GERD-induced mucosal edema, or secondary aspiration. These data suggest that in children with severe laryngomalacia, evaluation of GERD with video swallow studies or a 24-hour pH probe should be considered.

Treatment of laryngomalacia usually is unnecessary, and reassurance to parents is all that is required. Approximately 90% of children will experience a slow resolution of their stridor over the course of time without intervention. Indications for intervention in the remaining 10% of the population with laryngomalacia include significant respiratory compromise and failure to thrive. Respiratory compromise is considered when children demonstrate severe stridor as well as retractions with evidence of desaturations by oximetry. Failure to thrive sometimes can result from the significant increase in the overall work of breathing these children require. All children with laryngomalacia should be monitored closely for appropriate weight gain, and those failing to obtain target gains should be returned to their consulting otolaryngologist for treatment.

Surgical therapy for laryngomalacia can be directed at removing the redundant supraglottic tissue (endoscopic, often laser-assisted, ablation of excess supraglottic tissue, a so-called supraglottoplasty) or bypassing the larynx (tracheotomy). The former intervention has come to the forefront and is 70% to 90% effective in resolving airway obstruction and obviating a tracheotomy. Postoperative complications are minimal, and no long-term morbidity has been reported. Tracheotomy is the treatment of choice for supraglottoplasty failures as well as for those children with concomitant disorders such as cardiovas-

cular anomalies, pulmonary disease, or other airway lesions that require airway stabilization.

LARYNGEAL STENOSIS

Laryngeal stenosis is a term used to describe the presence of airway compromise involving the glottic or subglottic larynx. Although it is rare, supraglottic laryngeal stenosis also can occur. In most instances, glottic and subglottic stenoses result from prolonged intubation; however, some children who never have been intubated have subglottic stenosis secondary to a congenitally small airway. Congenital subglottic stenosis can be diagnosed with certainty only before any attempt at intubation. Although no one knows the proportion of intubated neonates who have laryngeal stenosis because of a preexisting subglottic stenosis, the size of the subglottis does vary. In approximately 1% of children, the larynx is one endotracheal tube size (1 mm) smaller than predicted; in 0.06%, the larynx is three tube sizes (1.5 mm) too small. Doubtless, some intubated infants have a smaller-than-normal larynx and therefore a greater risk for sustaining damage from an endotracheal tube. Although endoscopy is required to assess the larynx properly and to determine its size, preintubation laryngoscopy is not practiced; instead, the intubating physician must use gentle pressure to size the larynx with the selected endotracheal tube. If the fit seems tight, a smaller tube should be used. Ideally, the endotracheal tube should allow an audible leak at or below a pressure of 20 cm H_2O. Cuffed endotracheal tubes can obscure measurements of leak pressure and rarely are required in small children. Congenital stenosis at the subglottic level usually is secondary to a cartilaginous abnormality. Typically, the cricoid circumference is smaller than normal and somewhat flattened (Box 234.2). Another common finding is telescoping of the first

---

| **BOX 234.2** | **Differential Diagnosis of Glottic and Subglottic Stenosis** |

Glottic stenosis
Anterior or posterior web or scar
Vocal fold fixation
Tumor (papillomas, hemangiomas)
Saccular cysts
Bilateral vocal cord paresis
Postintubation granulation tissue

Subglottic stenosis
Firm stenosis (cartilaginous)
   Cricoid cartilage
      Normal configuration, small size
      Deformed cartilage
         Flattened anterior or posterior lamina
         Cleft (submucous, partial, complete)
         Oval
         Generalized thickening
         Ossified or obliterated lumen
      Trapped first tracheal ring
Soft stenosis
   Ductal cysts
   Submucosal fibrosis
   Glandular hyperplasia
   Granulation tissue

Modified from Chen J, Holinger LD. Acquired laryngeal lesions: pathologic study using serial macrosections. *Arch Otolaryngol Head Neck Surg* 1995;121:542, with permission.

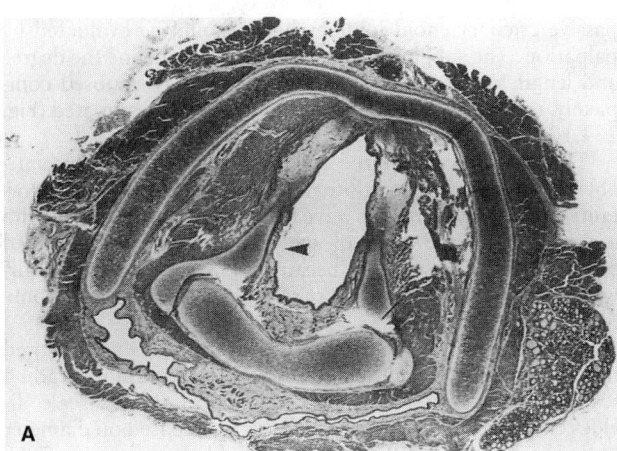
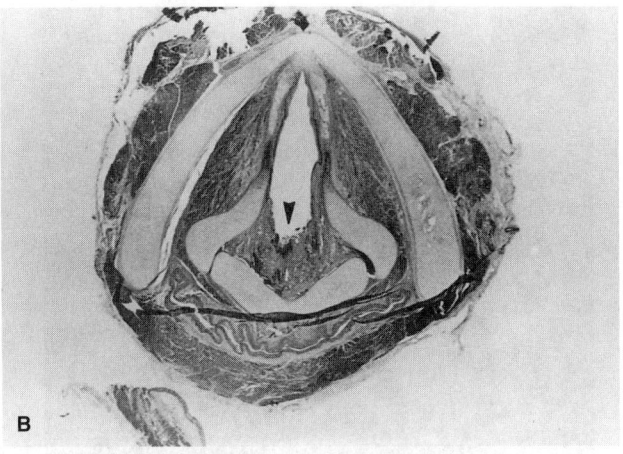

FIGURE 234.7. A: Intubation trauma of the left vocal fold with loss of epithelial continuity (*arrowhead*). **B:** Posterior glottic trauma with loss of the overlying epithelium and submucosal fibrosis (*arrowhead*). (Reproduced with permission from Liu H, Chen J, Holinger LD, Gonzalez-Crussi F. *Pediatric pathology and laboratory medicine*, vol 15. Washington, DC: Taylor & Francis, 1995:659. All rights reserved.)

tracheal ring within the cricoid cartilage and, as a consequence, narrowing of the airway. In addition, compromise of the soft tissue airway occurs if increased amounts of connective tissue or numerous hyperplastic-dilated mucous glands encroach on the subglottic lumen.

Minimal stenosis rarely causes problems except in association with upper–respiratory tract infections. In contrast, marked subglottic stenosis produces nearly constant biphasic stridor and sternal retractions. Pulmonary secretions are cleared ineffectively, and a barking cough and recurrent pulmonary infections are common occurrences.

However, most neonates with congenital subglottic stenosis respond to conservative therapy and can be treated with antibiotics and steroids during episodes of upper–respiratory tract infection and increased respiratory stridor. Fewer than 50% require a tracheotomy, which frequently can be removed as the airway cross-sectional area increases with growth and development. A weight increase from 2 to 10 kg is associated with an increase in the area of the airway at the cricoid from 20 to 60 mm². This tripling results in a ninefold decrease in airway resistance and, in many instances, obviates the need for major surgery.

Usually, however, glottic and subglottic stenoses are the sequelae of prolonged intubation. In 1965, long-term intubation was recognized as a safer alternative than is tracheotomy for treating upper airway problems in neonates. Many neonates sustained airway damage as a sequela, with the incidence of chronic subglottic stenosis in the late 1960s and early 1970s ranging from 12% to 20%. This figure has dropped significantly, reflecting the improved care these critically ill children now receive.

Damage develops because the mucosa of the larynx is highly reactive and vulnerable to injury. Inappropriately large tubes or repeated or traumatic attempts at intubation cause extensive tissue damage, with mucosal changes occurring almost immediately. In the first few hours after intubation, edema develops in the laryngeal mucosa. Within days, the epithelium becomes eroded, and mucosal necrosis occurs (Fig. 234.7). At the sites of injury, granulation tissue forms and often can be seen around the endotracheal tube if a direct laryngoscopy is performed. Attempted extubation at this time often is unsuccessful because the granulation tissue further narrows an already compromised airway. If the endotracheal tube is not withdrawn, full-thickness injury to the overlying mucosa may expose the cricoid perichondrium, leading to perichondritis, with possible

involvement of the arytenoid cartilages. Generally, progressive damage does not continue, and by the end of the first week of intubation, early signs of healing at the margins of the ulcers are present. Reepithelialization with metaplastic, squamous epithelium begins despite the continued presence of the endotracheal tube. By 4 weeks, fibrous tissue and squamous epithelium mark the site of the old ulcer (Fig. 234.8).

In itself, prolonged intubation probably is not followed by subglottic stenosis. Rather, associated risk factors (e.g., the respirator piston-action on the endotracheal tube, irritation from chemical constituents of the endotracheal tube, and concomitant bacterial infections) lead to increased injury and greater subsequent fibrosis. The reported incidence of subglottic stenosis as a complication of intubation ranges from 0.23% to 8.00%. In many instances, surgery is required before extubation can be achieved. Treatment possibilities that must be

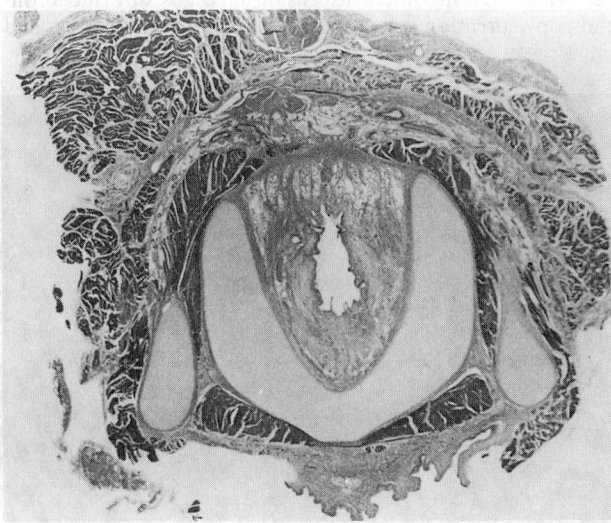

FIGURE 234.8. Subglottic stenosis resulting from extensive circumferential submucosal fibrosis. (Reproduced with permission from Liu H, Chen J, Holinger LD, Gonzalez-Crussi F. *Pediatric pathology and laboratory medicine*, vol 15. Washington, DC: Taylor & Francis, 1995:671. All rights reserved.)

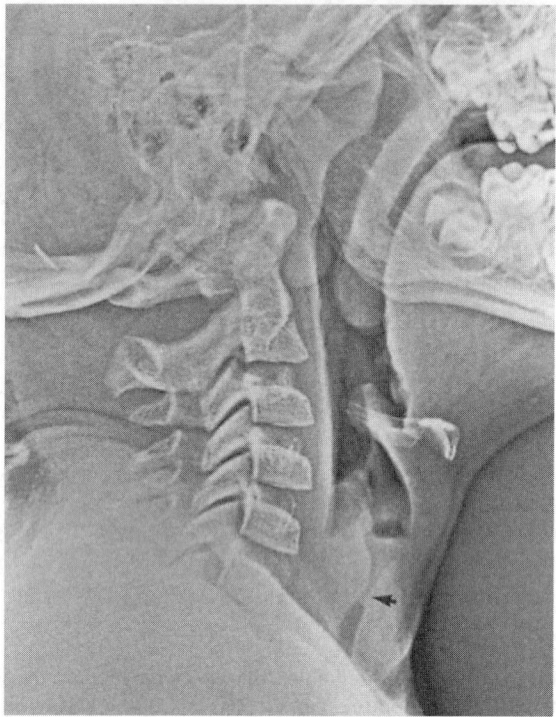

FIGURE 234.9. Xerography of the neck in a child with subglottic stenosis (*arrow*). The tract for the tracheotomy can be seen inferiorly.

considered in the presence of failed attempts to remove the endotracheal tube range from endoscopic laser surgery to cricoid-splitting procedures. If these therapeutic techniques are unsuccessful, a tracheotomy is required.

To assess the location, extent, and severity of the laryngeal stenosis accurately, several steps must be taken. Soft tissue roentgenography of the neck can delineate the length and severity of the stenosis (Fig. 234.9), but in-office flexible fiberoptic examination always should be performed to visualize the endolaryngeal dynamics. Mobility of the vocal cords must be assessed carefully, and the presence of interarytenoid fixation must be considered. An endoscopic examination also should be performed. During microsuspension laryngoscopy and bronchoscopy, attention is focused on the interarytenoid area, and

passive cricoarytenoid joint mobility should be evaluated by palpation. The subglottic area is examined to define the degree and length of stenosis; if the glottic lumen is stenosed completely, the degree of inferior extension must be estimated (Fig. 234.10).

The severity of acquired laryngeal stenosis is highly variable, but most patients ultimately require intervention. Mortality rates of 11% to 24% have been reported in children who are younger than 3 years of age and who have been treated conservatively, presumably because the reserve laryngeal airway is not adequate to support respiration if the tracheotomy tube becomes occluded.

Current approaches to surgical intervention are tailored to the severity of the stenosis. The most common grading scale used today is the Cotton classification. This scale divides children with stenosis into four grades based on diameter of narrowing: grade 1 encompasses children with up to 70% stenosis, grade 2 with between 70% and 90% stenosis, grade 3 with greater than 90% stenosis, and grade 4 with complete obstruction. Grade 1 and selected grade 2 stenoses often can be treated with endoscopic therapies that include lysis or laser ablation of scar tissue. These approaches have become more common with the use of the scar-inhibiting drug mitomycin-C. This drug, an antibiotic that initially was found to have intravenous chemotherapeutic uses, is used topically in the ophthalmology and otolaryngology fields to inhibit fibroblast activity and therefore scar formation.

Higher-grade stenoses are not amenable to endoscopic techniques and require "open" reconstructive methods. The stenotic segment can be resected and airway continuity can be restored by end-to-end anastomosis, techniques referred to as "cricotracheal" or "tracheal" resections, based on the tissue removed. Alternatively, a vertical laryngotracheal fissure procedure can be performed. Tissue is interposed in the fissure to increase the circumference of the trachea and the size of the airway. Sources of tissue include rib or thyroid cartilage. Occasionally, the spring of the cricoid ring is too unyielding, or posterior stenosis is present, and the posterior cricoid plate must be divided. A free autogenous graft can be interposed between the halves of the posterior cricoid plate, although usually this procedure is not necessary. This reconstructive technique is referred to as single-stage laryngotracheal reconstruction (Fig. 234.11). The operation is successful in 70% to 80% of cases, with the average time from the date of surgery to that of extubation being 5 to 10 days. Younis and Lazar showed that immediate extubation after laryngotracheal reconstruction may be

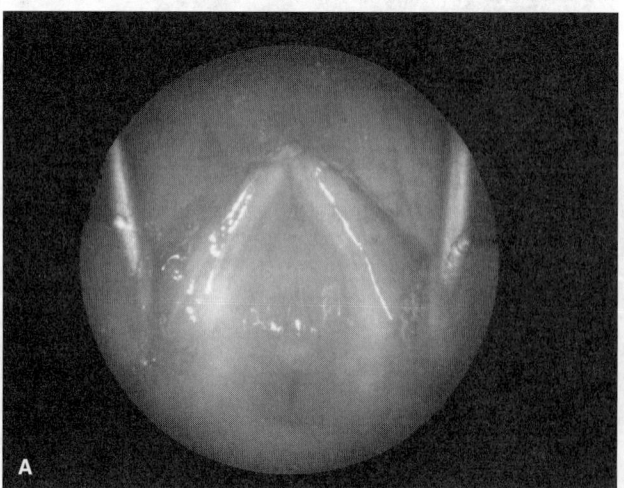

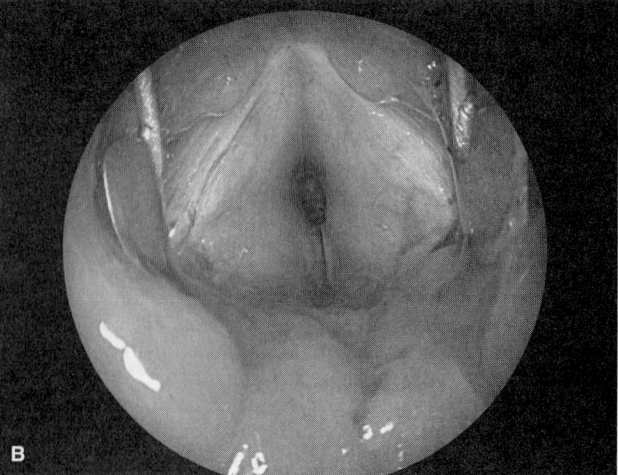

FIGURE 234.10. Two examples of nearly total laryngeal stenosis, one at the glottic level (**A**) and the other in the subglottic area (**B**).

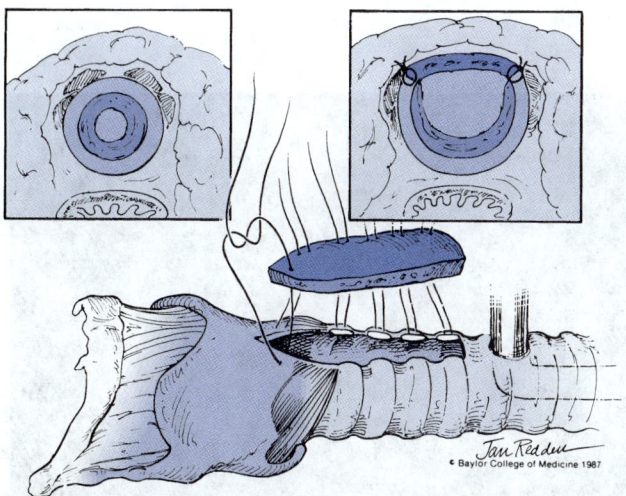

FIGURE 234.11. Illustration of a method of repair of laryngotracheal stenosis using costal cartilage.

appropriate for selected cases. When a stent has been placed in the laryngeal lumen and the tracheotomy tube is left in place, the operation is referred to as a two-stage procedure, and the average time from the date of surgery to that of removal of the tube is 3 months.

LARYNGEAL PAPILLOMA

Tumors of the larynx are uncommon in the pediatric population. Nearly all tumors are benign, and squamous papillomas are by far the most common. Hemangiomas, the second most common tumor of the larynx, typically are located in the subglottis. Various other tumors, including neurofibromas, lymphangiomas, chondromas, fibromas, and rhabdomyomas, have been reported. Malignant tumors, which are distinctly uncommon, include rhabdomyosarcoma (most common), angiosarcoma, fibrosarcoma, chondrosarcoma, neurofibrosarcoma, and squamous cell carcinoma.

Squamous papillomas account for more than 80% of laryngeal growths. Although benign, they tend to recur, can be difficult to cure, and can cause fatal airway obstruction. These characteristics are reflected in their common nomenclature,

recurrent respiratory papillomatosis (RRP). RRP is induced virally, most frequently by human papillomavirus subtypes 6 and 11. Most affected individuals are children presenting between the ages of 2 and 4 years, although papillomas do occur in individuals of all ages. Two of the three risk factors for papillomas—vaginal delivery, birth order (firstborn), and maternal age (teenage mothers)—are found in approximately 75% of affected children. An estimated 6,000 children in the United States have the disease, and health care costs reach nearly $110 million annually.

Because of the differences in initial manifestations and clinical courses, both adult and juvenile forms are described. The adult form has a male predilection, usually presents in the third decade, tends to have solitary papilloma, and usually does not spread to other sites. Often, a single surgical procedure is curative. In contrast, juvenile laryngeal papillomatosis tends to be extremely aggressive and resists treatment. Because the papillomavirus shows a predilection for epithelial transition zones, the structures most frequently involved are the true and false vocal cords. Exuberant growth can cover normal anatomy, and spread to contiguous areas can lead to involvement of the vallecula, hypopharynx, esophagus, trachea, and bronchi. Treatment can be difficult because recurrences are common, even after apparently complete removal. Additionally, the clinical course is unpredictable, and spontaneous regressions are seen occasionally at puberty.

The most common presenting symptom of RRP reflects the most frequent site of involvement. Slowly progressive hoarseness or stridor, voice change or complete aphonia, weak cry, and respiratory distress may occur. The average time from onset of symptoms to establishment of diagnosis is approximately 1 year. The diagnosis of RRP is made easily by visual examination of the larynx, using either a laryngeal mirror or a flexible fiberoptic laryngoscope used in the office setting. The histologic picture is pathognomonic. Papillary lesions with long, finger-like projections of connective tissue covered with acanthotic and hypoplastic, ingrowing epithelium abound. Enlarged stromal vessels lie contiguous to hypoplastic epithelium and immediately adjacent to the basement membrane, without apparent intervening stroma (Fig. 234.12).

In almost all cases, surgery is the primary treatment modality. In the past, cryosurgery, ultrasonography therapy, and cauterization were popular, but current techniques most often use either laser ablation or surgical shaving devices known as microdébriders. Both techniques are performed using a direct laryngoscope and a surgical microscope with the patient under

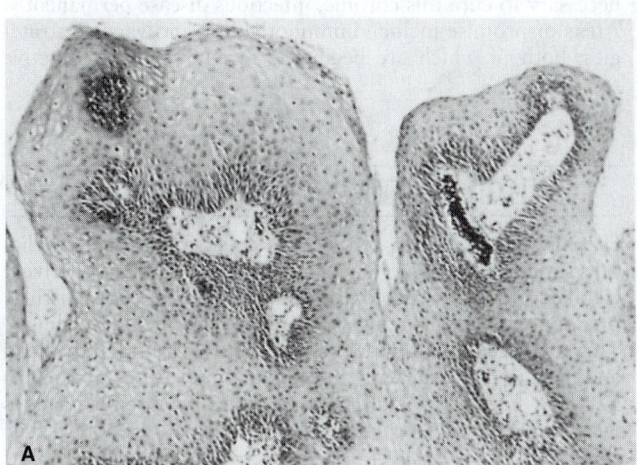
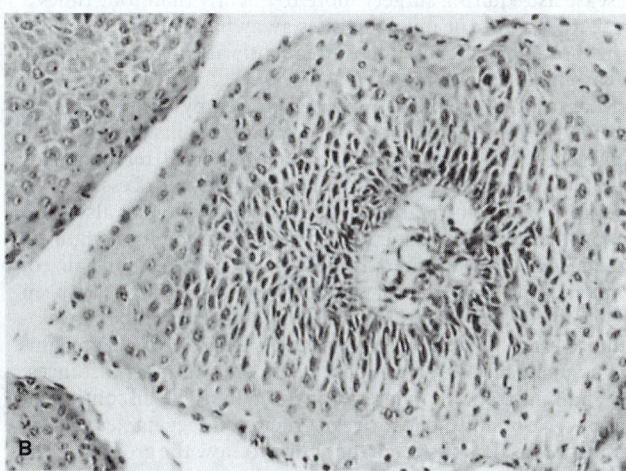

FIGURE 234.12. Histologic appearance of a papilloma. **A:** Fibrovascular cores and acanthosis. **B:** Under higher power, focal koilocytosis.

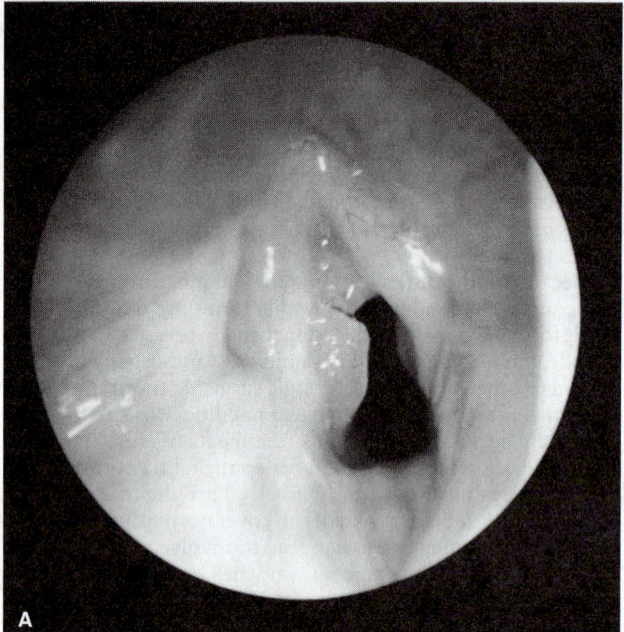
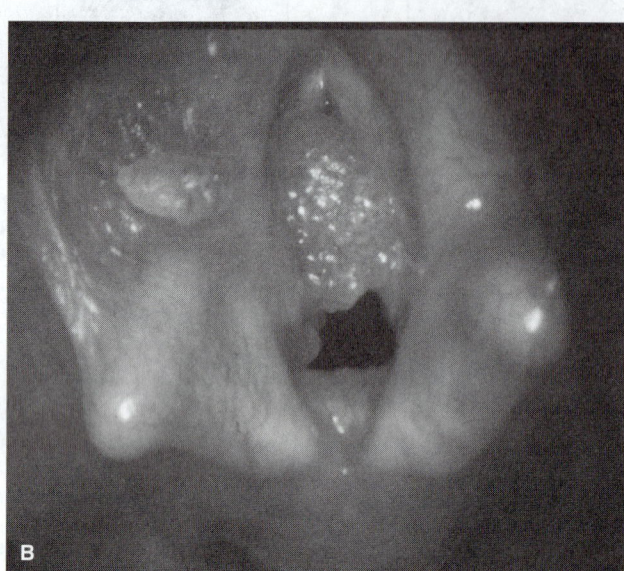

FIGURE 234.13. Marked laryngeal papillomatosis, mild disease (A) and bulky disease (B).

general anesthesia. Initially, papilloma bulk may be so great that normal laryngeal landmarks are obscured. With precise surgical resection, papillomas can be removed carefully, normal laryngeal anatomy can be preserved, and small underlying vessels can be cauterized easily (Fig. 234.13). Even with complete surgical excision of gross disease, recurrence is common, and children often need repeat surgical interventions at intervals ranging from 2 weeks to 1 year. Occasionally, the degree of papillomatosis is so severe that a tracheotomy must be performed. However, a tracheotomy increases the likelihood of development of tracheal and bronchial disease because it creates a new epithelial transition zone and often leads to distal spread of the virus. This step is taken only when the airway compromise is life-threatening. RRP involvement of the lower airways is the harbinger of a particularly poor prognosis.

No current medical therapy has shown a level of effectiveness sufficient to be considered as a primary treatment modality. Instead, available medications are reserved for adjuvant use in aggressive cases. General consensus now classifies aggressive disease as requiring surgery more frequently than four times a year for 2 years, or involving sites away from the endolarynx. The three adjuvants used most frequently are interferon, indol-3-carbinol, and cidofovir.

Large trials of alpha$_{2A}$ interferon therapy have been performed in several centers, and dramatic results occasionally have been seen. Several authors have reported regression or complete disappearance of papillomas, but, with cessation of therapy, exuberant regrowth can occur. Papillomas also tend to proliferate with reduction of dose. No definite length or standardized role of interferon treatment has been formalized, and the long-term role of this form of therapy has not been determined. Side effects include fever, malaise, fatigue, myelosuppression, nausea, vomiting, and elevation of serum glutamic oxaloacetic transaminase levels, but, in most instances, the administration of interferon need not be discontinued. Indol-3-carbonol, a derivative of cruciferous vegetables such as cabbage, has demonstrated the ability to slow the growth of papillomas in an animal model by altering estrogen metabolism. It is now available as a food supplement and is undergoing active clinical investigation. Finally, cidofovir, an antiviral drug

currently approved for the treatment of cytomegalovirus retinitis in patients with human immunodeficiency virus, has shown promise in small clinical trials involving direct injection of the lesions at the time of surgery. This drug also is undergoing randomized clinical studies to define its role in this disease process further.

Malignant degeneration of RRP to squamous cell carcinoma has been reported in 20 pediatric cases, with a 100% mortality rate. Unlike adult victims of malignant degeneration, which typically involves the larynx, pediatric patients are more prone to develop cancer in the bronchopulmonary tree. Human papillomavirus subtypes 6 and 16 appear to demonstrate the highest oncogenic potential. Careful monitoring for malignant degeneration in children with significant bronchopulmonary papillomas and high-risk subtypes is essential.

Optimal treatment of RRP requires serial surgical ablations with the use of adjuvant therapy in selected cases. Children with this disease require close monitoring and long-term care. Advances in medical rather than surgical therapy will be necessary to cure this chronic, infectious disease permanently. Areas of promise include immunotherapy and vaccine strategies, both of which are beginning to enter phases of active research.

SUBGLOTTIC HEMANGIOMA

Hemangiomas are hamartomatous collections of endothelial cells similar to those from which the vascular system is derived. Capillary loops, sinusoidal spaces, or arteriovenous fistulas predominate, and hemangiomas are subclassified accordingly. They are the benign tumors most commonly found in the head and neck in children, with an estimated prevalence of 10% to 12% in whites. This figure increases to 22% in preterm babies weighing less than 1,000 g. The female-to-male preponderance is 3:1.

Most commonly, hemangiomas appear in the skin, usually as a single tumor, although multiple cutaneous lesions can occur and involve other organ systems. If the hemangioma is

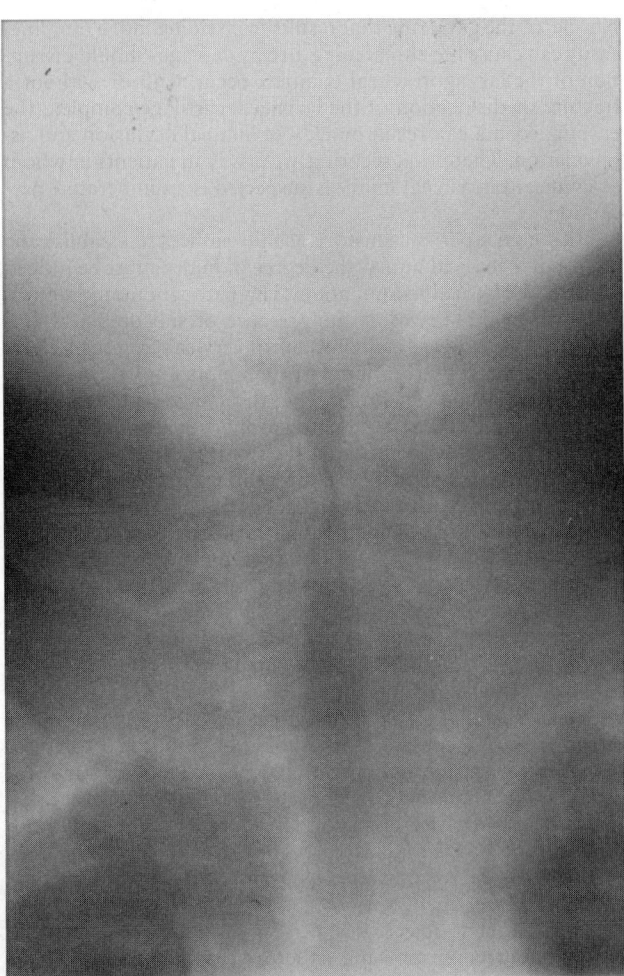

FIGURE 234.14. Soft tissue roentgenogram of the airway, showing encroachment of the tracheal air column by a subglottic hemangioma.

present in the subglottic area, the lesion can be life-threatening. Usually, subglottic hemangiomas are capillary, submucosal, and unencapsulated; in contrast, rarer supraglottic hemangiomas are more likely to be cavernous. Similar to hemangiomas in general, subglottic hemangiomas occur more commonly in female patients and are associated with concomitant cutaneous lesions in 50% of affected children. Sites of predilection for these associated hemangiomas are the head and neck.

Subglottic hemangiomas are present at birth, but they typically go unnoticed for several weeks or months. Varying degrees of airway distress develop, bringing affected infants to the attention of their pediatricians. The continuum of respiratory problems ranges from mild biphasic stridor that is troublesome only when it is associated with an upper respiratory tract infection to marked, acute stridor that results in dyspnea, failure to thrive, and cyanosis. The natural history is one of progressive enlargement of the hemangioma during the first 12 months of life, followed by spontaneous involution in the ensuing years. Not infrequently, croup can be the initial presenting symptom, and recurrent episodes should alert the physician to the possibility of an anatomic airway problem such as subglottic hemangioma.

Plain film roentgenograms of the neck can reveal an asymmetric subglottic mass (Fig. 234.14), and such supplemental studies as a cineesophagram can show the extent of invasion of the common tracheoesophageal wall. The definitive diagnosis is made by direct laryngoscopy under controlled conditions. A biopsy is not required because the appearance of the pink to bluish compressible mass in the lateral or posterolateral subglottic space is pathognomonic (Fig. 234.15).

Small, subglottic hemangiomas do not cause airway compromise and may not require treatment; however, with larger, life-threatening hemangiomas, a tracheotomy often must be performed to secure the airway for further intervention. Local compression is thought to hasten the regression of hemangiomas, and some lesions respond to a 10- to 14-day period of intubation. Systemic steroids may be administered concomitantly, although proof of their efficacy is lacking and their mechanism of action on hemangiomas is not clear. Presumably,

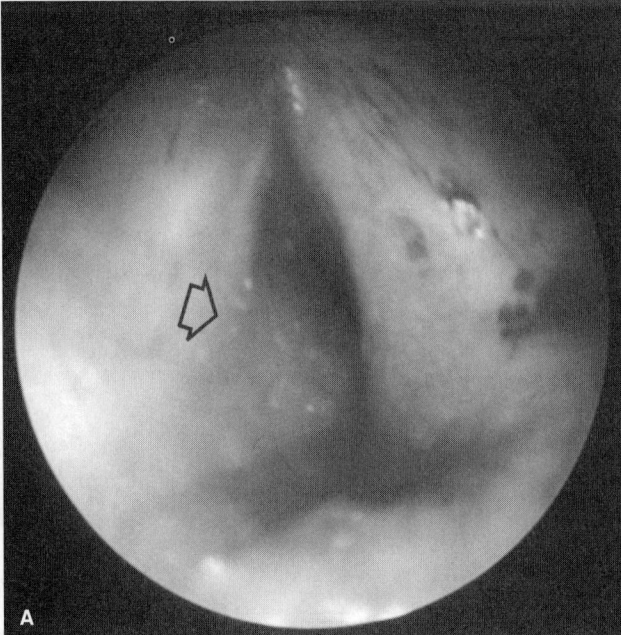

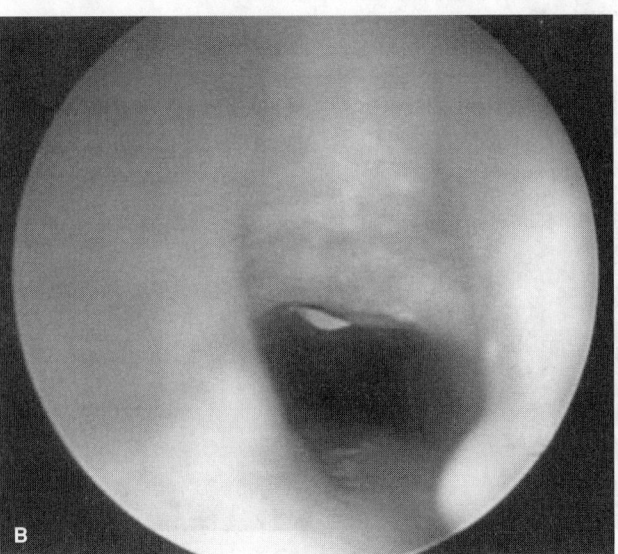

FIGURE 234.15. Endoscopic view of a left posterolateral subglottic hemangioma. **A:** Before laser therapy (*arrow*). **B:** After laser therapy.

steroids enhance the sensitivity of endothelial cells to endogenous circulating vasoconstrictors. However, when used alone, they usually are unsuccessful at relieving obstruction and afford only transient improvement in the airway condition.

Radiotherapy was recommended in the past, but its effect on hemangiomas is questionable. Possible treatment complications also are not inconsequential, and the known association of cervical irradiation with thyroid malignancies renders use of this technique unjustifiable. In some countries, gold grains have been inserted into hemangiomas, and, although regression occurs, the possible deleterious effects on tracheal and laryngeal cartilages require additional study.

Surgical treatment options include the injection of sclerosants, laser therapy, and excisional surgery. Of these choices, the carbon dioxide laser is especially applicable to endolaryngeal surgery because of the level of precision that is possible and the limited area of tissue damage that results. Usually, hemangiomas must be treated several times before sufficient intralesional scarring and fibrosis form to restore the airway to an adequate size (see Fig. 234.15).

Studies have also suggested that interferon-alpha$_{2A}$ may be effective in treating hemangiomas. Bauman and associates reported that 60% of children with massive or life-threatening hemangiomas demonstrated a marked response to therapy. Ohlms and colleagues reported that 4 of 11 children (36%) with airway hemangiomas in whom conventional therapy failed responded to interferon-alpha$_{2A}$. Initially developed as an antiviral agent, interferon-alpha$_{2A}$ has been observed to cause regression of pulmonary hemangiomatosis and life-threatening hemangiomas in infants. After initiating treatment at 1 million U/m^2, sustained therapy at a dose of 3 million U/m^2 for 9 to 14 months appears necessary because early withdrawal is followed by the regrowth of lesions. The association of interferon-alpha$_{2A}$ with the development of spastic diplegia mandates close neurologic follow-up if therapy is initiated in infancy.

LARYNGEAL TRAUMA

Injuries to the neck resulting in laryngeal trauma are relatively rare in children. The inherent degree of compressibility in the laryngeal cartilaginous framework affords some degree of protection; however, trauma (e.g., a blow to the neck from a baseball, injury sustained by falling against the handlebars of a bicycle, or the garroting that results from riding into a taut line) easily can cause life-threatening airway damage. Should disruption of the laryngotracheal complex occur, with or without a fracture or dislocation of the laryngeal cartilage complex, the ensuing edema can result quickly in luminal occlusion and asphyxiation. Therefore, securing an airway in patients in whom a significant laryngeal injury is suspected is an imperative precaution.

Although a patient's history usually suffices to establish the nature of a cervical injury, the degree of injury must be judged by careful physical examination. The pathognomonic sign of a breach in the airway is the presence of subcutaneous emphysema. Usually, a small amount of cervical crepitus reflects hypopharyngeal perforation; large amounts imply laryngotracheal injury. Symptoms of laryngeal damage include stridor, dyspnea, and dysphagia, often disproportionate to the degree of anterior cervical contusion and swelling. Concomitant injuries to adjacent structures can occur, and the great vessels, esophagus, and cervical spine must be evaluated. However, initial therapeutic steps mandate that the airway be protected.

To avoid development of long-term morbidity, an accurate assessment of the degree of injury must be made. Standard lateral and anteroposterior neck roentgenograms can confirm the presence of subcutaneous emphysema and can permit evaluation of the cervical spine, and computed tomography can delineate fractures clearly and should be performed on all patients with significant laryngeal trauma (Fig. 234.16). If possible, indirect or flexible laryngoscopy should be performed to assess the extent of laryngeal injury and vocal cord mobility. If vocal cord paralysis is found, the prognosis for ultimate return of function is poor. After an affected patient has been stabilized, direct laryngoscopy and bronchoscopy should be performed to establish the degree of endolaryngeal injury and to determine appropriate treatment options.

The treatment objective is to reestablish a mucosa-lined lumen without compromising either arytenoid motion or neuromuscular function. Severe injuries require tracheotomy and surgical repair through a laryngofissure. Fractured cartilages are reapproximated, and mucosal lacerations are closed to minimize the likelihood of development of future dysfunction. In minor injuries, after an adequate airway has been established, the larynx can be reassessed with fiberoptic laryngoscopy when the edema has resolved. Initial management should include a minimum of 24 hours of close observation, elevation of the head of the bed, humidification, and institution of steroids. If an

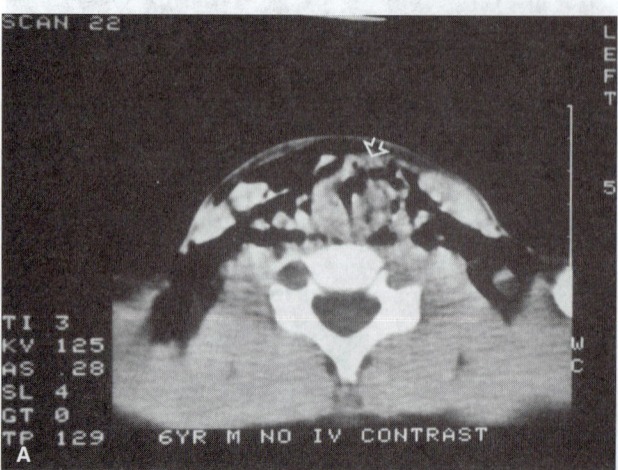
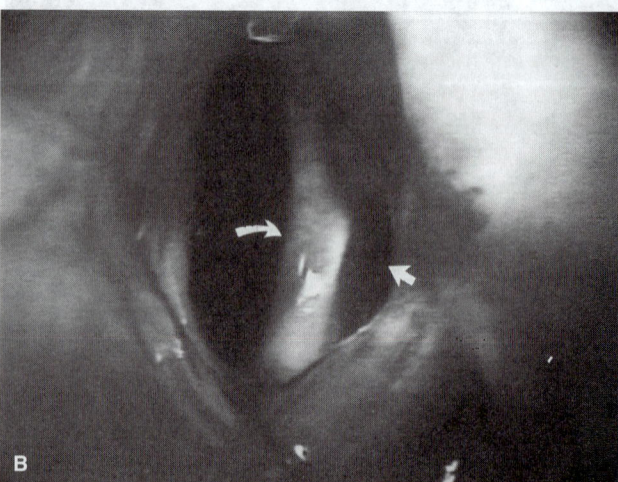

FIGURE 234.16. Computed tomographic scan. **A:** A fracture of the thyroid cartilage (*arrow*), with air in the adjacent soft tissue. **B:** Flexible fiberoptic examination showing an avulsed right true vocal fold (*curved arrow*) with a hematoma in the laryngeal ventricle (*straight arrow*).

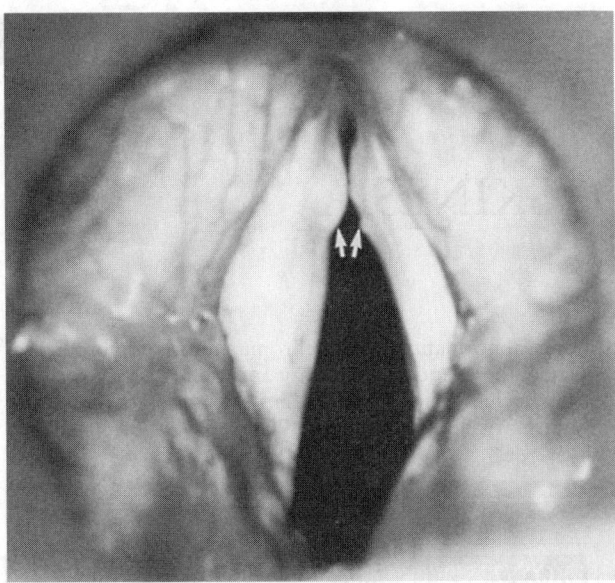

FIGURE 234.17. Vocal nodules present in the anterior one-third of the vocal folds (*arrows*).

affected patient demonstrates hoarseness, airway compromise, or swallowing dysfunction, radiographic and endoscopic evaluation is necessary.

Occasionally, seemingly trivial cervical trauma can cause laryngeal injury. Such symptoms as vague tenderness, pain, intermittent hoarseness, or intermittent dysphasia may reflect the presence of a small endolaryngeal hematoma. These symptoms will resolve in the ensuing weeks, and, as fibrosis and healing occur, an asymmetry of the laryngeal cartilages may develop. Years later, phonatory dysfunction can recur, and the past endolaryngeal injury may be detected as a deformity of the endolarynx at endoscopy.

More common than external cervical trauma is trauma secondary to voice abuse. The anterior two-thirds of the vocal cords vibrate synchronously during normal speech, and studies of mucosal dynamics with high-speed videostroboscopy have demonstrated that the vocal cords clearly collide during each cycle of vibration. If vibration is either too forceful or too prolonged, vascular congestion with edema results at the point of maximum trauma. In instances of acute abuse or overuse, only accumulation of fluid develops; however, with long-term overuse, hyalinization and fibrous tissue growth occur (Fig. 234.17). The altered mucosal mass and vocal cord thickness prevent complete glottic closure, a change that is evident on vocalization. Voice timbre and resonance are lowered, and the husky, breathy, and harsh quality of the voice is appreciated easily.

Aptly called *screamer's nodules*, these changes typically occur in loud and boisterous children. A noteworthy exception are children with a cleft palate or velopharyngeal insufficiency. Unable to maintain velopharyngeal closure, these children compensate by learning poor and damaging voice habits: glottal stops and abnormal lingual articulation that are used in an attempt to stop escape of nasal air. However, glottal stops cause trauma to the vocal cords, leading to formation of nodules; incorrect lingual articulation results in speech mechanics that can render language unintelligible.

Although auditory clues may suggest the presence of vocal nodules, visualizing the vocal cords with a mirror or a flexible fiberoptic laryngoscope is essential to confirm the diagnosis. Nodules are located at the junction of the anterior one-third and posterior two-thirds of the vocal cords and may vary in size, contour, and color depending on the duration and de-

gree of voice abuse. Papillomas, intracordal cysts, vocal cord polyps, and Reinke edema may mimic nodules; however, these possibilities are eliminated easily by direct visual examination.

Voice therapy is the cornerstone of treatment, and, because nodules are caused by voice overuse, misuse, or abuse, therapy alone may result in a complete cure, especially in acute cases. However, surgical removal is an option if nodules remain and the voice continues to be unacceptable despite an adequate period of voice therapy. Precise removal can be achieved with endoscopic microflap techniques. After surgery, a short period of voice rest is necessary, and a continued period of speech therapy is essential to prevent the recurrent development of nodules.

Suggested Readings

Infant Larynx

Pracy R. The infant larynx. *J Laryngol Otol* 1983;97:933.
Sasaki CT, Isaacson G. Functional anatomy of the larynx. *Otolaryngol Clin North Am* 1988;1:595.
Too-Chung MA, Green JR. The rate of growth of the cricoid cartilage. *J Laryngol Otol* 1974;88:65.

Laryngeal Papilloma

Bauman NM, Smith RJH. Recurrent respiratory papillomatosis. *Pediatr Clin North Am* 1996;43:1385.
Derkay CS. Recurrent respiratory papillomatosis. *Laryngoscope* 2001;111:57.
Green GE, Bauman NM, Smith RJH. Pathogenesis and treatment of juvenile onset recurrent respiratory papillomatosis. *Otolaryngol Clin North Am* 2000;33:187.
Shapiro AM, Rimell FL, Shoemaker D, et al. Tracheotomy in children with juvenile-onset recurrent respiratory papillomas: a Children's Hospital of Pittsburgh experience. *Ann Otol Rhinol Laryngol* 1996;105:1.

Laryngeal Stenosis

Bauman NM, Oyos TL, Murray DJ, et al. Postoperative care following single-stage laryngotracheoplasty. *Ann Otol Rhinol Laryngol* 1996;105:317.
Cotton RT. Management of subglottic stenosis. *Otolaryngol Clin North Am* 2000;33:111.
Lesperance MM, Zalzal GH. Assessment and management of laryngotracheal stenosis. *Pediatr Clin North Am* 1996;43:1413.
Lui H, Chen J, Holinger LD, et al. Histopathologic fundamentals of acquired laryngeal stenosis. *Pediatr Pulmonol Lab Med* 1995;15:655.
Monnier P, Lang F, Savary M. Cricotracheal resection for pediatric subglottic stenosis. *Int J Pediatr Otorhinolaryngol* 1999;5:S283.
Smith RJH. Laryngotracheal stenosis: a 5-year review. *Head Neck* 1991;13:140.

Laryngeal Trauma

Bent JP, Silver JR, Porubsky ES. Acute laryngeal trauma: a review of 77 new patients. *Otolaryngol Head Neck Surg* 1993;109:441.
Kadish H, Schunk J, Woodward GA. Blunt pediatric laryngotracheal trauma: case reports and review of the literature. *Am J Emerg Med* 1994;12:207.
Schaefer SD. The acute management of external laryngeal trauma. *Arch Otolaryngol Head Neck Surg* 1992;118:598.

Laryngomalacia

Little JP, Matthews BL, Glock MS, et al. Extraesophageal pediatric reflux: 24-hour double-probe pH monitoring in 222 children. *Ann Otol Rhinol Laryngol* 1997;106(suppl):1.
Mancuso RF, Choi SS, Zalzal GH, et al. Laryngomalacia: the search for the second lesion. *Arch Otolaryngol Head Neck Surg* 1996;122:302.
Olney DR, Greinwald JH Jr, Smith RJH, Bauman NM. Laryngomalacia and its treatment. *Laryngoscope* 1999;109:1770.
Toynton SC, Saunders MW, Bailey CM. Aryepiglottoplasty for laryngomalacia: 100 consecutive cases. *J Laryngol Otol* 2001;115:35.

Subglottic Hemangioma

Bauman NM, Burke DK, Smith RJH. Treatment of massive or life-threatening hemangiomas with recombinant alpha2A-interferon. *Otolaryngol Head Neck Surg* 1997;117:99.
Kveton JF, Pillsbury HC. Conservative treatment of infantile subglottic hemangioma with corticosteroids. *Arch Otolaryngol* 1982;108:117.
Ohlms LA, Jones DT, McGill TJI, et al. Interferon alfa-2A therapy for airway hemangiomas. *Ann Otol Rhinol Laryngol* 1994;103:1.
Wiatrak BJ, Reilly JS, Seid AB, et al. Open surgical excision of subglottic hemangiomas in children *Int J Pediatr Otorhinolaryngol* 1996;34:191.

CHAPTER 235 ■ CILIARY DYSKINESIA

M. JOHN HICKS

Mucociliary clearance from the respiratory tract depends on normal function and structure of cilia lining the mucosa along the nasal cavity and from the larynx to the sixteenth division of the bronchial tree. Cilia transport mucus from the bronchi to the hypopharynx and from the anterior nasal cavity to the oropharynx utilizing a synchronized beating motion. Mucus is propelled from the anterior nasal cavity at 4 to 7 mm/minute and from the depth of the bronchial tree at 4 to 5 mm/minute. Most debris and mucus are cleared from the ciliated airways in 6 to 24 hours. Disruption in ciliary motility caused by alterations in function or structure leads to ineffective mucociliary clearance, which, in turn, may result in sinusitis, otitis media, bronchiectasis, and sinopulmonary infections. As early as 1901, an association among sinusitis, bronchiectasis, and dextrocardia was noted. This triad was described more completely in the 1930s as chronic sinusitis, bronchiectasis, and *situs inversus* and became known as Kartagener syndrome (KS). In the late 1950s, infertility in men with this triad also was discovered, but not until the mid 1970s did ultrastructural examination reveal ciliary abnormalities. Immotile cilia syndrome became the accepted term for this condition. Later, researchers noted that many of those patients with KS and those with mucociliary clearance abnormalities alone (chronic sinusitis and bronchiectasis) had aberrant ciliary motility and ineffective mucociliary clearance. This finding led to the implementation of the current term, primary ciliary dyskinesia (PCD).

BOX 235.1 Molecular Genetics in Ciliary Dyskinesia

Most mutated genes are associated with axonemal and ciliary dynein chains (*DNAH5* chromosome 5p, *DNAI1* chromosome 9p13-21, *DNAH1* chromosome 3p21.3, *DNAH9* chromosome 17p12, *DNAH10*, *DNAH7p*, *DHC7*). Dynein arms are encoded by several genes in humans, and mutations may be numerous and quite variable in primary ciliary dyskinesia (PCD). In fact, cilia are composed of some 200 different proteins and polypeptides, thus rendering it likely that many mutated genes may be found in PCD and Kartagener syndrome (KS). The association of PCD with *situs inversus* (KS) may result from dynein mutations in the cilia with embryonic nodal cells. The embryonic nodal cell has a single cilium that directs leftward directional flow of extraembryonic fluid, creating a left-right gradient that leads to normal lateralization of organ systems. If a ciliary dynein mutation resulting in lack of directional flow is present, there will be no left-right gradient. By chance alone, then, 50% of affected individuals would have normal lateralization, and the other 50% would have *situs inversus*; this could explain why 50% of PCD is represented by KS (PCD with *situs inversus*). Several animal models with dynein gene mutations are being studied to understand better the molecular basis of PCD and laterality. Defining the role of dynein mutations may provide avenues for novel gene therapy in the future.

BOX 235.2 Diagnostic Tests Useful in Ciliary Dyskinesia

Muciliary Clearance Studies

The saccharin test uses a small particle of saccharin placed on the inferior turbinate. It is transported by the cilia posteriorly and should reach the tongue in 20 to 30 minutes with normal ciliary motility, where it elicits a sweet-taste sensation. In contrast, elicitation of the taste sensation in patients with PCD will take longer than 1 hour. A technetium-labeled albumin droplet also can be placed on the inferior turbinate and followed by nuclear scanning methods for clearance. In patients with PCD, this radiolabeled droplet fails to be transported from the inferior turbinate. Alternatively, a saline aerosol containing radiolabeled albumin can be inhaled, with lung clearance evaluated by nuclear scintillation. Patients who have PCD retain more than 75% of the radiolabeled albumin at 2 hours, compared with less than 40% for physiologically normal persons. Nitric oxide levels also may be used to assess mucociliary clearance. Nitric oxide in exhaled air from adults and children with PCD (less than 250 ppb) is reduced significantly compared with physiologically normal individuals. The reason for this difference is uncertain; however, exhaled nitric oxide levels may provide a noninvasive screening method for PCD in the near future.

Evaluation of Ciliary Motility

The motility of cilia located at the apical ends of respiratory mucosal epithelial cells may be assessed by using phase-contrast or differential interference-contrast light microscopy. Normal cilia have coordinated and directional motion that has been divided into three events. The effective stroke propels mucus forward and is followed by a resting phase of short duration. The third event is the recovery stroke that returns the cilia to its original position without allowing retrograde mucus movement. The beating frequency of normal cilia is between 11 and 16 Hz. Abnormal, uncoordinated ciliary motion and decreased beating frequency lead to ineffective mucociliary clearance. A beating frequency of less than 10 Hz is associated with PCD. Approximately 10% of patients with PCD have normal beating frequencies but dyskinetic beating patterns. Ciliary beating frequencies and patterns may be assessed using high-speed video, stroboscopic, laser, and photoelectric multiplier systems; however, most of these systems are unavailable in clinical laboratories and have been utilized primarily in research settings.

BOX 235.3   Ultrastructural Examination of Cilia

Ultrastructural examination of cilia requires evaluation of a minimum of 50 adequately oriented cross sections of cilia.

Normal structure/ultrastructure: More than 200 cilia are located on each ciliated epithelial cell. Cilia vary from 3 to 7 μm in length and from 0.2 to 0.3 μm in width. The ultrastructure of cilia is well defined (Figs. 235.1 and 235.2), with nine peripheral microtubule doublets (A and B tubules) and two central microtubules. The central microtubules are surrounded by a central sheath, and radiating from the sheath to the nine peripheral microtubule doublets are radial spokes. Each of the peripheral doublets is connected to its neighboring doublets by thin strands, referred to as nexin links. Extending from one of the peripheral microtubules (A tubule) are the outer and inner dynein arms. These dynein arms, via ATP hydrolysis of heavy dynein chains, propagate the beating motion and motility of the cilia by sliding the A tubule of the peripheral microtubule doublet along the B tubule. Abnormalities in these structures comprising the cilia lead to immotility, dyskinesia, and altered beating frequency.

Abnormal ultrastructure: The most common abnormalities found in PCD are absent, reduced numbers of, or markedly shortened outer and inner dynein arms (Fig. 235.3). Other abnormalities in PCD include absent or reduced radial spokes, absent central microtubule pairs, supernumerary microtubule doublets, loss of microtubule doublets, and transposition of peripheral microtubule doublets to the center of the cilia. Complete ciliary aplasia is found in 5% of cases of PCD. Defects in the orientation of the cilia with lack of alignment of adjacent cilia also may be present, resulting in random, noncoordinated beating motions. In secondary or acquired PCD, complex or compound cilia and edematous swollen cilia are found more commonly. In particular, deficiencies of the dynein arms and alterations in the central microtubule are more indicative of PCD than is a secondary or acquired process.

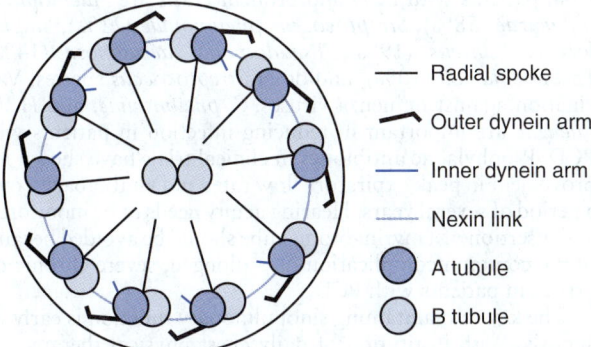

- —— Radial spoke
- ⌐ Outer dynein arm
- —— Inner dynein arm
- —— Nexin link
- 🔵 A tubule
- 🔵 B tubule

BOX 235.3. FIGURE 1. Diagram of a cilium in cross section from respiratory mucosal epithelial cells: ultrastructural components. (Reprinted by permission of Wiley-Liss Inc, a subsidiary of John Wiley & Sons, Inc.: Meeks M, Bush A. Primary ciliary dyskinesia (PCD). *Pediatr Pulmonol* 2000;29:307.)

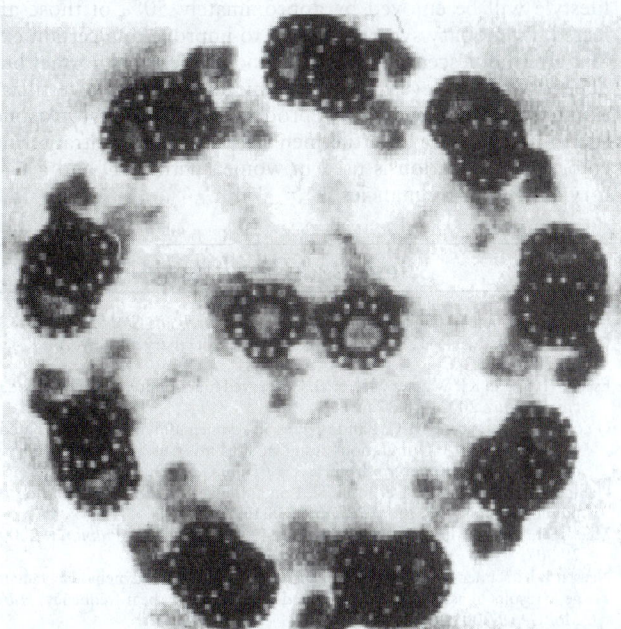

BOX 235.3. FIGURE 2. Normal cilium in cross section from a respiratory mucosal cell demonstrating nine peripheral microtubule doublets connected by radial spokes to the two central microtubules. The inner and outer dynein arms are seen readily. Nexin links connect the peripheral doublets to their adjacent neighbors. (Reprinted by permission of Wiley-Liss Inc, a subsidiary of John Wiley & Sons, Inc.: Meeks M, Bush A. Primary ciliary dyskinesia (PCD). *Pediatr Pulmonol* 2000;29;307.)

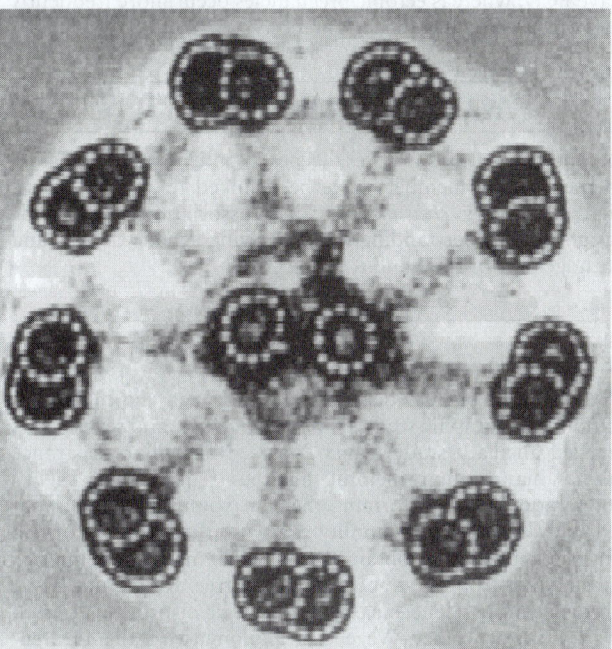

BOX 235.3. FIGURE 3. Abnormal cilium in cross section from a respiratory mucosal cell in a patient with primary ciliary dyskinesia. Note the lack of both outer and inner dynein arms. The nine peripheral microtubule doublets, two central microtubules, and radial spokes are present. (Reprinted by permission of Wiley-Liss Inc, a subsidiary of John Wiley & Sons, Inc.: Meeks M, Bush A. Primary ciliary dyskinesia (PCD). *Pediatr Pulmonol* 2000;29:307.)

EPIDEMIOLOGY AND CLINICAL PRESENTATION

The prevalence of PCD is based largely on clinical and radiographic studies. Overall, PCD prevalence is estimated to be 1 in 15,000 to 20,000, with approximately 50% having *situs inversus*. Ciliary aplasia also may occur and represents approximately 5% of cases of PCD. However, many individuals go undiagnosed, and the true prevalence is not known. A definite familial predilection with an autosomal recessive pattern of inheritance exists. Modes of transmission to offspring that have been proposed in isolated reports include X-linked, autosomal dominant, and autosomal dominant with incomplete penetrance.

PCD usually is manifested early in life. Shortly after birth, rhinitis, nasal congestion, neonatal tachypnea, and neonatal respiratory distress of unknown cause may occur. A common finding is a persistent moist cough in the neonatal period. Rare associations that may be detected in the neonatal period or on prenatal ultrasound are hydrocephalus caused by abnormal function and structure of ciliated ependymal cells lining the ventricles and spinal cord canal, complex congenital heart disease, esophageal disease or atresia, and biliary atresia. As mentioned previously, *situs inversus* occurs in approximately 50% of cases of PCD and will be evident with prenatal ultrasound and neonatal radiographic studies. If PCD is not identified early in life, sinopulmonary symptoms will progress, with the development of a chronic productive cough, chronic sinusitis with nasal polyps, chronic secretory otitis media (glue ear) with hearing loss, bronchitis, bronchiectasis (especially middle lobes and lingula), pneumonia, digital clubbing, and gastroesophageal reflux. In adulthood, infertility in both men and women may occur because of a lack of proper ciliary motility in the vas deferens and oviduct and axonemal dysfunction with sperm. Infertility is a more common problem in men who have PCD, whereas ectopic pregnancies occur more frequently in women who have PCD.

MOLECULAR GENETICS

Recently, mutations in several genes in patients with PCD and in their family members have been linked to PCD and left-right asymmetry (*situs inversus*). This association may provide insight into understanding the underlying genetic defects and pathogenesis of PCD and KS (Box 235.1).

DIAGNOSIS

The diagnosis of PCD depends on a thorough clinical examination, radiographic studies for *situs inversus*, and several specialized ancillary studies (Box 235.2). Mucociliary clearance studies may be quite helpful, but they require the patient's cooperation, and performing them in young children is not feasible. Direct ciliary motility evaluation may be performed on nasal brushings obtained from the middle or inferior turbinate or from the tracheobronchial tree. Ruling out cystic fibrosis, immunodeficiencies, immunologic disorders, alpha-1-antitrypsin deficiency, Wegener granulomatosis, allergies, environmental toxins, medications, chemical irritants, tobacco smoke, gastric secretions, and infections as possible causes of secondary or acquired ciliary dyskinesia is essential.

Ultrastructural examination of cilia using transmission electron microscopy remains the "gold standard" in the diagnosis of PCD. Box 235.3 describes the ultrastructure of normal cilia and common ultrastructural abnormalities.

TREATMENT AND PROGNOSIS

Therapy for PCD is identical to that for bronchiectasis secondary to other causes. Lung physical therapy, mucolytic (mesna, acetylcysteine) and bronchodilating agents, and appropriate antibiotic coverage in the presence of infection are the mainstays of treatment. The most common organisms isolated from patients with PCD and bronchiectasis are *Haemophilus influenzae* (58%), *Streptococcus pneumoniae* (21%), *Staphylococcus aureus* (19%), *Pseudomonas aeruginosa* (14%), *Escherichia coli* (10%), and other *Streptococcus* species. Vaccination against influenza viruses, *S. pneumoniae*, and *H. influenzae* are important in reducing infection in patients with PCD. Prophylactic antibiotics in clinical trials have shown improvement in peak expiratory flow rates and vital capacity over a period of several years. Hearing acuity needs to be monitored, and insertion of a myringotomy tube should be avoided because of the common complication of prolonged, severe chronic otorrhea in patients with PCD.

The key to maintaining sinopulmonary function is early diagnosis. With institution of daily chest physical therapy and twice-daily mucolytic agents, lung function can be maintained without a decrease in vital capacity, forced expiratory volume, or total lung capacity. Typically, a certain degree of airway resistance is present that is only partially reversible with physical therapy and routine follow-up.

Only limited longitudinal studies have assessed prognosis in PCD. In general, patients with PCD fare much better than do those afflicted with cystic fibrosis. Approximately 10% of patients with PCD will have disabling lung disease. Normal lifestyle will be enjoyed by approximately 50% of those affected. Pulmonary symptoms tend to improve to a certain extent after adolescence. Life expectancy typically is normal but depends on the severity of bronchiectasis. *In vitro* fertilization techniques provide for reproduction via intracytoplasmic sperm injection for infertile men with PCD, and intrauterine embryo implantation is used in women with PCD and a history of ectopic pregnancies.

Suggested Readings

Bush A, O'Callaghan C. Primary ciliary dyskinesia. *Arch Dis Child* 2002;87:363.

Cowan MJ, Gladwin MT, Shelhamer JH. Disorders of ciliary motility. *Am J Med Sci* 2001;321:3.

Essner JJ, Vogan KJ, Wagner MK, et al. Conserved function for embryonic nodal cilia. *Nature* 2002;418:37.

Guichard C, Harricane M-C, Lafitte J-J, et al. Axonemal dynein intermediated-chain gene (*DNAI1*) mutations result in situs inversus and primary ciliary dyskinesia (Kartagener syndrome). *Am J Hum Genet* 2001;68:1030.

Hellinckx J, Demedts M, De Boeck K. Primary ciliary dyskinesia: evolution of pulmonary function. *Eur J Pediatr* 1998;157:422.

Meeks M, Bush A. Primary ciliary dyskinesia (PCD). *Pediatr Pulmonol* 2000; 29:307.

Neesen J, Kirschner R, Ochs M, et al. Disruption of an inner dynein heavy chain gene results in asthenozoospermia and reduced ciliary beat frequency. *Hum Mol Genet* 2001;10:1117.

Noone PG, Zariwala M, Sannuti A, et al. Mutations in *DNAI1 (IC78)* cause primary ciliary dyskinesia. *Chest* 2002;121:97S.

Olbrich H, Haffner K, Kispert A, et al. Mutations in *DNAH5* cause primary ciliary dyskinesia and randomization of left-right asymmetry. *Nat Genet* 2002;30:143.

CHAPTER 236 ■ CYSTIC FIBROSIS

BERYL J. ROSENSTEIN

Cystic fibrosis (CF) is the most common life-shortening genetic disease affecting populations of European origin. The triad of chronic obstructive pulmonary disease, pancreatic exocrine deficiency, and abnormally high sweat electrolyte concentrations is present in most patients. CF is the major cause of chronic debilitating pulmonary disease and pancreatic exocrine deficiency in patients in the first three decades of life and accounts for a significant number of cases of neonatal intestinal obstruction. The name of the disease is derived from the characteristic histologic changes seen in the pancreas.

GENETICS

Estimates of the incidence of CF vary according to the population studied, but a reasonable figure for whites is 1 in 3,300 live births. The incidence in blacks in the United States is 1 in 16,300; in Asian Americans, it is 1 in 32,100. Transmission is autosomal recessive. On the basis of incidence figures, 1 in 29 whites in the United States is estimated to be a carrier (heterozygote) of a CF mutation. A heterozygote advantage has been postulated but never documented.

The gene responsible for CF spans 250,000 base pairs of genomic DNA located on the long arm of chromosome 7. It encodes a protein of 1,480 amino acids called the *cystic fibrosis transmembrane conductance regulator* (CFTR). A three-base deletion removing a phenylalanine residue at position 508 of CFTR (delta F508 mutation) is present on approximately 70% of CF chromosomes. The remaining cases are explained by more than 1,200 mutations, none of which accounts for more than 2% of the cases. The ability to detect CF mutations by direct DNA analysis allows for prenatal diagnosis, newborn screening, and heterozygote detection. Mutation analysis also can be used to confirm a diagnosis of CF. Genotype predicts pancreatic function, but, with rare exception, it does not predict the severity of pulmonary disease or overall clinical course. Evidence indicates that environmental factors and genes other than CFTR modify the severity of the disease.

PATHOPHYSIOLOGY

The CFTR protein is part of the ABC transporter family of membrane-bound glycoproteins involved in the transport of small molecules across cell membranes. CFTR functions as a cyclic adenosine monophosphate (cAMP)-activated chloride channel on the apical surface of epithelial cells and also regulates other membrane conductance pathways. The CFTR protein contains two nucleotide-binding folds with adenosine triphosphate-binding sites, a regulatory region with many phosphorylation sites, and two hydrophobic regions that probably interact with cell membranes. Functional expression of the CF defect reduces the ability of epithelial cells in the airways and pancreas to transport chloride in response to cAMP-mediated stimuli. Abnormal transport of sodium and chloride across the airway epithelium is thought to lead to water or

volume-depleted periciliary fluid, increased viscosity of airway mucus, and the abnormal mucociliary clearance seen in patients with CF. Complementation of the CF defect has been accomplished in CF airway epithelial cells *in vivo* and in animal models using viral and cationic liposome vectors.

When first descibed, CF was thought to involve primarily the pancreas, but many of the clinical and pathologic findings can be explained by a generalized defect in mucus secretion. Discovery of the sweat gland defect made it apparent that abnormalities exist in all exocrine glands. Glands are affected in varying distribution and degrees of severity and fall into three types: those obstructed by viscid or solid eosinophilic material in the lumen (pancreas, intestinal glands, intrahepatic bile ducts, gallbladder, submaxillary glands), those that produce an excess of histologically normal secretions (tracheobronchial and Brunner glands), and those that are histologically normal but secrete excessive electrolytes (sweat, parotid, and small salivary glands). The high concentration of electrolytes in sweat is the result of decreased transductal reabsorption of chloride and sodium.

CLINICAL FEATURES

Box 236.1 is a summary of clinical features consistent with a diagnosis of CF.

Pulmonary System

The respiratory tract almost always is involved, and pulmonary complications usually dominate the clinical picture. However, manifestations may not appear until weeks, months, or even years after birth. Autopsy studies suggest that the lungs are normal at birth. The initial pulmonary lesion is obstruction of the small airways by abnormally thick mucus secretions. Secondary to obstruction, bronchiolitis and mucopurulent plugging of the airways occur. Bronchial changes are more common findings than are parenchymal changes. Bronchiectasis is present in almost all patients older than 18 months of age. It progresses with age and is especially striking in older patients. Emphysema is not a common finding. Figure 236.1 shows a proposed mechanism for the pathophysiology of lung disease in CF.

Infection

Secondary bacterial infection, caused initially by *Staphylococcus aureus* and then by *Pseudomonas aeruginosa*, initiates a cycle of airway obstruction, chronic infection and inflammation leading to tissue damage, and eventual ventilatory failure. More than 80% of patients with advanced disease consistently harbor strains of *P. aeruginosa*, most of which are heavy slime producers known as *mucoid variants*. These variants rarely are found in other diseases. The susceptibility of patients with CF to infection with mucoid *Pseudomonas* strains may be related to a defect in phagocytosis in the lung or increased adherence

BOX 236.1

Clinical Features Consistent with a Diagnosis of Cystic Fibrosis

Chronic Sinopulmonary Disease Manifestations
Persistent colonization or infection with typical cystic fibrosis pathogens, including *Staphylococcus aureus*, nontypeable *Haemophilus influenzae*, mucoid and nonmucoid *Pseudomonas aeruginosa*, and *Burkholderia cepacia*
    Chronic cough and sputum production
    Persistent chest radiograph abnormalities (e.g., bronchiectasis, atelectasis, infiltrates, hyperinflation)
    Airway obstruction (wheezing and air trapping)
    Nasal polyps; radiographic or computed tomographic abnormalities of the paranasal sinuses
    Digital clubbing

Gastrointestinal and Nutritional Abnormalities
Intestinal: meconium ileus; distal intestinal obstruction syndrome; rectal prolapse
    Pancreatic: pancreatic insufficiency; recurrent pancreatitis
    Hepatic: chronic hepatic disease manifested by clinical or histologic evidence of focal biliary cirrhosis or multilobular cirrhosis
    Nutritional: failure to thrive (protein-calorie malnutrition), hypoproteinemia and edema, complications secondary to fat-soluble vitamin deficiency

Salt Loss Syndromes (Acute Salt Depletion; Chronic Metabolic Alkalosis)

Male Urogenital Abnormalities Resulting in Obstructive Azoospermia

Pathophysiologic Cascade

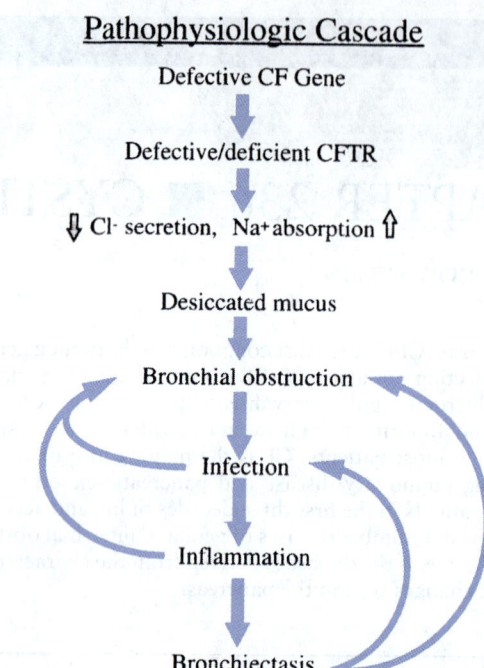

FIGURE 236.1. Proposed pathophysiologic cascade of cystic fibrosis lung disease. CF, cystic fibrosis; CFTR, cystic fibrosis transmembrane conductance regulator. (Reprinted with permission from Davis, PB, Drumm M, Konstan MW. Cystic fibrosis. *Am J Respir Crit Care Med* 1986;154:1229.)

of *P. aeruginosa* to respiratory tract receptors or mucins. The possibility of progression in the airways from intermittent colonization with nonmucoid strains to chronic colonization with nonmucoid strains and then chronic colonization with mucoid strains has been proposed. On initial acquisition, eradication of transient *Pseudomonas* may be possible, but once established in the airways, *Pseudomonas* is virtually impossible to eradicate. Systemic defense mechanisms appear to be intact, and infection tends to be localized to the respiratory tract. Septicemia and extrapulmonary infections are rare occurrences.

During the 1990s, the incidence of *Burkholderia cepacia* colonization among adolescent and adult patients was increased. Risk factors for colonization include increasing age and severity of underlying disease and recent hospitalization. Person-to-person transmission has been documented. Acquisition of this organism, especially by patients with moderate or advanced pulmonary disease, may be followed by an unexpectedly rapid decline. In some patients, the course is characterized by recurrent episodes of fever and bacteremia termed *Cepacia* syndrome. Colonization of the airways with methicillin-resistant *S. aureus* and with several gram-negative organisms, including *Stenotrophomonas maltophilia* and *Achromobacter xylosoxidans*, is seen in 5% to 10% of patients. If patients do not respond as expected to antimicrobial therapy, infection with unusual organisms such as *Mycobacterium tuberculosis*, nontuberculous mycobacteria (present in up to 10% of older patients), and *Aspergillus* should be considered.

Inflammatory Lung Damage

Inflammation contributes significantly to lung damage in patients with CF. Recruitment and activation of neutrophils in the airways lead to high levels of DNA, interleukin-8, and free neutrophil elastase in bronchoalveolar lavage fluid. Increased elastolytic activity secondary to the release of proteases is associated with breakdown of the lung matrix and with cleavage and inactivation of a variety of opsonins, thereby contributing to the persistence of *Pseudomonas* in the lung. An exaggerated and prolonged inflammatory response to bacterial and viral pathogens occurs. Significant lung inflammation has been documented in early infancy and in older patients before the onset of clinically apparent pulmonary disease. Immune complex formation is present in 20% to 100% of patients and may contribute to inflammatory lung damage. The presence of immune complexes correlates with disease severity and prognosis.

Signs and Symptoms

Half of all patients present with pulmonary manifestations usually consisting of chronic cough and wheezing along with recurrent or chronic infections. Infants can present with atelectasis, often involving the right upper lobe, or a severe bronchiolitic syndrome. The most prominent and constant feature of pulmonary involvement is chronic cough. At first the cough may be dry, but with progression of disease, it becomes paroxysmal and productive. Older patients expectorate mucopurulent sputum, particularly in association with pulmonary exacerbations. Often, wheezing is a prominent feature, especially in association with pulmonary exacerbations, but whether it reflects inflammation and bronchial obstruction or coincidental atopy remains unclear. As many as 5% of patients develop allergic bronchopulmonary aspergillosis. Physical findings include a barrel-chest deformity, kyphosis, use of accessory muscles of respiration, growth retardation, digital clubbing, pulmonary hypertrophic osteoarthropathy, and cyanosis.

Radiographic Changes

Chest radiographic and CT findings are not pathognomonic but can help to suggest a diagnosis of CF. Hyperinflation and bronchial wall thickening are the earliest findings. Subsequent changes include areas of infiltrate, atelectasis, and hilar adenopathy. With advanced disease, segmental or lobar atelectasis, cyst formation, bronchiectasis, and enlargement of the pulmonary arteries and right ventricle are seen. Characteristic branching, fingerlike opacifications representing mucoid impaction of dilated bronchi strongly suggest CF. In patients with mild disease and normal chest radiograph findings, bronchial wall thickening and bronchiectasis may be evident on high-resolution CT.

Pulmonary Function

Airway obstruction, air trapping, and ventilation-perfusion inequalities are the most important functional changes in CF. Usually, ventilation-perfusion scans demonstrate focal areas of inequality. Pulmonary function tests reveal the following: hypoxemia; reduction in forced vital capacity (FVC), in forced expiratory volume over 1 second (FEV_1), and in the ratio of FEV_1 to FVC; and an increase in residual volume and in the ratio of residual volume to total lung capacity. Flow-volume loops demonstrate a characteristic scooped-out appearance, indicative of small-airways disease (Fig. 236.2) and flow limitation at lower lung volumes. Airway reactivity, based on bronchoprovocative challenges, is present in 50% of patients and may be associated with accelerated progression of pulmonary disease. The response to bronchodilators is unpredictable and varies over the course of time and with changes in underlying pulmonary status.

Pneumothorax

In patients with advanced lung disease, pneumothorax, hemoptysis, and cor pulmonale are frequent complications. Pneumothorax occurs secondary to rupture of subpleural blebs. The cumulative incidence is 2% to 10% and, in adults, may be as high as 16%. Typically, patients present with acute onset of chest pain and respiratory distress. Spontaneous pneumothorax generally is a poor prognostic sign. After having a pneumothorax on one side, the patient has an increased risk of having an pneumothorax on the contralateral side within 6 to 12 months, and the median survival is approximately 48 months.

Hemoptysis

Often, patients experience blood streaking of their sputum. Bleeding is caused by erosion of abnormal bronchial arteries into a bronchus, often in association with an exacerbation of the underlying pulmonary infection. Massive hemoptysis (greater than 240 mL/24 hours) occurs in 1% of cases each year and is associated with significant mortality and high recurrence rates. The site of bleeding may be suggested by chest radiograph or CT findings and may be localized by bronchoscopy.

Cor Pulmonale

Cor pulmonale, manifested by hypertrophy of the right ventricle, is seen in 70% of patients dying with CF and occurs in 50% of patients surviving past age 15 years. Chronic alveolar hypoxia and hypoxemia serve as stimuli to vasoconstriction and medial hypertrophy of the pulmonary arteries. Severe cor pulmonale is associated with P_aO_2 values of less than 50 mm Hg. Clinical recognition of cor pulmonale may be difficult. Peripheral edema is present in only two-thirds of cases and often is a late manifestation. Liver tenderness may be an early clue. Electrocardiography does not correlate consistently with the presence of right ventricular hypertrophy. Echocardiography is the most practical and reliable way of documenting cor pulmonale and of following its course.

Upper Respiratory Tract

The upper respiratory tract is affected secondary to hyperactive mucus-secreting glands and hyperplasia and edema of mucous membranes. Symptoms of sinonasal disease are common and include nasal obstruction, rhinorrhea, headache, and mouth breathing. Nasal polyps occur in 6% to 48% of patients. They occur at a much younger age in patients with CF compared with those with underlying atopy, can be differentiated histologically, and tend to recur. On examination, the patient may have congestion and erythema of the nasal mucosa, abundant secretions, and broadening of the nasal bridge. Radiography and CT may be helpful in diagnosing CF because almost all patients with CF have opacification of the paranasal sinuses. Other findings include lack of development or hypoplasia of the frontal and sphenoid sinuses, demineralization of the medial walls, destruction of the lateral walls of the maxillary sinuses, and formation of mucoceles. CT scans can be helpful in selecting patients for surgery. The microbial flora (including *Pseudomonas*) of the sinuses tends to mirror that of the lower respiratory tract.

These patients have an increased incidence of sensorineural hearing loss for high-frequency sounds consistent with aminoglycoside-induced ototoxicity.

Course

The pulmonary course is characterized by chronic suppurative endobronchial infection with recurrent pulmonary exacerbations, often after viral respiratory infections. Infection with respiratory syncytial virus may be an important cause of significant respiratory morbidity in young infants. By age 10 years, 90% of patients have intermittent sputum production; by age 15 years, 90% have daily sputum production. Progressive shortness of breath and exercise intolerance occur. Pulmonary involvement advances at a variable rate, usually faster in female than in male patients, and eventually leads to respiratory failure, cardiac failure, or both.

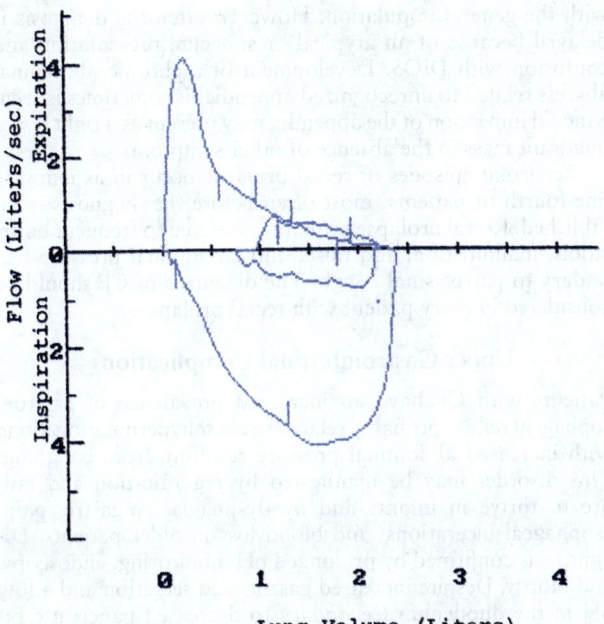

FIGURE 236.2. Flow-volume loop from a 23-year-old patient showing decreased flow at all lung volumes. The scooped-out appearance is indicative of small-airways disease.

Gastrointestinal System

Pancreatic Exocrine Deficiency

The most common gastrointestinal manifestations result from loss of pancreatic enzyme activity and consequent intestinal malabsorption of fats, proteins and, to a lesser extent, carbohydrates. Complete loss of enzyme activity is seen in 85% to 90% of patients. Loss of function may be progressive. Clinical manifestations include the following: poor weight gain; abdominal distention; deficiency of subcutaneous fat and muscle tissue; rectal prolapse; and frequent passage of pale, bulky, malodorous, and often oily stools. Steatorrhea and azotorrhea may be pronounced. Secondary to pancreatic insufficiency, patients have low serum lipid levels and may be deficient in fat-soluble vitamins and linoleic acid. Although some patients have a voracious appetite, often caloric intake is deficient. In adolescent patients, absence of a pubertal growth spurt and delayed maturation may occur. In general, growth retardation correlates closely with the degree of pulmonary involvement. Patients with pancreatic sufficiency tend to have lower sweat chloride values, less severe pulmonary involvement, better nutritional status, and better survival. They may have episodes of pancreatitis, sometimes as their presenting manifestation of CF.

Evaluation of Pancreatic Function

Exocrine pancreatic function can be evaluated by direct and indirect methods. The most direct measure involves analysis of duodenal fluid before and after the intravenous injection of pancreozymin and secretin. In patients with CF, volume and bicarbonate secretion (ductular activity) are reduced grossly, regardless of the presence of steatorrhea. In patients with steatorrhea, enzyme secretion (acinar activity) is virtually absent. However, this procedure is technically difficult and generally is used only in research studies.

Indirect and less invasive measures of pancreatic exocrine function include serum immunoreactive trypsin (IRT) levels, 72-hour fecal fat excretion, stool levels of trypsin and chymotrypsin, and the fecal elastase-1 test. The elastase-1 test is particularly useful because a normal test result has 99% predictive value for ruling out pancreatic insufficiency.

Carbohydrate Intolerance

In addition to experiencing pancreatic exocrine dysfunction, as many as 40% of patients show carbohydrate intolerance that progresses to chronic insulin-requiring diabetes in 15% to 20% of patients older than 18 years of age. The average age of onset of diabetes is between 18 and 21 years, but it can occur at any age. Diabetes in patients with CF is characterized by insidious onset, mild clinical course, and virtual absence of ketoacidosis. Deterioration in nutritional and pulmonary status may occur several years before CF-related diabetes is diagnosed. Retinopathy, nephropathy, and neuropathy may occur, with an adverse effect on survival. The mild course in patients with CF may result from preservation of some insulin secretion, decreased glucagon release, and compensatory enhancement of peripheral tissue sensitivity to insulin. Beginning in adolescence, annual glucose tolerance testing should be performed.

Meconium Ileus

Meconium ileus (MI), which occurs secondary to obstruction of the distal ileum by inspissated, tenacious meconium, occurs in 18% of newborns with CF. The presence of echogenic bowel on a prenatal ultrasound scan may be an early clue to the diagnosis. With rare exception, MI always is associated with CF. MI most likely is related to *in utero* deficiency of proteolytic enzymes, along with secretion of abnormal mucoproteins by the goblet cells of the small intestine. Infants present with evidence of intestinal obstruction. Abdominal radiography shows distended bowel loops and a "bubbly" pattern of inspissated meconium in the terminal ileum. Contrast enema shows a microcolon from disuse secondary to intrauterine obstruction. Associated intestinal complications, including small bowel atresia, volvulus, and perforation or peritonitis, are present in 40% to 50% of cases. MI tends to recur in patients' families. A delay in the passage of meconium and distal colonic obstruction secondary to the meconium plug syndrome also may be presenting manifestations of CF.

Late Intestinal Complications

The intestinal contents tend to be abnormally thick and puttylike as a result of abnormal intestinal gland secretions, abnormal chloride and water movement across the colonic epithelium, deficiency of pancreatic enzymes, and prolonged intestinal transit time. This condition may lead to a variety of late intestinal complications. Recurrent episodes of partial or complete obstruction of the small or large bowel, often preceded or accompanied by crampy abdominal pain, distention, anorexia, and a palpable mass in the right lower quadrant may occur. This symptom complex is called *distal intestinal obstruction syndrome* (DIOS) and occurs in as many as 15% of patients. Episodes may be precipitated by dehydration, change in diet, or inadequate enzyme supplementation. The incidence of severe obstruction in the immediate postoperative period following lung transplantation is high. Precipitated by the abnormal intestinal contents, episodes of small bowel volvulus or intussusception also may occur. The latter complication occurs in 1% of older patients and may be the presenting manifestation of CF. Episodes tend to recur and may be associated with chronic symptoms.

The diagnosis of CF can be suggested by the histologic features of the appendix. Goblet cells are increased in number and are distended with mucus, and eosinophilic casts may fill the crypts and extend into the lumen. The incidence of acute appendicitis probably is lower in patients with CF as compared with the general population. However, often the diagnosis is delayed because of an atypical or subacute presentation and confusion with DIOS. Development of a chronic abdominal abscess related to unrecognized appendicitis sometimes is seen. Mucoid impaction of the appendix may present as a right lower quadrant mass in the absence of other symptoms.

Recurrent episodes of rectal prolapse occur in as many as one-fourth of patients, most often before the diagnosis is established. Rectal prolapse probably is related to frequent bulky stools, malnutrition, and raised intraabdominal pressure secondary to paroxysmal cough. The diagnosis of CF should be considered in every patient with rectal prolapse.

Upper Gastrointestinal Complications

Patients with CF have an increased prevalence of gastroesophageal reflux, probably related to chest hyperinflation along with increased abdominal pressure resulting from coughing. This disorder may be manifested by regurgitation and failure to thrive in infants and by dysphagia, epigastric pain, esophageal ulcerations, and blood loss in older patients. Diagnosis is confirmed by prolonged pH monitoring, endoscopy, and biopsy. Despite increased gastric acid secretion and a low pH in the duodenum (secondary to decreased pancreatic bicarbonate output), duodenal ulcers infrequently have been diagnosed antemortem. A high incidence of peptic ulcer disease, however, has been reported in black adolescents. Radiographically, duodenal abnormalities consisting of thickened mucosal folds, nodular filling defects, and mucosal smudging are present in 80% of patients. Because of these abnormalities, diagnosing peptic ulcer disease radiographically may be difficult. In patients with signs and symptoms suggestive of peptic ulcer disease, endoscopy is the preferred diagnostic procedure.

Miscellaneous Gastrointestinal Complications

Crohns disease, giardiasis, *Clostridium difficile*-associated colitis, and celiac disease have been reported in patients with CF, and evidence suggests that patients may be at increased risk for developing these conditions. A significantly increased risk of development of digestive tract (colon, small intestine, biliary tract) cancers exists in adult patients. The risk is even more pronounced among patients who have had an organ transplant. This possibility must be considered in adult patients with intestinal obstruction, chronic abdominal pain, and gastrointestinal bleeding.

Nutrition and Metabolism

Vitamin and Mineral Deficiencies

Secondary to pancreatic achylia, malabsorption of fat-soluble vitamins occurs. Low-serum vitamin A levels result from steatorrhea and a reduction of retinol-carrier protein and retinol-binding protein. Xerophthalmia and night blindness occur rarely, usually in association with hepatic involvement. A bulging fontanelle secondary to vitamin A deficiency may be the presenting manifestation in infants. Overt rickets is a rare finding, but a significant reduction in vitamin D biologic activity with associated secondary hyperparathyroidism, reduced bone mineral content, and delayed bone maturation is seen commonly. Significant demineralization is present in half of all patients. Severe bleeding in association with hypoprothrombinemia and deficiency of clotting factors II, VII, IX, and X secondary to vitamin K deficiency may occur in infants. Hypoprothrombinemia is especially likely to occur in association with hepatic involvement or prolonged antibiotic administration. All patients with pancreatic achylia show a marked reduction in plasma alpha-tocopherol levels. Histologic evidence of vitamin E deficiency consists of focal necrosis of striated muscle and ceroid pigment deposition in intestinal smooth muscle. Red blood cells show a moderate decrease in survival that, on occasion, may result in hemolytic anemia. A progressive spinocerebellar syndrome consisting of ataxia, areflexia, and proprioceptive loss is seen in patients with prolonged vitamin E deficiency. Clinical problems secondary to deficiency of water-soluble vitamins are rare occurrences, but angular stomatitis may develop secondary to riboflavin deficiency.

Symptomatic hypomagnesemia has been reported in patients receiving prolonged aminoglycoside therapy and in those being treated for DIOS. Low plasma levels of zinc have been reported in 30% of young infants identified by newborn screening, and infants may present with signs and symptoms (acrodermatitis enteropathica) of severe zinc deficiency. Selenium levels may be low but do not correlate with clinical manifestations of deficiency. Iron deficiency anemia is seen in one-third of patients. Probably, it is related to inadequate iron intake, impairment of iron absorption, and chronic infection.

Edema and Hypoproteinemia

The syndrome of edema and hypoproteinemia, secondary to pancreatic enzyme deficiency, may be the presenting manifestation in as many as 8% of patients. Most often, it is seen in infants who are between ages 1 to 6 months and are breast-fed or receiving soy-based formula. Associated findings include hepatomegaly, elevation of liver enzymes, skin rash (acrodermatitis enteropathica), and anemia. False-negative sweat test results can be seen in the presence of edema.

Salt Loss

The sweat gland abnormality has important clinical implications. Patients may have a "salty taste" or salt crystal formation on the skin, findings that are highly suggestive of CF. Patients also may develop dehydration with massive salt depletion, especially in association with gastrointestinal losses or thermal stress. Profound hypoelectrolytemia, not accounted for by gastrointestinal losses, particularly suggests CF. In arid climates, chronic salt loss can lead to metabolic alkalosis and depletion of electrolytes without appreciable dehydration and is a common presenting manifestation of CF.

Hepatobiliary System

Liver

The liver is involved extensively in CF, and in some patients, liver complications may be the predominant and, at times, presenting features. Liver complications, which are seen almost exclusively in patients with pancreatic insufficiency, may have a familial pattern of occurrence.

Focal biliary cirrhosis, characterized by the inspissation of amorphous, granular material in the intrahepatic bile ducts, bile duct proliferation, inflammatory infiltrate, a variable degree of fibrosis, and focal distribution, is pathognomonic of CF. It is associated with and probably caused by an excessive accumulation of biliary mucus. Release of inflammatory mediators in the obstructed bile ducts leads to progressive liver damage. This lesion is present in 25% of patients and may appear as early as age 3 days. Usually, it produces no clinical manifestations, but, secondary to intrahepatic bile stasis, prolonged neonatal jaundice may be present. Half of such cases occur in association with MI and may predispose to later liver complications. In 4% to 6% of patients, focal biliary cirrhosis progresses to multilobular biliary cirrhosis that consists of groups of normal-appearing lobules surrounded by dense fibrous septa containing proliferating bile ducts with eosinophilic concretions. This lesion is specific for CF. Features of primary sclerosing cholangitis may be present in one-third of adult patients. Portal hypertension manifested by esophageal varices and hypersplenism develops in 1% to 2% of all patients, with a peak incidence of 2.7% in those between ages 16 and 20 years. Thrombocytopenia may be an early clinical clue. Liver failure is a rare finding. CF-related liver disease usually is slowly progressive and may remain asymptomatic over many years. The diagnosis often is problematic in that many patients have elevations of liver enzymes and ultrasound abnormalities in the absence of significant liver disease, whereas others have only mild enzyme elevations in the presence of severe cirrhosis. Liver biopsy results may be helpful but can be misleading because of the focal nature of the process.

Gallbladder

Abnormalities of the gallbladder are common findings, occurring in 60% of adult patients. Often, the gallbladder is hypoplastic and filled with thick, colorless mucus (white bile). Radiolucent stones, composed of calcium bilirubinate and protein, are present in as many as 33% of adult patients, and symptoms referable to gallbladder disease are seen in 5% to 10% of patients.

Reproductive System

Male Patients

Obstructive azoospermia and infertility are seen in 98% of male adults with CF. Histologically, the testes show active but decreased spermatogenesis. However, mechanical obstruction of sperm transport is present, secondary to absence or atresia of the vas deferens, along with associated abnormalities of the epididymis and seminal vesicle. The prostate is normal. All postpubescent boys with CF should have their semen analyzed for purposes of counseling. Defects of the wolffian duct structures appear to be related specifically to CF and are a consistent pathologic feature. An increased incidence of abnormalities associated with testicular descent (i.e., hernia, hydrocele, and undescended testes) also has been reported. Of particular interest are individuals with congenital bilateral absence of the vas deferens and other forms of obstructive azoospermia, usually without evidence of respiratory tract or pancreatic abnormalities. Many such individuals have CF mutations of one or both *CFTR* genes or an incompletely penetrant mutation (5T) in a noncoding region (intron 8) of *CFTR* that leads to missplicing of exons. Sweat chloride values may be normal, intermediate, or raised. Whether such individuals should be given a diagnosis of CF still is controversial.

Female Patients

In adult patients, fertility is decreased secondary to plugging of the cervical os by inspissated, dehydrated mucus and absence of a normal midcycle increase in water content, which probably acts as a barrier to sperm penetration. The ovaries and endometrium are normal. Among women who become pregnant, an increased incidence of premature labor and delivery and low birth weight (possibly related to maternal hypoxemia) may occur. Favorable pregnancy outcomes correlate with good nutritional status (greater than 85% ideal body weight) and good pulmonary function (FEV_1 greater than 60% predicted). Except for women with severe disease or diabetes mellitus, pulmonary function and 3-year survival are not affected adversely by pregnancy. In contemplating pregnancy, women with CF need to consider the potential health risk to themselves, the genetic risk to their children, and child care responsibility associated with impaired health and shortened life expectancy. Oral contraceptives have been shown to be safe.

Skeletal System

Pulmonary Hypertrophic Osteoarthropathy

Hypertrophic osteoarthropathy, manifested by arthralgias, long-bone pain, stiffness, joint swelling, effusion, and radiographic evidence of periostitis is present in as many as 15% of adolescent and adult patients and correlates with severity of the underlying pulmonary disease. The knees, ankles, and wrists are affected most frequently; usually, involvement is bilateral and symmetric. The course is one of chronicity with intermittent exacerbations. Nonsteroidal antiinflammatory agents provide symptomatic relief.

Rheumatoid Arthritis

Chronic seropositive arthritis has been reported in patients with CF. The finding probably is coincidental.

Back Pain and Spinal Deformity

Back pain not associated with trauma is present in most patients. Usually, it affects the middle and lower back, may be exacerbated by coughing, and often interferes with exercise, coughing, daily activities, and airway clearance treatments. Associated features include decreased range of motion and muscle strength, a "hunched-over" posture, and a high incidence of vertebral wedging. Treatment consists of exercise and postural counseling.

Episodic Arthritis

Unrelated to the severity of affected patients' lung disease, recurrent, transient episodes of nondisabling, seronegative, polyarticular arthritis may occur. Associated findings include erythematous and purpuric rashes, erythema nodosum, hypergammaglobulinemia, and elevated levels of circulating immune complexes. Large and small joints are affected; episodes tend to last less than 1 week and may recur at intervals of several weeks to longer than a year. Residual joint limitation and joint deformity do not occur. Usually, nonsteroidal antiinflammatory agents provide relief.

Osteopenia and Osteoporosis

Decreased bone mineralization is a frequent finding. Men and women are affected equally. Results of dual-energy x-ray absorptiometry scans are consistent with a reduction in both cortical and trabecular bone. Likely, both increased bone resorption and decreased bone formation are present. Potential contributing factors are reduced intestinal absorption of calcium and vitamin D, delayed puberty, use of glucocorticoids, reduced weight-bearing activity, and increased levels of circulating osteoclast-activating factors. Clinically, adults and young girls with CF have an increased incidence of traumatic fractures, and adults have a high incidence of kyphosis and unrecognized vertebral compression and rib fractures. Preventive measures include maintaining good nutrition, minimizing glucocorticoid use, encouraging regular exercise and activity, and providing calcium and vitamin D supplementation. In patients with CF who have received a lung transplant, bisphosphonates significantly increase bone mineral density.

Other Organ Systems

Ocular abnormalities in CF include visual field defects, venous engorgement and tortuosity, hyperemia, and blurring of the nerve head. Acute hemorrhagic retinopathy may occur at high altitude. Optic atrophy and neuritis have been observed in patients receiving long-term chloramphenicol therapy. Increased intracranial pressure, manifested by a bulging fontanelle, is seen in infants with severe respiratory distress, in association with vitamin A deficiency, and during recovery from malnutrition. Brain abscesses have been reported in young adults. Posterior column degeneration, in most cases limited to the fasciculus gracilis, is seen in patients dying after age 5 years. Its occurrence has been related to vitamin E deficiency. In the thyroid gland, excessive accumulation of lipofuscin pigment in the follicular epithelial cells is present. In patients treated with iodide, a high incidence of goiter occurs, often in association with clinical or laboratory evidence of hypothyroidism. Puberty is delayed in both boys and girls by an average of 1 to 4 years. Skeletal maturation progresses slowly, but most patients attain near-normal adult height. Maturational delays correlate with affected patients' underlying pulmonary and nutritional status. In male adolescents, growth acceleration can be achieved with a brief course of testosterone. Isolated growth hormone deficiency has been documented in several patients, probably as a coincidental finding. In general, growth hormone levels are normal.

The mucus-secreting salivary glands (i.e., submaxillary, sublingual, and submucosal) show morphologic changes similar to those seen in the pancreas, including dilated ducts with inspissated secretions and eventually atrophy of the acini and fibrosis. The serous-secreting parotid gland shows no morphologic changes. Enlarged submaxillary glands are palpable in more than 90% of patients, but no important clinical problems are related to the salivary glands.

Renal complications include microscopic nephrocalcinosis in a high percentage of young patients and, rarely, progressive renal insufficiency secondary to renal amyloidosis, immunoglobulin A nephropathy, use of ibuprofen, or diabetic nephropathy. Patients are at high risk of developing calcium oxalate stones secondary to low urine volume, hypocitraturia, and hyperoxaluria.

Psychosocial Implications

Impact on Family

CF is accompanied by a series of psychological crises from the time of diagnosis to the affected patient's death. The impact on the family is related to the severity of the disease, the rate of progression, the stability and mental health of the family before diagnosis, and the availability of support systems. Initially, parents may be frustrated and angry by medical delays in reaching the diagnosis of CF. After the diagnosis is confirmed, resultant shock and disbelief are accompanied by the guilt associated with the transmission of a genetic disease. Eventually, parents accept the diagnosis, but denial is used as the overriding defense mechanism. If adaptive, denial enables families to cope; if maladaptive, it can lead to denial of the diagnosis by the patient and family and to noncompliance with the treatment program. Usually, the impact on family functioning is significant. Hardest to accept by families is the concept of intensive, long-term care carried out with no guarantee of success. Often, a breakdown in intrafamilial communication and a withdrawal from the community occur. Psychosomatic complaints and depression are common occurrences. Siblings often resent the extra care and time required by the patient with CF but generally function fairly well. The occupational goals of the parents may have to be modified, and the financial burden can be considerable.

Impact on Patient

The reaction of affected patients to the diagnosis of CF varies with age and parental response. Often, denial of symptoms is the primary reaction, and maladaptive use of fantasy, repression, and regression may ensue. Feelings of anxiety and depression can lead to psychosomatic complaints and problems with discipline and academic achievement. Well-adjusted children are not embarrassed about having CF, discuss it openly with friends, and readily take medications and treatments in the presence of others. Adolescence is a critical period for patients, and psychological problems are prominent. Patients are dissatisfied with their appearance and have to cope with a delay in physical development and maturation. They may be forced to accept a realistic compromise of their academic and vocational goals. The extended dependency caused by CF interferes with the normal process of separation from parents. Often, conflicts during adolescence are manifested by social withdrawal, noncompliance with medical regimens, and risk-taking behavior.

Terminally Ill Patients

Terminally ill patients' responses to impending death vary with age, developmental level, family support systems, and openness of communication. In younger patients, loneliness and fear of abandonment may be present, whereas older patients usually experience feelings of anxiety and depression. Open communication decreases feelings of isolation, alienation, and the perception that the dying process is too terrible to discuss. Often, death is a lingering process with repeated "final episodes" from which the patient rebounds. The accompanying anger, confusion, and guilt challenge the coping abilities of most families.

DIAGNOSIS

Clinical Presentation

Physicians should remain vigilant for CF and should consider this diagnosis in a wide range of clinical situations. Although two-thirds of cases are diagnosed by the time the child reaches age 1 year, 10% of cases escape detection until adolescence or adulthood. Overall, 18% to 20% of patients present with neonatal intestinal obstruction secondary to MI or meconium plug syndrome. In the remaining patients, the diagnosis is suggested because of pulmonary manifestations or steatorrhea, often associated with failure to thrive, a positive family history, or a variety of miscellaneous manifestations related to salt depletion or deficiencies of vitamins, protein, minerals, or calories. In some patients, a single clinical feature (e.g., electrolyte abnormalities, pancreatitis, liver disease, sinusitis or nasal polyps) predominates. The types and severity of CF manifestations somewhat reflect genotypic heterogeneity. Pancreatic sufficiency (15% of cases) is seen in those patients who carry one or two mild CF mutations. The spectrum of clinical features is so varied and symptoms may be so minimal that one cannot exclude the possibility of CF even with a normal growth pattern, absence of pulmonary disease, or normal pancreatic exocrine function. Patients should not be deprived of an evaluation because of "looking too well to have CF."

Sweat Testing

The diagnosis of CF is confirmed almost always by documenting an elevated sweat electrolyte concentration. Indications for a sweat test are outlined in Box 236.2. The standard sweat test method is the quantitative pilocarpine iontophoresis sweat test (Gibson-Cooke) in which localized sweating is stimulated by the iontophoresis of pilocarpine into the skin, a sufficient volume of sweat (more than 75 mg) is collected, and the electrolyte concentration is measured. An alternative sweat testing procedure involves collecting sweat (more than 15 μL) with the Macroduct sweat collection system (Wescor, Logan, UT) and then measuring sweat electrolyte concentrations. Usually, the chloride concentration is measured because it discriminates better between physiologically normal individuals and those with CF. A chloride concentration greater than 60 mmol/L is consistent with the diagnosis of CF (Fig. 236.3). In infants younger than 3 months of age, a sweat chloride concentration greater than 40 mmol/L is highly suggestive of CF. The diagnosis should not be based solely on an elevated sweat electrolyte concentration but should be made only when it is associated with pancreatic exocrine deficiency, chronic pulmonary disease, MI, or a positive family history. The sweat electrolyte abnormality is present from birth and persists throughout life. However, obtaining a volume of sweat sufficient for analysis may be difficult in the neonatal period.

BOX 236.2   Indications for Performing Sweat Testing

Pulmonary and Upper Respiratory Tract
Chronic cough
Recurrent or chronic pneumonia
Wheezing*
Hyperinflation*
Tachypnea*
Retractions*
Atelectasis (especially of the right upper lobe)
Bronchiectasis
Hemoptysis
Pseudomonas colonization, especially with a mucoid
  strain
Nasal polyps
Pansinusitis
Digital clubbing

Gastrointestinal
Meconium ileus
Meconium plug syndrome
Prolonged neonatal jaundice
Steatorrhea
Rectal prolapse
Mucoid impacted appendix
Late intestinal obstruction
Intussusception, recurrent or at an atypical age
Cirrhosis and portal hypertension
Portal hypertension
Recurrent pancreatitis

Metabolic and Miscellaneous
Acrodermatitis enteropathica
Family history of cystic fibrosis
Failure to thrive
Salty taste on skin
Salt crystals on skin
Salt-depletion syndrome
Metabolic alkalosis
Vitamin K deficiency (hypoprothrombinemia and
  bleeding)
Vitamin A deficiency (bulging fontanelle, night blindness)
Vitamin E deficiency (hemolytic anemia)
Obstructive azoospermia
Absent vas deferens
Scrotal calcification
Hypoproteinemia and edema

*If persistent or refractory to usual therapy.

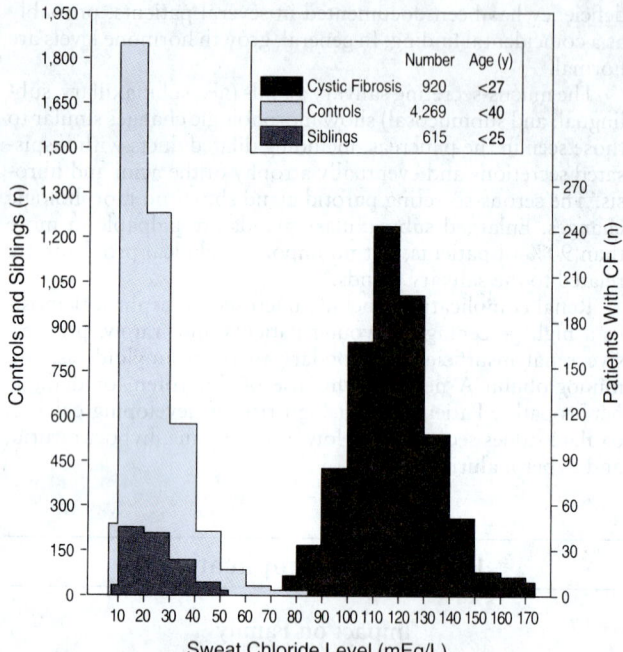

FIGURE 236.3. Sweat chloride concentrations in patients with cystic fibrosis (CF), in healthy persons, and in healthy siblings of patients with CF. (Reprinted with permission from Shwachman H, Mahmoodian A. Pilocarpine iontophoresis sweat testing: results of 7 years' experience. In: Rose E, Stoll E, eds. *Modern problems in pediatrics*. New York: Karger, 1967:158.)

The magnitude of the sweat gland abnormality does not correlate with the severity of pulmonary manifestations. Significantly lower, but still abnormal, sweat electrolyte concentrations are seen in patients with CF and pancreatic sufficiency. Elevated concentrations of sweat electrolytes have been reported in other conditions, including adrenal insufficiency, ectodermal dysplasia, nephrogenic diabetes insipidus, type I glycogen storage disease, anorexia nervosa, hypoparathyroidism, Mauriac syndrome, familial cholestatic syndromes, malnutrition, hypothyroidism, mucopolysaccharidoses, and fucosidosis. Most of these disorders can be differentiated by characteristic clinical features. Transient elevation of sweat electrolyte concentrations has been observed in children with evidence of abuse and neglect. In patients for whom a diagnosis is "confirmed" but whose disease does not follow a typical course, carrying out mutation analysis and repeating the sweat test are crucial. Normal sweat electrolyte concentrations have been reported in some patients with CF in the presence of edema and hypoproteinemia. Values become abnormal with resolution of the edema. Most false-positive and false-negative results are the result of technical errors, including inadequate sweat collection, sample contamination, and failure to interpret test results correctly. Physiologic variables, such as sweating rate, salt intake, and acclimatization, may affect the concentration of sweat electrolytes, but usually they do not interfere with the diagnostic value of the test. Although sweat electrolyte concentrations increase slightly with increasing age, they remain excellent discriminants for CF in adults. The sweat test is not useful in diagnosing CF heterozygotes.

Mutation Analysis

Because of its ability to detect CF mutations, DNA testing may substitute for the sweat test in certain situations. The presence on each *CFTR* gene of a mutation known to cause CF predicts with a high degree of certainty that an individual has CF. To date, more than 1,200 CF mutations have been identified, but only limited numbers of them are included in most currently available CF mutation panels. Thus, although specificity is high, the inability to detect two mutations does not exclude a diagnosis of CF.

Nasal Potential Difference Measurement

The active transport of ions across epithelial surfaces generates an electrical potential difference (PD) that can be measured *in vivo*. Abnormalities in ion transport in the respiratory epithelia of CF patients are associated with a different pattern of nasal PD as compared with normal epithelia and provide a basis for the use of nasal PD as a diagnostic aid in patients who present with atypical clinical features and nondiagnostic results on sweat testing and mutation analysis.

The ability to detect CF mutations and to measure nasal PD has expanded greatly the identification of clinical variation in CF. Approximately 2% of patients demonstrate an atypical phenotype that consists of chronic sinopulmonary disease, pancreatic sufficiency, and borderline (40 to 60 mmol/L) or normal (less than 40 mmol/L) sweat chloride concentrations. Patients with an atypical phenotype should undergo a comprehensive clinical, radiographic, genetic, and laboratory evaluation for features known to be consistent with the CF phenotype or for alternative diagnoses. Ancillary findings, such as radiographic and CT evidence of sinusitis, obstructive azoospermia, or the isolation of mucoid *Pseudomonas* from the respiratory tract, may be diagnostically helpful.

Newborn Screening

Newborn screening for CF has been possible since 1979. Initially, it was performed by measuring immunoreactive trypsinogen (IRT) in dried blood spots and performing a sweat test on infants with persistently elevated values. Immunoreactive trypsinogen is elevated both in pancreatic-insufficient and pancreatic-sufficient newborns with CF. Currently, there are two screening strategies. The first is an IRT/IRT protocol in which serial elevated IRT values at birth and at 2 weeks are followed by a sweat test. The second is an IRT/DNA protocol in which an elevated IRT value at birth is followed by direct mutation analysis for delta F508 or a pool of common mutations. Infants with two CF mutation are referred to a CF center, and those with one identified mutation are referred for sweat testing and further evaluation. The role of population-based newborn screening is now firmly established with plans in place to implement screening throughout the United States. Demonstrated benefits of screening include decreased early morbidity, better nutritional and cognitive outcomes, less deterioration in lung function, timely genetic counseling, a reduction in the anxiety associated with delayed diagnosis, and improved survival.

Prenatal Diagnosis

An *in utero* diagnosis of CF based on the detection of two CF mutations in the fetus is possible. Usually, testing is performed in a family in which a child born previously was affected or because of the detection of fetal echogenic bowel on routine ultrasonography. Although somewhat controversial, population-based CF carrier screening now is offered in the United States. The recommendation is that preconception and prenatal carrier testing *be offered to* all couples in whom one or both partners are white and are planning a pregnancy or seeking prenatal care and *be made available to* couples in other racial and ethnic groups who are at lower risk and in whom the testing may be less sensitive. These recommendations have led to a significant increase in prenatal CF diagnoses. An alternative for at-risk couples is the use of preimplantation diagnosis to screen the embryo for mutations before implantation.

MANAGEMENT

Because of multisystem involvement, frequency of complications, psychosocial burden, and uncertain prognosis, implementation of a comprehensive, intensive therapy program is essential. Affected patients should be followed regularly by a multidisciplinary team of specialty physicians, nurses, nutritionists, physical-respiratory therapists, and counseling personnel who can provide continuity of care over an extended period. The Cystic Fibrosis Foundation in Bethesda, Maryland, supports a nationwide network of centers involved in patient care, teaching, and clinical and basic research. Services provided by the centers include diagnostic testing, evaluation and provision of a therapeutic plan, continuity of outpatient and inpatient services, patient and family education, nutrition counseling, instruction in physical and respiratory therapy, psychosocial support including individual counseling and family education-support groups, financial counseling, genetic counseling, subspecialty consultative services, and an opportunity to participate in clinical research projects. Vocational, educational, financial, and premarital counseling can help the increasing number of adult patients to make a smooth transition to independent living. Optimal patient management involves coordination of services between the CF center and the primary-care provider, who can provide ongoing psychosocial support, offer general medical care, and coordinate home, community, and educational services. The goals of therapy are to maintain adequate nutrition and normal growth, to prevent or slow the decline in pulmonary function, to encourage appropriate physical activity, and to promote a reasonable quality of life.

Pulmonary Therapy

Antimicrobial Therapy

Aggressive antimicrobial therapy is a key component in the management of patients with CF, but great variation in treatment strategies exists. Options include the following: short-term treatment of acute exacerbations with oral, aerosol, or intravenous antibiotics; chronic suppressive therapy with oral or aerosol antibiotics; and long-term intermittent treatment with quarterly courses of intravenous antibiotics. Ideally, antibiotic choice should be based on the results of respiratory tract (oropharyngeal, sputum, bronchoalveolar lavage fluid) culture and sensitivity testing. However, *in vitro* susceptibility testing does not always correlate with clinical response. Patients with mild to moderate acute pulmonary exacerbations usually are treated with a 2- to 4-week course of oral or aerosol antibiotics, or both. Coverage against *Haemophilus influenzae* and *S. aureus* can be achieved with a beta-lactamase–stable penicillin or cephalosporin, trimethoprim-sulfamethoxazole, or a macrolide antibiotic. For patients colonized with *P. aeruginosa*, an oral fluoroquinolone or aerosol aminoglycoside (tobramycin) used alone or in combination may be effective. Patients who do not respond to oral or aerosol therapy and those with more severe exacerbations are candidates for a 10- to 21-day course of intravenous antibiotics, usually consisting of an antipseudomonal beta-lactam (ticarcillin, piperacillin, ceftazidime) in combination with an aminoglycoside (tobramycin, gentamicin) chosen on the basis of susceptibility test results. For patients who are allergic to beta-lactams, the carbapenem meropenem and the monobactam aztreonam may be useful alternatives. Patients may require high doses (approximately 10 mg/kg/day) of aminoglycosides to achieve acceptable serum concentrations. Serum drug levels should be monitored, and dosage should be adjusted to achieve a postinfusion peak level of 8 to 10 μg/mL and a trough value of less than 2 μg/mL. Patients also have increased renal clearance of penicillins and may require high doses to achieve adequate serum levels. Data suggest that a single daily intravenous dose of aminoglycoside, equivalent to the total daily dose, may be as effective as are multiple daily doses. Patients who have an acute pulmonary exacerbation, are otherwise clinically stable, and meet well-defined selection criteria often are candidates for home intravenous antibiotic therapy.

Chronic suppressive antibiotic therapy is used in patients of all ages to improve quality of life, slow decline in pulmonary function, and increase the interval between pulmonary exacerbations. The oral agents used most commonly are trimethoprim-sulfamethoxazole, amoxicillin-clavulanate, and beta-lactamase-stable cephalosporins. In patients colonized with *P. aeruginosa*, chronic alternate-month aerosol administration of high-dose tobramycin (300 mg twice daily) has been shown to decrease sputum density of *P. aeruginosa*, decline in pulmonary function, and frequency of acute pulmonary exacerbations. This form of therapy is tolerated well because little systemic drug absorption occurs. Although not supported by controlled trials, long-term aerosol colistin sometimes is substituted for or alternated with tobramycin in patients colonized with tobramycin-resistant strains of *P. aeruginosa*. Among patients who are older than 6 years of age and colonized with *P. aeruginosa*, long-term administration of the macrolide antibiotic azithromycin is associated with improved pulmonary function and nutritional status and a decrease in the frequency of pulmonary exacerbations. A common treatment strategy is to administer 250 mg (patient weighing less than 40 kg) or 500 mg (patient weighing more than 40 kg) on a Monday, Wednesday, Friday schedule, usually in conjunction with alternate-month administration of aerosol tobramycin. Because of the rapid emergence of antibiotic-resistant isolates, fluoroquinolones should not be used for chronic suppressive therapy. For patients colonized with more virulent organisms, such as *B. cepacia, S. maltophilia,* and multidrug-resistant strains of *P. aeruginosa,* the choice of an antibiotic therapy should be based on special susceptibility and synergy testing.

In recent years, a significant change has occurred in the management of initial airway colonization with *P. aeruginosa*. Aggressive treatment results in at least transient eradication of *Pseudomonas* in a high percentage of cases and may be associated with improved clinical outcomes. Treatment options include aerosol tobramycin or colistin alone or in combination with an oral quinolone, or a course of intravenous antibiotics. In the United States, a 1- to 2- month course of aerosol tobramycin, often in association with an oral quinolone, is the preferred regimen.

Airway Clearance Techniques

Airway clearance techniques enhance the removal of bronchial secretions and should be performed by all patients. They usually are recommended at the time of diagnosis or at the first indication of lower respiratory tract involvement. In infants, toddlers, and young children, chest physiotherapy consisting of postural drainage, manual or mechanical percussion, vibration, and assisted coughing is carried out several times each day. In infants, the head-down position should be avoided to reduce episodes of gastroesophageal reflux. In older children, adolescents, and adults, useful methods of secretion removal include autogenic drainage, active cycle of breathing techniques, use of a high-frequency chest compression vest, or positive expiratory pressure maneuvers using a mask or oscillating device (Acapella, Flutter). The choice of technique should be based on the preference of the patient and family. A regular exercise program should be encouraged to complement, but not replace, airway clearance techniques. Exercise has no demonstrable short-term effect on lung function, but it can improve cardiorespiratory conditioning, muscle strength, exercise tolerance, sense of well-being, and self-image. Supplemental oxygen therapy may allow patients with severe disease to exercise safely and with benefit.

Mucolytic Agents

Recombinant human DNase (dornase alfa) ezymatically degrades DNA, which is present in high concentration in purulent airway secretions, and decreases sputum viscoelasticity. In patients older than age 5 years of age, long-term daily nebulization of dornase alfa at a dose of 2.5 mg/day can delay decline in pulmonary function and reduce the frequency of pulmonary exacerbations. These benefits are seen in patients with a wide range of clinical severity, including children who show only mild impairment of lung function. It can be used in conjunction with all other usual therapies. Nebulization of hypertonic (7%) saline twice a day leads to improvement in pulmonary function in patients with moderate to severe pulmonary disease. No data document the efficacy of oral expectorants. Cough suppressants are contraindicated.

Bronchodilator Therapy

Over the course of time, most patients demonstrate bronchodilator responsiveness during pulmonary function testing. However, responses tend to be inconsistent and to vary widely with time and with the degree of illness. Patients with advanced disease and unstable airways may show a paradoxic decrease in pulmonary function after using an inhaled bronchodilator. In short-term trials, inhalation of a short-acting (albuterol) or long-acting (salmeterol) beta agonist is associated with improvement in pulmonary function. However, a long-term benefit has not been demonstrated. In clinical practice, most patients use a beta agonist before carrying out airway clearance. Nebulization and metered-dose inhalation (MDI) probably are equally effective, but ease of administration favors MDI use.

Antiinflammatory Agents

Antiinflammatory agents are playing an increasingly important role in the treatment of patients with CF. Long-term daily use of ibuprofen at a dose sufficient to achieve a peak plasma concentration between 50 and 100 μg/mL has been shown to slow the rate of decline in pulmonary function significantly and to decrease the need for intravenous antibiotics in young patients (ages 5 to 13 years) with mild pulmonary involvement. Although therapy appears to be tolerated well, patients need to be monitored closely for adverse effects. In several long-term controlled trials, alternate-day glucocorticoid therapy at a dose of 1 to 2 mg/day has been shown to slow the expected rate of decline in pulmonary function and to decrease serum immunoglobulin G levels. However, treatment for longer than 24 months has been associated with retardation of linear growth, development of glucose abnormalities, and formation of cataracts. Systemic glucocorticoids are indicated for infants with a severe bronchiolitic syndrome, patients with severe airway obstruction unresponsive to conventional bronchodilators, patients with allergic bronchopulmonary aspergillosis, and those with evidence of hypersensitivity characterized by recurrent episodes of fever, rash, and joint pain. Inhaled glucocorticoids are used frequently, but in controlled studies a significant clinical benefit has not been demonstrated. Their use probably should be restricted to infants and young children with wheezing and to older patients whose course is complicated by asthma or allergic bronchopulmonary aspergillosis. Cromolyn sodium administered by nebulization or MDI has not been shown to be of clinical benefit.

Miscellaneous Therapies

Tracheobronchial lavage has been used to remove impacted bronchial secretions, but it is no more effective than is conventional therapy. Therapeutic bronchoscopy has been performed in patients with lobar and segmental atelectasis, but results are no better than those obtained with intensified medical therapy. Intermittent positive-pressure breathing may worsen chest overinflation and usually is contraindicated. Intravenous infusion of gamma globulin enriched with *P. aeruginosa* mucoid exopolysaccharide antibody has not been shown to be beneficial. The antioxidant glutathione sometimes is administered as an aerosol, but efficacy has not been documented, and its use is highly controversial. Surgical treatment of pulmonary complications is undertaken infrequently because involvement of the lungs usually is generalized, but lobectomy or segmental resection may be useful in some cases of persistent atelectasis, localized bronchiectasis, or hemoptysis.

Treatment of Pneumothorax

Every patient with a newly diagnosed pneumothorax, even if it is asymptomatic, should be hospitalized and observed for a minimum of 24 hours. Active intervention is indicated for a pneumothorax greater than 10%. The goals are to achieve resolution of the leak and reexpansion of the lung and to prevent recurrence. Conventional therapy consists of closed thoracostomy drainage via a chest tube. Patients with persistent air leak can be treated by resection-stapling of blebs and localized pleural abrasion via an open thoracotomy or thoracoscopy procedure. Chemical pleurodesis using sclerosing agents such as quinacrine and tetracycline is highly effective but leads to marked pleural fibrosis and may complicate subsequent lung transplantation. Pleurodesis should be reserved for patients in whom chest tube drainage fails and whose condition is such that the risk of surgery outweighs its benefits. In many cases, a pneumothorax will occur in association with a pulmonary exacerbation. In such instances, intensive antibiotic therapy is used in conjunction with the aforementioned measures. To prevent pneumothorax, patients should avoid engaging in such activities as power weight lifting, intensive isometric exercise, and scuba diving, which lead to marked fluctuations in intrapleural pressure.

Treatment of Hemoptysis

Usually, heavy blood streaking of sputum and episodes of hemoptysis reflect advanced bronchiectasis and increased pulmonary infection. The site of bleeding (often right upper lobe) may be suggested by localized symptoms, chest radiographs, or CT. In cases in which the site is not clear, bronchoscopy may be helpful.

In patients with heavy blood streaking, intensive antibiotic therapy alone may be sufficient. With massive hemoptysis (greater than 240 mL/24 hours) or with protracted or recurrent episodes of moderate bleeding, treatment options include intravenous antibiotics, discontinuation of drugs that interfere with coagulation, correction (vitamin K, fresh-frozen plasma) of identified coagulation defects, replacement of acute blood loss, and intravenous administration of vasopressin (Pitressin). For patients who do not respond to these measures, percutaneous catheter embolization of the involved bronchial arteries is the procedure of choice. Bleeding immediately ceases in more than 80% of patients. After the procedure, however, repeat bleeding often occurs, and one-third to half of affected patients require repeat embolization. In rare cases in which embolization is not successful, localized pulmonary resection may be indicated.

Treatment of Cor Pulmonale

The management of right ventricular failure includes therapy of the underlying pulmonary obstruction and infection along with diuretics, salt restriction, and oxygen, but the response often is unsatisfactory. Generally, digitalis is not useful. Overall, results are not favorable. In adults with non-CF chronic obstructive pulmonary disease, pulmonary hypertension may be reversed by long-term continuous oxygen therapy. This achievement has not been demonstrated in patients with CF, however, and the role of oxygen therapy remains poorly defined. Usually, it is prescribed to relieve hypoxemia and dyspnea and to improve tolerance for exercise.

Treatment of Respiratory Failure

Patients who have obstructive pulmonary exacerbations complicated by respiratory failure should receive intensive standard care for CF, preferably in an intensive care unit. For those patients who have refractory hypercapnia, a short course of intravenous methylprednisolone may be helpful. Mechanical ventilation may play a useful role in infants and young children with acute respiratory failure, in patients who have acute and potentially reversible complications such as hemoptysis and pneumothorax, and in patients for whom lung transplantation is an imminent option. Results are especially promising in children younger than age 5 years. For patients who have progressive respiratory failure and who are not candidates for transplants, ventilatory support of longer than 2 weeks duration is associated with poor outcomes and should be discouraged.

For patients who have chronic stable respiratory failure, noninvasive positive-pressure ventilation provided via a tight-fitting nasal or face mask can play an important role. This type of support is associated with improvements in gas exchange, sleep efficiency, respiratory muscle strength, and reductions in dyspnea and work of breathing. It can play an especially valuable role in patients awaiting transplantation.

Lung Transplantation

Bilateral lung transplants can be performed successfully in carefully selected patients with end-stage lung disease. Results are similar to those seen in patients who do not have CF, with 75% to 80% survival at 1 year, 60% at 3 years, and 40% at 5 years after transplantation. Overall, survival is comparable for children and adults. Bilateral lobar transplantation from living donors is offered at some centers as an alternative to cadaveric transplantation, with similar results. Patients colonized with *B. cepacia* may have less favorable outcomes but are considered for transplantation at some centers. After successful transplantation, pulmonary function and exercise performance rapidly return toward normal. Airways of the transplanted lungs have normal transepithelial ion transport. Early complications include rejection, bleeding, and infection, whereas infection and chronic rejection (bronchiolitis obliterans) are the leading late complications. Daily monitoring of lung function allows early detection of infection and rejection episodes, with confirmation of the diagnosis by transbronchial biopsy. Wider application of lung transplantation is limited by donor organ availability.

Immunoprophylaxis

Recommended vaccination schedules should be followed, especially for pertussis, varicella, *H. influenzae* type b, and measles. Patients should be immunized against pneumococcus starting in infancy and against influenza starting at age 6 months and followed by a yearly booster. Household contacts also should be immunized. A live intranasal influenza virus vaccine is approved for healthy individuals ages 5 to 49 years but not for individuals with CF. Antiviral drugs are not a substitute for influenza immunization, but, when given after exposure, the neuraminidase inhibitors zanamivir and oseltamivir are effective both in prevention and in treatment of influenza A and B. Palivizumab is safe and well tolerated in infants and young children with CF, but efficacy has not been established. *Pseudomonas* vaccines have been used investigationally but are not available for clinical use.

Treatment of Upper Airway Problems

Patients with symptomatic sinusitis should be treated with a 4- to 6-week course of antibiotics. For patients who do not respond and for those with chronic or recurrent symptoms, functional endoscopic sinus surgery to improve sinus drainage is indicated. Patients with chronic symptoms and colonization with *P. aeruginosa* may benefit from intermittent lavage of the sinuses with an aminoglycoside.

For patients with nasal polyps, intranasal steroids, hypertonic saline irrigations, and oral antihistamines and decongestants may provide transient symptomatic relief but rarely are curative. Antibiotics and immunotherapy are not helpful. Patients with distressing symptoms require polypectomy combined with functional endoscopic sinus surgery.

Gastrointestinal Therapy

Treatment of Pancreatic Exocrine Deficiency

Pancreatic enzyme supplements, derived from hog pancreas, constitute the primary therapy of the pancreatic enzyme deficiency. The most effective preparations consist of capsules containing pancrelipase in pH-sensitive enteric-coated microspheres or microtablets. The enteric coating prevents gastric acid inactivation of the enzyme. Powdered preparations are available for use in young infants. Enzyme supplements are given with all meals and snacks; the dosage is determined by the frequency and character of the patient's stools and the patient's growth pattern. Usually, infants are started at a dose of 2,000 to 4,000 lipase units per 120 mL of formula or per breast-feeding. Beyond infancy, weight-based dosing is used, starting at 1,000 lipase U/kg per meal for children younger than age 4 years of age and at 500 lipase U/kg per meal for those older than age 4 years. Usually, half the standard dose is given with snacks. Doses of more than 2,500 lipase U/kg per meal or 10,000 lipase U/kg/day should be avoided because high enzyme dosages have been associated with the development of fibrosing colonopathy. Manifestations of this disorder include intestinal obstruction, bloody diarrhea, chylous ascites, or the combination of abdominal pain, ongoing diarrhea, and poor weight gain. Strictures can be suggested by contrast enema, and the diagnosis can be confirmed by biopsy. Often, development of constipation while a patient is taking enzymes is an indication for more rather than less enzyme. A misguided reduction in dosage of enzymes in this situation may precipitate an episode of DIOS.

After enzyme supplementation has been initiated, amounts of fat and nitrogen are reduced in stools, although the values do not return to normal. Persistence of significant steatorrhea after initiation of enzyme therapy may result from inactivation of enzymes by gastric acid or a low duodenal pH. In such cases, a pancreatic enzyme preparation that combines pancrelipase and bicarbonate or addition of a histamine (H_2) receptor antagonist or proton pump inhibitor may help. Complications of enzyme therapy other than fibrosing colonopathy rarely occur. Irritation of the skin and mucous membranes may be seen in infants. Hypersensitivity reactions can occur in family members exposed to powdered extracts but are rare findings in patients themselves.

Nutrition Therapy

The goal of nutrition therapy is to promote normal growth. Contrary to earlier anecdotal reports of a voracious appetite in patients with CF, most patients have grossly deficient caloric intake. Because of incomplete correction of steatorrhea and increased metabolic demands, the recommendation is that patients receive 30% to 50% more calories than usual daily allowances, which usually can be achieved by a well-balanced, high-protein diet with liberal fat. Restriction of fats no longer is recommended. Infants can be breast-fed if they are receiving enzyme supplements, but weight gain must be monitored closely. For most formula-fed infants, predigested formulas containing medium-chain triglycerides offer no advantage over standard formulas, but they may be useful in infants with liver involvement and persistent steatorrhea and after intestinal resection.

Older patients should be provided with an unrestricted-fat, high-protein, high-calorie diet consistent with food preferences and lifestyle. Supplements with medium-chain triglycerides and glucose polymers can boost caloric intake. For patients who have poor growth and inadequate caloric intake despite nutritional counseling and oral supplementation, enteral supplementation may be useful. It is accomplished by nightly infusion of high-calorie elemental formulas via a nasogastric, gastrostomy, or jejunostomy tube. This type of supplementation, when provided over an extended period of time, may stabilize or even improve pulmonary function. Parenteral hyperalimentation can be used for short-term support in patients with specific problems, but it is costly and associated with complications of prolonged central-line infusions. It is not appropriate for long-term energy supplementation. No evidence strongly supports the use of artificial elemental diets or supplements with essential fatty acids.

In adolescents and adults with malnutrition and poor appetite, short-term use of the synthetic progesterone derivative megestrol acetate can lead to significant increases in lean body mass and body fat and improved pulmonary function. Long-term use is limited by a number of complications including nausea, vomiting, insomnia, mood changes, diabetes, and adrenal insufficiency.

Although patients with CF are not growth hormone deficient, daily administration of growth hormone over the course of 6 to 12 months is associated with improved height and weight velocities, lean body mass, respiratory muscle strength, and exercise tolerance. The effect on pulmonary function is variable. It is not used routinely, probably because of the cost and complexity added to the patient's treatment regimen.

Vitamin and Mineral Supplementation

Vitamin deficiencies can be prevented by daily administration of a water-miscible vitamin preparation. Patients with steatorrhea should receive a daily supplement of a water-miscible alpha-tocopherol preparation at a dose of 5 to 10 U/kg up to a maximum daily dose of 400 units. Routine supplementation with vitamin K is not recommended but may be indicated in patients with extensive liver involvement, at times of surgery, and in patients with demonstrated coagulation problems. To monitor compliance with and response to therapy, serum levels of vitamin A, D, and E should be checked at least annually. Iron deficiency is a common finding. Iron status should be evaluated periodically, and appropriate supplementation should be provided to patients with anemia or low serum ferritin levels. Iron absorption may be impaired in patients with CF, and response to therapy should be monitored closely. With pancreatic enzyme supplementation, supplementation with other trace metals should not be needed. Additional dietary salt should be provided at times of thermal stress, including increased activity in hot weather. Usually, administration of salt tablets is not indicated.

Treatment of Carbohydrate Intolerance

Diabetes is managed by adequate caloric intake, consistent timing of meals and snacks, and insulin. Insulin requirements are based on results of daily blood glucose monitoring and periodic glycosolated hemoglobin values. Generally, oral hypoglycemic agents are not useful. With improved survival, patients should be monitored closely for retinal and renal vascular complications.

Treatment of Meconium Ileus

In uncomplicated cases of MI, the meconium can be removed nonoperatively by isoosmolar enemas administered under hydrostatic pressure. Multiple doses may be required. In patients in whom this procedure is unsuccessful and in those experiencing such complications as volvulus and perforation, resecting the involved segment of bowel may be necessary. In some cases, mucolytics are used intraoperatively to liquefy the inspissated meconium and may eliminate the need for performing intestinal resection. Patients who survive the newborn period have worse lung function beginning at 8 to 10 years of age.

Treatment of Distal Intestinal Obstruction Syndrome

In patients with DIOS who have no evidence of complete obstruction, oral administration of polyethylene glycol or administration of a cleansing electrolyte solution, either orally or by nasogastric tube, is the treatment of choice. On evidence of significant obstruction, enemas with isoosmolar contrast material may be both diagnostic and therapeutic. Most episodes can be managed without surgical intervention. For patients with recurrent episodes, helpful measures include optimization of pancreatic enzyme dosing, increased fluid intake, and administration of a stool-wetting agent, high-fiber diet, and lactulose. In patients with intussusception, hydrostatic reduction should be attempted, although surgery may be necessary. Surgery is indicated for episodes of volvulus.

Miscellaneous Complications

Treatment of esophageal reflux needs to be tailored to the individual patient and may include frequent small feedings, thickened feeds, an acid blocker, metoclopromide, and avoidance of caffeine, theophylline, and head-down tilting during chest physiotherapy. For patients who have severe disease that is not controlled by medical management, performing a fundoplication procedure may be indicated.

Hepatobiliary Therapy

Although no specific therapy exists for CF-related liver complications, long-term administration of the hydrophilic bile acid ursodeoxycholic acid is indicated. It results in dramatic improvement in biochemical indices of liver disease and improves hepatic function in patients with nodular biliary cirrhosis. It may reverse the early sonographic findings suggestive of focal biliary cirrhosis and arrest progresssion from focal biliary cirrhosis to multinodular biliary cirrhosis. In patients with portal hypertension and varices, endoscopic injection sclerotherapy or esophageal variceal ligation can be used to control acute or recurrent episodes of bleeding. The transjugular intrahepatic postcaval shunt procedure is very effective in lowering portal pressure and controlling acute variceal bleeding. It can be used as a short-term method of portal decompression in patients awaiting liver transplantation. Portosystemic shunting should be considered for the long-term management of portal hypertension in patients who are not candidates for liver transplantation. In patients with severe liver disease and good pulmonary status, liver transplantation is a treatment option.

Posttransplant survival rates after 1 year (90%) and 5 years (75%) are comparable to the results of transplants performed for other indications. Although gallbladder abnormalities, including cholelithiasis, are common findings, affected patients usually are asymptomatic. Laparoscopic or surgical cholecystectomy should be reserved for symptomatic patients.

Psychosocial Therapy

Psychosocial support for affected patients and their families is especially important at the time of diagnosis, with exacerbations, and during the terminal phase of the disease. As with any chronic illness, consistency of medical care providers is essential. Members of the health care team should allow patients to develop close relationships with them and should provide ongoing support throughout life. Importantly, such team personnel should know the entire family medically and psychosocially and should be sensitive to individual needs and coping mechanisms. Open communication is essential from the time of diagnosis. Questions should be answered honestly and directly but within a framework of guarded optimism.

Part of every visit should be devoted to a discussion of psychosocial issues. Parents should be encouraged to talk about CF rather than acting as though it does not exist. Involvement of extended family members should be encouraged. Parents constantly should be encouraged to treat affected children normally and to avoid overprotection. Giving special treatment and privileges to these children should be discouraged. Working with adolescents to promote independence and to encourage making realistic academic and vocational goals is important. Families can be helped by being introduced to a CF-affected family that is coping well, educational and support groups, and individual counseling. The health care team should make appropriate referrals to and interface with mental health consultants, interact with the patients' teachers, ensure that families avail themselves of all appropriate community and financial resources, arrange for vocational counseling, and, in the case of adolescents, plan for a smooth transition to adult care. With appropriate support, most patients can make an age-appropriate adjustment at home and school.

COURSE AND PROGNOSIS

The course of disease varies from patient to patient, probably in relation to mutation heterogeneity, gene modifiers, intensity of treatment, and environmental factors. Prognosis is determined largely by the degree of pulmonary involvement. Some patients retain near-normal lung function over the course of many years but, in general, experience an exponential decline in pulmonary function of approximately 2% per year. The FEV_1 adjusted for age and gender is the best predictor of prognosis. Early colonization with mucoid *Pseudomonas* is associated with a more rapid decline in pulmonary function. Exposure to cigarette smoke is associated with a more rapid decline in clinical status and should be avoided. Patients who are pancreatic sufficient generally have milder pulmonary disease and better survival. Other factors associated with improved longevity are male gender, absence of colonization with mucoid *Pseudomonas*, presentation with predominantly gastrointestinal symptoms, balanced family functioning and coping, and compliance with treatment regimens. Clinical scoring systems are available for longitudinal assessment of patients, prognosis counseling, and classifying patients in clinical studies.

A steady improvement in prognosis has occurred over the course of the last 5 decades. In 1950, survival past infancy was unusual. By 2004, median predicted survival age was 35 years

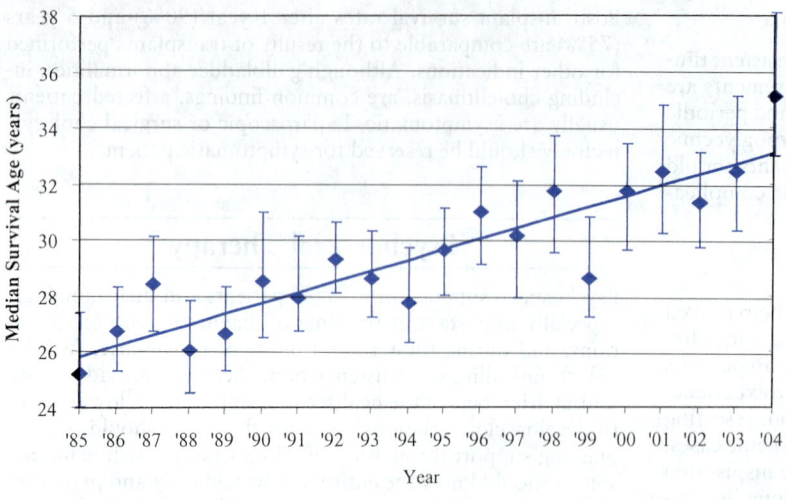

FIGURE 236.4. Survival curve and 95% confidence intervals for cystic fibrosis care center patients in 2004. (Courtesy of the Cystic Fibrosis Foundation, Bethesda, MD.)

(Fig. 236.4). Approximately 42% of all patients under care at specialized CF centers are older than 18 years of age, and survival into the fourth and fifth decades no longer is a rare occurrence. For reasons that are not clear, survival of male patients is better than that of female patients, but the gap has narrowed.

Suggested Readings

Borowitz DS, Grand RJ, Durie PR, and the Consensus Committee. Use of pancreatic enzyme supplements for patients with cystic fibrosis in the context of fibrosing colonopathy. *J Pediatr* 1995;127:681.

Cystic Fibrosis Genotype-Phenotype Consortium. Correlation between genotype and phenotype in patients with cystic fibrosis. *N Engl J Med* 1993;329:1308.

Davis PB, Byard PJ, Konstan MW. Identifying treatments that halt progression of pulmonary disease in cystic fibrosis. *Pediatr Res* 1997;41:161.

Farrell PM, Mischler EH. Newborn screening for cystic fibrosis. *Adv Pediatr* 1992;39:35.

Fuchs HJ, Borowitz DS, Christiansen DH, et al. Effect of aerosolized recombinant human DNase on exacerbations of respiratory symptoms and on pulmonary function in patients with cystic fibrosis. *N Engl J Med* 1994;331:637.

Kerem E, Reisman J, Corey M, et al. Prediction of mortality in patients with cystic fibrosis. *N Engl J Med* 1992;326:1187.

Konstan MW, Byard PJ, Hoppel CL, et al. Effect of high-dose ibuprofen in patients with cystic fibrosis. *N Engl J Med* 1995;332:848.

Konstan MW, Hilliard KA, Norvell TM, et al. Bronchoalveolar lavage findings in cystic fibrosis patients with stable, clinically mild lung disease suggest ongoing infection and inflammation. *Am J Respir Crit Care Med* 1994;150:448.

Kotloff RM, FitzSimmons SC, Fiel SB. Fertility and pregnancy in patients with cystic fibrosis. *Clin Chest Med* 1992;13:623.

LeGrys VA. Sweat testing for the diagnosis of cystic fibrosis: practical considerations. *J Pediatr* 1996;129:892.

Lewin LO, Byard PJ, Davis PB. Effect of *Pseudomonas cepacia* colonization on survival and pulmonary function of cystic fibrosis patients. *J Clin Epidemiol* 1990;43:125.

Ramsey BW, Dorkin HL, Eisenberg JD, et al. Efficacy of aerosolized tobramycin in patients with cystic fibrosis. *N Engl J Med* 1993;328:1740.

Schidlow DV, Taussig LM, Knowles MR. Cystic Fibrosis Foundation Consensus Conference report on pulmonary complications of cystic fibrosis. *Pediatr Pulmonol* 1993;15:187.

Smith JJ, Travis SM, Greenberg EP. Cystic fibrosis airway epithelia fail to kill bacteria because of abnormal airway surface fluid. *Cell* 1996;85:229.

Stern RC. The primary care physician and the patient with cystic fibrosis. *J Pediatr* 1989;114:31.

Stern RC. The diagnosis of cystic fibrosis. *N Engl J Med* 1997;336:487.

Sweet SC, Spray TL, Huddleston CB, et al. Pediatric lung transplantation at St. Louis Children's Hospital, 1990–1995. *Am J Respir Crit Care Med* 1997;155:1027.

Tsui LC. The spectrum of cystic fibrosis mutations. *Trends Genet* 1992;8:392.

Wilcken B, Wiley V, Sherry G, et al. Neonatal screening for cystic fibrosis: a comparison of two strategies for case detection in 1.2 million babies. *J Pediatr* 1995;127:965.

Williams MT. Chest physiotherapy and cystic fibrosis: why is the most effective form of treatment still unclear? *Chest* 1994;106:1872.

CHAPTER 237 ■ PULMONARY HEMOSIDEROSIS

MARIANNA M. SOCKRIDER

Pulmonary hemosiderosis is a rare condition characterized by an abnormal accumulation of hemosiderin in the lungs. Deposition of hemosiderin results from bleeding into the lungs with diffuse alveolar hemorrhage, rather than from hemorrhage from larger arteries. In chronic pulmonary hemosiderosis, bleeding usually is low-grade, repetitive, or persistent, often with superimposed episodes of brisk hemorrhage. Pulmonary hemosiderosis is classified as isolated, associated with other organ dysfunction, or secondary, depending on the pathogenesis (Box 237.1).

Idiopathic pulmonary hemosiderosis occurs at any age, but it usually is seen in childhood. Familial occurrence has been reported. No gender difference in incidence exists. Most cases in infancy and childhood are isolated and idiopathic, with no identifiable etiology. Often, the idiopathic form is more episodic and may be exacerbated by viral illness. Pulmonary hemosiderosis resulting from hypersensitivity to cow's milk has been described in young infants, but this relationship is questionable. Associated gastrointestinal or upper respiratory symptoms may occur. A few cases of pulmonary capillary

---

BOX 237.1 — Classification of Pulmonary Hemosiderosis

Isolated
Idiopathic
Cow's milk hypersensitivity (Heiner syndrome)
Pulmonary capillary hemangiomatosis
Pulmonary capillaritis

Associated with Other Organ Dysfunction
Nephritis
    Goodpasture syndrome
    Nephritis with immune complexes
    Nephritis without immune complexes
Myocarditis
Celiac disease
Diabetes
Collagen-vascular disease
Wegener granulomatosis
Henoch-Schönlein purpura and other systemic vasculitides
Lymphangioleiomyomatosis
Tuberous sclerosis

Secondary
Mitral stenosis
Congestive heart failure
Venoocclusive disease
Clotting disorders
Malignancy
Immunosuppression
Diffuse alveolar injury
Chemicals (penicillamine, nitrofurantoin, trimellitic anhydride, toxic hydrocarbons, cytotoxic agents)
Insecticides

---

hemangiomatosis have been reported in children and young adults. This condition is characterized by a proliferation of capillaries that can result in significant alveolar hemorrhage, hemosiderosis, and pulmonary hypertension. Pulmonary capillaritis, a small vessel vasculitis has been reported to cause diffuse alveolar hemorrhage in children.

Usually, Goodpasture syndrome occurs in young men, and development of pulmonary hemosiderosis may precede renal involvement. Diffuse pulmonary hemorrhage with other forms of nephritis is an unusual occurrence in children. Acute pulmonary hemorrhage and hemosiderosis are rare features of numerous collagen-vascular diseases, such as systemic lupus erythematosus in children, but they may precede other systemic manifestations. Systemic vasculitis, such as that seen in Wegener granulomatosis and Henoch-Schönlein purpura, may cause diffuse pulmonary hemorrhage. Selected drug and chemical exposures have been associated with diffuse pulmonary hemorrhage. Reports of case clusters have suggested an association with exposure to environmental factors such as contaminants from water damage or environmental tobacco smoke. A series of infant cases in Cleveland, Ohio suggested an association with exposure to the toxigenic fungus *Stachybotrys atra* (*Stachybotrys chartarum*) in infants' homes. Further epidemiologic review has raised doubt regarding the possible relation to mold exposure in these cases. One case of a child with pulmonary hemorrhage with a positive bronchoalveolar lavage culture for *Stachybotrys* and home exposure has been reported. Analysis of this isolate and isolates from Cleveland case and control homes suggest that some *Stachybotrys* strains are more pathogenic, by producing siderosphores and hemolysin.

Pulmonary hemosiderosis may mimic other chronic pulmonary conditions of childhood, including asthma, cystic fibrosis, and alveolar filling diseases. Acute bleeding episodes may be confused with bacterial pneumonia. Hemoptysis may be seen in bronchiectasis and tuberculosis.

CLINICAL FINDINGS

The most helpful clinical features are iron deficiency anemia, recurrent pulmonary symptoms, and characteristic abnormalities on chest radiography. Any of these features may be the first sign of pulmonary hemosiderosis. Hemoptysis is a helpful clue, although discerning the source of bleeding in young children may be difficult. Hemoptysis should be distinguished from hematemesis or bleeding from the nasopharyngeal airway. Pulmonary hemosiderosis should be considered when unexplained hematemesis occurs. Usually, the clinical picture is characterized by recurrent episodes of acute pulmonary bleeding. Associated fever, tachycardia, tachypnea, and leukocytosis also may occur. Sometimes, only long-term observation leads to establishing the correct diagnosis. Occasionally, pallor and fatigue symptomatic of iron deficiency anemia may be the initial clinical observations.

Physical findings vary according to clinical status. Pallor or cyanosis may be present, although cyanosis is not seen in severely anemic children. Lung findings include bronchial or suppressed breath sounds, wheezing, crackles, and productive or repetitive cough. Transient hepatosplenomegaly occurs in 20% of cases. Recurrent episodes of pulmonary bleeding may cause signs of chronic respiratory disease, including dyspnea, finger clubbing, and pulmonary hypertension. Poor weight gain and easy fatigability are common findings in more severe disease.

LABORATORY FINDINGS

Microcytic hypochromic anemia is present with a low serum iron concentration despite accumulated iron in the lungs. Reticulocytosis is variable and may be seen during active bleeding, depending on available iron stores. Anemia may improve during periods of remission. The total white blood cell count may be elevated moderately, with a shift to the left. Eosinophilia can occur and suggests cow's milk hypersensitivity or an autoimmune process. Often, stool hematesting is positive, owing to blood swallowed during active bleeding. Bleeding studies usually are normal. Transient elevation in serum bilirubin may occur with acute bleeding. Some patients have a positive direct Coombs test and circulating cold agglutinins. All serum immunoglobulin levels may be increased. Conversely, associated deficiency of immunoglobulin A (IgA), of IgG4, or of both has been observed. No consistent pattern of immunologic abnormalities across patients exists. Renal function testing and urinalysis should be performed for evidence of nephritis. In autoimmune diseases, antinuclear antibodies, rheumatoid factor, and erythrocyte sedimentation rate (ESR) may be elevated. Patients with pulmonary capillaritis tend to have lower hematocrit and higher ESR. Serum antibodies to basement membrane are seen in patients with Goodpasture syndrome. Serum antinuclear cytoplasmic antibodies suggest Wegener granulomatosis. Gliadin antibodies are associated with celiac disease.

Iron-laden macrophages (siderophages) provide good presumptive evidence of the presence of pulmonary hemosiderosis. Siderophages may be found in gastric fluid, sputum, bronchial washings, or lung biopsy specimens with Prussian blue staining. Usually, gastric fluid contains siderophages from the lungs, even when no obvious hemoptysis is present. Bronchial lavage is the most direct and reliable method for recovering macrophages containing hemosiderin. Between 2 and 3 days are required for hemosiderin to appear in macrophages after introduction of blood into the lungs.

ADDITIONAL EVALUATIONS

Chest radiographic findings, which often change with clinical course, include transient infiltrates, atelectasis, and hilar adenopathy. Chronically, a reticulonodular pattern and diminished aeration of the lungs are noted, chiefly involving the lower lobes. Diffuse, soft, perihilar infiltrates are common findings and may mimic other processes. Serial chest radiography may show progression, clearing, or even migratory infiltrates. Evaluation of pulmonary function is important to establish the extent of involvement typically demonstrating restrictive changes and impaired diffusion. Occasionally, an obstructive component is present. Changes are most marked during and immediately after acute bleeding episodes occur. A diminished Po_2 with a variable change in Pco_2 during acute episodes occurs. Cardiac evaluation should be done to exclude possible cardiac or vascular-related causes. Lung biopsy should be strongly considered.

PATHOLOGY

Pathologic findings include alveolar epithelial hyperplasia and degeneration. The characteristic feature is presence of large numbers of siderophages in alveolar spaces and interstitium. Iron content of the lung is increased. Amounts of interstitial fibrosis and mast cell accumulation vary. Vasculitis may be observed. Electron microscopy and immunofluorescent staining may be helpful in cases of Goodpasture syndrome and connective tissue disorders.

CLINICAL COURSE

The clinical course varies and may include periods of remission. Establishing prognosis is difficult because of the disease's rarity and variability. Most deaths are caused by acute respiratory failure or shock with massive intrapulmonary bleeding. Usually, repeated exacerbations lead to development of chronic pulmonary disease, with interstitial fibrosis, pulmonary hypertension, and right-sided heart failure. In cases of cow's milk hypersensitivity, a good prognosis is associated with dietary restriction of cow's milk. Goodpasture syndrome carries a poor prognosis, with death occurring from renal failure. One series of 17 children with idiopathic pulmonary hemosiderosis reported an 86% 5-year survival rate. Another series of 15 pediatric patients followed from 10 to 36 years found that 80% had mild or no respiratory problems. The presence of antineutrophil cytoplasm antibodies or other autoantibodies was associated with a poor prognosis.

THERAPY

Appropriate therapy should be initiated for other primary diseases, when identified, or factors that could help to cause or aggravate pulmonary hemosiderosis. An attempt can be made to reintroduce milk every 1 to 2 years. Acute episodes of bleeding should be treated with oxygen. Use of intermittent positive-pressure ventilation may improve delivery of oxygen. Respiratory failure or persistent bleeding occasionally are reversed with mechanical ventilation using positive end-expiratory pressure. Blood transfusions are indicated to correct severe anemia or shock. Superimposed bronchospasm resulting from irritative bronchitis with acute bleeding may respond to bronchodilators.

Acute bleeding in pulmonary hemosiderosis may respond to high-dose corticosteroids. Adrenocorticotropic hormone (10 to 25 U/day), methylprednisolone (1 mg/kg every 6 hours), or hydrocortisone (4 to 8 mg/kg/day) administered intravenously is recommended initially, followed by maintenance oral methylprednisolone, 1 to 2 mg/kg/day. Once remission is achieved, steroids should be tapered gradually until discontinued or until symptoms recur. Little evidence exists to corroborate the efficacy of long-term steroid therapy in preventing relapse. If maintenance steroids are needed, the minimal dose required to suppress symptoms should be used. Use of inhaled corticosteroids for maintenance has been reported, but no clinical trials have been conducted.

In cases showing an inadequate response to corticosteroids, other immunosuppressant drugs have been used. Lung biopsy should be obtained if not done previously to assess for capillaritis. Azathioprine (Imuran) is used most frequently, and success is reported in using 1.2 to 5.0 mg/kg/day, usually in combination with prednisone. Other drugs reported to have some success include cyclophosphamide, chlorambucil, and hydroxychloroquine. An attempt should be made to stop all drugs after 1 year of clinical remission. Intravenous gamma globulin replacement therapy may be considered in subjects with symptomatic immunoglobulin deficiencies. Splenectomy has uncertain value. If other measures fail or in the presence of chronic severe disease, iron chelation with deferoxamine has been suggested, but its effects are largely undocumented. Close follow-up is important to monitor disease activity. Transplantation has been done with severe lung disease, and a case of recurrent hemosiderosis after transplantation has been reported.

Suggested Readings

Boat TF. Pulmonary hemorrhage and hemoptysis. In: Chernick V, Boat TF, eds. *Kendig's disorders of the respiratory tract in children,* 6th ed. Philadelphia: WB Saunders, 1998:623.

Calabrese F, Giacometti C, Rea F, et al. Recurrence of idiopathic pulmonary hemosiderosis in a young adult patient after bilateral single-lung transplantation. *Transplantation* 2002;74:1643.

Centers for Disease Control and Prevention (CDC). Update: pulmonary hemorrhage/hemosiderosis among infants—Cleveland, Ohio, 1993–1996. *MMWR Morb Mortal Wkly Rep* 2000;49:180.

Dearborn DG, Smith PG, Dahms BB, et al. Clinical profile of 30 infants with acute pulmonary hemorrhage in Cleveland. *Pediatrics* 2002;110:627.

Elidemir O, Colasurdo GN, Rossmann SN, Fan LL. Isolation of *Stachybotrys* from the lung of a child with pulmonary hemosiderosis. *Pediatrics* 1999; 104:64.

Fullmer JJ, Langston CC, Dishop MK, et al. Pulmonary capillaritis in children: a review of eight cases with comparison to other alveolar hemorrhage syndromes. *J Pediatr* 2005;146:376–81.

Kiper N, Gocmen A, Ozcelik U, Dilber E, et al. Long-term clinical course of patients with idiopathic pulmonary hemosiderosis (1979–1994): prolonged survival with low-dose corticosteroid therapy. *Pediatr Pulmonol* 1999;27: 180.

LeClainche L, LeBourgeois M, Fauroux B, et al. Long-term outcome of idiopathic pulmonary hemosiderosis in children. *Medicine (Baltimore)* 2000;79:318.

Levy J, Wilmott RW. Pulmonary hemosiderosis. *Pediatr Pulmonol* 1986;2:384.

Milman N, Pedersen FM. Idiopathic pulmonary haemosiderosis: epidemiology, pathogenic aspects and diagnosis. *Respir Med* 1998;92:902.

Montana E, Etzel RA, Allan T, et al. Environmental risk factors associated with pediatric idiopathic pulmonary hemorrhage and hemosiderosis in a Cleveland community. *Pediatrics* 1997;99:1.

Saeed MM, Woo MS, MacLaughlin EF, et al. Prognosis in pediatric idiopathic pulmonary hemosiderosis. *Chest* 1999;116:721.

Vesper SI, Dearborn DG, Elidemir O, Haugland RA. Quantification of siderophore and hemolysin from *Stachybotrys chartarum* strains, including a strain isolated from the lung of a child with pulmonary hemorrhage and hemosiderosis. *Appl Environ Microbiol* 2000;66:2678.

CHAPTER 238 ■ OBSTRUCTIVE SLEEP APNEA SYNDROME

CAROLE L. MARCUS

Obstructive sleep apnea syndrome (OSAS) is an important cause of morbidity in children. If left untreated, it can result in cor pulmonale, neurologic impairment, and failure to thrive. Pediatric OSAS was rediscovered when it was described in detail by Christian Guilleminault and colleagues in 1976. However, descriptions of this syndrome date back to the writings of William Osler, more than a century ago.

Obstructive apnea is defined as the cessation of airflow at the nose and mouth, despite continued respiratory effort, secondary to upper airway obstruction. This is distinct from central apnea, in which cessation of airflow is associated with absent respiratory effort. Many children with OSAS exhibit continuous partial airway obstruction, associated with hypoxemia and hypoventilation, rather than complete airway obstruction; this has been termed obstructive hypoventilation.

EPIDEMIOLOGY

The prevalence of OSAS in the pediatric age group is estimated to be 2% of preschool children, as reported by Redline and colleagues. The peak incidence is between approximately 2 to 6 years of age. However, OSAS can occur at any age, from the neonatal period through adolescence. In prepubertal children, in contrast to adults, OSAS occurs equally among boys and girls.

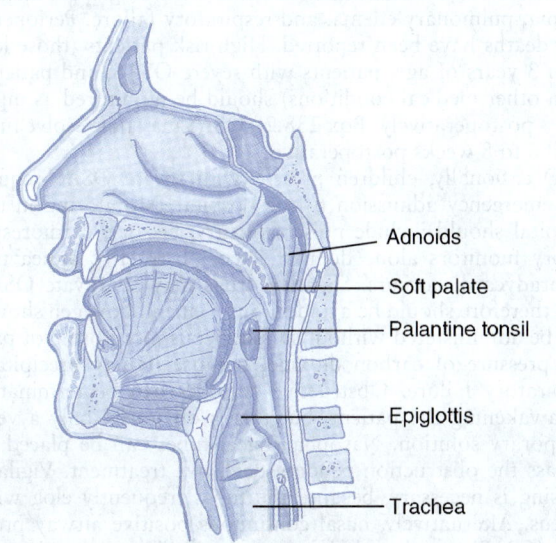

FIGURE 238.1. Diagram of the upper airway. (Reprinted from Moore KL, Augur AMR. *Essential clinical anatomy,* 2nd ed. Baltimore: Lippincott Williams & Wilkins, 2002.)

Labels: Adnoids, Soft palate, Palantine tonsil, Epiglottis, Trachea

PATHOLOGY

The upper airway above the level of the epiglottis (i.e., the nasopharynx, oropharynx and hypopharynx) is a hollow, neuromuscular tube (Fig. 238.1). It is usually patent, but it has the potential to collapse to facilitate speech and swallowing. In patients with OSAS, the upper airway collapses abnormally during sleep.

OSAS results from a combination of abnormal neuromuscular control and anatomic narrowing of the upper airway. During wakefulness, the patient with a narrow airway can compensate by augmenting upper airway muscle tone; thus, OSAS does not occur. During sleep, there is a decrease in ventilatory drive and in neuromuscular tone that facilitates upper airway collapse. In contrast, patients with obstruction in the cartilaginous portion of the upper airway have fixed obstruction during both wakefulness and sleep. This is associated with stridor rather than snoring.

In children, the anatomic narrowing of the upper airway is usually the result of adenotonsillar hypertrophy. Other common causes of structural narrowing include craniofacial anomalies and obesity. Patients with neuromuscular disorders resulting in hypotonia (e.g., muscular dystrophy) or incoordination of the upper airway musculature (e.g., cerebral palsy) are also at increased risk for OSAS. Children with syndromes encompassing developmental delay, hypotonia, obesity, and upper airway narrowing (e.g., children with trisomy 21) are at very high risk for OSAS (Box 238.1).

CLINICAL MANIFESTATIONS AND COMPLICATIONS

Most children present with a history of snoring and difficulty with breathing during sleep. The onset is usually insidious. Children with OSAS have persistent, loud snoring that can often be heard outside the bedroom. During sleep, the child has labored breathing, retractions, and paradoxical inward motion of the chest wall during inspiration. During periods of complete obstruction, the child can be observed to be making respiratory efforts, but no snoring is heard and no airflow is detected. Obstructive episodes are usually terminated by gasping, movements, or arousal from sleep. The child sleeps restlessly and may adopt unusual sleeping positions, such as sleeping in a seated position or with the neck hyperextended. Diaphoresis, pallor, or cyanosis may be present. The appearance of the child during sleep can be so alarming that it is not unusual for parents to maintain bedside vigils or to stimulate or reposition the child continually throughout the night. Nevertheless, many parents do not volunteer a history of their child's sleep symptoms unless specifically asked. In the clinic, it is useful to ask parents to mimic their child's snoring and breathing pattern.

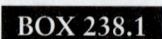

BOX 238.1 — Conditions Commonly Associated with Obstructive Sleep Apnea Syndrome*

Primarily Structural
Adenotonsillar hypertrophy
Obesity
Craniofacial anomalies
Sickle cell disease
Mucopolysaccharidosis

Primarily Neuromotor
Hypotonia (e.g., muscular dystrophy)
Spasticity (e.g., cerebral palsy)

Combination of Structural and Neuromotor
Genetic syndromes (e.g., Down syndrome)
Hypothyroidism

---

*This is only a partial list of medical conditions associated with obstructive sleep apnea syndrome. Most of these conditions involve both structural and neuromotor factors, in varying proportions.

During wakefulness, the child breathes normally. Nonspecific symptoms of adenotonsillar hypertrophy may be present. These include mouth breathing, rhinorrhea, dysphagia, and recurrent otitis media. Excessive daytime sleepiness may be present, but it is unusual in young children. There may be a family history of snoring or OSAS.

Physical Examination

In the majority of children with OSAS, the physical examination during wakefulness is entirely normal. This commonly leads to a delay in diagnosis, because the physician often does not have the opportunity to see the child asleep.

Physical examination should include an assessment of the child's growth. Failure to thrive or, conversely, obesity may be present. Allergic stigmata, mouth breathing, adenoidal facies, midfacial hypoplasia, and retrognathism or micrognathia or other craniofacial abnormalities may be present. The patency of the nares should be assessed. The pharynx should be evaluated for tongue size, pharyngeal integrity, oropharyngeal diameter, redundant palatal mucosa, palatal length, and size of the tonsils and uvula. The lungs are usually clear to auscultation. Cardiac examination may reveal signs of pulmonary hypertension, such as an increased pulmonic component of the second heart sound. A neurologic examination should be performed to evaluate muscle tone and developmental status.

Complications

The trend to earlier diagnosis has resulted in a decrease in the rate of complications. Patients with severe OSAS can have failure to thrive, but even patients in the normal growth range often have accelerated growth after treatment. Growth abnormalities are probably the result of a combination of increased work of breathing and decreased growth hormone production. Severe OSAS can result in pulmonary hypertension. This can progress to cor pulmonale and congestive heart failure. This resolves following successful treatment of OSAS. Systemic hyper-

tension may occur. Neurobehavioral complications result from sleep fragmentation and nocturnal hypoxemia. These include hyperactivity, personality changes, poor school performance, and developmental delay. Enuresis, especially secondary enuresis, may result from OSAS. Seizures, asphyxial brain damage, and coma have been reported.

DIAGNOSIS

According to the American Academy of Pediatrics, the diagnosis of OSAS should be established by polysomnography (sleep study). This can be performed in children of any age, provided experienced pediatric personnel are present. History alone is inadequate for diagnosis, because it cannot distinguish between OSAS and primary snoring or other causes of sleep-related symptoms, as noted by Goldstein and associates. In addition, polysomnography provides objective measures of severity and a baseline for those children whose condition does not resolve postoperatively. During polysomnography, noninvasive monitoring of sleep architecture, chest and abdominal wall motion, airflow, oxygenation, and carbon dioxide tension is performed. Polysomnography should be performed in a laboratory used to studying children, because techniques and normative values differ widely between children and adults.

THERAPY

Most children are cured by adenotonsillectomy. OSAS results from the relative size and structure of the upper airway components, rather than the absolute size of the tonsils and adenoids. Therefore, both the tonsils and adenoids should usually be removed, even if one or the other appears to be the primary abnormality. By the same logic, adenotonsillectomy should usually be the initial treatment of OSAS in children with other predisposing factors (e.g., obesity, Down syndrome), although further treatment may be necessary. Even though adenotonsillectomy is frequently considered minor surgery, it can be associated with significant complications. Therefore, snoring without OSAS is not an indication for surgery. Children with OSAS are at risk for postoperative complications, including upper airway edema, pulmonary edema, and respiratory failure. Perioperative deaths have been reported. High-risk patients (those less than 3 years of age, patients with severe OSAS, and patients with other medical conditions) should be monitored as inpatients postoperatively (Box 238.2). OSAS may not resolve fully until 6 to 8 weeks postoperatively.

Occasionally, children present with severe OSAS requiring emergency admission to the hospital. Monitoring in the hospital should include pulse oximetry, because cardiorespiratory monitors alone do not detect obstructive apnea until bradycardia occurs. Sedative drugs may aggravate OSAS and therefore should be avoided. Supplemental oxygen should *not* be administered without simultaneous monitoring of partial pressure of carbon dioxide, because it may precipitate respiratory failure. Obstructive episodes can be terminated by awakening the patient, but this is obviously only a very temporary solution. Nasopharyngeal tubes can be placed to bypass the obstruction pending definitive treatment. Vigilant nursing is necessary, because the tubes frequently clog with mucus. Alternatively, nasal continuous positive airway pressure (CPAP) may be administered. Intubation is occasionally necessary.

A few patients with OSAS do not respond to adenotonsillectomy. Nasal CPAP can be used successfully in most children, provided the parents and child are motivated and the care providers are well versed in pediatric CPAP use. Behavioral and psychological support may be necessary. Other treatments are useful in individual cases. When applicable, specific craniofacial surgery may be useful (e.g., lip-tongue adhesion procedures in patients with Pierre Robin sequence). Seid and colleagues noted that uvulopharyngopalatoplasty has been shown to be helpful in children with cerebral palsy. Obese patients should be encouraged to lose weight, but they require treatment (e.g., CPAP) pending weight loss. With the advent of nasal CPAP, tracheotomy is rarely necessary for sleep apnea.

PROGNOSIS

Most children experience a dramatic resolution of their symptoms following adenotonsillectomy. However, the natural course and the long-term prognosis of pediatric OSAS are unknown. Some evidence suggests that children with treated OSAS are at risk for recurrence during adulthood, as reported by Guilleminault and associates.

Acknowledgments

Supported in part by grant National Institute of Health (NIH) RO1HL58585.

Suggested Readings

American Academy of Pediatrics. Clinical practice guideline: diagnosis and management of childhood obstructive sleep apnea syndrome. *Pediatrics* 2002;109:704.
American Thoracic Society. Standards and indications for cardiopulmonary sleep studies in children. *Am J Respir Crit Care Med* 1996;153:8668.
Arens R, McDonough JM, Costarino AT, et al. Magnetic resonance imaging of the upper airway structure of children with obstructive sleep apnea syndrome. *Am J Respir Crit Care Med* 2001;64:698.
Goldstein NA, Sculerati N, Walsleben JA, et al. Clinical diagnosis of pediatric obstructive sleep apnea validated by polysomnography. *Otolaryngol Head Neck Surg* 1994;111:611.
Guilleminault C, Eldridge FL, Simmons FB, et al. Sleep apnea in eight children. *Pediatrics* 1976;58:23.
Guilleminault C, Partinen M, Praud JP, et al. Morphometric facial changes and obstructive sleep apnea in adolescents. *J Pediatr* 1989;114:997.
Marcus CL, Ward SL, Mallory GB, et al. Use of nasal continuous positive airway pressure as treatment of childhood obstructive sleep apnea. *J Pediatr* 1995;127:88.
McColley SA, April MM, Carroll JL, et al. Respiratory compromise after adenotonsillectomy in children with obstructive sleep apnea. *Arch Otolaryngol Head Neck Surg* 1992;118:940.
Redline S, Tishler PV, Schluchter M, et al. Risk factors for sleep-disordered breathing in children: associations with obesity, race, and respiratory problems. *Am J Respir Crit Care Med* 1999;159:1527.
Seid AB, Martin PJ, Pransky SM, et al. Surgical therapy of obstructive sleep apnea in children with severe mental insufficiency. *Laryngoscope* 1990;100:507.

CHAPTER 239 ■ CENTRAL HYPOVENTILATION SYNDROMES

CAROLE L. MARCUS

Central alveolar hypoventilation is defined as an increase in arterial carbon dioxide tension (greater than 45 mm Hg during wakefulness) due to a decrease in central nervous system ventilatory drive. It is usually associated with hypoxemia. Patients with central hypoventilation fail to breathe adequately, despite having normal lungs, upper airway, and chest wall. Central hypoventilation may be congenital or acquired, and primary or secondary. Some causes of central hypoventilation are listed in Box 239.1.

Sleep is associated with a decrease in central ventilatory drive and upper airway neuromotor tone. Thus, the P_{CO_2} is increased during sleep even in normal subjects, and a P_{CO_2} greater than 50 mm Hg for up to 10% of sleep time is normal

in children. For this reason, all patients with central hypoventilation will breathe worse during sleep than during wakefulness. Some patients, particularly those with congenital central hypoventilation syndrome, may hypoventilate only during sleep.

CLINICAL MANIFESTATIONS AND COMPLICATIONS

Patients with congenital central hypoventilation usually present in the neonatal period with cyanosis or apnea.

BOX 239.1   Causes of Central Hypoventilation

Primary
  Congenital central hypoventilation syndrome (CCHS)
  Late-onset central hypoventilation syndromes
    associated with hypothalamic/endocrine
    dysfunction
  Prader-Willi syndrome

Secondary
  Obesity-hypoventilation syndrome
  CNS abnormalities or increased intracranial pressure
    Arnold-Chiari malformation
    Hydrocephalus
    Ventriculoperitoneal shunt malfunction
    Achondroplasia
    Hypoxic-ischemic encephalopathy
    CNS trauma
    CNS hemorrhage
    CNS tumor
    CNS congenital anomalies
    Moebius syndrome
    Meningoencephalitis
    Poliomyelitis
  Other neurologic syndromes
    Autonomic neuropathies (familial dysautonomia)
    Mitochondrial defects, including subacute necrotiz-
      ing encephalomyelopathy (Leigh's Disease)
    Neurodegenerative syndromes
  Miscellaneous
    Drugs
    Hyperthermia
    Hypothyroidism
    Metabolic dysfunction; inborn errors of metabolism

BOX 239.2   Diagnostic Evaluation of Suspected Hypoventilation

Establishing the Presence and Severity of Hypoventilation
  Arterial blood gas
  Polysomnography
Determining the Etiology*
  Chest radiograph
  Pulmonary function tests
  Ventilatory responses to hypoxia and hypercapnia
  Genetic testing
  Evaluation of diaphragmatic function (fluoroscopy,
    ultrasound)
  Evaluation of ventilatory muscle strength
  Fiberoptic laryngoscopy
  Magnetic resonance imaging of the brainstem
  Brainstem auditory evoked potentials
  Endocrine evaluation
  Serum glucose, ammonia, pyruvate, lactate
  Serum and urinary amino acids, organic acids
Assessing Complications
  Hematocrit/hemoglobin
  Serum bicarbonate
  ECG, echocardiogram
  Neurodevelopmental evaluation

---

*Selected tests should be used on an individual basis.

Although they may rarely present at a later age, symptoms usually are traceable to infancy. Patients with acquired central hypoventilation can present at any age. Patients may initially have nonspecific symptoms, such as lethargy, poor sleep, irritability, or morning headaches. These subtle signs are frequently overlooked, and it is not unusual for patients to be diagnosed only following catastrophic events, such as apparent life-threatening events (ALTE), seizures, or congestive heart failure resulting from cor pulmonale.

Patients with central hypoventilation do not have signs of respiratory distress or increased respiratory effort, even when severely hypoxemic or hypercapnic. The term "happy hypoxia" has been applied. This is in marked contrast to patients with respiratory failure secondary to pulmonary mechanical abnormalities, who will have subjective distress, tachypnea, and retractions. Patients with central hypoventilation usually have shallow, slow breathing rather than frank central apnea. The patient may be able to transiently breathe adequately voluntarily when instructed to do so.

The physical examination in children with central hypoventilation is usually normal. Growth failure or signs of pulmonary hypertension (such as an increased pulmonic component of the second heart sound) may be present. In children with secondary central hypoventilation, the underlying condition or associated neurologic abnormalities are usually evident.

DIAGNOSIS

Laboratory tests are necessary to (a) establish the presence of hypoventilation, and (b) investigate the cause. The presence of hypoventilation is established by arterial blood gas analysis. However, a single arterial blood gas does not reflect adequately the patient's ventilation, particularly during sleep. Thus, serial blood gas monitoring via an arterial line, or continuous noninvasive capnometry and oximetry monitoring during polysomnography, is preferable. It is essential to assess gas exchange during both wakefulness and sleep.

Potential diagnostic tests are shown in Box 239.2; the choice of tests must be individualized for each patient. Pulmonary and neuromuscular causes of hypoventilation must be excluded. In particular, isolated diaphragmatic paralysis should be excluded. The hypoventilation can be assumed to be central in origin if tests of pulmonary function and ventilatory muscle strength are normal, and metabolic abnormalities are excluded. Magnetic resonance imaging of the brainstem is recommended for all patients with central hypoventilation of undetermined etiology. The diagnosis of congenital central hypoventilation syndrome (CCHS) is made primarily by exclusion, according to the following criteria: (a) persistent hypoventilation during sleep (PCO_2 consistently greater than 60 mm Hg during sleep), (b) onset of symptoms from birth or early infancy, and (c) absence of primary pulmonary, cardiac, central nervous system, neuromuscular, or metabolic dysfunction. Recently, generic confirmation become available.

THERAPY

The aim of treatment is to prevent respiratory failure, cor pulmonale, and hypoxic neurologic damage. Whenever possible, the primary cause of the hypoventilation should be treated. The mainstay of treatment, for those in whom the primary cause of hypoventilation cannot be successfully treated, is ventilatory support. A number of different ventilator modalities have been used. The most common modality is positive pressure ventilation via either tracheostomy or nasal mask. Great care must be taken with nasal mask ventilation, particularly in infants and young children, because mask displacement or other technical problems can result in inadequate ventilation. It is crucial to prevent intermittent episodes of hypoxemia, particularly early in life, in order to optimize neurocognitive development. For this reason, many experts recommend positive pressure ventilation via tracheotomy during infancy, with a possible transition to face mask ventilation when the child is older, in order to prevent episodes of inadequate ventilation due to factors such as mask displacement. Diaphragm pacemakers have been used in those children with CCHS who require ventilatory support 24 hours a day, because the pacers allow the child to be ambulatory.

Pharmacologic therapy is rarely efficacious after infancy. Supportive care includes the prompt treatment of respiratory tract infections, avoidance of sedative medications, nutritional support, and economic and psychosocial support for the family.

PROGNOSIS

Prognosis depends on the underlying cause of the hypoventilation. With modern techniques for home ventilation, children with CCHS and other forms of hypoventilation can lead fulfilling lives. Many of these patients attend normal schools and participate in sporting and social events. To date, children with CCHS who receive ventilatory support have been followed into early adulthood, and no indications suggest that they are at risk for early mortality. However, the older literature demonstrates that untreated patients with central hypoventilation have a high mortality. Patients usually died from cor pulmonale rather than from respiratory failure or apnea.

SPECIFIC DISEASE CONDITIONS

Congenital Central Hypoventilation Syndrome

Congenital central hypoventilation syndrome (CCHS) is a rare condition in which patients have intact voluntary control of ventilation, but lack automatic control. Previously, this syndrome was named "Ondine's curse" after a German fable; this term is no longer used due to its negative connotations. Classically, children with CCHS were described as having normal breathing during wakefulness, but severe hypoventilation during sleep. It is now recognized that many patients with CCHS cannot breathe adequately even when awake. Some require ventilatory support 24 hours a day; others are asymptomatic during wakefulness but demonstrate subclinical abnormalities, such as desaturation during exercise. Patients with CCHS have normal cognitive function if hypoxemic episodes are prevented. Associated abnormalities that may be present include autonomic dysfunction, Hirschsprung disease (approximately 16% of patients) and tumors of neural crest origin (such as neuroblastoma, ganglioneuroma).

Recently, it was discovered that CCHS is due to a mutation in the homeobox gene *PHOX2B*. In most cases, this is due to a *de novo* mutation, which is dominant Clinical testing, including prenatal diagnostic testing, now is available. CCHS

has been reported in siblings and twins, and at least four cases have been documented of children with CCHS born to parents with CCHS. Normal births also have been reported.

The exact pathophysiology of CCHS is unknown, and specific pathologic lesions have not been found. It has been speculated that the primary physiologic defect in CCHS is in the brainstem, where afferent impulses from the central and peripheral chemoreceptors are integrated. Mechanoreceptors in the limbs appear to play a role in stimulating breathing during wakefulness in these patients.

The older literature described substantial morbidity and mortality in children with CCHS. Death usually resulted from cor pulmonale, aspiration, or sepsis. However, recent reports describe prolonged survival, with a good quality of life. Children continue to need ventilatory support, and do not "outgrow" their disease.

Late-Onset Central Hypoventilation

A syndrome of late-onset central hypoventilation associated with hypothalamic abnormalities has been described. These patients typically present at approximately 1 to 5 years of age with morbid obesity due to an uncontrollable appetite, central hypoventilation, and hypothalamic endocrine abnormalities (e.g., growth hormone deficiency, diabetes insipidus). Similar to CCHS, they may have neural tumors. The cause of this condition is unknown. The cranial MRI is normal.

Arnold-Chiari Malformation

Children with Arnold-Chiari malformations have central hypoventilation secondary to abnormal central chemoreceptor function. The type I Arnold-Chiari malformation consists of caudal herniation of the cerebellar tonsils through the foramen magnum. The type II malformation consists of caudal displacement of the cerebellar vermis, brainstem, and fourth ventricle, and is associated with brainstem compression and/or dysplasia. The type II Arnold-Chiari malformation is present in the vast majority of patients with spina bifida; it is this population that the pediatrician is most likely to encounter. It has been estimated that as many as two-thirds of children with spina bifida have abnormal breathing during sleep, although in many patients this may be subclinical. Patients with Arnold-Chiari malformation and severe ventilatory control dysfunction may have normal intellectual function. Clinical manifestations of ventilatory control dysfunction include central apnea, cyanotic spells, prolonged breath-holding spells, respiratory failure, and sudden death. Sleep-disordered breathing has been estimated to be the cause of death in 13% of patients with spina bifida, and is of particular concern in young infants. In addition to central hypoventilation, children with spina bifida are predisposed to other pulmonary problems, such as restrictive lung disease secondary to ventilatory muscle weakness, scoliosis, and aspiration. Bilateral vocal cord paralysis can occur as a result of traction on the vagus nerve roots. An increase in apnea or stridor indicates an increase in intracranial pressure, and "croup" in children with Arnold-Chiari malformation should always be regarded as a sign of increased intracranial pressure until proven otherwise. Patients with Arnold-Chiari malformation and hypoventilation or vocal cord paralysis may improve following ventriculoperitoneal shunting or posterior fossa decompression. However, many patients have either permanent brainstem damage or brainstem dysplasia, and require chronic ventilatory support.

Obesity-Hypoventilation Syndrome

The obesity-hypoventilation syndrome (Pickwickian syndrome) occurs in morbidly obese patients. These patients have a decreased ventilatory drive, resulting in hypercapnia and hypoxemia during both wakefulness and sleep. Cor pulmonale is a frequent complication. Additional pulmonary problems that may be present include restrictive lung disease and the obstructive sleep apnea syndrome. The pathophysiology of the obesity-hypoventilation syndrome is not fully understood. Patients with the syndrome have a decreased ventilatory drive in response to hypoxia and hypercapnia. It is hypothesized that obese patients have chronic hypoxemia and hypercapnia due to mechanical limitation of ventilation, and therefore develop a secondary blunting of their ventilatory drive. This can be reversed by weight loss. However, weight loss can be notoriously difficult to achieve. In the interim, patients can be supported by mechanical ventilation (via face mask or tracheotomy).

Prader-Willi Syndrome

Prader-Willi syndrome (PWS) is a congenital disorder typified by hypothalamic obesity, mental retardation, hypotonia, and hypogonadism. The vast majority of patients have abnormalities of chromosome 15. Although patients with PWS do not have classic central hypoventilation, they are included here, because physiologic testing has shown abnormalities of ventilatory control. When evaluating patients with PWS, it is difficult to separate the effects of obesity from the effects of the underlying syndrome (Fig. 239.1). Obstructive sleep apnea and desaturation during rapid eye movement sleep are seen com-

monly. Patients tend to have restrictive lung disease due to hypotonia and obesity, which can explain the tendency to desaturate. Excessive daytime sleepiness is common, and it has not been established whether this is due to sleep-disordered breathing or to central nervous system abnormalities. Physiologic studies in PWS have shown blunted hypercapnic ventilatory responses secondary to obesity; patients in whom weight has been controlled have a normal hypercapnic drive. The hypoxic ventilatory drive is abnormal, suggesting carotid body dysfunction. Recently, several case reports have described death during sleep in patients with PWS receiving exogenous growth hormone. Because many children with PWS now receive growth hormone therapy, it is not known whether these deaths are truly related to the medication (e.g., by exacerbating obstructive sleep apnea). Interestingly, one study showed an increase in ventilatory drive following growth hormone administration in this population, despite an unchanged body mass index.

Miscellaneous Causes of Central Hypoventilation

Central hypoventilation can result from any congenital or acquired central nervous system lesion that results either in severe and diffuse neurologic damage, or selective brainstem damage (Box 239.1). In patients with hypoventilation secondary to severe, generalized central nervous system dysfunction, quality of life should be considered before instituting invasive therapy, and palliative treatment may be an appropriate option.

Acknowledgments

Supported in part by grant RO1 HL58585.

Suggested Readings

Amiel J, Laudier B, Attie-Bitach T, et al. Polyalanine expansion and frameshift mutations of the paired-like homeobox gene *PHOX2B* in congenital central hypoventilation syndrome. *Nat Genet* 2003;33:459.

Katz ES, McGrath S, Marcus CL. Late-onset central hypoventilation with hypothalamic dysfunction: a distinct clinical syndrome. *Pediatr Pulmonol* 2000;29:62.

Kirk VG, Morielli A, Brouillette RT. Sleep-disordered breathing in patients with myelomeningocele: the missed diagnosis. *Dev Med Child Neurol* 1999;41:40.

Lindgren AC, Hellstrom LG, Ritzen EM, et al. Growth hormone treatment increases Co2 response, ventilation and central inspiratory drive in children with Prader-Willi syndrome. *Eur J Pediatr* 1999;158:936.

Marcus CL. Sleep-disordered breathing in children. *Am J Respir Crit Care Med* 2001;164:16.

Marcus CL, Omlin KJ, Basinki DJ, et al. Normal polysomnographic values for children and adolescents. *Am Rev Respir Dis* 1992;146:1235.

Marcus CL, Jansen MT, Poulsen MK, et al. Medical and psychosocial outcome of children with congenital central hypoventilation syndrome. *J Pediatr* 1991;119:888.

Nixon GM, Brouillette RT. Sleep and breathing in Prader-Willi syndrome. *Pediatr Pulmonol* 2002;34:209.

Sugar O. In search of Ondine's curse. *JAMA* 1978;240:236.

Swaminathan S, Paton JY, Ward SL, et al. Abnormal control of ventilation in adolescents with myelodysplasia. *J Pediatr* 1989;115:898.

Waters KA, Forbes P, Morielli A, et al. Sleep-disordered breathing in children with myelomeningocele. *J Pediatr* 1998;132:672.

Weese-Mayer DE, Silvestri JM, Menzies LJ, et al. Congenital central hypoventilation syndrome: diagnosis, management, and long-term outcome in thirty-two children. *J Pediatr* 1992;120:381.

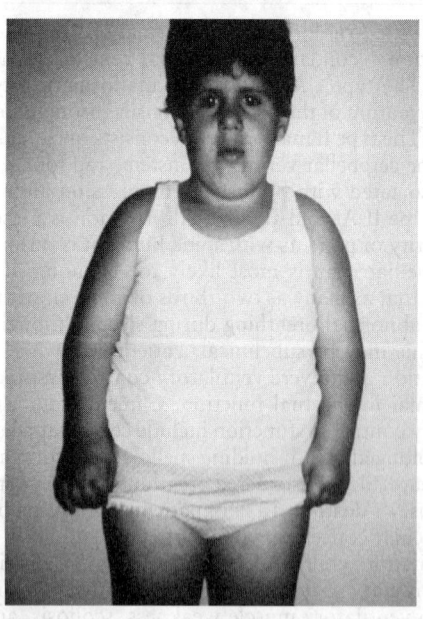

FIGURE 239.1. Prader-Willi syndrome in a 7-year-old patient. The features include truncal obesity and a round face with almond-shaped eyes. (Reproduced with permission from Morrissy RT and Weinstein SL. *Lovell and Winter's pediatric orthopaedics*, 5th ed. Philadelphia: Lippincott Williams & Wilkins, 2000.)

CHAPTER 240 ■ CHRONIC DIFFUSE INTERSTITIAL LUNG DISEASE IN CHILDHOOD

ILEY BROWNING AND CLAIRE LANGSTON

Chronic diffuse interstitial lung disease in children includes a heterogeneous group of pathologic states characterized by a diffuse inflammatory process that involves the interstitium or supporting structures of the lung as opposed to the alveolar spaces. Interstitial pneumonia is a nonspecific reaction to injury that can be a manifestation of infection, drugs, toxic inhalants, collagen vascular disease, or a variety of genetic, metabolic, or inflammatory disorders.

ETIOLOGY

Diffuse interstitial lung disease in children can be classified in numerous ways. Classification by etiology and by age at presentation is particularly useful (Box 240.1). Age at presentation is an important factor when considering the diagnostic possibilities because a group of conditions exist that are seen only in newborns and infants but not in older children. Newborns and near-term infants who present with early respiratory failure and fail to respond to conventional therapies should be assessed for developmental and genetic disorders, including deficiency of surfactant proteins B and C and abnormality

of ABCA3, a transporter protein thought to be involved in surfactant secretion, the structural abnormality known as alveolar capillary dysplasia with misalignment of pulmonary veins, congenital alveolar dysplasia, and other abnormalities of intrauterine lung growth. The disease processes that present exclusively in infants include persistent tachypnea of infancy (also known as neuroendocrine hyperplasia of infancy), infantile cellular interstitial pneumonitis (also known as pulmonary interstitial glycogenosis), and chronic pneumonitis of infancy (now widely thought to be the histologic appearance of some surfactant dysfunction mutations, more often surfactant C protein deficiency). Most cases of pulmonary alveolar proteinosis seen in children, as well as the histologic appearance of some of surfactant dysfunction mutations, also present in infants.

CLINICAL MANIFESTATIONS AND COMPLICATIONS

These diseases are all uncommon occurrences, and many are poorly understood. The usual clinical presentation is insidious

---

| **BOX 240.1** | **Pediatric Interstitial Lung Disease—Etiologic Classification*** |

Known Etiology
  Aspiration syndromes
  Chronic infection in immunocompetent and immuno-
    compromised host
    Viral (EBV, CMV, adenovirus, others)
    Bacterial (chlamydia, mycoplasma, mycobacteria,
      others)
    Fungal (aspergillosis, histoplasmosis, pneumocystis,
      others)
    Parasitic
  Bronchopulmonary dysplasia
  Environmental/physical agents
    Hypersensitivity pneumonitis
    Drug induced
    Radiation induced
    Oxygen induced
    Chemical fumes
    Mineral dusts
  Lipid storage diseases
  Pulmonary alveolar proteinosis with genetic deficiency of
    surfactant protein B
Unknown Etiology
  Actual interstitial pneumonia (AIP)
  Usual interstitial pneumonia (UIP)
  Desquamative interstitial pneumonia (DIP)

Lymphocytic interstitial pneumonia (LIP) and related disorders
ILD associated with autoimmune disorders
ILD associated with malignancies
Pulmonary hemosiderosis
Pulmonary histiocytosis (eosinophilic granuloma)
Pulmonary infiltrates with eosinophilia
Pulmonary vascular disorders (hemangiomatosis, veno-occlusive disease, etc)
Pulmonary lymphatic disorders (lymphangiomatosis, lymphangiectasis)
Sarcoidosis
Bronchiolitis obliterans
Bronchiolitis obliterans with organizing pneumonia
Neurocutaneous syndromes
Cellular interstitial pneumonitis
Infantile cellular interstitial pneumonitis
Chronic pneumonitis of infancy
Persistent tachypnea of infancy
Nonspecific

AMV, cytomegalovirus; EBV, Epstein-Barr virus; ILD, interstitial lung disease.
Modified with permission from Fan LL, Langston C. Chronic interstitial lung disease in children. *Pediatr Pulmonol* 1993;184:16.

onset and minimal early findings, although acute fulminate presentation can occur. Tachypnea is the hallmark physical finding and may be the only early finding, although occasionally acute presentation with tachypnea, hypoxemia, and fever may occur. Older children may present with dyspnea, with or without wheezing, whereas infants and toddlers more frequently present with tachypnea without respiratory distress. Fine crackles often are present with progression of disease. Symptoms overlap with those of common respiratory infections, but the prolonged course, lack of response to initial therapies, and imaging findings will separate these processes from the more common acute pulmonary infections. The chest radiograph may be normal initially, but later it often shows a diffuse interstitial pattern of reticulonodular infiltrate. Chest computed tomography (CT) scan generally is a more sensitive indicator of disease activity and shows better correlation with symptoms than does chest radiograph. Separating the various disease processes that produce chronic diffuse interstitial lung disease may be difficult using clinical, laboratory, and radiologic findings, and frequently lung biopsy is necessary to define the pathologic process.

LUNG DISEASE PRESENTING IN NEWBORNS

Genetic Deficiency of Surfactant Protein B

Lung disease on the basis of a genetic abnormality of surfactant protein B is a rare, chronic, diffuse lung disease seen in young infants. Affected infants generally present soon after birth with hypoxia and respiratory distress; chest radiographs shows a ground-glass appearance; investigations for infectious etiologies are negative. The diagnosis can be made by performing appropriate studies on blood (for the genetic abnormality) and lavage fluid (for the surfactant protein B deficiency) and lung biopsy. Surfactant replacement is not a viable therapy. Some affected infants have been treated with lung transplantation with good results. The picture on lung biopsy varies, with some infants having the classic picture of pulmonary alveolar proteinosis, whereas others have less prominent proteinosis and instead have a picture of alveolar epithelial hyperplasia with relatively limited amounts of proteinosis material, and still others have conditions that resemble chronic pneumonitis of infancy.

Infants with genetically based abnormalities of the transporter protein ABCA3, located on the lamellar body membrane, have a clinical picture that is identical to that for genetic deficiency of surfactant protein B. Diagnosis is established similarly, through evaluation for the genetic defect. Lung biopsy also shows features similar to those of surfactant-B deficiency, although electron microscopy may reveal absent or abnormally small lamellar bodies with eccentric dense inclusions.

Genetic Deficiency of Surfactant Protein C

Infants with genetic abnormalities of surfactant protein C often present somewhat later in life and with somewhat milder disease than do those with a deficiency of surfactant protein B. Diagnosis is established by analysis of the surfactant protein C gene for typical mutations. Lung biopsy often has the appearance of "chronic pneumonitis of infancy" and may have a prominent lipoid component. Occasionally, presentation is delayed until later in childhood or even in adult life.

Alveolar Capillary Dysplasia with Misalignment of Pulmonary Veins

Infants with this abnormality are term or near-term and present with respiratory failure. Persistent pulmonary hypertension is a major finding, and the infants do not respond to conventional therapy. The clinical presentation is variable, with chest radiographic findings that can vary from clear lung fields to diffuse radiologic abnormalities. The family history of an affected sibling may help with establishing the diagnosis. Lung biopsies are characterized by abnormalities of both the pulmonary vasculature and the lobular parenchyma, with striking medial thickening and peripheral extension of arterial smooth muscle into the tiny intralobular vessels, dilated veins that accompany hyperplastic arteries throughout their course, and deficient capillary development within the lobar parenchyma. Approximately one-third of affected infants have pulmonary lymphangiectasis, and many have developmental abnormalities of other organ systems, usually minor, but sometimes major. No specific gene defect has been identified for this disease, but the disorder is familial, probably autosomal recessive.

Congenital Alveolar Dysplasia

Congenital alveolar dysplasia is another of the rare abnormalities of lung development that may be seen in the term infant who presents with respiratory and sometimes cardiac insufficiency. Some, but not all, affected infants have persistent pulmonary hypertension. Such infants may survive for weeks to months with supportive measures and assisted ventilation, but ultimately they cannot be removed from supportive measures and die of respiratory failure. Lung biopsy shows arrest of lung development in the late canalicular or early saccular stage, although few cases have been well-characterized. Some reports of alveolar capillary dysplasia without vein misalignment may be examples of congenital alveolar dysplasia.

Intrauterine Lung Growth Abnormalities

Fetal lung development is affected by numerous intrauterine factors including amniotic fluid adequacy, available thoracic space, and neuromuscular function. Infants with abnormal intrauterine environments or other abnormalities limiting thoracic volume may be born with severely hypoplastic lungs that never will be capable of supporting normal function. Oligohydramnios, those related to both renal abnormalities and other conditions, and congenital diaphragmatic hernia are well-known examples of these conditions. Although, for many of these infants, the presence of another condition clearly is responsible for the lung dysfunction, sometimes the intrauterine condition is subtle and not associated with another malformation, and those patients who do not respond to standard supportive therapies may require a lung biopsy. These patients' lungs show features of deficient alveolarization, usually accompanied by pulmonary arterial changes. Similar changes also may be seen in very premature infants after receiving long-term supportive care.

DISEASES PRESENTING IN INFANCY

Neuroendocrine Hyperplasia of Infancy

This condition, initially known as persistent tachypnea of infancy, and now termed *neuroendocrine hyperplasia of infancy*

(NEHI), presents with tachypnea and often hypoxemia; imaging findings are minimal, and the lung biopsy appears near normal. Increased numbers of neuroendocrine cells in distal airways and often increased numbers of neuroendocrine bodies in the lobular parenchyma have been reported in this condition. Symptoms may continue for months to years, but they usually resolve slowly with time.

Pulmonary Interstitial Glycogenosis/Infantile Cellular Interstitial Pneumonitis

A histologically identical condition has been reported as *infantile cellular interstitial pneumonitis* and as *pulmonary interstitial glycogenosis*. Controversy exists regarding the etiology of this condition. Some researchers consider it to be a developmental abnormality, whereas others suggest that it is a nonspecific reactive process in the infant lung. It may be seen as an isolated condition, but it is seen more often in association with other well-defined pulmonary diseases, particularly lung growth abnormalities and new bronchopulmonary dysplasia. Infants present with tachypnea and often hypoxemia; chest radiographs show a hazy ground-glass pattern. Lung biopsy shows widening of the lobular interstitium by increased numbers of cells, initially thought to be histiocytes, but now widely thought to be proliferated structural cells and not infiltrating cells. The prognosis for infants with this process is that of the underlying disease process. In the absence of other pulmonary disease, most infants do well and eventually recover completely with supportive therapy only.

Chronic Pneumonitis of Infancy

Chronic pneumonitis of infancy is a recently described histologic pattern of lung disease in infants now thought to be a manifestation of surfactant dysfunction mutation, more often surfactant C deficiency. Infants present with tachypnea and hypoxemia; their imaging studies show a diffuse interstitial process. Lung biopsy shows several changes that vary in their severity from case to case. Generally, the patient has thickening of the alveolar wall, with moderate epithelial cell hyperplasia and a mild infiltrate of mononuclear cells. Cellular proliferation similar to that of infantile cellular interstitial pneumonitis commonly is found, as is an alveolar exudate of macrophages and eosinophilic debris and globules. Occasionally, cholesterol clefts also are present. Similar changes have been described in the lungs of infants and older children in association with gastroesophageal reflux disease, lysinuric protein intolerance, and other conditions. Although some of the affected infants recovered, many did not respond to therapy, consisting of high-dose steroids, and died of their respiratory disease.

PEDIATRIC INTERSTITIAL LUNG DISEASE

The diffuse interstitial lung diseases that affect older children also may be seen in infants. These diseases are unusual findings in both adults and children, and they are seen more commonly in the setting of immunocompromise in children. They can, however, be seen without underlying disease. Interstitial lung disease (ILD) in children encompasses a wide variety of specific conditions. And, although many of the disease entities seen in children also are seen in adults, the common adult condition, usual interstitial pneumonia (UIP), does not occur in children. In infants, desquamative interstitial pneumonia (DIP) may be

a manifestation of surfactant dysfunction mutation. Lymphocytic interstitial pneumonia (LIP) in children and adults now is considered to be in the spectrum of lymphoproliferative disease and is seen in the setting of congenital and acquired immune deficiency, including solid organ transplant and pediatric acquired immunodeficiency syndrome (AIDS). Giant cell interstitial pneumonia (GIP) has not been described in children; it now is thought to be a hard-metal pneumoconiosis. A rapidly progressive form of diffuse ILD with a characteristic histologic picture that has been called by various terms, including acute interstitial pneumonia (AIP), rapidly progressive interstitial pneumonia, and Hamman-Rich syndrome, does occur in children and shows features similar to those of the disease in adults.

The frequency of diagnosis of DIP has decreased in adults, in whom it is associated most often with the use of nonfiltered cigarettes, but it has remained constant in childhood. Familial cases that present in infancy and early childhood now are thought to be a manifestation of surfactant dysfunction mutations. The age of onset for DIP in children is divided evenly between those younger than 1 year and older children. No difference in mortality rate exists between the two groups; the overall mortality rate is 35%. The disease is characterized histologically by a hyperplasia of the alveolar epithelial cells and the filling of alveoli with numerous macrophages, with only mild alveolar septal thickening and generally sparse inflammatory infiltrates.

The most common of the ILDs seen in childhood are those associated with infectious agents. Of the noninfectious conditions, nonspecific interstitial pneumonia appears to be the most common. It has been seen in adults with a wide variety of underlying conditions including hypersensitivity pneumonia, therapeutic drug reactions, and collagen vascular disease. In adults, nonspecific interstitial pneumonia has been divided into cellular and fibrotic subtypes, with the cellular subtype having a better response to immunomodulatory therapy and often going into remission, whereas the fibrotic subtype is progressive. Studies have not been done in children to define the prognosis associated with more cellular or more fibrotic histologic pictures.

DIAGNOSIS

Some or potentially all of the infectious etiologies may be diagnosed on the basis of serologic studies and bronchoscopy with bronchoalveolar lavage. Transbronchial biopsy may add somewhat to establishing the potential diagnosis in a small number of cases, but it is of less usefulness than in adults, in whom tumors and granulomas are being sought more frequently by biopsy. Sarcoidosis is the only diagnosis under the listing of ILD from unknown etiologies that may be diagnosed definitively from transbronchial biopsy, particularly when combined with appropriate laboratory studies and evaluation of lavage fluid for lymphocytosis. The remaining diseases usually require open-lung biopsy to establish the diagnosis. To differentiate clearly among these entities, proper handling by the pathologist, including inflation of the biopsy, should occur. Communication with the pathologist often is helpful in assuring that the specimen is handled properly.

THERAPY

The treatment of pediatric ILD is quite variable. For some diseases associated with compromised immunity, immune modulation may be appropriate; for those associated with human immunodeficiency virus (HIV) infection, modulation of antiretroviral therapy may be important. For other conditions, high-dose steroids given daily or as monthly pulses may be appropriate. Cyclosporin, hydroxychloroquine, and cyclophosphamide have been used in several of these entities with variable response. Response to therapy is variable and unpredictable, ranging from complete recovery to progression to respiratory failure and death.

Suggested Readings

Bokulic RE, Hillman BC. Interstitial lung disease in children. *Pediatr Clin North Am* 1994;41:543.

Canakis A, Cutz E, Manson D, O'Brodovich H. Pulmonary interstitial glycogenosis: a new variant of neonatal interstitial lung disease. *Am J Respir Crit Care Med* 2002;165:1557.

Churg A. An inflation procedure for open lung biopsies. *Am J Surg Path* 1988;7:69.

Deterding RR, Fan LL, Morton R, et al. Persistent tachypnea of infancy (PTI). A new entity. *Pediatr Pulmonol* 2001;23:72.

Fan LL, Langston C. Chronic interstitial lung disease in children. *Pediatr Pulmonol* 1993;184:16.

Fan LL, Lung MCI, Wagener JS. The diagnostic value of bronchoalveolar lavage in immunocompetent children with chronic diffuse infiltrates. *Pediatr Pulmonol* 1997;23:8.

Fisher M, Roggli V, Merten D, et al. Coexisting endogenous lipoid pneumonia, cholesterol granulomas, and pulmonary alveolar proteinosis in a pediatric population. *Pediatr Pathol* 1992;12:365.

Galambos C, Vargas SO, Arnold J, et al. Congenital alveolar dysplasia. *Mod Pathol* 2003;16:3P.

Gianoulis M, Chan N, Wright JL. Inflation of lung biopsies for frozen section. *Mod Pathol* 1988;1:357.

Hilman BC. Diagnosis and treatment of ILD. *Pediatr Pulmonol* 1997;23:1.

Katkin JP, Hansen TN, Langston C, Hiatt PW. Pulmonary manifestations of AIDS in children. *Semin Pediatr Infect Dis* 1990;1:40.

Katzenstein AL, Gordon LP, Oliphant M, Swender PT. Chronic pneumonitis of infancy. A unique form of interstitial lung disease occurring in early childhood. *Am J Surg Pathol* 1995;19:439.

Langston C. Misalignment of pulmonary veins and alveolar capillary dysplasia. *Pediatr Pathol* 1991;11:163.

Langston C. Pediatric lung biopsy. In: Cagle P, ed. *Diagnostic pulmonary pathology*. New York: R Marcel Dekker, Inc., 2000:19.

MacMahon HE. Congenital alveolar dysplasia. *Am J Pathol* 1948;24:919.

Nogee LM, deMello DE, Dehner LP, Colten HR. Brief report: deficiency of pulmonary surfactant protein B in congenital alveolar proteinosis. *N Engl J Med* 1993;328:406.

Nogee LM, Dunbar AE, Wert SE, et al. A mutation in the surfactant protein C gene associated with familial interstitial lung disease. *N Engl J Med* 2001;344:573.

Schroeder SA, Shannon DC, Mark EJ. Cellular interstitial pneumonitis in infants. A clinicopathologic study. *Chest* 1992;10:1065.

Shulenin S, Nogee LM, Annilo T, et al. ABCA3 gene mutations in newborns with fatal surfactant deficiency. *N Engl J Med* 2004;350:1296.

CHAPTER 241 ■ PULMONARY ALVEOLAR MICROLITHIASIS

CAROL L. ROSEN

ETIOLOGY

Pulmonary alveolar microlithiasis is a rare disorder of unknown etiology recognized by the characteristic radiographic appearance of widespread intraalveolar accumulation of calcific concretions. Despite the striking calcifications, no metabolic abnormalities of calcium or vitamin D have been identified.

EPIDEMIOLOGY

No consistent epidemiologic pattern or exposure history to environmental toxins or infectious agents has been established, and autosomal recessive inheritance has been suggested. Onset can occur in childhood, although most cases are reported in adults. Approximately one-half of cases are familial, identified among asymptomatic siblings after diagnosis of the incident case. Excluding the secondary cases, more than 400 cases have been reported worldwide.

CLINICAL PRESENTATION

Frequently, the illness is discovered in asymptomatic patients when a chest roentgenogram is taken for an unrelated illness. When symptoms develop, cough often is the chief complaint.

DIAGNOSIS

The characteristic chest roentgenogram shows fine bilateral diffuse, "sandlike" micronodulation, most prominent in the bases, often obliterating the diaphagmatic, mediastinal, and cardiac borders (Fig. 241.1). An unusual feature of this disease is the striking radiographic changes in contrast to the relative paucity of physical findings. High-resolution computed tomography more precisely defines the extent and severity of the disease. Bronchoalveolar lavage and open lung biopsy show calcispherites in recovered fluid and in the alveolar spaces, respectively. In children, the differential diagnosis of this miliary pattern includes disseminated tuberculosis, healed disseminated histoplasmosis, and other conditions associated with diffuse calcification such as chronic renal failure, hyperparathyroidism, or vitamin D intoxication. Pulmonary function tests show restrictive lung disease, the severity of which correlates with the degree of interstitial lung disease. Histologically, numerous laminated calcispherites (average diameter 1 mm) are found within the alveolar spaces with either normal or thickened fibrotic interstitium. This appearance is distinct from other disorders associated with metastatic and dystrophic calcification in which calcification occurs in the interstitial or vascular components. Although additional evaluations (bronchoalveolar lavage, 99m-technetium bone scintigraphy, computed tomography, and transbronchial or open lung biopsy)

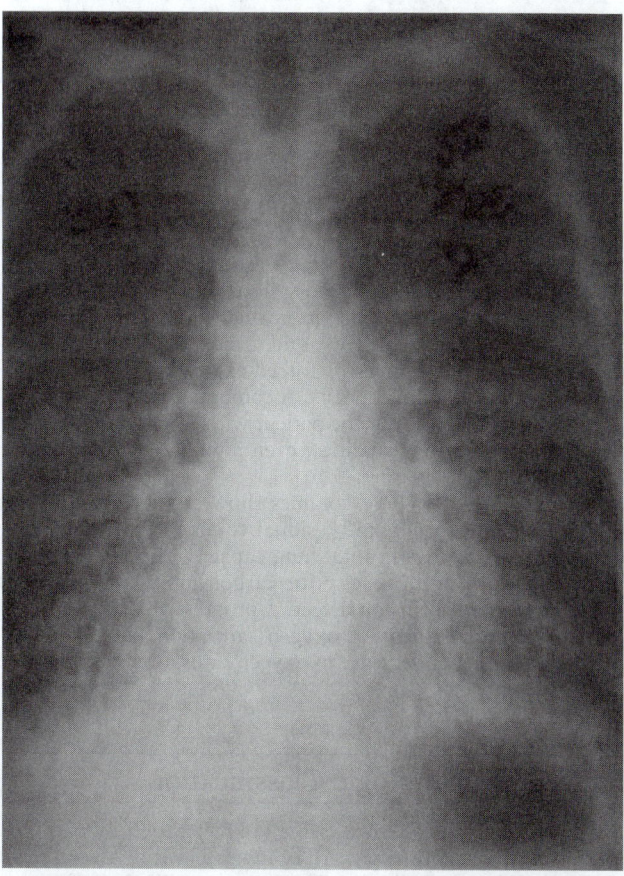

FIGURE 241.1. Pulmonary alveolar microlithiasis. (Reprinted from Brandenburg VM, Schubert H. Images in clinical medicine. Pulmonary alveolar microlithiasis. *N Engl J Med* 2003;348:1555, with permission.)

have been performed, none usually provides more diagnostic information than do the clinical history and plain-film roentgenogram of the chest.

THERAPY

No specific treatment is known, and care is supportive. Corticosteroids, chelating agents, and repeated bronchial alveolar lavage have not demonstrated benefit, and the evidence for bisphosphonates is conflicting. Siblings of affected patients should be screened for the disease with chest radiography because of the increased familial incidence and the paucity of initial symptoms. Because patients are healthy except for this cardiopulmonary problem, lung transplantation has been used successfully for treatment of end-stage disease.

PROGNOSIS

Patients can remain asymptomatic for years, but most die in middle adulthood of progressive interstitial fibrosis with hypoxemia, respiratory failure, and cor pulmonale.

Suggested Readings

Castellana G, Gentile M, Castellana R, et al. Pulmonary alveolar microlithiasis: clinical features, evolution of the phenotype, and review of the literature. *Am J Med Genet* 2002;111:220.

Castellana G, Lamorgese V. Pulmonary alveolar microlithiasis: world cases and review of the literature. *Respiration* 2003;70:549.

Chan ED, Morales DV, Welsh CH, et al. Calcium deposition with or without bone formation in the lung. *Am J Respir Crit Care Med* 2002;165:1654.

Helbich TH, Wojnarovsky C, Wunderbaldinger P, et al. Pulmonary alveolar microlithiasis in children: radiographic and high-resolution CT findings. *AJR Am J Roentgenol* 1997;168:63.

Jankovic S, Pavlov N, Ivkosic A, et al. Pulmonary alveolar microlithiasis in childhood: clinical and radiological follow-up. *Pediatr Pulmonol* 2002;34:384.

Lauta VM. Pulmonary alveolar microlithiasis: an overview of clinical and pathological features together with possible therapies. *Respir Med* 2003;97:1081.

CHAPTER 242 ■ EMPHYSEMA

BRUCE G. NICKERSON

Emphysema is an uncommon but serious problem in pediatrics. It is under-recognized and may masquerade as refractory asthma, or it may be a component of other lung diseases. Usually, emphysema is recognized by clinical suspicion in a patient with a hyperinflated chest, prolonged expiratory phase, and wheezing that responds poorly to bronchodilators. Emphysema is diagnosed by chest roentgenogram or computed tomography (CT) scan with the findings of hyperinflation, dark lung fields, and diaphragms below the tenth or eleventh posterior ribs. Diagnosis can be confirmed by measuring lung volumes, flow rates, and compliance in the pulmonary function laboratory. A lung biopsy shows a deficiency of elastic tissue and simplification of alveolar septation.

DEFINITIONS

The pathologist defines emphysema as the abnormal, permanent enlargement of air spaces distal to the terminal bronchioles, accompanied by destruction of alveolar walls. The physiologist defines emphysema as the permanent loss of elastic recoil of the lungs. The clinician defines emphysema as overexpansion of a region of the lungs that is not reversible with maximal bronchodilator therapy.

Enlargement of air spaces without destruction of their walls is termed *overinflation*. The term *emphysema* seldom is used in pediatrics. Although many children have lungs that fit the preceding descriptions, few come to lung biopsy or autopsy for definitive diagnosis. Furthermore, the rapid increase in the number of alveoli until a child reaches the age of 8 years allows for a dramatic improvement in the clinical status of children who experience even severe emphysematous changes in the first year of life. Several clinical syndromes and common pediatric respiratory diseases have significant components of emphysema.

NORMAL DEVELOPMENT OF THE LUNGS

All airways down to the terminal bronchioles are present by 16 weeks of postconceptional age. Thus, the full complement of airways is developed in the most premature infants who are viable.

An acinus is the unit distal to the terminal bronchiole that includes the alveolar ducts and alveoli ventilated by a single terminal bronchiole. Adjacent acini are separated by fibrous septa. Alveoli develop by budding from alveolar ducts. They increase in number until the child reaches approximately 8 years of age. After that, the alveoli continue to expand until the lungs reach adult size, at approximately 17 years in girls and 20 years in boys. From then on, the alveoli gradually simplify, and the alveolar surface area decreases by approximately 4% per decade through adult life.

PATHOPHYSIOLOGY

At the end of expiration, all respiratory muscles usually are relaxed, and the volume of the lungs is determined by the balance between elastic recoil of lung tissue and compliance of the thoracic cavity. Normally, a network of elastic fibers runs throughout the lungs in the interstitial spaces that provide the elastic recoil of the lungs. Disruption or destruction of this elastic network occurs in emphysema. Recoil decreases, diminishing the normal tendency for the lungs to shrink, and the functional residual capacity (i.e., the lung volume at the end of passive expiration) increases. This process causes numerous secondary changes. The diaphragms do not ascend to their normal position at the end of expiration, so they are at a mechanical disadvantage for developing negative pressure in the chest for inspiration. Phrenic muscle fibers are shorter, so they develop less tension. Consequently, the diaphragms pull less air into the lungs. Also, because of decreased driving pressure, expiratory flows decrease, causing a decrease in forced expiratory volume over 1 second (FEV_1) and a consequent decrease in maximum minute ventilation, which reduces exercise capacity. With severe emphysema, loss of alveolar surface area decreases the surface area available for gas exchange. It can be measured either as a low diffusion capacity for carbon monoxide or as a decrease in oxygen saturation during exercise.

Elastic recoil of the lung can be determined by measuring pulmonary compliance. Almost all pediatric patients with emphysema have regional defects, however, and other regions of the lungs may exhibit restrictive processes. Compliance measured in the pulmonary function laboratory reflects the conflicting effects of these two opposing abnormalities. Because of this difficulty, and because measurement of pulmonary compliance requires swallowing an esophageal balloon, this test seldom is performed in children.

In clinical practice, useful tests for a patient with emphysema include a forced expiratory flow volume loop that typically shows a mild decrease in normal forced vital capacity, a moderate decrease in FEV_1, and a more severe decrease in flows at low lung volumes or forced expiratory flow between 25% and 75% of vital capacity. A component of bronchoconstriction may coexist, but the patient with emphysema has significant residual abnormalities, even after the administration of potent bronchodilators.

Measurements of lung volumes show an increase in functional residual capacity and residual volume. With severe emphysema, an increase in total lung capacity also is present. A test of the diffusion capacity for carbon monoxide can help to quantitate the diffusion defect. A progressive exercise stress test, with measurement of oxygen saturation, often demonstrates a significant decrease in oxygen saturation with moderate exercise.

Pathologic Classification

Four distinct types of emphysema are recognized by pathologists on the basis of the pattern of involvement of alveoli relative to terminal bronchioles. They are panacinar, centriacinar, paraseptal, and irregular emphysema (Table 242.1).

Panacinar Emphysema

In panacinar emphysema, all alveoli, from those close to the bronchioles to those in the lobar septum, are involved, with overextension and destruction of their walls. This type of emphysema typically occurs in adults with alpha$_1$-antitrypsin deficiency. Approximately 1 in 3,500 individuals in the North American population has a homozygous deficiency of the enzyme alpha-1-antitrypsin, with levels less than 20% of normal. Alpha-1-antitrypsin protects elastic fibers of the lungs from digestion by proteolytic enzymes released by polymorphonuclear leukocytes and alveolar macrophages.

Panacinar emphysema develops over the course of many years. Most children with an alpha-1-antitrypsin deficiency have no respiratory symptoms and normal pulmonary function. They are more likely to have prolonged neonatal jaundice and symptoms caused by liver involvement. Thus, measurement of alpha-1-antitrypsin levels seldom is indicated in

TABLE 242.1

PATHOLOGY OF EMPHYSEMA

Pathologic Type	Involvement	Clinical Setting
Panacinar emphysema	All alveoli involved	Alpha-1-antitrypsin deficiency
Centriacinar emphysema	Overdistention of the alveoli near the terminal bronchi	Long-time cigarette smokers
Paraseptal emphysema	Most distal alveoli	Tall, thin young adults with spontaneous pneumothoraces
Irregular emphysema	Alveoli near areas of scar tissue	Bronchopulmonary dysplasia or after necrotic pneumonia

the work-up of the pediatric pulmonary patient unless a positive family history exists or the child has unexplained liver disease or irreversible overinflation of the lungs.

Individuals with alpha-1-antitrypsin deficiency should be counseled to avoid cigarette smoking because nearly all smokers with this defect develop emphysema in young adulthood, whereas more than one-half of nonsmokers escape this complication.

Centriacinar Emphysema

Centriacinar emphysema is characterized by overdistention and destruction of the alveoli near the terminal bronchiole, with relatively normal alveoli at the periphery of the acinus. It is seen commonly in adults with a long history of cigarette smoking but seldom is seen in pediatric patients. This disease, which accounts for disability and premature mortality in adults, is preventable. Because most cigarette smokers begin the smoking habit in adolescence, pediatricians can be instrumental in preventing this disease by helping their patients avoid developing the smoking habit.

Paraseptal Emphysema

Paraseptal emphysema involves the alveoli most distant from the terminal bronchioles, near the septa between adjacent acini. It is seen most often in tall male adolescents and young adults who develop spontaneous pneumothoraces. Generally, these individuals do well with decompression of the pneumothorax by tube thoracostomy. Occasionally, an individual with recurrent pneumothoraces requires sclerosis of the pleural surfaces to prevent recurrence. It can be accomplished by instilling agents such as sterile talcum through the chest tube. Occasionally, surgical abrasion of the pleural surfaces is necessary and can be performed endoscopically without a thoracotomy.

Irregular Emphysema

Irregular emphysema—the overdistention of alveoli near scar tissue—can be seen in many patients with pulmonary scarring or chronic atelectasis. Overdistention of the alveoli appears to be caused by local traction from the scarred area. Areas of irregular emphysema may be seen in many pediatric patients, with processes that cause scarring, including bronchopulmonary dysplasia, necrotizing pneumonias, cystic fibrosis, and residually after mechanical ventilation using high pressures for acute respiratory distress syndrome.

CLINICAL MANIFESTATIONS AND COMPLICATIONS

Clinicians encounter emphysema in numerous clinical syndromes that occur in patients of different age groups. Medical treatment of emphysema is outlined in Box 242.1.

Congenital Lobar Emphysema

Congenital lobar emphysema actually represents lobar hyperinflation and may present in the first few hours or days of life with increasing tachypnea, respiratory distress, and cyanosis. The chest radiograph shows dramatic overinflation of one or two lobes. The disease most commonly involves the left upper lobe, but it may involve any lobe. If the respiratory distress is significant and of rapid onset and if the overdistended lobe becomes larger and compresses adjacent structures, a surgical emergency exists. The infant should be referred to an experienced pediatric chest surgeon for prompt bronchoscopy to rule out a ball-valve obstruction in the bronchus of the affected

---

BOX 242.1	Treatment of Emphysema

1. Provide adequate oxygenation at rest and during exercise.
2. Provide adequate nutrition for growth, particularly in the first 8 years when alveolar formation is occurring.
3. Use bronchodilators to treat reversible airway obstruction.
4. Use diuretics to treat interstitial pulmonary edema.
5. Consider anticholinergic bronchodilators for some patients.
6. Use inhaled steroids if there is ongoing inflammation.
7. Consider alpha-1-antitrypsin replacement if there is deficiency of this enzyme.
8. Prevent viral infections by avoidance of day-care centers or exposure to others with respiratory infections.
9. Provide vaccination against influenza and respiratory syncytial virus when appropriate.
10. Use agents to thin mucus if it is sticky and a nidus for infection.
11. Consider surgical lobectomy in cases of extreme localized disease.

---

lobe and, possibly, for thoracotomy and removal of the lobe. In a child with a rapidly deteriorating condition, diagnostic tests such as CT, magnetic resonance imaging (MRI), and ventilation perfusion scans may become superfluous. They should be omitted if they do not contribute to the surgical decision-making and involve unnecessary delay, which may cause further respiratory compromise. In the more stable patient, these tests may be useful in demonstrating the exact locations of the lesions and their blood supply. Congenital lobar emphysema may be confused with congenital cystic adenomatoid malformation of the lung, polyalveolar lobe, and, sometimes, a large pneumothorax.

Giant Blebs or Cavitary Lung Lesions

Occasionally, infants develop giant blebs, which may be congenital or may occur after necrotizing pneumonia or after receiving mechanical ventilation using high inspiratory pressures. Most of these infants do well with conservative therapy. Alternative therapies, such as selective intubation of the opposite main stem bronchus and surgical obliteration of large or multiple smaller blebs, have been described. Occasionally, infants with severe overextension of a bleb that compresses more normal lung tissue can benefit from a lobectomy. This surgery results in permanent loss of lung tissue, however, and should be performed only if all options are exhausted.

Bronchopulmonary Dysplasia

Infants with bronchopulmonary dysplasia commonly have emphysematous changes that combine focal hyperinflation and destructive remodeling of lung tissue. Older infants with severe respiratory failure requiring mechanical ventilation with high inspiratory pressures caused by pneumonia, aspiration, acute respiratory distress syndrome, or other causes may have a similar picture. Some areas of the lungs show alveolar destruction and loss of elastic recoil and are overinflated. Other areas may have scarring, bronchiolar obstruction, and atelectasis that increases local elastic recoil. The incidence of severe hyper-inflation seems related to the use of high inspiratory pressures and has decreased in the last decade.

Infants with bronchopulmonary dysplasia and severe lung hyperinflation often have a more prolonged recovery period than do other infants with this disease. During recovery, they are prone to recurrent exacerbations with viral infections. If gas exchange is marginal, the infants may develop cor pulmonale. The meticulous management of pulmonary status with treatment of reversible airway obstruction using bronchodilators, treatment of interstitial edema using diuretics, prevention of acquisition of respiratory syncytial virus, and close attention to good oxygenation are essential. These infants require increased caloric intake to compensate for the metabolic needs of the chronic inflammation in their lungs. Because the resolution of symptoms depends on the development of new alveolar growth and repair of damaged airways, excellent nutrition and steady weight gain in the first 2 years is essential.

Interstitial Emphysema

Premature infants with respiratory distress syndrome may develop interstitial emphysema, which is the dissection of air into the interstitial spaces of the lungs. Premature infants who develop this lesion have a high incidence of progression to bronchopulmonary dysplasia. Treatment involves lowering the inspiratory pressure for good oxygenation. Encouraging results have been reported in some, but not all, studies using high-frequency ventilation to lower the maximal inspiratory pressures and still obtain adequate gas exchange.

Unilateral Emphysema

Occasionally, a child is found to have unilateral emphysematous changes after having a severe viral infection. This syndrome is called the *MacLoud* or *Swyer-James syndrome*. It generally occurs in children younger than 8 years old during the period of rapid increase in alveolar number. Biopsy studies have shown that these children suffer from a decrease in alveolar number, but no true destruction of alveolar walls occurs.

Thus, this entity fits the radiographic but not the pathologic definition of emphysema. Generally, these children do well as they grow older, although occasionally they have recurrent infections in the involved area.

Stevens-Johnson Syndrome

Edell and associates reported on an 8-year-old girl with emphysema after having Stevens-Johnson syndrome. I am aware also of several other girls who developed severe emphysema after having Stevens-Johnson syndrome. Biopsy tests revealed severe loss of alveolar septa, and pulmonary function tests showed severe obstructive changes. Long-term follow-up shows that these changes may be irreversible.

Emphysema Changes with Asthma

Some children with severe undertreated asthma (see Chapter 420, Asthma) may develop chronic hyperinflation of the lungs, with loss of elastic recoil, significant deformity of the chest wall, and irreversible pulmonary function changes. These individuals appear to have a form of emphysema, although lung biopsy seldom has been performed in them. More aggressive treatment of chronic asthma to prevent overinflation might prevent this illness.

Suggested Readings

American Thoracic Society. Chronic bronchitis, asthma, and pulmonary emphysema. Statement by the Committee on Diagnostic Standards for Nontuberculous Respiratory Disease. *Am Rev Respir Dis* 1962;85:762.

Coalson JJ. Pathology of new bronchopulmonary dysplasia. *Semin Neonatol* 2003;8:73.

Edell DS, Davidson JJ, Muelenaer AA, Majure MM. Unusual manifestations of Stevens-Johnson syndrome involving the respiratory and gastrointestinal tract. *Pediatrics* 1992;89:429.

Kraemer R, Meister B, Schaad UB. Reversibility of lung function abnormalities in asthma. *J Pediatr* 1983;102:347.

Nickerson BG. An overview of bronchopulmonary dysplasia: pathogenesis and current therapy. In: Lund CH, ed. *Bronchopulmonary dysplasia: strategies for total patient care*. Petaluma, CA: Neonatal Network, 1990.

CHAPTER 243 ■ DISEASES OF THE PLEURA

JAMES S. KEMP AND TERRENCE W. CARVER, JR.

STRUCTURE AND PHYSIOLOGY OF THE NORMAL AND INFLAMED PLEURA

The embryonic coelomic cavity is lined by mesothelial cells and fibroelastic tissue. This embryonic mesothelial lining gives rise to the pleura and peritoneum. The parietal and visceral pleural mesothelia each is a single cell layer thick and forms a stretchable serous membrane over the lung and chest wall. The visceral

pleura also is composed of collagen and elastin connective elements, through which travels its vascular supply, rendering it thicker than the parietal pleura. Once formed, the visceral pleura adheres tightly to the lung parenchyma and interlobar fissures. The parietal pleura also is firmly anchored to the ribs, intercostal muscles, and central diaphragm, and it is tightly adherent as it reflects over the descending aorta, esophagus, and pericardium. Because of the structures that the pleura invests, pressures within the pleural space are important determinants of the transmural pressure of the heart, esophagus, and lungs.

Normally no communication occurs between the left and right pleural cavities, but fluid may enter the pleural space from the peritoneal cavity in some children through pores in the diaphragm. In healthy children, fluid enters the pleural space from the capillaries, lymphatics, and interstitial spaces of both pleurae. Approximately 0.01 mL/kg/hour of fluid enters the space. In the healthy state, this fluid amounts to approximately 0.25 mL/kg body weight per pleural space and creates a film 10 μm thick between the parietal and visceral pleurae. The fluid lining allows for direct mechanical coupling between the lungs and the diaphragm, intercostal muscles, and other muscles of the chest wall. Mechanical coupling via the pleural space transmits to the lungs the forces generated by the diaphragm and other muscles of inspiration. Any widening of the pleural space reduces the efficiency of the inspiratory muscles. In addition to coupling to inspiratory-force generators, fluid in the pleural space permits the pleurae to slide over one another during the respiratory cycle. Glycoproteins within the matrix formed by microvilli on mesothelial cells also reduce friction during breathing.

Research on animals with pleurae similar in thickness to those of humans shows that the visceral pleura, because of its relative thickness, plays a limited role in fluid resorption in both health and disease. The parietal pleura, though more leaky, also plays a larger role in fluid uptake. Most of the fluid is resorbed by lymphatics in the parietal pleura, with an apparent maximal rate of absorption of 0.20 mL/kg/hour, which tends to minimize the amount of fluid in the pleural space. The fluid equilibrium for the pleural space is defined by permeability of pleural mesothelial cells, hydrostatic pressure differences between the parietal and visceral capillaries and lymphatics, and the oncotic pressure of blood compared with pleural fluid.

The normal cell population within the pleural space is small—1,500 to 4,500/μL—and is composed of 75% percent macrophages, with the balance lymphocytes. Mesothelial macrophages are active phagocytes and may have enhanced antigen-presenting capacity.

Free radicals of nitric oxide (NO), produced from activity of inducible NO synthase within mesothelial cells, likely are the first line of defense against infection of the pleural surfaces. Mesothelial cells also secrete proinflammatory (tumor necrosis factor-alpha) and antiinflammatory (interleukin-10) cytokines in abundance when stimulated. During inflammation, neutrophils enter the pleural space under the "direction" of mesothelial cells via mechanisms similar to those described for vascular endothelial cells and involving intercellular adhesion models, selectins, and integrins, whose production is upregulated within the mesothelial cells. Early in inflammation, all types of cells aggregate around openings in the parietal lymphatics to form "pleural tonsils," called Kampmeir foci. During inflammation, these foci are found most commonly on the dorsal, caudal, and mediastinal parietal pleura. The foci appear on scanning electron microscopy as mounds of lymphocytes, histiocytes, neutrophils, plasma cells, and swollen and metabolically active mesothelial cells.

Three clinically recognized stages occur during inflammation. First, dry or plastic pleurisy reflects ingress of inflammatory cells, with minimal fluid. Second, pleurisy with effusion indicates that the inflammatory process has increased the permeability of the mesothelial cells, and fluid enters the pleural space at rates exceeding its removal. Third, organizing pleural disease is reached only with bacterial or fungal parapneumonic effusions. The effusion becomes fibrinous, and the accumulating pleural fluid no longer flows freely in the space. Instead, pockets of fluid are loculated between gelatinous adhesions. If frank pus is present in the pleural space, the effusion can correctly be called an *empyema*. Because of widespread confusion about the correct meaning of the term *empyema*, it should be used only after a clear statement of the intended meaning is made.

CLINICAL FINDINGS IN DISEASES OF THE PLEURA

Findings Caused by Excess Fluid and Inflammation

Regardless of cause, excess fluid accumulates in the pleural space when production exceeds resorption. Systemic diseases increasing visceral fluid hydrostatic pressures or decreasing plasma oncotic pressure cause thin, transudative pleural effusions. Thicker, exudative effusions (protein concentrations greater than or equal to 50% of serum) result from diseases, usually inflammatory, involving the pleural surfaces themselves. Inflammation increases the permeability of mesothelial cells and the permeability of pleural capillaries to protein, and may decrease parietal lymph resorption.

Underlying cardiac, hepatic, or renal diseases usually cause transudative effusions. Ventilatory function may be impaired directly by the underlying disease (e.g., pulmonary edema). A large pleural effusion also partially uncouples the lung from the muscles of inspiration, deforms the diaphragm and chest wall, and compresses the lung. Consequently, worsening tachypnea, cyanosis, and retractions with diminished breath sounds and dullness to percussion usually accompany large transudative effusions (see Hydrothorax). Dyspnea associated with transudation into the pleural space, in the absence of inflammation, may be related to mechanical inefficiencies caused by mechanical uncoupling of the lungs and the muscles of respiration and by compression of lung neurogenic receptors connected to vagal and sympathetic fibers within the lung.

Classic findings of early pleuritis are pain in the chest or shoulder (implying that the parietal pleura of the central diaphragm is involved), guarding of the affected side, upper quadrant abdominal pain (pleura on costal diaphragm involved), a pleural friction rub, and grunting, shallow respirations. Pain fibers are present in the parietal but not the visceral pleura. Therefore, pleuritic pain reflects extension of inflammation to the chest wall early in the course of the thoracic process. Because inflammatory effusions cause pain and are exudative, the presence of pain indicates that the effusion quite likely is an exudate. An inflammatory effusion that is becoming large reduces these signs quickly, except for cough and rapid, shallow respirations and, occasionally, chest wall hyperesthesia. Later, the child has fever, cough, and dyspnea. Thus, a child with a large inflammatory effusion appears ill, with fever and dyspnea. Children with immunodeficiencies and those on corticosteroids may have large pleural effusions with few clinical findings. In immunocompetent children, if the inflammation is triggered by an infection with anaerobic bacteria, the findings of pleural involvement may be less dramatic than is typical for infections caused by pathogens such as *Streptococcus pneumoniae*, *Staphylococcus aureus*, *Haemophilus influenzae*, or *Streptococcus pyogenes* (group A beta-hemolytic streptococcus). Whether the effusion is exudative or transudative, intercostal spaces may bulge outward and the mediastinum may be pushed to the contralateral side, if the effusion is massive. There can be "e" to "a" changes on auscultation; breath sounds are diminished in intensity and often are "tubular" or resembling the sound of a drummer's brush sliding across a drum.

Important conditions in the differential diagnosis of pleuritic chest pain in children include costochondritis, chest pain associated with asthma or gastroesophageal reflux, herpes zoster, and occult trauma.

Air in the Pleural Space

If the air leak is small and the child has little antecedent lung disease, the only symptom of a pneumothorax may be chest pain. The mechanism for this pain is unclear. If the pneumothorax is large or the child has severe underlying disease, pain, cough, dyspnea, and cyanosis may be present. Breath sounds usually are reduced on the side of accumulation of air in the pleural space. If very large, the trachea and cardiac impulse are displaced contralaterally. In a small infant, a large pneumothorax causes subcostal fullness.

Imaging of the Pleura and Pleural Space

The most common and important process involving the pleura in children, a pleural effusion, usually is detected first on the chest radiograph. Skillful use of chest radiography, with occasional help from thoracic ultrasound and computed tomography (CT), allows identification of pleural disease, characterization of an effusion as free or loculated, and distinction between intrapleural processes and peripheral parenchymal disease of the lung.

The usual chest radiographic projections used to evaluate pleural disease are the posteroanterior or anteroposterior, lateral and lateral decubitus (Box 243.1).

Ultrasound has proven to be the imaging modality of choice in pediatrics in localizing pleural fluid and in evaluating peripheral densities abutting the pleura. If a pleural effusion likely is present but decubitus views suggest that it is not free in the pleural space, thoracic ultrasound may identify a loculation that can be aspirated under direct ultrasound guidance. Even when a CT image suggests that a pleural fluid accumulation is homogeneous, the ultrasound often correctly shows that the pleural process is variegated and that large quantities of fluid cannot be removed from one thoracentesis. In these cases, the ultrasound image may show areas of pleural thickening, with

fibrinous adhesions separating areas containing relatively thin fluid from others filled with thick pus. Other advantages of ultrasound for use in children are that it is portable and that it does not require separation from parents or a controlled breathing pattern.

If the hemithorax is partially opacified, obtaining lateral decubitus radiographs is preferable first. If the entire hemithorax is opacified, ultrasound is the first imaging choice.

CT scan images offer the promise of more precise portrayal of pleural disease. However, they can be misleading when used to image inflammatory processes like parapneumonic effusions. They show the effusion in worrisome detail that often hastens consideration of unnecessary invasive remedies (see Fibrothorax). CT scans do help in distinguishing between lung abscesses touching the visceral pleura and loculated pus in the pleural space. Lung abscesses rarely require more than antibiotic therapy, and not tube thoracostomy or débridement. Pus in the pleural space, which often requires drainage or débridement, makes an obtuse angle with the chest wall, and an abscess makes an acute angle. CT scans also help detail parenchymal and hilar adenopathy and calcifications accompanying pleural inflammation and may, therefore, help clarify the etiology of the effusion in puzzling cases. High resolution CT scanning should provide more detailed images of how pleural processes affect the parietal pleura and intercostal muscles. Magnetic resonance imaging (MRI), though useful in other aspects of thoracic imaging, particularly of the mediastinum, usually is not required to evaluate pediatric pleural disease because primary and metastatic malignancies of the pleura are such uncommon findings in children. Digitally stored images, created using x-rays because of their image enlargement and clarification capabilities, should prove useful when evaluating pneumothoraces, in particular.

PNEUMOTHORAX

Free air in the pleural space is detected on chest radiography when bronchovascular markings end at the visceral pleural line and do not extend to the chest wall (Box 243.2). (Fig. 243.1). Air can enter the pleural space by a primary tear in the pleura; by dissection along the bronchovascular sheath after alveolar or airway rupture, with formation and rupture of subpleural blebs; and directly, after rupture of the esophagus or extraparenchymal bronchi. Clinical findings are described previously.

A pneumothorax always is a serious complication in children with underlying severe lung disease, but its importance in otherwise healthy patients depends on its size. Plain radiographs yield relatively poor estimates of the size of the pneumothorax, compared with CT. Children with small primary pneumothoraces should be observed carefully. If they develop respiratory distress, the pneumothorax should be evacuated. In children without significant underlying lung disease, a pneumothorax that occupies 15% or more of the hemithorax can be managed with needle aspiration. Patients with a secondary pneumothorax and those receiving mechanical ventilation usually are treated with tube thoracostomy. Breathing 100% oxygen hastens resorption of free air by four- to sixfold, but hyperoxia should not be maintained for more than a few hours and must be avoided completely in the premature infant.

Recurrent primary pneumothorax causes anxiety and pain but is almost never life-threatening because tension pneumothoraces appear to be quite rare after a primary pneumothorax develops. Pleurodesis should be considered in any patient with recurrent primary pneumothorax and in patients whose underlying lung disease is unremitting. Effective pleurodesis, causing lasting adherence of the parietal to the visceral pleura, can be accomplished with talc. Surgical pleurodesis or

---

BOX 243.2 | **Common Causes of Pneumothorax**

Primary
Congenital subpleural blebs
Familial spontaneous pneumothorax
Catamenial
Idiopathic

Secondary
Cystic fibrosis
Asthma
Hyaline membrane disease
Trauma—pleural tear, esophageal or bronchial rupture
Bacterial pneumonia with pyopneumothorax or abscess
Acquired immunodeficiency syndrome with or without
    Pneumocystis jiroveci or tuberculosis
Tuberculosis
Chronic interstitial pneumonitis
Histiocytosis X or eosinophilic granuloma of lung
Marfan syndrome
Ehlers-Danlos, type IV

Iatrogenic
Mechanical ventilation
Thoracentesis
Bronchoscopy, especially with transbronchial biopsy
Cardiopulmonary resuscitation
Subclavian vein catheterization

local pleurectomy with oversewing of subpleural blebs also can be used as a primary approach and has become the approach of first choice since the advent of video-assisted thoracoscopic surgery. Previous pleurodesis can increase the amount of pleural bleeding dramatically when diseased and adherent lungs are removed at the time of transplantation. Pleural bleeding can cause important morbidity after transplantation, but previous pleurodesis no longer is an absolute contraindication for performing transplantation in some centers.

Primary pneumothoraces are surprisingly common findings among adolescents seen in a referral practice. A high-resolution CT scan, including both lung apices, should be obtained in all previously healthy children and adolescents with a primary pneumothorax, and the radiologist should be asked to focus attention on the apices. As many as 80% have five or more subpleural blebs, usually in the ipsilateral or contralateral apex, despite having a normal plain chest radiograph. A third of these patients, who usually are adolescents, will have recurrent pneumothorax. Because they are entering a time in their lives of less adult supervision, travel, and other changes, surgical pleurodesis with oversewing or marsupialization of blebs should be considered early in this group of patients. Thoracoscopic surgery with video assistance has been particularly successful in the treatment of this type of idiopathic pneumothorax.

Serious blunt chest trauma can cause tears in the trachea or large bronchi, with a pneumothorax that persists despite closed-chest tube drainage. These tears should be suspected in a victim of thoracic crush injury. After bronchoscopic inspection, proximal tears must be repaired surgically.

A tension pneumothorax results when a large accumulation of intrapleural air leads to hypoxemia, impaired venous return, and shock. In an emergency, needle aspiration with a large-bore needle, with or without a three-way stopcock, should be done before tube thoracostomy is performed. The needle should be inserted over the second or third rib anteriorly, and the air should be aspirated with a syringe.

A pneumothorax may persist for several days without causing tension. If a pneumothorax causing symptoms has been present for longer than 3 days, particularly in patients with primary pneumothorax, a small risk exists for reexpansion pulmonary edema. Ipsilateral pulmonary edema can be significant, and the chance of its occurring may be reduced by draining the chest tube to water seal only.

PNEUMOMEDIASTINUM

A pneumomediastinum is free air within the mediastinum and may come from traumatic rupture of the trachea or esophagus, from the neck after facial or dental surgery, from the retroperitoneum after abdominal surgery or penetrating trauma, and from the lung after the development of pulmonary interstitial emphysema. Additional causes are listed in Box 243.3. Trauma,

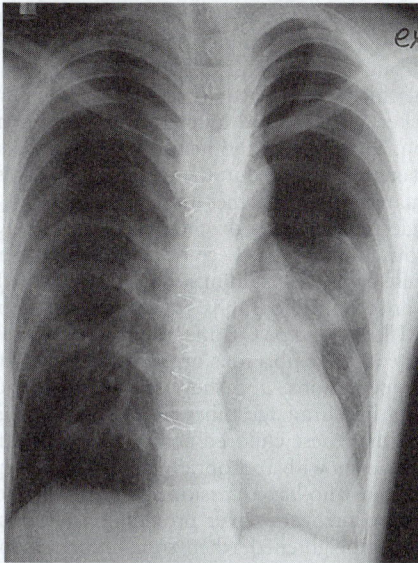

FIGURE 243.1. This chest radiograph of a 16-year-old patient shows a large left pneumothorax. (Courtesy of Dr. Mark Waltzman; used with permission from Fleisher GR, Ludwig S, Baskin MN, eds. *Atlas of pediatric emergency medicine.* Philadelphia: Lippincott Williams & Wilkins, 2004:71.)

BOX 243.3 | **Common Causes of Pneumomediastinum**

Intrathoracic airway obstruction caused by asthma, cystic
    fibrosis, bronchiolitis, or foreign body aspiration
Trauma with tracheal or esophageal rupture, or rupture
    of subpleural blebs
Screaming
Vigorous playing of brass or woodwind musical
    instruments
Violent emesis
Surgery of the head and neck, thorax, or abdomen
    (including laparoscopic)
Spontaneous
Illicit drug use, including Valsalva maneuver when
    smoking marijuana, cocaine, ecstasy, or heroin

either sharp or blunt, and the Valsalva maneuver against an imposed elastic or resistive load (such as coughing or vomiting) are particularly likely to cause pneumomediastinum. A clinical diagnosis based on a triad of chest pain, dyspnea, and subcutaneous emphysema can be made. Additional symptoms of pneumomediastinum include cough, dysphagia, sore throat, facial and neck swelling, and a muffled voice. Signs on physical examination include chest wall and cervical crepitus, distant heart sounds, a crunching sound with cardiac systole (Hamman sign), and, rarely, signs of low cardiac output. The diagnosis can be confirmed by anterior and lateral chest radiographs showing subcutaneous air in the neck, streaks of free air in the mediastinum, "highlighting" by air of the heart and mediastinal vessels, and an increase in size of the retrosternal airspace.

Evacuation of a pneumomediastinum generally is unnecessary, and it typically resolves over the course of 7 to 10 days with rest. However, treatment of a large pneumomediastinum that compromises cardiac output, particularly in a neonate, sometimes is needed.

HYDROTHORAX

The term *hydrothorax* refers to a large transudative pleural effusion. Congestive heart failure, nephrotic syndrome, glomerulonephritis, and hepatic cirrhosis are the most common causes of hydrothorax. Transudative effusions usually are bilateral with heart failure, unilateral or bilateral with nephrosis, or right-sided with cirrhosis. Effusions clearly associated with cardiac, renal, or hepatic disease need not be sampled by thoracentesis unless the child is febrile or respiration is compromised by a large effusion. In the absence of venous hypertension, most children with low serum osmolarity secondary to cirrhosis do not develop an effusion based on low osmolarity alone. Rather, in a small percentage of cirrhotic children, ascitic fluid leaks across the diaphragm through small pores.

The febrile child with cardiac, renal, or hepatic disease and with a pleural effusion usually has an intercurrent infection not involving the pleural space. If another source of fever is not apparent after a period of observation, however, the effusion should be sampled to be certain that the fluid has not become infected. Of the three groups of patients prone to hydrothorax, those with cirrhosis and ascites may be most likely to develop an infected transudative effusion, caused by *Escherichia coli*, *Klebsiella pneumoniae*, *Enterococci*, or group A streptococci.

Children with malignancies may have large pleural effusions caused by parietal pleural metastases and, more commonly, by lymphatic obstruction in the mediastinum with high back pressure through the parietal lymphatics. Children with large transudative effusions but little primary cardiopulmonary disease may have surprisingly few symptoms, except for a "heaviness" in their chest. Minimal changes in arterial blood gases may occur. Draining such a large transudative effusion usually is elective and may have a surprisingly small relative impact on the vital capacity. In adults, the vital capacity increases, on average, only 20 mL for each 100 mL of fluid drained from the pleural space.

If thoracentesis to completely remove fluid is done after the transudative effusion has been present for several days, the protein content may be equal to serum as a result of osmotic equilibration. To treat or prevent circulatory collapse, removal of large quantities of pleural fluid should be performed with an adequate intravenous infusion in place. Reexpansion pulmonary edema can complicate removal of large quantities of fluids that have compressed the lung. Closed chest tube drainage may be indicated if the effusion recurs rapidly.

FIBROTHORAX AND COMPLICATED PARAPNEUMONIC EFFUSIONS

A fibrothorax occurs when a thick layer of fibrous tissue replaces the visceral pleura after an inflammatory process. Fibrothorax, with an associated "trapped lung," developing after a complicated parapneumonic effusion occurred much more commonly in the preantibiotic era. Other processes that rarely can cause fibrothorax include hemothorax, tuberculous pleuritis, pancreatitis or uremia with effusion, and collagen vascular disease. The histologic picture in fibrothorax shows fibroblasts in a dense fibrous stroma that covers the lung. The chest radiograph, on posteroanterior projection, shows lateral separation of the lung from the chest wall and a thin pleural density, representing thickening.

In advanced cases of fibrothorax, which now are exceedingly rare in pediatric patients, narrowing of the ipsilateral intercostal spaces and calcification within the fibrous "peel" that encapsulates the lung can occur. This condition is associated with reduction in ipsilateral lung volume and, in severe cases, exercise intolerance that is out of proportion to the changes seen on the chest radiograph. This physical limitation may be due to marked reduction in ipsilateral lung perfusion. Treatment of fibrothorax is surgical removal of the fibrous "peel" from the lung. Surgical débridement should be done if the restrictive process is unchanged for 6 months or longer (fixed) or progressive, the patient has exertional dyspnea, and the underlying parenchyma appears normal when imaged. In these selected cases, even when the lung has been "trapped" for months or years, function appears to return to near-normal levels after surgery.

Because fibrothorax is so uncommon after a parapneumonic effusion in children, in the antibiotic era, the early management of these effusions is quite controversial and often different from that used in adults. The controversy relates to management within the first several days and weeks of the effusion. We recommend thoracentesis for all but the smallest parapneumonic effusions, particularly if the history suggests that the pleural process is less than 24 to 48 hours old. If the effusion is fresh, large, and freely flowing, the response to tube thoracostomy drainage may be gratifying to the patient and physician. Recently, tissue plasminogen activator (TPA) has been instilled through the tube to enhance drainage of fluid that has become thicker and partially loculated, sometimes resulting in quicker recovery and avoidance of additional surgical intervention. However, if the history suggests that the pleural space has been involved in the pneumonic process for several days, management becomes more challenging, as treatment with a single thoracentesis or chest tube is unlikely to drain proteinaceous fluid that has become gelatinous and more loculated. In these cases, the child may have been febrile for 5 days or longer, and the radiographs suggest extensive pleural involvement. Ultrasound or CT images should be obtained; they often reveal extensive fibrinous organization with fronds, septation, and loculations, and they may help in placement of single or multiple drainage tubes. Retrospective studies have reminded us that these children can remain ill and febrile for several weeks, even with appropriate antibiotic therapy, in contrast to children who have effusions that are relatively homogeneous. The controversy over providing additional surgical management is heightened when some experts contend that decortication, usually meaning removal of gelatinous adhesions, never is needed in children. Further confusion is added when other writers define decortication to include stripping away of large areas of visceral pleura with additional risk of hemorrhage.

Obviously, the intended meaning of decortication must be stated carefully when surgical intervention is discussed. Retrospective studies suggest, but do not confirm, that either video-assisted thoracoscopic surgery (VATS) or limited thoracotomy with débridement of the pleural space, without extensive pleural stripping, hastens defervescence and hospital discharge, particularly in children with prolonged symptoms from pleural inflammation that has progressed to fibrinous organization on radiographic images. Clinical improvement commonly occurs within 48 hours of débridement of the pleural space. We suggest performing surgical débridement and adhesiolysis, either through a thoracoscope or small thoracotomy, in children who have failed a trial of TPA or remain ill with fever and inanition for more than 7 to 14 days, in the presence of a complicated parapneumonic effusion.

The predominate causes of parapneumonic effusions in children are *S. pneumoniae*, *S. aureus*, and *S. pyogenes*. Penicillin-nonsusceptible *S. pneumoniae* is more likely to be the cause in younger children and more often causes bacteremia. *S. aureus* sensitivity to semisynthetic penicillins has decreased with time. The reappearance of pneumonia with effusions caused by group A beta-hemolytic streptococci (*S. pyogenes*) may present new and acute challenges for clinicians unfamiliar with disease caused by this pathogen. *S. pyogenes* long has been known for its propensity to cause necrotizing pneumonia just beneath the visceral pleura. Unlike patients whose pleural space has been invaded by the usual organisms noted previously, with effusions that cause morbidity but with an indolent clinical course, those with *S. pyogenes* are more likely to have secondary sepsis with shock when it invades the pleural space. Therefore, the surveillance within the first 24 hours of appearance of effusions in patients with effusions caused by *S. pyogenes* should be much more expectant, with early use of chest tube drainage or surgical débridement in unstable patients with true sepsis arising from pneumonia with effusion.

A common and predictable sequela of a parapneumonic effusion is fusion, or symphysis, of the parietal and visceral pleurae without restriction of the lung. These pleural adhesions prevent the pleural surfaces from sliding over one another during respiration, but unlike fibrothorax, are not associated with reduction in breathing capacity or P_aO_2.

HEMOTHORAX

Bleeding into the pleural space is an unusual occurrence in children and occurs most commonly after thoracic trauma or insertion of a central venous catheter. In adults, but rarely in children, hemothorax without trauma raises the possibility of malignancy metastatic to the pleurae, or a pulmonary embolus. Other causes of hemothorax in children include coagulopathies, rupture of a ductus arteriosus, a coarctation or a pulmonary arteriovenous malformation, and bleeding from aberrant vessels serving a sequestered lobe of the lung. Pleural endometriosis is a cause of nontraumatic hemothorax in young females.

Hemothorax often is associated with a pneumothorax, and clinical findings are those of both fluid and air in the pleural space. The diagnosis of hemothorax is supported by a chest radiograph and confirmed by thoracentesis. Aspirated fluid is red and has a hematocrit that is either at least 50% of the peripheral blood or is increasing on serial thoracenteses. Pink-tinged fluid is seen commonly without pleural bleeding and is of no diagnostic significance. Because red pleural fluid may have a hematocrit less than or equal to 5%, a hematocrit assay should be used to confirm the diagnosis of hemothorax in puzzling cases.

Hemothorax should be suspected after trauma associated with a pneumothorax. Because blood may not be apparent for 24 hours, another chest radiograph should be taken 1 day after serious chest trauma causing a pneumothorax. Blood in the pleural space may come from the diaphragm, chest wall, lung, and great vessels of the thorax. Hemothorax should be treated with a chest tube to drain the pleural space and to allow tamponade of the vessels leaking into the thorax. If sustained bleeding is greater than 10 mL/kg/hour, the thorax should be explored surgically.

Four important complications of hemothorax are retained blood clots, empyema, pleural effusion after chest tube removal, and fibrothorax. Retained blood clots are thought to be important if they occupy more than 30% of the hemithorax and compress the lung. Empyema is more likely to occur if the pleural space is contaminated at the time of trauma and if the chest tube is left in for many days. Pleural effusion that occurs after removal of the chest tube usually is benign, although a thoracentesis should be done to rule out pus or recurrent hemothorax. Fibrothorax occurs in fewer than 1% of hemothoraces and is more likely to occur with associated empyema.

CHYLOTHORAX

Chyle is a milky, opalescent, bacteriostatic fluid that may accumulate in the pleural space, usually on the right, but it may be on the left or bilateral, depending on the site of abnormality in the thoracic duct. The amount of chyle and its turbidity are dependent on ingestion of fat. Chyle is clear and scant in a newborn that has not been fed. Chyle contains triglycerides and usually 400 to 6,800 lymphocytes/mL.

Many potential causes of chylothorax are listed in Box 243.4. The thoracic duct is fragile and subject to leak with stretch or even mild blunt trauma. Nonetheless, the overall incidence of chylothorax after thoracic surgery is less than 1%; it may occur more commonly after surgery on the esophagus. Thrombosis of large central veins and obstruction by malignancy can cause chylothorax. In neonates in particular, the cause is presumed to be some malformation of the thoracic duct, and in many cases the cause is unknown and, thus, idiopathic.

Symptoms from chylothorax first arise from accumulation of fluid and compression of the lung. Because chyle is bacteriostatic and not irritative, dyspnea, rather than fever or pleuritic pain, is seen. Traumatic or surgical chylothorax may appear rapidly, with respiratory embarrassment and shock. Usually, though, surgical chylothorax appears over the course of many days because the postoperative patient is not fed and therefore has minimal chyle flow.

BOX 243.4 **Common Causes of Chylothorax**

Neonatal "idiopathic" chylothorax
Left thoracotomy, especially for cardiac or great vessel surgery
Penetrating chest trauma
Surgery involving the neck, vertebrae, or mediastinum (especially the esophagus)
Lymphoma and other mediastinal tumors
Thrombosis of the superior vena cava or subclavian veins
Hilar lymphadenopathy associated with tuberculosis

The diagnosis of chylothorax is confirmed when milky opalescent fluid is obtained by thoracentesis and the fluid has the requisite components. If a nonchylous effusion is present for several weeks, it may be milky and have a high triglyceride level (greater than 110 mg/dL) and very high levels of cholesterol. This condition is termed a *pseudochylothorax* and should be considered in any patient with no clear risk factors for chylothorax. Lipoprotein electrophoresis of chyle shows chylomicrons and the various lipoproteins distinguishing a true chylothorax from a pseudochylothorax.

Chyle contains electrolytes in concentrations similar to those of serum and usually 3 g/dL of protein, 0.4 to 0.6 g/dL of lipid, and fat-soluble vitamins. If chyle is drained from the pleural space in appreciable quantities, these nutrients should be replaced. Other important treatment modalities include a diet containing medium-chain triglycerides and, if necessary, total parenteral nutrition (TPN). If dietary manipulations and TPN fail, particularly if sustained lymphopenia occurs, performing ligation of the thoracic duct occasionally is necessary. Chemical pleurodesis and pleuroperitoneal shunts have been used with success in selected cases when ligation of the thoracic duct would not be tolerated.

PLEURAL COMPLICATIONS OF THE ACQUIRED IMMUNODEFICIENCY SYNDROME

Pleural disease, including pleural effusion and pneumothorax, though still a rare occurrence, has been described with increasing frequency in children with acquired immunodeficiency syndrome (AIDS). Although bacterial parapneumonic effusions and empyema caused by the usual pathogens (*S. pneumoniae, S. aureus, H. influenzae, S. pyogenes*) remain the most common causes for effusions, other causes must be considered. *Pneumocystis jiroveci* can cause pleural effusions in children with AIDS, and a silver stain or antibody study for *P. jiroveci* should be done on all pleural fluid from these patients. Tuberculous pleural effusions with negative purified protein derivative (PPD) skin test results are unusual findings in children, but not in children with AIDS; atypical mycobacteria also can cause effusions; acid-fast bacilli (AFB) smears and cultures from pleural effusions and sputum appear to be more helpful in identifying organisms in patients with AIDS than they have been in the past for children with mycobacterial effusions and intact immune systems. Adults with AIDS and Kaposi sarcoma have effusions, but this malignancy is a rare occurrence in children. Pulmonary nocardiosis, cryptococcosis, aspergillosis, histoplasmosis, and lymphoma, as well as hypoalbuminemia and cardiac and renal problems, occur in patients with AIDS and cause effusions.

Pneumothorax may occur with increased frequency in children with AIDS. Pulmonary disease caused by *P. jiroveci*, patients treated with aerosolized pentamidine, and those with lymphoid interstitial pneumonitis are specifically at risk for pneumothoraces. Heimlich valves and surgical intervention with excision of subpleural blebs and/or pleurodesis may be needed more often in these patients because the pneumothorax may not heal with tube thoracostomy alone.

Suggested Readings

Braman SS, Donat WE. Explosive pleuritis: a manifestation of group A beta-hemolytic streptococcal infection. *Am J Med* 1986;81:723.

Buckingham SC, King MD, Miller ML. Incidence and etiologies of complicated parapneumonic effusions in children, 1996–2001. *Pediatr Infect Dis J* 2003;22:499.

Carver TW Jr, Smith TF. Pulmonary manifestations of pediatric AIDS. *Immunol Allergy Clin North Am* 1995;15:355.

Chinnock BF. Chylothorax: case report and review of the literature. *J Emerg Med* 2003;24:259.

Heller RM, Hernanz-Schulman M. Applications of new imaging modalities to the evaluation of common pediatric conditions. *J Pediatr* 1999;135:632.

Hardie WD, Roberts NE, Reising SF, Christie CDC. Complicated parapneumonic effusions in children caused by penicillin-nonsusceptible *Streptococcus pneumoniae. Pediatrics* 1998;101:388.

Lee YCG, Lane KB. Cytokines in pleural disease. In: Light RW, Lee YCG, eds. *Textbook of pleural diseases.* London: Arnold, 2003:63.

Light RW, Hamm H. Pleural disease and acquired immune deficiency syndrome. *Eur Respir J* 1997;10:2638.

Naunheim KS, Mack MJ, Hazelrigg SR, et al. Safety and efficacy of video-assisted thoracic surgical techniques for the treatment of spontaneous pneumothorax. *J Thorac Cardiovasc Surg* 1995;109:1198.

Ramnath RR, Heller RM, Ben-Ami T, et al. Implications of early sonographic evaluation of parapneumonic effusions in children with pneumonia. *Pediatrics* 1998;101:68.

Ray TL, Berkenbosch JW, Russo P, Tobias JD. Tissue plasminogen activator as an adjuvant therapy for pleural empyema in pediatric patients. *Pediatr Crit Care Med* 2003; in press.

CHAPTER 244 ■ RECURRENT OR PERSISTENT LOWER RESPIRATORY TRACT SYMPTOMS

PETER W. HIATT

Cough and wheeze are common symptoms in children. When they persist or recur, they raise parental and physician concerns that an underlying chronic lung disease is present. When confronted with this situation, physicians need to distinguish between multiple unrelated acute respiratory infections and a significant chronic pulmonary disease. The history and physical examination are extremely important in making this distinction and cannot be overemphasized.

DISTINGUISHING ACUTE AND CHRONIC DISEASE

Although cough and wheeze commonly are found in children with serious pulmonary problems, they also are manifestations of acute self-limited illness. The presence of other signs and symptoms is useful in identifying children with an underlying

---

BOX 244.1 — History and Physical Findings Suggesting Chronic Lung Disease

History
Chronic cough
Recurrent wheeze
Decreased activity
Malabsorption symptoms
Fever for longer than 3 weeks
Weight loss
Recurrent pneumonia
Chronic sputum production
Multiple serious bacterial infections
Interstitial pneumonia in first 3–6 weeks of life

Physical findings
Poor growth and nutritional status
Tachypnea
Dyspnea (head bobbing, flaring of alae nasi, use of
    accessory muscles of respiration, wheezing, grunting,
    retractions)
Hypoxia
Signs of allergy ("allergic shiners," nasal mucosal
    swelling, crease across nasal bridge)
Deviated trachea
Increased anteroposterior diameter of chest
Wheezing, crackles (rales)
Clubbing
Neurologic delay

---

chronic disorder. Box 244.1 lists signs and symptoms that suggest chronic pulmonary disease.

Generally, the closer to birth that symptoms first appear, the greater the chance is that they are secondary to a congenital malformation or the manifestation of an inherited disease.

Such malformations as tracheoesophageal fistula, laryngeal webs, and vascular rings may present shortly after birth, whereas inherited diseases may present a few months after delivery. Table 244.1 lists inherited lung diseases; the most likely candidate from this list is cystic fibrosis.

Affected children's histories should include such specific important points as the presence of fever, noisy breathing, snoring, grunting, sputum production, and environmental exposure. If acute infection is present, it usually is accompanied by fever, purulent secretions, and an overall toxic appearance of affected children. Fever accompanied by grunting often represents a pneumonic process with frequent pleural involvement. Often, noisy breathing or snoring during sleep is associated with enlarged adenoids, nasal polyposis, choanal narrowing, nasal foreign body, or Pierre Robin syndrome.

Sputum production varies in children. Generally, children younger than 5 years old are unable to expectorate their sputum; they swallow their secretions after mobilization from the lung. School-aged children begin to expectorate, and attendant physicians should ask about volume, color, viscosity, and odor of the sputum. Often, clear or white secretions are observed in children with asthma, whereas yellow-green sputum is more consistent with a bacterial infection. Blood-tinged mucus can be a sign of tuberculosis, although it can have more benign causes as well. Purulent sputum can be observed with bronchiectasis and lung abscess or can be confused with postnasal drainage from sinusitis. Environmental exposure, with a special emphasis on passive smoke inhalation, should be investigated in all children with chronic or recurrent pulmonary symptoms. Passive smoke exposure may contribute to chronic airway irritation and increase airway reactivity. Other environmental irritants to consider are wood-burning stoves, unvented gas stoves or heaters, pesticides, and airborne allergens (animal dander, molds, pollens).

The physical examination can help to confirm the presence of underlying lung disease, but normal findings in the examination do not exclude the possibility of significant abnormalities. The physical examination should begin with an evaluation of the overall nutritional status of affected children. This assessment, together with analysis of the growth curve, gives a good indication of such children's recent health. The physical examination should determine the pattern of respiration and adequacy of oxygenation and note specific signs.

First, the rate of respiration should be determined. Respiratory rate decreases with age and is measured best in infants and young children by observing with them in their mother's arms and with the children's clothing removed. Rapid rates are observed in the presence of anxiety, fever, exercise, anemia, and metabolic and respiratory disease. Slow rates can be seen with metabolic alkalosis and respiratory acidosis (central nervous system [CNS] depression). An elevated resting respiratory rate should prompt attendant physicians to look for a significant illness because tachypnea in such children is a sensitive indicator of lung disease. The ease of respiration can be determined by

TABLE 244.1
HEREDITARY DISEASES OF THE LUNGS

Agammaglobulinemia (Bruton disease)	Sex-linked recessive
	Autosomal recessive
Ataxia-telangiectasia syndrome	Autosomal recessive
Chronic granulomatous disease	Sex-linked recessive
	Autosomal recessive
Cystic fibrosis	Autosomal recessive
Familial dysautonomia	Autosomal recessive
Homozygous deficiency of alpha$_1$-antitrypsin	Autosomal recessive
Familial interstitial fibrosis	Autosomal dominant
Familial pulmonary alveolar microlithiasis	Autosomal recessive
Familial spontaneous pneumothorax	Autosomal dominant
Hunter syndrome	Sex-linked recessive
Hurler syndrome	Autosomal recessive
Kartagener syndrome	Autosomal recessive
Lung in Marfan syndrome	Autosomal dominant
Tuberous sclerosis	Autosomal dominant

observation. Usually, dyspnea represents obstructive lung disease and is observed readily in children resting in their mother's lap. Head bobbing in sleeping infants is a sign of dyspnea. The phenomenon probably is explained by use of accessory muscles during respiration. Variously, flaring of the alae nasi, use of accessory muscles of respiration, wheezing, grunting, and retractions are signs of dyspnea and indicators of respiratory disease in affected children.

Assessing adequacy of gas exchange is more difficult. An observer's ability to detect hypoxia varies, and determining hypoxia is difficult, even for experienced physicians. Most observers cannot detect hypoxia in children until oxygen saturation is 80% or less at sea level. Often, hypercapnia is associated with hypoxemia, and determining it by examination alone also is difficult; generally, an arterial blood gas is required to measure the level of carbon dioxide. Pulse oximeters allow easy noninvasive determination of oxygen saturation even in infants and young children. Although this instrument works well for measuring oxygenation, a comparable device is not readily available for easy, noninvasive measurement of carbon dioxide or acid-base balance.

The head, neck, chest, and extremities should be inspected closely. Commonly, "allergic shiners" under the eyes, nasal mucosal swelling, or a crease across the bridge of the nose is observed in children with allergic disease. Enlarged palatine tonsils are observed in some children with obstructive sleep apnea. The position of the trachea can be determined by palpating the neck. Normally midline, the trachea may be shifted to the right or left in the presence of volume loss in one lung, severe unilateral gas trapping, or a space-occupying lesion. An increase in the anteroposterior diameter of the chest is consistent with severe obstructive lung disease. Auscultation of the chest can reveal crackles, wheezes, or suppression of breath sounds. Clubbing of the extremities is an uncommon finding in children and rarely occurs in asthmatic individuals. If present, an

extensive evaluation should be undertaken to rule out chronic liver, heart, and gastrointestinal disease. Clubbing can be familial. When a pulmonary disorder is suspected, however, a search should be made for such diseases as bronchiectasis, cystic fibrosis, immotile cilia syndrome, and disorders causing interstitial fibrosis.

If a serious respiratory disorder is suspected after completion of the history and physical examination, evaluation should proceed on the basis of an age-dependent differential diagnosis.

DIFFERENTIAL DIAGNOSTIC FEATURES OF CHRONIC COUGH BY AGE

Cough clears secretions and foreign materials from the lungs. The cough reflex is composed of three parts: the afferent limb, the central cough center, and the efferent limb. The afferent portion of the cough reflex is composed of sensory fibers located in the ciliated epithelium from the pharynx to the small bronchioles. Sensory receptors are responsive to both mechanical and chemical stimuli. Impulses generated from these receptors are transmitted to the brain via the vagus nerve. Such an impulse from the lungs is received in the central cough center, which is located in the upper brainstem and pons and probably is the site of action for pharmacologic cough suppressants. Efferent impulses are initiated by the cough center and are carried by the phrenic, vagus, and spinal motor nerves to the muscles of the larynx, chest, abdominal wall, diaphragm, and pelvic floor. A complex set of muscular contractions results in a cough.

Cough is a symptom of both upper and lower airway illness, and the disease responsible for its presence must be diagnosed carefully. A chronic cough is defined as a persistent cough lasting 3 weeks or longer; Table 244.2 lists characteristics of

---

TABLE 244.2

GENERAL CHARACTERISTICS OF CHRONIC COUGH AND THEIR POTENTIAL SIGNIFICANCE

Characteristic	Significance
Nonproductive	Asthma, foreign-body aspiration, vascular ring, environmental irritants
Productive	
Clear or white	Asthma
Blood-tinged	Tuberculosis, bronchiectasis, cystic fibrosis, hemosiderosis, nasopharyngeal irritation
Purulent	Bronchiectasis, cystic fibrosis
Paroxysms	Foreign-body aspiration, pertussis
Timing of cough	
Nocturnal	Bronchospasm, postnasal discharge
On awakening	Bronchospasm, cystic fibrosis
Absent with sleep	Psychogenic cough
Shortly after lying down	Chronic sinusitis
Seasonal	Allergies, asthma
Associated activity	
Feeding	Aspiration
Exercise	Bronchospasm, bronchiectasis
Excitement	Asthma, reactive airway disease
Stress or attention	Psychogenic cough
Sleep	Asthma, reactive airway disease
Sound	
Dry and hacking	Asthma, reactive airway disease
Staccato, harsh	*Chlamydia trachomatis* acquired at birth
Posttussive whoop	Pertussis (may be absent), postviral syndrome
Honking, seal-like	Psychogenic cough, Tourette syndrome
Worsens over 2 weeks	*Mycoplasma pneumoniae* infection with headache, malaise, fever, sore throat

---

BOX 244.2   Differential Diagnosis of Chronic Cough in Children

Infants
Infection
    Adenoviruses (postviral syndrome)
    Human metapneumovirus
    Influenza virus (postviral syndrome)
    Parainfluenza virus type 3 (postviral syndrome)
    Respiratory syncytial virus (postviral syndrome)
    Rubella (congenital)
    Cytomegalovirus
    Chlamydia trachomatis (interstitial pneumonia)
    Bordetella pertussis (whooping cough)
    Lung abscess
    Tuberculosis
Aspiration
    Congenital malformation (tracheoesophageal fistula, laryngeal cleft, vascular ring)
    Neuromuscular weakness or pharyngeal incoordination
    Gastroesophageal reflux
Asthma or reactive airway disease
Environmental irritants (e.g., environmental tobacco smoke)
Cystic fibrosis
Acquired immunodeficiency syndrome
Congenital heart disease with congestive failure
Immotile cilia syndrome

Toddlers and preschool-aged children
Infection
    Adenoviruses (postviral syndrome)
    Human metapneumovirus
    Influenza virus (postviral syndrome)
    Parainfluenza virus type 3 (postviral syndrome)
    Respiratory syncytial virus (postviral syndrome)
    Bordetella pertussis (whooping cough)
    Lung abscess
    Tuberculosis

Asthma or reactive airway disease
Environmental irritants (e.g., environmental tobacco smoke)
Foreign-body aspiration
Chronic sinusitis
Cystic fibrosis
Aspiration
    Neuromuscular weakness or pharyngeal incoordination
Bronchiectasis
Congenital heart disease with congestive failure
Acquired immunodeficiency syndrome
Auricular nerve stimulation

School-aged and adolescent children
Asthma
Chronic sinusitis
Pneumonia (*Mycoplasma pneumoniae*)
Smoking, drug use
Infection
    Postviral syndrome
    Histoplasmosis, other mycotic infections
    Tuberculosis
    Lung abscess
Psychogenic or habit cough
Cystic fibrosis
Bronchiectasis
Hypersensitivity pneumonitis
Use of angiotensin-converting enzyme inhibitors
Tourette syndrome
Kartagener syndrome
Sarcoidosis
Auricular nerve stimulation

---

chronic cough and their potential associations with disease. Children's ages are important in developing a differential diagnosis, and Box 244.2 lists potential causes of chronic cough by age group. Some of the more common causes are discussed later.

Infancy

If symptoms of recurrent cough begin at birth, a congenital malformation should be suspected. Tracheoesophageal fistula and laryngeal cleft, congenital anomalies first noted in the neonatal period, lead to aspiration of milk during feedings. Affected children have symptoms of chronic aspiration, cough, and recurrent pneumonia. Vascular anomalies also can cause chronic cough and feeding disorders. Vascular rings are an assortment of large-blood-vessel abnormalities that partially obstruct the trachea and esophagus. Airway or esophageal obstruction results in respiratory distress, cough, and swallowing dysfunction. Vascular anomalies can become symptomatic shortly after birth or during the first year of life. For all these congenital anomalies, a careful barium esophagogram with special attention given to swallowing can reveal the diagnosis by illustrating esophageal compression, aspiration, or tracheoesophageal fistula. If a vascular anomaly is suspected, then a magnetic resonance imaging (MRI) scan of the chest should be obtained to demonstrate visualization of the vascular anatomy.

Similarly, disorders that affect coordination of swallowing are associated with chronic cough and wheeze because of recurrent aspiration. Swallowing dysfunction found during the neonatal period probably represents early symptoms of neuromuscular disease, severe developmental delay, or an esophageal motility problem. If a neurologic disorder exists, such associated findings as muscle tone alteration, abnormal deep-tendon reflexes, weakness, or delayed social adaptive skills can be found.

Generally, an interstitial pneumonia and cough in babies in their first 4 to 6 weeks of life represent congenital viral infection or chlamydial pneumonia. Both rubella and cytomegalovirus (CMV) can cause an interstitial pneumonia but differ in their effects on other organ systems. CMV infection acquired postnatally produces pneumonitis and hepatosplenomegaly, but it is a self-limited disease in most infants. Lung infection from *Chlamydia trachomatis* is acquired from an infected genitourinary tract in affected mothers at the time of birth. By 3 to 4 weeks after delivery, affected infants can develop conjunctivitis, interstitial pneumonia, and cough. The cough has a characteristic staccato, harsh sound and is accompanied by tachypnea and crackles that appear on examination. The chest radiography shows hyperinflation with diffuse interstitial or patchy infiltrates. Both CMV and *Chlamydia* infections can be diagnosed by culture. Antigen detection methods are the preferred test for conjunctivitis and pneumonia with *Chlamydia* infections.

The therapy of choice for the treatment of chlamydia, conjunctivitis, and pneumonia in infants is erythromycin for 2 to 3 weeks. The efficacy has been reported to range from 80% to 90% (see Chapter 86 for further information on treatment).

A paroxysmal cough in infants younger than 12 months suggests infection with *Bordetella pertussis*. Pneumonia, feeding difficulties, and choking spells from thick, tenacious mucus in the upper airway are present during pertussis infection. If secretions are not cleared well by the infant, airway obstruction and hypoxia occur repeatedly. These episodes are potentially life-threatening to the infant, who may require hospitalization for supportive care. The posttussive whoop can be absent or can appear later during the course of illness. A pertussis-like syndrome also has been reported after adenovirus and influenza virus infection. The first choice for treatment of *B. Pertussis* is a macrolide, which, if given early in the course of the illness, eliminates the organism from the respiratory tract. (For further details on treatment, see Chapter 168.)

Reactive airway disease (RAD) in infants is characterized by chronic cough, which typically is dry and hacking. The cough worsens with excitement and when the infant is asleep at night. The cough represents the first symptom of lower airway disease and may become prominent after viral respiratory infections. When RAD is suspected, a trial of symptomatic bronchodilator therapy is reasonable. If affected children respond to treatment, a presumptive diagnosis of RAD can be made. If an inadequate response occurs, additional clinical features should be reviewed to exclude other diagnoses.

As with RAD, bronchiolitis in infants usually presents with cough or wheeze. Bronchiolitis is caused most commonly by respiratory syncytial virus (RSV) occurring in yearly epidemics in the late fall and winter months. Prodromal symptoms of fever and rhinorrhea are followed by increasing lower airway symptoms of cough, wheezing, or respiratory distress. Using nasal secretions, an enzyme-linked immunosorbent assay confirms a diagnosis of RSV bronchiolitis. Usually, distinguishing clinically between RAD and bronchiolitis is difficult, particularly during affected infants' first episode of cough. A careful history and laboratory investigation are important factors in establishing the correct diagnosis. Frequently, infants who have been hospitalized with RSV bronchiolitis have recurrent cough and wheeze, with subsequent respiratory viral infections.

Several respiratory viruses can cause lower respiratory tract disease. Commonly known viruses in this group include RSV, parainfluenza virus, adenovirus, and influenza virus. Human metapneumovirus is a new RNA virus first isolated in 2001 by researchers in the Netherlands. Recent studies suggest that human metapneumovirus is a major cause of bronchiolitis and croup in children. Lower respiratory infections with this virus were similar to RSV, occurring in the winter season during the first year of life. Hospitalization rates are similar to RSV infections for lower respiratory tract disease. Rapid diagnostic tests to identify human metapneumovirus are not currently available; however, the virus can be identified by cell culture inoculation.

In infants, cystic fibrosis usually presents with recurrent respiratory symptoms or failure to thrive. In the lungs, abnormally thick mucus predisposes to infection presenting as cough, wheezing, or fever. In children with respiratory symptoms, particularly those associated with an abnormal chest radiograph and poor growth, the diagnosis of cystic fibrosis should be considered. Infants also may present with only failure to thrive as a result of malabsorption caused by pancreatic insufficiency. With either presentation, a pilocarpine iontophoresis quantitative sweat test or serum to determine the presence of two cystic fibrosis mutations should be performed to diagnose cystic fibrosis. (Refer to Chapter 236 for treatment of cystic fibrosis.)

Toddlers and Preschool-Aged Children

Asthma and postnasal drip syndrome are the most common diagnoses for preschool-aged children with chronic cough. Asthma is the respiratory disorder that occurs most frequently in children, estimated to occur in 5% of the general population. The cough in asthma occurs from both irritation of the airways and excessive production of mucus. This cough may be triggered by a variety of environmental stimuli, but in young children, most asthma episodes are precipitated by respiratory infections.

Acute cough caused by an upper respiratory tract infection usually resolves in 10 to 14 days. If a viral infection seems most likely to be the cause of these symptoms, then no further therapy is usually necessary. Although symptoms associated with these infections are problematic, there is little evidence for the effectiveness of over-the-counter cough medicines. These medications can be divided into several groups consisting of antitussives, mucolytics, and antihistamine-decongestant combinations. Very few prospective placebo-controlled trials are available that support the use of these medications in diminishing symptoms; therefore, they are not recommended for routine treatment.

Foreign-body aspiration is a common cause of chronic cough in toddlers and preschool-aged children and should be considered even if a history of choking is not obtained. Peanuts and small plastic objects are materials commonly seen in foreign-body aspiration. The cough that follows the aspiration event is sudden, violent, and sometimes followed by cyanosis. Conversely, if the obstructive object is small and does not obstruct the airway, minimal cough occurs. The cough after aspiration may resolve after 1 or 2 days, only to recur after the buildup of secretions, movement of a foreign body, or development of atelectasis. This period of time between the foreign-body aspiration and recurrence of cough may be days, weeks, or months. A chest radiograph helps in establishing the diagnosis if a radiopaque object is found or hyperinflation is noted. Inspiratory and expiratory chest radiographs can demonstrate unilateral hyperinflation. However, a normal chest radiograph does not rule out foreign-body aspiration. Lateral decubitus films may simulate expiratory radiographs in young children who are uncooperative or tachypneic. Fluoroscopy of the chest is a more sensitive, noninvasive method of assessing the dynamics of breathing in children suspected of having foreign-body aspiration; it should be used if radiographs are nondiagnostic but a high index of suspicion exists. Subtle air trapping in a particular lobe of the lung and mediastinal shift are significant. If foreign-body aspiration is suspected, a rigid bronchoscopy performed with the child under general anesthesia is indicated for evaluation and removal.

Chronic sinusitis can cause a long-standing cough. Nasal discharge and postnasal drip precipitate cough throughout the day and shortly after the child lies down at night. In allergic children, one may see only clear secretions, yet frank mucopus may be observed in other children. Upset stomachs and vomiting may be the result of swallowing drainage from the nose to the posterior pharynx; the secretions also can cause an unpleasant taste or a burning sensation in the throat. Older toddlers may convey the idea of "head hurt." Allergic disorders associated with chronic sinusitis should be treated with antihistamines and/or topical steroids once the specific allergen is identified. Nasal washes help loosen secretions and enhance mucociliary clearance. Antibiotic therapy should be based on culture and sensitivity information. If antibiotics are used, then treatment should be prescribed for at least 3 weeks.

No widely accepted definition of childhood chronic bronchitis is available; because of the strong overlap between airway reactivity with excessive production of mucus and bronchitis, separating the two conditions is difficult. In the presence of an apparent history of chronic bronchitis, other causes for this symptom complex should be entertained. Asthma, cystic fibrosis, bronchiectasis, foreign-body aspiration, infection, and immunodeficiency variously should be considered as possible underlying causes.

School-Aged Children and Adolescents

Asthma and postnasal drip syndrome are the principal causes of chronic cough in school-aged children. As such children experience fewer viral infections with increasing age, other environmental triggers become more important causes of asthma episodes. Environmental tobacco smoke is a common trigger, and often parents who smoke are the source. Older children and teenagers should be questioned in a separate interview about their own use of tobacco, marijuana, or cocaine.

With chronic sinusitis, drainage of secretions from the nose to the posterior pharynx results in a sensation of dryness or burning at the back of the nose and an unpleasant taste in the mouth. Morning headaches also may be reported.

Generally, an insidious cough that worsens over the course of 2 weeks and is accompanied by headache, malaise, fever, and sore throat is observed with infection caused by *Mycoplasma pneumoniae*. The peak incidence for this illness is between ages 10 and 15 years. During epidemics, however, older groups commonly are infected. The approach most widely used to establish a diagnosis of *M. pneumonia* is serologic demonstration of IgM (predominately) or IgG antibody by complement fixation test. Clinically, the occurrence of pneumonia in adolescents and findings of a single titer of greater than or equal to 1:32 support the diagnosis. Isolation of the organism by culture or demonstration of specific antibodies (a fourfold rise in titer in paired sera) helps to confirm the diagnosis. The treatment of choice in children with *M. pneumonia* is with a macrolide antibiotic. Azithromycin and clarithromycin offer the advantage of less frequent dosing, fewer gastrointestinal side effects, and a shorter duration of therapy compared to erythromycin.

A honking or seal-like cough in adolescents may represent a psychogenic or habit cough. Usually, it occurs after a respiratory illness and persists when other clinical symptoms of disease resolve. The cough worsens when affected children are under stress or are the focus of attention but is absent at night after such children are asleep. Usually, production of sputum is absent, and a paucity of clinical findings is present on examination. Treating such children is difficult; the intervention of psychologists or psychiatrists may help with management of these children's cough. Although rare, a similar barking cough can be seen in children with Gilles de la Tourette syndrome, but often verbal or motor tics accompany the cough. Treatment with haloperidol reportedly decreases the severity and frequency of cough in Tourette syndrome.

DIFFERENTIAL DIAGNOSTIC FEATURES OF WHEEZING BY AGE

A wheeze is a high-pitched musical sound produced by rapid vibration of a large bronchial wall. It indicates airflow obstruction from isolated or multiple sites of airway narrowing. High rates of air movement produce bronchial wall vibration, which is achieved only in large airways. Wheeze occurs when expiratory effort exceeds the pressure necessary to achieve maximal flow. Pulmonary disorders that obstruct the airway, whether caused by inflammation, mucosal edema, or bronchospasm, reduce the pleural pressure required to reach maximum flow limitation. Any greater expiratory effort produces a wheeze and

fails to improve flow in the obstructed airway. Box 244.3 lists potential causes of chronic or recurrent wheezing by different age groups. Asthma is the most common diagnosis associated with wheezing. According to the National Asthma Education and Prevention Program, the hallmarks of asthma are chronic inflammation of the airways; recurrent episodes of wheezing, breathlessness, chest tightness, and coughing; widespread but variable airflow obstruction that is reversible; and bronchial hyperresponsiveness to a variety of stimuli. These stimuli can be environmental irritants, allergens, respiratory virus infection, or exercise.

Infancy

Lower airway disease associated with respiratory viral infection is the most common cause of wheezing in infancy. Such environmental irritants as tobacco smoke or air pollution may precipitate wheezing and should be controlled whenever possible. Allergen-induced asthma becomes more prominent when children reach 3 to 4 years of age. Recurrently wheezing infants who do not respond well to initial bronchodilator medication should be considered for sweat testing because these symptoms may be the early manifestations of cystic fibrosis or gastroesophageal reflux disease.

Bronchiolitis is a common cause of wheezing in infants younger than 12 months. Most commonly, it is caused by RSV, but it has been reported after infection with human metapneumovirus, adenovirus, influenza, and parainfluenza virus. After 3 days of having cold-like symptoms, infants with RSV develop increasing respiratory distress and wheezing. Generally, bronchiolitis resolves with supportive therapy over the course of 4 to 5 days, but a high incidence of future recurrent wheezing is reported in children who require hospitalization.

In infants, recurrent aspiration of food (primarily milk) due to poor swallowing coordination can result in wheezing. Choking or cough is reported during feedings, and chest radiography demonstrates streaky infiltrates, most often in the right upper lobe or right lower lobe. Gastroesophageal reflux with aspiration has a similar radiographic appearance, but generally the history is one of frequent vomiting during or shortly after feedings. Aspiration of formula caused by tracheoesophageal fistula is associated with wheezing in infancy, but these episodes characteristically are accompanied by sudden cough and cyanosis. Often, a barium esophagogram reveals the mechanical or structural abnormality leading to aspiration events. A swallow study with a speech pathologist in attendance can be instrumental in determining abnormalities of swallowing.

Typically, vascular anomalies externally compress the tracheobronchial tree and cause wheezing during the child's first weeks of life. Both inspiratory and expiratory wheezing can be heard on auscultation, depending on the severity of airway compression. A pulmonary sling results when an anomalous left pulmonary artery compresses the right main stem bronchus, causing obstruction and hyperinflation of the right lung. A double aortic arch can cause wheezing and swallowing difficulties by compressing the trachea bilaterally and the esophagus posteriorly. A barium swallow demonstrates both bilateral and posterior indentation of the esophagus. A right aortic arch and a ligamentum ductus produce clinical symptoms similar to those of a double arch; on plain chest roentgenography, however, the trachea tends to be deviated to the right, and an esophagogram demonstrates greater indentation on the right side of the esophagus than on the left. Other radiographic findings are similar to those observed with the double aortic arch. A magnetic resonance image of the chest will define the vascular anatomy and identify the presence of a vascular ring.

Other infants who have wheezing in the first month of life are those with congenital heart disease or bronchopulmonary

BOX 244.3   Differential Diagnosis for Recurrent Wheezing in Children

Infants
Viral infection, postviral syndrome
    Respiratory syncytial virus
    Human metapneumovirus
    Parainfluenza virus type 3
    Adenoviruses
    Influenza viruses
Asthma or reactive airway disease
Cystic fibrosis
Congenital heart disease with large left-to-right shunt
Bronchopulmonary dysplasia
Acquired immunodeficiency syndrome
Aspiration
    Pharyngeal incoordination
    Gastroesophageal reflux
    Tracheoesophageal fistula
    Laryngotracheoesophageal cleft
Congenital malformation
    Vascular anomalies
    Tracheobronchial anomalies
    Lung cyst
    Mediastinal lesions (e.g., thymus hyperplasia)
Tuberculosis
Histoplasmosis, other mycotic infections
Hypocalcemia

Toddlers and preschool-aged children
Asthma or reactive airway disease
Environmental irritants (e.g., environmental tobacco smoke)
Viral infection, postviral syndrome
    Respiratory syncytial virus
    Human metapneumovirus
    Adenoviruses
    Parainfluenza virus type 3
    Influenza viruses

Foreign-body aspiration
Gastroesophageal reflux
Tuberculosis
Histoplasmosis, other mycotic infections
Cystic fibrosis
Tumor
    Leukemia
    Lymphoma
    Lymphosarcoma
Visceral larva migrans
Congenital heart disease with left-to-right shunt
Aspiration (less common)
Pulmonary hemosiderosis
Acquired immunodeficiency syndrome

School-aged and adolescent children
Asthma
Smoking, drug use
Viral infection
    Adenoviruses
    Influenza
Gastroesophageal reflux
Tuberculosis
Histoplasmosis, other mycotic infections
Tumor
    Leukemia
    Lymphoma
    Lymphosarcoma
Cystic fibrosis
Kartagener syndrome
Hypersensitivity pneumonitis
Vocal cord dysfunction
Angioneurotic edema

---

dysplasia. Airway compression caused by an enlarged heart and pulmonary congestion caused by large left-to-right shunts are responsible for the wheeze observed in infants with cardiac defects. Bronchospasm and fibrosis lead to wheezing in babies with bronchopulmonary dysplasia.

Toddlers and Preschool-Aged Children

Toddlers or preschool-aged children presenting with acute onset of wheezing should be suspected of having a foreign-body aspiration, regardless of an existing history of a choking episode. The differential diagnosis should make use of both radiography and fluoroscopy (see Differential Diagnostic Features of Chronic Cough by Age).

Acute onset of cough and wheezing usually is the result of a new viral infection. Antibiotics are used by some physicians to prevent bacterial complications of viral infections. A meta-analysis of trials in adults using prophylactic antibiotics to prevent bacterial disease following viral infections concluded that the frequency and severity of bacterial complications were not reduced. Fever is a common sign in the first 2 days of viral infection and therefore is not helpful in determining the presence of bacterial infection early in the course of infection. Wheezing bronchitis is another common finding with viral respiratory

infection and usually is not observed in children with bacterial pneumonia. Cough and wheezing illnesses that are less than 10 days in duration secondary to viral respiratory infection usually do not require antimicrobial treatment.

The principal cause of chronic wheezing in this age group is asthma. Asthma can worsen with viral respiratory infections or such environmental irritants as tobacco smoke or air pollution. The underlying cause should be identified and removed whenever possible.

Wheeze in this age group can be caused also by cystic fibrosis, bronchopulmonary dysplasia, or congenital heart disease, although generally children with these problems become symptomatic in the first 12 months of life. Wheeze associated with aspiration, whether from swallowing dysfunction or gastroesophageal reflux, also occurs less commonly in preschool-aged children unless a degenerative neurologic disease or neuromuscular disorder is present.

Disease processes that cause enlargement of the hilar and mediastinal lymph nodes can present symptomatically with wheezing by compression of a major bronchus. Enlarged lymph nodes on chest radiography should suggest an infectious disease or tumor. Tuberculosis, histoplasmosis, and other mycotic diseases are common infectious agents responsible for enlargement of lymph nodes. Generally, hilar adenopathy from tuberculosis occurs with progressive disease and is associated with symptoms of fever, anorexia, and poor weight gain. A tuber-culin skin test, with appropriate controls, aids in establishing the diagnosis of an active tuberculosis infection. Usually, histo-plasmosis is either a mild self-limited illness or an asymptomatic infection. A more severe illness can occur with malaise, weight loss, hepatosplenomegaly, and hilar adenopathy. Because of the high incidence of positive skin-test reactions in endemic areas, antigen detection in the urine, complement fixation titers, and gel diffusion studies are more helpful in making the diagnosis of histoplasmosis disease.

Enlargement of hilar and mediastinal lymph nodes can rep-resent the presence of primary or secondary tumors in affected children. Variously, leukemia, lymphoma, and lymphosarcoma can cause enlargement of hilar nodals. All children with hi-lar lymphadenopathy should receive a careful examination for other signs of malignancy, such as anemia, splenomegaly, bone pain, and fever. In children with mediastinal tumor, a diagno-sis may be established by the examination of peripheral blood smears, by biopsy of lymph nodes, or by examination of bone marrow.

Visceral larva migrans is a clinical syndrome seen in young children with a history of pica, eating of dirt, or exposure to dogs. The disease is produced by *Toxocara canis* and occurs after ingestion of ova from contaminated soil. The larvae make their way from the intestine to the lung, where they induce eosinophilic granulomas. Clinically, children have wheezing, bronchitis, hepatomegaly, and eosinophilia on peripheral blood smear. A diagnosis is made from the history, physical findings, and an elevated titer to *Toxocara* antigen (by means of enzyme-linked immunosorbent assay).

School-Aged Children and Adolescents

Most school-aged children or adolescents who wheeze have asthma. Wheezing can be triggered by respiratory allergens, by food allergens, or by respiratory irritants. Among the latter, en-vironmental tobacco smoke is a frequent culprit, and often the source is caregivers who smoke. Older children and teenagers should be questioned in a separate interview about their to-bacco or marijuana use. Respiratory infection can trigger an asthma exacerbation. Influenza virus infection is a common cause of acute respiratory illness in this age group. The disease can be prevented with yearly immunization using the trivalent inactivated vaccine and is recommended yearly for children with asthma, neuromuscular disease, and chronic lung disease.

Children with neuromuscular disease become weaker with age, losing their ability to protect their airway from secretions. Weakness then predisposes them to aspiration and pneumo-nia. Typically, other causes of wheezing, such as immotile cilia syndrome, cystic fibrosis, and congenital heart disease, are di-agnosed at an earlier age. Almost always, congenital malfor-mations have their first onset of symptoms early in life.

Suggested Readings

Castro-Rodriguez JA, Holberg CJ, Wright AL, Martinez FD. A clinical index to define risk of asthma in young children with recurrent wheezing. *J Respir Crit Care Med* 2000;162:1403.

Chang AB. Cough, cough receptors, and asthma in children. *Pediatr Pulmon* 1999;28:59.

Corrao WM. Chronic persistent cough: diagnosis and treatment update. *Pediatr Ann* 1996;25:162.

Couriel J. Assessment of the child with recurrent chest infections. *Br Med Bull* 2002;61:115.

Levison H, Tabachnik E, Newth CJL. Wheezing in infancy, croup and epiglottitis. *Curr Probl Pediatr* 1982;12:7.

Morton RL, Sheikh S, Corbett ML, Eid NS. Evaluation of the wheezy infant. *Ann Allerg Asthma Immunol* 2001;86:251.

National Heart, Lung, and Blood Institute (National Institutes of Health), National Asthma Education and Prevention Program. *Guidelines for the diagnosis and management of asthma. Expert panel report 2: clinical practice guidelines. Update on Selected Topics 2002* [NIH publ. no. 02-50741]. Bethesda, MD: National Institutes of Health, 2002.

O'Brien KL, Dowell SF, Schwartz B, et al. Cough illness/bronchitis—principles of judicious use of antimicrobial agents. *Pediatrics* 1998;101:178.

Owayed AF, Campbell DM, Wang EEL. Underlying causes of recurrent pneu-monia in children. *Arch Pediatr Adolesc Med* 2000;154:190.

Schroeder K, Fahey T. Should we advise parents to administer over the counter cough medicines for acute cough? Systematic review of randomised con-trolled trials. *Arch Dis Child* 2002;86:170.

Vaughan D, Katkin JP. Chronic and recurrent pneumonias in children. *Semin Respir Infect* 2002;17:72.

Williams JV, Harris PA, Tollefson SJ, et al. Human metapneumovirus and lower respiratory tract disease in otherwise health infants and children. *N Engl J Med* 350;5:443.

CHAPTER 245 ■ THE COMMON COLD

SARAH S. LONG

Respiratory tract illness annually accounts for more than one-half of all acute disabling conditions in U.S. adults and for an equal percentage of child outpatient visits to health care providers. The common cold, almost always caused by a virus, is the most frequent of the specific disorders. Most of the med-ical science regarding the common cold derives from studies performed in adults, with additional occasional reports in chil-dren providing the modest basis for extrapolation. All respi-ratory pathogens can cause undifferentiated upper respiratory tract illness. The term common cold should be used only for an acute illness with nasal stuffiness, rhinitis, no objective evidence of pharyngitis, and no or minimal fever.

EPIDEMIOLOGY

Peak age of occurrence is the second 6 months of life. Incidence does not fall significantly until the second decade of life. The number of colds increases during group child-care exposure in infancy. Exposure to viruses in schools and child-care centers serves to introduce viruses into the family. Boys have symp-tomatic respiratory tract illnesses more frequently than do girls. Usually, adults are victims rather than sources of common cold viruses; primary caregivers and infants have the highest rates of secondary illness.

Viruses causing the common cold spread from person to person by means of virus-contaminated respiratory secretions. Studies in adult volunteers suggested that rhinoviruses are spread by small airborne particles, by inhalation or impalement of large particles when transmitters and recipients are at very close range, and through self-inoculation after direct hand contact with a transmitter's infected nasal secretions or indirect contact with contaminated objects. Direct contact is the primary means for the spread of the common cold. Compared with adults, infected children have higher concentrations of virus in secretions and longer duration of shedding. Coughing, talking, drooling, and kissing are not highly contagious behaviors. Sneezing, nose blowing and wiping, and hand transfer of secretions from paper tissues or environmental surfaces to nose or conjunctiva are more contagious behaviors.

PATHOGENESIS

Etiologic Agents

Initially believed to be caused by either a single virus or a group of viruses, the common cold now is recognized to be associated with more than 200 viruses, occasional bacteria, protozoa, and *Mycoplasma*. Metapneumovirus, coronaviruses, and *Chlamydophila pneumoniae* are recent additions whose relative importance is not yet clear. Table 245.1 provides an abbreviated list of etiologic agents and their relative prevalence in children. Rhinoviruses and coronaviruses have even more importance in adults, in whom symptoms of the common cold are the classic manifestations of infection.

Although rhinoviruses are the most frequent cause of the common cold overall, the role of other agents can be suggested by consideration of factors related to the host and the setting

TABLE 245.1

ETIOLOGIC AGENTS OF THE COMMON COLD IN CHILDREN

Agent	Prevalence
Viruses	
Rhinoviruses	+++
Parainfluenza viruses	++
Respiratory syncytial virus	+
Coronaviruses	+
Adenoviruses	+
Enteroviruses	+
Influenza viruses	+
Reoviruses	+
Other	
Mycoplasma pneumoniae	+
Bordetella pertussis	+

+, occasional cause; ++, prevalent cause; +++, most prevalent cause.

of the illness (Table 245.2). Season (Box 245.1), age, and prior immunologic experience are the most important influences on cause. For example, disease resulting from respiratory syncytial virus and parainfluenza viruses is most common and most severe in patients who are younger than age 3. Infection occurs less commonly and with milder symptoms (frequently those of the common cold) with increasing age.

Rhinoviruses belong to the family of picornavirus, included among enteroviruses. They are RNA viruses with a diameter of 15 to 50 nm. They are ether-stable but, unlike other enteroviruses, are inactivated in 3 to 4 hours by a pH level of 3. Although serotypes are stable antigenically and type-specific immunity accrues after infection, more than 100 distinct serotypes exist, accounting for lifelong susceptibility.

TABLE 245.2

USE OF HISTORICAL INFORMATION TO DIFFERENTIATE AMONG CAUSES OF NONSPECIFIC UPPER RESPIRATORY TRACT ILLNESSES

Factor	Typical for Rhinovirus	Examples of Factors Typical for Other Etiologies	
Age	School-aged	Toddler	Parainfluenza viruses
		School-aged	*Mycoplasma pneumoniae*
Season	Fall, spring	Winter	RSV, influenza
		Summer	Adenoviruses
Immunization status	Any	Incomplete	*Bordetella pertussis*
		Incomplete	Mumps
Sibling	School-aged	Infant	RSV
		Adolescent	Adenoviruses
		Toddler	Parainfluenza viruses
Illness in contacts	Common cold	Bronchiolitis	RSV
		Croup	Parainfluenza viruses
		Conjunctivitis	Adenoviruses
		Exudative pharyngitis	Adenoviruses, Epstein-Barr virus
		Ulcerative enanthem	Enteroviruses
Incubation period	3–5 d	2 wk	*M. pneumoniae, B. pertussis*
Acquisition	Home	Hospital	RSV, influenza viruses
		Day care	All agents
Community epidemic	Common cold	Parotitis	Mumps
		Hand-foot-and-mouth disease	Enteroviruses
		Aseptic meningitis	Enteroviruses
		Febrile upper respiratory tract infection	Influenza viruses, adenoviruses

RSV, respiratory syncytial virus.

BOX 245.1 Seasonal Peaks of Respiratory Tract Pathogens

Fall
Rhinoviruses
Parainfluenza viruses
Group A streptococcus

Winter
Respiratory syncytial virus
Adenoviruses
Influenza viruses
Coronaviruses

Spring
Rhinoviruses
Parainfluenza viruses
Group A streptococcus

Summer
Adenoviruses
Bordetella pertussis
Enteroviruses

Rhinoviruses are found in nasal secretions in greater density than in oral secretions and are not found in stool specimens. Peculiar requirements for growth limit attempts at isolation to research laboratories. Most serotypes grow only in human cell lines, and some fastidious strains grow only in organ explant cultures of human tracheal or nasal epithelium. No rapid test for antigen detection is available.

Viral Pathobiology

Site of viral inoculation, cytopathic effects, and degree and mode of spread vary with the many viruses that cause common cold symptoms and the immunologic naiveté of hosts. Generally (and specifically for rhinoviruses), during primary infection, virus is inoculated onto the nasal or conjunctival mucosa. Replication follows and, within 2 days, cellular damage to respiratory epithelium leads to increased nasal secretions, with elevated protein content. Local extension causes the symptoms of nasal stuffiness, sneezing, rhinitis, and throat irritation. Frequently, paranasal sinuses are affected. Ciliary epithelium is denuded. Viral shedding peaks at 2 to 7 days in uncomplicated upper respiratory tract illness but persists at lower quantities for as long as 3 weeks. Frequently, extension to the tracheobronchial area occurs in adult volunteers after aerosol inoculation but apparently occurs to a lesser extent in natural infection.

Mucociliary dysfunction is present maximally during the acute phase of illness but can persist for weeks after recovery. Studies of pulmonary function conducted during periods in which symptomatology is confined to the upper respiratory tract suggest that occult lower respiratory tract involvement occurs. Viremia is unusual during the common cold.

Host response to infection with rhinovirus is noted by day 2 after inoculation, when nasal discharge becomes mucoid and then mucopurulent. Leukocytes, including neutrophils, are recruited to the site of viral replication and cellular damage. Interferon is produced locally by days 3 to 5 and plays an important role in halting viral replication for weeks after recovery. Specific serum-neutralizing antibody peaks on days 14 to 21, and secretory antibody peaks 1 to 2 weeks later.

Studies of adults artificially inoculated with rhinoviruses have shown that psychological stress (but not exposure to cold) increases risk of infection and that having social ties is associated with less clinical illness if a person is infected.

CLINICAL MANIFESTATIONS

The common cold syndrome has been defined as that which most typically follows rhinovirus infection. Throat irritation, sneezing, and nasal stuffiness are the primary complaints on the first and second days of illness; rhinitis, watering eyes, and sometimes hoarseness and cough follow on the second to fourth days of illness. Fever is absent or low-grade. Chilliness, headache, and achiness can be present early in the illness. Cough and nasal discharge are the most persistent complaints. Typically, illness caused by rhinoviruses lasts for 6 to 7 days. Nasal symptoms tend to be more prominent, and throat and systemic symptoms tend to be less prominent in upper respiratory tract illness caused by rhinovirus as compared with that caused by other viruses. The large number of rhinovirus types is associated predictably with variable symptoms and degrees of discomfort.

The symptoms described are typical for older children and adults. Infants are more likely to exhibit a temperature of 38°C or 39°C, fussiness, and restlessness. Nasal obstruction can interfere with sleeping and eating.

Infection with rhinovirus and other common cold viruses can extend to cause viral otitis media, sinusitis, and pneumonia or can predispose to secondary bacterial infections. Rhinoviruses cause exacerbation of bronchitis in adults and, alone or in consort with other viruses, occasionally cause pneumonia. In children with hyperreactive airways, mild viral upper respiratory tract illnesses can incite episodes of asthma or can induce pulmonary decompensation in infants with bronchopulmonary dysplasia.

THERAPY

Treatment of the common cold is supportive. No antiviral agent effective against rhinovirus is available. Use of interferon is not practical or cost-effective and has significant side effects. Recent educational initiatives aimed at health care professionals and parents have curbed inappropriate use of antibiotics. Although annual sales of proprietary cold remedies total more than $1 billion in the United States, these preparations have been shown to have no (or modest) benefit and can be harmful in children. Performing clinical trials in children is difficult, as potentially beneficial outcomes rely on subjective assessments of severity of symptoms or objective measurements that require considerable cooperation of involved subjects. On the other hand, studies of cold remedies showing benefit in adults can be misleading when symptoms are due to allergic rather than to infectious illnesses. In blinded, placebo-controlled studies in adults, rhinorrhea and sneezing improved modestly (though statistically significantly) with use of a first-generation antihistamine, as did cough with use of an antihistamine–decongestant combination. Using objective measurements, a topical adrenergic decongestant did not improve abnormal middle-ear pressure in infants with nasal congestion during the common cold. Pharmacokinetics of orally administered cold remedies given to children have been subjected to little or no study or have been shown to vary from those in older individuals. Such side effects as sedation, hypertension, and dystonic reactions are especially common in children. Considering the data (albeit imperfect) and potential benefit versus safety of cold remedies for symptoms of the common cold, nasal or oral decongestants and antihistamines should not be given to children younger than age 6 months and should be given infrequently and after individual consideration to older infants and children.

Aspirin should not be given to children with symptoms of viral illness because of its association with Reye syndrome. Acetaminophen or ibuprofen should be used infrequently for the common cold (and rarely in those younger than age 6 months) to relieve discomfort. Hepatotoxicity, hepatic failure, and deaths have occurred from inadvertent overdosing of acetaminophen, especially in infants. In adults challenged intranasally with rhinovirus, these agents were associated with suppressed antibody response and increased nasal signs and symptoms as compared with placebo.

Although in some studies vitamin C apparently reduced severity and duration of symptoms, the large doses used cannot be recommended for use in children; whether effective or not, zinc lozenges would not be practical for younger patients because of metallic taste; aromatic rubs cannot be subjected to placebo-controlled study; results of hot mist are conflicting; hot chicken soup temporarily may increase velocity of nasal mucus, but hypernatremia must be avoided; and adequate study of homeopathic and most herbal remedies has not been performed. Echinacea has been found to have no effect in placebo-controlled trials in adults and children.

Antibiotics have no place in the therapy for the common cold and have been shown to be ineffective in altering the course of attendant purulent rhinorrhea. Expected changes in character of nasal secretions during uncomplicated rhinovirus infection are progression from clear to mucoid, mucopurulent (opaque white, yellow, or green), and clear over a 7- to 10-day period.

The relief of nasal obstruction is the most important focus of supportive care. Comfortable environmental temperature and humidity should be maintained. Humidification soothes irritated nasopharyngeal mucosa and helps to prevent drying of nasal secretions, thus promoting their elimination. A placebo-controlled study in adults demonstrated no beneficial effect of steam inhalation on common cold symptoms. Use of isotonic saline nasal drops and gentle aspiration or, occasionally, higher-volume nasal saline flush can provide temporary relief for young infants.

PREVENTION

Meticulous hand washing by staff should be practiced in hospitals and other facilities where small children are located. Personal hygiene should be taught to children. Phenol-alcohol solution (Lysol) is an effective environmental disinfectant, as are tincture of iodine and povidone-iodine.

Interest in the development of a vaccine against the common cold viruses waned when continual antigenic drift of rhinoviruses was considered the best explanation for the multiple serotypes, conventional parenteral routes of vaccine administration did not provide protection against nasal challenge, and nasal inoculation provided only short-term benefit. The task of developing an attenuated nasal vaccine seems less formidable now that the serotypes of rhinovirus appear to be multiple but stable and the number of serotypes causing the majority of disease may be only 30.

Suggested Readings

Bauchner H, Besser RE. Promoting the appropriate use of oral antibiotics: there is some very good news. *Pediatrics* 2003;111:668.

Cohen S, Doyle WJ, Skoner DP, et al. Social ties and susceptibility to the common cold. *JAMA* 1997;277:1940.

De Smet P. Herbal remedies. *N Engl J Med* 2002;347:2046.

Falck G, Gnarpe J, Gnarpe H. Prevalence of *Chlamydia pneumoniae* in healthy children and in children with respiratory tract infections. *Pediatr Infect Dis J* 1997;16:549.

Graham NMH, Burrell CJ, Douglas RM, et al. Adverse effects of aspirin, acetaminophen, and ibuprofen on immune function, viral shedding, and clinical status in rhinovirus-infected volunteers. *J Infect Dis* 1990;162:1277.

Heikkinen T, Järvinen A. The common cold. *Lancet* 2003;361:51.

Heubi JE, Barbacci MB, Zimmerman HJ. Therapeutic misadventures with acetaminophen: hepatotoxicity after multiple doses in children. *J Pediatr* 1998; 132:22.

Mainous AG III, Hueston WJ, Eberlein C. Colour of respiratory discharge and antibiotic use. *Lancet* 1997;350:1077.

Musher DM. How contagious are common respiratory tract infections? *N Engl J Med* 2003;348:1256.

Nokso-Koivisto J, Pitkäranta A, Blomqvist S, et al. Viral etiology of frequently recurring respiratory tract infections in children. *Clin Inf Dis* 2002;35:540.

Schwartz RH. The nasal saline flush procedure [letter]. *Pediatr Infect Dis J* 1997;16:725.

Taylor JA, Weyler W, Standisk L, et al. Efficacy and safety of echinacea in treating upper respiratory tract infections in children: a randomized controlled trial. *JAMA* 2003;290:2824.

Turner RB, Darden PM. Effect of topical adrenergic decongestants on middle ear pressure in infants with common colds. *Pediatr Infect Dis J* 1996;15:621.

Turner RB, Sperber SJ, Sorrentino JV, et al. Effectiveness of clemastine fumarate for treatment of rhinorrhea and sneezing associated with the common cold. *Clin Infect Dis* 1997;25:824.

van Elden LJ, van Loon AM, van Alphen F, et al. Frequent detection of human coronaviruses in clinical specimen from patients with respiratory tract infection by use of a novel real-time reverse-transcriptase polymerase chain reaction. *J Infect Dis* 2004;189:652.

Wolf DG, Zakay-Rones Z, Fadeela A, et al. High seroprevalence of human metapneumovirus among young children in Israel. *J Inf Dis* 2003;188:1865.

CHAPTER 246 ■ PARANASAL SINUSITIS

ELLEN R. WALD

Acute infection of the paranasal sinuses is a common complication of allergic or infectious inflammation of the upper respiratory tract. Approximately 5% of upper respiratory infections are complicated by acute sinusitis. Because adults average two to three colds per year and children experience six to eight, sinusitis is a problem seen commonly in clinical practice.

Of the four paired paranasal sinuses—ethmoid, maxillary, sphenoid, and frontal—all but the frontal sinuses are present at birth. The frontal sinuses develop from the anterior ethmoid sinuses and become clinically important after the tenth birthday. The maxillary and ethmoid sinuses are the principal sites of sinus infection in young children.

ANATOMY

The anatomic relationship between the nose and the paranasal sinuses is shown in Fig. 246.1. The nose is divided in the midline by the nasal septum. From the lateral wall of the nose emerge three shelf-like structures: the inferior, middle, and superior turbinates. Beneath the middle and the superior turbinates is a natural meatus that drains two or more of the paranasal sinuses. The posterior ethmoid sinus and the sphenoid sinuses drain into the superior meatus, and the anterior ethmoid sinuses, the frontal sinuses, and the maxillary sinuses drain into

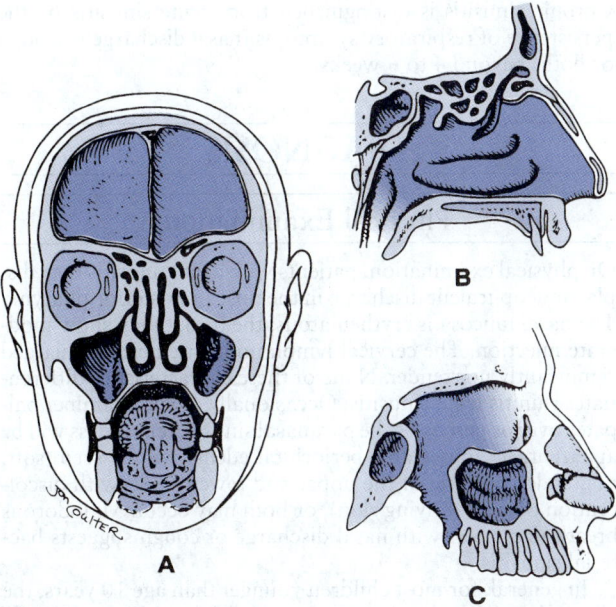

FIGURE 246.1. Anatomy of the paranasal sinuses. **A:** Coronal section demonstrating the relationship between the nose and the ethmoid and maxillary sinuses. **B:** Sagittal section showing the nasal turbinates as well as the frontal, ethmoid, and sphenoidal sinus. **C:** Parasaggital section shows the body of the maxillary and sphenoid sinus.

the middle meatus; only the lacrimal duct drains into the inferior meatus. The position of the outflow tract of the maxillary sinus, high on the medial wall of the sinus cavity, impedes gravitational drainage of secretions and accounts for the frequency of involvement of the maxillary sinuses when upper respiratory tract inflammation becomes complicated by bacterial superinfection.

PATHOPHYSIOLOGY AND PATHOGENESIS

Three elements are important to the normal physiology of the paranasal sinuses: the patency of the ostia, the function of the ciliary apparatus, and, integral to the latter, the quality of secretions. Retention of secretions in the paranasal sinuses is caused by one or more of the following: obstruction of the ostia, reduction in the number (or impaired function) of the cilia, or overproduction or change in the viscosity of the secretions.

Ostial Obstruction

The ostia of the paranasal sinuses are the key to disorders in the sinus area. The ostia of the maxillary sinuses are small, tubular structures having a diameter of 2.5 mm (cross-sectional area, approximately 5 mm) and a length of 6 mm. The diameter of the ostium of each of the individual ethmoid air cells that drains independently into the middle meatus is even smaller, measuring 1 to 2 mm. The narrow caliber of these individual ostia sets the stage for obstruction to occur easily and often.

The factors predisposing to ostial obstruction can be divided into those that cause mucosal swelling and those that result from mechanical obstruction (Box 246.1). Although many conditions may lead to ostial closure, viral upper respiratory infection and allergic inflammation are by far the most common and most important.

BOX 246.1   Factors Predisposing to Sinus Ostial Obstruction

Mucosal Swelling
Systemic disorder
　Viral upper respiratory infection
　Allergic inflammation
　Cystic fibrosis
　Immune disorders
　Immotile cilia
Local insult
　Facial trauma
　Swimming, diving
　Rhinitis medicamentosa
Mechanical Obstruction
Choanal atresia
Deviated septum
Nasal polyps
Foreign body
Tumor

Alternation in Ciliary Number or Function

In the posterior two-thirds of the nasal cavity and within the sinuses, the epithelium is pseudostratified columnar, in which most of the cells are ciliated. Usually, the normal motility of the cilia and the adhesive properties of the mucous layer protect the respiratory epithelium from bacterial invasion. However, certain respiratory viruses (influenza, adenovirus) may have a direct cytotoxic effect on the cilia. The alteration of cilia number, morphology, and function may facilitate secondary bacterial invasion of the nose and the paranasal sinuses.

Microbiology

Maxillary sinus aspiration in children with acute bacterial sinusitis has shown the microbiologic features of sinus secretions to be similar to those found in acute otitis media. The predominant organisms are *Streptococcus pneumoniae*, *Moraxella catarrhalis*, and nontypeable *Haemophilus influenzae*. Both *H. influenzae* and *M. catarrhalis* may produce beta-lactamase and, consequently, may be resistant to amoxicillin. In addition, a dramatic increase has been seen in the frequency of *S. pneumoniae* isolates not susceptible to penicillin. As many as 50% of maxillary sinus isolates have a minimum inhibitory concentration of more than 0.1 μg/mL for penicillin. The risk factors that predispose to penicillin-nonsusceptible isolates of *S. pneumoniae* are recent receipt of antimicrobials, attendance at day care, and age less than 2 years. Anaerobic isolates and staphylococci rarely are recovered. Several viruses, including adenoviruses, influenza viruses, parainfluenza viruses, and rhinoviruses, have been isolated from maxillary sinus aspirates. Summary figures for the prevalence of various bacterial species in children with acute sinusitis are shown in Table 246.1. The performance of nasal, throat, or nasopharyngeal cultures is of no value in patients with acute sinusitis, because the results are not predictive of the bacterial isolates within the maxillary sinus cavity. The microbiology of chronic sinusitis differs slightly from that of acute sinusitis. Anaerobes of the respiratory tract, viridans streptococci, and, occasionally, *Staphylococcus aureus* are found in addition to the aerobes of acute sinusitis.

TABLE 246.1

BACTERIOLOGY OF ACUTE SINUSITIS

Bacterial species	Prevalence (%)
Streptococcus pneumoniae	25–30
Moraxella catarrhalis	15–20
Haemophilus influenzae	15–20
Streptococcus pyogenes	2–5
Anaerobes	2–5
Sterile	20–35

CLINICAL MANIFESTATIONS

In most children with acute or chronic sinusitis, the respiratory symptoms of nasal discharge, nasal congestion, and cough are prominent. During the course of an apparent viral upper respiratory tract infection, two common clinical presentations suggest a diagnosis of acute sinusitis.

The first, most common clinical situation raising suspicion of sinusitis is the presence of persistent signs and symptoms of a cold. Nasal discharge and daytime cough that continue beyond 10 days and are not improving are the principal complaints. Most uncomplicated upper respiratory tract infections last for 5 to 7 days; although patients may not be asymptomatic by the tenth day, usually their condition has improved. The persistence of respiratory symptoms without appreciable improvement beyond the 10-day mark suggests that a complication has developed. The nasal discharge may be of any quality (thin or thick, clear, mucoid, or purulent), and usually the cough (which may be dry or wet) is present in the daytime, although often it is noted to be worse at night. Cough occurring only at night is a common residual symptom of an upper respiratory tract infection. When it is the only residual symptom, usually it is nonspecific and does not suggest a sinus infection; it is more likely to represent reactive airways disease. Conversely, the persistence of daytime cough frequently is the symptom that brings affected children to medical attention. Such children may not appear ill; usually, if fever is present, it will be low grade. Often, malodorous breath is reported by parents of affected preschoolers. The complaint of malodorous breath accompanied by respiratory symptoms (in the absence of exudative pharyngitis, dental decay, or nasal foreign body) is a clue to the presence of a sinus infection. Facial pain rarely is present, although intermittent, painless, periorbital swelling (present in the morning and resolving later in the day) may have been noted by observant parents. In this case, the persistence, not the severity, of the clinical symptoms calls for attention.

The second, less common presentation is a cold that seems more severe than usual. The fever is high (greater than 39°C), the nasal discharge is purulent and copious, and associated periorbital swelling or facial pain may be present. The periorbital swelling may involve the upper or lower eyelid; it is gradual in onset (evolving over hours to days) and most obvious in the morning after awakening. The swelling may decrease and actually disappear during the day, only to reappear the following day. A less common complaint is headache (a feeling of fullness or a dull ache either behind or above the eyes), reported most often in children older than 5 years. Occasionally, such children complain of dental pain, either from infection originating in the teeth or from pain referred from the sinus infection.

Headache is not a common complaint in children with acute sinusitis. When headache is a symptom of acute sinusitis, it is almost always accompanied by prominent respiratory complaints. Usually, the headache is most severe on awakening and is relieved partially when affected patients are up and about.

Chronic sinusitis is distinguished from acute sinusitis by the persistence of respiratory symptoms (nasal discharge or cough or both) beyond 4 to 6 weeks.

DIAGNOSIS

Physical Examination

On physical examination, patients with acute sinusitis may display mucopurulent discharge in the nose or posterior pharynx. The nasal mucosa is erythematous; the throat may show moderate injection. The cervical lymph nodes are neither enlarged significantly nor tender. None of these characteristics differentiates rhinitis from sinusitis. Occasionally, as the examiner palpates over or percusses the paranasal sinuses, tenderness will be apparent, or appreciable periorbital edema will be seen (soft, nontender swelling of the upper and lower eyelid with discoloration of the overlying skin), or both may occur. Malodorous breath in concert with nasal discharge or cough suggests bacterial sinusitis.

In general, for most children younger than age 10 years, the physical examination is not very helpful in making a specific diagnosis of acute sinusitis. However, if the mucopurulent material can be removed from the nose and the nasal mucosa is treated with topical vasoconstrictors, pus may be seen coming from the middle meatus. The latter observation, the presence of periorbital swelling, or a combination is the most specific finding in acute sinusitis.

Radiography

Traditionally, radiography has been used to determine the presence or absence of sinus disease. Standard radiographic projections include an anteroposterior, a lateral, and an occipitomental view. The anteroposterior view is optimal for evaluation of the ethmoid sinuses, and the lateral view is best for viewing the frontal and sphenoid sinuses. The occipitomental view, taken after tilting the chin upward 45 degrees from the horizontal, allows evaluation of the maxillary sinuses. The radiographic findings most diagnostic of bacterial sinusitis are the presence of an air-fluid level in, or complete opacification of, the sinus cavities (Fig. 246.2). However, an air-fluid level is an uncommon radiographic finding in children with acute sinusitis who are younger than 7 or 8 years old. In the absence of an air-fluid level or complete opacification of the sinuses, measuring the degree of mucosal swelling may be useful. If the width of the sinus mucosa is 5 mm or greater in adults or 4 mm or greater in children, the sinus aspirate likely will contain pus or will yield a positive bacterial culture. When clinical signs and symptoms suggesting acute sinusitis are accompanied by abnormal maxillary sinus radiographic findings, bacteria will be present in a sinus aspirate 70% of the time. A normal radiograph is strong evidence that a sinus is free of disease.

Computed tomographic (CT) scans are superior to plain film radiography in the delineation of sinus abnormalities. However, such scans are not necessary in children with uncomplicated acute sinusitis and should be reserved for the evaluation of children with recurrent, chronic, or complicated sinus infections.

Sinus Aspiration

To establish the precise cause of a sinus infection, aspiration of the maxillary sinus (the most accessible of the sinuses) can be performed in children who are older than 2 years. Puncture

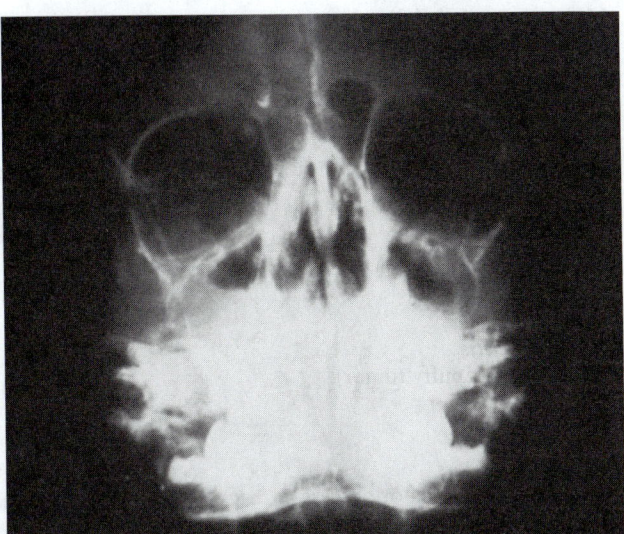

FIGURE 246.2. Maxillary sinusitis. This radiograph demonstrates bilateral maxillary sinusitis. There is an air-fluid level present in the right maxillary sinus and an example of mucosal swelling demonstrated in the left maxillary sinus.

is performed best by the transnasal route, with the needle directed beneath the inferior turbinate through the lateral nasal wall. This route is preferred to avoid injury to the natural ostium and to permanent dentition. Careful sterilization of the puncture site is essential to prevent contamination by nasal flora. Indications for sinus aspiration in patients with suspected sinusitis include clinical unresponsiveness to conventional therapy, sinus disease in an immunosuppressed patient, such severe symptoms as intense and unremitting headache or facial pain, and such life-threatening complications as intraorbital or intracranial suppuration at the time of clinical presentation.

Differential Diagnosis

The major symptoms that prompt consideration of the diagnosis of acute sinusitis are persistent or purulent nasal discharge and persistent cough. Alternative diagnoses to consider for patients with purulent nasal discharge are simple viral upper respiratory infection, group A streptococcal infection, adenoiditis, and nasal foreign body. In simple upper respiratory infection, usually the purulent nasal discharge is accompanied by low-grade fever and other elements of upper respiratory inflammation, such as pharyngitis and conjunctivitis. The symptoms commonly begin to improve after a few days. Streptococcal infection in children younger than 3 years, so-called streptococcosis, may present with such persistent respiratory symptoms as nasal discharge, low-grade fever, lassitude, and poor appetite. The diagnosis can be excluded by culturing the nasopharynx or throat for group A streptococci. Adenoiditis is suggested when purulent nasal discharge persists without improvement beyond 10 days in patients with normal sinus radiographic findings. Usually, a nasal foreign body is characterized by unilateral nasal discharge, which is purulent and often bloody. Most strikingly, the nasal discharge is very foul-smelling, a fact that often can be noted from the doorway of the examining room.

Patients who have persistent cough as the most troublesome symptom prompt the consideration of several diagnoses, including reactive airways disease, *Mycoplasma pneumoniae*

bronchitis, cystic fibrosis, whooping cough, and gastroesophageal reflux. Reactive airways disease triggered by upper respiratory infection may cause dramatic cough without accompanying wheezing. Occasionally, this condition occurs in conjunction with acute sinusitis, but more often it is a residual symptom after an upper respiratory infection and substantially prolongs the clinical course of the illness.

Usually, *Mycoplasma* bronchitis occurs in children between the ages of 5 and 15 years. The illness begins with a prominent sore throat and fever. As the upper respiratory symptoms subside, cough begins and becomes prominent and persistent. Infection with *Bordetella pertussis* begins with nasal discharge. Soon the cough becomes the prominent symptom. If the cough is paroxysmal, the diagnosis may be recognized quickly. In partially immune children, the cough may not be characteristic. Cystic fibrosis should be considered in children with persistent cough, although it is unlikely to explain the symptom in previously thriving children who present with an intercurrent illness. Gastroesophageal reflux may be responsible for pulmonary and neurologic symptoms and for failure to thrive. It should be considered most seriously in children who have nighttime coughing only or in those who have had poorly controlled asthma or previous episodes of pneumonia.

THERAPY

The objectives of antimicrobial therapy for acute sinus infection are achievement of a rapid clinical cure, sterilization of the sinus secretions, prevention of suppurative orbital and intracranial complications, and prevention of chronic sinus disease.

Antimicrobial Agents

The relative frequency of occurrence of the various bacterial agents suggests that a combination of amoxicillin and potassium clavulanate (Augmentin) at 90 and 6.4 mg/kg/day, respectively, in two divided doses, is an appropriate drug regimen for most cases of acute sinusitis in children (Table 246.2). This dose of amoxicillin will result in a concentration of antimicrobial within the paranasal sinuses that will exceed the minimum inhibitory concentration of all isolates of *S. pneumoniae* that are susceptible and intermediate in susceptibility to penicillin. The minimum inhibitory concentration of some but not all highly resistant *S. pneumoniae* will also be exceeded. This small amount of potassium clavulanate will be sufficient

TABLE 246.2

ANTIMICROBIALS AND DOSAGE SCHEDULES FOR THE TREATMENT OF SINUSITIS IN CHILDREN

Antimicrobial Agent	Dose
Amoxicillin	60–90 mg/kg/day in two divided doses
Amoxicillin-potassium	90/6.7 mg/kg/day in two divided doses
Trimethoprim-sulfamethoxazole	8/40 mg/kg/day in two divided doses
Cefuroxime axetil	30 mg/kg/day in two divided doses
Cefprozil	30 mg/kg/day in two divided doses
Cefpodoxime proxetil	10 mg/kg/day once daily
Cefdinir	14 mg/kg/day in a single daily dose
Azithromycin	10 mg/kg/day on day 1; 5 mg/kg/day on days 2 to 5 in a single daily dose

to inhibit the growth of all beta-lactamase–producing *H. influenzae* and *M. catarrhalis*. Potassium clavulanate irreversibly binds the beta-lactamase, if it is present, and thereby restores amoxicillin to its original spectrum of activity. Most alternative therapies for patients who cannot tolerate or who fail to respond to amoxicillin and potassium clavulanate are not as potent as high-dose amoxicillin and clavulanate. Cefuroxime axetil (Ceftin), 30 mg/kg in two divided doses, cefdinir (Omnicef), 14 mg/kg once daily, cefprozil (Cefzil), 30 mg/kg in two divided doses, and cefpodoxime (Vantin), 10 mg/kg given once daily are available but inferior substitutes. For patients with serious hypersensitivity reactions to beta-lactams, azithromycin (Zithromax) is a reasonable alternative, although it has not been approved for this indication by the Food and Drug Administration. When emesis precludes oral therapy but does not mandate admission to the hospital, intramuscular ceftriaxone (50 mg/kg/once daily) can be used until oral therapy is tolerated. Patients with acute sinusitis may require hospitalization because of systemic toxicity or inability to take oral antimicrobial agents. These patients may be treated with either ceftriaxone, at a dosage of 80 to 100 mg/kg/day, or cefotaxime, at 200 mg/kg/day intravenously, in two and four divided doses, respectively.

Clinical improvement is prompt in nearly all children treated with an appropriate antimicrobial agent. Patients febrile at the initial encounter will become afebrile, and a remarkable reduction in nasal discharge and cough takes place within 48 hours. If affected patients do not improve or worsen in 48 hours, clinical reevaluation is appropriate. If the diagnosis is unchanged, sinus aspiration may be considered for precise bacteriologic information.

Usually, the antimicrobial regimens recommended to treat acute sinusitis are prescribed for 10 to 14 days. If affected patients are improved but not recovered completely by 10 or 14 days, continuing treatment for another week is reasonable. In patients with chronic sinusitis, antimicrobial therapy should be maintained for 3 to 4 weeks.

The effectiveness of antihistamines or decongestants, or combinations thereof, applied topically (by inhalation) or administered by mouth in patients with acute or chronic sinus infection has not been studied adequately. Because appropriate antimicrobial therapy results in prompt clinical improvement within 48 to 72 hours, usually additional pharmacologic agents are not necessary.

Irrigation and Drainage

Irrigation and drainage of infected sinuses may result in dramatic relief of pain for patients with acute sinusitis. Usually, drainage procedures are reserved for those who fail to respond to medical therapy with antimicrobial agents, for immunosuppressed patients who may be infected with unusual microbiologic species, or for those who have a suppurative intraorbital or intracranial complication. If an episode of acute sinusitis cannot be treated effectively by medical therapy alone or by medical therapy and simple sinus puncture, more radical surgery may become necessary.

Surgical Therapy

Surgical therapy in children with chronic sinusitis initially focused on creating a nasoantral window, or fistula, in the maxillary sinus to facilitate gravitational drainage. However, these fistulas proved to be relatively ineffective, in part because the cilia that line the maxillary sinus still transport secretions toward the natural meatus.

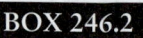

| **BOX 246.2** | **Major Complications of Sinusitis** |

Orbital
Inflammatory edema (preseptal or periorbital cellulitis)
Subperiosteal abscess
Orbital abscess
Orbital cellulitis
Optic neuritis

Osteomyelitis
Frontal (Pott puffy tumor)
Maxillary

Intracranial
Epidural abscess
Subdural empyema or abscess
Cavernous or sagittal sinus thrombosis
Meningitis
Brain abscess

At present, the focus of surgical therapy is the ostiomeatal unit. Most current surgical efforts involve using an endoscope to enlarge the natural meatus of the maxillary outflow tract by excising the uncinate process and the ethmoidal bullae and performing an anterior ethmoidectomy. Endoscopic surgery in children requires further systematic study. It may be helpful for patients with cystic fibrosis or for those with specific anatomic abnormalities. Unclear is which other patients will benefit more from surgical therapy than from medical therapy alone.

COMPLICATIONS

Complications of sinus disease may cause both substantial morbidity and occasional mortality. Major complications result from either contiguous spread or hematogenous dissemination of infection. A complete list of the major complications of sinusitis is provided in Box 246.2.

Orbital Complications

Clinical Manifestations and Diagnosis

Orbital complications are the most common serious complications of acute sinusitis and, despite antimicrobial therapy, may lead to loss of vision and severe morbidity. The usual presenting feature of sinus-related orbital complications is a swollen eye. A classification useful in establishing the severity of the orbital cellulitis is shown in Table 246.3. Clinical establishment of the severity of the cellulitis is essential so appropriate decisions can be made regarding specific therapy and the need for surgical drainage. With early involvement (stage I), the inflammatory edema is confined to the medial aspect of the upper or lower eyelid. Gradual onset of lid swelling, minimal skin discoloration, and low-grade or no fever are present. No proptosis, visual impairment, or limitation of extraocular movement is observed. This condition is not an actual infection of the orbit but, rather, swelling caused by impedance of the local venous drainage. As such, it must be distinguished from a much more virulent form of periorbital or so-called preseptal cellulitis caused by bacteremic infection with either *H. influenzae* type b or *S. pneumoniae*. The septum is a connective tissue

TABLE 246.3

CLINICAL STAGING OF ORBITAL CELLULITIS

Stage	Clinical Features
I: Inflammatory edema	Inflammatory edema, beginning in medial aspect of upper or lower eyelid; nontender erythema may be prominent; no induration, visual impairment, or limitation of extraocular movement
II: Subperiosteal abscess	Abscess beneath the periosteum of the ethmoid or frontal bone; proptosis down and out, varying degrees of chemosis, and limitation of extraocular movement
III: Orbital abscess	Abscess within the fat or muscle cone in the posterior orbit; severe chemosis and proptosis; complete ophthalmoplegia and moderate to severe vision loss (globe displaced forward or down and out)
IV: Orbital cellulitis	Edema of orbital contents with varying degrees of proptosis, chemosis, limitation of extraocular movement, or vision loss
V: Cavernous sinus	Proptosis, globe fixation, severe loss of thrombophlebitis visual acuity, prostration, signs of meningitis; progresses to proptosis, chemosis, and vision loss in the contralateral eye

Modified from Chandler JR, Langenbrunner DJ, Stevens ER. The pathogenesis of orbital complications in acute sinusitis. *Laryngoscope* 1970;80:1414.

reflection of periosteum that inserts into the eyelid and provides an anatomic barrier protecting the orbit. Both inflammatory edema and *H. influenzae* type b preseptal infection involve tissues anterior to the orbital contents. *H. influenzae* type b periorbital cellulitis, however, is characterized by an abrupt onset, rapid progression, and severe systemic toxicity. The markedly swollen and tender periorbital tissue has a violaceous, almost hemorrhagic discoloration, the texture of the skin is altered, and the subcutaneous tissue is indurated. *H. influenzae* type b is recovered frequently (and *S. pneumoniae* less often) from blood cultures and tissue aspirates. Because most *H. influenzae* organisms isolated from sinus aspirates are nontypeable, the relationship, if any, of these acute bacteremic *H. influenzae* type b infections to sinusitis is unclear. Other entities to distinguish from inflammatory edema include an infected periorbital or blepharal laceration, insect bite, contact allergy, conjunctivitis, dacryocystitis, and eczematoid dermatitis.

When proptosis and ophthalmoplegia are present, stages II to V of orbital complications must be considered (see Box 246.2). When infection tracks backward into the cavernous sinus, affected patients will have signs of meningitis, focal or generalized seizures, deterioration of consciousness, and, usually, involvement of the opposite eye by way of the circumfundibular communicating conduits between the two cavernous sinuses.

When eye swelling is the result of inflammatory edema, plain film radiography of the sinuses will disclose partial or complete opacification, mucous membrane thickening, or an air–fluid level. Most commonly, the ethmoid and maxillary sinuses are involved together, but in patients with a history of chronic sinus disease, pansinusitis is the usual finding. In early and late stages, the orbit, the paranasal sinuses, and the intracranial dural venous sinuses can be studied simultaneously with contrast-enhanced CT. Thin CT cuts of the orbit, using the multiplanar imaging technique, also are helpful in detecting and defining the extent of subperiosteal and orbital abscesses.

Therapy and Prognosis

Occasionally, children with stage I disease can be treated carefully as outpatients by the usual regimen for acute sinusitis, provided their parents are cooperative and can return for reevaluation readily. The antimicrobial agent selected must provide an antibacterial spectrum that includes beta-lactamase–producing *H. influenzae* and *M. catarrhalis*. Careful follow-up is essential to detect progression of infection and the need for hospitalization. If the infection has progressed beyond stage I, hospitalization and intravenous antibiotics are mandatory. The choice of antibiotics is guided by knowledge of the usual bacteriology of acute sinusitis. Ceftriaxone, 80 to 100 mg/kg/day intravenously in one or two doses, or cefotaxime, 200 mg/kg/day in four divided doses, is an appropriate selection. Ampicillin-sulbactam

(Unasyn), 200 mg/kg/day intravenously in four divided doses, likewise is a reasonable combination. Blood and sinus aspirates should be obtained and cultured aerobically and anaerobically; appropriate antimicrobial agents should be added if unsuspected organisms are isolated or observed on Gram staining of purulent material obtained from the sinus cavity or orbit. Surgical drainage is required for many subperiosteal or orbital abscesses depending on their size and clinical presentation, but orbital cellulitis may respond to antimicrobial agents without surgical intervention. Usually, the prognosis for patients with stage I and stage II disease is excellent if diagnosis and appropriate therapy are carried out promptly, but residual loss of vision as a result of infection of the optic nerve may complicate orbital abscesses. Severe neurologic sequelae or death may follow cavernous sinus thrombophlebitis.

Intracranial Complications

Intracranial extension of infection is the second most common complication of acute sinusitis. Although the incidence of suppurative intracranial disease in patients with sinusitis is unknown, paranasal sinusitis is the source of 35% to 65% of subdural empyemas.

Clinical Manifestations

Four groups of symptoms and signs may be recognized:

- *Signs of pansinusitis*: Approximately 50% to 60% of patients with subdural empyema secondary to sinusitis have symptoms of acute frontal sinusitis or an acute exacerbation of chronic pansinusitis. They have low-grade fever, malaise, frontal headache, and marked forehead and maxillary tenderness to digital pressure. Occasionally, subperiosteal pus overlying the anterior wall of the frontal sinus results in dramatic epicranial edema and a painful fluctuation called *Pott puffy tumor*.
- *Signs of increased intracranial pressure*: With increased intracranial pressure, an initial headache worsens despite repeated doses of analgesic and oral antibiotic agents. Vomiting becomes intractable, and the level of consciousness deteriorates gradually. High intracranial pressure results from local cerebral edema in the area adjacent to the subdural pus, and it may progress rapidly to cause stupor and coma. With an isolated extradural empyema, cortical involvement is less extensive, and affected patients generally remain alert.
- *Signs of meningeal irritation*: During the stage of depressed sensorium, usually nuchal rigidity and photophobia are seen. This condition reflects an intense

inflammatory response in the leptomeninges in contact with a subdural abscess, rather than septic leptomeningitis.

- *Focal neurologic deficits*: These deficits are caused by a combination of local brain compression (by the empyema), edema, and infarction. A frontoparietal convexity subdural empyema causes contralateral brachiofacial weakness, contralateral conjugate gaze palsy, and expressive dysphasia. Usually, lower limb involvement occurs late. Focal seizures involving the arm and face occur in more than 60% of patients with dorsolateral lesions. With parafalcine empyema, often Jacksonian seizures begin in the foot and march upward and include the trunk, arm, and face. Weakness also affects primarily the leg, with sparing of speech and facial musculature. Bilateral parafalcine collections may present with paraplegia, simulating thoracic spinal cord compression. In the disease's terminal stage, affected patients are comatose and hemiplegic, have evidence of generalized and meningeal sepsis, and, finally, show signs of uncal or tonsillar herniation.

Diagnosis

Intracranial infection should be suspected if signs of systemic toxicity and headache do not improve after an adequate course of oral antibiotics has been given for the original sinusitis. Diagnostic tests must be arranged immediately if the headache becomes excruciating, if systemic toxicity worsens, or if intractable vomiting or visual blurring develops. Whenever meningeal signs develop in patients with sinusitis, attendant clinicians may be tempted to obtain cerebrospinal fluid by lumbar puncture. They must remember, however, that pure meningitis rarely occurs with sinusitis and that all the other intracranial suppurative complications are mass lesions likely to cause brain herniation with lumbar puncture. Therefore, this procedure should be deferred until the CT scan has ruled out empyema and abscess.

CT scanning is recognized now as the most definitive test for the diagnosis of intracranial suppuration secondary to sinusitis; it virtually has eliminated the need for cerebral angiography, radionuclide scanning, and electroencephalography. This noninvasive procedure defines and localizes even small purulent collections exactly, delineates associated cerebral edema, assesses the amount of brain shift, and detects concomitant brain abscess or bilateral empyema that often was missed by angiography in the era before CT. The extent of sinus disease also can be evaluated concurrently by low axial cuts that include the ethmoid, sphenoid, and maxillary sinuses. Characteristically, a parenchymal abscess shows up as a low-density center with an intensely enhancing capsule and surrounding edema. Extracerebral empyema always possesses an enhancing inner membrane, and often the underlying cerebral edema causes an impressive midline brain shift that cannot be explained by the amount of pus present. This combination of a small extracerebral collection and a disproportionate degree of brain shift distinguishes subdural empyema from chronic subdural hematoma, in which the severity of brain shift is determined primarily by the size of the clot.

Therapy and Prognosis

The treatment of sinusitis-related intracranial suppuration requires antimicrobial agents, drainage, and excellent supportive care. Rarely, brain abscess or highly selected cases of subdural empyema may be treated nonoperatively. More commonly, aspiration rather than excision is the operative procedure performed. Because either acute sinusitis or an acute exacerbation of chronic sinusitis may precede intracranial complications, the antibiotics selected must be appropriate to include activity against *S. pneumoniae*, *H. influenzae*, *M. catarrhalis*, respiratory anaerobes, streptococci, and *S. aureus*. The newer carbapenem, meropenem, 40 mg/kg every 8 hours (not to exceed 2 g/dose), is an excellent choice because of its very broad antibacterial spectrum. Vancomycin, 15 mg/kg every 6 hours, may be added if infection was suspected or proved to be caused by methicillin-resistant *S. aureus* or highly penicillin-resistant *S. pneumoniae*. Alternatively, a combination of aqueous penicillin G, 200 to 300 U/kg/day intravenously in four to six divided doses, and cefotaxime, 200 to 300 mg/kg/day intravenously in four divided doses, is used frequently. If cultures or Gram-stained smears of purulent material reveal a predominance of gram-positive cocci in clusters, nafcillin (150 mg/kg/day intravenously in four divided doses) may be substituted for penicillin G. Additional drugs, such as metronidazole for fastidious anaerobes, may be prescribed if unexpected bacterial flora are seen on Gram staining or are recovered by culture.

Hyperosmolar agents should be given if high intracranial pressure threatens brain herniation. Systemic steroids should be prescribed with caution because of their theoretic suppressive effect on granulocytic and immune functions. Anticonvulsant agents should be given prophylactically to protect against a high incidence of associated seizures.

Extradural and subdural empyemas should be drained through a generous craniotomy. An underlying brain abscess is handled best by intracapsular evacuation and catheter drainage to avoid unnecessary brain damage associated with radical excision of deep-seated lesions within eloquent areas of the brain. In some cases of subdural empyema, the underlying brain is so swollen that the bone flap must be left out for external decompression.

Postoperatively, intravenous antibiotics should be maintained for a minimum of 2 to 3 weeks. The shrinking of the abscess or empyema can be observed accurately by serial CT scans. Despite modern diagnostic and surgical capabilities, the mortality associated with subdural empyema and brain abscess is more than 20%. Early diagnosis remains the most effective way of improving survival.

Suggested Readings

American Academy of Pediatrics, Subcommittee on Management of Sinusitis and Committee on Quality Improvement. Clinical practice guideline: management of sinusitis. *Pediatrics* 2001;108:798.

Chandler JR, Langenbrunner DJ, Stevens EF. The pathogenesis of orbital complications in acute sinusitis. *Laryngoscope* 1975;80:1414.

Gwaltney JM Jr. Computed tomographic study of the common cold. *N Engl J Med* 1994;330:25.

Gwaltney JM Jr. Weisinger BA, Patric JT. Acute community-acquired bacterial sinusitis: the value of antimicrobial treatment and the natural history. *Clin Infect Dis* 2004;30:326–8.

Kovatch AL, Wald ER, Ledesma-Medena J, et al. Maxillary sinus radiographs in children with nonrespiratory complaints. *Pediatrics* 1986;73:306.

Wald ER. Chronic sinusitis in children. *J Pediatr* 1995;127:339.

Wald ER. Sinusitis in children. *N Engl J Med* 1992;326:319.

Wald ER, Chiponis D, Ledesma-Medina J. Comparative effectiveness of amoxicillin and amoxicillin–clavulanate potassium in acute paranasal sinus infections in children: a double-blind, placebo-controlled trial. *Pediatrics* 1986;77:795.

Wald ER, Milmoe GJ, Bowen A, et al. Acute maxillary sinusitis in children. *N Engl J Med* 1981;304:749.

CHAPTER 247 ■ OROFACIAL INFECTIONS

THOMAS R. FLYNN, JOSEPH F. PIECUCH, AND RICHARD G. TOPAZIAN

Most infections of the oral cavity and face in children are odontogenic in origin and often are responsive to local treatment. Occasionally, spread to adjacent or distant fascial spaces or to the maxilla and mandible may result in life-threatening complications.

ODONTOGENIC INFECTIONS

Pathogenesis

Normal Flora of the Oral Cavity

The oral cavity provides an environment favorable to the growth of microorganisms. Bacterial counts in the range of 108 to 1,011/mL of saliva have been reported. Normally, more than 30 species of bacteria can be identified in saliva in varying proportions, depending on a dynamic interaction of different microbial ecosystems, including the tongue, the gingival crevice, and the presence of bacterial plaque. Variously, factors that can modify the microbial population include age, anatomic relationships, eruption of teeth, presence of decayed teeth, diet, oral hygiene, antibiotic therapy, systemic disease, and hospitalization. The estimated ratio of anaerobic to aerobic organisms in the oral cavity ranges from 3:1 to 10:1. Even the edentulous person may have a preponderance of anaerobes, because such areas as the buccal vestibule, when the cheek is approximated against the teeth or alveolar ridges, may have greatly reduced oxygen tension.

The flora of children is fairly similar to that of adults, with several exceptions. At birth, the oral cavity is sterile, but colonization with a wide variety of microbes occurs within hours. Although many sources of oral microbial colonization exist, a predominant source has been shown to be the oral flora of infants' mothers. Interestingly, the bacterial strains found in fathers' mouths are not found routinely in children's oral cavity. *Streptococcus salivarius* has been found in 80% of cultures taken from 1-day-old infants. The percentage of *Streptococcus* species decreases from 98% on the day after birth to 70% at age 4 months as other organisms become established. *Staphylococcus* species, *Neisseria*, *Veillonella*, *Actinomyces*, *Nocardia*, *Fusobacterium*, *Bacteroides*, *Corynebacterium*, *Candida*, and a variety of coliforms gradually become established by age 1 year. As eruption of the primary dentition occurs, anaerobic organisms become well established in the gingival crevice, yet spirochetes and the *Bacteroides melaninogenicus* group (now known as the *Prevotella* and *Porphyromonas* genera and commonly associated with the gingival crevice in adults) appear to be present in fewer numbers before ages 13 to 16 years.

Pathogenic Organisms

Most odontogenic infections, whether they are carious, periodontal, or periapical, are polymicrobial, with a mixed aerobic-anaerobic flora averaging four to six isolates per case. A combination of an oral streptococcus and an anaerobe is involved in the majority of these infections. Early in the course of an infection, the streptococci predominate, invading tissue and spreading infection by elaborating enzymes, such as hyaluronidases, that break down the ground substance of connective tissue. This process generates necrotic tissue and a reduced oxygen environment and provides such nutrients as vitamin K, hemin, and succinate that favor the growth of oral anaerobes, including *Prevotella*, *Porphyromonas*, *Fusobacterium*, and anaerobic streptococci. As the infection matures, the anaerobes cause tissue liquefaction via collagenases, producing an abscess with a mixed flora. Late infections, with chronic encapsulated abscesses, often yield a purely anaerobic culture. The primary pathogens in orofacial odontogenic infections are identified in Table 247.1.

The taxonomy of the oral flora is changing. Clinical isolates from orofacial infections still may be identified by the laboratory as *Streptococcus viridans* or *B. melaninogenicus*; however, research involving genetic analysis of the various strains of these species has resulted in a rapidly changing classification and nomenclature for these organisms, with the acceptance of several new genera and species within these older classifications. Current classifications are summarized in Table 247.2. As molecular diagnostic methods develop, our understanding of the roughly 60% of oral species that cannot be cultured will change significantly.

Anatomic Considerations

Most severe orofacial infections develop as a result of periapical, periodontal, or pericoronal dental infection (the latter surrounding the crown of an erupting tooth), with spread occurring along the anatomic pathways of least resistance. Generally, periodontal and pericoronal infections drain through the gingival sulcus into the oral cavity and rarely have major sequelae; the exception is pericoronal infections involving erupting third molar teeth, which can spread into deeper anatomic

TABLE 247.1

MOST FREQUENT PATHOGENS ISOLATED IN OROFACIAL INFECTIONS IN TWO STUDIES

Microorganism	Percentage of Cases per Study	
	Lewis	Heimdahl
Streptococcus milleri	50	31
Peptococcus species	64	31
Other anaerobic streptococci	8	38
Bacteroides oralis	40	9
Bacteroides gingivalis	28	—*
Bacteroides melaninogenicus	24	26
Fusobacterium species	14	45

*This organism was not reported in this study.
Reprinted from Flynn TR. Odontogenic infections. *Oral Maxillofac Surg Clin North Am* 1991;3:311.

TABLE 247.2

TAXONOMIC CHANGES IN SELECTED ORAL PATHOGENS

Older Terminology	Current Terminology
Streptococcus viridans	*Streptococcus anginosus*
	Streptococcus intermedius
	Streptococcus constellatus
	Streptococcus mutans
	Streptococcus sanguis
	Streptococcus mitis
	Streptococcus salivarius
	Streptococcus vestibularis
Streptococcus milleri	*Streptococcus anginosus*
	Streptococcus intermedius
	Streptococcus constellatus
Bacteroides melaninogenicus	*Prevotella melaninogenica*
	Prevotella intermedia
	Porphyromonas asaccharolyticus
	Porphyromonas gingivalis
	Porphyromonas endodontalis
	Capnocytophaga species
Streptococcus faecalis	*Enterococcus faecalis*
Streptococcus faecium	*Enterococcus faecium*
Peptococcus species	*Peptostreptococcus* species

spaces because of their posterior location in the oral cavity. Conversely, usually infections associated with root apices are confined within the bony alveolar process. Should spontaneous intraoral drainage occur through either the periodontium or the pulp chamber, further spread through marrow spaces is unlikely. If such drainage does not occur, spread through bone (osteomyelitis) or perforation of the cortical plate of the affected jaw may take place. Once penetration of the cortical plate occurs, infection will involve the adjacent soft tissues and may manifest either as cellulitis or as a soft tissue abscess that eventually may perforate mucous membrane or skin as a sinus tract (Fig. 247.1).

Usually, perforation of periapical infections through bone follows a typical pattern stemming from the position of the root apices in relation to the bony cortex and to muscle attachments (Fig. 247.2). Abscesses associated with anterior teeth and the buccal roots of maxillary posterior teeth tend to perforate labially or buccally (into the cheek) because the tooth roots are close to that cortical plate. Abscesses associated with mandibular posterior teeth may perforate either the buccal or the lingual cortical plate. When the spread of a mandibular infection occurs lingually, the relationship of the tooth apex to the mylohyoid muscle origin is significant. If the roots are superior to the mylohyoid muscle, infections will localize intraorally in the floor of the mouth (sublingual space). Usually, apices of the second and third molars are located inferior to

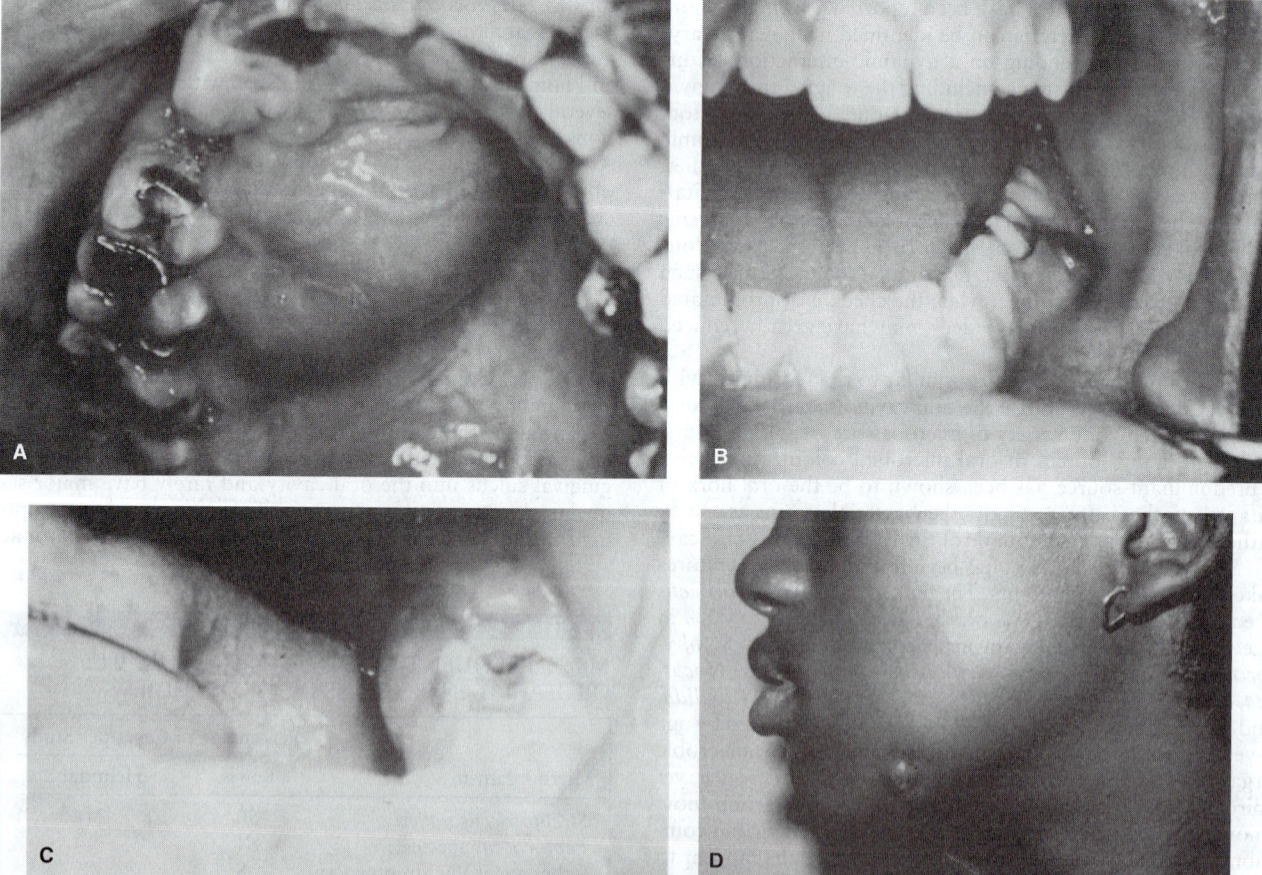

FIGURE 247.1. Spread of odontogenic infection. **A:** Palatal abscess resulting from an infected first premolar. **B:** Intraoral mucosal sinus tract from periapical abscess of mandibular first molar. **C:** Pericoronitis. **D:** Extraoral draining sinus from mandibular first molar infection in an adolescent. (A, Reprinted from Piecuch JF. Odontogenic infections. *Dent Clin North Am* 1982;26:135. B,C, Reprinted from Simos C, Flynn TR, Piecuch JF, et al. Infections of the oral cavity. In: Feigin RD, Cherry JD, eds. *Textbook of pediatric infectious diseases,* 5th ed. Philadelphia: WB Saunders, 2004:149. D, Reprinted from Waite DE. *Textbook of practical oral and maxillofacial surgery.* Philadelphia: Lea & Febiger, 1987:289.)

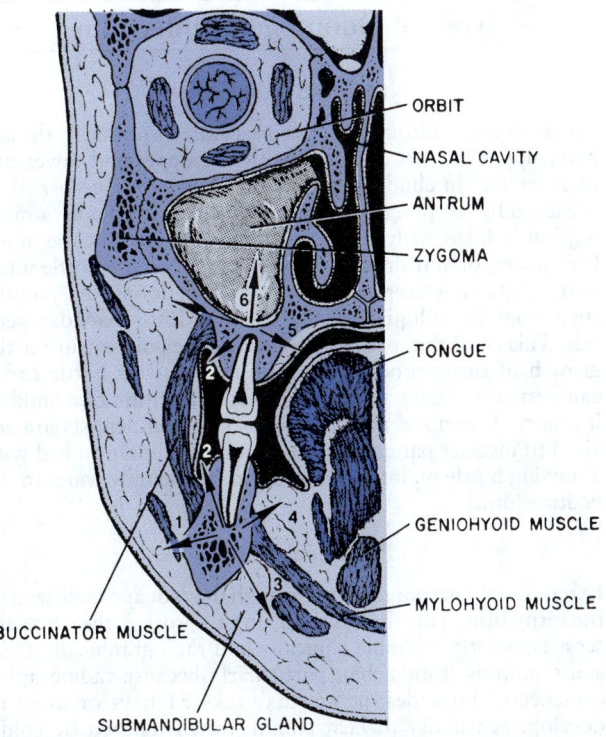

ORBIT

NASAL CAVITY

ANTRUM

ZYGOMA

TONGUE

GENIOHYOID MUSCLE

MYLOHYOID MUSCLE

BUCCINATOR MUSCLE

SUBMANDIBULAR GLAND

FIGURE 247.2. Possible pathways of spread of periapical infection. (Adapted from Goldberg MH, Topazian RG. Odontogenic infections and deep fascial space infections of dental origin. In: Topazian RG, Goldberg MH, eds. *Oral and Maxillofacial Infections*, 3rd ed. Philadelphia: WB Saunders, 1994:206.)

the mylohyoid muscle; consequently, the submandibular space will be involved, with extraoral localization.

In children, often the maxillary and mandibular root apices are located superior and inferior, respectively, to the attachment of the buccinator muscle. Consequently, dental infections in younger patients may have a greater tendency to spread into the facial soft tissues and to localize extraorally.

Two fascial spaces commonly associated with odontogenic infections are the submandibular and masticator spaces. The submandibular space is formed by a splitting of the superficial layer of deep cervical fascia, superficial to the mylohyoid muscle and inferior to the mandible. Anteriorly and posteriorly, it is limited by the digastric muscle. Within this space lie the submandibular gland and portions of the facial artery and anterior facial vein. This space is approximated closely to the sublingual and lateral pharyngeal spaces. Often, infections of the submandibular space originate from lower molar teeth, and submandibular space infections either may spread to or arise from infections in the sublingual, lateral pharyngeal, or masticator spaces.

The masticator space also is formed by a splitting of the superficial layer of deep cervical fascia to surround the muscles of mastication and the lower jaw. Its contents include the masseter muscle, the internal and external pterygoid muscles, the temporal muscle, and the mandibular ascending ramus. The temporal and infratemporal spaces are the superior extensions of the masticator space. Adjacent are the submandibular, lateral pharyngeal, and retropharyngeal spaces. Infections of the masticator space may originate in adjacent spaces or can spread to it from periapical or pericoronal infections of the mandibular second and third molars and the maxillary third molar.

Diagnosis

Patients with odontogenic infections may have symptoms ranging from minor to life-threatening. Patients with an orofacial infection should receive thorough systemic and extraoral head and neck evaluations; importantly, the intraoral examination for a possible odontogenic cause must not be overlooked. Thorough intraoral evaluation begins with assessing the degree of mandibular opening. The interincisal distance on wide opening may be 40 mm or more, even in young children. Painful limitation of opening, or trismus, is associated with inflammation of the muscles of mastication and indicates spread of the infection to the masticator space. Teeth are inspected visually for caries, by percussion for tenderness, and by electric or hot and cold stimulation for pulpal involvement. Gingival tissues are probed for periodontal defects, and salivary glands are palpated for tenderness and are milked to observe for purulent discharge from the duct orifices.

Therapy

New treatment concepts for caries and periodontal disease, the most common oral infections, are evolving. These infections are coming to be viewed as a pathologic colonization of the oral cavity by specific normally nonresident pathogens. Traditional dental therapy for caries and periodontal disease aimed at suppressing the growth of a polymicrobial flora and repairing the damage that it causes. Instead, the goal of treatment would not be to control the growth of *Streptococcus mutans* (the primary agent of caries) or of a variety of periodontal pathogens by oral hygiene measures alone, but rather to eliminate *S. mutans* entirely.

Strategies for eradicating such organisms include the elimination of colonization sites for *S. mutans* by sealing the pits and fissures of the teeth with acrylic resins, use of such topical antiseptics as chlorhexidine, oral hygiene measures, and periodic culturing of saliva for this caries-producing organism. Similarly effective, especially in adults, may be elimination of periodontal pathogens by periodontal surgical débridement of the entire dentition at one visit and by a course of antibiotics effective against these organisms, followed by oral hygiene measures and topical fluoride therapy. Treatment protocols using these strategies are being tested. As with infections elsewhere in the body, the principles of treatment of orofacial infections involve surgical drainage and antibiotics. In a review of serious pediatric head and neck inpatient infections, Dodson and colleagues found that infections located above the upper lip originated most frequently in the sinuses or upper respiratory tract, whereas lower facial infections were primarily odontogenic. Almost always, odontogenic infections required surgical intervention, probably owing to the abscess-producing flora of odontogenic infections and the deep intrabony portal of entry afforded to those organisms by the roots of the teeth. Dental infections treated only with antibiotics almost always recur in a manifestation worse than the previous. Surgical drainage, preferably intraoral, may include standard incision and drainage of cellulitis or abscess or, in the case of localized periapical infection, endodontic drainage through the pulp (root canal therapy) or extraction of the offending tooth. Antibiotic therapy, although not necessary for minor, well-localized periapical lesions in noncompromised patients, is indicated if cellulitis or abscess, infections of adjacent bone (osteomyelitis), systemic signs (fever, dehydration, lymphadenopathy), trismus, or immunocompromise are present.

Generally, antibiotic selection for odontogenic infections, although based ultimately on Gram stain and aerobic and anaerobic cultures, is begun empirically before culture results are available. Penicillin is the logical first choice for oral therapy of outpatient odontogenic infections because of its lack of toxicity, its bactericidal nature, and the sensitivity of most streptococci and oral anaerobes to this drug. Such aminopenicillins as ampicillin and amoxicillin with or without clavulanate have not demonstrated significantly better clinical success than that of penicillin V. If clinical signs or Gram stain results suggest the presence of *Staphylococcus aureus*, a penicillinase-resistant drug, such as oxacillin or dicloxacillin, may be added to the penicillin until the culture results are available. Alternately, a first- or second-generation cephalosporin, such as cephalexin or cefuroxime, may be used. In the case of penicillin allergy, clindamycin may be substituted, but it remains the drug of second choice for outpatient infections because of its greater toxicity. The macrolide antibiotics should be considered as tertiary selections for orofacial infections because of the high rate of resistance found among the oral streptococci and anaerobes. Among the macrolides, azithromycin would be the best choice, because of its ability to concentrate above serum levels in phagocytes. Tetracycline may result in severe staining of teeth in children younger than age 12 years and should be avoided, except when given specifically for *Actinobacillus actinomycetem-comitans* in cases of severe juvenile periodontitis. Similarly, the safety of using metronidazole in children has not been established, even though it is highly effective against obligate anaerobic bacteria. The fluoroquinolones are chondrotoxic in children, and their bacterial spectrum is not highly effective against most oral pathogens. Among the fluoroquinolones, however, moxifloxacin appears to have the optimum antimicrobial spectrum for odontogenic infections. However, orofacial infections severe enough to warrant hospital admission may differ microbiologically from less severe infections. Resistance to penicillin among the oral pathogens is increasing. In one study in the United Kingdom, 55% of the strains isolated were resistant to penicillin. Therefore, parenteral clindamycin, which remains highly effective against oral pathogens, is the antibiotic of first choice in severe odontogenic infections.

Types of Odontogenic Infections

Nursing-Bottle Caries

An identified syndrome of tooth decay affects primarily the primary upper incisors and frequently the upper and lower primary molars in children of bottle-feeding age (Fig. 247.3). It is caused by the practice of putting a child to bed with a nursing bottle filled with a sugar-containing drink, such as milk, fruit juices, or soft drinks. The child sucks on the bottle intermittently during sleep, when salivary secretion is low, and the sugar-containing liquids stay in the mouth for extended periods. This condition provides an excellent environment for the growth of caries-producing organisms. Nursing-bottle caries can destroy virtually the entire primary dentition of a child as it erupts. Therefore, pediatric physicians and dentists are advised to instruct parents to avoid putting children to bed with a nursing bottle or, if they must do so, to use only water in the bedtime drink.

Periapical Abscess

Extension of microorganisms through the root apex will lead to the formation of an abscess. Early in this process, the acute abscess is indistinguishable clinically and radiographically from acute pulpitis (toothache), particularly because radiographic evidence of bone destruction may take 21 days or more to develop. Sensitivity to heat stimuli (often relieved by cold), exquisite sensitivity to percussion, and tenderness to finger pressure on the alveolar process are indications that a tooth has become abscessed. Chronic abscesses are diagnosed more easily by observing looseness of the tooth, the presence of suppuration from draining sinuses or from the gingival crevice, and the presence of a periapical radiolucency on the radiograph (Fig. 247.4). Depending on the path of least anatomic resistance, tender swellings may be noted in the buccal or lingual mucosa. The classic presentation of swollen face or neck, pain, elevated

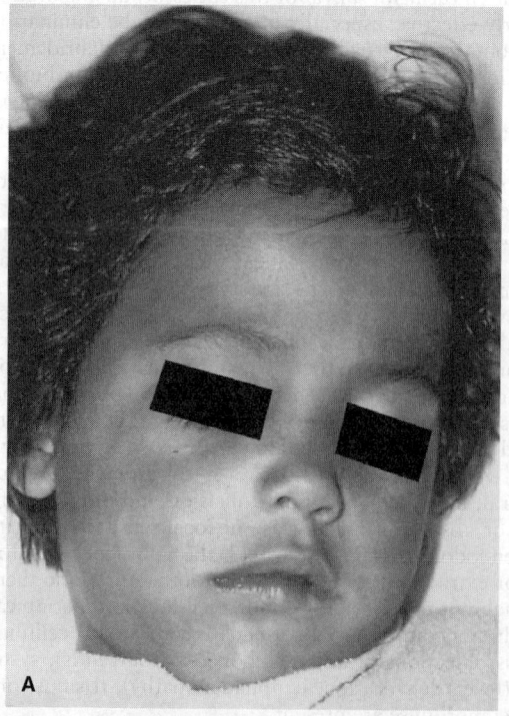
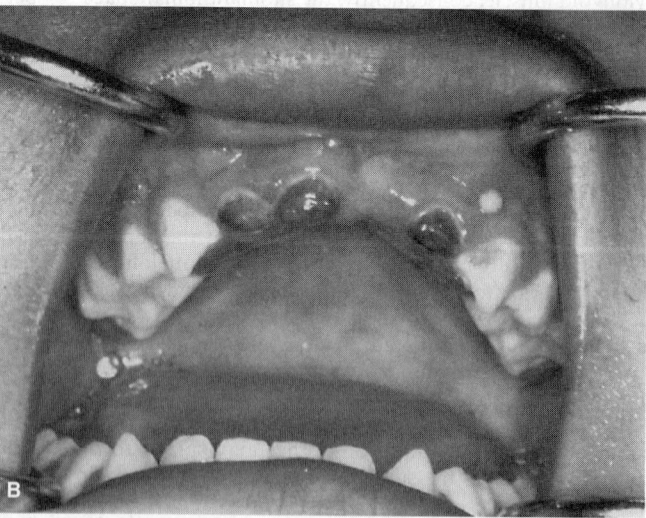

FIGURE 247.3. **A:** Four-year-old boy with a right infraorbital space infection resulting from nursing-bottle caries. Note the swelling of the infraorbital region, elevating the ala of the nose and protruding the upper lip. **B:** Intraoral view of the same patient. Note the darkened stumps of the carious upper primary incisors and the draining sinus tract *(white dot)* near the upper lateral incisor.

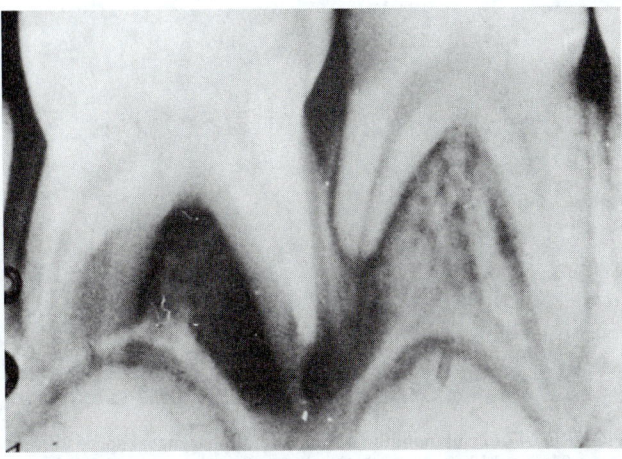

FIGURE 247.4. Radiolucency representing a chronic periapical abscess involving the mesial root of the primary second molar and the distal root of the primary first molar. The developing mandibular bicuspids are seen inferior to the primary roots. The cause of the abscess is the deep carious lesion in each tooth, which appears to have penetrated the pulp chambers.

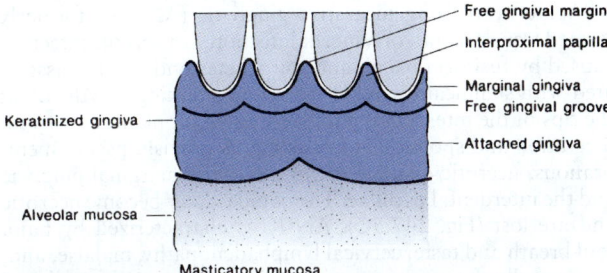

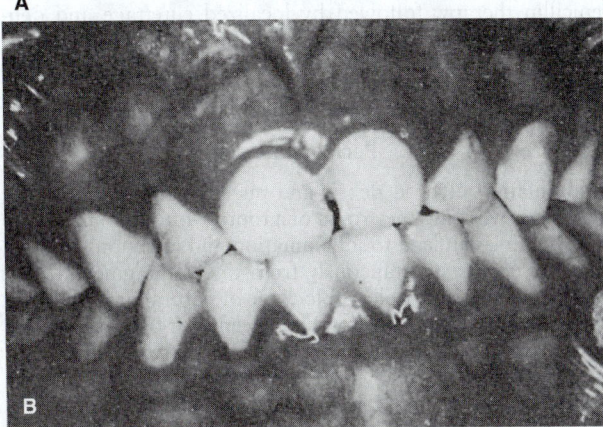

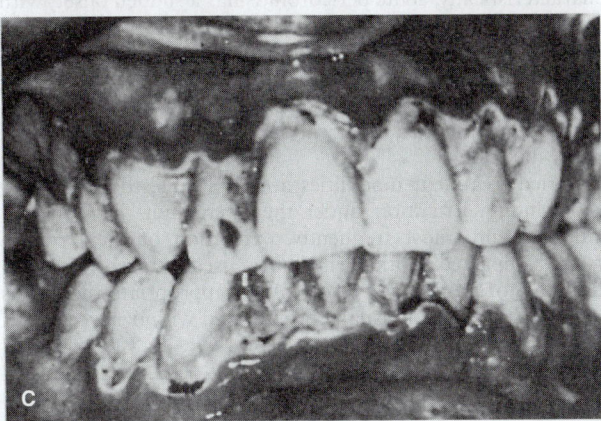

FIGURE 247.5. Normal and abnormal gingiva. **A:** Normal gingiva. **B:** Gingivitis. Interdental papillae are swollen, and accumulations of white plaque are present on teeth. **C:** Acute necrotizing ulcerative gingivitis. (Reprinted from Lesco B, Brownstein M. Recognition of periodontal disease in children. *Pediatr Clin North Am* 1982;29:457.)

temperature, and malaise should direct clinicians to suspect an odontogenic infection. Adequate surgical drainage is the key principle in the treatment of periapical abscesses and may be accomplished by endodontic (root canal) therapy, extraction of the tooth, or incision and drainage, as necessary. Antibiotic therapy should be considered an adjunctive rather than a primary therapeutic modality, because antibiotics alone will not remove the cause of the infection.

Extraction of unsalvageable abscessed teeth soon after the diagnosis has been made has been found to be curative in approximately 96% of cases. Early extraction has also been shown to be associated with a decreased requirement for extraoral incision and drainage procedures, as compared with treatment only with antibiotics.

Periodontal Infections

Surrounding the teeth is a distinctive, coral-pink keratinized mucosa known as the gingiva. Normal gingiva is attached firmly to the alveolar bone and extends between the teeth as the interdental papilla. A thin cuff of free (unattached) gingiva surrounds each tooth, and normally the resulting crevice between the free gingiva and the tooth is approximately 3 mm deep (Fig. 247.5A).

The accumulation of food deposits and bacteria (dental plaque) in the gingival crevice may result in gingivitis, a localized inflammation of the free gingiva presenting as an erythematous, painless edema of the interdental papillae, accompanied by deepening of the gingival sulcus. In severe cases (Fig. 247.5B), the gingival architecture may become distorted, and accumulations of plaque are evident. Bleeding on toothbrushing and probing is characteristic. Gingivitis is prevalent at all ages and, in some studies, has been shown to affect more than 60% of children at age 5 years and almost all adults. Often, it is most severe in compromised hosts, including diabetic patients and otherwise immunosuppressed patients. However, poor oral hygiene is the usual cause, and generally this condition responds well to dental prophylaxis (cleaning) and improved home care. Chlorhexidine gluconate mouth rinse (Peridex) has been shown to be effective in gingivitis and is recommended for routine use in immunocompromised patients as an adjunct to good oral hygiene and regular professional care.

In both adolescents and adults, gingivitis may progress to periodontitis, a progressively severe infection characterized by inflamed gingivae, tooth mobility caused by resorption of alveolar bone, and a purulent gingival exudate. Notably, this insidious condition generally is painless and may progress for years before being recognized. Usually, periodontal treatment and meticulous oral hygiene arrest the condition.

A rare variant—juvenile periodontitis—is localized to the molar and incisor regions of otherwise healthy children. A predisposing factor, however, may be repeated episodes of tonsillitis in earlier childhood, with the infected tonsillar crypts acting as a reservoir for *A. actinomycetemcomitans*. The cause is thought to be the relative predominance of this facultative gram-negative organism, which produces leukotoxin, an enzyme capable of killing leukocytes locally. Deep gingival pocketing and severe bone resorption are characteristic of this disease and may result in loss of the dentition in these areas. Tetracycline has been shown to be useful in combination with periodontal surgery and meticulous home care.

Acute necrotizing ulcerative gingivitis (ANUG), formerly termed trench mouth or Vincent infection, is a specific infection caused by fusiform bacilli and spirochetes and is often associated with significant psychic stress and smoking. Erythema at the tips of the interdental papillae soon is supplanted by frank ulceration and spontaneous bleeding. A grayish, pseudomembranous, necrotic exudate forms along the marginal gingivae and the interdental papillae. The papillae later become necrotic and are lost (Fig. 247.5C). ANUG is characterized by pain, foul breath and taste, cervical lymphadenopathy, malaise, and, occasionally, fever. Treatment consists of 3 to 5 days of oral penicillin therapy, followed by localized curettage and dental scaling combined with oral rinses of 0.12% chlorhexidine (Peridex). With treatment, resolution should occur within 6 to 10 days.

Pericoronitis

Accumulation of food debris and microorganisms under the soft tissue overlying the crown of a tooth—often a mandibular third molar—can lead to inflammation and infection. Usually, drainage occurs spontaneously from under the gingival flap, thus localizing the problem. Blockage of natural drainage may lead to spread of the infection to adjacent soft tissues and deep fascial spaces. Therefore, prompt definitive treatment is indicated.

Pericoronitis may be classified into acute and chronic forms. Characteristically, acute pericoronitis has a sudden onset, with severe pain, trismus, swelling, and dysphagia. Fever may be present, as well as tender enlargement of ipsilateral lymph nodes. Purulent material may be drained from beneath the erythematous, edematous flap (see Fig. 247.1C). Chronic pericoronitis presents as a recurrent discomfort of several days' or longer duration.

Varied treatment modalities are applicable to pericoronitis, including irrigation under the operculum, incision and drainage, and, most frequently, extraction of the partially erupted impacted tooth. Penicillin is used if fever, lymphadenopathy, or trismus is present. After appropriate therapy is begun, resolution can usually be expected within 1 week.

Complications

Fascial Space Infections

Spread of infection to the fascial spaces may result in dramatic facial swelling, high temperature, and, if the infection is untreated, respiratory embarrassment. The characteristics of the more common fascial space infections are described later.

Generally, infraorbital space infections are connected with maxillary anterior teeth and are well localized to the infraorbital region by the levator labii superioris and levator anguli oris muscles. Facial swelling lateral to the nose is prominent, as is weakness of the upper lip resulting from inflammation of these muscles. Generally, intraoral incision and drainage, with placement of a small Penrose drain for 1 to 2 days, comprise sufficient treatment. Antibiotics are indicated for all such fascial space infections. Figure 247.3 illustrates an infraorbital space infection in a 4-year-old boy that was caused by nursing-bottle caries affecting the upper anterior teeth. It was treated by incision and drainage and by extraction of the unsalvageable carious incisors.

Trismus is the classic sign of masticator space infection. Because this space is located both medial and lateral to the mandibular ramus, swelling may occur in either direction, and resultant abscesses may point either extraorally or toward the lateral pharyngeal wall. Usually, both intraoral and extraoral incision and drainage are required for masticator space infections. Clinicians must maintain a high level of suspicion of

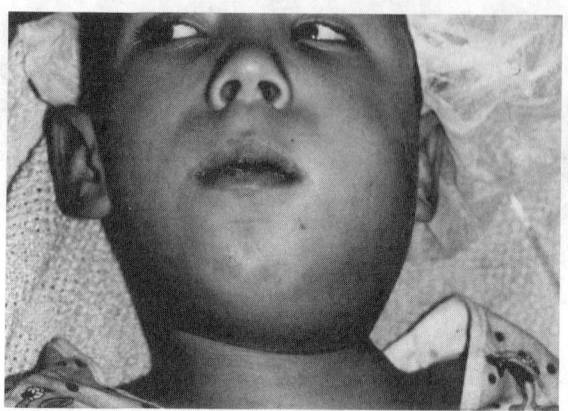

FIGURE 247.6. Submandibular and lateral pharyngeal space abscess in an 8-year-old boy. Note the swelling of the left upper lateral neck and the lateral deviation of the head to the right. This maneuver helps to position the upper airway over the deviated larynx and trachea. (Reprinted from Simos C, Flynn TR, Piecuch JF, et al. Infections of the oral cavity. In: Feigin RD, Cherry JD, eds. *Textbook of pediatric infectious diseases*, 5th ed. Philadelphia: WB Saunders, 2004:155.)

masticator space infection if trismus is present. Infection of the pterygomandibular portion of the masticator space causes no external swelling, yet trismus hinders visualization of the swelling of the tonsillar pillar. This common sequela of pericoronitis of the lower third molar (wisdom tooth) can spread easily to the lateral pharyngeal and deeper spaces if it is left untreated.

Infections of the submandibular space or pterygomandibular portion of the masticator space can spread easily to the lateral pharyngeal space. Figure 247.6 illustrates a submandibular and lateral pharyngeal space abscess caused by an infected lower primary molar. (Note that the patient is deviating the head laterally away from the infected side to position the upper airway over the deviated larynx and tracheal airway.)

First described in 1836, Ludwig angina consists of infection of the sublingual, submental, and submandibular spaces bilaterally and is characterized by hard, brawny cellulitis and a minimum of suppuration. Often, the tongue is edematous and is raised to the roof of the mouth, with little mobility (Fig. 247.7). Airway obstruction is impending; indeed, the greatest

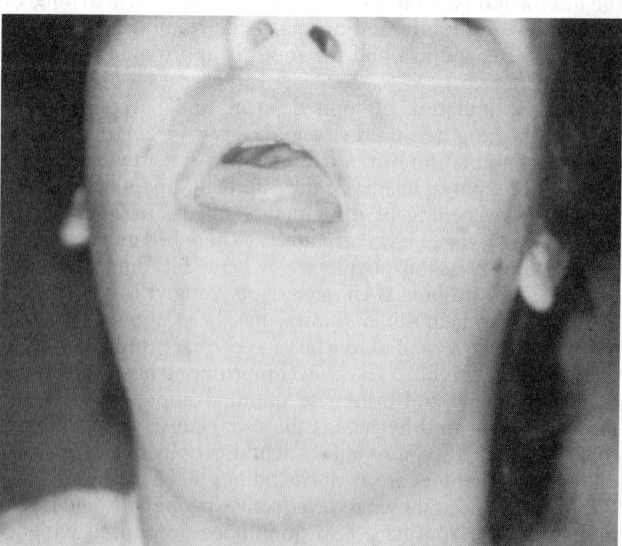

FIGURE 247.7. Ludwig angina. (Reprinted from Flynn TR, Topazian RG. Infections of the oral cavity. In: Waite D, ed. *Textbook of practical oral and maxillofacial surgery*. Philadelphia: Lea & Febiger, 1987:302.)

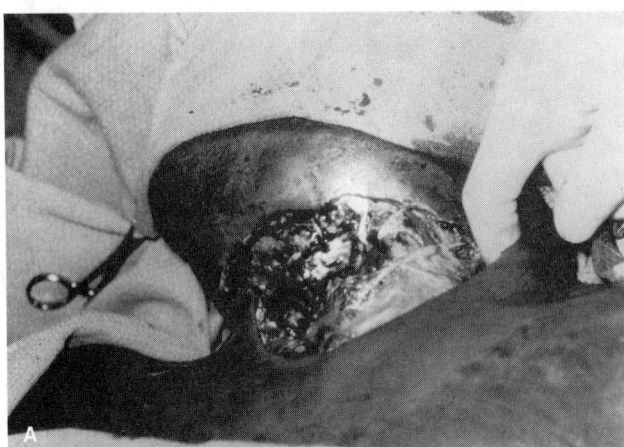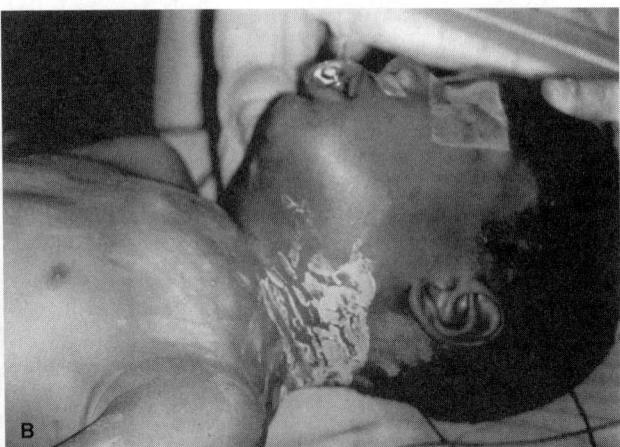

FIGURE 247.8. Necrotizing fasciitis. **A:** Surgical débridement of cervicofacial necrotizing fasciitis. A large portion of the skin of the left side of the neck was necrotic and had to be removed. Note that the skin is undermined by the infection and is dissected easily by finger pressure alone. **B:** An 8-year-old boy with cervicofacial necrotizing fasciitis secondary to an infected lower primary molar. Note the swelling extending from the cheek to the anterior chest wall. The chalky material on his neck is calamine lotion placed by his mother, thinking that the vesicles on the skin were poison ivy. (Reprinted from Simos C, Flynn TR, Piecuch JF, et al. Infections of the oral cavity. In: Feigin RD, Cherry JD, eds. *Textbook of pediatric infectious diseases,* 5th ed. Philadelphia: WB Saunders, 2004:156.)

cause of death with this affliction is hypoxia, which occurred in more than 50% of patients before antibiotics were available. Today, death is rare, although the need for tracheotomy or prolonged endotracheal intubation is common. Often, this infection is odontogenic, but it may result also from a laceration of the floor of the mouth or a fracture of the mandible. Usually a disease of young men, it is rare in children but may occur in greater frequency in those who are immunologically compromised. Surgical drainage of all infected spaces is indicated, accompanied by high-dose parenteral antibiotic therapy.

Necrotizing Fasciitis

Necrotizing fasciitis is rapidly spreading superficial cellulitis that can cause necrotic loss of the platysma muscle and the overlying skin. It may begin as painful, reddened swelling (often with vesicles) that soon becomes violaceous, then dusky, and then black and necrotic. Often, cervicofacial necrotizing fasciitis is odontogenic and typically follows the platysma muscle from the cheek down the entire neck to the anterior chest wall (Fig. 247.8A). Figure 247.8B illustrates such a swelling in an 8-year-old boy. The presumptive cause was odontogenic infection of the primary molars, which caused a high fever and a rapidly progressive swelling. Often, the cause of these infections is group A beta-hemolytic streptococci, but a wide variety of microorganisms, including anaerobes associated with dental infections, may be involved. Therefore, broad-spectrum antibiotic therapy is indicated empirically, along with hydration, transfusions if necessary, and support of electrolyte balance, especially with calcium, which may be sequestered by necrotic fat molecules.

Odontogenic Sinusitis

Odontogenic sinusitis may result from infection of a tooth adjacent to the maxillary sinus, or it may occur after extraction of a tooth that has roots close to that sinus. Usually, the diagnosis can be made on the basis of pain, tenderness to percussion over the sinus facially, purulent intranasal discharge, and radiopacity of the sinus on a Waters view plain radiograph or computed tomography (CT) scan. Initial treatment includes oral antibiotics and decongestants to promote drainage through the ostium. Occasionally, nasal antrostomy or functional endoscopic sinus surgery may be necessary to reestablish normal pathways of sinus drainage. Of course, appropriate dental treatment of the offending tooth or teeth is also indicated.

Figure 247.9 illustrates the case of a 9-year-old boy with an infected upper primary molar, left infraorbital swelling, and upper eyelid ptosis with displacement of the optic globe. His CT scan shows opacified left maxillary and ethmoid sinuses, a subperiosteal orbital abscess, and forward and lateral displacement of the globe. He was treated by dental extraction, incision and drainage of the infraorbital and orbital spaces, and endoscopic débridement and drainage of the maxillary and ethmoid sinuses.

Haemophilus Influenzae Buccal Cellulitis

Occasionally, children will present with acute cellulitis of the buccal space but no clinically apparent odontogenic cause. Usually, a history of recent upper respiratory infection or sinusitis is revealed. Sometimes, pathogenic sinus flora, especially *Haemophilus influenzae,* has been cultured from these infections, which may have inoculated the cheek by following venous channels through the bone overlying the lateral surface of the maxillary sinus. Unless the infection is severe, incision and drainage are not usually necessary, and treatment with antibiotics directed to the flora of sinusitis, such as amoxicillin-clavulanate or a second-generation cephalosporin, is successful.

Orbital and Intracranial Complications

Orbital and intracranial complications of odontogenic infections are rare. They may occur by direct extension, through the sinuses, and by hematogenous spread through the ophthalmic vein system. Probably no more than 5% to 10% of all cases of orbital cellulitis are odontogenic. Generally, this infection is unilateral and is characterized by proptosis, chemosis, eyelid edema, and restriction of extraocular movement secondary to the edema. No nerve palsies or visual changes are present. Treatment includes surgical drainage, antibiotics, and appropriate dental therapy.

Cavernous sinus thrombosis, which may be difficult to differentiate clinically from orbital cellulitis, is considerably more serious because microorganisms proliferate intracranially. The

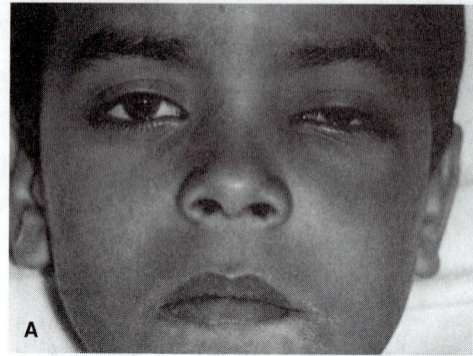

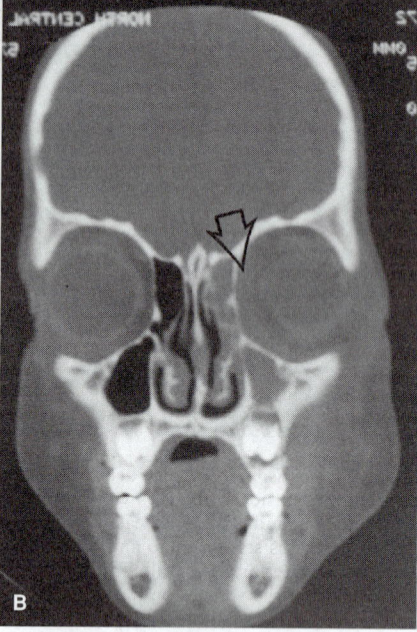

FIGURE 247.9. Odontogenic sinusitis and orbital infection. **A:** A 9-year-old boy with an infected upper primary molar, left infraorbital swelling, and upper eyelid ptosis with displacement of the optic globe. **B:** His computed tomographic scan shows opacified left maxillary and ethmoid sinuses, a subperiosteal orbital abscess (*arrow*), and forward and lateral displacement of the globe. (Reprinted from Simos C, Flynn TR, Piecuch JF, et al. Infections of the oral cavity. In: Feigin RD, Cherry JD, eds. *Textbook of pediatric infectious diseases,* 5th ed. Philadelphia: WB Saunders, 2004:157.)

risk of death or serious morbidity is high. Characteristics include bilateral ophthalmic involvement (because of rapid progression from one eye to the other), proptosis, chemosis, and eyelid edema. Extraocular movements are limited owing to inflammation of the third, fourth, and sixth cranial nerves. Systemic signs of meningeal irritation and funduscopic evidence of obstruction of the retinal veins also are present. Treatment includes high doses of parenteral antibiotics.

Subdural empyema and brain abscess complicating odontogenic infection are exceedingly rare today, compared with several decades ago. CT may be helpful in establishing the diagnosis, and intracranial drainage may be necessary.

HERPES SIMPLEX INFECTIONS

Commonly, herpes simplex infections are manifested as a herpetic gingivostomatitis. Five stages of infection have been identified: primary mucocutaneous infection, acute infection of ganglia, establishment of latency, reactivation, and recurrent infection.

Primary infection is established by direct contact either with a person who has draining lesions or with an asymptomatic carrier who may continue to shed the virus despite lack of symptoms. The highest incidence of primary infection appears to occur from ages 2 to 4 years. In large series of children with gingivostomatitis, no cases were seen in children younger than 6 months; such infants are protected by maternal antibodies. No seasonal variation or male-female difference in incidence is apparent.

The incubation period of the disorder is thought to be approximately 6 days, followed by the development of small vesicles that may coalesce to form larger lesions or ulcers. In severe cases, the lips, gingivae, oral mucosa, and pharynx variously may be involved (Fig. 247.10). Healing occurs in 1 to 2 weeks, with gradual crusting of the lesions followed by reepithelialization. However, many patients with primary herpes infection may remain asymptomatic.

Latency is thought to continue throughout life, with reactivation occurring at various times, possibly triggered by

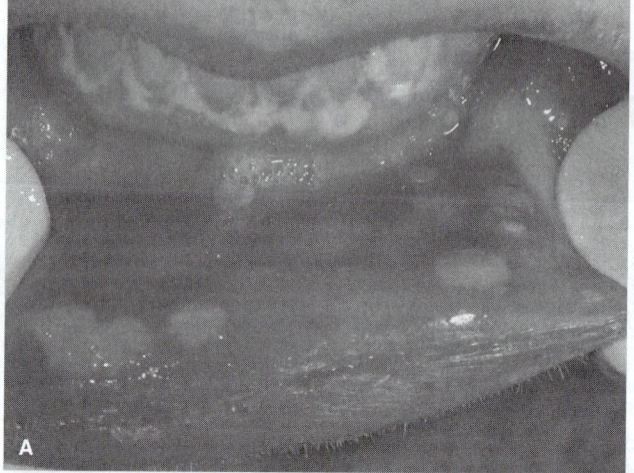

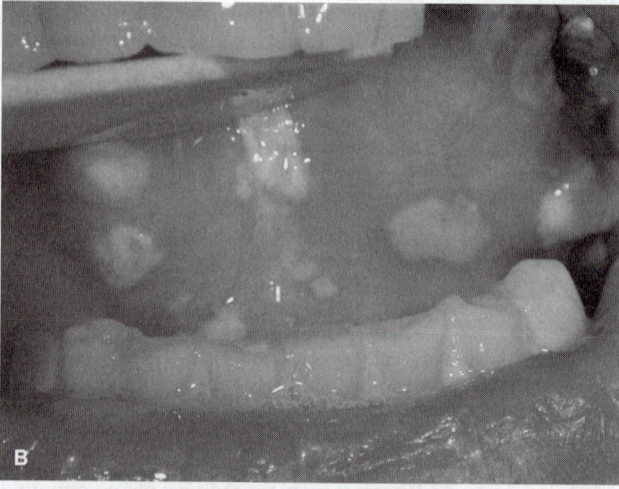

FIGURE 247.10. Herpetic gingivostomatitis. **A:** Lesions of the labial mucosa. **B:** Lesions of the ventral surface of the tongue.

emotional and physical stress or sunlight. Recurrent disease is manifested by vesicles at the mucocutaneous border of the lip or on the attached gingivae or palate that are painful for approximately 2 days, followed by crusting and complete healing in 7 to 10 days.

Recurrent aphthous ulcers (canker sores) are not caused by the herpes simplex virus. They are seen on the unkeratinized oral mucosa, and usually secondary herpetic lesions are seen on the keratinized oral mucosa, such as the gingiva and palate, and on the lips.

Therapy

Treatment of primary and recurrent lesions is palliative and supportive. Lesions should be kept clean and dry, and analgesic and antipyretic medications should be given as needed. Small children with severe primary gingivostomatitis may be subject to dehydration. Studies with acyclovir and other antiviral agents have not shown a reduction in duration of symptoms when the agents are used topically for recurrent lesions, but they may decrease the severity of the manifestations. Oral and intravenous therapy has shown some benefit in the compromised host for the reduction of pain and systemic symptoms.

Prognosis

As many as 50% of the adult population in industrialized countries, and a higher percentage in developing nations, may have recurrent herpes labialis. Surprisingly, many (if not most) adults who develop recurrent "cold sores" are not aware that they can transmit the disease, and they should be counseled in this regard. Likewise, medical, dental, and nursing personnel also should be advised that the occurrence of cutaneous lesions (herpetic whitlow) is not unknown after direct contact of practitioners' fingers with lesions during physical examination.

ORAL LESIONS ASSOCIATED WITH HUMAN IMMUNODEFICIENCY VIRUS

Human immunodeficiency virus (HIV) infection first was recognized in children in 1983. Since then, research has clarified that the oral manifestations of this infection are frequent and protean and that they differ significantly from those in adults.

Similarities of symptoms in adults and children with HIV infection include failure to thrive, fever, lymphadenopathy, opportunistic infections with atypical pathogens, and persistent oral candidiasis. In contrast to affected adults, children infected with HIV have a greater susceptibility to bacterial infections, especially with such encapsulated organisms as *Streptococcus pneumoniae* and *H. influenzae*. Septicemia from an oral focus of infection can become a life-threatening problem in HIV-infected children; therefore, optimal oral health must be established and should be maintained vigorously in such children. Children with HIV also have a much greater incidence of persistent diffuse parotitis, in which the gland may become large and disfiguring. Usually, parotid enlargement is caused by lymphocytic infiltration and intraparotid lymphadenopathy, rather than by infection of the gland.

The oral lesions associated with HIV seropositivity can be classified as fungal, bacterial, viral, neoplastic, and idiopathic. The most common oral manifestation is persistent candidiasis, which is common in children, especially in neonates. It has also been reported in children born to intravenous drug–abusing mothers who are not infected with HIV. Oral can-

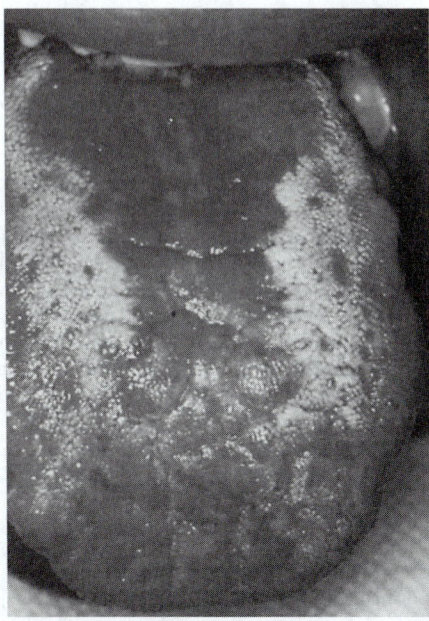

FIGURE 247.11. Oral candidiasis. Pseudomembranous and erythematous candidiasis of the dorsum of the tongue. Note the white candidal lesions (pseudomembranous type) on the filiform papillae laterally and the patchy red areas with loss of filiform papillae producing a bald tongue centrally (erythematous type).

didiasis may progress to esophageal candidiasis, a marker for the acquired immunodeficiency syndrome; therefore, oral candidiasis should be treated aggressively in children suspected of having HIV infection.

Candidal lesions in the mouth may take four forms: pseudomembranous, erythematous, hyperplastic, and angular cheilitis. The pseudomembranous form is the classic manifestation, with white, curd-like mucosal colonies that leave a raw, red underlying surface when the colonies are wiped off. The erythematous variant presents as reddened oral mucosa that may vary from fiery red to pink, without the presence of creamy white colonies. On the tongue, it causes loss of the filiform papillae, leaving bald patches resembling geographic tongue (Fig. 247.11). The hyperplastic form is characterized by a papillary mucosal hyperplasia, especially in the palate. Angular cheilitis can be recognized by red, tender patches at the corners of the mouth, from which *Candida albicans* may be identified. Treatment is accomplished with antifungal agents, the preparation of which becomes very important in establishing compliance with therapy in children. Sucrose-containing antifungal preparations, however, have been associated with the onset of rampant caries in children.

The most common oral bacterial infections seen in HIV-seropositive children are HIV gingivitis and ANUG. HIV gingivitis is characterized by linear erythema of the gingival margins surrounding the teeth, and it is unresponsive to improved oral hygiene. The progression of this lesion to the rapid destruction of periodontal bone and soft tissue seen in adults has not been reported in children. ANUG, recognized by necrotic loss of the interdental gingival papillae with pain and malodor, has not been reported in HIV-positive children in the United States but is common in malnourished, immunosuppressed children from developing countries.

As described, herpes simplex virus infection can be particularly severe in HIV-infected children, leaving large, crater-like painful ulcers with a gray-white pseudomembrane. This infection is treated with acyclovir or other antivirals orally or intravenously as necessary.

Oral neoplasms associated with HIV infection in adults, such as non-Hodgkin lymphoma and Kaposi sarcoma, have not been reported in children. Similarly, the persistent aphthous ulcerations common in HIV-positive adults are infrequent in children.

For preventing life-threatening infections and improving the quality of life in HIV-infected children, the maintenance of optimal oral health holds great significance. Such children should have regular pediatric oral and dental examinations and care consisting of excellent oral hygiene, frequent dental prophylaxis (cleanings) and fluoride treatments, and early and aggressive treatment of such oral infections as caries, gingivitis, candidiasis, and herpetic gingivostomatitis. Routine use of chlorhexidine (Peridex) may help to minimize gingivitis, candidiasis, and bacterial superinfections of the oral cavity.

OSTEOMYELITIS OF THE JAWS IN CHILDREN

Usually, osteomyelitis of the jaws in children results from the spread of odontogenic infection. Open fracture of the jaws with delayed treatment is also a significant cause of osteomyelitis. Extension from such contiguous infections as otitis, parotitis, and mastoiditis occurs much less often.

Osteomyelitis of the jaws in children must be viewed with great concern, because it may result in the following problems: loss of primary and permanent teeth; sequestration of segments of the jaws; such jaw growth deformities as mandibular hypoplasia, asymmetry, and ankylosis of the temporomandibular joint; disfiguring facial scars and cutaneous fistulas; and lesions suggesting malignancy, which require open biopsy. For these reasons, osteomyelitis of the jaws in children should be diagnosed rapidly and should be treated aggressively.

Predisposing Factors

Preexisting systemic diseases, including diabetes, leukemia, and febrile illnesses, with accompanying alteration of host resistance, play a major role in the initiation of osteomyelitis of the jaws. Conditions that alter the vascularity of bone and thus the ability to combat infections, including sickle cell anemia, bone tumors, fibrous dysplasia, Paget disease, and radiation to the jaws, also are important predisposing conditions. Major maxillofacial injuries resulting in open fractures of the jaws, especially those that are not treated immediately or that undergo inadequate fixation, are an important cause of osteomyelitis. Osteomyelitis involves the mandible far more frequently than the maxilla because the relatively poor blood supply to the mandible comes primarily from one major endosteal vessel and the periosteum.

Microbiology

Because osteomyelitis of the jaws is not always odontogenic, the bacterial spectrum is broad. Most cases of osteomyelitis of the jaws are caused by those organisms found commonly in odontogenic infections. These organisms include aerobic and facultative streptococci *(S. viridans)*, anaerobic streptococci, and other anaerobes, particularly *Peptostreptococcus, Fusobacterium, Prevotella,* and *Porphyromonas.* Occasionally, such gram-negative organisms as *Klebsiella, Pseudomonas,* and *Proteus* are found. Specific forms of osteomyelitis are caused by *Actinomyces* species, *Treponema pallidum,* and *Mycobacterium tuberculosis.* Unlike in long-bone osteomyelitis,

---

BOX 247.1	Osteomyelitis of the Jaws

Suppurative Osteomyelitis
Acute suppurative osteomyelitis
Chronic suppurative osteomyelitis
    Primary
    Secondary
Infantile osteomyelitis

Nonsuppurative Osteomyelitis
Chronic osteomyelitis
    Focal sclerosing osteomyelitis
    Diffuse sclerosing osteomyelitis
    Recurrent multifocal osteomyelitis
Garré sclerosing osteomyelitis
Actinomycotic osteomyelitis
Radiation osteomyelitis and necrosis

---

staphylococci rarely are a cause, except when external trauma involving the skin has been a contributing factor.

Classification

A useful classification of osteomyelitis of the jaws is provided in Box 247.1. Four major forms of the disease may be distinguished clinically: (a) acute suppurative osteomyelitis; (b) secondary chronic osteomyelitis, the form that begins as acute osteomyelitis and then becomes chronic; (c) primary chronic osteomyelitis, the form that has no acute phase and always has appeared to be a low-grade infection; and (d) nonsuppurative osteomyelitis. Those forms seen most often in children are the acute suppurative, the secondary chronic, and one nonsuppurative form known as Garré sclerosing osteomyelitis.

Suppurative Osteomyelitis

Usually, suppurative osteomyelitis begins with deep, intense pain in the jaws, intermittent high fever, and an obvious cause: most often a fracture of the mandible or a deeply carious or infected tooth. Occasionally, in the early stages, mental nerve paresthesia is present. Facial swelling develops over the course of several days, and teeth begin to loosen, pus exudes from the gingival sulcus, and multiple mucosal or cutaneous sinuses form after 10 to 14 days. Firm cellulitis is present in the soft tissues, accompanied by trismus and cervical lymphadenopathy. Bone scintigraphy with technetium, gallium, and indium are very sensitive tools for diagnosing osteomyelitis of the jaws, but false-positive results can be caused by tooth extraction within the past year, trauma, growth, and minor inflammation.

Leukocytosis occurs, typically ranging from 8,000 to 15,000 cells/mm^3, although ordinarily it does not reach the levels seen in acute osteomyelitis of the long bones. The erythrocyte sedimentation rate may be elevated, but, unlike that in long-bone disease, this value rarely is a valid indicator of the extent or course of osteomyelitis of the jaws. After 10 to 21 days, radiography may show scattered areas of bone destruction with a moth-eaten appearance (Fig. 247.12); periosteal reaction characterized by the laying down of new bone also is common. Smears of specimens and cultures should be taken whenever possible, including cultures of bone sequestra.

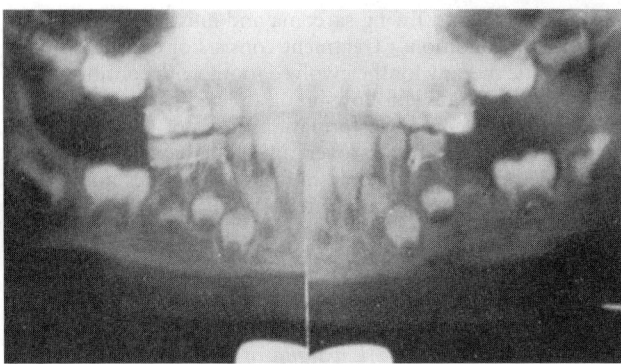

FIGURE 247.12. Radiograph of the jaws of a 4-year-old girl with suppurative osteomyelitis of the left mandible. The film shows marked destruction of the midbody and ramus of the mandible. (Reprinted from Simos C, Flynn TR, Piecuch JF, et al. Infections of the oral cavity. In: Feigin RD, Cherry JD, eds. *Textbook of pediatric infectious diseases*, 5th ed. Philadelphia: WB Saunders, 2004:158.)

Interpretation of cultures must be made with caution because of the possibility of skin and oral contaminants in the specimen.

Initially, intravenous antibiotics should be given empirically. As results from smears and culture are obtained, antibiotics may be changed as appropriate. Involved teeth should be removed as early as possible to allow for drainage and to remove a source of continuous bacterial inoculation of the bone. A change from intravenous to oral antibiotics is permissible after affected patients have been afebrile for 48 hours and all draining sinus tracts have closed.

A belief possibly retained from the preantibiotic era is that teeth must not be extracted in the presence of infection. Several well-conducted studies have shown that tooth extraction in the acute stage of infection hastens resolution and minimizes complications.

Antibiotic therapy should be continued for at least 2 to 4 weeks after all symptoms subside. If an infection persists, repeated cultures should be obtained, and the antibiotic should be changed, as indicated. Consideration should be given to sequestrectomy and saucerization, which involve removal of teeth in the immediate area and removal of the overlying cortical plate of bone, thus allowing access to the medullary portion and sequestra that may be present. Occasionally, placing catheters via an extraoral approach for continuous irrigation is necessary. This procedure permits the instillation of antibiotics in close contact with bone. Hyperbaric oxygen treatment may be considered in patients with chronic cases refractory to antibiotic treatment.

Infantile Osteomyelitis

Osteomyelitis of the jaws in the newborn is uncommon, but, because of its serious sequelae, is worthy of special mention. This type of osteomyelitis occurs most often a few weeks after birth and usually involves the maxilla. It is not odontogenic, but is thought to arise from neonatal trauma to oral tissues, from hematogenous spread from the skin, middle ear, mastoid process, or tonsils, or from maternal mastitis during nursing. Clinically, the patient has facial cellulitis centered about the orbit (Fig. 247.13). Irritability and malaise precede cellulitis and are followed by marked elevation in temperature, anorexia, and dehydration. Intercanthic swelling, palpebral edema with closure of the eye, conjunctivitis, and proptosis, and a purulent discharge from the nose or inner canthus may ensue.

Oral examination reveals swelling of the maxilla on the infected side, extending to both the buccal and the palatal regions, with fluctuant areas often present with multiple drain-

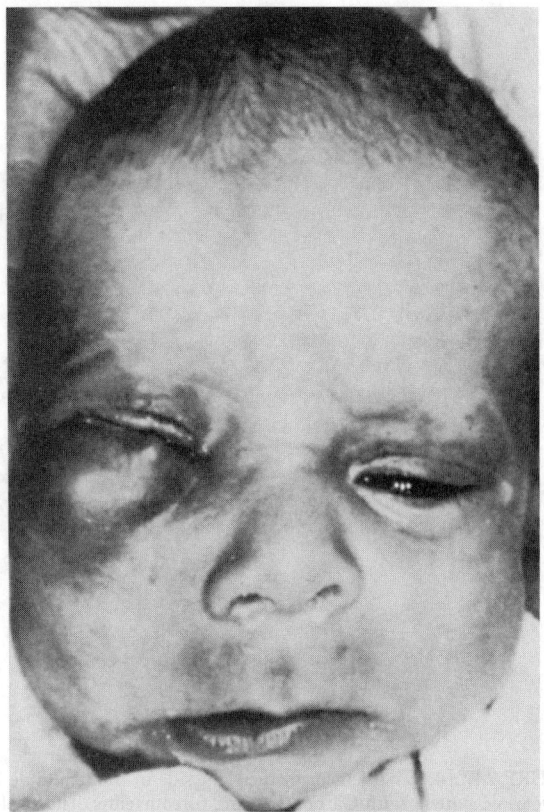

FIGURE 247.13. A 3-week-old child with infantile osteomyelitis. (Reprinted from Simos C, Flynn TR, Piecuch JF, et al. Infections of the oral cavity. In: Feigin RD, Cherry JD, eds. *Textbook of pediatric infectious diseases*, 5th ed. Philadelphia: WB Saunders, 2004:159. Original image courtesy of M. Michael Cohen, Sr., D.D.S.)

ing sinuses. *S. aureus* is the usual organism found. Aggressive, prompt treatment must be undertaken to prevent permanent optic damage, neurologic complications, loss of tooth buds in the bone, and extension to the dural sinuses. Initial antibiotic treatment includes intravenous vancomycin, pending results of Gram stain, culture, and sensitivity testing. Fluctuant areas must be drained. Antibiotics should be continued orally for 2 to 4 weeks after all signs of the infection have disappeared. If sequestra form, they should be removed conservatively. Notably, tooth buds may be lost, and surviving teeth may be deformed or discolored after eruption.

Chronic Recurrent Multifocal Osteomyelitis of Children

An uncommon form of osteomyelitis of the jaws that has been described affects children at an average age of 14 years and is characterized by unpredictable periods of exacerbation and remission. It is called chronic recurrent multifocal osteomyelitis of children. Its cause is as yet unclear. Mandibular lesions are bilateral, irregular, mottled, and multilocular. Antibiotics and débridement appear to have little effect on the prolonged course of this disease.

Garré Sclerosing Osteomyelitis

Garré sclerosing osteomyelitis, also known as chronic nonsuppurative sclerosing osteomyelitis and proliferative osteomyelitis of Garré is notable because of the similarity of some of its characteristics to those of other neoperiostoses. It is characterized by a localized, hard, nontender swelling of the mandible

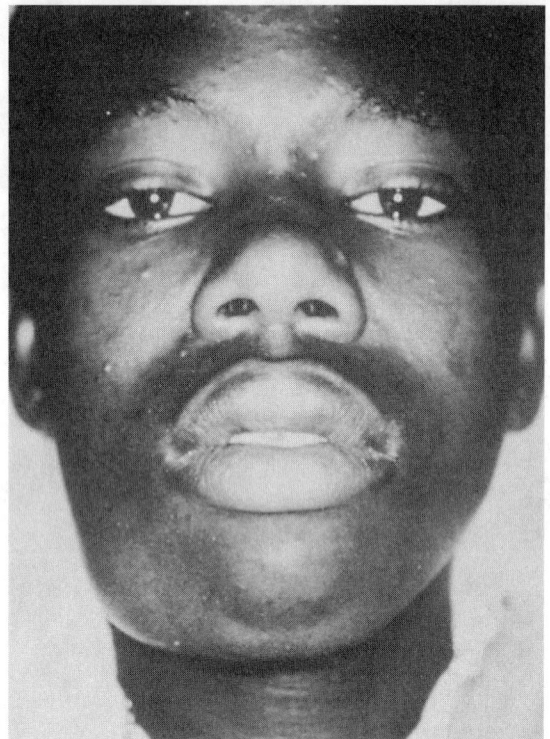

FIGURE 247.14. Enlargement of the right side of the mandible in a 12-year-old patient with Garré sclerosing osteomyelitis. The swelling is hard and nontender. (Reprinted from Simos C, Flynn TR, Piecuch JF, et al. Infections of the oral cavity. In: Feigin RD, Cherry JD, eds. *Textbook of pediatric infectious diseases,* 5th ed. Philadelphia: WB Saunders, 2004:159.)

(Fig. 247.14). Lymphadenopathy, fever, and leukocytosis are not present. Commonly, the disorder is associated with a carious tooth, usually the lower first molar, with a history of a toothache that may have resolved. It may be associated also with a recent dental extraction or with pericoronitis of an erupting tooth. Radiography is fairly impressive, showing a focal area of well-calcified bone proliferation that is smooth and often has a laminated or onion-peel appearance (Fig. 247.15). Garré osteomyelitis is thought to be a response to a low-grade stimulus, such as a dental infection, that influences the potentially active periosteum of young individuals. Its appearance resembles that of infantile cortical hyperostosis (Caffey disease),

osteosarcoma, and Ewing sarcoma and must be distinguished from these conditions. Treatment consists of extraction of or endodontic therapy for the involved tooth, with continued clinical and radiographic follow-up of affected patients to ensure that abnormal new bone formation does not progress. Ordinarily, remodeling occurs over time, but biopsies should be performed to rule out neoplasm if the lesion does not regress. No antibiotic therapy is indicated.

Acknowledgments

The authors thank Lisa Lavargna of the Harvard School of Dental Medicine for her editorial input.

Suggested Readings

Anderson MH, Bales DJ, Omnell KA. Modern management of dental caries: the cutting edge is not the dental bur. *J Am Dent Assoc* 1993;124:37.

Balcerak RJ, Sisto JM, Bosack RC. Cervicofacial necrotizing fasciitis: report of three cases and literature review. *J Oral Maxillofac Surg* 1988;46:450.

Benca PG, Mostofi R, Kuo P. Proliferative periostitis (Garré's osteomyelitis). *Oral Surg* 1987;63:258.

Dodson TB, Perrott DH, Kaban LB. Pediatric maxillofacial infections: a retrospective study of 113 patients. *J Oral Maxillofac Surg* 1989;47:327.

Flynn TR. Anatomy of oral and maxillofacial infections. In: Topazian RG, Goldberg MH, Hupp JR, eds. *Oral and maxillofacial infections,* 4th ed. Philadelphia: WB Saunders, 2002:188.

Flynn TR. Surgical management of orofacial infections: atlas. *Oral Maxillofac Surg Clin North Am* 2000;8:77.

Flynn TR. The swollen face. *Emerg Med Clin North Am* 2000;15:481.

Flynn TR. The timing of incision and drainage. In: Piecuch JF, ed. *Oral and maxillofacial surgery knowledge update 2002.* Rosemont, IL: American Association of Oral and Maxillofacial Surgeons, 2002.

Flynn TR. Update on the antibiotic therapy of oral and maxillofacial infections. In: Piecuch JF, ed. *Oral and maxillofacial surgery knowledge update 2002.* Rosemont, IL: American Association of Oral and Maxillofacial Surgeons, 2002.

Flynn TR, Halpern LR. Antibiotic selection in head and neck infections. *Oral Maxillofac Surg Clin North Am* 2003;15:17.

Gilmore WC, Jacobus NV, Gorbach SL, et al. A prospective double-blind evaluation of penicillin versus clindamycin in the treatment of odontogenic infections. *J Oral Maxillofac Surg* 1988;46:1065.

Hall HD, Gunter JW, Jamison HC, et al. Effect of time of extraction on resolution of odontogenic cellulitis. *J Am Dent Assoc* 1968;77:626.

Heimdahl A, VonKonow L, Satoh T, et al. Clinical appearance of orofacial infections of odontogenic origin in relation to microbiological findings. *J Clin Microbiol* 1985;22:299.

Leggott PJ. Oral manifestations of HIV infection in children. *Oral Surg Oral Med Oral Pathol Oral Radiol Endod* 1992;73:187.

Lewis MAO, MacFarlane TW, McGowan DA. Quantitative bacteriology of acute dentoalveolar abscesses. *J Med Microbiol* 1986;21:101.

Lewis MAO, Parkhurst CL, Douglas CW, et al. Prevalence of penicillin-resistant bacteria in acute suppurative oral infection. *J Antimicrob Chemother* 1995; 35:785.

Mampalam TJ, Rosenblum ML. Trends in the management of bacterial brain abscesses: a review of 102 cases over 17 years. *Neurosurgery* 1988;23:451.

Marx RE. Chronic osteomyelitis of the jaws. *Oral Maxillofac Surg Clin North Am* 1991;3:367.

O'Ryan F, Diloreto D, Barber HD, et al. Orbital infections: clinical and radiographic diagnosis and surgical treatment. *J Oral Maxillofac Surg* 1988; 46:991.

Scully C, McCarthy G. Management of oral health in persons with HIV infection. *Oral Surg Oral Med Oral Pathol Oral Radiol Endod* 1992;73:215.

Simos C, Flynn TR, Piecuch JF, Topazian RG. Infections of the oral cavity. In: Feigin RD, Cherry JD, eds. *Textbook of pediatric infectious diseases,* 5th ed. Philadelphia: WB Saunders, 2004:147.

Straus SE, Rooney JF, Sever JL, et al. NIH conference. Herpes simplex virus infection: biology, treatment, prevention. *Ann Intern Med* 1985;103:404.

Topazian RG, Goldberg MH, eds. *Oral and maxillofacial infections,* 4th ed. Philadelphia: WB Saunders, 2002.

Trieger N. Periodontal infections. In: Kelly JPW, ed. *OMS knowledge update,* vol 1, part II. Rosemont, IL: American Association of Oral and Maxillofacial Surgeons, 1995:65.

Tuite-McDonnell M, Griffen AL, Moeschberger MC, et al. Concordance of *Porphyromonas gingivalis* colonization in families. *J Clin Microbiol* 1997; 35:455.

Watanabe K. Prepubertal periodontitis: a review of diagnostic criteria, pathogenesis, and differential diagnosis. *J Periodont Res* 1990;25:31.

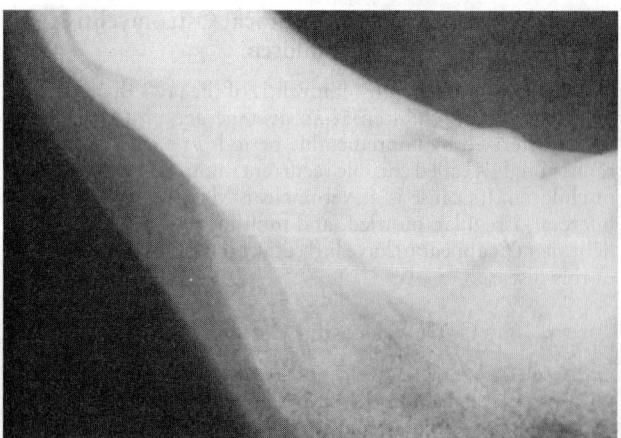

FIGURE 247.15. Characteristic radiograph of Garré osteomyelitis, showing the laminated or onion-peel appearance of the mass.

CHAPTER 248 ■ PHARYNGITIS

MARGARET R. HAMMERSCHLAG

Children and young adults visit physicians for sore throats more often than for any other problem or symptom. Technically, pharyngitis is an inflammatory illness of the mucous membranes and underlying structures of the throat. Although the symptom of sore throat invariably is present with pharyngitis, it should not be used as the sole criterion for diagnosis. Sore throat can be a common complaint in children with colds when no evidence of pharyngeal inflammation is present.

Pharyngitis can be subdivided into two categories: illness with and illness without nasal symptoms. This division has important etiologic implications. Almost always, nasopharyngitis has a viral cause, whereas illness without nasal symptoms (pharyngitis or tonsillopharyngitis) can have diverse causative agents, including bacteria, viruses, and fungi (Table 248.1).

ETIOLOGY

Most often, the etiologic agents involved in nasopharyngitis are viruses, with adenovirus types 7a, 9, 14, and 15 being the most common. Influenza, parainfluenza, and Epstein-Barr virus are the other major viral agents. Rhinovirus and respiratory syncytial virus infections are not often associated with objective pharyngeal findings.

Pharyngitis (including tonsillitis and tonsillopharyngitis) can be caused by a diversity of infectious agents, ranging from group A beta-hemolytic streptococci to more obscure agents, such as *Corynebacterium diphtheriae* and *Francisella tularensis*. As with other infections, the probability that any one agent is the cause of pharyngitis depends on the age and immune status of affected patients, the season, and the environment. In normal, healthy children, more than 90% of all cases of pharyngitis are caused by the following organisms, listed in order of decreasing frequency of occurrence: group A beta-hemolytic streptococci; adenoviruses; influenza viruses A and B; parainfluenza viruses 1, 2, and 3; Epstein-Barr virus; enteroviruses; and *Mycoplasma pneumoniae*. Pharyngitis and sore throat may be present also in 44% of patients with acute human immunodeficiency virus type 1 infection.

Other beta-hemolytic streptococci, especially groups C and G, have also been isolated from children and young adults with pharyngitis. Other, less common bacterial sources of pharyngitis include *Arcanobacterium haemolyticum*, formerly called *C. hemolyticum*. The genus *Arcanobacterium* currently includes six species. *A. haemolyticum* has also been isolated from chronic skin ulcers, soft tissue infections, and brain, peritonsillar, paravertebral, and intraabdominal abscesses. The organism has also been associated with pneumonia, sinusitis, and orbital cellulitis in children. *A. haemolyticum* has been identified in 0.5% to 9.3% of children and adolescents with pharyngitis in three studies from Canada, Greece, and Finland. In one study, 50% of the patients with *A. haemolyticum* also had group A streptococci isolated from their throat cultures. The organism has been found infrequently in individuals without pharyngitis. A study of Finnish army conscripts found *A. haemolyticum* in 0.4% of asymptomatic individuals. Children

in the 15- to 18-year-old age group were most likely to be affected. Clinically, pharyngitis due to *A. haemolyticum* closely resembles that caused by group A beta-hemolytic streptococci, and a significant number of patients may also have a scarlatiniform rash. There are no population-based studies on the role of

TABLE 248.1

CAUSES OF PHARYNGITIS

Organism	Percentage of Cases	Associated Disorders or Symptoms
Bacteria		
Group A streptococcus	5–20	Tonsillitis, scarlet fever, ARF
Beta-hemolytic streptococci group C or G	6	Tonsillitis, scarlatiniform rash
Neisseria gonorrhoeae	Rare	Tonsillitis
Arcanobacterium haemolyticum	0.5–9.3	Scarlatiniform rash
Corynebacterium diphtheriae	Rare	Diphtheria
Francisella tularensis	Rare	Tularemia (oropharyngeal form)
Virus		
Adenovirus, types 7a, 9, 14, 15	19	Pharyngoconjunctival fever, acute respiratory disease including pneumonia
Epstein-Barr virus	7–15	Infectious mononucleosis
Rhinovirus	?	Common cold
Coronavirus	?	Common cold
Respiratory syncytial virus	1	Bronchiolitis, URI
Parainfluenza virus	5	Cold and croup
Coxsackie A	?	Herpangina, hand-foot-and-mouth disease
Influenza A and B virus	?	Influenza
Cytomegalovirus	?	CMV mononucleosis
Herpes simplex virus types 1, 2	?	Gingivostomatitis
Human immunodeficiency virus	?	Primary HIV infection
Other		
Mycoplasma pneumoniae	10–13	Pneumonia, bronchitis, otitis, erythema multiforme
Chlamydia pneumoniae	?	Pneumonia

ARF, acute rheumatic fever; CMV, cytomegalovirus; HIV, human immunodeficiency virus; URI, upper respirator infection.

A. haemolyticum in pharyngitis from the United States. *Neisseria gonorrhoeae* should be considered in adolescents who are sexually active or are known to have been exposed and possibly should be considered in abused children. Most abused children from whom *N. gonorrhoeae* has been isolated from the nasopharynx are asymptomatic.

Among viral causes, adenovirus is the most prevalent. One study has found viruses to be responsible for 42% of all cases of pharyngitis in a group of children who were between ages 6 months and 17.9 years and who had acute exudative tonsillitis. Adenovirus was responsible for 19% of the cases, followed by Epstein-Barr virus. Two children (1.8%) had infections with herpes simplex virus, and five children had infections with *M. pneumoniae*.

CLINICAL MANIFESTATIONS AND COMPLICATIONS

Nasopharyngitis tends to be more common in younger children. The presentation can vary, depending on the agent. Usually, fever is present. Infection with adenovirus may be associated with conjunctivitis and exudative pharyngitis, whereas infection with influenza A or B frequently is associated with more severe systemic complaints. The onset of pharyngitis can be acute, with fever and the complaint of sore throat. Affected children also may have headache, nausea, vomiting, and, occasionally, abdominal pain. Usually, physical examination reveals moderate to severe pharyngeal erythema and tonsillar enlargement and varying degrees of cervical adenitis. The erythema can be associated with follicular, ulcerative, and petechial lesions and with areas of exudate. Follicular tonsillitis is fairly characteristic of adenoviral infections, and ulcerative lesions usually are observed with enteroviral infections. The presence of exudate has been thought in the past to be most common or characteristic of group A streptococcal infection or infectious mononucleosis. A prospective, 1-year study of acute febrile exudative tonsillitis, however, found that 42% of the cases had a viral cause, predominantly adenovirus. The only clinical clues to the nature of the infecting agent were cough and rhinitis, both of which were observed in 45% of patients with viral disease and in only 10% of children with beta-hemolytic streptococci. Pharyngitis in children is almost entirely acute and self-limited, lasting from 4 to 10 days, depending on the cause.

Streptococcal pharyngitis can have significant suppurative complications, including peritonsillar abscess and bacteremia. Postanginal sepsis is a clinical syndrome that usually occurs in adolescents or young adults after an oronasopharyngeal infection (frequently infectious mononucleosis). After a latency period of several days, contiguous or lymphatic spread of local infection, septicemia, and septic metastases can be observed. Usually, septicemia in these cases is attributed to thrombophlebitis in small and large vessels of the face and neck. The organisms involved most frequently in this syndrome are anaerobes, including *Fusobacterium* species and *Bacteroides* species. Streptococcal toxic shock syndrome is usually not associated with streptococcal pharyngitis. An uncommon recently recognized complication of streptococcal pharyngitis is the PANDAS syndrome: pediatric autoimmune neuropsychiatric disorder associated with group A streptococci. PANDAS is an entity characterized by five working criteria: presence of obsessive-compulsive disorder (OCD) and/or tic disorder, pediatric onset, abrupt onset and episodic course of symptoms, association with group A streptococcal infections, and association with neurologic abnormalities, such as hyperactivity, choreiform movements, or tics. Most knowledge about PANDAS to date has been obtained by studying patients with known tic disorder or long-standing OCD.

One prospective study of children in a primary care practice over a 3-year period identified 12 with PANDAS, all of whom had documented group A streptococcal tonsillopharyngitis. Antibiotic therapy resulted in improvement of the OCD symptoms in all of the patients; four patients resolved their symptoms in 5 to 21 days without recurrence. Recurrent symptoms developed in six cases associated with a new episode of tonsillopharyngitis; a repeat course of antibiotics again ameliorated symptoms.

DIAGNOSIS

Differential Diagnosis

Because of the numerous organisms that can cause pharyngitis and the significant overlap among them in clinical presentation and findings, making a specific diagnosis on the basis of physical findings alone (e.g., the presence of exudate) is difficult. The age and clinical status of affected patients and the time of year should be taken into account. Age may be the most important factor in predicting the causative agent, with viral tonsillitis being most common in patients younger than age 3 and group A beta-hemolytic streptococci being found most often in children aged 6 or older. The presence of rhinitis also is more suggestive of a viral infection. In adolescents and adults, viral infection or infection with *M. pneumoniae* is more likely. Although pharyngitis and sore throat are frequent in patients with lower respiratory tract infection due to *Chlamydia pneumoniae*, the role of this organism as an etiologic agent of pharyngitis in children is unknown.

Pharyngeal Culture

Because infection with group A streptococci can have significant suppurative and nonsuppurative complications, streptococcal disease must be excluded in all instances of acute pharyngitis. If affected children are younger than 3 years old or have obvious viral infection, such as pharyngoconjunctival fever (adenovirus) or herpangina, antibiotic therapy is not needed and, therefore, cultures are not indicated.

The definite diagnosis of group A streptococcal infection remains identification of the organism in the pharynx by culture. Confirmation that early treatment of severe streptococcal pharyngitis hastens recovery has rendered rapid diagnosis of this condition desirable. However, even "routine" culture methods may have problems with sensitivity. If done correctly, the sensitivity of culture of a single throat swab for the detection of group A streptococci is 90% to 95%. The manner in which the throat swab is obtained can also affect the accuracy of throat culture results. The specimen should be obtained from the surface of both tonsils and the posterior pharyngeal wall. Duration of incubation can also affect the yield of the throat culture. An additional incubation of the plate overnight at room temperature will identify a sizable number of positive cultures that were not identified after the initial 18- to 24-hour incubation at 35°C to 37°C.

A number of rapid, nonculture antigen detection kits are available for the diagnosis of streptococcal pharyngitis. The earlier tests used latex agglutination methods that were relatively insensitive. The majority of currently available tests are based on enzyme immunoassay techniques that offer increased sensitivity and more sharply defined endpoints. These tests all detect the group A cell wall carbohydrate by an antibody-antigen reaction. Overall, the tests appear to be very specific (95% to 99%) compared with blood agar plate culture. This means that false-positive test results are uncommon and therapeutic decisions can be made with confidence on the basis of a positive test. However, the sensitivities range from 53% to 97%, when compared with blood agar plate culture. Two approved tests using novel technologies, molecular biology–based methods (direct DNA probe and a one-rapid-cycle real-time polymerase chain reaction [PCR]) and an optical immunoassay, are highly specific, but the sensitivities have also been found to have a considerable range, from 86% to 95% for the DNA probe and PCR and 75.5% to 98.9% for the optical immunoassay. It has been suggested that false-negative rapid test results might be due to low concentration of organisms in the throat swab specimen, and that these patients are only chronic carriers. However, several studies have demonstrated little correlation between the degree of positivity (number of colonies) and changes in streptococcal antibody titers. In one study, 45% of the children who had false-negative throat antigen test results using a rapid test kit had significant changes in their streptococcal antibody titers. If the prevalence of infection also is low (less than 50%) in a particular population, the positive predictive value of these tests may be 56% or less. Neither conventional throat culture nor sensitive rapid tests accurately differentiate acutely infected persons from asymptomatic streptococcal carriers with an intercurrent viral infection. The currently available rapid tests will not identify groups C and G streptococci. The DNA probe and real-time PCR are not point-of-service tests that can be performed in the clinician's office.

Current recommendations regarding the use of rapid tests for detection of group A streptococci in throat swabs are based on the performance characteristic of high specificity, which means that one is unlikely to get a false-positive tests, and lower sensitivity, which requires confirmation of negative rapid test by culture. One should obtain duplicate specimens, one for the rapid test and one for standard culture. If the rapid test is positive, no further testing is indicated (positive results do not need to be confirmed by culture). If the test is negative, the second swab should be processed for culture. Recommendations for the clinical use of rapid tests should reflect the clinical setting in which they are performed, whether it be hospital, private office, or clinic, as well as cost issues and the availability and expense of standard throat cultures. If the clinician wishes to rely on a rapid test, he or she should establish that the specific rapid test to be used performs satisfactorily compared with throat cultures in his or her own practice.

For identification of other bacteria, such as *A. haemolyticum* or *N. gonorrhoeae*, the laboratory must be informed specifically so that appropriate media are used. Examination of Gram stains of the exudate does not appear to be an accurate way to identify group A streptococci, *N. gonorrhoeae*, or *A. haemolyticum*.

THERAPY

Because the majority of pharyngitis episodes are viral and self-limited, specific therapy is not indicated except for streptococcal pharyngitis and infections due to *N. gonorrhoeae*. Intramuscular benzathine penicillin or a 10-day course of oral penicillin remains the treatment of choice because of the proven efficacy (greater than 90%), safety, narrow spectrum, and low cost. Erythromycin is a suitable alternative for patients sensitive to penicillin. First- or second-generation cephalosporins also are acceptable for treating patients who do not exhibit immediate hypersensitivity to beta-lactam antibiotics. Most oral antibiotics must be administered as a 10-day course to achieve maximal eradication of group A streptococci from the pharynx. Some of the newer cephalosporins and macrolides, including azithromycin, clarithromycin, and telithromycin, have been reported to achieve comparable clinical and bacteriologic cure rates when these drugs were given for 5 days or less. How-

ever, data still are limited, and these shorter courses cannot be recommended unequivocally at this time. In addition, these antibiotics have spectrums much broader than those of penicillin and are more expensive. Although azithromycin has been found to be effective in a short course regimen for eradication of oropharyngeal group A streptococci, it was found that treatment also selected for macrolide-resistant strains of *Streptococcus pneumoniae*. Resistance of group A streptococci to erythromycin and other macrolides can develop with extensive use of these agents. Although the overall rate of resistance to erythromycin among group A streptococci in the United States is not more than 5%, there have been recent outbreaks among schoolchildren where the rates of resistance exceeded 40%. None of these isolates was resistant to clindamycin. Molecular typing in one outbreak that occurred in Pittsburgh in 2001 indicated that the outbreak was due to a single strain of group A streptococci. Recent treatment studies evaluating 5-day courses of clarithromycin have found failures when used in areas where macrolide-resistant group A streptococci are common. Studies have suggested that some clinical and bacteriologic treatment failures after therapy with penicillins may have been caused by the presence of beta-lactamase–producing bacteria, especially *Bacteroides fragilis* and *B. melaninogenicus*. Subsequent treatment with an antibiotic resistant to beta-lactamase, such as clindamycin, or with a cephalosporin frequently was effective.

The importance of accurate diagnosis and appropriate therapy of pharyngitis cannot be emphasized too strongly. A resurgence of acute rheumatic fever has been seen in several parts of the United States, including Utah, Pennsylvania, and Ohio. In an outbreak in Akron, Ohio, the patients generally were not indigent and had good access to medical care. Approximately 80% of the patients had had an illness suggesting pharyngitis within 1 month of the onset of acute rheumatic fever; of these, 39% either had failed to receive a full 10-day course of antibiotics or had received no antibiotics at all.

Suggested Readings

Alpert JJ, Pickering MR, Warren RJ. Failure to isolate streptococci from children under the age of 3 years with exudative tonsillitis. *Pediatrics* 1966;38:663.

Bisno AL. Acute pharyngitis: etiology and diagnosis. *Pediatrics* 1996;97:949.

Bisno AL, Gerber MA, Gwaltney JM, et al. Practice guidelines for the diagnosis and management of group A streptococcal pharyngitis. *J Infect Dis* 2002;35:113.

Brook I. Beta-lactamase-producing bacteria recovered after clinical failures with various penicillin therapies. *Arch Otolaryngol* 1984;110:228.

Brook I, Leyva F. Discrepancies in the recovery of group A beta-hemolytic streptococci from both tonsillar surfaces. *Laryngoscope* 1991;101:795.

Carlson P, Kontiainen S, Renkonen OV, Sivonen A, Visakorpi R. *Arcanobacterium haemolyticum* and streptococcal pharyngitis in army conscripts. *Scand J Infect Dis* 1995;27:17.

Carlson P, Renkonen OV, Kontiainen S. *Arcanobacterium haemolyticum* and streptococcal pharyngitis. *Scand J Infect Dis* 1994;26:283.

Chapin KC, Blake P, Wilson CD. Performance characteristics and utilization of rapid antigen test, DNA probe and culture for detection of group A streptococci from an acute care clinic. *J Clin Microbiol* 2002;40:4207.

Congeni B, Rizzo C, Congeni J, et al. Outbreak of acute rheumatic fever in northeast Ohio. *J Pediatr* 1987;111:176.

Gerber MA, Schulam ST. Rapid diagnosis of pharyngitis caused by group A streptococci. *Clin Microbiol Rev* 2004;17:571.

Gieseker KE, Roe MH, MacKenzie T, et al. Evaluating the American Academy of Pediatrics Diagnostic Standard for *Streptococcus pyogenes* pharyngitis: backup culture versus repeat rapid antigen testing. *Pediatrics* 2003;111:e666.

Houvonen P, Lahtonen R, Ziegler T, et al. Pharyngitis in adults: the presence and coexistence of viruses and bacterial organisms. *Ann Intern Med* 1989;110:612.

Kaplan EL. Recent evaluation of antimicrobial resistance in beta-hemolytic streptococci. *Clin Infect Dis* 1997;24:S89.

Kaplan EL, Hill HR. Return of rheumatic fever: consequences, implications and needs. *J Pediatr* 1987;111:244.

Karpathios T, Drakonaki S, Zervoudaki A, et al. *Arcanobacterium haemolyticum* in children with presumed streptococcal pharyngotonsillitis or scarlet fever. *J Pediatr* 1992;121:735.

Limjoco-Antonio AD, Janda WM, Schreckenberger PC. *Arcanobacterium haemolyticum* sinusitis and orbital cellulitis. *Pediatr Infect Dis J* 2003; 22:465.

Mackenzie A, Fuite LA, Chan FT, et al. Incidence and pathogenicity of *Arcanobacterium haemolyticum* during a 2-year study in Ottawa. *Clin Infect Dis* 1995;21:177.

Martin JM, Green M, Barbadora KA, et al. Erythromycin resistant group A streptococci in schoolchildren in Pittsburgh. *New Engl J Med* 2002;346:1200.

McIsaac WJ, Kellner JD, Aufricht P, Vanjaka A, Low DE. Empirical validation of guidelines for the management of pharyngitis in children and adults. *JAMA* 2004;291:1587.

Miller RA, Brancato F, Holmes KK. *Corynebacterium hemolyticum* as a cause of pharyngitis and scarlatiniform rash in young adults. *Am J Med* 1986; 105:867.

Morita JY, Kahn E, Thompson T, et al. Impact of azithromycin on oropharyngeal carriage of group A streptococcus and nasopharyngeal carriage of macrolide-resistant *Streptococcus pneumoniae. Pediatr Infect Dis J* 2000;19:41.

Murphy ML, Pichichero ME. Prospective identification and treatment of children with pediatric autoimmune neuropsychiatric disorder associated with group A streptococcal infection (PANDAS). *Arch Pediatr Adolesc Med* 2002; 156:356.

Putto A. Febrile exudative tonsillitis: viral or streptococcal. *Pediatrics* 1987; 80:6.

Turner JC, Hayden GF, Kiscelica D, et al. Association of group C beta-hemolytic streptococci with endemic pharyngitis among college students. *JAMA* 1990;264:2644.

Van Cauwenberge PB, Vander Mijnsbrugge AM. Pharyngitis: a survey of the microbiologic etiology. *Pediatr Infect Dis J* 1991;10:S39.

CHAPTER 249 ■ DEEP NECK ABSCESSES

NIRA A. GOLDSTEIN AND MARGARET R. HAMMERSCHLAG

A deep neck abscess is a collection of pus in a potential space bounded by fascia. These potential spaces are areas of least resistance to the spread of infection. An infection may begin with a minimal area of cellulitis and progress to a deep neck abscess, which then may extend to invade adjacent potential spaces; these spaces frequently encompass vital structures in the neck. Destruction and dysfunction of these structures represent the major complications of deep neck infections.

PERITONSILLAR ABSCESS (QUINSY)

A peritonsillar abscess (quinsy) is circumscribed medially by the fibrous wall of the tonsil capsule and laterally by the superior constrictor muscle. Peritonsillar abscesses rarely occur in young children. They most commonly occur in patients in late adolescence and in the early part of the third decade. One series from Pittsburgh, Pennsylvania, reported the mean age of the children with peritonsillar infection to be 11 years. The cause of peritonsillar abscesses is not constant; they may follow any "virulent" case of tonsillitis, with extension through the fibrous tonsil capsule.

Clinical Manifestations

The recent history may include a sore throat with unilateral pain, malaise, low-grade pyrexia, chills, diaphoresis, dysphagia, reduced oral intake, trismus, and a muffled "hot potato voice." Trismus results from irritation and reflex spasm of the internal pterygoid muscle. Impaired palatal motion from edema contributes to the muffled voice. Physical examination reveals minimal to moderate toxicity, dehydration, and drooling. Inspection of the oropharynx may be compromised by trismus. The soft palate is displaced toward the unaffected side, is swollen and red, and is frequently palpably fluctuant. The edematous uvula is pushed across the midline. The displaced tonsil and its crypts are rarely coated with exudate. The breath is fetid, and ipsilateral, tender, cervical adenopathy is present.

The white blood cell count is elevated, with a predominance of polymorphonuclear leukocytes. Brodsky and associates attempted to identify the clinical signs that could distinguish peritonsillar abscess from peritonsillar cellulitis in a group of 21 children admitted to the Children's Hospital of Buffalo, New York, from 1985 through 1987. No significant difference in age, duration of sore throat, fever, or white blood cell count was noted, although a greater degree of pharyngotonsillar bulge and muffled voice was found in the patients with abscess. However, patients with peritonsillar cellulitis improved after receiving 24 hours of intravenous antibiotics, whereas patients with peritonsillar abscess had no change or worsening of symptoms. Blotter and colleagues confirmed these findings in a group of 102 patients admitted to Children's Hospital of Columbus, Ohio, between 1995 and 1998.

Therapy

Traditionally, management of peritonsillar abscess in children involved hospital admission for intravenous hydration, antibiotic therapy and analgesia, and either intraoral incision and drainage of the abscess or "acute quinsy tonsillectomy" with removal of the medial wall of the abscess. Acute tonsillectomy was often performed to prevent future recurrence of the peritonsillar abscess.

Studies have suggested that many peritonsillar abscesses can be managed by simple needle aspiration combined with antibiotic therapy on an outpatient basis. An extensive metaanalysis by Herzon of 10 previous studies conducted from 1961 through 1994 involving 496 patients with peritonsillar abscesses found an overall success rate of needle aspiration of 94% (range, 85% to 100%). This success rate compares favorably with the success rate reported for incision and drainage. Weinberg and associates successfully performed needle aspiration in 41 of 43 children, aged 7 to 18 years, with a mean age of 13.9 years. All were admitted for intravenous antibiotic therapy, two (5%) required repeat aspiration for resolution, and five (12%) did not respond and required acute tonsillectomy. Other studies, which have included both adults and children with peritonsillar abscesses, have reported that 0% to 14% of patients required hospitalization, although the ages of the patients requiring hospitalization was not reported. Younger children often require admission to correct dehydration. Younger children are also more likely than older children to respond to intravenous antibiotics alone and to have negative findings at surgical drainage. The use of conscious sedation has been reported to be a safe and effective approach for the drainage of peritonsillar abscesses in children.

A suggested approach to the management of children with peritonsillar abscess is as follows. Cooperative children should undergo needle aspiration of the abscess and treatment with antibiotics. Children who can tolerate liquids orally may be managed as outpatients, and the remainder should be admitted for hydration and intravenous antibiotics. Approximately 4% of children will require a repeated aspiration for resolution. Children who remain symptomatic after undergoing needle aspiration require incision and drainage or acute quinsy tonsillectomy depending on the prior history of recurrent tonsillitis. Children who cannot tolerate needle aspiration on initial presentation are admitted for administration of intravenous antibiotics. If no response occurs within 24 hours, incision and drainage or acute tonsillectomy is performed depending on the prior history of recurrent tonsillitis. Delayed tonsillectomy is reserved for children who recover from the peritonsillar abscess without general anesthesia but have a history of recurrent tonsillitis or prior peritonsillar abscess.

Untreated peritonsillar abscess may point, with spontaneous rupture, or may extend to the parapharyngeal space with potentially fatal complications. Upper airway obstruction, septicemia, and vascular catastrophe may occur. Necrotizing fasciitis has also been reported in adults with peritonsillar abscess.

RETROPHARYNGEAL ABSCESS (POSTERIOR VISCERAL SPACE, RETROVISCERAL SPACE, AND RETROESOPHAGEAL SPACE ABSCESSES)

The anterior wall of the retropharyngeal space is the middle layer of the deep cervical fascia, which abuts the posterior esophageal wall (the superior pharyngeal constrictor muscle). The deep layer of the deep cervical fascia circumscribes the posterior wall of this potential space. Inferiorly, these two fasciae fuse to limit the depth of this pocket at a level between the first and second thoracic vertebrae. A retropharyngeal abscess can erode inferiorly through the junction of these fasciae to extend posteriorly into the prevertebral space. Subsequently, pus in the prevertebral space can descend inferiorly below the diaphragm to the psoas muscles.

The retropharyngeal space contains two paramedial chains of lymph nodes that receive drainage from the nasopharynx, adenoids, posterior paranasal sinuses, middle ear, and eustachian tube. These structures are prominent in early childhood and atrophy at puberty. Retropharyngeal abscesses have been reported to occur more frequently in young children with a mean age of presentation of 4 years and are thought to be secondary to suppurative adenitis of these retropharyngeal nodes. Other sources of infection are penetrating foreign bodies, endoscopy, trauma, pharyngitis, vertebral body osteomyelitis, petrositis, dental procedures, and branchial cleft anomalies.

Clinical Manifestations

The symptoms of retropharyngeal abscess frequently begin insidiously after mild antecedent infection. No trismus occurs, but a stiff neck secondary to muscle tenderness may be present along with an ipsilateral tender cervical adenopathy. Although classic teaching described stridor and upper airway obstruction in children with retropharyngeal abscesses, more recent reviews have shown that these symptoms are uncommon in children, most likely because children are presenting earlier in the course of the disease. Early in the course, midline or unilateral swelling of the posterior pharynx occurs. Later, gentle palpation may demonstrate a large, fluctuant mass in the posterior pharynx. Posterior mediastinitis can result from the spread of infection from the retropharyngeal area into the prevertebral space. Other complications may be seen when the abscess extends to the parapharyngeal space and involves the great vessels and cranial nerves.

As with other abscesses, the white blood count is increased, with a predominance of granulocytes. Plain films of the neck are often the initial radiologic study performed but must be taken with the patient in a true lateral position, with the neck in extension, and on inspiration, or the child's retropharyngeal soft tissues may appear abnormally thickened. Widening of the prevertebral soft tissues exceeding the anteroposterior diameter of the contiguous vertebral bodies or thickening of the retropharyngeal space greater than 7 mm at C2 in both children and adults, or 14 mm at C6 in children or 22 mm at C6 in adults, suggests retropharyngeal inflammation.

Computed tomography (CT) scanning has made the diagnosis and management of deep neck space infections more precise. In contrast to conventional radiologic studies, the CT scan distinguishes cellulitis of the neck, which usually does not require surgical treatment, from a deep neck abscess, which requires surgical drainage. With its ability to define differences in tissue density, CT scanning permits accurate determination of the extent of the abscess and its extension and involvement of adjacent spaces. An abscess is distinguished from cellulitis by a low-attenuation homogeneous area surrounded by a ring enhancement of contrast material. Kirse and Roberson reported scalloping of the abscess wall to be a more useful predictor of the presence of pus than ring enhancement (Fig. 249.1).

A 10-year retrospective study from the Massachusetts Eye and Ear Infirmary compared preoperative CT scans with intraoperative findings in 38 patients who underwent surgical exploration of the parapharyngeal or retropharyngeal space within 48 hours after the scans were performed. Overall, the intraoperative findings confirmed the CT scan interpretation in 76.3% of the patients. Of the 38 patients, 5 (13.2%) had CT scans indicative of abscesses that were not confirmed at surgery. Exploration of the parapharyngeal or retropharyngeal space revealed cellulitis. The false-negative rate was 10.5%. The sensitivity of CT scanning for detection of parapharyngeal or retropharyngeal space abscess was 87.9%.

Therapy

Treatment consists of administration of intravenous antibiotics and incision and drainage through a peroral incision with the patient in the Rose position (supine with the neck hyperextended). Some reports have documented that patients with small retropharyngeal abscesses may respond to treatment with intravenous antibiotics alone. Broughton described the experience at the University of Kentucky Medical Center, in which 8 (57%) of 14 patients with deep neck infections seen during a 9-year period were treated successfully by antibiotics alone. All were reported to have small abscesses on CT scan. However, possibly some had only cellulitis. Craig and Schunk described the successful treatment of 10 (38%) of 27 patients with retropharyngeal abscesses on CT by intravenous antibiotics alone. Close clinical follow-up is mandatory for children

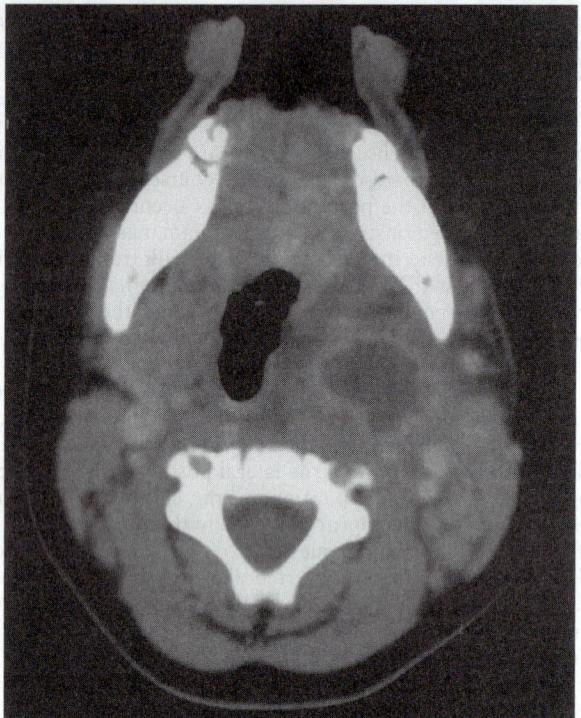

FIGURE 249.1. Appearance on a computed tomography scan of a focal, ring-enhancing retropharyngeal abscess with a scalloped contour to the abscess wall. (Reprinted from Kirse DJ, Robersin DW. Surgical management of retropharyngeal space infections in children. *Laryngoscope* 2001;111:1413.)

treated with intravenous antibiotics alone. Children who do not improve within 24 to 48 hours require surgical drainage.

PARAPHARYNGEAL ABSCESS (PTERYGOMAXILLARY, PHARYNGOMAXILLARY, LATERAL, AND PHARYNGEAL SPACE ABSCESSES)

The potential parapharyngeal space is an inverted conical cavity lying along an oblique axis roughly parallel to the ramus of the mandible. The base of the skull at the jugular foramen forms the base of the "cone," and its apex is at the hyoid bone. The parapharyngeal space is contiguous with the peritonsillar, submandibular, and retropharyngeal spaces, all of which are potential avenues of egress for an extending parapharyngeal space abscess. The posterior portion of the cone contains the contents of the carotid sheath (carotid artery and internal jugular vein), cranial nerves IX through XII, and the cervical sympathetic chain. Anterior are the internal pterygoid muscle and fatty connective tissue.

By the time a patient with an abscess seeks medical attention, the source of the parapharyngeal space infection may be unclear. Reports indicate variable causes: incompletely or inadequately treated bacterial pharyngitis, tonsillitis, peritonsillar abscess, dental infections, bacterial parotitis, otitis, mastoiditis (Bezold abscess from a mastoid tip infection traveling along the digastric muscles), petrositis, cervical adenitis with suppuration, cervical vertebral tubercular adenitis in the adult, foreign bodies, trauma, intravenous drug abuse, branchial cleft

anomalies, and cat-scratch disease. Parapharyngeal abscesses in children tend to occur in later childhood and in adolescence.

Clinical Manifestations

Presenting complaints include tender cervical swelling, induration and erythema of the side of the neck, torticollis, sore throat, dysphagia, trismus, hoarseness, malaise, chills, and diaphoresis. Variable low-grade pyrexia with occasional temperature spikes occurs. Examination discloses variable toxicity, medial displacement of the lateral pharyngeal wall and inferior tonsil pole, trismus, and, infrequently, drooling, respiratory tract distress, and laryngeal edema. Palpation of the neck reveals a tender, high cervical mass, initially diffuse and later fluctuant.

The complications of parapharyngeal abscesses are related to the structures involved: involvement of the carotid artery can produce hemiplegia from emboli; internal jugular vein thrombosis with cephalad extension may lead to a cavernous sinus thrombosis, whereas inferior extension leads to internal jugular vein thrombosis. Internal jugular vein thrombosis is characterized by spiking temperature, toxicity with intense diaphoresis, headaches, and increased intracranial pressure. Septic pulmonary emboli are occasionally present. Extension into the retropharyngeal region by a parapharyngeal abscess may lead to posterior mediastinitis. Airway obstruction secondary to laryngeal edema and aspiration pneumonia from suppuration of the abscess into the pharynx have been reported. Initially, the parapharyngeal abscess may be difficult to differentiate from a peritonsillar abscess, but the patient with a peritonsillar abscess is usually less toxic and there is a distinct, soft palate fluctuance.

As described for the diagnosis of retropharyngeal abscess, CT is an extremely useful tool for distinguishing parapharyngeal abscess from cellulitis and for localizing the abscess for surgical planning. In a review of 47 children who presented with a deep neck infection to the Children's Hospital of Buffalo over a 5½-year period, CT scan demonstrated that 34 (77%) of 44 patients who underwent CT scan had involvement of both the parapharyngeal and retropharyngeal spaces. The involvement of both spaces had implications for the approach to surgical drainage.

Therapy

Intravenous antibiotic therapy with incision and drainage is the primary treatment. The incision should be external, with sufficient exposure to provide immediate access to the common carotid artery for ligation, should there be carotid artery erosion. An intraoral drainage and incision procedure has traditionally been condemned because rapid access to the vital structures of the neck is not possible with this approach. However, Nagy and associates successfully treated 21 of 22 children with either parapharyngeal or combined parapharyngeal and retropharyngeal abscesses through an intraoral approach. The authors emphasized that CT with intravenous contrast enhancement demonstrated that all the abscesses were located medial to the great vessels and were adjacent to the pharyngeal wall.

The use of CT has made it possible for some patients with parapharyngeal abscesses to be managed with intravenous antibiotics. However, the number of reported cases is small and has usually been analyzed with cases of retropharyngeal abscess. Nagy and associates treated 3 (13%) of 24 children with small parapharyngeal abscesses, and Sichel and associates treated 7 (14%) of 11 children with abscesses limited to the parapharyngeal space by intravenous antibiotics alone. Close clinical follow-up is necessary in children with parapharyngeal cellulitis or small parapharyngeal abscesses who are treated conservatively with intravenous antibiotics. Surgical drainage should be performed in children who do not improve within 24 to 48 hours.

MICROBIOLOGY OF DEEP NECK ABSCESSES

Group A streptococci (Streptococcus pyogenes) and Staphylococcus aureus have been considered to be the organisms most frequently associated with pharyngeal space infections. However, studies have demonstrated the presence of oral anaerobes in these infections; these organisms may be responsible for the gas seen on lateral neck radiographs. This is not surprising because the main portals of entry for pharyngeal space infections are the nasopharynx, oropharynx, paranasal sinuses, mastoid, and lower molars, all areas that are colonized with anaerobes. Some studies published since the mid-1980s, primarily of peritonsillar abscesses, showed that most are polymicrobial, with the predominant aerobes being S. pyogenes and S. aureus and a variety of anaerobic species, including Prevotella, Fusobacterium, Peptostreptococcus species, Bacteroides species, and Porphyromonas (Table 249.1). Generally, the number of anaerobic species outnumber aerobes. The pathogenic role of anaerobic bacteria in peritonsillar abscesses has been reinforced by reports of complications resulting from fusobacterial infection in children. Fusobacterium and Bacteroides species have been associated with septic thrombophlebitis and pulmonary emboli from the jugular veins.

Data on the microbiology of retropharyngeal and parapharyngeal abscesses in children are more limited. However, and not surprisingly, the organisms isolated are similar to those found in peritonsillar abscesses, but with a higher number of anaerobic species. Brook examined aspirated pus from 14 children 1 to 6 years of age (median age, 3 years and 2 months) with retropharyngeal abscesses. Anaerobes were isolated from all patients, and they were the only organisms isolated in two patients (14%) and were mixed with aerobes in the remainder (86%). The predominant anaerobic species were Bacteroides, Peptostreptococcus, and Fusobacterium. The predominant aerobic species were alpha- and gamma-hemolytic streptococci, S. aureus, Haemophilus species, and group A beta-hemolytic streptococci. Seventy-one percent of the isolates were beta-lactamase positive, including all isolates of S. aureus, 6 of 18 of the B. melaninogenicus group (33%), and 2 of 3 of the Bacteroides oralis group.

Dodds and Maniglia reported the results of cultures from nine retropharyngeal and three parapharyngeal abscesses from children and adolescents. The organisms isolated were similar to those reported by Brook, but the microbiology was not as complete because this was a retrospective study and all specimens may not have been processed for anaerobic culture. Streptococcal species were the most frequent isolates, followed by S. aureus and H. influenzae. There was one isolate each of Fusobacterium necrophorum, Escherichia coli, and Klebsiella pneumoniae. Asmar performed cultures on material from 17 children with retropharyngeal abscesses; viridans streptococci were isolated from 11 of the abscesses, followed by S. aureus (8) and group A streptococci (6). The most frequently identified anaerobes were Peptostreptococcus species. Overall, there were 45 aerobic and 18 anaerobic species identified. A recent report by Coticchia and colleagues found some very striking age- and site-specific differences in the organisms isolated from deep neck abscesses in children. Children less than 1 year of age were more likely to have S. aureus isolated, 79% versus 6% for S. pyogenes, compared with 16% and 29% in children older than 1 year, respectively.

Rarely, retropharyngeal abscess may result from anterior extension from cervical osteomyelitis. This has been described with tuberculosis and atypical mycobacteria causing a retropharyngeal abscess in a similar clinical setting. Because a large variety of organisms can be found in pharyngeal space infections, obtaining adequate cultures is of the greatest importance. The optimal material for culture is an aspirate of the pus obtained at operation. Throat swabs or swabs of the abscess obtained after drainage usually are inadequate because of contamination with normal oropharyngeal flora. The pus, when obtained, can be transported in a capped syringe if anaerobic transport media are not available. Most pathogenic obligate anaerobes can survive in a purulent exudate, despite extended periods of air exposure. A Gram stain of the exudate will provide important clues to the bacterial origin. A Gram stain showing a mixture of organisms suggests a mixed aerobic-anaerobic infection.

Although use of a beta-lactamase–resistant antibiotic may be necessary in the treatment of deep neck abscesses because of the presence of beta-lactamase–producing bacteria, including S. aureus, H. influenzae, and Bacteroides species, results of two studies from 1998 and 1999 suggested that penicillin alone was equivalent to broad-spectrum antibiotics for treatment of peritonsillar abscesses. Yilmaz and associates compared procaine penicillin with intramuscular ampicillin-sulbactam in outpatient treatment in 40 patients with peritonsillar abscesses who underwent peroral drainage procedures. There was no statistical difference in duration of symptoms and clinical recovery between the two groups. Kieff and colleagues retrospectively evaluated 103 patients with peritonsillar abscesses who were treated with incision and drainage. Fifty-eight patients were treated with broad-spectrum antibiotics, alone and in combination, including ampicillin-sulbactam, clindamycin, cephalosporins, and metronidazole; 45 patients were treated with penicillin alone. All patients were hospitalized after drainage, and comparison of the clinical outcomes including duration of hospitalization and fever did not differ significantly between the two groups. There was no significant difference in the organisms isolated, and failure and complication rates also did not differ.

There are no comparative treatment studies for retropharyngeal or parapharyngeal abscesses. Treatment in these cases

TABLE 249.1

BACTERIA ISOLATED FROM DEEP NECK ABSCESSES IN CHILDREN

Organism	Frequency
Aerobic and facultative isolates	
Streptococcus pyogenes	6%–29%
Staphylococcus aureus	11%–79%
Haemophilus influenzae	7%
Eikenella corrodens	5%
Gram-negative bacilli	10%
Viridans streptococci (S. milleri)	11%–27%
Anaerobic isolates	
Anaerobic cocci (Peptostreptococci)	20%
Fusobacterium species	~30%
Prevotella species	~30%
Bacteroides species	~30%
Porphyromonas species	~5%

Data from Brook I. Microbiology and management of peritonsillar, retropharyngeal and parapharyngeal abscesses. *J Oral Maxillofac Surg* 2004;62:1545; and Coticchia JM, Getnick GS, Yun RD, et al. Age-, site-, and time-specific differences in pediatric deep neck abscesses. *Arch Otolaryngol Head Neck Surg* 2004;130:201.

should be based on the results of cultures, as stated earlier. Drugs that may be effective include ampicillin-sulbactam, expanded-spectrum cephalosporins such as ceftriaxone, oxacillin or nafcillin, ticarcillin-clavulanic acid, and piperacillin-tazobactam. The cephalosporins may need to be used in combination with clindamycin or metronidazole for adequate anaerobic coverage. Erythromycin is less satisfactory because it has less activity against *Bacteroides fragilis* and *Fusobacterium*. Erythromycin is also frequently inactive against *S. aureus*. New trends in antibiotic resistance may also influence the choice of antibiotics. Coticchia and colleagues also noted an increase in resistance to clindamycin of *S. aureus*, from 100% susceptible in 1989 to 1994 to 10% resistant in 1994 to 1999. None of the *S. aureus* isolates were methicillin resistant during both periods. Attention to clindamycin resistance will be important because the drug is used frequently for treatment of community-acquired methicillin-resistant *S. aureus*. The routine use of aminoglycoside antibiotics is not indicated because aerobic gram-negative enteric rods rarely are found in these infections. Antibiotic therapy, however, is effective only in conjunction with adequate surgical drainage.

Suggested Readings

Asmar BI. Bacteriology of retropharyngeal abscess in children. *Pediatr Infect Dis J* 1990;9:595.

Barratt GE, Koopmann CF, Coulthard SW. Retropharyngeal abscess: a ten year experience. *Laryngoscope* 1984;94:455.

Bauer PW, Lieu JEC, Suskind DL, Lusk RP. The safety of conscious sedation in peritonsillar abscess drainage. *Arch Otolaryngol Head Neck Surg* 2001;127:1477.

Blotter JW, Yin L, Glynn M, Wiet GJ. Otolaryngology consultation for peritonsillar abscess in the pediatric population. *Laryngoscope* 2000;110:1698.

Brodsky L, Sobie SR, Korwin D, Stanievich JF. A clinical prospective study of peritonsillar abscess in children. *Laryngoscope* 1988;98:780.

Brook I. Microbiology and management of peritonsillar, retropharyngeal and parapharyngeal abscesses. *J Oral Maxillofac Surg* 2004;62:1545.

Brook I, Frazier EH, Thompson DH. Aerobic and anaerobic microbiology of peritonsillar abscess. *Laryngoscope* 1991;101:289.

Broughton RA. Nonsurgical management of deep neck infections in children. *Pediatr Infect Dis J* 1992;11:14.

Coticchia JM, Getnick GS, Yun RD, Arnold JE. Age-, site-, and time-specific differences in pediatric deep neck abscesses. *Arch Otolaryngol Head Neck Surg* 2004;130:201.

Craig FW, Schunk JE. Retropharyngeal abscess in children: clinical presentation, utility of imaging, and current management. *Pediatrics* 2003;111:1394.

Dodds B, Maniglia AJ. Peritonsillar and neck abscesses in the pediatric age group. *Laryngoscope* 1988;98:956.

Flödstrom A, Hallander HO. Microbiological aspects of peritonsillar abscesses. *Scand J Infect Dis* 1976;8:157.

Friedman NR, Mitchell RB, Pereira KD, et al. Peritonsillar abscess in early childhood: presentation and management. *Arch Otolaryngol Head Neck Surg* 1997;123:630.

Herzon FS. Peritonsillar abscess: incidence, current management practices, and a proposal for treatment guidelines. *Laryngoscope* 1995;105:1.

Jokipii AMM, Jokipii L, Sipila P, Jokinen K. Semiquantitative culture results and pathogenic significance of obligate anaerobes in peritonsillar abscesses. *J Clin Microbiol* 1988;26:957.

Jousimies-Somer H, Savolainen S, Makitie A, Ylikoski J. Bacteriologic findings in peritonsillar abscesses in young adults. *Clin Infect Dis* 1993;16:S292.

Kieff DA, Bhattacharyya N, Siegel NS, Salman SD. Selection of antibiotics after incision and drainage of peritonsillar abscesses. *Otolaryngol Head Neck Surg* 1999;120:57.

Kirse DJ, Robersin DW. Surgical management of retropharyngeal space infections in children. *Laryngoscope* 2001;111:1413.

Kronenberg J, Wolf M, Leventon G. Peritonsillar abscess: recurrence rate and the indication for tonsillectomy. *Am J Otolaryngol* 1987;8:82.

Lazor JB, Cunningham J, Eavey RD, Weber AL. Comparison of computed tomography and surgical findings in deep neck infections. *Otolaryngol Head Neck Surg* 1994;111:746.

de Marie S, Tjon A, Tham RT, et al. Clinical infections and nonsurgical treatment of parapharyngeal space infections complicating throat infection. *Rev Infect Dis* 1989;11:975.

Morrison JE Jr, Pashley NR. Retropharyngeal abscess in children: a 10-year review. *Pediatr Emerg Care* 1988;4:9.

Nagy M, Pizzuto M, Backstrom J, Brodsky L. Deep neck infections in children: a new approach to diagnosis and treatment. *Laryngoscope* 1997;107:1627.

Oleske JM, Starr SE, Nahmias AJ. Complications of peritonsillar abscess due to *Fusobacterium necrophorum*. *Pediatrics* 1976;57:570.

Ophir D, Bawnik J, Poria Y, et al. Peritonsillar abscess: a prospective evaluation of outpatient management by needle aspiration. *Arch Otolaryngol* 1988;114:661.

Sichel J-V, Dano I, Hocwald E, et al. Nonsurgical management of parapharyngeal space infections: a prospective study. *Laryngoscope* 2002;112:906.

Stringer, SP, Schaefer SD, Close LG. A randomized trial for outpatient management of peritonsillar abscess. *Arch Otolaryngol* 1988;114:278.

Ungkanont K, Yellon RF, Weissman JL, et al. Head and neck space infections in infants and children. *Otolaryngol Head Neck Surg.* 1995;112:375.

Weinberg E, Brodsky L, Stanievich J, Volk M. Needle aspiration of peritonsillar abscess in children. *Arch Otolaryngol Head Neck Surg* 1993;119:169.

Yilmaz T, Ünal ÖF, Figen G, et al. A comparison of procaine penicillin with sulbactam-ampicillin in the treatment of peritonsillar abscesses. *Eur Arch Otolaryngol* 1998;255:163.

CHAPTER 250 ■ OTITIS EXTERNA

MARK W. KLINE

Under normal circumstances, the external auditory canal is protected from infection by a physical barrier of squamous epithelium and a chemical barrier provided by the acidic pH of cerumen. Factors that disrupt these barriers, such as trauma, excessive cleansing or wetting, and high temperature and humidity, predispose to development of otitis externa.

CLINICAL MANIFESTATIONS

A history of swimming or diving or of repetitive ear cleansing with soapy water and cotton-tipped swabs often is elicited. Most patients are seen for evaluation of ear pain, itching, and fullness. Pain is exacerbated by manipulation of the pinna or tragus, a feature useful in differentiating between otitis externa and otitis media. Purulent discharge may be present in the external auditory canal. The canal walls are diffusely erythematous and edematous. Ipsilateral cervical lymph node enlargement may be noted, but usually fever is absent.

DIAGNOSIS

Otitis externa is a clinical diagnosis. The historical features and physical findings are sufficiently characteristic so most patients present no real diagnostic dilemma. Conversely, several other conditions mimic external otitis in some cases. Furunculosis is, in a sense, a focal form of otitis externa. Symptoms and signs resemble those of the diffuse condition, but otoscopy reveals a discrete furuncle or pustule with surrounding erythema in the outer portion of the external auditory canal. Otitis media causes ear pain that is not exacerbated by manipulation of the pinna. Usually, perforation of the tympanic membrane results in symptomatic improvement, although the external canal may fill with purulent debris. Cleansing the canal permits otoscopic detection of the perforated tympanic membrane. A foreign body, usually visible in the external canal, may cause inflammation and discharge closely mimicking diffuse external otitis.

A microbiologic diagnosis helps to guide antibiotic therapy for otitis externa. A nasopharyngeal calcium alginate swab is used to obtain purulent material from the auditory canal for routine bacterial cultures and Gram stain. Special stains and cultures for fungi, mycobacteria, or viruses may be indicated under unusual circumstances. The most common causative agents are *Staphylococcus aureus*, *Pseudomonas aeruginosa*, and other gram-negative bacilli and group A streptococci. Frequently, infections are polymicrobial. Fungi, such as *Aspergillus niger* and *Candida albicans*, occasionally are isolated as the sole or predominant organisms. Varicella-zoster virus may produce external otitis with ipsilateral oral vesicles and facial nerve paralysis.

THERAPY

After cultures are obtained, the auditory canal can be flushed with 3% saline or 2% acetic acid and can be dried with a cotton-tipped applicator. A combination drug containing polymyxin B–neomycin-hydrocortisone has been used for many years in the treatment of otitis externa. Available in a variety of formulations, it generally is instilled in the canal three or four times daily for 10 to 14 days. Initial swelling may be so severe that drops will not enter the auditory canal. In these cases, antibiotic cream may be placed in the canal on a wick and removed in approximately 24 hours (when inflammation has subsided). Cutaneous sensitivity to neomycin, with local signs and symptoms mimicking those of otitis externa, is a potential complication of therapy with this combination drug. The fluoroquinolone drugs ofloxacin and ciprofloxacin, both available in topical formulations for otitis externa, are alternatives to the use of polymyxin B–neomycin-hydrocortisone. The approved otic formulation of ciprofloxacin contains hydrocortisone, whereas the approved formulation of ofloxacin does not. Topical clindamycin and vancomycin have been used to treat otitis externa caused by methicillin-resistant *S. aureus*. Prevention of recurrent otitis externa may be accomplished by use of 2% acetic acid eardrops after swimming.

Systemic antibiotic therapy for otitis externa is indicated if affected patients are febrile or exhibit associated cervical adenitis or cellulitis of adjacent tissues. Appropriate oral antibiotics for initial therapy include trimethoprim-sulfamethoxazole, cefuroxime axetil, or amoxicillin-clavulanate.

Generally, malignant otitis externa, a particularly aggressive form of the disease, is diagnosed in elderly patients with diabetes. It occurs rarely in immunocompromised children and is characterized by extensive destruction of soft tissues, cartilage, bone, and nerves around the external auditory canal. Granulation tissue may be seen in the canal itself. The causative organism is *P. aeruginosa*. Effective therapy combines surgical débridement with intravenous antibiotics that are active against *Pseudomonas*.

Suggested Readings

Brook I. Treatment of otitis externa in children. *Paediatr Drugs* 1999;1:283.
Dohar JE. Evolution of management approaches for otitis externa. *Pediatr Infect Dis J* 2003;22:299.
Hwang JH, Tsai HY, Liu TC. Community-acquired methicillin-resistant *Staphylococcus aureus* infections in discharging ears. *Acta Otolaryngol* 2002; 122:827.
Roland PS, Stroman DW. Microbiology of acute otitis externa. *Laryngoscope* 2002;112:1166.

CHAPTER 251 ■ OTITIS MEDIA

HEIDI SCHWARZWALD AND MARK W. KLINE

Otitis media is a general term denoting inflammation of the middle ear. *Acute otitis media* refers to suppurative middle-ear infection of relatively sudden clinical onset. The term *chronic otitis media* encompasses several entities of insidious onset, the differentiation of which by clinical or pathologic criteria is difficult. Chronic suppurative conditions include tubotympanitis (e.g., permanent perforation syndrome), atticoantral disease (e.g., Shrapnell disease or cholesteatoma), and end-stage disease (e.g., atelectatic ear, adhesive otitis media, or tympanosclerosis). Otitis media with effusion (secretory otitis media) is a chronic condition characterized by the persistence of fluid in the middle ear. Temporally, usually otitis media with effusion follows an episode of acute otitis media. Extension of inflammation beyond the mucoperiosteal lining of the middle ear constitutes a complication of otitis media (e.g., mastoiditis, epidural abscess).

OVERVIEW

Epidemiology

Otitis media is one of the most common infectious diseases of childhood. One large study revealed that 33% of pediatric office visits for illness of any kind were attributable to disease of the middle ear (acute otitis media or otitis media with effusion). Infants and young children are at highest risk for the development of otitis media, with a peak prevalence between 6 and 36 months of age. Two of every three children have at least one episode of otitis media before their first birthday. By age 3, 80% of children have had at least one episode of acute otitis media, and nearly 50% have had three or more episodes. After an initial episode of acute otitis media, 40% of children have middle-ear effusion that persists for at least 4 weeks, and 10% have persistent effusion after 3 months. Children in whom otitis media with effusion develops early in life are at increased risk of recurrent acute or chronic middle-ear disease. The overall childhood prevalence of otitis media with effusion is estimated to be 15% to 20%. The incidence and prevalence of otitis media decline after approximately age 6.

Otitis media occurs more commonly in boys than in girls and is particularly prevalent among Inuit and Native Americans and among children with cleft palate or other craniofacial defects. A familial predisposition to otitis media may exist in some cases. Other implicated predisposing factors include lower socioeconomic status, bottle-feeding with the baby supine, bottle-feeding versus breast-feeding, day-care center attendance, and atopy. In general, the highest rates of otitis media are observed in the winter months, coinciding with the peak incidence of respiratory viral infections.

Pathogenesis

Abnormal eustachian tube function underlies most cases of otitis media. Normally, the eustachian tube permits equilibration of middle-ear pressure with atmospheric pressure, protects the middle ear from reflux of nasopharyngeal secretions, and drains secretions from the middle ear into the nasopharynx. Either obstruction or abnormal patency of the eustachian tube may lead to the development of otitis media. Intrinsic (e.g., inflammation secondary to infection or allergy) and extrinsic (e.g., tumor or adenoid enlargement) types of mechanical eustachian tube obstruction are recognized. Functional obstruction, caused by persistent collapse of an abnormally compliant eustachian tube, an abnormal active opening mechanism, or both, is common in young children and individuals with cleft palate. An abnormally patent, or patulous, eustachian tube, commonly found among Native American populations, permits reflux of nasopharyngeal secretions into the middle ear. Reflux, aspiration, or insufflation of nasopharyngeal bacteria into the middle ear on any basis leads to mucoperiosteal inflammation and otitis media.

Complications

Serious complications of otitis media are uncommon when appropriate medical therapy is initiated promptly. Extracranial complications include serous or purulent labyrinthitis, mastoiditis, osteomyelitis of the temporal bone, and facial nerve paralysis. Intracranial complications are subdivided into meningeal and extrameningeal complications. Epidural and subdural abscess, meningitis, lateral sinus thrombosis, and otitic hydrocephalus are reported as meningeal complications of otitis media. Lateral sinus thrombosis is characterized by high temperature, chills, signs and symptoms of increased intracranial pressure, and septicemia with embolization. The mortality is approximately 25%. Otitic hydrocephalus may follow acute otitis media by several weeks and usually is associated with impaired intracranial venous drainage. Commonly, hydrocephalus subsides spontaneously. Extrameningeal complications of otitis media include brain abscess and petrositis.

ACUTE OTITIS MEDIA

Clinical Manifestations

The classic description of acute otitis media is of children who have upper respiratory tract infection and suddenly develop fever, otalgia, and hearing loss. A classic presentation, however, may be the exception rather than the rule. Fever and hearing loss are inconstant features of the disease, and otalgia may be present but not be reported. In many young children in particular, otitis media must be inferred on the basis of nonspecific symptoms (e.g., fretfulness or irritability, anorexia, loose stools) and subtle findings suggestive of middle-ear disease (e.g., scratching or tugging at the ear). Otitis media must be excluded before children are labeled as having fever without localizing signs or having fever of undetermined origin. Unfortunately, overdiagnosis of acute otitis media is common, especially in uncooperative patients.

The appearance of the tympanic membrane is key to the diagnosis of acute otitis media. Evidence of middle-ear effusion and inflammation should be present. All wax and debris must be removed from the external canal before examination. Usually, otoscopy reveals a hyperemic, opaque tympanic membrane with distorted or absent light reflex and indistinct landmarks. A red appearance of the drum may be noted if affected children are agitated or if inadequate illumination is provided; this condition is not evidence of otitis media in the absence of other findings. Adequate assessment of tympanic membrane mobility requires pneumatic otoscopy, using an ear speculum large enough to occlude the external canal completely. Mobility may be further evaluated by tympanometry and/or acoustic reflectometry. Decreased mobility of the drum may result from either eustachian tube dysfunction or middle-ear effusion.

Usually, the diagnosis of acute otitis media is apparent, but if examination is difficult, diagnosis can be elusive as well. Referred otalgia may be associated with infections and other conditions of the tonsils, adenoids, teeth, or pharynx, however. The tympanic membrane should appear normal in these conditions. Purulent otorrhea may indicate otitis media with tympanic membrane perforation, but otitis externa must be excluded. In diseases of the external canal, frequently pain is elicited by manipulation of the pinna.

Diagnosis

Bacteria may be isolated from middle-ear fluid in approximately two-thirds of patients with acute otitis media. The approximate prevalence rates of various bacterial agents of otitis media beyond the neonatal period are shown in Table 251.1. Substantial percentages of *Streptococcus pneumoniae* isolates are resistant to penicillin and amoxicillin; resistance to other oral penicillins and cephalosporins also has been observed. With increased use of the heptavalent pneumococcal vaccine, the incidence of otitis media caused by *S. pneumoniae* has been decreasing. Many untypeable *Haemophilus influenzae* strains and almost all strains of *Moraxella catarrhalis*

TABLE 251.1

BACTERIAL ETIOLOGY OF ACUTE OTITIS MEDIA IN CHILDREN*

Bacterial Isolate	Prevalence (%)
Streptococcus pneumoniae	31
Haemophilus influenzae, untypeable	22
Moraxella catarrhalis	7
Group A streptococcus	2
Enteric gram-negative bacteria	1
Staphylococcus aureus	1
Other	3
No bacterial isolate	33

*Findings based on cultures obtained by needle tympanocentesis.

TABLE 251.2

ANTIMICROBIAL THERAPY FOR ACUTE OTITIS MEDIA

	Nonsevere Illness	Severe Illness	Penicillin Allergy (Non-Type I)	Penicillin Allergy (Type I)
First-line therapy	Amoxicillin	Amoxicillin-clavulanate	Cefdinir, cefuroxime, cefpodoxime (for severe illness, consider ceftriaxone, 1 or 3 days)	Azithromycin, clarithromycin
Second-line therapy	Amoxicillin-clavulanate	Ceftriaxone, 3 days	Ceftriaxone, 3 days	Clindamycin

produce beta-lactamase and therefore also are resistant to penicillin and amoxicillin. Bacterial cultures of middle-ear fluid are sterile in approximately one-third of patients with acute otitis media. Studies assessing the role of viruses have found a low rate of isolation from middle-ear fluid, with respiratory syncytial virus and influenza viruses being most common. *Chlamydia trachomatis* and *Mycoplasma pneumoniae* probably are infrequent causes of otitis media. These organisms are not necessarily associated with bullous myringitis, as is commonly thought.

Other than the more frequent occurrence of disease caused by enteric gram-negative bacteria (approximately 20% of cases), and occasional recovery of usual neonatal pathogens (e.g., group B streptococci), the cause of otitis media in neonates is similar to that in older children. Diagnosis of the specific causative agent is desirable in unusual or complicated cases of otitis media. Qualitative nasopharyngeal cultures correlate poorly with cultures obtained from middle-ear fluid. Therefore, when the diagnosis of otitis media is in doubt or an unusual pathogen is suspected, aspiration of middle-ear fluid should be performed. Specific indications for needle tympanocentesis or myringotomy include the following: serious illness or toxicity; suppurative complications (e.g., mastoiditis or meningitis); otitis media in neonates, immunocompromised patients, or patients receiving mechanical ventilation; and otitis media developing in spite of, or failing to respond to, antimicrobial therapy. Discordance in middle-ear cultures may be found in 20% of cases of bilateral otitis media.

Therapy

In the era before antibiotics, frequently otitis media resolved spontaneously, but tympanic membrane perforation and suppurative sequelae were common. Antibiotic therapy has changed the clinical course of otitis media dramatically, by arresting infection before complications develop. However, the rise of bacterial resistance to antibiotics has prompted more judicious use of antibiotics for otitis media. As a rule, children younger than 1 month old who have otitis media should be admitted to the hospital. Cultures of blood, cerebrospinal fluid, and middle-ear fluid should be obtained, and parenteral antibiotic therapy should be initiated. If blood and cerebrospinal fluid cultures are sterile after 72 hours and affected infants appear well, with disease limited to the middle ear, therapy may be completed with an oral antibiotic active against the middle-ear isolate.

For children between the ages of 6 months and 12 years, the clinician's treatment options include providing the family with treatment for the patient's pain and watching the patient closely for 48 to 72 hours to determine whether the infection resolves without antibiotics. This approach of watchful waiting should only be used in certain circumstances. First, the practitioner determines whether or not the diagnosis is certain. Then, he or she must determine whether the illness is severe or not. The illness is considered severe if the child has fever greater than 39°C, or moderate to severe otalgia. In children between the ages of 6 months and 2 years, observation should only be employed if the practitioner is uncertain of the diagnosis of otitis media and the patient's illness is considered nonsevere. In children more than 2 years of age, observation may be considered for the nonseverely ill child (even if the diagnosis is certain), or if the diagnosis is uncertain. If observation is the treatment of choice, there must be a caregiver who can observe the child, readily reach the practitioner, and return for reexamination if the child does not improve in 48 to 72 hours. Finally, the child can have no other medical conditions.

The choice of an antibiotic for acute otitis media must take into account many factors, including the local antibiotic susceptibility patterns of common bacterial isolates, compliance of the patient population with various antibiotic regimens, and the cost of the various antibiotics under consideration. A list of possible antibiotic choices can be found in Table 251.2, and dosages are found in Table 251.3. High-dose oral amoxicillin is a reasonable first choice for the treatment of otitis media in older infants and children. An alternative agent may be needed

TABLE 251.3

DOSAGE OF ANTIMICROBIAL THERAPY FOR ACUTE OTITIS MEDIA

Drug	Daily Dosage
Amoxicillin	80–90 mg/kg PO in two or three divided doses × 10 days
Amoxicillin-clavulanate Amoxicillin-clavulanate ES	90 mg/kg amoxicillin with PO in two divided doses × 10 days
Azithromycin	10 mg/kg PO daily day 1, 5 mg/kg PO daily days 2–5. Or 30 mg/kg PO single dose
Cefdinir	14 mg/kg/day PO in one or two divided doses × 10 days
Cefpodoxime proxetil	10 mg/kg PO in two divided doses
Ceftriaxone	50 mg/kg IM once daily × 10 days
Cefuroxime axetil	30 mg/kg PO in two divided doses
Clarithromycin	30 mg/kg PO in two divided doses × 10 days
Clindamycin	30 mg/kg PO in four divided doses × 10 days

IM, intramuscularly; PO, orally.

in the absence of response to therapy in 48 to 72 hours or if a resistant organism is cultured from middle-ear fluid. Antibiotic ear drops are of no value in treating acute otitis media.

Diverse opinions surround indications for myringotomy in acute otitis media. Therapeutic myringotomy should be considered for relief of persistent severe pain or persistent conductive hearing loss. Nasal and oral decongestants, sometimes administered in combination with an oral antihistamine, have been advocated for relief of nasal and eustachian tube obstruction in children with otitis media. In clinical trials, these preparations have had equivocal, and sometimes contradictory, results in affecting rates of treatment failure, recurrence, or persistence of middle-ear effusion. At present, the efficacy of these preparations is unproven, and their routine use cannot be recommended. Antihistamine use during acute otitis media actually may prolong the duration of middle-ear effusion. Perforation of the tympanic membrane associated with acute otitis media requires no treatment and usually heals in several days. If chronic perforation develops, observation is the treatment of choice for several months. If resolution does not occur, referral to an otolaryngologist is recommended.

Supportive therapy, including acetaminophen, topical anesthetics (as long as no perforation is present) and local heat, may be helpful in treating children with acute otitis media. Sedation should be avoided.

Caregivers should be counseled that if the child's symptoms persist 48 to 72 hours after antibiotics are initiated, they should contact the health provider. At that time, the child should be reexamined for the possibility of other illnesses, and second-line therapy should be considered. The usual duration of oral antibiotic therapy in uncomplicated cases of acute otitis media is 10 days, but both longer and shorter therapy courses have been proposed. Studies have shown that for children 6 years of age or older, with mild to moderate disease, a 5- to 7-day course of antibiotics is acceptable. A single intramuscular dose of ceftriaxone was found to be comparable in clinical efficacy to 10 days of oral trimethoprim-sulfamethoxazole for treatment of acute otitis media. Every child should be examined at the end of therapy to document resolution of tympanic membrane inflammation. Complete resolution of middle-ear effusion may require 2 to 3 months.

RECURRENT ACUTE OTITIS MEDIA

Recurrence of episodes of acute otitis media is common. Underlying susceptibility to middle-ear infection is important in the development of recurrent otitis media; recurrences represent reinfection more often than recrudescence or relapse. Early development of otitis media caused by *S. pneumoniae* seems particularly likely to predispose to recurrent otitis media.

Several strategies have been used for the prevention of recurrent acute otitis media. Antibiotic prophylaxis with amoxicillin (20 mg/kg once daily) or sulfisoxazole (75 mg/kg/day in two divided doses) is reasonable in children who have at least three episodes of acute otitis media within 6 months or four episodes in 1 year. Generally, prophylaxis is continued for 3 to 6 months, at which time the antibiotic is discontinued, and affected children are observed. Pneumococcal conjugate vaccine may provide moderate protection against acute otitis media and may reduce the risk of recurrent otitis media. Myringotomy with tympanostomy tube insertion is an option for patients who fail to respond to antibiotic prophylaxis. Results of studies of adenoidectomy for prevention of recurrent otitis media have been equivocal. Adenoidectomy at the time of insertion of tympanostomy tubes may reduce the subsequent likelihood of hospitalizations and additional surgeries related to otitis media.

The relative efficacies of the various strategies for prophylaxis, alone and in combination, are largely unknown.

OTITIS MEDIA WITH EFFUSION

After an episode of acute otitis media, 10% of children have middle-ear effusion that persists for 3 months or longer (chronic otitis media with effusion). Clinically, otitis media with effusion is characterized by a sensation of fullness in the ears, muffled hearing, and tinnitus. Usually, pneumatic otoscopy reveals an opaque tympanic membrane with decreased mobility. Frequent acute otitis media, catarrh, exposure to cigarette smoke, and atopy may increase the risk of persistent effusion. Language, behavioral, and learning deficits may result, particularly for children of lower socioeconomic status.

Bacteria are recovered from one-third to one-half of all middle-ear fluid specimens obtained at myringotomy in cases of otitis media with effusion. The bacteriologic features closely mimic those of acute otitis media. Not known is whether the bacteria have a direct pathogenic role, but an initial course of antibiotic therapy similar to that used for acute otitis media seems warranted. Oral decongestant-antihistamine combinations and corticosteroids have not been found effective in the treatment of persistent middle-ear effusion. Evaluation for respiratory allergy, obstructive adenoid enlargement, immune deficiency, or such anatomic abnormalities as submucous cleft palate may be necessary in patients whose disease does not respond to treatment.

For patients whose condition fails to respond to medical therapy, myringotomy with tympanostomy tube insertion may prevent subsequent accumulation of middle-ear fluid and can improve hearing. However, tympanostomy tubes do not measurably imrpove developmental outcome in children less than 3 years of age with persistent middle-ear effusion. Tympanostomy tubes are used also to prevent structural middle-ear damage and cholesteatoma in selected cases. Tonsillectomy is not efficacious in the treatment of otitis media with effusion.

Suggested Readings

American Academy of Pediatrics Subcommittee on Management of Acute Otitis Media. Diagnosis and management of acute otitis media. *Pediatrics* 2004; 113:1451.

Bluestone CD. Efficacy of ofloxacin and other ototopical preparations for chronic suppurative otitis media in children. *Pediatr Infect Dis J* 2001;20:111.

Chonmaitree T, Saeed K, Uchida T, et al. A randomized, placebo-controlled trial of the effect of antihistamine or corticosteroid treatment in acute otitis media. *J Pediatr* 2003;143:377.

Coyte PC, Croxford R, McIsaac W, et al. The role of adjuvant adenoidectomy and tonsillectomy in the outcome of the insertion of tympanostomy tubes. *N Engl J Med* 2001;344:1188.

Fireman B, Black SB, Shinefield HR, et al. Impact of the pneumococcal conjugate vaccine on otitis media. *Pediatr Infect Dis J* 2003;22:10.

Garbutt J, Jeffe DB, Shackelford P. Diagnosis and treatment of acute otitis media: an assessment. *Pediatrics* 2003;112:143.

Leibovitz E. Acute otitis media in pediatric medicine: current issues in epidemiology, diagnosis, and management. *Pediatr Drugs* 2003;5(suppl 1):1.

Paradise JL, Dollaghan CA, Campbell TF, et al. Otitis media and tympanostomy tube insertion during the first three years of life: developmental outcomes at the age of four years. *Pediatrics* 2003;112:265.

Paradise JL, Feldman HM, Campbell TF, et al. Effect of early or delayed insertion of tympanostomy tubes for persistent otitis media on developmental outcomes at the age of three years. *N Engl J Med* 2001;344:1179.

Piglansky L, Leibovitz E, Raiz S, et al. Bacteriologic and clinical efficacy of high dose amoxicillin for therapy of acute otitis media in children. *Pediatr Infect Dis J* 2003;22:405.

Sagraves R. Increasing antibiotic resistance: its effect on the therapy for otitis media. *J Pediatr Health Care* 2002;16:79.

Straetemans M, Sanders EA, Veenhoven RH, et al. Review of randomized controlled trials on pneumococcal vaccination for prevention of otitis media. *Pediatr Infect Dis J* 2003;22:515.

Weber SM, Grundfast KM. Modern management of acute otitis media. *Pediatr Clin North Am* 2003;50:399.

CHAPTER 252 ■ MASTOIDITIS

MARK W. KLINE

Inflammation of the mucoperiosteal lining of the mastoid air cells usually accompanies otitis media. Clinically evident suppurative infection, or *mastoiditis*, develops when inflammation causes progressive swelling and obstruction to drainage of exudative materials from the mastoid. Mastoiditis is uncommon in this era of effective antibiotic therapy for otitis media, but it remains a potentially life-threatening disease requiring prompt recognition and appropriate treatment.

CLINICAL MANIFESTATIONS

Almost invariably, children with mastoiditis have otitis media concomitantly. Classically, children with acute mastoiditis present with fever, otalgia, and postauricular swelling and redness. Typically, swelling occurs over the mastoid process, pushing the earlobe superiorly and laterally (Fig. 252.1); in infancy, it may occur above the ear, displacing the pinna inferiorly and laterally. The clinical presentation of acute mastoiditis may be fairly subtle, particularly in children who have received oral antibiotic therapy for otitis media (so-called masked mastoiditis). Mastoiditis should be considered in patients with otitis media unresponsive to antibiotic therapy.

Generally, chronic mastoiditis develops in individuals with long-standing middle-ear disease. The clinical course is indolent. Fever and local signs referable to the mastoid may or may not be present. Chronic purulent drainage from the ear and conductive hearing loss may occur.

DIAGNOSIS

In some cases, the diagnosis of mastoiditis can be made with confidence on clinical grounds alone. Plain-film roentgenography may show coalescence of mastoid air cells and loss of nor-

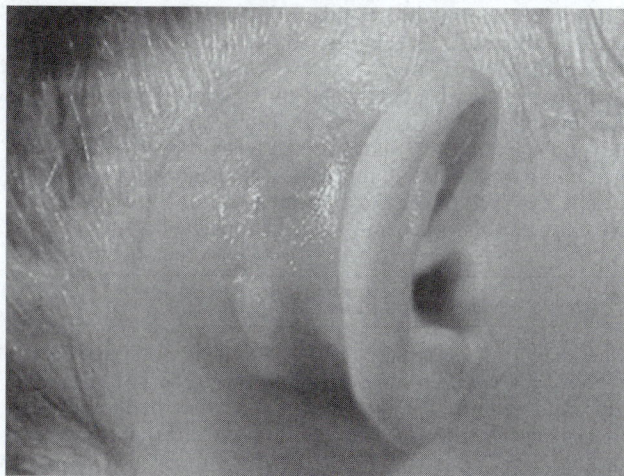

FIGURE 252.1. Mastoiditis.

mal bony trabeculations. If osteomyelitis develops, sometimes sclerosis or destruction of adjacent bone is noted. Abnormalities on roentgenography of the mastoid bone do not necessarily imply mastoiditis, however; conversely, normal study results do not exclude the diagnosis. Sometimes, computed tomography is helpful in cases in which clinical findings and plain-film roentgenography are equivocal or nonspecific.

A bacteriologic diagnosis is highly desirable in cases of mastoiditis. Tympanocentesis obtained through an intact tympanic membrane yields bacteriologic information that correlates well with specimens obtained from the mastoid bone itself. Common causative agents of acute mastoiditis include *Streptococcus pneumoniae*, group A streptococcus, *Staphylococcus aureus*, and *Haemophilus influenzae*. In chronic mastoiditis, prevalent isolates include anaerobic bacteria, such as *Peptococcus* species, *Actinomyces* species, or *Bacteroides* species, and aerobic gram-negative bacilli (including *Pseudomonas aeruginosa*). Frequently, chronic mastoiditis is polymicrobial. *Mycobacterium tuberculosis* rarely causes chronic mastoiditis today, but it should be considered in the presence of suggestive epidemiologic or historical features in the case.

In all cases of mastoiditis, specimens from the middle ear or mastoid should be cultured aerobically and anaerobically, and a Gram stain should be performed. Special fungal and mycobacterial stains and cultures may be indicated in some cases. A skin test for tuberculosis should be performed in all cases of chronic mastoiditis or with a history of exposure to tuberculosis.

THERAPY

Usually, patients with acute onset of symptoms and no evidence of intracranial or local extracranial complications of mastoiditis are treated initially with myringotomy and parenteral antibiotics alone. Signs of increased intracranial pressure or meningeal irritation signal such complications of mastoiditis as meningitis, brain abscess, epidural abscess, subdural empyema, or venous sinus thrombosis. A postauricular fluctuant area implies subperiosteal abscess formation. Because of proximity to the mastoid bone, other local structures may be involved by infection, producing facial-nerve paralysis, jugular venous thrombosis, or internal carotid artery erosion and hemorrhage. Lack of appropriate response to medical therapy or development of complications necessitates mastoidectomy and possibly other surgical interventions. The initial selection of specific antibiotic therapy is made empirically, with some guidance provided by Gram stain of specimens from the middle ear or mastoid. In acute mastoiditis, a combination of vancomycin (to provide coverage against penicillin-resistant *S. pneumoniae* and oxacillin-resistant *S. aureus*) and one of the third-generation cephalosporins (e.g., cefotaxime or ceftriaxone) is reasonable. In chronic mastoiditis, an aminoglycoside with activity against *Pseudomonas* (e.g., amikacin or tobramycin) may be used initially, usually in combination with an antipseudomonal penicillin (e.g., ticarcillin-clavulanate) that is active against many anaerobic bacteria and *S. aureus*. Eventual antibiotic therapy is determined by the bacteriology of the process. Provided complications have not occurred and if it is feasible on the basis of the organisms' susceptibility to oral agents, the course of therapy can be completed orally once signs of acute inflammation have subsided. The minimum course of therapy for mastoiditis is 21 days, and it may be longer if complications of infection have occurred. For patients discharged on oral antibiotic therapy, careful monitoring of compliance and documentation of bactericidal activity in serum are desirable.

Suggested Readings

Ghaffar FA, Wordemann M, McCracken GH Jr. Acute mastoiditis in children: a seventeen-year experience in Dallas, Texas. *Pediatr Infect Dis J* 2001;20:376.
Go C, Bernstein JM, de Jong AL, Sulek M, Friedman EM. Intracranial complications of acute mastoiditis. *Int J Pediatr Otorhinolaryngol* 2000;52:143.
Luntz M, Brodsky A, Nusem S, et al. Acute mastoiditis—the antibiotic era: a multicenter study. *Int J Pediatr Otorhinolaryngol* 2001;57:1.
Zapalac JS, Billings KR, Schwade ND, Roland PS. Suppurative complications of acute otitis media in the era of antibiotic resistance. *Arch Otolaryngol Head Neck Surg* 2002;128:660.

CHAPTER 253 ■ UVULITIS

ELLEN R. WALD

Infections of the uvula have been reported infrequently in the medical literature. When the uvula is the most inflamed structure in the posterior pharynx of febrile children, acute infection should be suspected.

ETIOLOGY

The bacterial agents that cause most cases of uvulitis in children are *Haemophilus influenzae* type b and *Streptococcus pyogenes*. Uvulitis caused by *H. influenzae* may occur concurrently with epiglottitis or as an isolated site of infection. Uvulitis caused by *S. pyogenes* appears to occur always in concert with pharyngitis. Two cases of uvulitis and associated epiglottitis caused by *Streptococcus pneumoniae* have been reported in adults. Two cases of uvulitis caused by anaerobic bacteria have been reported: One was caused by *Fusobacterium nucleatum* and the other by *Prevotella intermedia*. Another cause of uvulitis in children is *Candida albicans*. Two cases occurred in immunocompetent infants.

EPIDEMIOLOGY

The epidemiology of uvulitis is the epidemiology of its two etiologic agents: *S. pyogenes* and *H. influenzae* type b. As such, it can be seen in the school-aged child of between 5 and 15 years (the so-called streptococcal age group) in association with pharyngitis. Similarly, it was seen in the "*H. influenzae* age group" of 3 months to 5 years before universal immunization with conjugate vaccines for *H. influenzae* type b. Cases of uvulitis in association with epiglottitis have been reported in the United States as well as in England. Virtually all cases of bacteremic illness caused by *H. influenzae* type b, including uvulitis and epiglottitis, have disappeared since universal immunization of infants in 1991. Infections caused by *S. pyogenes* and *H. influenzae* occur primarily in winter and spring, but both can occur throughout the year.

PATHOPHYSIOLOGY

Uvulitis is an acute cellulitis characterized by dramatic swelling and erythema. Infection of the uvula probably arises from direct invasion by *S. pyogenes* or *H. influenzae* type b, both recognized as normal nasopharyngeal flora. With the latter, epiglottitis may arise also by direct extension, and the bacteremia may result secondarily from either the uvula or the epiglottis as a primary site of infection. Alternately, the pathogenesis of most *H. influenzae* type b infections is by hematogenous spread from the nasopharynx as a portal of entry.

CLINICAL MANIFESTATIONS

In a review of five patients with streptococcal uvulitis, all were reported to have associated pharyngitis. The patients had low-grade fever and sore throat. Three of the five experienced a choking or gagging sensation in the pharynx, which induced coughing and spitting; one of these patients also experienced drooling. Although pharyngitis was noted on physical examination, the swelling and erythema of the uvula were most dramatic. None of the patients had evidence of respiratory distress.

In patients with uvulitis and epiglottitis, the presentation usually is typical for epiglottitis, with sudden onset of high temperature, dysphagia, and increasing respiratory distress. Rapkin, however, reported a case of uvulitis-epiglottitis in which the epiglottitis initially was unsuspected. The lateral neck radiograph, performed to evaluate the possibility of retropharyngeal abscess, belatedly alerted attendant clinicians to the correct diagnosis.

In patients with uvulitis and no epiglottitis, the presentation may be similar to that of epiglottitis (acute onset of fever, odynophagia, and drooling) or can be less specific (fever and irritability or decreased appetite). The diagnosis in the latter case is apparent on physical examination of the oropharynx, which shows a swollen and erythematous uvula.

DIAGNOSIS

The diagnosis of streptococcal uvulitis is suspected when school-aged children are seen with low-grade fever, pharyngitis, and uvulitis. The diagnosis is confirmed by the recovery of *S. pyogenes* from a surface culture of the throat, the uvula, or both.

The diagnosis of uvulitis caused by *H. influenzae* is suspected in highly febrile infants or in preschool children who have uvular inflammation on physical examination and have not received a conjugate vaccine for *H. influenzae* type b. A lateral neck radiograph must be performed to evaluate the possibility of epiglottitis unless signs of upper respiratory obstruction are obvious, in which case immediate endoscopy is warranted. If epiglottitis is discovered, the airway must be secured, and appropriate parenteral antimicrobial agents must be initiated after blood and surface cultures are obtained. Any surface culture that is obtained to search for *H. influenzae* must be plated onto chocolate agar. After appropriate cultures are obtained, parenteral antimicrobial agents should be initiated, as in other bacteremic *H. influenzae* infections.

DIFFERENTIAL DIAGNOSIS

The differential diagnosis of patients with acute onset of fever, dysphagia, and drooling includes herpes simplex gingivostomatitis, uvulitis, epiglottitis, severe pharyngitis, and peritonsillar or retropharyngeal abscess. Although extreme caution is appropriate in examining the pharynx of any patient with suspected epiglottitis, some children tolerate attempted visualization of the oral cavity without undue upset. Instrumentation with a tongue blade should be avoided. If the examination does not show gingivostomatitis or peritonsillar abscess, a lateral neck radiograph should be performed. If epiglottitis or retropharyngeal abscess is confirmed, airway management and antimicrobial agents or incision and drainage combined with antimicrobial agents are indicated, respectively. If the lateral neck is normal and the uvula is inflamed, uvulitis with or without pharyngitis is confirmed.

Noninfectious inflammation of the uvula may be caused by allergy (as in angioedema), irritants (as in marijuana abuse), trauma, and vasculitis (an early manifestation of Kawasaki disease).

THERAPY

The treatment of uvulitis is guided primarily by the associated pharyngitis or epiglottitis, if either is present. In the case of streptococcal pharyngitis, penicillin therapy for 10 days is most appropriate; oral penicillin V, 250 to 500 mg two to three times daily, will suffice. Clinical improvement of the uvular and pharyngeal inflammation should occur within 24 to 48 hours after the initiation of treatment.

In the case of uvulitis-epiglottitis, management of the airway is most important. It can be accomplished by nasotracheal intubation or tracheotomy. Appropriate parenteral antibiotic therapy should be initiated.

In the case of uvulitis without epiglottitis, antimicrobial therapy appropriate for bacteremic *H. influenzae* type b is necessary. In geographic areas where beta-lactamase–producing *H. influenzae* is prevalent, an advanced-generation cephalosporin is appropriate (e.g., cefuroxime, 150 mg/kg/day in three divided doses, or cefotaxime, 200 mg/kg/day in four divided doses). In patients with serious penicillin hypersensitivity, a carbapenem (meropenem) or a monobactam (aztreonam) may be used. After the fever has subsided and an affected patient has improved clinically, an oral antimicrobial agent can be substituted. Clinical improvement can be expected within 24 to 48 hours. The results of blood and surface cultures can be used to guide therapy.

For an ampicillin-sensitive *H. influenzae* organism, amoxicillin, 40 to 45 mg/kg/day in two to three divided doses, should be prescribed to complete a 7- to 10-day course of treatment. For beta-lactamase–producing *H. influenzae*, a variety of oral agents can be prescribed, including the following: cefixime, 10 mg/kg/day in a single dose; ceftibuten, 9 mg/kg/day in a single dose; trimethoprim-sulfamethoxazole (trimethoprim, 8 mg/kg/day, and sulfamethoxazole, 40 mg/kg/day) in two divided doses; and amoxicillin–potassium clavulanate, 45 mg/kg/day of the amoxicillin component in two divided doses.

COMPLICATIONS

Obstruction of the oral airway may occur in extreme cases of uvulitis. When uvulitis is associated with epiglottitis, airway obstruction may be complete. The latter should be managed with nasotracheal intubation or tracheostomy. In isolated uvulitis, if obstruction is present, a nasopharyngeal airway will suffice until medical therapy results in clinical improvement.

Suggested Readings

Boyce SH, Quigley MA. Uvulitis and partial airway obstruction following cannabis inhalation. *Emerg Med* 2002;14:106.
Brook I. Uvulitis caused by anaerobic bacteria. *Pediatr Emerg Care* 1997;13:221.
Kotloff KL, Wald ER. Uvulitis in children. *Pediatr Infect Dis J* 1983;2:392.
Krober MS, Weir MR. Acute uvulitis apparently caused by *Candida albicans*. *Pediatr Infect Dis J* 1991;10:73.
Li KI, Kiernan S, Wald ER. Isolated uvulitis due to *Haemophilus influenzae* type b. *Pediatrics* 1984;74:1054.
Rapkin RH. Simultaneous uvulitis and epiglottitis. *JAMA* 1980;43:1843.

CHAPTER 254 ■ LIFE-THREATENING UPPER AIRWAY OBSTRUCTION

FERNANDO STEIN AND JORGE M. KARAM

Children with unstable airways deserve the utmost attention because most cardiac arrests in children are the result of respiratory failure, frequently in conjunction with some sort of upper airway obstruction. Clinicians should identify immediately children who are in respiratory distress or failure as a result of upper airway obstruction and should institute the preventive and interventional procedures to maintain and secure the airway to guarantee appropriate delivery of oxygen and gas exchange.

TABLE 254.1

CLINICAL FINDING IN UPPER AIRWAY OBSTRUCTION

Clinical Finding	Supraglottic Disorder	Subglottic Disorder
Crying, speech	Muffled	Hoarse
Cough	Absent	Barking
Position	Tripod, upright, protective, "strange"	Not specific
Swallow	Drooling, dysphagia	Able to swallow

TABLE 254.2

CHARACTERISTICS OF SUBGLOTTIC STENOSIS

Feature	Congenital Birth–Few Months	Acquired 2 Weeks–10 Years
Patient presentation	Stridor	Usually inspiratory
	Occasional hoarseness	Stridor after extubation
	Weak/unusual cry	
Physical examination	Stridor	Dyspnea
	Occasional dyspnea	Respiratory distress
	Normal growth	Normal growth
Radiograph findings	Narrow subglottic area on lateral	Narrow subglottic area on lateral
Bronchoscopy	Marked soft tissue swelling	Severe stenosis possibly circumferential
Management	Expectant watching	Racemic epinephrine
		Steroids
	Periodic bronchoscopy	Tracheostomy
		Tracheoplasty
	Dilatation	
	Tracheostomy	
	Tracheoplasty	

@ http://www.vh.org, pending response from Greg Johnson, greg@vh.org, who is contacting authors for permission. They are: Donna M. Santer, M.D., Assistant Professor of Pediatrics at the Children's Memorial Hospital, Northwestern University Medical School, Chicago; Michael P. D'Alessandro, M.D., Department of Radiology, University of Iowa, ???, michael-dalessandro@uiowa.edu, Children's Virtual Hospital; and Lauren D. Holinger, M.D., Children's Memorial Hospital, Northwestern University Medical School, Chicago. http://www.vh.org/pediatric/provider/pediatrics/ElectricAirway/Text/SubStenosis.html

The four common sites where stenotic lesions of the airway are found are as follows: the nose; the nasopharynx; the larynx in the supraglottic, glottic, or subglottic areas; and the tracheobronchial tree. Supraglottic and subglottic airway obstructions are the simplest way to classify the anatomic nature of the obstruction. The subglottic region of the larynx is the narrowest point of the pediatric airway and is the most common site of life-threatening upper airway obstruction.

The origin of subglottic obstruction is stenosis caused by congenital, acquired, or idiopathic lesions. Congenital subglottic stenosis is defined as subglottic stenosis present at birth, in the absence of a history of intubation, extrinsic compression (e.g., double aortic arch), or laryngeal trauma. A congenital lesion should be high in the differential diagnosis. Acquired subglottic stenosis is caused by laryngeal trauma, intubation, previous airway surgery, foreign body, infection, neoplasia, or chemical irritation (thermal or caustic).

Other causes of life-threatening acquired laryngeal abnormalities obstruction are autoimmunity, infection (epiglottitis, diphtheria, and laryngotracheobronchitis), gastroesophageal reflux, inflammatory diseases, laryngeal papillomatosis, neoplasms, and inhaled foreign body.

Generally, the approach to the differential diagnosis of upper airway obstruction is limited to three areas: (a) Is the airway maintainable with or without an endotracheal tube? (b) Is the disorder supraglottic or subglottic? (c) Is the insertion of an endotracheal tube urgent and possible outside the operating room? Table 254.1 illustrates the clinical features that differentiate supraglottic from subglottic upper airway obstruction.

In ideal circumstances, when affected patients have been identified with a life-threatening upper airway obstruction, a quick decision must be made about whether such patients can wait under expert supervision for the time necessary to align the operating room, an anesthesiologist, and an ear, nose, and throat surgeon to perform the intubation of the trachea. If the clinical assessment is that such children cannot wait, they must be intubated as described in Chapter 445. However, because patients with acute and life-threatening upper airway obstruction may or may not have a full stomach, the technique called *blitz intubation* should be used. This technique avoids having to use the 2 to 3 minutes of bag-and-mask ventilation prescribed in the standard intubation procedure and uses a rapid sequence of medications for the purposes of intubation. The sequence of medications used is described in Chapter 445.

Patients with life-threatening upper airway obstruction should be managed medically as long as they are able to tolerate it (see Chapters 229 and 255). Of crucial importance in such patients is avoidance of painful or distressing procedures or situations, such as needlesticks, forceful separation from parents, and abrupt manipulations by medical personnel. Af-

fected children should be observed closely and connected to cardiorespiratory monitoring and pulse oximetry. Physicians should request assistance without leaving the bedside of the child and, as assistance arrives, should assemble the necessary equipment for intubation of the trachea. The intubation equipment (see Table 254.1) must be pulled out, and endotracheal tubes, blades, stylet, and accessories of appropriate size must be prepared as if the intubation is to take place immediately. The chosen drugs in their appropriate doses also need to be drawn. Then, with the equipment and medications in place, the next steps are taken.

If the airway is unstable without a tube, undertaking diagnostic studies is inadvisable. After the airway is secured, the appropriate diagnostic procedures can be performed.

In general, subglottic airway obstruction is easier to handle than is supraglottic airway obstruction. The appropriate management of supraglottic life-threatening airway obstruction is accomplished in the operating room by appropriate personnel, including an anesthesiologist, an otolaryngologist, or a pediatric surgeon able to perform rigid bronchoscopy or urgent tracheostomy. Table 254.2 illustrates an easy guide for the characteristics and management of subglotic stenosis.

The main complications in the management of life-threatening upper airway obstruction are, obviously, obstruction or hypoxia (or both) and related consequences. Management begins with diagnosis of the physiologic consequences of the obstruction and the assessment of its urgent treatment under safe conditions.

CHAPTER 255 ■ CROUP

ELLEN R. WALD

The term *croup* describes a clinical syndrome characterized by a barking cough, hoarseness, and inspiratory stridor. This discussion of infectious nondiphtheritic croup is divided into four sections: (a) acute infectious laryngitis, (b) laryngotracheitis, (c) laryngotracheobronchitis (bacterial tracheitis), and (d) spasmodic croup.

ACUTE INFECTIOUS LARYNGITIS

Acute infectious laryngitis is experienced primarily by older children, adolescents, and adults during the respiratory virus season. The principal symptom of infection is hoarseness, which may be accompanied by variable upper respiratory symptoms (coryza, sore throat, nasal stuffiness) and constitutional symptoms (fever, headache, myalgias, malaise). The presence of associated complaints varies with the infecting virus: adenoviruses and influenza viruses may cause more systemic disease; parainfluenza viruses, rhinoviruses, and respiratory syncytial virus most often cause mild illness.

Diagnosis

The diagnosis of acute laryngitis is made on clinical grounds, and laboratory evaluation is unnecessary. In febrile, school-aged children who experience hoarseness, complain of sore throat, and have tender anterior cervical adenopathy, a throat culture to detect *Streptococcus pyogenes* may be appropriate. Hoarseness without any other respiratory symptoms may represent voice abuse.

Therapy

Acute infectious laryngitis virtually always is self-limited. Treatment consists of symptomatic therapy with fluids and humidified inspired air. Voice rest is beneficial. Protracted episodes of hoarseness (no improvement after 7 to 10 days) suggest an underlying anatomic abnormality.

ACUTE LARYNGOTRACHEITIS

Usually, *croup* refers to acute laryngotracheitis, a respiratory disease prevalent in preschool children. Acute laryngotracheitis is seen in children of any age but is most common between the first and third years of life; boys are affected more often than are girls. The causative agents are respiratory viruses exclusively, and frequently the illness occurs in epidemic patterns. Most frequently, the viruses implicated are parainfluenza types 1 and 3, but influenza A and B, respiratory syncytial virus, parainfluenza 2, adenoviruses, and herpes simplex virus have been cited as other causes. *Mycoplasma pneumoniae* also may cause croup. In areas in which measles is endemic, severe croup may dominate the clinical picture. In summertime croup, the en-teroviruses (coxsackievirus A and B and echovirus) or parainfluenza type 3 are the usual cause.

Pathophysiology

The causative virus is transmitted by the respiratory route, either via direct droplet spread or hand-to-mucosa inoculation. After acquisition, primary viral infection involves the nasopharynx. Viral replication ensues, producing nasal symptoms, and infection spreads locally and involves the larynx and trachea. Endoscopically, the mucosa is erythematous and swollen. Histologic evaluation reveals mucosal edema with cellular infiltration of the lamina propria, submucosa, and adventitia. The cellular constituents include lymphocytes, histiocytes, and polymorphonuclear leukocytes.

Clinical Manifestations and Complications

The usual onset of croup is with the signs and symptoms of a common cold: coryza, nasal congestion, sore throat, and cough, with variable fever. The cough becomes prominent, with a barking quality (akin to that of a puppy or seal), and the voice becomes hoarse. Many children with this syndrome never visit a physician. Such children may begin to have evidence of respiratory distress, however, with the onset of tachypnea, stridor (when agitated or crying), nasal flaring, and suprasternal and intercostal retractions. The increase in respiratory distress prompts a visit to the physician or emergency department. Usually, the illness peaks in severity over 3 to 5 days and then begins to resolve. Most characteristically, the signs and symptoms worsen in the evening.

Diagnosis

In typical cases of acute laryngotracheitis, the diagnosis is made easily on clinical grounds, and no radiography or blood tests are required. If anteroposterior radiography is performed, a so-called steeple sign may be seen as a consequence of subglottic swelling (Fig. 255.1). Usually, the blood count is fewer than 10,000 cells per cubic millimeter, with a predominance of lymphocytes. Indications for hospitalization, undertaken in approximately 10% of children with laryngotracheitis, include the presence of stridor, anxiety or restlessness, cyanosis, retractions at rest, or hypoxemia. In addition, children with a history of croup or previous airway intubation may benefit from hospitalization. Children for whom close follow-up cannot be arranged or whose families cannot provide the necessary observation and care also should be admitted to the hospital.

Therapy

As laryngeal inflammation increases and secretions accumulate, respiratory distress increases, and complete obstruction may occur. Almost always, this progression is gradual and is

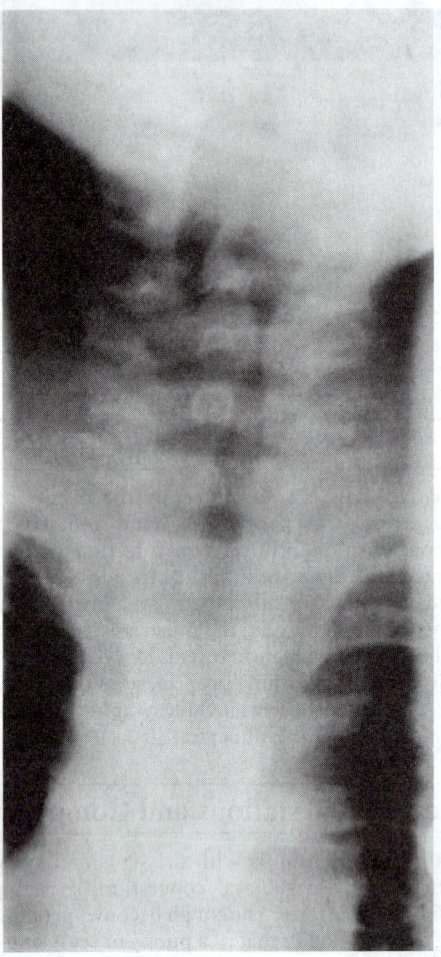

FIGURE 255.1. Steeple sign. This radiograph shows the characteristic narrowing of the subglottis indicative of acute laryngotracheobronchitis. (Reproduced with permission from Cotton RT, Myer CM. *Practical pediatric otolaryngology.* Philadelphia: Lippincott Williams & Wilkins, 1999.)

signaled by slowly increasing respiratory rate and effort, increased stridor at rest, and pallor or cyanosis. Agitation increases and air entry is poor. In approximately 5% of hospitalized patients, intubation is required to overcome the respiratory obstruction. Children who have a deteriorating respiratory status should be monitored in an intensive care unit by staff skilled in the care of pediatric patients.

One of the most important principles of treatment in patients with croup or other upper airway problems is minimal disturbance. Any stimulus that upsets affected children will result in crying, which causes hyperventilation and an increase in respiratory distress. The parents should be encouraged to hold and comfort such children whenever possible, and invasive procedures should be kept to a minimum.

Treatment strategies for acute infectious laryngotracheitis have included mist, racemic epinephrine, and corticosteroids. Although not subjected to study until recently, mist therapy has been considered standard management. Several investigations have suggested that mist is of no demonstrable benefit; however, this remedy still is used frequently. Racemic epinephrine, in use since 1971, is a potentially life-saving therapy in croup patients who are in moderate to severe respiratory distress. Racemic epinephrine is an equal mixture of the D- and L-isomers of epinephrine. The dose is 0.5 mL of a 2.25% solution diluted with 3.5 mL of water (1:8), delivered via a nebulizer with a mouthpiece held in front of the child's face. Administration results in rapid clinical improvement; by its beta-adrenergic vasoconstrictive effects on mucosal edema,

racemic epinephrine increases the airway diameter. The peak effect is observed in 2 hours. Accumulating evidence substantiates that patients who receive a single dose of epinephrine do not necessarily require hospitalization (as was the practice in the 1980s). Affected children may be discharged to home if, in addition to receiving epinephrine, they were treated simultaneously with dexamethasone and remain improved during a 3-hour observation period. The dosing interval for epinephrine in hospitalized patients depends on the severity of the laryngotracheitis; it can be administered every 20 to 30 minutes in the intensive care unit, where monitoring is possible, but usually is spaced 3 to 4 hours apart when such patients are in a regular hospital unit.

The use of corticosteroids in acute laryngotracheitis has been controversial for three decades. However, the efficacy of glucocorticoids for hospitalized children with croup now has been accepted as the standard of care, consequent to the accumulation of a consistent body of evidence from prospective, randomized, controlled trials. Corticosteroids have been shown to be effective when given by the oral route (0.15 mg/kg of dexamethasone), the parenteral route (0.3 to 0.5 mg/kg per dose), or as nebulized budesonide. The oral route is most convenient (unless the child is vomiting) and is least expensive. In general, the corticosteroid dose is given only once, although it can be repeated. In addition to the acceptance of corticosteroid therapy in hospitalized patients, enthusiasm is increasing for the use of nebulized budesonide or oral dexamethasone in patients who are seen in the emergency department and for whom admission may not be necessary. Routine use of oral steroids in the primary care setting has not been endorsed yet. Nebulized budesonide results in acute improvement in croup symptoms, shortens stays in the emergency department, and significantly reduces admission rates. However, nebulized drugs are more difficult to deliver than are oral medications. Antibiotics are not indicated in the routine treatment of children with this croup syndrome.

Most patients who are hospitalized for acute laryngotracheitis are treated with supportive therapies (occasionally oxygen and intravenous fluids) and can be discharged in a few days. Patients treated with corticosteroids recover more quickly than do those who are not given corticosteroids; intubated children can be extubated earlier, and those with severe disease may avoid intubation. If intubation is required, frequently the nasotracheal tube must remain in place for 3 to 4 days until an air leak develops around it, reflecting subsidence of the inflammation. Hospitalization for several days after extubation is desirable to ensure respiratory stability and the reintroduction of oral feeding.

SEVERE LARYNGOTRACHEOBRONCHITIS (BACTERIAL TRACHEITIS)

Bacterial tracheitis is a recently redescribed example of upper airway obstruction that was recognized more regularly in the era before antibiotics. Initial reports, in 1979, emphasized the clinical presentation and bacterial component of the infectious process. More recent investigations, which have had the benefit of more complete microbiologic evaluation, indicate convincingly that the process represents a secondary bacterial infection of a primarily viral process.

Epidemiology

Bacterial tracheitis occurs principally during the respiratory virus season, overlapping the seasonal occurrence of laryngotracheitis: fall and winter. This pathologic entity affects all age groups, from young infants to school-aged children, with a predominance in 1- to 2-year-olds. Boys and girls are affected equally.

Pathophysiology

The consensus holds that bacterial tracheitis represents a secondary bacterial infection of viral laryngotracheitis. The specific agents that have been implicated in the etiology of the viral tracheitis include parainfluenza and influenza viruses and enteroviruses. Most often, the secondary bacterial invaders are coagulase-positive staphylococci. Group A streptococci, viridans streptococci, *Haemophilus influenzae*, gram-negative enteric bacteria, and anaerobes also have been implicated.

The site of infectious inflammation is the mucosa of the subglottic area and upper trachea. In some cases, autopsy material reveals a necrotizing inflammatory reaction, with mucosal ulceration and microabscess formation. In other cases, a thick pseudomembrane is described. The membrane is attached loosely, and removal without hemorrhage is easy. The membrane may become detached from the mucosa spontaneously, leading to further obstructive symptoms. The purulent exudate that frequently is suctioned from patients with bacterial tracheitis shows abundant polymorphonuclear leukocytes. Usually, Gram stain reveals the involved bacterial species. Bacteremia is absent in these cases, but pneumonia is a frequent accompaniment.

Clinical Manifestations and Complications

The onset of croup varies. Some children become ill acutely and have severe respiratory distress within hours of onset of the illness. Others exhibit a 1- to 5-day prodromal period of mild upper respiratory symptoms and the onset of cough, stridor, and hoarseness characteristic of typical croup; then, within just a few hours, higher temperature, a toxic appearance, and a remarkable increase in respiratory distress develop. Notably, as distress becomes apparent, such patients do not respond to the inhalation of racemic epinephrine. Typically, high temperature, prominent cough, and stridor are noted at the time of clinical presentation. Clinical differentiation of this illness from epiglottitis may be helped by the usual absence of dysphagia and drooling in bacterial tracheitis. When signs of airway obstruction escalate, however, the key issue, as in cases of suspected epiglottitis, is securing the airway.

Complications of croup occur before and after intubation. The most serious is complete respiratory obstruction leading to respiratory arrest. A number of cases of severe hypoxia and, ultimately, death have occurred in patients with bacterial tracheitis. Pneumomediastinum and pneumothorax also may be seen as complications of intubation. Pneumonia occurs in approximately 50% of cases. Rarely, a toxic shock syndrome has accompanied bacterial tracheitis due to *Staphylococcus aureus*.

Diagnosis

The diagnosis of bacterial tracheitis may be suspected clinically, but it is confirmed endoscopically. At the time of intubation or bronchoscopy, the epiglottis is found to be normal. The pathologic process involves the subglottic area, with extension into the trachea. Abundant purulent exudate and pseudomembranes may be present. If radiographic studies have been performed, the anteroposterior radiograph will show the steeple sign and, occasionally, the detached pseudomembrane may be seen as a soft tissue shadow or shadows of irregular configuration in the upper trachea. Frequently, pneumonia is a com-

plication in cases of bacterial tracheitis. Leukocytosis may be prominent, but blood culture results are negative.

Therapy

The appropriate treatment of bacterial tracheitis includes securing the airway and instituting antimicrobial therapy. Tracheal intubation is recommended for patients in whom bacterial tracheitis has been diagnosed. This procedure can be accomplished with nasotracheal intubation or tracheostomy. In either case, observation in an intensive care unit is essential. The copious and thick secretions may lead to blockage of the artificial airway, thus necessitating meticulous respiratory toileting. Because the *Staphylococcus* species has been implicated most commonly, nafcillin therapy is indicated in patients in whom gram-positive cocci or no organisms at all have been seen on a smear. In cases suspected to be caused by methicillin-resistant stephyloccus aureus, vancoinycin may be initiated until suspectibility data are available. In patients in whom gram-negative rods or mixed flora are observed, an advanced-generation cephalosporin (cefotaxime, ceftriaxone, or cefepime) or an advanced-generation penicillin (piperacillin/tazobactam) is appropriate. Parenteral therapy should be continued for the duration of intubation or for several days after the patient's fever has abated. Oral antimicrobial agents may be used to complete a 10-day course of therapy in patients in whom the clinical improvement has been prompt. Typically, the clinical course of bacterial tracheitis is longer than that of uncomplicated croup or epiglottitis and requires an average of 10 days of hospitalization.

SPASMODIC CROUP

Acute spasmodic croup is a clinical entity seen in the same season and caused by the same viruses as acute infectious laryngotracheitis. Typically, children experiencing an episode of acute spasmodic croup go to sleep well or with the mildest of upper respiratory infections. They awaken in the night with a barking cough, hoarseness, inspiratory stridor, and variable degrees of respiratory distress. They always are afebrile. Most patients respond to mist therapy, provided by the bathroom shower or a cool-water vaporizer. Occasionally, the night air inhaled en route to the hospital is sufficient to reduce the dyspnea. Although most episodes are mild to moderate, occasionally airway support is required. Recurrences may be observed during the same evening or on the subsequent 2 to 3 nights.

Spasmodic croup may be differentiated from infectious laryngotracheitis endoscopically. Whereas examination of the mucosa in infectious laryngotracheitis reveals an erythematous, inflamed, velvety appearance, the mucosa is pale and boggy in acute spasmodic croup. Although viral cultures yield the same agents as those found in laryngotracheitis, the mucosal appearance and clinical course suggest an allergic component of the pathophysiologic process. Usually, this group of patients benefits from racemic epinephrine if the degree of respiratory distress mandates its use. Likewise, these patients may do well with corticosteroid therapy, reflecting either the allergic nature of the process or the natural history of a self-limited disease.

DIFFERENTIAL DIAGNOSIS OF UPPER AIRWAY OBSTRUCTION

The differential diagnosis in patients who have upper airway obstruction includes both infectious and noninfectious problems. The noninfectious causes are foreign-body aspiration and angioneurotic edema. Foreign-body aspiration occurs most

TABLE 255.1

DIFFERENTIAL DIAGNOSIS OF ACUTE INFECTIOUS OBSTRUCTION IN THE REGION OF THE LARYNX

Feature	Epiglottitis	Acute Laryngotracheitis	Laryngotracheobronchitis	Spasmodic Croup
Prodrome	Usually none or mild upper respiratory infection	Usually upper respiratory symptoms	Usually upper respiratory symptoms	None or minimal coryza
Age	1–8 yr	3 mo to 3 yr	3 mo to 3 yr	3 mo to 3 yr
Onset	Rapid (4–12 hr)	Gradual	Variable	Sudden, always at night
Fever	High (39.5°C)	Variable	Usually high	None
Hoarseness, barking cough	No	Yes	Yes	Yes
Dysphagia	Yes	No	No	No
Toxic appearance	Yes	No	Yes	No
Microbiology	Blood culture positive for *Haemophilus influenzae* type b	Viral infection	Viral infection with bacterial superinfection	Viral infection with allergic component

Adapted from Cherry JD. Croup. In: Feigin RD, Cherry ID, eds. *Textbook of pediatric infectious diseases*, 2nd ed. Philadelphia: Saunders, 1987.

often in children aged 2 to 4 years. If aspiration is observed, the diagnosis is straightforward. However, ambulatory preschoolers often are unobserved when such aspiration occurs. They experience an initial choking and gagging episode, usually followed by a "silent" period during which they are asymptomatic. The recurrence of symptoms may include the acute onset of cough, wheezing, stridor, or dysphagia in variable combinations. Usually, such children have no upper respiratory symptoms or fever. Auscultation of the lungs may reveal differential aeration and wheezing. Most aspirated foreign bodies are vegetable matter (e.g., peanuts, carrots, corn); therefore, plain-film radiography may not reveal their presence. The sudden onset of upper respiratory tract obstruction in previously well children always should arouse concern about foreign-body aspiration. Endoscopy is diagnostic and therapeutic in this situation.

Angioneurotic edema may cause sudden respiratory obstruction in previously well children of any age. Such children may have a history of allergies or previous episodes of respiratory tract obstruction. The angioneurotic edema may be based on a hereditary C1 esterase deficiency; in these patients, a positive family history may be found. Alternatively, a sudden allergic reaction to ingested material or inhalants may cause swelling of the tongue, epiglottis, or larynx. In any case, if severe reactions do not respond to injected or inhaled epinephrine, endoscopy and airway intubation may be necessary.

In addition to laryngitis, laryngotracheitis, laryngotracheobronchitis, and spasmodic croup, the infectious causes of upper airway obstruction include laryngeal diphtheria. Currently, this infection is rare in the United States, occurring in limited geographic regions. Fully immunized individuals should be immune. Partially immunized or nonimmunized children will have symptoms of low-grade fever and sore throat. The illness is slowly progressive, but toxicity is out of proportion to the degree of fever. Respiratory difficulty develops over 2 to 3 days and usually is characterized by hoarseness and barking cough, as in the usual case of croup. However, dysphagia commonly is present in diphtheria, in contrast to viral croup. Physical examination of the throat reveals a membranous exudative pharyngitis; the membrane is tightly adherent to the underlying tissue, and removal is difficult. Smear and culture of the membrane will disclose the infecting *Corynebacterium diphtheriae*.

The remaining causes of acute infectious obstruction in the region of the larynx are contrasted in Table 255.1. Laryngitis is not included, because it rarely presents difficulty in differential diagnosis. Acute epiglottitis is a medical emergency that must be differentiated from the remaining croup syndromes to enable appropriate airway management. Severe laryngotracheobronchitis (bacterial tracheitis) may require immediate airway placement. In both situations, affected children are highly febrile, appear to be in a toxic condition, and are in marked respiratory distress. Immediate endoscopy is diagnostic and allows proper airway management.

Suggested Readings

Ausejo M, Saenz A, Pham B, et al. Glucocorticoids for croup. *Cochrane Acute Respiratory Infections Group Cochran Database of Systemic Reviews* 1:2003.

Donnelly BW, McMillan JA, Weiner LB. Bacterial tracheitis: report of eight new cases and review. *Rev Infect Dis* 1990;12:729.

Geelhoed GC. Croup. *Pediatr Pulmonol* 1997;23:370.

Kaditis AG, Wald ER. Viral Croup: current diagnosis and treatment. *Pediatr Infect Dis J* 1998;17:827.

Kairys SW, Olmstead EM, O'Connor GT. Steroid treatment of laryngotracheitis: a meta-analysis of the evidence from randomized trials. *Pediatrics* 1989; 83:683.

Klassen TP, Feldman ME, Watters LK, et al. Nebulized budesonide for children with mild to moderate croup. *N Engl J Med* 1994;331:285.

Neto GM, Kentab O, Klassen TP, Osmond MH. A randomized controlled trial of mist in the acute treatment of moderate croup. *Acad Emergency Med* 2002; 9:873.

CHAPTER 256 ■ CERVICAL LYMPHADENITIS

C. MARY HEALY AND CAROL J. BAKER

Cervical adenitis is inflammation of one or more lymph nodes of the neck. In children, the most common causes of cervical lymph node enlargement exceeding 10 mm are reactive hyperplasia in response to an infectious stimulus in the head or neck and infection of the node itself. Self-limited cervical lymph node inflammation occurs in association with upper respiratory tract infection because the lymphatic channels drain proximally affected sites. In 80% of children with acute cervical adenitis, the submaxillary, submandibular, and deep cervical nodes are inflamed because these are the routes by which much of the lymphatic drainage of the head and neck proceeds. Malignancy is the second most common cause of lymph node enlargement in children, but neoplasia and infiltrative disorders constitute a minority of neck masses. Children with malignant lesions tend to have systemic complaints and firm, nontender nodes located characteristically in the posterior triangle or supraclavicular regions.

EPIDEMIOLOGY

The epidemiology of infectious cervical adenitis is that of its etiologic agents. Although often it is a manifestation of focal viral infection involving the upper respiratory tract, it also may be part of a generalized reticuloendothelial response to systemic infection. Viruses commonly associated with prominent cervical lymph node enlargement include Epstein-Barr virus (EBV), cytomegalovirus (CMV), and the human immunodeficiency virus (HIV). Age, geographic location, and socioeconomic status affect the incidence and clinical features of cervical adenitis. As a general principle, younger urban dwellers of lower socioeconomic status have a higher incidence of infection. Geographic location also may be important in some children—for example, those residing in the southwestern United States, where *Yersinia pestis* has become endemic.

Although patients at any age may be affected, most children with cervical adenitis are 1 to 4 years old. This age restriction and the peak in incidence reflect the prevalence of infections caused by viral agents, *Staphylococcus aureus*, group A streptococci, and atypical mycobacteria. The increasing incidence of nosocomial and community-acquired methicillin-resistant *S. aureus* (MRSA) infections noted in the United States and elsewhere, especially in children, requires that this organism be strongly considered as a possible cause. The genders are affected equally by cervical adenitis, with two exceptions. Some studies indicate a female predominance for granulomatous lymphadenitis caused by atypical mycobacteria, and young infants with the cellulitis-adenitis syndrome caused by group B streptococci are predominantly male. Droplet-borne and direct contact transmission are the routes of acquisition for most viral causes of cervical adenitis and for bacterial disease caused by group A streptococci and *Mycobacterium tuberculosis*. The remaining bacterial agents are normal inhabitants of the mouth, oropharynx, and nose or are bacteria inoculated by trauma to the skin with secondary spread to regional nodes. No ethnic predilection avails for acute bacterial cervical adenitis (Table 256.1). In contrast, adenitis caused by atypical mycobacteria occurs commonly in whites, whereas that caused by *M. tuberculosis* tends to have a greater incidence in African American and Hispanic populations. For children living in temperate climates, an increase in incidence occurs during the winter and spring months. A history of dog or cat contact, bite, or scratch may be a helpful clue in suggesting specific causative agents, such as *Pasteurella multocida*, *Bartonella henselae*, or *Toxoplasma gondii*. Similarly, a history of a minor inoculation wound of the skin proximal to affected cervical lymph nodes should suggest the possibility of such soil organisms as *Nocardia brasiliensis*, atypical mycobacteria, or gramnegative enteric organisms. Finally, HIV should be added to the list of agents causing cervical adenopathy, and, because most HIV-infected children are infected perinatally, the epidemiology reflects that of the mothers.

TABLE 256.1

DIFFERENTIATION OF BACTERIAL AND MYCOBACTERIAL CERVICAL ADENITIS

Clinical Characteristics	Bacteria	Atypical Mycobacteria	*Mycobacterium tuberculosis*
Onset	Acute (<1 wk)	Subacute to chronic	Subacute to chronic
Age (yr)	1–4*	1–6	All
Ethnic origin	All	White	Black or Hispanic
Regional node distribution	Unilateral	Unilateral	Unilateral or bilateral
Focal tenderness	Mild to marked	Often absent	Usually absent
Exposure to adult with tuberculosis	Absent	Absent	Present
Abnormal chest radiograph appearance	Never	Rare	Often
Tuberculin skin test result >15 mm induration	Never	Uncommon	Often

*Constitutes 70% to 80% of cases.
Adapted from Healy CM, Baker CJ. Cervical Lymphadenitis. In: Feigin RD, Cherry JC, Demmler GJ, Kaplan SL, eds. *Textbook of pediatric infectious diseases*, 5th ed. Philadelphia: Saunders, 2004:187.

PATHOGENESIS AND PATHOLOGY

The pathogenesis of cervical adenitis is elucidated poorly. Apparently, a microorganism first must infect asymptomatically the upper respiratory tract, anterior nares, mouth, or skin of the head or neck before spreading to the cervical lymph nodes. Overt infection of the skin, teeth, or oropharynx may occur in association with cervical adenitis, but clinically evident infection proximal to the affected nodes is not a requisite. For example, asymptomatic colonization of the anterior nares routinely precedes the development of cervical adenitis resulting from *S. aureus*. The common occurrence of group A streptococcal adenitis in children younger than 2 years old, in contrast to the infrequency with which streptococcal pharyngitis is observed in infants, suggests that adenitis may result when host defense mechanisms are insufficient to limit this organism to mucous membrane sites in the pharynx. Some investigators consider group A streptococci to be responsible for invasion of the nodes, with *S. aureus* playing a secondary role in patients from whose infected cervical lymph nodes both agents have been isolated. Dental caries or abscesses may predispose to the development of anaerobic cervical adenitis. However, when proper culture techniques are used, mixed aerobic-anaerobic infections frequently are diagnosed. This outcome suggests that elaboration of extracellular enzymes by mixed mouth flora may have a role in the pathogenesis of these infections. Certain infections are characterized by direct inoculation of skin proximal to regional lymph nodes (e.g., group A streptococci, *Nocardia*, *B. henselae*). Finally, viral cervical adenitis may reflect either a local response to a virus invading the oropharynx or respiratory tract (e.g., adenovirus) or a more generalized reticuloendothelial response to systemic viral infection (e.g., EBV). Some have stated that in considering the pathogenesis of cervical adenitis in children, physicians should consider the three Ts: tonsils, teeth, and areas of skin trauma.

The increased size of lymph nodes (greater than 1.0 cm) in response to infection is the result of an increase in the number of cells. While the lymph node is filtering pyogenic microorganisms, chemoattraction of neutrophils to the lymph node may result in the formation of microabscesses and small areas of necrosis or in frank suppuration. Rapid, extensive reactions almost always are caused by pyogenic organisms, notably *S. aureus* or group A streptococci. Granuloma formation with a delayed cellular immune response leading over a period of weeks or months to a "cold" abscess is characteristic of infection caused by mycobacteria, fungi, or *B. henselae* (Fig. 256.1). Tuberculous cervical lymphadenopathy occurs through pulmonary infection and involvement of the regional and more distant lymph nodes. Nontuberculous mycobacteria are ubiquitous in the environment; oropharyngeal acquisition followed by local infection leads to lymph node involvement. With both *M. tuberculosis* and atypical mycobacteria, biopsy material usually reveals extensive replacement of normal architecture by caseating granulomas surrounded by epithelioid cells and giant cells, and acid-fast organisms are demonstrable in sections that are appropriately stained in approximately 50% of cases. Epithelioid granulomas infiltrated with neutrophils, forming large pus-filled sinuses, are characteristic of the lymph nodes excised from children with cat-scratch adenitis. Once infection has resolved, destruction of nodal tissue sometimes leads to healing with fibrous tissue proliferation, most often in the submandibular group, and this may persist indefinitely.

CLINICAL MANIFESTATIONS

Cervical adenitis may be classified according to its mode of presentation as *acute*, in which symptoms are of less than 2 weeks'

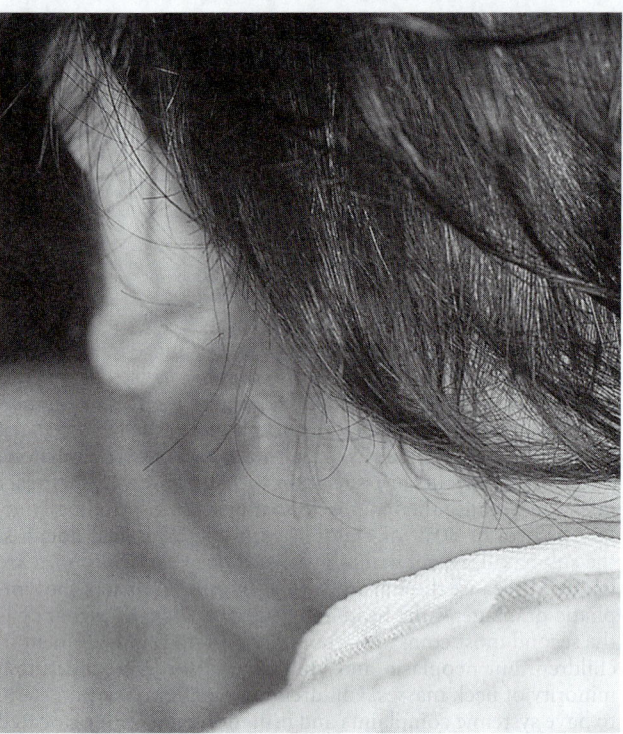

FIGURE 256.1. Mycobacterial lymphadenitis. This young girl, who had recently returned from India, presented with an inflamed lymph node and additional signs of systemic disease. An excisional biopsy showed caseating granulomas. (Reprinted from Fleisher GR Ludwig W, Baskin MN. *Atlas of pediatric emergency medicine*. Philadelphia: Lippincott, Williams & Wilkins, 2004.)

duration, or as *subacute to chronic* (Table 256.2). The causative agents tend to fall into one of these two categories, although they may overlap. Overall, approximately three-fourths of all the infections have an acute presentation. The duration of lymph node swelling is less than 3 days in one-half of all children with acute adenitis and less than 1 week in the majority. Generally, acute bilateral cervical adenitis is associated with upper respiratory tract viral infection, including EBV and CMV, or with acute streptococcal pharyngitis. Lymph nodes may be tender, but no other signs of inflammation are found. The appearance of such an enanthem as gingivostomatitis or of such an exanthem as scarlatina should suggest either a viral or a streptococcal cause.

Generally, children with acute unilateral cervical lymphadenitis have a paucity of systemic manifestations. A history of upper respiratory tract symptoms, such as sore throat, earache, coryza, or impetigo, can be elicited from one-fourth to one-third of patients. Usually, the diameter of an infected node (or nodes) ranges from 2.5 to 6.0 cm; the nodes are tender and exhibit varying degrees of warmth and erythema. *S. aureus* and group A streptococci are the causative agents in approximately 50% to 90% of infections. Less commonly, other bacteria residing in the oropharynx are implicated (see Table 256.2). Streptococcal adenitis occurs in younger children, is accompanied more often by generalized adenopathy, has a shorter duration of symptoms (less than 5 days), and is less likely to suppurate than are nodes infected by *S. aureus*. Overall, one-fourth to one-third of involved nodes suppurate, and 90% of these become fluctuant within 2 weeks of onset. Concomitant lymphadenopathy at other sites is observed in as many as one-third of children with acute unilateral cervical adenitis, most commonly in association with a generalized viral process or a group A streptococcal infection in very young children.

TABLE 256.2

INFECTIOUS AGENTS OR DISEASES ASSOCIATED WITH CERVICAL ADENITIS

Agent of Disease	Frequency	Onset	Generalized Adenopathy
Bacterial			
Staphylococcus aureus	+++	A	–
Group A. streptococcus	+++	A	+
Anaerobes	+++	A/S	–
Bartonella henselae	+++	S	–
Atypical mycobacteria	+++	S	–
Mycobacterium tuberculosis	++	S	±
Nocardia brasiliensis	++	S	–
Gram-negative enteric organisms	++	A	–
Group B streptococcus*	++	A	–
Pasteurella multocida	++	A	+
Haemophilus influenzae	+	A	–
Yersinia pestis	+	A	+
Actinomyces israelii	+	A	–
Diphtheria	+	A	–
Tularemia	+	A	–
Brucella	+	S	+
Syphilis	+	S	+
Anthrax	+	A	–
Viral			
Epstein-Barr virus	+++	A/S	+
Herpes simplex virus	+++	A	–
Cytomegalovirus	+++	A/S	+
Adenovirus	+++	A	–
Varicella	++	A	+
Enterovirus	+++	A	+
Human herpesvirus type 6	+	S	+
Measles	+	A	+
Mumps	+	A	–
Rubella	+	A	+
Human immunodeficiency Virus	+	S	+
Fungal			
Histoplasmosis	+	S	+
Cryptococcus	+	S	–
Aspergillosis	+	S	–
Candida	+	S	–
Coccidioides	+	S	–
Sporotrichosis	+	A	–
Parasitic			
Toxoplasma gondii	+	S	+

–, not found; +, rare; ++, uncommon; +++, common; A, acute onset; S, subacute to chronic onset.
*Neonates and young infants only.
Adapted from Healy CM, Baker CJ. Cervical Lymphadenitis In: Feigin RD, Cherry JC, Demmler GJ, Kaplan SL, eds. *Textbook of pediatric infectious diseases*, 5th ed. Philadelphia: Saunders, 2004;191.

Hepatomegaly or splenomegaly is rare, however; if found, either condition should suggest a generalized process (e.g., EBV, CMV, or HIV infection, tuberculosis, reticuloendotheliosis, lymphoma). Kawasaki disease may present as a febrile illness associated with bilateral or unilateral cervical lymphadenopathy.

In infants, *S. aureus* is the agent most commonly grown from unilaterally infected cervical lymph nodes. The presentation is similar to that in older infants and children, except irritability and other systemic signs may be observed more frequently. Infants at ages 1 to 2 months with facial or submandibular adenitis, particularly male infants with ipsilateral otitis me-

dia, may have the cellulitis-adenitis syndrome that is caused by group B streptococci. In contrast to infants with staphylococcal adenitis, those with group B streptococcal infection have a high likelihood (greater than 90%) of concomitant bacteremia.

The most common causes of subacute to chronic cervical adenitis are EBV, atypical mycobacteria, cat-scratch disease caused by *B. henselae*, and *Nocardia*. Uncommonly, toxoplasmosis, fungal infections, or syphilis may present as subacute or chronic cervical lymphadenitis (see Table 256.2). The features that aid in differentiating atypical mycobacterial adenitis from that caused by *M. tuberculosis* are found in Table 256.1. Nontuberculous adenitis exhibits an age distribution similar to that of acute bacterial adenitis and almost invariably is unilateral and localized to a single submandibular or tonsillar node. Although marked erythema may develop, these masses may be "cold" and demonstrate less tenderness than would be expected, given the degree of erythema.

Some geographic variation pertains, but *Mycobacterium avium-intracellulare* is the species isolated most often from affected nodes. Some of the apparent increase in incidence of nontuberculous mycobacterial infections most likely results from improvements in diagnostic methods. The regional findings are similar in atypical mycobacterial and *M. tuberculosis* adenitis, but the latter is distinguished by bilateral involvement in 10% of patients, by almost invariable exposure to a household adult contact with tuberculosis, and by abnormalities on chest radiography in approximately 30% of cases. Tuberculin skin testing is a helpful discriminator, because usually the diameter of the reaction exceeds 15 mm when infection is caused by *M. tuberculosis*, whereas reactions of smaller diameter are found commonly in children with infection caused by atypical mycobacteria. However, clinicians should remember that more than 40% of children with cervical adenitis caused by atypical mycobacteria may have tuberculin skin tests with greater than a 15-mm diameter of induration, and lymph node biopsy culture is the only precise method of assigning causation in these patients.

Cat-scratch disease is a lymphocutaneous syndrome in which regional lymph nodes proximal to the subcutaneous inoculation of *B. henselae* become inflamed. The interval between the cat scratch (or bite) and the development of adenitis ranges from 1 week to 2 months. Sixty percent of patients or parents describe a small papular lesion (2 to 3 mm) at the inoculation site, but this may have resolved at the time the adenitis is most severe. Lymph nodes of the head or neck were involved in 58% of the 548 patients described in one large series. Fever with a mean duration of 7 days occurs in 25% of children, but constitutional symptoms of malaise, anorexia, and headache are mild or absent in the majority. In approximately 25% of children, the lymph nodes suppurate. Uncommon manifestations include oculoglandular syndrome of Parinaud, encephalopathy, osteolytic lesions, and prolonged fever with hepatosplenic granulomas. Usually, adenitis resolves after 2 to 6 weeks, but it may persist for a more protracted interval in some children (up to 20%).

Another lymphocutaneous syndrome that may present as subacute cervical adenitis is caused by *Nocardia brasiliensis*. Traumatic introduction of this soil organism on the face or head produces a pustule or localized cellulitis, followed several days later by cervical or preauricular lymph node enlargement. Typically, these nodes are moderately inflamed, and mild systemic symptoms may accompany the early phase of illness. Clues to causation include the presence of an inoculation lesion and failure of the inflammation to resolve when antibiotics usually prescribed for cervical adenitis are administered.

Lymphadenitis is the most common form of acquired toxoplasmosis. It may present with generalized adenopathy (see Table 256.2), but, in approximately one-half of the cases, it appears as regional adenitis, typically restricted to a single nontender node in the posterior cervical chain. Usually, contact with cats or their litter or with undercooked meat is elicited in the history. In most children, the disease is asymptomatic, resolution is complete, and specific therapy is not required.

Chronic, recurrent cervical adenitis is part of the periodic fever, apthous stomatitis, pharyngitis, cervical adeuitis (PFAPA) syndrome, a chronic syndrome characterized by periodic episodes of high fever (less than 39°C) lasting 3 to 6 days and recurring every 3 to 8 weeks in association with apthous ulcers, pharyngitis, and cervical adenitis. Most affected children are greater than 5 years of age. The syndrome is self-limited, and recovery without long-term sequelae is the rule. Oral steroids effectively abort an attack.

A rare disorder of unknown cause that may present as painless cervical adenopathy is necrotizing lymphadenitis or Kikuchi-Fijimoto disease. Typical patients are female adolescents or young women, and usually the course is benign, with resolution occuring over 3 to 4 months. Some patients have associated autoimmune phenomena. Characteristic histopathologic findings in the lymph node biopsy confirm this diagnosis.

DIFFERENTIAL DIAGNOSIS

Cervical swellings are common in pediatric practice, and most represent lymph nodes that are infected. Noninfectious causes of cervical adenitis include a variety of benign and malignant entities (Table 256.3). Their duration is an aid to diagnosis because most tumors and miscellaneous conditions that cause cervical adenitis are characterized by chronicity. Usually, these lymph nodes are painless, are not inflamed, and exhibit a firm consistency. Location also is a helpful distinguishing feature because approximately one-half of all masses located in the posterior triangle are malignant tumors, whereas masses found

TABLE 256.3

NONINFECTIOUS CAUSES OF CERVICAL ADENITIS

Causes	Frequency	Associated with Generalized Adenopathy
Neoplasm		
Hodgkin's disease	++	+
Lymphosarcoma, rhabdomyosarcoma	++	−
Non-Hodgkin's lymphoma	++	+
Neuroblastoma	++	+
Leukemia	+	+
Metastatic carcinoma	+	+
Thyroid tumor	+	−
Collagen-vascular disease		
Lupus erythematosus	+	+
juvenile rheumatoid arthritis	+	+
Miscellaneous		
Kawasaki disease	+++	+
Drug-associated disease	++	+
Sarcoidosis	+	+
Histiocytosis X	+	+
Reticuloendotheliosis	+	+
Sinus histiocytosis with massive lymphadenopathy	+	+
PFAPA syndrome	+	−

−, not found; +, rare; ++, uncommon; +++, common.
Adapted from Healy CM, Baker CJ. Cervical Lymphadenitis. In: Feigin RD, Cherry JC, Demmler GJ, Kaplan SL, eds. *Textbook of pediatric infectious diseases*, 5th ed. Philadelphia: Saunders, 2004:191.

in the anterior triangle, with the exception of those involving the thyroid, tend to be benign. Masses that extend across the sternocleidomastoid muscle and involve both the anterior and the posterior triangles should be viewed as potentially malignant. Finally, age is a discriminator to some extent because lymphoreticular malignant tumors are more frequent occurrences in older children, in contrast to the infectious causes that predominate in children younger than 6 years old.

Lymphoid neoplasms and neuroblastoma constitute two-thirds of all malignant neck masses seen in children (see Table 256.2). Lymphomas, both Hodgkin's and non-Hodgkin's types, are more common findings than is neuroblastoma in older children, whereas neuroblastoma is the malignant lesion most common in young children. With the exception of thyroid tumors and metastatic carcinoma, which may present as isolated cervical masses, the conditions included in the differential diagnosis of cervical adenitis have generalized adenopathy or other systemic features. Other lesions include parotid tumors and benign tumors. Kawasaki disease deserves special mention because it is a common cause of unilateral anterior cervical adenitis for which the causative agent is undefined. Clinical criteria that include persistence of fever for 5 days or longer, and the presence of other major features—conjunctivitis, truncal exanthem, oral manifestations, and involvement of the hands and feet—are diagnostic of this syndrome. An enlarged lymph node (greater than 1.5 cm) in the cervical chain is one clinical feature of this disease that is noted in one-half to two-thirds of affected patients.

A rare but important cause of cervical lymphadenitis in association with generalized lymphadenopathy or hepatosplenomegaly is infection-associated or virus-associated hemophagocytic syndrome. This diagnosis should be considered if the foregoing features occur with prolonged fever, cytopenia, and high ferritin and triglyceride levels. The diagnosis is confirmed by demonstrating hemophagocytosis on bone marrow or lymph node biopsy.

Congenital lesions of the neck may simulate cervical adenitis. The most common of these is the thyroglossal duct cyst, which may be distinguished by its midline location and movement with tongue protrusion. These cysts may become infected secondarily and even may progress to frank suppuration. The existence of a pit, dimple, or draining sinus along the anterior margin of the sternocleidomastoid muscle serves to differentiate between branchial cleft cyst and cervical adenitis, although the distinction may be difficult if the cyst becomes infected secondarily. Cystic hygromas are soft masses that transilluminate, thereby aiding in their differentiation from inflammatory or malignant neck masses.

DIAGNOSIS

A detailed history to ascertain the duration of the illness (acute or subacute to chronic), the presence or absence of associated systemic symptoms, animal exposures, preceding trauma, contact with an adult with tuberculosis, the presence of maternal risk factors for HIV infection, drug usage (especially phenytoin), ingestion of unusual substances (i.e., undercooked meat, unpasteurized milk), or recent travel may yield important diagnostic clues regarding the cause of cervical adenitis. The physical examination reveals the location of the adenitis (anterior or posterior triangle); the presence of dental disease, noncervical lymphadenopathy, or oropharyngeal or skin lesions; and evidence of generalized or localized involvement. Radiologic evaluation of adenitis is unnecessary in most mild to moderate cases. Ultrasonography is performed when the presenting neck mass is very large, is increasing in size, or has not responded to initial antibiotic therapy. It is useful in diagnosing suppuration and expediting incision and drainage. Contrast-enhanced computer tomography scans or magnetic resonance imaging should be reserved for more severe cases in which the cervical mass may be impinging on other structures in the neck or when the diagnosis is not clear from the history and physical examination.

In children with acute infection, needle aspiration of the largest or most fluctuant affected node is the best method for establishing a specific cause. In 60% to 88% of patients with acute cervical adenitis caused by aerobic agents or mycobacteria, a causative agent is recovered by this diagnostic maneuver. Only inflamed nodes should be aspirated, however. They need not be fluctuant. Of course, clinicians should ensure that the cervical mass is not a vascular structure. The skin should be cleansed and anesthetized, and an 18- or 20-gauge needle attached to a 10- to 20-mL syringe should be used for aspiration. If no material is aspirated, 0.5 to 1 mL of sterile, nonbacteriostatic saline should be injected into the node, and it should be aspirated again. Gram and acid-fast bacillus stains of the aspirated material should be performed in addition to aerobic and anaerobic cultures. If *Nocardia* is suspected, the laboratory should be informed and asked to hold blood agar plates for up to 7 days. If mycobacterial or fungal infection is suspected, processing of the aspirate in appropriate culture media should be requested. Cultures of infected skin lesions or exudates on tonsils (if present) also should be performed.

If purulent material is not obtained, cultures for aerobic bacteria fail to yield a pathogen, and an affected patient does not respond to antibiotics active against staphylococci and streptococci, the following laboratory evaluation should be considered: throat culture; Mantoux intradermal purified protein derivative test; complete blood cell count; and serologic tests for EBV, CMV, *Bartonella* (performed by the Centers for Disease Control and Prevention or by state health department laboratories), *Toxoplasma*, HIV, *Francisella tularensis*, and *Brucella*. Tuberculin skin testing for *M. tuberculosis* always should be performed in patients with subacute or chronic adenitis. Induration greater than 15 mm is suggestive of infection with *M. tuberculosis*, whereas smaller reactions are more consistent with atypical mycobacterial infection. Patients with tuberculin skin test induration exceeding 10 mm should undergo chest radiography and be subjected to further questioning about recent exposure to tuberculosis.

If the foregoing evaluation does not reveal the cause of the adenopathy and it persists, enlarges, or is hard or fixed to adjacent structures, excisional biopsy should be considered strongly. Pathologists should be aware of affected patients' clinical history before receiving the surgical specimen. Excision of *the entire node* should be performed, if possible, because atypical mycobacterial infection is so common in children, and this surgical procedure is optimal for outcome. Biopsy material should be submitted for the microbiologic studies listed and for routine histology, Ziehl-Neelsen or auramine O, Giemsa, Fite, and methenamine silver stains. In select cases only, viral cultures can be requested. Sarcoidosis involving the lymph nodes has a similar histologic appearance to the noncaseating granulomata found on biopsy in cat-scratch disease, but this illness is rare in children.

Older children are more likely to be candidates for excisional lymph node biopsy. They also are the patients more likely to have lymphomas or other malignant lesions. Therefore, a biopsy of the appropriate node must be performed, and the specimen must be removed intact for proper fixation, cutting, and staining. The largest node should be chosen, and if several sites of involvement are present, specimens from the lower neck and supraclavicular area should be removed because they have the highest diagnostic yield. Other areas, including the upper cervical, submandibular, axillary, and parotid nodes, are more likely to exhibit reactive hyperplasia that may or may not be related to the underlying process. Reactive hyperplasia is the final diagnosis in approximately one-half of all cases. In these children, particularly when no improvement is noted, a repeat biopsy performed at a later time may offer additional information. For example, the lymphocyte-predominant variety of Hodgkin's lymphoma, which readily is confused histologically with reactive hyperplasia, may become apparent. If lymphoma is suspected, needle biopsies or frozen sections are useless for diagnosis.

THERAPY

Many infants and children with cervical lymphadenopathy accompanying viral infections of the respiratory tract never see a physician because of the self-limited nature of these infections. In others, cervical adenitis resolves during the course of antimicrobial therapy given for a primary diagnosis of otitis media, streptococcal pharyngitis, or impetigo of the face or scalp. In another group of children, the primary site of infection is acute inflammation of cervical lymph nodes. In these patients, empiric antimicrobial therapy without prior needle aspiration may be given. If no clinical response occurs within 48 hours, however, aspiration should be performed. Empiric antibiotic therapy should be directed against *S. aureus* and group A streptococci, and it should include such agents as cephalexin (50 mg/kg/day) or, for penicillin-allergic patients, clindamycin (30 mg/kg/day) or cefprozil (30 mg/kg/day). A combination of amoxicillin and clavulanic acid (45 mg/kg/day), provides good activity for staphylococci and streptococci and for oral anaerobic bacteria, if a dental focus of infection is suspected. This expanded activity and palatability render amoxicillin-clavulanic acid a good alternative to penicillinase-resistant penicillins. However, in areas where community-acquired MRSA is common, clindamycin (30 mg/kg/day) is appropriate empiric therapy because to date most community-acquired MRSA isolates are clindamycin-susceptible, and clindamycin also has activity against streptococci, anaerobes, and methicillin-susceptible *S. aureus*. Trimethoprim-sulfamethoxazole (10 mg/kg/day of the trimethoprim component) is an alternative choice for oral therapy of community-acquired MRSA infections but should not be used initially because it is not active against group A *Streptococcus*. Third-generation cephalosporins or newer macrolides have no place in empiric therapy for presumed bacterial adenitis.

In children with acute suppurative cervical adenitis, surgical drainage is key to appropriate resolution. Some patients have progression of local inflammation and persistence of systemic symptoms despite receiving oral antimicrobial therapy. Such children require parenteral therapy, and nafcillin (100 to 150 mg/kg/day) is recommended. In the penicillin-allergic patient, cefazolin (100 mg/kg/day) or clindamycin (30 mg/kg/day) may be substituted. Clindamycin also is appropriate when community acquired MRSA is a likely pathogen. In the severely ill child with signs of airway compromise, vancomycin (45 mg/kg/day) in combination with other agents against potential bacterial pathogens is appropriate until cultures results are available. Antimicrobial therapy should be modified once a causative agent is identified (e.g., group A streptococcal infection should be treated with penicillin G or V) and may need to be modified for an obvious primary infectious focus, such as a dental abscess, when therapy for anaerobes is mandatory. In the latter circumstance, penicillin V (50 mg/kg/day), clindamycin, or amoxicillin-clavulanic acid are useful agents.

Adenitis caused by group A streptococci should be treated for a minimum of 10 days or approximately 5 days after signs of local inflammation and systemic symptoms have disappeared. If affected children are penicillin-allergic, erythromycin ethylsuccinate (40 mg/kg/day) or cephalexin can be used. Warm, moist dressings over the inflamed area give symptomatic relief but probably do not aid in the localization process. If abscess formation occurs late in the first or early in the second week of antibiotic therapy, incision and drainage are indicated, and therapy should be continued for another 5 to 7 days.

Clinical improvement in bacterial adenitis is expected within 48 to 72 hours of the initiation of treatment, but usually the size of the node or nodes does not regress at this stage, and low-grade fever may persist. Regression of lymph node enlargement is slow. As a general guideline, significant enlargement that persists beyond 6 to 8 weeks demands exclusion of an underlying disorder and consideration of an excisional biopsy.

When organisms other than staphylococci or streptococci are involved or when lymph node enlargement is the result of noninfectious processes, rational therapy for cervical lymphadenitis depends on the cause of the condition. Disease caused by *M. tuberculosis* requires antituberculous chemotherapy and family-contact tracing for the infected adult. Disease caused by atypical mycobacteria is treated optimally by complete surgical excision of affected lymph nodes without medical therapy. However, clarithromycin monotherapy and combination therapy with clarithromycin and ethambutol or rifampin may be a valuable adjunct when surgery is not feasible or is refused. *Nocardia* infections are treated with trimethoprim-sulfamethoxazole orally, but often therapy for as long as 3 or 4 weeks is required for resolution. Usually, *Bartonella* infections are benign, and resolution without specific therapy occurs. In certain patients, however, ongoing local discomfort may be an indication for aspiration to hasten resolution and to relieve discomfort. Surgical excision is reserved for occasional patients who have ongoing systemic symptoms, persistence of significant adenopathy, or development of draining sinuses. Reports suggest that oral trimethoprim-sulfamethoxazole, rifampin, azithromycin dihydrate or (in older children) ciprofloxacin, and parenteral gentamicin sulfate are effective in *Bartonella* infections and should be strongly considered in immunocompromised patients or if uncommon manifestations of disease such as hepatosplenic granulomas are present.

COMPLICATIONS

Generally, cervical adenitis resolves without complication when the infection is caused by bacteria (e.g., staphylococci and streptococci) susceptible to antimicrobial therapy. Delay in establishing the diagnosis or initiating therapy, however, may prolong the clinical course. In this situation, complications or sequelae, including sinus tracts (mycobacteria and *B. henselae*), abscess formation, cellulitis and bacteremia (*S. aureus* and group A streptococci), acute glomerulonephritis (group A streptococci), and disseminated infection (*M. tuberculosis*), may occur. Usually, untreated suppurative cervical adenitis drains exteriorly; rarely, this process may extend internally, producing thrombosis of the jugular vein, rupture of the carotid artery, mediastinal abscess, or purulent pericarditis. Compression of the esophagus or larynx also has been described.

These complications, with the exception of abscess formation, are rare. In children with abscess, appropriate drainage and specific antimicrobial therapy result in prompt resolution of signs and symptoms, and relapse is rare. In unusual patients with repeated adenitis caused by *S. aureus*, chronic granuloma-

tous disease should be excluded. Moreover, this white blood cell disorder should be suspected in children who have cervical adenitis caused by *Serratia*, *Candida*, or *Aspergillus* species.

The availability of effective antibacterial and antituberculous agents has resulted in an excellent prognosis for almost all children with cervical adenitis. With surgical excision early in the course of lymphadenitis caused by atypical mycobacterial infection, resolution can be anticipated. Persistent and recurrent disease is the most frequent complication encountered. Clarithromycin monotherapy or combination therapy is useful in ameliorating these complications or when surgery is not feasible.

PREVENTION

The elimination of such predisposing conditions as dental caries or abscesses, group A streptococcal upper respiratory infection, bacterial otitis media, and impetigo of the scalp or face should reduce the incidence of adenitis. Minimizing the exposure of infants and young children to adults with active tuberculosis is an obvious means of preventing this extrapulmonary manifestation of tuberculosis. Likewise, lack of exposure to dogs and cats has been hypothesized by some as a means by which reduction in infections resulting from zoonoses may be achieved, but corroborating data are lacking. Clearly, our poor understanding of the pathogenesis of many of the causative agents of cervical adenitis limits insight concerning prevention.

Suggested Readings

Bass JW, Freitas BC, Freitas AD, et al. Prospective randomized double blind placebo-controlled evaluation of azithromycin for treatment of cat-scratch disease. *Pediatr Infect Dis J* 1998;17:447.

Debley JS, Rozansky DJ, Miller ML, et al. Histiocytic necrotizing lymphadenitis with autoimmune phenomena and meningitis in a 14-year-old girl. *Pediatrics* 1996;98:130.

Hazra R, Robson CD, Perez-Atayde AR, Husson RN. Lymphadenitis due to nontuberculous mycobacteria in children: presentation and response to therapy. *Clin Infect Dis* 1999;28:123.

Healy CM, Baker CJ. Cervical lymphadenitis. In: Feigin RD, Cherry JD, Demmler GJ, Kaplan SL, eds. *Textbook of pediatric infectious diseases*, 5th ed. Philadelphia: WB Saunders, 2004:185.

Huebner RE, Schein MF, Cautheu GM, et al. Usefulness of skin testing with mycobacterial antigens in children with cervical lymphadenopathy. *Pediatr Infect Dis J* 1992;11:450.

Lai KK, Stottmeier KD, Sherman JH, et al. Mycobacterial cervical lymphadenopathy: relation of etiologic agents to age. *JAMA* 1984;251:1286.

Marcy SM. Infections of lymph nodes of the head and neck. *Pediatr Infect Dis J* 1983;2:397.

Margileth AM, Chandra R, Altman RP. Chronic lymphadenopathy due to mycobacterial infection: clinical features, diagnosis, histopathology, and management. *Am J Dis Child* 1984;138:917.

Montoya JG, Remington JS. Studies on the serodiagnosis of toxoplasmic lymphadenitis. *Clin Infect Dis* 1995;20:781.

Naimi TS, LeDell KH, Boxrud DJ, et al. Epidemiology and clonality of community-acquired methicillin-resistant *Staphylococcus aureus* in Minnesota, 1996–1998. *Clin Infect Dis* 2000;33:990.

Palazzi DL, McClain KL, Kaplan SL. Hemophagocytic syndrome in children: an important diagnostic consideration in fever of unknown origin. *Clin Infect Dis*. 2003;36:306.

Sattler CA, Mason EO, Kaplan SL. Prospective comparison of risk factors and demographic and clinical characteristics of community-acquired, methicillin-resistant *versus* methicillin-susceptible *Staphylococcus aureus* infection in children. *Pediatr Infect Dis J* 2002;21:910.

Slap GB, Brooks JS, Schwartz S. When to perform biopsies of enlarged lymph nodes in young patients. *JAMA* 1984;252:1321.

Thomas KT, Feder HM Jr, Lawton AR, Edwards KM. Periodic fever syndrome in children. *J Pediatr* 1999;135:15.

CHAPTER 257 ■ HERPANGINA

SARAH S. LONG

Herpangina is a common, specific, acute febrile viral illness that usually occurs in epidemic form in young children in the summer and fall in temperate climates. Although the clinical symptoms and signs were mentioned in 1906, Zahorsky introduced the name *herpangina* in 1924, to distinguish the clinical entity.

ETIOLOGY

At least 24 enteroviral agents have been isolated in epidemic or sporadic cases of herpangina. Group A coxsackieviruses were associated definitively in the early 1950s with summer epidemics of herpangina, when suckling mice were inoculated for virus isolation; nine different group A coxsackieviruses have been documented to cause epidemic herpangina. With use of serology, tissue-culture, and molecular diagnostic techniques, multiple echoviruses, group B coxsackieviruses, and enterovirus 71 also have been associated with epidemic or sporadic cases of herpangina. Other viruses, such as herpes simplex virus (HSV) and polioviruses, are occasional causes of nonepidemic herpangina. Group A coxsackieviruses probably continue to be the most common cause of herpangina, although confirmation is lacking because some group A viruses are recovered only after the inoculation of suckling mice.

Coxsackieviruses are 30-nm particles composed of a single strand of RNA with a protein coat of icosahedral symmetry. Morphologically, they are indistinguishable from each other and from other enteroviruses, are stable at a pH of 3, and are resistant to inactivation by ether. Assignment of a virus to group A or group B is based on its chemical properties, ability to grow in tissue cultures, pathogenicity for laboratory animals, and serologic reactivity.

EPIDEMIOLOGY

Enteroviruses have a worldwide distribution, and they produce disease in both sporadic and epidemic forms, particularly during summer in temperate climates. Sporadic cases occur throughout the year. Humans are the only known natural host. The majority of enteroviral infections cause either no symptoms or mild nonspecific febrile illnesses. Illness is reported most commonly in children of 1 to 4 years of age. In a family study of enterovirus 71, the transmission rate to household contacts was 52%, with 53% of infected adults but only 6% of children remaining asymptomatic. In epidemic enteroviral disease, all age groups can be symptomatic.

PATHOPHYSIOLOGY

In experimental infection with coxsackievirus A4 in rhesus monkeys, oropharyngeal lesions typical of herpangina developed 2 to 7 days after inoculation. The data suggest that, regardless of the site of inoculation, oropharyngeal lesions occur and represent the secondary site of infection after viremia, rather than the primary site of viral replication.

In humans, the transmission of the viruses that cause herpangina is predominantly fecal-oral or oral-oral. Airborne transmission probably occurs, but is less common. Viruses can be isolated from throat and fecal specimens in the acute phase of illness and from fecal specimens for several weeks after recovery. Infection elicits the production of type-specific humoral and secretory antibody. The role of cellular immune responses is not well-defined. Infection appears to elicit life-long protection from clinical illness caused by the same agent. Local reinfection with a brief period of viral replication occurs.

CLINICAL MANIFESTATIONS AND COMPLICATIONS

The diagnosis of herpangina is suggested by the presence and character of lesions in the oropharynx. With no prodrome, or only a few hours of anorexia or listlessness, herpangina begins suddenly with the onset of fever. Temperature varies from normal to 41°C, and onset can be accompanied by a seizure. High fever, listlessness, and vomiting are more common in children younger than 5 years. Headache, backache, sore throat, and dysphagia are noted by older patients. Usually, the oropharyngeal lesions are present at the onset of fever or occur in the subsequent 24 hours. The characteristic lesion evolves from a small papule to a 1- to 2-mm vesicle with surrounding erythema and then to an ulcer. Lesions enlarge to only 3 to 4 mm over the cause of 3 days and remain discrete (i.e., do not coalesce, as do ulcers of HSV infection, mucositis, and Stevens-Johnson syndrome). The average number of lesions is five, with more than 20 being distinctly unusual. Characteristically, lesions involve the anterior tonsillar pillars, tonsils, soft palate, uvula, and pharyngeal wall. Occasionally, posterior buccal surfaces and the tip of the tongue are involved. The diagnosis of herpangina should be made only when the enanthem on the posterior oral cavity is obvious. Usually, other diseases associated with enanthems can be distinguished by careful attention to the number, size, and nature of the lesions involved. Features differentiating herpangina from other diseases with enanthems are shown in Table 257.1. Depending on the enterovirus circulating, epidemic aseptic meningitis can accompany herpangina. Enterovirus 71 is unduly complicated by poliomyelitis-like syndrome, encephalomyelitis, and cardiopulmonary failure.

DIAGNOSIS

The diagnosis of herpangina is made on clinical grounds. Delineation of a specific cause is helpful to define an epidemic, confirm an unusual case, or prove an unusual cause. Throat and stool specimens are the best source of viruses. Some group A coxsackieviruses will be missed unless suckling mice are inoculated. An increase in specific serum antibody can be demonstrated between acute and convalescent serum samples. The

TABLE 257.1

FEATURES DIFFERENTIATING HERPANGINA FROM OTHER DISEASES WITH ENANTHEMS

Disease	Etiology	Occurrence	Character of Oral Lesions	Site of Oral Lesions	Number of Lesions	Size of Lesions	Other Features
Herpangina	Coxsackieviruses, echoviruses	Acute	Vesicles, ulcers with erythema	Anterior pillars, posterior palate, and pharynx	1–5	1–2 mm	Dysphagia
Herpetic stomatitis	Herpes simplex virus type 1	Acute	Vesicles, shallow ulcers	Gingival and buccal mucosa, tongue, lips	Any	>5 mm, coalescent	Drooling, lymphadenopathy
Hand-foot-and-mouth disease	Coxsackieviruses, enterovirus 71	Acute	Vesicles, shallow ulcers	Tonsillar fauces, buccal mucosa, tongue	Any	1–3 mm, coalescent	Vesicles on hands and feet, maculopapular rash
Aphthous stomatitis	Unknown	Acute, recurrent	Ulcers with rim of erythema, gray exudate	Buccal and lingual mucosa, lateral tongue	1–2	>5 mm	Pain, no fever
Behcet syndrome	Unknown	Chronic, recurrent	Ulcers with rim of erythema, gray exudate	Any	1–5	>5 mm	Ulcers of genital mucosa, uveitis
Stevens-Johnson syndrome	Many, unknown	Acute	Ulcers, hemorrhagic ulcers, pseudomembranes	All, lips	Confluent	Confluent	Systematic illness, rash, drug history
Mucositis (ulcerative gingivitis)	Neutropenia, chemotherapy, bacteria	Acute, recurrent, chronic	Ulcers, exudate, pseudomembranes	Gingival, buccal mucosa	Confluent	Confluent	Fetid breath, pain, other gastrointestinal mucosal lesions
Kawasaki disease	Unknown	Acute	Erythema, strawberry tongue	Diffuse	—	—	Prolonged fever, rash, conjunctival hyperemia, cracked lips
Toxin-mediated syndromes	Staphylococcus aureus and group A streptococcus toxins	Acute	Erythema, strawberry tongue	Diffuse	—	—	Erythroderma and scarlatina, conjunctival hyperemia, hypotension
Streptococcal pharyngitis	Group A streptococcus	Acute	Erythema, exudates, strawberry tongue, palatal petechiae	Tonsils, pharynx	—	—	Sore throat, dysphagia, lymphadenitis
Adenoviral pharyngitis	Adenoviruses	Acute	Follicles, erythema, exudate	Tonsils, pillars, pharynx	—	—	Dysphagia, lymphadenopathy, conjunctivitis
Epstein-Barr virus pharyngitis	Epstein-Barr virus	Acute	Exudate, palatal petechiae	Tonsils	—	—	Lymphadenopathy, fatigue, splenomegaly

lack of a common enteroviral antigen and the large number of serotypes that are etiologic possibilities render serologic confirmation of the pathogen feasible only when a virus is isolated concurrently from the patient.

THERAPY AND PREVENTION

No specific antiviral therapy is available for the treatment of herpangina caused by enteroviruses. Pleconaril, which has *in vitro* and clinical activity against enteroviruses, is no longer available even for compassionate release. Acyclovir and ganciclovir have no role. Treatment is focused on maintaining comfort and adequate hydration and on observing patients for the involvement of other organ systems. The usual duration of signs and symptoms is 3 to 6 days. The prognosis is excellent, except in rare instances when herpangina is associated with hepatitis, meningitis, encephalitis, or myocarditis or with disseminated disease in the neonate.

Oral secretions and feces are infectious during acute phases of the illness, and virus can be recovered from feces for weeks after symptoms abate. Asymptomatically infected individuals probably are the primary sources for the spread of infection. Care in handling diapers, good hand-washing practices, and attention to personal hygiene limit the spread of these viruses.

Suggested Readings

Chang L-Y, Tsao K-C, Hsia S-H, et al. Transmission and clinical features of enterovirus 71 infections in household contacts in Taiwan. *JAMA* 2004; 291:222.

Pichichero ME, McLinn S, Rotbart HA, et al. Clinical and economic impact of enterovirus illness in private pediatric practice. *Pediatrics* 1998;102:1126.

Rotbart HA, McCracken GH, Whitley RJ, et al. Clinical significance of enteroviruses in serious summer febrile illnesses of children. *Pediatr Infect Dis J* 1999;18:869.

Sawyer MH. Enterovirus infections: diagnosis and treatment. *Pediatr Infect Dis J* 1999;18:1033.

CHAPTER 258 ■ PHARYNGOCONJUNCTIVAL FEVER

SARAH S. LONG

Pharyngoconjunctival fever is an acute viral illness defined by the presence of fever, conjunctivitis, and pharyngitis. It occurs in epidemic and sporadic fashion. Soon after adenoviruses were first isolated in tissue culture by Rowe in the 1950s, several distinct serotypes of adenovirus were confirmed as causative agents of pharyngoconjunctival fever worldwide, and swimming pools were identified as a major site for communicability.

ETIOLOGY

Approximately 50 immunologically distinct types of adenoviruses have been recovered from humans, with type-specific variability in epidemiology, communicability, clinical manifestations, and severity (see Chapter 187, Adenoviruses). Some have estimated that adenoviruses are responsible for 2% to 24% of viral respiratory illnesses in children. They are the sole cause of epidemic pharyngoconjunctival fever and the usual cause of sporadic cases. Epidemic disease has been associated most often with adenovirus type 3, with adenovirus type 7 second in prevalence; one or more epidemics have been caused by adenovirus types 2, 4, 7a, 11, and 14. Sporadic pharyngoconjunctival fever has been associated with these and with types 1, 4, 5, 6, 8, 19, and 13/30 (an intermediate type).

EPIDEMIOLOGY

Pharyngoconjunctival fever occurs in large community epidemics (usually associated with public swimming facilities), in local outbreaks (e.g., hospitals, clinics, child-care centers, schools, and camps), and sporadically. Infection can occur at any age. The circumstances of inoculation are most important. Close contact probably is necessary for person-to-person spread (by aerosolized droplets to the conjunctiva and upper respiratory tract) or self-inoculation (after hand contact with contaminated secretions from infected individuals and fomites). This last factor probably was the mode of transmission in an outbreak in a child-care center. Direct inoculation of eyes occurs from contaminated swimming pool water. The increase in frequency noted in outbreaks that occur in the summer and at camps probably reflects the risk of conjunctival inoculation in swimming pools. Inadequately chlorinated water was implicated in one epidemic of adenovirus disease. Direct inoculation of patients' conjunctivae from improperly sterilized ophthalmologic tools or the contaminated hands of staff has been responsible for multiple outbreaks of keratoconjunctivitis caused by adenovirus. Hospital-associated outbreaks otherwise have occurred primarily in intensive-care settings, where injury of the conjunctivae, direct inoculation, or both may predispose to infection. Nosocomial neonatal infection can be fatal.

Usually, conjunctival infection is the result of direct inoculation. The same serotypes of adenovirus that cause the pharyngoconjunctival fever associated with swimming-pool outbreaks rarely cause sporadic cases of conjunctivitis. Volunteer studies have documented that pharyngoconjunctival fever occurs after conjunctival, but not after nasopharyngeal, inoculation.

PATHOPHYSIOLOGY

The route of inoculation of adenoviruses causing pharyngoconjunctival fever determines the pathophysiologic sequence.

Biopsies of conjunctivae in infected volunteers reveal, predominantly, infiltration of lymphocytes in the submucosa. Biopsy material from tonsils and involved lymph nodes reveals hypertrophy and hyperplasia of the lymphoid tissue, with congestion and edema of connective tissue. Primary infection, regardless of the clinical syndrome, generally confers protection against clinical illness caused by that strain. Adenoviruses do not destroy the cells they infect *in vivo*. Virus can persist in the nuclei of cells and can replicate intermittently to detectable levels. Although adenoviruses are most communicable during the first few days of acute illness, shedding can persist for long periods, even months.

CLINICAL MANIFESTATIONS AND COMPLICATIONS

The incubation period of swimming pool-associated infections is 5 to 7 days. Although individuals infected with the same adenovirus type can have variable manifestations of primary infection, by definition, patients with pharyngoconjunctival fever exhibit pharyngitis (hoarseness, sore throat, cough, or local signs of pharyngeal inflammation) and conjunctivitis (eye pain, itching, excessive tearing, hyperemic conjunctivae, sticky discharge) in addition to fever. Fever onset is abrupt, and the temperature is greater than 39.2°C (102.6°F) in more than 50% of cases. Throat complaints range from mild irritation to severe pain and dysphagia. Usually, tonsils are enlarged, and approximately one-third of patients have follicular exudates. Conjunctival abnormalities are more severe than are symptomatic complaints. Symptoms frequently begin in one eye and then become bilateral. Itching, aching, and soreness are common; photophobia, exudate, and keratitis occur less frequently. Conjunctivae are erythematous and edematous. The palpebral conjunctiva appears granular, and 1- to 3-mm yellow-gray collections of lymphocytes on hyperemic epithelium sometimes are visible (so-called follicles). During epidemics or school or family outbreaks, not all infected individuals have the triad of signs and symptoms. Common additional symptoms and signs include nasal complaints related to adenoidal infection and hypertrophy (coryza, stuffiness, epistaxis), posterior nasal discharge causing cough, systemic complaints (headache, malaise, achiness, anorexia), tender anterior and posterior cervical lymph node enlargement, and flushed appearance of the face.

Compared with other viral upper respiratory tract illnesses, adenoviral infections are more severe and protracted. Generally, high fever is sustained for 4 to 5 days. In children younger than 2 years of age, adenoviral conjunctivitis can mimic preseptal and orbital cellulitis, with striking eyelid edema and erythema and periorbital ecchymosis. An inflammatory membrane on the palpebral conjunctiva (a pseudomembrane) was a consistent and relatively specific finding in one report. Although eye findings improve by the end of the first week of illness, symptoms of burning or irritation, dryness of the throat, and general malaise persist into the second week. Frequently, the peripheral white blood cell count is elevated, with an increase in polymorphonuclear leukocytes.

DIAGNOSIS

Diagnosis can be confirmed by direct antigen detection in conjunctival scraping using immunofluorescence or enzyme immunoassay. Investigations of polymerase chain reaction tests are promising. The isolation of virus in tissue culture is relatively easy because viruses replicate in a variety of commonly used tissue-culture systems. Characteristic cytopathic effect and intranuclear inclusions can be seen both in tissue-culture cells

---

BOX 258.1   Differential Diagnosis of Pharyngoconjunctival Fever

- Conjunctivitis caused by coxsackievirus A24, enterovirus 70, herpes simplex virus.
- Viral infections (Epstein-Barr virus, parainfluenza viruses, and influenza viruses)
- Bacterial infections of the conjunctiva (e.g., *Haemophilus influenzae*, *Streptococcus pneumoniae*, *Neisseria gonorrhoeae*, *Chlamydia trachomatis*, *Mycoplasma pneumoniae*)
- Kawasaki disease
- Toxic shock syndrome
- Tularemia
- Leptospirosis
- Psittacosis
- Cat-scratch disease
- Newcastle disease
- Allergic conjunctivitis

---

and in infected human tissue. A routine histologic examination of conjunctival scrapings does not provide a sensitive means of establishing the diagnosis. Rapid antigen-detection methods are used routinely to confirm isolates in culture. Conjunctival specimen is a better source than is throat or stool specimen to confirm specific etiology. Acute and convalescent serum samples are expected to show a rise in group-specific antigen, but this confirmation is impractical and infrequently necessary.

Differential Diagnosis

The differential diagnosis of pharyngoconjunctival fever is not problematic because the triad that leads to the appellation is unique (Box 258.1). Epidemic hemorrhagic conjunctivitis, caused by coxsackievirus A24 and enterovirus 70, is associated with subconjunctival hemorrhages ranging in size from small petechiae to large blotches. Chemosis and hyperemia of the bulbar conjunctivae, serous discharge, and fine corneal erosions also can be observed; preauricular lymphadenitis occurs commonly, but high fever and pharyngitis do not. Conjunctivitis caused by herpes simplex virus is much more serious and usually is distinguished by its unilateral involvement, vesicular eyelid lesions, corneal involvement, and preauricular lymphadenopathy. Eye complaints also occur during a variety of illnesses characterized by fever and pharyngitis, such as those due to Epstein-Barr virus, parainfluenza viruses, and influenza viruses. However, conjunctival abnormalities are minimal, and other findings predominate the clinical constellation in these disorders. The hallmark of bacterial infections of the conjunctivae, such as those caused by *Haemophilus influenzae*, *Streptococcus pneumoniae*, and *Neisseria gonorrhoeae*, is purulent exudate. In these infections, involvement of other body sites frequently is present. An exceptional outbreak on a college campus was caused by an unencapsulated *S. pneumoniae*. Infection caused by *Chlamydia trachomatis* causes nonspecific conjunctival abnormalities and cannot be diagnosed on the basis of clinical findings alone. The predilection of *C. trachomatis* conjunctivitis for infants younger than 4 months, the lack of associated fever and systemic illness, and the accessibility of highly sensitive diagnostic tests help to establish a diagnosis of *Chlamydia* infection. The distinctive systemic manifestations of Kawasaki disease, toxic shock syndrome, tularemia, and leptospirosis aid in differentiating these disorders that may be associated with conjunctival hyperemia or suffusion from the inflammatory conjunctivitis that is caused by adenoviruses. The degree of lower respiratory tract involvement noted in patients with psittacosis or infection caused by *Mycoplasma pneumoniae* helps to suggest infection with these agents when they cause conjunctivitis. The history and physical examination should separate patients with pharyngoconjunctival fever from those with cat-scratch disease, Newcastle disease, or allergic conjunctivitis.

THERAPY AND PREVENTION

No specific form of therapy shortens the course of pharyngoconjunctival fever. Topical application of the antiviral agent cidofovir is under study. The prophylactic use of antibiotics administered topically has no proven efficacy. Corticosteroid-containing ophthalmic ointments should not be used. If purulent conjunctival discharge appears, culture should be performed to exclude a bacterial cause for which topical antibiotic is indicated. The prognosis for complete recovery is excellent. Even when keratitis occurs, permanent scarring is rare. Neonatal infection can include pneumonia and visceral dissemination.

Swimming pools are the predominant sources of epidemics of pharyngoconjunctival fever. Appropriate chlorination, adequate water filtration systems, avoidance of shared towels, and exclusion of infected individuals can eliminate this source. Care in handling the secretions of infected individuals, scrupulous hand washing, and careful personal hygiene habits should be practiced to reduce transmission in hospitals and clinics, within families, and in camps. Ophthalmologic instruments must be sterilized properly, and single-dose topical medications should be used. No adenovirus vaccine is available for nonmilitary use.

Suggested Readings

Bisno AL. Acute pharyngitis. *N Engl J Med* 2001;344:205.
Cheung D, Bremner J, Chan JT. Epidemic kerato-conjunctivitis—do outbreaks have to be epidemic? *Eye* 2003;17:356.
Faden H, Wynn RL, Campagna L, et al. Outbreak of adenovirus 30 in a neonatal intensive care unit. *J Pediatr* 2005;146:523.
Faix DJ, Houng HS, Gaydos JC, et al. Evaluation of a rapid quantitative diagnostic test for adenovirus type 4. *Clin Infect Dis* 2004;38:391.
Leibowitz HM. The red eye. *N Engl J Med* 2000;343:345.
Martin M, Turco JH, Zegans ME, et al. An outbreak of conjunctivitis due to atypical *Streptococcus pneumoniae*. *N Engl J Med* 2003;348:1112.
Pacini DL, Collier AM, Henderson FW. Adenovirus infections and respiratory illnesses in children in group day care. *J Infect Dis* 1987;156:920.
Ruttum MS, Ogawa G. Adenovirus conjunctivitis mimics preseptal and orbital cellulitis in young children. *Pediatr Infect Dis J* 1996;15:266.
Wald ER, Greenberg D, Hoberman A. Short term oral cefixime therapy for treatment of bacterial conjunctivitis. *Pediatr Infect Dis J* 2001;20:1039.

CHAPTER 259 ■ PAROTITIS

ELLEN R. WALD

Inflammation of the parotid gland may result from infectious or noninfectious causes. In children, most single attacks of parotitis result from viral infection of the gland. This chapter is divided into considerations of viral parotitis, suppurative parotitis, and recurrent parotitis.

VIRAL PAROTITIS

Before the availability of the Jeryl Lynn vaccine, licensed in 1967, the most common cause of parotitis in children was infection with mumps virus, a myxovirus categorized in the same group of RNA viruses as that listing influenza and parainfluenza viruses. After vaccine licensure, it became apparent that other viruses—parainfluenza types 1 and 3, influenza A and B, coxsackieviruses A and B, echoviruses, Epstein-Barr virus, and lymphocytic choriomeningitis virus—could cause parotitis. Parotitis may be seen also as one of the protean manifestations of infection with the human immunodeficiency virus (HIV).

Pathogenesis

A myxovirus is transmitted by the respiratory route. After it is acquired, the virus replicates in the epithelial cells of the nasopharynx; subsequently, a viremia occurs, with ultimate localization of virus in the parotid gland.

Clinical Manifestations and Complications

In typical cases of viral parotitis, preschool or school-aged children may have a brief prodrome of such constitutional symptoms as fever, headache, anorexia, and malaise. The initial local complaint is ear pain located near the lobe of the ear and accentuated by chewing movements. Initially, when the parotid gland begins to swell, the sulcus between the mastoid and the mandible is obliterated. The gland enlarges symmetrically in front of and behind the ear, obscuring the angle of the mandible and displacing the lobe of the ear upward and outward (Fig. 259.1). The entire parotid gland becomes swollen in a uniform fashion. The gland peaks in size in 1 to 3 days and can be fairly tender and painful. Visually, the swelling is impressive. On occasion, the swelling is boggy to the touch, and delineating the parotid gland precisely by palpation is difficult. In other patients, the gland is firm and indurated, with a well-demarcated posterior edge. The skin overlying the gland is neither erythematous nor warm, remaining nearly normal in appearance. The orifice of Stensen duct opposite the second molar may be prominent as a consequence of erythema and swelling. Expressed secretions appear clear. Generally, the parotid on one side swells first and then, in several days, the contralateral gland also becomes involved. Unilateral involvement is seen in 25% of cases. Pain, trismus, and dysphagia are common manifestations leading to poor oral intake. The swelling may take 7 to 10 days to subside.

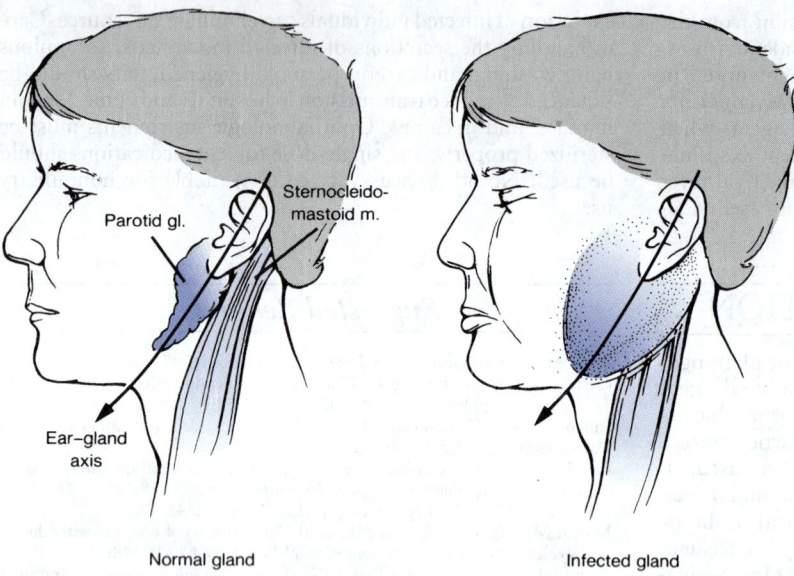

FIGURE 259.1. Parotid gland infected with virus (*right*), compared with normal gland (*left*). An imaginary line bisecting the long axis of the ear divides the parotid gland equally. These anatomic relationships are not altered in the enlarged gland.

Diagnosis and Therapy

Usually, the diagnosis of viral parotitis is clinical. Culturing the throat for virus may allow a delineation of the precise causative agent. Surprisingly, the amylase level is not always elevated in cases of parotitis. Treatment of viral parotitis is symptomatic. Analgesics may be prescribed. A fluid or soft diet is preferable when the parotid swelling is maximal.

SUPPURATIVE PAROTITIS

Suppurative parotitis is an unusual clinical problem in the pediatric age group. It is most common in neonates, and occurs sporadically in children older than 10 years. The usual predisposing cause is stasis of secretions in the parotid gland. This condition may be secondary to dehydration or to an abnormality of Stensen duct, either a congenital or an acquired malformation, including a sialolith (stone).

Pathogenesis

The most common bacterial isolate in cases of suppurative parotitis is *Staphylococcus aureus*. Other bacterial species that have been implicated include *Streptococcus pneumoniae*, alpha- and beta-hemolytic streptococci, enteric gram-negative bacilli, and *Haemophilus influenzae*. An important role for anaerobic bacterial species (*Bacteroides melaninogenicus* and *Peptostreptococcus* species) has been emphasized. The path of infection is thought to be the ascending route; the oral flora gain access to Stensen duct, and stasis of secretions prevents further washing out of organisms. Although cases occasionally occur by the hematogenous route, this process is much less common.

Clinical Manifestations and Complications

Clinically, affected children are highly febrile (temperature of 40.5°C) and toxic, and the gland becomes swollen, hot, and very tender to the touch. The overlying skin is erythematous. Purulent secretions can be expressed through Stensen duct by milking the gland.

Therapy

Treatment of suppurative parotitis consists of providing appropriate parenteral antibiotics and such supportive therapies as fluids and analgesics. Gram stain of parotid secretions, in addition to ultimate culture and sensitivity tests, should direct the selection of an antimicrobial agent. If gram-positive cocci are observed in clusters, nafcillin, 150 mg/kg/day in four divided doses, is appropriate initial treatment. Alternatively, clindamycin, 30 mg/kg/day in four divided doses, provides excellent coverage for staphylococci, streptococci, and respiratory anaerobes. If methicillin-resistant S. aurens is a concern, vancomycin, at 40 mg 1 kg/day in 4 divided doses, may be initiated until susceptibility data are available. Rarely, incision and drainage of the parotid gland is required if medical management does not result in a clinical cure. Response to therapy should occur in approximately 48 hours. Treatment of neonates should be extended for 10 to 14 days. Treatment of the older child may be completed with an oral antimicrobial agent for a total course of 7 to 10 days.

RECURRENT PAROTITIS

Recurrent parotitis of childhood, which is characterized by rapid and repeated swelling of one or both parotid glands, is accompanied by constitutional symptoms of fever and malaise and by local symptoms of pain and tenderness. The episodes may last for 3 to 7 days. The usual age of onset is between ages 3 and 6. Attacks recur at variable intervals but typically take place every 3 to 4 months. Frequently, recurrent juvenile parotitis appears in multiple members of a single family. Most individuals experience spontaneous remission of episodes in late adolescence.

Because the duration of attacks appears to be independent of antibiotic therapy, it is presumed that this condition is noninfectious. Often, the first and second episodes are thought to be examples of suppurative parotitis and, accordingly, are treated with antimicrobial agents. In the past, when cultures of the parotid saliva were performed in cases of recurrent parotitis, the usual isolates were alpha-hemolytic streptococci, which were presumed to be normal flora. More recently, *S. pneumoniae* and *H. influenzae* in high density have been recovered from quantitative cultures of parotid secretions obtained from children with recurrent juvenile parotitis. This finding again raises the question of whether a bacterial component exists that is related to the recurrent inflammation.

In cases of recurrent parotitis, sialography is an appropriate step to perform. Before this examination is undertaken, a scout film should be performed to scan for the presence of a stone. If a stone is found, sialography is not indicated. Most often, stones in the parotid duct are located close to the orifice of the duct; usually, they can be removed by milking the gland and duct. Surgical incision made through the ostium of the duct may be required. If no stone is found in the scout film, sialography should be performed. The sialogram will demonstrate diminished acinar components of the gland, partial destruction of the ductal system, and impaired clearance of contrast material. Follow-up studies performed when attacks remit ultimately may show improvement in the glandular elements and the ductal system. The sialogram appears to exert a therapeutic effect in some patients; fewer recurrences may be seen after the procedure. An alternative noninvasive method for imaging the parotid gland ductal system is with magnetic resonance sialography. Using special techniques, this method provides excellent visualization of the main duct and primary branching ducts. Recently, ultrasonography has become popular for the diagnosis of recurrent parotitis. Sonography shows hypoechoic, heterogenous internal echoes.

DIFFERENTIAL DIAGNOSIS

When the parotid gland swells initially, the diagnosis of either viral or suppurative disease is made on the basis of the findings of the physical examination (Table 259.1). The presence of systemic toxicity and overlying cutaneous changes suggests a suppurative process. Microscopic examination of the drainage emerging from Stensen's duct should clarify the process further: Purulent material consisting of polymorphonuclear leukocytes is seen in suppurative parotitis.

Occasionally, distinguishing acute suppurative lymphadenitis from suppurative parotitis may be difficult. When the lymph node in the parotid or buccinator area becomes inflamed, the distinction may be impossible. Identifying a site of drainage from the oral cavity, teeth, facial skin, eyes, or external auditory canal may help to clarify the issue. In suppurative submandibular lymphadenitis, the swelling is firm and tender. The overlying skin is erythematous, and the swollen lymph node is delineated easily. Approximately one-half of affected patients demonstrate fever and an obvious focus of infection being drained by the node. The peak age group is 2 to 4 years.

Other causes of persistent salivary gland swelling include amyloidosis, sarcoidosis, disseminated lupus erythematosus, Sjögren syndrome, and Mikulicz syndrome. Infectious causes of persistent parotitis include actinomycosis, *Mycobacterium*, toxoplasmosis, melioidosis, and cat-scratch disease. Otherwise, asymptomatic salivary gland swelling may accompany

TABLE 259.1

DIFFERENTIAL DIAGNOSIS OF PAROTID SWELLING

Infectious	Noninfectious
A. Viral	A. Bulimia
Parainfluenza 1 and 3	B. Autoimmune
Influenza A and B	Sjögren's
Mumps	Recurrent parotitis in
Coxsackie A and B	children (?)
Echovirus	Lupus
Epstein-Barr Virus	
Lymphocytic chori-	C. Granulomatous disease
omeningitis	Wegener granulomatosis
HIV	Sarcoid
B. Bacterial	D. Neoplastic disease lym-
Staphylococcus aureus	phoma
Streptococcus pneumo-	E. Drug-induced
niae	Potassium iodide
Streptococci (α- and	Thiouracils
β-hemolytic)	
Haemophilus influenzae	F. Heavy metal exposure
Gram negative enteric	Copper
bacilli	Lead
Anaerobic bacterial	Mercury
species	
Bartonella henselae	
Actinomycosis	
Mycobacterium	

drug therapy with supersaturated potassium iodide or the thiouracils. It may be a manifestation also of pneumoparotitis, a condition caused by forcing air through Stensen's duct. This condition may result from playing a wind instrument or voluntarily by purposely blowing with a closed mouth. Symptomatic parotitis may accompany high-dose etoposide, the use of L-asparaginase, and autologous bone marrow transplantation. Toxic parotitis may occur secondary to copper, lead, or mercury poisoning.

Suggested Readings

Brook I. Acute bacterial suppurative parotitis: microbiology and management. *J Craniofacial Surg* 2003;04:37.

Ericson S, Zetterlund B, Ohman J. Recurrent parotitis and sialectasis in childhood. *Ann Otol Rhinol Laryngol* 1991;100:527.

Fischbach R, Kugel H, Erast S, et al. MR sialography: initial experience using a T2-weighted fast SE sequence. *J Comput Assist Tomogr* 1997;21:826.

Giglio MS, Landaeta M, Pinto ME. Microbiology of recurrent parotitis. *Pediatr Infect Dis J* 1997;16:381.

Isaacs D. Recurrent parotitis. *J Paediatr Child Health* 2002;38:92.

SECTION III ■ DISEASES OF THE CARDIOVASCULAR SYSTEM

CHAPTER 260 ■ ECHOCARDIOGRAPHY AND ELECTROCARDIOGRAPHY

JAMES C. HUHTA

ECHOCARDIOGRAPHY

Since the early 1980s, echocardiography (i.e., ultrasonic imaging) of the heart and cardiovascular system has provided a major advance in pediatric cardiology and has allowed imaging of anatomy, appraisal of ventricular function, and assessment of peripheral blood velocities in both arteries and veins. This noninvasive modality has altered the assessment of fetal and neonatal congenital heart disease. Early in pediatric cardiology, the electrocardiogram (ECG) was the major tool for the exploration of the intracardiac anatomy, whereas the chest radiograph was the screening tool used for signs of congestive heart failure and for extracardiac anatomy such as the pulmonary artery size and vascularity. No assessment could be made of the fetus because the fetus ECG had not, and still has not, been developed. Now, a complete anatomic and physiologic assessment can be obtained of the neonate and of the fetus at 20 weeks' gestation.

The technique has changed the practice of pediatric cardiology slowly by replacing cardiac catheterization for the diagnosis of congenital malformations, and combined with the use of prostaglandin for maintaining the patency of the ductus arteriosus, echocardiography has dramatically reduced the need for emergency cardiac catheterization in neonates. Most patients with congenital heart disease detected in the neonatal period can have palliative surgery without cardiac catheterization, and most definitive surgical repairs can be performed successfully without the risks of invasive studies. Pulsed, continuous-wave, color, and tissue Doppler studies have added important capabilities for anatomic and functional assessment. The intraoperative and postoperative management of congenital heart defects has been aided by the addition of transesophageal echocardiography (TEE). This mode can add improved resolution in neonates and older patients for whom performing transthoracic imaging is difficult, and it greatly aids the surgeon by providing feedback about the quality of the repair before separating the patient from the heart-lung machine. Higher-resolution imaging systems continue to evolve and lead to improvements in echocardiography equipment. Made possible by new multielement transducer technology and high-speed computer advances, three-dimensional real-time imaging, color Doppler, and, today, tissue Doppler techniques can be used for an advanced approach to the assessment of systolic and diastolic function of the myocardium.

Diagnosis of Congenital Heart Disease

Echocardiography will continue to be the mainstay of the diagnosis of congenital heart disease in neonates, infants, and children and will become more important as additional experience is accumulated. Pioneered by Van Praagh in 1972 for describing congenital cardiac defects at the autopsy table, the segmental approach has been applied to cardiovascular diagnosis using various methods, including echocardiography. A logical analysis of cardiovascular anatomy requires a step-by-step segmental approach. This segmental approach is used for assessing complex congenital malformations in which some portions of the heart may be absent or malpositioned and for the angiographic delineation of cardiac anatomy. The segmental approach is based on the condition that all aspects of abnormal cardiovascular morphology can be broken down into discrete, mutually exclusive descriptors, allowing any complex congenital malformation to be described unambiguously. The schema must include information on the presence, position, and connection of each cardiac segment. Classically, three segments have been recognized: atria, ventricles, and great arteries. In complex malformations, a detailed approach to segmental diagnosis that can be used for noninvasive examination in any setting is necessary.

By describing the anatomic segments and indicating the normality or abnormality of each, a complete description of the cardiac anatomy can be made. Data are obtained by combining the findings from several echocardiographic windows. A complete, step-by-step approach to cardiac diagnosis includes atrial situs diagnosis; identification of the chambers and their interconnections; and a systematic assessment of valves, septa, coronary arteries, systemic and pulmonary veins, and aortic anatomy. Coding of cardiac anatomic abnormalities now has been implemented by the collaboration of many surgical and cardiology groups.

Cardiac Function Assessment

Echocardiography is a tomographic anatomic tool, but it also provides dynamic information about cardiac function and structure. Doppler echocardiography can provide functional information that is not available from any other method. For example, atrioventricular (AV) valve regurgitation can be diagnosed, and the severity, which depends on many technical and physiologic factors, can be estimated. In addition to seeing a ventricular septal defect, the jet of a left-to-right shunt can be detected by pulsed Doppler, the pressure gradient quantitated by continuous-wave Doppler (using the simplified Bernoulli equation: pressure gradient = four times the peak velocity squared), and the defect spatially oriented by color Doppler. Using the continuity equation and the PISA concept, the flow area and volume can be calculated in left-to-right shunts, and the regurgitant volume and area in AV valve regurgitation can be calculated. The pulmonary artery pressure can be estimated using the peak velocity of the tricuspid regurgitation jet, and the severity of semilunar stenosis or coarctation can be estimated using the peak and mean gradients. These hemodynamic findings can be integrated into this segmental approach using the anatomic segment as the finding and the functional aspect as the modifier. For example, the morphologic mitral valve is the anatomic site and location, and the regurgitation is the modifier.

Structure-Oriented Approach

Adult-oriented, two-dimensional echocardiographic reports usually take a view approach to the cardiac anatomy, which usually is highly predictable. The investigators describe the appearance of a given cardiac lesion in a standard parasternal, apical, or subcostal scan. However, this approach can lead to diagnostic errors when it is applied to congenital heart disease. For example, a scan of an aortopulmonary window from the right ventricular outflow tract can simulate the origin of the aorta from the right ventricle (i.e., transposition of the great arteries). In congenital heart disease, the various views must be integrated, scanning from one to another echocardiographic window to perform a complete anatomic examination. Although the echocardiographic examiner with experience learns to identify the normal appearances of the heart without congenital defects from various echo windows, a structure-oriented or anatomic approach always is superior to one based on standardized views.

The diagnostic accuracy of two-dimensional echocardiographic imaging in children has been proven in several prospective studies, including that of Gutgesell and colleagues. In 250 consecutive children with congenital heart disease treated at Texas Children's Hospital, Houston, Texas, only one surgically significant error in diagnosis occurred. This standard requires a compulsive approach to detect rare variations in anatomy that can have importance to the surgeon. For example, coronary artery anomalies such as a coronary originating from the pulmonary artery can be detected using a standardized approach to defining the origins and courses of the coronary branches.

Situs Diagnosis

The diagnosis of cardiac position and atrial-visceral situs using echocardiographic signs is a standard part of the assessment of congenital heart disease and is the foundation of the segmental approach. Atrial situs and atrial morphology are diagnosed together, and possibilities are described in Box 260.1 (Fig. 260.1).

Atrioventricular Connection

The diagnosis of a connection of the atria and ventricles (i.e., AV connection) requires knowledge of the atrial and ventricular morphology. The echocardiographic criteria for a morphologic left ventricle include insertion of the mitral valve at the crux of the heart farther from the cardiac apex than from the tricuspid valve, two normally placed left ventricular papillary muscles, mitral semilunar continuity, a typical elliptic, smooth wall septum, and a fish-mouth appearance of the mitral valve with two commissures. In the absence of the typical offsetting of the AV valves and with cardiac malposition, the trabecular pattern of the ventricles sometimes can be recognized: a smooth wall pattern of the left ventricle and coarser, more heavily trabeculated pattern of the right ventricle. The appearance of the ventricular outflow tracts may aid in establishing ventricular morphologic diagnosis and should be observed as part of the segmental approach. Normally, a continuity between the mitral valve of the left ventricle and the aortic valve is present, but muscle separates the tricuspid and the pulmonary valves in the right ventricular outflow tract. The most reliable criterion for identification of the morphologic right ventricle is tricuspid valve chordal attachments to the septum. With an atrial septal defect of the primum type, the valves are at the same

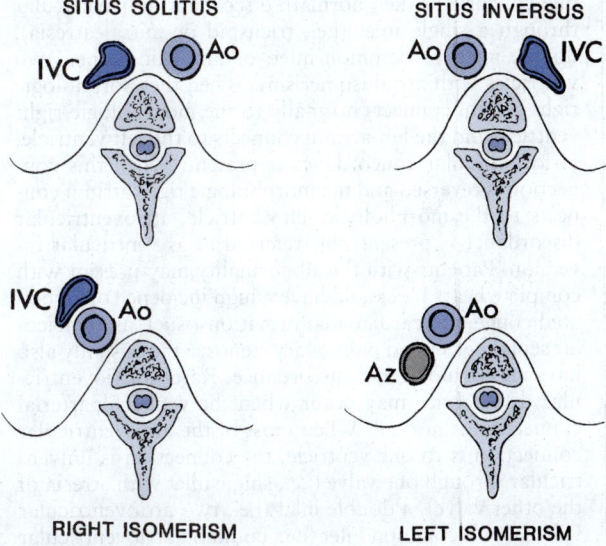

FIGURE 260.1. Situs by echocardiography. Situs solitus is normal and the aorta (Ao) and inferior vena cava (IVC) are positioned symmetrically adjacent to the spine. In situs inversus, a mirror-image relationship is present. In right atrial isomerism, the IVC and the Ao run together on either side of the spine. In left isomerism, there is azygos continuation of the IVC(Az) located retroperitoneally with the Ao.

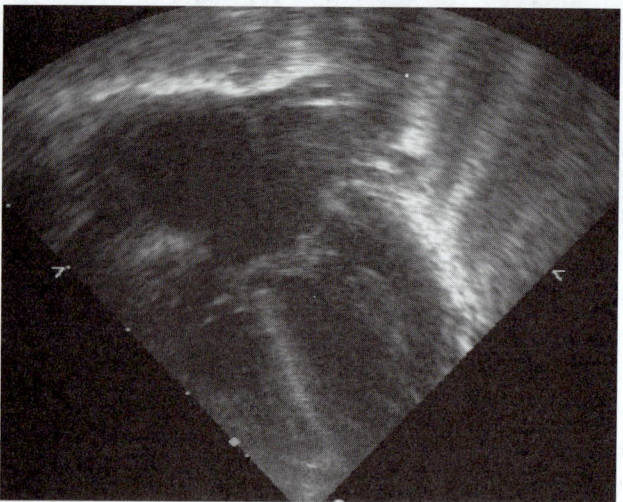

FIGURE 260.2. Atrioventricular (AV) canal defect with a large primum atrial septal defect. Note the mitral and tricuspid valves are at the same level.

level (Fig. 260.2). Four types of AV connection are described in Box 260.2.

The accuracy of echocardiographic imaging in the diagnosis of AV connection is unsurpassed by other modalities. Occasionally, an inexperienced observer may confuse a common inlet with a common (four-leaflet) valve with a single inlet. After experience with imaging the variations of AV septal defect, this differentiation should not present problems. Identification of the lower atrial septum unequivocally identifies the crux of

---

Atrioventricular Connections Seen on Echocardiography

Atrioventricular connections may be any of the following: concordant (i.e., normal); discordant; univentricular through a single inlet (i.e., tricuspid or mitral atresia), double inlet, or common inlet; or ambiguous (i.e., two ventricles with atrial isomerism). When the morphologic right atrium connects normally to the morphologic right ventricle and the left atrium connects to the left ventricle, atrioventricular concordance is present. When this connection is reversed and the morphologic right atrium connects to the morphologic left ventricle, atrioventricular discordance is present; this referred to as ventricular inversion. Patients with this abnormality may present with complete heart block and have a high incidence of associated congenital cardiac malformations, such as ventricular septal defect and pulmonary stenosis; they usually also have ventriculoarterial discordance. Rarely, atrioventricular discordance may occur when the ventriculoarterial connection is normal. When most of the atrioventricular connection is to one ventricle, the connection is univentricular through one valve (i.e., single inlet with atresia of the other valve), a double inlet (i.e., two atrioventricular valves), or a common inlet (i.e., common atrioventricular valve). A common inlet ventricle is part of the spectrum of atrioventricular septal defect (i.e., atrioventricular canal) in which hypoplasia of one of the ventricular chambers occurs and the atrioventricular connection is predominantly to the other.

---

the heart and points to a single inlet with atresia of the other valve. The general consensus is that echocardiography in experienced hands is the best method for assessing AV connection and for assessing abnormalities of the cardiac valves.

Ventriculoarterial Connection

Ventriculoarterial connection is the manner in which the great arteries and semilunar valves connect to the ventricular outflow tracts. Normally, the morphologic right ventricle connects to the pulmonary valve, and the morphologic left ventricle connects to the aortic valve. Four types of AV connection are described in Box 260.3.

Reports of neonates with abnormalities of ventriculoarterial connection and children with transposition of the great arteries show that echocardiography can detect accurately these abnormalities (Fig. 260.3). A newborn with cyanosis caused by transposition can be diagnosed without catheterization, and most neonates now have surgery without catheterization.

Atrial and Ventricular Septa

Atrial Septum. Before birth, the atrial septum usually bows toward the morphologic left atrium because of the significant

---

Types of Ventriculoarterial Connections Seen on Echocardiography

Ventriculoarterial connections may be concordant (i.e., normal), discordant (i.e., right ventricle to the aorta and left ventricle to the pulmonary trunk), double outlet (usually the right ventricle), or single outlet (i.e., aortic or pulmonary atresia or truncus arteriosus). When the morphologic right ventricle connects to the pulmonary valve and the morphologic left ventricle connects to the aortic valve, concordance is present. When the morphologic right ventricle gives rise to the aorta and the morphologic left ventricle gives rise to the pulmonary trunk (i.e., ventriculoarterial discordance), transposition of the great arteries, the most common type of abnormality of ventriculoarterial connection, occurs (see Fig. 260.3). To diagnose this abnormality, the great vessels must be identified. The pulmonary artery is identified by its branching pattern into left and right pulmonary arteries and ductus arteriosus, and the aorta is identified by the coronary, carotid, and subclavian arteries. Both great vessels may originate from either ventricle (usually the morphologic right ventricle), creating a double-outlet right ventricle. If the aortic or pulmonary valve is atretic, a single-outlet ventricle is the result. When a single truncal valve originates from the ventricular mass but overrides the ventricular septum, truncus arteriosus, another example of a single-outlet abnormality, occurs. The ventriculoarterial connection is designated as a single outlet with an overriding truncal valve. In complex malformations, including right atrial isomerism with the asplenia syndrome, the atrioventricular septal defect often is associated with a double-outlet right ventricle. In tetralogy of Fallot, overriding of the aortic valve often is present so that almost one-half of the valve annulus appears to arise from the right ventricle. Mitral aortic continuity is present, and, except for the rare circumstance in which more than 50% overriding of the aortic valve occurs, the ventriculoarterial connection in tetralogy of Fallot is concordant.

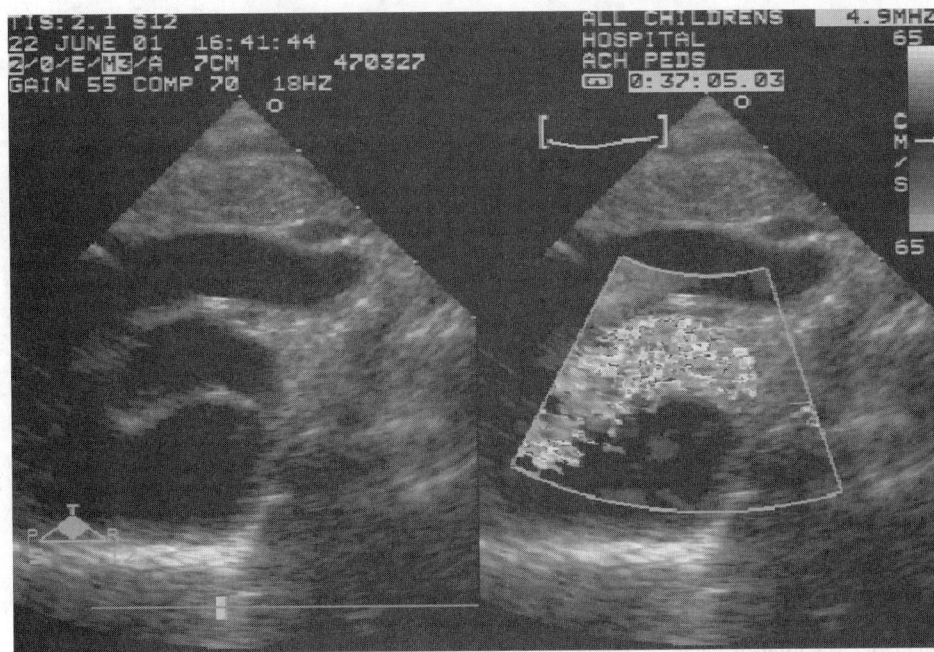

FIGURE 260.3. Transposition of the great arteries (discordant ventriculoarterial connection). Note the parallel exit of the anterior aorta and the posterior pulmonary artery.

blood flow to the left side of the heart through the fossa ovalis. This aneurysmal bowing of the atrial septum after birth may be a clue to right-to-left or left-to-right intraatrial shunting if it is bowing toward the right atrium. Color Doppler studies have confirmed that left-to-right shunting through a patent foramen ovale is a normal finding soon after birth, particularly if the ductus arteriosus has not closed. After the infant reaches 6 weeks of age, persistent shunting at the atrial level is considered abnormal if the color diameter of the shunt is greater than 3 mm.

The results of echocardiographic imaging of atrial septal defects are good. Detailed analysis of the venous connections is needed to exclude partial anomalous pulmonary venous return, for example. In the prospective study of Gutgesell and associates, one false-positive and one false-negative result for diagnosing sinus venosus defects occurred. Since then, the triage of patients with an atrial defect requires detailed measurements of the rims of the defect to determine whether the patient is a candidate for the device closure of the defect in the catheterization laboratory. The popular Amplatzer device straddles the hole and effectively closes it permanently. Another practical application of echocardiography is the evaluation of the atrial defect created by balloon atrial septotomy or blade and balloon techniques.

A thin strand of tissue in what appears to be a common atrium suggests right atrial isomerism. The upper atrial septum, where a sinus venosus defect may occur, can be difficult to evaluate in an older child, but color flow mapping has improved the ability to evaluate all forms of atrial septal defect.

Ventricular Septum. Defects of the ventricular septum can be analyzed using multiple tomographic imaging approaches, and defects can be separated into those that are perimembranous, muscular, or subarterial. An inlet perimembranous defect (i.e., AV canal-type defect) can be differentiated from the AV canal by the presence of the central fibrous body at the internal crux of the heart. Small muscular ventricular septal defects and even a significant defect in the perimembranous region may be missed by imaging alone, but color Doppler has improved substantially the ability to detect muscular defects. With multiple ventricular septal defects, color may be crucial for detection. The sensitivity in older children with smaller muscular ventric-

ular septal defects and another large ventricular septal defect was only 72% in one study. The details of complicated interventricular communications in the trabecular septum may be aided by angiography or a detailed evaluation by TEE. Echocardiography with color Doppler appears to be adequate to evaluate these patients by using the transesophageal approach, especially in older patients. Three-dimensional echocardiography offers the promise of improved spatial orientation and delineation of the defect.

Valves

Atrioventricular Valves. A wide variety of malformations may involve the left or right AV valves. The mitral or tricuspid valve may be abnormally positioned, stenotic, regurgitant, or hypoplastic, or the valve may have a cleft or exhibit prolapse, straddling, or Ebstein malformation. The pattern of opening on real-time imaging is augmented by the Doppler or M-mode functional assessment. Virtually all forms of congenital abnormalities of the mitral valve can be recognized immediately by imaging alone, with the possible exception of supravalvar mitral ring, in which the ring may adhere to the valve tissue. The normal papillary muscles in this disorder differentiate it from most other congenital forms of mitral stenosis. Color flow mapping and continuous-wave Doppler more effectively evaluate the hemodynamics of AV valve stenosis than do invasive techniques. Regurgitation of AV valves can be detected with excellent sensitivity, and color Doppler scans can enable the examiner to grade the severity of regurgitation of the AV and semilunar valves.

Semilunar Valves. Semilunar valves (either pulmonary or aortic valves) are described by their size after adjustment for age, the morphology of the cusps, and the pattern of opening of the valve. Because the size of a valve annulus reflects the flow through it, hypoplasia of the valve annulus usually is associated with severe stenosis, and echocardiographic imaging may detect this condition, the doming of a stenotic valve, or the muscular hypertrophy of infundibular stenosis. The abnormal coaptation of the semilunar valve cusps also correlates with regurgitation of the valve. In assessing congenital heart disease, echocardiography alone detected pulmonary stenosis with a sensitivity of 77% and a specificity of 97%. Sensitivity and specificity approach 100% with the application of color, pulsed, and continuous-wave techniques. Because of the variability of cardiac output through a stenotic valve, the flow-independent method, known as the continuity equation, may be more useful for looking at the ratio of the mean velocity at the valve to below the valve for assessing stenosis and the effective subvalve-to-valvular area ratio. Prosthetic valves may be present in the pediatric population and require a combination of transthoracic and echocardiography and TEE.

Systemic Veins

Systemic Venous Connections. A segmental diagnosis of systemic venous connection can be established by echocardiography before and after birth. Systemic venous return may be typical of the atrial situs (e.g., azygos continuation with left atrial isomerism). Systemic venous return that is abnormal in situs solitus may be normal if the situs is not solitus. Normal inferior and superior vena cavae connecting to the right atrium indicate a normal systemic venous connection to the morphologic right atrium. Identifying the inferior vena cava connecting to the heart and extending into the abdomen is important so that hepatic veins connecting separately are not mistaken for it. Each of the systemic venous segments, including the right superior vena cava, the left superior vena cava, the inferior vena cava, coronary sinus, and hepatic veins, should be examined individually. A prospective assessment of this approach showed a sensitivity of more than 95% for assessing each segment, with the exception of the smaller, bridging innominate veins.

Systemic Venous Anomalies. A persistent left superior vena cava is present in as many as 10% of patients with congenital heart disease and can be detected by echocardiography and confirmed by contrast studies. It is the most common venous defect and is present is 0.5% of patients without congenital cardiac defects. Rarely does this minor defect require attention, except to document its presence in case surgical management is needed for other forms of congenital heart disease. If the persistent left superior vena cava appears to be connected to the left atrium or drain to this site because of unroofing of the coronary sinus, cyanosis results, and an echo-contrast injection in the left arm will show immediate opacification of the left atrium. A sinus venosus atrial septal defect can direct superior vena caval drainage to the left atrium, causing cyanosis of mild degree in an otherwise normal child.

Pulmonary Veins

Each pulmonary vein connecting to the morphologic left atrium must be imaged in a sequential fashion. A four-chamber view often reveals at least two pulmonary veins connecting to the left-sided morphologic left atrium. The suprasternal scan may demonstrate all four pulmonary veins connecting to the left atrium. Total anomalous pulmonary venous connection can be detected with high sensitivity, depending on the experience of the examiner. Although accurate diagnosis of isolated total anomalous pulmonary venous connection can be made in neonates and infants, the ability of any noninvasive tool to exclude an isolated partial anomalous connection of one vein has not been tested. Color Doppler can confirm pulmonary venous flow in the location where the vein is thought to be connecting. Detection of pulmonary venous obstruction and variations depends on Doppler imaging. Direct visualization of all four pulmonary veins is mandatory before corrective surgery is performed for any defect, especially for atrial septal defect or anomalous pulmonary venous connection. Any deviation from the usual anatomy should prompt a complete angiographic study, or a detailed study by magnetic resonance imaging (MRI) in experienced hands can clarify the defect. Severely cyanotic neonates with atrial isomerism usually have abnormalities of

pulmonary venous connection and may require angiography before undergoing palliative surgery.

Coronary Arteries

If intracardiac repair is contemplated, the origin of the coronary vessels must be visualized using a segmental approach. With the exception of aneurysm detection in Kawasaki disease or the abnormal origin of the common left or right coronary artery, ultrasonography is limited in the definition of the abnormalities of the coronary circulation. Use of TEE can significantly improve the ability to diagnose the intramural course of coronary arteries. In the case of fistula, the enlargement of one of the coronary arteries usually can be detected, and pulmonary atresia with a significant fistula can be diagnosed. Anomalous origin of one or both coronary arteries from the pulmonary trunk can be detected with high specificity by using high-frequency two-dimensional color Doppler and a low peak repetition frequency. Any ECG evidence of coronary insufficiency (see later) should prompt performing immediate coronary angiography if surgical intervention is contemplated. Imaging studies of the coronary artery anatomy in tetralogy of Fallot and transposition should be successful with experience. All patients with tetralogy of Fallot should have an assessment made of the coronaries to define the origin of the left anterior descending branch before a right ventriculotomy is performed. In our experience, an isolated coronary fistula can be repaired without bypass, and the entry site can be defined with color Doppler imaging.

Aorta

Segmental analysis of the aorta and congenital abnormalities that affect it includes assessment of the ascending aorta, aortic arch branching, the aortic isthmus, and the descending aorta. Echocardiography is highly accurate (i.e., sensitivity of 95%, specificity of 99%) for diagnosing abnormalities of the aorta in neonates, infants, and children. Each segment of the aorta is in a slightly different tomographic plane, requiring a sequential, segmental approach. Normal branching of the right innominate artery indicates a left aortic arch with normal branching. Branching to the left indicates a right aortic arch with mirror-image branching. A patent ductus arteriosus is the most common abnormality of the aorta. Color and continuous-wave Doppler echocardiography are indicated in every study to detect ductal shunting (Fig. 260.4).

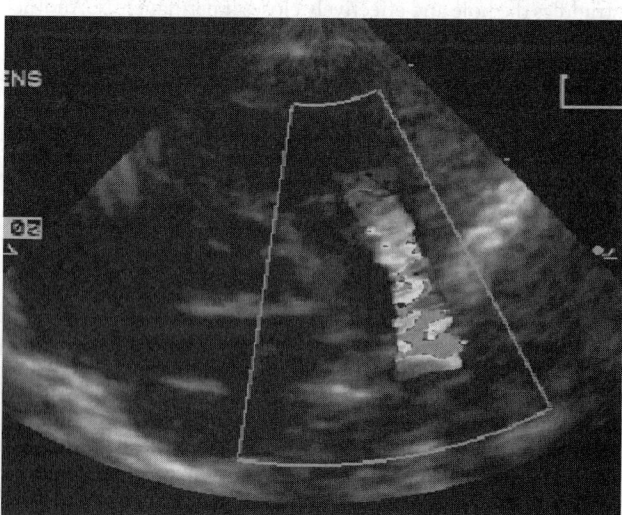

FIGURE 260.4. Patent ductus arteriosus in a neonate. Left-to-right shunt is seen by color Doppler. See Color Figure 260.4 in color section.

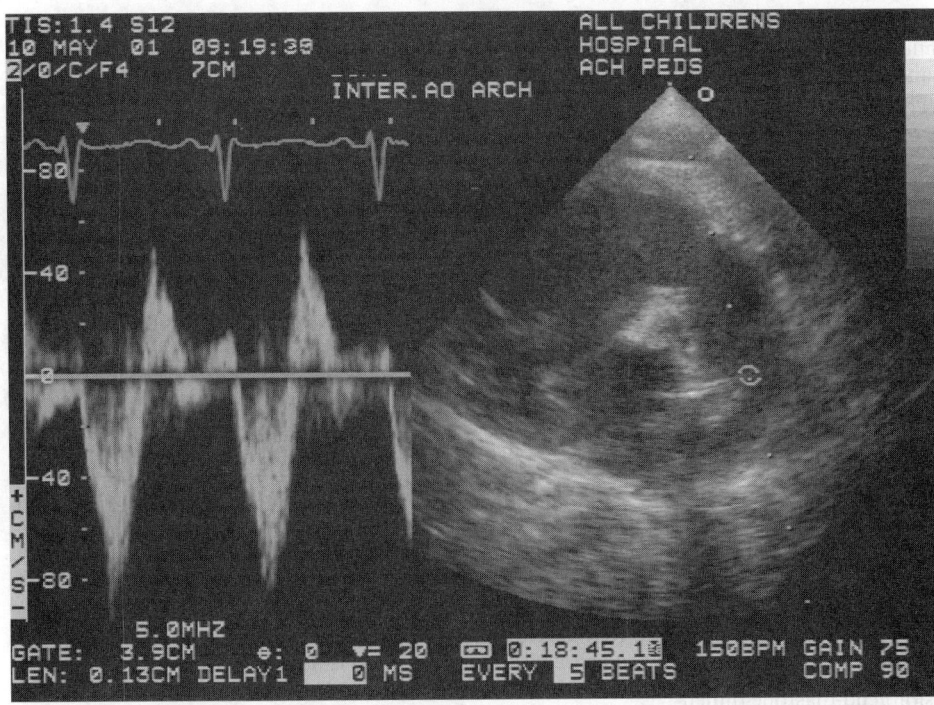

FIGURE 260.5. Bidirectional shunting by pulsed Doppler in the ductus arteriosus of a neonate with interrupted aortic arch and a large patent ductus arteriosus.

Coarctation of the aorta, which has a typical appearance in the neonatal period that includes hypoplasia of the transverse aortic arch and right ventricular enlargement, can be diagnosed by echocardiography. The typical Doppler pattern confirms the diagnosis if the ductus has closed. The presence of a posterior ledge and a transverse arch that is similar in size to the left subclavian artery establishes the diagnosis. With an open ductus, the flow pattern may be mildly turbulent without gradient. In patients with a large ventricular septal defect, the status of the aorta always should be investigated to exclude coarctation. In hypoplastic left heart syndrome with aortic atresia, the patent ductus arteriosus has bidirectional shunting similar to that seen in interrupted aortic arch (Fig. 260.5). In hypoplastic left heart syndrome, the ascending aorta is small, with reversed flow in the arch (Fig. 260.6).

In adults, the segmental analysis of the aorta is less reliable, but Doppler techniques have significantly improved the ability to detect aortic obstruction in cases for which imaging was poor, and the use of TEE can allow detection of the presence and size of internal mammary branches.

Systemic Arteriovenous Fistulas

Systemic arteriovenous fistulas cause enlargement of the artery feeding the fistula and generalized enlargement of the aorta. Sequestration and hepatic and cerebral fistulas are the most common. Sequestration of the lung and other fistulas causing an obligatory shunt can be detected by careful technique. The defect may simulate coarctation of aorta because of the aortic isthmus morphology. Angiography is required for defining the small vessel anatomy preoperatively.

Pulmonary Arteries

The most common abnormality of the pulmonary arteries that indicates congenital heart disease is hypoplasia. The pulmonary arteries normally are confluent in the midline, and this detail of anatomy has importance in planning a palliative approach to cyanotic congenital heart disease. Abnormalities of the origin or size of the pulmonary arteries may occur. In severe right ventricular outflow tract obstruction in neonates, pulmonary artery hypoplasia is associated with a reciprocal increase in the size of the aorta, and the ratio of size of the pulmonary arteries to the aorta may be useful in establishing the diagnosis of this abnormality and in making surgical decisions when the ability of the pulmonary vascular bed to carry the total combined cardiac output is in question. Assessment of the details of the distal arteries requires angiography or MRI. A patient with pulmonary arteriovenous fistula presents with cyanosis and enlargement of the pulmonary arteries and veins on echocardiography, and the diagnosis should be confirmed by angiography and pulmonary venous oxygen saturation measurements.

Tetralogy with pulmonary atresia with major aortopulmonary artery collaterals may be difficult to evaluate. The neonate with this condition can be differentiated from one with ductal-dependent pulmonary supply by the oxygen saturation

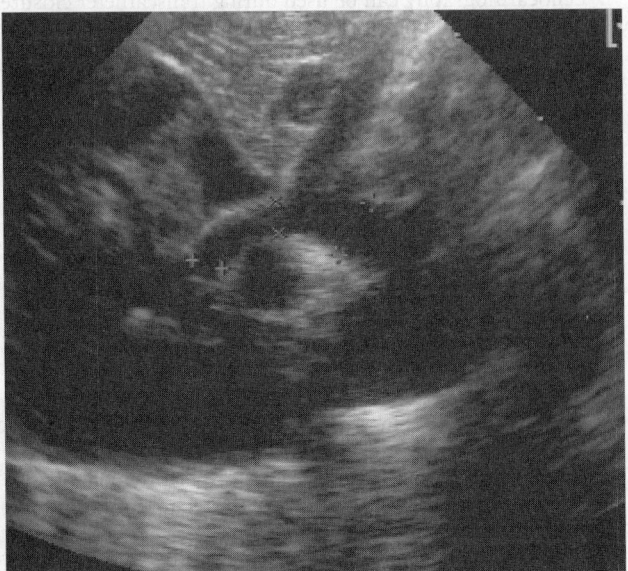

FIGURE 260.6. Small ascending aorta in a neonate with aortic atresia (hypoplastic left heart syndrome).

when the child is not receiving prostaglandin and by imaging the ductus and poorly developed confluent pulmonary arteries. All patients with collateral arteries and multifocal pulmonary supply must have complete angiographic evaluation before undergoing surgery.

Ventricular Function Assessment

The temporal resolution of two-dimensional echocardiography is limited by the scanning rate limits of the equipment. M-mode techniques, conversely, interrogate the heart at a much higher rate (800 to 1,500 times/second) and allow tracking of the ventricular wall and valves at rapid rates of movement. The most useful application of M-mode echocardiography is the measurement of absolute cardiac chamber dimensions and wall thicknesses and their dynamic changes. Normal values for the systolic and diastolic dimensions of the left atrium and ventricle increase with increasing age and body size, and comparisons of right and left heart measurements with normal ranges should be part of every echocardiogram. M-mode parameters from the left ventricle can be used to estimate the wall stress of the left ventricle and its dynamic changes, as well as the rate of relaxation. Systolic function can be estimated using the concept of shortening fraction, as follows: shortening fraction = (end-diastolic dimension—systolic dimension)/end-diastolic dimension. In the case of normovolemia, the dimensional shortening of the left ventricular endocardial cavity correlates well with the stroke volume.

Diastolic function can be assessed using tissue Doppler techniques and may be useful in establishing the diagnosis of cardiac transplant rejection. Tissue Doppler refers to the new technique that examines the low-velocity, high-intensity signal from the valve annuli, and the cardiac walls are examined to assess contraction and relaxation of the myocardium.

New advances in the calculation of segmental wall strain are being studied. An easily obtained parameter that is nongeometric and useful for assessment of right and left ventricular performance is the myocardial performance index. This so-called myocardial performance index is the ratio of the isovolumic times to the ejection time of the ventricle. This nongeometric index is useful for detecting abnormalities of systolic or diastolic function when the ventricular shape is altered, such as in the morphologic right ventricle.

Those patients with valvular regurgitation allow measurement of the first derivative of the pressure change in the ventricle by taking the slope of the pressure change curve on the continuous-wave Doppler waveform. Practically, it can be calculated by measuring the time in seconds from the waveform at the 1- and 3-m/second points and dividing it into 32, which gives the dP/dt in millimeters of mercury/second.

Contrast Echocardiography

An ultrasonic contrast agent is a substance that stabilizes microbubbles in solution, which are large enough to reflect ultrasound but small enough that they disappear rapidly and are physiologically safe. The agent may be as simple as an injection of saline into the circulation during two-dimensional echocardiographic imaging or as complex as precision-engineered microbubbles of polysaccharide that dissolve in the circulation after injection. New advances in bubble technology allow the myocardial capillary perfusion to be imaged. Contrast also can be useful in defining the identity of a structure that is imaged. For example, a structure under the aortic arch may be confusing but can be confirmed to be the innominate vein by an echocardiographic contrast injection in a left arm vein. In congenital

heart disease, the major application of contrast echocardiography is for evaluating the postoperative patient with residual shunts or for excluding congenital heart disease. Systemic venous injection of contrast fills the right side of the heart sequentially, and the site of residual right-to-left shunting can be defined. In the neonatal intensive care unit, contrast injections using agitated saline can detect right-to-left interatrial shunting in cases of persistent pulmonary hypertension.

A catheter can be advanced retrograde into the left ventricle after closure of a ventricular septal defect, and a contrast injection can enable to examiner to diagnose the presence and severity of residual left-to-right shunts. Newer agents will cause opacification of the left-sided heart circulation after injection.

Transesophageal Echocardiography

The indications for TEE in congenital heart disease are expanding as a result of the excellent aid that this technique gives to intracardiac imaging. TEE is a technique that pediatric cardiologists cannot be without in a surgical practice. As with any new technique, it has a learning curve, but the methods are now well developed and useful. Use of training guidelines and frequent continuing education is desirable. Biplane probes are of a size now that even in neonates weighing only 2.5 to 5 kg, a biplane probe can be passed safely in the operating room with the patient under general anesthesia, with minimal hemodynamic compromise. Multiplane probes for pediatrics are progressing slowly, and current technology allows use of such a probe in infants weighing as little as 5 kg or more.

The reproducibility of quantitative measurements with TEE is good, in the range of 5% for multiple examiners. Added value comes from TEE in pediatric practice. This value has been demonstrated in the lesions of left ventricular outflow obstruction and in AV and semilunar valve assessment. Assessment of mitral regurgitation is important after repair or rerepair of an AV canal defect. TEE can identify the type and severity of mitral regurgitation and is superior to transthoracic echocardiography or cineangiography.

Complications with TEE are more common in smaller patients. Failure to pass the probe occurs in about 0.8% of children with congenital heart disease, and airway obstruction occurs in approximately 1%.

Echocardiography can be used during transcatheter closure for precise positioning of a device or coil. During ductal closure, the TEE is useful as well. Intraoperatively, ductal patency can be monitored during minimally invasive procedures. For example, in neonates with critical aortic stenosis, the positioning of the balloon can be monitored using TEE. Guidance of radiofrequency ablation catheters can be facilitated with TEE, particularly when single ventricle anatomy is present.

Cardiac output can be estimated using TEE by measuring the minute distance (time-velocity integral) in the descending aorta. The assessment of ventricular function using Doppler techniques and calculating the first derivative of the pressure change in the left ventricle (dP/dt) has been shown to be useful for predicting which patients are in need of inotropic support.

Use of TEE in the intensive care unit both preoperatively and postoperatively is increasing. Critically ill infants and children and those on assisted circulatory devices can be evaluated optimally this way. The average time for performance of TEE includes approximately 42 minutes of the technician's time and 32 minutes of the physician's time.

Adults with congenital heart disease can be analyzed optimally with TEE. Reviews of the use of TEE in pediatrics have confirmed that increased utilization of this technique will occur in the future.

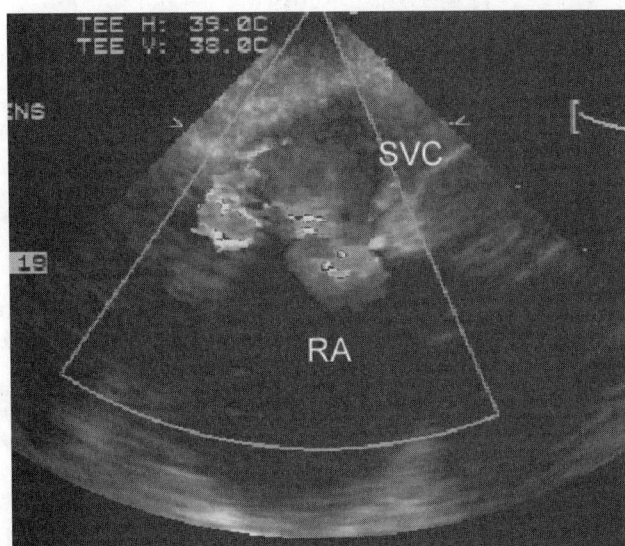

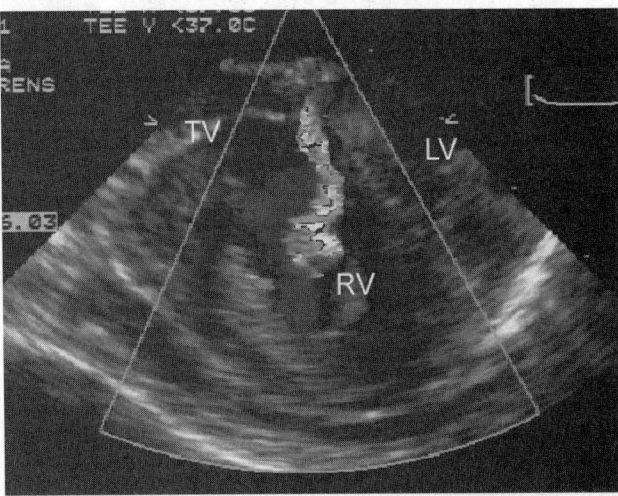

FIGURE 260.8. Color Doppler of shunt transesophageal echocardiography from the left ventricle (LV) to the right ventricle (RV) through a ventricular septal defect (VSD). The VSD is perimembranous because of its proximity to the tricuspid valve (TV).

Complex Heart Defects. Complex congenital heart defects require a segmental approach exactly as with transthoracic imaging. For example, with a single AV valve, the situs, AV connection, and ventriculoarterial connection must be defined. With hypoplastic left heart syndrome, the function of the tricuspid valve is important. Assessment of the atrial septum should be performed at each preoperative examination because of the possibility of late constriction. The details of AV canal defect can be defined, and the commitment of the valves and the valvular function can be seen (Fig. 260.9).

Left Heart Lesions. Left ventricular outflow obstruction can be defined with great accuracy by TEE. Details of the aortic valve, subvalvar region, and mitral valve can be seen easily. Three-dimensional imaging is slow to perform but may add significantly to the armamentarium in the future. The presence of subaortic stenosis can be defined. The structure and the function of the aortic valve are defined precisely with TEE. No other imaging tool is as good at examining the fine structure of the cusps and the presence of regurgitation. After the Ross procedure, whereby the pulmonary valve has been transplanted into

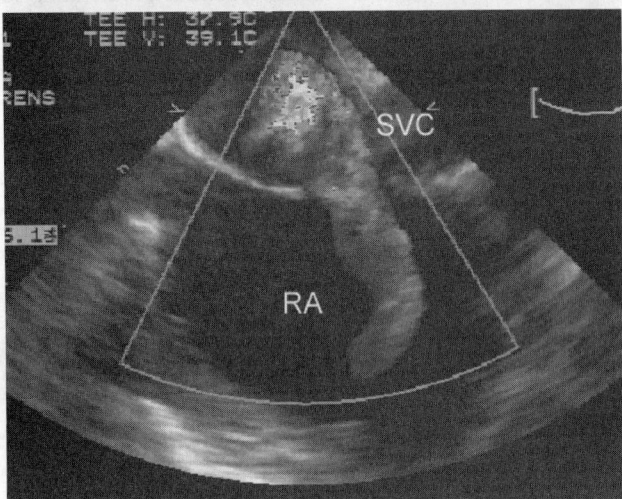

FIGURE 260.7. Sinus venosus atrial septal defect in a sagittal scan by transesophageal echocardiography with left-to-right shunting shown by color Doppler. RA, right atrium; SVC, superior vena cava. See Color Figure 260.7 in color section.

Specific Lesions

Shunts. Shunting lesions are seen well from the multiple-view possibilities that TEE offers. Atrial level shunts, for example, are defined most accurately with TEE. In older patients, TEE is mandatory for establishing accurate diagnoses. Defects at fossa ovalis can be quantitated by size and shunt. The higher sinus venosus defect can be seen readily, and the associated anomalies of pulmonary venous drainage can be detailed (Fig. 260.7).

Ventricular septal defects can be analyzed without difficulty, and multiple holes can be distinguished. The most common defect is the perimembranous ventricular septal defect and often is associated with partial closure by tricuspid valve tissue. The larger defects in this position may extend into either the inlet or outlet septum. Defining both size and position is possible after significant experience is gained (Fig. 260.8) and shunt is defined by color Doppler imaging.

Shunting through the patent ductus arteriosus can be seen with high positions of the probe. After the descending aorta in sagittal planes is found, the area of the main pulmonary artery and that of the left pulmonary artery are identified. Use of color Doppler may be necessary because the imaging is marginal.

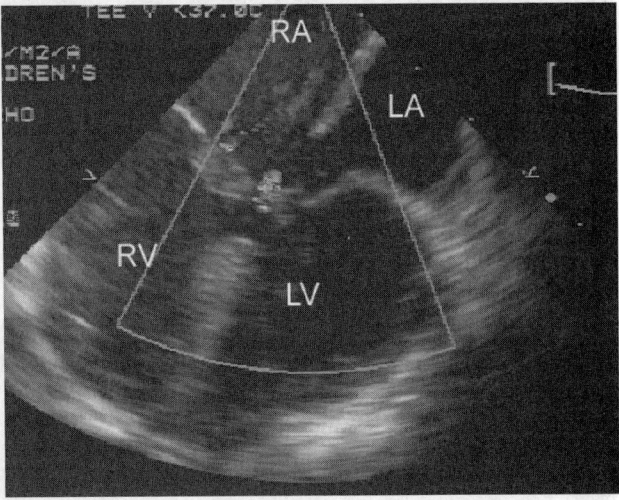

FIGURE 260.9. Complete atrioventricular (AV) canal with a trace of valvular regurgitation directed from the left ventricle (LV) to the right atrium (RA).

the left ventricular outflow tract, neoaortic valve function can be evaluated without difficulty.

Right Heart Lesions. In general, the right ventricular outflow tract is more difficult to evaluate with TEE because it is farther away from the transducer. Nonetheless, the details of tetralogy of Fallot can be seen and communicated to the surgeon in the operating room. The presence of complicating lesions also can be defined. Assessment of tetralogy of Fallot before and after surgery can be accomplished accurately. The right ventricul-to-pulmonary artery gradient can be assessed using continuous-wave Doppler. The best angle may be from the subgastric views with probe flexion or from the high probe position aiming back at the right ventricular outflow tract.

The tricuspid valve can be seen well, and the details of its leaflets, chordal attachments, and function can be assessed. This ability is particularly important in infants with pulmonary atresia with intact septum and hypoplasia of the valve. More than absolute measurements, the diastolic and systolic function and the structure of the valve best predict the potential for growth.

Regurgitation of the mitral valve can be diagnosed, but the current approach to the assessment of this valve demands making conclusions about the mechanism of the regurgitation. A posteriorly directed jet is consistent with mitral valve prolapse. Doppler imaging can be used to assess the hemodynamics, including the rate of change of the velocity to calculate the dP/dt. More complex types of abnormality may be associated with anomalies of the left ventricular outflow tract (Fig. 260.10). Use of TEE in the infant and child with congenital heart disease can enhance significantly the quality of care. When the patient is under general anesthesia, either immediately preoperatively or in preparation for surgery, the information gained by TEE often will change the management plan. Further advances in three-dimensional imaging and probe technology promise to extend this valuable technique to many more patients.

Safety of Ultrasound

Significant adverse effects from the use of ultrasound for imaging, M-mode, or Doppler evaluation have not been reported. The potentially negative bioeffects of ultrasound can be classified as those caused by cavitation and those caused by heating. Cavitation refers to the development of tiny, gas-filled bubbles that resonate at the ultrasonic frequency and induce neighboring particles of liquid to vibrate, potentially damaging the ultrasound-transmitting medium. Practically, the intensities for echocardiography (typically 10 W/cm^2) are almost an order of magnitude less than those known to produce cavitation. Thermal effects may result from heat generated in the tissue. To reach the thermal threshold for damage using modern ultrasonic intensities, an average intensity of 1,000 W/cm^2 must be applied for many hours.

Diagnostic ultrasound used at the pulse intensity levels used in diagnostics does not constitute a risk or hazard to the patient. Higher intensities with pulsed Doppler have the potential to cause cavitation, and concerns about the use of Doppler for first-trimester fetal assessment are being investigated.

Costs and Benefits

One of the major reasons that ultrasound is proliferating so rapidly in pediatrics is that it is noninvasive and painless in most examinations. Ultrasound equipment is less expensive than is radiographic equipment, and the indications for cardiac catheterization are being reassessed. The development of echocardiography as an extension of the clinician's other assessment skills has decreased the use of catheterization, especially in neonatal patients. If catheterization can be avoided completely, echocardiography has the potential to decrease the cost of medical care for these patients.

For the most effective cardiovascular application of ultrasound, the physician should be involved in the study and its interpretation. A more physician-intensive diagnostic process may benefit the patient, but it may become more expensive than comparable tests that can be performed by technicians.

ELECTROCARDIOGRAPHY

The ECG (previously EKG) continues to be a basic tool in the clinical assessment of the neonate and child with congenital cardiac malformations. Standard 12-lead tracing can give information concerning the rhythm, the cardiac chamber sizes

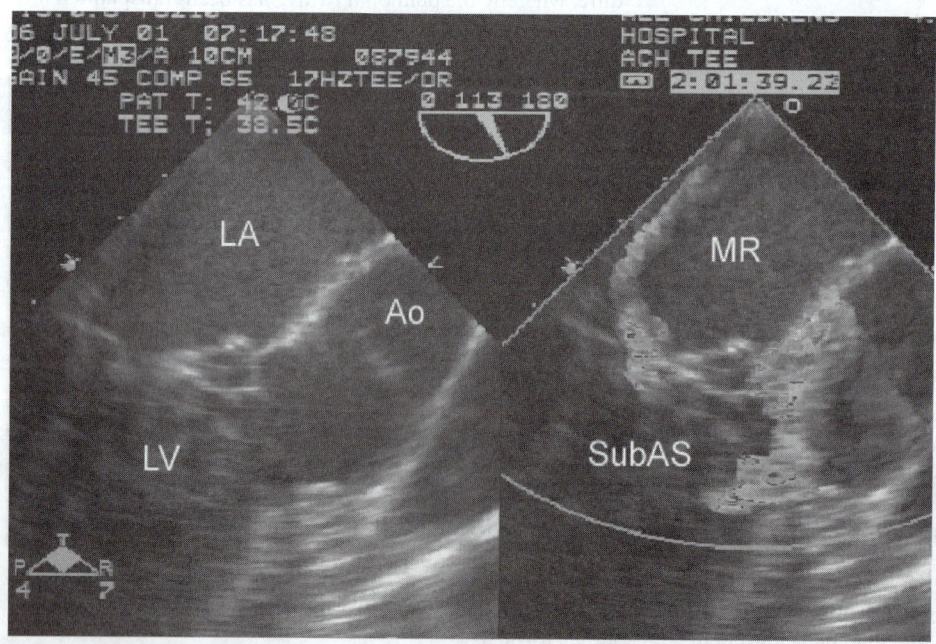

FIGURE 260.10. Complex left ventricular (LV) outflow defect with mitral regurgitation (MR) and subaortic stenosis (SubAS). Ao, ascending aorta; LA, left atrium.

BOX 260.4 Neonatal ECG Interpretation

Lead V_1 reflects right ventricular pressure, and the T wave normally will be upright for 48 hours after birth and then invert. Persistent upright T wave in lead V_1 is a good sign of right ventricular hypertrophy (actually persistent elevation of right ventricular pressure). A qR pattern in V_1 always is indicative of congenital heart disease, usually complex.

Lead aVL reflects the pattern of QRS activation of the ventricles. The normal pattern at any age is a rS wave that reflects the normal clockwise pattern of depolarization in the frontal plane. A qR pattern reflects a counterclockwise depolarization pattern and left axis deviation. A qR pattern in the neonate always is present with two types of congenital heart disease: atrioventricular canal defect and tricuspid atresia.

Sinus bradycardia with a prolonged QT interval (corrected QT interval of greater than 0.5 seconds) is abnormal and requires evaluation for electrolyte abnormalities and inherited prolonged QT syndrome.

---

and masses, the electrical relaxation properties of the heart, and the electrical properties of abnormal pathways in the heart. The screening of the neonate with possible heart disease can be summarized for the beginner in a few simple rules of thumb (Box 260.4).

Rhythm Abnormalities

Simple ladder diagrams can be constructed to aid in establishing the diagnosis of the rhythms abnormalities that occur in childhood. Normal rhythm is a P wave from the atrial contraction followed within 0.16 seconds by the QRS complex that represents the electrical activation of the His bundle and the left and right bundle branch and the myocardium. The sinus node is located in the high right atrium and initiates the atrial activation. This wave travels to the AV node that slows conduction and then activates the bundle of His and the ventricles.

Heart Block

Failure of conduction from the upper to the lower chambers is known as heart block and can be mild with prolongation of the PR interval (first-degree AV block), can involve failure of each atrial contraction to conduct through the AV node (second-degree block), or can involve failure of any AV conduction (third-degree block or complete heart block). Common natural causes of complete heart block in pediatrics are AV discordance and left atrial isomerism.

Tachycardia

Rapid repetitive beating of the atria or ventricles is known as tachycardia. Ventricular tachycardia is a rare occurrence in pediatrics and usually is an unstable rhythm needing cardioversion. Atrial tachycardia is rapid beating of the upper chambers and may manifest as atrial flutter, reentrant atrial tachycardia (e.g., Wolf-Parkinson-White syndrome), or automatic tachycardia. Wolf-Parkinson-White syndrome can be cured with ab-

lation therapy in the catheterization laboratory and is the first type of treatment of this type of supraventricular tachycardia in children older than 2 years of age.

ST Changes

Elevation of the ST portion of the ECG is indicative of ischemia when it is in the typical distribution of a coronary artery abnormality. However, in pediatrics, the more common cause of ST elevation is pericarditis or pericardial effusion.

Electrolyte Abnormalities

ST-segment and T-wave abnormalities are common findings in the presence of abnormalities of the serum electrolytes. The QT interval, for example, can be prolonged in the presence of hypocalcemia at any age. Hypokalemia shows ST-segment abnormalities in all leads.

Hypertrophy

Thickening of a cardiac chamber or increased voltage from an increased flow through the chamber will lead to increased voltages on the ECG. The most common type of left ventricular hypertrophy is that resulting from hypertension, aortic stenosis, or cardiomyopathy and causing the sum of the R wave in lead V_6 and the S wave in lead V_1 to total more than 45 mm.

TRENDS

Technology has been changing so rapidly that predicting which technique will be optimal in 5 years for evaluation of a given lesion is difficult. The rapid development of nuclear MRI and spectroscopy is beginning to show potential for the field. Rapid computed tomography has the potential to create high-quality three-dimensional images in pediatric patients. Positron emission tomography can be used to assess myocardial perfusion and rarely is used in pediatrics at this time. The emerging areas in echocardiography include the following: the development of contrast agents, some of which allow myocardial blood flow assessment by ultrasonography; tissue characterization techniques; automated cardiac function assessment; three-dimensional real-time imaging and color Doppler display; invasive imaging probes for intracardiac imaging; TEE in neonates for intraoperative functional assessment; and three-dimensional reconstruction of cardiac images from ultrasound data. One thing is certain: continued reevaluation of the roles of the various diagnostic modalities used in assessing congenital heart disease will be needed.

Suggested Readings

Andropoulos DB, et al. The effects of transesophageal echocardiography on hemodynamic variables in small infants undergoing cardiac surgery. *J Cardiothorac Vasc Anesth* 2000;14:133.

Aronson S. Adherence to physician training guidelines for pediatric transesophageal echocardiography affects the outcome of patients undergoing repair of congenital cardiac defects. *J Am Soc Echocardiogr* 1999;12:1008.

Daubeney PE, et al. Relationship of the dimension of cardiac structures to body size: an echocardiographic study in normal infants and children. *Cardiol Young* 1999;9:402.

Drant SE, et al. Guidance of radiofrequency catheter ablation by transesophageal echocardiography in children with palliated single ventricle. *Am J Cardiol* 1995;76:1311.

Frommelt PC, et al. Prospective echocardiographic diagnosis and surgical repair of anomalous origin of a coronary artery from the opposite sinus with an interarterial course. *J Am Coll Cardiol* 2003;42:148.

Frommelt PC, Whitstone EN, Frommelt MA. Experience with a DICOM-compatible digital pediatric echocardiography laboratory. *Pediatr Cardiol* 2002;23:53.

Frommelt MA, Frommelt PC. Advances in echocardiographic diagnostic modalities for the pediatrician. *Pediatr Clin North Am* 1999;46:427.

Goldberg SJ, et al. The time required to perform pediatric transthoracic echocardiographic studies. *J Am Soc Echocardiogr* 1995;8:739.

Gutgesell HP, Huhta JC, Latson LA, Huffines D. Accuracy of 2-dimensional echocardiography in the diagnosis of congenital heart disease. *Am J Cardiol* 1985;55:514.

Hijazi Z, et al. Transcatheter closure of atrial septal defects and patent foramen ovale under intracardiac echocardiographic guidance: feasibility and comparison with transesophageal echocardiography. *Cathet Cardiovasc Interv* 2001;52:194.

Ho AC, et al. The use of multiplane transesophageal echocardiography to evaluate residual patent ductus arteriosus during video-assisted thoracoscopy in adults. *Surg Endosc* 1999;13:975.

Huhta JC, Gutgesell HP, Nihill MR. Two-dimensional echocardiographic diagnosis of total anomalous pulmonary venous connection. *Br Heart J* 1985; 53:525.

Huhta JC, Smallhorn JF, MaCartney FJ. Two dimensional echocardiographic diagnosis of situs. *Br Heart J* 1982;48:97.

Huhta JC, Smallhorn JF, MaCartney FJ, Anderson RH. Cross-sectional echocardiographic diagnosis of systemic venous return. *Br Heart J* 1982;48:388.

Humpl T, McCrindle BW, Smallhorn JF. The relative roles of transthoracic compared with transesophageal echocardiography in children with suspected infective endocarditis. *J Am Coll Cardiol* 2003;41:2068.

Joyce JJ, et al. Reliability of intraoperative transesophageal echocardiography during tetralogy of Fallot repair. *Echocardiography* 2000;17:319.

Kavanaugh-McHugh A, et al. Transesophageal echocardiography in pediatric congenital heart disease. *Cardiol Rev* 2000;8:288.

Kececioglu D, et al. Morphologic characterization and assessment of mitral regurgitation after repair of atrioventricular defects in children. *Thorac Cardiovasc Surg* 1997;45:70.

Kececioglu D, et al. Reproducibility of quantitative pediatric transesophageal echocardiography. *J Am Soc Echocardiogr* 1995;8:735.

Lam J, et al. The use of transesophageal echocardiography monitoring of transcatheter closure of a persistent ductus arteriosus. *Echocardiography* 2001;18:197.

Matitiau A, et al. Transcatheter closure of secundum atrial septal defects with the Amplatzer septal occluder: early experience. *Isr Med Assoc J* 2001;3:32.

Miller-Hance WC, Silverman NH. Transesophageal echocardiography (TEE) in congenital heart disease with focus on the adult. *Cardiol Clin* 2000;18:861.

Marianeschi SM, McElhinney DB, Reddy VM. Pulmonary arteriovenous malformations in and out of the setting of congenital heart disease. *Ann Thorac Surg* 1998;66:688.

Marx GR, Sherwood MC. Three-dimensional echocardiography in congenital heart disease: a continuum of unfulfilled promises? No. A presently clinically applicable technology with an important future? Yes. *Pediatr Cardiol* 2002; 23:266.

Miller-Hance WC, Silverman NH. Transesophageal echocardiography (TEE) in congenital heart disease with focus on the adult. *Cardiol Clin* 2000;18: 861.

Mizelle KM, Rice MJ, Sahn DJ. Clinical use of real-time three-dimensional echocardiography in pediatric cardiology. *Echocardiography* 2000;17:787.

O'Leary PW. Intracardiac echocardiography in congenital heart disease: are we ready to begin the fantastic voyage? *Pediatr Cardiol* 2002;23:286.

Phoon CK, Divekar A, Rutkowski M. Pediatric echocardiography: applications and limitations. *Curr Probl Pediatr* 1999;29:157.

Pignatelli RH, et al. Role of echocardiography versus MRI for the diagnosis of congenital heart disease. *Curr Opin Cardiol* 2003;18:357.

Rhodes J, et al. Evaluation of ventricular dP/dt before and after open heart surgery using transesophageal echocardiography. *Echocardiography* 1997;14:15.

Rice MJ, et al. Pediatric echocardiography: current role and a review of technical advances. *J Pediatr* 1996;128:1.

Rubay JE, et al. The Ross operation: mid-term results. *Ann Thorac Surg* 1999;67:1355.

Sahn DJ, Vick GW 3rd. Review of new techniques in echocardiography and magnetic resonance imaging as applied to patients with congenital heart disease. *Heart* 2001;86(suppl 2):II41.

Silverman MH. An ultrasonic approach to the diagnosis of cardiac situs, connections, and malpositions. In: Friedman WF, Higgins CB, eds. *Pediatric cardiac imaging*. Philadelphia: WB Saunders, 1984.

Simpson IA, et al. Current status of flow convergence for clinical applications: is it a leaning tower of "PISA"? *J Am Coll Cardiol* 1996;27:504.

Singh GK, et al. Diagnostic accuracy and role of intraoperative biplane transesophageal echocardiography in pediatric patients with left ventricle outflow tract lesions. *J Am Soc Echocardiogr* 1998;11:47.

Sloth E, et al. Pediatric multiplane transesophageal echocardiography in congenital heart disease: new possibilities with a miniaturized probe. *J Am Soc Echocardiogr* 1996;9:622.

Smallhorn JF. Intraoperative transesophageal echocardiography in congenital heart disease. *Echocardiography* 2002;19:709.

Stanger P, Silverman NH, Foster E. Diagnostic accuracy of pediatric echocardiograms performed in adult laboratories. *Am J Cardiol* 1999;83:908.

Stevenson JG. Incidence of complications in pediatric transesophageal echocardiography: experience in 1650 cases. *J Am Soc Echocardiogr* 1999;12:527.

Tibby SM, Hatherill M, Murdoch IA. Use of transesophageal Doppler ultrasonography in ventilated pediatric patients: derivation of cardiac output. *Crit Care Med* 2000;28:2045.

Tworetzky W, et al. Echocardiographic diagnosis alone for the complete repair of major congenital heart defects. *J Am Coll Cardiol* 1999;33:228.

Van Der Velde ME, Perry SB. Transesophageal echocardiography during interventional catheterization in congenital heart disease. *Echocardiography* 1997;14:513.

Van Praagh R. The segmental approach to diagnosis in congenital heart disease. In: Bergsma D, ed. *Birth defects*. Baltimore: Williams & Wilkins, 1972.

Weber HS, Mart CR, Myers JL. Transcarotid balloon valvuloplasty for critical aortic valve stenosis at the bedside via continuous transesophageal echocardiographic guidance. *Cathet Cardiovasc Interv* 2000;50:326.

Wolfe LT, Rossi A, Ritter SB. Transesophageal echocardiography in infants and children: use and importance in the cardiac intensive care unit. *J Am Soc Echocardiogr* 1993;6:286.

CHAPTER 261 ■ HYPERTENSION

J. TIMOTHY BRICKER

PATHOGENESIS

Artifacts in Blood Pressure Measurement

Physicians who care for children monitored by indwelling arterial lines must understand how to zero out, calibrate, and prevent artifacts in the system. An artifact from an underdamped indwelling arterial line is a common source of apparent hypertension in the critically ill child. Inaccurate calibration or inappropriate zeroing of a manometer may result in artifactual hypertension. An overdamped system, a partially occluded arterial line, or an arterial spasm may cause a low measured arterial blood pressure, with the diagnosis of an acute increase in blood pressure when the arterial line is discontinued and cuff measurements are begun. Periodic cuff pressures should be recorded for the patient being monitored with an indwelling arterial line.

Oscillometric methods of pressure measurement have been shown to correlate well with other methods, including indwelling arterial lines, and have come into general use on many pediatric inpatient units. The patient's motion can cause artifactual hypertension when the motion artifact is confused with pulse-wave oscillation by the pressure measurement device. Another common cause of artifactual hypertension is a cuff that is too small for the patient. The width of the cuff bladder should be approximately 40% to 50% of the circumference of the child's upper arm at its midpoint. This principle applies to both oscillometric and auscultatory methods of determining blood pressure.

The missed auscultatory gap is another type of artifact with auscultatory measurement of the systemic arterial pressure. The auscultatory gap is a silent pressure interval between the onset of Korotkoff sounds and their final disappearance or muffling. Failure to inflate the cuff to a sufficient pressure (i.e., 20 mm Hg above the point at which Korotkoff sounds are heard on the first measurement, confirmed by the disappearance of the radial pulse) or failure to listen for Korotkoff sounds all the way down to zero can result in the appearance of a sudden increase or decrease in blood pressure when it is measured accurately.

CLINICAL MANIFESTATIONS AND COMPLICATIONS

Effects of Systemic Arterial Blood Pressure Elevation

Systemic arterial hypertension can be an acute pediatric emergency because of the effect of a severely elevated pressure on vital organ systems. The most prominent effects of severe, acute hypertension involve the neurologic and the cardiovascular systems.

Neurologic Complications

Neurologic abnormalities caused by hypertension can include lethargy, headache, confusion, stupor, focal motor deficits, vision loss, seizures, and coma. In a retrospective study of hypertension with neurologic complications, convulsions were the initial feature in 42% of the children. Two of the patients had altered consciousness alone, and two had cranial nerve findings. Nausea and vomiting may be present in the early stages.

Physical findings often include advanced hypertensive retinopathy with papilledema, retinal hemorrhages, and retinal exudates, as well as abnormalities on neurologic examination.

Evidence of cerebral edema is likely to be seen on computed tomographic (CT) scanning. If features such as a stiff neck and fever mandate a lumbar puncture, both the cerebrospinal fluid (CSF) pressure and protein content probably will be elevated. Most cases of hypertensive encephalopathy can be managed without a lumbar puncture, and the risk of undergoing a lumbar puncture in the presence of an elevation in intracranial pressure (ICP) is increased.

The treatment of the hypertension typically results in rapid improvement in the neurologic signs and symptoms, although some findings may require several days to resolve. Pathologic features include swelling of the brain, hemorrhages (punctate to massive), and microinfarctions. In some cases, swelling of the brain may be sufficient for herniation to be apparent.

The specific diagnosis of hypertensive encephalopathy (Box 261.1) is important to pursue because treatment for hypertensive encephalopathy (i.e., abruptly lowering the blood pressure to normal) can be detrimental in some patients with chronic hypertension. For example, the patient with severe renal artery stenosis may have diminished flow distal to the obstruction, which may result in renal ischemia if the arterial pressure is lowered abruptly by a systemic arteriolar dilator.

The diagnosis of hypertensive encephalopathy should be viewed with some skepticism in the setting of hypertension that is chronic and not extremely severe, and if a plausible alternative explanation of the encephalopathy exists. Lowering the systemic arterial blood pressure in many of the chronically

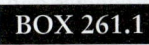

BOX 261.1 | Conditions that May Be Confused with Hypertensive Encephalopathy*

Illicit or therapeutic drugs
Uremic encephalopathy
Encephalitis or meningoencephalitis
Hypoglycemia
Hypocalcemia
Trauma
Low cerebral blood flow
Hepatic causes
Reye syndrome
Diabetic ketoacidosis
Seizure disorder
Hyperthyroidism or hypothyroidism
Psychosis
Cerebritis

---

*Hypertensive encephalopathy is defined as a hypertensive state with alternative (superimposed) explanation of encephalopathic features.

hypertensive patients admitted to the intensive care unit (ICU) may be necessary, but it is not safe to do so as abruptly as one would with those acutely hypertensive patients who usually are normotensive.

Children who recover from hypertensive encephalopathy can be expected to do well. In a 10-year study of 45 children with neurologic complications of hypertension, no neurologic or cognitive sequelae were noted on long-term follow-up.

Another neurologic problem associated with severe hypertension is the development of intracranial hemorrhage. Massive hemorrhage caused by hypertension may occur in a child with a berry aneurysm of the circle of Willis or who recently has undergone a neurosurgical procedure. Systemic hypertension in profoundly premature infants is thought to put them at risk for having subependymal bleeding from the germinal matrix.

Cardiopulmonary Complications

Acute and severe hypertension can be associated with cardiac dilation, elevation of the left ventricular end-diastolic pressure, and symptomatic pulmonary edema. The normal myocardium handles the acute increase in left ventricular afterload relatively well. Children with acute glomerulonephritis typically do not have findings of a low cardiac output state as a result of increased afterload, and typically symptomatic pulmonary edema resolves rapidly without residual cardiac abnormality when the excessive intravascular blood volume associated with acute glomerulonephritis is lowered through diuretic therapy.

Some children have a limited cardiac reserve because of severe prematurity, congenital cardiac disease, or acquired cardiac disease. Under these circumstances, a hypertensive crisis may result in cardiovascular decompensation. An abrupt lowering of the systemic arterial pressure is required in this setting. Cardiovascular decompensation with hypertensive crisis occurs more commonly in adults than in children because of the prevalence of overt or subclinical coronary artery atherosclerotic disease among adults with hypertension. Most children with hypertension have a hyperdynamic apex impulse, a dilated heart with an apex impulse displaced laterally, and a diastolic filling sound during a hypertensive crisis. Chronic hypertension is a risk factor for the development of atherosclerosis later in

Hypertensive Emergencies and Urgencies in the Pediatric Intensive Care Patient

Hypertensive Emergencies
Hypertension causing neurologic symptoms
Hypertension causing congestive heart failure
Hypertension associated with aortic dissection

Hypertensive Urgencies
Hypertension in the postoperative cardiac patient
Hypertension in the postoperative neurosurgery patient
Hypertension after renal transplantation
Hypertension in the profoundly premature infant
Hypertension in the child who must be taken to the operating room for a surgical emergency
Extreme asymptomatic hypertension
Severe hypertension in the patient with risk of bleeding (e.g., after renal biopsy)

life. Chronic hypertension may be associated with left ventricular hypertrophy and arterial abnormalities. Acute aortic dissection has occurred in severely hypertensive children who did not have features of Marfan syndrome or other abnormalities of connective tissue. The degree of left ventricular hypertrophy ascertained by electrocardiography and echocardiography can give a clue to the chronicity of hypertension. Left ventricular mass, as measured by echocardiography, is associated with long-term cardiovascular risk.

Complications in Other Organ Systems

Renal abnormalities may develop or progress in the child with extremes of hypertension. Ophthalmic abnormalities may be related to severe hypertensive retinopathy. Non-neurologic manifestations of the effects of severe, acute hypertension in children are lower in frequency and severity compared with effects on the brain. Urgent therapy for hypertension might be considered in the child whose hypertension is associated with bleeding after cardiac surgery or whose hypertension might compromise the success of a renal transplant (Box 261.2).

Blood Pressure Elevation of Diagnostic Importance in the Pediatric Intensive Care Unit

In many pediatric patients in the ICU, hypertension is neither an emergency nor of urgent significance, but it provides insight into the patient's disease process and assists the astute clinician in diagnosing and treating the patient.

A common cause of hypertension in the pediatric ICU is pain or agitation. An example is the child who requires neuromuscular junction blocking agents for adequate mechanical ventilation and who is not well sedated. Hypertension may be noted before the next dose of sedatives is due, and the hypertension responds to an increase in dose or in frequency of administration. The child who has a physiologic narcotic dependency caused by a prolonged need for sedation in the ICU may manifest withdrawal through hypertension. Hypertension may also be associated commonly with an increase in intracerebral pressure. The concomitant findings of sinus bradycardia and irregular breathing may give the clue to the etiology of hypertension in this setting. Hypertension may be present in the early phase of

septic shock and may be noted as a response to chronic ventilatory insufficiency. The child with a hypertensive emergency is more likely to have a renal or renovascular etiology than is the case with mild hypertension presenting as an outpatient. Various diagnostic modalities that are of potential use in this setting include renal angiography, renal vein renin assay, ultrasound, Doppler analysis of renal artery and vein flow, magnetic resonance imaging (MRI), spiral CT, and captopril-enhanced radionuclide angiography. The choice of imaging modalities depends on the presentation, the stability of the patient, and the experience of the imaging staff. The differential diagnosis of hypertension in children is given in Box 261.3.

THERAPY

Nitroprusside is an arteriolar dilator that lowers blood pressure by dropping the systemic vascular resistance. A nitroprusside infusion acts rapidly to lower the pressure and can be titrated to the arterial pressure desired. Blood pressure usually does not need to be decreased into the normal range to treat a hypertensive emergency. This is particularly true if chronic hypertension has been present before the hypertensive emergency. Nitroprusside must be used carefully because of the tendency of this drug to lower blood pressure below desired limits. Continuous measuring of blood pressure with an indwelling arterial line is optimal during nitroprusside infusions. The usual dose ranges from 0.5 to 8.0 μg/kg/minute. High doses and prolonged infusions are associated with toxicity from cyanide and thiocyanate (Table 261.1).

In the past, diazoxide has been a standard agent for lowering blood pressure in patients with hypertensive encephalopathy. An advantage is that this drug is less likely than is nitroprusside to "bottom out" the blood pressure, but titration of effect is more difficult. The usual range in the dose is 3 to 5 mg/kg intravenously; however, a dose of 1 to 2 mg/kg has been found to be adequate in many cases, so an initial dose in the lower range is recommended. A dose of 10 mg/kg may be required in some cases. Diazoxide must be given in a rapid bolus because slow intravenous infusions result in binding of the drug by plasma proteins and loss of effect. Although diazoxide is unlikely to lower the blood pressure to an excessive degree, monitoring the pressure immediately after a bolus dose is wise. The appropriate management of excessive hypotension includes a volume infusion (e.g., 10 mL/kg of normal saline). Hyperglycemia is a side effect of diazoxide and is of particular concern when repeated doses are required.

Treating cerebral edema with an osmotic agent, such as mannitol or glycerol, and with hyperventilation sufficient to maintain the arterial P_{CO_2} in the low 30 mm Hg range may be necessary in some cases of hypertensive encephalopathy associated with profound brain swelling. Lowering blood pressure alone is sufficient in the vast majority of cases.

The use of nitroprusside to abruptly lower the blood pressure in the setting of a hypertensive crisis with congestive heart failure is reasonable. Volume reduction through diuretic therapy alone may ameliorate the findings of pulmonary edema in some of these cases. Diuretic therapy should be included for most patients with a hypertensive crisis that includes pulmonary edema. Patients in renal failure with a hypertensive crisis may not be responsive to diuretics. If substantial volume overload occurs, patients with renal impairment and cardiac dysfunction or cardiogenic pulmonary edema may need dialysis or plasmapheresis. Pericardial effusion is a common cause of radiographic cardiomegaly in the uremic patient. Cardiac tamponade in the uremic patient should be kept in mind as a possible cause of the symptoms of heart failure. Abrupt volume reduction without treatment of cardiac tamponade in this setting is likely to result in further hemodynamic deterioration.

BOX 261.3 Differential Diagnosis of Hypertension in Children

Iatrogenic, Factitious, Accidental

Acute Na overload: $NaHCO_3$, glucose and electrolyte mixtures, Scholl antibiotics (Na-penicillin or Na-carbenicillin), sodium polystyrene sulfonate (Kayexalate), phosphate replacements, contrast media (Hypaque, 786 mEq/L), intravenous fluids

Licorice and related compounds (similar to aldosteronism)

Exogenous corticosteroids

Nonsteroidal antiinflammatory drugs: mineralocorticoid-like effect, probably mediated by prostaglandins

Antidepressant drugs: monoamine oxidase inhibitors (with other drugs), tricyclics, lithium

Other sympathomimetics (direct and indirect): phenylephrine eye or nose drops, appetite suppressants, cold medicines, thyroid medications

Drug abuse: cocaine, amphetamines

Immunosuppressive agents

Erythropoietin

Anesthetics: ketamine, cyclopropane, local anesthetics, pancuronium, narcotics (especially naloxone [Narcan])

Ergot alkaloids (for migraines, in obstetrics, from plants)

Antihypertensive drug therapy (beta blockers, saralasin, clonidine, postganglionic blockers, methyldopa) with catecholamine excess or rebound

Poisons: heavy metals, spider bites, drugs, plants

Accidents: burns, orthopedic accidents, trauma

Cardiovascular Etiology

Coarctation of the aorta: preoperative, acute postoperative, residual, recurring

Causes of diastolic runoff (systolic hypertension with a wide pulse pressure): patent ductus arteriosus, arteriovenous fistula, aortic regurgitation, anteroposterior window, ruptured sinus of Valsalva aneurysm, large aorticopulmonary anastomosis

Infective endocarditis (renal mechanism)

Arteritis (radiation, Takayasu disease, connective tissue disease)

Peripheral atherosclerosis (systolic only with wide pulse pressure)

Renovascular Hypertension

Intrinsic renal artery disease

Intimal fibrosis (postinjury, idiopathic)

Medial (fibromuscular dysplasia, muscular hyperplasia)

Subadventitial (fibrosis or dysplasia)

Arteritis
   Sequela of Kawasaki disease
   Moyamoya disease

Thrombotic

Embolic

Aneurysms, dissecting aneurysms

Fistulas

Neurofibromatosis

Associated with other congenital defects

Renal artery stenosis with coarctation

Uteropelvic junction obstruction

William syndrome

Atherosclerotic lesions

Alagille syndrome

Extrinsic compression

Renal parenchymal tumors

Paraaortic tumors

Neurofibroma

Pheochromocytoma

Ganglioneuroma

Paraaortic lymphatics

Lymphoma

Chronic granulomatous disease

Ectopic kidney position

Iatrogenic (ligature involving a normal or aberrant renal artery)

Renal Parenchymal and Structural Disease

Cystic disease

Infantile polycystic kidneys

Adult polycystic kidneys

Medullary sponge kidney (juvenile nephronophthisis) with Zellweger, Jeune, Goldenhar, trisomies D and E, and orofacial digital syndromes; short rib polydactyly; Ehlers-Danlos syndrome; various chromosome translocations

Segmental hypoplasia (Ask-Upmark kidney)

Renal myofibromatosis

Hydronephrosis

Pyelonephritis

Glomerulonephritis

Renal vein thrombosis (uncommon)

Trauma

Page kidney (cellophane), resultant parenchymal compression

Transient hypertension after blunt abdominal trauma

Nephrotic syndrome

Hemolytic-uremic syndrome

Sickle cell disease

Endocrine Causes

Congenital adrenal hyperplasia

11-Hydroxylase deficiency

17-Hydroxylase deficiency

Cushing syndrome

Iatrogenic

Hyperaldosteronism

Primary

Exogenous

Secondary

Tumors

Pheochromocytoma, neuroblastoma, ganglioneuroblastoma, argentaffinoma, Wilms tumor, juxtaglomerular apparatus tumors

Thyrotoxicosis

Hyperparathyroidism

Turner syndrome patients taking estrogens

Oral contraceptives, syndrome of inappropriate antidiuretic hormone excess

Central Nervous System Hypertension

Elevated intracranial pressure, ischemia

Riley-Day syndrome (familial dysautonomia)

Quadriplegia, polio, Guillain-Barré syndrome

Absent corpus callosum, increased antidiuretic hormone–hypertension syndrome

Other Causes

Volume excess from polycythemia

Stevens-Johnson syndrome

Cyclic vomiting with dehydration

Intussusception

Femoral nerve traction

TABLE 261.1

DRUGS AND DOSAGES FOR USE IN THE TREATMENT OF HYPERTENSIVE EMERGENCIES IN CHILDREN

Drug	Dose	Comments
Diazoxide	1–10 mg/kg per dose IV	Should start at lower range; rapid infusion; watch for hypotension and hyperglycemia
Hydralazine	0.2–0.8 mg/kg per dose IV 1.05–5.00 mg/kg/day PO	Concerns about development of lupus-like phenomenon
Nifedipine	0.25 mg/kg IV	
Nitroprusside	0.5–8.0 μg/kg/minute infusion	Cyanide and thiocyanate toxicity with prolonged high-dose therapy
Propranolol	0.1–2.0 mg/kg per dose IV	Use with slow infusion and with capability to pace if bradycardia is excessive
Verapamil	0.1–0.2 mg/kg per dose	Should not be used if patient is younger than 6 months, is on beta blockers, or has congestive heart failure
Hydrochlorothiazide	0.5–2.0 mg/kg/day PO	More often for chronic therapy
Methyldopa	10–40 mg/kg/day	More often for chronic therapy
Esmolol	50–300 μg/kg/minute infusion	Beta blocker with extremely rapid onset and termination of effect
Phentolamine	2.5–15.0 μg/kg/minute infusion	Direct alpha blocker
Labetalol	0.5–3.0 mg/kg/hour infusion	Both alpha and beta blockade; little effect on cardiac output
Thorazine	0.5–1.0 mg/kg per dose IV	Sedative effects predominate; alpha-blockade side effect makes this agent useful after coarctation repair
Phenoxybenzamine	0.5–1.0 mg/kg IV	Investigational pediatric use as a vasodilator after heart surgery

An abrupt onset of severe hypertension immediately after repair of coarctation of the aorta can result in neurologic and cardiovascular complications, increase the risk of postoperative bleeding, and lead to other findings of post coarctectomy syndrome. Numerous antihypertensives have been used over the years. Our standard initial approach is to give a single dose of chlorpromazine (Thorazine, 0.5 to 1.0 mg/kg per dose intravenously), which lowers the blood pressure because of the side effect of alpha blockade, in addition to providing mild sedation. A single dose often is effective in lowering the blood pressure after coarctation surgery. Lowering pressure to the range of the preoperative pressure in the upper extremities is adequate.

Hydralazine is a common choice for the management of a hypertensive crisis after emergency treatment. Hydralazine can be given at a dose of 0.2 to 0.8 mg/kg intravenously or 1 to 5 mg/kg/day orally. A lupus-like syndrome occurs in some patients given hydralazine, but it typically is reversible when the drug is discontinued. Hydralazine is used commonly for patients who have hypertension associated with systemic lupus erythematosus, including a hypertensive crisis.

Beta blockers may be useful adjuncts in the treatment of chronic hypertension. Intravenous beta-blocker therapy rarely is required for pediatric hypertension. If such therapy is needed, an agent with rapid onset and termination of action, such as esmolol, is the optimal choice.

Alpha blockade using phentolamine is useful in treating hypertension occurring with hypercatecholamine states. Phentolamine treatment of pheochromocytoma cases and prophylaxis for pheochromocytoma at the time of surgery is standard practice. Phenoxybenzamine is an alpha blocker used in lowering systemic vascular resistance and systemic arterial pressure after an infant has undergone heart surgery. Prazosin is an alpha$_1$ blocker used in chronic antihypertensive therapy but not in hypertensive emergencies.

Calcium channel blockers have been useful in the treatment of chronic hypertension. Short-acting nifedipine, at initial doses of 0.25 mg/kg or less, has been useful for severe hypertension in the pediatric intensive care setting, without causing a precipitous lowering of the blood pressure. Angiotensin-converting enzyme (ACE) inhibitors are valuable in the chronic treatment of hypertension, but they have little role in emergency management.

Renovascular hypertension may respond to operative or catheter intervention, but such intervention generally is not needed in the management of acute cases.

Suggested Readings

Blaszak RT, Savage JA, Ellis EN. The use of short-acting nifedipine in pediatric patients with hypertension. *J Pediatr* 2001;139:34.

Falkner B, Sadowski RH. Hypertension in children and adolescents. *Am J Hypertens* 1995;8:106.

Fivish B, Neu A, Furth S. Acute hypertensive crises in children: emergencies and urgencies. *Curr Opin Pediatr* 1997;9:233.

Hohn AR. Diagnosis and management of hypertension in childhood. *Pediatr Ann* 1997;26:105.

Inglefinger J. *Hypertension in childhood*. Philadelphia: Saunders, 1982.

National High Blood Pressure Education Program Working Group on Hypertension Control in Children and Adolescents. National High Blood Pressure Education Program. *Pediatrics* 1996;98:649.

Park MK, Menard SM. Accuracy of blood pressure measurement by the Dinamap monitor in infants and children. *Pediatrics* 1987;79:907.

Trompeter RS, Smith RL, Hoare RD, et al. Neurologic complications of arterial hypertension. *Arch Dis Child* 1982;57:913.

Wells TG, Belshea CW. Pediatric renovascular hypertension. *Curr Opin Pediatr* 1996;8:128.

CHAPTER 262 ■ TRANSPOSITION OF THE GREAT ARTERIES

WILLIAM H. NECHES, SANG C. PARK, AND JOSE A. ETTEDGUI

Transposition of the great arteries, or complete transposition, is a common form of cardiac abnormality found in approximately 5% of all patients with congenital heart disease. The distinguishing anatomic feature of transposition is the discordant ventriculoarterial connection of the great arteries whereby the aorta originates from the morphologic right ventricle and the pulmonary artery from the morphologic left ventricle. The consequence of this anatomic arrangement is that unoxygenated systemic venous blood returning to the heart passes through the right atrium and right ventricle and is ejected into the aorta. Similarly, oxygenated pulmonary venous blood reaches the left side of the heart and is returned to the pulmonary artery. The clinical situation that results from this cardiac anomaly is characterized by severe, life-threatening hypoxemia early in life. The presence or absence of associated cardiac abnormalities dictates the presentation, clinical course, and surgical approach to the management of the three main categories of patients with transposition:

1. Transposition with an intact interventricular septum (complete transposition). These patients may or may not have left ventricular outflow tract obstruction (subpulmonary stenosis).
2. Transposition with ventricular septal defect. This is complete transposition and an interventricular communication but without narrowing in the left ventricular outflow tract.
3. Complex transposition, which is complete transposition, ventricular septal defect, and varying degrees of left ventricular outflow tract obstruction. These patients usually have significant subpulmonic stenosis and equal right and left ventricular pressures. This category includes patients with pulmonary atresia.

Other major associated cardiac lesions include patent ductus arteriosus and coarctation of the aorta.

Before the modern era of cardiac catheterization and cardiac surgery, more than 90% of patients with transposition died in infancy. This lesion was one of the most common causes of death from congenital heart disease in the first year of life. In recent years, advancements in cardiac catheterization and cardiac surgery have transformed the devastating natural history of this anomaly so that today more than 90% of patients with this lesion are expected to survive into adulthood.

PHYSIOLOGY AND HEMODYNAMICS

In the normal heart, the circulation is connected in series. Systemic venous return passes into the pulmonary artery, while pulmonary venous return passes into systemic arterial circulation. In the heart with transposition of the great arteries, the result of the abnormal arterial connection is that the individual has two parallel circulations (Fig. 262.1). Systemic venous

return passes through the right heart and is ejected into the aorta, whereas pulmonary venous return passes through the left heart and is again ejected into the pulmonary artery. This physiologic arrangement is incompatible with life unless blood can be mixed between the two circulations. In the neonate with transposition of the great arteries and an intact interventricular septum, a foramen ovale or atrial septal defect usually is present and facilitates exchange of blood at atrial level. A patent ductus arteriosus enhances this exchange. The ductus arteriosus is usually a transient neonatal structure, however, and tends to close physiologically within a few days after birth. Closure of the duct precipitates a dramatic change in the clinical appearance of an apparently healthy newborn to one with intense cyanosis.

The patient with transposition of the great arteries and a significantly sized ventricular septal defect presents an entirely different clinical picture. These patients often have adequate exchange of blood, with a combination of mixing at atrial and ventricular levels. As a result, only mild cyanosis is present in the early neonatal period, and, therefore, a significant cardiovascular anomaly often is not suspected until a few weeks later. As a result of this large ventricular septal defect, patients

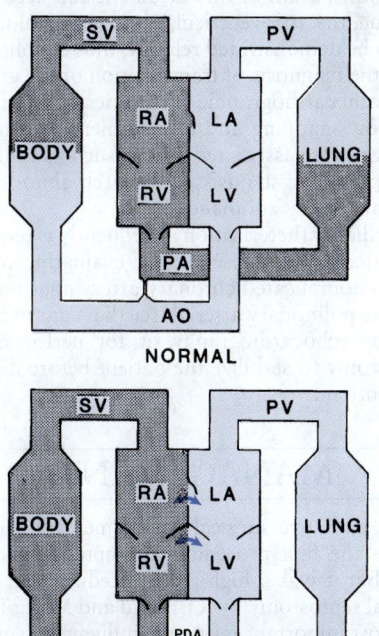

FIGURE 262.1. Circulatory pathways in transposition of the great arteries. Ao, aorta; LA, left atrium; LV, left ventricle; PA, pulmonary artery; PDA, patent ductus arteriosus; PV, pulmonary veins; RA, right atrium; RV, right ventricle; SV, systemic veins.

present with congestive heart failure toward the end of the first month of life and are at risk for subsequent development of pulmonary vascular disease.

The physiologic features in patients with complex transposition (transposition with ventricular septal defect and pulmonary stenosis) differ from those of either of the other two clinical forms. Patients with complex transposition have a large ventricular septal defect, and the balance between pulmonary and systemic blood flow depends on the degree of pulmonary stenosis. When severe pulmonary stenosis or pulmonary atresia is present, the patient presents with cyanosis and reduced pulmonary blood flow early in life. If pulmonary stenosis is less severe, then clinical presentation results from the presence of cyanosis or detection of a heart murmur and may occur even later in infancy.

DIAGNOSIS

Cyanosis, with or without associated heart murmur, is the most common presenting manifestation of transposition of the great arteries. As previously stated, associated lesions temporarily may provide adequate blood mixing, so the infant may be only mildly cyanotic or have significant cyanosis only during exercise (feeding or crying). Patients with transposition and an intact interventricular septum often have no murmur; other than cyanosis, the only abnormalities on physical examination may be a loud, single second heart sound and a prominent right ventricular impulse. In other patients, a murmur may be related to a ventricular septal defect or patent ductus arteriosus, or it may be caused by pulmonary stenosis.

The electrocardiogram shows right axis deviation and right ventricular hypertrophy, which is a normal pattern in a newborn. Although the classic "egg-on-a-string" radiographic pattern may be seen in approximately one-third of patients, usually the chest roentgenogram is normal in the first few days of life.

Cross-sectional echocardiography provides the noninvasive diagnostic information of this cardiac lesion accurately. With this technique, the atrioventricular and ventriculoarterial connections can be demonstrated reliably, thus enabling the establishment of the diagnosis of transposition of the great arteries. Additional echocardiographic modalities, including Doppler and color flow mapping and three-dimensional imaging, are able to demonstrate associated lesions such as ventricular septal defects, pulmonic stenosis, aortic arch abnormalities, and some coronary artery anomalies.

Thus, cardiac catheterization infrequently is required in this group of patients and is reserved for evaluating certain situations such as complicated coronary artery anatomy or abnormalities of the pulmonary arterial tree that cannot be evaluated accurately by echocardiography or for performing balloon atrial septostomy to stabilize the patient before definitive surgical intervention.

MANAGEMENT

Historically, palliative surgical enlargement of the interatrial opening was the first procedure attempted (Blalock-Hanlon operation), but it was a high-risk procedure. Introduction of balloon atrial septostomy by Rashkind and Miller in 1966 was the single most important milestone influencing survival of infants with transposition of the great arteries. Balloon atrial septostomy was extremely effective in providing immediate palliation for the critically cyanotic and hypoxic infant with this lesion by enabling adequate mixing at the atrial level. Subsequently, the blade atrial septostomy technique was introduced by Park and colleagues in 1975 for use in the patient with an unusually thickened atrial septum for which an adequate inter-

atrial opening could not be created effectively by the balloon technique.

Several types of atrial redirection operations were introduced by Senning in 1959 and Mustard in 1964. These atrial baffle procedures redirect the venous inflow to the heart by channeling systemic venous drainage to the mitral valve, whereas the pulmonary venous drainage is channeled to the tricuspid valve and, eventually, out into the aorta. In the years before the use of profound hypothermia and circulatory arrest, the Mustard procedure generally was performed in children between 1 and 3 years of age.

Despite good early postoperative results with these atrial baffle procedures, increasing problems, including systemic or pulmonary venous obstruction, right ventricular dysfunction, and atrial arrhythmias, became apparent. In addition, concerns about long-term systemic right ventricular function led to the use of the definitive surgical procedure, of switching the great arteries, that was introduced by Jatene and colleagues in 1976. Technically, to divide the transposed great arteries and to reanastomose the vessels to provide a concordant ventriculoarterial connection is relatively easy. However, the coronary arteries arise from the sinuses of the semilunar valve that is connected to the right ventricle. These arteries must be transferred to their respective new aortic sinuses, thus requiring transplantation of both coronary arteries into the reconnected aorta (Fig. 262.2). Although this procedure was associated with high mortality rates during the early experience, the recent mortality rate is at an acceptable level, and this anatomic repair now is a worldwide standard.

LATE RESULTS

Although most patients have good functional results, many long-term problems have been identified in patients who have undergone atrial baffle procedures. Approximately 10% to 20% of patients who underwent a Mustard or Senning operation developed systemic venous obstruction postoperatively. A few cases were severe enough to require reoperation. Pulmonary venous obstruction was found less frequently, in approximately 5% to 10% of survivors, often occurring as a late complication. These complications commonly consisted of more severe degrees of obstruction that required reoperation.

Atrial arrhythmias (atrial flutter, supraventricular tachycardia, and sick-sinus syndrome) are important problems in patients who have undergone a Mustard or Senning operation. Modifications of the operative technique to avoid injury to the sinoatrial node or its artery were successful in reducing the incidence of early postoperative rhythm disturbances before the use of the arterial switch procedure. Despite the reduction in the number of early arrhythmias, the percentage of atrial arrhythmias in patients who have had these atrial redirection procedures continues to increase in frequency with increasing length of postoperative follow-up.

Tricuspid valve incompetence also has been reported to occur after atrial baffle operations. It may be caused by the inability of the tricuspid valve to function as the systemic atrioventricular valve over a long period of time. In some series, tricuspid incompetence was seen most often in patients who had closure of a ventricular septal defect through the tricuspid valve, a finding suggesting that injury to the valve structure, or its support apparatus, at the time of operation also may play a role. These problems are present with both types of atrial baffle repair.

The arterial switch procedure results in an anatomic as well as physiologic correction, and physicians theorize that this procedure will provide a better functional result over the course of many years as compared with the atrial baffle procedures. With current, improved surgical techniques, the immediate surgical

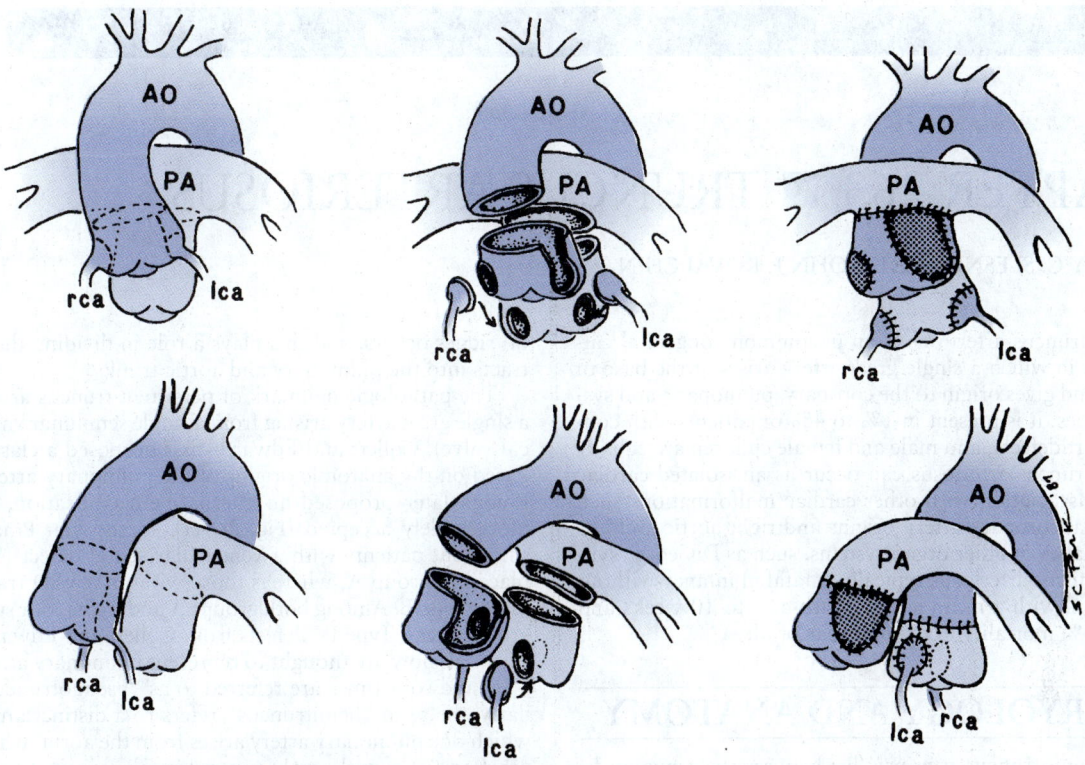

FIGURE 262.2. Diagram illustrating the arterial switch operation. **Top:** Frontal view. **Bottom:** Sagittal view. AO, aorta; PA, pulmonary artery; lca, left coronary artery; rca, right coronary artery.

results generally are excellent. Long-term results of patients who undergo an arterial switch repair for transposition of the great arteries are still unknown. However, most survivors of the arterial switch procedure seem to be doing well. Maintenance of normal coronary artery blood flow is of major importance, and the long-term effects related to growth are unknown. The initial surgical challenge is the effective transfer of both coronary arteries without any compromise in flow. However, some surgical limitations exist in the case of an unusual origin or course of the coronary arteries. Another concern is the occurrence of stenosis at the site of anastomosis of the great arteries, mostly occurring in the pulmonary artery. When it occurs, some patients have required reoperation to correct this problem. Progressive dilation of the aorta, which previously was the proximal pulmonary artery, also may occur in some patients. Despite the lack of long-term follow-up to decide questions such as the growth of anastomotic sites and the fate of transplanted coronary arteries, the arterial switch repair is the preferred procedure for surgical management of the patient with transposition of the great arteries.

Suggested Readings

Hutter PA, Kreb DL, Mantel SF, et al. Twenty-five years' experience with the arterial switch operation. *J Thorac Cardiovas Surg* 2002;124:790.

Jatene AD, Fontes VF, Paulista PP, et al. Anatomic correction of transposition of the great vessels. *J Thorac Cardiovasc Surg* 1976;72:364.

Kanter RJ, Papagiannis J, Carboni MP, et al. Radiofrequency catheter ablation of supraventricular tachycardia substrates after Mustard and Senning operations for D-transposition of the great arteries. *J Am Coll Cardiol* 2000;35:428.

Kreutzer C, De Vive J, Oppido G, et al. Twenty-five-year experience with Rastelli repair for transposition of the great arteries. *J Thorac Cardiovasc Surg* 2000;120:211.

Mustard WT. Successful two-stage correction of transposition of the great vessels. *Surgery* 1964;55:469.

Park SC, Neches WH, Mathews RA, et al. Hemodynamic function after the mustard operation for transposition of the great arteries. *Am J Cardiol* 1983;51:1514.

Park SC, Neches WH, Mullins CE, et al. Blade atrial septostomy: collaborative study. *Circulation* 1982;66:258.

Quaegebeur JM, Rohmer J, Brom AG, et al. Revival of the Senning operation in the treatment of transposition of the great arteries. *Thorax* 1977;32:517.

Rashkind WJ, Miller WW. Creation of an atrial septal defect without thoracotomy: a palliative approach to complete transposition of the great arteries. *JAMA* 1966;196:991.

Rastelli GC, Wallace RB, Ongley PA. Complete repair of transposition of the great arteries with pulmonary stenosis: a review and report of a case corrected by using a new surgical technique. *Circulation* 1969;39:83.

Senning A. Surgical correction of transposition of the great vessels. *Surgery* 1959;45:966.

Shaher R. *Complete transposition of the great arteries.* New York: Academic Press, 1973.

Williams WG, McCrindle BW, Ashburn DA, et al. Outcomes of 829 neonates with complete transposition of the great arteries 12–17 years after repair. *Eur J Cardiothorac Surg* 2003;24:1.

CHAPTER 263 ■ TRUNCUS ARTERIOSUS

TIMOTHY C. SLESNICK AND JOHN P. KOVALCHIN

Persistent truncus arteriosus is an uncommon congenital cardiac defect in which a single great artery arises at the base of the heart and gives origin to the coronary, pulmonary, and systemic arteries. It is present in 1% to 4% of patients with congenital heart defects, and male and female children are equally affected. Truncus arteriosus can occur as an isolated cardiac defect, in association with other cardiac malformations such as abnormal coronary artery origins and right aortic arch, or with anomalies of other organ systems, such as DiGeorge syndrome. Truncus arteriosus typically is fatal in infancy without intervention, with a mean age of death at 5 to 10 weeks and 70% to 85% mortality in the first year of life.

EMBRYOLOGY AND ANATOMY

The embryonic truncus arteriosus lies between the conus cordis and aortic sac, and at approximately week 4 to 5 of fetal development, it begins separating into the aorta and pulmonary artery. This separation is thought to occur through fusion of two spiral ridges to form the conotruncal septum between the two great arteries and is influenced by the primary looping of the ventricles. An immigration of neural crest cells into the distal ridges occurs, and this plays a role in dividing the outflow tracts into the pulmonary and aortic trunks.

The pathologic hallmark of persistent truncus arteriosus is a single great artery arising from a single semilunar valve (truncal valve). Collett and Edwards first proposed a classification based on the anatomic origins of the pulmonary arteries. Van Praagh later proposed an alternative classification, which is more widely accepted (Fig. 263.1). In the Van Praagh classification, patients with a ventricular septal defect (VSD) are placed in group A, whereas those without a VSD (rare) comprise group B. Among both groups A and B, the four subgroups are identical. Type IV defects from Collett and Edwards' classification now are thought to represent pulmonary atresia with VSD and sometimes are referred to as "pseudotruncus." Similarly, the term "hemitruncus" refers to a distinct anomaly in which one pulmonary artery arises from the aorta, whereas the other arises from the right ventricle with a distinct pulmonary valve. Both these defects have a clearly different embryologic basis than that of persistent truncus arteriosus, and, therefore, both terms are misnomers.

The truncal valve has a variable number of leaflets, which often are abnormal in morphology. Approximately 65% of patients have tricuspid valves, 23% have quadricuspid valves,

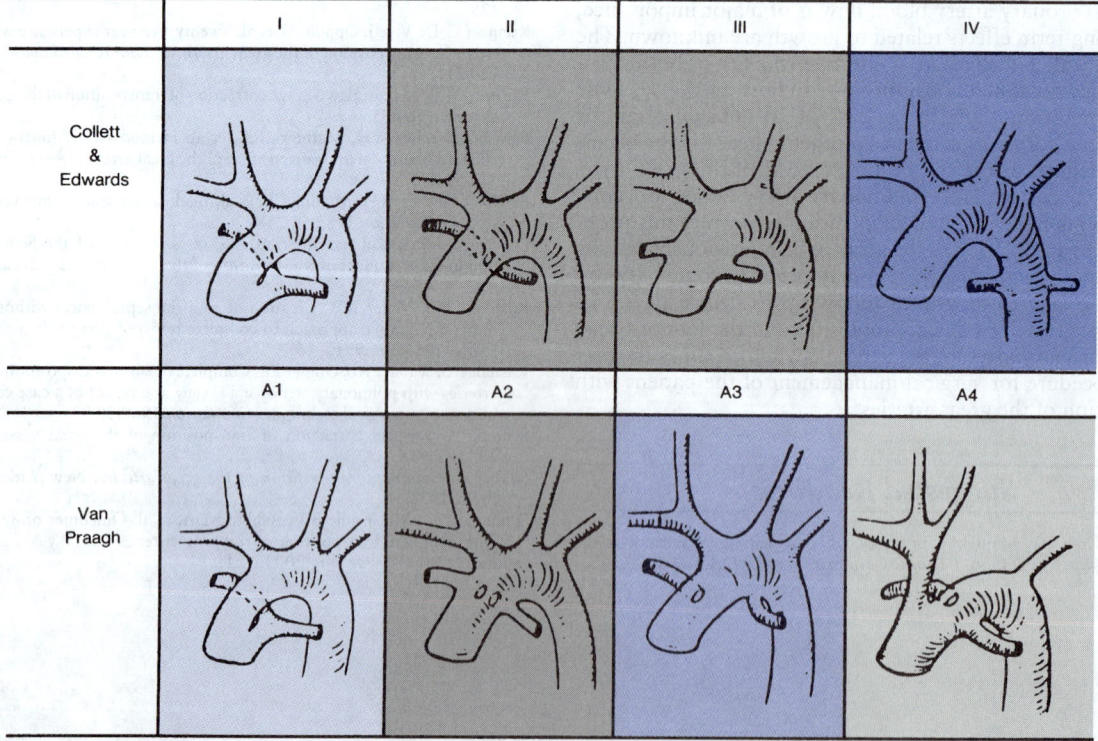

FIGURE 263.1. Classic Collett and Edwards' classification of truncus arteriosus compared with the Van Praagh classification. Type I is the same as A1. Types II and III are grouped as a single type, A2. Type IV commonly is referred to as pseudotruncus. Type A3 denotes unilateral pulmonary artery atresia with collateral supply to the affected lung. Type A4 denotes truncus associated with an interrupted aortic arch.

9% have bicuspid valves, and occasionally unicuspid or greater than four cusps can occur. The truncal valve usually has fibrous continuity with the mitral valve, but it is rarely continuous with the tricuspid valve. Truncal valve insufficiency is present in one-half of patients with truncus arteriosus and is moderate to severe in up to one-fourth of cases. Truncal valve stenosis also has been reported in up to 30% of patients. Either regurgitation or stenosis can be caused by a variety of mechanisms, but most commonly it occurs when the valve leaflets and cusps are thickened or dysplastic. The truncal root typically straddles the VSD, with a biventricular origin in up to 80% of patients. Among the remaining patients, isolated truncal origin from the right ventricle is more common than from the left ventricle.

The most commonly associated cardiac malformations with truncus arteriosus are coronary artery anomalies, occurring in one-third to one-half of patients. Aortic arch anomalies also are common findings with one-third of cases having a right arch. An interrupted aortic arch (Van Praagh type A4) is seen in 11% to 19% of patients, and conversely 12% of patients with an interrupted arch also have truncus arteriosus. Unilateral absence of a branch pulmonary artery (Van Praagh type A3) can be seen in one-sixth of patients and is ipsilateral to the side of the arch in 75% of cases.

Extracardiac anomalies also are common, seen in as many as 30% of cases, and include skeletal, renal, intestinal, and systemic defects. An association with DiGeorge syndrome has been established, such that 35% of patients with truncus arteriosus also have DiGeorge syndrome. Conversely, 9% to 11% of patients with DiGeorge syndrome have truncus arteriosus. Patients with truncus arteriosus should undergo fluorescence *in situ* hybridization screening for the microdeletion of chromosome 22q11, which is present in up to 90% of patients with DiGeorge syndrome.

CLINICAL MANIFESTATIONS

Most patients with truncus arteriosus present during early infancy, often in the first month of life. Fetal echocardiography allows diagnosis prenatally, although outflow tract anomalies can be difficult to visualize in the standard four-chamber view. Prenatal diagnosis allows delivery and evaluation to occur in a center experienced in surgical correction of the defect. Patients not diagnosed prenatally typically present with congestive heart failure, and symptoms depend on the volume of pulmonary blood flow and severity, if any, of truncal valve regurgitation. Infants with large volumes of pulmonary blood flow may have no visible cyanosis from birth, but the persistence of elevated pulmonary resistance in the first few weeks of life may cause mild cyanosis. As pulmonary resistance drops, however, pulmonary blood flow increases with greater mixing of saturated than of desaturated blood, and the cyanosis becomes less apparent. Tachypnea, tachycardia, difficulty with feedings, and irritability may be the first clinical signs of heart failure resulting from excessive blood flow through the pulmonary circulation. Symptoms usually occur within the first few days of life, but they may take several weeks to become apparent, secondary to delayed decrease in pulmonary vascular resistance.

On physical examination, patients typically have a normal first heart sound, a loud systolic ejection click, a loud, single second heart sound, and sometimes a third heart sound heard best at the apex. Peripheral pulses may be bounding, and the pulse pressure often is widened, primarily because of pulmonary artery runoff and truncal valve regurgitation when present. A loud, often holosystolic murmur is heard best at the left sternal border and sometimes is accompanied by a thrill. Additionally, an apical low-pitched diastolic murmur from increased flow across the mitral valve or a high-pitched early diastolic murmur of truncal regurgitation can be heard.

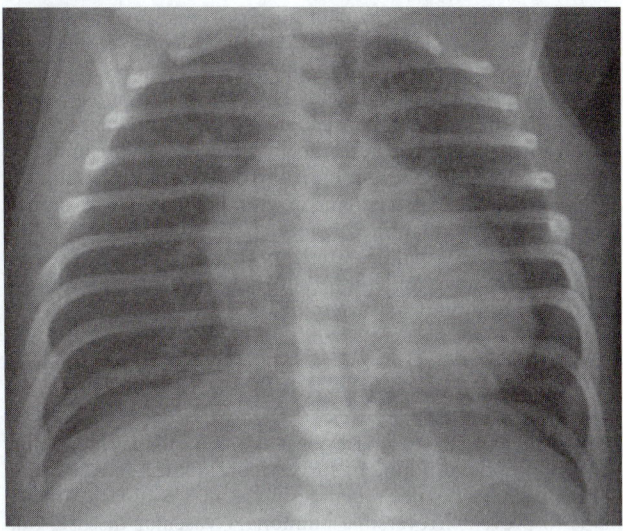

FIGURE 263.2. Chest radiograph of a neonate with truncus arteriosus and a right aortic arch. Cardiomegaly and increased pulmonary vascular markings are evident, and the trachea is deviated to the left.

The electrocardiogram typically shows a normal QRS axis with biventricular hypertrophy. Isolated right or left ventricular hypertrophy is less common. Occasionally, left ventricular ischemic changes caused by coronary insufficiency may be seen.

The chest radiograph shows cardiomegaly after the first 1 to 2 days of life. The aortic arch is right-sided in one-third of patients, and presence of a right arch with increased pulmonary vascularity strongly suggests truncus arteriosus (Fig. 263.2). As the pulmonary vascular resistance decreases and pulmonary overcirculation worsens, heart size continues to increase. If atresia of one of the pulmonary arteries is present (Van Praagh type A3), asymmetry of the pulmonary vascularity may be seen.

IMAGING MODALITIES

Improvements in imaging quality have allowed echocardiography to become the primary imaging modality for diagnosing truncus arteriosus, and now most children are sent to surgery based on echocardiographic imaging information alone. Two-dimensional and Doppler echocardiography are used to define the anatomy and any associated hemodynamic abnormalities, such as truncal valve stenosis or regurgitation. The common trunk, including the origins of the pulmonary arteries, can be visualized arising from a single semilunar valve. Tetralogy of Fallot, pulmonary atresia with VSD, and aortopulmonary window may appear similar to truncus arteriosus, but only in truncus arteriosus can the pulmonary arteries be seen arising directly from the posterolateral aspect of the truncal root. The aortic arch must be fully imaged to determine whether there is an interrupted arch with a ductal dependent descending aorta. Visualization of the coronary arteries, including their relationships with the truncal valve and pulmonary arteries, is also possible. Additional imaging may be required when echocardiography is unable to provide sufficient anatomic information preoperatively, and in these cases cardiac magnetic resonance imaging is a useful noninvasive alternative because of its ability to provide excellent visualization of the pulmonary arteries, aortic arch, and coronary arteries.

Cardiac catheterization was formerly recommended in all or most patients with truncus arteriosus to define the anatomy and to measure pulmonary arteriolar resistance, because patients with resistances greater than 8 Wood units/m^2 were not considered operable candidates. However, echocardiography currently allows excellent delineation of anatomy, and early surgical correction in the first 6 months of life helps to prevent irreversible pulmonary vascular disease, such that preoperative cardiac catheterization is usually not necessary in most young infants. Preoperative cardiac catheterization is now largely reserved for patients in whom the anatomic features cannot be defined noninvasively, or for patients whose condition is not diagnosed until they are older and in whom pulmonary resistance levels need to be quantified before considering surgery. Additionally, interventional catheterization is occasionally used in patients who have undergone surgical correction for procedures such as pulmonary artery dilation or stenting.

THERAPY

Management of truncus arteriosus is essentially surgical, and debate on optimal timing of surgery continues. The consensus is that primary repair sometime in the first 6 months of life helps to prevent irreversible pulmonary vascular disease, but whether to perform the repair in the early neonatal period or to allow infants to grow for several months before the repair is not as well-established. Over the years, the trend for surgery in congenital heart disease has been for earlier and complete repairs and extends to surgical intervention for truncus arteriosus. At our institution, these children generally undergo repair procedures in the neonatal or early infant period, usually within the first 6 weeks of life. Initially, however, medical therapy is indicated to manage pulmonary overcirculation, by using digoxin and diuretics. Prostaglandin E_1 may be required when an interrupted aortic arch is present. Maximizing caloric intake to facilitate growth also is thought to be beneficial. Medical management is largely unsuccessful at controlling heart failure, however, and it is only a temporizing effort until surgical correction can be performed.

Before 1967, the only surgical palliation available for truncus arteriosus was pulmonary artery banding, but early mortality rates still approached 50%, and the band frequently migrated or was ineffective. Definitive repair for truncus arteriosus was performed first by McGoon and associates, who used a valved homograft to connect the right ventricle and pulmonary arteries, a modification of a technique first described by Rastelli for use in pulmonary atresia with VSD. Ebert and colleagues were the first to advocate primary repair in infancy, and they demonstrated an early mortality rate of only 11% in their patients.

Repair of truncus arteriosus consists of removal of the pulmonary arteries from the truncal root with primary or patch closure of the defect, closure of the VSD so the left ventricle empties through the truncal valve, and establishment of continuity between the right ventricle and the pulmonary arteries, typically using a valved homograft conduit (Fig. 263.3). When significant truncal valve insufficiency is present, surgical valvar repair or replacement with a homograft valve also is performed. Risk factors for mortality after repair include later age at repair, the presence of significant truncal insufficiency, interrupted aortic arch, or coronary abnormalities. Over the decades since McGoon first described complete repair of truncus arteriosus, advances in surgical techniques and postoperative management have allowed trends toward earlier age at surgery and improved survival rates, with in-hospital mortality rates now lower than 5% to 10% at some institutions. Long-term outcome studies are difficult to perform with truncus arteriosus because of the significant advances in surgical techniques, intraoperative myocardial protection, and postoperative care over the last 30 years. Reddy and associates reported an 83% survival rate at 15 years for the 165 patients who survived the initial hospitalization following complete surgical repair at their institution.

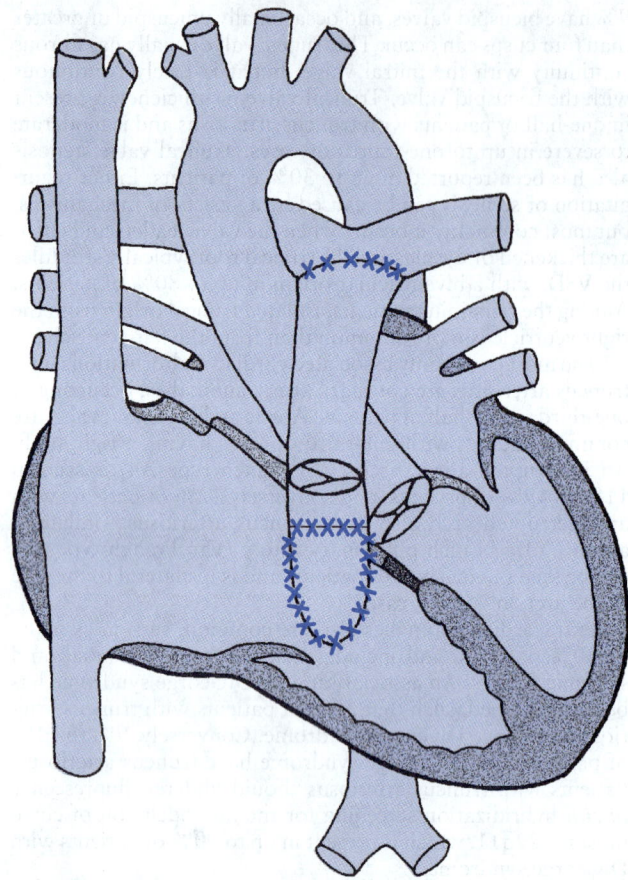

FIGURE 263.3. Illustration of a repaired truncus arteriosus. The pulmonary arteries have been removed from the aorta and brought into continuity with the right ventricle using a valved conduit. The ventricular septal defect has been patched closed, directing the left ventricular outflow to the aorta.

SUMMARY

The infant with persistent truncus arteriosus presents many challenges to general pediatricians and cardiologists alike. Timing of surgical intervention is critical, and until then optimizing growth and maintaining stable hemodynamics can be challenging. These children have the potential for rapid cardiac deterioration, and over time almost all develop pulmonary hypertension if the defect is not repaired. Surgery performed during the first 6 months of life helps to prevent irreversible pulmonary vascular disease, and most children undergo repair procedures within the first few months. After surgical correction, careful follow-up to monitor for signs of truncal valve disease, conduit stenosis, and branch pulmonary artery stenosis is essential because nearly all children will need future interventions, primarily conduit replacement. Continued advances in surgical therapy for truncus arteriosus since the 1960s allow a lesion previously considered inoperable to be corrected surgically, and the diagnosis and treatment continue to be refined.

Suggested Readings

Collett RW, Edwards JE. Persistent truncus arteriosus: a classification according to anatomic types. *Surg Clin North Am* 1949;29:1245.

Duke C, Sharland GK, Jones AM, Simpson JM. Echocardiographic features and outcome of truncus arteriosus diagnosed during fetal life. *Am J Cardiol* 2001; 88:1379.

Ebert PA, Turley K, Stanger P, et al. Surgical treatment of truncus arteriosus in the first 6 months of life. *Ann Surg* 1984;200:451.

Goldmuntz E, Clark BJ, Mitchell LE, et al. Frequency of 22q11 deletions in patients with conotruncal defects. *J Am Coll Cardiol* 1998;32: 492.

Marcelletti C, McGoon DC, Danielson GK, et al. Early and late results of surgical repair of truncus arteriosus. *Circulation* 1977;55:636.

Marino B, Digilio MC, Toscano A, et al. Anatomic patterns of conotruncal defects associated with deletion 22q11. *Genet Med* 2001;3:45.

McGoon DC, Rastelli GC, Ongley PA. An operation for the correction of truncus arteriosus. *JAMA* 1968;205:69.

Reddy VM, Hanley F. Late results of repair of truncus arteriosus. *Semin Thorac Cardiovasc Surg Pediatr Card Surg Annu* 1998;1:139.

Rice MJ, Seward JB, Hagler DJ, et al. Definitive diagnosis of truncus arteriosus by two-dimensional echocardiography. *Mayo Clin Proc* 1982;57:476.

Tometzki AJ, Suda D, Kohl T, et al. Accuracy of prenatal echocardiographic diagnosis and prognosis of fetuses with conotruncal anomalies. *J Am Coll Cardiol* 1999;33:1696.

Van Praagh R, Van Praagh S. The anatomy of common aorticopulmonary trunk (truncus arteriosus communis) and its embryologic implications: a study of 57 necropsy cases. *Am J Cardiol* 1965;16:406.

Webb S, Qayyum SR, Anderson RH, et al. Septation and separation within the outflow tract of the developing heart. *J Anat* 2003;202:327.

Williams JM, de Leeuw M, Black MD, et al. Factors associated with outcomes of persistent truncus arteriosus. *J Am Coll Cardiol* 1999;34:545.

CHAPTER 264 ■ TRICUSPID ATRESIA

DAVID J. DRISCOLL

Tricuspid atresia, the third most common form of cyanotic congenital heart disease, consists of complete agenesis of the tricuspid valve and absence of direct communication between the right atrium and the right ventricle (Fig. 264.1). The prevalence of tricuspid atresia in clinical series of patients with congenital heart disease ranges from 0.3% to 3.7%. The prevalence rate in autopsy series is 2.9%. Tricuspid atresia occurs in one in 10,000 to one in 17,857 live births.

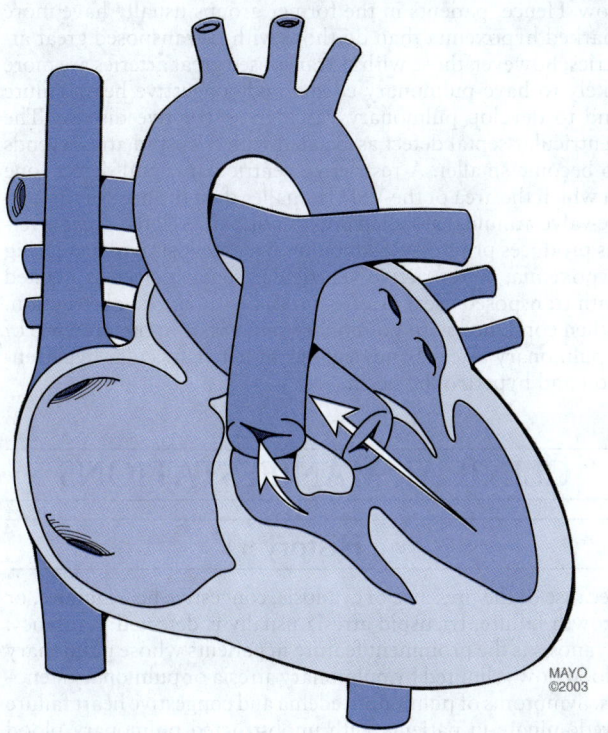

e1064437-010-0

FIGURE 264.1. Diagrammatic representation of tricuspid atresia with normally related great arteries.

PATHOLOGY

Tricuspid atresia is divided into three types on the basis of the great artery relationship: I, normally related great arteries; II, D-transposed great arteries; and III, L-transposed great arteries (Table 264.1). The three types are subclassified according to the presence or absence and size of the ventricular septal defect and the presence or absence of pulmonary atresia or stenosis. Approximately 70% of cases are type I, 23% are type II, and 7% are type III.

An opening in the atrial septum allows egress of blood from the right atrium. The interatrial communication can be (or can become) restrictive. Additional cardiovascular abnormalities occur in 18% of patients with normally related great arteries and in 63% of patients with transposed great arteries. These abnormalities include coarctation of the aorta, patent ductus

TABLE 264.1

CLASSIFICATIONS OF TRICUSPID ATRESIA

Type	Description	Relative Frequency (%) Clinical	Relative Frequency (%) Autopsy
I	Normally related great arteries	70	69
I-A	No VSD; pulmonary atresia		9
I-B	Restrictive VSD; pulmonary stenosis		51
I-C	Large VSD; no pulmonary stenosis		9
II	D-transposition of great arteries	23	28
II-A	VSD; pulmonary atresia		2
II-B	VSD; pulmonary stenosis		8
II-C	VSD; no pulmonary stenosis		18
III	L-transposition of great arteries	7	3

VSD, ventricular septal defect.
Adapted from Rosenthal A, Dick M. Tricuspid atresia. In: Adams FH, Emmanouilides GC, eds. *Moss's heart disease in infants, children, and adolescents*, 3rd ed. Baltimore: Williams & Wilkins, 1983:271, with permission.

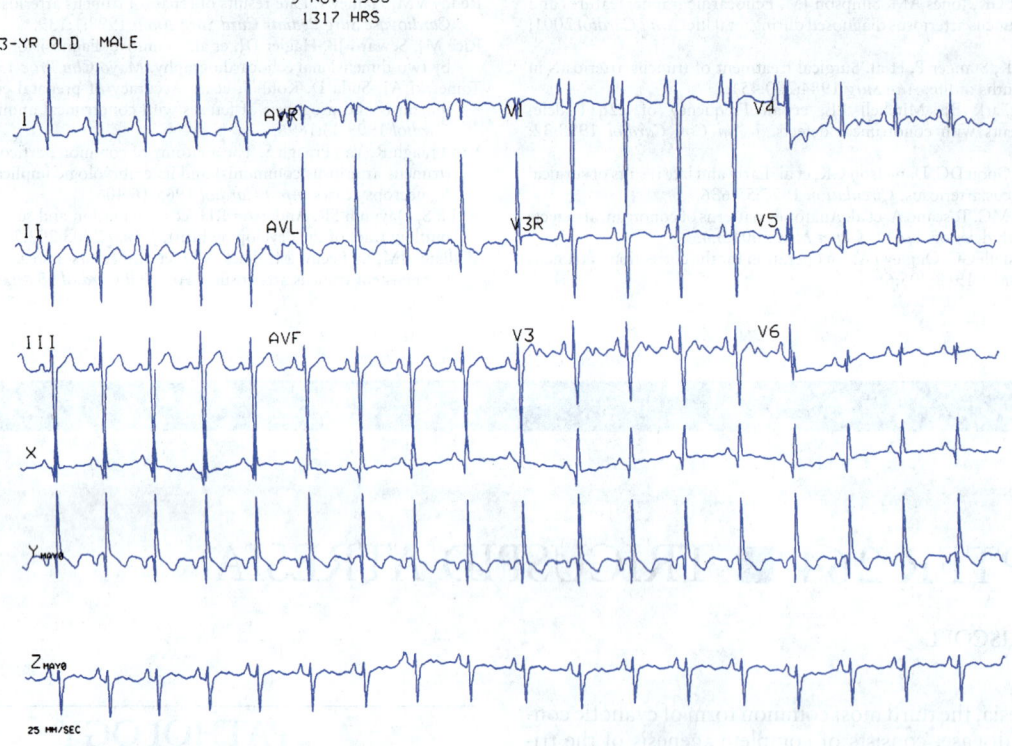

FIGURE 264.2. Typical electrocardiographic recording from a patient with tricuspid atresia and normally related great arteries. Note the left axis deviation with a counterclockwise frontal plane loop (Q waves in leads I and aVL), atrial enlargement, and left ventricular hypertrophy.

arteriosus, and right aortic arch. Extracardiac anomalies occur in 20% of cases.

In tricuspid atresia, the left bundle of the cardiac conduction system originates early from the bundle of His and is unusually posterior and short. Presumably, this anatomic malformation of the conduction system accounts for the leftward or superior frontal plane axis of the electrocardiogram in patients with tricuspid atresia (Fig. 264.2).

HEMODYNAMICS

In tricuspid atresia, hemodynamic features depend on the presence or absence of pulmonary atresia, the degree of pulmonary stenosis, the presence of normally related or transposed great arteries, and the presence or absence of subpulmonary or subaortic stenosis. Because all systemic venous return (blood oxygen saturation low) and pulmonary venous return (blood oxygen saturation high) mix in the left atrium, the level of blood oxygen saturation reaching the left ventricle (and subsequently the aorta) depends on the relative volumes of pulmonary venous return and systemic venous return. Patients with tricuspid atresia and increased pulmonary blood flow (i.e., no pulmonary or subpulmonary stenosis) have a volume of pulmonary venous return relatively larger than that of systemic venous return and have relatively high systemic arterial blood oxygen saturation. In contrast, patients with relatively low pulmonary blood flow (caused by pulmonary or subpulmonary stenosis or pulmonary atresia) may have marked systemic arterial hypoxemia. The volume of pulmonary blood flow and the clinical characteristics may change. Patients with pulmonary stenosis may depend on patency of the ductus arteriosus for pulmonary blood flow, and, as the ductus closes, pulmonary blood flow may decrease significantly.

In general, pulmonary obstruction or subpulmonary obstruction (at the level of the ventricular septal defect [VSD])

is present or occurs during the first year of life in most patients with tricuspid atresia and normally related great arteries. In contrast, most patients with tricuspid atresia and D-transposed great arteries (type II-C) have unobstructed pulmonary blood flow. Hence, patients in the former groups usually have more marked hypoxemia than do those with D-transposed great arteries; however, those with D-transposed great arteries are more likely to have pulmonary edema and congestive heart failure and to develop pulmonary vascular obstructive disease. The ventricular septal defect associated with tricuspid atresia tends to become smaller. A restrictive ventricular septal defect (one in which the area of the VSD is smaller than the area of the aortic valve annulus) associated with normally related arteries produces progressive subpulmonary stenosis and increasing hypoxemia. A restrictive ventricular septal defect associated with transposed great arteries produces subaortic obstruction. When combined with pulmonary stenosis or in the presence of a pulmonary artery band, significant left ventricular hypertension and hypertrophy occur.

CLINICAL MANIFESTATIONS

History

Because of the presence of cyanosis, congestive heart failure, or growth failure, tricuspid atresia usually is detected in infancy. Cyanosis is the prominent feature in patients whose pulmonary blood flow is limited by pulmonary atresia or pulmonary stenosis. Symptoms of pulmonary edema and congestive heart failure predominate in patients with unobstructed pulmonary blood flow; cyanosis also can be apparent. If pulmonary blood flow depends on the patency of the ductus arteriosus and that vessel closes, the degree of cyanosis and arterial hypoxemia may increase dramatically. If pulmonary atresia is present, closure of the ductus can produce profound hypoxemia, acidosis, and death. In patients with unobstructed pulmonary blood flow, as the pulmonary vascular resistance decreases and pulmonary blood flow increases, signs and symptoms of congestive heart failure and pulmonary edema can increase.

Without surgical intervention, significant pulmonary vascular obstructive disease occurs in patients with unrestricted pulmonary blood flow (types I-C and II-C; see Table 264.1). Pulmonary vascular obstructive disease in patients with tricuspid atresia and normally related great arteries occurs much less commonly than it does in patients with transposed great arteries because most of the former have or will have (at perhaps 1 year of age) pulmonary or subpulmonary stenosis. Bacterial endocarditis and brain abscess are recognized complications of tricuspid atresia. Neurologic complications also can result from cerebrovascular accidents secondary to polycythemia and iron deficiency or to intravascular thrombosis or embolic phenomena.

Physical Examination

Cyanosis is the most common clinical feature of tricuspid atresia. Infants with tricuspid atresia and normally related great arteries may have excessive pulmonary blood flow and little cyanosis, but the degree of cyanosis may increase as the ventricular septal defect becomes progressively restrictive, causing subpulmonary stenosis and decreasing blood flow.

The intensity of the second heart sound usually is normal if the great arteries are related normally (i.e., pulmonary artery anterior) and the pulmonary artery pressure is normal. Because the aorta is nearer to the anterior chest wall when great arteries are transposed (i.e., the aorta is anterior to the pulmonary artery), the second heart sound may be more intense despite normal pulmonary artery pressure.

Cardiac murmurs are present in 80% of patients with tricuspid atresia. A low-frequency holosystolic (or, at times, a crescendo-decrescendo) murmur is produced by the flow of blood through the ventricular septal defect. A systolic midfrequency crescendo-decrescendo murmur is present in patients with pulmonary stenosis. Patients with pulmonary atresia and a systemic–to–pulmonary collateral blood supply and patients who have had a surgical systemic arterial–to–pulmonary arterial anastomosis have a continuous murmur. A diastolic mitral murmur may be audible in patients who have excessive pulmonary blood flow.

Electrocardiography

First-degree atrioventricular block occurs in 15% of cases and presumably is caused by prolonged atrial conduction, because atrioventricular node function usually is normal. Because of the early origin of the left bundle from the common bundle, the frontal plane QRS axis usually is leftward or superior, and the frontal plane electrocardiographic loop is counterclockwise. Rarely, the frontal plane QRS axis is normal, a finding that suggests the presence of transposed great arteries. The right ventricular electrocardiographic forces are diminished, and left ventricular hypertrophy is evident, as are frequently discordant QRS and T waves.

Chest Radiography

Usually, the heart is enlarged. The right border of the heart may be prominent, reflecting enlargement of the right atrium. The pulmonary vascular markings are increased when the pulmonary blood flow is excessive. In 80% of patients with tricus-

pid atresia, however, the pulmonary blood flow is diminished, and the pulmonary vascular markings are decreased.

Echocardiography

Basic anatomy, size of the atrial septal defect, size of the ventricular septal defect, ventricular function, great artery relationships, and valvular function can be ascertained by using M-mode, two-dimensional, Doppler, and color-flow echocardiography.

Cardiac Catheterization

In infants, cardiac catheterization is used mainly to determine sources and reliability of pulmonary blood flow. Administration of prostaglandin E_1 to maintain ductal patency has improved the safety of cardiac catheterization for babies with decreased or duct-dependent pulmonary blood flow. Cardiac catheterization may be necessary in infants (2 to 6 months old) to measure pulmonary artery pressure and resistance. This information can serve as a guide to the need for pulmonary artery banding to prevent development of pulmonary vascular obstructive disease. In adolescents and adults, cardiac catheterization and angiography define anatomic and hemodynamic details important in surgical management.

CLINICAL MANAGEMENT

Infants

Three major considerations should guide the management of infants with tricuspid atresia:

1. The need for manipulating the amount of pulmonary blood flow, either to decrease hypoxemia and polycythemia by increasing pulmonary blood flow or to decrease symptoms of congestive heart failure by decreasing pulmonary blood flow.
2. The need for preserving myocardial function, pulmonary vascular integrity, and the pulmonary vascular bed to optimize conditions for a future Fontan operation.
3. The need for reducing risks of associated cardiovascular complications, such as bacterial endocarditis and thromboembolism.

Babies with severe hypoxemia and acidosis should be treated promptly with an infusion of prostaglandin E_1 to maintain patency of the ductus arteriosus, thereby improving pulmonary perfusion. Echocardiography and, sometimes, cardiac catheterization and angiography are used to establish sources of pulmonary blood flow and provide help in planning for the type of surgical systemic-to–pulmonary artery anastomosis.

Infants with transposed great arteries and unrestricted pulmonary blood flow have signs and symptoms of pulmonary edema and congestive heart failure. Such infants benefit from treatment with digitalis and diuretics. Traditionally, these patients have had a pulmonary artery band surgically placed to decrease the pulmonary blood flow. Some investigators suggest, however, that pulmonary artery banding may accelerate ventricular septal defect closure. In patients with tricuspid atresia with transposed great arteries, this procedure would create subaortic obstruction and could lead to marked ventricular hypertrophy. Because marked ventricular hypertrophy is an adverse risk for a subsequent successful Fontan operation, surgical procedures to reduce pulmonary blood flow and to bypass potential areas of subaortic obstruction have been recommended.

Children and Adolescents

Before 1971, palliative procedures to control pulmonary blood flow (pulmonary artery banding, systemic-to–pulmonary artery anastomoses, or superior vena cava–to–pulmonary artery anastomoses) were the mainstays of surgical treatment for patients with tricuspid atresia. In 1971, Fontan and associates described a unique procedure for separating the systemic and pulmonary venous returns to eliminate the right-to-left intracardiac shunt and thereby reduce the volume of ventricular overload. These surgeons constructed a Glenn anastomosis to direct superior vena caval systemic venous return to the right lung and directed inferior vena caval systemic venous return to the pulmonary artery with a valve-containing conduit connection placed between the right atrium and the pulmonary artery. They also inserted a valve into the inferior vena cava, closed the interatrial communication, and obliterated the connection between the pulmonary artery and the ventricle. Since its original description, the procedure has been modified considerably, but the concept of directing systemic venous return directly to the pulmonary artery retains the eponymic label *modified Fontan procedure* (Fig. 264.3).

Tricuspid Atresia After Fontan Operation

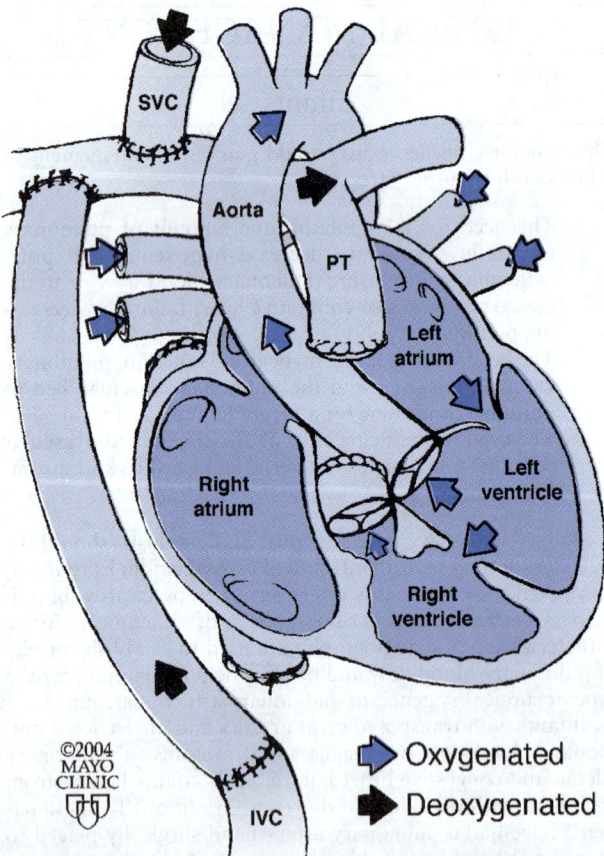

©2004
MAYO
CLINIC

▶ Oxygenated
▶ Deoxygenated

FIGURE 264.3. Diagrammatic representation of a modified ("extracardiac") Fontan operation. The superior vena cava (SVC) has been disconnected from the right atrium and connected directly to the right pulmonary artery ("bidirectional Glenn anastomosis"). The main pulmonary artery has been divided. The inferior vena cava (IVC) has been connected to the right pulmonary artery with an interposition graft that is exterior to the right atrium.

Ten guidelines for performing relatively low-risk operations described by Choussat and colleagues are listed in Box 264.1. Additional criteria include the absence of ventricular hypertrophy, more recent calendar year of operation, the absence of subaortic obstruction, shorter operative ischemic time, and the absence of incorporation of prosthetic valves into the repair. Although most of these criteria are relative, clearly, as more of them are violated, operative mortality increases, and the chances of achieving excellent long-term results decrease.

In a follow-up study of 125 patients who underwent a modified Fontan operation between 1973 and 1985, the 30-day, 6-month, and 1-, 5-, and 10-year survival rates were 90%, 84%, 84%, 80%, and 70%, respectively. Quality of life and tolerance for exercise improved after the operation. Preliminary data suggest that the operation prolongs life. However, a relatively high incidence of atrial arrhythmias occurs in survivors of the Fontan operation. In addition, 5% to 10% of survivors may develop protein-losing enteropathy, a complication that has a 5-year 50% mortality rate.

Suggested Readings

Choussat A, Fontan F, Bosse P, et al. Selection criteria for Fontan's procedure. In: Anderson RH, Shinebourne EA, eds. *Paediatric cardiology 1977*. Edinburgh: Churchill Livingstone, 1978:559.

Dick M, Fyler DC, Nadas AS. Tricuspid atresia: clinical course in 101 patients. *Am J Cardiol* 1975;36:327.

Driscoll DJ, Danielson GK, Puga FJ, et al. Exercise tolerance and cardiorespiratory response to exercise after the Fontan operation for tricuspid atresia or functional single ventricle. *J Am Coll Cardiol* 1986;7:1087.

Driscoll D, Offord K, Feldt R, et al. Five- to fifteen-year follow-up after the Fontan operation. *Circulation* 1992;85:469.

Fontan F, Mounicot F, Baudet E, et al. "Correction" de l'atresie tricuspidienne; rapport de deux cas "corrigés" par l'utilisation d'une technique chirurgicale nouvelle. *Ann Chir Thorac Cardiovasc* 1971;10:39.

Gentles T, Gauvreau K, Mayer J, et al. Functional outcome after the Fontan operation: factors influencing late morbidity. *J Thorac Cardiovasc Surg* 1997;114:392.

Gentles T, Mayer J, Gauvreau K, et al. Fontan operation in five hundred consecutive patients: factors influencing early and late outcome. *J Thorac Cardiovasc Surg* 1997;114:376.

Rao PS. *Tricuspid atresia*. Mount Kisco, NY: Futura, 1982:13.

Rosenthal A, Dick M. Tricuspid atresia. In: Adams FH, Emmanouilides GC, eds. *Moss's heart disease in infants, children, and adolescents,* 3rd ed. Baltimore: Williams & Wilkins, 1983:271.

Tandon R, Edwards JE. Tricuspid atresia: a reevaluation and classification. *J Thorac Cardiovasc Surg* 1974;67:530.

Vlad P. Tricuspid atresia. In: Keith JD, Rowe RD, Vlad P, eds. *Heart disease in infancy and childhood*, 3rd ed. New York: Macmillan, 1978:518.

CHAPTER 265 ■ TETRALOGY OF FALLOT

WILLIAM H. NECHES, SANG C. PARK, AND JOSE A. ETTEDGUI

Tetralogy of Fallot refers to a spectrum of anatomic abnormalities that have in common a large, unrestrictive ventricular septal defect and right ventricular outflow tract obstruction—the two major features of the condition, although right ventricular hypertrophy and overriding of the aorta are additional features that complete the tetralogy (Fig. 265.1). Clinical presentation varies from the asymptomatic acyanotic child with a heart murmur to the severely hypoxic newborn infant. Severity of presentation depends largely on the nature and degree of the outflow obstruction. The anatomic hallmark of tetralogy of Fallot is the anterocephalad deviation of the outlet portion of the interventricular septum. The severity of the infundibular stenosis ranges from mild to severe pulmonary stenosis and to pulmonary atresia. Further obstruction to pulmonary blood flow often occurs at other levels. Pulmonary valve stenosis is a common finding, and stenoses often are found also in the supravalvar region, at the bifurcation of the pulmonary artery branches, or in the distal pulmonary arteries.

The typical ventricular septal defect in tetralogy of Fallot is large and unrestrictive and is the result of malalignment of the outlet portion with the rest of the interventricular septum. Muscular ventricular septal defects, an inlet defect, or a complete atrioventricular septal defect also may be present.

Other possible associated abnormalities include an atrial septal defect (so-called *pentalogy of Fallot*) or coronary artery abnormalities such as a left anterior descending coronary artery arising from the right coronary artery, which may limit the surgical approach. Approximately 25% of patients with tetralogy of Fallot have a right-sided aortic arch, an important consideration if a patient undergoes a systemic–to–pulmonary artery anastomosis. Severity of presentation depends largely on the nature and degree of the outflow obstruction.

Tetralogy of Fallot occurs in approximately 6% of infants born with congenital heart disease. The etiology is obscure. Although tetralogy of Fallot and most other forms of congenital heart disease generally occur as isolated abnormalities, children with tetralogy of Fallot are afflicted with additional major extracardiac malformations significantly more often (15.7%) than are patients with other congenital heart defects (6.8%). In addition, the extracardiac malformations may be more serious in patients with tetralogy of Fallot and include cleft lip and palate, hypospadias, and skeletal malformations. Although tetralogy of Fallot commonly is not part of specific hereditary malformation syndromes or chromosomal abnormalities, it often is found in many malformation associations, including cardiofacial, VACTERL (vertebral, anal, cardiac, tracheal, esophageal, renal, limb), and CHARGE (coloboma, heart disease, atresia choanae, retarded growth and development and/or central nervous system anomalies, genital hypoplasia, and ear anomalies and/or deafness) associations, and 22q11 deletion, as well as De Lange, Goldenhar, and Klippel-Feil syndromes.

PHYSIOLOGY AND HEMODYNAMICS

Equalized right and left ventricular pressures, along with normal or reduced pulmonary artery pressure, are the hemodynamic features produced by anatomic abnormalities in patients with tetralogy of Fallot. Because the ventricular septal defect is large and unrestrictive and the right and left ventricles contract simultaneously, the end result is, in effect, a common ventricular chamber ejecting into systemic and pulmonary circulations. Pulmonary and systemic blood flows therefore depend on the relation between pulmonary and systemic resistances. Normally, pulmonary resistance is approximately 10% of systemic resistance, and these resistances are determined by their respective distal arteriolar beds. In tetralogy of Fallot, however, pulmonary vascular (arteriolar) resistance usually is normal or less than normal, and resistance to right ventricular ejection into the pulmonary vascular bed is related instead to pulmonary stenosis.

The presenting symptoms and severity of clinical manifestations in patients with tetralogy of Fallot depend on the relation between the resistances to systemic and pulmonary outflow. When the total right ventricular outflow obstruction is such that pulmonary outflow resistance is less than systemic resistance, a net left-to-right shunt is present, and clinical manifestations are similar to those of patients with a ventricular septal defect of small to moderate size. When pulmonary and systemic resistances are similar, there is a balanced shunt with nearly equal pulmonary and systemic blood flows at rest. Finally, when resistance to pulmonary outflow exceeds systemic resistance, a net right-to-left shunt is seen, and systemic flow is greater than pulmonary flow.

Cyanosis may be mild or undetectable at rest in patients with tetralogy of Fallot but usually becomes apparent or increases with physical activity. With exercise, increased cardiac output and decreased systemic arteriolar resistance result in a considerable increase in the degree of right-to-left shunting.

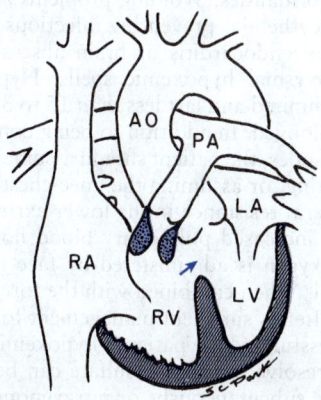

FIGURE 265.1. Anatomic abnormalities in tetralogy of Fallot. Ao, aorta; LA, left atrium; LV, left ventricle; PA, pulmonary artery; RA, right atrium; RV, right ventricle. Note the ventricular septal defect (*arrow*), the infundibular pulmonary stenosis (*stippled area*), and the overriding aorta.

Although effective cardiac output is maintained, right-to-left shunting produces a rapid decrease in systemic arterial oxygen saturation and results in exertional dyspnea and decreased tolerance for exercise. In contrast to episodes of paroxysmal hypoxemia (tetralogy spells), the systemic desaturation is limited by the duration of exercise and improves as soon as activity ceases.

Squatting is a common posture in patients with tetralogy of Fallot, particularly in young children who easily assume the more comfortable knee-chest position. Squatting often is seen in children after exercise. They also frequently are seen to assume this position while playing quiet games with their peers who are sitting. Squatting likely results in an increase in systemic arterial resistance caused by kinking and compression of the major arterial circulation to the lower extremities. This increase in peripheral resistance, in the presence of relatively fixed pulmonary outflow resistance, decreases the degree of right-to-left shunting and increases pulmonary blood flow. The result is an immediate increase in systemic arterial oxygen saturation.

Episodes of paroxysmal hypoxemia, also called *hypercyanotic* or *tetralogy spells*, often are seen in infants and children with tetralogy of Fallot and other cardiac malformations with similar physiologic features. These spells usually are self-limited and last less than 15 to 30 minutes, although they may be longer. The spells are seen more often in the morning but may occur during the day and may be precipitated by activity, a sudden fright, or injury, or they may occur spontaneously without any apparent cause. The spell is characterized by increasing cyanosis and an increased rate and depth of respiration. The physiologic change that produces a hypoxemic spell is an increase in right-to-left shunting and concomitant decrease in pulmonary blood flow. The exact mechanism by which this phenomenon occurs is unknown.

DIAGNOSIS

The presentation of patients with tetralogy of Fallot ranges from the small infant with severe hypoxemia to the asymptomatic child with "pink tetralogy." The severity of symptoms is related to the degree of pulmonary stenosis. Cyanosis usually is present in the neonate with severe tetralogy of Fallot or with associated pulmonary atresia. Another relatively common presentation is the asymptomatic infant with a heart murmur. These patients may seem to have only a ventricular septal defect because the murmur of the right ventricular outflow obstruction in the infant with tetralogy of Fallot may be indistinguishable from that of an isolated ventricular septal defect. The presence of significant right ventricular hypertrophy on the electrocardiogram may be a clue to the nature of the underlying abnormality.

Cyanosis and clubbing may be present on physical examination of the child with tetralogy of Fallot. An increased left parasternal impulse, indicating right ventricular hypertrophy, may be seen. The first heart sound usually is normal, whereas the second sound is single because the pulmonary closure sound is very soft. An ejection systolic murmur is heard at the midupper left sternal border and may radiate toward the back. Loudness of the murmur depends on the volume of blood crossing the right ventricular outflow tract. As infundibular stenosis becomes more severe, less blood flows through the right ventricular outflow, and the murmur becomes softer and shorter. The child having a hypoxemic spell has much less antegrade flow into the pulmonary arteries, and the murmur disappears.

The chest radiograph in older children with tetralogy of Fallot exhibits the classically described "boot-shaped" heart. It is caused by mild enlargement of the right ventricle and concavity of the upper left heart border caused by absence of the main pulmonary artery segment. In infants, the chest radiograph may be normal or may show only decreased pulmonary vascular markings.

The anatomic features of tetralogy of Fallot are identified by echocardiography. The large ventricular septal defect is visualized easily, and the aorta overriding the ventricular septal defect is apparent. The infundibular narrowing of the right ventricular outflow tract, or a thickened and abnormal pulmonary valve, usually can be demonstrated. Doppler echocardiography demonstrates an increased velocity of blood flow in the main pulmonary artery and is useful in estimating the gradient across the right ventricular outflow tract. Echocardiography has replaced cardiac catheterization and angiocardiography as the single most important modality in the diagnosis and preoperative assessment of tetralogy of Fallot.

Cardiac catheterization and angiocardiography continue to have value in complementing the information obtained by echocardiography. These invasive tools are important in the assessment of the preoperative patient who has a poor echocardiographic window or in the presence of associated abnormalities such as multiple ventricular septal defects, pulmonary arterial abnormalities, or coronary artery abnormalities that could adversely affect the success of surgical repair. In the postoperative patient with residual defects, cardiac catheterization provides an assessment of the hemodynamic result, ventricular function, severity of residual anatomic abnormalities, and electrophysiologic status.

MEDICAL MANAGEMENT

Although many patients with tetralogy of Fallot are acyanotic in early infancy, the subpulmonary stenosis tends to be progressive and usually results in the appearance of cyanosis during infancy or early childhood. Before the development of systemic to pulmonary artery anastomoses in the mid 1940s, approximately 50% of patients with tetralogy of Fallot died in the first year of life, and seldom did a patient survive past the third decade. Mortality usually was a consequence of hypoxia, secondary hematologic changes, or problems such as infective endocarditis or brain abscess. With palliative surgical procedures and complete repair, the outlook for patients with this anomaly has improved dramatically. Today, complete repair is performed commonly during infancy, and 90% or more of patients with tetralogy of Fallot are expected to survive to adulthood.

Treatment of significant resting hypoxia or hypercyanotic spells is surgical. Medical management in patients with tetralogy of Fallot therefore is directed toward treating associated noncardiac abnormalities, avoiding problems associated with anemia or polycythemia, preventing infectious complications such as bacterial endocarditis or brain abscess, and acutely managing paroxysmal hypoxemic spells. Hypoxemic spells usually are self-limited and last less than 15 to 30 minutes, but they can be prolonged. In addition to being comforted during one of these episodes, the patient should assume the knee-chest position. Squatting, or assuming the knee-chest position, may increase peripheral resistance in the lower extremities that, in turn, promotes increased pulmonary blood flow. In a hospital situation, oxygen is administered by face mask during a hypoxemic spell. When combined with the foregoing physical maneuvers, it often is sufficient management for a short spell. If it is not successful and the patient's hypoxemic episode does not appear to resolve, morphine sulfate can be administered intramuscularly, subcutaneously, or intravenously (as a single dose) of 0.1 mg/kg of body weight. The effectiveness of morphine sulfate in treating hypoxemic spells has been known for many years, but its exact mechanism of action is unclear. Because this drug can be administered intramuscularly, it is valuable to use morphine for initial management of a hypoxemic spell when an intravenous route is unavailable. Once an intravenous line is placed, the dose of morphine sulfate can be repeated. Because metabolic acidosis appears quickly after the onset of a hypoxemic spell, sodium bicarbonate in a dose of 1.0 mEq/kg can be given empirically as soon as intravenous access is available. If these measures are unsuccessful, a beta-adrenergic blocking agent such as propranolol is valuable in managing a hypoxemic spell. This drug is given intravenously to a maximum total dose of 0.1 mg/kg of body weight. The total calculated dose should be diluted with 10 mL of fluid in a syringe, and no more than half of the calculated dose should be given initially as an intravenous bolus. The remainder can be given slowly over the course of the next 5 to 10 minutes if necessary. Propranolol also has been used in the long-term nonoperative management of paroxysmal hypoxemic spells. It is administered orally in a dose of 1 to 4 mg/kg of body weight/day in four divided doses.

SURGICAL MANAGEMENT

Surgical management of patients with tetralogy of Fallot consists of either palliative systemic–to–pulmonary artery anastomoses (shunts) or complete repair. Because palliative procedures do not require cardiopulmonary bypass, they can be performed in very small infants or in patients with anatomic features that are unfavorable for complete repair. In most centers, primary repair is performed electively during infancy if the anatomy is suitable.

Surgical palliation became possible in the 1940s with the development of the Blalock-Taussig shunt, an end-to-side anastomosis between the subclavian artery and the pulmonary artery. Other forms of systemic–to–pulmonary artery anastomoses such as the Potts procedure (between the descending aorta and the left pulmonary artery) and the Waterston shunt (between the ascending aorta and the right pulmonary artery) have either been abandoned or seldom are performed. Currently, a modified Blalock-Taussig shunt is performed when needed. It consists of interposition of a synthetic tube between the subclavian artery and the pulmonary artery, thus preserving blood flow to the arm.

Total correction is preferred, if possible, and consists of patch closure of the ventricular septal defect and relief of the right ventricular outflow tract obstruction. Occasionally, infundibular resection alone relieves the subpulmonary stenosis, but placement of a patch of synthetic material to widen the right ventricular outflow tract further may be necessary, especially when complete repair is performed in early infancy. In patients with severe pulmonary stenosis, this patch may need to be extended across the pulmonary valve annulus onto the main pulmonary artery and even out onto the branches, when pulmonary artery hypoplasia is present. In some of these patients, homograft conduits are used instead of synthetic material. When reconstruction of the right ventricular outflow tract is not possible, such as when an anomalous coronary artery is crossing this area, a palliative procedure may be performed initially, thus delaying definitive repair until the patient is older and surgery is technically easier.

LATE RESULTS

In most centers, more than 90% of patients who undergo complete repair of tetralogy of Fallot will survive to adulthood and have a good functional long-term result. Postoperative hemodynamic abnormalities such as residual ventricular septal defects, or some degree of right ventricular outflow tract obstruction, often are present, but they usually are not severe enough to require reoperation. Some pulmonary regurgitation often is present, especially in patients who have required a transannular right ventricular outflow tract patch. Even significant pulmonary regurgitation, however, usually is well tolerated in early life. However, some patients with significant pulmonary regurgitation become symptomatic in their second or third decade of life with right-sided heart failure and may have associated atrial and/or ventricular arrhythmias.

Arrhythmias, particularly ventricular ectopy, are of concern in patients who have undergone repair of tetralogy of Fallot. Sudden, unexpected death occurs in a small percentage of postoperative patients and may be caused by a ventricular arrhythmia. The combination of ventricular ectopy and hemodynamic abnormalities, especially residual pulmonary stenosis with high right ventricular pressure and right or left ventricular dysfunction, presents an increased risk for mortality. In these patients, further surgical intervention may be performed to preserve the ventricular function by correcting the residual right ventricular outflow obstruction, relieving pulmonary artery stenosis, and restoring pulmonic valve competency. Several options to achieve the task are available and include a prosthetic valve, homograft valve, or heterograft valve. Recently, valve placement has been achieved using transcatheter techniques. Even after complete repair, patients with tetralogy of Fallot still are at risk of developing subacute bacterial endocarditis and should receive appropriate antibiotic prophylaxis. Preservation of good right and left ventricular function and the possible effects of coronary artery disease in a heart with a repaired congenital defect are potential long-term problems.

Suggested Readings

Anderson RA, Allwork SP, Ho SY, et al. Surgical anatomy of tetralogy of Fallot. *J Thorac Cardiovasc Surg* 1981;81:887.

Bonchek LI, Starr A, Sunderland CO, et al. Natural history of tetralogy of Fallot in infancy: clinical classification and therapeutic implications. *Circulation* 1973;48:392.

Castaneda AR, Freed MD, Williams RG, et al. Repair of tetralogy of Fallot in infancy. *J Thorac Cardiovasc Surg* 1977;74:372.

Daily PO, Stinson EB, Griepp RB, et al. Tetralogy of Fallot: choice of surgical procedure. *J Thorac Cardiovasc Surg* 1978;75:338.

Duncan BW, Mee RB, Prieto LR, et al. Staged repair of tetralogy of Fallot with pulmonary atresia and major aortopulmonary collateral arteries. *J Thorac Cardiovasc Surg* 2003;126:694.

Fuster V, McGoon DC, Kennedy MA, et al. Long-term evaluation (12 to 22 years) of open heart surgery for tetralogy of Fallot. *Am J Cardiol* 1980;46:635.

Garson A Jr, Randall DC, Gillette PC, et al. Prevention of sudden death after repair of tetralogy of Fallot: treatment of ventricular arrhythmias. *J Am Coll Cardiol* 1985;6:221.

Ghai A, Silversides C, Harris L, et al. Left ventricular dysfunction is a risk factor for sudden cardiac death in adults late after repair of tetralogy of Fallot. *J Am Coll Cardiol* 2002;40:1675.

Gupta A, Odim J, Levi D, et al. Staged repair of pulmonary atresia with ventricular septal defect and major aortopulmonary collateral arteries: experience with 104 patients. *J Thorac Cardiovasc Surg* 2003;126:1746.

Kramer H, Majewski F, Trampisch HJ, et al. Malformation patterns in children with congenital heart disease. *Am J Dis Child* 1987;141:789.

Moulton AL, Brenner JI, Ringel R, et al. Classic versus modified Blalock-Taussig shunts in neonates and infants. *Circulation* 1985;72(suppl):II-35.

Nollert GD, Dabritz SH, Schmoeckel M, et al. Risk factors for sudden death after repair of tetralogy of Fallot. *Ann Thorac Surg* 2003;76:1901.

Poirier RA, McGoon DC, Danielson GK, et al. Late results after repair of tetralogy of Fallot. *J Thorac Cardiovasc Surg* 1977;75:900.

Shinebourne EA, Anderson RA, Bowyer JJ. Variations in clinical presentation of Fallot's tetralogy in infancy. *Br Heart J* 1975;37:946.

Therrien J, Siu SC, Harris L, et al. Impact of pulmonary valve replacement on arrhythmia propensity late after repair of tetralogy of Fallot. *Circulation* 2001;103:2489.

CHAPTER 266 ■ DOUBLE-OUTLET RIGHT VENTRICLE

MICHAEL J. SILKA

Double-outlet right ventricle (DORV) refers to a diverse group of congenital heart defects characterized by common origin of both the aorta and the pulmonary artery above the morphologic right ventricle. DORV specifies the anatomic relationship of the great arteries to the right ventricle; however, it does not specify circulatory physiology, which is determined largely by the combination of associated congenital heart defects. Historically, various terms, including *Taussig-Bing* complex, origin of both great vessels from the right ventricle, and partial transposition, have been applied to this malformation and subtypes.

DORV is an uncommon finding, representing 1.5% of all congenital heart defects, with a predicted incidence of 1 case per 15,000 live births. Although associations with trisomy 18 and maternal diabetes are recognized, most cases of DORV occur in infants with no other congenital anomalies. The embryologic basis of DORV involves failure of rotation and shift of the truncus arteriosus from above the primitive right ventricle (bulbus cordis) to a more leftward position, which aligns the future aorta above the morphologic left ventricle. Varying degrees of arrest of conoventricular rotation and leftward truncal shift result in the spectrum of congenital heart defects grouped as DORV.

ANATOMY AND PHYSIOLOGY

DORV is a specific malformation representing one of the types of malposition of the great arteries. A ventricular septal defect (VSD), which provides the only outlet for the left ventricle, is located beneath either the pulmonary artery or the aorta or, rarely, remote from both great arteries (Fig. 266.1). Associated subpulmonic stenosis, which restricts pulmonary blood flow, is present in more than 50% of patients with DORV.

The relationship of the VSD to the great arteries and the presence or absence of pulmonic stenosis are the primary determinants of the circulatory physiology in DORV. When the VSD is related closely to the aorta (see Fig. 266.1A), the physiologic features are similar to those of a large VSD with left-to-right shunt and pulmonary hypertension. In this setting, symptoms of congestive heart failure dominate after the anticipated decrease of pulmonary vascular resistance occurs, with little or no cyanosis. Conversely, when the pulmonary artery overrides the VSD, without associated pulmonic stenosis (see Fig. 266.1B), the hemodynamics simulate those of transposition of the great arteries with a large VSD. Frequently called the *Taussig-Bing complex*, clinical features of this condition include both cyanosis and congestive heart failure. Coarctation of the aorta and variable degrees of hypoplasia of the subaortic outflow tract often occur in this form of DORV. In either of these subsets of DORV, the clinical course is determined by pulmonary vascular resistance and the presence or absence of left heart obstructive lesions. Severe subpulmonic or pulmonary valvar stenosis occurs most frequently when the VSD is subaortic (see Fig. 266.1C). The resultant physiology and clinical manifestations are indistinguishable from tetralogy of Fallot, with cyanosis and pulmonary oligemia.

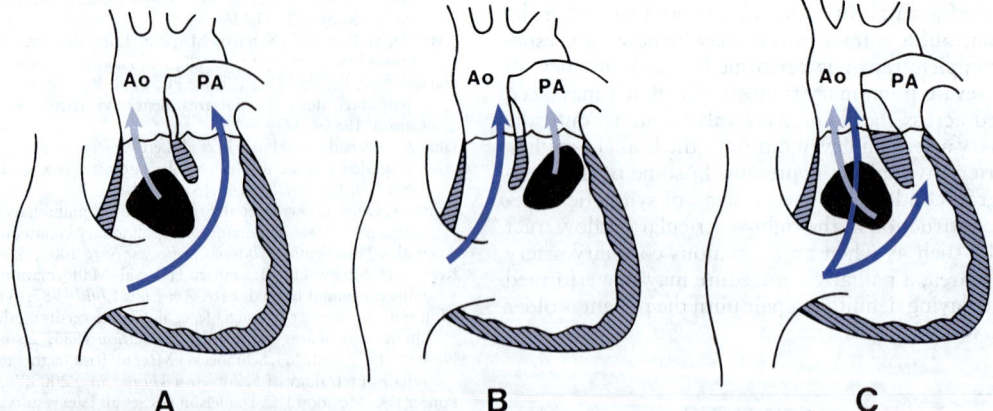

FIGURE 266.1. The three major forms of double-outlet right ventricle, illustrated with the anterior free wall of the right ventricle removed. **A:** The ventricular septal defect (VSD) is subaortic, and oxygenated blood (*light blue arrow*) from the left ventricle (LV) is directed preferentially to the aorta (Ao), whereas the deoxygenated systemic venous return (*dark blue arrow*) is directed to the pulmonary artery (PA). **B:** The VSD is subpulmonic and results in preferential flow of the oxygenated blood from the LV to the PA, whereas deoxygenated systemic venous return is directed to the Ao, resulting in cyanosis. **C:** Subpulmonic stenosis results in restricted pulmonary blood flow with mixing of both oxygenated and deoxygenated blood in the Ao. The subaortic VSD directs the limited pulmonary venous return to the Ao, resulting in variable degrees of cyanosis.

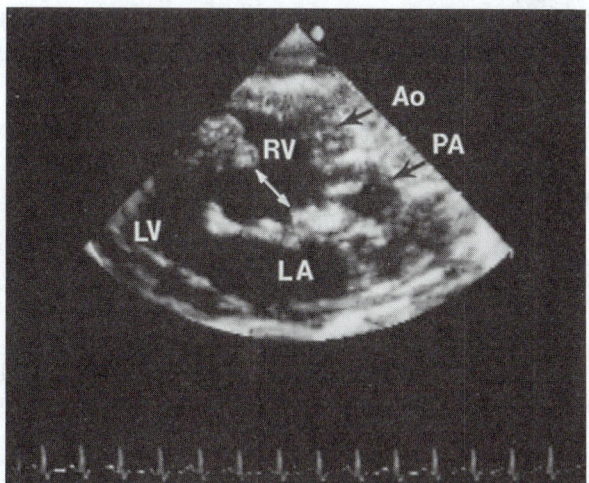

FIGURE 266.2. Echocardiographic features of double-outlet right ventricle (RV). Parasternal long-axis view demonstrating origin of both great arteries above the RV, with the ventricular septal defect (*white arrow*) as the only outlet for the left ventricle (LV). The aorta (Ao) is anterior and remote from the ventricular septal defect compared with the pulmonary artery (PA). LA, left atrium.

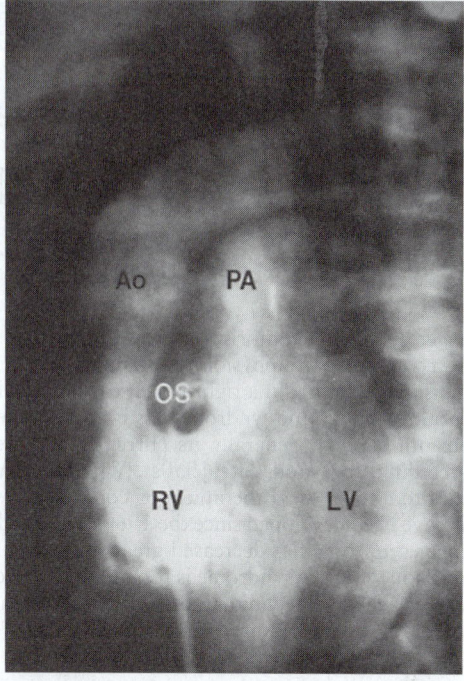

FIGURE 266.3. The angiographic features of double-outlet right ventricle. Lateral view right ventriculogram demonstrating the origin of both great arteries above the right ventricle (RV) with an outlet septum (OS) separating the two outflow tracts. The aorta (Ao) is anterior to the pulmonary artery (PA). The left ventricle (LV) is remote from either great artery.

DIAGNOSTIC CONSIDERATIONS

Clinical features of the forms of DORV reflect variations of circulatory physiology and, on physical examination, cannot be differentiated from an isolated large VSD, transposition of the great arteries with a VSD, or tetralogy of Fallot with similar hemodynamics. The chest roentgenogram and electrocardiogram may contain subtle features suggestive of DORV, but they cannot be considered diagnostic. Accurate diagnosis in each type of DORV is established with two-dimensional echocardiography. The combination of parasternal and apical imaging demonstrates the origin of both great arteries above the right ventricle, the relationship of the VSD to the great arteries, and the presence or absence of pulmonic stenosis and other associated cardiac anomalies (Fig. 266.2).

In most infants, cardiac catheterization is not required before intracardiac repair of DORV is performed. However, in more complex forms of this defect or in the older child with unrepaired DORV, cardiac catheterization with selective angiography remains useful in establishing morphologic details of the intracardiac anatomy, along with determining the pulmonary vascular resistance and coronary artery anatomy (Fig. 266.3).

with institutional protocols used in patients with a large VSD or tetralogy of Fallot. Experience suggests that long-term survival rates exceed 95%, with excellent function.

The surgical approach to DORV with a subpulmonic VSD evolved with the development of arterial switch techniques. Ninety to 95% of operative survival rates and excellent late functional status are reported when the VSD is baffled to the left semilunar valve, followed by arterial switch and coronary artery translocation. This technique represents a significant improvement over earlier repairs based on atrial switch procedures in conjunction with an intraventricular baffle.

Although short-term surgical results may be excellent, long-term evaluation and follow-up are required for these patients. Stenosis of the outflow tract or conduit may require reoperation in some patients, whereas others may develop cardiac arrhythmias years or decades after surgery. Bacterial endocarditis prophylaxis is indicated at times of risk.

SURGICAL PALLIATION AND REPAIR

In newborns with severe cyanosis caused by stenosis of the pulmonary outflow tract in association with DORV, placement of a systemic-pulmonary anastomosis provides effective palliation until elective intracardiac repair can be performed when the child reaches 6 to 12 months of age. In the forms of DORV with unrestricted pulmonary blood flow, primary intracardiac repair is advocated whenever a biventricular repair can be performed.

Surgical repairs of most variants of DORV now are performed during the first year of life. When the VSD is subaortic, an intraventricular baffle establishes continuity between the left ventricle and the aorta. When pulmonic stenosis is present, similar repair is performed, along with additional resection of the infundibular stenosis or placement of a homograft conduit to establish right ventricular-pulmonary artery continuity. These forms of DORV currently are managed in accordance

Suggested Readings

Aoki M, Forbess JM, Jonas RA, et al. Result of biventricular repair of double outlet right ventricle. *J Thorac Cardiovasc Surg* 1994;107:338.

Bostrom MPG, Hutchins GM. Arrested rotation of the outflow tract may explain double-outlet right ventricle. *Circulation* 1988;77:1258.

Ferencz C, Rubin JD, McCarter RJ, Clark EB. Maternal diabetes and cardiovascular malformations: predominance of double-outlet right ventricle and truncus arteriosus. *Teratology* 1990;41:319.

Kleinert S, Sano T, Weintraub RG, et al. Anatomic features and surgical strategies in double-outlet right ventricle. *Circulation* 1997;96:1233.

Lev M, Bharati S, Meng CCL, et al. A concept of double-outlet right ventricle. *J Thorac Cardiovasc Surg* 1972;64:271.

Macartney FJ, Rigby ML, Anderson RH, et al. Double outlet right ventricle cross sectional echocardiographic findings: their anatomical explanation and surgical relevance. *Br Heart J* 1984;52:164.

Monro JL, Alexiou C, Salmon AP, Keeton BR. Reoperations and survival after primary repair of congenital heart defects in children. *J Thorac Cardiovasc Surg* 2003;126:511.

Rogers TR, Hagstrom JCW, Engle MA. Origin of both great vessels from the right ventricle with the trisomy-18 syndrome. *Circulation* 1965;32:802.

CHAPTER 267 ■ EISENMENGER SYNDROME

STEPHEN M. PARIDON

Eisenmenger syndrome comprises a group of cardiac defects that share a common pathophysiology: pulmonary vascular obstructive disease resulting in a right-to-left cardiac level shunting of blood. Although the syndrome has been described since the nineteenth century, generally its currently accepted definition is credited to Wood (late 1950s). With the diagnostic approaches to and surgical therapies for congenital heart defects that have been developed since the 1960s, the incidence of Eisenmenger syndrome has decreased greatly. However, a certain population with this syndrome is too old to have benefited from the newer medical techniques or is the result of failure of current medical understanding.

ETIOLOGY AND PATHOPHYSIOLOGY

Eisenmenger syndrome is not a discrete cardiac defect. Rather, it is a group of cardiac defects with the common components of a large cardiac defect that allows the intracardiac shunting of blood with superimposed obstructive pulmonary vascular disease.

Lesions most likely to lead to Eisenmenger syndrome are those that allow high pulmonary-to-systemic flow ratios to occur in the presence of high pulmonary pressures, such as large defects of the ventricular septum, atrioventricular canal lesions, and patent ductus arteriosus. The presence of hypoxemia, such as occurs in D-transposition of the great arteries with a ventricular septal defect or truncus arteriosus, hastens the development of pulmonary vascular disease. Generally, defects with low pulmonary pressures, such as atrial septal defects, are much less likely to lead to Eisenmenger syndrome. Usually, despite their high rate of pulmonary blood flow, these lesions are tolerated well for decades, whereas high-pressure defects may result in changes in the pulmonary vascular bed that occur within several years or, occasionally, months.

As obstructive pulmonary vascular disease develops, resistance increases in the pulmonary vascular bed. Systemic venous blood, following the course of least resistance, is shunted away from the pulmonary arteries and through the cardiac defect into the systemic circulation. The result is systemic hypoxemia, the degree of which depends on the relative pulmonary-to-systemic vascular resistance. The more severe the pulmonary resistance or the lower the systemic resistance, the greater is the right-to-left shunting.

Generally, at the time diagnosis of heart disease is made, the clinical presentation is that of pulmonary overcirculation, which results from a high rate of pulmonary blood flow caused by large cardiac defects with low pulmonary vascular resistance. In lesions that result in hypoxemia and a high pulmonary blood flow rate, such as D-transposition of the great arteries with ventricular septal defect, cyanosis is superimposed on pulmonary congestion.

As pulmonary vascular resistance increases, signs and symptoms of pulmonary congestion decrease. The duration of this change varies from months to decades, depending on the pre-

senting cardiac defect and the rate at which vascular changes occur. When pulmonary resistance exceeds systemic resistance, hypoxemia ensues and then progresses as pulmonary vascular resistance rises.

CLINICAL MANIFESTATIONS AND COMPLICATIONS

Physical Findings

Findings on physical examination of patients with Eisenmenger syndrome vary depending on the severity of pulmonary obstructive disease. In advanced stages, cyanosis is pronounced. Usually, clubbing of the extremities is present. In early cases, cyanosis may be mild or absent, or it may become noticeable only when systemic resistance drops, such as with exercise.

Findings of the cardiovascular examination are typical of patients with pulmonary hypertension. The precordium is hyperdynamic, and a right ventricular lift may occur in patients with defects that include a normal right ventricle. The second heart sound is very loud and frequently is palpable at the left upper sternal border because of the pulmonary (P_2) component of the second sound. Generally, splitting of the second sound is absent or very narrow as a result of the decreased ejection time of the right ventricle in the presence of high pulmonary resistance.

Usually, murmurs are soft because the intracardiac defects are large, with little pressure gradient present between the chambers, and most of the right-to-left shunting of blood in these defects occurs during diastole, a period of relatively low pressure. The findings typical of left ventricular failure, such as rales caused by pulmonary edema, are absent. In severe cases, evidence of right ventricular failure may be present. Hepatomegaly and peripheral edema may occur in end-stage disease.

Laboratory Findings

The chest radiograph in Eisenmenger syndrome varies with the clinical course. Early in life, before the onset of increased pulmonary vascular resistance, the size of the heart usually is larger, with increased pulmonary vascular markings. Flooded pulmonary vasculature and pulmonary edema are evident (Fig. 267.1A). The classic chest radiograph for Eisenmenger syndrome develops after the onset of elevated pulmonary vascular resistance. The cardiac silhouette is small to normal. Proximal pulmonary arteries are dilated and tortuous. Generally, a diminished distal pulmonary vasculature occurs, giving the lung fields a black appearance in the periphery (Fig. 267.1B). Late in the clinical course, cardiomegaly also can be seen in which right-sided cardiac decompensation has occurred. Pulmonary vasculature, however, remains sparse and tortuous (Fig. 267.1C).

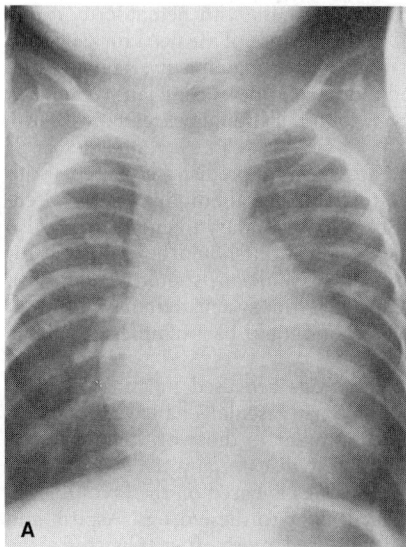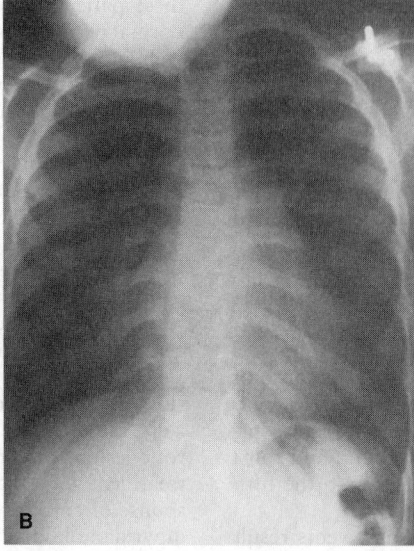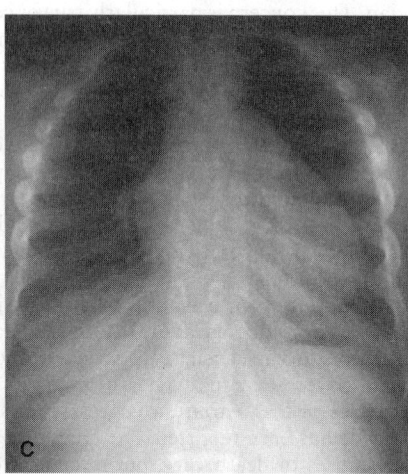

FIGURE 267.1. Progressive changes observed with pulmonary vascular obstructive disease in a series of chest radiographs from a patient with an unrepaired complete atrioventricular canal. **A:** At age 6 months, cardiomegaly with increased pulmonary vascular markings caused by pulmonary overcirculation is noted. **B:** At age 4 years, cardiac size is only slightly enlarged, with prominent main pulmonary arteries but diminished peripheral lung field vasculature. **C:** At age 15 years, cardiomegaly is caused by dilated, poorly functioning ventricles. The main pulmonary arteries are prominent, but the peripheral vasculature remains sparse.

Findings on electrocardiography are nonspecific and generally reflect the underlying lesion rather than identify specific pulmonary vascular disease. Ventricular enlargement, usually of both chambers if they are present, is a common finding. Enlargement of the atria, especially the right atrium, may occur with the onset of significant atrioventricular valve regurgitation.

Two-dimensional echocardiography is useful in delineating the anatomy of the underlying cardiac defects. Generally, Doppler echocardiography allows accurate prediction to be made of the pulmonary artery pressures. Pulmonary vascular resistance cannot be measured accurately by noninvasive means. In select cases, however, evidence of right-to-left shunting through such structures as the ductus arteriosus may be highly suggestive of elevated pulmonary vascular resistance.

In early mild cases, cardiac catheterization frequently is required to establish the diagnosis of obstructive pulmonary vascular disease. This diagnosis is crucial because very few cardiac lesions cannot be corrected or palliated surgically in the absence of advanced pulmonary vascular disease. Pulmonary vascular resistance and reactivity of the pulmonary bed to conditions that result in vasodilatation or constriction must be assessed carefully.

Generally, polycythemia is found after the onset of significant right-to-left shunt and increases as hypoxemia worsens. As a result, the hematocrit frequently increases to the 60% to 70% range. Because of increased production of red blood cells and high iron demands, indices of red cells frequently show indications of a relative iron deficiency anemia, despite an overall polycythemia.

Clinical Course

The onset of significant vascular changes occurs from as early as several months to as late as many years after birth. Large atrial septal defects, for example, seldom result in pulmonary obstructive disease until the patient is well into the adult years, whereas a child with Down syndrome and an atrioventricular canal defect may have significant disease as early as 2 or 3 months of age.

In patients who initially have large left-to-right shunt lesions, a period of hemodynamic stability follows the onset of obstructive pulmonary vascular disease. During this time, the amount of left-to-right shunting decreases, and symptoms of pulmonary congestion improve. The size of the heart usually decreases, and tolerance for exercise may improve, as does general well-being. Initially, the predominance of cardiac shunting remains from left to right, with evidence of occasional bidirectional flow.

As pulmonary vascular changes progress, the left-to-right shunting decreases, and the right-to-left shunting begins to predominate. With the onset of clinically evident hypoxemia, the patient's hemodynamic status usually deteriorates at an accelerated pace. Complications of systemic hypoxemia begin to arise. The effects of polycythemia and hypoxemia on pulmonary vascular resistance further compromise pulmonary blood flow.

Studies examining polycythemia and blood viscosity have found that the viscosity increases exponentially with the hematocrit. The crucial value appears to be the 70% to 75% range. At this hematocrit level, blood viscosity increases dramatically. In addition, studies indicate that both systemic vascular resistance and, especially, pulmonary vascular resistance increase exponentially with hematocrit as a result of the increase in viscosity. Coronary artery blood flow also decreases significantly as the hematocrit increases, although the degree of decrease in delivery of oxygen to the myocardium appears to be less than that to systemic tissues.

Generally, the presence of a mild degree of polycythemia resulting in a modest increase in hematocrit to the 55% to 65% range results in increased systemic oxygen delivery. When the hematocrit rises above approximately the 70% range, the blood viscosity rises dramatically, resulting in decreased delivery of oxygen because of decreased cardiac output, despite an increase in the oxygen-carrying capacity of the blood.

Clinically, the manifestations of polycythemia vary. Some patients may complain only of headaches or general malaise. Anorexia, dyspnea, and visual disturbances have been seen frequently. More severe problems, such as thrombi or embolic events, are less common occurrences, but they occur often enough to be a significant source of concern to the clinician. This concern is particularly true of central nervous system events, which may present initially with manifestations seen more commonly in polycythemia than as a frank focal deficit.

Causes of these findings are not known, although hyperviscosity and red blood cell aggregation seem to play a major role. In addition, abnormalities of platelet function are noted in these patients. Platelet half-life often appears to be reduced, and absolute thrombocytopenia is not an uncommon finding. Because of these abnormalities, the incidence of hemorrhage, especially postoperatively, is high in patients with polycythemia and hypoxemia.

Long-term survival rates in these patients vary because of both the patient's age at onset for pulmonary changes and complicating factors, such as Down syndrome, that may affect survival adversely. Usually, death occurs in the second and third decades of life. Variation is great, and survival into the fifth decade has been reported.

Causes of death vary, but often the terminal events result from a combination of hypoxia and arrhythmias. The occurrence of acute hypoxemic episodes during medical procedures (e.g., phlebotomy) that terminate in intractable ventricular arrhythmias lends credence to the notion that sudden death in these patients probably is the result of this mechanism; this cause is particularly likely if exercise-related sudden death occurs.

Complications of endocarditis, brain abscess, and cerebrovascular accidents also are causes of death related to the patient's hypoxemia and polycythemia. Changes in the pulmonary vascular bed result in an increased incidence of hemoptysis and pulmonary hemorrhage. Large pulmonary hemorrhage resulting in increasing hypoxemia, as well as systemic hypotension, can be rapidly fatal in these patients.

THERAPY

The use of heart-lung transplantation, lung transplantation, and repair of cardiac defects has been increasing in frequency since the 1980s. Problems with rejection (specifically bronchiolitis obliterans) and frequent occurrences of respiratory infections in this immunocompromised population have limited the success of these procedures. The current 2-year survival rate after undergoing bilateral lung transplantation is slightly more than 50%. In addition, the paucity of donor organs and mismatching of donor-recipient size frequently result in the death of patients awaiting transplantation. This problem has led to the use of partial living-donor lung transplantation in certain cases.

Because of morbidity and mortality that occur after transplantation, the long-term outcome is uncertain. Generally, transplantation should be reserved for patients with severe symptoms. In patients who do not warrant immediate consideration for transplantation or when transplantation is not a therapeutic option, care should consist of monitoring and treating the sequelae of chronic hypoxemia and the pulmonary vascular changes.

The hemoglobin status of patients should be monitored closely. An increased blood hemoglobin content is required to maintain systemic oxygen delivery in the normal range as hypoxemia increases. This level is beneficial as long as the hematocrit does not rise above the 60% to 65% range. Above this level, blood viscosity increases dramatically, and phlebotomy should be performed to lower the hematocrit to a safe range.

Of equal importance, anemia should not be tolerated because it seriously compromises delivery of oxygen. Anemia in these patients is relative and occurs with hematocrits in the normal to high-normal range because of the need for increased hemoglobin to expand oxygen-carrying capacity. Regular monitoring of indices of red blood cells alerts clinicians to any evidence of iron deficiency; if found, it should be treated with iron supplements.

An intracardiac right-to-left shunt predisposes patients with Eisenmenger syndrome to paradoxical embolization and endocarditis. Septic embolization secondary to endocarditis also may occur. Any significant infection should be evaluated for the possibility of endocarditis. Clinicians should be alert also to any changes in the central nervous system that may appear to be caused by polycythemia but could be a manifestation of a cerebral embolus or abscess.

Frequently, antiplatelet drugs are used in an attempt to slow progression of pulmonary vascular changes. Histologically, these changes appear similar to those of the atherosclerotic lesions of coronary artery disease, and the rationale for treatment with antiplatelet drugs is based on the favorable response of coronary artery lesions to these drugs. Aspirin and dipyridamole are the drugs used most often. Generally, the dosage is similar to that for adults with coronary artery disease, but it remains controversial. Long-term benefits of this therapy have not been proven.

Vasodilators of many types have been tried in patients with obstructive pulmonary vascular disease. They have produced limited results, partly because of the lack of responsiveness of the pulmonary bed, which has a relatively fixed obstruction, and partly because these vasodilators have the same or more vasodilating effect on the systemic vascular bed. Calcium channel blockers are the vasodilators used most widely; they have significant effect in less than 15% to 20% of the patient population.

Newer pulmonary vasodilative agents have been introduced during the last decade. Prostacyclin is the agent that has been used with the greatest frequency. It requires a continous intravenous infusion and may result in a life-threatening pulmonary hypertensive crises if administration is disrupted acutely. Trials of an inhaled form of prostacyclin are ongoing. Inhaled nitric oxide may be useful in certain short-term cases. Nitric oxide is a potent pulmonary vasodilator. It generally can be administered in only an intensive care setting, thus severely limiting its use as a long-term agent. Sildenafil stimulates release of endogenous nitric oxide. Studies of the effects of oral Sildenafil on pulmonary hypertension are ongoing.

Bosentan is a endothelin receptor antagonist. It blocks the effects of endothelin-1 on the pulmonary vasculatures smooth muscle. It has the advantage of oral adminstration and has been shown to be beneficial in improving symptoms and tolerance for exercise in patients with primary pulmonary hypertension. Its usefulness in patients with congenital heart disease and in children has not been demonstrated.

Finally, physicians should exercise care in performing any medical procedure on patients with Eisenmenger syndrome. This period can be a time of high risk for cardiac decompensation. Procedures such as phlebotomy and cardiac catheterization, which decrease circulating volume and systemic vascular resistance, can result in increased hypoxemia and tissue hypoxia if circulating volume is not maintained carefully. Surgical procedures and use of general anesthetic agents can result in vascular volume shifts and in an increased incidence of ventricular arrhythmias. Hypoventilation and resultant acidosis should be avoided during medical procedures. Embolic events, especially air emboli from intravenous lines, should be avoided because of the presence of right-to-left shunt in these patients. Careful monitoring as outlined herein can maximize the chances of an uneventful medical procedure in these very labile patients.

Suggested Readings

Anyanwu AC, Rogers CA, Murday AJ, Steering Group. Intrathoracic organ transplantation in the United Kingdom 1995–99: results from the UK cardiothoracic transplant audit. *Heart* 2002;87:449.

Beekman RH, Turi DT. Acute hemodynamic effects of increasing hemoglobin concentration in children with a right-to-left ventricular shunt and relative anemia. *J Am Coll Cardiol* 1985;5:357.

Boerboom LE, Olinger GN, Bonchek LI, et al. Aspirin or dipyridamole individually prevents lipid accumulation in primate vein bypass grafts. *Am J Cardiol* 1985;55:556.

Clabby ML, Canter CE, Moller JH, Bridges ND. Hemodynamic data and survival in children with pulmonary hypertension. *J Am Coll Cardiol* 1997;30: 554.

Olschewski H, Simoneau G, Nazzareno G, et al. Inhaled Lloprost for severe pulmonary hypertension. *N Engl J Med* 2002;323:347.

Lewis JR, Badesch DB, Barst RJ, et al. Bosentan therapy for pulmonary arterial hypertension. *N Engl J Med* 2002;896:346.

Nihill MR. The pathogenesis of pulmonary arteriosclerosis: propophylaxis with drugs that affect platelet aggregation. *Cardiovasc Dis Bull Texas Heart Inst* 1974;1:137.

Rosenthal A, Nathan DG, Marty AT, et al. Acute hemodynamic effects of red cell volume reduction in polycythemia of cyanotic congenital heart disease. *Circulation* 1970;42:297.

Steele P, Ellis JH, Weily HS, Genton E. Platelet survival time in patients with hypoxemia and pulmonary hypertension. *Circulation* 1977;55:660.

Stoica SC, McNeil KD, Perreas K, et al. Heart-lung transplantation for Eisenmenger syndrome: early and long-term results. *Ann Thorac Surg* 2001;72: 1887.

Wessel DL, Adatia I, Thompson JE, Hickey PR. Delivery and monitoring of inhaled nitric oxide in patients with pulmonary hypertension. *Crit Care Med* 1994;22:930.

Wood P. The Eisenmenger syndrome, or pulmonary hypertension with reversed central shunt. *BMJ* 1958;2:701.

CHAPTER 268 ■ SINGLE VENTRICLE

EDWARD V. COLVIN

A univentricular atrioventricular (AV) connection is present when both atria are connected to a single chamber within the ventricular mass. Even though most hearts so constituted have two chambers within the ventricular mass, *single ventricle* is the term used most often for this anomaly.

NOMENCLATURE

The segmental approach to nomenclature is used to describe single-ventricle hearts (Fig. 268.1). This nomenclature is presented in Box 268.1.

ANATOMY

Hearts with univentricular AV connection are subdivided according to ventricular morphology into three basic types: dominant left, dominant right, or indeterminate ventricular morphology. Dominant left or dominant right ventricular morphology can occur with D-loop or L-loop (Fig. 268.2).

The most common type is called *double-inlet left ventricle*, or *single left ventricle*. Usually, the nondominant ventricle is located anteriorly and to the left and gives rise to one or both of the great vessels.

Hearts in which the dominant chamber possesses an apical trabecular portion of right ventricular type are called *double-inlet right ventricle*, or *single right ventricle*. The nondominant ventricle is located posteriorly. Usually, this chamber has neither inlet nor outlet components.

Hearts in which only one abnormally trabeculated ventricle is found are termed hearts with *univentricular AV connection* and *indeterminate ventricular morphology*, or *single-ventricle with morphologically undetermined myocardium*.

Certain hearts have been described as having a ventricular mass containing a trabecular pattern typical of a right ventricle on one side and of a left ventricle on the other, with only a tiny

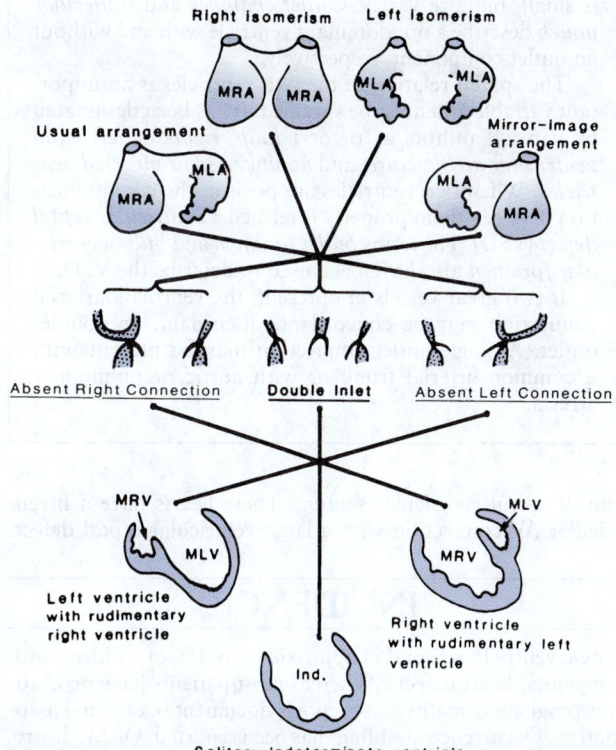

FIGURE 268.1. Atrial situs, modes of atrioventricular connection, and types of ventricular morphology. LA, left atrium; LV, left ventricle; M, morphologic; RA, right atrium; RV, right ventricle. (Reprinted from Becker AE, Anderson RH, Penkoske PA, Zuberbuhler JR. Morphology of double inlet ventricle. In: Anderson RH, Crupi G, Parenzan L, eds. *Double inlet ventricle.* Tunbridge Wells, UK: Castle House Publications, 1987:36, with permission.)

| BOX 268.1 | Terms Used to Describe Single-Ventricle Hearts |

Atrial situs may be solitus, inversus, or ambiguus with bilateral right or left morphology. The type of atrioventricular (AV) connection is, by definition, univentricular. The mode of connection may be double-inlet, absent left, or absent right AV connection. In double-inlet connection, the two atria may be connected to the ventricle by two separate AV valves or via a common valve. Usually, the two AV valves do not have typical characteristics of mitral and tricuspid valves and therefore are termed *right* and *left* on the basis of the anatomic location of the atrium to which they are connected.

In descriptive morphologic terms, a complete ventricle may have inlet, apical trabecular, and outlet components. Usually, the apical trabecular portion can be used to classify a chamber as being of right or left morphology. In the morphologically right ventricle, the apical component has characteristic coarse trabeculations. In contrast, the apical component of the morphologically left ventricle has much finer crisscrossing trabeculations and a smooth septal surface.

When two chambers are found within the ventricular mass, one has a right and the other a left ventricular apical trabecular component. Usually, the ventricle receiving the AV valve or valves is larger and is termed the *dominant ventricle*. The other ventricle is described as *nondominant*, or *rudimentary*. Usually, the nondominant ventricle is small, but size varies. *Outlet chamber* and *trabecular pouch* describe a nondominant ventricle with and without an outlet component, respectively.

The spatial relation of the two ventricles is an important variable and must be specified. It has been designated by various authors as D- or L-*loop*, *right-* or *left-hand ventricular architecture*, and *noninverted* or *inverted ventricles*. When two ventricles are present, the communication between them properly is termed a *ventricular septal defect* (VSD). The terms *outlet foramen* and *bulboventricular foramen* also have been used to describe the VSD.

If two great vessels are present, the ventriculoarterial connection may be concordant, discordant, or double-outlet. A single-outlet connection may be present with a common arterial trunk or with aortic or pulmonary atresia.

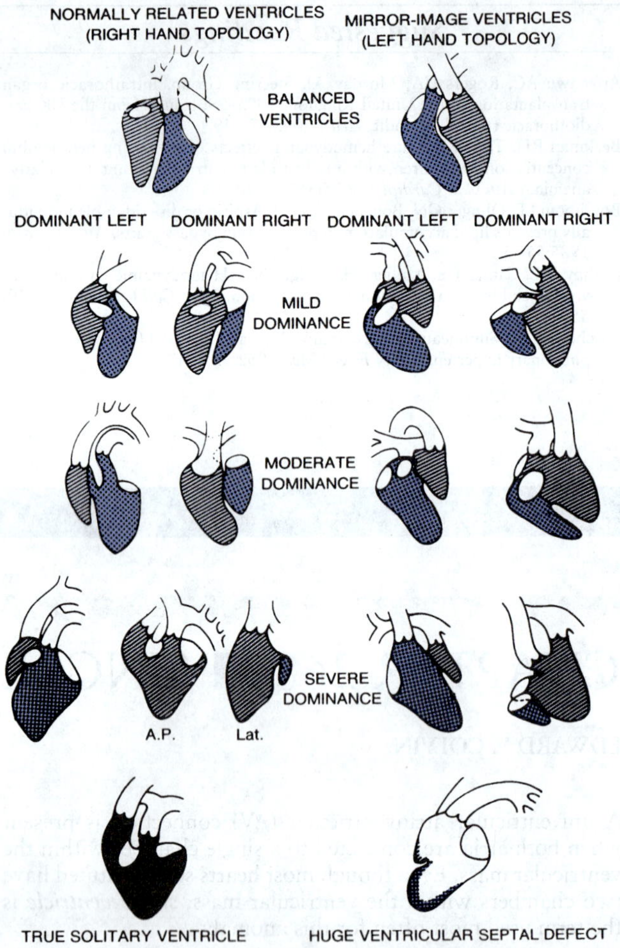

FIGURE 268.2. Spectrum of hearts with one large and one small ventricle. Hearts are traced from angiograms. A.P., anteroposterior; Lat., lateral. (Reprinted from Bargeron LM. Angiography of double inlet ventricle. In: Anderson RH, Crupi G, Parenzan L, eds. *Double inlet ventricle*. Tunbridge Wells, UK: Castle House Publications, 1987:146, with permission.)

rim of apical ventricular septum. These hearts have a biventricular AV connection with a large ventricular septal defect.

INCIDENCE

Single ventricle is found in approximately 1% of children with congenital heart defects. Whereas most patients have no chromosomal abnormality, case reports document occasional association. Occurrence in siblings has been reported. Of 237 hearts in one series, 140 had a dominant left ventricle, 34 had a dominant right ventricle, and 41 had indeterminate morphology. Associated cardiovascular anomalies are common.

CLINICAL MANIFESTATIONS

Most patients present early in life with cyanosis or congestive heart failure. A few children who are naturally balanced early in life present later in childhood with asymptomatic murmur and mild clinical cyanosis. A few neonates with left outflow obstruction have onset of poor perfusion when the ductus closes in the first few days of life.

Pulmonary stenosis is present in approximately 67% and atresia in 5% of cases. In earlier series, patients with atresia died without coming to surgery. More recently, the widespread availability of prostaglandin E_1 allows more of these patients to survive until they can undergo surgical correction. With stenosis, a harsh ejection-quality murmur at the base of the heart is present. With atresia, a continuous murmur from ductal patency is present.

Patients without pulmonary stenosis may present with a murmur or gallop in the first few days of life, but clinical symptoms usually do not become apparent until they reach the age of 3 to 6 weeks, when the fall in pulmonary vascular resistance allows excessive pulmonary blood flow. The findings at that time are those of congestive heart failure with tachypnea, subcostal retraction, poor feeding, hepatomegaly, and splenomegaly.

In patients with left AV valve atresia or severe stenosis and nearly intact interatrial septum, symptoms of pulmonary venous hypertension may develop as arteriolar resistance falls and pulmonary blood flow increases.

Subaortic obstruction may become manifest early. If present, the fetal circulation pattern usually is quite abnormal, and often a reduction in the size of the ascending aorta and severe coarctation or interruption of the aortic arch are present. If associated coarctation is present and the ductus closes, femoral pulses decrease. If the ductus is patent, palpable lower-extremity pulses in the presence of severe coarctation or interruption may occur.

DIAGNOSIS

Chest Radiography and Electrocardiography

Findings on chest radiography depend on the degree of pulmonary outflow obstruction. With moderately restricted pulmonary blood flow, generally the heart size is near normal and pulmonary vascular markings are normal. When pulmonary blood flow is obstructed severely, the pulmonary vascular markings are decreased. When little or no pulmonary stenosis is present, cardiomegaly with increased pulmonary vascular marking occurs. If pulmonary venous return is obstructed severely, the lung fields exhibit a reticular pattern.

Electrocardiographic findings vary. Usually, sinus rhythm occurs and the PR interval is normal, although first-degree heart block is present in approximately 30% of patients. Patients with first-degree heart block are not likely to progress to complete heart block during follow-up. Congenital complete heart block is present in a few patients. Efforts to relate findings on scalar electrocardiogram or the vectorcardiogram with the morphologic type of ventricular mass have been disappointing.

Two-Dimensional and Doppler Echocardiography

Two-dimensional echocardiography greatly reduces the time required to make a diagnosis. Pulsed range-gated Doppler sampling enables detection of any flow in the ductus and differentiation of venous from arterial structures in complicated cases. Insufficiency of AV valves can be detected and can be semiquantitated. Color flow mapping provides similar information more quickly. Continuous-wave Doppler enables quantitation of gradients.

Usually, structure and physiology are demonstrated well by these techniques, and catheterization can be directed to obtaining information not available by echocardiography. In many cases, catheterization can be postponed safely until the child is larger and less fragile.

Catheterization and Angiography

Timing of the catheterization may be dictated by the need in the newborn period for balloon atrial septostomy, shunting, or banding. Catheterization may demonstrate streaming of arterial and venous blood within the heart, so pulmonary and aortic oxygen saturations may differ significantly. The primary determinant of the systemic oxygen saturation is the amount of pulmonary arterial blood flow relative to the systemic blood flow ($\dot{Q}_p/\dot{Q}_s$).

Angiography has played a major role in the understanding of hearts with univentricular AV connection. Axial angiography enables clearer demonstration of the anatomy. Often, in fragile newborns, interest is in the anatomy crucial to planning a shunt procedure, and some injections may be deferred for later catheterizations.

NATURAL HISTORY

Case reports document survival into adulthood, and female patients have experienced successful pregnancy. Most patients exhibit exercise intolerance and cyanosis. Causes of death include dysrhythmia or sudden unexplained death, congestive heart failure, thrombotic occlusion of the pulmonary valve, brain abscess, pancreatitis, cerebral infarction, cerebral embolus and hemorrhage, and pulmonary embolus.

SURGERY

The dismal natural history for this group of patients has motivated development of numerous palliative procedures and two more radical "definitive" procedures: Fontan-type operations and septation. Palliative procedures include systemic–to–pulmonary artery shunts, pulmonary artery banding, atrial septectomy, atrial switch procedures, superior vena cava–to–right pulmonary artery anastomosis, and numerous procedures to relieve subaortic obstruction. The goal of these palliative procedures is to relieve symptoms and to allow survival to an age when a more "definitive" procedure can be performed. Deciding early in the life of the patient which definitive operations are possible, to establish the goals of early palliative surgery, is important.

Subaortic stenosis is an ominous finding in this group of patients. When subaortic stenosis is present with or without previous banding, numerous operations, including enlargement of the ventricular defect, placement of a left ventricular-to-descending aorta conduit, and anastomosis of the pulmonary artery to the ascending aorta with placement of a shunt (Damus-Kaye-Stansel operation), have been attempted to achieve palliation.

Fontan and Kreutzer devised an operation that used the single ventricle in tricuspid atresia to generate systemic blood flow while allowing pulmonary flow to occur directly from the right atrium to the pulmonary artery. This concept was extended to treatment of other forms of univentricular AV connection. For optimal candidates, the risk of operation is 2% to 10%. Presence of a significant subaortic gradient is associated with a high operative mortality rate. For the Fontan procedure in general, death seldom occurs, early after hospital dismissal. Late problems include ventricular dysfunction, AV valve insufficiency, atrial arrhythmia, and protein-losing enteropathy. Exercise performance in survivors is subnormal, although most patients carry on lives with minimal limitation on exercise.

In some centers, the Fontan operation is performed as a two-step procedure, with an initial cavopulmonary anastomosis and subsequent secondary operation performed to divert the inferior vena caval (IVC) flow to the pulmonary artery. The IVC flow may be directed to the pulmonary arteries by use of a lateral tunnel, an intraatrial tube, or an extracardiac tube. Fontan modifications also may include an initial fenestration in the IVC–to–pulmonary artery pathway, which may be closed later. Fenestration has allowed survival of patients who otherwise would be considered poor candidates for the Fontan operation.

When two AV valves are present, a septation operation may be considered. The single ventricle is divided by a large patch. Initially, operative mortality rates were high. Postoperative complete heart block was universal, and late postoperative sudden deaths occurred. A better outcome has been described for an ideal set of patients. More recently, a two-stage approach to septation has been reported. In early infancy, a patch is placed at the apex, and a second patch is placed between the AV valves. Widely spaced sutures are used to avoid the conduction system. A pulmonary artery band is placed. A second stage is undertaken 6 to 18 months later, at which time the opening between the two patches is closed and the band is removed. This approach has not been applied widely.

Improved operative risk after the Fontan-Kreutzer–type operation and the reasonable midterm results render this operation the current choice for patients to whom either operation could be applied.

For the newborn with pulmonary atresia or severe stenosis, a modified Blalock-Taussig shunt is placed. As the patient grows, cyanosis progresses, requiring a second intervention. A superior vena cava–to–right pulmonary artery anastomosis (bidirectional Glenn shunt) may be performed as an initial step toward a Fontan operation. If early evaluation reveals no pulmonary stenosis and the anatomy seems unlikely to lead to development of subaortic stenosis, pulmonary artery banding may be undertaken. For the patient with subaortic stenosis, a Damus-Kaye-Stansel operation and a systemic–to–pulmonary artery shunt are performed. If ventricular function, AV valve competency, and pulmonary vascular structures are acceptable, an elective Fontan operation is planned for the period when the patient is between 1.5 and 5.0 years of age.

Currently, septation is reserved as an option for older patients who have optimal internal anatomy and moderate elevation in pulmonary artery resistance and for whom Fontan repair is not possible. Cardiac transplantation is the only option for some of these patients.

Suggested Readings

Anderson RH, Becker AE, Tynan M, et al. The univentricular atrioventricular connection: getting to the root of a thorny problem. *Am J Cardiol* 1984;54: 822.

Becker AE, Anderson RH, Penkoske PA, Zuberbuhler JR. Morphology of double inlet ventricle. In: Anderson RH, Crupi G, Parenzan L, eds. *Double inlet ventricle*. Tunbridge Wells, UK: Castle House Publications, 1987:36.

Colvin EV. Single ventricle. In: Garson A Jr, Bricker JT, McNamara DG, eds. *The science and practice of pediatric cardiology*. Philadelphia: Lea & Febiger, 1988.

Crupi G, et al. Palliative surgery. In: Anderson RH, Crupi G, Parenzan L, eds. *Double inlet ventricle*. Tunbridge Wells, UK: Castle House Publications, 1987:165.

Danielson GK. Surgical management of double inlet ventricle. In: Anderson RH, Crupi G, Parenzan L, eds. *Double inlet ventricle*. Tunbridge Wells, UK: Castle House Publications, 1987:174.

Ebert PA. Staged partitioning of single ventricle. *J Thorac Cardiovasc Surg* 1984; 88:908.

Freedom RM. The dinosaur and banding of the main pulmonary trunk in the heart with functionally one ventricle and transposition of the great arteries: a saga of evolution and caution. *J Am Coll Cardiol* 1987;10:427.

Huhta JC, Seward JB, Tajik AJ, et al. Two-dimensional echocardiographic spectrum of univentricular atrioventricular connection. *J Am Coll Cardiol* 1985; 5:149.

Kopf GS, Kleinman CS, Hijazi ZM, et al. Fenestrated Fontan operation with delayed transcatheter closure of atrial septal defect. *J Thorac Cardiovasc Surg* 1992;103:1039.

Pacifico AD, Stefanelli G, Kirklin JW, Kirklin JK. Septation operation. In: Anderson RH, Crupi G, Parenzan L, eds. *Double inlet ventricle*. Tunbridge Wells, UK: Castle House Publications, 1987:183.

Van Praagh R, Ongley PA, Swan HJC. Anatomic types of single or common ventricle in man: morphologic and geometric aspects of 60 necropsied cases. *Am J Cardiol* 1964;13:367.

CHAPTER 269 ■ HYPOPLASTIC LEFT HEART SYNDROME

BENJAMIN W. EIDEM

First described by Lev in 1952, hypoplastic left heart syndrome (HLHS) is a constellation of congenital cardiac anomalies characterized by hypoplasia of the left ventricle (LV), left atrium, aortic and mitral valves, and ascending aorta. In 1958, Nadas and Noonan coined the term *hypoplastic left heart syndrome* and described the pathophysiology and clinical implications of this continuum of cardiovascular abnormalities.

EPIDEMIOLOGY AND GENETICS

HLHS is the fourth most common congenital heart lesion to present within the first year of life, accounting for 1.4% to 3.8% of congenital heart disease. With a birth prevalence described by the New England Regional Infant Cardiac Program of 0.163 per 1,000 live births, more than 1,000 infants with HLHS are expected to be born in the United States each year.

As many as 28% of patients with HLHS may have a definable genetic or extracardiac abnormality. Both autosomal recessive and multifactorial inheritance patterns have been suggested. HLHS has been reported in siblings, with a recurrence rate of 0.5% for HLHS and 2.2% for any congenital heart lesion. First-degree relatives have a 12% prevalence of cardiac

abnormalities, with a particularly high incidence of bicuspid aortic valves. Many syndromes, including Turner syndrome, Noonan syndrome, Smith-Lemli-Opitz syndrome, and Holt-Oram syndrome, have a known association with HLHS. Numerous chromosomal abnormalities have been and continue to be reported in children with HLHS and include the following: trisomy 9, 13, 18, and 21; duplication of 12p and 16q; chromosomal deletions 2q-, 4p-, 4q-, 7q-, 11q-, 18p-, and 22q11-; and balanced 3:7 translocation. Abnormalities of the central nervous system are the most common extracardiac malformation, with one series reporting a 29% incidence of major or minor neurologic abnormalities, including microcephaly, microencephaly, abnormal cortical mantle, agenesis of the corpus callosum, and holoprosencephaly.

ANATOMY AND PATHOLOGY

HLHS is characterized by significant hypoplasia of left heart structures, including the left atrium, LV, mitral and aortic valves, and ascending aorta. Most (85%) neonates with HLHS have a combination of aortic and mitral valve atresia or stenosis. The remainder (15%) typically present with a right ventricle

(RV)–dominant complete atrioventricular canal defect with malalignment of the ventricular septum, aortic atresia, and significant LV hypoplasia. Infrequently, patients with HLHS may have other associated cardiac lesions, including ventricular inversion or double-outlet RV. The degree of LV hypoplasia in HLHS is variable depending on the relative patency of the aortic and mitral valves. The LV cavity may be slit-like or absent, severely hypoplastic with prominent endocardial fibroelastosis, or even normal or nearly normal in size. The size of the ascending aorta varies depending on the patency of the aortic valve. An additional discrete juxtaductal coarctation often is found in 70% to 80% of infants with HLHS.

Right-sided heart structures, including the right atrium, RV, and pulmonary arteries characteristically are dilated. The left atrium in neonates with HLHS is significantly hypoplastic with thickened endocardium. A mildly restrictive interatrial communication typically is present, with a patent foramen ovale or small secundum atrial septal defect most commonly identified. An intact atrial septum is found in 10% of patients with HLHS and likely represents premature closure of the fossa ovalis *in utero* or a congenitally absent fossa ovalis. Pulmonary venous return to the hypoplastic left atrium usually is normal; however, anomalous pulmonary venous connections often occur in neonates with a significantly restrictive interatrial communication.

PATHOPHYSIOLOGY

Although HLHS has a heterogeneous anatomic substrate, the pathophysiologic manifestations are similar. Because oxygenation occurs in the placenta and the RV provides systemic output, fetuses with HLHS typically have normal *in utero* development. After birth, survival depends on the continued patency of intracardiac shunts at both atrial and ductal levels to maintain adequate systemic oxygenation and perfusion. Pulmonary venous return is shunted from the hypoplastic left atrium to the right atrium via a patent foramen ovale, where it mixes with systemic venous return. Systemic cardiac output from the RV must traverse a patent ductus arteriosus to provide antegrade blood flow to the body and vital organs via the descending aorta and retrograde blood flow to the aortic arch to supply the brachiocephalic vessels, ascending aorta, and coronary arteries.

Shortly after birth, normal physiologic changes can result in severe hemodynamic compromise. In the infant with HLHS, the systemic and pulmonary circulations run in parallel rather than in series. The proportion of systemic versus pulmonary blood flow is dependent on the relative resistances between the two circuits. The typical fall in neonatal pulmonary vascular resistance occurring after birth predisposes the infant with HLHS to increased pulmonary blood flow at the expense of adequate peripheral systemic perfusion. Improved oxygen saturation may obscure the underlying hemodynamic implications of this fall in pulmonary vascular resistance, leading to worsening systemic perfusion, metabolic acidosis, and congestive heart failure. Subsequent constriction of the ductus arteriosus further impairs systemic output, leading to profound metabolic acidosis, tissue hypoxemia, shock, and eventual death.

CLINICAL MANIFESTATIONS

Neonatal Presentation and Physical Examination

Infants with HLHS often appear normal at birth, with normal birth weight and Apgar scores. Male infants are affected more commonly than female infants (60% to 70%). Clinical presentation occurs in 40% of neonates by the time they are 2 days of age, in 75% by 6 days of age, and in 86% by 2 weeks of age.

The most common clinical presentation is one of respiratory distress secondary to increased pulmonary blood flow, with resultant congestive heart failure and worsening systemic perfusion. Symptoms generally appear on the second or third day of life and include progressive tachypnea, tachycardia, diminished peripheral pulses, hypothermia, and gradually increasing cyanosis. This early clinical presentation may be mistaken for sepsis, thus delaying diagnosis. The cardiac examination is significant for a prominent RV impulse with diminished LV impulse, a gallop rhythm, a single second heart sound, and often a soft systolic ejection or holosystolic murmur along the left sternal border. Because mixing occurs at the atrial level, systemic oxygen saturation is mildly, but symmetrically, decreased in all four extremities.

After significant constriction of the ductus arteriosus occurs, typically within the first few days of life, infants with HLHS may present with cardiovascular collapse. These neonates have profoundly decreased systemic perfusion with resultant severe myocardial dysfunction and typically present with concomitant metabolic acidosis, renal failure, seizures, and eventual death. Severe cyanosis presenting shortly after birth is the least common neonatal presentation of HLHS. Profound cyanosis most commonly results from inadequate intracardiac mixing at the atrial level caused by a restrictive atrial septum and typically necessitates prompt surgical intervention.

Electrocardiogram

The electrocardiogram in neonates with HLHS is nonspecific. Sinus tachycardia is a common occurrence, with a normal or rightward QRS axis in most infants (+90 to +210 degrees). A leftward QRS axis suggests an atrioventricular canal-type defect with LV hypoplasia. Both right atrial enlargement and RV hypertrophy are typical findings in HLHS. Decreased LV forces may be present (36%) but are not universal findings. Diffuse ST–segment–T-wave changes may reflect underlying coronary insufficiency. Subsequent electrocardiographic changes become more apparent postnatally and are related to both LV hypoplasia and concomitant RV volume and pressure overload.

Chest Radiography

Similar to electrocardiography, no specific radiologic pattern is diagnostic of HLHS, and findings may be normal in the immediate neonatal period. Cardiomegaly often is a prominent finding, with a globular cardiac contour described in one-third of neonates. Pulmonary vascular markings at birth also are variable. Increased vascular markings become more prominent after the first day of life. In infants with a restrictive atrial communication, a reticular pattern consistent with pulmonary venous obstruction often is evident radiographically.

DIAGNOSIS

Fetal Echocardiography

Fetal echocardiography has become the primary diagnostic modality for the early identification of HLHS. Fetal echocardiography provides accurate diagnosis as early as 16 weeks' gestation and also offers valuable insight into the natural

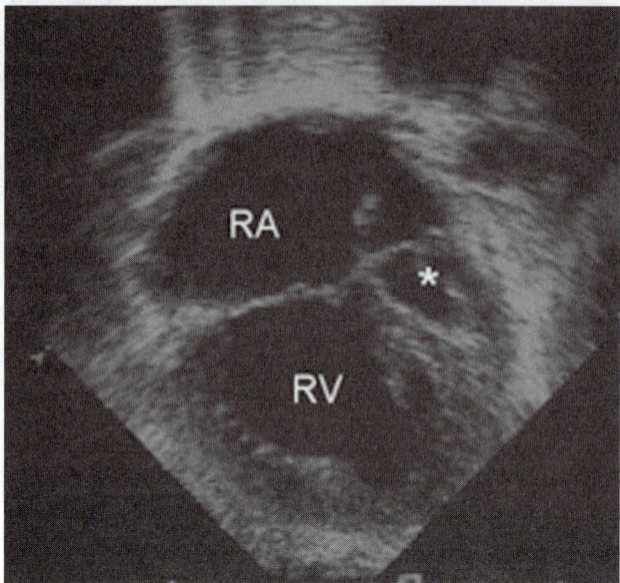

FIGURE 269.1. Apical four-chamber view demonstrating hypoplastic left heart syndrome in a neonate. Note the significant left ventricular (LV) hypoplasia (asterisk) and the dilated right heart chambers. RA, right atrium; RV, right ventricle.

progression of left heart hypoplasia *in utero*. Early identification of this congenital heart lesion *in utero* facilitates family counseling, allows evaluation for other fetal extracardiac and chromosomal abnormalities, enables coordination of perinatal and postnatal care, and has been shown to improve neonatal survival. Early fetal intervention strategies, including balloon dilatation of the fetal aortic valve, offer hope in the improvement of left heart hemodynamics and promotion of LV growth during pregnancy.

Postnatal Echocardiography

Postnatal echocardiography establishes the diagnosis of HLHS and is instrumental in defining the anatomic heterogeneity of the lesion as well as the overall clinical prognosis (Fig. 269.1). Classic features of HLHS readily defined by echocardiography include (a) marked hypoplasia of the left atrium and LV, (b) variable hypoplasia of the ascending and transverse aortic arch, (c) atresia or severe stenosis of the aortic valve, (d) severe hypoplasia or atresia of the mitral valve, (e) atrial septal morphology and communication (patent foramen ovale or atrial septal defect), and (f) the presence of significant coarctation of aorta. Of particular clinical importance, the patency of the ductus arteriosus, connection of the pulmonary veins, and size of the atrial communication all can be defined confidently. Assessment of global RV function, as well as of the anatomy and function of the tricuspid and pulmonary valves, also is indicated. Color Doppler echocardiography is useful to quantify the degree of tricuspid regurgitation, the presence of which is one of the important preoperative risk factors associated with poor outcome in these neonates. Finally, echocardiography can identify variants of HLHS, including unbalanced complete atrioventricular septal defects. Common features in this defect include the presence of a large primum atrial septal defect, inlet ventricular septal defect, and malalignment of the ventricular septum, resulting in significant LV hypoplasia.

Cardiac Catheterization

Preoperative cardiac catheterization rarely is indicated for the diagnosis of HLHS. Catheterization, however, often is helpful in the evaluation of complex systemic and pulmonary venous anomalies, evaluation of pulmonary arterial anatomy, and assessment of LV outflow tract obstruction and aortic arch anatomy. In neonates with restrictive atrial communications or recurrent postoperative aortic arch obstruction, interventional catheterization procedures may be helpful to relieve significant obstruction. In addition, cardiac catheterization remains routine in the preoperative evaluation before the second and third staged palliative procedures.

THERAPY

Without treatment, HLHS is an almost uniformly lethal lesion. Isolated case reports have documented survival of well-balanced unoperated patients into the third decade of life. However, the mortality in infants with HLHS is 95% during the first month of life.

Medical Management

Management strategies of infants born with HLHS classically have been divided into three basic approaches: (a) staged palliative reconstruction, (b) cardiac transplantation, and (c) supportive care only.

When considering either a staged palliative pathway or cardiac transplantation, immediate medical management is centered on maintaining ductal patency and optimizing the balance between systemic and pulmonary vascular resistance. Intravenous prostaglandin E_1 is effective in maintaining patency of the ductus arteriosus and enables the neonate to have optimized cardiac hemodynamics and a normalized acid-base balance before surgical intervention. Oxygen administration, hyperventilation, and high-dose inotropic agents should be avoided if possible so as not to alter the tentative balance between the pulmonary and systemic vascular beds.

Staged Palliative Reconstruction

Initial surgical palliation of the infant with HLHS, first described by Norwood and colleagues in 1980, usually is performed during the infant's first week of life. The goals of the Norwood operation are to ensure unobstructed systemic blood flow to the ascending and descending aorta, to provide a stable source of pulmonary blood flow, and to create a large nonrestrictive interatrial communication. These goals are achieved surgically by the following: (a) creating a large anastomosis between the proximal main pulmonary artery and the diminutive ascending aorta; (b) performing an extensive patch augmentation of the ascending aorta, transverse aortic arch, descending aorta, and pulmonary artery bifurcation; (c) extensively excising the septum primum to create a large atrial septal defect; and (d) placing a systemic-to-pulmonary artery shunt (Blalock-Taussig shunt) from the base of the innominate artery or subclavian artery to the proximal pulmonary artery bifurcation (typically a 3.0- to 3.5-mm Gore-Tex graft). Immediate and long-term surgical survival have improved dramatically following the Norwood procedure, with current 30-day hospital survival reported as high as 91% compared with just 63% perioperative survival 1 decade ago.

The second stage of palliation, the bidirectional Glenn anastomosis or hemi-Fontan procedure, typically is performed when the child is between 4 and 6 months of age. In this procedure, deoxygenated blood is directed from the superior vena cava into the proximal pulmonary artery, and the Blalock-Taussig shunt is ligated. This second stage of palliation has many advantages, including decreased RV volume overload, preservation of global RV function, and protection of the pulmonary vascular bed from pulmonary hypertension and pulmonary artery distortion. Perioperative survival for the bidirectional Glenn procedure is excellent and has been reported to be as high as 95% in many surgical series.

The final stage of the palliative reconstructive approach is the Fontan procedure, performed typically when the child is between 18 and 24 months of age. This surgical procedure involves creation of a tunnel, either within the right atrium or external to the heart, that directs systemic venous return from the inferior vena cava to the pulmonary artery. The creation of a small communication, or fenestration, between the Fontan tunnel and the systemic atrium also may be performed to allow gradual accommodation of systemic venous pressure within the Fontan circuit. Similar to the bidirectional Glenn anastomosis, perioperative survival for the Fontan operation is excellent, often exceeding 90% to 95% in most recent reported series.

Cardiac Transplantation

First attempted by Yacoub in 1984 and successfully performed by Bailey and colleagues in 1985, cardiac allotransplantation has become the preferred method of surgical intervention in some medical centers for neonates with HLHS. Although it provides a "biventricular repair" with more normal cardiac hemodynamics and physiology, cardiac transplantation continues to be associated with many challenges in the long-term palliation of neonates with HLHS. The most significant issue limiting cardiac transplantation is donor availability, with some series reporting mortality rates as high as 20% to 40% among those awaiting an available donor organ. However, neonates who undergo cardiac transplantation have excellent perioperative survival, reportedly 82% to 88%, and long-term survival at 5 years is improving. Long-term challenges primarily stem from the need of lifelong immunosuppression and include chronic organ rejection, renal dysfunction, hypertension, infection, and risk of development of both graft coronary artery disease and lymphoproliferative disease.

Compassionate Care

Once viewed as an acceptable management approach in infants with HLHS, compassionate care only no longer is an encouraged treatment strategy in most medical centers. With 5-year survival approaching 70% and the presence of major extracardiac malformations relatively low, the outcome of infants with HLHS currently rivals that of infants with many other commonly repaired congenital heart lesions.

OUTCOME

What once was an almost uniformly fatal congenital heart lesion with greater than 95% mortality rate at 1 month of age has become a surgically treatable lesion with improving long-term survival. Recent studies report 5-year survival rate in neonates with HLHS as high as 73% for staged palliation and 75% for cardiac transplantation. Although surgical mortality continues to improve, potential long-term morbidity in these patients becomes a significant consideration. Sudden cardiac death, most notably after the Norwood procedure, is not uncommon. Significant tricuspid regurgitation, RV dysfunction, and recurrent anatomic obstruction of either the pulmonary arteries or aortic arch also portend poor long-term outcome in these children.

Neurodevelopmental outcome is one of the greatest concerns facing physicians and families of infants with HLHS. Both congenital and acquired neurologic abnormalities are reported in as many as 40% of neonates with HLHS. In addition, the cumulative affects of persistent cyanosis and cardiopulmonary bypass with circulatory arrest also raise concerns for long-term developmental outcome. Studies in childhood survivors of HLHS report that most children have normal intelligence with low normal mean verbal and performance scores. These scores, however, are lower compared with children with other repaired congenital heart lesions. In addition, motor skills have been noted to lag behind concomitant verbal skills in these children.

Suggested Readings

Bauer J, Thul J, Kramer U, et al. Heart transplantation in children and infants: short-term and long-term follow-up. *Pediatr Transplant* 2001;5:457.

Brenner JI, Berg KA, Schneider DS, et al. Cardiac malformations in relatives of infants with hypoplastic left-heart syndrome. *Am J Dis Child* 1989;143:1492.

Chiavarelli M, Gundry SR, Razzouk AJ, et al. Cardiac transplantation for infants with hypoplastic left heart syndrome. *JAMA* 1993;270:2944.

Douglas WI, Goldberg CS, Mosca RS, et al. Hemi-Fontan procedure for hypoplastic left heart syndrome: outcome and suitability for Fontan. *Ann Thorac Surg* 1999;68:1361.

Gaynor JW, Mahle WT, Cohen MI, et al. Risk factors for mortality after the Norwood procedure. *Eur J Cardiothorac Surg* 2002;22:82.

Ikle L, Hale K, Fashaw L, et al. Developmental outcome of patients with hypoplastic left heart syndrome treated with heart transplantation. *J Pediatr* 2003;142:20.

Mahle WT, Clancy RR, Moss EM, et al. Neurodevelopmental outcome and lifestyle assessment in school-aged and adolescent children with hypoplastic left heart syndrome. *Pediatrics* 2000;105:1082.

Mahle WT, Spray TL, Wernovsky G, et al. Survival after reconstructive surgery for hypoplastic left heart syndrome: a 15-year experience from a single institution. *Circulation* 2000;102(suppl 3):III136.

Norwood WI Jr. Hypoplastic left heart syndrome. *Ann Thorac Surg* 1991;52:688.

Tweddell JS, Hoffman GM, Mussatto KA, et al. Improved survival of patients undergoing palliation of hypoplastic left heart syndrome: lessons learned from 115 consecutive patients. *Circulation* 2002;106(suppl 1):I82.

Tworetzky W, McElhinney DB, Reddy VM, et al. Improved surgical outcome after fetal diagnosis of hypoplastic left heart syndrome. *Circulation* 2001;103:1269.

CHAPTER 270 ■ CARDIAC MALPOSITION AND HETEROTAXY

HOWARD P. GUTGESELL

CARDIAC MALPOSITION

The term *cardiac malposition* implies location of the heart anywhere other than in its usual position in the left hemithorax, or it may describe location of the heart in the left hemithorax when other organs are in abnormal positions, as in situs inversus viscerum. *Dextrocardia*, *levocardia*, and *mesocardia* are general terms that indicate the cardiac position only and do not describe intracardiac anatomy. Dextrocardia denotes a right-sided heart, levocardia a left-sided heart, and mesocardia a midline heart. Situs solitus is the normal or usual arrangement of organs (i.e., heart on left, liver on right, stomach on left). Situs inversus is the mirror image of normal (i.e., heart on right, liver on left, stomach on right). The term *heterotaxy* designates abnormal arrangements of body organs that differ from the orderly arrangements of situs solitus or situs inversus. Typically, duplication or absence of normally unilateral structures occurs (especially the spleen). The terms *situs ambiguus* and *indeterminate situs* are synonymous with heterotaxy. Isomerism indicates presence of paired, mirror-image sets of normally unilateral structures, such as the lungs and atria. Left isomerism refers to the presence of two anatomic left lungs and two left atria, whereas right isomerism implies bilateral right lungs and atria.

Dextrocardia

The incidence of situs inversus is 1 in 8,000 to 1 in 7,000 living persons. Dextrocardia with situs solitus (isolated dextrocardia) occurs less commonly. Incidence estimates are as low as 1 in 29,000.

Dextroversion, dextrorotation, and pivotal dextrocardia describe dextrocardia with situs solitus. Often, the heart appears as if the apex has been swung from the left side of the chest to the right side. The term *isolated dextrocardia* similarly connotes that the other organs are in their normal locations and that dextrocardia is an isolated finding. Generally, *mirror-image dextrocardia* is applied to more or less normal hearts in subjects with situs inversus. Dextrocardia resulting from displacement of the heart into the right hemithorax by external causes (pneumothorax, diaphragmatic hernia, or hypoplasia of the right lung) is termed *secondary dextrocardia* or *dextroposition*.

Although dextrocardia can be diagnosed by physical examination, usually it is detected by chest roentgenography. The clinical presentation may be that of a newborn with cyanosis, respiratory distress, or heart murmur. In cases of secondary dextrocardia, a chest roentgenogram may be the only diagnostic test necessary (e.g., in pneumothorax). In the absence of such an obvious cause, the initial step in evaluating dextrocardia is to determine the situs of the other viscera. Frequently, a chest roentgenogram is useful in showing the location of the liver and stomach. The situs of the lungs may be inferred from chest films. On the electrocardiogram (ECG), a P vector directed leftward and inferiorly suggests situs solitus of the atria, whereas a rightward P axis suggests situs inversus. The details of visceral situs and intracardiac anatomy can be determined by echocardiography, supplemented by magnetic resonance imaging or angiocardiography.

Frequently, dextrocardia in the presence of situs solitus is associated with major intracardiac abnormalities (Fig. 270.1). The most common findings are summarized in Table 270.1. Often, atrioventricular discordance (L-loop ventricles), single ventricle, transposition, and pulmonary stenosis or atresia are present.

The *scimitar syndrome* is an uncommon but well-described constellation of cardiopulmonary anomalies consisting of dextrocardia, situs solitus of the atria and viscera, hypoplasia of the right lung, anomalous systemic arterial blood supply to the right lung, and anomalous pulmonary venous connection of the right lung to the inferior vena cava. Often, the anomalous pulmonary vein is visible on the chest roentgenogram as a curvilinear shadow in the right lung and resembles a Turkish sword or scimitar (Fig. 270.2).

The incidence of congenital heart disease in subjects with dextrocardia and situs inversus is much lower than that in

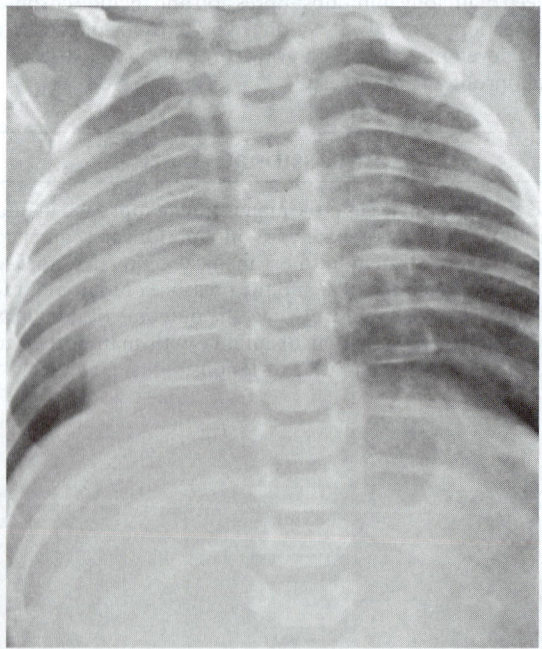

FIGURE 270.1. Chest roentgenogram in a neonate with dextrocardia. Echocardiography revealed situs solitus and normal intracardiac anatomy. The heart has shifted to the right, a process probably related to hypoplasia of the right lung.

TABLE 270.1

INCIDENCE OF INTRACARDIAC ABNORMALITIES IN PATIENTS WITH DEXTROCARDIA

Dextrocardia with situs solitus
Normal heart 5%
Congenital heart disease 95%
  Common lesions
  AV discordance
  Single ventricle or VSD
  "Corrected" TGA
  PS/PA

Dextrocardia with situs inversus
Normal heart >95%
Congenital heart disease <5%
  Common lesions
  VSD, DORV
  PS/PA
  "Complete" TGA
  Right aortic arch

AV, Antrioventricular; DORV, double-outlet right ventricle; PS/PA, pulmonary stenosis or atresia; TGA, transposition of the great arteries; VSD, ventricular septal defect.

subjects with dextrocardia and situs solitus. Although precise determination is not available, the incidence of congenital heart disease may not differ from that in the general population (approximately 8 in 1,000). Cardiac abnormalities found in dextrocardia with situs inversus are summarized in Table 270.1. Atrioventricular discordance and transposition complexes are common findings but occur less frequently than in dextrocardia with situs solitus. Double-outlet right ventricle, pulmonary stenosis or atresia, and ventricular septal defect are present in one-third to two-thirds of reported cases. Usually, the aortic arch is right-sided.

As many as 15% to 25% of patients with situs inversus have chronic respiratory disease. The most notable is Kartagener syndrome. In 1933, Kartagener described four patients with situs inversus, chronic sinusitis, nasal polyposis, and bronchiectasis. The ultrastructural basis for the respiratory disease and for the male infertility found in this syndrome subsequently was shown to be an abnormality on the dynein arms on the microtubules of the cilia and spermatozoa, with resultant immotility of the spermatozoa and decreased mucociliary transport.

Levocardia

Almost invariably, levocardia occurring in the presence of situs inversus or heterotaxy is associated with major intracardiac anomalies. The most common lesions include atrioventricular canal, transposition complexes, and pulmonary stenosis or atresia. The likelihood of occurrence of asplenia or polysplenia is high (80%).

Mesocardia

Mesocardia, or midline heart, is found in fewer than 1% of autopsied cases of congenital heart disease, but clinicians viewing large numbers of roentgenograms have a somewhat different perspective. Many tall, slender adolescents and adults have an almost vertical heart, a condition that may be termed *mesocardia*. Thus, the setting in which mesocardia occurs is important; cyanotic newborns with a murmur and a midline heart are likely to have serious heart disease, whereas a midline heart probably is of no concern in asymptomatic children with no murmur.

Summary

Four generalizations apply to hearts in abnormal locations within the thorax. First, dextrocardia with situs solitus (isolated dextrocardia) almost always is associated with major intracardiac defects. Scimitar syndrome should be considered even in the absence of obvious intracardiac abnormalities. Second, in dextrocardia with situs inversus, the incidence of congenital heart disease probably is the same as that in the general population. The Kartagener syndrome is present in 15% to 25% of patients with situs inversus. Third, isolated levocardia almost invariably is associated with major intracardiac abnormalities. Fourth, approximately one-third of patients with dextrocardia and at least two-thirds of those with isolated levocardia have either asplenia or polysplenia.

HETEROTAXY

Heterotaxy, or situs ambiguus, represents a defect in laterality. A genetic basis is likely, and familial cases indicate abnormalities of both autosomal and X-linked genes with both dominant and recessive expression. Although some overlap occurs, patients tend to have features of either right isomerism (so-called asplenia syndrome) or left isomerism (polysplenia syndrome).

Asplenia Syndrome

The usual presentation in asplenia syndrome is that of cyanotic newborns, often with respiratory distress. The first and second heart sounds are single. An ejection systolic murmur, a continuous murmur, or the absence of murmur may be exhibited. Often, a midline liver is identifiable by palpation. Clues to the presence of asplenia syndrome often are found on chest roentgenography (Fig. 270.3), and this condition should be considered when the cardiac position is discordant with that of

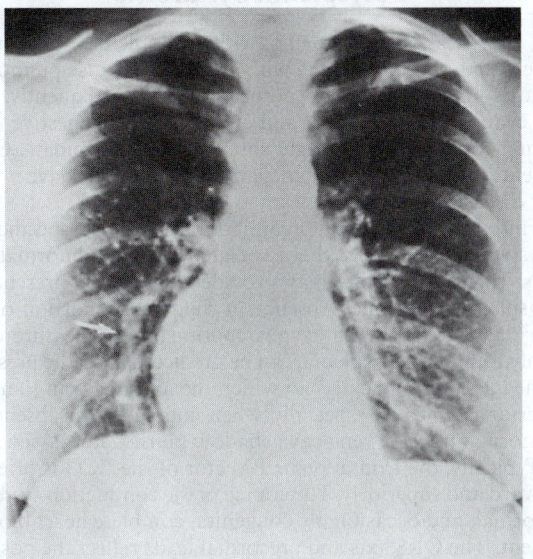

FIGURE 270.2. Scimitar syndrome in young adult with mild dextrocardia (actually mesocardia). Note in the right lung the vertical shadow (*arrow*) created by the anomalous right pulmonary vein's descent toward the diaphragm to join the inferior vena cava.

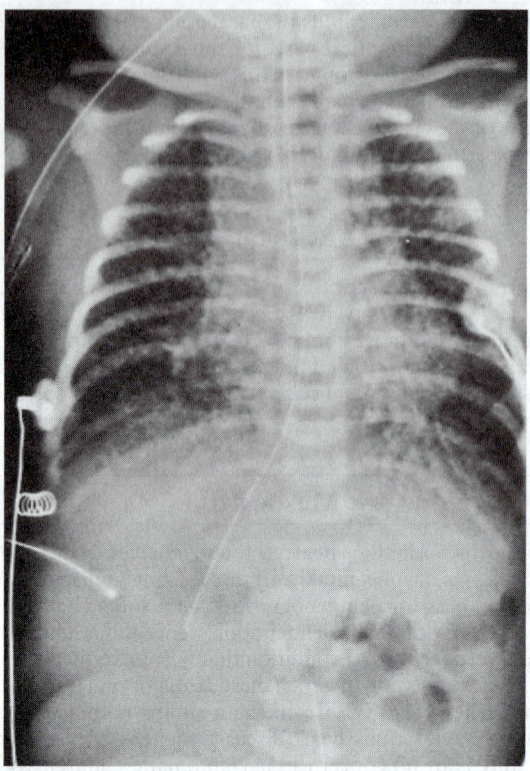

FIGURE 270.3. Chest roentgenogram of a neonate with asplenia syndrome. Although the heart is on the left, the stomach is on the right. Prominent pulmonary venous markings are the result of the obstructed form of the total anomalous pulmonary venous connection. Intracardiac anomalies included complete atrioventricular canal, transposition of the great arteries, and pulmonary atresia.

the stomach and liver, especially if pulmonary vascular markings are very diminished (owing to pulmonary atresia) or if pulmonary edema (obstructed pulmonary veins) is evident.

Generally, the ECG is abnormal, but the findings are not specific for asplenia. The P-wave axis may be either leftward and inferior (normal) or rightward and inferior because of the frequency of bilateral sinus nodes. Occasionally, congenital complete heart block is present. The QRS axis and morphology reflect the cardiac position and intracardiac anatomy; the QRS axis tends to be superior in the presence of two ventricles and inferior in patients with a single ventricle.

Details of intracardiac anatomy and systemic and pulmonary venous connections can be established by two-dimensional echocardiography, magnetic resonance imaging, and angiocardiography. The presence of Howell-Jolly bodies in the red blood cells in a peripheral blood smear suggests asplenia, although occasionally these bodies are present in physiologically normal infants in the first week of life. Absence of the spleen can be documented by ultrasonography, computed tomography, or radionuclide scans.

Major intracardiac abnormalities are present in nearly all subjects with congenital asplenia (Table 270.2). Atrioventricular canal, transposition of the great arteries, and pulmonary stenosis or atresia are present almost invariably, and approximately 75% of cases have total anomalous pulmonary venous connection. Typically, patients with asplenia syndrome have two "right" lungs (i.e., three-lobed) and two anatomic "right" atria, giving the impression of bilateral right-sidedness, or right isomerism.

Patients with asplenia are at increased risk for acquisition of overwhelming bacterial infection, and administration of prophylactic antibiotics is recommended. In the first 6 months of

TABLE 270.2

COMPARISON OF ASPLENIA AND POLYSPLENIA SYNDROMES

Asplenia (Right Isomerism)	Polysplenia (Left Isomerism)
Incidence of CHD	
>95%	90–95%
Common cardiac lesions	
AV canal	AV canal
TGA	VSD
PS/PA	DORV
TAPVC	PAPVC
	Absent IVC
Dextrocardia in 40%	Dextrocardia in 40%
Other	
Howell-jolly bodies on blood smear	Malrotation of bowel
Predisposition of sepsis	Biliary atresia
Malrotation of bowel	

AV, Antrioventricular; CHD, congenital heart disease; DORV, double-outlet right ventricle; IVC, inferior vena cava; PAPVC, partial anomalous pulmonary venous connections; PS/PA, pulmonary stenosis or atresia; TAPVC, total anomalous pulmonary venous connections; TGA, transposition of the great arteries; VSD, ventricular septal defect.

life, coverage against gram-negative and gram-positive organisms is advised; amoxicillin is used most frequently. Generally, penicillin is sufficient for older infants and children. Likewise, administration of pneumococcal and *Haemophilus influenzae* vaccines is recommended. Serologic testing confirms that an adequate response has been achieved.

Many of the cardiac anomalies associated with the asplenia syndrome are amenable to palliative surgery or to intracardiac repair using modifications of the Fontan technique. Because of the complexity of the intracardiac lesions and the decreased immune function, the prognosis for infants with the asplenia syndrome is guarded, but it has been improved by advances in the surgical management of cardiac abnormalities.

Polysplenia Syndrome

The presentation of patients with polysplenia varies more widely than that of patients with asplenia. Because pulmonary stenosis and transposition occur relatively infrequently, usually cyanosis is not severe, and symptoms of congestive heart failure from large left-to-right shunts may predominate. Other patients may be asymptomatic, and some patients have no cardiac disease at all.

Findings on physical examination are not specific for polysplenia and reflect the associated cardiac abnormalities. Chest roentgenography may provide clues to the presence of polysplenia syndrome. Absence of the hepatic portion of the inferior vena cava with azygos continuation, a feature commonly found in polysplenia, can be predicted from the presence of mediastinal "knuckle," in which the azygous vein joins the superior vena cava, especially when coupled with absence of the normal inferior vena cava shadow on the lateral view.

Typically, the frontal plane P vector of the ECG is oriented leftward and superiorly. The course of the conduction system is abnormal, and occasionally congenital complete heart block is present. The QRS axis and precordial leads reflect the position of the heart in the thorax and the nature of the intracardiac lesion. A superiorly oriented frontal plane QRS axis reflecting atrioventricular canal defect is common.

The intracardiac and vascular abnormalities occurring in the polysplenia syndrome are summarized in Table 270.2.

Despite considerable overlap, certain features occur with much higher frequency in either asplenia or polysplenia, a finding fostering the notion that these conditions represent syndromes. Atrioventricular canal defect is found commonly in both conditions. In polysplenia, the absence of the hepatic portion of the inferior vena cava is a common finding, as is partial anomalous pulmonary venous connection. Pulmonary stenosis or atresia is uncommon in polysplenia, and normally related great arteries are seen more commonly than is transposition.

Many of the cardiac abnormalities associated with polysplenia are amenable to surgical correction. Unlike its incidence in asplenia, overwhelming bacterial infection is not a risk factor.

ECTOPIA CORDIS

Ectopia cordis is the rarest and most dramatic of the cardiac malpositions. The heart is either partially or totally outside the thorax. The thoracic type is the classic form of ectopia cordis. The entire heart lies outside the thorax, uncovered by pericardium. Attempts to place the heart into the thorax have been difficult because of cardiorespiratory insufficiency resulting from compression of the heart and lungs within the small thoracic cavity.

The thoracoabdominal form of ectopia cordis occurs as part of a constellation of associated anomalies, including midline supraumbilical abdominal defect, defect in the distal sternum, deficiency of the diaphragmatic pericardium, deficiency of the anterior diaphragm, and intracardiac defect.

Intracardiac abnormalities occur commonly but not invariably in patients with ectopia cordis. The most frequently seen abnormalities are atrial and ventricular septal defect, tetralogy of Fallot, and tricuspid atresia. Additionally, a diverticulum protruding from the apex of the left ventricle is present in 20% of patients with a thoracoabdominal defect.

Suggested Readings

Anderson C, Devine WA, Anderson RH, et al. Abnormalities of the spleen in relation to congenital malformations of the heart: a survey of necropsy findings in children. *Br Heart J* 1990;63:122.

Aylsworth AS. Clinical aspects of defects in the determination of laterality. *Am J Med Genet* 2001;101:345.

Azakie A, Merklinger SL, Williams WG, et al. Improving outcomes of the Fontan operation in children with atrial isomerism and heterotaxy syndromes. *Ann Thorac Surg* 2001;72:1636.

Gikonyo DK, Tandon R, Lucas RF Jr, Edwards JE. Scimitar syndrome in neonates: report of four cases and review of the literature. *Pediatr Cardiol* 1986;6:193.

Ivemark BI. Implications of agenesis of the spleen in the pathogenesis of conotruncus anomalies in childhood: an analysis of the heart malformations in the splenic agenesis syndrome, with fourteen new cases. *Acta Paediatr* 1955;44 (suppl 104):1.

Peoples WM, Moller JH, Edwards JE. Polysplenia: a review of 146 cases. *Pediatr Cardiol* 1983;4:129.

Stanger P, Rudolph AM, Edwards JE. Cardiac malpositions: an overview based on study of sixty-five necropsy specimens. *Circulation* 1977;56:159.

Van Mierop LHS. Asplenia and polysplenia syndrome: original article series. *Birth Defects* 1972;8:74.

Webber SA, Sandor GGS, Patterson MWH, et al. Prognosis in asplenia syndrome: a population-based review. *Cardiol Young* 1992;2:129.

CHAPTER 271 ■ DEFECTS OF THE ATRIAL SEPTUM, INCLUDING THE ATRIOVENTRICULAR CANAL

G. WESLEY VICK III AND LOUIS I. BEZOLD

Congenital defects of the atrial septum are common occurrences. They may be located in different anatomic portions of the atrial septum, and the location of the defect generally reflects the abnormality of embryogenesis that led to the anomaly (Fig. 271.1) Atrial septal defect (ASD) may be isolated or may be associated with other congenital cardiac abnormalities. ASD sizes vary greatly, and functional consequences are related to the anatomic location of the defect, the size of the defect, and the presence or absence of other cardiac anomalies.

Developmental defects resulting from abnormalities in partitioning of the embryologic atrioventricular (AV) canal and in the endocardial cushions often lead to a communication between the right and left atria. Most AV canal (endocardial cushion) malformations demonstrate major anomalies of the AV valves in addition to an intraatrial communication. Defects of the ventricular septum often are present.

Interatrial communications can be considered in two groups. The first group results from abnormal development of the septa that normally partition the atrial portion of the developing heart into right and left atria. The second group includes interatrial communications that result primarily from maldevelopment of the partitioning of the AV canal and endocardial cushions. The first group may be viewed as isolated ASDs and the second group as AV canal defects.

ISOLATED ATRIAL SEPTAL DEFECTS

Isolated ASDs include patent foramen ovale, ASD at the fossa ovalis (secundum ASD), defects superior to the fossa ovalis (superior sinus venosus type ASD, superior vena caval defect), defects inferior to the fossa ovalis (inferior sinus venosus type ASD, inferior vena caval defect), and coronary sinus defects. AV canal defects include complete forms, incomplete forms, and common atrium. Pathophysiologic features of ASDs are described in Box 271.1.

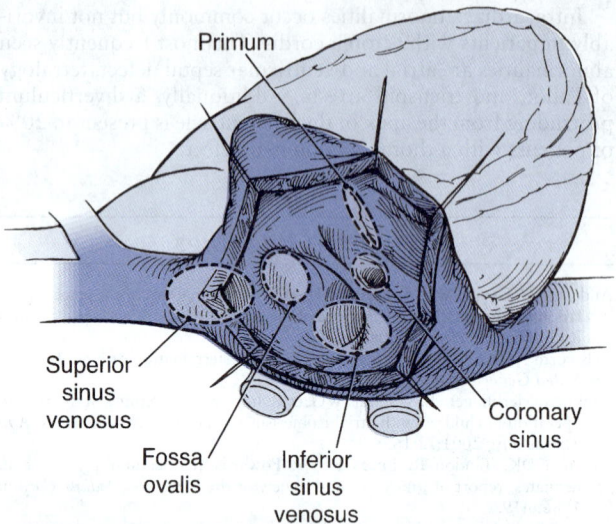

FIGURE 271.1. Atrial septal defects. Only defects within the fossa ovalis are true defects of the interatrial septum, although all the defects permit interatrial shunting.

Associated Cardiac Defects

ASDs often occur in conjunction with other congenital cardiac anomalies. In many of these anomalies, the associated defects are the lesions of primary importance; however, the ASD may play a major role in the physiologic features of the condition. For example, in complete transposition of the great arteries, an ASD permits mixing between the pulmonary and systemic circulations necessary to sustain life. Another example is tricuspid atresia, in which the entire cardiac output must pass across the ASD.

Effect on Intrauterine and Postnatal Cardiac Physiology

Because pulmonary blood flow is relatively minimal before birth, nearly all blood reaching the left atrium does so by passage across the foramen ovale. When the lungs expand after birth, pulmonary venous return to the left atrium increases substantially, concomitant with a fall in pulmonary vascular resistance and an increase in systemic vascular resistance. As a result, left atrial pressure normally rises above the right atrial pressure, and functional closure of the foramen ovale occurs. When an ASD is present, intrauterine physiology is largely unchanged. However, after birth, the normal hemodynamic changes result in left-to-right shunting at the atrial level. In some patients with elevated pulmonary pressures, right-to-left shunting via the ASD also may occur and may be associated with mild cyanosis in the neonatal period.

Significance of Atrial Septal Defects

Small Defects

Small ASDs are defined as those with a pulmonary-to-systemic flow ratio ($\dot{Q}_p : \dot{Q}_s$) of less than 2:1 in the absence of significant associated cardiovascular anomalies. The presence of a small ASD does not cause major changes in cardiac hemodynamics, although these defects may allow paradoxical embolism whenever the right atrial pressure rises above the left atrial pressure.

| BOX 271.1 | Pathophysiologic Features of Atrial Septal Defects |

Patent Foramen Ovale

If the flap valve of the foramen ovale (the remnant of the embryonic septum primum) is competent, shunting at the atrial level cannot occur as long as left atrial pressure remains higher than right atrial pressure. However, even in physiologically normal individuals, the right atrial pressure may rise transiently above the left atrial pressure. In this circumstance, right-to-left interatrial shunting may occur if the valve of the foramen ovale is not sealed anatomically or is insufficient to close the foramen ovale. Similarly, blood clots or other emboli may cross the atrial septum from right to left in such circumstances (paradoxical embolism). In patients with pulmonary vascular disease or pulmonary stenosis, right-to-left shunting across a patent foramen ovale may be sufficient to cause systemic arterial desaturation.

Approximately 30% to 40% of normal adult hearts have a patent, valve-incompetent foramen ovale that usually is not considered a true atrial septal defect. This valve incompetence may be congenital or may be acquired by stretching of the right or left atrium in conditions in which those chambers are enlarged.

Defects at the Fossa Ovalis (Secundum Defects)

Typical defects in the fossa ovalis are contained within the area bordered by the limbus of the fossa ovalis. Sizes of these defects vary greatly. In addition, the floor of the fossa ovalis (valve of foramen ovale) in this region may be fenestrated, so multiple defects can occur. Secundum defects may be associated with or confluent with other defects of the atrial septum, such as a sinus venosus defect or an ostium primum defect.

Sinus Venosus Defects

Superior sinus venosus defects (sometimes called *superior vena caval defects*) are located in the part of the atrial septum immediately below the superior vena caval orifice. The right upper- and middle-lobe pulmonary veins often connect to the superior vena caval and right atrial junction, resulting in a partial anomalous pulmonary venous connection.

Inferior sinus venosus defects (sometimes called *inferior vena caval defects*), which are less common than superior defects, are located in the part of the atrial septum immediately above the inferior vena caval orifice. Frequently, inferior sinus venosus defects also are associated with partial anomalous connection of the right pulmonary veins.

Coronary Sinus Defect

Coronary sinus defects are characterized by absence of part or all of the common wall between the coronary sinus and the left atrium. A persistent left superior vena cava also is present in many cases.

Moderate and Large Defects

Moderate and large ASDs are defined as those associated with a $\dot{Q}_p : \dot{Q}_s$ greater than 2:1 in the absence of significant associated cardiovascular anomalies. The direction of the atrial level shunt is determined by the relative pressures in the right and left atria. The atrial pressures are determined principally by the resistances to filling of the respective ventricles. Thus, with large defects, the volume of the shunting does not depend solely on the size of the defect, but rather on the relative compliance of the right and left ventricles.

Natural History

Isolated secundum ASDs typically do not cause major symptoms during infancy and childhood. In the absence of unrelated problems, more than 99% of patients with isolated secundum defects will live beyond the first year of life. Although unusual, mild cyanosis sometimes is evident during the neonatal period. Children and infants with these defects tend to be somewhat smaller than normal, but failure to thrive on the basis of an ASD alone is a rare occurrence. Exercise intolerance may develop in some patients as early as the second decade of life, whereas others may remain asymptomatic for several more decades.

Left-to-right shunting tends to increase with age in many patients. Thus, the frequency of congestive heart failure with attendant fluid retention, hepatomegaly, and elevated jugular venous pressure increases with the age of the patient. The large shunts present in many older patients cause stretching of the atria, which presumably predisposes to atrial arrhythmias, including atrial flutter, fibrillation, and tachycardia. These arrhythmias are a major cause of morbidity and mortality in older patients with ASDs. Pulmonary vascular disease does develop occasionally in older patients with isolated ASD, but this complication is a rare finding in children and adolescents.

A recent natural history study on the growth of secundum ASDs reported growth in the size of the defect in 65% of children at a mean rate of 0.8 mm/year. Although defects greater than 12 mm in diameter tended to have a higher rate of growth than did smaller defects, this study demonstrated the potential for even initially small defects (less than 6 mm) to enlarge to the point that transcatheter closure may be difficult (larger than 20 mm).

Conversely, what has become apparent is that a substantial number of ASDs detected during infancy will close spontaneously. Radzik and colleagues observed a closure rate of 87% in 101 patients with secundum ASDs identified before 3 months of age using two-dimensional and Doppler echocardiography over a follow-up period of 265 ± 190 days. All defects less than 3 mm (n = 32) closed spontaneously; however, no defect larger than 8 mm (n = 4) was observed to close spontaneously in this study. Spontaneous closure of an ASD also has been documented by cardiac catheterization. Cockerham and colleagues detected the presence of an isolated secundum ASD by cardiac catheterization and cineangiography in 54 patients younger than 2 years of age. Of these patients, 14 were documented to have complete closure of their ASD at a subsequent cardiac catheterization. Other investigators also have described spontaneous complete closure of ASDs in early childhood.

Thus, either enlargement or spontaneous closure of ASDs may occur with time. The substantial rate of spontaneous closure in the first 2 years of life suggests that performing secundum ASD closure is not warranted in infants and young children in the absence of substantial symptoms. The propensity of some defects to enlarge supports the common practice of electively closing moderate size defects in childhood, before they have a chance to enlarge beyond the size at which performing transcatheter closure is feasible.

Pregnancy

Pregnancy places additional demands on the cardiovascular system and may cause patients with previously occult ASDs to become symptomatic. In particular, exercise intolerance and congestive heart failure may become apparent during pregnancy. Venous thrombosis secondary to venous stasis in pregnancy may lead to paradoxical embolism in the presence of an ASD. When pulmonary vascular disease is present, pregnancy carries a substantial health risk for the mother and often results in miscarriage.

Diagnosis

Physical Examination

Inspection and Palpation. As mentioned earlier, children with ASDs may be slightly smaller than normal, but failure to thrive is rare. A precordial bulge may be present in those with a large left-to-right shunt, and Harrison grooves (transverse depressions along the sixth and seventh costal cartilages at the site of attachment of the anterior part of the diaphragm) may be apparent. The presence of a hypoplastic thumb, radius, or phocomelia should cause suspicion of Holt-Oram syndrome, an autosomal dominant disorder in which an upper limb deformity is found with congenital heart disease (most often an ASD in association with prolonged AV conduction). Cyanosis may be present in infants, particularly those with right ventricular outflow obstruction or elevated pulmonary artery pressures.

In patients with a thin body habitus and a large atrial left-to-right shunt, a hyperdynamic right ventricular impulse may be observed. Palpation along the left sternal border and in the subxiphoid area will demonstrate this impulse, often termed a *right ventricular heave*. When pulmonary vascular disease or obstruction to right ventricular outflow exists, the right ventricular impulse is less dynamic and has more of a tapping or thrusting quality, suggesting the presence primarily of pressure rather than volume overload. An enlarged and pulsatile pulmonary trunk may be palpated at the second left intercostal space in many patients and is even more prominent and may be associated with a palpable second heart sound if pulmonary hypertension is present.

Arterial Pulse. The arterial pulse is normal at rest in patients with uncomplicated ASDs. In large ASDs, palpation of the arterial pulse during the straining phase of a Valsalva maneuver may fail to demonstrate the usual pulse amplitude decrease because the large volume of blood pooled in the lungs permits left ventricular output to be maintained.

Jugular Venous Pulse. Patients with isolated and nonrestrictive ASDs have a normal amplitude jugular venous pulse. However, as the two atria are connected by a nonrestrictive channel, the A and V waves of the venous pulse attain equal height. When pulmonary vascular disease supervenes, the right atrium contracts more forcefully, causing large A waves to form.

Auscultation. In patients with ASDs, the first heart sound—best heard at the apex and lower left sternal edge—may be single or split with an intensified second (tricuspid) component. The classic characteristic auscultatory finding in ASD is wide, fixed splitting of the second sound. This finding is present in patients with large left-to-right shunts and normal pulmonary artery pressure. Additional details about this split second heart sound are presented in Box 271.2.

ASDs with moderate to large left-to-right shunts are associated with a pulmonary systolic ejection murmur that begins shortly after the first heart sound, peaks in early to mid systole, and ends before the second heart sound. A palpable thrill is usually absent and when present suggests either a very large shunt or pulmonic stenosis. Rapid flow through the peripheral pulmonary arteries may cause systolic crescendo-decrescendo murmurs that are most prominent in the peripheral lung fields rather than the second intercostal space. Because the pressure gradient across the atrial septum seldom is large, audible

BOX 271.2 ### Second Heart Sound in Patients with Atrial Septal Defects

The fixed splitting of the second sound results from a combination of factors. In physiologically normal individuals, inspiratory splitting of the second sound results primarily from increased pulmonary capacitance during inspiration. With expiration in normal persons, pulmonary capacitance decreases, and splitting of the second sound decreases. In contrast, in patients with atrial septal defects (ASDs) and significant left-to-right shunts, the capacitance of the pulmonary bed is increased, resulting in wide splitting between the first and second components of the second heart sound. Because of less respiratory variation in the pulmonary capacitance, little variation in splitting of the second sound occurs in patients with an ASD. When the left-to-right shunt is small or negligible, as it is in most neonates with ASDs, fixed splitting of the second sound does not occur. Because relatively wide (but not truly fixed) splitting of the second sound occurs commonly in supine patients, evaluation of the second sound is better performed with the patient sitting or standing. The intensities of the pulmonic and aortic components of the second sound are equal in most patients with uncomplicated ASDs. Patients with pulmonary hypertension have an accentuated pulmonic component of the second sound. Occasionally, in a patient with normal pulmonary pressures, the pulmonic component of the second sound is intensified because of the proximity of the dilated pulmonary artery to the chest wall.

murmurs from flow across the ASD itself are rare findings (although intracardiac phonocardiography can demonstrate them).

The diastolic murmur most commonly associated with ASD is a middiastolic murmur resulting from the high flow across the tricuspid valve. This murmur becomes apparent when the left-to-right shunt is greater than 2:1. The murmur is of low to medium frequency and does not increase with inspiration. Another diastolic murmur sometimes associated with ASD is a low-pitched murmur of pulmonic regurgitation, probably a consequence of dilatation of the pulmonary artery.

In the occasional patient with ASD and right-to-left shunting caused by pulmonary hypertension, auscultatory findings differ greatly from those usually found in ASDs. A right ventricular fourth heart sound may be present. The midsystolic pulmonic murmur is softer and shorter, and the tricuspid diastolic flow murmur is absent as a result of the relatively normal right ventricular stroke volume because of lack of significant left-to-right atrial shunting. The pulmonic component of the second sound is increased in intensity, but the fixed splitting characteristic of ASD is not present. If a murmur of pulmonic insufficiency is present, it is high pitched. A holosystolic murmur of tricuspid insufficiency also may be present.

Electrocardiography

Sinus rhythm is customary in young patients with uncomplicated secundum ASDs. Prolongation of the PR interval is a common finding and sometimes has a familial association. Beyond the third decade of life, patients with ASD have a high frequency of atrial arrhythmias, particularly atrial fibrillation, but including atrial flutter and supraventricular tachycardia.

Patients with secundum ASDs usually have normal P waves. Often, sinus venosus ASDs are associated with a leftward frontal plane P-wave axis (i.e., negative in leads III and aVF and positive in lead aVL), usually caused by an ectopic pacemaker that occurs near the usual anatomic location of the sinus node.

The QRS complex in patients with secundum ASDs often has a slightly prolonged duration and a characteristic rSr′ or rsR′ pattern, thought to result from disproportionate thickening of the right ventricular outflow tract, which is the last portion of the ventricle to depolarize. Often, the term *incomplete right bundle branch block* is used to describe this QRS pattern, but that term is a misnomer because the pattern is a consequence of hypertrophy and not a conduction disturbance. With increasing degrees of pulmonary hypertension, patients with secundum ASDs tend to lose the rSr′ pattern in lead V_1 and develop a tall monophasic R wave with a deeply inverted T wave. Right axis deviation of the frontal plane QRS axis (ranging from +95 degrees to +135 degrees) is often present. A northwest axis or left axis deviation of the QRS axis suggests the presence of an AV canal defect, but such deviation can occur with uncomplicated secundum ASD as well.

Chest Radiography

The chest radiograph in patients with secundum ASD and sizable left-to-right shunts characteristically shows cardiac enlargement (particularly the right atrial shadow) and increased pulmonary vascularity (Fig. 271.2). Typically, increased pulmonary vascularity extends to the periphery of the lung fields, with a dilated pulmonary trunk and central branches. Enlargement of the pulmonary arteries prevents the aortic shadow from forming the border of the cardiac silhouette creating a characteristic "triangular" cardiac shape. Right atrial and right ventricular enlargement are usually present, but the left atrium and ventricle are typically normal size.

Echocardiography

M-Mode Echocardiography. The M-mode echocardiogram in patients with isolated moderate to large secundum ASDs shows right ventricular enlargement with paradoxical motion of the interventricular septum often present. Diastolic movement of

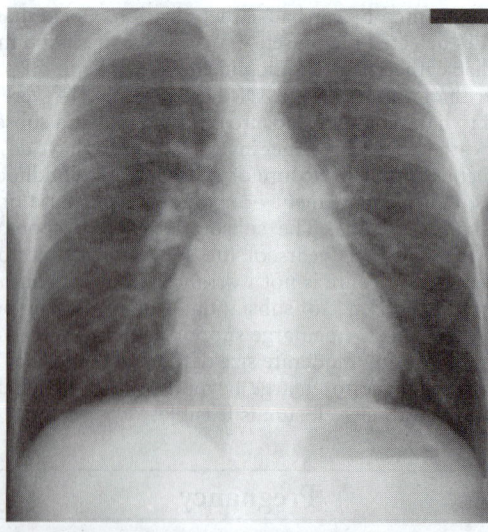

FIGURE 271.2. Chest radiograph of a patient with a secundum atrial septal defect. Note the cardiomegaly and increased pulmonary vascular markings. The main pulmonary artery is enlarged, and the aortic knob is small.

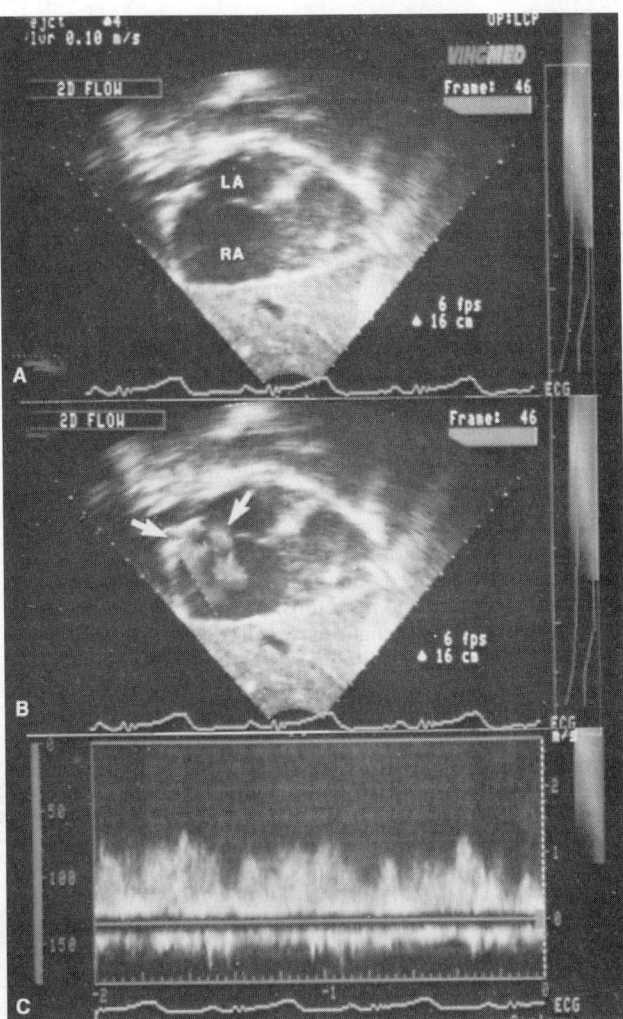

FIGURE 271.3. Two-dimensional echocardiogram demonstrating a fossa ovalis atrial septal defect. **A:** Note the opening in the fossa ovalis region of the septum between the left atrium (LA) and the right atrium (RA). **B:** Color Doppler study demonstrating flow across the atrial septum from left to right through the secundum atrial septal defect. **C:** Pulsed Doppler study demonstrating low-velocity flow from left to right across the defect.

the anterior mitral valve leaflet stops short of the level of the ventricular septum. In contrast, in patients with AV canal defects, the M-mode echocardiogram shows apparent diastolic motion of the mitral valve through the plane of the ventricular septum.

Two-Dimensional Echocardiography. Two-dimensional echocardiography enables direct noninvasive visualization of all types of ASDs (Fig. 271.3). Reliability of the two-dimensional echocardiogram in demonstrating characteristic dropout in the atrial septum is greatest when the axis of the echo beam is perpendicular to the atrial septum, which for most defects is obtained from subcostal views. Additional views, such as suprasternal or parasternal windows, may be useful depending on the location of the defect. ASDs often can be seen in the apical four-chamber view, but, as a consequence of the parallel angle of the echo beam to the atrial septum and the thinness of the fossa ovalis, false echo dropout often occurs, resulting in overdiagnosis.

In addition to direct visualization of the ASD, two-dimensional echocardiography also may demonstrate enlargement of

the right atrium, right ventricle, and pulmonary arteries, and it often confirms the paradoxical ventricular septal motion noted on M-mode. In many cases, the pulmonary and systemic venous connections also can be demonstrated.

Doppler Echocardiography. Abnormal flow across the atrial septum can be detected reliably by pulsed Doppler echocardiography. The accuracy of Doppler identification of flow across the atrial septum can be improved greatly by two-dimensional direction of the Doppler sampling. Characteristically, a shunt across the ASD shows turbulent flow in the direction of the shunt and minimal flow in the opposite direction. Continuous-wave Doppler echocardiography can be particularly helpful in evaluating the gradient across the atrial septum in patients with left atrial hypertension and restrictive ASDs and in evaluating patients for obstruction to pulmonary venous return. Color Doppler imaging allows for the direct visualization of the flow across the ASD and is particularly helpful in distinguishing normal right superior vena caval flow from left-to-right shunting across the atrial septum.

If additional confirmation of diagnosis is desired, contrast echocardiography using agitated saline or indocyanine green is effective in demonstrating the presence of an ASD. A right-to-left shunt can be detected by direct visualization of microcavitation bubbles in the left atrium and left ventricle. A left-to-right shunt can be detected as a negative contrast washout effect in the right atrium if good opacification of the atrium is achieved.

Transesophageal Echocardiography. Transthoracic echocardiography is limited by the ability of ultrasonography to penetrate to regions of interest. Particularly in older patients and in patients with chest wall deformities and lung disease, transthoracic echocardiographic windows may be so poor that the atrial septum cannot be visualized clearly in its entirety. In such instances, transesophageal echocardiography often is helpful. Two-dimensional anatomic visualization of the atrial septum from the transesophageal approach generally is excellent. Additionally, two-dimensionally directed pulsed, color, and even continuous-wave Doppler studies of blood flow can be performed from the transesophageal approach with appropriate equipment. In addition to its diagnostic role in selected cases, transesophageal echocardiography is especially useful for guiding catheter placement of atrial septal occlusion devices.

Intracardiac Echocardiography. Ultrasound transducers mounted on cardiac catheters now are available and provide high-quality direct intracardiac imaging of the atrial septum (Fig. 271.4). Although it is not indicated for routine diagnostic purposes because of its invasive nature, this technique is particularly useful during placement of a transcatheter atrial septal occlusion device. Catheter-based intracardiac imaging can eliminate the need for endotracheal intubation, which frequently is necessary for transesophageal imaging during device placement in the catheterization laboratory.

Three-Dimensional Echocardiography. Since the mid-1990s, investigational three-dimensional echocardiographic devices have been used to evaluate the atrial septum. Three-dimensional displays can facilitate more precise sizing of ASDs. These displays can demonstrate also the relation of an ASD to fossa ovalis superior and inferior limbic band tissue and to the AV valves. This information is potentially important for therapeutic planning.

At present, three-dimensional echocardiographic evaluation is relatively time-consuming and has been confined to application by a few skilled investigators. Continued improvements in three-dimensional equipment, including real-time scanning, potentially will speed and simplify acquisition and processing of data so the use of three-dimensional echocardiography will become more routine.

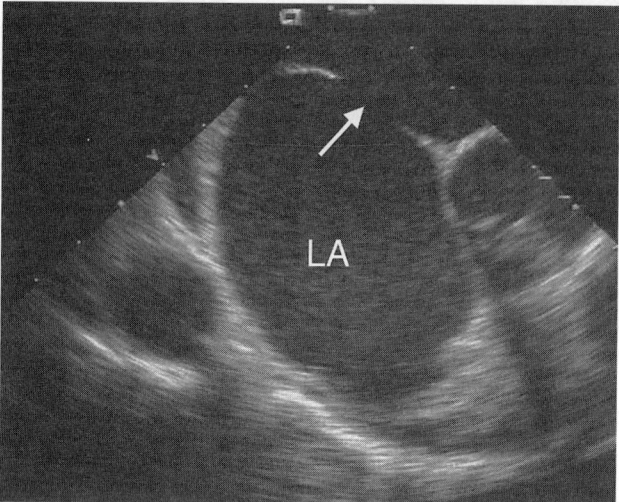

FIGURE 271.4. Intracardiac echocardiogram in patient with secundum atrial septal defect. The *arrow* points to location of atrial septal defect. Note the high quality of structure definition of the intracardiac echocardiogram. This patient had poor transthoracic acoustic windows. LA, left atrium.

Magnetic Resonance Imaging

Isolated ASDs can be identified clearly by noninvasive magnetic resonance imaging (MRI) methods. These methods may have a role in sizing and anatomically defining ASDs before catheter or surgical closure, particularly in patients with poor acoustic windows. At present, MRI is used usually for defining extracardiac structures, such as anomalous pulmonary and systemic veins that may be demonstrated poorly by echocardiography because of surrounding lung tissue. Particularly interesting are the recently developed cineangiographic methods that facilitate visualization and quantitation of intracardiac and extracardiac blood flows.

Cardiac Catheterization

Cardiac catheterization rarely is indicated for diagnostic purposes in uncomplicated ASDs. Secundum ASDs sometimes can be differentiated from sinus venosus and AV canal defects because characteristic high or low catheter courses across the atrial septum are seen with the latter two defects, respectively. In secundum ASDs, the catheter passes across the middle portion of the atrial septum.

Left-to-right shunting across the atrial septum causes an increase in oxygen saturation in the right atrium in patients with ASDs. An increase of 5% to 10% over superior vena caval blood saturation generally indicates the presence of a left-to-right shunt at the atrial level.

Cineangiography

The presence of an ASD with left-to-right shunting can be demonstrated in the anteroposterior and lateral projections by injecting contrast medium into the main pulmonary artery. After passing through the lungs, contrast material passes into the right atrium and ventricle in the presence of an ASD. Pulmonary artery injection also is a good method for evaluating the pulmonary venous return and usually demonstrates any abnormal pulmonary venous connections. Although this technique is useful for revealing the presence of an ASD, it does not provide good visualization of the size and location of the ASD. For optimal direct visualization, an injection just outside the orifice of the right upper pulmonary vein in a four-chamber

view is the most appropriate approach. In the four-chamber view, secundum ASDs are demonstrated in the middle of the atrial septum, sinus venous defects appear at the top of the atrial septum, and AV canal defects are shown at the inferior aspect of the atrial septum.

Treatment

Isolated secundum ASDs associated with a large left-to-right shunt and either symptoms or significant cardiomegaly should be closed electively in childhood. Most physicians consider that when the findings from a comprehensive noninvasive evaluation demonstrate a classic isolated secundum ASD, cardiac catheterization for diagnosis is not essential. The noninvasive studies should be of good technical quality, however, so pulmonary hypertension, as well as such associated anatomic defects as anomalous pulmonary and systemic venous connections, can be excluded.

When pulmonary hypertension is present or the atrial shunt is small, recommendations regarding closure are more controversial. When advanced pulmonary vascular disease is present, operative mortality and morbidity are high, and closure of the ASD may worsen the prognosis. Small ASDs cause only a minimal increase in cardiopulmonary stress. Therefore, the hemodynamic gain from closing them may not be worth the hazard of the procedure. However, the risk of a paradoxical embolism occurring through a small atrial defect or valve-incompetent patent foramen ovale is uncertain. This risk may justify closure in selected patients, such as those with a history of cryptogenic stroke. Further clinical studies are required to assess the benefits of intervention more definitely in such cases.

Successful catheter closure of secundum ASDs has been performed using occlusion devices (Fig. 271.5). Various devices in various stages of investigation and approval are available, and the use of such devices for closure of small to moderate defects in the fossa ovalis region is now routine and is expected to increase. Large secundum defects substantially greater than 20 mm generally are addressed surgically, although defects greater than 30 mm reportedly have been closed successfully via a transcatheter approach. Catheter closure has the advantage of avoiding the need to perform thoracotomy, cardiopulmonary bypass, and atriotomy with their attendant potential problems. Initial and intermediate-term results with catheter ASD occlusion are promising, but long-term follow-up studies subsequent to catheter ASD closure are not yet available. Surgical closure typically is performed with the aid of cardiopulmonary bypass. Patch closure with either pericardium or Dacron is preferred for all but small defects because closure of larger defects by primary suture can distort the atrium. Limited or minimally invasive approaches to surgical closure, including the use of robotics, are becoming available, promising the potential for improved cosmetic results and shorter recovery times.

Prognosis

Surgical results in uncomplicated secundum ASD are good. Short- and intermediate-term results of catheter ASD closure also are good. Mortality and morbidity rates are increased with advanced age and congestive heart failure at the time of closure. After operation, the left-to-right shunt and its consequent cardiac volume overload are eliminated. Without closure, patients with moderate and large secundum ASDs generally do well until the third decade of life, after which they tend to become progressively more symptomatic, with a substantially higher mortality rate than that of the general population.

With the exception of a possible increased incidence of stroke, the prognosis of small ASDs seems to be excellent in

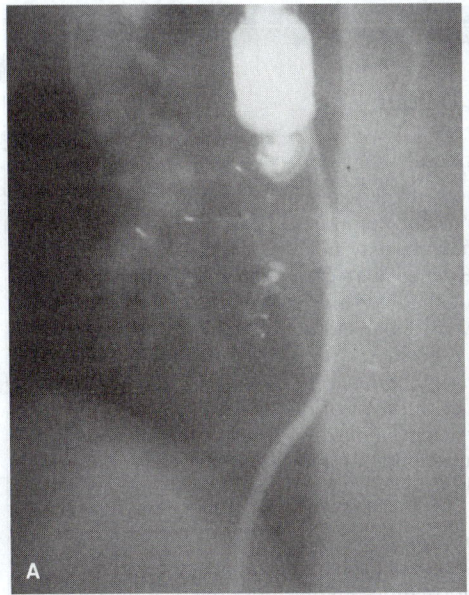 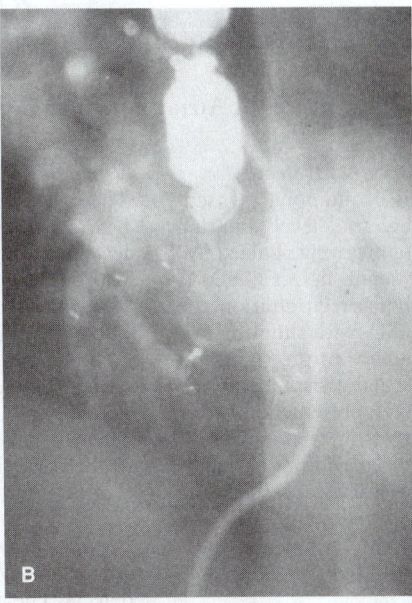

FIGURE 271.5. **A:** Atrial septal defect occlusion device in place. Note transesophageal echocardiographic probe positioned immediately superior to the device. **B:** Left atrium opacified by pulmonary artery angiogram. No contrast is seen in right atrium, demonstrating closure of atrial septal defect by the device. (Courtesy of Charles E. Mullins, M.D.)

most cases without specific therapy. Because these defects are difficult to detect, their incidence probably is clinically underestimated. Some data indicate that scuba divers and possibly aviators with small ASDs may be at risk for development of paradoxical systemic embolism of venous gas bubbles after hyperbaric or altitude decompression. Preliminary studies have suggested an association of migraine headaches and small ASDs.

PERSISTENT COMMON ATRIOVENTRICULAR CANAL DEFECTS

AV canal defects include a range of malformations, a central feature of which is an ASD of the ostium primum type. Because these defects involve deficiency of the AV septum, abnormalities of one or both AV valves are usual and ventricular septal defects may also occur. Numerous terms, including *endocardial cushion defect*, *AV septal defects*, and *persistent common AV canal*, have been applied to these malformations.

In view of the variety of types of AV canal defects, different classifications exist. In this discussion, the term *complete AV canal defect* indicates the presence of both atrial and ventricular septal defects and a common AV orifice with a common AV valve (Fig. 271.6); all other forms that are parts of the spectrum are termed *partial* or *incomplete* forms. Pathophysiologic features of AV canal defects are described in Box 271.3.

Natural History

The natural history of AV canal defects depend primarily on the pathologic anatomy of the malformation. In patients with only an ostium primum ASD and minimal regurgitation of the mitral valve, the clinical course is similar to that for patients with a large secundum ASD. Generally, these patients do well without treatment during infancy, childhood, and adolescence. During adulthood, they have an increasing tendency to develop congestive heart failure, particularly as atrial arrhythmias develop and with the increasing mitral regurgitation that occurs with time.

Patients with ostium primum ASDs and moderate to severe mitral valve regurgitation develop congestive heart failure in early life, with consequent high morbidity and mortality rates that relate primarily to the severity of the AV valve insufficiency.

Generally, patients with complete AV canal defects develop severe symptoms of congestive heart failure in early infancy. They have frequent respiratory infections and poor weight gain. If they survive infancy untreated, generally they develop pulmonary vascular disease with fixed pulmonary hypertension as an additional major deleterious factor.

Diagnosis

Physical Examination

Appearance. Patients with partial AV canal defects and minimal mitral regurgitation usually appear normal in infancy and

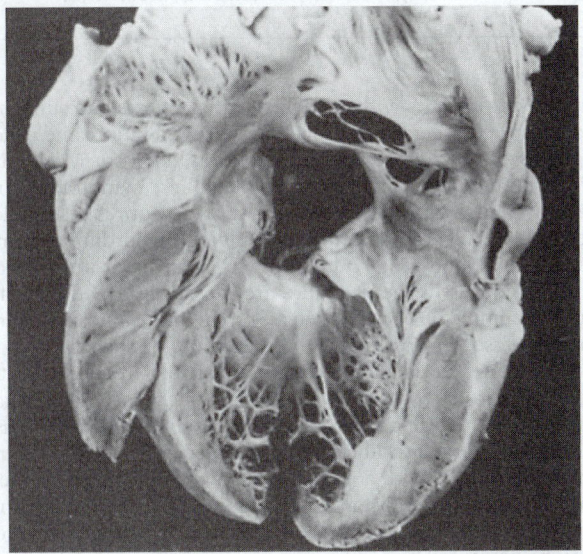

FIGURE 271.6. Complete atrioventricular canal defect. This view is from the opened left atrium and left ventricle. Note the large cleft in the anterior mitral leaflet. (Courtesy of Debra Kearney, M.D.)

| BOX 271.3 | Pathophysiologic Features of Atrioventricular Canal Defects |

Partial (Incomplete) Atrioventricular Canal Defect

In the absence of pulmonary stenosis or pulmonary vascular disease, predominant left-to-right atrial level shunting is present in patients with incomplete atrioventricular (AV) canal defects. When only the atrial septal defect (ASD) is present without substantial mitral valvular regurgitation, the physiology is identical to that of an ASD, with shunting primarily determined by relative compliance of the right and left ventricles and the pulmonary vascular resistance. When significant mitral valvular regurgitation is present, additional left-to-right shunting can occur directly from left ventricle to right atrium, via the cleft mitral valve. This additional high-pressure to low-pressure left-to-right shunt causes volume overload of both the left and right ventricles and is associated with heart failure early in life.

Complete Atrioventricular Canal Defects

When a large interventricular communication is present in a complete AV canal defect, additional left-to-right shunting occurs at the ventricular level. Such shunts generally are associated with systemic pulmonary artery pressures unless significant pulmonary stenosis is present. Regurgitation of the left component of the common AV valve compounds the ventricular volume overload in these patients, who often have symptoms caused by pulmonary congestion. When pulmonary vascular disease develops (as is likely in unrepaired defects), patients may initially improve symptomatically; however, when advanced pulmonary vascular disease ensues in later life, the physiology is the same as that in patients with Eisenmenger syndrome (reversal of the intracardiac shunt as a result of suprasystemic pulmonary artery pressures), with the additional volume overload imposed by left AV valve regurgitation.

Atrial Septum

Virtually all AV canal defects include an interatrial communication called an *ostium primum ASD*. These defects lie at the lowest part of the atrial septum and vary in size but usually are large in relation to cardiac size. Characteristically, the superior margin of the primum ASD is concave.

Ventricular Septum

The basal portion of the ventricular septum is deficient in hearts with persistent common AV canal, but ventricular level shunting may or may not be present. In those hearts without an interventricular communication (*partial or incomplete forms*), the AV valve tissue attaches to the crest of the deficient ventricular septum such that interventricular communication is occluded. In hearts with an interventricular communication (*complete AV canal*), AV valvular tissue does not attach to the crest of the deficient septum, leaving a ventricular level communication between the undersurface of the valve tissue superiorly and the crest of the ventricular septum inferiorly.

Atrioventricular Valves

Abnormal AV valves are the hallmarks of persistent AV canal defects. The abnormalities involve both the overall configuration and orientation of the valve apparatus and the local structure of the AV valves. Usually, in partial AV canal defects, there are two separate AV valve annuli. The anterior (septal) leaflet of the mitral valve is composed of two components that usually are of approximately equal size and are separated by a gap (cleft) with resultant varying degrees of mitral regurgitation. In complete AV canal defects, a common AV valve exists. Both an ostium primum ASD and a ventricular septal defect of the AV canal type are present and are confluent. The common AV valve has anterior and posterior common leaflets that bridge across the ventricular septum and relate to both ventricles (also called *anterior* and *posterior bridging leaflets*). Regurgitation of the common valve is the rule.

Common Atrium

Like other persistent AV canal defects, these uncommon ASDs almost always are associated with a cleft anterior leaflet of the mitral valve, mitral regurgitation, and a deficient crest of the ventricular septum. The entire atrial septum is almost absent. Often, a band of muscular tissue crosses the atrium, suggesting a vestigial atrial septum.

---

childhood. Patients with partial AV canal defects and substantial mitral regurgitation may manifest growth failure and other signs of chronic congestive heart failure. In contrast, patients with complete AV canal defects typically are symptomatic in early infancy, with manifestations such as poor physical development, hyperinflated thorax, bulging precordium, Harrison grooves, and mild or intermittent cyanosis. If no signs of chronic congestive heart failure are present in a patient with known complete AV canal defect, pulmonary stenosis or pulmonary vascular obstructive disease should be suspected.

Complete AV canal defects are associated frequently with Down syndrome (trisomy 21), which has a characteristic facial appearance including a flat facial profile, oblique palpebral fissures, and a large protuberant tongue. Generally, the hands are short and broad, with a palmar simian crease, a short, curved fourth finger, and a distal axial triradius. The skin is dry and distinctively pale or mottled. Two distinctive ocular features may be present. The most frequent is an inner epicanthic skin fold that inserts on the lower eyelid; the second is the presence of Brushfield spots (speckled iris). When Down syndrome is seen in conjunction with the physical signs of chronic con-

gestive heart failure, the coexistence of complete common AV canal should be suspected, although other types of congenital heart disease also occur in Down syndrome.

Arterial and Jugular Venous Pulse. In partial AV canal defect, mitral regurgitation may be associated with a water-hammer pulse caused by the rapid ejection of a large left ventricular stroke volume. Alternatively, patients with congestive heart failure may have a small pulse volume. When a left ventricle to right atrial shunt is present, the jugular venous pulse may have a dominant V wave because the right atrium receives left ventricular systolic flow.

Precordial Movement and Palpation. When mitral regurgitation is present in patients with partial AV canal defect, a systolic thrill radiating toward the sternum often is present. When a large left-to-right shunt is present, a palpable impulse in the second and third left intercostal spaces frequently is noted, reflecting the presence of a dilated, pulsatile pulmonary artery trunk. The pulmonic component of the second heart sound may be palpable. The right ventricular volume and pressure overload associated with complete AV canal defects causes a prominent systolic impulse or heave at the left sternal border and in the subxyphoid area.

Auscultation. Complete AV canal defects may be associated with a variety of auscultatory manifestations, depending on the nature of the underlying pathologic physiology. Because one common AV valve is present, usually the first heart sound is single. When the AV conduction time is prolonged (as is often the case), the first heart sound tends to be relatively soft. Fixed splitting of the second sound usually occurs, although when severe pulmonary hypertension is present, the splitting will be narrow. Pulmonary hypertension may be associated also with a loud pulmonic component of the second sound. Frequently, a murmur of AV valve incompetence is present. This murmur typically is maximal at the left ventricular apex and may radiate toward the sternum rather than toward the left axilla, reflecting the predominance of left ventricular–to–right atrial shunting over left ventricular–to–left atrial shunting. When the ventricular septal defect is restrictive, a separate murmur of ventricular septal defect may be present, most prominently heard at the lower left sternal border.

The auscultatory findings in ostium primum ASD are similar to those found in fossa ovalis defects (pulmonic flow murmur in the second left intercostal space, and wide, fixed splitting of the second heart sound), with the addition of an apical holosystolic murmur, secondary to mitral valve insufficiency, that may radiate toward the sternum.

Electrocardiography

The most characteristic ECG abnormality of an AV canal defect is a superiorly oriented QRS frontal plane axis with a counterclockwise depolarization pattern (so-called northwest axis). The mechanism of alteration of the frontal plane QRS axis in these patients is not caused by ventricular hypertrophy but by abnormally positioned conduction tissue, which causes abnormal sequences of cardiac activation. AV conduction delay often exists as evidenced by a prolonged PR interval. ECG manifestations of right ventricular hypertrophy may be present. Findings consistent with biventricular or left ventricular hypertrophy may also occur, particularly if mitral or common AV valve insufficiency is severe.

Chest Radiography

Cardiomegaly is common finding on chest radiography in patients with ostium primum or complete AV canal defects, particularly involving right atrial and right ventricular enlargement. The enlarged right heart may displace the left ventricle, rendering evaluation of left ventricular size difficult. Usually, the main pulmonary artery is prominent, and, if a large left-to-right shunt is present, increased pulmonary vascular markings are typical. With severe pulmonary vascular disease, the distal pulmonary vessels may have a lucent, pruned appearance. Severe enlargement of the pulmonary trunk and left atrium may compress the left main stem bronchus and cause atelectasis of parts of the left lung.

Echocardiography

M-Mode Echocardiography. In most cases, M-mode echocardiograms of patients with AV canal defects characteristically demonstrate apparent diastolic movement of the mitral valve through the plane of the ventricular septum. M-mode echocardiography also shows an enlarged right ventricle and paradoxical motion of the interventricular septum in many patients.

Two-Dimensional Echocardiography. Two-dimensional echocardiography is highly reliable in identifying AV canal defects. The hallmark of the diagnosis is demonstration of an absent AV septum. In ostium primum ASDs, the AV valve leaflets appear to originate from the crest of the ventricular septum. In complete AV canal defects, the bridging leaflets of the common AV valve are observed to cross the ventricular septum.

Doppler Echocardiography. Doppler echocardiography can contribute substantially to the evaluation of AV canal defects. Pulsed Doppler is especially useful in detecting left and right ventricular outflow obstruction and the presence of associated lesions such as a ductus arteriosus. Pulsed Doppler examination also facilitates detection and quantification of AV valve regurgitation. Continuous-wave Doppler is useful in estimating pressure gradients and cardiac chamber pressures in these patient using the modified Bernoulli formula. Color Doppler studies are particularly helpful in determining the location and roughly quantitating the degree of AV valve insufficiency.

Transesophageal Echocardiography. Excellent images of the AV septum and of the AV valves and their attachments can be obtained with transesophageal echocardiography. Generally, Doppler color flow mapping of AV valve flow from the transesophageal approach also is excellent. The most extensive use of transesophageal imaging in patients with AV canal is intraoperatively to evaluate postoperative AV valve regurgitation, to check for residual atrial and ventricular septal defects, to rule out ventricular outflow tract obstruction, and to assess cardiac function.

Magnetic Resonance Imaging

MRI can demonstrate defects in the AV septum, but the ability of this modality to characterize the AV valves is limited by the relatively low temporal resolution of current systems. MRI is helpful as an adjunct to echocardiography to demonstrate extracardiac anatomy and organ situs in patients who have complex anomalies, such as heterotaxy syndrome in association with AV canal defects.

Cardiac Catheterization

AV canal defects can be suspected at cardiac catheterization when the catheter course across the atrial septum is low. Oxygen saturation and hemodynamic data obtained at cardiac catheterization can provide definitive assessment of pulmonary pressures, of left-to-right and right-to-left shunting, and of pulmonary vascular resistance.

Cineangiography

Selective left ventricular angiography in the anteroposterior projection demonstrates an elongated left ventricular outflow tract, with an abnormally low insertion of the anterior leaflet of the left AV valve, deficiency in the diaphragmatic wall of the left ventricle, and a disproportionately short inlet septum as compared to the outlet septum. This combination of characteristics is diagnostic of an AV canal defect and is termed the *gooseneck deformity* (Fig. 271.7).

Treatment

Medical Therapy

When heart failure and associated pulmonary congestion are present, such anticongestive measures as diuretics, afterload reduction, and digoxin are indicated. Long periods of fluid restriction are counterproductive because the patients in distress usually are small infants, and such restriction deprives them of calories needed for growth. Hydralazine has been shown to reduce the magnitude of left-to-right shunting on a short-term basis in these patients, but no long-term experience with the drug in complete AV canal defects has been reported. Most

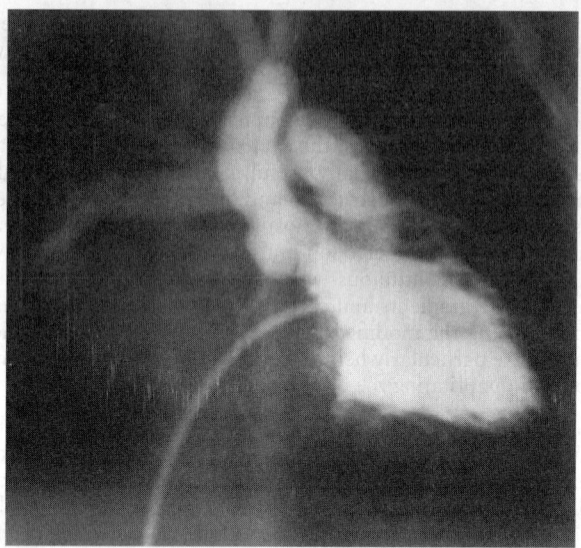

FIGURE 271.7. Frontal view of left ventriculogram in patient with complete atrioventricular canal defect. The "gooseneck" deformity of the left ventricular outflow tract is clearly demonstrated.

cardiologists do not favor prolonged medical therapy in affected patients if symptoms are refractory, but instead refer these patients for surgical treatment.

Surgical Therapy

Recommendations for surgical treatment depend on the anatomic characteristics of the defect and on associated anomalies. Generally, patients with an ostium primum ASD, separate AV valves, no ventricular defect, and minimal AV valve insufficiency are asymptomatic during infancy and childhood. Because repair of ostium primum ASD is associated with greater morbidity and mortality rates than is repair of a secundum ASD, some cardiologists do not recommend surgery at any age if cardiomegaly is absent, which usually is the case when AV valve insufficiency is mild and the pulmonary-to-systemic flow ratio is less than 2:1. In most cases, however, asymptomatic patients with ostium primum ASDs who do exhibit cardiomegaly are referred for elective surgical repair when they are near school age. Almost invariably, infants who have partial AV canal defects and are symptomatic have severe AV valve regurgitation. Generally, pulmonary artery banding does not help these patients. Therefore, corrective surgery with mitral valvuloplasty and closure of the ASD is recommended.

For patients with uncomplicated complete AV canal defects, most centers advocate performing corrective surgery in early infancy. Palliative procedures, such as pulmonary artery banding, may be more appropriate in patients who have AV canal defects in association with other anomalies, such as hypoplasia of the left ventricle. When pulmonary pressures are near systemic, as they generally are in patients who have complete AV canal defects but do not have associated right ventricular

outflow obstruction, pulmonary vascular disease usually develops after the first year of life (although can develop sooner). Therefore, performing either corrective surgery or a palliative procedure to protect the pulmonary circulation during infancy is recommended in such patients.

Prognosis

Long-term results of surgical therapy depend greatly on the degree of preoperative pulmonary vascular disease and on the extent of residual left AV valve regurgitation. In many cases, the left AV valve regurgitation is reduced substantially, and the left-to-right shunt is abolished or is reduced to minimal levels by corrective surgery. However, when pulmonary vascular disease is present preoperatively, hospital morbidity and mortality rates are high, and little improvement occurs in the late follow-up period for those patients who survive surgery. Postoperative arrhythmias, including complete heart block, can occur and may increase in frequency as patients grow older. With advancing age, patients may require mitral valve replacement.

Suggested Readings

Cockerham JT, Martin TC, Gutierrez FR, et al. Spontaneous closure of secundum atrial septal defect in infants and young children. *Am J Cardiol* 1983;52:1267.
Craig RJ, Selzer A. Natural history and prognosis of atrial septal defect. *Circulation* 1968;37:805.
Di Tullio M, Sacco RL, Gopal A, et al. Patent foramen ovale as a risk factor for cryptogenic stroke. *Ann Intern Med* 1993;117:461–465.
Edwards JE. Congenital malformations of the heart and great vessels: A. Malformations of the atrial septal complex. In: Gould SE, ed. *Pathology of the heart,* 2nd ed. Springfield, IL: Charles C Thomas, 1960:260.
Feldt RH, Edwards WD, Puga FJ, et al. Atrial septal defects and atrioventricular canal. In: Moss AJ, Adams FH, Emmanouilides GC, eds. *Heart disease in infants, children, and adolescents,* 5th ed. Baltimore: Williams & Wilkins, 1990:118.
McMahon CJ, Feltes TF, Fraley JK, et al. Natural history of growth of secundum atrial septal defects and implications for transcatheter closure. *Heart* 2002;87:256.
Moss AJ, Siassi B. The small atrial septal defect: operate or procrastinate? *J Pediatr* 1971;79:854.
Mullins CE. Pediatric and congenital therapeutic cardiac catheterization. *Circulation* 1989;79:1153.
Murphy JG, Gersh BJ, McGoon MD, et al. Long-term outcome after surgical repair of isolated atrial septal defect: follow-up at 27 to 32 years. *N Engl J Med* 1990;323:1645.
Nadas AS, Fyler DC. *Pediatric cardiology.* Philadelphia: WB Saunders, 1972:317.
Perloff JK. *The clinical recognition of congenital heart disease.* Philadelphia: Saunders, 1987:272.
Radzik D, Davignon A, van Doesburg, et al. Predictive factors for spontaneous closure of atrial septal defects diagnosed in the first 3 months of life. *J Am Coll Cardiol* 1993;22:851.
Rudolph AM. *Congenital diseases of the heart.* Chicago: Year Book Medical, 1974:239.
Silverman N, Levitsky S, Fisher E, et al. Efficacy of pulmonary artery banding in infants with complete atrioventricular canal. *Circulation* 1983;68(suppl 2):148.
Studer M, Blackstone EH, Kirklin JW, et al. Determinants of early and late results of repair of atrioventricular septal (canal) defects. *J Thorac Cardiovasc Surg* 1982;84:523.
Titus JL, Rastelli GC. Anatomic features of persistent common atrioventricular canal. In: Feldt RH, ed. *Atrioventricular canal defects.* Philadelphia: WB Saunders, 1976.

CHAPTER 272 ■ VENTRICULAR SEPTAL DEFECT

CARL H. GUMBINER

Ventricular septal defect (VSD) is the most common cardiac abnormality in children, with a prevalence of 1.5 to 2.5 per 1,000 live births. One-third of children with congenital heart disease have VSD. The evaluation and management of this common and comparatively "simple" abnormality have evolved since the 1960s in steps that exemplify many of the advances in the field of pediatric cardiology as a whole.

ANATOMY

The ventricular septum separates the left ventricle from the right ventricle and, to a small extent, from the right atrium. It consists of a membranous and muscular portion and is subdivided into inflow, trabecular, and outflow regions. Defects in the septum may occur in each region. They range in size from pinhole defects of 1 mm or less to virtual absence of the septum.

The location of a defect within the ventricular septum is not of great hemodynamic consequence, but it is a critical surgical consideration and an important determinant of natural history. Perimembranous defects are bounded by a portion of the membranous septum and a portion of muscular septum. Muscular defects, bounded entirely by muscle, frequently are multiple and tend to close spontaneously. Doubly committed subarterial defects (formerly designated *supracristal* or *type I defects*) lie in the outflow portion of the muscular septum beneath the pulmonary and aortic valves. They often are associated with development of aortic regurgitation and, although relatively rare among white children constitute up to 30% of VSDs in Asian children. Malalignment defects, in which the crest of the septum lies in a plane different from the anterior portion of the aortic root, are found in many complex lesions but also occasionally constitute an isolated VSD. Progressive left ventricular outflow tract obstruction is a common finding with such defects.

PHYSIOLOGY

VSD allows a communication to exist between the systemic and pulmonary circulations. The hemodynamic effect of this communication depends on the size of the left-to-right shunt, which, in turn, is a function of the anatomic size of the defect and the relative pulmonary and systemic vascular resistances. Left-to-right shunting at the ventricular level results in increased pulmonary blood flow and increased volume work of the left ventricle. Consequently, left atrial and pulmonary venous pressures are increased. The combination of increased pulmonary blood flow and elevated pulmonary venous pressure produces increased oncotic pressure within the pulmonary capillary bed and accumulation of pulmonary interstitial fluid. Decreased pulmonary compliance with increased work of breathing accounts for the early manifestations of congestive heart failure (CHF). More profound heart failure, causing alveolar fluid collection, also can interfere with pulmonary gas exchange.

Pulmonary vascular resistance is elevated in the fetus and newborn. Normally, resistance falls during the infant's first several days of life, but it may remain high for several months in the presence of large interventricular communication. Hence, the hemodynamic manifestations of a left-to-right shunt are not evident at birth and may not appear until later in infancy. Elevated pulmonary artery pressure that invariably is present with large or "unrestrictive" VSD produces characteristic changes in the pulmonary arteriolar bed. Pulmonary vascular obstructive disease (PVOD) with marked, irreversibly elevated resistance may develop when a child is as young as 2 years old. It usually occurs after a period of low resistance (hence, high pulmonary blood flow with CHF), but it may develop progressively in children whose pulmonary vascular resistance never declines postnatally. The later stages of progressive PVOD in these patients, in which cyanosis is caused by reversed shunting through a large interventricular communication, is termed *Eisenmenger syndrome*. This well-known late chapter in the natural history of VSD with pulmonary hypertension has made customary the surgical repair of large defects before the child reaches 6 months of age, even in the absence of severe symptoms.

CLINICAL MANIFESTATIONS

Small VSDs seldom cause significant symptoms and usually come to the attention of a physician because of the associated heart murmur. Whereas the murmur is not present in the immediate newborn period, it may be audible as early as the second day of life and usually is heard at the routine 2-week checkup. It characteristically is a high-pitched, harsh, holosystolic murmur, well localized along the left sternal border. A small VSD may produce a murmur of low pitch, but a high-pitched murmur strongly suggests that the defect is not large. The precordium is quiet, but a localized thrill may be palpable. The first and second heart sounds are normal, and seldom is a diastolic murmur present. Except for mild tachypnea in small infants, other physical findings are normal. Small defects, sometimes called *maladie de Roger*, do not interfere with normal growth. A significant number, estimated to be in the range of 30% to 70%, will undergo spontaneous closure, usually in the child's first 2 years of life. Certain types of defects, regardless of size, however, may predispose to development of secondary conditions, especially aortic regurgitation and left ventricular outflow tract obstruction. For this reason, children with physical findings of small VSD should undergo echocardiographic examination to confirm the diagnosis and to localize the defect.

Large defects may come to the attention of a physician later than do small defects because elevated pulmonary vascular resistance may delay the appearance of a murmur. When present, symptoms are those of CHF. They include irritability, increased respiratory effort, poor feeding, and poor weight gain. Recurrent respiratory infections are common occurrences, and pneumonia often is the preliminary diagnosis.

Signs of CHF include tachycardia, tachypnea, increased work of breathing, pallor, diaphoresis, and failure to thrive.

Pulmonary rales are a late finding. The precordium is hyperactive, and a thrill often is palpable. The second heart sound is single or narrowly split. When audible, it usually is accentuated, but often it is obscured by a loud, low-pitched, harsh, holosystolic murmur. The murmur is loudest along the left sternal border but is much less well localized than is the murmur of a small VSD. It may radiate to the right of the sternum but radiates poorly to the back. A diastolic murmur or rumble heard at the lower left sternal border is related to increased mitral flow. Its presence implies a pulmonary–to–systemic flow ratio exceeding 2:1. Pulses may be diminished with severe CHF, but they are symmetric. The liver and sometimes the spleen are enlarged.

Moderate defects may produce physical findings suggestive of small defects, although rarely does one detect a murmur of high pitch. Usually, some degree of tachypnea and increased respiratory effort is present. Because of increased volume load of the left ventricle, the precordial impulse is hyperactive, and often a thrill is present. When associated with low pulmonary vascular resistance and high pulmonary blood flow, a moderate defect may produce findings similar to those of a large defect, including CHF.

Large defects with high resistance and thus little increase in pulmonary blood flow may cause no symptoms or growth failure in a small child. Although the precordial impulse is hyperactive and the pulmonic closure sound is accentuated, an absent or subtle murmur may allow this defect to pass undetected. Older children with more advanced PVOD exhibit resting cyanosis, exercise intolerance, and nail-bed clubbing. A murmur of VSD flow usually is not heard, but a systolic murmur of tricuspid regurgitation or a diastolic murmur of pulmonic regurgitation may be present.

DIAGNOSTIC STUDIES

Radiographic findings generally reflect the size of the left-to-right shunt. Small defects may produce mild cardiac enlargement on a plain chest roentgenogram, but usually size of the heart is normal. Moderate defects are associated with cardiomegaly, usually of a predominant left ventricular type. The left atrium may be enlarged on lateral projection. Pulmonary blood flow is increased. Large defects produce a more diffuse cardiomegaly, increased pulmonary vascular markings, and, often, signs of pulmonary edema. In patients with a large VSD and PVOD, only mild cardiomegaly is demonstrated on the chest roentgenogram. The main pulmonary artery segment usually is prominent, and peripheral vascular markings are normal or diminished.

Electrocardiographic changes with small VSD are minimal. Moderately sized defects usually produce some degree of left ventricular hypertrophy, whereas large defects commonly produce combined ventricular hypertrophy. Large defects with PVOD may show right ventricular hypertrophy.

Echocardiography and Doppler echocardiography are the primary modalities for anatomic and physiologic assessment of VSD. Real-time two-dimensional echocardiographic imaging in the standard views discloses the presence, location, and size of nearly all defects (Fig. 272.1), as well as the presence of associated lesions. Color-flow Doppler investigation increases the sensitivity of standard imaging, particularly for small or multiple defects. Pulsed continuous-wave Doppler studies facilitate the assessment of right ventricular pressure and the difference in pressure between the ventricles.

Magnetic resonance imaging and magnetic resonance angiography are sensitive and specific modalities for the diagnosis and anatomic assessment of VSD (Fig. 272.2) and are particularly useful for evaluating associated extracardiac vascular malformations such as coarctation of the aorta.

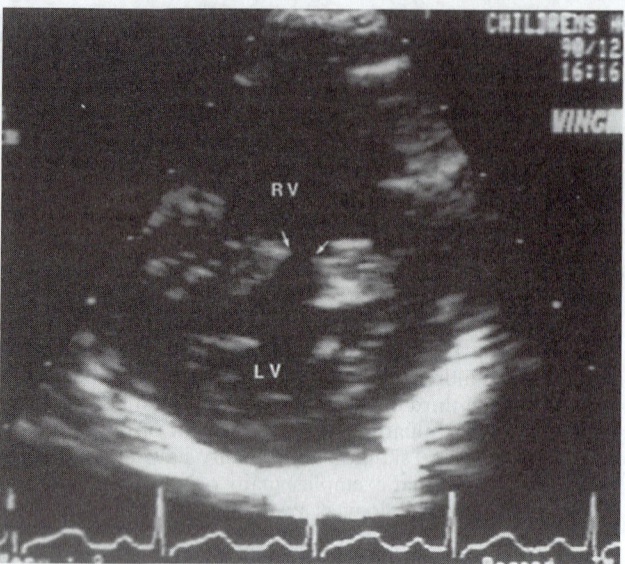

FIGURE 272.1. Short-axis two-dimensional echocardiographic view of a large muscular ventricular septal defect. The *arrows* point to the margins of the defect. LV, left ventricle, RV, right ventricle.

Cardiac catheterization and angiography (Fig. 272.3) play a role in evaluating patients with VSD, but these techniques are reserved for patients with unusual or complex anatomy and for patients who require precise investigation of pulmonary blood flow or pulmonary vascular resistance. Such evaluation also may entail assessment of response to intervention such as administration of oxygen or nitric oxide.

MANAGEMENT

The therapeutic approach to an infant or child with VSD depends on the patient's age, the size of the defect, the severity of symptoms, and the anatomy of the defect itself. Infants with small VSDs seldom require treatment. They should be evaluated during the first 6 months of life, when pulmonary vascular resistance is expected to decline. Physical examinations and noninvasive studies should be employed to ascertain the expected minimal increase in pulmonary blood flow and the

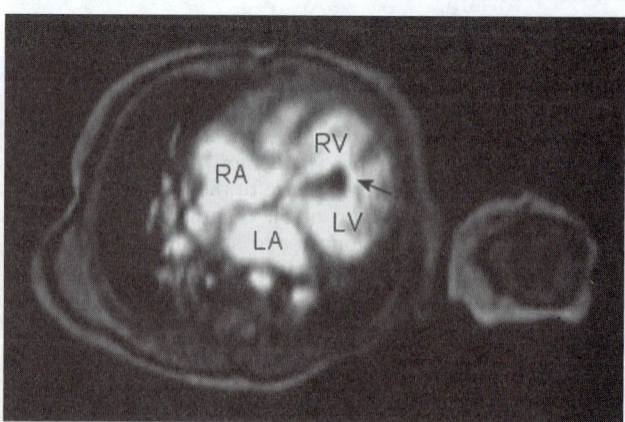

FIGURE 272.2. Single frame from a cine-magnetic resonance imaging series (horizontal long-axis four-chamber projection) demonstrating a muscular ventricular septal defect (VSD). LV, left ventricle, RV, right ventricle, LA, left atrium, RA, right atrium. The *arrow* points to the VSD.

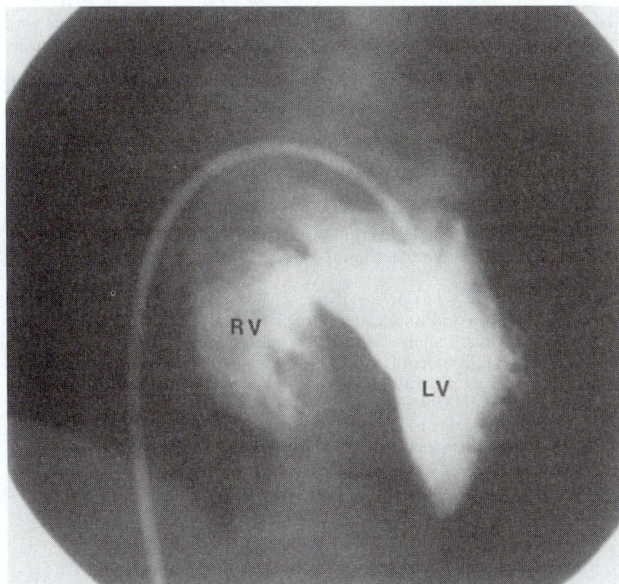

FIGURE 272.3. Left ventriculogram demonstrating flow of contrast across a moderately sized perimembranous ventricular septal defect. LV, left ventricle; RV, right ventricle.

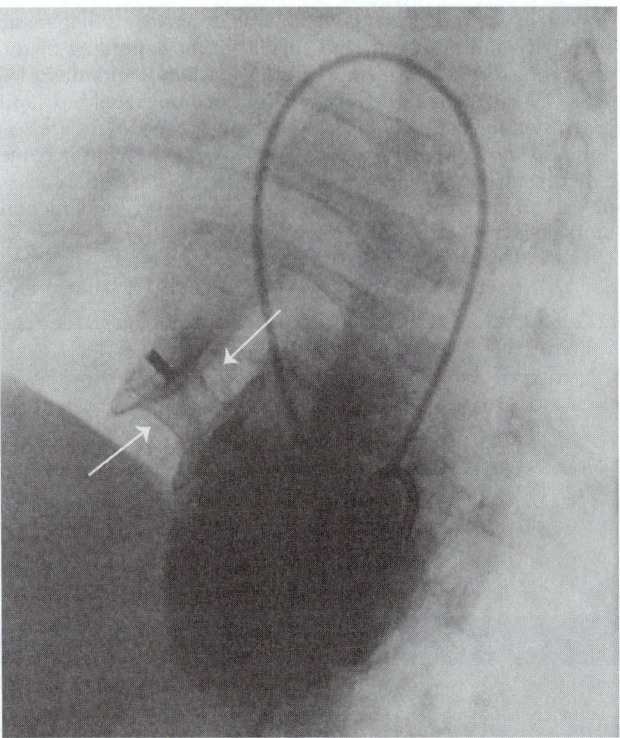

FIGURE 272.4. Left ventriculogram performed following placement of an AMPLATZER Muscular VSD (ventricular septal defect) Occlusion device. The *arrows* point to the device, which is positioned in the muscular trabecular septum. (Courtesy of AGA medical corp.)

absence of pulmonary hypertension. Many defects, especially those in the muscular septum, close spontaneously.

Infants with moderate or large VSDs often have symptoms associated with significant left-to-right shunting. CHF caused by an isolated VSD can be treated with conventional medical therapy, including diuretics, afterload reduction, and digoxin. The usual initial choice of a diuretic is furosemide, 1 to 2 mg/kg twice daily, or chlorothiazide, 10 to 20 mg/kg twice daily. Afterload reduction with an angiotensin-converting enzyme inhibitor (captopril, 0.1 to 0.5 mg/kg three times daily, or enalapril, 0.08 mg/kg twice daily) may improve symptoms significantly, especially in patients with low pulmonary vascular resistance. Digoxin, 0.01 mg/kg/day, remains part of the therapeutic regimen in many centers, but its use has decreased considerably since the mid 1990s. It should not be used in lieu of afterload reduction.

Even with aggressive medical therapy, infants with excessive pulmonary blood flow may gain weight poorly. Caloric requirements often in excess of 140 kcal/kg/day, fluid restriction, and poor feeding combine to render achieving adequate nutrition a challenge. Caloric supplementation and, occasionally, nasogastric feeding, may be required.

The goals of medical therapy are relief of symptoms and normal growth. When these goals are not achieved, early surgical repair should be considered strongly. Perimembranous defects associated with uncontrolled symptoms or failure to thrive should be repaired promptly, usually in the first 4 to 6 months of life. Large muscular defects, because of their tendency to become smaller and the technical difficulty associated with the surgical approach to apical defects, may be managed medically for longer periods of time.

Transcatheter closure of certain VSDs in selected patients has become a reasonable alternative to the conventional surgical approach in recent years. Large or multiple defects in the muscular septum can be difficult for the surgeon to correct, or they may require left ventriculotomy. These defects have been closed successfully with occlusion devices in the catheterization laboratory (Fig. 272.4) and, in some cases, in the operating room using a transventricular approach. The technology is advancing further with the development of specially designed devices for closure of perimembranous defects.

Patients whose pulmonary artery pressure remain elevated despite sucessful medicial therapy should undergo surgical repair by the time they are 6 to 12 months of age. When pulmonary artery pressure is normal, the decision whether to repair the defect is largely dependent on its location. Most subarterial defects, because of their high association with development of aortic regurgitation, are repaired by the time the child reaches school age. Perimembranous defects can be associated with aortic valve insufficiency, subaortic obstruction, right ventricular outflow tract obstruction, and left ventricle–to–right atrial shunting. For these reasons, many centers advocate repairing most perimembranous defects before the child reaches school age, regardless of the size of the defect. Small muscular defects are benign and require little cardiology follow-up after the child is 1 year of age.

ENDOCARDITIS PROPHYLAXIS, PREGNANCY, SPORTS, AND INSURABILITY

Older children and adults with VSD should continue receiving antimicrobial prophylaxis against bacterial endocarditis. A small VSD does not interfere with normal pregnancy. Children and adults with small or repaired VSDs need not be restricted from sports and should be eligible for health and life insurance with standard premiums.

FUTURE DIRECTIONS

The approach to VSD has changed in the past few decades as a result of continued improvement in surgical results (especially for small infants), improved noninvasive diagnostic sensitivity and precision, and enhanced understanding of the natural history of perimembranous, subarterial, and muscular defects. Diagnostic catheterization for uncomplicated VSD and protracted medical therapy for the symptomatic infant are seldom used now, whereas transcatheter intervention has become a therapeutic reality. Future work will help to clarify the causes of VSD and its treatment and prevention at a more fundamental biologic level.

Suggested Readings

Dickinson DF, Arnold R, Wilkinson JL. Ventricular septal defect in children born in Liverpool 1960 to 1969. *Br Heart J* 1981;46:47.

Frontera-Izquierdo P, Cabezuelo-Huerta G. Natural and modified history of isolated ventricular septal defect: a 17 year study. *Pediatr Cardiol* 1992;13:193.

Gabriel HM, Heger M, Innerhofer P, et al. Long-term outcome of patients with ventricular septal defect considered not to require surgical closure during childhood. *J Am Coll Cardiol* 2002;39:1066.

Gumbiner CH, Takao A. Ventricular septal defect. In: Garson A, Bricker JT, eds. *The science and practice of pediatric cardiology*. Baltimore: Williams & Wilkins, 1998.

Helmcke F, deSouza A, Nanda NC, et al. Two-dimensional and color Doppler assessment of ventricular septal defect of congenital origin. *Am J Cardiol* 1989;63:1112.

Hijazi ZM, Hakim Ff, Al-Fodley F, et al. Transcatheter closure of single muscular ventricular septal defects using the AMPLATZER Muscular VSD Occluder: initial results and technical considerations. *Cathet Cardiovasc Interv* 2000;49:167.

Lewis DA, Loffredo CA, Correa-Villasenor A, et al. Descriptive epidemiology of membranous and muscular ventricular septal defects in the Baltimore-Washington Infant Study. *Cardiol Young* 1996;6:281.

Van Den Heuval F, Timmers T, Hess J. Morphological haemodynamic, and clinical variables as predictors for management of isolated ventricular septal defect. *Br Heart J* 1995;73:49.

Weintraub RG, Menahem S. Early surgical closure of a large ventricular septal defect: influence on long term growth. *J Am Coll Cardiol* 1991;18:552.

Wu M, Wu JM, Chang CI, et al. Implication of aneurysmal transformation in isolated perimembranous ventricular septal defect. *Am J Cardiol* 1993;72:596.

CHAPTER 273 ■ PATENT DUCTUS ARTERIOSUS

CHARLES E. MULLINS

The patent ductus arteriosus (PDA) occurs normally as an essential structure in the fetus and becomes abnormal only when it persists after birth. In the term infant, the *persistent* patent ductus probably represents a structural abnormality in the ductus tissues present at birth. The persistent patency of the ductus in the premature infant is a more common problem and usually is a result of immaturity of ductal tissues. The ductus in the premature infant is covered in Chapter 53, Cardiovascular Disease in the Newborn, and is not discussed here. Persistent PDA is the second most common congenital heart defect, accounting for approximately 10% of all congenital heart defects in full-term infants.

The walls of the ductus arteriosus are composed of thick, spiraling elastic fibers and smooth muscles, which, when they contract, cause constriction of the lumen of the ducts. In the fetal circulation, the ductus allows right ventricular blood to bypass the nonexpanded and nonventilated lungs. Both the low Po_2 of the blood and a high level of circulating prostaglandins in the fetus inhibit constriction of the ductus. In the normal newborn, lung expansion occurs immediately with delivery. As a result, most of the right heart blood and, in turn, pulmonary artery blood is diverted immediately to the now lower-resistance pulmonary vascular bed. This obligatory flow through the lungs allows circulating prostaglandins in the fetus to be cleared by the most effective clearing system, the lungs, and immediately allows oxygenation of the blood, thereby increasing the circulating Po_2. Both the decreased prostaglandins and the increased blood Po_2 contribute to the normal constriction of the ductus. Normally, the ductus of a newborn functionally is closed by, at most, 72 hours of age and structurally is sealed by 3 months of age.

All factors resulting in persistent patency of the ductus are not understood. Factors such as high altitude or severe pulmonary disease, which cause persistent hypoxia, predispose to persistent patency of the ductus. Continued high prostaglandin levels, in the presence of a compromised or inefficient pulmonary clearing function (found in premature infants or in the marked decrease pulmonary flow occurring in some pulmonary atresia patients), contribute to the persistent patency of the ductus. Rubella (and possibly other viral infections) that occurs during the first trimester of pregnancy frequently results in patency of the ductus. Some evidence shows that a lower socioeconomic status, probably resulting in inadequate perinatal nutrition, may predispose to persistent patency of the ductus.

PATHOPHYSIOLOGY

When the ductus remains open and, with normal lungs, pulmonary resistance drops further, blood flows from the aorta through the ductus into the pulmonary arteries. Eventual flow to the lungs from the ductus depends on the size and shape of the ductus and on how close to normal levels the pulmonary vascular resistance drops. With normal pulmonary resistance, the flow through the ductus begins during mid to late systole and continues through diastole. This flow pattern corresponds to the timing of the maximal pressure gradient between the aorta and the pulmonary artery during the various phases of the cardiac cycle.

In the usual patient with a left aortic arch, the ductus arteriosus connects the junction of the main and left pulmonary artery to the descending thoracic aorta at a point just distal to the origin of the left subclavian artery. The persistent ductus varies in shape from very short and broad-based at both ends to long and tortuous. The diameter of the clinically detectable ductus ranges from less than 1 mm to more than 1 cm at the narrowest diameter and is independent of the shape of the ductus. Clinical finding depends on the final net flow through the lungs into the left atrium, left ventricle, aorta, and back through the ductus.

The uncomplicated patent ductus places a pure volume workload on the left heart with little or no effect on the right heart. The blood from the aorta flows through the ductus into the pulmonary arteries, through the pulmonary vascular bed into the left atrium, into the left ventricle, and back into the aorta. The total additional workload on the left ventricle depends directly on the size of the persistent ductus arteriosus and the magnitude of the resultant flow through the ductus. The additional blood from the ductus does mix with the blood ejected from the right ventricle into the pulmonary artery; however, in the absence of increased pulmonary resistance, the extra blood does not add significantly to the work of the right ventricle. As a result, in the absence of increased pulmonary resistance, little or no additional volume or pressure work is placed on the right ventricle, and no physical or clinical laboratory signs are present to suggest any right-sided involvement.

CLINICAL MANIFESTATIONS AND COMPLICATIONS

The clinical histories of patients with persistent patent ductus range from florid heart failure in the young infant to the presence of an incidental murmur in an otherwise perfectly healthy child or occasionally, even, in an adult. Occasionally, a patent ductus is discovered coincidentally on an echocardiogram with no associated symptoms or signs, thus suggesting a patent ductus—the so-called "silent ductus." The patient with a patent ductus presents as early as the newborn period and anytime thereafter, including into late adulthood. The most common presentation of the patient with a persistent patent ductus is a heart murmur discovered incidentally in an asymptomatic young child being examined for some other reason. The infant or child with a moderate-to-large patent ductus may be prone to, or more susceptible to, secondary lower respiratory tract infections after an initial upper airway respiratory infection. This susceptibility presumably is due to the decreased compliance of the lungs associated with the significantly increased pulmonary blood flow.

The murmur and associated clinical finding of a patent ductus usually are characteristic and often pathognomonic of the defect. The typical murmur of a patent ductus is continuous (sounding like machinery) and is maximal in intensity in the first and second left intercostal spaces in the left midclavicular line. The murmur begins with the first heart sound, then crescendos throughout systole until the second heart sound. The murmur peaks in intensity at the second sound before trailing off during diastole. Depending on the shape and size of the ductus, the intensity of the murmur varies from grade 1 to grade 6, and the quality ranges from high-pitched and blowing to low-frequency and rough.

The pulmonary component of the second sound is increased in intensity and delayed in occurrence, which widens the splitting and increases the overall intensity of the second sound, giving it a "slapping sail" quality. The second sound is maximal in intensity in the second and third left intercostal spaces. In the larger ductus with a significant increase in pulmonary flow, an associated left ventricular lift and an apical diastolic flow rumble occur, both of which are caused by the increased volume flow across an otherwise normal mitral valve.

Peripheral pulses are bounding in quality as a result of both the increased left ventricular stroke volume and the diastolic runoff through the ductus into the lungs. This combination generates a wide pulse pressure. In the patient with a large persistent ductus, pulses often are visible in the suprasternal, carotid, axillary, and femoral areas.

Several situations with an isolated ductus exist in which physical findings of the ductus are atypical. In the patient with higher pulmonary resistance, the diastolic runoff into the lungs is decreased or stopped entirely, so the clinical findings resulting from this runoff are not present. The diastolic component of the murmur, in particular, decreases or disappears, the bounding pulses no longer are present, and no mitral flow murmur occurs. These atypical findings may occur in the presence of significant bronchospastic disease or a superimposed severe lower respiratory tract infection.

At the other extreme, in the young infant with a very large ductus and low pulmonary resistance, much of the flow through the ductus into the pulmonary arteries occurs during systole, or the ejection phase of the blood, with little continued flow occurring during diastole. In these patients, the murmur is localized further down the left sternal border, and the diastolic component is decreased markedly or is absent. The tip-off to the presence of a patent ductus in these patients is the persistence of the split and "slapping" second sound and the bounding pulses caused by the wide pulse pressure. The atypical persistent patent ductus requires an accurate echocardiogram and/or, often, a detailed cardiac catheterization for confirmation of the diagnosis.

The electrocardiogram in the patient with the uncomplicated ductus is normal or, in the larger ductus, shows left ventricular hypertrophy and left atrial enlargement. The chest radiograph shows cardiomegaly proportionate to the flow through the ductus, with a prominent main pulmonary artery segment, large ascending aorta and arch, increased pulmonary vascular markings, and a "left ventricular" contour to the heart shadow, with possible left atrial enlargement.

DIAGNOSIS

The diagnosis is supported by the echocardiogram. The ductus usually is seen on two-dimensional echocardiogram. Turbulent flow by Doppler interrogation in the main pulmonary artery supports the echocardiographic findings. Intracardiac lesions other than persistent ductus are ruled out by the echocardiogram, as are lesions that can be confused with the ductus. Continuous-wave Doppler can detect very small streams of abnormal flow in the pulmonary artery. Even the very tiny ductus (the so-called silent ductus), which is too small to be audible or visualized by echocardiogram, can be detected by continuous-wave Doppler, and/or the flow can be seen using color Doppler.

When all clinical findings of the ductus are assimilated and are absolutely characteristic, the diagnosis is established without further study. If even one atypical feature in any part of the clinical assessment is present, then the diagnosis should be established by cardiac catheterization. A cardiac catheterization for a patent ductus should be performed only in a catheterization laboratory capable of treating, as well as diagnosing, the ductus in the catheterization laboratory.

During the catheterization of an isolated patent ductus, the hemodynamic information demonstrates an increase in the oxygen saturation of the mixed venous blood, which is maximized in the main pulmonary artery. Usually, this step-up in saturation is higher in the main pulmonary artery than in the more distal branch pulmonary arteries as a consequence of the direct stream of blood flowing through the ductus directly toward the main pulmonary artery and pulmonary valve. During the cardiac catheterization, the cardiac catheter often passes preferentially from the main pulmonary artery through the ductus into the descending aorta. Although it adds support to the diagnosis, the catheter passage alone cannot be used to confirm the diagnosis. Similar, if not identical, hemodynamics and catheter course are observed when the catheter passes from the right ventricle through a ventricular septal defect into the ascending aorta and then around the arch to the descending aorta, or when the catheter passes from the pulmonary artery through an aortopulmonary window into the ascending aorta and then around the arch. The presence of a ductus arteriosus is confirmed by an angiocardiogram recorded, preferentially, in the lateral view with the contrast injected into the descending aorta immediately adjacent to the usual entrance site of the ductus. This same angiocardiogram provides details about the size and exact shape of the ductus. When a catheterization is performed, it definitively rules out defects that may be confused with a ductus and/or establishes the presence of other defects that may be associated incidentally with the ductus.

Differential Diagnosis

The venous hum is the murmur most often confused with the patent ductus arteriosus; it is the most benign and easiest to differentiate clinically. When carefully examined, the venous hum is a continuous sounding murmur; however, it usually is a softer, more distant continuous murmur. Most important, the venous hum crescendos or peaks in intensity during diastole. The venous hum usually is maximal in intensity in the first and second right intercostal spaces. It varies in intensity, or actually is eliminated by changes in body position, respirations, or neck rotation. The murmur of the venous hum can be stopped by placing the patient in the supine position and simultaneously applying gentle compression over the right jugular vein in the right supraclavicular area. With the auscultatory characteristics of the venous hum and the maneuvers to eliminate it, no further diagnostic studies are necessary to differentiate this murmur.

Potentially, the lesion that is the most difficult to differentiate from the persistent ductus is the aortopulmonary window. The aortopulmonary window is a very rare, window-like communication between the proximal ascending aorta and the main pulmonary artery that allows systemic blood to flow directly from the ascending aorta into the pulmonary artery. The hemodynamics are virtually identical to those of the ductus, with the site of the abnormal "window" communication anatomically close to that of the ductus; thus, many clinical findings are similar, if not identical, to those of the patent ductus.

The aortopulmonary (A-P) window usually is a large communication and results in a very large systemic-to-pulmonary shunt. Consequently, patients with this condition usually present early in infancy with significant respiratory distress and signs of pulmonary congestion and "heart" failure. Because of the large size of the defect and the proximal location on the aorta, most of the runoff of the blood into the pulmonary artery from the aorta occurs during systole. As a result, the murmur may be only systolic and usually is located more over the left sternal border than in the infraclavicular area. Because of the proximal location of the communication in the ascending aorta, a blood steal from the more peripheral circulation and vessels, including the brachiocephalic and the descending aorta, occurs. As a consequence, in the presence of a large A-P window, all the palpable pulses may be decreased rather than bounding. The rarer, small aortopulmonary window, on the other hand, has findings indistinguishable from those of a small persistent ductus. Confirmation of the diagnosis is established by echocardiogram and/or, more usually, high-quality angiography.

A more common lesion that can be confused with a patent ductus, particularly when the physical examination is not precise, is the combination of ventricular septal defect with associated aortic valve insufficiency. The murmur in these patients is to-and-fro rather than continuous. A plateau pansystolic murmur, which ends at the second heart sound as a result of the ventricular septal defect, is heard. It is followed by a higher-pitched, decrescendo, diastolic murmur of the aortic regurgitation. Other physical findings, electrocardiogram, and radiographs may be similar to those of a patent ductus, but the lesions should be distinguishable by astute auscultation on the physical examination; if not, it is diagnosed by echocardiogram and/or cardiac catheterization.

A sinus of Valsalva fistula creates a murmur and clinical findings similar to those of a patent ductus. On close auscultation, however, the murmur, like the murmur of the ventricular septal defect with aortic insufficiency, is more to-and-fro, with separate systolic and diastolic components. Also, the murmur of a sinus of Valsalva fistula frequently is localized and/or maximal over the lower left or right sternal border.

Any intrathoracic systemic-to-pulmonary artery or systemic-to–venous fistula can generate a continuous murmur, which possibly could be confused with a persistent patent ductus. In virtually all these lesions, however, the continuous murmur has a markedly different location, depending on the site of the fistulous communication. Over the location of maximum intensity, the murmur of a fistula often has an almost superficial or "close" sounding quality, which is a particularly common finding with a coronary artery camera fistula. This fistula is the most likely fistulous lesion to be localized close to the location of the ductus and, in turn, the most likely to mimic the ductus murmur.

All other lesions with continuous murmurs (e.g., truncus arteriosus, pulmonary atresia/ventricular septal defect with systemic collaterals, and stenosed anomalous pulmonary veins) have cyanosis and markedly different associated physical findings, electrocardiograms, and roentgenograms.

Complicated Ductus

When a ductus is present in association with other congenital heart lesions, it may be difficult to detect. The physical signs, radiographic appearance, and electrocardiographic findings of the associated lesion usually overshadow the characteristic murmur and radiographic findings of the ductus. In the absence of the classical continuous murmur of the persistent ductus, the one finding on physical examination that should cause the examiner to suspect a patent ductus is the presence of full, bounding pulses, which would not be expected with an *intra*cardiac shunt lesion. The associated defects and the persistent ductus usually are visualized by a carefully performed echocardiogram. When combination lesions are suspected, however, they are confirmed by a detailed cardiac catheterization. Catheterization documents the presence of the ductus as well as determines the relative hemodynamic importance of each lesion in these cases.

In two categories of congenital heart lesions the associated patent ductus is essential to the survival of the patient—the ductus-dependent lesions. In the first category are severe left-heart obstructive lesions. In patients with severe mitral and/or aortic stenosis, most of the systemic flow is from the right ventricle through the ductus. In patients with severe coarctation of the aorta or interruption of the aortic arch, the blood flow to the lower body depends on the ductus. With the coarctation, the dilated aortic end of the open ductus allows additional blood flow around or adjacent to the obstruction in the aorta. With complete interruption of the aorta, the blood flow is from the pulmonary artery through the ductus into the descending aorta, with the lower-body blood flow coming solely from this route.

The second category of ductus-dependent lesions are those with a severely restricted, or even totally obstructed, pulmonary valve. In patients with this condition, most, or even total pulmonary blood flow is through the patent ductus. These ductus-dependent lesions must be recognized early, and efforts must be made to keep the ductus open until an appropriate interventional procedure can be performed to maintain or replace the ductus.

Another complicated ductus arteriosus is the ductus with pulmonary hypertension and associated pulmonary vascular disease. In patients with this condition, none of the characteristic findings of the ductus is present. Because of the high pulmonary resistance, little or no flow occurs from the aorta into the pulmonary artery and, in turn, all the physical findings of flow through the ductus are absent. Usually, a right ventricular lift is present, and the second heart sound is single, very loud, and often palpable. No murmur or only a short nonspecific systolic murmur is present. With very high resistance, the desaturated pulmonary artery blood flows from the pulmonary artery into the descending aorta. This latter phenomenon produces the pathognomonic clinical finding of a cyanotic lower trunk and lower extremities with, at the same time, normal coloration of the upper trunk, head, and upper extremities. These patients have right ventricular hypertrophy on electrocardiogram. Radiographs reveal a normal to slightly enlarged heart size with a very prominent main pulmonary artery segment and proximal right and left pulmonary arteries, yet normal or decreased peripheral pulmonary vascular markings. The patient with the pulmonary hypertensive ductus should be studied by cardiac catheterization to unequivocally exclude the possibility of any other cause of increased total pulmonary resistance.

Bacterial endocarditis is a potential complication of any patent ductus arteriosus. Since the advent of early surgical correction of the ductus and the use of prophylactic antibiotics in patients with congenital heart lesions, the incidence of this complication has decreased markedly. Of all isolated congenital heart defects, the incidence of endocarditis in patients now occurs least in the patent ductus arteriosus, whereas the prevention of this complication now is the major indication for correcting most of the small ductus.

THERAPY

Therapy for a PDA is supportive until definitive therapy is possible. The supportive therapy is treatment of symptoms resulting from the patent ductus. Patients with a large persistent ductus have signs and symptoms of pulmonary over circulation, with shortness of breath, dyspnea, and, even, overt pulmonary edema. Symptoms are treated with digoxin and vigorous diuretic therapy. Occasionally, the young infant with a large patent ductus requires intubation and ventilation with end-expiratory positive pressure to control the pulmonary overcirculation. These medical measures help control symptoms but do not treat the underlying anatomic defect. Definitive intervention is indicated when supportive therapy does not support the infant or child or does not allow normal growth, development, and activity.

When no therapy is necessary, or when supportive therapy is required but satisfactorily maintains the patient without symptom or signs, then elective definitive repair is considered anytime after the patient reaches 2 to 3 years of age, but usually before the child enters school. The primary urgency for providing very early repair of the asymptomatic ductus is the anxiety of the child's physician, which often is relayed to the parents. Definitive therapy for the ductus is to interrupt blood flow through the ductus completely and permanently. In the past, this interruption was achieved by performing an operative ligation and division of the ductus through a thoracotomy, but now it is accomplished in the cardiac catheterization laboratory.

Surgical repair of the ductus requires a thoracotomy or, at least, very sophisticated thoracoscopy; however, it does not require cardiopulmonary bypass and is considered a minor cardiac surgical procedure. Nonetheless, it is a surgical procedure with the inherent discomfort and morbidity of such. The thoracic surgical patient requires deep general anesthesia, intubation, a thoracotomy, and a one-day stay in the recovery ward with a period of continued intubation or with a chest tube in place. The postoperative surgical patient has 3 to 5 days of hospitalized recovery and a further 4- to 8-week convalescence before returning to full normal physical activity. The patient undergoing thoracoscopic ligation of the ductus does have a decreased duration of intensive care and hospitalization and postoperative convalescence.

In addition to the acute risks of surgery and recovery from surgery, rare, but possibly permanent complications, which may be associated even more commonly with thoracoscopic repairs, can occur. They include vocal cord or diaphragmatic paralysis from intrathoracic nerve injury or even the ligation of the wrong vessel or structure within the chest. In addition to the morbidity of the surgery, a small, finite rate of mortality is associated with surgical repair of the patent ductus.

One year after the ligation and division surgery, the ductus is considered cured. By then, complete healing is ensured, and the risk of developing endocarditis is considered eliminated. After ligation-only at the time of surgery, recanalization of the ductus occurs in as many as 10% of cases. Data accumulated from other ductus occlusion techniques and from high-resolution Doppler studies show that the recanalization of the ductus after surgical ligation usually, if not always, is a residual tiny ductus following the initial attempted ligation.

Several alternative, nonsurgical definitive techniques and devices can be used for the elective correction of the patent ductus in the cardiac catheterization laboratory. These devices and the associated techniques for the nonsurgical repair of the ductus have evolved over the course of almost four decades, beginning with the report by Dr. Porstmann in 1967, when a catheter-delivered Ivalon plug was used for the occlusion of the ductus. The delivery of this plug required a very large introductory system and involved a very complex arteriovenous catheterization. A much smaller, hooked umbrella and then a double-umbrella PDA device, both developed by Rashkind, were introduced shortly after the Porstmann device. The Rashkind double umbrellas proved to be very effective and safe in an extensive clinical trial performed in the United States. The Rashkind umbrellas were accepted throughout the rest of the world as standard therapy in the 1980s, and they had a very widespread use for the occlusion of the ductus. The Rashkind umbrellas never were approved for routine use in the United States and, with the absence of that market, were withdrawn from production and availability. In spite of their disappearance, the Rashkind devices did demonstrate unequivocally that the patent ductus could be cured in the catheterization laboratory both safely and effectively. With the lack of availability in the United States and then the relatively sudden, total withdrawal of a demonstrated safe and effective nonsurgical correction of the ductus, the modification and development of other devices for transcatheter PDA occlusion was stimulated, and at an almost frantic pace.

The first "new" device to be modified for the ductus was the standard Gianturco coil, which already had been approved for decades for the treatment of vascular occlusions. Moore and Cambier showed that the coil could be teetered on the narrow area of the ductus and would effectively occlude the PDA. The implant of the coils was somewhat precarious and did lead to coil embolization, with the subsequent need to retrieve the iatrogenic foreign body. Numerous devices and techniques were developed to control the delivery and implant of the coil, with the result that, by the mid 1990s, coil occlusion of the PDA was accepted everywhere by medical professionals as the standard of care for the correction of the patent ductus.

In addition to modifications and additions to the Gianturco coils, entirely new devices and procedures for the transcatheter occlusion of the PDA were developed. The most effective of which was the Amplatzer PDA Occluder. The Amplatzer PDA occluders are specifically shaped, basket-like plugs made of a mesh of many fine Nitinol memory wires. Each plug, at its resting and body temperature configuration, is a small, short, slightly tapered cylinder with a small flange circumferentially around the larger end of the cylinder. To stop flow through the mesh initially, several polyester disks are present within each plug. The Amplatzer PDA devices are available in multiple sizes to fit the different-sized ductus. The mesh is stretched into a long thin strand for delivery. The device is delivered to the ductus through a long sheath with a small diameter and fixes in the ductus by re-expanding to its resting configuration.

The Amplatzer PDA device has had extensive use outside of the United States; underwent a detailed, controlled Food and Drug Administration (FDA) IDE trial in the United States and, in 2003, received FDA approval for PDA occlusion in the catheterization laboratory by specifically trained physicians. With the use of either coils or the Amplatzer PDA device, the PDA in all patients past the newborn period now are closed in the cardiac catheterization laboratory as the accepted standard of care throughout the world, including the United States. Although the patent ductus in the premature infant still requires surgical closure, surgical correction of the ductus beyond early infancy now seldom is performed and then usually only in the very unusual or complex ductus or in very sick patients, so that it no longer represents a simple operation.

Suggested Readings

Alzamora V, Rotta A, Gattilana G, et al. On the possible influence of great altitudes on the determination of certain cardiovascular anomalies. *Pediatrics* 1953;12:259.

Cambier PA, Kirby WC, Moore JW, et al. Percutaneous closure of the small (<2.5 mm) patent ductus arteriosus using coil embolization. *Am J Cardiol* 1992;69:815.

Gittenberger-De Groot AC, Van Ertbruggen I, Moulaert AJMG, et al. The ductus arteriosus in the preterm infant: histologic and clinical observations. *J Pediatr* 1980;96:88.

Heymann MA, Rudolph AM. Control of the ductus arteriosus. *Physiol Rev* 1975;55:62.

Mansura J, Walsh KP, Hijazi ZM, et al. Catheter closure of moderate to large-sized paten ductus arteriosus using the new Amplatzer Duct Occluder: immediate and short term results. *J Am Coll Cardiol* 1998;31:878.

Portsmann W, Wierny L, Warnke H. Der verschluss des D.A.P. ohne thorakotomie (1 Mitteilung). *Thoraxchirurgie* 1967;15:199.

Rashkind WJ, Cuaso CC. Transcatheter closure of patent ductus arteriosus: successful use in a 3.5 kilogram infant. *Pediatr Cardiol* 1979;1:3.

Rashkind WJ, Mullins CE, Hellenbrand WE, et al. Nonsurgical closure of patent ductus arteriosus: clinical application of the Rashkind PDA Occluder system. *Circulation* 1987;75:583.

Rudolph AM, Drorbaugh JE, Auld PA, et al. Studies on the circulation in the neonatal period: the circulation in the respiratory distress syndrome. *Pediatrics* 1961;27:551.

Swan C, Tostevin AL, Black GHB. Final observations on congenital defects in infants following infectious diseases during pregnancy with special reference to rubella. *Med J Aust* 1946;2:889.

Thibeault DW, Emmanouilides GC, Nelson RJ, et al. Patent ductus arteriosus complicating the respiratory distress syndrome in preterm infants. *J Pediatr* 1975;86:120.

CHAPTER 274 ■ PULMONARY STENOSIS

JOHN P. CHEATHAM

Obstruction of pulmonary blood flow may occur within the right ventricle, at the valve, or anywhere in the pulmonary arterial system. In general terms, pulmonary stenosis occurs in approximately 20% to 30% of all patients with congenital heart disease. In approximately one-half of these patients, the ventricular septum is intact.

PULMONARY VALVE STENOSIS

Epidemiology

Pulmonary valve stenosis constitutes approximately 7% to 12% of all congenital heart disease and as many as 80% to 90% of all lesions causing obstruction of right ventricular output. The defect originally was described in 1761 by Morgagni. The exact pathogenetic mechanism for its development is unclear. Several authors suggest that an abnormality of the distal bulbus cordis leads to valvar obstruction with sparing of the proximal bulbus, which participates in closure of the ventricular septum. Fetal endocarditis also is implicated in the etiology of this defect. Genetic factors may play an equally important role because pulmonary valve stenosis often is found in various syndromes.

Pathology

The gross and microscopic features of pulmonary valve stenosis are classified into six categories: domed (42%); tricuspid (6.5%); bicuspid (10%); unicommissural (16%); hypoplastic annulus (6.5%); and dysplastic (19%). The pathologic processes affecting the remaining portion of the right-sided cardiac structures involve changes secondary to the valve obstruction (i.e., right ventricular hypertrophy, fibrosis, and tricuspid valve abnormalities).

Clinically, pulmonary valve stenosis with intact ventricular septum is described best as mild, moderate, or severe. *Mild stenosis* is defined here as a systolic transvalvular gradient of less than 40 mm Hg or right ventricular pressure of less than one-half of systemic arterial pressure. *Moderate obstruction* is considered to be present when the systolic gradient across the pulmonary valve is greater than 40 mm Hg or right ventricular pressure is greater than one-half of, but still less than, systemic arterial pressure. *Severe stenosis* is defined as a systolic gradient of more than 80 mm Hg or the presence of suprasystemic right ventricular pressure.

Clinical Manifestations and Complications

Patients with mild stenosis are asymptomatic, exhibiting normal growth and development and no cyanosis. The jugular venous pulse is normal, and no sign of congestive heart failure is present. Children with moderate stenosis and an intact ventricular septum may develop mild dyspnea with exertion, but frequently they are asymptomatic. Cyanosis with exertion may be noted occasionally if an atrial septal defect is present. Individuals with severe valvular stenosis usually demonstrate symptoms, although as many as 25% of these patients are asymptomatic. Frequently, dyspnea and fatigue with only a moderate amount of exertion are present. Central cyanosis is one of the most important signs in patients with an atrial communication; it may be present at rest or with minimal exercise. Some evidence indicates that the degree of cyanosis increases with age. When "squatting" is seen in a cyanotic child suspected of having pulmonary valve stenosis, the diagnosis of tetralogy of Fallot must be considered. Growth and development in infants with severe stenosis usually are normal, without evidence of wasting. "Moon facies" in conjunction with a chubby phenotype has been described as characteristic of young children with pulmonary valve stenosis, but it is not pathognomonic and is present in fewer than 50% of infants with severe obstruction.

Diagnosis

The cardiovascular examination aids in establishing the diagnosis of pulmonary valve stenosis. The precordial activity is quiet with mild obstruction, but it may be increased with a palpable right ventricular tap in patients with moderate or severe stenosis. A systolic thrill over the pulmonary valve area may be present as the severity increases. The striking auscultatory feature of pulmonary valve stenosis is a prominent systolic ejection murmur. The murmur may vary in length and intensity, but it usually ends before the aortic valve closes. The maximum intensity of the murmur is at the upper left sternal border radiating to the back, but it also is heard along the precordium and the neck. As the severity increases, the systolic ejection murmur lengthens, and the peak in intensity occurs later. The murmur of pulmonary valve stenosis increases in duration and intensity after amyl nitrate inhalation, whereas the opposite is true in children with tetralogy of Fallot.

A high-pitched ejection sound or systolic click usually is audible along the left upper sternal border. The click probably originates from the sudden opening and doming of the thickened pulmonary valve leaflets. As the severity of the obstruction increases, the systolic ejection click occurs earlier until, in severe stenosis, it may be indistinguishable from the first heart sound. The second heart sound usually is split and of normal intensity in mild stenosis. The degree of splitting is directly proportional to the severity of obstruction. An inverse relationship exists between the severity of stenosis and the intensity of the pulmonary component of the second heart sound. In severe stenosis, therefore, a wide splitting of the second heart sound is present, with a very soft pulmonary component that often is heard as a single second sound.

The electrocardiogram frequently is normal in patients with mild stenosis, whereas it is normal in only 10% of children with moderate obstruction, and it is uniformly abnormal in cases of severe stenosis. Right axis deviation frequently is seen, with right ventricular hypertrophy noted in the anterior precordial leads. In patients with moderate stenosis, the magnitude of the R wave in V_1 usually is less than 20 mm, whereas an upright T wave in V_1 is present approximately 50% of the time. A qR or a pure R wave of more than 20 mm is present in patients with severe stenosis. In some children, ST or T waves may suggest ischemia.

The most consistent and distinctive radiographic feature is prominence in the main pulmonary artery segment secondary to poststenotic dilation of the pulmonary trunk and the proximal left pulmonary artery (Fig. 274.1). This finding is present in as many as 90% of patients, but it does not correlate with the severity of obstruction. In patients with severe stenosis, the cardiac apex may be tilted upward, and generalized cardiomegaly and right atrial prominence may be present, especially if right-sided failure is present. The aortic arch usually is left-sided.

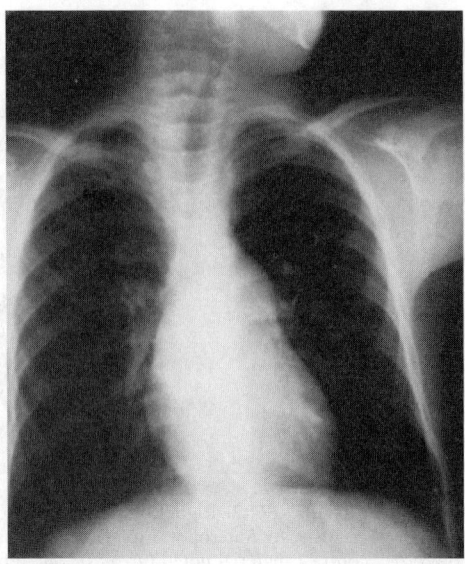

FIGURE 274.1. Chest roentgenogram from an 8-year-old boy with mild stenosis of the pulmonary valve. Heart size usually is normal. Pulmonary vascular markings are unremarkable. The most distinctive radiographic feature of this disease is poststenotic dilation of the pulmonary trunk, as depicted in this chest film. The degree of dilation is unrelated to the severity of stenosis.

Presence of a right arch should lead the physician to consider the diagnosis of tetralogy of Fallot.

The noninvasive evaluation of abnormalities of the pulmonary valve by M-mode and two-dimensional echocardiography has been less than satisfactory. Doppler echocardiography with color flow mapping techniques increases both the sensitivity and specificity of the diagnosis of pulmonary valve stenosis. Two-dimensional echocardiography enables visualization of the thickened and domed pulmonary valve leaflets, pulmonary annulus, dilated pulmonary trunk, hypertrophic right ventricle, and other associated congenital heart defects. Pulsed and continuous-wave Doppler echocardiography enable accurate estimation to be made of the location and severity of pulmonary stenosis without using invasive procedures. The recorded peak flow velocity on spectral display is converted to an estimated transvalvular pressure gradient using the modified Bernoulli equation: $PG = 4V^2$, where PG equals instantaneous pressure gradient (mm Hg) and V equals peak Doppler velocity (m/second). Color-coded Doppler echocardiography may provide additional hemodynamic information about patients with pulmonary valve stenosis.

The role of cardiac catheterization and angiography in the diagnosis and treatment of pulmonary valve stenosis has changed significantly since the early 1980s. In the past, information obtained in the catheterization laboratory was a prerequisite for selecting patients for surgical valvotomy. Since the initial use of percutaneous, transluminal balloon pulmonary valvuloplasty in 1982, the catheterization laboratory has become the location for the "treatment" of moderate and severe pulmonary valve stenosis. The most important hemodynamic information obtained during cardiac catheterization is the measurement of right ventricular pressure simultaneously with left ventricular or aortic pressure and the systolic gradient across the pulmonary valve. Defining any associated cardiac defects at this time also is important. The use of biplanar angiocardiography with high-resolution video disks, recorders, and monitors has helped greatly in the use of therapeutic techniques during interventional pediatric cardiac catheterization. Angiographic features of pulmonary valve stenosis include thickening and doming of valve leaflets with poststenotic dilation of the pulmonary trunk (Fig. 274.2).

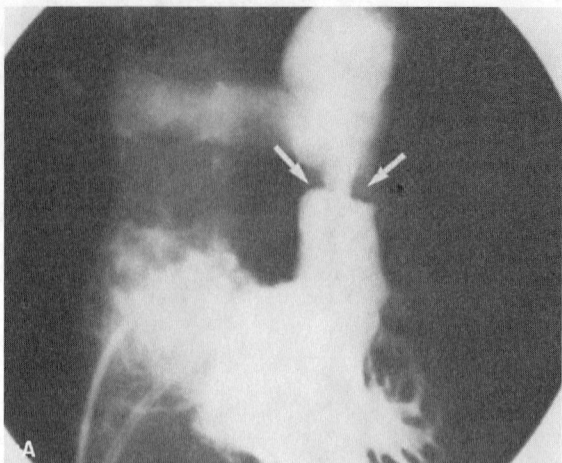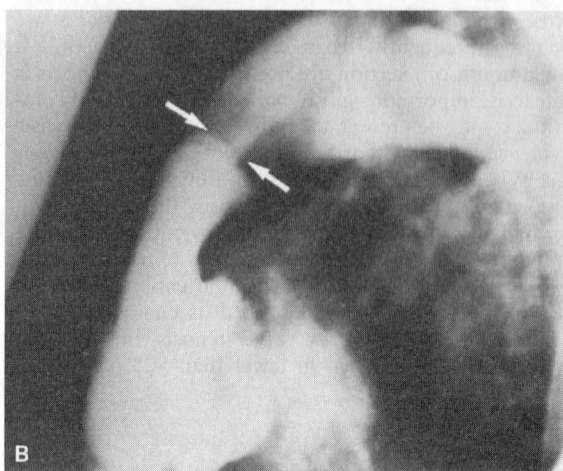

FIGURE 274.2. Right ventriculogram in a patient with typical features of moderate pulmonary valve stenosis. **A:** Anteroposterior view demonstrating systolic doming of the stenotic leaflets with a "jet" of contrast material noted (*arrows*). The infundibulum is widely patent, and the main pulmonary artery is dilated. **B:** Lateral projection shows the systolic jet that passes through the thickened leaflets (*arrows*).

Some studies demonstrate hemodynamic abnormalities during exercise in children and adults with pulmonary valve stenosis. In both children and adults with severe stenosis, myocardial performance during exercise was altered (i.e., decreased stroke and cardiac index and increased right ventricular end-diastolic pressure). Adults, however, had a disproportionately lower cardiac index and heart rate at rest and during exercise than did children with obstruction of the same magnitude. Evidence exists of myocardial fibrosis in uncorrected moderate to severe pulmonary valve stenosis in adults, which suggests the need for aggressive treatment of this condition during childhood.

The differential diagnosis of pulmonary valve stenosis with intact ventricular septum includes atrial septal defect, pulmonary artery stenosis, ventricular septal defect (VSD), idiopathic dilation of the main pulmonary artery, straight-back syndrome, mitral valve prolapse, aortic valve stenosis, and innocent pulmonary flow murmurs. When cyanosis is present, tetralogy of Fallot and pulmonary valve atresia with intact ventricular septum should be considered. The correct diagnosis usually can be made by physical examination, but echocardiography may help distinguish among various congenital heart defects. Pulmonary valve stenosis may be associated with various systemic diseases and syndromes (e.g., glycogen storage disease, neurofibromatosis, gout, neoplasm, carcinoid bowel disease, and Noonan, Williams, Watson, and Leopard syndromes).

The natural history of mild pulmonary valve stenosis is benign. Little improvement in severe obstruction occurs, however, and often the transvalvular gradient increases with age. A definite risk of right-sided congestive heart failure, myocardial fibrosis, and sudden death in these patients exists. The clinical course and prognosis of moderate pulmonary valve stenosis is debated, but exercise studies demonstrating right ventricular dysfunction in adults are alarming. The risk of infective endocarditis developing in patients with pulmonary valve stenosis is low, but all individuals, regardless of the severity of stenosis or whether intervention has taken place, should receive selected antibiotics for infective endocarditis prophylaxis during indicated dental or surgical procedures.

Therapy

Medical treatment of children with pulmonary valve stenosis usually is confined to neonates with critical obstruction. These newborns present with cyanosis, right-sided congestive heart failure, and cardiomegaly. Because adequate pulmonary blood flow depends on patency of the ductus arteriosus, intravenous infusion of prostaglandin E_1 (0.05 to 0.10 μg/kg/minute) is life-saving. Anticongestive medications (e.g., digoxin, furosemide, dopamine) also may be necessary. The treatment of choice in these neonates, as well as in children with moderate to severe stenosis, is transcatheter balloon pulmonary valvuloplasty performed in the cardiac catheterization laboratory.

Since its initial description in 1982, balloon dilation of the thickened pulmonary valve has evolved into a fairly standard treatment performed by the pediatric cardiac interventionalist. After hemodynamic measurements are obtained and right ventriculography is performed, a properly sized balloon catheter is chosen (1.2 to 1.4 times the size of the angiographically measured annulus). The balloon catheter is positioned over a guidewire through the stenotic pulmonary valve, and the balloon is inflated (by use of a handheld gauge) to the recommended burst pressure (measured in atmospheres) or until the balloon "waist" disappears (Fig. 274.3). The introduction of larger-diameter balloon catheters (20 to 40 mm) allows a single catheter to be used in most instances. Occasionally, two balloon catheters are required.

In the neonate with critical pulmonary valve stenosis, the transcatheter dilation of the valve is considerably more difficult to perform and requires that the operator have expertise. The right ventricular cavity and tricuspid valve diameter may be very small, with significant tricuspid regurgitation. The opening of the pulmonary valve frequently is less than 1 mm and requires that a 0.014-in. floppy-tip coronary guidewire be passed through the orifice by use of a 5 Fr. right coronary artery guiding catheter. The guidewire is aimed through the patent ductus arteriosus into the descending aorta, where it is snared through the umbilical artery catheter to form a "transductal rail." This maneuver facilitates passage of the balloon catheter over the guidewire across the very abnormal and thickened pulmonary valve.

Balloon valvuloplasty produces relief of obstruction by commissural splitting of the valve but sometimes may cause avulsion of leaflets. Typically, immediate relief of the transvalvar gradient occurs in moderate pulmonary valve stenosis after successful balloon valvuloplasty (Fig. 274.4). In patients with severe stenosis, and certainly in the neonate with critical obstruction, the right ventricular pressure falls significantly but seldom is normal. Dynamic infundibular subpulmonary

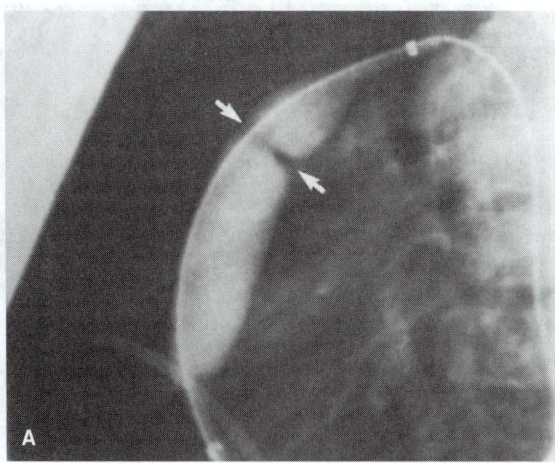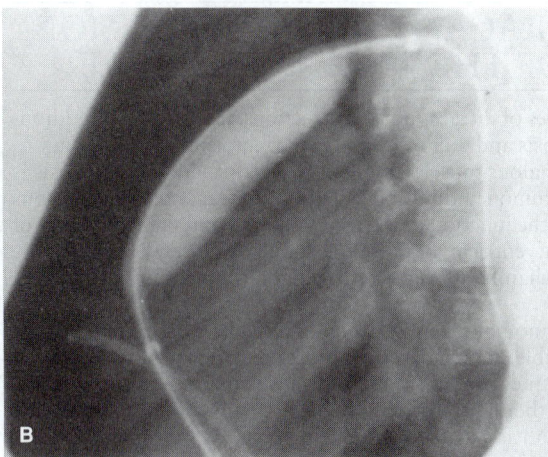

FIGURE 274.3. Proper positioning of the balloon catheter for pulmonary valvuloplasty via the lateral view under fluoroscopy. A: A guidewire passes through the catheter from the right ventricular outflow tract into the left pulmonary artery. The balloon is inflated with diluted contrast material (20%) until a "waist" is seen that corresponds to the stenotic valve leaflets (*arrows*). Attempts to maintain the waist at the midportion of the balloon should be made while the catheter is positioned. In this case, the waist is toward the distal one-third of the balloon. B: The balloon is repositioned more distally and is completely inflated using a handheld manometer. Note that the hourglass waist has disappeared.

stenosis accounts for the residual gradient initially, but it has a tendency to improve with time as the right ventricular hypertrophy regresses.

The response of dysplastic pulmonary valves to balloon dilation varies but, in general, is less than that of nondysplastic valves. This type of valvar stenosis is present in approximately 50% of children with Noonan syndrome. Valve leaflets are

FIGURE 274.4. Pressure recordings obtained at cardiac catheterization before and after balloon valvuloplasty for moderate pulmonary valve stenosis. A: The right ventricular (*RV*) systolic pressure is somewhat greater than 70 mm Hg before balloon valvuloplasty. Note the triangular appearance of the RV pressure curve, which is indicative of significant stenosis. B: The RV systolic pressure decreases to 30 mm Hg with a completely normal pressure curve. Aortic (*Ao*) pressure remained unchanged during the procedure.

unfused and excessively thick and demonstrate little motion during the cardiac cycle. Both balloon valvuloplasty and surgical valvotomy usually are inadequate procedures to relieve the obstruction completely. Partial or total surgical valvectomy may be required to relieve the valvar gradient in these children, but balloon valvuloplasty should be attempted initially using a high-pressure balloon catheter.

According to the Valvuloplasty and Angioplasty of Congenital Anomalies (VACA) Registry, the overall risk of a major complication occurring during balloon pulmonary valvuloplasty is 0.6% and includes death (0.2%), cardiac perforation with tamponade (0.1%), and severe tricuspid insufficiency (0.2%). Minor complications occur in 1.3% of patients, whereas 2.6% experience an incident defined as arrhythmia, hypoxemia, or venous bleeding. The incidence of complications is related inversely to age, being substantially higher in neonates who exhibit critical narrowing of the pulmonary valve.

Although surgical pulmonary valvotomy is a relatively low-risk procedure (3% to 4% mortality), seldom is this procedure necessary because balloon valvuloplasty is available and effective. When surgery is required, inflow occlusion with transarterial valvotomy or "open" valvotomy with cardiopulmonary bypass is the method usually used. The incidence of pulmonary insufficiency postoperatively varies from 57% to 90%, whereas an incidence of 13% to 45% has been reported after balloon valvuloplasty. However, Doppler echocardiography and color-flow mapping are sensitive methods for detecting valvar insufficiency and suggest that a small amount of regurgitation is present in most patients after surgical or balloon valvotomy.

A special task force committee composed of members of the American Heart Association who specialize in cardiovascular diseases of the young recommends that physical activity in patients with treated or untreated mild pulmonary valve stenosis remain unrestricted. Light exercise (e.g., nonstrenuous team games, recreational swimming, jogging, cycling, and golf) is recommended for patients with moderate stenosis. Moderate limitation of physical activities (e.g., attending school but not participating in physical education classes) is recommended for children with severe pulmonary valve stenosis. A general guideline is to treat the underlying stenosis rather than to restrict physical activity.

INTRACAVITARY OBSTRUCTION OF THE RIGHT VENTRICLE

Two types of intracavitary obstructions are primary infundibular stenosis and double-chambered right ventricle secondary to an anomalous muscle bundle. Primary infundibular stenosis is an uncommon finding and usually occurs secondary to a fibrous band at the junction of the infundibulum and the main body of the right ventricle. Because this anomaly closely resembles the double-chambered right ventricle, only the latter is discussed here.

The anomalous muscle bundles dividing the right ventricle into double chambers probably are a secondary outcome of the arrested incorporation of the primitive bulbus cordis into the body of the right ventricle, which explains the common occurrence of an associated VSD, present in as many as 93% of cases. A subaortic valve membrane also is seen in association with these defects. The proximal inlet chamber has high pressure, whereas the distal outflow chamber has low pressure that is equal to the pulmonary arterial pressure. Physical examination reveals a systolic ejection murmur lower along the left sternal border than is usual with pulmonary valve stenosis. No systolic ejection click is heard, and the murmur often is confused with a VSD. The electrocardiogram demonstrates right ventricular hypertrophy, depending on the severity of the obstruction. The chest radiograph is unremarkable; however, echocardiography usually defines the intracavitary obstruction sufficiently to determine the need for therapy. Cardiac catheterization and angiography may be used to obtain precise hemodynamic and anatomic information in selected patients but usually is unnecessary in this era.

Natural history studies indicate that the severity of intracavitary obstruction is progressive. Treatment of significant obstruction by an anomalous right ventricular muscle bundle consists of surgical resection of the bundle, with care being taken to avoid injury to the tricuspid valve apparatus. Associated VSD and subaortic valve membrane may require closure and resection, respectively. Balloon dilation of the intracavitary obstruction usually is ineffective and is not recommended. Infective endocarditis prophylaxis is recommended for all patients, regardless of treatment.

PULMONARY ARTERY STENOSIS

Pathology

Obstruction of pulmonary blood flow along the pulmonary arterial tree may occur at many sites. The overall incidence of pulmonary arterial stenosis is 2% to 3% of cases of congenital heart disease. Isolated or "native" pulmonary artery stenosis occurs in one-third of the cases, but associated cardiac defects occur in two-thirds of the patients. The most common associated defects are pulmonary valve stenosis and VSD (i.e., tetralogy of Fallot). Multiple peripheral pulmonary artery stenoses commonly are present in rubella and in Williams syndrome. Several other syndromes, including Noonan, Alagille, Ehlers-Danlos, cutis laxa, and Silver-Russell, also have this associated defect.

Clinical Manifestations and Complications

Clinical features of pulmonary artery stenosis may be masked easily by associated defects. Close inspection and auscultation, however, reveal a systolic ejection murmur that is heard over the pulmonary area but is particularly loud in the back

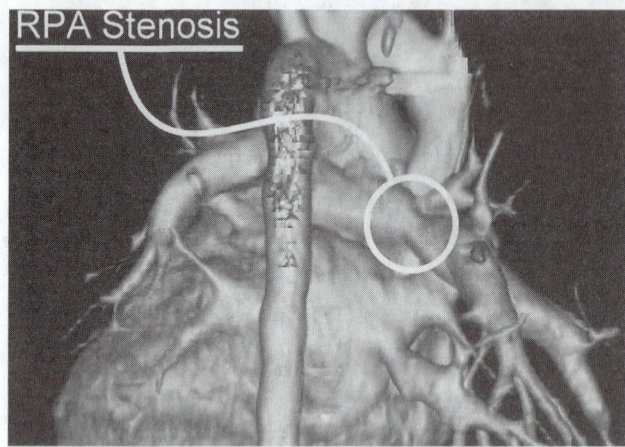

FIGURE 274.5. Three-dimensional volume-rendered multislice computed tomography scan performed on a 3-year-old with tetralogy of Fallot repair using breath-hold technique. Note the right pulmonary artery stenosis secondary to a previous right Blalock-Taussig shunt.

and lateral lung fields. A systolic ejection click is absent. A continuous murmur may be present in as many as 10% of patients, indicating a significant diastolic as well as systolic gradient. The degree of right ventricular hypertrophy visible on the electrocardiogram depends on the severity of the obstruction. The chest roentgenogram usually is normal. Whereas the echocardiogram may be helpful in defining associated intracardiac defects, it is not reliable in imaging the sites of pulmonary artery stenosis. More recently, magnetic resonance imaging (MRI) and breath-hold multislice computed tomography (MSCT) have been extremely helpful in evaluating the proximal as well as distal pulmonary arteries. With three-dimensional, volume-rendered MSCT, planning of transcatheter and/or surgical management strategies are made (Fig. 274.5). Cardiac catheterization and angiography continue to be used in these children. Selective right ventriculography and pulmonary arteriography are necessary to define precisely the areas of stenosis.

In "native" pulmonary artery stenosis, the natural history may be benign, but progressive increase in severity with subsequent death in early infancy and childhood has been reported. Because of the poor surgical results in the treatment of "native" and complicated pulmonary artery stenosis, the use of balloon angioplasty began in 1980. Initial balloon diameters three to four times the diameter of the stenotic vessel were chosen when only low-pressure balloons (4 to 6 atm) were available. However, newer materials allow high-pressure balloon inflation (8 to 18 atm), with improved results of gradient reduction using balloon diameters of only two to three times the stenotic pulmonary artery diameter. Histopathologic and, more recently, intravascular ultrasound studies have demonstrated intimal disruption with extension of a medial tear in successful balloon pulmonary artery angioplasty. At times, the tear may extend to the level of the adventitia. Therefore, the mechanism of successful balloon angioplasty also plays a role in the potential complication of vessel disruption leading to hemorrhage. For this reason, surgical backup and blood availability are arranged when this procedure is to be performed.

The VACA Registry reports a 3% risk of death occurring during balloon pulmonary artery angioplasty. In addition, complications such as vessel perforation, hemorrhage, and arrhythmias occur in 10% of patients. Success for dilation was defined arbitrarily as (a) an increase in stenosis diameter equal to or greater than 50% of predilation diameter, (b) an increase of more than 20% of blood flow to the affected lung, or (c) a decrease of at least 20% in the ratio of systolic right ventricular

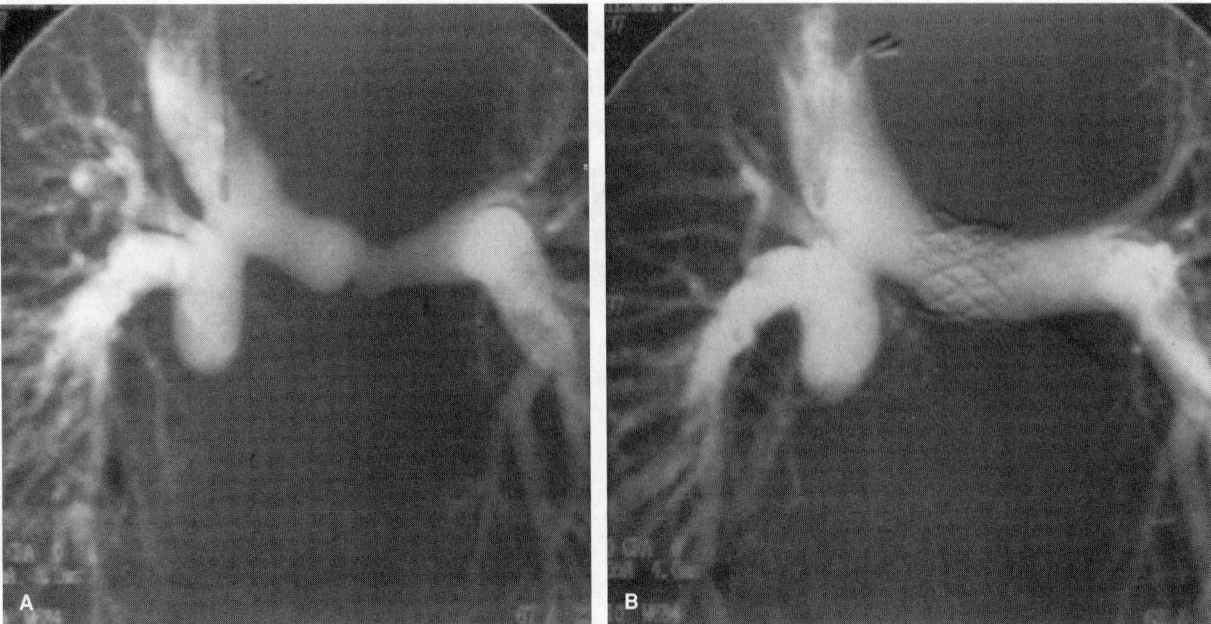

FIGURE 274.6. Pulmonary angiogram from a patient with a bidirectional Glenn shunt as a staged repair for single-ventricle physiology. **A:** Note the discrete stenosis of the left pulmonary artery. **B:** After intravascular stent placement, the left pulmonary artery appears normal.

to aortic pressure. The success rate using low-pressure balloons (4 to 8 atm) was a disappointing 55%. However, using high-pressure balloons, the rate increased to 80% in the vessels dilated, with only a 2% mortality risk and an overall 13% complication rate.

Since 1991, the use of the balloon expandable Palmaz intravascular stent has improved dramatically the results of transcatheter therapy for pulmonary artery stenosis. The intravascular stent overcomes the natural "recoil" of the artery and significantly reduces the pressure gradient and increases vessel diameter. In addition, the balloon expandable characteristic of the stent allows for future redilation to a larger diameter as the child grows. The addition of intravascular stents in the treatment of pulmonary artery stenosis has improved the overall results significantly in more than 95% of stenotic lesions. The average systolic gradient after balloon angioplasty alone decreased to 37 mm Hg, compared to a 50 mm Hg gradient before treatment. A further decrease to a 14 mm Hg gradient after stent implantation and only an 8 mm Hg gradient after later stent redilation clearly demonstrates the superiority of the intravascular stent over balloon angioplasty alone (Fig. 274.6).

The operator's expertise and skill required to implant intravascular stents successfully in children with pulmonary artery stenosis is high. Therefore, this procedure should be performed only by appropriately trained pediatric cardiac interventionalists. The risks of the procedure are no different from those of balloon angioplasty alone, except for the possibility of stent migration or embolization. Antiplatelet therapy (aspirin, dipyridamole) usually is recommended after intravascular stent implantation to decrease the incidence of thrombosis. Regardless of therapy, infective endocarditis prophylaxis is recommended for all patients with this cardiac defect.

Suggested Readings

Edwards BS, Lucas RV Jr, Lock JE, et al. Morphologic changes in the pulmonary arteries after percutaneous balloon angioplasty for pulmonary arterial stenosis. *Circulation* 1985;71:195.

Fogelman R, Nykanen D, Smallhorn JF, et al. Endovascular stents in the pulmonary circulation: clinical impact on management and medium-term follow-up. *Circulation* 1995;92:881.

Gallucci V, Scalia D, Thiene G, et al. Double-chambered right ventricle: surgical experience and anatomical considerations. *J Thorac Cardiovasc Surg* 1980;28:13.

Gentles TL, Lock JE, Perry SB. High pressure balloon angioplasty for branch pulmonary artery stenosis: early experience. *J Am Coll Cardiol* 1993;22:867.

Gikonyo BM, Lucas RV, Edwards JE. Anatomic features of congenital pulmonary valvar stenosis. *Pediatr Cardiol* 1987;8:109.

Hanley FL, Sade RM, Freedom RM, et al. Outcomes in critically ill neonates with pulmonary stenosis and intact ventricular septum: a multiinstitutional study. *J Am Coll Cardiol* 1993;22:183.

Hayes CJ, Gersony WM, Driscoll DJ, et al. Second natural history study of congenital heart defects. *Circulation* 1993;87:I28.

Kan JS, Marvin WJ, Bass JL, et al. Balloon angioplasty-branch pulmonary artery stenosis: results from the Valvuloplasty and Angioplasty of Congenital Anomalies Registry. *Am J Cardiol* 1990;65:798.

Lock JE, Castaneda-Zuniga WR, Fuhrman BP, et al. Balloon dilatation angioplasty of hypoplastic and stenotic pulmonary arteries. *Circulation* 1983;67:962.

Moller JH. Exercise responses in pulmonary stenosis. *Prog Pediatr Cardiol* 1993;2:8.

O'Laughlin MP, Perry SB, Lock JE, et al. Use of endovascular stents in congenital heart disease. *Circulation* 1991;83:1923.

O'Laughlin MP, Slack MC, Grifka RG, et al. Implantation and intermediate-term follow-up of stents in congenital heart disease. *Circulation* 1993;88:605.

Stanger P, Cassidy SC, Girod DA, et al. Balloon pulmonary valvuloplasty: results of the Valvuloplasty and Angioplasty of Congenital Anomalies Registry. *Am J Cardiol* 1990;65:775.

Trant CA, O'Laughlin MP, Ungerleider RM, et al. Cost-effectiveness analysis of stents, balloon angioplasty, and surgery for the treatment of branch pulmonary artery stenosis. *Pediatr Cardiol* 1997;18:339.

CHAPTER 275 ■ PULMONARY VALVE ATRESIA WITH INTACT VENTRICULAR SEPTUM

DONALD A. RIOPEL

Pulmonary valve atresia with intact ventricular septum (PA:IVS) results in varying degrees of hypoplasia of the right ventricle and tricuspid valve. The clinical course of severe hypoplasia of the right ventricle can be almost as devastating as that of severe hypoplasia of the left side of the heart. Infants with moderate or mild hypoplasia, however, have a more favorable clinical course.

INCIDENCE

The defect is estimated to occur in 0.1 to 0.4 per 10,000 births. No distinct gender preference exists.

ETIOLOGY

At stage 15 of embryologic development, four mounds of endocardial cushion tissue, which eventually form the thin aortic and pulmonary valve cusps, are present in the outflow channel of the developing heart tube. Abnormalities of one valve without abnormalities of the other suggest that the cause of the condition occurs after the valve cusps are formed. The association of pulmonary artery obstruction with rubella infection is one indication that a fetal inflammation may be causative.

PATHOLOGY

The pulmonary valve obstruction is complete. The valve tissue is a membrane, usually with fused commissures depicted by raphes and with three formed cusps. The right ventricular cavity ranges in size from tiny to larger than normal, although it is smaller than normal in most cases.

Communications between the right ventricle and the coronary artery system via myocardial sinusoids frequently are seen. They are unique to this lesion and carry an unfavorable prognosis.

The tricuspid valve, by definition, is patent in all cases, and the size of the tricuspid orifice appears to be proportional to the right ventricular cavity. The deformity of the tricuspid valve results in varying degrees of severity of stenosis or insufficiency. The size of the right atrium depends on the degree of tricuspid insufficiency and on the presence and size of the communication between the atria.

PHYSIOLOGY

Fetal

With no outlet of the right ventricle, the fetus with PA:IVS directs all systemic venous blood to the left side of the heart through a communication in the atrial septum. Therefore, the blood flow through the entire left side of the heart is greater than that in the physiologically normal fetus.

Postnatal

Systemic venous blood enters the right atrium from the vena cavae. With no exit possible through the pulmonary valve, the blood must cross the atrial septum through the foramen ovale or an atrial septal defect. Systemic saturation depends on the amount of pulmonary blood flow, which, in turn, depends on the size and patency of the ductus arteriosus. As the ductus undergoes a natural tendency to close, oxygen tension decreases and symptoms of hypoxia occur.

The presence of communications between the coronary artery system and the right ventricle via right ventricular sinusoids affects coronary blood flow and causes ischemia and subendocardial fibrosis of both ventricles.

CLINICAL MANIFESTATIONS

Symptoms

Most of these infants are born at term, have not had growth retardation *in utero*, and are vigorous. Symptoms of cyanosis occur within a few hours to several days after birth and are dependent on ductal flow. Cyanosis may be intermittent and associated only with the stress of feedings or may be sudden and severe because of sudden closure of the ductus arteriosus. Infants with severe cyanosis also have accompanying acidosis and deep compensatory respirations in an attempt to correct the metabolic acidosis. Hypoxia, acidosis, or hypoglycemia, singly or in combination, can lead to seizure activity.

Signs

In the symptomatic infant, severe cyanosis of the mucous membranes and nail beds occurs, with paleness of the skin occurring secondary to a low cardiac output and peripheral vasoconstriction. Hyperpnea is present, and no rales are heard on auscultation of the lungs. Cardiac auscultation may reveal only the single second heart sound of aortic closure with no murmur. When tricuspid insufficiency is present, a long systolic murmur is heard along the lower left sternal border. Rarely is a continuous murmur heard. The liver may be engorged and pulsatile because of passive congestion, such as occurs with tricuspid atresia. Pulses are weak and thready. Cyanosis of the nail beds and clubbing occurs in infants older than 4 months of age.

LABORATORY FINDINGS

Arterial blood gases in severely cyanotic infants who are not receiving prostaglandins have a low pH, a very low Po_2 (often

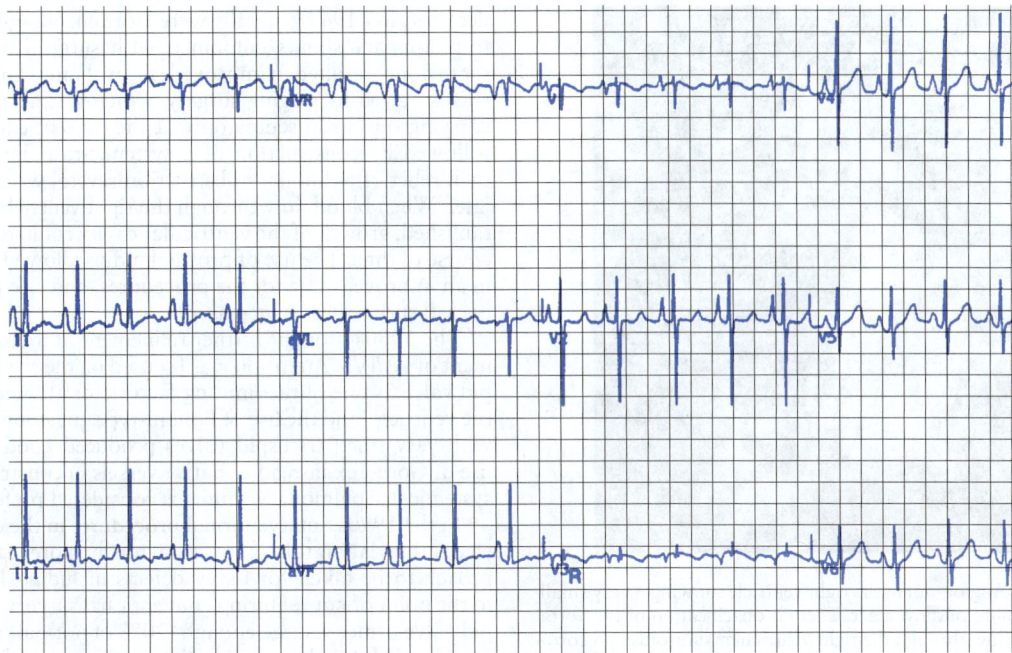

FIGURE 275.1. Twelve-lead electrocardiogram of a neonate with pulmonary atresia and intact ventricular septum. The tall P waves in lead II indicate right atrial enlargement, and the relative lack of R waves in lead V_1 represents the absence of right ventricular forces.

in the teens), and a somewhat low PCO_2 with a negative base deficit. In infants receiving prostaglandins, arterial blood gas values may approach normal.

Electrocardiographic findings in PA:IVS depend on the anatomy of the defect. The rhythm is sinus with normal time intervals, and the P wave often is tall and peaked. The QRS frontal plane vector tends to be in the lower left quadrant in cases of a small right ventricle, whereas it usually is rightward (greater than 120 degrees) in cases with a normal or a large right ventricle. With a severely hypoplastic right ventricle, the R-to-S ratio in the horizontal plane favors the posterior forces, a finding suggesting absent or diminished right ventricular forces (Fig. 275.1). The T wave usually is normal, except when ischemia of ventricles is present, whereupon discordant T vectors are seen and ST changes of strain are present.

Chest roentgenography results in PA:IVS vary with anatomic types. In cases involving a tiny right ventricle and little or no tricuspid insufficiency, the heart is normal in size. The vascularity is reduced but may appear to be normal, depending on the patency of the ductus arteriosus. With tricuspid insufficiency, a large right atrium is present, giving considerable convexity to the right heart border.

Two-dimensional echocardiography, especially in four-chambered views, shows the relative sizes of the ventricles and the atria. The patency and size of the tricuspid valve are seen clearly, and function of the ventricles can be evaluated. In short-axis views, the pulmonary valve membrane and the size of the valve ring can be seen, and the distance of the proximal main pulmonary artery from the distal right ventricular outflow tract can be measured. Color-flow Doppler shows the presence and degree of tricuspid insufficiency, the right-to-left shunt across the atrial septum, and the flow into the main pulmonary artery through the ductus.

Cardiac Catheterization

Because of the clarity of today's echocardiographic technology, cardiac catheterization usually is not necessary. If catheteri-

zation is needed, administration of prostaglandins allows the catheterization to proceed at a more opportune time and allows time for the infant to recover from the catheterization before undergoing surgery.

Usually, only a venous catheter is necessary for catheterization because most infants have an umbilical artery monitoring catheter. The left atrium is entered through a patent foramen ovale or septal defect. Manipulation into the left ventricle is possible from the left atrium. Right atrial pressures are elevated, with tall A waves of 15 to 20 mm Hg. Right ventricular systolic pressures often attain suprasystemic values, with a peaked configuration of the pressure curve, and may achieve levels of 200 mm Hg. Left ventricular pressures have normal newborn values, unless severe hypoxia, acidosis, and hypoglycemia occur, all of which decrease contractility. Oxygen saturations invariably are very low in infants who are not receiving prostaglandins. Because of the large intracardiac right-to-left shunt, administration of oxygen increases systemic saturations very little, if at all.

Balloon septostomy should be performed if a good communication between the atria does not exist. Angiography in the right ventricle establishes the diagnosis, shows the size of the right ventricle, and allows the defect to be classified. Communications with the coronary artery system via myocardial sinusoids (Fig. 275.2), as well as the degree of tricuspid hypoplasia and insufficiency, may be demonstrated.

A left ventricular injection shows the size and function of the left ventricle and eliminates the possibility of a ventricular septal defect. Good opacification of the aorta occurs, and the pulmonary arteries opacify via the ductus arteriosus or other collateral circulation.

DIFFERENTIAL DIAGNOSIS

Other lesions to be considered in newborns with severe cyanosis include tetralogy of Fallot with pulmonary atresia, severe pulmonary stenosis with intact ventricular septum,

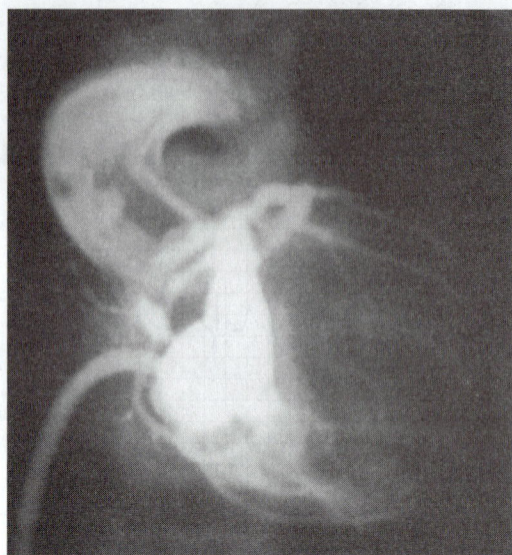

FIGURE 275.2. Angiogram in the right ventricle showing a very small ventricle and a blind outflow tract. There is opacification of the aorta from retrograde flow through the right ventricular sinusoids and coronary arteries.

tricuspid atresia, and total anomalous pulmonary venous return with obstruction of pulmonary veins.

THERAPY

Medical Treatment

The use of prostaglandin E_1 to dilate the ductus arteriosus and maintain pulmonary blood flow in these infants has enhanced the safety of catheterization greatly. The infant changes from being blue, pale, and acidotic to being pink and well perfused within minutes of starting an infusion of prostaglandin E_1 at the rate of 0.05 to 0.10 μg/kg/minute. The infusion is effective given through any vessel. The improved state is maintained as long as the prostaglandins are infused. Treatment of PA:IVS begins in the neonatal period with the onset of symptoms. As soon as the diagnosis of heart disease with decreased pulmonary blood flow is made, access to the vascular system should be established and an infusion of prostaglandin started to reestablish pulmonary blood flow. This procedure restores a normal acid-base balance. An arterial line then should be established, most readily in the umbilical artery, because frequent determinations of arterial blood gas levels will need to be made, especially during and after surgery. Abnormalities in glucose or calcium levels should be corrected.

Surgical Treatment

Analysis of the anatomy delineated by the catheterization dictates the mode of surgical intervention. The general goal of surgery is to establish adequate pulmonary blood flow by a systemic-to-pulmonary shunt, to create a communication between the right ventricle and pulmonary artery, or both. The order and timing of these interventions have varied over the years.

Historically, the concept of systemic-to-pulmonary shunting of blood advanced by Blalock and Taussig in 1945 remains an integral part of the treatment of PA:IVS. Publications from the decades after 1945 generally were more encouraging. Systemic-to-pulmonary shunts combined with surgical atrial balloon septostomy resulted in improved survival rates. Greater success was achieved by staging surgery, which was accomplished by carrying out atrial septostomy at the time of catheterization, followed by construction of a systemic-to-pulmonary shunt, then relief of pulmonary obstruction several weeks or months later. When blood flow through the right ventricle could be established, growth of the ventricular cavity could occur over the course of time. The use of prostaglandins allowed infants to be in an improved state for the procedures, and late in the 1970s, overall survival rates increased.

The 1980s brought further refinement of the surgical treatment of PA:IVS. Attention was focused on the size of the tricuspid valve as one of the limiting factors for allowing growth of the ventricle, and the use of Fontan-type anastomoses in hearts with very small tricuspid valves produced good results. The use of Gore-Tex instead of native vessels in construction of the systemic–to–pulmonary shunts is considered preferable.

In the 1990s, interventional procedures in the cardiac catheterization laboratory allowed a much more aggressive approach to be taken for many defects including PA:IVS, even to the point of not requiring conventional surgery. If the tricuspid valve orifice is large enough (70% of normal) and the right ventricle is favorable, the atretic membrane can be perforated by wire, laser, or radiofrequency energy, and the orifice can be dilated with a balloon. This approach may allow blood to flow freely through the right ventricle and allow it to grow larger. Later, the atrial septal defect can be closed with a catheter-delivered device.

If the right ventricle and tricuspid valve are marginal, then decompression by surgery together with a shunt may allow eventual growth of the right ventricle, the shunt can be closed with catheter-delivered coils, and the atrial septal defect can be closed at the same time with an occluder device. For those defects with unfavorable tricuspid valve and right ventricle, a surgical shunt and eventual series of surgeries leading to a complete Fontan are the procedures required, sometimes with thromboexclusion of the right ventricle.

PROGNOSIS AND FUTURE DEVELOPMENT

Although some patients with PA:IVS have lived into early adulthood without having to undergo surgical treatment, the prognosis for patients who have this lesion, even with surgery, is somewhat guarded. Results continue to improve, but the eventual outcome appears to depend on the presence or absence of sinusoid–coronary communications and on the size of the tricuspid valve and right ventricle. Patients who have undergone a Fontan procedure who have the left ventricle as their systemic ventricle (e.g., those with PA:IVS) generally seem to have a better prognosis than do those with hypoplastic left hearts whose right ventricle becomes the systemic ventricle.

Suggested Readings

Blalock A, Taussig HB. The surgical treatment of malformations of the heart in which there is pulmonary stenosis or pulmonary atresia. *JAMA* 1945; 128:189.

Bull C, de Leval MR, Mercanti C, et al. Pulmonary atresia and intact ventricular septum: a revised classification. *Circulation* 1982;66:266.

De Leval MR, Bull C, Stark J, et al. Pulmonary atresia and intact ventricular septum: surgical management based on a revised classification. *Circulation* 1982;66:272.

Freedom RM, Dische MR, Rowe RD. The tricuspid valve in pulmonary atresia and intact ventricular septum: a morphological study of 60 cases. *Arch Pathol Lab Med* 1978;102:28.

Freedom RM, Wilson G, Trusler GA, et al. Pulmonary atresia and intact ventricular septum. *Scand J Thorac Cardiovasc Surg* 1983;17:1.

Fyfe DA, Edwards WD, Driscoll DJ. Myocardial ischemia in patients with pulmonary atresia and intact ventricular septum. *J Am Coll Cardiol* 1986;8:402.

Gibbs JL, Blackburn ME, Uzun O, et al. Laser valvotomy with balloon valvoplasty for pulmonary atresia with intact ventricular septum: five years' experience. *Heart* 1997;77:225.

Humpl T, Söderberg B, McCrindle BW, et al. Percutaneous balloon valvotomy in pulmonary atresia with intact ventricular septum. *Circulation* 2003;108:826.

Justo RN, Nykanen DG, Williams WG, et al. Transcatheter perforation of the right ventricular outflow tract as initial therapy for pulmonary valve atresia and intact ventricular septum in the newborn. *Cathet Cardiovasc Diagn* 1997;40:408.

Najm HK, Williams WG, Coles JG, et al. Pulmonary atresia with intact ventricular septum: results of the Fontan procedure. *Ann Thorac Surg* 1997;63:669.

O'Conner WN, Cotrill CM, Johnson GL, et al. Pulmonary atresia with intact ventricular septum and ventriculocoronary communications: surgical significance. *Circulation* 1982;65:805.

CHAPTER 276 ■ COARCTATION OF THE AORTA

MARY J. H. MORRISS

Coarctation of the aorta is a congenital malformation characterized by a constriction of a segment of the aorta. Usually, an abrupt narrowing of the lumen of the vessel occurs in the thoracic descending aorta, producing obstruction to blood flow (Fig. 276.1) A localized shelflike thickening of the media protrudes into the lumen just beyond the origin of the left subclavian artery, leaving an eccentric orifice displaced toward the usual site of insertion of the vestigial ligamentum arteriosus. To be clinically significant, the narrowing must be marked and must reduce effectively the diameter of the aorta by at least 50%. To maintain flow and adequate perfusion pressure to the kidneys and lower body, blood pressure proximal to the obstruction becomes elevated.

OCCURRENCE

Coarctation of the aorta is a common congenital defect occurring in frequency just after ventricular septal defect and patent ductus arteriosus in most series. It has a striking male-to-female preponderance in excess of 2:1. Patients with the full XO Turner syndrome with ovarian agenesis and short stature have a high incidence of coarctation in 20% of cases. A more extreme anomaly with complete interruption of the aortic arch in a slightly different location, proximal to the origin of the left subclavian artery, has a high association with DiGeorge syndrome, with deletion in the critical region of chromosome 22q11, and is functionally analogous to severe coarctation with a reverse ductus arteriosus.

CLASSIFICATION

A clear anatomic distinction can be made between an isolated, discrete coarctation (referred to by some investigators as *adult* or *postductal coarctation*) and a more diffuse, long-segment narrowing. The latter usually is part of a coarctation syndrome with other more complicated heart defects, resulting in a systemic right ventricle and right-to-left shunting through a persistently patent ductus arteriosus (preductal or infantile coarctation). Rarely, multiple sites of coarctation or an atypical location, such as abdominal coarctation, thought by many to be an acquired disease in association with nonspecific arteritis, may occur.

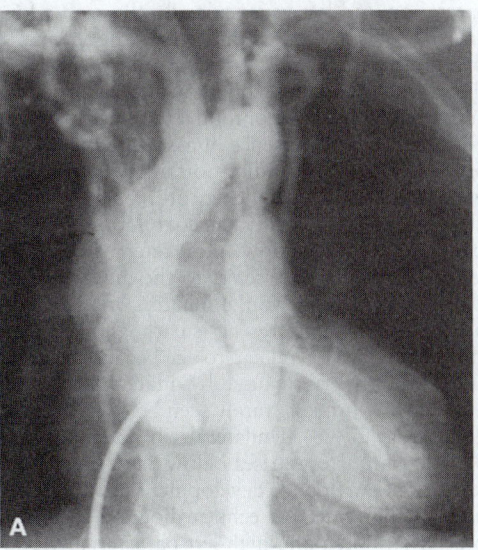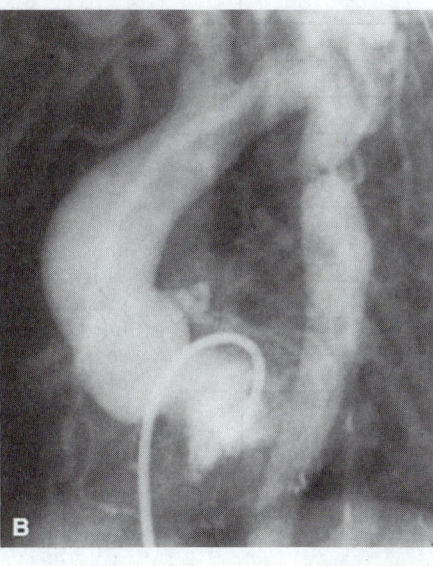

FIGURE 276.1. Anteroposterior (A) and lateral (B) frames from left ventricular angiography. Discrete coarctation is seen in the descending thoracic aorta. Well-developed collateral vessels are evident.

EMBRYOLOGY

The Skodaic theory of causation is based on an observation that smooth muscle from the ductus arteriosus extends into the aorta, and, when ductal constriction occurs after birth, traction on the aorta can narrow the lumen and cause coarctation of the aorta. The general agreement is that ductal closure can unmask a coarctation lesion, but the theory does not explain the location of the shelflike protrusion of the aorta arising from the wall opposite the ductal insertion. Conceptually, an explanation easier to accept is that alterations in intrauterine flow patterns promote diffuse narrowing in the isthmic region between the origin of the left subclavian artery and the ductus arteriosus, which postnatally is recognized as coarctation. Coexistence of a large ventricular septal defect, or even bicuspid aortic valve with mild obstruction, may divert flow from the aorta into the pulmonary artery, with resultant reduction in the amount of flow crossing the isthmus, the point at which natural separation occurs between flow to the upper body and flow to the lower body *in utero.*

PHYSIOLOGY

The major physiologic burden imposed by coarctation of the aorta is an increase in afterload of the left ventricle. By the time the aortic lumen is moderately constricted, an increase in systolic pressure occurs above the obstruction, and a lesser degree of elevation is noted in diastolic pressure, with widening of the pulse pressure. Below the coarctation is a narrowed pulse pressure, with decreased systolic and diastolic pressure (Fig. 276.2). These alterations in wave form are reflected by a tactile sensation of delay between radial and femoral pulses. Hypertension is not related directly to the severity of obstruction and may not be extreme. Left ventricular hypertrophy develops, and stimulation for development of collateral vessels to bypass the obstruction occurs.

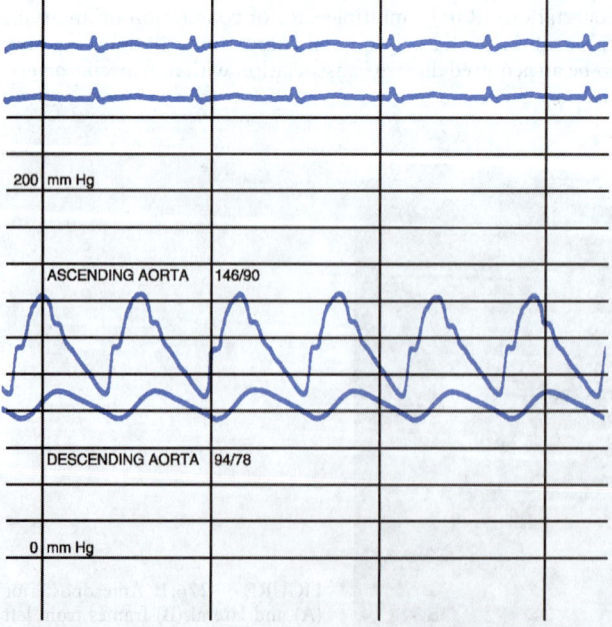

FIGURE 276.2. Pressure recordings simultaneously obtained at catheterization from ascending aorta above coarctation and from descending aorta below coarctation in a 5-year-old child.

CLINICAL FEATURES

Coarctation Beyond Infancy

Coarctation of the aorta beyond infancy is recognized clinically when blood pressure recordings are obtained from all four extremities; its hallmark is hypertension in the upper extremities and decreased blood pressure in the lower extremities. The discrepancy in blood pressure, rather than an absolute level of proximal blood pressure elevation, is the most striking finding; however, evaluation of any patient with hypertension should exclude coarctation as a cause. Most individuals with isolated coarctation have no cardiac symptoms, although minor complaints of cold feet, leg cramps, and nose bleeds often are volunteered. Unilateral headaches, particularly of unusual severity, rarely point to an associated cerebral aneurysm, but they may be worrisome enough to prompt performing a full neurologic evaluation. Physical examination shows striking inequality between the strength of pulses from vessels arising proximal to the obstruction and those distal to the obstruction. Simultaneous palpation of brachial and femoral pulses is recommended; in the presence of well-developed collateral vessels, femoral pulses can be felt easily despite the presence of a coarctation, and the discrepancy in timing and pulse volume should be sought. Auscultation should be performed systematically in an attempt to explain the auscultatory findings, rather than with a prejudice that a particular murmur always is found with coarctation. A systolic murmur generated from the coarctation site may be heard best in the left infraclavicular area, in the axilla, or over the left posterior chest. The murmur may seem to originate after the first heart sound, accentuate in later systole, and extend into diastole. The murmur reflects an apparent lag between cardiac systole and flow through the coarctation site, as well as the persistence of a coarctation gradient in early diastole.

True continuous murmurs may be generated by collateral vessels. The presence of an aortic ejection click and an ejection murmur in the aortic area may raise suspicion of an additional bicuspid aortic valve, which is found with high frequency in as many as 85% of patients with aortic coarctation. A thrill at the right upper sternal border or suprasternal notch may accompany significant aortic stenosis, but it also can be found with coarctation alone because of rapid ejection into the dilated proximal aorta.

Despite the presence of a significant aortic coarctation, the results of the electrocardiogram may be normal in older children. When changes occur, they are manifested chiefly by voltage criteria for left ventricular hypertrophy. The rare patient with severe coarctation and left ventricular dysfunction additionally may have ST-T wave changes indicative of ischemia.

The typical radiologic examination of an older child reveals normal heart size, with less common findings of mild enlargement and left ventricular contour. Pulmonary vascular markings are normal in the absence of associated intracardiac defects. Dilatation of the ascending aorta may be present. In some patients, radiographic evidence of the prestenotic and poststenotic dilatations resulting from coarctation appears along the left paramediastinal shadow and is referred to as the *3 sign. Reversed 3 sign,* or *E sign,* refers to the mirror-image prestenotic and poststenotic dilatations impinging on a barium-filled esophagus. Rib notching, if present, is pathognomonic of coarctation of the aorta, but it is related to age because erosion of the inferior portion of the ribs caused by dilated intercostal collateral vessels is a slow process, rarely seen before a patient reaches school age (Fig. 276.3). Unilateral rib notching suggests that one subclavian artery arises below the coarctation in the low-pressure zone, with poor development of collaterals and rib notching on that side. An echocardiogram, particularly when suprasternal notch and high left parasternal views

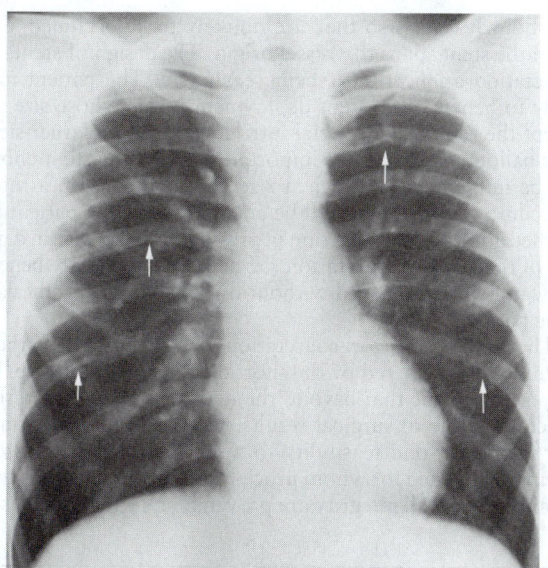

FIGURE 276.3. Posteroanterior chest film with rib notching (*arrows*) and a 3 sign identified in a 7-year-old child.

are used, may enable recognition of coarctation, but difficulties in examining the entire aorta throughout its course are well described. The principal values of echocardiography are that associated defects can be assessed, left ventricular function and hypertrophy can be quantitated, and, if visualization of the coarctation site is possible, a more confident recommendation can be made to the surgeon that a typical coarctation is present. Parameters of Doppler flow, including peak velocity and, in particular, striking pandiastolic flow, are useful in supporting echocardiographic recognition of coarctation. Coexistence of coarctation with a persistently patent ductus in the neonate further challenges echocardiographic accuracy.

Magnetic resonance imaging has application in the prospective identification and follow-up of patients with coarctation of the aorta, and testing of this method's contribution is ongoing. Catheterization and angiography, with detailed visualization of the anatomy of the coarctation area, can confirm the diagnosis, thus directing therapy.

Coarctation in Infancy

Coarctation syndrome in infancy is characterized by a high association with other defects that result in systemic right ventricle, reversed flow from right to left through the ductus arteriosus, and more severe hypoplasia of a greater portion of the aortic arch, although discrete coarctation may be present. Infants with coarctation can appear to be well at birth, but cardiac failure, respiratory distress, and cardiogenic shock may appear rapidly as the ductus constricts. Because of the severe impairment of cardiac output, a murmur may not be detected until the infant is stabilized and treated. The pulse discrepancy may not be apparent in the infant because the widely patent ductus serves as a route for flow to the descending aorta, so coarctation is not excluded even if normal pulses are felt on a routine newborn examination. Differential cyanosis can exist potentially, with shunting of the blood with a lower saturation to the lower body from the pulmonary artery via the ductus. However, the high frequency of associated defects, particularly left-to-right shunts, may allow pulmonary saturations to be only slightly lower than aortic saturations, masking this difference clinically. Marked benefit can be obtained by dilating the ductus arteriosus with prostaglandin infusion, thus enabling

improved renal perfusion and reversal of acidosis and cardiogenic shock.

The electrocardiogram of infants with coarctation of the aorta is normal less frequently because it reflects coexistent anatomic defects. Isolated coarctation of the aorta in infancy is accompanied by electrocardiographic evidence of right ventricular hypertrophy, but additional left ventricular hypertrophy or rare left ventricular strain also can be present.

The chest film of the ill infant generally correlates with the clinical state, showing dilatation of the heart with congestive heart failure and an increase in pulmonary vascular markings caused by either an associated left-to-right shunt or passive venous congestion.

The echocardiogram helps outline additional defects of the heart, enables assessment of left ventricular function and possibly shows the area of coarctation, but with testing confounded in the presence of a widely patent ductus arteriosus.

Response to prostaglandin therapy also has been evaluated with echocardiography to assess ductal patency. Catheterization is undertaken at increased risk in a moribund infant with coarctation, so noninvasive recognition is pursued more urgently.

TREATMENT

Surgical Treatment

Coarctation of the aorta has been considered a congenital defect amenable to surgical repair since the mid-1940s. The expected result is complete relief of the obstruction so flow to the distal aorta remains unobstructed. Best results are obtained by elective resection and end-to-end anastomosis in a young child, with the single operation providing immediate and long-term relief of hypertension without the need for reoperation. Surgery is performed from a posterolateral thoracotomy incision, made by spreading the ribs to allow access to the thorax. Mobility of the aorta is improved by performing ligation and division of a ductus arteriosus or a ligamentum arteriosum. In the presence of well-developed collaterals, the aorta is safely cross-clamped just above and below the coarctation site, and cardiopulmonary bypass usually is not used. No one method of repair is ideal for all patients (Fig. 276.4). Because of the high rate of restenosis when resection and end-to-end procedures were used in infants, with a reoperation rate of up to 60%, a repair using a flap of the subclavian artery was popularized. This vascular flap enables bridging of a long-segment hypoplasia, with the presumption that growth will be permitted. Patch angioplasty and interposition grafts are techniques that can be used when more complex anatomy dictates the need. Complications of surgery include the following: injury to the recurrent laryngeal nerve, with resulting hoarseness; diaphragmatic injury from phrenic nerve trauma; bleeding from high-pressure suture lines; chylothorax; and, rarely, spinal cord injury, which is less likely to occur when well-developed collateral circulation is present.

A special postoperative syndrome of mesenteric arteritis may be related to the duration of preoperative hypertension, the presence of postoperative rebound hypertension, and the introduction of feeding too early postoperatively. Typically, this postcoarctectomy syndrome is recognized by hypertension, abdominal pain and tenderness, vomiting, and, in severe cases, a progression to bowel necrosis. The exact mechanism is unknown, but it appears to be related to vasoconstriction of mesenteric vessels reintroduced to pulsatile flow after successful repair of the coarctation. Because of this described problem, postoperative hypertension is treated vigorously, and nothing-by-mouth status is continued for 72 hours, with slow introduction of feeding in these patients.

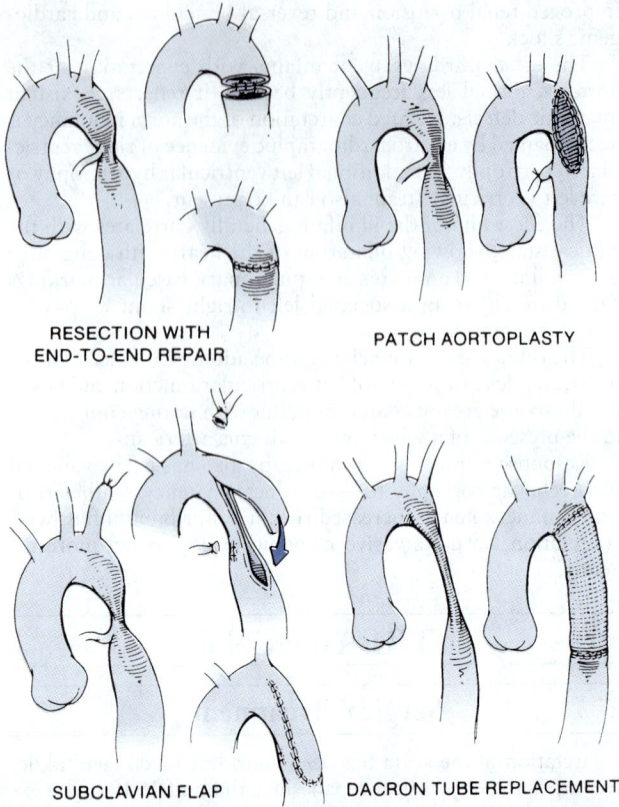

RESECTION WITH
END-TO-END REPAIR

PATCH AORTOPLASTY

SUBCLAVIAN FLAP

DACRON TUBE REPLACEMENT

FIGURE 276.4. Techniques of repair commonly used for coarctation.

An infant requiring early repair of a coarctation also may require pulmonary artery banding because of associated defects, although enthusiasm for cardiopulmonary bypass even in very young patients has led to a preference for complete, definitive repair.

Therapeutic Catheterization

Interventional catheterization techniques for nonsurgical treatment of aortic coarctation are being developed rapidly and compared with operation. Balloon angioplasty and intravascular stents are the transcatheter therapies on trial. Choice of therapy relates to patient age, size, anatomy of obstruction and associated defects, and whether the coarctation site is native or is a restenosis lesion that occurred after previous treatment.

The mechanism of relief from obstruction using balloon dilation involves vascular injury with a tear of intima and part of the media. The procedure has been judged to be safest and most effective in postsurgical recoarctation when scarring and adhesions contribute to support of the vessel wall. Risks and unsatisfactory results may be greater in infants and when treating native coarctation. Limitations in its use relate to concern for elastic recoil of the vessel with unsustained luminal enlargement and infrequent procedural consequences of dissection of the aorta with potential for rupture or formation of an aneurysm. Short-term palliation and good long-term results justify this choice of treatment in children who have been selected appropriately.

Stenting of coarctation lesions can be used as an alternative to balloon angioplasty to avoid causing major transmural tears and vessel recoil. Small tears in the wall are splinted by the expanded stent, and the open strut design of the stent allows flow

into branch vessels so they are unlikely to be occluded, even when the stent spans the vessel origin. The design of stents for coarctation application is being evaluated. The patient most likely to benefit from stent deployment is one whose size will accept the retrograde arterial introduction of the larger stent-over-balloon assembly. Of importance is that the stent chosen can be implanted at sufficient size or redilated with a future procedure to a size that will be adequate after the patient has reached adulthood. Reduction in pressure and increase in diameter of the narrow coarctation segment are immediate benefits and can be accomplished without use of general anesthesia in some patients.

The enthusiasm for coarctation treatment with catheter techniques is tempered by the short duration of follow-up, but proponents argue that beyond the newborn period the results are comparable to surgical results. Catheterization treatment may evolve beyond feasibility to preferred therapy if patient groups are defined for whom procedural safety, lack of restenosis, and vessel wall integrity are proven long-term outcomes.

NATURAL HISTORY AND FOLLOW-UP

The former natural history of coarctation of the aorta, with an estimated 75% rate of mortality by midadult years, has been altered by surgical treatment. Endocarditis with the potential for formation of a mycotic aneurysm is a lifelong threat, and endocarditis prophylaxis should be observed by all patients, both preoperatively and postoperatively. The reversibility of hypertension is thought to be favored by repair in early childhood, thus avoiding long-standing preoperative hypertension as well as permitting complete relief of the obstruction. Considerations based on normal growth of the aorta and concern about reversibility of preoperative hypertension have led pediatric cardiologists to recommend elective repair of aortic coarctation for patients before they reach school age.

A high incidence of congenital berry aneurysms is described, estimated to occur in as many as 10% of patients with coarctation. The risk of intracranial hemorrhage occurring may be reduced by successful coarctation repair. Follow-up of patients with coarctation for restenosis, recurrent or residual hypertension, endocarditis, ascending aorta dilation, and surveillance of formation of an aneurysm at sites of repaired coarctation continues to be appropriate.

Suggested Readings

Aluquin VP, Shutte D, Nihill MR, et al. Normal aortic arch growth and comparison with isolated coarctation of the aorta. *Am J Cardiol* 2003;91:502.

Becker AE, Becker MJ, Edwards JE. Anomalies associated with coarctation of the aorta: particular reference to infancy. *Circulation* 1970;41:1067.

Campbell M. Natural history of coarctation of the aorta. *Br Heart J* 1970;32:633.

Carvalha JS, Redington AN, Shinebourne EA, et al. Continuous wave Doppler echocardiography and coarctation of the aorta: gradients and flow patterns in the assessment of severity. *Br Heart J* 1990;64:133.

Cheatham JP. Stenting of coarctation of the aorta. *Cathet Cardiovasc Interv* 2001;54:112.

Gupta T, Wiggers CJ. Basic hemodynamic changes produced by aortic coarctation of different degrees. *Circulation* 1951;3:17.

Ho ECK, Moss AJ. The syndrome of "mesenteric arteritis" following surgical repair of aortic coarctation. *Pediatrics* 1972;49:40.

Morriss MJH, McNamara DG. Coarctation of the aorta and interrupted aortic arch. In: Garson AJ, Bricker JT, Fisher DJ, Neish SR, eds. *The science and practice of pediatric cardiology*, 2nd ed. Baltimore: Williams & Wilkins, 1998.

Ovaert C, McCrindle BW, Nykanen D, et al. Balloon angioplasty of native coarctation: clinical outcomes and predictors of success. *J Am Coll Cardiol* 2000;35:988.

Ramaciotti C, Chin AJ. Noninvasive diagnosis of coarctation of the aorta in the presence of a patent ductus arteriosus. *Am Heart J* 1993;125:179.

Rothman A. Coarctation of the aorta: an update. *Curr Prob Pediatr* 1998;2:33.

Rudolph AM, Heymann MA, Spitznas U. Hemodynamic considerations in the development of narrowing of the aorta. *Am J Cardiol* 1972;30:514.

Ryan AK, Goodship JA, Wilson DI, et al. Spectrum of clinical features associated with interstitial chromosome 22q11 deletions: a European collaborative study. *J Med Genet* 1997;34:798.

Toro-Salazar OH, Steinberger J, Thomas W, et al. Long-term follow-up of patients after coarctation of the aorta repair. *Am J Cardiol* 2002;89:541.

Van Mierop LH, Kutsche LM. Interruption of the aortic arch and coarctation of the aorta: pathogenetic relations. *Am J Cardiol* 1984;54:829.

CHAPTER 277 ■ ANOMALOUS PULMONARY VENOUS CONNECTIONS

KENT E. WARD

Partial anomalous pulmonary venous connection (PAPVC) occurs when one or more, but not all, pulmonary veins connect anomalously to the right atrium, either directly or through a systemic venous tributary. PAPVC, which often is found in association with an atrial septal defect (ASD), demonstrates hemodynamic findings of an acyanotic cardiac lesion with increased pulmonary blood flow similar to that observed in an ASD alone.

When all pulmonary veins connect anomalously to the systemic venous circulation, total anomalous pulmonary venous connection (TAPVC) is defined. TAPVC is associated with total mixing of pulmonary and systemic venous blood at the level of the right atrium and, as such, is defined as a cyanotic form of cardiac disease that may demonstrate increased or decreased pulmonary blood flow. Increased pulmonary blood flow is usual. Decreased pulmonary blood flow may occur when severe obstruction in the anomalous pulmonary venous channel is present. In addition, TAPVC always is associated with an interatrial communication, usually a patent foramen ovale.

EMBRYOLOGY

A review of the embryologic development of the systemic and pulmonary venous systems is necessary to understand fully the abnormalities observed in this spectrum of cardiac defects. In the developing embryo, the primitive foregut gives rise to the lungs, larynx, and tracheobronchial tree. The primordial lung buds share a common vascular plexus (splanchnic plexus) with other derivatives of the foregut and, early on, drain through the paired common cardinal and umbilicovitelline veins. As development proceeds, this splanchnic plexus differentiates into the primitive pulmonary vascular bed, thus becoming committed to draining pulmonary venous blood. This pulmonary vascular bed, however, remains in communication with the cardinal and umbilicovitelline system of veins until later in development. At 27 to 29 days of gestation, a small endothelial outgrowth arises from the posterior superior wall of the primordial left atrium. This outgrowth, called the *common pulmonary vein*, merges with the splanchnic plexus and begins to drain blood from this region. If development proceeds normally, the pulmonary portion of the splanchnic plexus loses connections with the cardinal and umbilicovitelline venous systems. Tributaries to the common pulmonary vein coalesce to form two pulmonary

veins that drain each lung. If the right or left portion of the common pulmonary vein becomes atretic or loses connection with the pulmonary plexus, persistence of the primitive pulmonary venous–systemic venous connection on that side leads to PAPVC. If the common pulmonary vein–left atrium connection is disrupted totally, TAPVC occurs (Fig. 277.1).

PARTIAL ANOMALOUS PULMONARY VENOUS CONNECTION

PAPVC is a relatively common occurrence and is found in 0.6% of all autopsy studies. The relatively high incidence of this defect observed in autopsy specimens supports the contention that many cases of PAPVC do not produce symptoms and thus are not diagnosed during life. In order of decreasing frequency, the most common types of PAPVC encountered are right pulmonary veins to right superior vena cava, right pulmonary veins to right atrium, right pulmonary veins to inferior vena cava, and left pulmonary veins to the left innominate vein. Connection from the right lung anomalously occurs approximately twice as often as does that from the left lung.

Clinically apparent PAPVC usually is found in association with other cardiac defects, most commonly an ASD of the secundum or sinus venosus type. PAPVC from the right lung to the inferior vena cava occurs in the scimitar syndrome, a complex of anomalies that includes pulmonary hypoplasia or sequestration, diaphragmatic abnormalities, and anomalous systemic arterial supply to the right lung. Both scimitar syndrome and isolated PAPVC have been diagnosed prenatally using fetal echocardiography and Doppler color flow imaging as early as 20 weeks of gestation.

Hemodynamics and Clinical Features

The basic hemodynamic alteration that occurs in PAPVC is that of a pretricuspid left-to-right shunt in which fully oxygenated blood is recirculated through the lungs via the right atrium, right ventricle, and pulmonary artery. The increased pulmonary blood flow leads to enlargement of the right atrium, enlargement and hypertrophy of the right ventricle, and dilatation of

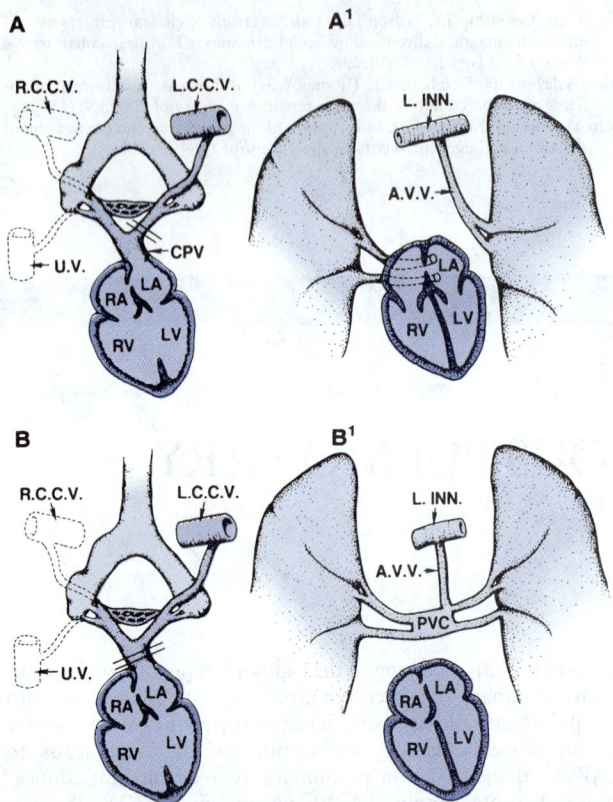

FIGURE 277.1. Embryology of anomalous pulmonary venous connections. **A:** The primitive left atrium (LA) is connected to the pulmonary venous plexus via the common pulmonary vein (CPV). Partial interruption of this connection early in gestation leads to persistence of ipsilateral systemic venous channels, resulting in partial anomalous pulmonary venous connection (A^1). **B:** Complete interruption of the common pulmonary vein results in total anomalous pulmonary venous connection (B^1). A.V.V., anomalous vertical vein; L.C.C.V., left common cardial vein; L. INN., left innominate vein; LV, left ventricle; PVC, pulmonary venous confluence; RA, right atrium; R.C.C.V., right common cardinal vein; RV, right ventricle; U.V., umbilicovitelline vein. (Adapted with permission from Lucas RV. Anomalous venous connections, pulmonary and systemic. In: Adams FH, Emmanouilides GC, eds. *Heart disease in infants, children, and adolescents*, 3rd ed. Baltimore: Williams & Wilkins, 1983:458.)

the pulmonary artery. The left heart chambers are not affected, and systemic cardiac output is normal. Most patients with PAPVC, with or without an interatrial communication, do not exhibit symptoms in early life. These patients often are referred with a cardiac murmur or an abnormal chest roentgenogram. When symptoms are elicited at this age, the most common complaint is mild intolerance for exercise. Progressive symptoms, if they appear, usually begin when the patient is in the mid-thirties or early forties. They consist of dyspnea, recurrent bronchitis, hemoptysis, chest pain, and palpitations associated with supraventricular arrhythmias. Physical examination in patients with isolated PAPVC may be normal if only a single lobe connects anomalously. When multiple lobes are involved or when an associated ASD is present, the findings are typical of an uncomplicated ASD. Occasionally, a low-frequency continuous murmur may be heard over the base, representing flow through an anomalous venous channel. The electrocardiogram usually demonstrates right ventricular hypertrophy, although it may be normal in patients without associated cardiac defects. Atrial arrhythmias are rare occurrences in the infant and child, but they may occur in the third and fourth decade of life and usually are associated with an ASD or mitral stenosis.

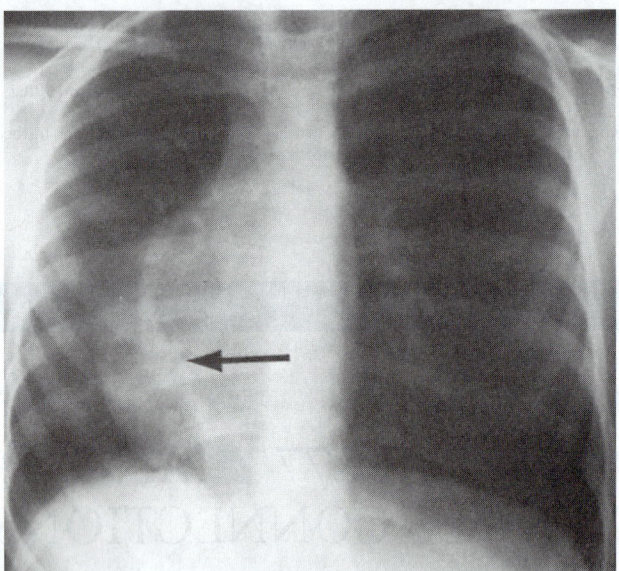

FIGURE 277.2. Scimitar syndrome. Chest radiograph in a patient with dextrocardia and partial anomalous pulmonary venous connection from the right lung to the inferior vena cava. The *arrow* points to the anomalous scimitar vein. (Courtesy of Dr. Teresa Stacy.)

In the presence of an ASD, the chest roentgenogram often shows evidence of right atrial and right ventricular enlargement in addition to increased pulmonary vascularity. Specific radiographic findings related to the insertion or drainage of the anomalous pulmonary vein or veins are described well, the scimitar sign being a classic example (Fig. 277.2).

PAPVC with or without an ASD has echocardiographic findings similar to those reported for ASDs, including mild to moderate dilatation of the right atrium and ventricle and, usually, paradoxical interventricular septal motion. The anomalous venous connection may be visualized directly in the infant and small child by color flow Doppler mapping. In the older child or teenager, transesophageal echocardiographic imaging or cine-magnetic resonance imaging (cine-MRI) may be required to delineate the course of the anomalous veins, as well as any associated ASD. Cardiac catheterization with selective angiography is the definitive diagnostic procedure for most patients with suspected PAPVC with or without associated cardiac defects. Intracardiac pressures usually are normal in patients with PAPVC when fewer than 50% of the pulmonary veins connect anomalously. Exceptions include patients older than 40 years with an associated ASD or mitral stenosis and younger patients with the scimitar syndrome. In these circumstances, moderate or marked elevation of right atrial, right ventricular, and pulmonary artery pressures may be observed.

Treatment

Surgical treatment of PAPVC should be considered in the following circumstances:

- In the presence of a hemodynamically significant left-to-right shunt (pulmonary–to–systemic flow ratio greater than 2:1, cardiomegaly on chest radiograph, right ventricular hypertrophy by electrocardiography), including most patients with isolated PAPVC, in whom 50% or more of pulmonary veins connect anomalously
- When recurrent pulmonary infections are associated with scimitar syndrome
- In conjunction with surgical repair of other major cardiac lesions (ASD, mitral stenosis)

■ When the anomalous connection affects surrounding structures by compression or obstruction

Surgical technique involves routing the anomalous pulmonary venous blood to the left atrium, either by performing transection and direct anastomosis of the anomalous channel or by use of an intracardiac baffle through the right atrium.

Operative results in asymptomatic patients are good, and the prognosis is similar to that observed after closure of an ASD. Late complications developing after surgery are rare; they include atrial arrhythmias and obstruction of systemic or pulmonary venous return.

TOTAL ANOMALOUS PULMONARY VENOUS CONNECTION

TAPVC affects 2% to 5% of all patients with congenital heart disease. In all cases, systemic blood flow is maintained by way of right-to-left shunting through an interatrial communication, usually a patent foramen ovale. The male-to-female ratio is equal in most types of TAPVC, except for a strong male predominance (3:1) in infants with TAPVC of the infradiaphragmatic type. In the group of patients with this abnormality, approximately one-third have other significant major cardiac malformations, including single ventricle, atrioventricular canal defect, hypoplastic left heart, patent ductus arteriosus, and transposition of the great vessels. Many patients in this group have abnormalities of atrial and visceral situs associated with the heterotaxy syndromes (asplenia and polysplenia). Most cases of TAPVC are sporadic and are not associated with syndromes or chromosomal abnormalities.

Anatomy

TAPVC can be classified according to the site of insertion of the anomalous channel. The four types and their frequency of occurrence are as follows: type 1, supracardiac connection (55%); type 2, cardiac connection (30%); type 3, infracardiac (infradiaphragmatic) connection (13%); and type 4, mixed connection (2%) (Fig. 277.3).

Obstruction of pulmonary venous return may occur at many sites along the anomalous venous pathway. Obstruction occurs less often in supracardiac and cardiac TAPVC, but it is almost universal in connection with the infracardiac type because pulmonary venous blood returning through the portal venous system must traverse the hepatic sinusoids.

Hemodynamics

The primary physiologic derangement in patients with TAPVC is a pretricuspid left-to-right shunt with mixing of both pulmonary venous and systemic venous blood in the right atrium, resulting in cyanosis of a variable degree. Factors that determine blood flow distribution in the systemic and pulmonary venous circuits, thus the predominant clinical symptoms, include the presence and severity of obstruction in the extracardiac pulmonary venous channels and the relative size of the interatrial communication.

When obstruction occurs in the pulmonary venous channels, pulmonary venous pressures become elevated, leading to pulmonary edema, reflex pulmonary vasoconstriction, and pulmonary hypertension. Pulmonary blood flow diminishes because of right-to-left shunting through the foramen ovale and ductus arteriosus. Progressive systemic hypoxemia leads to metabolic acidosis, multisystem organ failure, and death within a few days if the obstruction is not relieved.

In infants without significant extracardiac obstruction, the size of the interatrial communication plays a critical role in the development of symptoms after the neonatal period. A patent foramen ovale is found in most infants with uncomplicated TAPVC and results in impedance of left ventricular filling and decreased cardiac output in the first few months of life. The result is massive pulmonary overcirculation, pulmonary hypertension, and congestive heart failure. Surgical or transvenous atrial septostomy relieves both pulmonary hypertension and congestive heart failure in most patients. Unless they undergo septostomy or total surgical correction, most patients die before they are 1 year of age.

Clinical Features

Total Anomalous Pulmonary Venous Connection with Obstruction

Infants born with obstruction in the anomalous pulmonary venous channels develop symptoms shortly after birth and demonstrate severe cyanosis and respiratory distress. Physical examination reveals a prominent right ventricular impulse, accentuation of the second heart sound, and, at times, a gallop rhythm over the left lower sternal border. Murmurs are infrequent findings. Hepatomegaly usually is present and often is dramatic in APVC to the portal venous system. The electrocardiogram may demonstrate right ventricular hypertrophy and a paucity of left ventricular forces.

The chest radiograph at times is diagnostic in TAPVC with obstruction. The cardiac size usually is normal. Pulmonary vascular markings are striking, characterized by a diffuse, linear reticular pattern radiating from the hilar regions (Fig. 277.4). Overt pulmonary edema with Kerley B lines may be present. Hyperinflation of the lungs may be seen, which should differentiate this cardiac anomaly from early hyaline membrane disease. Increased pulmonary vascularity helps to distinguish this entity from persistent fetal circulation syndrome.

Total Anomalous Pulmonary Venous Connection with a Restrictive Interatrial Communication

Infants born with a restrictive interatrial communication usually are asymptomatic at birth and during the first few weeks of life; then they develop respiratory distress, feeding difficulties, and poor weight gain. Physical examination reveals tachypnea with perioral duskiness, a hyperdynamic precordium, and hepatomegaly. Auscultation demonstrates a pulmonary systolic murmur, fixed splitting of the second heart sound, and, often, a diastolic murmur over the left lower sternal border. Occasionally, a continuous venous hum may be detected in an area overlying the anomalous venous connection. The electrocardiogram demonstrates right axis deviation, right atrial enlargement, and right ventricular hypertrophy. The chest roentgenogram reveals cardiomegaly, dilatation of the pulmonary artery, and increased pulmonary vascularity. Distinctive radiographic features may be observed, reflecting the course of the anomalous pulmonary venous channel (Fig. 277.5).

Total Anomalous Pulmonary Venous Connection with a Nonrestrictive Interatrial Communication

Infants with a large ASD or who have undergone an atrial septostomy may have minimal symptoms in the first year of life. These patients often can undergo elective surgery after they are 1 year of age, with a low chance of mortality.

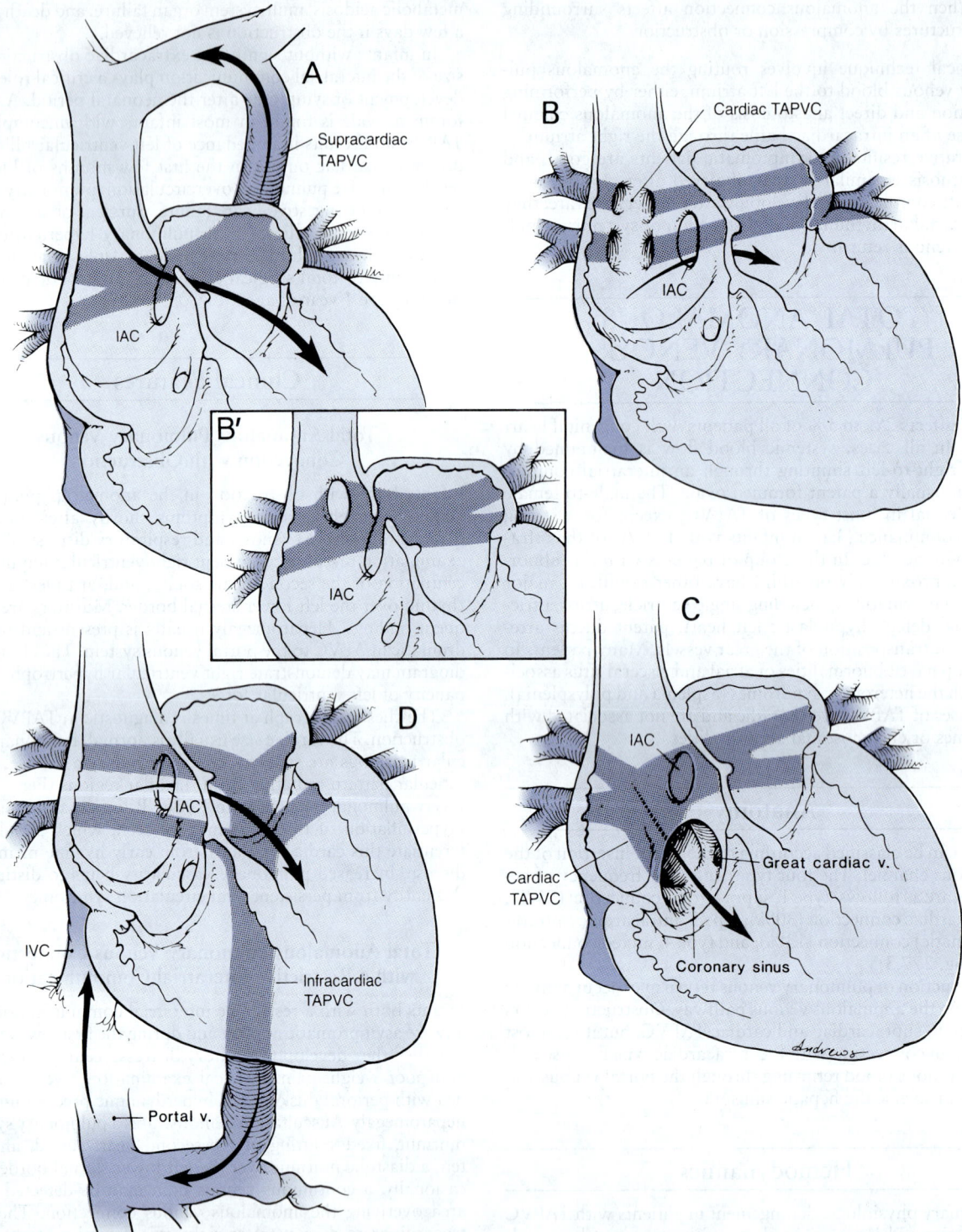

FIGURE 277.3. Types of total anomalous pulmonary venous connection (TAPVC). **A:** Supracardiac connection to left innominate vein. **B:** Cardiac connection via four separate veins. **B′:** Cardiac connection via single common orifice. **C:** Cardiac connection to coronary sinus. **D:** Infracardiac (subdiaphragmatic) connection to portal system. IAC, interatrial communication. (Adapted with permission from Ward KE, Mullins CE. Anomalous pulmonary venous connections. In: Garson A Jr, Bricker JT, Fisher DJ, Nelsh SR, eds. *The science and practice of pediatric cardiology.* Baltimore: Williams & Wilkins, 1998:1442.)

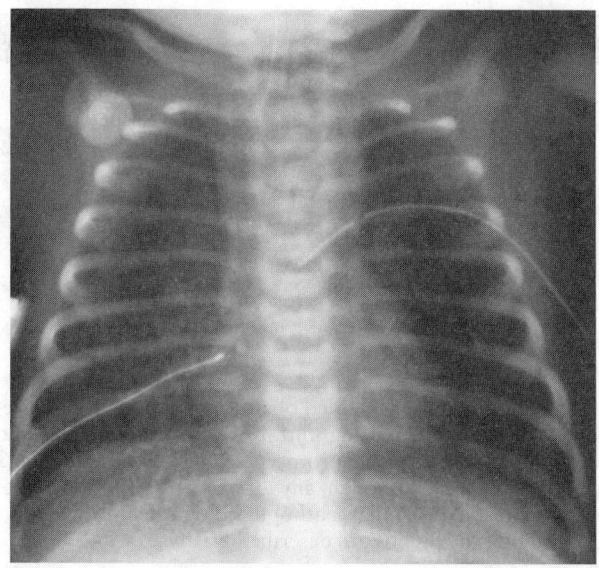

FIGURE 277.4. Total anomalous pulmonary venous connection with obstruction. The heart size is normal, and the lungs are hyperinflated. Pulmonary vascularity demonstrates a diffuse, linear reticular pattern radiating from the hilum, representing pulmonary venous engorgement.

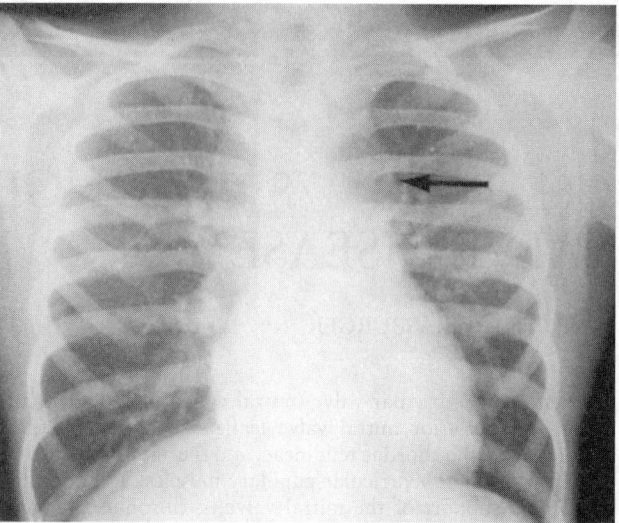

FIGURE 277.5. Supracardiac total anomalous pulmonary venous connection. Chest radiograph in a child with connection to the left innominate vein demonstrating figure-of-eight or "snowman" appearance. The *arrow* points to an anomalous vertical vein. (Courtesy of Dr. Teresa Stacy.)

Diagnostic Studies

Echocardiography and cardiac catheterization are the diagnostic procedures of choice in patients with TAPVC. Cine-MRI has been shown to be comparable in diagnostic accuracy, especially in the older infant. Although surgery may be performed based on two-dimensional and color Doppler echocardiography alone, catheterization and selective angiography often are required to delineate the anatomy in patients with complex cardiac defects or in mixed-type TAPVC. In addition, atrial septostomy can be performed during catheterization if the infant is *in extremis* with pulmonary hypertension and low systemic cardiac output.

Treatment

In infants with TAPVC who present with marked cyanosis, pulmonary edema, and cardiovascular collapse in the first few days of life, the presence of severe obstruction in the extracardiac pulmonary venous channel must be assumed. Intubation with adequate sedation and muscle paralysis is mandatory early after diagnosis is established to minimize demands for oxygen. Surgery should be undertaken immediately after diagnostic studies are performed. Alternatively, extracorporeal membrane oxygenation has been used in some infants to stabilize their cardiovascular system rapidly before surgical repair is undertaken. Prostaglandin E₁ has been reported to dilate the ductus venosus in patients with TAPVC below the diaphragm to enhance pulmonary venous return and relieve severe obstruction.

Operative mortality rates have improved to as low as 14%, but still they remain relatively high in these patients when compared with those without obstruction. Survival has been enhanced by the use of inhaled nitric oxide for postoperative pulmonary hypertensive crises.

Infants without obstruction who have an adequate atrial septal communication (either native or acquired) usually can undergo semielective surgery within 2 to 4 weeks after diagnosis is established and anticongestive medication (digitalis and diuretics) has been instituted. The operative mortality rate in these patients is 6% to 8%. The surgical technique involves performing an anastomosis of the pulmonary venous confluence to the left atrium with ligation of the anomalous channel.

The long-term outlook after surgery generally is excellent, although a few patients may require reoperation for obstruction because of inadequate growth of the pulmonary venous anastomosis or native pulmonary vein stenosis. The late development of atrial and ventricular arrhythmias has been reported to occur in as many as 25% of patients, although these developments usually are well controlled with medication and/or catheter-based ablation therapy.

Suggested Readings

Allan LD, Sharland GK. The echocardiographic diagnosis of totally anomalous pulmonary venous connection in the fetus. *Heart* 2001;85:433.

Burroughs JT, Edwards JE. Total anomalous pulmonary venous connection. *Am Heart J* 1960;59:913.

Edwards JE. Pathologic and developmental considerations in anomalous pulmonary venous connection. *Mayo Clin Proc* 1953;28:441.

Huhta J, Gutgesell HP, Nihill MR. Cross-sectional echocardiographic diagnosis of total anomalous pulmonary venous connection. *Br Heart J* 1985;53:525.

Kirklin JW, Ellis FH, Wood EH. Treatment of anomalous pulmonary venous connection in association with interatrial communications. *Surgery* 1956;39:389.

Mathey J, Galey JJ, Logeais Y, et al. Anomalous pulmonary venous return into inferior vena cava and associated bronchovascular anomalies (the scimitar syndrome): report of three cases and review of the literature. *Thorax* 1968;23:398.

Michielon G, DiDonato RM, Pasquini L, et al. Total anomalous pulmonary venous connection: long-term appraisal with evolving technical solutions. *Eur J Cardiothorac Surg* 2002;22:184.

Lupinetti FM, Kulik TJ, Beekman RH, et al. Correction of total anomalous pulmonary venous connection in infancy. *J Thorac Cardiovasc Surg* 1993;106:880.

Ward KE, Mullins CE. Anomalous pulmonary venous connections. In: Garson A Jr, Bricker JT, Fisher DJ, Neish SR, eds. *The science and practice of pediatric cardiology*. Baltimore: Williams & Wilkins, 1998.

Ward KE, Mullins CE, Huhta JC, et al. Restrictive interatrial communication in total anomalous pulmonary venous connection. *Am J Cardiol* 1986;57:1131.

CHAPTER 278 ■ CONGENITAL MITRAL VALVE DISEASE

JANETTE F. STRASBURGER

The left atrioventricular valve (mitral valve) includes the anterior and posterior mitral valve leaflets separated by their commissures, the chordae tendineae, and the anteromedial and posterolateral left ventricular papillary muscles. The annulus, or skeletal support of the mitral valve, is fibromuscular and contracts with the heart. The mitral valve permits egress of blood during diastole and atrial systole from the left atrium to the left ventricle and prevents reflux of blood into the left atrium during ventricular systole. Thus, closure of the mitral valve is the earliest component of the first heart sound. Abnormalities in the development of the mitral valve apparatus can result in hemodynamic alterations in blood flow, which can present with either congestive heart failure or pulmonary edema during fetal, neonatal, or later development.

Most abnormalities of the mitral valve are associated with other congenital cardiac defects, such as atrioventricular septal defects, and are not isolated mitral abnormalities. When isolated mitral abnormalities occur in the pediatric age group, they usually are acquired as the result of rheumatic carditis, myocardial ischemia or infarction, hypertension, Marfan syndrome, mitral valve prolapse syndrome, bacterial endocarditis, myocarditis, or cardiomyopathy. Congenital mitral valve abnormalities are much rarer. Because of the severity of obstruction of flow across the valve, valvular regurgitation, or associated cardiac defects, patients with congenital mitral abnormalities often present during infancy. Congenital lesions of the mitral valve are listed in Table 278.1.

Other abnormalities of the pulmonary veins or left atrium also can cause obstruction of left ventricular filling or pulmonary venous egress proximal to the mitral valve. They include the following: cor triatriatum, a perforated fibromuscular membrane that subdivides the left atrium; supravalvar stenosing mitral ring, a fibrous, shelflike ridge just above the mitral valve that encroaches on its orifice; left atrial tumor; and unilateral or common pulmonary venous stenosis or atresia. All these lesions can result in pulmonary edema and right-sided cardiac failure secondary to obstructed left-sided flow and pulmonary hypertension.

The physiology of left-sided obstructive and regurgitant lesions is discussed here using mitral valvular insufficiency and mitral valvular stenosis as prototypes (Figs. 278.1 and 278.2 and Table 278.2), although any of the aforementioned defects can result in similar pathophysiologic features. Differences among the lesions are described briefly.

CONGENITAL MITRAL STENOSIS

Mitral valve stenosis presents clinically with right-sided cardiac failure and pulmonary hypertension. The age at presentation depends on the degree of obstruction of left atrial emptying. Because exercise demands greater cardiac output, initial symptoms often are related to exercise. In infants, feeding requires increased cardiac output, and babies often present with dyspnea or cyanosis during feeding and with failure to grow. Because of pulmonary edema, infants and children are at risk for having recurring respiratory infections. Tachypnea, hemoptysis, respiratory distress, low cardiac output, and atrial fibrillation can be associated findings of mitral stenosis. Atrial fibrillation and left atrial thrombi are relatively uncommon occurrences in children; however, if atrial fibrillation is observed, the presence of intracardiac thrombi must be excluded before cardioversion.

The physical examination in mitral stenosis is characterized by a right ventricular lift at the left lower sternal border and by an increased pulmonary component of the second heart sound caused by pulmonary hypertension. A fourth heart sound sometimes is audible secondary to enhanced atrial systolic contraction. A long pandiastolic murmur often is audible

TABLE 278.1

CONGENITAL ABNORMALITIES OF THE MITRAL VALVE APPARATUS

Congenital Mitral Stenosis	Congenital Mitral Insufficiency
Parachute mitral valve	Cleft mitral valve
Double-orifice mitral valve	Congenital mitral valve regurgitation
Mitral valve stenosis or hypoplasia	Double-orifice mitral valve
	Intrauterine rupture of the chordae tendineae or papillary muscle

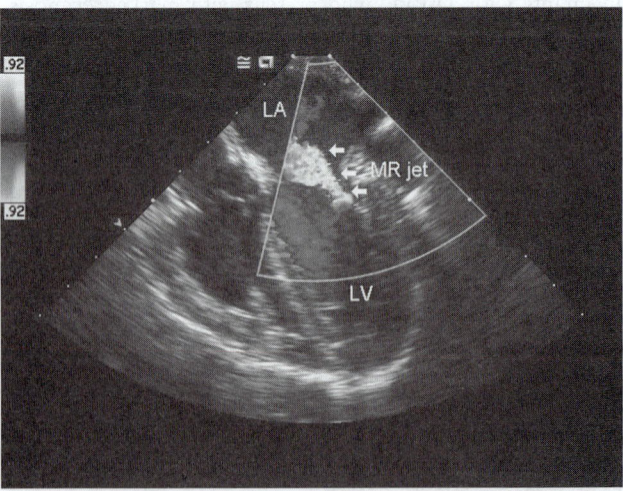

FIGURE 278.1. Mitral regurgitation. The mitral regurgitation jet (MR jet, *arrow*) is noted as a light colored flame directed into the left atrium (LA) from the left ventricle (LV) during systole.

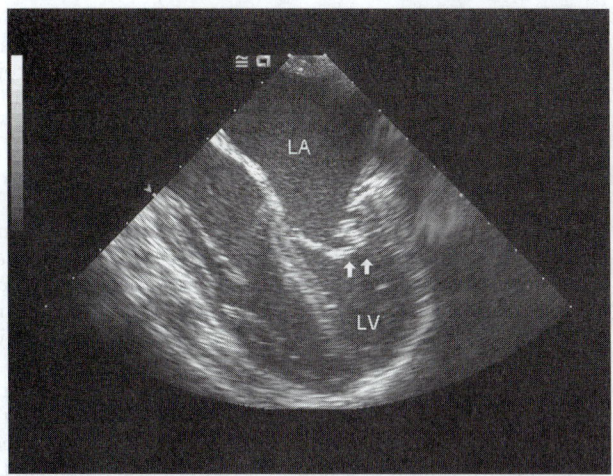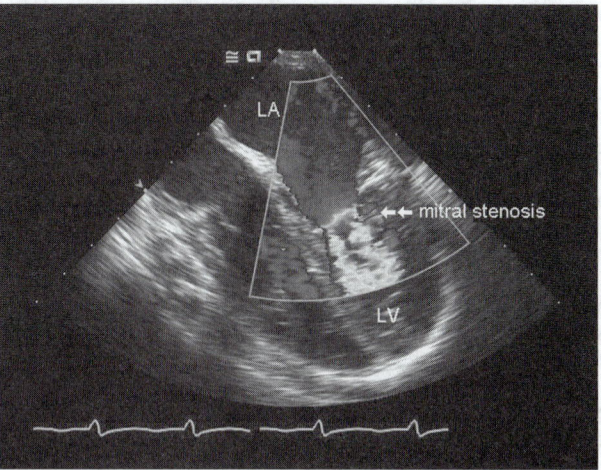

A B

FIGURE 278.2. Mitral stenosis. **A:** Note the thickened mitral valve leaflets *(arrows),* left atrial enlargement (LA), and orientation of the mitral valve toward the single "parachute" papillary muscle along the lateral left ventricular (LV) wall in this patient with mitral stenosis. **B:** The light color jet (labeled mitral stenosis) during diastole is projected toward the left ventricle (LV). The diameter of the valve is reduced compared with normal.

at the cardiac apex. The chest radiograph usually shows left atrial enlargement, with widening of the angle between the left and right main bronchi. In older children, a redistribution of blood flow can be seen, with increased flow to the upper lobes. Kerley B lines and pulmonary edema also are present. Generally, the electrocardiogram shows left atrial or biatrial enlargement during sinus rhythm, and, rarely, atrial fibrillation is present. Right ventricular hypertrophy with right axis deviation generally is seen. Two-dimensional and Doppler echocardiography studies determine the presence of mitral stenosis by measuring the cross-sectional area of the valve and its flow gradient, and they detect structural abnormalities of the mitral valve or supporting apparatus. The left atrial size often is enlarged, but the left ventricular volume usually is 70% to 100% of normal. Transesophageal echocardiography, which allows excellent imaging of the left atrium and mitral valve when the

patient is under sedation or general anesthesia, frequently is used to provide specific anatomic and Doppler detail and can be an adjunct to cardiac catheterization and surgical valvuloplasty procedures or before cardioversion. Cardiac catheterization usually is reserved for situations in which the echocardiographic diagnosis is unclear or associated defects are present. Cardiac catheterization demonstrates elevation in pulmonary arterial pressure and right ventricular systolic pressure. A gradient between the left atrial A wave and the left ventricular end-diastolic pressure exists. Often, estimating the left atrial pressure using pulmonary capillary wedge pressure or entering the left atrium via transseptal puncture is necessary. Injections in the pulmonary artery or left atrium usually demonstrate abnormalities of the mitral valve or adjacent structures.

Mild or moderate mitral stenosis can be managed by diuretic therapy, supplemental nutrition, and aggressive management

TABLE 278.2

CLINICAL CHARACTERISTICS ASSOCIATED WITH CONGENITAL MALFORMATIONS OF THE MITRAL VALVE

Findings in Severe Disease	Congenital Mitral Stenosis	Congenital Mitral Insufficiency
Prevalent clinical symptoms	Tachypnea, exercise intolerance, poor weight gain	Tachypnea, exercise intolerance, poor weight gain
Physical findings	RV lift, fourth heart sound, pandiastolic murmur at apex, increased S_2P_2	LV lift, palpable cardiomegaly, decreased S_1, normal to increased S_2P_2, Pansystolic murmur and diastolic flow rumble at apex
Electrocardiographic findings	LAE or Bi-AE, RVH, with or without atrial fibrillation	LAE, LVH, or BVH, with or without atrial fibrillation
Radiographic findings	LAE, splayed left and right bronchi, pulmonary edema, with or without right heart enlargement	Cardiomegaly, splayed bronchi, increased pulmonary vascular markings, LAE and LVE
Echocardiographic findings	LAE, small mitral valve orifice with increased diastolic flow velocity, abnormal valve appearance, mildly reduced LV size, pulmonary hypertension, RV enlargement and RVH, diastolic color Doppler jet directed toward the LV	LAE, LVE, abnormal mitral valve appearance, normal to increased LV function, broad color Doppler systolic jet directed toward the LA and pulmonary veins
Catheterization findings	Increased LA pressure, LA-to-LV diastolic gradient, pulmonary hypertension	Increased LA pressure, with or without LV end-diastolic pressure, LAE and LVE and with or without LV dysfunction, pulmonary hypertension

Bi-AE, biatrial enlargement; BVH, biventricular hypertrophy; LA, left atrial; LAE, left atrial enlargement; LV, left ventricular; LVE, left ventricular enlargement; LVH, left ventricular hypertrophy; RVH, right ventricular hypertrophy, S_2P_2, pulmonic component of the second heart sound.

of respiratory infections. Usually, use of digoxin therapy is not helpful for right ventricular failure, although it sometimes is used for arrhythmias. Atrial fibrillation may complicate mitral stenosis in older children. Transesophageal echocardiography is indicated before cardioversion of atrial fibrillation to exclude atrial thrombi that may not be evident on precordial echocardiography. Anticoagulation is necessary before cardioversion when thrombi are suspected. Long-term anticoagulation with warfarin (Coumadin) is indicated in patients for whom recurrence of atrial fibrillation is likely. Rarely, the addition of quinidine, procainamide, sotalol, or amiodarone to digoxin therapy is necessary to maintain sinus rhythm. Arrhythmias seen early postoperatively, within 3 months after surgery, usually improve as the hemodynamic features stabilize.

Balloon mitral valvuloplasty to enlarge the mitral valve orifice during cardiac catheterization has lost favor for pediatric patients with congenital mitral valve disease, but it is still used in postrheumatic mitral stenosis. The greatest experience with this technique has been gained in the adolescent patient. Five-year follow-up after balloon mitral valvuloplasty has shown that restenosis rates vary from 2% to 30%, depending on the technique used. Complications have included thromboembolism, endocarditis, atrial septal injury, and mitral regurgitation.

Surgery is indicated for children with low cardiac output, severe symptoms with exercise, and severe pulmonary hypertension. The preferred treatment is surgical commissurotomy, which is open heart surgery consisting of incision along the mitral commissure. The operation must be considered palliative because patients often have either annular hypoplasia or abnormalities in the supports of the mitral valve. When obstruction is caused by a fibromuscular ridge or cor triatriatum, these structures must be removed. Whenever possible, mitral valve replacement should be avoided in young children because anticoagulation is necessary for metallic prosthetic valves in the mitral position. During the last decade, surgeons have become more adept at repair of the mitral valve. Prognosis for survival after undergoing mitral valve surgery is 95% or better in the short term, but the mortality rates are higher in younger patients and in those with associated defects.

Unlike isolated mitral stenosis, parachute mitral valve, double-orifice mitral valve, and mitral hypoplasia usually occur with other cardiac defects, not as isolated defects. These defects can cause mitral stenosis, mitral regurgitation, or both. Because of the complexity of associated defects, they are less amenable to surgical repair. Shone complex consists of parachute mitral valve, subaortic stenosis, and coarctation of the aorta with or without a ventricular septal defect when mitral annular hypoplasia is present. The type of surgical intervention is strongly dependent on the size of the left ventricle. When the left ventricle is hypoplastic, the left side of the heart is circumvented with the Norwood operation.

CONGENITAL MITRAL REGURGITATION

During mitral regurgitation, the left ventricle decompresses into the left atrium, and one-half of the regurgitant volume during ventricular systole occurs before the opening of the aortic valve. When the regurgitant volume exceeds the stroke volume of a single systole, cardiac output decreases, resulting functionally in an increase in left atrial and left ventricular volume and cardiomegaly. Pulmonary edema develops because of pulmonary venous congestion.

Clinical symptoms of mitral regurgitation are related to the severity of the regurgitation, associated cardiac defects, left ventricular function, pulmonary artery pressure, and rate of development of the regurgitation. Acute mitral regurgitation of moderate or severe degree is tolerated poorly and leads rapidly to acute pulmonary edema and low cardiac output. Chronic mitral regurgitation of mild or moderate degree may be asymptomatic. With increasing severity, symptoms in infants and children include diaphoresis, recurrent respiratory infections, tachypnea, exercise intolerance, and failure to grow because of high caloric requirements.

Children with mitral regurgitation generally have a diffuse left ventricular lift and a palpably enlarged heart. The first heart sound is normal or decreased, and the pulmonary component of the second heart sound is either normal or increased. Mitral regurgitation causes a high-pitched, blowing, apical pansystolic murmur; it must be differentiated from the murmur of a ventricular septal defect, which usually is audible near the left sternal border rather than at the apex. During diastole, the increased flow across the mitral valve results in a low-pitched diastolic flow rumble and sometimes a third heart sound at the apex.

The radiographic appearance of mitral regurgitation consists of cardiomegaly of moderate degree, with increased pulmonary vascular markings. Enlargement of the left atrial and left ventricular contours of the heart is present. The electrocardiogram generally shows left atrial enlargement and left ventricular hypertrophy. Atrial fibrillation is an uncommon finding. Two-dimensional echocardiography detects abnormalities of valve appearance, motion, and attachments. The left ventricular systolic function is normal or increased because of Frank Starling forces. Decreased left ventricular contractility, especially in the presence of cardiomegaly, suggests cardiomyopathy in association with mitral regurgitation.

Color flow mapping is useful in qualitative assessment of the amount of regurgitation. Severe regurgitation occurs over a broad area of the annulus and refluxes far into the left atrium, whereas in mild mitral regurgitation, only a small narrow jet is noted. Reversal of flow velocities in the pulmonary veins also is indicative of severe regurgitation.

Mild or moderate mitral insufficiency generally can be managed by diuretic and digoxin therapy. Afterload reduction with nitroprusside has been lifesaving in acute mitral regurgitation. Oral afterload-reducing agents, such as captopril and enalapril, are used as adjuvant therapy in patients with congestive heart failure or cardiomyopathy associated with mitral regurgitation.

Cardiac catheterization is reserved for presurgical evaluation and may be used to assess the severity of the regurgitation, as well as the degree of pulmonary hypertension and left ventricular dysfunction.

Surgical intervention is necessary for congestive heart failure and pulmonary edema secondary to mitral regurgitation, which is poorly controlled by medical management, or for progressive left ventricular dysfunction and cardiomegaly. The surgical treatment of choice is mitral valvuloplasty (repair of the mitral valve) or annuloplasty (plication of the mitral annulus). The mortality rate for valvuloplasty surgery is approximately 4% for patients in stable condition, but it may exceed 10% when a child has low cardiac output, systemic infection, multiple cardiac defects, or severe pulmonary edema, or if the child requires more than one valve replacement. Dr. Carpentier has defined the anatomy and surgery for the mitral valve. Techniques used include annulus adjustment, leaflet repair, commissurotomy, and chordal or papillary muscle splitting to allow a valve of adequate size for the body surface area of the patient. When a mechanical mitral valve is placed for recurrent mitral regurgitation, it generally is a low-profile tilting disk valve. A metallic prosthetic valve requires long-term anticoagulation therapy. An international normalized ratio of 3.0 to 3.5 is recommended at all times, and low-molecular-weight subcutaneous heparin may be used as a substitute when dental extractions or surgery are anticipated. The smallest valve available is a 17-mm valve that can be implanted in a child at a minimum age of 1 to 2 years. Surgical correction of other mitral defects, such as double-orifice mitral valve and parachute mitral valve, rarely is required alone and operation depends on associated cardiac defects. Pulmonary hypertension secondary to either mitral regurgitation or mitral stenosis generally is relieved by surgery because venous congestion usually does not result in irreversible pulmonary vascular disease.

Suggested Readings

Banerjee A, Kohl T, Silverman NH. Echocardiographic evaluation of congenital mitral valve anomalies in children. *Am J Cardiol* 1995;76:1284.

Buck ML. Anticoagulation with warfarin in infants and children. *Ann Pharmacother* 1996;30:1316.

Carpentier A. Mitral valve reconstruction in operative surgery. In: Jamieson SW, Shumway NE, eds. *Operative surgery,* 4th ed. Stoneham, MA: Butterworth-Heinemann 1986:405.

Carpentier A. Branchini B, Cour JC, et al. Congenital malformations of the mitral valve in children. *J Thorac Cardiovasc Surg* 1976;72:854.

Hirsh J, Fuster V, Ansell J, Halperin JL. AMA/ACC foundation guide to warfarin therapy. *Circulation* 2003;107:1692.

Moore P, Adatia A, Spevak PJ, et al. Severe congenital mitral stenosis in infants. *Circulation* 1994;89:2099.

Oakley CM. Management of valvular stenosis. *Curr Opin Cardiol* 1995;10:117.

Roberts WC, Perloff JK. Mitral valvular disease: a clinicopathologic survey of the conditions causing the mitral valve to function abnormally. *Ann Intern Med* 1972;77:939.

Solymar L, Rao PS, Mardini MK, et al. Prosthetic valves in children and adolescents. *Am Heart J* 1991;121:557.

Zias EA, Mavroudis C, Basker CL, et al. Surgical repair of the congenitally malformed mitral valve in infants and children. *Ann Thorac Surg* 1998;66:1551.

CHAPTER 279 ■ MITRAL VALVE PROLAPSE

VICTORIA E. JUDD

Mitral valve prolapse (MVP) is the most common cardiac disorder diagnosis, with childhood prevalence estimates of 0.5% to 17%. The overall prevalence in the general population is 2% to 4%, with no gender difference. Early studies, which used less specific echocardiographic criteria, had the estimated incidence much higher, particularly for young women.

MVP occurs most frequently as a primary condition characterized by myxomatous degeneration of the leaflets. Primary MVP usually is sporadic. Familial clustering of MVP of autosomal dominant inheritance has been reported. MVP may occur in association with other conditions such as Marfan syndrome, Ehlers-Danlos syndrome, and other diseases that affect connective tissue.

Secondary MVP refers to the MVP that does not have myxomatous valvular changes. It may occur with leaner body mass index and smaller left ventricle cavity size.

CLINICAL MANIFESTATIONS AND COMPLICATIONS

Associated conditions are described in Box 279.1.

Clinical Presentation

Most children with MVP are asymptomatic and initially are referred for cardiac evaluation because a click and/or a murmur is detected during a routine examination. Numerous studies report a high incidence of symptoms with MVP, but they probably are due to selection bias. Small subgroups of patients may be highly symptomatic. However, little direct evidence links these symptoms with MVP. Symptoms may include chest pain, fatigue, weakness, palpitations, dyspnea, dizziness, near syncope, syncope, anxiety, and orthostatic hypotension.

Abnormalities on physical examination include thoracic and skeletal abnormalities, such as a tall slender habitus, pectus excavatum, pectus carinatum, scoliosis, or kyphosis. A high arched palate, increased joint laxity, or abnormal dermatoglyphics patterns also may be present.

MVP is characterized by a midsystolic click or a late systolic murmur. The click and murmur vary, depending on an affected patient's position, and may vary in auscultatory findings at different times in different patients. The change in the click and murmur is caused by alterations in left ventricular volume. Such maneuvers as moving from a sitting to a supine position or from a standing to a squatting position, passive leg raising, and maximal isometric exercise increase left ventricular volume and decrease the degree of MVP and mitral regurgitation. The click and murmur move toward the second heart sound, and the murmur is shorter.

Left ventricular size and left ventricular volume are decreased by administration of amyl nitrate; a Valsalva maneuver; sudden change from a supine to a sitting position, from a sitting

---

BOX 279.1   Associated Conditions

Mitral valve prolapse (MVP) occurs with increased frequency in patients with Marfan syndrome, Ehlers-Danlos syndrome, and other heritable disorders of connective tissue disease that increase the size of mitral valve leaflets and apparatus. It is seen also with higher frequency in patients with myotonic dystrophy, hyperthyroidism, Turner syndrome, fragile X syndrome, anorexia nervosa, systemic lupus erythematosus, polyarteritis nodosa, secundum atrial septal defects, acute rheumatic heart disease, and adult polycystic kidney disease. It is seen also in patients with thoracic abnormalities, such as straight-back syndrome, pectus excavatum, scoliosis, and thin body habitus.

to a standing position, and from a squatting to a standing position; and inspiration. MVP and mitral valve regurgitation increase; thus, the click and murmur move toward the first heart sound, and the murmur becomes longer. Because of the changing intensity or timing with different body positions, auscultation should be performed with the patient in many positions.

The high-pitched, low-intensity, nonejection midsystolic click is heard best at the apex of the heart. It may occur from just after the first heart sound to just before the second heart sound. Multiple clicks may be present in certain patients. Usually, the crescendo, late systolic murmur of MVP, is preceded by a click and is heard best at the apex. Occasionally, the murmur is described as having a honking or whooping quality and may be heard without a stethoscope.

The murmur of MVP may be confused with the murmur of hypertrophic cardiomyopathy. During the strain of the Valsalva maneuver, the murmur of hypertrophic cardiomyopathy increases in intensity and the murmur of MVP becomes longer but not louder.

Usually, the chest radiograph is normal unless associated cardiac or skeletal defects are present. If a routine chest roentgenogram shows thoracic spine and chest-wall abnormalities, such as scoliosis, pectus excavatum, or straightened thoracic spine, an evaluation for MVP is indicated.

The electrocardiogram usually is normal. Three types of abnormalities are reported: ST-T–wave depression or T-wave inversion in leads II, III, and aV_F; prolongation of the QT interval; and arrhythmias. The ST-T depression is seen more commonly with exercise.

Usually, the exercise test is normal. Arrhythmias and ST-T–wave changes have been reported.

Echocardiography is useful in defining MVP. M-mode echocardiography should not be used to diagnose MVP; two-dimensional echocardiography should be used. M-mode echocardiography may overdiagnose or underdiagnose MVP. The apical four-chamber view in two-dimensional echocardiography is too sensitive and not specific for the diagnosis of MVP. Many patients who have a normal auscultatory examination may have MVP as documented by the apical four-chamber view. The mitral valve annulus is not flat but is saddle-shaped. The four-chamber view may show superior displacement of the mitral valve leaflets, but it may not be true MVP. The long axis view is the most specific view to determine the presence or absence of MVP.

Echocardiographic evaluation of patients with possible MVP should include evaluation for mitral annulus dilation, dysplasia of the mitral valve, mitral valve regurgitation, presence or absence of ruptured chordae and vegetations, and coexistent cardiovascular abnormalities. Prolapse of the tricuspid valve and aortic valve occurs more often in patients with MVP.

Stress radionuclide scintigraphy aids in establishing the differential diagnosis between MVP (associated with atypical chest pain and electrocardiogram abnormalities) and primary coronary artery disease associated with MVP. A negative test may confirm the diagnosis of primary MVP without coronary artery disease. A false-positive test, however, may occur in patients with MVP without associated coronary artery disease.

Although diagnostic cardiac catheterization with angiography rarely is needed in patients with isolated MVP, if needed, it is used to assess the severity of associated cardiac abnormalities.

Complications

Usually, the prognosis of MVP in children is benign. Such complications as endocarditis, significant arrhythmias, sudden death, progressive mitral regurgitation, stroke, and cerebral ischemia occur infrequently.

Chest Pain

If patients with MVP have symptoms, the most common presenting symptom is disabling chest pain. The exact mechanism of chest pain is unknown. In some patients with MVP, esophageal motility disorders account for chest pain.

Infective Endocarditis

Patients with MVP and mitral regurgitation have an increased incidence of infective endocarditis. Antibiotic prophylaxis should be used in the presence of a systolic murmur.

Cerebral Vascular Events

Cerebral vascular events in patients with MVP are caused by conditions other than MVP. Evidence of an association between MVP and stroke is lacking.

Arrhythmias

Patients with MVP without mitral regurgitation do not have increased incidence of arrhythmias.

Sudden Death

Sudden death is a rare complication postulated to be secondary to a lethal arrhythmia. Patients who may be at increased risk of sudden death may have complex ventricular arrhythmias, severe mitral regurgitation, left ventricular dysfunction, prolonged QT interval, a history of syncope, or a family history of sudden death.

Mitral Regurgitation

Progressive mitral regurgitation is a rare complication. Severe mitral valve regurgitation occurs more frequently in men who are older than 50 years and have higher systolic pressures and body weight.

DIAGNOSIS

The diagnosis of MVP may be made by auscultatory, echocardiographic, angiocardiographic, and pathologic criteria. Perloff et al. proposed specific clinical criteria for the diagnosis of MVP. The midsystolic click and the late systolic murmur best heard at the apex are diagnostic auscultatory criteria of MVP. Echocardiographic diagnostic criteria are two-dimensional echocardiography showing 2 mm above the mitral annulus and superior systolic displacement of the mitral leaflets either in the apical or parasternal long axis view. The diagnosis may not be made on the basis of symptoms, physical appearance, electrocardiographic abnormalities, chest radiograph abnormalities, or nonspecific echocardiographic abnormalities.

THERAPY

Patients who have no symptoms need no special treatment other than subacute bacterial endocarditis (SBE) prophylaxis.

A resting electrocardiogram is recommended in all patients to look for evidence of ST-T–wave changes, prolonged QT interval, or an arrhythmia. If coexisting cardiac defects are not present, a CXR is not needed. A 24-hour Holter monitor or exercise treadmill is indicated in patients with palpitations, lightheadedness, dizziness, syncope, arrhythmias on resting electrocardiogram, family history of sudden death, or a prolonged QT interval on resting electrocardiogram. Angiography may be indicated if other cardiac defects coexist.

An asymptomatic patient with an isolated midsystolic click, no evidence of mitral regurgitation, or dysplastic mitral valve should be reassured of the benign nature of MVP and should be followed up every 3 years.

Patients with mitral valve regurgitation on examination or echocardiogram or with a dysplastic mitral valve should observe SBE prophylaxis.

Indications for mitral valve replacement are severe mitral regurgitation with or without severe life-threatening arrhythmias unresponsive to medical management.

Patients with MVP should not participate in competitive athletics if they have a history of syncope with exertion, complex ventricular arrhythmias, significant mitral regurgitation with left ventricular enlargement and dysfunction, prolongation of the QT interval, Marfan syndrome, or a family history of sudden death.

Suggested Readings

Bisset GS III, Schwartz DC, Meyer RA, et al. Clinical spectrum and long-term follow-up of isolated mitral valve prolapse in 119 children. *Circulation* 1980; 2:62.

Boudoulas H, Kolibash AJ, Baker P, et al. Mitral valve prolapse and the mitral valve prolapse syndrome: a diagnostic classification and pathogenesis of symptoms. *Am Heart J* 1989;118:796.

Cheng TO. Mitral valve prolapse. *Annu Rev Med* 1989;40:201.

Committee on Sports Medicine and Fitness, 1994 to 1995. Mitral valve prolapse and athletic participation in children and adolescents. *Pediatrics* 1995; 95:789.

Devereux RB, Kramer-Fox R, Kligfield P. Mitral valve prolapse: causes, clinical manifestations, and management. *Ann Intern Med* 1989;4:111.

Devereux RB, Kramer-Fox R, Shear MK, et al. Diagnosis and classification of severity of mitral valve prolapse: methodologic, biologic, and prognostic considerations. *Am Heart J* 1987;113:1265.

Freed LA, Benjamin EJ, Levy D, et al. Mitral valve prolapse in the general population. *J Am Coll Cardiol* 2002;40:1298.

Gilon D, Buonanno FS, Joffe MM, et al. Lack of evidence of an association between mitral valve prolapse and stroke in young patients. *N Engl J Med* 341:8.

Kavey RA, Blackman MS, Sondheimer HM, et al. Ventricular arrhythmias and mitral valve prolapse in childhood. *J Pediatr* 1984;105:885.

Krivokapich J, Child JS, Dadourian BJ, et al. Reassessment of echocardiographic criteria for diagnosis of mitral valve prolapse. *Am J Cardiol* 1988;61:131.

Perloff JK, Child JS, Edwards JE. New guidelines for the clinical diagnosis of mitral valve prolapse. *Am J Cardiol* 1986;57:1124.

Savage DD, Garrison FJ, Devereux RB, et al. Mitral valve prolapse in the general population. I. Epidemiologic features: the Framingham study. *Am Heart J* 1983;106:571.

Warth DC, King ME, Cohen JM, et al. Prevalence of mitral valve prolapse in normal children. *J Am Coll Cardiol* 1985;5:5.

CHAPTER 280 ■ AORTIC ARCH AND PULMONARY ARTERY ABNORMALITIES

W. ROBERT MORROW

Anomalies of the aortic arch and pulmonary arteries constitute a diverse group of malformations. The range of possible deviations from normal morphology of the aortic arch and pulmonary artery is broad. Vascular rings are formed when one or more aortic arch anomalies, with or without a patent ductus arteriosus or ligamentum, produce a ring that completely encircles the trachea and esophagus, leading to symptoms of tracheal or esophageal constriction. A vascular sling, produced by an abnormal origin and course of the left pulmonary artery or left ductus arteriosus, does not encircle the trachea and esophagus completely but usually produces severe symptoms of tracheal and bronchial compression.

PATHOGENESIS

Most anomalies of the aortic arch can be described by postulating the regression of a segment of the arch that normally persists or, conversely, the persistence of a segment of the arch that normally regresses. In this concept, the normal left aortic arch develops by regression of the eighth segment of the embryonic right dorsal aorta. The remaining elements of the right aortic arch contribute to development of the right innominate artery and the primitive right subclavian artery. Normally, the right ductus arteriosus regresses, eliminating continuity of the right sixth aortic arch with the aorta. A double aortic arch is postulated to result from the persistence of both paired dorsal aortic arches.

A right aortic arch may form by one of two mechanisms, giving rise to a right aortic arch with or without mirror-image branching. A right aortic arch with mirror-image branching occurs when the left eighth dorsal aortic arch segment regresses. When regression of the left arch occurs between the left carotid artery and the left subclavian artery (left fourth primitive aortic arch), the latter arises from the descending aorta and courses posterior to the esophagus. In this situation, the ductus arteriosus arises from the descending aorta at the base of the left subclavian artery or from a retroesophageal diverticulum and produces a vascular ring completely encircling the esophagus and trachea. Regression may occur between the right carotid artery and the right subclavian artery, giving rise to an anomalous origin of the right subclavian artery from the descending aorta. A cervical aortic arch probably results from the persistence of the third primitive aortic arch, with regression of the contralateral arch between the carotid artery and the subclavian artery (fourth primitive arch).

An anomalous origin of the left pulmonary artery, unilateral absence of one pulmonary artery, and unilateral origin of one pulmonary artery from the ascending aorta result from the abnormal regression of the left proximal sixth arch. The unilateral origin of one pulmonary artery from the ascending aorta may result from a malalignment of the conotruncal ridges. With septation of the truncus arteriosus, one pulmonary artery maintains connection with the ascending aorta, and the other is connected to the main pulmonary artery.

Aortic Arch Anomalies

Left Aortic Arch with Anomalous Right Subclavian Artery

Left aortic arch with anomalous origin of the right subclavian artery is the most common aortic arch malformation noted on postmortem examination. The incidence of this abnormality in the general population is approximately 0.5%. The left arch has a normal course to the left and anterior to the trachea, but the right subclavian artery arises as the last branch of the arch and courses posterior to the esophagus. Most patients with anomalous right subclavian artery are asymptomatic, and the abnormality is discovered incidentally at esophagography or at catheterization. Often, an anomalous right subclavian artery is seen in patients with tetralogy of Fallot and left aortic arch and, therefore, has a significant bearing on which systemic-to-pulmonary artery shunt is chosen for palliation of cyanosis. In addition, an anomalous right subclavian artery may be present in patients with coarctation of the aorta, and it often arises distal to the site of coarctation. In these patients, blood pressure in the right arm and legs does not reflect the coarctation gradient. It is necessary, then, to determine blood pressure in both arms and in the legs during the examination of patients with suspected coarctation.

Although most patients with an anomalous right subclavian artery are asymptomatic, some older children and adults may experience dysphagia. Routine chest radiography does not demonstrate this anomaly, but barium esophagography is diagnostic. The oblique course of the anomalous vessel posterior to the esophagus in the anteroposterior projection and the posterior indentation of the esophagus in the lateral or left anterior oblique projection usually are diagnostic (Fig. 280.1). The diagnosis of an anomalous right subclavian artery may be made using two-dimensional echocardiography when the first branch of the aorta is to the right, but the normal bifurcation into a right carotid artery and right subclavian artery cannot be demonstrated. An anomalous right subclavian artery may be noted incidentally when aortography is performed in patients with congenital heart disease.

If symptoms of a vascular ring (e.g., stridor, wheezing, cough) are present in a patient with an anomalous right subclavian artery, an alternative diagnosis, such as laryngomalacia or tracheomalacia, should be considered. Rarely, an anomalous right subclavian artery in association with a left aortic arch, retroesophageal descending aorta, and right ductus arteriosus or ligamentum produces a symptomatic vascular ring. The retroesophageal descending aorta in these patients results in a large, rounded, posterior indentation on barium esophagogram, which usually is distinguished readily from the more shallow indentation produced by an anomalous right subclavian artery without a retroesophageal descending aorta. The diagnosis should be confirmed by magnetic resonance imaging (MRI).

Double Aortic Arch

The double aortic arch is the most common clinically recognized form of vascular ring. The ascending aorta divides anterior to the trachea into left and right arches, which then pass on either side of the trachea. Usually, the right arch is larger than is the left, and it passes posterior to the esophagus to join the descending aorta to the left of the midline. Uncommonly, the left arch is atretic. A complete vascular ring is formed by the arches on each side of the trachea and esophagus, with the ascending aorta anterior and the retroesophageal arch or descending aorta posterior. Usually, the ductus arteriosus is left-sided and is not an essential component of the vascular ring, but the length of the ductus arteriosus or ligamentum may affect significantly the severity of symptoms. Usually, associated congenital heart disease is not present, but it may occur in as many as 22% of patients. Cyanotic congenital heart disease, including tetralogy of Fallot and transposition of the great arteries, predominates.

Usually, patients with a double aortic arch are severely symptomatic in infancy, with stridor, dyspnea, cough, and recurrent respiratory infections. Infants feed poorly because of severe respiratory distress and may prefer to assume an opisthotonic posture. Life-threatening episodes of apnea with cyanosis may occur. The diagnosis of a double aortic arch, like almost all vascular rings, often is suggested by the presence of a right aortic arch on routine chest radiography. In patients with a double aortic arch, both arches sometimes are seen, and evidence of hyperinflation of either or both lungs caused by obstruction of the lower trachea and mainstem bronchi may be present.

Barium esophagography often demonstrates bilateral indentations of the esophagus in the anteroposterior projection (Fig. 280.2) but may show only a prominent right-sided indentation. When two indentations are seen, usually the right arch produces the larger and more superior indentation. In the lateral or left anterior oblique projection, a large posterior indentation is seen and represents the retroesophageal component of the arch. Also present is an anterior and more inferior indentation of the arch produced by posterior deviation of the trachea. Although surgery may be performed without additional imaging studies, confirmation of the diagnosis can be obtained by MRI, echocardiography, or angiography. MRI provides sufficient anatomic detail to perform surgery and may even demonstrate tracheal compression (Fig. 280.3).

Usually, stridor and respiratory distress are severe, and affected infants will die without early surgical intervention. The mortality rate from surgery is low, and usually eventual

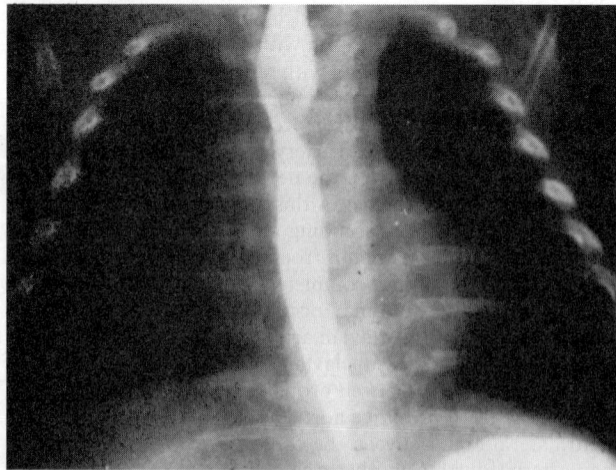

FIGURE 280.1. Anteroposterior projection of a barium esophagogram obtained from a patient with tetralogy of Fallot, left aortic arch, and anomalous right subclavian artery. The retroesophageal course of the anomalous right subclavian artery produces an oblique indentation of the esophagus. (Courtesy of Dr. Michael Nihill, Baylor College of Medicine, Houston, TX.)

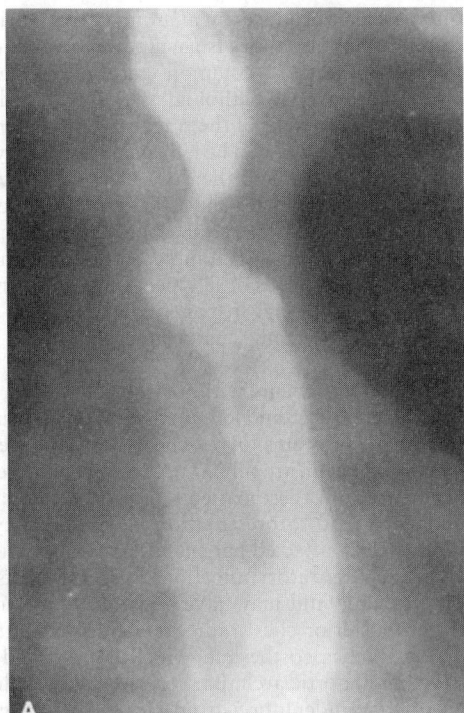
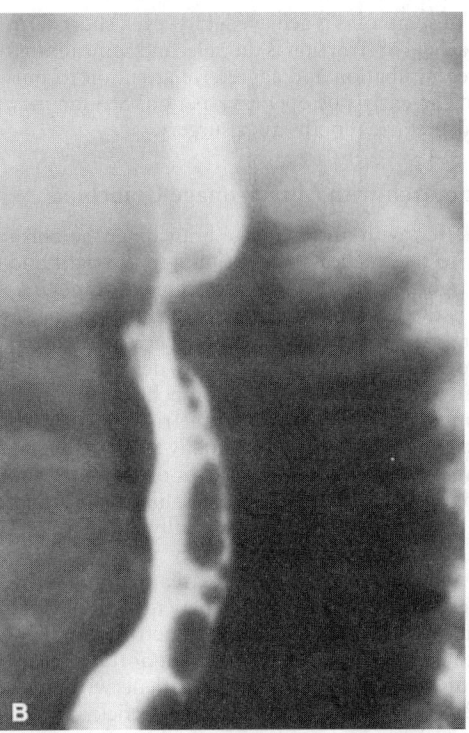

FIGURE 280.2. A double aortic arch. **A:** Bilateral indentation of the esophagus is characteristic in the anteroposterior projection. **B:** In addition, a deep posterior indentation on the lateral projection is produced by the retroesophageal portion of the arch. The larger and more superior indentation in the anteroposterior projection—in this case, on the right of the esophagus—usually is produced by the dominant arch. (Courtesy of Dr. Michael Nihill, Baylor College of Medicine, Houston, TX.)

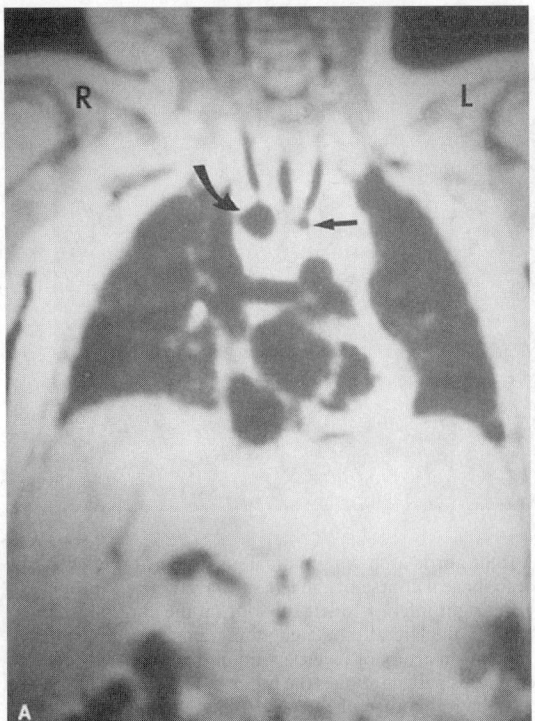
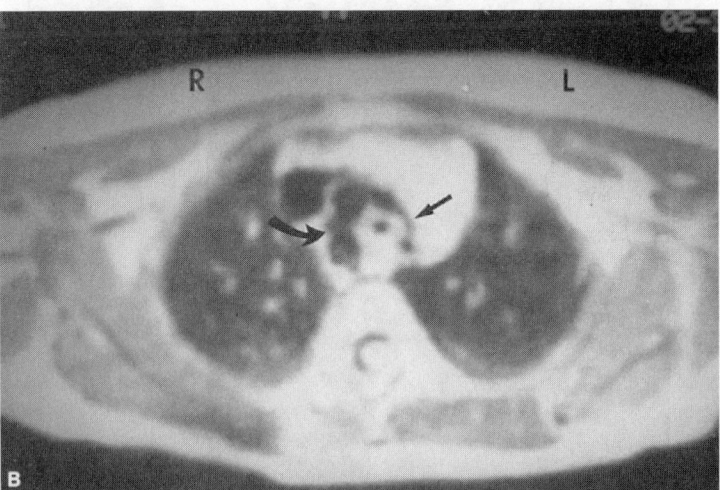

FIGURE 280.3. T1-weighted gated magnetic resonance imaging in a patient with a double aortic arch. **A:** Coronal images demonstrate both the major arch on the right (*curved arrow*) and the minor arch on the left (*straight arrow*). **B:** In the axial plane, the vascular ring is demonstrated partially, and the major arch on the right (*curved arrow*) and the minor arch on the left (*straight arrow*) are seen clearly. The position of the trachea in the center of this ring is seen as the small, dark, circular area of signal loss. (Courtesy of Dr. Gary Hedlund, The Children's Hospital, Birmingham, AL.)

long-term relief of symptoms is achieved. However, short-term postoperative tracheal obstruction is the rule, and some infants require prolonged intubation and aggressive attention to pulmonary toilet in the early postoperative period. Stridor may persist to some degree for months after surgery.

Right Aortic Arch with Mirror-Image Branching

In a right aortic arch with mirror-image branching, the aorta ascends anterior to the trachea and continues to the right and posteriorly. In a right aortic arch with mirror-image branching, the first branch is the left innominate artery, which pursues a course to the left and anterior to the trachea. The continuation of the arch to the right of the trachea produces deviation of the trachea to the left. The second and third branches of the arch are the right common carotid artery and the right subclavian artery. The descending aorta continues initially to the right and anterior to the vertebral bodies, then courses obliquely to the left, exiting from the thorax through the aortic hiatus. In a right aortic arch with mirror-image branching, usually the ductus arteriosus arises from the left innominate artery at the origin or near the bifurcation. Congenital heart disease, predominantly cyanotic, is present in as many as 98% of patients with a right aortic arch and mirror-image branching. With tetralogy of Fallot, from 13% to 34% of patients have a right aortic arch. A right aortic arch also is relatively common in patients with truncus arteriosus (36%) and double-outlet right ventricle (20%), but it is uncommon in patients with transposition of the great arteries (3%). A right aortic arch with mirror-image branching does not produce a vascular ring and usually is asymptomatic.

Right Aortic Arch with Anomalous Left Subclavian Artery

A right aortic arch with anomalous left subclavian artery and left ductus arteriosus is the most common type of aortic arch anomaly that produces an anatomic vascular ring. Usually, this group of abnormalities is asymptomatic and, therefore, ranks as the second most common cause of symptomatic vascular ring. The essential pathologic features include the course of the arch to the right of the trachea, with the first branch being the left carotid artery. The left subclavian artery arises from the descending aorta, and the ductus arteriosus, which originates from a retroesophageal diverticulum of the descending aorta, courses to the left and connects to the pulmonary artery. Unlike the condition in a double aortic arch, the presence of a left ductus arteriosus or ligamentum is an essential component of the vascular ring. In patients with a right aortic arch and anomalous branching, associated congenital heart disease is uncommon.

Although patients with a right aortic arch, anomalous left subclavian artery, and left ductus arteriosus usually are asymptomatic. Symptoms of tracheal or esophageal obstruction, when they occur, are similar to those encountered with a double aortic arch. In these patients, however, symptoms are milder and often lead to presentation later in infancy or childhood. Nonetheless, affected patients present with stridor, cough, and recurrent respiratory infections. Older patients may complain of dysphagia and may have a history of stridor or wheezing. Anteroposterior chest radiographs demonstrate the deviation of the trachea to the left, which is produced by the density of the right aortic arch. Barium esophagography demonstrates an oblique indentation from right to left (Fig. 280.4) in the anteroposterior projection and a large posterior indentation of the esophagus in lateral views. In symptomatic patients, MRI confirms the presence of a retroesophageal diverticulum and left subclavian artery and may demonstrate tracheal compression (Fig. 280.5). Anatomic features can be demonstrated also using echocardiography and angiography. Surgery is indicated for patients with symptomatic tracheal or esophageal compression. As for a double aortic arch, the surgical mortality rate is low, and long-term relief of symptoms is the rule.

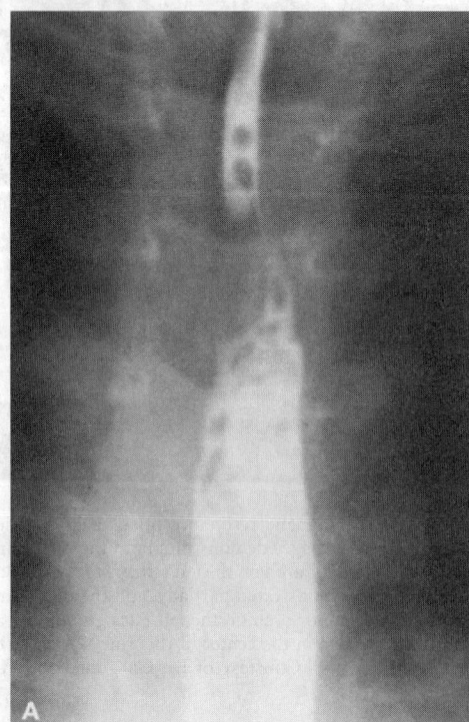
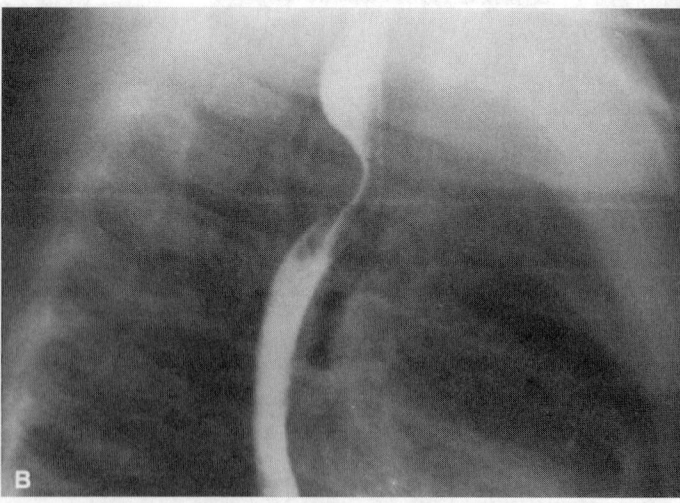

FIGURE 280.4. A: In a right aortic arch with anomalous origin of the left subclavian artery, the retroesophageal course of the left subclavian artery produces an oblique impression from right inferior to left superior on the anteroposterior barium esophagogram. **B:** On the lateral esophagogram, a posterior impression is produced by the left subclavian artery or diverticulum of the descending aorta. The large posterior defect in this patient implies the presence of a retroesophageal diverticulum or a retroesophageal course of the descending aorta. (Courtesy of Dr. Albert Schlesinger, Wilford Hall Air Force Medical Center, San Antonio, TX.)

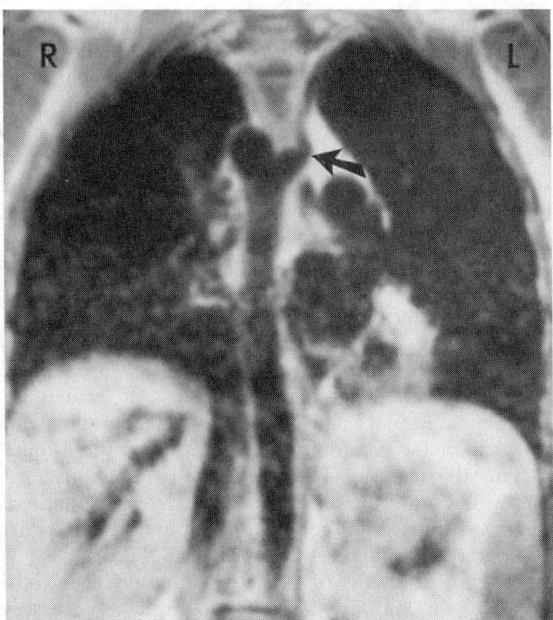

FIGURE 280.5. Gated magnetic resonance imaging study in a patient with a right aortic arch and an anomalous left subclavian artery. A T1-weighted coronal image is shown, demonstrating the descending aorta with origin of a large Kommerell diverticulum and left subclavian artery (*arrow*). The point of constriction between the Kommerell diverticulum and left subclavian artery indicates the point of origin of the ligamentum arteriosus. (Courtesy of Dr. Gary Hedlund, The Children's Hospital, Birmingham, AL.)

Symptoms may persist for weeks or months after surgical correction.

Cervical Aortic Arch

A cervical aortic arch is a rare anomaly characterized by a cervical position of the aorta, separate origin of the carotid artery contralateral to the arch, and an anomalous origin of the subclavian artery on the side contralateral to the arch. In addition, a separate origin of the internal carotid, external carotid, and subclavian arteries on the side of the arch usually is present. A ductus arteriosus or ligamentum originating from the descending aorta on the side contralateral to the arch, producing a vascular ring, also may be present. Associated congenital heart disease is uncommon.

Most patients with cervical aortic arch are asymptomatic. When present, symptoms range from mild dysphagia to significant respiratory distress. The latter occurs when a coexisting vascular ring is present. A pulsatile mass always is noted in the neck. Compression of the mass produces a palpable reduction in leg pulses and in the arm pulse on the side opposite the arch. This physical finding is pathognomonic for a cervical aortic arch. In addition, a thrill and a murmur are present over the mass.

Routine chest radiography demonstrates loss of the normal aortic knob on the left, widening of the upper mediastinum, and an aortic density in the apex of the hemithorax on the side of the arch. A large posterior indentation of the esophagus in the lateral projection on esophagography is present. Variations in arterial branching patterns render angiography a prerequisite to surgical repair. In a typical case, aortography reveals an elongated ascending aorta and the apex of the aortic arch above the clavicle. Surgery is reserved for patients with symptoms of tracheal or esophageal compression and for patients with aneurysm formation or coarctation.

Anomalous Innominate Artery

Stridor and respiratory distress associated with anterior compression of the trachea have been described in infants, with both symptoms and compression of the trachea being attributed to an anomalous origin and course of the innominate artery. However, the role of innominate artery compression in producing symptoms is disputed. The high incidence of coexisting tracheomalacia in affected infants, and the frequent finding of anterior tracheal indentation in asymptomatic children undergoing bronchoscopy, cast doubt on the primary role of vascular compression in producing symptoms. In addition, Swischuk (1971) emphasized the role of anterior mediastinal crowding, commonly seen on lateral chest radiographs in infancy, in producing apparent anterior tracheal compression. This finding is seen in both asymptomatic and symptomatic infants and, apparently, it resolves with age.

Symptoms ascribed to innominate artery compression are basically the same as those caused by tracheomalacia. Affected infants have cough, stridor, and dyspnea and may have episodes of apnea and cyanosis. Infants who experience apnea and cyanosis have a relatively poor prognosis. In addition to the findings on chest radiograph and bronchoscopy, echocardiography shows a normal left aortic arch, with the first branch being the innominate artery to the right. Barium esophagography is normal, excluding vascular rings and vascular slings. Usually, careful bronchoscopic examination demonstrates either local or diffuse tracheomalacia, in addition to varying degrees of anterior indentation produced by the innominate artery.

Most affected infants improve without surgical intervention. The indication for surgery in both tracheomalacia and an anomalous innominate artery is the severity of symptoms. The innominate artery, the aorta, or the anterior mediastinal fascia is sutured to the posterior sternal periosteum to relieve compression. Likely, the primary diagnosis in most patients is tracheomalacia, and the effect of surgery is to reduce the extrinsic compression of the trachea produced by "anterior mediastinal crowding."

Pulmonary Artery Anomalies

Anomalous Left Pulmonary Artery–Pulmonary Artery Sling

An anomalous origin of the left pulmonary artery is a rare congenital anomaly that produces severe tracheobronchial obstruction in most affected patients. A normal left pulmonary artery is absent, and the left lung is supplied by an anomalous left pulmonary artery arising from the distal right pulmonary artery. Tracheal and bronchial compression are produced as this artery courses posterior and caudal to the right mainstem bronchus and then to the left, posterior to the trachea and anterior to the esophagus. The course of the vessel to the right of the trachea produces a deviation of the lower trachea to the left. The resulting compression of the right mainstem bronchus and lower trachea leads to airway obstruction, primarily affecting the right lung. However, obstruction of the lower trachea and left mainstem bronchus may occur, resulting in bilateral obstruction.

Associated congenital anomalies are common occurrences and are present in 58% to 83% of patients. Anomalies of the trachea, bronchi, and lung parenchyma are common findings

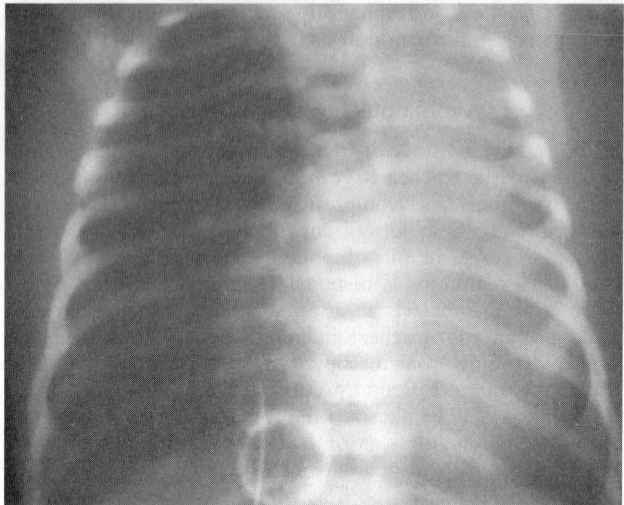

FIGURE 280.6. Posteroanterior radiograph demonstrating loss of volume (atelectasis) with opacity of the left lung field in a patient with a pulmonary artery sling. Often, the course of the left pulmonary artery posterior to the trachea and left bronchus produces compression, with resulting atelectasis of the left lung or hyperinflation of the right. (Courtesy of Dr. Gary Hedlund, The Children's Hospital, Birmingham, AL.)

and include complete cartilaginous rings, tracheomalacia, abnormal pulmonary lobulation, and bronchus sinus. Congenital heart defects are present in approximately 40% to 50% of patients and include persistent left superior vena cava, atrial septal defect, patent ductus arteriosus, and ventricular septal defects, among others.

Symptoms caused by an anomalous left pulmonary artery occur early in most patients. Two-thirds of affected infants are symptomatic by the age of 1 month. Symptoms include severe respiratory distress with stridor, wheezing, cyanosis, and recurrent pneumonitis. Obstructive apnea may occur and can be fatal. Unlike aortic vascular rings, dysphagia is rare because the anomalous left pulmonary artery passes anterior to the esophagus without significant esophageal compression. Although the majority of patients are severely symptomatic, asymptomatic and mildly affected patients have been observed.

On anteroposterior chest radiographs, hyperinflation of the right or left lung caused by tracheal and bronchial compression is observed often. Obstruction of the left bronchus also may produce varying degrees of volume loss (atelectasis) of the left lung (Fig. 280.6). Usually, barium esophagography demonstrates a characteristic anterior indentation of the esophagus on the lateral projection. The diagnosis of anomalous left pulmonary artery and of associated cardiac defects is made readily using two-dimensional echocardiography. Pulmonary artery sling also may be recognized by MRI (Fig. 280.7).

Although the presence of a vascular sling can be established noninvasively, pulmonary artery angiography is necessary to delineate the anatomic detail necessary for surgical correction. Catheterization is indicated also to assess the severity of associated cardiac defects. Survival of symptomatic infants is unlikely without early surgical intervention; surgery should be performed early in infants suffering from severe respiratory obstruction. Although many reports have described the successful treatment of this anomaly by surgery, the mortality rate after surgical procedures is high, at 40% to 50%. Coexisting tracheal or bronchial stenosis is disproportionately prevalent and severe in nonsurvivors and undoubtedly is a major contributing factor in postoperative death.

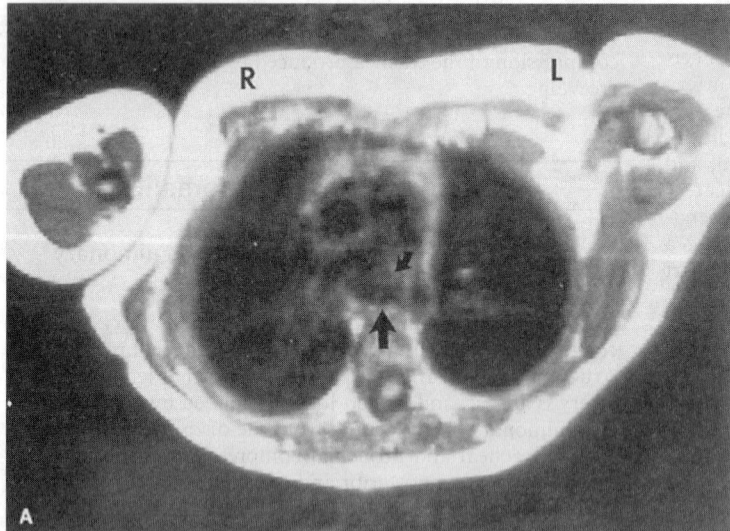
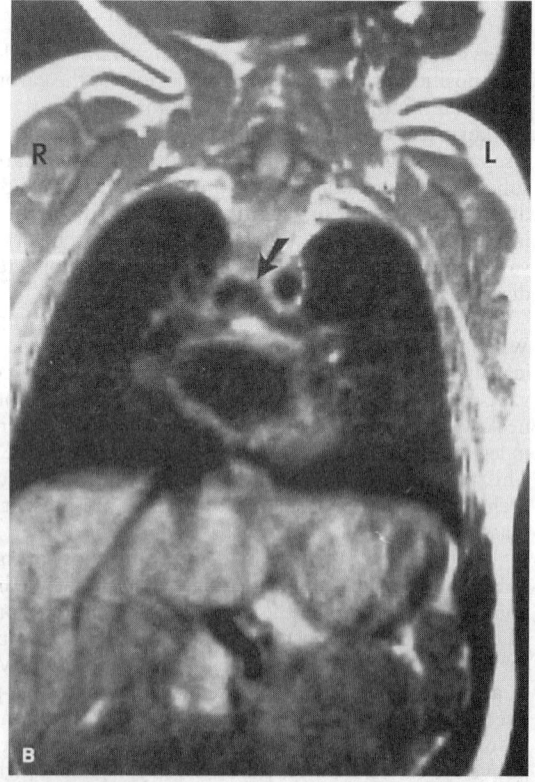

FIGURE 280.7. Coronal and axial T1-weighted magnetic resonance imaging study demonstrating a pulmonary artery sling. **A:** The axial image demonstrates origin of the left pulmonary artery from the posterior aspect of the right pulmonary artery. The left pulmonary artery (*straight arrow*) courses posterior to the trachea, which is demonstrated by signal loss (*curved arrow*). **B:** In the coronal imaging plane, the left pulmonary artery (*arrow*) originates from the right pulmonary artery to the right of the trachea.

Unilateral Absence of One Pulmonary Artery

The unilateral absence of one pulmonary artery is an uncommon congenital defect. Forty percent of cases occur without associated cardiac defects, whereas the remaining patients usually have tetralogy of Fallot, patent ductus arteriosus, or ventricular septal defect. Usually, the absent pulmonary artery is opposite the side of the aortic arch. Often, patients with an isolated unilateral absence of one pulmonary artery are asymptomatic, but they may experience recurrent pneumonitis, bronchiectasis, or hemoptysis. When associated congenital heart disease is present, generally symptoms are those of the associated defect. Patients with left-to-right shunts, however, may experience more severe symptoms of pulmonary congestion because both the normal cardiac output and the left-to-right shunt must perfuse the normally connected lung. Likewise, no specific physical findings indicate the unilateral absence of a pulmonary artery, although most patients have a nonspecific systolic murmur at the left sternal border. Patients with coexisting cardiac defects have compatible physical findings.

The differential perfusion of the lungs, with reduced vascular markings in infants, may not be apparent on chest radiographs. In older children and adults, chest radiographs demonstrate increased vascular markings on the side with normal pulmonary artery connection and decreased markings on the affected side. The unilateral absence of one pulmonary artery is readily apparent by two-dimensional echocardiography. In addition, associated cardiac defects and the side of the descending aortic arch are identified by two-dimensional echocardiography. Right ventricular or pulmonary artery angiography demonstrates the absent pulmonary artery and the normally connected pulmonary artery. Aortography is useful also in identifying the source of systemic arterial supply to the affected lung. In addition, cardiac catheterization enables an assessment of pulmonary artery pressure and resistance in the normally connected lung to be established. Approximately 20% of patients without associated left-to-right shunts demonstrate evidence of pulmonary hypertension, whereas 90% of those with left-to-right shunts have pulmonary hypertension.

Although patients without associated heart defects may escape early recognition, usually those with coexisting left-to-right shunts are recognized in infancy and should undergo early surgical repair to prevent the development of irreversible pulmonary hypertension. Older patients with pneumonitis should be treated medically. If severe recurrent lung infection or hemoptysis occurs, however, pneumonectomy of the affected lung should be considered.

Unilateral Origin of One Pulmonary Artery from the Ascending Aorta

The unilateral origin of one pulmonary artery from the ascending aorta is a rare finding, occurring in 0.05% of patients with congenital heart disease. In most patients, the right pulmonary artery arises from the ascending aorta and usually is the same size as or larger than the left pulmonary artery. The vessel connects to the aorta just above the aortic valve and on the right of or posterior to it, and it courses directly to the right hilum. Most patients with an origin of one pulmonary artery from the ascending aorta have an associated patent ductus arteriosus to the unaffected pulmonary artery. Cardiac defects associated with origin of the right pulmonary artery from the ascending aorta include ventricular septal defect, coarctation of the aorta, interrupted aortic arch, atrial septal defects, and contralateral pulmonary vein stenosis. Tetralogy of Fallot often is present when the left pulmonary artery arises from the ascending aorta, and usually it is accompanied by a left aortic arch.

Characteristically, patients in whom one pulmonary artery originates from the ascending aorta but who do not exhibit tetralogy of Fallot present in early infancy with severe congestive heart failure and cyanosis. Cyanosis results from a right-to-left shunt at the ductal level due to pulmonary hypertension. Often, the heart is enlarged massively on chest radiographs, and the pulmonary vascular markings either are increased symmetrically or are greater on the affected side. The diagnosis may be made using two-dimensional echocardiography. In addition to demonstrating the origin of the affected pulmonary artery to be from the aorta, echocardiographic examination demonstrates two arterial valves, thus excluding truncus arteriosus.

Without surgical intervention, most patients either die or develop significant pulmonary vascular obstructive disease by the age of 6 months. Therefore, early surgical repair is indicated once a pulmonary artery originating from the ascending aorta is diagnosed.

Suggested Readings

Barry A. The aortic derivatives in the human adult. *Anat Rec* 1951;111:221.

Congdon ED. Transformation of the aortic arch system during the development of the human embryo. *Contrib Embryol* 1922;1:47.

Huhta JC. *Pediatric imaging. Doppler ultrasound of the chest: extracardiac diagnosis.* Philadelphia: Lea & Febiger, 1986.

Kirklin JW, Barratt-Boyes BG. *Cardiac surgery.* New York: Wiley, 1986.

Knight L, Edwards JE. Right aortic arch. Types and associated cardiac anomalies. *Circulation* 1974;50:1047.

Moes CAF. Vascular rings and anomalies of the aortic arch. In: Keith JD, Rowe RD, Vlad P, eds. *Heart disease in infancy and childhood,* 3rd ed. New York: Macmillan, 1978.

Morrow WR, Huhta JC. Anomalies of the aortic arch and pulmonary arteries. In: Garson A Jr., Bricker JT, Fisher DJ, Neish SR, eds. *The science and practice of pediatric cardiology,* 2nd ed. Philadelphia: Lea & Febiger, 1998.

Shuford WH, Sybers RG. *The aortic arch and its malformations, with emphasis on the angiographic features.* Springfield, IL: Charles C Thomas, 1974.

Stewart JR, Kincaid OW, Edwards JE. *An atlas of vascular rings and related malformations of the aortic arch system.* Springfield, IL: Charles C Thomas, 1964.

Swischuk LE. Anterior tracheal indentation in infancy and early childhood: normal or abnormal? *Am J Roentgenol Radium Ther Nucl Med* 1971;112:12.

CHAPTER 281 ■ CONGENITAL CORONARY ARTERY ABNORMALITIES

DAVID J. DRISCOLL

NORMAL CORONARY ANATOMY

The left main coronary artery divides into the left anterior descending (LAD) coronary artery and the circumflex coronary artery (Fig. 281.1). Branches of the LAD coronary artery include the left conus, septal, and diagonal arteries. Branches of the circumflex coronary artery may include the sinus node artery, the Kugel artery, marginal arteries, and the left atrial circumflex artery.

Branches of the right coronary artery (RCA) include the right conal branch, the sinus node artery, an atrial branch, the right ventricular muscle branches (including the acute marginal branch), the posterior descending coronary artery, the atrioventricular node artery, and septal branches (Fig. 281.2).

MAJOR CORONARY ANOMALIES

Anomalous Origin of the Left Coronary Artery from the Pulmonary Artery

Anomalous origin of the left coronary artery (ALCA) from the pulmonary artery may be the most common important coronary anomaly with which pediatricians and pediatric cardiologists must deal. A patient with ALCA may present with signs and symptoms of myocardial infarction and congestive heart failure in infancy or be detected serendipitously in adulthood or at autopsy. Subjects with well-developed collateral connections between the RCA and left coronary artery (LCA) systems may not develop myocardial infarction and may do well, but subjects with poor collateral circulation may have myocardial infarction and present in infancy. In the immediate newborn period, pulmonary artery resistance and pressure are increased,

flow through the anomalously arising LCA is antegrade from the pulmonary artery, and myocardial perfusion is adequate. As pulmonary resistance and pressure decrease, antegrade flow of blood from the pulmonary artery through the LCA decreases, and myocardial infarction can occur. Clinical features of ALCA in infancy are similar to those of myocarditis and cardiomyopathy, and the diagnosis of ALCA must be considered in the differential diagnosis of unexplained congestive heart failure in infancy. In teenagers and adults, the presence of ALCA may be suspected in the presence of unexplained cardiomegaly, mitral insufficiency, or continuous cardiac murmur. Angina may occur. The ideal treatment of ALCA is to detect the presence of the anomaly before myocardial infarction occurs and to establish a coronary system that prevents myocardial infarction. However, most cases in infancy come to medical attention only after myocardial ischemia and infarction have occurred. Treatment consists of surgically establishing a two-coronary artery system originating from the aorta. Several techniques to accomplish this system have been described. Infants with evidence of acute myocardial infarction should be treated with oxygen, sedation, rest, digitalis, and diuretics while awaiting definitive operation.

Anomalous Origin of the Left Coronary Artery from the Right Sinus of Valsalva

ALCA from the right sinus of Valsalva or from the proximal RCA is a rare but important malformation because it is

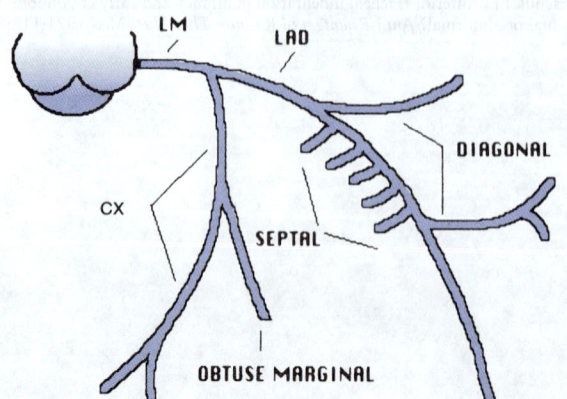

FIGURE 281.1. Normal left coronary artery system. CX, circumflex; LAD, left anterior descending; LM, left main.

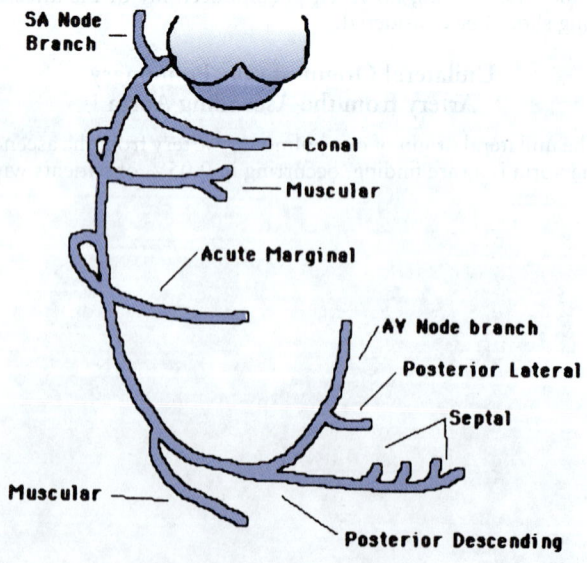

FIGURE 281.2. Normal right coronary artery system. AV, atrioventricular; SA, sinuatrial.

associated with sudden death. Patients in whom the aberrantly arising LCA passes between the aorta and the pulmonary artery appear to be at the greatest risk for sudden death. Usually, patients are asymptomatic until sudden death occurs, although some patients may have symptoms of angina or coronary insufficiency. Symptoms may include syncope or lightheadedness associated with exercise. This diagnosis must be considered in children and adolescents with angina-like chest pain or syncope/presyncope associated with exercise.

Usually, echocardiograph, CT scanning and/or coronary angiography must be performed to establish or exclude the diagnosis. Particularly when the LCA passes between the aorta and the pulmonary artery, operative repair is indicated to prevent sudden death.

Anomalous Origin of the Right Coronary Artery from the Left Sinus of Valsalva

Anomalous origin of the RCA from the left sinus of Valsalva is detected less often than is anomalous origin of the LCA from the right sinus of Valsalva. This anomaly can be associated with sudden death. Operative repair is indicated if signs and symptoms of myocardial ischemia are present without any other apparent causes. Some clinicians believe that operation should be performed even in the absence of symptoms.

Congenital Coronary Ostial Web

A rare but important cause of coronary insufficiency is the presence of a membrane covering the orifice of a coronary artery. Usually, it involves the left coronary ostia and is associated with a dysplastic aortic valve. This diagnosis must be considered in the differential diagnosis of angina pectoris.

Single Coronary Artery

Single coronary artery occurs in approximately 2 of every 1,000 patients. It is associated with transposition of the great arteries, coronary artery fistula, and bicuspid aortic valve.

The clinical significance of a single coronary artery is unclear. A patient in whom the single coronary artery arises from the right coronary sinus—with a connecting branch that travels between the aorta and the pulmonary artery, then distributes in the location of a normal LCA—may be at risk for sudden death caused by acute angulation of the connecting branch. This condition is similar to the situation in which the LCA originates from the right sinus of Valsalva.

CORONARY ARTERY FISTULA

Coronary artery fistula constitutes 0.2% to 0.4% of congenital cardiac defects. Fistulas originate equally from the RCA and LCA systems. Usually, the fistula connects to the right ventricular cavity. The right atrium is the second most common terminus, and two-thirds of fistulas draining into the right atrium originate from the RCA. A fistula can terminate also in the pulmonary artery, left atrium, left ventricle, superior vena cava, coronary sinus, or a persistent left superior vena cava. Usually, the involved coronary artery is dilated, and the chamber into which the fistula terminates may be enlarged. In a child or adolescent, usually the fistula does not produce symptoms, but signs and symptoms of congestive heart failure can occur secondary to a large left-to-right shunt. Usually, the presence of a fistula is detected by finding a continuous precordial murmur. A precordial thrill, decreased diastolic blood pressure,

and widened pulse pressure may occur. Physical findings may be confused with those of patent ductus arteriosus, but usually the murmur of a patent ductus arteriosus is heard best in the left infraclavicular area and that of a coronary artery fistula at the midleft sternal border. Except for very small fistulas, the presence of a coronary artery fistula is the indication for its surgical obliteration.

CORONARY ARTERY PATTERNS ASSOCIATED WITH CONGENITAL HEART DEFECTS

Tetralogy of Fallot

Although only 4% to 5% of patients with tetralogy of Fallot have associated coronary artery anomalies, these abnormalities must be recognized so that damage to essential coronary arteries is avoided during surgery. The origin of the LAD coronary artery from the RCA occurs in 4% of patients with tetralogy of Fallot. A single coronary artery is the second most common coronary anomaly associated with this condition. Forty percent of patients with tetralogy of Fallot have a long and large right conus artery that distributes to a significant mass of myocardium.

D-Transposition of the Great Arteries

Two major coronary artery patterns occur in D-transposition of the great arteries (also known as *complete* or *simple transposition of the great arteries*). Usually, the RCA arises from the posterior aortic sinus, and the LCA arises from the left coronary sinus and divides into a circumflex and an anterior descending coronary artery. The right aortic sinus of Valsalva is the noncoronary cusp. In the second coronary artery pattern, the RCA arises from the posterior aortic sinus and gives rise to the circumflex coronary artery, which passes posterior to the pulmonary artery. The anterior descending coronary artery arises from the left coronary sinus, and the right aortic sinus of Valsalva is the noncoronary sinus.

L-Transposition of the Great Arteries

The aorta is anterior to and left of the pulmonary artery in L-transposition of the great arteries (also known as *corrected transposition of the great arteries* or *ventricular inversion*). One aortic sinus of Valsalva is oriented anteriorly (anterior sinus of Valsalva), one posterior and rightward (right sinus of Valsalva), and one posterior and leftward (left sinus of Valsalva). The RCA originates from the right aortic sinus of Valsalva and divides into an anterior descending branch that follows the course of the interventricular sulcus. The RCA continues to follow a course in the right atrioventricular sulcus. The LCA originates in the left aortic sinus of Valsalva and follows the course of the circumflex coronary artery in the left atrioventricular sulcus. The LCA (circumflex) produces a marginal branch and continues as the posterior descending coronary artery.

Suggested Readings

Baltaxe H, Wixson D. The incidence of congenital anomalies of the coronary arteries in the adult population. *Radiology* 1977;122:47.

Cheitlin M, DeCastro C, McAllister H. Sudden death as a complication of anomalous left coronary origin from the anterior sinus of Valsalva, a not-so-minor congenital anomaly. *Circulation* 1974;50:780.

Driscoll D, Nihill M, Mullins C, et al. Management of symptomatic infants with anomalous origin of the left coronary artery from the pulmonary artery. *Am J Cardiol* 1981;47:642.

Elliott L, Amplatz K, Edwards J. Coronary arterial patterns in transposition complexes. *Am J Cardiol* 1966;17:362.

Hurwitz R, Caldwell R, Girod D, et al. Clinical and hemodynamic course of infants and children with anomalous left coronary artery. *Am Heart J* 1989; 118:1176.

Roberts W. Major anomalies of coronary arterial origin seen in adulthood. *Am J Cardiol* 1986;111:941.

Schwartz M, Jonas R, Colan S. Anomalous origin of the left coronary artery from pulmonary artery: recovery of left ventricular function after dual coronary repair. *J Am Coll Cardiol* 1997;30:547.

Taylor A, Rogan K, Virmani R. Sudden cardiac death associated with isolated congenital coronary artery anomalies. *J Am Coll Cardiol* 1992;20:640.

Vlodaver Z, Neufeld H, Edwards J. *Coronary arterial variations in the normal heart and in congenital heart disease.* New York: Academic Press, 1975.

CHAPTER 282 ■ MYOCARDITIS

RICHARD A. FRIEDMAN AND JEFFREY A. TOWBIN

The term *myocarditis* refers to an inflammation of the muscular walls of the heart. In 1984, a group of pathologists meeting in Dallas Texas, tried to define this broad term as "a process characterized by inflammatory infiltrate of the myocardium with necrosis and/or degeneration of adjacent myocytes not typical of the ischemic damage associated with coronary artery disease." This section deals with proven and presumed infectious causes of myocarditis and describes the clinical presentation and etiology when known. In general, this disease may go unrecognized in many patients whose illness resolves spontaneously, or it may lead to fulminant disease, with a rapid downhill course or to a chronic state, possibly resulting in dilated congestive cardiomyopathy.

EPIDEMIOLOGY

Studies show that myocarditis is a relatively uncommon occurrence in children (Box 282.1). Myocarditis generally is a sporadic disease, although epidemics have been reported. In a significant number of cases, manifestations may be subclinical and recognized either through other findings (e.g., electrocardiographic changes) or, perhaps, not at all.

Myocarditis also may be only one component of a generalized disease and, if the cardiac dysfunction is mild, may be completely overlooked, which could explain the discrepancy between the clinical and the autopsy series. Myocarditis may be secondary to many of the common infectious illnesses that affect children and infants. Various causes are listed in Box 281.2. Alternatively, myocarditis may occur as a manifestation of hypersensitivity or as a toxic reaction to drug administration.

Until the early 1990s, coxsackievirus B was the most frequently reported cause of epidemics in children. This organism was found to be associated with myocarditis during a nursery epidemic in southern Rhodesia. Reports from Holland, the United States, Singapore, and South Africa have followed. Infections secondary to coxsackieviruses occur commonly throughout the general population. Target organs include the upper respiratory tract, gastrointestinal tract, liver (hepatitis), lung (pneumonia), central nervous system (meningoencephalitis), lymph nodes (infectious mononucleosis-like syndrome), kidney (hemolytic uremic syndrome), and heart (carditis). Significant titers of type-specific protective antibodies are present in most adults in the United States. After birth, spread occurs by the fecal-oral or airborne route. The coxsackievirus B organ-

isms use receptors that are not shared with other enteroviruses to attach to their target cells. These receptors are thought to be an element essential for viral replication and may help determine tissue tropism. Infections caused by coxsackievirus B or enteroviruses are subclinical in 50% of cases. During an outbreak of coxsackievirus B in Europe, in 1965, cardiac manifestations were noted in 5% of patients. A much higher percentage (12%) of patients in similar outbreaks of the disease that same year in Scotland, Finland, and Austria developed some evidence of myocardial dysfunction. Whereas myocarditis is associated with coxsackievirus B serotypes 1 to 6, the most serious disease is attributed to types 3 and 4. Coxsackievirus B antigens have been demonstrated with the use of an immunofluorescent technique in 41% of 29 infants and children who were found at routine autopsy to have had interstitial myocarditis. Another study found 1,299 cases of unexpected death in an autopsy series of 2,427 patients; 20 cases of viral myocarditis were identified. Of the 20, nearly one-half had positive serologic evidence for coxsackievirus B infection. One investigator found a 9% incidence of myocarditis in 67 verified cases of influenza infection during a 1978 epidemic in Sweden. Although much less common, coxsackievirus A and echoviruses also are suspected etiologies.

Rubella virus, a teratogen present during the first trimester of pregnancy, also is implicated in myocarditis. Persistence of the virus in the fetus has been shown to produce severe cases of myocarditis. One study found 10 of 47 infants with congenital rubella to have evidence of myocarditis. Seven of these infants had active disease, and four died with severe myocardial failure. Morbidity secondary to chronic cardiac dysfunction was thought to be severe in the survivors. A significant reduction in the number of cases of congenital rubella has occurred because of aggressive immunization programs, and only 28 cases were recorded in 1975.

More recently, adenovirus has emerged as a major cause of this disease in children. The identification of this agent has been aided greatly by use of modern molecular biologic techniques, including *in situ* hybridization and polymerase chain reaction (PCR). PCR has been used to examine autopsy specimens of patients with myocarditis and a previously unidentified etiology. In those cases, adenovirus emerged as the major organism, placing it second in importance to the enteroviruses as the etiologic agent responsible for myocarditis.

Herpes simplex virus results in infections of newborns at a rate of 1 in 7,500 deliveries. Type 2 virus is found most commonly and usually is acquired from the genital tract.

BOX 282.1 Reports of Myocarditis in Children

Myocarditis was found in only 0.3% of 14,322 patients seen in the cardiology service at Texas Children's Hospital between 1954 and 1977, findings similar to those for a group at the Toronto Children's Hospital between 1951 and 1964. Not all cases of myocarditis are recognized by the clinician, however, and a much higher incidence is noted in autopsy series. During the same two decades at Texas Children's Hospital, an autopsy incidence of 1.15% was found. This figure is in contrast to the report by Saphir and colleagues, who noted an incidence of 6.83% among 1,420 autopsies on children. In that series, nearly one-third of the patients were thought to have had rheumatic carditis.

One study of 138 cases attempted to estimate the evidence of myocarditis in children who died suddenly and children who died unexpectedly (violently). The control group consisted of 48 children who died violent deaths with no history suggestive of myocarditis; the other 90 children died suddenly. The study found that 17 cases (12.3%) revealed evidence of active or healing myocarditis and that 15 of these cases occurred in children who died suddenly. In contrast, only 4.2% of children dying a violent death had histologic evidence suggestive of myocarditis. Because this study was retrospective, viral cultures and serologic studies were not obtained routinely at the time of autopsy. Another series found evidence of interstitial myocarditis in 29 of 50 infants and young children who had undergone routine postmortem examination.

Several investigations found that a significant number of patients undergoing endomyocardial biopsy for unexplained myocardial dysfunction had histologic findings suggestive of myocarditis. Likewise, patients being investigated for occult ventricular arrhythmias for which no etiology could be proved also were found to have evidence of interstitial lymphocytic infiltrates suggestive of myocarditis. A potential for the overdiagnosis of myocarditis exists, and one investigator notes that approximately 5% of "normal" hearts may be found to have minor foci of inflammatory cells. The investigator determined that a normal finding was 25 to 30 interstitial lymphocytes per square millimeter. In that study, the number of lymphocytes per square millimeter in endomyocardial biopsy specimens was lower than that found in autopsy specimens (3.5 versus 7.2 cells per square millimeter).

BOX 282.2 Etiologic Agents of Myocarditis

Viral
Coxsackievirus A
Coxsackievirus B
Echoviruses
Rubella virus
Measles virus
Adenoviruses
Polioviruses
Vaccinia virus
Variola virus
Mumps virus
Herpes simplex virus
Epstein-Barr virus
Cytomegalovirus
Rhinoviruses
Hepatitis viruses
Arboviruses
Influenza viruses
Varicella virus

Rickettsial
Rickettsia rickettsii
Rickettsia tsutsugamushi

Bacterial
Meningococcus
Klebsiella
Leptospira
Diphtheria
Salmonella
Clostridia
Tuberculosis
Brucella
Legionella pneumophila
Streptococcus

Protozoal
Trypanosoma cruzi
Toxoplasmosis
Amebiasis

Other Parasites
Toxocara canis

Schistosomiasis
Heterophyiasis
Cysticercosis
Echinococcus
Visceral larva migrans

Fungi and Yeasts
Actinomycosis
Coccidioidomycosis
Histoplasmosis
Candida

Toxic
Scorpion (diphtheria)

Drugs
Sulfonamides
Phenylbutazone
Cyclophosphamide
Neomercazole
Acetazolamide
Amphotericin B
Indomethacin
Tetracycline
Isoniazid
Methyldopa
Phenytoin
Penicillin

Hypersensitivity/ Autoimmune Reactions
Rheumatoid arthritis
Rheumatic fever
Ulcerative colitis
Systemic lupus erythematosus

Other
Sarcoidosis
Scleroderma
Idiopathic
Cornstarch inhalation

Herpesvirus has been found in the myocardium of autopsy specimens, documenting its association with myocarditis.

During a 1-year period, investigators found a 5.8% incidence of myocarditis in 312 cases of varicella. In that study, patients who complained of skeletal myalgia seemed to have a significantly higher risk of developing cardiac involvement.

With the appearance of recent bioterrorism threats, the U.S. Department of Defense initiated a Smallpox Vaccination Program in December of 2002. In little more than 2 years, they had immunized 615,000 personnel, representing the largest smallpox vaccination program in 25 years. Within a cohort of 540,824 people vaccinated, 67 developed a myopericarditis as evidenced by symptoms of chest pain and enzymatic (troponin) as well as echocardiographic and electrocardiographic evidence of disease. These cases all developed within 30 days of receiving vaccination and fortunately, all recovered. This information may be important should any further initiatives be needed in the future.

PATHOGENESIS

Immunology

Microscopic and immunologic changes seen in humans with viral myocarditis have been well described. To examine the immunopathogenesis of this disease, animal models have been necessary, the most thoroughly studied of which is the murine model. Studies using coxsackievirus B and encephalomyocarditis viruses have been used extensively. Box 282.3 provides more information on the immunopathogenesis of viral myocarditis.

BOX 282.3	Immunopathogenesis of Viral Myocarditis

After infection with coxsackievirus B, a viremia exists for between 24 and 72 hours, with maximum growth occurring in the tissues at between 72 and 96 hours. Shortly thereafter, virus titers decline, and essentially no organism can be found as early as 7 to 10 days after inoculation. As virus titers decline, antibody concentrations increase, implying an active role by antibodies in viral clearance. Macrophages appear at between 5 and 10 days after infection in the coxsackievirus B model of myocarditis.

Factors that affect the severity of myocarditis in the murine model include age, strain of mouse, viral variant, and gender. Several mechanisms are active in the production of myocarditis in this model. Viruses are associated directly with the destruction of the myofiber. The greatest damage, however, probably is caused by an interaction between the myofiber and T cells. Virally induced changes of the myocardial cell produce a neoantigen that is recognized by cytotoxic T lymphocytes that preferentially destroy the myocardial cell. In addition, coxsackievirus may induce cytotoxic T lymphocytes that are autoreactive against antigens on infected myocytes. Mice that are pretreated with antithymocyte serum, thus lacking a normal immunologic response, develop a less extensive myocardial necrosis compared with animals similarly infected and treated with normal rabbit serum. Animals deficient in T cells clear their viremia normally but develop significantly less myocardial injury. The implication is that T cells are not required in elimination of virus but do play a delayed role in the major inflammatory response. Mice that are pretreated with neutralizing antibody fail to develop myocarditis; thus, a combination of macrophages and antibodies appears to suppress viral infection.

Another type of cell known as the *natural killer* (NK) cell is important in the pathogenesis of this disease. Animals depleted of NK cells before acquiring infection with coxsackievirus develop a more severe myocarditis. Murine skin fibroblasts demonstrate the antiviral activity of activated NK cells. NK cells are activated by interferon, which is an indirect modulator of myocardial injury. When murine skin fibroblasts served as target cells for coxsackievirus B–sensitized cytotoxic T cells, the NK cells limited the nonenveloped virus infection specifically by killing the virally infected cells. This finding has important implications in host immunity and may help explain why female mice develop a less severe myocarditis than do their male counterparts. Male mice are less efficient in activating NK cells. Presumably, the more efficient viral clearance is, the less opportunity exists for virally induced neoantigen production and recognition by cytotoxic T lymphocytes to occur.

The different ways in which T cells effect injury include the accumulation of activated macrophages, production of antibody and antibody-dependent cell-mediated cytotoxicity, direct lysis by antibody and complement, and direct action of cytotoxic T cells. The primary importance of cytotoxic T cells in direct myocardial-cell injury was demonstrated in BALB/c mice infected with coxsackievirus B3. Both virus-infected and noninfected myocytes are destroyed in T cell-deficient animals. Infected host cells stimulate the production of a subset of cytotoxic T cells responsible for injury. These cells then recognize virus-specific and major histocom-

patibility antigens (modified H-2 antigens) present on the cell surface and directly interact, resulting in myocytolysis.

This ongoing injury is considered an autoimmune-type process. To support this concept, investigators studied the CD1 mouse infected with coxsackievirus B3 and demonstrated a KC1 extractable antigen in the hearts of mice previously infected with this virus that was specifically immunoreactive with immune mouse peritoneal-exudate cells (i.e., stimulated production of a migration-inhibitory factor). Investigators were unable to demonstrate viral activity in animals that had this extractable antigen. In addition, antigen responsible for cytotoxic T-cell activity cannot be detected by using antiserum-containing antibodies directed at the structural components of the viral capsid. The ineffectiveness of antiviral serum in preventing myocarditis also has been demonstrated.

Susceptibility variation of the BALB/c mouse to coxsackievirus B3 also has been studied. The age of greatest susceptibility was found to be between 16 and 18 weeks, with male mice having a maximal rate of myocarditis greater than that seen in female mice. Enhanced myocardial inflammation was seen in older female mice and was eliminated when they were treated with estradiol, implying that sex hormones play a key role in host susceptibility. Studies both *in vitro* and *in vivo* have shown that testosterone seems to increase the cytolytic activity in male more than in female mice. Either a preferential stimulation of T-helper cells or an inadequate stimulation of T-cytolytic/suppressor cells could explain why antibody responses to various antigens frequently are enhanced and cellular immune responses are depressed in female mice. Host genetic composition not only affects the severity of disease but also plays a role in the pathogenic mechanisms involved. With use of coxsackievirus B3 to induce myocarditis in the BALB/c mouse and the DBA/2 mouse, important differences have been found. The BALB/c mouse develops myocarditis in response to cytolytic T cells. Two distinct cytolytic T-cell populations are formed: one that recognizes virus-infected cells and produces direct myocytolysis and one that destroys uninfected myocytes and probably is an autoreactive lymphocyte. Complement depletion increases the amount of inflammation in this species, and no reactive immunoglobulin G (IgG) antibody is found in the myocytes. In the DBA/2 mouse, however, T-helper cells mediate the course of disease indirectly, and complement depletion reduces inflammation. Cytolytic T cells are produced but apparently are not pathogenic, and IgG antibody is found in the myocytes.

Several other viral agents have been used to produce experimental myocarditis. The induction of myocarditis using influenza A virus (H2N2) in mice has been studied. In one study, mice that were pretreated with radiation or depleted of T lymphocytes did not develop disease. Encephalomyocarditis virus has been used to develop models of acute and chronic myocarditis in mice. This virus is a picornavirus that is similar to the coxsackievirus group. Studies demonstrate a progression from acute myocarditis to dilated cardiomyopathy similar to that seen in humans.

Several studies also have been performed in humans. Antibody-mediated cytolysis has been demonstrated in 30%

(Continued)

BOX 282.3   (Continued)

of 144 patients with suspected myocarditis, as well as in 18 of 19 patients with proven viral infections caused by coxsackievirus B, influenza A, or mumps. A muscle-specific antimyolemmal antibody was found in these patients and correlated with the degree of *in vitro*-induced cytolysis of rat cardiocytes. Another study used complementary DNA (to coxsackievirus B2 RNA) cloning techniques to develop a coxsackievirus B-specific cDNA "hybridization probe" that detected virus nucleic acid sequences in patients diagnosed as having active or healed myocarditis or dilated cardiomyopathy. Patients with unrelated disorders served as the control group, and no virus-specific sequences were found in those patients. This study suggests that, in patients with congestive cardiomyopathy or healing myocarditis, viral particles persist although viral culture results almost always are negative. Thus, a continual viral replication in cells may conceal the antigenicity by an immunologic process that prevents correct posttranslational processing of capsid proteins. Adult patients with myocarditis have been found to have been exposed to a greater number of coxsackievirus B1 to B6 organisms, as demonstrated by the number of positive and negative responses to neutralizing antibodies of those viruses. Some authors suggest that immunization against several types of coxsackievirus B is essential in the development of myocarditis. Although they have postulated this cross-immunization theory, a few cases of myocarditis in their patients involved exposure to only one type of coxsackievirus B, thus casting some doubt on the validity of this theory. A defect in cell-mediated immunity has been shown, with a finding of a reduction in suppressor cell (concanavalin A-induced) activity in some patients with myocarditis and congestive cardiomyopathy.

After viral clearance has occurred, autoantibodies to various cellular elements can be found. They include antimyosin,

adenine nucleotide, and translocator proteins. Inflammatory cytokines, including tumor necrosis factor and interleukin-1, have been demonstrated in a rat model of myocarditis. The administration of antitumor necrosis factor to rats prior to inoculating them with encephalomyocarditis virus improved survival and diminished the pathologic response usually seen. Specific molecules such as intercellular adhesion molecule-1 (ICAM-1) may be involved with progressive inflammation that develops after infection. The appearance of this molecule is up-regulated by cytokines such as interleukin-1 and tumor necrosis factor alpha. Treatment with anti-ICAM-1 monoclonal antibody has been shown to reduce the amount of inflammation seen in the animal model. Finally, recent data suggest that matrix metalloproteinases (MMPs) and tissue inhibitors of matrix metalloproteinases (TIMPs) that regulate the former require a critical balance that may be severely altered as a result of cytokines present in the tissue resulting from viral infection and inflammation. This condition may lead directly to dilation of the heart and ventricular dysfunction.

In summary, the pathogenesis of this disease can be viewed as follows: Infection of the mouse with coxsackievirus B3 induces a viremia and replication within the myocardial cells of this virus. Direct viral myocytolysis ensues, with production in other cells of neoantigen in response to viral infection. Cytotoxic T cells directed at both infected and noninfected (autoimmune) cells produce further injury. NK cells attack the virally infected cells only and are responsible for viral clearance. Antibody binding and complement-mediated cell destruction also occur in the delayed immunologic response. Host factors including age, gender, and immunocompetence play key roles in modulating these processes (Fig. 282.1).

Gross and Microscopic Findings

Pathologic findings usually are nonspecific, with similar gross and microscopic changes noted regardless of the causative agent. Grossly, the weight of the heart is increased. The muscle appears flabby and pale, with petechial hemorrhages often seen on the epicardial surfaces. A bloody pericardial effusion, related to the often combined finding of pericarditis, also may be seen. The ventricular wall frequently is thin, although hypertrophy may be found as well. The valves and endocardium usually are spared; however, they may appear glistening white in cases of chronic myocarditis, suggesting to some investigators that the disease process known as *endocardial fibroelastosis*, which may present with similar clinical findings, could represent an end result of viral myocarditis, possibly induced *in utero*. See Box 282.4 for further details concerning pathologic findings in myocarditis.

Pathophysiology

Myocardial function usually is reduced in the presence of extensive interstitial inflammation or injury, which results in cardiac enlargement and an increase in the end-diastolic volume. Normally, this increase in volume results in an increase in the force of contraction, ejection fraction, and cardiac out-

put, as described in the Starling mechanism. However, in the disease state, reduced cardiac output results from the inability of the heart muscle to respond to these stimuli. Congestive heart failure usually ensues, with progression of the disease or with intercurrent infections, resulting in fever or anemia that further stress the myocardial reserve. The progressive increase in end-diastolic volume and pressure results in increasing left atrial pressure that is transmitted into the pulmonary venous system. The resulting hydrostatic forces overcome the colloid osmotic pressure, which normally prevents transudation of fluid across the capillary membranes. Congestive heart failure with pulmonary edema and systemic venous engorgement is a common occurrence in more acute forms of myocarditis. Echocardiographic examination may demonstrate severe left ventricular dilatation, and a decreased ejection fraction usually is found. Evaluation of ventricular function using M-mode echocardiography helps establish a baseline at the time of presentation and provides a way to as monitor function during therapeutic interventions.

During the healing stages of myocarditis, normal myofibers are replaced with fibroblasts, with resultant formation of scar tissue. Reduced elasticity and ventricular performance can result in continuing congestive heart failure. Ischemia may be exacerbated by attempts to preserve cardiac output, with sinus tachycardia further worsening the supply-demand ratio for oxygen in the heart muscle.

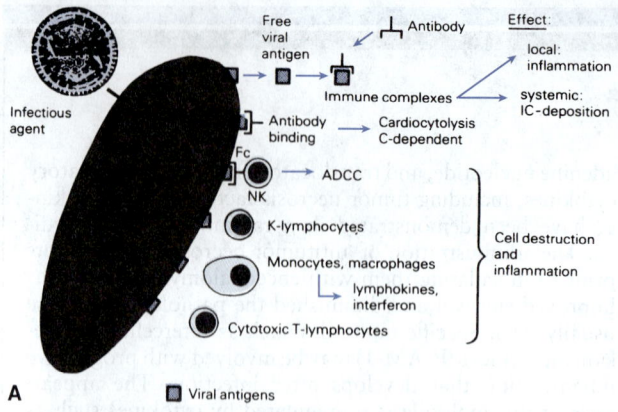

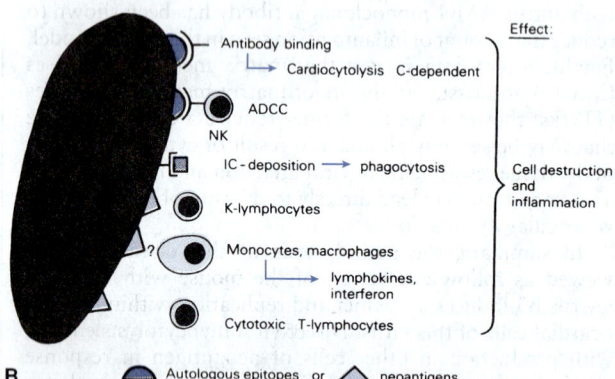

FIGURE 282.1. **A:** Early immunopathogenesis. The cell cycle is altered by viral infection. Viral proteins then are expressed on the surface of the cell and become targets of various immunologic effectors. They include the monocytes and macrophages, which release mediators; cytotoxic T lymphocytes and K cells, which lyse the myocardial cell; and natural killer (*NK*) cells, which together with antibodies also effect cell lysis. Complement-activated, antibody-mediated cell destruction also occurs with the production of antiviral antibodies. Formation of immune complexes (*IC*) may occur when circulating viral antigen is coupled with viral antibodies, resulting in local or systemic reactions. **B:** Delayed immunopathogenesis. In addition to the mechanisms described in early immunopathogenesis, modulation of the inflammatory response by T cells (helper and suppressor types) against autologous heart cells occurs. Complement-activated, antibody-mediated cell destruction is more important than is antibody-dependent cellular cytotoxicity (*ADCC*) in this phase of the injury process. The presence of viral antigens during this phase is negligible compared with that in the early phase of injury. (Reprinted with permission from Maisch B, et al. Immunological cellular regulator and effector mechanisms in myocarditis. *Herz* 1985;10:11.)

CLINICAL MANIFESTATIONS AND COMPLICATIONS

The clinical presentation of myocarditis varies in response to host factors, including age and immunocompetence. Although most cases probably are not noticed, with no apparent clinical illness, a rapidly fatal illness may occur. Newborn infants are susceptible to infection with coxsackievirus B, which may result in the severe form of myocarditis. Infections with rubella, herpes simplex, and toxoplasmosis also may result in a severe form of illness in infants.

Myocarditis may be merely one component of a more severe generalized illness, with coexisting hepatitis or encephalitis. Myocardial involvement may be only a mild clinical disturbance in these cases. One study found a nursery epidemic of coxsackievirus B5 infection in preterm infants during a virologic survey in one institution. The disease was unnoticed clinically and discovered by chance during this survey. No instance of severe myocarditis was seen, and all infants recovered fully from infection. The major symptoms were lethargy, failure to gain weight, and aseptic meningitis. In a review of 25 infants with myocarditis caused by coxsackievirus B, other symptoms of lethargy and anorexia heralded the onset of severe disease. Fever was recorded in more than 50% of the cases, although hypothermia also was noted. Cyanosis, respiratory distress or tachycardia, cardiomegaly, or electrocardiographic changes were present in 19 of 23 infants; vomiting was noted in four. Initial symptoms in infants include irritability and periodic episodes of pallor, which may precede sudden onset of cardiorespiratory symptoms.

Clinical manifestations of myocarditis generally are less severe in older infants and children than in newborns. Rapidly fatal illness has been reported in association with myocarditis of unknown etiology, enteroviruses, adenoviruses, mumps, varicella, cytomegalovirus, and diphtheria. The usual clinical picture is either an acute or a subacute illness, often beginning with a mild respiratory infection and low-grade fever.

The child usually is anxious and apprehensive, although some children appear apathetic and listless. Pallor and mild cyanosis may be present, with the skin cool to the touch and mottled in appearance. Respirations usually are rapid and sometimes labored; grunting may be prominent. The pulse is thready, although blood pressure may be normal or slightly reduced unless the patient is in shock. Palpation of the chest demonstrates a quiet precordium. Tachycardia usually is present. Heart sounds may be muffled, especially in the presence of pericarditis, and a gallop rhythm frequently is heard. With severe ventricular dysfunction, mitral regurgitation with a pansystolic murmur at the apex may be heard. Auscultation of the lungs reveals scattered rhonchi and fine crepitations in the lung bases. Peripheral edema is a rare finding, but hepatomegaly is found almost uniformly. Some infants may have only mild congestive heart failure, without evidence of peripheral circulatory compromise, whereas others have such a mild illness that the only abnormal finding may be a conduction disturbance visible on surface electrocardiography.

DIAGNOSIS

The diagnosis of myocarditis often is difficult to establish but should be suspected in any infant or child who presents with unexplained congestive heart failure. Fever is a common occurrence in children, and the frequency of viral illness may be so high as to invalidate the causal relationship in the history of recent illness in the child who presents with congestive heart failure. If this relationship is found, however, it should be documented for epidemiologic purposes.

A sinus tachycardia out of proportion to the level of fever and in association with a quiet precordium and a gallop rhythm should strongly suggest the diagnosis. A third heart sound, which is a common finding in healthy children, usually is associated with a relatively hyperdynamic precordium with heart sounds that are increased or crisp. When a prominent third heart sound exists without these findings, a significant disturbance in ventricular compliance usually is present and deserves further investigation by chest radiography, electrocardiography, and echocardiography. Children with myocarditis and congestive heart failure usually show cardiomegaly and pulmonary edema on chest radiography.

In newborn infants whose first sign of illness is acute circulatory collapse, the cardiac size may be normal, as may be the case in children who present with an arrhythmia secondary to myocarditis. Stokes-Adams attacks secondary to complete

---

| BOX 282.4 | Pathologic Findings in Myocarditis |

Coxsackievirus B3 has been found in the myocardium of 13 of 28 infants with endocardial fibroelastosis, and echovirus 9 has been found in a 5-month-old infant with myocarditis and severe congestive heart failure who also had histologic findings consistent with endocardial fibroelastosis. Virus was isolated not only in the heart and lungs but also in the liver and lymph nodes. Of interest is that the clinical appearance of endocardial fibroelastosis in newborns without any co-existing congenital heart disease is a distinctly uncommon occurrence today. This "disappearance" may be linked to the near elimination of mumps virus as a result of successful immunization programs. This linkage was made from a PCR analysis performed on autopsy specimens of newborns who died from secondary severe congestive heart failure and who had a pathologic descriptive diagnosis of endocardial fibroelastosis.

Mural thrombi have been described in the left ventricles of some patients with myocarditis. Small emboli have been seen in the coronary and cerebral vessels. Coronary emboli, although rare findings, may produce areas of ischemia or injury, with the resultant production of the cardiac arrhythmias that sometimes occur during the acute disease.

The typical microscopic picture of acute myocarditis is that of a focal or diffuse interstitial collection of mononuclear cells, including lymphocytes, plasma cells, and eosinophils. Polymorphonuclear types are noted rarely, except in cases of bacterial myocarditis.

Extensive necrosis of the myocardium, with loss of cross-striation in the muscle fibers and edema, is seen in severe infections. A perivascular accumulation of lymphocytes and plasma cells is described with coxsackievirus B myocarditis, but it usually is a minor finding. In disease caused by *Rickettsia*, varicella, trypanosomes, or other parasites, and in reactions to sulfonamides, a much more prominent finding exists.

Myocarditis secondary to diphtheria infection frequently is complicated with arrhythmias, especially complete atrioventricular block. Diphtheria exotoxin has a particular affinity for the specialized conduction tissue in the heart. The toxin interferes with protein synthesis by inhibition of a translocating enzyme in the delivery of amino acids. Triglyceride accumulation occurs as a result of induction of abnormal carnitine metabolism, and fatty changes in the myofibers occur. Myocarditis caused by bacterial agents usu-

ally presents with a different picture than that seen in disease caused by viral agents. Microabscesses and patchy focal suppurative changes may be seen. *Trichinella* usually causes a focal infiltrate with lymphocytes and eosinophils. Larvae usually are not identified.

A severe myocarditis may develop in response to *Trypanosoma cruzi*, with the development of Chagas disease. This disease, which can affect as much as 50% of the population in an endemic region, most commonly is found in South America and seldom in North America. Protracted heart failure and death may ensue after an acute infection. Microscopic examination may demonstrate the presence of the organism as well as neutrophils, lymphocytes, macrophages, and eosinophils.

Sudden infant death syndrome occurs in as many as 1 in 500 children and could be caused by cardiac arrhythmias that may result from myocardial inflammation. One study of cases of infants who died in northern Ireland described a resorptive, degenerative process in the His bundle and at the left margin of the atrioventricular node, with the absence of inflammatory cells. The investigator postulated that lethal arrhythmias or conduction disturbances could be caused by developmental histologic changes in these critical regions of the heart. Lymphocytic infiltrates were demonstrated in the region of the His bundle and left fascicle in a 3-month-old child who died suddenly. No degenerative changes were seen in this heart; thus, the significance of these findings is speculative. Giant cell myocarditis is diagnosed when giant cells are found, with or without granulomas. Patients with tuberculosis, syphilis, rheumatoid arthritis, rheumatic heart disease, sarcoidosis, and certain fungal or parasitic infections all may have granulomas found within the myocardium. Giant cells also have been described in idiopathic or Fiedler myocarditis. In many cases, however, giant cells are found but no specific etiology is discovered. Two types of giant cells are postulated, one of which is myogenic in origin and thought to represent transitional forms of myocardial cells. Granulomas usually are not found with this type. The more characteristic type of giant cell probably is derived from interstitial histiocytes and usually is found in patients with myocarditis not caused by viral agents. Similar cells have been noted in patients who received neomercazole therapy, and granulomatous myocarditis associated with ingestion of phenylbutazone has been reported.

---

atrioventricular block also may be a presenting sign of myocarditis in children. A not uncommon scenario is an infant or toddler who appears ill and who has not been taking fluids normally for 1 to 2 days. A diarrheal illness also may exacerbate the infant's volume status. The initial chest radiograph may not demonstrate cardiomegaly, only to change rapidly once fluid rehydration takes place. The dysfunctional ventricle may not be able to keep up with the augmented fluid volume and only then may cardiomegaly and pulmonary edema become evident.

When an arrhythmia occurs after a febrile illness, the clinician should suspect the diagnosis and look for other signs of disease. One study found significant arrhythmias in five infants with isolated myocarditis. Four of the five infants died, and three of them had paroxysmal atrial tachycardia. Paroxysmal atrial tachycardia also has been reported in patients with

viral myocarditis. Atrial ectopic-focus tachycardia may mimic sinus tachycardia and should be suspected in a child with persistent sinus tachycardia and congestive heart failure. Careful inspection of the P-wave axis and morphology in a 15-lead electrocardiogram and a 24-hour Holter monitor to observe the variance in rate are essential in establishing the diagnosis. Complete atrioventricular block secondary to idiopathic myocarditis, rubella, coxsackievirus, and respiratory syncytial virus has been described. Some of these patients developed permanent atrioventricular block and required permanent pacing, whereas the finding was transitory in others.

Ventricular tachycardia, when present, usually is poorly tolerated and should be treated aggressively. Our initial approach is to use lidocaine and, if it is unsuccessful, to administer amiodarone intravenously. Despite this intervention, infants

BOX 282.5   Electrocardiographic Studies in Myocarditis

Electrocardiograms of 87 conscripts, 28 of whom had myocarditis, were examined in one study. The most common finding was that of T-wave changes consisting of reduced amplitude or inversion in the left chest leads. Sinus tachycardia was the most common arrhythmia, followed by uniform premature ventricular contractions. Another study described four patterns of electrocardiograms in patients with proven viral myocarditis: normalization even in the presence of severe myocardial damage during the acute stage, "pseudoinfarction" patterns with pathologic-appearing Q waves and poor R wave progression in the precordial leads, conduction disturbances possibly requiring pacemaker support, and chronic arrhythmias consisting of ventricular tachycardia and supraventricular tachycardia.

Animal studies have been performed to investigate the electrophysiologic effects of myocarditis. In one study, coxsackievirus B3 myocarditis was produced in hamsters. ST- or T-wave changes on the surface electrocardiogram were seen in 80% of the animals. Peak changes were seen between days 2 and 4, when mortality rates were highest. Histologic examination demonstrated that the inner third of the endocardium was involved primarily, suggesting that the subendocardial injury corresponded to the ST- and T-wave changes found on the surface electrocardiogram. In another study, myocarditis was induced in DBA/2 mice with encephalomyocarditis virus. Advanced atrioventricular block, premature atrial contractions, and premature ventricular contractions all were seen acutely. The chronic stage was characterized by sinus tachycardia and low voltage of the QRS complex. In the late chronic stages, QRS voltages returned toward normal, possibly reflecting diminished myocardial edema or compensatory ventricular hypertrophy.

ST-segment and T-wave changes are sensitive indices of myocardial ischemia, but they also appear to be nonspecific findings. This is a true prolonged PR segment, which is a common occurrence during fever.

One study found a 1.49% prevalence of ST- and T-wave changes and prolonged PR segments in a group of 737 infants and children with respiratory tract infections. In another study, the prolongation of PR segment and changes in T wave also were demonstrated in infants and children with pneumonia and no signs of myocarditis. Another nonspecific finding, prolonged QT interval, has been noted in acute myocarditis, as well as in measles and poliomyelitis without myocardial involvement.

---

who present with hemodynamically unstable ventricular tachycardia have a mortality rate exceeding 50%.

The electrocardiographic pattern classically described in myocarditis is that of low-voltage QRS complexes (less than 5 mm of total amplitude in all limb leads), with low-amplitude or slightly inverted T waves and a small or absent Q-wave in leads V_5 and V_6. The low voltage also may be present in the precordial leads. Additional information about electrocardiographic evidence of myocarditis is presented in Box 282.5.

Echocardiography is essential in establishing the diagnosis of myocarditis. Pericardial effusion, as a cause of cardiomegaly, can be determined using either single-crystal or two-dimensional techniques. Depressed ventricular function with dilatation of one or more chambers in the absence of any structural abnormality helps establish the diagnosis.

Although not used much today, nuclear imaging has been used in the past as a screening test to help establish the diagnosis of myocarditis. Screening of patients with dilated cardiomyopathy using ^{67}gallium (^{67}Ga) may help in selecting a subgroup of patients who could benefit from endomyocardial biopsy. The biopsy sample would be used to confirm the presence of active inflammation and might aid in guiding therapy. In one study, 68 patients with a diagnosis of dilated cardiomyopathy underwent 71 parallel studies with ^{67}Ga scanning and endomyocardial biopsy. A dense gallium uptake was found in five of six patients for whom biopsy samples showed active inflammation. Only nine of 65 negative biopsy test results had equivocally positive scan results. A 36% incidence of myocarditis was noted on biopsy test results with positive scan results, whereas only a 1.8% incidence of myocarditis was found on the biopsy test results with negative scan results. This technique has not been used in children, and we do not advocate its use today.

Acutely ill patients with myocarditis should be stabilized before undergoing cardiac catheterization. Infants may require study to exclude anomalous origin of the left coronary artery, although advances in two-dimensional echocardiography and magnetic resonance imaging have helped to determine the origins and course of the coronary arteries.

Since the 1980s, endomyocardial biopsy has become a relatively safe and effective means of sampling heart muscle. The widest application is in patients who have undergone cardiac transplantation and who require repeated samples to assess the degree of allographic rejection. Endomyocardial biopsy helps to establish the diagnosis of myocarditis and possibly to classify the phase of disease (acute, healed, chronic). Histologic classification is difficult and, at times, controversial. The sampling of small areas precludes establishing an accurate diagnosis, especially if the inflammation is focal. In most patients, multiple samples (at least three) should be obtained from the right ventricular septum or apex.

Sampling from other areas of the heart (i.e., the left ventricle) is considered by some physicians to be more sensitive, but this technique is not applied widely. Sampling error during endomyocardial biopsy has confounded establishing an accurate diagnosis of this disease. One study used autopsy specimens from patients who died from myocarditis. These hearts then were subjected to biopsy tests using the same bioptome that would have been used in the patient during an actual biopsy procedure. The investigators found only a 63% incidence in these autopsy-proven myocarditis hearts (i.e., one-third of the cases would have been improperly diagnosed as normal). They concluded that when myocarditis is diagnosed using only the biopsy technique, then only positive findings should be considered diagnostic. One study reported the findings of normal myocardium examined with hematoxylin-eosin stain and compared this process to staining with monoclonal antibodies. The findings supported those of previous studies, that fewer than five lymphocytes per high-power field (400 ×) was normal. No correlation was found between the peripheral lymphocyte count and the lymphocyte count in the myocardium. Specifically, B cells and killer T cells were uncommon findings, whereas the helper-type T cell (OKT4) predominated over the suppressor/cytotoxic type of T cell (OKT8) in a ratio similar to that found in the peripheral circulation (1:44).

As mentioned, the technique of gene amplification using PCR may aid in establishing the diagnosis of myocarditis, especially in borderline cases that have significant inflammatory cells but no concomitant myocyte destruction. PCR uses an enzyme known as *Taq DNA polymerase* that is added to the following: a solution of target DNA to be amplified; primers,

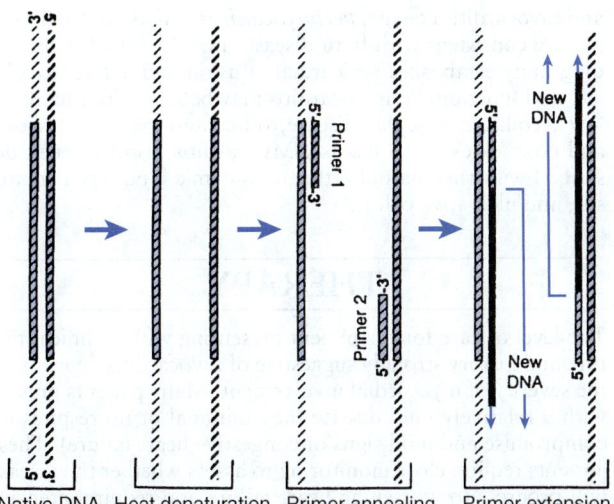

Native DNA Heat denaturation Primer annealing Primer extension

FIGURE 282.2. First round of the polymerase chain reaction. The basic polymerase chain reaction cycle consists of three steps performed in the same closed container but at different temperatures. The elevated temperature in the first step melts the double-stranded DNA into single strands. As the temperature is lowered for the second step, the two oligonucleotide primers that are oppositely directed anneal to complementary sequences on the target DNA, which acts as a template. During the third step, also performed at a lower temperature, the *Taq* polymerase enzymatically extends the primers covalently in the presence of excess deoxyribonucleoside triphosphates, the building blocks of new DNA synthesis. The native DNA target sequences, which will be massively amplified as "short products" in the ensuing cycles, are boxed. The vector of action of the DNA polymerase is denoted by the arrows projecting from the newly synthesized DNA (*dark bars*). (Reprinted with permission from Eisenstein BI. The polymerase chain reaction: a new method of using molecular genetics for medical diagnosis. *N Engl J Med* 1990;3:179.)

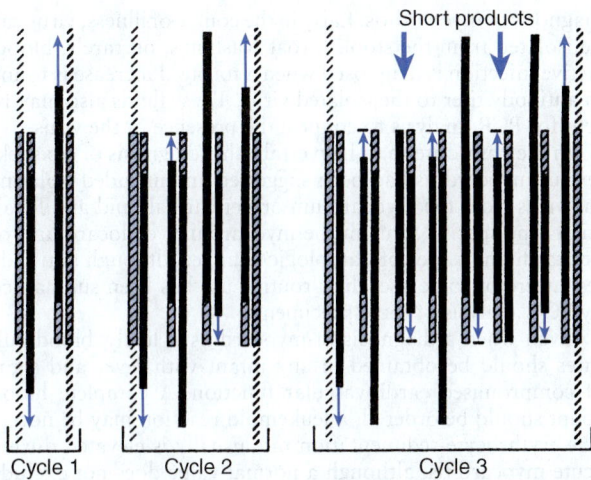

Cycle 1   Cycle 2   Cycle 3

FIGURE 282.3. Products at the end of the initial polymerase chain reaction cycles. A key element of the polymerase chain reaction is the repetitive thermo cycling of the steps shown in Figure 282.2. At each cycle, dark bars denote accumulated DNA that has been synthesized; currently synthesized DNA is indicated by arrows that project in the direction of active DNA polymerization. Because the synthesized products of all previous cycles act as templates for all ensuing cycles, the number of short products increases geometrically at the completion of each cycle. After approximately 30 cycles, the ratio of short products to other DNA entities is so large that they appear to be the only detectable DNA in the reaction mixture. (Reprinted with permission from Eisenstein BI. The polymerase chain reaction: a new method of using molecular genetics for medical diagnosis. *N Engl J Med* 1990;322:179.)

which are two single-stranded oligonucleotides produced to complement known sequences in the target DNA; and excess deoxyribonucleoside bases. This mixture is heated and cooled many times to cycle the following reaction: (a) during heating, the target DNA separates into single strands, each of which acts as a template for producing a new double-stranded DNA that (b) when cooled, incorporates the primer that is complementary to the heat-denatured strands of target DNA, and (c) finally, with further cooling, the *Taq* polymerase catalyzes the synthesis of the remainder of the strand in the presence of excess base. When performed 30 to 50 times, a geometric amplification of the original target DNA occurs. Identification of the target DNA with a specific viral agent then can proceed (Figs. 282.2 and 282.3). Several reports have linked the presence of viral RNA in patients with dilated cardiomyopathy, thus implicating viral myocarditis as a precursor illness.

Investigators using PCR analysis have shown that adenovirus is an important cause of myocarditis in patients with a diagnosis of endocardial fibroelastosis. Using fixed tissue samples, viral genome was seen in 21% of specimens with this diagnosis. Moreover, in one study of patients with presumed myocarditis, adenoviral genome was found in 58% followed by enterovirus (29%), the latter traditionally thought to be the most common etiologic agent.

Although current diagnostic modalities are an improvement over those of the past, they still lack the sensitivity to identify all cases of myocarditis. Several new approaches, including the use of *in situ* PCR and recognition of inflammatory mediators, will improve the diagnostic yield in the future.

Some studies used endomyocardial biopsy to investigate patients who present with occult ventricular arrhythmias and a clinical picture of dilated cardiomyopathy. In these cases, the establishment of a diagnosis helped tailor therapy, with resulting improvement of the arrhythmias in some patients.

In one study, endomyocardial biopsy was used to establish the diagnosis of myocarditis in 34 patients who presented with dilated cardiomyopathy. The disease of these patients was classified on the basis of clinical and histologic findings in an attempt to stratify patients who might benefit from immunosuppressive therapy. Three groups—acute, rapidly progressive, and chronic—were formed. Immunosuppressive therapy was beneficial in only those patients with chronic disease.

Subsequently, 27 patients referred for endomyocardial biopsy with the diagnosis of dilated cardiomyopathy were studied. Although two-thirds of the patients had a biopsy consistent with myocarditis, no correlation was found between histologic classification and outcome. More important, no difference in outcome between the group receiving immunosuppressive therapy and those who did not receive the drugs was noted. The biopsy result was negative in 30% of patients who had the clinical criteria of myocarditis and was positive in two of five patients without any clinical evidence of myocarditis.

One investigator reviewed 1,200 biopsy specimens from patients with a clinical diagnosis of dilated cardiomyopathy and found that approximately 25% had a diagnosis of myocarditis based on the critical evaluation of tissue specimens. No large series of pediatric patients with myocarditis exist to help clarify this issue.

Laboratory Tests

Although rarely successful, an attempt should be made to identify the offending organism for each child with the suspected diagnosis of myocarditis. Early in the course of illness, virus can be isolated from the stool, throat washings, or, rarely, blood. Active infection is diagnosed when a fourfold increase is found in antibody titer to the isolated virus. These fluids also may be sent for PCR analysis to confirm the presence of the virus.

In the past, criteria to help establish a diagnosis of coxsackievirus myocarditis had been suggested and included isolating the virus from the myocardium or pericardial fluid and localizing type-specific virus in the myocardium, endocardium, or pericardium at sites of pathologic change. Although antibody tests were of some use, their routine use has been supplanted by PCR analysis of these specimens.

Even when a diagnosis of myocarditis is likely, blood cultures should be obtained in any infant with fever and signs of compromised cardiovascular function. A complete blood count should be ordered; a leukemoid reaction may be noted. The erythrocyte sedimentation rate usually is elevated during acute myocarditis, although a normal value does not exclude the diagnosis. Elevated levels of serum glutamic-oxaloacetic and glutamic-pyruvic transaminase can occur as the result of a generalized viral infection, although they also may be seen during episodes of diphtheritic myocarditis. Creatine phosphokinase and lactate dehydrogenase enzymes also should be measured. One study found that elevation of isozyme 1 of lactate dehydrogenase was a specific finding in patients with idiopathic myocarditis.

Differential Diagnosis

Any cause of acute circulatory failure may mimic the presentation of acute myocarditis. Hypoxia, hypoglycemia, and hypocalcemia in newborns may be seen with heart failure. Circulatory collapse with shock frequently occurs in cases of overwhelming sepsis in this age group. Serum measurements of glucose and calcium, as well as blood cultures, should be obtained in infants presenting with heart failure if sepsis is suspected.

Many infants with significant structural defects of the heart (e.g., hypoplastic left-heart syndrome, critical aortic valve stenosis) have no audible murmur when severely ill because of extremely low cardiac output. When cardiac function is improved, however, murmurs may be apparent, as may be hyperactive precordium and clear, not muffled, heart sounds. Echocardiographic diagnosis is essential in the evaluation of these patients to rule out structural abnormalities.

Beyond the immediate neonatal period, many other etiologies are possible. An anomalous left coronary artery arising from the pulmonary artery should be investigated by echocardiography and angiography. Endocardial fibroelastosis, type II glycogen storage disease (Pompe disease), medial necrosis of the coronary arteries, and left atrial myxoma are among the many diseases that can present a clinical picture similar to that of myocarditis. Murmurs may be audible with anomalous left coronary artery or endocardial fibroelastosis. They usually are apical in location, rarely more than grade 3 (of 6), and usually secondary to mitral insufficiency. Endocardial fibroelastosis is impossible to differentiate from myocarditis by clinical presentation. Endomyocardial biopsy and angiographic changes of the left ventricle help establish this diagnosis. Electrocardiography in the anomalous left coronary artery may show a pattern of myocardial infarction, with abnormal q waves in the anterolateral precordial leads. A qR pattern with inverted T waves in limb leads I and aVL also may be noted.

Pericarditis, which may be secondary to viral illness, usually occurs in children rather than infants. The clinical history may be similar to that in patients with myocarditis. Cardiovascular function, however, usually is less severely compromised for the degree of apparent cardiomegaly because of the amount of pericardial effusion. Cardiac tamponade may occur in severe cases and present with circulatory collapse. When pericarditis

and myocarditis coexist, *perimyocarditis* results, and a clinical picture consistent with both diseases may be found. Echocardiography establishes pericardial effusion and left ventricular size and function. Perimyocarditis may be seen with rheumatic fever, collagen vascular disease, other autoimmune diseases, and coxsackievirus B disease. Myocarditis also has been described with rheumatoid arthritis, systemic lupus erythematosus, and ulcerative colitis.

THERAPY

The level of care for the patient presenting with a clinical picture and history strongly suggestive of myocarditis depends on the severity of myocardial involvement. Many patients present with a relatively mild disease (i.e., minimal or no respiratory compromise and mild signs of congestive heart failure). These patients require close monitoring to assess whether the disease will progress to worsening heart failure and require intensive medical care. Experimental studies in animals suggest that bed rest may prevent an increase in intramyocardial viral replication during the acute stage; therefore, to place patients under this restriction at the time of diagnosis is prudent.

Although no specific therapy aimed at reversing myocardial injury is recommended widely, maintenance of cardiac output at levels that supply adequate tissue perfusion and prevent metabolic disturbance is essential. In cases of congestive heart failure, digitalis may be used, and it has effected dramatic improvement in some instances. During periods of acute inflammation, the myocardium may be overly sensitive to digitalis; thus, rapid administration to achieve therapeutic levels should be avoided. Generally, the oral route is preferred, and a dose of 0.03 mg/kg rather than 0.04 mg/kg should be used as a total digitalizing dose. One-half of this dose should be given initially and the remaining half given in two divided doses at 8-hour intervals. Maintenance therapy should be tailored to achieving adequate serum therapeutic levels.

Diuretics frequently are administered in conjunction with digitalis. Although no direct beneficial effect on the myocardium is achieved, removal of excess extracellular fluid volume may help improve cardiac function. These agents should be administered cautiously; shock may result if extracellular volume is removed too rapidly. Excessive loss of potassium ion secondary to induced diuresis may exacerbate digitalis toxicity and should be avoided. Furosemide should be administered in a dosage of 1 mg/kg per dose. The frequency of administration depends on the clinical state of the patient and may require the addition of spironolactone, a potassium-sparing diuretic agent, if dosing three times a day is required (total daily dose more than 2 mg/kg/day).

Newborn infants may present initially in shock. Blood pressure usually is maintained at or near normal levels until late in the course and is not a sensitive indicator of the severity of illness. Rather, close attention to the adequacy of peripheral perfusion, heart rate, and urine output gives the clinician a better picture of the hemodynamic status of the infant. Although the hearts of these infants and children generally respond poorly to volume loading, selected patients may respond temporarily to boluses of 5 mL/kg of 5% albumin in Ringer's lactated solution or a transfusion of packed red blood cells if a concomitant anemia exists. High central venous filling pressures of 12 to 18 mm Hg may be required to sustain adequate cardiac output, in contrast to 5 mm Hg in a child with a normally functioning heart.

When these measures fail to reestablish an adequate cardiac output, a positive inotropic agent is administered. Dopamine in doses of 2 to 10 μg/kg/minute is recommended to support blood pressure and effect some degree of dilation of the renal vasculature. As the dose increases toward 20 μg/kg/minute, dopamine exerts an increasingly dominant alpha-adrenergic effect and may increase systemic peripheral vasculature resistance;

therefore, avoiding doses of more than 15 μg/kg/minute usually is wise. Dobutamine, a sympathomimetic amine that stimulates beta$_1$-, beta$_2$-, and alpha-adrenergic receptors, is used frequently in combination with dopamine. This agent exerts significant positive inotropy, while reducing left ventricular filling pressure. Its chronotropic response is not as positive as is dopamine's, and it seems to result in less ventricular ectopy during administration. When used in combination with dopamine at low doses (more than 10 μg/kg/minute), dobutamine, in doses of 10 μg/kg/minute or more, may result in a significant increase in ventricular contractility while avoiding a sinus tachycardia that may compromise cardiac output. For this reason, isoproterenol is best avoided in these patients because the resultant sinus tachycardia, which in other patients may improve cardiac output, may be affected adversely in this circumstance.

Because of its afterload-reducing effects, sodium nitroprusside has been used extensively in children. Cardiac output is improved by a reduction of systemic arterial resistance and, thus, ventricular filling pressure. In patients with myocarditis, this agent may be used in conjunction with dopamine or dobutamine, if hypotension does not coexist. Although bedside assessment of cardiac output using thermodilution techniques after placement of a Swan-Ganz catheter can aid in the pharmacotherapy of the altered hemodynamic profiles, it may be arrhythmogenic and rarely is used today. When chronic oral therapy can be given, an afterload-reducing drug such as captopril, an angiotensin-converting enzyme (ACE) inhibitor, may be used with digitalis and diuretics. More recently, the use of low-dose beta blockers has been used successfully to manage heart failure. We routinely use in combination metoprolol or carvedilol, in addition to the ACE inhibitors or angiotensin converting blockers (ACBs) and diuretics noted above.

Arrhythmias should be treated vigorously. Supraventricular tachyarrhythmias often are suppressed with digitalis, which usually has been administered previously for the treatment of congestive heart failure. Other agents may be used acutely through the intravenous route. Procainamide has been useful in suppressing atrial tachycardias if hemodynamic compromise is present. Beta blockers, which are concomitantly used for the management of heart failure, also may be useful in suppressing these arrhythmias. Chronically, sotalol may be used as both a beta blocker and antiarrhythmic in some patients. Ventricular arrhythmias may be responsive to lidocaine, given in a loading dose of 1 mg/kg (up to 50 mg total bolus dose), followed by a continuous infusion adequate to maintain a therapeutic serum concentration (1 to 5 mg/mL). If lidocaine fails to control the ventricular tachycardia adequately, then amiodarone is

---

BOX 282.6   **Some Reports of Use of Immunosuppressive Therapy in Myocarditis**

Using endomyocardial biopsy to diagnose myocarditis, some investigators followed the inflammatory response to immunosuppressive therapy with follow-up biopsy tests in a series of ten patients. Eight patients received both prednisone and azathioprine, whereas two received only prednisone. Clinical and histologic improvements were seen in four patients. Two patients who had their medications discontinued suffered relapses, which were reversed by reinstituting therapy. One patient worsened while on therapy and died. Although it was an uncontrolled study, the authors noted that the reversal of congestive heart failure in the two patients who resumed therapy was highly suggestive of the beneficial effect of immunosuppressive therapy. Another study found definite hemodynamic and histologic improvement in seven of nine patients treated with a combination of prednisone and azathioprine. After discontinuing therapy for 4 months, however, only four of seven patients still showed improvement. One patient improved with reinstitution of therapy, whereas two patients deteriorated.

The results of the Myocarditis Trial were published in 1995. A total of 111 patients were assigned randomly to one of three treatment groups. One group received azathioprine and prednisone, a second group received cyclosporine and prednisone, and the third group received conventional supportive therapy. The results showed that, after 24 weeks of therapy, no difference among the groups was found in their left ventricular performance or survival. The authors concluded that no beneficial effect was associated with the routine use of corticosteroids in these patients with myocarditis.

One study illustrates the problem of biopsy-directed treatment in myocarditis. Nine patients were treated with single or combined immunosuppressive therapy after a biopsy sample showed evidence of inflammation. Improvement was seen in four of nine patients; however, 6 of 18 patients who did not receive therapy also improved, nullifying any statistically significant difference between the two groups.

Another study attempted to use a clinicopathologic description to categorize myocarditis into types that might respond to immunosuppressive treatment. The categories mimicked those of postviral hepatitis syndromes (i.e., fulminant, acute, chronic active, and chronic persistent). The only patients who seemed to respond to immunosuppressive agents were those with acute myocarditis, although some of them went on to develop congestive cardiomyopathy despite the absence of inflammatory cells on their follow-up biopsy samples. Other studies have shown that patients with borderline myocarditis respond better (improved left ventricular contractile function) than do patients with unequivocally positive biopsy samples.

A tabulation of results from most studies showing the effects of immunosuppressive therapy revealed that 60% of 82 biopsy-proven cases of myocarditis improved with therapy. Patients who had lower-grade changes apparently did better than did those with greater involvement. Complications of immunosuppressive therapy, including opportunistic infections and a cushingoid state, should be considered before the administration of these drugs. Controlled studies are under way in the adult population to address the usefulness of immunosuppressive therapy, including cyclosporine; a similar study in children should be undertaken before firm recommendations can be given to clinicians. The prognosis for acute myocarditis in newborns is poor. A 75% mortality rate was found in 25 infants with suspected coxsackievirus B myocarditis. The highest rate of mortality occurred in the first week of illness. The six infants who survived showed no apparent sequelae, although long-term follow-up was not reported. Older infants and children have a better prognosis, with a mortality rate of between 10% and 25% in clinically recognizable cases. Adult patients who recover may be asymptomatic at rest or with light exertion, but they may demonstrate a reduced working capacity with exercise stress testing.

administered intravenously. We begin with a loading regimen of between 10 and 15 mg/kg, given in 2- to 5-mg/kg aliquots over the course of 15 to 20 minutes, and then start an infusion of between 10 and 15 mg/kg/day. Rarely, higher doses of up to 20 mg/kg may be required. If complete atrioventricular block occurs, a temporary transvenous pacemaker should be inserted. The patient must be observed over the course of 10 to 14 days (in an intensive care unit) for the return of normal atrioventricular conduction. A permanent pacing device should be implanted if complete atrioventricular block persists beyond that time. Implantation can be done as an elective procedure when the patient's condition is stable.

Antibiotic agents should not be given unless a bacterial infection is suspected and cultures are obtained before initiating therapy.

Previous editions of this text have noted that a promising therapy for acute myocarditis was the use of intravenous gamma globulin, usually given as a 2 g/kg dose over the course of 6 to 12 hours, depending on the patient's tolerance to volume loading. Continued reports in the literature demonstrate some good outcomes following this therapy, and for all practical purposes, it has become standard therapy in many institutions. Unfortunately, the use of immunosuppressive agents in suspected or proven viral myocarditis remains controversial, and we must report that there still exists no multicenter, prospective, randomized clinical trial to justify the formal recommendation for this therapy. The initial study, reported in 1994, showed that 21 of 46 children treated with this agent soon after initial presentation had better left ventricular performance at 1-year follow-up and a trend to better survival. Most importantly, a larger multicenter study still is needed to help further analyze whether this promising therapy is worthwhile. Some animal studies suggest an exacerbation of virus-induced cytotoxicity in the presence of immunosuppressive drugs, possibly caused by interference with interferon production. Additional information about the use of immunosuppressive therapy in myocarditis is presented in Box 282.6.

The etiology of the disease may affect prognosis. Patients who develop conduction abnormalities or arrhythmias with diphtheritic myocarditis have a poor prognosis. Some investigators report a 100% mortality rate in those patients with conduction disturbances or supraventricular tachycardia.

Finally, during the past few years, the development of left ventricular and biventricular assist devices has progressed remarkably. The devices have been downsized and now can be applied successfully to infants and small children. Studies now suggest that, in severe cases, early intervention with these extracorporal or implantable assist devices may allow time for the acute inflammatory process to pass and for early healing to begin. Unloading the myocardium from the metabolic demands of maintaining an adequate cardiac output for a short time may permit time for the reversal of acute injury and improved survival to occur. Complications including stroke, bleeding, and infection still are significant but may be justified easily in extreme cases. One recent series included 19 children with body surface area of less than 1.3 square-meters. Mean duration of support was 43 days (range 1 to 120 days) with a survival rate of 72%. As the devices continue to diminish in size, and as surgical techniques are perfected, even the most severely affect infants and young children may be able to survive with this novel therapy.

Suggested Readings

Daly K, et al. Acute myocarditis: role of histological and virological examination in the diagnosis and assessment of immunosuppressive treatment. *Br Heart J* 1984;51:30.

Dery P, Marks MI, Shapera R. Clinical manifestations of coxsackievirus infections in children. *Am J Dis Child* 1974;128:464.

Drucker NA, et al. Gamma globulin treatment of acute myocarditis in the pediatric population. *Circulation* 1994;89:252.

Eckart RE, et al. Incidence and follow-up of inflammatory cardiac complications after smallpox vaccination. *J Am Coll Cardiol* 2004;44:201.

Edwards WD, Holmes DR, Reader GS. Diagnosis of active lymphocytic myocarditis by endomyocardial biopsy: quantitative criteria for light microscopy. *Mayo Clin Proc* 1982;57:419.

Fenoglio JJ, et al. Diagnosis and classification of myocarditis by endomyocardial biopsy. *N Engl J Med* 1983;308:12.

Griffin LD, et al. Analysis of formalin fixed and frozen myocardial autopsy samples for viral genome in childhood myocarditis and dilated cardiomyopathy with endocardial fibroelastosis using polymerase chain reaction. *Cardiovasc Pathol* 1995;4:3.

Hauck AJ, et al. Evaluation of postmortem endomyocardial biopsy specimens from 38 patients with lymphocytic myocarditis: implication for rule of sampling error. *Mayo Clin Proc* 1989;64:1235.

Lerner AM, Wilson MF. Virus myocardiopathy. *Prog Med Virol* 1973;15:63.

Lyden D, Olazewski J, Huber S. Variation in susceptibility of BALB/c mice to coxsackievirus group B type 3-induced myocarditis with age. *Cell Immunol* 1987;105:332.

Maisch B, et al. Diagnostic relevance of humoral and cell-mediated immune reactions in patients with acute viral myocarditis. *Clin Exp Immunol* 1982;48:533.

Mason J, et al. A clinical trial of immunosuppressive therapy for myocarditis. *N Engl J Med* 1995;333:270.

McManus BM, Kandolf R. Evolving concepts of cause, consequence, and control in myocarditis. *Curr Opin Cardiol* 1991;6:418.

Pauschinger M et al. Myocardial remodeling in viral heart disease: Possible interactions between inflammatory mediators and MMP-TIMP system. *Heart Failure Rev* 2004;9:21.

Reifhartz O et al. Thoratec ventricular assist devices in children with less than 1.3 m^2 of body surface area. *ASAIO J* 2003;49:727.

Saphir O, Simon WA, Reingold MI. Myocarditis in children. *Am J Dis Child* 1944;67:294.

Woodruff JF. Viral myocarditis: a review. *Am J Pathol* 1980;101:427.

Zee-Cheng CS, et al. High incidence of myocarditis by endomyocardial biopsy in patients with idiopathic congestive cardiomyopathy. *J Am Coll Cardiol* 1984;3:63.

CHAPTER 283 ■ CARDIOMYOPATHY

JEFFREY A. TOWBIN AND NEIL E. BOWLES

Cardiomyopathies in children are major causes of morbidity and mortality, and since the late 1980s, limited improvements in outcome have been reported. However, on the basis of improvements in the understanding of several of the major forms of cardiomyopathy in adults, as well as the treatment of these disorders, numerous concepts have been tested (or are currently being tested) in childhood forms of these disorders. In addition, various forms of cardiomyopathy commonly present early in childhood, and these disorders are being described in detail by pediatric cardiologists.

The major classifications of the forms of cardiomyopathies include (a) dilated cardiomyopathy (DCM), which includes approximately 55% of all cardiomyopathies; (b) hypertrophic cardiomyopathy (HCM), which accounts for approximately 35% of all cardiomyopathies; (c) restrictive cardiomyopathy (RCM), an uncommon form accounting for fewer than 5% of cases; and (d) arrhythmogenic right ventricular cardiomyopathy (ARVC), an uncommon form of disease as well, particularly in children. An unclassified form of cardiomyopathy, left ventricular noncompaction (LVNC), is considered to be quite rare, but recent evidence suggests that this disorder actually is relatively common but only rarely diagnosed.

These classified and unclassified disorders generally are considered diseases affecting primarily systolic function (DCM affecting the left ventricle, ARVC affecting the right ventricle), diastolic function (HCM and RCM), or both (LVNC). Based on these functional considerations, therapies have been devised that focus on affecting systole or diastole directly or indirectly.

Since the late 1980s, advances made in molecular genetics and mouse modeling efforts have resulted in modifications of our understanding of these disorders, as well as in therapies designed to treat these disorders. In this chapter, the clinical description, therapies, molecular basis, and functional abnormalities of these disorders are discussed. The goal of this chapter is to acquaint the reader with these disorders and a variety of new considerations regarding form and function of the heart and the potential new diagnostic and therapeutic horizons of the future for these potentially devastating diseases.

EPIDEMIOLOGY

The cardiomyopathies are heart muscle disorders associated with significant rates of morbidity and mortality. These disorders are classified by the World Health Organization (WHO) into four forms: (a) DCM, (b) HCM, (c) RCM, and (d) ARVC. More recently, another cardiomyopathy, LVNC, has gained attention, although it does not meet criteria for a separate classification currently.

The most common cardiomyopathy is DCM, accounting for approximately 55% of cases. HCM is second most common, accounting for approximately 35%, with the remaining forms accounting for approximately 5% or less in each case. The importance of these disorders lies in that they are responsible for a high proportion of cases of congestive heart failure (CHF) and sudden death, as well as the need for cardiac transplantation. The mortality rate in the United States from cardiomyopathy is greater than 10,000 deaths/year, with DCM being the major contributor to this death rate. The total cost of health care in the United States focused on cardiomyopathies is in the billions of dollars, and only limited success has been achieved. To achieve improved care and outcomes in children and adults, understanding of the causes of these disorders has been sought in earnest during the past decade.

PATHOGENESIS AND PATHOPHYSIOLOGY

HCM and RCM are primarily diastolic disorders, whereas DCM and ARVC are primarily systolic disorders. LVNC is a combination overlap disorder with evidence of both systolic and diastolic dysfunction. The molecular basis of HCM has been well studied since the early 1990s, and to date, 11 genes have been identified as being causes of disease. Nearly all

TABLE 283.1

DILATED CARDIOMYOPATHY GENETICS

CHR Locus	Gene	Protein
Xp21.2	DYS	Dystrophin
Xq28	G4.5	Tafazzin
1q21	LMNA	Lamin A/C
1q32	TNNT2	Cardiac troponin T
1q42–43	ACTN	alpha-Actinin
2q31	TTN	Titin
2q35	DES	Desmin
5q33	SGCD	delta-Sarcoglycan
6q22.1	PLN	Phospholamban
10q22.3–23.2	ZASP/Cypher	ZASP
10q22–q23	VCL	Metavinculin
11p11	MYBPC3	Myosin-binding protein C
11p15.1	MLP	Muscle LIM protein
14q12	MYH7	beta-Myosin heavy chain
15q14	ACTC	Cardiac actin
15q22	TPM1	alpha-Tropomyosin

these genes encode proteins comprising the sarcomere, including beta-myosin heavy chain, alpha-tropomyosin, cardiac troponin T, cardiac troponin I, myosin-binding protein C, myosin essential light chain, myosin regulatory light chain, actin, muscle LIM protein, and titin. Hence, the disease now is considered a disease of the sarcomere. One recently identified gene appears to question whether the sarcomere is the only region of the heart causing HCM when altered. This gene, called *adenosine monophosphate (AMP)-kinase (AMPK)*, is important in metabolic regulation, participating in energy utilization, and its function appears to be similar to that seen in a glycogen storage disease.

DCM has become a popular target of research during the past 7 to 8 years, with multiple genes identified during that period (Table 283.1). These genes appear to encode two major subgroups of proteins, cytoskeletal and sarcomeric. The cytoskeletal proteins identified to date include dystrophin, desmin, lamin A/C, delta-sarcoglycan, metavinculin, muscle LIM protein, and alpha-actinin. In the case of sarcomere-encoding genes, the same genes identified for HCM appear to be implicated in select patients. A new gene, *cypher/ZASP*, a Z-line protein, has been identified recently as well. In addition, two genes with uncertain mechanisms (including *phospholamban* and *G4.5/Tafazzin*) also are reported. Another form of DCM, the acquired disorder viral myocarditis, has the same clinical features as DCM, including heart failure, arrhythmias, and conduction block. The most common causes of myocarditis are viral and include the enteroviruses (coxsackieviruses and echovirus), adenoviruses, parvovirus B19, and other cardiotropic viruses. Evidence suggests that viral myocarditis and DCM (genetic) have similar mechanisms of disease based on the proteins targeted.

RCM, ARVC, and LVNC recently were recognized scientifically, but progress is being made in unraveling the underlying mechanisms of these disorders. Once the cardiomyopathies are understood at the molecular and cellular levels, targeted therapies can be developed in addition to current strategies, with the hope for improved outcomes. In this chapter, we review the clinical and scientific characteristics of these disorders and describe potential novel therapeutic approaches for future consideration. To understand the mechanisms responsible for the development of the clinical phenotype, an understanding of normal cardiac anatomy is necessary (Box 283.1 and Fig. 283.1). In addition, it is necessary to understand how other factors contribute to cardiomyopathy.

BOX 283.1   Normal Cardiac Structure

Cardiac muscle fibers are composed of separate cellular units (myocytes) connected in series. In contrast to skeletal muscle fibers, cardiac fibers do not assemble in parallel arrays but bifurcate and recombine to form a complex three-dimensional network. Cardiac myocytes are joined at each end to adjacent myocytes at the intercalated disc, the specialized area of interdigitating cell membrane (see Fig. 283.1). The intercalated disc contains gap junctions (containing connexins) and mechanical junctions, composed of adherens junctions (containing N-cadherin, catenins, and vinculin) and desmosomes (containing desmin, desmoplakin, desmocollin, and desmoglein). Cardiac myocytes are surrounded by a thin membrane (sarcolemma), and the interior of each myocyte contains bundles of myofibrils arranged longitudinally. The myofibrils are formed by repeating sarcomeres, the basic contractile units of cardiac muscle composed of interdigitating thin (actin) and thick (myosin) filaments (see Fig. 283.1) that give the muscle its characteristic striated appearance. The thick filaments are composed primarily of myosin but additionally contain myosin binding proteins C, H, and X. The thin filaments are composed of cardiac actin, alpha-tropomyosin (alpha-TM), and troponins T, I, and C (cTnT, cTnI, cTnC). In addition, myofibrils contain a third filament formed by the giant filamentous protein, titin, which extends from the Z-disc to the M-line and acts as a molecular template for the layout of the sarcomere. The Z-disc at the borders of the sarcomere is formed by a lattice of interdigitating proteins that maintain myofilament organization by cross-linking antiparallel titin and thin filaments from adjacent sarcomeres (see Fig. 283.1). Other proteins in the Z-disc include alpha-actinin, nebulette, telethonin/T-cap, capZ, microsomal lipoprotein (MLP), myopalladin, myotilin, Cypher/ZASP, filamin, and FATZ.

Finally, the extrasarcomeric cytoskeleton, a complex network of proteins linking the sarcomere with the sarcolemma and the extracellular matrix (ECM), provides structural support for subcellular structures and transmits mechanical and chemical signals within and between cells. The extrasarcomeric cytoskeleton has intermyofibrillar and subsarcolemmal components, with the intermyofibrillar cytoskeleton being composed of intermediate filaments, microfilaments, and microtubules. Desmin intermediate filaments form a three-dimensional scaffold throughout the extrasarcomeric cytoskeleton, with desmin filaments surrounding the Z-disc, allowing for longitudinal connections to adjacent Z-discs and lateral connections to subsarcolemmal costameres. Microfilaments composed of nonsarcomeric actin (mainly gamma-actin) also form complex networks linking the sarcomere (via alpha-actinin) to various components of the costameres. Costameres are subsarcolemmal domains located in a periodic, grid-like pattern, flanking the Z-discs and overlying the I-bands, along the cytoplasmic side of the sarcolemma. These costameres are sites of interconnection between various cytoskeletal networks linking sarcomere and sarcolemma and are thought to function as anchor sites for stabilization of the sarcolemma and for integration of pathways involved in mechanical force transduction. Costameres contain three principal components: the focal adhesion-type complex, the spectrin-based complex, and the dystrophin/dystrophin-associated protein complex (DAPC). The focal adhesion-type complex, composed of cytoplasmic proteins (i.e., vinculin, talin, tensin, paxillin, zyxin), connects with cytoskeletal actin filaments and with the transmembrane proteins alpha-, beta-dystroglycan, alpha-, beta-, gamma-, delta-sarcoglycans, dystrobrevin, and syntrophin. Several actin-associated proteins are located at sites of attachment of cytoskeletal actin filaments with costameric complexes, including alpha-actinin and the muscle LIM protein, MLP. The C-terminus of dystrophin binds beta-dystroglycan (see Fig. 283.1), which, in turn, interacts with alpha-dystroglycan to link to the ECM (via alpha-2-laminin). The N-terminus of dystrophin interacts with actin. Also notable, voltage-gated sodium channels colocalize with dystrophin, beta-spectrin, ankyrin, and syntrophins, and potassium channels interact with the sarcomeric Z-disc and intercalated discs. Because arrhythmias and conduction system diseases are common occurrences in children and adults with dilated cardiomyopathy, this factor could play an important role. Hence, disruption of the links from the sarcolemma to ECM at the dystrophin C-terminus and those to the sarcomere and nucleus via N-terminal dystrophin interactions could lead to a domino-effect disruption of systolic function and development of arrhythmias.

Role of Cytokines in Myocarditis and Dilated Cardiomyopathy

During the last few years, considerable interest has been shown in the role of cytokines in the pathogenesis of myocarditis and DCM. Animal studies have suggested that a relationship may exist between subclinical viral infection and later development of DCM. This process is presumed to occur by an autoimmune-like mechanism triggered by the initial viral insult. Several murine models have been studied that suggest that cytokine-mediated modulation of the immune response to viral infection may lead to induction of chronic autoimmune myocarditis.

Among their many immunomodulatory activities, cytokines contribute to regulation of antibody production and maintenance of "self-tolerance." Certain susceptible murine strains, when infected with coxsackievirus B3, are known to develop myocyte necrosis and an acute inflammatory response consisting mainly of neutrophils and macrophages within the heart. After the initial viral infection, resolution of inflammation eventually occurs. In other strains, however, a second autoimmune phase of myocarditis appears later with findings of diffuse mononuclear cell infiltrates within the heart. These mononuclear cells are a significant source of the cytokines interleukin-1 (IL-1) and tumor necrosis factor-alpha (TNF-alpha), and work by Henke and associates demonstrated that release of large amounts of TNF-alpha and IL-1beta by human monocytes exposed to coxsackievirus B3 occurs. Both these cytokines are known to participate in leukocyte activation, which may be beneficial in promoting a specific lymphocyte response to viral infection. However, these cytokines also may promote cardiac fibroblast activity, and, therefore, researchers have speculated that local secretion of cytokines in the myocardium perpetuates the inflammatory process, which secondarily leads to the fibrosis associated with DCM and resultant deterioration of cardiac function. Studies by Gulick and associates

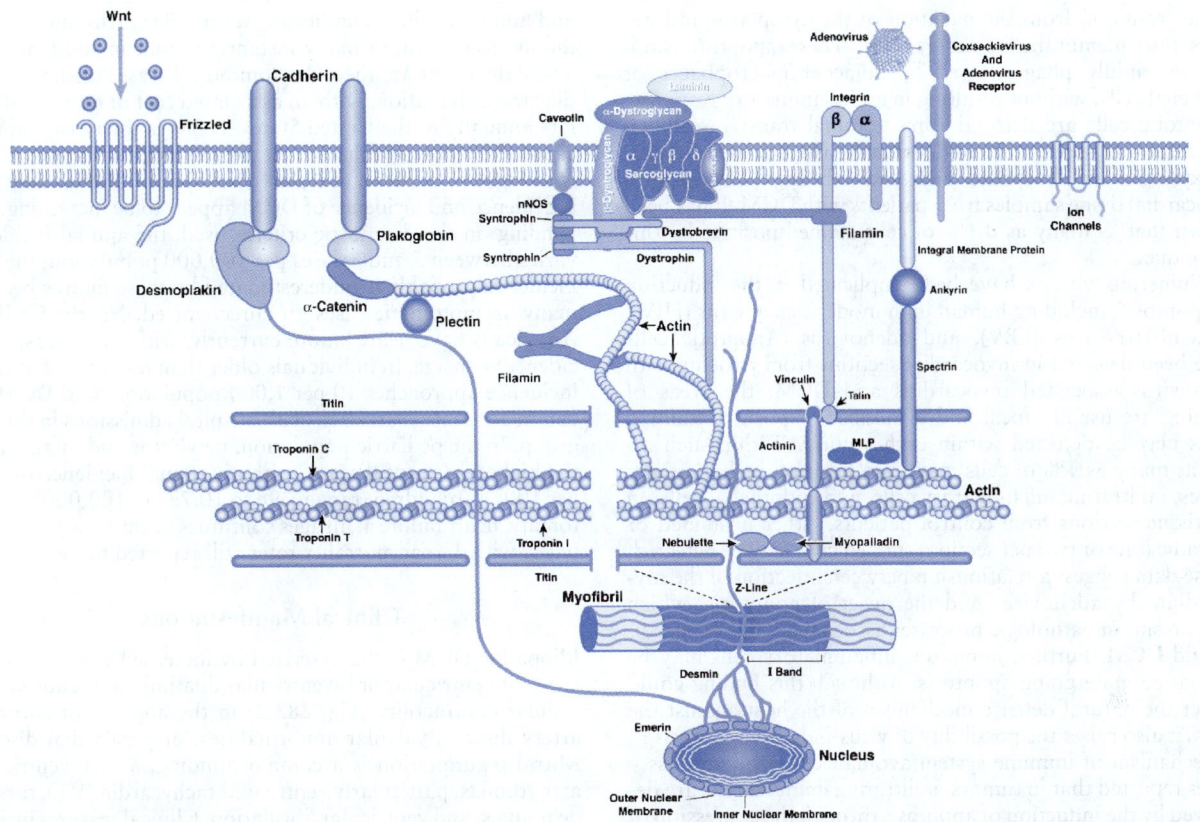

FIGURE 283.1. Cardiac myocyte cytoarchitecture. Schematic of the interactions between dystrophin and the dystrophin-associated proteins in the sarcolemma and intracellular cytoplasm (dystroglycans, sarcoglycans, syntrophins, dystrobrevin, sarcospan) at the C-terminal end of the dystrophin. The integral membrane proteins interact with the extracellular matrix via alpha-dystroglycan-laminin alpha-2 connections. The N-terminus of dystrophin binds actin and connects dystrophin with the sarcomere intracellularly, the sarcolemma, and the extracellular matrix. N, amino terminus; C, carboxy terminus; MLP, muscle LIM protein.

initially implicated IL-1 and TNF-alpha as potential inhibitors of cardiac myocyte beta-adrenergic responsiveness, and further studies showed IL-1 and TNF-alpha to be the macrophage factors mediating this effect. In particular, TNF-alpha has been studied in some detail, resulting in reports of elevated TNF-alpha levels in the serum of patients with chronic heart disease, including a subset of patients with myocarditis or DCM. TNF-alpha is able to potentiate the immune response and induce apoptosis in cells, both of which appear to hold special importance in the pathogenesis of myocarditis. Other inflammatory mediators, including IL-1 and granulocyte colony-stimulating factor, also are elevated in patients with myocarditis and have received attention as well. Other studies have suggested that inflammatory cytokines actually may cause a direct negative inotropic response.

Role of Cell Adhesion Molecules in Myocarditis and Dilated Cardiomyopathy

Molecules now known to play major roles in many processes of inflammation, the distinct classes of cell adhesion molecules (CAMs), also may play roles in the pathogenesis of myocarditis. One molecule that is well known to play a major role in cell-cell adhesion, particularly leukocyte adherence and transendothelial migration, is intercellular adhesion molecule-1 (ICAM-1). ICAM-1 is a member of the immunoglobulin su-

pergene family of CAMs and is a single-chain glycoprotein of 80 to 115 kDa with an extracellular domain composed of five immunoglobulin-like repeats. ICAM-1 is expressed predominantly on endothelial cells but also on fibroblasts, epithelial cells, mucosal cells, lymphocytes, monocytes, and cardiac myocytes after inflammatory injury. Expression of ICAM-1 on endothelial cells is known to be upregulated by cytokines such as IL-1 and TNF-alpha. A well-established binding ligand of ICAM-1 is lymphocyte function-associated antigen-1 (LFA-1), a molecule that is part of the beta-2 integrin family and consists of a 180-kDa alpha subunit (CD11a) and a 95-kDa beta subunit (CD18). LFA-1 is expressed on virtually all leukocytes, including monocytes. The adhesive interaction between LFA-1 and ICAM-1 is known to mediate adhesion-dependent helper T-cell, cytotoxic T-cell, and NK cell functions. Antibody to LFA-1 has been used for therapy in animal models of myocarditis, with resultant blockade of the inflammatory response.

Apoptosis

Apoptosis, or programmed cell death, has an important role in embryogenesis, tissue homeostasis, and regulation of immunologic responses, among normal physiologic processes, and it is associated with the growth and regression of tumors. Cells undergoing apoptosis exhibit characteristic morphologic and biochemical features, including chromatin aggregation, nuclear and cytoplasmic aggregation, and formation of apoptotic bodies resulting from the partition of the cytoplasm and nucleus into membrane bound-vesicles. These apoptotic bodies are rapidly phagocytosed by adjacent macrophages or epithelial cells, without resulting in an inflammatory response. Apoptotic cells are detectable by terminal transferase labeling (terminal deoxynucleotide transferase-mediated biotin-deoxyuridine triphosphate nick end labeling [TUNEL]) in myocardial tissue samples from patients with DCM. It has been shown that as many as 0.1% of cells stained positive by this technique.

Numerous viruses have been implicated in the induction of apoptosis, including human immunodeficiency virus (HIV), Epstein-Barr virus (EBV), and adenovirus. Apoptotic cells have been detected in myocardial sections from patients with adenovirus-associated myocarditis and DCM, the areas of staining are usually focal and a number of positive-staining areas may be detected within each section. Within such areas, as many as 1% of cells may stain positive, including myocytes, infiltrating inflammatory cells, and endothelial cells. In the tissue sections from control patients, either unstained or sporadic (one or two per section) stained cells may be detected. These data suggest a relationship between infection of the myocardium by adenovirus and the onset of apoptosis, which could result in pathologic processes associated with myocarditis and DCM. Further, numerous inflammatory cells may be seen to be undergoing apoptosis. Although this finding could reflect the natural defense mechanism of the host against the virus, it also raises the possibility of virus-induced apoptosis as a mechanism of immune system avoidance. Strand and associates reported that in tumors, infiltrating immune cells are destroyed by the induction of apoptosis through the expression of Fas ligand on the tumor cell that binds Fas on the lymphocyte.

DISORDERS OF VENTRICULAR SYSTOLIC DYSFUNCTION

Dilated Cardiomyopathy

Epidemiology

CHF caused by myocardial dysfunction is a serious malady that is a major cause of morbidity and mortality in children and adults. In these conditions, ventricular arrhythmias commonly occur and, in many instances, result in sudden death. These disorders are the most common diseases leading to cardiac transplantation, with an associated cost of billions of dollars annually in the United States. DCM is the most common cause of CHF, and, although the overall incidence varies, DCM is thought to occur in at least 40 of 100,000 population. The prevalence and incidence of DCM appear to be increasing. Depending on the diagnostic criteria used, the annual incidence varies between 5 and 8 cases per 100,000 population; the true incidence probably is underestimated by these figures because many asymptomatic cases go unrecognized. Nearly 5 million Americans have heart failure currently, with an increasing incidence with age. In individuals older than 65 years of age, the incidence approaches 10 per 1,000 population, and DCM accounts for more than 20% of all hospital admissions in this age group. In the pediatric population, newborns and infants have the highest rates of disease, with an annual incidence of 4.58 per 100,000 children (range 5.98 to 10.72 per 100,000). Symptomatic heart failure at all ages continues to confer a poor prognosis, with 1-year mortality rates still reported to be 45%.

Clinical Manifestations

Idiopathic DCM is characterized by increased ventricular size (i.e., left ventricular or biventricular dilation) and reduced ventricular contractility (Fig. 283.2) in the absence of coronary artery disease, valvular abnormalities, or pericardial disease. Mitral regurgitation is a common finding, as are ventricular arrhythmias, particularly ventricular tachycardia (VT), torsade de pointes, and ventricular fibrillation. Clinical features include the signs and symptoms of CHF, which include breathlessness, fatigue, orthopnea, diaphoresis, chest pain, palpitations, exercise intolerance, and syncope. On physical examination, tachypnea, tachycardia, diaphoresis, an S_3 or summation of S_3 and S_4 gallop, and hepatomagly are seen commonly with or without peripheral edema or ascites. Supportive data include radiographic evidence of cardiomegaly (with or without pulmonary edema) and reduced cardiac contractility with (or without) ventricular dilation on echocardiography. In adults, the condition is seen more frequently in men (2.5:1) and in African Americans (2.5:1), but the causes of these differences are not well understood. In children, it appears to be different, with the male-to-female ratio being 60% males, 40% females. The

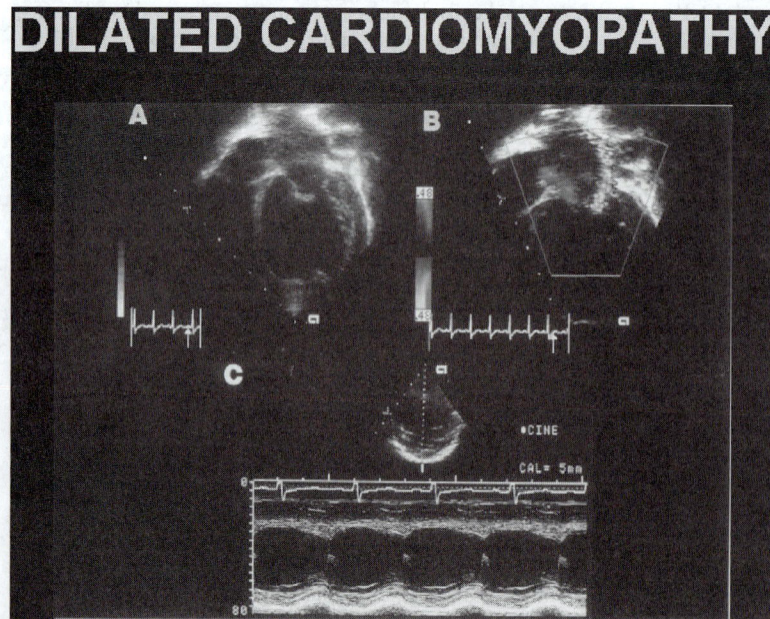

FIGURE 283.2. Echocardiography in dilated cardiomyopathy. **A:** Apical four-chamber view demonstrating a dilated left ventricle. **B:** Similar view showing mitral regurgitation. **C:** M-mode image showing poor systolic function.

clinical course of DCM, almost regardless of origin, may be progressive, with approximately 50% of individuals reported to die within 5 years of diagnosis without cardiac transplantation. The cause of death is divided evenly between sudden death and pump failure. Longer survival has been accomplished more recently with improved medical therapies (i.e., angiotensin-converting enzyme [ACE] inhibitors, beta blockers) and interventions (i.e., implantable defibrillators, ventricular assist devices).

Diagnostic Evaluation

The usual evaluation includes chest radiography, electrocardiography (ECG), echocardiography, and Holter monitoring. Exercise testing and cardiac catheterization, with or without endomyocardial biopsy (EMB), also may be performed. Blood and urine testing, particularly in young children, is mandatory to define an underlying cause.

Chest Radiography. Chest radiographs typically identify cardiomegaly and pulmonary edema with increased pulmonary vascular markings and Kerley B lines. In patients with a dilated left atrium, tracheal narrowing and atelectasis may occur. In some cases, pleural effusions are notable.

Electrocardiography. Sinus tachycardia occurs most commonly. In patients with a dilated left atrium, left atrial enlargement may occur. Ventricular arrhythmias and, on occasion, preexcitation may be identified, as may bundle branch block or atrioventricular block (AVB).

Echocardiography. Classic features include a dilated left ventricle with poor ventricular function. Doppler and color Doppler interrogation may demonstrate atrioventricular valve regurgitation (particularly mitral regurgitation). A pericardial effusion also may be seen, along with atrial dilation.

Holter Monitoring. The purpose of 24-hour ECG monitoring is to identify episodes of ventricular arrhythmias or bradycardia/AVB.

Cardiac Catheterization. Cardiac catheterization typically is not used as a diagnostic modality except to obtain EMB specimens to evaluate for possible myocarditis or, rarely, for mitochondrial abnormalities. Hemodynamic evaluation may identify elevated left ventricular end-diastolic pressure and pulmonary wedge pressures; in some cases, pulmonary vascular resistance may be elevated substantially. If endomyocardial biopsies are obtained, polymerase chain reaction (PCR) analysis for viral genome should be considered.

Metabolic Studies. In children, the underlying cause of DCM may include mitochondrial or metabolic derangement. For this reason, urine analysis for lactate, amino acids, and organic acid elevations may be useful and in some cases, such as Barth syndrome, may help to narrow the differential diagnosis. In Barth syndrome, for instance, elevated 3-methyl-glutaconic acid in a male patient with neutropenia would be diagnostic. Blood studies, including complete blood count, acylcarnitine profile (for fatty acid oxidation defects), pyruvate dehydrogenase complex, electrolyte profile, creatine kinase (with isoform analysis if elevated), plasma amino acids, and blood for genetic testing, all are reasonable. Elevation of creatine kinase muscle isoform (CK-MM) is useful to identify associated skeletal myopathy and may lead to identification of dystrophin (or other) mutations. Viral serologic studies may or may not be helpful. In some patients, particularly young children, skeletal muscle biopsy for microscopy, electron microscopy, and electron transport chain biochemistry can be useful and, if abnormal, should suggest the need for performing blood studies to evaluate for mitochondrial DNA mutations.

Arrhythmias and Conduction System Disease

The rate of sudden cardiac death in individuals with heart failure was reported by Stevenson and Stevenson to be six to nine times that seen in the general population. The basis of this sudden demise is thought to be the presence of ventricular tachyarrhythmias or severe bradyarrhythmias in children. The cause of these rhythm disturbances currently is unknown, but researchers have speculated that myocardial irritability caused by remodeling and fibrosis is a common inciting event. In addition, the myocardial conduction system is likely to be vulnerable to the same pathologic processes affecting the myocytes and interstitial elements, resulting in altered conduction. Furthermore, patients with DCM develop atrial stretching resulting from elevated end-diastolic ventricular pressure caused by poor systolic function and from mitral regurgitation, with electrical instability ensuing. In adults, this condition leads to atrial fibrillation, a decidedly uncommon event in children. However, abnormal myocardial conduction also may lead to ventricular conduction delays and bundle branch block, leading in some patients to worsening mechanical coupling, ventricular activation and contraction, ventricular dyssynchrony, abnormal diastolic function, and significant hemodynamic consequences that could trigger ventricular arrhythmias. These arrhythmias dramatically increase the risk of sudden death and currently are treated with internal defibrillators and/or antiarrhythmic drugs. In adults, left bundle branch block is a significant predictor of sudden death and a common finding in adults with heart failure; however, this does not appear to be the case in children.

Heart Failure with Preserved Systolic Function

The usual teaching regarding heart failure specifies the need for either systolic dysfunction (pump failure) or volume overload. However, another form of heart failure has become increasingly common in adults (20% to 50% of patients with heart failure) and is beginning to crop up in a small number of children with heart failure. In this patient cohort, the usual systolic function indices (shortening fraction, ejection fraction) are preserved. Despite normal contractility, diastole (relaxation) is impaired, and cardiac output is therefore limited by the abnormal filling characteristics of the ventricles, particularly during exercise. For a given ventricular volume, ventricular pressures are elevated, leading to pulmonary congestion, dyspnea, and edema. These symptoms are identical to those of patients with pump failure. This disorder is an unusual occurrence in children and is seen most commonly in elderly, usually female, patients with obesity, hypertension, and diabetes. Mortality is similar to that of typical CHF.

Syndrome of Heart Failure

Traditionally, the syndrome of heart failure has been viewed as a constellation of clinical findings resulting from inadequate systolic function ("pump function"). However, since the early 1990s, this view has been altered by a variety of clinical and basic data, including the continued poor outcomes of patients despite treatment with therapies designed to improve systolic function. In addition, information regarding inflammatory mediators, apoptosis, structure-function studies, and genetics has resulted in a concept that the syndrome of heart failure occurs as a result of a complex interaction of structural, functional, and biologic disturbances of the heart.

The current concepts regarding the syndrome of heart failure integrate a series of models of heart failure, including the hemodynamic model, neurohormonal model, structural model, and autocrine-paracrine model of heart failure. In the hemodynamic model, alterations in load on the failing ventricle are central to the hypothesis, which relies heavily on pump dysfunction as the key contributor. Based on this model, therapies were developed that focused on inotropic agents and vasodilators, with a goal of improving contractility. In distinction to this model, the neurohormonal model focused on the importance of the renin-angiotensin-aldosterone system and the sympathetic nervous system as central to the development of heart failure and resulted in attempts to pharmacologically antagonize the effect of circulating norepinephrine and angiotensin II. The autocrine-paracrine model was developed because of the findings that norepinephrine, angiotensin II, and other vasoactive substances such as brain natriuretic peptide (BNP) also are synthesized within the myocardium, thereby having actions in an autocrine and paracrine manner in addition to their actions in the circulation. Finally, the structural model focuses on the necessity of proper interactions between the sarcomere and sarcolemma via cytoskeletal and other proteins. These interactions, as well as models relying on inflammatory mediators and apoptosis, all have been used to explain the features of heart failure; likely each plays a role in the clinical disorder.

Despite the probable complexity of interactions resulting in heart failure, a major abnormality at the center of the disorder and its reversal is the process of remodeling. Improved outcomes appear to be linked to the ability to reverse this process ("reverse-remodeling"). Remodeling of the left ventricle is a process in which ventricular size, shape, and function are altered because of mechanical, genetic, and neurohormonal factors that lead to hypertrophy, myocyte loss, and interstitial fibrosis. In DCM, the process of progressive ventricular dilation and morphologic ventricular change to a more spheric shape, associated with changes in ventricular function and/or hypertrophy, occurs without known initiating disturbance except in patients with myocardial infarction. Because of this remodeling event, mitral regurgitation may develop as the geometric relations among the mitral valve apparatus, mitral ring, and papillary muscles are altered. The presence of mitral regurgitation results in increasing volume overload on an already compromised ventricle, further contributing to remodeling, symptoms, progression of disease, and left atrial dilation.

Clinical Genetics

DCM initially was thought to be inherited in a small percentage of cases until Michels and associates showed that approximately 20% of probands had family members with echocardiographic evidence of DCM when family screening was performed. More recently, inherited, familial DCM (FDCM) has been shown to occur in more than 30% of cases. In the remaining cases, many are acquired, with viral myocarditis playing a significant role.

As noted, more than 30% of patients with DCM have a familial form of disease. Autosomal dominant inheritance is the predominant pattern of transmission, with X-linked, autosomal recessive, and mitochondrial inheritance being less common. Mitochondrial inheritance is seen most commonly in childhood forms of FDCM, whereas X-linked and autosomal recessive forms probably are evenly mixed between childhood and adult forms of disease. During the past decade, progress has been made in the understanding of the genetic origin of FDCM. Initial progress was made studying families with X-linked forms of DCM, with the autosomal dominant forms of DCM beginning to unravel during the past few years. Box 283.2 gives additional information concerning the genetics of DCM.

Muscle Is Muscle: Cardiomyopathy and Skeletal Myopathy Genes Overlap

Nearly all the genes identified for inherited DCM also are known to cause skeletal myopathy in humans and/or mouse models. In the case of *dystrophin*, mutations cause Duchenne muscular dystrophy and Becker muscular dystrophy, whereas *delta-sarcoglycan* mutations cause LGMD2F. *Lamin A/C* has been shown to cause autosomal dominant Emery-Dreifuss muscular dystrophy and LGMD1B, whereas actin mutations are associated with nemaline myopathy. *Desmin*, *G4.5*, *alpha-dystrobrevin*, *Cypher/ZASP*, *MLP*, *alpha-actinin-2*, *titin*, and *beta-sarcoglycan* mutations also have associated skeletal myopathy, a finding suggesting that cardiac and skeletal muscle function is interrelated and that possibly the skeletal muscle fatigue seen in patients with DCM with and without CHF may result from primary skeletal muscle disease and not solely cardiac dysfunction. It also suggests that the function of these muscles has a "final common pathway," and cardiologists and neurologists should consider evaluation of both sets of muscles.

Further support for this concept comes from studies of animal models. Mutations in *delta-sarcoglycan* in hamsters result in cardiomyopathy, and mutations in all sarcoglycan subcomplex genes in mice cause skeletal and cardiac muscle disease. Mutations in other DAPC genes as well as *dystrophin* in murine models also consistently demonstrate abnormalities of skeletal and cardiac muscle function. Arber and associates also produced a mouse deficient in muscle MLP, a structural protein that links the actin cytoskeleton to the contractile apparatus. The resultant mice develop severe DCM, CHF, and disruption of cardiac myocyte cytoskeletal architecture. Murine mutations in titin, cypher, alpha-dystrobrevin, desmin, and other all demonstrate cardiac and skeletal muscle disease. Finally, Badorff and colleagues showed that DCM that develops after viral myocarditis has a mechanism similar to that of the inherited forms. Using coxsackievirus B3 infection of mice, the authors showed that the coxsackievirus B3 genome encodes for a protease (enteroviral protease 2A) that cleaves dystrophin at the third hinge region of dystrophin, resulting in force transmission abnormalities and DCM. In addition, Xiong and associates showed that abnormal dystrophin increases susceptibility to viral infection and resultant myocarditis. As reported previously by our laboratory, a similar dystrophin mutation affects the first hinge region of dystrophin in patients with X-linked cardiomyopathy, demonstrating a consistent mechanism of DCM development, abnormalities of the cytoskeleton/sarcolemma, and sarcomere. In addition, we have shown that N-terminal dystrophin is reduced or absent in hearts of patients with all forms of DCM (ischemic, acquired, genetic, idiopathic) and that reduction of mechanical stress by use of left ventricular assist devices (LVADs) results in reverse remodeling of dystrophin and of the heart itself.

Treatment

The therapy for DCM has changed since the early 1990s from focusing on improving systolic function to improving cardiac efficiency. In the past, inotropic therapy was a mainstay of therapy, whereas today it is less popular. We tend to avoid using inotropic medications as much as possible and instead use combinations of medication aimed at avoiding arrhythmias. Low-dose (renal dose) dopamine, in addition to milrinone and diuretics, has been useful. More recently, neseritide, a BNP synthetic, has been useful in improving urine output and cardiac function. In children requiring intubation and mechanical ventilation, calcium infusion with or without vasopression has worked well in selected patients. In some centers, dobutamine and epinephrine remain mainstays of treatment.

In patients in whom these therapies are ineffective, mechanical assist device therapies using an LVAD device or extracorporeal membrane oxygenator (ECMO) has been lifesaving. We have hypothesized that LVAD treatment reduces mechanical stress on the myocardium, thus enabling reverse remodeling via dystrophin to occur. We previously showed that the

| BOX 283.2 | Genetics of Dilated Cardiomyopathy |

X-Linked Cardiomyopathies
X-Linked Dilated Cardiomyopathy

X-linked dilated cardiomyopathy (XLCM) was described first in 1987 by Berko and Swift as DCM occurring in male patients in the teen years and early 20s with rapid progression from congestive heart failure (CHF) to death resulting from ventricular tachycardia/ventricular fibrillation (VT/VF) or cardiac transplantation. Patients with this condition are distinguished by elevated serum CK-MM. Female carriers tend to develop mild to moderate DCM in the fifth decade of life, and the disease is slowly progressive. In 1993, Towbin and colleagues were the first to identify the disease-causing gene and to characterize the functional defect. In this report, the dystrophin gene was shown to be responsible for the clinical abnormalities, and protein analysis by immunoblotting demonstrated severe reduction or absence of dystrophin protein in the heart of these patients. These findings were confirmed later by Muntoni and associates when a mutation in the muscle promoter and exon 1 of *dystrophin* was identified in another family with XLCM. Subsequently, multiple mutations have been identified in dystrophin in patients with XLCM.

Dystrophin is a cytoskeletal protein that provides structural support to the myocyte by creating a lattice-like network to the sarcolemma. In addition, dystrophin plays a major role in linking the sarcomeric contractile apparatus to the sarcolemma and extracellar matrix. Furthermore, dystrophin is involved in cell signaling, particularly through its interactions with nitric oxide synthase. When mutated, the *dystrophin* gene also is responsible for Duchenne and Becker muscular dystrophy (DMD/BMD). These skeletal myopathies present early in life (DMD is diagnosed in patients younger than age 12 years, whereas BMD is seen in male teenagers older than 16 years of age) and most patients develop DCM before reaching their twenty-fifth birthday. In most patients, CK-MM is elevated similar to that seen in XLCM; in addition, manifesting female carriers develop disease late in life, similar to those with XLCM. Furthermore, immunohistochemical analysis demonstrates reduced levels (or an absence) of dystrophin, similar to that seen in the hearts of patients with XLCM.

Murine models of dystrophin deficiency demonstrate abnormalities of muscle physiology based on membrane structural support abnormalities. In addition to the dysfunction of dystrophin, mutations in dystrophin secondarily affect proteins that interact with dystrophin. At the amino-terminus (N-terminus), dystrophin binds to the sarcomeric protein actin, a member of the thin filament of the contractile apparatus. At the carboxy-terminus (C-terminus), dystrophin interacts with alpha-dystroglycan, a dystrophin-associated membrane-bound protein that is involved in the function of the dystrophin-associated protein complex (DAPC), which includes beta-dystroglycan, the sarcoglycan subcomplex (alpha, beta, gamma, delta, and ε sarcoglycan), syntrophins, and dystrobrevins (see Fig. 283.1). In turn, this complex interacts with alpha-2-laminin and the extracellular matrix. As with dystrophin, mutations in these genes lead to muscular dystrophies with or without cardiomyopathy, a finding supporting the contention that these proteins are important to the normal function of the myocytes of the heart and skeletal muscles. In both cases, mechanical stress appears to play a significant role in the age-onset dependent dysfunction of these muscles. The information gained from the studies on XLCM, DMD, and BMD led us to hypothesize that DCM is a disease of the cytoskeleton/sarcolemma that affects the sarcomere. We also have suggested that dystrophin mutations play a role in idiopathic DCM in male patients. Recently, we showed that 3 of 22 boys with DCM studied for dystrophin mutations using a rapid DNA mutation screening method had mutations and all had elevated CK-MM as well. In addition, eight families with DCM and possible X-linked inheritance also were screened; in three of eight families, dystrophin mutations were noted. Again, CK-MM was elevated in all subjects carrying mutations.

Barth Syndrome

Initially described as X-linked cardioskeletal myopathy with abnormal mitochondria and neutropenia by Neustein and Barth and their colleagues, this disorder typically presents in male infants as CHF associated with neutropenia (cyclic) and 3-methylglutaconic aciduria. Mitochondrial dysfunction is noted on electron microscope and electron transport chain biochemical analysis. Recently, abnormalities in cardiolipin have been noted. Echocardiographically, these infants typically have left ventricular dysfunction with left ventricular dilation, endocardial fibroelastosis, or a dilated hypertrophic left ventricle. In some cases, these infants die of CHF/sudden death VT/VF, or sepsis caused by leukocyte dysfunction. Most of these children survive infancy and do well clinically, although DCM usually persists. In some cases, cardiac transplantation has been performed. Histopathologic evaluation typically demonstrates the features of DCM, although endocardial fibroelastosis may be prominent, and the mitochondria are abnormal in shape and abundance.

The genetic basis of Barth syndrome was described first by Bione and colleagues, who cloned the disease-causing gene, *G4.5*. This gene encodes a novel protein called tafazzin, whose function is not currently known. Researchers have speculated, however, that the gene product is an acyltransferase based on the cardiolipin abnormalities. Mutations in *G4.5* result in a wide clinical spectrum, which includes apparent classic DCM, hypertrophic DCM, endocardial fibroelastosis, or left ventricular noncompaction (LVNC). In the latter case, the LVNC is characterized by deep trabeculations giving the appearance of a "spongiform" myocardium (see Fig. 283.11). The mechanisms responsible for this clinical heterogeneity are not known. More detail is provided regarding LVNC in the section on this disorder.

Autosomal Dominant Dilated Cardiomyopathy

The most common form of inherited DCM is the autosomal dominant form of disease. These patients present as classic "pure" DCM or DCM associated with conduction system disease (CDDC). In the latter case, patients usually present in their 20s with mild CDDC that can progress over the course of decades to complete heart block. DCM usually presents late in the course but is out of proportion to the degree of CDDC. The echocardiographic and histologic findings in both subgroups are classic for DCM, although the conduction system may be fibrotic in patients with CDDC. In both groups of patients with DCM, VT, VF, and torsade de pointes occur and may result in sudden death.

(Continued)

BOX 283.2   (Continued)

Genetic heterogeneity exists for autosomal dominant DCM, with 15 loci mapped for pure DCM and 5 loci for CDDC. In the case of pure DCM, 10 genes have been identified to date and include 3 by our group (delta-sarcoglycan, alpha-actinin-2, ZASP), as well as actin, desmin, troponin T, beta-myosin heavy chain, titin, metavinculin, myosin binding protein C, alpha-tropomyosin, MLP, and phospholamban (see Table 283.1).

Most of the genes identified to date encode either cytoskeletal or sarcomeric proteins. In the case of cytoskeletal proteins (desmin, delta-sarcoglycan, metavinculin, MLP), defects of force transmission are considered to result in the DCM phenotype, whereas defects of force generation have been speculated to cause sarcomeric protein-induced DCM.

Cardiac actin is a sarcomeric protein that is part of the sarcomeric thin filament interacting with tropomyosin and the troponin complex. As previously noted, actin plays a significant role in linking the sarcomere to the sarcolemma via its binding to the N-terminus of dystrophin. Interestingly, the mutations in actin that resulted in DCM as described by Olson and associates appear to be involved directly in the binding of dystrophin, whereas mutations in the sarcomeric end of actin result in hypertrophic cardiomyopathy (HCM). The DCM-causing mutations are thought to result in DCM by causing force transmission abnormalities. Further, actin interacts in the sarcomere with TnT and beta-MHc, two other genes resulting in either DCM or HCM depending on the position of the mutation. In the case of TnT and beta-MHC, force generation abnormalities have been speculated as the responsible mechanism.

Desmin is a cytoskeletal protein that forms intermediate filaments specific for muscle. This muscle-specific 53-kDa subunit of class III intermediate filaments forms connections between the nuclear and plasma membranes of cardiac, skeletal, and smooth muscle. Desmin is found at the Z-lines and intercalated disc of muscle; its role in muscle function appears to involve attachment or stabilization of the sarcomere. Mutations in this gene appear to cause abnormalities of force and signal transmission similar to those thought to occur with actin mutations.

Another DCM-causing gene, *delta-sarcoglycan*, encodes a member of the sarcoglycan subcomplex of the DAPC. This gene encodes for a protein involved in stabilization of the myocyte sarcolemma, as well as signal transduction. Mutations identified in familial and sporadic cases resulted in reduction of the protein within the myocardium. In the absence of delta-sarcoglycan, the remaining sarcoglycans (delta, beta, gamma, epsilon) cannot assemble properly in the endoplasmic reticulum. Mouse models of delta-sarcoglycan deficiency demonstrate dilated, HCM, sarcolemmal fragility, and disrupted vasculin smooth muscle that leads to vascular spasm, including coronary spasm. In addition, mutations in this gene lead to the phenotype of the cardiomyopathic Syrian hamster. Other human mutations in *delta-sarcoglycan* cause a form of autosomal recessive limb girdle muscular dystrophy (LGMD2F) that rarely is associated with heart disease.

The final cytoskeletal protein-encoding gene, *metavinculin*, encodes vinculin and its splice variant metavinculin. Vinculin is expressed ubiquitously, and metavinculin is co-expressed with vinculin in heart, skeletal, and smooth muscle, with this protein complex localized to subsarcolemmal costameres in the heart, where they interact with alpha-actinin, talin, and gamma-actin to form a microfilamentous network linking cytoskeleton and sarcolemma. In addition, these proteins are present in adherens junctions in intercalated discs and participate in cell-cell adhesion. Mutations in metavinculin have been shown to disrupt the intercalated discs and alter actin filament cross-linking.

As previously noted, mutations in the sarcomere may produce HCM or DCM. In the latter case, abnormalities in force generation or transmission are thought to contribute to the development of this phenotype. In addition to mutations in the thin filament protein actin, mutations in the thick filament protein-encoding gene beta-myosin heavy chain have been shown to cause DCM with associated sudden death in at least one infant, as well as DCM in older children and adults. Mutations in this gene are thought to perturb the actin-myosin interaction and force generation or alter cross-bridge movement during contraction. Mutations in cardiac troponin T, a thin filament protein, have been speculated to disrupt calcium-sensitive troponin C binding. Mutations in phospholamban also have been identified that further support calcium handling as a potentially important mechanism in the development of DCM. Interestingly, Haghighi and associates identified homozygous mutations causing DCM and heart failure, whereas heterozygoes had cardiac hypertrophy. Recessive mutation in *troponin I* is thought to impair the interaction with troponin T. alpha-Tropomyosin mutations also have been identified and were predicted to alter the surface charge of the protein leading to impaired interaction with actin.

A recent area of interest for evaluation at the molecular level is the Z-disc. Knoll and colleagues identified mutations in *muscle MLP* and demonstrated that these mutations result in defects in the interaction with telethonin. Using mouse models, these investigators also demonstrated that MLP acts as a stretch sensor and that mutant MLP causes defects in this activity. More recently, Mohapatra and associates demonstrated mutations in MLP in families and sporadic cases and identified abnormalities in the T-tubule system and Z-disc architecture by electron microscopy, which correlates with the histopathology seen in MLP-knockout mice. This finding was supported further by the finding of reduced expression of MLP in chronic human heart failure. In addition, mutations in *alpha-actinin-2*, which is involved in crosslinking actin filaments and shares a common actin binding domain with dystrophin, also were identified in FDCM, which disrupts its binding to MLP. Finally, Vatta and colleagues identified mutations in the Z-band alternatively spliced PDZ-motif protein *ZASP*, the human homolog of the mouse cypher gene, which when disrupted leads to DCM. Multiple mutations in this gene were identified in families and sporadic cases of DCM and with LVNC. This protein, which interacts with alpha-actinin-2, disrupts the actin cytoskeleton when mutated. Another gene, *titin*, which encodes the giant sarcomeric cytoskeletal protein titin that contributes to the maintenance of the sarcomere organization and myofibrillar elasticity, interacts with these proteins at the Z-disc/I-band transition zone. Mutations have been identified in FDCM as well.

(Continued)

| **BOX 283.2** | **(Continued)** |

As seen in pure autosomal dominant DCM, genetic heterogeneity also exists for CDDC. To date, CDDC genes have been mapped to chromosomes 1p1-1q1, 2q14-21, 3p25-22, and 6q23. The only gene thus far identified was reported initially by Fatkin and colleagues and Brodsky and associates to be *lamin A/C* on chromosome 1q21, which encodes a nuclear envelope intermediate filament protein.

The lamins are located in the nuclear lamina at the nucleoplasmic side of the inner nuclear membrane, and lamin A and C are expressed in heart and skeletal muscle. Mutations in this gene initially were reported to cause the au-

tosomal dominant form of Emery-Dreifuss muscular dystrophy, which has skeletal myopathy associated with DCM and conduction system disease. It also has been found to cause a form of autosomal dominant limb girdle muscular dystrophy (LGMD1B), which also is associated with conduction system disease. Multiple mutations have been identified in patients with DCM and conduction system disease, which, in some patients, had mildly elevated CK. This gene defect appears to be a relatively common occurrence in patients with CDDC. The mechanisms responsible for the development of DCM and conduction system abnormalities are unknown.

N-terminus of dystrophin is lost in DCM, and, after weeks of LVAD treatment, reversal occurs, resulting in relinkage of the sarcolemma and sarcomere at the actin-binding domain of dystrophin. More recently, we demonstrated similar findings in the right ventricle as well and showed biventricular reversal using either pulsatile or continuous-flow LVADs. In patients well enough to be treated as outpatients, ACE inhibitors and beta blockers have been shown to be efficacious. The use of diuretics also may be useful. The certainty of efficacy of digoxin has come into question, and controversy also exists regarding the use of "vitamins" such as coenzyme Q10, carnitine, thiamin, riboflavin, and others. In the latter case, these medications usually are reserved for patients with mitochondrial or metabolic-based disease.

Other novel approaches currently undergoing investigation include biventricular pacing (also known as resyndronization therapy). In those patients with AVB, a pacemaker also is appropriate, whereas patients with VT currently are considered for use of internal defibrillators.

Myocarditis

Myocarditis is a process characterized by inflammatory infiltrate of the myocardium with necrosis and/or degeneration of adjacent myocytes not typical of the ischemic damage associated with coronary artery disease. This definition does not account for the underlying cause.

Etiology

Most cases of myocarditis in the United States and Western Europe result from viral infections. The most common viral causes include adenovirus (particularly serotypes 2 and 5) and enterovirus (coxsackieviruses A and B, echovirus, poliovirus), particularly coxsackievirus B (Table 283.2). However, many other viral causes of myocarditis in children and adults, including influenza, cytomegalovirus, herpes simplex virus, parvovirus, hepatitis C, rubella, varicella, mumps, EBV, HIV, and respiratory syncytial virus, among others, have been described. Other nonviral causes include the following: other infectious agents such as rickettsiae, bacteria, protozoa and other parasites, fungi, and yeasts (Table 283.3); various drugs including antimicrobial medications; hypersensitivity, autoimmune, or collagen-vascular diseases such as systemic lupus erythematosus, mixed connective tissue disease, rheumatic fever, rheumatoid arthritis, and scleroderma; toxic reactions to infectious agents (e.g., diphtheria); or other disorders such as Kawasaki disease and sarcoidosis (see Table 283.3). In most cases, however, "idiopathic" myocarditis is encountered.

Epidemiology

Myocarditis is a disorder that is underdiagnosed, but the incidence of the usual lymphocytic form of myocarditis has been reported to be from 4% to 5% (as obtained from reports of young men dying of trauma) to as high as 16% to 21% (as found

TABLE 283.2			

VIRAL POLYMERASE CHAIN REACTION (PCR) ANALYSIS OF MYOCARDITIS AND DILATED CARDIOMYOPATHY (DCM): THE DETECTION OF VIRUSES BY PCR IN MYOCARDIAL SAMPLES

Diagnosis	Samples (n)	PCR-Positive Samples (n)	PCR Amplimer (n)
Myocarditis	624	239 (38%)	Adenovirus 142 (23%)
			Enterovirus 85 (14%)
			Cytomegalovirus 18 (3%)
			Parvovirus 6 (<1%)
			Influenza A 5 (<1%)
			Herpes simplex virus 5 (<1%)
			Epstein-Barr virus 3 (<1%)
			Respiratory syncytial virus 1 (<1%)
DCM	149	30 (20%)	Adenovirus 18 (12%)
			Enterovirus 12 (8%)
Controls	215	3 (1.4%)	Enterovirus 1 (<1%)
			Cytomegalovirus 2 (<1%)

TABLE 283.3

CAUSES OF MYOCARDITIS

Viral	**Other Parasitic**
Coxsackievirus A	*Toxocara canis* (visceral larva
Coxsackievirus B	migrans)
Echoviruses	*Schistosoma*
Rubella virus	*Heterophyes*
Measles virus	*Cysticercus*
Parvovirus	*Echinococcus*
Adenovirus	**Fungi and Yeasts**
Polioviruses	*Actinomyces* and *Arachnia*
Vaccinia virus	*Coccidioides*
Mumps virus	*Echinococcus*
Herpes simplex virus	*Histoplasma*
Epstein-Barr virus	*Candida*
Cytomegalovirus	**Toxic**
Rhinoviruses	Scorpion
Hepatitis viruses	Diphtheria
Arboviruses	**Drugs**
Influenza viruses	Sulfonamides
Varicella virus	Phenylbutazone
Rickettsial	Cyclophosphamide
Rickettsia rickettsii	Neomercazole
Rickettsia tsutsugamushi	Acetazolamide
Bacterial	Amphotericin B
Neisseria meningitidis	Indomethacin
(meningococcus)	Tetracycline
Klebsiella	Isoniazid
Leptospira	Methyldopa
Corynebacterium diphtheriae	Phenytoin
(diphtheria)	Penicillin
Salmonella	**Hypersensitivity/Autoimmune**
Clostridium	Rheumatoid arthritis
Mycobacterium tuberculosis	Rheumatic fever
Brucella	Ulcerative colitis
Legionella pneumophila	Systemic lupus erythematosus
Streptococcus	**Other**
Protozoal	Sarcoidosis
Trypanosoma cruzi	Scleroderma
Toxoplasma gondii	Idiopathic
Entamoeba histolytica	Cornstarch

in autopsy series of children dying suddenly). In adults with unexplained DCM, the reported incidence varies between 3% and 63%, although the large multicenter Myocarditis Treatment Trial, which was strictly based on the "Dallas criteria," reported a 9% incidence.

Usually sporadic, viral myocarditis also can occur as an epidemic. Epidemics usually are seen in newborns, most commonly in association with coxsackievirus B. Intrauterine myocarditis also has been seen during epidemics, as well as sporadically. Postnatal spread of coxsackievirus is via the fecal-oral or airborne route. The WHO reports that this ubiquitous family of viruses results in cardiovascular sequelae in less than 1% of infections, although this incidence increases to 4% when coxsackievirus B3 is considered. Other important viral causes, such as adenovirus and influenza A, are transmitted through the air. Although the disease can occur equally throughout the year, the exact cause probably is season-dependent [in other words, certain viral causes are seasonal (e.g., coxsackievirus) whereas others are year-round conditions (e.g., adenovirus)].

Clinical Manifestations

Differences in presentation are seen depending on the age of the child (i.e., newborn or infant versus child or adolescent), thus rendering establishing the diagnosis challenging. Adults present with findings similar to those of adolescents. In general, myocarditis should be considered in all children and adults with new-onset CHF in whom no other cause is found. In many cases, an antecedent, nonspecific flu-like illness or episode of gastroenteritis may precede the manifestation of symptoms of CHF. The younger the child, the poorer the prognosis, with death reported in more than 50% of neonates and infants (18 months or younger). In a study by Bowles and colleagues, 81% of newborns (78 of 93) with symptomatic myocarditis referred for molecular diagnosis died, with death occurring in 71% (108 of 152) of infants between 1 month and 12 months of age and in 58% (11 of 18) of those 12 to 18 months of age.

Newborns and Infants. Newborns or infants typically present with fever, irritability or listlessness, periodic episodes of pallor (which may precede the sudden onset of cardiorespiratory symptoms including tachypnea or respiratory distress), and diaphoresis. Poor appetite or vomiting also can be seen frequently. Sudden death may occur in this subgroup of children. On physical examination, pallor and mild cyanosis commonly are noted. The skin usually is cool and mottled (and sometimes clammy), consistent with poor perfusion resulting from decreased cardiac output. Respirations usually are rapid and labored; grunting may be prominent, but rales are uncommon findings (in fact, if rales are auscultated, one should strongly consider pneumonia with or without sepsis as the diagnosis). The cardiovascular examination is consistent with CHF and includes resting tachycardia and a gallop rhythm, muffled heart sounds, and frequently an apical systolic murmur caused by mitral regurgitation. In some of these young children, particularly newborns, a tricuspid regurgitation murmur may also be identified. The pulses are usually thready, and hepatomegaly is usually obvious. Depending on the underlying origin, splenomegaly also may be prominent, but it is very uncommon when myocarditis is the cause of heart failure. Arrhythmias (supraventricular tachycardia or VT) or AVB also may occur.

An important point is that the younger the child, the more likely that intrauterine myocarditis occurred and that the findings may be associated more with chronic disease than otherwise expected in acute disease. In addition, as noted, this patient group has the worst prognosis.

Children, Adolescents, and Adults. Older children, adolescents, and adults commonly report a recent history of viral disease, generally 10 to 14 days before presentation. Initial symptoms include lethargy, low-grade fever, and pallor; the child usually has decreased appetite and may complain of abdominal pain. Diaphoresis, palpitations, rashes, intolerance for exercise, and general malaise are common signs and symptoms. Later in the course of illness, respiratory symptoms become predominant; syncope or sudden death may occur as a result of cardiac collapse. Findings on physical examination are consistent with CHF. Unlike in newborns, jugular venous distention and pulmonary rales may be found, and resting tachycardia may be prominent. Arrhythmias, including atrial fibrillation, supraventricular tachycardia, or VT, as well as AVB, may occur.

Diagnostic Evaluation

The diagnosis of myocarditis often is difficult to establish but should be suspected in any infant or child who presents with unexplained CHF or VT. Appropriate diagnostic studies include the following:

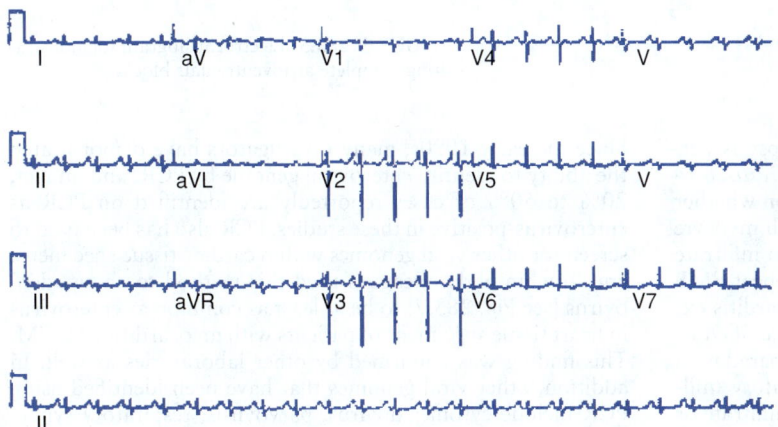

FIGURE 283.3. Electrographic features classically seen in myocarditis. Note the low-voltage QRS complexes.

Chest Radiography. Cardiomegaly with prominent pulmonary vascular markings suggestive of pulmonary edema, possibly consistent with CHF, is notable. Comparisons over the course of time may demonstrate significant improvement or normalization of the chest radiograph within a few months of presentation, a finding suggesting transient disease state (most typically myocarditis).

Electrocardiography. Sinus tachycardia with low-voltage QRS complexes (less than 5 mm total amplitude in all limb leads) with or without low-voltage or inverted T waves classically are described (Fig. 283.3). A pattern of myocardial infarction with wide Q waves (longer than 35 milliseconds) and ST-segment changes also may be seen. VT (Fig. 283.4), supraventricular tachycardia, atrial fibrillation, or AVB occurs in some children (Fig. 283.5).

Echocardiography. A dilated and dysfunctional left ventricle consistent with DCM (i.e., left ventricular end-diastolic and end-systolic dimensions are increased, and shortening and ejection fractions are decreased) is seen on two-dimensional and M-mode echocardiography. Segmental wall motion abnormalities are relatively common findings, but global hypokinesis is predominant. Pericardial effusion frequently occurs. Doppler and color Doppler images commonly demonstrate mitral regurgitation. Dilation of other chambers also may be seen. Cardiac output calculations also may be obtained and typically are reduced. Coronary artery or structural abnormalities, which could result in these features, should be excluded.

Endomyocardial Biopsy. Cardiac catherization and EMB may be performed to obtain cardiac output and intracardiac pressure measurements. Low cardiac output is seen commonly along with elevated end-diastolic ventricular pressures. EMB, usually obtained from the right ventricle, is used to evaluate the myocardium directly for evidence of inflammation histologically (Fig. 283.6). Usually, five tissue specimens are obtained for analysis (as outlined by the Dallas criteria) because the inflammatory infiltrate usually is patchy and scattered in the ventricular myocardium. Evidence of significant mononuclear cell infiltrate is diagnostic of myocarditis, although it does not delineate the cause. Unfortunately, the results of EMB commonly are nondiagnostic, with the incidence of biopsy-proven myocarditis in patients presenting with new-onset CHF and DCM ranging from 3% to 63% of cases. This lack of sensitivity was shown clearly by Hauck and associates, Chow and colleagues, Lie, and others; in fact, using the usual number of specimens (i.e., five biopsy specimens) outlined by the Dallas criteria, only approximately 50% of all true cases of myocarditis will be identified. To identify 80% of cases, 17 or more specimens must be obtained. Because risk is associated with EMB, particularly in young children or those with severe ventricular dilatation, many centers have abandoned this procedure.

Dallas Criteria. This standardized histopathologic definition and classification scheme was devised to minimize the discrepancy or disagreement in diagnosis. It defines myocarditis as "a process characterized by an inflammatory infiltrate of the myocardium with necrosis and/or degeneration of adjacent myocytes not typical of ischemic damage" caused by coronary

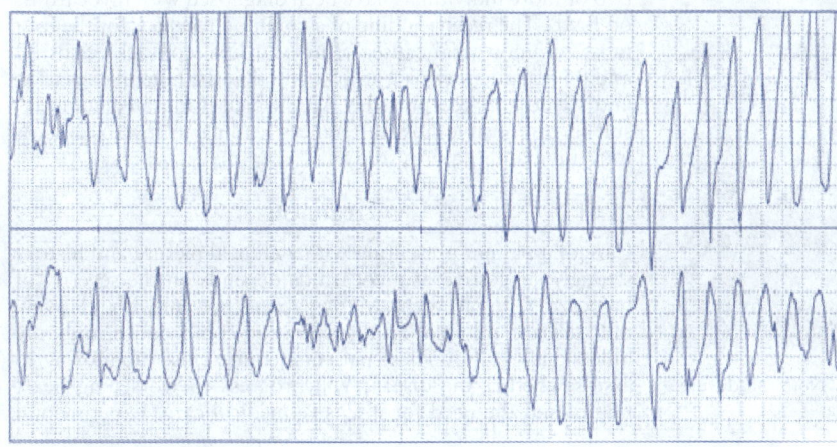

FIGURE 283.4. Electrocardiogram demonstrating ventricular tachycardia.

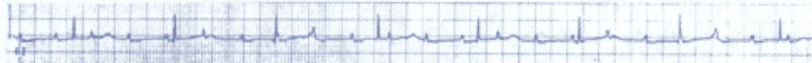

FIGURE 283.5. Electrocardiogram demonstrating complete atrioventricualr block.

artery or other disease. At the time the initial biopsy is performed, a specimen may be classified as *active myocarditis, borderline myocarditis,* or *no myocarditis,* depending on whether an inflammatory infiltrate occurs in association with myocyte degeneration or necrosis (*active*) or too sparse of an infiltrate or no myocyte degeneration occurs (*borderline*). Repeat EMB may be appropriate when strong suspicion of myocarditis exists clinically; on repeat EMB, histology may be classified as *ongoing myocarditis* (similar or worse findings compared with the initial biopsy), *resolving myocarditis* (inflammatory infiltrate diminished), or *resolved myocarditis* (cellular infiltrate or myocyte necrosis no longer present).

Viral Studies. The diagnostic "gold standard" of the viral origin is positive viral culture from the myocardium; this finding is rare, however. Viral cultures of peripheral specimens, such as blood, stool, or urine, are performed commonly but are unreliable at identifying the causative infection. Other studies used to delineate the viral cause include serologic studies in which a fourfold rise in antibody titer is required. Antibody studies commonly performed include type-specific neutralizing, hemagglutination inhibiting, or complement-fixing antibody studies. However, these studies are nonspecific, because prior infection with the causative virus is commonplace. Molecular analysis using *in situ* hybridization has been used to identify coxsackievirus B sequences in myocardial samples, but this method never gained popularity. Currently, PCR has been used to amplify viral sequences rapidly and specifically from cardiac tissue samples (see the following section).

Molecular Diagnostics. In 1986, the first molecular diagnostic approach was reported by Bowles and associates; *in situ* hybridization was performed on myocardial tissue using probes for coxsackievirus. Subsequently, other reports noted the utility of this method in identifying coxsackievirus RNA within cardiac tissue specimens. However, the difficulty of using this technique in the hospital-based setting reduced the interest in pursuing this technique. In 1990, Jin and colleagues first reported the use of PCR in identifying viral genome within the myocardium. This amplification process allows for specific portions of the viral genome of interest to be identified on an agarose gel after electrophoresis and is quite sensitive and specific (Fig. 283.7).

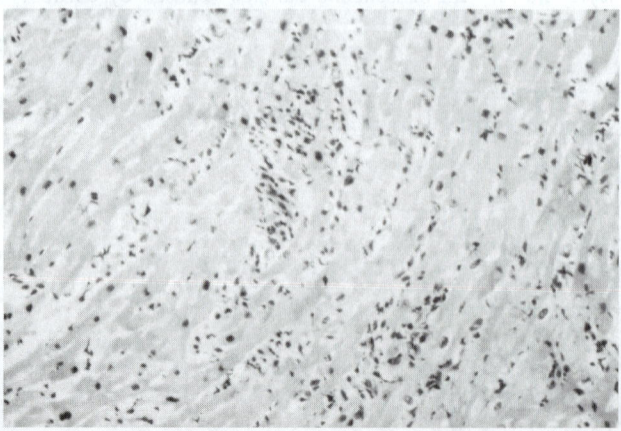

FIGURE 283.6. Histologic findings in myocarditis. Note the diffuse inflammatory infiltrate, myocyte necrosis, and edema.

Since the early 1990s, many investigators have demonstrated the ability to identify enteroviral genome by PCR, and, in fact, 20% to 50% of cases reportedly are identified on PCR as enterovirus-positive in these studies. PCR also has been used to screen for other viral genomes within cardiac tissue specimens, and Towbin and colleagues used this method to show adenovirus (see Fig. 283.7) to be at least as common as enterovirus in heart tissue specimens of patients with myocarditis or DCM. This finding was confirmed by other laboratories as well. In addition, other viral genomes that have been identified using PCR include cytomegalovirus, parvovirus, respiratory syncytial virus, EBV, herpes simplex virus, and influenza A virus. Further, this method has been used to identify mumps virus as the responsible agent in endocardial fibroelastosis, a previously important cause of heart failure in children that has disappeared since the mid-1980s.

PCR analysis usually does not identify viral genome in peripheral blood of patients with myocarditis; however, Akhtar and colleagues demonstrated the ability of this method to identify viral genome in tracheal aspirates of intubated children with myocarditis, thus potentially reducing the need for EMB.

Long-Term Sequelae

When resolution of cardiac dysfunction does not occur, chronic DCM results. What the underlying cause of these long-term sequelae could be has been unclear, but viral persistence and autoimmunity have been speculated widely. Badorff and colleagues demonstrated that enteroviral protease 2A directly cleaves the cytoskeletal protein dystrophin, resulting in dysfunction of this protein (Fig. 283.8). Because mutations in dystrophin are known to cause an inherited form of DCM, as well as the DCM associated with the neuromuscular diseases Duchenne and Becker muscular dystrophy, these mutations are likely responsible to a large extent for the chronic DCM seen in enteroviral myocarditis. Other viruses, such as adenoviruses, also have enzymes that cleave membrane structural proteins or result in activation or inactivation of transcription factors, cytokines, or adhesion molecules to cause chronic DCM. Therefore, a complex interaction between the viral genome and the heart appears to occur and and to result in the long-term outcome of affected patients.

Some reports suggest that myocarditis could be inherited. Support for this suggestion includes the frequent finding of myocardial lymphocytic infiltrate in patients with FDCM and sporadic DCM, as well as the few reports of families in which two or more individuals have been diagnosed with myocarditis on EMB. The recent finding of a common receptor for the four most common viral causes of myocarditis (coxsackievirus B3 and B4 and adenovirus 2 and 5), and that the human coxsackie and adenovirus receptor (HCAR), which if mutated could result in responsible host differences leading to myocarditis, is intriguing and requires study.

Treatment

Care of a patient presenting with a clinical picture and history strongly suggestive of myocarditis depends on the severity of myocardial involvement. Many patients present with relatively mild disease, minimal or no respiratory compromise, and only mild signs of CHF. These patients require close monitoring to assess whether the disease will progress to worsening heart failure and the need for intensive medical care. Experimental

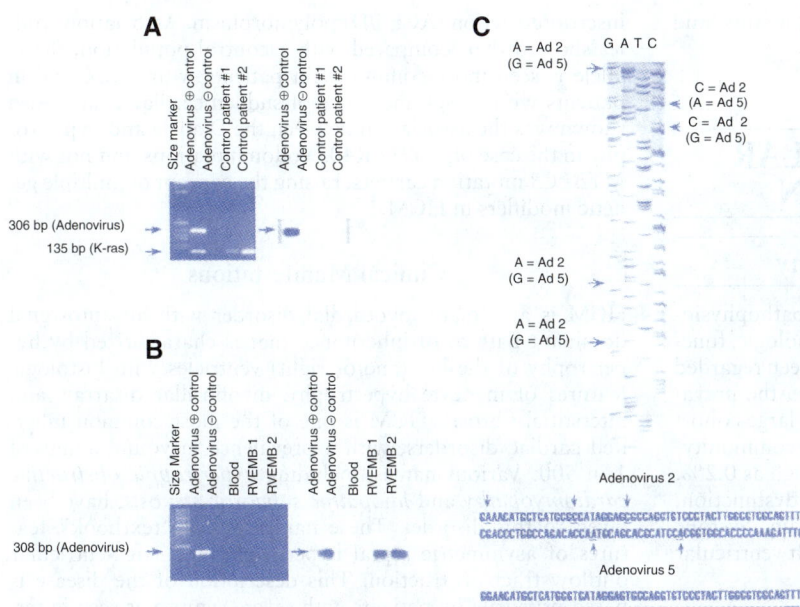

FIGURE 283.7. Adenoviral polymerase chain reaction. **A:** Note the band at 308 base pairs (bp), the size of the expected band for adenovirus as seen in the adenovirus control lane only and confirmed by radioactive blotting. **B:** Note the same 308-bp bands in the control lane and two patients (RV1, RV2). Again, this is confirmed by radioactive blotting. **C:** The sequencing analysis demonstrates type 2 adenovirus.

animal studies suggest that bed rest may prevent an increase in intramyocardial viral replication in the acute stage; thus, to place patients under this restriction at the time of diagnosis appears prudent. Normal arterial blood oxygen levels should be maintained for any patient with compromised hemodynamics resulting in hypoxemia. Although no specific therapy aimed at reversing myocardial injury currently is recommended widely, maintenance of cardiac output at levels that supply adequate tissue perfusion and prevent metabolic disturbances is essential. In cases of CHF, the same general approaches to supportive care as described for heart failure associated with DCM are relevant.

The use of immunosuppressive agents in suspected or proven viral myocarditis is controversial. Some animal studies have suggested an exacerbation of virus-induced cytotoxicity in the presence of immunosuppressive drugs, possibly caused by interference with production of interferon.

Another potential therapeutic option is the use of intravenous gamma-globulin in children with myocarditis. This use is based on the early results of Drucker and colleagues, who investigated the use of this agent in 21 of 46 children with myocarditis. Patients who received this drug had better left ventricular function at follow-up. In addition, survival tended to be higher at 1 year, although the data did not reach statistical significance because of the small number of patients in the study. Whether this approach proves to be beneficial or whether these early results mirror the early published experience with corticosteroids remains to be seen.

LVADs and aortic balloon pumps have been used to support the cardiovascular system in some cases, and ECMO therapy has been used in others. When necessary, the devices may be lifesaving and should be considered as options in children large enough to allow successful placement of the devices. In some circumstances, cardiac transplantation becomes necessary.

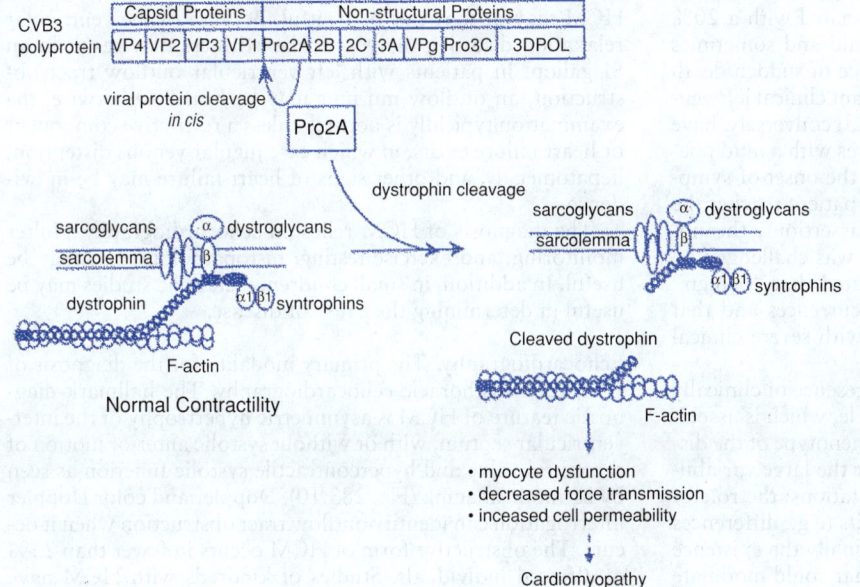

FIGURE 283.8. Coxsackievirus B3 protease 2A cleaves dystrophin, resulting in dilated cardiomyopathy in viral myocarditis.

The prognosis of acute myocarditis in newborns, infants, and children, however, remains poor.

DISEASES OF VENTRICULAR DIASTOLIC FUNCTION

Hypertrophic Cardiomyopathy

HCM is a complex cardiac disease with unique pathophysiologic characteristics and a great diversity of morphologic, functional, and clinical features. Although HCM has been regarded largely as a relatively uncommon cardiac disease, the prevalence of echocardiographically defined HCM in a large cohort of apparently healthy young adults selected from a community-based general population was reported to be as high as 0.2%. The disorder is considered to result from diastolic dysfunction, a disease of relaxation of the ventricular myocardium. Systolic function is preserved or is hypercontractile, and left ventricular outflow tract obstruction may occur.

Genetics of Familial Hypertrophic Cardiomyopathy

The genetics of HCM are described in Box 283.3, Table 283.4, and Figure 283.9.

Genotype-Phenotype Relations. The pattern and extent of left ventricular hypertrophy in patients with HCM vary greatly even in first-degree relatives, and a high incidence of sudden death is reported in selected families. An important issue therefore is to determine whether the genotype heterogeneity observed in HCM accounts for the phenotypic diversity of the disease. However, the results must be seen as preliminary because the available data relate to only a few hundred individuals, and although a given phenotype may be apparent in a small family, examining large or multiple families with the same mutation is required before drawing unambiguous conclusions. Several concepts have been published for mutations in the *MYH7, TNNT2,* and *MYBPC3* genes. For *MYH7,* the prognosis for patients with different mutations has been shown to vary. For example, the R403Q mutation was thought to be associated with markedly reduced survival, whereas some others, such as V606M, appeared more benign. The disease caused by *TNNT2* mutations reportedly was associated with a 20% incidence of nonpenetrance, a relatively mild and sometimes subclinical hypertrophy, but a high incidence of sudden death that occurred even in the absence of significant clinical left ventricular hypertrophy. Mutations in *MYBPC3,* conversely, have been characterized by specific clinical features with a mild phenotype in young subjects, a delayed age at the onset of symptoms, and a favorable prognosis before the patient reaches the age of 40 years. However, despite these assertions, the notion of mutation-specific clinical outcomes was challenged by Van Driest and colleagues, who demonstrated that "benign" mutations were uncommon (5 of 253) occurrences and that the mutations studied all were associated with severe clinical disease.

Genetic studies also have revealed the presence of clinically healthy individuals carrying the mutant allele, which is associated in first-degree relatives with a typical phenotype of the disease. Several mechanisms could account for the large variability of the phenotypic expression of the mutations: the role of environmental differences and acquired traits (e.g., differences in lifestyle, risk factors, and exercise) and finally the existence of modifier genes and/or polymorphisms that could modulate the phenotypic expression of the disease. Significant results have been obtained thus far regarding the influence of the ACE

insertion/deletion (ACE I/D) polymorphism. Association studies showed that, compared with a control population, the D allele is seen more commonly in patients with HCM and in patients with a high incidence of sudden cardiac death. Also shown was the association between the D allele and hypertrophy in the case of *MYH7* R403 codon mutations, but not with *MYBPC3* mutation carriers, raising the concept of multiple genetic modifiers in HCM.

Clinical Manifestations

HCM is a primary myocardial disorder with an autosomal dominant pattern of inheritance that is characterized by hypertrophy of the left (and/or right) ventricles with histologic features of myocyte hypertrophy, myofibrillar disarray, and interstitial fibrosis. HCM is one of the most common inherited cardiac disorders, with a prevalence in young adults of 1 in 500. Various names, including *hypertrophic obstructive cardiomyopathy* and *idiopathic subaortic stenosis,* have been given to this disorder. These names reflect "textbook" features of asymmetric septal hypertrophy and left ventricular outflow tract obstruction. This description of the disease is based primarily on patients with severe symptoms seen in tertiary hospital referral centers. Epidemiologic studies now suggest that a wide spectrum of clinical manifestations of varying severity and prognosis is present in community populations. The first clinical description of HCM was reported in 1869 in France, and HCM was recognized to be a genetic disorder in the late 1950s. Since then, numerous clinical and pathologic studies of HCM have been performed. Since 1990, molecular genetic studies have given important insights into the pathogenesis of HCM and have provided a new perspective for the diagnosis and management of patients with this disorder.

Diagnostic Evaluation

Affected individuals with HCM exhibit significant variability in their clinical presentation. They may be asymptomatic or may present with symptoms ranging from palpitations and dizziness to syncope and sudden death. The age of onset of symptoms varies, with some children presenting at birth or during childhood and others presenting late in life, such as the fifth or sixth decade. Most commonly, patients present in the first 2 decades of life. The physical examination in subjects with HCM may or may not be fruitful. Because of the ventricular relaxation disorder, the ventricular stiffness may result in an S_4 gallop. In patients with left ventricular outflow tract obstruction, an outflow murmur may be heard. Otherwise, the examination typically is normal unless a restrictive component or heart failure exists, in which case jugular venous distention, hepatomegaly, and other signs of heart failure may be in evidence.

The diagnosis of HCM relies on echocardiography, Holter monitoring, and exercise testing; histopathology also may be useful. In addition, in small children, metabolic studies may be useful in determining the cause of disease.

Echocardiography. The primary modality for the diagnosis of HCM is transthoracic echocardiography. The hallmark diagnostic feature of HCM is asymmetric hypertrophy of the interventricular septum, with or without systolic anterior motion of the mitral valve and hypercontractile systolic function as seen by M-mode imaging (Fig. 283.10). Doppler and color Doppler interrogation can identify outflow tract obstruction when it occurs. The obstructive form of HCM occurs in fewer than 25% of affected individuals. Studies of kindreds with HCM have shown that the distribution and severity of left ventricular hypertrophy may vary considerably, that asymmetric hypertrophy

BOX 283.3   Genetics of Familial Hypertrophic Cardiomyopathy

The first gene for familial hypertrophic cardiomyopathy (FHC) was mapped to chromosome 14q11.2-q12 using genome-wide linkage analysis in a large Canadian family. Soon afterward, FHC locus heterogeneity was reported and subsequently was confirmed by the mapping of the second FHC locus to chromosome 1q3 and of the third locus to chromosome 15q2. Carrier and associates mapped the fourth FHC locus to chromosome 11p11.2. Multiple other loci, including loci on chromosomes 7q3, 3p21.2-3p21.3, 12q23-q24.3, 19p13.2-q13.2, and 15q14, subsequently were reported (see Fig. 283.9). Several other families are not linked to any known FHC loci, indicating the existence of additional FHC-causing genes (see Table 283.4).

All the disease-causing genes identified to date code for proteins that are part of the sarcomere (see Fig. 283.9), which is a complex structure with an exact stoichiometry and multiple sites of protein–protein interactions. These interactions include the following: three myofilament proteins—the beta-myosin heavy chain (beta-MyHC), the ventricular myosin essential light chain 1 (MLC-1 s/v), and the ventricular myosin regulatory light chain 2 (MLC-2 s/v); four thin filament proteins: cardiac actin, cardiac troponin T (cTnT), cardiac troponin I (cTnI), and alpha-tropomyosin (alpha-TM); and one myosin-binding protein, the cardiac myosin-binding protein C (cMyBP-C) (see Table 283.4). Each of these proteins is encoded by multigene families that exhibit tissue-specific, developmental, and physiologically regulated patterns of expression. The giant protein titin and its interactive Z-disc protein, MLP, also have been identified. In addition, the gene located on chromosome 7q3 associated with HCM and Wolff-Parkinson-White syndrome was identified as AMPK, which has been suggested to play a role in energy metabolism and cause infiltration of a glycogen-like substance similar to that seen in Pompe disease.

Thick Filament Proteins
Myosin Subunits

Myosin is the molecular motor that transduces energy from the hydrolysis of ATP into directed movement and that, by doing so, drives sarcomere shortening and muscle contraction. Cardiac myosin consists of two heavy chains (MyHC) and two pairs of light chains (MLCs), referred to as essential (or alkali) light chains (MLC-1) and regulatory (or phosphorylatable) light chains (MLC-2), respectively. The myosin molecule is highly asymmetric, consisting of two globular heads joined to a long, rod-like tail. The light chains are arranged in tandem in the head-tail junction. Their function is not fully understood. Neither MLC type is required for the adenosine triphosphatase activity of the myosin head, but they probably modulate it in the presence of actin and contribute power stroke. Mutations have been found in the heavy chains and in the two types of ventricular light chains.

Concerning the heavy chains, the beta isoform (beta-MyHC) is the major isoform of the human ventricle and of slow-twitch skeletal fibers. It is encoded by *MYH7*. This gene appears to be the HCM gene most commonly mutated, and hot spots for mutations have been identified. Most mutations are missense mutations located either in the head or in the head-rod junction of the molecule. Based on their structural location in the myosin head, most mutations are likely to disrupt both mechanical and catalytic components of actin-myosin interactin, resulting in reduced force gen-

eration. Sarcomere assembly also is likely to be disrupted. Mutations in the light meromyosin domain also have been identified, and Blair and colleagues speculated that HCM develops in this case as a result of abnormalities of myosin filament assembly or interactions with thick filament binding proteins.

The MLC isoforms are expressed in the ventricular myocardium and in the slow-twitch muscles and are the so-called ventricular myosin regulatory light chains (MLC-2 s/v) encoded by *MYL2*, and the ventricular myosin essential light chain (MLC-1 s/v) encoded by *MYL3*. The MLCs are thought to influence the mechanical efficiency of cross-bridge cycling and speed of contraction. These proteins are thought to regulate power output via a calcium-dependent mechanism, and disruption leads to the HCM phenotype.

Myosin-Binding Protein C

MyBP-C is part of the thick filaments of the sarcomere, located at the level of the transverse stripes, 43 nm apart, seen by electron microscopy in the sarcomere A band. Its function is uncertain, but, for more than a decade, evidence has existed to indicate both structural and regulatory roles. Partial extraction of cMyBP-C from rat skinned cardiac myocytes and rabbit skeletal muscle fibers alters calcium-sensitive tension, and it has shown that phosphorylation of cMyBP-C alters myosin cross-bridges in native thick filaments, findings suggesting that cMyBP-C can modify force production in activated cardiac muscles. The cardiac isoform is encoded by the *MYBPC3* gene.

Thin Filament Proteins

The thin filament contains actin, the troponin complex, and tropomyosin. The troponin complex and tropomyosin constitute the calcium-sensitive switch that regulates the contraction of cardiac muscle fibers. Mutations have been found in alpha-TM and in two of the subunits of the troponin complex: cTnI, the inhibitory subunit, and cTnT, the tropomyosin-binding subunit.

alpha-TM is encoded by *TPM1*. The cardiac isoform is expressed both in the ventricular myocardium and in fast-twitch skeletal muscles. It shares the overall structure of other tropomyosins that are rod-like proteins that possess a simple dimeric, alpha-coiled coil structure of other tropomyosins that are rod-like proteins that possess a simple dimeric, alpha-coiled coil structure in parallel orientation along their entire length. Researchers suggest that some mutations in this gene could alter tropomyosin binding to actin.

cTnT is encoded by *TNNT2*. In human cardiac muscle, multiple isoforms of cTnT have been described that are expressed in the fetal, adult, and diseased heart and that result from alternative splicing of the single gene *TNNT2*. The precise physiologic relevance of these isoforms remains poorly understood. Mutations in this gene are predicted to influence the inhibitory regulatory effect of the tropomyosin-troponin complex.

cTnI is encoded by *TNNI3*. The cTnI isoform is expressed only in cardiac muscles. Cooperative binding of cTnI to actin-tropomyosin is a unique property of the cardiac variant; mutations are thought to disrupt the calcium-sensitive switch mediated by this protein, resulting in increased calcium sensitivity and reduced maximum tension.

(Continued)

BOX 283.4   (Continued)

alpha-Cardiac actin (ACTC) mutations also cause of FHC. Mogensen and colleagues identified mutations in a family with heterogeneous phenotypes, ranging from asymptomatic with mild hypertrophy to pronounced septal hypertrophy and left ventricular outflow tract obstruction. Mutations in titin and MLP also have been identified, suggesting the Z-disc to be important in the development of HCM, although the mechanism is uncertain.

---

no longer is an essential requirement for the diagnosis of this disorder, and that the features may differ even within the same family. The diagnosis of HCM generally requires exclusion of secondary causes of hypertrophy, such as hypertension or aortic stenosis; however, in some individuals, particularly in older age groups, these conditions may coexist. Differentiating HCM from physiologic left ventricular hypertrophy may be difficult, particularly in competitive athletes. The extent of left ventricular hypertrophy also may vary depending on different mutant genes. For example, individuals with beta-MHC gene mutations usually develop moderate or severe hypertrophy with a high disease penetrance, whereas those with cardiac troponin T gene mutations reportedly have only mild or clinically undetectable hypertrophy. Unusual forms of hypertrophy, localized to the left ventricular apex (cardiac troponin I mutations) or midcavity (cardiac actin and MLC gene mutations), have been reported. The extent of left ventricular hypertrophy also may vary among members of a single family with the same gene mutation, as previously noted. These observations may be explained by a modifying role of additional genetic and environmental factors, such as blood pressure, exercise, diet, and body mass.

Electrocardiography. The ECG tracing may be normal in HCM or may have associated left ventricular hypertrophy or biventricular hypertrophy. Giant QRS complexes are common findings in patients with Pompe disease or LVNC. Preexcitation also may be noted in patients with HCM. Ventricular, atrial, or supraventricular arrhymias may be seen on surface ECG as well. Patients with restrictive physiology may demonstrate atrial enlargement. Holter monitoring also may demonstrate arrhythmias.

Exercise Testing. Risk stratification has been reported with the use of exercise testing, with blunting or reduction of blood pressure and/or blunting of heart rate response to exercise associated with increased risk. In particular, reduction of blood pressure by more than 15 mmHg or failure to increase blood pressure more than 25 mmHg is associated with increased risk. Other associated risk factors include syncope, nonsustained VT, severe left ventricular hypertrophy on echocardiography (more than 3 cm in adults), and a family history of premature death.

Histopathology. The classic features of HCM include myocyte hypertrophy, myofiber disarray, and patchy fibrosis. In some patients, mitochondrial proliferation or morphologic abnormalities with or without inclusion material, glycogen stores, vacuolization, or desmin deposits may be seen.

Metabolic Studies. As in DCM, metabolic and mitochondrial abnormalities may be causative, and, therefore, the same blood, urine, and muscle studies should be obtained. In addition, using fibroblasts for alpha-1, 4-glycosidase (acid maltase) deficiency to diagnose Pompe disease should be considered.

Natural History

The natural history of HCM is variable; some individuals remain asymptomatic throughout life, and others may develop progressive symptoms with or without heart failure or experience sudden death. Longitudinal echocardiographic studies have documented left ventricular remodeling with age. Progressive increases of the thickness of the left ventricular wall have been reported in individuals during adolescence and early adult life. In some individuals, the thickness of the left ventricular wall may increase in later life. Age-related reductions in thickness of the left ventricular wall, associated with myocyte loss and fibrosis, also have been described in individuals with long-standing disease ("burnt out" HCM). From 10% to 20% of individuals with HCM may develop DCM; 10% to 16% of affected adult individuals develop atrial fibrillation, and this risk of atrial fibrillation is increased in those with left atrial enlargement.

HCM is a frequent cause of sudden death, particularly in young individuals and competitive athletes. Estimates of the prevalence of sudden death vary according to the population studied, ranging from less than 1% in the general community to 3% to 6% in tertiary care hospital referral centers. Various mechanisms for sudden death have been proposed and include ventricular bradyarrhythmias caused by sinus node and atrioventricular conduction abnormalities and tachyarrhythmias triggered by reentrant depolarization pathways related to myofibrillar disarray and fibrosis, abnormal calcium homeostasis, myocardial ischemia, left ventricular diastolic dysfunction, or left ventricular outflow tract obstruction. Various risk stratification algorithms based on clinical parameters have been proposed to identify individuals with an increased predisposition to sudden death. Given the complexity of mechanisms that may precipitate sudden death, one is not surprised that no single risk factor has been identified. Conflicting results have been found for the positive predictive value of young age at diagnosis, history of syncope, severity of symptoms, left ventricular wall thickness, left ventricular outflow tract gradient,

TABLE 283.4

HYPERTROPHIC CARDIOMYOPATHY GENETICS

CHR Locus	Gene	Protein
1q32	TNNT2	Cardiac troponin T
2q31	TTN	Titin
3p21.2	MLC-1	Myosin essential light chain
7q31	PRGKγ	AMP kinase
11p11	MYBPC3	Myosin-binding protein C
11p15.1	MLP	Muscle LIM protein
12q2.3	MLC-2	Myosin regulatory light chain
14q12	MYH7	beta-Myosin heavy chain
15q14	ACTC	Cardiac actin
15q22	TPM1	alpha-Tropomyosin
19p13.2	TNNI3	Cardiac troponin I

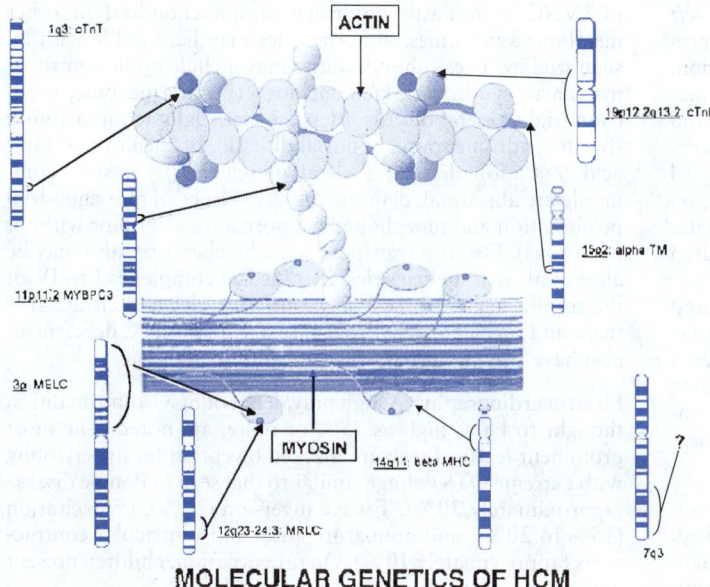

MOLECULAR GENETICS OF HCM

FIGURE 283.9. Genetics of hypertrophic cardiomyopathy. Shown are the chromosomal regions, genes, and proteins causing hypertrophic cardiomyopathy. All affected genes encode sarcomeric proteins.

left atrial size, atrial fibrillation, exercise response of blood pressure, and heart rate. Genotype also has been suggested to predict outcome. The mechanisms whereby HCM gene mutations influence prognosis are unknown. Although some HCM mutations that alter the charge of the encoded amino acid have been associated with a poor outcome, other mutations that alter the charge have a good prognosis. Genetic studies and animal model studies, including electrophysiologic studies in mouse models, may provide important insights into the differential propensity for sudden death among different HCM gene mutations.

Treatment

The mainstay of therapy in children with HCM has been pharmacologic approaches. The two major medication classes used are beta blockers and calcium channel blockers. In small children, we have used propranolol as our drug of choice because of its ease of access, liquid formulation, and low side effect profile. Therapy in these children is monitored by heart rate response, with the goal being approximately 80 to 100 beats/minute. Therapy typically ranges in dosage from 2 to 5 mg/kg/day, divided three times daily. Verapamil has been popular in some institutions and reportedly results in good outcomes. In older children, we typically treat with atenolol; in children with excessive hypertrophy and severe outflow tract obstruction, we occasionally consider use of combination therapy (beta blocker plus calcium channel blocker), although this approach is not

without risk. However, the risk-to-benefit ratio must be determined for each patient.

When standard pharmacologic therapy fails, options are limited, although the size of the child plays a role. In small children, myomectomy is the only proven option. Again, this option is not without risk. In older patients, pacing protocols have been used, but that approach is controversial. In adults, alcohol septal ablation has been utilized, but it has not been championed in children yet because of the long-term uncertainties associated with creating an infarct in a young individual.

In patients with syncope, ventricular arrhythmias, or other presumed high-risk factor, internal defibrillator implantation should be considered. In some patients, pacing is necessary as well.

Finally, in children with metabolic or mitochondrial dysfunction underlying the HCM, metabolic therapies have been successful on occasion. Similar to the therapy in DCM caused by these deficiencies, carnitine, coenzyme Q10, riboflavin, and thiamin may be considered.

OVERLAP DISORDERS

Left Ventricular Noncompaction

This disorder has been considered to be a rare disease and has been identified by a variety of names including *spongy*

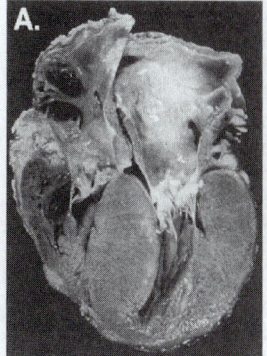
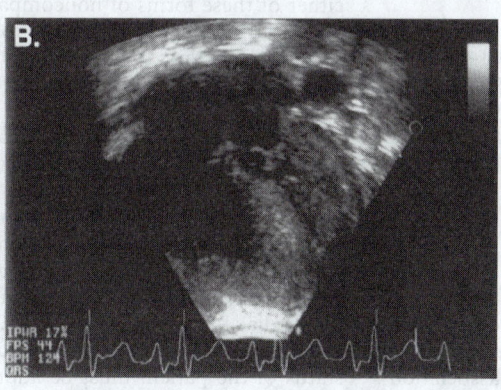

FIGURE 283.10. Hypertrophic cardiomyopathy. Anatomic (**A**) and echocardiographic (**B**) features of hypertrophic cardiomyopathy with a thickened interventricular septum and left ventricular posterior wall.

myocardium, fetal myocardium, and *noncompaction of the left ventricular myocardium.* The abnormality is thought to represent an arrest in the normal process of myocardial compaction, the final stage of myocardial morphogenesis, resulting in persistence of multiple prominent ventricular trabeculations and deep intertrabecular recesses. This cardiomyopathy is somewhat difficult to diagnose unless the physician has a high level of suspicion during echocardiographic evaluation. In fact, on careful review of echocardiograms and other clinical data, LVNC appears to be a relatively common finding in children and is also seen in adults.

Two forms of LVNC occur: (a) isolated noncompaction and (b) noncompaction associated with congenital heart disease such as septal defects (ventricular and/or atrial septal defect), pulmonic stenosis, and hypoplastic left heart syndrome, among others. In the isolated form and the form associated with congenital heart disease, metabolic derangements may be notable.

Genetics

When LVNC is inherited, it can be transmitted as an X-linked, mitochondrial, autosomal recessive or autosomal dominant trait. In approximately 20% to 30% of cases, familial inheritance has been identified. The X-linked form usually is associated with isolated noncompaction and a mutation in the G4.5 (tafazzin) gene located on chromosome Xq28. This gene also has been identified in patients with Barth syndrome.

In autosomal dominant inherited cases, mutations in the Z-line protein encoding ZASP, located on chromosome 10q22, have been identified in isolated noncompaction, and mutations in the gene encoding alpha-dystrobrevin, a cytoskeletal protein located on chromosome, have been identified in patients with noncompaction associated with congenital heart disease. No genes have been identified thus far for autosomal recessive inherited noncompaction, but mutations in mitochondrial DNA have been seen in patients with noncompaction.

Clinical Manifestations

LVNC most commonly presents in infancy with signs and symptoms of heart failure, but some patients are identified during later childhood, adolescence, or adulthood. Pignatelli and associates recently reported the findings on 36 children identified over the course of a 5-year period, with the median age at presentation being 90 days (range, 1 day to 17 years). In this study, 40% of the children presented with low cardiac output or CHF, and only one child (3%) presented with syncope. The most common presenting symptom other than heart failure was asymptomatic ECG or radiographic abnormalities, with 42% asymptomatic. In addition, 14% of children had associated dysmorphic features, and 19% of affected children had first-degree relatives with cardiomyopathy. One of the children with dysmorphic features was diagnosed with DiGeorge syndrome, and another one had congenital adrenal hyperplasia.

Diagnostic Evaluation

The usual evaluation includes an ECG, chest radiograph, and echocardiogram, as well as Holter monitoring, blood and urinary studies, and skeletal muscle biopsy. These studies, in addition to the clinical evaluation and a high degree of suspicion, should lead to a higher likelihood of establishing the correct diagnosis.

Chest Radiography. Chest radiographs commonly demonstrate cardiomegaly (20%) or signs of heart failure such as increased pulmonary vascular markings (40%).

Metabolic Testing. Blood and urine studies, as well as muscle biopsy with biochemical analysis, are important diagnostic tests in patients with LVNC. Because of the association

of LVNC with Barth syndrome or mitochondrial or other metabolic syndromes, abnormalities may be notable with all such studies. These abnormalities may include cyclic neutropenia (Barth syndrome), lactic acidosis (Barth syndrome, mitochondrial or metabolic disorders), 3-methylglutaconic aciduria (Barth syndrome, mitochondrial disease), of carnitine or fatty acid oxidation defects; skeletal muscle biopsy results commonly are abnormal, demonstrating evidence of mitochondrial proliferation and morphologic abnormalities (with or without inclusions). Electron transport chain biochemistry also may be abnormal, with deficiencies identified in complexes I to IV of the respiratory chain in association with elevated citrate synthase and succinate dehydrogenase. Cytochrome C deficiencies also have been reported.

Electrocardiography. A high prevalence of ECG abnormalities, thought to be as high as 75% or more, are noted. The most prominent features seen are marked biventricular hypertrophy with extreme QTS voltage similar to that seen in Pompe disease (approximately 30%), T-wave inversion (20%), preexcitation (15% to 20%), and premature atrial and ventricular contractions (approximately 10%). On rare occasion, children present with supraventricular tachycardia or VT.

Echocardiography. Two-dimensional echocardiography demonstrates the classic features of noncompaction including noncompaction morphology of deep trabeculations and intertrabecular recesses and ventricular hypertrophy (especially apical hypertrophy) with or without dilation (Fig. 283.11). In nearly 90% of patients, systolic dysfunction is noted at presentation. Most commonly, the left ventricle alone is affected (80%), whereas biventricular noncompaction occurs in approximately 20% of children. Congenital heart disease occurs in 10% to 20% of children and should be evaluated specifically. Doppler interrogation identifies abnormal mitral inflow velocities consistent with restrictive physiology (decreased E/A ratio) in approximately half of the cases. Interestingly, several children demonstrate increased hypertrophy, and systolic function normalizes (or becomes hypercontractile) before reverting to the initial phenotype. In rare instances, thrombi (particularly in the intertrabecular apical recesses) are noted.

Treatment

The specific therapy depends on the clinical and echocardiographic findings. In patients with systolic dysfunction and heart failure, anticongestive therapy identical to that used in patients with DCM is appropriate. In particular, ACE inhibitors such as captopril (in young children) and enalapril (in older children capable of swallowing pills), as well as beta-adrenergic blocking agents such as metoprolol or carvedilol are useful. Diuretics also may be needed. However, in those patients exhibiting findings more consistent with an HCM or diastolic dysfunction physiologic phenotype, beta-blocker therapy alone with propranolol or atenolol is more appropriate. In patients with either of these forms of noncompaction with associated mitochondrial or metabolic dysfunction, some investigators add a "vitamin cocktail" to the cardiac therapy, with coenzyme Q10, carnitine, riboflavin, and thiamin commonly used alone or in combination.

In patients having associated congenital heart disease, appropriate therapeutic approaches may include simple pharmacologic therapy with diuretics for volume overload associated with left-to-right shunts, more complex pharmacologic therapy for patients with restrictive physiology and pulmonary hypertension, or invasive therapy with catheter intervention or surgical repairs, depending on the lesions. Intimate understanding of the cardiac function abnormalities, evidence of thrombi (which should be treated with anticoagulation), and the metabolic status of the patient must be addressed by the interventional

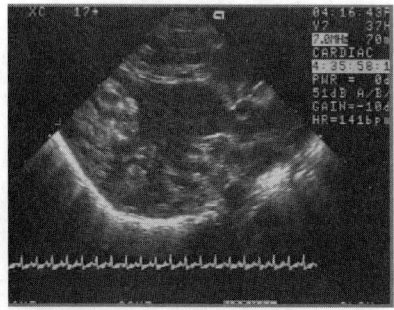

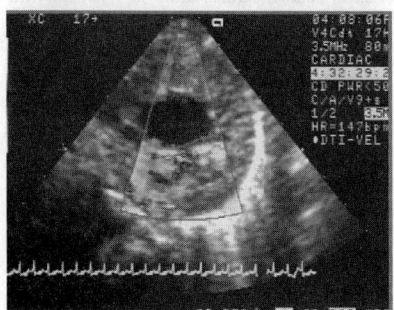

LV NONCOMPACTION

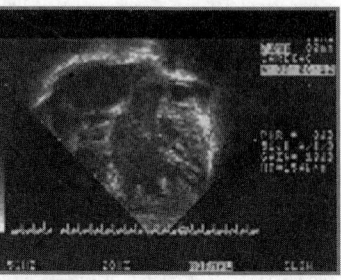

FIGURE 283.11. Left ventricular noncompaction. Echocardiogram with Doppler tissue imaging. Note the highly trabeculated left ventricle with deep recesses in the free wall creating the appearance of holes in the myocardium in left ventricular noncompaction or "spongy myocardium" (**top left**). The trabeculations are well seen by color, with blood noted in some of the trabeculations. In the apical four-chamber view (**right**), the hypertrophic, trabeculated, dilated left ventricule is well seen. LA, left atrium; LV, left ventricle; RA, right atrium; RV, right ventricle.

cardiologist, cardiac anesthesiologist, and surgeon in approaching these patients invasively. In addition, cardiac rhythm disturbances need to be identified, and therapies such as pacemakers, implantable defibrillators, and intracardiac ablations need to be considered.

The clinical outcome of patients with noncompaction has been reported to be poor, with death resulting from heart failure or sudden death, presumably related to arrhythmia or stroke, caused by embolization of left ventricular thrombi. However, Pignatelli and colleagues demonstrated a 5-year survival rate of 86%; when patients who had undergone cardiac transplantation were added, the 5-year survival free of death or cardiac transplantation was 75%.

Suggested Readings

Aaronson KD, Schwartz JS, Chen TM, et al. Development and prospective evaluation of a clinical index to predict survival in ambulatory patients referred for cardiac transplant evaluation. *Circulation* 1997;95:2660.

Abelman WH, Lorrell BH. The challenge of cardiomyopathy. *J Am Coll Cardiol* 1989;13:1219.

Ainger LE, Lawyer NG, Fitch CW. Neonatal rubella myocarditis. *Br Heart J* 1966;28:691.

Akhtar N, Ni J, Langston C, et al. PCR diagnosis of viral pneumonitis from fixed-lung tissue in children. *Biochem Mol Med* 1996;58:66.

Arad M, Benson DW, Perez-Atayde AR, et al. Constitutively active AMP kinase mutations cause glycogen storage disease mimicking hypertrophic cardiomyopathy. *J Clin Invest* 2002;109:357.

Araishi K, Sasaoka T, Imamura M, et al. Loss of the sarcoglycan complex and sarcospan leads to muscular dystrophy in beta-sarcoglycan-deficient mice. *Hum Mol Genet* 1999;8:1589.

Arber S, Hunter JJ, Ross J Jr, et al. MLP-deficient mice exhibit a disruption of cardiac cytoarchitectural organization, dilated cardiomyopathy, and heart failure. *Cell* 1997;88:393.

Archard LC, Bowles NE, Olsen EGJ, et al. Detection of persistent coxsackie B virus in dilated cardiomyopathy and myocarditis. *Eur Heart J* 1987;8:437.

Archard LC, Khan MA, Soteriou BA, et al. Characterization of coxsackie B virus RNA in myocardium from patients with dilated cardiomyopathy by nucleotide sequencing of reverse transcription-nested polymerase chain reaction products. *Hum Pathol* 1998;29:578.

Aretz HT, Billingham ME, Edwards WD, et al. Myocarditis: a histopathologic definition and classification. *Am J Cardiovasc Pathol* 1987;1:3.

Arola A, Touminen J, Ruuskanen O, et al. Idiopathic dilated cardiomyopathy in children: prognostic indicators and outcome. *Pediatrics* 1998;101:369.

Badorff C, Lee GH, Lamphear BJ, et al. Enteroviral protease 2A cleaves dystrophin: evidence of cytoskeletal disruption in an acquired cardiomyopathy. *Nat Med* 1999;5:320.

Baig MK, Goldman JH, Caforio ALP, et al. 1998. Familial dilated cardiomyopathy: cardiac abnormalities are common in asymptomatic relatives and may represent early disease. *J Am Coll Cardiol* 31:195.

Banergee P, Banergee T, Khand A, et al. Diastolic heart failure: neglected or misdiagnosed? *J Am Coll Cardiol* 2001;39:138.

Barbaro G, Di Lorenzo G, Grisorio B, et al. Incidence of dilated cardiomyopathy and detection of HIV in myocardial cells of HIV-positive patients. *N Engl J Med* 1998;339:1093.

Barresi R, Di Blasi C, Negri T, et al. Disruption of heart sarcoglycan complex and severe cardiomyopathy caused by beta sarcoglycan mutations. *J Med Genet* 2000;37:102.

Barth AL, Nathke IS, Nelson WJ. Cadherins, catenins and APC protein: interplay between cytoskeletal complexes and signaling pathways. *Curr Opin Cell Biol* 1997;9:683.

Barth PG, Scholte HR, Berden JA, et al. An X-linked mitochondrial disease affecting cardiac muscle, skeletal muscle and neutrophil leukocytes. *J Neurol Sci* 1983;62:327.

Begley D, Mohiddin S, Fananapazir L. Dual chamber pacemaker therapy for mid-cavity obstructive hypertrophic cardiomyopathy. *Pacing Clin Electrophysiol* 2001;24:1639.

Benjamin EJ, Wolf PA, D'Agostino RB, et al. Impact of atrial fibrillation on the risk of death: the Framingham Heart Study. *Circulation* 1998;78:946.

Bergelson JM, Cunningham JA, Drouguett G, et al. Isolation of a common receptor for coxsackie B viruses and adenoviruses 2 and 5. *Science* 1997;275:1320.

Berko BA, Swift M. X-linked dilated cardiomyopathy. *N Engl J Med* 1987;316:1186.

Berkovich S, Rodriguez-Torres R, Lin JS. Virologic studies in children with acute myocarditis. *Am J Dis Child* 1968;115:207.

Bione S, D'Adamo P, Maestrini E, et al. A novel X-linked gene, G4.5, is responsible for Barth syndrome. *Nat Genet* 1996;12:385.

Blair E, Redwood C, Ashrafian H, et al. Mutations in the α2 subunit of AMP-activated protein kinase cause familial hypertrophic cardiomyopathy: evidence for a central role of energy compromise in disease pathogenesis. *Hum Mol Genet* 2001;10:1215.

Blair E, Redwood C, de Jesus Oliveira M, et al. Mutations of the light meromyosin domain of the β-myosin heavy chain rod in hypertrophic cardiomyopathy. *Circ Res* 2002;90:263.

Bleyl SB, Mumford BR, Thompson V, et al. Neonatal, lethal noncompaction of the left ventricular myocardium is allelic with Barth syndrome. *Am J Hum Genet* 1997;61:868.

Bonne G, Carrier L, Bercovici J, et al. Cardiac myosin binding protein-C gene splice acceptor site mutation is associated with familial hypertrophic cardiomyopathy. *Nat Genet* 1995;11:438.

Bonne G, DiBarletta MR, Varnous S, et al. Mutations in the gene encoding lamin A/C cause autosomal dominant Emery-Dreifuss muscular dystrophy. *Nat Genet* 1999;21:285.

Bowles NE, Bowles KR, Towbin JA. The "Final Common Pathway" hypothesis and inherited cardiovascular disease: the role of cytoskeletal proteins in dilated cardiomyopathy. *Herz* 2000;25:168.

Bowles NE, Ni J, Kearney DL, et al. Detection of viruses in myocardial tissues by polymerase chain reaction: evidence of adenovirus as a common cause of myocarditis in children and adults. *J Am Coll Cardiol* 2003;42:466.

Bowles NE, Richardson PJ, Olsen EGJ, et al. Detection of coxsackie-B virus specific RNA sequences in myocardial biopsy samples from patients with myocarditis and dilated cardiomyopathy. *Lancet* 1986;1:1120.

Bowles NE, Rose ML, Taylor P. End-stage dilated cardiomyopathy: persistence of enterovirus RNA in myocardium at cardiac transplantation and lack of immune response. *Circulation* 1989;80:1128.

Bowles NE, Towbin JA. Molecular aspects of myocarditis. *Curr Opin Cardiol* 1998;13:179.

Bowles NE, Towbin JA. Molecular aspects of myocarditis. *Curr Infect Dis Rep* 2000;2:134.

Bowles NE, Vallejo J. Viral causes of cardiac inflammation. *Curr Opin Cardiol* 2003;18:182.

Braunwald E. Expanding indications for beta-blockers in heart failure. *N Engl J Med* 2001;344:1711.

Brodsky GL, Muntoni F, Miocic S, et al. Lamin A/C gene mutation associated with dilated cardiomyopathy with variable skeletal muscle involvement. *Circulation* 2000;101:473.

Burridge K, Chrzanowska-Wodnicka M. Focal adhesions, contractility, and signaling. *Annu Rev Cell Dev Biol* 1996;12:463.

Calabrese F, Rigo E, Milanesi O, et al. Molecular diagnosis of myocarditis and dilated cardiomyopathy in children: clinicopathologic features and prognostic implications. *Diagn Mol Pathol* 2002;11:212.

Campbell KP. Three muscular dystrophies: loss of cytoskeleton-extracellular matrix linkage. *Cell* 1995;80:675.

Capetanaki Y. Desmin cytoskeleton: a potential regulator of muscle mitochondrial behaviour and function. *Trends Cardiovasc Med* 2002;12:339.

Carrier L, Hengstenberg C, Beckmann JS, et al. Mapping of a novel gene for familial hypertrophic cardiomyopathy to chromosome 11. *Nat Genet* 1993;4:311.

Chan KY, Iwahara M, Benson LN, et al. Immunosuppressive therapy in the management of acute myocarditis in children: a clinical trial. *J Am Coll Cardiol* 1991;17:458.

Chang SM, Lakkis NM, Franklin J, et al. Predictors of outcome after alcohol septal ablation therapy in patients with hypertrophic obstructive cardiomyopathy. *Circulation* 2004;109:824.

Chang WJ, Iannaccone ST, Lau KS, et al. Neuronal nitric oxide synthase and dystrophin-deficient muscular dystrophy. *Proc Natl Acad Sci USA* 1996;93:9142.

Channer KS, McLean KA, Lawson-Matthew P, et al. Combination diuretic treatment in severe heart failure: randomized controlled trial. *Br Heart J* 1994;71:146.

Charron P, Dubourg O, Desnos M, et al. Clinical features and prognostic implications of familial hypertrophic cardiomyopathy related to cardiac myosin binding protein C gene. *Circulation* 1998;97:2230.

Chaudary S, Jaski BE. Fulminant mumps myocarditis. *Ann Intern Med* 1989;110:569.

Chen R, Tsuji T, Ichida F, et al. Mutation analysis of the G4.5 gene in patients with isolated left ventricular noncompaction. *Mol Genet Metab* 2002;77:319.

Chin TK, Perloff JK, Williams RG, et al. Isolated noncompaction of left ventricular myocardium: a study of eight cases. *Circulation* 1990;82:507.

Chow LH, Radio SJ, Sears TD, et al. Insensitivity of right ventricular biopsy in the diagnosis of myocarditis. *J Am Coll Cardiol* 1989;14:915.

Codd MB, Sugrue DD, Gersh BJ, et al. Epidemiology of idiopathic dilated and hypertrophic cardiomyopathy: a population-based study in Olmsted County, Minnesota, 1975–1984. *Circulation* 1989;80:564.

Cohen JJ. Apoptosis. *Immunol Today* 1993;14:126.

Cohn JN, Bristow MR, Chien KR, et al. Report of the National Heart, Lung, and Blood Institute Special Emphasis Panel on Heart Failure Research. *Circulation* 1997;95:766.

Coral-Vazquez R, Cohn RD, Moore SA, et al. Disruption of the sarcoglycan-sarcospan complex in vascular smooth muscle: a novel mechanism for cardiomyopathy and muscular dystrophy. *Cell* 1999;98:465.

Coughlin SS, Szklo M, Baughman K, et al. The epidemiology of idiopathic dilated cardiomyoypathy in a biracial community. *Am J Epidemiol* 1990;131:48.

Cox GF, Kunkel LM. Dystrophies and heart disease. *Curr Opin Cardiol* 1997;12:329.

D'Adamo P, Fassone L, Gedeon A, et al. The X-linked gene G4.5 is responsible for different infantile dilated cardiomyopathies. *Am J Hum Genet* 1997;61:862.

Dalakas MC, Park K-Y, Semino-Mora C, et al. Desmin myopathy a skeletal myopathy with cardiomyopathy caused by mutations in the desmin gene. *N Engl J Med* 2000;342:770.

Dec GW, Fallon JT, Southern JF, et al. "Borderline" myocarditis: an indication for repeat endomyocardial biopsy. *J Am Coll Cardiol* 1990;15:283.

Dec GW, Palacios IF, Fallon JT, et al. Active myocarditis in the spectrum of acute dilated cardiomyopathies: clinical features, histologic correlates, and clinical outcome. *N Engl J Med* 1985;312:885.

Di Barletta R, Ricci E, Galluzzi G, et al. Different mutations in the LMNA gene cause autosomal dominant and autosomal recessive Emery-Dreifuss muscular dystrophy. *Am J Hum Genet* 2000;66:1407.

Doiuchi J, Hamada M, Ito T, et al. Comparative effects of calcium-channel blockers and beta-adrenergic blocker on early diastolic time intervals and A-wave ratio in patients with hypertrophic cardiomyopathy. *Clin Cardiol* 1987;10:26.

Drucker NA, Colan SD, Lewis AB, et al. Gamma-globulin treatment of acute myocarditis on the pediatric population. *Circulation* 1994;89:252.

Emery AE. The muscular dystrophies. *Lancet* 2002;359:687.

Fatkin D, Graham RM. Molecular mechanisms of inherited cardiomyopathies. *Physiol Rev* 2002;82:945.

Fatkin D, MacRae C, Sasaki T, et al. Missense mutations in the rod domain of the lamin A/C gene as causes of dilated cardiomyopathy and conduction-system disease. *N Engl J Med* 1999;34:1715.

Feng J, Yan J, Buzin CH, et al. Comprehensive mutation scanning of the dystrophin gene in patients with nonsyndromic X-linked dilated cardiomyopathy. *J Am Coll Cardiol* 2002;40:1120.

Feng J, Yan J, Buzin CH, et al. Mutations in the dystrophin gene are associated with sporadic dilated cardiomyopathy. *Mol Genet Metab* 2002;77:119.

Ferlini A, Galie N, Merlini L, et al. A novel Alu-like element rearranged in the dystrophin gene causes a splicing mutation in a family with X-linked dilated cardiomyopathy. *Am J Hum Genet* 1998;63:436.

Francis GS, Wilson-Tang WH. Pathophysiology of congestive heart failure. *Rev Cardiovasc Med* 2003;4(suppl 2):S14.

Franz W-M, Muller M, Muller AJ, et al. Association of nonsense mutation of dystrophin gene with disruption of sarcoglycan complex in X-linked dilated cardiomyopathy. *Lancet* 2000;355:1781.

French WJ, Criley JM. Caution in the diagnosis and treatment of myocarditis. *Am J Cardiol* 1984;54:445.

Frenneaux MP. Assessing the risk of sudden cardiac death in a patient with hypertrophic cardiomyopathy. *Heart* 2004;90:570.

Friedman RA, Schowengerdt KO, Towbin JA. Myocarditis. In: Bricker JT, Garson A Jr, Fisher DJ, et al., eds. *The science and practice of pediatric cardiology*, 2nd ed. Philadelphia: Williams & Wilkins, 1998:1777.

Friman G. The incidence and epidemiology of myocarditis. *Eur Heart J* 1999;20:1063.

Frishman W, Kraus ME, Zabkar J, et al. Infectious mononucleosis and fatal myocarditis. *Chest* 1977;72:535.

Furukawa T, Ono Y, Tsuchiya H, et al. Specific interaction of the potassium channel beta-subunit minK with the sarcomeric protein T-cap suggests a T-tubule-myofibril linking system. *J Mol Biol* 2001;313:775.

Gaffney TE, Braunwald EB. Importance of the adrenergic nervous system in the support of circulatory function in patients with congestive heart failure. *Am J Med* 1963;34:320.

Gardner AJS, Short D. Four faces of acute myopericarditis. *Br Heart J* 1973;35:433.

Garvey SM, Rajan C, Lerner AP, et al. The muscular dystrophy with myositis (mdm) mouse mutation disrupts a skeletal muscle-specific domain of titin. *Genomics* 2002;79:146.

Geier C, Perrot A, Ozcelik C, et al. Mutations in the human muscle LIM protein gene in families with hypertrophic cardiomyopathy. *Circulation* 2003;107:1390.

Geisterfer-Lowrance AA, Kass S, Tanigawa E, et al. A molecular basis for familial hypertrophic cardiomyopathy: a β-cardiac myosin heavy chain gene missense mutation. *Cell* 1990;62:999.

Gerber TC, Nishimura RA, Holmes DR Jr, et al. Left ventricular and biventricular pacing in congestive heart failure. *Mayo Clin Proc* 2001;76:803.

Gerul B, Gramlich M, Atherton J, et al. Mutations of TTN encoding the giant muscle filament titin, cause familial dilated cardiomyopathy. *Nat Genet* 2002;30:201.

Goldfarb LG, Park K-Y, Cervenakova L, et al. Missense mutations in desmin associated with familial cardiac and skeletal myopathy. *Nat Genet* 1998;19:402.

Gollob MH, Green MS, Tang ASL, et al. Identification of a gene responsible for familial Wolff-Parkinson-White syndrome. *N Engl J Med* 2001;344:1823.

Graber HL, Unverferth DV, Baker PB, et al. Evolution of hereditary cardiac conduction and muscle disorder: a study involving a family with 6 generations affected. *Circulation* 1986;74:21.

Grady RM, Grange RW, Lau KS, et al. Role for α-dystrobrevin in the pathogenesis of dystrophin-dependent muscular dystrophies. *Nat Cell Biol* 1999;1:215.

Granzier H, Labeit S. The grant protein titin: a major player in myocardial mechanics, signaling, and disease. *Circ Res* 2004;94:284.

Gregorio CC, Antin PB. To the heart of myofibril assembly. *Trends Cell Biol* 2000;10:355.

Griffin LD, Kearney D, Ni J, et al. Analysis of formalin-fixed and frozen myocardial autopsy samples for viral genome in childhood myocarditis and dilated cardiomyopathy with endocardial fibroelastosis using polymerase chain reaction (PCR). *Cardiovasc Pathol* 1995;4:3.

Grist NR, Reid D. General pathogenicity and epidemiology. In: Bendinelli M, Friedman H, eds. *Coxsackieviruses: a general update*. New York: Plenum Press, 1962:241.

Grogan M, Redfield MM, Bailey KR, et al. Long-term outcome of patients with biopsy-proven myocarditis: comparison with idiopathic dilated cardiomyopathy. *J Am Coll Cardiol* 1995;26:80.

Grunig E, Tasman JA, Kucherer H, et al. Frequency and phenotypes of familial dilated cardiomyopathy. *J Am Coll Cardiol* 1998;31:186.

Gulick T, Chung MK, Pieper SJ, et al. Interleukin-1 and tumor necrosis factor inhibit cardiac myocyte β-adrenergic responsiveness. *Proc Natl Acad Sci USA* 1989;86:6753.

Hack AA, Cordier L, Shoturma DI, et al. Gamma-sarcoglycan deficiency leads to muscle membrane defects and apoptosis independent of dystrophin. *J Cell Biol* 1999;142:1279.

Hackman P, Vihola A, Haravuori H, et al. Tibial muscular dystrophy is a titinopathy caused by mutations in TTN, the gene encoding the grant skeletal muscle protein titin. *Am J Hum Genet* 2002;71:492.

Haghighi K, Kolokathis F, Pater L, et al. Human phospholamban null results in lethal diliated cardiomyopathy revealing a critical difference between mouse and human. *J Clin Invest* 2003;111:869.

Hauck AJ, Kearney DL, Edwards WD. Evaluation of postmortem endomyocardial biopsy specimens from 38 patients with lymphocytic myocarditis: implication for role of sampling error. *Mayo Clin Proc* 1989;64:1235.

Heart Failure Society of American (HFSA) Practice Guidelines. HFSA guilde-lines for management of patients with heart failure caused by left ventricular systolic dysfunction-pharmacological approaches. *J Card Fail* 1999;5:357.

Henke A, Nain M, Stelzner A, et al. Induction of cytokine release from human monocytes by coxsackievirus infection. *Eur Heart J* 1991;12(suppl D):134.

Herskowitz A, Wu T-C, Willoughby SB, et al. Myocarditis and cardiotropic vi-ral infection associated with severe left ventricular dysfunction in late-stage infection with human immunodeficiency virus. *J Am Coll Cardiol* 1994; 24:1025.

Hilton DA, Variend S, Pringle JH. Demonstration of coxsackie virus RNA in formalin-fixed tissue sections from childhool myoarditis by in situ hybridiza-tion and the polymerase chain reaction. *J Pathol* 1993;170:45.

Hirschman ZS, Hammer SG. Coxsackie virus myopericarditis: a microbiological and clinical review. *Am J Cardiol* 1974;34:224.

Hobs RE, Pelegrin D, Ratliff NB, et al. Lymphocytic myocarditis and dilated cardiomyopathy: treatment with immunosuppressive agents. *Cleve Clin J Med* 1989;56:628.

Hoffman EP, Brown RH, Kunkel LM. Dystrophin: the protein product of the Duchenne muscular dystrophy locus. *Cell* 1987;51:919.

Hofmann PA, Hartzell HC, Moss RL. Alterations in Ca^{2+} sensitive tension due to partial extraction of C-protein from rat skinned cardiac myocytes and rabbit skeletal muscle fibers. *J Gen Physiol* 1991;97:1141.

Huber SA. Autoimmunity in myocarditis: relevance of animal models. *Clin Im-munol Immunopathol* 1997;83:93.

Hunkeler NM, Kullman J, Murphy AM. Troponin I isoform expression in human heart. *Circ Res* 1991;69:1409.

Hunt SA, Baker DW, Chin MH, et al. ACC/AHA guidelines for the evaluation and management of chronic heart failure in the adult: Executive Summary: a Report of the American College of Cardiology/American Heart Association Task Force on Practice Guidelines. *J Am Coll Cardiol* 2001;38:2101.

Hutchins GM, Vie SA. The progression of interstitial myocarditis to idiopathic endocardial fibroelastosis. *Am J Pathol* 1972;66:483.

Ichida F, Hamamichi Y, Miyawaki T. Clinical features of isolated noncom-paction of the ventricular myocardium: long-term clinical course, hemo-dynamic properties, and genetic background. *J Am Coll Cardiol* 1999;34: 233.

Ichida F, Tsubata S, Bowles KR, et al. Novel gene mutations in patients with left ventricular noncompaction or Barth syndrome. *Circulation* 2001;103:1256.

Jarcho JA, McKenna W, Pare JAP, et al. Mapping a gene for familial hypertrophic cardiomyopathy to chromosome 14q1. *N Engl J Med* 1989;321:1372.

Jessup M, Brozena S. Heart failure. *N Engl J Med* 2003;348:2007.

Jin O, Sole M, Butany J. Detection of enterovirus RNA in myocardial biopsies from patients with myocarditis and cardiomyopathy using gene amplification by polymerase chain reaction. *Circulation* 1990;82:8.

Johnston J, Kelley RI, Feigenbaum A, et al. Mutation characterization and genotype-phenotype correlation in Barth syndrome. *Am J Hum Genet* 1997;61:1053.

Jung D, Duclos F, Apostal B, et al. Characterization of delta-sarcoglycan, a novel component of the oligomeric sarcoglycan complex involved in limb-girdle muscular dystrophy. *J Biol Chem* 1996;271:32321.

Jung M, Poepping I, Perrot A, et al. Investigation of a family with autosomal dom-inant dilated cardiomyopathy defines a novel locus on chromosome 2q14-q22. *Am J Hum Genet* 1999;65:1068.

Kamisago M, Sharma SD, DePalma SR, et al. Mutations in sarcomere protein genes as a cause of dilated cardiomyopathy. *N Engl J Med* 2000;343:1688.

Kaprielian RR, Stevenson S, Rothery SM, et al. Distinct patterns of dystrophin organization in myocyte sarcolemma and transverse tubules of normal and diseased human myocardium. *Circulation* 2000;101:2586.

Karjalainen J, Nieminen MS, Heikkila J. Influenza A1 myocarditis in conscripts. *Acta Med Scand* 1980;20:27.

Karjalainen J, Viitasalo M, Kala R, et al. 24-hour electrocardiographic recordings in mild acute infectious myocarditis. *Ann Clin Res* 1984;16:34.

Kasper EK, Agema WR, Hutchins GM, et al. The causes of dilated cardiomy-opathy: a clinicopathologic review of 673 consecutive patients. *J Am Coll Cardiol* 1994;23:586.

Kass S, MacRae C, Graber HL, et al. A gene defect that causes conduction sys-tem disease and dilated cardiomyopathy maps to chromosome 1p1-1q1. *Nat Genet* 1994;7:546.

Katz AM. Cytoskeletal abnormalities in the failing heart. Out on a LIM? *Circu-lation* 2000;101:2672.

Kaye DM, Lefkovits J, Jennings GL, et al. Adverse consequences of high sympa-thetic nervous activity in the failing human heart. *J Am Coll Cardiol* 1995; 26:1257.

Keeling PJ, McKenna WJ. Clinical genetics of dilated cardiomyopathy. *Herz* 1994;19:91.

Kelley RI, Cheatham JP, Clark BJ, et al. X-linked dilated cardiomyopathy with neutropenia, growth retardation, and 3-methylglutaconic aciduria. *J Pediatr* 1991;119:738.

Khand A, Gemmel I, Clark AL, et al. Is the prognosis of heart failure improving? *J Am Coll Cardiol* 2000;36:2284.

Kimby AG, Sodermark T, Volpe U, et al. Stokes-Adams attacks requiring pace-maker treatment in three patients with acute nonspecific myocarditis. *Acta Med Scand* 1980;207:177.

Kimura A, Harada H, Park JE, et al. Mutations in the cardiac troponin I gene associated with hypertrophic cardiomyopathy. *Nat Genet* 1997;16:379.

Kleinert S, Weintraub RG, Wilkinson JL, et al. Myocarditis in children with dilated cardiomyopathy: incidence and outcome after duel therapy immuno-suppression. *J Heart Lung Transplant* 1997;16:1248.

Klietsch R, Ervasti JM, Arnold W, et al. Dystrophin-glycoprotein complex and laminin colocalize to the sarcolemma and transverse tubules of cardiac mus-cle. *Circ Res* 1993;72:349.

Knoll R, Hoshijima M, Hoffman HM, et al. The cardiac mechanical stretch sensor machinery involves a Z disc complex that is defective in a subset of human dilated cardiomyopathy. *Cell* 2002;11:943.

Koenig M, Hoffman EP, Bertelson CJ, et al. Complete cloning of the C (DMD) cDNA and preliminary genomic organization of the DMD gene in normal and affected individuals. *Cell* 1987;50:509.

Konno S, Sakakibara S. Endomyocardial biopsy. *Chest* 1963;44:345.

Konstam MA. Progress in heart failure management? Lessons from the real world. *Circulation* 2000;102:1076.

Konstam MA, Rousseau MF, Kroneberg MW, et al. Effects of the angiotensin converting enzyme inhibitor enalapril on the long-term progression of left ventricular dysfunction in patients with heart failure. *Circulation* 1992; 86:431.

Kroemer G, Martinez AC. Cytokines and autoimmune disease. *Clin Immunol Immunopathol* 1991;61:275.

Kubota T, McTiernan CF, Frye CS, et al. Cardiospecific overexpression of tumor necrosis factor-alpha causes lethal myocarditis. *J Card Fail* 1997;3:117.

Kucera JP, Rohr S, Rudy Y. Localization of sodium channels in intercalated disks modulates cardiac conduction. *Circ Res* 2002;91:1176.

Kyu BS, Matsumori A, Sato Y. Cardiac persistence of enteroviral RNA detected by polymerase chain reaction in a murine model of dilated cardiomyopathy. *Circulation* 1992;86:522.

Lane JR, Neumann DA, Lafond-Walker A, et al. Interleukin 1 or tumor necrosis factor can promote coxsackie B3–induced myocarditis in resistant B10.A mice. *J Exp Med* 1992;175:1123.

Lane JR, Neumann DA, Lafond-Walker A, et al. Role of IL-I and tumor necro-sis factor in coxsackie virus–induced autoimmune myocarditis. *J Immunol* 1993;151:1682.

Lees-Miller JP, Helfman DM. The molecular basis for tropomyosin isoform di-versity. *Bioessays* 1991;13:429.

Lejemtel TH, Sonnenblick EH, Frishman WH. Diagnosis and management of heart failure. In: Fuster V, Alexander RW, O'Rourke RA, eds. *Hurst's the heart*, 10th ed. Philadelphia: McGraw-Hill, 2001:687.

Li D, Tapscott T, Gonzalez O, et al. Desmin mutations responsible for idiopathic dilated cardiomyopathy. *Circulation* 1999;100:461.

Lie JT. Myocarditis and endomyocardial biopsy in unexplained heart failure: a diagnosis in search of a disease (editorial). *Ann Intern Med* 1988;109:525.

Lipshultz SE, Easley KA, Orav EJ. Left ventricular structure and function in children infected with human immunodeficiency virus. *Circulation* 1998; 97:1246.

Lipshultz SE, Sleeper LA, Towbin JA, et al. The incidence of pediatric cardiomy-opathy in two regions of the United States. *N Engl J Med* 2003;348:1647.

Lorber A, Zonis A, Maisuls E, et al. The scale of myocardial involvement in varicella myocarditis. *Int J Cardiol* 1988;20:257.

Lorell BH. Use of calcium channel blockers in hypertrophic cardiomyopathy. *Am J Med* 1985;78:43.

Lowry PJ, Thompson RA, Little WA. Humoral immunity in cardiomyopathy. *Br Heart J* 1983;50:390.

Lozinski GM, Davis GC, Krous HF, et al. Adenovirus myocarditis: retrospec-tive diagnosis by gene amplification from formalin-fixed, paraffin-embedded tissues. *Hum Pathol* 1994;25:831.

Lurie PR, Fujita M, Neustein HB. Transvascular endomyocardial biopsy in in-fants and small children: description of a new technique. *Am J Cardiol* 1978; 42:453.

MacRae CA, Ghaisas N, Kass S, et al. Familial hypertrophic cardiomyopathy with Wolff-Parkinson-White syndrome maps to a locus on chromosome 7q3. *J Clin Invest* 1995;96:1216.

Maeda M, Holder E, Lowes B, et al. Dilated cardiomyopathy associated with deficiency of the cytoskeletal protein metavinculin. *Circulation* 1997;95:17.

Maron BJ. Appraisal of dual-chamber pacing therapy in hypertrophic cardiomy-opathy: too soon for a rush to judgment? *J Am Coll Cardiol* 1996;27:431.

Maron BJ. Hypertrophic cardiomyopathy and sudden death: new perspective on risk stratification and prevention with the implantable cardioverter-defibrillator. *Eur Heart J* 2000;21:1979.

Maron BJ. Hypertrophic cardiomyopathy: a systemic review. *JAMA* 2002; 287:1308.

Maron BJ, Carney KP, Lever HM, et al. Relationship of race to sudden cardiac death in competitive athletes with hypertrophic cardiomyopathy. *J Am Coll Cardiol* 2003;41:974.

Maron BJ, Gardin JM, Flack JM, et al. Prevalence of hypertrophic cardiomyopa-thy in a general population of young adults: echocardiographic analysis of 411 subjects in the CARDIA study. *Circulation* 1995;92:785.

Martin AB, Webber S, Fricker FJ, et al. Acute myocarditis: rapid diagnosis by PCR in children. *Circulation* 1994;90:330.

Mason JW. Distinct forms of myocarditis. *Circulation* 1991;83:1110.

Mason JW, O'Connell JB, Herskowitz A, et al. A clinical trial of immunosup-pressive therapy for myocarditis. *N Engl J Med* 1995;333:269.

Matsumori A, Yamada T, Suzuki H, et al. Increased circulating cytokines in patients with myocarditis and cardiomyopathy. *Br Heart J* 1994;72:561.

McKenna WJ, Behr ER. Hypertrophic cardiomyopathy: management, risk strat-ification, and prevention of sudden death. *Heart* 2002;87:169.

Meng H, Leddy JJ, Frank J, et al. The association of cardiac dystrophin with myofibrils/Z-discs regions in cardiac muscle suggests a novel role in the contractile apparatus. *J Biol Chem* 1996;271(21):12364.

Mesnard L, Logeart D, Taviaux S, et al. Human cardiac troponin T: cloning and expression of new isoforms in the normal and failing heart. *Circ Res* 1995;76:687.

Messina DN, Speer MC, Pericak-Vance MA, et al. Linkage of familial dilated cardiomyopathy with conduction defect and muscular dystrophy to chromosome 6q23. *Am J Hum Genet* 1997;61:909.

Mestroni L, Miani D, DiLenarda A, et al. Clinical and pathologic study of familial dilated cardiomyopathy. *Am J Cardiol* 1990;65:1449.

Michels VV, Driscoll DJ, Miller FA, Jr. Familial aggregation of idiopathic dilated cardiomyopathy. *Am J Cardiol* 1985;55:1232.

Michels VV, Moll PP, Miller FA, et al. The frequency of familial dilated cardiomyopathy in a series of patients with idiopathic dilated cardiomyopathy. *N Engl J Med* 1992;326:77.

Milasin J, Muntoni F, Severini CM, et al. A point mutation in the 5′ splice site of the dystrophin gene first intron responsible for X-linked dilated cardiomyopathy. *Hum Mol Genet* 1996;5:73.

Mogensen J, Klausen IC, Pederson AK, et al. α-Cardiac actin is a novel disease gene in familial hypertrophic cardiomyopathy. *J Clin Invest* 1999;103:T39.

Mohapatra B, Jimenez S, Lin JH, et al. Mutations in the muscle LIM protein and α-actinin-2 genes in dilated cardiomyopathy and endocardial fibroelastosis. *Mol Genet Metab* 2003;80:207.

Molander N. Sudden natural death in later childhood and adolescence. *Arch Dis Child* 1982;57:572.

Monrad ES, Matsumori A, Murphy JC, et al. Therapy with cyclosprine in experimental murine myocarditis with encephalomyocarditis virus. *Circulation* 1986;73:1058.

Moolman JC, Corfield VA, Posen G, et al. Sudden death due to troponin T mutations. *J Am Coll Cardiol* 1997;29:549.

Moran AM, Colan SD. Verapamil therapy in infants with hypertrophic cardiomyopathy. *Cardiol Young* 1998;8:310.

Muchir A, Bonne G, van der Kooi AJ, et al. Identification of mutations in the gene encoding lamin A/C in autosomal dominant limb girdle muscular dystrophy with atrioventricular conduction disturbance (LGMD1B). *Hum Mol Genet* 2000;9:1453.

Muntoni F, Cau M, Ganau A, et al. Brief report: deletion of the dystrophin muscle-specific promoter region associated with X-linked dilated cardiomyopathy. *N Engl J Med* 1993;329:921.

Murphy RT, Mogensen J, Shaw A, et al. Novel mutation in cardiac troponin I in recessive idiopathic dilated cardiomyopathy. *Lancet* 2004;363:371.

Nagueh SF, Ommen SR, Lakkis NM, et al. Comparison of ethanol septal reduction therapy with surgical myectomy for the treatment of hypertrophic obstructive cardiomyopathy. *J Am Coll Cardiol* 2001;38:1701.

Nakajima-Taniguchi C, Matsui H, Fujio Y, et al. Novel missense mutation in cardiac troponin T gene found in Japanese patient with hypertrophic cardiomyopathy. *J Mol Cell Cardiol* 1997;29:839.

Neumann DA, Lane JR, Allen GS, et al. Viral myocarditis leading to cardiomyopathy: do cytokines contribute to pathogenesis? *Clin Immunol Immunopathol* 1993;68:181.

Neuspiel DR, Kuller LH. Sudden and unexpected natural death in childhood and adolescence. *JAMA* 1985;254:1321.

Neustein HD, Lurie PR, Dahms B, et al. An X-linked recessive cardiomyopathy with abnormal mitochondria. *Pediatrics* 1979;64:24.

Neuwald AF. Barth syndrome may be due to an acyltransferase deficiency. *Curr Biol* 1997;7:R465.

Ni J, Bowles NE, Kim Y-H, et al. Viral infection of the myocardium in endocardial fibroelastosis: molecular evidence for the role of mumps virus as an etiological agent. *Circulation* 1997;95:133.

Nielsen CD, Killip D, Spencer WH 3rd. Nonsurgical septal reduction therapy for hypertrophic obstructive cardiomyopathy: short-term results in 50 consecutive procedures. *Clin Cardiol* 2003;26:275.

Nigro V, de Sa Moreira E, Piluso G, et al. Autosomal recessive limb-girdle muscular dystrophy, LGMD2F, is caused by a mutation in the delta-sarcoglycan gene. *Nat Genet* 1996;14:195.

Nigro V, Okazaki Y, Belsito A, et al. Identification of the Syrian hamster cardiomyopathy gene. *Hum Mol Genet* 1997;6:601.

Nimura H, Bachinski LL, Sangwatanaroj S, et al. Mutations in the gene for cardiac myosin-binding protein C and late-onset familial hypertrophic cardiomyopathy. *N Engl J Med* 1998;338:1248.

Noren GR, Adams P Jr, Anderson RC. Positive skin reactivity to mumps virus antigen in endocardial fibroelastosis. *J Pediatr* 1963;62:604.

Noren GR, Staley NA, Bandt CM, et al. Occurrence of myocarditis in sudden death in children. *J Forensic Sci* 1977;22:188.

Novak KJ, Wattanasikichaigood D, Goebel HH, et al. Mutations in the skeletal muscle alpha-actin gene in patients with actin myopathy and nemaline myopathy. *Nat Genet* 1999;23:208.

Nugent AW, Danbeney PEF, Chondros P, et al. The epidemiology of childhood cardiomyopathy in Australia. *N Engl J Med* 2003;348:1639.

O'Connell JB, Bristow MR. Economic impact of heart failure in the United States: time for a different approach. *J Heart Lung Transplant* 1994;13:S107.

O'Connell JB, Fowles RE, Robinson JA, et al. Clinical and pathologic findings of myocarditis in two families with dilated cardiomyopathy. *Am Heart J* 1984;167:127.

Okabe M, Fukuda K, Arakawa K, et al. Chronic variant myocarditis associated with hepatitis C virus infection. *Circulation* 1997;96:22.

Olson TM, Doan TP, Kishimoto NY, et al. Inherited and de novo mutations in the cardiac actin gene cause hypertrophic cardiomyopathy. *J Mol Cell Cardiol* 2000;32:1687.

Olson TM, Illenberger S, Kishimoto NY, et al. Metavinculin mutations alter actin interaction in dilated cardiomyopathy. *Circulation* 2002;105:431.

Olson TM, Keating MT. Mapping a cardiomyopathy locus to chromosome 3p22-p25. *J Clin Invest* 1996;97:528.

Olson TM, Kishimoto NY, Whitby FG, Michels VV. Mutations that alter the surface charge of alpha-tropomyosin are associated with dilated cardiomyopathy. *J Mol Cell Cardiol* 2001;33:723.

Olson TM, Michels VV, Thibodeau SN, et al. Actin mutations in dilated cardiomyopathy, a heritable form of heart failure. *Science* 1998;280:750.

Ommen SR, Nishimura RA. Hypertrophic cardiomyopathy. *Curr Probl Cardiol* 2004;29:239.

O'Rourke RA. Cardiac pacing: an alternative treatment for selected patients with hypertrophic cardiomyopathy and adjunctive therapy for certain patients with dilated cardiomyopathy. *Circulation* 1999;100:786.

Ortiz-Lopez R, Li H, Su J, et al. Evidence for a dystrophin missense mutation as a cause of X-linked dilated cardiomyopathy. *Circulation* 1997;95:2434.

Ortlepp JR, Vosberg HP, Reith S, et al. Genetic polymorphisms in the renninangiotensin-aldosterone system associated with expression of left ventricular hypertrophy in hypertrophic cardiomyopathy: a study of five polymorphic genes in a family with a disease causing mutation in the myosin binding protein C gene. *Heart* 2002;87:270.

Osama SM, Krishnamurti S, Gupta DN. Incidence of myocarditis in varicella. *Ind Heart J* 1979;31:315.

Ozawa E, Yoshida M, Suzuki A, et al. Dystrophin-associated proteins in muscular dystrophy. *Hum Mol Genet* 1995;4:1711.

Parillo JE, Cunnion RE, Epstein SE, et al. A prospective, randomized, controlled trial of prednisone for dilated cardiomyopathy. *N Engl J Med* 1989;321:1061.

Park TH, Lakkis NM, Middleton KJ, et al. Acute effect of nonsurgical septal reduction therapy on regional left ventricular asynchrony in patients with hypertrophic obstructive cardiomyopathy. *Circulation* 2002;106:412.

Pauschinger M, Bowles NE, Fuentes-Garcia FJ, et al. Detection of adenoviral genome in the myocardium of adult patients with idiopathic left ventricular dysfunction. *Circulation* 1999;99:1348.

Perez-Atayde A, Pulido S. Acute and subacute myocarditis. *Cardiovasc Rev Rep* 1984;5:912.

Petrof BJ, Shrager JB, Stedman HH, et al. Dystrophin protects the sarcolemma from stresses developed during muscle contraction. *Proc Natl Acad Sci USA* 1993;90:3710.

Pignatelli RH, McMahon CJ, Dreyer WJ, et al. Clinical characterization of left ventricular noncompaction in children: a relatively common form of cardiomyopathy. *Circulation* 2003;108:2672.

Pitt B, Zannad F, Remme WJ, et al. The effect of spironolactone on morbidity and mortality in patients with severe heart failure. *N Engl J Med* 1999;341:709.

Poetter K, Jiang H, Hassanzadeh S, et al. Mutations in either the essential or regulatory light chains of myosin are associated with a rare myopathy in human heart and skeletal muscle. *Nat Genet* 1996;13:63.

Poole-Wilson PA, Swedberg K, Cleland JFG, et al. Comparison of carvedilol and metoprolol on clinical outcomes in patients with chronic heart failure in the Carvedilol vs. Metoprolol European Trial (COMET): randomized controlled trial. *Lancet* 2003;362:7.

Puchkov GF, Minkovich BM. A case of respiratory syncytial virus infection in a child by interstitial myocarditis with lethal outcome. *Arkh Patol* 1972;34:70.

Pyle WG, Solaro RJ. At the crossroads of myocardial signaling: the role of Z-discs in intracellular signaling and cardiac function. *Circ Res* 2004;94:296.

Regitz-Zagrosek V, Daehmlow S, Knueppel T, et al. Novel mutations in the β-myosin heavy chain and myosin binding protein C gene are associated with dilated cardiomyopathy. *Circulation* 2001;104(suppl 2):II572.

Reinlib L, Abraham W. Recovery from heart failure with circulatory assist: a working group of the National Heart, Lung, and Blood Institute. *J Card Fail* 2003;9:459.

Report of the 1995 World Health Organization/International Society and Federation of Cardiology Task Force on the Definition and Classification of Cardiomyopathies. *Circulation* 1996;93:841.

Ribaux P, Bleicher F, Couble ML, et al. Voltage-gated sodium channel (SkM1) content in dystrophin-deficient muscle. *Pflugers Arch* 2001;441:746.

Rosenberg HS, McNamara DG. Acute myocarditis in infancy and childhood. *Prog Cardiovasc Dis* 1964;7:179.

Sakamoto A, Abe M, Masaki T. Delineation of genomic deletion in cardiomyopathic hamster. *FEBS Lett* 1999;447:124.

Sakamoto A, Ono K, Abe M, et al. Both hypertrophic and dilated cardiomyopathies are caused by mutation of the same gene, delta-sarcoglycan, in hamster: an animal model of disrupted dystrophin-associated glycoprotein complex. *Proc Natl Acad Sci USA* 1997;94:13873.

Schiaffino S, Reggiani C. Molecular diversity of myofibrillar proteins: gene regulation and functional significance. *Physiol Rev* 1996;76:371.

Schlame M, Kelley R, Feigenbaum A, et al. Phospholipid abnormalities in children with Barth syndrome. *J Am Coll Cardiol* 2003;42:1994.

Schlame M, Towbin JA, Heerdt PM, et al. Deficiency of tetralinoleoyl-cardiolipin in Barth syndrome. *Ann Neurol* 2002;51:634.

Schmitt JP, Kamisago M, Asahi M, et al. Dilated cardiomyopathy and heart failure caused by a mutation in phospholamban. *Science* 2003;299:1410.

Schonian U, Crombach M, Maser S, et al. Cytomegalovirus associated heart muscle disease. *Eur Heart J* 1995;16(suppl):46.

Schowengerdt KO, Ni J, Denfield SW, et al. Parvovirus B19 infection as a cause of myocarditis and cardiac allograft rejection: diagnosis using the polymerase chain reaction (PCR). *Circulation* 1997;96:3549.

Schwartz SM, Duffy JY, Pearl JM, et al. Cellular and molecular aspects of myocardial dysfunction. *Crit Care Med* 2001;29:S214.

Seidman JG, Seidman C. The genetic basis for cardiomyopathy: from mutation identification to mechanistic paradigms. *Cell* 2001;108:557.

Seko Y, Matsuda H, Kato K, et al. Expression of intercellular adhesion molecule-1 in murine hearts with acute myocarditis caused by coxsackievirus B3. *J Clin Invest* 1993;91:1327.

Senni M, Redfield MM. Heart failure with preserved systolic function: a different natural history? *J Am Coll Cardiol* 2001;38:1277.

Shanes JG, Ghali J, Billingham ME, et al. Inter-observer variability in the pathologic interpretation of endomyocardial biopsy results. *Circulation* 1987;75:401.

Shapiro LM, Rozkovec A, Cambridge G, et al. Myocarditis in siblings leading to chronic heart failure. *Eur Heart J* 1983;4:742.

Shimizu C, Rambaud C, Cheron G, et al. Molecular identification of viruses in sudden infant death associated with myocarditis and pericarditis. *Pediatr Infect Dis J* 1995;14:584.

Smith SC, Allen PM. Neutralization of endogenous tumor necrosis factor ameliorates the severity of myosin-induced myocarditis. *Circ Res* 1992;70:856.

Solomon SD, Jarcho JA, McKenna WJ, et al. Familial hypertrophic cardiomyopathy is a genetically heterogeneous disease. *J Clin Invest* 1990;86:993.

Springer TA. Adhesion receptors of the immune system. *Nature* 1990;346:425.

Squire JM. Architecture and function in the muscle sarcomere. *Curr Opin Struct Biol* 1997;7:247.

Sterner G. Adenovirus infections in childhood: an epidemiological and clinical survey among Swedish children. *Acta Paediatr* 1962;142:1.

Stevens PJ, Underwood Ground KE. Occurrence and significance of myocarditis in trauma. *Aerospace Med* 1970;41:770.

Stevenson WG, Stevenson LW. Prevention of sudden death in heart failure. *J Cardiovasc Electrophysiol* 2001;12:112.

Stewart M. Intermediate filament structure and assembly. *Curr Opin Cell Biol* 1993;5:3.

Stollberger C, Finsterer J. Left ventricular hypertrabeculation/noncompaction. *J Am Soc Echocardiogr* 2004;17:91.

Stollberger C, Finsterer J, Blazek G. Left ventricular hypertrabeculation/noncompaction and association with additional cardiac abnormalities and neuromuscular disorders. *Am J Cardiol* 2002;90:899.

Strand S, Hofmann WJ, Hug H, et al. Lymphocyte apoptosis induced by CD95 (APO-1/Fas) ligand-expressing tumor cells: a mechanism of immune evasion? *Nat Med* 1996;2:1361.

Straub V, Campbell KP. Muscular dystrophies and the dystrophin-glycoprotein complex. *Curr Opin Neurol* 1997;10:168.

Stuurman N, Heins S, Aebi U. Nuclear lamins: their structure, assembly and interactions. *J Struct Biol* 1998;122:42.

Sutton MGSJ, Sharpe N. Left ventricular remodeling after myocardial infarction: pathophysiology and therapy. *Circulation* 2000;101:2981.

Tazalaar HD, Billingham ME. Myocardial lymphocytes: fact, fancy or myocarditis? *Am J Cardiovasc Pathol* 1986;1:47.

Tesson F, Dufour C, Moolman JC, et al. The influence of the angiotensin I converting enzyme genotype in familial hypertrophic cardiomyopathy varies with the disease gene mutation. *J Mol Cell Cardiol* 1997;29:831.

Thierfelder L, MacRae C, Watkins H, et al. A familial hypertrophic cardiomyopathy locus maps to chromosome 15q2. *Proc Natl Acad Sci USA* 1993;90:6270.

Thierfelder L, Watkins H, MacRae C, et al. α-Tropomyosin and cardiac troponin T mutations cause familial hypertrophic cardiomyopathy: a disease of the sarcomere. *Cell* 1994;77:701.

Tiula E, Leinikki P. Fatal cytomegalovirus infection in a prevously healthy boy with myocarditis and consumption coagulopathy as a presenting sign. *Scand J Infect Dis* 1972;4:57.

Tomko RP, Xu R, Philipson L. HCAR and MCAR: the human and mouse cellular receptors for subgroup C adenoviruses and group B coxsackieviruses. *Proc Natl Acad Sci USA* 1997;94:3352.

Torre-Amione G, Kapadia S, Lee J, et al. Tumor necrosis factor-alpha and tumor necrosis factor receptors in the failing human heart. *Circulation* 1996;93:704.

Towbin JA. Familial dilated cardiomyopathy. In: Berul CI, Towbin JA, eds. *The molecular and clinical genetics of cardiac electrophysiological disease.* Kluwer Academic Publishers, 2000:195.

Towbin JA. Molecular genetic aspects of cardiomyopathy. *Biochem Med Metab Biol* 1993;49:285.

Towbin JA. Myocarditis. In: Finberg L, Kleinman R, eds. *Saunders manual of pediatric practice.* 2nd ed. Philadelphia: WB Saunders, 2002:660.

Towbin JA. Pediatric myocardial disease. *Pediatr Clin North Am* 1999;46:289.

Towbin JA. The role of cytoskeletal proteins in cardiomyopathies. *Curr Opin Cell Biol* 1998;10:131.

Towbin JA, Bowles KR, Bowles NE. Etiologies of cardiomyopathy and heart failure. *Nat Med* 1999;5:266.

Towbin JA, Bowles NE. The failing heart. *Nature* 2002;415:227.

Towbin JA, Griffin LD, Martin AB, et al. Intrauterine adenoviral myocarditis presenting as non-immune hydrops fetalis: diagnosis by polymerase chain reaction. *Pediatr Infect Dis J* 1994;13:144.

Towbin JA, Hejtmancik JF, Brink P, et al. X-linked dilated cardiomyopathy (XLCM): molecular genetic evidence of linkage to the Duchenne muscular dystrophy gene at the Xp21 locus. *Circulation* 1993;87:1854.

Towbin JA, Lipshultz SE. Genetics of neonatal cardiomyopathy. *Curr Opin Cardiol* 1999;14:250.

Townsend P, Barton P, Yacoub M, et al. Molecular cloning of human cardiac troponin T isoforms: expression in developing and failing heart. *J Mol Cell Cardiol* 1995;27:2223.

Tsubata S, Bowles KR, Vatta M, et al. Mutations in the human delta-sarcoglycan gene in familial and sporadic dilated cardiomyopathy. *J Clin Invest* 2000;106:655.

Valentine HA, Hunt SA, Fowler MB, et al. Frequency of familial nature of dilated cardiomyopathy and usefulness of cardiac transplantation in this subset. *Am J Cardiol* 1989;63:959.

Van den Veyver IB, Ni J, Bowles N, et al. Detection of intrauterine viral infection using the polymerase chain reaction (PCR). *Mol Genet Metab* 1998;63:85.

Van Driest SL, Ackerman MJ, Ommen SR, et al. Prevalence and severity of "benign" mutations in the β-myosin heavy chain, cardiac troponin T, and α-tropomyosin genes in hypertrophic cardiomyopathy. *Circulation* 2002;106:3085.

Vasan RS, Levy D. Defining diastolic heart failure: a call for standardized diagnostic criteria. *Circulation* 2000;101:2118.

Vatta M, Mohapatra B, Jimenez S, et al. Mutations in cypher/ZASP in patients with dilated cardiomyopathy and left ventricular non-compaction. *J Am Coll Cardiol* 2003;42:2014.

Vatta M, Stetson SJ, Jimenez S, et al. Molecular normalization of dystrophin in the failing left and right ventricle of patients treated with either pulsatile or continuous flow-type ventricular assist devices. *J Am Coll Cardiol* 2004;43:811.

Vatta M, Stetson SJ, Perez-Verdra A, et al. Molecular remodeling of dystrophin in patients with end-stage cardiomyopathies and reversal for patients on assist device therapy. *Lancet* 2000;359:936.

Vignola PA, Aonuma K, Swaye PS, et al. Lymphocytic myocarditis presenting as unexplained ventricular arrhythmias: diagnosis with endomyocardial biopsy and response to immunosuppression. *J Am Coll Cardiol* 1984;4:812.

Vigoreaux JO. The muscle Z band: lessons in stress management. *J Muscle Res Cell Motil* 1994;15:237.

Vikstrom KL, Leinwand LA. Contractile protein mutations and heart disease. *Curr Opin Cell Biol* 1996;8:97.

Vreken P, Valianpour F, Nijtmans LG, et al. Defective remodeling of cardiolipin and phosphatidyl-glycerol in Barth syndrome. *Biochem Biophys Res Commun* 2000;279:378.

Vulpian A. Contribution à l'étude des rétrécissements de l'orifice ventriculo-aortique. *Arch Physiol* 1868;3:220.

Watkins H. Genetic clues to disease pathways in hypertrophic and dilated cardiomyopathies. *Circulation* 2003;107:1344.

Watkins H, Conner D, Thierfelder L, et al. 1995. Mutations in the cardiac myosin binding protein-C gene on chromosome 11 cause familial hypertrophic cardiomyopathy. *Nat Genet* 2003;11:434.

Watkins H, MacRae C, Thierfelder L, et al. A disease locus for familial hypertrophic cardiomyopathy maps to chromosome 1q3. *Nat Genet* 1993;3:333.

Watkins H, McKenna WJ, Thierfelder L, et al. Mutations in the genes for cardiac troponin T and α-tropomyosin in hypertrophic cardiomyopathy. *N Engl J Med* 1995;332:1058.

Watkins H, Rosenzweig T, Hwang DS, et al. Characteristic and prognostic implications of myosin missense mutations in familial hypertrophic cardiomyopathy. *N Engl J Med* 1992;326:1106.

Weller AH, Hall M, Huber SA. Polyclonal immunoglobulin therapy protects against cardiac damage in experimental coxsackievirus-induced myocarditis. *Eur Heart J* 1992;13:115.

Wheeler MT, Allikian MJ, Heydemann A, et al. Smooth muscle cell-extrinsic vascular spasms arise from cardiomyocyte degeneration in sarcoglycan-deficient cardiomyopathy. *J Clin Invest* 2004;113:668.

White E. Regulation of apoptosis by the transforming genes of the DNA tumor virus adenovirus. *Proc Soc Exp Biol Med* 1993;204:30.

Woodruff JF. Viral myocarditis: a review. *Am J Pathol* 1980;101:427.

Wynn J, Braunwald E. The cardiomyopathies and myocardities. In: Braunwald E, ed. *Heart disease: a textbook of cardiovascular medicine.* Philadelphia: WB Saunders, 1997:1404.

Xiong D, Lee GH, Badorff C, et al. Dystrophin deficiency markedly increases enterovirus-induced cardiomyopathy: a genetic predisposition to viral heart disease. *Nat Med* 2002;8:872.

Yonega K, Okamoto H, Machida M, et al. Angiotensin-converting enzyme gene polymorphism in Japanese patients with hypertrophic cardiomyopathy. *Am Heart J* 1995;130:1089.

Yoshida K, Nakamura A, Yazak M, et al. Insertional mutation by transposable element, L1, in the DMD gene results in X-linked dilated cardiomyopathy. *Hum Mol Med* 1998;7:1129.

Zee-Cheng CS, Tsai CC, Palmer DC, et al. High incidence of myocarditis by endomyocardial biopsy in patients with idiopathic congestive cardiomyopathy. *J Am Coll Cardiol* 1984;3:63.

Zhou Q, Chu PH, Huang C, et al. Ablation of cyipher, a PDZ-LIM domain Z-line protein, causes a severe form of congenital myopathy. *J Cell Biol* 2001;155:605.

Zile MR, Brutsaert DL. New concepts in diastolic dysfunction and diastolic heart failure. II. Causal mechanisms and treatment. *Circulation* 2002;105:1503.

Zolk O, Caroni P, Bohm M. Decreased expression of the cardiac LIM domain protein MLP in chronic human heart failure. *Circulation* 2000;101:2674.

CHAPTER 284 ■ INFECTIVE ENDOCARDITIS

RICHARD A. FRIEDMAN AND JEFFREY R. STARKE

Infective endocarditis (IE) refers to a condition in which an organism or organisms infect the endocardium, valves, or related structures that have been injured previously by surgery, trauma, or disease. The infecting organism may be bacterial, fungal, chlamydial, rickettsial, or viral. In the first half of the twentieth century, many patients with IE had had prior rheumatic heart disease. In the latter part of the century, most children with IE have complex congenital heart defects.

Previous classifications divided cases between acute bacterial endocarditis (i.e., rapid, fulminant course with death occurring within 6 weeks) and subacute bacterial endocarditis (i.e., slow, indolent course, usually taking several months). The acute form usually was caused by *Staphylococcus aureus, Streptococcus pyogenes,* or *Streptococcus pneumoniae,* and the subacute form most commonly involved the viridans streptococci. The newer classification is based on a microbiologic cause rather than a description of the course of disease, and the general term *IE* is the name more widely accepted.

EPIDEMIOLOGY

Widely divergent figures are reported for the incidence of IE in children. Most large series are retrospective and do not report the total number of admissions to a given institution during the study period. From 1952 to 1962, 1 of 4,500 pediatric admissions to the Hospital for Sick Children in Toronto was for endocarditis. At Boston Children's Hospital, 1 of 1,800 admissions from 1963 to 1972 was for endocarditis, but between 1933 and 1963, the incidence was only 1 in 4,500. Between 1972 and 1982, 1 of 1,280 pediatric admissions to Case Western Reserve–Rainbow Babies Hospital was a child with endocarditis. A recent review indicates that endocarditis accounts for approximately 1 in 1,280 pediatric admissions per year.

The mean age of children with endocarditis is increasing, probably because of increases in longevity after corrective or palliative surgery. Between 1930 and 1950, the average age at the time of hospital admission was approximately 5 years, but between 1960 and 1980, it increased to 8.5 to 13.0 years of age. However, a large retrospective study comparing operated and unoperated children with congenital heart disease (CHD) who developed IE demonstrated no difference in the mean ages of these groups of patients.

The increased incidence of IE among neonates without congenital heart defects seems to be associated with advances in life support in this population and the frequent use of indwelling catheters for nutritional or pharmacologic support.

Virtually any congenital defect may predispose to the development of IE. The lifetime risk of developing IE in a patient with an unrepaired, simple ventricular septal defect is between 3.2% and 13.0%. In a large, cooperative study of the natural history of aortic stenosis, pulmonic stenosis, and ventricular septal defect, the risk of developing endocarditis by 30 years of age was determined to be 9.7% for unoperated patients; if the patient had undergone surgical repair, the incidence of IE was much lower. For aortic stenosis, the risk (1.4%) was slightly increased after surgical intervention, and patients with pulmonic stenosis had a 0.9% risk of developing IE.

In other studies, tetralogy of Fallot accounted for the largest percentage of patients with CHD who developed IE. Ventricular septal defect was the second most common lesion, followed by aortic stenosis (8%), patent ductus arteriosus (7%), and transposition of the great vessels (4%). The most common lesions in patients with CHD who developed endocarditis after surgery were tetralogy of Fallot and transposition of the great vessels with pulmonary stenosis; both occurred in patients who had received systemic-pulmonary shunts. Several other patients had had complex cyanotic CHD with shunts, and 70% of this group developed IE 1 to more than 5 years after surgery. Of patients requiring prosthetic valves, 79% developed infections more than 3 months after surgery. Events predisposing the patient to bacteremia were identified in approximately one-third of these cases. Details concerning the unoperated patients with underlying heart disease were not described well, but apparently most had congenital valve deformities or valve disease secondary to rheumatic fever.

A smaller series from the Yale–New Haven Hospitals showed a higher incidence of IE in patients with CHD who had not undergone surgery than in those who had. Acyanotic lesions occurred more commonly in the unoperated group, and cyanotic lesions predominated in the postoperative group. Dacron patches and Gore-Tex grafts were more common sites of infection than were prosthetic valves. Apparently, patients with complete correction of tetralogy of Fallot have a low incidence of endocarditis compared with patients who remain palliated. In a large series of patients followed for a mean of 23.7 years, only one patient (1%) developed IE. Tricuspid atresia with diminished pulmonary artery flow commonly is palliated with a shunt procedure; these patients may have an incidence of IE approaching 25%.

A retrospective study looked at the differences in the underlying defects between pediatric patients diagnosed with endocarditis between 1970 and 1990 and those in earlier studies. As expected, almost one-half of the patients had undergone surgery for their defects, and many of them had artificial valves inserted at the time of operation. Mitral valve prolapse seems to have become a major risk factor, presenting in 29% of patients with IE.

IE associated with prosthetic materials, especially valves and valved conduits, has increased. Prosthetic valve endocarditis has been categorized as early onset (i.e., within 3 months of implant) or late onset. The incidence of infection after implantation ranges from less than 1% to 10%. Neither the type of valve nor the site of implant significantly affects the incidence of prosthetic valve endocarditis. *Staphylococcus* spp. predominate in early-onset prosthetic valve endocarditis, and *Streptococcus* spp. are the most common cause of infection in late-onset disease, probably a reflection of intraoperative contamination. The overall incidence of early-onset prosthetic valve endocarditis has been reduced greatly since the standard administration of perioperative antibiotics was instituted.

PATHOPHYSIOLOGY

Animal studies and clinical and autopsy investigations have shown that a series of events creates an environment suitable for the establishment of IE. Hemodynamic factors that predispose to turbulence of blood flow and subsequent endothelial damage have been shown to be primary in the development of a nidus of infection in the heart and great vessels. Studies have shown that a Venturi effect is responsible for the fact that the highest yield of bacteria can be found on the low-pressure sink side of a high-pressure jet (i.e., left atrial surface of mitral valve in mitral regurgitation, right ventricular side of ventricular septal defect). As a consequence of turbulent blood flow, endothelial damage occurs and initiates the formation of platelet and fibrin deposition. This series of events is similar to that seen in the course of primary plug formation with vascular injury. Exposure to cold, high cardiac output states, hormonal manipulations, high altitude, and passage of a sterile catheter across a heart valve in animals also have caused this lesion.

Growth in fibrin and platelet deposition results in the formation of a nonbacterial thrombotic vegetation (NBTV) that is essential in the pathogenesis of endocarditis. Transient bacteremias that occur as a normal part of daily life may cause colonization of the NBTV. As the NBTV grows in size and bacteria adhere, infected vegetation develops. The virulence of different bacteria may be related directly to their ability to adhere to the NBTV. A factor that may be important in increased virulence is the ability of certain streptococci found in the oral cavity to produce dextran; the amount of dextran produced by the bacterial strain also may correlate with virulence. Another substance that may be a receptor for certain organisms is fibronectin, a substance found on the surface of NBTV in polyethylene catheter-induced IE. Organisms such as *S. aureus*, *Candida albicans*, *Streptococcus sanguis*, and *Streptococcus faecalis* adhere to fibronectin, but nonadherence is the rule for organisms rarely found to cause IE.

After the NBTV is colonized, the size of the vegetation grows by increasing numbers of bacteria and by additional deposition of platelets and fibrin. The colonized NBTV produces a constant bacteremia, and reseeding of the vegetation occurs by adherence of circulating organisms to the already enlarging vegetation. Three zones in the vegetation have been described: necrotic endocardium; a broad zone of bacteria, pyknotic nuclear debris, and fibrin; and a thin surface coat of fibrin and leukocytes. Proliferation of bacteria in the protected middle zone is relatively unchecked because the normal host defense mechanisms are unable to penetrate into the vegetation, and penetration of any circulating antimicrobial agent is diminished. Because the internal environment of the middle zone of the NBTV depresses bacterial metabolism, the action of any antimicrobial agent that does penetrate is attenuated.

Pathologic changes observed in the heart are produced by local extension of the infection. Vegetations may be single or multiple, ranging from less than 1 mm to several centimeters. Large lesions may resemble tumors and cause hemodynamically significant stenosis. Certain organisms, such as *Candida* spp., *Haemophilus* spp., and *S. aureus,* may produce friable lesions that can embolize. Ulceration of tissue, especially heart valves, may result in perforation and produce the onset of sudden congestive heart failure (CHF). Other complications include rupture of chordae tendineae, abscesses of the valve ring, fistula formation with the development of pericardial empyema and tamponade, aneurysms of the sinus of Valsalva or ventricle, and myocardial infarction secondary to emboli.

Distant organ involvement secondary to emboli may occur. One necropsy review of endocarditis in children found the most common site of distant organ involvement to be the lungs; the kidney was the organ most frequently involved on the systemic side of the circulation. In other studies, cerebral emboli have been found in 30% of adults and children who had IE, with subsequent development of infarction, abscess, mycotic aneurysm, subarachnoid hemorrhage, and acute hemiplegia of childhood. Microemboli in the cerebral circulation may cause a confused mental state. Strokes usually are secondary to emboli in the middle cerebral artery. Aortic valve infection probably has the highest incidence of embolic complications.

Immunologic mechanisms during subacute IE play an important role in the pathogenesis and sequelae. Cell-mediated and humoral immunity are active in this disease process. A hypergammaglobulinemic state that usually exists is caused by polyclonal and antigen-specific B-cell activation. Part of the hypergammaglobulinemia is caused by circulating rheumatoid factors. Levels of rheumatoid factor may decrease with successful therapy and increase with relapse of disease. Antibody responses directed at the infecting organism and nonspecific responses have been demonstrated. Possibly, C3b in conjunction with circulating immune complexes may bind to the surface of B cells and initiate production of antibodies not directed primarily at the infecting organism. Circulating immune complexes are found with increased frequency in patients with long-standing illness, right-sided disease, hypocomplementemic states, and extravalvular manifestations. One study of 29 patients with culture-proven IE found that almost all of them had levels of circulating immune complexes higher than 12 fg/mL. A mixed-type cryoglobulinemia occurs in 90% of patients with IE. Renal involvement with focal and diffuse glomerulonephritis has been described, and immune complex deposition is found in both. Other autoantibodies, including antiendocardial, antisarcolemmal, antimyolemmal, and antinuclear, are detected during the course of IE.

CLINICAL MANIFESTATIONS

The clinical manifestations of IE depend on the underlying pathophysiologic processes of the disease. The extent of local involvement of the myocardium or valves, embolization from vegetations, and activation of immunologic mechanisms play essential roles in clinical expression. Patients with acute IE may present in shock and with clinical pictures consistent with overwhelming sepsis. In some cases, confirmation of endocarditis may be found only at autopsy. The subacute form of the disease may follow an indolent course, and a diagnosis may not be established for weeks or months. Because endocarditis frequently occurs in children with underlying heart disease, subtle changes in their physical examination may be missed unless the examiner is discerning and alert. Table 284.1 lists the major clinical manifestations of IE and their relative frequency of occurrence in children.

The most common finding in IE is fever, although approximately 10% of patients have no fever. Fever usually is low-grade and shows no specific pattern, especially in the subacute form. Other nonspecific complaints include malaise, anorexia, weight loss, fatigue, and sleep disturbances. Involvement of the large joints, with arthralgias or arthritis, occurs in 24% of patients. Nausea, vomiting, and nonspecific abdominal pains are found in 16% of patients. Chest pains, which usually are related to myalgias but sometimes are secondary to pulmonary embolism, especially with tricuspid valve involvement, occur in as many as 10% of older children.

Heart murmurs in patients with IE have been accepted as a classic finding. They occur in as many as 90% of affected children, but most of these patients have underlying congenital defects and initially present with murmurs specific for their lesions. A new or changing murmur occurs in approximately 25% of children. CHF may affect as many as 30% of children

TABLE 284.1

SYMPTOMS AND PHYSICAL FINDINGS IN INFECTIVE ENDOCARDITIS

Symptom/finding	Incidence (%)
Fever	56–100
Anorexia/weight loss	8–83
Malaise	40–79
Arthralgias	16–38
Gastrointestinal problems	9–36
Chest pain	5–20
Heart failure	9–47
Splenomegaly	36–67
Petechiae	10–50
Embolic events	14–50
New/changing murmur	9–44
Clubbing	2–42
Osler nodes	7–8
Roth spots	0–6
Janeway lesions	0–10
Splinter hemorrhages	0–10

with IE, and it is especially common in patients who develop a new murmur of valvular insufficiency. Exacerbation of CHF in children with rheumatic or congenital lesions should alert the clinician to consider the diagnosis of IE for patients who previously had been controlled well on medical therapy for their chronic condition.

Signs and symptoms of neurologic involvement are seen in approximately 20% of children with IE. The sudden development of a clinical picture consistent with cerebral infarction in a child with an underlying heart defect should suggest the diagnosis. Acute hemiplegia, seizures, ataxia, aphasia, focal neurologic defects, sensory loss, and changing mental status may occur as presenting features or even years after the disease process has been treated.

Splenomegaly occurs in approximately 55% of children with IE, usually in those with subacute disease and activated immune systems. On palpation, the spleen is not tender. Hepatomegaly also is observed in many patients. Infarction of the spleen or abscess formation should be suspected in patients with left upper quadrant pain and tenderness that radiates to the shoulder area. A pleural friction rub or pleural effusion may be observed.

Specific skin lesions associated with IE occur more commonly in adults than in children. Petechiae are seen in approximately one-third of the children, especially in those with a more chronic course. Common sites of involvement are the mucous membranes of the mouth, the conjunctivae, and the extremities. Petechiae are the most common skin manifestations in IE, occurring in as many as 40% of patients; purpura is a rare finding. Osler nodes, which also have been described in systemic lupus erythematosus and in extremities distal to the sites of prolonged arterial catheterization, are exquisitely tender lesions. They are found most commonly on the pads of the fingers and toes, the thenar and hypothenar eminences, the sides of the fingers, and the skin on the lower part of the arm. Much controversy exists regarding whether they represent an immunologic response to infection manifesting as a vasculitis or are septic emboli. Janeway lesions are nontender, hemorrhagic plaques that occur frequently on the palms and the soles and represent septic emboli with bacteria, neutrophils, and subsequent necrosis with subcutaneous hemorrhage. Roth spots are small, pale retinal lesions with areas of hemorrhage that usually are located near the optic disc. Osler nodes, Janeway lesions, splinter hemorrhages, and Roth spots occur in only 5% to 7% of children with endocarditis.

Although accounting for a small percentage of cases of endocarditis, *S. pneumoniae* carries a high risk of mortality. Two recent reviews of this disease noted that the presence of "Osler triad"—pneumonia, meningitis, and endocarditis—is not as prevalent in children as it is in the adult population. However, some of these patients did have concomitant meningitis, and experts cautioned that this additional diagnosis should be eliminated in these patients.

Infants and neonates may present with a clinical picture less specific than that seen in older children. The onset is more acute and clinically mimics overwhelming sepsis. The diagnosis rarely is suspected before death occurs. The use of indwelling vascular catheters has increased the incidence of endocarditis in neonates. Persistent bacteremia associated with a deterioration in pulmonary function, coagulopathies, thrombocytopenia, and the appearance of murmurs should arouse suspicion of the possible presence of endocarditis in a neonate.

The clinical presentation of IE in intravenous drug abusers has several distinctive features. Previous underlying heart disease is found in one-third of these patients. The tricuspid valve is the site most commonly affected, and these patients often have pulmonary complications, including infarction, abscess formation, and signs and symptoms of pleural effusion. Extracardiac sites of infection are found in approximately two-thirds of these patients. Tricuspid insufficiency with findings of a murmur of tricuspid regurgitation, a pulsatile liver, and a gallop rhythm are found in 33% of patients.

DIAGNOSIS

Laboratory Investigation

Table 284.2 summarizes the most common laboratory findings in children with IE. Blood cultures are the single most important diagnostic tool for establishing the diagnosis of IE. Because bacteremia usually is continuous and low-grade, the timing and site of collection do not affect the yield. In approximately 66% of all cases of IE, the blood cultures grow the infecting organism and, in 90%, the results of the first two blood cultures are positive. If a patient has received antibiotics before the culture is tried, the chance of obtaining a positive culture may be reduced from between 95% and 100% to 64%. If pretreatment has occurred, placing the blood sample in hypertonic media may enhance the chance of isolating the organism. Patients with fungal endocarditis may have only intermittently positive blood culture results, and the organism may take a week or longer to grow in culture.

Ideally, three to five sets of blood cultures should be obtained within the first 24 hours. The commonly practiced simultaneous drawing of blood for culture with fever is not supported by any studies. Bacteremia in endocarditis usually is continuous and thus can be drawn at any time. In children in whom drawing large volumes of blood would be contraindicated, blood should be cultured in aerobic conditions because endocarditis caused by an anaerobic organism is an extremely rare event.

TABLE 284.2

LABORATORY FINDINGS IN INFECTIVE ENDOCARDITIS

Finding	Incidence (%)
Elevated erythrocyte sedimentation rate	71–94
Positive rheumatoid fever	25–55
Anemia	19–79
Positive blood culture result	68–98
Hematuria	28–47

Specimens should be taken from different sites and should contain 3 to 5 mL of blood. Thioglycolate broth should be used, and the bottles should be kept for 3 weeks to detect slow-growing organisms. Nutritionally variant streptococci should be suspected if a gram-positive coccus is isolated in broth but fails to grow in subculture. The organism then should be subcultured onto media enriched with pyridoxal phosphate or L-cysteine.

Blood culture results may be negative in 10% to 15% of cases of suspected endocarditis because of prior administration of antibiotics; endocarditis caused by rickettsiae, chlamydiae, or viruses; slow-growing organisms (e.g., *Candida* spp., *Haemophilus* spp., *Brucella* spp.) or nutritionally variant streptococci; infections caused by anaerobic organisms; NBTV endocarditis; mural endocarditis; right-sided endocarditis; fungal endocarditis (especially *Aspergillus* spp.); or an incorrect diagnosis. Additional sites, including urine, sputum, cerebrospinal fluid, synovial fluid, bone marrow, and lymph nodes, may be infected concomitantly, and cultures of these additional sites should be included if blood culture results fail to demonstrate an infecting agent.

Necessary adjunctive laboratory tests include measurement of the erythrocyte sedimentation rate, which is elevated in as many as 90% of patients and correlates with the hypergammaglobulinemia found in this disease. An artifactually low erythrocyte sedimentation rate may be found with renal disease, severe CHF, or polycythemia. The erythrocyte sedimentation rate should decrease toward normal if therapy has been successful, and serial measurements may be helpful in monitoring therapy. A positive rheumatoid factor has been found in one-fourth to one-half of pediatric patients with IE and may be supportive evidence for the diagnosis in cases of culture-negative endocarditis. Immune complex–mediated glomerulonephritis, although not a common finding, may result in hypocomplementemia. Anemia, usually caused by a chronic disease state, is found in 40% of patients. Because children with cyanotic CHD frequently develop IE, the finding of a normal or slightly high hemoglobin level should suggest the possibility of anemia. Although leukocytosis is not an uncommon occurrence, leukopenia may occur in acute cases with overwhelming sepsis. Microemboli and consequent microinfarcts in the kidney produce hematuria with or without proteinuria, casts, and bacteremia in 25% to 50% of patients.

Circulating immune complexes as measured by the Raji cell radioimmune assay or the ^{123}I-C1q-binding assay are present in most adults with IE, although they may be conspicuously absent in acute disease. Immune complexes may be found in septicemic patients and in as many as 10% of normal adult controls. Although few studies have reported on circulating immune complex levels in children with IE, elevated levels have been found in some patients.

Serologic testing for specific organisms may be helpful in cases of culture-negative endocarditis. Antibodies against teichoic acids, which are major components of the cell wall in *S. aureus,* may be present in 85% of adults with IE, although the false-positive rate may be as high as 10%. A teichoic acid antibody titer of greater than 1:1 in a bacteremic adult patient correlates with deep-seated infections, including but not restricted to endocarditis. However, teichoic acid antibody levels do not differentiate the types of deep-seated infection. As with circulating immune complexes, serial measurements of teichoic acid antibody levels may correlate with successful therapy. Unfortunately, no data exist concerning teichoic acid antibody levels in children with IE.

Echocardiography

The role of echocardiography in helping to establish the diagnosis of IE has grown considerably because the technology has improved vastly since single-crystal M-mode techniques were introduced. M-mode echocardiography uses a single, narrow ultrasound beam, and the reflected ultrasound echoes are recorded on moving paper. Two-dimensional (2D) echocardiography uses multiple echo beams and provides a cross-sectional moving image of the heart, which can be recorded from several angles. The 2D technique usually is superior to the M-mode technique in investigating vegetative lesions. Some areas of the heart, such as the pulmonary valve, are visualized better using 2D imaging, and the increased sensitivity of this technique in detecting pulmonary valve endocarditis has been documented. The value of 2D echocardiography in prosthetic valve endocarditis also is superior to that of M-mode echocardiography. An echo-free space found in more than one tomographic plane has aided in establishing the diagnosis of perivalvular abscess, which may complicate 30% of the native valve endocarditis cases and even more cases of prosthetic valve endocarditis. Adjunctive use of the Doppler technique to diagnose prosthetic valve regurgitation before it becomes apparent clinically may aid in earlier establishment of the diagnosis. The sensitivity of echocardiography in detecting vegetative lesions in suspected endocarditis in adults ranges from 13% to 83%, with a greater sensitivity exhibited in the more recently published series using the 2D technique. Several studies have concluded that patients with a "positive echo" were twice as likely to develop serious complications (usually emboli, more commonly cerebral than peripheral) and that patients were at higher risk for death or development of severe CHF if the vegetation were larger than 1 cm^2. However, the risk of embolization does not appear to correlate with the size of the vegetation.

Transesophageal echocardiography (TEE) has become important in evaluating patients for vegetations. TEE takes advantage of the proximity of the heart, especially the left atrium to the esophagus. This technique also eliminates the inability to image transthoracically in some patients who do not have good "echo windows" from that approach. The quality of the image is better, rendering diagnosis more certain. Although this technique can be accomplished using light sedation, our experience has been that heavy sedation administered by an anesthesiologist is preferable.

One study in adults with endocarditis using the transesophageal approach yielded the following conclusions: When combined with a high clinical suspicion of endocarditis, TEE offers a high sensitivity for properly diagnosing IE, and TEE is significantly better than is transthoracic echocardiography (TTE) in imaging vegetations in these patients. Our clinical experience has confirmed these conclusions, and we now routinely use TEE if the TTE result is equivocal or negative for a patient who we suspect has the disease.

In a study using M-mode and 2D techniques for 15 children with IE, vegetations were detected in ten (66%) of the patients. Of the ten, three had systemic emboli and two died, but none of the patients without an echocardiography-proven vegetation had an embolic complication. This finding suggested that echocardiography may help identify a high-risk population that could benefit from surgical intervention. Some studies have suggested that the size and mobility of a vegetation may be useful in differentiating bacterial from fungal endocarditis. In our experience, however, this claim probably is not valid because large vegetations are seen frequently in bacterial or fungal endocarditis.

Several recent studies have addressed the role for TEE versus TTE in evaluating patients for endocarditis. Generalizing the results, these investigators found that TEE should be reserved for patients in whom TTE has been technically unfeasible, such as in patients who are very obese, are overly muscular, or have concomitant pulmonary disease, all of which result in poor "acoustic windows." Moreover, as a "screening tool," any type of echocardiographic study should be reserved for those patients in whom a high index of suspicion exists as outlined by either the clinical criteria of von Reyn or the so-called "Duke criteria." In the absence of a moderate to high suspicion of risk, echocardiographic studies are not cost-efficient. TEE also has the potential risks involved with general anesthesia and endotracheal intubation in order to accomplish the study.

A negative echocardiographic study result does not rule out the presence of vegetations. The resolution on most equipment limits the detection of vegetations to those larger than 2 to 3 mm. Poor technique also may hinder evaluation. Rheumatic heart disease with preexisting valve disease, mitral valve prolapse (MVP) with thickened leaflets, marantic vegetations, Löffler endocarditis, Chiari networks in the right atrium, and valve ring abscesses pose interpretive problems to the echocardiographer. After a vegetation is detected, it may show no significant change during therapy, and a recurrence of disease cannot be diagnosed unless a noticeable increase in size occurs or a new vegetation appears. Attempts to estimate serially the size of a vegetation are fraught with technical and interpretive errors and probably are of little value. However, continued growth of a vegetation coexistent with persistent bacteremia or evidence of further endocardial infiltration may indicate a treatment failure or the need for surgical intervention. One study attempted to define risk factors involved with an echocardiographically demonstrable vegetation in adult patients with IE. Significant complications included peripheral and central nervous system (CNS) embolization, failure to respond to therapy, CHF, need for surgery, and death. Using univariate analysis in patients with native left-sided valve endocarditis, the investigators found that vegetation's size, extent, mobility, and consistency all were significant predictors of complications. Multivariate analysis demonstrated that size, extent, and mobility could be used to score a patient into a high-risk group. An echocardiographic examination performed at the time of hospital discharge of a patient after an apparently successful course of antibiotic therapy can be used as a baseline for further evaluation.

Electrocardiography

Numerous electrocardiographic abnormalities may be found throughout the course of IE. Ventricular ectopy in patients with hemodynamic compromise may be life-threatening. Atrial fibrillation in adults and children may be secondary to atrioventricular valve regurgitation. Extension of abscess formation or an inflammatory response may cause direct injury to the conduction system. Complete right bundle branch block, left anterior or posterior fascicular block, and complete atrioventricular block have been reported. The onset of complete atrioventricular block may be an indication for surgical intervention, especially if it occurs during the course of appropriate antibiotic therapy. Abscess formation in the perivalvular aortic region may cause direct injury to the atrioventricular node because of its proximity to that structure, which may result in sudden death unless temporary and eventually permanent pacing is instituted.

PROPHYLAXIS

The use of antibiotics before and during any procedure that induces a transient bacteremia has become standard medical practice for the prevention of IE. Numerous failures, with subsequent development of endocarditis, have been reported. Although failure often is related to inappropriate drug regimens, infection occasionally develops despite adherence to published guidelines. In 1997, significant revisions were made

---

TABLE 284.3

CARDIAC CONDITIONS ASSOCIATED WITH ENDOCARDITIS

Endocarditis prophylaxis recommended

High-risk category
  Prosthetic cardiac valves, including bioprosthetic and homograft valves
  Previous bacterial endocarditis
  Complex cyanotic congenital heart disease (e.g., single ventricle states, transposition of the great arteries, tetralogy of Fallot)
  Surgically constructed systemic pulmonary artery shunts or conduits

Moderate-risk category
  Most other congenital cardiac malformations (other than those listed previously or that follow)
  Acquired valvar dysfunction (e.g., rheumatic heart disease)
  Hypertrophic cardiomyopathy
  Mitral valve prolapse with valvar regurgitation, thickened leaflets (men older than 45 even without regurgitation, exercise-induced regurgitation), or both

Endocarditis prophylaxis not recommended

Negligible-risk category (no greater risk than general population)
  Isolated secundum atrial septal defect
  Surgical repair of atrial septal defect, ventricular septal defect, or patent ductus arteriosus (without residua beyond 6 months)
  Previous coronary artery bypass graft surgery
  Mitral valve prolapse without regurgitation
  Physiologic, functional, or innocent heart murmurs
  Previous Kawasaki disease without valvular dysfunction
  Previous rheumatic fever without valvular dysfunction
  Cardiac pacemakers (intravascular and epicardial) and implanted defibrillators

---

in the guidelines for endocarditis prophylaxis. This report emphasized that, in fact, most cases of endocarditis are not attributable to an invasive procedure. Cardiac conditions were stratified into high, moderate, and negligible risk categories to help the clinician assess risk based on potential morbidity and mortality. These conditions are summarized in Table 284.3. In addition, further elaboration on the types of procedures that are associated with a relatively higher risk of bacteremia is given. No longer are two doses of antibiotics recommended for oral procedures. Rather, only one dose, with a maximum of 2 g (50 mg/kg), is given, and either cephalexin (50 mg/kg, maximum dose of 2 g) or, for patients with immediate-type hypersensitivity reactions to penicillins, azithromycin or clarithromycin (15 mg/kg, maximum 500 mg) should be given 1 hour before the procedure. Finally, prophylaxis for genitourinary and gastrointestinal procedures was simplified. These changes are shown in Tables 284.4 to 284.6.

Perhaps not a surprise, several recent studies have demonstrated that antibiotic prophylaxis frequently is not given because of both the patient *and physician's* failure to either understand the need for or to educate the parents about proper prophylaxis regimens. Most clinics have and routinely distribute a card published by the American Heart Association to the parents and/or patients with congenital heart disease outlining the appropriate conditions for and dosage of antibiotics. Unfortunately, these wallet cards often are misplaced and not replaced at subsequent visits. These studies highlight the need to reiterate and document, at least yearly, the need for prophylaxis in patients at risk.

TABLE 284.4

DENTAL PROCEDURES AND ENDOCARDITIS PROPHYLAXIS

Endocarditis prophylaxis recommended[a]

Dental extractions

Periodontal procedures, including surgery, scaling and root planning, probing, and recall maintenance

Dental implant placement and reimplantation of avulsed teeth

Endodontic (root canal) instrumentation or surgery only beyond the apex

Subgingival placement of antibiotic fibers or strips

Initial placement of orthodontic bands but not brackets

Intraligamentary local anesthetic injections

Prophylactic cleaning of teeth or implants where bleeding is anticipated

Endocarditis prophylaxis not recommended

Restorative dentistry[b] (operative and prosthodontic) with or without retraction cord[c]

Local anesthetic injections (nonintraligamentary)

Intracanal endodontic treatment; postplacement and buildup

Placement of rubber dams

Postoperative suture removal

Placement of removable prosthodontic or orthodontic appliances

Taking of oral impressions

Fluoride treatments

Taking of oral radiographs

Orthodontic appliance adjustment

Shedding of primary teeth

[a]Prophylaxis is recommended for high- and moderate-risk cardiac conditions.
[b]This includes restoration of decayed teeth (filling cavities) and replacement of missing teeth.
[c]Clinical judgment may indicate antibiotic use in selected circumstances that may create significant bleeding.

TABLE 284.5

OTHER PROCEDURES AND ANTIBIOTIC PROPHYLAXIS

Endocarditis prophylaxis recommended

Respiratory tract

Tonsillectomy, adenoidectomy, or both

Surgical operations that involve the respiratory mucosa

Bronchoscopy with a rigid bronchoscope

Gastrointestinal tract[a]

Sclerotherapy for esophageal varices

Esophageal stricture dilation

Endoscopic retrograde cholangiography with biliary obstruction

Biliary tract surgery

Surgical operations that involve the intestinal mucosa

Genitourinary tract

Prostatic surgery

Cysioscopy

Ureteral dilation

Endocarditis prophylaxis not recommended

Respiratory tract

Endotracheal intubation

Bronchoscopy with flexible bronchoscope, with or without biopsy[b]

Tympanostomy tube insertion

Gastrointestinal tract

Transesophageal echocardiography[b]

Endoscopy with or without gastrointestinal biopsy

Genitourinary tract

Vaginal hysterectomy[b]

Vaginal delivery[b]

Cesarean section

Infected tissue caused by urethral catheterization, uterine dilation and curettage, therapeutic abortion, sterilization procedures, insertion or removal of intrauterine devices

Other

Cardiac catheterization, including balloon angioplasty

Implanted cardiac pacemakers, implanted defibrillators, and coronary stents

Incision or biopsy of surgically scrubbed skin

Circumcision

[a]Prophylaxis is recommended for high-risk patients and is optional for medium-risk patients.
[b]Prophylaxis is optional for high-risk patients.

Numerous theories attempt to explain how antibiotics given prophylactically prevent development of endocarditis. Two possibilities are that the magnitude of a bacteremia associated with a procedure is reduced by the antibiotic or that bacterial adherence mechanisms are altered such that a nidus of infection would be unlikely to develop. The latter hypothesis is supported by a study in which the effects of single-dose amoxicillin and erythromycin administered after the development of sterile aortic vegetations were evaluated in rats. In this model, periodontally diseased teeth were extracted to produce a bacteremia similar to the conditions that might occur in humans during dental manipulation. Endocarditis developed in 89% of the control group (i.e., vegetations but no prophylaxis). The organisms cultivated from the rats' dental plaque were identical to those found in blood culture, confirming the relation between extraction and seeding of the vegetation. The incidence of bacteremia was almost the same for the control and the treated groups, but almost none of the treated groups developed endocarditis.

Special circumstances can affect the use of antibiotic prophylaxis. Table 284.7 lists various conditions and procedures and the infecting organisms responsible for the development of IE in children and adults. In patients requiring multiple dental procedures who recently have received antibiotic prophylaxis, oral streptococci with reduced susceptibility may flourish, possibly resulting in ineffective prophylaxis. Although 3 g of amoxicillin given once per week does not result in a high incidence of resistant streptococci, erythromycin given at the same frequency may result in a significant number of resistant organisms. If prophylaxis is required twice in 1 month, amoxicillin can be given as recommended. In penicillin-allergic patients who require erythromycin, the interval between dental procedures should be increased if possible. If a dental abscess is found in a patient undergoing treatment for IE, it should be drained surgically.

Patients who develop a condition that must be treated surgically and who are being treated for IE should receive additional prophylaxis specific to the area of surgical interest and in accord with the published recommendations. Patients receiving penicillin prophylaxis for rheumatic fever should receive additional prophylaxis as previously described. Elective surgery, for whatever reason, should be postponed until the treatment of active IE is completed. Prophylaxis should be instituted for patients with permanent transvenous pacing leads, cerebral ventriculoatrial shunts, and arteriovenous shunts.

The use of antibiotic prophylaxis in patients with MVP is controversial. This condition exists in approximately 5% of the population in the United States. A case-control study comparing persons with MVP with normal controls found that the odds for the association of IE with MVP was 8.2; it increased to 15.2 when a murmur of mitral regurgitation was present. Another study attempted to define the absolute risk (i.e., chances of developing IE over the course of a time period) rather than

TABLE 284.6

PROPHYLACTIC REGIMENS FOR SURGICAL PROCEDURES

Situation	Agent[a]	Regimen[b]
Dental, oral, respiratory tract, or esophageal procedures		
Standard general prophylaxis	Amoxicillin	Adults: 2 g; children: 50 mg/kg Orally 1 hour before procedure
Unable to take oral medications	Ampicillin	Adults: 2 g IM or IV; children: 50 mg/kg IM or IV Within 30 minutes before procedure
Allergic to penicillin	Clindamycin *or*	Adults: 600 mg; children: 20 mg/kg Orally 1 hour before procedure
	Cephalexin or cefadroxil *or*	Adults: 2 g; children: 50 mg/kg Orally 1 hour before procedure
	Azithromycin or clarithromycin	Adults: 500 mg; children: 15 mg/kg Orally 1 hour before procedure
Allergic to penicillin and unable to take oral medications	Clindamycin *or*	Adults: 600 mg; children: 20 mg/kg IV Within 30 minutes before procedure
	Cefazolin	Adults: 1 g; children; 25 mg/kg IM or IV Within 30 minutes before procedure
Genitourinary/gastrointestinal procedures (excluding esophageal)		
High-risk patients	Ampicillin plus gentamicin	Adults: ampicillin, 2 g IM or IV, plus gentamicin, 1.5 mg/kg (not to exceed 120 mg), within 30 minutes of starting procedure; 6 hours later, ampicillin, 1 g IM or IV, or amoxicillin, 1 g orally Children: ampicillin, 50 mg/kg IM or IV (not to exceed 2 g), plus gentamicin, 1.5 mg/kg, within 30 minutes of starting procedure; 6 hours later, ampicillin, 25 mg/kg IM or IV, or amoxicillin, 25 mg/kg orally
High-risk patients allergic to ampicillin/amoxicillin	Vancomycin plus gentamicin	Adults: vancomycin, 1 g over 1 to 2 hours, plus gentamicin (as previously mentioned); complete injection/infusion within 30 minutes of starting procedure Children: vancomycin, 20 mg/kg IV over 1 to 2 hours, plus gentamicin (as previously mentioned); complete injection/infusion within 30 minutes of starting procedure
Moderate-risk patients	Amoxicillin or ampicillin	Adults: amoxicillin, 2 g orally 1 hour before procedure, or ampicillin, 2 g IM or IV, within 30 minutes of starting procedure Children: amoxicillin, 50 mg/kg orally 1 hour before procedure, or ampicillin, 50 mg/kg IM or IV within 30 minutes of starting procedure
Moderate-risk patients allergic to ampicillin/amoxicillin	Vancomycin	Adults: vancomycin, 1 g IV over 1 to 2 hours; complete infusion within 30 minutes of starting procedure Children: vancomycin, 20 mg/kg IV over 1 to 2 hours; complete infusion within 30 minutes of starting procedure

[a]Total children's dose should not exceed adult dose.
[b]No second dose of vancomycin or gentamicin is recommended.

the relative risk. The group with MVP and no mitral regurgitation had an absolute risk for the development of IE of 0.0046% (1 person in 21,950 per year), compared with 0.520% (1 person in 1,920 per year) for the group with MVP and mitral regurgitation. During a 50-year period, 26 of 1,000 patients with MVP and mitral regurgitation will develop IE; only 2 of 1,000 patients with MVP but without mitral regurgitation will develop IE, which is not significantly greater than the risk to the general population. This analysis suggests that routine prophylaxis should be used only in patients with MVP and mitral regurgitation. This study also showed that male gender and an age greater than 45 years were independent risk factors for the development of IE in patients with MVP, suggesting that they would receive added benefit from taking routine antibiotic prophylaxis.

Unfortunately, reports on the natural history of MVP in children that address the risk of developing IE are sparse. None of the 30 children with MVP followed in one study for an average of 4 to 5 years developed IE, indicating no additional risk for this lesion. However, the relatively short duration of follow-up should preclude such a firm conclusion. A prospective analysis of 300 patients with MVP with a mean follow-up period of 6.1 years found a 6% incidence of IE, which accounted for 15% of all serious complications in these patients.

An algorithm specific for MVP was adopted recently. If a patient has a murmur of mitral regurgitation, subacute bacterial endocarditis prophylaxis definitely is recommended. If regurgitation is not determined or unknown, the patient is referred for further evaluation. In this scenario, if regurgitation is documented on examination or echocardiographically,

TABLE 284.7

TABLE 284.7

PROCEDURES ASSOCIATED WITH BACTEREMIA IN CHILDREN AND ADULTS

Procedure	Associated Organism	Positive Blood Cultures (%)
Dental extraction	*Streptococcus*, diphtheroids	30–65
Chewing gum, candy	*Streptococcus, Staphylococcus epidermidis*	0–51
Brushing teeth	*Streptococcus*	0–26
Tonsillectomy	*Streptococcus, Haemophilus,* diptheroids	28–38
Bronchoscopy (rigid scope)	*Streptococcus, S. epidermidis*	15
Bronchoscopy (flexible scope)		0
Nasotracheal intubation/suctioning	*Streptococcus*, aerobic gram-negative rods	16
Orotracheal intubation		0
Sigmoidoscopy/colonoscopy	Enterococci, aerobic gram-negative rods	0–9.5
Upper gastrointestinal endoscopy	*Streptococcus, Neisseria, S. epidermidis*, diphtheroids, other	8–12
Percutaneous liver	Pneumococci, aerobic gram-negative rods, *Staphylococcus aureus*, other	3–14
Urethral catheterization	Not stated	8
Manipulation of *S. aureus* suppurative foci		54

Reprinted with permission of Everett ED, Hirschmann JU. Transient bacteremia and endocarditis prophylaxis. A review. *Medicine (Baltimore)* 1977;56:61.

subacute bacterial endocarditis prophylaxis is warranted. TEE may pose a risk similar to that of orotracheal intubation (i.e., no prophylaxis required). One case of endocarditis that developed after an apparently uncomplicated procedure has been reported. However, a large study looking at the incidence of transient bacteremia after performing TEE did not demonstrate a significant increase in the rate of transient bacteremia and recommended no administration of prophylaxis for this type of echocardiography. The recommendations addressed this topic specifically and concluded that subacute bacterial endocarditis prophylaxis is indicated for the high-risk patient but is optional for those at medium risk.

A recent report worthy of mention here is the use of prophylaxis in patients, including those considered at moderate risk, who are being evaluated in the emergency department for urinary tract infection. Although current guidelines indicate the need to administer antibiotics, this study evaluated the cost-effectiveness of providing prophylaxis versus performing the urinary catheterization without giving antibiotics. As a randomized, controlled study to perform this analysis was not possible, they used a theoretical construct to do the analysis. Their analysis was that prophylaxis would prevent seven cases of endocarditis for every 1 million children treated. The cost of providing the prophylaxis was $10 million per Quality Adjusted Life Year (QALY) when amoxicillin was used or $70 million per QALY when vancomycin was used in penicillin-allergic patients. Unfortunately, the concepts about cost-effectiveness and the use of QALYs, although well accepted by many, are not used routinely in clinical practice. Nonetheless, this important study deserves review by clinicians who care for these patients.

MICROBIOLOGY

Many different organisms have been associated with IE in humans. Table 284.8 lists the most common causative agents responsible for the development of IE. Gram-positive cocci are the etiologic agents in 90% of cases in which an organism is isolated. Streptococci, especially of the viridans group, remain the bacteria isolated most frequently. Because of the increasing role of surgery and prosthetic material in the correction and palliation of CHD, the percentage of cases caused by staphylococci, gram-negative bacilli, and fungi have increased. Identification of the causative agent is the single most important procedure involved in confirming the diagnosis, directing therapy, and predicting outcome and possible complications.

Streptococci

Streptococci are a heterogenous group of organisms. Different systems of classifications depend on several features, including patterns of hemolysis observed on blood agar plates, biochemical reactions, growth characteristics, antigenic reaction, and

TABLE 284.8

CAUSATIVE AGENTS IN PEDIATRIC INFECTIVE ENDOCARDITIS

Organism	Incidence (%)
Streptococci	
Viridans	17–72
Enterococci	0–12
Pneumococci	0–21
beta-Hemolytic	0–8
Staphylococci	
Staphylococcus aureus	5–40
Staphylococcus epidermidis	0–15
Gram-negative aerobic bacilli	0–15
Fungi	0–12
Miscellaneous	0–10
Culture negative	2–32

serologic relatedness. The least discriminating system is based on the type of hemolysis produced by a strain of streptococcus when grown on a blood agar plate. In beta-hemolysis, a clear zone caused by complete blood cell lysis surrounds each colony; in gamma-hemolysis, no detectable hemolysis exists; and in alpha-hemolysis, an inner layer of unhemolyzed cells and an outer layer of hemolyzed cells produce a greenish discoloration in the medium. The term *viridans streptococci* refers to most strains that are alpha-hemolytic, although other strains such as the pneumococcus also may be alpha-hemolytic. The group of viridans streptococci is made up of many different species that vary considerably in biochemical properties and biologic behaviors. For instance, the viridans streptococcus *S. milleri* is especially virulent and causes a high incidence of suppurative intracardiac and extracardiac complications in patients with endocarditis. When a viridans streptococcus is isolated in a patient with endocarditis, it may be valuable for species determination to be performed by the laboratory. The most common viridans streptococci isolated from adults with IE are *S. sanguis, S. bovis, S. mutans,* and *S. mitior.*

The Lancefield typing system was devised to differentiate beta-hemolytic streptococci into serogroups by means of antigenic differences in cell-wall carbohydrates. Certain alpha- and gamma-hemolytic strains also contain group-specific antigen, such as enterococci, which contain group D cell-wall carbohydrates. Viridans streptococci may be Lancefield typable or nontypable.

The viridans streptococci are the most common etiologic agents in childhood IE, accounting for approximately 40% of cases. These organisms are part of the indigenous flora of the mouth and gastrointestinal tract. Any procedure that disrupts the mucosal integrity in these areas, such as dental surgery or extraction, predisposes to bacteremia with viridans streptococci. These streptococci commonly cause endocarditis in patients with underlying heart disease, but they are less common causes of postoperative infection. Although viridans streptococci usually are associated with a more indolent, subacute clinical presentation, they can cause acute, rapidly progressive disease. Most strains of viridans streptococci are exquisitely susceptible to penicillin, although prior antibiotic administration may promote infection with resistant strains. Recurrences and treatment failures are rare events.

Nutritionally variant viridans streptococci are being recognized increasingly as the etiologic agent of IE in children. The organisms grow in broth, but they do not grow in subculture unless L-cysteine or pyridoxine is added to the media. These organisms must be looked for in every case of culture-negative endocarditis.

The enterococcus is an unusual strain of streptococci because it is much less susceptible to penicillin; successful treatment requires use of an additional antibiotic, usually gentamicin, in children. Enterococcal endocarditis occurs less commonly in children than in adults, accounting for only 4% of pediatric cases. This strain of organisms inhabits the gastrointestinal and genitourinary tracts and may enter the bloodstream after instrumentation to these areas. Although 40% of adult patients with enterococcal endocarditis have no underlying heart disease, affected children rarely have previously normal hearts. Endocarditis should be considered in all infants and children with unexplained enterococcal bacteremia.

The pneumococcus is an alpha-hemolytic streptococcus, but the clinical presentation of pneumococcal endocarditis usually is very different from that of endocarditis carried by viridans streptococci. In the preantibiotic era, the pneumococcus accounted for 10% to 15% of cases of endocarditis, but it now causes fewer than 5% of cases. Approximately one-half of these infections occur in persons without underlying heart disease. The clinical course usually is acute and fulminant, with valvular dysfunction and cardiac decompensation occurring frequently.

Generally, in children, the mitral valve is affected predominantly. Early surgical intervention usually is required because the mortality with medical management alone may be as high as 50% to 75%.

Endocarditis caused by beta-hemolytic streptococci also occurred more commonly in the preantibiotic era than it does today. Most cases are caused by Lancefield groups B and G strains; groups C and A strains rarely cause endocarditis.

Staphylococci

Staphylococci are associated with 20% to 30% of the pediatric cases of IE, and the incidence is increasing. Most cases are caused by coagulase-positive *S. aureus,* but coagulase-negative staphylococci are causing an increased number of infections after cardiac surgery. *S. aureus* may attack previously normal heart valves and normal cardiac structures. *S. aureus* is the most likely cause of acute endocarditis in a previously normal child. The course often is fulminant, with frequent suppurative complications in the heart (e.g., myocardial abscess, pericarditis, valve ring abscess) and in other organs. *S. aureus* causes more than 50% of cases of endocarditis among intravenous drug abusers, but their disease tends to be less severe. The origin of the infecting strain is thought to be the addict's own nose or skin, not the injection paraphernalia. Endocarditis associated with indwelling vascular catheters or prosthetic heart valves frequently is caused by *S. aureus* bacteremia, even if a peripheral focus of infection exists. Treatment of *S. aureus* endocarditis has been complicated by the emergence of methicillin-resistant strains, which may require synergistic antibiotic combinations such as vancomycin and rifampin for cure.

The incidence of endocarditis caused by coagulase-negative staphylococci, usually *S. epidermidis,* is increasing rapidly. These organisms rarely cause IE in persons without underlying heart disease, but they are common etiologic agents of endocarditis after cardiac surgery. Coagulase-negative staphylococci are the major agents in prosthetic valve endocarditis, causing 25% to 67% of early cases and 25% to 33% of late cases. These organisms can be locally invasive. The mortality rate for adults with *S. epidermidis* prosthetic valve endocarditis and no valve replacement may approach 75%.

Gram-Negative Organisms

Gram-negative bacteria are the etiologic agents in 4% to 5% of pediatric cases of endocarditis. However, the percentage of children with gram-negative bacteremia who develop endocarditis is very low. Burn patients, immunosuppressed hosts, recipients of prosthetic heart valves, and narcotics addicts are at increased risk for development of gram-negative enteric bacteremia. Many species of gram-negative enteric organisms have caused IE in children, but no clear pattern has emerged because data are limited to case reports and general medicine reviews. Morbidity and mortality rates are high, with frequent development of large vegetations, embolic complications, and cardiac decompensation. Endocarditis should be suspected in patients with gram-negative infection if bacteremia persists despite administration of appropriate antibiotic therapy, especially if an unexplained heart murmur and anemia develop. In the early postoperative period after cardiac surgery, sustained gram-negative bacteremia commonly is secondary to other foci of infection (e.g., urinary tract) and does not imply the presence of endocarditis.

Pseudomonas spp. endocarditis is especially difficult to treat and has a high mortality rate. Most patients with this disease abuse intravenous drugs. Major embolic complications and CHF are common occurrences.

Other gram-negative organisms associated with IE are the HACEK coccobacilli (i.e., *Haemophilus* spp., *Actinobacillus* spp., *Cardiobacterium* spp., *Eikenella* spp., and *Kingella* spp.). Endocarditis caused by *Haemophilus influenzae* has been reported in several children, but cases caused by *H. aphrophilus* and *H. parainfluenzae* occur more commonly. A similar organism, *Streptobacillus moniliformis,* has been linked to endocarditis. All HACEK organisms are fastidious and may require 2 to 3 weeks for primary isolation, needing subculture onto chocolate agar in 5% to 10% carbon dioxide for optimal growth. These organisms should be considered in all presentations of culture-negative endocarditis.

In the preantibiotic era, *Neisseria gonorrhoeae* was responsible for 10% of IE cases. Since 1942, fewer than 40 cases have been reported. The onset usually is acute. It tends to attack previously normal valves, and valve replacement frequently is necessary. Nonpathogenic *Neisseria* spp. are isolated more frequently in endocarditis than are gonococci, but they usually attack abnormal or prosthetic valves.

Gram-Positive Bacilli

Corynebacterium organisms are unusual agents of IE, but they may be found on normal and abnormal heart valves. Both toxigenic and nontoxigenic strains of *Corynebacterium diphtheriae* cause endocarditis in children. *Listeria monocytogenes* endocarditis is a rare finding in children and has a high mortality rate. Unlike other forms of listeriosis, it is not seen frequently in immunocompromised hosts, and it has not been associated with listeriosis in neonates. Fewer than 30 cases of *Lactobacillus* spp. endocarditis have been described. This infection usually develops after dental manipulation in a person with underlying heart disease. Embolic phenomena are common occurrences, but treatment usually is successful if appropriate antibiotics are used.

Fungi

The most common predisposing conditions for fungal endocarditis in children are cardiovascular surgery, prolonged antibiotic usage, and an indwelling intravenous catheter. Most infections are caused by *Candida albicans,* but other *Candida* species, including *C. tropicalis, C. stellatoides, C. krusei, C. parapsilosis,* and *C. guilliermondi,* have been implicated. Endocarditis caused by intravenous drug abuse is caused more frequently by species other than *C. albicans.* The clinical course usually is subacute. Embolic phenomena are extremely common findings and may be the first clinical indication of infection. Large, friable vegetations occur frequently. Ocular and cutaneous manifestations may aid in establishing the diagnosis. The prognosis for *Candida* endocarditis is poor because of the propensity for septic emboli to major organs, the tendency for invasion into the myocardium, and the poor penetration of antifungal agents into the vegetations. Diagnosis may be delayed by the tendency for blood culture results to be negative or positive only intermittently. Successful therapy usually requires surgical intervention.

Aspergillus organisms are the second most common cause of fungal endocarditis in children. Most patients have had underlying heart disease and recent cardiac surgery, although normal valves can be affected. The manifestations seen most frequently are fever and emboli, especially to the CNS. Only four cases in children have been diagnosed antemortem, three by culture of peripheral emboli. Blood culture results usually are negative. Surgical removal of all infected material is recommended, although only one child has been treated successfully.

Other fungi that rarely cause IE include *Histoplasma capsulatum, Coccidioides immitis, Cryptococcus neoformans, Torulopsis glabrata, Hormodendrum* spp., *Mucor* spp., *Paecilomyces* spp., *Phialophora* spp., and *Chrysosporium* spp.

Other Organisms

Anaerobic bacilli cause 1% of IE in adults, but reports of anaerobic endocarditis in children are exceedingly rare.

IE caused by *Coxiella burnetii* (i.e., Q fever) has been documented in more than 100 patients, including several children. Clinical manifestations, including anemia, hepatosplenomegaly, fever, and intracardiac vegetations, are similar in children and adults. The diagnosis is confirmed by serologic and immunohistologic investigation. Although Q fever has been documented in the United States, it occurs much more commonly in England, Australia, and France.

TREATMENT

Several general principles provide the basis for treatment of IE. The preferable route of antibiotic administration is intravenous. Oral antibiotics may be absorbed poorly or erratically, especially in infants, which may result in treatment failure. A course of at least 4 and up to 6 weeks or longer is required to sterilize vegetations and prevent relapse. Bacteriostatic agents are contraindicated and may lead to failure or relapse if used. Synergism between certain agents may produce a rapid bactericidal effect and allow smaller doses of each drug to be administered, thereby reducing possible toxic side effects. However, certain drug combinations, such as penicillin and chloramphenicol, may be antagonistic.

After therapy has been initiated, daily blood cultures should be obtained. Although negative blood culture results may not correlate necessarily with therapeutic success, continued positive blood culture results usually indicate a need for investigation of the serum concentration of the drug in the patient, for the addition of another agent, or for a change in therapy. If the patient has not responded clinically to initial antibiotic therapy within several days, more blood cultures should be obtained. In addition, attention to the patient's clinical course is essential. Patients usually begin to improve within a few days of the initiation of appropriate therapy, although persistent fever may occur occasionally in patients who eventually have a good outcome.

Electrocardiographic monitoring should be performed in the early stages to assess for the presence of arrhythmias or the development of conduction disturbances that may require immediate attention. If second-degree atrioventricular block develops during an episode of endocarditis, temporary transvenous pacing should be considered. Pacing always should be instituted for third-degree atrioventricular block. Physical examination to assess for development of regurgitant murmurs or embolic events also is mandatory.

Current recommendations for optimal therapy in pediatric IE are based largely on studies from adult patients. These regimens usually are more successful and less toxic in children than in adults (Tables 284.9 to 284.14).

The timing of therapy generally depends on the clinical condition of the patient. In a case of suspected IE in a seriously ill child, empiric therapy should begin immediately after the appropriate blood cultures have been obtained. In patients in whom *S. aureus* is probable (e.g., acute presentation, intravenous drug abusers), a penicillinase-resistant penicillin should be added to the usual regimen of penicillin G and an aminoglycoside. The latter two agents would be used in a patient with a subacute presentation and would be appropriate

TABLE 284.9

SUGGESTED INTRAVENOUS ANTIBIOTIC DOSES AND SCHEDULES FOR INFECTIVE ENDOCARDITIS IN CHILDREN

Antibiotic	Daily Dose/kg	Divided Doses Every
Aqueous crystalline Penicillin G sodium	200,000–300,000 U	4 hr
Ampicillin sodium	200–300 mg	4–6 hr
Cefazolin	100 mg	6–8 hr
Ceftriaxone	75–100 mg	12–24 hr
Gentamicin sulfate	3.0–7.5 mg	8 hr
Nafcillin sodium	100–200 mg (max., 12 g)	4–6 hr
Oxacillin sodium	100–200 mg (max., 12 g)	4–6 hr
Rifampin	20 mg	8–12 hr
Vancomycin Hydrochloride	30–60 mg	6–12 hr

for viridans streptococci, enterococci, and most gram-negative organisms. Patients who have recently undergone cardiac surgery would receive vancomycin in addition to an aminoglycoside because of the high incidence of hospital-acquired *S. epidermidis,* which may be resistant to methicillin or nafcillin. Once the blood cultures are examined for sensitivity to various antibiotic agents, therapy may be tailored appropriately for the patient.

Several tests are available to determine how sensitive an organism is to treatment with antimicrobials. The minimal inhibitory concentration (MIC) is defined as the lowest concentration of the agent that prevents visible growth, usually in broth, after incubation for 18 to 24 hours. The minimal bactericidal concentration is defined as the lowest concentration resulting in either sterilization or a decline in bacterial count of 99.9%. Monitoring the inhibitory and bactericidal activity of the patient's serum is controversial. The Schlichter test is an *in vitro* determination of the maximal serum inhibitory and serum bactericidal levels specific for an infecting organism. However, standardization of this test is poor among different laboratories, which creates problems for interpretation. Studies in rabbits who have experimentally induced endocarditis show that bactericidal titers of 1:8 or greater usually correlate with therapeutic success. In humans with IE, no similar correlation was seen at titers of 1:8. Although no formal recommendation exists, prospective studies suggest that therapy should be tailored to achieve peak titers of 1:64 or greater and trough titers equal to or greater than 1:32. The Kirby-Bauer disc sensitivity test is neither reliable nor quantitative and should not be used to guide therapy. Most viridans streptococci, *S. pyogenes, S. pneumoniae,* and nonenterococcal group D streptococci have an MIC for penicillin of less than 0.2 fg/mL in broth. Resistance, as defined by organisms with an MIC of greater than or equal to 0.2 fg/mL, occurs in approximately 15% to 20% of viridans streptococci. Tolerance occurs when growth of the organism is inhibited to an MIC to penicillin of less than 0.1 fg/mL along with a minimal bactericidal concentration greater than eight times the MIC. Treatment failure may result because of organisms that become tolerant to therapy when penicillin is used as the sole agent. Streptomycin and gentamicin each act synergistically with penicillin or vancomycin *in vitro* and have been effective in eradicating vegetations in experimentally induced endocarditis in rabbits.

In adults with IE caused by penicillin-sensitive viridans streptococci, an unacceptable relapse rate is obtained if penicillin is used alone for 2 weeks. However, if intramuscular procaine penicillin and streptomycin are given together for 2 weeks, 99% of patients are cured, a rate identical to that for a 4-week course of penicillin agents alone or penicillin for 4 weeks with streptomycin administered concomitantly during the first 2 weeks. However, streptomycin is not synergistic for strains with high-level streptomycin resistance; gentamicin is the preferred second drug for these rare isolates. A 2-week regiment of penicillin–gentamicin is the least expensive and is the preferred therapy in uncomplicated cases of penicillin-susceptible streptococcal endocarditis in young adults. In patients with a high risk of developing gentamicin-induced ototoxicity or those in renal failure, 4 weeks of penicillin alone is recommended. Vancomycin or ceftriaxone is recommended for 4 weeks in those with penicillin allergy and penicillin-susceptible viridans streptococcal infection. Adults with a complicated course should receive 4 weeks of penicillin and 2 weeks of gentamicin during the initial 2 weeks of therapy. Patients with a streptococcal infection of a prosthetic valve or other material should receive a 6-week course of penicillin with the addition of an aminoglycoside.

Most strains of enterococci have an MIC-to-penicillin value greater than or equal to 0.4 μg/mL and a minimal bactericidal concentration greater than or equal to 6.25 μg/mL. Penicillin alone is ineffective and requires the addition of an aminoglycoside to act synergistically to effect a cure. Penicillin plus gentamicin is the preferred initial treatment because of a 20% to 50% resistance rate (MIC greater than 2,000 μg/mL) for streptomycin among enterococcal strains. Streptomycin-resistant strains have responded to the synergistic effect of penicillin and gentamicin *in vitro*. Since some resistance to gentamicin has been seen in some isolates, all aminoglycosides should be tested because of selective resistance to this class of drugs.

TABLE 284.10

SUGGESTED REGIMENS FOR TREATMENT OF NATIVE-VALVE ENDOCARDITIS CAUSED BY PENICILLIN-SUSCEPTIBLE VIRIDANS *STREPTOCOCCI* AND *STREPTOCOCCUS BOVIS* (MIC ≤1 μg/mL) IN ADULTS

Antibiotic(s)	Duration (wks)	Comments
Aqueous crystalline penicillin G sodium Or	4	Preferred for patients with impairment of the eighth cranial nerve or renal function
Ceftriaxone sodium	4	
Aqueous crystalline penicillin G sodium ceftriaxone Plus	2	Gentamicin peak serum concentration of approximately 3 μg/mL is desirable
Gentamicin sulfate	2	
Vancomycin hydrochloride	4–6	Recommended for patients allergic to β-lactam antibiotics

From Wilson WR, Karchmer AW, Dajani AS, et al. Antibiotic treatment of adults with infective endocarditis due to streptococci, enterococci, staphylococci, and HACEK microorganisms. *JAMA* 1995;274:1706.

TABLE 284.11

SUGGESTED THERAPY FOR NATIVE-VALVE ENDOCARDITIS CAUSED BY STRAINS OF VIRIDANS *STREPTOCOCCI* AND *STREPTOCOCCUS BOVIS* RELATIVELY RESISTANT TO PENICILLIN G (MIC, 0.1 AND 0.5 μg/mL) IN ADULTS

Antibiotic(s)	Duration (wks)	Comments
Aqueous crystalline penicillin G sodium	4	Cefazolin or other first-generation cephalosporins may be substituted for penicillin in patients whose penicillin hypersensitivity is not of the immediate type
Or		
Ceftriaxone sodium		
Plus		
Gentamicin sulfate	2	
Vancomycin hydrochloride	4–6	Recommended for patients allergic to β-lactam antibiotics

From Wilson WR, Karchmer AW, Dajani AS, et al. Antibiotic treatment of adults with infective endocarditis due to streptococci, enterococci, staphylococci, and HACEK microorganisms. *JAMA* 1995;274:1706. Copyright 1995. American Medical Association.

For patients with IE caused by *S. aureus,* a semisynthetic penicillinase-resistant penicillin is given for 6 weeks. A penicillin-susceptible strain (MIC less than 0.1 μg/mL) is encountered occasionally, and penicillin G can be used. Usually, semisynthetic penicillinase-resistant penicillin given for 4 to 6 weeks is the recommended therapy. Although *in vitro* and animal studies have demonstrated enhanced killing of these organisms when gentamicin is added to nafcillin, no real value has been found for most patients, and this combination usually is reserved for seriously ill patients. Vancomycin is used in penicillin-allergic patients or for methicillin resistance. However, a prospective study of adults with methicillin-resistant *S. aureus* endocarditis demonstrated a delayed response compared with patients with a methicillin-sensitive strain. The addition of rifampin did not appear to improve the response time or to be more effective than was vancomycin alone. Vancomycin is used in patients with hospital-acquired infection caused by *S. epidermidis* because of the high rate of methicillin-resistant organisms found in this infection. Its bactericidal activity may be increased by the addition of gentamicin or rifampin, and it is recommended in prosthetic valve endocarditis caused by *S. epidermidis.*

Infectious endocarditis caused by gram-negative organisms requires individualized therapy determined by the findings of *in vitro* susceptibility testing. If *Klebsiella* or *Pseudomonas* are involved, a total of 6 to 8 weeks of therapy with two or more agents may be necessary, and surgical therapy frequently is necessary. Infections caused by *Haemophilus* organisms usually respond to ampicillin administered for 4 weeks, although the addition of an aminoglycoside may improve the outcome. Most anaerobes are sensitive to penicillin alone, but if resistant *Bacteroides fragilis* organisms are found, treatment with metronidazole is recommended.

Fungal endocarditis presents the clinician with several difficult problems. The overall survival rate is only 20%, and only rarely is medical therapy reported to be successful in eradicating the disease. A delay in establishing the diagnosis is encountered frequently because of slow growth in blood culture media. Embolic events often are the first serious sign of fungal endocarditis that may necessitate immediate surgical intervention. The primary antifungal agent used is amphotericin B, alone or in combination with 5-fluorocytosine. Amphotericin B is given at a dose of 0.5 to 1.0 mg/kg/day. Although usually less severe in children than in adults, toxic reactions may necessitate altering the usual regimen. Fevers, chills, phlebitis, anemia, nephrotoxicity, renal tubular acidosis, hypocalcemia, and thrombocytopenia are the toxic effects reported most commonly. Although the optimal dose of amphotericin B is unknown, total doses of 20 to 50 mg/kg usually are used. Adults should not receive more than 50 mg/day. Therapy usually continues for at least 8 weeks and, over the course of a long time, the physician should look for evidence of recurrence because relapses have been observed as long as 2 years after a presumed cure. Amphotericin B penetrates vegetations poorly and may not prevent continued growth of the fungal organism. Reseeding of the vegetation from distant metastatic sites may occur, further complicating attempts at cure. Most physicians agree that the combination of antifungal agents and surgery is the treatment of choice in fungal endocarditis.

In patients with culture-negative endocarditis, empiric therapy with two or more agents is used for 6 weeks, during which time continuing efforts to identify an organism are pursued. In

TABLE 284.12

SUGGESTED THERAPY FOR ENDOCARDITIS CAUSED BY ENTEROCOCCI AND OTHER SELECTED STREPTOCOCCI* IN ADULTS

Antibiotic(s)	Duration (wks)	Comments
Aqueous crystalline penicillin G sodium	4–6	Four-week therapy recommended for patients with symptoms <3 mo in duration. Six-week therapy recommended for patients with symptoms >3 mo in duration
Plus		
Gentamicin sulfate	4–6	
Ampicillin sodium	4–6	
Plus		
Gentamicin sulfate	4–6	
Vancomycin hydrochloride	6	Recommended for patients allergic to β-lactam antibiotics
Plus		
Gentamicin sulfate	6	

*This table is for endocarditis caused by gentamicin- or vancomycin-susceptible enterococci viridans streptococci with an MIC greater than 0.5 μg/mL, Abiotrophia species, or prosthetic-valve endocarditis to viridans streptococci or Streptococcus bovis.
MIC, minimal inhibitory concentration.
From Wilson WR, Karchmer AW, Dajani AS, et al. Antibiotic treatment of adults with infective endocarditis due to streptococci, enterococci, staphylococci, and HACEK microorganisms. *JAMA* 1995;274:1706.

TABLE 284.13

SUGGESTED THERAPY FOR ENDOCARDITIS CAUSED BY STAPHYLOCOCCI IN THE ABSENCE OF PROSTHETIC MATERIAL IN ADULTS

Antibiotic(s)	Duration	Comments
Methicillin-Susceptible Staphylococci*		
Nafcillin sodium or oxacillin sodium	6 wk	Benefit of additional aminoglycoside
Optional addition of Gentamicin sulfate	3–5 days	has not been established
Cefazolin or other first-generation Cephalosporin	6 wk	For patients with non-immediate-type hypersensitivity to penicillin
Optional addition of Gentamicin sulfate	3–5 days	
Vancomycin hydrochloride	6 wk	Recommended for patients allergic to penicillin
Methicillin-Resistant Staphylococci		
Vancomycin hydrochloride	≥6 wk	
Plus		
Rifampin	≥6 wk	
Gentamicin	2 wk	

*If *Staphylococcus* is penicillin-susceptible (minimal inhibitory concentration ≤0.1 μg/mL), aqueous crystalline penicillin G sodium can be used for 6 weeks instead of nafcillin or axacillin.
Data from Wilson WR, Karchmer AW, Dajani AS, et al. Antibiotic treatment of adults with infective endocarditis due to streptococci, enterococci, staphylococci, and HACEK microorganisms. *JAMA* 1995;274:1706 and Ferrieri P, Gewitz MH, Gerber MA, et al. Unique features of endocarditis in children. *Pediatrics* 2002;109:931.

a study of culture-negative endocarditis in 52 adult patients, survival was correlated with the clinical response to the initial choice of antibiotics, and most deaths were attributable to CHF or systemic embolic events.

Surgery has been a valuable adjunct to medical therapy for IE in certain circumstances. Many studies of the role of surgery recruited mostly adult patients and included a few pediatric patients. In one review of 139 patients who underwent surgical therapy for the treatment of IE, the most common reason for referral was CHF, alone or combined with other conditions (e.g., embolization, persistent infection). Aortic valve involvement predominated over mitral valve disease. The early mortality rate was 25%, and the late mortality (more than 30 days) rate was 8.6%. Only 1.6% of the patients had residual infection, despite the fact that 10% had had a positive valve culture result at the time of surgery. One review found that

the most common indication for surgical intervention was severe CHF, alone (84%) or combined with other factors (12%). The early and late mortality were 30% and 7%, respectively. The most significant factor affecting survival was severe cardiac failure. In the cases of fungal endocarditis included in the study, recurrent emboli and persistent infection were found more commonly than was severe CHF as the indication for surgery.

When aortic valve disease alone is considered, unstable hemodynamics may be the primary reason to perform surgery. Placement of a prosthetic valve during active infection seems to contradict classic surgical techniques. However, a surprisingly low incidence of recurrent infection occurs when valve replacement is performed in patients other than intravenous drug abusers. No difference in the reinfection rates of bioprosthetic valves and prosthetic valves has been reported. Human

TABLE 284.14

SUGGESTED THERAPY FOR ENDOCARDITIS CAUSED BY STAPHYLOCOCCI IN THE PRESENCE OF A PROSTHETIC VALVE OR OTHER PROSTHETIC MATERIAL IN ADULTS

Antibiotic(s)	Duration (wks)	Comments
Methicillin-Susceptible Staphylococci		
Nafcillin sodium or oxacillin Sodium	≥6	First-generation cephalosporins or vancomycin should be used in
Plus		patients allergic to β-lactam antibiotics
Rifampin	≥6	Rifampin plays a unique role in eradication of staphylococci from prosthetic material
Plus		
Gentamicin sulfate	2	
Methicillin-Resistant Staphylococci		
Vancomycin hydrochloride	≥6	
Plus		
Rifampin	≥6	
Plus		
Gentamicin sulfate	2	

From Wilson WR, Karchmer AW, Dajani AS, et al. Antibiotic treatment of adults with infective endocarditis due to streptococci, enterococci, staphylococci, and HACEK microorganisms. *JAMA* 1995;274:1706.

allograft valves also have been used with success, even in high-risk patients. Double valve replacement (i.e., aortic and mitral) has been performed with success when the infection has involved both structures. Extravalvular aortic root infection can be managed successfully with aortic valve replacement, alone or with a Teflon patch attached.

A study of surgical treatment of IE that included 11 patients with CHD (seven with ventricular septal defect, two with patent ductus arteriosus, one with transposition of the great vessels, and one with secundum atrial septal defect) found that the primary indications for intervention were heart failure secondary to valve destruction, removal of a newly leaking prosthetic valve, persistent or recurrent infection, and large, left-sided, mobile vegetations, regardless of the occurrence of embolism. Overall, the patients with CHD had the lowest mortality rate, which the researchers attributed to the primary involvement of the right side of the heart and the low incidence of embolic events. The mortality rate was dramatically lower for surgical therapy for prosthetic valve endocarditis than for native valve endocarditis (10% versus 32%). The investigators concluded that surgery should be considered earlier when medical treatment is failing; when large, mobile vegetations are observed on echocardiographic study; and when fungal endocarditis is encountered. Operative intervention can be performed, even during active infection, with good results.

A large series of patients from South Africa was studied prospectively to establish the safety and efficacy of early surgical intervention in native left-sided endocarditis. These patients were referred for surgery if they had CHF from valve dysfunction and vegetations seen on an echocardiographic examination. Despite heart failure and abscess formation, only a 4% hospital mortality and a 10% late mortality occurred. These exceptionally low mortality figures in this high-risk group make a strong case for early intervention after CHF develops rather than following a more conventional, medical approach. Unfortunately, no similar studies of the pediatric group with congenital heart disorders have been performed. Patients with infected or contaminated (e.g., skin breakdown over the pacemaker site with no evidence of inflammation) endocardial pacemaker or pacemaker leads must have these leads removed and temporary pacing instituted. Permanent pacing leads can be placed safely after successful therapy has been administered. Patients who have been treated successfully for endocarditis and who have prosthetic material in the heart should *not* receive chronic oral suppressive therapy in an attempt to prevent a relapse.

PROGNOSIS

The course and prognosis of patients depend on many underlying factors, including the severity of the primary cardiac lesion, the presence of prosthetic material, the infecting organism, the duration of illness before diagnosis, initiation of appropriate therapy, and the clinical condition at the time of diagnosis (e.g., degree of respiratory, neurologic, and cardiovascular or renal compromise). IE was fatal almost 100% of the time in the pre-antibiotic era. The rate of mortality is now between 20% and 30% because of improved methods of diagnosis and treatment with appropriate antibiotics. The mortality rate is somewhat higher in patients with acute staphylococcal infection, fungal infection, and prosthetic valve endocarditis. Sudden cardiac decompensation caused by CHF remains the single most important factor affecting mortality. Several studies of the adult population have correlated directly mortality and uncontrolled CHF. Death may be the result of sudden perforation of the aortic valve with severe aortic insufficiency, chordal rupture with resultant mitral regurgitation, and myocardial necrosis with resultant intracardiac shunting through a ventricular or atrial septal defect or through an atrioventricular communication. Intramyocardial abscess formation with the development of myocarditis may be an important factor determining the ultimate prognosis.

Patients who survive always will be at risk for future development of IE. After an apparently successful course of therapy, the disease may recur early (within 3 months of completion of therapy) or late (3 to 6 months after completion of therapy), and it should be suspected if fever or other symptoms recur shortly after antibiotics are discontinued. The organism found at relapse may be identical to or different from the organism identified initially.

Suggested Readings

Awadallah SM, Kavey RE, Byrum CJ, et al. The changing pattern of infective endocarditis in childhood. *Am J Cardiol* 1991;68:90.

Blieden LC, et al. Bacterial endocarditis in the neonate. *Am J Dis Child* 1972;124:747.

Caviness AC, Jones JL, Deguzman MA, et al. A cost-effectiveness analysis of bacterial endocarditis prophylaxis for febrile children who have cardiac lesions and undergo urinary catheterization in the emergency room. *Pediatrics* 2004;113:1291.

Choi M, Mailman TL. Pneumococcal endocarditis in infants and children. *Pediatr Infect Dis J* 2004;23:166.

Clemens JD, Horwitz RI, Jaffe CC, et al. A controlled evaluation of the risk of bacterial endocarditis in persons with mitral valve prolapse. *N Engl J Med* 1982;307:776.

Dajani AS, Taubert KA, Wilson W, et al. Prevention of endocarditis. Recommendations by the American Heart Association. *JAMA* 1997;277:1794.

Ferrieri P, Gewitz MH, Gerber MA, et al. Unique features of infective endocarditis in childhood. *Circulation* 2002;105:2115.

Givner LB, Mason ED, Jr, Wald ER, et al. Pneumococcal endocarditis in children. *CID* 2004;38:1273.

Humpl T, McCrindle BW, Smallhorn JF, et al. The relative roles of transthoracic compared with transesophageal echocardiography in children with suspected infective endocarditis. *J Am Coll Cardiol* 2003;41:2068.

Ivert TS, Dismukes WE, Cobbs CG, et al. Prosthetic valve endocarditis. *Circulation* 1984;69:223.

Johnson DH, Rosenthal A, Nadas A. A forty-year review of bacterial endocarditis in infancy and childhood. *Circulation* 1975;51:581.

Kaplan EL, Rich H, Gersony W, et al. A collaborative study of infective endocarditis in the 1970s. Emphasis on infections in patients who have undergone cardiovascular surgery. *Circulation* 1979;59:327.

Karl T, Wensley D, Stark J, et al. Infective endocarditis in children with congenital heart disease: comparison of selected features in patients with surgical correction or palliation and those without. *Br Heart J* 1987;58:57.

Knirsch W, Hassberg D, Beyer A, et al. Knowledge, compliance and practice of antibiotic endocarditis prophylaxis of patients with congenital heart disease. *Pediatr Cardiol* 2003; 24:344.

Michelfelder EC, Ochsner JE, Khoury P, et al. Does assessment of pretest probability of disease improve the utility of echocardiography in suspected endocarditis in children? *J Pediatr* 2003;142:263.

Rubinstein E, Noriega ER, Simberkoff MS, et al. Fungal endocarditis: analysis of 24 cases and review of the literature. *Medicine (Baltimore)* 1975;54:331.

Sande MA, Scheld WM. Combination antibiotic therapy of bacterial endocarditis. *Ann Intern Med* 1980;92:390.

Van Hare GF, Ben-Shachar G, Liebman J, et al. Infective endocarditis in infants and children during the past 10 years: a decade of change. *Am Heart J* 1984;107:1235.

Weinstein L, Schlesinger JJ. Pathoanatomic, pathophysiologic, and clinical correlations in endocarditis. *N Engl J Med* 1974;291:832.

CHAPTER 285 ■ RHEUMATIC FEVER

GALAL M. EL-SAID, YASSER M. K. BAGHDADY, AND HOWAIDA G. EL-SAID

Rheumatic fever (RF) is a delayed, nonsuppurative sequela to upper respiratory infection with group A beta-hemolytic streptococci. It is a diffuse inflammatory disease of the connective tissue that involves principally the heart, blood vessels, joints, central nervous system, and subcutaneous tissues.

The term *acute RF* is a misnomer because it may not be acute, rheumatic, or febrile. Although the term emphasizes involvement of the joints, the disease owes its importance to involvement of the heart. As early as 1884, Lasegue described this feature: "Rheumatic fever is a disease that licks the joints but bites the heart."

EPIDEMIOLOGY

Numerous investigators have documented the declining incidence of RF, even before the introduction of penicillin (Fig. 285.1). In Rochester, Minnesota, the age-adjusted annual incidence per 100,000 persons was 20 from 1939 to 1949, 12 from 1950 to 1964, and 3 from 1965 to 1978. Several more recent outbreaks in military and civilian populations in the United States correlated with the reappearance of virulent M-protein strains belonging to the M serotype associated with previous RF epidemics.

In contrast to trends in the United States, the incidence of RF has not decreased in developing countries. Worldwide, an estimated 5 to 30 million children and young adults have chronic rheumatic heart disease (RHD), and 90,000 patients die of this disease each year.

Several factors predispose to development of RF: age, family history, season, recurrent streptococcal infections, and host factors affecting susceptibility. The first attack usually occurs in patients between 5 and 15 years of age. RF is a a rare occurrence in children younger than 4 years of age. No gender preference exists unless chorea is included, in which case the incidence is slightly greater among girls.

RF may affect more than one member in the same family. The same housing conditions possibly predispose several persons to recurrent streptococcal infections. Constitutional susceptibility may be a factor, but no evidence for genetic markers in rheumatic patients exists, and HLA genotypes do not correlate with the development of RF. Like streptococcal pharyngitis, RF occurs more commonly in the winter and spring.

Recurrent streptococcal infections are the most important predisposing factor in the occurrence and recurrence of RF. Approximately 1% to 5% of streptococcal throat infections are followed by development of RF. The most important factors that may be related to the attack rate of RF after streptococcal pharyngitis are the magnitude of the immune response to the antecedent infections and the duration of convalescent carriage of the organisms. Skin infections are unlikely to produce the disease.

Because RF develops after streptococcal pharyngitis in a relatively small percentage of patients, host predisposition probably is a factor (Fig. 285.2). After RF is acquired, its reactivation after subsequent streptococcal infections is much more likely to occur. The recurrence rate per infection is approximately 50% during the first year after the initial attack; it decreases sharply after that. The rate levels off after several years to

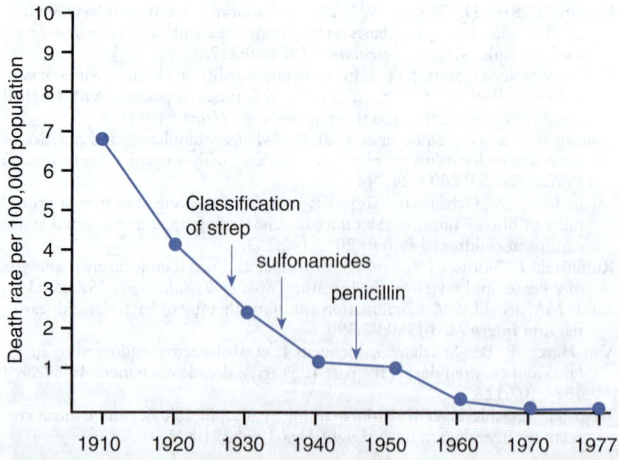

FIGURE 285.1. Diseases often "disappear" before they should. Here is the reported mortality rate for rheumatic fever in the United States, seemingly unrelated to discoveries as the classification of streptococci, sulfonamides, and penicillin. (Reprinted from Gordis L. The virtual disappearance of rheumatic fever in the United States: lessons in the rise and fall of disease. T. Duckett Jones Memorial Lecture. *Circulation* 1985;72:1155.)

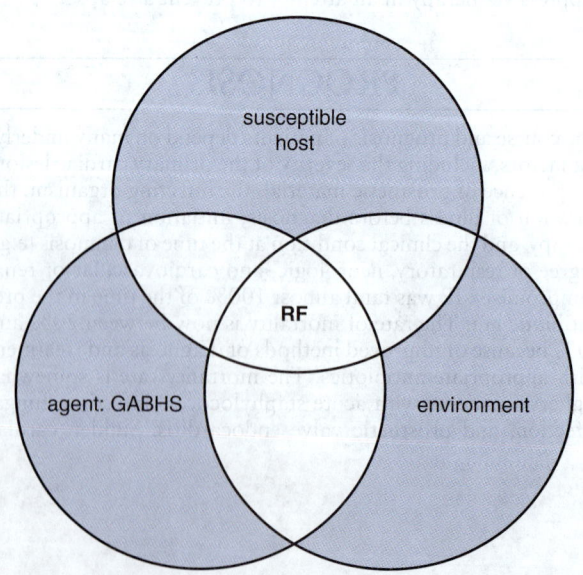

FIGURE 285.2. Epidemiologic triad of rheumatic fever (RF). GABHS, group A beta-hemolytic streptococci.

approximately 10%. This persistently high attack rate after RF suggests acquired hyperreactivity.

ETIOLOGY

Streptococci

Streptococci are a large group of gram-positive microorganisms that are distributed widely in nature. When cultured, they are arranged in chains. Their ability to hemolyze erythrocytes to various degrees is an important basis for their classification. The alpha-hemolytic streptococci form colonies surrounded by an ill-defined, greenish halo in which hemolysis is incomplete. The beta-hemolytic streptococci produce a clear zone of hemolysis on blood agar; gamma-streptococci do not have any effect on blood-containing media. The streptococcus (Fig. 285.3) is composed of a core of cytoplasm surrounded by three layers: a cytoplasmic membrane, a cell wall, and a capsule that constitutes the external surface of the organism. The capsule is composed of hyaluronate, which is nonantigenic. The cell wall is composed of three layers: the outermost protein, the middle carbohydrate, and the innermost mucopeptide protoplast. The middle layer of the cell wall, the carbohydrate layer, provides the group specification, given as the alphabetic classification (e.g., A through H) of Lancefield. The outer protein layer and its fimbriae, which are attached to the surface of the organism, contain the proteins designated M, T, and R. The M protein is the most important because it determines the virulence of the organism, stimulates formation of opsonizing and precipitating antibodies, and may impede phagocytosis. Lancefield and colleagues further classified group A streptococci into serologic types on the basis of the M protein. RF can result from infection by many of the serotypes of group A beta-hemolytic streptococci, but glomerulonephritis is associated with only a limited number of these serotypes. The cytoplasmic membrane is an antigenic lipoprotein that cross-reacts with several mammalian tissue antigens, including the glomerular basement membrane and sarcolemmal antigen.

The streptococcus produces several extracellular products, some of which are involved in the diseases produced by the microorganism. Erythrogenic toxin is responsible for the rash of scarlet fever. Streptolysin O, which is active only in the reduced state, is cardiotoxic and leukotoxic, is responsible for hemolysis of erythrocytes, and elicits an antibody response, antistreptolysin O (ASO), which is the basis for a useful assay of streptococcal infections. The antigenicity of streptolysin O is inhibited by lipid extracts (probably cholesterol) of skin, and this property may be responsible for the lack of association between streptococcal skin infections and RF. Streptolysin S, an oxygen-stable product, produces the hemolysis characteristic of beta-hemolytic streptococci when cultured on sheep blood agar. Streptokinase converts plasminogen to plasmin, an active proteolytic enzyme that digests fibrin. Diphosphopyridine nucleotidase, which determines the ability of the organism to kill leukocytes, elicits an antibody response (i.e., antidiphosphopyridine nucleotidase). There are four deoxyribonucleases (i.e., A, B, C, D), all of which are antigenic. Deoxyribonuclease B, known as *streptodornase*, is produced in the largest quantities in response to group A streptococcal infections and is the most consistent of the deoxyribonucleases.

RF develops when children or adolescents develop pharangitis with group A beta-hemolytic streptococcal infection. The organism attaches itself on the epithelium of the upper respiratory tract and invades the tissues. The incubation period is 2 to 4 days, and the invading organism elicits an acute inflammatory response resulting in sore throat, fever, malaise, headache, and an elevated leukocyte count that last for 3 to 5 days. RF occurs in a small percentage of these patients after resolution of the sore throat. Only infections of the pharynx initiate or reactivate RF.

Direct contact with respiratory secretions transmits the organism, and crowding enhances transmission. Patients remain infected for weeks after symptomatic resolution of pharangitis and may serve as a reservoir for infecting others.

Mechanism Producing Rheumatic Fever

RF is thought to be an autoimmune disease. The requirements for its development include group A beta-hemolytic streptococcal infection in the throat with an antibody response indicative of recent infection and persistence of the organism in the pharynx for a period sufficient to produce an immunologic

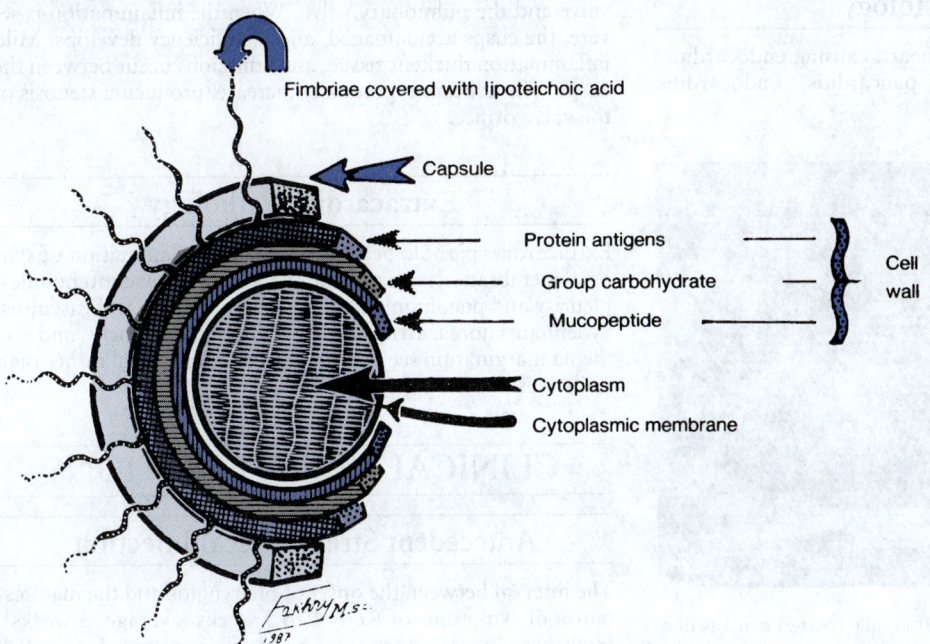

Fimbriae covered with lipoteichoic acid

Capsule

Protein antigens

Group carbohydrate — Cell wall

Mucopeptide

Cytoplasm

Cytoplasmic membrane

FIGURE 285.3. With one end embedded in the protein layer of the streptococcal cell wall, fimbriae covered with lipoteichoic acid help the organism adhere to the throat epithelium (i.e., adherence factor). These fimbriae contain M protein (i.e., virulence factor). Each of the layers of the cell wall and the cytoplasmic membrane cross-reacts with several antigens.

response. The magnitude of the antibody response is a major factor determining the attack rate of RF after streptococcal infection. The predisposing organism has antigens immunologically similar to proteins in the human heart, and the antibodies produced against the streptococci react with the heart (i.e., cross-reactive immunity). A plethora of streptococcal cellular components cross-reacting with various mammalian tissues has been described. The hyaluronate capsule is identical to human hyaluronate. Antibodies to the cell wall polysaccharide cross-react with glycoproteins of heart valves. Membrane antigens cross-react with the sarcolemma and smooth muscles of endocardial and myocardial arteries. Antibody to the streptococcal group A polysaccharide persists in the serum of patients with rheumatic valvular disease, in contrast to its more rapid decline in patients with RF without cardiac involvement. As with other possible autoimmune diseases, the difficulties of differentiating cause from effect of injury have rendered this hypothesis unprovable.

Conclusion

Although the precise pathogenetic mechanisms of RHD remain elusive, a mounting body of evidence is emerging to support the concept of an abnormal, autoimmune host response following exposure of susceptible individuals to group A streptococcal antigens. Abnormalities in both cellular and humoral immune responses have been documented in affected patients.

PATHOLOGY

General Pathology

Nonspecific lesions result from fibrinoid degeneration of the connective tissue, inflammatory edema, and inflammatory cell infiltration. Specific lesions result from a proliferative reaction that forms Aschoff nodules (Fig. 285.4). Aschoff nodules are paravascular nodules consisting of a center of fibrinoid degeneration surrounded by Aschoff cells, lymphocytes, and fibroblasts.

Cardiac Pathology

RF affects the three layers of the heart, causing endocarditis, myocarditis, and pericarditis (i.e., pancarditis). Endocarditis

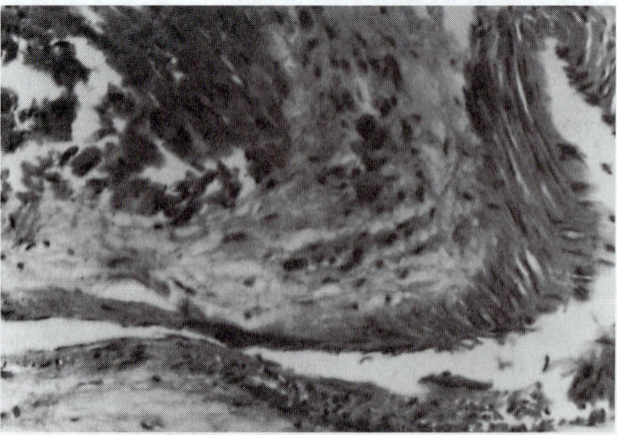

FIGURE 285.4. A paravascular Aschoff nodule *(center)* consists of a central area of fibrinoid change and an Aschoff giant cell surrounded by edematous intermyocardial connective tissue. (Courtesy of Dr. Soheir Mahfouz, Pathology Department, Cairo University, Cairo, Egypt.)

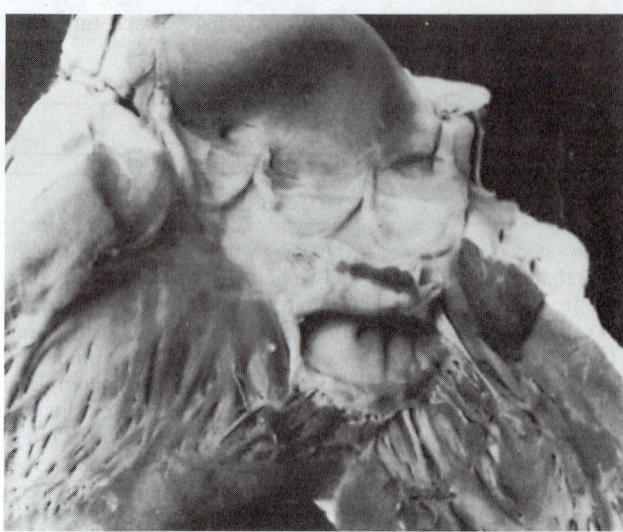

FIGURE 285.5. An opened left ventricle displays the mitral and aortic valves of a patient with acute rheumatic fever. The mitral valve shows small (1- to 2-mm) linear vegetations on the atrial surface of the anterior and posterior mitral leaflet margins. The aortic valve appears to be unaffected. (Courtesy of Dr. Soheir Mahfouz, Pathology Department, Cairo University, Cairo, Egypt.)

affects the mitral and aortic valves and rarely affects the tricuspid or pulmonary valves. In the active phase, the valves become edematous and the endocardium is damaged along the contact margins 2 or 3 mm from the free edges. At this site, tiny vegetations consisting of platelet thrombi are formed (Fig. 285.5). After inflammation subsides, fibrosis and contracture occur. Similar changes cause shortening of the chordae tendineae. The site of the lesions, at the contact points of the cusps, suggests that trauma determines the position of the damage. The degree of trauma determines the frequency with which the valves are involved. The mitral valve, closing at the highest pressure (greater than120 mm Hg), is subjected to the greatest stress and is the valve most frequently affected. The aortic valve, which closes by systemic diastolic pressure of 80 mm Hg, is the valve next most often involved, followed by the tricuspid valve and the pulmonary valve. When the inflammation is severe, the cusps are damaged, and insufficiency develops. Mild inflammation thickens tissue, and adhesions occur between the cusps. The adhesions gradually increase, producing stenosis of the valve orifice.

Extracardiac Pathology

Extracardiac pathologic features include inflammation of synovial membranes, subcutaneous collections of Aschoff nodules, pleurisy and pneumonitis, meningoencephalitis, and vasculitis. Sydenham chorea, atrioventricular conduction blocks, and erythema marginatum seem to be related to functional rather than visible lesions.

CLINICAL MANIFESTATIONS

Antecedent Streptococcal Infection

The interval between the onset of pharyngitis and the manifestation of symptoms of RF is 1 to 5 weeks (average, 3 weeks). However, clinical evidence for a preceding streptococcal infection may be lacking. Approximately one-third of patients have had no apparent illness during the preceding month.

Polyarthritis

Inflammation affects the large joints and moves from one to another. The affected joint is hot, red, tender, and swollen. The arthritis characteristically leaves the joints without any sequelae and responds almost immediately to salicylates. The severity of joint involvement is inversely proportional to the severity of cardiac involvement.

Carditis

In contrast to the seriousness of its prognosis, rheumatic carditis, unless it causes heart failure or pericarditis, produces no symptoms of its own and usually is diagnosed during examination of a patient with arthritis or chorea.

The development of an apical systolic murmur that is propagated to the axilla accompanied by a muffled first sound and a third sound indicates the development of mitral insufficiency. A systolic murmur over the apex without these characteristics may be caused by fever and not by mitral valvulitis.

The occurrence of a middiastolic murmur over the apex is a definite sign of mitral valvulitis. The diastolic apical murmur is caused by narrowing of the mitral orifice by the thickened, edematous cusps. The murmur may persist, indicating permanent damage, but it frequently disappears for a variable period, followed later by the appearance of the diastolic murmur of stenosis caused by the development of adhesions between the valve cusps.

The occurrence of a high-pitched, early diastolic murmur over the base indicates aortic valvulitis. As in mitral valvulitis, the occurrence of a systolic murmur over the base may be caused by fever or aortic valvulitis.

The murmurs of mitral and aortic valvulitis may disappear or may be followed by the establishment of valve regurgitation, stenosis, or both, according to the pathologic process occurring in the valve. Regurgitation, the result of damage, takes a short time to develop, but stenosis, the result of union between mobile cusps, takes years to decades to occur.

Myocarditis usually is accompanied by valvulitis and leads to tachycardia (especially if it persists during sleep) that is disproportionate to the patient's fever and can lead to gallop rhythm, rapid cardiac enlargement, and heart failure. Pericarditis accompanies valvulitis in approximately 5% to 10% of patients. The degree of effusion in pericarditis varies from none to moderate.

Electrocardiographic changes characteristically include prolongation of the PR and QT intervals. Second-degree or a complete atrioventricular block may occur in response to inflammation of the conduction system. ST-segment and T-wave changes of pericarditis or myocarditis may occur.

With the advent of echocardiography, patients with rheumatic carditis were found to have, most commonly, involvement of the mitral valve, with the development of mitral regurgitation. Mitral regurgitation in rheumatic carditis is related to ventricular dilatation, restriction of leaflet mobility, or both. A significant elongation of the anterior chordae of the mitral valve and the annulus also was found, and the mitral regurgitation jet usually is posteriorly directed (Figs. 285.6 and 285.7). Approximately one-fourth of patients with rheumatic carditis have valve nodules (over the valve) that may represent the echocardiographic equivalent of rheumatic verrucae. Rheumatic carditis does not result in congestive heart failure in the absence of hemodynamically significant valve lesions.

Chorea

Rheumatic or Sydenham chorea, a late manifestation of RF, occurs more commonly among female than male patients. Chorea

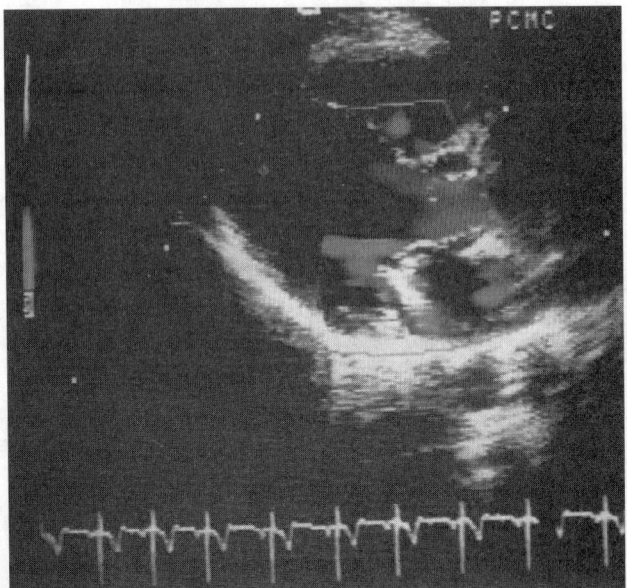

FIGURE 285.6. Posterolateral direction of the jet of rheumatic mitral regurgitation. Parasternal long-axis view from a patient with no audible murmur showing color Doppler interrogation of the mitral valve. The typical jet of rheumatic mitral regurgitation is directed towards the posterolateral left atrial wall.

may last from 1 week to longer than 2 years. Chorea is not seen simultaneously with arthritis, but it may coexist with carditis. If no carditis is present, the sedimentation rate is not elevated. In such cases, the ASO and other streptococcal antibody titers may not be increased, probably because chorea appears only after a latent period as long as 6 months after the streptococcal infection, and by that time, the acute-phase reactants and the streptococcal antibody titer may have returned to normal.

Involuntary, incoordinate, jerky movements are present and are accompanied by hypotonia and emotional disturbances, with abrupt alterations between laughter and tears. Flexion at the wrist and dorsiflexion of the fingers occur in the outstretched hands. Objects often fall from the hands (Fig. 285.8). After protruding the tongue for inspection, the patient may withdraw it rapidly, snapping the jaws over it.

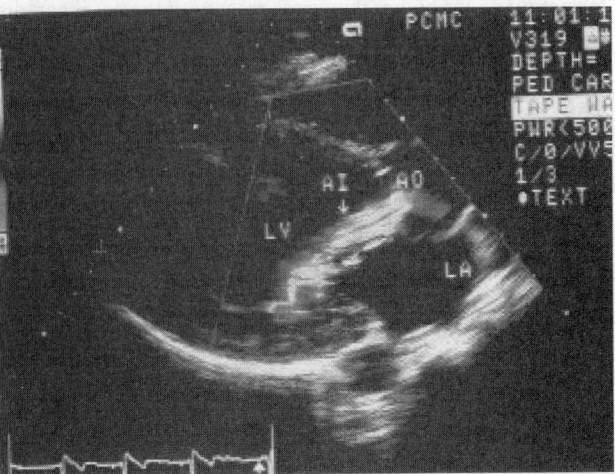

FIGURE 285.7. Parasternal long-axis view from a patient with no audible diastolic murmur. Color Doppler interrogation of the aortic valve demonstrates a high-velocity, regurgitant diastolic jet characteristic of rheumatic aortic valvulitis.

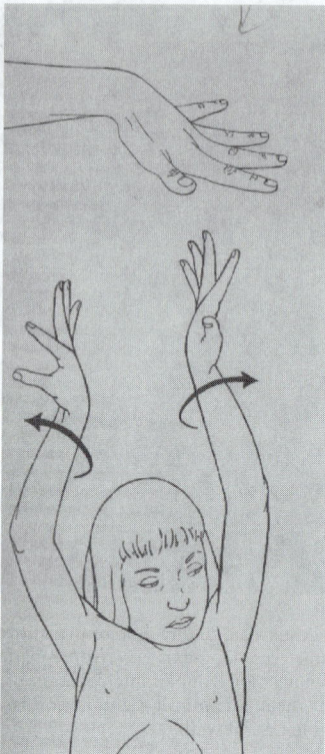

FIGURE 285.8. Chorea. **Top:** "Spooning" of the hands in a patient with chorea. Notice the flexion of the wrists, the hyperextension of the metacarpophalangeal joints, the straightening of the fingers, and the abduction of the thumb. **Bottom:** Pronator sign in a patient with chorea. When the patient raises her hands above her head, she also tends to pronate her hands. (Reprinted from Taranta A. Rheumatic fever: clinical aspects. In: Hollander L, McCarty DJ Jr, eds. *Arthritis and allied conditions.* Philadelphia: Lea & Febiger, 1972:764.)

The PANDAS disorder may be associated with chorea. Children have been identified in whom streptococcal infection appears to have triggered a relapsing-remitting symptom complex characterized by obsessive-compulsive personality disorder and/or a tic disorder and neurologic abnormalities (e.g., cognitive defects, motoric hyperactivity). The symptoms may include emotional lability, separation anxiety, and oppositional behaviors, and they are prepubertal in onset. Some experts have proposed that the streptococcal infection triggers the formation of antibodies that cross-react with the basal ganglia of genetically susceptible hosts in a manner similar to the proposed mechanism for Sydenham chorea and causes the symptom complex.

Subcutaneous Nodules

Now rarely seen, subcutaneous nodules usually indicate severe carditis. The nodules are attached to the tendon sheaths and occur on the extensor surfaces and bony prominences of the arms and legs and on the scapula and the mastoid processes. Histologically, they consist of collections of Aschoff bodies.

Erythema Marginatum

The rash of erythema marginatum generally appears as an area of erythema. The margins progress as the center clears. The rash occurs chiefly over the trunk and the proximal parts of the limbs (Fig. 285.9).

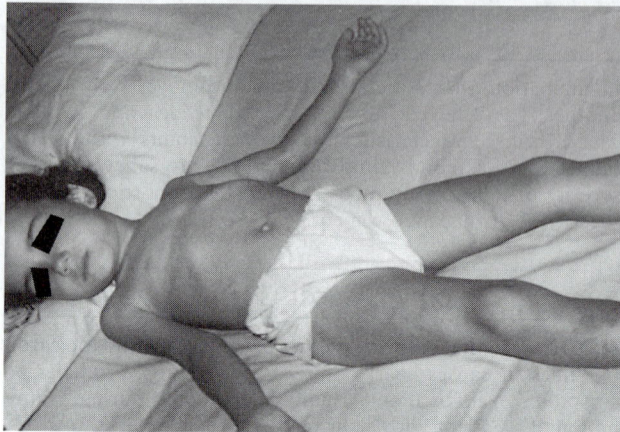

FIGURE 285.9. A 6-year-old girl with erythema marginatum has acute rheumatic fever with severe carditis. (Courtesy of Dr. Samir Kassem, Alexandria Medical School, Alexandria, Egypt.)

Signs of Inflammation

Pallor, epistaxis, elevated temperature (greater than 39°C; it may be low-grade, less than 38°C in children with mild carditis, or absent in patients with chorea), tachycardia, anorexia, and weight loss are signs of inflammation. They indicate rheumatic activity in a patient already diagnosed as having RF. Pleurisy, pneumonia, and abdominal pain (simulating appendicitis) caused by vasculitis have the same significance.

DIAGNOSIS

Laboratory tests typically show a high erythrocyte sedimentation rate, anemia, leukocytosis, and positive C-reactive protein. The ASO antibody is elevated abnormally in 70% to 85% of patients with RF. A single value of 500 units indicates recent streptococcal infection, and a value of 333 units is of borderline significance. If the ASO titer is 333 units or less, additional antistreptococcal antibody assays should be obtained. ASO and anti-DNase are used most often for establishing the diagnosis, and antihyaluronidase is a third choice.

The lack of unique clinical features of streptococcal throat infection has led to the use of the throat culture to distinguish streptococcal from viral pharyngitis. With traditional throat culture methods, the inherent waiting period of 24 to 48 hours for results has led to initiation of antibiotic therapy before final results are ready. Therefore, large numbers of children receive unnecessary antibiotic therapy. Conversely, some patients who initially are not treated are lost to follow-up and do not receive appropriate therapy. Although the advent of newer, commercially available, rapid streptococcal tests have allowed physicians to diagnose streptococcal pharyngitis with greater speed and results are ready while the patient waits at the physician's office, some epidemiologic concerns still remain (Table 285.1).

The diagnosis of RF is important because serious cardiac disease can be prevented or minimized by long-term antistreptococcal therapy. No single diagnostic test for RF exists. The laboratory tests indicate recent streptococcal infection, but the diagnosis of RF rests on the ability to satisfy the Duckett Jones criteria (Table 285.2). It is mandatory to demonstrate recent streptococcal infection (usually by elevation of ASO titer) and to find one major and two minor criteria or to identify two major criteria. The minor manifestations are less specific for the illness.

TABLE 285.1

BENEFITS AND DRAWBACKS OF THE USE OF RAPID DETECTION TESTS FOR STREPTOCOCCAL THROAT INFECTION

Benefits	Prompt diagnosis allows early administration of antibiotics:
	    To prevent sequelae
	    To shorten duration of illness
	    To shorten period of communicability
	Provides improved diagnostic accuracy over clinical diagnosis
	Could be valuable in areas where culture methods are not available

Drawbacks	Has moderate sensitivity and specificity Predictive values are poor Reliability is decreased when performed by poorly trained personnel

RF should be differentiated from juvenile rheumatoid arthritis, innocent murmur with a febrile illness, bacterial arthritis, systemic lupus erythematosus, Schönlein-Henoch purpura, acute leukemia, sickle cell anemia, and mucocutaneous lymph node syndrome.

The diagnosis of a recurrent attack of RF has been suggested if evidence exists of recent group A streptococcal infection and a patient with RHD has one major or two minor Duckett Jones criteria. A presumptive diagnosis of recurrent attacks of RF may be made when a patient presents with one minor criterion and several other manifestations, such as anemia, abdominal pain, rapid sleeping pulse rate, tachycardia out of proportion to fever, malaise, epistaxes, precordial pain, and an elevated level of immunoglobulin G (IgG), IgA, C3 complement component, and circulating immune complexes.

COURSE AND PROGNOSIS

RF usually follows a characteristic clinical course. The latent period is short for disease complicated by arthritis and erythema marginatum, longest for RF with chorea, and midlength

TABLE 285.2

DUCKETT JONES CRITERIA FOR THE DIAGNOSIS OF RHEUMATIC FEVER

Requirements for diagnosis
Two major criteria
or
One major plus two minor criteria
plus
Evidence of previous streptococcal infection (e.g., elevated anti-streptolysin O titer)

Major criteria	Minor criteria
Carditis	Previous rheumatic fever
Arthritis	Arthralgia
Chorea	Fever
Erythema marginatum	Elevated erythrocyte sedimentation rate
Subcutaneous nodules	Elevated leukocyte count
	Prolonged PR interval
	C-reactive protein

for RF with carditis and subcutaneous nodules. The duration of active disease usually is less than 3 months. Fewer than 5% of patients with RF have disease that remains active for longer than 6 months, a condition known as *chronic active carditis*. The prognosis is excellent for the patient who does not develop carditis during the initial attack. The prognosis becomes poorer with increasing severity of initial carditis.

Over the course of years, changes have occurred in the epidemiology of RF and in its severity, presentation, and clinical manifestations. RF is seen less commonly in developed countries, and, when it occurs, it tends to be mild. In tropical and subtropical countries, RF and RHD occur commonly and assume more malignant forms (Fig. 285.10). In areas where RF is still a common occurrence, the course of the disease is subacute or chronic. Joint involvement is less conspicuous. Rheumatic nodules and erythema marginatum are seen less frequently, but chorea occasionally is part of the clinical picture.

TREATMENT

RHD seems in many ways emblematic of an older era in medicine, without any prospects of new development or change.

Prophylactic Therapy

Prevention of RF is achieved by improving socioeconomic circumstances and sanitation. The aim of primary prophylaxis is to prevent initial attacks of RF by promptly and accurately recognizing and treating streptococcal pharyngitis or by providing antibiotic prophylaxis using benzathine penicillin intramuscularly for members of a susceptible population. Modern outbreaks in the United States were blamed in part on diminished adherence to conventional recommendations for penicillin, which is highly effective in preventing RF caused by pharyngeal infections.

Secondary prophylaxis is the prevention of recurrences of RF by continuous chemoprophylaxis. The most effective method is a single monthly intramuscular injection of 600,000 to 1,200,000 units of benzathine penicillin. RF recurs in approximately 0.45% of individuals who use benzathine penicillin prophylaxis, compared with 11.5% of those who do not comply with treatment. In areas where RF is endemic, twice-monthly (or once every 3 weeks, as advised by the World Health Organization) benzathine penicillin prophylaxis was found to decrease significantly the recurrence rate of RF, compared with monthly injections. The incidence of allergic reactions is approximately 3%, but anaphylaxis occurs after only in 10,000 injections. Oral penicillin prophylaxis can be provided by 500 to 1,000 mg of penicillin G administered twice daily. If the patient is allergic to penicillin, prophylaxis can be achieved by administering 250 mg of erythromycin given twice daily. The injectable form of prophylaxis is more effective than are the oral forms because patient compliance is superior and the medication is not affected by variations in intestinal absorption. The duration of secondary prophylaxis depends on the variables that influence the recurrence rate and the degree to which the heart has been affected. The risk of recurrence declines with age and with an increased RF-free interval from the last rheumatic attack after 10 years. The American Heart Association currently recommends that patients with RF without carditis receive prophylactic antibiotics for 5 years or until the age of 21 years, whichever is longer. Patients with RF with carditis but no valve disease should receive prophylactic for 10 years or well into aduthood, whichever is longer. Finally, patients with RF with carditis and valve disease should receive antibiotics at least 10 years or until the age of 40 years,

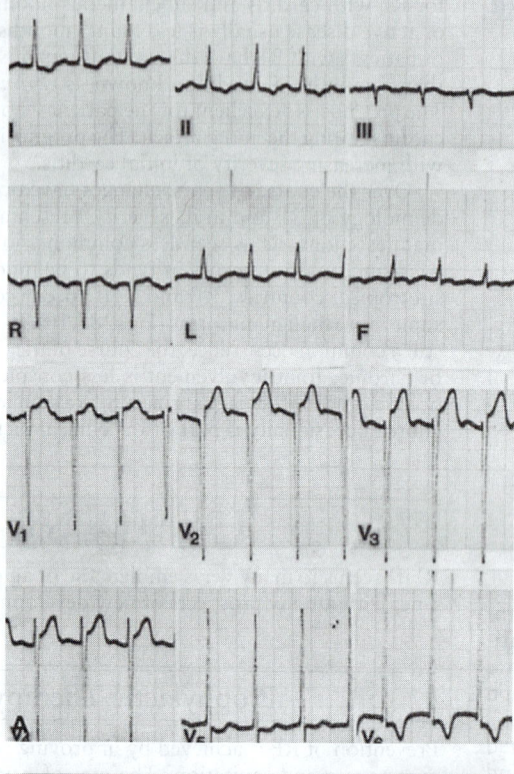

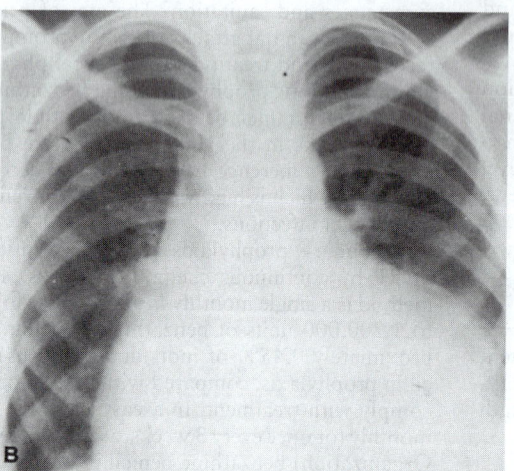

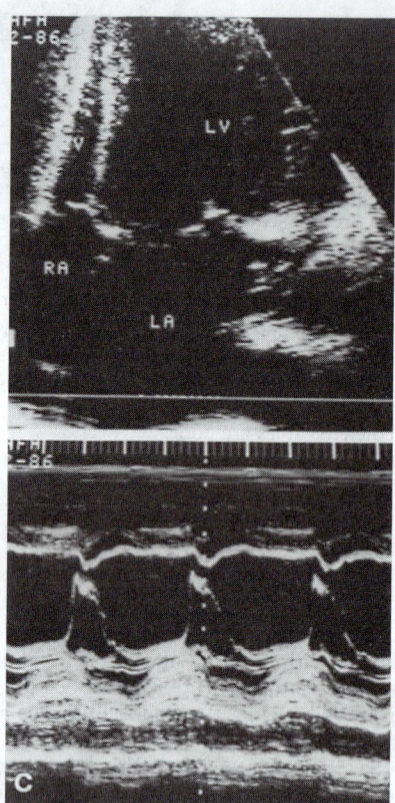

FIGURE 285.10. The electrocardiogram (ECG), roentgenogram, and echocardiogram are from an underdeveloped 11-year-old patient with recurrent rheumatic fever with mitral and aortic rheumatic valve disease. **A:** The ECG shows sinus tachycardia, a prolonged PR interval, and left ventricular hypertrophy and strain. **B:** The roentgenogram shows gross cardiomegaly. **C:** The apical four-chamber echocardiographic view shows a dilated left ventricle (LV) and left atrium (LA) and a thickened mitral valve. The M-mode echocardiogram shows a thickened mitral valve and small pericardial effusion. RA, right atrium, RV, right ventricle.

whichever is longer. Indefinite antibiotic prophylaxis can be considered for patients at high risk (e.g., health care workers, teachers, day-care workers).

No vaccine is available, but conserved regions of the M protein have been shown to contain both T-cell and B-cell helper epitopes, which will be the target of group A streptococcal vaccine development.

Curative Therapy

Bed rest is required until the signs and symptoms of acute inflammation disappear. Salt is restricted if signs of heart failure are observed.

A course of antibiotics should be initiated after a throat culture has been obtained. Antibiotics should be administered even in the absence of positive throat culture results. One

intramuscular injection of benzathine penicillin (600,000 to 1,200,000 units) or a 10-day course of oral penicillin G (500 to 1,000 mg, four times daily) is recommended. Patients who are allergic to penicillin should receive erythromycin (250 to 500 mg, four times daily) or a first-generation cephalosporin for 10 days. Other options include clarithromycin for 10 days or azithromycin for 5 days. Do not use tetracyclines and sulfonamides to treat streptococcal infection.

In general, antimicrobial therapy is not indicated for pharyngeal carriers of group A streptococci, except for the follows:

- Outbreaks of RF or poststreptococcal glomerulonephritis
- Family history of RF
- Outbreaks of pharyngitis in a closed community
- When tonsillectomy is considered for chronic streptococcal carriage

- When multiple episodes of documented streptococcal pharyngitis occur within a family despite receiving appropriate therapy
- Following group A streptococcal toxic shock syndrome or necrotizing fasciitis in a household contact

The selection of an antirheumatic drug is not critical to the outcome of RF. Salicylates and corticosteroids are valuable symptomatic drugs, but they are not curative and actually may prolong the course of the disease.

Acetylsalicylic acid (aspirin) is analgesic and antipyretic and reduces malaise. It causes such dramatic improvement of the arthritis that it can be given as a therapeutic test, but it has no effect on carditis. Aspirin is given to patients with or without mild carditis, if side effects or contraindications to corticosteroids are present, and during and after withdrawal from corticosteroids. Side effects include tinnitus, gastric irritation, bleeding caused by inhibition of platelet function, metabolic acidosis, hyperventilation that may lead to respiratory alkalosis, and hypoglycemia. The dosage is 60 to 120 mg/kg/day, given in six divided doses and administered until a satisfactory clinical response is obtained. The dosage then is reduced by one-third and is continued until all laboratory findings return to normal, which usually requires 6 to 9 weeks. The dosage is decreased gradually to avoid the rebound that occurs if the drug is stopped abruptly.

Corticosteroids do not shorten the course of illness markedly or diminish the likelihood of cardiac damage. Corticosteroids do produce prompt control of the subcutaneous nodules, erythema marginatum, fever, and arthritis. Corticosteroids are indicated for patients with severe carditis. The dosage of prednisone or prednisolone is 2 mg/kg/day (not to exceed 60 mg/day) for 3 to 4 weeks. Shortly before or at the time corticosteroid therapy is discontinued, aspirin (90 to 120 mg/kg/day) should be given, and it should be continued for 1.5 to 6.0 months, probably until active inflammation subsides.

Chorea

The patient with chorea should be maintained in a quiet atmosphere, protected from self-injury, and given a tranquilizer such as phenobarbitone or chlorpromazine. Haloperidol (butyrophenone), a centrally acting drug, is the most effective in controlling chorea, but severe, adverse extrapyramidal reactions have been reported. Patients with concomitant rheumatic activity should be given salicylates.

Heart Failure

Heart failure may be an indication for the use of corticosteroids or diuretic agents. Operative repair or replacement of a severely compromised cardiac valve may be necessary during acute RF if signs and symptoms of severe congestive heart failure are unresponsive to medical therapy.

Suggested Readings

Annegers JF, Pillman NL, Weidman WH, et al. Rheumatic fever in Rochester, Minnesota, 1935–1978. *Mayo Clin Proc* 1982;57:753.

Committee Report of the American Heart Association. Jones criteria (revised) for guidance in the diagnosis of rheumatic fever. *Circulation* 1965;32:664.

Feldman J. Rheumatic heart disease. *Curr Opin Cardiol* 1996;11:126.

Huang C. An approach to the diagnosis of recurrent attack of rheumatic fever in patients with rheumatic heart disease. *Chung Hua Nei Ko Tso Chih* 1995;34:L687.

International Rheumatic Fever Study Group. Allergic reactions to long-term benzathine penicillin for rheumatic fever. *Lancet* 1991;337:1308.

Kassem A, Madkour A, Zaher S. Benzathine penicillin G for RF prophylaxis: 2 weekly versus 4 weekly regimens. *Indian J Pediatr* 1992;59:741.

Narula J, Virmani R, Reddy K, et al. *Rheumatic fever.* Washington, DC: American Registry of Pathology, Armed Forces Institute of Pathology, 1999.

Pruksakorn S. *Molecular immunological approach to rheumatic fever vaccine development.* Thesis submitted in the Tropical Health Program. University of Queensland, Australia, 1994.

Stollerman GH. Rheumatogenic group A streptococci and return of rheumatic fever. *Adv Intern Med* 1990;35:1.

Stollerman GH. Rheumatic fever and other rheumatic diseases of the heart. In: Braunwald E, ed. *Heart disease: a textbook of cardiovascular medicine.* Philadelphia: Saunders, 2002.

Vasan R, Shirvastava S, Vijayakumar M, et al. Echocardiographic evaluation of patients with acute rheumatic fever and rheumatic carditis. *Circulation* 1996;94:73.

Volga H, Pinto M, Carrinho M, et al. Clinical and echocardiographic study of mitral valve in children with severe rheumatic carditis: aspects of prolapse or rupture. *Arq Bras Cardiol* 1996;66:125.

CHAPTER 286 ■ RHEUMATIC HEART DISEASE

GALAL M. EL-SAID, YASSER M. K. BAGHDADY, AND HOWAIDA G. EL-SAID

Rheumatic heart disease (RHD), like rheumatic fever, is seen more commonly in areas where the standard of living is low. RHD remains one of the leading causes of heart disease in developing countries, where rheumatic fever occurs commonly. It assumes malignant and chronic forms that can lead to significant valvular heart disease in childhood, often accompanied by significant pulmonary hypertension, and may require surgery at an early age (Figs. 286.1 and 286.2). In children and adolescents with RHD, the mitral valve is involved in 85% of the cases, the aortic valve in 55%, and the tricuspid and pulmonary valves in fewer than 5%.

RHEUMATIC MITRAL INSUFFICIENCY

Mitral insufficiency is the most common cardiac defect in children and adolescents with RHD. As the left ventricle (LV) contracts, part of its stroke volume regurgitates into the left atrium (LA) through the incompetent mitral valve. Because of the difference in pressure between the LV and LA, regurgitation starts during the isometric contraction phase.

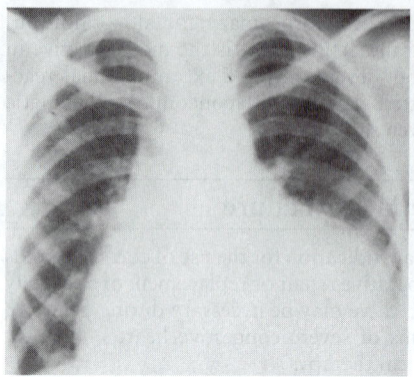
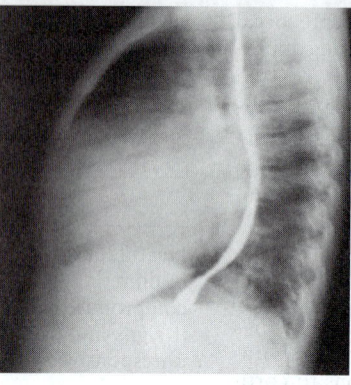

FIGURE 286.1. Posteroanterior and lateral chest radiographs show gross cardiac enlargement.

Compensation begins with dilation of the LV to accommodate the increased blood volume. In chronic mitral insufficiency, the increase in LV end-diastolic volume usually is not accompanied by increased end-diastolic pressure because of increased LV compliance. The increase in LV end-diastolic volume (i.e., increased preload) brings the Frank-Starling mechanism into play, which permits a large stroke output. Because the regurgitant mitral orifice is in parallel with the aortic orifice, the resistance to LV emptying is reduced (i.e., decreased afterload) (Fig. 286.3).

The compensatory mechanisms of increased compliance, increased preload, decreased afterload, and increased wall thickness are not sufficient to overcome persistent mitral insufficiency. Myocardial contractility becomes impaired because of the chronic volume overload. Symptoms of low cardiac output are followed by symptoms of lung congestion caused by LV failure (see Fig. 286.3).

Clinical Manifestations

Because symptoms usually do not develop until the LV is compromised, the interval between acquiring rheumatic fever and the development of symptoms of mitral insufficiency tends to be longer than that for mitral stenosis (MS), often exceeding 2 decades. Unlike MS, symptoms of low cardiac output (e.g., weakness, fatigue) are more prominent and appear before symptoms of lung congestion (e.g., exertional, nocturnal, or resting dyspnea; recurrent chest infections; hemoptysis).

The cardiac impulse is diffuse, forceful, and displaced downward and laterally. The first heart sound usually is diminished. A loud apical third heart sound usually is audible and is caused by the increased transmitral volume flow that occurs during the rapid filling phase. The characteristic murmur of mitral insufficiency is a high-pitched holosystolic murmur, beginning with the soft first sound and continuing to the second sound. The second heart sound sometimes is obscured by the murmur. The murmur is loudest at the apex, with radiation to the axilla and left infrascapular area.

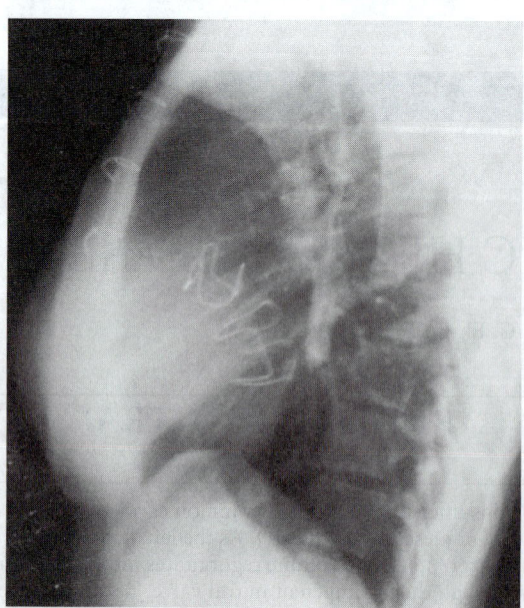

FIGURE 286.2. A lateral chest radiograph shows the mitral and aortic valve stents that were placed at a young age.

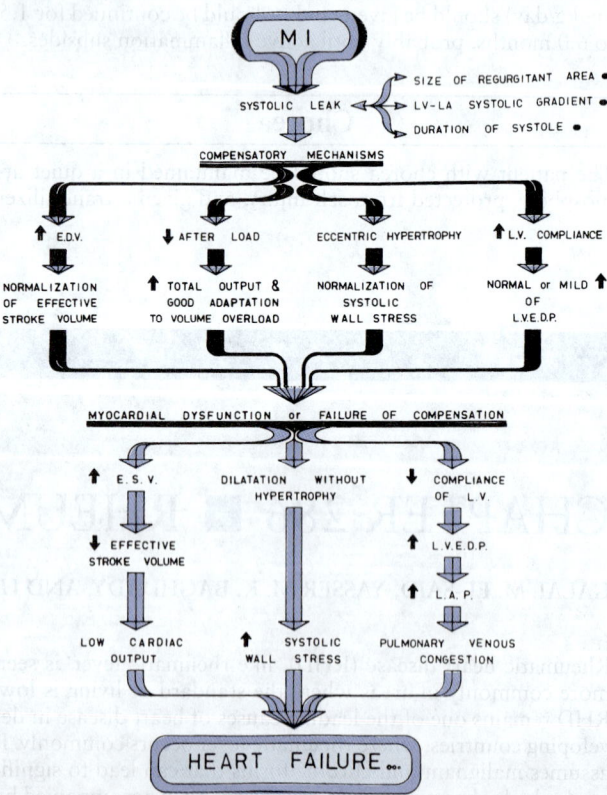

FIGURE 286.3. The diagram depicts factors that determine the degree of regurgitation, compensation, and decompensation in mitral insufficiency. EDP, end-diastolic pressure; EDV, end-diastolic volume; ESV, end-systolic volume; LA, left atrium; LAP, left atrial pressure; LV, left ventricle; MI, mitral insufficiency.

Laboratory Findings

In chronic mitral insufficiency, the electrocardiogram exhibits evidence of enlargements of the LV and LA. Radiologically, the cardiac shadow is normal early in the course of the disease; later, LA and LV enlargements become evident.

Echocardiography is useful for identifying the cause and degree of mitral insufficiency and for evaluating LV function. M-mode echocardiography can show an increase in the LV diastolic dimension and a significant decrease in LV diameter during the preejection phase. The two-dimensional echocardiographic criteria for the diagnosis of rheumatic mitral insufficiency include thickened mitral valve leaflets, incomplete closure of the mitral valve, a relatively immobile posterior mitral leaflet, a dilated LA with systolic expansion, and a dilated LV with hyperdynamic septal and posterior wall motion. The degree of mitral insufficiency can be assessed using Doppler echocardiography, by determining the extension and intensity of the Doppler signal of the regurgitant jet in the LA. Color-flow Doppler and pulsed techniques correlate well with angiographic methods of estimating the severity of mitral insufficiency. Transesophageal echocardiography (TEE), especially color mapping, is superior to transthoracic echocardiography in assessing the degree of mitral regurgitation. Although slight overestimation may occur, TEE also is useful in delineating the anatomy of the mitral valve and thus is useful for determining whether the mitral valve can be repaired or whether mitral valve replacement will be necessary.

Cardiac catheterization demonstrates elevated LA pressure (particularly the v wave). The diagnosis can be established by left ventriculography. Mitral insufficiency is indicated by the appearance of contrast material in the LA after LV injection through a retrograde aortic catheter.

Management Strategy

Medical therapy for asymptomatic patients with chronic mitral insufficiency is controversial. No long-term study supports any benefit of reducing preload or afterload by the use of vasodilators in these patients.

In patients who develop symptoms but with preserved LV function, surgery is the treatment option of choice. If atrial fibrillation develops, control of rate by digitalis, beta blockers, rate-lowering calcium channel blockers, and/or amiodarone will be necessary. Anticoagulation achieved by warfarin, maintaining an international normalized ratio between 2 and 3, also will be necessary to reduce embolic complications.

Surgery for mitral insufficiency is by mitral valve repair, mitral valve replacement with preservation of the subvalvular apparatus, or mitral valve replacement without preservation of the subvalvular apparatus. Each of the treatment options has its own advantages and disadvantages. Asymptomatic patients with severe mitral regurgitation should undergo surgery if deterioration of the LV function is present during serial follow-up or if the ejection fraction is 0.6 or less, or if the end-systolic diameter is 45 mm or greater. Other compelling causes for performing surgery in the asymptomatic patient with mitral insufficiency include the development of atrial fibrillation and/or the development of pulmonary hypertension (pulmonary artery systolic pressure 50 mm Hg at rest or 60 mm Hg during exercise).

RHEUMATIC MITRAL STENOSIS

Stenosis of the mitral valve usually is secondary to rheumatic carditis. Other causes include congenital MS, atrial myxoma, infective endocarditis with bulky vegetations, and mu-

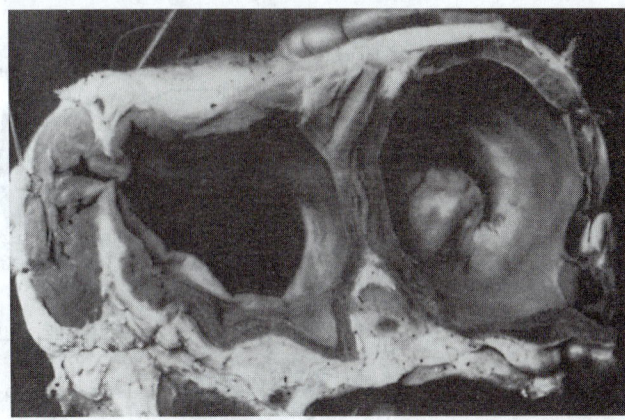

FIGURE 286.4. The cross section shows a stenosed mitral valve (*right*), giving a buttonhole appearance. The tricuspid valve on the *left* is grossly insufficient. Insufficiency occurs in the later stages of mitral stenosis after long-standing, severe secondary pulmonary hypertension. (Courtesy of Dr. Soheir Mahfouz, Pathology Department, Cairo University, Cairo, Egypt.)

copolysaccharidosis of the Hunter-Hurley phenotype. The combination of MS and secundum atrial septal defect frequently is referred to as *Lutembacher syndrome*, but the MS almost always is rheumatic, and the association is fortuitous.

Rheumatic fever causes MS through fusion of the commissures, cusps, or chordae tendineae of the mitral valve apparatus (Fig. 286.4). Obstruction of flow across the narrowed mitral valve produces a diastolic gradient between the LA and LV. Serious circulatory disturbances, with consequent clinical symptoms, occur when the area of the mitral opening is less than 1 cm². As narrowing proceeds, the LA pressure increases, as does the pressure in the pulmonary veins and capillaries, leading to lung congestion. Pulmonary arteriolar vasoconstriction occurs to protect the lungs against congestion, but the protection is at the expense of developing pulmonary hypertension, which produces right ventricle (RV) hypertrophy and possible RV failure (Fig. 286.5).

Clinical Manifestations

The symptoms of MS may appear insidiously within 3 to 4 years after the attack of acute rheumatic fever, or they may be delayed for as long as 50 years. The onset of symptoms sometimes is abrupt, and acute pulmonary edema, systemic embolism, or atrial fibrillation may be the initial manifestations. The symptoms depend on the state of the disease. No symptoms may be present in mild cases. If the lungs are congested, dyspnea, orthopnea, nocturnal dyspnea or pulmonary edema, recurrent chest infections, and hemoptysis will occur. As pulmonary hypertension develops, symptoms caused by lung congestion decrease, and low cardiac output symptoms (mainly exertional fatigue) begin to appear. Symptoms caused by systemic congestion appear if the RV fails.

In a patient with MS, the pulse usually is normal unless atrial fibrillation supervenes. The apical impulse is felt at the normal location as a "hurried, slapping" impulse. A characteristic diastolic or presystolic thrill ending in a palpable accentuated first sound can be detected over the apex. The first mitral sound is loud, short, and snappy. The accentuation of the first sound is caused by the open position of the cusps in the LV at the end of diastole as a result of the high LA pressure and the incomplete emptying of the LA. An opening snap occurs, which is a sharp, clicky sound separated from the second sound by the isovolumic relaxation phase. The snap is caused by the sudden opening

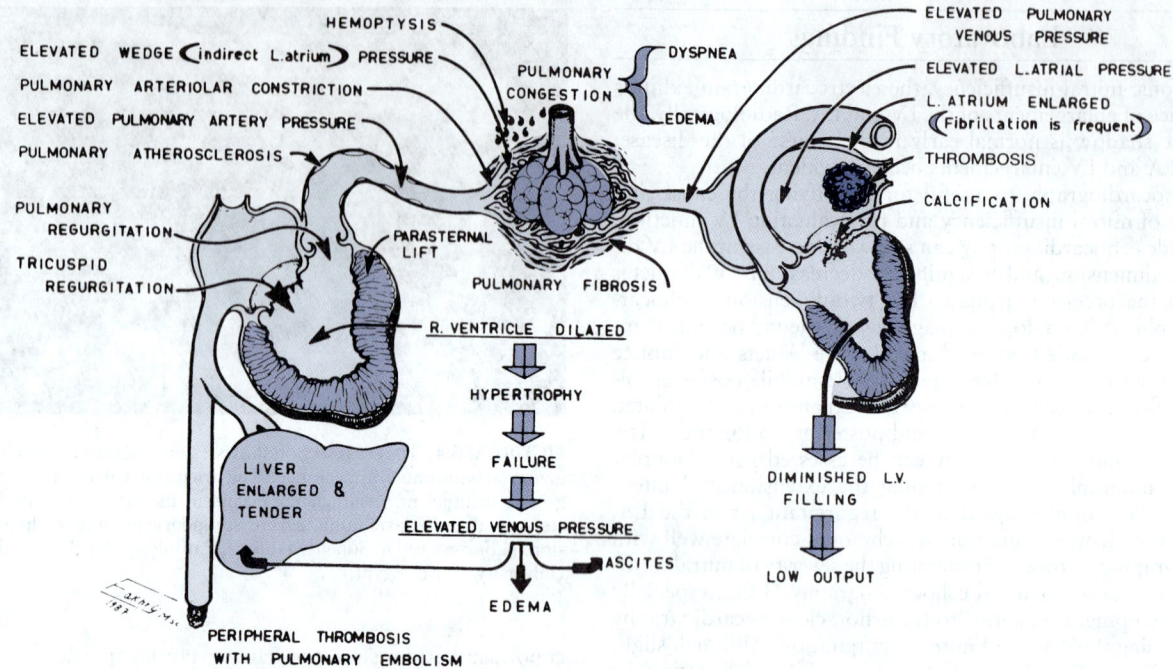

FIGURE 286.5. The diagram depicts the hemodynamic alterations and complications that occur because of mitral stenosis. LV, left ventricle.

of the rigid mitral valve by the high LA pressure. The murmur characteristic of MS is a middiastolic or presystolic murmur. Developing pulmonary hypertension produces an accentuated pulmonary second sound.

Laboratory Findings

The electrocardiographic and cardiac silhouettes are normal in patients with mild cases. In patients with moderate or severe obstruction, the principal feature is enlargement of the LA. RV hypertrophy is seen when pulmonary hypertension develops.

The feature diagnostic of MS in a two-dimensional echocardiographic study is doming of the anterior leaflet in diastole (i.e., the body of the leaflet separates more widely than do the edges). The posterior leaflet frequently is immobile or severely restricted in diastolic movement (Fig. 286.6). The mitral valve area derived by two-dimensional echocardiography often compares favorably with that measured directly at surgery. A Doppler echocardiographic study provides information about the flow of blood across the mitral valve and can estimate the gradient and the mitral valve area reasonably well. TEE, which provides images superior to those seen by transthoracic echocardiography, can show a detailed anatomy of the mitral valve apparatus and thus is useful in evaluation before using balloon valvuloplasty in determining the presence of an LA thrombus (Fig. 286.7), the thickness of the interatrial septum, and the degree of associated mitral regurgitation.

Cardiac catheterization and angiography usually are unnecessary for evaluating isolated MS, but they may be performed in patients with atypical cases. Pressure measurements show elevated LA and pulmonary wedge pressures. In patients with severe stenosis and those in whom pulmonary vascular resistance is increased, pulmonary arterial pressure is elevated.

Differential Diagnosis

Conditions that may mimic MS include LA myxoma, cor triatriatum, and pulmonary venoocclusive disease. The auscul-

tatory findings of the Austin Flint murmur (found in aortic regurgitation) and the Carey-Coombs murmur (found in acute rheumatic mitral valvulitis) may mimic true MS.

Management Strategy

In the patient with MS, the major problem is mechanical obstruction to inflow at the level of the mitral valve, and no medical therapy will specifically relieve the fixed obstruction. The LV is protected from a volume or pressure overload, and thus no specific medical therapy is required in the asymptomatic patient

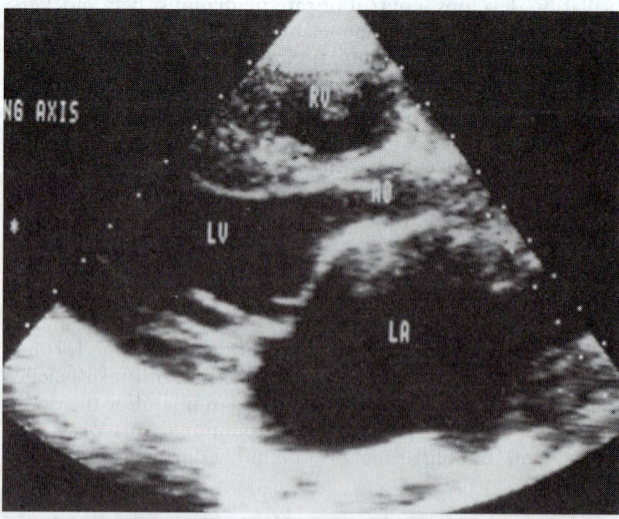

FIGURE 286.6. The two-dimensional echocardiogram from a patient with mitral stenosis shows an incomplete opening of the mitral valve. The anterior leaflet is domed, and the posterior leaflet is restricted. The left atrium (LA) is markedly enlarged. AO, aorta; LV, left ventricle; RV, right ventricle.

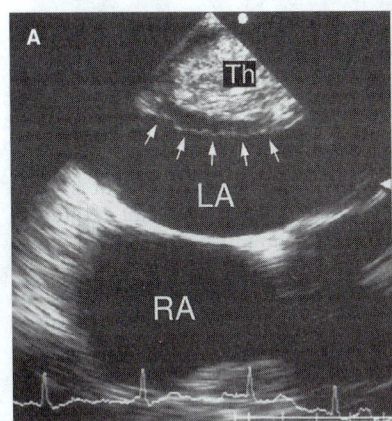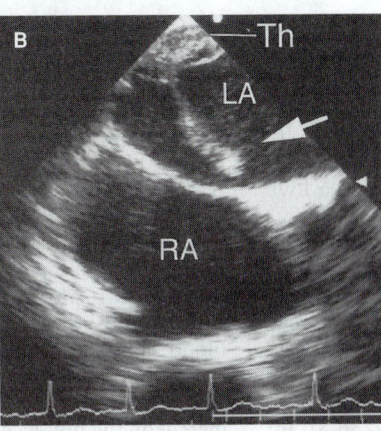

FIGURE 286.7. A: Transesophageal echocardiogram 35 cm from the incisors. There was a large thrombus covered with thin membrane *(arrows)*. **B:** Transesophageal echocardiogram 40 cm from the incisors showing a mobile, string-like echo *(arrow)* attached to the thrombus. LA, left atrium; RA, right atrium; Th, thrombus.

who has normal sinus rhythm and mild MS. Because rheumatic fever is the primary cause of MS, prophylaxis against rheumatic fever is recommended. Infective endocarditis is an uncommon finding but does occur in isolated MS, and appropriate endocarditis prophylaxis also is recommended. In the patient who has more than a mild degree of MS, counseling on avoidance of unusual physical stresses is advised. Increased flow and a shortening of the diastolic filling period by tachycardia increase LA pressure against an obstructed mitral valve. Agents with negative chronotropic properties such as beta blockers or calcium channel blockers may be of benefit in patients in sinus rhythm who have exertional symptoms if these symptoms occur with high heart rates. Restriction of salt and intermittent administration of a diuretic are useful if evidence of pulmonary vascular congestion is present. Digitalis does not benefit patients with MS in sinus rhythm unless they have LV and/or RV dysfunction. If atrial fibrillation occurs, the patient will need either rhythm or rate control and full anticoagulation.

Balloon Mitral Valvotomy

Dilation of a stenosed mitral valve by a balloon valvuloplasty catheter can relieve mitral obstruction. This procedure is used in patients who have pliable, noncalcified mitral leaflets. LA thrombi must be excluded, the best means for which is TEE studies, especially in patients with atrial fibrillation. The balloon technique is an ideal way for children (who usually have pliable, noncalcified leaflets) to avoid having to undergo thoracotomy. The patients should be symptomatic (functional class II or more), with moderate to severe MS (with a mitral valve area of 0.8 cm^2/m^2 of body surface area). If balloon mitral valvotomy is not feasable, surgical valvotomy (open or closed) or mitral valve replacement can be performed.

RHEUMATIC AORTIC VALVE DISEASE

Aortic valvulitis, which may develop during rheumatic carditis, may cause aortic insufficiency or stenosis. Aortic insufficiency, which results from damage of the aortic leaflets, may occur relatively early in the course of the disease and may be exaggerated over time by fibrosis, thickening, and contracture of the aortic leaflets. Aortic stenosis, which results from fusion of the commissures, takes a long time to develop. As a result, in children and adolescents, aortic valve disease caused by rheumatic conditions presents usually as isolated or dominant aortic insufficiency with mild or no stenosis. Dominant stenosis at a young age, with or without insufficiency, usually is congenital.

The inability of the scarred and shortened aortic leaflets to coapt and close the aortic orifice completely during ventricular diastole causes diastolic regurgitation of blood from the aorta to the LV because the normal aortic diastolic pressure approximates 80 mm Hg, and the normal LV diastolic pressure is 0 to 12 mm Hg.

With chronic aortic insufficiency, the LV dilates with an increasing volume of blood for many years. The increased LV diastolic volume is not accompanied by an increase in end-diastolic pressure, probably because of an increase in the LV diastolic compliance. The increased LV end-diastolic volume, according to the Frank-Starling principle, results in increased stroke volume (i.e., preload reserve). The stroke volume also is maintained by reduced aortic impedance, which occurs with peripheral vasodilation (i.e., decreasing afterload) (Fig. 286.8).

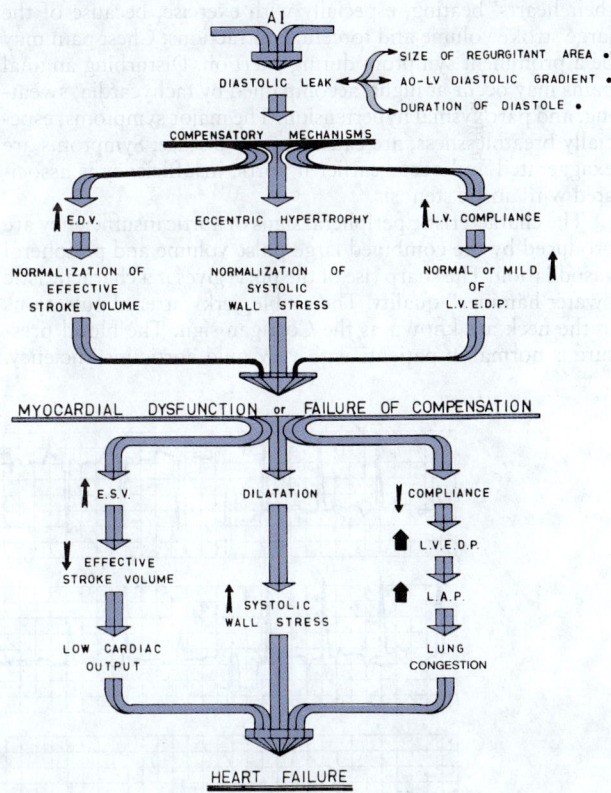

FIGURE 286.8. The diagram depicts factors that determine the amount of regurgitation, compensation, and decompensation in aortic insufficiency. AI, aortic insufficiency; AO, aorta; EDP, end-diastolic pressure; EDV, end-diastolic volume; ESV, end-systolic volume; LAP, left atrial pressure, LV, left ventricle.

The increased LV stroke volume, with consequent elevation in the systolic blood pressure accompanied by a decrease in the diastolic blood pressure (caused partly by regurgitation of a part of the stroke volume and partly by peripheral arteriolar vasodilation), increases the pulse pressure. The classic peripheral arterial pulses of aortic insufficiency have a rapid increase to a high peak, with a collapsing descending limb and a low diastolic pressure.

Because the major portion of coronary flow occurs during diastole, when arterial pressure is lower than normal, coronary perfusion may be reduced. The increased oxygen demand caused by hypertrophy in the presence of reduced coronary flow may lead to myocardial ischemia, especially with exercise.

Exhaustion of the compensatory mechanisms (i.e., preload reserve, increased contractility, diminished afterload) and myocardial ischemia may result in LV failure (see Fig. 286.8). In chronic aortic insufficiency, these compensatory changes occur before the onset of symptoms. Symptoms usually start only after the high LV end-diastolic pressure is reflected in the LA and pulmonary capillary pressures.

Associated aortic stenosis causes significant deleterious alterations in pathophysiology. The increased stroke volume produced by aortic insufficiency causes a corresponding increase in the pressure gradient across the stenotic valve. At the same time, the decreased compliance of the LV secondary to hypertrophy produced by the aortic stenosis prevents the LV from accommodating the regurgitant blood of aortic insufficiency.

Clinical Manifestations

Early symptoms are unusual, except in patients with gross aortic insufficiency. Patients may complain that they are aware of their hearts' beating, especially with exercise, because of the large stroke volume and forceful contractions. Chest pain may be a prominent symptom during exertion. Disturbing anginal pains may occur at night, accompanied by tachycardia, sweating, and paroxysmal hypertension. The major symptoms, especially breathlessness, are caused by LV disease. Symptoms are exaggerated and occur earlier if aortic insufficiency is associated with aortic stenosis.

The characteristic peripheral signs of aortic insufficiency are produced by the combined large pulse volume and peripheral vasodilation. The sharp rise of the pulse gives it a characteristic "water hammer" quality. The visible, jerky arterial pulsations in the neck are known as the Corrigan sign. The blood pressure is normal in patients with very mild aortic insufficiency.

With increasing severity of aortic insufficiency, the systolic pressure increases and the diastolic pressure decreases. The apical impulse in aortic valve disease is diffuse and hyperdynamic, and it may be displaced laterally and inferiorly.

The typical murmur of aortic insufficiency is an early diastolic, high-pitched, blowing, decrescendo murmur over the base, which begins with the second sound. The murmur is heard best with the diaphragm of the stethoscope in full expiration while the patient is sitting and leaning forward. The duration, rather than the quality or the loudness, of the aortic diastolic murmur correlates with the severity of the aortic insufficiency. An ejection systolic murmur at the base, caused by increased blood flow across the aortic valve in systole, is heard in almost all cases of aortic insufficiency of more than mild degree. The diagnosis of associated aortic stenosis cannot be based merely on the presence of this systolic murmur. A middiastolic or presystolic rumble over the mitral area, the Austin Flint murmur, usually is heard in patients with moderate or severe aortic insufficiency without associated organic MS. The Austin Flint murmur may be caused by relative MS secondary to improper opening of the anterior leaflet of the mitral valve by the regurgitant bloodstream or by the high LV diastolic pressure. Echocardiography is the most sensitive way to differentiate an Austin murmur from an organic apical diastolic murmur.

Laboratory Findings

The electrocardiogram is normal in mild cases of aortic insufficiency. LV hypertrophy develops in severe cases (Fig. 286.9). As the severity of aortic insufficiency increases, more dilation and enlargement of the LV occur radiologically. Typically, the LV enlarges in an inferior and leftward direction and can be seen below the diaphragmatic level.

The most common and characteristic M-mode echocardiographic finding in chronic aortic insufficiency is fine diastolic fluttering of the mitral valve, more frequently the anterior leaflet. The echocardiographic study has an important role in the clinical assessment and evaluation of changes in LV function in patients suffering from aortic insufficiency. Serial echocardiographic studies can reveal early changes in LV functions. Deterioration is indicated if a progressive increase in end-systolic and end-diastolic dimensions accompanied by gradual reduction in LV shortening is present. Doppler imaging is the most sensitive noninvasive method for detecting aortic insufficiency. Color Doppler flow mapping of the regurgitant jet offers a more precise approach to quantitation of the severity of the aortic

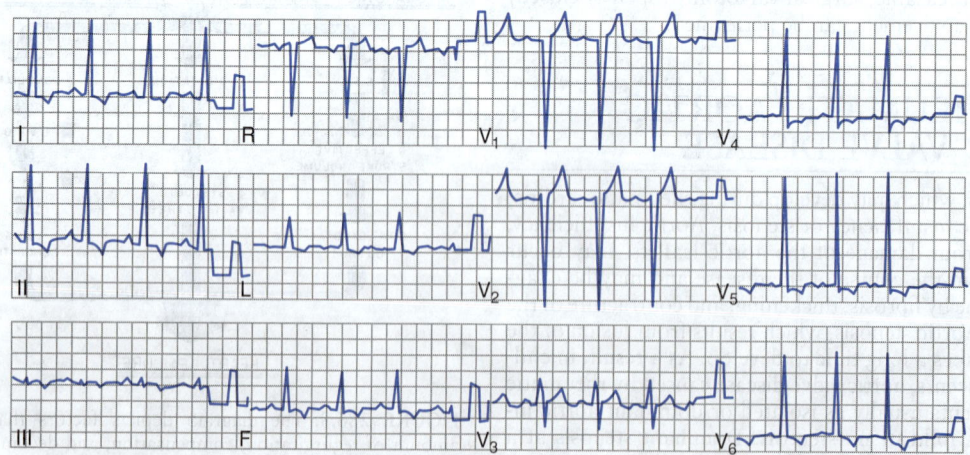

FIGURE 286.9. The electrocardiogram shows severe left ventricular hypertrophy and strain in a patient with gross aortic insufficiency.

insufficiency. Aortography enables establishing the diagnosis of aortic insufficiency and grading of its severity, but it rarely is needed.

Differential Diagnosis

Establishing the diagnosis of aortic insufficiency usually is not difficult if the characteristic murmur is detected. After the murmur is heard, its cause must be differentiated from other causes of left parasternal diastolic murmurs, such as the Graham Steell murmur. The Graham Steell murmur is a soft, early diastolic, left parasternal murmur caused by functional pulmonary incompetence secondary to dilatation of the pulmonary artery as a result of severe pulmonary hypertension. Aortic insufficiency should be differentiated from other causes of aortic runoff, including patent ductus arteriosus, ruptured sinus of Valsalva, systemic arteriovenous fistula (e.g., coronary), and aortic LV tunnel.

After the diagnosis of aortic valve disease is established, a search for the cause is necessary. A history of rheumatic fever or evidence of organic mitral valve disease favors a rheumatic origin. If evidence of associated significant aortic stenosis—supravalvular, valvular, or discrete subvalvular—is present, the cause of aortic insufficiency usually is congenital. Isolated congenital aortic insufficiency is rare, but it can occur in patients with aneurysms of the sinus of Valsalva. Aortic insufficiency at a young age also can occur with coarctation of the aorta, ventricular septal detect, or Marfan syndrome. An important element in the differential diagnosis is infective endocarditis on a congenitally deformed aortic valve.

Management Strategy

Aortic Regurgitation

Medical treatment of patients with aortic regurgitation involves the use of vasodilatory drugs. Therapy with vasodilating agents is designed to improve forward stroke volume and reduce regurgitant volume. These effects should translate into reductions in LV end-diastolic volume, wall stress, and afterload, resulting in preservation of LV systolic function and reduction in LV mass.

Vasodilating agents have three potential uses in chronic aortic regurgitation, but these criteria apply only to patients with severe aortic regurgitation. The first is long-term treatment of patients with severe aortic regurgitation who have symptoms and/or LV dysfunction and who are considered poor candidates for surgery because of additional cardiac or noncardiac factors. The second is improvement in the hemodynamic profile of patients with severe heart failure symptoms and severe LV dysfunction with short-term vasodilator therapy before proceeding with aortic valve replacement. In such patients, vasodilating agents with negative inotropic effects should be avoided. The third is prolongation of the compensated phase of asymptomatic patients who have a volume-loaded LV but normal systolic function.

Aortic Stenosis

An optimal schedule for repeated medical examinations has not been defined; many physicians perform an annual history and physical examination on patients with mild aortic stenosis. Patients with moderate and severe aortic stenosis should be examined more frequently.

Physical activity is not restricted in asymptomatic patients with mild aortic stenosis; these patients can participate in competitive sports. Patients with moderate aortic stenosis should

avoid competitive sports that involve high dynamic and static muscular demands. Other forms of exercise can be performed safely, but such patients should be evaluated with an exercise test before they begin an exercise or athletic program. Patients with severe aortic stenosis should be advised to limit their activity to relatively low levels.

Surgery should be considered only in the asymptomatic patient with severe aortic stenosis. One should adjust the valve area to the body surface area, the threshold for severity being less than 0.6 cm/m^{-2} body surface area. Even if the benefit is not proven definitely, surgery is recommended in the following circumstances:

- Patients with an abnormal response to exercise: development of symptoms, fall in blood pressure, inadequate rise in blood pressure, markedly impaired tolerance for exercise
- Patients with moderate to severe calcification, a peak jet velocity more than 4 m/second, and with an accelerated rate of progression of peak velocity (0.3 m/second/year or greater) because of their fast progression towards symptoms
- Patients with LV dysfunction (LV ejection fraction less than 50%). This situation is rare, however, in asymptomatic aortic stenosis.

Even if a lower level of evidence is present, surgery probably can be considered in the following situations:

- Severe LV hypertrophy (greater than 15 mm wall thickness) unless it is aused by hypertension
- Severe ventricular arrhythmias for which no cause other than severe aortic stenosis can be identified

RHEUMATIC TRICUSPID VALVE DISEASE

Rheumatic tricuspid valve disease develops in 5% to 10% of patients with RHD and is almost invariably associated with mitral or mitral and aortic valve disease. Organic tricuspid insufficiency can occur alone or with organic tricuspid stenosis as a result of rigidity of the valve edges, shrinkage of leaflet tissue, annular dilation, or a combination of these abnormalities. Functional tricuspid incompetence is the result of annular dilation and malalignment of papillary muscles secondary to RV failure complicating pulmonary hypertension.

Tricuspid insufficiency permits blood to regurgitate into the right atrium (RA), diminishing the forward flow by the same amount. The larger volume of blood in the RA increases the RA pressure. When the RV relaxes, it is subjected to a higher filling pressure and dilates more to accommodate this extra blood. RV dilation intensifies the leak and magnifies the heart failure.

The cardinal feature in tricuspid stenosis is a diastolic pressure gradient across the tricuspid valve with elevation in RA pressure. Tricuspid valve disease is rare in childhood.

CONCOMITANT TREATMENTS IN PATIENTS WITH RHEUMATIC HEART DISEASE

Effective prevention of RHD includes prophylaxis against rheumatic fever and its recurrence and against the occurrence of infective endocarditis. For asymptomatic patients with mild or moderate valvular disease and with a normal heart size or insignificant cardiomegaly, normal school activity should be encouraged. Restriction of activity is unnecessary. For symptomatic patients, activities should be limited to those that do not produce symptoms of fatigue, dyspnea, or excessive palpitation. Weight lifting and other isometric exercises should be discouraged. Competitive sports are not encouraged because individuals tend to ignore symptoms in the excitement of a contest.

Anemia and Infections

Patients with chronic RHD have diminished cardiac reserves. Cardiac decompensation can be precipitated by anemia or minor infections, which should be treated promptly and aggressively. Because chest infections may be precipitated by pulmonary congestion, a diuretic usually is needed.

Arrhythmias

In rheumatic mitral valve disease, frequent atrial premature contractions often presage atrial fibrillation, and the administration of antiarrhythmic drugs may be effective in preventing this complication. Atrial fibrillation, flutter, and tachycardia can complicate these cases. The immediate treatment for atrial fibrillation should be directed toward reducing the ventricular rate and, if possible, reestablishing sinus rhythm by pharmacologic therapy and cardioversion, singly or in combination. After reversion to the sinus rhythm, administration of quinidine or a similar antiarrhythmic agent should be continued indefinitely to diminish the likelihood of recurrence.

Thromboembolic Complications

If surgery is not performed, oral anticoagulants should be administered to patients with mitral valve disease who have had systemic emboli and to patients who are at high risk of embolization, such as those who are in atrial fibrillation, have a greatly enlarged LA, or have LA thrombus demonstrated by transthoracic echocardiography and TEE.

Infective Endocarditis

The cause, diagnosis, and treatment of infective endocarditis are discussed in Chapter 284.

Heart Failure

Digitalis should be administered to patients with significant valvular lesions who begin to develop effort fatigue or dysp-

nea, with or without frank evidence of left-sided or right-sided heart failure. However, if a patient with isolated MS does not have right-sided heart failure or atrial fibrillation or flutter, little hemodynamic benefit can be expected from the use of digitalis. Fluid retention in such conditions responds well to treatment with diuretics. A low-sodium diet is advised, especially if the diuretics are not completely effective. The measures designed to reduce pulmonary venous pressure, including sedation, assumption of upright posture, and aggressive diuresis, are used to treat the hemoptysis of lung congestion. Patients with overt cardiac failure are treated in the usual way. Uncontrollable heart failure in children suggests the possibility of severe valvular afflictions, rheumatic activity, infective endocarditis, or electrolyte imbalance.

For patients with isolated MS, administration of betablocking agents may increase exercise tolerance by reducing the heart rate and increasing the diastolic time.

The response to vasodilator therapy, which diminishes the afterload, is impressive in patients with mitral and aortic insufficiency. Reducing the impedance to ejection in the aorta reduces the volume of regurgitating blood. Hemodynamic studies have shown beneficial effects of intravenous sodium nitroprusside in acute mitral insufficiency and oral angiotensin-converting enzyme inhibitors and prazosin in chronic cases. This therapy may be helpful in stabilizing patients who are waiting to undergo surgery. Agents such as sublingual nitroglycerin may be effective in relieving dyspnea brought on by exercise and may permit the same exercise to be undertaken with the pulmonary artery pressure lowered because of venous dilatation, arteriolar dilatation, or both.

Suggested Readings

American College of Cardiology/American Heart Association Task Force on Practice Guidelines, Committee on Management of Patients with Valvular Heart Disease. ACC/AHA guidelines for the management of patients with valvular heart disease: a report of the American College of Cardiology/American Heart Association Task Force on Practice Guidelines (Committee on Management of Patients With Valvular Heart Disease). *J Am Coll Cardiol* 1998;32:1486.

Bach D, Deeb G, Bolling S. Accuracy of intra-operative trans-esophageal echocardiography for estimating the severity of functional mitral regurgitation. *Am J Cardiol* 1995;76:508.

Braunwald E. Valvular heart disease. In: Braunwald E, ed. *Heart disease: a textbook of cardiovascular medicine,* 4th ed. Philadelphia: WB Saunders, 1997.

Dalen JE, Alpert JS, eds. *Valvular heart disease,* 2nd ed. Boston: Little, Brown, 1987.

Recommendations on the management of the asymptomatic patient with valvular heart disease. *Eur Heart J* 2002;23:1253.

Shaff HV, Danielson GK. Current status of valve replacement in children. In: Frankl WS, West AN, eds. *Valvular hear disease: comprehensive approach and management.* Philadelphia: FA Davis, 1986:427.

Wood P. An appreciation of mitral stenosis. *BMJ* 1954;1:1051.

CHAPTER 287 ■ ABNORMALITIES OF RATE AND RHYTHM

BRYAN CANNON

NORMAL SINUS RHYTHM

The sinus node is located in the upper portion of the heart at the junction of the superior vena cava and the right atrium. Impulses that begin atrial contraction typically come from this position. For this reason, the normal P-wave axis is between 0 and 90 degrees (i.e., positive P waves in leads I and aVF). The sinus node is not a discrete structure but rather is an oblong structure along the lateral wall of the right atrium. Therefore, for normal subjects to have P waves with two different origins is not unusual. The P-wave axis and morphology may change such that the P wave varies from positive to negative in lead aVF. For the pacemaker to originate in the left atrium, rendering the P wave negative in lead I, is extremely rare, and an abnormal tachycardia focus must be excluded in this situation.

In *sinus arrhythmia* (also known as *respiratory sinus arrhythmia*), the P-wave axis remains normal, but the interval between P waves increases with inspiration and decreases with expiration. This phenomenon is related to changes in vagal tone and is entirely normal. This variation in rate rarely exceeds 100% (e.g., from a rate of 60 to 120 beats per minute); if it does, it may signify a pathologic process.

Sinus bradycardia is defined as a heart rate below the normal limits for age. The normal values for heart rate are listed in Table 287.1. Sinus bradycardia typically is associated with increased vagal tone and only rarely is related to a primary cardiac cause. The most common reason for sinus bradycardia is the athletic heart, a condition that may cause bradycardia in adolescents and requires no further workup if the patient is asymptomatic. Other reasons for sinus bradycardia include the presence of increased intracranial pressure, anorexia nervosa, gastric distention, pharyngeal stimulation, and drugs that potentiate bradycardia (e.g., digoxin, beta blockers, sedatives).

In an otherwise asymptomatic patient, sinus arrhythmia and sinus bradycardia require no further evaluation. However, excessive variation in the rate or constant sinus bradycardia even with activity may indicate an underlying abnormality.

TABLE 287.1

HEART RATES IN NORMAL INFANTS AND CHILDREN

Age (Years)	Resting Awake Low	Resting Awake High	Asleep (Low)	Agitated (High)
<1	90	180	70	210
1–4	70	150	50	200
4–10	60	130	45	190
10–18	50	130	35	190

ABNORMALITIES IN SINUS RHYTHM: WOLFF-PARKINSON-WHITE SYNDROME AND LONG QT INTERVAL

On any routine electrocardiogram (ECG), the tracing should be examined for the possible presence of two disorders: Wolff-Parkinson-White syndrome and long QT interval. Automated pediatric ECG analysis programs often can miss these abnormalities. Both disorders may cause syncope or seizure-like activity in a previously well child. An ECG to evaluate for these disorders should be a part of the workup of a patient who presents with syncope or a nonfebrile seizure.

Wolff-Parkinson-White syndrome involves the constellation of three findings: a PR interval shorter than normal for age, a slurred upstroke of the QRS complex (i.e., a delta wave), and a QRS complex longer than normal for age (Fig. 287.1). There are frequently changes in the ST or T waves. These findings may not be present in all leads, and the midprecordial leads (V_2 to V_4) may be the most sensitive. Other clues to the presence of Wolff-Parkinson-White syndrome are left axis deviation, the absence of Q waves in lead V_6, and abnormally wide Q waves in the limb leads. Patients with Wolff-Parkinson-White syndrome usually have structurally normal hearts, but the syndrome can be associated with congenital heart disease such as Ebstein anomaly of the tricuspid valve, corrected transposition of the great arteries, and hypertrophic cardiomyopathy. For this reason, an echocardiogram is indicated in patients with this disorder.

A prolonged QT interval is diagnosed when the corrected QT interval, or QTc, (i.e., QT interval in seconds divided by the square root of the previous RR interval in seconds) is longer than 0.44 in a child and 0.45 in an adolescent female patient. Patients with a prolonged QT interval may have *prolonged QT syndrome*. The T waves in these patients frequently appear flattened or abnormal. Patients with prolonged QT syndrome are at risk for having ventricular arrhythmias (particularly a form of polymorphic ventricular tachycardia called torsade de pointes) and sudden death. Patients with prolonged QT syndrome may have sinus bradycardia and occasionally have T-wave alternans (upright T wave alternating with a negative T wave in the same lead of an ECG tracing; Fig. 287.2). Treatment with beta blockers has been shown to decrease the risk of sudden death occurring in patients with prolonged QT syndrome. A number of medications (including erythromycin) can prolong the QT interval and should be avoided by these patients. Implantable cardioverter-defibrillator placement is indicated in those patients with ventricular tachycardia, recurrent syncope, or resuscitated sudden death. Prolonged QT syndrome frequently is familial, and several different ion channel defects have been identified. A prolonged QT interval also can result from medications or electrolyte imbalances, and these patients also may be predisposed to having ventricular arrhythmias.

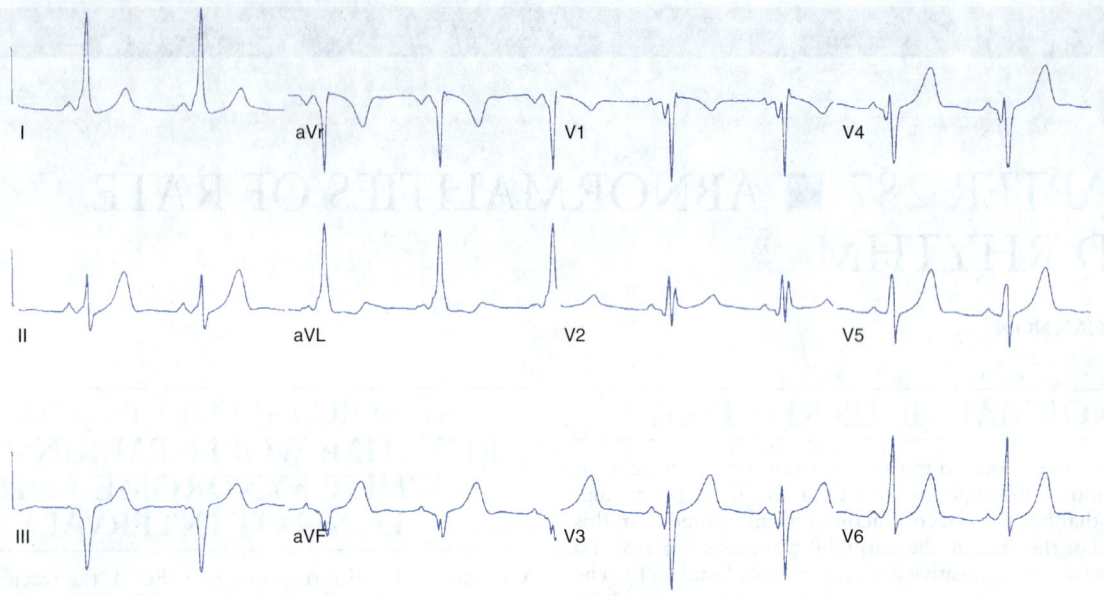

FIGURE 287.1. Electrocardiographic evidence of Wolff-Parkinson-White syndrome is seen on this strip. A shortened PR interval, widened QRS complex, and delta wave are seen. There is no Q wave in V₆ and left axis deviation. A bizarre QRS morphology and an abnormal Q wave in leads III and aVF are seen. Not all patients with Wolff-Parkinson-White have a delta wave that is this prominent, and some patients may be only intermittently preexcited.

ATRIOVENTRICULAR BLOCK

First-degree atrioventricular (AV) block is diagnosed when the PR interval is above normal limits for age. Normal PR intervals are less than 0.14 for children younger than 2 months of age, less than 0.16 for children between 2 months and 8 years, less than 0.18 in children older than 8 years of age, and less than 0.2 in older adolescents and adults. First-degree AV block typically is a benign condition resulting from increased vagal tone. It rarely progresses to a higher degree of block. No further evaluation is necessary in the asymptomatic patient.

Four types of *second-degree AV block* exist. The first type is Mobitz type I, also known as Wenckebach, which results in a progressive lengthening of the PR interval until a P wave is not conducted to the ventricle. It also may result from increased vagal tone. During sleep, this block can be a normal phenomenon. It does not require further evaluation unless it occurs while the patient is awake or it is associated with symptoms. Mobitz type II is failure to conduct to the ventricle with no associated progressive lengthening of the PR interval. This type of block always is abnormal and requires additional testing. Another form of second-degree AV block is 2:1 AV block, which occurs when every other P wave is not conducted. The final type is high-grade second-degree AV block, in which two or more consecutive P waves do not conduct to the ventricle but still some evidence of AV conduction exists.

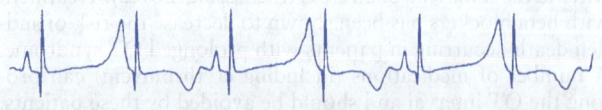

FIGURE 287.2. Congenital prolongation of the QT interval with T-wave alternans is shown on this tracing. This tracing is from a 6-week-old infant who presented with seizure-like episodes that were caused by ventricular tachycardia with resultant syncope. The corrected QT measures 680 milliseconds. The T waves have a bizarre morphology and at times may be mistaken for P waves.

In *complete AV block*, the P waves are entirely dissociated from the QRS complexes (Fig. 287.3). The P and QRS complexes typically are regular, but small variations in both can occur. Complete AV block can be congenital or acquired. Congenital complete AV block typically is associated with maternal collagen-vascular disease, but it also can be associated with congenital heart disease. Mothers with collagen-vascular disease frequently are asymptomatic, although some may have systemic lupus erythematosus or a similar disease. Women with clinical or subclinical disease have a high titer of anti-Ro (ss-A) or anti-La (ss-B) antibodies that cross the placenta and preferentially attack the AV node. Affected infants usually do not have other signs of collagen-vascular disease. Despite a low antibody titer, the complete AV block does not reverse in these infants. Some infants born with second-degree AV block may develop complete AV block within the first year of life, a finding implying that congenital AV block may be an evolving process.

Children with congenital complete AV block may not require immediate pacemaker therapy. As long as the ventricular rate consistently is greater than 55 beats per minute and no symptoms of congestive heart failure exist, these infants and children fare quite well. If congenital heart disease coexists in these patients, pacing often is instituted earlier. Patients with complex ventricular ectopy or a ventricular escape rhythm also may require consideration for early pacing. As children with congenital complete AV block grow, they may exhibit subtle symptoms such as frequent napping, mild growth failure, night terrors, or intolerance for exercise. They also may develop dilation of their left ventricle. If these findings occur, pacemakers typically are implanted. Because of a risk for late development of complications, these children all will require pacemakers sometime before they reach adulthood.

Complete AV block outside the newborn period often is associated with congenital heart disease, most commonly corrected transposition of the great arteries. It also may occur secondary to infectious causes such as Chagas or Lyme disease, with rheumatic diseases, or acutely in the setting of electrolyte disturbances.

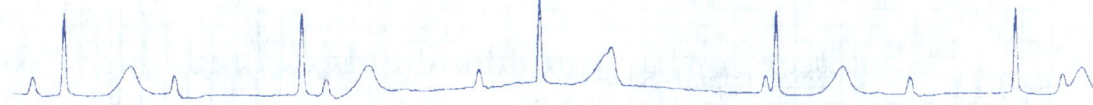

FIGURE 287.3. Complete atrioventricular block in a 6-year-old child is demonstrated on this strip. The atrial rate is 71 beats per minute. The ventricles are controlled by a narrow complex junctional rhythm at a rate of 45 beats per minute. The P waves have no relation to the QRS complexes. The atrial rate is faster than the ventricular rate, excluding sinus bradycardia with junctional escape or accelerated junctional rhythm. The P waves occurring after the end of the T waves should conduct to the ventricles, but they do not.

Patients with prolonged QT syndrome can have congenital high-grade or complete AV block. Patients with the combination of long QT syndrome with second- or third-degree AV block are at high risk for sudden death. Implantation of a pacemaker or implantable cardioverter-defibrillator is indicated in these patients.

Complete AV block also can occur after cardiac surgery. These patients are at higher risk for sudden death and frequently have a very slow underlying escape rhythm. For this reason, implantation of pacemakers is indicated in these patients.

SUPRAVENTRICULAR ARRHYTHMIAS

Premature Atrial Contractions

A premature atrial contraction (PAC) is defined on an ECG as a premature P wave. In most instances, it has a different morphology and axis from those of the sinus P waves. Most PACs are conducted to the ventricles with a normal QRS. When the premature P wave occurs early, conduction to the ventricles may occur with a different QRS morphology than that of sinus rhythm (i.e., aberrantly conducted PAC). This occurrence may simulate a premature ventricular contraction (PVC). For any early QRS complex that has a morphology different from that of the sinus beats, the preceding T wave should be examined carefully for a hidden P wave. Occasionally, a premature P wave may occur so early that it does not conduct to the ventricles at all (i.e., block). This situation may simulate sinus bradycardia because the premature P wave may reset the sinus node, delaying the next expected sinus impulse. In situations of paroxysmal bradycardia, especially those in which conducted PACs are on the same tracing, the T wave should be searched carefully for the presence of hidden P waves. This phenomenon is an especially common finding in newborn infants. Many tracings similar to the one in Fig. 287.4 are interpreted as multiform PVCs with PACs and sinus bradycardia, when in fact most of these patients have only PACs, some of which conduct aberrantly and some of which block. Isolated PACs are benign and do not require further evaluation. If frequent PACs are noted on an ECG or on monitoring strips, a 24-hour Cardio Scan monitor should be considered to exclude episodes of atrial tachycardia.

Atrial Flutter

Atrial flutter is an uncommon arrhythmia in the pediatric population. It typically occurs in newborn infants and postoperatively in patients with congenital heart disease. Newborn infants present with tachycardia and typical "saw-toothed" flutter waves on ECG. The atrial rate can be between 300 and 600 beats per minute with variable conduction to the ven-

tricles. If the ECG is difficult to interpret, adenosine can be given intravenously to block the AV node and reveal the flutter waves. Treatment is direct-current synchronized cardioversion with 0.5 to 1 watt-second/kg. Atrial overdrive pacing also can be used to terminate atrial flutter. Newborns who have atrial flutter typically have no structural heart disease and have no further problems after returning to normal sinus rhythm. A 24-hour Cardio Scan should be placed after cardioversion because rarely reentrant tachycardias or atrial tachycardias will initiate atrial flutter. If the patient has no recurrence of the atrial flutter or evidence of other arrhythmias, no further evaluation is necessary. Patients with atrial flutter after surgery for congenital heart disease (also know as intraatrial reentrant tachycardia) typically require long-term treatment to control their arrhythmias. The atrial rate typically is slower (100 to 250 beats per minute), and the ECG baseline may return to normal between successive P waves. Therefore, to examine the T wave and QRS complex for evidence of a hidden P wave in patients with congenital heart disease and tachycardia is important.

Supraventricular Tachycardia

Supraventricular tachycardia (SVT) is defined as an abnormally rapid rhythm that originates proximal to the bifurcation of the bundle of His, that is caused by an abnormal mechanism

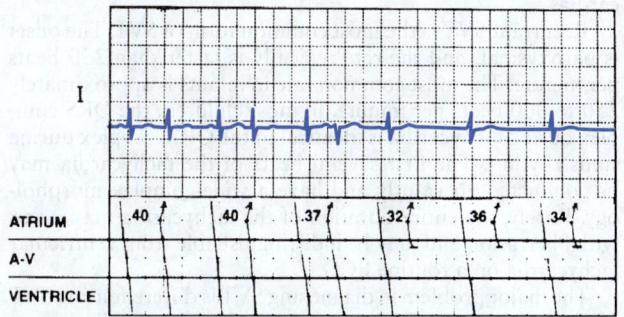

FIGURE 287.4. Premature atrial contractions (PACs) in a 1-day-old infant are shown in this tracing. The first beat is of sinus origin and is followed by a PAC conducted normally to the ventricles. The baseline is completely flat immediately after the sinus T wave, after which a slight change in the baseline occurs. This deflection represents the P wave of a PAC that occurs 0.40 seconds after the preceding P wave. The fifth beat is of sinus origin and is followed by an earlier PAC (0.37 seconds after the preceding sinus P wave). This beat conducts to the ventricle with a different QRS morphology, indicating QRS aberration (aberrantly conducted PAC). In the last three beats on the tracing, the sinus T wave has a different shape than that of the other sinus T waves, a finding indicating that a P wave is buried in the T wave. Because these premature beats occur earlier than do the previous ones, they do not conduct to the ventricles, and the P wave is not followed by a QRS complex. This pattern of "blocked premature atrial contractions" simulates sinus bradycardia. A-V, atrioventricular.

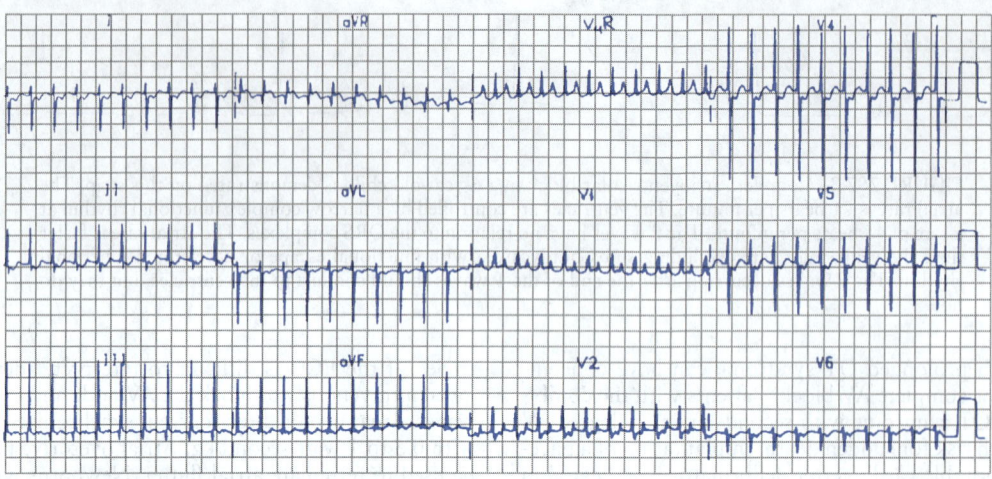

FIGURE 287.5. This tracing was taken from an infant during an episode of supraventricular tachycardia. The ventricular rate is 250 beats per minute. In this patient, who has Wolff-Parkinson-White syndrome demonstrated during sinus rhythm, the QRS complex during supraventricular tachycardia is normal. P waves occur after the QRS complex and are seen best in lead V2.

(specifically excluding sinus tachycardia), and that does not have flutter waves on the surface ECG (Fig. 287.5). The two basic mechanisms for SVT are automatic focus and reentry. Automatic tachycardias such as atrial ectopic tachycardia result from abnormal impulse generation in the atria and are a rare cause of SVT. This arrhythmia often is incessant and may present with an abnormal P-wave axis and prolonged PR interval on ECG. The atrial rate in atrial ectopic tachycardia may vary with catecholamine state and frequently displays periods or "warming up" and "cooling down" rather than a paroxysmal onset and termination. Adenosine typically blocks the AV node with no effect on the atrial rate and does not terminate the tachycardia. Cardioversion and overdrive pacing may suppress the atrial ectopic tachycardia temporarily, only to have it quickly resume its initial rate. Atrial ectopic tachycardia may be controlled with antiarrhythmic medication or may be eliminated using cardiac catheterization with ablation techniques. The remainder of the discussion focuses on reentrant tachycardias.

Reentrant SVT is the most common form of SVT. The onset is paroxysmal, and the rate typically is faster than 230 beats per minute. The most common rate in infants is approximately 250 to 300 beats per minute. In most children, the QRS complex during tachycardia is identical to the QRS complex during sinus rhythm. The first several beats of the tachycardia may be conducted aberrantly and have a wide-complex morphology. Rarely, the entire duration of the tachycardia may occur with aberration and may be indistinguishable from ventricular tachycardia on a routine ECG.

The major problem in diagnosing SVT is differentiating SVT from sinus tachycardia because both rhythms usually have a normal QRS complex. If the rate is faster than 230 beats per minute, the rhythm virtually always is SVT. If the rate is slower, the disorder could be SVT or sinus tachycardia. If the P waves are clearly visible and positive in leads I and aVF (normal P-wave axis), it likely is sinus tachycardia. In approximately one-half of patients with SVT, P waves may be found, but the P waves typically have an abnormal P-wave axis and usually are seen in the T wave. The condition of the patient also may be helpful. Most infants or children with very rapid sinus tachycardia have fever, sepsis, irritability, or another reason for this finding. Most children with SVT are well otherwise. In addition, most patients with SVT have a rapid onset and offset of their tachycardia.

The initial treatment of paroxysmal SVT involves assessing whether the patient has any signs of compromised cardiac out-

put (e.g., decreased peripheral pulse volume, decreased blood pressure, diaphoresis, lethargy). In this situation, quick conversion to sinus rhythm is essential. If intravenous access is quickly available, adenosine, 100 to 300 μg/kg, may be given by a rapid bolus with continuous ECG monitoring during the infusion. Equipment for defibrillation should be readily available because significant atrial and ventricular arrhythmias may result after administration of adenosine. If intravenous access or adenosine is not readily available, DC cardioversion at a dose of 0.5 to 1.5 watt-second/kg is used. The cardioversion must be synchronized to the QRS.

Many infants with less severe circulatory embarrassment present with mild irritability, decreased feeding, tachypnea, and hepatomegaly. In these infants, administration of adenosine at a dose of 100 to 300 μg/kg should be the first line of therapy. It is important to have a large-bore IV as close to the heart as possible when administering adenosine. Because the half-life of adenosine is extremely short, the bolus should be given rapidly over the course of 1 to 2 seconds. A three-way stopcock with an adenosine syringe in one port and a normal saline flush syringe in the other may aid in administration. Alternatively, two syringes may be placed into a single intravenous line at one time, thus allowing rapid administration of adenosine followed by normal saline flush. It is important to record an ECG tracing continuously because tachycardia termination may give important clues to the mechanism of the tachycardia. If adenosine is unavailable, the diving reflex may be initiated by placing a wet washcloth in crushed ice or filling a rubber glove with crushed ice and placing it over the infant's mouth and nose for as long as 15 to 30 seconds. This procedure always should be done with continuous ECG recording. Although rare, ventricular fibrillation or asystole has been reported with the dive reflex, so resuscitation equipment should be readily available when performing this maneuver. In older patients, having the patient perform the Valsalva maneuver or cough may break the tachycardia. Other vagal maneuvers such as ocular pressure, carotid sinus massage, and gagging are not recommended in children.

After conversion to sinus rhythm occurs, antiarrhythmic therapy generally is initiated. The efficacy of digoxin alone is highly controversial. The practice at our institution is to begin a beta blocker as first-line therapy. Propranolol is used, in a dose of 4 mg/kg/day divided every 6 hours in newborns and divided every 8 hours in infants older than 6 months of age. Atenolol, 1 mg/kg/day divided twice daily, is used in patients able to swallow pills. If control is not achieved using propranolol alone, sotalol, at a dose of 120 to 150 mg/body surface area in meters squared divided twice daily (three times daily in infants), or another antiarrhythmic drug such as amiodarone, is used.

With the improvement in ultrasound technology, arrhythmias frequently can be identified and characterized *in utero* with fetal echocardiography. Antiarrhythmics, including digoxin, flecainide and sotalol, then can be given to the mother during careful monitoring to control the tachycardia in the fetus.

Significant numbers of patients who present with SVT in the newborn period have spontaneous resolution of their tachycardia by the time they reach 1 year of age. Around this time, medications often are discontinued in these patients, although a few patients will have a recurrence, typically when they are between 6 and 7 years of age or during early adolescence. Patients who present with SVT who are older than 1 year of age are unlikely to have spontaneous resolution of their tachycardia. In patients older than 4 years of age, cardiac catheterization with catheter ablation can be used safely and effectively to eliminate the mechanism of tachycardia in more than 90% of patients. Catheter ablation can be performed earlier if the tachycardia cannot be controlled medically and is resulting in a compromise in ventricular function.

VENTRICULAR ARRHYTHMIAS

Premature Ventricular Contractions

A PVC is a premature QRS complex that does not have the same morphology as that of the sinus complex and is not preceded by a premature P wave. Especially in infants, PVCs may not have a broad QRS complex, but they have a morphology different from that of the sinus QRS. If all PVCs have similar shapes, they are referred to as *uniform*, and if they have more than one morphology, they are called *multiform*. A *couplet* is two PVCs in a row, and *bigeminy* is an alternating rhythm in which every other beat is a PVC.

Most children with uniform PVCs have normal hearts. If the heart is completely normal, the prognosis for the child with uniform PVCs (even those frequent enough to present as bigeminy) is good, and the condition is entirely benign. Although less well studied, uniform ventricular couplets probably have the same prognosis as that for isolated PVCs. If the history, physical examination, ECG (other than the rhythm), and echocardiogram are normal and the 24-hour Cardio Scan monitor shows only uniform PVCs and/or couplets, institution of medical therapy is not necessary in these patients. To repeat the Cardio Scan once after the initial evaluation to ensure that no change or progression of the ectopy has occurred is prudent. If a patient wishes to participate in competitive sports, an exercise treadmill may be useful to determine the response of the ectopy to exercise.

Occasionally, PVCs are associated with long QT syndrome, myocarditis, hypertrophic cardiomyopathy, and congenital heart disease before or after surgery. Often in these patients, the resting ECG is abnormal, the ectopy is frequent (more than 1,000 PVCs/hour), or the PVCs are multiform. Closer surveillance is required in these patients, and they may require further workup or evaluation.

Ventricular Tachycardia

Ventricular tachycardia is defined as three or more PVCs in a row at a rate faster than 180 beats per minute in infants and young children and 120 beats per minute in older children and adolescents (Fig. 287.6). Slower rates, within approximately

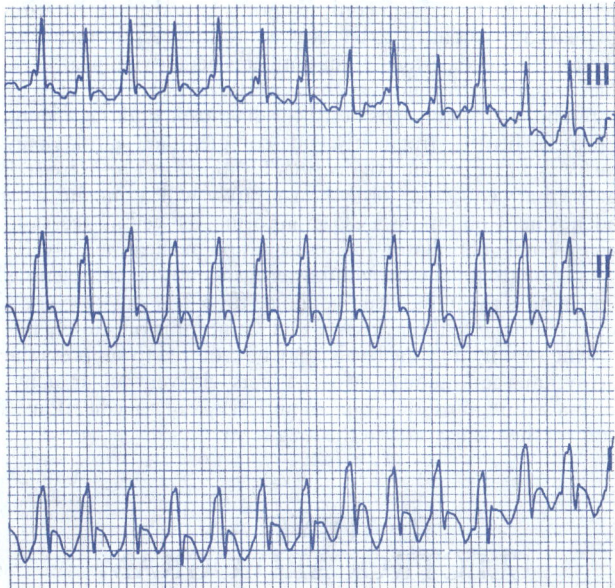

FIGURE 287.6. This strip demonstrates ventricular tachycardia in a newborn. The ventricular rate is 263 beats per minute. The QRS complex is wide with a notched morphology and is completely different from the QRS in sinus rhythm. Small changes in the T wave can be seen sporadically in lead III, which represent P waves. The atrial rate is slower, and no relationship exists between the P waves and the tachycardia (ventriculoatrial dissociation).

20% of the sinus rate, are referred to as *accelerated ventricular rhythms*. The QRS complex in ventricular tachycardia is different from that of the sinus QRS complex. The QRS complex does not necessarily have to be wide. In children younger than 2 years of age, the QRS duration may be between 0.06 and 0.11 seconds and the rate can be as fast as 400 beats per minute. Although ventricular tachycardia is an unusual diagnosis for an infant or a child, it must be suspected whenever the QRS complex is different from the sinus QRS complex.

Ventricular tachyarrhythmias in young infants may be associated with myocarditis, prolonged QT syndrome, severe electrolyte disturbances, or small hamartomas within the ventricular myocardium. In older children, ventricular tachycardia may be associated with myocarditis, prolonged QT syndrome, medication overdose or toxicity, various forms of cardiomyopathy, arrhythmogenic right ventricular dysplasia (a form of cardiomyopathy with fatty infiltrates in the myocardium), coronary artery abnormalities, and congenital heart disease both before and after surgery.

Additional diagnostic studies, including an electrophysiology study in the cardiac catheterization laboratory, may be required to help risk stratify patients with ventricular tachycardia and to determine therapy for their arrhythmias. During this procedure, it may be possible to localize the abnormal tachycardia focus and to eliminate it with radiofrequency or another type of energy (ablation procedure). Patients with sustained or hemodynamically unstable ventricular arrhythmias or resuscitated sudden death episodes generally require placement of an implantable cardioverter-defibrillator, a device similar to a pacemaker that can detect abnormal rhythms and then deliver pacing therapy or a shock to terminate abnormal rhythms. This therapy can be implemented in children, including patients as young as 1 year of age, at specialized centers.

The initial management of an acute presentation of ventricular tachycardia depends on the hemodynamic stability of the patient. Any patient with compromised blood pressure and perfusion should receive synchronized direct-current cardioversion (1 to 2 watt-second/kg). Synchronized cardioversion may terminate the tachycardia only temporarily, and administration of medications is likely to be necessary to suppress the tachycardia for extended periods. If the patient is hemodynamically stable, a dose of intravenous adenosine (100 to 300 µg/kg given by rapid bolus) may be considered for diagnostic and therapeutic purposes because frequently wide-complex tachycardias may be SVTs with aberrant conduction. Caution must be exercised, given that ventricular arrhythmias rarely will terminate with adenosine. Continuous ECG monitoring, as well as access to an external defibrillator and resuscitation medications, always should be secured before administering adenosine. Intravenous lidocaine is the initial drug of choice for VT (1 mg/kg every 5 minutes for up to three doses). A lidocaine infusion, closely following serum lidocaine levels, may be required to suppress the arrhythmia continuously. Most patients with ventricular tachycardia will require some type of antiarrhythmic medication to control the tachycardia in the long term.

READING AN ELECTROCARDIOGRAM

An entire book could be filled with all the subtleties of reading an ECG. This chapter focuses on only the basic principles of reading an ECG. Before beginning to read an ECG, one should understand some basic principles about how the ECG is set up.

Leads

The limb leads consist of I, II, III, aVR, aVL, and aVF. These measure forces in a coronal plane. Each of these leads is assigned a position (Fig. 287.7). Forces directed toward these leads are represented on the ECG by upward (positive) deflec-

tions. Forces away from the lead are represented by downward (negative) deflections.

The precordial or chest leads consist of V_1 to V_6 and measure cardiac forces in a transverse plane. Once again, forces toward these leads are represented by positive deflections, and forces away from the leads are represented by negative deflections.

Basic Setup

The ECG is a measure of the electrical forces in the heart over the course of time. The ECG typically is recorded on paper containing 1- by 1-mm squares and larger boxes that are 5 mm by 5 mm. Horizontal squares represent time. At a standard paper speed of 25 mm/second, each small (1- by 1-mm) box is equal to 0.04 seconds (40 milliseconds). Vertical squares represent ECG voltages. They are important in determining atrial enlargement and ventricular hypertrophy. Each small box represents 0.1 mV. However, by standard, vertical deflections are recorded in millimeters rather than millivolts (Fig. 287.8).

Wave Morphologies

The ECG consists of multiple deflections, all of which are named (Fig. 287.9). The P wave represents depolarization of the atria. The QRS complex represents depolarization of the ventricles. The first initial downward deflection (if present) is called the Q wave. The upward deflection above the baseline following the Q wave is the R wave. The downward deflection below the baseline following the R wave is the S wave. The T wave represents repolarization of the ventricles. An additional smaller deflection after the T wave, which is called a U wave, also may be present.

Intervals

The PR interval is measured from the start of the P wave to the beginning of the QRS complex. This measurement represents the time for atrial depolarization and conduction through the AV node. The QT interval is measured from the *beginning* of the QRS complex to the *end* of the T wave. It represents the time from ventricular depolarization to ventricular repolarization. Because the QT varies with heart rate, this interval must be corrected (Fig. 287.10) by dividing the QT interval (in seconds) by the square root of the previous RR interval

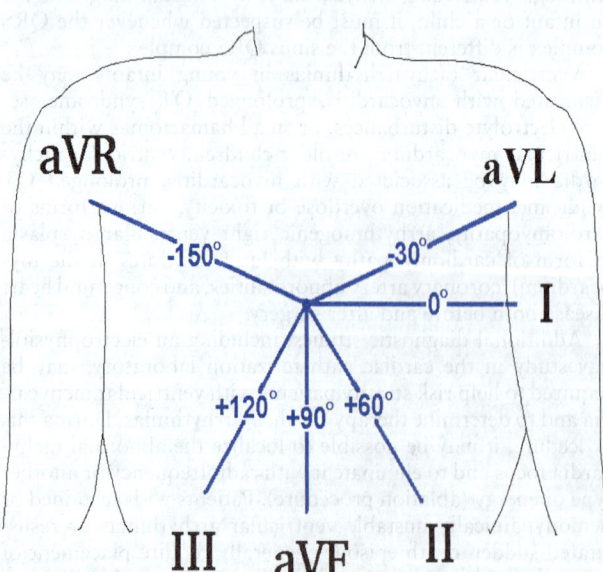

FIGURE 287.7. This diagram represents the hexaxial reference scheme viewed from the patient's front. Forces toward any of the leads are represented by positive deflections on the tracing. Forces away from the leads are represented by negative deflections. For example, because the sinus node usually is located in the upper right corner of the heart at the junction of the superior vena cava and the right atrium, electrical depolarization occurs with a wave downward and to the left. Therefore, the P wave in sinus rhythm would be upright in leads I, II, and aVF and is negative in aVR.

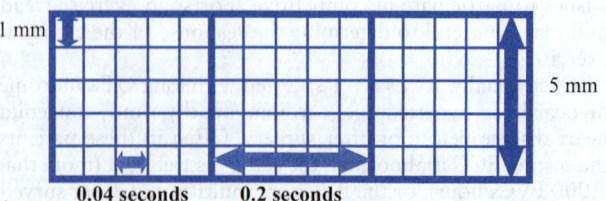

FIGURE 287.8. This diagram shows a standard electrocardiographic (ECG) layout. Each small square is 1 by 1 mm, and each large square is 5 by 5 mm. Vertical deflections represent voltages of the myocardium (by convention measured in millimeters and not millivolts), and horizontal calibrations represent time. At a standard paper speed, each small horizontal square is 0.04 seconds (40 milliseconds). If vertical voltages are too large, the ECG can be run at "half-standard," with all the deflections recorded at one-half their actual height rather than "full standard"; determining which setting has been used when interpreting an ECG is important.

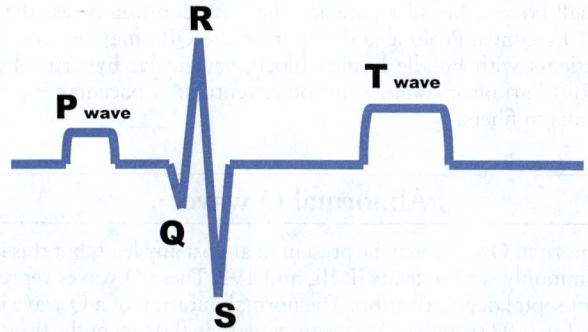

FIGURE 287.9. This figure demonstrates usual deflections on the electrocardiogram. The initial deflection is the P wave, which represents atrial depolarization. The next initial downward deflection, if present, is called the Q wave. The R wave is the next upward deflection above the baseline, followed by a downward deflection known as the S wave. If an additional upward deflection above the baseline following the S wave occurs, it is known as R′ (R prime). The QRS complex represents ventricular depolarization. The next deflection is the T wave, which represents ventricular repolarization. The PR interval is from the start of the P wave to the beginning of the QRS complex. The ST segment is from the termination of the QRS complex to the beginning of the T wave. The TP segment stretches from the end of the T wave to the next P wave and is a time during which measurable electrical activity in the heart is minimal (isoelectric baseline).

(in seconds). A second small deflection following the T wave, known as a U wave, also may occur. The U wave is important only in calculating the QT interval. If the U wave is less than one-half the height of the T wave, it can be ignored. If the U wave is greater than one-half the height of the T wave, it should be used in calculating the QT interval.

Heart Rate

Heart rate can be estimated on the ECG and typically is measured in beats per minute. There are two methods of determining heart rate. The first method is to count the number of QRS complexes in a 10-second period (the typical length of a standard ECG) and then multiply this number by 6. Alternatively, if only a rhythm strip is available, the number of QRS complexes can be counted in a 6-second period (30 large boxes)

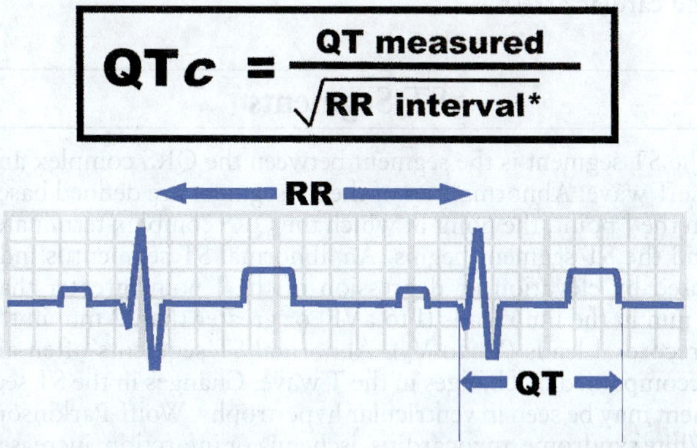

$$QTc = \frac{QT\ measured}{\sqrt{RR\ interval^*}}$$

FIGURE 287.10. Because the QT interval varies with heart rate, the measured QT interval should be corrected using a standard formula. The QT interval is measured from the *onset* of the QRS complex to the *end* of the T wave. The formula for the QT interval is the measured QT interval in seconds divided by the square root of the RR interval in seconds. *The RR interval used in calculation is the RR interval immediately preceding the QT measured.

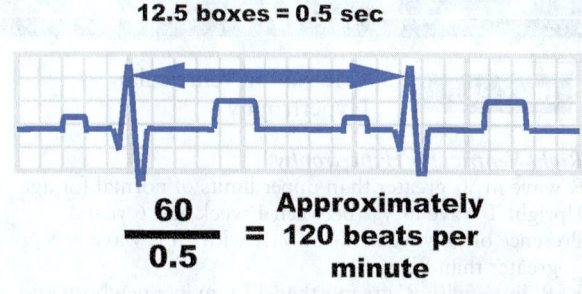

FIGURE 287.11. This figure shows a method for estimating heart rate. The distance between two consecutive RR intervals is measured in seconds. This number then is divided into 60 to obtain an estimated heart rate (120 beats per minute in this example). This method is only an estimation and is not accurate if the heart rate is irregular.

and multiplied by 10. If the heart rate is regular, a shortcut can be employed to estimate the heart rate. First, determine the amount of time in seconds between two consecutive RR intervals, remembering that each small box represents 0.04 seconds. Then, divide this number into 60 (Fig. 287.11).

Cardiac Rhythm

In most patients, atrial contractions are initiated by the sinus node that is located at the junction of the superior vena cava and the right atrium. To call a rhythm sinus, it must meet three criteria. First, a P wave must be present before every QRS complex. Second, a QRS complex must be present after every P wave. Third, a normal P-wave axis (upright P wave in leads I and aVF) must be present.

Axis

The QRS axis gives information about the relationship of forces in the heart. The normal range for an axis varies with age. The limb leads (I, II, III, aVR, aVL, and aVF) are used to calculate an axis. An axis may be affected by ventricular hypertrophy, bundle branch block, or other conduction disturbances. The specifics for determining axis are beyond the scope of this chapter. Right ventricular hypertrophy most commonly is the cause of right axis deviation. In contrast, left ventricular hypertrophy only rarely causes left axis deviation. Common causes of left axis deviation include partial or complete AV canal, tricuspid atresia, and Wolff-Parkinson-White syndrome. In a child with an axis less than zero, an echocardiogram probably is indicated to rule out congenital heart disease.

ABNORMALITIES ON THE ELECTROCARDIOGRAM

Atrial Enlargement

Because the right atrium is in close proximity to the sinus node, right atrial enlargement results in *tall* peaked P waves. P waves taller than 3 mm (three small boxes) in any lead are suggestive of right atrial enlargement. These changes are seen most commonly in leads II or V_1 but may be seen in any lead.

Because the left atrium is distant from the sinus node, left atrial enlargement results in *wide* P waves. P waves longer than 0.10 seconds (2.5 small boxes) are suggestive of left atrial

BOX 287.1	Criteria for Ventricular Hypertrophy

Right Ventricular Hypertrophy
R wave in V_1 greater than upper limits of normal for age
Upright T wave in V_1 (between 1 week and 6 years)
Presence of Q wave in V_1 or V_3R with an R wave in V_1 greater than 8 mm
RSR' in V_1 with R' greater than 15 mm in a newborn and R' greater than 10 mm in a child
Pure R wave (no S wave) in V_1 after 6 months
S in V_6 greater than upper limits of normal for age
R/S ratio in V_1 greater than upper limits of normal for age
Right axis deviation

Left Ventricular Hypertrophy
R wave in V_6 greater than upper limits of normal for age
S wave in V_1 greater than upper limits of normal for age
R/S ratio in V_6 greater than upper limits of normal for age
Asymmetric T wave inversion in leads V_5 or V_6
Q wave in III greater than upper limits of normal for age

Biventricular Hypertrophy
R wave plus S wave in any lead greater than 60 mm

enlargement. It is seen most commonly in leads II and V_1, and lead V_1 may have a broad notched or biphasic P wave with a negative terminal segment.

Ventricular Hypertrophy

Thickening of one or both of the ventricles may be suggested by findings on the ECG. Although the ECG is fairly good at indicating right ventricular hypertrophy, it is a poor predictor of left ventricular hypertrophy. ECG findings suggesting right and left ventricular hypertrophy are listed in Box 287.1. Extremely large voltages (so large that containing them on the ECG paper is difficult) can be seen in patients with glycogen storage disease (most commonly Pompe disease, also known as *acid maltase deficiency* or *glycogen storage disease type II*) or other storage diseases.

Low-Voltage QRS Complex

Low-voltage QRS complexes are diagnosed if the R wave plus the S wave is less than 5 mm in the limb leads (I to aVF) *and* less than 8 mm in the precordial leads (V_1 to V_6). Low-voltage QRS complexes may be seen in patients with myocarditis, pericarditis, pneumothorax, or hypothyroidism, in normal newborns (especially premature neonates), and in individuals with a thick chest wall.

QRS Complex Duration

The duration of the QRS complex varies with age. Similar to almost all other ECG intervals, the QRS duration is shorter in younger patients. The QRS duration in patients younger than 1 year of age typically is less than 0.08 seconds (two

small boxes). In older patients, the QRS duration is less than 0.10 seconds. Prolonged duration of the QRS may be seen in patients with bundle branch block, ventricular hypertrophy, Wolff-Parkinson-White syndrome, ventricular pacemakers, or Mahaim fibers.

Abnormal Q waves

A normal Q wave may be present in almost any lead, but this is commonly seen in leads II, III, and aVF. These Q waves represent septal depolarization. The normal duration of a Q wave is 0.01 to 0.02 seconds. Q waves greater than 0.03 seconds (three-fourths of a small box) always are abnormal. Wide Q waves may be seen in patients with myocardial infarction, myocardial fibrosis, hypertrophic cardiomyopathy, Wolff-Parkinson-White syndrome, or left ventricular noncompaction (a type of cardiomyopathy). Deep, wide Q waves in leads I and aVL (infarction pattern) are classic ECG findings for anomalous left coronary artery and should prompt immediate referral to a pediatric cardiologist. In patients with anomalous left coronary artery, the left coronary originates from the pulmonary artery, thus causing an infarction of the myocardium supplied by the artery (resulting in the Q waves in leads I and aVL). The infarction typically occurs when the patient is approximately 2 to 4 months of age as the pulmonary pressures normally drop. Deep, but not wide, Q waves may indicate ventricular hypertrophy, but they also may be normal variants.

T-Wave Changes

Because ventricular repolarization is not as organized as is ventricular depolarization, T-wave changes are nonspecific. The T wave in lead V_1 is upright at birth and then inverts during the first week of life. The T wave once again becomes upright around adolescence. An upright T wave between these two time frames is indicative of right ventricular hypertrophy. Tall peaked T waves may be seen in hyperkalemia, left ventricular hypertrophy, and myocardial infarctions. In hyperkalemia, T waves begin to increase in size at a serum potassium level of approximately 6 mmol/L. As the serum potassium level increases, the QRS duration is prolonged followed by prolongation of the PR interval then disappearance of the P wave. As the potassium level continues to rise, a wide-complex QRS with loss of distinction between the QRS and T wave results (often called a "sine wave" pattern). It is followed by ventricular fibrillation and cardiac arrest.

ST Segments

The ST segment is the segment between the QRS complex and the T wave. Abnormalities of the ST segment are defined based on the J point, the point at which the QRS complex terminates and the ST segment begins. An abnormal ST segment is indicated by elevation or depression of the J point greater than 1 mm in the limb leads (I to aVF) or greater than 2 mm in the precordial leads (V_1 to V_6). Abnormal ST segments often are accompanied by changes in the T wave. Changes in the ST segment may be seen in ventricular hypertrophy, Wolff-Parkinson-White syndrome, myocarditis, ischemia or infarction, increased intracranial pressure, or electrolyte disturbances. Diffuse ST-segment elevation is a classic finding in pericarditis but may not be present in all cases and should not be used as the sole method for eliminating pericarditis from a differential diagnosis. Nonpathologic ST segment changes may be seen in a condition called early repolarization. In this condition, ST segments are elevated in leads with an upright T wave and are depressed in leads with a negative T wave. In addition, the slope of the ST segment is in the same direction as the T wave.

Ischemia

Ischemia may be manifested in many different ways on the ECG. Changes may include ST-segment elevation, ST-segment depression, left or right axis deviation, T-wave inversion, hyperacute T waves, abnormal Q waves, widening of the QRS, and arrhythmias. The specifics about ECG findings in ischemia are beyond the scope of this chapter.

Right-Sided Chest Leads

Many pediatric ECGs will include right-sided chest leads (V_3R and V_4R). These leads are placed in the same chest position as are leads V_3 and V_4, but on the right side of the chest. These leads are helpful in determining right ventricular hypertrophy (as mentioned earlier) and dextrocardia. If the combined voltages of the R wave and S wave are greater in leads V_3R and V_4R than in leads V_3 and V_4, the heart is positioned on the right side of the chest and the diagnosis of dextrocardia or dextroposition of the heart can be made. Some pediatric ECGs will also display lead V_7, which has no well-defined use.

Suggested Readings

Etheridge SP, Judd VE. Supraventricular tachycardia in infancy: evaluation, treatment and follow-up. *Pediatrics* 1997;100:439.

Garson A Jr. The electrocardiogram. In: Garson A Jr, Bricker JT, Fisher DJ, Neish SR, eds. *The science and practice of pediatric cardiology.* Baltimore: Williams & Wilkins, 1998.

Garson A Jr, Gillette PC, McNamara DG. Supraventricular tachycardia in children: clinical features, response to treatment, and long-term follow-up in 217 patients. *J Pediatr* 1981;98:875.

Jacobsen J, Garson A Jr. Irregular heartbeat. In: Garson A Jr, Bricker JT, Fisher DJ, Neish SR, eds. *The science and practice of pediatric cardiology.* Baltimore: Williams & Wilkins, 1998.

Task Force of the Working Group on Arrhythmias of the European Society of Cardiology. The Sicilian gambit: a new approach to the classification of antiarrhythmic drugs based on their actions on arrhythmogenic mechanisms. *Circulation* 1991;84:1831.

CHAPTER 288 ■ THERAPEUTIC CARDIAC CATHETERIZATION

CHARLES E. MULLINS

Although very few procedures and/or specific devices are "approved" for use in pediatric and congenital heart lesions in the United States by the Food and Drug Administration (FDA), therapeutic catheterization procedures now not only are accepted worldwide by knowledgeable physicians but also represent the primary indication for performing cardiac catheterizations in congenital heart patients. For more than five decades, cardiac catheterizations have been the definitive diagnostic tool for all cardiac diseases. The diagnostic cardiac catheterization allows establishment of the hemodynamic quantification of normal and abnormal physiologies of the heart. With the addition of selective biplane angiography to the diagnostic catheterization, the anatomic defects can be defined very precisely. Catheterization has been particularly important in establishing the diagnosis of and managing complex congenital cardiac defects. As more complex techniques for the surgical correction of congenital heart defects have been developed, a detailed catheterization with accurate angiography has become a prerequisite to performing surgery. In the last two decades, a proliferation of "noninvasive" diagnostic techniques have been developed and have enabled many patients now to be sent to surgery without having to undergo catheterization. Despite the many noninvasive diagnostic technologies, cardiac catheterization still remains the gold standard and is absolutely essential for many of the fine details of the complex anatomy and the hemodynamics in congenital heart lesions.

Techniques for treating intracardiac and intravascular defects definitively in the cardiac catheterization laboratory were introduced more than four decades ago. From the very first introduction of a diagnostic cardiac catheter, cardiologists envisioned the concept of correcting cardiac defects using the cardiac catheterization laboratory. Use of therapeutic procedures in the pediatric cardiac catheterization laboratory first became a reality with the innovative and courageous development of the balloon atrial septostomy catheter and procedure by Dr. William Rashkind in 1966. This procedure was a lifesaving palliation for critically ill infants and, equally as important, it demonstrated the feasibility of performing therapeutic procedures for congenital heart disease in the catheterization laboratory. The balloon atrial septostomy procedure paved the way for all subsequent catheterization procedures aimed at therapy. This particular procedure has served the test of time and still is an essential procedure in the care of infants with complex congenital heart disease. Porstmann (1967) reported the closure of the patent ductus using a large and complex delivery system requiring a combined venous and arterial approach. The Porstmann procedure was the first "corrective" procedure performed in the catheterization laboratory, but it now rarely is used.

Additional therapeutic catheterization procedures of major importance for congenital heart lesions, particularly in pediatric patients, were slow in developing. Although the procedures that were developed were unique for the congenital heart patients, most of the equipment used was (and is!) developed for, and in turn represents "hand me downs" from, adult therapeutic catheterization procedures. During the last two decades, development of new procedures proliferated, and several specific new devices were developed, until the therapeutic procedures for congenital heart lesions now represent the most revolutionary developments in the management of congenital heart disease since the introduction of surgery for these patients.

The numerous therapeutic catheterization procedures available for the pediatric cardiac patients are divided arbitrarily into seven main categories: septostomies, catheter removal of intravascular foreign bodies, valve dilations, vessel dilations, vessel dilation with intravascular stent implant, valve and vessel perforations/recanalizations, and occlusion/closure procedures. Each of these categories contains well-established procedures as well as many procedures that remain investigational. All of the therapeutic catheterization procedures require special equipment and special skills. The success and safety of the procedures correlate with the skill and experience of the operators and the centers performing the procedures. For these reasons, not every pediatric cardiologist or every pediatric cardiac center should attempt every therapeutic catheterization procedure.

ATRIAL SEPTOSTOMIES

The oldest, one of the most established, and still used therapeutic catheterization procedures is the balloon atrial septostomy. The balloon septostomy is most effective in infants younger than 1 month of age. It is the one therapeutic catheterization procedure that should be available in *all* centers caring for infants with congenital heart disease. The balloon septostomy is lifesaving in newborn infants with transposition of the great arteries in whom no other intracardiac communication exists and in infants with hypoplastic left heart syndrome with a restrictive atrial communication. It provides some immediate mixing of the totally separated systemic and pulmonary venous blood and/or "venting" of the left atrium. This mixing is required urgently to correct hypoxemia and acidosis and to stabilize these infants, even if performing an arterial switch or a "Norwood"-type surgical procedure is anticipated within hours or days.

An atrial septostomy is indicated in many other infants with a variety of other cyanotic lesions in whom an adequate, pre-existing, interatrial septal communication is not present, but, at the same time, the continuity of the circulation depends on such a lesion. For example, a septostomy is performed in infants with hypoplastic right heart syndromes, such as pulmonary or tricuspid atresia, in which all of the systemic venous blood must pass from the right atrium through the atrial septum to return to the effective systemic circulation. In patients with total anomalous pulmonary venous return, the only access of both the systemic and pulmonary venous returns back to the systemic circulation is through the atrial septal defect. If the atrial septal defect is at all restrictive in any of these lesions, a septostomy is indicated.

Although improvements have been made in the balloon catheters available for the balloon septostomy, the balloon atrial septostomy procedure is essentially the same as originally described by Rashkind and Miller (1966). An inflatable, spherical balloon attached at the distal end of a catheter is used to tear an opening in the interatrial septum. The deflated balloon is advanced from the right atrium into the left atrium, and the balloon is inflated in the left atrium and then rapidly and forcefully pulled (i.e., jerked) through the atrial septum into the right atrium, which, in turn, tears an opening in the interatrial septum. The hole created allows free mixing or passage of blood across the atrial septum.

Some patients with these cyanotic defects and/or even more complex lesions live for months or years before requiring enlargement of an atrial septal defect or further surgery. When one of these patients older than 1 month of age does require a further opening of the atrial septum, the *balloon* septostomy procedure alone merely stretches the atrial septal tissues and does not create a permanent opening because of the thickened, tougher septa. Dr. Sang Park extended the use of the septostomy procedure for these older patients with the introduction of the blade septostomy catheter in 1975.

The blade septostomy procedure is accomplished using a catheter with a small retractable blade at its distal end. The catheter, with the blade retracted, is advanced through a long sheath into the left atrium. The blade is opened carefully in the left atrium, and the blade catheter is withdrawn forcefully, but slowly and with careful control, through the atrial septum, which, in turn, incises an opening in the septum. This procedure is repeated, changing the side-to-side angle of the blade with each withdrawal. After the multiple incisions with the blade are completed, a balloon septostomy is performed to further increase the septal opening.

In much older patients with septae, which are extremely resistant to further tearing by the septostomy balloon, a dilation balloon is used after the blade incision to open the atrial septum further. A deflated "angioplasty" balloon catheter is advanced over a wire until the balloon is centered across the atrial septum. The dilation balloon is inflated, further extending the previous blade cuts. As with other dilation procedures, two smaller dilation balloons used simultaneously are as effective as or more effective than is one balloon, but they cause less trauma to the venous system.

As an alternative to the blade atrial septostomy, particularly in patients with a very small left atrium, intravascular stents now are placed across the septal opening to maintain the patency of the atrial septal defect. A balloon expandable intravascular stent is expanded in a small interatrial communication on a dilation balloon. The expanded stent remains at the final diameter of the balloon, fixing the opening in the septum at the expanded diameter, preventing "recoil" or late closure of the atrial defects.

The balloon, blade, and balloon and/or stented septostomies are palliative procedures, but often they are the only procedures available or required for many of the extremely complex congenital heart lesions. Although the patients often are extremely ill, the catheter septostomies, when performed cautiously and with meticulous attention to the technical details of the procedures, are effective and safe procedures.

CATHETER REMOVAL OF INTRAVASCULAR FOREIGN BODIES

Since they were first introduced purposefully into the vascular system, pieces of indwelling intravenous lines, cardiac catheters, or implantable intravascular devices occasionally have broken off, come loose, or otherwise gone astray in the circulation. The most common of these foreign bodies are pieces of indwelling "catheters" from hyperalimentation or chronic chemotherapy lines, which have been sheared off during attempted removal. Most of these loose pieces and devices are in the systemic venous side of the circulation and end up migrating to the right heart and/or, more often, to the pulmonary arteries. These foreign bodies originally required surgical removal and occasionally even an open heart procedure.

Early in the development of cardiac catheterization, devices were modified from urologic devices and/or fabricated by cardiologists for the purpose of catching and retrieving the errant objects. Multiple, commercially manufactured catheter devices, which are miniaturized in order to pass through small catheters or sheaths, now are available specifically for the removal of foreign bodies in the cardiac catheterization laboratory. These devices include a variety of wire loop snares, collapsible wire baskets, and small grasping forceps. With the use of these tools and biplane fluoroscopy to localize the errant object, physicians can grasp essentially any item within the heart or pulmonary artery and withdraw it from the circulation through a sheath without requiring even a cutdown over the exit vessel. Removal of intravascular foreign bodies performed in the catheterization laboratory is the accepted therapy for most intravascular foreign bodies, although some very large, dislodged, intravascular devices still must be removed surgically.

BALLOON DILATIONS

The development, manufacture, and use in the 1970s of tiny, cylindrical, fixed-diameter, high-pressure balloons for dilating renal and coronary arteries began a revolution in the treatment of cardiovascular disease. These balloons inflate to a predetermined, fixed diameter when inflated to a specified pressure, and, at that diameter, the surface becomes very hard and rigid. The extension of this technology to similar but larger balloons in the early 1980s opened the way to the dilation of stenotic valves and larger vessels in patients with congenital heart disease. Techniques using the larger balloons initially were described for the dilation of pulmonary veins, pulmonary valves, recoarctations of the aorta, pulmonary branch stenoses, and aortic valves. The very long-term results of the balloon dilation procedures still are being determined, however, in a large initial collaborative study, and now, after 20 years of use, the dilation procedures have been demonstrated to be immediately effective, to be safe for the patient, to produce much less morbidity, and also to have sustained results equal to comparable surgical procedures. The balloon dilation procedures are accepted as the standard therapy for most obstructive congenital heart lesions.

VALVULOPLASTY (VALVE DILATIONS)

A double balloon technique is recommended for virtually all valve dilations. The advantages of the double balloon technique are multiple. The greatest advantage is that two smaller balloons with a much lower profile of each deflated balloon are easier and less traumatic to introduce into the peripheral vessels than is a single, larger deflated balloon that would be required for the same annulus size. Additionally, because two "lumens" always persist between and adjacent to the two inflated balloons within a "circular" orifice, blood flow through the lesion being dilated never is obstructed totally as it is with a single balloon. In turn, systemic cardiac output is not reduced as drastically while the balloons are being inflated. The two balloons make the dilation of much larger valves possible when single balloons of adequate size are not available and/or are too massive in their deflated profile.

The pulmonary valve was the first valve to be dilated successfully and is the valve with which the most extensive and valid experience has been accumulated. Shortly after the introduction of the technique in 1982, a voluntary collaborative registry from 27 pediatric cardiology centers was established. By the end of 1986, data on the experience with more than 800 patients who had pulmonary valve dilation established the procedure as safe and effective. Longer-term data just now are becoming available. The 20-year or longer follow-up data continue to demonstrate the acute success of dilation of valvular pulmonary stenosis, with no recurrence of the stenosis after an initial successful dilation. Pulmonary valve regurgitation is created, but it appears to be tolerated very well for at least the two decades of follow-up.

Before a dilation of the pulmonary valve is performed, the hemodynamics and exact anatomy are established by cardiac catheterization and selective angiography. From previous echocardiograms and/or the angiocardiograms, an accurate measurement is made of the diameter of the valve annulus. Two long exchange guidewires are passed through two separate catheters previously introduced and maneuvered from the right and left femoral veins into distal pulmonary arteries. The catheters are removed, leaving the two wires in place. The appropriate balloons are passed over the separate wires, positioned side by side in the valve, with the balloon centers located exactly within the stenotic orifice. The combined diameter of the two balloons that are used is 1.5 to 1.8 times the diameter of the annulus of the pulmonary valve. The balloons are inflated simultaneously and rapidly to the maximal recommended pressure of the balloons and/or until the circumferential indentation in the balloons created by the stenotic valve disappears; then they are deflated rapidly. To ensure that the balloons were in the optimal position, the positioning of the balloons is changed slightly and the inflation and deflation process is repeated several times. After dilation, the hemodynamics and angiograms are repeated. Pulmonary valve dilation using these techniques is safe, effective, and probably curative. It is the accepted standard therapy for pulmonary valve stenosis.

Valvular aortic stenosis was the next congenital valvular lesion to be treated with balloon dilation. Enthusiasm for aortic valve dilation initially was limited because of the expected difficulties and dangers of performing extensive manipulations in the arteries and in the systemic circulation and the fear that significant aortic regurgitation would be created. Eventually, several major centers began dilating valvular aortic stenosis on carefully controlled protocols. With success and complication rates, which were comparable to surgical results, reported from the investigating centers, the procedure gained a wider acceptance. In many centers, it is now the treatment of choice. Like the surgery for valvular aortic stenosis, dilation of the aortic valve still is a palliative procedure.

Balloon dilation of aortic valve stenosis is indicated for patients with pure aortic valvular stenosis that is severe enough to indicate treatment using the same criteria used for surgical intervention. The goal in the dilation of the aortic valve is not to "cure" the patient but to reduce the obstruction from a critical level to a mild degree without producing significant aortic regurgitation. After hemodynamic parameters have been recorded and accurate measurements of the aortic annulus diameter have been obtained, end-hole catheters are introduced from both femoral arteries. Each catheter is passed retrograde across the stenotic aortic valve into the left ventricle. Exchange length guidewires are passed through the catheters and positioned securely in the left ventricle. The catheters are removed, leaving the wires in place. Two balloon dilation catheters with long balloons are advanced over the wires until the balloons are centered in the stenotic valve orifice. The combined diameters of the two balloons are equal to or no more than 10% larger than the diameter of the aortic annulus. The balloons simultaneously and rapidly are inflated and deflated, splitting the stenotic valve. If a single balloon is used for aortic valve dilation, an even longer balloon is used, and the diameter of the single balloon should be no larger than the diameter of the valve annulus.

The double balloon technique, the use of much longer dilation balloons, and the very accurate measurement of the annulus with strict attention to the precise balloon-to-annulus ratio have rendered aortic valve dilation safer and more successful. However, even these techniques and precautions have not eliminated all the risks nor improved the predictability of the procedure. Although aortic valve dilation is used widely and no longer is considered an investigational procedure, its use should be limited to centers with adequate equipment and expertise and centers where long-term data on the technique and results of the procedure are being accumulated.

In the Middle East, Far East, and in less developed Western countries, rheumatic fever with resultant rheumatic mitral stenosis remains rampant. In those areas of the world where rheumatic heart disease exists, experience with the dilation of rheumatic mitral valve stenosis has been extensive and successful. Because of the control of rheumatic fever, rheumatic mitral valve stenosis is a rare problem in children and adults in the developed nations of the world, and congenital mitral stenosis is the major form of mitral disease encountered in developed countries. Congenital mitral stenosis usually results in a grossly deformed mitral valve and valve apparatus. The congenital stenotic mitral valves are poor candidates for any type of intervention except valve replacement, and little enthusiasm exists for, and there is even less experience with, dilation of the congenitally stenotic mitral valve. The techniques for dilation of the stenotic rheumatic mitral valves have been applied with satisfactory results to some of the more severe congenital mitral stenoses. These patients otherwise require surgical mitral valve replacement.

The technique for dilating the mitral valve in children involves making two separate transseptal punctures through the atrial septum. Then, two catheters are advanced from the left atrium across the mitral valve and into the left ventricle. Two exchange guidewires are advanced through the catheters and carefully looped in the left ventricle. Two dilation balloons are used with a combined diameter equal to, or slightly exceeding, the diameter of the mitral annulus or chosen according to the normal estimated valve diameter for the patient's body surface area. The balloon dilation catheters are advanced through the atrial septum and into the left atrium. From there, the balloons are advanced across the mitral valve and simultaneously inflated to the maximal recommended pressures and diameters and then deflated as rapidly as possible. The inflation and deflation procedure is repeated until the operator is satisfied that no residual indentations remain in the balloons or until the gradient across the valve is abolished.

The dilation procedure for the mitral valve has evolved into a reliable and safe procedure if performed meticulously. The early and medium-term results of rheumatic mitral valve dilations and the early experience with congenital mitral stenosis dilation have been encouraging. Because of the limited experience and technical difficulties associated with dilating congenital mitral valves, the dilation of this lesion remains investigational and should be performed only by institutions that technically are experienced and are accumulating longitudinal data on each case.

Tricuspid valve stenosis of any type is an extremely rare lesion, but it can be dilated successfully and relatively easily using a double balloon technique. Two exchange guidewires are passed from the femoral veins into the apex of the right ventricle or into the distal pulmonary arteries. Long dilating balloons are advanced over these wires, centered on the stenosed tricuspid valve, and inflated to their maximal pressure or until the balloon's "waist" disappears. Meaningful data on the effectiveness of this technique are lacking, but considering the surgical alternative and the relative ease and safety of this dilation procedure, dilations of stenotic tricuspid valves are attempted as the first line of therapy.

ANGIOPLASTY (DILATION) OF VASCULAR STENOSIS

Many congenital and surgically acquired vascular stenoses are amenable to balloon dilation by a catheter technique, and most stenoses do respond acutely to dilation. However, in many (most!) of these stenotic lesions, the obstruction is not relieved completely by dilation alone and/or there is a "rebound" of the stenosis. These residual and/or recurrent problems can be overcome by the adjunct use of intravascular stents, which are covered subsequently.

The first congenital vascular stenosis to be dilated successfully was recoarctation of the aorta after previous surgical repair. This lesion seemed ideally suited for a dilation procedure. Recoarctation of the aorta usually is discrete, the area of the recoarctation is surrounded by dense (i.e., supportive) scar tissue from the original surgery, and the lesion is difficult to re-repair surgically. These considerations, coupled with the reported first successful cases, generated enthusiasm for dilation of recoarctation, and many cases were performed in numerous centers, allowing data on coarctation dilation to be accumulated rapidly in the collaborative Valvuloplasty and Angioplasty of Congenital Anomalies Registry.

The procedure usually is effective in reducing immediately the obstruction to a minimal residual resting gradient. During follow-up as long as 20 years, the residual obstruction does not seem to progress, although it can be "outgrown." Early complications occurred, mostly involving arterial damage. In the registry, two deaths were reported to be related to the procedure. They appeared to be exaggerated vagal-like reactions. With the development of improved equipment and techniques and more precise measurements, dilation is an accepted standard procedure for postoperative residual or recoarctation. In the older (larger) patient, dilation with primary intravascular stent implant is replacing dilation alone for this and many other vascular lesions.

The procedure for the dilation of recoarctation is relatively straightforward. The site and size of the coarctation and the adjacent proximal and distal aortic diameters in the area of the coarctation are visualized and measured accurately on an aortogram. A balloon is chosen with a diameter equal to the narrowest adjacent "normal" aortic diameter. A guidewire is passed retrograde through the coarctation and into a distal subclavian artery. The balloon dilation catheter is passed over the guidewire to the site of the coarctation, and the deflated balloon is centered exactly at the narrowing of the coarctation. The balloon is inflated to its maximal diameter at the recommended pressure for the particular balloon. The waist in the balloon usually disappears with the first inflation and is not apparent on subsequent inflations. Follow-up pressures and aortograms are recorded.

After the success of dilating recoarctation was achieved, the same procedure was extended to the dilation of native coarctation of the aorta. The immediate results of these dilations were even more satisfactory than were those for recoarctation, and very few immediate complications were encountered. However, occasional cases of aneurysms developing at the site of the dilated coarctation were reported during follow-up. Although, so far, neither acute nor long-term major events have developed from these aneurysms, their presence in the few cases caused some concern and prompted a reappraisal of angioplasty alone for coarctation. An attempt is being made to determine the exact cause and the natural history of the few cases of aneurysm. Overdilation of the adjacent aorta in an attempt to overcome any "rebound" stenosis seems to be a common denominator, but not the only factor. With the significantly decreased morbidity and with results apparently equal to those of surgical repair, the dilation of native coarctation in many centers continues with carefully controlled long-term monitoring of each patient until the complete information on the long-term results is available. Dilation still is not the universally accepted standard therapy for native coarctation of the aorta and, like recoarctation, is being replaced by primary stent implant in larger patients.

Neither congenital nor acquired pulmonary artery branch stenosis following previous surgery is relieved successfully by surgical intervention because of the nature of the vessels involved and the location of the obstructions deep within the lung parenchyma. The surgery usually provides no benefit and/or worsens the situation. Initially, these lesions seemed ideal for a balloon dilation technique. Most pulmonary artery branch stenoses can be dilated acutely up to the normal or greater than normal vessel diameter by significant overdilation of the vessel compared to the nominal vessel size. However, 80% (100%!) of the dilated pulmonary arteries are stretched only temporarily and/or incompletely opened. The dilated pulmonary vessels usually return to their predilation stenotic diameter, configuration, and hemodynamics. Complications are significant and are as serious as is pulmonary artery rupture (with a few deaths). The large, rough, oversized dilation balloons can result in total obstruction of the entry site vein. Dilation by itself of pulmonary artery branch stenosis has fallen into disfavor and now is reserved for very small patients with severe obstruction, deteriorating hemodynamics, and vessels that are too small to accommodate the primary implant of intravascular stents that eventually can be dilated to adult diameters.

Dilation of systemic venous stenosis is successful acutely, but, like the dilation of most other vascular stenoses, the long-term patency of these lesions is very disappointing. In the venous switch type of repair for transposition of the great arteries (i.e., Mustard or Senning procedures), venous obstruction frequently is created within the baffle. Surgical repair of baffle obstruction requires a complete takedown and re-do of the baffle, with the inherent risks and morbidity of repeat open heart surgery. Acute dilation of these stenoses is possible, and a few of these areas remain open after they initially are dilated to a diameter much wider than (twice) the adjacent normal vessels. These lesions are suited for a double balloon technique because of the small size of the patients and the introductory veins and the need for dilations to large diameters. Two separate guidewires are passed across the stenosis from separate entry veins. Two balloons passed over these wires are inflated simultaneously in the area of the stenosis. The inflations are repeated until the waists in the balloons disappear. Although usually acutely successful, a high rate of restenosis occurs in these lesions. Dilation is recommended for all systemic venous stenoses, but now, similar to the dilation of most other vascular stenoses, in conjunction with the primary implant of intravascular stents to ensure patency.

DILATION WITH CONCURRENT IMPLANT OF INTRAVASCULAR STENTS FOR VASCULAR OBSTRUCTIONS

Catheter-delivered, balloon-expandable, intravascular stents provide a definitive correction of most vascular stenoses. The implanted stents support the lesions permanently at the diameter of the implanted stents. After very favorable results were achieved in an animal trial of the use of stents in pulmonary arteries and systemic veins, in 1989 the use of intravascular stents in these same lesions was begun in an FDA Investigational Device Exemption (IDE) clinical trial in patients with congenital heart disease. The results in humans were even more favorable and led to the eventual acceptance of stents as the standard of care for most obstructive vascular lesions in congenital heart patients, although no stent is "approved" by the FDA for congenital use.

No matter how small the patient is at the time of implant, when an intravascular stent is implanted in a congenital heart patient, the stent must be capable of dilation to the eventual adult diameter of that particular vessel in order not to create a future stenosis. The vascular stents are mounted on a dilation balloon of the precise diameter of the "normal" vessel adjacent to the area to be stented at the time of the implant. The balloon/stent combination is delivered to the area of stenosis over an exchange wire and through a very long, relatively large diameter sheath. The sheath is withdrawn from the stent/balloon combination, and the balloon is inflated, which expands the stent within the stenosed vessel. The balloon then is deflated, leaving the expanded stent in place and supporting the vessel at the full open dimension of the stent.

In a single-center series at Texas Children's Hospital (TCH), Houston, Texas, intravascular stents were used successfully in more than 700 patients and in more than 1,000 vessels, with continued extremely favorable results. The results after follow-up for 4 years were reported for the first 215 of these patients in the IDE protocol study. Particularly, when the extremely severe underlying disease in the patients being treated in that series are considered, relatively minimal complications occurred. In the entire experience at TCH, five deaths occurred, all of which were related more to the underlying disease than to the stent implant. With as long as 14 years follow-up, when a stent is implanted ideally within the vessel, no recurrence of the stenosis or significant endothelial proliferation occurred within the stents in the pulmonary arteries, systemic veins, or the aorta. Stents were tried in pulmonary vein stenosis, but, like dilation of pulmonary veins, they failed almost universally in this location. Intravascular stents are ideal for the primary and definitive therapy of congenital and/or acquired pulmonary branch stenoses, systemic venous stenosis, and systemic arterial stenoses, including all forms of coarctation. Intravascular stents currently are approved for use in humans and, although not specifically approved by the FDA for any congenital lesions or any pediatric patient, intravascular stents now represent the standard of care throughout the world in the treatment for most vascular stenoses in congenital heart disease.

PERFORATIONS/ RECANALIZATIONS

Occasionally, valvular atresia or total occlusions of vessels are encountered in the congenital heart patient. Attempts at perforating atretic pulmonary valves and long segment vascular occlusions with various stiff wires and/or even transseptal needles were attempted in the past and still are used occasionally. Now, preferentially, a controlled, radio frequency (RF) energy is delivered to the tip of a special wire to accomplish a more controlled and safer perforation of the atretic pulmonary valves and some selected vascular occlusions. The tip of a small catheter is positioned against the atretic valve or the obstructed area of a vessel. The RF wire is passed through the catheter until it is firmly against the obstructing tissues. The controlled RF energy is delivered until the RF wire advances through the atretic/obstructed tissue into the lumen distal to the obstruction. A very small balloon is passed over the wire, and the lesion is dilated sequentially with larger and larger balloons. In vascular obstructions, the opened vessel is maintained open with the implant of an intravascular stent.

OCCLUSION/CLOSURE PROCEDURES

Cardiologists have attempted closing existing abnormal openings, communications, and/or vessels by catheter techniques for as long as the procedures have existed for opening structures in the catheterization laboratory. However, the development and miniaturization of closure devices and the technical problems of delivering and implanting these devices were more difficult to overcome. The first clinically successful occlusion technique for a congenital lesion was a device and technique used for the closure of patent ductus developed by Dr. Werner Portsmann in 1967. His technique was complex, required a large delivery catheter, and used a combined arterial and venous approach. As a consequence, it never was applicable to infants and small children, it never gained widespread popularity, and, although the technique is still in use in a few centers, it is useful for only larger patients. King and Mills developed and used a unique double umbrella device and delivery technique for the closure of atrial defects in 1974. It was successful in several patients, but, again, the technique required a large delivery system and, in turn, it never achieved popularity or any continued use.

Dr. Rashkind, while still perfecting the balloon septostomy technique, also developed several umbrella-type devices and techniques for closing intracardiac defects. The first clinical use of one of these devices was reported in 1979, with the successful closure of a patent ductus in a 3.5-kg infant. His device and procedure demonstrated that miniaturization of a catheter-delivered intracardiac device was possible. Although his original device had significant inherent problems, it led to development of modifications, which resulted in the Rashkind Double Umbrella Patent Ductus Arteriosus (PDA) Occluding Device. The Rashkind PDA device was a miniature, double umbrella with a stainless steel frame and polyurethane foam disks. The two umbrella components of the device folded away from each other so that when positioned in the ductus, one umbrella was positioned on the aortic end of the ductus and the opposing umbrella was on the pulmonary side. A central spring mechanism held the two umbrellas together in the open position and in place in the ductus. The umbrellas were delivered from the venous or the arterial route through a very long, relatively large sheath.

The device was tested in a controlled FDA IDE clinical trial in the United States for 11 years. The trial demonstrated it to be very safe and relatively effective for the closure of ductus in older infants, children, and adults. It received approval from the Medical Device Panel of the FDA in February 1989; however, after 6 more years, the Rashkind PDA device never made it through the paper process to be released for clinical use in the United States and was abandoned permanently for introduction into the U.S. market by the manufacturer. The device was approved in almost all countries outside of the United States and had extensive and successful use in more than 8,000 patients. The Rashkind PDA device did have 10% to 15% persistent leaks after successful implant. Although the leaks usually did not create an immediate problem and could be corrected with a second device, because of this problem and the lack of the U.S. market, the Rashkind device was abandoned by the manufacturer and no longer is available anywhere. However, the widespread and very successful use of the Rashkind PDA device and then its sudden withdrawal from availability led to an almost frantic proliferation in the development of new techniques and "devices" for use in the catheterization laboratory for closing the patent ductus.

Other catheter techniques, devices, and combinations of devices already in use and approved to occlude abnormal vascular communications included persistent systemic-to-pulmonary collateral vessels to the lungs, arterial-to-venous shunts, pulmonary arteriovenous fistulas, and some surgically created systemic-to-pulmonary shunts. The device of this type most commonly used is the Gianturco coil, which has been in use for closure of abnormal vascular communications for several decades. It is a small coil of a spring guidewire with fine fabric threads embedded within the coils of the wire. The coil is delivered through a catheter as a short, straight segment of spring wire, which, as it is extruded out of the delivery catheter, coils to its predetermined size in the vessel at the site of the vessel to be occluded. As thrombus forms within the coil, the abnormal vessel is occluded. These catheter-delivered embolization devices are the standard accepted treatment for most aortopulmonary or arteriovenous lesions.

The frustration from the combination of finally being able to successfully and safely correct a PDA nonsurgically with a catheter-delivered device and then abruptly having that device withdrawn from any availability led to alternate methods of nonsurgically closing the PDA. The first of these attempts was not with the development of a new device, but rather with the utilization of the existing, approved, Gianturco coil, but for the closure of the PDA. Drs. Moore and Cambier demonstrated that these same coils could be "teetered" on the narrow area of the ductus relatively easily and safely to produce an effective closure, albeit with a relatively high rate of dislodgement and embolization of the coils. Multiple different delivery techniques were developed and still are in use to add control to the release of the coil and to overcome the problem of distal embolization. Outside the United States, the Jackson coil, which is a commercially manufactured screw-type, attach/release mechanism for a Gianturco coil, is in standard use for PDA occlusions. In the United States, attach/release mechanisms are fashioned using a snare, a specially modified catheter, or a small bioptome. One and/or several of these modifications provided a secure and relatively safe means of delivering a Gianturco coil to the ductus to a degree that transcatheter closure of a patent ductus, once again, is accepted as the standard of care in the management of PDA.

While modifications for the delivery of coils to the PDA were being refined, entirely different devices designed for other lesions and/or specifically for PDA occlusion were developed. The most successful of these to date is the Amplatzer PDA Occluder Device, which is a "mesh" or tiny "basket" of fine Nitinol "memory" wires that is shaped to fit specifically within the conical shape of the ductus arteriosus. Each device contains several disks of polyester material to help block blood flow until the PDA thrombosis. Multiple sizes of the Amplatzer PDA device are available to fit the different-sized ductus, although even the very smallest Amplatzer device is not applicable for the very small and/or very short PDA. The "basket" is stretched into a long, thin strand for delivery and, like most of the occlusion devices, is delivered through a long sheath to the lesion. Almost 100% occlusion occurs within 24 hours of implant. The Amplatzer PDA device is the only device that has FDA approval for occlusion of a PDA and represents the standard accepted care for the moderate- to large-sized PDA.

PDA was not the only congenital defect considered for nonsurgical closure. There have been rapid and exciting developments of devices and techniques specifically for the closure of atrial septal defects (ASDs). King and Mills introduced the concept in 1976. This was followed in 1981 by the Rashkind ASD Device, which had a slightly smaller delivery system and a single umbrella, which attached to the septum by tiny hooks at the distal ends of the arms of the umbrella. The hooks created problems during delivery and resulted in a very limited use of the device. The larger double umbrella (Rashkind PDA) device was used for the closure of small atrial septal defects, and that success led to the development of an even larger double umbrella device for the larger atrial septal defects. Problems with apposition against the atrial septum with the Rashkind devices led to the addition of hinges to each leg of the device, known as the Clamshell ASD device. The Clamshell device entered a multicenter FDA IDE clinical trial in 1989. Very satisfactory results were achieved in selected small- to moderate-sized ASDs with minimal complications related to the device; however, incidental fractures of the legs of the device were noted. Although no clinical sequelae developed from the fractures, the device was withdrawn totally from use, redesigned, and reintroduced as the CardioSEAL ASD device.

The CardioSEAL is similar in design except that it has an additional hinge on each leg and is manufactured from a more flexible alloy. The CardioSEAL device was effective for the smaller sized ASD but had no "centering" mechanism, so it could not be used in defects over 20 mm in diameter. Fine Nitinol coil spring wire centering wires were added as part of the STARFlex ASD device but still did not allow the use of this device in the larger ASD. While Clamshell was being modified into the CardioSEAL and then the STARFlex device, multiple other atrial septal defect occluders were developed and introduced into clinical trials throughout the United States and Europe. These devices included the Button, the ASDOS, the Angel Wings, the Helix, and the Amplatzer ASD devices.

The most exciting and successful of all of the ASD occlusion devices is the Amplatzer ASD Occluder. The Amplatzer ASD Occluder was the predecessor of the Amplatzer PDA Occluder and, like the PDA device, is a "basket" or mesh of fine Nitinol "memory" wires with several polyester disks incorporated within the "baskets." In its "relaxed" state at room (and body) temperature, the ASD devices form into double, flat, opposing disks with a large diameter, but a short, connecting waist, or hub. The diameter of the *waist* represents the size of the device. Unlike all of the other ASD devices, the Amplatzer ASD occluder relies on the central hub of the device stretching into the circumference of the atrial defect for fixation and for most of the "occlusion" of the defect. The Amplatzer ASD devices are available and capable of occluding atrial defects from 4 to 38 mm in stretched diameter. Like the Amplatzer PDA and other devices, the ASD device stretches into a long, thin strand for delivery to the ASD through a relatively long sheath with a small diameter. The Amplatzer ASD Occluder had very successful extensive use in Europe and in one equally successful U.S. FDA IDE trial. It is the first device approved by the FDA for permanent implant specifically for a congenital and/or a pediatric patient and now represents the accepted standard treatment for most secundum atrial septal defects.

As occurred with the PDA devices, additional uses for the ASD devices became apparent and, either in their existing form or with modifications, proved superior to the surgical occlusion techniques for those additional defects. The CardioSEAL ASD device and a specially modified Amplatzer Muscular VSD device are available and approved for the closure of muscular interventricular septal defects. The CardioSEAL ASD device and a special Amplatzer PFO (patent foramen ovale) device have FDA humanitarian use approval for the closure of a PFO in patients who have had cerebral vascular accidents and for the closure of fenestrations purposefully left in the baffle during caval pulmonary (i.e., Fontan) repairs of complex congenital heart defects. All of these uses of the various occlusion devices are effective, are safer, and result in less morbidity than does the alternative surgical approach, and they now are used routinely in the cardiac catheterization laboratory.

A unique, eccentric, Amplatzer VSD (ventricular septal defect) device presently is in use in Europe and in an FDA IDE clinical trial in the United States for closure of the more common perimembranous VSD. Hopefully, with its continued successful usage and with the Amplatzer ASD, PFO, PDA, and muscular VSD devices as "predicate devices," this VSD device will be available for use in the United States for the far more common perimembranous VSD by the time of this publication.

CONCLUSION

Therapeutic procedures, which can be accomplished by a catheterization technique rather than by a surgical procedure, have numerous advantages for the pediatric and congenital heart patients as well as for society. The most obvious advantage is the elimination of the physical pain and discomfort of the surgical procedure. The recovery from the catheterization procedure and return to full activity is 1 to 2 days, compared to a 1-week hospitalization plus 6 or more weeks of convalescence to recover from a thoracic surgical procedure. The actual risk of the therapeutic catheterization procedure is far less than the risk of the surgical procedure, which includes the thoracotomy, the associated deeper anesthesia, intubation, respiratory support, cardiopulmonary bypass, chest tube(s), blood transfusion, and greater risk of development of wound and/or systemic infections. Although the catheterization devices and procedures themselves are expensive, significant financial savings are realized from the therapeutic catheterization procedure compared to a surgical procedure for the same defect when the expenses of the surgical procedure, the required anesthesia, recovery room/intensive care time, the longer duration of hospitalization, and much longer convalescence are calculated.

In 2006, the standard of care for the treatment of the PDA, the secundum ASD, muscular VSDs, and miscellaneous intracavitary/intravascular communications; stenosis of systemic veins and pulmonary and systemic arteries; and stenosis of the pulmonary valve and some aortic and mitral valves primarily is in the cardiac catheterization laboratory. Additional defects are being and will be added to this list of lesions, which will be treated in the catheterization laboratory in the ensuing years.

Suggested Readings

Abele JE. Balloon catheters and transluminal dilatation: technical considerations. *AJR* 1980;135:901.

Allen HD, Mullins CE. Results of the Valvuloplasty and Angioplasty of Congenital Anomalies Registry. *Am J Cardiol* 1990;65:772.

Cambier PA, Kirby WC, Moore JW, et al. Percutaneous closure of the small (<2.5 mm) patent ductus arteriosus using coil embolization. *Am J Cardiol* 1992;69:815.

Chuang VP, Wallace S, Gianturco C. A new improved coil for tapered tip catheter for arterial occlusion. *Radiology* 1980;135:507.

Grifka RG, O'Laughlin MP, Nihill MR, et al. Double transseptal, double balloon valvuloplasty for congenital mitral stenosis. *Circulation* 1992;85:123.

Gruntzig A. Die perkutane Rekanalisation chronischen arterieller Verschlusse (Dotter-Prinzip) mit einem neuen doppellumigen Dilations kateter. *Fortschr Rontgenstr* 1976;124:80.

Hellenbrand WE, Allen HD, Golinko RJ, et al. Balloon angioplasty for aortic recoarctation: results of the Valvuloplasty and Angioplasty of Congenital Anomalies Registry. *Am J Cardiol* 1990;65:793.

Hijazi ZM, Hakim F, Haweleh AA, et al. Catheter closure of perimembranous ventricular septal defects using the new Amplatzer membranous VSD occluder: initial clinical experience. *Catheter Cardiovasc Interv* 2002;56:508.

Justo RN, Nykanen DG, Williams WC, et al. Transcatheter perforation of the right ventricular outflow tract as initial therapy for pulmonary valve atresia and intact ventricular septum in the newborn. *Catheter Cardiovasc Diagn* 1997;40:408.

Kan JS, White RI Jr, Mitchell SE, et al. Percutaneous balloon valvuloplasty: a new method for treating congenital pulmonary valve stenosis. *N Engl J Med* 1982;307:540.

Kan JS, White RI Jr, Mitchell SE, et al. Treatment of restenosis of coarctation by percutaneous transluminal angioplasty. *Circulation* 1983;68:1087.

King TD, Mills NL. Nonoperative closure of atrial septal defects. *Surgery* 1974;75:383.

Labadidi Z, Wu RJ, Walls TJ. Percutaneous balloon aortic valvuloplasty: results in 23 patients. *Am J Cardiol* 1984;53:194.

Lock JE, Bass JL, Amplatz K. Balloon dilatation angioplasty of aortic coarctation in infants and children. *Circulation* 1983;68:109.

Lock JE, Bass JL, Castaneda-Zuniga W, et al. Dilation angioplasty of congenital or operative narrowings of venous channels. *Circulation* 1984;709:457.

Lock JE, Castaneda-Zuniga WR, Fuhrman BP. Balloon dilation angioplasty of hypoplastic and stenotic pulmonary arteries. *Circulation* 1983;67:962.

Lock JE, Cockerham J, Keane J, et al. Transcatheter umbrella closure of congenital heart defects. *Circulation* 1987;75:593.

Lock JE, Khalilullah M, Shrivastava S, et al. Percutaneous catheter commissurotomy in rheumatic mitral stenosis. *N Engl J Med* 1985;313:1515.

Lock JE, Rome JJ, Davis R. Transcatheter closure of atrial septal defects: experimental studies. *Circulation* 1989;79:1091.

Mansura J, Gavora P, Formanek A, et al. Transcatheter closure of secundum atrial septal defects using the new self-centering Amplatzer septal occluder; initial human experience. *Catheter Cardiovasc Diagn* 1997;42:388.

Mansura J, Walsh KP, Thanopoulos BV, et al. Catheter closure of moderate to large-sized patent ductus arteriosus using the new Amplatzer Duct Occluder: immediate and short term results. *J Am Coll Cardiol* 1998;31:878.

Marvin WJ, Mahoney LT, Rose EF. Pathologic sequelae of balloon dilation angioplasty for unoperated coarctation of the aorta in infants and children. *J Am Coll Cardiol* 1986;7:117A.

Mullins CE, Latson LA, Neches WH. Balloon dilation of miscellaneous lesions: results of the Valvuloplasty and Angioplasty of Congenital Anomalies Registry. *Am J Cardiol* 1990;65:802.

Mullins CE, Nihill MR, Vick GW III, et al. Double balloon technique for dilation of valvular or vessel stenosis in congenital and acquired heart disease. *J Am Coll Cardiol* 1987;10:107.

Mullins CE, O'Laughlin MP, Vick III GW, et al. Implantation of balloon expandable intravascular grafts by catheterization in pulmonary arteries and systemic veins. *Circulation* 1988;77:188.

O'Laughlin MP, Perry SB, Lock JE, et al. Use of endovascular stents in congenital heart disease. *Circulation* 1991;83:1923.

Palmaz JC, Windeler SA, Garcia F, et al. Atherosclerotic rabbit aortas: expandable intraluminal grafting. *Radiology* 1986;160:723.

Park SC, Neches WH, Mullins CE, et al. Blade atrial septostomy: collaborative study. *Circulation* 1982;66:258.

Park SC, Zuberbuhler JR, Neches WH, et al. A new atrial septostomy technique. *Catheter Cardiovasc Diagn* 1975;1:195.

Portsmann W, Wierny L, Warnke H. Der Verschluss des D.a.p. ohne Thorakotomie (1 Mitteilung). *Thoraxchirurgie* 1967;15:199.

Rashkind WJ, Cuaso CC. Transcatheter closure of atrial septal defects in children. *Proc Assoc Eur Pediatr Cardiol* 1977;13:49.

Rashkind WJ, Cuaso CC. Transcatheter closure of patent ductus arteriosus: successful use in a 3.5 kilogram infant. *Pediatr Cardiol* 1979;1:3.

Rashkind WJ, Miller WW. Creation of an atrial septal defect without thoracotomy: a palliative approach thoracotomy: palliative approach to complete transposition of the great arteries. *JAMA* 1966;196:991.

Rashkind WJ, Mullins CE, Hellenbrand WE, et al. Nonsurgical closure of patent ductus arteriosus: clinical application of the Rashkind PDA Occluder system. *Circulation* 1987;75:583.

Ring JC, Bass JL, Marvin W, et al. Management of congenital branch pulmonary artery stenosis with balloon dilation angioplasty: report of 52 procedures. *J Thorac Cardiovasc Surg* 1985;90:35.

Rocchini AP, Beekman RH, Shachar GB, et al. Balloon aortic valvuloplasty: results of the Valvuloplasty and Angioplasty of Congenital Anomalies Registry. *Am J Cardiol* 1990;65:784.

Rosenthal E, Qureshi SA, Chan KC, et al. Radiofrequency-assisted balloon dilation in patients with pulmonary valve atresia and an intact ventricular septum. *Br Heart J* 1993;69:347.

Sharafuddin MJA, Gu X, Titus J, et al. Transvenous closure of secundum atrial septal defects: preliminary results with a new self-expanding nitinol prosthesis in a swine model. *Circulation* 1997;95:2162.

Stanger P, Cassidy SC, Girod DA. Balloon pulmonary valvuloplasty: results of the Valvuloplasty and Angioplasty of Congenital Anomalies Registry. *Am J Cardiol* 1990;65:775.

Tynan M, Finley JP, Fontes V, et al. Balloon angioplasty for the treatment of native coarctation: results of the Valvuloplasty and Angioplasty of Congenital Anomalies Registry. *Am J Cardiol* 1990;65:790.

Waldman JD, Waldman J, Jones MH, et al. Failure of balloon dilation in mid-cavity obstruction of the systemic venous atrium after Mustard operation. *Pediatr Cardiol* 1983;4:151.

Zaibag AM, Kasab AS, Ribeiro AP, et al. Percutaneous double-balloon mitral valvotomy for rheumatic mitral valve stenosis. *Lancet* 1986:756.

SECTION IV ■ DISEASES OF THE BLOOD

CHAPTER 289 ■ NUTRITIONAL ANEMIAS

PAUL L. MARTIN

The important nutritional anemias result from dietary deficiencies of iron, folic acid, or vitamin B_{12}. Deficiencies of other nutrients such as vitamins B_6 and E may be associated with anemia, but they are unusual in pediatric practice (Table 289.1).

IRON DEFICIENCY ANEMIA

Iron deficiency anemia is defined as anemia caused by inadequate availability of iron to sustain bone marrow erythropoiesis. Anemia caused by iron deficiency is the most common hematologic disease of infancy and childhood. The body of the newborn infant contains 0.3 to 0.5 g of iron; the body of an adult contains up to 5 g. To make up the 4.5-g difference, an average net increase of 0.5 mg of iron must be absorbed each day during the first 15 years of life. In addition to this requirement for growth, a small amount of iron is necessary to balance normal losses, estimated at 0.5 to 1 mg/day. To maintain a positive iron balance during childhood, 0.8 to 1.5 mg of iron must be absorbed each day from the diet. Because less than 10% of dietary iron is absorbed from the average mixed diet, 8 to 15 mg of iron daily is necessary for optimal nutrition. During the first years of life, when relatively small quantities of iron-rich food are ingested, it is difficult to attain these amounts. An infant's diet should include iron-fortified foods, such as cereals or iron-supplemented formulas, by 6 months of age.

Pathophysiology

Most of a newborn's iron is contained in the circulating hemoglobin. As the high hemoglobin concentration of the newborn decreases during the first 2 to 3 months of life, iron is reclaimed and stored. These stores are usually sufficient for the first 6 to 9 months of life. In low-birth-weight infants or in those with perinatal blood loss, the transplacental iron may be depleted earlier.

Although abundant, iron's relative insolubility makes its bioavailability extremely low. Most environmental iron exists as insoluble salts. Gastric acidity assists conversion to absorbable forms, but the efficiency of this process is limited. Any medication that affects the gastric pH, such as histamine$_2$ blockers and acid pump blockers, impedes this process, and impaired iron absorption can result. Heme is the most readily absorbed form of iron. Uptake occurs independently of gastric pH. Heme iron is derived primarily from animal tissue. The relative absence of meat from much of the world's diet is one of the leading causes of iron deficiency anemia.

Other environmental factors that share iron's absorption machinery can cause iron deficiency anemia. Metals that interfere with the gastrointestinal absorption of iron include lead, cobalt, and strontium. Of these, only lead is a significant problem. Iron deficiency increases the rate of uptake of both iron and lead from the gastrointestinal tract.

TABLE 289.1

NUTRITIONAL ANEMIAS

Deficiency	Prevalence	Associated Laboratory Findings	Treatment
Iron	Common	Low reticulocyte count Low MCV Low serum ferritin Low iron/total iron-binding capacity	Replace iron PO, or IM 6 mg/kg of elemental iron
Folic acid	Uncommon	Low reticulocyte count Elevated MCV Low serum folate levels Normal serum vitamin B_{12} levels	Replace folic acid
Vitamin B_{12}	Uncommon	Low reticulocyte count Elevated MCV Low serum vitamin B_{12} levels Normal serum folate levels	Replace B_{12} PO or IM depending on results from Schilling test

MCV, mean corpuscular volume.

Blood loss is the world's leading cause of iron deficiency anemia. Blood loss caused by gastrointestinal lesions commonly causes iron deficiency. The most frequent congenital defect in the gastrointestinal tract is Meckel diverticulum. Other causes of occult gastrointestinal bleeding include peptic ulcer disease, polyps, or hemangiomas. Arteriovenous malformations involving the superficial blood vessels along the gastrointestinal tract occur with hereditary hemorrhagic telangiectasia. Whole cow's milk contains proteins that may irritate the lining of the gastrointestinal tract in infants. Although cow's milk contains iron at approximately the same concentration as does human milk, the bioavailability of iron in human milk is much greater.

The world's leading cause of gastrointestinal blood loss is parasitic infestation. Hookworm infection, caused primarily by *Necator americanus* or *Ancylostoma duodenale*, is endemic to much of the world and is often asymptomatic. Microscopic blood loss leads to iron deficiency in more than 1 billion people. Once prevalent in the southeastern United States, hookworm infection has declined with better sanitation and the routine wearing of footwear when outside.

Clinical Manifestations

Anemia solely caused by inadequate dietary iron is unusual during the first 4 to 6 months of life, but it becomes more common from 9 to 24 months of age. The usual dietary pattern of infants with iron deficiency anemia is the consumption of large amounts of milk and carbohydrates not supplemented with iron. Pallor is the most frequent sign of iron deficiency anemia. In mild to moderate deficiency (i.e., hemoglobin level of 7 to 10 g/dL), few symptoms of anemia are seen. As the anemia progresses, tachycardia, cardiac dilation, and systolic murmurs occur. The spleen is palpable in 10% to 15% of patients. The child with iron deficiency anemia may be obese or overweight. Often other evidence of undernutrition is present.

Some children with iron deficiency anemia have pica. Iron deficiency anemia and even iron deficiency without significant anemia may adversely affect the attention span, behavior, and performance of affected children.

Laboratory Findings

Because iron is essential for hemoglobin synthesis, erythrocyte production is among the first casualties of iron deficiency. *Prelatent* iron deficiency occurs when stores are depleted without a change in hemoglobin or serum iron levels. This stage is rarely detected. *Latent* iron deficiency occurs when the serum iron level decreases and the total iron-binding capacity increases without a change in the hemoglobin. The level of serum ferritin provides a biochemical estimate of body iron stores. Serum ferritin levels in the range of 10 to 20 ng/mL indicate depletion of iron stores; levels of less than 10 ng/mL are diagnostic of iron deficiency. *Frank* iron deficiency anemia is associated with serum iron levels of less than 30 ng/dL, an increased serum iron-binding capacity, and a resulting serum transferrin saturation of less than 15%. As iron deficiency progresses, the erythrocytes become smaller than normal, with decreased hemoglobin content (microcytic and hypochromic) and abnormal shapes (poikilocytosis). The mean corpuscular volume (MCV) decreases to less than normal for age. The reticulocyte count is normal or minimally elevated, and the leukocyte counts are normal. Elevated platelet counts (greater than $600,000/\mu L$) often are seen, although occasionally thrombocytopenia may be present.

Iron deficiency must be differentiated from other hypochromic, microcytic anemias (Fig. 289.1). In lead poisoning, the erythrocytes are morphologically similar, but coarse basophilic

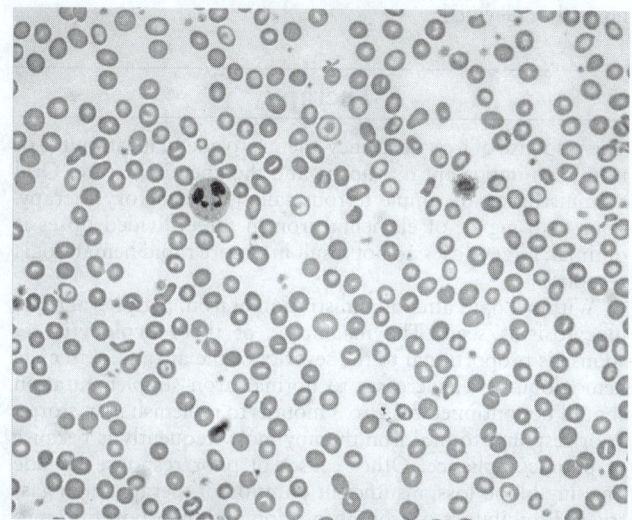

FIGURE 289.1. Microcytosis. Note both the small size of these red cells as well as the increased central pallor of the cells (hypochromia). This is consistent with iron deficiency anemia, although other causes are possible, especially if a trial of iron fails to improve the anemia. (Courtesy of Susan J. Neblett, M.T., Beverly Williams, M.T., and Donald Beam, M.D.)

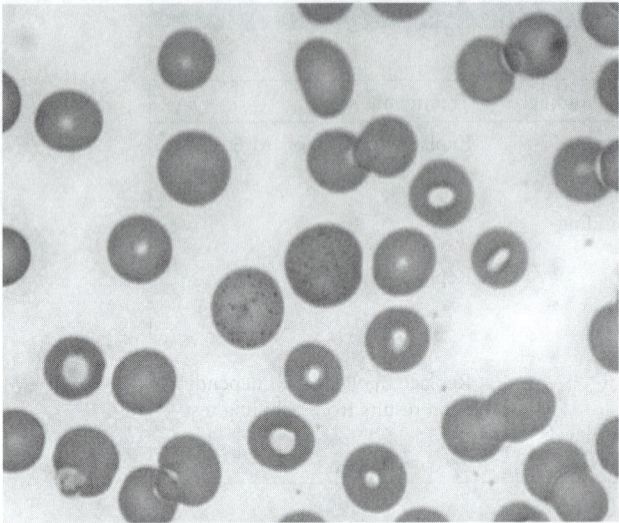

FIGURE 289.2. Basophilic stippling. Note the small, fine dark granules in several of the red cells present in this photomicrograph. These granules represent aggregates of ribosomes in an active young red cell. They can be seen in iron deficiency, lead poisoning, red cell enzyme deficiencies, thalassemia, and many other causes of significant anemia. (Courtesy of Susan J. Neblett, M.T., Beverly Williams, M.T., and Donald Beam, M.D.)

stippling is prominent (Fig. 289.2). Evaluation reveals elevations of blood lead and marked elevation of free erythrocyte protoporphyrins. As described previously, many children with lead poisoning have concomitant iron deficiency anemia. Thalassemia trait (alpha- or beta-thalassemia) is sometimes confused with iron deficiency anemia. Alpha-thalassemia trait occurs in approximately 3% of blacks and in many people of Southeast Asian origin. Beta-thalassemia major with its organomegaly, erythroblastosis, and hemolytic component is usually clinically apparent. Beta-thalassemia trait is common in individuals of Mediterranean descent. The erythrocyte morphology of chronic inflammatory or infectious conditions may be microcytic. In these conditions, the serum iron and iron-binding capacity is reduced, and the serum ferritin levels are normal or elevated.

Therapy

The response of iron deficiency anemia to adequate amounts of iron is an important diagnostic and therapeutic feature. Oral administration of simple ferrous salts is satisfactory therapy. Four to 6 mg/kg of elemental iron in three divided doses is optimal; larger doses do not result in a more rapid hematologic response.

Within 4 days after administration of iron, peripheral reticulocytosis is seen. The magnitude of the reticulocytic response is proportional to the severity of the anemia. After the hemoglobin level increases to normal, iron supplementation should be continued for 2 to 3 months to replenish iron stores. Poor response to oral iron therapy most frequently is because of poor compliance. Other causes of poor response include ongoing blood loss, insufficient duration of therapy, high gastric pH, inhibitors of iron absorption and incorporation into hemoglobin (e.g., plumbism, chronic inflammation, or neoplasia), or an incorrect diagnosis. A simple test may differentiate poor compliance from these rarer causes of iron malabsorption. In an iron-deficient patient, if iron is being absorbed, 2 to 4 mg/kg of iron administered orally will cause a sharp increase in serum iron levels after only 30 minutes.

Parenteral iron replacement is indicated when oral iron is poorly tolerated, rapid replacement of iron stores is needed, or gastrointestinal iron absorption is compromised. Iron dextran, in which iron is bound to a high-molecular-weight complex for stabilization, can be administered by intramuscular or intravenous injection.

Because a rapid hematologic response can be predicted confidently in typical iron deficiency anemia, blood transfusion is indicated only when the anemia is severe or if infection may interfere with response. Packed red blood cells should be administered to increase the hemoglobin to only approximately 7 g/dL, rather than attempting complete correction of the anemia. Often, it is advisable to split the packed red blood cell transfusion into two aliquots, with a dose of diuretic between the administration of each aliquot to avoid fluid overload in the patient. In patients with frank congestive heart failure, exchange transfusion with packed red blood cells may be indicated.

RARE HYPOCHROMIC MICROCYTIC ANEMIAS

More unusual cases of hypochromic, microcytic anemia with other abnormalities of iron absorption and metabolism have been described. Some patients have had defects in iron mobilization or reuse. Siblings have been described with iron deficiency anemia without evidence of reduced iron intake or gastrointestinal blood loss who failed to respond to oral iron therapy and who had a partial but incomplete response to parenteral iron dextran. No evidence suggested other well-defined causes of hypochromic, microcytic anemia or a generalized disorder of intestinal absorption (Buchanan syndrome). Congenital absence of the iron-binding protein (i.e., atransferrinemia) is associated with severe hypochromic anemia, which requires lifelong transfusions. Iron is absorbed normally but is deposited in the visceral organs rather than in the bone marrow. Several patients have had refractory hypochromic anemia associated with massive lymphatic tumors or lymphoid hyperplasia (Castleman disease). Correction of the anemia follows removal of the lymphatic tissue in these children.

MEGALOBLASTIC ANEMIAS

The megaloblastic anemias are uncommon disorders characterized by abnormal red blood cell morphology and maturation. In megaloblastic anemia, erythroid precursors have a normal DNA content together with an elevated RNA content. For this reason, they have more cellular RNA per unit of DNA and thus have nuclear to cytoplasmic dissociation. These anemias are usually caused by deficiencies of folate or, more rarely, vitamin B_{12} (Fig. 289.3).

Folic Acid Deficiency

Because folic acid is absorbed throughout the small intestine, diffuse inflammatory or degenerative disease of the intestine may impair folate's absorption. Both tropical and nontropical sprue, chronic infectious enteritis, or enteroenteric fistulas may lead to folic acid deficiency. Many patients have low serum levels of folic acid during therapy with anticonvulsant drugs because malabsorption of folic acid appears to be induced by these drugs. Drugs such as methotrexate prevent the use of folic acid by inhibiting reduction to its active coenzymatic forms. Megaloblastic anemia can be seen in some adolescent girls and women taking oral contraceptives. Deficiency of folate also

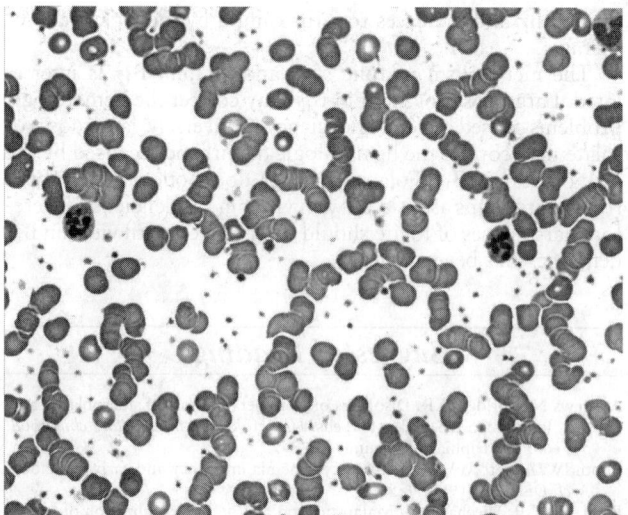

FIGURE 289.3. Hypersegmentation of polymorphonuclear neutrophils. Presence of both large red cells (macrocytosis) and increased numbers of hypersegmentation of neutrophils (more than five lobes) is consistent with macrocytic anemia, most commonly caused by vitamin B$_{12}$ or folate deficiency. (Courtesy of Susan J. Neblett, M.T., Beverly Williams, M.T., and Donald Beam, M.D.)

can occur for the following reasons: defects of absorption (inherited defects of absorption, infiltrative diseases of the small bowel), inadequate nutrition (insufficient diet, maternal deficiency affecting the fetus and breast-fed infant), and inherited defects in folate metabolism (methylenetetrahydrofolate reductase deficiency and methionine synthase deficiency) and folate transfer.

A rare megaloblastic anemia of infancy is caused by a deficient intake or malabsorption of folic acid often aggravated by infection. Goat's milk and powdered cow's milk are poor sources of folic acid. The presence of an allergy to cow's milk also can cause malabsorption of folic acid. Vitamin C deficiency impairs folic acid absorption. This megaloblastic anemia has a peak incidence at 4 to 7 months of age. In addition to being pale, these children are irritable, fail to gain weight, and often have chronic diarrhea.

Vitamin B$_{12}$ Deficiency

To be absorbed, dietary vitamin B$_{12}$ must combine with intrinsic factor that is secreted by the parietal cells of the gastric fundus. The vitamin B$_{12}$–intrinsic factor complex passes to the terminal ileum, where specific absorptive receptors exist. Vitamin B$_{12}$ deficiency can result from inadequate dietary intake, lack of secretion of intrinsic factor, disruption of the vitamin B$_{12}$–intrinsic factor complex, or abnormalities or absence of the receptor sites in the terminal ileum. Vitamin B$_{12}$ deficiency also can be caused by a variety of other factors, including defects in absorption, gastritis, total gastrectomy, intrinsic factor gene mutations, diseases of the small intestine, surgical resection or bypass of the terminal ileum, Crohn disease, competition by parasites, or transcobalamin II deficiency. In children with transcobalamin II deficiency, cobalamin is malabsorbed, leading to severe megaloblastic anemia that occurs within the first few months of life.

Vitamin B$_{12}$ is present in many foods. Pure dietary deficiency is rare. Deficiency may be seen in children eating diets containing no milk, eggs, or animal products (i.e., vegans). It is reported also in breast-fed infants whose mothers are deficient

in vitamin B$_{12}$ because of a vegan diet or pernicious anemia. Because the vitamin occurs in so many foods, most cases of vitamin B$_{12}$ deficiency are a consequence of a failure to absorb the vitamin.

Juvenile Pernicious Anemia

Juvenile pernicious anemia is a rare disease caused by a genetically determined inability to secrete intrinsic factor. Unlike adult cases of anemia, patients with juvenile pernicious anemia have normal stomach acidity and histology. Consanguinity often is found in parents of affected children, a finding suggesting a recessive inheritance pattern.

Symptoms develop at 1 to 5 years of age, a time consistent with exhaustion of the vitamin B$_{12}$ stores acquired transplacentally from the mother. Progressive irritability, anorexia, and listlessness occur. The tongue is smooth and red. Neurologic manifestations include ataxia, hyporeflexia, and Babinski responses.

The anemia is macrocytic (MCV greater than 95 fL), with prominent macroovalocytosis. The neutrophils are hypersegmented. Neutropenia and thrombocytopenia may develop. Serum vitamin B$_{12}$ levels are reduced. Serum lactate dehydrogenase activity is increased markedly. Large amounts of methylmalonic acid are excreted in the urine. Unlike in pernicious anemia in adults, serum antibodies against parietal cells or intrinsic factor cannot be detected in these children. The gastric mucosa is histologically normal, but intrinsic factor is absent in the gastric secretions. Vitamin B$_{12}$ malabsorption is indicated by an abnormal Schilling test result and is corrected by exogenous intrinsic factor.

A prompt hematologic response follows parenteral administration of vitamin B$_{12}$. If evidence of neurologic involvement is found, 1 mg should be given intramuscularly daily for several weeks. Maintenance therapy consists of monthly intramuscular administration of 1 mg of vitamin B$_{12}$. Oral therapy is ineffective and contraindicated.

Laboratory Findings

Megaloblastic anemia is macrocytic (MCV greater than 95 fL). The reticulocyte count is low, but nucleated red blood cells demonstrating megaloblastic morphology may be seen in the blood. Children with severe disease may have thrombocytopenia and neutropenia. Many of the neutrophils are hypersegmented (Fig. 289.3). In folate deficiency, serum folate levels are usually reduced, but low levels of red cell folate are a better indication of chronic deficiency. Serum lactate dehydrogenase activity is markedly elevated. The bone marrow is hypercellular because of erythroid hyperplasia and shows prominent megaloblastic changes. Large, abnormal neutrophilic forms (giant metamyelocytes) with cytoplasmic vacuolization may be seen.

Therapy

Successful treatment of children with folate deficiency involves correction of the deficiency; improvement of the underlying disorder if possible, improvement of the diet by increasing folate intake, and follow-up evaluation. In cases of suspected folate deficiency, a therapeutic trial can be started with 50 to 100 μg of oral folate/day. This dose produces a prompt response in folate deficiency but has no effect on vitamin B$_{12}$ deficiency. Once the diagnosis is proved, it is usual to treat patients with up to 1 mg of folate/day. In most patients, 7 to 14 days of oral treatment induces a maximal hematologic response and significant replenishment of body stores. Within 1 to 2 days, the patient's appetite improves, and a sense of well-being returns. An increase in reticulocytosis is seen in 2 to 4 days that reaches a peak in 4 to 7 days. Hemoglobin levels return to normal in 2 to 6 weeks. The neutropenia and thrombocytopenia improve with the reticulocytosis. The duration of therapy depends on the underlying disorder, but folic acid is given for several months until a new population of red blood cells has been formed.

Children with suspected vitamin B_{12} deficiency are given a therapeutic trial with 25 to 100 μg of vitamin B_{12}. This dose corrects the hematologic problem caused by this vitamin deficiency, but it does not correct the defect in folate-deficient children. The reticulocyte response to this therapy is similar to that noted in folate deficiency. Once the diagnosis is firmly established, daily doses of 25 to 100 μg may be used to initiate therapy. Alternatively, maintenance therapy can be started with monthly intramuscular injections in doses between 200 and 1,000 μg. Patients with defects affecting the intestinal absorption of vitamin B_{12} respond to parenteral vitamin B_{12}, which completely bypasses the defective step in vitamin B_{12} metabolism. Reticulocytosis is seen by the third or fourth day of therapy and increases to a maximum by the eighth day of therapy.

The metabolism of folic acid and vitamin B_{12} is interrelated. Large doses of vitamin B_{12} may correct the hematologic problems caused by folate deficiency. Conversely, large doses of folate may correct the hematologic disturbances caused by the lack of vitamin B_{12}. Folate, however, does not correct the neurologic problems associated with vitamin B_{12} deficiency. Therefore, large doses of folate should not be given until vitamin B_{12} deficiency has been excluded.

Suggested Readings

Andrews NC, Bridges KR. Disorders of iron metabolism and sideroblastic anemia. In: Nathan DB, Orkin SH, eds. *Hematology of infancy and childhood*, 5th ed. Philadelphia: WB Saunders, 1997.

Booth IW, Aukett MA. Iron deficiency anaemia in infancy and early childhood. *Arch Dis Child* 1997;76:549.

Buchanan GR, Sheehan RG. Malabsorption and defective utilization of iron in three siblings. *J Pediatr* 1981;98:723.

Davenport J. Macrocytic anemia. *Am Fam Physician* 1996;53:155.

CHAPTER 290 ■ HEMOGLOBINOPATHIES AND THALASSEMIAS

PAUL L. MARTIN

The genetic, molecular, and biochemical characteristics of human hemoglobin are well known. The genes for the polypeptide chains of hemoglobin are located on chromosomes 11 and 16, and their DNA sequences have been determined. Each of the alpha and beta chains of adult hemoglobin consists of approximately 150 amino acids. The single amino acid substitution in these chains that causes each abnormal hemoglobin syndrome can be identified and located. Although more than 400 types of abnormal human hemoglobins have been characterized, only a few of them are prevalent.

Hemoglobin variants are identified by hemoglobin electrophoresis, a technique that usually permits a specific genotypic diagnosis. The thalassemias are associated with decreased production of the normal polypeptide chains of hemoglobin. The thalassemias are quantitative rather than qualitative abnormalities of hemoglobin.

SICKLE CELL DISEASE AND TRAIT

The gene for sickle cell hemoglobin (Hb S) is not exclusively African, although a broad periequatorial sickle cell belt is found in Africa. The sickle gene was introduced into the Western Hemisphere from Africa by the slave trade during the sixteenth through the eighteenth centuries. In the United States, sickling disorders are particularly prevalent in the South and in the urban North, reflecting the demographics of the African American population. In Latin America, relatively high frequencies are seen in the Caribbean, Panama, Guyana, and Brazil, but not in Mexico and most of South America. A high incidence of sickle genes, apparently resulting from independent mutational events, is found in Italy, Greece, the Middle East, and India.

Pathophysiology

In Hb S, a valine residue is substituted for the usual glutamic acid in the chains of the hemoglobin molecule. When Hb S becomes deoxygenated, polymerization occurs, with the formation of long, crystalline tactoids. These ultimately form elongated, sickled erythrocytes. Sickled erythrocytes have markedly shortened survival, and they can obstruct small blood vessels and can cause distal tissue ischemia and necrosis.

Heterozygosity for a sickle gene has a benign clinical course. Approximately 8% of African Americans have the trait. The sickle gene is thought to confer a degree of resistance to falciparum malaria during infancy in endemic areas. The erythrocytes in sickle trait contain only 30% to 40% Hb S, and sickling does not occur under physiologic conditions. Rarely, hypoxia resulting from shock or from flying at high altitudes in an unpressurized aircraft may produce vasoocclusive phenomena. Unexpected death has also been observed in military recruits during the extreme exertion of basic training. Spontaneous hematuria, usually from the left kidney, and mild hyposthenuria also occur. Anemia or hemolysis should not be attributed to the sickle trait.

In persons homozygous for the sickle gene, sickle cell anemia is a severe, chronic hemolytic anemia. The clinical course is marked by episodes of pain caused by occlusion of small blood vessels by the spontaneously sickled erythrocytes. These events have traditionally been called crises (Table 290.1).

TABLE 290.1

CLINICAL CRISES SEEN IN PATIENTS WITH SICKLE CELL DISEASE

Crisis Designation	Cause	Treatment
Pain crisis	Vaso-occlusion of small vessels, frequently	Hydration, narcotics
Hand-foot syndrome (dactylitis)	Infarcts of small bones in hands, frequently seen in infancy	Hydration, narcotics
Sequestration crisis	Acute trapping of red cells in spleen, causing an abrupt fall in blood volume and red cell mass	Transfusion, often exchange transfusion, oxygen and splenectomy as last resort
Acute chest crisis	Vasoocclusion of pulmonary vessels leading to an often severe pulmonary process	Hydration, oxygen, narcotics, antibiotics, positive-pressure ventilation if necessary
Acute hemolytic crisis	Rapid and unpredictable increase in hemolysis leading to rapid fall in hemoglobin	Transfusion, oxygen, exchange transfusion may be necessary
Aplastic crisis	Infection with parvovirus B19 causing severe reticulocytopenia	Transfusion if necessary

Clinical Manifestations

Manifestations of sickle cell disease usually do not appear until the second 6 months of life, coincident with the postnatal decrease in fetal hemoglobin (Hb F) and an increase in Hb S. The hemolytic process is evident by 6 months of age.

The painful or vasoocclusive crises are the most frequent clinical symptoms. Symmetric, painful swelling of the hands and feet (i.e., hand-foot syndrome) caused by infarction of the small bones of the hands and feet may be the initial manifestation of sickle cell anemia in infancy. Older patients may have painful involvement of the larger bones and joints and severe abdominal pain resembling acute surgical conditions. Strokes may leave permanent paralysis as well as more subtle neurologic damage. Extensive pulmonary consolidation occurs, and it is difficult to differentiate infarction from pneumonia. Vasoocclusive crises usually are not associated with changes in the hematologic picture at baseline.

A second type of crisis, seen only in young infants and children, is called the sequestration crisis. Large amounts of blood become pooled in the abdominal organs. The spleen becomes massively enlarged, and signs of circulatory collapse develop rapidly. If volume replacement is given, much of the sequestered blood is remobilized. The sequestration crisis is an important cause of death in infants with sickle cell disease.

The third well-characterized type of crisis is the aplastic crisis, which results from erythroblast maturation arrest caused by parvovirus B19 infection (see Chapter 192). Parvovirus B19 causes generally a brief, self-limited illness in patients with sickle cell disease. Rarely, it can persist for weeks, but generally it resolves in a few days, although the reticulocytopenia may persist for several weeks in some patients.

In addition to these acute crises, various clinical signs and symptoms result from chronic severe hemolytic anemia and vasoocclusive disease. Impairment of liver function contributes to the jaundice of these patients. Gallstones can occur in children as young as 3 years. Renal function is progressively impaired by diffuse glomerular and tubular fibrosis, resulting in hyposthenuria and polyuria.

As many as 30% of children with sickle cell anemia develop pneumococcal sepsis during the first 5 years of life. The increased risk is a result of functional hyposplenia and low levels of specific serum antibodies. Increased susceptibility to *Salmonella* osteomyelitis is also a feature of sickle cell disease.

By middle childhood, most patients are underweight, and puberty is delayed, particularly in boys. Chronic leg ulcers are common in adolescence and early adult life. The median life span for patients with sickle cell disease ranges from 40 to 60 years. Causes of death include infection, acute chest crisis, and stroke.

Laboratory Findings

Hemoglobin levels range from 5 to 9 g/dL. Peripheral blood smears show irreversibly sickled cells, a finding almost diagnostic of homozygous sickle cell disease (Fig. 290.1). The reticulocyte count ranges from 5% to 15%, and nucleated erythrocytes and Howell-Jolly bodies are usually observed. The total leukocyte count is elevated (12,000 to 20,000/μL), with a predominance of neutrophils. The platelet count is increased, and the sedimentation rate is slow. Other changes include abnormal liver function test results, hyperbilirubinemia, and diffuse hypergammaglobulinemia. The bone marrow shows erythroid hyperplasia.

Diagnostic studies to demonstrate Hb S include the sickle cell preparation and hemoglobin solubility studies. However, hemoglobin electrophoresis is more conclusive and is necessary for a precise diagnosis. After infancy, the erythrocytes of patients with sickle cell anemia contain approximately 90% Hb S, 2% to 10% Hb F, and a normal amount of Hb A$_2$; they do not contain Hb A.

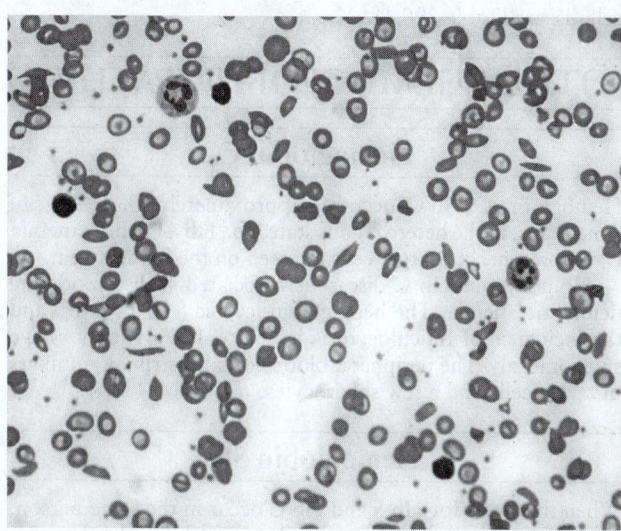

FIGURE 290.1. Photomicrograph of peripheral blood from a patient with sickle cell anemia. Note both the elongated sickle forms and an increased number of target cells and microcytes. (Courtesy of Susan J. Neblett, M.T., Beverly Williams, M.T., and Donald Beam, M.D.)

Therapy

No antisickling pharmacologic agent has proved safe or of consistent value. For mild or moderately painful crises, analgesics are indicated. Parenteral narcotics are often necessary for severe pain. Dehydration and acidosis should be corrected. Bacterial infections require appropriate antibiotic therapy. The risk of sepsis from encapsulated organisms is high enough to justify the use of prophylactic penicillin in all patients with sickle cell disease from 6 months to at least 6 years of age. Immunization with conjugated pneumococcal vaccine as recommended for all infants in the United States should be followed by immunization with pneumococcal polysaccharide vaccine at age 2 and again at age 7 years. The value of prophylaxis after 6 years of age is being studied. Blood transfusions are unnecessary for the usual painful crises but are indicated for prolonged or extreme pain, for extensive involvement of lungs or central nervous system, and as preparation for general anesthesia. When the homozygous patient's circulating Hb S erythrocytes can be diluted to less than 40% by transfusions of normal blood, vasoocclusive symptoms usually abate. Partial exchange transfusion can be done to lower the percentage of erythrocytes rapidly.

Exchange transfusion should be done only in consultation with a pediatric hematologist because volume overload, hyperviscosity, the reason for the exchange, and the initial percentage of Hb S present must all be factored into the amount of blood to be exchanged.

A promising investigational treatment for sickle cell anemia is the use of hydroxyurea to cause "stress" erythropoiesis, which can increase the percentage of Hb F. Use of hydroxyurea in young children appears to have acceptable toxicity, and preliminary results show a decrease in sickle cell crises. Bone marrow transplantation from human leukocyte antigen (HLA)—identical siblings has been performed in a number of children with sickle cell disease. The risk of death from toxicity of the transplant and the risk of chronic graft-versus-host disease appear to be 5% to 10%. Until the toxicity of bone marrow transplantation can be reduced, parents and physicians will face the difficult task of weighing the risk of early death from transplantation with the risk of death from long-term complications of sickle cell disease.

Newborn screening for sickle hemoglobinopathies is mandated in nearly all states. Medical counseling of affected families and initiation of prophylactic penicillin for affected infants have been effective in decreasing early mortality from sickle cell disease (Table 290.1).

OTHER HEMOGLOBINOPATHIES

Hemoglobin C

Hemoglobin C (Hb C) occurs in approximately 2% of African Americans. In the heterozygous state (i.e., Hb AC trait), anemia is not present, but target cells are seen on the blood smear.

Homozygous Hb C disease is associated with a moderate hemolytic anemia. The hemoglobin level is 8 to 11 g/dL, and the incidence of reticulocytosis is 5% to 10%. Patients have splenomegaly. The peripheral blood contains striking numbers of target cells and a few spherocytes.

Hemoglobin SC

When the genes for Hb S and Hb C occur in the same person, moderately severe anemia with splenomegaly results. Vasoocclusive episodes are usually less frequent and milder than in sickle cell disease. Aseptic necrosis of the femoral head is an occasional complication, and severe retinal damage also occurs.

Hemoglobin SC (Hb SC) disease usually does not affect growth and is compatible with extended survival. The hemoglobin concentration averages 9 to 10 g/dL. Target cells are seen in large numbers on blood smears. Hemoglobin electrophoresis reveals an almost equal mixture of Hb S and Hb C, with a slight elevation of Hb F.

Hemoglobin D

The hemoglobin D (Hb D) syndromes include several varieties of abnormal hemoglobin with electrophoretic mobilities at an alkaline pH similar to that of Hb S, but they do not have the biochemical and physical properties of Hb S. Sickling does not occur in Hb D syndromes. The homozygous state (i.e., Hb DD) is characterized by a mild hemolytic anemia with splenomegaly. Hemoglobin D occurs in white populations and has a relatively high prevalence in northwest India.

Hemoglobin E

Hemoglobin E (Hb E), an electrophoretically slow variant, is prevalent in persons from Southeast Asia, particularly Thailand and Cambodia. The Hb E heterozygote (i.e., Hb AE) has increased numbers of target cells on blood smears. Homozygous Hb E disease is characterized by a mild or moderate hemolytic anemia and by prominent target cells, microcytosis, and splenomegaly.

Unstable Hemoglobin Syndromes

Approximately 50 varieties of abnormal hemoglobins are characterized by molecular instability and are associated with the precipitation of hemoglobin (i.e., Heinz bodies) within the erythrocytes, causing chronic hemolysis. These anemias are inherited as autosomal dominant traits. Hemolysis is manifested during the first 6 months of life. Patients usually have jaundice and splenomegaly. The abnormal hemoglobin accounts for 30% to 40% of the total, but it may not be detected by electrophoresis. Heating of the hemolysate at 50°C for 1 hour usually results in a heavy precipitate of the abnormal hemoglobin. Splenectomy sometimes improves mild or moderately severe hemolytic disease, but severe hemolysis may not be improved by surgery.

Hemoglobinopathies Causing Cyanosis

A group of abnormal hemoglobins, designated hemoglobin M (Hb M), is associated with dominantly transmitted familial cyanosis. Because the characteristic amino acid substitutions are strategically located near the heme groups, internal oxidation of heme iron to the trivalent (i.e., ferric) form occurs. The Hb M diseases are characterized by cyanosis and mild polycythemia and have sometimes been mistaken for cyanotic congenital heart disease. Hb M can be differentiated from other forms of methemoglobinemia by characteristic changes in the spectral absorption patterns of hemoglobin solutions and by normal levels of erythrocyte methemoglobin reductase (i.e., diaphorase). No therapy is indicated.

Hemoglobinopathies with Altered Oxygen Affinity

More than 20 abnormal hemoglobins are associated with an increase in oxygen affinity, which is indicated by a shift to the left of the oxygen dissociation curve and a low partial pressure of oxygen at which hemoglobin is half saturated (P_{50}). Because of the increased affinity for hemoglobin, the decreased release of oxygen to the tissues leads to tissue hypoxia. This condition accelerates production of erythropoietin and secondary polycythemia.

Six hemoglobin variants with markedly reduced affinity for oxygen have been reported and are associated with familial chronic cyanosis or pseudoanemia. The oxygen dissociation curve is shifted to the right, with P_{50} values greater than 30 mm Hg.

THALASSEMIAS

The thalassemias are a group of hereditary hypochromic anemias associated with defective synthesis of one of the polypeptide chains of hemoglobin. In the United States, they chiefly affect persons of Mediterranean and Southeast Asian ethnic backgrounds. In the heterozygous state, thalassemia genes produce mild anemia. In the homozygous form, they are associated with severe hematologic disease.

Pathophysiology

More than 40 separate genetic variants of thalassemia have been identified. These result in quantitative deficiencies of the mRNA of the alpha- or beta-polypeptide chains of hemoglobin. Unbalanced polypeptide chain synthesis results in formation of unstable hemoglobin complexes within the erythrocyte that lead to erythrocyte death, much of which occurs in the bone marrow. The pathophysiology of thalassemia reflects ineffective erythropoiesis with severe hemolysis and compensatory hypertrophy of erythroid tissue in medullary and extramedullary sites.

Clinical Manifestations

Heterozygous thalassemia of the beta-chain variety (i.e., thalassemia minor) is a mild familial hypochronic microcytic anemia. Hemoglobin levels are 2 to 3 g/dL less than age-appropriate normal values. The mean corpuscular volume averages 68 fL (range, 58 to 75 fL). The erythrocytes are hypochromic and microcytic, with target cells, ovalocytes, and basophilic stippling. Elevation of Hb A_2 levels (greater than 3.5%) establishes the diagnosis. No therapy is effective or necessary.

Homozygous beta-thalassemia (i.e., thalassemia major, Cooley anemia) usually becomes symptomatic in the first year of life. The anemia is so profound that regular blood transfusions are necessary to sustain life; if untreated, life expectancy is only a few years. However, approximately 10% of homozygous patients are able to maintain hemoglobin levels of 6 to 8 g/dL without regular transfusions (i.e., thalassemia intermedia). In the untransfused or poorly transfused patient, massive splenomegaly and progressive bone changes become evident during the first few years of life.

Laboratory Findings

The erythrocyte changes of thalassemia major are extreme. In addition to severe hypochromia and microcytosis, many poikilocytes and target cells are seen. Large numbers of nucleated erythrocytes circulate, especially after splenectomy. Typically, the hemoglobin level decreases progressively to less than 5 g/dL unless transfusions are given. The unconjugated serum bilirubin level is elevated. The serum iron level is high, with increasing saturation of iron-binding capacity. Lactate dehydrogenase activities are very high, reflecting ineffective erythropoiesis. Large amounts of Hb F are contained in the erythrocytes. The level of Hb F exceeds 70% during the early years of life but tends to decline with increasing age.

Therapy

Transfusions of packed erythrocytes are given to maintain the hemoglobin level at more than 10 g/dL. This hypertransfusion has a striking clinical benefit. It permits normal activity with comfort and prevents progressive marrow expansion and its attendant cosmetic problems and osteoporosis. Transfusions are necessary every 4 to 5 weeks.

Hemosiderosis is an inevitable and fatal consequence of prolonged transfusion therapy, because each 200 mL of erythrocytes contains approximately 200 mg of iron that cannot be physiologically excreted. The iron burden can be reduced with iron-chelating agents, especially desferrioxamine, which must be given parenterally, administered subcutaneously at night over 8 to 12 hours using a battery-driven pump. In many patients, a negative iron balance is possible. A chronic chelation program can reverse the poor prognosis of this disease if the patient complies with the demanding regimen. Iron-chelating drugs, especially those that can be taken orally, are undergoing clinical testing. If efficacious and safe, these new drugs will improve compliance with chelation therapy and will significantly reduce the incidence of hemosiderosis in chronically transfused patients. Deferasirox has recently been approved for use as an oral iron-chelating medication.

Splenectomy is often necessary because of the size of the organ or because of secondary hypersplenism, but it has no effect on the basic hematologic disease. Immunization with pneumococcal vaccine is indicated, and prophylactic penicillin therapy is advocated by some authorities.

Bone marrow transplantation from HLA-identical and partly mismatched siblings has been performed in more than 400 children with thalassemia. Early death from toxicity and graft-versus-host disease is low (less than 10%) in young patients without hepatic dysfunction. The risk of death is considerably higher for older patients, especially if liver function is already compromised by hemosiderosis. If an HLA-matched, healthy sibling is available, bone marrow transplantation should be considered, especially in a patient who has not yet developed symptoms of hemosiderosis. Introduction of an abnormal beta-globin gene using gene therapy remains an area of active research.

Other Thalassemias

Thalassemia Intermedia

Thalassemia intermedia is a term assigned to patients with thalassemia syndromes intermediate in severity between major and minor. They have jaundice and moderate splenomegaly. The hemoglobin level is maintained at 7 to 8 g/dL. Regular transfusions are unnecessary, but transfusion therapy may be indicated to prevent severe osseous abnormalities. Even without regular blood transfusions, these patients absorb large amounts of iron, and hemosiderosis ultimately occurs.

Hemoglobin S–Thalassemia Disease

The combination of a beta-thalassemia and Hb S gene results in a clinical disease more severe than with either trait alone. Hb S–thalassemia disease is a moderately severe, microcytic, hemolytic anemia with vasoocclusive symptoms. The proportion of Hb S ranges from 60% to 90%; the remainder is Hb A and variable amounts of Hb F and Hb S–beta-thalassemia. Sometimes no Hb A can be detected (Hb Sβ^+ thalassemia). Family studies reveal one parent to have thalassemia trait and the other to have a sickle cell syndrome.

alpha-Thalassemias

A group of diseases, especially prevalent in Southeast Asians, results from genetic deletions of alpha-chain genes. Five percent of African Americans have an alpha-thalassemia trait associated with deletion of two alpha-chain genes. Clinically, the disorder is characterized by microcytic anemia that is unresponsive to iron. Three and four alpha-chain deletions are rare among African Americans. The diagnosis is made by excluding other causes of anemia. Hemoglobin electrophoresis is not helpful after the immediate postnatal period since it is only in the newborn period, that electrophoresis shows 3% to 6% hemoglobin Barts (γ_4 instead of the normal Hb F ($\alpha_2\gamma_2$)). Patients are asymptomatic but should be counseled so they may prevent well-meaning health providers from prescribing iron for presumed iron deficiency or from performing a workup for anemia.

In Asians, the four distinct alpha-thalassemia syndromes are the silent carrier state, alpha-thalassemia trait, hemoglobin H (Hb H) disease, and fetal hydrops syndrome. These result from increasing numbers of alpha-thalassemia gene deletions, from one to four. Deletion of four alpha-thalassemia genes produces the clinical picture of hydrops fetalis *in utero*. The predominant hemoglobin is Barts (gamma-4). This variant has abnormal oxygen dissociation properties that make oxygen unavailable to the tissues, thus causing fetal death.

Deletion of three alpha-thalassemia genes causes the less severe Hb H disease, which is moderately severe anemia that resembles thalassemia major or intermedia. It is characterized by 5% to 10% of unstable Hb H (gamma-4).

Hereditary Persistence of High Fetal Hemoglobin

Hereditary persistence of high Hb F is associated with high levels of normal Hb F but few hematologic abnormalities. It occurs predominantly in black and Mediterranean people. The erythrocytes contain 15% to 30% Hb F. An even distribution of Hb F is found in the erythrocyte population, in contrast to the thalassemias, in which Hb F content varies from cell to cell. The hereditary persistence of high Hb F homozygote has 100% Hb F but no significant anemia. If hereditary persistence of high Hb F and a sickle gene affect the same person, only Hb S and Hb F are found. However, the even distribution of Hb F in the erythrocyte population prevents sickling, and hematologic and clinical symptoms are minimal.

Suggested Readings

Bunn HF, Forget BG, Ranney HM. *Human hemoglobins.* Philadelphia: WB Saunders, 1977.
Charache S, Lubin B, Reid CD. *Management and therapy of sickle cell disease.* Publication No. 85–2115. Bethesda, MD: National Institutes of Health, 1985.
Kirkpatrick DV, Barrios NJ, Humbert JH. Bone marrow transplantation in sickle cell anemia. *Semin Hematol* 1991;28:240.
Lucarelli G, Galimberti M, Polchi P, et al. Bone marrow transplantation in thalassemia: the experience of Pesaro. *N Engl J Med* 1990;322:417.
Pearson HA. Sickle cell diseases: diagnosis and management in infancy and childhood. *Pediatr Rev* 1987;9:121.
Serjeant GR. *Sickle cell disease.* Oxford: Oxford University Press, 1985.
Walters MC, Patience M, Leisenring W, et al. Collaborative multicenter investigation of marrow transplantation for sickle cell disease: current results and future directions. *Biol Blood Marrow Transplant* 1997;3:310.
Weatherall DJ. Bone marrow transplantation for thalassemia and other inherited disorders of hemoglobin. *Blood* 1992;80:1379.
Weatherall DJ, Cligg JB. *The thalassemia syndromes,* 3rd ed. Oxford: Blackwell Scientific, 1981.
Zimmerman SA, Schultz WH, Davis JS, et al. Sustained long-term hematologic efficacy of hydroxyurea at maximum tolerated dose in children with sickle cell disease. *Blood* 2004;103:2039.

CHAPTER 291 ■ HEMOLYTIC ANEMIAS

PAUL L. MARTIN

After release from the bone marrow, mature, nonnucleated erythrocytes survive for 100 to 120 days in the circulation. In the steady state, 1% of the senescent erythrocytes is destroyed daily and replaced by an equal number of new erythrocytes released from the bone marrow. The basic pathophysiology of the hemolytic anemias is a reduced erythrocyte life span, ranging from nearly normal to remarkably shortened. In compensation, the bone marrow increases its output of erythrocytes, a response mediated by increased production of erythropoietin. In adults with hereditary spherocytosis (HS), the bone marrow can increase output of erythrocytes sixfold to eightfold. With this maximal response, erythrocyte survival can be reduced to only 20 to 30 days without the onset of anemia (i.e., compensated hemolysis). The limits of erythrocyte production in some hemolytic states have not been determined, particularly in infants and children.

A hemolytic process can be measured directly by erythrocyte survival rates or indirectly by the presence of increased levels of the metabolic products of hemolysis. Alternatively, a hemolytic process may be inferred by documentation of the increase in erythrocyte production that usually accompanies hemolytic states.

In response to shortened survival of erythrocytes, the activity of bone marrow increases, and the reticulocyte count exceeds 2%. Sustained reticulocytosis is presumptive evidence of hemolysis. Hyperplasia of the erythropoietic marrow elements occurs, with reversal of the myeloid-to-erythroid ratio from the normal 3:1. In the severe, chronic hemolytic processes of childhood, hypertrophy of the marrow may expand the medullary spaces and produce bone changes, particularly in the skull and hands.

Elevations of unconjugated bilirubin often occur in children with hemolytic anemias. However, overt jaundice may be absent. Bilirubin levels in excess of 5 mg/dL are unusual if liver function is normal. Chronic hemolysis is associated with increased excretion of bilirubin pigments leading to pigmented gallstones that may develop in early childhood.

In any hemolytic state, hemoglobin is released into the plasma, where it combines irreversibly with serum haptoglobin. The large complex is rapidly cleared from the circulation. When haptoglobin use exceeds synthesis, serum levels are decreased (less than 20 mg/dL).

Besides these indirect indicators of hemolysis, isotopic techniques can measure erythrocyte survival directly. Sodium chromate is most often used as an erythrocyte tag. A shortened erythrocyte survival is likely when the chromium half-time is reduced to less than 20 days. Such survival studies are rarely needed in clinical practice.

The hemolytic disorders may be conveniently and fairly accurately classified according to whether the shortened erythrocyte survival is a result of an intrinsic abnormality of the erythrocyte or an extrinsic abnormality acting on a normal erythrocyte. Intrinsic hemolytic anemias generally result from inherited abnormalities of the erythrocyte membrane, intracellular enzymes, or hemoglobin. Extrinsic disorders usually are acquired and result from forces or agents that immunologically, chemically, or physically damage the erythrocyte. These two categories are not mutually exclusive, and some hemolytic disorders are caused by a combination of intrinsic and extrinsic mechanisms (Table 291.1).

INTRINSIC HEMOLYTIC ANEMIAS

Hereditary Spherocytosis

HS occurs predominantly in people of northern European ancestry, although it has been found in patients of many ethnic groups. The typical features are a familial hemolytic anemia of various degrees of severity, splenomegaly, and spheric erythrocytes found on the blood smear.

In approximately three-fourths of patients, pedigree analysis indicates an autosomal dominant transmission. Sporadic dominant mutations have been invoked, and autosomal recessive transmission is present in some cases. The gene for some patients with HS is located on chromosome 8.

Pathophysiology

A deficiency or abnormality of the erythrocyte membrane structural protein spectrin appears to affect most patients with HS. Other erythrocyte membrane structural proteins that have been demonstrated to play a role in this disease include ankyrin, band 3, and protein 4.2. They all have in common the relative deficiency of spectrin. This deficiency is associated with an accelerated loss of the erythrocyte membrane, which reduces the erythrocyte surface area. Because no concomitant loss of cellular volume occurs, the erythrocytes become spheric.

The spleen is intrinsically involved in the hemolytic process. The splenic circulation imposes a metabolic stress on spherocytic cells. The spherocyte is relatively rigid and passes with difficulty through the splenic cords and sinuses. This results in their sequestration and destruction. The hemolytic process regresses after splenectomy, although biochemical and morphologic abnormalities persist.

Clinical Manifestations

The disease may present in the neonatal period with anemia and hyperbilirubinemia that may require phototherapy or exchange transfusion. The anemia varies considerably in severity but tends to be similar within the same family. The patient usually has slight jaundice. Expansion of the marrow cavity occurs to a lesser extent than in thalassemia. The spleen is almost always palpably enlarged after 2 or 3 years of age. Pigmentary gallstones have occurred as early as 4 years of age. Aplastic crises associated with parvovirus infections are the most serious complications during childhood. Other complications have been reported and are less common, including gout, leg ulcers, and growth retardation.

Laboratory Findings

Indicators of hemolysis include reticulocytosis, anemia, and hyperbilirubinemia. The hemoglobin level ranges from 6 to 10 g/dL, and the reticulocyte count ranges from 5% to 20% (average, 10%). The mean corpuscular hemoglobin concentration usually is elevated (greater than 36%). The spherocytic erythrocytes are smaller than normal erythrocytes and lack the central pallor of the biconcave disc, but only relatively small proportions of the cells are spherocytic. Erythroid hyperplasia occurs in the marrow, but erythrocyte precursors are not spherocytic.

Abnormality of the erythrocyte can be demonstrated by osmotic fragility studies. This test measures the ability of red blood cells to swell and increase their volume when they are subjected to varying degrees of hypotonic environments.

TABLE 291.1

CAUSES AND TREATMENTS OF HEMOLYTIC ANEMIAS

Disorder	Cause of Anemia	Treatment
Hereditary spherocytosis (HS)	Defect in spectrin	Splenectomy if severe disease
Hereditary elliptocytosis	Defect in spectrin in some	Splenectomy if severe disease
Paroxysmal nocturnal hemoglobinuria (PNH)	Abnormal surface protein anchor	Supportive care; stem cell transplant if aplastic anemia develops
Hereditary stomatocytosis	Increased cation permeability	Splenectomy may help if hemolysis is severe
Pyruvate kinase deficiency	Absent or decreased pyruvate kinase	Supportive care and transfusions as needed; splenectomy may help symptoms in severe cases
Glucose-6-phosphate dehydrogenase (G6PD) deficiency	Decreased amounts or decreased half-life of G6PD	Avoid oxidative medications (i.e., sulfa drugs) and oxidative dietary items (fava beans)
Autoimmune hemolytic anemia (AIHA)	Auto antibodies directed against the patient's own red cell antigens	Immunosuppression, transfusions as needed with least incompatible donor red cells

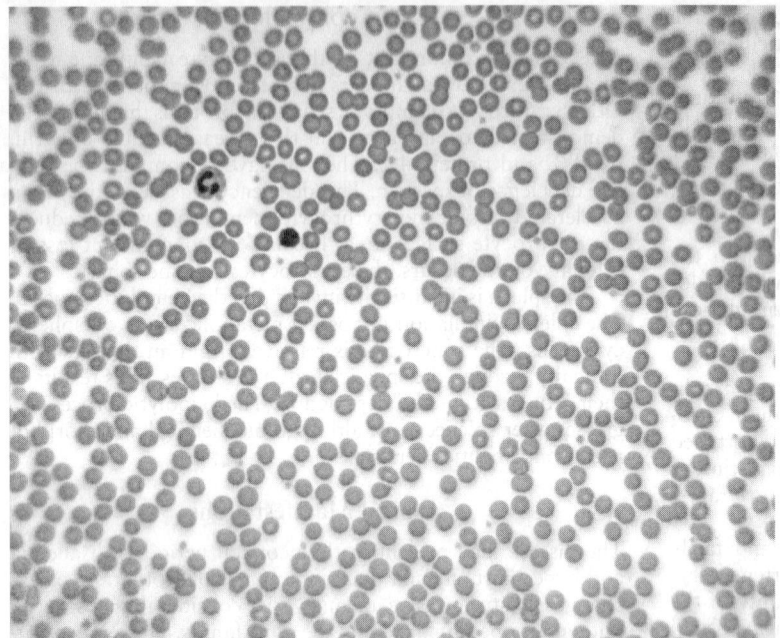

FIGURE 291.1. Normal blood. Note the size of the red cell is approximately equal to the size of the lymphocyte and smaller than the neutrophil. (Courtesy of Susan J. Neblett, M.T., Beverly Williams, M.T., and Donald Beam, M.D.)

Because of their decreased surface-to-volume ratio, spherocytes have a limited capability of doing so and will be lysed at a higher salt concentration than normal cells. In 10% to 20% of patients with HS, the osmotic abnormality can be demonstrated only if the blood is incubated at 37°C for 24 hours.

HS must be differentiated from other congenital hemolytic states. Family history, blood smear, and osmotic fragility studies offer the most diagnostic value. Acquired spherocytosis of the erythrocytes is seen in autoimmune hemolytic anemias (AIHAs), in which the spherocytosis is often more pronounced than in HS, and the direct Coombs test result is positive (Figs. 291.1 and 291.2). It may be difficult to differentiate HS from hemolytic disease caused by ABO incompatibility in the newborn infant. A period of observation may be necessary to clarify the diagnosis.

Therapy

Splenectomy almost invariably produces a clinical cure, although in a few instances of severe HS with recessive transmission, the operation is not curative. Splenectomy should be deferred if possible until the patient is at least 5 or 6 years of age. Immunization with conjugated pneumococcal and *Haemophilus influenzae* type b vaccine as recommended for all infants in the United States should be provided. In addition, polyvalent pneumococcal vaccine should be given at 2 years of age, with a boost at age 7 years. If anemia is severe enough to impair growth or normal activity, the operation can be considered earlier, after a period of observation. Splenectomy prevents further gallstone formation and eliminates the threat of aplastic crises.

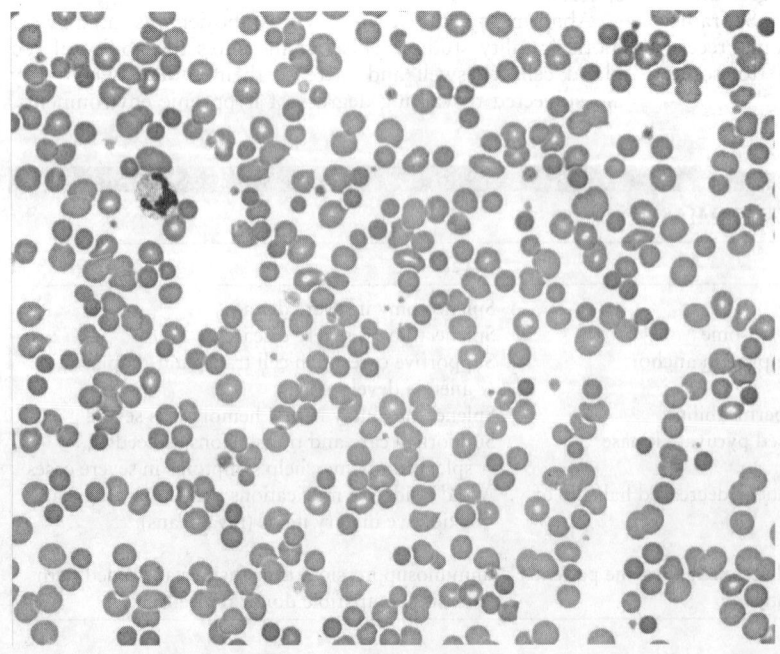

FIGURE 291.2. Spherocytosis. Note the small red cells with less or absent central pallor. This is most commonly associated with hereditary red cell membrane defects or acquired autoimmune anemias. The red cells become spheric as a result of the loss of membrane surface area. (Courtesy of Susan J. Neblett, M.T., Beverly Williams, M.T., and Donald Beam, M.D.)

After splenectomy, jaundice and reticulocytosis disappear. The hemoglobin level becomes normal, although the spherocytosis and osmotic fragility abnormalities become more pronounced. Overwhelming sepsis after splenectomy occurs infrequently if the surgical procedure is delayed until the child is 5 or 6 years of age, but the febrile child must be carefully evaluated for sepsis. Polyvalent pneumococcal, *H. influenzae* type b, and perhaps meningococcal vaccines should be given at least 2 weeks before splenectomy if possible. Prophylactic penicillin therapy after splenectomy is mandatory if the operation is done before the child is 6 years of age.

Hereditary Elliptocytosis

Some oval or elliptic erythrocytes may be seen in a number of conditions, especially thalassemia and iron deficiency; however, they occur in much larger numbers as a dominantly inherited trait in hereditary elliptocytosis (HE; hereditary ovalocytosis). Fifteen percent to fifty percent of the circulating erythrocytes of these patients are elongated. In most patients, no associated hemolysis occurs, and the hematologic values, including reticulocyte counts, are normal. However, in approximately 10% of patients with elliptic cells, evidence of hemolysis exists, with hemoglobin levels averaging 8 to 10 g/dL and reticulocytes comprising 5% to 15% of the cells.

Pathophysiology

A structural abnormality of spectrin has been described in erythrocytes from some patients with HE with or without hemolysis. The bases for hemolytic HE and HE without hemolysis are unclear. In most family studies of hemolytic HE, one parent has elliptic erythrocytes without hemolysis, and the other parent is hematologically normal.

Clinical Manifestations

HE with hemolysis may be associated with neonatal jaundice, but characteristic elliptocytosis may not be evident at birth. The blood smear instead shows bizarre poikilocytes and pyknocytes. The usual features of chronic hemolytic process, including anemia, jaundice, splenomegaly, and osseous changes, may be seen later. Cholelithiasis occurs in later childhood, and aplastic crises have been reported.

Laboratory Findings

The morphology of the erythrocytes is the most important diagnostic feature. Elliptic cells characterized by a length more than 1.5 times the diameter account for 15% to 70% of the erythrocytes (Fig. 291.3). In hemolytic HE, the reticulocyte count is increased. Erythroid hyperplasia is evident in the bone marrow, but the erythrocyte precursors are not elliptic. Increased erythrocyte osmotic fragility and increased thermal instability occur in hemolytic HE, which has sometimes led to designating cases of hemolytic HE as pyropoikilocytosis (Fig. 291.4).

Therapy

If significant hemolysis exists, splenectomy is usually beneficial. Erythrocyte morphology is not changed after the operation, and it may become even more abnormal.

Paroxysmal Nocturnal Hemoglobinuria

Paroxysmal nocturnal hemoglobinuria (PNH) is a rare chronic anemia with prominent intravascular hemolysis that may have its onset in late childhood. Hemolysis is characteristically worse during sleep, and morning hemoglobinuria is usual.

The primary defect in PNH resides in an abnormal surface protein anchor to the red blood cell membrane. This extracellular anchor, or glycosylphosphatidyl-inositol, is missing from all cells in those patients affected with PNH. This abnormality renders erythrocytes susceptible to hemolysis by serum complement. PNH is a clonal abnormality, with the *PIGA* gene mutated in affected patients. The hemoglobinuria is explainable because red blood cells no longer express CD55 and CD59, both of which are required for clearance of randomly deposited complement factors from the erythrocyte membrane, which allows chronic, complement-mediated intravascular hemolysis. In addition to chronic hemolysis, thrombocytopenia and

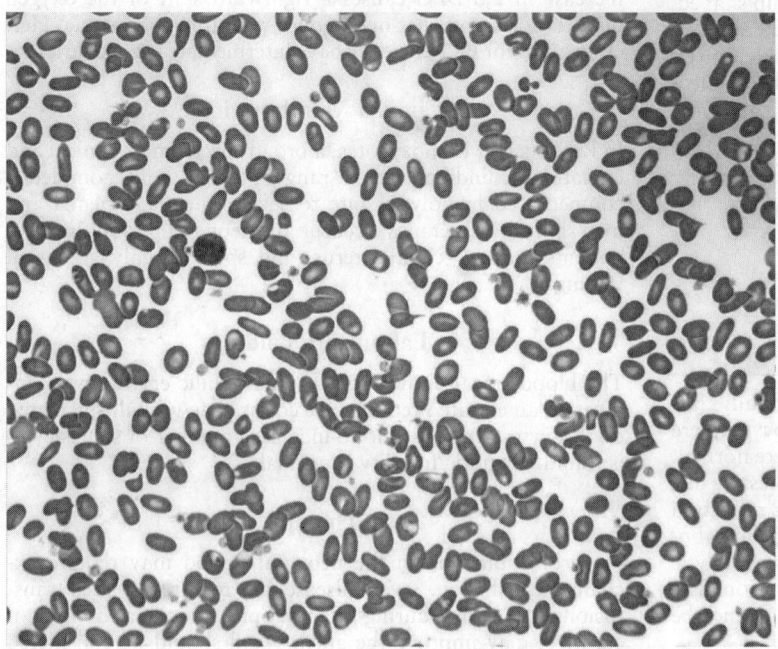

FIGURE 291.3. Elliptocytosis. Elongated red cells are associated with inherited red cell membrane defects as well as thalassemia, sickle cell disease, and other less common conditions. Elliptocytes can be found in asymptomatic patients as well as in patients with serious medical conditions. (Courtesy of Susan J. Neblett, M.T., Beverly Williams, M.T., and Donald Beam, M.D.)

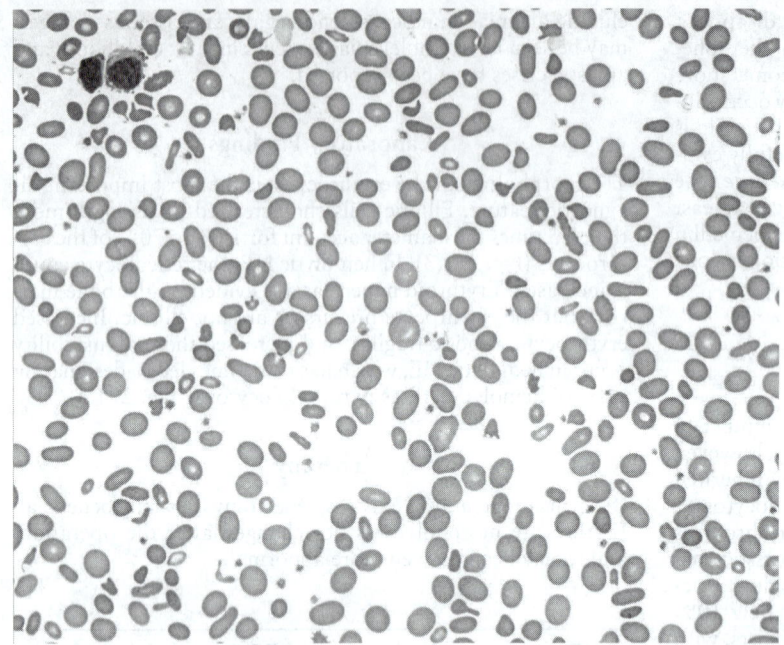

FIGURE 291.4. Pyropoikilocytosis. Hereditary pyropoikilocytosis is a rare type of hemolytic anemia characterized by extreme variation in red blood cell size and shape. It is caused by defects in spectrin, an important membrane protein in the red cell. (Courtesy of Susan J. Neblett, M.T., Beverly Williams, M.T., and Donald Beam, M.D.)

leukopenia may develop. Some cases have been followed by aplastic anemia.

The diagnosis is established by flow cytometry of the patient's red cells. Absence of CD59 establishes the diagnosis. Infections tend to trigger hemolysis, although frequently no identifiable reason exists. Therapy is supportive and symptomatic; however, oral corticosteroids at a dose of 1 to 2 mg/kg have shown some effectiveness at limiting the duration of the hemolysis. Bone marrow transplantation has been successful in some cases.

Hereditary Stomatocytosis

Hereditary stomatocytosis is a rare type of hemolytic anemia associated with erythrocytes that are swollen and cup shaped. On stained smears, the erythrocytes have a mouth-like slit (i.e., stoma) in place of the usual circular central pallor. Hemolytic anemia is associated with extreme permeability of the erythrocyte membrane to cations. Splenectomy may be indicated.

HEMOLYTIC ANEMIAS RESULTING FROM ABNORMALITIES OF ERYTHROCYTE GLYCOLYTIC ENZYMES

This group of congenital hemolytic anemias was originally classified as nonspherocytic because spherocytic erythrocytes were not found and results of the osmotic fragility test were normal. Most of these anemias are inherited as autosomal recessive disorders. A diagnosis is established by demonstrating reduction of the enzyme as well as decreased levels of glycolytic metabolites distal to the deficient enzyme. Deficiencies of glycolytic enzymes compromise adenosine triphosphate generation. The metabolic energy requirements of the erythrocytes cannot be met, and the erythrocyte life span is shortened.

Pyruvate Kinase Deficiency

An inherited deficiency of pyruvate kinase (PK) is the most frequent of the erythrocyte glycolytic enzyme deficiencies. PK activity, measured in the erythrocytes, is reduced markedly, but the enzyme activity in other blood cells and tissues is normal.

Pathophysiology

The disease is caused by homozygosity for an autosomal recessive gene, which results in markedly decreased production of a mutant PK isoenzyme. The PK-deficient erythrocytes are depleted of adenosine triphosphate, and their survival is compromised. Levels of glycolytic intermediates, especially 2,3-diphosphoglycerate (2,3-DPG), are increased greatly. The increase in 2,3-DPG causes a rightward shift of the oxygen dissociation curve that may reduce symptoms of anemia. Heterozygotes for PK deficiency have intermediate enzyme levels.

Clinical Manifestations

In PK-deficient homozygotes, a broad spectrum of clinical and hematologic findings occurs, ranging from a mild, completely compensated hemolytic state to severe anemia. Anemia and hyperbilirubinemia may occur in the neonatal period. In older patients, pallor, scleral icterus, and splenomegaly are usual findings.

Laboratory Findings

The blood smear shows polychromatophilic erythrocytes, indicating an elevated reticulocyte count. A few small spiculated erythrocytes are seen, but no increased number of spherocytes is found. Osmotic fragility is normal.

Therapy

Hyperbilirubinemia in the neonatal period may require exchange transfusion. Severe disease may require repeated transfusions for anemia during infancy. Splenectomy, although not curative, may improve the anemia and should be considered in patients with severe disease. Marked reticulocytosis occurs after splenectomy.

Glucose-6-Phosphate Dehydrogenase Deficiency Syndromes

Glucose-6-phosphate dehydrogenase (G6PD) deficiency results in two kinds of hematologic problems: a common, acute condition manifested by hemolytic episodes induced by infection or certain drugs, and a rare chronic, nonspherocytic hemolytic anemia. The G6PD gene is on the X chromosome. In the hemizygous affected male subject, the condition results from inheritance of one abnormal G6PD gene. In the affected homozygous female subject, two abnormal genes are inherited. The normal G6PD enzyme found in most white populations is designated *G6PD B+*. A normal isoenzyme designated *G6PD A+* is common in blacks. More than ten distinct enzyme variants of G6PD have been documented.

Pathophysiology

Thirteen percent of black men and 2% of black women have a mutant enzyme called *G6PD A−* that is unstable and is associated with reduced erythrocyte enzyme activity (5% to 15% of normal). Affected persons of Mediterranean, Arabic, and Asian ethnic groups have relatively high frequencies of G6PD deficiency because of a variant designated *G6PD B−*. The enzyme activity of the homozygous female or the hemizygous male subject is less than 5% of normal.

G6PD, the rate-limiting enzyme of the pentose phosphate pathway, is crucial for protection of the erythrocytes from oxidant stress. In G6PD deficiency, oxidant metabolites of a number of drugs produce denaturation and precipitation of hemoglobin, thereby causing erythrocyte injury and rapid hemolysis. Hemolysis occurs only if the patient is exposed to oxidant drugs, such as antipyretics, naphthalene, sulfonamides, antimalarials, and naphthaquinolones, or to the fava bean. The degree of hemolysis varies with the drug's antioxidant effect, the amount ingested, and the severity of the enzyme deficiency in the patient.

Laboratory Findings

Hemoglobinemia and hemoglobinuria occur 24 to 48 hours after the ingestion of an oxidant substance. The hemoglobin level may decrease to as low as 2 to 5 g/dL. Heinz bodies are not visible on stained blood smears. They can be demonstrated initially on supravital preparations, but they disappear after 3 or 4 days. Spontaneous recovery is usual and is heralded by reticulocytosis and an increase in hemoglobin concentration, starting 4 or 5 days after the acute hemolytic episode.

Diagnosis depends on direct or indirect demonstration of reduced G6PD activity in erythrocytes. By direct measurement, enzyme activity in affected persons is less than 15% of normal. The reduction of enzyme activity is more extreme in whites and Asians than in G6PD-deficient blacks. Shortly after a hemolytic event, G6PD activity may be normal, secondary to reticulocytosis. A repeat examination several weeks later may be necessary to prove the diagnosis.

Therapy

Prevention of hemolysis by avoiding oxidant drugs is important. Men and boys belonging to ethnic groups in which a significant incidence of G6PD deficiency occurs should be tested for the defect before drugs that are known to be potent oxidants are given. After hemolysis has occurred, supportive therapy is indicated, including blood transfusions if the anemia is severe and the patient is symptomatic.

Chronic Nonspherocytic Hemolytic Anemia Associated with Glucose-6-Phosphate Dehydrogenase Deficiency

Instances of chronic hemolytic anemias not associated with oxidant drug ingestion have been associated with profound deficiencies of G6PD caused by several enzyme variants. These have occurred predominantly in people of northern European ancestry. For this X-linked disease, splenectomy has been of minimal value.

Other Inherited Abnormalities of Erythrocyte Glycolytic Enzymes

Deficiencies of several other glycolytic erythrocyte enzymes have been described in patients with congenital nonspherocytic hemolytic anemias. These include deficiencies of hexokinase, glucose-6-phosphate isomerase, phosphofructose kinase aldolase, triosephosphate isomerase, glyceraldehyde-3-phosphate isomerase, and phosphoglycerate kinase. Most of these diseases are transmitted as autosomal recessive traits.

Chronic hemolysis, often manifested in infancy, is a common feature. Specific erythrocyte morphologic abnormalities are not seen. Diagnosis depends on demonstration of reductions of the specific erythrocyte enzyme. No specific therapy exists, but splenectomy may reduce the rate of hemolysis.

Deficiencies of Other Enzymes of the Pentose Phosphate Pathway

The most important function of the pentose pathway is to provide the reduced nicotinamide-adenine dinucleotide phosphate (NADPH) necessary for maintaining glutathione in the reduced state. This is essential for the physiologic inactivation of oxidant compounds. Without adequate levels of glutathione, when oxidant drugs are ingested, hemoglobin becomes denatured and precipitates into erythrocyte inclusions called *Heinz bodies*. These damage the erythrocyte membrane and cause acute hemolysis.

EXTRINSIC HEMOLYTIC ANEMIAS

Agents that damage erythrocytes may lead to their premature destruction. The most clearly defined of these agents are the antibodies associated with immune hemolysis. Antibodies directed against specific intrinsic membrane antigens damage the erythrocytes and produce hemolysis. The most important feature of these diseases is the positive Coombs antiglobulin test, which detects immunoglobulins or components of complement on the erythrocyte surface.

Autoimmune Hemolytic Anemias

In AIHAs, the patient's antibodies are directed against the patient's own erythrocytes. The factors evoking such an autoimmune response are unknown, but they include viral infections and occasionally specific drugs.

Pathophysiology

AIHAs associated with an underlying disease process such as lymphoma, lupus erythematosus, or immunodeficiency are said to be secondary. In idiopathic AIHA, no such underlying disease exists. Drugs such as penicillin, cephalosporins, and alpha-methyldopa evoke the formation of antibodies in some patients.

Clinical Manifestations

AIHAs occur in two clinical patterns. The first type, a fulminant variety that occurs in infants and young children, is frequently preceded by a respiratory infection. The onset is acute, with pallor, jaundice, and hemoglobinuria. The spleen is enlarged. A consistent response to corticosteroid therapy, low mortality, and complete recovery are characteristic. No underlying disease is found. A second type of AIHA has a prolonged course and a significant mortality. Underlying diseases are frequently found.

Laboratory Findings

The anemia may be severe, with hemoglobin levels of less than 6 g/dL. Spherocytosis and polychromasia are prominent. Reticulocytosis and nucleated erythrocytes are found, and leukocytosis is common. The platelet count usually is normal; occasionally, concomitant immune thrombocytopenic purpura occurs (i.e., Evans syndrome).

The direct and indirect Coombs test results are positive, indicating the presence of antibodies attached to the erythrocytes or free in the serum. These antibodies belong to the immunoglobulin G (IgG) class. They are often nonspecific panagglutinins, but they may have specificity for ubiquitous antigens of the Rh system (e.g., E, LW). Because of spontaneous erythrocyte agglutination, the patient may be mistakenly typed as blood group AB, Rh positive. In acute, transient cases, only complement is found on the erythrocytes, chiefly the C3 and C4 components. In chronic AIHA, a pure IgG Coombs test result often is found.

Therapy

Transfusion may be required, but it offers only transient benefit. Completely compatible blood is difficult to find, and giving blood that is "incompatible" as judged by the crossmatch often is necessary. Prednisone should be administered in a dose of 2 to 4 mg/kg every 24 hours. Treatment should be continued until hemolysis decreases. The dose can then be gradually reduced. The acute form of the disease usually remits spontaneously within a few weeks or months, but the Coombs test result may remain positive for an extended period. Splenectomy may be beneficial in several refractory cases. Immunosuppressive agents, including recently available monoclonal antibodies to proteins found on the surface of mature, antibody-producing B lymphocytes, have been used in patients refractory to conventional therapy. In AIHA secondary to lymphoma or lupus erythematosus, the disease tends to be chronic, and the course of the underlying disease determines the ultimate prognosis.

Hemolytic Anemias Associated with Cold Antibodies

Low levels of cold antibodies may exist normally, but after some viral or mycoplasmal infections, they may increase to very high levels. These high titers of cold antibodies induce intravascular hemolysis with hemoglobinemia. The antibodies often have specificity for the I antigen and react poorly with human cord blood cells possessing the i antigen. The antibodies are of the IgM class and require complement for activity. Spontaneous agglutination and rouleau formation are seen on the blood smear. Patients with infectious mononucleosis may develop acute hemolytic anemia. The antibodies in these cases have anti-I specificity.

Paroxysmal Cold Hemoglobinuria

Paroxysmal cold hemoglobinuria is a rare condition associated with a specific type of cold antibody, the Donath-Landsteiner hemolysin, which has anti-P specificity. Intravascular hemolysis is precipitated by low environmental temperature. Approximately one-third of cases are associated with congenital or acquired syphilis.

Suggested Readings

Austin RF, Deforges JI. Hereditary elliptocytosis: an unusual presentation of hemolysis in the newborn period associated with transient morphological abnormalities. *Pediatrics* 1969;44:196.

Beutler E. G6PD deficiency. *Blood* 1994;84:3613.

Buchanan GR, Boxer LA. The acute and transient nature of idiopathic immune hemolytic anemia in childhood. *J Pediatr* 1976;88:780.

Gallagher PG, Ferriera JDS. Molecular basis of erythrocyte membrane disorders. *Curr Opin Hematol* 1997;4:128.

Habibi B, Homberg JC. Autoimmune hemolytic anemia in children. A review of 80 cases. *Am J Med* 1974;56:61.

Hassoun H, Palek J. Hereditary spherocytosis: a review of the clinical and molecular aspects of the disease. *Blood Rev* 1996;10:129.

Izui S. Autoimmune hemolytic anemia. *Curr Opin Immunol* 1994;6:926.

Miwa S, Kanno H, Fujii H. Concise review: pyruvate kinase deficiency: historical perspective and recent progress of molecular genetics. *Am J Hematol* 1993;42:31.

Rosse WF, Ware RE. The molecular basis of paroxysmal nocturnal hemoglobinuria. *Blood* 1995;86:3277.

Trucco JI, Brown AK. Neonatal manifestations of hereditary spherocytosis. *Am J Dis Child* 1967;113:263.

Valentine WN, Paglia DE. Erythrocytic enzymopathies, hemolytic anemia, and multisystem disease. *Blood* 1984;64:583.

Young LE. Hereditary spherocytosis. *Am J Med* 1955;18:480.

CHAPTER 292 ■ HYPOPLASTIC AND APLASTIC ANEMIAS

PAUL L. MARTIN

HYPOPLASTIC ANEMIAS

The hypoplastic anemias (i.e., pure erythrocyte anemias, aregenerative anemias) constitute an uncommon group of congenital or acquired blood disorders characterized by anemia, reticulocytopenia, and a paucity of erythroid precursors in otherwise normal cellular bone marrow. Unlike the aplastic anemias (i.e., pancytopenias), the other formed elements of the blood usually are present in normal or increased numbers.

Pathophysiology

An understanding of the pathophysiology of the hypoplastic anemias requires a brief review of cellular aspects of erythropoiesis. Insight into the understanding of the nature and interactions of erythropoietic primordial cells has been possible because of the development of techniques for *in vitro* culture of bone marrow in media such as plasma clots, methylcellulose, and agar. Early committed erythroid progenitor cells can be inferred by their ability to form colonies of erythroid cells using these techniques. Two classes of progenitor cells have been identified: so-called colony-forming units, erythroid (CFUs-E), which give rise to compact colonies containing 10 to 100 hemoglobinized erythroid cells after 48 hours of culture; and more primitive erythroid progenitor cells, designated as burst-forming units, erythroid (BFUs-E), recognized by their capacity to form large colonies containing as many as 30,000 erythroid cells after 7 to 9 days of culture. Colony formation by CFUs-E requires the presence of erythropoietin, the glycoprotein hormone that regulates erythrocyte formation in the intact animal. BFU-E development does not require the presence of erythropoietin. BFUs-E and CFUs-E are present in small numbers in the normal bone marrow and morphologically resemble mature lymphocytes.

The next phases of erythrocyte development are represented by cells that can be morphologically identified as belonging to the erythroid series. These include the pronormoblast and the basophilic, polychromatophilic, and acidophilic normoblasts. In the latter stages of maturation of the erythrocyte, nuclear condensation and extrusion occur, resulting in the reticulocyte and finally the mature erythrocyte.

The hypoplastic anemias are a heterogenous group; both congenital and acquired varieties are recognized (Box 292.1). Factors that contribute to hypoplastic anemia are listed in Box 292.2.

Congenital Hypoplastic Anemia

At the 1938 meeting of the American Pediatric Society, Diamond and Blackfan described four children with severe aregenerative anemia that developed during the first year of life and required regular transfusions for survival. Only approximately 300 cases of congenital hypoplastic anemia (CHA) have been described in the literature, but many more cases have been recognized.

A familial recurrence in some families suggests that genetic factors may be operative occasionally but, in most cases, no inherited pattern is evident. Approximately 25% of the patients have physical abnormalities of various kinds, including short stature and facial, cardiac, and renal abnormalities. A subset of patients has thumbs with three rather than the usual two phalanges (i.e., Wranne syndrome).

Clinical Presentation

Anemia at or shortly after birth is the presenting manifestation of CHA. Approximately one-fourth of the patients are pale at birth. Sixty-five percent are anemic by 6 months of age, and almost all are anemic by 1 year of age. CHA described in older infants, particularly those reported before 1970, must be viewed with some skepticism because the cases may have represented transient erythroblastopenia of childhood.

Laboratory Findings

At the time of diagnosis, hemoglobin levels may be as low as 2.5 g/dL. The erythrocytes are macrocytic and have biochemical properties of fetal erythrocyte (i.e., increased levels of fetal hemoglobin for the patient's age, presence of the i erythrocyte antigen, and increased levels of age-dependent erythrocyte enzymes such as glucose-6-phosphate dehydrogenase [G6PD]). These findings may be of limited diagnostic value in early infancy when fetal cells are still present.

The reticulocyte count is characteristically very low, even in the presence of severe anemia. The remainder of the peripheral blood count is usually normal, although elevated platelet counts and modest neutropenia have been found occasionally.

Serum bilirubin levels are normal. Serum iron levels usually are elevated with increased transferrin saturation. Plasma and urinary levels of erythropoietin are elevated.

BOX 292.1   **Hypoplastic Anemias**

Congenital
Congenital hypoplastic anemia (Diamond-Blackfan syndrome)

Acquired
Transient erythroblastopenia of childhood
Parvovirus-induced aplastic crises of hemolytic anemias

BOX 292.2   **List of Drugs, Infections, and Environmental Toxins that Can Contribute to Hypoplastic Anemia or Other Blood Dyscrasias**

Medications

Antibiotics
Sulfonamides
Chloramphenicol
Ganciclovir
Cidofovir

Thyroid Mediations
Propylthiouracil
Methimazole

Anticonvulsants
Dilantin
Carbamazepine
Valproic acid

Other
Phenothiazines
Indomethacin
Quinidine

Infections
Parvovirus
Cytomegalovirus
Epstein-Barr virus
Hepatitis B
Hepatitis C
Human herpesvirus-6

Insecticides
Chlordane
DDT
Lindane
Organophosphates

Organic Solvents
Benzene
Toluene
Carbon tetrachloride

Radiation
Accidental
Environmental-radon
Therapeutic

In most patients with CHA, erythrocyte adenine deaminase levels are elevated two to three times higher than normal values. However, elevations also have been seen in some cases of acute leukemia, and the enzyme elevation may be an indicator of disordered erythropoiesis rather than a specific marker for CHA.

The most important diagnostic features are found in the bone marrow. The marrow in patients with CHA is normally cellular with normal numbers of megakaryocytes, lymphocytes, and myeloid precursors. However, erythrocyte precursors at every level of development are absent or markedly reduced. The proportion of myeloid-to-erythroid precursors in the bone marrow (M:E ratio), normally 3:1, is markedly increased (10:1 to 200:1). In some patients, a few primitive pronormoblasts can be recognized, but no more mature erythroid precursors are seen. Bone marrow erythroid cultures consistently have few BFUs-E and CFUs-E.

Therapy

The degree of anemia is often so profound at presentation that erythrocyte transfusions are necessary. Approximately 10% to 20% of patients are refractory to therapy and continue to require regular transfusions. Transfusions with packed, leukocyte- poor erythrocytes are given to maintain a hemoglobin level compatible with normal activity and comfort, usually more than 8 g/dL.

When chronic transfusion therapy is necessary, transfusional hemosiderosis inevitably occurs. Serum ferritin levels should be monitored periodically, and chelation therapy should be begun when evidence exists of tissue iron overload (see Chapter 290, Hemoglobinopathies and Thalassemias).

The use of adrenocorticotropic hormone and corticosteroids in CHA was suggested as early as 1949, but it was not until 1961 that a relatively large number of corticosteroid-treated patients were reported. Between 60% and 70% of patients respond to corticosteroid therapy. The mechanism of corticosteroid action may involve an enhancement of the ef-

fect of erythropoietin on CFU-E proliferation and maturation. Corticosteroids, such as prednisone, are administered at an initial dose of 2 mg/kg. Response is heralded by the appearance of erythropoietic precursors in the bone marrow within 1 to 2 weeks, followed by reticulocytosis and an increase in the hemoglobin level. The full dose of prednisone is continued until the hemoglobin attains a normal level. The dose can then be gradually decreased until a minimal effective dose is attained, which is often as little as 0.5 to 1.0 mg/day. In many instances, corticosteroids can be administered on alternate-day schedules that further decrease corticosteroid side effects. Some patients do not respond to the usual dose of corticosteroids and should be given a trial with larger doses (4 to 6 mg/kg). Approximately 20% to 30% of these children are nonresponsive to corticosteroids and require regular blood transfusions.

Children refractory to corticosteroids usually have not responded to other forms of therapy including androgenic and immunosuppressive agents. Bone marrow transplantation has been effective for patients with acceptable donors.

Transient Erythroblastic Anemia of Childhood

Transient erythroblastic anemia of childhood (TEC) is a striking syndrome of temporary failure of erythropoiesis, which is increasingly encountered in clinical practice. TEC is characterized by moderate to severe aregenerative anemia in an otherwise healthy child. The condition is self-limited and usually does not recur.

Pathophysiology

TEC seems to have an autoimmune basis. A circulating immunoglobulin that inhibits growth of CFUs-E or BFUs-E in tissue culture has been found in most of these patients. The stimulus that evokes this antibody has not been defined, and the inhibitor disappears from the serum as recovery occurs. TEC has not been associated with parvovirus infection.

Clinical Manifestations

TEC occurs in children older than 1 year, but it has been seen as early as 4 months of age. Pallor and symptoms of anemia are the usual presenting manifestations. Because the anemia reflects a complete cessation of erythropoiesis without increased hemolysis, the anemia develops very slowly.

If a patient has a hemoglobin level of 5 g/dL on presentation, it can be assumed that erythrocyte production has been minimal for at least 2 months. Because the anemia develops insidiously, pallor or symptoms may not be noticed by the parents. Except for the features of anemia, the remainder of the physical examination is normal.

Laboratory Findings

The degree of anemia may be severe, as low as 2.5 g/dL, with a low reticulocyte count. The leukocyte count is normal. The platelet count is usually normal but may be elevated. Other laboratory findings include a high serum iron level reflecting decreased use. The bone marrow shows a paucity of erythrocyte precursors with a high M:E ratio. The other marrow elements are normal.

Recovery occurs spontaneously within a few weeks and is accompanied by a brisk reticulocytosis and rapid increase in hemoglobin level.

The major differential diagnosis of TEC is CHA, particularly in the infant younger than 1 year. In contrast to CHA, in TEC the erythrocyte population at presentation has age-appropriate characteristics; a mean corpuscular volume of 70 to 80 fL; fetal hemoglobin less than 2% to 5%; normal levels of erythrocyte age-dependent enzymes (G6PD); and the usual adult I erythrocyte antigen. Erythrocyte adenine deaminase levels are not elevated.

A patient first seen in the recovery state of TEC may be erroneously considered to have a hemolytic process because of the concomitant low hemoglobin and high reticulocyte count. Observation can clarify the diagnosis.

Therapy

No specific therapy is necessary. Corticosteroid therapy is not indicated. If the anemia is severe, a small erythrocyte transfusion may be considered to sustain the child until recovery occurs. Most children have no recurrence of this disease.

Aplastic Crisis of Hemolytic Anemias Associated with Parvovirus Infection

Episodes of exaggerated anemia and reticulocytopenia in patients with various kinds of hemolytic anemias have been recognized for many years. Such episodes usually occur in the wake of viral infections and often affect several family members.

A correlation between aplastic crises patients in sickle cell disease and infection by the parvovirus was established in 1981 by the demonstration of virus particles in the blood of these patients. Most severe aplastic crises in patients with hemolytic anemias are likely caused by the parvovirus, an organism that also has been established as the cause of erythema infectiosum (i.e., fifth disease). Intrauterine parvovirus infection, detected by molecular technique, has been shown to be associated with some cases of nonimmunologic hydrops fetalis.

Pathophysiology

The parvovirus directly infects CFUs-E, damaging the cells and inhibiting their ability to proliferate. This causes a virtual cessation of erythrocyte production. The inhibition lasts for only 1 to 2 weeks until the virus is cleared. In a normal person whose erythrocyte survival is 100 days, 10 days of erythrocyte aplasia result in an insignificant decrease of the hemoglobin level. However, in patients with hemolytic anemia, whose erythrocyte lifespan is reduced to 10 to 30 days, even 1 week of aplasia results in profound anemia.

During other viral infections, patients with hemolytic anemias may have decreased numbers of reticulocytes, suggesting some degree of marrow suppression. The resultant decrease in hemoglobin is not as severe as that caused by the parvovirus.

Clinical Manifestations

During aplastic crises, the degree of anemia worsens and jaundice decreases. Profound reticulocytopenia occurs and no erythrocyte precursors exist in the bone marrow. Early in the aplastic crisis, parvovirus particles can be found in the serum by electron microscopic examination. Later evidence of infection can be documented by changes in antibody titers in acute and convalescent sera.

Therapy

Supportive blood transfusions are indicated if the degree of anemia is severe or if the patient is symptomatic. Because parvovirus infections evoke protective levels of circulating antibodies, aplastic crises do not recur in the same patient.

APLASTIC ANEMIAS

The aplastic anemias have diverse causes whose common features are varying degrees of peripheral pancytopenia accompanied by marked hypocellularity of the bone marrow.

Acquired Aplastic Anemia

Pathophysiology

In many instances, aplastic anemia is believed to be a result of destruction or dysfunction of the pluripotential stem cell (CFU-S) that is the progenitor of erythrocytes, platelets, monocytes, and granulocytes. An environmental toxin or agent is believed to cause the stem cell damage, but in as many as one-third of patients, aplastic anemia appears to be an autoimmune disorder mediated through an inhibitory process involving T lymphocytes. Other mechanisms, such as an abnormal microenvironment for bone marrow proliferation, have been postulated.

Many drugs, infections, and environmental factors have been associated with the development of aplastic anemia. Some of these agents are directly toxic to the bone marrow and regularly produce marrow hypoplasia in a dose-dependent manner. Such obligate marrow suppressors include ionizing radiation, a variety of chemicals, and many antineoplastic agents.

Another group of drugs produces marrow hypoplasia in only a small proportion of patients who receive them, so that the disease is considered to represent an idiosyncratic reaction. These include a variety of antibiotics, antiinflammatory agents, and anticonvulsants. Chloramphenicol has been the drug most frequently associated with aplastic anemia. It has been estimated that only approximately 1 in 20,000 to 50,000 persons taking chloramphenicol develops aplastic anemia, but in as many as 50% of the cases of drug-related aplastic anemia, chloramphenicol has been implicated. A particularly serious form of aplastic anemia occurs in the wake of viral hepatitis. In approximately one-half of these patients, no causative factor can be implicated, and their disease is designated *idiopathic*, although an environmental factor cannot be excluded.

Clinical Manifestations

The signs and symptoms of aplastic anemia reflect the degree of pancytopenia at presentation. The most common initial manifestations are petechiae and bruising as a consequence of thrombocytopenia. Pallor and bacterial infections develop as anemia and neutropenia ensue. The spleen, liver, and lymph nodes are not enlarged.

Laboratory Findings

A variable degree of pancytopenia is found at diagnosis. Platelet counts are moderately to severely reduced (5,000 to 50,000/μL). A moderate to severe, usually macrocytic anemia (hemoglobin of 3 to 10 g/dL; mean corpuscular volume greater than 90 fL) with low reticulocyte counts (less than 0.1%) and neutropenia (absolute neutrophil count less than 1,500/μL) are observed at the time of diagnosis or develop within a few months.

Diagnosis is established by examination of the bone marrow by aspiration and biopsy. The marrow is hypocellular because of a loss of hematopoietic elements. Megakaryocytes are reduced and fat is increased. Bone marrow cultures reveal a marked reduction of progenitor cells of erythroid, granulocytic, and megakaryocytic lines.

The disease is classified as severe if two of the following three peripheral blood value abnormalities occur in combination with severe hypocellularity of the marrow biopsy: neutrophil count of less than 500/μl, platelet count of less than 20,000/μL, and a corrected reticulocyte count of less than 1%.

Therapy

Anemia and thrombocytopenia may require transfusions of erythrocytes and platelets. These should be used sparingly to prevent isoimmunization that could compromise future bone marrow transplantation. If an HLA-compatible sibling is available, bone marrow transplantation is the preferred treatment. The survival rate after bone marrow transplantation for young, untransfused patients with aplastic anemia is between 85% and 95%. Because the patient is already aplastic, reduction in the conditioning before bone marrow transplantation has allowed most patients to avoid serious long-term side effects, including infertility. Clinical trials with various hematopoietic colony-stimulating factors have been unsuccessful. The use of HLA-incompatible marrow transplantation has been attempted with success in a few patients.

In patients who do not have an HLA-compatible sibling as a donor, various forms of immunosuppressive therapy have been used, including injections of horse or sheep antithymocyte or antilymphocyte globulin, high-dose methylprednisone, granulocyte colony-stimulating factor (G-CSF), and cyclophosphamide. Response rates as high as 50% to 60% have been reported. Androgens have been ineffective in severe aplastic anemia but may produce a degree of hematologic improvement in patients with moderate disease. However, there is a significant risk of myelodysplasia developing years after successful immunosuppressive therapy in these patients.

Congenital Aplastic Anemia

Congenital aplastic anemia (CAA) (Fanconi syndrome, constitutional aplastic anemia) was first described by Professor Fanconi in Switzerland in 1927. More than 600 cases have been reported in many ethnic groups. Although CAA is genetically determined and transmitted as an autosomal recessive disorder, it is not usually hematologically evident during infancy and early childhood. Clinical CAA is characterized by severe pancytopenia, hypoplasia of the bone marrow, and a constellation of physical abnormalities. Some patients do not have obvious physical anomalies.

Pathophysiology

CAA is believed to be caused by an ill-defined defect in DNA that renders the patient's cells susceptible to damage by environmental agents. This sensitivity may predispose the patient to bone marrow failure.

The cells of these patients demonstrate abnormal mitotic divisions in tissue culture, which is evident in phytohemagglutinin-stimulated lymphocyte cultures. Structural abnormalities include chromatid breaks, exchanges, and gaps and endoreduplication. These occur in more than 10% of metaphases. Other cell culture lines from these patients, including skin fibroblasts, show similar changes, making prenatal diagnosis possible.

Clinical Manifestations

Short stature and generalized hyperpigmentation affect most patients. Approximately one-half of the patients with CAA have congenital skeletal anomalies. The most striking of these includes bilateral absence or hypoplasia of the thumb, sometimes accompanied by abnormalities of the radii. Approximately one-third of patients have renal abnormalities, including unilateral aplasia and horseshoe kidney. Approximately 50% of patients have no gross anatomic abnormalities.

The onset of progressive bone marrow failure is initially manifested by petechiae and ecchymosis secondary to thrombocytopenia between 2 and 22 years of age (mean age, 7). Anemia and neutropenia develop somewhat later than does thrombocytopenia.

Laboratory Findings

Disordered erythropoiesis is manifested by macrocytosis (mean corpuscular volume greater than 90 fL) and elevated levels of fetal hemoglobin before the onset of marrow failure. Ultimately, severe pancytopenia develops. Serial bone marrow examinations show progressive hypocellularity and ultimately frank aplasia. The peripheral blood lymphocytes, when cultured in the presence of diepoxybutane, an alkylating agent, consistently show chromosomal abnormalities. This is a useful test when the physical stigmata of Fanconi anemia are absent.

Treatment

Supportive therapy, including transfusions of erythrocytes and platelets, offers only temporary benefit. In the past, approximately three-fourths of these patients died within 2 years of the onset of marrow failure.

Therapy with pharmacologic doses of androgenic hormones produces a hematologic improvement in more than two-thirds of patients. The response to these agents may be sustained for several years, but maintenance therapy is usually necessary. Complications of androgen therapy, including masculinization and liver dysfunction, are common. Ultimately, most patients become refractory to androgens and again require transfusions. Bone marrow transplantation using HLA-compatible siblings who do not themselves have CAA has been successful in many patients.

Long-term complications of the disease and its therapy include androgen-associated hepatic disease and tumors and an increased risk of acute myeloid leukemia and other malignancies.

Suggested Readings

Congenital Hypoplastic Anemia

Alter BP. Childhood red cell aplasia. *Am J Pediatr Hematol Oncol* 1980;2:121.
Glader BE, Backer K. Elevated erythrocyte adenosine deaminase activity in congenital hypoplastic anemia. *N Engl J Med* 1986;309:1486.
Nathan DG, Clark BJ. Erythroid precursors in congenital hypoplastic (Diamond-Blackfan) anemia. *J Clin Invest* 1978;61:489.

Transient Erythroblastic Anemia of Childhood

Wang NC, Mentzer NC. Differentiation of transient erythroblastopenia of childhood from a congenital hypoplastic anemia. *J Pediatr* 1976;88:784.
Wranne L. Transient erythroblastopenia in infancy and childhood. *Scand J Haematol* 1970;7:76.

Aplastic Crisis of Hemolytic Anemias Associated with Parvovirus Infection

Brow T, Anan H. Intrauterine parvovirus infections associated with hydrops fetalis. *Lancet* 1984;2:1033.
Serjeant GR, Topley JM. Outbreak of aplastic crises in sickle cell anemia associated with parvovirus-like agent. *Lancet* 1981;2:595.
Young NS. Parvovirus infection and its treatment. *Clin Exp Immunol* 1996;104:26.

Aplastic Anemias

Brodsky RA, Jones RJ. Aplastic anemia. *Lancet* 2005;365:1647.
Camita BM, Stork R, Thomas ED. Acquired aplastic anemia. *N Engl J Med* 1982;306:645.

Congenital Aplastic Anemia

Alter AP. The bone marrow failure syndromes. In: Nathan DG, Oski FA, eds. *The hematology of infancy and childhood*. Philadelphia: Saunders, 1987:159.
Auerback AD, Adler B, Chaganti RSK. Prenatal and postnatal diagnosis and carrier detection of Fanconi anemia by a cytogenetic method. *Pediatrics* 1981;67:128.
Halperin DS, Grisaru D, Freedman MH, et al. Severe acquired aplastic anemia in children: 11-year experience with bone marrow transplantation and immunosuppressive therapy. *Am J Pediatr Hematol Oncol* 1989;11:304.
Sanders JE, Whitehead J, Storb R, et al. Bone marrow transplantation experience for children with aplastic anemia. *Pediatrics* 1986;77:179.

CHAPTER 293 ■ POLYCYTHEMIA

YVES D. PASTORE AND C. PHILIP STEUBER

Polycythemia is an excess of erythrocytes in relation to blood volume (i.e., erythrocytosis). As blood volumes and hemoglobin levels vary with age, the diagnosis of polycythemia is made when hemoglobin and hematocrit values are greater than two standard deviations above normal, on two independent sets of measures. At any age, if the hematocrit persistently exceeds 60%, the person should be evaluated for polycythemia and its complications.

Traditionally, polycythemic patients are grouped into those with an absolute increase in erythrocytes and those whose hemoglobin or hematocrit values are elevated but who have a normal erythrocyte mass and decreased plasma volume (i.e., relative or spurious polycythemia). Absolute polycythemias can either be primary or secondary. In primary polycythemias, a molecular defect results in an increased sensitivity to circulating cytokines and leads to a proliferation of the erythroid progenitors. In secondary polycythemia, the increased production of red blood cells results from an increase in circulating cytokines, mostly erythropoietin (Epo). Primary and secondary polycythemias can either be congenital or acquired. Box 293.1 lists conditions associated with absolute polycythemias.

PRIMARY POLYCYTHEMIAS

Primary polycythemias are defined as those conditions resulting from acquired or inherited mutations within the hematopoietic progenitors that lead to an increased sensitivity to circulating cytokines.

Polycythemia Vera

Polycythemia vera (PV) is an acquired hematologic stem cell disorder of clonal origin. It is rare in the pediatric population, and very few cases have been described. Common presenting complaints include itching, headache, weakness, and dizziness. Patients appear plethoric and often have elevated blood pressures. Enlargement of the spleen and liver is common. Patients are at risk for thrombosis and hemorrhage. In addition to increased hemoglobin and hematocrit values, peripheral blood findings include moderate thrombocytosis and leukocytosis. These findings, along with an increase in the red blood cell mass, are part of diagnostic criteria developed by the Polycythemia Vera Study Group. Bone marrow specimens are usually hypercellular with increased megakaryocytes. Although there have been a variety of nonrandom cytogenetic abnormalities detected in a few patients at diagnosis, none of them is specific for PV, and their incidence increases with time from diagnosis. Erythropoietin levels are typically low and do not increase in response to phlebotomy. Demonstration of the growth of erythroid progenitors *in vitro* in the absence of erythropoietin (or endogenous erythroid progenitors [EECs]) is considered a hallmark of the disease.

Therapy is directed toward the reduction of the erythrocyte mass through phlebotomy. Hydroxyurea or interferons are currently preferred above radioactive phosphorus or the use of alkylating agents. Phlebotomy to reduce the hematocrit to 45% should be the initial approach for pediatric patients, unless complicating factors contribute to hyperviscosity and vasoocclusive events. The literature on PV patients has suggested that iron deficiency in adults induced by repeated phlebotomies may increase the long-term risk for thrombosis.

BOX 293.1 **Causes and Classification of Polycythemia**

A. Primary polycythemia
   1. Polycythemia vera
   2. Primary familial congenital polycythemia (PFCP)[AD]
B. Secondary polycythemia
   1. Appropriate erythropoietin response
      1.1 Pulmonary disease
      1.2 Congenital heart disease with right-to-left shunt
      1.3 Hemoglobins with increased oxygen affinity[AD]
      1.4 Reduced erythrocyte 2,3-diphosphoglycerate levels[AR or AD]
      1.5 Pickwickian syndrome
      1.6 High-altitude residence
   2. Inappropriate erythropoietin production
      2.1 Tumors
         a. Kidney
         b. Liver
         c. Adrenal gland
         d. Cerebellum
         e. Uterus
         f. Ovary
      2.2 Other renal problems
         a. Cysts
         b. Obstructive uropathy
         c. Bartter syndrome
         d. After renal transplantation
      2.3 Primary or secondary endocrine imbalance
         a. Excess adrenocorticoids
         b. Excess androgens
         c. Growth hormone therapy
      2.4 Abnormal hypoxia response
         a. Chuvash polycythemia[AR]
         b. Von Hippel Lindau disease (some)[a]

AD, autosomal dominant inheritance; AR, autosomal recessive inheritance; a, some patients with Von Hippel-Lindau (VHL) syndrome, an autosomal dominant cancer-predisposition syndrome, develop polycythemia in association with the development of tumors. Some patients with apparently congenital sporadic polycythemias have been found to be homozygous or compound heterozygous for *VHL* mutations.

For this reason, along with the possible consequences of iron deficiency on child development, iron supplementation may be considered in polycythemic pediatric patients requiring regular phlebotomies. Acute myeloid leukemia may develop during the patient's course, and its incidence may be increased by therapy with alkylating agents. Myeloid fibrosis is another possible complication of PV and bone marrow transplantation should be considered for these patients.

Primary Familial Congenital Polycythemia

Primary familial congenital polycythemia (PFCP) is an uncommon cause of polycythemia, but it is still more prevalent than other congenital polycythemic disorders of autosomal dominant inheritance, such as high oxygen affinity hemoglobin disorders. PFCP patients are usually asymptomatic, and the polycythemia is often found incidentally; some complain of mild headache and more rarely of erythromelalgia (paroxysmal burning pain in the skin, accompanied by dusky mottled redness, affecting mostly extremities).

Although recognized as a benign condition, an increased incidence of cardiovascular problems in early adulthood has been observed in some PFCP families. Characteristics for PFCP are (a) autosomal dominant inheritance, (b) an increase in the red blood cell mass without an increase in platelets or leukocytes counts, (c) an absence of splenomegaly, (d) normal vitamin B_{12} levels, (e) normal oxygen dissociation, (f) low serum erythropoietin levels that do not increase after phlebotomy, and (g) in vitro hypersensitivity of erythroid progenitors to erythropoietin. In up to 15% of PFCP families, mutation-causing truncation of the distal, intracytoplasmic portion of the erythropoietin receptor has been found. Phlebotomy may be indicated to relieve symptoms, particularly when the hematocrit exceeds 65%. Other therapeutic interventions typically used in PV have no place in the treatment of PFCP patients.

SECONDARY POLYCYTHEMIA

In secondary polycythemia, the increase in erythrocyte mass is secondary to an increase in circulating cytokines, mostly erythropoietin. Leukocytosis and thrombocytosis do not occur. The increased erythropoietin production may be physiologically appropriate or inappropriate.

Appropriate or compensatory increases in erythrocyte mass are seen in conditions that cause tissue hypoxia and are most often associated with cardiac or pulmonary abnormalities. Chronic sleep apnea can also lead to polycythemia, although it may be more rarely observed in children than in adults. A relative tissue hypoxia may be secondary to decreased oxygen delivery as a result of increased hemoglobin oxygen affinity. Such elevated oxygen affinity is observed in rare congenital disorders such as 2,3 bisphosphoglycerate (2,3 BPG) deficiency, methemoglobinemias, and high oxygen affinity hemoglobin mutants. An increase in P_{50}, corresponding to the oxygen pressure at which the hemoglobin is 50% saturated, is diagnostic of such disorders. P_{50} can be estimated using the oxygen saturation and the oxygen tension of a venous blood gas. With the exception of very rare cases of 2,3 BPG deficiency, most conditions associated with increased P_{50} are of autosomal dominant inheritance.

Inappropriate secretion of erythropoietin has been associated with a variety of benign and malignant tumors, renal abnormalities, and endocrine imbalances caused by exogenous excess of various hormones. Erythrocytosis is a complication observed in up to 14% of patients after renal transplantation. Intoxication with cobalt is a rare cause of polycythemia with increased serum erythropoietin. Congenital abnormalities in the hypoxia-sensing pathway may also lead to an inappropriately increased erythropoietin production. For example, Chuvash polycythemia is an autosomal recessive polycythemic disorder endemic in the Chuvash Republic in Russia. It is characterized by a normal to high serum erythropoietin, which typically increases after phlebotomy. A high mortality due to thrombosis is observed. This disorder is caused by a homozygous mutation in the Von Hippel-Lindau (VHL) tumor suppressor gene. Homozygosity or compound heterozygosity mutations in the VHL gene also have been found in patients with apparently sporadic congenital polycythemia and elevated serum erythropoietin, and may represent the most common genetic defect for congenital polycythemia. Therefore, VHL mutations should be sought in cases of polycythemia and elevated serum erythropoietin without apparent explanation.

The physical examination of patients with secondary polycythemia reveals a ruddy complexion, some conjunctival suffusion, and sporadic optic vein enlargement. In contrast to polycythemia vera, enlargement of the spleen and liver is not a common feature, except in some patients with congestive heart failure.

After the elimination of easily recognizable causes, the evaluation of the child with polycythemia should include measurement of the erythrocyte mass, Po_2, determination of the oxygen pressure at which the hemoglobin is 50% saturated (P_{50}), serum and urine erythropoietin levels, and a radiologic assessment of the genitourinary tract. Efforts to obtain blood count on first-degree relatives should also be made, as the finding of other affected family members should point to inherited conditions. If the erythrocyte mass is elevated for the patient's age, a reduced arterial oxygen pressure reading should prompt a search for causes of hypoxemia. If the P_{50} is decreased, a hemoglobin profile should be performed, as well as measurement of 2,3 BPG. By definition, patients with secondary polycythemia have elevated erythropoietin levels, although in patients with high oxygen affinity hemoglobin, the erythropoietin level may normalize.

Because renal abnormalities are a common cause of increased erythropoietin production, anatomic investigation is warranted early in the evaluation using ultrasonography, computed tomography, magnetic resonance imaging, or intravenous pyelography. An evaluation of the brain by magnetic resonance imaging should also be considered, as polycythemia may be observed in association with intracranial lesions, such as cerebellar hemangioblastomas.

Treatment of secondary polycythemia is directed at elimination or correction of the primary or underlying cause. When this is not possible, prevention of vasoocclusive episodes may be accomplished by periodic phlebotomy designed to keep the hematocrit level at less than 60%. Phlebotomies should be performed with caution in patients with high oxygen affinity hemoglobin though, as they may result in decreased exercise tolerance and anaerobic threshold. Iron deficiency is a complication of chronic phlebotomy and should be prevented or treated.

Relative Polycythemia

Relative polycythemia is a term applied to conditions with elevated hemoglobin and hematocrit values but a normal erythrocyte mass. The apparent or spurious polycythemia is a result of diminished plasma volume. In pediatrics, this loss of fluid (i.e., hemoconcentration) could be associated with decreased fluid intake or increased fluid loss, such as in dehydration secondary to diarrhea or extensive burns. Such polycythemias are usually transient, and are resolved upon appropriate fluid and colloid replacement.

Suggested Readings

Kralovics R, Prchal JT. Congenital and inherited polycythemia. *Curr Opin Pediatr* 2000;12:29.

Pastore YD, Prchal JT. Classification and consequences of polycythemias (erythrocytoses). In: Jelkmann W, Jelkmann W, eds., *Erythropoietin: molecular biology and clinical use.* Johnson City, TN: FP Graham Publishing Co., 2002:245.

Pearson TC, Messinezy M, Westwood N, et al. A polycythemia vera updated: diagnosis, pathobiology, and treatment hematology. *Am Soc Hematol Educ Program* 2000:51.

CHAPTER 294 ■ QUANTITATIVE GRANULOCYTE DISORDERS

DONALD H. MAHONEY, JR.

NEUTROPENIAS

Neutropenia is defined as an absolute decrease in the number of circulatory neutrophils in the blood. The age and race of the child are important variables for the definition of normal values. In the normal newborn, the neutrophil accounts for approximately 60% of the differential count. However, by 2 weeks of age, lymphocytes assume predominance and retain this predominance until approximately 4 years of age. For normal white infants between 2 weeks and 1 year of age, the lower limit of normal for the absolute neutrophil count (ANC) including neutrophils and bands is 1,000 cells/μL. After infancy, an ANC of 1,500 cells/μL is the lower limit. For African American children, the lower limits of normal are 200 to 400 cells/μL less than those for white children. Technical factors such as excessive leukocyte clumping or lengthy delays in performance of leukocyte counts may cause falsely low values.

Classification

The classification of the neutropenias on a pathophysiologic basis has been problematic. Kinetic, biochemical, and functional studies are difficult to perform because of an insufficiency of circulating neutrophils. Most neutropenia states are transient, and some discretion in the choice of investigations is indicated. Chronic neutropenia is defined as having an ANC of less than 500 for more than 6 months. Chronic neutropenia syndromes are rare and are largely characterized on the basis of their clinical features.

As a first step, individual cases may be characterized by the severity of neutropenia. Mild neutropenia may be defined as an ANC of 1,000 to 1,500 cells/μL, moderate neutropenia as an ANC of 500 to 1,000 cells/μL, and severe neutropenia as an ANC of less than 500 cells/μL. This is a functional classification based on a recognized susceptibility for life-threatening infections, especially in children with persistent, severe neutropenia. For the neutropenic child, infection with *Staphylococcus* or with a gram-negative enteric organism is the greatest danger. However, any organism may become a pathogen. Stomatitis, gingivitis, perirectal inflammation, recurrent otitis media, cellulitis, pneumonia, and septicemia are potential clinical complications. On the other hand, these patients do not have an increased susceptibility to viral or parasitic infections.

Using a functional classification scheme, neutropenia of childhood may be categorized as either intrinsic disorders of myeloid production and proliferation or acquired disorders resulting from extrinsic factors, such as infections, drugs, or immune-mediated mechanisms.

Disorders of Production and Proliferation

Reticular dysgenesis is a rare defect of the committed stem cell compartment and is characterized by thymic agenesis, severe neutropenia and lymphopenia, and agammaglobulinemia. Early in life, infants are vulnerable to fatal bacterial and viral infections.

Cyclic neutropenia is a sporadic or autosomal dominant disorder characterized by regular, periodic oscillations in the numbers of circulating neutrophils and is associated with cyclic clinical manifestations. The disease affects both genders. The underlying defect has been shown to be due to a mutation in the neutrophil elastase gene, mapped to chromosome 19p13.3. The mutation appears to increase apoptosis of neutrophil precursors. Cyclic oscillations in bone marrow function result in neutropenia with nadirs at intervals of 19 to 21 days. The specific periodicity is regular and constant for each patient and may be as short as 14 days or as long as 28 to 36 days. A 21-day cycle has been observed in more than 70% of patients. The neutropenia is severe with an ANC of less than 200 cells/μL and may persist for 3 to 10 days, followed by increasing neutrophil counts and normal physical findings. For some patients, neutrophil oscillations may not exceed 1,000 cells/μL and the patient may have the appearance of chronic neutropenia. Oscillations of monocytes, platelets, and reticulocytes also may occur. During the neutropenic phase, patients may suffer with fever, malaise, oral ulcers, stomatitis, pharyngitis, and lymphadenopathy. More serious infections such as mastoiditis, pneumonia, and sepsis have occurred, and an estimated 10% of patients have died from complications of infectious diseases.

The diagnosis is established by serial neutrophil counts obtained over a 6- to 8-week period to establish the periodicity. Bone marrow examinations during periods of neutropenia may show granulocytic hypoplasia or an apparent arrest of maturation. Treatment is symptomatic. Recombinant human granulocyte colony-stimulating factor (G-CSF) produces marked benefits for patients by reducing the duration of neutropenia and substantially decreasing the risk of infection. However, some patients may still experience neutropenic cycles, but of shorter duration.

Severe congenital neutropenia (i.e., infantile genetic agranulocytosis of Kostmann) is a rare autosomal recessive disorder characterized by a failure of terminal differentiation of the myeloid precursor. The ANC is usually less than 200 cells/μL. Monocytosis and eosinophilia are commonly observed. The bone marrow morphology reveals a developmental arrest at the promyelocyte or myelocyte stage. Studies of bone marrow *in vitro* colony-forming units reveal a capacity to produce neutrophilic colonies, but with aberrant cells exhibiting bizarre nuclei, excessive cytoplasm, and decreased granules. Mutations in the neutrophil elastase gene (*ELA-2*) have been observed in more than two-thirds of studied patients, but are more diverse than those observed with cyclic neutropenia.

The clinical presentation is usually one of an acute, life-threatening infection occurring within the first few months of life. Fever, cellulitis, omphalitis, pneumonia, perianal and urinary tract infections, and sepsis have been associated with this disease. Common pathogens include *Staphylococcus aureus, Escherichia coli,* and *Pseudomonas.* Recombinant G-CSF is effective treatment, leading to increased numbers of neutrophils and decreased infectious complications. However, with continued follow-up, the cumulative risk for myelodysplasia and acute myeloid leukemia is 13% at 8 years of G-CSF treatment. Bone marrow transplantation has resulted in partial or complete correction of this disorder.

The Shwachman-Diamond-Oski Syndrome is a rare autosomal recessive disorder characterized by multiorgan dysfunction. The gene locus has been mapped to the centromeric region of chromosome 7. Onset is during infancy with failure to thrive, pancreatic exocrine insufficiency, metaphyseal dysostosis, and eczema. Neutropenia is seen in all patients, but may be intermittent in two-thirds of patients. Anemia, thrombocytopenia, and progressive bone marrow failure are common, and transformation to leukemia has been reported in 12% to 25%.

Several additional clinical syndromes have evidence of ineffective granulopoiesis as a common pathophysiologic characteristic. Nutritional deficiencies of vitamin B_{12} or folic acid, in addition to causing megaloblastic anemia, may be associated with neutropenia. Advanced states of malnutrition, such as anorexia nervosa, marasmus in infants, and copper deficiency, may be complicated by neutropenia. Ineffective myelopoiesis is an important element in the *Chédiak-Higashi syndrome* and in a rare condition described as *myelokathexis.* Increased intramedullary destruction of neutrophils with elevated serum lysozyme levels is part of the clinical spectrum.

Dyskeratosis congenita is an X-linked recessive disease characterized by hyperpigmentation, leukoplakia, nail dystrophy, and, in approximately 35% of the cases, mild neutropenia. *Cartilage-hair hypoplasia* is an autosomal recessive condition associated with short-limbed dwarfism, fine hair, and moderate neutropenia. This condition has been identified frequently in Asian populations. Increased infections and impaired immunologic functions are common complications.

Disorders of immunoglobulin production have been associated with neutropenia syndromes. Patients with X-linked agammaglobulinemia may experience neutropenia during the course of their illness. Dysgammaglobulinemia type I (i.e., no IgA and IgG, normal to elevated IgM) may be associated with periodic or persistent neutropenia. Bacterial infections, failure to thrive, and hepatosplenomegaly may complicate this condition. A syndrome of neutropenia, eczema, polyarthralgia, eosinophilia, and increased IgA levels has been reported. Depressed cellular immunity and an increased risk for infection, including devastating varicella, have been observed with this disease.

Neutropenia may complicate a number of metabolic disorders. Children with hyperglycinemia, isovaleric academia, and methylmalonic academia may have significant neutropenia. High concentrations of these metabolites have been proposed as the causative mechanism for impaired myeloid proliferation. Myelofibrosis may be associated with Gaucher disease. Glycogenesis Ib is an inherited disorder of glycogen metabolism asso-

---

TABLE 294.1

FREQUENTLY RECOGNIZED CAUSES OF ACQUIRED NEUTROPENIA

I. Infection
   A. Viral: hepatitis A and B, varicella, influenza A, measles, rubella, herpes simplex virus, respiratory syncytial virus, cytomegalovirus, infectious mononucleosis, human immunodeficiency virus, parvovirus
   B. Bacterial: overwhelming sepsis, especially group B streptococci, typhoid, paratyphoid, tularemia, brucellosis, tuberculosis
   C. Rickettsial: rickettsialpox, epidemic typhus, scrub typhus, Rocky Mountain spotted fever
   D. Protozoan: malaria, toxoplasmosis
II. Drugs
   A. Antibiotics: penicillins, aminoglycosides, sulfa, trimethoprim-sulfamethoxazole, cephalosporins, amphotericin, dapsone, griseofulvin, streptomycin, nitrofurantoins, chloroquine
   B. Anticonvulsants: trimethadione, phenytoin, barbiturates, valproic acid, clonazepam, carbamazepine, ethosuximide
   C. Antiinflammatory agents: gold, indomethacin, phenylbutazone, ibuprofen, naproxen, aspirin, penicillamine
   D. Miscellaneous: imipramine, thiazides, acetazolamide, quinidine, procaine amide, propranolol, antithyroid agents, phenothiazines
III. Chemical or environmental toxins
   Benzol, benzene, arsenic, thiocyanate, carbon tetrachloride, insecticides (e.g., DDT, chlordane)
   Radiation exposure
IV. Anticancer chemotherapy
V. Bone marrow infiltration
   Leukemia, lymphoma, neuroblastoma, rhabdomyosarcoma, retinoblastoma, primitive neuroectodermal tumor, myelofibrosis, storage disease

DDT, dichlorodiphenyltrichlorothane.

---

ciated with variable neutropenia, abnormal neutrophil motility, and recurrent life-threatening infections. Supportive medical care is the only available therapy for these patients.

Many acquired conditions may be associated with periods of neutropenia (Table 294.1). Infectious diseases are the most common cause of neutropenia in children. The mechanisms responsible for neutropenia include direct marrow suppression, exhaustion of marrow reserves, redistribution of neutrophils from circulating to marginating pools, and neutrophil aggregation and sequestration after complement activation. Increased destruction of neutrophils may occur as a direct result of interactions with pathogens or indirectly as the result of the formation of antineutrophil antibodies. Enterovirus infections, respiratory syncytial virus, influenza A, measles, rubella, varicella, hepatitis A and B, and Epstein-Barr virus are just a few of the more common causes of transient neutropenia. Leukopenia and neutropenia also may be seen with human immunodeficiency virus, typhoid and paratyphoid, tuberculosis, brucellosis, and tularemia. Inflammatory-mediated accelerated destruction of neutrophils may cause neutropenia. Overwhelming bacterial sepsis, especially in the neonate, may directly affect the marrow pool. Depletion of precursor and neutrophil pools and degenerative changes in myelopoiesis may occur. Several investigators have suggested that granulocyte transfusions or recombinant G-CSF in the face of overwhelming bacterial sepsis and profound neutropenia may be lifesaving.

Drug-induced neutropenias are probably the second most common cause of acquired neutropenia in childhood.

Mechanisms of action include direct toxic effects of drugs or metabolites on the bone marrow or the committed stem cells. Induction of an immune response directed at neutrophils also has been implicated.

To list all medications with a potential for producing neutropenia would be an exhaustive exercise. The physician should refer to the product information supplied by the pharmaceutical company when evaluating a neutropenic patient receiving a medication. Idiosyncratic reactions are uncommon but can produce severe neutropenia (ANC less than 500 cells/μL). More commonly, neutropenia may follow extended dosing periods and may be aggravated by underlying genetic or metabolic factors. Certain drugs are conspicuous for their frequency of use and are associated more commonly with episodes of neutropenia. These include antimicrobials, particularly the penicillins, trimethoprim-sulfamethoxazole, and certain classes of cephalosporins; anticonvulsants, such as barbiturates, phenytoin, valproic acid, carbamazepine, clonazepam, and ethosuximide; antiinflammatory agents; cardiovascular agents; and antirheumatic agents. Certain drugs may act in combination to produce myelosuppression. The onset of drug-induced neutropenia is unpredictable, but after neutropenia occurs, the most important therapeutic action is to withdraw all drugs that are not essential, especially those with a significant risk for myelosuppression.

The immune-mediated neutropenias may present as primary disorders or in association with other disorders (secondary). The two classic primary immune neutropenias in childhood are the isoimmune and the autoimmune neutropenias. Isoimmune neutropenia is observed in the neonate and is analogous to Rh sensitization. During gestation, fetal neutrophil antigens, most frequently NA1 and NB1, immunize the mother, resulting in an IgG antibody, which crosses the placenta and destroys the infant's neutrophils. At birth, severe neutropenia, monocytosis, and, occasionally, eosinophilia are observed. Although usually asymptomatic, infants may suffer from cutaneous infections or more serious complications such as sepsis. By 6 to 7 weeks, the neutrophil counts usually have returned to normal. Treatment varies according to symptoms. Some responses to high doses of intravenous gammaglobulin have been seen and G-CSF has been used in selected cases where there has been a heightened concern for infection.

Autoimmune neutropenia (AIN), also recognized as chronic benign neutropenia of infancy and childhood, is the most common cause of chronic neutropenia in young children. The disorder frequently presents in the 6- to 36-month-old child and frequently may be confused with idiopathic chronic neutropenia. Antibodies of IgG, IgM, or IgA class, directed against specific neutrophil antigens (e.g., NA1, NA2, NB1), can be detected by direct or indirect immunofluorescent assays in most patients and are proposed mediators of peripheral destruction of circulatory neutrophils. Patients may generate these autoantibodies for no apparent reason or in response to certain infections (e.g., mononucleosis), drugs (e.g., penicillins), or in association with certain inflammatory diseases (e.g., rheumatoid arthritis, systemic lupus erythematosus, chronic active hepatitis). The clinical presentation frequently follows a blood count performed in a febrile but otherwise asymptomatic child. Hemoglobin and platelet counts are normal. Some children may experience an increased incidence of otitis media or minor skin infections. Less than 12% of children may have more serious infections. Bone marrow examinations may show maturation arrest. Treatment is primarily supportive care. Corticosteroids and high-dose intravenous gammaglobulin have been of value in selected cases. Most children with autoimmune neutropenia require no intervention and recover without specific therapy. Occasional patients may benefit from G-CSF.

As compared to AIN, *chronic idiopathic neutropenia* is a nonfamilial disorder of variable clinical and laboratory presentation. This condition usually presents in the older child.

The total leukocyte count is usually normal. However, the neutrophil numbers fluctuate between fewer than 500 cells and 1,000 cells/μL. The risk of infection is proportional to the degree of neutropenia. Bone marrow morphology usually reveals an adequate number of myeloid precursors associated with an apparent arrest at the metamyelocyte or band stage. Studies of bone marrow *in vitro* colony-forming units have suggested decreased or ineffective production of neutrophils in some patients. In the mild form of disease, a neutrophilic response may be observed in the peripheral blood during the course of infection or in response to an endotoxin challenge. Children with the mild form generally do not experience serious complications with infection. Spontaneous remissions have been reported to occur in children 2 to 4 years after presentation.

Familial benign chronic neutropenia is an autosomal dominant disorder characterized by mild to moderate degrees of neutropenia and minimal symptoms. This disorder has been observed in successive generations of Yemenite Jews and in families from Germany, France, the United States, and South Africa. The illness is usually benign, and treatment usually is not indicated.

Evaluation

A complete history and physical examination are the essential first steps in the evaluation of a child presenting with neutropenia. The history should include a summary of the recent infections, medications, and possible toxic exposures for the child; race and ethnic background, including phenotypic abnormalities; and family medical history for any member with recurrent infections or unexplained deaths in infants younger than 1 year. The physical examination should include an assessment of nutritional status and a search for signs of skin or mucous membrane infections, gingival inflammation, lymphadenopathy, and hepatosplenomegaly. Evaluation for skeletal or cutaneous phenotypic abnormalities is important. The initial laboratory examination should include a complete blood count, with platelets and reticulocytes, to exclude other cytopenias.

In the acutely ill child with fever, severe neutropenia (ANC less than 500 cells/μL), and/or anemia and thrombocytopenia, a bone marrow aspirate and biopsy may aid in the diagnosis by establishing the extent of marrow neutrophil reserves and by excluding the possibility of a malignant infiltration or marrow failure syndromes. In the asymptomatic patient, clinical observation is appropriate with a bone marrow examination pursued at a later date. In patients with a persistent neutropenia, a leukocyte count should be obtained at twice-weekly intervals for 6 to 8 weeks to determine the periodicity. Further evaluation beyond this point should be dictated by the clinical impression. In infants, quantitative immunoglobulins, T- and B-cell functions, exocrine pancreatic function tests, and specific antineutrophil antibody assays may help in differentiating the more common causes of chronic neutropenia. In the older child, screening for collagen-vascular disorders, paroxysmal nocturnal hemoglobinuria (PNH), folate, vitamin B_{12}, copper, and metabolic deficiency states are appropriate.

Treatment

The management of children with neutropenia must be linked to the presumed diagnosis. Children with fever (with or without specific presenting signs of infection) and with acute-onset (i.e., primary) neutropenia of unknown cause or associated with the diagnosis or treatment of a malignant condition or bone marrow failure syndrome require immediate medical attention. In these circumstances, a substantial risk exists of acute, overwhelming bacterial sepsis. Hospitalization with cultures of blood, urine, and respiratory secretions and prompt initiation of broad-spectrum intravenous antibiotics are indicated. If cultures fail to yield a pathogen and clinical investigations fail to document evidence of bacterial infection, antibiotics may be discontinued 3 days after the patient has become afebrile.

For the child with AIN and adequate marrow reserves, management recommendations are less clear. The asymptomatic patient requires no specific medical intervention. Good oral hygiene and skin care are important preventive measures. For an ill-appearing child with sustained fever greater than 101°F or chills or both, our usual practice is to examine the child for signs of infection, repeat the leukocyte count, and, if the ANC value is less than 500 cells/μL, obtain a blood culture and administer a dose of parenteral broad-spectrum antibiotics. If the patient appears toxic, hospitalization is recommended; otherwise, cautious follow-up as an outpatient is appropriate. For the patient with an ANC of 500 to 1,000 cells/μL, clinical discretion must be exercised.

Symptomatic patients with severe chronic neutropenia may benefit from a trial of recombinant G-CSF. Prophylactic trimethoprim-sulfamethoxazole schedules may be of some value in patients with severe congenital neutropenia or in patients undergoing cancer chemotherapy, but can also be myelosuppressive when used over long time periods.

NEUTROPHILIA

Neutrophilia may result from an increased mobilization of neutrophils from marrow storage compartments or marginating pools, from impaired egress of neutrophils into tissue, or from accelerated proliferation of myeloid progenitor cells.

Increased mobilization of neutrophils from marrow compartments may follow acute stress events, such as acute infection, anesthesia, electrical shock, abrupt temperature changes, hypoxia, or endotoxin exposure. Endogenous release of epinephrine and glucocorticoids under stress conditions mediates the release of neutrophils from storage sites. The administration of pharmacologic doses of glucocorticoids mimics this state.

Increased granulopoiesis and neutrophilia are most frequently the result of acute infections, especially by pyogenic organisms. Profound neutrophilia with a shift to the left involving immature myeloid cells (i.e., a leukemoid reaction) may occur with infections and with other conditions (Table 294.2).

EOSINOPHILIA

Eosinophilia is usually defined as an absolute eosinophil count in excess of 500 cells/μL. Allergy is the most common cause of eosinophilia in children in the United States. Children with bronchial asthma, recurrent urticaria, infantile eczema, serum sickness, and angioneurotic edema often have evidence of eosinophilia. However, symptoms do not directly correlate with the degree of eosinophilia. Children with allergic rhinitis have eosinophils in their nasal secretions.

Eosinophilia may be associated with chronic inflammatory diseases of the bowel, including Crohn disease; tumors such as Hodgkin disease; and immune deficiency syndromes, especially Wiskott-Aldrich syndrome.

Parasitic infections are the most common cause of eosinophilia outside of the United States. Careful examination of freshly collected feces for evidence of ova or larval forms confirms the diagnosis in most cases. Visceral larva migrans, secondary to *Toxocara canis* or *T. cati*, is probably the most common cause for hypereosinophilic syndromes in children. Patients are usually asymptomatic, but some may have fever, occasional wheezing, hepatomegaly, anemia, and hyperglobulinemia. Retinal lesions may be indistinguishable from

TABLE 294.2

DISORDERS ASSOCIATED WITH LEUKEMOID REACTIONS

Infections
Pyogenic bacteria
Tuberculosis
Brucellosis
Toxoplasmosis
Leptospirosis
Viral (acute phase): herpes simplex, varicella, rabies, poliomyelitis, mononucleosis
Kawasaki disease

Chronic inflammatory conditions
Rheumatoid arthritis
Polyserositis

Tumor invasion
Lymphoma
Rhabdomyosarcoma
Neuroblastoma
Retinoblastoma

Drug reaction
Lithium
Glucocorticoids

Others
Acute glomerulonephritis
Acute liver failure
Functional asplenia
Diabetic acidosis
Disorders of neutrophil motility [LFA-1 deficiency (associated with the leukocyte adhesion deficiency syndrome)]
Transient myeloproliferative syndrome in neonatal Down syndrome

LFA-1, lymphocyte function–associated antigen 1.

retinoblastoma lesions. A leukemoid reaction with counts of 100,000 cells/μL and 80% to 90% mature eosinophils may occur. The diagnosis cannot be established from stool analysis. Increased isohemagglutinins directed against group A and B substances on erythrocytes and specific serologic tests are necessary to confirm the diagnosis. Specific treatment is usually not

TABLE 294.3

CAUSES OF EOSINOPHILIA IN CHILDREN

Allergic disorders
Asthma, atopic eczema, urticaria, hay fever, drug reactions

Infections
Parasitic infections: *Ascaris*, trichinosis, *Echinococcus*, bookworm, *Strongyloides*, filariasis, *Toxocara*, *Pneumocystis carinii*, malaria, amebiasis
Nonparasitic infections: scarlet fever, tuberculosis, histoplasmosis

Skin disorders
Pemphigus, toxic epidermal necrolysis

Tumors
Hodgkin disease, myeloproliferative syndromes

Hereditary causes
Idiopathic hypereosinophilic syndrome

Miscellaneous disorders characterized by chronic inflammation
Chronic hepatitis, regional enteritis, rheumatoid arthritis, periarteritis nodosa, peritoneal dialysis

needed. Numerous conditions that also may produce transient eosinophilia are outlined in Table 294.3.

MONOCYTOSIS AND BASOPHILIA

Monocytosis is an unusual finding in children. Absolute monocyte numbers in normal persons range from 300 to 800 cells/μL. Infection with intracellular microorganisms or parasites is the most common cause of monocytosis. Infections include malaria, trypanosomiasis, leishmaniasis, rickettsial disease, and *Listeria monocytogenes*. Persistent monocytosis with abnormal forms may precede a variety of lymphoproliferative and histiocytic disorders, such as Hodgkin disease and juvenile myelomonocytic leukemia. Monocytosis is associated frequently with granulocytopenic states.

Suggested Readings

Bux J, Behrens G, Jaeger G, et al. Diagnosis and clinical course of autoimmune neutropenia in infancy: analysis of 240 cases. *Blood* 1998;91:181.

Dale DC, Bolyard AA, Aprikyan A. Cyclic neutropenia. *Semin Hematol* 2002; 39:89.

Dale DC, Cottle TE, Fier CJ, et al. Severe chronic neutropenia: treatment and follow-up of patients in the severe chronic neutropenia international registry. *Am J Hematol* 2003;72:82.

Dale DC, Person RE, Bolyard AA, et al. Mutations in the gene encoding neutrophil elastase in congenital and cyclic neutropenia. *Blood* 2000;96: 2317.

Dinaur MC. The phagocytic system and disorders of granulopoiesis and granulocyte function. In: Nathan DG, Orkin SH, Ginsburg D, et al., eds. *Nathan and Oski's hematology of infancy and childhood*, 6th ed. Philadelphia: Saunders, 2003;923.

Dror Y. Shwachman-Diamond syndrome: a review. *Brit J Hematol* 2002;118: 701.

CHAPTER 295 ■ THE SPLEEN AND LYMPH NODES

RICHARD H. SILLS

The spleen and lymph nodes are the major components of the mononuclear-phagocyte system (MPS), serving as a filter removing damaged cells and particulate matter, and delivering antigens to the immune system. The MPS, originally called the reticuloendothelial system, consists of fixed phagocytic cells in different organs. These cells share a common derivation from circulating blood monocytes. Functionally, these phagocytes interact locally with lymphocytes and play an essential role in the recognition of antigens and their interaction with immunocompetent cells. The MPS constitutes a crucial component of our immunologic defense mechanisms.

Although components of the MPS occur in most tissues, they are particularly dense in the spleen and lymph nodes. The specialized filtering capabilities of these organs provide ideal locations for contact between antigens and the immune system. Macrophages perching on endothelial cells and reticulum fibers assume the role of immunologic sentries and are vital in initiating host response.

THE SPLEEN

Anatomy

The spleen is the largest lymph node in the body. Its anatomy provides for uniquely close contact between its immunologic tissues and blood. The splenic tissue consists of red and white pulp lying within a capsule (Fig. 295.1). The white pulp, rich in T- and B-cell lymphocytes, is supplied by central arterioles. These vessels tend to branch at right angles, resulting in the preferable skimming of plasma into the white pulp for antigen processing. The main terminal splenic arteries, which contain the remaining hemoconcentrated blood, continue directly forward into the contiguous red pulp.

The red pulp is the majority of splenic tissue, consisting of splenic cords that interdigitate between splenic venous sinusoids. At least 90% of the hemoconcentrated blood reaching

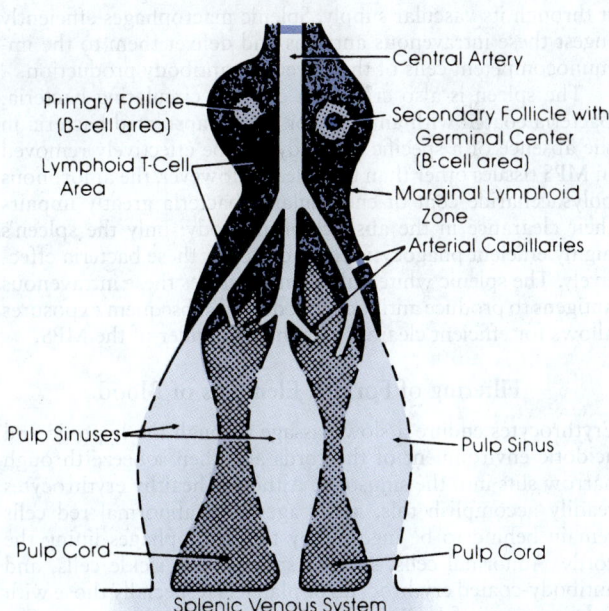

FIGURE 295.1. The spleen is composed of multiple units of red and white pulp surrounding small branches of the splenic artery called *central arteries*. The white pulp areas of the spleen are lymphoid. Within the white pulp, B cells primarily occupy the follicular zones, and T cells predominate around the follicles and the arterial capillaries. Antigenic stimulation causes primary follicles to become secondary follicles with germinal centers. Most of the circulation to the red pulp enters the pulp cords and reaches the pulp sinuses through the basement membrane fenestrations. (Modified from Hayes B. Enlargement of lymph nodes and spleen. In: Braunwald E, Isselbacher KJ, Petersdorf RG, et al., eds. *Harrison's principles of internal medicine.* New York: McGraw-Hill, 1987:276.)

the red pulp enters these splenic cords, which contain a fibrous network of mononuclear-phagocyte tissue. The circulation in the cords is designated as *open* because there is no well-defined endothelial lining. The cords lie between and share a basement membrane with the adjacent splenic venous sinuses. To exit the cords, blood must pass through 1- to 5-μm slits in this fenestrated basement membrane to reach the sinuses. The circulation through the cords is slow and congested because the blood reaching the red pulp is hemoconcentrated, and erythrocytes require additional time to pass through the small and limited number of slits that must be traversed to reach the sinuses. This delay provides prolonged exposure of blood cells, bacteria, and particulate matter to the dense mononuclear-phagocyte elements within the red pulp. This anatomic arrangement and the fact that the spleen (with an average weight of only 180 g in adults) receives approximately 6% of cardiac output provide a tremendous filtration capability.

After blood reaches the sinuses, it passes into the splenic venous system. Blood from the sinuses enters trabecular veins and eventually the hepatic portal vein; there are no valves in this system, which remains at the same pressure as the hepatic portal vein.

Physiology

Although none of the spleen's individual cells is unique, its distinctive anatomic arrangement provides it with characteristic functional capabilities.

Resistance to Infection

The spleen plays a major role in the processing of small doses of intravenous particulate and polysaccharide antigens that reach it through its vascular supply. Splenic macrophages efficiently ingest these intravenous antigens and deliver them to the immunocompetent cells of the spleen for antibody production.

The spleen is also critical in clearing circulating bacteria. Bacteria coated with antibody or nonencapsulated bacteria in the absence of a specific antibody can be effectively removed in MPS tissues other than the spleen. However, the amorphous polysaccharide coat of encapsulated bacteria greatly impairs their clearance in the absence of antibody; only the spleen's highly efficient phagocytic cords can clear these bacteria effectively. The splenic white pulp then processes these intravenous antigens to produce antibody that during subsequent exposures allows for efficient clearance by the remainder of the MPS.

Filtering of Formed Elements of Blood

Erythrocytes endure a slow passage through the hypoxic and acidotic environment of the cords and then squeeze through narrow slits into the sinusoids. Although healthy erythrocytes readily accomplish this, many aged and abnormal red cells remain behind to be ingested by the macrophages lining the cords. Abnormal cells, such as spherocytes, sickle cells, and antibody-coated erythrocytes or platelets (especially those with light coatings of IgG), are mainly cleared by the spleen. The splenic cords are also uniquely capable of removing erythrocytic inclusions, such as nuclear remnants (i.e., Howell-Jolly bodies) or precipitated globin (i.e., Heinz bodies), without destroying the cell.

Other Functions of the Spleen

Other splenic functions include remodeling of reticulocytes, hematopoiesis during early fetal development, and a reservoir function for platelets and plasma proteins such as factor VIII. Its function as a reservoir for erythrocytes is insignificant except in pathologic states such as hypersplenism.

Physical Examination of the Spleen

The spleen is best palpated by standing on the right side of the child and examining the left side of the abdomen with the right hand. The child should be examined in the supine or right lateral decubitus position with the knees up. Only light pressure should be used in small children because the spleen can easily be pushed out of the way without feeling its edge.

A palpable spleen is not unusual in normal children. A 1- to 2-cm spleen tip is palpable below the left costal margin in 30% of full-term neonates and in as many as 10% of normal children. Almost 3% of healthy college freshman have palpable spleens. The normal, palpable spleen tip is soft and nontender. A spleen tip enlarged beyond 1 to 2 cm should be considered abnormal.

The spleen can usually be differentiated from other left upper quadrant masses by the absence of overlying bowel and its movement with respiration. It may occasionally be confused with the left lobe of the liver or a left upper quadrant tumor such as Wilms tumor or neuroblastoma. In the presence of any doubt, ultrasonography can usually define the anatomy.

Excessive Splenic Function

Splenomegaly

Splenomegaly is the most frequent and important clinical problem involving the spleen. The most common causes of splenic enlargement are listed in Box 295.1. Splenomegaly in children usually results from hyperplasia of the MPS, which can be categorized as excessive antigenic stimulation, disorders of immunoregulation, or excessive destruction of abnormal blood cells. The spleen is rarely the primary site of disease, usually being affected by a systemic process involving lymphoid tissues.

Excessive antigenic stimulation is usually the result of infection, which causes most splenomegaly in children. Viral infections do this most frequently, and the associated splenomegaly is usually transient and only mild to moderate in severity. Although Epstein-Barr virus and cytomegalovirus are the best known viral agents to cause splenomegaly, the more routine viral illnesses of childhood cause it more frequently. A less common but important cause of splenic enlargement is acquired immune deficiency syndrome. Other common infectious causes include bacterial, protozoal, and fungal infections. In endemic areas, malaria and schistosomiasis are routine causes of splenomegaly. Concomitant generalized lymphadenopathy is common in many of these infectious causes.

Disorders that result in the effective destruction of blood cells or that affect immunoregulation are less common causes of splenomegaly.

Neoplastic disorders may also present with splenomegaly. One-half of children with acute lymphoblastic leukemia have splenomegaly, which also occurs in the lymphomas (both Hodgkin disease and non-Hodgkin lymphoma) and acute myeloblastic leukemia. Metastatic involvement of the spleen, which is uncommon in children, is most often caused by neuroblastoma. The spleen can also be infiltrated by histiocytes, a condition in children that usually is caused by Langerhans cell histiocytosis.

Impaired venous blood flow in the splenic or portal venous system can cause splenomegaly. The most common causes include cavernous transformation of the portal vein, hepatic cirrhosis, and congestive heart failure. Children with extrahepatic portal venous obstruction, such as cavernous transformation, often present with splenomegaly as the primary manifestation of their disease.

BOX 295.1	Causes of Splenomegaly in Children

Hyperplasia of the monocyte-phagocyte system
Excessive antigenic stimulation
  Viral infections
    Infectious mononucleosis
    Cytomegalovirus
    Acquired immunodeficiency syndrome
  Bacterial infections
    Septicemia
    Endocarditis
    Salmonella
  Protozoal infections
    Toxoplasmosis
    Malaria
  Fungal infections
    Histoplasmosis
Disorders of immunoregulation
    Juvenile rheumatoid arthritis
    Systemic lupus erythematosus
    Serum sickness
Excessive destruction of blood cells
    Hereditary spherocytosis
    Sickle cell disease
    Neonatal Rh or ABO incompatibility

Neoplastic infiltration
    Acute leukemias
    Hodgkin disease
    Non-Hodgkin lymphoma
    Neuroblastoma
    Histiocytoses
    Benign tumors

Disordered splenic blood flow
    Cavernous transformation of the portal vein
    Hepatic cirrhosis
    Congestive heart failure

Infiltration with abnormal material
    Gaucher disease
    Niemann-Pick disease

Space-occupying lesions
    Hematomas
    Pseudocysts
    Congenital cysts

Extramedullary hematopoiesis
    Thalassemia major
    Osteopetrosis

Storage diseases such as Gaucher or Niemann-Pick disease are associated with splenomegaly because of the accumulation of abnormal lipids in splenic macrophages. Splenomegaly may be the first clinical manifestation of these disorders.

After trauma, palpable subcapsular hematomas may develop in the spleen. These hematomas may eventually develop into clinically palpable pseudocysts. Congenital splenic cysts usually present with asymptomatic splenomegaly.

Although normally only found during early fetal development, extramedullary hematopoiesis may occur in diseases associated with intense demand on the bone marrow for cell production. Thalassemia major and osteopetrosis are examples of this rare cause of splenomegaly.

Hypersplenism

Hypersplenism is a clinical syndrome in which splenic function becomes excessive as the spleen and its MPS tissues enlarge. It is defined by the following criteria: splenomegaly, a deficiency of at least one or more of the peripheral blood cell lines, normal or increased levels of bone marrow precursors, and an expectation that splenectomy will resolve the cytopenias. As the spleen enlarges, it can sequester erythrocytes, leucocytes, and platelets, resulting in decreases in some or all of these cell lines.

The most common cause of hypersplenism is venous obstruction. Because of the absence of valves in the portal venous system, an increase in portal pressure is reflected immediately in the splenic venous sinuses. This impairs blood flow out of the cords and results in the sequestration of blood cells and hypersplenism. Hypersplenism in children most often is caused by portal hypertension due to extrahepatic venous obstruction, often secondary to thrombosis of the portal vein caused by umbilical venous catheterization, septic omphalitis, or thrombosis because of dehydration or shock. Intrahepatic venous obstruction is usually due to cirrhosis. Schistosomiasis and malaria are important causes in endemic areas.

Children with hypersplenism can present with simple fatigue, pallor, and irritability or with unexplained splenomegaly. Portal hypertension increases flow through minor collateral vessels between the portal and systemic circulation. This can result in recognizable dilation of the superficial abdominal veins as well as esophageal varices. These varices may present with sudden and catastrophic gastrointestinal hemorrhage. Esophagoscopy is the most accurate means for confirming esophageal varices.

Therapy of hypersplenism depends on the site, nature, and severity of the vascular obstruction. Splenectomy cures the pancytopenia, but it is usually not indicated because the pancytopenia rarely causes serious problems. However, vascular shunts may be necessary to prevent esophageal variceal bleeding.

Hypersplenism occurs less frequently as a result of splenomegaly in the absence of venous obstruction, as in infections such as malaria and storage diseases such as Gaucher disease.

The splenic sequestration crisis is a distinct form of acute hypersplenism in young children with sickle cell disease. These children may develop sudden and massive splenic enlargement with sequestration of large portions of blood volume. They present with sudden weakness, dyspnea, left-sided abdominal pain, and increasing splenomegaly. So much blood can be trapped within the spleen that death due to hypovolemia can rapidly result. Treatment consists of restoration of blood volume and transfusion. To prevent recurrences, splenectomy may be indicated.

Impairment of Splenic Function

Causes

Hyposplenism may be anatomic (e.g., absence of splenic tissue), functional (e.g., impaired function despite an intact spleen), or a combination of both. The most common causes of hyposplenism in children are surgical splenectomy, sickle cell disease, and congenital absence of the spleen. The functional hyposplenism of sickle cell disease is readily understood in physiologic terms. The hypoxic and acidotic conditions in the splenic cords are ideal for inducing sickling. Once sickled, the erythrocytes are less able to pass from the cords to the sinuses. Splenic circulation becomes so obstructed that splenic function is gradually lost in most patients in the first 2 to 3 years of life.

Conditions associated with acquired hyposplenism include inflammatory bowel disease, systemic lupus erythematosus, immune complex glomerulonephritis, splenic irradiation, graft-versus-host disease, and adult celiac disease. Normal neonates may demonstrate impaired splenic function as a developmental phenomenon, although its clinical significance is not known.

Diagnosis

Hyposplenism is usually suspected because of the occurrence of a disorder known to cause it. Less commonly, it is detected because of the incidental recognition of erythrocyte inclusions that accumulate in the absence of normal splenic clearance. These inclusions, which include Howell-Jolly bodies, nucleated erythrocytes, and Heinz bodies, are not pathognomonic of hyposplenism. The best studies to specifically evaluate splenic function are technetium (Tc)-99m sulfur colloid radionuclide scanning, which readily labels a functioning spleen, and the observation of increased erythrocytic vesicles using interference contrast microscopy.

Consequences and Treatment

The primary consequence of impaired splenic function is overwhelming bacterial septicemia. In the absence of effective splenic clearance, intravascular bacteria reproduce so rapidly that overwhelming septicemia results. The causative encapsulated bacteria are most often *Streptococcus pneumoniae*, followed in frequency by *Haemophilus influenzae* and *Neisseria meningitidis*.

The overall risk of septicemia in asplenic patients averages 2%, but is very variable. Very young children are at the greatest risk for hyposplenia-related septicemia because they have had less prior exposure to these bacteria and are less likely to produce protective antibody when exposed. The risk of septicemia is twice as great for children younger than 4 years of age, and is 30% or higher in the first year of life. The risk is also increased when there are concurrent immunologic or MPS deficits, as with sickle cell anemia, thalassemia major, or Hodgkin disease. The risk of septicemia in these groups is 7% or more, compared with a risk of less than 2% for those undergoing splenectomy for trauma.

Affected children most often present with high fever without an obvious source of infection. They quickly appear ill and become confused and irritable. Meningitis, purpura, and disseminated intravascular coagulation are common. Septic shock and death can occur within 4 to 6 hours from the onset of symptoms. The mortality rate is 30% to 50%. Unfortunately, initially differentiating overwhelming septicemia from the routine febrile viral illness of childhood is usually impossible.

The most important aspect of treatment is prevention, which includes prophylactic penicillin, immunization against *S. pneumoniae* and *H. influenzae*, and education. Significant febrile episodes should be urgently treated with high-dose intravenous antibiotics. If treatment of febrile episodes is withheld until the patient looks very ill, the chance of death is very high. The family must understand the importance of complying with antibiotic prophylaxis and seeking immediate medical attention when the child is febrile.

Structural Abnormalities of the Spleen

Congenital Malformations

Accessory Spleens. One or more accessory spleens are found in 15% of the population. Averaging only 1 to 2 cm in diameter, they are identified with radionuclide scanning using Tc-99m sulfur colloid. Accessory spleens are inconsequential except when they are not removed during splenectomy to treat disorders requiring this procedure. Postoperative hypertrophy

of the accessory spleen can then result in a recurrence of the underlying disorder.

Congenital Asplenia. The spleen is the only organ arising on the left side of the body. Congenital asplenia is usually part of a clinical complex that results from a pathologic tendency toward symmetric development of normally asymmetric organs. In this instance, the abnormality is bilateral right-sidedness; the spleen is absent, the lungs are trilobed, and the liver is symmetric and centrally located. Dextrocardia is usually evident, and a high risk of other severe congenital cardiac anomalies exists. Overwhelming septicemia is a common complication because of the absence of the spleen during infancy.

Polysplenia. Polysplenia represents bilateral left-sidedness. Multiple small spleens are found along the greater curvature of the stomach in association with bilateral bilobed lungs and a high incidence of intrahepatic biliary atresia. Congenital heart disease is less frequent and severe than in congenital asplenia. The total volume of splenic tissue in polysplenia may rarely be small enough to be associated with a risk of sepsis.

Splenic Cysts. Splenic cysts are relatively uncommon. They are usually identified as smooth, nontender, left upper quadrant masses. The diagnosis can be established using ultrasonography or computerized tomography. Clinical consequences include rupture with associated hemorrhage and infection. Larger cysts are usually removed surgically to avoid these complications, but normal surrounding splenic tissue is left intact if possible.

Acquired Disorders

Tumors. Most neoplastic disorders of the spleen are malignant. Benign tumors of the spleen are rare; they are usually hemangiomatous and may be associated with similar tumors of other organs.

Splenic Trauma and Rupture. Splenic injury usually results from direct trauma to the left side of the abdomen or the left flank during motor vehicle accidents or contact sports. Splenic rupture occurs more readily when the spleen is enlarged and friable because of disorders such as infectious mononucleosis. Neonates are particularly susceptible to splenic trauma after difficult deliveries or during cardiopulmonary resuscitation. Trauma often ruptures the splenic capsule and produces intraperitoneal bleeding. If the capsule remains intact, subcapsular hematomas may occur.

Symptoms include left shoulder, left upper quadrant, or generalized abdominal pain, with signs of peritoneal irritation and hypovolemic shock possible. When subcapsular hematomas develop, symptoms may be overlooked until sudden rupture occurs days to months later. In the neonate, evidence of shock and abdominal rigidity may be the only clinical signs of splenic rupture. The diagnosis is probably best established with computerized tomography, although radionuclide scanning is helpful.

Splenectomy is avoided if possible to prevent the risk of postsplenectomy septicemia. Surgery is often unnecessary because many hemorrhages from a lacerated spleen stop spontaneously in children. If the child's vital signs are stable and transfusion requirements are moderate (less than 25 mL/kg), careful observation is reasonable as long as a surgical team is readily available. If the hemorrhage is severe enough to result in deterioration in blood pressure, surgical intervention is indicated. Splenic repair, rather than splenectomy, can often be performed to preserve splenic function. Splenectomy is performed only if safe repair is judged to be hazardous or technically impossible.

Splenosis. During the course of splenic rupture or subsequent surgical intervention, splenic tissue may autotransplant onto the peritoneal surface. This process, called *splenosis*, occurs more commonly in children than adults. When the spleen has been removed, these implants enlarge. Splenosis has no serious consequences. It is not yet known whether splenosis confers adequate protection against overwhelming septicemia.

Indications for Splenectomy

Surgical Indications

Splenic trauma has been the most common indication for splenectomy. Splenic cysts, tumors, and vascular lesions may also require surgical removal. In many instances, adequate normal splenic tissue may be preserved, but total splenectomy is occasionally necessary. Splenectomy may be necessary in disorders such as Gaucher disease and thalassemia major when splenomegaly is so massive that relief from the mechanical stress is necessary. Laparoscopic splenectomy is becoming the standard of care for children who require spleen removal.

Medical Indications

Splenectomy may be helpful in several medical conditions, including congenital anemias such as hereditary spherocytosis or elliptocytosis, autoimmune disorders such as immune thrombocytopenic purpura and autoimmune hemolytic anemia, Gaucher disease, thalassemia major, and hypersplenism. Splenectomy is no longer used in the routine staging of Hodgkin disease because of the high risk of postsplenectomy sepsis in these patients.

LYMPH NODES

Anatomy and Physiology

The MPS tissue in the spleen, liver, and bone marrow serves as an immunologic filter for circulating blood and for these organs themselves. However, most foreign antigens enter the body through the skin, gastrointestinal tract, and respiratory tract and then reach the lymphoid circulation rather than blood. Lymph nodes, with their widespread peripheral locations, provide the most common initial site of contact between antigens and the MPS.

Lymph nodes are individual encapsulated anatomic units of the MPS distributed along lymph vessels throughout the body. Their anatomic arrangement (Fig. 295.2) allows circulating lymph to be filtered throughout the node. The cortical follicles are centers of B-cell activity. Antigenic stimulation causes the primary follicles to become secondary follicles by enlarging and developing pale-staining germinal centers containing B lymphocytes in various stages of activation, helper T cells, macrophages, and reticulum cells. The surrounding paracortical areas between the primary and secondary follicles and the inner medullary region are centers of T-cell activity. This structure provides ideal conditions for delivering antigens to the immune system, optimizing antigen recognition, and the subsequent activation of the cellular and humoral components of the immune response. The node therefore acts as a protective barrier to local infection and as a facilitator of the immune response. The ability of lymph nodes to proliferate under immunologic stimulation can be impressive; the nodes can enlarge 15 times their normal size within 5 to 10 days of antigenic exposure.

Lymph nodes undergo important developmental changes. At birth, there is considerable lymphoid activity throughout the body, but individual lymph nodes usually are not palpa-

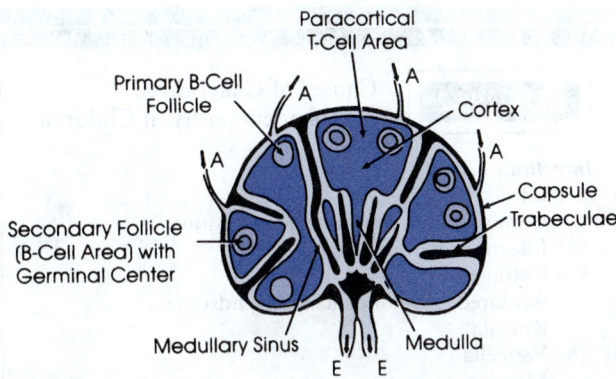

FIGURE 295.2. Lymph node. Lymph flows into the nodes through afferent lymphatics (A) and enters the cortex. Flow continues through the medulla, and lymph exits the node through the efferent lymphatics (E). B-cell activities are concentrated in the primary and secondary follicles in the cortex, and T cells are concentrated in the paracortical and medullary regions. (Modified from Hayes B. Enlargement of lymph nodes and spleen. In: Braunwald E, Isselbacher KJ, Petersdorf RG, et al., eds. *Harrison's principles of internal medicine.* New York: McGraw-Hill, 1987:276.)

ble. After birth, exposure to environmental antigens results in a steady increase in the mass of lymphoid tissue until 8 to 12 years of age. During puberty, lymphoid tissue begins to undergo a progressive atrophy, which continues throughout life. Children respond to new antigens more rapidly and with more exaggerated hyperplastic lymphoid responses than do adults. Palpable lymph nodes are therefore much more common in children, especially in the cervical, axillary, and inguinal regions. In contrast, supraclavicular, popliteal, and mediastinal nodes rarely enlarge, even in children.

Lymphadenopathy

By adult standards, almost all children have lymphadenopathy. Absence of palpable cervical or inguinal nodes in children is unusual and even may provide a clinical clue to an underlying immune deficiency. Common viral or bacterial illnesses of childhood often result in lymphadenopathy, which can be dramatic. These factors explain the difficulty in determining whether palpable lymph nodes in children represent a normal finding, transient hyperplasia in response to a simple viral illness, or more serious underlying pathology. This decision is based on clinical experience and judgment, but general guidelines are useful. Normal nodes usually do not exceed 2.5 cm in diameter and do not demonstrate warmth, tenderness, fluctuance, overlying erythema, or any tendency to mat together into less well-defined masses. The groups of nodes involved are important. Palpable cervical, axillary, and inguinal nodes are expected; however, supraclavicular nodes, if present at all, should be barely palpable.

Lymphadenopathy can be caused by an increase in normal lymphocytes and macrophages during a response to an antigen (e.g., viral illness), nodal infiltration by inflammatory cells in response to an infection localized to the nodes themselves (e.g., lymphadenitis), proliferation of neoplastic lymphocytes or macrophages (e.g., lymphoma), or infiltration of nodes by metabolite-laden macrophages in storage diseases (e.g., Gaucher disease).

Lymphadenopathy is the most common clinical problem related to lymph nodes and a frequent diagnostic challenge in pediatrics. The differential diagnosis of lymphadenopathy has much in common with that of splenomegaly, which is not surprising in view of the common MPS functions of the two

---

BOX 295.2 · **Causes of Generalized Lymphadenopathy in Children**

Infections
Viral
   Common upper respiratory infections
   Infectious mononucleosis
   Cytomegalovirus
   Acquired immunodeficiency syndrome
   Rubella
   Varicella
   Measles
Bacterial
   Septicemia
   Typhoid fever
   Tuberculosis
Protozoal
   Toxoplasmosis
Fungal
   Coccidioidomycosis

Autoimmune disorders and hypersensitivity states
   Juvenile rheumatoid arthritis
   Systemic lupus erythematosus
   Serum sickness
   Drug reactions (phenytoin, allopurinol, isoniazid)

Abnormal Proliferation of Cells
   Acute leukemias
   Non-Hodgkin lymphoma
   Hodgkin lymphoma
   Neuroblastoma
   Histiocytoses

Storage diseases
   Gaucher disease
   Niemann-Pick disease

---

organs. Most children with lymphadenopathy have benign disorders, but a few will have serious and even life-threatening diseases.

Generalized Lymphadenopathy

Generalized lymphadenopathy involves enlargement of two or more noncontiguous lymph node regions. Disorders causing generalized lymphadenopathy are usually associated with other findings in the history, physical examination, and laboratory data that assist in establishing a diagnosis (Box 295.2). Hepatosplenomegaly often is an associated finding.

Infection. Viral infections are the most common cause of generalized lymphadenopathy. This most often results from transient responses to common viral upper respiratory infections. Infectious mononucleosis and cytomegalovirus infections are common and may be associated with more impressive lymphadenopathy. Acquired immunodeficiency disease is an important cause of lymphadenopathy. Viral infections are usually associated with soft and minimally tender nodes. Bacterial infections are associated with more tender, warm, and sometimes fluctuant nodes with overlying erythema. In some cases, the bacterial infection is acute and associated with toxic symptoms, as with septicemia and typhoid fever. In contrast, systemic symptoms are much less severe in more chronic diseases such as tuberculosis.

Autoimmune Disorders and Hypersensitivity States. Many immunologic disorders are associated with lymphadenopathy. Enlarged nodes are common findings during the acute phases of juvenile rheumatoid arthritis, although other manifestations usually dominate the clinical picture.

Abnormal Proliferation of Cells in Lymph Nodes. Although malignancies are not a frequent cause of lymphadenopathy, they must be considered because of the importance of rapidly establishing a diagnosis and instituting therapy. Malignant adenopathy is usually nontender and not associated with overlying erythema; the nodes may have a rubbery texture, and groups of nodes may become matted together, losing their individual character. Diffuse adenopathy is commonly associated with acute lymphoblastic leukemia and non-Hodgkin lymphoma.

Storage Diseases. Storage diseases are rare causes of lymphadenopathy. The primary manifestations of these diseases are hepatosplenomegaly or neurologic deterioration.

Regional Lymphadenopathy

The involvement of a single or multiple contiguous nodal regions constitutes regional lymphadenopathy (Box 295.3). Understanding the normal pattern of lymph drainage is crucial to identifying the cause of adenopathy. Establishing a diagnosis for regional, and particularly cervical, lymphadenopathy often is difficult. Infections are the most common cause of regional adenopathy, but more serious underlying diseases remain a concern.

Occipital Nodes. Occipital nodes at the back of the head drain the posterior scalp. These nodes are palpable in approximately 5% of normal children. Although often enlarged as part of generalized lymphadenopathy, regional enlargement is almost always infectious in cause and often related to pediculosis capitis, tinea capitis, or seborrheic dermatitis. Roseola infantum and rubella cause enlargement in this region.

Preauricular Nodes. Preauricular nodes drain the lateral portions of the eyelid, conjunctiva, and the skin of the temporal region and cheek. They are not normally palpable. Their enlargement is most often caused by local skin infections, chronic ophthalmic infections (e.g., *Chlamydia*, adenovirus), and cat-scratch fever.

Tonsillar Nodes. The tonsils undergo the same physiologic hypertrophy as other lymph nodes, reaching a peak size at approximately 7 years of age. Isolated tonsillar hypertrophy, which has often resulted in unnecessary tonsillectomy, is an important example of the physiologic lymphoid hyperplasia of childhood. Superimposed viral or bacterial infections (especially simple upper respiratory infections or streptococcal pharyngitis) frequently cause additional, but usually transient, tonsillar enlargement. Bacterial infections can localize to the tonsil and produce a peritonsillar abscess.

Cervical Nodes. Cervical nodes drain the tongue, external ear, parotid gland, and deeper structures of the neck. They are normally palpable in all children beyond early infancy. This region is also the most common site of abnormal lymph node enlargement. Common viral infections of the upper respiratory tract are the most frequent cause of such enlargement. Posterior cervical involvement is especially common in infectious mononucleosis and rubella. During viral illness, nodes tend to be soft, are minimally tender, and are usually enlarged bilaterally. Beta-hemolytic streptococcal pharyngitis often is associated with bilateral cervical lymphadenopathy, in which the nodes are usually more tender.

Acute lymphadenitis is a common disorder resulting from localization of a regional infection to a node or group of nodes.

| BOX 295.3 | Causes of Regional Lymphadenopathy in Children |

Occipital
Pediculosis capitis
Tinea capitis
Secondary infection of seborrheic
   dermatitis and eczema
Roseola infantum
Rubella

Preauricular
Local skin infections
Chronic ophthalmic infections
Cat-scratch disease

Tonsillar
Viral upper respiratory infection
Streptococcal pharyngitis
Tonsillar abscess

Cervical
Viral upper respiratory infection
Infectious mononucleosis
Rubella
Cat-scratch disease
Streptococcal pharyngitis
Mycobacterial infection
Toxoplasmosis
Acute lymphadenitis
Acute leukemias
Neuroblastoma
Non-Hodgkin lymphoma
Hodgkin disease
Rhabdomyosarcoma
Kawasaki disease

Submaxillary and submental
Local infections of teeth and mouth
Acute lymphadenitis

Supraclavicular
Tuberculosis
Histoplasmosis
Coccidiomycosis
Hodgkin disease
Non-Hodgkin lymphoma

Axillary
Local bacterial infections
Cat-scratch disease
Reactions to immunizations
Juvenile rheumatoid arthritis
Non-Hodgkin lymphoma

Mediastinal
Tuberculosis
Histoplasmosis
Coccidioidomycosis
Acute lymphoblastic leukemia
Hodgkin disease
Non-Hodgkin lymphoma
Cystic fibrosis
Sarcoidosis

Abdominal
Acute mesenteric adenitis
Hodgkin disease
Non-Hodgkin lymphoma

Inguinal/Iliac
Local infections/inflammation

The cause is usually a bacterial infection in the upper respiratory tract, teeth, gums, and skin. Cervical nodes are most commonly involved, although any region can be affected. The affected nodes are usually unilateral, enlarged, warm, and tender. Abscess formation, acute periadenitis, and inflammation of the overlying skin often develop. Fever, malaise, and leukocytosis are common. Antibiotic therapy is indicated and is directed at the two usual etiologic agents, staphylococcus and beta-hemolytic streptococci. If suppuration occurs, surgical drainage may be necessary. Chronic cervical lymphadenitis is much less common and is most often caused by cat-scratch disease, *Mycobacterium tuberculosis*, and atypical mycobacteria.

Kawasaki disease is associated with nonsuppurative cervical adenopathy in 75% of patients. It can be marked and is often unilateral.

Approximately one-quarter of childhood malignancies present in the head and neck, and the cervical nodes are the most common site of involvement. During the first 6 years of life, acute leukemias, neuroblastoma, non-Hodgkin lymphoma, and rhabdomyosarcoma are most common. In older children, the lymphomas predominate. Cervical adenopathy is the presenting manifestation of 80% to 90% of children with Hodgkin disease; the enlargement is usually unilateral, and the nodes are firm and painless. Approximately 40% of patients with non-Hodgkin lymphoma present with cervical adenopathy, which is usually bilateral.

Nonlymphoid cervical masses may be mistaken for lymph nodes, including cervical ribs, cysts, branchial sinuses, and benign tumors.

Submaxillary and Submental Nodes. The areas drained by the submaxillary and submental nodes include the teeth, gums, tongue, and buccal mucosa. Adenopathy is usually caused by localized infection, including dental abscess, pharyngitis, and herpetic gingivostomatitis.

Supraclavicular Nodes. The supraclavicular nodes drain the head and neck, arms, superficial thorax, lungs, mediastinum, and abdomen. The right supraclavicular nodes drain the mediastinum and lungs. Mediastinal adenopathy, which is often not otherwise identifiable on physical examination, should be suspected if the patient has right supraclavicular lymphadenopathy. The left supraclavicular nodes are closely related to the thoracic duct. Intraabdominal processes associated with abdominal adenopathy often spread to the thoracic duct and cause enlargement of the left supraclavicular nodes. Although splenomegaly may be observed, left supraclavicular adenopathy may be the only clinical manifestation of this type of abdominal process.

Chest radiography should be obtained on patients with supraclavicular adenopathy to exclude both pulmonary and mediastinal disease. Lymphomas are common causes of supraclavicular adenopathy, and early biopsy is indicated in the absence of an easily documented pulmonary infection. Thoracic or abdominal computerized tomographic scans may be indicated, particularly with left-sided involvement.

Axillary Nodes. Axillary nodes drain the hand, arm, lateral chest wall, lateral abdominal wall, and lateral portion of the breast. They may be palpated in 90% of children. Cat-scratch disease often results in adenopathy here. Recent immunizations in the arm, especially with bacilli Calmette-Guérin vaccine, commonly result in axillary adenopathy. Of the malignancies, non-Hodgkin lymphoma most commonly presents here.

Mediastinal Nodes. Mediastinal nodes drain the thoracic viscera, including the lungs, heart, thymus, and esophagus. Because mediastinal nodes are not directly demonstrable on physical examination, they must be examined radiologically. The most common indirect clinical evidence of mediastinal adenopathy is supraclavicular adenopathy; direct effects of mediastinal node enlargement include cough, wheezing, respiratory distress, dysphagia, and obstruction of the great vessels; the latter is manifested by superior vena cava syndrome.

Malignancies are a common cause of mediastinal lymphadenopathy. Bilateral hilar adenopathy is also associated with cystic fibrosis, fungal infection, and sarcoidosis. Unilateral hilar adenopathy is often caused by tuberculosis. Common viral or bacterial infections of the lungs are rarely associated with lymphadenopathy in this region. Nonlymphoid structures that may be mistaken for mediastinal adenopathy include the thymus (which can be quite large during early childhood), cysts, teratomas, substernal thyroid gland, abnormalities of the great vessels, and neuroblastoma.

Abdominal Nodes. Abdominal nodes drain the lower extremities and all pelvic and abdominal organs. Adenopathy here can cause abdominal pain, backache, constipation, increased urinary frequency, and intestinal obstruction because of intussusception. Any disorder causing local abdominal or generalized adenopathy may produce these symptoms. Local disorders include typhoid fever, ulcerative colitis, and acute mesenteric adenitis of childhood. Mesenteric adenitis is probably viral in cause. It is characterized by right lower quadrant abdominal pain caused by enlarged mesenteric nodes in the region of the ileocecal valve and may be difficult to differentiate from appendicitis. Abdominal adenopathy is also a manifestation of the lymphomas.

Inguinal and Iliac Nodes. The lower extremities, genitalia, perineum, buttocks, and lower abdominal wall are drained by the inguinal and iliac nodes. They are normally palpable in children and their enlargement is usually caused by infection. Readily overlooked causes include diaper dermatitis and insect bites. Nonlymphoid masses that may be mistaken for nodes include hernias, ectopic testes, lipomas, and aneurysms.

Lymph Node Biopsy

The evaluation of regional or generalized lymphadenopathy often raises the question of when to consider biopsy. The answer depends on the group of nodes involved, the clinical circumstances, laboratory studies, and the appraised relative risk of malignancy or other serious disease. Signs of acute infection, such as tenderness, warmth, erythema, and a site of primary infection, support delaying biopsy and treating with antibiotics.

If biopsy is indicated, it is important to choose a large node that has been recently enlarging, to try to avoid a biopsy of the inguinal nodes because their architecture is frequently distorted by chronic infection, and to avoid choosing a node primarily because of its surgical accessibility. Following these precautions can decrease the risk of obtaining an unrepresentative or reactive node and missing the actual underlying diagnosis.

Lymph Vessels

The lymphatic vessels collect lymph from almost all tissues except the central nervous system, striated muscle, cartilage, and the cornea. Lymph is essentially colorless extracellular fluid containing large numbers of lymphocytes and material too large to be absorbed into blood capillaries. This fluid and its contents are delivered to thin-walled transparent lymph vessels and then to regional lymph nodes. Large numbers of lymphocytes are added to the lymph, which exits the nodes through efferent lymphatics and eventually reaches the thoracic duct and the right lymphatic duct. At this point in the base of the neck, the lymph enters the venous circulation.

Acute Lymphangitis

A regional bacterial infection that cannot be localized may involve the lymphatic vessels in an acute lymphangitis. Erythematous streaks that are a few millimeters to several centimeters wide may be seen extending from the primary site of infection to regional nodes. Painful swelling of regional nodes usually follows, and peripheral edema may occur as a result of lymphatic obstruction. Bacteremia may follow as soon as 24 to 48 hours from the onset of the initial lesion. Antibiotic treatment is indicated for local control and to prevent bacteremia.

Lymphedema

Lymphedema is a diffuse edema that results from obstruction of the lymphatic flow. It most commonly involves the lower extremities and may be complicated by verrucous hypertrophy of the skin and recurrent infections. The edema may or may not demonstrate pitting. Lymphedema is most often acquired as a result of inflammatory processes or of surgical or radiologic obliteration of lymphatic channels; it may have no identifiable cause. Treatment is ineffective.

Suggested Readings

Chapman WC, Newman M. Disorders of the spleen. In: Lee GR, Foerster J, Lukens J, et al., eds. *Wintrobe's clinical hematology*. Philadelphia: Lea & Febiger, 1999:1969.

Chesney PJ. Cervical adenopathy. *Pediatr Rev* 1994;15:276.

Grossman M, Shiramizu B. Evaluation of lymphadenopathy in children. *Curr Opin Pediatr* 1994;6:68.

Lane PA. The spleen in children. *Curr Opin Pediatr* 1995;7:36.

Morland B. Lymphadenopathy. *Arch Dis Child* 1995;73:476.

Pearson HA. The spleen and disturbances of splenic function. In: Nathan DG, Orkin SH, eds. *Hematology of infancy and childhood*. Philadelphia: WB Saunders, 1998:1051.

Stockman JA. Splenomegaly. In: Stockman JA, ed. *Difficult diagnoses in pediatrics*. Philadelphia: WB Saunders, 1990:301.

Twist CJ, Link MP. Assessment of lymphadenopathy in children. *Pediatr Cl NA* 2002;49:1009.

CHAPTER 296 ■ GENERAL APPROACHES TO COAGULOPATHIES

CLIFFORD M. TAKEMOTO AND JAMES F. CASELLA

INTRODUCTION

Abnormalities of the hemostatic system are encountered commonly in hospitalized children, because primary diseases of hemostasis often require hospitalization, and systemic diseases severe enough to require hospitalization often produce abnormalities of hemostasis. In addition, pediatricians are frequently called on to evaluate coagulation abnormalities before or after surgery.

Coagulation disorders can be divided into conditions with abnormal bleeding (i.e., hypocoagulable states) and those associated with the development of thromboses (i.e., hypercoagulable states). Current knowledge of factors necessary for normal clotting to occur and for maintaining blood in a fluid state is sufficiently complex that a full understanding of all the mechanisms involved is a challenge even for an experienced hematologist. New information is being acquired rapidly, especially in the area of hypercoagulability. Despite this surge of new information, most abnormalities of hemostasis can still be approached in an orderly fashion, beginning with a detailed history and physical examination, the evaluation of readily available laboratory tests, and a general overview of hemostatic mechanisms.

Coagulopathies may be secondary to abnormalities of the blood vessels, platelets, or plasma clotting factors, and some hemostatic defects involve more than one of these systems. The result of the history, including the family pedigree, physical examination, and screening laboratory testing, should provide information about which system is responsible for the bleeding abnormality. The following paragraphs summarize the basic functions of each component of the hemostatic mechanism and provide a background for understanding the mechanisms underlying clinical abnormalities. The relative contributions of the history, physical examination, and laboratory testing are then discussed.

NORMAL PHYSIOLOGY

Coagulation Mechanisms

The primary response to bleeding includes a vascular response, platelet activation, and the coagulation cascade. Within seconds of injury, damaged blood vessels demonstrate a vasoconstrictive response. During this vasoconstriction phase, platelets begin to adhere to the damaged endothelium, where collagen, a potent activator of platelet adhesion and von Willebrand factor (vWF) ligand, are exposed. Adherence and aggregation of platelets appear to be mediated through the action of specific platelet membrane receptors, including glycoprotein Ib (the major vWF receptor) and glycoprotein IIb/IIIa (the fibrinogen receptor). Adherent platelets then release platelet-stimulatory

agents, such as thromboxane and adenosine diphosphate, and mediators of platelet interaction, such as fibrinogen and vWF, promoting adherence and activation of more platelets, with the resulting formation of an *unstable hemostatic plug*. Serotonin released from platelet granules further constricts the large vessels. Platelet factor 4, a substance released from platelet granules, neutralizes heparin. Receptors for activated factors V (FVa) and VIII (FVIIIa) are also expressed on the phospholipid membranes of activated platelets.

Coincident with these events, the coagulation system is activated, leading to the activation of thrombin and the subsequent deposition of an insoluble fibrin clot. This system has traditionally been modeled as a linear cascade of events activated at two levels ("extrinsic and intrinsic") (Fig. 296.1) resulting in clot formation; however, the emerging picture is one of an interacting set of enzyme complexes that coordinate the initiation, amplification, and dissolution of the fibrin clot. These complexes consist of serine proteases and cofactors that are activated by proteolysis and require calcium and a phospholipid surface for full activity. The initial activation of this system *in vivo* begins through the extrinsic pathway with the exposure of tissue factor (TF) from damaged tissue. TF forms a complex with the serine protease, activated factor VII (FVIIa). This complex (TF/FVIIa), also called the *extrinsic tenase*, then activates factor X (FX) in the presence of calcium and phospholipid on the surface of cell membranes. Activated FX (FXa) assembles with its cofactor, FVa on the surface of activated platelets to form the prothrombinase complex. This prothrombinase complex, in turn, cleaves prothrombin to thrombin, and thrombin then cleaves soluble fibrinogen to fibrin, which polymerizes into a fibrin gel. In addition, thrombin further potentiates clotting by activating both platelets and factor XIII (FXIII), a transglutaminase that stabilizes the clot by covalently cross-linking fibrin.

Thus, clot formation *in vivo* initiates through the TF/FVIIa complex and the extrinsic pathway. However, TF/FVIIa can also activate the intrinsic pathway to a lesser degree by cleaving factor IX (FIX) to activated FIX (FIXa). The intrinsic pathway is important for the propagation of the clot by a positive feedback loop in which thrombin activates components of the intrinsic system (FIX, FVIII, and FV) and thus amplifies thrombin production. FVIIIa and FVa combine to form the intrinsic tenase complex that cleaves FX on a phospholipid surface in the presence of calcium. The distinction of the "intrinsic" versus the "extrinsic" system is useful in understanding the components that affect the prothrombin time (PT) and activated partial thromboplastin time (aPTT). Deficiencies of factors of the extrinsic system result in PT prolongation, whereas deficiencies of factors of the intrinsic system lead to aPTT elevation. However, PT and aPTT measurements do not faithfully predict physiologic bleeding. Patients with deficiencies of factor XII, (FXII) prekallikrein, or high-molecular-weight kininogen have prolongation of the aPTT, but no bleeding symptoms. Similarly, soluble factors, such as a lupus anticoagulant, can prolong

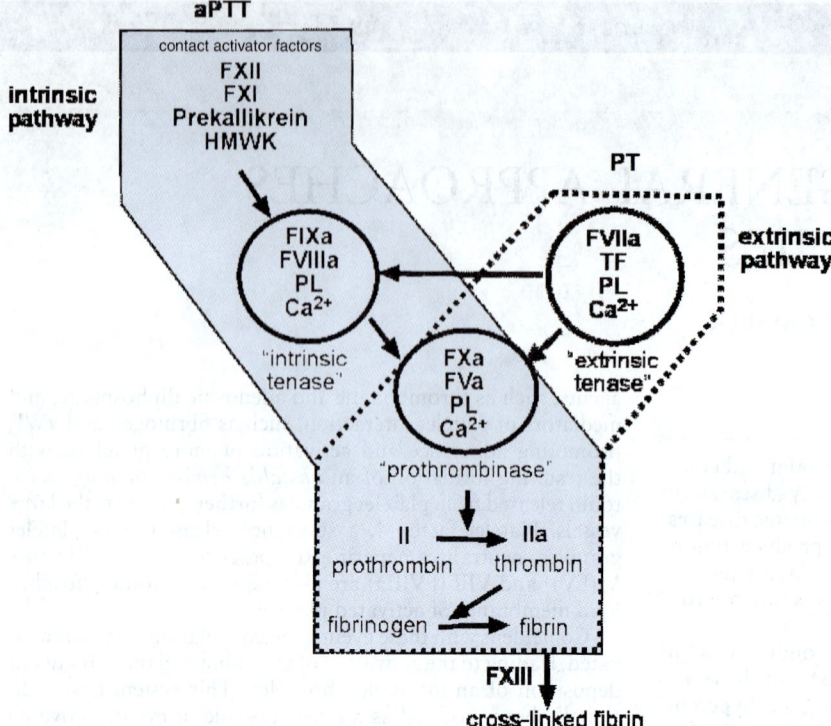

FIGURE 296.1. The coagulation cascade. The major enzyme systems that regulate the intrinsic and extrinsic pathway are depicted. The "prothombinase" complex contains activated factors X and V (FXa and FVa) and requires calcium (Ca^{2+}) and a phospholipid surface (PL). The prothrombinase complex activates prothrombin (II) to thrombin (IIa), which subsequently converts soluble fibrinogen to the fibrin clot. Factor XIII (FXIII) cross-links fibrin monomers to stabilize the clot. The prothrombinase complex is activated in two ways, by either the "intrinsic" tenase (FIXa and FVIIIa) or the "extrinsic" tenase (activated factor VII [FVIIa] and tissue factor [TF]). The intrinsic tenase can be activated by FVIIa/TF and by the contact activation factors (factor XII (FXII), factor XI (FXI), prekallikrein, and high-molecular-weight kininogen [HMWK]). The factors that are known to affect the activated partial thromboplastin time (aPTT) are within the *shaded area*, whereas the factors that are known to affect the prothrombin time (PT), are contained within the area outlined with the *dotted lines*.

the aPTT, but they may infer a risk of thrombosis rather than hemorrhage. FXII and factor XI (FXI), prekallikrein, and high-molecular-weight kininogen can be activated on negatively charged surfaces, and together they comprise what is termed the *contact activation pathway* of coagulation.

Anticoagulation Mechanisms

The presence of such an elegant system for the formation of blood clots implies that an equally sophisticated system must be in place to prevent the inadvertent formation of blood clots and to provide for their removal and remodeling once formed. Three major systems inhibit the coagulation system: (a) the protein C/S system, (b) antithrombin, and (c) the TF pathway inhibitor (TFPI). In addition, removal of the thrombus through fibrinolysis is mediated by the plasminogen system. Protein C, an anticoagulant protein, plays a primary role in inhibiting the clotting cascade and inducing the dissolution of clots. Like some of the procoagulant factors (e.g., factor II [FII], FVII, FIX, and FX), protein C is a vitamin K–dependent factor synthesized in the liver. Unlike the procoagulant factors, activated protein C possesses anticoagulant activity, which is achieved primarily through cleavage and inactivation of FVa and FVIIIa. Activated protein C also stimulates fibrinolysis.

Paradoxically, the activation of protein C depends on cleavage of protein C zymogen by thrombin, one of the final products of the clotting cascade. The activation of protein C by thrombin is catalyzed by an endothelial-bound receptor, thrombomodulin, a reaction that requires the essential cofactors, protein S, which is also a vitamin K–dependent factor, and intact factor V. Protein C and protein S deficiencies are inherited disorders associated with predispositions to thromboses. Thrombin appears to play a pivotal role in both coagulation and anticoagulation; it serves as a procoagulant by cleaving fibrinogen and activating platelets and as an anticoagulant by activating protein C in the presence of thrombomodulin. Thrombin activity, in the presence or absence of thrombomodulin, is, in turn, modulated by antithrombin. Antithrombin forms a 1:1 complex with activated serine proteases, such as thrombin, FIX, and FX, and thus inhibits their activity. The affinity of antithrombin for thrombin is enhanced 1,000-fold in the presence of heparin, and this accounts at least in part for the anticoagulant activity of heparin. Deficiencies of antithrombin have been reported to result in a tendency toward hypercoagulability. Inhibition of the extrinsic system is achieved primarily through TFPI. TFPI binds FXa and inhibits the activity of the FVIIa/TF complex. Recombinant TFPI has been shown promise as an anticoagulant in animal models.

As is the case with thrombin, FV also has both procoagulant and anticoagulant activities. Activation of FV is an essential step in the coagulation cascade and the formation of fibrin (procoagulant activity), whereas intact FV functions as a cofactor for activated protein C (anticoagulant activity). An abnormality of FV (FV Leiden) has been described that causes a significant defect in anticoagulant activity because of reduced activation of protein C and persistence in plasma of abnormal FVa with reduced sensitivity to inactivation by protein C.

Fibrinolysis can be induced by the enzyme plasmin, which is a cleavage product of plasminogen. Plasmin formation is catalyzed by several factors, including urokinase and tissue plasminogen activator. Cleavage of fibrin or fibrinogen by plasmin results in the formation of soluble fibrin degradation products, also referred to as *fibrin-split products*. Proteolysis of the fibrin matrix after cross-linking by FXIII releases dimers of cross-linked protein domains (the D-domains) of fibrin (D-dimers). Activated protein C appears to stimulate fibrinolysis by reducing the activity of both plasminogen activator inhibitor-1 (PAI-1) and thrombin activatable fibrinolysis inhibitor (TAFI). In addition to PAI-1 and TAFI, alpha-2-antiplasmin also functions as a major inhibitor of plasmin *in vivo*. Regulation of the coagulation system can be achieved by other means. Most of the factors in the procoagulant scheme and some of the anticoagulant proteins (e.g., protein C) are serine proteases and can therefore be inhibited by a wide variety of serine protease inhibitors in plasma (e.g., alpha-2-macroglobulin, alpha-1-antitrypsin).

The coagulation and anticoagulation mechanisms are delicately balanced and interdependent systems, possessing

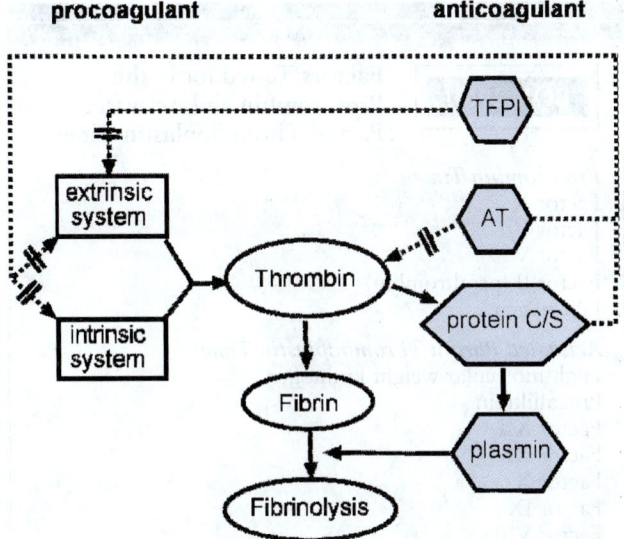

procoagulant   **anticoagulant**

FIGURE 296.2. Interactions among the major factors in the procoagulant and anticoagulant scheme. The major procoagulant arms are depicted in the *white boxes* and *ovals*. Prothrombin conversion to thrombin is driven by the intrinsic and extrinsic coagulation cascades. Thrombin converts fibrinogen to fibrin, the major constituent of clots. The major anticoagulant arms are depicted in the shaded hexagons; these factors include tissue factor pathway inhibitor (TFPI), antithrombin (AT), protein C and S, and plasmin. Inhibitory interactions between anticoagulant and procoagulant factors are illustrated by *dotted lines*. Thrombin regulates the anticoagulant arm by activating protein C in the presence of protein S, which neutralizes the intrinsic and extrinsic systems. Activated protein C also promotes fibrinolysis by indirectly upregulating plasmin activity. Antithrombin antagonizes activated thrombin (IIa) as well as factors of the intrinsic and extrinsic pathways. TFPI is a selective inhibitor of the extrinsic system, by inactivating activated factor VII. Plasmin promotes fibrinolysis by degrading the fibrin clot.

numerous redundancies, checks, and counterbalances that maintain the blood in fluid phase under normal circumstances, yet allow for the rapid formation of clots and their ultimate dissolution in pathologic circumstances. Important interactions among these procoagulant and anticoagulant factors are illustrated in schematic form in Fig. 296.2.

History

Although the search for a possible bleeding disorder is often initiated by an abnormal laboratory test result, the history and physical examination remain the most useful approaches for defining the presence and type of hemorrhagic diathesis. For example, purpura and mucosal bleeding are common presentations of platelet disorders. Abnormalities of the plasma clotting factors are much more likely to present with deep soft tissue bleeding or hemarthrosis. The history may indicate that the coagulation abnormality is a secondary phenomenon and may lead to the recognition of an underlying systemic illness.

In obtaining a history of abnormal bleeding, the clinician should ask specific rather than general questions. The question, "Do you or does your child bruise easily?" is answered affirmatively by so many parents that a positive answer is often of little value. The examiner should use specific questions, using recognizable childhood events as a trigger for the parents' memories. Was separation of the umbilical cord or circumcision associated with abnormal bleeding? Approximately one-half of patients with hemophilia have a history of bleeding in the neonatal pe-

riod, a fact that is often overlooked or unsolicited in the history. Patients with FXIII deficiency may experience delayed bleeding after umbilical cord separation. Did the child bleed at the sites of immunization? Did the child bleed during eruption of teeth or after minor trauma to the mouth (e.g., from falling into furniture)? Prolonged bleeding from a torn frenulum suggests FVIII deficiency. Does the child bleed after minor trauma, such as falling from playground equipment? How frequent are epistaxes, and how long do they last? These questions are useful in gaining positive and negative information. For example, the complaint of frequent nosebleeds often raises concern about a possible coagulation disorder, but nosebleeds that predictably stop within minutes are encountered rarely in patients with significant bleeding disorders. How long does the child bleed from minor cuts? Does the wound heal normally? Finding a scar is useful, because it often jogs the parents' memory about a forgotten laceration.

Previous surgical procedures are an extremely important source of information about potential coagulation abnormalities. The child who has had a tonsillectomy or dental extractions without unusual bleeding is less likely to have a serious coagulopathy. In questioning parents about dental procedures, it should be remembered that bleeding for 24 to 48 hours after dental extractions may occur even in physiologically normal persons and should not cause undue alarm.

Trauma, stasis, or overuse syndromes are often antecedents of thromboses. A history of diseases associated with a predisposition to thrombosis (e.g., nephrotic syndrome, systemic lupus erythematosus, inflammatory bowel disease, liver disease) should be pursued.

A detailed history of drug administration is essential. Many substances (e.g., aspirin or other nonsteroidal antiinflammatory drugs [NSAIDs] such as ibuprofen) are available in over-the-counter medications and are not reported by parents unless specifically mentioned by the examiner. A history of prolonged antibiotic administration, especially in exclusively breast-fed infants, or use of drugs that antagonize or interfere with the absorption of vitamin K (e.g., anticonvulsants) may prompt a diagnosis of vitamin K deficiency. Certain foods have been associated with platelet dysfunction, such as omega-3 fatty acids (found in fish oils), Chinese food (black tree fungus), and the spices cumin and turmeric. Ingestion of rodent poisons containing coumarins may cause coagulopathy. Oral contraceptives and L-asparaginase are associated commonly with thrombosis.

A careful family history often provides important information. The finding of a sex-linked pattern of transmission of a bleeding tendency may be the first clue to deficiencies of FVIII (i.e., classic hemophilia A) or FIX (i.e., classic hemophilia B). Discovery of an autosomal dominant mode of transmission is characteristic of von Willebrand disease. Idiopathic thrombocytopenic purpura is commonly encountered in families in which other immunoregulatory abnormalities, such as lupus erythematosus and thyroid disease, are prevalent. When considering hypercoagulable states, a family history of cerebrovascular accidents, myocardial infarctions, or venous or arterial thromboses by the third or fourth decades of life may be indicative of a hereditary prothrombotic disorder. In addition, obstetric complications such as late fetal loss, preeclampsia, and fetal growth retardation have been associated with maternal thrombophilia.

Physical Examination

The physical examination can provide important diagnostic clues. Petechiae, easily overlooked, are an important indication of reduced platelet number or function. Bruises with firm nodular or indurated centers are seen commonly in hemophilia and may be the first sign of a congenital factor deficiency. Poorly healed scars may be seen in patients with FXIII deficiency. The finding of an enlarged liver may be an indication of a systemic illness or a coagulation disturbance that is secondary to a primary hepatic disorder. An enlarged spleen may reflect significant portal hypertension with consequent hypersplenism and thrombocytopenia. The finding of characteristic angiomatous skin and mucous membrane lesions in a child with gastrointestinal bleeding may lead to a diagnosis of hereditary hemorrhagic telangiectasia. Patients with the stigmata of Ehlers-Danlos syndrome also may manifest purpura. Livido reticularis may be seen in patients with antiphospholipid syndromes and thromboses.

Laboratory Evaluation

Excellent screening procedures and tests for specific abnormalities are available for evaluating the patient with a possible coagulation disorder. The physician should first consider whether any laboratory testing is required. The approach advocated by Rapaport is worthy of review. To paraphrase, after the history and physical examination, the physician should be able to reach one of the following conclusions:

- The history and physical examination contain sufficient information to conclude that hemostatic function is normal.
- The history and physical examination do not contain sufficient information to conclude that hemostatic function is normal.
- The history and physical examination suggest the possibility or likelihood of a hemostatic defect.

Appropriate laboratory testing (or no laboratory testing) can then be obtained. A tabulation of all the available tests of coagulation is beyond the scope of this chapter, but some of the commonly used screening procedures can be discussed. Automated counting of platelets is readily available. Numeration and sizing of platelets by this method are routine and inexpensive. A stained blood smear prepared directly from peripheral blood by finger puncture should be examined to confirm the platelet count and size and to search for platelet dysmorphology. This allows an independent crosscheck of platelet number, using the rule that an average of one platelet per high-power field on a thin smear viewed with a $10\times$ ocular and a $100\times$ microscope objective indicates the presence of 10,000 to 15,000 platelets/μL. The aPTT measures functional activity of all the soluble factors in the classic intrinsic cascade in addition to those involved in the extrinsic cascade, with the exception of FVII (Box 296.1). Prolongation of the aPTT therefore can be secondary to an abnormality of one of the contact activation factors, of FX, FIX, FVIII, FV, or FII, or of fibrinogen. An abnormality of PT occurs with abnormalities of FX, FVII, FV, FII, or fibrinogen. Abnormalities of PT or aPTT also can be caused by ingested or endogenous circulating anticoagulants (e.g., warfarin, antiphospholipid antibodies) or liver disease.

Circulating inhibitors of anticoagulation, such as antiphospholipid antibodies, are readily detected by the failure of correction of a prolonged PT or aPTT after addition of normal

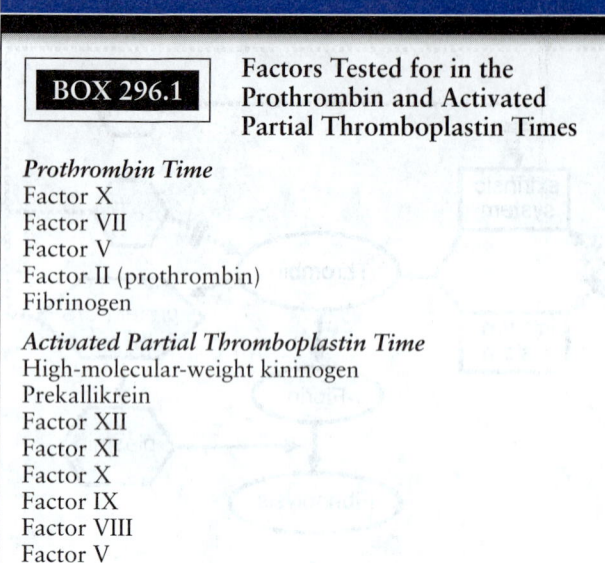

plasma (mixing study). More sophisticated tests for the detection of circulating anticoagulants (e.g., the Russell viper venom test) also are available.

Bleeding times may be abnormal in diseases of platelet function or number or in diseases affecting vascular integrity. Although the bleeding time often is recommended as a general screening procedure, several points should be recognized when considering its use. The bleeding time is extremely sensitive to platelet number; its use should be restricted to instances in which the platelet count has been determined previously. A history of recently ingested drugs, particularly aspirin or other NSAIDs, should be obtained before performing the bleeding time. Bleeding times, especially in inexperienced hands, often show considerable test-to-test variability, even when these tests are performed with calibrated templates. Citing these and other factors, several authoritative reviews have called into question the usefulness of the bleeding time as a preoperative screen.

Suggested Readings

Andrew M. Developmental hemostasis: relevance to thromboembolic complications in pediatric patients. *Thromb Haemost* 1995;74:415.

Burk CD, Miller L, Handler SD, Cohen AR. Preoperative history and coagulation screening in children undergoing tonsillectomy. *Pediatrics* 1992;89:691.

Jenny NS, Mann KG. Coagulation cascade: an overview 1. In: Loscalzo J, Schafer AI, eds. *Thrombosis and hemorrhage*. Philadelphia: Lippincott Williams & Williams, 2004:1.

Rapaport SI. Preoperative hemostatic evaluation: which tests, if any? *Blood* 1983; 61:229.

Rosendaal FR. Venous thrombosis: a multicausal disease. *Lancet* 1999;353:1167.

CHAPTER 297 ■ DISORDERS OF PLATELETS

JAMES F. CASELLA, MARIA A. PELIDIS, AND CLIFFORD M. TAKEMOTO

Abnormalities of platelets may be quantitative (i.e., caused by reduced platelet number) or qualitative (i.e., caused by an intrinsic defect that diminishes platelet function).

QUANTITATIVE CONGENITAL ABNORMALITIES OF THE PLATELETS

Thrombocytopenia with Absent Radius Syndrome

The thrombocytopenia with absent radius (TAR) syndrome is perhaps the most striking and most easily recognized of the congenital thrombocytopenias. Clinical recognition of the disorder occurs soon after birth in the infant with purpura and characteristic limb deformities. Although absence of the radius is the most consistent finding in this condition, cardiac, renal, and other skeletal malformations (e.g., complete or partial agenesis of other bones or joints, bony synostoses) also may occur. Leukoerythroblastic responses, often associated with severe diarrhea, often are observed in the neonatal period and infancy. The inheritance pattern appears to be autosomal recessive. Bone marrow specimens exhibit reduced numbers of megakaryocytes, which often appear dysplastic. Transfused platelets survive normally, and many patients can be maintained on weekly platelet transfusions for long periods. The risk of platelet allosensitization with chronic transfusions is low with modern blood banking methods; however, if allosensitization does occur, patients can be managed with human leukocyte antigen (HLA)–matched platelets. The thrombocytopenia tends to remit spontaneously in the second and third years of life.

Amegakaryocytic Thrombocytopenia

Patients with amegakaryocytic thrombocytopenia may present without radial or other congenital abnormalities. These patients generally present with isolated thrombocytopenia. Associations with neurologic defects and generalized bone marrow dysfunction developing later in life have been documented. Mutations in the thrombopoietin receptor (Mpl) have been identified in patients with amegakaryocytic thrombocytopenia.

Other Causes of Inherited Thrombocytopenia

Other syndromes associated with marrow failure or aplastic anemias that may present with thrombocytopenia include Fanconi aplastic anemia, Shwachman syndrome, and dyskeratosis congenita. Both Fanconi aplastic anemia and Shwachman syndrome can present in the neonatal period, whereas dyskeratosis congenita usually manifests in the second decade of life. Although all three syndromes can be associated with congenital abnormalities, Shwachman syndrome is differentiated by

exocrine pancreatic insufficiency, bony dysostoses, and neutropenia in most cases. Mutations in a gene of unclear function, SBDS, has been identified in the majority of these patients.

In Fanconi syndrome, a variety of congenital abnormalities may exist in addition to pancytopenia. Many patients have absent radii, mimicking the TAR syndrome, but in all reported cases of Fanconi syndrome, absence of the radius is associated with absence of the thumb. In the TAR syndrome, invariably the thumb is present despite the absence of the radius. The phenotype of patients with Fanconi syndrome often varies within the same family. Some patients exhibit no detectable congenital abnormalities, but the syndrome can be detected on the basis of characteristic chromosomal abnormalities. Chromosomes of patients with Fanconi syndrome are more susceptible to damage by DNA cross-linking agents such as diepoxybutane and mitomycin C and have more chromosomal breakages than healthy control subjects when they are exposed to these agents. To date, eight complementation groups (A, B, C, D1, D2, E, F, G) for Fanconi anemia have been described, and each complementation group is thought to represent a distinct Fanconi anemia gene. These genes appear to cooperate in a cellular pathway that participates in DNA repair. Patients with Fanconi syndrome are susceptible not only to bone marrow failure, but also to malignant diseases, particularly leukemias and squamous cell carcinomas.

Dyskeratosis congenita presents with the triad of hyperpigmentation of the skin, dystrophic nails, and oral leukoplakia. This syndrome is inherited in autosomal dominant, autosomal recessive, and sex-linked recessive patterns. Patients with dyskeratosis congenita have been found to have mutations in hTERC and DKC1; these genes are important for the function of the enzyme telomerase and thus chromosomal stability. As in Fanconi anemia, patients with dyskeratosis congenita are at risk to develop malignant diseases, especially epithelial cancers.

Certain chromosomal abnormalities have also been associated with thrombocytopenia. Patients with trisomy 13 and 18 can exhibit thrombocytopenia, as can patients with Down syndrome. Deletions of chromosome 22q11 are found in patients with velocardiofacial syndrome; many of these patients are also thrombocytopenic. Paris-Trousseau syndrome is characterized by clinodactyly, hypertelorism, mental retardation, and thrombocytopenia. These patients have deletions of chromosome 11q23.

Thrombocytopenias transmitted as autosomal dominant traits with and without normal platelet survival have been described. Autosomal recessive inheritance of thrombocytopenia has also been reported. These syndromes may be easily confused with idiopathic thrombocytopenic purpura. Several familial giant platelet syndromes with thrombocytopenia, such as May-Hegglin anomaly, Fechner syndrome, Sebastian syndrome, and Epstein syndrome, result from mutations in the nonmuscle heavy chain of myosin 9 (MYH9). Other inherited conditions associated with giant platelets and thrombocytopenia include Bernard-Soulier and gray platelet syndrome; Bernard-Soulier syndrome arises from defects in the platelet receptor (GPIb/IX) for von Willebrand factor (vWF), whereas gray platelet syndrome results from a deficiency of platelet alpha granules. In contrast, small platelets are one of the most consistent findings in the Wiskott-Aldrich syndrome; this finding can be very helpful in the differential diagnosis of inherited thrombocytopenias, particularly when a sex-linked recessive inheritance pattern is elicited.

Patients with Wiskott-Aldrich syndrome have been found to have mutations in the WASP gene. A sex-linked recessive form of thrombocytopenia without the severe immunodeficiency of Wiskott-Aldrich syndrome has also been shown to result from WASP mutations. Another sex-linked recessive syndrome with thrombocytopenia has been described in families with mutations in the transcription factor, GATA1. These patients also have dyserythropoietic anemia. Noonan syndrome is often inherited in an autosomal dominant fashion and can be associated with mild thrombocytopenia. Thrombocytopenia also occurs in the Tn-polyagglutination syndrome, a rare clonal disorder caused by an abnormality in glycosylation of the MN blood group antigen.

QUALITATIVE CONGENITAL ABNORMALITIES OF THE PLATELETS

Platelet disorders may arise because of a defect in platelet function despite adequate numbers of platelets. These syndromes are characterized by purpura, abnormal platelet aggregation, and prolonged bleeding times. In some cases, platelet morphology is abnormal.

Glanzmann Thrombasthenia

Glanzmann thrombasthenia is a prototype of the qualitative platelet disorders. This abnormality is inherited as an autosomal recessive trait. Although the number and morphology of the platelets are normal, life-threatening hemorrhagic complications may be encountered. The spectrum of severity of bleeding symptoms is broad, ranging from mild to severe. Platelets from patients with Glanzmann disease do not aggregate *in vitro* in response to adenosine diphosphate, collagen, epinephrine, and thrombin, but they do agglutinate in the presence of ristocetin and vWF. Clot retraction may be abnormal. These abnormalities are caused by the partial or complete absence of a cytoadhesive protein, glycoprotein IIb/IIIa (the platelet fibrinogen receptor), from platelet membranes. The ability of these platelets to agglutinate in the presence of ristocetin and vWF can be attributed to the presence of normal amounts of another cytoadhesive membrane protein, glycoprotein Ib, the major vWF receptor. Transfusion of platelets is an effective therapy for severe bleeding, but in a minority of cases it may result in the development of antibodies directed against the glycoprotein IIb/IIIa complex and resistance to further platelet transfusions. Larger than predicted platelet transfusions may be required, presumably because of interference of abnormal platelets with transfused platelets. Epsilon-aminocaproic acid can be extremely helpful for oral or nasal hemorrhage.

In the past several years, growing experience has suggested that recombinant factor VIIa is effective treatment for bleeding in patients with Glanzmann thrombasthenia and other platelet dysfunctions. Patients with Glanzmann thrombasthenia are at high risk for iron deficiency anemia secondary to frequent bleeding episodes; in particular, iron supplementation should be considered for infants and adolescent female patients with Glanzmann thrombasthenia. Numerous mutations in both glycoprotein IIb and IIIa have been described that result in Glanzmann phenotypes.

Bernard-Soulier Syndrome

In Bernard-Soulier syndrome, another autosomal recessive disease resulting in severe hemorrhagic complications, platelets aggregate *in vitro* in the presence of adenosine diphosphate, collagen, epinephrine, and thrombin. However, agglutination does not occur in the presence of ristocetin, even with vWF. Platelets are often described as large and bizarre. Platelet number is often reduced, sometimes out of proportion to the number observed on peripheral blood smear. Underestimation of platelet counts by electronic techniques can be caused by their abnormal size and density. The primary defect in Bernard-Soulier syndrome appears to be an absence of glycoproteins Ib, V, and IX from the platelet surface. The deficiency of glycoprotein Ib results in the inability to bind vWF or respond to ristocetin. As in Glanzmann thrombasthenia, platelet transfusion is the preferred therapy for severe bleeding, but adjunctive measures such as epsilon-aminocaproic acid may be useful in specific instances, such as mouth bleeding. Development of antibodies against the glycoprotein Ib in transfused platelets may render patients refractory to platelet transfusions. In these cases, recombinant factor VIIa may be useful therapy.

Several mutations, involving both subunits of glycoprotein Ib, have been identified as causing Bernard-Soulier syndrome. Atypical Bernard-Soulier disease caused by mutations of glycoprotein IX has also been described.

Gray Platelet Syndrome

Abnormalities of the platelet granules have been described. In the gray platelet syndrome, washed-out or gray-appearing platelets are seen on Wright-stained peripheral blood smears, and a bleeding diathesis occurs that usually is apparent at birth. A specific deficiency of alpha granules has been implicated as the cause of this disorder. A reduction occurs in platelet levels of alpha-granule constituents, such as fibrinogen, vWF, factor V, high-molecular-weight kininogen, fibronectin, thrombospondin, beta-thromboglobulin, platelet factor 4, and platelet-derived growth factor.

Storage Pool Disorders

Deficiencies of the adenine nucleotide-containing dense granules or their contents have been reported in a heterogeneous group of patients. These abnormalities often are referred to collectively as the *storage pool disorders*. Bleeding symptoms usually are not severe. The defect can be demonstrated *in vitro* by a diminished response of platelets to agonists such as collagen, which depend on release of endogenous platelet nucleotides (i.e., second phase of platelet aggregation) for completion of the aggregatory response or by electron microscopy. Dense body deficiencies have been described as part of Hermansky-Pudlak syndrome (i.e., large, bizarre platelets associated with oculocutaneous albinism and accumulation of ceroid in bone marrow macrophages), TAR syndrome, Chédiak-Higashi syndrome, Ehlers-Danlos syndrome, Wiskott-Aldrich syndrome, and osteogenesis imperfecta.

Abnormalities of the Platelet Release Reaction

In addition to the storage pool disorders, several abnormalities associated with the defective release of platelet granular contents have been reported. Abnormalities of arachidonic acid metabolism affect some patients, and defects of calcium metabolism have been postulated for others.

Other Congenital Disorders Associated with Platelet Dysfunction

Abnormalities of platelet function occur in other congenital disorders, such as type I glycogen storage disease, cyanotic congenital heart disease, and pseudoxanthoma elasticum. Platelet dysfunction also can be seen with megathrombocyte disorders, such as Epstein syndrome.

QUANTITATIVE ACQUIRED ABNORMALITIES OF PLATELETS

The acquired disorders of platelets encompass a diverse spectrum of illnesses, including those occurring primarily as disorders of the platelets and a larger group secondary to systemic illnesses. An important diagnostic question is whether thrombocytopenia is occurring as an isolated cytopenia or is accompanying a more generalized marrow failure disorder or systemic illness. One should consider whether the thrombocytopenia is caused by increased destruction or decreased production or is the result of sequestration of platelets. The acquired thrombocytopenic disorders then can be subdivided into immunologic and nonimmunologic processes.

Immunologic Causes of Thrombocytopenia

Idiopathic (Immune) Thrombocytopenic Purpura

Idiopathic thrombocytopenic purpura (ITP), sometimes referred to as *immune* or *autoimmune thrombocytopenic purpura*, is perhaps the most commonly encountered acquired platelet disorder of childhood.

Etiology and Pathogenesis. Although abundant evidence indicates an immunologic basis for this disease, in most cases the cause of the immunologic aberration is not clear, and the term *idiopathic* is preferred. Clinically, the disease is recognized in acute and chronic forms, and a multitude of pathogenetic mechanisms are probably involved. The immunologic basis of the disease has been suggested by classic experiments demonstrating that homologous and autologously transfused platelets are rapidly removed from the circulation, that the illness in adults can be passively transmitted from one person to another by administration of serum from an affected patient, that platelets from patients with ITP typically show increased amounts of immunoglobulin G (IgG) associated with the platelet membrane in several *in vitro* tests, that in some cases specific antiplatelet antibodies can be demonstrated by Western blotting techniques and other assays, and that the disease can be produced in infants by passive transplacental transfer of antiplatelet antibodies from the mother to the fetus. The reticuloendothelial system of the spleen is the major site of destruction of platelets in ITP, with a less important contribution from the reticuloendothelial system of the liver, bone marrow, and lungs.

Although the concept that an immunologic basis exists for ITP is well accepted, the inciting cause for antibody production often remains obscure. Acute ITP in childhood often is preceded by a viral illness, and it has been postulated that viral antigens may trigger the production of antibodies that cross-react with the platelet membrane. The most convincing evidence for this hypothesis is the finding that postinfectious sera from some patients with varicella contain an antibody that cross-reacts with specific platelet membrane glycoproteins. Specific antiglycoprotein IIb/IIIa antibodies have been demonstrated in the chronic forms of ITP, which often occur in the set-

ting of other known autoimmune illnesses. However, the exact significance of the autoantibodies demonstrated in ITP remains the subject of debate. Some studies suggest that much of the platelet-associated IgG (PAIgG) in ITP is not directed against specific platelet antigens. Other serum proteins are associated with platelet membranes in increased amounts, possibly as a nonspecific response to platelet injury. Studies have shown decreased production of platelets in otherwise classic cases of ITP, a finding suggesting that the thrombocytopenia may be the consequence of decreased production and increased destruction in some cases.

Clinical and Laboratory Features. The acute and chronic ITPs tend to vary considerably in their initial presentations. In acute ITP, preceding viral illnesses are common, and the onset of petechiae and ecchymosis (Fig. 297.1) is typically abrupt, so much so that parents can often recount the exact hour that they became aware of the problem. In chronic ITP, antecedent illnesses are less common, and the onset of purpura is often much more insidious. Acute ITP most often presents in previously healthy children, whereas chronic ITP is more common in patients with other underlying immunoregulatory abnormalities, such as systemic lupus erythematosus, IgA deficiency, autoimmune endocrinopathy, common variable immunodeficiency, or autoimmune hemolytic anemia (i.e., Evans syndrome), or with family histories of these disorders. Immunologic destruction of platelets associated with human immunodeficiency virus (HIV) infection is often chronic as well. Acute ITP tends to occur equally in both genders, whereas chronic ITP is more common in female patients. Acute ITP is predominately a disease of early childhood. Chronic ITP is much more common in children older than 10 years.

In acute and chronic ITP, purpura and mucosal bleeding are the most prominent symptoms. The finding that the children generally appear well except for the purpuric lesions is helpful in excluding other illnesses associated with severe thrombocytopenia. Large submucous hemorrhages in the mouth (Fig. 297.2) are thought to be associated with an increased risk for serious hemorrhage. Hepatomegaly, splenomegaly, and lymphadenopathy are notably absent, and their presence

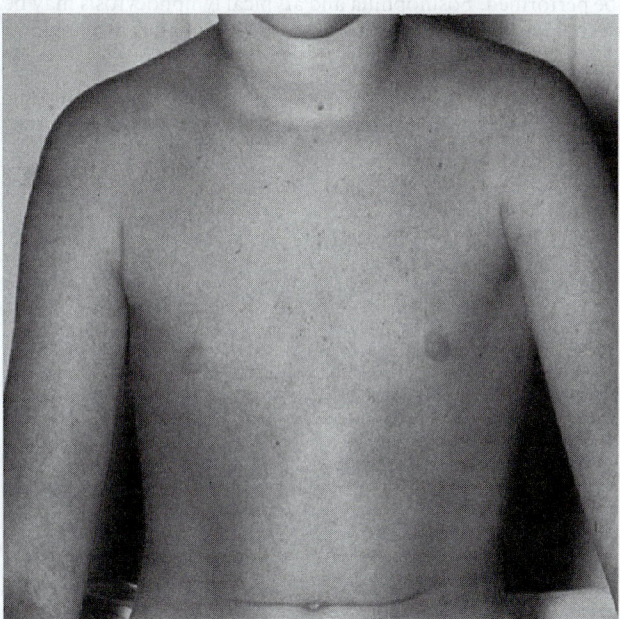

FIGURE 297.1. Petechiae in a patient with idiopathic thrombocytopenic purpura.

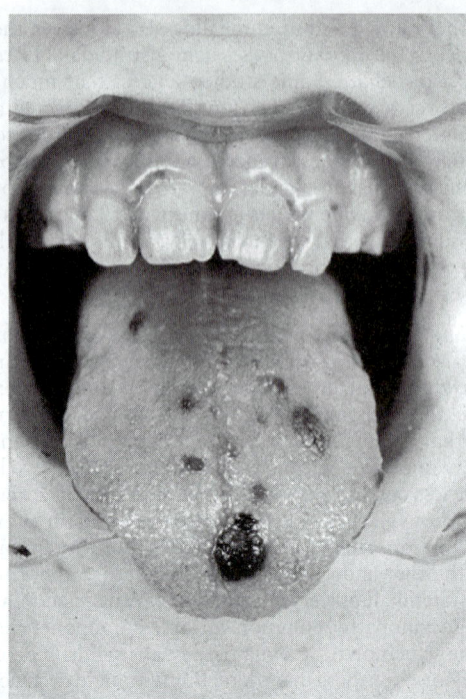

FIGURE 297.2. Submucous hemorrhages in a patient with idiopathic thrombocytopenic purpura.

should initiate an investigation for other possible underlying illnesses associated with thrombocytopenia. Gastrointestinal and renal hemorrhages sometimes occur. Central nervous system bleeding (Fig. 297.3) is the most feared complication of ITP, but it occurs in fewer than 1% of these patients, usually early in the course of the illness. Such hemorrhages are often, but not invariably, fatal.

Platelet counts vary from normal (in a compensated phase) to undetectable, but they tend to be lower in acute ITP than in chronic ITP. The rest of the complete blood count should be normal, unless bleeding sufficient to cause anemia has occurred. A careful review of the peripheral blood smear should be performed. Eosinophilia and atypical lymphocytosis may be seen, but other abnormalities, including immature white blood

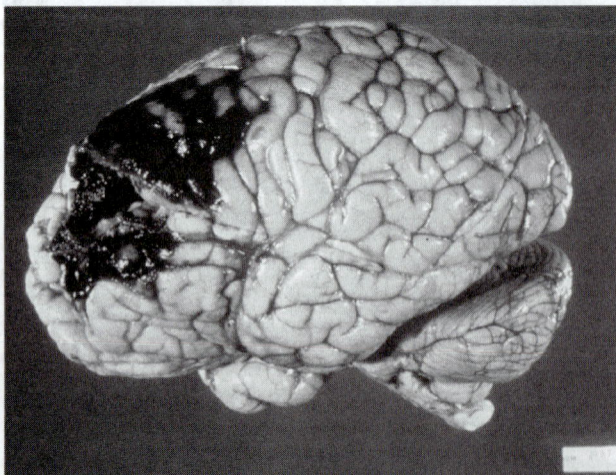

FIGURE 297.3. Intracranial hemorrhage in a patient with idiopathic thrombocytopenic purpura.

cells, are inconsistent with this disorder. Particular attention should be given to identifying red cell morphology consistent with microangiopathic hemolysis, which occurs in thrombotic thrombocytopenic purpura (TTP), a much more serious disorder that can be associated with severe thrombocytopenia. Bone marrow aspirates should exhibit normal to increased numbers of megakaryocytes. In most cases of ITP, however, bone marrow biopsy or aspiration is not necessary, unless signs and symptoms exist of possible bone marrow disease, such as an abnormally low or high white blood cell count, immature white blood cell forms on the peripheral blood smear, red blood cell macrocytosis, systemic symptoms, or organomegaly on physical examination. PAIgG on the platelet surface (i.e., the direct test) is usually positive if sufficient platelets can be obtained for study, but the patient's serum may or may not increase the amount of IgG on the surface of control platelets (i.e., the indirect test). The prothrombin time and activated partial thromboplastin time should be normal. However, no definitive test exists for ITP. The diagnosis remains one of exclusion.

ITP in young children frequently has a benign course with an excellent prognosis. More than 50% of untreated children with ITP recover within 4 weeks without treatment, and more than 80% spontaneously recover within 6 months. The resolution of symptoms and the thrombocytopenia occur in a variety of patterns, from abrupt to slow with frequent relapses. ITP is generally not considered chronic unless symptoms persist for more than 6 months. Relapses are common in chronic ITP. Acute ITP tends not to recur, but relapses have been reported. Improvement of symptoms often precedes a detectable increase in the platelet count.

Treatment. The incidence of serious complications of ITP is very low. Mortality and morbidity are most often associated with intracranial hemorrhage. Given the low incidence of intracranial hemorrhage, no prospective, randomized trials have been carried out that can truly estimate the likelihood that this complication can be prevented. The goal of treatment for most practitioners is to reduce the likelihood of bleeding during periods of maximal risk. Because the spontaneous remission rate for acute ITP is extremely high, a waiting period is usually warranted before attempting therapy at presentation if the disease is mild (i.e., platelet count greater than 20,000/μL, no bleeding other than purpura). Platelet counts of less than 20,000/μL and extensive mucosal hemorrhage may indicate a higher risk for internal hemorrhage, and treatment should be considered. If serious complications are present or suspected or if a protective environment cannot be guaranteed, treatment should be initiated. Historically, corticosteroid administration had been the most commonly used therapy, but now intravenous immune globulin (IVIG) and anti-D immunoglobulin therapy have gained widespread acceptance. The effectiveness of various treatments in this disease is still debated, but the following statements are generally considered to be true:

- Treatment with IVIG or anti-D therapy rapidly increases platelet counts in most patients; treatment with corticosteroids generally increase platelet counts more slowly.
- Treatment does not change the natural history of the disease; that is, treatment does not induce a true remission or shorten the duration of the disease.
- Serious bleeding is rare, seen in about 3% or less of patients.
- Intracranial hemorrhage is rare (less than 1%), but occurs most often with platelet counts lower than 20,000/μL.
- It is not proven that treatment reduces morbidity or mortality with ITP.

Intravenous gamma globulin (IVIG) is a useful modality in the treatment of ITP. The mechanism of action of this agent is not clear, but the best evidence to date suggests that it may act by causing a reticuloendothelial blockade, as evidenced by the reduced splenic clearance of sensitized erythrocytes after administration. Recent animal models of ITP demonstrate that IVIG may inhibit phagocytosis of platelets by upregulation of the inhibitory receptor, $Fc\gamma RIIb$. Other animal models suggest that IVIG promotes clearance of antiplatelet antibodies. Modulation of T- or B-cell function has also been postulated, and it has been speculated that the clearance of infection or antigenemia may play a role. Commonly used treatment regimens vary from 0.8 to 2.0 g/kg divided over 1 to 5 days. The most commonly used dose is 1 g/kg in a single administration. Responses are usually rapid and transitory and should not be expected in all patients. Although this therapy is quite efficacious, up to 34% of patients may experience transient complications manifested by severe headache, nausea and, rarely, aseptic meningitis. Premedication with corticosteroids or acetaminophen and diphenhydramine may decrease the frequency of these side effects. As with all plasma-derived products, some risk of transmission of infection exists, although modern products appear to be quite safe. In addition, IVIG therapy is extremely expensive.

Anti-D immunoglobulin is a relatively new therapy, but it is emerging as the most commonly used treatment for ITP in the United States. Although the mechanism of action is incompletely understood, antibody-coated red cells are hypothesized to compete with antibody-coated platelets for destruction in the reticuloendothelial system. Patients who are Rh negative have no response to anti-D immunoglobulin. Splenectomized individuals may respond suboptimally, but responses have been seen. Treatment regimens vary from 25 μg/kg/dose on 1 or 2 consecutive days to 50 to 75 μg/kg intravenously in a single administration and can be infused within half an hour. Intramuscular use also has been reported. Response rates appear to be similar to that of IVIG, with perhaps a slightly longer delay in response; however, this finding may be dose related. The major toxicity associated with anti-D immunoglobulin is a predictable decrease in hemoglobin (mean hemoglobin decrease, 1.3 g/dL). Severe anemia as a result of therapy with anti-D immunoglobulin appears to be rare. However, this therapy is not recommended for patients with significant anemia. Given its ease of use, the outstanding safety record of anti-D immunoglobulin for other indications, and its significantly lower protein load and expense, use of this therapy has gained widespread acceptance. As with all plasma-derived products, caution is indicated in its use, because of potential infectious risks and the possibility of allergic reactions.

Prednisone is usually administered at an initial dosage of 2 mg/kg/day orally, but higher or intravenous dosages up to 30 mg/kg/day of methylprednisolone for very short periods may be more effective. In addition, high-dose Decadron (40 mg/day for 4 days) has been used with some success in adult patients with ITP and chronic ITP. Although prednisone will increase the platelet count in the majority of patients with ITP, the response is somewhat slower than that of IVIG and anti-D immunoglobulin. Corticosteroids are commonly used at stable initial doses for 1 to several weeks, followed by a tapering schedule. Corticosteroid toxicity limits long-term use at high doses; however, relapse is common after a taper that is too rapid, and responsive patients may tolerate low daily or alternate-day therapy remarkably well over long periods, even years.

Platelet transfusions are generally eschewed in ITP, because of the shortened survival of transfused platelets. However, platelet transfusions may be effective in immediately reducing serious bleeding. Splenectomy is effective in resolving the thrombocytopenia in approximately two-thirds of patients,

but generally it is used only in emergencies or in extremely resistant cases. Other therapeutic approaches, such as *Vinca*-loaded platelets or vincristine infusions, other immunosuppressive agents such as azathioprine, cyclosporine, and cyclophosphamide, and miscellaneous agents such as interferon, ascorbic acid, or danazol have been used in chronic ITP. Recently, an intriguing association with *Helicobacter pylori* infection and patients with chronic ITP has been described; the ITP has improved in some patients treated for the infection. The significance of these early findings and the indications for treatment for *Helicobacter pylori* infection remain to be clarified, especially in children. In general, success rates tend to be low with all these therapies and should be used after more conventional modes of therapy have failed. Newer therapies have shown promise in the treatment of refractory ITP. Rituximab, which is a monoclonal antibody directed against the CD20 antigen of B lymphocytes, is emerging an effective treatment in selected patients.

Drug-Induced Immune Thrombocytopenia

Acute thrombocytopenia caused by the development of specific antibodies has been attributed to a variety of drugs. These antibodies may be directed against a specific platelet antigen–drug (i.e., hapten) complex or may result from absorption of antigen–antibody complexes onto the platelet surface (i.e., "innocent bystander" phenomenon). In rare instances, they may represent true autoantibodies that recognize platelet antigens in the absence of the drug. Clinically, the onset of thrombocytopenia tends to be abrupt, within hours after the ingestion or administration of the drug, and ceases with clearance of the drug. The thrombocytopenia is frequently severe enough to be life-threatening and tends to recur with repeated administration of the drug. Rechallenge with the offending drug should not be undertaken unless the drug in question is indispensable. *In vitro* testing to determine whether a drug is responsible for an immune-mediated thrombocytopenia is available. If postrecovery serum from the patient increases PAIgG on the patient's or the control's platelets *in vitro* only in the presence of the drug, it can be assumed that the drug tested is the causative agent.

Drugs that have been convincingly demonstrated to be causes of drug-induced thrombocytopenia include the penicillins, trimethoprim-sulfamethoxazole, digoxin, quinine, quinidine, cimetidine, benzodiazepine, stibophen, novobiocin, and allylisopropylacetylurea (Sedormid). Many other agents have the potential for causing immune-mediated thrombocytopenia. Withdrawal of the potential offending drug and *in vitro* testing should be considered in equivocal cases.

Heparin-induced thrombocytopenia (HIT) is well recognized in adults and is becoming a more frequently appreciated complication in pediatric patients. Two forms of HIT have been described. Mild, nonimmune-mediated thrombocytopenia can occur within 1 to 2 days in the course of heparin therapy and is benign. In other cases, more severe thrombocytopenia develops 4 to 10 days after initiation of heparin. This form of HIT is immune mediated and may be paradoxically associated with both arterial and venous thrombosis. In this severe form of HIT, antibodies are formed against a complex of heparin and the platelet factor 4 hapten antigen. Antibodies bound to heparin–platelet factor 4 complex then bind and activate platelets via the Fc portion of the antibodies. The activated platelets and platelet microparticles may lead to thrombotic events; the platelets are cleared more quickly, resulting in thrombocytopenia. If this type of HIT is diagnosed, further exposure to all forms of heparin, including both unfractionated and low-molecular-weight heparin, is contraindicated.

Neonatal Immune Thrombocytopenia

Severe thrombocytopenia in the neonatal period may occur because of transplacental transfer of antibody from a mother who has ITP (i.e., passive autoimmune thrombocytopenia). In these cases, PAIgG usually can be detected on the mother's platelets (i.e., direct PAIgG test) and often in the mother's serum (i.e., indirect PAIgG test). The mother's platelet count is not a good predictor of thrombocytopenia in the infant. Mothers with normal platelet counts, especially those who have undergone splenectomy for ITP, may deliver severely thrombocytopenic infants. However, thrombocytopenic mothers with ITP often deliver infants with normal platelet counts. In some cases, the platelet count may decrease over the first few days of life. The thrombocytopenia may persist for days to months, paralleling the disappearance of maternal antibody from the infant's circulation.

Neonatal thrombocytopenia may occur in infants born to mothers who have been sensitized to antigens on the infant's platelets that are absent from her platelets (i.e., alloimmune or isoimmune thrombocytopenia). Five well-known human platelet alloantigen systems (HPA 1 through 5) exist, each a result of a single amino acid substitution in the gene for the glycoprotein on which the antigen resides. The frequency of the platelet antigens varies among different ethnic groups. The most common platelet antigen incompatibility involves the Pl^{A1} system, or HPA 1. In this system, three phenotypes are possible: HPA(1a/1a) (i.e., homozygous Pl^{A1} positivity), HPA(1a/1b) (i.e., heterozygous Pl^{A1} positivity), and HPA(1b/1b) (i.e., homozygous Pl^{A1} negativity). Approximately 98% of the population of the United States is HPA(1a/1a) or HPA(1a/1b). If the mother is HPA(1b/1b), the father is likely to be HPA(1a/1a) or HPA(1a/1b), and the infant will be a candidate for alloimmune disease. Certain platelet antigens belonging to systems HPA 2 through 5, such as Bak, Pen (Yuk), Ko, Pl^t, and Br, less commonly implicated as a cause of alloimmune thrombocytopenia have been described, as well as other minor platelet antigens capable of causing alloimmune disorders. The mother's platelet count is normal in these disorders. *In vitro* testing should demonstrate that the direct test result for PAIgG on the mother is negative. However, her serum should increase the amount of PAIgG on the father's or the infant's platelets and control antigen-positive platelets (i.e., indirect test). Alloimmune thrombocytopenia most often resolves within a few weeks, but it can persist for longer. As with erythrocyte sensitization, a high risk of recurrence exists with future pregnancies.

Cesarean section should be considered for any delivery in which the child is at risk for alloimmune-mediated thrombocytopenia, because the risk of intracranial hemorrhage at the time of delivery is high; platelets should be available in the delivery room. However, because of the low risk of intracranial hemorrhage in neonates of mothers with ITP, many obstetricians prefer vaginal delivery. Neonatal immune thrombocytopenia has been treated successfully with transfusion of platelets and exchange transfusion. Corticosteroids may be useful if administered to the mother before delivery or to the infant after delivery. Intracranial hemorrhages may occur *in utero* in some infants, most commonly in cases of alloimmune thrombocytopenia resulting from HPA 1 sensitization. Several therapies have been proposed to prevent these hemorrhages, and what constitutes optimal therapy is still controversial. The administration of IVIG to mothers prenatally appears to reduce the incidence of intracranial hemorrhage. *In utero* transfusions of maternal platelets have also been used to prevent intracranial hemorrhage in alloimmune disease. The use of a corticosteroid preparation that is not inactivated by the placenta, such as dexamethasone, is controversial. Postnatally, IVIG for autoimmune thrombocytopenia appears to be equally effective as in other forms of ITP. Intravenous gamma globulin also may increase the platelet count in alloimmune thrombocytopenia; however, transfusion of mother's platelets represents optimal therapy postnatally, because they do not possess the sensitizing antigen and therefore have normal survival.

Posttransfusion Purpura

A few patients, usually adults, respond to erythrocyte transfusions by developing severe thrombocytopenia. The lowering of the platelet count typically occurs abruptly approximately 1 week after the erythrocyte transfusion. Affected patients are typically HPA(1b/1b) (i.e., Pl^{A1} negative) women with a history of one or more pregnancies, who have been transfused with blood from an HPA(1a/1a) or HPA(1a/1b) (i.e., Pl^{A1} positive) donor. Some studies suggest that the thrombocytopenia is secondary to passive absorption of soluble HPA 1a antigen from the donor's plasma onto the recipient's platelets, but the pathophysiology may be more complex.

Nonimmune Causes of Thrombocytopenia

Infectious Thrombocytopenia

Thrombocytopenia may be associated with a variety of infections, viral infections being the most common offenders. The thrombocytopenia may occur during the active infection or as a postinfectious manifestation of the illness. In congenital rubella, for example, the thrombocytopenia can persist for months and often follows a course similar to that of ITP. Viruses and viral infections associated with thrombocytopenia include varicella, Epstein-Barr virus, cytomegalovirus, other herpesviruses, and measles. In some cases, thrombocytopenia may be caused by generalized marrow suppression that sometimes occurs after Epstein-Barr viral infections and hepatitis. The mechanism of the thrombocytopenia is not always clear, but in the case of rubella and cytomegalovirus, the virus can be cultured from the marrow. Thrombocytopenia may accompany a number of other systemic infections, including toxoplasmosis, ehrlichiosis, malaria, syphilis, tuberculosis, and overwhelming bacterial or rickettsial sepsis.

Infection with HIV is an increasingly common cause of thrombocytopenia. Features of immune and nonimmune causes of thrombocytopenia are encountered. Thrombocytopenia can be seen early in the course of HIV infection as the only hematologic abnormality in patients who are otherwise asymptomatic or later in the disease as part of a more generalized bone marrow suppressive process associated with overt acquired immunodeficiency syndrome. The opportunistic infections of these patients, or the administration of antiviral therapy, can cause thrombocytopenia. HIV infection has been postulated to cause thrombocytopenia by a variety of mechanisms, including immune destruction of platelets, direct viral invasion of megakaryocytes, and inhibition of stem cells. Increased levels of PAIgG often occur with normal numbers of megakaryocytes, producing a clinical syndrome compatible with ITP. In addition, hemolytic uremic syndrome (HUS) and TTP have been reported in association with HIV.

Administration of IVIG or anti-D immunoglobulin is often effective in reversing thrombocytopenia in HIV infection. In many cases, corticosteroids and splenectomy are effective in elevating the platelet count, but they are less preferred therapies. Antiviral therapy may improve the platelet count. This result may be mediated by direct antiviral effects or an effect on the underlying aberrant immune response. Attention should be directed toward treatment of possible associated opportunistic infections. Therapies specific to the particular disorder should be considered if the symptoms suggest HUS or TTP.

Microangiopathic Causes of Thrombocytopenia

Thrombocytopenia is a hallmark feature of HUS and TTP. HUS typically presents with bloody diarrhea, followed by the onset of renal failure, thrombocytopenia, and anemia. Central nervous system involvement, often manifested by seizures, is common. Other extrarenal manifestations include myocarditis, pancreatitis, hepatitis, intussusception, and colitis, which may be followed by colonic strictures. Bacterial and viral infections, toxins, drugs, and prostaglandin abnormalities have been implicated in the pathogenesis of HUS. A verotoxin-producing *Escherichia coli* (*E. coli* O157:H7) identified in several outbreaks of HUS is an important etiologic agent in the epidemic form of the syndrome. Thrombin is activated, and fibrin degradation products are often elevated, but disseminated intravascular coagulation (DIC) is generally not seen. In addition, patients have evidence for impaired fibrinolysis. Platelet survival is shortened, presumably secondary to a local microangiopathic process involving fibrin deposition. As discussed elsewhere in this book in more detail (see Chapter 457), typical HUS is treated generally with supportive care, often including peritoneal dialysis. Red blood cell transfusions are given only to prevent cardiac failure. Platelet transfusions generally are not needed and should be given only in the event of serious hemorrhage caused by thrombocytopenia or as prophylaxis for invasive procedures.

The syndrome of TTP overlaps significantly with HUS, to the point that the two syndromes may be different parts of the same spectrum. TTP tends to occur in adults and is more commonly associated with fever than HUS. Neurologic symptoms and microangiopathic hemolytic anemia are prominent, but renal dysfunction is less common and less severe than in HUS. Vascular lesions in HUS show a predominance of fibrin, but platelet aggregates predominate in the vessels of patients with TTP. Recently, molecular mechanisms underlying TTP have been elucidated, revealing a biochemical distinction between these syndromes. Patients with TTP have significantly depressed activity of a protease that cleaves high-molecular-weight multimers of vWF, called ADAMTS13. It is postulated that deficiency of this activity leads to increased high-molecular-weight vWF multimers and platelet clumping. Congenital deficiencies have been described, and acquired cases are often the result of inhibitory antibodies to this enzyme. TTP is usually fatal if treated with supportive care alone, but dramatic improvements in survival have been produced using corticosteroids and plasma exchange as primary therapies. Platelet transfusions should be avoided if possible, because they may exacerbate central nervous system and cardiac symptoms.

Hemangiomas may result in thrombocytopenia (i.e., Kasabach-Merritt syndrome). The pathogenesis of this phenomenon involves platelet sequestration and destruction in the hemangiomatous lesion. Often, evidence exists of fibrin consumption. The pathologic features of the lesions that result in Kasabach-Merritt syndrome are usually those of kaposiform hemangioendotheliomas. Various treatments have been proposed, including corticosteroid administration, platelet and cryoprecipitate transfusions, epsilon-aminocaproic acid, radiation therapy, aspirin, dipyridamole, and surgery. Promising results have been reported with the use of interferon-alpha-2a, however this treatment carries the risk of spastic diplegia. Vincristine has been shown to be effective in a number of refractory cases. Newer antiangiogenic factors show promise, but they are still experimental therapies. The ultimate usefulness of each therapy is not clear. Conservative treatment is indicated when possible, because the lesions tend to regress spontaneously. Thrombocytopenia may be a manifestation of DIC, which is discussed later in this chapter.

Drug-Induced Thrombocytopenia

Several drugs cause thrombocytopenia in the absence of an identifiable immune mechanism. In the pediatric population, valproic acid is a common offender. Heparin administration can be complicated by an immune and a nonimmune form of HIT, as described in the section on drug-induced immune thrombocytopenia. Chloramphenicol may produce thrombocytopenia as an isolated finding or as part of a more generalized marrow aplasia. Other agents suppressing megakaryopoiesis and thrombopoiesis include the thiazide diuretics, alcohol, chemotherapeutic drugs, anticonvulsants, antibiotics, and ionizing radiation.

Miscellaneous Thrombocytopenias

Many other clinical conditions may be associated with significant thrombocytopenia. Hypersplenism of any cause, including congestive (e.g., Banti syndrome), infiltrative (e.g., Gaucher disease), sequestrative (e.g., sickle cell disease), or rheumatologic (e.g., Felty syndrome) can cause thrombocytopenia. Thrombocytopenia is seen commonly in cyanotic congenital heart disease with polycythemia. Severe liver disease of almost any cause may be associated with a low platelet count. Severe hypothermia or anoxia, as well as respiratory distress syndrome, may induce thrombocytopenia in the neonate. Thrombocytopenia may be a manifestation of severe iron deficiency or deficiencies of folate or vitamin B_{12}. Placement of large-vessel catheters, cardiopulmonary bypass, cardiac prostheses, rejection phenomena, and severe allergic reactions can lower the platelet count. Myeloproliferative and myelodysplastic disorders, leukemia, congenital and acquired aplastic anemia are commonly associated with thrombocytopenia (Fig. 297.4).

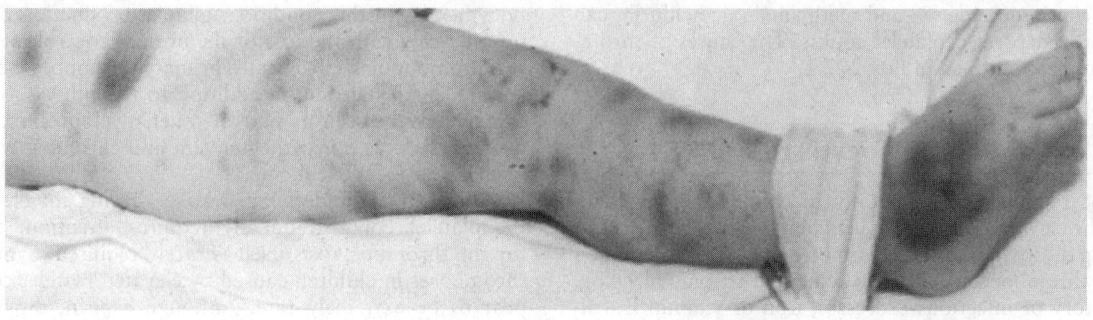

FIGURE 297.4. Extensive ecchymosis in a patient with leukemia and thrombocytopenia.

BOX 297.1   Causes of Thrombocytopenia

Immune
Idiopathic (Immune) Thrombocytopenia Purpura
Idiopathic
Associated with viral infections
    Epstein-Barr virus
    Cytomegalovirus
    Measles
    Varicella
    Human immunodeficiency virus
Associated with autoimmune disease or immunodeficiency
    Systemic lupus erythematosus
    Common variable immunodeficiency
Posttransfusion purpura
Tn-polyagglutination syndrome

Drug-Induced Thrombocytopenia
Heparin-induced thrombocytopenia
Penicillin
Quinine
Other drugs

Neonatal Thrombocytopenia
Neonatal alloimmune thrombocytopenia
Neonatal autoimmune thrombocytopenia

Nonimmune
Congenital Thrombocytopenia
Syndromes associated with ineffective platelet production and/or bone marrow failure
    Thrombocytopenia with absent radius syndrome
    Amegakaryocytic thrombocytopenia
    Associated with WASP mutations
        Wiskott-Aldrich syndrome
        Sex-linked recessive thrombocytopenia
    Fanconi aplastic anemia
    Shwachman syndrome
    Dyskeratosis congenita
Chromosomal abnormalities
    Trisomy 13, 18
    Down syndrome
    Chromosome 11q23 deletion (Paris-Trousseau)
    Chromosome 22q11 deletion (velocardiofacial syndrome)

Familial giant platelet syndromes
    Associated with MYH9 mutations
    May-Hegglin anomaly
    Fechtner syndrome
    Sebastian syndrome
    Epstein syndrome
Bernard-Soulier syndrome
Gray platelet syndrome

Acquired Thrombocytopenia
Myelosuppression
    Infection-associated
    Drug-associated
Bone marrow infiltration
    Leukemia
    Storage disease
Bone marrow failure
    Acquired aplastic anemia
    Myelodysplastic syndrome
    Vitamin B_{12}/folate deficiency
Microangiopathic hemolytic anemia
    Hemolytic-uremic syndrome
    Thrombotic thrombocytopenia purpura
    Disseminated intravascular coagulopathy
    Hemangioma (Kasabach-Merritt syndrome)

Miscellaneous Etiologies
Hypersplenism
Liver disease
Polycythemia with cyanotic heart disease
Associated with deep venous thrombosis
Associated with intravascular catheters
Severe iron deficiency
Osteopetrosis
Graft-versus-host disease
Asphyxia
Respiratory distress syndrome
Severe allergic reactions
Type 2B von Willebrand disease
Noonan syndrome
Sex-linked thrombocytopenia with *GATA1* gene mutations
Inborn errors of metabolism

Osteopetrosis causes the obliteration of the bone marrow cavity, with resulting thrombocytopenia and bone marrow failure. Graft-versus-host disease is another cause of thrombocytopenia, which is seen after bone marrow transplantation, or if can be transfusion associated. Several inborn errors of metabolism, such as proprionicacidemia and methylmalonic aciduria, can also result in depressed platelet counts. The causes of thrombocytopenia are outlined in Box 297.1.

Thrombocytosis

Thrombocytosis occurs commonly in children. In most instances, the elevation of the platelet count is attributable to an underlying disorder associated with thrombocytosis. Common causes of thrombocytosis include acute and chronic bleeding, inflammatory or infectious processes, iron or vitamin E deficiency, hemolytic anemia, and asplenia. Thrombocytosis may occur as a result of neoplastic processes, drug administration

(e.g., vinca alkaloids, epinephrine), nephrotic syndrome, graft-versus-host disease, or during treatment of megaloblastic anemias. Kawasaki disease is frequently associated with extremely high platelet counts. Rarely, thrombocytosis is the result of a primary myeloproliferative syndrome, such as essential thrombocythemia. In this condition, platelet production occurs autonomously, with the loss of the normal control mechanisms for thrombopoiesis. Ironically, primary thrombocythemia is associated with bleeding in addition to thrombosis. Thrombocytosis may be seen as part of other myeloproliferative syndromes, such as polycythemia vera and chronic myelogenous or megakaryocytic leukemia.

Although an underlying disease causing an elevation of the platelet count frequently requires attention, treatment for the thrombocytosis itself is rarely required. Symptomatic thromboses in children caused by elevated platelet counts appear to be extremely rare. Although aspirin, dipyridamole, or other platelet antagonists are sometimes prescribed for extreme thrombocytosis, their efficacy in preventing thrombotic complications in children has not been demonstrated. The natural history of thrombocythemia is poorly understood, and the value of treatment of this disorder with chemotherapeutic agents has not been documented.

QUALITATIVE ACQUIRED ABNORMALITIES OF PLATELETS

Acquired abnormalities of platelet function occur most commonly after the ingestion of drugs that inhibit platelet function. Although large numbers of drugs inhibit platelet function *in vitro*, exposure to aspirin-containing compounds or other cyclooxygenase inhibitors is by far the most common cause of drug-induced platelet dysfunction. Some semisynthetic penicillins, carbenicillin in particular, and valproic acid cause a prolongation of the bleeding time that may be attributable to impaired platelet function. Acquired abnormalities of platelet function have been demonstrated in uremia and severe liver disease. The exact mechanism of the abnormality in platelet function in these patients is not well characterized but presumably relates to the accumulation of toxins. Interference with platelet function may occur in DIC because of the accumulation of fibrin degradation products. Platelet function may be abnormal in several myeloproliferative disorders. In rare instances, platelet dysfunction may be secondary to the development of antibodies against specific platelet-surface glycoproteins (e.g., acquired or pseudo-Bernard-Soulier disease caused by antiglycoprotein Ib antibodies). Antibody-induced platelet dysfunction may be present in some cases of ITP.

Acknowledgments

The authors gratefully acknowledge William Zinkham, M.D. for supplying patient photographs.

Suggested Readings

Ancona KG, Parker RI, Atlas MP, Prakash D. Randomized trial of high-dose methylprednisolone versus intravenous immunoglobulin for the treatment of acute idiopathic thrombocytopenic purpura in children. *J Pediatr Hematol Oncol* 2002;24:540.

Blanchette V, Imbach P, Andrew M, et al. Randomised trial of intravenous immunoglobulin G, intravenous anti-D, and oral prednisone in childhood acute immune thrombocytopenic purpura. *Lancet* 1994;344:703.

Blanchette VS, Carcao M. Childhood acute immune thrombocytopenic purpura: 20 years later. *Semin Thromb Hemost* 2003;29:605.

Blanchette VS, Price V. Childhood chronic immune thrombocytopenic purpura: unresolved issues. *J Pediatr Hematol Oncol* 2003;25(suppl 1):S28.

Bussel JB. Fetal and neonatal cytopenias: what have we learned? *Am J Perinatol* 2003;20:425.

Coyle TE. Hematologic complications of human immunodeficiency virus infection and the acquired immunodeficiency syndrome. *Med Clin North Am* 1997;81:449.

Geddis AE, Kaushansky K. Inherited thrombocytopenias: toward a molecular understanding of disorders of platelet production. *Curr Opin Pediatr* 2004;16:15.

Handin RJ. Blood platelets and the vessel wall. In: Nathan DG, Orkin SH, Ginsberg D, Look AT, eds. *Hematology of Infancy and Childhood*. Philadelphia: WB Saunders, 2004:1457.

Kuhne T, Buchanan GR, Zimmerman S, et al. A prospective comparative study of 2540 infants and children with newly diagnosed idiopathic thrombocytopenic purpura (ITP) from the Intercontinental Childhood ITP Study Group. *J Pediatr* 2003;143:605.

Parise LV, Smyth SS, Coller BS. Platelet morphology, biochemistry and function. In: Beutler E, Lichtman MA, Coller BS, et al, eds. *Williams hematology*. New York: McGraw-Hill, 2000:1357.

CHAPTER 298 ■ DISORDERS OF COAGULATION FACTORS

JAMES F. CASELLA, CLIFFORD M. TAKEMOTO, AND MARIA A. PELIDIS

CONGENITAL ABNORMALITIES OF COAGULATION FACTORS

Abnormalities of the Factor VIII Complex

Classically, two major congenital disorders have been attributed to abnormalities of the factor VIII molecule: hemophilia A, also referred to as *factor VIII deficiency*, and von Willebrand disease. Hemophilia A represents a defect in factor VIII procoagulant activity in which platelet function is normal, whereas von Willebrand disease involves a defect in platelet function associated with a variable abnormality of factor VIII procoagulant activity. The abnormality of platelet function in von Willebrand disease is caused by decreased or defective von Willebrand factor (vWF), a substance necessary for platelet adhesion to damaged blood vessel walls and maintenance of a normal bleeding time.

In the past, the relation of factor VIII procoagulant activity to vWF was poorly understood. Advances in the molecular biology and protein biochemistry of factor VIII have demonstrated that circulating factor VIII is a complex of two different proteins: the factor VIII procoagulant protein (i.e., factor VIII:C) and vWF. These proteins are products of separate genes, and each has unique antigenic sites. vWF is a macromolecular structure (i.e., multimer) composed of multiple smaller subunits and appears to act as a carrier protein for the factor VIII procoagulant molecule. Therefore, factor VIII procoagulant activity is likely to be reduced when vWF is not present in sufficient quantities. The designation *vWF:Ag* refers to the major antigen on vWF that is recognized by heterologous antisera against the factor VIII complex; the designation *vWF:RCo* (i.e., ristocetin cofactor) indicates one of the activities of vWF *in vitro* (i.e., the ability of the molecule to support ristocetin-induced agglutination of platelets). An appreciation of these relationships is essential to understanding the clinical disease states.

Factor VIII Deficiency

Etiology and Pathogenesis. Factor VIII deficiency (i.e., hemophilia A) is a sex-linked disorder, occurring in approximately 1 in 5,000 male newborns. The disease results from a deficient or abnormal factor VIII procoagulant molecule (factor VIII:C). More than 200 discrete mutations or deletions in the factor VIII gene that result in hemophilia A have been described. However, inversions at the end of the X chromosome appear to be responsible for 35% to 45% of the cases of severe factor VIII deficiency. Spontaneous mutations are common and occur at "hot spots" in the factor VIII gene that are prone to mutations. Factor VIII levels in affected persons vary from less than 1% to approximately 25% of normal activity. Levels of vWF are normal. Female carriers of the disease are usually asymptomatic and generally have factor VIII levels between 25% and 75% of normal, with normal vWF assays. However, a carrier may have factor VIII:C activity levels higher than 100% of normal (normal range, 50% to 200%); thus, the carrier state cannot be identified in all women by use of functional assays of factor VIII:C alone. However, measurements of factor VIII:C and vWF with determinations of DNA polymorphisms among family members can detect more than 95% of the carriers of the abnormal X chromosome. Clinical severity of the disease varies with the degree of deficiency of factor VIII activity and tends to be consistent among affected male subjects in a given kindred; however, significant variations in factor VIII activity among siblings with the same mutation have been reported, a finding suggesting that the severity of the disease can be modified by other genetic factors.

Clinical and Laboratory Features. Factor VIII deficiency is characterized by a lifelong tendency toward serious and often life-threatening hemorrhage. Whereas surface bleeding and purpura can occur, deep soft tissue bleeding and hemarthrosis are the hallmarks of the disease. Patients with hemophilia can be divided into three groups based on clinical severity of the disease and the level of factor VIII activity: severe (less than 1% factor VIII activity), moderate (1% to 5% factor VIII activity), and mild (5% to 25% factor VIII activity). Patients with severe hemophilia are subject to spontaneous bleeding into joints or soft tissue sites. Those with moderate hemophilia classically develop severe bleeding only after trauma, but patients with mild hemophilia may be symptomatic only after surgery or major trauma. Life-threatening bleeding can occur in all groups. Patients with severe hemophilia may not bleed excessively immediately after small lacerations or venipunctures because of lack of impairment of platelet function; however, delayed bleeding at such sites is common, particularly if sutures have been placed.

The symptoms tend to vary with age. Approximately 50% of patients with hemophilia escape detection in the neonatal period, even if circumcisions are performed. Serious hemorrhages, including intracranial, are not uncommon in the neonatal period. Mucous membrane bleeding in the mouth and bruises, particularly palpable subcutaneous hematomas, are much more common in infancy than later life. The frequency of hemarthrosis tends to increase as the child becomes ambulatory. The age of first bleeding varies considerably. In one study, approximately 10% of patients with hemophilia suffered at least one joint hemorrhage by 11 months of age (none before 30 days of age), 27% by 18 months of age, and 33% by 30 months of age.

Although bleeding may occur at virtually any anatomic site, the most common serious bleeding encountered in hemophilia is hemarthrosis, with knees, elbows, and ankles representing the most commonly affected joints; shoulders, wrists, and hips are less frequently involved. The onset of hemarthrosis is often marked by development of pain without other objective findings, followed by acute swelling, warmth, and tenderness of the joint, sometimes accompanied by erythema or discoloration. Bleeding into soft tissues and bursae around the joint may occur. Repeated bleeding into the same joint results in synovial damage and hypertrophy, and produces secondary cartilaginous and bony abnormalities. The development of muscular atrophy and contraction of ligamentous structures around such target joints is common. The combination of soft tissue, bony, and cartilaginous abnormalities results in an anatomically abnormal joint that is more susceptible to successive bleeding episodes. Disruption of the epiphyseal structures may result in growth abnormalities. The development of bony cysts represents a late complication of hemarthrosis. Rarely, erosive pseudotumors of bone may be seen.

Central nervous system bleeding is one of the most feared complications of hemophilia and is usually the result of trauma. Symptoms may be minimal immediately after the traumatic event, and the seriousness of the bleeding may not become evident until several days after the initial incident. Even minor episodes of head trauma may be followed by intracranial bleeding, and spontaneous intracranial hemorrhage may occur.

Hemorrhage with dental procedures can be severe; preferably, patients should seek treatment from dentists who are familiar with the management of hemophilia. Lip or tongue lacerations occur frequently in toddlers and younger children and can be quite troublesome, possibly because of the high level of fibrinolytic activity of saliva. Excessive bleeding from a torn frenulum can indicate hemophilia, as does the development of a large fleshy clot (Fig. 298.1). Other gastrointestinal bleeding can occur and is usually associated with some type of structural abnormality. Bleeding into retroperitoneal spaces occurs with some frequency and can sometimes be mistaken for an intraabdominal process. Hematuria is relatively common and can be persistent. Bleeding into muscles or soft tissue can occur at any site. The seriousness of these bleeding episodes is dictated usually by their anatomic location. Entrapment of nerves or blood vessels can be particularly problematic. Bleeding in

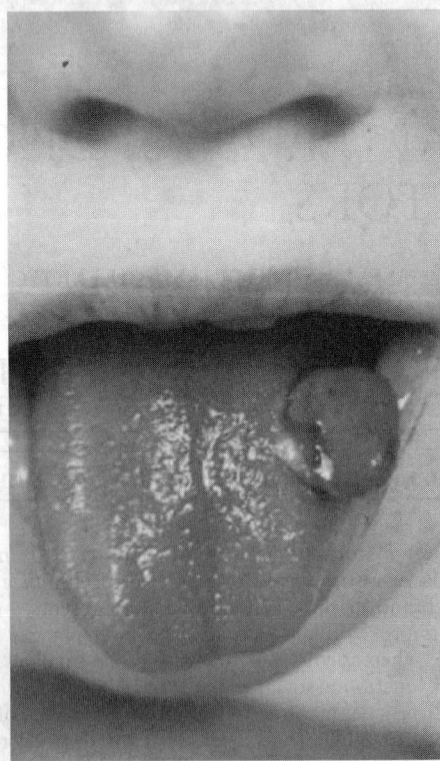

FIGURE 298.1. Granuloma formation after tongue laceration in a patient with hemophila.

the area of the airway should be managed as a life-threatening event. Severe hemorrhage may be experienced after surgery if adequate replacement therapy is not administered.

Diagnosis of hemophilia A requires demonstration of low factor VIII:C activity in the presence of a normal vWF assay. The activated partial thromboplastin time (aPTT) usually is prolonged, and the prothrombin time (PT) is normal; however, in some mild forms of factor VIII deficiency, the aPTT result may be normal. Test results of platelet function usually are normal, although abnormal template bleeding times have been observed in some patients with hemophilia. A family history may reveal a sex-linked pattern of inheritance; however, the family history may be negative because of a predominance of female family members in successive generations or the high rate of spontaneous mutations.

Treatment, Prevention, and General Care. Prevention of bleeding should be a major goal of treatment, with care taken to avoid overprotecting the patient. Infants should be provided with padded cribs and playpens. The beneficial effects of regular exercise in strengthening muscles and protecting joints from injury should be stressed. Most practitioners recommend against contact sports, but nontraumatic sports such as swimming should be encouraged. How restrictive recommendations about sports should be is a subject of considerable debate. Blanket recommendations are often of little use, and family and patient lifestyle preferences and acceptance of risk should be taken into account in these decisions. Platelet-inhibitory substances such as aspirin and nonsteroidal antiinflammatory drugs should be avoided. Immunizations should be administered after replacement with factor VIII or should be given intradermally rather than intramuscularly to avoid hemorrhagic complications. Vaccination against hepatitis B should be given in infancy as part of the current routine immunizations; in older children who were not vaccinated, hepatitis B immunization should be administered as soon as possible. In addition, hepatitis A vaccination is recommended for all patients with hemophilia. Prophylactic dental treatment should be encouraged. Invasive procedures such as lumbar puncture should be performed only under coverage with factor VIII.

Replacement therapy with factor VIII remains the most important part of the care of the patient with hemophilia. Home therapy has gained widespread acceptance and offers the opportunity for earlier treatment of bleeding episodes and increased autonomy for the patient. Such programs require close physician supervision. Prophylactic therapy has gained wider acceptance and should be offered to all patients with hemophilia. The goal of this therapy is to provide replacement therapy frequently enough to maintain a trough level of factor VIII greater than 1% at all times (as discussed in a following section) and to reduce long-term joint morbidity. Although expensive, this therapy can result in a significant improvement in quality of life.

Bloodborne infections such as hepatitis and acquired immunodeficiency syndrome have been major complications of therapy in hemophilia. Most patients with hemophilia who were exposed to factor VIII replacement between 1979 and 1984 are seropositive for human immunodeficiency virus (HIV). After introduction of screening procedures in 1985, the rate of HIV seroconversion in previously uninfected patients decreased dramatically. Improved methods of viral inactivation further enhanced the safety of plasma-derived factor concentrates; since 1987, there have been no documented cases of HIV transmission with these products. Recombinant factor products have been available since 1992, thus providing an extra margin of safety.

Dosage and Schedule of Factor VIII Replacement. The level and duration of replacement with factor VIII depend on the severity of bleeding. Replacement. doses can be calculated using the rule that 1 U of factor VIII/kg of body weight increases circulating factor VIII levels by 2%. For minor soft tissue bleeding, replacement to 20% of normal levels is often sufficient. For hemarthroses or more extensive soft tissue bleeding, at least 40% replacement should be achieved and may be required for several days. Levels of 70% or greater may be required for extensive dental work. Replacement of 80% to 100% is essential in the event of central nervous system bleeding or for surgical procedures. Treatment for 10 to 14 days may be required for surgical procedures or head injury.

With the first dose in a given series, factor VIII has a half-life of approximately 8 hours. Thereafter, the biologic half-life approximates 12 hours, and doses should be given at that interval to maintain a trough level one-half of the initial increment. A steady state can be achieved also by continuous infusion of factor VIII when adequate hemostasis at all times is essential (e.g., after major surgery or head injury). In these instances, a loading dose of factor VIII sufficient to raise the factor VIII level to between 50% and 100% should be given. A dosage of 3 or 4 U/kg/hour thereafter should maintain a level of approximately 50%. Considerable variation in the biologic half-life of factor VIII may be seen from patient to patient. In the event of surgery, serious hemorrhage or prolonged or continuous therapy, levels of factor VIII after infusion should be measured to determine the adequacy of replacement.

For prophylactic treatment, factor is administered on a routine schedule, usually 20 to 25 U/kg three times per week (e.g., Monday, Wednesday, and Friday, or Tuesday, Thursday, and Saturday) or every other day. Trough levels of factor VIII and the frequency of hemorrhages are useful to monitor the effectiveness of the program. Prophylactic treatment is generally considered to be optimal therapy for children with severe factor VIII or IX deficiency. The disadvantages of this approach include use of greater quantities of clotting factor concentrates, which are quite expensive. In addition, frequent venous access may be difficult for some patients, and central venous access lines such as subcutaneous ports may be required to administer the therapy. Preliminary cost-to-benefit analyses suggest that the cost of the clotting factor may be offset by the reduced arthropathy and its associated health care costs.

Preparations of Factor VIII. Recombinant factor is now considered by most practitioners to be optimal therapy for factor deficiencies and is the preferred therapy for patients with hemophilia who are naive to clotting factor replacement. Recombinant Factor VIII is purified from hamster-derived cell lines engineered to produce human Factor VIII protein. These products have virtually no risk of human bloodborne infectious agents; however, the risk of possible contamination by infectious agents still exists during production or processing. In addition, many recombinant factor VIII products are stabilized with human serum albumin, although several albumin-free products are now available. Initial concerns about the high incidence of inhibitors to factor VIII in early trials of recombinant factor VIII appear not to have been borne out, and these products have attained widespread use.

Several commercial preparations of concentrated plasma-derived factor VIII are also available. Each administration results in exposure of the recipient to tens of thousands of donors, increasing the risk of transmission of bloodborne infections. The risk of transmission of these infections has been minimized by newer techniques of preparation of factor VIII concentrates, such as detergent and wet-heat treatment. Purification and concentration of factor VIII through use of monoclonal antibodies and other techniques have resulted in production of high-purity factor VIII concentrates with low infectious risks.

Several plasma preparations contain enough factor VIII to provide at least some replacement. Fresh-frozen plasma contains approximately 1 U/mL of factor VIII, but volume considerations and infectious risks limit its usefulness. Cryoprecipitate prepared in most blood banks contains approximately 80 to 120 U of factor VIII per bag, which can be resuspended in 10 to 20 mL of plasma or saline. Currently available methods for virus inactivation are not applicable to cryoprecipitate, and it carries a higher risk for transmission of bloodborne infections than factor VIII concentrates. For practical purposes, cryoprecipitate is of historical interest only in the treatment of hemophilia, and its use has been supplanted by factor VIII concentrates.

Adjunctive Measures for Specific Bleeding Problems

Joint Bleeding. Aspiration with irrigation of joints is not routinely done, but may be useful, especially if extreme distention of the joint capsule is encountered. If aspiration is required, coverage with factor VIII should be instituted before the procedure. Strict aseptic technique must be adhered to, because blood-filled joints may be easily infected. Prompt removal of blood from an affected joint, especially in severe bleeding, may reduce the likelihood of subsequent damage to the joint and development of target joints; however, this procedure generally requires a surgeon experienced with hemophilia. The combination of factor replacement therapy with a short course of corticosteroids (1 to 2 mg/kg/day for 3 to 5 days) may be beneficial in the event of recurrent or intractable hemorrhage or for joints in which synovial hypertrophy and synovitis have developed. Cold compresses may be applied, and brief immobilization of affected joints may provide comfort. Prolonged splinting should be avoided to prevent the development of disuse atrophy and contractures. Physical therapy should be instituted as soon as possible.

Hematuria. Although hematuria may be dramatic in hemophilia, a discrete anatomic source for the bleeding is usually not found. Administration of factor VIII is usually not effective in treating hematuria, and the administration of epsilon-aminocaproic acid is probably contraindicated because of the risk of clot formation in the ureters. Hematuria usually resolves without specific treatment. Administration of prednisone may be effective in reducing the duration and degree of spontaneous hematuria.

Dental Procedures and Mouth Bleeding. Although coverage with factor VIII remains the mainstay of therapy, epsilon-aminocaproic acid or tranexamic acid therapy may inhibit clot lysis in the mouth. Epsilon-aminocaproic acid usually is given in an oral dose of 75 to 100 mg/kg every 4 to 6 hours to a daily maximum of 24 g. Tranexamic acid is given orally at 25 mg/kg on the same schedule.

Alternative Treatments for Mild and Moderate Hemophilia. Desmopressin acetate (DDAVP), administered intravenously or intranasally, usually increases factor VIII levels two- to fivefold in patients with detectable baseline factor VIII levels. This type of increment may be sufficient to treat minor bleeding episodes in patients with significant levels of factor VIII, but it is not useful in patients with severe hemophilia A. The usual dose for intravenous administration is 0.3 μg/kg. For intranasal administration, the dose is 150 μg (for patients less than 50 kg) or 300 μg (for patients greater than 50 kg). DDAVP may be administered every 12 to 24 hours. Tachyphylaxis may occur with repeated administrations. In some patients, danazol therapy has the same effect, but its use has been limited by a high frequency of side effects and unpredictable responses.

Inhibitors. Development of circulating inhibitors against factor VIII is a major therapeutic problem. High titer inhibitors are most problematic and affect 10% to 15% of patients with hemophilia. Failure to reach the expected level of factor VIII activity after infusion of factor VIII or a shortening of the biologic half-life of transfused factor VIII may be the first sign that an inhibitor is present. These inhibitors are immunoglobulin G (IgG) antibodies and often show species specificity. Their frequency does not appear to be related directly to the number of transfusions of factor VIII. Affected patients may be "low responders," who do not increase their inhibitor level significantly with each administration of exogenous factor VIII, or "high responders," who experience a true anamnestic response to factor VIII infusion. Low responders usually can be treated with higher doses of factor VIII. High responders may be treated at least transiently with porcine factor VIII, if their antibodies do not cross-react significantly with porcine factor VIII *in vitro*. Massive transfusions of human factor VIII concentrates often can overwhelm the inhibitor initially if the titer is low. Plasmapheresis may transiently lower the titer of inhibitor. Use of human and porcine factor VIII in high responders is generally restricted to instances of life-threatening emergencies or essential surgery; administration of either preparation may produce within days high titers of inhibitors that persist for long periods.

Prothrombin concentrates and activated products such as FEIBA (factor VIII inhibitor bypassing activity; Immuno-US, Inc., Rochester, MN) and Autoplex (Baxter Healthcare Corp., Glendale, CA) have had some therapeutic effect in controlled, double-blind studies and do not increase inhibitor levels. These products may be helpful in treating non–life-threatening bleeding, but the best results with these products do not approach the effectiveness of factor VIII in patients without inhibitors. Trials of NovoSeven (recombinant factor VIIa, Novo Nordisk, Princton, NJ) have demonstrated efficacy and safety in the treatment of patients with inhibitors and may become the treatment of choice for patients with high-titer inhibitors; however, this product has a short half-life requiring frequent intravenous administration as well as high cost.

Considerable progress has been reported in the use of "immune-tolerance" regimens in children with high titers of inhibitors. In many cases, tolerance to factor VIII infusions can be achieved without use of cytotoxic therapy. Continued administration of factor VIII to these patients several times each week appears to be required to prevent reappearance of the inhibitor in most cases. Considerable effort and even greater expense are involved. Whether these patients actually achieve immune tolerance instead of temporary suppression or absorption of their inhibitor is not clear. At this time, this therapy cannot be recommended for all patients with inhibitors but should be considered for patients with recent development of inhibitors, recurrent life-threatening hemorrhage, or excessive morbidity caused by an inhibitor. Treatment of inhibitors promises to continue to be one of the most vexing problems of hemophilia.

von Willebrand Disease

The term *von Willebrand disease* encompasses a heterogeneous group of disorders resulting from either deficiency or dysfunction of vWF. The two major functions of vWF are (a) to mediate platelet adhesion at sites of tissue injury and (b) to act as a carrier protein for factor VIII in the plasma. Abnormalities of vWF result in decreased platelet adhesiveness, impairment of agglutination of platelets in the presence of ristocetin, and prolongation of the bleeding time. Deficiency or dysfunction of vWF also results in variably decreased levels of factor VIII procoagulant activity that contribute to the coagulation disturbance. Von Willebrand disease has been classified into three major forms (Table 298.1). Mild quantitative deficiencies of vWF are referred to as *type 1* or *classic* von Willebrand disease, which is by far the most common form, accounting for 80% to 85% of people with von Willebrand disease. Qualitative abnormalities are classified as type 2, of which four subtypes are identified (2A, 2B, 2M and 2N). Severe quantitative

TABLE 298.1

CLASSIFICATION OF VON WILLEBRAND DISEASE

	Type 1 (Partial Deficiency)	Type 2 (Qualitative Deficiency)	Type 3 (Severe Deficiency)
Inheritance	Autosomal dominant	Usually autosomal dominant	Autosomal recessive
Ristocetin cofactor activity (vWF function)	Decreased	Decreased (except type 2N)	Decreased
vWF antigen	Decreased	Normal to decreased	Severely decreased
Multimer analysis	Mild decrease in all multimers	Usually loss of high molecular weight multimers (for type 2A and 2B, but not type 2N and 2M)	Severe decrease in all multimers
Ristocetin-induced platelet aggregation	Normal to decreased	Usually decreased; increased in type 2B	Severely decreased
Treatment	DDAVP usually effective	vWF concentrates (DDAVP usually not effective; can be detrimental in 2B)	vWF concentrates

DDAVP, desmopressin; vWF, von Willebrand factor.

deficiencies of vWF are classified as type 3. Most patients with von Willebrand disease have a mild to moderate bleeding tendency, usually involving mucocutaneous surfaces. Epistaxis, increased bruisability, and hemorrhage after dental extraction are common manifestations. Melena and menorrhagia may occur. Excessive bleeding after trauma or surgery can develop. Hemarthroses are unusual, except in type 3 disease or after significant trauma. Studies suggest that 0.8% to 1.6% of the general population shows biochemical abnormalities consistent with von Willebrand disease, thus making von Willebrand disease the most common of the inherited coagulation disorders. However, many persons with these biochemical abnormalities report no bleeding symptoms.

In contrast to hemophilia A and B, type 1 von Willebrand disease is inherited in an autosomal dominant fashion, although there may be considerable variability in symptoms and von Willebrand levels among affected family members. The mutations resulting in type 1 von Willebrand disease are largely undefined. Type 2 abnormalities are also inherited in an autosomal dominant fashion and can be subcategorized into four types (2A, 2B, 2M and 2N) on the basis of abnormalities of vWF subunit and multimer structure, as demonstrated by immunoelectrophoretic techniques, decreased or increased responsiveness to ristocetin in platelet aggregation studies, or DNA analysis. Type 2A von Willebrand disease is characterized by a deficiency of large-molecular-weight multimers that is associated with decreased platelet adhesion. Bleeding in this group of patients can be severe, because the largest multimers appear to be the most functional. In type 2B, the abnormal multimers have increased affinity for platelet glycoprotein Ib. This type of von Willebrand disease can be associated with thrombocytopenia. Patients with type 2M von Willebrand disease exhibit markedly decreased platelet-dependent vWF function, despite a relatively normal multimer distribution. The *M* in the designation 2M stands simply for *multimer*. This type is caused by mutations that reduce the ability of vWF to bind to platelet receptors. The last type 2 variant—2N—is defined by the inability of vWF to bind factor VIII. This interaction is necessary for the normal survival of factor VIII in the circulation; these patients have factor VIII deficiency associated with normal platelet adhesion. The *N* in the designation 2N

derives from Normandy, France, where one of the first families with this disorder was identified. It is important to distinguish this autosomal disorder from X-linked factor VIII deficiency to provide appropriate counseling and therapy for these patients. Quantitative deficiencies of vWF and factor VIII:C may or may not be found in type 2 disorders. Patients with type 3 von Willibrand disease have severely decreased levels of vWF and factor VIII:C activity. Most patients with type 3 disease are thought to be homozygotes or compound heterozygotes.

Diagnosis of von Willebrand disease is complicated by the finding that results of laboratory testing sometimes vary, not only within families, but for the same person on repeated determinations. Five tests are used to screen for the diagnosis of von Willebrand disease: (a) von Willebrand antigen, (b) von Willebrand activity (ristocetin cofactor activity), (c) factor VIII:C activity, (d) aPTT, and (e) bleeding time or other platelet function assay (such as PFA-100). Two other tests are useful in further classifying the type of von Willebrand disease: (a) von Willebrand multimer analysis and (b) ristocetin-induced platelet aggregation. Type 1 von Willebrand disease results in proportionate reductions of both vWF antigen and activity owing to a quantitative deficiency. In type 3 von Willebrand disease, the reductions in vWF:Ag and factor VIII:C are also proportionate, but severe. This is in contrast to type 2 disease, which typically results in discordance between low activity levels and normal or near-normal antigen levels. The aPTT is prolonged in some, but not all, patients with von Willebrand disease. The reason for the prolongation of the aPTT is not always clear. In many cases, the factor VIII:C level is low and may be the cause. In others, this prolongation occurs despite normal levels of VIII:C. Similarly, the bleeding time is often prolonged in patients with von Willebrand disease, but this is an insensitive screen. More recently, the PFA-100, an *in vitro* assay of platelet function, has been purported to be prolonged in the majority of patients with von Willebrand disease; however, the utility of this test in clinical practice is yet to be determined. vWF normally circulates in the plasma as multimers; in the multimer analysis, the size distribution of multimers and the banding pattern is assessed by agarose gel electrophoresis. In some variants of type 2 disease (2A and 2B) multimer analysis shows a loss of high molecular weight multimers. Ristocetin-induced platelet aggregation can identify the rare type 2B variants that show hyperresponsiveness to low doses of ristocetin and are therefore at risk for *in vivo* platelet aggregation and thrombocytopenia.

The treatment of choice for mild to moderate bleeding episodes in type 1 von Willebrand disease is DDAVP. Administration of DDAVP will result in a two- to fivefold increase in von Willebrand levels in the majority of patients by stimulating release of endogenous stores from vascular endothelium. This therapy is often sufficient for surgical procedures, but adjunctive therapy with plasma products may be required for extensive surgery or serious hemorrhagic episodes. DDAVP should not be given to patients who show increased responsiveness to ristocetin in platelet aggregation studies, unless they have been studied and demonstrated to benefit from this therapy, because they may be at risk for significant thrombocytopenia. DDAVP may lack effectiveness in some patients with type 2 disease. The effect of DDAVP on bleeding time is transient, approximately 3 to 4 hours, and tachyphylaxis may occur. DDAVP can be administered intravenously (0.3 μg/kg/dose, every 12 to 24 hours) or intranasally (150 μg for patients weighing less than 50 kg and 300 μg for patients weighing more than 50 kg). Patients should be tested for efficacy before DDAVP is used as a therapeutic agent because 10% to 15% of patients do not respond. In very mild cases of von Willebrand disease, specific treatment is often not required.

For severe bleeding, extensive surgery, or for patients non responsive to DDAVP, intermediate-purity factor VIII concentrates are effective therapy. These products (such as Humate-P, Aventis, King of Prussia, PA) contain a nearly normal complement of vWF multimers and have fixed ratios of factor VIII to vWF activity (as measured by ristocetin cofactor activity). Although these products are derived from blood donor pools, they undergo antiviral treatment and carry low infectious risks.

Cryoprecipitate also contains intact vWF of all molecular weights and is effective in treating most subtypes of von Willebrand disease. However, cryoprecipitate does not undergo antiviral treatment; hence, the use of the intermediate concentrates is preferred when infusion of vWF is required.

Platelet-Type or Pseudo–von Willebrand Disease

A disorder closely related to von Willebrand disease is platelet-type or pseudo–von Willebrand disease, in which the primary defect appears to reside in the platelet receptor (i.e., glycoprotein Ib) for vWF. Increased amounts of vWF are bound to the platelet membrane because of an abnormally high affinity of the receptor for vWF. This results in depletion of the highest-molecular-weight multimers from plasma. As in type 2B von Willebrand disease, in which the high-molecular-weight multimers show an increased affinity for the platelet surface, increased responsiveness to ristocetin and thrombocytopenia may be seen. This syndrome is easily confused clinically and biochemically with type 2B von Willebrand disease. The two syndromes can be differentiated by the finding that infusion of vWF causes increased aggregation of platelets in pseudo–von Willebrand disease but not in type 2B von Willebrand disease or by studying the differential binding of the patient's vWF to formalin-fixed platelets.

Other Inherited Coagulation Abnormalities

Factor IX Deficiency

Like factor VIII deficiency, factor IX deficiency (i.e., hemophilia B, Christmas disease) is inherited as a sex-linked trait of variable severity. Clinically, factor IX deficiency is virtually indistinguishable from factor VIII deficiency. The diagnosis is made in the same way as factor VIII deficiency, except a factor IX assay is used to confirm the diagnosis. Very low levels of factor IX are occasionally seen in female carriers of factor IX deficiency, in some cases caused by abnormality of the chromosomal homologue, such as a deletion in the region of the factor IX gene. Inhibitors occur much less frequently than in factor VIII deficiency. A relationship between anaphylaxis with administration of factor IX and the development of inhibitors to factor IX has been observed.

Recombinant factor IX became available in 1997 and has become standard therapy for factor IX replacement. This product, created in the absence of human or animal proteins and which functions in coagulation in a manner that is indistinguishable from native factor IX, is effective and safe in the treatment of factor IX deficiency. Clinical studies have demonstrated that recovery of recombinant factor IX is reduced compared with plasma-derived products; however, availability of this safe and potentially infection-free product provides an important therapeutic option for patients with factor IX deficiency. Certain plasma-derived products are also available. Intermediate-purity concentrates contain all the other vitamin K–dependent factors at variable levels; higher-purity products, isolated with antibody affinity columns to factor IX, contain only factor IX similar in purity to those used for factor VIII deficiency. Treatment with plasma is effective, but larger doses are required than in hemophilia A to achieve the same level of factor replacement.

A dose of 1 U of plasma-derived factor IX/kg of body weight generally increases factor IX levels by 1.0% to 1.5% (0.8% for recombinant factor IX), as opposed to the approximate 2% increase seen with factor VIII. This difference is compensated for by a relatively longer biologic half-life of factor IX when compared with factor VIII. After an initial loading dose, a subsequent dose is usually given in 4 to 12 hours to account for the shorter initial half-life and every 24 hours thereafter. Individual patients should be studied to assess recovery and half-life of recombinant factor IX before relying on this product for routine use.

Factor XI Deficiency

Factor XI deficiency (hemophilia C) is characterized by an autosomal recessive inheritance pattern and a mild bleeding tendency. Heterozygotes also manifest reduced levels of factor XI. The disease occurs most often in persons of Ashkenazi Jewish descent. Symptoms include increased bruisability, epistaxis, menorrhagia, and postoperative bleeding. Hemarthroses and deep soft tissue bleeding are unusual. Hemorrhagic symptoms in severely deficient patients usually can be controlled with small doses of plasma.

Other Uncommon Specific Factor Abnormalities

Selective abnormalities of fibrinogen, factors II, V, VII, X, XII, XIII, prekallikrein, and high-molecular-weight kininogen have been described.

Congenital afibrinogenemia may present with hemorrhagic complications in the neonatal period and is associated with a lifelong bleeding abnormality. The spectrum of symptoms seen in this disorder is similar to that of hemophilia A, but the disease is usually much less severe. Patients with a variety of dysfibrinogenemias have been described. Most of these patients are asymptomatic, but increased bruisability, menorrhagia, wound dehiscence, posttraumatic and surgical bleeding, and thrombosis have been reported. Congenital afibrinogenemia appears to be an autosomal recessive disorder, whereas dysfibrinogenemia is autosomal dominant in most cases. Therapy with plasma, cryoprecipitate, and fibrinogen concentrates is effective in both disorders.

Congenital prothrombin (factor II) deficiency and dysprothrombinemia result in mild bleeding disorders that usually do not require therapy and are inherited in an autosomal recessive fashion. If necessary, the defect can be corrected with fresh-frozen plasma or prothrombin complex concentrates.

Factor V deficiency is associated also with a mild, autosomal recessively inherited bleeding disorder. Replacement with fresh plasma is preferred, because of the extreme instability of factor V with storage. Factor V deficiency is sometimes associated with renal, cardiovascular, and skeletal abnormalities and with the development of inhibitors.

Factor VII deficiency is potentially symptomatic in the heterozygous and homozygous forms. Symptoms include mucosal bleeding, gastrointestinal hemorrhage, menorrhagia, and intracranial hemorrhage. Factor VII deficiency should be suspected in patients in whom the aPTT result is normal and the PT result is significantly prolonged. Fresh-frozen plasma or prothrombin complex concentrates have been effective replacement therapies; however, this situation is now complicated by the depletion of factor VII in many newer prothrombin complex concentrates. NovoSeven (recombinant factor VIIa, Novo Nordisk, Princeton NJ) has been used successfully for the treatment of factor VII deficiency with doses much lower than those used for treatment of hemophilia with inhibitors.

Factor X deficiency is similar to factor VII deficiency in its inheritance pattern and symptoms. The aPTT result is abnormal, as is the PT result. Fresh-frozen plasma or vitamin K–dependent factor concentrates are used for treatment.

Factor XII (i.e., Hageman factor), prekallikrein (i.e., Fletcher factor), and high-molecular-weight kininogen (i.e., Fitzgerald factor) deficiencies are associated with prolongation of the aPTT, but they do not cause a significant bleeding abnormality. These abnormalities should be recognized to differentiate them from other causes of a prolonged aPTT that are associated with bleeding symptoms. The Passovoy defect causes prolonged aPTT, and it is associated with variable degrees of bleeding. Hemorrhage after surgery has been described in patients with the Passovoy defect. In these four disorders, the diagnosis can be made by showing that the patient's plasma does not correct the defect in plasma from a patient known to have the disorder; however, no specific "Passovoy factor" has yet been isolated, and some of these patients have been found to have alternative causes of bleeding and aPTT elevation, such as von Willebrand disease. The diagnosis of prekallikrein deficiency is confirmed when the prolonged aPTT is corrected by 10-minute preincubation of the plasma with a glass surface. Physicians should understand that routine screening with aPTT testing will uncover patients with these disorders, many of whom have no symptoms of clinical significance.

Factor XIII deficiency is a heterogeneous disorder associated with instability of fibrin clots. Delayed bleeding from the umbilical stump or after trauma is a classic presentation of the disease. Purpura and poor wound healing may be seen. Patients appear to be at higher risk for intracranial hemorrhage and spontaneous abortion. Routine coagulation study results are normal. The diagnosis is established by the relative instability of the patient's clots in urea. Treatment with plasma or cryoprecipitate is effective.

Alpha-2-antiplasmin deficiency has been reported as a cause of bleeding diathesis in several families. The results of routine coagulation tests are normal. Bleeding occurs as a result of excessive fibrinolytic activity. Homozygotes have suffered hematomas, hemarthroses, and muscular and central nervous system bleeding; in addition, some patients have been reported to suffer unusual intramedullary osseous bleeding. Heterozygotes may show increased bruisability and postsurgical or dental bleeding.

Inherited Coagulation Factor Abnormalities Caused by Deficiencies of More Than One Factor

Several patients have been described who have a deficiency of multiple vitamin K–dependent factors. These patients have simultaneous deficiencies of factors II, VII, IX, X, protein C, and protein S, and they have been shown to have a defect resulting from gamma-carboxylation of the vitamin K–dependent clotting factors. The hemorrhagic symptoms are consistent with vitamin K deficiency.

Several kindreds have been described in which multiple persons have deficiencies of two or more clotting factors. Combined factor V and factor VIII deficiency is the most commonly reported hereditary combined deficiency of clotting factors and has been identified in more than 60 kindreds. Levels of factors V and VIII as low as 5% and 4%, respectively, have been observed in patients, but levels of approximately 15% for both factors seem to be more common. In most of the families, the dual deficiency is thought to be based on single or closely linked genetic defects. Molecular abnormalities that result in this combined deficiency (mutations in the endoplasmic reticulum–Golgi intermediate-compartment protein ERGIC-53, a gene product distinct from factors V and VIII) have been described.

Inherited Coagulation Abnormalities Resulting in Hypercoagulability

The contribution of genetic risk factors to the occurrence of thrombosis has become increasingly clear. This discovery has been driven by advances in the understanding of the molecular basis of thrombosis. Many children who develop thrombosis have definable genetic abnormalities; in fact, the occurrence of multiple genetic or acquired risk factors in children with thromboses is more the rule than the exception. The discovery of the anticoagulant properties of protein C was a key step in these developments.

Protein C is a vitamin K–dependent factor, which is converted to its activated form by thrombin in the presence of protein S. This reaction is catalyzed by a surface receptor, thrombomodulin, which binds thrombin and increases its affinity for protein C. Protein C is the most potent anticoagulant protein known. Inherited protein C deficiency has been described in heterozygous and homozygous states. Homozygotes usually have no protein C activity, and the condition is detected shortly after birth. Purpura fulminans is usually the first recognized symptom. Venous thromboses in the central nervous system and kidneys are common. Thrombosis of the retinal vessels tends to occur early in life, followed by secondary vitreous bleeds, resulting in fibrosis and blindness. The disease is fatal if untreated. Patients with apparently homozygous protein C deficiency presenting later in life have been described, but they have detectable levels of protein C activity. Transmission of the disease appears to be autosomal recessive in most kindreds with homozygous protein C deficiency.

Treatment with heparin was previously thought to be ineffective, but there have been reports of successful treatment with low-molecular-weight heparin. Sufficient protein C can be administered with fresh-frozen plasma to reverse the clinical symptoms. Long-term management can be achieved with warfarin (Coumadin) administration, by at least partially restoring the balance between procoagulant and anticoagulant forces. Infusions of purified plasma-derived protein C concentrates as well as human recombinant activated protein C have been used to treat this disorder. Successful correction of homozygous protein C deficiency by hepatic transplantation has been accomplished in at least two patients.

Heterozygous protein C deficiency can be associated with thrombotic disease. Heterozygotes typically manifest levels of activity between 35% and 65% of normal. Patients with levels of antigenic protein C higher than their activity levels have been described, indicating a qualitative defect of protein C. Most heterozygotes in the best studied kindreds do not become symptomatic until the third decade of life, but children with symptomatic disease in the first and second decades are recognized with increasing frequency. Symptomatic individuals with heterozygous protein C deficiency commonly have other associated genetic or acquired risk factors.

Deep venous thrombosis and central nervous system thrombosis are among the most common findings. Patients with heterozygous protein C deficiency may manifest skin necrosis shortly after warfarin administration. This unusual reaction to warfarin is attributed to the short half-life of protein C relative to some of the vitamin K–dependent procoagulant proteins. Because all the vitamin K–dependent proteins are reduced after warfarin therapy, very low levels of protein C may develop quickly in patients with lower than normal levels of protein C at the initiation of therapy, resulting in a procoagulant-anticoagulant imbalance favoring thrombosis.

Transmission of symptomatic heterozygous protein C deficiency appears to be autosomal dominant, but asymptomatic heterozygotes are detected commonly in families of homozygous patients. Asymptomatic heterozygotes have been detected by random screening of blood bank donors. Various mutations in the protein C gene have been associated with protein C deficiency, but the clinically dominant and recessive forms of the disease cannot be segregated on the basis of these mutations. Symptomatic heterozygous patients can be treated with warfarin, but this agent should be administered simultaneously with heparin until adequate anticoagulation with warfarin is achieved.

A single point mutation in the coagulation factor V gene (nucleotide position 1691 resulting in a Gln for Arg substitution at codon 506) has been identified as one of the most common known genetic risk factors for thrombosis. This mutation results in the production of a mutant factor V protein, factor V Leiden. Factor V Leiden has normal procoagulant activities; however, the mutation renders the factor V protein resistant to inactivation by activated protein C. In addition, normal factor V serves as a cofactor for activated protein C function; factor V Leiden functions as an inefficient cofactor. The combination of these effects (resistance to inactivation and reduced protein C activation) produces a hypercoagulable state. Factor V Leiden is quite prevalent and has been found in 2% to 11% of the general population. This mutation is most commonly found in white people and less commonly in those of African or East Asian origin. Screening for the factor V Leiden mutation can be performed by testing for relative resistance of the abnormal factor V molecule to inactivation by activated protein C (activated protein C resistance). In addition, this mutation can be genetically determined using polymerase chain reaction assays. Up to 60% of adults with venous thrombosis and a family history of thrombosis are heterozygotes for this mutation. Although few in number, similar pediatric studies have reported that up to 30% of children with venous thrombosis are heterozygotes for the factor V Leiden mutation.

Heterozygous protein S deficiency results in recurrent thromboses with a pattern similar to that of heterozygous protein C deficiency.

Antithrombin deficiency is inherited as an autosomal dominant trait. The occurrence of thromboses usually begins in the second decade of life. Heparin resistance can be a feature of antithrombin deficiency, because antithrombin is a cofactor for heparin. Anticoagulation can be achieved with warfarin. In addition, available antithrombin concentrates can be used for those who have antithrombin deficiency and present with an acute thrombotic event.

Another recognized genetic risk factor for thrombophilia is a point mutation in the 3'-untranslated region of the prothrombin gene. A single nucleotide change occurs (position 20210, G to A), and this mutation is known as the *G20210A prothrombin variant*. Heterozygotes with this mutation have elevated prothrombin levels and are at threefold risk for venous thrombosis when compared with normal control subjects.

Thrombosis has been associated with qualitative and quantitative abnormalities of plasminogen, impaired plasminogen activator release, increased plasminogen activator inhibitor-1, dysfibrinogenemias, and reduced levels of heparin cofactor II. The inheritance pattern in these cases is less clear.

Patients with the rare metabolic disease homocystinuria caused by cystathionine beta-synthase deficiency are at increased risk for arterial and venous thrombotic episodes. These episodes, which occur in up to one-third of these patients, are likely to occur before the age of 30 years and include deep vein thrombosis, pulmonary embolism, and arterial thrombosis involving cerebral, peripheral, and coronary vessels. Therapies aimed at decreasing the plasma levels of homocysteine, such as folate, pyridoxine, betaine, and hydroxocobalamin, may reduce the risk of cardiovascular disease. A strong correlation between the presence of factor V Leiden and the occurrence of thromboses in patients with homocystinuria has been reported in an Israeli population.

Mild to moderate hyperhomocysteinemia also is emerging as an important hereditary risk factor for cardiovascular disease. This disorder is most commonly attributed to a specific polymorphism (position 677 C to T) in the gene for methylenetetrahydrofolate reductase (MTHFR), an enzyme that is important for homocysteine metabolism. This condition is relatively common in the Northern American population; approximately 12% of individuals are homozygous and 35% are heterozygous for this polymorphism. Some studies suggest that presence of this genetic defect alone is not associated with a risk for thrombosis unless homocysteine levels are elevated. Supplementation with folate, pyridoxine, and vitamin B_{12} can decrease the plasma homocysteine levels, but whether this supplementation reduces cardiovascular risks in these individuals remains to be seen.

ACQUIRED ABNORMALITIES OF COAGULATION FACTORS

Vitamin K Deficiency

Vitamin K is an essential substrate for the synthesis of procoagulant and anticoagulant proteins, including factors II, VII, IX, and X, protein C, and protein S. Identical clinical states can be produced by absence of vitamin K or interference with its action by pharmacologic means. Dietary vitamin K consists mainly of vitamin K_1, a fat-soluble naphthoquinone found in leafy vegetables. Intestinal bacteria also synthesize vitamin K compounds. Therapeutically and physiologically, the fat-soluble forms of vitamin K appear to be most useful, and toxicity has resulted from the administration of water-soluble analogues. True dietary deficiency of vitamin K appears to be unusual, except in early infancy or in the setting of prolonged intravenous feedings without supplemental administration of vitamin K. Most cases of apparent dietary insufficiency in older children are caused by malabsorptive syndromes, such as pancreatic insufficiency, biliary obstruction, prolonged diarrhea affecting absorption of vitamin K in the upper small intestine, or the administration of drugs. Drugs that antagonize or interfere with the metabolism of vitamin K include phenobarbital, phenytoin, some cephalosporins, rifampin, isoniazid, and coumarin. Vitamin K deficiency caused by antibiotic suppression of intestinal flora appears to be unusual without a dietary deficiency of vitamin K. However, vitamin K deficiency has been noted in thriving infants after relatively brief bouts of diarrhea, particularly if these infants are breast-fed.

Uncomplicated vitamin K deficiency is characterized by bleeding symptoms (e.g., bruising, oozing from puncture sites of the skin, visceral hemorrhage) with an acquired prolongation of the PT and aPTT and a normal fibrinogen level. Often, a disproportionate prolongation of the PT occurs, which can be helpful in diagnosis. Other clotting factors that are produced in the liver but are not vitamin K dependent (e.g., factors V, VIII, XI, XII) are normal; however, the clinical and laboratory picture is often affected by a primary disorder that produces liver disease and malabsorption or decreased utilization of vitamin K, such as biliary atresia, cystic fibrosis, hemolytic anemia with obstructive jaundice, hepatitis, alpha-1-antitrypsin deficiency, or abetalipoproteinemia. In the absence of severe hepatic disease or antagonists, response to vitamin K is rapid, usually occurring within 6 hours. Anaphylactoid reactions may occur with parenteral administration of vitamin K, but they are unusual. Infusion of plasma is effective in emergencies.

Hemorrhagic disease of the newborn appears to represent a special case of vitamin K deficiency. As classified by Hathaway, hemorrhagic disease of the newborn can occur in early, classic, and late forms. Early hemorrhagic disease of the newborn often occurs in the setting of maternal ingestion of vitamin K antagonists (e.g., anticonvulsants, antituberculous drugs) but may be unassociated with known risk factors. Early disease presents in the first 24 hours of life, often with catastrophic bleeding. Classic hemorrhagic disease of the newborn occurs after the first day of life, usually within the first week. Purpura, oozing from the umbilical cord or circumcision site, hematemesis, hematuria, and gastrointestinal and vaginal bleeding are common symptoms, but intracranial hemorrhage is rare. Premature infants are at increased risk for developing hemorrhagic symptoms. Late-onset disease occurs 1 to 3 months after birth and is associated with a high incidence of central nervous system hemorrhage and mortality. Exclusive breast-feeding without vitamin K supplementation and failure to administer parenteral vitamin K at birth appear to be at least contributing, and probably causative, factors in classic and late disease. Some cases of early disease may not respond to parenteral vitamin K at birth, but virtually all cases of classic disease can be prevented by oral or parenteral vitamin K administration. The practice of oral vitamin K administration has been adopted by some countries other than the United States; however, this route of administration appears to be less effective than intramuscular vitamin K in preventing late hemorrhagic disease. In addition, earlier concerns about a possible causal link between parenteral vitamin K administration and cancer do not appear to be justified. For this reason, a single intramuscular dose of vitamin K for all infants is still recommended by the American Academy of Pediatrics.

Liver Disease

The liver is the major site of production of most coagulation factors and is important for the clearance of activated factors and fibrin degradation products. In pathologic states, reduced synthesis of clotting factors is common and often affects vitamin K–dependent factors most severely. In addition, consumption of clotting factors and platelets occurs frequently in liver disease. Essentially all the laboratory abnormalities seen in disseminated intravascular coagulation (DIC) may occur in severe liver disease, including prolonged PT and aPTT, increased fibrin degradation products, and thrombocytopenia. Factor VIII appears to be relatively spared in liver disease because of significant extrahepatic synthesis; simultaneous measurements of factor VIII and one or more factors made primarily in the liver (e.g., factor VII and IX) can help to differentiate hepatic disease from DIC, in which factor VIII levels usually are depressed. Studies have shown that protein C and antithrombin are reduced in many forms of liver disease, and this may explain some of the thrombotic complications observed in hepatic diseases.

Treatment of the coagulopathy associated with liver disease usually involves administration of vitamin K to protect against deficiency or impaired utilization of vitamin K caused by hepatocellular disease, fresh-frozen plasma to replace factors synthesized in the liver, and platelets as necessary. If volume considerations become important, fibrinogen levels can be raised by administration of cryoprecipitate. Rarely, replacement with vitamin K–dependent factor concentrates may be indicated in patients with life-threatening disease, but administration of these factors to patients with liver disease carries a high risk of thrombotic complications. Activated FVIIa has also been used effectively to treat bleeding associated with liver disease.

Disseminated Intravascular Coagulation

DIC describes a constellation of clinical and laboratory abnormalities associated with activation of the coagulation system with subsequent fibrin deposition in the microvasculature, often leading to organ dysfunction; this process is manifested by a combination of accelerated fibrinogenesis and fibrinolysis. Rather than being considered a disease in and of itself, DIC should be thought of as a secondary phenomenon that occurs in response to a variety of stimuli. DIC may be triggered by local or systemic factors. Examples of local problems that can result in systemic DIC include hemangiomas (i.e., Kasabach-Merritt syndrome), in which a localized vascular lesion results in consumption of fibrinogen and platelets and in which elevations of fibrin degradation products can be massive, and brain injury, in which release of thromboplastic substances may initiate systemic clotting. Abruptio placentae and massive pulmonary emboli also may produce systemic signs of DIC. Systemic causes of DIC include sepsis, shock of any cause, transfusion of incompatible blood, and injection of snake venom. DIC is encountered in toxemia of pregnancy, respiratory distress syndrome, malignant diseases, burns, hypothermia, heat stroke, postoperative states, and any situation in which massive tissue damage is encountered. Severity of DIC varies widely, from transient and insignificant to overwhelming. Patients with DIC manifest purpura, and oozing from incisions or venipuncture sites is common. Circulatory collapse may occur.

Purpura fulminans is a syndrome of DIC associated with hemorrhagic necrosis of the skin. This rare disorder is characterized at its onset by purpura and DIC, usually in association with viral (e.g., varicella), bacterial (e.g., meningococcal, streptococcal), or rickettsial infections or severe hypernatremia. Pathologically, this disease is characterized by widespread microthrombi in the vascular beds of a variety of organs. Renal failure is common. The purpuric lesions are often symmetric and show sharply demarcated borders with a surrounding inflammatory reaction. Scarring of the skin and loss of extremities are common, and the fatality rate is high. Rarely, purpura fulminans may be seen as a manifestation of protein C deficiency.

No single laboratory test is diagnostic for DIC; however, common laboratory findings in DIC include thrombocytopenia, prolongation of the PT and aPTT, and a reduction of clotting factors, particularly fibrinogen and factor II, V, and VIII. The activities of anticoagulant proteins (protein C, protein S, and antithrombin) are also reduced. Microangiopathic changes in the erythrocytes may be seen in the peripheral blood smear. Plasma levels of fibrin degradation products usually are elevated and may play a pathogenetic role by inhibiting clotting and platelet function. Measurement of fibrinopeptide A, a cleavage product of fibrinogen, and fibrinogen turnover studies increase the diagnostic sensitivity, but these assays are not routinely available.

Treatment of DIC should be aimed primarily at correcting the inciting cause. Concern has been raised about the possibility of "feeding the fire" by administering clotting factors and platelet concentrates. However, the risks of allowing severe thrombocytopenia or hypofibrinogenemia to develop are not warranted on the basis of what are mostly theoretic concerns, and replacement therapy should be given if consumption has been severe. Heparin may be helpful in some cases if the underlying defect cannot be corrected, but its usefulness is still a matter of debate. Some authors believe that heparin is an effective therapy for purpura fulminans if initiated early in the illness. Protein C concentrates may be beneficial in the treatment of this devastating condition. A few reports exist of successful treatment of purpura fulminans with recombinant tissue plasminogen (t-PA) activator, and the usefulness of antithrombin replacement is being investigated. Epsilon-Aminocaproic acid, in general, is not considered to be effective in most cases of DIC. However, cases of DIC associated with acute promyelocytic leukemia and Kasabach-Merritt syndrome have reportedly been treated successfully with epsilon-aminocaproic acid.

Circulating Anticoagulants

Circulating anticoagulants are usually IgG molecules that prolong the aPTT. These conditions can be distinguished from a factor deficiency as a cause of aPTT prolongation by persistence of aPTT inhibition after mixing with normal plasma. Circulating anticoagulants often occur in otherwise healthy children after administration of antibiotics or after viral infections. Most of these patients have no bleeding symptoms or other clinical complications; thus, the term "anticoagulant" describes its *in vitro* effect on the aPTT rather than its *in vivo* effect. Furthermore, these anticoagulants usually disappear spontaneously in several weeks to months. Often, they are detected during routine preoperative screening using the aPTT. The true incidence of circulating anticoagulants is difficult to assess, because most patients do not have symptoms. However, in a study of more than 1,600 patients in which aPTTs were used as a preoperative screen, 11 patients (0.7%) had circulating anticoagulants.

In the minority of cases, circulating inhibitors are associated with bleeding symptoms. In these patients, antibodies that target prothrombin often can be demonstrated. This results in prolongations of both the aPTT and PT and low thrombin (factor IIa) activity. In other patients, anti–factor V antibodies can be demonstrated. The development of inhibitors sometimes can be explained by prior sensitization to clotting factors from other species; this exposure typically occurs when clotting agents are applied topically during surgery (e.g., fibrin glue). Rarely, patients develop acquired antibodies to other factors, such as factor VIII. These conditions appear more commonly in adults, and the bleeding disorder can mimic the deficiency state for that factor. Many of these patients have underlying immunoregulatory abnormalities or malignant diseases. Specific antifactor antibodies that develop after administration of factor replacement in patients with hemophilia are covered in the section on hemophilia and inhibitors.

Circulating anticoagulants directed against protein-phospholipid complexes are also called *lupus anticoagulants*. Although they are seen in some patients with systemic lupus erythematosus, they can also be demonstrated in many other diseases, such as HIV infection, as well as in healthy individuals. In contrast to what the name suggests, these antiphospholipid antibodies can be associated with thromboembolic events and are discussed in the section on hypercoagulability.

The presence of circulating anticoagulants can be documented by lack of correction of the aPTT after mixing with normal plasma (mixing study) or a positive dilute Russell Viper venom test. Anticardiolipin antibody testing is often positive as well. Circulating anticoagulants should be looked for in any patient with an unexplained prolongation of the PT or aPTT.

Miscellaneous Acquired Coagulation Abnormalities

Low levels of clotting factors and elevated fibrin-split products have been reported in children with cyanotic congenital heart disease and polycythemia. Many of these abnormalities are probably explained by concomitant hepatic dysfunction. A variety of coagulation disturbances may be seen after cardiac surgery, including reduced clotting factors and elevations of fibrin-split products, sometimes as a manifestation of DIC. These defects occur most commonly as a result of cardiopulmonary bypass or deep hypothermia, but their exact nature is poorly understood.

Depressions of factors VIII and IX have been described in hypothyroidism. The depressions disappear after restoration of the euthyroid state. Amyloidosis has been associated with deficiencies of factors V, VII, IX, and X. L-Asparaginase therapy depresses many coagulation factors, including antithrombin and protein C. These abnormalities may explain the thromboses that occur in children after the use of L-asparaginase therapy. Low levels of free protein S have been noted during infectious or inflammatory episodes. Variable depressions and elevations of specific clotting factors have been described in the nephrotic syndrome, including antithrombin deficiency. Hypofibrinogenemia has been reported after administration of valproate, and dysfibrinogenemias have been associated with tumors, liver disease, and pseudotumor cerebri.

Hypercoagulability

Numerous acquired clinical states have been associated with a predisposition to thrombosis. Venous stasis caused by immobilization, hyperviscosity, polycythemia, congestive heart failure, vascular damage or occlusion secondary to sickle cell disease, or other conditions is a major etiologic factor of thrombosis. Similarly, abnormal intravascular surfaces caused by indwelling catheters, artificial heart valves, arteritides (e.g., Kawasaki disease, polyarteritis), or homocystinemia may result in thromboses. A thrombotic tendency may be seen in the setting of malignant disease, liver disease, renal disease, infection, inflammatory disease (e.g., ulcerative colitis, regional enteritis), diabetes mellitus, paroxysmal nocturnal hemoglobinuria, contraceptive use, or pregnancy. Hypercoagulability may be seen in patients with nephrotic syndrome or after the administration of coagulation factors or drugs such as L-asparaginase, warfarin, epsilon-aminocaproic acid, or heparin. Lupus anticoagulants and anticardiolipin antibodies are antiphospholipid antibodies associated with both venous and arterial thrombosis. These antibodies are directed against complexes of phospholipid bound to proteins such as beta-2-glycoprotein, prothrombin, and cardiolipin, but how they promote thrombosis is not clear.

Even in patients with hereditary defects predisposing to thromboses, additional factors are often the trigger to clinically evident thromboses. Numerous insights into the possible mechanisms by which other clinical states may result in thromboses are available. Protein C levels, for example, are low in liver disease, in DIC, and after L-asparaginase therapy, and they have been shown to decrease after surgery at about the time that deep venous thromboses are found. Low free protein S levels have been reported in inflammatory states. These depressions are attributed to an increase in the protein S–binding protein (C4BP), which is generated as part of the acute-phase response. Thus, the free (active) form of the protein is reduced. Antithrombin levels are depressed in nephrotic syndrome, pregnancy, DIC, liver disease, oral contraceptive use, and after administration of heparin or L-asparaginase. Although it is tempting to assume causality in these instances, other coagulation factors are dramatically affected in these situations, and the expression of hemorrhage or thrombosis is the result of a complicated interplay among multiple factors.

Thrombotic complications such as deep venous thromboses and pulmonary emboli, once considered rare in children, are now recognized with increasing frequency. Much of this increase can be attributed to the growing use of invasive procedures in infants and children, particularly central venous catheters. Cardiac surgery remains one of the more common indications for anticoagulation in children. The recognition of deep venous thrombosis in infants and children always demands a rigorous search for underlying genetic and acquired factors that predispose to thrombosis. As mentioned previously, the identification of a single risk factor should not deter the search for others, because multiple predisposing factors are more the rule than the exception. The decision to anticoagulate and for how long is often complicated and should be individualized. There remains a paucity of information on the treatment of thrombosis that is specific to children. Unfortunately, decisions must often be made on the basis of extrapolation from data derived from experience with adult patients.

A detailed explanation of indications and methods for anticoagulation is beyond the scope of this chapter; if possible, anticoagulants, particularly thrombolytics, should be administered with advice from a clinician experienced in their use. The following information regarding anticoagulation may be helpful to the general pediatrician. Although heparinization remains a mainstay in the acute treatment of thrombosis, the availability of thrombolytic therapy provides a useful additional tool for treatment. Use of thrombolytic therapy such as urokinase, t-PA, or streptokinase early in the occurrence of thrombosis appears to reduce the incidence of long-term complications of thromboses, such as postphlebitic syndrome after deep venous thrombosis in the leg, which is caused by residual venous insufficiency and can result in recurrent painful swelling of the leg and ulceration of the skin. Use of this therapy carries a higher risk of serious and even fatal hemorrhage. Intracranial lesions such as tumors, arteriovascular malformations, or hemorrhages are currently considered absolute contraindications to using fibrinolytics. Preliminary studies have demonstrated that these agents can be used with safety and efficacy in infants for nonintracranial thromboses, as well as in children. Urokinase often is preferred to streptokinase because of a lower rate of adverse reactions, especially with repeated use. Urokinase is generally administered as a bolus of 4,400 U/kg, followed by a continuous infusion at a rate of 4,400 U/kg/hour for 1 to 3 days. The fibrinogen level and platelet count should be monitored during its use, in addition to the PT and aPTT. Thrombin times can be adjusted to 1.5 to 5.0 times their baseline values. The usual dose of t-PA is 0.1 to 0.5 mg/kg/hour for 1 to 3 days, and it is monitored like urokinase. t-PA has also been used in infants, and relatively lower doses (0.06 mg/kg/hour) appear to be safe and effective. Catheter-directed administration of thrombolytics directly into the thrombus carries the theoretic advantage of using smaller effective doses with potentially less bleeding risk; however, a larger experience will be needed to

demonstrate whether this is true. Heparin is recommended by some clinicians as adjunctive therapy with thrombolysis. If this is undertaken, bolus administration of heparin should probably be avoided. Heparin also interferes with use of the thrombin time for monitoring. If no response is seen to thrombolytic therapy, plasminogen concentration should be measured and plasma infusions given if the level is low.

Standard heparin is still valued for its relatively short half-life, reversibility by protamine, low cost, and proven efficacy. Heparin's activity is dependent on antithrombin, and heparin resistance can be seen in antithrombin-deficient individuals. Standard heparin is usually administered at a dose of 50 to 75 U/kg, given as a bolus, followed by 10 to 25 U/kg/hour (average, 20 U/kg) by continuous infusion. Infants generally require higher doses of heparin, and the initial rate of infusion should be higher (average, approximately 28 U/kg/hour). Therapy should be monitored with aPTT evaluations every 6 to 8 hours until a steady-state value is achieved; the usual therapeutic range is 1.5 to 2.0 times the control aPTT. Platelet counts should also be monitored. Introduction of low-molecular-weight heparin offers an alternative to the use of standard heparin. Low-molecular-weight heparin has the advantage of more predictable pharmacokinetics and thus less need for frequent monitoring. It is administered subcutaneously and does not require venous access. However, it has a much longer half-life than standard heparin (in the range of 8 to 12 hours compared with 45 minutes for standard heparin), and it is not fully reversed by protamine sulfate. Large metaanalyses in adults show that low-molecular-weight heparin is at least as effective as standard heparin, with possibly less bleeding risk. Although low-molecular-weight heparin has not been as extensively studied in infants and children, its use is becoming widespread in this population. Growing experience suggests that it is a safe and effective alternative to standard heparin. Enoxaparin, one of the most commonly used preparations, is given every 12 hours at a dose of 1 mg/kg subcutaneously. Higher doses are required in infants (average, 1.5 mg/kg); use of the intravenous route has not been studied to date in infants. Lower doses (one-half the full treatment dose) are used for prophylaxis. The aPTT often is not elevated, and therapy is monitored by measuring anti-factor Xa activity; however, many clinicians believe that monitoring low-molecular-weight therapy in adults is not necessary, except in certain conditions such as renal dysfunction, morbid obesity, or pregnancy. In pediatric patients, because of less extensive experience, occasional monitoring is advisable. The usual therapeutic range is 0.6 to 1.0 U of anti–factor Xa activity/mL of plasma for full anticoagulation, and 0.2 to 0.4 for prophylactic dosing, measured on samples obtained 4 hours after administration of the agent. With prolonged (longer than 3 months) therapy with either standard or low-molecular-weight heparin, a propensity exists for development of osteoporosis, and bone density should be monitored.

Warfarin is most often used for long-term anticoagulation. Because long-term treatment with warfarin carries a significant risk of morbidity and mortality from bleeding, the decision to undertake this therapy should be made with great care. Warfarin exerts its effect by antagonizing vitamin K, and it has a very long and variable half-life, measured in days. The majority of warfarin remains protein bound, and only the unbound form is active. Numerous drugs can enhance the effectiveness of warfarin by interfering with protein binding, thereby increasing the fraction of warfarin that is free and active. Drugs also can affect the activity of warfarin by competing for degradation in the liver or inducing activity of enzymes involved in its metabolism. Warfarin activity also can be affected by fluctuations in the amount of available vitamin K in the diet or administered parenterally. Careful dietary counseling also should be provided for patients receiving long-term warfarin therapy. Warfarin usually is administered at a loading dose of 0.1 to 0.2 mg/kg/day for 2 to 3 days, followed by a daily dose sufficient to maintain the international normalized ratio (INR) in the desired range, usually 2.0 to 3.0. During the initiation of warfarin therapy, heparin is used concomitantly until the INR is therapeutic. The reason for this practice is that a relative prothrombotic state can result during first few days of warfarin initiation; this is the result of the relatively rapid drop in the activity of the anticoagulants protein C and S compared with other procoagulant factors. Infants often require higher daily doses of warfarin. Introduction of the INR for monitoring warfarin treatment is an attempt to standardize the monitoring of warfarin from institution to institution. This effort was undertaken in recognition of the fact that activities of the thromboplastins used in the determination of PTs vary greatly, and the formula used to calculate the INR mathematically corrects for this effect. In most patients, fairly frequent monitoring of warfarin therapy (every 1 to 2 weeks) is required to avoid inadvertent overcoagulation or underanticoagulation, even after an apparently stable dose has been achieved. Home devices for monitoring warfarin therapy are available and can simplify treatment. If necessary, warfarin's effect can be reversed by administering oral or parenteral vitamin K or plasma.

All anticoagulated patients should be protected from trauma as much as is feasible. Intramuscular injections are contraindicated. Arterial punctures carry a great deal of risk and should be avoided, if at all possible. The use of platelet antagonists should be avoided. Excellent manuals addressing the details and practical applications of anticoagulants are available from the American Heart Association, the American College of Chest Physicians, and the Canadian Children's Thrombophilia Society.

Suggested Readings

American Academy of Pediatrics, Committee on Fetus and Newborn. Controversies concerning vitamin K and the newborn. *Pediatrics* 2003;112:191.

Bolton-Maggs PH, Pasi KJ. Haemophilias A and B. *Lancet* 2003;361:1801.

Carcao MD, Aledort L. Prophylactic factor replacement in hemophilia. *Blood Rev* 2004;18:101.

Centers for Disease Control and Prevention. Perspectives in disease prevention and health promotion safety of therapeutic products used for hemophilia patients. *MMWR Morb Mortal Wkly Rep* 1988;37:441.

Cochran JB, Panzarino VM, Maes LY, Tecklenburg FW. Pneumococcus-induced T-antigen activation in hemolytic uremic syndrome and anemia. *Pediatr Nephrol* 2004;19:317.

Lee R, Frenkel EP. Hyperhomocysteinemia and thrombosis. *Hematol Oncol Clin North Am* 2003;17:85.

Levi M, de Jonge E, Meijers J. The diagnosis of disseminated intravascular coagulation. *Blood Rev* 2002;16:217.

Monagle P, Michelson AD, Bovill E, Andrew M. Antithrombotic therapy in children. *Chest* 2001;119:344S.

Sadler JE, Gralnick HR. Commentary: a new classification for von Willebrand disease. *Blood* 1994;84:676.

Selhub J, Andrew M. Low molecular weight heparin in children. *Eur J Pediatr* 2002;161:71.

Streif W, Andrew M, Marzinotto V, et al. Analysis of warfarin therapy in pediatric patients: a prospective cohort study of 319 patients. *Blood* 1999; 94:3007.

SECTION V ■ NEOPLASTIC DISEASES

CHAPTER 299 ■ GENERAL CONSIDERATIONS OF NEOPLASTIC DISEASES

C. PHILIP STEUBER

By any measure, cancer in children is a rare disease, accounting for approximately 8,600 cases annually among children younger than 14 years in the United States and 3,700 cases annually in the 15- to 19-year-old age group. The annual incidence is approximately 17 cases per 100,000 individuals at risk. Nevertheless, cancer remains the leading cause of death from disease in children between 1 and 18 years of age. In contrast, more than 1.2 million new cases of cancer are diagnosed annually among adults. This disparity in numbers is not wholly attributable to the relative size of the populations of adults and children but reflects the significant role of chronic environmental exposures in adult cancer. Although more than 85% of adult malignant neoplasms are carcinomas, carcinomas are rare in children. The most common cancers in children are the acute leukemias (30%) and central nervous system tumors (18%). Environmental factors do play a role in pediatric carcinogenesis, but the associations are different for pediatric patients than for adults. Some pediatric neoplasms are associated with developmental defects, anomalies, or cytogenetic or molecular aberrations and can be anticipated on the basis of preexisting immunologic deficiency states, genetic and chromosomal disorders, and congenital anomalies (Box 299.1 and Tables 299.1 to 299.3). When identified, such patients require careful observation and regular evaluation to enable early detection and optimal management. Environmental factors may play a role by triggering neoplastic transformation or activating preexisting defects. In general, however, the incidence of childhood cancers attributable to a defined inherited or congenital predisposition or environmental factor is low. A family history of a high incidence of cancer is an important consideration. Some of the syndromes described may not manifest fully until the individual is older and need not be considered in the very young infant or child.

Except for these uncommon circumstances and conditions, the detection of cancer in children requires the caregiver to be alert to the possibility. Early diagnosis of childhood cancer often is delayed because of the nonspecific nature of the initial signs and symptoms, the relative rarity of pediatric cancers, and a low index of suspicion. The seven warning signs of cancer in adults are of limited help in evaluating the pediatric patient. Warning signs in children can include fever, persistent headache, pain, a mass, purpura, pallor, and changes in gait, balance, personality, and the eyes (e.g., squint, retinal reflections), all of which may evolve insidiously. Some of these are

BOX 299.1	Immune Deficiency Diseases Predisposing to Neoplastic Disease

X-linked lymphoproliferative disease
Bruton agammaglobulinemia
Severe combined immunodeficiency
Wiskott-Aldrich syndrome
IgA deficiency
Common variable immunodeficiency
DiGeorge syndrome
Ataxia-telangiectasia
Chédiak-Higashi syndrome

common nonspecific pediatric complaints with common explanations, but the alert primary physician can quickly sort out the unusual from the usual problems.

Fever is a universal pediatric complaint that brings children to the physician. In the absence of infection, unrelenting or recurring fever may reflect an occult lymphoma or may be secondary to necrosis within a tumor, such as neuroblastoma or Wilms tumor. Recurrent or Pel-Ebstein fever, seen in adults with Hodgkin disease, is rarely seen in children. In Langerhans cell histiocytosis, persisting fever may be the only presenting complaint. Peripheral blood counts can often be helpful in identifying the problem underlying the fever. Neutropenia associated with fever may suggest a disease with marrow involvement such as leukemia. On the surface, the infection may appear to be routine, except for the failure to respond to appropriate therapy. However, although neutropenia may predispose patients to infection, the converse is more often true in children with neutropenia. In any event, peripheral blood counts are a good starting point in evaluating patients with unexplained fever and, in cases of leukemia, blast cells often may be seen on the peripheral blood smears. When indicated, a bone marrow examination can immediately confirm or rule out a disorder of the bone marrow in a patient with fever.

Headache is another common pediatric complaint. Morning headaches, especially associated with morning vomiting, suggest increased intracranial pressure possibly caused by brain tumor. In infants, open cranial sutures may permit a natural decompression and mask early symptoms of increasing intracranial pressure. Unusual irritability may be a symptom of intracranial disease in the very young child. Persistent pain in any joint or bone is a common complaint of children with leukemia or neuroblastoma.

TABLE 299.1

GENETIC INSTABILITY AND DNA REPAIR DISORDERS ASSOCIATED WITH CHILDHOOD CANCER

Disorders	Cancers
Xeroderma pigmentosum	Basal cell carcinoma, squamous cell carcinoma, melanoma
Bloom syndrome	Leukemia, lymphoma, gastrointestinal cancers
Fanconi anemia	Leukemia, hepatoma, squamous cell carcinoma
Ataxia-telangiectasia	Lymphoma, leukemia, Hodgkin disease, and brain, gastric, ovarian, and other epithelial cancers

TABLE 299.2

CONSTITUTIONAL CHROMOSOME DISORDERS ASSOCIATED WITH CHILDHOOD CANCERS

Disorders	Cancers
Down syndrome	Leukemia, testicular cancer, retinoblastoma
Turner syndrome	Neurogenic, gonadal, and endometrial cancers
Klinefelter syndrome	Leukemia, germ cell tumors
Other sex aneuploidy	Retinoblastoma
XY gonadal dysgenesis	Gonadoblastoma, dysgerminoma
Trisomy 13	Teratoma, leukemia, neurogenic cancer
Trisomy 18	Neurogenic cancer, Wilms tumor
XYY, XYY mosaic	Osteosarcoma, medulloblastoma

Any mass always deserves prompt attention. Regardless of the child's age, all masses in the abdomen should be considered to be malignant until proven otherwise. Computed tomography, magnetic resonance imaging, and real-time sonography are effective diagnostic clinical aids that may identify the problem quickly. Persistent lymphadenopathy is yet another common pediatric complaint. Any large asymptomatic node that increases in size after 2 weeks or fails to regress after 4 to 6 weeks should be considered for biopsy. Nontender, firm lymph nodes should raise the suspicion of malignant disease, as should any swollen lymph node in an unusual location such as in the supraclavicular area, and should lead to early biopsy. Thrombocytopenia and anemia with resultant purpura and pallor usually reflect bone marrow failure. A bone marrow examination may be diagnostic.

Changes in gait or balance or other neurologic abnormalities such as head tilt are common complaints in children with posterior fossa tumors. A variety of neurologic problems can result from brain tumors, and some of them may be subtle, such as personality changes in children with supratentorial tumors. Some of these subtle problems may be recognized only by a parent at first. More than a few parents have complained about difficulty in convincing physicians that something was wrong with their child. Fortunately, imaging studies of the head (computed tomography and magnetic resonance imaging) are widely available, are of tremendous diagnostic value, and have enhanced the ability of physicians to make an early diagnosis of intracranial lesions. These modalities have proven invaluable not only in diagnosing but also in monitoring the course of these patients.

Retinoblastoma may cause changes of vision and may be accompanied at first by squinting and later by an obvious leukocoria (i.e., cat's eye reflex). Neuroblastomas, rhabdomyosarcomas, and occasionally myeloid leukemias may cause complaints

TABLE 299.3

CONGENITAL MALFORMATIONS ASSOCIATED WITH TUMORS

Malformations	Tumor
Aniridia	Wilms tumor
Hemihypertrophy	Wilms tumor
Cryptorchidism	Testicular tumors
Gonadal dysgenesis	Gonadoblastoma
Enchondromatosis (Ollier disease)	Chondrosarcoma

about the eye and orbit that usually warrant an ophthalmologic examination, even if no obvious physical abnormality exists. This often requires sedation or anesthesia in the young child.

Once a malignant neoplasm is suspected, the application of modern imaging techniques can be most helpful in specifying the location and extent of the problem and in identifying the best area to biopsy. The approach to the diagnosis should be based on the type of tumor suspected. Many of the lymphomas and solid tumors such as neuroblastoma and rhabdomyosarcoma metastasize early. Metastatic disease involving the bone marrow may lead to a quick diagnosis of cancer and, coupled with the use of histochemical staining and electron microscopy, may provide a specific tissue diagnosis, eliminating the need for a major surgical procedure. If the marrow examination is not diagnostic, then the appropriate surgical procedure can be performed.

Knowledge of the precise histologic diagnosis and extent of the disease (i.e., staging) is essential before planning any type of intervention. Ideal management usually involves a team approach, which may include surgeons, pediatric oncologists, radiologists, pathologists, radiotherapists, and other specialists, depending on the diagnosis and the complications at the time. The management should consider the effect of the diagnosis on all family members, so that provisions can be made for social service and psychological counseling as needed. Children with probable or proven cancer must be immediately referred to the proper pediatric facility for complete diagnosis and therapy assignment. Errors or omissions at diagnosis seldom can be rectified at a later date.

In general, pediatric tumors are much more responsive to therapy than are adult cancers. Progress since the early 1970s has resulted in a dramatic improvement of the overall 5-year survival rate, which is approximately 75% for all children with cancer (Surveillance, Epidemiology and End Results Program [SEER] data). Because of the dramatic success with treatment and subsequent reduction of mortality, each child suspected of or found to have cancer should be given a chance to receive the optimal available therapy. Such therapy should be focused not only on cure but also on minimization of late effects. Although for some specific entities, such as Wilms tumor, therapy is close to being standardized (survival rate exceeds 90%), most therapies for newly diagnosed childhood cancer are not standardized and are administered in the setting of a clinical trial program. Participation in such trials is considered to be the standard of care in pediatric oncology. Optimal therapy for any of the childhood cancers is most likely to be found in pediatric cancer centers.

Suggested Readings

Smith MA, Gloeckler Ries LA. Childhood cancer: incidence, survival, and mortality. In: Pizzo PA, Poplack DG, eds. *Principles and practice of pediatric oncology,* 4th ed. Philadelphia: Lippincott Williams & Wilkins, 2002.
Vietti TJ, Steuber CP. Clinical assessment and differential diagnosis of the child with suspected cancer. In: Pizzo PA, Poplack DG, eds. *Principles and practice of pediatric oncology,* 4th ed. Philadelphia: Lippincott Williams & Wilkins, 2002.

CHAPTER 300 ■ ACUTE LYMPHOBLASTIC LEUKEMIA

DONALD H. MAHONEY, JR.

EPIDEMIOLOGY AND ETIOLOGY

Acute leukemia is the most common malignancy diagnosed in children. An estimated 3,000 cases of leukemia in children younger than 15 years occur in the United States each year. Based on mortality statistics, the overall incidence is estimated between 35 and 49 per million children younger than 15 years. Approximately three-fourths of the cases are acute lymphoblastic leukemia (ALL), and most of the remaining cases of leukemia are acute nonlymphocytic leukemia. In the United States, childhood ALL has a peak incidence approaching 80 per million among white children between 2 and 5 years of age, with a less prominent peak approaching 35 per million in black children. The highest rates have been reported among Hispanics, Filipinos, and Chinese, and the lowest rates among African-Americans. The reason for this difference is unexplained. Childhood ALL occurs more frequently in boys than in girls, and the difference increases with age. Geographic variation in incidence, rates, and subtype of leukemia (i.e., leukemic clusters) has been reported in the United States and worldwide.

The molecular basis for leukemic transformation in humans is unknown. In normal bone marrow, undifferentiated pluripotent *progenitor* cells with a capacity for self-renewal give rise to committed progenitor cells. These are morphologically recognizable cells that give rise to the erythroid, myeloid, megakaryocytic, eosinophilic, and monocytic-macrophage series. In the clonal expansion theory, leukemia arises from a damaged progenitor cell that has the propensity for unlimited self-renewal or has lost the ability to differentiate along the lines of normal committed progenitor cells. Proposed molecular mechanisms for leukemic induction include activation of a protooncogene or the creation of a fusion gene with oncogenic properties, or the loss or inactivation of genes whose proteins suppress leukemia.

A variety of environmental, genetic, viral, and immunologic factors may contribute to the development of disease (Table 300.1). Of the possible environmental factors, ionizing radiation has been the most extensively studied. The increased incidence of leukemia in survivors within 1,000 meters of the atomic bomb explosions during World War II has

TABLE 300.1

RISK ESTIMATES FOR DEVELOPING CHILDHOOD LEUKEMIA

Population at Risk	Estimate Risk	Time Interval (Years)
U.S. white children	1:2,800	10
Siblings of child with leukemia	1:700	10
Identical twin of a child with leukemia	1:5	Weeks to months
Children with Down syndrome	1:75	10
Children with Fanconi syndrome	1:12	21
Children with Bloom syndrome	1:8	26
Children with ataxia-telangiectasia	1:8	25
Exposures		
Atom bomb within 1,000 m	1:60	12
Ionizing radiation	?	10–25
Benzene	1:960	12
Alkylating agents	1:2,000?	10–20

been well documented. ALL developed most frequently in those younger than 15 years at the time of exposure. Exposure to radiation *in utero*, usually from diagnostic examinations, has been associated with a small but statistically significant risk for development of childhood leukemia. Radiation dose and inherited susceptibility play contributing roles in the development of radiation-associated malignancies. The relative risk of contracting leukemia or other forms of cancer in persons exposed to electromagnetic fields has been investigated in several studies, but no definitive cause and effect association has been established.

Several chemical agents are known to induce or promote leukemia in animals. Except for benzene exposure, however, little is known about the importance of such agents in humans. With the exception of second malignancies in children previously treated with chemotherapy, usually including alkylating agents or epipodophyllotoxins, with or without radiation therapy, no clear association for chemical carcinogenesis has been established in children.

Based on studies in monozygotic twins, a prenatal origin of childhood leukemia has been proposed. Using neonatal blood spots from Guthrie cards, investigators were able to demonstrate the presence of $t(12;21)(p13;q22)$ *TEL/AML1* fusion sequences from six of nine infants and a pair of twins who subsequently developed lymphoblastic leukemia. This important leukemic-associated clonal mutation has now been demonstrated to occur prenatally; however, postnatal events are required to promote clonal expansion to the clinical disease state.

Several hypotheses have been proposed to suggest a role for infection, particularly *in utero* or during early infancy as a leukemogenic risk factor. No single infectious agent emerges as a clear risk factor. Socioeconomic status, geographic isolation with sudden shifts in population mix or density, and other community characteristics have been suggested as cofactors contributing to abnormal patterns of infection that lead to an increase risk for leukemia.

An unusual susceptibility to leukemia has been associated with certain heritable diseases, chromosomal disorders, and constitutional syndromes. Children with trisomy 21 (i.e., Down syndrome) have at least a 10- to 15-fold increased risk

for developing leukemia compared with normal children. The greatest risk period for leukemia in children with Down syndrome is before the age of 5 years. Before 3 years of age, acute nonlymphoblastic leukemia predominates. Increased chromosomal fragility may predispose these patients to leukemic transformation. Cases of childhood leukemia have been associated with several heritable syndromes, including Klinefelter syndrome, Rubinstein-Taybi syndrome, Poland syndrome, Shwachman syndrome, neurofibromatosis, and Kostmann congenital agranulocytosis. The relation between these syndromes and leukemia and other childhood cancers requires further definition.

Several immunodeficiency states have an associated increased risk for lymphoma and leukemia. These conditions include the syndromes of Wiskott-Aldrich, X-linked agammaglobulinemia, severe combined immune deficiency, and ataxia-telangiectasia. The loss of cellular immune surveillance capability for tumor antigens and the inability to self-regulate lymphoproliferative processes may contribute to malignant transformation in these patients. When a child with an identical twin develops leukemia, the risk for leukemia in the other twin is approximately 20%, but the risk diminishes with age. Fraternal twins and siblings of children with leukemia have an estimated fourfold greater risk for leukemia than children in the general population. However, an annual risk that increases from 4 per 100,000 to 16 per 100,000 is not of major clinical significance and should not be a cause for alarm for parents. Epidemiologic studies do not indicate an increased frequency of leukemia in children of leukemic parents, in children breast-fed by mothers who subsequently develop leukemia, in recipients of blood products from donors who develop leukemia, or in households with pets with leukemia.

CLASSIFICATION AND CYTOGENETIC ASPECTS

Childhood leukemia is a heterogenous disease. Morphologic, immunologic, biochemical, and cytogenetic features are used to characterize the disease, estimate prognosis, and develop successful therapeutic strategies. Under normal conditions, less than 5% of the nucleated marrow is composed of blast forms. Blasts are primitive, undifferentiated-appearing precursor cells not normally seen in the peripheral circulation, except in unusual circumstances. With the Wright-Giemsa stain, blasts can be recognized by their large size and high nuclear-to-cytoplasmic ratio. The nuclear membrane is round or clefted, and the nuclear chromatin appears fine and homogeneous with an occasional small nucleolus. The leukemic lymphoblast frequently reacts with the periodic acid-Schiff stain but not with myeloperoxidase and Sudan black.

Using a morphologic classification system developed by a French-American-British (FAB) collaboration, approximately 85% of the children with ALL have lymphoblasts of L1 morphology. Fewer than 15% of the patients have lymphoblasts of L2 morphology. Lymphoblasts with L3 morphology are identical to Burkitt lymphoma cells, ordinarily possess surface immunoglobulin, and are associated with a distinct karyotypic abnormality. Specific immunologic phenotypes have not otherwise been associated with L1 or L2 morphology. The FAB classification may have some prognostic value. Childhood ALL with L1 morphology has a high remission induction rate and more prolonged survival, whereas patients with L3 disease have a worse prognosis.

Immunologic marker analysis has allowed lineage assignment and maturational staging of the lymphoid leukemias and has offered some insight into the pathology of these diseases (Table 300.2). Approximately 65% of the children with ALL

TABLE 300.2

IMMUNOLOGIC CLASSIFICATION OF CHILDHOOD ACUTE LYMPHOBLASTIC
LEUKEMIA IMMUNOPHENOTYPES

Characteristic	Early Pre–B Cell	Pre–B Cell	T Cell	B Cell
Percent of patients	63–65%	18–20%	13–15%	1%
FAB	L1, L2	L1, L2	L1, L2	L3
TdT	+	+	+	–
Monoclonal antibodies (CD)				
CD2, 5, 7	–	–	++++	–
CD10	90	90	15–30	+++
CD19	+++	+++	–	+++
CD20	++	++	++	
CD22/24	++	++	++	
Immunoglobulin	–	cIg+	–	sIg+
HLA-DR	97–98%	97–98%	12–17%	94%
Heavy-chain gene rearrangement	++	++	–	++
Light-chain gene rearrangement	±	±	–	+
Glucocorticoid receptors	++++	++	++	+
Cytogenetics	t(12;21)	t(1;19)	t(11;14)	t(8;22)

–, absent; ±, observed infrequently; +, observed; ++, observed sometimes; +++, observed frequently; ++++, observed in most patients; CD, cluster of differentiation antigen; FAB, French-American-British classification; HLA-DR, human leukocyte differentiation antigen; TdT, terminal deoxynucleotidyl transferase.

have early pre–B lymphoblasts. Using monoclonal antibodies directed at specific antigen sites defined as clusters of differentiation (CD), these lymphoblasts were found to express CD10, CD19, CD20, CD22, and the HLA-DR antigen (Ia). These lymphoblasts lack surface (sIg) and cytoplasmic (cIg) immunoglobulins, and do not react with monoclonal antibodies directed at T-cell antigens.

Pre–B-cell ALL represents approximately 18% to 20% of the new cases of ALL. Morphologic and immunologic features are similar to the early pre–B-cell ALL, except for the presence of heavy-chain (cIg) immunoglobulin within the cytoplasm.

B-cell ALL (B-ALL) is rare in children, representing 1% of all cases. The lymphoblasts are characterized by their Burkitt-like appearance and express sIg.

T-cell phenotypes represent 13% to 15% of childhood ALL. Monoclonal antibodies corresponding to different stages of intrathymic differentiation are used to identify these patients, with one-third to one-half of T-ALL cases reacting with antigens of the early thymocyte state (i.e., CD2, CD5, CD7).

Approximately 1% to 3% of patients fail to react with any antigen test system and are classified as undifferentiated, null, or stem cell leukemias.

The immunologic subtypes may be important for predicting response to conventional therapy. Patients with early pre–B-ALL experience an increased remission induction rate and prolonged remission and survival. Patients with pre–B-ALL and the t(1;19)(q23;p13) translocation may not enjoy the same degree of long-term disease control as patients with early pre–B-ALL. Patients with T-cell disease are frequently older (average age, 8 to 12 years) and are boys (male-to-female ratio, 4:1). They frequently present with a leukocyte count of more than 100,000/μL, a mediastinal mass, normal hemoglobin concentration, hepatosplenomegaly, and adenopathy. This disease is more difficult to treat and cure than other forms. Children with B-ALL have an aggressive leukemia (cell doubling time, 24 hours) and require very intensive therapies to achieve a cure. Infants (less than 1 year of age) frequently fail to express reactivity to any lymphoid antigens, are CD10 negative, and have a poor prognosis.

Approximately two-thirds of the patients with ALL have karyotypic abnormalities involving the leukemic cell. These alterations are broadly defined as changes in chromosome number (i.e., ploidy) or chromosome structure (i.e., translocations, deletions, inversions). Ploidy can be determined by classic enumeration of chromosome number from metaphase preparations or by analysis of DNA content by flow cytometry. Prognostic significance has been suggested for certain cytogenetic subgroups. Patients with hyperdiploidy (more than 53 chromosomes per cell) without structural abnormalities and patients with trisomy of chromosomes 4, 10, and/or 17 have a more favorable prognosis with conventional therapy than other groups. Most newly diagnosed ALL patients have a diploid or near diploid chromosome complement. Patients with pseudodiploid or hypodiploid chromosome numbers have a poor prognosis. Multiple leukemic stem lines occur in approximately 9% to 15% of patients. The significance of these complex chromosome combinations is not understood.

Several specific chromosome translocations have been recognized in childhood ALL and have significance for disease ontogeny and clinical outcome (Table 300.3). The genetic basis for ALL is presented in Box 300.1.

DIAGNOSIS AND PROGNOSIS

Clinical Presentation and Initial Laboratory Findings

In ALL, an uncontrolled proliferation of immature lymphoid cells produces bone marrow failure and may be associated with extramedullary infiltration. The presenting signs and symptoms are a reflection of these events (Table 300.4). The most common presenting symptoms are fever, pallor, purpura, and pain. The onset may be abrupt or insidious. The evolution of symptoms may occur over a few days, weeks, or months. At first, symptoms may be nonspecific and may mimic other nonmalignant conditions. Fever, although a nonspecific complaint,

TABLE 300.3

CHROMOSOMAL TRANSLOCATIONS IN CHILDHOOD ACUTE LYMPHOBLASTIC LEUKEMIA

Translocation	Genes	Frequency (%)	Features
t(12;21)(p13;q22)	TEL/AML1	21–25	B-cell lineage; favorable prognosis
t(1;19)(q23;p13)	E2A/PBX1	5–6	Pre–B cell; increased white blood cells
t(4;11)(q21;q23)	MLL/AF4	4–8	Mixed lineage; CD10⁻; infants
t(9;22)(q34;q11)	BCR/ABL	3–4	B-cell lineage; older age; poor prognosis
t(1;14)(p34;q11)	TAL1/TCR	3	T cell; male; increased white blood cells
t(8;14)(q24;q32)	MYC/IGH	1	B cell; FAB L3 morphology

FAB, French-American-British classification.

is a significant symptom in the child with ALL. Fever, particularly if coupled with other nonspecific complaints, may mimic more common pediatric illnesses. Of the first 400 children with ALL treated at Texas Children's Hospital, 6% presented with fever of unknown origin and no other clinical or laboratory evidence for leukemia. The diagnosis was established by bone

---

BOX 300.1

Chromosome Translocations in Acute Lymphoblastic Leukemia

The t(12;21)(p13;q22) translocation produces the *TEL/AML1* fusion gene and is the most common genetic rearrangement in childhood acute lymphoblastic leukemia (ALL), accounting for up to 25% of all cases. However, this frequent gene rearrangement is best detectable by molecular probes. The t(1;19) abnormality has been observed in approximately 30% of the children with pre–B-ALL. The t(9;22)(q34;q11) abnormality (i.e., Philadelphia chromosome) is most commonly associated with the adult form of chronic myelogenous leukemia. However, approximately 6% of the children with ALL present with this abnormality. A rearrangement of the *abl* protooncogene, distinct from the *abl/bcr* rearrangement described in the adult form of chronic myelogenous leukemia, has been described. These patients tend to present with higher leukocyte counts and have a poor prognosis.

The t(8;14), t(2;8), and t(8;22) are immunophenotype-specific translocations observed in B-ALL. These translocations produce a rearrangement of the *myc* protooncogene located on chromosome 8, with the immunoglobulin heavy-chain genes located on chromosome 14 or the immunoglobulin light-chain genes located on chromosomes 2 and 22. The aberrant expression of these translocated genes is postulated as a critical mechanism in the malignant transformation of B-ALL. The t(4;11)(q21;q23) translocation occurs in approximately 5% of childhood ALL and is associated with high leukocyte counts (greater than 150,000/(L) and often with a CD10 negative phenotype. Cytochemical studies of these leukemic cells frequently reveal monocytic features, suggesting a mixed-lineage or pluripotent leukemic stem cell as the cause of this disease. Infants presenting with ALL demonstrate translocations involving the 11q23 region in up to 75% of cases; this finding is associated with a very poor prognosis. Translocations involving breakpoints at 14q11, 7q35, and 7p15, which contain the T-cell receptor genes, are detected in 30% to 40% of children with T-ALL. Other random translocations have been reported in approximately 7% to 10% of pediatric ALL cases.

---

marrow examination. Because many of these children have absolute neutropenia (neutrophil count less than 500/μL) secondary to bone marrow failure, they are at extreme risk for bacterial sepsis.

Anemia occurs in 76% of patients. Anemia is gradual in onset, normocytic, and rarely associated with significant symptoms. In a rare patient, tachycardia, air hunger, apprehension, and restlessness may signal acute blood loss secondary to thrombocytopenia-associated hemorrhage with impending hypovolemic shock.

Petechiae and bruising are frequently noticed on physical examination and are related to the high incidence (71%) of thrombocytopenia. Epistaxis is not uncommon, especially when thrombocytopenia is severe (platelets less than 20,000/μL). Under such conditions, the child may swallow blood and experience gastrointestinal irritation, nausea, and vomiting with hematemesis, followed by melena or bloody diarrhea. All of these symptoms have a profound psychological effect on the child, parents, and unsuspecting physician.

Symptoms of anorexia and vague abdominal pains are common. Children may present with bone, hip, or joint pain. Arthralgias and refusal to walk may reflect leukemic infiltrations of the bony cortex or the joint compartment. Lymphadenopathy is common, and some degree of hepatosplenomegaly occurs in more than one-half of the patients. Massive infiltrations can occur but are uncommon.

Clinical laboratory data often reveal a broad spectrum of abnormal findings. In addition to anemia and thrombocytopenia, the leukocyte counts and morphology may be abnormal. Approximately 20% of children present with leukocyte counts greater than 50,000/μL (range, 100 to 1 million/μL). Approximately 44% of children have leukocyte counts less than 10,000/μL. Occasionally, hypereosinophilia has been observed and is thought to be a reactive phenomenon. Leukemic blasts may or may not be seen on peripheral smears.

The diagnosis of leukemia can rarely be established from peripheral blood examination alone. Osteopetrosis, myelofibrosis, granulomatous infections, sarcoid, Epstein-Barr virus (EBV) infection in the very young, other acute viral infections,

---

TABLE 300.4

FREQUENCY OF PRESENTING COMPLAINTS IN CHILDHOOD ACUTE LYMPHOBLASTIC LEUKEMIA

Symptoms	Frequency (%)
Fever	43–61
Pallor	39–55
Bleeding	24–55
Bone/joint pain	31–38
Abdominal pain	9–19
Anorexia	17–33
Fatigue	30

and metastatic tumor are conditions that can result in the release of immature-appearing blasts into the circulation.

The diagnosis of ALL is established by bone marrow examination. In children, the bone marrow specimen usually is obtained from the posterior iliac crest rather than by sternal or pretibial puncture. Diagnostic aspirations may be technically difficult to perform because of the density of blast forms or the presence of marrow fibrosis or necrosis. A Jamshidi needle biopsy may be required for diagnosis. For patients for whom the diagnosis of ALL is strongly suspected, we recommend that the diagnostic bone marrow biopsy be performed by an experienced pediatric hematologist with the aid of appropriately monitored sedation. This will minimize patient discomfort, avoid the necessity for repeat procedures, and maximize the bone marrow sample yield necessary for smears, electron microscopy, cytogenetic studies, and immunophenotype investigations. These studies and special experimental projects that use marrow leukemic blasts usually are required by pediatric leukemic therapeutic protocols.

The normal bone marrow contains less than 5% blasts. A minimum of 25% lymphoblasts on differential examination of the bone marrow aspirate is necessary for the diagnosis of ALL. Most children with ALL have hypercellular marrow with 60% to 100% of the cells as blasts. The presenting characteristics of childhood ALL are outlined in Table 300.5.

Differential Diagnosis

Because children with ALL present with a variety of nonspecific symptoms, several pediatric nonmalignant conditions may be confused with leukemia. Idiopathic thrombocytopenic purpura is a common cause of bruising and petechiae in children. Anemia, leukocyte disturbances, and significant hepatosplenomegaly are not typical findings. Bone marrow examinations reveal normal or increased numbers of megakaryocytes and no increase in blast forms in children with thrombocytopenic purpura. Children with infectious mononucleosis (i.e., EBV) or other acute viral illnesses may present with fever, malaise, adenopathy, splenomegaly, rash, and lymphocytosis. In the young child with EBV, lymphocytosis may be extreme (80,000 to 100,000/μL) and thrombocytopenia and immunohemolytic anemia may further confuse the diagnosis. The atypical lymphocytes characteristic of these diseases are larger and pleomorphic, have more abundant pale blue cytoplasm, and may resemble the leukemic lymphoblast. Specific viral serologies can establish the diagnosis, but a bone marrow examination sometimes is necessary.

Leukemoid reactions may be observed in bacterial sepsis, acute hemolysis, granulomatous diseases, vasculitis, and metastatic tumor to the bone marrow. In these circumstances, underlying clinical events may offer some clues to the differential diagnosis. A bone marrow aspirate usually reveals myeloid hyperplasia. The leukemoid reaction resolves as the underlying disease is managed successfully. Isolated neutropenia also may be observed in asymptomatic infants after the use of certain medications for overwhelming bacterial sepsis. In this case, the bone marrow examination may reveal a maturational arrest of the granulocytic precursors, but increased blast forms are not usually seen.

Children with ALL presenting with fever, arthralgias, arthritis, or a limp frequently may be confused with juvenile rheumatoid arthritis (JRA). Anemia, leukocytosis, and mild splenomegaly, all of which may be observed in JRA, can be misleading. Of the first 400 children with ALL treated at Texas Children's Hospital, 4.5% presented with a diagnosis of osteomyelitis or JRA. Several of these patients were receiving antiinflammatory agents for several weeks before the diagnosis of ALL. Until a reliable positive test for JRA becomes available, a bone marrow

TABLE 300.5

PRESENTING CHARACTERISTICS OF CHILDREN WITH ACUTE LYMPHOBLASTIC LEUKEMIA

Characteristic	Frequency (%)*
Age (years)	
<1.5	6–8
>1.5–10	72–80
>10	15–22
Gender (male)	54–57
Race (white)	80–89
Leukocyte count	
<10,000/μL	44
10,000–50,000/μL	34
>50,000/μL	22
Platelets	
<20,000/μL	20
20,000–100,000/μL	51
>100,000/μL	29
Hemoglobin	
<7.5 g/dL	46
7.5–10 g/dL	30
>10 g/dL	24
Hepatomegaly (below umbilicus)	8–13
Splenomegaly (below umbilicus)	11–14
Lymphadenopathy	
None/minimal	73
Moderate/marked	28
Mediastinal mass	8
CNS symptoms	4
Immunoglobulin abnormalities (one or more)	9
FAB	
L1	82
L2	17
L3	1
Karyotype abnormality	70–75

CNS, central nervous system; FAB, French-American-British classification.
*Percentages are estimates based on accumulated data from large numbers of patients treated by the Pediatric Oncology Group and the Children's Cancer Study Group.

examination to exclude ALL should be strongly considered as part of the diagnostic evaluation of patients with atypical presentations of JRA.

Pancytopenia and fever are presenting symptoms for both aplastic anemia and ALL in children; however, lymphadenopathy and hepatosplenomegaly are unusual findings in aplastic anemia. The bone marrow aspirate and biopsy usually clarify the diagnosis. Patients with aplastic anemia have a hypocellular marrow with cellularity usually less than 10%, no normal marrow precursors, and only small lymphocytes seen on smears. Occasionally, the bone marrow in children with ALL is initially hypocellular, and multiple aspirates and biopsies from additional sites are necessary to establish the diagnosis. Myeloproliferative syndromes and preleukemic conditions are rare in childhood but must be considered in the differential diagnosis whenever a disturbed or dysmyelopoietic bone marrow examination is observed.

Leukemia is a small, blue, round cell malignancy. Other small, blue, round cell malignancies can present in childhood and may produce bone marrow invasion, with the resulting signs and symptoms of fever, pain, petechiae, bruising, and pancytopenia. Neuroblastoma is the most common pediatric solid tumor associated with a high frequency (70%) of bone marrow invasion in children older than 2 years at diagnosis. The pattern of bone marrow infiltration, including discrete clumps or rosettes, the usual presence of a retroperitoneal mass, and elevated urinary catecholamine levels help to differentiate this disease from ALL. Other small, blue, round cell tumors that may produce bone marrow infiltration include rhabdomyosarcoma, non-Hodgkin lymphoma, retinoblastoma, medulloblastoma, and Ewing sarcoma. Other significant clinical abnormalities characteristic for these diseases help to establish the correct diagnosis.

TREATMENT

The treatment of childhood ALL has become progressively complex. Curative therapy for ALL has not been established, and investigational therapy is the treatment of choice. These therapeutic programs recognize that ALL is a heterogeneous disease, that certain risk factors may have importance for response to therapy, that optimal scheduling and delivery of effective chemotherapeutic agents have not been defined, that factors leading to relapse are unknown, and that answers to these and other questions can be obtained only through carefully conducted and critically evaluated cooperative clinical trials. Consequently, the best therapy for the child newly diagnosed with ALL is offered by pediatric cancer centers participating in ongoing clinical therapeutic trials.

Combination chemotherapy is the principal therapeutic modality for childhood ALL. The therapy can be divided into four phases:

- Remission induction and consolidation (i.e., intensification)
- Presymptomatic central nervous system (CNS) therapy (i.e., prophylaxis)
- Maintenance
- Elective discontinuation of therapy and long-term, late-effects follow-up

Remission Induction and Consolidation Therapy

The objectives of remission induction are to eliminate as many leukemic cells as biologically tolerable and to reestablish a normal clinical and hematologic state for the patient. Most pediatric cancer centers use three to four drugs to achieve remission: vincristine, prednisone, and L-asparaginase, with or without doxorubicin or daunorubicin. Rapid cytoreduction is associated with a decreased likelihood of emergence of resistant leukemic clones and increased relapse-free survival. The assessment of prognostic factors at diagnosis becomes useful at this point. Patients with high-risk leukemia (i.e., patients with high leukocyte counts, unfavorable immunophenotypes such as T-ALL, slow early responders to induction therapy, or unfavorable biologic characteristics such as the Philadelphia translocation) are assigned to more intensive induction and consolidation regimens at diagnosis. The morbidity of aggressive therapy is counterbalanced by the need for more intensive cytoreductive therapies for biologically more aggressive leukemias. The estimated remission induction rate with this therapy is 98%. Patients who fail to achieve a remission at the end of 4 weeks of induction therapy have a shorter survival even if remission is obtained eventually.

Intensification is the phase of therapy that immediately follows remission induction. This consolidation phase of treatment is designed to deliver multiple chemotherapeutic agents in a relatively short period. The objective of treatment is to further reduce residual leukemia and minimize the develop-

ment of cross-resistance. This approach has resulted in improved overall survival, as reported by several large clinical trials. Patients with very high leukocyte counts at presentation, hypodiploid leukemic karyotype, Philadelphia chromosome karyotype, or infants with the 11q23/MLL gene rearrangement continue to have a poor prognosis. Bone marrow transplantation therapy is under investigation for these subsets of patients.

Presymptomatic Central Nervous System Therapy

Presymptomatic CNS prophylaxis therapy is an integral component of ALL therapy. Effective CNS treatment programs have decreased the incidence of CNS leukemia as a primary site of relapse from 50% to between 3% and 6%. Several regimens have been investigated and include intrathecal methotrexate and cranial irradiation (2,400 cGy); intrathecal triple therapy with methotrexate, hydrocortisone, and ARA-C; and intrathecal methotrexate alone or coupled with high-dose intravenous methotrexate.

In early studies from St. Jude Children's Research Hospital, cranial irradiation and intrathecal methotrexate were established as effective in preventing CNS leukemia. Subsequent investigations by the Children's Oncology Group suggested that lower radiation doses (1,800 cGy) coupled with intrathecal therapy were as effective and potentially less toxic. Three consecutive studies reported by the Pediatric Oncology Group demonstrated equivalent disease control with triple intrathecal therapy without cranial irradiation in patients with B-progenitor ALL. Potential delayed effects after cranial irradiation include growth delay, intellectual impairment, and occasional brain tumors. Recent investigations of intensive intravenous methotrexate schedules with intrathecal therapy without cranial radiation have shown that a risk exists for leukoencephalopathy and intellectual impairment.

Maintenance Therapy

The rationale for extended treatment during remission is based on historic evidence that patients discontinuing therapy after less than 6 months after achieving remission relapsed rapidly. The common element in all maintenance or continuation schedules has been the use of weekly methotrexate and daily 6-mercaptopurine. Pharmacologic investigations suggest marked variability in the bioavailability of orally administered methotrexate and 6-mercaptopurine. Several current protocols seek evidence about whether delayed reinduction or intensification pulse therapy, when combined with conventional maintenance, is more effective for prevention of late relapse. These pulse therapies may include vincristine and prednisone, epipodophyllotoxins, cytarabine, cyclophosphamide, anthracyclines, or dexamethasone.

The minimal duration for effective chemotherapy has not been established, in part because of an inability to recognize or treat minimal residual disease. The standard duration of therapy is 2 to 3 years. Improved disease-free survival has not been clearly established for therapy schedules extending beyond 3 years of remission. Historically, of the children with ALL who discontinue therapy after 3 years, 5% to 15% relapsed. The risk of relapse was greatest within the first year off therapy, with virtually no relapses occurring 4 years after cessation. Unfortunately, isolated cases of relapsed leukemia have been reported as late as 10 to 15 years after cessation of therapy.

For children who remain in continuous complete remission for 2 to 3 years on therapy, it has been the practice to discontinue therapy and to observe closely during the first 2 years off therapy for evidence of relapse. Because of the risk for late recurrence, these children will require periodic monitoring indefinitely. Whether children will continue to experience this rate of relapse after discontinuation of current protocols remains to be determined.

Discontinuation of Therapy and Long-Term, Late Therapeutic Effects

As with all children with cancer, the management of the child with ALL requires a team approach. Pediatric nurse specialists, psychologists, play therapists, dietitians, and other hospital and clinic personnel play an important role in the total care of these patients. The stresses that frequently are faced by families of a child with ALL include concerns about the discomfort or disfigurement (especially alopecia) associated with chemotherapy; the financial pressures of medical care or disruption of family employment schedules; school performance and peer relationships, particularly for the older child; communication about fears and apprehensions among parents, the patient, and siblings; and anxiety preceding the elective cessation of therapy.

With prolonged survival, monitoring for late effects of antileukemic therapy assumes increasing importance. The areas of interest include monitoring for specific organ dysfunction, impaired genetic or immunologic mechanisms, and second malignancies. Several long-term problems have been associated with CNS prophylaxis. These may include up to 50% incidence of cranial computed tomographic scan abnormalities for children treated with cranial irradiation and intrathecal methotrexate, seizures, neuropsychological deficits that result in school problems, and endocrine disturbances (e.g., growth hormone deficiency). These problems are remediable and are insufficient reasons for altering a successful treatment program. Current leukemia protocols are seeking to obviate some of these complications by the use of high-dose systemic chemotherapy and intrathecal therapy without irradiation. The success of these programs remains to be established.

Delayed sexual maturation may be observed in children receiving irradiation to gonadal tissue, such as boys with testicular leukemia. Male adolescents may be at risk for spermatogenic dysfunction after cyclophosphamide therapy. Successful parenthood in long-term survivors has been reported, but the progeny of survivors of childhood leukemia are few. The data from cooperative late effects studies do not indicate an excess of congenital abnormalities or cancer in the offspring.

Clinical and laboratory-based research for childhood ALL is proceeding along two principal lines. First, an increased understanding of the molecular and genetic events that regulate normal cellular proliferation and differentiation is essential. By recognizing normal regulatory events in bone marrow and lymphoreticular tissues, it should be possible to identify abnormal regulatory mechanisms and devise strategies for treatment. An increased understanding of the genetic mechanisms that offer the leukemic cell-specific and nonspecific resistance advantages against antileukemic therapy will be necessary before the problem of leukemic relapse can be solved. Second, refinements in antileukemic therapy should proceed along more pharmacologically oriented schedules. Early antileukemic therapy was based principally on empiric data. Advances in the technologies of drug pharmacology, immunology, and cell kinetics will contribute to more effective treatment combinations that target specific mechanisms of leukemic proliferation or differentiation, minimize the risk for toxicity, and increase the patient's chance for long-term survival.

COMPLICATIONS OF THERAPY AND SUPPORTIVE CARE

At diagnosis, the critical issues of management relate directly to complications of the leukemic burden. Patients with high leukocyte counts at diagnosis, massive organomegaly, or immunophenotypes such as T- or B-ALL are at greatest risk for these complications (Box 300.2).

Hyperleukocytosis in leukemia is associated with early morbidity and mortality because of complex metabolic complications and leukostasis in the vertebral and pulmonary vasculature. Early introduction of cytoreductive chemotherapy is essential. Exchange transfusion and leukapheresis also may be useful. Life-threatening metabolic complications may result from spontaneous or chemotherapy-induced leukemic cell lysis. Hyperuricemia, hyperkalemia, and hyperphosphatemia with secondary hypocalcemia may develop within hours of the diagnosis and treatment. Careful hydration, alkalinization of the urine, allopurinol, and urate oxidase are useful for managing hyperuricemia. A progressive increase in blood urea nitrogen and creatinine, phosphorous, or potassium levels requires

---

BOX 300.2

Potential Complications of Childhood Acute Lymphoblastic Leukemia and its Therapy

Metabolic complications
  Hyperuricemia
  Hyperkalemia
  Hyperphosphatemia
  Syndrome of inappropriate antidiuretic hormone
  Hyponatremia
Hemorrhage (platelets <20,000/μL)
  Skin; mucous membranes; occasional gastrointestinal, CNS
Hyperleukocytosis (WBCs >100,000/μL)
  Infarction: pulmonary, CNS hemorrhage
Infection
  Agranulocytic: bacterial (staphylococcus, enteric organisms)
  Lymphocytic: *Pneumocystis*, fungal, viral (herpes simplex virus, cytomegalovirus, varicella)
Extravasation burns: vincristine, doxorubicin, daunorubicin
Anaphylaxis: L-asparaginase, VP-16, VM-26
Myelosuppression: doxorubicin, daunorubicin, cyclophosphamide, cytosine arabinoside, 6-mercaptopurine, methotrexate, etoposide, nitrogen mustard, procarbazine, dactinomycin
Emetic: high-dose methotrexate, cytosine arabinoside, cyclophosphamide, doxorubicin, daunorubicin, VP-16, VM-26
Dysuria: cyclophosphamide
Mucositis: high-dose methotrexate, cytosine arabinoside, doxorubicin
Hypertension: prednisone
Hepatic dysfunction: methotrexate 6-mercaptopurine, cytosine arabinoside
Pancreatic dysfunction: L-asparaginase, cytosine arabinoside

CNS, central nervous system; WBC, white blood cell.

early intervention with hemodialysis. Drugs such as cyclophosphamide and vincristine may induce a syndrome of inappropriate antidiuretic hormone secretion.

Hemorrhage in children with ALL usually is caused by thrombocytopenia. The skin and mucous membranes are the usual sites of involvement. Significant visceral bleeding is unusual. Intracranial hemorrhages are rare but life-threatening events. Hemorrhagic complications are associated more commonly with acute nonlymphocytic leukemia. Patients with platelet counts of less than $20,000/\mu$L are at the greatest risk for hemorrhage. The condition of the patient, evidence of active bleeding, and anticipated course of therapy should be used as guidelines for platelet transfusion. The recommended dose of platelet concentrates is 6 U/m². All blood products should be irradiated before transfusion. Whenever possible, screening serologies for cytomegalovirus, hepatitis, and human immunodeficiency virus should be obtained before starting transfusion therapy. Prophylactic platelet transfusion therapy in the absence of overt bleeding has not been established as necessary care for all patients. Frequent transfusions of platelets may induce alloimmunization to HLA antigens and may reduce the effectiveness of this therapy. Bleeding secondary to a vitamin K–dependent coagulopathy also may occur in patients requiring prolonged broad-spectrum antibiotic support.

Transfusions of packed red blood cells are used frequently in the management of children with ALL, although the indications are not clear. The child who presents with signs or symptoms of acute blood loss clearly requires packed red blood cells and platelet transfusion support. However, guidelines for transfusion of children with anemia without overt bleeding are not established. Some investigators have suggested transfusions at hematocrits less than 20%. Patients without overt bleeding have been managed successfully through the remission induction schedule without packed red blood cell support, even with gradual hemoglobin concentration declines to less than 3 g/dL. The final decision for transfusion should be based on the condition of the patient, anticipated problems associated with the induction program, degree of anemia and reticulocytopenia, and presence or absence of bleeding.

Infection associated with granulocytopenia is a potentially life-threatening complication for the child with ALL. Any break in the skin, insect bite, blister, sore, gingival or mucous membrane irritation, or perianal fissure may serve as a portal for bacterial penetration, agranulocytic cellulitis, and sepsis. Overwhelming bacterial sepsis is the greatest threat to the child with ALL receiving intensive antileukemic therapy. Any child who presents with fever of 101°F or higher and an absolute granulocyte count of less than $500/\mu$L must be assumed to have sepsis. This is a medical emergency. These children should be hospitalized immediately; cultures of blood, urine, and respiratory secretions obtained; and broad-spectrum intravenous antibiotics initiated without delay. The principal pathogens include *Pseudomonas, Escherichia coli,* and *Staphylococcus.* With increased use of central venous catheters, cutaneous types of organisms (i.e., skin contaminants) may be the pathogens.

In addition to bacterial infections, a variety of nonbacterial, opportunistic infections can cause devastating illness in these patients. Varicella-zoster, herpes zoster, and herpes simplex may cause serious systemic complications, including pneumonitis, hepatitis, and cerebritis. Treatment with acyclovir has been successful in controlling these infections. *Pneumocystis jiroveci* pneumonia is a protozoan infection that occurs in the severely immunosuppressed patient. This illness may present as unexplained fever. The patients are usually lymphopenic but not granulocytopenic. The infection may rapidly progress to cause life-threatening interstitial pneumonia. A program of prophylaxis involving trimethoprim-sulfamethoxazole administered twice daily for 3 days per week is effective in prevention of this disease. Invasive fungal infections continue to be observed in patients receiving intensive immunosuppressive therapy, with prolonged neutropenia and concomitant use of broad-spectrum antibiotics. The major pathogens are *Candida* and *Aspergillus.* Amphotericin B remains the treatment of choice for invasive infections.

Miscellaneous complications related to the choice of chemotherapy agents and routes of administration may be observed. Vincristine, doxorubicin, and daunorubicin are vesicants; care must be taken to avoid extravasation, or serious chemical burns may result. High doses of cyclophosphamide may induce cystitis, with symptoms of dysuria and hematuria. L-Asparaginase and the epipodophyllotoxins (i.e., VP-16, VM-26) have associated risks for allergic reactions; appropriate medications should be available at the patient's bedside or within the physician's office to deal with an allergic crisis. High doses of methotrexate, 6-mercaptopurine, and cytosine arabinoside, alone or in combination with other agents, are emetogenic. Hepatic dysfunction also may be associated with these agents. Severe mucositis may be associated with methotrexate and with the anthracyclines.

BONE MARROW AND EXTRAMEDULLARY RELAPSE AND TRANSPLANTATION

The most serious complication of ALL treatment is bone marrow relapse. Although reinduction of remission is possible, most patients relapse again and eventually succumb to their disease. Patients who relapse while receiving continuation therapy have the worst prognosis. This event usually signals the emergence of resistant leukemic clones. Patients who relapse more than 24 months from diagnosis have a somewhat more favorable prognosis.

Bone marrow transplantation (BMT) is the treatment of choice for patients with hematologic relapse. Allogeneic-matched BMT is the optimal approach; matched-related and unrelated donor and autologous transplants are reasonable alternatives but remain investigational in their design. Treatment schedules, bone marrow processing, and posttransplant support measures are undergoing continual refinement. The procedure is risky, with increased mortality and morbidity associated with nonallogeneic approaches. Acute and chronic graft-versus-host disease, interstitial pneumonitis, and relapse of leukemia are some of the many significant complications that may follow the transplantation procedure. The overall outcome for patients treated with BMT, as reported by large registries (i.e., International Bone Marrow Transplant Registry), is greater than 40% disease-free survival with a plateau from 2.5 to 10 years in follow-up.

The CNS and testes are the most common sites of extramedullary relapse. However, these isolated events should be considered as localized manifestations of recurrent systemic disease; aggressive systemic chemotherapy is an essential part of the management.

Although fewer than 10% of the children with ALL have CNS leukemia at diagnosis, it remains the most common site of extramedullary relapse. Patients with T-ALL or high leukocyte counts at diagnosis have the greatest risk for this event. The clinical signs and symptoms of CNS leukemia may include headache, nausea, and vomiting secondary to increased intracranial pressure; diplopia or blurred vision; nuchal rigidity or hemiparesis with cord involvement; or even hyperphagia and pathologic weight gain. The diagnosis is established by lumbar puncture and analysis of cerebrospinal fluid cytopreparations for leukemic blasts. Symptoms of increased intracranial pressure are not a contraindication for a lumbar puncture.

Treatment for overt CNS leukemia has included intrathecal methotrexate, intrathecal triple therapy, cranial irradiation, craniospinal radiation, intraventricular methotrexate by way of an Ommaya reservoir for resistant disease, high-dose methotrexate, or a combination of these therapies. Significant chronic neurotoxicity is associated with schedules using more than two modalities. Children who develop overt CNS leukemia after adequate presymptomatic CNS therapies have an increased risk for hematologic relapse. These children must be treated with intensive systemic reinduction, consolidation, and maintenance chemotherapy schedules together with a combination of intrathecal methotrexate and cranial or craniospinal irradiation if there is to be any hope for survival and cure.

Isolated testicular leukemia occurs in less than 5% of male subjects receiving modern therapy. Patients usually present with a painless swelling; ultrasound examination may be helpful in excluding other causes of testicular swelling. Testicular infiltration may be occult. The diagnosis is confirmed by bilateral testicular wedge biopsies. Patients diagnosed with testicular leukemia should receive radiation therapy to a dose of 2,400 cGy to both testes, followed by systemic chemotherapy. The long-term prognosis for these patients remains good. Other sites of extramedullary infiltration with ALL have been observed in children. Renal infiltrates are found in 40% of the children at diagnosis and may contribute to metabolic complications and hypertension during induction therapy. Isolated ovarian involvement has been reported occasionally and may extend to the fallopian tubes, uterus, and pelvic nodes. Radiographic changes in the skeleton, with or without associated symptoms, may be seen in as many as 30% of the patients at diagnosis. Leukemic infiltrates have been observed in the lower gastrointestinal tract, oral and gingival regions, retina and iris, heart, lungs, and skin.

PROGNOSIS

The single most important prognostic factor in childhood ALL is effective therapy. Before 1970, the likelihood for long-term survival was less than 10%, but by 2000, the estimated 5-year event-free survival (EFS) rate was in excess of 80%. During the 1970s, a poor outcome was documented for a certain subset of patients (i.e., patients with high leukocyte counts, older patients, patients with T- or B-ALL) compared with other patients managed on a common chemotherapy protocol. These observations led to the development of clinical prognostic risk categories. Categorizing patients in good-risk and poor-risk groups was an attempt to recognize biologically different forms of ALL and has resulted in the development of more aggressive forms of chemotherapy tailored for the different patient populations. As time progressed, many of the unfavorable factors were found to overlap (i.e., mediastinal disease and T-ALL) or lost some of their independent significance as therapeutic regimens improved. By administering the most intensive therapy that is biologically tolerable for the patient, some therapeutic programs (e.g., West German BFM [Berlin-Frankfurt-Munster] studies) have attempted to cancel the prognostic factors as significant variables for survival.

For childhood ALL, the patient's age at diagnosis and the initial leukocyte count have been the two most reliable indicators for response to therapy. In 1996, the National Cancer Institute, together with the large cooperative pediatric cancer treatment groups, devised a consensus risk classification with children presenting at ages between 1.0 and 9.9 years and with a leuko-

TABLE 300.6

PROGNOSTIC FACTORS FOR CHILDHOOD ACUTE LYMPHOBLASTIC LEUKEMIA AT DIAGNOSIS

Factor	Favorable	Unfavorable
Cell type	FAB L1	FAB L3
Leukocyte count	$<50,000/\mu L$	$\geq 50,000/\mu L$
Age (years)	1.0–9.99	<1 or ≥10
Ploidy	>1.16	≤1.16
Cytogenetics	Hyperdiploid	Hypodiploid
	t(12;21)	t(9;22)
	Trisomies 4 and 10	11q23
Cell lineage	CD10$^+$	CD10$^-$
	Early pre–B cell	B>T>pre–B cell
Race	White	Black
Gender	Female	Male
Central Nervous System Involvement	Absent	Present

FAB, French-American-British classification.

cyte count of less than 50,000/μL as the minimal criterion for lower-risk ALL; all other cases are considered as higher risk. Using these criteria, it has been estimated that 60% to 70% of B-precursor ALL would be classified as lower risk, with an estimated EFS rate of 80%; the remainder of cases would be higher risk, with an estimated EFS rate of 60% to 65% with modern therapy. Additional biologic factors associated with favorable prognosis include leukemic DNA hyperdiploidy, leukemic trisomies 4 and 10, and t(12;21) with the *TEL/AML1* fusion gene. Biologic features associated with poor prognosis include the presence of t(9;22) Philadelphia chromosome, the 11q23/*MLL* gene rearrangement, overt central nervous system disease, and leukemic hypodiploidy. Two additional factors have recently been reported as predictors of outcome. Rapidity of response to induction chemotherapy is highly predictive for outcome. Persistence of blasts in bone marrow or peripheral blood by day 7 or 14 of induction correlates with poor outcome. Levels of minimal residual disease, detected by molecular techniques early in the course of treatment, also predict outcome. The commonly recognized prognostic factors for childhood ALL are listed in Table 300.6. Prognostic factors will continue to be defined and redefined as therapeutic interventions improve.

Suggested Readings

Bhatia S and Robinson LL. Epidemiology of leukemia in childhood. In: Nathan DG, Orkin SH, Ginsburgy D, Look AT, eds. *Nathan and Oski's hematology of infancy and childhood*, 6th ed. Philadelphia: WB Saunders, 2003:1081.

Greaves MF, Alexander FE. An infectious etiology for common acute lymphoblastic leukemia in childhood? *Leukemia* 1993;7:349.

Margolin JF, Steuber CP, Poplack DG. Acute lymphoblastic leukemia. In: Pizzo PA, Poplack DG, eds. *Principles and practice of pediatric oncology*, 4th ed. Philadelphia: Lippincott-Raven, 2002:489.

Nachman J, Sather HN, Gaynon PS, et al. Augmented Berlin-Frankfurt-Munster therapy abrogates the adverse prognostic significance of slow response to induction chemotherapy for children and adolescents with acute lymphoblastic leukemia and unfavorable presenting features: a report from the Children's Cancer Group. *J Clin Oncol* 1997;15:2222.

Pui CH. Acute lymphoblastic leukemia. *Pediatr Clin North Am* 1997;44:831.

Silverman LB, Sallan SE. Acute lymphoblastic leukemia. In: Nathan DG, Orkin SH, Ginsburg D, Look AT, eds. *Nathan and Oski's hematology of infancy and childhood*, 6th ed. Philadelphia: WB Saunders, 2003:1135.

Wiemels JL, Cazzaniga G, Daniotti M, et al. Prenatal origin of acute lymphoblastic leukemia in children. *Lancet* 1999;354:1499.

CHAPTER 301 ■ ACUTE MYELOID LEUKEMIA

GLADSTONE E. AIREWELE AND C. PHILIP STEUBER

EPIDEMIOLOGY

Acute myeloid leukemia (AML) represents approximately 20% of all leukemia diagnosed in children. In the United States, about 500 new cases are diagnosed annually in children less than 15 years old. Unlike acute lymphoid leukemia (ALL), the incidence of AML remains stable from birth until 10 years of age, and the disease occurs with equal frequency in boys and girls and in the various ethnic groups. The factors that lead to the development of AML are unknown in the overwhelming majority of cases, but certain conditions and exposures are known to predispose to AML (Box 301.1). In general, AML cells are more resistant to chemotherapy compared to ALL, and the therapy for childhood AML has not reached the degree of success achieved for ALL. Nevertheless, major therapeutic improvements have occurred in the last 20 years, and the overall long-term survival now approaches 50% to 60% in some studies. This improvement has been due largely to clinical trials conducted by various childhood cancer treatment groups and also to improvement in general supportive-care capabilities.

PATHOPHYSIOLOGY

AML is the result of a clonal proliferation of a hematopoietic precursor cell. The abnormal proliferation results in an accumulation of immature myeloid cells that are incapable of differentiating into mature cells. Although the precise pathophysiology of AML development is not completely understood, as in other malignancies, this abnormal proliferation results from a series of mutations affecting genes that are responsible for regulating the proliferation and differentiation of the hematopoietic stem cell. The term AML includes a variety of leukemia subtypes that are designated by apparent cell of origin (Table 301.1).

Chromosomal aberrations involving the leukemia blast cells are demonstrable in the majority of children with AML. Many of these aberrations are recurring, and some are AML-subtype–specific. Many of the recurring chromosomal aberrations in AML have been shown to enhance the activity of oncogenes and/or silence the activity of tumor suppressor genes. The recognized nonrandom disease and genotype associations are listed in Table 301.2. Children with AML-related abnormal cytogenetic findings usually lose those chromosomal changes when they are in complete remission and regain them on relapse.

Classification

The French-American-British (FAB) classification scheme for AML describes eight subtypes of AML (i.e., M0 through M7) based on morphologic and histochemical criteria. The characteristics and relative frequencies of the FAB subtypes in children are shown in Table 301.1.

A newer classification scheme proposed by the World Health Organization (WHO) attempts to incorporate clinical, genetic, and biologic features in addition to morphology to define specific AML subtypes. It is hoped that this revised approach will provide more clinically relevant information compared with the FAB classification system. Immune phenotyping uses a panel of monoclonal antibodies directed against the surface antigens that are expressed at different times during hematopoiesis. In general, AML blasts exhibit patterns of myeloid antigen expression that often are inconsistent with the defined stages of normal maturation. Myeloid markers that are usually expressed on AML blasts include CD13, CD15, CD33, and CD34 (where CD represents *cluster designation*). Additional markers for monocyte lineage are CD11b and CD14. AML blasts may also express T-lineage markers (CD2, CD4, and CD7) but not B-lineage markers (CD10, CD19, and CD20). Acute erythroleukemia (M6) blasts usually express erythrocyte glycoprotein (glycophorin A), and acute megakaryoblastic leukemia (M7) is distinguished by the expression of platelet-associated antigens such as CD41/61 and CD42.

CLINICAL MANIFESTATIONS AND COMPLICATIONS

As with ALL, children with AML most often present with symptoms of bone marrow failure and infiltration. Pallor, bone pain, fever, infection, and bleeding are the most common complaints at diagnosis. Consumptive coagulopathy, particularly in patients with the promyelocytic (M3) or monocytic (M4, M5) forms sometimes contributes to the bleeding.

Enlargement of the liver and spleen affects approximately one-half of the children, particularly younger children with

---

BOX 301.1 | **Conditions Associated with an Increased Incidence of Childhood Acute Myeloid Leukemia**

Blackfan-Diamond syndrome
Bloom syndrome
Chemotherapy for previous malignancy
Down syndrome
Familial myeloproliferative syndromes
Fanconi anemia
Klinefelter syndrome
Kostmann syndrome
Li-Fraumeni syndrome
Neurofibromatosis
Paroxysmal nocturnal hemoglobinuria (PNH)
Radiation exposure
Wiskott-Aldrich syndrome

TABLE 301.1

THE FAB CLASSIFICATION SYSTEM WITH TYPICAL IMMUNOPHENOTYPING

FAB Type	Morphologic Designation	Relative Frequency	Histochemistry	Typical Immunophenotyping [CD, Cluster Designation]
M0	Myeloblastic leukemia–minimally differentiated	<5%	MPO⁻ SB⁻ NSE⁻ PAS⁻	Myeloid markers: [CD13, CD33, CD34]⁺ T-cell markers: [CD2, CD3, CD7]⁺ or ⁻ B-cell markers: [CD10, CD19, CD20]⁻
M1	Myeloblastic leukemia–without maturation	15–20%	MPO⁺ SB⁺ NSE⁻ PAS⁻	Myeloid markers: [CD13, CD33, CD34]⁺ T-cell markers: [CD2, CD3, CD7]⁺ or ⁻ B-cell markers: [CD10, CD19, CD20]⁻
M2	Myeloblastic leukemia–with maturation	25–30%	MPO⁺ SB⁺ NSE⁻ PAS⁻	Myeloid markers: [CD13, CD33, CD34]⁺ T-cell markers: [CD2, CD3, CD7]⁺ or ⁻ B-cell markers: [CD10, CD19, CD20]⁻
M3	Promyelocytic leukemia	5–10%	MPO⁺ SB⁺ NSE⁻ PAS⁻	Myeloid markers: [CD13, CD33, CD34, CD117]⁺ T-cell markers: [CD2, CD3, CD7]⁺ or ⁻ B-cell markers: [CD10, CD19, CD20]⁻
M4	Myelomonocytic leukemia	25–30%	MPO⁺ SB⁺ NSE⁺ PAS⁻	Myeloid markers: [CD11b, CD13, CD14, CD33, CD34]⁺ T-cell markers: [CD2, CD3, CD7]⁺ or ⁻ B-cell markers: [CD10, CD19, CD20]⁻
M5	Monocytic leukemia	15–20%	MPO⁺ SB⁺ NSE⁺ PAS⁻	Myeloid markers: [CD 11b, CD13, CD14, CD33, CD34]⁺ T-cell markers: [CD2, CD3, CD7]⁺ or ⁻ B-cell markers: [CD10, CD19, CD20]⁻
M6	Erythroleukemia	<5%	MPO⁻ SB⁻ NSE⁺ PAS⁺	Myeloid markers: [CD13, CD33, CD34]⁺ T-cell markers: [CD2, CD3, CD7]⁺⁻ B-cell markers: [CD10, CD19, CD20]⁻ Erythroid marker: Glycophorin A ⁺
M7	Megakaryoblastic	5–10%	MPO⁻ SB⁻ NSE⁺ PAS⁻ Platelet peroxidase⁺	Myeloid markers: [CD13, CD33, CD34]⁺ T-cell markers: [CD2, CD3, CD7]⁺⁻ B-cell markers: [CD10, CD19, CD20]⁻ Megakaryocytic markers: [CD41/61, CD42]⁺

MPO, myeloperoxidase; SB, Sudan black; NSE, nonspecific esterase; PAS, periodic acid-Schiff.

M4 or M5 subtypes. Extramedullary manifestations such as chloromas or granulocytic sarcomas, particularly of the orbit and skin, or gingival hyperplasia may occur in a small percentage of patients, especially in children whose disease has a monocytic component (i.e., M4, M5). Lymphadenopathy is not usually a prominent feature. Testicular involvement at any stage of disease is infrequent. The initial leukocyte count is usually less than 50,000 per microliter, but extreme leukocytosis (greater than 100,000 per microliter) is recorded in one of five AML patients.

TABLE 301.2

ASSOCIATIONS OF NONRANDOM CYTOGENETIC ABNORMALITIES AND LEUKEMIC SUBTYPE

Cytogenetic Abnormality	FAB Subtype
t(8;21) t(6;9)	Acute myelogenous (MI, M2)
t(15;17) t(11;17)	Acute promyelocytic (M3)
inv (16) t(16;16) t(9;11) t(6;9)	Acute myelomonocytic (M4)
t(9;11) t(1;11) t(10;11) t(8;16)	Acute monocytic (M5)
t(11q23)	Acute myelomonocytic (M4) and monocytic (M5)
t(1;22)	Acute megakaryoblastic (M7)
−7/del(7) −5/del(5) +8	All AML subtypes

DIAGNOSIS

The diagnosis of AML most often is based on the finding of an excess of blasts on bone marrow examination. Although ALL blasts may resemble AML blasts, a definitive diagnosis of AML is usually possible after consideration of histochemical stains, immunophenotyping, and cytogenetics (Tables 301.1 and 301.2). Cerebrospinal fluid studies demonstrate leukemic involvement in 5% to 10% of patients at diagnosis. These cerebrospinal fluid findings are usually asymptomatic.

THERAPY

As in ALL, the major initial treatment objective is the rapid reduction of the leukemia clone and the reestablishment of normal bone marrow function. Chemotherapy regimens to achieve this objective generally are more toxic compared with those used in treating ALL, and early death occurs in 5% to 15% of patients. Most of these deaths are due to bleeding and/or infection.

Complete initial remissions in childhood AML are obtained in over 80% of newly diagnosed patients. Initial remission induction treatment in AML commonly utilizes a combination of an anthracycline (most commonly daunomycin), plus cytosine arabinoside (Ara-C), with or without additional drugs such as etoposide and 6-thioguanine. Postremission therapy typically consists of three to six courses of intensive chemotherapy; it utilizes drugs similar to those used in induction therapy and results in a total treatment duration of about 4 to 6 months. The subgroup of patients with M3 AML (promyelocytic) benefit from the addition of all-*trans* retinoic acid (ATRA), which is a differentiation agent. Unlike ALL, maintenance therapy (i.e. continuing low-dose chemotherapy over a prolonged period) has not been shown to definitely improve long-term results in children with AML who received aggressive initial therapy.

PROGNOSIS

Agreement is not universal about prognostic factors in childhood AML because of the generally poor outcome and the relatively small number of cases per year. Certain factors have been identified as associated with better outcomes. These include cytogenetic abnormalities of t(15;17), t(8;21), and inv16. Also, patients with Down syndrome and AML (commonly FAB M7) have a good prognosis using chemotherapy alone. Poor prognosis factors include the finding of deleted chromosomes 5 or 7, complex cytogenetic abnormalities, or FLT3 gene abnormalities. In addition to cytogenetic abnormalities, other factors that have been suggested as poor prognostic factors include age less than 2 years, hyperleukocytosis, poor response to induction chemotherapy, and FAB types M6 or M7. Many of these prognostic factors have not been found consistently across the different treatment protocols. This underscores the fact that risk factors may not be fully independent, but rather are dependent on specific treatment protocols, and their importance may change as the general therapy of AML improves.

The 5-year overall survival rate for children with AML is about 50% using current therapy, and rates as high as 65% have been reported for certain good prognosis subsets, such as those with t(15;17), t(8;21), and inv16 cytogenetic abnormalities.

The role of allogeneic stem-cell transplantation as an alternative post-remission therapy is controversial. Clinical outcome information from U.S. leukemia trials supports the use of allogeneic grafts during first remission in patients who have matched siblings. Continuing improvements in chemotherapy regimens may alter this recommendation, especially in patients with a good prognosis, such as those with cytogenetic finding

of t(8;21), and inv16. Patients with Down syndrome or those with M3 AML (promyelocytic) respond well to chemotherapy regimens and should not undergo transplantation in first remission. Stem-cell transplantation using matched unrelated donors has been advocated for patients with poor prognosis factors, such as secondary AML, cytogenetic finding of deleted chromosomes 5 or 7, complex cytogenetic abnormality, FLT3 gene abnormalities, poor response to induction chemotherapy, and FAB types M6 or M7.

Central nervous system (CNS) prophylaxis or the therapy of occult CNS disease usually is accomplished by the intrathecal administration of single or multiple agents (Ara-C, methotrexate) combined with high doses of drugs that penetrate the blood–brain barrier, such as Ara-C. The effect of CNS therapy on ultimate disease-free survival is unknown, because marrow remissions are of short duration in most patients. Refinements of CNS therapy principles in AML await improvements in systemic therapy.

New drugs and drug combinations are being evaluated for use in induction and postinduction therapy, with the purpose of improving disease-free survival. They include newer anthracyclines (such as mitoxantrone and idarubicin), antimetabolites (such as 2-chlorodeoxyadenosine and gemcitabine), molecularly targeted therapy (farnesyl transferase and tyrosine kinase inhibitors), antibodies such as gemtuzumab ozogamicin, and tumor vaccines. The final role and relative value of these agents remains undefined.

New molecular techniques to detect minimal residual disease (MRD) are available, although the meaning of MRD in the setting of morphologic remission presently is unknown. These technologies promise to refine our definitions of remission in the future and potentially guide therapy. It also is likely that, as in ALL, AML therapy will become increasingly risk adapted.

Suggested Readings

Creutzig U. Treatment of acute myeloid leukemia in children. In: Pui C, ed. *Treatment of acute leukemias: new directions for clinical research*, 1st ed. Totowa, NJ: Humana Press Inc., 2003:237.

Glolub TR, Arceci RJ. Acute myelogenous leukemia. In: Pizzo PA, Poplack DG, eds. *Principles and practice of pediatric oncology*, 4th ed. Philadelphia: Lippincott Williams & Wilkins, 2002:545.

CHAPTER 302 ■ CHRONIC MYELOPROLIFERATIVE DISORDERS

C. PHILIP STEUBER

The chronic myeloproliferative disorders in children are rare conditions accounting for 1% to 2% of all childhood malignancies and 3% to 5% of all childhood leukemias. As with the acute myeloid leukemias (AML), these disorders are the result of the uncontrolled clonal proliferation of one or more marrow-cell lineages. Each entity listed in Box 302.1 is designated according to the predominant type of cell involved. The term *chronic* is somewhat deceptive in that the prognosis for these disorders is generally worse than that for the acute leukemias.

JUVENILE MYELOMONOCYTIC LEUKEMIA

Juvenile myelomonocytic leukemia (JMML), formerly designated as juvenile chronic monomyelogenous leukemia (JCML), is a clonal panmyelopathy most often presenting in children younger than 2 years. Boys predominate (by more than 2:1). The children present with lymphadenopathy that is often suppurative and fever. They frequently exhibit a chronic

---

BOX 302.1
BOX 302.1   Chronic Myeloproliferative
Disorders Seen in Childhood

Juvenile monomyelogenous leukemia (JMML)
Chronic myelogenous leukemia (CML)
Myelodysplastic syndromes (MDS)
Polycythemia vera
Thrombocythemia
Myelofibrosis

BOX 302.2   Proposed Clinical and
Laboratory Criteria for the
Diagnosis of JMML

Clinical Features
  Fever
  Hepatomegaly
  Lymphadenopathy
  Pallor
  Rash
Laboratory Features
  Peripheral blood monocyte count greater than
    1×10^9/L
  Less than 20% blasts in the bone marrow
  Absence of Philadelphia chromosome and BCR/AML
    rearrangement
Additional Features (minimum of two elements required)
  Elevated fetal hemoglobin
  Circulating immature myeloid cells on peripheral
    blood smear
  Leukocytosis (WBC count over 10×10^9/L)
  Cytogenetic abnormalities (commonly involving
    chromosomes 7 and 8)
  Hypersensitivity of myeloid progenitors to GM-CSF
    in cultures

---

eczematoid facial rash and moderate organomegaly. Hematologic abnormalities include a mild anemia, symptomatic thrombocytopenia, and moderate leukocytosis (usually less than 100,000 cells per microliter). The leukocytosis is caused by circulating immature monocytes and myelocytes, which are identifiable histochemically and in cell culture. Circulating nucleated erythrocytes also can be seen. Fetal hemoglobin levels are markedly elevated. Bone marrow specimens are hypercellular, with elevated numbers of myeloid and monocytoid forms. Dyserythropoietic changes are observed, and megakaryocytes are diminished. Although erythroid, myeloid, and megakaryocytic cell lines are involved, abnormal monocyte forms usually predominate. Characteristically, marrow cultures are considered the diagnostic study, and demonstrate predominantly monocytic differentiation, with granulocyte-macrophage colony-forming unit growth occurring spontaneously in the absence of growth factors. Marrow cultures demonstrate a marked growth response when exposed to granulocyte-macrophage colony stimulating factor (GM-CSF). Polyclonal elevations of immunoglobulins have been described, and an association with chronic Epstein-Barr virus infection has been reported. Specific cytogenetic patterns have not been associated with JMML. When chromosomal abnormalities are detected, they most often involve chromosomes 7 and 8. However, most patients studied have normal karyotypes. Diagnostic criteria for JMML have been proposed; these are listed in Box 302.2.

Children with JMML respond poorly to therapy. Younger patients (less than 1 year of age) generally fare better. Transient responses have been reported with various low- and high-dose chemotherapy regimens. Radiation therapy and splenectomy usually are not helpful. The use of isotretinoin (13-*cis*-retinoic acid) alone or in combination with chemotherapy regimens to induce maturation of the monocytes and myelocytes is reported to be transiently effective. It has been suggested that aggressive therapy, similar to that effective in acute forms of myeloid and monocytic leukemia, should be used, and that subsequent allogeneic bone marrow transplantation should be considered as the primary therapeutic option. Improved survivals after transplantation have been reported. Most children with JMML die within 1 to 2 years of diagnosis, regardless of therapy.

ADULT CHRONIC MYELOGENOUS LEUKEMIA

The incidence of adult chronic myelogenous leukemia (ACML) in the pediatric age group is approximately twice that of JMML. ACML is uncommon before 3 years of age, and usually is diagnosed between the ages of 10 and 14. As with JMML, males predominate. Common chief complaints include fever, weakness, pain, weight loss, and increasing abdominal girth. Respiratory system complaints are common. Marked splenomegaly is evident.

Peripheral blood counts demonstrate extreme leukocytosis (greater than 100,000 cells per microliter), usually with thrombocytosis and mild anemia. The circulating leukocyte differential reveals cells at all levels of myeloid differentiation, including eosinophils and basophils. Bone marrow specimens show marked myeloid hyperplasia, increased numbers of megakaryocytes, eosinophilia, and basophilia. Bone marrow blast counts do not exceed 25%.

Using classical cytogenetic methods, most ACML patients (greater than 90%) demonstrate the Philadelphia chromosome (Ph) in the malignant cells. This usually results from a reciprocal translocation between the long arms of chromosomes 9 and 22, t(9;22)(q34;q11). In this translocation, the *abl*-1 oncogene from chromosome 9 is fused to the breakpoint cluster region (*bcr*) of chromosome 22. The resultant fusion gene (*bcr/abl*) plays an integral part in the development of ACML by encoding an abnormal deregulated tyrosine kinase with augmented activity. This results in excessive proliferation of myeloid progenitor cells. The *bcr/abl* fusion gene is easily and rapidly detectable using fluorescent *in situ* hybridization (FISH) methodology. In a few cases, the Ph abnormality involves chromosomes other than 9. Approximately 5% to 10% of ACML patients do not have evidence of the Ph chromosome or *bcr/abl* and they respond less well to therapy. Multiple reports attest to the clonal nature of the proliferative disorder in ACML.

The natural history of ACML is separated into two phases. The initial or chronic phase persists for a limited period (median, 2.5 years) and is followed by an accelerated phase. The accelerated phase is characterized by deteriorating blood counts, progressive neutrophil dysfunction, increasing splenomegaly, and the development of additional chromosomal abnormalities. This phase usually evolves over several months and terminates in acute blastic leukemia. In children, approximately 25% to 30% of the cases of acute leukemia have lymphoid characteristics and patterns of drug response, and the remainder are myeloid. Occasionally, the transformation phase takes place abruptly and is referred to as a *blastic crisis*. After transformation occurs, subsequent response to therapy is poor, and most patients die within a few months, regardless of morphologic classification.

Until recently, management of the chronic phase has consisted of the administration of agents singly or in combination (i.e., hydroxyurea, cytarabine, interferon-alpha or busulfan) to control leukocytosis. Without the use of bone marrow transplantation, the disease was considered to be incurable and acute leukemic transformation inevitable. Efforts at more aggressive drug therapies to eliminate the malignant clone were largely failures. The prolonged use of interferon-alpha has been the initial therapeutic choice for many patients. Interferon-alpha is capable of suppressing the Ph-positive clone, at least temporarily, in adults and children with chronic monomyelogenous leukemia. Reports indicate that interferon therapy may prolong the chronic phase but does not prevent ultimate blastic transformation.

Recently, the development of a selective tyrosine kinase inhibitor, imatinib mesylate, has dramatically altered initial therapy for ACML. The agent inhibits proliferation and induces apoptosis in *bcr/abl* positive cells. It is administered orally and has minimal toxicities. It is the initial therapy of choice for most cases of ACML. Resistance to imatinib mesylate does occur, and it is unlikely that its use as a single agent will be curative.

Hematopoietic stem cell transplantation, if an appropriate donor exists, remains the only truly curative therapy, but the optimal application of such grafts has not been determined. The best results have been observed when the graft is done early in the course of the disease, usually in the first year after diagnosis. However, the timing of the transplant may be impacted by the availability of imatinib mesylate.

Alternative therapies for ACML have included the use of autologous marrow cryopreservation. Marrow is harvested early during the chronic phase, and after the disease accelerates, the patient receives myeloablative therapy followed by reinfusion of the stored marrow. Restoration of the chronic phase in this fashion has had only limited success.

MYELODYSPLASTIC SYNDROMES

The myelodysplastic syndromes are a group of loosely defined clinical and laboratory syndromes that often precede the diagnosis of acute leukemia. They have been called *preleukemia*. The French-American-British (FAB) classification categorizes these entities into five subsets: refractory anemia, refractory anemia with ringed sideroblasts, refractory anemia with excess blasts, refractory anemia with excess blasts in transformation, and chronic myelomonocytic leukemia. These entities are characterized by progressive cytopenia and marrow abnormalities. Patients usually present with problems related to marrow failure. The findings at physical examination, with the exception of pallor and bleeding, usually are unremarkable. Circulating bizarre erythrocyte granulocyte (Fig. 302.1) and platelet forms usually are detected. A mild elevation in fetal hemoglobin may occur, probably reflecting ineffective erythropoiesis. Several defects in granulocytic function have been reported.

Cytogenetic abnormalities, particularly involving deletions of all or part of chromosomes 5 or 7, and trisomy 8 have been reported for many of these patients. The hematologic abnormalities may persist for months.

Management primarily involves transfusion support and the treatment of opportunistic infections. The developing malignancy is usually AML, and response to therapy is poor. Marrow growth factors and other biologic response modifiers are undergoing trials. Bone marrow transplantation has been successful in selected patients and, where possible, should be considered the treatment of choice in the pediatric patient with a myelodysplastic syndrome.

POLYCYTHEMIA VERA AND PRIMARY THROMBOCYTHEMIA

Polycythemia vera and primary or essential thrombocythemia rarely have been reported in children. As with other malignant myeloproliferative syndromes, they are clonal disorders of the affected progenitors. Children with polycythemia vera have complications related to hyperviscosity (see Chapter 293, Polycythemia), and those with thrombocythemia have problems with vascular occlusion secondary to massive platelet numbers. Splenomegaly is a prominent feature in both entities. Bone marrow cell cytogenetic studies occasionally may be abnormal in polycythemia vera but are always normal in thrombocythemia. Because of the rarity of these disorders in pediatric patients, the causes of secondary polycythemia

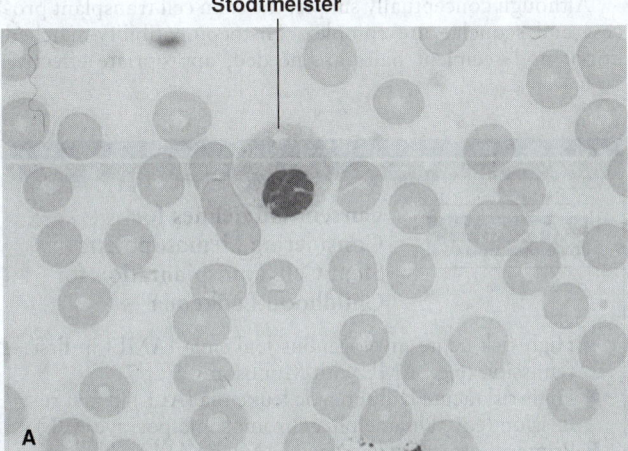

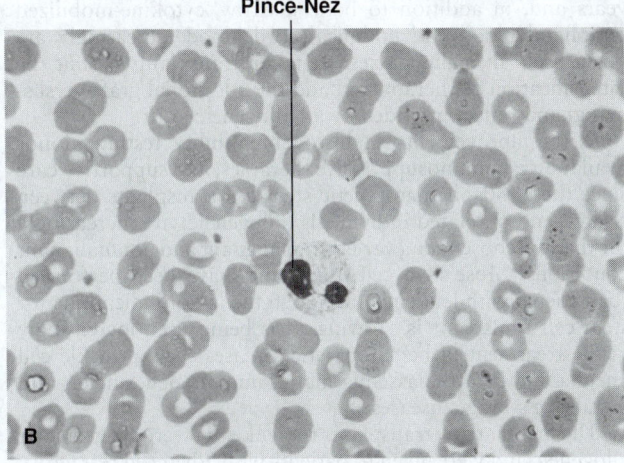

FIGURE 302.1. Photomicrographs of the **A:** unilobed, or Stodtmeister and **B:** bilobed, or Pince-Nez nuclear forms characteristic of the Pelger-Huet anomaly seen in the granulocytes of patients with myelodysplastic disease. These cells can also be seen as a familial trait, inherited in an autosomal dominant fashion, without pathologic significance. (Reprinted with permission from Anderson SC, Poulsen KB. Anderson's Atlas of Hematology. Philadelphia: Lippincott Williams & Wilkins, 2003:76.)

and thrombocythemia must be investigated carefully. The management guidelines are the same as those used for adult patients.

PRIMARY MYELOFIBROSIS

Myelofibrosis is characterized by a fibrotic proliferation within marrow spaces. Pediatric cases are rare. Splenomegaly is common. Hematologic manifestations include bizarre circulating erythrocytes (especially teardrop cells) and platelets and immature myeloid cells, including Pelger-Huët cells (Fig. 302.1). Multiple immunologic defects have been observed. Bone marrow aspiration is not diagnostic, and a biopsy is necessary to confirm the diagnosis. Possible causes of secondary marrow fibrosis, malignant and nonmalignant, must be considered. In years past, many cases previously diagnosed as primary or acute myelofibrosis in children were probably instances of acute megakaryocytic leukemia.

Management is primarily by transfusion and infection control. Occasionally, splenectomy is indicated to control symptoms secondary to mechanical dysfunction (e.g., hypersplenism, portal hypertension). Corticosteroids have been effective rarely, and the role of aggressive chemotherapy or bone marrow transplantation has not been established.

Suggested Readings

Aaltman AJ. Chronic leukemias of childhood. In: Pizzo PA, Poplack DG, eds. *Principles and practice of pediatric oncology.* Philadelphia: Lippincott Williams & Wilkins, 2002:591.

Bennett C, Hsu K, Look AT. Myeloid leukemia, myelodysplasias, and myeloproliferative disease in children. In: Nathan DG, Orkin SH, Ginsberg D, Look AT eds. *Hematology of infancy and childhood,* 6th ed. Philadelphia: Saunders, 2003:1167.

CHAPTER 303 ■ HEMATOPOIETIC STEM CELL TRANSPLANTATION FOR CHILDHOOD LEUKEMIAS

INGRID KUEHNLE AND C. PHILIP STEUBER

Hematopoietic stem cell transplantation (HSCT or SCT) is the process of replacing or substituting a patient's diseased, defective, or damaged bone marrow elements with healthy donor stem cells. A basic requirement is that the host's defect be correctable by hematopoietic stem cell-derived cells. Potential sources of hematopoietic stem cells have increased in recent years and, in addition to bone marrow, cytokine-mobilized peripheral blood and umbilical cord blood increasingly are being used. In malignancies, stem cell transplants permit the intensification of therapy and add the additional graft-versus-malignancy effect provided by an allogeneic graft.

With improvements in histocompatibility testing, donor availability, immunosuppressive therapies, and supportive care since the 1980s, hematopoietic stem cell transplants between related and unrelated individuals (allogeneic) are increasingly the therapy chosen for a variety of malignant and nonmalignant conditions. Most stem cell transplants have been performed for patients with leukemia, although the list of indications for stem cell transplant is growing. It is being used increasingly in the treatment of hematopoietic diseases such as sickle cell anemia and beta-thalassemia major, immunodeficiencies, and metabolic storage diseases.

The first marrow transplants for leukemia were syngeneic or allogeneic and were given to patients with advanced refractory disease to rescue them from myeloablative therapies. The few successes (5% to 10%) observed at that time outnumbered those seen with other therapies and led investigators to explore the indications for and optimal applications of the transplant procedure.

Although HSCT is indicated unequivocally for diseases for which no other curative therapy exists, such as severe combined immunodeficiency, the value of transplant for many malignant diseases remains controversial. Current guidelines for considering hematopoietic stem cell transplantation for childhood leukemia include the diagnoses found in Box 303.1.

Although conceptually simple, the stem cell transplant process and sequelae are complex. Histocompatibility-matched donor and recipient pairs are needed, appropriate effective

---

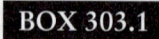

BOX 303.1

Current Guidelines for Considering Hematopoietic Stem Cell Transplantation for Childhood Leukemia

- High risk acute myelogenous leukemia (AML) in first remission (e.g., AML with Monosomy 5 or 7)
- High-risk acute lymphocytic leukemia (ALL) in first remission (e.g., Philadelphia chromosome-positive ALL)
- Primary refractory leukemia (AML or ALL)
- Adult and juvenile forms of chronic myelogenous leukemia during the chronic phase
- Recurrent leukemia of any type
- Myelodysplastic syndromes

preparative programs are required, and the extensive capabilities must be available to support a lengthy period of marrow aplasia, immunosuppression, and graft-versus-host disease (GVHD) after transplantation.

DONOR SELECTION

Initially, allogeneic hematopoietic stem cell donors were full siblings who inherited the same genes determining class I (HLA A and B), and class II (HLA DR, DP, and DQ) antigens. Historically however, only 30% to 40% of patients have an HLA-genotype matched-sibling donor available. Recent progress in graft manipulation, immunosuppressive strategies, and post-transplant supportive therapies has shown improved results using mismatched family members such as parents (i.e., haploidentical), and HLA-matched or partially matched unrelated donors. For pediatric patients with acute leukemias, the outcome after an unrelated matched donor stem cell transplant is approaching that after a matched-sibling donor transplant.

In comparison to HLA-identical sibling donor transplants, stem cell transplants from matched/mismatched unrelated or mismatched related donors increase the risk of posttransplant complications, particularly GVHD. GVHD is caused by immunocompetent donor T cells transferred to the patient with the donor stem cell infusion. To reduce the incidence and severity of GVHD under HLA-disparate conditions, methods are used to purge the donor stem cells of immunocompetent T cells. Reduction of donor T cells can be achieved using either *in vivo* or *in vitro* T cell-depleting antibodies or by targeted selection of CD34+ hematopoietic stem cells. These methods are effective in reducing the GVHD-related problems, but the incidence of graft rejection, infectious complications, and recurrent leukemia increases. These observations underscore the contribution of immunocompetent donor T cells to engraftment and to disease control.

Since it was established in 1986, the National Marrow Donor Program (NMDP) has facilitated more than 15,000 unrelated transplants and now has an ethnically diverse database with 5 million potential stem cell donors and more than 25,000 umbilical cord blood units. The probability of identifying a suitably matched donor through the NMDP is currently 80%.

PREPARATIVE REGIMENS

Conditioning regimens administered in preparation for stem cell transplantation for leukemia serve not only to eradicate the host immune system in order to permit engraftment but also to eradicate malignant cells, or to eradicate abnormal host hemopoiesis. The transplant procedure permits an intensification of therapy, with a corresponding curative potential. For this reason, preparative regimens used to treat malignancies are more intense than those administered for nonmalignant conditions. A multitude of different preparatory regimens currently are employed. When total body irradiation (TBI) is included, it is combined with one or more chemotherapeutic agents, of which cyclophosphamide has been most extensively used. Other regimens add or substitute agents such as cytosine arabinoside, busulfan, and etoposide in an effort to reduce the relapse rate after transplant. Although TBI regimes vary in total dose, dose rate, schedule, and sequence, fractionated irradiation generally is preferred to reduce the incidence of possible interstitial pneumonitis and cataracts. Regardless of the schedule, however, TBI increases the risk of growth failure, sterility, pulmonary fibrosis, and second malignancy. Patients who are not irradiated usually receive a combination of busulfan and cyclophosphamide. T cell-depleting antibodies, such as antithymocyte globulin or alemtuzumab, often are added to prevent graft rejection for patients receiving transplants from HLA-disparate donors. The patient or recipient is rescued from the results of these myelotoxic therapies by the infusion of healthy donor hematopoietic stem cells. The best results are seen in younger patients who are transplanted early in the course of their disease.

The recognition that a graft versus leukemia effect plays a major part in the eradication of certain hematopoietic malignancies after allogeneic transplant recently has led to the concept of using less intensive, so-called non- or submyeloablative conditioning therapies. By reducing the intensity of the conditioning regimen, regimen-related side effects are fewer, and the treatment may be offered to patients who previously were not candidates for stem cell transplant.

COMPLICATIONS

Obstacles to the ultimate success of stem cell transplantation include acute and chronic GVHD, recurrent disease, fatal infection (particularly in patients with GVHD), lethal toxicity from the conditioning regimen, and failure to engraft.

Alloreactivity between donor and recipient may lead to graft rejection (host versus graft disease) or GVHD. These responses are mediated primarily by alloreactive T lymphocytes. In engraftment failure, the recipient's immune system dominates, whereas in GVHD, donor T lymphocytes prevail. In GVHD, donor-derived T cells produce injury in host tissue, particularly the skin, liver, and gastrointestinal tract. The severity of GVHD correlates to some extent with laboratory measures of histocompatibility, but GVHD occurs even in HLA-matched donor–recipient pairs, reflecting the limitations of current histocompatibility assessment. Acute GVHD usually occurs within 3 months of grafting. It develops in approximately 25% of patients younger than 18 years receiving matched sibling allografts. In contrast, the incidence of acute GVHD is approximately 50% to 70% in patients receiving unrelated donor grafts that have not been T cell–depleted. All patients undergoing allogeneic stem cell transplant require GVDH prophylaxis. The GVHD prophylactic regimens are designed to deplete T cells or inhibit their expansion, consequently maintaining their numbers below the threshold sufficient to incite clinical GVHD. Methotrexate, usually administered with prednisone, was the predominant GVHD-preventive therapy prior to the availability of cyclosporine. More recently, tacrolimus in combination with methotrexate has been shown to further decrease the risk of severe GVDH in patients receiving unrelated donor transplant.

As an alternative or adjunct to the pharmacologic approach to GVHD prevention, donor T cells may be removed from the donor stem cell product through a variety of methods. Although T-cell depletion reduces the incidence and severity of GVHD, it may not be accompanied by improved disease-free survival. Recipients of T cell–depleted stem cell products appear to have a higher risk of nonengraftment, and relapse rates are higher in some hematologic malignancies, for example chronic myelogenous leukemia (CML). Once acute GVHD occurs, high-dose prednisone becomes the treatment of choice.

The incidence of chronic GVHD is 20% to 40% in patients after HLA-identical sibling donors transplants, and it is much higher in recipients of alternative donor stem cell grafts. It often occurs in patients who have experienced acute GVHD, but it may develop independently, usually more than 3 months after the graft. The onset may be earlier after alternative donor stem cell grafts. Chronic GVHD has many features similar to autoimmune diseases, targeting the skin, eyes, intestinal tract, liver, lungs, and, by definition, the immune system. Extensive chronic GVHD affecting most or all of these sites often is fatal. Prolonged corticosteroids, cyclosporine, tacrolimus, or azathioprine administration is the primary treatment. Thalidomide has reduced the severity of chronic GVHD in some patients, and skin involvement may respond to extracorporeal photopheresis. Many novel therapies, such as antibodies directed against inflammatory cytokines or newer immunosuppressant agents (i.e., rapamycin or mycophenolate mofetil), are being explored as alternative therapies for chronic GVHD.

Many transplant investigators recognize a beneficial antileukemic effect from the reaction of the recipient's tissue to the donor T cells, known as the *graft-versus-leukemia (GVL) effect*. They cite the improved disease-free survival of allogeneic grafts over that of autologous, syngeneic, or T cell–depleted grafts as verification. Data show that patients experiencing some degree of GVHD have a lower relapse rate than those who experience none.

In addition to extensive transfusion requirements and the need for parenteral nutrition support, the prevention and treatment of infection is a universal component of the transplant process, because the conditioning regimens destroy the recipient's own immune and hematopoietic systems. Recovery depends on engraftment and the development of donor-derived immune and hematopoietic systems. Until recovery occurs, various strategies to prevent infectious complications, such as prophylactic antibacterial, antiviral, and antifungal regimens and isolation procedures, commonly are used. The degree and nature of the risk depends on the type of transplant and the development of GVHD. The risk also changes with time after transplant.

Hematopoietic growth factors (e.g., granulocyte colony-stimulating factor or granulocytes macrophage colony-stimulating factor) can be given to hasten marrow recovery and shorten the period of risk for infection.

PROGNOSIS

Despite these complicating factors and unsettled issues, the successes of stem cell transplant are substantial. For children with acute myeloid leukemia (AML) in first remission, the disease-free survival rate is approximately 65% to 80% after allogeneic transplants. These figures are reduced if the grafting takes place in second or subsequent remission or at the time of overt relapse. In patients transplanted for AML, most failures are caused by transplant-related causes, and the relapse rate appears to be less than 15%. However, advances in the characterization of prognostic factors for the drug treatment for childhood AML may require a reevaluation of the timing of stem cell transplantation for some patients.

The responses of children with acute lymphoid leukemia (ALL) to transplant have been somewhat less gratifying. Because approximately 70% to 75% of the newly diagnosed patients with ALL respond to chemotherapy regimens, stem cell transplantation usually is reserved for patients who fail initial therapy and are in second or subsequent remission. Under such circumstances, long-term, disease-free survivals have been of the magnitude of 55% to 70%, with relapse accounting for the largest number of failures. Selected patients with ALL in first remission whose curability with intensive front-line chemotherapy is considered less than 50% may benefit from early allogeneic hematopoietic stem cell transplant. A widely accepted high-risk feature is the presence of t(9;22), or the Philadelphia chromosome; for those patients, in first remission, the use of alternative donors is an appropriate treatment option. Stem cell transplants are not recommended for patients with ALL in frank relapse or with primary refractory disease, because previous attempts have not been successful. After a relapsed patient is in second remission, however, every consideration should be given to the possibility of expeditious stem cell transplant.

It generally is accepted that allogeneic stem cell transplant can cure selected patients with CML in the chronic phase, and it remains the preferred treatment for younger patients (less than 21 years of age) who have an HLA-matched sibling. Since the introduction of imatinib, considerable controversy has arisen regarding the optimal timing of stem transplant for patients who lack a sibling donor. Frequently, patients are treated initially with imatinib and are offered transplant when this therapy fails. Although most data reported give the results of treating adult patients, sufficient pediatric information exists to suggest that most affected children can be cured by transplant if a suitable donor is available. The information is sparser for children with juvenile chronic myelogenous leukemia (JCML), but case reports and small series demonstrate that stem cell transplantation is the only curative therapy for the vast majority of children with this disorder. Long-term follow-up information for patients transplanted for chronic leukemia is forthcoming.

The use of autologous stem cell transplants for leukemia patients in remission who do not have matched donors provides another approach to leukemia therapy. Autografting allows for higher-dose chemoradiotherapy without the limitations imposed by marrow-suppressive toxicity, and it enables hematopoietic recovery without the risk of GVHD that is seen in allografts. Autografting has disadvantages. If the marrow obtained during remission is contaminated with undetected leukemic cells, the patient may have disease recurrence as a result of the reinfusion of malignant cells. The cytoreductive preparative regimens used to treat autograft patients are similar to those used in allogeneic transplants, but autografts do not have the added benefit of the GVL effect. No accurate method exists to definitively determine if relapse under these circumstances reflects reinfusion of disease, inadequate systemic conditioning therapy, or lack of the GVL effect, although gene marking experiments have shown that reinfused leukemic cells participate in disease recurrence.

Suggested Readings

Guinan EC. Stem cell transplantation in pediatric oncology. In: Pizzo PA, Poplack DG, eds. *Principles and practices in pediatric oncology*, 4th ed. Philadelphia: Lippincott Williams & Wilkins, 2002.

The National Marrow Donor Program: http://www.marrow.org/index.html.

CHAPTER 304 ■ HODGKIN DISEASE

KENNETH L. McCLAIN

EPIDEMIOLOGY

Lymphomas (Hodgkin disease [HD] and non-Hodgkin lymphomas) together make up the third largest group of malignant diseases in children 0 to 19 years of age. The annual incidence of HD per million children is 5.7 for those less than 15 years of age and 34.7 for 15 to 19 year olds. Lymphomas occur more often in white than in black children (1.5:1).

PATHOGENESIS

The pathologic Reed-Sternberg cell (Fig. 304.1) in HD is a B lymphocyte as defined by the immunophenotype and molecular studies of Carbone and associates. In HD lesions, the Reed-Sternberg cell is accompanied by varying amounts of fibrosis and lymphocytic infiltration described in the systems of typing for HD. Because more patients are from better socioeconomic conditions, delayed exposure to a common infectious agent, such as Epstein-Barr virus (EBV), may be relevant, as reported by Razzouk and colleagues. Patients with HD have a higher titer against the EBV viral capsid antigen than most children do years after infectious mononucleosis. However, this finding may be secondary to abnormalities of the immune system in HD. Data supporting the contagion theory of HD are controversial. Reported clusters of HD have been discounted on the basis of flawed statistical analysis. Molecular studies have identified EBV RNA and viral proteins in Reed-Sternberg cells. Molecular evidence of EBV DNA in 58% of all HD cases was reported from one institution. Of the nodular sclerosis cases studied, 42% tested positive for EBV, and in the mixed cellularity cases, 65% were positive. Seventy-six percent of cases from children younger than 10 years had positive test results, but only 22% of those from children older than 10 years had EBV in the tumor cells.

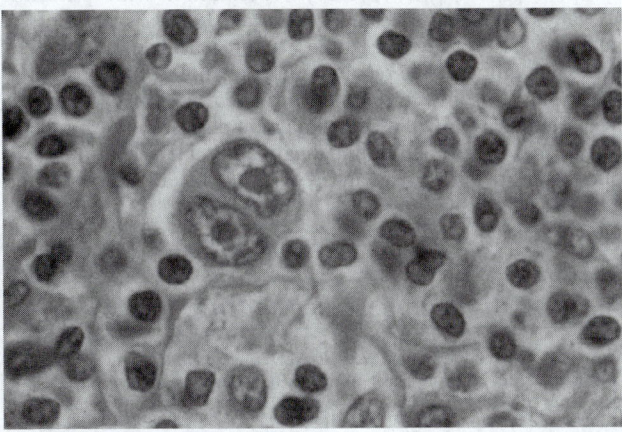

FIGURE 304.1. Reed-Sternberg cell.

CLINICAL MANIFESTATIONS AND DIAGNOSIS

Presenting Signs and Symptoms

Most children present with painless lymphadenopathy in the cervical, supraclavicular, axillary, or inguinal nodes. Splenic or hepatic enlargement is infrequently found in early stages of HD. Fewer than 20% of patients have the systemic (B-symptoms) of fever, night sweats, or weight loss of more than 10%.

A mediastinal mass is seen on chest radiographic films in 17% to 40% of patients and is found more often in children older than 12 years with enlargement of low cervical or supraclavicular nodes. Nearly 30% have mediastinal masses greater than one-third of the chest diameter that may cause dysphagia, dyspnea, cough, or the superior vena cava syndrome.

Differences exist in the histologic type and the stage of disease in children younger than and older than 7 years. Almost 75% of the older group has the nodular sclerosing type of HD, compared with 50% of the younger group. The younger group has more cases of lymphocyte predominance and mixed-cellularity histology. Almost 60% of the younger and 33% of older children have limited-stage disease (i.e., stage I or IIA). Conversely, 38% of the older group and 12% of the younger group have stage IIIB or IV disease.

Staging

A complete evaluation (staging) of patients with suspected HD is mandatory before beginning chemotherapy treatment so radiotherapy (RT) can be appropriately directed to sites of disease. Evaluation and treatment of these diseases should be undertaken at a center that has a team of pediatric oncologists, pathologists, surgeons, radiotherapists, nurses, and social workers experienced in the diagnosis and care of children with cancer. Prompt and efficient care of the child in this setting is the only way to guarantee optimal treatment and the best outcome. This is especially true for the 15- to 19-year-old group of patients. Studies have shown that they are the least likely to be enrolled on clinical trials in which the most up to date therapy is available. Consequently, their overall survival is much lower than that of patients placed in the appropriate Children's Oncology Group trials.

Routine evaluation of a patient with suspected HD should include a complete history, with emphasis on constitutional symptoms such as fever and weight loss, previous infections, family exposures to toxins, parental occupational hazards, and evidence for underlying immune deficiencies and familial cancer. A complete physical examination means assessment of general health, height and weight, size and location of lymphadenopathy, liver and spleen size, skin infiltrations, pulmonary findings, and neurologic signs. Laboratory evaluation should include a complete blood count, erythrocyte sedimentation rate, renal and liver function tests (including lactate

TABLE 304.1

ANN ARBOR SYSTEM FOR STAGING OF HODGKIN DISEASE*

Stage	Features
Stage I	Involvement of a single lymph node region (I) or a single extralymphatic organ or site (I_E)
Stage II	Involvement of two or more lymph node regions on the same side of the diaphragm (II) or extension to an extralymphatic site and one or more lymph node regions on the same side of the diaphragm (II_E)
Stage III	Involvement of lymph node regions on both sides of the diaphragm (III), localized involvement by extension to an extralymphatic organ or site (III_E), or involvement of the spleen
Stage IV	Diffuse or disseminated involvement of one or more extralymphatic organs or tissues with or without associated lymph node enlargement

*All stages are further classified as A or B to indicate the absence or presence, respectively, of systemic symptoms: unexplained fever, night sweats, or weight loss greater than 10% of normal body weight. If laparotomy and histologic review show that disease is limited to spleen, splenic, celiac, or portal nodes, the classification is substage IIIA1. Involvement of the lower abdominal nodes, such as paraaortic, iliac, and inguinal nodes, designates substage IIIA2.
Reprinted from Carbone PP, Kaplan HS. Report of the committee on Hodgkin's disease staging classification. *Cancer Res* 1971;31:1860.

dehydrogenase levels), urinalysis, anteroposterior and lateral chest radiographic films, and computed tomographic scans of the abdomen and chest with oral and intravenous contrast. Positron emission tomography scans may provide additional sensitivity to identifying pathologic lymph nodes or infiltration of other organs. Because of increased resolution of computed tomographic scans and new treatment regimens, bipedal lymphangiography has largely been abandoned. Gallium-67 (^{67}Ga) scans also can be helpful in defining the disease activity of mediastinal HD. Eighty percent of patients have uptake of ^{67}Ga in their mediastinal masses at the time of diagnosis. After therapy, a patient with a residual mediastinal mass that continues to absorb ^{67}Ga is likely to have active HD. Bone marrow biopsies have long been recommended as part of the routine evaluation of all patients with HD. However, data from our institution suggest that patients with clinical evidence of low-stage (I to IIIA) disease do not need these tests routinely. Of 110 patients, only two had bone marrow trephine biopsies with evidence of HD in them. Both these patients had clinical stage IIIB disease.

Historically, staging had two aspects: clinical and pathologic (surgical). However, combined-modality (chemotherapy and RT) treatments can now "sterilize" areas of hidden disease. Table 304.1 outlines the Ann Arbor staging system for HD in children or adults.

THERAPY AND PROGNOSIS

Current treatment protocols based on the careful analysis of previous studies have allowed oncologists to optimize results (cure rates of more than 90% for most patients) and to minimize the secondary complications of chemotherapy and RT (see later). As of 2003, chemotherapy protocols for all children with HD were based on four basic chemotherapy agents: doxorubicin hydrochloride (Adriamycin), bleomycin (Blenoxane), vincristine (Oncovin), and etoposide (VePesid), a regimen abbreviated ABVE, with two additional drugs (prednisone and cyclophosphamide [Cytoxan]), a regimen abbreviated PC, given

for higher-risk patients and another set of four agents applied for patients with a slow response. The number of chemotherapy cycles is tailored to response such that patients with a rapid early response receive a lower total dose of chemotherapy. Patients receive RT only to enlarged lymph nodes, lung, or splenic nodules.

The patients with the best prognosis (stages IA and IIA) are given two courses of ABVE and are reevaluated by physical examination and diagnostic imaging. If the HD is no longer visible (complete response), they have involved-field RT and are evaluated at regular intervals for disease recurrence and side effects of the therapies. These patients have essentially a 100% chance of cure, according to Donaldson and associates. Patients in the intermediate-risk group (stage IB, IIB, IA or IIA with lymph node masses greater than 6 cm in diameter and stage IIAE, IIIA, or IVA) receive three courses of ABVE-PC and are evaluated. Those with a rapid response receive one more course of chemotherapy and are randomized to receive or not receive involved-field RT. Those with a slow response are randomized to receive another course of ABVE-PC and RT or two augmented chemotherapy treatments with dexamethasone, etoposide, cisplatin (Platinol), and cytosine arabinoside (Cytosar) and ABVE-PC with RT. Previous combined-therapy regimens for this group of patients resulted in cure rates of 85% to 95%. Therapy for patients with stage IIIB and IVB disease is currently three to five courses (based on response) of ABVE-PC followed by RT. These patients have cure rates of about the same as those of the intermediate-risk group.

LATE EFFECTS

All patients have alopecia, weight loss, transient pancytopenia, and extreme susceptibility to infections while receiving therapy. RT may stunt bone growth and cause thyroid dysfunction. This event is dose dependent and usually causes compensated hypothyroidism, with as many as one-third of patients needing thyroid replacement therapy.

Patients may suffer pulmonary or mucous membrane damage from RT, and some male patients have decreased fertility from the chemotherapy. For female patients, delay and alteration of menstrual cycles was reported, especially after pelvic irradiation. Cardiotoxicity from doxorubicin may cause defective cardiac wall motion in children many years after having received chemotherapy, as reported by Krischer and colleagues. This and other long-term effects of treatments and the disease make it essential that such patients be followed in "late effects" clinics to monitor their outcomes.

Patients with HD are at increased risk of infections because of their underlying immune deficiency and from the cytopenias caused by therapy. Vaccination with pneumococcal, *Haemophilus influenzae*, and *Neisseria meningitidis* antigens should be done routinely before splenectomy. Prophylactic penicillin also is recommended for life in these patients. Varicella-zoster infections have occurred in as many as 75% of patients with HD. Second malignant diseases occur in 7.6% of patients by 20 years after diagnosis of HD. The most frequent tumors are breast cancer, thyroid cancer, and soft tissue sarcomas.

Suggested Readings

Carbone A, Gloghini A, Gattei V, et al. Reed-Sternberg cells of classical Hodgkin's disease react with the plasma cell-specific monoclonal antibody B-B4 and express human syndecan-1. *Blood* 1997;89:3787.

Donaldson SS, Whitaker SJ, Plowman PN, et al. Stage I–II pediatric Hodgkin's disease: long-term follow-up demonstrates equivalent survival rates following different management schemes. *J Clin Oncol* 1990;8:1128.

Hudson MM, Donaldson SS. Hodgkin's disease. In: Pizzo PA, Poplack DG, eds. *Principles and practice of pediatric oncology,* 4th ed. Philadelphia: Lippincott Williams & Wilkins, 2002:637.

Krischer JP, Epstein S, Cutherbertson DD, et al. Clinical cardiotoxicity following anthracycline treatment for childhood cancer: the Pediatric Oncology Group experience. *J Clin Oncol* 1997;15:1544.

Mahoney DH, Schreuders LC, Gresik MV, McClain KL. Role of staging bone marrow examination in children with Hodgkin disease. *Med Pediatr Oncol* 1998;30:175.

Razzouk BI, Gan YJ, Mendonca C, et al. Epstein-Barr virus in pediatric Hodgkin's disease: age and histiotype are more predictive than geographic region. *Med Pediatr Oncol* 1997;28:248.

CHAPTER 305 ■ NON-HODGKIN LYMPHOMA

KENNETH L. McCLAIN

EPIDEMIOLOGY

Non-Hodgkin lymphomas (NHLs) represent 6% of all tumors in the pediatric age group and are the fifth most frequent. The incidence per million children is 8.5 for those less than 15 years and 17.1 for children 15 to 19 years of age, with a slight male predominance and 1.5 times as many white patients as black. Three major histologic varieties exist—lymphoblastic lymphoma (LL), Burkitt lymphoma (BL), and large cell lymphomas—most of which are considered high grade. Patients with congenital or acquired immunodeficiency (including those with human immunodeficiency virus infection and transplant recipients) are at higher risk for developing lymphomas than the physiologically normal population. There is a statistically significant association for all subtypes of NHL with maternal pesticide exposure when the patient with lymphoma was *in utero*.

CLINICAL MANIFESTATIONS

Lymphoblastic Lymphoma

LLs make up 30% to 35% of childhood NHLs. For a child with lymphomatous features of massive lymphadenopathy and hepatosplenomegaly, an arbitrary distinction between leukemia and lymphoma is made by evaluating the bone marrow aspirate. If fewer than 25% lymphoblasts exist in the marrow, the diagnosis is lymphoma; if more than 25%, the diagnosis is acute lymphoblastic leukemia. The cell of origin usually is a T lymphoblast, especially in patients with stage III or IV disease (Table 305.1). Frequent cytogenetic abnormalities are found in the T-cell receptor gene on the long arm (q11.2) of chromosome 14. The B-precursor immunophenotype is found in one-third of patients with stage I and II disease, but in fewer than 5% of patients with a higher stage.

Most children present with painless cervical lymphadenopathy, a mediastinal mass, and moderate hepatosplenomegaly. Fevers and weight loss are less common than in Hodgkin disease, but they are an unfavorable prognostic sign if present. An anterior mediastinal mass with or without a pleural effusion may cause respiratory compromise or the superior vena cava syndrome, and either can be a true medical emergency. These patients should not be forced to lie flat because their airway may obstruct. A high incidence of central nervous system involvement and leukemic transformation exists in patients with LL.

Burkitt Lymphoma

BL is the most common of NHL in childhood (40% to 50%). Patients usually present with an abdominal mass that may originate in the bowel, kidneys, or gonads and may be accompanied by massive ascites. BL is a particularly dangerous form of childhood cancer because it is a rapidly growing tumor that masquerades as an apparently benign case of tonsillitis or as an intussusception from a leading enlargement of cecal, ileal, or mesenteric nodes (Fig. 305.1). Bone marrow involvement may show the L3 variety of lymphoblast, containing many vacuoles.

Immunophenotyping studies reveal tumor cells of a mature B-cell phenotype with surface immunoglobulin. The classic translocation of chromosomes 8 and 14 juxtaposing the

TABLE 305.1

STAGING OF CHILDHOOD NON-HODGKIN LYMPHOMA

Stage	Features
Stage I	Single tumor in a node or extralymphatic site, excluding the mediastinum or abdomen
Stage II	Single extranodal tumor with regional node positive
	Two or more nodal areas on the same side of the diaphragm
	Two extranodal tumors on the same side of the diaphragm regardless of nodal involvement
	Primary gastrointestinal tract tumor with or without associated mesenteric nodes, grossly completely excised
Stage III	Two single extranodal tumors on opposite sides of the diaphragm
	Two or more nodal areas above and below the diaphragm
	All tumors originating in mediastinum, pleura, or thymus
	All extensive primary intraabdominal disease (usually many implants, not totally resectable); often ascites
Stage IV	Any of previously mentioned stages with initial central nervous system, bone marrow, or both central nervous system and bone marrow involvement

Adapted from Murphy SB. Childhood non-Hodgkin's lymphoma. *N Engl J Med* 1978;299:1446.

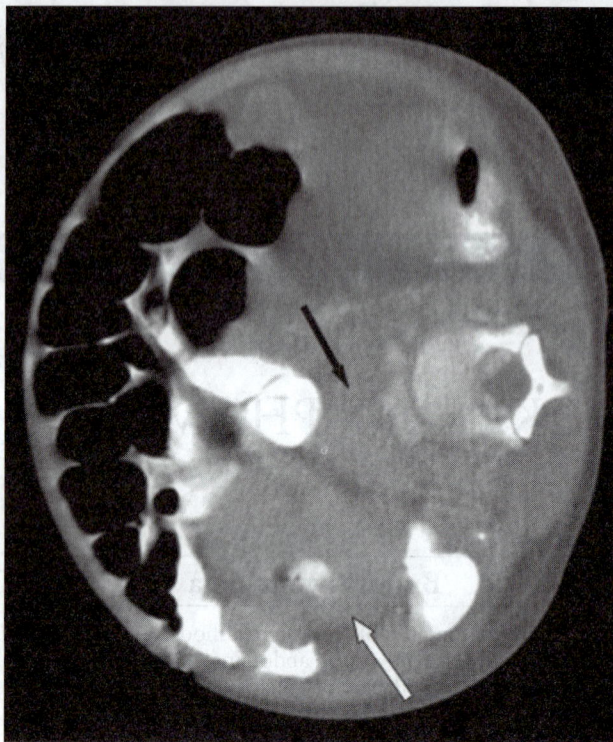

FIGURE 305.1. Abdominal computed tomographic scan of a patient with Burkitt lymphoma showing a mass surrounding the cecum (*white arrow*) and massive periaortic lymphadenopathy (*black arrow*). (Courtesy of Robert P. Guillerman M.D., Singleton Department of Radiology, Texas Children's Hospital, Houston, TX.)

c-myc oncogene (8q24.1) and an immunoglobulin heavy-chain promoter (14q32) are found in more than 80% of cases. Alternative immunglobulin light-chain-*myc* transolocations t2;8 or t8;22 account for nearly 20% of cases. Additional cytogenetic abnormalities including duplications of chromosome 1, especially bands q21-23, are found in 30% of cases.

Large Cell Lymphoma

The third type of childhood NHL is large cell lymphoma, previously called *histiocytic lymphoma*. This disease often presents in lymphoid tissue of the tonsils, adenoids, Peyer patches, or anterior mediastinum. Extranodal disease in the skin, bone, and soft tissue is more often found with this type of lymphoma than with the other two, but bone marrow and central nervous system involvement is less frequent. These patients frequently have fevers, night sweats, and weight loss. The cells of origin in these diffuse lymphomas are usually B lymphocytes associated with t8;14 or additional copies of chromosome 1q. A particularly interesting subtype, the CD30$^+$ anaplastic large cell lymphomas, comprises T-lineage cells with a t(2;5) chromosome translocation. The resulting fusion of a tyrosine kinase (ALK, chromosome 2) with a nucleophosphoprotein (NPM, chromosome 5) acitvates several cellular growth factors.

PATIENT EVALUATION AND DIAGNOSIS

Evaluation of patients with NHL begins with a thorough history and physical examination. Laboratory investigations should include a complete blood count, urinalysis, chest radiography, lumbar puncture, and bone marrow biopsy and aspirate, with samples sent for chromosome and cell marker analysis. Requisite blood chemistry evaluation includes serum electrolytes, including calcium and phosphate, liver function tests, blood urea nitrogen, creatinine, uric acid, and serum lactate dehydrogenase (LDH) levels. Because of the rapid turnover of these cells and tumor lysis from chemotherapy (or before), the physician must know whether cell breakdown has resulted in dangerously increased levels of uric acid, potassium, or phosphate as well as hypocalcemia. Hyperkalemia may cause cardiac dysrhythmias. Renal damage results from precipiatates of uric acid or calcium phosphate in the kidney. This complication usually is preventable by vigorous hydration, cautious alkalinization, and allopurinol or, more recently, use of urate oxidase (rasburicase) before treatment is begun.

If the serum LDH level is more than 1,000 units/L, the patient is considered to be in the highest risk category and requires the most vigorous treatment schedule for the B-cell lymphomas. Chest radiographic and abdominal computed tomographic examinations are necessary for determining the extent of intracavitary disease. Skeletal films and bone scans are indicated when symptoms in patients with LL or BL indicate the need. These studies should be routinely done in patients with anaplastic large cell lymphomas because bone involvement is quite frequent.

Biopsy of abdominal or tonsillar masses or biopsy of mediastinal nodes is required to make the diagnosis, but extensive surgery is not indicated. Tissue samples should be sent for cell surface marker studies, chromosome analysis, and special molecular studies to improve understanding of tumor biology. The clinical staging categories are listed in Table 305.1.

THERAPY AND PROGNOSIS

Lymphoblastic Lymphoma

Localized LL (i.e., stages I and II) historically responded well to short induction and consolidation with vincristine (Oncovin), doxorubicin hydrochloride (Adriamycin), prednisone, cyclophosphamide (Cytoxan), intrathecal medications, and a 33-week maintenance program, but many late relapses occurred. Now more intensive treatment lasting 2 years is used that includes L-asparaginase (Elspar), mercaptopurine (Purinethol), cytosine arabinoside (Cytosar), and methotrexate (Mexate).

Patients with stage III and IV LL present more challenging problems because the type of therapy depends on the immunologic identification of cell type. Current therapy with 13 drugs lasts approximately 2 years, with an expected survival rate of 90%. Granulocyte colony-stimulating factor is used to prevent extreme neutropenia and sepsis.

Burkitt Lymphoma

Patients with stage I and II BL have been treated with vincristine (Oncovin), doxorubicin hydrochloride (Adriamycin), cyclophosphamide (Cytoxan), prednisone, and intrathecal medications as induction and consolidation therapy lasting only 9 weeks. A 91% to 99% complete remission rate has been reported. Increased intensity of treatment is also curative in 91% of patients with stage III BL and in 87% of those with stage IV BL. These patients represent an especially challenging group, because the high metabolic turnover of their tumor puts them at risk for renal and electrolyte complications (i.e., tumor lysis syndrome) before and during induction therapy.

Generous prehydration, alkalinization, and allopurinol treatment are necessary. Many patients have life-threatening infections during the initial stages of treatment. Patients who present with a serum LDH less than twice the upper limit of normal have a 94% event-free survival (EFS) versus those with an LDH more than twice the upper limit of normal whose EFS is 89%. If a patient has a poor response to the initial week of treatment, the chance of EFS is 70%.

Large Cell Lymphoma

Most large cell lymphomas are of the B-cell phenotype and are currently treated with the same protocols as for limited (stages I and II) or extensive (stages III and IV) BL regimens. Patients with anaplastic large cell lymphomas have been treated with separate protocols because of the unique biology of this disease. The extent of treatment is based on stage and on whether the lymph nodes (or bone lesion) can be completely resected. Poor prognostic characterisitics are involvement of the spleen, liver, lung, and mediastinal nodes, multiple bones, or skin infiltration or sytemic symptoms. The overall survival ranges from 65% to 89%, with EFS 59% to 80%.

Suggested Reading

Magrath IT. Malignant non-Hodgkin's lymphoma in children. In: Pizzo PA, Poplack DG, eds. *Principles and practice of pediatric oncology*, 4th ed. Philadelphia: Lippincott Williams & Wilkins, 2002:661.

CHAPTER 306 ■ MALIGNANT BRAIN TUMORS

MURALI M. CHINTAGUMPALA

Primary brain tumors are the second most common type of cancer reported in children and adolescents. In the United States, the annual incidence of primary brain tumors in children younger than 15 years is approximately 1,200 new cases each year. Unfortunately, progress in the field of pediatric neuro-oncology has been slow compared with that in other childhood malignancies.

Surgery and radiation therapy traditionally constituted the standard therapeutic approach. The tendency has been to manage these children within the general medical community, contrary to the now common practice of referral to a pediatric cancer center for definitive diagnosis and treatment. Pessimism has followed failure to excise the tumor completely, and chemotherapy has been viewed as noxious, with little justification. However, progress in the comprehensive care of children with malignant brain tumors under the direction of experienced pediatric neuro-oncology teams has provided a rational basis for a departure from a previously gloomy scenario. Tumor heterogeneity, the relatively small numbers of patients with a specific tumor type available for investigation, the limitations of drug delivery across the blood–brain barrier, and the relative biologic resistance to therapy in certain tumors, such as gliomas, are unique technical and theoretical challenges that can be resolved only by continued collaborative clinical and laboratory research.

CLINICAL MANIFESTATIONS AND COMPLICATIONS

Early symptoms of central nervous system (CNS) tumors frequently are nonspecific. In infants with open sutures, these may consist of increased head circumference, irritability, head tilt, and loss of developmental milestones. Older children may present with headache. This symptom usually increases in frequency, becomes more severe in the morning, and is typically followed by vomiting. Approximately 85% of the children with malignant brain tumors have abnormal findings on neurologic or ocular examinations within 2 to 4 months of the onset of headaches.

Children who report an unchanging pattern of headaches without focal neurologic findings for more than 12 months have a low probability for CNS tumors. Specific neurologic symptoms such as ataxia, somnolence, hemiparesis, seizures, head tilt, cranial nerve palsies, diencephalic syndrome, and diabetes insipidus may occur later in the illness and may suggest localization of the CNS tumor.

The differential diagnosis for CNS tumors in children is extensive and includes brain abscesses, hemorrhage, nonneoplastic hydrocephalus of any cause, arteriovenous malformations or aneurysm, and indolent virus infections.

Classification

Traditionally, CNS tumors of childhood have been classified on the basis of location (e.g., infratentorial versus supratentorial) and histology. In children between the ages of 4 and 11 years, infratentorial (posterior fossa) tumors predominate. These include cerebellar tumors and brainstem tumors. Supratentorial tumors occur more frequently during the first years of life and during late adolescence and young adulthood. Approximately 45% of the childhood brain tumors arise in the cerebellum. Cerebellar astrocytomas and medulloblastomas are the tumors diagnosed most frequently in this region. Ependymomas that arise in and around the fourth ventricle represent between 3% and 14% of all childhood tumors and have been included as cerebellar tumors by some authorities.

The cerebrum is the next most common site of involvement in children, accounting for 20% to 27% of all brain tumors. The most frequent tumors include astrocytomas, glioblastomas, and ependymomas. Brainstem neoplasms account for 9% to 15% of all intracranial neoplasms. Approximately 75% of all brainstem tumors occur in children younger than 10 years. Midline tumors, which include a mix of germ-cell tumors, craniopharyngiomas, pinealomas, optic gliomas, and pituitary adenomas, account for another 10%.

The traditional practice of classifying CNS tumors on the basis of location is being reevaluated. An international panel of neuropathologists has proposed a revision of the World Health Organization (WHO) classification system to classify tumors on the basis of histopathologic features alone. For example, medulloblastoma, a highly malignant, poorly differentiated, "small, blue, round cell" tumor was said to arise only within the cerebellum. The revised classification system recognizes this tumor as a primitive neuroectodermal tumor (PNET), with or without elements of astrocytic, neuronal, or ependymal differentiation. Tumors of this identical histologic type arising anywhere within the brain are classified as PNETs. The pinealoblastoma arising in the pineal region, or the ependymoblastoma or classic PNET arising within the supratentorial regions, are identified by the new classification schema as PNETs. However "medulloblastoma" is still retained for PNET of the cerebellum. PNETs arising from different areas of the brain display similar histology but appear to be biologically different, with different cytogenetic abnormalities and different outcomes when treated in a similar manner. This classification system recognizes the heterogeneity of tumors arising within a single site, and it may be useful for future prognostic staging and for the design of new therapeutic strategies.

DIAGNOSIS

Computed tomographic (CT) scanning, with and without contrast enhancement, had been the standard noninvasive diagnostic tool. The unenhanced CT scan can suggest whether a lesion is cystic or solid and whether calcifications, hemorrhage, edema, and hydrocephalus exist. After intravenous contrast, enhancement of the tumor occurs because of a disruption of the blood–brain barrier. This improves detection of small tumors, definition of isodense or hypodense regions within the tumor, and differentiation of areas of edema surrounding the tumor mass. Subarachnoid and leptomeningeal seeding of tumor also may be detected with enhanced scans. Cranial CT scans have a sensitivity of greater than 94% for primary brain tumors, but certain limitations of resolution must be recognized. Small lesions within the posterior fossa, especially within the brainstem, and small midline cystic structures near the base of the skull occasionally escape detection.

Magnetic resonance imaging (MRI) with gadolinium enhancement is a sensitive neuroimaging technology for the diagnosis of CNS tumors and is now perceived as the standard diagnostic modality in the diagnosis and management of primary brain tumors. MRI scans are superior to CT scans in the detection and definition of low-grade glial tumors and of lesions at the vertex, within the posterior fossa (especially within the brainstem), near the wall of the middle fossa, and at the base of the skull (Fig. 306.1). MRI myelogram with gadolinium enhancement is the best method for detecting spinal cord tumors or delineating leptomeningeal tumor invasion. MRI scans use no ionizing radiation and have no calvarium artifact. Limitations include increased cost, longer scan times and duration of sedation in the young patient, an inability to detect calcifications, and limited access to the patient during the actual scan time.

The child with a positive scan result may benefit from additional diagnostic procedures. Angiography gives information about blood supply and may occasionally assist the neurosurgeon in planning the operative approach. Cerebrospinal fluid (CSF) examination is of great importance in patients presenting with PNETs, germinomas, ependymomas, and high-grade glial tumors, but it must be performed with great care in patients with increased intracranial pressure. Lumbar puncture for CSF may be safely performed 14 to 21 days after the initial operation and intracranial decompression. When CSF is obtained immediately after surgery for the primary tumor, it appears to be of limited value. Standard radionuclide scans no longer are used routinely. Spectroscopy, perfusion/diffusion studies, and positron emission tomography (PET) studies have the potential to provide additional information with respect to diagnosis and management of these children with brain tumors. These studies may help differentiate viable from necrotic tumor after therapy.

Electroencephalography, visual evoked potential, and brainstem auditory evoked potential may be useful at diagnosis and in the management of complications of the disease (e.g., seizures) or of certain therapeutic strategies (e.g., cisplatin-associated ototoxicity). Tumor markers are also important

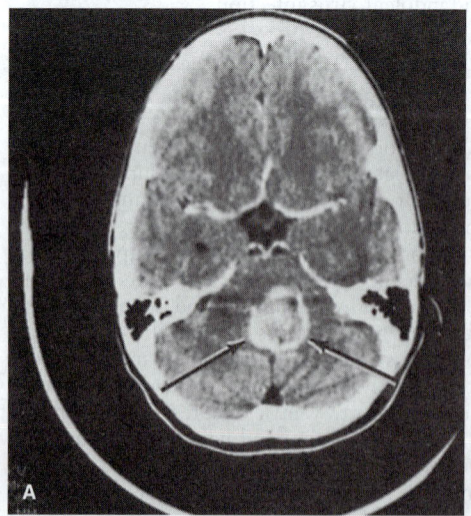
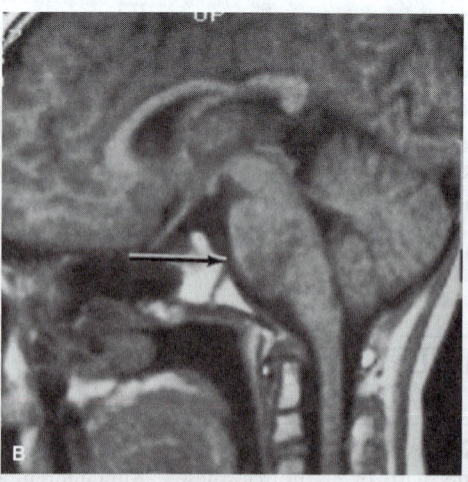
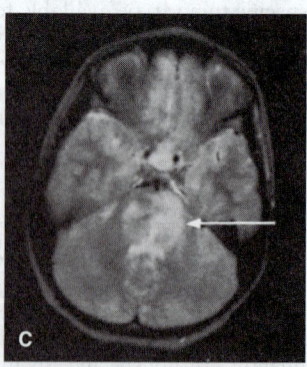

FIGURE 306.1. Computed tomographic (CT) scan and magnetic resonance imaging (MRI) study of a brainstem glioma. **A:** CT scan demonstrating a ringlike enhancing mass (*arrows*) involving the mid pons. **B:** Six months after the diagnosis and radiotherapy, the MRI sagittal view (T1 weighted) reveals an enlarging mass in the mid pons (*arrows*). **C:** The axial T2-weighted scan reveals abnormal signal intensity (*arrow*) extending into the left brachium pontis.

in selected malignant conditions. Alpha-fetoprotein and beta-chorionic gonadotropin are useful markers of malignant germ-cell tumors that may arise in the pineal or suprasellar regions. Investigations of tumor cytogenetics, monoclonal antibody characterization of specific tumor antigens, and oncogene expression are becoming important aspects of the ongoing studies of the biology of CNS tumors in children, and their use highlights the importance of neurosurgical care at established pediatric cancer centers. Fresh tumor tissue, obtained at the time of surgery, is essential for these biologic studies. Because neuropsychologic testing and endocrine surveillance make up a critical aspect of the management of long-term survivors, base-line examinations are important.

THERAPY

Published treatment results for various childhood malignant brain tumors vary widely and should be interpreted with caution. The number of patients with specific tumor histologies available for clinical investigations is small, and studies may report results from trials with limited patient entries. Despite this caveat, progress has been made in the treatment of several pediatric CNS tumors. Continued efforts must be made to enroll these patients in prospective, multimodal, cooperative treatment studies, and to accelerate the development of more effective therapeutic strategies.

Cerebellar Astrocytomas

Cerebellar astrocytomas account for approximately 20% of all brain tumors in children. Boys and girls are affected equally, and the mean age at diagnosis is 6 years. Two histologic variants occur. The juvenile pilocytic astrocytoma accounts for 80% to 85% of the cases. With complete surgical excision, which is usually possible in this location, 10-year survival rates of 80% to 95% have been reported. Recurrence may follow a partially excised tumor, but retreatment is usually possible. Diffuse astrocytomas make up approximately 15% of the cases. Radiation therapy may be considered in older patients with incomplete resections who show evidence of progression. In children younger than 5 years, with residual tumor after surgery, who have progression of the tumor or become symptomatic, chemotherapy has proven effective for some patients, thereby preventing the adverse effects of radiotherapy on the developing brain.

Medulloblastomas

Medulloblastomas are highly malignant primitive neuroectodermal tumors, usually arising in the roof of the fourth ventricle and cerebellar vermis. They occur more frequently in boys, primarily affect children between 4 and 8 years of age, and account for 20% of all brain tumors in children. Diagnostic studies of these patients should include cranial MRI scans with and without enhancement, cerebrospinal fluid cytology, MRI myelogram, and radionuclide bone scan. Metastatic disease or diffuse subarachnoid involvement may be apparent at diagnosis. Bone marrow examinations are not performed unless clinical or laboratory evidence suggests bone marrow involvement.

It is highly recommended that a patient with the diagnosis of medulloblastoma be referred to a pediatric facility where the multidisciplinary approach to a child with a brain tumor is well established. The standard of care for children with medulloblastomas is postoperative craniospinal radiotherapy followed by chemotherapy. The goals of neurosurgery are to establish a tissue diagnosis, relieve intracranial pressure, and debulk or totally excise gross tumor, as clinical conditions per-

mit. Complete tumor excision is achievable in more than 50% of the patients and may offer a survival advantage.

A preoperative staging system developed by Chang et al., based on a grading scale of T0 to T4 for extent of local tumor and M0 to M4 for metastatic disease, has had prognostic value in several studies. Medulloblastoma is a radiosensitive and chemosensitive tumor. The conventional radiation therapy schedule depends on the initial stage of the disease. Patients who had complete resection of the tumor, with no evidence of tumor in the CSF obtained by lumbar puncture 14 to 21 days after surgery, and with no evidence of leptomeningeal spread (standard-risk), receive approximately 2,400 cGy to the craniospinal axis and a total of more than 5,000 cGy to the posterior fossa. Patients who have local residual tumor greater than 1.5 cm^2, or those with evidence of tumor spread (high-risk) receive 3,600 cGy to the craniospinal axis, with a dose to the posterior fossa of over 5,000 cGy. All patients receive chemotherapy, which usually consists of cisplatin, vincristine, cyclophosphamide, or lomustine (CCNU). The reduction in the dose of radiation to the craniospinal axis, along with the use of effective chemotherapy in patients who are at standard-risk, has not compromised the disease-free survival rates seen with higher doses of radiation to the craniospinal axis with no chemotherapy. More important, preliminary evidence suggests that patients who receive a lower radiation dose to the craniospinal axis have fewer detrimental neuropsychologic sequelae. Using current therapies, the 5-year disease-free survival rates are between 70% and 80% for patients at standard-risk and 60% to 70% for those at high-risk for recurrences.

Current efforts are directed towards identifying groups of patients with medulloblastoma who have a better prognosis and for whom the dose of radiation to the craniospinal axis can be further reduced, thereby further reducing the neuropsychologic sequelae, especially in children less than 8 years of age.

Brainstem Tumors

Brainstem gliomas have the worst prognosis of all pediatric CNS tumors, with an estimated median survival rate after local irradiation of less than 12 months and a 5-year disease-free survival rate of 15% to 18%.

Progressive cranial nerve dysfunctions and gait disturbances, coupled with an intrinsic mass in the brainstem, as demonstrated by CT or MRI scan, are the hallmarks of this disease (Fig. 306.2). The staging and surgical management of this disease are controversial. The surgical approach to brainstem lesions is hazardous. Patients with inoperable lesions involving the pons or medulla have a poor prognosis. Patients with operable exophytic components, lower-grade histology, or lesions arising in higher brainstem regions may experience longer survival.

Conventional therapy has included high-dose corticosteroids and local posterior fossa irradiation to 5,500 cGy over 6 weeks. More than 50% of the patients respond, but the tumor invariably recurs. Adjuvant chemotherapy trials have failed to demonstrate any survival advantage for patients. Hyperfractionation radiation techniques with and without concomitant chemotherapy as radiosensitive agents did not improve survival. Current efforts are directed towards identifying those biologic agents that target specific molecules within the tumor that contribute to the malignant potential of the tumor.

High-Grade Astrocytomas

High-grade astrocytomas (i.e., anaplastic astrocytoma or glioblastoma) represent approximately 25% of childhood tumors.

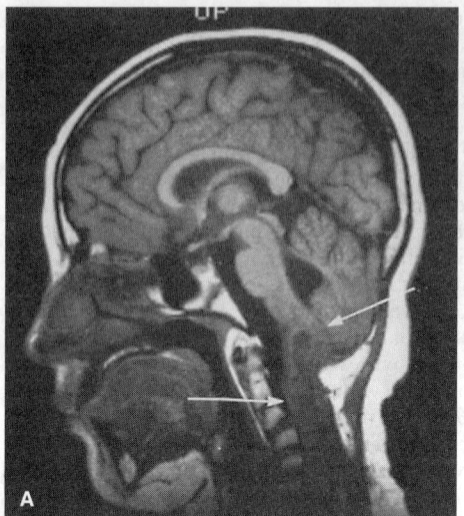
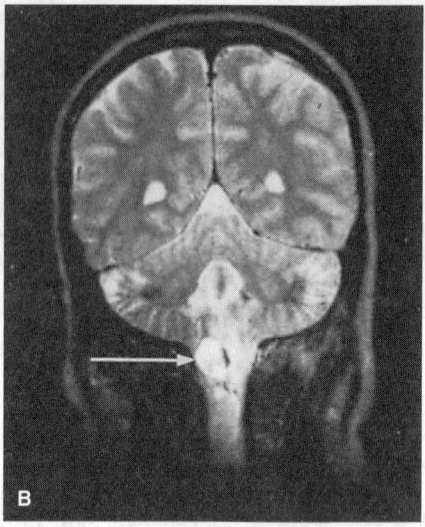

FIGURE 306.2. Magnetic resonance imaging study of a brainstem and cervical tumor. **A:** Sagittal view (T1-weighted) reveals enlargement of the caudal brainstem, extending below the foramen magnum to the level of C5 to C6 (*arrows*). **B:** Coronal view (T2-weighted) reveals an increased signal intensity highlighting the cystic component of this lesion as it extends into the cervical cord (*arrow*).

These tumors develop in the cerebral hemisphere (51%), brainstem (37%), and cerebellum (Fig. 306.3).

The conventional management of high-grade astrocytomas includes aggressive surgical excision, whenever possible, and radiation therapy to 5,500 cGy or greater. The 5-year disease-free survival rate is less than 25%. Adjuvant chemotherapy has been of marginal benefit. In a randomized trial, the Children's Cancer Study Group (CCSG) reported a survival advantage for patients treated with CCNU, vincristine, and prednisone after surgery and radiation therapy, compared with patients treated without chemotherapy (45% versus 13% 5-year disease-free survival rates). Subsequent trials to establish the benefit of chemotherapy have not been successful. Current chemotherapy regimens appear to be of marginal benefit and do not significantly improve upon the results obtained with surgical resection and involved-field radiotherapy. Current trials are aimed at identifying effective chemotherapy agents and biologic agents that can target specific molecules in the tumor cells.

Ependymomas

Ependymomas represent only 9% of all brain tumors in children. These tumors are locally invasive, may be cystic, and demonstrate a spectrum of histologic appearances. Ependymomas occur equally among boys and girls. Intracranial lesions typically occur in children between the ages of 2 and 6 years, but spinal tumors occur more often during the teenage years. In children, most ependymomas arise in the posterior fossa, near the fourth ventricle. Large supratentorial tumors in paraventricular regions also may occur (Fig. 306.4). The incidence of spinal cord seeding at diagnosis has been reported as 10% to 11%, although the actual incidence varies with the location and histology of the primary tumor. Conventional treatment includes aggressive surgery, with the goal of gross total excision, followed by radiation therapy. In children with localized disease, radiation therapy is limited to the tumor and a margin around it. When evidence of leptomeningeal spread is present, craniospinal radiation is recommended. Complete resection of the tumors followed by radiation therapy usually carries a good prognosis. Recent evidence suggests that, regardless of the

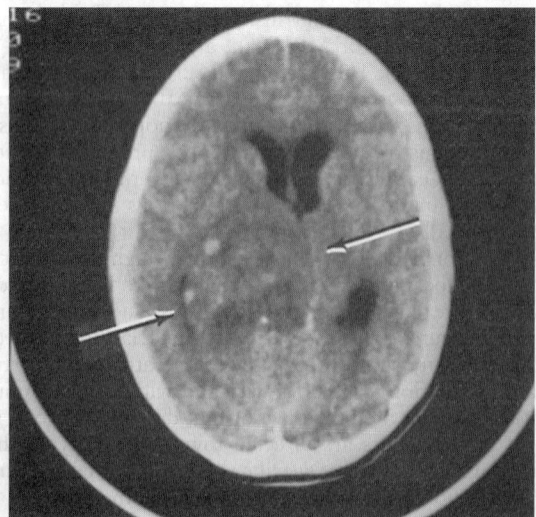

FIGURE 306.3. An unenhanced computed tomographic scan demonstrates a large, inhomogeneous mass (*arrows*) involving the right parietal lobe, with a midline shift. Partial excision revealed an anaplastic astrocytoma. Dye sensitivity prevented a contrast study, a problem not encountered with magnetic resonance imaging techniques.

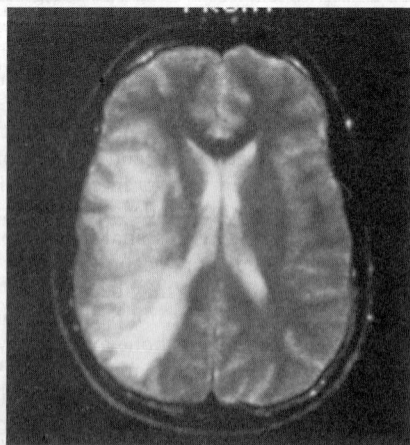

FIGURE 306.4. A T2-weighted magnetic resonance imaging scan in the axial projection reveals a large right frontal-parietal mass, with the central component representing neoplasm (ependymoma) and the peripheral component probably representing edema.

degree of resection, anaplastic histology carries a poor prognosis. The role of chemotherapy is unclear. Several chemotherapy agents elicit responses but do not appear to contribute to a better disease-free survival rates. Chemotherapy is likely to be used to reduce the size of the tumors and make them more amenable to complete surgical resection and thereby improve disease-free survival.

Preirradiation Chemotherapy in Young Children

Effective preirradiation chemotherapy combinations are being investigated for children younger than 3 years with malignant brain tumors. Thirteen percent of all brain tumors occur in children younger than 2 years, and the standard therapy of surgery and irradiation has produced a dismal 5-year disease-free survival rate of only 18%. Moreover, the quality of life in the few survivors has been poor. Neurotoxicity among survivors has been profound, leaving almost one-half of the patients retarded or handicapped.

Preliminary experience with postoperative chemotherapy and delayed irradiation for infants has been encouraging. The M. D. Anderson Cancer Center has reported successful management of children younger than 36 months with medulloblastoma, treating them with mechlorethamine (Mustargen), vincristine (Oncovin), procarbazine, and prednisone chemotherapy alone for 2 years. The projected 5-year survival rate was 77%. Neuropsychologic assessment of survivors not receiving radiation therapy indicated average or above-average performance scores. The Pediatric Oncology Group completed a multi-institutional study of infants younger than 3 years. After surgery, the children with malignant brain tumors were treated with high-dose cyclophosphamide, vincristine, cisplatin, and VP-16, and radiation therapy was deferred. Overall, the 2-year progression-free survival rate was 37%. Many patients received no radiation therapy. The long-term disease-free survival for these young children continues to be poor. The delayed use of radiation therapy, because of concerns about the deleterious effects of radiation on the developing brain, is one reason for the poor survival rates. However, current efforts to improve survival in these patients include the early use of focal radiation therapy (conformal radiation therapy) to treat the tumor bed in an effort to prevent local recurrence and the use of intrathecal chemotherapy to prevent leptomeningeal spread.

Suggested Readings

Gajjar A, Hernan R, Kocak M, et al. Clinical, histopathologic, and molecular markers of prognosis: toward a new disease risk stratification system for medulloblastoma. *J Clin Oncol* 2004;22:984.
Merchant TE. Current management of childhood ependymoma. *Oncology* 2002;16(5):629.
Packer RJ, Goldwein J, Nicholson HS, et al. Treatment of children with medulloblastomas with reduced-dose craniospinal radiation therapy and adjuvant chemotherapy: a Children's Cancer Group Study. *J Clin Oncol* 1999;17:2127.
Strother DR, Pollack IF, Fisher PG et al. Tumors of the central nervous system. In: Pizza PA, Poplack DG, eds. *Principles and practice of pediatric oncology.* Philadelphia: Lippincott Williams & Wilkins, 2002:751.
Thomas PRM, Deutsch M, Kepner JL, et al. Low-stage medulloblastoma: final analysis of trial comparing standard-dose with reduced-dose neuraxis irradiation. *J Clin Oncol* 2000;18:3004.

CHAPTER 307 ■ WILMS TUMOR

MURALI M. CHINTAGUMPALA

Wilms tumor is a malignant embryonal neoplasm of the kidney of mixed cellular histology. The incidence remains remarkably constant, with 8.1 cases per million white children younger than 15 years reported annually. Wilms tumor is diagnosed only slightly less often than neuroblastoma, and like neuroblastoma, it is a tumor of young children: Eighty percent of these tumors occur in children younger than 5 years, and more than 98% of cases present by 7 years. The incidence peaks in children between the ages 3 and 4 years, with a median of 42 months for girls and 35 months for boys with unilateral disease. The tumors associated with congenital anomalies and synchronous bilateral tumors occur at an earlier age. Worldwide, the gender ratio is close to 1:1, but in the United States, the rate of unilateral tumor in girls is 22% higher than in boys.

ETIOLOGY

Wilms tumor occurs in hereditary and nonhereditary forms. The hereditary form is autosomal dominant, may be multifocal in presentation, and may be associated with other congenital anomalies. Tumors in multiple family members have been reported but are extremely rare.

A variety of congenital abnormalities can occur in association with Wilms tumor. Children with Wilms tumor, aniridia, genitourinary abnormalities, and mental retardation (WAGR syndrome) have a constitutional deletion at chromosome 11p13, where the Wilms tumor gene *WT1* has been located. These patients have a 30% probability of developing Wilms tumor. A second Wilms tumor gene (*WT2*), located at 11p15.5, was strongly suggested by tumor-specific loss of heterozygosity and linkage studies in familial Beckwith-Wiedemann syndrome, which is characterized by gigantism and macroglossia. The risk of developing Wilms tumor in Beckwith-Wiedemann syndrome is in the range of 3% to 5%.

Most patients with sporadic isolated aniridia have some degree of 11p13 deletion with a significant risk of Wilms tumor. Isolated hemihypertrophy also is associated with an increased risk for the development of Wilms tumor. Other syndromes that have an increased risk for the development of Wilms tumor include Perlman syndrome, Sotos syndrome, and Denys-Drash syndrome. The most common genitourinary anomalies associated with Wilms tumor are hypoplasia, fusion and ectopia of the kidney, duplications in the collecting systems, hypospadias, and cryptorchidism.

PATHOLOGY

Wilms tumor is thought to arise from abnormalities in the development of metanephric blastema. Persistent metanephric blastemal cells in the postnatal period are termed *nephrogenic rests* and are regarded as precursor lesions for Wilms tumor.

Histologically, the tumor is composed of mixed mesenchymal elements in different stages of maturity. Renal blastema denotes epithelial elements that form abortive or embryonic glomerulotubular structures. These structures appear in an undifferentiated stroma, which also may contain differentiated mesenchymal structures such as striated muscles, cartilage, adipose tissue, and bone. The tumors have been referred to so as to denote the involvement of blastemal, epithelial, and stromal elements. Individual tumors may have a monomorphic pattern that can be mistaken for a hamartoma.

The use of the terms *favorable histology* and *unfavorable histology* was derived from the National Wilms' Tumor Study (NWTS). Initially, three types of unfavorable histology were identified, which accounted for 10% to 14% of all Wilms tumors and for more than 60% of mortality. These are as follows: focal or diffuse anaplastic tumors; clear cell sarcoma, often called the *bone-metastasizing tumor*; and rhabdoid tumor, which often metastasizes to the brain. The rhabdoid histologic type is a highly malignant tumor similar in structure to sarcomatous tumors that occur outside the kidney. This tumor and clear cell sarcoma are no longer considered Wilms tumor variants by the NWTS. They account for a small proportion of all tumors that have been registered as Wilms tumors but a disproportionately high percentage of the fatalities.

The classic, congenital mesoblastic nephroma is a benign tumor that sometimes resembles a clear cell sarcomatous form of Wilms tumor. Approximately 60% of these tumors are diagnosed in the first 3 months and 90% during the first year of life.

CLINICAL AND DIAGNOSTIC FEATURES

The classic Wilms tumor appears as a silent mass in the abdomen in almost two-thirds of patients. The tumor often is detected accidentally by the patient's parents or incidentally during the course of a physical examination performed for other medical reasons. Abdominal pain occurs in approximately one-third of the patients. The mass is usually hard, smooth, and confined to the flank or one side of the abdomen. Occasionally, a patient with Wilms tumor experiences a sudden hemorrhage into the tumor and presents with rapid abdominal enlargement and anemia. Hematuria has been observed in 12% to 25% of patients, and hypertension has been reported in 25% of cases. Nonspecific symptoms such as fever, malaise, constipation, and anorexia may be reported, but weight loss is an uncommon association.

The diagnosis of Wilms tumor must be suspected in any child who has an abdominal mass. The evaluation includes complete blood counts, liver and kidney function studies, a skeletal survey, chest radiography, ultrasonography, and a computed tomographic (CT) scan of the abdomen. Areas of hemorrhage and calcification are less common than in neuroblastoma, but intratumoral necrosis does occur and is probably responsible for many of the spills during surgery. A CT scan of the lungs may identify metastasis not seen on routine chest films and is recommended if the tumor appears to arise in the kid-

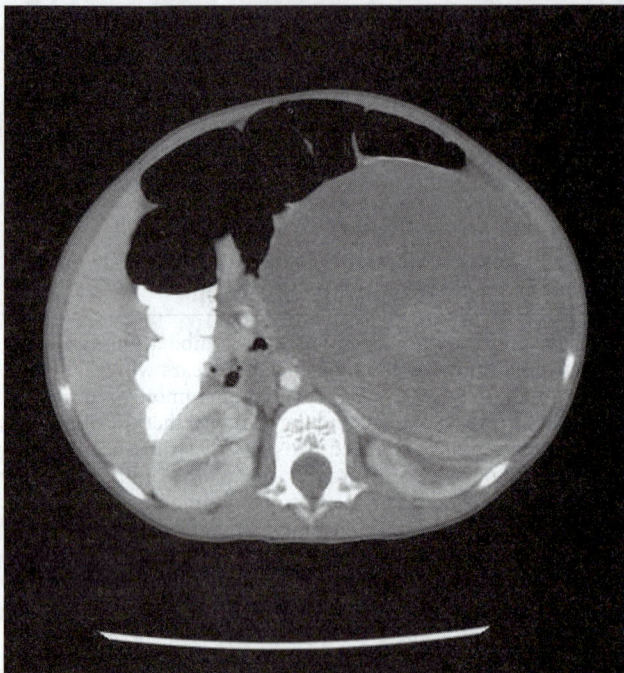

FIGURE 307.1. Wilms tumor arising from the left kidney. The right kidney is normal.

ney. A few patients have normal chest radiographic results but demonstrate pulmonary nodules by CT scan. The true nature of these nodules is uncertain, and biopsy is encouraged before considering them to be metastatic disease. Imaging studies (usually CT scans) obtained to evaluate the possibility of hepatic parenchymal involvement enable the surgeons to judge how aggressive their attempts should be to excise the disease completely in all locations.

The differential diagnosis includes neuroblastoma, rhabdomyosarcoma, leiomyosarcoma, renal cell sarcoma, fibrosarcoma, hypernephroma, polycystic kidneys, adrenal hemorrhage, renal vein thrombosis, dysplastic kidney, and renal carbuncle—almost anything that can cause a mass in the upper abdomen. The final diagnosis depends on a biopsy or a complete excision of the tumor and subsequent histologic examination.

Rarely, syndromes of polycythemia, acquired von Willebrand disease, and hypercalcemia have been associated with Wilms tumor. Wilms tumor occurs rarely in adults, who have a much poorer prognosis than pediatric patients.

Staging

Surgical exploration should be made through a transabdominal approach and should include samples of hilar, periaortic, and other lymph nodes, regardless of their gross appearance. Liver biopsies are performed if any unusual hepatic lesions exist. Exploration of the opposite kidney after opening Gerota fascia is essential to rule out synchronous bilateral disease.

The staging system developed by the NWTS has been adopted widely with minor variations (Table 307.1). The criteria are determined by the anatomic extent of the disease discovered at surgery and by the results of histopathologic examination. The system incorporates the key prognostic variables, which have changed from time to time according to the results of improved therapy. The major factors in staging are

TABLE 307.1

STAGING SYSTEM DEVELOPED BY THE THIRD NATIONAL WILMS' TUMOR STUDY

Stage	Features
Stage I	Tumor is limited to kidney and is completely excised. Capsular surface intact; no tumor rupture; no residual tumor apparent beyond margins of excision
Stage II	Tumor extends beyond the kidney but is completely excised. Regional extension of tumor; vessel infiltration; tumor biopsied or local spillage of tumor confined to the flank; no residual tumor apparent at or beyond the margins of excision
Stage III	Residual nonhematogenous tumor is confined to the abdomen. Lymph node involvement of hilus, periaortic chains, or beyond; diffuse peritoneal contamination by tumor spillage; peritoneal implants of tumor; tumor extending beyond surgical margins microscopically or macroscopically; tumor not completely removable because of local infiltration into vital structures
Stage IV	Deposits beyond stage III (e.g., lung, liver, bone, brain)
Stage V	Bilateral renal involvement at diagnosis

distant metastatic disease, involvement of the lymph nodes or other residual disease, and histologic type of tumor (i.e., favorable or unfavorable). Other less important factors involved in prognosis have changed somewhat since the initial NWTS. Favorable histology and early stage are the crucial factors for a good prognosis. Preliminary evidence suggests that patients who had tumor-specific loss of heterozygozity of 16q had worse relapse-free and overall survival rates. Because of a significant number of misdiagnoses after preoperative treatment with radiation therapy or chemotherapy in the European trials (Société Internationale d'Oncologie Pediatrique), clinical investigators in the United States have preferred to establish a tissue diagnosis first. However, for tumors considered to be inoperable based on size or invasion and in patients with bilateral tumors, pretreatment with chemotherapy after initial biopsies of the unilateral or bilateral tumors (to establish diagnosis and local staging) can produce successful results. Continued refinements in therapy in the United States and Europe have brought the results of the two groups closer together.

TREATMENT

Wilms tumor is sensitive to chemotherapy and radiation therapy. Nevertheless, the first line of therapy is complete surgical excision of the tumor whenever possible. The NWTS confirmed the value of combined vincristine and dactinomycin therapy and subsequently showed the significant benefit contributed by adding doxorubicin to vincristine and dactinomycin for patients with advanced-stage disease with favorable histology.

NWTS-3 was the first study in which therapy was stratified according to histology and clinicopathologic staging. The results of the study can be summarized as follows: Postoperative radiation is unnecessary in patients with stages I and II favorable histology and stage I anaplasia when treated with chemotherapy postoperatively. Patients with stage III favorable histology benefit from doxorubicin therapy in addition to vincristine and dactinomycin (actinomycin D) and do not require more than 1,000 cGy to the abdomen. The addition of cyclophosphamide did not improve the survival of patients with stage IV favorable histology who also received doxorubicin, vincristine, and actinomycin D with radiation therapy to the whole abdomen and both lungs. However, the addition of cyclophosphamide to the other three drugs appeared to benefit patients with stages II through IV anaplastic histology.

Results from NWTS-4 indicate that actinomycin D given in a pulse-intensive manner as a single dose was found to be as effective as a standard dose of actinomycin D given daily over 5 days without greater toxicity and with fewer physician and hospital encounters. Therefore, pulse-intensive actinomycin D is recommended as the new standard.

Bilateral tumors can be synchronous or metachronous. The NWTS experience identified 4.2% of patients with synchronous disease and 1.6% with metachronous disease. By use of combined chemoradiotherapy and surgical or multiple surgical procedures, the survival rate of children with bilateral Wilms tumor has risen impressively. Only in rare instances has it been necessary to perform bilateral nephrectomies, subsequent dialysis, and eventual renal transplantation.

An aggressive approach to metastatic disease has resulted in the salvage of many patients. Pulmonary irradiation and chemotherapy with multiple agents have achieved survival rates of more than 50%. Many institutions excise liver or lung metastases if the lesions are surgically accessible and then administer chemotherapy or combined chemoradiotherapy. The prognosis is poorer for patients with metastatic lesions that develop during the initial therapy, but the prognosis is reasonably good for patients who are not taking chemotherapy who develop metastatic disease.

The late effects of therapy are being reviewed continuously by the NWTS. The most prominent effects are bone and muscle changes secondary to radiation therapy. Significant among these are degrees of muscle atrophy and impairment of vertebral bone growth, which result in a high incidence of scoliosis. The younger the patient, the more profound is the subsequent damage, and many of these children have required corrective surgery, back braces, and long-term physical therapy. Irradiation to the chest can damage mammary tissue in young patients. The incidence of second malignant diseases is low, and the risk is increased in a dose-dependent manner among irradiated patients and is further increased in those who were treated with doxorubicin in addition to irradiation. Cardiac, renal, and hepatic dysfunction also have been described secondary to radiation, chemotherapy, or both.

Suggested Readings

Coppes MJ, Ritchey ML, D'Angio GJ, eds. The path to progress in medical science: a Wilms tumor conspectus. *Hematol Oncol Clin North Am* 1995;9:xiii.

D'Angio GJ, Breslow N, Beckwith JB, et al. Treatment of Wilms' tumor: results of the Third National Wilms' Tumor Study. *Cancer* 1989;64:349.

Green DM, Beckwith JB, Breslow NE, et al. Treatment of children with stage II to IV anaplastic Wilms' tumor: a report from the National Wilms Tumor Study Group. *J Clin Oncol* 1994;12:2126.

Grundy PE, Green DM, Coppes MJ, et al. Renal tumors. In: Pizzo PA, Poplack DG, eds. *Principles and practice of pediatric oncology*, 4th ed. Philadelphia: Lippincott Williams & Wilkins, 2002.

Seibel NL, Li S, Breslow NE, et al. Effect of duration of treatment on treatment outcome for patients with clear-cell sarcoma of the kidney: a report from the National Wilms' Tumor Study Group. *J Clin Oncol* 2004;22:468.

CHAPTER 308 ■ NEUROBLASTOMA

DOUGLAS R. STROTHER AND HEIDI V. RUSSELL

Neuroblastic tumors, which include neuroblastoma, ganglioneuroblastoma, and ganglioneuroma, develop from neural crest tissue. They cover a spectrum from highly malignant to benign in both histologic appearance and clinical behavior. The most common presentation of the disease spectrum, disseminated neuroblastoma, has distinctly different behavior in children under 1 year of age (infants) compared with histologically identical disease in older children. Particularly in infants, the regression of primary and metastatic disease may occur spontaneously or after surgical resection of the primary tumor. In the older child, metastatic neuroblastoma usually is fatal, despite sensitivity to chemotherapy and radiation therapy. Newborn screening for disease through the measurement of urinary catecholamines has failed to reduce the mortality associated with advanced-stage neuroblastoma.

EPIDEMIOLOGY

Neuroblastoma is the most common extracranial solid tumor in children and is the most common malignancy in the first year of life. It is slightly more common in boys, and its incidence is 10.4 per 1 million white children per year and 8.3 per 1 million black children per year. The median age at diagnosis is 17.3 months; approximately one-third of cases are diagnosed by the age of 1 year, 80% by 4 years, and 97% by 10 years. Overall, approximately 600 new cases of neuroblastoma are diagnosed each year in the United States.

The cause of neuroblastoma is unknown; environmental exposures have not been shown to be causative. Genetic predisposition through mutation of a germinal cell may play a role in approximately 20% of all cases. In addition, multiple cases of neuroblastoma have been described within families, and in these patients, tumors occur at a younger age and are more often multifocal.

PATHOLOGY

Derivatives of neural crest tissue include the adrenal medullae and sympathetic nervous system ganglia. The different histologic patterns of neuroblastoma, ganglioneuroblastoma, and ganglioneuroma correlate with normal patterns of differentiation of these tissues (Fig. 308.1).

Neuroblastoma is one of the pediatric small, blue, round-cell tumors, and is the most primitive appearing of the spectrum of neural crest tumors. Differentiation is either lacking altogether or present in less than one-half of tumor cells. Electron microscopy may reveal neurosecretory granules, microfilaments, and microtubules. Tumors with more than 50% of cells showing gangliocytic differentiation are called *ganglioneuroblastoma*. The degree of differentiation may vary within a tumor, and histologic examination of the entire tumor is required to distinguish this tumor from the other histologic extremes. The benign form of neuroblastic tumors is called *ganglioneuroma*. These tumors are comprised of mature ganglion cells,

neuropil, and Schwann cells. Tumors may originate as ganglioneuromas or, alternatively, evolve through spontaneous or therapy-induced differentiation of more malignant disease.

CLINICAL MANIFESTATIONS AND COMPLICATIONS

Neuroblastic tumors may arise from anywhere in the sympathetic nervous system (Fig. 308.2). Two-thirds of cases arise in the abdomen, nearly evenly distributed between the adrenal glands and paraspinal sympathetic ganglia. Tumors in the chest and neck are more common in infants. Tumor may metastasize to lymph nodes, liver, bone, bone marrow, and skin. Brain and lung parenchyma rarely are involved at diagnosis. Symptoms of neuroblastoma result most commonly from mass effect at sites of involvement. Nonmetastatic disease may present with pain or a palpable mass. Intrathoracic disease commonly is diagnosed incidentally during an evaluation for trauma or possible infectious disease. Manifestations of metastatic disease include fever, pain, periorbital ecchymoses and proptosis, abdominal distention, lymph node enlargement, pallor, weight loss, and failure to thrive. Metastatic skin nodules occur in infants and are bluish, palpable, and nontender. Compression of the spinal cord at any level by extension of tumor through neural foramina may result in pain, paresis, or paralysis. Less common but classic manifestations of neuroblastoma include Horner syndrome, obstruction of the superior or inferior vena cava, and paraneoplastic syndromes that result in secretory diarrhea or opsoclonus-myoclonus. Symptoms secondary to production of catecholamines are uncommon.

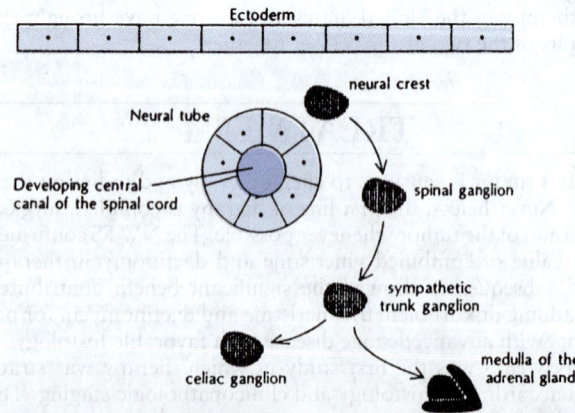

FIGURE 308.1. Migration of the neural crest in the human embryo. (Reproduced with permission from Matthay KK, Haas-Kogan D, Constine LS. Neuroblastoma. In: Halperin EC, Constine LS, Tarball NJ, Kun LE, eds. *Pediatric radiation oncology,* 4th Edition. Philadelphia: Lippincott Williams & Wilkins, 2005:180.)

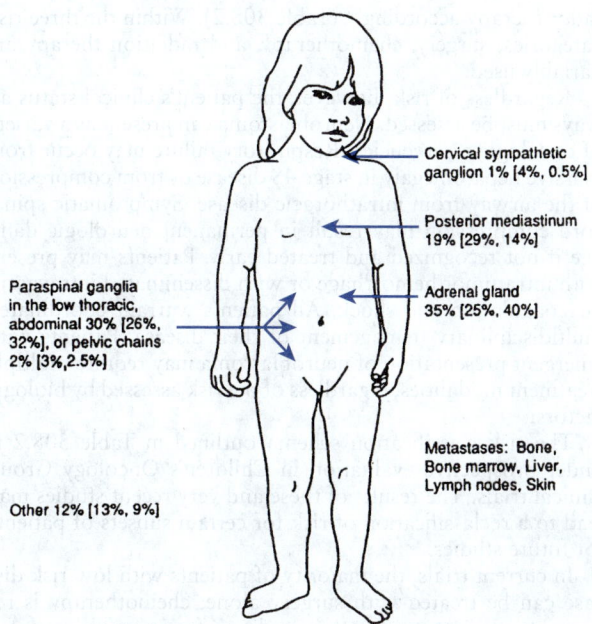

Cervical sympathetic
ganglion 1% [4%, 0.5%]

Posterior mediastinum
19% [29%, 14%]

Paraspinal ganglia
in the low thoracic,
abdominal 30% [26%,
32%], or pelvic chains
2% [3%,2.5%]

Adrenal gland
35% [25%, 40%]

Metastases: Bone,
Bone marrow, Liver,
Lymph nodes, Skin

Other 12% [13%, 9%]

FIGURE 308.2. Common locations of neuroblastoma. The first percentage is the overall proportion of cases at the site. The numbers in parentheses are the percentages of cases at a given site in children 1 year of age or younger and older than 1 year of age. (Data used with permission from Bernstein ML, Leclerc JM, Bunin G, et al. A population-based study of neuroblastoma incidence, survival, and mortality in North America. *J Clin Oncol* 1992;10:323; and from J. Shuster, PhD, Pediatric Oncology Group Statistical Office and Matthay KK, Haas-Kogan D, Constine LS. Neuroblastoma. In: Halperin EC, Constine LS, Tarball NJ, Kun LE, eds. *Pediatric radiation oncology,* 4th Edition. Philadelphia: Lippincott Williams & Wilkins, 2005:180.)

DIAGNOSIS

Neuroblastoma usually can be suspected by the clinical presentation. Histologic confirmation is required, however, and can be accomplished from biopsies of either primary or metastatic disease. In addition to a histologic analysis of tumor, assessing tumor for various indicators of biologic behavior is helpful (see section, Tumor Biology) so that appropriate therapy can be assigned.

More than 90% of neuroblastomas produce the measurable urinary catecholamines homovanillic acid (HVA) and vanillylmandelic acid (VMA). Levels can be assessed accurately on a few milliliters of urine. When the histologic assessment of tumor is impossible, the diagnosis of neuroblastoma may alternatively be made by the finding of cells compatible with neuroblastoma in the bone marrow of a patient with radiographic evidence of disease and urine levels of HVA and VMA that are elevated to more than three standard deviations above the mean values for age.

Staging

Staging of disease should include an evaluation of the primary tumor and all possible metastatic sites. Computed tomography (CT) or magnetic resonance imaging (MRI) of the chest, abdomen, and pelvis usually is done at diagnosis, although plain chest radiography and abdominal ultrasonography are used occasionally. The skeletal system is evaluated through nuclear bone scanning and bone radiography. Bilateral bone marrow aspirates and biopsies complete staging. Spinal MRI

is useful when compression of the spine is suspected. More centers are using whole-body imaging with radiolabeled ^{131}I-meta-iodobenzylguanidine to evaluate all sites of disease.

Until the late 1980s, a variety of staging systems were used throughout the world to designate the extent of disease. Although comparable in many aspects, variations among them made direct comparison of clinical trial outcomes very difficult. In 1987 and 1990, representatives from around the world met to formulate and revise, respectively, a uniform staging system based on clinical, radiographic, and surgical evaluations of children with neuroblastoma. The International Neuroblastoma Staging System (INSS) resulted (Box 308.1). Use of the INSS will greatly aid in the development of new clinical trials and in the analysis of potential new prognostic variables.

BOX 308.1 **International Neuroblastoma Staging System***

Stage 1 Localized tumor with complete gross excision, with or without microscopic residual disease; representative ipsilateral lymph nodes negative for tumor microscopically (nodes attached to and removed with the primary tumor may be positive)

Stage 2A Localized tumor with incomplete gross resection; representative ipsilateral nonadherent lymph nodes negative for tumor microscopically

Stage 2B Localized tumor with or without complete gross excision, with ipsilateral nonadherent lymph nodes positive for tumor; enlarged contralateral lymph nodes must be negative microscopically

Stage 3 Unresectable unilateral tumor infiltrating across the midline,[†] with or without regional lymph node involvement; or localized unilateral tumor with contralateral regional lymph node involvement; or midline tumor with bilateral extension by infiltration (unresectable) or by lymph node involvement

Stage 4 Any primary tumor with dissemination to distant lymph nodes, bone, bone marrow, liver, skin, and/or other organs (except as defined for stage 4S)

Stage 4S Localized primary tumor (as defined for stage 1, 2A, or 2B) with dissemination limited to skin, liver, and/or bone marrow[‡] (limited to infants less than 1 year of age)

---

*Multifocal primary tumors (e.g., bilateral adrenal primary tumors) should be staged according to the greatest extent of disease, as defined, and followed by a subscript M (e.g., 3$_M$).
[†]The midline is defined as the vertebral column. Tumors originating on one side and crossing the midline must infiltrate to or beyond the opposite side of the vertebral column.
[‡]Marrow involvement in stage 4S should be minimal (i.e., less than 10% of total nucleated cells identified as malignant on bone marrow biopsy or marrow aspirate). More extensive marrow involvement would be considered to be stage 4. The ^{131}I-meta-iodobenzylguanidine scan result (if performed) should be negative in the marrow.
From Brodeur GM, Pritchard J, Berthold F, et al. Revisions of the international criteria for neuroblastoma diagnosis, staging, and response to treatment. *J Clin Oncol* 1993;11:1466.

Tumor Biology

Indicators of inherent tumor behavior, or tumor biology, now complement the historically most important clinical prognostic factors of patient age and stage of disease at diagnosis. Biologic factors that affect risk classification and therapy include tumor-cell DNA content, *MYCN* protooncogene amplification, and tumor histopathology.

Tumor-cell DNA content is expressed in terms of the DNA index. Hyperdiploid tumors, those with a DNA index of greater than one, are associated with favorable outcome in infants. The increased DNA content generally contains few chromosomal rearrangements. In children older than 1 year, the DNA index is not prognostically useful. *MYCN* protooncogene number is determined most commonly by fluorescence *in situ* hybridization. An amplification of *MYCN* number is associated with aggressive, advanced-stage disease and a poor prognosis, regardless of patient age and stage of disease. Tumor histology, when combined with patient age, appears to reflect the biology of disease as well. Two different systems devised by Shimada and Joshi for distinguishing favorable and unfavorable biology were used in the past. In 1999, an international panel of pediatric pathologists formulated the International Neuroblastoma Pathology Classification system (Table 308.1). In evaluations to date, this classification system has shown a distinct difference in event-free survival between favorable and unfavorable histology tumors (90% versus 27%, respectively; $P < .0001$).

The relative importance of other indicators of tumor biology are under investigation. These include expression of the neurotrophic factors TRK-A and TRK-B, loss of chromosome 1p heterozygosity, and gain of chromosome 17.

THERAPY

Contemporary treatment protocols use clinical and biologic factors to assign a risk of relapse category to patients and to tailor therapy accordingly (Table 308.2). Within the three risk categories, surgery, chemotherapy, and radiation therapy are variably used.

Regardless of risk, however, the patient's clinical status always must be assessed. Neuroblastoma can present as a variety of oncologic emergencies. Respiratory failure may occur from massive hepatomegaly in stage 4S disease or from compression of the airway from intrathoracic disease. Symptomatic spinal cord compression may result in permanent neurologic damage if not recognized and treated early. Patients may present with intratumor hemorrhage or with disseminated intravascular coagulation and shock. All patients warrant coordinated multidisciplinary management of their disease. Patients with emergent presentation of neuroblastoma may require multiple treatment modalities, regardless of the risk assessed by biologic factors.

The risk classification schema outlined in Table 308.2 is under prospective evaluation in Children's Oncology Group clinical trials. The results of these and very recent studies may lead to a reclassification of risk for certain subsets of patients for future studies.

In current trials, the majority of patients with low-risk disease can be treated with surgery alone; chemotherapy is reserved for patients with emergent disease at presentation or for those with unresectable or recurrent disease. Survival rates are expected to exceed 95% using this approach.

Intermediate-risk disease is treated with surgery and multiagent chemotherapy, with or without radiation therapy. Many chemotherapy agents with activity against neuroblastoma exist, but the platinum compounds in combination with epipodophyllotoxins, and cyclophosphamide in combination with doxorubicin, are among the most active. Radiation therapy may be useful in controlling disease that remains unresectable after chemotherapy. Treatment for these patients is predicted to result in a survival rate of more than 90%.

High-risk disease remains a therapeutic challenge. Despite the incorporation and continued study of new agents, and an intensification of chemotherapy utilizing stem-cell rescue, the long-term survival rate remains generally less than 30%.

TABLE 308.1

INTERNATIONAL NEUROBLASTOMA PATHOLOGY CLASSIFICATION

		Prognostic Group
Neuroblastoma	(Schwannian stroma-poor)	
Favorable		Favorable
<1.5 years	Poorly differentiated or differentiating and low or intermediate MKI tumor	
1.5–5 years	Differentiating and low MKI tumor	
Unfavorable		Unfavorable
<1.5 years	a. undifferentiated tumor	
	b. high MKI tumor	
	c. undifferentiated or poorly differentiated tumor	
1.5–5 years	a. undifferentiated or poorly differentiated tumor	
	b. intermediate or high MKI tumor	
>5 years	All tumors	
Ganglioneuroblastoma	(Schwannian stroma-rich)	Favorable
Ganglioneuroblastoma, nodular	(Composite Schwannian stroma-rich/ stroma-dominant and stroma-poor)	Unfavorable
Ganglioneuroma	(Schwannian stroma-dominant)	Favorable
Maturing		
Mature		

Adapted with permission from Shimada H, Ambros IM, Dehner LP, et al. The international neuroblastoma pathology classification (the Shimada system). *Cancer* 1999;86:364.

TABLE 308.2

CHILDREN'S ONCOLOGY GROUP RISK ASSIGNMENT STRATA

INSS Stage	Age	MYCN Status	Pathology Classification	DNA Ploidy	Risk Group Assignment
1	0–21 years	Any	Any	Any	Low
2	<365 days	Any	Any	Any	Low
	>365 days–21 years	Non-Amp	Any	—	Low
		Amp	Fav	—	Low
	>365 days–21 years	Amp	Unfav	—	High
	>365 days–21 years				
3	<365 days	Non-Amp	Any	Any	Intermediate
	<365 days	Amp	Any	Any	High
	>365 days–21 years	Non-Amp	Fav	—	Intermediate
		Non-Amp	Unfav	—	High
	>365 days–21 years	Amp	Any	—	High
	>365 days–21 years				
4	<365 days	Non-Amp	Any	Any	Intermediate
	<365 days	Amp	Any	Any	High
	>365 days–21 years	Any	Any	—	High
4S	<365 days	Non-Amp	Fav	>1	Low
	<365 days	Non-Amp	Any	=1	Intermediate
	<365 days	Non-Amp	Unfav	Any	Intermediate
	<365 days	Amp	Any	Any	High

However, short-term survival rates have been improved with intensive, multimodality regimens. The use of differentiating and immunomodulating agents after autologous transplant therapy are under investigation. Still, new agents and treatment approaches are badly needed for these children.

Suggested Readings

Bowman LC, Castleberry RP, Cantor AB, et al. Genetic staging of unresectable or metastatic neuroblastoma in infants: a Pediatric Oncology Group study. *J Natl Cancer Inst* 1997;89:373.

Brodeur GM, Maris JM. Neuroblastoma. In: Pizzo PA, Poplack DG, eds. *Principles and practice of pediatric oncology*, 4th ed. Philadelphia: Lippincott Williams & Wilkins, 2002:895.

Brodeur GM, Maris JM, Yamishiro DJ, et al. Biology and genetics of human neuroblastomas. *J Pediatr Hematol Oncol* 1997;19:93.

Brodeur GM, Pritchard J, Berthold F, et al. Revisions of the international criteria for neuroblastoma diagnosis, staging, and response to treatment. *J Clin Oncol* 1993;11:1466.

Evans AE, Silber JH, Shpilsky A, et al. Successful management of low-stage neuroblastoma without adjuvant therapies: a comparison of two decades, 1972 through 1981 and 1982 through 1992, in a single institution. *J Clin Oncol* 1996;14:2405.

Gurney JG, Davis S, Severson RK, et al. Trends in cancer incidence among children in the US. *Cancer* 1996;78:532.

Look AT, Hayes FA, Shuster JJ, et al. Clinical relevance of tumor cell ploidy and n-*myc* gene amplification in childhood neuroblastoma: a Pediatric Oncology Group study. *J Clin Oncol* 1991;9:581.

Matthay KK, Villablanca JG, Seeger RC, et al. Treatment of high-risk neuroblastoma with intensive chemotherapy, radiotherapy, autologous bone marrow transplantation, and 13-cis-retinoic acid. Children's Cancer Group. *N Engl J Med* 1999;341:1165.

Shimada H, Ambros I, Dehner LP, et al. The international neuroblastoma pathology classification (the Shimada system). *Cancer* 1999;86:364.

Woods WG, Gao R-N, Shuster JJ, et al. Screening of infants and mortality due to neuroblastoma. *N Engl J Med* 2002;346:1047.

CHAPTER 309 ■ SOFT-TISSUE SARCOMAS

MURALI M. CHINTAGUMPALA

The soft-tissue sarcomas form a diverse group of malignant neoplasms that arise from embryonal mesenchyma. As a group, these tumors are rare in children, and most of the information known about these diseases is derived from treating adults. The exception is rhabdomyosarcoma (RMS), a tumor of embryonal mesenchyma that gives rise to striated skeletal muscle. This malignancy is the most common soft-tissue sarcoma of children, and it accounts for 5% to 15% of all malignant solid tumors in patients younger than 15 years. Since the early 1980s, successful treatment regimens have been developed, especially for localized disease, using a combination of surgery, irradiation, and chemotherapy.

RHABDOMYOSARCOMA

The first recorded description of RMS was by Weber in 1854, and the histology of these muscle tumors was described by

Rakov in 1937. Series of patients, mostly adults, were presented by Stout in 1946 and by Pack and Eberhart in 1952. The histology of these tumors was pleomorphic, a type we now know is rare in children. In 1950, Stobbe and Dargeon described the embryonal form of RMS, the most common histologic variety in pediatric patients. In 1958, Horn and Enterline described the four currently recognized histologic subtypes of this malignancy: pleomorphic, embryonal, alveolar, and botryoid.

Surgical removal of the primary tumor was the original therapy, and this resulted in some long-term survival. It was found, however, that the malignancy recurred frequently and early in the course of the disease. Survival varied by the site of the primary disease: Head and neck, excluding orbit, had survival rates of 7% to 14%; orbit, 21% to 48%; trunk or extremity, 22%; bladder, 73%; and vagina, 40%. In retrospect, it was evident that, in most cases, the metastases had occurred before the diagnosis could be made.

In 1950, Stobbe and Dargeon reported that at least some RMSs were radiosensitive. In 1959, D'Angio et al. observed a synergistic effect using radiation and dactinomycin. Edland (in 1965) and Sagerman (in 1972) showed that a fractionated total dose of 6,000 cGy could locally control this tumor.

During the same time, reports surfaced that chemotherapeutic agents used singly were successful in producing complete or partial responses in some patients, but the duration of improvement was short. Combined treatment regimens were increasingly more successful. Pinkel and Pickren suggested a coordinated approach to the treatment of RMS using surgery, irradiation, and chemotherapy. The utility of this approach has been confirmed repeatedly.

Because RMS is such a rare disease, the three pediatric groups studying cancer in children pooled their patients and resources to form the Intergroup Rhabdomyosarcoma Study (IRS). The results from the IRS studies have greatly advanced our knowledge of and success in dealing with this disease.

Epidemiology

RMS is the most common of the soft-tissue sarcomas in children, accounting for 4% to 8% of all malignant diseases in children younger than 15 years. RMS is the third most common neoplasm among the extracranial solid tumors of childhood after neuroblastoma and Wilms tumor. The annual incidence is between 4 and 7 cases per 1 million children, with approximately 250 new cases diagnosed in the United States each year. This tumor is 1.4 times more common in boys than in girls. The incidence of RMS appears to be lower in most of Asia than in the white populations of the Western industrialized countries. Relatives of children with RMS have a high frequency of carcinoma of the breast and of brain tumors. RMS has been associated with certain familial syndromes, such as neurofibromatosis and the Li-Fraumeni syndrome, which is associated with germline mutations of the p53 gene. The use of marijuana, cocaine, or any other recreational drug by one or both parents has been shown to be associated with an increased risk of RMS in the child.

Clinical Manifestations and Complications

RMS can occur anywhere in the body. The percentage of cases presenting at each anatomic location is depicted in Table 309.1. The head and neck (including the orbit) are the most common sites of primary occurrence, with 38% of the cases presenting in this region. The orbit accounts for 10% of the total presentations. The genitourinary tract is next in order of frequency, followed by the extremities, trunk, retroperitoneum, and other sites.

TABLE 309.1

PRIMARY SITES OF RHABDOMYOSARCOMA

Site	Frequency (%)
Orbit	10
Head and neck	28
Trunk	7
Extremities	18
Genitourinary tract	21
Intrathoracic tissues	3
Gastrointestinal and hepatic systems	3
Perineum and anus	2
Retroperineum	7
Other sites	1

Approximately two-thirds of the tumors occur in children 6 years or younger, with a peak incidence between the ages of 2 and 5 years. The signs and symptoms relate to the primary site of the tumor or the metastases. Usually a painless, enlarging mass is noticed.

Tumors in the orbit can produce proptosis, chemosis, and ocular paralysis. These tumors can begin as a mass in the conjunctiva or eyelid. Tumors in the nasopharynx can cause a nasal voice, dysphagia, airway obstruction, epistaxis, or pain. Tumors in the paranasal sinuses cause swelling, pain, discharge, sinusitis, obstruction, or epistaxis. Laryngeal tumors cause hoarseness. Tumors in the middle ear are associated with a polypoid tumor in the external auditory canal that can causes pain, chronic otitis media, and a facial nerve palsy. RMS may present as a painless facial or parotid mass. Patients with neck masses may present with hoarseness or dysphagia. Parameningeal tumors may extend into the central nervous system (CNS), resulting in meningeal symptoms, cranial nerve palsies, or respiratory paralysis.

Tumors arising from the trunk, extremities, or paratesticular region usually occur as painless masses that are noticed by the child or parents. Tumors in the retroperitoneum usually are asymptomatic or are found as large masses that may cause gastrointestinal or urinary tract symptoms. Bladder and prostate tumors usually produce urinary tract symptoms. Tumors from the perineum may involve the bowel or bladder. Botryoid tumors appear as grapelike clusters of clear tissue protruding from the uterus or cervix.

The tumor characteristically grows with indistinct margins along fascial planes and infiltrates into surrounding tissues. Metastases spread hematogenously and by lymphatics to the lung, bone, bone marrow, lymph nodes, CNS, heart, and breast.

Diagnosis

Open biopsy of the tumor is the definitive diagnostic procedure for an unexplained mass. Certain tests are performed before the surgical procedure to assess the extent of the disease for staging and therapeutic purposes.

Preoperative assessment should include a complete blood count, urinalysis, measurement of electrolytes (including calcium and phosphorus), liver and renal function tests, and a uric acid determination. Computed tomography (CT) or magnetic resonance imaging (MRI) of the primary tumor should be performed to delineate the involvement of adjacent structures and to aid in the surgical management of the patient. A CT scan of the chest, bone marrow examination, bone scan or skeletal survey, and liver scan should be performed to look for metastases. Patients with cranial parameningeal tumors also should

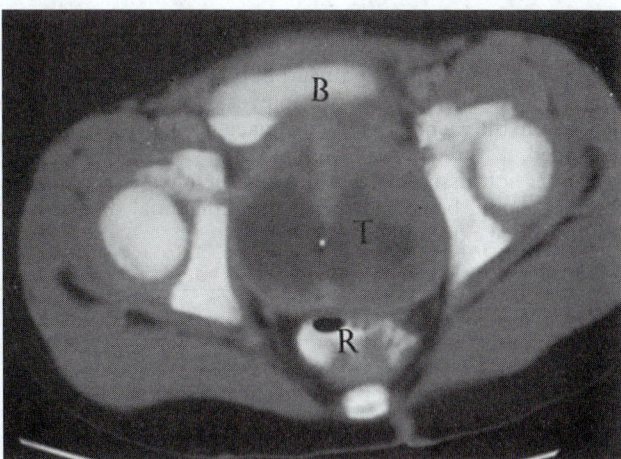

FIGURE 309.1. In the computed tomographic scan of a patient with a pelvic mass that was shown to be rhabdomyosarcoma after a surgical biopsy, the large pelvic tumor (*T*) is possibly associated with the prostate, displacing the rectum (*R*) posteriorly and the bladder (*B*) anteriorly, and extending to the side walls bilaterally. Notice the Foley catheter in the center of the tumor and the central area of necrosis depicted by the darker region of the mass.

have a CT scan and/or MRI of the head and an examination of the cerebrospinal fluid (CSF) to look for evidence of meningeal seeding with CSF pleocytosis, elevation in protein, and reduction of glucose. A CT scan may be used to assess retroperitoneal lymph node involvement in patients with lower extremity and genitourinary tumors. Figure 309.1 shows a solid tumor in the pelvis that was demonstrated to be RMS after surgical biopsy.

Histology

Histologically proven RMS on gross examination does not differ from other malignant soft tissue tumors and, with the exception of the grapelike clusters of sarcoma botryoides, the tumors do not differ from each other. The tumors are firm, nodular, and grossly well circumscribed but not encapsulated, and they aggressively invade adjacent tissues.

Four histologic variations have been described. The most common form is the embryonal type, which consists of spindle-shaped myoblasts and small round cells. This type accounts for 57% of RMSs and 75% of the tumors arising from the head and neck and genitourinary tract. Patients with this histologic variant have a relatively favorable prognosis.

The alveolar type is the second most common type of tumor, accounting for approximately 20% to 30% of the cases. The alveolar type is seen more commonly in children older than 6 years and occurs most often in the trunk, extremities, and perianal region. These tumor cells grow in cords that often have cleftlike spaces resembling alveoli. Patients with this tumor have a poorer prognosis than those with the embryonal type.

The botryoid type is most often seen in the genitourinary tract. This tumor accounts for approximately 6% of cases and is seen more commonly in children younger than 6 years. A deep, compact zone of spindle-shaped cells resembling myoblasts is found under a layer of myxoid stroma with a layer of small round cells at the periphery. This tumor is associated with a prognosis similar to the embryonal type.

The pleomorphic cell type is found more commonly in adults and is associated with only 1% of all the cases of RMS in children. When found, the disease is associated more often with primary tumors of the trunk and extremity. As the name suggests, the cells are large and pleomorphic, and they often contain multiple giant nuclei with cytoplasmic tails.

Other histologic varieties of mesenchymal tumors have been identified and often were included as RMS variants. These tumors arise in the soft tissue adjacent to the bone, carry a characteristic chromosomal t(11;22) anomaly, and currently are classified under the Ewing sarcoma family of tumors; they have a treatment approach different from that used in RMS.

The histologic type frequently is difficult to determine, and mixtures of the various types may occur in the same tumor. Cross-striations are not always found under light microscopy and are not necessary to make the diagnosis. Electron microscopy may be of value in cases that are difficult to diagnose. Thin myosin filaments and primitive Z bands may be seen and are helpful in making the diagnosis, but the lack of these findings in the presence of other characteristic observations does not preclude the diagnosis of RMS.

Characteristic genetic alterations recognized in the embryonal and alveolar subtypes can aid in the diagnosis. The alveolar subtype has a characteristic translocation: (2;13)(q35;q14). This translocation involves the juxtaposition of the PAX3 gene and the FKHR gene, a member of the forkhead family of transcriptions factors, and this fusion transcription factor presumably activates a gene or genes that results in malignant transformation. Rarely the PAX7 gene located at 1p36 may be involved. Involvement of PAX7 or PAX3 appears to be of prognostic significance in patients with metastatic disease, and those patients having tumors with PAX7-FKHR having a better prognosis. Embryonal tumors show a consistent loss of heterozygosity for multiple closely linked loci at chromosome 11p15.

Clinical Staging

The IRS Clinical Grouping Classification used in the IRS I, II, and III studies is shown in Table 309.2. This Clinical Group Staging system relies on surgical judgment and has had historic utility. Two problems are associated with this system. First, no surgically defined therapeutic questions can be asked, because the extent of surgery defines the clinical stage. One surgeon may perform a biopsy of a tumor, classifying the patient as having clinical group III disease, and a second surgeon may perform aggressive resection, classifying a similar patient clinical group I or II. The biologic role of the particular tumor or the aggressive surgical management of the similar tumor in patient outcome cannot be assessed. The second shortcoming of this staging

---

TABLE 309.2

INTERGROUP RHABDOMYOSARCOMA STUDY CLINICAL CLASSIFICATION SYSTEM

Group I	Localized disease, can be completely removed; regional nodes not involved
	1. Confined to muscle or organ of origin
	2. Contiguous involvement with infiltration outside the muscle or organ of origin
Group II	1. Grossly removed tumor with microscopical residual diseases, no evidence of gross residual tumor, no evidence of regional node involvement
	2. Regional disease, completely removed (regional nodes involved or extension of tumor into an adjacent organ, no microscopical residual disease)
	3. Regional disease with involved nodes, grossly removed but with evidence of microscopical residual disease
Group III	Incomplete removal or biopsy with gross residual disease
Group IV	Distant metastatic disease present at initial diagnosis

TABLE 309.3

STAGING CRITERIA

Stage I	Primary tumors found at sites considered to be of favorable prognosis without distant metastases
Stage II	All other primary tumors less than 5 cm in diameter without metastases
Stage III	1. All other tumors greater than 5 cm in diameter 2. All other tumors with adjacent nodal involvement
Stage IV	All tumors with distant metastases at diagnosis

system was discovered after analysis of the patient survival curves from IRS I and II. A clear difference in survival is found in patients with metastatic disease (less than 20% long-term survival rate) compared with those without metastatic disease (approximately 70% long-term survival rate). The difference between the other stages is less significant and less useful in defining treatment-related questions.

Several attempts have been made to correct the two inadequacies of the IRS system. By analyzing the same patient survival data from the previous IRS studies, four criteria were found to have statistically significant prognostic implications: primary site of tumor, size of tumor at diagnosis, evidence for tumor invasiveness at the time of diagnosis, and the presence or absence of metastases. A staging system incorporating these criteria is shown in Table 309.3. Patients with tumors arising from favorable sites (e.g., orbit, head and neck, genitourinary tract excluding bladder and prostate) and without evidence of metastases are grouped together as stage I. Stage II accounts for small tumors from unfavorable primary sites, stage III includes large tumors from unfavorable sites, and stage IV includes all metastatic tumors regardless of the primary site. A further subdivision of stage III includes patients found to have lymph node involvement associated with unfavorable primary disease. A second staging proposal substitutes the degree of tumor invasiveness for the tumor size in patients having primary malignancies in unfavorable sites (i.e., stage II and stage III disease).

Either staging proposal enables an assessment of the extent of disease independently from the surgical procedure used, thus allowing surgical treatment questions to be addressed. The patient survival data from IRS II have been reassessed using these staging criteria in a retrospective approach and were found to have statistically significant differences between each stage. The two objections to the current system have been addressed, and a modification of the staging system presented in Table 309.3 was used in the IRS IV study.

Differential Diagnosis

The differential diagnosis of RMS reflects the presenting complaint. With orbital tumors, it includes infection (i.e., orbital cellulitis), proptosis secondary to hyperthyroidism, hemangioma, metastatic neuroblastoma, optic nerve glioma, retinoblastoma, granuloma, lymphoma, granulocytic sarcoma, fibrous dysplasia of bone, and Langerhans histiocytosis.

Other tumors that can arise in the nasopharynx and paranasal sinus include inflammatory granulomas, lymphoma, other soft-tissue sarcomas, carcinomas, and juvenile nasopharyngeal angiofibroma. Tumors in the neck must be differentiated from inflammatory lesions, branchial cleft cyst, lymphoma, carcinoma, sinus histiocytosis, and Langerhans histiocytosis.

An intraabdominal mass must be differentiated from a mesenteric cyst, intestinal duplication, Wilms tumor, neuroblastoma, hepatoma, hemangioma, lymphoma, teratoma, carcinoma, the Ewing sarcoma family of tumors, and other soft-tissue sarcomas. A paratesticular mass could be a benign tumor,

including a varicocele or hydrocele, a seminoma, teratoma, embryonal carcinoma, lymphoma, or a rare tumor of the spermatic cord. In the bladder, neurofibroma, hemangioma, and transitional-cell carcinoma or leiomyosarcoma should be considered. In the vagina, rhabdomyoma, a benign lesion, must be excluded.

Other soft-tissue sarcomas can occur on the trunk. Bone tumors should be considered in the differential diagnosis of tumors of an extremity.

Therapy

The therapy for RMS consists of a coordinated approach using surgery, radiation therapy, and chemotherapy. The surgeon provides tissue for diagnosis and attempts a total resection of the primary tumor, without radical extirpative procedures if possible. A reduction in tumor burden is achieved if total resection is not possible. Initial aggressive excision surgery is not indicated in treating these children. Following initial surgery, chemotherapy is given in an attempt to eradicate systemic disease in all patients and reduce the size of the local residual tumor in patients with gross residual disease. After several weeks of chemotherapy, either surgery or radiotherapy or combination of surgery and radiotherapy is pursued in all patients with residual disease following initial surgery. Based on recent data, for patients with alveolar rhabdomyosarcoma who undergo complete resection at initial surgery, the recommendation is to provide local radiation therapy.

Radiation therapy is used to lessen the chance of recurrence of the primary tumor and to aid in the control of metastases. Relatively high doses are recommended (4,000 to 5,500 cGy). Vital structures such as the lung, liver, and kidney need appropriate shielding to prevent excessive radiation to these organs. Irradiation should be administered using appropriate high-energy equipment by radiotherapists skilled in treating children.

All children with RMS receive multiagent, intensive chemotherapy in an attempt to eradicate microscopic residual disease and to reduce macroscopic bulk disease. This approach has improved survival for patients with this malignancy.

Prognosis

Several significant prognostic variables exist. Based on these prognostic factors, patients can be divided into those with excellent, very good, intermediate, and poor prognosis. The presence or absence of metastases, favorable versus unfavorable site (e.g., orbit versus parameningeal), extent of surgical resection (clinical group), histology, and age are specific prognostic factors used in current rhabdomyosarcoma studies in North America. Outcome was best among patients with primary tumors of the orbit or nonbladder, nonprostate genitourinary tract; intermediate among patients with tumors in other head and neck sites and in the bladder or prostate; and worst among patients with extremity, cranial, parameningeal, and other sites. Alveolar histology is an adverse prognostic factor. Patients with completely resected tumors fare better than those with clinical group II disease. Patients with gross residual disease (clinical group III) at diagnosis have a poorer prognosis than groups I and II. The prognosis for patients with metastases at diagnosis remains grim, although patients less than 10 years of age with embryonal histology and those with alveolar histology with PAX7-FKHR seem to have a better prognosis. Local or distal recurrence carries a grave prognosis. Occasionally, a prolonged remission can be attained, especially if the tumor recurs after the completion of chemotherapy in a site amenable to surgery. Relapses, when they do occur, usually are seen within 2 years of institution of therapy, although a relatively small risk of late recurrences has been reported.

OTHER SOFT-TISSUE SARCOMAS

The other soft-tissue sarcomas make up a histologically heterogeneous group of tumors that arise from undifferentiated mesenchymal cells. These tumors occur in fibrous, connective, lymphatic, or vascular tissue and tend to recur locally. Using a combined therapeutic approach, control of local disease is attainable, and prevention of the development of metastases may be possible. Current treatment regimens are testing whether chemotherapy has a role in the treatment of these diseases in children. Preliminary trials suggest that chemotherapy and radiation therapy probably do not have a role in the management of grossly resected, non-RMS soft-tissue sarcomas in children (i.e., groups I and II). Clinical trials are evaluating the role of these treatment regimens in nonresectable (i.e., group III) and metastatic (i.e., group IV) tumors. Biopsy of the mass is the means to a diagnosis, and the differential diagnosis includes malignant and benign tumors at the site of origin. Because these tumors are rare in children, the diagnosis of a soft-tissue sarcoma other than RMS is not high on a list of differential diagnoses. A brief description of these sarcomas follows.

Synovial Sarcoma

Synovial sarcoma is a tumor resembling synovial tissue histologically, but it usually occurs far from a joint. The tumor presents as a painless mass, usually in the extremities in adults. Approximately 31% of cases occur in patients less than 20 years of age, according to one large series. The most common site of involvement is the lower extremity. The most common site of metastases is the lung. The tumor also tends to metastasize to regional lymph nodes and bone. Histologically, the tumor is biphasic, with a spindle-cell fibrous stroma often indistinguishable from fibrosarcoma and a glandular component with absolute epithelial differentiation. Synovial sarcoma is characterized by the translocation t(X;18)(q11;Xp11), which results in fusion of the *SYT* gene located on chromosome 18q11 and one of three closely related genes *SSX1, SSX2,* or *SSX4* located on Xp11 breakpoint. Treatment consists of surgical removal with a wide excision, irradiation to control local microscopic disease if normal function and normal growth can be maintained, and chemotherapy in the presence of bulky disease. The best outcome is associated with patients with group I disease.

Alveolar Soft-Part Sarcoma

Alveolar soft-part sarcoma occurs as a slow-growing asymptomatic mass usually involving the extremities. In children, the head and neck region are the more common sites. Chromosomal analyses have shown an abnormality at 17q25. Therapy has included local surgery and irradiation; response to chemotherapy has been poor. The tumor commonly recurs locally, and most patients develop metastatic disease. Although 60% of the patients in one study were surviving at 5 years, all the patients had died within 20 years after diagnosis.

Fibrosarcoma and Congenital or Infantile Fibrosarcoma

Fibrosarcoma is a tumor of fibrous tissue that has a tendency toward local recurrence but infrequently develops widespread metastases. This tumor has been reported to occur congenitally. Fibrosarcoma tends to occur in the muscles of the extremities. Treatment includes surgery of the primary tumor. Irradiation and chemotherapy have been used with some success.

Congenital or infantile fibrosarcoma occurs in children of less than 1 year of age. These tumors display t(12;15) translocation, with a novel fusion gene ETV6. This abnormality is not found in infantile myofibromatosis, hemangiopericytoma, or other childhood fibromatoses. The treatment of choice is local wide excision without significant loss of function. These tumors are chemosensitive, as indicated by several reports. One approach in patients with large tumors can be chemoreduction followed by conservative surgical procedures. Chemotherapy has no established role after surgical removal of the tumor.

Dermatofibrosarcoma Protuberans

Dermatofibrosarcoma protuberans is a slow-growing fibrous tumor of the skin characterized by a high recurrence rate locally but with a low incidence of metastases. The condition usually begins as one or more small, firm nodules in the skin, which often have a bluish or reddish color and blanch with pressure. The tumors develop slowly but may suddenly grow rapidly. The tumors are found most often on the trunk, arms, or thighs. Surgery is the primary treatment. Chemotherapy has been used with some success in patients with disseminated disease. Because metastases are rare, this disease has a good prognosis.

Malignant Fibrous Histiocytoma

Malignant fibrous histiocytoma (MFH) are tumors that are more common in adults. The presence of a storiform pattern of tumor cells with radiating fascicles of tumor cells at right angles to one another is diagnostic of the tumor. Angiomatoid MFH, the common form of MFH in children, is a unique soft-tissue sarcoma with an unusually favorable prognosis in children. Surgery is the primary therapeutic modality. Radiation therapy and chemotherapy have been used to control metastases. Although this is a chemosensitive tumor, the optimal regimen has not been established.

Liposarcoma

Liposarcoma is a malignant tumor of adipose tissue. The tumor is rare in children but must be differentiated from the histologically similar lipoblastomatosis, which is a benign disorder occurring in infants and children and which seldom recurs after local excision. Liposarcomas in children have a male preponderance. The liposarcomas occur wherever adipose tissue exists, but the thigh is the most common site. Local recurrence after surgery and metastases have been reported. Surgery and radiation therapy are used most often in the therapy of this tumor; the role of chemotherapy is unclear. The prognosis for children is significantly better than that for adults.

Hemangiopericytoma

Hemangiopericytoma is a vascular tumor of the cells that surround blood vessels. The most common site of origin is the lower extremity. In infants, these tumors arise most commonly in the tongue and sublingual region. Local recurrence after surgery and metastases are not uncommon. Surgery, radiation therapy, and chemotherapy all are recommended in the treatment of this disease. Late recurrences of the disease are not unusual.

Leiomyosarcoma

Leiomyosarcoma is a rare tumor of the smooth muscle in children. It also has been seen in association with the acquired immunodeficiency syndrome (AIDS) in children. Presenting symptoms depend on the site of the primary tumor. Gastrointestinal tumors may present with abdominal pain, hemorrhage, and associated anemia, but they may be asymptomatic. Intestinal obstruction may occur, especially in the neonatal period. Respiratory tract tumors may cause chest pain, cough, or hemoptysis, although patients may be asymptomatic at presentation. Dysuria and urinary retention may be the presenting symptoms of genitourinary lesions. Pain or swelling can be the symptoms of a patient with leiomyosarcoma of the blood vessels in the extremities. Surgery with wide local excision is the treatment of choice. The roles of radiation therapy and chemotherapy have not been established in children.

Suggested Readings

Crist W, Gehan EA, Ragab AH, et al. The third Intergroup Rhabdomyosarcoma Study. *J Clin Oncol* 1995;13:610.

Ensinger PM, Weiss SW, eds. *Soft tissue tumors*. St. Louis: Mosby, 1983.

Horowitz ME, Pratt CB, Webber BL, et al. Therapy for childhood soft-tissue sarcomas other than rhabdomyosarcoma: a review of 62 cases treated at a single institution. *J Clin Oncol* 1986;4:559.

Miser JS, Pappo AS, Triche TJ, et al. Other soft-tissue sarcomas of childhood. In: Pizzo PA, Poplack DG, eds. *Principles and practice of pediatric oncology,* 4th ed. Philadelphia: Lippincott Williams & Wilkins, 2002:1017.

Pappo AS, Shapiro DN, Crist WM, Maurer HM. Biology and therapy of pediatric rhabdomyosarcoma. *J Clin Oncol* 1995;13:2123.

Pratt CB, Pappo AS, Gieser P, et al. Role of adjuvant chemotherapy in the treatment of surgically resected pediatric nonrhabdomyosarcomatous soft-tissue sarcomas: a Pediatric Oncology Group study. *J Clin Oncol* 1999;17:1219.

Raney BR, Anderson JR, Barr FG, et al. Rhabdomyosarcoma and undifferentiated sarcoma in the first two decades of life: a selective review of Intergroup Rhabdomyosarcoma Study Group experience and rationale for Intergroup Rhabdomyosarcoma study V. *J Ped Hematol Oncol* 2001;23:215.

Sorensen PHB, Lynch JC, Qualman SJ, et al. PAX3-FKHR and PAX7-FKHR Gene fusions are prognostic indicators in alveolar rhabdomyosarcoma: a report from the Children's Oncology Group. *J Clin Oncol* 2002;20:2672.

Wexler LH, Crist WM, Helman LJ. Rhabdomyosarcoma and the undifferentiated sarcomas. In: Pizzo PA, Poplack DG, eds. *Principles and practice of pediatric oncology,* 4th ed. Philadelphia: Lippincott Williams & Wilkins, 2002:939.

CHAPTER 310 ■ RETINOBLASTOMA

MURALI M. CHINTAGUMPALA

EPIDEMIOLOGY

Retinoblastoma is a rare, highly malignant tumor of the retina of young children. Retinoblastoma is the seventh most common pediatric malignancy in the United States. The worldwide incidence of retinoblastoma is relatively stable at 1 case per 18,000 to 30,000 live births. No significant difference in incidence exists between sexes or among races. The average age at presentation ranges between 13 and 18 months; more than 90% of the cases are diagnosed before age 5 years. Retinoblastoma is a relatively slow-growing tumor that usually remains confined to the eye for months or even years. With early diagnosis, the overall 5-year survival rate exceeds 90%.

Retinoblastoma occurs unilaterally in 70% to 75% of cases. In more than 70% of cases, the tumor originates from a single focus and, when clinically detected, involves more than one-half of the retina, with extension into the vitreous chamber. Multifocal involvement may be observed with unilateral retinoblastoma, but is more common with bilateral disease. Although multiple tumor foci usually present simultaneously, in as many as 25% of cases, new foci may develop within weeks to months after the original diagnosis. The potential for metachronous occurrence of retinoblastoma warrants careful follow-up examination, even of the previously unaffected retina. Bilateral disease is detected at an earlier age (median, 13 months) than unilateral disease (median, 24 months). The long-term outlook for bilateral disease is significantly worse than for unilateral disease because of an increased incidence of second, nonocular malignant tumors in bilaterally affected cases.

Genetics

Retinoblastoma occurs in both hereditary (germinal) and nonhereditary (nongerminal) forms. Knudson has postulated a "two-hit" mutational event as being necessary for the development of disease. The retinoblastoma gene locus resides on human chromosome 13 at band q14. This retinoblastoma gene has been further characterized, mapped, and cloned and is the prototype for a class of recessive human cancer genes (tumor suppressor genes) in which a loss of activity of both normal alleles is thought to be associated with tumor genesis. Retinoblastoma gene mutations also have been found in some osteosarcomas, soft-tissue sarcomas, breast carcinomas, small cell carcinomas of the lung, and prostatic carcinomas.

Between 85% and 90% of the patients have no family history of retinoblastoma and represent the first mutational event within the family. All patients with bilateral retinoblastoma (25% of all patients with retinoblastoma) and approximately 15% of the patients with unilateral retinoblastoma harbor a germinal mutation. According to Knudson's hypothesis, a somatic mutation after the germinal mutation is necessary for malignant transformation to occur. Approximately 85% of sporadic unilateral cases are nongerminal; according to Knudson's hypothesis, two somatic mutations are required to produce the disease in these patients. When patients with either bilateral or unilateral retinoblastoma have the germinal mutation, 50% of their offspring will be affected by the disease, and 1 in 100 will harbor a gene but not express the disease. Direct analysis of the genetic defect in the genomic DNA is available to predict familial predisposition to retinoblastoma.

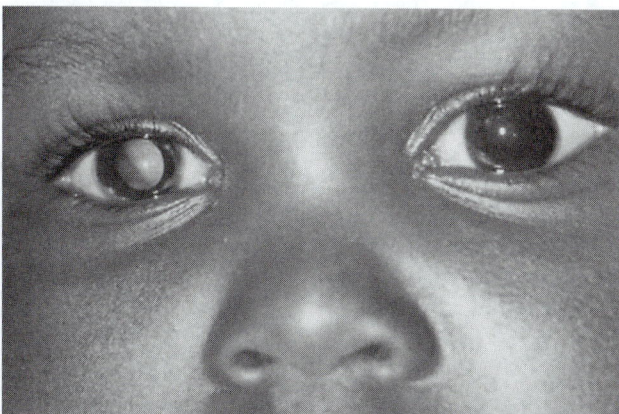

FIGURE 310.1. Abnormal white reflex, leukokoria, in a 7-month-old child with unilateral retinoblastoma.

Perhaps 5% of patients with retinoblastoma present with additional abnormalities, including developmental delay, abnormal dermatoglyphics, imperforate anus, and failure to thrive. Constitutional deletions of the long arm of chromosome 13 have been found in these patients.

CLINICAL MANIFESTATIONS AND COMPLICATIONS

In the United States, most children with retinoblastoma are first identified by their parents. The most common presenting sign is a white pupillary reflex called *leukokoria* (Fig. 310.1 and Box 310.1). This abnormal reflex, present in 60% of patients, is the result of a centrally located tumor at the posterior pole. Replacement of the vitreous with tumor or retinal detachment also may be noted.

The second most common sign is strabismus, present in 20% of patients. In children younger than 4 years, strabismus is usually the result of esotropia. With retinoblastoma, both esotropia and exotropia may occur and usually indicate tumor involvement of the macular area. Other signs include a red, painful eye with glaucoma (7%), poor vision (5%), unilateral dilated pupil, heterochromia (different-colored irises), or nystagmus. Children with advanced stages of disease may present with signs of lethargy, anorexia, failure to thrive, neurologic defects, orbital mass, proptosis, or blindness.

DIAGNOSIS

The well-child examination during the first 2 years of life should include an assessment for strabismus and, at minimum, the demonstration of a normal red reflex as a screen for retinoblastoma or other intraocular pathology. If the previously mentioned signs or symptoms are observed, the infant should undergo an examination by an experienced ophthalmologist using an indirect ophthalmoscope, under general anesthesia and with the pupils dilated.

The most common clinical classification schema for intraocular extent of disease is the Reese-Ellsworth system. At an early stage, the retinoblastoma appears as a hemispheric, localized retinal lesion that is usually pink but may appear gray or white. Larger lesions become pinker with increased vascularization. Tumors originating in the outer nuclear layer may cause retinal detachment. Alternatively, tumors arising from the inner nuclear layers may present as a localized mass or masses. These tumors are friable and may produce vitreous seeding. Intraocular calcifications may be noted with larger tumors. The presence of massive tumor, extensive retinal detachment, or vitreous seeds (group V in the Reese-Ellsworth system) is associated with a poor prognosis for salvage of the affected eye.

Metastatic extension occurs via the systemic circulation, through choroidal blood vessels into the orbit, or directly through the optic nerve tract into the central nervous system. Sites of metastases include the orbit, central nervous system, bone, bone marrow, and occasionally the lung. Ancillary noninvasive examinations, including computed tomographic (CT) scanning and ultrasonography, may help the clinician to make a diagnosis and may be useful in defining extraocular extension of disease (Fig. 310.2). Pineal involvement also may be documented with CT. Magnetic resonance imaging (MRI) may be more useful in determining extension into the optic nerve or the ocular coats.

Differential Diagnosis

The differential diagnosis for retinoblastoma depends on whether the tumor presents as a solitary mass or underlies an area of retinal detachment. When the tumor presents as a mass, two principal considerations are astrocytic hamartomas and granulomas of *Toxocara canis*. If the eye contains a retinal detachment, three diagnoses should be considered: coats disease, retrolental fibroplasia, and persistent hyperplastic

---

BOX 310.1	Presenting Signs and Symptoms of Retinoblastoma

Clinical Finding	Frequency at Presentation
Unilateral disease	75%
Leukocoria	60%
Strabismus	20%
Red, painful eye (glaucoma)	7%
Poor vision	5%

Other signs at presentation include unilateral dilated pupil, heterochromia, hyphema, nystagmus, and hyphema.

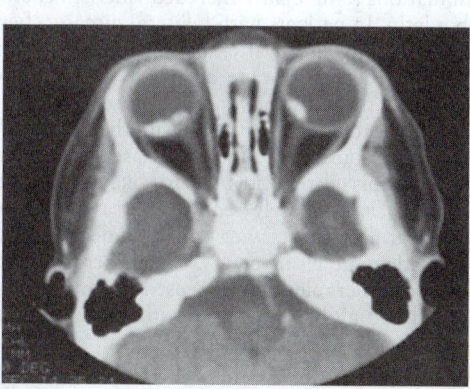

FIGURE 310.2. Computed tomographic scan of the orbits, revealing bilateral, calcified orbital masses arising from the posterior aspect of the retina and confined to the globe.

primary vitreous. The patient's age, past medical history (i.e., oxygen exposure for retrolental fibroplasia, tuberous sclerosis for astrocytic hamartomas), and presentation help the experienced ophthalmologist to distinguish between these disorders.

THERAPY

The priorities in treatment for retinoblastoma are to preserve life, retain vision, and ensure favorable cosmetic results. Modalities in current use are enucleation, radiation (external beam and localized radioactive plaques), photocoagulation, cryotherapy, and systemic chemotherapy.

The following indications have been proposed for enucleation: advanced group V disease with no expectation of vision preservation with therapy, early neovascular glaucoma, and failure of conservative treatment to control disease. Most children with unilateral retinoblastoma present with advanced disease and little hope of vision preservation. At surgery, care must be taken to avoid rupture at tumor insertions, and attempts must be made to remove a long stump of optic nerve.

External beam radiation has been the mainstay of treatment for retinoblastoma. Lateral portal radiation therapy, using a high energy of 6 meV or more for a total dose up to 3,600 cGy, produces tumor regression in virtually all tumors. With three-dimensional planning, one can deliver conformal radiation therapy and minimize dose to normal tissues, including the bony orbit. Radioactive applicators, surgically attached to the sclera (plaque radiotherapy) and left in place for 2 to 6 days, have produced successful tumor regression in small solitary tumors in 90% of cases and, with more advanced retinoblastoma, have salvaged more than one-half of the eyes.

Photocoagulation, using lasers applied through the pupil under anesthesia, is a highly effective means for treating small tumors that appear after radiation or for treating tumors unresponsive to irradiation. Cryotherapy also may be used to treat isolated lesions. The limiting factor for success for both of these measures is size and location: Tumors larger than 3 to 4 DD respond poorly to these treatments.

The role for chemotherapy is increasing in patients with retinoblastoma. Several agents, including nitrogen mustard, vincristine, cyclophosphamide, doxorubicin, cisplatin, carboplatin, and the epipodophyllotoxins, have produced objective responses in patients with retinoblastoma. Several reports support the effectiveness of new chemotherapeutic combinations for the treatment of intraocular retinoblastoma. The most effective combinations to date have included vincristine, etoposide, and carboplatin. In patients with bilateral disease, chemotherapy is used initially in an attempt to reduce the tumors in both eyes and thereby salvage as much vision as possible. The globe with the most advanced disease and least vision is usually enucleated and further chemotherapy, along with focal therapies, is used to control disease in the remaining eye. Such attempts also contribute to delaying radiotherapy if this modality is ultimately required to save the globe and cure the patient. In patients with unilateral disease, with small tumors and adequate visual acuity, chemotherapy in conjunction with focal therapies often is used to salvage vision in that eye and the globe. However, with advanced unilateral disease, enucleation is recommended. Attempts are underway to develop a staging system that will reflect more accurately the prognosis and better determine effective therapies using all treatment modalities available. Histopathologic evaluation after enucleation may reveal that ocular coats (e.g., choroid) are involved with tumor or that extension of the tumor has progressed into the optic nerve beyond lamina cribrosa. Pa-

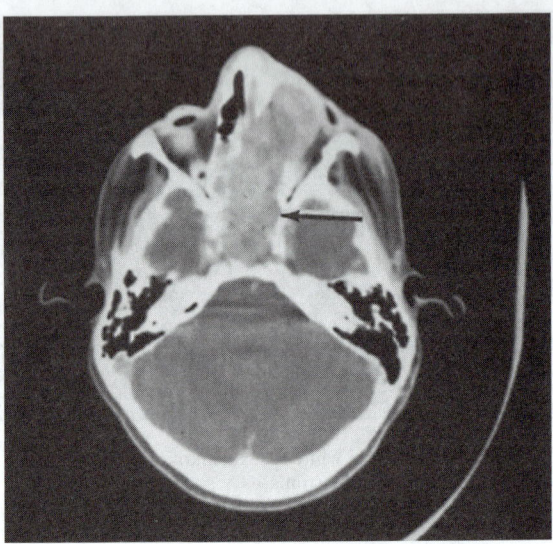

FIGURE 310.3. Computed tomographic scan of face, sinuses, and orbits of a 14-year-old child with bilateral retinoblastoma, treated 12 years before. Note the large destructive osteosarcoma involving the left ethmoid and sphenoid area.

tients with these findings are at a higher risk for metastases and require prophylaxis with chemotherapy. Extraocular extension or metastatic disease is relatively uncommon, but is associated with a poor prognosis. Trials using intensive combination chemotherapy with autologous bone marrow rescue have resulted in some significant improvement in longer-term outcome for these patients. Future studies may include gene transduction techniques to treat and eradicate intraocular disease.

Second Tumors

Patients who have the germinal mutation for retinoblastoma, and who survive the ocular tumor, have a high risk for developing other malignancies. The incidence increases with time and has been estimated to range from 30% to 50% at 20 years from diagnosis and up to 90% at 30 years from diagnosis. Tumors appear both within and outside the field of radiation. Tumors within the field include osteogenic sarcoma, fibrosarcoma, soft-tissue sarcoma, neuroblastoma, and meningioma. Osteosarcoma of the skull occurs 2,000 times more frequently in survivors of bilateral retinoblastoma than in the general population (Fig. 310.3). Patients with primitive neuroectodermal tumors involving the pineal region have been described as having *trilateral* retinoblastoma. The most common tumor outside the radiation field is osteosarcoma. The retinoblastoma gene commonly is identified in these nonocular tumors. The mortality associated with advanced second malignancies is high.

Suggested Readings

Abramson DH, Frank CM. Second nonocular tumors in survivors of bilateral retinoblastoma: a possible age effect on radiation-related risk. *Ophthalmology* 1998;105:573.

Fontanesi J, Pratt CB, Kun LE, et al. Treatment outcome and dose-response relationships in infants younger than 1 year treated for retinoblastoma with primary irradiation. *Med Pediatr Oncol* 1996;26:297.

Gallie BL, Budning A, DeBoer G, et al. Chemotherapy with focal therapy can cure intraocular retinoblastoma without radiotherapy. *Arch Ophthalmol* 1996;114:1321.

Honavar SG, Singh AD, Shields CL, et al. Post-enucleation adjuvant therapy in high risk retinoblastoma. *Arch Ophthalmol* 2002;120:923.

Hurwitz RL, Shields CL, Shields JA, Chevez Barrios P, et al. In: Pizzo PA, Poplack DG, eds. *Principles and practice of pediatric oncology,* 4th ed. Philadelphia: Lippincott Williams & Wilkins, 2002:825.

Shields CL, DePotter P, Himelstein BP, et al. Chemoreduction in the initial management of intraocular retinoblastoma. *Arch Ophthalmol* 1996;114:1330.

Shields CL, Shields JA, Baez KA, et al. Choroidal invasion of retinoblastoma: metastatic potential and clinical risk factors. *Br J Ophthalmol* 1993;77:544.

Shields CL, Mashayekhi A, Demirci H et al. Practical approach to management of retinoblastoma. *Arch Ophthalmol* 2004;122:729.

Uusitalo MS, Van Quill KR, Scott IU, et al. Evaluation of chemoprophylaxis in patients with unilateral retinoblastoma with high-risk features on histopathologic examination. *Arch Ophthalmol* 2001;119:41.

CHAPTER 311 ■ MALIGNANT BONE TUMORS

MURALI M. CHINTAGUMPALA

The optimal management for malignant bone tumors arising in children involves a multidisciplinary approach using surgery, chemotherapy, radiation therapy, and rehabilitative therapy. Early diagnosis and prompt referral to an experienced pediatric cancer center results in a significantly improved clinical outcome in patients presenting with these aggressive tumors. The two most common malignant bone tumors in children and adolescents are osteogenic sarcoma and Ewing sarcoma.

OSTEOGENIC SARCOMA

Epidemiology

Osteogenic sarcoma is a malignant spindle-cell sarcoma of bone in which the tumor cells directly form neoplastic osteoid. Osteogenic sarcoma, or osteosarcoma, is the most common primary malignancy of bone in children. The estimated incidence is 11 cases per 1 million adolescents. The male-to-female ratio is approximately 1.5:1.0. The peak incidence occurs within the second decade, during periods of rapid growth spurts, and gradually declines thereafter.

The etiology of osteosarcoma is unknown, but several associations with underlying medical conditions have been reported. Patients who have the germinal mutation for retinoblastoma and who survive the ocular tumor have a 2,000-fold increased risk for osteosarcoma in irradiated craniofacial bones. These patients have a 500-fold increased risk for osteosarcoma at any site, regardless of prior radiation exposure. This risk appears to be linked to the expression of the retinoblastoma gene, located on chromosome 13 at band q14. Radiation-induced osteosarcoma also is being diagnosed with increased frequency in long-term survivors of childhood cancer. Pediatric cancer groups studying late effects estimate a 40-fold risk for bone cancer in survivors who have received more than 6,000 rad to the bone. The median time to onset is 10 years. An increased risk is associated with alkylating agents, proportional to cumulative doses. In older patients with Paget disease, an increased risk exists for osteosarcoma involving the affected bone. Occasional cases also have been reported in association with chondroma, osteochondromatosis, and nonossifying fibroma. Two recessive oncogenes, *p53* and *RB*, appear to be involved either individually or in cooperation in both osteosarcoma development and progression.

Clinical Manifestations and Complications

The metaphyseal portion of the long bone is the site of predilection. Almost one-half of all new cases present with involvement in the region of the knee. In order of presentation, the most common sites are the distal femur, proximal tibia, and proximal humerus. However, any membranous bone may be involved, and even cases of extraosseous osteosarcoma have been reported.

Pain, which initially may be intermittent, and swelling of the extremity, which may evolve over several weeks, are the cardinal symptoms. Because these symptoms are nonspecific, adolescents presenting with pain in the area of the knee without a history for trauma should undergo a radiographic examination. Pathologic fractures are uncommon. However, minor trauma with disproportionate symptoms of pain may cause these patients to present for evaluation and lead to the recognition of a preexisting pathologic lesion.

Diagnosis

The diagnosis of osteosarcoma may be suspected from good-quality radiographs; tumors may appear as lytic, sclerotic, or mixed lesions. Irregular periosteal new-bone formation in the metaphyseal region may be an initial observation. In more advanced cases, cortical destruction, sclerosis, a sunburst pattern of periosteal new-bone formation, and contiguous, calcified soft tissue extensions may be noted (Fig. 311.1). Submicroscopic extension along the diaphysis can produce "skip" metastases some distance from the primary lesion.

The diagnosis is best made by incisional biopsy and permanent section. A carefully performed needle biopsy also may provide material sufficient for diagnosis. Extreme care must be taken in the biopsy of these lesions, because an incorrectly directed biopsy may produce an inadequate or misleading diagnosis or may leave a track that complicates possible consideration for limb salvage therapy. Ultimately, the biopsy track must be excised *en bloc* with the tumor at the time of definitive surgery. In view of the rarity of these tumors, and because of developments in the multimodal management of these patients, referral to a pediatric cancer center for definitive biopsy and diagnosis is in the patient's best interest.

Staging of the disease should include chest radiography and computed tomography (CT) of the chest. Osteosarcoma may

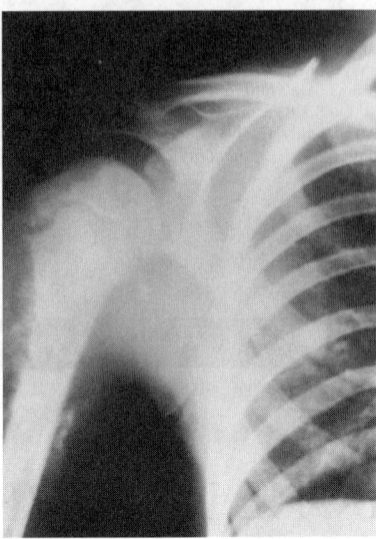

FIGURE 311.1. A large permeating lesion of the proximal right humerus, representing osteosarcoma beginning at the metaphyseal plate, with soft tissue extension and calcifications caused by osteosarcoma.

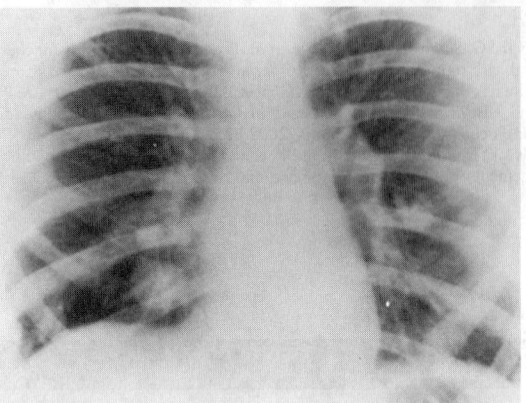

FIGURE 311.2. Chest radiograph demonstrating multiple, bilateral pulmonary nodules of metastatic osteosarcoma.

spread by hematogenous routes; metastases involving the lungs or bone are detected at the time of diagnosis in 10% to 20% of the cases (Fig. 311.2). Radionuclide scans are more sensitive for detecting the foci of osseous disease distant from the primary site. Approximately 2% to 3% of all childhood or adolescent cases of osteosarcoma are multifocal. This rare type, called *multifocal sclerosing osteogenic sarcoma*, presents with simultaneous or synchronous metastases at multiple metaphyseal regions and has a rapidly lethal outcome.

Patients considered for limb preservation (see below) require magnetic resonance imaging (MRI) examinations of the tumor-bearing bone and occasionally angiography. MRI scans are very accurate in the assessment of intraosseous extension of tumor and are the preferred examination for patients undergoing limb salvage procedures.

Approximately 60% of adolescent cases have elevated alkaline phosphatase levels, but this does not appear to have prognostic significance.

Histologic examination permits a division of osteosarcoma into two broad categories. Patients with low-grade osteosarcomas, including juxtacortical or periosteal and low-grade central osteogenic sarcoma, have a survival rate of approximately 70% with amputation or wide local excision alone. High-grade osteosarcomas include fibroblastic, chondroblastic, osteoblastic, telangiectatic, and small cell osteosarcoma. Patients presenting with these lesions require more aggressive treatment.

Therapy

Before the 1970s, the prognosis for children with osteosarcoma of the extremity was dismal. Despite control of the primary tumor with amputation, distant metastases developed in most patients, and survival was approximately 20% at 5 years from diagnosis. Current multimodal treatment strategies for osteosarcoma have reversed this trend, and approximately 60% to 65% of patients with nonmetastatic disease of the extremities are surviving their disease. Both surgery and high-dose chemotherapy play a significant part in achieving this result.

Surgery has an established role in the treatment of osteosarcoma. Ablative procedures usually involve amputation through the bone above the affected bone. The general opinion is that the amputation should be several cm beyond the most proximal limits of the lesion to minimize the risk for local recurrence. Large lesions involving the proximal femur or humerus occasionally require a disarticulation procedure.

With the availability of more effective chemotherapy programs, limb salvage surgery, after *en bloc* tumor excision and endoprosthetic replacement, has become a viable and more frequently used alternative in patients with osteosarcoma of the extremities (Fig. 311.3). Several factors are assessed before patients are considered eligible for the limb salvage procedure, including the extent of the tumor within the medullary cavity of the involved bone, the relationship of the soft tissue component of the tumor to the major blood vessels and nerves, and evidence of joint involvement influence the type of definitive surgery to be undertaken.

Patients and the parents should be fully aware of the nature of the procedure (limb-salvage procedure or amputation), reasonable expectations for functional outcome, and estimated

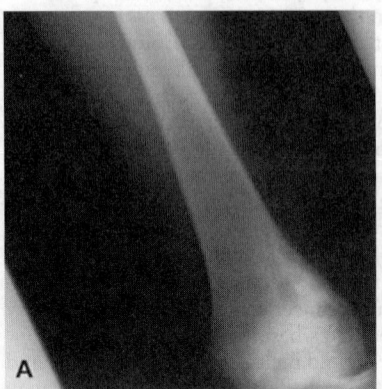
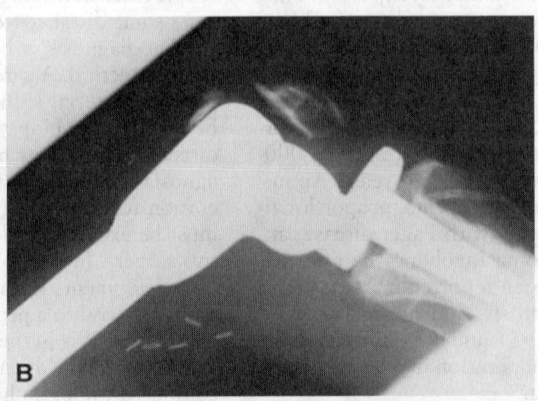

FIGURE 311.3. A: A 14-year-old girl with a small sclerotic osteosarcoma involving the distal left femur. B: Three months after receiving preoperative chemotherapy, she underwent *en bloc* resection and placement of an endoprosthesis, with proximal insertion into the femur and distal insertion into the tibia.

risks for complications, local recurrence, and possible failure of the procedure.

Limb salvage may be performed by immediate *en bloc* resection or may follow a brief course of chemotherapy (neoadjuvant chemotherapy).

The potential advantages of preoperative chemotherapy are that it allows for planning and acquisition of a custom prosthesis, and the antitumor effects may enhance the safety of the surgical procedure. More important, the response of the tumor (degree of tumor necrosis) to the preoperative chemotherapy provides the single most important prognostic factor for outcome. A potential disadvantage in using preoperative chemotherapy is that the tumor is *in-situ* and can metastasize or the tumor can develop cells that become chemoresistant. Most pediatric cancer centers use preoperative treatment in all osteosarcoma patients. No difference in survival outcome is apparent between patients who undergo amputation at the time of diagnosis and those who had limb-salvage surgery after several courses of chemotherapy.

Since the 1970s, nonrandomized multicenter chemotherapy trials have established unequivocally the value of high-dose adjuvant chemotherapy for increased relapse-free survival for patients with nonmetastatic osteosarcoma of the extremities. The first successful demonstration of adjuvant chemotherapy was a study by the Pediatric Division of the Southwest Oncology Group in 1970. The COMPADRI-I program, with more than 15 years of follow-up, produced an overall 49% disease-free survival rate. Studies conducted at the Dana-Farber Cancer Center in the 1970s and early 1980s, using high-dose methotrexate and doxorubicin, produced an overall disease-free survival rate of more than 55%.

In the early 1980s, randomized studies by the Pediatric Oncology Group (POG 8107) and the University of California–Los Angeles clearly established that postoperative adjuvant chemotherapy improved the disease-free survival rate of patients with nonmetastatic osteosarcoma of the extremities when compared with surgery alone (64% versus 19%). Since that study, several chemotherapeutic programs have produced long-term disease-free survival rates in excess of 60% (Table 311.1). Common features of these programs include the use of high doses of methotrexate, doxorubicin, ifosfamide, or cisplatin. Investigations of tumor histology after preoperative chemotherapy suggest that patients who experience tumor necrosis of more than 90% are more likely to remain free of disease. Changes in postoperative chemotherapy regimens to improve the survival in patients with less than 90% tumor necrosis have not been successful.

TABLE 311.1

SUMMARY OF CHEMOTHERAPY TRIALS IN OSTEOSARCOMA, 1979–1992

Protocol	Disease-free Survival ≥3 yr (%)	Cancer Programs
COSS-80, -82	68	German Pediatric Oncology Group
HDMTX, IA DDP, ADR	80	Instituto Rizzoli Osteosarcoma study 2
IFOS, ADR, HDMTX	82	Mayo
ADR, IA DDP	76	M. D. Anderson Hospital
T-10	76	Memorial Sloan-Kettering

ADR, Adriamycin (doxorubicin); HDMTX, high-dose methotrexate; IA DDP, intraarterial cisplatin; IFOS, ifosfamide.

These chemotherapy programs are potentially toxic and require considerable expertise in management. Cisplatin may produce difficulties with renal function and hearing. High cumulative doses of doxorubicin may be associated with cardiotoxicity. All patients require extensive rehabilitation support to resume normal activities.

Pulmonary metastases remain the major obstacle to cure for patients with osteosarcoma. The number and time of presentation of metastases may have clinical significance: Early-appearing, multiple lesions may be associated with drug-resistant disease and poor prognosis. Aggressive surgical treatment, including multiple and occasionally bilateral thoracotomies, coupled with intensive chemotherapy, may salvage 25% to 50% of newly diagnosed patients with metastatic lesions to the lungs. Complete removal of all metastatic tumor at the time of the initial thoracotomy may have the greatest importance for long-term survival.

Prognosis

The further refinement of limb-salvage techniques will increase the number of children who might enjoy a more functionally and cosmetically satisfying result from the primary surgical treatment.

Efforts to improve outcome in patients with osteosarcoma are now focused on identifying possibly prognostic molecular markers at the time of diagnosis. Treatment efforts are directed toward the intensification of therapy using alkylating agents and the targeting of cellular receptors with biologic agents.

EWING SARCOMA

Epidemiology

Ewing sarcoma is an uncommon primary sarcoma of nonosseous origin that usually arises in children or adolescents. James Ewing is credited with the first description of this tumor in 1921. Ewing sarcoma represents approximately 1% of all cancers reported in children, but approximately 30% of all bone tumors in this age group. The estimated incidence is 2 per 1 million white individuals younger than 20 years in the United States; Ewing sarcoma is rare in the nonwhite population. The male-to-female ratio is 1.54:1.00.

The etiology for Ewing sarcoma is unknown. Unlike osteosarcoma, ionizing radiation exposure does not represent a significant risk factor.

Pathology

Ewing sarcoma is a small round-cell tumor. Because of a poorly differentiated or undifferentiated histology, it may be confused with other undifferentiated round-cell tumors of childhood. The Ewing tumor typically is composed of a uniform population of small polygonal cells with scant cytoplasm and hyperchromatic nuclei. The cytoplasmic borders may be indistinct. Glycogen granules may be present but are not pathognomonic for the disease. The diversity of light microscopical patterns in Ewing sarcoma makes the diagnosis a challenge for even the most experienced pathologist. Investigations have demonstrated a cytogenetic abnormality [t(11;22) (q24;q12)], with fusion genes EWS-FLI1 in this tumor. This translocation is present in 90% to 95% of tumors within the Ewing's sarcoma family. The second most common translocation is EWS-ERG [t(21;22)(q22;q12)], which occurs in 5% to 10% of tumors. The presence of these translocations confirm the diagnosis in

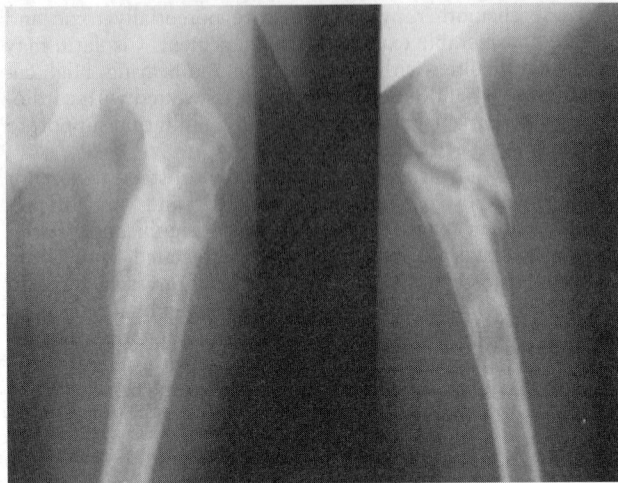

FIGURE 311.4. Two radiographic views of the left femur demonstrating a diffuse, destructive process caused by Ewing sarcoma, involving the intertrochanteric region and extending to the midshaft. A pathologic fracture is seen.

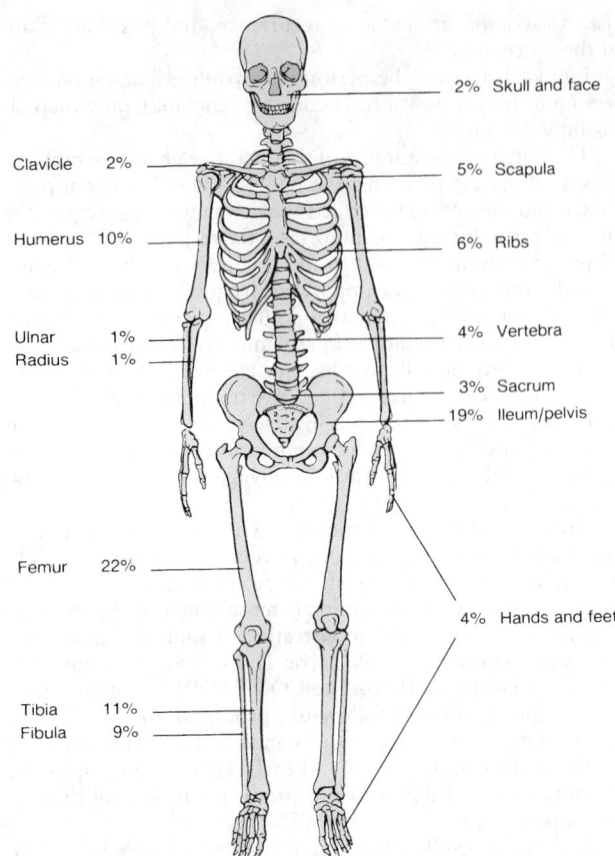

FIGURE 311.5. Anatomic distribution of Ewing sarcoma, based on 836 cases. (Reproduced with permission from Nesbit ME, Robison LL, Dehner LP. Round cell sarcoma of bone. In: Sutow WW, Fernbach DJ, Vietti TJ, eds. *Clinical pediatric oncology.* St. Louis: Mosby, 1984:710.)

patients with Ewing sarcoma and peripheral primitive neuroectodermal tumors, neuroepitheliomas, and Askin tumors. The distinctions among these tumors are related more to their primary sites and extent than to their histologic differences. All these tumors are generally referred to as *Ewing sarcoma family of tumors* (ESFT).

Other round-cell tumors to be considered in the differential diagnosis include non-Hodgkin lymphoma, rhabdomyosarcoma, neuroblastoma, small cell osteosarcoma, metastatic medulloblastoma, and the acute leukemias of all types.

Clinical Manifestations and Complications

Pain is the most common first symptom in Ewing sarcoma, occurring in more than one-half of patients. Swelling associated with a soft-tissue mass may become evident weeks to months thereafter. Fever and an elevated erythrocyte sedimentation rate may develop in time and may confound the diagnosis. Pathologic fractures are uncommon.

The femur is the bone most commonly involved, but any bone of the body may be involved (Figs. 311.4 and 311.5). The classic radiographic feature is a diffuse, mottled, lytic lesion affecting the medullary cavity and cortical bone. Regions of increased density may be found and are associated with new bone formation. Tumor that penetrates the cortex and extends into the periosteum may produce elevations characterized by multiple layers of reactive new-bone formation, creating an onion-skin appearance on radiographic examination. The tumor may expand the affected bone and resemble a cystic malformation. A soft-tissue mass, rarely including calcifications, may be associated with the primary bone tumor. Although these radiographic features have been described clearly with Ewing tumors, several conditions can produce similar features, including acute and chronic osteomyelitis, eosinophilic granuloma, osteosarcoma, metastatic sarcomas, and lymphoma. An MRI scan of the affected bone gives the best assessment of intramedullary tumor extension. Ewing sarcoma primarily affecting the soft tissues is called *extraosseous Ewing sarcoma.*

An open biopsy is the procedure of choice to establish the diagnosis of Ewing sarcoma. In general, needle biopsies do not provide sufficient material for interpretation and have on occasion produced confusing information. The two conditions most often mistaken for Ewing sarcoma are eosinophilic granuloma and osteomyelitis. The presence of necrosis or inflammatory cells within the tumor can be misleading if the biopsy material is inadequate. Biopsy of cortical lesions should be as small and round as possible, avoiding the tension side of the bone if possible, and should include touch preparations and material for electron microscopy. If a malignant bone tumor is suspected in a child or adolescent, referral to a pediatric cancer center for the definitive diagnosis ensures the most experienced surgical assessment and optimal biopsy for these patients.

Once the diagnosis of Ewing sarcoma is established, clinical staging is essential, including chest radiography, CT of the chest, MRI of the bone bearing the primary lesion, radionuclide bone scanning, and bone marrow aspiration and biopsy. These investigations are pursued because the lungs and bones are the most common sites of metastases (90% of the cases). Other baseline studies also are recommended, including serum lactate dehydrogenase, alkaline phosphatase, and erythrocyte sedimentation rate. These tests may reflect the extent of tumor activity. Urinary catecholamines may be helpful to rule out neuroblastoma in the younger patient.

Therapy

Ewing sarcoma is a highly malignant tumor with a great propensity for metastatic spread before diagnosis. Before the 1960s, surgery and radiotherapy were the mainstays of therapy. Local control was adequate, but long-term disease-free survival was only 9%. A multidisciplinary approach is now the recognized treatment of choice.

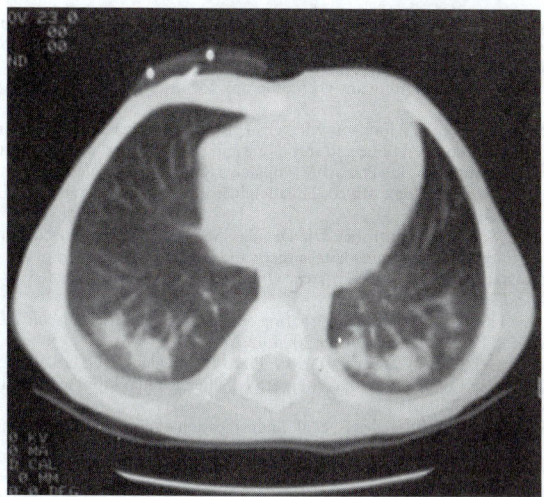

FIGURE 311.6. Computed tomographic scan of the chest, revealing bilateral pulmonary metastasis in a child initially treated for a Ewing sarcoma of the femur.

No uniform staging system exists for Ewing sarcoma. Tumor size, location, and the presence of metastases at diagnosis have been considered as prognostic factors. Patients with pelvic or proximal primary tumors had the least favorable outcome, whereas the most favorable sites were distal lesions, usually in expendable bones. Patients with large soft-tissue extensions did less well with therapy because of an increased risk for distant, usually pulmonary, metastases (Fig. 311.6). Modifications in current therapy may alter the significance of these risk factors.

Most treatment regimens include an initial phase of chemotherapy followed by local disease control measures followed by further chemotherapy. Surgery or radiotherapy are effective modalities for local tumor control. In every patient, decision regarding local control is best made with a discussion involving the medical oncologist, radiation oncologist, and the orthopedic surgeon. The recommendations then are discussed with the family and patient, and the potential advantages and disadvantages of the methods for local control are outlined.

In general, surgery is recommended for lesions in expendable bones in which resulting disability is acceptable (i.e., lesions in the foot, fibula, rib, forearm bone, clavicle, or scapula). Amputation may be recommended for extremity lesions that have huge destructive components, pathologic fractures, or involvement of distal femoral epiphysis in children younger than 6 years. Debulking of large pelvic primary tumors after initial tumor reduction with chemotherapy also may increase

chances for long-term survival. Some of the patients with large pelvic tumors may require radiotherapy in addition to surgery and chemotherapy. The risk of second malignancies is minimal when surgery is the only modality used for local tumor control along with chemotherapy.

Radiation therapy plays a major role in the control of local disease. Most investigations suggest that doses of 5,000 to 5,500 cGy divided over 5.5 weeks, when coupled with adjuvant chemotherapy, will achieve local control in more than 90% of patients with extremity lesions. A small but definite risk for the development of second malignancies exists when radiation therapy is used. In addition, radiation therapy could result in major growth and functional deficits.

Since the early 1970s, adjuvant chemotherapy has played an important role in the improved survival of patients with Ewing sarcoma. The principal agents of established value include vincristine, dactinomycin, cyclophosphamide, and doxorubicin. Patients with nonmetastatic disease with primary lesions in an extremity have a projected 3-year survival rate of more than 60% and a local recurrence rate of less than 10% with modern therapy (Table 311.2). Ifosfamide and etoposide (VP-16) are new agents with activity against this tumor. One clinical trial showed that patients who received ifosfamide and VP-16 in addition to vincristine, cyclophosphamide, and doxorubicin had a higher relapse-free survival rate (69%) than those who received vincristine, cyclophosphamide, and doxorubicin (50%). This study included patients with extremity and pelvic lesions and patients with Ewing sarcoma and peripheral primitive neuroectodermal tumors. Current efforts are directed towards studying the effects of intensified chemotherapy (combination chemotherapy given every 2 weeks) on disease-free survival.

The presence of metastatic disease at diagnosis has been reported in 14% to 35% of patients and is associated with a poor prognosis. Historically, the median disease-free survival rate for patients with metastatic disease at diagnosis has been 75 weeks. Patients developing distant metastases while receiving therapy have resistant disease and an expected median survival of 37 weeks.

Prognosis

For survivors of Ewing sarcoma, several late consequences of treatment may have a significant effect. Pathologic fractures may occur at primary tumor sites involving lower extremities at periods of 6 months to 3 years from diagnosis. This complication may be related to impaired bone remodeling after

TABLE 311.2

SUMMARY OF SELECTED THERAPEUTIC TRIALS IN NONMETASTATIC EWING SARCOMA

Institution	Study Period	Local Radiation to Primary	Chemotherapy	Disease-free Survival >2 yr (%)
Memorial Sloan-Kettering	1970–1979	+	T-2/T-6/T-9*	79
Intergroup Ewing Sarcoma Study-II	1973–1978	+	V, A, C + ADR	74
Intergroup Ewing Sarcoma Study-I	1978–1983	+	V, A, C + ADR	>70
National Cancer Institute	1983–1986	+	V, C + ADR	70
St. Jude	1978–1981	+ (delayed)	V, A, C	>70

A, actinomycin D (dactinomycin); ADR, Adriamycin (doxorubicin); C, cyclophosphamide; V, vincristine.
*Combination therapy with four, six, and nine agents, including V, A, C + ADR.

radiation and chemotherapy. Demineralization and radiation-associated delayed healing may aggravate this situation by causing nonunion of the fracture site. Other potential complications of radiation therapy include retarded bone growth, limb-length discrepancy, fibrosis, sclerosis, and functional limitations. The combination of radiation and chemotherapy has carcinogenic potential. The estimated rate for second cancers is 72 times the expected value in the normal population. Other potential complications include sterility associated with prolonged use of cyclophosphamide and cardiotoxicity associated with doxorubicin.

Suggested Readings

Link MP, Goorin AM, Horowitz, et al. The effect of adjuvant chemotherapy on relapse-free survival in patients with osteosarcoma of the extremity. *N Engl J Med* 1986;314:1600.

Burgert EO, Nesbit ME, Garnsey LA, et al. Multimodal therapy for the management of nonpelvic localized Ewing's sarcoma of bone: Intergroup Study IESS-II. *J Clin Oncol* 1990;8:1514.

Eilber FR, Rosen G. Adjuvant chemotherapy for osteosarcoma. *Semin Oncol* 1989;16:312.

Ginsberg JP, Woo SY, Johnson ME, et al. Ewing sarcoma family of tumors: Ewing's sarcoma of bone and soft tissue and the peripheral primitive neurectodermal tumors. In: Pizzo PA, Poplack DG, eds. *Principles and practice of pediatric oncology*, 4th ed. Philadelphia: Lippincott Williams & Wilkins, 2002:973.

Goorin AM, Schwartzentruber DJ, Devidas M, et al. Presurgical chemotherapy compared with immediate surgery and adjuvant chemotherapy for nonmetastatic osteosarcoma: Pediatric Oncology Group Study POG 8651. *J Clin Oncol* 2003;21:1574.

Hosalkar HS, Dormans JP. Limb sparing surgery for pediatric musculoskeletal tumors. *Pediatr Blood Cancer* 2004;42:295.

Link MP, Gebhart MC, Meyers PA. In: Pizzo PA, Poplack DG, eds. *Principles and practice of pediatric oncology*, 4th ed. Philadelphia: Lippincott Williams & Wilkins, 2002:1051.

Meyers PA, Gorlick R, Heller G, et al. Intensification of preoperative chemotherapy for osteogenic sarcoma: results of the Memorial-Sloan Kettering (T12) protocol. *J Clin Oncol* 1998;16:2452.

CHAPTER 312 ■ MALIGNANT TUMORS OF THE GASTROINTESTINAL TRACT, LIVER, AND ENDOCRINE SYSTEM

VICTOR A. LEWIS AND DOUGLAS R. STROTHER

Whereas metastases from pediatric tumors to sites within gastrointestinal (GI) tract are relatively common, primary GI neoplasms are exceedingly rare in children. Because of this rarity, their treatment has been adapted from that of adults with similar tumors.

HEPATIC NEOPLASMS

Hepatoblastoma (HB) and hepatocellular carcinoma (HCC) are the most common hepatic malignant diseases. Much less commonly, *undifferentiated sarcoma* of the liver (known also as *embryonal sarcoma* or *malignant mesenchymoma* of the liver), *hemangiosarcoma*, and *cholangiocarcinoma* may occur. Rhabdomyosarcoma and undifferentiated sarcomas arising from the biliary tract are discussed elsewhere.

HB and HCC occur as a right upper quadrant mass. Both diseases are associated with a male preponderance, whereas HB clearly occurs in younger children, with a median age of 16 months at diagnosis. Associations with overgrowth syndromes, such as the Beckwith-Wiedemann syndrome, and with hemihypertrophy and isosexual precocity have been described with HB. Patients may present with thrombocytosis and anemia. Although osteopenia occurs commonly with HB, it is not indicative of metastatic disease. Alpha-Fetoprotein is a tumor marker for HB that is usually elevated at diagnosis. Patients with HCC generally are older, with a median age of onset of 12 years, and they appear more ill at diagnosis. They commonly present with nausea, vomiting, fever, and abdominal pain. Multifocal liver involvement with metastasis to extrahepatic sites is common

at diagnosis. HCC is associated with hepatitis B, but cirrhosis may or may not be present.

Ultrasound examination of the abdomen is useful in identifying both types of hepatic tumors. Computed tomography, or, for better detail, magnetic resonance imaging, is necessary to define the intrahepatic extent of disease; both are useful for surgical management of disease. Computed tomography and nuclear medicine imaging are used to identify extrahepatic metastases.

Although complete removal of primary HB and HCC is necessary for cure, this can be accomplished in only in one-half of HB and one-third of HCC cases. Neoadjuvant chemotherapy can help to decrease the size of HB to allow later complete excision. Postsurgical chemotherapy is not required after complete excision of HB with purely fetal histology. In cases of embryonal, anaplastic, and macrotrabecular HB, postsurgical chemotherapy reduces the risk of recurrence. Cisplatin, vincristine, doxorubicin, and 5-fluorouracil are among the most active drugs for HB.

Metastatic disease at time of diagnosis diminishes ultimate survival rates. Repeat operations are warranted for children with advanced or recurrent disease. If surgical excision of the primary tumor is achieved, metastatic disease can be controlled with chemotherapy. Surgical control of metastatic disease has also contributed to long-term survival.

Although HCC is sensitive to chemotherapy, responses are less durable than in patients with HB. Platinum compounds, cyclophosphamide, doxorubicin, etoposide, and 5-fluorouracil have shown activity against HCC. Chances of survival are increased with adjuvant chemotherapy after complete resection of HCC. Residual or metastatic disease carries an extremely poor prognosis. Radiation therapy only helps to control microscopic residual disease.

The role of stem cell rescue after high-dose chemotherapy is controversial, and newer drugs, such as irinotecan, are being tested actively in recurrent and high-risk cases.

OTHER TUMORS OF THE GASTROINTESTINAL TRACT

Oropharyngeal Tumors

Carcinoma of the oropharynx has been observed in older children. These tumors are primarily mucoepidermoid carcinomas involving the salivary glands. Rare cases of squamous cell carcinoma of the lip or tongue in childhood also have been reported. Esophageal carcinoma has been found in patients as young as 15 years.

Gastric Tumors

Malignant gastric tumors in children are usually lymphomas or sarcomas, but gastric adenocarcinomas have been documented. Most primary tumors found in the stomach are benign, and surgical resection is curative. For malignant gastric disease, surgery is the initial therapy, with postoperative radiation therapy or chemotherapy as indicated.

Gallbladder Tumors

Primary gallbladder tumors are exceedingly rare. They are highly malignant and unresponsive to all forms of therapy. Metastatic disease to the liver and lymph nodes is usually present at diagnosis. The most common childhood cancer to involve the gallbladder is rhabdomyosarcoma.

Small Bowel Tumors

Finding primary small bowel tumors is unusual at any age, but particularly so in children. These patients usually present with some manifestations of partial or complete intestinal obstruction. Occasionally, small bowel tumors cause ulceration, intestinal bleeding, and, rarely, perforation. The most frequently diagnosed small bowel tumor is lymphoma. Therapy after surgery is dictated by the histologic classification and staging of the primary tumor.

Appendiceal Tumors

Carcinoid tumors are the appendiceal tumors recognized most often in children. These tumors usually are detected early before they have spread, because they present with signs and symptoms of appendicitis. Appendectomy is the only therapy indicated.

Pancreatic Tumors

Pediatric pancreatic tumors fall into three categories: exocrine and ductal tumors, endocrine tumors, and mesenchymal tumors. Most pancreatic tumors in children are benign and are

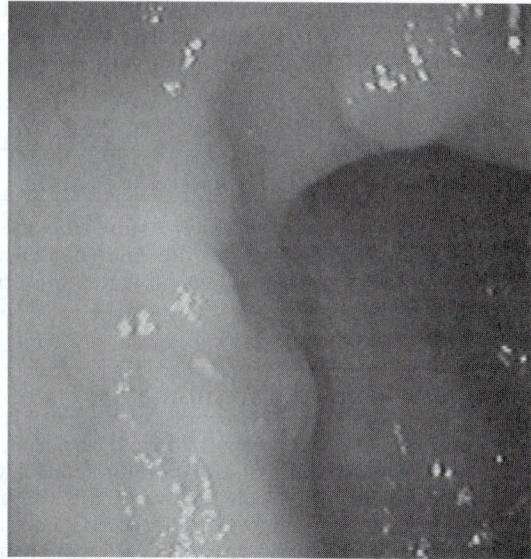

FIGURE 312.1. Endoscopic view demonstrating familial adenomatous polyposis.

treated by excision. Pancreatic carcinoma, however, is highly malignant. Pancreatic carcinoma requires radical surgery. Because it has often spread to the liver and lung at the time of diagnosis, disease usually cannot be resected. Presenting features include an abdominal mass and pain, GI disturbances, and, rarely, obstructive jaundice. Chemotherapy and radiation therapy are ineffective.

Large Bowel Tumors

The most common colonic tumors in children are benign polyps that manifest as rectal bleeding. The hamartomatous type of polyp can involve the GI tract either as a major manifestation or as a secondary feature of a syndrome. These syndromes include juvenile polyposis syndrome, Peutz-Jeghers syndrome, Cowden disease, and Ruvalcaba-Myhre-Smith syndrome. Although extremely rare, these syndromes (except Ruvalcaba-Myhre-Smith syndrome) are associated with an increased risk of GI and extra-GI malignant disease. Other preexisting conditions predispose children to colon cancer. These conditions include ulcerative colitis and the variants of familial adenomatous polyposis coli syndromes (Fig. 312.1), autosomal dominantly inherited conditions characterized by multiple colonic polyps, and lesions of other soft tissues or the central nervous system. Infections such as with *Helicobacter pylori* may also increase the risk of future malignant diseases of the GI tract. Immunocompromised patients, especially recipients of liver, kidney, heart, and allogeneic hematopoietic stem cell transplants have an increased risk of developing lymphoma related to primary infection with or reactivation of Epstein-Barr virus infection. These posttransplant lymphoproliferative processes can also affect the GI tract.

Despite these many predisposing conditions, colon cancer in childhood is rare; most cases occur in the second decade of life. The malignant disease may manifest as a change in bowel habits or the passage of bloody or tarry stools. Signs and symptoms vary according to the portion of bowel affected. Early detection is important. The disease is usually more extensive at diagnosis compared with adults. The tumor may metastasize throughout the abdomen and to lungs, bone, and brain. The value of carcinoembryonic antigen determination in childhood colon cancer has not been established. Aggressive surgery is the mainstay of treatment. Effective chemotherapy has not been established for colon cancer. Radiation therapy may be helpful for rectosigmoid lesions. Long-term survival rates remain dismal.

ENDOCRINE TUMORS

Most endocrine-related tumors in children arise from the gonads or central nervous system; these are covered elsewhere. Cancers of the thyroid gland and adrenal cortex are briefly discussed here.

Thyroid Carcinoma

Thyroid carcinoma is uncommon in children. Its incidence has decreased with diminished use of radiation for children with tonsillitis and adenoid hypertrophy. However, the use of radiation and chemotherapy for pediatric cancer is associated with the development of thyroid carcinoma, as is environmental radiation exposure. Iodine deficiency, immune disorders involving the thyroid gland, and genetic factors are associated with an increased risk of thyroid cancer as well. Localized thyroid cancer may be palpable as one or more thyroid nodules. More commonly, the disease presents with anterior cervical lymphadenopathy. Metastases to bone and lung also may occur. Metastatic disease does not necessarily portend a poorer chance of survival.

Therapy for thyroid carcinoma consists of surgical extirpation or the administration of iodine[131] if distant metastases exist. External radiation and chemotherapy are not indicated in the management of thyroid cancer in children. Although the overall survival figures appear favorable, a notable incidence of late relapses occurs, and patients must be followed for a prolonged time.

Adrenal Cortex Tumors

Tumors of the adrenal cortex are either benign adenomas or malignant carcinoma. Both tumor types may be hormonally active or inactive. Virilism and Cushing syndrome are the most common presenting manifestations. Feminizing or aldosterone-secreting tumors are extremely rare. Adenomas are localized tumors but may be present in both adrenal glands. Carcinomas may spread locally, regionally, or to distant sites such as lung and bone.

For a patient with an adenoma, surgical removal of the tumor generally is curative. Carcinomas are much more aggressive tumors. Chemotherapy may be helpful, but surgical removal of primary, metastatic, and recurrent disease appears to offer the best chances for long-term survival. Nevertheless, chances for survival are poor. Endocrine symptoms associated with unresectable carcinomas usually can be managed medically.

Suggested Readings

Behel CA, Bhattacharyya N, Hutchinson C, et al. Alimentary tract malignancies in children. *J Pediatr Surg* 1997;32:1004.

Douglas EC, Pratt CB. Management of infrequent cancers of childhood. In: Pizzo PA, Poplack DG, eds. *Principles and practice of pediatric oncology,* 3rd ed. Philadelphia: Lippincott–Raven, 1997:977.

Fabre M, Yilmaz F, Buendia MA. Hepatic tumors in childhood: experience on 245 tumors and review of literature. *Ann Pathol* 2004;24:536.

Hameed R, Parkes S, Davies, P, Morland BJ. Paediatric malignant tumors of the gastrointestinal tract in the West Midland, UK, 1957–2000: a large population based survey. *Pediatr Blood Cancer* 2004;43:257.

Katzenstein HM, Krailo MD, Malogolowkin MH, et al. Hepatocellular carcinoma in children and adolescents: results from the Pediatric Oncology Group and the Children's Cancer Group intergroup study. *J Clin Oncol* 2002;20:2789.

Stratakis CA, Chrousos GP. Endocrine tumors. In: Pizzo PA, Poplack DG, eds. *Principles and practice of pediatric oncology,* 3rd ed. Philadelphia: Lippincott–Raven, 1997:947.

CHAPTER 313 ■ GONADAL AND GERM CELL NEOPLASMS

VICTOR A. LEWIS AND DOUGLAS R. STROTHER

Germ cell tumors (GCT) constitute 1% of cancers in children less than 15 years of age. Located mostly close to the vertical midline, they can be gonadal or extragonadal. As precursors of sperm and egg cells, germ cells have the ability to produce a multiplicity of tumors with varying histology and anatomic distribution (Box 313.1). The peak incidence of extragonadal GCT is in early childhood, and the peak incidence of gonadal GCT is in adolescents.

EMBRYOLOGY

Several hypotheses have been proposed to explain the occurrence of GCT in extragonadal sites. During the migration of the germ cells from the yolk sac wall to the hindgut and to the gonadal ridge, some cells may be left behind or stray from the normal path and come to rest at various midline sites in the embryo. Viable cells may later undergo a transformation and give rise to tumors in those locations. Alternatively, GCT may arise from pluripotent embryonal cells that failed to develop along normal differentiation pathways and undergo cancerous transformation.

Histologically, GCT can have benign and malignant elements. Although their locations may vary, their histology remains the same. They are classified based on the malignant potential of the cancer cells as well as the stage at which this development occurs. Multipotential germ cells may differentiate into unipotential primitive germ cells from which the ovaries and testes develop. Germinomas are a cancerous development of the unipotential primitive germs cells. *Seminomas* refer to

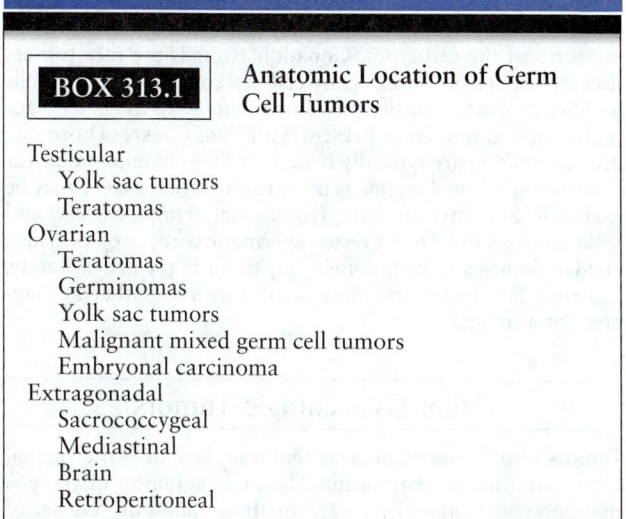

GCT of the testes, whereas similar tumors of the ovary are called *dysgerminomas*. The multipotential germ cell also may undergo embryonal differentiation. Tumors arising from this early stage are called *embryonal carcinoma*. Further differentiation of the multipotential germ cells gives rise to embryonal and extraembryonal structures. Tumors from the former are called *teratomas* and may be mature, immature, or malignant. Extraembryonal structures include the yolk sac and placenta. Tumors arising from the cells forming those structures are called *yolk sac tumors* or *endodermal sinus tumors*, and *choriocarcinomas*, respectively (Fig. 313.1).

PATHOLOGY

Histologic variations exist between and within GCT. Because treatment is determined by the most malignant component, a meticulous histologic assessment of the whole tumor is necessary. Germinomas are composed entirely of malignant germ cell elements. They are the most common pure GCT of the ovary and central nervous system. Embryonal carcinoma rarely occurs as a single histologic subtype and is seen much more commonly as a component of a mixed GCT. Embryonal carcinoma is characterized histologically by anaplasia, necrosis, and frequent mitoses; these tumors are highly malignant. Teratomas contain elements from at least two of the three germ cell layers: endoderm, mesoderm, and ectoderm. In a mature teratoma, elements are fully differentiated, and the tumor may contain teeth, bone, hair, and skin. Immature teratomas contain elements more reminiscent of fetal or embryonal structures. Malignant teratomas most commonly contain yolk sac tumor elements but also may have elements of neuroblastoma or medulloepithelioma. Yolk sac tumors are the most common malignant GCT of the young child and the most common type of malignant GCT of the testes of infant and young boys. The most common histologic patterns of yolk sac tumor contain Schiller-Duval bodies. Choriocarcinoma microscopically resembles the chorion layer of the placenta, with multinucleated syncytiotrophoblasts and cytotrophoblasts. It may arise from the nongestational pluripotent germ cell or from the gestational placenta in a pregnant woman.

Alpha-fetoprotein (α-FP) and the beta subunit of human chorionic gonadotropin (β-HCG) can be used as diagnostic and clinical markers for GCT. First produced by the yolk sac and later by the liver and gastrointestinal tract, α-FP also may be produced by yolk sac tumors and, less commonly, by choriocarcinomas. Serial measurements of this marker in serum can be used to monitor disease and effects of treatment. β-HCG is produced by the syncytiotrophoblasts of the placenta. Choriocarcinomas, germinomas, and, less commonly, embryonal carcinomas show positive histologic staining. This marker is used to monitor disease status similar to α-FP.

Anatomic Distribution

Two percent of all malignant cancers in boys are testicular tumors. The majority of these tumors occur in children less than 5 years of age or in the postpubertal period. Three-quarters of testicular tumors in boys are GCT, and two-thirds of those are yolk sac tumors. Teratomas constitute about 10% of all testicular tumors. Undescended testes remain a significant risk factor for the development of testicular cancer.

In girls, 20% of GCT occur in the premenarchal age group. Ovarian neoplasms are predominantly GCT, and the majority of those are teratomas. The risk of malignancy is highest in the younger age groups. Germinomas are the most common germ cell malignancy of the ovary followed by yolk sac tumor, malignant mixed GCT, and embryonal carcinoma.

Sacrococcygeal tumors represent 75% of extragonadal GCT (EGCT); tumors in the mediastinum, brain, and retroperitoneum comprise the remaining 25%. A female preponderance exists for EGCT. Tumors diagnosed in the first month of life tend to be benign, whereas those occurring later are commonly malignant. Intrathoracic GCT affect boys more than girls, tend to occur mostly in the anterior mediastinum, and are teratomas

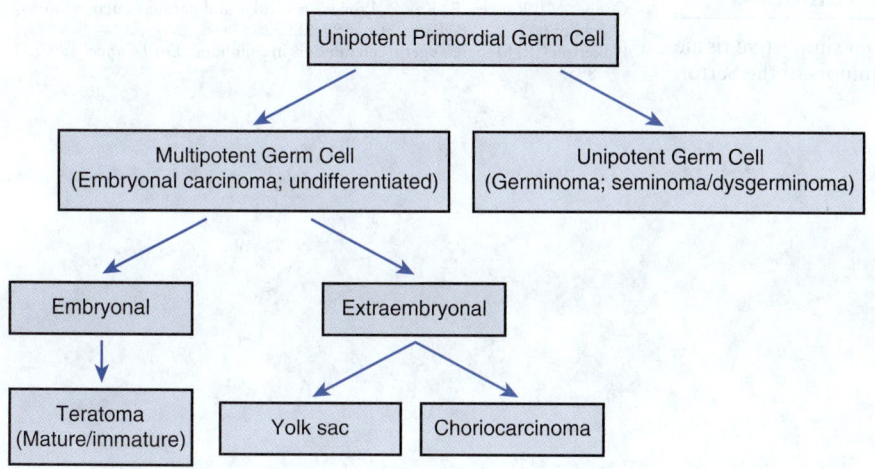

FIGURE 313.1. Differentiation of germ cell tumors.

in a majority of cases. In the brain, GCT are twice as frequent in the pineal gland as they are in the suprasellar region, and they occur much more commonly in boys. Although mostly germinomas, they may be malignant mixed GCT.

CLINICAL MANIFESTATIONS AND COMPLICATIONS

Extracranial GCT are relatively asymptomatic unless they press on vital structures and affect their function. They may present with pain or as nontender masses. Intrathoracic GCT often are discovered as incidental findings while evaluating other illnesses. Testicular tumors present as painless masses, unlike the swelling seen from infection, trauma, and torsion. There may be accompanying inguinal hernias and hydrocele. Positive transillumination may mask the tumor. Ovarian tumors present with pain, distention, and a palpable mass in the belly. Constipation, enuresis, vaginal bleeding, and amenorrhea may be other presenting features. Precocious puberty tends to suggest a nongerminomatous GCT. For all patients with GCT, an evaluation of metastatic spread using chest radiography, computed tomography (CT) scanning of the chest, abdomen and pelvis, as well as technetium bone scanning is necessary to assess the extent of disease. Intracranial lesions should be assessed with cranial CT or magnetic resonance imaging (MRI). MRI of the spinal cord, along with a lumbar puncture, also should be included in the work-up. Spinal fluid should be examined for the presence of tumor markers as well as malignant cells.

THERAPY

GCT are treated primarily with chemotherapy, with or without radiation. Radiation also is used to treat most types of intracranial GCT. Cooperative groups in pediatric oncology are presently focusing on defining good and bad features in the tumors of patients with GCT so that treatment may be optimized and long-term effects minimized. Where possible, the tumor should be completely excised without sacrificing vital structures. This approach may be curative for benign tumors. Chemotherapy is beneficial when tumors cannot be completely removed, have spread, or contain malignant elements. Cisplatin-based regimens tend to show the best activity against the tumors, but other drugs are also effective. Importantly, children with GCT should be treated at centers having pediatric subspecialty care, where cooperative group guidelines and protocols are available.

Non–Germ Cell Gonadal Tumors

Sex cord and stromal tumors may arise from supportive tissue within the gonads. In the testes, these are tumors of the Sertoli and Leydig cells, and in the ovary, they are tumors of the granulosa and theca cells. Tumors may exist in boys and girls as mixtures of the cell types. Gonadoblastomas are rare tumors that represent a mixture of germ cell, sex cord, and stromal cells and are characteristically seen in patients with dysgenetic gonads. These tumors may present with signs of excess hormone production and are typically benign. If they contain malignant elements, treatment regimens that are effective for GCT may be useful. Rhabdomyosarcoma, lymphoma, neuroblastoma, and leukemia may involve the testes, spermatic cord, or epididymis. Hemangiomas and lymphomas may occur in the penis. Rarely, leukemia and lymphoma may involve ovaries, either at diagnosis or at relapse.

Other Gynecologic Tumors

Tumors of the lower female genital tract including the vagina, cervix, and uterus may occur. The most common of these is rhabdomyosarcoma of the sarcoma botryoides, or "cluster of grapes," type seen in cavitary organs of young children. The management of rhabdomyosarcoma is discussed in Chapter 309, Soft-Tissue Sarcomas. The prognosis for these patients is very good. Adenocarcinoma of the vagina and cervix may be seen in adolescent girls, particularly those who were exposed to diethylstilbestrol (DES) during gestation. Young girls with vaginal symptoms, with or without a history of DES exposure, should undergo a complete pelvic examination. This should include cytologic smears and biopsy of suspicious lesions. Primary treatment for carcinoma includes surgery and radiation therapy. Chemotherapy has shown variable success when used in the treatment of metastatic disease.

Although primary malignant tumors of the breast have been seen in girls as young as 3 years, the majority of these tumors in children are benign. Fibroadenomas are the most common tumors. They may be bilateral and massive. Differentiation of these lesions from virginal hypertrophy early in their growth may be difficult. Malignant infiltration of the breast can occur in acute leukemia, especially in the postpubertal child, and in lymphoma and rhabdomyosarcoma. Less than 0.1% of all breast cancer occurs in women younger than 20 years. Juvenile carcinoma of the breast is treated with surgical excision. Metastases are unlikely, but when they exist, management similar to that used with adult women should be considered.

Suggested Readings

Castleberry RP, Cushing B, Perlman E, et al. Germ cell tumors. In: Pizzo PA, Poplack DG, eds. *Principles and practice of pediatric oncology,* 3rd ed. Philadelphia: Lippincott–Raven, 1997:921.

Coppes MJ, Rackley R, Kay R. Primary testicular and paratesticular tumors of childhood. *Med Pediatr Oncol* 1994;22:329.

Pinkerton CR. Malignant germ cell tumours in childhood. *Eur J Cancer* 1997;33: 895.

CHAPTER 314 ■ HISTIOCYTIC PROLIFERATIVE DISEASES

KENNETH L. McCLAIN

LANGERHANS CELL HISTIOCYTOSIS

Epidemiology

The incidence of Langerhans cell histiocytosis (LCH) is approximately 5 per million children or 1 in 25,000 live births. Based on the U.S. census for 2000, this would mean approximately 300 new cases diagnosed each year in this country. LCH is the preferred term instead of the histiocytosis X syndromes (Letterer-Siwe disease, Hand-Schüller-Christian syndrome, and eosinophilic granuloma) because the proliferative cell associated with this disease is a bone marrow–derived dendritic histiocyte called the *Langerhans cell*. It contains characteristic pentalaminar Birbeck granules seen by electron microscopy. These cells also stain with monoclonal antibodies to the CD1a antigen and a newly recognized antigen, langerin, the protein of the Birbeck granules.

Pathogenesis

The Langerhans cell diseases are not malignant, despite the presence of clonal proliferations of the Langerhans cells in solitary or diffuse lesions. Current etiologic theories revolve around immunologic dysregulation, because no viral or other infectious cause has been identified. Like other antigen-processing cells, the Langerhans cells produce and receive cytokines to or from T lymphocytes and macrophages, including tumor necrosis factor-alpha, granulocyte-macrophage colony-stimulating factor, interleukin-1, interferon-gamma, and interleukin-10. Somewhere in the interactive cycle, regulatory elements are lost such that the histiocytes proliferate locally or diffusely along with lymphocytes, macrophages, and eosinophils.

Clinical Manifestations and Diagnosis

Many patients present with a seborrheic rash of the scalp and periauricular regions similar to cradle cap or eczema (Box 314.1). Others have a diffuse erythematous, papular rash that may resemble a *Candida* diaper rash (Fig. 314.1). Copious white material draining from ears mimics chronic otitis externa. Most patients have painful lesions of the skull (Fig. 314.2), ribs, femurs, vertebra or mandible, skin, or lymph node involvement (low-risk disease). Hepatosplenomegaly, anemia, thrombocytopenia, and pulmonary disease with organ dysfunction occur in patients with the high-risk disease. Of the children presenting with generalized LCH, involvement of various organ systems is found in bone (100%), skin (88%), liver (71%), lung (54%), lymph nodes (42%), spleen (25%), bone marrow (18%), and central nervous system (CNS; pituitary or parenchymal lesions)

(16%). Organ dysfunction includes evidence of hepatic failure by a total protein less than 5.5 g/dL, albumin less than 2.5 g/dL, total bilirubin of more than 1.5 mg/dL, edema, and ascites. Hematologic dysfunction is defined by a hemoglobin less than 10 g/dL, leukocyte count less than 4,000/μL, neutrophils less than 1,500/μL, and platelets less than 100,000/μL. Pulmonary dysfunction includes tachypnea, dyspnea, cyanosis, cough, pneumothorax, and pleural effusion.

Patient evaluation should include a complete history and physical examination with complete blood count, bone marrow aspirate and biopsy when an abnormal blood count is found, radiographic survey of the complete skeleton, skull survey, and chest radiography, as well as radionucleotide bone scan. A high-resolution chest computed tomography scan is done if abnormalities are seen by plain chest radiography or if respiratory distress is present. A magnetic resonance imaging (MRI) scan of the brain is indicated when CNS symptoms are present. If there are symptoms of diabetes insipidus, careful monitoring of liquid intake and output, serum, and urine osmolality and a water deprivation test are needed. The biopsy material from an affected site should be sent for immunocytochemistry evaluation with anti-langerin and CD1a stains and sometimes for electron microscopy to look for Birbeck granules.

Treatment

It is critical that patients be registered on the most current treatment protocols of the Histiocyte Society so advances in the knowledge and treatment of these diseases can be achieved. (Contact the Histiocytosis Association of America for protocol information: 1-856-589-6606.)

BOX 314.1 **Signs and Symptoms of Langerhans Cell Histiocytosis**

Fever
Skin rash: eczematoid scalp rash; erythematous, papular (*Candida*-like) anywhere, but especially in the diaper area and lower abdomen; ulcers in the groin, axillae, or mouth
Gingival hypertrophy, loose teeth
Chronic otitis externa with white discharge
Bone lesions: swelling, tenderness
Protuberant abdomen: hepatosplenomegaly
Lymphadenopathy
Diarrhea
Tachypnea: may mimic viral pneumonia or present with a mediastinal mass
Polydipsia/polyuria

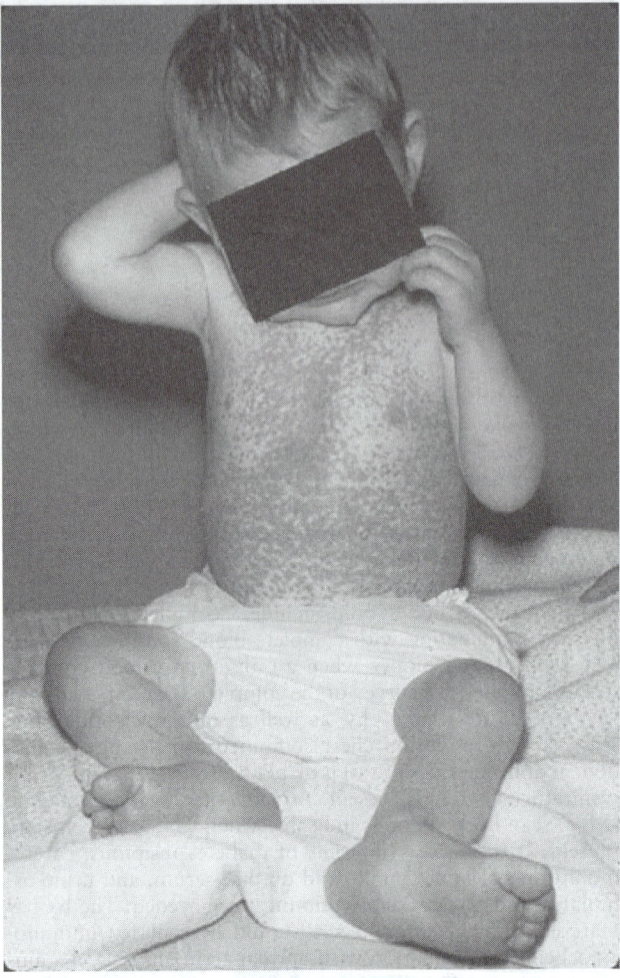

FIGURE 314.1. Diffuse erythematous-papular rash of Langerhans cell histiocytosis.

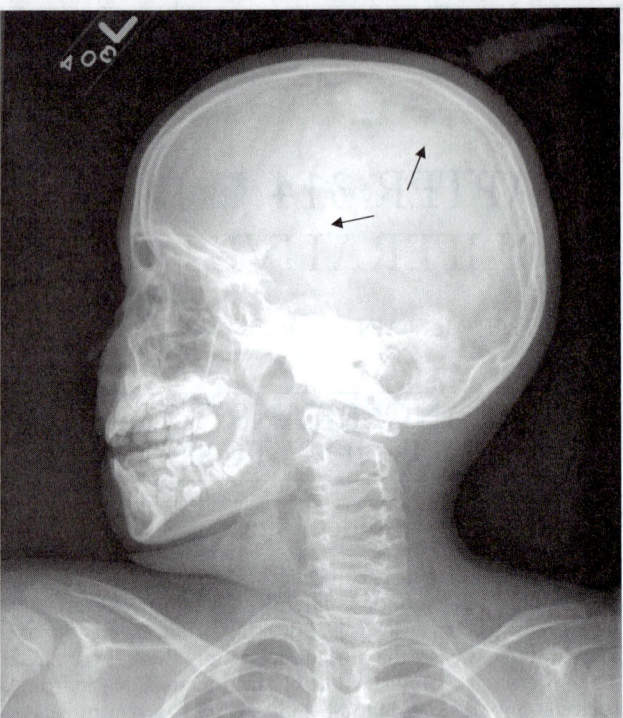

FIGURE 314.2. Lateral skull radiograph of Langerhans cell histiocytosis patient showing lytic lesions in the temporal and parietal bones.

Although some solitary skull lesions can be treated with curretage alone, steroid injections, or radiotherapy, these are not the correct approaches for patients with lesions of the orbits, mastoid, sphenoid, or temporal bones. Patients with involvement of these sites have a markedly increased chance of developing diabetes insipidus or parenchymal brain disease. When single-agent therapy is applied to these disease sites, 40% of the patients will develop diabetes insipidus, as compared with fewer than 20% of patients treated with 6 months of vinblastine (Velban) and prednisone.

According to Gadner and colleagues, patients with low-risk disease are currently randomized between 6 and 12 months of treatment with vinblastine and prednisone and are essentially all cured. High-risk patients with organ dysfunction receive 1 year of therapy. Currently all receive 1 year of vinblastine, prednisone, and mercaptopurine. Half of the patients are randomized to receive methotrexate also to determine whether more patients can be cured. Those who do not respond by the sixth week of treatment should be switched to another protocol. Patients who respond by the sixth or twelfth week of therapy have a much better prognosis than those who do not respond by that time. Various chemotherapy combinations and anti–tumor necrosis factor-alpha therapy are being investigated. A few patients have been successfully treated with high-dose chemotherapy and rescue by bone marrow transplantation. *Pneumocystis carinii* infection, a constant threat to patients receiving chemotherapy, is prevented by prophylactic treatment with trimethoprim-sulfamethoxazole during therapy and for 6 months after completing therapy.

Late Effects of Disease and Treatment

LCH is a chronic disease with a waxing and waning nature that tries the patience of all involved. Many patients have diabetes insipidus, growth failure, intellectual impairment, neurologic deficit, emotional or orthopedic problems, chronic lung disease, or hearing deficits. Up to 50% of patients with diabetes insipidus will develop other endocrinopathies as late as 10 years after the onset of LCH. Of greater concern are recent data showing that for patients with diabetes insipidus who were followed-up for 5 years, 50% developed signs of neurologic involvment on MRI (mass lesions or T_2-weighted enhancement of the cerebellum, pons, or basal ganglia (Fig. 314.3). Symptoms of neurologic LCH (ataxia, dysarthria, dysmetria, or learning problems) occur in one half of the 50% who have MRI findings of LCH. These data further support the need to treat patients with mastoid, orbiatal, or temporal bone lesions, as noted before. Patients with LCH also have an increased incidence of malignant diseases, mostly lymphomas and leukemias.

HEMOPHAGOCYTIC LYMPHOHISTIOCYTOSES: FAMILIAL OR SPORADIC

Epidemiology

The incidence of the hemophagocytic lymphohistiocytosis (HLH) is thought to be 1 to 2 per million based on a survey done in the Nordic countries. However, underrecognition

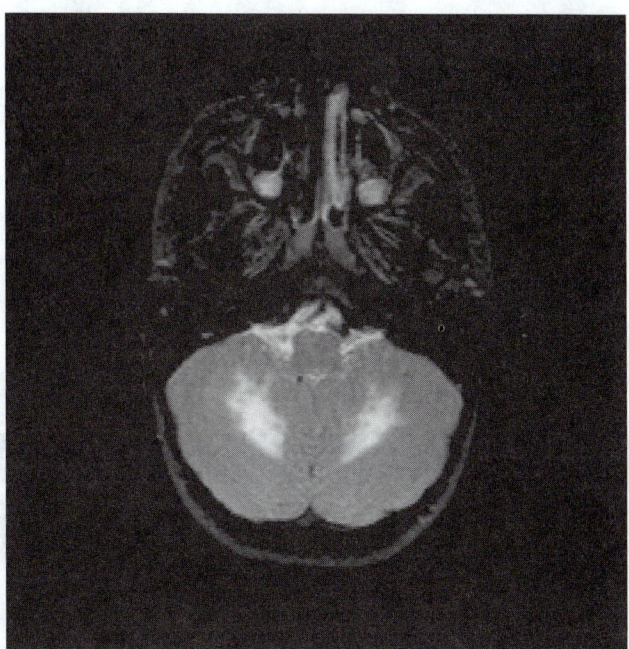

FIGURE 314.3. Magnetic resonance imaging scan of a patient with Langerhans cell histiocytosis with neurodegenerative disease showing T_2-weighted enhancement of white matter in the cerebellum.

of this entity is common, and it is likely that many children die without a proper diagnosis. As reported by Palazzi and associates and Rooms and colleagues, many patients are thought to have fever of unknown origin, hepatitis, sepsis, or even to be victims of abuse when presenting with only CNS findings.

Pathogenesis

HLH is caused by aggressive proliferation of macrophages in the bone marrow, lymph nodes, spleen, liver, and CNS, most often accompanied by hemophagocytosis of other blood cells. This proliferation is promoted by a "cytokine storm" of interferon-gamma, interleukin-10, tumor necrosis factor, and other cytokines in the context of several types of immune dysregulation. Among familial cases, defects on chromosome 10 (the perforin gene) chromosome 9 (unknown gene), and the X-linked lymphoproliferative gene have been identified. Evidence for viral infections as causes of HLH may be difficult to obtain and requires molecular as well as serologic tests. Bacteria and other organisms also may cause HLH, or it may be malignancy associated. The macrophage activation syndrome in patients with rhematoid arthritis has many of the same features, but it may be treated with slightly less aggressive therapy. Familial syndromes are distinct because of the high rate of consanguinity and occurrence in identical twins or siblings. Identical clinical and laboratory features occur in the familial and sporadic cases.

Clinical Manifestations and Laboratory Diagnosis

Patients present with high spiking fevers, splenomegaly, lymphadenopathy, rashes, and often CNS findings of somnolence, seizures, bradycardia, or even respiratory depression (Box 314.2). Key laboratory findings include cytopenias of at least two lines, coagulopathy with decreased fibrinogen, hypertriglyceridemia, elevated liver enzymes, and extraordinarily

---

BOX 314.2	Signs and Symptoms of Hemophagocytic Lymphohistiocytosis

Fever
Hepatosplenomegaly
Pallor
Petechiae
Lymphadenopathy
Seizures, somnolence, coma
Cytopenia in two cell lines
Hyperbilirubinemia and elevated liver enzymes
Elevated ferritin or triglycerides
Low fibrinogen
Prolonged prothrombin time and partial thromboplastin time
Hemophagocytosis in bone marrow or lymph node
Decreased natural killer (NK) cell activity and decreased perforin staining in NK and T cells
Elevated interleukin-2 receptor (soluble CD25) greater than 2,400 U/mL
Mutations in perforin or *MUNC-13* gene

---

elevated serum ferritin levels (more than 10,000 ng/mL, but a value greater than 500 ng/mL is considered one of the diagnostic criteria). Up to 40% of patients have defective natural killer (NK) cell function. It is important to assay the cytotoxic T lymphocytes and NK cells for perforin because defects in this gene are critical to NK activity.

Treatment

Therapy for children with HLH had been frustratingly ineffective until 1994, when the Histiocyte Society initiated the HLH treatment protocol (see contact information in the section on LCH), as reported by Henter and associates. Before then, nearly all patients died of coagulopathy or secondary infections. Patients are treated with dexamethasone (Decadron), etoposide (VePesid), and cyclosporine. For young children with absent NK cell activity and markedly decreased perforin staining of NK cells or cytotoxic T lymphocytes, or proven cases of familial HLH, bone marrow transplantation is necessary and is curative in more than 60% of patients. Older children who have the infection-associated form and who regain normal NK function may be cured with only 8 weeks of treatment.

SINUS HISTIOCYTOSIS WITH MASSIVE LYMPHADENOPATHY

Children with sinus histiocytosis with massive lymphadenopathy present with a marked enlargement of cervical lymph nodes, fever, elevated erythrocyte sedimentation rate, neutrophilia, and eosinophilia. Other sites include the orbit and other bones, nose, pharynx, lungs, and skin. Some patients with fatal cases have underlying immune deficiency such as Wiskott-Aldrich syndrome or autoimmune phenomena. Approximately 7% of these patients die of secondary infections, bleeding, or malignant disease. Therapies have included surgery alone for isolated lymph node masses and oral prednisone or mercaptopurine (Purinethol) and methotrexate (Mexate) for systemic disease.

OTHER SYNDROMES

Other rare syndromes include monocytic leukemia, chronic myelomonocytic leukemia, "true histiocytic lymphoma," and benign xanthogranuloma.

Suggested Readings

Gadner H, Grois N, Arico M, et al. A randomized trial of treatment for multi-system Langerhans cell histiocytosis. *J Pediatr* 2001;138:728.

Henter J-I, Samuelsson-Horne AC, Arico M, et al. Treatment of hemophagocytic lymphohistiocytosis with HLH-94 immunochemotherapy and bone marrow transplantation. *Blood* 2002;100:2367.

Ladisch S, Jaffe ES. Histiocytoses. In: Pizzo PA, Poplack DG, eds. *Principles and practice of pediatric oncology*, 4th ed. Philadelphia: Lippincott Williams & Wilkins, 2002:733.

Palazzi DK, McClain KL, Kaplan SL. Hemophagocytic syndrome in children: an important diagnostic consideration in fever of unknown origin. *Clin Infect Dis* 2003;36:306.

Rooms L, Fitzgerald N, McClain KL. Hemophagocytic lymphohistiocytosis (HLH) masquerading as child abuse: presentation of three cases and review of central nervous system findings in HLH. *Pediatrics* 2003;111:e636.

CHAPTER 315 ■ VASCULAR MALFORMATIONS

DENISE W. METRY AND MARY L. BRANDT

The nomenclature used to describe vascular birthmarks has long been a source of confusion in the medical literature. A biologic classification system proposed by Mulliken and Glowacki led to the current understanding of vascular birthmarks. This classification system, the most widely accepted standard for categorizing vascular birthmarks today, is the official classification system of the International Society for the Study of Vascular Anomalies. It is based on clinical behavior and cellular dynamics, and it divides vascular birthmarks into two main categories: vascular tumors (VTs) and vascular malformations (VMs).

VTs are dynamic lesions, sometimes present at birth, that are characterized by endothelial cell hyperplasia and demonstrate proliferation in infancy. In contrast, VMs almost always are present at birth (although they may not manifest until later in childhood), arise from dysmorphogenesis, exhibit normal cellular turnover, and are static or undergo slow expansion over time. VMs can be subdivided further on the basis of flow rate (fast or slow) and resemblance to vessel type (capillary, lymphatic, venous, or arteriovenous), and they can occur alone or in combination (Box 315.1). Using this classification system, more than 90% of vascular birthmarks can be distinguished from one another based on careful history and physical examination, without the need for performing ancillary studies. Accurate classification is important for understanding prognosis, potential complications, and appropriate patient management. Although most vascular anomalies are sporadic, mendelian inheritance has been observed in some families. Several causative genes, which primarily seem to affect endothelial cells, have been identified recently and have shed light on the pathophysiologic pathways involved.

CAPILLARY MALFORMATIONS

Capillary malformations (CMs) ("port-wine stains") are present at birth as bright red patches that may occur in any cutaneous location (Fig. 315.1). Histologically, they are composed of dilated capillary- to venule-sized vessels in the

---

BOX 315.1   **Classification of Vascular Malformations**

Slow-Flow
    Capillary (port-wine stain)
    Lymphatic
    Venous
Fast-Flow
    Arteriovenous
Combined (Klippel-Trenaunay Syndrome; Parkes-Weber Syndrome)

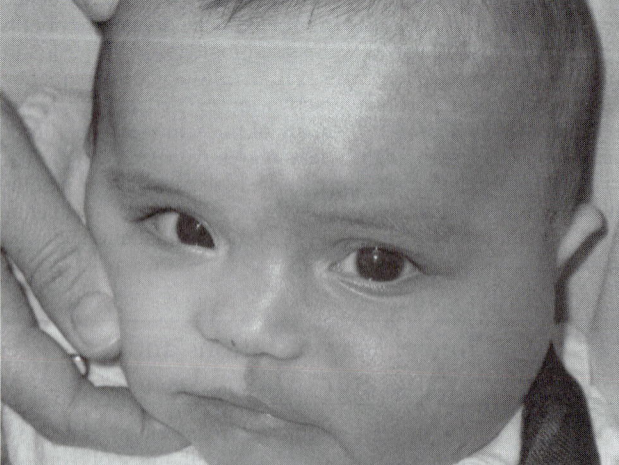

FIGURE 315.1. Capillary malformation (port-wine stain). See Color Figure 315.1 in color section.

superficial dermis, which have a reduced number of normal, surrounding nerve fibers. CMs often lighten deceptively in the first year of life, but persist thereafter. Facial CMs show a tendency to thicken, darken, and develop fibrovascular nodules, sometimes as early as during adolescence. For unknown reasons, such changes rarely occur in CMs affecting nonfacial locations. However, cutaneous CMs in any location may be associated less commonly with underlying soft tissue and skeletal hypertrophy. For example, facial CMs that involve the trigeminal V3 dermatome may result in a number of dental complications, including gingival hyperplasia, maxillary or mandibular overgrowth, and open bite deformity. Midline spinal or scalp CMs, especially those associated with other midline developmental abnormalities such as hypertrichosis, cutaneous dimples, or sinuses, can be a clue to occult spinal or cranial dysraphism.

In most cases, CMs pose predominantly cosmetic concerns. The flashlamp-pumped, pulsed-dye laser is a well-established and safe treatment for CMs. Laser treatments may be more effective when initiated earlier in childhood, before significant vascular dilatation or hypertrophic changes occur, but other factors such as location, size, and skin pigmentation also may affect response. Individual response to therapy and the number of treatment sessions required are variable; the lateral face and trunk tend to respond better than do the extremities or central face. Treatment is safe, with minimal postprocedure discomfort and a low risk of scarring, but most CMs lighten rather than disappear completely. Because the depth of flashlamp-pumped, pulsed-dye laser penetration is less than 1.2 mm, soft tissue and skeletal hypertrophy and fibrovascular proliferation still may develop, necessitating use of other forms of intervention.

Sturge-Weber syndrome (SWS) is the association of a facial CM with ipsilateral ocular and leptomeningeal vascular anomalies. Affected children nearly always have a CM that involves the trigeminal V1 dermatome, although fewer than 10% of infants who present with this distribution have SWS. Leptomeningeal involvement, which generally can be detected by T_1-weighted, gadolinium-enhanced magnetic resonance imaging (MRI), often leads to early-onset seizures, generally by the time the child reaches 2 years of age. Without prompt pharmacologic management, brain hypoxia and psychomotor deterioration may ensue. Regular ophthalmologic examinations are required for children at risk for development of SWS because increased choroidal vascularity can cause retinal detachment, glaucoma, and blindness. The Sturge-Weber Foundation is a well-established support network for affected patients and their families and for research.

Common types of vascular birthmarks that often are confused with the CM are popularly known as the "angel kiss" (forehead, eyelids, glabella, nose, and upper lip) and "stork bite" (on the nape). These birthmarks represent a minor dilatation of superficial dermal vessels, and most of them fade by the time the child is 1 to 2 years of age, although lesions of the nape often persist.

VENOUS MALFORMATIONS

VMs are structural anomalies of the venous vasculature. They generally involve the skin, subcutaneous tissues, or mucosa as soft, deep-blue masses that are easily compressible and slowly refill on release. They are present, although not always evident, at birth and can involve virtually any anatomic site. VMs swell with dependency or activity and may undergo slow expansion over time. Extensive VMs, especially those involving an extremity, can cause localized intravascular coagulopathy (LIC) owing to the chronic consumption of clotting factors,

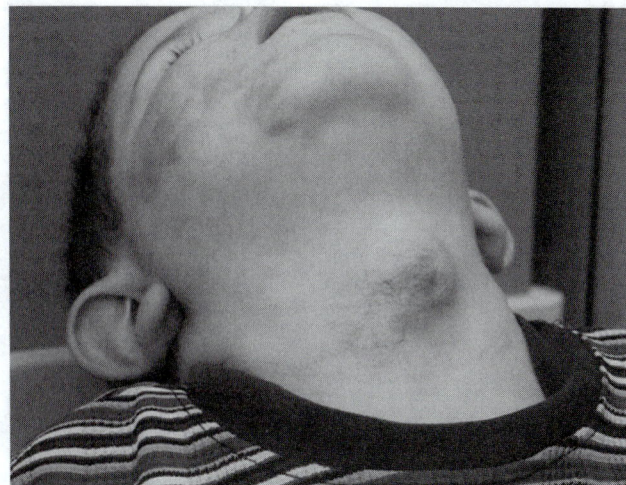

FIGURE 315.2. Venous malformation.

evidenced by low fibrinogen, elevated D-dimers, and a normal or moderately low platelet count. LIC also can cause the formation of phleboliths, which are a characteristic feature of VMs, even early in childhood, and are a common source of localized pain. Pain and stiffness at the site of a VM on morning awakening and dull aching are other common complaints. LIC also can lead to bleeding, which can be especially problematic when a VM involves the joint synovium.

Most VMs are solitary and localized, although multiple and extensive lesions also can occur. VMs of the head and neck, usually unilateral, can lead to progressive distortion of facial features as well as dental malalignment, open bite deformity, enlargement of the orbit, or obstructive sleep apnea, depending on the location (Fig. 315.2). Patients with craniofacial VMs also have up to a 25% incidence of developmental venous anomalies (DVAs) in the brain; these DVAs consist of dilated intramedullary veins converging into a large draining vein and are not true cerebral VMs. DVAs generally cause no symptoms or complications, including cerebral hemorrhage. VMs of the limb can involve the skin alone or extend into muscles, bone, and/or joints, causing swelling, functional impairment, and limited motility. Intraosseous VMs can lead to fractures, and lesions of the joint synovium, especially those associated with LIC, can lead to painful hemarthroses and progressive degenerative arthritis.

Although most VMs occur sporadically, multifocal lesions may be familial, such as occurs in the autosomal dominant, familial cutaneous-mucosal VM syndrome, characterized by small, dome-shaped lesions. Blue-rubber bleb nevus syndrome is a rare, autosomal dominant or sporadic disorder characterized by skin (most commonly trunk, palms, and soles) and bowel VMs that commonly lead to chronic gastrointestinal bleeding. Intussusception and, more rarely, volvulus also may occur. Another VM subtype, the glomuvenous malformation (GVM), also known as glomangioma or glomus tumor, also frequently is inherited. GVM differs from classic VM by its bluish-purple, "cobblestone," and/or hyperkeratotic appearance, its lack of tendency to mucosal or deep muscle involvement, and its frequent tenderness to palpation (Fig. 315.3).

Magnetic resonance imaging (MRI) is the most informative imaging study for VMs; MR venography is particularly useful for extremity lesions. Ultrasound is the imaging study of choice if intussusception or volvulus is being considered, because the lesions usually originate in the small bowel. Treatment of VMs is reserved for those lesions causing significant functional

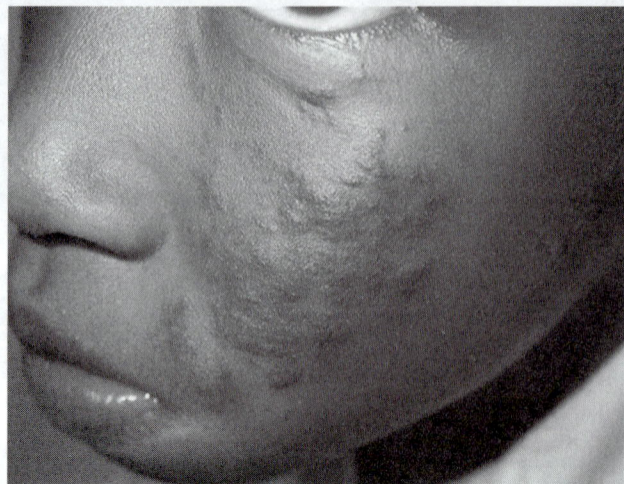

FIGURE 315.3. Glomuvenous malformation.

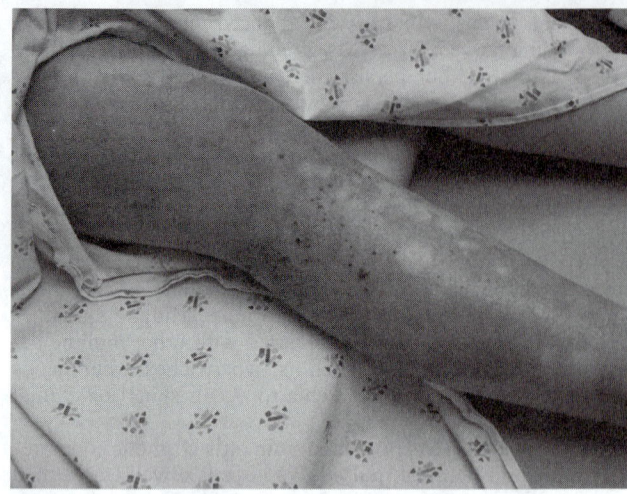

FIGURE 315.4. Lymphatic malformation.

compromise or cosmetic deformity. Protective measures, such as elastic compression stockings, are vital for patients with VMs of the extremities, although achieving correct fitting and using these stockings can be challenging in younger patients. Compression serves to decrease pain, minimize swelling, and improve coagulopathy. Whereas low-dose aspirin minimizes the pain associated with phlebothromboses, heparin often is required to minimize the painful hematoma or hemarthrosis associated with LIC. Sclerotherapy and surgical resection, performed alone or in combination, are other therapeutic options for VMs. However, multiple treatments over the course of years often are required, and cure is difficult to achieve, save for the small, best-localized lesion. For most actively treated VMs, eventual recanalization and recurrence are to be expected. In contrast to true VMs, GVMs show no response to elastic compression, which only serves to increase pain, or to aspirin, because such lesions have no associated coagulopathy.

LYMPHATIC MALFORMATIONS

Lymphatic malformations (LMs) usually are evident at birth or early childhood and may be localized, diffuse, or multiple in distribution. LMs can be characterized as microcystic, macrocystic, or combined. Previous nomenclature included the terms *lymphangioma* for primarily microcystic and *cystic hygroma* for primarily macrocystic lesions. LMs most commonly occur in the axilla/chest, cervicofacial, mediastinal, retroperitoneal, buttock, and anogenital regions. The overlying skin may be normal or may have a well-defined, patterned, or "geographic" red stain (Fig. 315.4). Microcystic LMs in the skin manifest as small, clear, fluid-filled vesicles that may turn dark red with intralesional bleeding (Fig. 315.5). Congenital lymphedema (Milroy disease), transient localized lymphedema with puffiness of the dorsal feet (as seen in Turner and Noonan syndromes), and intestinal lymphangiectasia also are included as types of LMs.

Common complications of LMs are intralesional bleeding (spontaneously or after trauma) and infection, both of which can result in episodic enlargement of the lesion, bruising, and pain. Swelling can occur indirectly with infection elsewhere in the body, a generally harmless occurrence. However, bacterial cellulitis within an LM can be a potentially dangerous situation, depending on the location. As with any vascular malformation,

slow expansion over time is the rule. Spontaneous involution of LMs has been reported, but it is rare.

A variety of other complications can result from LMs, depending on the location. Craniofacial LMs, which most commonly are combined microcystic and macrocystic, lead to progressive asymmetry and distortion of facial features. Pressure on the periodontal tissue may result in loss of teeth and/or enlargement and deformity of the mandible. Intraorbital LMs can cause orbital enlargement, exophthalmia, and visual axis occlusion; sudden proptosis and even visual loss can result from intralesional bleeding. Bulky involvement of the tongue impairs speech, and cervical LMs may result in airway obstruction; tracheostomy occasionally must be performed in young infants (Fig. 315.6). In extreme situations, performing an EXIT procedure to maintain the infant on placental "bypass" may be necessary to control the airway safely. Cervical and axillary lesions, often accompanied by mediastinal LMs, may cause recurrent chylothorax and chylopericardium. Limb LMs result in lymphedema, skeletal changes, distortion, and hypertrophy, sometimes leading to gigantism. Pelvic LM manifests with vaginal chylous discharge, bladder outlet obstruction,

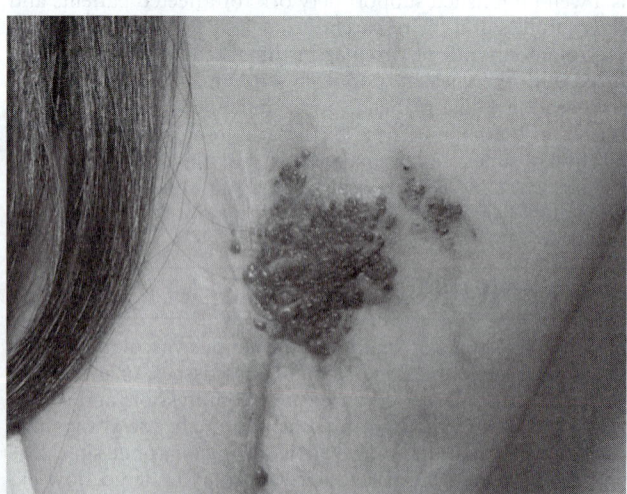

FIGURE 315.5. Recurrent microcystic lymphatic malformation superimposed on a previous surgical scar.

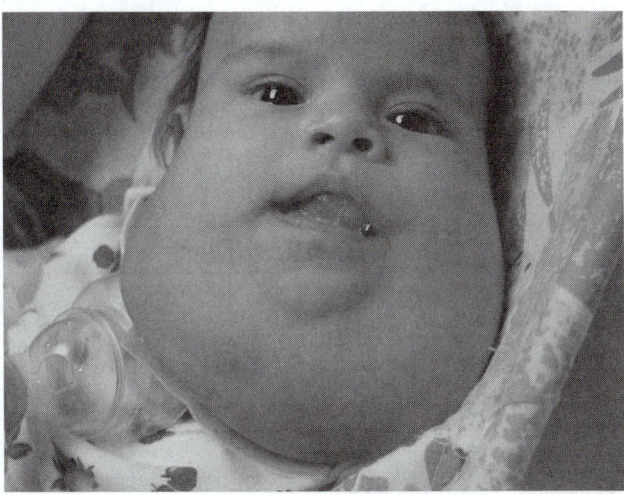

FIGURE 315.6. Macrocystic lymphatic malformation.

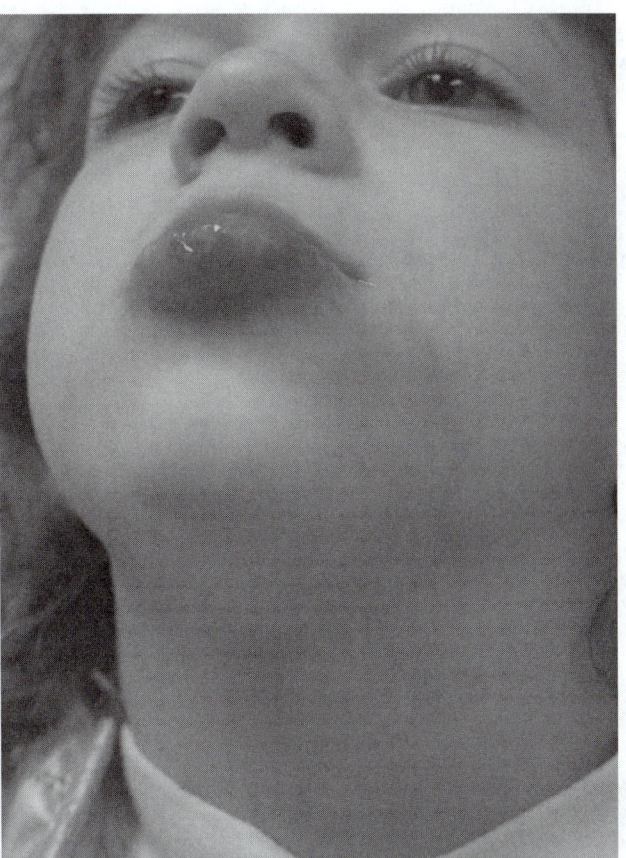

FIGURE 315.7. Arteriovenous malformation.

constipation, and/or recurrent infection. Abdominal LM with involvement of the gut, often accompanied by multiorgan involvement (lymphangiomatosis), may cause protein-losing enteropathy and hypoalbuminemia. Rupture may lead to chylous ascites. Similar to VMs, extensive LMs also may result in chronic LIC. Finally, a rare disorder, known as vanishing bone disease, Gorham syndrome, or phantom bone syndrome, is a disorder of diffuse soft tissue and skeletal LM. In this progressive, osteolytic process, bone is gradually replaced by capillaries and lymphatic clefts. Pain, bleeding, fractures, severe chronic disseminated intravascular coagulation, and sometimes death result.

MRI is the best means of determining the extent of the lesion; MR lymphangiography is especially useful for extremity lesions. Prenatal diagnosis of macrocystic LMs often is made by ultrasonography. Treatment of LMs, like that of VMs, is reserved for functional compromise or cosmetic deformity. For intralesional bleeding and cellulitis, symptomatic treatment generally suffices. Bacterial cellulitis occurring within cervicofacial LMs is potentially dangerous because of the risks of airway compromise. In such instances, systemic antibiotics should be administered at the first sign of swelling, pain, redness, or systemic toxicity. Also as for VMs, the mainstay of therapy for LMs includes surgery and/or sclerotherapy, although cure rarely is achieved except for the smallest, best-localized lesion. Attempts at surgical resection often are accompanied by a variety of intraoperative and postoperative complications, including recurrence. Aspiration, often followed by sclerotherapy with agents such as absolute ethanol, sodium tetradecylsulfate or OK-432 (a killed strain of group A *Streptococcus pyogenes*), is not effective for microcystic lesions but can be used as a temporizing measure for macrocystic LMs, alone or in conjunction with surgical techniques. Microcystic LMs of the skin can be treated with laser photocoagulation, but again this approach is a temporary measure reserved for patients who desire treatment for recurrent bleeding or pain. Elastic compression stockings, pneumatic compression devices, and massage all have proved useful in controlling the progressive lymphedema that often occurs with limb LMs.

ARTERIOVENOUS MALFORMATIONS

Arteriovenous malformations (AVMs) are fast-flow vascular anomalies that, when extensive, represent the most dangerous type of vascular anomaly. They are composed of microscopic and macroscopic arteriovenous fistulas. Early cutaneous AVMs may appear as a faint vascular stain that often is mistaken for a CM. However, an AVM eventually will manifest itself, often after trauma or with the onset of puberty, as a warm, pulsatile mass with draining, tortuous veins and deepening of color (Fig. 315.7). Chronic skin manifestations are those of ischemia, with recalcitrant ulceration, pain, bleeding, and disfigurement. High-output cardiac failure can occur with an extensive AVM.

Diagnosis may be confirmed by color Doppler ultrasonography or MRI/MR angiography. Most experts agree that in all but the best-localized lesions, intervention should not be considered until significant symptoms develop because treatment always is complex and difficult. In most cases, angiography is performed just before embolization and/or sclerotherapy. Although complete surgical excision is desirable for well-localized AVMs, as with other VMs, most lesions are so extensive and permeating that surgery cannot be performed. Furthermore, partial embolization or resection of an AVM invariably leads to a more ominous and symptomatic lesion, sometimes with severe disfigurement, limb amputation, or death resulting from visceral extension of a cephalic or truncal lesion.

COMBINED/COMPLEX VASCULAR ANOMALIES

Combined VMs are described by numerous eponyms that are best replaced by the use of the current classification system

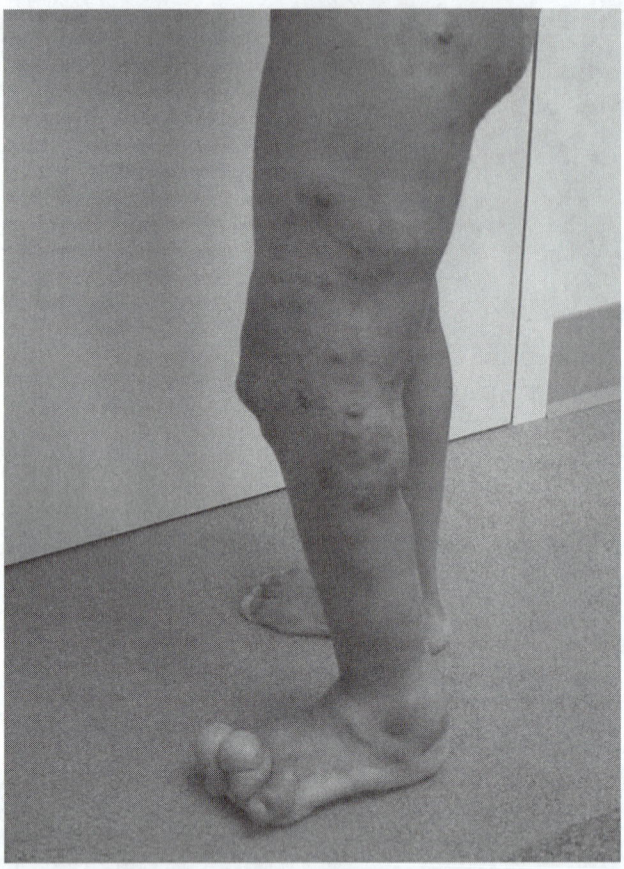

FIGURE 315.8. Combined capillary-lymphatic-venous malformation with soft tissue and skeletal overgrowth (Klippel-Trenaunay syndrome).

describing the abnormal vessels involved. For example, Klippel-Trenaunay syndrome is a combined CM-LM-VM, generally of the extremity, that often is accompanied by soft tissue and skeletal overgrowth (Fig. 315.8). Parkes-Weber syndrome is a combined, fast-flow CM-AVM, generally of the limb and proximal trunk.

Suggested Readings

Brouillard P, Vikkula M. Vascular malformations: localized defects in vascular morphogenesis. *Clin Genet* 2003;63:340.

Enjolras O, Garzon MC. Vascular stains, malformations, and tumors. In: Eichenfield L, Esterly N, Frieden I, eds. *Textbook of neonatal dermatology*. Philadelphia: WB Saunders, 2001:473.

Enjolras O, Mulliken JB. Vascular tumors and vascular malformations (new issues). *Adv Dermatol* 1998;13:375.

Enjolras O, Mulliken JB. Vascular malformations. In: Harper J, Oranje A, Prose N, eds. *Textbook of pediatric dermatology*. Oxford: Blackwell Science, 2000:975.

Mulliken J, Young A. *Vascular birthmarks: hemangiomas and malformations*. Philadelphia: WB Saunders, 1988.

Mulliken JB, Fishman SJ, Burrows PE. Vascular anomalies. *Curr Probl Surg* 2000;37:517.

Mulliken JB, Glowacki J. Hemangiomas and vascular malformations in infants and children: a classification based on endothelial characteristics. *Plast Reconstr Surg* 1982;69:412.

CHAPTER 316 ■ HEMANGIOMAS AND OTHER VASCULAR TUMORS OF INFANCY

DENISE W. METRY

The most common tumors of infancy are benign vascular lesions. Before 1982, the term "hemangioma" was used to encompass a wide range of vascular growths, independent of clinical manifestations, natural history, or embryologic origin. Subsequently, Mulliken and Glowacki proposed the first biologic classification for vascular birthmarks. Their landmark article was the first to distinguish a hemangioma, characterized by a growth phase during infancy and an involutional phase during childhood, from a vascular malformation, a structural anomaly derived from arteries, veins, or lymphatics. In 1997, this classification was broadened to include two additional vascular entities: kaposiform hemangioendothelioma (KHE) and tufted angioma (TA). Box 316.1 presents the revised classification system.

In most cases, the correct classification of a vascular birthmark can be made based on history and clinical evaluation alone. For challenging lesions, imaging (most commonly magnetic resonance imaging [MRI]) may be a helpful diagnostic tool. However, one must emphasize that if any question of malignancy exists, obtaining a tissue biopsy is imperative. Rarely, malignant tumors such as infantile fibrosarcoma can mimic benign vascular tumors and generally cannot be differentiated on the basis of imaging studies alone.

HEMANGIOMAS OF INFANCY

Epidemiology

Hemangiomas of infancy (HOI) are the most common tumors of childhood, estimated to occur in as many as 10% of infants.

BOX 316.1 — Classification of Vascular Birthmarks

Vascular Tumors

Hemangiomas of infancy (HOI)
  Localized, segmental, multifocal
  Visceral hemangiomas
    Multiple (five or more)
    Significance in terms of organ involvement:
      liver >gastrointestinal >brain
  Developmental anomalies
    PHACE(S) syndrome (*posterior fossa
      malformations, HOI, arterial anomalies,
      coarctation of the aorta/cardiac defects, eye
      anomalies, sternal clefting/supraumbilical raphe*)
    Other: spinal dysraphism, genitourinary and
      anorectal anomalies

Other Vascular Tumors

"Congenital" hemangiomas
  Rapidly involuting
  Noninvoluting
Kasabach-Merritt phenomenon
  Kaposiform hemangioendothelioma
  Tufted angioma
Malignant tumors (e.g., infantile fibrosarcoma)

Vascular Malformations

BOX 316.2 — Origin of Hemangiomas

Recent evidence points to shared immunoreactivity between hemangioma tissue and several placental vascular-specific antigens, an interesting discovery because a greater than 20% incidence of hemangiomas of infancy (HOI) exists among mothers who undergo chorionic villous sampling. However, HOI are not simply a result of ectopic placental tissue, because they do not demonstrate placental villous architecture on histopathology, nor do they express known trophoblastic placental markers. Researchers have postulated that cells of placental origin may embolize to receptive fetal tissues during gestation. Recently, an immunohistochemical stain (GLUT-1) was recognized as a specific marker for HOI in all growth phases. GLUT-1 is a glucose transporter normally expressed in blood-tissue barriers, but not normal skin. Positive staining for GLUT-1 will occur only with HOI and not with any other vascular tumor or malformation.

The several known risk factors for their development are female gender (in at least a 3 to 5:1 female-to-male ratio), prematurity (low gestational age and/or weight), and white ethnicity. For reasons unknown, more than 60% of HOI are located on the head and neck, although they may develop anywhere in the skin and/or viscera. Most HOI are inherited sporadically, although autosomal dominant transmission has been reported in a few families.

Pathogenesis

Although the life cycle of hemangiomas is known to result from an imbalance between proliferative and apoptotic angiogenic factors, their precise origin remains elusive. Additional information concerning the origin of hemangiomas is presented in Box 316.2.

Clinical Features

Most HOI are not present at birth, but they become visible in the first few weeks to months of life. Early lesions may be subtle and mistaken by caregivers as a "scratch" or "bruise." A telangiectatic patch surrounded by a vasoconstricted halo also is a typical early presentation. Proliferation of HOI subsequently occurs for approximately 6 to 18 months until a plateau phase is reached, and then involution begins. Involution is a slow process, which occurs over the course of 2 to 12 years at an estimated rate of 10% per year, leading to the following often-quoted percentages of complete HOI involution: 50% of children by age 5 years, 70% by age 7 years, and 90% by age 9 years.

HOI most commonly are superficial in presentation and less commonly are deep or combined. Superficial HOI are raised, bright-red papules, nodules, or plaques (Fig. 316.1), whereas deep HOI are soft, flesh-colored nodules or tumors that may show a bluish hue and/or central telangiectasias (Fig. 316.2). Occasionally, deep HOI are not recognized until several months after birth as a result of their sometimes subtle appearance. The historical, yet still commonly used, descriptors "strawberry" and "cavernous" should be discarded because they incorrectly imply that superficial and deep HOI are behaviorally and histologically distinct. Involution of superficial HOI manifests as a change of color from bright red to darker red, and grayish discoloration often is noted centrally as the tumors soften and flatten. Deep HOI undergo involution as do their superficial counterparts, although such changes generally are not visible clinically.

Risks of Scarring

When discussing the prognosis for HOI, one must recognize that complete involution eventuates in normal-appearing skin in only half of the cases. Thus, explaining to a caregiver that

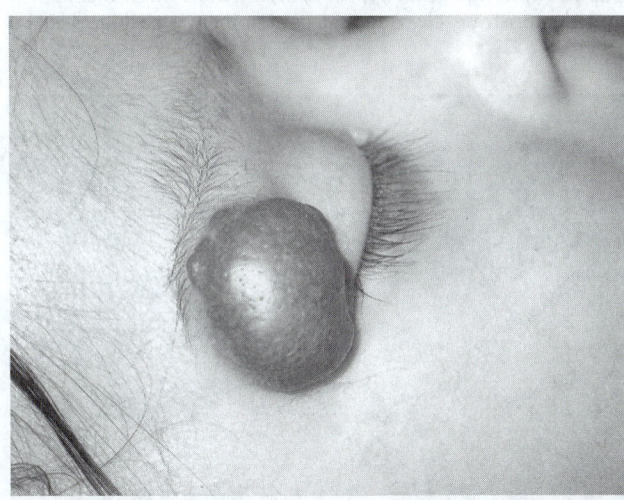

FIGURE 316.1. Superficial, localized hemangioma of infancy in the early proliferative phase.

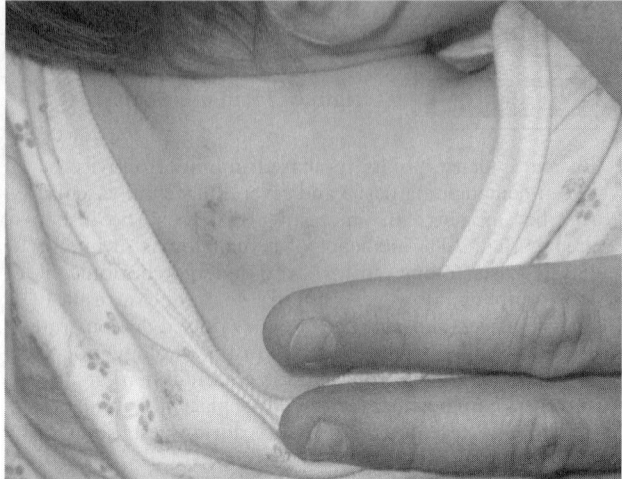

FIGURE 316.2. Deep hemangioma of infancy.

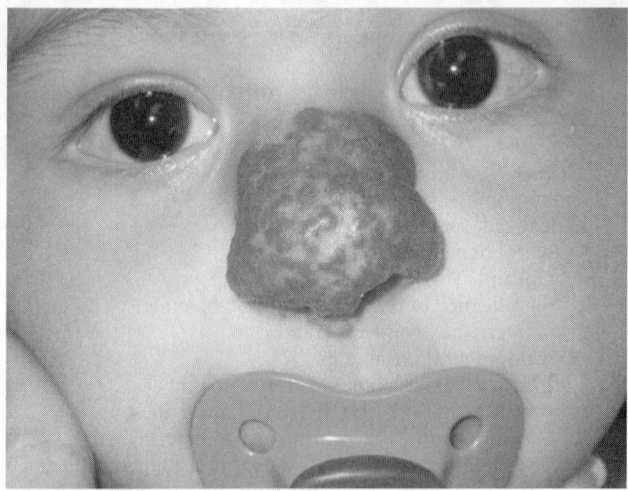

FIGURE 316.4. Superficial hemangioma of infancy of the nose in a patient at risk for permanent disfigurement.

HOI will "go away" is not always accurate. Potential residual damage includes fibrofatty tissue (especially with very raised and/or pedunculated, superficial HOI), atrophy, yellowish discoloration, and/or telangiectasias (Fig. 316.3). Locations especially at risk for a suboptimal cosmetic outcome are the lip (particularly when HOI cross the vermilion border) and the cartilaginous regions of the ear and nose (Fig. 316.4). Ulceration, the most common overall complication of HOI, also inevitably results in scarring in addition to potential infection, bleeding, and pain (Fig. 316.5). Ulceration generally occurs during the proliferative phase in locations subject to trauma, especially the perineum and lip. The precise cause of ulcer development is unknown; however, given the characteristic locations, maceration and frictional stress are probable contributing factors.

Morphology and Complications

Although most HOI remain inconsequential, some may cause or be associated with significant complications. The clinical appearance of a lesion often provides an important clue to identifying worrisome cases. A recently developed classification system divides HOI into *localized*, *segmental*, or *multifocal* types, based on morphology.

Localized HOI, by far the most common, are defined as papules or nodules that appear to arise from a single focal point and demonstrate clear spatial containment (see Fig. 316.1).

Localized lesions are not random in distribution but occur near lines of mesenchymal or mesenchymal-ectodermal embryonic fusion. Furthermore, most (more than 60%) localized HOI occur within a relatively small area of the central face, of which the midcheek, lateral portion of the upper lip, and upper eyelid are the most common locations.

Segmental HOI are plaque-like in morphology and show a linear and/or geographic pattern over a specific cutaneous territory (Fig. 316.6A). In comparison with localized HOI, segmental lesions are much more likely to be associated with

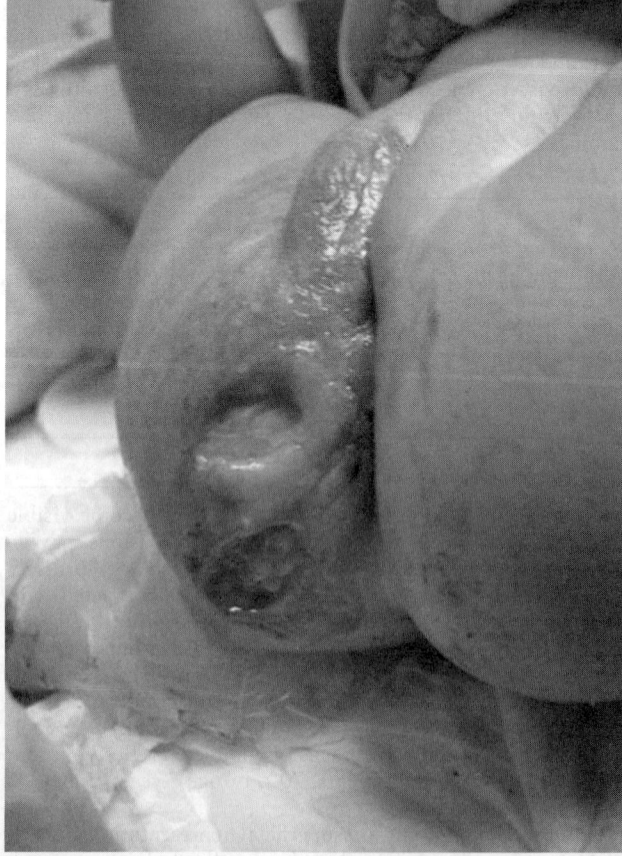

FIGURE 316.5. Segmental perineal hemangioma of infancy complicated by deep ulceration.

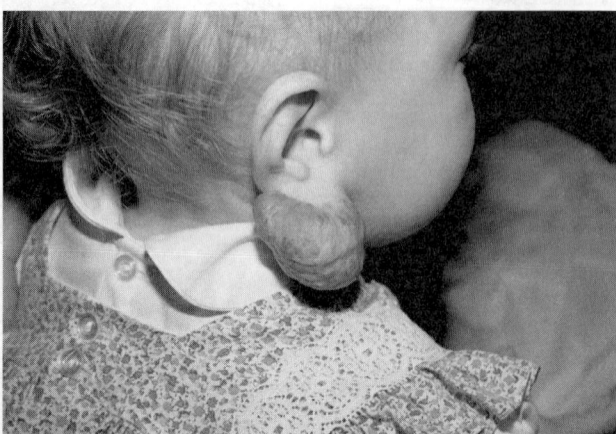

FIGURE 316.3. Residual fibrofatty mass of the earlobe after involution.

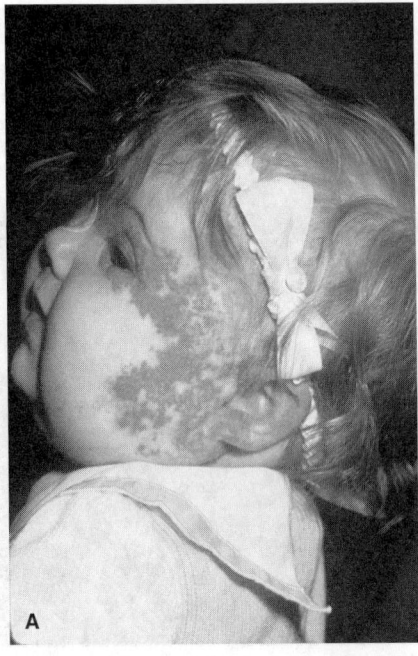
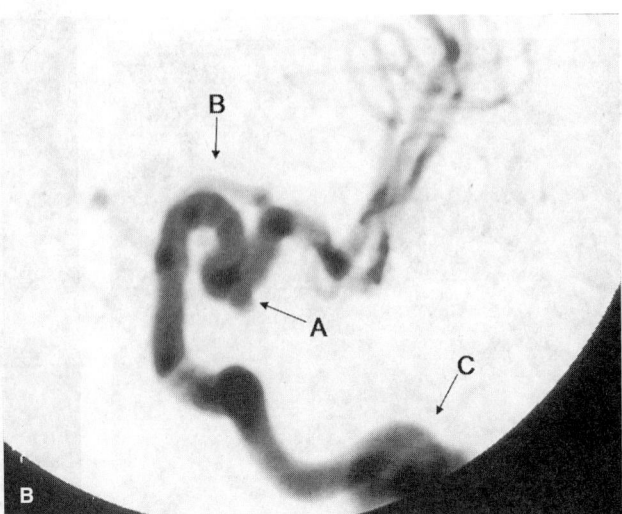

FIGURE 316.6. A: Nine-month-old infant with PHACE syndrome who developed severe, left-sided migraine headaches at age 8 years. **B:** Magnetic resonance angiogram of the brain (from child shown in A) showing aneurysm formation (A), redundant dysplasia (B), and tortuosity of the cervico-petrous portion (C) of the left internal carotid artery.

complications such as ulceration and developmental defects to require more intensive and prolonged therapy, and to have a poorer overall outcome. Although speculative, HOI morphology and potential complications may reflect the timing of HOI etiopathogenesis, with earlier events (between 6 and 8 weeks' gestation) resulting in segmental lesions and later events in localized ones.

Multiple HOI, generally defined as five or more lesions, usually are limited to the skin but rarely can be associated with symptomatic visceral hemangiomatosis.

Vital Organ Compromise

Both morphology and location must be considered when deciding whether HOI may result in compromise of a vital organ. Best known is the potential for periorbital HOI to impair

visual development. Upper eyelid HOI are of greatest concern because of the potential for gravity-induced ptosis (Fig. 316.7), although lesions of the lower eyelid also may prove problematic. Amblyopia can occur from stimulus deprivation when the visual axis is directly obstructed, or astigmatism can result from insidious distortion of the growing cornea. Evaluation by an experienced ophthalmologist is necessary.

An association also exists between segmental HOI in a cervicofacial, mandibular, or "beard" distribution and simultaneous airway HOI (Fig. 316.8). Infants at risk should be followed for the development of stridor, which generally occurs early in infancy concomitant with rapid HOI proliferation. Endoscopic evaluation performed by an otolaryngologist is the best means of establishing confirmation.

Finally, visceral HOI can occur in the presence or absence of cutaneous HOI. The association of multiple (five or more), small, cutaneous HOI with potential visceral involvement is

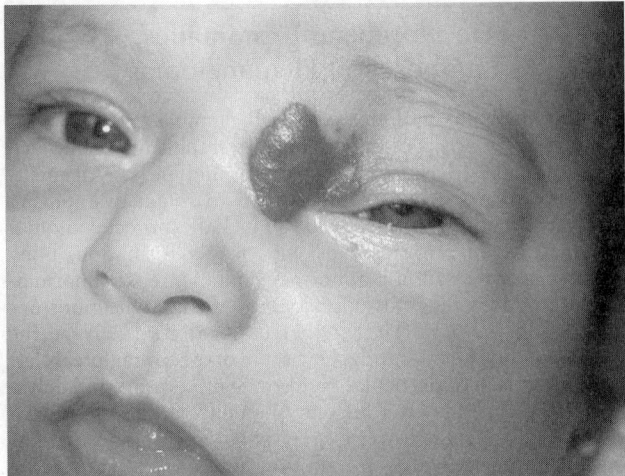

FIGURE 316.7. Combined periocular hemangioma of infancy in a patient at risk for stimulus-deprivation amblyopia.

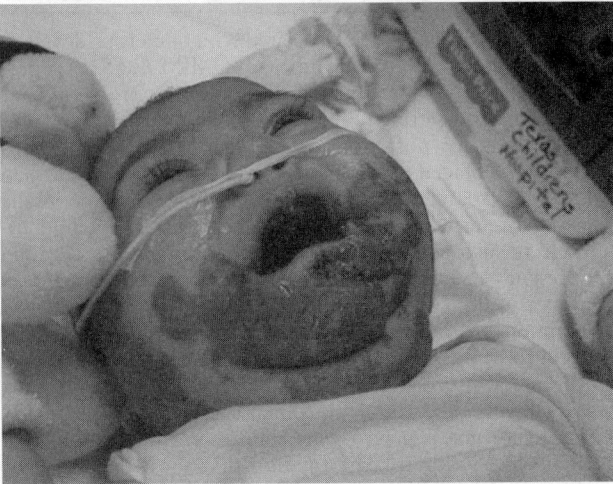

FIGURE 316.8. Segmental mandibular or "beard" hemangioma of infancy in association with hemangioma of infancy of the upper airway.

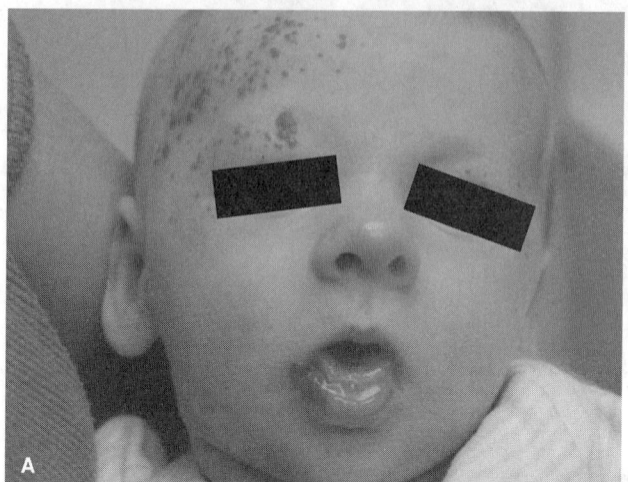

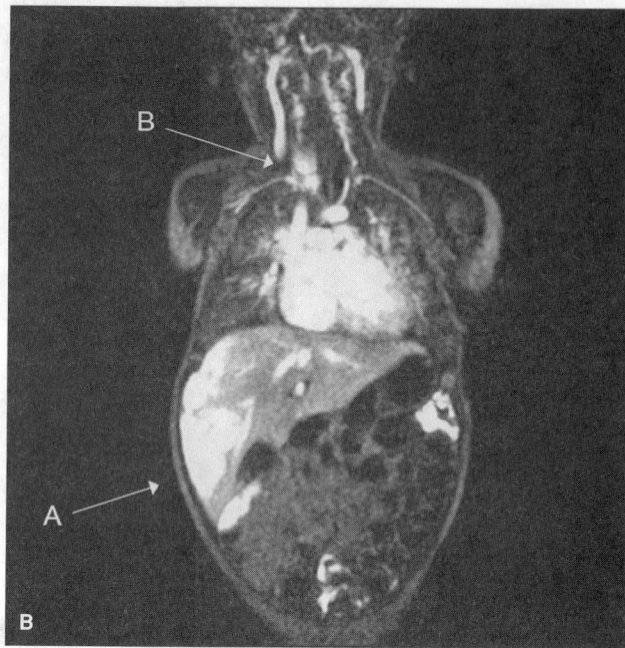

FIGURE 316.9. A: Multiple facial hemangiomas present in a segmental distribution in an infant with a large ventricular septal defect and cerebrovascular anomalies as manifestations of PHACE syndrome. **B:** Magnetic resonance angiogram of the chest/abdomen (from child shown in A) showing multiple hepatic (A) and paratracheal (B) hemangiomas.

well known. However, solitary, segmental cutaneous HOI recently have been recognized to be risk factors for visceral involvement (Fig. 316.9). Visceral HOI are most worrisome when they involve the liver, gastrointestinal tract, and brain. Symptomatic multifocal intrahepatic HOI generally manifest in early infancy with a triad of congestive heart failure, hepatomegaly, and anemia, while diffuse lesions cause massive hepatomegaly with abdominal compartment syndrome. Gastrointestinal HOI can lead to significant bleeding, whereas involvement of the brain can lead to mass effects and a variety of neurologic sequelae, depending on location. Whereas routine ultrasound can be used to screen for visceral involvement, MRI is the most sensitive means of establishing the diagnosis. Overall, visceral HOI probably occur much more commonly than realized, but they remain undetected because asymptomatic infants are not evaluated otherwise.

Developmental Anomalies: PHACE Syndrome

Segmental HOI also can be associated with numerous developmental anomalies. PHACE syndrome (OMIM 606519) represents the best-known example of the variety of problems that can occur in this setting (Table 316.1). The PHACE acronym, which stands for *p*osterior fossa brain malformations, *s*egmental cervicofacial *h*emangiomas, *a*rterial anomalies, *c*ardiac defects and *c*oarctation of the aorta, and *e*ye anomalies, is sometimes referred to as PHACE(S) when ventral developmental defects such as *s*ternal clefting and supraumbilical raphe are present (see Figs. 316.6A and 316.9A). PHACE syndrome is now a well-recognized neurocutaneous association that is uncommon but not rare. In fact, PHACE syndrome now is thought to be possibly even more common than Sturge-Weber syndrome, a disorder with which PHACE sometimes is confused. However, the vascular birthmark associated with Sturge-Weber syndrome is a port-wine stain that, unlike HOI, is a capillary-like vascular malformation that shows no signs of proliferation during infancy, and does not regress.

The diagnosis of PHACE syndrome requires the presence of the characteristic HOI and only one other extracutaneous find-

ing because most infants affected do *not* manifest the complete spectrum of anomalies. Structural cerebral and cerebrovascular anomalies are the most common and potentially devastating features of the syndrome, which may result in neurologic sequelae, including developmental delay and acute ischemic stroke during infancy. Infants most at risk for developing brain anomalies have HOI involving the upper half of the face (see Fig. 316.6). In contrast, patients with mandibular involvement alone are at higher risk for developing ventral developmental defects, airway HOI, and possibly cardiac defects. Children presenting with segmental, cervicofacial HOI should undergo careful cutaneous, ophthalmologic, cardiac, and neurologic assessment, with additional imaging assessment (echocardiogram, MRI/MR angiography imaging of the head and neck) performed for those patients deemed at highest risk. Long-term outcome data from children with PHACE syndrome is necessary before further diagnostic and therapeutic guidelines can be established.

Developmental Anomalies: Lumbosacral Hemangiomas

Finally, segmental HOI located over the lumbar or sacral spine carry their own risks of occult spinal dysraphism or genitourinary anomalies. Lesions that span the midline, are of greatest concern (Fig. 316.10). In addition to spinal dysraphism, anomalies reported with sacral HOI include anorectal anomalies such as imperforate anus with fistula formation, bony anomalies of the sacrum, abnormal genitalia, renal abnormalities, and lipomeningomyelocele. Of all the complications underlying lumbosacral HOI, tethered spinal cord may be the most potentially devastating. Deviation of the supragluteal cleft is a clinical sign of particular concern. Symptoms of spinal dysraphism, which may not arise until a child reaches 3 years of age or older, include lower extremity paresis, muscle atrophy, and incontinence. Early recognition and surgical release are imperative because failure to do so may result in permanent neurologic sequelae. MRI is the most sensitive means for establishing the diagnosis.

TABLE 316.1

TABLE 316.1

MANIFESTATIONS OF PHACE SYNDROME (DESCENDING ORDER OF FREQUENCY)

PHACE Anomaly	Incidence (%)	Specific Manifestations
Structural brain malformations	44 (56/128)	Dandy-Walker (posterior fossa) malformation Hypoplasia or agenesis of cerebellum or cerebellar vermis, corpus callosum, cerebrum, septum pellucidum Solitary reports of absent foramen lacerum, frontal lobe calcification, microcephaly, transverse sinus thrombosis
Cerebrovascular anomalies	29 (37/128)	Aneurysmal dilatations and anomalous branches of the internal carotid artery Cerebral arterial stenosis/occlusion and aneurysm formation "Moya-moya" phenomenon (arterial occlusion with dilated basal collaterals) Retroorbital and parasagittal arteriovenous malformations "Angiomatous malformations" at both carotid siphons and the hypothalamic zone
Neurologic sequelae*	44 (32/72)	Developmental delay Stroke Seizures Contralateral hemiparesis Migraine headaches Solitary reports of apnea, "head bobbing," hypotonia, intention tremor and "disturbed coordination," mental retardation (severe), opisthotonos, unexplained vomiting
Ventral developmental defects	33 (42/128)	Sternal clefting Supraumbilical raphe

Eye anomalies	19 (24/128)	Ipsilateral
		  Microphthalmos
		  Optic atrophy
		  Iris vessel hypertrophy
		  Iris hypoplasia
		  Optic nerve hypoplasia
		  Solitary reports of congenital cataracts, congenital third nerve palsy, exophthalmos, Horner syndrome, lens coloboma, monocular blindness, "morning-glory" deformity of the retina, ocular motor apraxia, sclerocornea, strabismus
		Contralateral
		  Solitary reports of esotropia, glaucoma, optic nerve hypoplasia

Cardiac defects	16 (20/128)	Patent ductus arteriosus Ventricular septal defects Atrial septal defects Pulmonary stenosis Solitary reports of atrial enlargement, cor triatriatum, patent foramen ovale, tetralogy of Fallot, tricuspid atresia, tricuspid stenosis, ventricular hypertrophy
Aortic anomalies	12 (15/128)	Coarctation Aberrant origin of the subclavian artery Subclavian or innominate artery aneurysms Ascending aorta or aortic arch aneurysms and/or dilatation Anomalous left superior vena cava Congenital valvular aortic stenosis "Steal" syndrome Solitary reports of absent right aortic arch, cervical aortic arch, double aortic arch and double aortic coarctation, hypoplastic descending aorta
Miscellaneous	2 reports 1 report 3 reports 2 reports	Congenital hypothyroidism Lingual ectopic thyroid Micrognathism Auricular hypoplasia or agenesis

*Among patients with structural and/or cerebrovascular brain anomalies.

Treatment Overview

Although the decision to treat ulcerated HOI or those that are causing vital organ compromise usually is straightforward, the decision to treat a lesion that may result in a poor cosmetic outcome or is causing significant psychosocial distress for the patient and/or parent can be challenging. In such instances, one must carefully weigh the risks and benefits of available treatment options against a policy of waiting for natural involution. Although most HOI are uncomplicated and require no intervention, a decision not to treat is not necessarily passive.

The psychosocial implications of HOI, especially those involving the face, deserve special mention. Parents commonly are subject to inappropriate comments from strangers, including accusations of child abuse. Television programs or Web sites may contribute to parental anxiety because parents often lack the education to know where their child fits within the HOI spectrum and that their child's lesion will not develop into the dramatic photographs often depicted in such programs. Addressing the psychosocial aspects of care and providing the parents anticipatory guidance, emotional support, and reassurance are essential for effective management.

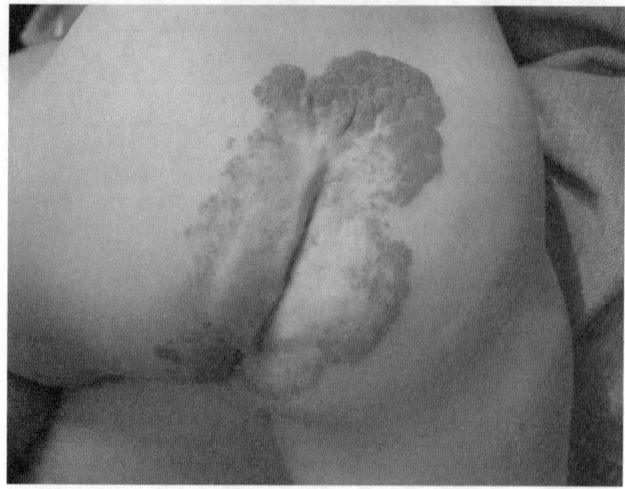

FIGURE 316.10. Segmental lumbosacral hemangioma of infancy in an infant with a tethered spinal cord.

Ulceration Therapy

Local wound care is the mainstay of ulcer therapy and is especially important for lesions in locations subject to trauma and infection, such as the perineum. Commonly used therapies include topical and oral antibiotics, barrier pastes such as zinc oxide, and bioocclusive dressings. Local wound care not only provides a barrier against secondary infection but also reduces pain. A variety of additional modalities, including corticosteroids (CSs; topical, intralesional, and systemic) and pulsed-dye laser therapy, also may provide benefit.

Becaplermin 0.01% gel (Regranex, Ortho-McNeil Pharmaceutical, Raritan, NJ) has emerged recently as a potential therapeutic option for ulcerated HOI refractory to standard therapy. Composed of recombinant platelet-derived growth factor, becaplermin is approved by the U.S. Food and Drug Administration for the treatment of lower extremity, diabetic, neuropathic ulcers. My colleagues and I recently reported a small case series of eight infants treated successfully with becaplermin gel for ulcerated, segmental HOI of the perineum. Becaplermin was applied in a thin layer, once daily, and was covered with a thick application of a barrier paste and nonstick dressing when possible. Rapid healing of the ulcers occurred in all patients within 3 to 21 days (average, 10.25 days), allowing a reduction in the risk of development of secondary infection, pain, and need for hospitalization, as well as the costs that often accumulate from multiple follow-up visits and long-term therapy. Proliferation of HOI, a potential risk of using a growth factor product on a vascular tumor, was not seen in any of our cases. A larger study evaluating the efficacy of becaplermin for ulcerated HOI is in progress. Before the ulcer heals, it is important to address associated pain, which may be relieved with topical lidocaine hydrochloride 2% gel. To avoid the risk of the child developing lidocaine toxicity, parents should be instructed to apply only a pea-sized amount of lidocaine to the affected area no more than four times daily.

Pharmacotherapy

Systemic Corticosteroids

Systemic CSs often are first-line therapy for patients with HOI who are at risk for vital organ compromise or a poor cosmetic outcome, although the exact mechanism of CS action still is not well understood. CSs generally are used to inhibit further proliferation, and thus they are most effective when initiated as early as possible in the growth phase. CS-induced HOI involution ideally, but not always, occurs. The typical starting dose is 2 to 3 mg/kg/day of the 3 mg/mL prednisolone suspension, which generally is continued for 2 to 4 weeks or until a response is seen. The medication then can be tapered slowly over the course of the proliferative phase to minimize rebound growth.

Systemic CSs should be administered in a one-time, morning dose to minimize side effects. Studies of infants treated for HOI with systemic CSs show minor, transient side effects (e.g., cushingoid facies, gastrointestinal upset, insomnia) to be fairly common, whereas serious and/or long-term complications (aseptic necrosis of the femoral head, hypertension, osteoporosis, cataracts) are extremely rare. Delayed skeletal growth may be seen, resulting from a temporary inhibition of collagen synthesis, but virtually all affected children catch up to their normal growth curve on discontinuation of CSs. Because of immunosuppression, vaccines composed of live virus should not be administered to infants receiving supraphysiologic CS doses.

Intralesional and Topical Corticosteroids

CSs also can be administered intralesionally, which can be beneficial for patients with small, localized HOI or ulceration. However, intralesional therapy should be performed cautiously, especially in the periocular location, where rare but serious side effects, including eyelid necrosis and central retinal artery occlusion, have been reported. Topical, superpotent (class 1) CSs for relatively thin, superficial HOI plaques also may provide benefit in select cases.

Interferon

Interferon, administered at an initial dose of 3 million U/m^2/day, often is an effective alternative for treating infants with life-threatening HOI that have not responded to systemic CSs. However, use of interferon in infants has been limited by reports of neurotoxicity, specifically, spastic diplegia, which has proved in some cases to be irreversible despite withdrawal of the drug. Although neurotoxicity appears to be dose- and duration-dependent, the precise cause remains unknown. Infants should receive close neurologic follow-up while undergoing treatment with interferon. Vincristine, which interferes with mitotie spindle microtubles and induces apoptosis in tumor cells in vitro, is another option for patients who have failed or cannot tolerate other medical therapies, and is currently under investigation.

Laser and Surgical Therapy

Other therapeutic options for HOI include laser and surgical therapy. The flashlamp-pumped, pulsed-dye laser may be a useful modality for lightening superficial lesions, but it cannot be expected to affect HOI with deeper involvement because the depth of laser penetration is only 1.2 mm. The most widely accepted use of flashlamp-pumped, pulsed-dye laser for HOI is for postinvolution erythema and/or telangiectasias. In contrast to its use for port-wine stains, use of pulsed-dye laser therapy for early HOI is controversial because of concerns regarding potential hypopigmentation, textural changes, and the promotion of ulceration. For significantly raised (especially pedunculated), localized HOI at risk for significant fibrofatty residuum, early consultation with an experienced surgeon is reasonable. However, the risks and benefits of surgical intervention, especially the resultant scar, require careful consideration.

For children in whom the risks of a poor cosmetic outcome are relatively minor, we advise waiting as long as possible for natural involution, until approximately 2 to 4 years of age, a time when the development of self-esteem and social awareness

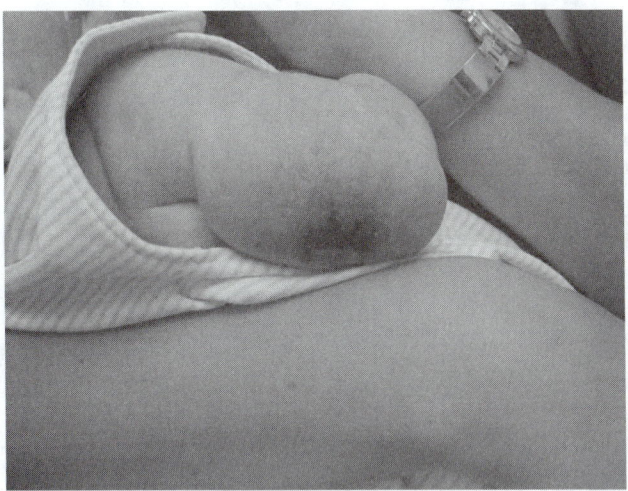

FIGURE 316.11. Rapidly involuting "congenital hemangioma" of the arm.

begins. This rationale provides the chance of needing *no* intervention and if ultimately treatment is decided, theoretically it will be less than that required before involution.

OTHER VASCULAR TUMORS

"Congenital" Hemangiomas: Noninvoluting and Rapidly Involuting

The differential diagnosis of HOI includes several, relatively rare vascular tumors, all of which are glucose transporter 1 (GLUT-1)-negative. Fully developed, hemangioma-like lesions, previously known as "congenital" hemangiomas, now are recognized to be distinct vascular tumors that may either undergo rapid involution in infancy (Rapidly Involuting Congenital Hemangioma or RICH) or persist over time (NonInvoluting Congenital Hemangioma or NICH). Clinically, a RICH presents as a gray-violaceous nodule or tumor that, unlike true HOI, most commonly is located on an extremity (Fig. 316.11). Rapid involution generally occurs within the first year of life, with characteristic atrophy. In contrast, a NICH most commonly presents on the trunk as an oval to round plaque with coarse, central

telangiectasias and a surrounding rim of pallor (Fig. 316.12). A NICH often feels warm to palpation and may have a slight bruit. The pathologic features of a NICH are a hybrid between a vascular tumor and malformation.

Kasabach-Merritt Phenomenon: Kaposiform Hemangioendothelioma and Tufted Angioma

Kasabach-Merritt phenomenon (KMP) refers to the development of life-threatening thrombocytopenia as a result of platelet trapping within a vascular tumor. Infants presenting with large HOI once were monitored closely for the development of KMP. However, in 1997 researchers recognized that KMP is not associated with HOI but with two other, clinically and immunohistochemically distinct vascular entities: KHE and TA.

KHE, although benign histologically, carries a significant mortality risk if left untreated. This lesion most commonly affects children younger than 2 years of age, often is present at birth, and affects male and female children equally. KHE generally is solitary and favors the skin (particularly the trunk or extremities) or retroperitoneum. To our knowledge, hepatic involvement does not occur. Early lesions may mimic HOI but with maturity develop a distinctive violaceous color resulting from underlying KMP. Further examination of the skin also may reveal the presence of telangiectasias and/or ecchymoses. KHE demonstrates an infiltrative, nodular growth pattern that closely mimics a malignant tumor (Fig. 316.13).

Further evaluation of suspected KHE requires MRI and tissue for pathologic examination. Characteristic MRI findings include ill-defined tumor margins with the involvement of

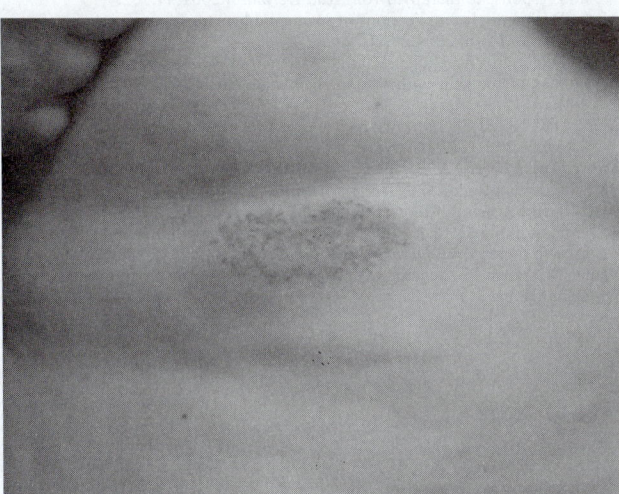

FIGURE 316.12. Noninvoluting "congenital hemangioma" of the trunk.

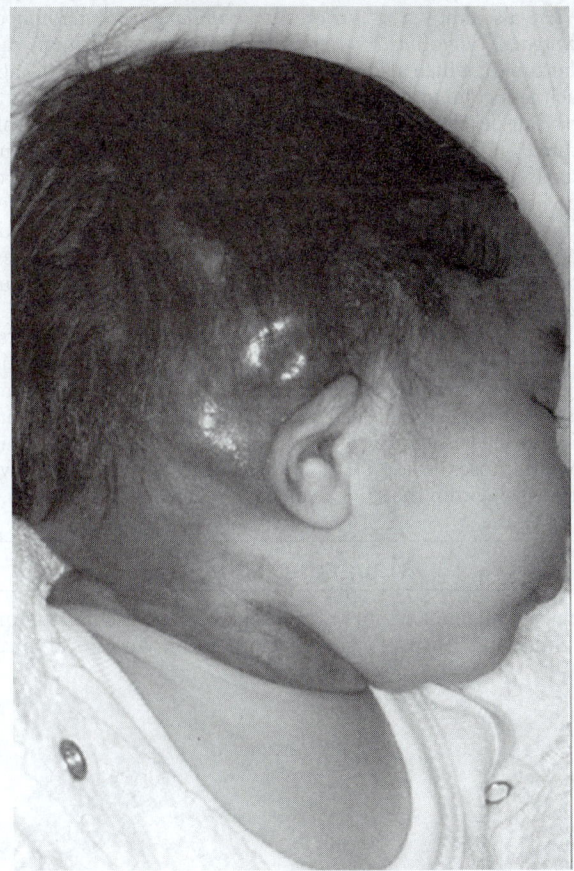

FIGURE 316.13. Kaposiform hemangioendothelioma.

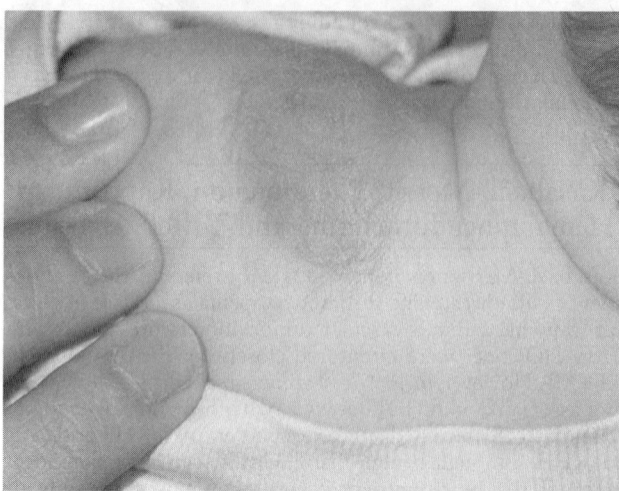

FIGURE 316.14. Tufted angioma.

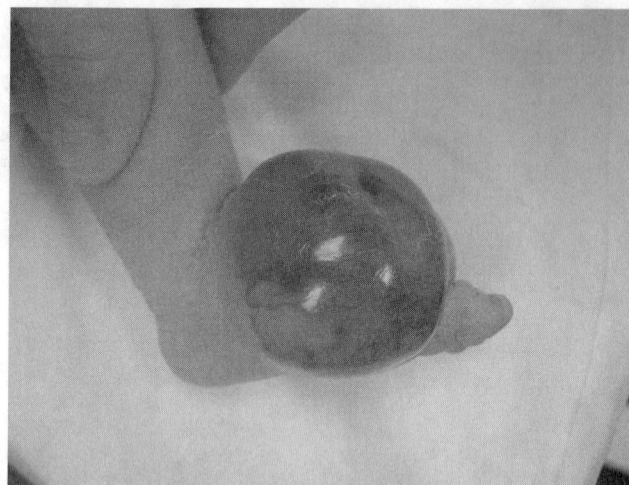

FIGURE 316.15. Infantile fibrosarcoma.

multiple tissue layers. The feeding or draining vessels within KHE tend to be small and few in number relative to size, in contrast to HOI. Another distinguishing feature is the presence of signal voids without flow-related enhancement, indicative of hemosiderin, other blood products, or fibrosis. Histologically, KHE shows a lobular infiltrate of benign endothelial cells. Thrombosed capillaries, slit-like vascular spaces, and scattered epithelioid cells are seen frequently. The pathologic features is similar to those of Kaposi sarcoma, hence the term kaposiform. The evaluation of an infant with a suspected or confirmed KHE also should include a complete blood count and coagulation studies to detect coexisting KMS.

TA, also known as *progressive capillary hemangioma* or *Nakagawa angioblastoma*, is a rare, histologically benign vascular tumor, which also may be complicated by KMP, although much less commonly than KHE. Most TAs are not present at birth but develop within the first year of life. Most commonly located on the upper trunk or proximal extremity, TA manifests as a subcutaneous plaque or nodule with a dusky red to blue hue. Lesions may be tender to palpation, with increased vellus hair growth and hyperhidrosis of the surrounding skin (Fig. 316.14). Slow, lateral extension continues for a few months to several years. Spontaneous regression may occur, and may be more common to congenital lesions.

On low microscopic power, numerous lobules or "tufts" of capillaries are present within the middle to lower dermis. Higher magnification reveals that the capillary tufts are composed of benign spindle cells, which may show protrusion into neighboring vessels. The histologic features of the TA may overlap with those of the KHE, a finding suggesting that these two entities lie within the same neoplastic spectrum.

Malignant Tumors

Finally, malignant tumors may mimic benign vascular tumors of childhood. Suspect lesions include those with an atypical clinical appearance and/or infiltrative growth pattern. For example, infantile fibrosarcoma may present at birth or shortly thereafter as a firm, rapidly growing tumor. Sometimes, lesions have a shiny transparent surface, under which prominent underlying vessels may be seen (Fig. 316.15). Deep growths that fail to show any of the cutaneous clues typical of a deep HOI also should be held suspect. Imaging generally cannot distinguish between benign and malignant vascular tumors, and, if clinically indicated, obtaining tissue biopsy is imperative.

Suggested Readings

Batta K, Goodyear HM, Moss C, et al. Randomised controlled study of early pulsed dye laser treatment of uncomplicated childhood haemangiomas: results of a 1-year analysis. *Lancet* 2002;360:521.

Boon LM, MacDonald DM, Mulliken JB. Complications of systemic corticosteroid therapy for problematic hemangioma. *Plast Reconstr Surg* 1999;104:1616.

Chiller KG, Passaro D, Frieden IJ. Hemangiomas of infancy: clinical characteristics, morphologic subtypes, and their relationship to race, ethnicity, and sex. *Arch Dermatol* 2002;138:1567.

Enjolras O, Wassef M, Mazoyer E, et al. Infants with Kasabach-Merritt syndrome do not have "true" hemangiomas. *J Pediatr* 1997;130:631.

Kim HJ, Colombo M, Frieden IJ. Ulcerated hemangiomas: clinical characteristics and response to therapy. *J Am Acad Dermatol* 2001;44:962.

Metry D. Potential complications of segmental hemangiomas of infancy. *Semin Cutan Med Surg* 2004;23:107.

Metry D, Hawrot A, Altman C, et al. Association of solitary, sequential hemangiomas of the skin with visceral hemangiomatosis. *Arch Dermatol* 2004;140:591.

Metry DW, Dowd CF, Barkovich AJ, et al. The many faces of PHACE syndrome. *J Pediatr* 2001;139:117.

Metry DW, Hebert AA. Benign cutaneous vascular tumors of infancy: when to worry, what to do. *Arch Dermatol* 2000;136:905.

Metz BJ, Rubenstein MC, Levy ML, et al. Response of ulcerated perineal hemangiomas of infancy to be caplermin gel, a recombinant human platelet-derived growth factor. *Arch Dermatol* 2004;140:867.

Waner M, North PE, Scherer KA, et al. The nonrandom distribution of facial hemangiomas. *Arch Dermatol* 2003;139:869.

CHAPTER 317 ■ THYMOMAS

JED G. NUCHTERN

EPIDEMIOLOGY

Thymic tumors are rare occurrences in children. These masses account for 18% of mediastinal tumors in adults but only 3% in children. Tumors involving the thymus include cysts and hamartomas, thymomas and thymic adenomas, thymolipomas, germ cell tumors, and carcinoids, as well as leukemia and lymphoma. Thymomas are primary neoplasms of the thymic epithelium. Fewer than 10% of thymomas occur in children and adolescents.

Although thymomas are found in 8% to 15% of adult patients with myasthenia gravis, only two cases of thymoma in children with this autoimmune disease have been reported, suggesting that the neoplasm plays a lesser role in the pathophysiology of myasthenia gravis in younger patients. Red cell aplasia and hypogammaglobulinemia also are associated with thymoma.

DIAGNOSIS

Thymomas are slow-growing tumors that often are diagnosed as incidental findings on routine chest roentgenography. Approximately 50% of patients will present with symptoms including cough, dysphagia, dyspnea, and vague chest pain. Computed tomographic (CT) scans are useful in defining the characteristics of the mass and to assess the involvement of contiguous mediastinal structures. The center of the mass usually is where the normal thymus would be located, below the innominate vein and apposing the posterior surface of the sternum. These masses normally are of soft tissue density but may contain calcifications. Vascular invasion, encasement, and pleural deposits are associated with malignancy.

The differential diagnosis of anterior mediastinal masses includes lymphoma and germ cell tumors. The typical appearance of lymphoma on CT is an ill-defined lobulated mass, often with associated regional or distant lymphadenopathy. Benign germ cell tumors normally have well-defined margins and may contain cystic, calcified, and adipose tissue. Nonseminomatous germ cell tumors tend to have large, diffuse appearance on CT imaging, with areas of necrosis and hemorrhage. The latter also will have diagnostic elevations of alpha-fetoprotein and beta-human chorionic gonadotropin.

The initial approach to a pediatric patient with an anterior mediastinal mass is based on the clinical, imaging, and laboratory findings. Small, well-encapsulated masses with CT characteristics of thymoma or benign germ cell tumor may be resected primarily through a median sternotomy. Larger masses, and those with an uncertain histology, should undergo initial incisional biopsy through an anterior mediastinotomy on the side of the sternum overlying the greater bulk of tumor. Prior to undergoing any surgical procedure, all patients with large anterior mediastinal masses should be evaluated for potential airway obstruction on induction of general anesthesia.

Although progress is being made, no histologic grading scheme has emerged that is more robust than clinical staging for thymomas. Masaoka et al. have proposed the most broadly utilized clinical staging system, based on the degree of invasiveness: Stage I lesions do not extend beyond the capsule; pericapsular growth into mediastinal fat defines stage II; stage III involves invasion into surrounding organs; and stage IV has distant metastases (pleural, pericardial, lymphogenous, or hematogenous). Therapy is aimed at achieving a complete surgical resection, which is the single most important predictor of survival. Thymomas generally are quite sensitive to radiation. All patients with invasive tumors should be treated with radiation therapy postoperatively. Chemotherapy with cisplatin, doxorubicin, and cyclophosphamide is reserved for those with bulky tumors with incomplete resections and those with stage III and IV disease. Preoperative chemotherapy and radiotherapy can be effective in shrinking large, invasive masses before definitive surgical resection is performed, provided that a histologic diagnosis is made beforehand. Based on recent series (mostly adults), the 5-year survival rates for patients with thymomas range from 100% for encapsulated stage I tumors to less than 70% for stage III and IV disease.

Thymic cysts usually are asymptomatic. They normally are unilocular and may present as a cervical or anterior mediastinal mass along the embryonic route of descent of the thymus. Usually, they can be resected without difficulty.

Suggested Readings

Masaoka A, Monden Y, Nakahara K, et al. Follow-up study of thymoma with special reference to their clinical stages. *Cancer* 1981;48:2485.

Park HS, Shin DM, Lee JS, et al. Thymoma: a retrospective study of 87 cases. *Cancer* 1994;73:2491.

Pokorny WJ, Sherman JO. Mediastinal masses in infants and children. *J Thorac Cardiovasc Surg* 1974;5:869.

Shamberger RC, Holzman RS, Griscom NT, et al. Prospective evaluation by computed tomography and pulmonary function tests of children with mediastinal masses. *Surgery* 1995;118:468.

Thomas CR, Wright CD, Loehrer PJ. Thymoma: state of the art. *J Clin Oncol* 1999;17:2280.

CHAPTER 318 ■ SPLENIC CYSTS

TOM JAKSIC AND SID JOHNSON

EPIDEMIOLOGY

Splenic cysts are uncommon occurrences. They may be found incidentally or may be associated with left upper-quadrant pain, infection, hemorrhage, and unexplained splenomegaly. Splenic cysts are classified as "true" or "pseudo" cysts, in relation to the presence or absence of an epithelial lining. True cysts can be subdivided into paracytic and nonparacytic or "epithelial" cysts. In endemic regions, hydatid cystic disease caused by *Echinococcus granulosus* is the most frequent etiologic agent, with the spleen being the third most affected organ after the liver and lung. Epithelial cysts usually are considered to be congenital in nature and constitute approximately 25% of nonparacytic cysts in the United States. Pseudocysts are the most common type of cysts, accounting for 75% of nonparacytic splenic cysts in the United States. These pseudocysts of the spleen are thought to evolve as a consequence of splenic trauma. Malignancy within splenic cysts is an extremely rare event.

CLINICAL MANIFESTATIONS AND COMPLICATIONS

Large splenic cysts manifest clinically as progressively enlarging masses in the left upper quadrant, with approximately one-third being associated with pain or discomfort. Hemorrhage, secondary infection, and spontaneous rupture are infrequent complications but may be associated with repeat trauma. In neonates, spontaneous resolution of incidentally discovered splenic cysts has been reported.

Most splenic cysts are found by abdominal computed tomography (CT) scan or abdominal ultrasound examination. Plain films of the abdomen may reveal displacement away from the spleen of the stomach, splenic flexure of the colon, and left kidney. Calcification outlining the splenic cyst suggests hydatid disease. Doppler ultrasound is a sensitive and cost-effective means to diagnose and locate splenic lesions. CT scanning provides the most accurate anatomic detail for preoperative planning.

THERAPY

The treatment of splenic cysts is surgical. Traditionally, the treatment of splenic cysts was splenectomy. However, in children, because of concerns of postsplenectomy sepsis, surgical treatment now favors splenic conservation. Large nonparasitic cysts are managed by unroofing the extrasplenic component of the cyst, thereby preserving the spleen and obviating the risk of developing postsplenectomy sepsis. A laparoscopic approach is well suited for this operation. Hydatid cysts require laparotomy, with great care being taken to avoid spillage of the cyst contents and resultant peritoneal seeding. Splenic salvage often is not possible with hydatid disease.

Suggested Readings

De Caluwé D, Phelan E, Puri P. Pure alcohol injection of a congenital splenic cyst: a valid alternative? *J Pediatr Surg* 2004;38(4):629.

MacKenzie RK, Youngsona GG, Mahomed AA. Laparoscopic decapsulation of congenital splenic cysts: A step forward in splenic preservation. *J Pediatr Surg* 2004;39(1):88.

Safioleas M, Misiakos E, Manti C. Surgical treatment for splenic hydatidosis. *World J Surg* 1997;21:374.

Targarona EM, Martinez J, Ramos C, Becerra JA, Trias M. Conservative laparoscopic treatment of a posttraumatic splenic cyst. *Surg Endosc* 1995;9:71.

Touloukian RJ, Maharaj A, Ghoussoub R, Reyes M. Partial decapsulation of splenic epithelial cysts: studies on etiology and outcome. *J Pediatr Surg* 1997; 32:272.

Tsakayannis DE, Mitchell K, Kozakewich HP, Shamberger RC. Splenic preservation in the management of splenic epidermoid cysts in children. *J Pediatr Surg* 1995;30(10):1468.

SECTION VI ■ DISEASES OF THE GENITOURINARY SYSTEM

CHAPTER 319 ■ MORPHOLOGIC DEVELOPMENT OF THE KIDNEY

LAURA S. FINN

The development of the kidney is a complex and well-coordinated process relying on the integration of cellular proliferation, programmed cell death, migration, morphogenesis, and differentiation. Through the regulated expression of various transcription factors, adhesion molecules, and growth factors, nephrogenesis proceeds in an orderly fashion; aberration of the systematic progression can lead to a wide spectrum of renal disorders that manifest in children and adults.

The mature human kidney and ureters are the third set of renal organs derived sequentially from intermediate mesoderm. The first paired organs, the most cranially oriented pronephroi (singular, pronephros), appear early in the fourth week of gestation and consist of primitive tubules that attach to a ductal system that empties into the cloaca. These temporary organs do not function in the human embryo, and they degenerate as soon as they are formed, being replaced late in the fourth week of gestation by the second kidney, the mesonephros. The mesonephroi develop primitive glomeruli and tubules that connect to the excretory ducts of the pronephroi. These ducts, renamed *mesonephric* or *Wolffian ducts*, connect with the cloaca. The mesonephroi are known to function in some lower animals and may do so transiently in humans. They slowly degenerate as the third set of paired organs, the metanephroi, evolve.

The development of the metanephros, the definitive kidney in mammals, begins during the fifth week of gestation. Signals from the nephrogenic mesenchyme (metanephric blastema), a specialized region of the intermediate mesoderm, induce outgrowth of the *ureteric bud* from the caudal mesonephric duct. The glial-derived neurotrophic factor (GDNF)–RET signaling pathway is a crucial initiator, as targeted *Gdnf* deletions can result in bilateral renal agenesis with failure of ureteric bud development. Early stages of development also are dependent on the activity of WT1 that is expressed in metanephric blastema but not in the Wolffian duct or ureteric bud. Upon invasion of the blastema, reciprocal inductive signals promote the elongation and branching of the tip (*ampulla*) of the ureteric bud to form the collecting system, as well as proliferation of the metanephric blastema, which acquires a stem-cell phenotype and will differentiate into nephrons. The caudal portion of the ureteric bud will lengthen eventually to form the ureter.

The advancing ampulla of the ureteric bud undergoes a rapid sequence of dichotomous divisions, with each branch forming a new ampulla. This branching is under the control of a host of growth factors that induce (e.g., epidermal growth factor) or inhibit (e.g., transforming growth factor–beta) the process. Remodelling of the first three to five generations, by a process of distension and coalescence, forms the major calyces. Subsequent generations of branches form the minor calyces, into which 10 to 20 papillary collecting ducts will drain. The development of the pelvicaliceal system is complete by the tenth to twelfth week of gestation.

Further divisions of the ampullae are dedicated to nephrogenesis. A stimulus from the advancing ampulla induces metanephric blastema to condense, migrate, and proliferate. *PAX2* activation and subsequent *WNT4* signaling derived from the aggregating mesenchyme are required for the epithelial conversion that results in the formation of the *renal vesicle*. Changes in the expression patterns of various other transcription factors, protooncogenes, growth factors, and adhesion molecules occur at all steps of nephron formation.

The renal vesicle, with its slit-like cavity, elongates and folds to form an S-shaped structure, the proximal end of which joins the lumen of the associated ampulla, destined to become the collecting duct. The midportions of the S-shaped vesicle lengthen and bend to form the proximal and distal convoluted tubules and the loop of Henle (Fig. 319.1). The distal portion of the S-shaped structure becomes concave, to form Bowman capsule and the visceral epithelial cells of the glomerulus, which encase the emerging capillary tuft. The strict developmental delineation of ureteric bud-to-collecting system and metanephric blastema-to-nephron has been challenged by lineage tracing studies that have demonstrated ureteric bud cells in proximal tubules and metanephric blastema in presumed collecting ducts, thus highlighting the plasticity of embryogenesis. Mesangial cells, too, may originate from the nephrogenic mesenchyme.

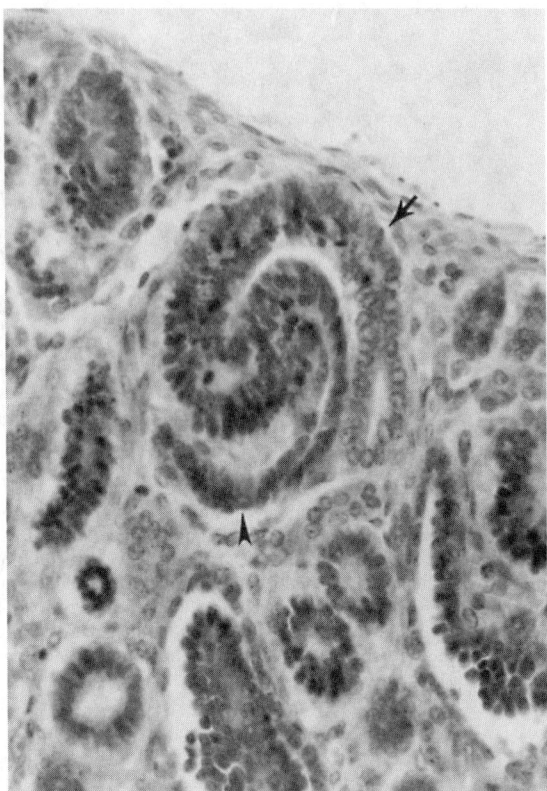

FIGURE 319.1. A small segment of the subcapsular nephrogenic zone. The proximal portion of the S-shaped structure in the center has made connection (*arrow*) with the ureteric bud. The epithelial portions of the glomerulus will form from the distal end (*arrowhead*) (hematoxylin and eosin, magnification 400×).

The blood supply to the developing metanephros originates in lateral sacral branches of the aorta. As the kidneys are relocated to their final position, the branches arise at progressively higher levels, with the definitive renal arteries branching from the aorta near the second lumbar vertebra. The development of the glomerular capillaries remains incompletely understood but is commensurate with nephrogenesis. Both angiogenesis (recruitment of nearby vascular endothelial cells) and vasculogenesis (differentiation of vascular endothelium from "angioblasts" derived from mesenchyme) appear to have roles. These processes are regulated by vascular endothelial growth factor (VEGF) and its receptors, platelet-derived growth factor (PDGF), Eph receptors, and ligands, as well as the angiopoietin/Tie system.

The metanephric kidney becomes functional between 11 and 13 weeks of gestation and begins to contribute significantly to the amniotic fluid after the eighteenth week. The subcapsular *nephrogenic zone* of blastema induction disappears between the thirty-fifth and thirty-sixth weeks of gestation, when nephrogenesis is completed. No new nephrons develop postnatally, but the tubules continue to elongate through childhood.

The mature kidneys are paired, bean-shaped structures composed of an inner medulla and an outer cortex, containing approximately 1 million functioning glomeruli. The medulla consists of 8 to 18 cone-shaped structures, called *renal pyramids*, that contain segments of the loops of Henle and the inner portions of the collecting ducts, which drain into the minor calyces through several pores at the tips of the pyramids. The minor calyces empty into the major calyces, which then empty into the renal pelvis.

Microscopically, the mature glomerulus consists of a capillary network derived from the afferent arteriole (Fig. 319.2).

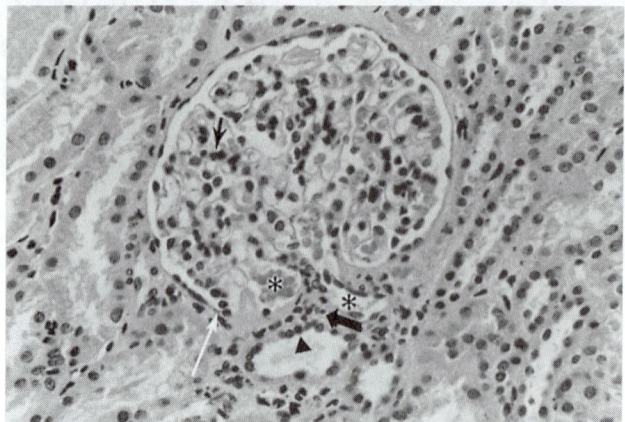

FIGURE 319.2. The glomerulus in this section has wide open capillary loops covered by visceral epithelial cells that are in continuity with the parietal epithelial cells lining Bowman capsule (*white arrow*). The loops are separated by mesangial cells and mesangial matrix (*small arrow*). Both afferent and efferent arterioles (*asterisks*) are seen at the hilum. The modified epithelial cells (macula densa) of the thick ascending limb of Henle (*arrowhead*) are seen adjacent to the afferent arteriole. The renin-producing cells (a component of the juxtaglomerular apparatus) are present in the interstitium (*large arrow*) (hematoxylin and eosin, magnification 315×).

The capillaries are covered by epithelium and separated by mesangial cells embedded in a basement membrane-like matrix. They rejoin to form the efferent arteriole, which supplies the remainder of the nephron and associated collecting duct via thin-walled capillaries called *vasa recti*. The visceral epithelium is continuous with the parietal epithelium lining Bowman capsule. This epithelium is, in turn, continuous with the epithelium of the proximal convoluted tubule.

The juxtaglomerular apparatus, which regulates glomerular hemodynamics, is a specialized region at the glomerular hilum composed of arteriolar smooth muscle cells, extraglomerular mesangium (lacis cells), and modified tubular epithelial cells of the most distal segment of the thick limb of the loop of Henle, the macula densa. Renin is produced in the juxtaglomerular granular cells.

Suggested Readings

Burrow CR. Regulatory molecules in kidney development. *Pediatr Nephrol* 2000;14:240.

Glassberg KI. Normal and abnormal development of the kidney: a clinician's interpretation of current knowledge. *J Urol* 2002;167:2339.

Piscione TD, Rosenblum ND. The molecular control of renal branching morphogenesis: current knowledge and emerging insights. *Differentiation* 2002;70:227.

Risdon RA, Woolf AS. Development of the kidney. In: Jennette JC, Olson JL, Schwartz MM, Silva FG, ed. *Heptinstall's pathology of the kidney*, 5th ed., vol. 1. Philadelphia: Lippincott-Raven, 1998:67.

Robert B, Abrahamson DR. Control of glomerular capillary development by growth factor/receptor kinases. *Pediatr Nephrol* 2001;16:294.

CHAPTER 320 ■ DISORDERS OF RENAL DEVELOPMENT AND ANOMALIES OF THE COLLECTING SYSTEM, BLADDER, PENIS, AND SCROTUM

DAVID R. ROTH AND EDMOND T. GONZALES

DISORDERS OF RENAL DEVELOPMENT

Abnormalities of Position

Simple Ectopia

Simple renal ectopia is a condition in which a kidney is located in an abnormal position but remains on its own side of the midline. Often, associated incomplete rotation of the renal unit occurs. The most common position is in the true pelvis; less common locations are the iliac fossa or the thorax. Ectopia occurs in 1 in 500 to 1,200 live births; is more common on the left side; and most often is discovered as part of an evalua-

tion for other abnormalities, the most common of which are other urologic, musculoskeletal, cardiovascular, gastrointestinal, and otolaryngologic anomalies. Treatment, if any, should address pathologic factors (primarily ureteral obstruction or vesicoureteral reflux) but not the position of the renal unit.

Simple Malrotation

During embryogenesis, the kidney rotates from a position in which the renal pelvis faces anterior to its usual postnatal position, which is with the renal pelvis facing medially. Disorders of renal ascent often are associated with persistence of the original orientation. A better term would be *incomplete rotation* rather than *malrotation*. Unless problems associated with this abnormality of rotation exist, such as ureteropelvic obstruction, no treatment is needed.

Fusion Anomalies

In patients with fusion anomalies, the two renal units may remain in the true pelvis and be connected by a large mass of parenchyma (cake kidney) in the midline, or they may be partially ascended and connected by a thin isthmus of tissue below the inferior mesenteric artery connecting the lower poles (horseshoe kidney). In crossed fused ectopia, one renal unit crosses the midline and fuses to the normally positioned contralateral kidney; the ureters arise from the appropriate sides of the bladder, but one crosses the midline to enter the lower segment of the fused renal units. The anomaly is seen slightly more commonly in boys than in girls, and the kidneys reside on the right side twice as often as on the left. No treatment is needed, although an increased incidence of reflux and ureteral obstruction that might require surgery is associated with this entity.

Horseshoe kidney is the most common fusion anomaly, accounting for approximately 90% of these abnormalities. It often is discovered incidentally during an evaluation of associated anomalies or urinary infection, or at autopsy. The kidneys are positioned lower than normal, with their lower poles joined by an isthmus of tissue. They are incompletely rotated, and their axes are more vertical than normal, a consistent and characteristic sign on intravenous urography (Fig. 320.1). The isthmus usually crosses the midline anterior to the great vessels below the inferior mesenteric artery, which blocked further ascent of the kidneys during fetal development. The ureters may be somewhat dilated superior to the isthmus, which they cross; however, the need for surgical repair is unusual. Associated anomalies are common findings but usually are less serious than are those related to crossed renal ectopia. Urologic evaluation should include voiding cystourethrography because reflux is a common finding. Treatment decisions are based on the same criteria as those for a normal kidney: infection, pain, and deterioration of renal function. The abnormal location of the kidneys, as well as the isthmus, which crosses the spinal column, increases the possibility of renal injury occurring in these patients. Thus, parental counseling concerning the risks of contact sports is appropriate.

Anomalies of Renal Parenchyma

Agenesis

Unilateral renal agenesis is present in 1 in 450 to 1,800 live births. Its etiology is related to maldevelopment of the metanephric duct (primitive ureter) and renal blastema. Often, the ipsilateral ureter and vas deferens are absent because their embryologic origins are similar. Compensatory hypertrophy of the solitary kidney is a common finding but not specific for this lesion. Diagnosis often is made during an investigation of other anomalies (cardiovascular, gastrointestinal, musculoskeletal). No treatment is needed, but the child and parents should be cautioned that activities that put the single kidney at undue risk of injury (e.g., organized football, rugby, riding motorcycles) should be avoided.

Bilateral renal agenesis is a rare entity that is incompatible with life. A high incidence of associated anomalies and developmental abnormalities of the bladder, urethra, and ureters occurs. Pulmonary hypoplasia is a common occurrence and generally is the immediate cause of demise. The infants have typical features, described by Potter, that include increased distance between the eyes, flattening or broadening of the nose, a prominent inner canthal fold, spade-like hands, and amnion nodosum. These findings, characteristic of Potter syndrome, are the result of severe oligohydramnios, which is caused by the absence of intrauterine urine production. This syndrome is not specific for bilateral renal agenesis, however, because any condition in which markedly decreased amniotic fluid volume occurs would produce similar findings.

Renal Hypoplasia

Renal hypoplasia is an unusual condition in which the number of renal lobules is reduced, thereby producing a kidney that is small but with normal nephron differentiation. The number of calyces is decreased, and the renal weight is diminished. If the condition is bilateral, the total nephron mass is deficient, and the result is progressive renal insufficiency with its typical complications of growth arrest and developmental delay. Patients may require renal dialysis or transplantation at any time from shortly after birth until early adulthood. Unilateral hypoplasia, on the other hand, does not cause any problems or require intervention.

Other, more common causes of small kidneys must be considered before hypoplasia is diagnosed. They include atrophy secondary to reflux nephropathy, atrophic pyelonephritis, vascular ischemia, renal vein thrombosis, and dysplasia.

Renal Dysplasia

Renal dysplasia is caused by abnormal metanephric differentiation and is a histologic rather than a clinical diagnosis. Dysplastic kidneys may involve both cystic and hypoplastic changes, although both elements not always are present. Histologically, primitive glomerular and tubular elements, cartilage, smooth muscle, and cysts are seen in the parenchyma. The dysplasia may be segmental or involve the entire renal unit. Affected parts of the kidney generally do not function. The kidney may be reniform in shape, or the dysplasia may be so severe that the unit has little resemblance to a normal kidney. Urinary tract obstruction may be associated with dysplasia and contribute to its formation.

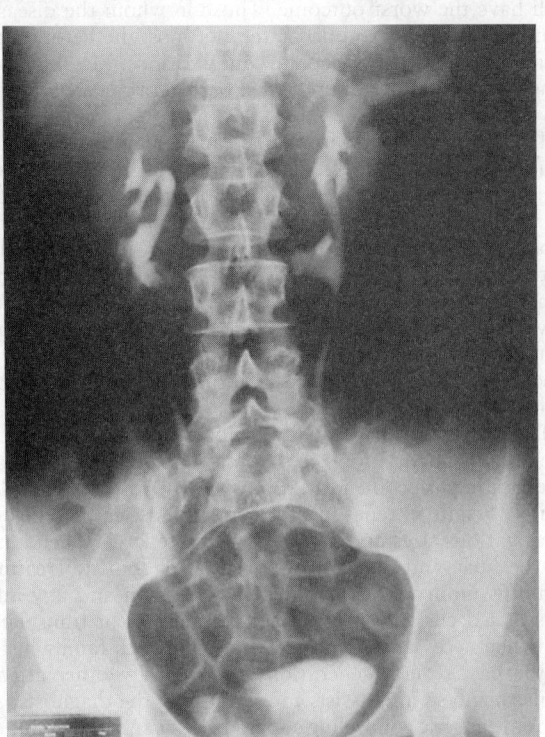

FIGURE 320.1. Intravenous pyelography of a horseshoe kidney. Note the axis deviation and incomplete rotation of the kidneys.

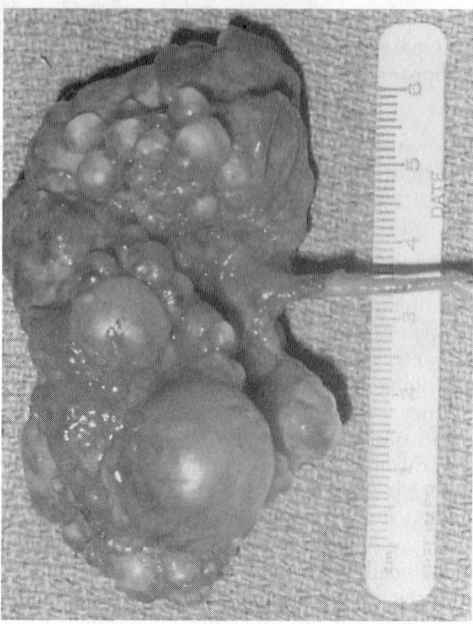

FIGURE 320.2. A gross photograph of a multicystic kidney. (Reprinted with permission from Gonzales ET Jr. Genitourinary disorders in the neonate. In: Whitaker RH, Woodard JR, eds. *Paediatric urology.* London: Butterworth, 1985.)

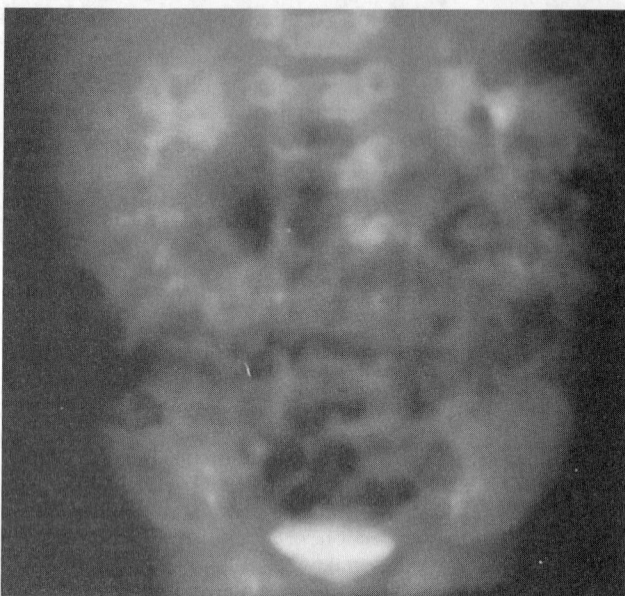

FIGURE 320.3. In this intravenous pyelogram of a child with recessive polycystic kidney disease, note the massive enlargement of the kidneys, good excretion, and linear streaking of the contrast material. (Reprinted with permission from Gonzales ET Jr. Genitourinary disorders in the neonate. In: Whitaker RH, Woodard JR, eds. *Paediatric urology.* London: Butterworth, 1985.)

The most common and well-known dysplastic disorder is the multicystic kidney, which consists of numerous fluid-filled cysts that do not communicate (Fig. 320.2). It is one of the two most common renal masses in the newborn (the other is ureteropelvic junction obstruction), and its diagnosis usually is suggested by ultrasound, performed either prenatally or later for evaluation of an abdominal mass. The presence of a multicystic kidney generally is confirmed by the absence of any function on a renal scan. Voiding cystourethrography should be obtained because reflux is associated in 10% of these cases. Rarely, complications occur and include urinary tract infection (UTI), rupture of renal cysts, and hypertension. The question of malignant degeneration has been raised, but the incidence of cancers is very small. Whether these lesions require nephrectomy remains controversial. Most urologists follow these children with ultrasound because, with time, almost all multicystic kidneys involute and do not seem to cause problems. Fewer physicians remove these kidneys to avoid the long-term, limited risk of development of complications and the necessity of following the children for an extended time with repeated studies.

Polycystic Kidney

Polycystic kidney disease is an inherited disorder, either autosomal recessive (infantile polycystic disease) or autosomal dominant (adult polycystic disease). The two entities are distinct and should not be confused. The recessive form is found in homozygotes, the dominant form in heterozygotes. Other organs, especially the liver, are involved; in the dominant form, cerebral aneurysms are common findings.

In the recessive form, the kidneys retain their reniform configuration but are enlarged. The parenchyma is filled with dilated renal collecting tubules that appear as small radial cysts. The collecting system (renal pelvis and ureter) is normal, as is the renal pedicle. All children with recessive polycystic kidney disease have involvement of the liver consisting of dilation and proliferation of the bile duct, with varying amounts of periportal fibrosis. Areas of uninvolved parenchyma are interspersed

among these involved segments. The degree of renal and hepatic involvement appears to be inversely related, with younger children having more renal but less hepatic involvement. Children who are older when they present usually have more severe hepatic impairment, with marked periportal fibrosis. Prognosis is related to age at diagnosis; those children diagnosed at birth have the worst outcome. Those in whom the disease is found late in childhood do better, but most die before reaching adulthood, often of hepatic complications. Renal and liver transplantations have offered these patients a chance for longer survival.

The recessive disease in infants can be identified prenatally by ultrasound and suspected in a family with a history of polycystic kidney disease or early childhood death from renal or unknown causes. In the neonate, the diagnosis usually is made as part of an evaluation for palpable renal masses noted on routine examination. An ultrasound shows enlarged kidneys with increased, diffuse echogenicity. Intravenous urography shows typical radial streaking of the dilated collecting tubules. Although the kidneys function, they do so poorly; without delayed films, visualization of dye in the renal pelvis, ureter, or bladder is unusual (Fig. 320.3).

The dominant form usually is noted in adults with a positive family history for renal cystic disease and is a completely different problem. It, too, is slowly progressive and ultimately results in renal insufficiency in most cases. The cysts are of various sizes and may become quite large. The kidneys may be huge and fill almost the entire abdomen. Treatment usually is limited to controlling hypertension and any infections that occur and intervening with dialysis or transplantation when necessary. A complete and thorough family history for the past several generations may identify other affected family members and assists in establishing the diagnosis. Appropriate genetic counseling should be done. Although this disorder rarely causes symptoms during childhood, small renal cysts often can be identified by renal ultrasound in affected children.

ANOMALIES OF THE COLLECTING SYSTEM

Ureteropelvic Junction Obstruction

Obstruction at the ureteropelvic junction is the most common cause of hydronephrosis in children and one of the two most common etiologies for a renal mass in neonates (the other is a multicystic kidney). The obstruction often is caused by an intrinsic fibrosis at the junction of the renal pelvis and ureter that disrupts the peristaltic wave across that region. Less common etiologies include a crossing renal vessel, kinking of the ureter, stenosis of the junction, and adhesions or extrinsic fibrosis at the ureteropelvic junction. The obstruction leads to increased intrapelvic pressure, which causes dilation of the pelvis and calyces. This obstruction predisposes to urinary stasis, infection, hematuria, pain, and gradual destruction of renal parenchyma.

The diagnosis often is suggested by prenatal ultrasound and confirmed by postnatal studies. Other signs and symptoms include UTI, pyelonephritis, abdominal or flank pain, sepsis, palpable masses, nausea, failure to thrive, or an incidental finding during the evaluation of associated congenital anomalies. Investigations should include a renal ultrasound, intravenous pyelography, or renal scan. These studies demonstrate pyelocaliectasis and late emptying of the renal pelvis (Fig. 320.4). Because intravenous pyelography often shows poor excretion, films delayed up to 24 hours may be necessary. The renal scan can estimate the relative contribution of the obstructed kidney to overall renal function, and the addition of diuresis (with furosemide) may show a prolonged washout period that suggests obstruction. Voiding cystourethrography is necessary because high-grade vesicoureteral reflux can mimic a ureteropelvic junction obstruction or cause a secondary ureteropelvic junction obstruction, as a result of the large volume of refluxed urine. In both of these cases, control of the reflux resolves the upper tract difficulties. Additionally, 10% of children with a hydronephrosis have associated reflux.

A pyeloplasty is the surgical repair of a ureteropelvic junction obstruction. Its goal is to provide a funneled and dependent pelvis leading to the ureter. Reduction of pelvic size may be necessary to facilitate renal emptying. Improvement in radiographic appearance and renal function usually occurs after relief of obstruction, although it may take years to do so.

Many patients with ureteropelvic junction obstruction are identified on prenatal ultrasound. Some of them demonstrate severe renal damage and need early surgery. The trend, though, is toward observation of neonatal hydronephrotic kidneys with good function on renal scan. Many of these kidneys improve over the course of time without surgery, demonstrating stable renal function and less hydronephrosis. Close monitoring of the renal status is necessary because occasionally a kidney deteriorates quickly and requires surgical repair. If significant hydronephrosis is present after several years, most urologists proceed to surgical correction. Neonates tolerate the surgery quite well, and, with the use of optical magnification, the procedure is overwhelmingly successful in even the youngest children. Long-term follow-up is necessary both for confirmation of an adequate postoperative anatomic result and for final assessment of renal function.

Megaureter

Ureters that are wide and dilated are called *megaureters*. They are divided into primary and secondary megaureters.

The primary megaureter (ureterovesical junction obstruction) is dilated, usually more distally than proximally, to the level of the ureterovesical junction, where a stenotic region, or distal inert (aperistaltic) segment, is encountered. Histologic evaluation has shown a deficiency of muscle fibers in this area that disrupts the peristaltic wave and causes functional obstruction. The usual presentations include hydronephrosis that is discovered on prenatal ultrasound or incidentally at the time of evaluation for other congenital anomalies, UTI, flank pain, or hematuria. Pyelography or ultrasound generally suggests the diagnosis. Confirmation of true obstruction usually requires that the patient undergo a diuretic renogram or, rarely, a percutaneous nephrostomy with pressure flow measurements. Voiding cystourethrography should be obtained because reflux can give the same picture on upper-tract imaging. Ureteroneocystostomy is required if obstruction is confirmed. Ureteral narrowing by tapering or tailoring may be required for an adequate repair. Generally, prognosis is good, but it depends on the extent of renal damage present at the time of surgery.

Secondary megaureters are divided into refluxing and nonrefluxing units. Those that reflux are either developmentally dysplastic or have become dilated by the volume of urine

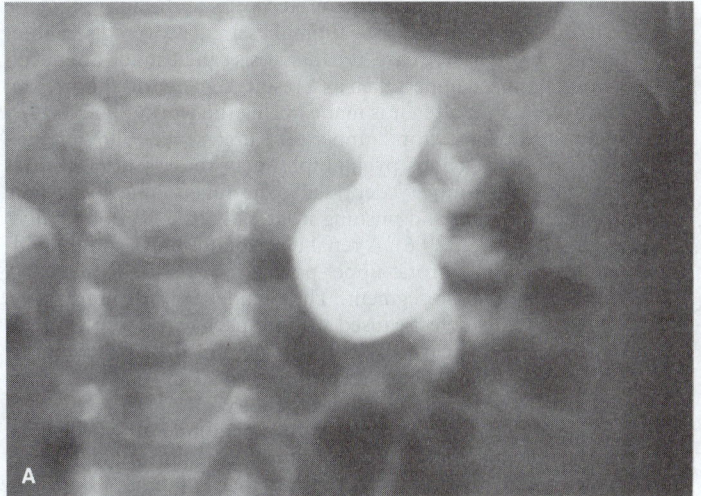
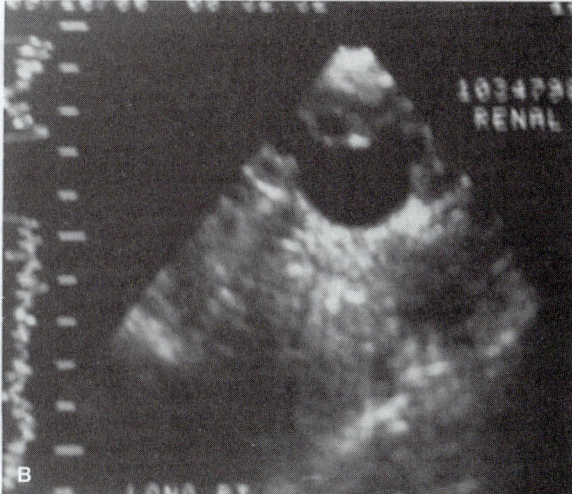

FIGURE 320.4. Ureteropelvic junction obstruction demonstrated by A: intravenous pyelography and B: renal ultrasound.

propelled retrograde by the bladder contraction. In either case, the ureterovesical junction is incompetent and allows the reflux to occur. In most cases, surgical control of the reflux resolves the problem; however, the surgical complication rate for refluxing megaureters exceeds that for obstructed megaureters, implying that an intrinsic ureteral abnormality contributes to the ureterectasis in some cases.

The nonrefluxing secondary megaureter is dilated secondary to urinary obstruction at a level distal to the ureterovesical junction. The most common causes are posterior urethral valves, urethral strictures, neuropathic bladders, and dysfunctional voiding. Establishing the diagnosis may be difficult, and, because the treatments are completely different, care must be taken not to confuse the primary obstructed megaureter with the secondary form. The most reliable methods of distinguishing one from the other are diuretic renograms with a catheter in the bladder and pressure flow studies involving a percutaneous nephrostomy. In nonrefluxing secondary megaureters, control of the distal obstructive process usually solves the problem, and attention should be directed there rather than to the ureterovesical junction.

A final group of patients are those with nonobstructive, nonrefluxing megaureters. This group consists of boys with prune belly syndrome (see following discussion) and children with transient megaureters associated with endotoxins from an acute UTI. Neither condition requires treatment for the megaureter itself and, thus, an accurate diagnosis must be made to avoid unnecessary intervention.

Simple Ureterocele

A simple ureterocele is a cystic dilation of the intravesical segment of the ureter. A simple ureterocele subtends a single (nonduplicated) renal unit. These anomalies are thought to develop if incomplete dissolution of the Chwalla membrane occurs. Many simple ureteroceles are small and asymptomatic, but they can be large and obstruct the ureter or bladder neck. They usually are found when upper-tract imaging (usually a renal ultrasound) is performed to evaluate a UTI. Many are recognized on prenatal ultrasound. The radiographic findings are pathognomonic, showing a "cobra head" deformity within the bladder (Fig. 320.5). If obstruction is not present, no treatment is necessary. A transurethral incision of the ureterocele or, less commonly, ureteroneocystostomy may be required to relieve ureteral obstruction or prevent recurrent infections.

Retrocaval Ureter

The retrocaval ureter is a rare congenital anomaly in which the right ureter passes posterior and medial to the vena cava. Its etiology is related to the persistence of the subcardinal vein ventral to the developing ureter. The ureter then hooks around the future vena cava. The condition rarely is seen in children and is significant only if obstruction of the right kidney is diagnosed. Treatment consists of dividing the ureter and reanastomosing it anterior to the great vessels. Prognosis generally is excellent, with relief of the obstruction and resolution of the symptoms.

Ureteral Duplication, Ureteral Ectopia, and Ureteroceles

Complete Duplication

Ureteral duplication is the most common congenital urologic anomaly; it affects approximately 1 in 150 individuals. Duplication results when two ureteral buds arise from a single

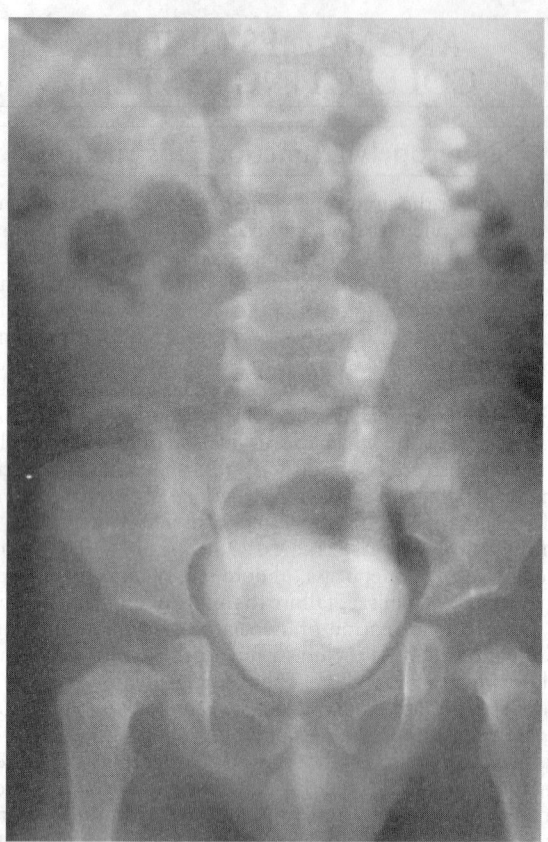

FIGURE 320.5. A simple ureterocele is shown in this intravenous pyelogram. Note the ureteral dilation and swelling of the distal ureter.

Wolffian duct. Both buds reach the developing metanephros and stimulate renal differentiation. The ureter to the lower segment is absorbed into the developing bladder earlier and, therefore, travels further along the trigone, finally resting lateral and cephalad to the upper pole ureter, which lies medial and caudal. This relationship is known as the *Weigert-Meyer law*. The lower-pole ureter is prone to reflux, whereas the upper-pole ureter (medial and inferior) is associated more often with obstruction from either ectopia or an ectopic ureterocele.

A full spectrum of renal involvement has been observed, ranging from the child with severe bilateral lower-pole reflux and bilateral obstructing ureteroceles to the asymptomatic adult in whom duplication anomalies are discovered serendipitously. In the severe case, the diagnosis can be made after evaluation has been undertaken as a result of an abnormal prenatal ultrasound, but often it is made during the workup of a UTI or symptoms of an ectopic upper-pole ureter (see following discussion). Intravenous pyelography may show a nonfunctioning upper-pole moiety depressing the functioning lower-pole collecting system and pushing it laterally (the "drooping lily" deformity) (Fig. 320.6). A renal ultrasound shows similar findings: a hydronephrotic upper-pole cap of tissue depressing a normal lower-pole segment. The bladder may demonstrate a negative filling defect caused by nonopacification of the ureterocele. A renal scan can estimate the functional capacity of each segment, and voiding cystourethrography is required for assessment of possible lower-pole reflux.

Treatment is as varied as is the presentation. Often, when the upper pole has no function, an upper-pole partial nephroureterectomy is performed. If, on the other hand, good function exists in that segment, a transurethral incision of the ureterocele can be performed. This procedure usually relieves the obstruction, but it may cause the development of upper-pole reflux. At other times, a ureteropyelostomy connecting the upper-pole

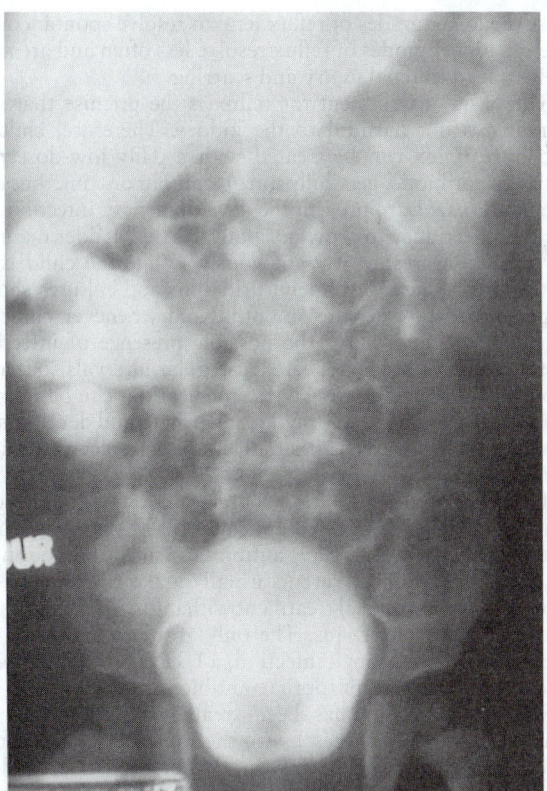

FIGURE 320.6. Intravenous pyelogram of a neonate with a right duplication anomaly. Nonvisualization of the right upper pole with the "drooping lily" deformity of the lower pole moiety is seen. (Reprinted with permission from Gonzales ET Jr. Genitourinary disorders in the neonate. In: Whitaker RH, Woodard JR, eds. *Paediatric urology*. London: Butterworth, 1985.)

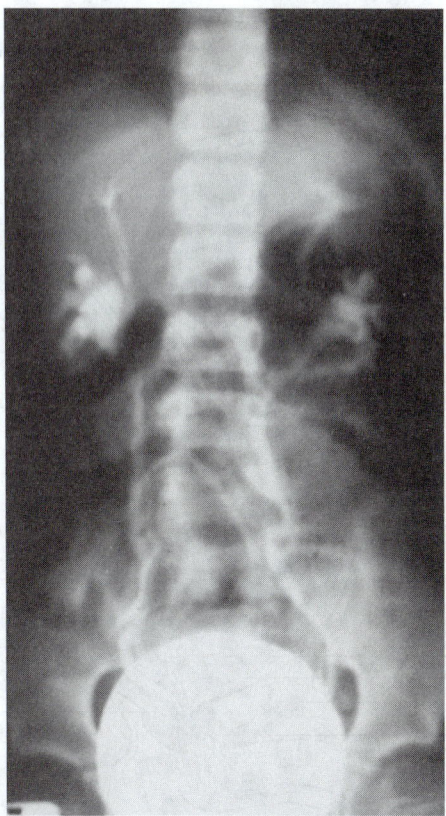

FIGURE 320.7. This voiding cystourethrogram shows bilateral partial duplication anomalies without hydronephrosis or obstruction.

ureter to the lower-pole renal pelvis, in conjunction with partial resection of the distal upper-pole ureter, is preferred. If lower-pole reflux is present with an upper-pole ureterocele, some surgeons reimplant the ureters at the same time the upper systems are addressed. Other surgeons delay performing any bladder surgery for several months or years, in the hope that the reflux may resolve once the ureterocele, which has been distorting the bladder, has been decompressed. When reflux to the lower pole is present without upper-pole obstruction, a common sheath ureteroneocystostomy usually is all that is required.

The prognosis depends on the degree of renal damage present at the time of intervention. However, renal function generally is adequate, and further problems seldom occur.

Incomplete Duplication

Division of the ureteral bud after it originates from the Wolffian duct causes incomplete ureteral duplication. Two ureteral buds thus promote adjacent renal differentiation but arise from a single ureteral orifice. This condition generally is asymptomatic and does not need attention (Fig. 320.7).

Ureteral Ectopia

Ureteral ectopia occurs when the ureteral orifice lies medial and inferior to its normal location. This condition can be related to either a single or duplicated drainage system. Its developmental etiology is related to the anomalous development of the terminal segment of the Wolffian duct. The origin of the ureteral bud is more cephalad than normal on the mesonephric

system, precluding the usual incorporation into the trigone. In boys, the ureter can terminate along the vas deferens, seminal vesicle, prostatic urethra, or distal trigone. Because all these locations are proximal to the external sphincter, urinary continence is preserved. In girls, the analogous structures of the Wolffian duct and urogenital sinus are the bladder neck, urethra, vestibule, and Gartner duct, some of which are distal to the urinary sphincter. Ureters draining at those locations generally are associated with constant urinary leakage (Fig. 320.8), a typical presenting symptom.

The clinical features of this disorder depend on the location of the ureteral orifice and the degree of developmental renal dysplasia. The symptoms usually are those of infection or incontinence. In girls, a history of lifelong constant wetness despite a normal voiding pattern suggests ureteral ectopia. In boys, the diagnosis of ureteral ectopia should be considered whenever a mass is found in the seminal vesicle or epididymitis or prostatitis is encountered. Radiographic studies may show either a nonfunctioning renal unit or ureteral dilation, depending on the degree of developmental abnormality. Cystoscopy can be helpful, especially if bilateral ectopia or a hemitrigone is found.

Treatment generally consists of a nephroureterectomy of the involved renal unit because renal function usually is poor. However, if kidney function is good, or in the case of bilateral ureteral ectopia, reimplantation is appropriate.

VESICOURETERAL REFLUX

Vesicoureteral reflux is the retrograde regurgitation of urine from the bladder toward the kidney. Reflux is either primary or acquired; in children, primary reflux is more prevalent. Its etiology is embryologically related to the abnormal position

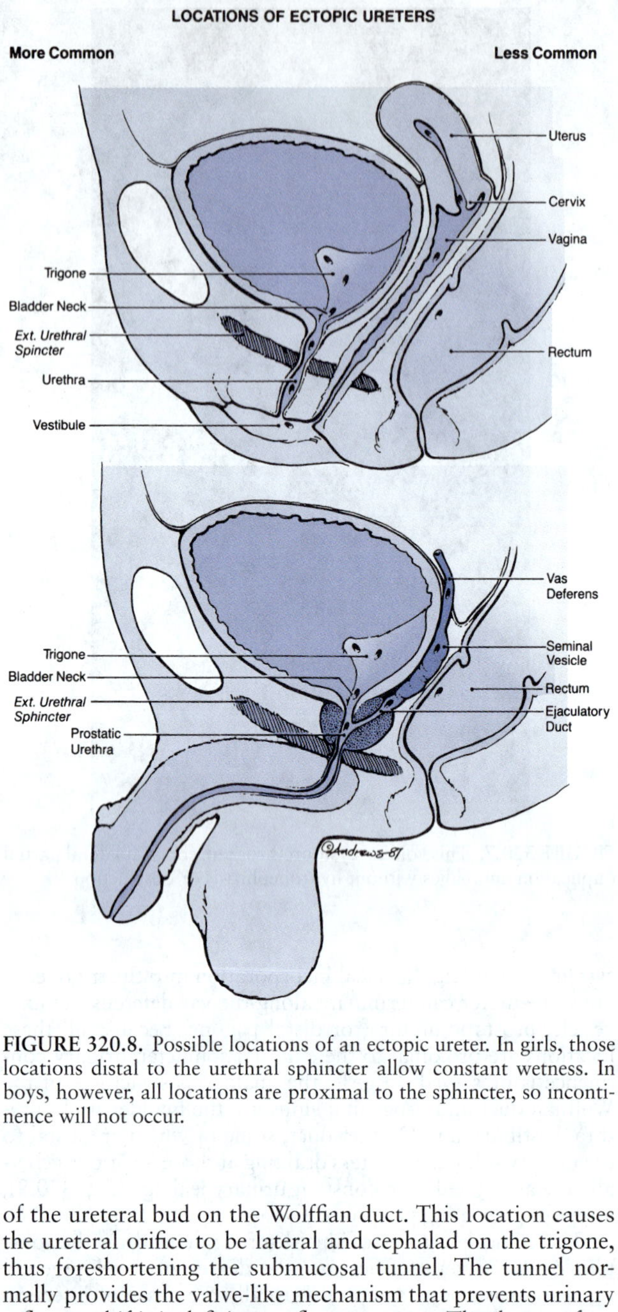

LOCATIONS OF ECTOPIC URETERS

More Common   Less Common

FIGURE 320.8. Possible locations of an ectopic ureter. In girls, those locations distal to the urethral sphincter allow constant wetness. In boys, however, all locations are proximal to the sphincter, so incontinence will not occur.

of the ureteral bud on the Wolffian duct. This location causes the ureteral orifice to be lateral and cephalad on the trigone, thus foreshortening the submucosal tunnel. The tunnel normally provides the valve-like mechanism that prevents urinary reflux, and if it is deficient, reflux can occur. The degree of reflux may range from very mild (when urine enters the ureter but does not reach the kidney) to very severe (when the ureters are widely dilated and tortuous, with gross pyelocaliectasis). An objective system using well-described criteria for grading reflux is used throughout the world and is based on voiding a cystourethrography (Fig. 320.9).

The diagnosis of reflux is best made through voiding cystourethrography. Generally, this radiologic study is performed initially because it provides reproducible quantification of the reflux (which allows prognostic determination), defines anatomic anomalies at the ureteral insertion area (paraureteral diverticula, ectopia), and also visualizes the urethra, which is imperative in boys to rule out the presence of urethral obstruction. In subsequent follow-up studies, nuclear cystography may be substituted for voiding cystourethrography. The main advantage of nuclear cystography is that radiation exposure is lower compared with standard contrast cystography; however, it does not define the anatomy well, rendering grading less precise. Quantification of the reflux is important for prognosis because the lower grades of reflux tend to resolve spontaneously, whereas higher grades of reflux resolve less often and are more likely to lead to renal injury and scarring.

The basis of treatment for reflux is the premise that sterile reflux is not harmful to the kidney. Therefore, children who have reflux can be treated with a daily low-dose prophylactic antibiotic, generally nitrofurantoin or trimethoprim-sulfamethoxazole, to prevent the development of infection and to allow the kidney to grow normally. As the bladder matures, the reflux may resolve spontaneously. While the child is receiving prophylactic treatment, urinalysis and cultures should be performed every 3 to 4 months, and whenever clinically indicated, to monitor for the possible presence of infection. Cystography should be repeated at regular intervals so that, if resolution of the reflux occurs, the medications can be stopped and the child observed. Normal renal growth and development should follow; however, further infections may occur, especially during pregnancy.

The other treatment option is ureteral reimplantation (ureteroneocystostomy). In uncomplicated cases, the success rate exceeds 98%. After surgery, antibiotics can be discontinued and the child watched. Parents usually make the decision for either medical or surgical treatment with information and guidance from their physicians. The only absolute indication for surgery is a breakthrough infection, a UTI that develops while the child is receiving appropriate antibiotic therapy.

Since 1986, reflux has been treated endoscopically (by means of cystoscopic access) with the subureteric injection of either Teflon or collagen. Teflon has not been approved by the U.S. Food and Drug Administration (FDA) for this procedure, and most of this experience comes from Europe. Collagen has not produced satisfactory long-term results because of degradation of the compound. More recently, Deflux (dextranomer/hyaluronic acid copolymer) has been approved by the FDA and currently is experiencing widespread use by pediatric urologists for the treatment of mild to moderate degrees of reflux. The technique of endoscopic injection is easy, has a very low complication rate, has minimal symptoms, and has an 80% success rate. At this time, it seems to be a very valuable addition to our treatment options for vesicoureteral reflux.

Several other factors, including age, gender, family situation, and presence of renal scarring, may play roles in determining treatment. Cystoscopy, which in the past was used to predict the likelihood of spontaneous resolution of reflux occurring, no longer is considered to be useful in evaluating a child with straightforward reflux. Because of an increased incidence of reflux in siblings (30%) and offspring (60%) of an index case, they also should be investigated. The most accurate screening test is cystography, but in the older asymptomatic child with no history of urinary infection, a renal ultrasound only may be adequate. If significant reflux is present, the renal ultrasound may uncover upper-tract dilation or scarring. If low-grade reflux is present and the ultrasound is normal, the older child is thought to be beyond the age when most renal damage secondary to reflux occurs, and treatment should not be needed. Generally speaking, such a child should receive the same treatment as anyone else with documented reflux.

BLADDER AND URETHRAL ANOMALIES

Posterior Urethral Valves

Posterior urethral valves are rare congenital obstructing leaflets in the region of the verumontanum in the prostatic urethra. No analogous structure or pathology occurs in girls. Their etiology is unclear, but they may be related to anomalous development

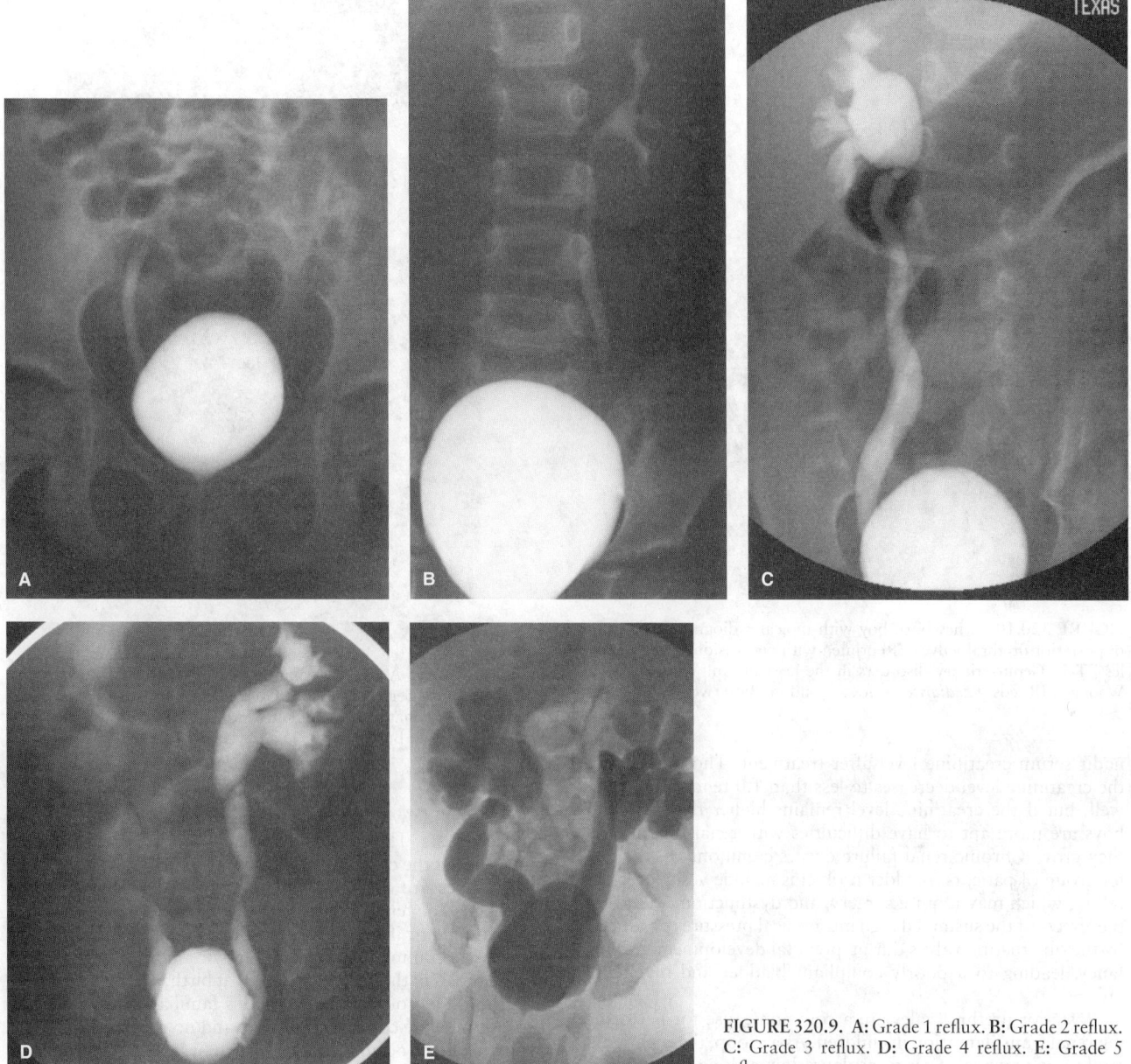

FIGURE 320.9. A: Grade 1 reflux. **B:** Grade 2 reflux. **C:** Grade 3 reflux. **D:** Grade 4 reflux. **E:** Grade 5 reflux.

of the plicae colliculi, normal folds in the urethra that define the migration pathway of the ducts of Cowper glands. Problems with posterior urethral valves stem from their narrowing of the bladder outlet, proximal to the external urethral sphincter. The obstruction causes increased voiding pressure with dilation of the prostatic urethra, hypertrophy of the bladder neck, bladder trabeculation, and saccule formation. Renal dysplasia and insufficiency are common findings and often associated with vesicoureteral reflux.

Clinical presentation is varied, but with the advent of prenatal ultrasonography, these children often are diagnosed before birth with the typical findings of bilateral hydroureteronephrosis, a thickened bladder, and a widened, elongated prostatic urethra. Neonatal discovery may be prompted by the findings of a distended bladder, palpable kidney, UTI, renal insufficiency, and a poor or dribbling urinary stream. Constitutional symptoms, such as failure to thrive, abdominal distention, and vomiting, may signal the presence of posterior urethral valves. In older boys, voiding problems may predominate and may be obvious. They vary from the expected (poor stream, urinary

retention, and bladder distention) to quite subtle (hematuria, enuresis, and hesitancy). The diagnosis is made on voiding cystourethrography (Fig. 320.10).

Treatment is directed toward relief of the obstruction. Initial therapy, especially in the neonate, is placement of a transurethral catheter, hemodynamic stabilization, normalization of electrolytes, and treatment of any existing infection. If the renal function is normal or near normal, transurethral ablation of the valves is performed within a few days. In neonates with increasing creatinine levels, uncontrollable infection, or a urethra too small to accept an infant cystoscope, a temporary vesicostomy is appropriate. The older boy can almost always undergo transurethral surgery because size is not a problem, and severe renal insufficiency is a rare occurrence.

Long-term difficulties from posterior urethral valves are seen in both renal and bladder function. Traditionally, the younger the child is when the diagnosis is made, the poorer the prognosis. This standard, however, has been modified by prenatal ultrasound because even mild cases may be discovered before birth. Currently, the best predictor of prognosis is the

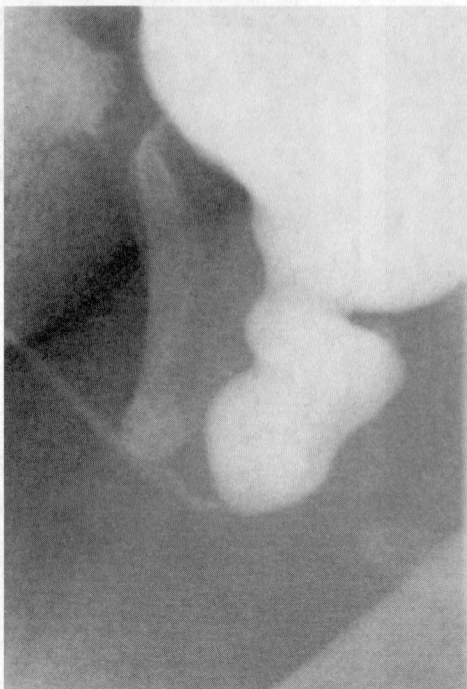

FIGURE 320.10. A newborn boy with typical radiographic findings of posterior urethral valves. (Reprinted with permission from Gonzales ET Jr. Genitourinary disorders in the neonate. In: Whitaker RH, Woodard JR, eds. *Paediatric urology*. London: Butterworth, 1985.)

nadir serum creatinine level after treatment. Those in whom the creatinine level decreases to less than 1.0 tend to do quite well, but if the creatinine level remains higher than 1.0, the boys are more apt to have difficulties with renal function as they grow. Chronic renal failure occurs commonly in the latter group of patients. Bladder problems include vesicoureteral reflux, which may require surgery, and dysfunction caused by the effects of the sustained high intravesical pressures produced by the obstructing valves during prenatal development and infancy, leading to a poorly compliant bladder and myogenic failure.

Posterior urethral vales are a common cause for performing renal transplantation in children. As a group, these patients tend to do very well after transplantation, as long as any bladder dysfunction is recognized and appropriately managed.

Exstrophy-Epispadias Complex

Classic exstrophy is a rare anomaly (1 in 30,000 to 40,000 individuals) of the lower abdominal wall. The cause of bladder exstrophy is not known but is thought to result from the persistence of the cloacal membrane, preventing the medial ingrowth of mesenchyme, which is necessary to form the musculature of the lower abdominal wall (Fig. 320.11). The fused layers of ectoderm and endoderm are unstable. When rupture of the membrane occurs, separation of the midline structures occurs, including the lower abdominal wall, rectus abdominis muscle and fascia, bladder, pubis, urethra, and genitalia.

The extent of the exstrophy defect depends on the size of the cloacal membrane and the time of its rupture. In the most common form, the bladder is open and exposed on the lower abdominal wall. The rectus muscles and fascia diverge around the bladder to insert on the laterally displaced pubic bones. The external genitalia are splayed; in girls, the clitoris is bifid, the labia lateral, and the vagina anterior. In boys, the penis is

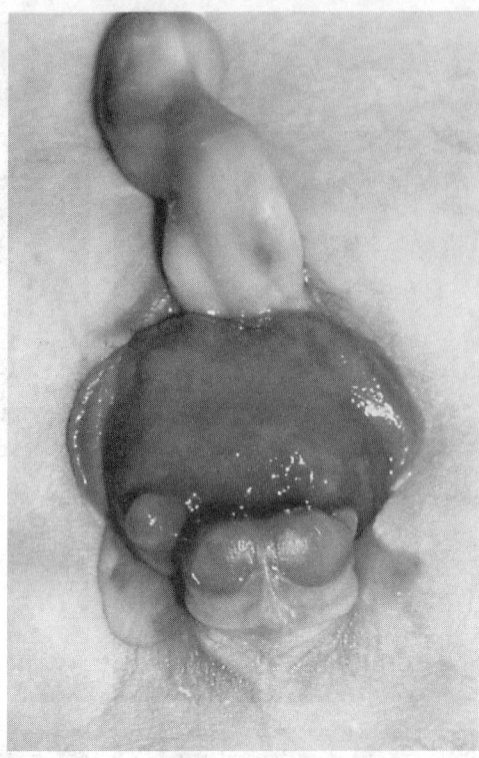

FIGURE 320.11. A typical example of classical bladder exstrophy. (Reprinted with permission from Gonzales ET Jr. Genitourinary disorders in the neonate. In: Whitaker RH, Woodard JR, eds. *Paediatric urology*. London: Butterworth, 1985.)

short and wide with a dorsal urethral strip. Significant dorsal chordee exists. The anus is displaced anteriorly, and the umbilicus lies at the cephalad portion of the exposed bladder. The pubic bones are divergent in the midline, leaving the pelvic ring open. The femoral heads are rotated externally and cause a waddling gait if not corrected. Both inguinal and umbilical hernias are common findings and may require surgery.

Diagnosis of the defect is obvious at birth, and prompt attention should be sought from surgeons familiar with such problems. Immediate care is supportive, and no recognized pattern of involvement occurs in other organ systems. Uroradiologic evaluation usually shows normally developed kidneys and collecting systems. With time, hypertrophy of the bladder mucosa and prolapse of the ureters may occur, leading to hydronephrosis. Initial management of the bladder requires covering the area with cellophane as a protective measure. The cover should remain in place until corrective surgery can be performed.

Currently, the goal of treatment is to provide a functioning bladder capable of social continence and functional genitalia. Although ambitious, these goals can be reached in most patients over a period of several years. The initial surgical procedure often is closure of the bladder and abdominal wall, leaving an open incontinent epispadiac bladder neck. If possible, this procedure should be undertaken within the first 48 to 72 hours of life. If not, consideration should be given to performing iliac osteotomies at the time of bladder closure. That orthopedic procedure allows the bladder to drop into the abdominal cavity and facilitates closure of the anterior abdominal wall. Several years after bladder closure is achieved, most urologists proceed with the second stage of the repair, which in girls is bladder neck reconstruction and ureteral reimplantation, to provide continence and eliminate reflux. Successful results are reported in as many as 80% of these children. In boys, epispadias repair, a combination of penile lengthening, release of dorsal chordee, and a urethroplasty, is undertaken before bladder neck surgery is performed. Currently, some surgeons experienced in the management of bladder exstrophy have begun to do total reconstruction of this defect in the neonatal period, with encouraging early results. Individuals whose bladder neck reconstruction has failed and who remain incontinent may be considered for a repeat procedure, placement of an artificial urinary sphincter, or urinary diversion. In some children with exstrophy, the exposed bladder is small and fibrotic. Occasionally, primary closure of the bladder cannot be achieved, and a continent urinary diversion to the skin may be necessary.

Cloacal exstrophy is a more complex and less common anomaly in which the cloacal membrane ruptures before complete descent of the urorectal septum. The resultant defect is much more severe than that of classic exstrophy. A strip of open gut splits the bladder plate on the abdominal wall. The proximal bowel leads to the ileum, and the distal opening leads to a blind-ending hindgut. The phallus is widely separated in both sexes. Because associated anomalies are common occurrences, a thorough evaluation of other organ systems is mandatory.

In the past, children with cloacal exstrophy rarely survived the neonatal period; however, advances in surgical techniques and parenteral alimentation have provided long-term survival for these babies. Initial management is directed toward stabilizing electrolyte losses from the short gut and meeting nutritional requirements. Diversion of both the fecal and urinary streams usually is required. Currently, enthusiasm exists for maintaining the rudimentary hindgut to extend the bowel and thus decrease the effects of the short bowel syndrome. Multiple surgeries can be expected to be performed in these patients to complete their genitourinary reconstruction.

Epispadias without exstrophy occurs less commonly than does exstrophy. In boys, epispadias is classified as balanitic, penile, or penopubic, and the urethral meatus, as well as any chordee, is dorsal (Fig. 320.12). Repair of epispadias involves correcting the chordee and constructing a neourethra. Female epispadias is more unusual and often goes undetected until a careful genital examination is performed on an older incontinent girl, in whom a bifid clitoris associated with a short

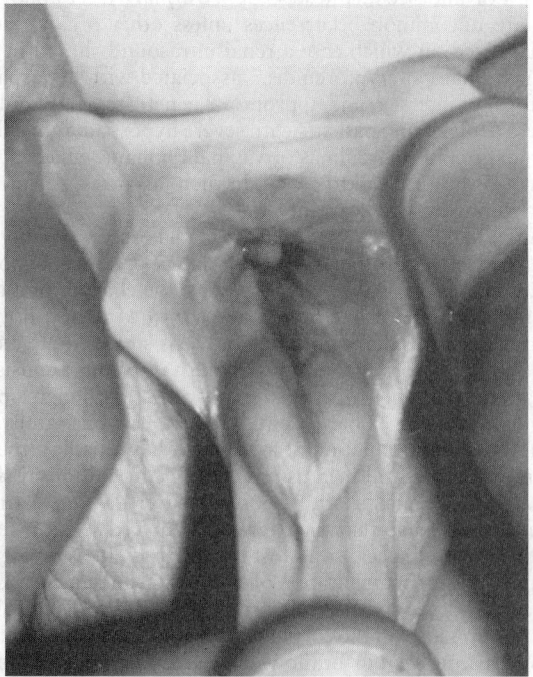

FIGURE 320.12. Penopubic epispadias with severe dorsal chordee.

and patulous urethra is discovered. If the epispadias extends through the bladder neck, surgery is required to provide continence and consists of either a bladder neck reconstruction or insertion of an artificial urinary sphincter, as is done for classical bladder exstrophy.

Anterior Urethral Pathology

Anterior Urethral Valves

Anterior urethral valves form a rare congenital obstruction of the penile urethra. The obstruction may be mild or very severe, similar to posterior urethral valves. Because voiding symptoms are common findings, this entity should be considered in boys complaining of urgency, frequency, or a poor stream. The diagnosis is made by voiding cystourethrography, which classically demonstrates a urethral diverticulum at the site of stenosis, with proximal urethral dilation. The distal edge of the diverticulum is the cause of the valvular obstruction. Treatment consists of transurethral destruction of the lesion or an open excision with reconstruction of the urethra. These patients require follow-up similar to that of patients with posterior urethral valves.

Anterior Urethral Strictures

Strictures of the penile urethra have several etiologies, the most common of which are traumatic, iatrogenic, and inflammatory. Currently, iatrogenic lesions are thought to account for many of the reported cases, although with better urethral catheters, the incidence seems to be decreasing. These lesions develop after urologic treatment for congenital anomalies or after long-term or traumatic urethral catheterization. Traumatic strictures also occur after direct injury to the perineum (a straddle injury). Inflammatory strictures are uncommon occurrences in children because they usually result from gonococcal urethritis. Whatever the cause, strictures may take years to develop after the initial urethral insult.

Symptoms of a stricture are the same as those associated with other forms of bladder outflow obstruction: strangury; hesitancy; small, thin stream with little pressure; and dribbling. Terminal hematuria may occur in conjunction with a stricture or with a nonspecific inflammation of the posterior urethra that may predispose to the subsequent formation of a stricture.

Treatment depends on the degree of narrowing, symptoms, and the length of the stricture. Endoscopic urethrotomy often is used. Open urethroplasty is an option usually reserved for patients with more severe strictures or those unresponsive to optical urethrotomy. Prognosis generally is excellent, but repeated operations occasionally are required.

Urethrorrhagia

Urethrorrhagia has been defined as the painless spotting of blood on a young boy's underwear. The urinalysis result is negative, without either hematuria or pyuria. The symptoms may last for months or even years and have a tendency to recur. Although urethrorrhagia is troublesome to parents, it has no long-term ill effects. Evaluation often includes an ultrasound, but it almost always will be normal. The ultrasound may be avoided if absolutely no evidence of hematuria exists. Cystoscopy, which occasionally is suggested, usually shows posterior urethritis. Antibiotic therapy often is prescribed, but it has no scientific basis. Because the process is self-limited, patience and reassurance alone probably provide the most appropriate therapy; however, follow-up is indicated because urethral strictures occasionally occur.

Megalourethra

An abnormally wide urethra with deficiency of the corpus spongiosum has been termed *megalourethra*. More severe cases may have absence of the corpora cavernosa. This rare entity is thought to be related to a developmental arrest that occurs during embryogenesis of the penis. A cystogram should be obtained to delineate urethral anatomy. Urethral obstruction is a rare development; however, other associated urologic anomalies are common findings, and upper-tract evaluation by renal ultrasound is indicated. Systemic anomalies often are more significant and may be life-threatening. A reduction urethroplasty may be required to reduce urinary stasis and improve both urethral emptying and cosmetic appearance.

Urethral Prolapse

Urethral prolapse is the protrusion of the female urethral mucosa and engorged corpus spongiosum through the external urethral meatus. The most prominent presenting symptom is bleeding, and physical examination suggests the diagnosis (Fig. 320.13). This condition is found primarily in preadolescent black girls and may be secondary to a transient increase in intraabdominal pressure. Various treatments have been proposed. Some authors suggest early primary excision as the modality with the fewest complications, lowest recurrence, and shortest hospital stay; however, an initial course of topical estrogens may provide significant improvement and avoid surgical excision. If left alone, the tissue will involute slowly and the problem will resolve. As this may take weeks to occur, medical or surgical treatment is preferred.

Urachal Anomalies

The urachus arises from the bladder dome and extends cephalad to the umbilicus. Its embryologic origin is either the anterior portion of the cloaca or the allantois. Normally, the urachus is a fibrous cord with an obliterated lumen; abnormalities of the urachus occur when this obliteration is incomplete. A continuum of involvement occurs, from a fully patent urachus to one in which extensive closure of the canal has occurred. The presentation of a patent urachus (communication between the bladder and umbilicus) usually is that of a wet or draining

umbilicus. Its presence should alert the clinician to possible bladder outlet obstruction, especially an atretic or obstructed urethra. Confirmation of the diagnosis can be made by voiding cystourethrography, fistulography through the draining umbilical site, cystoscopy, or instillation of methylene blue into the bladder and visualization of blue drainage from the umbilicus.

Another abnormality is an urachal cyst, which usually is located in the proximal third of the urachus, closest to the bladder. Intermittent infections most often occur in older children or adolescents. Symptoms are suprapubic pain, tenderness, swelling, a palpable mass, and drainage from the umbilicus. If an infected cyst drains to the umbilicus and a tract is formed, a urachal sinus develops. Persistent umbilical drainage and formation of granulation tissue at the umbilicus often are present.

Treatment for these conditions requires antibiotics for any acute infection and subsequent suprapubic exploration and excision of the infected urachal remnant. If not excised, recurrent infections, possibly with abscess formation, can occur.

ANOMALIES OF THE PENIS

Hypospadias

Hypospadias is a congenital penile deformity resulting from incomplete development of the distal or anterior urethra. The urethral meatus may be located at any point along the ventral shaft of the penis, the midline of the scrotum, or in the perineum. The more proximal the urethral meatus, the more likely the penis is to be curved because of inelasticity of the dysplastic urethral plate and a foreshortening of the ventrum of the paired corpora cavernosa. This curvature is termed *chordee* and may preclude intercourse if severe. The prepuce in a hypospadias patient is incompletely formed, with absence of the ventral foreskin but abundance of the dorsal skin, which drapes over the glans as a dorsal hood.

Hypospadias is the most common congenital anomaly of the penis, affecting approximately 3.5 per 1,000 male births. Associated anomalies consist mainly of inguinal pathology, either hernias or undescended testes. Upper urinary tract abnormalities are uncommon occurrences unless other organ systems are involved, in which case a renal ultrasound should be performed. Bilateral cryptorchidism associated with hypospadias is a form of intersex, and appropriate genetic testing should be done. Furthermore, patients with severe hypospadias may have a large utriculus masculinas or vaginal remnant, which can sequester urine and lead to a UTI. In such instances, performing cystography may be warranted.

A familial tendency toward hypospadias occurs. If a boy has hypospadias, his brother has a 14% chance of having hypospadias; if two brothers have hypospadias, the chances of a third brother having the same defect increase to 21%. If a boy has hypospadias, the chance that his father is similarly affected is 8%. A multifactorial inheritance pattern is the most consistent explanation for the incidence of hypospadias, although a point genetic mutation has been identified in at least one family.

In the initial evaluation of a boy with hypospadias, the position of the urethral meatus (glandular, coronal, distal shaft, midshaft, proximal shaft, penoscrotal, scrotal, or perineal) should be noted so that the degree of required surgical repair can be estimated. Because almost every hypospadias repair uses preputial skin, documentation of its position and amount is important, and neonatal circumcision is contraindicated. Slight perineal pressure on the corpora cavernosa mimics an erection by obstructing venous outflow. This erection should help the clinician to assess the degree (mild, moderate, severe) and location (glandular, distal shaft, midshaft, or proximal shaft) of

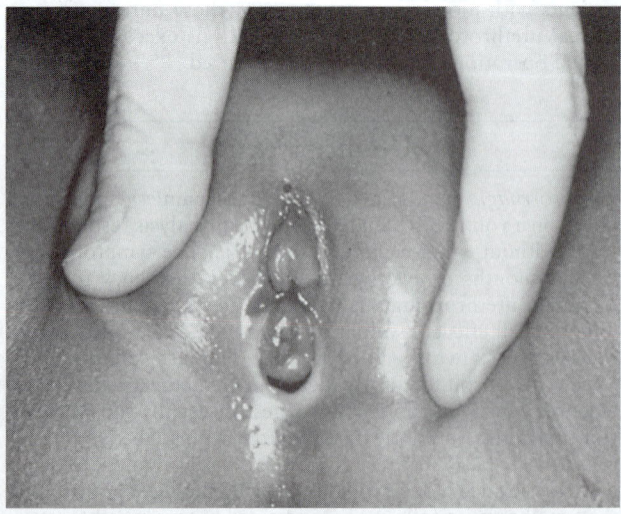

FIGURE 320.13. Urethral prolapse in a young girl.

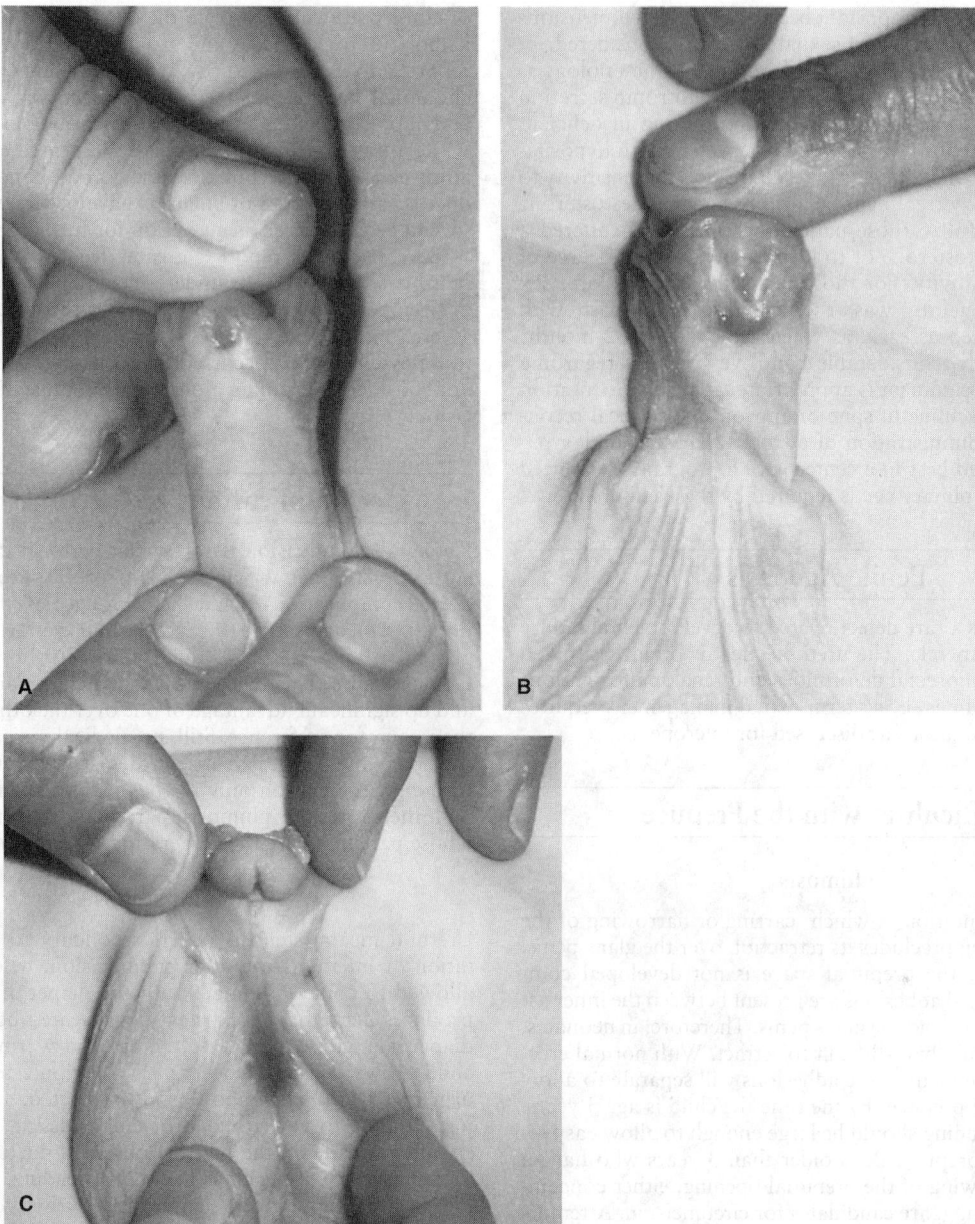

FIGURE 320.14. Three cases of hypospadias with varying degrees of involvement. **A:** A distal meatus without evidence of concomitant chordee. **B:** A more severe case in which severe chordee and deficiency of the ventral penile skin is seen. **C:** A perineal hypospadias with severe chordee.

chordee. In cases of severe hypospadias, an element of penoscrotal transposition may be present; the scrotal folds envelope or wrap around the proximal penile shaft. This abnormality can be addressed at the same time as are the hypospadias and chordee to improve the patient's appearance (Fig. 320.14).

The objectives of surgical repair of hypospadias are threefold. The first is to provide a straight penis that is adequate for intercourse; the second is to extend the urethral meatus to the tip of the glans penis; and the third is to improve the appearance of the penis to that of a normal circumcised phallus. Most pediatric urologists currently suggest that surgery be performed when the child is between ages 4 and 15 months. Sexual identification is not complete at this age, and the surgical procedure is less likely to be remembered. Today, a single surgical procedure is used to correct all but the most severe problems. In instances of penoscrotal or perineal defects, a two-stage procedure remains a reasonable option.

Generally, cosmetic results after hypospadias surgery are excellent, but a significant (15% to 40%) complication rate for patients with proximal defects remains. Distal repairs have a much lower complication rate (less than 5%). These problems consist mainly of fistulas, urethral strictures, and recurrent chordee. Any of these conditions could require a second procedure. Unfortunately, the occasional patient undergoes multiple procedures before an acceptable result is achieved.

Micropenis

Micropenis is a rare condition in which a small but normally developed phallus is present. A micropenis in a neonate is diagnosed if the stretched penile length from the pubic symphysis to the tip of the glans penis is less than 2.5 cm (less than 2 SD from the mean). Measurement of penile girth (diameter or circumference) also is important because corporeal dimensions will become important when sexual function is considered.

If the penis is normally formed but small, the etiology is thought to be related to a deficiency of gonadotropin secretion in the last two trimesters of gestation (resulting in deficient testosterone secretion). If micropenis is present with hypospadias, the problem more likely is a result of a local insensitivity to testosterone. Early treatment by local or systemic testosterone may prove helpful to those patients who *in utero* suffered a deficiency of testosterone or to identify boys with a degree of androgen insensitivity. For those with end-organ failure, sex reassignment generally was recommended in the past, with surgery performed as early as when the child was 2 months of age. Currently, considerable controversy exists regarding whether sex reassignment is appropriate, as sexual orientation may remain masculine in spite of appropriate surgical reconstruction and administration of estrogen. These complex patients are handled best in a center with a program committed to the multidisciplinary needs required by these children.

Penile Agenesis

Penile agenesis is a rare defect related to developmental failure of the genital tubercle. The urethral meatus often is situated near the anus. Anorectal deformities and renal malformations are common findings. Long-term sexual management requires the same considerations as discussed for micropenis.

Difficulties with the Prepuce

Phimosis

Phimosis is a condition in which scarring or narrowing of the preputial opening precludes its retraction over the glans penis. In the newborn, the preputial space is not developed completely, and normal adhesions are present between the inner aspect of the prepuce and the glans penis. Therefore, in neonates, the foreskin normally is difficult to retract. With normal erections and development, these adhesions will separate to allow retraction of the prepuce. By the time the child is age 3 years, the preputial opening should be large enough to allow easy retraction of the prepuce. Boys older than 3 years who have a persistent narrowing of the preputial opening, either congenital or from scarring, are candidates for circumcision. Attempts at blunt retraction and stretching of this opening may lead to tearing, bleeding, and edema and should be discouraged.

Paraphimosis

The occurrence of paraphimosis, as distinguished from phimosis, is an emergency that sometimes requires surgical reduction. In paraphimosis, the prepuce is incarcerated proximal to the glans penis, producing edema and swelling of the glans and prepuce. Local discomfort is universal and prompt reduction is mandatory. After the application of local anesthesia, pressure applied around the prepuce to reduce edema, followed by direct pressure to the glans in conjunction with counteraction on the prepuce, usually resolves the situation. If not, incision of the restricting band or circumcision is required. Patients and caregivers must be instructed in the proper care of the prepuce so that paraphimosis does not occur.

Infection

Balanitis is a fairly common infection of the prepuce (incidence, 6%). It usually responds to oral and topical antibiotics and warm baths. If simple measures are unsuccessful, parenteral antibiotics or circumcision may be required. Most often, mixed organisms are cultured from the exudate. Both group A beta-hemolytic streptococcus and group B streptococcus have been reported to cause balanitis. In sexually active teenagers, trichomonal balanitis and candidal infections are possibilities and, if present, should prompt investigation of sexual partners. Balanitis may become recurrent. Repeated episodes of balanitis can lead to preputial scarring and phimosis. Therefore, once several episodes of balanitis have occurred, circumcision should be considered as an option for further management.

Several studies report a greater frequency of UTIs in infant boys who have not undergone circumcision (1.8%) than in circumcised boys (0.2%). Generally, the infections were not severe, but they did require hospitalization and parenteral antibiotics when they occurred in neonates. Most surgeons do not consider this finding alone to be an indication for circumcision.

Complications of Circumcision

Neonatal circumcision is safe when performed by an experienced practitioner within the first several weeks of life. Reported complications include hemorrhage (less than 1%), infection (0.4%), dehiscence (0.16%), denudation of shaft (0.05%), glandular injury (0.02%), and urinary retention (0.02%). The Gomco clamp, Plastibell, and Mogen clamp are used widely, and no significant advantage of one over the other exists, other than operator preference. Still, no medical indication exists for the procedure. Most pediatric urologists currently suggest performing circumcision only for boys who have had difficulties with their foreskin (phimosis, paraphimosis, and balanitis) or whose parents desire the surgery for personal reasons.

Meatal Stenosis

Urethral meatal stenosis occurs secondary to glandular irritation or inflammation after circumcision, when the glans is allowed to come in contact with the diaper and this contact produces dermatitis. This meatitis is treated best by frequent diaper changes, exposure to the air, and warm baths. As the child grows, meatal stenosis may contribute to dysuria. The urinary stream is fine and dorsally deflected, at times rendering standing to void difficult or embarrassing. The diagnosis should be made on the basis of observed micturition because the appearance of the glans may be misleading. A narrow, slit-like meatus may stretch significantly during voiding to yield a quite satisfactory opening. If meatal stenosis is present, performing a meatotomy usually is indicated. This procedure can be performed easily in the office with topical anesthesia. Because meatal stenosis is a local effect from a limited dermatitis, further urologic investigations (including radiography and cystoscopy) are not indicated.

Unsightly Result

Significant complications from circumcision are uncommon occurrences, but parental dissatisfaction with the cosmetic result occurs much more frequently. Most often, the disappointment results from the appearance of excess skin left at the time of the neonatal circumcision. The parents may wish a revision of the circumcision, which must be performed under general anesthesia, preferably when the child is between 6 and 18 months old.

Circumcision and Hypospadias

Absolute contraindications for circumcision are the presence of hypospadias, epispadias, chordee, or anomalies of the penile skin. Therefore, before circumcision is performed, a careful inspection of the phallus is mandatory. In any anomaly of the penis, the presence of a redundant prepuce may be important to reconstructive efforts, and its absence may turn a rather simple operation into a major reconstruction requiring tissue grafts from distant sites.

Priapism

Priapism, an abnormal sustained erection, is a rare finding in healthy children, but it is not uncommon in boys with leukemia or sickle cell disease. In the first or second incident, resolution often is spontaneous, but with subsequent episodes, surgical decompression may be necessary. In cases of sickle cell priapism, initial efforts should be directed toward hydration, pain control, and exchange transfusion with packed normal red blood cells to decrease the hemoglobin S to less than 30% and the hematocrit to more than 30%. In boys with leukemia, chemotherapy and radiotherapy are the best initial courses of action in order to treat the underlying cause of the hemodynamic sludging. Priapism unresponsive to medical therapy is handled by a shunt between the engorged corpora cavernosa and flaccid corpus spongiosum. Impotence is not an uncommon development after priapism, whether or not surgical decompression is performed.

TESTICULAR AND SCROTAL ABNORMALITIES

Cryptorchidism

Testicular descent occurs late in fetal life and is regulated by many factors, including intraabdominal pressure, hormonal and neurologic influence, and presence of the gubernaculum. The absence of any one of these elements may contribute to cryptorchidism. The incidence of maldescent depends on fetal age, with as many as 30% of premature boys having either one or both testes undescended. In boys born at term, the incidence is between 3% and 4%. Shortly after birth, a transient increase in serum gonadotropin and testosterone occurs, which is responsible for spontaneous descent in more than one-half of boys with cryptorchidism at birth. After 1 year of life, testicles have descended in all but approximately 1% of boys. After that age, spontaneous testicular descent rarely occurs, and the incidence of cryptorchidism in untreated adults is approximately 1%.

True cryptorchidism must be distinguished from retractile testes, which are thought to be normal testes temporarily drawn into the inguinal canal by a hyperactive cremasteric muscle. With manipulation, these testes can be brought into the deep scrotum and will remain there for several moments after the examination. No treatment is needed because, with sexual maturation, the testes will remain in the scrotum spontaneously and function normally. Therefore, one must differentiate the retractile from the truly undescended testis accurately because the former needs no treatment.

The examination should take place in a relaxed, warm, and nonthreatening environment. The examiner should ensure that his or her hands are warm and should try to make the patient feel at ease. Repeated examinations with the patient in multiple positions (supine, sitting cross-legged, and squatting) may be beneficial. The history also is important, as a parent may remark that the testes are down during baths or diaper changes. The examination should be performed with two hands. One hand should start from the lateral area of the anterior superior iliac spine and sweep caudally along the inguinal canal, thereby trapping a testis so that it does not ascend into the abdomen.

The second hand should palpate the lower groin and scrotum to identify the gonad.

The position of the testis should be documented as either palpable (80%) or nonpalpable (20%). Palpable testes should be described further as inguinal, low inguinal, high scrotal, or ectopic. Even if the testes are not felt, it is often possible to identify testicular membranes on the spermatic cord; they should be documented for help in planning further therapy.

Several well-documented cases exist of a condition known as *ascending testis*, a gonad that at birth appears well descended into the scrotum but subsequently is found in the inguinal region. The cause for this condition has not been identified, and treatment should be instituted as for any other cryptorchid testis.

Treatment is suggested for several reasons. Progressive injury to the testis occurs as long as the testis remains in an extrascrotal position. Ultrastructural changes have been documented in children as young as 2 years of age, and impairment of sperm production has been reported after age 6 years. After puberty, hormonal production also may be affected adversely in a cryptorchid testis, and orchiectomy often is more appropriate than is orchiopexy. Fifty percent of adults with a history of unilateral cryptorchidism have oligospermia, but paternity rates approach normal. On the other hand, bilateral cryptorchidism is associated more often with both oligospermia (80%) and infertility. However, establishing that treatment at any age improves ultimate testicular function and fertility is difficult.

A second reason for relocating the testes in the scrotum is the increased incidence of malignant degeneration in testes with a history of maldescent. Testicular cancer, which is a rare occurrence before puberty, affects approximately 3 in 100,000 men. In men with a history of cryptorchidism, the incidence is from 4 to 40 times higher, yet no evidence exists that an orchiopexy provides protection against future malignancy. Ideally, a neoplasm in an orthotopic testis will be discovered and treated earlier than one in an inguinal or abdominal position, thus increasing the chance of survival because early, small-volume testicular cancer has a cure rate of better than 95%.

A further reason for treatment is so that the patient, like his friends, will have two intrascrotal testes, thereby improving self-image.

Currently, most pediatric urologists suggest treatment of cryptorchidism before the child is 2 years old, preferably when he is between 6 and 18 months. The modalities available are surgical or hormonal. Surgery is performed on an outpatient basis, and the results generally are excellent. An absent gonad is noted in approximately 20% of nonpalpable testes and can be a confirmed by finding a blind-ending vas deferens and testicular vessels, either at exploration or laparoscopy. Laparoscopy has been suggested for evaluation of nonpalpable testes, to document anorchia, to help plan the surgical approach, or, in some cases, to perform a laparoscopic orchiopexy.

Usually, an orchiopexy can relocate the cryptorchid testis into the scrotum without any problem; however, when the testis is intraabdominal or in a high inguinal position, division of the testicular artery and vein may be required so that the testis can reach the scrotum. In such an instance, the blood supply depends on the vasal artery and its supporting mesentery. The success rate in such a procedure drops from 99% to approximately 80%. Its main complications are those of any orchiopexy—atrophy and retraction. Autotransplantation of the testis (anastomosing the spermatic vessels to the inferior epigastric vessels) can be accomplished by microsurgical techniques, but whether this approach improves ultimate results over transfusion of the spermatic vessels alone remains unclear. A patent processus vaginalis (pediatric hernia), which occurs in association with 90% of cryptorchid testes, is repaired as part of the surgical procedure.

The other treatment modality is hormonal manipulation, based on the observation that increased testosterone may encourage testicular descent. In the United States, intramuscular human chorionic gonadotropin (hCG) is given in a series of injections at varying doses. Success rates with hCG are lower than those with an orchiopexy and, at best, reach 30%. In Europe, the trend is toward the use of intranasal gonadotropin-releasing hormone, given twice daily for 1 month. Success has been claimed in 80% of patients, although these data have been questioned. No long-term ill effects have been observed in association with this short-term hormonal therapy. For many patients and parents, however, orchiopexy is preferable to repeated injections of hCG.

When neither testicle is palpable, the question arises as to whether any testicular tissue is present and whether surgical intervention is necessary. Certain observations based on genital appearance and endocrinologic findings can assist in making this decision. The presence of adequate levels of fetal testosterone during the first trimester is necessary for normal penile formation. During the last two trimesters, fetal testosterone promotes phallic growth. If the boy has a normal-sized and normal-formed penis, one can deduce that he had functioning testicular tissue until late in gestation; however, the presence of hypospadias or micropenis raises further questions regarding testicular function and development.

Endocrine evaluation of bilateral anorchia consists of measuring serum gonadotropins (luteinizing hormone and follicle-stimulating hormone) and testosterone before gonadotropin stimulation and serum testosterone after administration of hCG. To ensure adequate stimulation, hCG should be given over the course of several days (usually 1,000 to 1,500 IU every day for four injections). For a diagnosis of anorchia, the boy should have normal-appearing anatomy, elevated luteinizing hormone and follicle-stimulating hormone levels, and no increase in prepubertal levels of testosterone after administration of hCG. When these rigid criteria are followed, the diagnosis of bilateral anorchia in this limited subgroup of patients can be made safely. Today, however, laparoscopy often is accomplished to confirm that both testes are absent.

Torsion

Spermatic Cord and Testes

Torsion of the testicle is one of the few true emergencies in pediatric urology and requires prompt intervention to avoid testicular necrosis. Testicular torsion must be differentiated from epididymitis and torsion of a testicular appendage because neither of these conditions requires surgery.

Testicular torsion occurs within the tunica albuginea (intravaginal) or includes the tunica albuginea (extravaginal). Intravaginal torsion occurs more commonly and most frequently in young adolescents. Intravaginal torsion is thought to result from the absence of posterior attachments between the tunica vaginalis and testis that normally stabilize the gonad within the scrotum. Signs of testicular torsion consist of the acute onset of severe scrotal pain, nausea, and vomiting. The attacks may be intermittent. Examination reveals an enlarged tender testis and frequently some degree of scrotal edema. The testis may be noted to have an unusual lateral lie. As time passes, the intrascrotal elements become confluent, and torsion may be difficult to differentiate from epididymitis. Additional investigations that are beneficial include a nuclear technetium scan of the testes or Doppler examination of the scrotum to assess testicular blood flow.

Prompt surgical exploration and detorsion are mandatory, as irreversible changes in the testis may occur within 4 hours. If treatment is not provided promptly, orchiectomy may be

required for a necrotic gonad. Because the abnormality (absence of posterior testicular attachment) often is bilateral, a contralateral scrotal orchiopexy should be performed whenever an intravaginal torsion is diagnosed.

Extravaginal torsion (torsion of the entire spermatic cord and testis, outside the tunica vaginalis) occurs almost exclusively in neonates and may occur before birth. Its etiology may be the lack of adhesions between the scrotum and the testicular membranes. It usually presents as a small, hard, nontender mass replacing the testis in a discolored hemiscrotum. Treatment is controversial because even prompt surgical exploration reveals a necrotic testis, and an orchiectomy is universal. Although evidence is lacking to show that the defect is bilateral, most surgeons fix the contralateral testis because the result of a subsequent torsion could be devastating (Fig. 320.15).

Torsion of a Testicular Appendage

Torsion of a testicular appendage must be distinguished from testicular torsion. Unless the diagnosis can be made with confidence, one must pursue a more thorough evaluation or surgically explore the acute scrotum. Often, but not always, the symptoms of a torsed appendage are less severe than those found with a testicular torsion. At times, the necrotic appendage is palpable in the upper aspect of the scrotum and can be seen through the thin scrotal skin as a pathognomonic blue dot. Diagnostic imaging tests, such as a doppler ultrasound, can help distinguish torsion of a testis from torsion of a testicular appendage. Appropriate treatment consists of limiting physical activity and nonsteroidal antiinflammatory agents; the natural course involves slow, steady improvement over the course of 10 to 14 days. Only rarely is surgical treatment needed to relieve severe pain.

Hydrocele and Hernia

In children, an inguinal hernia represents a persistent patent processus vaginalis, which normally obliterates before birth. This patency can result in a true hernia or only a communicating hydrocele (Fig. 320.16). Over the course of time, hydroceles become hernias as the patent processus dilates. Noncommunicating hydroceles, on the other hand, do not need emergency attention when present in the neonate; they tend to resolve spontaneously before the child reaches age 1 year, and intervention usually is delayed until that time. Reactive hydroceles secondary to infection, trauma, or torsion of an appendage resolve spontaneously and do not need separate attention. In general, the surgical approach to scrotal pathology is through the groin unless an obvious diagnosis of torsion of the testis or an appendage is made.

Varicoceles

Varicoceles are the pathologic dilation of the testicular vein and pampiniform plexus, most often on the left side. Their etiology is thought to be an absence of internal spermatic vein valves, which allows a continuous flow of a column of blood from the level of the renal vessels to the scrotum. The hydrostatic pressure causes the engorgement of the veins surrounding the testis. The resulting increase in scrotal temperature interferes with normal testicular development. The incidence of varicoceles has been reported to be as high as 15% in adolescent boys, but they are recognized much less commonly in children. Although varicoceles are the most common treatable cause of male infertility, not all men so afflicted will have difficulties with fecundity.

In the adolescent, indications for ligation of the internal spermatic vein, which corrects the varicocele, are pain,

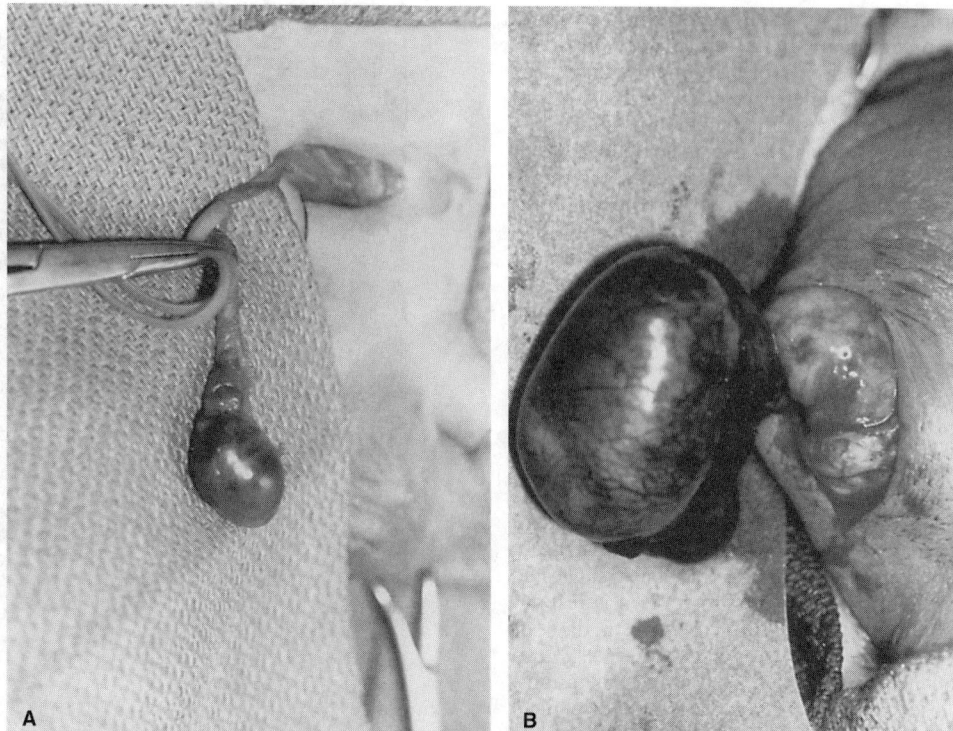

FIGURE 320.15. Testicular torsion. A: Neonatal torsion. Note that the cord twists proximal to the insertion of the tunica vaginalis (extravaginal torsion). (Reprinted with permission from Gonzales ET Jr. Genitourinary disorders in the neonate. In: Whitaker RH, Woodard JR, eds. *Paediatric Urology*. London: Butterworth, 1985.) B: Intravaginal torsion. The cord twists distal to the vaginal attachments.

ipsilateral testicular atrophy, or size. Some boys with varicoceles have normal-sized testicles but are found to have abnormalities in testicular hormone function on gonadotropin-releasing hormone stimulation testing. This condition is considered by

some surgeons to be another indication for performing elective repair. Ipsilateral testicular growth has been reported to increase in adolescents after repair of a varicocele, with subsequent testicular size matching or exceeding that of the contralateral side.

Epididymitis

Epididymitis is an unusual finding in a preadolescent boy, but its recognition is important because symptoms resemble those of testicular torsion. The treatment for the former is antibiotics and bed rest; for the latter, prompt surgical exploration is mandatory. The physical findings may be similar for the two entities: scrotal erythema, swelling, and pain. Laboratory data such as fever, leukocytosis, pyuria, and bacteriuria suggest a diagnosis of epididymitis. Furthermore, a testicular scan or Doppler ultrasound may assist in determining if testicular blood flow is absent (torsion) or increased (inflammation). If the diagnosis remains in question after examination and laboratory studies are performed, a scrotal exploration is appropriate.

Once epididymitis is confirmed in a prepubertal child, a renal ultrasound should be considered to identify any congenital anomalies. Positive findings (ureteral and vasal abnormalities predominate) have been reported in as many as one-fourth of the children. In these cases, correction of the problem often requires surgery.

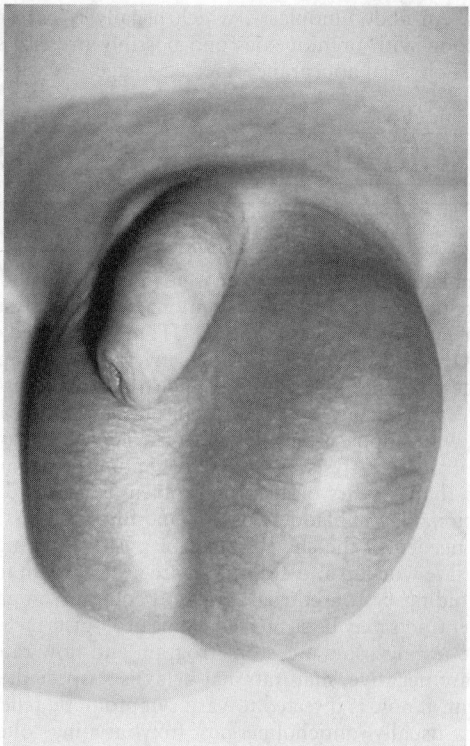

FIGURE 320.16. A large, tense hydrocele.

Prostatitis

Prostatitis, like epididymitis, is an unusual finding in the sexually inactive boy or man, and investigating for an anatomic etiology for the process is appropriate. Again, vasal and ureteral abnormalities predominate. In the sexually active adolescent, however, prostatitis is seen more commonly. Prostatitis is a general category and includes bacterial and nonbacterial prostatitis; bacterial prostatitis is either acute or chronic.

The diagnosis of prostatitis usually is made on clinical findings such as perineal pain, dysuria, urinary urgency, or urinary frequency. Fever, back pain, and chills are common symptoms in acute bacterial prostatitis but absent in the other forms. Rectal examination may reveal a tender, boggy prostate, and the expressed prostatic secretion often shows leukocytes and macrophages. Differentiating between chronic bacterial and nonbacterial prostatitis may be difficult, because the findings and symptoms are similar.

Antimicrobials are the mainstay of treatment for bacterial and nonbacterial prostatitis. Trimethoprim-sulfamethoxazole twice daily, or a quinolone in the older child, is the preferred therapy for bacterial prostatitis. Prolonged therapy (longer than 30 days) generally is the rule to prevent acute prostatitis from progressing to chronic prostatitis. The treatment of chronic prostatitis may require a course of the same agent for several months. Because chlamydia has been suggested as a causative agent, nonbacterial prostatitis often is responsive to a course of doxycycline (100 mg twice a day) or minocycline (100 mg twice a day) for several weeks. Warm baths may provide symptomatic relief. Zinc and megavitamins, which have been used in the past, have not shown clinical efficacy.

PRUNE BELLY SYNDROME

Prune belly syndrome is a rare (1 in 30,000 to 40,000) congenital absence of the abdominal musculature associated with severe nonobstructive urinary tract dilation and bilateral intraabdominal testes. Examination of the newborn usually reveals findings typical of the syndrome that makes the diagnosis obvious (Fig. 320.17). The spectrum of involvement is wide, ranging from minimal changes identifiable only radiographically to a full-blown case manifested as urethral atresia, pulmonary insufficiency, and renal dysplasia. Typical radiographic features include elongated and dilated ureters that cannot produce adequate peristalsis, a large-capacity bladder, and a urachal remnant that, in the presence of urethral atresia, remains open to form a patent urachus. The posterior urethra is dilated, and the prostate is either absent or hypoplastic. Often, a prominent posterior urethral lip is present, which is suggestive of posterior urethral valves, but it is not obstructive. The penis can be dysplastic, with deficient corpus spongiosum and resultant megalourethra. The kidneys may be dysmorphic, and renal function often is impaired.

The etiology of the prune belly syndrome is thought to be a generalized mesenchymal defect that contributes to the absence of musculature of both the body wall and the urinary tract. The associated cryptorchidism may result from decreased intraabdominal pressure *in utero*. Initial treatment is directed toward supportive care because, despite gross ureteral dilation, true obstruction is an uncommon occurrence and renal pelvic pressures are low.

Unless urethral atresia occurs, surgical intervention is not recommended in the infant. If infection occurs and is difficult to eradicate, providing a temporary urinary diversion may be appropriate. In the rare child with anatomic urinary obstruction, a vesicostomy or cutaneous ureterostomies should be considered. Some older boys require urinary tract reconstructive surgery, usually performed in an effort to reduce stasis and prevent recurrent urinary infections. These procedures may include ureteral reimplantation, reduction cystoplasty, and

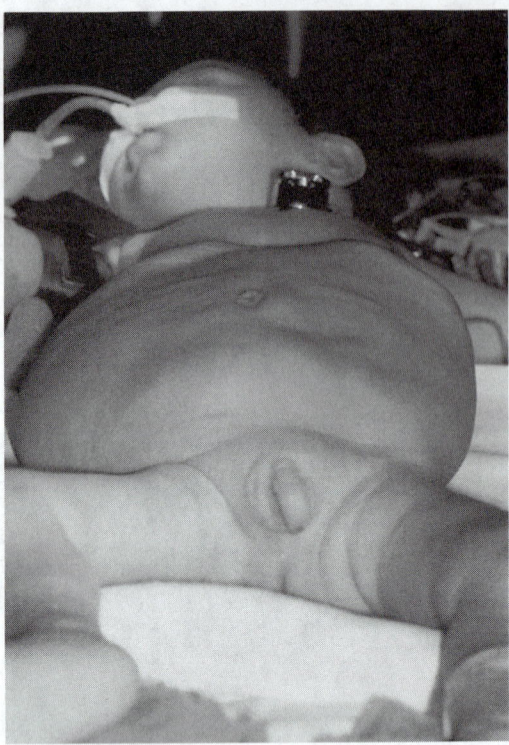

FIGURE 320.17. Typical appearance of a child with prune belly syndrome. (Reprinted with permission from Gonzales ET Jr. Genitourinary disorders in the neonate. In: Whitaker RH, Woodard JR, eds. *Paediatric Urology*. London: Butterworth, 1985.)

urethroplasty. Satisfactory orchidopexy usually can be accomplished if the procedure is done before the infant is 1 year of age. Although fertility is unlikely, hormonal function is normal. Testicular tumors have been reported, however, in these patients. An abdominoplasty, which usually is performed in conjunction with orchiopexies and possibly ureteral surgery, improves physical appearance and self-image.

DISORDERS OF MICTURITION

Voiding Dysfunction

Abnormal micturition in children is not an unusual finding and may take the form of urgency, retention, frequency, dysuria, incontinence, or perineal discomfort. UTI must be ruled out as a cause of these disturbances. Urologic investigation is appropriate in these settings and should include a thorough history, especially a voiding history; careful genitourinary physical examination, with emphasis on a possible neurologic etiology for the problem; and urinalysis. If no positive findings exist in a child younger than 5 years of age, the problem is assumed to be a maturational lag in bladder control, and further investigations are not needed. If the child is older or positive findings exist, appropriate workup and evaluation are necessary. In the older child, voiding cystourethrography and some investigation of the upper tracts may be suggested. Some urologists include urodynamic testing using a cystometrogram and flow rate. If the results are negative, maturational delay is suspected, and the treatment, if any, is directed toward symptomatic relief. Medications, usually anticholinergics (oxybutynin, tolterodine, hyoscyamine), have proved to offer significant help to some of these youngsters. Furthermore, because gradual improvement often occurs in these symptoms as the children get older, observation alone is a possible approach in the child who is not yet in school or who does not have problems at school.

For the rare older child with severe dysfunctional voiding associated with abnormalities revealed by radiographic and urodynamic testing, more involved therapy is indicated to relieve symptoms and to avoid renal damage. These youngsters may have an abnormal learned response in which the external sphincter contracts in conjunction with a detrusor contraction (bladder-sphincter dyssynergy). This condition has been termed a *non-neurogenic neurogenic bladder*. These children have normal innervation of the bladder and sphincter. The pattern may be difficult to eradicate and requires bladder retraining, usually by biofeedback. The prognosis may be good, but some children have severe hydroureteronephrosis and renal injury resulting from this disorder. Psychological evaluation and treatment may provide significant help.

Enuresis

Enuresis is the involuntary loss of urine. Generally, however, it has come to mean the loss of urine during sleep, more appropriately termed nocturnal enuresis. Enuresis may be either primary or secondary. Primary enuretics have never had a prolonged dry period, whereas secondary enuretics have had a period of at least several months during which they remained dry. Enuresis was documented in ancient times, and several unusual folk remedies can be found in early medical writings. Its incidence has been estimated to be 15% in 5-year-old children, with a natural resolution rate of approximately 15% per year. Therefore, by the time children are age 10 years, the incidence has fallen to 5% to 6%, and by age 15, to 1%. Boys are affected more frequently than are girls, and a correlation exists with a family history of enuresis and the child's developmental level at ages 1 and 3 years. However, factors such as the child's birth order, family's socioeconomic level, maternal and gestational age, changes in parents or residence, and family events have no significant influence on mean age of attaining nocturnal bladder control.

Various theories have been proposed to explain nocturnal enuresis. Traditionally, the most widely accepted was that of delayed maturational control; however, more recent data suggest that some of these patients have an inadequate level of antidiuretic hormone secretion during sleep. Explanations such as sleep disorder, psychological disturbances, transient negative reinforcement, and organic factors, including a small bladder, generally are discounted, although they may play a role in a specific case.

An appropriate evaluation requires a thorough history, which should include such topics as pattern of wetting, prior UTIs or unexplained high fevers, toilet training (bowel and bladder) history, emotional history, social interactions, and developmental milestones. Especially for boys, the physical examination should include an assessment of the child's urinary stream, either by observation or by a flow rate. The abdominal examination should include a check for the presence of palpable bladder or kidneys. The back examination should include a search for signs of neurologic involvement, such as scoliosis, a sacral dimple, or hairy nevus, that suggest occult spinal dysraphism. A neurologic examination is important; deep tendon reflexes and perineal sensation should be evaluated. During the rectal examination, sphincter tone, bulbocavernosus reflex, and the presence of a sacrum should be evaluated.

The purpose of initial laboratory tests usually is restricted to eliminating infection as a cause of the voiding problem. Therefore, a urinalysis often is the only test required. Diagnostic imaging usually is not performed when nocturnal enuresis is the only problem; however, for those children with refractory enuresis, a uroradiologic or urodynamic study may be necessary. Additionally, performing more involved tests for children older than 10 years has been suggested.

Many varied and unusual treatments have been proposed, but the first remedy with scientific basis was introduced in the late nineteenth century. Currently, several courses of management are accepted. The most successful of these tests are the use of desmopressin acetate, behavior modification, and tricyclic antidepressants. Each has advantages and disadvantages. Treatment with imipramine (25 to 50 mg at bedtime) has a success rate of 40% to 60%, but a fair degree of recidivism occurs. The physician must be alert for possible side effects: personality changes, gastrointestinal complaints, nervousness, and sleep disorders. Children are more sensitive than are adults to an overdose of this drug, especially with regard to cardiac toxicity; therefore, appropriate precautions must be taken to ensure that a younger sibling or patient does not have free access to the medication. If imipramine therapy is chosen, an adequate trial lasting several months should be given, but most patients respond within the first several days.

Desmopressin acetate is an analogue of vasopressin, whose efficacy is based on the data that some enuretics do not experience the normal nocturnal elevation of antidiuretic hormone. Accordingly, the child's night-time urine remains more dilute and of greater volume than that in nonenuretics. The increased volume simply overwhelms the capacity of the bladder, and wetting occurs. By taking an evening dose of desmopressin acetate, 70% of enuretics can remain dry overnight. The half-life of the drug is 2 hours, and it is gone by morning. Complications are uncommon occurrences, but fluids should be restricted after administering the medication to decrease the possibility of water intoxication. A prolonged treatment period of several months is required before attempting to taper the medication. If wetting recurs, desmopressin acetate can be restarted. Both intranasal and tablet forms of desmopressin are available in Europe and the United States.

The enuresis alarm is the most popular method of behavior modification and gives the best overall success (70% to 90%). It requires more parental support and involvement than does medical treatment; often the parent must sleep in the same room for the first week or two of use to ensure that the child is awakened by the alarm. The device consists of two components: the sensor and the sounder. The sensor must be small enough to be positioned near the urethral meatus so that when the child begins micturition the alarm will sound. Over a period of time (several weeks to months), a conditioned response should develop so that the child wakes as the bladder becomes full and before the onset of micturition. A course of treatment lasting several months often is necessary. As with medical treatment, a relapse rate occurs, but it is lower than that for pharmacologic therapy. Most failures seem to be related to the patient's sleeping through the alarm.

Other forms of therapy such as psychotherapy, motivational therapy, and bladder retention training are used, but treatment with the enuresis alarm, desmopressin acetate, or tricyclic antidepressants holds the greatest promise for individuals with nocturnal enuresis.

Suggested Readings

Daaboul J, Frader J. Ethics and the management of the patient with intersex: a middle way. *J Pediatr Endocrinol Metab* 2001;14:1575.

Gillenwater JY, Gray hack JT, Howards SS, Duckett JW, eds. *Adult and pediatric urology*, 3rd ed. St. Louis: Mosby-Year Book, 1996.

Gonzales ET Jr., Roth DR, eds. *Common problems in pediatric urology.* St. Louis: Mosby-Year Book, 1991.

Kelalis PP, King LR, Belman AB, eds. *Clinical pediatric urology,* 3rd ed. Philadelphia: WB Saunders, 1992.

King LR, ed. *Urologic surgery in infants and children.* Philadelphia: WB Saunders, 1998.

Kirsh AJ, Perez-Brayfield MR, Scherz HC. Minimally invasive treatment of vesicoureteral reflux with endoscopic infection of dextranomer/hyaluronic acid

copolymer: The Children's Hospital of Atlanta experience. *J Urol* 2003;170: 211.

O'Donnell B, Koff SA, eds. *Pediatric urology,* 3rd ed. Oxford: Butterworth-Heinemann, 1997.

Puri P, Chertin B, Velayudham M, et al. Treatment of vesicoureteral reflux by endoscopic infection of dextranomer/hyaluronic acid copolymer: preliminary results. *J Urol* 2003;170:1541.

Walsh PC, Retik AB, Vaughan EO Jr., Wein AJ, eds. *Campbell's urology,* 7th ed, vol 2. Philadelphia: WB Saunders, 1998.

CHAPTER 321 ■ URINARY TRACT INFECTION

EDMOND T. GONZALES AND DAVID R. ROTH

EPIDEMIOLOGY

During childhood, the urinary tract is second only to the upper respiratory tract as a source of morbidity from bacterial infection. Urinary tract infection (UTI) is predominantly a problem in girls. However, for the first few months after birth, the incidence of urinary infection in the male exceeds that of girls. An uncircumcised boy has approximately a 1% chance of developing an infection during childhood, mostly in the neonatal period. In male neonates, the incidence of asymptomatic bacilluria is 1.5%, but it decreases to 0.2% by the time boys are of school age. In circumcised boys, the incidence of urinary infection is about one-tenth that of the uncircumcised. This observation, though, is not considered to be an indication for routine circumcision in the newborn because complications from circumcision potentially negate the benefit of reducing the incidence of urinary infections. At this time, no data exist to suggest that remaining uncircumcised increases the risk of UTI developing in older boys. A girl's chance of developing an infection during childhood is close to 3%. Random screening of preschool and school-age girls has shown an incidence of asymptomatic bacilluria of 1%. The incidence peaks in children between age 3 and 5 years, the age that coincides with toilet training, and then returns to a baseline value of between 1% and 2%.

CLINICAL MANIFESTATIONS AND COMPLICATIONS

The signs and symptoms of UTI in an older child are those seen in the adult population, namely frequency, dysuria, hematuria, incontinence, suprapubic or flank tenderness, lethargy, and fever. In the young infant, though, symptoms are more subtle. Weight loss is a prominent symptom, followed by irritability, fever, lethargy, and cyanosis. Thus, nonspecific complaints or problems should raise the suspicion of a UTI in a newborn, although fewer than 20% of infants with nonspecific complaints and only 18% of children with specific voiding complaints will actually have a UTI.

Documentation of urinary infection requires that a specimen be properly obtained. Of the several ways to collect an aliquot of urine from a child, the easiest, once a child has been toilet trained, is the midstream clean-catch specimen. Before toilet training is complete, three methods remain, each with its

advantages and disadvantages. The simplest, but least reliable, is the U-bag. A negative culture from a U-bag is meaningful, but if the culture is positive, it is possible that the bacterium is a contaminant from the rectum, skin, or prepuce. Therefore, whenever this method produces a positive specimen, the culture should be repeated, utilizing a more accurate method. Two other procedures are available; both are somewhat more involved, but each should provide an uncontaminated aliquot of bladder urine. The first is a percutaneous bladder tap. In the neonate and infant, the bladder occupies an intraabdominal position, rendering suprapubic needle access easier than in older persons. However, if the bladder is not full, it can be difficult to locate. Occasionally, hematuria can result after a bladder tap. The second method is urethral catheterization. In the small girl, visualization of the urethra may be difficult, but with practice the procedure can be mastered easily. A small feeding tube (5 French or 8 French) is most appropriate for catheterization. Little risk of urethral trauma or introduction of bacteria into the bladder exists if standard care and antisepsis are used. Although routine urinalysis can suggest strongly that urinary infection is present, any treatment program should be based on an accurate culture and sensitivity. Consequently, obtaining the culture before antibiotics are started is imperative because a single dose of medication can give a false-negative result.

UTIs often are described based on the presumed location of the infection. Cystitis is a UTI that is confined to the bladder, whereas pyelonephritis involves the kidney. An accurate delineation between the two conditions is difficult to establish; however, clinical signs and symptoms do offer meaningful clues. High fever, nausea, vomiting, flank pain, and lethargy usually are associated with acute pyelonephritis, whereas dysuria, frequency, urgency, enuresis, suprapubic pain, and a low-grade fever are more common with cystitis. However, a crossover of symptoms does occur. Studies in adult patients with acute urinary infection, in which urine from the kidneys (obtained by ureteral catheterization after acquiring a bladder specimen) was negative, demonstrate that fever can be associated with cystitis. In fact, determining whether a patient with a positive culture from bladder urine also has bacteria in the renal pelvis or parenchyma is difficult. The traditional method used to obtain separate bladder and renal cultures involves ureteral catheterization, which requires anesthesia and is impractical in children. Currently, radionuclide renal imaging using dimercaptosuccinic acid (DMSA) is the most accurate and practical study available to demonstrate acute pyelonephritis. Decreased parenchymal uptake of the isotope has been shown in animals to correlate clearly with areas of experimental infection. In the clinical situation, however, focal decreased uptake of the isotope noted during a febrile urinary infection also could represent an old parenchymal scar and not necessarily a new lesion. Therefore, the routine use of DMSA scanning is not practical during the acute episode because the findings on DMSA scanning do not change initial therapy for the acute infection. Nonetheless, DMSA renal scanning remains the most sensitive and least invasive technique available to distinguish cystitis from apparent pyelonephritis. No recognized relationship exists between the location of the infection and the organism responsible for the infection.

THERAPY

Most UTIs can be treated adequately, on an outpatient basis, with a 7- to 10-day course of antibiotics. When shorter courses are used, the recurrence rate is higher. Initial treatment should begin after a urine specimen for culture and sensitivity has been obtained. A broad-spectrum agent such as amoxicillin (20 to 30 mg/kg/day, in three divided doses) or trimethoprim-sulfamethoxazole (dosing is based on the trimethoprim content, at 6 to 12 mg trimethoprim/kg/day, divided every 12 hours) then is begun empirically, with therapy being adjusted, if necessary, after the culture and sensitivity results are available. A repeat culture, to confirm eradication of the infection, should be obtained approximately 1 week after the completion of treatment. A child with severe symptoms accompanying pyelonephritis often requires hospitalization for parenteral antibiotics and control of nausea and vomiting. For the child with frequently recurring infections (at least four a year), a long-term, low-dose daily prophylactic antibiotic (usually nitrofurantoin or trimethoprim-sulfamethoxazole at one-fourth to one-half of the therapeutic dose) is appropriate. Usually, the medications are given for 6 to 12 months. Subsequent follow-up should include regular urinalyses and cultures when indicated.

All children with a documented UTI should undergo adequate studies to evaluate the anatomy of the urinary tract. Generally, studies to evaluate both the lower tract (the urethra and bladder) and upper tract are suggested. This recommendation is based on the clinical observation that the children most likely to sustain renal parenchymal damage from infection are those who have an anatomic defect of the urinary tract (Fig. 321.1). The positive yield from these evaluations is age- and sex-dependent and ranges up to 50% in young girls with pyelonephritis (primarily from discovery of vesicoureteral reflux). For the older girl with symptoms of only cystitis, one can argue that initially obtaining only an upper-tract study is sufficient because it will reveal any significant pathology. Any anatomic anomaly discovered might, of course, require additional work-up and individual treatment.

Imaging of the upper tracts nearly always is begun with the renal ultrasound. This study provides excellent anatomic detail, is independent of renal function, has no known untoward biologic effects, and is painless. Radionuclide renal scanning using DMSA is more sensitive at identifying focal scarring (Fig. 321.2), but seldom is used in the initial evaluation of a UTI. The intravenous urogram rarely is used today in the pediatric population. The diagnostic studies available to evaluate the lower

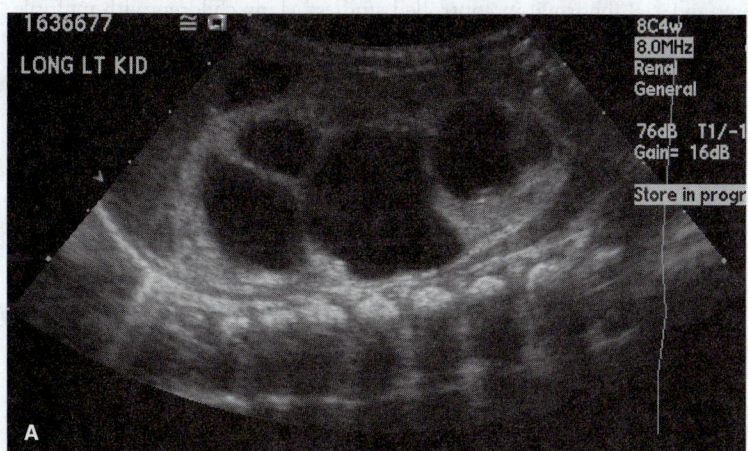

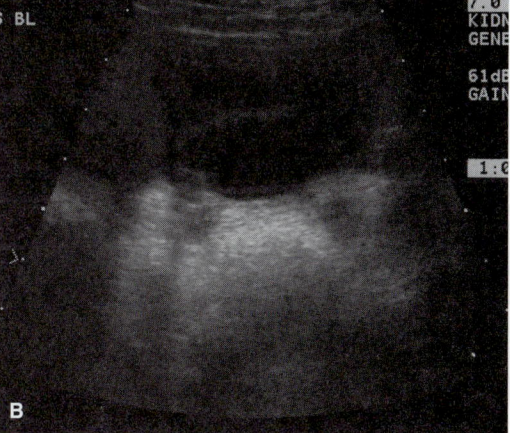

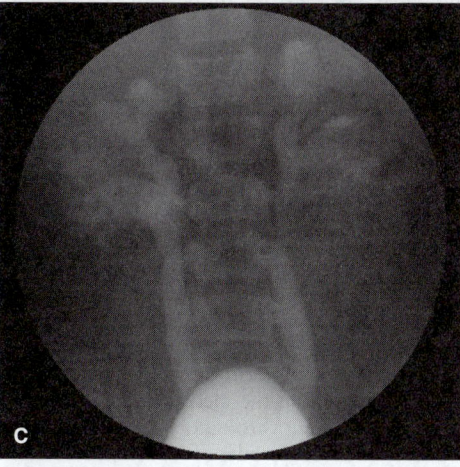

FIGURE 321.1. Examples of anomalies that might be recognized during diagnostic work-up for urinary infection. **A:** UPJ Obstruction seen on renal ultrasound; **B:** Ureterocele seen on bladder ultrasound; **C:** Vesicoureteral Reflux seen on VCUG.

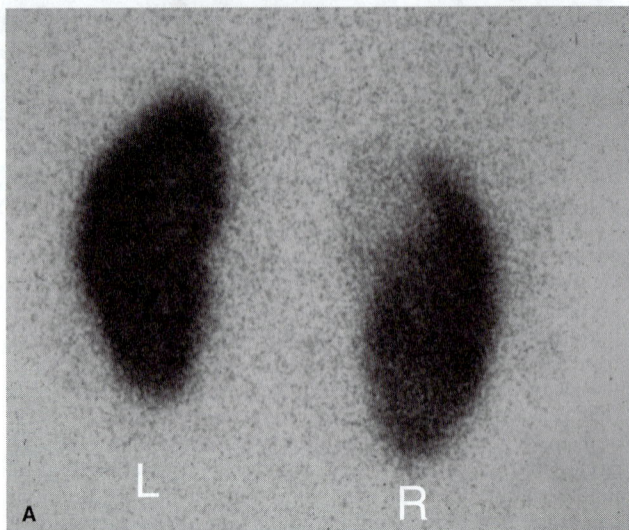 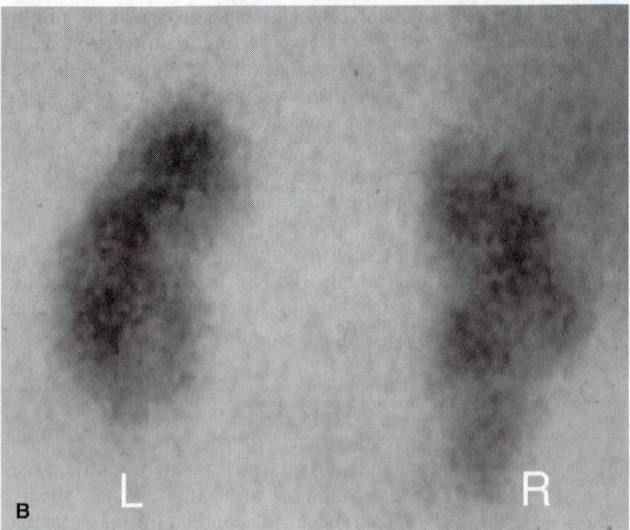

FIGURE 321.2. Examples of renal scarring seen on DMSA renal scan. **A:** Focal scar in upper pole of right kidney. The left kidney is normal. **B:** Extensive bilateral renal scarring. Note the patchy uptake in each kidney.

tract include either a voiding cystourethrogram (VCUG) or a nuclear cystogram. The VCUG provides optimal anatomic detail, allows for grading of reflux that may be present, and is the only study that delineates the male urethra. The nuclear cystogram is a sensitive test to identify the presence of reflux and results in somewhat less radiation exposure than the VCUG but offers poor anatomic detail. A nuclear cystogram is a better test to follow reflux over the long term. Cystoscopy and retrograde pyelography rarely are indicated in the work-up of a pediatric UTI.

The indications and timing for performing a VCUG remain somewhat controversial. Although several abnormalities may be identified when a VCUG is performed, by far, the primary reason for doing a VCUG is to identify the presence of vesicoureteral reflux. Vesicoureteral reflux is a common finding in children who present with febrile urinary infection, and the presence of reflux does correlate with an increased incidence of atrophic pyelonephritis. But, VCUGs are invasive and are not well accepted by older girls. Although complications are rare, occasionally UTIs or bladder rupture can occur because of the procedure. For these reasons, not every child who develops a urinary infection requires a VCUG. Indications for doing a VCUG would include all children with a febrile UTI, children with an abnormal renal ultrasound (renal scarring, pelviectasis, or ureterectasis), infants with UTI (less than 2 years old), and older boys with febrile UTI and voiding symptoms. Children with afebrile urinary infections and a normal renal ultrasound can be followed safely without having to undergo a VCUG.

CYSTITIS

Most urinary infections that occur in children with normal urinary tract anatomy remain limited to involvement of the bladder. Although symptoms are generally local (dysuria, frequency, urgency, lower abdominal pain), they can be socially disabling in older children. Fever can occur but usually is low-grade and not associated with systemic toxicity. The severity of symptoms varies widely, from debilitating frequency and dysuria in some to an apparent lack of symptoms in others. Some authors differentiate between infection (tissue invasion) and colonization (in which the organisms are limited to the urine), although clear clinical evidence for such a distinction is lacking. Recurrences

are common and, in some children, can develop within days of discontinuing antibiotics.

The causes for recurring lower-tract infections remain unknown and include both bacterial virulence factors and host defense deficiencies. Possible factors are an abnormal perineal flora or an abnormality in the glycosaminoglycan layer in the bladder. However, neither has been shown to be consistently abnormal in controlled studies. Many children with multiple, rapid recurrences also have symptoms of dysfunctional voiding even when they are not infected. These symptoms include urgency, frequency, precipitant voiding, and incontinence. When children with dysfunctional voiding are evaluated urodynamically, they commonly have been shown to generate abnormally high voiding pressures and may carry residual urine. In addition, they often also will have associated symptoms of constipation and/or fecal soilage. How these parameters might interrelate to cause urinary infections is unclear, but dysfunctional voiding currently is thought to be a primary cause for the development of bacilluria. The presence of large volumes of residual urine increases the chance that bacteria might establish urinary infection. Large bladder diverticula, neurogenic bladder dysfunction, vesicoureteral reflux, and perhaps some children with dysfunctional voiding are examples of problems in which significant voiding residual urine might be present. The consensus in the past that urethral obstruction in girls (socalled "Lyons ring") was a primary anatomic defect and a cause for urinary infection no longer is accepted, and routine urethral dilation is not appropriate.

From a urologic perspective, recurring lower-tract urinary infection often is viewed as a nuisance—a problem that interferes intermittently with day-to-day activities, but rarely, if ever, results in long-term impairment to renal or urinary tract function. Once it has been established that urinary tract anatomy is normal, one can anticipate normal renal growth despite numerous symptomatic episodes of cystitis. In most instances, oral antibiotics will resolve the symptoms promptly and sterilize the urine. Occasionally, though, a resistant organism might require parenteral therapy. The decision regarding the institution of prophylactic antibiotic therapy depends on many factors, but no data show that long-term treatment reduces the risk of recurrences after stopping the medications. A spontaneous resolution rate is apparent throughout childhood, with the cessation at puberty of most episodes of recurrent infection.

If the symptoms with each recurrence remain consistent with cystitis, no need exists for repeated, invasive evaluations. However, for the child with a persisting problem, it is prudent to repeat a renal ultrasound every 2 to 3 years to document normal renal growth.

UPPER-TRACT INFECTION

Tissue infection of the upper urinary tract is a much more serious problem. First, children with pyelonephritis tend to be very ill and appear toxic. They often require hospitalization for initial control of the fever and nausea and vomiting. Second, the ultimate outcome may be a focal "scar" in the renal parenchyma, with subsequent tissue atrophy and loss of segmental renal function.

The potential for bacteria to ascend into the upper urinary tract is a combination of decreased patient resistance as well as bacterial virulence. Whereas some bacteria are able to infect the kidney because of their intrinsic virulence, especially those that are P-fimbriated, all bacteria are more likely to cause pyelonephritis rather than cystitis when anatomic abnormalities are present. When children with urinary infection present with significant fever, 60% will be found to have structural abnormalities—most often vesicoureteral reflux. In addition, children with structural abnormalities are more likely to have pyelonephritis when they have a recurrence than are children who present with symptoms of pyelonephritis but whose diagnostic imaging evaluation was normal. However, the natural history and ultimate outcome of any episode of pyelonephritis does not seem to differ between children with normal anatomy and those with vesicoureteral reflux. An increased incidence and severity of scarring correlates with infection in younger children, with a delay in the initiation of appropriate chemotherapy, and in children with abnormally high voiding pressures—such as those with neurogenic bladder or true urethral obstruction.

Acute lobar nephronia is a radiologic diagnosis on the spectrum of renal parenchymal infections ranging from pyelonephritis to renal abscess and, ultimately, end-stage pyonephrosis. Lobar nephronia is a localized nonliquefactive infection that generally follows the lobular and lobar architecture of the kidney. Its histology is similar to that of pyelonephritis, with acute leukocytic infiltrate, hyperemia, and interstitial edema. Clinical suspicion should arise when a typical pyelonephritic fever curve is prolonged, or when the presence of a mass in the kidney is suggested by upper-tract studies. The intravenous pyelogram may suggest a mass by subtle distortion of the renal outline or renal collecting system; however, the ultrasound is more sensitive and may demonstrate a focal or poorly defined region that disrupts the corticomedullary junction. The best diagnostic tool is the computed tomography (CT) scan, which will show a wedge-shaped, nonhomogenous area with poor contrast enhancement. Treatment for lobar nephronia is prolonged antibiotic therapy, initiated with parenteral agents, and then followed by oral medication, with the drug of choice based on culture results. Inadequately treated lobar nephronia may progress to renal abscess.

Renal abscess is an unusual finding today. Historically, the most common organism causing a renal abscess has been the staphylococci, but, presently, the gram-negative rods predominate. As with lobar nephronia, the diagnosis requires a high degree of suspicion. Renal ultrasound and CT are the modalities best suited to confirm the diagnosis in a child who has continuing spiking fevers associated with infected urine, despite apparently adequate antibiotic treatment (Fig. 321.3). Once the entity is discovered, continuation of antibiotics, combined with drainage of the lesion, is necessary. Today, this treatment usually can be achieved by percutaneous access and only rarely is surgical exploration needed. Very small abscesses can be treated by prolonged, high-dose parenteral therapy in some cases. Rarely will nephrectomy be required, but in the severely ill child, unresponsive to antibiotics and with a poorly functioning kidney, that procedure should be considered. Once the abscess is controlled, the child should be evaluated for reflux or obstruction as an etiology for the infection.

VESICOURETERAL REFLUX

Of all the abnormalities associated with urinary infection in childhood, vesicoureteral reflux is by far the most common. Little doubt exists that the presence of vesicoureteral reflux contributes to the development of acute, ascending pyelonephritis, which may result in renal scarring. However, despite more than 50 years of intense clinical study, management of the individual child with reflux remains somewhat controversial.

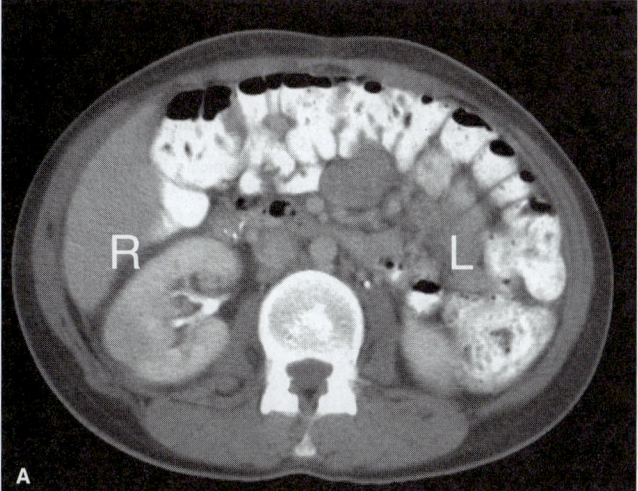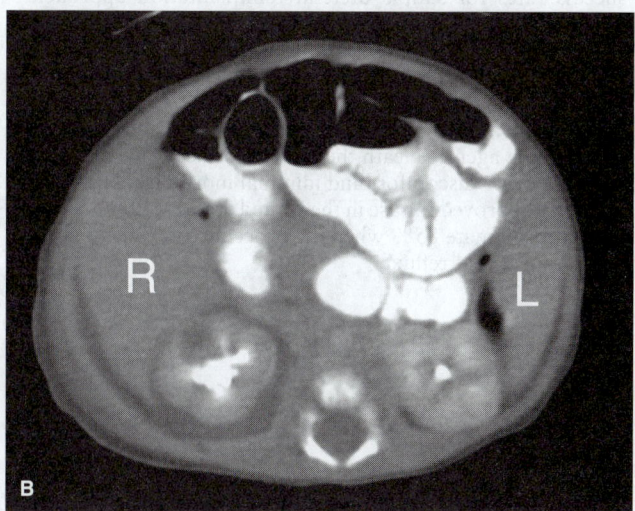

FIGURE 321.3. Examples of acute renal infection. **A:** Labor nephronia—right kidney. Note the "mass-like" effect on the lateral border. There is no liquefaction. **B:** Renal abscess—right kidney. Note the discrete, hypodense area in the anterior right renal cortex.

Not all children who develop pyelonephritis develop renal scars. Among children with vesicoureteral reflux, about 40% have renal scarring. However, most of these scars are noted on their initial evaluation; if additional infections occur, subsequent scarring often is minimal or does not seem to result, despite symptoms compatible with renal infection. These observations have resulted in the development of a theory that proposes that the risk of renal scarring depends on the anatomy of the renal papilla. Some papilla, termed *compound papilla*, are more likely to develop severe inflammatory atrophy, and some kidneys have a greater proportion of compound papilla than others. However, the likelihood of developing a renal scar also correlates with the number of episodes of pyelonephritis.

The treatment of reflux primarily is directed at preventing acute pyelonephritis. Correction of reflux does not prevent the development of recurring cystitis. The treatment of reflux can follow two separate paths:

- Nonoperative: Prevention of urinary infection
- Operative: Techniques to correct the reflux itself

Nonoperative Therapy

Nonoperative therapy can take two different approaches: initiation of maintenance antibiotics to prevent urinary infection or very careful observation (sometimes chosen in older girls) so as to promptly diagnose and treat any UTIs that may occur. In either case, the premise is that new scarring occurs only after UTI and that, if infection can be prevented or minimized, these patients can be followed safely for several years, with expectation that many of these children will outgrow their reflux. Seventy-five to 80% of grades 1 or 2 reflux can be expected to resolve with 5 years of medical management, whereas less than 25% to 30% of grade 4 reflux will resolve during that interval. Nonoperative therapy can require careful monitoring for years, multiple follow-up imaging studies, and long-term antibiotics.

Operative Therapy

The surgical correction of reflux has been available since the mid-1950s and has been imminently successful. Current success rates for simple ureteral reimplantation approaches 99%. However, it is an open surgical procedure that requires a short period of hospitalization and some morbidity from bladder spasms during convalescence—especially in older children.

A less invasive procedure involves the subureteric injection of a bulking agent beneath the ureteral orifice. This procedure has little or no discomfort and minimal morbidity. This procedure was approved for use in the United States in 2000. Success rates approximate 85% when the procedure is done in ureters with grade 2 to 4 reflux.

The choice of which therapy is most appropriate must consider several variables. These variables might include age and sex of the child, grade of reflux, extent of scarring, parental preferences, other associated anomalies, and other factors. In the past, open surgery often was avoided for many years in expectation that the reflux would resolve. Currently, though, great enthusiasm exists for subureteric Deflux injection. This minimally invasive procedure offers the opportunity to discontinue antibiotics at a much younger age, and it eliminates the need for repetitive VCUGs in most of these patients.

CONCLUSIONS

The recognition of urinary infection in children requires sufficient work-up to place children in categories of "at risk" or "minimal risk." The former are those with structural anomalies. These children are most likely to develop severe recurrences and renal atrophy. The latter may have multiple recurrences but with little or no risk of upper tract infection or damage. Their treatment is symptomatic and is driven by social as well as medical reasons.

Suggested Readings

Hannson S. Urinary incontinence in children and associated problems. *Scand J Urol Nephrol* 1992;141:47.

Hellerstein S. Antibiotic treatment for urinary tract infections in pediatric patients. *Minerva Pediatr* 2003;5:395.

Huland H, Busch R. Pyelonephritis scarring in 213 patients with upper and lower urinary tract infections: long-term follow-up. *J Urol* 1984;132:936.

Jodal U. The natural history of bacteriuria in childhood. *Infect Dis Clin North Am* 1987;1:713.

Kunin CM. Urinary tract infection in children. In: O'Donnell B, Koff SA, eds. *Pediatric urology*. Butterworth-Heinemann, 1997.

Madrigal G, Odio CM, Moks E, et al. Single-dose antibiotic therapy is not as effective as conventional regimens for management of acute urinary tract infections in children. *Pediatr Infect Dis J* 1988;7:316.

Majd M, Rushton HG, Jantausch B, Wiedermann BL. Relationship among vesicoureteral reflux, P-fimbriated *Escherichia coli*, and acute pyelonephritis in children with febrile urinary tract infection. *J Pediatr* 1991;119:578.

Parsons CL, Schrom SH, Hanno P, et al. Bladder surface mucin: examination of possible mechanism for its antibacterial effect. *Invest Urol* 1978;16:196.

Puri P, Chertin B, et al. Treatment of vesicoureteral reflux by endoscopic injection of dextranomer/hyaluronic acid copolymer: preliminary results. *J Urol* 2003;170:1541.

Ransley PG. Vesicoureteric reflux: continuing surgical dilemma. *Urology* 1978;12:246.

Rushton HG, Majd M, Jantausch B, Wiedermann B, Belman AB. Renal scarring following reflux and non-reflux pyelonephritis in children: evaluation with 99m technetium-dimercaptosuccinic acid scintigraphy. *J Urol* 1992;147:1327.

Shortliffe LMD. Urinary tract infections in infants and children. In: Walsh PC, Retik AB, Vaughn ED, Wein AJ, eds. *Campbell's urology*. Philadelphia: WB Saunders, 2002.

Smellie JM, Ransley PG, Normand ICS, et al. Development of new renal scars: a collaborative study. *Br Med J* 1985;290:1957.

Verber I, Meller S. Serial 99m Tc dimercaptosuccinic acid (DMSA) scans after urinary infections presenting before the age of 5 years. *Arch Dis Child* 1989;64:1533.

Wiswell T, Hackey W. Urinary tract infections and the uncircumcised state: an update. *Clin Pediatr* 1993;32:130.

CHAPTER 322 ■ CHRONIC RENAL FAILURE

EDWARD C. KOHAUT

During the late 1970s, whether any child was a candidate for any form of renal replacement therapy was questioned because the rigors of therapy were not thought to justify the potential benefit. Since that time, dialysis followed by renal transplantation has become routine therapy for the treatment of children with end-stage renal disease (ESRD). The decision rarely is whether to initiate renal replacement therapy but rather when to do so. Early intervention has become advantageous, placing even more responsibility on the pediatrician to recognize and participate in the treatment of children with renal insufficiency and failure.

The incidence of chronic renal disease (CRD) in children is unknown, but current data suggest that 1.5 to 3.0 children per 1 million population per year develop ESRD. In 1992, the North American Pediatric Renal Transplant Cooperative Study Group (NAPRTCS) initiated a registry of children treated with dialysis; as of 2003, 5,209 patients had been registered. NAPRTCS initiated a registry to collect data on children with chronic renal insufficiency (CRI) in 1994, and as of 2003, 5,381 patients have been registered.

SIGNS OF PROGRESSIVE LOSS OF RENAL FUNCTION

The databases mentioned previously have confirmed that children with chronic renal disease present in a different manner from similarly affected adults (Box 322.1). The adult patient with reduced renal function may develop hypertension, edema, and nocturia, but the uremic syndrome is the hallmark of renal failure in most adults. The uremic syndrome includes such nonspecific symptoms as lethargy, drowsiness, itching, nausea, vomiting, and paresthesias. Although at times the pediatrician sees these late symptoms, for the child with renal insufficiency, an earlier establishment of the diagnosis and initiation of therapy, when subtler symptoms occur, is advantageous.

The most common finding that should alert the pediatrician to the possibility of CRD is impairment of growth. The mean height of children entering the NAPRTCS CRI database is 1.49 standard deviations (SDs) below the mean. For the NAPRTCS dialysis database, mean height at entry is 1.69 SD below the mean. Short stature, particularly if associated with other symptoms, such as polyuria, frequent bouts of dehydration, salt craving, bone deformities, abnormal tooth development, or anemia, should suggest that the affected patient may have CRD. A previous history of urinary tract infections, nephrotic syndrome, or glomerulonephritis adds further support to this suspected diagnosis.

DEFINITIONS

The nomenclature describing stages of CRD is confusing. The currently accepted definitions are listed in Table 322.1. The term *impaired renal function* usually refers to an individual who is asymptomatic and has a residual renal function of 40% to 80% of normal. The term *CRI* is associated with a residual function of 25% to 50% of normal. At this level of renal function, distinct biochemical abnormalities may be present only when the patient is stressed. For example, the patient normally may maintain acid–base balance but, with stress, develop acidosis. Although serum calcium and phosphorous levels are normal, they remain so at the expense of an elevated serum parathyroid hormone. The child with CRI may develop dehydration early in the course of diarrhea because of reduced renal ability to retain sodium. With this degree of renal impairment, growth is slowed, and, although dialysis is not needed, aggressive therapy is indicated.

BOX 322.1   Symptoms of Renal Failure

Symptoms Seen in Adults and Children with Chronic Renal Failure
Hypertension
Edema
Nocturia, polyuria
Lethargy
Itching
Nausea, vomiting
Peripheral neuropathy
Encephalopathy

Symptoms Unique to Children with Chronic Renal Failure
Growth failure
Bone deformities
Abnormal tooth development
Unexplained dehydration
Craving of salt

TABLE 322.1

STAGES OF CHRONIC RENAL DISEASE

Stage	Residual Renal Function (%)	Symptoms or Metabolic Abnormality
Impaired renal function	40–80	None
Chronic renal insufficiency	25–50	Asymptomatic; short stature, increased parathyroid hormone
Chronic renal failure	<30	Acidosis, anemia, hypertension, lethargy
End-stage renal disease	Usually <10	Dialysis needed to maintain quality of life

The term *chronic renal failure* (CRF) is used to describe a patient who has residual renal function of less than 30%. The patient with CRF exhibits biochemical abnormalities even when not stressed. This patient usually has renal osteodystrophy, acidosis, and anemia; hypertension may be present. Vigorous therapeutic regimens may or may not successfully control these biochemical abnormalities.

ESRD is a term reserved for that stage of disease when renal replacement therapy, whether dialysis or transplantation, is required. The degree of renal function at which dialysis or transplantation is required varies and depends on many factors, including the cause of renal failure, age of the patient, and the patient's compliance with conservative therapy. Uremia is a symptom complex that includes anorexia, nausea, itching, neuropathy, and malaise. This complex is not associated with any specific concentration of urea in the blood, but it usually is considered to be the last stage of renal failure.

EPIDEMIOLOGY

The etiologies of CRF in children are listed in Box 322.2. The NAPRTCS registry confirms that different forms of obstructive uropathy (including reflux and dysplasia) account for almost 50% of the etiologies of renal failure in children. Other relatively common causes of ESRD in children that are rare in adults include renal hypoplasia and dysplasia, hereditary nephritis, infantile polycystic disease, cystinosis, and uremic medullary cystic disease. Focal glomerulosclerosis is the most common glomerulopathy leading to renal failure in young children (accounting for 14.8% of all children with ESRD), but older children may suffer from many forms of chronic glomerulonephritis.

Abnormalities Associated with Loss of Renal Function

With progressive loss of renal function, many metabolic changes occur (Box 322.3). The inability of patients with CRI to tolerate excess protein or nitrogen intake is well recognized. The level of blood urea nitrogen (BUN) is a function of dietary protein intake and renal clearance. Therefore, if intake of proteins remains constant as renal function declines, the BUN level increases. As blood urea concentration increases, urinary urea clearance increases until a steady state is achieved. Therefore, the patient with a BUN level of 60 mg/dL remains in nitrogen balance. However, the cost of achieving nitrogen balance is a high blood concentration of urea and other nitrogenous wastes. When these levels become excessive, uremic symptoms occur.

BOX 322.2 **Etiology of Chronic Renal Failure in Children in Order of Frequency**

Obstructive uropathy, including reflux nephropathy or renal dysplasia secondary to obstruction
Renal hypoplasia/dysplasia
Glomerulopathy/glomerulonephritis (all forms)
Hereditary disease, including hereditary nephritis or renal cystic diseases

---

BOX 322.3 **Metabolic Abnormalities Associated with Chronic Renal Failure**

Elevated blood urea nitrogen and protein intolerance
Decreased phosphate excretion
Decreased sodium excretion
Reduced ability to conserve sodium
Decreased hydrogen ion excretion
Decreased potassium excretion
Reduced production of 1,25-dihydroxycholecalciferol
Reduced production of erythropoietin

Uremia may lead to anorexia, with a subsequent reduction in the intake of proteins and a decrease in BUN. This change can lead less experienced physicians to think that the patient is improving when actually he is becoming malnourished, a condition that further complicates the disease process. The BUN level at which uremic symptoms occur depends on the patient's age, nutritional status, state of hydration, and the presence or absence of other metabolic abnormalities.

With further loss of renal function, the excretion of phosphorus decreases and may cause transient hyperphosphatemia and secondary hypocalcemia. The kidney produces 1,25-dihydroxycholecalciferol, the most active metabolite of vitamin D. Its synthesis is reduced in patients with renal insufficiency, resulting in reduced intestinal calcium absorption and hypocalcemia. Hyperphosphatemia associated with reduced calcium absorption results in low serum calcium. The relative contribution of these two is unknown; however, the net result of both is a lowered level of serum calcium, which then stimulates the secretion of parathyroid hormone. Increased serum parathyroid hormone (PTH) suppresses the proximal tubular reabsorption of phosphorus and normalizes serum phosphorus, but it also causes a reabsorption of calcium and phosphorus from bone. This effect, coupled with decreased calcification of bone caused by reduction in vitamin D activity, leads to renal osteodystrophy. Renal osteodystrophy in children is a combination of the pathologic changes seen with rickets and secondary hyperparathyroidism. Rickets occurs only in growing bone; hence, the ricketic component of renal osteodystrophy is present only in children.

As reduction in renal function progresses, the hydrogen ion balance becomes positive. Normally, more than one-half of the hydrogen ion excreted by the kidney is in the form of ammonium, which is produced by renal tubular cells and excreted into the tubular lumen. When hydrogen ion is available, ammonia (NH_3) becomes ammonium (NH_4). This positively charged polar molecule resists reabsorption and is excreted in the urine. With further loss of nephron mass, less and less NH_3 is produced, thereby decreasing excretion of hydrogen ion. Thus, early in the course of renal failure, the patient may maintain a urinary pH that is acid while having reduced excretion of hydrogen ion.

The second major buffer involved in acid excretion is phosphate. Because phosphate balance is maintained until relatively late in the course of renal failure, the excretion of hydrogen ion by this mechanism continues until the end-stage of the disease. As residual renal function decreases, a greater need to increase the excretion of sodium through the few remaining nephrons develops. This increase may be accomplished in some patients only by suppressing proximal tubular sodium reabsorption. If suppression occurs, reabsorption of bicarbonates from the proximal tubules also must be reduced, resulting in increased excretion of bicarbonates, an alkaline urine pH, and worsening of acidosis.

Sodium intolerance in patients with CRF is well-recognized. However, some children with CRF secondary to obstructive uropathy or cystic diseases may not be able to conserve sodium. Children with loss of renal function must maintain an intake of sodium within a narrow range. A normal adult may tolerate a dietary intake of 2 to 1,000 mEq of sodium per day. A patient with CRF and only 10% residual renal function may become depleted of sodium if dietary intake is less than 40 mEq/day. Conversely, the same patient may become hypertensive if intake of sodium exceeds 80 mEq/day.

Potassium balance can become positive in patients with CRF. Hyperkalemia usually is not seen until residual renal function is significantly less than 10% of normal. Hyperkalemia may be seen earlier in the course of CRF, if the patient is depleted of sodium. Hyperkalemia may occur with greater than 10% residual function in the rare patient who has defective renin release secondary to renal damage. Hypokalemia can occur in some patients with CRF because of renal potassium wasting, but it usually results from anorexia, emesis, and inadequate intake of potassium.

Anemia, a well-known consequence of CRF, is the result of defective erythropoietin production by the damaged kidney. Patients with renal failure also have reduced gastrointestinal absorption of iron. Therefore, when evaluating these patients, iron deficiency as a cause for anemia must be considered. Exogenous erythropoietin is available; through its use and the avoidance of iron deficiency, the anemia of CRF can be reversed. Many of the symptoms that previously were thought to be from uremia have been reversed by using erythropoietin and iron therapy to correct the anemia associated with CRI.

Neuropathy is a recognized part of the uremic syndrome. In children, especially infants, this consequence of CRF is of special importance. CRF that occurs early in life may delay brain development and lead to permanent neurologic impairment. Careful neurologic and frequent developmental evaluation of these children is required. Decisions concerning the timing of initiating dialysis or performing transplantation may depend on the results of these examinations.

THERAPY

Once CRF is recognized, and the physiology of lost renal function is understood, treatment is required. The nondialytic treatment of a child with renal insufficiency is in a state of flux. Numerous changes in recommended therapy have been made over the past few years and will continue to be made as more information becomes available about the metabolic abnormalities and the requirements for growth in these children (Box 322.4).

Changing dietary intake is one of the more important therapeutic interventions in children with CRF. However, these changes are difficult to implement and almost impossible to monitor. Two of the earliest signs of CRF are lethargy and reduced exercise tolerance. These symptoms may be a primary manifestation of retained uremic toxins or may result from anorexia, poor caloric intake, and an energy deficit. In children with CRF, differentiating the symptoms of uremia from those that may be secondary to malnutrition is difficult. Caloric intake of at least 100% of the recommended dietary allowance (RDA) for their ages should be provided to children with CRF. Dietary supplements may be required to reach this goal. Although increased caloric intake is recommended, it may not be used properly. Many dietary supplements used in the treatment of CRF contain glucose or simple carbohydrates. A relative glu-

---

BOX 322.4	Nondialytic Therapy of Chronic Renal Insufficiency or Chronic Renal Failure

Diet
Provide at least 100% recommended daily allowance of caloric intake
Protein intake; range 0.5–1.5 g/kg/day

Renal Osteodystrophy
1,25-Dihydroxycholecalciferol (dose variable)
Calcium carbonate (as a calcium supplement and PO_4 binder)

Anemia
May require iron
Erythropoietin

Hypertension
Control sodium intake
If hyperreninemic, consider angiotensin-converting enzyme inhibitor

Acidosis
May improve with reduced protein intake
Sodium citrate or $NaHCO_3$, 2–4 mEq/kg/day

---

cose intolerance, secondary to peripheral resistance to insulin, may develop as renal failure progresses. Early in the course of renal insufficiency, this defect is overcome by an enhanced production of insulin; thus, hyperglycemia is avoided at the expense of hyperinsulinemia. Later in the course of the disease, hyperglycemia may develop because even high levels of insulin cannot overcome the peripheral insensitivity to insulin. Serum glucose levels should be monitored when supplemental carbohydrates are given. This relative glucose intolerance also may cause hypertriglyceridemia.

Patients with CRF may develop hyperlipidemia if fats instead of glucose are used as a caloric supplement. Hyperlipidemia may be extreme in those patients who also are nephrotic. These patients should be evaluated and may benefit from lipid-lowering agents.

Dietary protein intake was the most controversial aspect of nutritional therapy of patients with CRD. In years past, protein intake was restricted. Patients with CRF do not use protein normally; therefore, to sustain normal growth and development, they require a greater intake of protein than do children without renal failure. The optimal dietary intake of protein for a child with renal failure has not been determined. Until studies provide answers to this dilemma, we recommend a diet containing proteins of high biologic value, providing at least 100% of the RDA for age. Providing an adequate intake of calories and protein to these children is challenging. Most of these patients require dietary supplements, and many will require nasogastric, transpyloric, or gastrostomy feedings.

The management of renal osteodystrophy in children with CRI is extremely important. If left untreated, these children will develop severe deformities in their limbs and certainly will grow poorly. They may develop symptomatic bone pain and metaphyseal fractures. Since the mid-1980s, significant advances in the understanding of how vitamin D is metabolized have been made. Two important steps in the synthesis of active vitamin D metabolites are known to occur in the kidney. Vitamin D can undergo hydroxylation at both the 1 and 24 positions in the renal interstitium. Renal hydroxylation leads to the formation of 1,25-dihydroxycholecalciferol, which has been synthesized and is available for use in patients with CRF. Its availability has rendered the treatment of renal osteodystrophy safer and more effective. In the past, both adults and children with CRI were treated with aluminum hydroxide gels to bind dietary phosphates and reduce absorption in an attempt to maintain phosphate balance. However, the intake of aluminum by children with renal insufficiency has been shown to cause severe neurologic and bone toxicity and never should be used. Many authors now recommend the use of calcium carbonate, which can serve both as a phosphate binder and a source of additional dietary calcium; the latter is deficient in the diets of most patients with CRF. With the timely initiation of therapy using 1,25-dihydroxycholecalciferol and calcium carbonate, many of the adverse effects of renal osteodystrophy can be minimized. Treatment requires careful monitoring because the use of too much calcium and active metabolites of vitamin D can oversuppress PTH, causing osteocyte hypoplasia and possible poor growth.

Treating the anemia associated with CRD is difficult but controllable. As stated before, many children with CRF become deficient in iron secondary to persistent microscopical blood loss in stools and to low dietary intake of iron. If iron deficiency is present, it should be corrected; however, the anemia usually persists despite the administration of iron therapy. One of the many functions of the kidney is to produce erythropoietin, which is reduced in patients with severe renal damage. Without this hormone, the production of erythrocytes is reduced and a hypoplastic anemia results. Recombinant human erythropoietin is available for the treatment of children with CRF. This agent corrects the anemia in patients with CRF and, thus, eliminates the need for costly and potentially dangerous blood transfusions.

Hypertension is a common sign of progressive renal function loss and most often results from excessive blood volume. The most effective treatment is to reduce sodium intake or to increase sodium excretion. Patients with renal failure become intolerant of both excessively high and low intakes of sodium. If restriction of sodium is too rigid, the patient may become hypovolemic, which can exacerbate other signs of CRF. The intake of sodium must be adjusted carefully to avoid both of these extremes. Occasionally, patients with CRF develop hypertension that is not related to volume but rather is caused by an excessive production of renin. These children can be treated successfully with an angiotensin-converting enzyme (ACE) inhibitor that blocks the conversion of angiotensin I to angiotensin II, lowers peripheral resistance, and normalizes blood pressure. The patient with CRF who develops hypertension, especially because of excessive blood volume, may require dialysis soon.

Patients with a progressive loss of renal function frequently develop metabolic acidosis. This event can occur early in the course, when obstructive uropathy is the cause of CRF. Acidosis may cause anorexia, vomiting, lethargy, growth failure, and other symptoms that mimic uremia. Correction with alkali therapy may reverse many of the previously mentioned symptoms and delay the need for renal replacement therapy. The base can be given as sodium bicarbonate or sodium citrate, usually in a dosage of 1 to 2 mEq/kg/day. Potassium salts may be used occasionally in the rare patient with CRF who also loses potassium. When the child with CRF no longer can tolerate the use of sodium buffers and, therefore, acidosis cannot be corrected, renal replacement therapy may be indicated.

Classic uremic neuropathy rarely is seen in children. If uremic neuropathy is noted, vigorous restriction of proteins may give temporary relief; however, this finding would surely indicate the need for renal replacement therapy.

Growth Failure

Growth failure is a common but now treatable consequence of CRF in children. Growth failure is particularly severe in children who develop renal insufficiency in the first year of life. Infants with CRF grow poorly between birth and age 2 years. Even if normal growth velocity can be achieved from age 2 onward, so much growth potential has been lost that dwarfism is the result. Growth retardation could be avoided if catch-up growth were achieved after successful renal replacement therapy. However, accelerated growth occurs only after the patient undergoes a successful renal transplantation, if that patient receives the transplant before the age of 6 years. To affect growth in this population, early recognition of CRF is essential.

To correct growth failure, one must attempt to correct all the metabolic abnormalities mentioned. Adequate dietary intake is important, especially in infants with renal failure. Several infants with CRF were identified early in life, and aggressive nutritional therapy was initiated. Dietary intake was given by tube feedings (either nasogastric or transpyloric) in an amount to provide at least 100% of the RDA for calories and 1 to 2 g/kg/day of protein. Although data are sparse, near-normal growth has been achieved in some patients. Providing adequate nutrition to older dialysis patients also has affected growth favorably.

Many children with CRF cannot conserve sodium. If sodium is restricted in these patients, poor growth may result; conversely, a greater intake of sodium by these patients improves growth. Acidosis often is a complication of CRF, and correction and control of the acidosis is essential to establish normal growth in this population. Early and aggressive therapy of renal osteodystrophy with vitamin D metabolites and calcium carbonate is required for optimal growth to occur in these children.

The anemia seen secondary to CRF may slow growth in these patients. Growth potential can be improved by giving careful attention to maintaining acid-base, electrolyte, and water balances in these patients. Treating renal osteodystrophy and providing adequate nutrition are essential in maintaining normal growth velocity. Although children with CRI and ESRD have growth hormone resistance, they respond favorably to supraphysiologic doses of growth hormone. The administration of recombinant human growth hormone has become the standard of care for the treatment of growth failure secondary to CRI and ESRD. However, its effect will be maximal only if all other metabolic abnormalities associated with renal failure are addressed.

Suggested Readings

Andreoli SP, Bergstein JM, Sheppard DJ. Aluminum intoxication from aluminum-containing phosphate binders in children with azotemia not undergoing dialysis. *N Engl J Med* 1984;310:1079.

Betts PR, McGrath G. Growth pattern and dietary intake in children with chronic renal insufficiency. *Br Med J* 1972;2:189.

Chantler C, Holliday M. Progressive loss of renal function. In: Holliday MA, Barratt TM, Vernier RL, eds. *Pediatric nephrology*, 2nd ed. Baltimore: Williams & Wilkins, 1987:773.

Chesney RW, Mehls O, Anast CS, et al. Renal osteodystrophy in children: the role of vitamin D, phosphorus, and parathyroid hormone. *Am J Kidney Dis* 1986;7:275.

Polinsky MS, Kaiser BA, Stover JB, et al. Neurologic development of children with severe chronic renal failure from infancy. *Pediatr Nephrol* 1987;1:157.

Rizzoni G, Broyer M, Guest G, et al. Growth retardation in children with chronic renal disease: scope of the problem. *Am J Kidney Dis* 1986; 7:256.

Seikaly, M, Ho PL, Emmett, Tejani. The 12th Annual Report of the North American Pediatric Transplant Cooperative Study. *Pediatr Transplant* 2001; 17:656.

Wassner SJ, Abitbol C, Alexander S, et al. Nutritional requirements for infants with renal failure. *Am J Kidney Dis* 1986;7:300.

CHAPTER 323 ■ END-STAGE RENAL DISEASE

EDWARD C. KOHAUT

DIALYSIS

Deciding when to initiate dialytic therapy in the child with chronic renal failure (CRF) often is difficult. No given level of serum creatinine or creatinine clearance is used as an absolute guide to the need for dialysis. Most children who require dialysis have residual renal functions of less than 10% of normal [a glomerular filtration rate (GFR) of less than 15 mL/minute/1.73M^2]. Even within this group, however, the need for dialytic therapy varies. When the child nearing end-stage renal disease (ESRD) no longer can function normally, is lethargic, cannot attend school, and has a poorer quality of life, dialytic therapy is indicated. Poor or absent growth once was an indication for considering dialysis, although growth may not normalize after dialysis is initiated. The use of supraphysiologic doses of recombinant human growth hormone has been shown to normalize growth velocity in children with chronic renal insufficiency (CRI), and, therefore, poor growth no longer is an indication for undergoing dialysis. Indications for infant dialysis may be different and are discussed separately.

Hemodialysis

Hemodialysis is a process by which blood is passed over an artificial semipermeable membrane, allowing the transfer of small molecules from the blood into surrounding dialysate. The rate of transfer of the solute depends on the concentration gradient of the solute, the blood flow over the membrane, and the permeability of the membrane to the solute. Movement of water across the membrane is a function of hydrostatic pressure. Hemodialysis is a relatively efficient process. Blood flows of 100 mL/minute through the dialyzer are possible, even in small patients. At that rate, using modern dialyzers, urea can be cleared at 70 to 80 mL/minute. Thus, during the treatment, the patient will have almost normal renal function. However, to hemodialyze a child for more than 4 to 5 hours, three times a week, is impractical. Aggressive hemodialysis performed for 15 hours a week would be equivalent to only 10% of normal renal function, which is an important point that should be stressed to children with renal failure and their parents. The expectation that once a child is placed on dialysis everything will return to normal is common, but that certainly is not the case.

Vascular Access

Vascular access always has been a particular problem for children undergoing hemodialysis. The blood vessel used must be large enough to permit the blood flow necessary for effective dialysis. In the small, frequently malnourished child with renal failure, femoral vessels often are the only option for vascular access.

Internal jugular catheters are used most often for semipermanent vascular access. This advance, coupled with the development of single-needle dialysis technology, has eliminated the need for using external shunts. Although the possibility of infection still is present, these newer catheters can be removed easily and a new one inserted at another site if infection is suspected. With this method, no loss of vascular integrity occurs. Many programs now use internal jugular catheters to hemodialyze infants. If the patient is thought to require long-term hemodialysis, a subcutaneous access should be created, which usually is accomplished by forming an arteriovenous fistula (the anastomosis of an artery directly to a vein) or by placing a graft (using a foreign material, usually polytetrafluoroethylene, to connect an artery to a vein). Either procedure usually provides long-term access for hemodialysis. Ideally, these procedures should be performed in the upper extremity, usually the forearm, but in smaller children, grafts may have to be placed in the femoral vessels to achieve adequate blood flow.

Some of the major complications of hemodialysis are related to access devices. Subcutaneous access devices can bleed from trauma, although trauma more often causes hematomas around the vessels, which may lead to compression and loss of flow or thrombosis. Infection was a common complication in patients with transcutaneous (Scriber) shunts, and it remains a problem with internal jugular catheter access. Infection seldom develops when subcutaneous access is used, but a strict sterile technique must be used when entering the vessels. These devices also may become infected when a patient becomes bacteremic. Administering prophylactic antibiotics before procedures when bacteremia can be expected (e.g., dental procedures) may be wise. Despite our best efforts, shunts and fistulas thrombose more frequently in children than in adults. This difference presumably is related to the smaller vessels and relatively lower blood flow in children. The pediatrician caring for these children always should examine these access devices and be aware of the frequent complications associated with them.

Procedure

The hemodialysis procedure itself is technically more demanding in children than in adults. The size of the dialyzer and blood tubing should be determined by the patient's blood volume. Ideally, no more than 10% of the child's blood volume should be in the extracorporeal circuit. Unfortunately, dialysis equipment and supplies are produced for the larger adult market, and compromises or innovations are required to meet the requirements for small children.

Another major complication of hemodialysis is a result of its efficiency. The child may begin dialysis with an elevated blood urea nitrogen (BUN) level that, with a large, efficient dialyzer, is lowered rapidly, leading to a sharp reduction in extracellular osmolality. If an equally rapid reduction in intracellular osmolality of brain cells does not follow, cerebral edema results; this event is termed dysequilibrium syndrome. This syndrome includes headache, abdominal pain, nausea, vomiting, and muscle cramps, followed by convulsions and coma. The syndrome can be avoided if clearances of urea are restricted to 3 or, at the most, 4 mL/kg/minute. Disequilibrium syndrome occurs more often in pediatric centers because of the availability of dialyzers that are more efficient than needed for the patient's size. Nonetheless, pediatric nephrologists have developed the required strategies to avoid the development of this syndrome in even the smallest patients.

Hypotension is a common complication of hemodialysis, and it occurs more frequently in children than in adults. During the hemodialysis procedure, excess fluid is removed from the extracellular fluid space, where it has accumulated since the last dialysis session. If the volume of blood is reduced rapidly and equilibration from the remaining extracellular fluid space is slow, hypovolemia usually results. Normally, an increase in peripheral vascular resistance would compensate, thus maintaining a normal blood pressure. However, vascular tone is deficient during dialysis, and hypotension often results. The lack of response of peripheral vessels to hypovolemia is thought to be caused by the activation of certain vasoactive substances by exposure of blood to the dialysis membrane. Less biologically active dialysis membranes are being studied. The incidence of hypotension can be limited by slow, regular removal of fluid.

Many other complications, including sudden death from many causes, occur with dialysis. The incidence of mechanical complications can be lowered by carefully maintaining equipment and having a vigilant nursing staff. This supervision is especially important when dialyzing small children, whose inquiring minds and busy fingers may not be aware of the dangers surrounding them.

At an experienced pediatric dialysis center, symptom-free dialysis of even the smallest child is possible. This goal is more difficult to achieve if interdialytic intake of salt and water has caused such excessive changes in body composition that vigorous dialysis cannot be avoided. Most centers limit the intake of protein in children treated with hemodialysis to 1 g/kg/day, with variability based on age and the needs of individual patients. The intake of sodium is restricted to less than 1.5 mEq/kg/day, which may be too low for some patients with residual function and salt wasting. High-potassium foods should be avoided, and specific restrictions of potassium sometimes are required. Some children treated with hemodialysis chronically have large intakes of water. They should be encouraged to limit fluids to 1.0 to 1.5 L/m²/day.

Adjunctive Therapy

Many of the therapeutic recommendations discussed in Chapter 322 for children with chronic renal failure (CRF) who do not yet require dialysis also apply to children treated with hemodialysis. As previously discussed, certain dietary restrictions are required in the management of these patients, but more of the chronic complications noted in these children are related to malnutrition than to dietary noncompliance. After undergoing vigorous hemodialysis treatments, children may be anorexic secondary to the disequilibrium syndrome; then, as the concentration of uremic toxins increases before the next dialysis, they may become anorexic from uremia. This anorexic cycle leads to malnutrition, which may perpetuate poor intake. Poor intake of dietary protein can cause a decrease in the BUN level, which may lead a less experienced physician to think that the patient is improving with dialysis, when actually the child is becoming malnourished. Malnutrition causes muscle wasting and a reduction in creatinine, which again can suggest the patient is improved, when actually the patient's health is failing. Careful and frequent dietary assessments must be made, and taking caloric dietary supplements should be encouraged if energy intake decreases to less than 100% of the recommended dietary allowance (RDA). Protein supplements occasionally are needed in severely anorexic patients. Too little intake of protein is as harmful as too much in children treated with hemodialysis. Increasingly, pediatric dialysis centers are using nasogastric tube or gastrostomy tube feedings in these patients to ensure they have adequate intake.

The intake of dietary phosphate also must be reduced. In the past, the absorption of phosphate was decreased through the use of aluminum hydroxide phosphate binders. This therapy now is contraindicated because patients receiving dialysis may develop aluminum toxicity, manifested by dementia or worsening of renal osteodystrophy. Calcium carbonate, now recommended as a replacement for aluminum hydroxide, acts as both a phosphate binder and a calcium supplement. Vitamin supplements, including 1,25-dihydroxycholecalciferol supplementation, are required by children with ESRD who are treated with hemodialysis. Folate and other water-soluble vitamins are removed by hemodialysis; therefore, the intake of a daily multivitamin supplement with folate is recommended.

Results

The treatment of the larger child with hemodialysis usually is successful. Dialyzing small infants remains difficult, although limited data suggest success. The mortality rate associated with hemodialysis is low in children weighing more than 15 kg who are treated at a pediatric dialysis center. However, this success does not mean that improvement is unnecessary. Children treated with hemodialysis rarely grow normally unless they also are treated with supraphysiologic doses of growth hormone, and they have great difficulty maintaining a reasonably normal lifestyle. Children have not been recommended for home hemodialysis treatment in the past, and hemodialysis performed in a specialized center results in a disrupted school schedule and reduced peer interaction. However, when this therapy is performed in a pediatric unit dedicated to the needs of chronically ill children, patients who for medical or social reasons cannot be treated with home therapy can thrive while being treated with hemodialysis.

Peritoneal Dialysis

The use of peritoneal dialysis as a renal replacement therapy for children has a relatively short history. In the 1950s and 1960s, peritoneal dialysis was used to treat acute renal failure. Treatment of CRF with peritoneal dialysis was unsuccessful until reliable peritoneal access was developed in the late 1960s. At that time, several pediatric programs using intermittent peritoneal dialysis were developed. Because of the parallel development of a more efficient therapy (hemodialysis), intermittent peritoneal dialysis never was used widely to treat CRF in either children or adults.

Continuous Ambulatory Peritoneal Dialysis and Continuous Cycling Peritoneal Dialysis

In 1976, a new form of peritoneal dialysis that later became known as continuous ambulatory peritoneal dialysis (CAPD) was described. CAPD overcomes the relative inefficiency of the peritoneal membrane by exposing it continually to dialysate. In the early 1980s, this form of dialysis was introduced as a form of therapy for children with CRF. In 1981, another form of continuous peritoneal dialysis was introduced and subsequently was named continuous cycling peritoneal dialysis (CCPD). CCPD has been adapted to children with ESRD. The descriptions of CAPD and CCPD have rekindled the interest of many pediatric nephrologists in peritoneal dialysis.

Both CAPD and CCPD are forms of dialysis that can be done at home. CAPD is a manual process. The patient or caretaker attaches a bag of sterile dialysate to a tube, and it enters the peritoneal cavity. This fluid remains there for 3 to 5 hours and then is drained into the same bag, which is discarded, and a new bag is aseptically attached to the tubing. This procedure is repeated three or four times a day, and a single 8-hour session is performed at night. CCPD is similar, except that the rapid filling and emptying is performed by a cycling device at night and a single long dwell is done during the day. The patient is fully ambulatory during the daytime with either procedure. Most children now treated with peritoneal dialysis are done so with variations of CCPD. This change has occurred because of the availability of cyclers adapted for small children and the fact that CAPD is very labor-intensive.

These forms of continuous peritoneal dialysis have been a major advance in the treatment of children with ESRD. They have provided forms of therapy that can be implemented at home, permitting the patient to attend school and have relatively normal peer interactions. Peritoneal dialysis is less costly than is in-center hemodialysis, and it can be used to treat even the smallest infant. The major disadvantage of CAPD is that it is labor-intensive. The caretaker, usually a parent, must be available to exchange a bag of dialysate every 4 to 5 hours during the day. Each bag exchange may take from 20 to 40 minutes, depending on how rapidly the fluid drains from the abdomen. Many parents may tire of this procedure after a period of time. CCPD is less demanding, and the caretaker must do only two procedures: at bedtime, attach the tubing from the patient's peritoneal cavity to the cycling device, and in the morning, disconnect the patient from the cycling device.

CAPD and CCPD are comparable in their efficacy of controlling the abnormal metabolic values associated with ESRD. The clearance of low-molecular-weight substances is similar with CAPD and CCPD. The clearance of middle molecules and higher-molecular-weight toxins may be slightly improved with CAPD. The major disadvantage of CCPD is that the patient must have a cycling device available, which decreases mobility because the device is not portable. Because CAPD and CCPD are so similar, no reason exists why both procedures cannot be taught to the same patient or parent. One may, on some days, take advantage of the decreased labor involved in CCPD and, on other days, use the mobility provided by CAPD. The remainder of this discussion treats these two forms of therapy as interchangeable because most of the complications and problems associated with them are similar.

Both therapies require peritoneal access, usually by the surgical placement of a Tenckhoff catheter. The catheter usually enters the peritoneal cavity at the lateral edge of the rectus muscle. A purse-string suture is placed around the peritoneal membrane, forming a seal as watertight as possible. A Dacron cuff is placed at the entrance site of the peritoneal membrane. The catheter is then tunneled under the skin, exiting through the skin at some distance from where the catheter enters the peritoneum. The catheter should be placed by a surgeon who understands the unique problems of children with ESRD because the procedure differs in many respects from that performed on adults.

As with other forms of dialysis, access is more of a problem in children than in adults. Children have more omentum than do adults. A possible complication resulting from this difference is outflow obstruction caused by a piece of omentum wrapping around the catheter. To avoid this complication, many pediatric programs advise performing partial or even total removal of the omentum at the time the catheter is placed. Dialysate leakage, another complication seen at a higher rate among children than adults, is thought to be caused by a relative decrease in the quantity of subcutaneous tissue in children. Leakage of dialysate has been minimized by using the peritoneal purse-string suture and by placing the catheter at the lateral edge of the rectus muscle.

Complications

Hernias may occur when patients begin therapy with continuous dialysis, or they may develop later in the course of therapy because of persistently increased intraabdominal pressure. These hernias usually can be repaired, and, although patients may need to receive hemodialysis for a short period, they can return to peritoneal dialysis. Some programs advise that the abdomen be left empty during the day if hernias recur, which causes a significant reduction in total clearance.

The most common complication of peritoneal dialysis is peritonitis. It usually is diagnosed by the caretaker, who notes cloudy effluent dialysate. Most often, the patient is infected with coagulase-negative staphylococcus, rarely is seriously ill, and is treated at home with intraperitoneal antibiotics. If peritonitis is not diagnosed and treated quickly, or if the patient is infected with a gram-negative organism, a more serious illness may result. If antibiotics cannot sterilize the peritoneal fluid, or if the patient develops recurrent infection, the peritoneal catheter may need to be removed. Frequent episodes of peritonitis may cause the patient to choose another form of dialysis. Some nephrologists may advise patients to seek another means of therapy if the incidence of peritonitis is high.

Adjunctive Therapy

Adjunctive therapy for the child treated with peritoneal dialysis is similar to that advised for patients treated with hemodialysis. One of the advantages of peritoneal dialysis is a relatively high clearance of middle- and high-molecular-weight toxins. Unfortunately, the peritoneal membrane is not selective, and loss of vital large molecules, such as protein, also occurs. Therefore, when patients are treated with peritoneal dialysis, intake of protein must be increased. Water-soluble vitamins and vitamin D metabolites are lost through the peritoneal membrane, and patients sustained by these forms of dialysis must supplement their diets with the active form of vitamin D and multivitamins.

Results

Many children have been treated with various forms of peritoneal dialysis. The advantages and disadvantages of each method are listed in Box 323.1. No one form of dialysis can be recommended for all patients, and each potential method of therapy must be judged according to how it can benefit each individual patient. The goal for every child with ESRD is to have a well-functioning renal allograft. The treatments described are both a means to reach that goal and a support when circumstances preclude performing transplantation.

BOX 323.1 | **Advantages of Continuous Ambulatory Peritoneal Dialysis and Continuous Cycling Peritoneal Dialysis**

Continuous ambulatory peritoneal dialysis
Mobility
No machine
Simple procedure
Less costly
Higher solute clearances

Continuous cycling peritoneal dialysis
Less time-consuming
No daytime pass
Reduced protein loss?
Reduced incidence of hernia and peritoneal leaks?

Treatment of the Small Infant with End-Stage Renal Disease

The aggressive treatment of a young infant with renal insufficiency may stimulate as many emotional, ethical, and economic issues as questions pertinent to medical therapy. Until the early 1980s, the approach to the young infant was to provide nondialytic therapy of variable aggressiveness until the infant survived to a certain age or size, when providing dialysis or renal transplantation was thought possible. Unfortunately, this approach has led to certain problems. The first one is that normal infants achieve 30% of their growth potential during the first 2 years of life. Infants with renal insufficiency, unless optimally treated, grow poorly during this critical period. If the patient is growth-retarded by age 2 years, and therapy is initiated, catch-up growth rarely occurs; the patient will never be of normal height. Of greater concern is that rapid brain growth also occurs during the first 2 years of life. Children with renal insufficiency during infancy may develop permanent and progressive neurologic complications. Because of the availability of CAPD, CCPD, and improved nutritional support, many investigators now consider that early and aggressive therapy of infants with CRI should be provided.

Infants should receive aggressive medical management even before dialysis is initiated. This treatment should include attempts to correct acid-base abnormalities, normalize calcium and phosphorus metabolism, and, most important, ensure adequate nutrition. The abnormalities seen in infants with renal insufficiency are similar to those seen in babies who have been malnourished during the first year of life. If patients will not or cannot ingest adequate calories because of the anorexia associated with CRI, nutritional supplements using enteral feedings may be indicated. If, despite receiving adequate nutrition and correction of metabolic abnormalities, the infant still fails to thrive, as indicated by poor linear growth, poor head growth, and poor weight gain, the use of dialysis should be considered.

One approach to this situation may be to treat the infant with hemodialysis, then perform a renal transplantation as soon as possible. Renal transplantation in infants is associated with a high mortality rate in most centers. Single-center data reported since the early 1990s have demonstrated success in a limited number of patients. This approach requires the use of specialized hemodialysis techniques and the involvement of well-motivated parents. Another approach to treating these patients may be to use peritoneal dialysis and then to perform renal transplantation when the patient is older and the procedure is better tolerated. This method now has been used by several groups with some success.

RENAL TRANSPLANTATION

Renal transplantation is the goal of therapy for children with ESRD. A well-functioning renal allograft is superior to dialysis in its ability to effect psychosocial and physical rehabilitation. However, successful transplantation may be difficult to achieve.

Criteria for Acceptance for Transplantation

The criteria for accepting a patient for transplantation are constantly changing. Until the 1990s, children younger than 5 years of age rarely were considered candidates for transplantation. The initial results in this age group were disappointing. However, more modern experience would indicate that children between ages 1 and 5 years old who received live related-

donor (LRD) renal allografts had acceptable outcomes. Most authors would not recommend transplantation for the infant younger than 1 year who is thriving while being treated with a form of peritoneal dialysis. If an LRD renal allograft is available, transplantation may be the best option for the child between ages 1 and 5 year old. If an LRD kidney is unavailable, and the child is thriving on dialysis, cadaveric transplantation might be delayed until the patient is older. Cadaveric transplantation may be the only option for the young child who fails to thrive while being treated with dialysis.

Uremia may cause severe neurologic complications, including developmental delay. This delay may be permanent, but it also may improve with treatment. Therefore, deciding whether a child is an acceptable candidate for transplantation based on mental function can be difficult. Parents of these children should be made fully aware of these complications and should be active participants in all decisions made concerning transplantation. If the decision is made not to pursue transplantation, then support from the renal program should be provided.

All children with chronic illness have some difficulty with psychosocial adaptation to their disease. This difficulty often is made most manifest during adolescence and results in rebellion and noncompliance. Nonadherence to treatment regimens by the transplant patient often results in rejection of the allograft. If predisposing factors for noncompliance are recognized in a patient, transplantation could be delayed until counseling is done to reduce this risk.

Malignancy is a contraindication to transplantation for many adult patients. In children with bilateral Wilms tumor, transplantation is considered if the patient is followed for 1 year on dialysis and no recurrence or metastasis is noted.

Obstructive uropathy is the most common single cause of ESRD in children. Many of these patients have abnormal bladders. Experience suggests that, in most cases, these bladders can be used for transplantation. Careful evaluation of the bladder is suggested, but only rarely is it found lacking. Even patients with neurogenic bladders can be transplanted, and the urine can be drained by intermittent catheterization.

Many immunologically mediated glomerulopathies that cause ESRD may recur in the transplanted kidney (Box 323.2). Although the rate of recurrent disease is significant, the number of grafts lost because of recurrent disease is small. Patients who develop renal failure secondary to these glomerulopathies still may be transplanted, but the risk of recurrence should be made clear to them and their families. If the patient were to lose a graft from recurrence of disease, a second transplant would not be recommended.

In summary, few absolute contraindications to transplantation exist. Any child with ESRD deserves to be evaluated for candidacy for renal transplantation.

BOX 323.2	Glomerulopathies That may Recur in a Transplanted Kidney

Focal glomerulosclerosis
Goodpasture syndrome (anti–glomerular basement membrane disease)
Membranoproliferative glomerulonephritis types I and II
Rapidly progressive glomerulonephritis
Henoch-Schönlein purpura, IgA nephropathy
Systemic lupus erythematosus
Membranous glomerulonephritis

Donor Selection

The best renal allograft survival rates are reached when an LRD, HLA-identical kidney is transplanted. When an HLA-identical sibling donates an organ, the graft survival rate at 1 year exceeds 90%. Unfortunately, many younger children do not have siblings old enough to be considered donors. Children often receive LRD renal allografts from a parent instead of a sibling. By definition, parents are a one-haplotype match with their children. The success of transplantation among one-haplotype-matched pairs exceeds 80% at 1 year. When an LRD kidney is unavailable, the use of a cadaveric donor is necessary. At this writing, both patient and graft survival rates are less than those quoted for LRD transplantation. The hope is that, as our knowledge of immunologic tolerance advances, cadaveric donor renal transplantation will become as successful as is LRD transplantation.

Always, patients waiting for cadaveric organs have been more numerous than the available organs. The formation of the national organ bank will increase the chances that a child will be offered an immunologically acceptable cadaveric renal allograft.

Immunosuppression

Current commonly used immunosuppressive drugs are listed in Box 323.3. Corticosteroids have been used to treat and prevent graft rejection. The exact mechanism of action is unknown. Prednisone is the corticosteroid used most commonly, but no data suggest that it is superior to other forms. Dosage regimens during the first few months after the transplant vary widely among transplant programs. Most dedicated pediatric transplant centers agree that a low-maintenance dose should be the goal. Some programs advise using very low daily doses of prednisone, but most prefer alternate-day corticosteroids at a dose of 0.3 to 0.5 mg/kg. A daily dose of prednisone of 8.5 mg/m^2 or greater causes growth failure. Other complications of the chronic use of corticosteroids include hypertension, hypercholesterolemia, cushingoid appearance, aseptic necrosis of the femoral head, and an increased incidence of specific infections. Large doses of corticosteroids (20 mg/kg/day) may be used for 3 or 4 days to reverse acute rejection. Newer immunosuppressive regimens are aimed at getting patients completely weaned from steroids.

Azathioprine (Imuran) may prevent, but will not reverse, rejection. It affects many functions within the immune system. The dose varies in the early posttransplant period, but most programs advise a maintenance dose of 1 to 2 mg/kg/day.

BOX 323.3   Commonly Used Immunosuppressants

Maintenance therapy
Azathioprine
Prednisone
Cyclosporine
Tacrolimus
Mycophenolate
Treatment of rejection
Methylprednisolone
Antilymphocyte globulin
OKT3, monoclonal antibody to T cells

Because the most common complication of azathioprine is myelosuppression, the white blood cell count, platelet count, and hematocrit should be monitored during therapy. This drug also may be hepatotoxic; the dose should be reduced if liver enzyme levels become elevated. Azathioprine contributes to the increased incidence of infection noted in these patients. Many programs are substituting mycophenolate mofetil for azathioprine in their immunosuppressive regimen. This new drug appears to be more immunosuppressive and is less hepatotoxic, but it often causes gastrointestinal side effects, including diarrhea.

Cyclosporine is an agent that is more specific in its effect on the immune system than are the drugs previously mentioned. Cyclosporine is only weakly suppressive to the bone marrow, but it is a potent inhibitor of many T-lymphocyte functions. It prevents the generation of cytotoxic T lymphocytes, thought to be the cells mainly responsible for acute rejection. The dose of cyclosporine varies from patient to patient, and drug levels must be followed to ensure effect and avoid toxicity. Unfortunately, cyclosporine is nephrotoxic. It appears to have an acute toxicity, associated with high serum drug levels, which is reversible when the dose is lowered. Tacrolimus has replaced cyclosporine in many programs. Its advantages and disadvantages in pediatrics are being studied.

Many pediatric programs now advise the use of all three drugs together. The use of azathioprine or mycophenolate mofetil with low-dose prednisone may allow the use of lower doses of cyclosporine or tacrolimus. The hope is that at these lower doses cyclosporine still will have an effect, but its toxicity will be minimal. New drugs constantly are being evaluated to treat these patients. The pediatrician caring for these patients is advised to be in communication with the transplant center and aware of the complications of the specific medications the patient is receiving.

Monitoring the Patient after Transplant

Follow-up of the child who has had a successful renal transplant can be a rewarding experience for the pediatrician. Often, the previously shy, lethargic, chronically ill patient emerges into an outgoing, energetic, "normal" child. We have the privilege to observe this rare transformation. At the same time, the patient's happy parents must be cautioned that rejection can occur. Without careful follow-up, many problems, including serious and life-threatening infections, may develop.

Classically, acute rejection of the renal allograft presents with systemic symptoms such as fever, lethargy, anorexia, chills, and joint pain. The graft should be tender and swollen. Unfortunately, with modern immunosuppressive protocols, acute rejection, especially if it occurs after the first month posttransplant, rarely is classic. Patients may have acute rejection made manifest only by an increasing serum creatinine level, a mildly elevated blood pressure, and a renal allograft that is slightly swollen. Obviously, careful and frequent observation of these patients is required to detect these changes. Sometimes the graft may need to be biopsied to confirm the diagnosis. If detected early, most episodes of acute rejection can be reversed. Acute rejection, if it occurs, usually is seen within 6 months of transplantation and rarely is diagnosed after that time. However, acute rejection can occur at any time if immunosuppressive therapy is discontinued by the noncompliant patient.

Chronic rejection can start anytime in the posttransplant patient. It usually is associated with a slowly increasing creatinine level accompanied by hypertension. Allograft biopsy is needed to confirm the diagnosis. Chronic rejection cannot be treated. However, with continued immunosuppression and, most important, control of hypertension, years may pass before the patient needs to return to using dialysis.

Blood pressure must be monitored in the posttransplant patient. Hypertension may be seen not only secondary to rejection, but also as a consequence of using prednisone or cyclosporine, or (rarely) stenosis at the anastomosis of the graft renal artery. Significant elevations in blood pressure must be evaluated and treated because hypertension from any cause may damage the allograft.

Fever in the immunosuppressed patient is an emergency that should alert the pediatrician to the possibility of a life-threatening infection. A complete evaluation is indicated, even if the patient does not appear very ill. Corticosteroids often mask symptoms of serious disease in these patients. The possibility of the presence of fungal and serious viral infections must be considered. Hospitalization may seem unnecessary but often is advised when the transplanted child develops fever.

Prognosis

Available data would suggest that at least 70% of children who receive LRD allografts and 60% of children who receive cadaveric transplants would be free of dialysis at 10 years posttransplant. However, graft survival curves have not yet flattened. A slow but constant incidence of graft failure occurs even 15 years posttransplant. The hope is that patients currently undergoing renal transplantation will have even higher long-term success rates.

The long-term outlook for the child with CRF is unfolding. Ideally, we hope to prevent the diseases and birth defects that cause the child to be devastated with CRF; until then, we must deal with these problems. Since the late 1970s, therapies have evolved that not only have lengthened the lives of these children but also have improved the quality of their lives.

Suggested Readings

Alliapoulos JC, Salusky JB, Hall T, et al. Comparison of continuous cycling peritoneal dialysis with continuous ambulatory peritoneal dialysis in children. *J Pediatr* 1984;105:721.

Baum M, Powell D, Calvin S, et al. Continuous ambulatory peritoneal dialysis in children: comparison with hemodialysis. *N Engl J Med* 1982;307:1537.

Diaz-Buxo JA, Walker PJ, Farmer CD, et al. Continuous cyclic peritoneal dialysis. *Trans Am Soc Artif Intern Organs* 1981;27:51.

Donckerwolcke RA, Chantler C. Hemodialysis. In: Holliday MA, Barratt TM, Vernier RL, eds. *Pediatric nephrology*, 2nd ed. Baltimore: Williams & Wilkins, 1987:799.

Ettenger RB, Fine RN. Renal transplantation. In: Holliday MA, Barratt TM, Vernier RL, eds. *Pediatric nephrology*, 2nd ed. Baltimore: Williams & Wilkins, 1987:828.

Kohaut EC, Whelchel J, Waldo FB, Diethelm AG. Aggressive therapy of infants with renal failure. *Pediatr Nephrol* 1987;1:150.

Neu AM, Ho PL, McDonald RA, Warady BA. Chronic dialysis in children and adolescents. The 2001 NAPRTCS annual report. *Pediatr Nephrol* 2002; 17:656.

Popovich RP, Moncrief JW, Nolph KD, et al. Continuous ambulatory peritoneal dialysis. *Ann Intern Med* 1978;88:449.

CHAPTER 324 ■ RENAL MALFORMATIONS

LAURA S. FINN

Developmental abnormalities of the kidney produce significant rates of morbidity and mortality and are the most common cause of renal failure in children. Malformations result from a failure of normal development: "primary" anomalies are caused by disordered induction, morphogenesis, growth, and migration; "secondary" anomalies ensue from alterations superimposed on apparently normally developed kidneys. The postulated influences include maternal disease, vascular compromise, teratogens, urinary tract obstruction, and genetic mutations. Morphologic classification of malformations is traditional, but new genetic insights will lead to refined classifications that reflect pathogenetic mechanisms.

Abnormalities in migration of the entire renal unit from the pelvis lead to renal ectopia, either unilateral or bilateral. Most commonly, the kidney remains in the pelvis or may cross the midline (crossed ectopia). *Fusion* of the kidneys, usually at their lower poles, results in "horseshoe" kidney, with complete fusion producing a pelvic "cake" kidney. *Abnormalities of ureteric branching* may lead to double ureters, crossed ectopia, or bilateral displacement of the vesicoureteral insertions. These anomalies generally are asymptomatic, but they may be associated with an increased incidence of infection and, occasionally, with obstruction.

ABNORMALITIES OF RENAL MASS

Renal agenesis is complete absence of one or both kidneys and usually is associated with absence of the corresponding ureter and bladder trigone; additional anomalies of mesonephric or paramesonephric duct derivates (testes, epididymis, vas deferens, and ejaculatory duct in male patients; uterus, fallopian tubes, ovaries, and vagina in female patients) are common occurrences. Renal agenesis is seen in transgenic mice with null mutations in *Wt1*, *Pax2*, and *Ret* and indicates a defect in the earliest stages of nephrogenesis. The incidence of unilateral agenesis is difficult to assess because most patients are asymptomatic with only compensatory hyperplasia of the single kidney, but the condition is estimated to occur in 1 in 350 to 1,000 births. Less common and incompatible with life, bilateral agenesis occurs in approximately 1 in 5,000 births. Affected infants are stillborn or die shortly after birth from respiratory failure. Oligohydramnios results from fetal anuria and the lack of fluid, and resulting constriction produces the constellation of features termed the *Potter syndrome*. The infants have low-set ears, prominent infracanthal folds, a flattened beaked nose, micrognathia, creased skin, and varying positional deformities of the limbs. Bilateral renal agenesis usually is sporadic but may be associated with hereditary renal adysplasia, a syndrome with probable autosomal dominant inheritance and variable expression, including unilateral and bilateral agenesis and dysplasia.

Hypoplasia refers to congenitally small kidneys and is an anomaly in which insufficient renal parenchyma is formed. Hypoplasia generally is sporadic, rarely familial. A decrease in the number of nephrons, frequently associated with a reduced number of renal lobes, suggests deficient ureteric bud branching or a decrease in epithelial morphogenesis. Renal hypoplasia has been associated with B-cell lymphoma-2 (BCL-2) and paired-box domain protein-2 (PAX-2) deficiencies. Hypoplasia is a rare malformation requiring morphologic confirmation. It often is confused clinically with atrophy, which can be differentiated by the presence of scarring or alterations in the architectural pattern of the kidney. Radiographic diagnosis is difficult to establish and is uncertain. Evidence of reflux or recurrent infection suggests atrophy rather than hypoplasia. Segmental renal hypoplasia (Ask-Upmark kidney) is considered to be an atrophic, rather than primary, developmental anomaly.

Bilateral renal hypoplasia ranks fourth as a cause of renal failure in children. The common form, *oligomeganephronia*, is an isolated and sporadic malformation characterized by extremely small kidneys that have decreased numbers of enlarged nephrons. The glomeruli are several times the norm in diameter, area, and volume, and the proximal tubules are dilated and lengthened. Oligomeganephronia occurs with a male-to-female ratio of 3:1. The major defect is in tubular concentration, leading to polyuria and dehydration. Growth retardation and moderate proteinuria are common findings when renal failure ensues. These children are good candidates for renal transplantation because the renal anomaly usually is an isolated malformation. A second, rare form of bilateral hypoplasia leading to renal failure is characterized by decreased numbers of normal nephrons.

ABNORMALITIES OF RENAL DIFFERENTIATION

Dysplasia is defined as altered differentiation of metanephric blastema. Dysplasia is seen with obstruction occurring before the completion of nephrogenesis, in association with several multiple malformation syndromes, or sporadically as an isolated event. The term is limited to kidneys showing the following characteristic histologic changes: collecting ducts lined by primitive epithelial cells with hyperchromatic nuclei; differentiated fibromuscular collars surrounding the ducts; and a loose, undifferentiated mesenchymal stroma. Metaplastic cartilage often is present in the cortex but is not an essential feature. Some metanephric differentiation always occurs, and primitive glomeruli and tubules are seen in varying numbers. Cysts, primarily involving tubules and ducts, are common findings (Fig. 324.1). Persistent fetal patterns of PAX2, BCL2, neural cell adhesion molecule (NCAM), and intercellular adhesion molecule expression (ICAM) in addition to altered growth factors and inflammatory mediators have been identified in multicystic dysplastic kidneys (MCDKs).

Renal dysplasia is associated with urinary tract malformations, particularly obstruction, in approximately 90% of cases; this finding contrasts with the lack of obstruction in hereditary and syndromal renal dysplasia. The most common of these anomalies is obstruction of the prostatic urethra in boys, a condition designated posterior urethral valves but more likely to be urethral stenosis of varying degrees of severity. When the obstruction is complete, severe bilateral dysplasia occurs. Lesser degrees of obstruction may not affect the kidney during the period of active nephrogenesis but may cause hydronephrosis

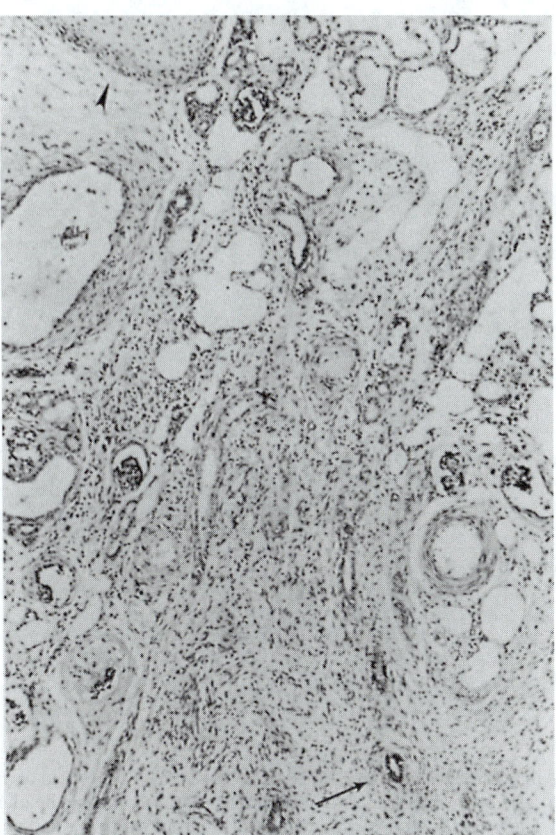

FIGURE 324.1. In this section from a cystic dysplastic kidney, primitive tubules surrounded by fibromuscular collars (*arrow*) are seen embedded in a loose mesenchymal stroma. Microscopic cysts and a few primitive glomeruli are present. One focus of metaplastic cartilage (*arrowhead*) also can be identified. (Masson trichrome, magnification 60×.)

or scarring later. Ureteral anomalies and malpositions, sometimes associated with ureteroceles, may cause bilateral, unilateral, or segmental dysplasia, depending on the location of the obstruction.

The most severe forms of dysplasia are *MCDK* and *aplastic kidney*, which are associated with complete ureteropelvic occlusion and ureteral atresia (Fig. 324.2). The MCDK is enlarged and has multiple cysts, has no reniform structure, and does not excrete urine. Bilateral complete disease is fatal, resulting in the Potter syndrome. Unilateral MCDK is estimated to occur in 1 in 4,300 births; most cases are sporadic. It appears to be related to obstruction occurring relatively late in nephrogenesis and usually has an inner core of more normal renal parenchyma. The aplastic-dysplastic kidney is quite small, with few cysts and little corticomedullary development. Microscopically, most of the tissue is dysplastic. This type of kidney seems to result from obstruction early in fetal development. The MCDK often is identified by prenatal ultrasonography and is the most common cause of an abdominal mass in the neonate. Lesser forms of unilateral or segmental dysplasia may remain asymptomatic for varying periods. A unilateral MCDK typically involutes, with compensatory hyperplasia of the contralateral kidney, and it may disappear, leading to a diagnosis of renal agenesis. Conservative management should include the evaluation of associated urinary tract abnormalities, particularly vesicoureteral reflux and contralateral ureteropelvic junction obstruction, which is estimated to occur in approximately 40%. In this setting, the kidneys have a higher incidence of infection. The development of hypertension may be alleviated by nephrectomy.

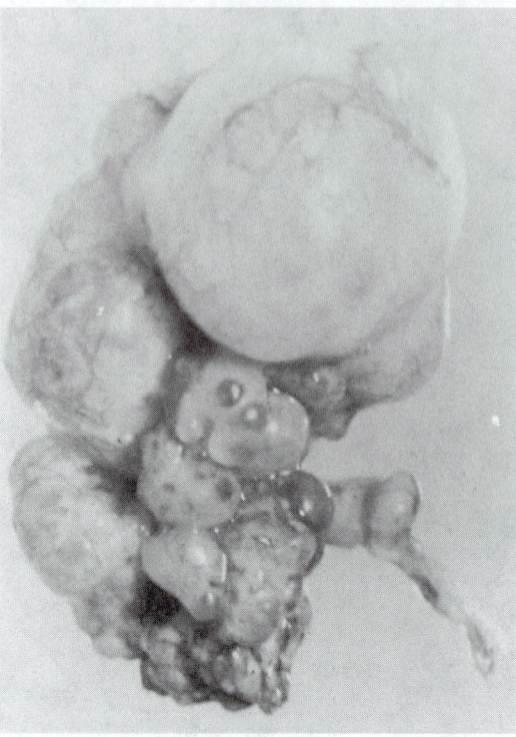

FIGURE 324.2. This multicystic dysplastic kidney is composed of multiple cysts of various sizes. No normal renal parenchyma can be identified. The ureter is cystically dilated at its junction with the renal pelvis and atretic distally.

Diffuse cystic dysplasia, unassociated with obstruction, varies in severity and typically is heritable and syndromal. The kidneys are large and may have few nephrons and limited medullary development. Cysts typically arise from primitive collecting ducts and can lie throughout the cortex. Infants have followed the same course as those with severe dysplasia related to obstruction.

Renal tubular dysgenesis is a form of deficient tubular differentiation associated with oligohydramnios and prematurity. The infants are stillborn with the Potter sequence, or they have postnatal anuria and die in the early neonatal period. Defects in skull ossification often accompany the renal anomalies. An autosomal recessive transmission is seen in some cases, whereas acquired forms have been associated with the maternal use of angiotensin-converting enzyme inhibitors. Similar tubular abnormalities have been described in the kidneys of the donor twin in the twin–twin transfusion syndrome and in less severe forms in fetuses exposed to nonsteroidal antiinflammatory drugs.

RENAL CYSTIC MALFORMATIONS

Polycystic Disease

Autosomal recessive polycystic kidney disease (ARPKD) has an estimated incidence of 1 in 20,000 live births. The clinical spectrum is variable, but all typical forms result from mutations in *PKHD1* localized on chromosome 6p12 that encodes polyductin. ARPKD always is accompanied by diffuse biliary dysgenesis (congenital hepatic fibrosis) and has three distinct presentations. Most commonly, infants present in the neonatal period with greatly enlarged, cystic, reniform kidneys (Fig. 324.3), but the mechanisms of cyst formation remain widely

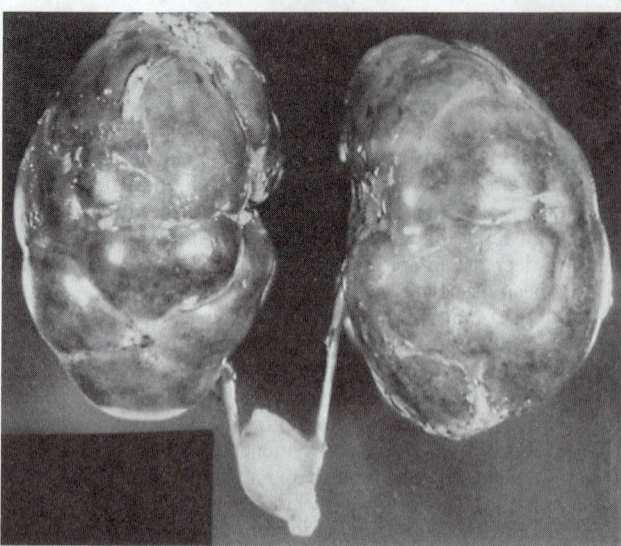

FIGURE 324.3. The massive enlargement of these kidneys from a neonate with autosomal recessive polycystic kidney disease can be appreciated when the kidneys are compared with the bladder, which is of normal size. Small cysts can be seen throughout both kidneys.

unknown. The cysts are fusiform dilations of the collecting ducts, which radiate from the medulla through the cortex to the subcapsular region. Normal renal parenchyma is present between cysts. Occasionally, the liver is enlarged, and each portal area has increased peripheral bile ducts that appear to ring the portal region and actually represent three-dimensional, flattened sacs. A slight increase in portal fibrous tissue also is present. The infants are oliguric and usually die within a few days of pulmonary insufficiency because of lung hypoplasia. Maternal oligohydramnios is considered to be the major factor contributing to the hypoplasia, although compression of the thoracic cage by the massively enlarged kidneys also has been suggested. A few infants survive and merge clinically and morphologically with the second type of presentation.

Infants past the neonatal period and young children with ARPKD present with flank masses and hepatosplenomegaly. The renal cysts are more rounded and less prominent than in the neonatal form of disease, and medullary duct ectasia is a constant and prominent feature. Portal fibrosis is increased, and varying degrees of bile duct ectasia are seen. Small pancreatic cysts may be present. Clinically, patients have a concentrating defect, which places them at risk for developing dehydration. They also may have renal tubular acidosis. The creatinine clearance usually is decreased somewhat for age, but renal function may remain stable for several years before progressing to renal failure. Renal transplantation is the treatment of choice because the disease does not recur in the transplanted kidney. Hypertension, which tends to develop early, is a common problem and requires aggressive therapy. Some children develop portal hypertension, which occasionally results in bleeding esophageal varices, but it responds to portacaval shunting.

A milder version of ARPKD is seen in a subset of children and young adults who present with portal hypertension and progressive hepatic fibrosis associated with biliary dysgenesis. This subset has mild renal involvement consisting of the same type of cystic dilation of collecting ducts and tubules as that seen with ARPKD in infants and young children.

Autosomal dominant polycystic kidney disease (ADPKD) is a systemic disorder primarily affecting the kidney. It has a prevalence of 1 in 1,000 and is present in approximately 10% of the adults who enter dialysis programs each year. Two genes responsible for ADPKD have been sequenced. *PKD1*, which localized to 16p13.3 and codes a transmembrane glycoprotein, polycystin-1, is responsible for approximately 85% of cases. An additional 10% to 15% of cases are the result of mutations in *PKD2*, mapped to 4q21-23, that encodes polycystin-2, which directly interacts with polycytin-1. Germline mutations are inherited in an autosomal dominant manner, but the slow development of cysts is caused by loss of heterozygosity of the second allele in an individual cell, resulting in clonally derived cysts.

ADPKD usually presents in the fourth or fifth decade of life, but a small number of children and infants also may develop symptomatic ADPKD. The clinical spectrum in the pediatric population ranges from the rare intrauterine presentation with Potter sequence to the ultrasound diagnosis of renal cysts in an asymptomatic child. The disease always is bilateral, but it may occur asynchronously in the two kidneys. The kidneys may be large and have variable numbers of cysts involving all portions of the nephron and collecting ducts (Fig. 324.4). Scattered cysts may be present in the liver and pancreas, but hepatosplenomegaly, portal fibrosis, and biliary dysgenesis usually are not features of ADPKD. The absence of these findings or the presence of berry aneurysms, which are rare occurrences in ARPKD, aids in the differentiation between ADPKD and ARPKD. Ultrasound scans of children with the dominant form of the disease occasionally may show medullary striations suggestive of the recessive form. The definitive diagnosis of ADPKD in childhood rests on molecular diagnostic studies in a child with a positive family history or the demonstration of asymptomatic cystic disease in one of the parents. Because *de novo* mutations occur in approximately 10% of families, a negative history does not rule out the diagnosis.

Children with ADPKD may have hematuria or recurrent urinary tract infections. Occasionally, patients require dialysis early in the course of the disease, but most maintain stable renal function for 10 years after the onset of symptoms before progressing to renal failure. Tubular defects are not seen. Hypertension tends to occur less often and later in children with ADPKD than in those with ARPKD, but aggressive control of blood pressure may be warrented to offset progression to end-stage renal disease. These children also are good candidates for renal transplantation.

Recent discoveries have localized polycystin-1, polycystin-2, and polyductin to the primary cilia of renal tubular epithelial cells, thus perhaps linking cilary dysfunction with cystic disease.

Glomerulocystic Disease

Glomerular cysts occur in several settings, some with a genetic basis. Human diseases associated with glomerular cysts include the following: (a) glomerulocystic disease, comprising sporadic and nonsydromic recessive and dominantly inherited forms; (b) glomerulocystic kidneys associated with malformation syndromes, such as oral facial digital syndrome type 1, tuberous sclerosis, renal-hepatic-pancreatic dysplasia, and glutaric acidemia type 2; and (c) glomerular cysts occurring in dysplastic kidneys, sometimes associated with intrauterine obstruction. In addition, glomerular cysts can predominate in fetal ADPKD. Mutations of the *HNF-1beta* gene have been described in some cases of glomerulocystic kidney disease. The kidneys may be grossly enlarged or small; those in patients with familial disease typically are small. Microscopically, cysts generally are only up to 2 to 3 mm across, and at least 5% of them contain a glomerular tuft identifying the cyst as Bowman space; they are particularly numerous in the subcortical region. Some patients have medullary fibrosis and varying degrees of collecting duct ectasia, suggesting intrarenal obstruction.

Infants with glomerulocystic disease usually present in the newborn period with abdominal masses and decreased renal function, and they frequently die of associated malformations. Infants who survive tend to have chronic but stable renal insufficiency, although a few may show improved renal function with time, and some may progress to renal failure.

Other Cystic Diseases

Nephronophthisis (NPHP) and medullary cystic kidney disease are hereditary forms of renal cystic malformation that share a similar histology of cysts, primarily at the corticomedullary junction and thickening and disintegration of the tubular basement membrane. Patients with medullary cystic kidney disease have an adult onset of renal failure, have an autosomal dominant inheritance, and lack extrarenal involvement. Hypercalciuria, urolithiasis, and concentrating defects are typical complications. Two genes, *MCKD1* on chromosome 1q23.1 and *MCKD2* on chromosome 16p12, have been identified.

The autosomal recessive form, NPHP, has an infantile, juvenile, or adolescent onset and is the most common genetic cause of progressive renal failure in children and young adults. Although it is most frequently isolated to the kidney, extrarenal involvement may occur. Two loci associated with the juvenile type (*NPHP1* on 2q12-13, *NPHP4* on 1p36) and one for the adolescent type (*NPHP3* on 3q21-22) encode *nephrocystin-1*, nephrocystin-4, and nephrocystin-3, respectively, whereas mutations in *INVS*, encoding inversin, are responsible for the infantile type (*NPHP2* on 9q22-31). Remarkably, these proteins interact and also localize to the primary cilia of renal tubular cells.

After the onset of symptoms, the kidneys are small and pale, and cysts are present in the medulla (Fig. 324.5). Late in the disease, impressive interstitial fibrosis and thinning of the cortex also occur. Clinically, children with NPHP exhibit

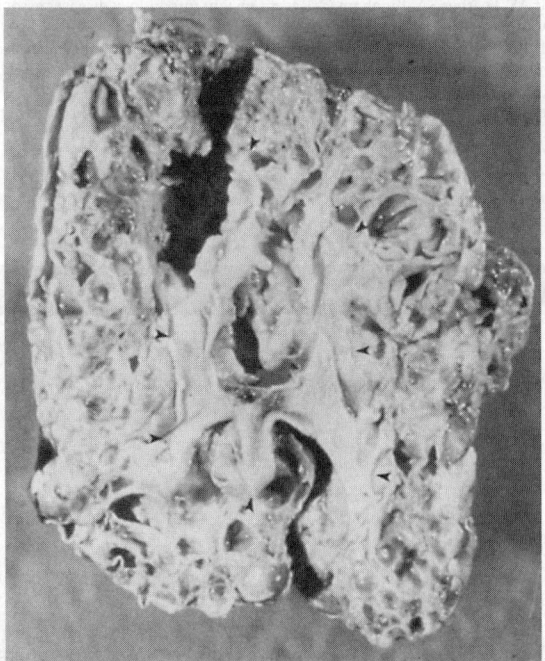

FIGURE 324.4. The cut surface of this bisected kidney from a patient with autosomal dominant polycystic kidney disease shows cysts of various sizes. These cysts are present throughout the parenchyma and obliterate normal renal architecture. No separation exists between the cortex and the medulla, and the usual reniform shape has been lost. The pelvis can be seen in the middle of the specimen (*arrowheads*).

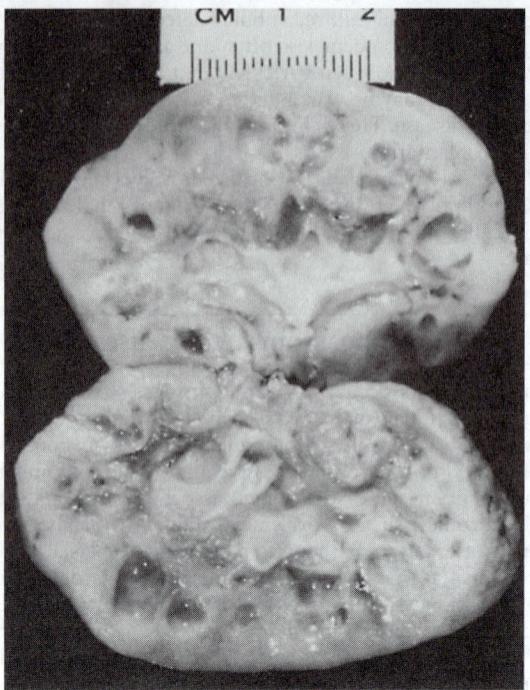

FIGURE 324.5. This kidney from an 11-year-old girl with juvenile nephronophthisis is small and pale. The cortex is somewhat thin, and multiple medullary cysts of various sizes can be seen.

a tubular defect characterized by inability to concentrate the urine, polyuria, polydipsia, growth retardation, and anemia, which may be greater than predicted from the extent of renal failure. Similar clinical and morphologic findings are seen in association with numerous malformation syndromes.

ASSOCIATED ANOMALIES

Many different renal anomalies are seen in association with malformation syndromes, and the list continues to increase. Liver, pancreas, and central nervous system anomalies fre-

quently accompany renal malformations. Renal dysplasia and cortical cysts are prominent in such syndromes as Meckel Gruber, Jeune, Zellweger, prune belly, and VATER (vertebral defects, imperforate anus, tracheoesophageal fistula, and radial and renal dysplasia). Small cortical cysts, alone or in association with dysplasia, occur with many of these syndromes, as well as with several of the trisomies. Medullary cysts and interstitial nephritis occur in Jeune, Laurence-Moon-Bardet-Biedl, and renal-retinal syndromes, and diffuse cysts may be seen in the syndromes of Ehlers-Danlos, tuberous sclerosis, and von Hippel–Lindau.

Suggested Readings

Bergmann C, Senderek J, Sedlacek B, et al. Spectrum of mutations in the gene for autosomal recessive polycystic kidney disease (ARPKD/PHKD1). *J Am Soc Nephrol* 2003;14:76.

Bernstein J, Risdon RA, Gilbert-Barness E. Renal system. In: Gilbert-Barness E, ed. *Potter's pathology of the fetus and infant.* St. Louis: Mosby-Year Book, 1997:863.

De Paepe ME, Stopa E, Huang C, et al. Renal tubular apoptosis in twin-to-twin transfusion syndrome. *Pediatr Dev Pathol* 2003;6:215.

Feldenberg LR, Siegel NJ. Clinical course and outcome for children with multicystic dysplastic kidneys. *Pediatr Nephrol* 2000;14:1098.

Fick-Brosnahan GM, Tran ZV, Johnson AM, et al. Progression of autosomal-dominant polycystic kidnye disease in children. *Kidney Int* 2001;59:1654.

Guay-Woodford LM, Desmond RA. Autosomal recessive polycystic kidney disease: the clinical experience in North America. *Pediatrics* 2003;111:1072.

Johnson CA, Gissen P, Sergi C. Molecular pathology and genetics of congenital hepatorenal fibrocystic syndromes. *J Med Genet* 2003;40:311.

Otto EA, Schermer B, Obara T, et al. Mutations in *INVS* encoding inversin cause nephronophthisis type 2, linking renal systic disease to the function of primary cilia and left-right axis determination. *Nat Genet* 2003;34:413.

Pohl M, Bhatnagar V, Mendoza SA, et al. Toward an etiological classification of developmental disorders of the kidney and upper urinary tract. *Kidney Int* 2002;61:10.

Salomon R, Tellier A, Attie-Bitach T, et al. PAX2 mutations in oligomeganephronia. *Kidney Int* 2001;59:457.

Watnick T, Germino G. From cilia to cyst. *Nat Genet* 2003;34:355.

Woolf AS. Clinical impact and biological basis of renal malformations. *Semin Nephrol* 1995;15:361.

Woolf AS, Feather SA, Bingham C. Recent insight into kidney diseases associated with glomerular cysts. *Pediatr Nephrol* 2002;17:229.

Woolf AS, Winyard PJD. Molecular mechanisms of human embryogenesis: developmental pathogenesis of renal tract malformations. *Pediatr Dev Pathol* 2002;5:108.

Zerres K, Rudnik-Schoneborn S, Steinkamm C, et al. Autosomal recessive polycystic kidney disease. *Neprhol Dial Transplant* 1996;11(suppl 6):29.

CHAPTER 325 ■ GLOMERULONEPHRITIS AND NEPHROTIC SYNDROME

EILEEN D. BREWER

OVERVIEW OF GLOMERULONEPHRITIS

Glomerulonephritis (GN) is the general name given to a heterogenous group of diseases that result from immunologic injury to glomeruli of the kidney. GN appears to be mediated primarily by immune mechanisms that invoke inflammatory changes in the glomerular capillaries, causing alteration of glomerular structure and function throughout both kidneys. Impairment of tubular function may occur, but it is not prominent and usually is the result of glomerular injury itself. GN may be a primary renal disease or one manifestation of a systemic disease, especially vasculitis.

Pathogenesis

Although the pathogenesis of GN has been studied actively since the 1950s, it is not fully understood. During the past decade, major advances in molecular biology and genetics have yielded important new insights into the immunopathogenic mechanisms that give rise to GN. Current evidence supports the concept that most GN results from an autoimmune response to a variety of different etiologic agents, some known and most still unknown. Loss of tolerance to self-antigens in the glomeruli either leads to immune complex formation *in situ* in glomeruli or elicits cell-mediated immune responses that affect glomerular permeability. Nephritogenic immune complexes themselves cause little tissue injury, but they trigger the release of many inflammatory mediators, including complement, cytokines, growth factors, and coagulation factors, which produce the functional and structural abnormalities of GN.

Formation of Immune Complexes

Antibodies that induce glomerular immune deposits may be directed against normal constituents of the glomeruli (e.g., antiglomerular basement membrane [anti-GBM] antibodies in Goodpasture disease), against nonrenal self-antigens localized in the glomeruli (e.g., DNA-nucleosome complexes in lupus), or against exogenous antigens that are trapped in the glomeruli by charge affinity or local precipitation (e.g., cryoglobulins in hepatitis C virus–associated membranoproliferative GN [MPGN]). The site at which glomerular immune deposits form dictates the degree of injury. Subendothelial deposits on the inner surface of the glomerular capillary walls easily recruit circulating neutrophils and macrophages as effector cells and induce more inflammation than do mesangial or subepithelial deposits, which are less accessible to the circulation. *In situ* immune complex formation results in local complement activation and is much more nephritogenic than is passive trapping of antibodies from the circulation. The character and quantity of immune deposits also affect the degree of tissue injury. Complement-fixing immunoglobulin G (IgG) subtypes cause more injury than do antibodies that do not activate complement as well. Larger quantities of immune deposits cause more tissue injury.

Mediators of Immune Complex Glomerular Injury

Immune complexes activate cellular and humoral mediators to induce glomerular injury. Glomerular immune deposits become an inflammatory focus that leads to generation of chemotactic factors that attract neutrophils, T cells, and macrophages to the site. Among the most important chemotactic factors are complement component C5a, interleukin-8, and glomerular endothelial cell adhesion molecules. Neutrophils attracted to the site of the deposits are activated by ingesting the immune complex aggregates and subsequently generate hydrogen peroxide and proteases, which, in turn, damage the locally surrounding tissue. Activated T cells play a less direct role in tissue injury by releasing chemokines to recruit macrophages to the site of injury. Macrophages, either recruited by T cells or attracted by local chemokines or adhesion molecules, release proteolytic enzymes and reactive oxygen species, which digest the immune deposits but also digest and injure the normal GBM. Macrophages also release transforming growth factor, induce fibrin formation, and initiate cellular crescent formation.

A secondary effect of immune mediators occurs in glomerular cells themselves, which respond in several ways, including cell proliferation, overproduction of oxidants and proteases, changes in cell phenotype, and overproduction of extracellular matrix. These changes in glomerular cells may herald a chronic phase of GN that progresses to glomerular sclerosis and permanent loss of renal filtration function.

IgG-containing immune complexes recruit humoral mediators, especially components of complement. The most important of these components is the complement membrane attack complex (C5b-9), which has membranolytic activity to damage glomerular cells directly and to alter glomerular permeability. C5b-9 also mediates an interstitial inflammatory response, especially in association with proteinuric forms of GN, such as membranous GN (MGN). Interstitial inflammation may progress to chronic interstitial fibrosis and may contribute to progressive renal scarring. The importance of C5b-9 as one of the mediators of tissue injury suggests a new avenue for future therapy to prevent chronic GN by altering the pathogenesis of GN at an early stage of the process before injury occurs. The use of molecularly engineered complement regulatory proteins to downregulate the generation of C5b-9 has the potential to ameliorate or completely prevent progression of some forms of GN.

Cellular Immunity

Less is known about the importance of cellular-mediated processes that contribute to the pathogenesis of GN. T cells and macrophages clearly play pathogenic roles in diseases such as MGN, minimal-change nephrotic syndrome (MCNS), and focal segmental glomerulosclerosis (FSGS). In these diseases, no significant antibody deposition, cellular infiltration, or glomerular cell proliferation is apparent by histologic examination of kidney tissue, but clinically dramatic increases occur in glomerular permeability, especially to protein. At least in MCNS and FSGS, a circulating permeability factor derived from T cells has been identified in experimental models as the likely mediator. The probable sites of action of this factor are the GBM and the glomerular epithelial cell (podocyte).

Coagulation Factors

Coagulation factors are important contributing factors to the pathogenesis of GN. In patients with rapidly progressive GN (RPGN), deposition of fibrin and its derivatives at sites of glomerular injury and gaps in the GBM is critical to the formation of glomerular crescents. Glomerular crescents are defined histologically by the presence of two or more layers of cells in Bowman's space that eventually may growth to obliterate that space. Platelet activation also appears to play a role in the pathogenesis of GN through elaboration of substances potentially injurious to the kidney. Platelet cationic proteins may neutralize the GBM-negative charge and allow proteins, which also are negatively charged, to be filtered freely instead of being repelled by the GBM negative-charge barrier. Platelet-activating factor (PAF) produces a decline in renal vascular resistance and mesangial cell contraction, which contributes to reduction of glomerular filtration rate (GFR). PAF also promotes glomerular macrophage accumulation, fibrin deposition, and crescent formation. Platelet-derived growth factor (PDGF), which has properties similar to those of PAF, also promotes glomerulosclerosis. Increased production of PDGF stimulates mesangial and endothelial cell proliferation in some proliferative forms of GN, including experimental nephritis, and the human diseases diffuse proliferative lupus nephritis, IgA nephropathy, mesangial proliferative nephritis, and antineutrophil cytoplasmic antibody-positive crescentic nephritis.

Toxic Factors

A few exogenous nephrotoxins cause GN. They include the drugs D-penicillamine, trimethadione, probenecid, and captopril and a few of the heavy metals, such as mercury and gold. The mechanism of injury depends on the toxin. D-Penicillamine induces immune complexes that indirectly injure the glomeruli. Trimethadione and mercury probably cause direct injury to the GBM. MGN is the histopathologic lesion most often induced by glomerular nephrotoxins.

Clinical Presentations

GN may present clinically in a variety of ways. Dividing the clinical presentation into a few main categories (Box 325.1) is useful to narrow the differential diagnosis and to direct the diagnostic evaluation.

The acute nephritic syndrome is the sudden onset of hematuria (either gross or microscopic) with or without proteinuria, decreased GFR, and retention of sodium and water. Reduced GFR and retention of sodium and water may result in edema, circulatory volume overload, and hypertension. The hallmark of nephritic syndrome is hematuria and red blood cell casts in the urine, with only minimal to moderate proteinuria. Acutely decreased GFR may result from decreased filtration surface area caused by a variety of factors, including cellular proliferation, endothelial cell swelling, neutrophil infiltration, locally induced vascular changes that decrease net filtration pressure, and obstruction of Bowman's space by fibrin deposition and crescent formation. The mechanism for sodium and fluid retention is understood incompletely and may occur without significant changes in serum albumin concentration. The degree of fluid overload often is out of proportion to the decrease in GFR. Volume overload leads to suppression of aldosterone and impaired potassium and hydrogen ion excretion, which contribute to the hyperkalemia and acidosis observed in some acutely nephritic patients.

Patients with chronic GN may have few overt symptoms. Asymptomatic hematuria or proteinuria discovered on routine urinalysis may be the only presenting sign. Likewise, malaise, fatigue, anemia, and failure to grow normally may be the only signs of slowly progressive chronic GN with chronic renal failure.

If the clinical course includes rapid decline of renal function to uremia, the presentation is termed RPGN. Rapid identification of RPGN by renal biopsy is very important if therapy is to be beneficial. Renal biopsies from affected patients show glomerular crescent formation alone or in addition to identifying characteristics of specific histopathologic types of GN. Sometimes, patients with RPGN do not present with symptoms until after permanent loss of renal function has occurred.

Patients with the nephrotic syndrome (NS) have massive proteinuria (more than 40 mg/m²/hour in children), hypoproteinemia, edema, and hyperlipidemia. Hematuria, either gross or microscopic, may be present but is not the prominent feature.

This chapter discusses many of the kinds of GN of children and adolescents under the headings of the main clinical presentations of GN. Because most of the disease entities that present with the acute nephritic syndrome also may have an insidious onset characteristic of chronic GN, acute and chronic GN are grouped together.

ACUTE AND CHRONIC CHILDHOOD GLOMERULONEPHRITIS

The disorders that present primarily with hematuria and red blood cells casts, whether in an acute or chronic fashion, include IgA nephropathy, Henoch-Schönlein purpura (HSP) nephritis, lupus nephritis, nephritis of chronic bacteremia, and MPGN. Because most patients with MPGN present with the NS or proteinuria, this disease entity is discussed later in this chapter (see the discussion of NS). Patients with acute poststreptococcal GN (APSGN) always present acutely, although occasionally the signs and symptoms may be so mild that patients do not seek medical attention.

Acute Poststreptococcal Glomerulonephritis

APSGN is the most common form of immune-mediated nephritis in children. It is by far the most common form of postinfectious nephritis, although infection with various other bacterial, viral, parasitic, rickettsial, and fungal agents may be followed by an acute nephritic syndrome similar to that experienced after infections with nephritogenic strains of group A beta-hemolytic streptococci. In contrast to "rheumatogenic" strains of group A streptococci, which cause acute rheumatic fever associated with pharyngeal infection, nephritogenic strains of group A streptococci may cause either pharyngeal or skin infections. Historically, most cases of APSGN were related to pharyngeal infections with type 12 group A streptococci, but the current list of nephritogenic types is large and includes types 1, 2, 3, 4, 18, 25, 31, 52, 56, 59, and 61. Types 2, 49 (Red Lake), 55, 57, and 60 are nephritogenic, but they are most often associated with a preceding pyodermal infection. APSGN may occur in epidemics but more often is encountered sporadically. The attack rate during epidemics has been estimated at approximately 10% to 12%. However, incidence figures are extremely unreliable because many cases of APSGN are mild and do not come to medical attention. In fact, APSGN may occur without any accompanying identifiable urinary abnormalities.

Susceptibility to APSGN may be determined genetically and depends on favorable host factors. Most often, the disease occurs in elementary school aged children (mean age, 7 years), is twice as common in male as in female patients, and is fairly rare in children younger than age 3 years old. An episode of group A streptococcal throat or skin infection precedes all cases of APSGN. In most instances, the interval between the infection and the onset of clinical GN is approximately 8 to 14 days, although both longer and shorter intervals have been reported.

Proof of the previous infection may not be available by bacterial culture, but serologic evidence of streptococcal infection is present at the time of presentation. Serum antistreptolysin O (ASO) titer is elevated in 80% of cases of patients who have had antecedent pharyngitis. The characteristic rise in the ASO titer is blunted by antimicrobial therapy, and the ASO titer seldom is elevated after skin infection occurs. When antihyaluronidase (AHT) and antideoxyribonuclease B (anti-DNase B) titers also are measured, proof of preceding infection nears 100%. The anti-DNase B titers are particularly important if the preceding infection was pyoderma. Elevation of serum antistreptococcal titers is essential to diagnose APSGN with certainty, but the magnitude of the titers holds no prognostic significance. The absence of serologic confirmation of a recent streptococcal infection renders the diagnosis of APSGN suspect, and other forms of nephritis should be considered (see the discussion of differential diagnosis).

Clinical Features

The clinical expression of APSGN is fairly variable and extends from a completely asymptomatic form to the most severe manifestations of acute renal failure, including edema, oliguria, congestive heart failure, hypertension, and encephalopathy. The most common presenting symptoms are hematuria, proteinuria, and edema, often accompanied by rather nonspecific findings of lethargy, anorexia, vomiting, fever, abdominal pain, or headache.

Gross hematuria is present in only 30% to 50% of children with APSGN. Usually, the urine is described as smoky, tea colored, cola colored, or, occasionally, dirty green. At least two-thirds of hospitalized patients have edema, which initially is mild and may be noted only periorbitally but can become fairly marked, especially if normal fluid intake occurs over the course of several days at the height of the disease. Evidence of circulatory congestion, including orthopnea, dyspnea, cough, auscultatory rales, and gallop heart rhythms, is apparent on physical examination in many children with edema. Usually, chest radiography shows cardiomegaly and pulmonary edema of varying degrees. Severe congestive heart failure is a very rare occurrence. Hypertension is seen fairly commonly in inpatients (50% to 90%), but hypertensive encephalopathy, characterized by headache, somnolence, convulsions, coma, confusion, aphasia, transient blindness, agitation, or combativeness, occurs in only a few (5%).

Laboratory Features

Laboratory investigation should begin with a careful analysis of the urine. The specimen may be yellow, slightly discolored, or grossly bloody and usually has a high specific gravity and a low pH. Microscopic hematuria with predominantly dysmorphic erythrocytes in the centrifuged urinary sediment is present in virtually all cases, and leukocyturia is almost as common. Red blood cell casts are found very often (60% to 85%) in centrifuged specimens in which the resuspended sediment is examined freshly and exhibits an acidic pH. Often, leukocyte casts in addition to hyaline and granular casts are seen. The presence of leukocytes and leukocyte casts should not be considered evidence of superimposed urinary tract infection but rather of glomerular inflammation. Proteinuria occurs in most cases and correlates qualitatively with the amount of blood in the urine, reaching nephrotic proportions in fewer than 5% of patients.

A laboratory evaluation for streptococcal infection is mandatory. Serum ASO and anti-DNase B titers (as described earlier) are most helpful for confirming previous recent infection of the throat or skin. AHT determinations have been discontinued in many laboratories because of difficulties in interpreting the test, which may be positive in other diseases. Throat and skin lesion cultures also may be positive at the time the patient has nephritis and should be treated with appropriate antibiotics. Because asymptomatic family members also may be affected, family screening for subclinical streptococcal disease and nephritis has been recommended.

One of the most important diagnostic laboratory findings in APSGN is a depressed serum concentration of C3. Activation of the alternate pathway of complement occurs in most cases, resulting in reduced serum C3 levels in at least 90% of patients examined in the early phase of nephritis. Occasionally, serum C4 also is depressed. In most cases, serum C3 returns to normal concentrations 10 days to 8 weeks after the onset of the nephritis. If the serum C3 is not measured within the first few days of presentation of the nephritis, the concentration may have returned to normal, and its depression will have been missed. Because prior treatment of the streptococcal infection with antibiotics may attenuate the period of serum C3 depression, the serum C3 may appear normal at the time of presentation of the nephritis. The degree of serum C3 depression bears no relationship to the severity of the disease. A follow-up serum C3 determination must be obtained 8 to 12 weeks after the onset of the acute episode to document the return of a normal concentration, which occurs in more than 90% of patients by this time interval. If the concentration remains low, other kinds of nephritis, such as MPGN or lupus, are more likely, and renal biopsy confirmation of the diagnosis should be sought.

Usually, GFR is depressed in hospitalized patients during the acute stage of moderate to severe nephritis. Serum urea nitrogen may be elevated disproportionately to serum creatinine. Even when GFR is normal or only slightly decreased, severe sodium and fluid retention may occur. Urine volume is reduced, but severe oliguria is uncommon. Urine-concentrating ability is well preserved. The fractional excretion of sodium is less than 1%, even in the presence of reduced GFR. The acutely inflamed kidney of APSGN retains sodium even in acute renal failure, unlike the high fractional excretion of sodium that occurs in acute tubular necrosis. If a child with APSGN is allowed free access to fluids, dilutional hyponatremia may develop. Acidosis and hyperkalemia may result from aldosterone suppression caused by extracellular volume expansion and from severe reduction in GFR.

Pathology

Although patients with APSGN rarely undergo renal biopsy today, many were assessed by biopsy in previous decades, thus giving us a comprehensive understanding of the histologic spectrum of the disease. By light microscopy, the glomeruli are seen to be enlarged and hypercellular, filling Bowman's space. The glomeruli are relatively bloodless because of the occlusion of capillary lumina by proliferating mesangial and endothelial cells accompanied by a variable amount of infiltration by neutrophils, macrophages, and eosinophils within the capillary lumina and mesangium. Crescents are uncommon findings but may be extensive and are associated with a poorer prognosis. The renal tubules appear normal. Interstitial edema may be prominent. Usually, the blood vessels are normal. Electron microscopy reveals typical electron-dense "humps" between the glomerular capillary basement membrane and the epithelial cells. The humps are present on immunofluorescence studies, showing up as bright granular deposits containing predominantly IgG and C3. Other immune reactants, such as IgM, IgA, fibrin, and other components of the alternate pathway of complement, may be found along the capillary walls and in the mesangium.

Pathogenesis

The precise mechanism of pathogenesis remains uncertain, despite widespread acceptance that APSGN is immune-complex mediated and is triggered by constituents of the nephritogenic strains of group A streptococci. Immune complexes containing IgG and C3 have been identified in the serum of affected patients. Attempts to identify streptococcal antigens within these complexes, either in the circulation or fixed in glomeruli, have been negative or inconclusive. Possibly, streptococcal antigens bind to the glomerular capillary wall and form the nidus for *in situ* immune complex formation. Additionally, direct complement activation by streptococcal antigens deposited in the glomeruli may induce local inflammatory changes that lead to glomerular injury.

Differential Diagnosis

At their onset, many types of GN mimic APSGN, but these occur less commonly. The absence of proof of a preceding streptococcal infection or the simultaneous occurrence of infection plus nephritis suggests other types of GN. GN caused by infectious agents other than streptococci (staphylococci, viruses) usually is coincident with the infection and often lacks the telltale sign of hypocomplementemia. Usually, the course of other infection-associated GN depends on the natural history of that infection rather than on the renal manifestations.

Other disorders frequently confused with APSGN include IgA nephropathy, hereditary nephritis (Alport syndrome), MPGN, HSP nephritis, idiopathic hypercalciuria, benign hematuria, and resolving episodes of previously undiagnosed postinfectious GN. Unlike in ASPGN, the episodic hematuria of IgA nephropathy occurs coincident with and not after an upper respiratory tract infection, and serum complement levels are normal. Previously unrecognized hereditary nephritis with microscopic or gross hematuria but no associated hypocomplementemia may first come to attention because of an abnormal urinalysis found during evaluation for ASPGN. In contrast, MPGN may present as an acute nephritic syndrome during or after a streptococcal infection but with hypocomplementemia that, when reassessed at a later date, does not resolve. The nephritis of HSP may mimic clinical APSGN precisely if it is associated with mild extrarenal manifestations and an evanescent rash. A careful history and physical examination may uncover the true diagnosis in such cases, and serum complement levels are normal. Idiopathic hypercalciuria may present as isolated hematuria but without proteinuria or hypocomplementemia. Benign hematuria is a diagnosis of exclusion after all other causes of hematuria have been eliminated and, like hypercalciuria, has no associated proteinuria or hypocomplementemia.

The exacerbation of chronic previously unrecognized GN also must be excluded. Patients with chronic GN may exhibit episodic gross hematuria, hypertension, or azotemia at the time of an intercurrent infection. A prior history of renal symptoms or features of chronic renal failure, such as growth retardation or renal osteodystrophy, should be sought carefully to help to distinguish forms of chronic GN from APSGN.

Therapy

No specific or general therapy is effective in ameliorating the inflammatory lesion of APSGN. All therapy is supportive and is directed toward treating the clinical manifestations of acute nephritis. Hypertension may be severe and require emergency treatment. Severe hypertension with encephalopathy demands immediate treatment. Fast-acting antihypertensive medication such as sublingual nifedipine or intravenous labetalol may be a suitable choice for initial therapy. If multiple doses are required, maintenance antihypertensive therapy should be started. Loop diuretics and fluid restriction are important adjunct therapies and usually suffice alone for mild hypertension and for relieving edema and circulatory congestion. Restricting fluid intake to an amount equal to insensible water loss may obviate the need for diuretic therapy. Conversely, the use of diuretics may allow affected patients to have a more palatable diet and to avoid the psychological tension associated with severe fluid restriction. Patients with oligoanuria may respond poorly to diuretics and may require strict fluid restriction for control of edema and hypervolemia. In such patients, hyperkalemia should be anticipated and treated with dietary potassium restriction, binding resins, or dialysis as needed.

Patients with evidence of ongoing throat or skin infection should receive a course of appropriate antistreptococcal antibiotics. This therapy in no way influences the course or prognosis of the nephritis. Bed rest has no therapeutic advantage but should be allowed as needed by the child. Dietary limitations of sodium, potassium, and fluid usually are necessary for the hospitalized child but are liberalized for the patient at discharge, when the peak of the disease has passed. Those who require maintenance antihypertensive therapy should continue dietary sodium restriction at home.

Prognosis

Overall, the prognosis of APSGN is excellent, with full recovery expected in more than 98% of affected children. The resolution must be documented at follow-up office visits over time. Most children spend no more than 5 days in the hospital, but the disease resolves fairly slowly over the course of many months. Few children develop chronic renal failure. Usually, hypertension and gross hematuria resolve within 3 weeks. Gross hematuria may recur at the time of future intercurrent infections during the recovery phase, but the reappearance holds no prognostic significance. Microscopic hematuria persists for many months and has been documented for as long as 3 years in a few patients. Proteinuria resolves within a few months; its persistence after 6 months should raise concern regarding the possibility of an incorrect diagnosis. The serum C3 concentration must be measured again 8 to 12 weeks after the acute episode occurs. Failure of C3 to increase into the normal range during this period, especially with persistent symptoms of hypertension, gross hematuria, or heavy proteinuria, strongly suggests the diagnosis of MPGN, and a renal biopsy should be performed for the appropriate diagnosis.

Immunoglobulin A Nephropathy

IgA nephropathy is the most common primary GN worldwide. It is characterized histologically by the presence of mesangial IgA deposits and clinically by chronic hematuria and normal renal function early in the course. Once considered a benign disease, IgA nephropathy now is known to progress to chronic renal failure in adulthood in as many as 40% of patients.

Clinical Features

IgA nephropathy may present at any age, but it most commonly occurs clinically in patients between the ages of 10 through 30 years. The prevalence is higher in boys, especially in North America and Europe. The disease occurs more frequently in Asians, whites, Native Americans in the southwestern United States, and Australian aborigines than in blacks in the United States and South Africa. Hematuria is the most common initial sign. Hematuria is microscopic in 100% and macroscopic in 85% of the children with biopsy-proven IgA nephropathy. Hematuria may occur for years without progression of disease. Gross hematuria often is episodic, usually in association with a febrile illness, most commonly of the upper respiratory tract. Proteinuria unrelated to gross hematuria occurs in approximately 40% to 50% of affected children, and it reaches the nephrotic range in some. Patients with moderate to severe proteinuria are at greater risk of developing renal insufficiency. Isolated proteinuria is not a sign of IgA nephropathy in children. Hypertension occurs in only approximately 10%; usually, its occurrence coincides with the development of chronic renal failure. Approximately 20% of patients experience a mild decrease in GFR during episodic gross hematuria. Complaints of fever, malaise, and loin or abdominal pain also are common findings at that time. Usually, renal function returns to normal after an acute episode.

Laboratory Features

A renal biopsy is necessary to confirm the diagnosis of IgA nephropathy. No other laboratory studies are specific. Serum

IgA levels are elevated in 50% to 70% of affected patients but appear to bear no relation to the severity or the activity of the disease. Serum IgG, IgM, and C3 concentrations seldom are abnormal.

Pathology

Immunofluorescence microscopy of a renal biopsy of a patient with IgA nephropathy characteristically shows dominant IgA or IgA codominant with IgG deposition in the mesangium. Light microscopy shows focal or diffuse mesangial cell proliferation and expansion of mesangial matrix. The renal lesion in HSP nephritis looks exactly the same and is distinguished from IgA nephropathy only by clinical symptoms. IgA may be found in the glomeruli in several other nephropathies, including systemic lupus erythematosus (SLE) or chronic liver disease, but it may be neither the dominant immune reactant nor confined to the mesangium. Often, IgM, C3, and properdin accompany IgA in the same pattern as the IgA distribution but with much less intensity. Electron microscopy confirms the presence of electron-dense deposits in the mesangium and rarely in adjacent subepithelial or intramembranous spaces of the GBM.

Although immunofluorescence defines the glomerulopathy, light microscopy predicts the prognosis. Biopsies have been classified into three groups according to the severity of glomerular proliferative changes. Approximately one-fourth of the biopsies show histologically normal glomeruli, with little or no interstitial disease. The other three-fourths are divided approximately evenly between those showing mesangial hypercellularity and those showing mesangial hypercellularity plus focal and segmental areas of necrosis, synechiae, crescent formation, or collapse of the glomerular capillary wall and sclerosis.

Pathogenesis

The pathogenesis of IgA nephropathy remains uncertain after 3 decades of investigation. The serum IgA immune response of patients with IgA nephropathy is increased in both antigen-specific and nonspecific assays. Systemic IgA may play a role in the pathogenesis of the disease. Lines of evidence to support this supposition include the presence of IgA in the mesangium, the recurrence of IgA nephropathy in renal allografts, and the observations that serum IgA concentrations are increased in some patients and that IgA-containing circulating immune complexes are found in nearly one-half the patients. The predominant form of IgA found in renal biopsies from affected patients is polymeric IgA1, reflecting the increased serum concentration of polymeric IgA1. Serum IgA1 has been found to have abnormal O-glycosylation in patients with IgA nephropathy and HSP nephritis but not in patients with other glomerulonephritides. A combination of polyclonal stimulation of IgA plus structural abnormalities of IgA may lead to mesangial deposition of IgA1 and glomerular injury, but has never been proven. Secretory IgA (IgA2) does not appear to play a major role in the immunogenesis of IgA nephropathy.

A genetic predisposition of some patients to IgA nephropathy is suggested by the association of human leukocyte antigen (HLA) types BW35, B27, DR1, and DR4 with IgA nephropathy and by the occurrence of the disease in multiple members of the same family and in HLA-identical twins.

Differential Diagnosis

Microscopic hematuria with or without mild proteinuria between episodes of gross hematuria also occurs in hereditary nephritis (Alport syndrome), in benign hematuria, in idiopathic hypercalciuria, occasionally in MPGN, and rarely in MGN. Hereditary nephritis can be distinguished from IgA nephropathy clinically by discovery of a positive family history or associated deafness. Usually, MPGN is associated with a decreased serum C3 level and heavier proteinuria, whereas MGN presents as NS with normal complement levels and microscopic or less often gross hematuria. Benign hematuria occurs without proteinuria or other signs or symptoms of renal disease. Proteinuria is absent in idiopathic hypercalciuria, which can be diagnosed by the presence of abnormally high calcium excretion in a 24-hour urine collection.

IgA nephropathy is easy to confuse with APSGN, especially if the initial presentation consists of an episode of gross hematuria and mild systemic complaints. Unlike patients with APSGN, patients with IgA nephropathy have no latent period between the development of infection and the onset of hematuria, and the serum C3 concentration is normal. Gross hematuria persists for only a few days in patients with IgA nephropathy and usually resolves when the fever remits.

Distinguishing the nephritis of HSP from IgA nephropathy is even more difficult. If the HSP rash is transient and is not obviously purpuric, and if the extrarenal manifestations of HSP are mild, the clinical syndrome is identical to IgA nephropathy. Furthermore, the renal biopsy findings of HSP nephritis are virtually identical to those of IgA nephropathy. These similarities have led some investigators to speculate that IgA nephropathy is a monosymptomatic form of HSP.

Therapy

No specific therapy is available for IgA nephropathy. The potential for progression to chronic renal failure and end-stage renal disease led to many uncontrolled trials of prednisone, cytotoxic drugs, platelet inhibitors, angiotensin-converting enzyme inhibitors, antioxidants, plasma exchange, and combination therapies. These studies were conducted mostly with patients who exhibited severe symptoms and signs of progressive disease, which may have been too late in the course of the disease to prove these therapies efficacious. Prednisone therapy has been shown to improve urinary findings and histopathologic lesions in subsequent renal biopsies in some children but not in others. In adult patients, daily fish oil supplementation for 2 years retarded the progression of renal failure in one controlled trial but not in others. No children were studied. A few multicenter randomized, controlled therapeutic trials for prednisone, fish oil, vitamin E, mycophenolate mofetil, and other therapeutic agents have been completed or are in progress, but they have shown no efficacy of any specific agent to date. More well-designed trials are needed before any guidelines for therapy of IgA nephropathy can be developed. In the meantime, attention should be paid to controlling hypertension and proteinuria to prevent progression of the disease. Angiotensin-converting enzyme inhibitors are the drugs of choice because of their antihypertensive and additional antiproteinuric effects.

Prognosis

Most children with IgA nephropathy have either a very slowly progressive or a completely benign course until adulthood; however, 5% to 10% of children develop end-stage renal disease in childhood or adolescence. IgA nephropathy recurs in a renal transplant at least 35% of the time but is slowly progressive and has not changed the 10-year renal transplant survival in these patients compared with other patients with end-stage renal disease. Predictors of poor prognosis in children are heavy proteinuria and the NS, hypertension, and the presence in the renal biopsy of glomerular proliferative lesions with crescents, sclerosis, or GBM alterations.

Henoch-Schönlein Purpura Nephritis

Henoch-Schönlein Purpura (HSP) is a systemic vasculitis that typically affects children and presents as a combination of purpuric rash, crampy abdominal pain, bloody diarrhea, and joint pain. Signs and symptoms of nephritis may not appear until days or several weeks into the course of the disease. Because of the unproven assumption in the past that these children are allergic to drugs, food, microorganisms, or some other unidentified antigens, the term *anaphylactoid purpura* has been applied to this disease. Although children with HSP do not appear to be more allergic than other children, the term has persisted.

HSP probably is mediated by IgA, which can be identified by immunofluorescence staining of renal and skin biopsies from affected patients. The renal lesion is identical to that seen in IgA nephropathy, a finding that raises the question whether IgA nephropathy and HSP may be within a spectrum of the same disease.

Clinical Features

Most affected children are boys between ages 3 and 10 years. Two-thirds of patients report the onset of an upper respiratory tract infection 1 to 3 weeks before the onset of purpura. The incidence of HSP is seasonal, with its peak in winter.

Usually, the disease begins with an acute erythematous macular rash, most often on the ankles and spreading to the dorsum of the legs, the buttocks, and occasionally the ulnar surfaces of the arms. The trunk is spared. Within a day, the lesions become purpuric and may coalesce. The skin lesions disappear in approximately 2 weeks, although in some children, the rash comes and goes over a period of days to weeks. Many patients with the rash experience edema of the scalp, face, and dorsum of the hands and feet. Joint pain with or without edema occurs in 60% to 75% of cases. Colicky abdominal pain with melena or bloody diarrhea occurs in one-half of affected children and mimics other gastrointestinal diseases. The incidence of abdominal pain is highest (90%) in children with HSP nephritis. Severe vasculitis of the bowel may result in gastrointestinal hemorrhage, perforation, or intussusception.

The renal manifestations of HSP are clinically mild and often silent. If the urine is examined over the duration of the disease, abnormalities will be found in almost every case. The spectrum of renal disease in HSP is broad, ranging from asymptomatic hematuria and proteinuria to full-blown acute nephritic syndrome with the NS. Hypertension is an uncommon finding.

Laboratory Features

No laboratory test is diagnostic of HSP. Leukocytosis occurs early in the course. Hemoglobin, hematocrit, and the peripheral blood smear are normal, as are the platelet count, bleeding time, and coagulation studies. The erythrocyte sedimentation rate may be elevated. Microscopic hematuria, red blood cell casts, and proteinuria are present in the urinalysis. Gross hematuria may be seen in 20% to 30% of cases. Azotemia occurs in as many as 20% of cases but usually is transient. Uremia requiring acute dialysis for a short time is very rare.

Serum IgA concentration is elevated in 50% of children with HSP. Often, the elevation occurs during the acute phase only, with levels returning to normal as symptoms resolve. Serum C3 concentration is normal, but breakdown products of complement are increased in the serum, a finding indicating complement activation, presumably by circulating immune complexes or cryoglobulins, which have been identified in many patients.

Pathology

If the clinical signs and symptoms of HSP are atypical, the diagnosis can be confirmed by microscopic examination of skin and renal biopsy specimens. Typically, skin lesions show leukocytoclastic vasculitis, characterized by transmural and perivascular infiltration with polymorphonuclear leukocytes, histiocytes, and sometimes eosinophils. The renal lesion is identical to that seen in IgA nephropathy (see foregoing) and ranges from no identifiable abnormalities by light microscopy to mesangial proliferation, focal and segmental proliferative lesions, and diffuse proliferative lesions with or without crescents. Brightly staining deposits of IgA always are found in the mesangium by immunofluorescence. Electron microscopic examination shows dense deposits in the same location.

Pathogenesis

The pathogenesis of HSP may involve a primary immune defect of IgA activity. The systemic nature of HSP, the appearance of IgA in extrarenal blood vessels, and the presence of IgA-containing circulating immune complexes in the serum of most patients suggest this possibility. An immune response has been assumed to be triggered by the presentation of offending antigen to the surface of either the respiratory or the gastrointestinal tract, which then leads to the production of IgA antibodies that may form immune complexes in the blood. Then the complexes make their way to various sites, including the kidney, where an inflammatory response ensues. For years, antigenic stimuli for the IgA response have been sought intensively, but specific relationships never have been substantiated, although many allergens have been implicated.

Differential Diagnosis

The purpuric nature and distribution of the skin lesions of HSP can be fairly characteristic. If the rash is atypical in distribution, other causes of purpura, such as leukemia, septicemia, hemolytic-uremic syndrome, SLE, and idiopathic thrombocytopenic purpura, must be considered. The abdominal symptoms mimic those of many infectious and inflammatory bowel diseases. HSP may cause an acute surgical emergency secondary to bowel perforation or intussusception. Pancreatitis is an uncommon development. Vasculitis of the testis may resemble torsion of the testis, orchitis, or incarcerated hernia. Distinguishing joint symptoms from those seen in rheumatoid arthritis, SLE, and acute rheumatic fever is difficult. The renal manifestations of HSP may appear identical to those seen in APSGN, bacterial endocarditis, SLE, polyarteritis, and MPGN.

Clinical Course and Therapy

The clinical course varies from very mild to severe. Most patients have several bouts of rash and abdominal pain during the first month of disease. Recurrences over the course of a longer period may be associated with a poorer prognosis. The main determinant of the overall prognosis is the persistence and severity of the renal disease. Children with minor urinary abnormalities have an excellent prognosis for complete recovery, whereas those who present with severe crescentic nephritis with acute renal failure or the NS are most likely to develop chronic renal failure and even end-stage renal disease. Patients who have renal disease should have long-term follow-up until the urinalysis is normal for several years. Those showing persistent urinary abnormalities or evidence of progressive renal failure should be seen by a pediatric nephrologist.

No drug therapy has been shown to be effective for severe HSP nephritis. Therapy usually is limited to supportive measures, when nephritis is mild or moderate. Careful monitoring to detect serious abdominal complications is of paramount importance in patients with abdominal pain. When abdominal pain is severe and incapacitating even after administration of analgesics, corticosteroids may provide relief. The use of analgesics and steroids is not without risk because they may mask symptoms of gastrointestinal perforation. No evidence corroborates that corticosteroids have any beneficial effect on the clinical course of the renal disease.

Lupus Nephritis

The full spectrum of disease caused by SLE is described in Chapter 434. Only the renal and urinary tract manifestations are described here under the name *lupus nephritis*.

Clinical and Laboratory Features

Like the extrarenal manifestations of SLE, lupus nephritis presents in various ways with varying levels of intensity. Rarely, patients with known SLE may have no symptoms of renal disease and a completely normal urinalysis but show an active renal lesion by renal biopsy. Some patients have only renal disease without extrarenal signs of SLE initially but later fulfill the diagnostic criteria for SLE.

Although SLE is more often a disease of young women (8:1 female-to-male ratio), 20% to 25% of cases are diagnosed in the first 2 decades of life, rarely even in infants. Nephritis occurs more commonly in childhood lupus and affects as many as 80% of patients. All World Health Organization (WHO) classes of nephritis occur in childhood (Table 325.1).

The laboratory diagnosis of SLE is reviewed in detail in Chapter 434. Usually, the serum C3 and C4 concentrations are severely decreased. Antinuclear antibody and antidouble-stranded DNA antibody titers are elevated at the time of diagnosis in 95% of patients with nephritis. Urinary abnormalities include hematuria, proteinuria, and casts (red cell, white cell, hyaline, or broad-waxy). Proteinuria may be mild or moderate or in the nephrotic range. Heavy proteinuria is associated with more severe disease. One-half of children with SLE nephritis have reduced renal function as noted by either an elevated serum creatinine level or decreased creatinine clearance.

Renal tubular disorders (e.g., type IV renal tubular acidosis or glucosuria) may occur, especially in patients with evidence of tubulointerstitial disease by renal biopsy. Ureteral vasculitis and noninfectious cystitis have been described and may be responsible for obstructive uropathy and lower urinary tract symptoms, respectively.

Pathology and Clinicopathologic Correlations

Over the years, several classifications of lupus nephritis have been proposed, but the most widely accepted today is that of the WHO (see Table 325.1). This classification is a useful investigational tool, but because not every biopsy fits neatly into one of the classes, the use of the WHO classification for predicting the prognosis for an individual patient is not as helpful. Serial biopsies often show transformation between classes during therapy and are useful to guide further therapy.

Biopsies from only approximately 5% of the patients show normal kidneys (class I). Minimal amounts of electron-dense deposits and immunofluorescent IgG and complement found exclusively in the mesangium are allowed in this class. Urinary abnormalities and renal failure hardly ever occur in this group of patients.

Mesangial proliferative lupus GN (class II) accounts for 20% of biopsies. Varying degrees of mesangial hypercellularity and mesangial deposition of IgG or IgM and C1q, C4, C3, and properdin are found in these biopsies. Clinically, urinalysis shows only mild asymptomatic hematuria or proteinuria in patients with class II disease.

Renal biopsies from patients with focal and segmental proliferative lupus GN (class III) are characterized by the finding

TABLE 325.1

WORLD HEALTH ORGANIZATION CLASSIFICATION OF SYSTEMIC LUPUS ERYTHEMATOSUS NEPHRITIS

Class	Histopathology	Description
Class I	Normal kidneys	Slight or no detectable changes by LM, EM, or IF
Class II	Mesangial changes	
IIA	Minimal alteration	Normal LM, mesangial deposits of immunoglobulin and complement by IF, mesangial deposits by EM
IIB	Mesangial glomerulitis	Same as IIA but also mesangial hypercellularity (>3 cells per mesangial area away from vascular pole in 2- to 4-μm sections) or increased mesangial matrix; minimal tubular or interstitial changes
Class III	Focal and segmental proliferative glomerulonephritis	In addition to any finding in class II, <50% of glomeruli involved with focal areas of intracapillary and extracapillary cell proliferation, necrosis, karyorrhexis, and leukocytic infiltration. EM and IF can show subendothelial and mesangial deposits. Tubular and interstitial changes usually are focal.
Class IV	Diffuse proliferative glomerulonephritis	Similar to class III but involving more glomerular surface area and >50% of the glomeruli. IF and EM often show abundant subendothelial deposits. Interstitial involvement is more marked. Membranoproliferative variant has prominent mesangial cell proliferation and capillary wall thickening by mesangial extensions.
Class V	Membranous glomerulonephritis	No mesangial, endothelial, or epithelial cell proliferation; capillary walls diffusely and uniformly thickened. IF and EM show mesangial and subepithelial deposits. Minimal interstitial involvement is seen, such as class II.
Class VI	Advanced sclerosing glomerulonephritis	>90% of glomeruli globally sclerosed

EM, electron microscopy; IF, immunofluorescence; LM, light microscopy.

of additional deposits of C1q, C4, C3, and properdin in the capillary walls but have fewer than 50% of glomeruli involved by the disease process. This lesion is similar to that found in severe IgA nephropathy and HSP nephritis. Hematuria and proteinuria are present in most patients, but the NS and renal failure are uncommon. Approximately 25% of biopsies are class III.

Diffuse proliferative GN (class IV) is found in 40% of biopsies. The pathologic features are similar to those of class III, but more than 50% of glomeruli are affected, rendering the lesion more severe and diffuse. Electron microscopic and immunofluorescence studies show heavy deposits of all immunoglobulins and complement, especially in the subendothelial space of the capillary wall. When these deposits are circumferential, the capillary loop has a "wire loop" appearance. Mesangial and epimembranous deposits are numerous. Crescent formation varies but may be severe, and it correlates clinically with the presence of RPGN. In class IV nephritis, hematuria and proteinuria almost always are present. Most patients who have the NS and/or renal failure also fall into this category. Class IV lupus nephritis is associated with progressive uremia and high mortality, if it is not aggressively treated with cytotoxic drugs such as cyclophosphamide as well as prednisone.

Membranous lupus GN (class V) accounts for 10% of renal biopsies, but in recent years the incidence appears to be increasing among pediatric patients. This lesion is characterized by subepithelial deposits of IgG and C3 in the GBM as well as mesangial hypercellularity and mesangial and subendothelial immune deposits. Membranous lupus nephritis may precede the extrarenal manifestations of SLE by years and may be diagnosed initially as idiopathic MGN.

A few patients have predominantly severe sclerosis (class VI), tubulointerstitial disease, or vascular disease. Tubulointerstitial disease often accompanies glomerular involvement in class III and IV nephritis but rarely occurs alone. When alone, interstitial inflammatory infiltrates are focal and are associated with interstitial fibrosis and tubular atrophy. Vasculitis involving the larger blood vessels of the kidney sometimes leads to vascular necrosis, hypertension, and renal failure.

Therapy and Prognosis

Although the beneficial effect of corticosteroid therapy for the extrarenal manifestations of SLE is well accepted, no controlled trial of this therapy for lupus nephritis in children has been performed. Long-term controlled studies of adults with various WHO classes of disease have demonstrated that a combination of prednisone and a cytotoxic drug, such as cyclophosphamide, results in better control of class IV lupus GN with fewer sclerotic lesions on follow-up renal biopsy and less progression to end-stage renal disease, as compared with patients receiving prednisone alone. Results suggest that intermittent-bolus intravenous cyclophosphamide in combination with corticosteroids is associated with the fewest side effects in adults. The optimal frequency and duration of cyclophosphamide pulse therapy have not been determined, but a regimen of at least monthly treatment for 6 to 9 months and quarterly treatment for a variable time thereafter has been clinically effective in many children. The well-known oncogenic potential of cyclophosphamide and its gonadal toxicity render it a drug for use in only the most serious forms of lupus nephritis (i.e., class IV and severe class III).

Overall, survival of children with SLE is good, with more than 80% alive at 10 years and 65% surviving 15 years after diagnosis. Most deaths are caused by infection or neurologic complications of lupus. With early aggressive therapy of class IV lupus nephritis, progression to end-stage renal disease seldom occurs.

Nephritis of Chronic Bacteremia

Immune complex–mediated proliferative GN may occur in the course of acute and subacute bacterial endocarditis, chronically infected ventriculoatrial shunts, and osteomyelitis. All these conditions have in common the presence of chronic bacteremia, usually with coagulase-positive or coagulase-negative staphylococci or streptococci. Rarely, patients with visceral abscesses (pulmonary, sinus, intraabdominal), with and without documented bacteremia, may present with a similar picture. Bacterial pathogens causing bacteremia in these patients usually are coagulase-positive staphylococci, but occasionally they are gram-negative organisms.

Clinical and Laboratory Features

The diagnosis should be suspected in patients who have a source of chronic bacteremia and who develop hematuria and proteinuria or red blood cell casts. Hydrocephalic children with "shunt nephritis" from chronically infected ventriculoatrial shunts have the NS at presentation in 30% to 50% of cases. Blood cultures are the best sources for identification of the inciting organism. Most patients have decreased serum C3 concentrations, positive rheumatoid factor, and the presence of circulating cryoglobulins and immune complexes. The serum levels of other components of complement (C4 and C1q) may be depressed. Acute renal failure with oliguria occurs, especially in patients with bacterial endocarditis or a visceral abscess that is occult for a long time before the diagnosis is established. The incidence of acute renal failure is high in intravenous drug abusers, who often present late for treatment and who may be infected with resistant organisms or have right-sided heart valvular disease with initially negative blood cultures.

Pathology and Pathogenesis

The renal lesion in affected patients is mesangial proliferation or mesangiocapillary proliferation, similar to type I MPGN. The lesion may be focal or diffuse and is more severe when the underlying illness is unsuspected and goes untreated for some duration. Affected patients may develop chronic pathologic changes, with focal or diffuse scarring of the glomeruli. Extensive crescent formation and the clinical course of RPGN occur rarely. Immunofluorescence staining shows granular deposits of IgG, IgM, and C3 in the mesangium and capillary loop. Soluble antigens of the infecting organism, with and without their specific antibodies, have been demonstrated in glomeruli, a finding suggesting a direct role for immune complexes in the pathogenesis of this lesion, either by deposition of circulating immune complexes or by antigen-induced *in situ* immune complex formation.

Prognosis and Therapy

Specific antibiotic therapy for the underlying infection results in resolution or inactivation of the GN over the course of a few weeks. In some cases, GN persists for years after apparent eradication of the infection has been achieved. As part of therapy, infected ventriculoatrial shunts should be removed and replaced later. Visceral abscesses should be drained surgically. If an infection is treated ineffectively, the GN may progress to chronic renal failure and end-stage renal disease, but this result rarely occurs with currently available antibiotic therapy.

RAPIDLY PROGRESSIVE GLOMERULONEPHRITIS

RPGN is the designation given to the group of glomerular diseases with rapid deterioration in renal function to uremia and

---

BOX 325.2   **Disorders Associated with Rapidly Progressive Glomerulonephritis and Usually Glomerular Crescent Formation**

Primary Renal Disorders
Immunoglobulin A nephropathy
Membranoproliferative glomerulonephritis type I and
    type II
Membranous glomerulonephritis
Alport syndrome (hereditary nephritis)
Idiopathic
    Type I (anti-GBM disease without pulmonary
        hemorrhage)
    Type II (immune complex disease)
    Type III (no immune complexes, ANCA-associated)

Disorders Associated with Infection
Poststreptococcal glomerulonephritis
Bacterial endocarditis
Hepatitis B

Other infection (pulmonary, sinus, or intraabdominal
    abscess)

Disorders Associated with Systemic Disease
Systemic lupus erythematosus
Henoch-Schönlein syndrome (anaphylactoid purpura)
ANCA vasculitis
Wegener granulomatosis
Pauciimmune polyarteritis nodosa (ANCA-positive)
Goodpasture syndrome (anti-GBM disease with
    pulmonary hemorrhage)
Mixed cryoglobulinemia
Neoplasm (lymphoma, carcinoma)

ANCA, antineutrophil cytoplasmic antibody; GBM, glomerular basement membrane.

---

often end-stage renal disease occurring within a few days to weeks of onset (Box 325.2). The term *RPGN* has been used to describe both the clinical course and the pathologic lesion of diffuse glomerular extracapillary crescent formation common to the disorders that cause clinical RPGN. The terms *crescentic GN* and *extracapillary proliferative GN* are used by many physicians to describe the pathologic lesion to avoid confusion between the clinical and pathologic aspects of the disease. Other pathologic lesions, such as the necrotizing GN of Wegener granulomatosis, also result in clinical RPGN. The term *RPGN* in this section includes all forms of clinical RPGN. The discussion of pathology and pathogenesis will focus only on crescent formation, the most common histopathologic lesion associated with clinical forms of RPGN.

Clinical and Laboratory Features

RPGN, either idiopathic or associated with any of the disorders listed in Box 325.2, occurs rarely. It affects adolescents more often than young children and adults more often than adolescents. Usually, RPGN presents with symptoms of acute GN, often gross hematuria, edema, hypertension, and oliguria or anuria. Most patients have severe anemia, out of proportion to their degree of azotemia or the apparent duration of their symptoms. Other symptoms may be those of the associated disorder, such as the purpuric rash of HSP or hemoptysis from the pulmonary hemorrhage associated with Goodpasture syndrome or Wegener granulomatosis. Goodpasture syndrome includes the triad of nephritis (usually RPGN), pulmonary hemorrhage, and anti-GBM antibody formation demonstrable in the circulation or in renal or lung tissue. Wegener granulomatosis is a systemic necrotizing vasculitis that involves the kidney, nasal mucosa, tracheobronchial tree, and lungs. Vasculitic skin lesions, sinusitis, serous otitis media, epistaxis, saddle-nose deformity, cough, eye lesions, and cardiac and neurologic symptoms may be present.

The antineutrophil cytoplasmic antibody (ANCA), with either cytoplasmic staining (C-ANCA) or perinuclear or nuclear staining (P-ANCA), is an important serologic marker for differentiating the underlying disease and assessing the activity of many forms of clinical RPGN. When ANCA is positive in the serum, the glomerular lesion always is pauciimmune necrotizing and crescentic GN. Ninety percent of patients with untreated active Wegener granulomatosis are C-ANCA positive,

and 80% of patients with pauciimmune polyarteritis nodosa are either C-ANCA or P-ANCA positive, whereas patients with immune complex-mediated polyarteritis are ANCA negative. Usually, patients with the pauciimmune subtype of idiopathic RPGN (type III) are P-ANCA positive. ANCA vasculitis occurs when other systemic symptoms of vasculitis are present along with ANCA-positive pauciimmune RPGN.

Pathology and Pathogenesis

Glomerular crescents are thought to derive from proliferation and epithelioid transformation of bloodborne macrophages that migrate from the glomerular capillary into the urinary space through breaks or "gaps" in an injured GBM. Leakage of fibrinogen and other intravascular contents through the pathologic gaps leads to fibrin polymerization, which probably acts as a nidus for the crescent formation. The increasing size of the proliferating crescent compresses the functional glomerulus to a smaller and smaller mass. Eventually, fibroblasts from the renal interstitium may migrate into the crescent and may convert the crescent into a sclerotic or fibrous scar. Predominance of fibrous crescents, global glomerular sclerosis, interstitial fibrosis, and tubular atrophy in a renal biopsy specimen portend a poor clinical prognosis. Unpredictably, some cellular crescents may resolve without sclerosis and permanent injury. The latter outcome occurs more commonly in RPGN associated with infectious disorders, such as poststreptococcal GN.

Multiple diseases can lead to severe GBM injury, with gaps and subsequent development of crescents and RPGN (see Box 325.2). Most of these disorders are discussed in detail elsewhere in this chapter.

When no other primary glomerular disease can be diagnosed and when crescents can be identified in 50% or more of the glomeruli sampled by a renal biopsy, the disorder is called *idiopathic RPGN*. Subtypes of idiopathic RPGN are classified according to the origin of the GBM injury. In type I, antibody to GBM antigen (anti-GBM) is formed secondary to an unknown stimulus and results in linear deposition of IgG along the GBM, readily identifiable by characteristic immunofluorescent staining of a renal biopsy. The glomerular endothelial cells show little if any proliferation. Most affected patients have measurable circulating anti-GBM antibody, although in some it is not detectable until after they have undergone nephrectomy.

In type II, circulating immune complexes of unknown origin are deposited in the mesangium and subendothelial portions of the GBM. These deposits are recognized by a granular pattern of IgG or IgM by immunofluorescence staining and as electron-dense deposits by electron microscopic examination of a renal biopsy. The circulating immune complexes may be measurable. Serum C3 may be decreased if it also is present in the deposits. Type III (pauciimmune) is characterized by sparsity or absence of any immune deposits, either linear or granular, in the glomeruli. Usually, the renal biopsy has features of necrotizing GN similar to those of Wegener granulomatosis or polyarteritis nodosa, a finding suggesting that type III may not be a distinct idiopathic RPGN subtype but a variant of a systemic necrotizing vasculitis limited to the kidney. In addition, because 80% of patients with type III RPGN are ANCA-positive, ANCA may participate directly in the pathogenesis of the glomerular lesion by activating neutrophils and macrophages within glomerular capillaries, resulting in necrotizing inflammatory injury and subsequent crescent formation.

Therapy

Therapy for RPGN has been aimed at stopping glomerular injury to prevent progression of crescent formation. RPGN is considered a medical emergency by nephrologists because therapy must be started as early as possible if it is to be of value. Pulse intravenous steroids may be started expectantly before diagnostic renal biopsy results are available, then discontinued within a day or so if the biopsy is not confirmative, so as not to miss the therapeutic window for treating RPGN. Because RPGN is a rare event and is associated with many disorders of diverse origin, no good, large, controlled therapeutic trials have been or ever may be performed to document the efficacy of a given drug regimen. However, high-dose steroids alone or in combination with cytotoxic agents, such as cyclophosphamide, have proved effective in improving renal function and in reducing dependence on dialysis in uncontrolled studies of adults and some children. Plasmapheresis in combination with high-dose steroids and cytotoxic agents is recommended for severely affected adults and also appears to be advantageous in the treatment of pediatric patients with anti-GBM disorders or vasculitis (ANCA, Wegener granulomatosis, or lupus), especially in the presence of pulmonary hemorrhage. Children with RPGN associated with poststreptococcal GN may need only supportive care because they often improve with or without drug therapy.

Prognosis

Duration of hospitalization may be prolonged for children with RPGN. Most of these children require dialysis and have severe complications, such as pulmonary hemorrhage or hypertension. Approximately one-half the children with crescentic GN and clinical RPGN progress to end-stage renal disease and require long-term dialysis or a renal transplant. The recurrence rate of RPGN in the transplanted kidney is 10% to 30%, depending on the underlying disorder, so renal transplantation usually is delayed for at least 1 year of dialysis therapy to allow the disease to become quiescent.

NEPHROTIC SYNDROME

The NS is a clinical condition resulting from the loss of large amounts of protein in the urine sufficient to cause hypoproteinemia and edema, if the serum albumin is less than 2.5 g/dL. Hyperlipidemia and lipiduria are part of the fully expressed NS.

The NS may be primary and a feature of any form of childhood GN or may be secondary to other systemic diseases, malignancies, allergic reactions, or injury from nephrotoxins (Box 325.3). The discussion in this section concentrates on primary NS, specifically those histopathologic types of GN that occur in children, whose clinical presentation is the NS itself and not the

---

BOX 325.3   Causes of the Nephrotic Syndrome

Primary Nephrotic Syndrome
Minimal-change disease
Diffuse mesangial proliferative glomerulonephritis
Focal segmental glomerulosclerosis
Membranoproliferative glomerulonephritis
Membranous glomerulonephritis

Secondary Nephrotic Syndrome
Other renal diseases
    Hemolytic-uremic syndrome, anti-GBM disease,
        immunoglobulin A nephropathy, idiopathic RPGN,
        diffuse mesangial sclerosis
Infectious diseases
    Bacterial (poststreptococcal, infective endocarditis,
        shunt nephritis, leprosy, syphilis), viral (hepatitis B,
        cytomegalovirus, Epstein-Barr, varicella, human
        immunodeficiency virus), protozoal (malaria,
        toxoplasmosis), parasitic (schistosomiasis,
        filariasis)
Neoplasia
    Lymphoma, leukemia, Wilms tumor,
        pheochromocytoma, others

Medications
    Mercurials, gold, penicillamine, trimethadione,
        mephenytoin
Systemic diseases
    Systemic lupus erythematosus, Henoch-Schönlein
        purpura, polyarteritis nodosa, Takayasu syndrome,
        dermatitis herpetiformis, sarcoidosis, Sjögren
        syndrome, amyloidosis, diabetes mellitus
Allergic reactions
    Insect stings, poison oak and ivy, serum sickness
Familial disorders
    Alport syndrome, Fabry disease, nail-patella
        syndrome, sickle cell disease, congenital nephrotic
        syndrome of the Finnish type
Circulatory disorders
    Constrictive pericarditis, congestive heart failure,
        renal vein thrombosis
Miscellaneous
    Chronic renal allograft rejection, preeclampsia,
        malignant hypertension

GBM, glomerular basement membrane; RPGN, rapidly progressive glomerulonephritis.

nephritic syndrome. Various names, including *lipoid nephrosis*, *idiopathic NS of childhood*, *childhood nephrosis*, *nil lesion syndrome*, and *foot process disease*, have been used historically to identify this condition, but none provides insight into the nature of the underlying pathogenesis. In this chapter, we have chosen to use the term *primary NS* instead of idiopathic NS or any of the other names to avoid confusion between clinical NS and the variety of pathologic entities associated with it. The specific disorders to be discussed are MCNS, diffuse mesangial proliferative GN, FSGS, MPGN, MGN, and the NS of infants.

Overview

The annual incidence of primary NS is approximately 2 to 4 cases per 100,000 children younger than 19 years old. These figures were determined in two major population studies: a 16-year survey in Erie County, New York, and a 17-year survey in Eastern Ontario, Canada. These and other studies show that in children younger than 10 years old, the most common diagnosis (65% to 80%) is MCNS, with most of these patients presenting between the ages of 2 and 6 years. MCNS is an uncommon finding in infants younger than age 1 year and accounts for only 30% of adolescent and 15% to 20% of adult cases of primary NS. The overall incidence of FSGS in pediatric patients ages 1 to 19 years has increased in the last decade and now approximates 15% to 25% of the cases of new-onset primary NS in childhood. The reason for this increase is uncertain, but it may be related to improvement in renal biopsy laboratory techniques, an increase in prevalence of childhood obesity, or genetic factors.

Because of the preponderance of MCNS in younger children, renal biopsy rarely is indicated for diagnosis in children younger than 10 years old, except in the presence of persistent hematuria, hypertension, renal failure, or failure to respond to at least a 4-week course of daily steroid therapy. Because older children are more likely to have underlying histopathologic types of GN other than MCNS, a diagnostic renal biopsy may need to be performed early in the disease course. The histopathologic type of GN, more than age at onset or any other feature of the NS, determines the clinical outcome and guides therapy. In cases of MCNS, the clinical course can be predicted most accurately by the response to the initial course of steroids and the frequency of early relapses.

Fewer than 5% of children with primary NS have affected siblings. Affected monozygotic (but not dizygotic) twins have been reported. Autosomal recessive congenital NS results from mutations in the nephrin gene (*NPHS1*). A rare, autosomal recessive form of FSGS is caused by mutations in the podocin gene (*NPHS2*). Both podocin and nephrin are important structural proteins of the glomerular podocyte slit diaphragm complex, which serves as the final barrier to loss of filtered protein into the urinary space. An autosomal dominant form of FSGS has been attributed to a mutation in the *ACTN4* gene, which encodes for the glomerular podocyte cytoskeletal protein alpha-actinin 4. Investigation of these rare forms of hereditary NS and the use of molecular genetics techniques, including high throughput genomic screening, are beginning to provide powerful new insights into the pathogenesis of all forms of primary NS in childhood. Associations of primary NS with specific HLA antigens, complement deficiencies, and atopy have been suggested but never substantiated, and their role in the pathogenesis of the NS is unlikely.

Structural Basis of Proteinuria

The GBM is composed of collagens, glycoproteins, and a variety of negatively charged glycosaminoglycans. Negative charge is enhanced by sialic acid residues on the visceral epithelial cells covering the GBM. The entire structure is an effective barrier to the passage of plasma proteins, which, for the most part, are too large and too negatively charged to cross into the urinary space. Using quantitative clearance studies of neutral, anionic, and cationic dextrans of differing molecular radii in normal humans, investigators have demonstrated that small molecules easily pass into the urine, large molecules are hindered, positively charged molecules pass by facilitated clearance, and negatively charged molecules are repelled and remain in the capillary blood.

Pathologic alterations of the glomerular barrier allow proteinuria to occur. Three types of alterations have been identified. The first is a loss of negative charge along the GBM and the epithelial cell surface, without obvious structural damage. Transmission electron microscopy using the tissue negative-staining method reveals small, round cavities and tunnels of uniform size and shape scattered throughout the GBM. This type of change occurs in MCNS and may be mediated by one or more soluble vascular permeability factors (VPFs) produced by lymphocytes that circulate in the plasma. A second type of change, commonly found in FSGS, is separation of the epithelial podocyte from the GBM. Genetic mutations in glomerular podocyte proteins, such as nephrin and podicin, may predispose some children to development of FSGS. The third type is the appearance of gaps in the GBM through which elements of blood, including cells, may pass. A combination of alterations occurs when immune proteins are deposited along the inner (subendothelial) or outer (subepithelial) aspect of the GBM, such as occurs in MPGN and MGN. Lesions that begin as negative-charge loss may progress to loss of structural integrity, activation of fibrosis and cell death, and eventually to sclerosis. Progressive sclerosis and subsequent loss of GFR may be sufficient to decrease protein excretion such that the NS appears to improve late in the course of the disease.

Clinical Consequences of Proteinuria

Many proteins appear in the urine of nephrotic patients, but albumin is found in greatest abundance. Albuminuria is the primary cause of hypoalbuminemia, the main determinant of reduced plasma colloid oncotic pressure in primary NS. Rapid reduction of oncotic pressure causes a shift of fluid from the intravascular compartment to the interstitial space, with consequent development of edema. In response to a rapid loss of vascular volume, the kidney increases its reabsorption of sodium and water and worsens the edema.

Historically, nephrotic patients were thought to reabsorb sodium avidly via the renin-angiotensin-aldosterone axis in response to decreased intravascular volume associated with low plasma oncotic pressure. Investigators have shown that nephrotic patients with stable, more chronic edema actually have increased or normal plasma volume and normal or suppressed levels of serum renin and aldosterone, a finding suggesting that retention of salt and water actually may be a primary renal disturbance, as in acute GN. Each explanation may be valid for patients with the NS, depending on their underlying renal disease, the stage of their disease at the time of study, and the rapidity of initial loss of protein.

Laboratory Features

Proteinuria is the hallmark of the NS. The urinalysis shows qualitatively large amounts of protein (2 to 4+ by dipstick), a high specific gravity, and hyaline and granular casts. To be classified as nephrotic-range proteinuria, the protein excretion rate should exceed 40 mg/m^2/hour in a 24-hour urine collection. In children, especially those who are not toilet trained or who have enuresis, obtaining reliable 24-hour urine collections is difficult. Alternative measurements, such as a random urine protein-to-creatinine ratio in excess of 2.0, may be substituted. A low serum albumin concentration, correlated with a series of strongly positive (2+ or more) dipstick tests for albumin in random urinalyses, may suffice.

Urinary protein selectivity (i.e., the relative clearance of albumin versus proteins of larger molecular weight) was useful to some clinicians for differential diagnosis in the past, but it rarely is used now that diagnostic renal biopsies are readily available. Patients with MCNS selectively excrete albumin; in contrast, patients with focal sclerosis or proliferative lesions excrete albumin and larger-molecular-weight proteins, such as IgG, equally. A comparison of albumin with IgG clearance can be calculated by the following formula:

$$\% \text{ Selectivity} = (U_{IgG})(P_{alb})/(P_{IgG})(U_{alb}) \times 100$$

where U_{IgG} and P_{IgG} = urine and plasma concentrations of IgG, and U_{alb} and P_{alb} = urine and plasma concentrations of albumin. Percentage selectivity less than 10% has been associated with a positive response to steroid therapy, and selectivity greater than 10% has been associated with a poor response. Neither is accurately predictive enough to justify the routine use of this test.

The massive proteinuria of the NS usually causes hypoalbuminemia, which becomes clinically significant when the serum albumin is 2.5 g/dL or less and edema occurs. Studies of hepatic albumin synthesis in patients with the NS have shown that an increase in albumin synthesis occurs but is insufficient to replace large ongoing albumin losses. The albumin synthesis rates in these patients, especially those with poor dietary protein intake, are considerably less than would be expected from the normal hepatic potential for increased albumin synthesis, which is approximately three times the baseline rate. Renal tubular catabolism of albumin also increases by three to five times the normal rate in patients with nephrotic diseases.

As with albumin, the concentration of other plasma proteins, such as coagulation inhibitors, thyroxine-binding globulin, and vitamin D–binding globulin (Box 325.4), are decreased because of increased urinary losses, decreased synthesis, or increased catabolism. Some plasma protein levels, including those of coagulation factors and lipoproteins, actually are increased in the NS. The increased levels probably result from increased and relatively unregulated hepatic production of protein in response to hypoalbuminemia. The clinical significance of these aberrations is discussed later (see the discussion of extrarenal complications and general management).

Serum cholesterol, triglycerides, and total lipids are elevated in most cases of primary NS of children. Serum concentrations of low-density lipoproteins, very-low-density lipoproteins, and apoproteins are increased, but high-density lipoproteins may be normal, increased, or reduced, depending on the severity of the proteinuria and the type of underlying renal lesion. Usually, total cholesterol levels are very elevated, exceeding 400 mg/dL in two-thirds of the children with MCNS. The degree of hypercholesterolemia is related inversely to the serum concentration of albumin. The serum concentration of triglycerides is more variable and may remain normal in some patients until the NS is fairly severe. The pathogenesis of hyperlipidemia is not understood completely. A marked increase in hepatic synthesis of lipoproteins and a reduction in catabolic removal occur in the NS. These abnormalities are correlated with the renal clearance of albumin, not the rate of albumin synthesis.

Lipids accumulate in renal tubular cells of nephrotic patients, especially in cells of the proximal renal tubule. Some of these lipid-laden renal tubular cells are sloughed into the urine and appear as "oval fat bodies" in the urinary sediment. When viewed with a polarizing microscope, the lipids are identified easily by their typical Maltese cross pattern.

Hematuria occurs in some children with primary NS. The presence of hematuria may be helpful in narrowing the differential diagnosis. Transient microscopic hematuria occurs in fewer than 25% of children with MCNS, and gross hematuria is rare. In children with other forms of primary NS, either gross hematuria or microscopic hematuria is present more than 50% of the time.

Renal function (GFR) measured by creatinine or inulin clearance is normal or increased in most patients with NS, although one-third of children with MCNS show transient depression of GFR at the onset of their disease, probably because of the rapid appearance of proteinuria and the rapid onset of hypovolemia with poor renal perfusion. If GFR remains low after the NS has been treated and improves clinically, an underlying diagnosis other than MCNS is likely, and the child should undergo further diagnostic evaluation, including renal biopsy. Renal tubular wasting of glucose, bicarbonate, amino acids, or phosphate, typical of partial or complete Fanconi syndrome, is an extremely uncommon finding and suggests the diagnosis of FSGS with renal tubular damage.

> **BOX 325.4**
>
> **Common Plasma Protein Concentration Derangements in Patients with the Nephrotic Syndrome**
>
> *Increased Levels*
> Alpha₂ globulins
> Beta globulins
> Coagulation factors
> Antifibrinolysins
> Most lipoproteins
>
> *Decreased Levels*
> Albumin
> Alpha₁ globulins
> Immunoglobulin G
> Coagulation inhibitors
> Transferrin
> Transcortin
> Thyroxine-binding globulin
> Vitamin D–binding globulin

Extrarenal Complications and General Management

Each protein abnormality of the NS causes specific clinical consequences. Hypoalbuminemia causes edema, which usually begins insidiously with unexpected weight gain and early morning periorbital swelling that shifts during the day to the lower legs and feet. In time, anasarca may occur, occasionally associated with an inability to open the eyes, respiratory distress from ascites pressing against the diaphagm or pleural effusions, and scrotal or labial edema that prevents walking. Therapy for severe edema includes intravenous or oral furosemide, alone or in combination with intravenous 25% albumin infusions or oral metolazone. These therapies should be used judiciously because they may produce profound electrolyte disturbances and cause hypovolemic shock or venous thromboses in patients already predisposed to these complications. Intravenous infusions of albumin should be reserved for children who experience severe hypovolemia with orthostatic hypotension, prerenal azotemia, or shock or for those with serum concentration of albumin less than 1.5 g/dL and severe and refractory edema.

Other potential adverse affects of hypoalbuminemia include enhanced platelet aggregability, increased stimulation of lipoprotein production, and enhanced drug toxicity caused by higher circulating free drug concentrations of drugs that normally are protein bound.

Protein-calorie malnutrition is a rare complication of chronic NS and is seen only in children with unremitting proteinuria. These children tend to eat poorly, thus preventing the compensatory production of protein that can occur in well-nourished nephrotic patients. Urinary losses of proteins other than albumin may lead to clinically significant problems in some patients with chronic, unremitting NS. Increased urinary losses of vitamin D-binding globulin and of the 25-hydroxyvitamin D bound to it may be a principal cause of the osteomalacia sometimes seen in these patients. Clinical hypothyroidism is a rare problem caused by loss of thyroid-binding proteins and free thyroxine, with resultant depression of serum total and free thyroxine and total triiodothyronine and a compensatory increase in serum thyroid-stimulating hormone.

Decreased serum concentrations of immunoproteins may be the basis of the predisposition of nephrotic patients to development of infection with encapsulated bacteria. The exact mechanism for serum IgG depression, an almost universal finding in patients with primary NS, is unknown and cannot be explained by urinary loss of IgG alone. Increased IgG catabolism and reduced synthesis have been established in human studies. The complement system is affected, with many patients showing low levels of C1q, C2, C8, C9, and factors B and I and sluggish activity of the alternate pathway. Low levels of factors B and I, which play a pivotal role in the regulation of C3b, the principal opsonin of *Escherichia coli*, *Streptococcus pneumoniae*, and *Haemophilus influenzae*, may predispose nephrotic patients to infections with these organisms. Bacterial peritonitis and sepsis are the main causes of death in nephrotic children. Approximately 6% of nephrotic children suffer at least one episode of primary peritonitis. Intravenous antibiotic therapy, including but not limited to specific coverage for the organisms noted earlier, should be given at the first suspicion of systemic or peritoneal infection after appropriate blood and peritoneal fluid cultures are obtained. Infection with *Pseudomonas* and other gram-negative organisms has become more common in the last decade and should be considered when choosing antibiotic therapy. Pneumococcal and *H. influenzae* type b vaccines may be effective long-term deterrents to infection in patients with the NS. To achieve an effective antibody response, however, vaccines should be given only when patients are in remission and are receiving minimal or no immunosuppressive medications. Ordinarily, patients with the NS tolerate viral infections well, unless they have been receiving high-dose immunosuppressive medications for long periods of time.

The incidence of thrombotic events in children with the NS is low (1.8%), but occasionally the consequences are fatal. Sites of thrombosis include the inferior vena cava, renal veins, hepatic veins, deep leg veins, pulmonary artery, pulmonary veins, femoral or iliac arteries, and the sagittal sinus. Arterial thromboses are seen more commonly in children than in adults with the NS. Renal vein thrombosis occurs more commonly in older children and adults with the NS of MGN.

Numerous defects in hemostasis occur in the NS. Alterations in almost every coagulation factor and clotting inhibitor, as well as thrombocytosis, increased platelet adhesiveness, and defects in the fibrinolytic system, have been reported. Systemic anticoagulation with low-molecular-weight heparin is indicated for all patients who develop thromboembolic disease and for those at high risk because of immobilization. Avoidance of bed rest, of volume depletion, of excessive diuretics, and of deep venous

or arterial punctures is important to lower the risk for thrombosis.

The clinical significance of hyperlipidemia in children with the NS is unknown. Epidemiologic studies of nonnephrotic patients who have decreased ratios of high-density to low-density cholesterol have shown an increased risk of developing arteriosclerotic coronary heart disease. Studies in a few children with chronic NS suggest that these patients are similarly at risk. Hyperlipidemia plays a role in the hypercoagulable state of patients with the NS and may play a role in the progression of glomerulosclerosis. When the NS goes into remission, lipid levels return to normal or near normal if steroid therapy is minimal. Treatment with cholesterol-lowering agents should be considered for children with prolonged and unremitting chronic NS and very high serum lipid levels.

Pathogenesis of Primary Nephrotic Syndrome

Diseases giving rise to primary NS are widely held to be immune-mediated. In MCNS, and perhaps mesangial proliferative GN and FSGS, abnormalities of immunoglobulin synthesis, lymphocyte function, and lymphokine production occur. In MPGN and MGN, immune complexes deposited in the GBM cause local damage, and massive proteinuria ensues. In chronic forms of the NS, massive amounts of filtered protein presented to the proximal tubular cells for recycling may cause injury to these cells and may contribute to tubulointerstitial injury associated with progression to chronic renal failure. Details of pathogenesis for each disease are reviewed later under the specific disease sections.

Minimal-Change Disease

MCNS is characterized by the onset of the NS without systemic disease, hypocomplementemia, or other serious signs of renal disease. Although nephritic features (hematuria, azotemia, and hypertension) occur in 10% to 25% of children with MCNS, these signs seldom occur together and hardly ever are severe or persistent. Two-thirds of the children with MCNS present for evaluation when they are between ages 2 and 6 years. For this reason, preadolescents who have the NS without nephritic signs, hypocomplementemia, or signs of systemic disease likely have MCNS and do not need to have a kidney biopsy for diagnosis before therapy is initiated. Steroid therapy effectively induces a remission in most patients. MCNS may occur in the presence of hematopoietic malignancies, especially Hodgkin lymphoma; MCNS in these patients remits with remission of the malignant disease. Clinical and laboratory features and pathophysiology are those of the NS as described earlier.

Pathology

Renal biopsies of patients with MCNS either appear normal by light microscopy or show no more than a mild, focal increase in mesangial cellularity and mesangial matrix. Tubular atrophy, interstitial fibrosis, and vascular changes are absent. Electron microscopic findings include effacement of epithelial cell foot processes, normal GBM thickness, and no more than an occasional small paramesangial electron-dense deposit. Immunofluorescence staining may be negative or slightly positive for IgM and, rarely, IgG and C3 in the mesangium.

Pathogenesis

In 1974, Shalhoub hypothesized that MCNS may be caused by an abnormal clone of T cells that produces a circulating lymphokine (VPF) that damages or alters the permeability of the GBM. His hypothesis was based on four well-recognized clinical observations indicative of T-cell activity: Remissions of the NS are induced by rubeola infection, patients with the NS have increased susceptibility to pneumococcal infection, remissions of the NS are induced by steroids and cyclophosphamide, and MCNS occurs in some patients with Hodgkin disease. For the last 30 years, many studies have focused on a potential role of circulating VPF and lymphocytes in the pathogenesis of MCNS. Only hemopexin, a heme-binding acute-phase reactant produced by lymphocytes that causes proteinuria when infused in experimental models, has been identified as a likely VPF in the pathogenesis of MCNS, but further confirmation is necessary. Genetic perturbations in glomerular podocyte proteins, such as nephrin, also may predispose patients with MCNS to the effects of VPF and may lead to the NS. Genetic screening studies of populations with MCNS are providing further incite into this possibility.

Although no consistent abnormalities of T- or B-cell numbers have been found, abnormalities of lymphocyte function are present in patients with MCNS. Serum from patients in relapse, but not those in remission, inhibits lymphocyte growth *in vitro*, either because the serum contains inhibitory substances or because it lacks certain factors necessary for growth. This finding may not be specific for MCNS, however, because serum from patients with FSGS and MGN also inhibits *in vitro* lymphocyte growth. Several experiments have shown that products of stimulated lymphocytes from nephrotic patients reduce the glomerular polyanionic charge of rat glomeruli. Foot process effacement was induced in some of the animals. Consistent production of proteinuria in these animals did not occur. Cellular immunity is altered in relapse, so affected patients have markedly reduced responses to tuberculin and other skin tests.

Although not specific for MCNS and apparently unrelated to glomerular injury, consistent abnormalities of immunoglobulins are found in the NS. Serum IgG concentrations are decreased in relapse but usually return to normal in remission. Often, serum IgM concentration is increased in relapse and may continue to be high or may return to normal in remission. Low serum levels of IgG result in part from urinary loss, but decreased production and increased catabolism also have been demonstrated. The mechanisms controlling the observed abnormalities of serum IgG and IgM are unknown.

Epithelial podocyte damage *per se* may contribute to proteinuria in MCNS. Decreased synthesis of heparan sulfate and other polyanions could disrupt the normal charge barrier to glomerular filtration of albumin. Relative preservation of pore size and the size-selective barrier of the GBM in the presence of loss of the normal charge barrier could explain the selectivity for albumin, and not large-molecular-weight proteins in the proteinuria of MCNS.

Differential Diagnosis

Differentiating MCNS from other disorders causing primary NS (see Box 325.3) was made easier by reports of the International Study of Kidney Disease in Children (ISKDC). By examining clinical and laboratory features of patients with biopsy-proven primary NS, these investigators identified certain clinical patterns suggesting the underlying renal histopathologic features. Usually, patients with MCNS present for evaluation before they reach age 6 years; those with MPGN rarely present before they are 8 years old. Hypertension occurs less commonly in MCNS (13%) than in FSGS (33%). Hematuria is transient and uncommon in MCNS (25%), but it occurs in more than one-half the patients with other diseases. Decreased serum C3 concentration occurs in three-fourths of patients with MPGN, but serum C3 almost always is normal in other forms of primary NS. Patients with MCNS usually respond to steroid therapy, so when the diagnosis of MCNS is suspected clinically but no remission of the NS is induced after 8 weeks of steroid therapy, another diagnosis is likely, and a diagnostic renal biopsy should be performed.

Therapy and Outcome

Usually, the diagnosis of the NS is suspected first in the outpatient setting. Hospitalization for a patient with newly diagnosed NS is recommended for dietary and, if needed, diuretic management of edema, for initiation of steroid therapy, and for parent and patient education about the disease and home monitoring of proteinuria. Before steroid therapy is begun in areas with a high incidence of tuberculosis, a tuberculin skin test should be performed, and if the result is negative at 24 hours, steroid treatment may be started safely.

Recommendations for steroid therapy have been made by the ISKDC and others. Usually, an adequate steroid regimen consists of prednisone, 60 mg/m^2/day (not exceeding a total dose of 80 mg/day) for 4 weeks, followed by 60 mg/m^2/day as a single dose given every other day in the morning for an additional 4 to 12 weeks. This standard approach was challenged by the German collaborative study, which showed that an initial 6-week course of daily prednisone followed by 6 weeks of alternate-day therapy resulted in a 50% reduction in relapse rate during the subsequent 12 months, as compared with the relapse rate of patients treated with a shorter course of steroids (36% versus 61%, respectively). Typically, responsive patients lose their proteinuria within the first 2 to 3 weeks of therapy. During the period of alternate-day prednisone after the first 4 to 6 weeks, the dose of prednisone is decreased gradually and is discontinued approximately 4 to 5 months after initiation of therapy. A recent randomized study of Japanese children with MCNS suggested that an even longer period of tapering prednisone is beneficial. When total time of therapy was extended to 6 months after initiation of steroids and reduction of dose made no more often than every 4 weeks, a significant decrease in frequently relapsing disease occurred, especially in children younger than 4 years old, who had 0% recurrence, compared with 60% recurrence within 2 years.

Relapses may occur in as many as 80% of affected children, often during the period of slow tapering of prednisone. While receiving steroid therapy, patients should check their urine routinely at home for protein by using a dipstick daily or at least three times weekly to screen for early signs of relapse, before the onset of edema. Patients who have fewer than two relapses in a 6-month period may be treated as described earlier for each relapse. Those who have more than two relapses in a 6-month period are called *frequent relapsers* and may do well on longer courses of alternate-day prednisone. Patients who cannot tolerate cessation of steroid therapy without a relapse are called *steroid dependent*. Steroid toxicity may become a major problem for either frequent relapsers or steroid-dependent patients who receive high doses of daily steroids for a long period of time.

Frequent relapsers and steroid-dependent patients may require a diagnostic renal biopsy. If the biopsy shows MCNS and additional therapy to control the NS is desirable, a 2-month course of chlorambucil (0.2 mg/kg/day) or cyclophosphamide (2.5 mg/kg/day) may produce a sustained remission. Patients with frequently relapsing NS have more prolonged remissions than do steroid-dependent patients after receiving cytotoxic therapy. During therapy, patients should have a weekly complete blood cell count to monitor for signs of bone marrow depression that may require altering the dosage or stopping the drug. Before beginning therapy with cytotoxic drugs, patients and parents also should be warned of other potential drug side effects, such as sterility in male patients after long-term cyclophosphamide therapy. Cyclosporine also has been effective in inducing a remission in steroid-dependent patients and in allowing tapering off prednisone, but the relapse rate after discontinuation of cyclosporine has been substantial, so continuous therapy for years is required.

Most patients with MCNS are hospitalized for a few days at the time of diagnosis, and most do not require hospitalization again. When feeling well, patients should attend school as usual, without any special physical restrictions. A sodium-restricted diet is mandatory during relapses and while the patient is taking prednisone, especially at high doses. Maintaining a relatively low-sodium diet during remissions may be helpful psychologically if the child is a frequent relapser. Usually, immunizations are withheld until the child is in remission and has been off steroids for at least 3 months. No live-virus vaccine should be given to a patient, siblings, or parents in the household while the patient is taking high-dose daily steroids or cytotoxic drugs.

The long-term prognosis for MCNS is excellent. Most patients (80%) enter a sustained remission during adolescence. The overall mortality in a large group of patients with MCNS followed by the ISKDC for 5 to 17 years was 2.5%.

Diffuse Mesangial Proliferative Glomerulonephritis

Only a few children (about 5%) presenting with primary NS have diffuse mesangial proliferative GN, which is characterized by diffuse mesangial hypercellularity with or without mesangial electron-dense deposits on renal biopsy. By immunofluorescence, any deposits present usually are identified as IgM, occasionally are associated with C3, and are located in the mesangium and rarely in the capillary loop. Biopsies showing predominantly IgM deposits have been classified by some physicians as IgM mesangial nephropathy, but patients with this lesion have been found to have no distinguishing clinical features compared with other children with primary NS. The significance of IgM deposits, like the pathogenesis of diffuse mesangial proliferation, is unknown. Some patients who have had serial biopsies later have developed FSGS, which heralds a poor prognosis.

Clinically, children with the NS and diffuse mesangial proliferative GN are more likely to have microscopic hematuria (90%), hypertension (50%), reduced renal function (25%), and poor initial response to steroid therapy (35% to 70%). Despite initial steroid resistance, most patients have a good prognosis, with some undergoing spontaneous remission of the NS and fewer than 10% progressing to severe renal failure and end-stage renal disease. For those who do progress to end-stage renal disease, the recurrence rate of diffuse mesangial proliferative GN after renal transplantation has been reported to be as high as 40%.

Focal Segmental Glomerulosclerosis

FSGS is a pathologic lesion with many causes (Box 325.5). This section will focus on the idiopathic form, which also may represent several different etiologic insults to the kidney that cannot be differentiated with our current knowledge.

Clinical and Laboratory Features

Approximately 15% to 25% of children presenting with primary NS have FSGS by renal biopsy evaluation. Not all patients with FSGS present with the NS. Twenty percent of cases are diagnosed after the appearance of asymptomatic proteinuria; these patients often develop the NS later. Microscopic hematuria occurs in more than 50% of affected children at presentation, but gross hematuria is a rare finding. Renal tubular dysfunction, including renal glucosuria, generalized am-

---

BOX 325.5	Etiology of Focal Segmental Glomerulosclerosis

Primary Renal
Idiopathic, with or without mesangial hypercellularity

Secondary
Reflux nephropathy
Reduced renal mass (single kidney, partial nephrectomy)
Heroin abuse nephropathy
Analgesic abuse nephropathy
Sickle cell disease
Alport syndrome
Late stage of nephritis of chronic bacteremia
Chronic rejection of renal transplant
Human immunodeficiency virus-associated nephropathy

---

moaciduria, renal tubular acidosis, partial or complete Fanconi syndrome, and concentrating defects, occasionally occurs as a result of tubulointerstitial injury and portends future progression to chronic renal failure. Patients who are hypertensive at presentation (40%) do not have a significantly worse prognosis for progression to renal failure.

Pathology

Early in the disease, the renal lesions of FSGS are focal and are located predominantly in the juxtamedullary glomeruli. Because of the focal presentation of FSGS in some glomeruli but not in others, affected glomeruli may not be obtained at the initial biopsy or even during one or two subsequent percutaneous renal biopsies, and establishment of definitive diagnosis may be delayed. Complete sectioning of renal biopsy material enhances the chance of encountering affected glomeruli. By light microscopy, affected and unaffected glomeruli are enlarged. Affected glomeruli may have segmental sclerotic lesions or just segmental capillary loop collapse and increased mesangial matrix. The visceral epithelial cells often are vacuolated and may be lifted off the GBM or may form caps over sclerotic areas. Foam cells, which are foamy-appearing lipid-laden macrophages, occasionally are associated with the segmental lesions. Mesangial hypercellularity occurs in 50% of the biopsies of affected children. Tubulointerstitial disease of varying degrees, especially disease in tubules of sclerosing glomeruli, almost always is present. IgM, often accompanied by C3, can be identified by immunofluorescence microscopy in the mesangium or focally along the GBM of affected capillary loops. Fibrin staining occurs in areas of sclerosis. Electron microscopic examination demonstrates endothelial cell swelling, effacement of epithelial podocytes, sclerosis, and scattered immune deposits.

Pathogenesis

The pathogenesis of primary FSGS is uncertain despite 3 decades of research. Cellular immunologic processes clearly play an important role, as suggested by the findings that renal biopsies show no significant antibody deposition or cellular infiltration or proliferation, that FSGS frequently recurs after transplantation, and that a circulating factor isolated from the blood of affected patients induces disease in experimental animals. This circulating FSGS factor occurs in some but not all patients with FSGS and has eluded researchers' attempts at purification and identification since the mid-1990s.

Clinical Course and Therapy

Regardless of whether the diagnosis of FSGS is made on the basis of the initial renal biopsy or a subsequent biopsy, affected children have a similar clinical course. Only 20% of children with FSGS respond initially to prednisone with a complete remission. Most of these patients subsequently experience a relapse. Approximately 20% to 30% of them progress to end-stage renal disease within 5 years, and by 10 years, almost 60% of these patients have end-stage renal disease. Cyclosporine, tacrolimus, and mycophenolate mofetil therapy have been used alone or in combination with steroids, with varying degrees of success in selected patients, in attempts to control severe NS. Pulse intravenous methylprednisolone therapy for 8 to 12 weeks in conjunction with alternate-day oral prednisone with or without an alkylating agent, either cyclophosphamide or chlorambucil, has been used successfully as well. In one series, 80% of patients treated with this regimen attained a sustained remission of the NS and maintained normal renal function for 1 to 12 years of follow-up. Every treatment regimen used to date has had untoward side effects. Comparative controlled trials in large groups of patients still are needed to determine which treatment combinations are preferable. A large multicenter trial of newer treatment regimens currently is in progress in the United States.

Persistent NS and an increase in globally sclerotic glomeruli noted in follow-up biopsies have been associated with progressive disease. No other clinical or pathologic markers of progressive disease have been confirmed. FSGS recurs in as many as 30% of initial renal transplants and in as many as 80% of subsequent transplants, sometimes with massive proteinuria and the NS within the first 24 hours and renal allograft loss within days to weeks. The NS has remitted without allograft loss in many children treated promptly with high-dose cyclosporine, alone or in combination with plasmapheresis.

Membranoproliferative Glomerulonephritis

Historically, MPGN has had a variety of names, including *hypocomplementemic GN*, *lobular* or *mixed membranous and proliferative GN*, and *mesangiocapillary GN*. In parts of the world outside the United States, MPGN still is referred to as *mesangiocapillary GN*. The name *membranoproliferative glomerulonephritis* is derived from the glomerular histopathologic lesion of patients with this disorder. Light microscopic examination of renal biopsy material shows a marked increase in mesangial cellularity and extension of mesangial cells into the capillary wall, causing the GBM to appear thickened and split or reduplicated. The proliferation of cells and the abnormal GBM give rise to the name *membranoproliferative*.

MPGN is a chronic disease of both children and adults that may be idiopathic or occasionally associated with other systemic diseases or infections, such as chronic hepatitis C. The age of onset in most patients is between 8 and 20 years. The male-to-female gender ratio is equal. A genetic predisposition to MPGN is suggested by the following: an association of MPGN with an inherited deficiency of several complement components; an association with the extended haplotype HLA-B8, DR3, SC01, GL02; the occurrence of the disease in some siblings; and the rarity of the disease in African Americans.

Clinical Features

Only 2% to 10% of cases of primary NS in childhood are caused by MPGN, and the incidence appears to be decreasing in childhood in many areas of the world during the last decade. The presentation is variable, with primary NS occurring in approximately 50%, asymptomatic proteinuria in 25%, and nephritis with hematuria and proteinuria in the other 25%. Many cases are identified initially by screening urinalysis for school, summer camp, or sports participation. Gross hematuria, hypertension, and azotemia each occur in 30% of patients. When these signs appear together acutely, MPGN may be confused with APSGN. Most patients have microscopic or gross hematuria at onset, and almost all have proteinuria. In those presenting without proteinuria, a low serum C3 may be the only clue to the diagnosis.

Laboratory Features

Besides the laboratory features of primary NS, the urine is positive for blood more than half the time and often contains red blood cell casts. Serum C3 concentrations are decreased in 60% to 75% of patients at the time of diagnosis. The absence of hypocomplementemia does not rule out the diagnosis of MPGN.

Pathology

Two well-defined subtypes of MPGN and a controversial third subtype are identified in children by their renal pathologic features. Type I is characterized by enlarged, lobular glomeruli with obliteration of capillary lumina and marked mesangial proliferation. Mesangial proliferation may be so marked that mesangial cells wedge between the GBM and the endothelium, resulting in an apparent reduplication of GBM material and a tram-track appearance. Electron microscopy shows mesangial and subendothelial deposits, which are positive for IgG and C3 by immunofluorescence staining.

Type II shares many of the same light microscopic findings as those of type I, but mesangial proliferation is less marked. Electron microscopy shows characteristic, very dense material within the GBM that gives type II MPGN its other common designation, *dense-deposit disease*. The origin of this dense material is unknown; it is not immune complex material. Positive immunofluorescence staining, mainly for C3, outlines the GBM around the dense deposits, but it does not occur within them. C3 occurs also in the mesangium and sparsely in the subendothelial and subepithelial spaces. Children with type III disease have mesangial, subendothelial, subepithelial, and transmembranous deposition of IgG and C3, with extensive disruption of the GBM.

Some investigators have described additional subtypes of MPGN in which the location and composition of the immune deposits differ slightly from those seen in type I. These additional subtypes have not proven to be useful classifications for the prediction of clinical outcomes because identical clinical disease has been associated with all the extra subtypes.

Pathogenesis

The morphologic diversity of renal biopsies from patients with MPGN suggests heterogeneity of pathogenesis. Immune complex deposition is a prominent feature of all types of MPGN. Circulating immune complexes have been measured in patients with all types of MPGN, but the presence of these complexes does not correlate with the severity of disease activity or with the degree of hypocomplementemia. The stimulus for immune complex formation is unknown.

Complement activation occurs by at least two mechanisms in MPGN. In type I MPGN, immune complexes stimulate the classic pathway, thus depleting serum concentration of C1q, C2, and C4 along with C3 and C5. Low serum C3 levels may retard the normal clearing of immune complexes from the circulation. As mentioned, inherited deficiencies of complement have been associated with MPGN type I and type III. In type II disease, alternate pathway activation by C3 nephritic factor (NF_a) reduces the serum concentration of C3, whereas C4 remains normal and C5 is normal or is depressed minimally. This type of C3 nephritic factor is an IgG autoantibody that increases alternate pathway degradation of C3. The presence of C3 nephritic factor does not appear to affect the outcome of patients with MPGN. Another nephritic factor, NF_t, causes complement activation in type III MPGN and results in markedly depressed serum C3 and C5 levels, with normal C4 concentration.

Course and Therapy

A few patients have spontaneous NS remissions that may last for years. The only evidence of activity of disease during this "silent phase" may be persistent hypocomplementemia. The natural history of patients with MPGN is to progress slowly toward end-stage renal disease. Approximately half of affected patients reach end-stage disease within 10 years of diagnosis. If the serum creatinine exceeds 2 mg/dL at presentation, dialysis probably will be required within 3 years. Hypertension, gross hematuria, and unremitting NS with edema portend a poor prognosis.

Historically, many treatments for MPGN, including steroids, other immunosuppressive agents, anticoagulants, and nonsteroidal antiinflammatory agents, have been tried. A double-blind, prospective, controlled trial of daily aspirin and dipyridamole therapy was associated with maintenance of a higher GFR, but the therapy had no effect on proteinuria in affected adults followed for many years. The ISKDC showed beneficial results of long-term, alternate-day prednisone for maintaining renal function in children with all types of MPGN. Aggressive management of steroid-induced hypertension was required in some cases.

Renal transplantation is successful in patients with MPGN, although type I and type II disease both recur in the allograft. The recurrence rate is only approximately 30% in type I disease but may be as high as 60% in type II MPGN. The clinical progression to graft loss from recurrent disease is quite slow and is an insufficient reason to withhold transplantation.

Membranous Glomerulonephritis

MGN is a rare disorder of children, accounting for fewer than 3% of the cases presenting with primary NS. The frequency of occurrence increases in adolescence (10% to 20%), and the disorder is common in adults with the NS (20% to 40%). MGN occurs as a primary renal disease (idiopathic MGN) in approximately 65% of affected children but is associated with systemic diseases, such as SLE or chronic hepatitis B infection, and rarely with exposure to drugs and toxins, in the remainder of patients (Box 325.6). The presentation of MGN may antedate the appearance of associated disorders, such as SLE, hepatitis B infection, or malignant disease, by months or years and may be confused with idiopathic MGN. MGN associated with malignant disease almost always occurs in adults with solid tumors, including those of lung and colon, and very rarely in children with non-Hodgkin lymphoma. MGN rarely recurs in renal transplants. For reasons that are unclear, MGN often arises *de novo* in patients with renal transplants.

Clinical and Laboratory Features

The onset of symptoms is gradual. Approximately one-third of MGN cases are discovered by the presence of proteinuria on routine screening urinalysis. The other two-thirds present with edema and the NS. Hypertension occurs in 30% or fewer cases and has no prognostic significance. Microscopic hematuria is a common finding in children (roughly 80% in some series), and gross hematuria occurs in as many as 20%. Usually, renal function is normal at presentation. Serum C3 is normal, ex-

---

BOX 325.6

Etiology of Membranous Glomerulonephritis

Primary Renal Disease
Idiopathic (no identifiable associated condition)

Associated with Infectious Disorders
Hepatitis B (chronic presence of hepatitis B surface antigen)
Syphilis (congenital or secondary)
Poststreptococcal disease
Hydatid disease
Leprosy
Malaria

Associated with Systemic Disorders
Systemic lupus erythematosus
Thyroiditis (with thyroglobulin antibodies)
Fanconi syndrome (with anti-tubular basement membrane or anti-renal tubular epithelial cell antibodies)
Sickle cell disease
Neoplasm (carcinoma, leukemia, Wilms tumor)
Other (Sjögren syndrome, Gardner-Diamond syndrome, Kimura disease, celiac disease, diabetes mellitus)

Associated with Drugs or Toxins
Heavy metals (gold, mercury, bismuth, silver)
D-Penicillamine
Trimethadione
Probenecid
Captopril

De novo *in Renal Transplantation*

---

cept in lupus- and hepatitis B-associated MGN, in which the level is low. Hepatitis B-associated MGN occurs primarily in children in endemic areas, who are asymptomatic chronic carriers of hepatitis B virus. Patients usually are younger than 10 years old, male, and African American or Asian. Serum aspartate aminotransferase levels tend to be normal or only mildly elevated. Serology is positive for hepatitis B surface antigen, anticore antibody, and e antigen and is negative for surface antibody. Liver biopsies may show evidence of chronic hepatitis. Hepatitis B antigens, especially e antigen, as well as anti-e antibody have been demonstrated in glomerular immune deposits in approximately 90% of patients. Appearance of hepatitis B core antibody in the serum has correlated positively with remission of the NS in a few patients.

Pathology

The characteristic pathologic lesion of MGN is diffuse thickening of the glomerular capillary wall caused by deposition of small immune complexes on the subepithelial side of the GBM without significant cellular proliferation. The deposits always contain IgG and often C3. Silver staining of light microscopic sections shows spikes of argyrophilic GBM material projecting like fingers around the subepithelial deposits toward the urinary space. With progression of MGN, the deposits become completely surrounded and incorporated into a very thickened GBM; the spikes then appear elongated, and some even join together to form silver-positive circles or domes around the nonstaining deposits. In advanced lesions, focal and segmental glomerular sclerosis may develop and is associated with a poor prognosis and progressive chronic renal failure.

Stages of MGN are classified by the light and electron microscopic appearance of the deposits in renal biopsy specimens. In stage I, deposits are subepithelial, small, and discrete, within a GBM of normal thickness. In stage II, deposits are larger, separated by intervening well-developed spikes of GBM material in a uniformly thickened capillary wall. In stage III, deposits are larger still, often completely engulfed by spikes, giving a railroad-track appearance on silver stain, in an irregularly thickened capillary wall with narrowed capillary lumen. In stage IV, deposits are almost entirely intramembranous and in various stages of dissolution; areas of glomerular sclerosis and tubular atrophy may be present. Stage V is a healing stage, noted in some patients with remitting NS and consisting of regression of the capillary wall changes and resorption of electron-dense deposits, with decreased intensity or disappearance of IgG by immunofluorescence staining. Different stages of MGN may be observed in one renal biopsy at any given time. Whether the stage of MGN correlates with the clinical severity and duration of illness in children is uncertain. In some cases, the lesions appear to remain stable over the course of years.

Pathogenesis

The pathogenesis of MGN is not understood completely, although it has been studied extensively in laboratory models. Two possibilities have emerged as most likely to initiate MGN. First, and most likely, is that circulating antibodies react with endogenous GBM antigens and result in formation of *in situ* immune complexes within the GBM, leading to the development of pathologic lesions described earlier. Second, deposition of preformed circulating immune complexes with an affinity for the GBM may be the initial event. These complexes may be induced from various stimuli, including autoimmune reactions, infectious agents, drugs, or toxins. The rarity of measurable circulating immune complexes in affected patients renders the second possibility less likely. Genetic factors also may be important. An association of HLA-DRW3 and DQA1 allele has been demonstrated for adults with MGN.

Prognosis and Therapy

The course of idiopathic MGN is slowly progressive over the course of years, resulting in chronic renal failure within a decade in only approximately 10% of children younger than 10 years old and in 20% of adolescents. Remissions of proteinuria are spontaneous in as many as 30% of pediatric patients. Because of the rarity of idiopathic MGN in children, determining the most appropriate therapy is difficult. Anecdotal experience has been reported, but no controlled trials in children or adolescents are available. Recommendations for therapy have been extrapolated from therapeutic trials in adults, who have the disease more often than do children. All children with proteinuria should be treated with an angiotensin-converting enzyme inhibitor or angiotensin II receptor blocker, or a combination of both, to reduce proteinuria, to control intraglomerular hypertension, and to prevent progression to chronic renal failure. Because of the benign course of MGN in many children, additional therapy is reserved for those with poorly controlled edema and the NS. A trial of 8 weeks of alternate-day, high-dose prednisone (60 mg/m^2/day), followed by slow tapering over the course of several months, has little risk of toxicity and may be efficacious in some patients. If a satisfactory response is not obtained with initial prednisone therapy for 8 weeks, a 6-month trial of a daily cytotoxic agent (cyclophosphamide or chlorambucil) or cyclosporine may be added. If that therapy is effective, the prednisone may be tapered rapidly. Cytotoxic agents have the potentially harmful side effects of sterility or late malignancy, so cyclosporine may be a better choice for children. Cyclosporine has the disadvantage of frequent relapse after discontinuation of therapy, so it may require long-term

administration for longer than 12 months. Clinical trials with mycophenylate mofetil are too premature to draw conclusions about its effectiveness. In the near future, more specific therapy directed against earlier steps in the pathogenesis of MGN may become available and may avoid the unwanted side effects of steroids and cytotoxic agents. A recent small adult clinical trial of rituximab, a monoclonal antibody directed against B cells to prevent their activation and subsequent antibody production, was successful in significantly reducing proteinuria, ameliorating edema, and stabilizing renal function without untoward side effects in eight patients with mild to moderate renal failure and MGN unresponsive to other therapies. Much more study is needed before therapies such as rituximab become accepted clinical strategies.

Treatment of patients with secondary MGN is dictated by the underlying disorder. MGN associated with SLE has been treated like idiopathic GN, if the other manifestations of SLE are in remission. Spontaneous remission of MGN associated with hepatitis B occurs commonly in children, so careful clinical observation is appropriate. Therapy with steroids should be avoided because of the possibility of worsening the viral infection. Antiviral therapy may be beneficial in children with unremitting NS. In children with MGN and congenital or secondary syphilis, early treatment with penicillin leads to rapid recovery. Usually, MGN associated with drugs or toxins is diagnosed after 6 to 12 months of exposure. Withdrawal of the inciting agent usually leads to recovery after several more months.

Nephrotic Syndrome in Infants

Onset of the NS within the first year of life is considered separately because the underlying disorders and clinical outcomes differ for infants compared with children and adolescents. The disorders leading to the NS in infancy may be primary or secondary, congenital or acquired, and often hereditary (Box 325.7). Congenital NS is a subset of this group and is defined as the NS occurring within the first 3 months of life, the most common form of which is congenital NS of the

---

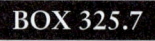

BOX 325.7   **Causes of Nephrotic Syndrome in Infants**

Primary Renal Diseases
Congenital nephrotic syndrome of the Finnish type
Diffuse mesangial sclerosis
Minimal-change nephrotic syndrome
Focal segmental glomerulosclerosis

Secondary to Other Disorders
Congenital infection (syphilis, toxoplasmosis, cytomegalovirus, rubella, hepatitis B, malaria)
Toxins (mercury, drugs)
Systemic lupus erythematosus
Neoplasm (Wilms tumor)
Denys-Drash syndrome (ambiguous genitalia, Wilms tumor, nephropathy)
Nephropathy associated with congenital brain malformation (Galloway-Mowat)
XY gonadal dysgenesis
Lowe syndrome
Nail-patella syndrome
Hemolytic-uremic syndrome

Finnish type (CNF). Diseases causing primary congenital NS almost always are hereditary and rarely are responsive to steroid therapy.

Primary Renal Disorders

The clinical presentation of primary NS of infants does not help to distinguish one disease from another. All patients have proteinuria, hypoalbuminemia, hyperlipidemia, hypogamma-globulinemia, and usually normal renal function. Edema may not occur initially but appears within a few weeks of onset of proteinuria. Hematuria is an uncommon finding. Renal biopsies are useful to distinguish MCNS and FSGS from other types, but pathologic features of CNF and diffuse mesangial sclerosis (DMS) may be so similar at some stages of the disease that differentiating by biopsy is difficult. Biopsies in both CNF and DMS show effacement of foot processes, diffuse epithelial cell proliferation, increased mesangial matrix, absence of electron-dense or immunofluorescent-positive deposits, persistence of fetal glomeruli, and glomerulosclerosis. Early in the course, biopsies from patients with DMS show no mesangial cell proliferation as compared with mild or moderate mesangial cell proliferation present in biopsies from patients with CNF. Late in the course of DMS, nonspecific trapping of IgM, C3, and C1q may appear as immune deposits within minimally affected glomeruli or around sclerosed glomeruli. Microcysts, which result from dilatation of Bowman's space in diseased glomeruli, once were thought to be a diagnostic feature of CNF but now are known to be a nonspecific finding of infants with the NS. Focal segmental sclerosis progressing to global sclerosis with tubular atrophy and interstitial fibrosis occurs with advancing age in patients with CNF, DMS, and FSGS.

Family history, clinical outcome, and response to immuno-suppressive therapy may be the only ways to arrive at a final diagnosis in infants with primary renal disease. MCNS is a rare event in early infancy but has been reported in infants as young as 3 weeks old, is quite responsive to steroid therapy, and does not progress to end-stage renal disease. MCNS should be suspected if the renal biopsy shows minimal changes and the family history is negative. FSGS, also rare, may be responsive to steroid therapy. Because of the rare occurrence of MCNS and FSGS as well the risk of development of severe infectious complications in infants with CNF, who have extremely low levels of circulating immunoglobulins, steroid therapy should not be undertaken routinely in infants younger than 3 months old before definitive diagnosis is established. DMS is a rare disorder that is clinically indistinguishable from CNF. It occurs in siblings but not in parents, a finding suggesting autosomal recessive genetic transmission; the defective gene has not been identified. DMS is not responsive to steroid therapy and progresses to end-stage renal disease before the child reaches 3 years of age. Early on, DMS is distinguishable pathologically from CNF by the predominance of mesangial matrix expansion without mesangial hypercellularity. Fibrillar increase in mesangial matrix and podocyte hypertrophy lead to thickening of the GBM, massive enlargement of the mesangium, crowding of the capillary lumina, and eventual sclerosis of the glomerular tuft, leaving a contracted sclerotic mass in a dilated Bowman's space (microcyst). DMS also is the pathologic lesion associated with the glomerulopathy of Denys-Drash syndrome (see later).

CNF is the most common form of the NS in infants. With or without known Finnish ancestry, CNF always is transmitted genetically in an autosomal recessive fashion. The incidence in Finland was as high as 1.2 cases per 10,000 births but decreased recently to 0.9 with widespread prenatal screening. Most patients seen in North America have no apparent Finnish ancestry, and the condition may occur in any ethnic group, but these patients have the same defective gene and clinical course.

The abnormal gene of CNF (*NPHS1*) is located on chromosome 19q13.1 and encodes for a transmembrane protein called *nephrin*, which is part of an immunoglobulin superfamily of cell adhesion molecules. Nephrin is an integral part of the slit diaphragm complex of glomerular podocytes. Patients with CNF have mutant nephrin protein and often lack identifiable slit diaphragms on renal biopsy. More than 60 mutations have been identified in affected families, but two mutations, Fin-major and Fin-minor, account for nearly 90% of all affected Finnish patients. The exact pathogenesis of mutant protein to clinical NS has not been elucidated, but it is the focus of much investigative activity. Insights into the pathogenesis of CNF are expected to yield important insights into the pathogenesis of many other forms of the NS, including MCNS.

CNF may be suspected *in utero* by elevation of amniotic fluid and maternal serum alpha-fetoprotein. Histopathologic evaluation of fetal renal tissue shows changes of CNF with foot process effacement and diffuse epithelial podocyte proliferation. Fetal proteinuria is manifest by week 15 and leads to a more than tenfold increase in amniotic fluid alpha-fetoprotein. Alpha-fetoprotein is not specific for CNF and can be falsely positive in heterozygous carriers for CNF who will not be clinically affected. Specific genetic testing is available and should be used to confirm prenatal diagnosis when needed after screening for elevation of alpha-fetoprotein.

Infants with CNF are small for gestational age and are born prematurely. The placenta is large, often weighing more than 25% of the infant's birth weight. Edema is present at birth in at least one-half of patients and always occurs by the time they have reached the age of 3 months. Even when edema is not present, patients have proteinuria sufficient to cause hypoalbuminemia and hypoimmunoglobulinemia. Infants with CNF are immunocompromised and are highly susceptible to severe bacterial infections. Supportive therapy includes supplemental immunoglobulin infusions and high suspicion for serious infection. Prophylactic antibiotics are not beneficial and should be avoided. Thyroxine is lost in the urine and usually leads to hypothyroidism that requires supplemental therapy. Newborn thyroid screening may detect low blood levels of thyroxine before the clinical diagnosis of CNF has been established. Thyroid-stimulating hormone concentration still may be normal at that time, but a decreased serum thyroid-binding globulin concentration (owing to its urinary loss) will suggest the correct diagnosis. Later in infancy, sufficient loss of transferrin and iron or protein-bound 25-hydroxyvitamin D may cause iron deficiency anemia or vitamin D deficiency, respectively. Thromboembolic complications may occur from the hypercoagulability associated with severe chronic NS.

Delayed growth and development and malnutrition from excessive protein losses, anorexia, and poor feeding occur in all affected infants. Gastric tube feedings and daily or alternate-day intravenous albumin infusions given through an indwelling central line usually are needed to promote adequate growth. Diuretics to control edema, immunoglobulin infusions, and anticoagulants (aspirin or dipyridamole) if indicated to control thromboembolism are important additional components of aggressive medical management. Renal function is normal initially but deteriorates progressively to end-stage renal disease, usually by the time the child is 3 to 8 years of age. If patients are poorly responsive to aggressive medical management, bilateral nephrectomy and dialysis may be indicated before the onset of end-stage renal disease, even when renal function remains greater than 50% of normal. The diagnosis of CNF should be certain before nephrectomy, dialysis, and renal transplantation are contemplated in the setting of normal renal function. A successful medical alternative to nephrectomy in some patients may be the combination of an angiotension-converting enzyme inhibitor and indomethacin to lower intraglomeular pressure and markedly reduce proteinuria.

Without aggressive management, untreated infants die before they reach 4 years of age. Good long-term survival (80%) has been attained by early initiation of aggressive medical management followed by dialysis and renal transplantation. Catch-up growth and development are common after the patient receives a renal transplant. CNF may recur in as many as 25% of patients after they have undergone renal transplantation. In these patients, introduction of a kidney with intact nephrin is recognized as a foreign protein, which induces production of antinephrin antibodies that damage the glomerular filtration barrier and lead to severe proteinuria and the NS.

Nephrotic Syndrome Secondary to Other Disorders

Secondary causes of the NS in infancy (see Box 325.7) may be identified by signs and symptoms of the underlying disorder (congenital syphilis or nail-patella syndrome), by a history of exposure to toxic drugs (mercury teething solution), or by specific diagnostic laboratory tests. The renal histopathologic lesions of secondary NS vary from classic membranous nephropathy associated with congenital syphilis to immune complex proliferative GN associated with other congenital infections and lupus to the unique GBM nephropathy associated with nail-patella syndrome. Therapy for secondary NS is directed at the underlying disorder. Recovery from the NS may be rapid in congenital syphilis treated with penicillin and in lupus treated with corticosteroids. Denys-Drash syndrome, a rare genetic disorder associated with mutations of the *WT1* gene on chromosome 11 and characterized by ambiguous genitalia, gonadoblastomas, Wilms tumor, and progressive glomerulopathy, has no specific therapy. The pathologic renal lesion is DMS, which is unresponsive to steroids and leads to progressive loss of renal function. Renal failure occurs early, usually reaching end-stage disease when the child is between ages 1 and 3 years. Dialysis and renal transplantation lead to successful long-term survival.

Suggested Readings

Acute Poststreptococcal Glomerulonephritis

Berrios X, Lagomarisino E, Solar E, et al. Post-streptococcal acute glomerulonephritis in Chile: 20 years of experience. *Pediatr Nephrol* 2004;19:306.

Clark G, White RHR, Glasgow EF, et al. Poststreptococcal GN in children: clinicopathologic correlations and long-term prognosis. *Pediatr Nephrol* 1988;2:381.

Dedeoglu I, Springate E, Waz WR, et al. Prolonged hypocomplementemia in poststreptococcal acute glomerulonephritis. *Clin Nephrol* 1996;46:302.

Potter EV, Lipschultz SA, Abidh S, et al. 12- to 17-year follow-up of patients with poststreptococcal acute GN in Trinidad. *N Engl J Med* 1982;307:725.

Congenital Nephrotic Syndrome

Kestila M, Lenkkeri U, Mannikko M, et al. Positionally cloned gene for a novel glomerular protein—nephrin—is mutated in congenital nephrotic syndrome. *Mol Cell* 1998;1:575.

Kovacevic L, Reif CJ, Rigden SP. Management of congenital nephrotic syndrome. *Pediatr Nephrol* 2003;18:426.

Papez KE, Smoyer WE. Recent advances in congenital nephrotic syndrome. *Curr Opin Pediatr* 2004;16:165.

Patrakka J, Kestila M, Wartiovaara J, et al. Congenital nephrotic syndrome (NPHS1) features resulting from different mutations in Finnish patients. *Kidney Int* 2000;58:972.

Schumacher V, Scharer K, Wuhl E, et al. Spectrum of early onset nephrotic syndrome associated with WT1 missense mutations. *Kidney Int* 1998;53:1594.

Diffuse Mesangial Proliferative Glomerulonephritis

Southwest Pediatric Nephrology Study Group. Childhood NS associated with diffuse mesangial hypercellularity. *Kidney Int* 1983;23:87.

Yang JY, Melvin T, Sibley R, et al. No evidence for a specific role of IgM in mesangial proliferation of idiopathic NS. *Kidney Int* 1984;25:100.

Focal Segmental Glomerulosclerosis

Andreoli SP. Racial and ethnic differences in the incidence and progression of focal segmental glomerulosclerosis in children. *Adv Renal Replace Ther* 2004;11:105.

Chishti AS, Sorof JM, Brewer ED, Kale AS. Long-term treatment of focal segmental glomerulosclerosis in children with cyclosporine given as a single daily dose. *Am J Kidney Dis* 2001;38:754.

Ingulli E, Singh A, Baqi N, et al. Aggressive, long-term cyclosporine therapy for steroid-resistant focal segmental glomerulosclerosis. *J Am Soc Nephrol* 1995;34:571.

Savin VJ, Sharma R, Sharma M, et al. Circulating factor associated with increased glomerular permeability to albumin in recurrent focal segmental glomerulosclerosis. *N Engl J Med* 1996;334:878.

Tune BM, Kirpekar R, Sibley RK, et al. Intravenous methylprednisolone and oral alkylating agent therapy of prednisone resistant pediatric focal segmental glomerulosclerosis: a long-term follow-up. *Clin Nephrol* 1995;43:84.

Waldo, FB, Benfield MR, Kohaut EC. Therapy of focal and segmental glomerulosclerosis with methylprednisolone, cyclosporine A and prednisone. *Pediatr Nephrol* 1998;12:397.

Henoch-Schönlein Purpura Nephritis

Davin J-C, Weening JJ. Henoch-Schönlein purpura nephritis: an update. *Eur J Pediatr* 2001;160:689.

Scharer K, Krmar R, Querfeld U, et al. Clinical outcome of Schönlein-Henoch purpura nephritis in children. *Pediatr Nephrol* 1999;13:816.

Tarshish P, Bernstein J, Edelmann CM. Henoch-Schönlein purpura nephritis: course of disease and efficacy of cyclophosphamide. *Pediatr Nephrol* 2004;19:51.

Immunoglobulin A Nephropathy

Donadio JV, Grande JP. IgA nephropathy. *N Engl J Med* 2002;347:738.

Friedman AL, Brewer E, Feld L, et al. Current concepts and controversies in IgA nephropathy. *Pediatr Nephrol* 1998;12:498.

Ponticelli C, Traversi L, Feliciani A, et al. Kidney transplantation in patients with IgA mesangial glomerulonephritis. *Kidney Int* 2001;60:1948.

Wyatt RJ, Hogg RJ. Evidence-based assessment of treatment options for children with IgA nephropathies. *Pediatr Nephrol* 2001;16:156.

Wyatt RJ, Kritchevsky SB, Woodford SY, et al. IgA nephropathy: long-term prognosis for pediatric patients. *J Pediatr* 1995;127:913.

Yoshikawa N, Tanaka R, Iijima K. Pathophysiology and treatment of IgA nephropathy in children. *Pediatr Nephrol* 2001: 16:446.

Immune Mechanisms

Couser WG. Glomerulonephritis. *Lancet* 1999;353:1509.

Couser WG. Complement inhibitors and glomerulonephritis: are we there yet? *J Am Soc Nephrol* 2003;14:815.

Eddy AA. Immune mechanisms of glomerular injury. In: Avner ED, Harmon WE, Niaudet P, eds. *Pediatric nephrology*, 5th ed. Philadelphia: Lippincott Williams & Wilkins, 2004:575.

Johnson RJ, Floege J, Couser WG, et al. Role of platelet-derived growth factor in glomerular disease. *J Am Soc Nephrol* 1993;4:119.

Rees AJ. Immunogenetics of renal disease. In: Neilson EG, Couser WG, eds. *Immunologic renal diseases,* 2nd ed. Philadelphia: Lippincott Williams & Wilkins, 2001.

Lupus Nephritis

Cameron JS. Lupus nephritis in childhood and adolescence. *Pediatr Nephrol* 1994;8:230.

McCurdy DK, Lehman JA, Bernstein B, et al. Lupus nephritis: prognostic factors in children. *Pediatrics* 1992;89:240.

Niaudet P. Treatment of lupus nephritis in children. *Pediatr Nephrol* 2000;14:158.

Sorof JM, Perez MD, Brewer ED, et al. Increasing incidence of childhood class V lupus nephritis. *J Rheumatol* 1998;25:1413.

Membranoproliferative Glomerulonephritis

Braun MC, West CD, Strife CF. Differences between membranoproliferative glomerulonephritis types I and III in long-term response to an alternate-day prednisone regimen. *Am J Kidney Dis* 1999;34:1022.

Habib R, Kleinknecht MC, Levy M. Idiopathic membranoproliferative GN in children: report of 105 cases. *Clin Nephrol* 1973;1:194.

Levin A. Management of membranoproliferative glomerulonephritis: evidence-based recommendations. *Kidney Int* 1999;70:S41.

Tarshish P, Bernstein J, Tobin J, et al. Treatment of mesangiocapillary GN with alternative day prednisone: a report of the International Study of Kidney Disease in Children. *Pediatr Nephrol* 1992;6:123.

West CD. Idiopathic membranoproliferative GN in childhood. *Pediatr Nephrol* 1992;6:96.

Membranous Glomerulonephritis

Cattran DC, Appel GB, Hebert LA, et al. Cyclosporine in patients with steroid-resistant membranous nephropathy: a randomized trial. *Kidney Int* 2001;59:1484.

Kerjaschki D. Molecular pathogenesis of membranous nephropathy. *Kidney Int* 1992;41:1090.

Makker SP. Treatment of membranous nephropathy in children. *Semin Nephrol* 2003;23:379.

Ponticelli C, Zucchelli P, Passerini P, et al. A 10-year follow-up of a randomized study with methylprednisolone and chlorambucil in membranous nephropathy. *Kidney Int* 1995;48:1600.

Reichert LJM, Koene RAP, Wetzels JFM. Prognostic factors in idiopathic membranous nephropathy. *Am J Kidney Dis* 1998;31:1.

Ruggenenti P, Chiurchiu C, Brusegan V, et al. Rituximab in idiopathic membranous nephropathy: a one year prospective study. *J Am Soc Nephrol* 2003; 14:1851.

Minimal-Change Nephrotic Syndrome

Abrass C. Clinical spectrum and complications of the nephrotic syndrome. *J Invest Med* 1997;45:143.

Hiraoka M, Tsukahara H, Matsubara K, Tsurusawa M. A randomized study of two long-course prednisolone regimens for nephrotic syndrome in children. *Am J Kidney Dis* 2003;41:1155.

Lahdenkari A-T, Kestila M, Holmberg C, et al. Nephrin gene (NPHS1) in patients with minimal change nephrotic syndrome (MCNS). *Kidney Int* 2004;65:1856.

Niaudet P, the French Society of Paediatric Nephrology. Comparison of cyclosporine and chlorambucil in the treatment of steroid-dependent idiopathic NS: a multicentre randomized controlled trial. *Pediatr Nephrol* 1992;6:1.

Orth SR, Ritz E. The nephrotic syndrome. *N Engl J Med* 1998;338:1202.

Tarshish P, Tobin JN, Bernstein J, et al. Prognostic significance of the early course of minimal change nephrotic syndrome: report of the International Study of Kidney Disease in Children. *J Am Soc Nephrol* 1997;8:769.

Nephritis of Chronic Bacteremia

Arze RS, Rashid H, Morley R, et al. Shunt nephritis: report of two cases and review of the literature. *Clin Nephrol* 1983;20:27.

Beaufils M, Morel-Maroger L, Sraer JD, et al. Acute renal failure of glomerular origin during visceral abscesses. *N Engl J Med* 1976;295:185.

Neugarten J, Gallo GR, Baldwin DS. GN in bacterial endocarditis. *Am J Kidney Dis* 1984;3:371.

Nephrotic Syndrome in Childhood

Bernare DB. Extrarenal complications of the NS. *Kidney Int* 1988;33:1184.

Filler G, Young E, Geier P, et al. Is there really an increase in non-minimal change nephrotic syndrome in children? *Am J Kidney Dis* 2003;42:1107.

Brenchley PEC. Vascular permeability factors in steroid-sensitive nephrotic syndrome and focal segmental glomerulosclerosis. *Nephrol Dial Transplant* 2003;18(suppl 6):VI21.

Rapidly Progressive Glomerulonephritis

Bolton KW. Rapidly progressive glomerulonephritis. *Semin Nephrol* 1996;16:517.

Gianviti A, Trompeter RS, Barratt TM, et al. Retrospective study of plasma exchange in patients with idiopathic rapidly progressive glomerulonephritis and vasculitis. *Arch Dis Child* 1996;75:186.

Jeanette JC. Rapidly progressive crescentic glomerulonephritis. *Kidney Int* 2003; 63:1164.

CHAPTER 326 ■ PROGRESSIVE HEREDITARY NEPHRITIS

EWA ELENBERG

Alport syndrome or *hereditary nephritis* is characterized by hematuria, proteinuria, progressive renal failure, sensorineural hearing loss, and ocular lesions. Affected male patients typically have severe disease, whereas the course in female patients tends to be mild. Alport syndrome at the molecular level results from inherited disorder of type IV collagen, a major constituent of basement membranes. To date, six chains of type IV collagen have been described: alpha1(IV) and alpha2(IV) collagens are products of the *COL4A1* and *COL4A2* genes located on chromosome 13; alpha3(IV) and alpha4(IV) collagens are products of the *COL4A3* and *COL4A4* genes located on chromosome 2; and alpha5(IV) and alpha6(IV) collagens are products of the *COL4A5* and *COL4A6* genes located on the X chromosome. The alpha1(IV) and alpha2(IV) chains form a collagen network in all basement membranes. In contrast, the alpha3(IV),

alpha4(IV), and alpha5(IV) chains appear to form a unique collagen network in only those basement membranes (glomerular, cochlear, and ocular) involved in the pathogenesis of Alport syndrome, consistent with the finding of *COL4A3*, *COL4A4*, or *COL4A5* collagen gene mutations in many patients with Alport syndrome.

GENETICS

Alport syndrome has three genetic forms of inheritance (Table 326.1). The most common, X-linked form, results from mutations of the *COL4A5* or *COL4A6* collagen gene; the less frequent, autosomal recessive form results from mutations of the *COL4A3* or *COL4A4* collagen gene. The third, very rare form

TABLE 326.1

MODES OF INHERITANCE OF ALPORT SYNDROME

Mode of Inheritance	Frequency of Inheritance	Chromosomal Localization of Affected Genes	Affected Gene	Affected Alpha Chain of Type IV Collagen
X-linked dominant	Most common	Xq22	*COL4A5*	alpha5(IV)
			COL4A6	alpha6(IV)
Autosomal recessive	Less common	2q35	*COL4A3*	alpha3(IV)
			COL4A4	alpha4(IV)
Autosomal dominant	Rare	2q35	*COL4A3*	alpha3(IV)
			COL4A4	alpha4(IV)

is the autosomal dominant, which has been linked to *COL4A3* and *COL4A4* genes.

Eighty-five percent of patients have the *X-linked dominant* form of Alport syndrome, caused by mutations in the *COL4A5* gene located in the Xq22 region that encodes for the alpha5(IV) chain of type IV collagen. Mutations of the *COL4A5* gene result in the loss of alpha5(IV) chain in basement membranes. More than 300 unique *COL4A5* mutations have been reported thus far. However, *COL4A5* mutations have been identified in only 50% of patients with X-linked Alport syndrome. Because of the X-linked dominant inheritance pattern, male patients are much more likely to develop severe disease, and affected male patients nearly always develop end-stage renal disease (ESRD). Male patients with mutations that significantly affect function of the alpha5(IV) chain develop ESRD and deafness by the third decade of life. However, male patients with mutations that have only a minor effect on the biology of the alpha5(IV) chain may not develop ESRD until later in life and may not develop deafness at all. In women, the risk of progression to ESRD is less than that in men. One specific mutation involving deletion of the 5′ ends of both the *COL4A5* and *COL4A6* genes is associated with development of leiomyomas of the esophageal tract, tracheobronchial tree, and female genital tract, in addition to early ESRD (Table 326.2).

Fifteen percent of patients have the *autosomal recessive* form caused by mutations in *COL4A3* or *COL4A4* collagen gene. Patients with *COL4A3* mutations appear to have sensorineural deafness and progress to ESRD before reaching age 30 years, regardless of gender. Autosomal recessive inheritance should be suspected when an individual exhibits typical and pathologic features of the disease but lacks a positive family history (see Table 326.2).

Fewer than 1% of patients have the *autosomal dominant* form, which is linked to *COL4A3* and *COL4A4* genes. Recently, a *COL4A3* mutation has been identified. ESRD and deafness appear to develop early. Some patients have thrombocytopenia with large platelets and impaired platelet aggregation (see Table 326.2).

TABLE 326.2

CLINICAL CHARACTERISTICS OF ALPORT SYNDROME

Mode of Inheritance	Genetic Features	Urinalysis	Clinical Characteristics
X-linked dominant	**Males** Males inherit disease from mother Father-to-son transmission not possible	Persistent proteinuria and microscopic hematuria with episodic gross hematuria	Males develop severe disease Deafness occurs early Ocular changes associated with more severe renal involvement HTN increases with age ESRD by fourth decade of life
	Females Females inherit disease from affected father or mother Females asymptomatic or with mild symptoms	Intermittent or no hematuria Proteinuria rare	Usually benign prognosis Deafness, ocular changes and HTN less frequent Low risk of progression to ESRD (increased risk of ESRD if gross hematuria, proteinuria, deafness, ocular changes) Mutation involving deletion of the 5′ ends of both the *COL4A5* and *COL4A6* genes associated with leiomyomas of the esophageal tract, tracheobronchial tree, and female genital tract, in addition to early ESRD
Autosomal recessive	History of consanguinity	Hematuria and proteinuria persistent in both male and female patients	Severe disease in affected females with mild or no symptoms in the parents Ocular changes, deafness, and HTN associated with more severe renal involvement Early onset of ESRD before age 30 years regardless of gender
Autosomal dominant	Father-to-son transmission possible	Hematuria and proteinuria	ESRD and deafness may develop early, although male patients have better prognosis than with X-linked inheritance Some families with Alport syndrome have thrombocytopenia with large platelets and deafness (Epstein syndrome)

ESRD, end-stage renal disease; HTN, hypertension.

PATHOGENESIS

Each type IV collagen molecule is composed of three alpha chains that fold ultimately into a triple helix. In Alport syndrome, mutations of *COL4A3*, *COL4A4*, or *COL4A5* can result in nonexpression of a chain or in expression of an abnormal collagen chain; in either case, the mutation does not allow that chain to associate with normal collagen chains to form the trimer. Likely, an abnormality of one alpha3(IV), alpha4(IV), or alpha5(IV) chain prevents formation of the normal network of alpha3(IV)/alpha4(IV)/alpha5(IV) collagen trimers, and the result is rapid degradation of unincorporated normal and abnormal chains. This mechanism would explain the absence of alpha3(IV), alpha4(IV), and alpha5(IV) chains, even though only one of the three genes is mutated.

CLINICAL MANIFESTATIONS

In the United States, Alport syndrome accounts for 3% of children with ESRD, and the incidence among adults with ESRD is 0.2%. Patients with Alport syndrome come from all geographic and racial backgrounds.

Hematuria is the cardinal feature at presentation of Alport syndrome, although rarely patients may present with deafness, hypertension, proteinuria, edema, or renal failure. Affected male patients have persistent microscopic hematuria and episodic gross hematuria during the first 2 decades of life. Episodes of gross hematuria occur frequently, usually appearing a few days after onset of an upper respiratory tract infection and rarely lasting longer than 2 weeks. Female patients, who are heterozygous for X-linked Alport syndrome, may have intermittent hematuria or no hematuria. Hematuria appears to be persistent in both male and female patients with the autosomal recessive form (see Table 326.2).

Proteinuria usually is absent during the first few years of life but develops eventually in male patients with the X-linked form and in both male and female patients with recessive disease, although it occurs infrequently in female patients who are heterozygous for the X-linked form. The onset of proteinuria is considered a poor prognostic sign because it usually is progressive and can culminate in the nephrotic syndrome. The risk of developing ESRD is higher in patients with proteinuria (see Table 326.2).

Hypertension also increases in incidence and severity with age. Like proteinuria, hypertension is much more likely to occur in affected male patients than in affected female patients in the X-linked form, although no gender difference exists in the autosomal recessive form.

Virtually all male patients with Alport syndrome develop chronic renal failure, which progresses steadily to ESRD over the course of a few years. Affected female patients are less likely to develop chronic renal failure and generally have a benign prognosis because the renal disease is milder. In male patients, the risk of developing ESRD by age 40 years is 90%, whereas in female patients, the risk of developing ESRD by age 40 years is 12%. Gross hematuria in childhood, the nephrotic syndrome, sensorineural deafness, anterior lenticonus, and diffuse glomerular basement membrane (GBM) thickening by observed electron microscopy are features suggestive of progressive nephritis in affected female patients.

Deafness occurs frequently, although it is not a universal finding in Alport syndrome: as many as 55% of affected male patients and 45% of female patients exhibit bilateral sensorineural deafness. In some families, deafness may occur late in life and may progress very slowly. Initially, hearing loss is detectable only by audiometry at frequencies between 2,000 and

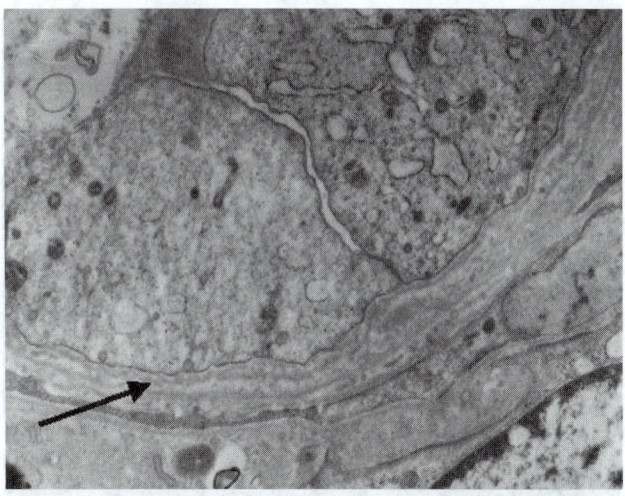

FIGURE 326.1. Electron micrograph of a segment of glomerular basement membrane (GBM) from a patient with Alport syndrome. The arrow points to thickened, split and reduplicated GBM (from Dr. John M. Hicks, Dept of Pathology, Texas Children's Hospital).

8,000 Hz. Hearing loss never is congenital, often is progressive, and always is accompanied by renal involvement. In patients with X-linked disease, hearing loss develops earlier and is more severe in male patients, who usually by adolescence have clinically apparent hearing loss extending to other frequencies. In female patients with X-linked Alport syndrome, hearing loss occurs less frequently and usually later in life. In the autosomal recessive form of Alport syndrome, no gender difference exists in the incidence or course of deafness.

Ocular defects are found in 15% to 30% of individuals with Alport syndrome. The spectrum of ocular lesions appears to be similar in X-linked and autosomal recessive forms. The ocular finding that is pathognomonic for Alport syndrome is lenticonus anterior, a protrusion of the central portion of lens into the anterior chamber, which can lead to significant visual impairment. The most common ocular lesion seen in Alport syndrome is perimacular spots, which are pigmentary changes consisting of whitish or yellowish spots surrounding the fovea (Fig. 326.1). Both perimacular spots and lenticonus anterior are associated with more severe renal involvement.

PATHOLOGY

Renal biopsy abnormalities usually are found in specimens from patients older than 5 years of age. Light microscopy and immunofluorescent findings usually are nonspecific. Electron microscopy reveals abnormalities of GBM typical for Alport syndrome. The pathognomonic features are thickening and splitting of the GBM. These thick areas have a characteristic split appearance formed by a crisscrossing network of bands of lamina densa. Lucent areas between these bands often contain multiple small, dark particles (Fig. 326.2). Some patients may have areas of thick (more than 350 nm) and thin (less than 150 nm) GBM. Heterozygous female patients may have normal-appearing GBMs or mild to moderate abnormalities.

By immunohistochemistry, the GBMs of individuals with X-linked Alport syndrome contain alpha1(IV) and alpha2(IV) collagen chains, but alpha3(IV), alpha4(IV), and alpha5(IV) chains usually are absent from the entire GBM in male patients and from stretches of the GBM in heterozygous female patients. Abnormalities also are found in other basement

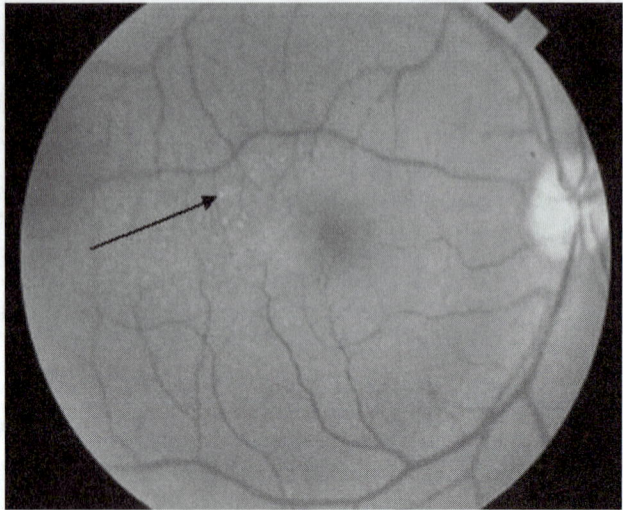

FIGURE 326.2. Perifoveal dot and fleck retinopathy (*arrow*) in a patient with Alport's syndrome. (Reprinted from *Br J Ophthalmol* 1997; 81:373.)

membranes. On the skin biopsy, the epidermal basement membrane of the normal individual expresses alpha5(IV) but not alpha3(IV) or alpha4(IV) chains; in male patients with X-linked Alport syndrome, alpha5(IV) chains are not detected, and female heterozygotes often demonstrate mosaicism. Individuals with autosomal recessive form also usually lack alpha3(IV), alpha4(IV), and alpha5(IV) collagen chains in their GBMs; however, alpha5(IV) collagen chains usually are present in the epidermis, in contrast to male patients with X-linked Alport syndrome.

Basement membranes in nonrenal tissues also are abnormal in affected individuals. In the cochlea, the stria vascularis shows changes similar to those seen in the glomerulus. In lenticonus anterior, the basement membrane forming the anterior lens capsule is thinned, allowing protrusion of the anterior lens.

DIAGNOSIS AND DIFFERENTIAL DIAGNOSIS

Diagnosis of Alport syndrome is based on findings of hematuria with or without proteinuria, hypertension, and renal failure in association with sensorineural hearing loss or ocular abnormalities and the history of familial hematuria and renal failure in at least one family member. A very detailed family history plays an essential role in establishing the diagnosis. Laboratory evaluation should search for proteinuria and renal failure. Patients suspected of having Alport syndrome should have their hearing and vision checked, and obtaining a skin biopsy may be considered, although a normal result does not exclude the diagnosis. Renal biopsy usually is reserved for individuals with proteinuria or renal insufficiency. The differential diagnosis is the same as that for other causes of hematuria, including thin basement membrane disease, immunoglobulin A nephropathy, familial idiopathic hypercalciuria, and acute poststreptococcal glomerulonephritis.

Patients with persistent hematuria but without evidence of familial involvement must be followed closely because the disease may have been transmitted by asymptomatic female carriers, or a new mutation may be present, which accounts for 18% of cases.

The genetic diagnosis is limited by the wide variety of mutations. At present, the diagnosis of asymptomatic carrier status or prenatal diagnosis is possible by linkage analysis or by direct characterization of a specific gene mutation in previously tested family members; however, few centers are performing such analyses.

THERAPY

No specific therapy is available for Alport syndrome. Angiotensin-converting enzyme inhibitors may be tried to decrease proteinuria. Chronic renal failure is treated with dialysis or renal transplantation. Overall graft survival in patients with Alport syndrome is good and is not different from that seen in other transplant recipients, even though 2% to 3% of patients irreversibly lose graft function owing to development of anti-GBM antibodies (the donor kidney contains a type IV collagen antigen that is absent in the host). In the future, gene therapy would be most optimal treatment.

Hearing aids temporarily benefit patients who have hearing loss. If the hearing loss is bilateral and extremely severe, cochlear implants should be considered. Retinal changes require no therapy because they do not interfere with vision.

Suggested Readings

Kashtan CE. Alport syndrome and thin glomerular basement disease. *J Am Soc Nephrol* 1998;9:1736.

Kashtan, CE. Alport syndrome: an inherited disorder of renal, ocular, and cochlear basement membranes. *Medicine (Baltimore)* 1999;78:338.

Jais JP, Knebelmann B, Giatras I, et al. X-linked Alport syndrome: natural history in 195 families and genotype-phenotype correlations in males. *J Am Soc Nephrol* 2000;11:649.

Jais JP, Knebelmann B, Giatras I, et al. X-linked Alport syndrome: natural history and genotype-phenotype correlations in girls and women belonging to 195 families. *J Am Soc Nephrol* 2003;14:2603.

CHAPTER 327 ■ BENIGN FAMILIAL HEMATURIA

EWA ELENBERG

Benign familial hematuria (BFH) also is known as *benign persistent hematuria, benign essential hematuria,* or *thin basement membrane disease* (TBMD). The term *benign* implies benign clinical course with good prognosis, and the term *familial* implies occurrence of hematuria in other family members.

BHF is a very common finding, occurring in more than 1% of the population. Affected individuals usually present with persistent or intermittent microscopic and occasionally gross hematuria. Hematuria usually is "dysmorphic" on phase contrast microscopy, with red cells of irregular size and shape. Proteinuria, progression to renal failure, or extrarenal symptoms such as hearing loss are not present. Physical examination is normal, and no abnormalities are noted with audiometric and ophthalmologic examinations. Laboratory studies reveal normal renal function and platelet count. Screening typically identifies hematuria in other family members, but these individuals fail to demonstrate hearing loss, renal failure, or proteinuria. Conversely, one-third of individuals with BFH may not have evidence of familial occurrence because the disease may be sporadic.

Renal biopsies from affected individuals are normal by light microscopy and immunofluorescence. Electron microscopy reveals the characteristic finding of focal or widespread thinning of the glomerular basement membrane (GBM), which is the hallmark of this disease, hence the term TBMD. However, these thin segments of GBM are not interspersed with segments of thick and split GBM typically seen in Alport syndrome.

The inheritance pattern of BFH is mostly autosomal dominant; however, in some cases, inheritance appears to be autosomal-recessive, or it occurs sporadically. Because recent reports have shown that both BFH and autosomally inherited Alport syndrome are linked to the *COL4A3/COL4A4* locus, some researchers have hypothesized that the pathogenesis of at least some cases of TBMD results from mutations similar to those of Alport syndrome. Many *COL4A3* and *COL4A4* mutations have been reported in BFH, although the detection rate of mutations is low. The studies suggest that BFH may represent the carrier state for autosomal recessive Alport syndrome or at least is affected by the same genes. BFH may be a phenotypic variant of Alport syndrome; if so, the definitions and the differential diagnoses of both these diseases may have to be revisited.

The two most important conditions in the differential diagnosis of BFH are immunoglobulin A nephropathy and Alport syndrome. The lack of proteinuria and progressive renal failure are the most suggestive features of BFH. All other causes of hematuria should be considered because BFH is a diagnosis of exclusion. The physical examination and laboratory investigations are normal. Because the transmission of BFH is mostly autosomal dominant, microscopic hematuria usually is found in the urine of parents, siblings, or other family members, despite the absence of a family history of renal disease. Obtaining a renal biopsy is not necessary, although when it is performed, it often reveals thinning of the GBM. However, in some patients, particularly children and heterozygous female members of families with otherwise typical features of Alport syndrome, isolated GBM attenuation also may be seen as a sole finding. Thus, diagnosis of Alport syndrome cannot be discarded based on clinical and morphologic features alone. In Alport syndrome, the progression to chronic renal failure may occur at a very late age. Patients with the diagnosis of TBMD should be followed on a regular basis because cases of patients with an initial diagnosis of TBMD who developed renal failure at later age and were found to have Alport syndrome have been reported.

The prognosis of BFH is very good; however, patients should be monitored yearly for the development of proteinuria, hypertension, or renal impairment that would necessitate the revision of the initial diagnosis of BFH. Moreover, the appearance of chronic renal failure in any family member requires careful reevaluation of the original diagnosis. Thus, the diagnosis of BFH should be made with caution.

Suggested Readings

Atkin CL, Gregory MC, Border WA. Alport syndrome. In: Schrier RW, Gottschalk CW, eds. *Diseases of the kidney,* 4th ed. Boston: Little, Brown, 1988:617.

Ozen S, Ertoy D, Heidet L, et al. Benign familial hematuria associated with a novel COL4A4 mutation. *Pediatr Nephrol* 2001;16:874.

Savige J, Rana K, Tonna S, et al. Thin basement membrane nephropathy. *Kidney Int* 2003;64:1169.

Yoshikawa N, Matsuyama S, Iijima K, et al. Benign familial hematuria. *Arch Pathol Lab Med* 1988;112:794.

CHAPTER 328 ■ FAMILIAL JUVENILE NEPHRONOPHTHISIS

EWA ELENBERG

Familial juvenile nephronophthisis (NPH), also termed *nephronophthisis type 1 (NPH1)*, is an autosomal recessive, progressive tubulointerstitial kidney disease. It is characterized clinically by polyuria, polydipsia, anemia, growth failure, and progressive renal failure. Pathologic characteristic features include chronic tubulointerstitial nephritis and medullary cysts. NPH is the most common genetic cause of end-stage renal disease (ESRD) in children; it accounts for 1% of cases of ESRD in the United States.

The renal pathologic features, clinical findings, and course are similar to those of medullary cystic kidney disease; however, the two are distinct syndromes. NPH is inherited as an autosomal recessive pattern, patients average 10 years of age at disease onset, ESRD develops early, and the disease often is associated with nonrenal anomalies. In contrast, medullary cystic kidney disease is inherited as an autosomal dominant pattern, patients average 28 years of age at onset of disease, ESRD develops late, and nonrenal anomalies are rare findings.

Juvenile NPH is caused by a defect in gene locus, *NPHP1*, which is mapped to chromosome 2q13. The *NPHP1* gene and its product, nephrocystin, a novel protein encoded by this gene, have been identified. The function of nephrocystin is unknown, but one hypothesis is that it may be involved in focal adhesion and/or adherens junction signaling.

PATHOLOGY

Kidney biopsy reveals a characteristic triad of disintegration of the tubular basement membrane (TBM), tubular atrophy with cyst development, and interstitial cell infiltration with fibrosis. Typically, the TBM has pronounced thickening and multilayering that represent the most characteristic histologic features of NPH. Small medullary cysts, located at the corticomedullary border, are found in as many as 75% of patients. Medullary cysts arise from both the distal convoluted and collecting tubules. The nature of the primary pathogenic mechanism leading to the NPH is unclear, although likely a defect in the TBM structure may be primarily responsible for cyst formation.

CLINICAL MANIFESTATIONS AND COMPLICATIONS

Children with NPH present with polydipsia, polyuria, anemia, and weakness and develop progressive azotemia. Fewer than one-half of children with NPH present with growth failure; edema and hypertension are rare findings. The tubular damage present in NPH usually causes a urine-concentrating defect with subsequent development of polyuria and polydipsia. The inability to concentrate urine maximally precedes development of azotemia and usually is the first sign of the disease, occurring in patients at around 4 years of age. Tubular damage also may lead to a salt-wasting state, which may explain the need for salt replacement and lack of hypertension and edema. Patients may be hypokalemic and have renal tubular acidosis. Urinalysis is unremarkable except for mild tubular proteinuria. Progressive renal failure often remains undetected until it has reached an advanced stage. Renal failure progresses to ESRD within 1 to 10 years and contributes to growth failure and anemia. The severity of anemia often is out of proportion to the degree of renal failure.

Patients with juvenile NPH also may have an extrarenal organ involvement including skeletal and ophthalmologic abnormalities, cerebellar ataxia, mental retardation, and hepatic fibrosis. The most common ophthalmologic disorders are tapetoretinal degeneration and retinitis pigmentosa associated with blindness. The combination of NPH1 and retinal abnormalities is known as the renal-retinal syndrome or Senior-Løken syndrome. NPH1 can occur in combination with Cogan syndrome, Joubert syndrome type B, and cone-shaped epiphyses in conorenal syndrome, also known as *Saldino-Mainzer syndrome*.

DIAGNOSIS

Patients presenting with typical signs and symptoms of NPH are diagnosed easily when siblings have NPH. However, a family history of sibling involvement is lacking in 50% of patients. In these cases, an ultrasound finding of hyperechogenic kidneys of smaller size with diminished corticomedullary differentiation and medullary cysts in a child with a chronic renal failure is highly suggestive of NPH, although the lack of cysts does not rule out the diagnosis of NPH.

Sporadic cases of medullary cystic disease occurring in younger patients may be indistinguishable from NPH unless the pattern of inheritance becomes clear. The sizes of the kidneys and cysts, as well as the locations of the cysts, usually enable one to distinguish between NPH (small kidneys with cysts at the corticomedullary junction) and polycystic kidney disease (large kidneys with uniform distribution of cysts); however, late-onset infantile polycystic kidney disease with hepatic fibrosis can be confused with NPH, and renal biopsy may be needed to establish the diagnosis. Large medullary cysts in a teenager suggest medullary sponge kidney, but these patients do not develop renal failure. The finding of medullary cysts renders the diagnosis of dysplastic or hypoplastic kidneys unlikely. Reflux nephropathy and chronic pyelonephritis can resemble NPH at presentation. Radiologic studies must be performed to rule out obstructive uropathy as a cause of tubular damage. Finally, the genetic diagnosis of a large deletion of the *NPHP1* locus on chromosome 2q13 is possible, but the lack of detection of mutations in the *NPHP1* gene does not exclude the diagnosis of NPH.

THERAPY

Therapy for patients with NPH is symptomatic. Salt wasting is treated with salt supplements, metabolic acidosis with alkali, hypokalemia with potassium, polyuria with free access to water, and chronic renal failure with the usual supportive therapy. Patients tolerate dialysis and renal transplantation well. The disease does not recur in patients with transplanted kidneys. Genetic counseling is recommended for all families of children with NPH.

Suggested Readings

Hildebrandt F, Omram H. New insights: nephronophthisis-medullary cystic kidney disease. *Pediatr Nephrol* 2001;16:168.

Hildebrandt F, Otto E. Molecular genetics of nephronophthisis and medullary cystic kidney disease. *J Am Soc Nephrol* 2000;11:1753.

Hildebrandt F, Strahm B, Nothwang HG, et al. Molecular genetic identification of families with juvenile nephronophthisis type 1: rate of progression to renal failure. *Kidney Int* 1997;51:261.

Konrad M, Saunier S, Calado J, et al. Familial juvenile nephronophthisis. *J Mol Med* 1998;76:310.

CHAPTER 329 ■ NEPHROPATHY OF DIABETES MELLITUS

L. LEIGHTON HILL

Diabetes mellitus is the leading cause of end-stage renal disease (ESRD) worldwide. In the United States, diabetic nephropathy accounts for approximately 40% of patients entering dialysis and transplantation programs. Thirty to 40% of patients with insulin-dependent diabetes mellitus (IDDM) eventually develop diabetic nephropathy, and most of these cases progress to ESRD unless preventive and therapeutic measures prove effective over the long term. ESRD from diabetes rarely is seen in the second decade of life, but it is a common development in the third, fourth, and fifth decades. Of great interest and at least partly unexplained at this time is the finding that more than one-half of patients with IDDM do not develop significant nephropathy, regardless of the duration and sometimes the degree of metabolic control. With the tremendous increase in obesity among children, adolescents, and young adults in this country, type 2 or non–insulin-dependent diabetes mellitus (NIDDM) is an emerging epidemic in the pediatric age group. Nephropathy appears to be at least as common in type 2 diabetes as in type 1, so a further significant increase in diabetic nephropathy and ESRD can be expected to occur during the next several decades.

NATURAL HISTORY

The development of significant dipstick-positive proteinuria (30 mg/dL or higher) usually is the first clinical sign of the nephropathy of diabetes mellitus (type 1 or type 2). However, before proteinuria develops, several hemodynamic and morphologic changes occur in the kidney. At the time of diagnosis of type 1 diabetes, increases in glomerular filtration rate, renal blood flow, and filtration fraction are present. Renal size often is increased, and microalbuminuria may be present. These early functional changes appear to be related to glycemic control because improvement in metabolic control is associated with a return of these parameters toward normal. The disappearance of microalbuminuria usually is followed by several years of normal albuminuria. By 5 to 15 years' duration, 30% to 40% of the patients with diabetes mellitus develop persistent microalbuminuria. The prevalence of hypertension, a condition that accelerates the progression of kidney disease, is greater in

diabetic patients with microalbuminuria. The definition of microalbuminuria varies, but the most widely accepted is that of Mogensen, who uses a rate between 20 and 200 μg/minute, with less than 20 μg/minute classified as normal albuminuria and more than 200 μg/minute classified as clinical or overt proteinuria. A value of 20 μg/minute equals approximately 30 mg/day, and 200 μg/minute equals just under 300 mg/24 hours. Random spot urines measuring albumin-to-creatinine ratios have been found to be reliable in the detection of microalbuminuria and overt proteinuria. An albumin-over-creatinine ratio of 0.5 or higher is indicative of clinical or overt proteinuria. Many investigators consider microalbuminuria a reliable predictor of later overt clinical proteinuria, chronic renal insufficiency, and other microvascular complications. However, because microalbuminuria can regress, a demonstration of persistence of microalbuminuria is important. Clinically detectable overt proteinuria in diabetic patients with nephropathy generally is found between 10 and 30 years after the diagnosis of IDDM has been established, with the peak incidence occurring 15 to 20 years after diagnosis. Azotemia usually occurs within 5 to 10 years of the onset of clinically significant proteinuria, and ESRD usually ensues within 1 to 2 years of the development of azotemia. Hypertension is present in approximately three-fourths of patients with significant nephropathy, and the nephrotic syndrome occurs in 5% to 10%. However, this sequence and the timing are not invariable, and extensive nephropathy can occur without proteinuria. The timing and sequence of changes in the kidney in type 2 diabetes in children and adolescents have not been studied as thoroughly, and because the onset of type 2 disease is not as abrupt and distinct, the duration of diabetes often is not as clear. Numerous therapeutic interventions apparently have been successful in altering the natural course of diabetic nephropathy.

PATHOLOGY

The most common pathologic lesion seen in diabetic nephropathy (in type 1 or type 2 diabetes) is diffuse glomerular sclerosis, a generalized widening of the glomerular mesangium with matrix material. The matrix material ultimately invades the subendothelial space, occludes the capillary lumina, and reduces filtration surface. Other pathologic changes include nodular glomerular sclerosis (Kimmelstiel-Wilson lesion), thickening of the glomerular basement membrane, afferent and efferent glomerular arteriolar hyalinosis, tubulointerstitial changes, and "capsular drops" in the parietal Bowman capsule. The structural progression of nephropathy appears to be similar in type 1 and type 2 diabetes.

PATHOGENESIS OF VASCULAR COMPLICATIONS

The pathogenesis of diabetic nephropathy is multifactorial. The preponderance of scientific data, especially those of the Diabetes Control and Complications Trial Research Group, indicates that insulin deficiency, with the associated metabolic, hormonal, and physiologic disturbances, is the principal cause of diabetic nephropathy and other microangiopathy in IDDM. Genetic susceptibility to nephropathy probably also is required, partly explaining why more than half of patients with diabetes do not develop significant nephropathy. Hyperglycemia from insulin deficiency (relative or absolute) appears to be clearly necessary for the development of nephropathy. Hormonal alterations (in growth hormone, glucagon, kinins, renin, angiotension, prostaglandins) also appear to be important. A correlation between nonenzymatic glycosylation of tissue and long-term complications in diabetes has been found. Diminution of fixed negative charges (e.g., glycosaminoglycans) in the basement membrane may reduce the repulsive electrostatic interaction with negatively charged plasma proteins and thereby increase the filtration and excretion of proteins. Over the years, evidence has accumulated that suggests a role for functional hemodynamic changes in the generation of diabetic nephropathy. Hostetter proposed that microvascular dilatation occurs in the diabetic kidney, with increased glomerular blood flow, glomerular hyperfiltration, and an increase in mean glomerular transcapillary hydraulic pressure difference. These investigators pointed out that the pathologic lesion of diabetic nephropathy (diffuse glomerular sclerosis) is the same lesion that occurs in other entities associated with whole-kidney and single-nephron hyperfiltration states, such as high-protein feeding and reduction in renal mass. Elevated glomerular capillary pressure may be the principal cause of the mesangial expansion and sclerosis. Probably, both hemodynamic factors and biochemical changes contribute to the development of renal damage in both type 1 and type 2 diabetes.

PREVENTION AND TREATMENT OF NEPHROPATHY

The studies of the Diabetes Control and Complications Trial Research Group demonstrated that meticulous metabolic control of IDDM, especially early in the course of the disease, is beneficial in preventing or at least postponing the microangiopathy in genetically susceptible patients with IDDM. Once nephropathy is manifest clinically by proteinuria, metabolic control is less likely to have an influence. Nonetheless, most clinicians experienced in the care of patients with diabetes mellitus continue to attempt to achieve excellent control of blood sugar, even in patients with established nephropathy and those with early to moderate renal insufficiency.

The American Diabetes Association recommends yearly testing for urinary protein in all patients with type 2 diabetes and for those with type 1 disease beginning 5 years after the onset of the disease or at puberty. Once proteinuria is discovered by dipstick testing (30 mg/dL or greater), it should be semiquantitated using early morning spot urinary protein-over-creatinine ratios, and these measurements then should be repeated two to three times a year along with serum creatinine determinations once a year. Postural or orthostatic proteinuria, a common finding in teenagers, should be excluded. A serum creatinine determination should be obtained yearly even in the absence of proteinuria after 10 years' duration of diabetes. Blood pressure should be measured routinely at each visit.

Control of blood pressure in the patient with diabetes is extremely important at any stage of renal involvement. Very strong evidence exists that progression of renal disease can be retarded by adequate control of blood pressure; therefore, good to excellent control of blood pressure is absolutely mandatory in the patient with IDDM or NIDDM. The target for control should be maximum systolic pressures in the 120 to 130 mm Hg range and diastolic pressures in the 75 to 80 mm Hg range. Several classes of antihypertensive agents have been used successfully, but the most efficacious are the angiotensin-converting enzyme (ACE) inhibitors. These drugs not only lower systemic blood pressure but also appear to reduce intrarenal hydrostatic pressures. Therefore, they seem to affect major factors in the progression of diabetic nephropathy directly. The ACE inhibitors produce a decrease in urinary protein excretion in diabetic patients with and without hypertension. Another category of drugs targeting the renin-angiotensin system are the angiotensin II receptor blockers (ARBs). The ARBs appear to have a renoprotective effect comparable to that of the ACE inhibitors in patients with type 1 diabetes. Studies are currently in progress to evaluate the use of ACE inhibitors and ARBs in the diabetic nephropathy of patients with type 2 disease. The data supporting the efficacy of ACE inhibitors in slowing the progression of renal disease in type 2 diabetes have been conflicting, but ARBs appear to delay progression in these patients. Combinations of ACE inhibitors and ARBs in preventing the progression of microalbuminuria to overt nephropathy and the progression of overt nephropathy to renal insufficiency have been proposed, but additional clinical trial data are needed. Other measures that should be taken in attempting to retard the progression of diabetic nephropathy include the use of antiplatelet agents, treatment of anemia, restriction of dietary protein and salt, lipid lowering, cessation of smoking, weight loss in the obese, and physical exercise.

The management of ESRD in patients with diabetes includes comprehensive medical management of renal failure, dialysis, and renal transplantation (see Chapter 323). If a renal transplant is undertaken, transplantation of pancreatic tissue also should be done to improve glycemic control. An additional problem that may be encountered with transplantation is the recurrence of diabetic nephropathy in the transplanted kidney.

Suggested Readings

American Diabetes Association and the National Kidney Foundation. Consensus development conference on the diagnosis and management of nephropathy in patients with diabetes mellitus. *Diabetes Care* 1994;17:1357.

Brenner BM, Cooper ME, de Zeeuw D, et al. Effects of losartan on renal and cardiovascular outcomes in patients with type 2 diabetes and nephropathy. *N Engl J Med* 2001;345:861.

Diabetes Control and Complications Research Group. Effect of intensive therapy on the development and progression of diabetic nephropathy in the Diabetes Control and Complications Trial. *Kidney Int* 1995;47:1703.

Fioretto P, Mogensen CE, Mauer SM. Diabetic nephropathy. In: Holliday MA, Barratt TM, Avner ED, eds. *Pediatric nephrology*, 3rd ed. Baltimore: Williams & Wilkins, 1994:576.

Hostetter TH. Mechanisms of diabetic nephropathy. *Am J Kidney Dis* 1994; 23:188.

Jacobsen P, Anderson S, Rossing K, et al. Dual blockade of the renin-angiotensin system versus maximal recommended dose of ACE inhibition in diabetic nephropathy. *Kidney Int* 2003;63:1874.

Mogensen CE. Microalbuminuria as a predictor of clinical diabetic nephropathy. *Kidney Int* 1987;31:673.

CHAPTER 330 ■ SICKLE CELL NEPHROPATHY

EWA ELENBERG

Children with sickle cell anemia, and often those with sickle cell trait, may present with a wide spectrum of significant urinary tract disorders, including hyposthenuria, acidosis, hematuria, proteinuria, nephrotic syndrome, chronic renal failure, and urinary tract infection (Box 330.1).

Hyposthenuria (inability to concentrate the urine maximally) is a common finding resulting from chronic damage to the renal medulla. Medullary environment, which is hyperosmolar, acidotic, and hypoxic, predisposes to sickling of red blood cells. Deformed sickled cells may obstruct blood flow in medullary vessels, thus leading to disruption of the normal concentrating mechanism. Hyposthenuria first appears in young children and is reversible by administration of multiple blood transfusions. However, hyposthenuria is irreversible in adolescents, and maximal urine concentration is approximately 450 mOsm/L. Clinically, children with hyposthenuria present with polyuria and often with enuresis; they are at greater risk for dehydration. Patients with sickle cell anemia also may have a mild defect in maximal urinary acidification (inability to decrease urine pH to less than 5.3) and potassium excretion by the distal tubule; however, clinically significant hyperchloremic metabolic acidosis and hyperkalemia are rare findings, even during sickle cell crises.

Microscopic or gross hematuria is a common finding, and episodes can last from days to months. The onset of hematuria usually is sudden and unprovoked, although some cases are associated with trauma, exercise, upper respiratory tract infection, or sickle cell crisis. Bleeding usually is painless, unless it is accompanied by papillary necrosis. The hematuria usually is unilateral, with the left kidney involved four times more frequently than the right. Most of the episodes are self-limited in children. However, massive, life-threatening, and prolonged periods of gross hematuria, which rarely occur in children, may be seen in men. The occlusion of blood flow in vasa recta may lead to papillary necrosis, a frequent complication of sickle cell nephropathy. Papillary necrosis presents usually as painless gross hematuria, although it may present in rare instances as renal colic secondary to the passage of blood clots or sloughed papillae. Intravenous pyelography is the method of choice for the radiographic demonstration of renal papillary necrosis. Membranoproliferative glomerulonephritis, renal artery thrombosis, and renal vein thrombosis are other complications of sickle hemoglobinopathy that can lead to hematuria.

Proteinuria is a frequent finding. It is seen in 20% to 30% of patients with sickle cell disease, who may develop persistent proteinuria or frank nephrotic syndrome. Glomerular capillary hypertension is thought to mediate proteinuria. Sudden edema or nephrotic-range proteinuria initially may suggest idiopathic nephrotic syndrome, but it is a rare finding. Renal vein thrombosis always should be excluded because of the predisposition of patients with hemoglobin SS to venous thrombosis.

Commonly, renal biopsy in patients with sickle cell nephropathy reveals glomerular hypertrophy and focal segmental glomerulosclerosis. Less common findings include membranoproliferative glomerulonephritis, isolated mesangial hypercellularity, membranous glomerulopathy, and minimal lesion nephrosis. In a few cases, immune complex nephropathy may be seen. Medullary lesions consist of edema, focal scarring, and atrophy. Renal papillary necrosis appears focally.

Patients with sickle cell disease are at higher risk for having acute renal failure secondary to dehydration, renal thrombosis, renal papillary necrosis, or myoglobinuria. Proteinuria, hypertension, severe anemia, and hematuria are predictors of chronic renal failure. Sickle cell disease is a rare cause of end-stage renal disease in pediatric patients and accounts for fewer than 1% of patients with end-stage renal disease. Children with sickle cell anemia or sickle cell trait also have increased susceptibility to urinary tract infections, likely related to altered immune response.

THERAPY

No specific treatment is available for sickle cell nephropathy. Episodes of dehydration, acidosis, hypoxia, infection, and severe anemia should be treated aggressively. Children with hyposthenuria should have free access to water. The use of angiotensin-converting enzyme inhibitors is recommended to decrease proteinuria and possibly to prevent the development of chronic renal failure. The use of corticosteroids may have beneficial effects in some patients, although most of patients are steroid resistant.

The gross hematuria usually is self-limited and resolves spontaneously; however, recurrences are common. Bed rest is recommended until significant bleeding stops (to avoid dislodging clots), followed by no participation in active sports for the next 3 to 4 weeks. The use of intravenous hydration in conjunction with diuretics can be attempted. Transfusions may be necessary for patients with excessive blood loss. Other therapies used less commonly, secondary to uncertain value, include urine alkalinization, hyperbaric oxygen inhalation therapy, administration of triglycyl vasopressin, oral urea to inhibit

---

| BOX 330.1 | Clinical and Laboratory Manifestations of Sickle Cell Nephropathy |

Enuresis
Hematuria
Urinary tract infection
Renal failure
Edema
Proteinuria
Acidosis
Hyposthenuria
Hypoalbuminemia

sickling, and epsilon-aminocaproic acid, which inhibits potentiators of urinary tract bleeding such as urokinase. Arteriographic localization and local embolization of the affected renal segment are indicated in patients with uncontrolled bleeding. Rarely, unilateral nephrectomy is required.

Patients with end-stage renal disease are treated with dialysis and renal transplantation. Short-term graft survival is similar to that of other patients; however, long-term graft survival tends to be lower in patients with sickle cell disease.

Suggested Readings

Falk RJ, Jennette JC. Sickle cell nephropathy. *Adv Nephrol* 1994;23:133.
Pham PTT, Pham PCT, Wilkinson AH, Lew SQ. Renal abnormalities in sickle cell disease. *Kidney Int* 2000;57:1.
Powars DR, Elliott-Mills DD, Chan L, et al. Chronic renal failure in sickle cell disease: risk factors, clinical course, and mortality. *Ann Intern Med* 1991;115:614.
Saborio P, Scheinman JI. Sickle cell nephropathy. *J Am Soc Nephrol* 1999;10: 187.

CHAPTER 331 ■ PRIMARY HYPEROXALURIA (OXALOSIS)

DAVID R. POWELL

EPIDEMIOLOGY

Primary hyperoxaluria (PH) encompasses two rare autosomal recessive disorders associated with excess production and urinary excretion of oxalic acid; often the result is progression to renal failure secondary to nephrocalcinosis or recurrent calcium oxalate nephrolithiasis. PH type I (PH1), with a prevalence of 1 to 2 per million individuals, is characterized by increased urinary oxalate and glycolate resulting from deficiency of hepatic alanine-glyoxylate aminotransferase (AGT). PH type II (PH2) is caused by deficiency of glyoxylate reductase/D-glycerate dehydrogenase, resulting in increased urinary oxalate and L-glycerate. Because PH2 is a much rarer form of PH, this discussion concentrates on PH1.

Patients with PH1 lack AGT activity in liver peroxisomes. Multiple phenotypes exist, including loss of AGT activity owing to intraperoxisomal aggregation or to impaired pyridoxine binding, loss of AGT protein from accelerated degradation, and mistargeting of active AGT to mitochondria instead of peroxisomes. More than 40 specific AGT mutations now are known, with each of the foregoing phenotypes linked to at least one mutation. In the absence of peroxisomal AGT, glyoxylate is metabolized inappropriately to oxalate and glycolate. Oxalate is removed from the body by renal excretion; in PH, the urine is oversaturated with oxalate in an attempt to compensate for excessive oxalate production. Calcium oxalate crystals then precipitate in renal tubules and collecting ducts, thus leading to chronic renal injury.

CLINICAL MANIFESTATIONS AND COMPLICATIONS

The onset and severity of renal involvement vary in patients with PH. Two-thirds of patients are symptomatic before reaching the age of 5 years, and most present with recurrent episodes of abdominal pain, gross hematuria, and other evidence of urolithiasis. Renal insufficiency, growth failure, and renal tubular acidosis may be present at the time of diagnosis. Abdominal radiography shows urolithiasis and nephrocalcinosis, and renal ultrasonography reveals diffuse, exaggerated echogenicity; kidney size usually is normal. Although more common causes than PH exist for urolithiasis in children, this diagnosis accounts for 1% to 2% of the total cases and must be considered. As many as 10% of patients with PH present in infancy, often with renal failure. The evaluation of any infant with renal failure should include abdominal radiographic and ultrasound studies, which demonstrate the same findings in infants with PH as found in older children, except urolithiasis is absent. In infants with cortical nephrocalcinosis and renal failure, possible causes are PH, chronic glomerulonephritis, and renal cortical necrosis.

DIAGNOSIS

Documenting the presence or absence of PH in patients with urolithiasis or nephrocalcinosis requires the collection of a 24-hour urine sample for oxalate or a spot urine sample for the oxalate-to-creatinine ratio in the younger child. High urinary oxalate levels in two collections confirm the diagnosis of hyperoxaluria. The diagnosis of PH1 may be established by demonstrating high urinary glycolate levels in the absence of secondary causes of hyperoxaluria, such as ethylene glycol ingestion or disease or resection of the distal ileum. In children presenting with chronic renal failure and oliguria or anuria, hyperoxaluria may be impossible to document, and serum oxalate assays may prove unreliable. However, oxalate and glycolate assays on whole spent dialysate may provide the diagnosis. The diagnosis is supported by demonstrating calcium oxalate deposits in kidneys and in extrarenal sites such as skin, retina, joints, and bone. Kidney biopsy can be striking when birefringent, pyramid-shaped crystals form rosettes within proximal tubular lumina; positive staining with alizarin red suggests that these are calcium oxalate crystals. Other kidney findings are nonspecific; glomeruli appear normal, but tubular epithelium is destroyed, and severe interstitial inflammation and fibrosis often are present. In most patients, the diagnosis of PH1 is best made or confirmed by molecular analysis of chromosomal DNA to identify specific mutations and/or by directly characterizing AGT abnormalities in liver tissue.

The natural history of untreated PH is gradual progression to a uremic death. In the past, more than 80% of patients with PH died of renal failure by age 20 years; 90% were dead within 10 years of diagnosis. The emphasis now is on establishing a diagnosis early, before significant renal damage has occurred, and on avoiding further renal injury by preventing calcium oxalate precipitation in kidneys. Diagnosis of affected siblings of a proband can be established early because urinary oxalate levels and renal echogenicity on ultrasonography may be increased in the first month of life. However, prenatal diagnosis is preferable. DNA isolated from chorionic villus or amniotic fluid samples obtained in the first trimester can be used to identify specific mutations or, if mutations are not identified, to perform DNA linkage analysis if DNA samples from family members and the proband also are available. In the absence of specific mutations or of family or proband DNA, fetal liver biopsy performed after 16 weeks' gestation can be used to test for the presence and activity of AGT.

PREVENTION

Certain measures may prevent formation of stones and renal damage in patients with PH who are not yet uremic. The most important measure is increasing urine output with liberal fluid intake. Usually, a fluid intake of 3 to 4 $L/m^2/day$ lowers the urinary oxalate level to less than the accepted target of 250 mmol/L. This intake should be divided equally throughout the day; in small children, administration of fluids by nasogastric tube may be required. Other important measures include ensuring that the patient has high intakes of citrate, orthophosphate, and magnesium, which inhibit formation of calcium oxalate crystals in urine. Treatment with pyridoxine, a cofactor for AGT activity, may increase glyoxalate metabolism by this enzyme in some patients with PH1; the resulting fall in production of oxalate can be recognized by detecting a fall in excretion of urinary oxalate over the course of weeks to months. Finally, the body oxalate burden can be lowered to a limited extent by avoiding oxalate-rich foods and ascorbic acid.

Patients with PH and chronic renal failure continue to overproduce oxalate. Because oxalate no longer is removed by the kidneys, the body burden increases. No single form of dialysis adequately removes oxalate from the body, so extrarenal deposits accumulate, leading to disabling bone disease, cardiac dysrhythmias, and peripheral vascular insufficiency. Renal transplantation can be successful in patients with PH and renal failure if the body oxalate burden is not too large at the time of transplantation, if episodes of graft rejection are minimized, and if ongoing calcium oxalate precipitation in the kidneys is minimized. Nonetheless, even patients with initially successful renal transplants are at great risk for developing long-term complications and loss of graft function because of their underlying PH. This risk has led to use of combined liver-kidney transplantation as a certain means to eliminate oxalate overproduction. To date, the results of this approach are encouraging. However, replacing the abnormal AGT gene is preferable to replacing the entire liver, which is otherwise normal; for this reason, strategies to treat PH1 with gene therapy are being studied. At present, aggressive management of children with PH and renal failure is justifiable, but therapy should be individualized and should take into account numerous factors including the specific mutation(s), residual AGT activity, pyridioxine responsiveness, and body oxalate burden.

Suggested Readings

Broyer M, Jouvet P, Niaudet P, et al. Management of oxalosis. *Kidney Int* 1996; 49:S93.

Danpure CJ, Purdue PE. Primary hyperoxaluria. In: Scriver CR, Beaudet AL, Sly SW, Valle D, eds. *The metabolic basis of inherited disease,* 7th ed. New York: McGraw-Hill, 1994:933.

Jamieson NV. The results of combined liver/kidney transplantation for primary hyperoxaluria (PH1) 1984 to 1997: the European PH1 transplant registry report. *J Nephrol* 1998;11:S36.

Pirulli D, Marangella M, Amoroso A. Primary hyperoxaluria: genotype-phenotype correlation. *J Nephrol* 2003;16:297.

Zhang X, Roe S, Hou Y, et al. Crystal structure of AGT and the relationship between genotype and enzymatic phenotype in primary hyperoxaluria type 1. *J Mol Biol* 2003;331:643.

CHAPTER 332 ■ NAIL-PATELLA SYNDROME (HEREDITARY ONYCHOOSTEODYSPLASIA)

DAVID R. POWELL

The cardinal features of nail-patella syndrome (NPS) are dysplastic nails and hypoplastic patellae; some patients have iliac horns, knee and elbow abnormalities, cataracts, and renal disease. NPS is inherited as an autosomal dominant disorder, probably with full penetrance but with variable expressivity. Affected individuals have heterozygous mutations in the transcription factor *LMX1B*. Impaired development of dorsal limb structures such as nails and patellae is consistent with an essential role for *LMX1B* in orchestrating normal dorsal-ventral limb patterning in vertebrates.

Renal disease aggregates in some kindreds with NPS while sparing others. In kindreds with a history of nephropathy, 50% of family members develop renal disease, and 15% progress to renal failure. The presence of nephropathy or renal failure in parents with NPS does not increase the risk of the same complication developing in their children. Most patients present with proteinuria, which may lead to nephrotic syndrome; occasionally, NPS is associated with congenital nephrosis. Chronic renal failure has been reported in children younger than 10 years, but usually it develops in teenagers and young adults, sometimes after they have had asymptomatic proteinuria for years.

Kidney biopsy specimens from patients with NPS have characteristic findings by electron microscopy; they include thickened and split glomerular basement membranes (GBMs), fibrillar or periodic collagen-like material in both GBM and mesangial matrix, and fused podocyte foot processes. The degree of abnormality revealed on electron microscopy does not correlate with a loss of kidney function in NPS, however, because changes have been present in biopsy specimens of patients with NPS who never developed renal dysfunction. *LMX1B* protein stimulates expression of the kidney-specific alpha-3 and alpha-4 chains of type IV collagen required for normal development of GBM and also stimulates expression of podocyte genes critical to the kidney's ultrafiltration barrier, a finding that may explain how mutations that impair *LMX1B* action can lead to the characteristic abnormalities of GBM and podocyte function found in NPS nephropathy.

Patients with NPS, especially those from kindreds with a history of renal disease, must be monitored periodically for the development of nephrosis and renal failure. Treatment of these complications is symptomatic. Renal transplantation is a good option for end-stage renal disease because the characteristic NPS renal lesions do not reappear in transplanted kidneys.

Suggested Readings

Dreyer SD, Zhou G, Baldini A, et al. Mutations in *LMX1B* cause abnormal skeletal patterning and renal dysplasia in nail patella syndrome. *Nat Genet* 1998;19:47.

Looij BJ Jr, Te Slaa RL, Hogewind BL, van de Kamp JJP. Genetic counseling in hereditary osteo-onychodysplasia with nephropathy. *J Med Genet* 1988; 25:682.

Miner JH, Morello R, Andrews KL, et al. Transcriptional induction of slit diaphragm genes by Lmx1b is required in podocyte differentiation. *J Clin Invest* 2002;109:1065.

Smeets HJM, Knoers VVAM, van de Heuvel LPWJ, et al. Hereditary disorders of the glomerular basement membrane. *Pediatr Nephrol* 1996;10:779.

CHAPTER 333 ■ RENAL TUBULAR ACIDOSIS

MYRA L. CHIANG AND L. LEIGHTON HILL

Renal tubular acidosis (RTA), a biochemical syndrome characterized by a persistent hyperchloremic (non–anion gap) metabolic acidosis, is caused by abnormalities in the renal regulation of bicarbonate concentration. The abnormality can be in the reabsorption of filtered bicarbonate or in the regeneration of bicarbonate by hydrogen ion secretion. The glomerular filtration rate (GFR) usually is normal but may be mildly depressed. In normal individuals, urinary net acid excretion (i.e., the hydrogen excreted as titratable acid and as ammonium ions minus urinary bicarbonate and urinary metabolizable organic anions) equals the quantity of acid added to extracellular fluids from the diet plus metabolism plus any fecal losses of alkali. RTA is caused by an upset in this hydrogen ion balance because of abnormal losses of bicarbonate in the urine, insufficient hydrogen ion excretion in the urinary buffers, or both. These RTA syndromes have a wide variety of pathogenetic mechanisms and causes.

PATHOGENESIS

RTA traditionally is classified as proximal or distal, based on the nephron segment that is thought to have an abnormal function (Table 333.1). A rare type 3 RTA has been described in infants with features of both distal (type 1) and proximal (type 2) RTA. This autosomal recessive syndrome (gene locus chromosome 8q22) is characterized by the additional findings of osteopetrosis and mental retardation, and it is caused by carbonic anhydrase II deficiency. Proximal RTA (often called *RTA type 2*) is a defect in the proximal tubular reabsorption of filtered bicarbonate. Ordinarily, approximately 85% (somewhat less in infants) of filtered bicarbonate is reabsorbed in the proximal tubule primarily by sodium-hydrogen ion exchange. In comparison, 15% is reabsorbed in the distal nephron primarily via hydrogen secretion by a proton pump (H-ATPase). In proximal

TABLE 333.1

PATHOPHYSIOLOGIC CLASSIFICATION OF RENAL TUBULAR ACIDOSIS

Type	Pathophysiology
Proximal RTA (type 2)	Impaired proximal tubular HCO₃ reabsorption
Distal RTA (type 1)	Impaired distal tubular H⁺ secretion
Secretory defect ("classic distal RTA")	H⁺ pump failure
Gradient defect	Increased back-leak of secreted H⁺
Voltage-dependent defect	Reduced luminal electronegativity
Hyperkalemic distal RTA (type 4)	Impaired ammoniagenesis
Hypoaldosteronism	
Primary	
Secondary	
Pseudohypoaldosteronism type 1	
Pseudohypoaldosteronism type 2 (chloride shunt)	Increased NaCl reabsorption in ascending loop of Henle

RTA, the renal threshold for bicarbonate reabsorption is abnormally low, so that at normal plasma levels of bicarbonate, more than 15% of filtered bicarbonate is delivered to the distal nephron for reabsorption, resulting in bicarbonate wasting and metabolic acidosis. Possible pathogenetic causes for proximal RTA include a defective sodium-potassium adenosinetriphosphatase (ATPase) activity in the basolateral membrane, which provides the energy for the luminal sodium-hydrogen antiporter by maintaining a low cell sodium concentration, hence a favorable gradient for passive sodium entry into the cell; a defect in the sodium-hydrogen antiporter itself; deficiency or inhibition of carbonic anhydrase activity; or impairment of the basolateral sodium bicarbonate cotransporter responsible for returning the reabsorbed bicarbonate into the systemic circulation.

Distal RTA (see Table 333.1) is seen in two major forms: type 1, usually associated with hypokalemia or normokalemia and rarely hyperkalemia, and type 4, always associated with hyperkalemia. Distal RTA type 1 results from a reduced rate of hydrogen ion secretion that normally occurs in the intercalated cells in the collecting tubules where luminal H-ATPase pumps are located. The most common cause of distal type 1 RTA is diminished H-ATPase pump (classic distal RTA). Mutations have been described in the genes encoding the B1 and alpha 4 subunits of the H-ATPase pump. In addition to metabolic acidosis, sensorineural deafness is seen in the B1 subunit mutation, suggesting that the pump is required for normal function of the inner ear. Other causes of distal type 1 RTA include increased luminal membrane permeability leading to back-leak of secreted hydrogen ions from lumen to cell (gradient defect). Amphoterium B causes RTA via this mechanism and impaired distal sodium transport, leading to reduced luminal electronegativity, and thereby inhibiting potassium and hydrogen ion secretion (voltage-dependent defect). The associated impairment of secretion of potassium leads to hyperkalemia, which renders it difficult to distinguish this type of distal type 1 RTA from that of hyperkalemic type 4 RTA.

Distal RTA type 1 may occur in an incomplete form. Patients with incomplete distal RTA type 1 have a persistent high urine pH and hypocitraturia, but in contrast to those with the complete form, they are able to maintain net acid excretion, and the plasma bicarbonate concentration remains in the normal range. Untreated, it can lead to recurrent urolithiasis or nephrocalcinosis.

In hyperkalemic RTA type 4, the acidification defect is caused mainly by impaired renal ammoniagenesis. Patients with this type cannot excrete the necessary amounts of hydrogen ion in urinary buffers to avoid a metabolic acidosis and cannot excrete potassium normally. However, the ability to lower urinary pH in response to systemic acidosis is maintained. RTA type 4 is observed most frequently in conditions associated with aldosterone deficiency or resistance.

RTA can be caused by a variety of disorders, most of which are rare (Boxes 333.1, 333.2, and 333.3). Hereditary RTA occurs most commonly in children. Recent advances in the molecular biology of acid-base transporters have allowed researchers to gain a better understanding of the different inherited forms. Proximal RTA can occur as an isolated abnormality; however, much more commonly, proximal RTA is seen as part of the Fanconi syndrome, with associated glycosuria, aminoaciduria, and phosphaturia.

CLINICAL MANIFESTATIONS AND COMPLICATIONS

RTA usually is suspected during the workup of patients with failure to thrive or unexplained acidosis. Children may have

---

BOX 333.1 Disorders Associated with Proximal RTA Type 2

Isolated Defect
Hereditary (persistent)
   Autosomal dominant (possibly due to mutations in Na$^+$/H$^+$ exchangers)
   Autosomal recessive with ocular abnormalities (caused by mutations in the Na$^+$/Hco$_3$$^+$ cotransporter, gene located in chromosome 4q21)
Sporadic (transient in infancy)

Fanconi Syndrome
Inherited
   Cystinosis / Galactosemia
   Tyrosinemia / Hereditary fructose intolerance
   Lowe syndrome / Glycogen storage disease type 1
   Wilson disease

Dysproteinemic states
   Multiple myeloma / Amyloidosis
   Light-chain disease

Drugs and Toxin
   Outdated tetracycline / Heavy metals (lead, cadmium, mercury, copper)
   Ifosfamide
   Carbonic anhydrase inhibitors

Miscellaneous
   Vitamin D deficiency / Renal transplantation
   Hyperparathyroidism / Congenital heart disease
   Medullary cystic disease / Leigh syndrome

BOX 333.2 Disorders Associated with Distal RTA Type 1

Primary
Hereditary (persistent)
   Autosoal dominant (caused by mutations in the basolateral Cl$^-$/Hco$_3^-$ exchanger, AEI gene located in chromosome 17q21-22)
   Autosomal recessive with deafness (caused by mutations in the B1 subunit of H$^+$-ATPase gene located in chromosome 2p13)
   Autosomal recessive without deafness (caused by mutations in the alpha 4 subunit of H-ATPase gene located in chromosome 7q33-34)
Sporadic (transient)

Secondary
Sjögren syndrome / Sickle cell disease
Cryoglobulinemia / Hypercalciuria
Rheumatoid arthritis / Renal transplantation
Hypergammaglobulinemia / Obstructive uropathy
Systemic lupus erythematosus / Amphotericin B
Chronic active hepatitis / Lithium
Hepatic cirrhosis / Toluene
Ehlers-Danlos syndrome

BOX 333.3   **Disorders Associated with Hyperkalemic RTA Type 4**

Aldosterone Deficiency
Primary
    Addison disease
    Congenital adrenal hyperplasia
    Isolated hypoaldosteronism
Hyporeninemic hypoaldosteronism
    Diabetic nephropathy
    Lupus nephropathy
    HIV nephropathy
    Acute glomerulonephritis
    Angiotensin converting enzyme inhibitors
    Cyclosporine
    Cyclo-oxygenase inhibitors
Aldosterone Resistance
Pseudohypoaldosteronism type 1
Pseudohypoaldosteronism type 2 (Gordon syndrome)
"Early childhood" hyperkalemia (transient)
Obstructive uropathy
Tubulointerstitial disease
Drugs (amiloride, spironolactone, triamterene, pentamidine)

---

histories of repeated episodes of dehydration and anorexia. Others may present with clinical manifestations of hypokalemia, such as polyuria, constipation, and profound weakness. In distal RTA type 1, the signs and symptoms of kidney stones may precede the establishment of the diagnosis of RTA. The physical examination may reveal only growth retardation or signs of dehydration. In some cases, the physical examination may suggest a secondary cause of proximal RTA, such as the finding of cystine crystals in cystinosis, mental retardation in Lowe syndrome, or evidence of liver involvement in Wilson disease. The presence of sensorineural deafness suggests the diagnosis of the autosomal recessive form of distal RTA type 1.

Laboratory Evaluation

Proximal Renal Tubular Acidosis Type 2

As with all types of RTA, the acidosis in proximal RTA is a hyperchloremic (non–anion gap) metabolic acidosis. Usually, at presentation, the patient is in a reasonably steady-state condition; the extent of lowering of the plasma bicarbonate is determined by the severity of the proximal tubular defect in bicarbonate reabsorption. This steady state has been reached because the filtered load of bicarbonate (glomerular filtration rate × plasma bicarbonate) has decreased to a point at which the amount that escapes reabsorption by the impaired proximal tubule is small enough to be reabsorbed completely by the distal nephron. Therefore, on presentation, usually no bicarbonate is present in the urine, and, because the distal acidification mechanisms are intact in proximal RTA, the urine is acid (pH level is less than 5.5). During the acidosis, total acid excretion (titratable acid plus ammonium minus bicarbonate) is elevated appropriately (greater than 60 μEq/1.73 m^2/minute) and the urine anion gap is negative (chloride greater than sodium plus potassium). If the patient is treated then with sufficient base, the plasma bicarbonate increases and the amount of bicarbonate filtered increases, which overwhelms the impaired proximal

tubules with bicarbonate and results in a large increase in the delivery of bicarbonate to the distal nephron. The urine, therefore, contains increasing amounts of bicarbonate as the plasma level increases, and the urine becomes alkaline (pH level greater than 5.5), even though the plasma bicarbonate still may be below normal. The fractional excretion of bicarbonate (F_{EHCO_3}) is increased (by greater than 10% to 15%).

Patients with proximal RTA type 2 often have hypokalemia, but serum potassium levels may be normal. The low potassium levels have been attributed to an increased delivery of sodium to the distal nephron, where, under the stimulus of aldosterone (aldosterone increases because of the sodium losses and mild volume depletion), sodium is reabsorbed in exchange for potassium ions, which then are excreted. Treatment with alkali may worsen hypokalemia by raising the filtered bicarbonate load. Patients with proximal RTA type 2 usually do not have hypercalciuria, and urinary citrate excretion is normal. Patients with this form of RTA seldom manifest the complications of nephrocalcinosis, nephrolithiasis, or bone disease that are common manifestations in patients with untreated distal RTA type 1.

Distal Renal Tubular Acidosis Type 1

The urine pH in distal RTA type 1 never is very acidic (pH of 5.5 or greater), the total acid excretion always is abnormally low, and the urine anion gap is positive despite the degree of acidosis. Hypokalemia occurs commonly and may be severe or life-threatening. Hypercalciuria also occurs commonly, and urinary citrate excretion is low. These abnormalities, along with the persistently alkaline urine, are instrumental in the development of nephrocalcinosis and nephrolithiasis. Acidemia enhances proximal citrate reabsorption, leading to low excretion of citrate. Citrate is a potent inhibitor of stone formation. Proximal tubular functions in patients with RTA type 1 are normal.

Hyperkalemic Distal Renal Tubular Acidosis Type 4

Hyperkalemic distal RTA (type 4) represents an abnormality of distal tubular function with regard to the renal handling of hydrogen and potassium ions. Hyperkalemia is the most distinctive clinical characteristic of this type of RTA when compared with types 1 and 2. Patients with RTA type 4 usually can make an acidic urine (pH level of less than 5.5), but total excretion of acid is low because of very low rates of ammonia excretion. The urine anion gap is positive, and the renal excretion of potassium is inappropriate to the serum concentration of potassium. The defects in the excretion of urinary potassium and hydrogen ion appear to be secondary to hypoaldosteronism or to end-organ resistance to aldosterone (pseudohypoaldosteronism). Hypoaldosteronism can be primary or secondary (Box 333.3).

Primary hypoaldosteronism is seen in patients with acute adrenal insufficiency, Addison disease, and salt-losing congenital adrenal hyperplasia. Patients may show all the signs of adrenal insufficiency, including salt wasting, tendency to low blood volume and low blood pressures, metabolic acidosis, hyponatremia, and hyperkalemia. Peripheral renin activity is increased, but circulating aldosterone virtually is absent. Renal function in these patients, including renal tubular function, is within normal limits.

Secondary hypoaldosteronism results from the decreased production or release of the active form of renin caused by destruction of the cells of the juxtaglomerular apparatus, as seen in patients with intrinsic renal disease, such as lupus nephropathy, and diabetic nephropathy. A reduction in overall renal function can be demonstrated, but the hyperkalemia and metabolic acidosis are out of proportion in severity to the degree of renal insufficiency. These patients do not demonstrate salt wasting.

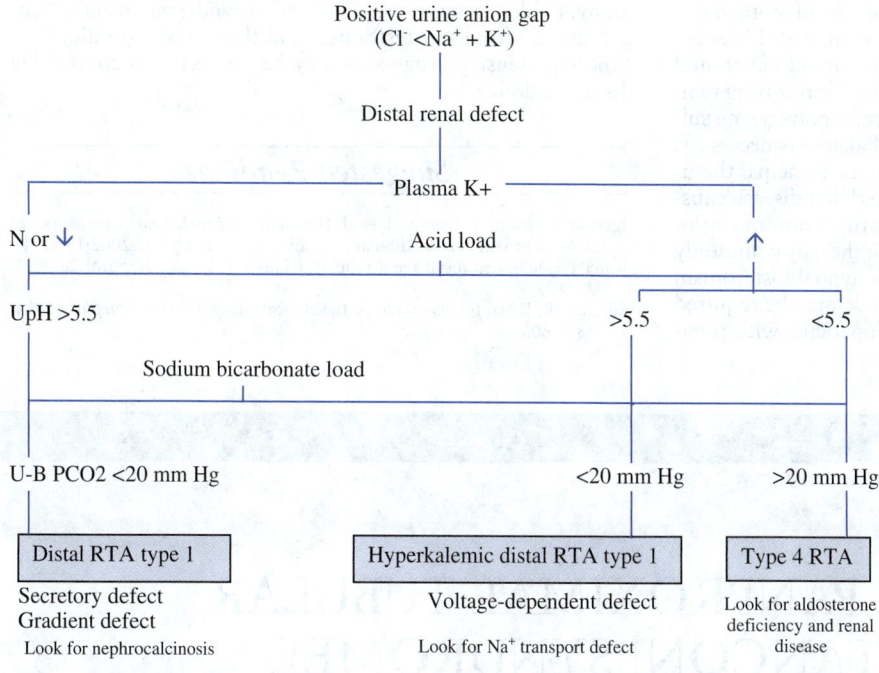

FIGURE 333.3. Diagnostic workup of a patient with hyperchloremic metabolic acidosis and a positive urine anion gap. RTA: renal tubular acidosis; U pH, urine pH; FE HCO_3^-, fractional excretion of bicarbonate; U-B PCO_2, urine-to-blood PCO_2 gradient. N, Normal; ↓, decreased; ↑, increased. (Adapted with permission from Rodriguez-Soriano J. Renal tubular acidosis: the clinical entity. *J Am Soc Nephrol* 2002;13: 2160.)

water. Because the carbon dioxide remains hydrated, it cannot diffuse back into the cells and blood and, therefore, is delivered to the urinary bladder as H_2CO_3; the voided urine then can be measured for PCO_2.

Patients with distal RTA type 4 have a positive urine anion gap and low total acid excretion (less than 60 $\mu Eq/1.73$ m²/minute), similar to those with distal RTA type 1. However, the presence of hyperkalemia and acid urine pH (less than 5.5) distinguishes type 4 from type 1 distal RTA (see Fig. 333.3 and Table 333.2).

Once the diagnosis of distal hyperkalemic RTA type 4 is established, the underlying pathophysiology should be determined if possible. A careful physical examination with regard to the status of the extracellular and blood vascular volume is essential, as are repeated measurements of the blood pressure. In addition, measurements of peripheral renin activity and plasma aldosterone are indicated in most instances. On the basis of these tests, plus a detailed history, the measurement of serum creatinine levels, ultrasound studies of the kidneys, and routine urine examinations, a diagnosis of the particular variety of RTA type 4 usually can be made.

THERAPY

General

The administration of alkali is a common therapy for almost all types of RTA. The alkalis used most frequently are sodium bicarbonate tablets (each gram provides 12 mEq) and sodium citrate in liquid form, available commercially as Bicitra. Each milliliter of Bicitra provides 1 mEq of sodium citrate. Liquid citrate also is available as Polycitra (each milliliter provides 1 mEq of sodium, 1 mEq of potassium, and 2 mEq of citrate) or Polycitra K (each milliliter provides 2 mEq of potassium and citrate). The latter two preparations are particularly helpful for patients with a hypokalemic type of RTA. Serum electrolyte studies should be performed every 2 to 4 days during adjustment of the alkali dosage. After the acidosis has been corrected, electrolytes should be measured monthly for several months. Ultimately, these determinations are done three to six times

a year, depending on the difficulty encountered in controlling the metabolic acidosis. Normal stature usually can be attained if the metabolic acidosis is well controlled over a prolonged period.

Proximal Renal Tubular Acidosis Type 2

Most patients with proximal RTA require a higher dose of alkali, beginning with 4 to 6 mEq/kg/day, and occasionally requiring up to 20 mEq/kg/day. The doses should be spread out over as much of the day as possible (four to six divided doses). Patients with Fanconi syndrome may require that a significant portion of the alkali be given as potassium citrate. Patients requiring very large amounts of base for correction of the acidosis may benefit from the administration of chlorothiazide (10 to 20 mg/kg/day), dietary sodium chloride restriction, or both. The thiazide diuretics tend to increase the proximal tubular reabsorption of bicarbonate by inducing a mild contraction of the extracellular fluid space.

Distal Renal Tubular Acidosis Type 1

In patients with distal RTA type 1, alkali therapy usually is initiated at a dose of 1 to 2 mEq/kg/day if no evidence of bicarbonate wasting exists and at 4 to 6 mEq/kg/day if bicarbonate wasting does exist. Type 1 patients with particularly severe problems with potassium homeostasis may require that up to 50% of the total base be given as potassium citrate. The successful correction of the acidosis results in normal urinary calcium and citrate excretions and greatly lessens the chances of developing complications such as nephrolithiasis, nephrocalcinosis, and bone disease.

Hyperkalemic Distal Renal Tubular Acidosis Type 4

For RTA type 4, doses of base in the range of 1 to 5 mEq/kg/day usually are sufficient to correct the acidosis and also may correct the hyperkalemia. Obviously, the use of potassium-containing alkali should be avoided. Furosemide also is effective in returning serum potassium levels to normal but should not be used in patients with salt wasting. Rarely, resorting temporarily to the use of exchange resins [sodium polystyrene sulfonate (Kayexalate)] to control the hyperkalemia is necessary. RTA type 4 has many etiologies, and often the principal therapeutic efforts are directed toward the underlying disease causing the RTA. If the problem results primarily from mineralocorticoid deficiency, hormonal replacement therapy commonly is quite effective. If the patient has pseudohypoaldosteronism type 1, large supplements of sodium chloride may be required for successful therapy. On the other hand, patients with pseu-

dohypoaldosteronism type 2 (Gordon syndrome) usually benefit greatly from salt restriction and the use of loop diuretics. Antihypertensive drugs also may be necessary to control the hypertension.

Suggested Readings

Igarashi T, Sekine T, Inatomi J, et al. Unraveling the molecular pathogenesis of isolated proximal renal tubular acidosis. *J Am Soc Nephrol* 2002;13:2171.

Karet FE. Inherited distal renal tubular acidosis. *J Am Soc Nephrol* 2002;13:2178.

Soriano JR. Renal tubular acidosis: the clinical entity. *J Am Soc Nephrol* 2002;13:2160.

CHAPTER 334 ■ PANPROXIMAL TUBULAR DYSFUNCTION (FANCONI SYNDROME)

EILEEN D. BREWER

Fanconi syndrome (FS) is the result of generalized transport dysfunction of the proximal renal tubule. It is characterized classically by excessive urinary losses of amino acids, glucose, bicarbonate, and phosphate but also by losses of calcium, magnesium, uric acid, and other organic acids, low-molecular-weight (tubular) proteins, sodium, potassium, and water. The urinary losses can result in metabolic acidosis, dehydration, hypokalemia, hypophosphatemia, rickets, and growth retardation in children. Many inherited and acquired disorders can lead to FS in adults and children (Box 334.1). When FS occurs in children, the cause usually is hereditary and is related to an inborn error of metabolism.

PATHOPHYSIOLOGY

Basic abnormalities underlying renal tubular transport dysfunction in FS are incompletely understood. Because a variety of inherited, acquired, and experimentally induced conditions can cause FS, specific pathologic mechanisms operative in one disorder may not be present necessarily in another, although each could lead to a final common pathway that results in the expression of FS. Suggested possibilities for a final common pathway include defective generation of energy to drive the transport processes, increased backleak of reabsorbed solutes across the cell membrane into the tubular lumen, and abnormal action or location of carriers that normally transport solutes across the cell membrane from the tubular lumen into the intracellular space. Recent advances in molecular genetics with identification of specific gene defects and their gene products are laying the foundation for a better understanding of the underlying pathophysiology of FS in each disorder.

CLINICAL MANIFESTATIONS AND LABORATORY FINDINGS

The general clinical manifestations of FS depend on the patient's age and on the type and chronicity of the underlying disease. Infants and children most often present with failure to thrive. Many features of FS, including chronic acidosis, volume contraction, hypokalemia, hypophosphatemia, and abnormal vitamin D metabolism, contribute to impaired linear growth. However, in some cases, especially in patients with cystinosis, these factors alone are not sufficient to explain the severity of the growth retardation. Rachitic bone changes may be a presenting or accompanying clinical sign in some children with FS. If the child has been walking, bowing deformities of the legs may be noticed first. A child who does not yet bear weight may have straight legs but noticeable metaphyseal widening at the wrists, knees, or ankles and radiographic changes classic for rickets at these sites. Infants younger than 5 months old rarely have the clinical findings of rickets.

Episodic vomiting, anorexia, polydipsia and polyuria, chronic constipation, and unexplained fevers are nonspecific symptoms of chronic FS. Constipation probably results from chronic depletion of volume associated with the polyuria, hypokalemia, and chronic metabolic acidosis of untreated FS. Unexplained fevers, which occur especially frequently in infants and young children with cystinosis, may reflect episodic dehydration.

The laboratory findings of FS reflect mostly abnormal proximal renal tubular function. In physiologically normal children, more than 98% of the filtered amino acids are reabsorbed in the proximal renal tubule. In FS, hyperaminoaciduria occurs in the presence of normal plasma amino acid levels and is an exaggeration of the normal excretory pattern of each amino acid, with the percentage of tubular reabsorption of each amino acid decreased below normal. Because urinary losses are trivial compared with intake, hyperaminoaciduria is not clinically significant, but it is an important clinical marker for FS. Plasma and urinary amino acids should be sampled simultaneously as part of the clinical evaluation of patients with FS.

Urinalysis often reveals characteristic abnormalities, including the following: glucosuria in the presence of a normal blood glucose concentration; abnormally high urine pH (greater than 5.5) in the presence of mild to moderate hyperchloremic metabolic acidosis but appropriately low pH with

| BOX 334.1 | Causes of Fanconi Syndrome |

Hereditary
Primary
  Idiopathic
Secondary
  Cystinosis
  Lowe syndrome (oculocerebrorenal syndrome)
  Galactosemia
  Hereditary fructose intolerance
  Fanconi-Bickel syndrome
  Tyrosinemia type I
  Wilson disease
  Dent disease
  Mitochondrial cytopathies (cytochrome C oxidase
    deficiency, Leigh syndrome, Kearns-Sayre syndrome)
  Metachromatic leukodystrophy
  Alport syndrome

Acquired
Intoxications
  Drugs
    Gentamicin and other aminoglycosides
    Outdated tetracycline
    Cephalothin
    Antiviral for human immunodeficiency virus infection
      (didanosine, cidofovir, adefovir, tenofovir)
    Valproic acid
    Streptozocin
    6-Mercaptopurine
    Azathioprine
    Cisplatin, carboplatin
    Ifosfamide
  Toxins
    Heavy metals (lead, mercury, cadmium, uranium,
      platinum)
    Glue (toluene) sniffing
    Paraquat
    Maleic acid (experimental in animals)
Diseases
  Nephrotic syndrome
  Sjögren syndrome
  Multiple myeloma
  Light-chain nephropathy
  Hypergammaglobulinemia
  Amyloidosis
  Interstitial nephritis with anti–tubular basement
    membrane antibody
  Renal vein thrombosis
  Malignancy (lymphoma, carcinoma)
  Renal transplantation

severe acidosis (type 2 renal tubular acidosis); specific gravity 1.010 to 1.015, even in the presence of dehydration; and mild albuminuria (1 to 2+, or 30 to 100 mg/dL) with normal serum protein and albumin.

Glucosuria, which often is intermittent, rarely exceeds 2+ (500 mg/dL) on the dipstick and is clinically insignificant except as a marker of FS, except in the Fanconi-Bickel syndrome, in which glucosuria and galactosuria are quite prominent as a result of the underlying genetic defect. Patients who present with severe hyperchloremic metabolic acidosis (plasma bicarbonate level 10 to 15 mEq/L) usually have a urinary pH less

than 5.5, characteristic of type 2 (proximal) renal tubular acidosis. When their acidosis is treated and the plasma bicarbonate concentration is kept in the normal range by supplemental alkali therapy, the excretion of bicarbonate exceeds 15% of the bicarbonate filtered by the glomerulus, a value typical of proximal renal tubular acidosis. The urinary pH usually exceeds 7.0. Fractional excretions of bicarbonate as high as 30% have been reported. If a patient has severe depletion of volume, paradoxical metabolic alkalosis actually can occur, but it changes to metabolic acidosis after volume expansion occurs. Depletion of volume in affected patients is the result of obligatory polyuria, which is caused mainly by the wasting of sodium, amino acids, glucose, and other osmotically active solutes from the proximal tubule. Polyuria may be worse in the presence of chronic hypokalemia, which can impair urinary concentration in the distal renal tubule and can stimulate thirst and polydipsia. In patients with FS, the urine specific gravity rarely exceeds 1.015 to 1.020, even in the presence of severe dehydration; thus, urine specific gravity should not be used as an indicator of the status of hydration.

Mild albuminuria (2+ or less, or 100 mg/dL or less by urinalysis dipstick) usually indicates tubular proteinuria. Tubular proteinuria is characterized not only by the predominance of low-molecular-weight species such as lysozyme (molecular weight 15,000 daltons) and beta-2-microglobulin (molecular weight 11,800 daltons) but also by albumin (molecular weight 40,000 daltons). Proteins of approximately 40,000 daltons or less, including a small amount of albumin, normally are filtered by the glomerulus and then are reabsorbed and catabolized in the proximal tubule. A receptor-mediated endocytic process in the first part of the proximal tubule normally reabsorbs these tubular proteins. In FS, dysfunction of proximal tubular transport results in tubular proteinuria. Like glucosuria and generalized aminoaciduria, tubular proteinuria appears to be of no clinical significance except as a marker of FS. Proteinuria may be more pronounced in the oculorenal syndrome of Lowe (OCRL), often exceeding 1 g/m^2/day, without causing nephrotic syndrome.

Serum chemistry studies often are abnormal in fully expressed FS. Besides having hyperchloremic metabolic acidosis with a normal anion gap, patients may have hyponatremia, hypokalemia, hypophosphatemia, and, in some cases, hypouricemia. Serum calcium and magnesium concentrations usually are normal, despite increased losses of calcium and magnesium in the urine. Excessive loss of sodium in the urine without sufficient sodium intake eventually can result in hyponatremia, although increased delivery of sodium to the distal renal tubule and high levels of renin and aldosterone caused by depletion of volume increase distal tubular sodium reabsorption to avoid hyponatremia. The preferential distal reabsorption of sodium worsens hypokalemia, especially in the presence of the proximal renal tubular acidosis of FS and delivery of excess bicarbonate to the distal nephron. During distal tubular reabsorption of sodium, sodium is exchanged for potassium, and potassium is secreted into the urine to become the primary cation to be excreted with the excess bicarbonate. The combination of excessive distal tubular secretion of potassium and increased proximal tubular rejection of potassium creates obligatory loss of large amounts of potassium in the urine, usually leading to hypokalemia and severe depletion of total body potassium. This depletion can cause weakness, poor growth, paralysis, and fatal cardiac arrhythmias. Treatment of acidosis with sodium bicarbonate without supplementation of potassium can result in death.

Hypophosphatemia results from excessive urinary wasting of phosphate and reduced tubular reabsorption of phosphate, even at low concentrations of serum phosphate. Serum parathyroid hormone concentration usually is normal. Serum levels of 1,25-dihydroxyvitamin D, which is made in the proximal renal tubule by 1-hydroxylation of 25-hydroxyvitamin D, often are reduced or are lower than expected for the degree of hypophosphatemia, which is a major stimulus for production of 1,25-dihydroxyvitamin D. Hypophosphatemia, impaired metabolism of vitamin D in the renal tubule, excessive urinary excretion of calcium, and chronic acidosis all contribute to the chronic bone disease (i.e., rickets and osteomalacia) of patients with FS.

Most patients with FS waste uric acid in the urine and have hypouricemia. Patients with hereditary fructose intolerance who are exposed to fructose have transient hyperuricemia instead because of the abnormal biochemical pathways underlying this disease.

Some affected patients, especially those with cystinosis and some with OCRL, may have decreased carnitine reabsorption in the proximal tubule and may be deficient in carnitine. Carnitine is required to transport free fatty acids into mitochondria for subsequent energy production. Deficiency in carnitine may contribute to muscle weakness and delayed development.

CAUSES

As previously stated, FS has many causes (see Box 334.1). Most of these disorders are discussed elsewhere in this text. This section focuses on diseases associated with FS that occur in children and lead to progressive chronic renal failure.

Cystinosis (Nephropathic Cystinosis)

Cystinosis is a rare lysosomal transport disorder in which intracellular accumulation of cystine is associated with FS, chronic renal failure, growth failure, corneal opacities, photophobia, and hypothyroidism. It is not related to the disease cystinuria, which is a genetically transmitted defect for transport of the dibasic amino acids in the renal tubule and intestine, resulting in massive urinary cystine and cystine nephrolithiasis. In cystinosis, plasma cystine concentration is normal, and urinary cystine concentration is elevated only to a degree consistent with the generalized hyperaminoaciduria of FS.

Three types of cystinosis are recognized based on age at onset and severity of symptoms: infantile nephropathic (MIM 219800), juvenile (MIM 219900), and ocular nonnephropathic (MIM 219750). All are autosomal recessive and monogenic, resulting from different mutations in the cystinosis gene *CTNS*, which is located on chromosome 17p13. Ocular nonnephropathic cystinosis is characterized by adult onset of mild photophobia without FS, glomerular disease, or retinal depigmentation; only cornea, bone marrow, and peripheral leukocytes exhibit significant cystine crystals. Intracellular cystine is increased only moderately (30 to 50 times normal, compared with 100 to 1,000 times normal for infantile nephropathic cystinosis). Juvenile cystinosis is similar to the infantile nephropathic form, except for a later age of onset in adolescence, usually between 12 and 15 years, and the absence of FS but the presence of proteinuria from glomerular injury, slower progression to end-stage renal disease, normal stature, photophobia, and late development of pigmentary retinopathy. Both the juvenile and ocular nonnephropathic forms of cystinosis are extremely rare and likely result from the combination of a severe nephropathic mutation of one allele and a mild mutation of the other allele for the *CTNS* gene. This discussion focuses on infantile nephropathic cystinosis, the most common and most severe presentation of this disease.

Nephropathic cystinosis occurs in approximately 1 in 200,000 live births in North America, but it has a higher prevalence in western France, the United Kingdom, and Germany and in French Canadians of Quebec. The carrier frequency approximates 1 in 225 people. This disease has been diagnosed in all ethnic groups, including children of northern European descent, African Americans, Hispanics, and Asians from the Middle East and India. The etiology of nephropathic cystinosis is described in Box 334.2.

Patients with infantile nephropathic cystinosis appear normal for the first 6 to 12 months of life and then develop symptoms of FS, including dehydration, electrolyte disturbances, failure to thrive, and rickets. An impaired ability to sweat contributes to frequent episodes of fever, flushing, and vomiting during excessive heat exposure. Hepatosplenomegaly may be noted before the patient reaches 5 years of age but is clinically insignificant. Characteristic corneal crystals are not present at birth but usually are evident by the time the child reaches 6 to 12 months of age. The crystals do not reduce visual acuity, but they cause photophobia, which begins within the first few years of life and worsens with age. Older patients may

---

BOX 334.2 **Etiology of Nephropathic Cystinosis**

The cystinosis gene *CTNS* encodes for cystinosin, which is an integral lysomal membrane protein specific for transporting L-cystine out of lysosomes into the cytoplasm. The activity of cystinosin is driven by the acid environment of the lysosome and the hydrogen ion electrochemical gradient across the lysosomal membrane. Deletion, missense, insertion, splice-site, and nonsense mutations of this gene lead to loss of the L-cystine transport function and accumulation of cystine in lysosomes of affected tissues all over the body. The most common mutation is a 57-kilobase deletion found in more than half of North American and European cystinotic patients. This mutation is detected easily by a multiplex polymerase chain reaction amplification assay, which has potential for use as a rapid molecular diagnostic test. Cystine is the disulfide of the amino acid cysteine and is very insoluble in water. Cystine transport out of lysosomes is greatly diminished in patients homozygous for cystinosis and is diminished by half in heterozygotic carriers. Accumulation of 100 to 1,000 times the normal amount of cystine in homozygote cells often leads to formation of crystals within affected cells. Birefringent, hexagonal, or rectangular crystals may be identified by slit-lamp examination of the cornea and conjunctiva or by microscopic examination of alcohol-fixed sections of kidney, rectal mucosa, thyroid follicles, liver, spleen, or bone marrow.

How intralysosomal accumulation of cystine results in FS is not understood. Cystinosin is abundant in proximal renal tubular cells, weakly present in distal tubular cells, and only faintly detectable in glomeruli. Accumulation of cystine begins at birth and increases with age, but lysomal accumulation of cystine alone does not result in FS in animal models. *In vitro* studies of rabbit proximal tubules and human proximal tubular cells that were intracellularly loaded with cystine by using cystine dimethyl ester have demonstrated that excess cystine decreases generation of energy (adenosine triphosphate) and inhibits sodium-dependent transporters. Reduction of adenosine triphosphate and dissipation of the sodium gradient necessary to drive transport processes could be the primary events leading to inhibition of transtubular transport in the proximal tubule in this disorder.

experience the continuous feeling of foreign-body irritation and may even develop corneal ulceration and blepharospasm. A generalized patchy depigmentation at the periphery of the retina, characteristic of cystinosis, has been identified in affected patients as early as age 5 weeks. Visual acuity remains unaffected by the retinopathy until the patient is at least 10 years of age. Blindness caused by retinal deterioration has occurred in several patients aged 13 to 35 years. Extensive accumulation of cystine has been identified in the retinal pigment epithelium.

In most patients, hypothyroidism occurs from destruction of the thyroid follicles by accumulation of cystine crystals. Screening with thyroid function studies reveals an elevated level of serum thyroid-stimulating hormone before symptoms of hypothyroidism occur. The mean age for initiation of thyroid supplementation is 10 years, but therapy has been necessary for untreated patients as young as 3 years old.

Renal manifestations of cystinosis are the most serious initially. In the patient's first years of life, electrolyte abnormalities resulting from FS may be quite severe and difficult to normalize with oral supplementation of alkali, potassium, phosphorus, and 1,25-dihydroxyvitamin D. Without cysteamine therapy, progressive renal failure, characterized by a slowly rising level of serum creatinine, usually is noticeable by the time the child is age 5 years. Virtually all patients not treated with cysteamine develop end-stage renal disease by age 10 years. Renal biopsy specimens show little change until renal failure appears, at which time light microscopy may reveal interstitial fibrosis and glomerular sclerosis, and electron microscopy may demonstrate characteristic crystals in the interstitium and proximal tubular cells.

As renal failure progresses, the electrolyte abnormalities of FS sometimes become easier to manage because of the reduced filtered load presented to the abnormal tubule. Successful renal transplantation from either a living related donor, including a heterozygotic parent, or a deceased donor is possible and has allowed patients to survive into the third and fourth decades of life. FS does not recur in the transplanted kidney. Cystine may accumulate in the interstitium and occasionally in the mesangium of the glomeruli of the transplanted kidney but not in the tubular cells.

After renal transplantation, cystine continues to accumulate in tissues other than the kidney. Of most concern is the finding that approximately 30% of patients older than 10 years have decreased visual acuity and 15% have corneal ulceration. Some patients also have developed pancreatic exocrine insufficiency and insulin-dependent diabetes mellitus. Almost all patients not treated with cysteamine continue to have growth failure and delayed sexual maturation. Cystine accumulates in testicular tissue, and, so far, no male fertility has been demonstrated in cystinosis. Primary ovarian failure has been described, but deliveries of normal, healthy infants to a few cystinotic women who have undergone renal transplantation also have been reported. Stunted height may remain an emotional and social problem for older adolescents and adults with cystinosis who have not had the benefit of receiving cysteamine or growth hormone therapy. Neurologic and muscular dysfunctions are important late manifestations of cystinosis in long-term survivors. Several cases of progressive neurologic and muscular problems, including dementia, spasticity, swallowing difficulty, and muscle wasting, have been reported. Postmortem examinations have shown extensive accumulation of crystals in dura, meninges, and perivascular spaces of the brain and in muscle.

The diagnosis of cystinosis can be made clinically by the presence of FS and the demonstration by slit-lamp examination of pathognomonic crystals in the cornea, but *in vitro* measurement of accumulated cystine in peripheral leukocytes or skin fibroblasts is the definitive way to establish the diagnosis. Prenatal diagnosis can be established by demonstrating increased levels of cystine in cultured amniotic cells obtained by amniocentesis at 16 weeks' gestation or in chorionic villus samples obtained as early as 9 weeks' gestation. Neonatal diagnosis can be made by measuring levels of cystine in placental tissue.

In addition to symptomatic treatment of FS and progressive renal failure, the most important treatment of cystinosis is directed at depletion of intracellular cystine in affected tissues. The most effective agent to date has been cysteamine, which can enter lysosomes and can react with cystine to form a mixed disulfide of cysteamine and cysteine. This compound is a structural congener of lysine that can be transported out of the lysosome by an unaffected lysine carrier-mediated mechanism. The result is a reduction in the accumulation of intracellular cystine all over the body. The preparation of choice since 1994 is cysteamine bitartrate capsules (Cystagon, Mylan Pharmaceuticals), started at a daily dose 10 mg free base/kg body weight (mg/kg) per day divided for oral administration every 6 hours. The dose is increased weekly by 10 mg/kg per day to a target dose of 60 to 90 mg/kg/day (1.3 to 1.95 g/m^2/day), which is adjusted as needed to maintain trough leukocyte cystine content of less than 1.0 nmol half-cystine per milligram protein. The capsule form avoids the foul odor and taste of the liquid and thus improves patients' compliance.

Oral cysteamine therapy is effective at any time in the clinical course of the disease, but it significantly alters the natural history of the disorder when treatment is initiated early in life. If therapy is started before the child is 2 years old, progression to renal failure is slowed or halted, hypothyroidism is prevented, and linear growth is improved to the normal range. In one study, for each month of early cysteamine therapy use before the child was age 2 years, at least 14 months of later renal function was preserved. Cysteamine therapy is important even after a patient has undergone renal transplantation, to attempt to preserve the function of extrarenal organs and to prevent complications, especially encephalopathy and myopathy, in long-term survivors. Oral cysteamine therapy has not been effective in reducing accumulation of corneal cystine crystals, but topical cysteamine applied 10 to 12 times daily has been effective in some patients after months of consistent therapy. Penetrating keratoplasty or corneal transplantation may be required in severe cases of corneal erosion.

In addition to cysteamine therapy, recombinant human growth hormone therapy has improved the severe short stature of cystinotic patients. Growth hormone is indicated for those children who continue to grow at less than the fifth percentile for height despite receiving adequate cysteamine treatment from early infancy or for those in whom renal failure prevents adequate growth.

Lowe Syndrome (Oculocerebrorenal Syndrome)

OCRL (MIM 30900) is an X-linked recessive disorder that characteristically occurs in male patients, who present in early infancy with dense congenital cataracts and glaucoma. Vision remains poor in many patients despite therapy, and it may be compromised later in childhood by corneal keloid formation. Renal tubular dysfunction, mental retardation, muscular hypotonia, and areflexia appear later in the first year of life. Seizures may be severe and occur early in life, may be mild and not appear until adolescence, or may never occur. Maladaptive behaviors, including temper tantrums, stereotypy, stubbornness, and obsessions or unusual preoccupations, are typical and specific to OCRL. Growth failure becomes evident in some patients after they reach age 1 year and usually in all by age 3 years. In surviving adults, final heights are less than the third percentile for physiologically normal men. Bone age lags behind height age after patients reach 3 years of age and until growth is complete. Noninflammatory arthritis has occurred in some patients after the first decade of life. Vellus hair cysts, skin rashes, and dental cysts may develop after the first decade.

The *OCRL1* gene is located on chromosome Xq26.1 and encodes for the protein phosphatidylinositol 4,5-biphosphate (PtdIns[4,5]P2) 5-phosphatase, which is a *trans*-Golgi network enzyme that plays an important role in regulation of Golgi vesicular transport and cytoskeletal assembly. Mutations in the gene lead to deficiency of PtdIns[4,5]P2 5-phosphatase activity in patients with OCRL, but how this deficiency causes the manifestations of the disease remains unknown. Prenatal diagnosis has been done using measurement of enzyme activity in cultured amniocytes.

The diagnosis of OCRL is made clinically, usually by the appearance of renal dysfunction during the first year of life in a male patient with congenital cataracts. Typical facies also may alert the experienced clinician to this disorder. Tubular proteinuria (including albuminuria identifiable by urinalysis), polyuria, and generalized hyperaminoaciduria appear first, usually within the first few months of life. Proteinuria may reach the nephrotic range in later childhood, but it does not lead to hypoalbuminemia and the nephrotic syndrome.

Other manifestations of FS are quite variable. Glucosuria is an intermittent, inconstant finding by urine dipstick evaluation and of small magnitude when evaluated quantitatively. Most patients have some degree of hyperphosphaturia, but not all develop hypophosphatemia or require phosphate supplementation. Rickets and osteomalacia may occur in early childhood and require therapy with 1,25-dihydroxyvitamin D and phosphate supplements. Type 2 renal tubular acidosis may occur within the first year of life, at a much later age in the first decade, or not at all. Potassium wasting, when present, has been mild and easy to treat with potassium supplements. Hypercalciuria is a frequent manifestation of FS but rarely is associated with nephrocalcinosis or nephrolithiasis except in OCRL and Dent disease. Some, but not many, boys with OCRL have significant nephrocalcinosis and symptomatic kidney stones diagnosed in the first decade of life.

Renal failure is a late manifestation, usually starting after the child reaches 5 to 10 years of age and not progressing to end stage until at least the third decade. Because few patients are older than 40 years, predicting the late renal course of most patients is difficult. Renal biopsies from young children with OCRL may be normal or may show tubular dilatation, atrophy, and interstitial fibrosis, with the earliest injury identified in the proximal tubules. Electron microscopy may reveal shortening of the brush border and disruption of mitochondria in the tubular cells. When the glomeruli become involved, the earliest findings are nodular thickening and splitting of the glomerular basement membrane and effacement of the foot processes. Renal biopsies from older children may show only nonspecific changes associated with chronic renal failure from any cause.

Other laboratory findings of OCRL include elevation of serum levels of creatine kinase, aspartate aminotransferase, and lactate dehydrogenase, probably related to direct muscle involvement by OCRL, as well as elevation of serum total and high-density lipoprotein cholesterol, with normal serum triglycerides. Urinary carnitine excretion is increased, but the level of plasma carnitine has been low only in some patients.

Therapy for OCRL is entirely symptomatic and involves the following: ophthalmologic intervention for cataracts and glaucoma; electrolyte and vitamin D metabolite supplementation as needed for FS; and physical therapy, anticonvulsants, behavioral medications, and special education for neurologic problems. Most boys with OCRL survive into adulthood. A few are able to live independently or in a group home. Several have undergone successful long-term peritoneal dialysis, hemodialysis, or renal transplantation for end-stage renal disease.

Idiopathic Fanconi Syndrome

The diagnosis of idiopathic FS is one of exclusion and no doubt includes cases with a variety of as yet unidentified causes. Idiopathic FS can develop at any age. Most cases are sporadic, but genetic transmission also has been identified, most often in an autosomal dominant fashion (MIM 134600), with linkage to chromosome 15q15.3 demonstrated in one large family. In some cases, only hyperaminoaciduria or tubular proteinuria appears in children, with complete FS not becoming manifest until as late as the third or fourth decade of life. Therapy is symptomatic. Patients with both the sporadic and familial forms of idiopathic FS are at risk for developing chronic renal failure within 10 to 30 years of diagnosis. Some progress to end-stage disease and require dialysis or transplantation. Recurrence of FS in the absence of allograft rejection has been reported in at least one case.

DIAGNOSIS

FS rarely is idiopathic, and an underlying condition always should be sought in children. The possibility of toxin exposure exists at any age, although toxins are a more common cause of FS in adults than in children. The patient's history of drug therapy should be reviewed, and the possibility of drug ingestion or of heavy metal contamination from the environment must be considered.

The age at which a child becomes symptomatic with FS often aids in correctly diagnosing the underlying disease. When a patient presents with FS in the first few months of life, an inborn error of metabolism should be suspected. Infants with galactosemia (MIM 230400) or hereditary fructose intolerance (MIM 229600) can be acutely symptomatic within the first few days of life if they are exposed to formula or foods containing galactose or fructose, respectively. Patients with galactosemia or the rare Fanconi-Bickel syndrome (MIM 227810) may be identified by high blood galactose levels on routine neonatal screening for inborn errors. Later in infancy or childhood, patients with galactosemia, hereditary fructose intolerance, Fanconi-Bickel syndrome, or tyrosinemia type I (MIM 276700) usually exhibit failure to thrive, vomiting, jaundice, and hepatomegaly. Except for those with Fanconi-Bickel syndrome, these patients exhibit only intermittent FS, depending on the severity of the disease or, in the case of galactosemia or hereditary fructose intolerance, on whether exposure to galactose or fructose is repeated but intermittent. The diagnosis of galactosemia is suggested by the findings of galactosuria and cataracts in an infant chronically fed lactose- or galactose-containing formulas. Punctate cataracts in the fetal lens nucleus may be identifiable at birth. A definitive diagnosis requires the demonstration of deficiency of galactose-1-phosphate uridyltransferase in red blood cells, fibroblasts, leukocytes, or hepatocytes. The abnormal gene is mapped to chromosome 9p13.

Symptoms of hereditary fructose intolerance, which include convulsions and coma, appear only after the introduction of foods containing fructose or sucrose, so exclusively breast-fed infants have no symptoms. Diagnosis is established by the results of an intravenous fructose tolerance test and by demonstration of deficiency of aldolase B activity in liver biopsy tissue, which is caused by mutation in the gene on chromosome 9q22.3. Patients with Fanconi-Bickel syndrome usually are diagnosed clinically by fasting hypoglycemia, postprandial hyperglycemia and hypergalactosemia, hepatomegaly, and abnormal glycogen storage in liver and kidney in the presence of FS. These abnormalities result from deficiency of the cell membrane monosaccharide transporter GLUT2, which is encoded by the gene on chromosome 3q26.1-26.3. Patients with tyrosinemia type I produce excess amounts of succinylacetone caused by reduced activity of fumarylacetoacetate hydrolase (FAH), the final enzyme in the degradation of tyrosine. Diagnosis is established by demonstrating large amounts of succinylacetone in the urine or blood and a deficiency of FAH in lymphocytes, fibroblasts, or liver biopsy tissue. The gene for FAH is mapped to chromosome 15q23-q25.

Infants and toddlers presenting with FS may have any of the foregoing illnesses, but they are most likely to have cystinosis. Children with nephropathic cystinosis generally do not show their first signs and symptoms before they are 6 months of age or after they are 2 to 3 years of age. The presence of corneal cystine crystals by slit-lamp examination and the measurement of increased levels of cystine in peripheral leukocytes or skin fibroblasts establish the diagnosis. If the patient is male and has congenital cataracts and developmental delay, he likely has OCRL. Partial or complete FS also may be associated with mitochondrial cytopathies, such as cytochrome C oxidase deficiency or Leigh syndrome, which are characterized by disrupted mitochondrial oxidative phosphorylation. The major clinical symptoms of cytochrome C oxidase deficiency are hypotonia and progressive weakness. The diagnosis is made by measuring reduced cytochrome C oxidase activity in muscle biopsy tissue.

In young children, some cases of FS are discovered incidentally when urinalysis obtained for another reason reveals dipstick-positive glucose in the presence of normal blood glucose concentrations. Dipstick-positive albuminuria in a patient with congenital cataracts may be the first sign of renal tubular dysfunction that leads to establishing the correct diagnosis of OCRL.

Older children presenting with FS usually have an acquired form of FS, although Wilson disease (MIM 277900), a rare inborn error of copper metabolism, may not be diagnosed until the end of the patients' first decade of life. These patients usually present with hepatic, neurologic, or psychiatric abnormalities rather than with FS, which may be found incidentally during the evaluation. Hepatic cirrhosis, Kayser-Fleischer rings (greenish brown deposits of copper in Descemet membrane of the cornea), and neurologic symptoms ranging from behavioral and psychiatric disorders to flapping tremors and dystonia are characteristic of Wilson disease. Concentration of serum ceruloplasmin is decreased to less than 20 mg/dL. Failure to incorporate radioactive copper into serum ceruloplasmin after an oral tracer dose establishes the definitive diagnosis. The gene for Wilson disease is located on chromosome 13q14.3-21.1 and encodes for a novel transporter P-type adenosine triphosphatase (*ATP7B*).

Acquired FS should be suspected in the presence of conditions such as nephrotic syndrome, renal transplantation, renal vein thrombosis, glue (toluene) sniffing, lead or other heavy metal intoxication, or exposure to drugs such as gentamicin, cisplatin, carboplatin, ifosfamide, valproic acid, or antiviral drugs used to treat human immunodeficiency virus infection (see Box 334.1). The dysproteinemias and amyloidosis occur almost exclusively in adults. Idiopathic FS is the diagnosis used when all other causes have been excluded.

THERAPY

Identification of the underlying cause for FS is crucial to direct therapy. In some cases, specific therapy or withdrawal of an offending substance may normalize the tubular dysfunction. When no specific therapy exists, symptomatic treatment of the electrolyte disturbances and of the bone disease of FS is the only alternative.

Proximal renal tubular acidosis may be severe, requiring large amounts of alkali therapy divided into four to six daily doses. Potassium supplementation almost always is necessary when alkali therapy is given. Administration of the potassium salt of citrate, bicarbonate, or acetate fulfills the dual purpose of treating acidosis and preventing hypokalemia. Mixtures of sodium and potassium citrate or potassium citrate alone are available commercially for oral use. Sodium wasting and dehydration are treated with combinations of sodium bicarbonate, citrate, and chloride, depending on the degree of acidosis. Prevention of dehydration from obligatory polyuria is handled best by allowing the patient free access to fluids. If the patient is vomiting and cannot readily ingest an adequate amount of fluids, dehydration may occur rapidly and requires early intervention with intravenous replacement therapy.

Hypophosphatemia and impaired renal vitamin D metabolism are the factors leading to rickets and other bone complications. Phosphate supplementation usually is given as neutral phosphate solution, 1 to 3 g divided into four to six daily doses. Diarrhea is a side effect of excessive oral phosphate therapy. The simultaneous administration of phosphate and alkali supplements may lead to tetany from acute hypocalcemia, so phosphate supplements should be added with caution in patients receiving alkali therapy. In some patients, supplementation with 1,25-dihydroxyvitamin D or dihydrotachysterol, neither of which requires further renal metabolism for biologic activity, is necessary to heal and sustain healing of rickets and osteomalacia. Hypercalciuria and transient hypercalcemia are toxic side effects of excessive vitamin D metabolite therapy.

Long-term dialysis and renal transplantation are viable alternatives for the management of end-stage renal disease in most patients. However, as patients with rare inborn errors of metabolism achieve prolonged survival through renal replacement therapy, important nonrenal late manifestations of these diseases are being revealed.

Suggested Readings

Brewer ED. Fanconi syndrome: clinical disorders. In: Gonick HC, Buckalew VM, eds. *Renal tubular disorders*. New York: Marcel Dekker, 1985:475.

Gahl WA. Early oral cysteamine therapy for nephropathic cystinosis. *Eur J Pediatr* 2003;162:S38.

Gahl WA, Thoene JG, Schneider JA. Cystinosis. *N Engl J Med* 2002;347:111.

Izzedine H, Launay-Vacher V, Isnard-Bagnis C, Deray G. Drug-induced Fanconi's syndrome. *Am J Kidney Dis* 2003;41:292.

Katalatzis V, Antignac C. New aspects of the pathogenesis of cystinosis. *Pediatr Nephrol* 2003;18:207.

Lowe Syndrome Association. *Living with Lowe syndrome: a guide for parents, friends and professionals*. Lowe Syndrome Association, www.lowesyndrome.org, 2000.

Santer R, Schneppenheim R, Suter D, et al. Fanconi-Bickel synrome: the original patient and his natural history, historical steps leading to the primary defect and a review of the literature. *Eur J Pediatr* 1998;157:783.

Suchy SF, Lin T, Horwitz JA, et al. First report of prenatal biochemical diagnosis of Lowe syndrome. *Prenat Diagn* 1998;18:1117.

Suchy SF, Nussbaum RL. The deficiency of PIP2 5-phosphatase in Lowe syndrome affects actin polymerization. *Am J Hum Genet* 2002;71:1420.

Wuhl E, Haffner D, Offner G, et al. Long-term treatment with growth hormone in short children with nephropathic cystinosis. *J Pediatr* 2001;138:880.

CHAPTER 335 ■ DISORDERS OF RENAL GLUCOSE TRANSPORT

L. LEIGHTON HILL

Primary renal glucosuria is a selective defect of proximal tubular glucose transport in which glucose is excreted in the urine at normal concentrations of blood glucose. The handling of all other filtered substances by the proximal tubules is normal, and the glucose transport defect is limited to the kidneys. The pattern of inheritance has been interpreted in some pedigrees to be autosomal dominant and in others to be autosomal recessive. Congenital renal glucosuria has been shown in at least one family with an autosomal recessive mode of inheritance to be a defect in the sodium glucose cotransporter gene (*SGLT2*). A defect in other sodium glucose cotransporter genes could be responsible for other types of primary renal glucosuria, such as the autosomal dominant varieties. At least two types of renal glucosuria are thought to occur, although establishing clinical differentiation sometimes is difficult. In one type, the maximum tubular reabsorptive capacity for glucose is low; that is, a reduced ability of almost all tubules to transport glucose occurs, resulting in reduction of both the minimal renal glucose threshold and the maximal tubular reabsorption. In another type, the maximum tubular reabsorptive capacity for glucose is normal, but a wide spectrum occurs in the ability of individual nephrons to reabsorb glucose, so the minimal renal glucose threshold is reduced despite the normal overall capacity of the proximal tubules to reabsorb glucose. A third and very rare type may involve abnormalities of several reabsorptive mechanisms and may result in very low rates of reabsorption of filtered glucose and a severe form of renal glucosuria. With the exception of this rare form, primary renal glucosuria almost always is clinically benign and asymptomatic and needs no therapy. However, it must be differentiated from diabetes mellitus by measuring glucose in blood and urine obtained nearly simultaneously via several random simultaneous tests or by performing a 3-hour glucose tolerance test. If the patient has renal glucosuria, the blood glucose concentrations should be within normal range, although the glucose tolerance curve may be somewhat flat if urinary glucose loss is considerable. The patient usually spills glucose in each urine specimen obtained, despite normal blood glucose levels.

Ensuring that the renal glucosuria is not an expression of panproximal tubular dysfunction (Fanconi syndrome) is important. Panproximal tubular dysfunction syndromes may be hereditary or acquired. Renal glucosuria also may be seen with other tubular defects that are not part of Fanconi syndrome such as the glucose-galactose malabsorption syndrome. In addition, transient renal glucosuria has been described in such conditions as acute pyelonephritis and exposure to renal toxins and also can be seen in the late stages of chronic renal insufficiency.

Suggested Readings

van den Heuvel LP, Assink K, Willemsen M, et al. Autosomal recessive renal glucosuria attributable to a mutation in the sodium glucose cotransporter (*SGLT2*). *Hum Genet* 2002;111:544.

Wright EM, Martin MG, Turk E. Familial glucose-galactose malabsorption and hereditary renal glycosuria. In: Scriver CR, Beaudet AL, Sly WS, Valle D, eds. *The metabolic and molecular bases of inherited disease,* 8th ed. New York: McGraw-Hill, 2001.

CHAPTER 336 ■ DISORDERS OF RENAL PHOSPHATE TRANSPORT

MYRA L. CHIANG

Phosphorus plays a critical role in skeletal development, mineralization, and cellular functions. The kidney regulates phosphate homeostasis by tubular reabsorption of filtered phosphates (TRP) and by 1-alpha-hydroxylation of calcidiol into the active form, 1,25-dihydroxyvitamin D_3 (calcitriol). Genetic defects that lead to renal phosphate wasting and abnormal vitamin D metabolism and function are the most common causes of inherited rickets (Table 336.1).

X-LINKED HYPOPHOSPHATEMIC RICKETS

X-linked hypophosphatemic rickets (XLHR) is the most common type of hereditary rickets, with an incidence of 1 in 20,000 births. It is characterized by rachitic bone disease, hypophosphatemia, phosphaturia caused by reduced activity of the

TABLE 336.1

HEREDITARY FORMS OF RICKETS

	Primary Defect	Gene Locus
Phosphopenic rickets		
X-linked hypophosphatemia	Mutations in *PHEX*	Chromosome Xp22.1
Autosomal dominant hypophosphatemia	Mutations in *FGF23*	Chromosome 12p13
Hereditary hypophosphatemic rickets with hypercalciuria	?	?
Calcipenic rickets		
Vitamin D–dependent type 1	Mutations in 1-alpha-hydroxylase	Chromosome 12q14
Vitamin D–dependent type 2	Mutations in vitamin D receptor	?

?, Unknown.

renal brush-border membrane sodium-phosphate cotransporter in the proximal tubule, and abnormal regulation of the renal 1-alpha-hydroxylase activity resulting in an inappropriately low serum concentration of 1,25-dihydroxyvitamin D_3, relative to the degree of hypophosphatemia. Although the disease is completely penetrant, substantial interfamilial and intrafamilial variations in severity of disease exist. Male and female patients appear to be affected similarly despite the X-linked dominant inheritance.

Pathogenesis

Functional studies indicate that the tubular defect and impaired synthesis of calcitriol in patients with XLHR are probably related to a circulating phosphaturic substance rather than an intrinsic defect in the kidney. A primary osteoblast abnormality also may exist. The gene responsible for XLHR was mapped to chromosome Xp22.1 and was named *PHEX* (phosphate regulating gene with homologies to endopeptidases on the X chromosome). *PHEX* is expressed predominantly in bones and teeth. Mutations in the *PHEX* gene cause decreased degradation of the hormone-like substances called phosphatonins,

leading to abnormally high circulating concentrations of these factors and consequent renal phosphate wasting and abnormal mineralization.

Clinical and Radiologic Findings

During early infancy, patients with XLHR appear to be clinically normal, although frontal bossing may be present. As the child begins to walk, bowing of the lower extremities becomes evident. Because of genu varum and coxa vara, patients walk with a waddling gait. Occasionally, genu valgum instead of genu varum is observed. Spontaneous periapical tooth abscesses associated with defective dentin formation develop with advancing age. Craniotabes, rachitic rosary, and deformity of the upper extremities occur less frequently than in vitamin D–deficient or vitamin D–dependent rickets. In addition, patients with XLHR do not have tetany and severe myopathy, which may occur in the other two forms of rickets. Growth retardation is marked in untreated male patients, who seldom reach a height of 5 feet. Bone pain, degenerative joint disease, and dental problems extend into the patient's adult life. Continuing treatment seems to ameliorate some of these symptoms.

Radiologic findings include the loss of provisional zone of calcification, metaphyseal widening, cupping, fraying, and coarse-appearing trabecular bone. All the radiologic findings are more pronounced in the lower extremities.

Laboratory Findings

The age at which hypophosphatemia first appears varies. Some patients have consistently low serum phosphorus values from birth, whereas others develop them at 6 to 8 months of age. This delay has been attributed to the normally low glomerular filtration rate (GFR) in newborns. The age-related variations in normal serum phosphate levels must be considered in interpreting abnormal values. Serum phosphate concentrations between 1.0 and 2.5 mg/dL are characteristic in older children with the disease, but levels may be as high as 4 mg/dL in infants with this condition. In contrast to the other forms of rickets (Table 336.2), serum calcium concentrations are normal or low normal. Parathyroid hormone (PTH) concentration usually is normal, and aminoaciduria is absent. The serum concentration of 25-hydroxyvitamin D_3 usually is normal and that of 1,25-dihydroxyvitamin D_3 (calcitriol) is slightly low or normal, despite the prevailing hypophosphatemia that normally is a stimulator of renal 1-alpha-hydroxylase.

TABLE 336.2

BIOCHEMICAL FINDINGS IN RICKETS

Type	Calcium	Phosphate	Alkaline Phosphatase	Parathyroid Hormone	25-(OH)D$_3$	1,25-(OH)$_2$D$_3$	Urine Calcium
Vitamin D–deficient	↓ or N	↓ or N	↑	↑	↓	↓ or N	↓ or N
Vitamin D–dependent type 1	↓	↓ or N	↑↑	↑	N	↓↓	↓
Vitamin D–dependent type 2	↓	↓ or N	↑↑	↑	N	↑↑	↓
X-linked hypophosphatemia	N	↓↓	↑	N	N	N or ↓	↓
Hereditary hypophosphatemic rickets with hypercalciuria	N	↓↓	↑	N or ↓	N	↑	↑

↑, increased; ↓, decreased; N, normal.

The main biochemical features of XLH are the low tubular reabsorption of filtered phosphate in the presence of a low serum phosphate and the absence of secondary hyperparathyroidism. The percentage of tubular reabsorption of phosphate (%TRP) can be calculated from the creatinine and phosphate concentrations on a near-simultaneously obtained random urine and serum sample:

$$\%TRP = 1 - \frac{UPO_4}{SPO_4} \times \frac{Scr}{Ucr} \times 100$$

Normal %TRP in children ranges from 80% to 95%. The mean %TRP in patients with XLHR is reduced to the 40% to 70% range. Because changes in GFR affect the TRP, a more appropriate measure of the maximum tubular phosphate transport (TmP) is TmP/GFR. The TmP can be obtained from Bijvoet nomogram by plotting the known values of TRP and creatinine clearance.

Treatment

The goals of treatment are to prevent development of or correct rickets or osteomalacia and for the patient to achieve normal adult height. Standard treatment consists of a combination of oral phosphate supplement (Neutra-Phos, 250 mg elemental phosphorus/tablet or Neutra-Phos powder, 250 mg elemental phosphorus/packet) starting at 40 mg of elemental phosphorus/kg/day, maximum of 4 g/day in five divided doses, and calcitriol (Rocaltrol, 0.25 μg/capsule or 1 μg/mL solution) at 20 to 50 ng/kg/day in two divided doses. High-dose oral phosphate can cause diarrhea; thus, starting with a lower dose and advancing slowly is advisable. The concomitant use of calcitriol enhances the intestinal absorption of calcium and phosphate. This enhanced calcium absorption prevents development of secondary hyperparathyroidism, which may occur with phosphate therapy alone. However, high-dose calcitriol can lead to hypercalcemia and hypercalciuria. When this problem is encountered, the dose of calcitriol must be decreased. Hydrochlorothiazide, at 2 mg/kg/day, may be added to decrease hypercalciuria. Amiloride hydrochloride, at 0.30 to 0.45 mg/kg/day, can be used in conjunction to compensate for the hypokalemic metabolic alkalosis induced by hydrochlorothiazide. Monitoring should include the following: checking serum calcium, phosphate, alkaline phosphatase, and creatinine concentrations, as well as urine calcium-to-creatinine ratio, at least every 3 months; checking the serum PTH level every 6 to 12 months; and performing renal ultrasonography and radiography of hands, wrists, and knees every 12 months.

Nephrocalcinosis as detected by renal ultrasonography is the major complication of treatment, with reported incidence as high as 50%. The long-term effect of nephrocalcinosis on renal function is not known. Isolated cases of renal insufficiency have been reported. Nephrocalcinosis appears to be related to the mean phosphate dose but not to the dose of calcitriol or the duration of therapy. Despite receiving long-term therapy with phosphate and calcitriol, few patients achieve expected adult height. Administration of recombinant growth hormone increases the serum phosphate level as a result of enhanced TRP and accelerates growth of children with XLHR, but whether therapy improves adult height remains to be seen.

AUTOSOMAL DOMINANT HYPOPHOSPHATEMIC RICKETS

Autosomal dominant hypophosphatemic rickets (ADHR) is characterized by low serum phosphate concentration, phosphaturia, inappropriately low or normal 1,25-dihydroxyvitamin D levels, and bone mineralization defects similar to those seen in XLHR. However, ADHR is far less common, exhibits male-to-male transmission, and is characterized by incomplete penetrance. The age of onset is variable. Patients with early-onset disease have phosphate wasting, rickets, and lower extremity deformities, but they may lose the phosphate-wasting defect after puberty. Patients who present after the epiphysis have fused may have bone pain, muscle weakness, and fractures but no lower extremity deformities. ADHR results from mutations in the fibroblast growth factor 23 (FGF23) gene on chromosome 12p13. FGF23 is a circulating phosphatonin. Mutations in the gene interfere with its cleavage, leading to elevated levels and phosphaturia. Whether the enzyme cleaving FGF is PHEX remains unknown. Therapy for ADHR consists of a combination of oral phosphate and vitamin D similar to that of XLHR.

HEREDITARY HYPOPHOSPHATEMIC RICKETS WITH HYPERCALCIURIA

Hereditary hypophosphatemic rickets with hypercalciuria (HHRH) was described first in a large Bedouin kindred. It is inherited in an autosomal dominant fashion. The pathogenesis and responsible gene remain unknown. Speculation of an impairment of the type 2 sodium-phosphate cotransporter in the proximal tubule was not validated. The clinical and radiologic findings of HHRH are similar to those of XLHR and ADHR. The outstanding difference between HHRH and the other two entities is that the impairment in HHRH is restricted to phosphate transport. Plasma calcitriol concentrations are elevated appropriately for the degree of hypophosphatemia. Elevated plasma calcitriol concentration leads to increased intestinal calcium absorption and hypercalciuria. Thus, in a patient presenting with hereditary rickets, urinary calcium excretion should be determined before treatment is initiated. Patients with HHRH should be treated with phosphorus supplementation alone, using the same dosing schedule as used in treatment for XLHR. Calcitriol is contraindicated because it may further increase intestinal absorption of calcium, thus raising the risk of nephrocalcinosis and renal damage.

VITAMIN D–DEPENDENT RICKETS

Vitamin D–dependent rickets is a rare inborn error of vitamin D metabolism transmitted by an autosomal recessive mode and is divided into types 1 and 2.

Type 1

Vitamin D–dependent rickets type 1, also called *pseudovitamin D deficiency rickets*, is secondary to inactivating mutations in the renal 1-alpha-hydroxylase responsible for the synthesis of 1,25-dihydroxyvitamin D_3 from 25-hydroxyvitamin D_3. The gene responsible for the disease has been mapped to chromosome 12q14. Symptoms usually begin within the child's first few months of life and include hypocalcemic tetany, convulsions, muscle weakness, and growth failure. A history of adequate vitamin D intake usually is obtained. Physical examination reveals a small, hypotonic child with findings similar to those in children with vitamin D deficiency rickets, including thickening of the wrists and ankles, frontal bossing with a wide anterior fontanelle, costochondral beading, and bowing of extremities. Severe tooth enamel hypoplasia is a common finding.

Trousseau and Chvostek signs frequently are positive. These children demonstrate the classic radiologic features of rickets, which are indistinguishable from those of vitamin D deficiency rickets. Hypocalcemia (often less than 8 mg/dL) is a cardinal feature. Serum phosphate usually is low but may be near normal. Alkaline phosphatase and PTH levels are elevated, and aminoaciduria is present. The diagnosis is made by demonstrating a normal serum level of 25-hydroxyvitamin D_3 and a low or undetectable serum level of 1,25-dihydroxyvitamin D_3 (see Table 336.2). Treatment with a relatively low dose of calcitriol at 1 to 2 μg/day is effective in most cases.

Type 2

Vitamin D–dependent rickets type 2 results from an end-organ resistance to calcitriol caused by mutations in the gene encoding the vitamin D receptor. Depending on the site of mutation, the abnormal receptors may not be able to bind calcitriol, may have defective nuclear localization, and may not be able to bind DNA or initiate gene transcription after DNA binding. The clinical findings are similar to those of type 1 disease, except total alopecia is observed in approximately half the patients with type 2 disease. This complete loss of hair is thought to be associated with abnormal vitamin D receptors in the hair follicle. Biochemically, type 2 disease differs from type 1 disease in that the level of 1,25-dihydroxyvitamin D_3 is very high. Although spontaneous remission may occur, treating this form of rickets is difficult. Most patients require a combination of calcium supplementation (1 to 3 g/day), which may have to be given as intravenous infusion into a central vein, and high doses of calcitriol (up to 30 μg/day).

OTHER CAUSES OF RICKETS

Dent disease (X-linked recessive nephrolithiasis) is a disorder of the proximal tubules that is characterized by low-molecular-weight proteinuria, hypercalciuria, nephrocalcinosis, recurrent renal stones, and progressive renal insufficiency. It is caused by mutations that inactivate a renal chloride channel, named CLC-5, and is encoded by a gene at chromosome Xp11.22. Some patients have phosphaturia and rickets that may present in infancy, polyuria, hematuria, glycosuria, and aminoaciduria. Symptomatic disease is confined exclusively to male patients. Treatment is directed at reducing calcium excretion by using a combination of increased fluid intake, a low-sodium diet, and thiazide diuretics.

Suggested Readings

DiMeglio LA, White KE, Econs MJ. Disorders of phosphate metabolism. *Endocrinol Metab Clin North Am* 2000;29:591.

Scheinman SJ. X-linked hypercalciuric nephrolithiasis: clinical syndromes and chloride channel mutations. *Kidney Int* 1998;53:3.

Tenenhouse HS, Murer H, Ritz E. Disorders of renal tubular phosphate transport. *J Am Soc Nephrol* 2003;14:240.

Thomas MK, Demay MB. Vitamin D deficiency and disorders of vitamin D metabolism. *Endocrinol Metab Clin North Am* 2000;29:611.

CHAPTER 337 ■ NEPHROGENIC DIABETES INSIPIDUS

ARUNDHATI S. KALE AND L. LEIGHTON HILL

Nephrogenic diabetes insipidus (NDI) is a hereditary or acquired disorder characterized by renal tubular resistance to the antidiuretic hormone arginine vasopressin (AVP). The inability to concentrate the urine because of this tubular disease leads to marked polyuria with compensatory polydipsia.

Inheritance of the *hereditary* forms of NDI may be X-linked or autosomal. Approximately 90% of congenital NDI cases are caused by mutations of the AVP receptor 2 gene (*AVPR2*), which codes for the vasopressin V2 receptor and occurs predominantly in males, consistent with an X-linked inheritance, with the locus at Xq28. Autosomal-recessive and, rarely, autosomal-dominant NDI is caused by mutations of the aquaporin 2 gene (*AQP2*), which has been localized to chromosome region 12q13. In the X-linked cases, at least 155 mutations have been identified that lead to the defective intracellular transport of receptors, thus resulting in the nonexpression of the receptors for binding AVP at the cell surface. Females usually show a limited tubular response to vasopressin, and even in males, the degree of severity of the defect varies; most males are diagnosed in early infancy because of a severe defect, but some escape detection until the second or third decade of life. Hereditary NDI in males with the severe defect usually is more severe than the *acquired* type, which has two general causes: loss of the concentration gradient in the medullary interstitial tissues or decreased responsiveness of the distal tubules and collecting ducts to AVP. The former occurs as a result of the tissue destruction occurring with obstructive uropathy, vesicoureteral reflux, sickle cell nephropathy, cystic disease, pyelonephritis, interstitial nephritis, or nephrocalcinosis. Decreased responsiveness of the distal tubules and collecting ducts to AVP can be caused by hypokalemia, hypercalcemia, amyloidosis, sarcoidosis, and various drugs that interfere with the action of AVP, such as lithium, demeclocycline hydrochloride, cisplatin, vinblastine sulfate, methoxyflurane, amphotericin B, and colchicine. Drug-induced NDI more closely resembles hereditary NDI than does NDI associated with the first group. NDI also can be seen as part of Fanconi syndrome, most likely because of the chronic hypokalemia that often occurs.

PATHOPHYSIOLOGY

AVP acts on at least two different types of receptors. The V1 (platelet/vascular/hepatic) receptors are present on nonrenal

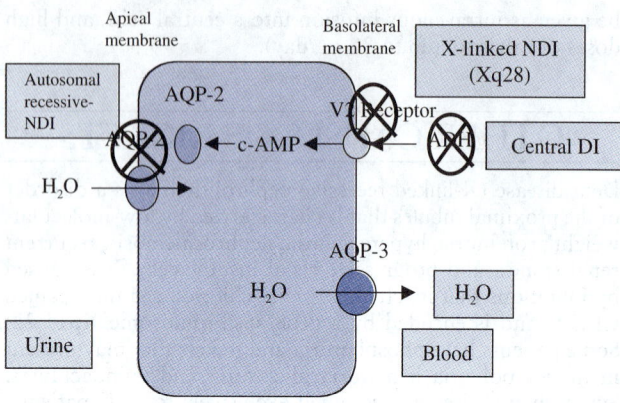

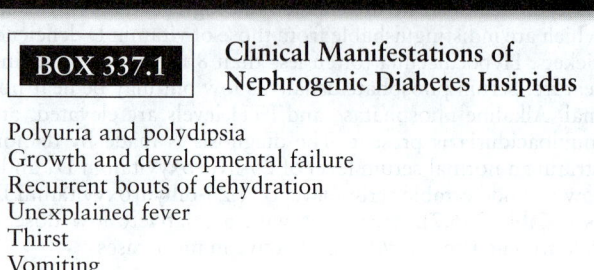

FIGURE 337.1. Schematic diagram of water transport in the principal cells of the collecting duct and genetic defects in different types of diabetes insipidus. AQP; aquaporins.

tissues, and the V2 or renal receptor is linked to adenylate cyclase and is phosphatidylinositol-independent. In normal individuals, the antidiuretic action of AVP begins with AVP binding to the V2 receptor, which leads to a cascade of events, including the activation of adenylate cyclase and the production of cyclic adenosine monophosphate (cAMP). The final step in the pathway is an increase in specific water channels (*AQP2*) on the luminal surface that facilitates water transport, as shown in Figure 337.1. Normal levels of AVP are found in patients with NDI as measured by radioimmunoassay, as opposed to low levels with central DI. Extrarenal vasopressin V2-like receptors also exist that mediate vasodilation, increase plasma renin activity, and stimulate the release of factor VIIIc and von Willebrand factor. In NDI, V1 receptor responses appear to remain intact, but renal V2 receptor responses are abnormal, having no antidiuretic response to the administration of either AVP or the V2-specific agonist desmopressin acetate (DDAVP) and no increase in plasma cAMP concentration. In hereditary NDI, the V2 abnormality may be generalized (renal and extrarenal) in the X-linked form or may be limited to the kidney, as in the autosomal recessive form. The two forms can be distinguished by clinical testing. DDAVP elicits normal extrarenal responses (increased levels of factor VIII, von Willebrand factor, and tissue plasminogen activator) in patients with autosomal recessive NDI but not in patients with X-linked NDI. The two forms also can be differentiated by molecular identification of *AVPR2* or *AQP2* mutations.

CLINICAL MANIFESTATIONS AND COMPLICATIONS

The most common clinical manifestations of NDI are shown in Box 337.1. Polyuria is constant, even during periods of dehydration. Elevated body temperature, a consequence of the dehydration, often leads to multiple investigations that attempt to identify a possible infectious cause. The large fluid ingestion may interfere with attaining adequate caloric intake, which, along with the deleterious effects of the chronic hypernatremia, leads to physical and mental retardation. The constant need for the intake of liquids interferes with normal sleep patterns. Chronic severe constipation is another result of the constant tendency toward negative water balance that characterizes NDI. With rehydration, a dramatic reversal in the condition is seen: The signs and symptoms of dehydration disappear; the fever abates; and the vomiting, irritability, and other manifestations disappear until dehydration recurs.

Laboratory Findings

Hypernatremia and hyperchloremia commonly are seen when the patient has been in negative water balance. The urinalysis usually is normal, except that the urine is inappropriately dilute, with the specific gravity being less than 1.006 and urine osmolality less than 200 mOsm/kg, despite evidence of dehydration. Small amounts of protein and a few red blood cells may be found in the urine, and the blood urea nitrogen (BUN) may be elevated during dehydration. Serum vasopressin levels are normal or high during periods of hypernatremia, distinguishing NDI from central DI. With rehydration, the sodium, chloride, BUN, and creatinine levels return to normal, and, although the urine remains dilute, the protein and red blood cells disappear. When the patient is in water balance, the glomerular filtration rate and all other renal function tests are normal, aside from the inability to conserve water. In the infant with NDI, the serum sodium level often is elevated early in the morning because of insufficient fluid intake during the night, but it may return to normal during the day with adequate fluid intake. Renal ultrasound may reveal marked dilatation of the urinary tract in NDI because of extremely high water turnover. This condition may not be apparent in very young infants but may worsen with age if control of water balance is not good. Marked dilatation of the urinary tract also may be seen in patients not identified as having NDI until later in childhood.

DIAGNOSIS

The diagnosis of NDI is suspected when polyuria, polydipsia, bouts of dehydration, hypernatremia, dilute urine, and a positive family history are noted. The differential diagnosis includes other causes of polyuria, such as central (AVP-deficient) diabetes insipidus, diabetes mellitus, psychogenic water drinking, and chronic renal insufficiency. Diabetes mellitus seldom presents in infancy, and patients have elevated blood and urine sugars and are not hypernatremic. Patients with primary polydipsia have normal to low-normal serum sodium concentrations. Patients with chronic renal insufficiency have azotemia even when hydrated, usually demonstrate isosthenuria rather than hyposthenuria, and generally have a much milder degree of polyuria than do patients with diabetes insipidus. The chief differential often is between central diabetes insipidus and NDI (vasopressin-resistant). Assessment and documentation of the magnitude of the polyuria and polydipsia by measuring intakes and outputs are essential. The most important test is a well-controlled water deprivation or concentration test performed in the hospital during the day under close medical supervision

BOX 337.2   Water Deprivation Test

1. Conduct the test in the hospital, during the day, under close observation.
2. Give breakfast or formula feeding early (e.g., 5:45 AM) with usual liquids.
3. At starting time (e.g., 6 AM), have the patient void and discard. With an infant, record time of spontaneous voiding and use this as the starting time.
4. Weigh the patient carefully at starting time and record.
5. Allow nothing by mouth from start time.
6. Obtain serum sodium and osmolality in vicinity of starting time.
7. Measure each urine voided for volume, specific gravity, and osmolality. Record time of each voiding.
8. Weigh, take temperature, and measure pulse rate every 2 hr × 3, then every hr × 6.
9. Repeat serum sodium and osmolality after 4 hours and then every 2 hr × 4 and also at conclusion of test.
10. Terminate the test when one or more of the following conditions is met:
    a. The specific gravity is 1.020 or more and urine osmolality is 600 mOsm/kg or more.
    b. The patient has lost 4% to 5% of body weight or has definite clinical signs of dehydration.
    c. The period of water deprivation reaches 6 hours for a young infant (less than 6 months), 8 hours for the child between 6 months and 2 years, and 12 hours for the child older than 2.
11. It is crucial to make the following observations at the time the test is stopped: body weight and vital signs, including temperature, serum sodium, serum osmolality, and urine specific gravity, osmolality, and volume.

(Box 337.2). The patient should not be allowed to lose more than 5% of body weight before the study is terminated. Careful monitoring of weight is essential, as are periodic observations of vital signs, urine and serum osmolalities, and sodium levels. A urine-to-plasma osmolality ratio of 2.0 or more is sufficient to rule out both NDI and central diabetes insipidus. If the polyuria continues, and the urine is not concentrated despite a 4% to 5% body weight loss or at the completion of the whole time course of the water deprivation test, then these two diagnoses remain strong possibilities. The serum vasopressin level can be measured at the end of the water deprivation test, before administering DDAVP.

The next step in the diagnostic process is to test the renal tubular response to antidiuretic compounds. The testing substance of choice is DDAVP, a synthetic analogue of 8-arginine vasopressin. DDAVP should be given intranasally at a dosage of 10 μg in infants and 20 μg in older children. Urine samples should be measured for volume and for concentration (specific gravity and osmolality) at 1- to 2-hour intervals after administration. If no response occurs (decrease in volume of urine and increase in osmolality of the urine), then a second dose should be given and additional urine samples collected and tested for volume and concentration. The serum sodium level and osmolality should be tested before and 4 hours after the administration of the DDAVP. The infant is allowed to take in fluid during this test. An alternative test is to give aqueous vasopressin USP (Pitressin) at a dosage of 2 U/m^2 body surface area intravenously over the course of a 1-hour period in 20 mL of isotonic saline. Urine samples should be obtained during the aqueous vasopressin infusion, at the conclusion of the infusion, and 1 hour and 2 hours after the infusion for measurement of volume, specific gravity, and osmolality. With either of these stimulation tests (DDAVP or aqueous vasopressin), a urine-to-plasma osmolality ratio of 1.5 or greater would indicate an adequate tubular response to antidiuretic compounds. If the patient fails to concentrate the urine during the water deprivation test and also after the administration of DDAVP or aqueous vasopressin stimulation, then a diagnosis of NDI is made. If the patient fails to concentrate with the water deprivation test but does respond to DDAVP or aqueous vasopressin stimulation by decreasing urine volume to less than 20 mL/m^2/hour and by raising the urine-to-plasma osmolality ratio to at least 1.5, then a diagnosis of central (AVP-deficient) diabetes insipidus is indicated.

Once a diagnosis of NDI is made, whether the defect is hereditary or acquired must be determined. Onset at an early age, a family history of polyuria, and bouts of dehydration in infancy strongly suggest that the defect is hereditary. Gene mutational analysis can be performed antenatally or in newborns with a strong family history of NDI and also in all patients with a definitive diagnosis of NDI. An early identification of newborns with the disease allows the prevention of episodes of dehydration, and early treatment with unrestricted water intake, low-sodium diet, and hydrochlorothiazide therapy may ensure normal physical and mental development. The workup also should include a thorough history of drug exposure; ultrasound studies of the kidneys and urinary tract; measurement of serum electrolyte, BUN, creatinine, and serum calcium levels; and possibly cystography. These studies should be sufficient to rule in or rule out the causes of secondary or acquired NDI mentioned above.

TREATMENT

The daily water turnover of infants and children with NDI can be enormous, equaling one-half or more of the patient's total body water each day. The intake of volumes of this magnitude may be very difficult to achieve purely from a mechanical point of view. Fluid intake as high as 300 to 400 mL/kg/day may be required just to maintain water balance. This high free-water intake should be spaced fairly evenly over the 24-hour period; water should be ingested even at night to prevent early-morning dehydration and hypernatremia. A diet that results in a low renal solute load is of major importance in reducing the obligatory renal water requirement. Such a diet is reasonably low in protein and sodium chloride. In the infant, breast milk is preferable, but if it is unavailable, a low-protein, low-electrolyte commercial formula suffices. Roughly 6% of the total calories should come from protein, and the daily sodium intake should not exceed 1 mEq/kg of body weight. In older children, the daily protein intake should be approximately 2 g/kg, and the total daily sodium content should be in the range of 1 to 2 g. The importance of a low renal solute load in determining the volume of obligatory urine water is shown in Table 337-1. Two disease states, chronic renal insufficiency and NDI, are compared with the normal state. The same diet is assumed for each of these three conditions (i.e., a diet yielding approximately 600 mOsm

TABLE 337.1

WATER TURNOVER RELATED TO INABILITY TO CONCENTRATE URINE

Disease	Solute Load (SL)[a]	Maximum Ability to Concentrate (C)	V = SL/C[b]	Obligatory Renal Water in Liters (V)	Degree of Polyuria
None	600	1,200 mOsm/kg	V = 600/1,200	0.5	None
Chronic renal failure	600	300 mOsm/kg	V = 600/300	2.0	Mild
NDI	600	100 mOsm/kg	V = 600/100	6.0	Severe
NDI	300	100 mOsm/kg	V = 300/100	3.0	Moderate

NDI, nephrogenic diabetes insipidus.

[a] Average diet might yield 600 mOsm of solute/m^2 to be excreted by kidney (principally urea, electrolytes, and other nitrogenous products).

[b] V = SL/C where V = obligatory urine volume in liters, SL = 24-hour renal solute load, and C = concentration of urine in mOsm/kg of water.

of solute for renal excretion per day). The normal child should be able to concentrate up to 1,200 mOsm/L of urine water, the patient with chronic renal failure usually can concentrate up to approximately 300 mOsm/L, and the patient with NDI can concentrate in the vicinity of 100 mOsm/L. The obligatory urine volume is determined by dividing the total solute load for excretion by the maximum ability to concentrate. As can be seen in this theoretic example, the person with no disease would have an obligatory renal water requirement of 0.5 L; the patient with chronic renal insufficiency would have a mild polyuria, with an obligatory water excretion of 2 L/day; and the patient with NDI would have severe polyuria, with an obligatory renal water excretion of 6 L/day. If the diet of the patient with NDI were reduced in protein and sodium chloride content so that the renal solute load was decreased to 300 mOsm/day, the obligatory renal water excretion would be only 3 L/day instead of 6 L/day, a 50% decrease. Thiazide diuretics can be used to further diminish the polyuria. The thiazide diuretics increase sodium excretion, thereby producing a borderline low blood volume. As a result, an increased proximal tubular reabsorption of salt and water occurs, and the delivery of water to the concentrating sites in the kidney is less. Thiazides also have shown to increase water permeability in the collecting duct, decreasing urine volume by as much as 20% to 40%. Therefore, these drugs are valuable in the very young infant who has a great physical problem in taking in the volume of free water required to stay in water balance. The decrease in urine volume also prevents or lessens dilatation of the urinary tract, which is almost inevitable at the high water turnover rates these patients experience when untreated. Because the effect of the thiazide is nullified almost completely by a high sodium intake, sodium restriction to the level previously recommended is vital. The other agents that appear to be helpful in the management of NDI are prostaglandin synthetase inhibitors (e.g., indomethacin). The effects of prostaglandins on renal function are quite complex

and appear to vary with the particular prostaglandin involved and the particular situation under which it is tested. In general, however, prostaglandin synthetase inhibitors usually inhibit water excretion. Obviously, the treatment of the acquired types of NDI varies depending on the therapy necessary to address the underlying disease causing the secondary tubular defect. However, many of the principles outlined for the therapy of hereditary NDI also apply to the treatment of patients with the acquired variety. In particular, these patients benefit from the provision of extra free water and a diet that yields a low renal solute load. With the identification of specific genes involved in hereditary NDI, gene therapy is being investigated. The experimental transfer of adenovirus-mediated genes, either by direct perfusion into the renal artery or by retrograde infusion into the renal pelvis in rats, resulted in expression of the gene in renal tissue. This result shows the promise of gene transfer therapy as a treatment modality in the future.

Suggested Readings

Bichet DG, Oksche A, Rosenthal W. Congenital nephrogenic diabetes insipidus. *J Am Soc Nephrol* 1997;12:1951.

Bichet DG, Razi M, Lonergan M, et al. Hemodynamic and coagulation responses to 1-desamino-8-D-arginine vasopressin in a patient with congenital nephrogenic diabetes insipidus. *N Engl J Med* 1988;318:881.

Brennan B, Seligsohn U, Aochberg Z. Normal response of factor VIII and von Willebrand factor to 1-desamino-8-d-arginine vasopressin in nephrogenic diabetes insipidus. *J Clin Endocrinol Metab* 1988;67:191.

Knoers NVAM, Deen PMT. Molecular and cellular defects in nephrogenic diabetes insipidus. *Ped Nephrol* 2001; 16:1146

Monn E. Prostaglandin synthetase inhibitors in the treatment of nephrogenic diabetes insipidus. *Acta Pediatr Scand* 1981;70:39.

Morello JP, Bichet DG. Nephrogenic diabetes insipidus. *Ann Rev Physiol* 2001; 63:607.

Williams RH, Henry C. Nephrogenic diabetes insipidus transmitted by females and appearing during infancy in males. *Ann Intern Med* 1947;27:84.

CHAPTER 338 ■ BARTTER SYNDROME

MYRA L. CHIANG

Hypokalemic salt-losing tubulopathies comprise a set of clinically and genetically distinct inherited renal disorders previously summarized under the designation Bartter syndrome (BS). Recent identification of mutations in four renal membrane proteins involved in electrolyte reabsorption have made

it possible to distinguish various subtypes of BS and the closely related Gitelman syndrome (GS), all of which follow autosomal recessive inheritance and share characteristic clinical features: renal salt wasting, hypokalemia, hypochloremia, metabolic alkalosis, and hyperreninemia with normal blood pressure.

TABLE 338.1

CLINICAL MANIFESTATIONS OF BARTTER SYNDROME AND GITELMAN SYNDROME

Bartter Syndrome (Types 1 and 2)	Bartter Syndrome (Type 3)	Gitelman Syndrome
Usually premature	Usually present between 6 months and 5 years of age	Usually diagnosed between 1 and 13 years of age
Maternal polyhydramnios	Polyuria less severe than in Bartter syndrome types 1 and 2	Asymptomatic hyporkalemia
Salt wasting	Nephrocalcinosis (rare)	
Polyuria	Short stature	Carpopedal spasm due to hypomagnesemia
Recurrent urinary tract infections and nephrocalcinosis may be present		

PATHOGENESIS

Active sodium chloride transport in the thick ascending limb of the loop of Henle requires the integrated function of different transporters and ion channels, namely the loop diuretic–sensitive sodium-potassium-chloride cotransporter (NKCC2) that allows sodium chloride entry into the tubular cells; the renal outer medullary potassium channels (ROMK) that permit reabsorbed potassium to leak back into the lumen; and the basolateral chloride channels (ClC-K) that permit the chloride that has entered the cell to exit and return to systemic circulation. Abnormalities in any of the three transporters result in impairment of sodium chloride reabsorption in the thick ascending limb, leading to volume depletion and activation of the renin-angiotensin-aldosterone system. The combination of increased sodium chloride in the distal tubule and hyperaldosteronism enhances secretion of potassium and hydrogen ion at the collecting tubules, leading to hypokalemia and metabolic alkalosis. Hypokalemia and volume contraction, in turn, stimulates the synthesis of vasodilator prostaglandins, which directly stimulates release of renin and synthesis of aldosterone, thereby exacerbating loss of potassium in the urine. The induced hypokalemia, along with the decreased medullary hypertonicity from the decreased reabsorption of sodium chloride in the ascending limb, explains the abnormal concentrating capacity seen in this disorder.

In the distal tubule, entry of sodium chloride into the cell is mediated by the thiazide-sensitive sodium chloride cotransporter (NCCT) located in the luminal membrane. At the basolateral membrane, reabsorbed sodium is pumped out of the cell by the Na-K-ATPase pump, while reabsorbed chloride exits via a chloride channel.

Loss-of-function mutations in the NKCC2 cotransporter (gene locus chromosome 15q15-21) and ROMK channel (gene locus chromosome 11q24) lead to neonatal BS types 1 and 2, respectively. Mutations in the ClC-K channel (gene locus chromosome 1p36) lead to classic BS (type 3). GS typically is caused by mutations in the NCCT cotransporter (gene locus chromosome 16q13), although mutations in the gene coding for the ClC-K channel also have been described. This finding accounts for overlap and confusion between BS and GS.

Another variant of neonatal BS invariably is associated with sensorineural deafness. Its recently identified gene, *Barttin*, is a beta subunit for chloride channels, which is crucial for reabsorption of renal chloride and secretion of inner ear potassium.

CLINICAL MANIFESTATIONS AND COMPLICATIONS

Most patients present with failure to thrive, dehydration, weakness, and constipation. Patients with neonatal BS types 1 and 2 commonly are born prematurely following severe polyhydramnios. They have pronounced salt wasting and massive polyuria due to impaired renal concentrating capacity. Fever, recurrent urinary tract infections, and nephrocalcinosis also may be present. Patients with classic BS (type 3) generally present when they are between ages 6 months and 5 years, are frequently short, have fewer abnormalities in concentrating capacity, and rarely have nephrocalcinosis.

Patients with GS often are diagnosed when they are between the ages of 1 and 13 years. Asymptomatic hypokalemia, and carpopedal spasm related to hypomagnesemia may be the initial presentation (Table 338.1).

LABORATORY FINDINGS

Characteristic laboratory abnormalities are hypokalemia with the serum potassium typically below 3.0 mEq/L, hypochloremia, metabolic alkalosis, and increased urinary potassium and chloride levels. Evidence of urinary sodium wasting frequently is present. Patients with neonatal BS (types 1 and 2) generally have hypercalciuria but no hypomagnesemia. In contrast, patients with GS have hypocalciuria and hypomagnesemia. Patients with classic BS (type 3) may have hypercalciuria or hypocalciuria. Elevated plasma renin activity consistently is present. Plasma aldosterone levels often are increased but may be normal due to the suppressive effect of hypokalemia. Patients with hypercalciuria may have nephrocalcinosis on renal ultrasound. Urinary prostaglandin E_2 excretion will be elevated in patients with BS but normal in those with GS.

DIAGNOSIS

The diagnosis is established when the following criteria are present: hypokalemia, hypochloremia, metabolic alkalosis with elevated urinary potassium and chloride, hyperreninemia in the presence of normal blood pressure, and exclusion of covert use of diuretics. Other differential diagnoses include familial chloride diarrhea, surreptitious vomiting, cystic fibrosis, and pyloric stenosis.

TREATMENT

Patients with neonatal BS (types 1 and 2) require immediate replacement of water and electrolyte losses, which may be life-threatening. The addition of indomethacin at 3 to 5 mg/kg/day divided into three doses often is necessary to correct the systemic effects of hyperprostaglandin. Restoration of normal potassium and magnesium often is difficult to achieve in classic BS (type 3) and in some patients with GS, despite high doses of potassium and magnesium supplementation and concomitant use of potassium-sparing diuretics such as spironolactone or amiloride.

PROGNOSIS

Some patients develop progressive renal insufficiency caused by severe tubulointerstitial nephritis or nephrotoxicity from prolonged indomethacin use. Deaths have been reported in infants as a result of hypokalemia, dehydration, and vascular collapse.

Most patients remain well when normal serum potassium concentration and hydration are maintained.

Suggested Readings

Peters M, Jeck N, Reinalter S, et al. Clinical presentation of genetically defined patients with hypokalemic salt losing tubulopathies. *Am J of Med* 2002; 112:3.

Shalev H, Ohali M, Kachko L, et al. The neonatal variant of Bartter syndrome and deafness: preservation of renal function. *Pediatrics* 2003;112:628.

CHAPTER 339 ■ RENAL HYPERTENSION

DANIEL I. FEIG, STUART L. GOLDSTEIN, AND L. LEIGHTON HILL

An abnormal activation of the renin-angiotensin-aldosterone system (RAAS) is a significant cause of hypertension in children. Intrinsic renovascular hypertension (RVH), which arises from a disturbance of the circulation to one or both kidneys, is considered the prototypical lesion leading to renin-mediated hypertension. However, other renal diseases associated with the obliteration of blood vessels within the renal parenchyma also are associated with renin-mediated hypertension, the most common of which is the hypertension caused by renal scarring that results from reflux and recurrent pyelonephritis. Renin-mediated hypertension also may be seen as a complication of renal vein thrombosis, renal dysplasia or hypoplasia, polycystic kidneys, obstructive uropathy, and radiation nephritis. Nephroblastomas, hamartomas, and arteriovenous malformations also can compress the renal artery, leading to ischemia and renin-mediated hypertension. Rarely, juxtaglomerular cell tumors and nephroblastomas may produce renin directly and cause hypertension without affecting the renal circulation.

PATHOPHYSIOLOGY

The importance of the RAAS in blood pressure control has been known since the 1930s, when experiments demonstrated that occlusion of the renal artery caused chronic hypertension. The decrease in renal perfusion caused by arterial occlusion leads to increased secretion of renin. Renin acts on the prohormone angiotensinogen and converts it to angiotensin I. Angiotensin I is converted by the lungs to the potent vasoconstrictor angiotensin II by the action of angiotensin-converting enzyme (ACE).

The acute hypertension seen from the increase in angiotensin II is a direct result of its vasoconstrictive properties. In addition, angiotensin II enhances secretion of aldosterone. Aldosterone acts on the distal nephron to promote sodium, chloride, and water reabsorption. Chronic elevation of angiotensin II leads to vascular smooth muscle hypertrophy. The combination of volume expansion and decreased vascular compliance results in the chronic renin-mediated hypertension. Recent studies in animal models and patients suggest that endothelial dysfunction, specifically impaired nitric oxide-mediated vasodilation, contributes to both acute and chronic RVH.

RENOVASCULAR HYPERTENSION

RVH is the second most common cause of surgically remediable hypertension in children. Obstruction of blood flow to the kidneys is either intrinsic (Box 339.1) or extrinsic (e.g., from paraaortic tumors, paraaortic lymph nodes). Of the intrinsic lesions, fibromuscular dysplasia occurs most often in children. Fibromuscular dysplasia often is limited to the renal arteries, but it has been known to occur in other locations. Renal artery stenosis has been associated with many connective tissue, inflammatory, and neuroendocrine disorders, including Marfan syndrome, Williams syndrome, abdominal coarctation of the aorta, Takayasu arteritis, Moya Moya, tuberous sclerosis, and neurofibromatosis. Clinically significant atherosclerotic vessel disease, the most common cause of RVH in adults, is a rare finding in children.

Clinical Manifestations

Box 339.2 lists clinical clues that suggest the presence of RVH. RVH should be considered in any severe case of hypertension

---

BOX 339.1   **Intrinsic Renal Artery Disease**

Fibromuscular lesions
  Intimal
  Medial
  Perimedial
Arteritic lesions
Thrombotic and embolic lesions
Aneurysms
Arteriovenous malformations (fistulas)
Neurofibromatosis (intimal lesion, nodular lesion)
Abdominal coarctation with renal artery involvement
Arteriosclerotic lesions

BOX 339.2   **Clinical Clues that Suggest Renovascular Hypertension**

Abrupt onset of severe hypertension
Epigastric, subcostal, or flank bruit
Progression to malignant-phase hypertension
Retinopathy
Hypokalemia
Plasma bicarbonate high-normal to elevated
Hypertension refractory to intensive antihypertensive regimen
Hypertension with unilateral small kidney
Excellent response to angiotensin-converting enzyme inhibitors
Transient impairment in renal function in response to angiotensin-converting enzyme inhibitor

---

(typically greater than 50 mm Hg systolic blood pressure or greater than 30 mm Hg diastolic blood pressure above the 95 percentile blood pressure) in a child whose condition is refractory to vasodilatory agents. An abdominal bruit, signs of secondary hyperaldosteronism (hypokalemia, mild alkalosis), and retinopathy suggest the presence of a chronic hypertensive disorder and should lead to a consideration of RVH. Finally, hypertension associated with a unilateral small kidney and an excellent response to ACE inhibitors is highly suggestive of RVH.

Diagnostic Studies

Renal arteriography remains the gold standard study for diagnosing RVH. Considerable effort has been expended during the 1990s to evaluate the sensitivity and specificity of less invasive modes of investigation to spare the patient from having to undergo unnecessary surgical investigation. Although many of these tests are useful in screening for RVH in adults, their effectiveness has not been studied extensively in children. Furthermore, these tests have a low predictive value when used to screen the general population. Because of the limitations of these tests, they should be used judiciously in patients in whom the suspicion is high for RVH interpreted only in their clinical context.

Peripheral Renin Activity

The measurement of peripheral renin activity (PRA) has not been of value in screening or as a diagnostic test for RVH. PRA has a sensitivity and specificity of less than 75% and may be elevated or suppressed by many medications. In addition, many unrelated conditions, including hyperthyroidism, congenital adrenal insufficiency, pheochromocytoma, and salt-wasting renal diseases, may elevate PRA.

Renal Ultrasonography

Renal ultrasonography should be performed as a screening test in all children with hypertension. Ultrasonography provides accurate and meaningful information regarding the size, location, architecture, and contour of the kidney. In newborns, it can detect vascular thrombosis secondary to umbilical artery catheters or dehydration. In adults, Doppler ultrasonographic imaging of renal arterial flow is nearly 90% sensitive for RVH. Unfortunately, the sensitivity in children likely is less than 50%. This difference may result from the differing causes of RVH in children and adults. In children, smaller vessels are involved more commonly and differences in renal blood flow cannot be resolved by Doppler imaging. In adults, RVH often is caused by atherosclerosis of larger vessels, which is more amenable to detection by Doppler imaging.

Other Radiologic Modalities

Magnetic resonance angiography (MRA) has been reliable in predicting stenosis of the main renal arteries in adults. Visualization of accessory renal arteries remains suboptimal; however, technologic improvements are expected to be made in the near future. Whereas MRA is used widely to evaluate cerebral circulation in children, its effectiveness in evaluating the renal circulation in children has not been studied. The current resolution limit for MRA is approximately 3 mm. Consequently, the MRA has limited sensitivity for mild to moderate stenosis in patients smaller than 35 kg. Computed tomographic renal angiography (CTRA) also has good sensitivity for renal artery stenosis but limited utility for branch artery stenosis. Its advantages over MRA are lower cost and the rapidity of the study.

Radionuclide Evaluation

ACE inhibitors have been used in conjunction with radionuclide imaging to diagnose RVH. Renal function in a kidney that has a stenotic artery is dependent on the high levels of renin produced by that kidney to maintain an elevated efferent arteriolar tone. This tone is depressed when an ACE inhibitor is given. When the kidney is visualized with radionuclide imaging after administration of an ACE inhibitor, a decreased uptake and clearance of the isotope from the affected kidney are present. This test has proved to be nearly 90% sensitive in diagnosing adults with suspected RVH. Studies in children have yielded conflicting results. Nonetheless, this study is helpful in identifying potential areas of disturbed renal circulation and is a valuable tool in the workup of suspected RVH. A negative test, however, should not preclude the diagnosis of RVH when the clinical picture is strongly suggestive of RVH.

Captopril Challenge Test

The captopril challenge test measures the rise in PRA after the administration of oral captopril. The positive predictive value of this test has been highly variable and should not be relied on for diagnosis of RVH.

Renal Arteriography

Renal arteriography with measurement of renal vein renin levels remains the gold standard in the diagnosis of RVH. These studies usually are performed simultaneously and provide both anatomic and functional information. The purpose of these studies is to visualize a functionally significant lesion (Fig. 339.1). The presence of collateral vessels with a stenotic lesion is considered significant. Differential renal vein renin levels are obtained from effluent venous blood from each renal vein and from the inferior vena cava. In unilateral RVH, the affected kidney should have a renal vein renin activity of at least 1.5 times that of the vein of the unaffected kidney. A renal-to-systemic renin index is calculated with the level from the inferior vena cava and when elevated is considered diagnostic for

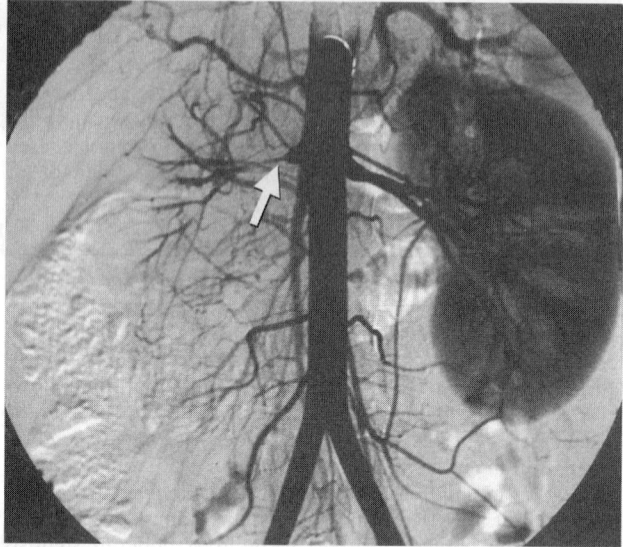

FIGURE 339.1. Direct renal arteriogram of a 15-year-old child with fibromuscular dysplasia leading to critical stenosis of the right renal artery. Balloon angioplasty was unsuccessful and unilateral nephrectomy was required to manage the child's severe hypertension.

renin-mediated hypertension, but is not unique to renal artery stenosis as differences in renin activity can be seen in reflux nephropathy and accentuated by depletion of sodium or administration of an ACE inhibitor. The presence of a significant difference in renal vein renin activity is 90% predictive of a benefit to be gained from surgical intervention; however, many patients with a negative study also benefit from surgery.

Clinical Management

The major objective of management of renin-mediated hypertension is to prevent the complications of hypertension by controlling blood pressure and preventing or slowing the loss of renal function. Control of moderate to severe hypertension is critical while the patient is undergoing evaluation. Long-term therapy may be medical, using pharmacologic agents, or surgical. Medical therapy has improved with the availability of ACE inhibitors since the 1980s. ACE inhibitors are the drugs of choice in children with renin-mediated hypertension. However, ACE inhibitors must be used with extreme caution in children with bilateral renal artery stenosis or evidence of a stenosis in a solitary kidney because they can cause renal failure in these circumstances. Thus, delaying initiation of ACE inhibitor therapy is prudent until these possibilities have been ruled out.

Surgical Options

Surgical options include nephrectomy, partial nephrectomy, revascularization by reconstructive vascular surgery, and au-

totransplantation. A minimally invasive surgical option is percutaneous transluminal renal angioplasty (PTRA). In PTRA, a balloon catheter is used to dilate the constricted portion of the renal artery. In children with fibromuscular dysplasia, PTRA provides a cure in 50% and significant clinical improvement in another 30%; however, the lesions associated with neurofibromatosis, developmental anomalies of the aorta, and lesions secondary to arteritis are less amenable to treatment with PTRA. The rates of restenosis vary from 10% to 30%. Often PTRA is performed at the time of renal arteriography. The advantages of PTRA over surgery include less anesthesia time, minimal patient morbidity, shorter hospital stays, and the ability to retain the affected kidney. This procedure should not be attempted without the availability of a vascular surgeon because possible complications include rupture of the renal artery, thrombus formation, and embolization.

Surgical Versus Medical Management

The appropriate surgical options listed previously should be considered strongly in children with RVH because otherwise these children would face a lifetime of medical therapy. These approaches often are curative and yield an acceptably low recurrence rate. Long-term medical therapy should be reserved for children whose vascular lesions are not amenable to surgical correction. In addition, medical therapy may be appropriate in young patients to allow for maturation of the renal vasculature to a stage that is more amenable to revascularization. Many clinicians are concerned that long-term ACE inhibitor therapy lowers blood pressure at the expense of perfusion to the stenotic kidney. Therefore, the patient should be monitored for evidence of azotemia and hyperkalemia after beginning ACE inhibitor therapy. If renal function does deteriorate, reconsideration must be given to surgical intervention or PTRA.

Suggested Readings

Chandar JJ, Sfakianakis GN, Zilleruelo GE, et al. ACE inhibition scintigraphy in the management of hypertension in children. *Pediatr Nephrol* 1999;13:493.

Estepa R, Gallego N, Orte L, et al. Renovascular hypertension in children. *Scand J Urol Nephrol* 2001;35:388.

Goonasekera CD, Shah V, Wade AM, et al. The usefulness of renal vein renin studies in hypertensive children: a 25-year experience. *Pediatr Nephrol* 2002;17:943.

Helenon O, Melki P, Correas JM, et al. Renovascular disease: Doppler ultrasound. *Semin Ultrasound CT MR* 1997;18:136.

Higashi Y, Sasaki S, Nakagawa K, et al. Endothelial function and oxidative stress in renovascular hypertension. *N Engl J Med* 2002;346:1954.

Lenz T, Kia T, Rupprecht G, et al. Captopril test: time over? *J Hum Hypertens* 1999;13:431.

McTaggart SJ, Gulati S, Walker RG, et al. Evaluation and long-term outcome of pediatric renovascular hypertension. *Pediatr Nephrol* 2000;14:1022.

Textor SC. ACE inhibitors in renovascular hypertension. *Cardiovasc Drugs Ther* 1990;4:229.

Vade A, Agrawal R, Lim-Dunham J, et al. Utility of computed tomographic renal angiogram in the management of childhood hypertension. *Pediatr Nephrol* 2002;17:741.

CHAPTER 340 ■ RENAL VASCULAR THROMBOSIS

STUART L. GOLDSTEIN AND L. LEIGHTON HILL

Renal vascular thrombosis is a rare condition in children that affects primarily neonates or children with a few select underlying conditions, such as nephrotic syndrome, or in the immediate postoperative renal transplant period. The newborn infant appears to be particularly at risk for the development of renal vascular thromboses. The vessels are small, renal blood flow is relatively low, the neonate is relatively polycythemic, vascular resistance is high, and fibrinolytic mechanisms may be immature. More than two-thirds of the children with renal vascular thrombosis are younger than 1 month old. The male-to-female ratio in reported series has ranged from 1.4:1.0 to 1.9:1.0 in the neonatal period.

RENAL VENOUS THROMBOSIS

Renal venous thrombosis (RVT) may be unilateral (most common) or bilateral. It is a rare condition in children past the neonatal period.

Etiology

In neonates and young infants, RVT is seen with dehydration, shock, increased tonicity of body fluids, and polycythemia. Infants with RVT frequently have experienced perinatal asphyxia, prenatal or postnatal stress, or septicemia. A high incidence of preceding diarrhea is present. Not uncommonly, these infants have been exposed to radiographic contrast media. Additional predisposing factors in the newborn period include congenital renal anomalies, congenital nephrosis, severe pyelonephritis, and maternal diabetes. RVT can be primary, first involving the veins of the kidney, or secondary, extending into the renal veins from a thrombus in the inferior vena cava.

RVT seen after infancy usually is associated with nephrotic syndrome or with cyanotic congenital heart disease (either spontaneously or after angiography). RVT does not cause nephrotic syndrome; rather, patients with active nephrotic syndrome have a predisposition for the development of RVT because they have low serum levels of proteins that counteract coagulation, including antithrombin III, protein C, and protein S, which are lost in the urine. RVT has been reported in 1% to 5% of patients in the immediate postoperative transplant period and seems to occur more frequently when kidneys from smaller cadaveric donors are used for transplantation or when patients are hypotensive in the recovery room.

Pathogenesis

During conditions of hypovolemia, hemoconcentration, hyperviscosity, hyperosmolarity, sepsis, and asphyxia, local microthrombi may occur peripherally in venous radicals, and the thrombus formation then may progress through the arcuate and interlobular veins toward the main renal vein. More rarely, the clotting process moves in the opposite direction.

RVT causes renal congestion and occasionally infarction. For signs and symptoms of RVT, see Box 340.1.

Laboratory Findings

Proteinuria occurs commonly, although in some instances it may be caused by the physical presence of gross blood in the urine. More than 50% of the infants with RVT demonstrate evidence of a microangiopathic hemolytic anemia with red blood cell fragmentation; thrombocytopenia; low levels of fibrinogen, factor V, and plasminogen; and an increase in fibrin degradation products. These findings may reflect the presence of active disseminated intravascular coagulation. Depending on the severity and whether the thrombosis is unilateral or bilateral, azotemia and other biochemical evidence of acute renal failure may be present.

Intravenous urography should not be performed. The most useful imaging studies include sonography of the urinary tract, which may reveal enlarged size, altered echogenicity, loss of corticomedullary definition, and a decrease in the size of the central sinus echo, and Doppler evaluation of renal arterial and renal venous blood flow. Isotope renography also may be useful. Selective venography may provide precise delineation of the vascular thrombosis but is considered risky and usually is unnecessary.

BOX 340.1 | **Signs and Symptoms of Renal Venus Thrombosis**

Sudden enlargement of one or both kidneys may occur.
Approximately 60% of the patients with RVT have a palpably enlarged renal mass.
Most patients have hematuria, which may be gross or microscopic, although hematuria also may be absent.
Renal enlargement may occur without other symptoms, but, more often, associated symptoms and signs are present. Associated symptoms include:
Pallor
Tachypnea
Vomiting
Abdominal distention
Shock
Fever
Oliguria or anuria
Many of the signs and symptoms noted are caused by the underlying disorder causing the RVT rather than by the vascular catastrophe itself.
Hypertension is an uncommon finding.

Differential Diagnosis

The many causes of hematuria must be considered. The common presence of a microangiopathic hemolytic anemia in RVT renders hemolytic-uremic syndrome an important differential diagnosis. Other causes of renal enlargement, such as perirenal hematoma, abscess, hydronephrosis, cystic renal disease, and renal tumors, also should be considered in the differential diagnosis.

Therapy

For the most part, therapy should be conservative and supportive. Correction of underlying pathophysiologic abnormalities should be attempted. If oliguria and azotemia occur with bilateral disease, medical management of acute renal failure may be required, and, in some instances, dialysis is needed. The efficacy of anticoagulant therapy (heparin sodium) has not been documented by controlled studies and should be considered only if laboratory evidence of continuing intravascular coagulation exists or if bilateral disease is present and the patient is at risk for developing chronic renal failure or end-stage renal disease. A surgical approach in the acute phase rarely is indicated, except in the immediate posttransplant period. Recovery of function in affected kidneys may occur, but progressive atrophy may result in small, scarred kidneys. Hypertension may be a late complication. Chronic renal failure can be the outcome in some patients who have bilateral RVT. Other patients may show predominantly tubular dysfunction as the sequela of RVT.

RENAL ARTERIAL THROMBOSIS

Renal arterial occlusions are more common findings than is RVT in the neonate, probably because of the extensive use of umbilical artery catheters. Many of the same etiologic and pathogenic factors at play in RVT also are important in renal artery thrombosis.

Obstruction of the renal arterial system may result from an embolus, and the ensuing renal infarction may be unilateral or bilateral, total or segmental, depending on the number and distribution of the emboli. Obstruction of the renal artery also may result from a large thrombus of the lumen of the aorta. The

kidney usually is enlarged, and abdominal distension and vomiting are common findings. Renin-related hypertension may be severe and difficult to control despite institution of aggressive pharmacologic therapy. Therapy with angiotensin-converting enzyme inhibitors or angiotensin II (A-II) receptor blockers should be instituted only in cases of unilateral disease because patients with bilateral disease may be dependent on A-II to preserve glomerular filtration. Congestive heart failure may occur. Hematuria and proteinuria frequently are seen, and the presence of renal failure often depends on whether the thrombosis is unilateral or bilateral. Color Doppler ultrasonography may demonstrate a decrease in renal blood flow, but diethylenetriaminepentaacetic acid (DPTA) renography is the method of choice to estimate renal blood flow and demonstrate perfusion defects. It also is useful in predicting outcome with regard to renal function. All patients receiving a renal transplant should receive a renal scan in the immediate postoperative period; a scan demonstrating no perfusion to the transplant indicates a renal vascular thrombosis and requires immediate surgical exploration to preserve the renal allograft.

Treatment largely is supportive and frequently is directed at the underlying pathophysiologic abnormalities. Heparinization, thrombolysis, or both may be considered in patients with massive thrombosis. Attempts at thrombectomy usually are contraindicated but may be entertained in unstable patients who are not responding to medical treatment. Acute or chronic management of renal failure, including dialysis, may be necessary. The renovascular hypertension may persist, requiring continued therapy; fortunately, in many instances, the hypertension resolves.

Suggested Readings

Adelman RD. Long-term follow-up of neonatal renovascular hypertension. *Pediatr Nephrol* 1987;1:35.

Brion LP, Bernstein J, Spitzer A. Kidney and urinary tract. In: Fanaroff AA, Martin RJ, eds. *Neonatal-perinatal medicine—diseases of the fetus and infant*, 6th ed. St. Louis: Mosby, 1997:1613.

McDonald RA, Smith JM, Stablein D, Harmon WE. Pretransplant peritoneal dialysis and graft thrombosis following pediatric kidney transplantation: a NAPRTCS report. *Pediatr Transplant* 2003;7:204.

Renfield ML, Kraybill EN. Consumptive coagulopathy with renal vein thrombosis. *J Pediatr* 1973;82:1054.

Stringer DA, Krysl J, Manson D, et al. The value of Doppler sonography in the detection of major vessel thrombosis in the neonatal abdomen. *Pediatr Radiol* 1990;21:30.

CHAPTER 341 ■ UROLITHIASIS

ARUNDHATI S. KALE AND L. LEIGHTON HILL

Marked variation exists in the incidence of urinary tract stones in children worldwide. In some countries, such as Turkey and Thailand, urolithiasis is endemic; bladder stones predominate, and dietary factors are postulated to play a causative role. In contrast, stones are uncommon findings in children in the United States, where fewer than 1% of all renal stones occur in children younger than 10 and fewer than 3% occur in children younger than 19 and most stones have a metabolic origin. In the United States, boys with stones outnumber girls by 2:1; stones are very uncommon findings in African American children; and bladder stones are seen much less commonly than are upper urinary tract stones. Children in the southeastern United States appear to have the greatest risk for formation of stones. A distinction should be made between urolithiasis or nephrolithiasis (stones in the urinary tract) and nephrocalcinosis (an increase in the calcium content within the renal tissue itself), although the two conditions may coexist.

FORMATION OF STONES

Urinary calculi consist of very small glycoprotein matrices with surrounding organic or inorganic crystals. Urinary crystalloids capable of being crystallized include calcium, phosphorus, oxalates, cystine, uric acid, xanthine, and ammonium. Supersaturation of the urine with various ionic species eventually leads to precipitation, with subsequent growth of crystals. Two products appear to be important in this process: the solubility product and the formation product. Below the solubility product for a given ionic pair (e.g., calcium and oxalate), the solution is undersaturated and formation of crystals does not occur. Above the formation product for a given ionic pair, the solution is supersaturated and spontaneous precipitation occurs. Between the solubility product and the formation product lies the metastable region in which precipitation does not occur unless the system is disturbed. Urine volume, through its effect on dilution and concentration, obviously plays a critical role in determining the degree of saturation. Urine pH is an important factor in determining solubility. Crystalline nuclei rarely form in free solution but rather on existing surfaces. Theoretically, any factor that increases the number of nuclei in tubular fluid or urine, such as epithelial injury, could lower the metastable limit, the supersaturation at which crystals first form. Also, certain inhibitor substances retard crystallization. Inhibitor absence has been suggested to explain calculus formation in patients with normal excretion of urinary crystalloids. Inhibitors are thought to include citrate, pyrophosphate, urinary glycoprotein crystallization inhibitors, Tamm-Horsfall mucoprotein, and magnesium-to-calcium and sodium-to-calcium ratios in the urine. Undoubtedly, many other inhibitors remain to be identified. The physicochemical principles underlying the formation of renal stones remain poorly defined. A classification of stones according to their composition is shown in Box 341.1. Calcium is a constituent of 90% of calculi. Calcium phosphate, the principal constituent of the calcium stones listed in part I of Box 341.1, also is found in struvite and other stones listed in the table. The struvite stones (magnesium ammonium phosphate) often are called infection stones.

CLINICAL FEATURES

The typical presentation with incapacitating renal colic is an unusual finding in children, especially young children and infants, and symptoms may be very nonspecific. Gross or microscopic hematuria may be the only manifestation, or hematuria may be accompanied by nonspecific abdominal pain or by fever, pyuria, and abdominal pain. Signs and symptoms might be those of a urinary tract infection (UTI). Typical renal colic may occur in older children. In some instances, the stone or gravel already has been passed spontaneously. Frequently, the patient has a family history of stones. Urinary stones can cause obstruction of the urinary flow, dilation of the urinary tract, and ultimately renal parenchymal damage. Stones can predispose to UTIs; conversely, UTIs can be important in the formation of stones.

| BOX 341.1 | Urolithiasis Classification Based on Stone Composition |

I. Calcium stones (calcium oxalate and calcium phosphate)
  A. Hypercalciuria
    1. Hypercalcemic hypercalciuria
       Hyperparathyroidism
       Thyrotoxicosis
       Vitamin D intoxication
       Idiopathic infantile hypercalcemia
       Sarcoidosis
       Neoplastic deposits in bones
       Immobilization
    2. Normocalcemic hypercalciuria
       Idiopathic or familial hypercalciuria
       Distal renal tubular acidosis type 1
       Acetazolamide use
       Loop diuretic use
       Immobilization
       Vitamin D excess
       Cushing syndrome
  B. Hyperoxaluria (calcium oxalate)
    1. Primary hyperoxaluria types I and II
    2. Secondary hyperoxaluria
       Inflammatory bowel disease
       Pyridoxine deficiency
       Massive doses of vitamin C
  C. Hyperglycinuria (calcium oxalate stones)
  D. Idiopathic urolithiasis
II. Magnesium ammonium phosphate (struvite) plus basic calcium phosphate (apatite)
  A. Urinary tract infection with urea-splitting organisms (mostly Proteus species)
  B. Foreign body plus urinary stasis plus infection
III. Uric acid stones*
  A. Hyperuricosuria
    1. Gout
    2. Lesch-Nyhan syndrome
    3. High purine diet
    4. Glycogen storage disease type I
    5. Leukemia-lymphoma
    6. Leukemia-lymphoma/chemotherapy
IV. Xanthine stones*
  A. Primary xanthinuria
  B. Allopurinol therapy
V. Dihydroxyadenine stones*
VI. Cystine stones
  A. Cystinuria

---

*Disorders of purine metabolism.

CLASSIFICATION

Calcium Stones

Hypercalciuria

Hypercalciuria is defined by a urinary calcium excretion of more than 4 mg/kg/day and may be associated with normal or high serum calcium. The diverse conditions causing hypercalcemia (see Box 341.1) are discussed elsewhere in the book. Hypercalcemia is more apt to cause nephrocalcinosis than urolithiasis.

Idiopathic or Familial Hypercalciuria. Idiopathic hypercalciuria is an inherited metabolic abnormality. In pediatric patients with nephrolithiasis, 73% had a family history of kidney stones in at least one first- or second-order relative. Urinary calcium excretion exceeds 4 mg/kg/day, or the calcium-to-creatinine ratio exceeds 0.21 in a child older than 2 years of age. Calcium excretion is greater in infancy; normal calcium-to-creatinine ratios are as high as 0.8 mg/mg in infants up to the age of 6 months and 0.6 mg/mg in children between 6 months and a 1 year of age. At least three mechanisms have been invoked to explain the hypercalciuria. The first—excessive intestinal absorption of calcium—can cause increased calcium excretion, and urinary calcium excretion returns to normal during fasting. A second type of hypercalciuria is called *renal hypercalciuria* because of apparently defective calcium reabsorption by the renal tubules. The renal loss of calcium results temporarily in a lower serum calcium level, which stimulates production of parathyroid hormone (PTH), bringing the serum calcium back to normal. Renal hypercalciuria is characterized by elevated levels of PTH, which stimulate increased production of 1,25-dihydroxycholecalciferol, which then enhances the intestinal absorption of calcium and increases the filtered load of calcium in the kidney. Children with renal hypercalciuria continue to put out calcium in abnormal amounts (more than 4 mg/kg/day) during fasting. A third type of hypercalciuria—1,25-dihydroxycholecalciferol–induced hypercalciuria—is recognized by some investigators. The defect may be a renal tubular leak of phosphate. The ensuing hypophosphatemia is thought to stimulate the renal synthesis of 1,25-dihydroxycholecalciferol, which then enhances intestinal absorption of calcium; this absorption in turn provides extra calcium for renal excretion. Many experts in calcium physiology argue that dividing the hypercalciurias into several pathogenetic entities is unjustified. They offer instead a unifying hypothesis that the various forms of hypercalciuria result from the same generalized defect, possibly a disordered regulation of 1,25-dihydroxycholecalciferol production. Children with idiopathic hypercalciuria also may have hematuria (either gross or microscopic), even though no stones have been detected, possibly from crystalluria. Hypercalciuria also should be in the differential diagnosis of isolated hematuria. The risk of developing stones in this population is approximately 15%. Many patients with biochemical evidence of hypercalciuria never experience problems with formation of stones. The genetic basis of this disorder is unknown.

Hyperoxaluria

Primary hyperoxaluria is a general term for two rare genetic disorders (types I and II) that result in recurrent calcium oxalate urolithiasis and nephrocalcinosis. Nephrocalcinosis is a greater problem than is urolithiasis because the deposition of calcium oxalate in the renal parenchyma ultimately leads to tissue destruction, fibrosis, and chronic renal failure. The renal calculi are extremely radiopaque and homogenous. Secondary hyperoxaluria with formation of stones also can occur, most often caused by chronic inflammatory bowel disease such as Crohn disease or by ileal bypass. Apparently, an increase in intestinal oxalate absorption occurs in enteric types of secondary hyperoxaluria. Other causes of acquired hyperoxaluria include renal tubular acidosis (RTA), hepatic cirrhosis, cystic fibrosis, and ethylene glycol poisoning.

Idiopathic Urolithiasis

Idiopathic urolithiasis refers to the finding of a stone in a patient whose workup, including urine cultures, urologic evaluation, and metabolic evaluation, is entirely negative. The number of children in this group is small, as a cause for stones usually can be found.

Struvite Stones

Struvite (magnesium ammonium phosphate) stones occur as a result of UTIs with urease-containing bacteria and account for approximately 13% of stones in children. These organisms, most commonly Proteus species, can split urinary urea into ammonia ions, which buffer hydrogen ions to form ammonium molecules, thereby producing a strongly alkaline urine loaded with ammonium compounds. The persistently alkaline urine favors the crystallization of calcium phosphate (apatite), and the increase in ammonium concentration raises the magnesium ammonium phosphate product. Seventy-five percent of struvite stones in children are seen before they reach age 5 years, and 80% are in boys. Children with struvite stones frequently have vesicoureteral reflux or other urologic abnormalities. The UTIs associated with struvite stones also may be caused by *Klebsiella*, *Pseudomonas*, *Candida*, and *Staphylococcus* and can be quite resistant to therapy, and organisms have been cultured from the interior of the stone. Despite advances in technology, most struvite stones still are removed surgically. Complete removal of these stones is mandatory.

Cystinuria

Cystine stones account for approximately 5% of pediatric urinary calculi. Cystinuria is a hereditary disorder of amino acid transport affecting the epithelial cells of both the renal tubule and the gastrointestinal tract. The gastrointestinal defect apparently causes no clinical problems. However, the renal tubular abnormality results in hyperexcretion in the urine of the neutral amino acid cystine and the cationic amino acids lysine, ornithine, and arginine. The diagnosis is suspected when cystine crystals are seen on urinalysis and proved by demonstrating abnormal quantities of these amino acids in a timed urine specimen. Patients with cystinuria often excrete more than 400 mg/1.73 m²/day of cystine, with normals being less than 60 mg/1.73 m²/day. The only clinical expression of cystinuria is urolithiasis; otherwise, individuals with this disorder can live a normal life. Whether urolithiasis eventually develops in every person with cystinuria is unknown. Genetic mutations have been identified in chromosomes 2 and 19 in different populations.

Uric Acid Stones

Uric acid stones constitute 3% to 4% of urinary calculi in children, and those resulting from primary gout are extremely rare findings in children. Hyperuricemia with uric acid calculi is seen as part of Lesch-Nyhan syndrome, a rare inborn error of metabolism. Uric acid stones also may occur as a consequence of the hyperuricosuria of glycogen storage disease type I. Hyperuricemia with uric acid stones or gravel in the urinary tracts of both kidneys occasionally is the presenting feature of leukemia. More commonly, the calculi occur after the patient has received cytotoxic chemotherapy for leukemia or lymphoma (tumor lysis syndrome). Urine flow may be blocked, resulting in acute renal failure. High uric acid levels also can be nephrotoxic and produce renal parenchymal damage directly. Uric acid excretion is extremely high in the neonatal period and remains fairly high during childhood. Total urate excretion, therefore, varies with age, but the amount of uric acid excreted per deciliter of glomerular filtrate does not vary with age. Normal excretion of uric acid is less than 0.56 mg per deciliter of GF after the child reaches the age of 2 years.

DIAGNOSIS

A high index of suspicion frequently is required to make the diagnosis of urolithiasis. Demonstration of the stone can be accomplished by imaging techniques such as a plain radiography of the abdomen, intravenous urography, ultrasound study of the urinary tract, or computed tomography. All stones containing calcium are radiopaque. Cystine stones are slightly radiopaque because of the sulfur present in cystine. Struvite stones also are radiopaque. The stones that most frequently are radiolucent are those resulting from disorders of purine metabolism (see Box 341.1). The diagnosis of urolithiasis also can be made by the proven passage of a stone, gravel, or sludge. Whenever urolithiasis is considered, any passed material must be saved, and the urine must be strained, whether at home or in the hospital, in an attempt to obtain a stone. The formation of a stone within the urinary tract is not a specific disease but instead is a complication of many highly varied disorders. The next step must be to determine which of the disorders caused the stone. Therefore, all passed stones or stone-like material must be tested completely for composition. The stone should be solubilized and analyzed qualitatively and quantitatively for its main contents. This analysis should be performed in a laboratory experienced in stone analysis. Children with the diagnosis of urolithiasis should undergo radiologic investigation of the urinary tract to evaluate for a possible anatomic abnormality of the genitourinary tract, to assess for the presence of and degree of obstruction caused by the stone, to search for other stones, and to determine if nephrocalcinosis also is present. This investigation usually includes either an ultrasound study of the urinary tract or an intravenous urogram and occasionally a cystourethrogram. The laboratory workup is suggested in Box 341.2. The metabolic evaluation of patients who form stones should begin 4 to 6 weeks after the stone has been diagnosed and passed because the passage itself may cause transient changes in the urinary chemistry. The patient then also would be free of the effects of obstruction and infection. The serum calcium level determines the possible presence of hypercalcemia. Serum phosphorus levels may be low in hyperparathyroidism, in one type of hypercalciuria, and in renal tubular acidosis, and they may be elevated in the tumor lysis syndrome. Serum creatinine estimates glomerular function. Electrolyte levels, pH, Pco_2, and urine pH are used to investigate the possible presence of RTA. All children with stones should undergo a spot chemical urine test for cystine to rule out cystinuria and a quantitative amino acid analysis if the spot test is positive. A timed urine sample (preferably 24 hours) is collected for quantitative measurement of calcium, citrate, oxalate, and uric acid. Quantitative urinary calcium excretion or a spot urine test for calcium-to-creatinine ratio provides information regarding the possible presence of hypercalciuria. Several determinations may be necessary. Hyperuricosuria can occur without hyperuricemia. These mostly routine tests frequently provide a diagnosis as to the cause of the stone. Sometimes leads from the routine tests may suggest performing more sophisticated studies. An accurate chemical analysis of the stone itself greatly enhances the possibility of establishing a correct diagnosis. Measurement of PTH may be indicated in some cases.

Imaging Modalities

Plain abdominal radiographs have only 62% sensitivity and 67% specificity. Plain films may be used to follow the progres-

---

| BOX 341.2 | Laboratory Workup for Urolithiasis |

Blood determinations
Calcium; repeat two or three times
Phosphorus
Alkaline phosphatase
Creatinine
Electrolytes
pH and pCO_2
Uric acid

Urine studies
Urinalysis, repeat two or three times
Urine culture
Spot urine for cystine (cyanide-nitroprusside test)
Urine pHs, repeat four to six times
Spot urine for calcium-to-creatinine ratio
24-hour urine for calcium, creatinine, citrate, oxalate, and uric acid: Add xanthine if patient has hypouricemia and quantitative amino acids if spot test for cystine is positive.

Other studies
Ammonium chloride loading test may be necessary to assess renal ability to acidify.

---

sion of stones after diagnosis. Ultrasound is highly sensitive in skilled hands. The use of the intravenous pyelogram has become almost obsolete and rarely is used. Noncontrast helical computed tomography scanning has become the standard of care in adults but has not been proven in children. Magnetic resonance imaging urography is another technique being investigated.

TREATMENT

One of the most important measures in preventing the formation or further growth of any stone regardless of cause is to increase urine volume, which reduces the urinary concentrations of calcium, phosphorus, oxalates, cystine, uric acid, and other possible constituents of stones. This dilution of the urine can be accomplished by raising the fluid intake to 1.5 to 2.0 times normal (2,400 mL/m^2/day or more). The high fluid intake should be distributed as much as possible throughout the 24 hours, including at bedtime and during the night if the patient awakens. Early morning urine should be kept at a specific gravity of less than 1.014. UTI, if present, must be treated, and a search for anatomic abnormalities completed. Any urologic abnormalities predisposing to infections or stones should be corrected.

Stone Removal

Many stones pass through and out of the urinary tract spontaneously. Others (e.g., uric acid stones) may dissolve slowly or at least not grow as a result of medical treatment. Some stones must be removed: struvite stones, stones causing prolonged blockage with obstructive nephropathy, and stones causing significant chronic pain or resistant UTI. In the past, the traditional surgical management of patients with calculus disease consisted of endoscopic manipulation with stone baskets or loops for stones in the lower part of the ureter (below the pelvic brim) or open surgical procedures for calculi higher in the urinary tract. These traditional methods of stone removal are being replaced by a variety of new modalities, including extracorporeal shock-wave lithotripsy, percutaneous nephrostolithotomy, and percutaneously placed endoscopes to fragment calculi with ultrasonic waves or lasers. These techniques, used first in adults, now are finding widespread application in children and represent a dramatic advance in medical therapy. With new-generation lithotriptors, infants as young as 3 to 4 months of age have benefited from extracorporeal shock-wave lithotripsy, with minimal side effects.

Specific Therapeutic Measures

The treatment for pediatric hypercalciuria and stones caused by hypercalcemia is elimination of the cause of the hypercalcemia, that is, parathyroidectomy (for patients with hyperparathyroidism), treatment of thyrotoxicosis or Cushing disease, withdrawal of vitamin D therapy, at least partial mobilization of immobilized patients, and so on. Distal RTA, a form of normocalcemic hypercalciuria, can be treated with appropriate amounts of sodium bicarbonate or sodium citrate plus potassium citrate in an effort to keep the serum bicarbonate concentration in the range of 22 to 28 mEq/L (see Chapter 333, Renal Tubular Acidosis). Treatment of urolithiasis caused by familial or idiopathic hypercalciuria is controversial. Trying to distinguish the various types of hypercalciuria for purposes of therapy probably no longer is necessary; rather, all patients with stones from idiopathic or familial hypercalciuria should be treated similarly, with increased fluid intake and a diet high in potassium and low in sodium. Thiazide diuretics, which enhance renal tubular reabsorption of calcium, are quite effective in reducing calcium excretion and preventing recurrent formation of stones. Because high intakes of sodium chloride tend to negate this effect of thiazides, restriction of sodium intake to a maximum of 2 mEq/kg/day is indicated. The addition of potassium citrate to this regimen (1 to 2 mEq/kg/day) is advised. Whether thiazide drugs should be used for long-term therapy depends on the number of recurrences of stones and the complications encountered. Restriction of dietary calcium is not recommended for children in light of reports of developing osteopenia. The use of phosphate compounds (cellulose phosphate, orthophosphate) in children is poorly tolerated and generally has been abandoned. Of these therapies for familial hypercalciuria, the thiazide diuretics have been the most successful, but long-term use of a thiazide would be considered only in patients with recurrent stones. Thiazides reduce formation of stones in patients with recurrent idiopathic urolithiasis, even though urinary calcium before treatment was normal.

No effective therapy for the primary hyperoxalurias exists. A few patients with type I appear to respond partially to pyridoxine therapy. Salts of phosphate, citrate, and magnesium, aimed at increasing the solubility of calcium oxalate, have been administered with some success. The ultimate therapy for primary hyperoxaluria is combined liver-kidney transplantation. All fragments of struvite stones must be removed because failure to do so may result in persistent infection and recurrence of stones. Complete eradication of infection and the correction of any anatomic abnormality causing urinary stasis are essential. Allopurinol therapy is very effective in patients with uric acid and dihydroxyadenine stones. A high urine output also is valuable in treating these two types of stones. Alkalinization of the urine to a pH of 6.5 with sodium bicarbonate or sodium citrate is important in treating and preventing uric acid calculi. Hemodialysis may need to be performed to control the extreme hyperuricemia seen in patients with tumor lysis syndrome. Dilution of the urine decreases the saturation of cystine, and alkalinization increases the solubility of cystine. The alkali therapy must be divided over the course of the entire day and night to ensure a pH above 7 (ideally above 7.4). Of these two treatments, increasing the fluid intake is much more important. Administration of tiopronin or penicillamine may be used. Both compounds interact with cystine to form a thiol–disulfide exchange with cystine, which is more soluble in urine.

Suggested Readings

Bleyer A, Angus ZS. Approach to nephrolithiasis. *Kidney* 1992;25:1.
Coe FL. Treatment of hypercalciuria. *N Engl J Med* 1984;311:116.
Coe FL, Parks JH, Asplin JR. The pathogenesis and treatment of kidney stones. *N Engl J Med* 1992;327:1141.
Hufnagle KG, Khan SN, Penn D, et al. Renal calcifications: a complication of long-term furosemide therapy in preterm infants. *Pediatrics* 1982;70:360.
Hulbert JC, Reddy PK, Gonzales R, et al. Percutaneous nephrostolithotomy: an alternative approach to the management of pediatric calculus disease. *Pediatrics* 1985;73:610.
Manthey DE, Teichman J. Nephrolithiasis. *Emerg Med Clin North Am* 2001;19:633.
Minevich E. Pediatric urolithiasis. *Pediatr Clin North Am* 2001;48:1571.
Mulley AG Jr. Shock-wave lithotripsy. *N Engl J Med* 1986;314:845.
Pak CYC, Peters P, Hurt G, et al. Is selective therapy of recurrent nephrolithiasis possible? *Am J Med* 1981;71:615.
Stapleton FB. Childhood stones. *Endocrinol Metab Clin North Am* 2002;4:1001.
Stapleton FB. Hematuria associated with hypercalciuria and hyperuricosuria: a practical approach. *Pediatr Nephrol* 1994;8:756.

SECTION VII ■ DISEASES OF THE GASTROINTESTINAL SYSTEM

CHAPTER 342 ■ NORMAL GASTROINTESTINAL FUNCTION

MARK A. GILGER

The gastrointestinal (GI) tract has many functions—digestion, absorption, and secretion, as well as endocrine and immunologic functions. This system can be thought of as a tube that extends from the mouth to the anus and is divided into three parts: the foregut (mouth to proximal duodenum), midgut (distal duodenum to colon), and hindgut (distal colon and rectum). Each part has a separate blood supply. The salivary glands, pancreas, liver, and gallbladder are outgrowths of the foregut and midgut. The *in utero* development of the human gut results in a digestive system that is nearly fully capable at birth.

DEGLUTITION

Swallowing, or deglutition, can be seen in the fetus by approximately 16 weeks of gestation. After birth, the normal swallow develops into three phases: oral, pharyngeal, and esophageal. The oral and pharyngeal phases are voluntary; the esophageal phase is reflexive. In feeding infants, sucking is accomplished by a rhythmic lowering of the tongue and compression of the nipple or areola. The bolus of milk is propelled backward by a rolling action of the tongue posteriorly. The nasopharynx then is sealed off by the soft palate, and the larynx is brought upward and forward as the epiglottis covers the trachea. The esophageal phase begins with a relaxation of the upper esophageal sphincter, allowing the bolus to enter the esophagus. A primary peristaltic wave is initiated, which then transports the bolus to the stomach. A secondary peristaltic wave within the body of the esophagus may be initiated by distention and frequently occurs as a result of esophageal reflux.

Peristalsis also is initiated in the esophagus by migrating motor complexes. These rhythmic involuntary complexes originate independently of swallow or distention and sweep through the entire GI tract, terminating in the rectum.

The ability to swallow solid foods, although partially present at birth, is completely functional by the time the child is age 4 to 6 months. Children who have not been fed solid foods by age 15 months have difficulty swallowing them. This fact suggests that infancy is a critical time in the development of the ability to handle solid foods.

ESOPHAGUS

The esophagus develops from the embryonic foregut. During elongation, the luminal surface differentiates into stratified squamous epithelium. The esophagus and respiratory tract begin as a single tube, which divides by 2 months' gestation. Incomplete division of the tube into two separate organs results in a variety of anomalies, such as a tracheoesophageal fistula.

The esophagus is a collapsed hollow tube lying posterior to the trachea. The esophageal mucosa is oriented into longitudinal folds that disappear when the esophagus is distended. Unlike the rest of the GI tract, the esophagus has no serosal surface. The upper third of the esophagus is striated or skeletal muscle, whereas the lower esophagus is smooth muscle. The luminal surface is covered with stratified squamous epithelium. Blood is supplied to the upper third of the esophagus by the inferior thyroid artery, whereas branches of the descending thoracic aorta supply the body. The left gastric artery supplies blood to the lower third of the esophagus. Venous drainage is to the superior vena cava superiorly, the azygos vein from the body, and the gastric veins from the lower esophagus. The gastric veins drain to the portal venous system. In cases of portal hypertension, venous flow can reverse, resulting in esophageal varices. The esophagus is innervated by the spinal accessory nerve and the vagus nerve.

Functionally, the esophagus is divided into three zones: the upper esophageal sphincter, the body, and the lower esophageal sphincter. The upper esophageal sphincter has a resting pressure of approximately 30 mm Hg and normally is closed. Swallowing results in relaxation and dilation of the upper esophageal sphincter and initiates a primary peristaltic wave that passes through the body of the esophagus. The lower esophageal sphincter has a resting manometric pressure of approximately 20 mm Hg and also normally is contracted. The primary peristaltic wave opens the lower esophageal sphincter

for approximately 7 seconds to allow passage of material into the stomach. The lower sphincter then returns to its resting state, which prevents reflux of acidic gastric contents into the esophagus.

STOMACH

The stomach develops from the primitive foregut and is evident by 4 weeks' gestation. Gastric glands appear by approximately 11 weeks' gestation. Structurally, the stomach is divided into four parts—the cardia, fundus, body, and antrum—terminating with the pyloric sphincter (Fig. 342.1). Gastric glands present in the lining of the stomach are composed of four cell types: chief cells (zymogen cells), which contain zymogen granules and secrete pepsinogen; parietal cells (oxyntic cells), which secrete hydrochloric acid and intrinsic factor; mucous neck cells; and endocrine-like cells (Fig. 342.2). Production of hydrochloric acid is measurable at 15 weeks' gestation and increases in amount until normal adult levels are reached at approximately 1 month after birth. Production of pepsin is evident at 16 weeks' gestation and reaches adult levels by the time the child is 2 years of age.

Blood supply is provided by the left and right gastric branches of the celiac artery (Fig. 342.3). Venous drainage is through the left and right gastric veins into the portal vein. The stomach is innervated by the vagus nerve and is completely autonomic.

The stomach has at least four major functions: storing meals, mixing and grinding foods, controlling the emptying of food into the duodenum, and acting as the initial barrier to pathogens and allergens entering the GI tract. At birth, the stomach has a capacity of approximately 30 mL (approximately 1 oz), but capacity increases to approximately 1,500 mL by adulthood. The fundus provides most of the storage capacity and responds to the ingestion of food by relaxing and increasing gastric volume. Mixing and grinding food are accomplished by the phasic gastric contractions and the cone shape of the

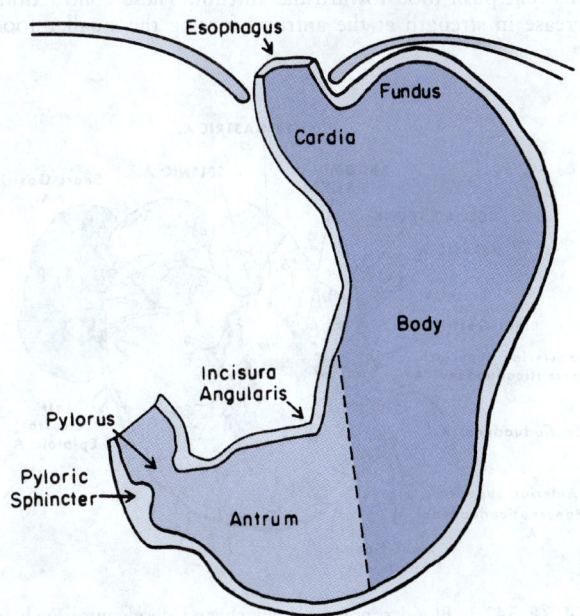

FIGURE 342.1. Anatomic regions of the stomach. (Reprinted with permission from Sleisenger MH, Fordtran JS. *Gastrointestinal disease: pathophysiology, diagnosis, and management,* 3rd ed. Philadelphia: Saunders, 1983:506.)

GASTRIC GLAND

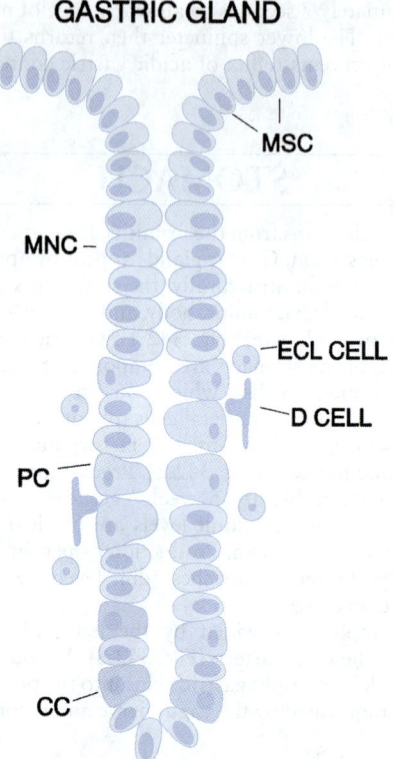

FIGURE 342.2. Schematic representation of a gastric gland indicating mucous surface cells (*MSC*), mucous neck cells (*MNC*), enterochromaffin-like cells (*ECL*), somatostatin-containing D cells, parietal cells (*PC*), and chief cells (*CC*). (Reprinted with permission from Lloyd KCK, Haile HT. Peripheral regulation of gastric acid secretion. In: Johnson LR, ed. *Physiology of the gastrointestinal tract,* 3rd ed. Philadelphia: Lippincott, 1994:1186.)

antrum. The gastric pacemaker, located in the body, generates three-per-second depolarization waves, which initiate contractions that push food toward the antrum. These contractions increase in strength at the antrum, forcing the smaller food

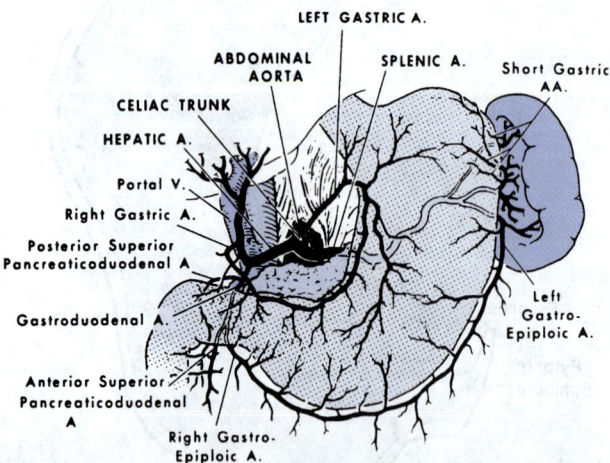

FIGURE 342.3. Blood supply to stomach and duodenum. Each of the three major branches of the celiac axis supplying the stomach and the anastomotic connections to the superior mesenteric artery near the duodenum is illustrated. (Reprinted with permission from Sleisenger MH, Fordtran JS. *Gastrointestinal disease: pathophysiology, diagnosis, and management,* 3rd ed. Philadelphia: Saunders, 1983:1544.)

particles, usually approximately 1 mm in size, into the duodenum. The emptying of food is controlled by the pylorus, which allows a relatively constant flow of nutrients into the duodenum. Liquids tend to empty more quickly (cool liquids faster than warm), and factors such as high fat content and high osmolarity of the meal tend to delay gastric emptying.

Gastric acid plays an important role in destroying or damaging intestinal pathogens. This acid barrier is the first of a series of nonimmunologic mechanisms that eradicate pathogens and other noxious agents.

SMALL INTESTINE

The small intestine develops from the midgut portion of the fetal archenteron or primitive gut. Initial growth occurs out of the abdominal cavity, within the vitelline stalk of the umbilicus. It returns into the abdominal cavity by 10 weeks' gestation due to the fixation of the cecum to the right lower quadrant of the abdomen. Failure of this fixation rotation results in the common malrotation syndromes. Villous formation is apparent first at 8 weeks' gestation and proceeds in a proximal to distal fashion. The entire small bowel has both villi and crypts by 12 weeks, and the enzymatic activities of pepsin, trypsin, and lipase have been documented by 18 weeks' gestation. The small intestine immune apparatus, M cells (membranous cells), and Peyer patches appear at 2 weeks' gestation. The number of Peyer patches increases until puberty, then decreases throughout adult life. The mucosa of the small intestine contains more immunocytes (plasma cells, lymphocytes, and so forth) than does any other organ in the body: 1 cm of small intestine contains approximately *ten* immunocytes (Box 342.1).

The small intestine is approximately 250 cm long in full-term infants and grows to between 2 and 3 m in the adult. The first 25 cm of small bowel or duodenum is fixed to the peritoneum. Beyond the ligament of Treitz, the intestine is freely mobile, supported only by the mesentery. The small intestine is covered by serosa (mesentery) beginning at the ligament of Treitz (Fig. 342.4). Beneath the serosa lie two muscular layers: an outer longitudinal and an inner circular layer, which act in concert to provide peristalsis. Within the submucosa, the next layer, lie numerous cellular elements, including lymphocytes, plasma cells, mast cells, eosinophils, and macrophages. Brunner glands are present in the submucosa of the duodenum (Fig. 342.4).

BOX 342.1   **Immunology of the Gut**

The immunologic cells of the gut commonly are called *gut-associated lymphoid tissue* (GALT). GALT has four basic components: intraepithelial lymphocytes, solitary lymphoid follicles, lamina propria lymphocytes and plasma cells, and Peyer patches. Peyer patches contain M cells. The M cell has no villi and is thought to be the prime site for antigen recognition and absorption. IgA in its dimeric form is the predominant antibody of the gut. It is produced locally by plasma cells in the lamina propria and secreted into the lumen after joining to the secretory component. Secretory IgA is unique in its ability to bind to foreign antigen and prevent absorption without causing a local inflammatory response; this phenomenon is known as *immune exclusion.*

Overall histologic organization of the digestive tube

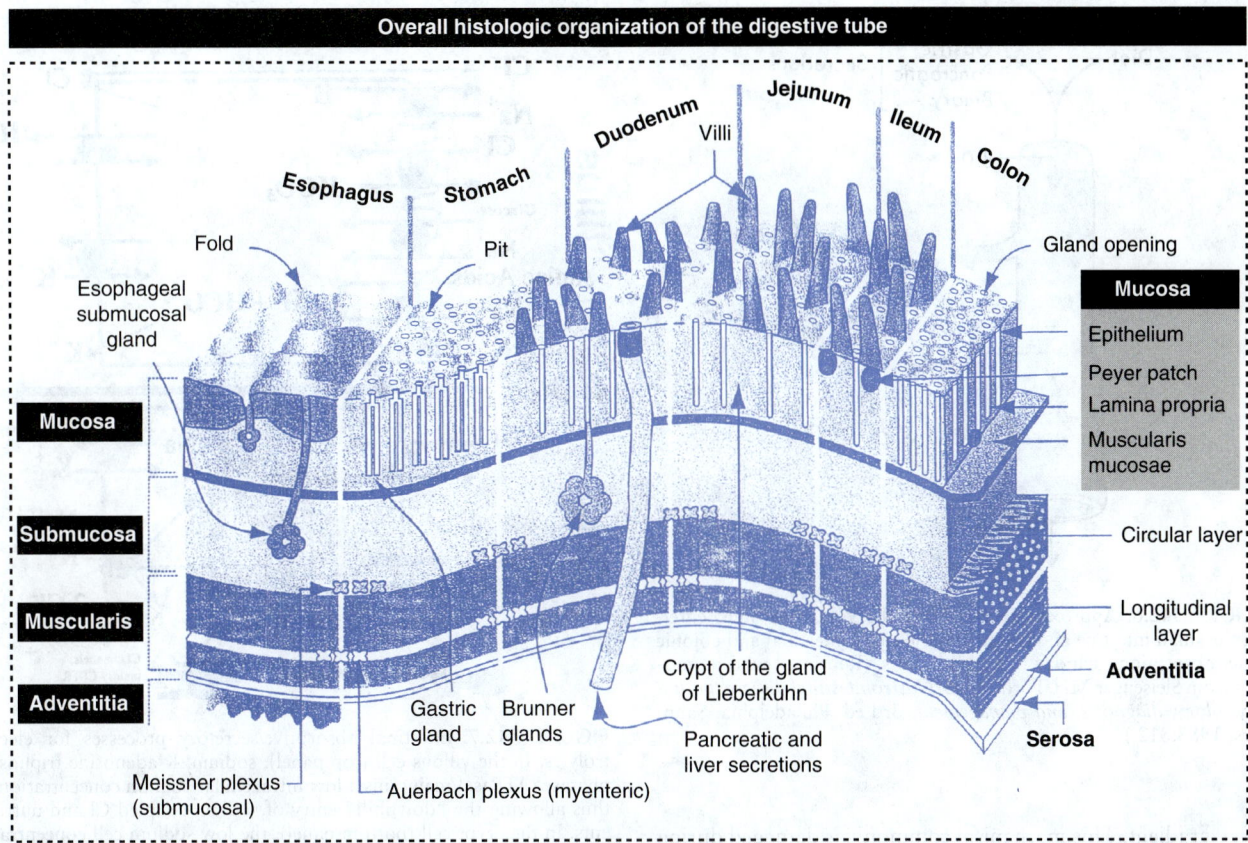

FIGURE 342.4. Schematic organization of the intestinal tract, illustrating the changes in histology from the esophagus to the colon. (Reprinted with permission from Kierszenbaum AL. *Histology and cell biology: an introduction to pathology.* St. Louis, MO: Mosby, 2002.)

The mucosal or luminal surface is covered with the villi and crypts, which increase the surface area available for digestion and absorption of nutrients (Fig. 342.4). The villi are composed of at least four cell types: absorptive cells; goblet cells, responsible for mucus production; endocrine cells; and the specialized M cells, the major site of antigen absorption and processing. Crypts are composed of four cell types: Paneth cells; goblet cells; undifferentiated or principal cells, responsible for cellular proliferation; and endocrine (argentaffin, enterochromaffin) cells, responsible for the production of gut hormones (Fig. 342.5).

The two major functions of the small bowel are to digest and absorb nutrients, water, vitamins, and minerals and to recognize and process antigenic and noxious substances. The small intestine absorbs 80% of the water ingested daily, and the colon absorbs the rest (Fig. 342.6). Minerals are absorbed either passively—by diffusion, convection, or solvent drag—or by active transport. The absorption of sodium is facilitated by electrogenic sodium absorption (Na^+, K^+-ATPase) (Fig. 342.7). Water is absorbed passively, always following a solute. In the small intestine, water is absorbed by three mechanisms: "neutral" sodium chloride absorption, "electrogenic" sodium absorption, and sodium cotransport (Fig. 342.7).

1. "Neutral" sodium chloride absorption occurs throughout the small intestine. This transport is mediated by two coupled systems; one exchanges sodium/hydrogen ions (cation exchanger) and the other exchanges chloride/bicarbonate ions (anion exchanger).
2. "Electrogenic" sodium absorption, previously known as active transport, occurs in both the small and large intestine. Sodium enters the cell via an electrochemical

Epithelial cells of the villus and crypt of Lieberkühn

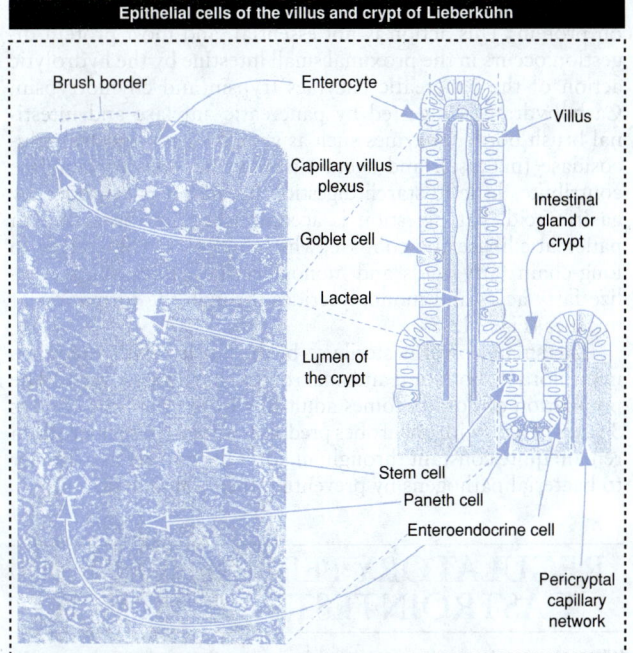

FIGURE 342.5. Diagram of a villus and crypt of Lieberkühn with histologic inserts of the brush border and crypt. (Reprinted with permission from Kierszenbaum AL. *Histology and cell biology: an introduction to pathology.* St. Louis, MO: Mosby, 2002.)

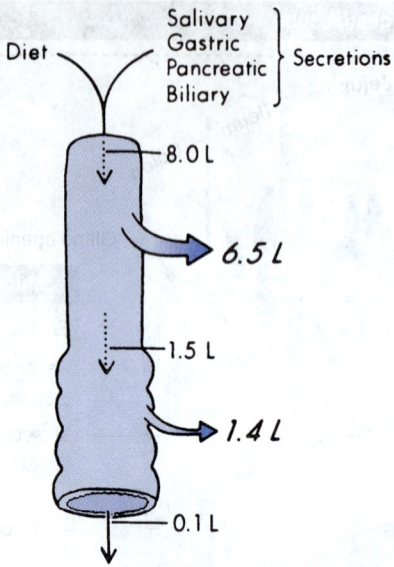

FIGURE 342.6. Approximate values for the volume of fluid entering the small intestine and colon, and the small intestinal and colonic water absorption each day in healthy adults. (Reprinted with permission from Sleisenger MH, Fordtran JS. *Gastrointestinal disease: pathophysiology, diagnosis, and management*, 3rd ed. Philadelphia: Saunders, 1983:812.)

gradient. This mechanism commonly is damaged during acute enteric infection, resulting in diarrhea.

3. Sodium cotransport operates only in the small intestine. Sodium absorption is coupled to the absorption of organic solutes such as glucose, many amino acids, and peptides. This mechanism remains intact during acute enteric infection and is the reason that oral rehydration is possible during acute diarrheal illness.

Digestion begins in the stomach with the action of pepsin on protein. This action is not essential, and most protein digestion occurs in the proximal small intestine by the hydrolytic action of the pancreatic enzymes trypsin and chymotrypsin. Carbohydrate is digested by pancreatic amylase and intestinal brush border enzymes such as galactosidase (lactase), glucosidase (maltase), and sucrase-isomaltase. Salivary amylase contributes little to starch digestion because it is degraded by gastric acid. Fat digestion is accomplished by the action of pancreatic lipase and colipase, which hydrolyze triglyceride to long-chain fatty acids and monoglycerides. Bile salts solubilize fatty acids and monoglycerides through the formation of micelles (Fig. 342.8).

The small bowel is sterile at birth, but it rapidly acquires microflora by both oral and anal routes shortly after birth. The population of flora becomes adult-like by the time the child is 3 years of age, with anaerobes predominating. These microflora remain quite constant throughout adult life and act as a barrier to bacterial pathogens by preventing their colonization.

REGULATORY PEPTIDES OF THE GASTROINTESTINAL TRACT

The GI tract is an important, although still poorly understood, endocrine organ. Historically, the discovery of secretin in the proximal jejunum by Starling in 1905 led to the modern science of endocrinology. The GI tract now is known to produce a variety of regulatory peptides that allow intercellular com-

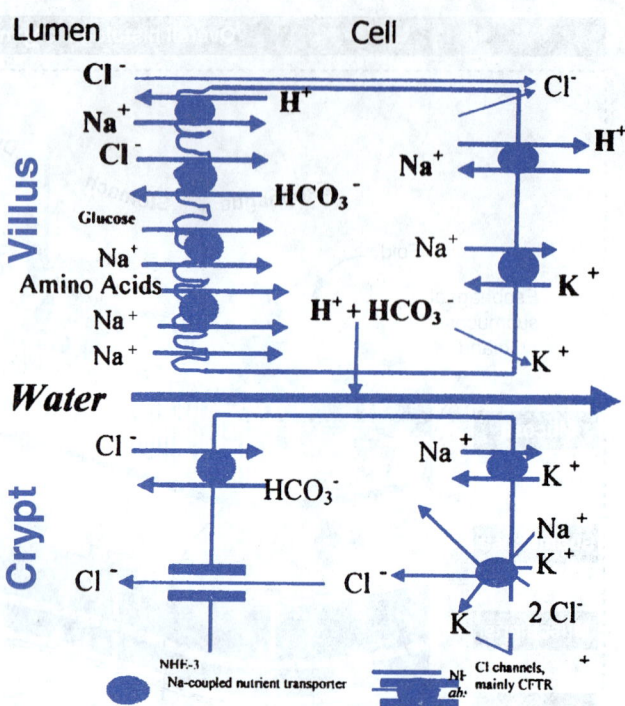

FIGURE 342.7. Intestinal absorptive/secretory processes for electrolytes. In the villous cell (top panel), sodium, K adenosine triphosphatase (ATPase) maintains a low intracellular sodium concentration, thus allowing the "downhill" entry of sodium-coupled Cl and nutrients. In the crypt cell (bottom panel), the low sodium cell concentration maintained by sodium, potassium, and adenosine triphosphatase builds a sodium gradient between the extracellular compartment and the cell. Energized by such a gradient, a carrier in the basolateral membrane (lower part of the figure) couples the flow of one Na, two Cl, and one K from the serosal compartment into the crypt cell. As a result, Cl accumulates above its electrochemical equilibrium and under physiologic circumstances leaks into the lumen across a semipermeable apical membrane. As the absorptive activity going on in the villous cell quantitatively far exceeds the minor secretion arising from the crypts (as suggested in the figure by the arrows' sizes), the net result is absorption of electrolytes and nutrients. Water absorption then passively follows, mainly through the intercellular tight junctions. Secretory changes are induced by second messengers. Cyclic AMP, cyclic GMP, and Ca^{++}/protein kinase C have similar effects. In the mature villous cell (above), they inhibit the coupled influx of sodium and Cl. In the undifferentiated crypt cell, cyclic AMP, cyclic GMP, and Ca^{++}/protein kinase C act by opening Cl channels (mainly CFTR) in the luminal membrane. As a consequence, Cl leaves the cell moving down its electrochemical gradient. Because the epithelium cannot secrete only anions, cations (Na) flow across the paracellular pathway, driven by the electrical gradient created by the secretory transport of Cl. Thus, antiabsorptive (in the villous cell) and prosecretory (in the crypt cell) forces combine to shift ions, and with them water, from absorption to secretion. The molecular identity of the transporters involved is illustrated in the figure. AMP, adenosine monophosphate; GMP, guanosine monophosphate; CFTR, cystic fibrosis transmembrane regulator. (Reprinted with permission from Guarino A, Albano F, Guandalini S, and the Working Group on Acute Gastroenteritis. Oral rehydration: toward a real solution. *J Pediatr Gastroenterol Nutr* 2001;33:S2.)

munication. More than 20 such peptides, or gut hormones, have been identified, and they are located in endocrine cells and in nerves (Table 342.1). These gastrointestinal hormones exert their action through the classic endocrine, neurocrine, paracrine, and autocrine pathways. Their functions are diverse, ranging from cell growth and differentiation for epidermal growth factor to the classic pancreatic bicarbonate secretion for secretin.

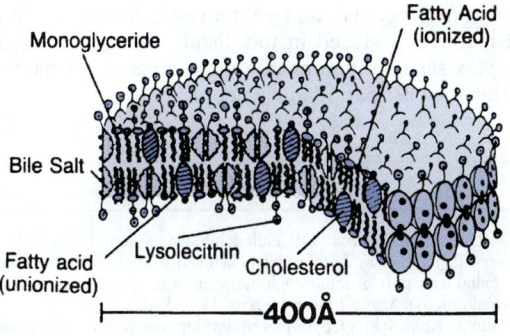

FIGURE 342.8. Proposed structure of the intestinal mixed micelle based on the light-scattering studies of Carey. The bilayered disc has a band of amphophilic bile salt at its periphery and other, more hydrophobic components (fatty acids, monoglyceride, phospholipids, and cholesterol) protected within its interior. (Reprinted with permission from Carey MC. Enterohepatic circulation. In: Arias AM, Popper H, Schacter D, et al., eds. *The liver: biology and pathology.* New York: Raven Press, 1982.)

COLON

The colon develops from both the midgut and the hindgut. To accommodate growth in length, it migrates with the small intestine into the vitelline duct of the umbilicus and returns to the abdominal cavity at 10 weeks' gestation. Haustra and teniae appear at 8 to 12 weeks' gestation. Villi are found at 10 to 12 weeks' gestation, but they disappear at 24 to 28 weeks, suggesting that the colon has the potential for nutrient absorption in fetal life.

The structure of the colon is similar to that of the small intestine, except that the villi are replaced by a flat columnar epithelium, and the outer longitudinal muscle is separated into three distinct bands, the teniae coli (Fig. 342.4). Between the teniae are outpouchings, termed *haustra*, separated by folds. The colonic mucosa is characterized by the crypts of Lieberkühn, lined with absorptive cells, goblet cells, and endocrine cells.

The blood supply to the colon is via branches of the superior and inferior mesenteric arteries, with associated venous and lymphatic structures (Fig. 342.9).

TABLE 342.1

GASTROINTESTINAL REGULATORY PEPTIDES: MAIN ANATOMIC SOURCES, LIKELY MODES OF ACTION, AND POSSIBLE PHYSIOLOGIC ROLES

Regulatory Peptide	Sources	Mechanisms	Actions
EGF	Salivary glands Brunner glands Paneth cells	Hormone/paracrine	Stimulates mucosal proliferation and differentiation Regulates GI secretion Has cytoprotective/ulcer-healing effects Stimulates hepatocyte proliferation
TGF-alpha	Villus enterocytes	Paracrine	Stimulates enterocyte proliferation and cell migration from crypts
TGF-beta	Villus enterocytes	Paracrine/autocrine	Inhibits enterocyte proliferation Maintains enterocyte differentiation Restores epithelial integrity
IGF-1	Gut and liver	Hormone/paracrine/autocrine	Stimulates crypt cell proliferation and enterocyte differentiation Promotes intestinal adaptation
HGF	Intestinal crypt cells	Hormone/paracrine	Stimulates liver cell and crypt cell proliferation and crypt cell migration
Gastrin	Gastric antrum	Hormone	Stimulates gastric acid secretion
Cholecystokinin	Proximal small intestine	Hormone/neurotransmitter	Stimulates gallbladder contraction and pancreatic and CNS enzyme secretion
Secretin	Proximal small intestine	Hormone	Stimulates pancreatic bicarbonate secretion
Pancreatic glucagon	Pancreas	Hormone	Stimulates hepatic glucose output
Enteroglucagon	Ileum and colon	Hormone	Stimulates gut mucosal growth Regulates gut motility
Pancreatic polypeptide	Pancreas	Hormone	Inhibits pancreatic enzyme secretion and gallbladder contraction
Gastric inhibitory	Proximal small intestine	Hormone	Enhances insulin secretion polypeptide
Motilin	Proximal small intestine	Hormone	Stimulates gastrointestinal motility
VIP	All tissues	Neurotransmitter	Promotes secretomotor, vasodilatation, and smooth muscle relaxation
Bombesin	Gut, CNS, and lung	Neurotransmitter/paracrine	Stimulates gut hormone release
Somatostatin	Gut and CNS	Paracrine/neurotransmitter	Inhibits hormone release and hormone target issues
Neurotensin	Ileum and CNS	Hormone/neurotransmitter	Inhibits gastric emptying and acid secretion
Substance P	Gut, CNS, and skin	Neurotransmitter	Is a sensory neurotransmitter (especially pain)
Leuenkephalin and metenkephalin	Gut and CNS	Neurotransmitter	Has opiate-like effects (endorphin system)
Peptide HI	Gut and CNS	Unknown	Unknown
Peptide YY	Gut and CNS	Hormone	Inhibits gastric acid secretion and gut motility

CNS, central nervous system; EGF, epidermal growth factor; GI, gastrointestinal; HGF, hepatocyte growth factor; IGF-1, insulinlike growth factor-1; TGF, transforming growth factor; VIP, vasoactive intestinal polypeptide.

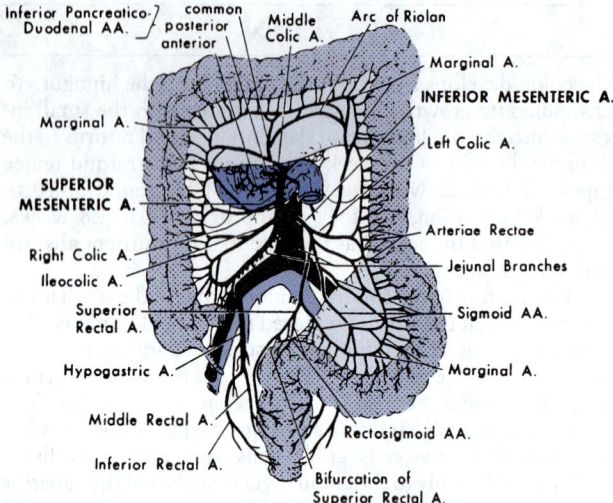

FIGURE 342.9. Blood supply to the small and large intestines. The figure shows anastomotic connections to the celiac axis in the region of the duodenum and between the superior and inferior mesenteric arteries. Illustrated here are those branches of the left and middle colic arteries that in many patients connect directly (and apart from the marginal artery) to form the arc of Riolan, or "meandering mesenteric" artery. (Reprinted with permission from Sleisenger MH, Fordtran JS. *Gastrointestinal disease: pathophysiology, diagnosis, and management*, 3rd ed. Philadelphia: Saunders, 1983:1544.)

The colon has two basic functions: the absorption of water and electrolytes and the storage and elimination of feces. The colon absorbs all but approximately 1% of the water left after passage through the small intestine (Fig. 342.6). Colonic microflora can metabolize unabsorbed nutrients, particularly carbohydrates, which then can be absorbed. This process, termed *colonic salvaging*, may represent a vestigial nutritive function. Fecal material is stored in the distal colon and excreted via a complex series of neural stimuli, addressed in Chapter 343, Functional Constipation and Encopresis.

Suggested Readings

Arey LB. *Developmental anatomy*. Philadelphia: Saunders, 1974.

Brandtzaeg P, Baklien K. Immunohistochemical studies of the formation and epithelial transport of immunoglobulins in normal and diseased human intestinal mucosa. *Scand J Gastroenterol* 1976;36:1.

Bustamante S, Koldovsky O. Synopsis of development of the main morphologic structures of the human GI tract. In: Lebenthal E, ed. *Textbook of gastroenterology and nutrition in infancy*. New York: Raven Press, 1981:49.

Christie DL. Development of gastric function during the first month of life. In: Lebenthal E, ed. *Textbook of gastroenterology and nutrition in infancy*. New York: Raven Press, 1981:118.

Estrada RL. *Anomalies of intestinal rotation and fixation*. Springfield, IL: Mosby, 1958.

Gray GM, Cooper HL. Protein digestion and absorption. *Gastroenterology* 1971;61:535.

Herbst JJ. Development of suck and swallow. *J Pediatr Gastroenterol Nutr* 1981; 2:131.

Hofmann AF, Small DM. Detergent properties of bile salts: correlation with physiological function. *Annu Rev Med* 1967;18:333.

Israel EJ, Walker WA. Host defense development in gut and related disorders. *Pediatr Clin North Am* 1988;35:1.

Koldovsky O. *Development of the functions of the small intestine in mammals and man*. Basel: S Karger, 1969.

Scammon RE, Kittleson JA. The growth of the GI tract of the human fetus. *Proc Soc Exp Biol Med* 1926;24:303.

Siegal M, Lebenthal E. Development of GI motility and gastric emptying during fetal and newborn periods. In: Lebenthal E, ed. *Textbook of gastroenterology and nutrition in infancy*. New York: Raven Press, 1981:136.

Sleisenger MH, Fordtran JS. *GI disease: pathophysiology, diagnosis, and management*, 3rd ed. Philadelphia: Saunders, 1983.

Solcia E, Capella C, Buffa R, et al. Endocrine cells of the digestive system. In: Johnson LR, Christensen J, Grossman MI, et al., eds. *Physiology of the GI tract*. New York: Raven Press, 1981:39.

Tomasi TB Jr. Mechanisms of immune regulation at mucosal surfaces. *Rev Infect Dis* 1983;5:784.

CHAPTER 343 ■ FUNCTIONAL CONSTIPATION AND ENCOPRESIS

WILLIAM J. KLISH

Chronic constipation is a common complaint in children. It accounts for 3% of office visits to a primary care physician and 20% to 25% of the referrals to a pediatric gastroenterologist. Because stool habits are a major concern of many parents, the physician or health care worker should become familiar with both normal and abnormal patterns of defecation to properly advise parents. Distinguishing functional constipation (i.e., without evidence of a pathologic cause) from constipation with an organic cause is important. Beyond the neonatal period, the most common cause of constipation is functional constipation.

Constipation is defined as a delay or difficulty with defecation, present for 2 or more weeks. Children with chronic constipation have infrequent bowel movements that are unusually large, hard, dry, and painful to pass. The frequency of defecation and the consistency of stool are related to the patient's age and diet. Infants have a mean of four stools per day during the first week of life. However, some infants have a bowel movement after each feeding because of an active gastrocolic reflex, and others, particularly breast-fed infants, can have stools every 2 to 3 days. Breast-fed infants usually have stools more frequently than do formula-fed infants. This frequency gradually declines to a mean average of 1.7 stools per day at 2 years of age and 1.2 stools per day at 4 years of age. After 4 years of age, the frequency of bowel movements remains unchanged. Less frequent stools should be of concern if they are hard, dry, unusually large, or difficult to pass.

Encopresis is involuntary fecal soiling or incontinence secondary to chronic constipation. Physiologic encopresis occurs most commonly and is manifested as overflow incontinence that occurs as a result of severe constipation, fecal impaction, and a dilated rectum. Children with encopresis frequently have related behavioral components, including active withholding of stool, fear, and embarrassment that frequently resolve with adequate treatment. A less common form of psychological encopresis usually is manifested as full bowel movements in the underwear. The diagnosis of psychogenic incontinence should be reserved for older and previously toilet-trained children who have full bowel movements in their underwear on a regular basis.

PATHOPHYSIOLOGY

For defecation to proceed, a normal rectum and puborectalis muscle, normal internal and external anal sphincters, and normal innervation of these structures through both the autonomic and somatic nervous systems must be present. The rectum functions not as a storage area for fecal material but rather as a sensing organ that initiates the process of defecation. When stool moves into the rectum from the sigmoid colon, pressure is put on the wall and the rectal valves. This pressure initiates an impulse within the intrinsic nervous system of the rectum resulting in relaxation of the internal anal sphincter, which is experienced as the urgency felt just before defecation. If defecation is inconvenient, contraction of the external sphincter is initiated, first by reflex and then intentionally. The external sphincter is assisted by contraction of the puborectalis muscle, which helps constrict and angulate the anal canal. If the external sphincter is held contracted long enough, the reflex to the internal sphincter wanes and the urge to defecate disappears. When defecation is convenient, the external sphincter is relaxed consciously, and stool is propelled by colonic peristalsis through the open anal canal. As stool enters the anal canal, a secondary reflex is initiated via the somatic nervous system that results in contraction of the abdominal musculature and assists in emptying the lower colon.

Many general causes exist for constipation. Often it is a familial complaint, and the parents of constipated children often report being constipated when they were children. This history implies a genetic component to constipation, which may be the result of increased efficiency of water extraction from fecal material caused by a congenitally long or hypomotile large bowel. Diet plays a role in the volume and hardness of fecal material throughout life. Some dietary residue, such as plant fiber, tends to make stools soft, whereas other residue, such as the calcium salts in cow's milk, tends to make stools firm. Elemental and chemically defined diets decrease dietary residue and thus decrease the frequency of having stools.

Hospitalized children may become constipated because of decreased stimulus for defecation resulting from inactivity. Diseases associated with fever may result in acute constipation. Some chronic diseases, such as hypothyroidism, are associated with constipation. The differential diagnosis of constipation is discussed later.

Children who develop functional constipation associate discomfort with defecation. The most common reason for discomfort is an anal fissure resulting from either hard stool or the use of suppositories, enemas, or a rectal thermometer. Occasionally, the sense of discomfort results from a bad toilet-training experience. Whatever the cause, the result is the same. Whenever the child feels the sensation associated with relaxation of the internal anal sphincter, he or she aggressively contracts the external sphincter to prevent expulsion of stool and the pain it is expected to bring. Increased amounts of stool collect in the rectum, and over a period of months, the rectum gradually dilates. As it enlarges, it becomes less capable of propulsive peristaltic activity, which results in more retention of stool. As the volume of the rectum increases, its sensory capacity diminishes, so that retention is easier. Eventually, the constipation becomes self-perpetuating.

Encopresis develops when the rectal vault enlarges sufficiently to exert pressure on the structures of the floor of the pelvis, including the levator muscle. This muscle interdigitates with the anal sphincters. As it is pushed downward, the anal sphincters become distorted and the anal canal is shortened. If the external anal sphincter is allowed to relax, it assumes a slightly open position. During activity, loose or mushy stool then can flow around firmer stool present in the rectum and can leak out. Affected children instinctively know they have little control over the leakage at this point, so they often adopt a casual attitude that is frustrating to parents. They constantly smell of fecal material, which may result in ridicule by their peers and secondary psychological problems.

CLINICAL FINDINGS

The most common symptom associated with constipation is chronic recurrent abdominal pain, which occurs in approximately 60% of patients. The pains are intermittent and localized to the periumbilical region and resemble functional abdominal pain. Enuresis is reported in approximately 30% of the children with encopresis. Many of them have daytime as well as nocturnal enuresis, which resolve when the constipation is treated. Urinary tract infection is a common complication in girls with chronic constipation.

Stools of very large caliber are another associated symptom. Parents often must break up stools mechanically to flush the toilet. The size of the stool is a function of the size of the colon.

In children with encopresis, fecal incontinence tends to occur in the late afternoon and early evening, but it can occur at any time of day or night. The pattern of incontinence tends to parallel the child's activity, with soiling occurring less frequently when the child is sedentary. Most children insist that they do not feel the stools coming and do not perceive the sensation of impending soiling until they actually feel stool in their underwear.

Poor appetite and poor growth occasionally are seen in association with constipation and may result from early satiety caused by the feeling of fullness of the colon. Parents frequently describe their constipated children as lethargic.

DIFFERENTIAL DIAGNOSIS

Functional constipation must be differentiated from Hirschsprung disease, anterior displacement of the anus, and sacral nerve abnormalities, which usually are associated with spina bifida occulta or a tethered cord. Other causes of constipation are listed in Box 343.1.

DIAGNOSIS

The diagnosis of functional constipation or encopresis is made from the history and physical examination. Stool often is palpable in the abdomen, particularly in the left lower quadrant. Rectal examination reveals a short anal canal associated with a large dilated rectum, full of stool. The external sphincter is intact, and the child can squeeze the examiner's finger. The anus should be positioned properly, approximately midway between the scrotum and the tip of the coccyx in boys and approximately one-third the distance from the vaginal fourchette to the coccyx in girls. It also should be centered within the perianal skin pigmentation. Normal contraction of the external anal sphincter (anal wink) should be elicited by stimulating the perianal skin to rule out abnormalities of sensory input.

> ### BOX 343.1   Causes of Constipation
>
> Functional constipation and encopresis
> Dietary causes
> Protracted vomiting
> Excessive intake of cow's milk
> Lack of bulk in diet
> Drugs that affect motility
> Structural defects of the anus or rectum
> Anterior displacement of the anus
> Anal or rectal stenosis
> Presacral teratoma
> Rectal prolapse
> Smooth muscle disease
> Scleroderma
> Dermatomyositis
> Systemic lupus erythematosus
> Primary chronic intestinal pseudoobstruction
> Abnormal myenteric ganglion cells
> Hirschsprung disease
> Chagas disease
> Von Recklinghausen disease
> Multiple endocrine neoplasia type II B
> Absence of abdominal musculature
> Spinal cord defects
> Spina bifida occulta
> Myelomeningocele
> Meningocele
> Diastematomyelia
> Paraplegia
> Cauda equina tumor
> Tethered cord syndrome
> Metabolic and endocrine disorders
> Hypothyroidism
> Hypoparathyroidism
> Renal tubular acidosis
> Diabetes insipidus
> Vitamin D intoxication
> Idiopathic hypercalcemia
> Hypokalemia
> Neurologic and psychiatric conditions
> Myotonic dystrophy
> Amyotonia congenital
> Mental retardation
> Psychosis

Evidence of fecal soiling at the anal opening may be present. Anal fissures often are present and consistent with the history of large, hard stools. The anus may be patulous, confirming a prolonged history of constipation and fecal impaction.

Occasionally further evaluation may be helpful. Abdominal radiograph of the abdomen may be helpful in the child who is obese with an incomplete abdominal examination, who refuses a rectal examination, or in whom other psychological factors (sexual abuse) are present or to rule out obstruction when the rectal examination finds no stool in the rectum. An unprepped barium enema, to evaluate for evidence of Hirschsprung disease, may be considered. Unprepped means no clean-out preparation of the colon (e.g., no enemas, no suppositories, and no rectal examinations or rectal stimulation for 48 to 72 hours prior to the study). If tethered cord or spinal abnormalities are suspected, radiographic study of the spinal cord may be

helpful. Laboratory studies, including thyroid function tests, serum calcium level, and celiac disease workup, may be helpful to rule out organic causes. Rectal manometry can be helpful in distinguishing functional constipation from Hirschsprung disease and sacral nerve abnormalities. Functional constipation is associated with normal relaxation of the internal anal sphincter and no contraction of the external anal sphincter in response to considerable distention of the rectal ampulla.

TREATMENT

Treatment depends on the age of the child. The basic goals of treating constipation include (a) promoting one to two daily soft stools, (b) allowing the dilated rectum to normalize in size, and (c) establishing a stooling pattern that encourages the child to pass the stool without fear or holding back. Simple constipation in the neonate is treated best with a nonabsorbable carbohydrate such as malt extract (Maltsupex) or lactulose. Malt extract usually is given at a dose of 1 tsp added to the formula three times a day. Lactulose is started at a dose of 2 to 3 mL and titrated upward until the desired effect is achieved. Dark corn syrup has been a traditional method to soften stools, but it is less reliable. Light corn syrup has no effect on the stools because it is absorbed totally. In older children and adolescents with simple constipation, stool softeners such as docusate sodium (Colace) or bulking agents are suggested.

In children with long-standing functional constipation or associated encopresis associated with a megarectum, a laxative program is required. If the child is significantly constipated or impacted with stool, the stool will have to be cleared. A large-volume enema preparation such as soapsuds or saline usually is more effective than is a small-volume enema such as phospho-soda (Fleet enema). A soapsuds enema is made by adding 1 tsp of dish detergent to 1 qt of water; saline is prepared by mixing 1 tsp of salt to 1 qt of water. The amount delivered as an enema should be approximately 20 mL/kg body weight to a maximum of approximately 1 L. No more than two enemas should be given in a single day; the routine use of soapsuds enemas can result in a detergent proctitis. If stool in the rectal vault is firm, a preliminary mineral oil enema acts as a softener and lubricant. Mineral oil may be given orally but it is not recommended in a child younger than 1 year of age because of the risk of aspiration and lipoid pneumonia occurring. It may be mixed with juice or a crushed popsicle/freezer pop, with the oil poured over the top and fed with a spoon.

Once the rectum has been cleared of stool, a program of daily administration of a laxative should be initiated to prevent reaccumulation of fecal material and to allow the rectum to return to normal size. Laxatives should be taken only once a day, preferably in the morning so that the day's activity can enhance the effect.

Preferred laxatives are polyethylene glycol electrolyte solution and powder (Miralax) or concentrated milk of magnesia. Miralax is a nonabsorbable electrolyte solution that can be taken orally or by nasogastric tube if used for disimpaction or cleaning before colonoscopy. It comes in a powdered form that dissolves in 4 to 8 oz of water or flavored beverage and is given once a day. In our experience, doses 0.5 to 1 tsp for children 18 months and younger, 2 to 3 tsp for children 18 months to 3 years of age, and 2 to 4 tsp for children 3 years and older are the preferred starting doses. Although used frequently for management of constipation, formal studies on Miralax have not been done to establish the safety of long-term maintenance in children. Milk of magnesia (concentrated) is administered starting at a dose of 0.5 tsp for children younger than 2 years of age, 1 tsp for children aged 2 to 5 years, and 2 tsp for children older than 5 years. For both of these laxatives, the dose is titrated up or down in increments of 0.5 tsp, depending on the daily response. If a bowel movement has not occurred in the previous 24 hours, the dose is decreased. If the child passes more than two normal-sized stools per day, the dose is decreased by 0.5 tsp. Adjustments are made daily until a dose is found that stimulates one or two normal bowel movements per day. Three to four weeks may be required to establish the proper dose of laxative. Other laxatives shown to be effective include senna (normally given in conjunction with mineral oil) and lactulose. Whichever laxative is used, the parents should be instructed on how to manage the dosage themselves.

Patients should be reexamined at 1- to 2-month intervals, and a rectal examination should be performed to determine rectal vault size. Laxatives can be tapered when the rectal vault returns to normal size, which may take 6 months to 1 year. At that time, parents and children should be instructed about proper diet and the use of bulking agents to avoid development of hard stools. During laxative therapy, attempts should be made to establish a bowel habit. Once the parent determines when the laxative begins to stimulate, the child should be asked to sit on the toilet at that time each day. This behavior should continue after the laxative has been discontinued. Usually, children withhold to avoid pain. Stool withholding behaviors often are eliminated or at least decreased when the pain is eliminated by the laxative program that produces painless bowel movements. Parents and caregivers need to be counseled to be supportive and to encourage children to relax with bowel movements, and not to punish the child for soiling.

Simple rewards like using a calendar or chart with stickers (e.g., "smiley faces") provide positive support to reinforce the child's progress.

Most children do not want to soil but frequently have developed tolerance to soiling and are not concerned about soiled clothing. Therefore, more effort may be required to get them to use the bathroom. Children with attention deficit and hyperactivity disorder tend to have more problems because they may be distracted easily. For some children, enlisting the aid of a behavioral psychologist to support the medical treatment plan may be helpful.

Suggested Readings

Baker SS, Liptak GS, Colletti RB, et al. Constipation in infants and children: evaluation and treatment. *J Pediatr Gastroenterol Nutr* 1999;29:612.

Bishop PR, Nowicki JM. Defecation disorders in the neurologically impaired child. *Pediatr Ann* 1999;28:322.

Blum NJ, Taubman B, Osborne ML. Behavioral characteristic of children with toileting refusal. *Pediatrics* 1997;99:50.

Buttross S. Encopresis in the child a behavioral disorder: when the initial treatment does not work. *Pediatr Ann* 1999;28:317.

Dautenhahn LW, Blumenthal BI. Functional constipation: a radiologist's perspective. *Pediatr Ann* 1999;28:304.

Davidson M, Kugler MM, Bauer CH. Diagnosis and management in children with severe and protracted constipation and obstipation. *J Pediatr* 1963;62:261.

Guerrero RA, Cavender CP. Constipation: physical and psychological sequelae. *Pediatr Ann* 1999;28:312.

Lemoh JN, Brooke OG. Frequency and weight of normal stools in infancy. *Arch Dis Child* 1979;54:719.

Lewis LG, Rudolph CD. Practical approach to defecation disorders in children. *Pediatr Ann* 1999;28:260.

Loening-Baucke V. Chronic constipation in children. *Gastroenterology* 1993;105:1557.

Loening-Baucke V. Urinary incontinence and urinary tract infection and their resolution with treatment of chronic constipation of childhood. *Pediatrics* 1997;100.

Lowe JR, Parks BR. Movers and shakers: a clinician's guide to laxatives. *Pediatr Ann* 1999;28:307.

North American Society for Pediatric Gastroenterology and Nutrition. Medical position statement on constipation in infants and children: evaluation and treatment.

Nowicki MJ, Bishop PR. Organic causes of constipation in infants and children. *Pediatr Ann* 1999;28:293.

Silverberg M. Constipation in infants and children. *Pract Gastroenterol* 1987;1143.

CHAPTER 344 ■ CHRONIC NONSPECIFIC DIARRHEA OF CHILDHOOD

WILLIAM J. KLISH

Chronic nonspecific diarrhea of childhood (also called *protracted diarrhea* or *irritable bowel syndrome*) is a common and often frustrating problem seen in children between 6 and 36 months of age. It is characterized by a pattern of two or more loose, voluminous stools per day lasting for more than 4 weeks, unassociated with other symptoms such as pain or growth failure. Children with this syndrome usually are not bothered by the diarrhea. Their parents, however, have difficulty dealing with this symptom because most of the affected children are still in diapers, and the stool volume is so great that the stool spills from the diapers, making a mess.

ETIOLOGY

Although chronic nonspecific diarrhea of childhood is the most common form of chronic diarrhea without failure to thrive in young children, the etiology remains unknown. Because malabsorption of nutrients is not a factor in this disease, the cause of the diarrhea is either enhanced secretion of fluid in the distal bowel or interference with absorption of water and electrolytes from the colon. Chronic nonspecific diarrhea frequently is initiated by an acute infection, which usually is treated with a broad-spectrum antibiotic such as ampicillin, so alteration of bacterial flora in the colon may play a role in the diarrhea.

Some investigators have thought that the diarrhea might be induced by the increased intake of fluids observed in these children. However, the increased thirst is more likely to be the effect rather than the cause of the diarrhea. Some children drink large amounts of fruit juice, such as apple or grape juice. This intake undoubtedly plays some role in the perpetuation of the diarrhea because these juices contain enough poorly absorbed carbohydrate, such as sorbitol or fructose, to induce colonic fermentation, resulting in the stimulus for diarrhea, as seen in other forms of carbohydrate intolerance.

A low dietary fat intake has been hypothesized to play a role in the persistence of the diarrhea, but this observation has not held up under scrutiny. However, because many of these children eventually are placed on strict elimination diets, dietary restriction of fiber and other residue may help perpetuate the loose stools.

One group of investigators has suggested that disordered small-intestine motility plays a role in chronic nonspecific diarrhea of childhood. They showed that the migrating motor complex of the duodenum was not suppressed as it normally should be with the introduction of glucose into the bowel, which implies that children with this disorder have relative hypermotility of the intestine during meals.

DIFFERENTIAL DIAGNOSIS

The diagnosis of chronic nonspecific diarrhea of childhood should be suspected if the following criteria are met: child's age is between 6 and 36 months; two or more loose, voluminous stools, frequently containing undigested food particles, are passed per day; the diarrhea lasts for more than 4 weeks; abdominal pain is absent; failure to thrive is absent; and no definable cause is found for the chronic diarrhea (Box 344.1).

Disaccharide intolerance, infection, protein hypersensitivity, and occasionally inflammatory bowel disease can mimic chronic nonspecific diarrhea in presenting symptoms. Carbohydrate intolerance can be diagnosed by placing the patient on a totally unrestricted diet with milk and testing several stools for the presence of sugar or acid. Unabsorbed disaccharide (lactose or sucrose) appears in the stool either unchanged or partially fermented to the monosaccharides, including glucose. Their presence can be determined through the use of Clinitest tablets or glucose test strips. Complete fermentation of sugars results in the production of organic acids such as acetic and butyric acids. Their presence can be found by testing the stool pH with Nitrazine paper. A pH of less than 5.5 is considered suggestive of carbohydrate intolerance.

Stools should be cultured for bacteria. Most pathogenic bacteria cannot produce diarrhea for longer than several weeks. However, *Campylobacter jejuni* has been implicated in several cases of chronic diarrhea and must be ruled out. The presenting symptoms of *Giardia lamblia* infection can be identical to those of chronic nonspecific diarrhea, and this infection also must be ruled out.

A complete blood count with differential, reticulocyte count, and stool guaiac test might give a clue to the presence of either protein hypersensitivity or inflammatory bowel disease.

BOX 344.1

Differential Diagnosis of Chronic Nonspecific Diarrhea

Disaccharide intolerance
Infection—bacterial, viral, parasitic
Protein hypersensitivity
Inflammatory bowel disease

Eosinophilia occasionally is present in protein hypersensitivity. If this diagnosis is suspected, a carefully constructed elimination diet should be initiated; the diet must provide adequate intake for the child to thrive.

TREATMENT

Before treatment is initiated, the clinician should stress that, although the diarrhea is hard for the parents to deal with, it does not threaten the child's well-being. Treatment fails in 10% to 20% of children, regardless of the form of therapy. The syndrome improves with age, and most children have outgrown it by the time they are 3 years of age.

Therapy should be initiated by placing the child on a diet normal for his or her age. If the diet has been restricted, many children normalize their stool pattern due to an increase in dietary residue. If large amounts of fruit juices are being given, attempts should be made to substitute other liquids.

Psyllium bulking agents are very effective at minimizing the diarrhea. A dose of 2 to 3 g of psyllium fiber should be given twice a day for 2 weeks. It can be mixed with other foods for palatability. If a good response is obtained, the psyllium usually can be discontinued without return of the diarrhea. If no response is seen in 7 to 10 days, persisting with psyllium therapy is not necessary. Other bulking agents do not appear to be as effective as is psyllium.

Cholestyramine has been used successfully to treat this syndrome. A dose of between 7.5 and 20.0 g/day, divided into four doses, should be given for 2 weeks. Because of some potential for side effects from cholestyramine, it should not be tried until after psyllium therapy fails.

Some children respond to a 7- to 10-day course of metronidazole. The recommended amount is 15 mg/kg/day, divided into three doses.

Suggested Readings

Boyne LJ, Kerzner B, McClung HJ. Chronic nonspecific diarrhea: the value of a preliminary observation period to assess diet therapy. *Pediatrics* 1985;79:557.

Burks AW, Vanderhoof JA, Mehra S, et al. Randomized clinical trial of soy formula with and without added fiber in antibiotic-induced diarrhea. *J Pediatr* 2001;139:578.

Cole CR, Rising R, Lifschitz F. Consequences of incomplete carbohydrate absorption from fruit juice consumption in infants. *Arch Pediatr Adolesc Med* 1999;153:1098.

Fenton TR, Harries JT, Milla PJ. Disordered small intestinal motility: a rational basis for toddlers' diarrhea. *Gut* 1983;24:897.

Hoekstra JH, van Kempen AA, Kneepkens CM. Apple juice malabsorption: fructose or sorbitol? *J Pediatr Gastroenterol Nutr* 1993;16:39.

Kneepkens CM, Hoekstra JH. Chronic nonspecific diarrhea of childhood: pathophysiology and management. *Pediatr Clin North Am* 1996;43:375.

Lebenthal-Bendor Y, Theuer RC, Lebenthal A, et al. Malabsorption of modified food starch (acetylated distarch phosphate) in normal infants and in 8–24-month-old toddlers with non-specific diarrhea, as influenced by sorbitol and fructose. *Acta Paediatr* 2001;90:1368.

Leung AK, Robson WL. Evaluating the child with chronic diarrhea. *Am Fam Physician* 1996;53:635.

Moukarzel AA, Lesicka H, Ament ME. Irritable bowel syndrome and nonspecific diarrhea in infancy and childhood-relationship with juice carbohydrate malabsorption. *Clin Pediatr (Phila)* 2002;41:145.

Smally JR, Klish WJ, Campbell MA, Brown MR. Use of psyllium in the management of chronic nonspecific diarrhea of childhood. *J Pediatr Gastroenterol Nutr* 1982;1:361.

Vanderhoof JA. Chronic diarrhea. *Pediatr Rev* 1998;19:418.

Walker WA. Benign chronic diarrhea of infancy. *Pediatr Rev* 1981;3:153.

CHAPTER 345 ■ INGUINAL HERNIA

CHARLES N. PAIDAS AND MARK L. KAYTON

Groin bulges, some of which represent inguinal hernias, are a common reason for visits to primary care physicians and emergency rooms and among the most frequent indications for surgical consultation. However, not all groin bulges are inguinal hernias. In this chapter we will present tactics to recognize, diagnose, and treat pediatric inguinal pathology. We will also discuss the complications of operations, a topic often minimized.

PATHOPHYSIOLOGY

The origin of inguinal hernias lies in the embryology that is common to both males and females. Fetuses of both sexes have a genitoinguinal ligament that connects the developing urogenital ridges with the labioscrotal swelling. This genitoinguinal ligament becomes, in males, the gubernaculum testis, which presumably serves to guide the testis in its descent. In females, the genitoinguinal ligament becomes the round ligament of the uterus. In both sexes a tubular extension of the peritoneal sac develops ventral to either the gubernaculum or round ligament; this tubular outpouching is the processus vaginalis. If the processus vaginalis fails to obliterate, the stage is set for an inguinal hernia.

A processus vaginalis that contains intestine is called an inguinal hernia. One containing fluid is called a hydrocele (Fig. 345.1). Thus, hernias and hydroceles share a common embryology, but their treatment differs, as will be discussed later. Most inguinal hernias seen by pediatricians are congenital, indirect hernias, meaning that they are due to a patent processus vaginalis. Acquired, direct hernias are less common in childhood and stem from an inherent weakness in the musculature forming the inguinal canal rather than from a patent processus vaginalis. The congenital, indirect hernia arises lateral to the

inferior epigastric vessels. The acquired, direct hernia arises medial to the inferior epigastric vessels (Fig. 345.2). In the clinical practice of pediatrics, this distinction is somewhat academic, because indirect and direct inguinal hernias may have the same outward appearance, and the indications for referral and treatment do not differ. Ordinarily, in children, the type of hernia cannot be discerned until the time of operative dissection.

CLINICAL MANIFESTATIONS

The clinical examination for hernia begins, in boys, with examination of the testes to determine whether both testes are descended into the scrotum. If not in the scrotum, the testicle itself, lying in the inguinal canal, may be the cause of the observed groin bulge.

Immobilizing the testicle in the scrotal sac with one hand, the examiner uses the other hand to palpate the external inguinal ring. A bulge may be detected. If not, efforts to make the child strain or cry or holding the baby in an erect upright position may produce a bulge. When a hernia can not be

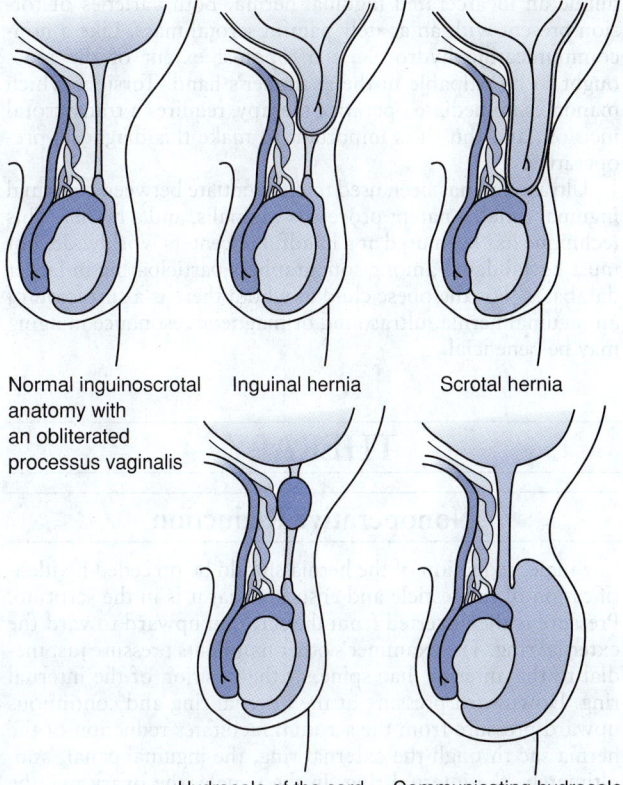

Normal inguinoscrotal anatomy with an obliterated processus vaginalis   Inguinal hernia   Scrotal hernia

Hydrocele of the cord   Communicating hydrocele

FIGURE 345.2. Diagram of typical positions and associated anatomic landmarks found with indirect and direct inguinal hernias.

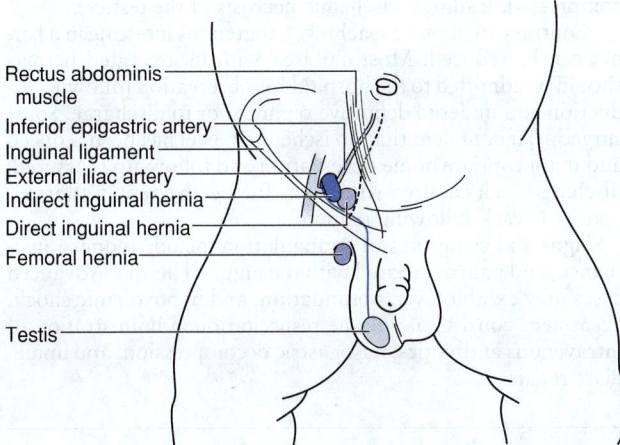

Rectus abdominis muscle
Inferior epigastric artery
Inguinal ligament
External iliac artery
Indirect inguinal hernia
Direct inguinal hernia
Femoral hernia

Testis

FIGURE 345.1. Inguinoscrotal anatomy, in normal presentation as well as in cases of inguinal and scrotal hernia, hydrocele, and communicating hydrocele.

discretely identified, sometimes the examiner will feel a thickened processus vaginalis, empty of intestine or other organs; this is referred to as the "silk glove sign" and is evidence of swelling of cord vasculature and is associated with freely reducible inguinal hernia.

DIFFERENTIAL DIAGNOSIS

An inguinal hernia can present with a bulge that extends to the external inguinal ring. This cranial extension prohibits the physician from fully grasping the neck of the hernia in his or her hand. A hydrocele, in contrast, may be wholly contained in the scrotum—the so-called noncommunicating hydrocele—and the examiner may be able to get around the top of the bulge with his or her fingers. This feature, when present, can help to distinguish some hydroceles from hernias. In many patients a noncommunicating hydrocele resolves without treatment, but most surgeons recommend surgery if the hydrocele persists at 12 to 18 months of age. A communicating hydrocele, in contrast, indicates that a continuous passage of fluid is occurring between the inguinal bulge and the peritoneal cavity, and it should be treated like a hernia.

Groin lymphadenopathy can be confused with an inguinal hernia. The relationship of the observed bulge to the external inguinal ring may help clarify the cause of swelling. Typically, if there are multiple inguinal groin nodes, they parallel the groin crease. Erythema or fluctuance of a groin mass may suggest presence of either abscess or strangulated inguinal hernia. Surgical referral should be made if the clinician is uncertain. Often, the history and clinical picture will help to differentiate the two, but operative exploration may be required if the diagnosis cannot be made clinically. If the swelling is determined to be an abscess, it should be drained under anesthesia.

Finally, torsion of the testis or of the appendix testis can mimic an incarcerated inguinal hernia. Both varieties of torsion present with an acutely painful scrotal mass. Like a noncommunicating hydrocele, the topmost extent of the mass ought to be palpable in the examiner's hand. Torsion, which mandates immediate operative therapy, requires a transscrotal incision, and thus it is important to make this diagnosis preoperatively.

Ultrasound has been used to differentiate between a normal inguinal canal, a patent processus vaginalis, and a hernia. This technique has been used at a handful of centers worldwide, but must be validated among sonographers participating in larger databases. For the obese child in whom there is a suspicion of an inguinal hernia, ultrasound or magnetic resonance imaging may be beneficial.

THERAPY

Nonoperative Reduction

In a male, reduction of the hernia should be preceded by identification of the testicle and ensuring that it is in the scrotum. Pressure is then exerted from the scrotum upward toward the external ring. The examiner's other hand puts pressure just medial to the anterior iliac spine, at the position of the internal ring. Downward pressure at the internal ring and continuous upward pressure from the scrotum facilitates reduction of the hernia sac through the external ring, the inguinal canal, and, ultimately, the internal ring. In the female, the ovary may be within the hernia sac. Thus, using this similar technique, reduction must include confirmation that hernia and ovary have been reduced.

Timing of Repair

For a premature infant with a clinically observed inguinal hernia, repair of the hernia may be undertaken after the infant reaches approximately 2 kg. If the infant is to remain in a neonatal intensive care unit under observation for other conditions, repair may be delayed until just before discharge, allowing for additional growth of the infant. The need for anesthesia for other conditions (e.g., gastrostomy or ventriculoperitoneal shunt) should prompt consideration for hernia repair at the same setting.

Infants that have been discharged from the hospital but develop clinical evidence of an inguinal hernia are scheduled for elective repair. Most undergo hernia repair as outpatients. Antibiotic prophylaxis is not needed in the absence of comorbid medical conditions. Young infants born prematurely are at significantly increased risk of postoperative apnea and bradycardia, and require a 24-hour hospital stay for cardiorespiratory monitoring. The postconceptual age at which premature infants can safely undergo repair as an outpatient has not yet been established and practice varies. Caudal analgesia is helpful if it can be administered. Effective treatment of postoperative pain is an important component of care.

The technique of open hernia repair has been challenged by laparoscopic herniorrhaphy in children. Either technique is safe, technically effective, and cosmetically adequate. Although some surgeons prefer the laparoscopic technique, prospective randomized trials are necessary to better compare the techniques. At present, the vast majority of inguinal hernias are repaired using the open technique (unilateral) or a combination of open and laparoscopic technique for discerning bilaterality.

Incarceration and Strangulation

An incarcerated hernia is one that cannot be reduced by spontaneous activity or gentle pressure. It presents without pain or fluctuance. Incarceration should prompt immediate medical attention. Avoidance of incarceration should be the primary goal in the management of inguinal hernia; once present, incarceration is itself a risk factor for future recurrence, because resulting tissue edema makes repair more technically difficult. Incarceration, if not treated promptly, can progress to strangulation within 6 to 8 hours. Pressure on the trapped organ, or on its vascular supply, may lead to ischemia and necrosis of the herniated organ, whether it is intestine, an ovary, a piece of bladder, or other tissue. Even the testicle is at risk. Though they are not within the hernia sac, the testicular vessels can be compressed, leading to ischemic necrosis of the testicle.

Contrary to popular teaching, gangrenous intestine in a hernia can be reduced. Most children with incarcerated hernias should be admitted to the hospital for observation following reduction and undergo definitive repair prior to discharge. Some surgeons, if confident that no ischemic bowel has been reduced and if appropriate home observation and follow-up is assured, discharge such children with plans for elective repair approximately 1 week following reduction.

Signs and symptoms of strangulation include redness, fluctuance, and pain associated with the inguinal hernia. Advanced cases may exhibit fever, obtundation, and hypovolemic shock. Treatment consists of volume resuscitation, administration of intravenous antibiotics, nasogastric decompression, and immediate repair.

Contralateral Exploration

There is controversy over the wisdom of contralateral exploration during the repair of a unilateral inguinal hernia. Part of the reason this issue is difficult to settle is that presence of contralateral patent processus vaginalis, whether detected by laparoscopy or by groin incision, does not uniformly predict progression to contralateral hernia. A prospective study by Tackett et al. found that only 8.8% of children manifested a contralateral hernia with a mean follow-up of 25.5 months. A more recent prospective study by Nassiri of equal number of male and female children who underwent a unilateral inguinal hernia repair (1 month to 12 years age) reported a 3.6% incidence of contralateral hernia with a follow-up of 4 to 10 years.

Connective tissue disease, history of prematurity, or conditions predisposing to fluid in the abdomen, such as ventriculoperitoneal shunts or peritoneal dialysis, are considered by most surgeons to be indications to explore the contralateral side and to ligate a patent processus vaginalis if found. Because in many cases the processes vaginalis will spontaneously obliterate during the first few years of life, the decision to perform contralateral exploration should be weighed against the risk of additional anesthesia.

Intersex Anomalies

Intersex anomalies may be discovered during repair of an inguinal hernia. A phenotypic female with a palpable gonad in the labia may actually be a male with testicular feminization syndrome due to androgen insensitivity or a true hermaphrodite. Usually, a true hermaphrodite has ambiguous genitalia, and thus the diagnosis is suspected preoperatively. If a gonad that appears to be a testicle is discovered during exploration of the female groin, it should be biopsied. Postoperatively, an ultrasound should delineate what gonadal tissue is present (normal ovaries may coexist with a testicle). Findings should guide counseling of the family. Formal orchiectomy, for a phenotypic female, can follow once evaluation and discussion have occurred. If ovaries are absent, future hormone replacement therapy should be considered.

COMPLICATIONS

Bleeding and infection are unusual complications of inguinal hernia repair. Recurrence occurs in approximately 0.5% of uncomplicated cases, but at a much greater rate following repair of an incarcerated hernia. Recurrence of any pediatric hernia may be indirect or direct. Postoperative scrotal edema or hematoma, while they are visually disturbing and painful complications, both resolve spontaneously in 2 to 3 months, and aspiration should not be attempted.

Infertility may result from inguinal hernia repair and may not become clinically manifest until decades have passed. Steigman and colleagues at Cardinal Glennon Children's Hospital, in a historical study of pathology reports from hernia sacs in over 7,000 boys, found that fragments of epididymis or vas deferens had been excised in 0.53% of patients. Data suggest that even unilateral occlusion of a vas can lead to high concentration of antisperm antibodies, which have been implicated as contributing to male infertility. Such problems are not exclusive to males. The fallopian tube, if present in a hernia sac, can be mistakenly ligated. Although the incidence of infertility related to prior inguinal hernia repair is low, knowledge of this complication should influence pediatric surgeons' discussions with parents and should foster a policy of contralateral groin explorations only in carefully selected patients.

Suggested Readings

Bhatia AM, Gow KW, Heiss KF, et al. Is the use of laparoscopy to determine presence of contralateral patent processus vaginalis justified in children greater than 2 years of age? *J Ped Surg* 2004;39:778.

Erez I, Rathause V, Vacian I, et al. Preoperative ultrasound and intraoperative findings of inguinal hernias in children: a prospective study of 642 children. *J Ped Surg* 2002;37:865.

Gorsler CM, Schier F. Laparoscopic herniorrhaphy in children. *Surg Endosc* 2003;17:571.

Graf JL, Caty MG, Martin DJ, Glick PL. Pediatric hernias. *Semin Ultrasound CT MR* 2002;23:197.

Hollinshead WH, Rosse C. *Textbook of anatomy,* 4th ed. Philadelphia: Harper & Row, 1985.

Jewett TC, Kuhn JP, Allen JE. Herniography in children. *J Ped Surg* 1976;11:451.

Nassiri SJ. Contralateral exploration is not mandatory in unilateral inguinal hernia in children: a prospective 6 year study. *Pediatr Surg Int* 2002;18:470.

Parkhouse H, Hendry WF. Vasal injuries during childhood and their effect on subsequent fertility. *Br J Urol* 1991;67:91.

Steigman CK, Sotelo-Avila C, Weber TR. The incidence of spermatic cord structures in inguinal hernia sacs from male children. *Am J Surg Pathol* 1999;23:880.

Steinau G, Treutner KH, Feeken G, Schumpelick V. Recurrent inguinal hernias in infants and children. *World J Surg* 1995;19:303.

Strauch ED, Voigt RW, Hill JL. Gangrenous intestine in a hernia can be reduced. *J Ped Surg* 2002;37:919.

Swanson JA, Chapler FK. Infertility as a consequence of bilateral herniorrhaphies. *Fertil Steril* 1977;28:1118.

Tackett LD, Breuer CK, Luks FI, et al. Incidence of contralateral inguinal hernia: a prospective analysis. *J Ped Surg* 1999;34:684.

Urman BC, McComb PF. Tubal occlusion after inguinal hernia repair: a case report. *J Reprod Med* 1991;36:175.

CHAPTER 346 ■ GASTROINTESTINAL BLEEDING

MARILYN R. BROWN

Gastrointestinal (GI) bleeding in children is a common and occasionally life-threatening occurrence. The physician first determines if the child has bled. If the child has bled a significant amount, therapy may need to be instituted before the site of bleeding is determined. The physician attempts to find out whether the bleeding is from the upper (originating above the ligament of Treitz) or lower GI tract. The cause and specific site of bleeding are determined, if possible (Box 346.1). Thirty years ago, a definite cause could be found in only approximately one-half of cases. Current diagnostic techniques, including fiberoptic endoscopy, radiography, scintography, angiography, and video endoscopy, allow

BOX 346.1 — Causes of Gastrointestinal Bleeding

First 4 weeks
Swallowed maternal blood
Hemorrhagic disease of the newborn
Anal fissure
Hemorrhagic gastritis
Stress ulcers
Infective enterocolitis
Protein-sensitive enterocolitis
Necrotizing enterocolitis
Hirschsprung enterocolitis
Duplication cysts
Midgut volvulus
Vascular malformations

First 6 months
Nonspecific colitis
Anal fissure
Esophagitis
Infective enterocolitis
Protein-sensitive enterocolitis
Intussusception
Lymphonodular hyperplasia
Duplication cysts
Hirschsprung enterocolitis
Vascular malformations

6 months to 5 years
Epistaxis
Esophagitis
Esophageal varices
Gastritis
Infective enterocolitis
Clostridium difficile colitis
Lymphonodular hyperplasia
Intussusception
Meckel diverticulum
Vascular malformations
Henoch-Schönlein purpura
Hemolytic uremic syndrome
Neutropenic typhlitis
Polyps
Anal fissure

5 to 18 years
Same as for 6 months to 5 years plus
   Tear in gastric mucosa (Mallory-Weiss syndrome)
   Gastritis
   Peptic ulcer
   Chronic ulcerative colitis
   Crohn disease
   Hemorrhoids

localization of the site of bleeding to be determined in most cases.

Some causes of bleeding are more likely to occur at certain ages, and some causes are associated with certain rates of bleeding, varying from slow loss of small amounts to rapid loss of large amounts. Minor bleeding may be caused by esophagitis, infective and allergic enterocolitis, Crohn disease, colonic polyps, and anal fissures. Slow chronic bleeding can result from chronic esophagitis, chronic inflammatory bowel disease, and sometimes colonic polyps. Acute significant losses

may be caused by esophageal varices, hemorrhagic gastritis, peptic and stress ulcers, Meckel diverticulum, chronic inflammatory bowel disease, and vascular malformations. The passage of a "currant jelly" stool (mixed blood and mucus, light red) often indicates an acute intestinal obstruction such as intussusception.

ESTABLISHMENT OF BLOOD LOSS

Whether or not blood loss has occurred must be determined first. Many substances ingested by children may be mistaken for blood. Red food coloring, fruit-flavored drinks, fruit juices, and beets may color the vomitus or stool reddish. Stools can acquire a black color from ingested iron, bismuth subsalicylate, grape juice, spinach, and blueberries. The vomitus or gastric aspirate is tested by Gastroccult (pH buffered) and the stool by guaiac, Hemoccult, or Hematest for the presence of blood. If a child presents in the office with anemia that has no clear explanation, several stools should be tested for occult blood.

TYPE OF BLEEDING

A description of the color, location, and amount of blood usually is helpful. Did the child cough up blood (hemoptysis) or vomit up blood (hematemesis) after epistaxis? Gastric acid turns the blood a brown color. Small amounts of bright red blood (hematochezia) or blood streaking in the stool most often is caused by polyps, proctitis, constipation with anal fissures, or hemorrhoids. Bright red blood on the outside of the stool accompanied by pain on passage of the stool usually is from an anal fissure. Bright red blood mixed with mucus in a loose stool is typical of chronic ulcerative colitis. The classic currant jelly stool occurs from ileocolic intussusception (prolapse of the ileum through the ileocecal valve into the colon) and may occur with midgut volvulus. Melena (black or dark maroon stool) suggests a lesion proximal to the right colon, such as a Meckel diverticulum, or an upper GI bleed. A bleeding duodenal ulcer can present with red bloody stools instead of melena because of rapid transit through the GI tract.

If the patient enters the emergency department with melena or hematochezia with evidence of anemia and tachycardia or hypotension, an aspiration of gastric contents must be obtained to look for evidence of upper GI bleeding.

The magnitude of the blood loss is important in formulating the therapeutic and diagnostic plan, as is the age of the patient. Severe life-threatening hemorrhage is a rare occurrence in children, but the cause usually is found; however, the cause of chronic slow blood loss sometimes is difficult to determine.

AGE-INDEPENDENT ETIOLOGIES

Certain causes of GI bleeding are seen more commonly in specific age groups, but considerable overlap exists. At all ages, stress (burns, central nervous system trauma) and ingestion of aspirin or nonsteroidal antiinflammatory drugs (NSAIDs) may lead to gastric or duodenal stress erosions and ulcerations. Thrombocytopenia and coagulopathies must be considered. Intestinal bleeding is not an uncommon occurrence in children with cancer who develop thrombocytopenia secondary to chemotherapy. Chemotherapy may be followed by esophagitis, gastritis, and enterocolitis. Although primary tumors of the GI tract are rare findings, they must be considered in the differential diagnosis at any age. Blood in the stool rarely accompanies giardiasis, whereas it is a common finding in amebiasis.

AGE-ASSOCIATED ETIOLOGIES

First 4 Weeks

In the first few days to months of life, a long list of causes of gastrointestinal bleeding include swallowed maternal blood, hemorrhagic disease of the newborn, irritation from a nasogastric tube, anal fissure, hemorrhagic gastritis, gastric or duodenal stress ulcers, necrotizing enterocolitis, Hirschsprung enterocolitis, and midgut volvulus. In the first few days of life, hematemesis or the passage of bloody stools in a healthy newborn most likely is caused by swallowed maternal blood, which can be differentiated from fetal hemoglobin by the Apt alkali denaturation test. If the red blood denatures with alkali to a brown color, the hemoglobin is of adult origin. Hemorrhagic disease of the newborn with prolongation of the prothrombin time must be considered when vitamin K has not been administered. Breast-fed infants are particularly susceptible to this complication. An anal fissure is a common cause of bleeding, usually initiated by the passage of a firm stool that makes a small tear along the anal canal. Significant bleeding in the neonate, particularly in the stressed newborn and premature infant, may occur from hemorrhagic gastritis, gastric erosions, or gastric stress ulcers. Necrotizing enterocolitis (ischemic damage to the bowel wall) may begin with mild diarrhea, which is positive for reducing substances, and with increased gastric residuals after feeding, followed by blood in the stool and the appearance of abdominal distension and pneumatosis intestinalis. Hirschsprung enterocolitis, midgut volvulus, and intestinal duplication cysts also may present with bleeding and must be kept in mind. Irritation from nasogastric tube feedings is a common cause of small amounts of blood in the gastric aspirate or stool.

First 6 Months

A little bit older infant may have protein-induced colitis, gastroesophageal reflux esophagitis, allergic gastritis, bacterial colitis, or malabsorption of vitamin K in cystic fibrosis. Nonspecific colitis and protein-induced colitis are frequent causes of hematochezia in infants younger than 6 months old. Gastroesophageal reflux is a very common occurrence in infants and occasionally will cause reflux esophagitis with blood loss.

Among bacterial causes, shigellosis or salmonellosis may cause blood in the diarrheal stool, but infection with *Campylobacter jejuni* is a more common cause of bloody diarrhea. Enteroinvasive, enterotoxic, and enteropathogenic *Escherichia coli* infections can cause bloody diarrhea, but tests for diagnosis are not readily available, except for *E. coli* O157:H7. Antibiotic-associated diarrhea is a frequent finding, but blood loss in the stool is not seen commonly. The presence of *Clostridium difficile* organisms and toxins are fairly common in the asymptomatic infant, but the association of antibiotic usage and subsequent diarrhea with blood in the stools may signify a causative role. Viral diarrheas are associated less commonly with blood in the stool.

Enterocolitis induced by milk, soy, or other proteins is a frequent cause of blood in the intestinal tract in the infant. Allergic gastritis can lead to bloody vomitus. Allergic enteritis can lead to protein-loss hypoalbuminemia and guaiac-positive stools. The most common allergic symptoms are related to colitis, which presents as blood-streaked mucousy stools early in infancy. It also may occur in infants who are breast-fed; in these cases, the mother may be tried on a diet free of milk, soy, or both. Lymphonodular hyperplasia of the colon occurs at all ages and is characterized by multiple tiny, yellowish nodules that are enlarged lymphoid follicles with mucosal inflammation and a thin epithelial lining overlying them. These nodules are thought to be secondary to infection and may be associated with the appearance of blood in the stool. Intestinal arteriovenous malformations, hemangiomas, or telangiectasias occasionally bleed. Also, cystic fibrosis with malabsorption of vitamin K may be the cause of bruising or GI bleeding in an infant.

6 Months to 5 Years of Age

Causes in this age group include epistaxis, reflux esophagitis, esophageal varices, intussusception, Meckel diverticulum, Henoch-Schönlein purpura, infection, and colonic polyps. Epistaxis always must be considered as a cause of blood in vomitus. The blood loss from esophagitis associated with gastroesophageal reflux may be associated with "coffee ground" (dark brown) emesis, but it often is occult and may cause chronic anemia.

Bleeding from esophageal varices usually is brisk and associated with significant hematemesis. Portal hypertension may occur from liver diseases or other causes of blockage of the portal venous system. Extrahepatic portal hypertension from extrahepatic blockage of the portal vein may occur early in life, and the associated esophageal varices may first bleed during the first few years of life.

Intussusception (the telescoping of a proximal portion of the intestine into the distal portion) occurs most commonly during the child's first 2 years of life and usually presents with brief, frequent episodes of severe abdominal pain. The process may progress to vomiting, lethargy, currant jelly stools, and complete intestinal obstruction. A sausage-shaped mass may be felt in the abdomen. Ileocolonic intussusception occurs most commonly. Diagnosis is confirmed by barium enema or ultrasonography; reduction with air, water, or barium under mild pressure is successful in most cases. In a child older than 2 years of age, a mass acting as a lead point often is present.

Meckel diverticulum, a remnant of the omphalomesenteric duct located in the ileum approximately 30 cm from the ileocecal valve, often is asymptomatic; however, when it contains gastric mucosa, secretion of acid can cause ulceration in either the diverticulum or the adjacent ileum, with subsequent painless bleeding presenting as black or maroon stools and anemia. The diagnosis is made by technetium (Tc)-99m pertechnetate radionuclide scan. A Meckel diverticulum also may act as a lead point for intussusception.

Henoch-Schönlein purpura is a systemic vasculitis in which abdominal cramps and intestinal bleeding may precede the purpuric skin manifestations. Ileoileal intussusception is not an uncommon occurrence. Hemolytic uremic syndrome may develop after a variety of infections such as *E. coli* O157:H7, which causes severe colitis with frequent bloody stools, usually before the onset of uremia and anemia. Neutropenic typhlitis is a necrotizing enterocolitis involving the cecum and right colon in immunosuppressed individuals.

Juvenile colonic polyps (inflammatory hamartomas) are a common cause of intermittent painless hematochezia in children 2 to 5 years of age. Most of these polyps are solitary and located within 30 cm of the anus. The diagnosis is made by digital rectal examination, barium enema, sigmoidoscopy, or colonoscopy. Snare cauterization polypectomy through the colonoscope is appropriate. Hereditary polyposes usually present a little later.

5 to 18 Years of Age

Although the following diagnoses may be made before the child reaches the age of 5 years, they are made more commonly afterward. They include epistaxis, Mallory-Weiss tear from vomiting, NSAID gastritis, *Helicobacter pylori*, chronic inflammatory bowel disease, hereditary polyposes, and vascular lesions.

Epistaxis is seen more commonly in older children. Repeated episodes of forceful vomiting may cause a small linear tear (Mallory-Weiss syndrome) at the gastroesophageal junction, with usually minimal blood loss. Ingestion of caustic materials may cause severe damage to the esophagus or stomach. Gastric erosions from ingestion of aspirin are seen less frequently today because of the decreasing use of aspirin in children. The increased use of NSAIDs has been associated with increased incidence of abdominal pain and evidence of gastritis and bleeding.

The spiral gram-negative organism *H. pylori* may inhabit the surface of mucosal epithelial cells of the stomach and occasionally the duodenum. Its presence is associated with local inflammation (chronic gastritis). Children with *H. pylori* gastritis may present with recurrent epigastric pain, nausea, vomiting, hematemesis, and occult blood in the stools. Children with duodenal ulcers may have *Helicobacter* infection. If the organism is eradicated, the relapse rate of the ulcer after treatment is 20%. If the organism is not eradicated, the relapse rate is approximately 80%. The organism can be detected by testing an endoscopic antral biopsy for urease activity or observing the organism microscopically in the antral biopsy specimen. A carbon 13 or carbon 14 urea breath test is available as a noninvasive diagnostic test for urease activity. More recently, the antigens of the organism have been detected in stool samples. Positive antibody titers indicate past or present infection. The organism is sensitive to bismuth, proton pump inhibitors, amoxicillin, clarithromycin, and metronidazole. The highest rate of eradication with drugs available in the United States is with combination therapy, usually amoxicillin, clarithromycin, and a proton pump inhibitor for 1 to 2 weeks. Studies have shown that in persons undergoing long-term treatment with NSAIDs, the incidence of GI bleeding is much higher in those who have *H. pylori* than in those who do not. Therefore, eradication of *H. pylori* is recommended before beginning long-term use of NSAIDs.

The chronic inflammatory bowel diseases, Crohn disease and chronic ulcerative colitis, are of unknown etiology and characterized by a remitting-relapsing symptom pattern. In mild stages of Crohn disease, chronic ulcerative colitis, or ulcerative proctitis, only occult or small amounts of visible blood in the stool may occur. Crohn disease that involves only the small intestine may be accompanied by only occult blood in the stool. The nearer the lesions are to the anus, the more likely hematochezia will occur. Tenesmus and urgency to stool are more common findings in ulcerative colitis, whereas Crohn disease may present with painless bright red bleeding. Severe blood loss is seen more frequently in ulcerative colitis, but it occurs in both conditions. Usually other signs and symptoms, including diarrhea, weight loss, fever, abdominal pain, anorexia, malaise, aphthous ulcers, joint pain, and decreased growth, are seen. Diagnosis is suspected by history, physical examination, presence of microcytic anemia, thrombocytosis, elevated erythrocyte sedimentation rate, and hypoalbuminemia; it is confirmed by intestinal radiography, colonoscopy, and biopsy. Sulfasalazine (or the newer acetyl salicylate derivatives) and corticosteroids are the mainstays of treatment. Other medications that are increasing in use include 6-mercaptopurine, azathioprine, metronidazole, cyclosporine, tacrolimus, methotrexate, and antitumor necrosis factor antibodies.

Peutz-Jeghers syndrome consists of diffuse GI hamartomas, most marked in the small bowel, associated with melanotic areas on the buccal mucosa and lips. Other chronic polyposes include juvenile polyposis coli, familial adenomatous polyposis, and Gardner syndrome (familial adenomatous polyposis associated with bony lesions, subcutaneous tumors, and cysts). These conditions have clear malignant potential, and colectomy may be indicated in children.

Vascular lesions take a variety of forms. Telangiectasias may be associated with Turner syndrome. Small angiodysplasias, hemangiomas, or arteriovenous malformations may occur, and arteriography may be helpful in establishing the diagnosis. Large hemorrhoids are relatively uncommon findings in children, so portal hypertension should be considered. A cause of monthly GI bleeding in an adolescent girl may be ectopic endometrium in the GI tract.

DIAGNOSIS AND THERAPY

A careful history and physical examination are helpful in most cases. The condition of the child determines the rapidity of the approach to diagnosis. If the child is pale and weak with tachycardia and hypotension, immediate stabilization of the child's cardiovascular status is paramount, and history, physical examination, diagnosis, and therapy must be performed rapidly.

Important elements of the history include age of the child; amount and character of the bleeding in vomitus or stool; presence of associated abdominal or rectal pain, diarrhea, drug ingestion, fever, and systemic symptoms such as joint pain or aphthous ulcerations; growth pattern; recent illnesses; foreign travel; and family history of GI or bleeding disorders.

Important components of the physical examination are evaluation of general appearance and vital signs; examination of skin for telangiectasias or purpura or melanotic spots on lips; examination for evidence of epistaxis, abdominal organomegaly, or tenderness or masses; and anorectal examination to verify the presence of blood in the stool and to identify fissures, fistulas, and distal polyps.

If upper GI bleeding is present on gastric aspiration, upper endoscopy is attempted when the gastric aspirate after lavage is almost clear. Small-diameter endoscopes allow examination of infants. If upper GI bleeding has stopped or has been minimal, an upper GI radiologic examination or upper endoscopy may be performed. Upper GI bleeding usually is accompanied by melena; however, if the bleeding has been abrupt, the stool guaiac still may be negative. Also, bleeding from a duodenal ulcer may result in red blood in the stools if the transit through the intestinal tract is rapid.

Upper GI bleeding is more likely to be massive than is lower GI bleeding. Massive lower GI bleeding is most likely from a Meckel diverticulum or arteriovenous malformation, but occasionally it occurs with the inflammatory bowel diseases. Currant jelly stool with abdominal pain and tenderness suggests infarction of the bowel secondary to intussusception. Similar findings may be present secondary to intestinal volvulus or an incarcerated internal hernia, which may occur in association with a tethered Meckel diverticulum.

Melena may signify upper or lower GI bleeding. Meckel diverticulum commonly presents as painless melena in a healthy 18- to 24-month-old child who has a significant decrease in hematocrit, but it may bleed at any age. When bleeding is ongoing, visualization through the colonoscope may be hindered by the blood. In these situations, a red blood cell scan or angiography with Tc-99m sulfur colloid labeling may be helpful in identifying a site of bleeding. If these procedures do not identify a lesion, colonoscopy can be attempted after the child has undergone a large-volume cleansing electrolyte lavage. Computerized axial tomography or magnetic resonance imaging is helpful when the bleeding is from an identifiable mass or large lesion.

If hematochezia is accompanied by diarrhea, a sigmoidoscopy is helpful in determining friability or visualizing the pseudomembranes associated with *C. difficile* infection.

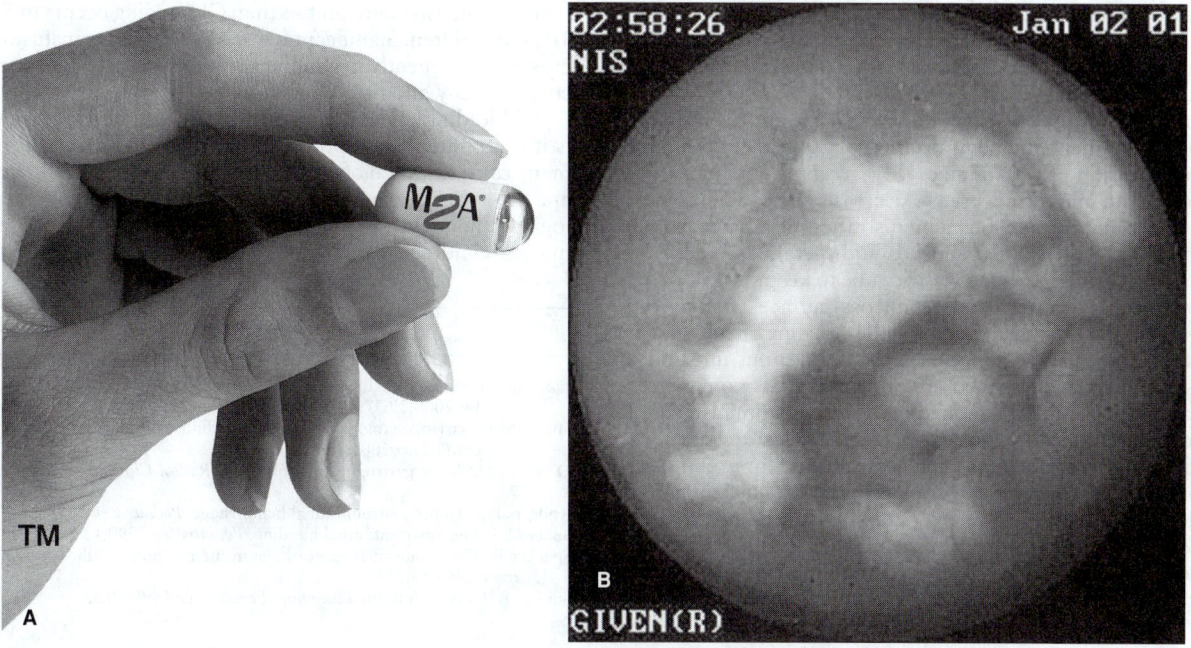

FIGURE 346.1. A: Given video capsule. **B:** Ulcer of Crohn disease in small bowel.

Biopsies may reveal amebae or distinguish between chronic and acute inflammatory changes. Stool cultures for *Shigella*, *Salmonella*, *C. jejuni*, and *Yersinia* should be obtained; tests also should be performed for *C. difficile* toxin and *E. coli* O157:H7.

Colonoscopy is most helpful in establishing the diagnosis of inflammatory bowel disease, arteriovenous malformations that are visible through the mucosal surface, lymphonodular hyperplasia, and polyps. The barium enema is valuable for detecting polyps, inflammatory bowel disease, lymphonodular hyperplasia, Hirschsprung disease, and colonic duplication and for making the diagnosis of and providing treatment for intussusception. A new form of endoscopy that may visualize a small bowel lesion not detected by other techniques is video capsule endoscopy (Fig. 346.1).

Therapy for a massive GI hemorrhage is aimed at resuscitating the patient, localizing the site of bleeding, and deciding on a treatment plan to stop the hemorrhage (Fig. 346.2). If orthostasis or frank hypotension is present, a large-bore intravenous catheter is inserted to obtain blood for laboratory studies and to infuse with normal saline or colloid until typed and cross-matched blood is available. Blood is sent for complete blood count, type, and cross-match, and for measurement of erythrocyte sedimentation rate, platelet count, clotting function, liver function, blood urea nitrogen, and serum electrolytes. A large-bore nasogastric tube is placed into the stomach, and gastric contents are aspirated. An aspirate of red blood or "coffee ground" material from the stomach indicates bleeding above the ligament of Treitz, although absence of blood does not rule out bleeding just distal to the pylorus. If fresh blood is

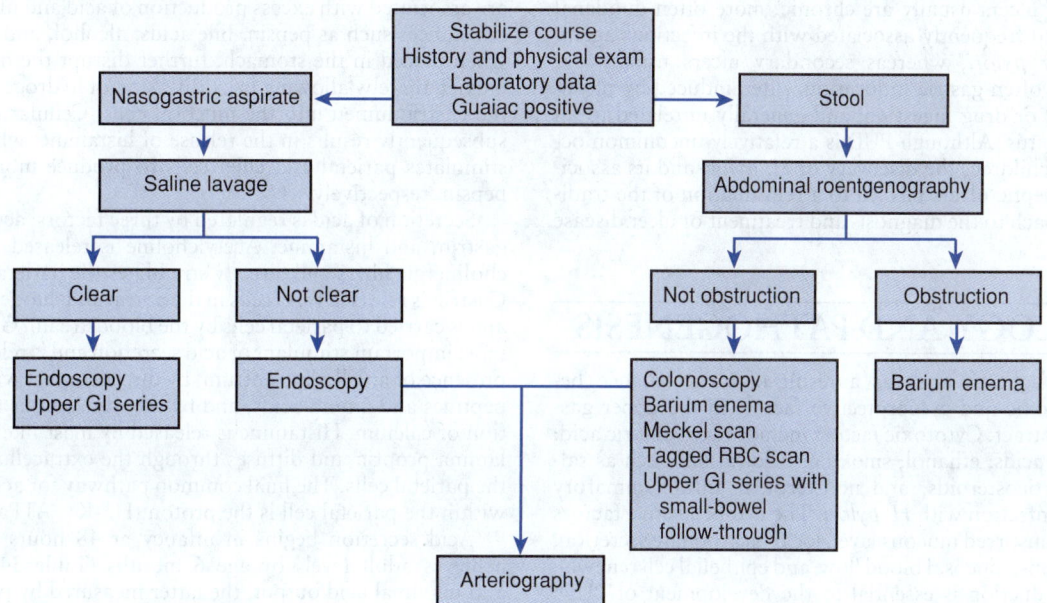

FIGURE 346.2. Approach to acute gastrointestinal bleeding. GI, gastrointestinal; RBC, red blood cell.

present, saline lavage may be carried out. Abdominal radiographs are taken in the upright, supine, and cross-table lateral positions to look for signs of obstruction and air outside the GI tract.

Further therapy for severe upper GI bleeding consists of blood replacement and neutralization of gastric acid. An intravenous infusion of a histamine$_2$ (H$_2$) receptor antagonist or a proton pump inhibitor is used to decrease gastric acidity. After endoscopy and intravenous administration of a proton pump inhibitor have been done, antacids and sucralfate may be administered through the nasogastric tube to keep the gastric pH above 5 and to coat the irritated mucosal surfaces. If nonbleeding esophageal varices are seen or the bleeding site cannot be identified and bleeding continues, an intravenous infusion of the somatostatin analogue octreotide acetate is commenced. Occasionally, a nitroglycerine compound is administered. If bleeding does not stop, the next step is sclerotherapy or rubber banding for varices, endoscopic heater probe (or argon laser) coagulation of bleeding sites, vasoconstrictive injections next to bleeding ulcers, selective angiography with embolization, or surgery. The placement of transjugular intrahepatic portosystemic shunts in children by interventional radiologists for the control of variceal bleeding is increasing in use gradually.

In an intensive care unit setting, GI bleeding occurs in 5% to 10% of children. Significant bleeding requiring transfusion occurs most frequently in children with respiratory failure and/or coagulopathy and thrombocytopenia.

GI bleeding is a common occurrence, but only occasionally is it a life-threatening problem in infants and children. It has many causes, several of which are age-related. A careful history and physical examination plus use of the endoscopic and radiologic techniques available can identify a source of hemorrhage in most children.

Suggested Readings

Fox VL. Gastrointestinal bleeding in infancy and childhood. *Gastroenterol Clin North Am* 2000;29:37.

Gilger MA. Gastroenterologic endoscopy in children: past, present and future. *Curr Opin Pediatr* 2001;13:429.

O'Hara SM. Acute gastrointestinal bleeding. *Radiol Clin North Am* 1997;35:879.

Rodgers BM. Upper gastrointestinal hemorrhage. *Pediatr Rev* 1999;20:171.

Silber G. Lower gastrointestinal bleeding. *Pediatr Rev* 1990;12:85.

Spencer R. Gastrointestinal hemorrhage in infancy and childhood: 476 cases. *Surgery* 1964;55:718.

Squires RH. Gastrointestinal bleeding. *Pediatr Rev* 1999;20:95.

CHAPTER 347 ■ PEPTIC ULCER DISEASE

KATHLEEN J. MOTIL

Peptic ulcer disease (PUD) is an ulcerative condition of the stomach or duodenum that may be accompanied by mucosal inflammation. PUD is classified as primary when it occurs in healthy children and as secondary when underlying disorders associated with injury, illness, or drug therapy coexists. Primary peptic ulcers usually are chronic, more often duodenal in origin, and frequently associated with the infectious agent, *Helicobacter pylori*, whereas secondary ulcers usually are acute, more often gastric in location, often induced by physiologic stress or drug ingestion, and generally unrelated to an infectious status. Although PUD is a relatively uncommon occurrence in children, the discovery of *H. pylori* and its association with peptic ulcers has led to a reevaluation of the traditional approach to the diagnosis and treatment of ulcer disease in children.

ETIOLOGY AND PATHOGENESIS

PUD is thought to arise as a result of an imbalance between cytotoxic and cytoprotective factors in the upper gastrointestinal tract. Cytotoxic factors include hydrochloric acid; pepsin; bile acids; ethanol; smoking; medications such as salicylates, corticosteroids, and nonsteroidal antiinflammatory drugs; and infection with *H. pylori*. The cytoprotective factors include the unstirred mucous layer, local bicarbonate secretion, prostaglandins, mucosal blood flow, and epithelial cell renewal.

Acid production is essential to the development of PUD. Oxidative phosphorylation of glucose and fatty acids within the parietal cells produces hydrogen ions that are secreted actively across a concentration gradient into the gastric lumen. When the concentration of intraluminal acid is twice the normal concentration, the gastric mucosal barrier may be broken. Entities such as Zollinger-Ellison syndrome and antral G-cell hyperplasia, both of which are rare events in children, are associated with excess production of acid and ulcer disease. Substances such as pepsin, bile acids, alcohol, and salicylates, when placed in the stomach, further disrupt the mucosal cell barrier, thereby allowing back diffusion of hydrogen ions from the gastric lumen into the mucosal cells. Cellular destruction subsequently results in the release of histamine, which further stimulates parietal and chief cells to produce more acid and pepsin, respectively.

Secretion of acid is regulated by three factors: acetylcholine, gastrin, and histamine. Acetylcholine is released from vagal cholinergic fibers and directly stimulates the parietal cell mass. Gastrin is released by G cells in the antral and duodenal mucosa and is carried to parietal cells by the bloodstream. Gastrin is the most important stimulant of acid secretion and is released in the presence of an alkaline antrum, by direct contact with ingested peptides and amino acids, and by the intravenous administration of calcium. Histamine is released by mast-like cells of the lamina propria and diffuses through the extracellular fluid to the parietal cells. The final common pathway for acid secretion within the parietal cell is the proton (H$^+$-K$^+$-ATPase) pump.

Acid secretion begins in infancy at 48 hours of life and achieves adult levels by age 6 months (Table 347.1). Basal and maximal acid output, the latter measured by pentagastrin stimulation, generally is higher in children with PUD than in healthy individuals, although overlap exists with normal values

TABLE 347.1

GASTRIC ACID SECRETION IN CHILDREN

Age	Acid Output (mEq/kg/hour)
4 weeks	0.02
12 weeks	0.10
24 weeks	0.17
4–9 years	0.24
>11 years	0.19

TABLE 347.3

SERUM GASTRIN LEVELS AFTER PROTEIN MEAL STIMULATION IN CHILDREN WITH PEPTIC ULCER DISEASE

Group	Serum Gastrin (pg/mL)		
	Basal	(1-hour Postprandial)	(2-hour Postprandial)
Ulcer disease			
Duodenal	40 ± 7	69 ± 11	57 ± 9
Gastric	44 ± 7	50 ± 7	46 ± 6
Healthy	34 ± 6	45 ± 6	39 ± 7

(Table 347.2). Serum gastrin concentrations are normal in children with primary or secondary gastric ulcers and may be normal or moderately elevated (100 to 120 pg/mL) in children with primary duodenal ulcers (Table 347.3). Hypergastrinemia may be seen in other disease entities, such as the Zollinger-Ellison syndrome, antral G-cell hyperplasia, long-standing pyloric obstruction, renal failure, short-gut syndrome, hyperparathyroidism, multiple endocrine neoplasias, pheochromocytoma, neurofibromatosis, primary pernicious anemia, and atrophic gastritis.

Mucous secretion by the epithelial mucous glands protects the stomach from ulceration by retarding the diffusion of acid from the lumen to the mucosal surface. Bicarbonate secretion from the stomach and duodenum serves as a buffer that minimizes the deleterious effect of a low pH. Prostaglandins bind to receptors in parietal cells and block acid secretion. Prostaglandins also stimulate mucosal blood flow, thereby providing an adequate supply of oxygen and nutrients for epithelial cell renewal.

EPIDEMIOLOGY

PUD is an uncommon occurrence in children. The prevalence is estimated to be less than 1% of pediatric hospital discharges and approximately 2% of children who undergo upper endoscopy for various complaints (Table 347.4). The median age of children with a diagnosis of primary ulcer disease is 9 years, but the age may range from infancy through adolescence. Most primary peptic ulcers occur in children older than 8 years of age, whereas secondary ulcers occur at all ages. The gender distribution of primary ulcer disease is 60% males and 40% females. In one report of primary peptic disease in children, duodenal ulcers occurred in 34% of cases and gastric ulcers occurred in 51%. *H. pylori* was found in 39% of children with duodenal ulcers and in 15% of those with gastric ulcers.

PATHOLOGY

Primary peptic ulcers usually are solitary lesions located in the duodenum and less commonly in the gastric antrum. The le-

sions are round or oval, are less than 2 cm in size, and have a sharp, punched-out defect. The ulcer may be superficial, may erode into the muscularis mucosa, or may penetrate the entire wall into adjacent organs. Chronic ulcers underlying scarred mucosa may cause puckering of the gastric folds and result in a spoke-like appearance on gross examination. The histologic appearance of PUD is that of active necrosis. The base and margins of the ulcer have fibrinoid debris overlying an acute inflammatory infiltrate. In the base of the ulcer, granulation tissue infiltrated with mononuclear cells is present and rests on a more solid collagenous scar. With reepithelialization, the glands of the mucosal margins become mucous-secreting, a change called *intestinalization*. In a large proportion of pediatric PUD, the spiral shaped, gram-negative, urease-producing bacterium *H. pylori* can be found within the mucosal inflammation and ulceration. However, 20% of pediatric cases may be negative for *H. pylori*.

Secondary peptic ulcers occur as single or multiple lesions and are found primarily in the stomach. The lesions tend to be circular, are less than 1 cm in diameter, and involve the mucosa or superficial epithelium. The ulcer base appears brown due to acid digestion of the blood within the superficial erosion, but the lesion is not indurated. An acute inflammatory infiltrate may be found in the margins and base of the ulcer, but scarring of blood vessel walls is absent. Reepithelialization is rapid and demonstrates many mitotic nuclei.

PREDISPOSING FACTORS

H. pylori has been associated causally with PUD (Box 347.1). However, although all children infected with *H. pylori* develop

TABLE 347.2

GASTRIC ACID PRODUCTION IN CHILDREN WITH PEPTIC ULCER DISEASE

Group	Acid Output (mEq/kg/hour)		
	Basal	Maximal	Peak
Peptic ulcer disease			
Duodenal	0.12 ± 0.04	0.51 ± 0.05	0.57 ± 0.04
Gastric	0.06 ± 0.02	0.47 ± 0.08	0.52 ± 0.10
Healthy	0.07 ± 0.02	0.30 ± 0.05	0.36 ± 0.05

TABLE 347.4

EPIDEMIOLOGY OF PEPTIC ULCER DISEASE IN CHILDREN

Feature	Occurrence
Prevalence (%)	
Pediatric hospital discharges	<1
Children undergoing endoscopy	2
Sex (male-to-female) ratio	1.5:1
Age distribution (%)	
Birth to 6 months	14
6 months to 2 years	8
2 to 5 years	17
5 to 10 years	30
10 to 15 years	31

| **BOX 347.1** | **Factors Predisposing to Peptic Ulcer Disease in Children** |

Helicobacter pylori
Alcohol, caffeine
Cigarette smoking
Drugs (corticosteroids, salicylates, nonsteroidal antiinflammatory agents)
Feeding devices (gastrostomy tubes)
Complications of systemic illness (sepsis, hypotension, respiratory distress)
Injury (burns, head injury)

---

chronic-active gastritis, most appear to have asymptomatic infections that may never lead to clinically evident disease. Only a minority of children develop peptic ulceration. The factors that result in formation of ulcers in this setting are unknown.

H. pylori disease is a chronic infection that typically is acquired in childhood. The prevalence of *H. pylori* is related inversely to socioeconomic status. Seroprevalence of *H. pylori* gradually increases with age, suggesting that the rate of acquisition decreases with age in successive generations of children as the standard of living improves. The human is the only known host for *H. pylori*. Clustering of *H. pylori* infection occurs within families, suggesting a common source of infection, person-to-person transmission, or a genetic predisposition to infection. Although the mode of transmission probably is person to person, the route of transmission is controversial. Genetic factors may influence the susceptibility to acquire *H. pylori* infection, but environmental factors are more important. Breast-fed children have a lower rate of *H. pylori* infection than do those who are not breast-fed, regardless of the educational status of the mother. Children with *H. pylori* gastritis often are asymptomatic. Symptoms such as abdominal pain and vomiting do not differentiate children with *H. pylori* colonization of the gastric mucosa from those who are not colonized. Treatment of *H. pylori* gastritis may not resolve abdominal symptoms unless patients also have duodenal ulcer disease. The eradication of *H. pylori* is associated with a pronounced reduction in the relapse rate of duodenal ulcers. Ulcer relapse is associated with either reinfection or recrudescence of *H. pylori* infection in medically noncompliant patients. Chronic gastric colonization with *H. pylori* may predispose the child to the development of mucosa-associated lymphoid tissue (MALT) lymphoma. *H. pylori* also is one of many risk factors that may lead to gastric carcinoma.

Exogenous factors such as alcohol and caffeine damage gastric mucosa and increase acid secretion, but evidence that these factors cause ulcer disease is inconclusive. Cigarette smoking not only leads to duodenal ulcer formation but also slows healing and increases recurrence rates. Drugs, feeding devices, and systemic illnesses have been associated with gastric ulcers. Corticosteroid therapy often is complicated by the appearance of gastric ulcers, presumably caused by the inhibition of phospholipase A and prostaglandin synthesis. Similarly, salicylates and nonsteroidal antiinflammatory agents inhibit synthesis of prostaglandin, thereby increasing the risk of gastric mucosal damage and formation of an ulcer. Gastrostomy tubes may injure the mucosa of the posterior gastric wall, resulting in recurrent bleeding from superficial erosions and frank ulcerations. Stress ulcers in children can occur in conjunction with systemic illnesses such as sepsis, hypotension, respiratory distress, extensive burns (Curling ulcer), and brain injury (Cushing

ulcer). These ulcers may result from a low-flow state (i.e., a shunting of blood from the superficial epithelium during stress), leading to a relative hypoxemia and depletion of nutrients necessary for cellular metabolism. Cystic fibrosis, Crohn disease, sickle cell disease, and insulin-dependent diabetes mellitus are associated with an increase in the frequency of ulcer disease in children.

CLINICAL MANIFESTATIONS

Recurrent abdominal pain, usually epigastric and less commonly periumbilical in location, is the hallmark symptom of primary PUD in children (Table 347.5). Symptoms such as nocturnal pain that awakens the child from sleep or abdominal pain that is exacerbated by or relieved by food are less common findings in children than in adults. Approximately one-third of children may present with hematemesis, occult blood in the feces, or frank melena. Nausea, vomiting, early satiety, anorexia, headache, and weight loss occur in a small proportion of children with PUD. The family history may be positive for ulcer disease, particularly among individuals previously treated for *H. pylori* disease. The medical history may reveal the use of potentially causative medications (e.g., nonsteroidal antiinflammatory drugs, corticosteroids), alcohol, tobacco, or inadequate dosing or frequency of administration of acid-suppressive medication. Despite the presence of typical complaints, the interval between the onset of symptoms and establishment of a diagnosis may exceed 1 year in primary ulcer disease.

Abdominal tenderness with overt upper gastrointestinal bleeding, melena, and anemia may be found on physical examination in children with PUD (Table 347.5). An acute abdomen with features of abdominal distention, decreased bowel sounds, and peritoneal irritation, consistent with the diagnosis of perforation or obstruction, occurs less commonly at presentation.

In the neonate, perforation of a gastric ulcer usually is the first manifestation of peptic disease, although bleeding commonly occurs. The neonate generally has a history of prematurity, respiratory distress, sepsis, hypoglycemia, or an intraventricular hemorrhage. Children younger than 3 years old are more likely to have an acute ulcer in conjunction with illness, surgery, or trauma and present with hematemesis,

TABLE 347.5

CLINICAL FEATURES OF PEPTIC ULCER DISEASE IN CHILDREN

Symptom	Frequency (%)
Abdominal pain	65
Epigastric	60
Periumbilical	6
Nocturnal awakening	12
Relief with food	4
Gastrointestinal bleeding	33
Vomiting	12
Family history positive for peptic ulcer disease	31
Sign	
Abdominal tenderness	58
Gastrointestinal bleeding	53
Acute abdomen	
Perforation	18
Obstruction	7
Anemia	11

melena, or perforation. Ulcers in this age group are located equally in the stomach or duodenum. In children between 3 and 6 years of age, periumbilical pain and vomiting are the more common presenting symptoms characteristic of primary ulcer disease. The stomach and duodenum are affected equally. In children older than 6 years old and in adolescents, the clinical findings are more comparable to those in adults with primary PUD.

LABORATORY, RADIOLOGIC, AND ENDOSCOPIC STUDIES

Laboratory studies in PUD generally are normal unless overt or occult bleeding is a prominent feature. Approximately 10% of children with PUD have an iron-deficiency anemia. Hemoglobin, hematocrit, serum iron, and ferritin levels may be low, whereas the reticulocyte count and total iron-binding capacity may be elevated with chronic blood loss. Red blood cell smears may show hypochromic and microcytic morphology, and stool smears may be positive for occult blood.

Gastric acid analysis shows higher maximal and peak acid outputs after pentagastrin stimulation in PUD, although an overlap exists with normal values (Table 347.2). Fasting serum gastrin levels in children with ulcers may be within the normal range or elevated; however, the response of serum gastrin levels to a protein meal is higher than normal in children with primary PUD (Table 347.3). Measurements of gastric acid output and serum gastrin levels are not performed routinely unless the diagnosis of antral G-cell hyperplasia or Zollinger-Ellison syndrome is entertained. In the presence of antral gastritis and PUD, *H. pylori* may be detected by an *H. pylori*-specific IgG antibody serologic test or a ^{13}C-urea breath test. Increased serum pepsinogen, previously thought to be a genetic marker of familial PUD because of its occurrence in conjunction with the familial clustering of *H. pylori*, represents a nonspecific response to ulcer formation and is not predictive of a genetic predisposition to PUD.

An upper gastrointestinal series radiograph may be the most readily available test for establishing the diagnosis of PUD in children. Roentgenographic signs of PUD in the duodenum are characterized by a filling defect or a deformity of the duodenal bulb (Fig. 347.1). In some instances, duodenal irritability may be the only finding because the barium moves too rapidly out of the bulb or a fibrin clot covers the ulcer. Ulcer craters also may be found in the pyloric region, leading to outlet obstruction. The diagnosis of PUD should not be made unless a persistent crater is demonstrated. Deformity of the duodenal bulb with formation of scar tissue suggests the presence of a previous ulcer and does not imply the presence of currently active disease.

Primary gastric ulcers usually are located on the lesser curvature of the stomach. The crater is sharply delimited and surrounded by edematous, radiating gastric folds that may obstruct the pyloric channel. In contrast, secondary ulcer craters are shallow and often multiple and may be present in both the stomach and duodenum.

Overall, upper gastrointestinal series radiographs detect PUD in 70% of the children who are studied. The frequency of detection for duodenal ulcer is 89%, compared with 50% for gastric ulcers. Air contrast imaging may enhance the features of PUD and lead to establishment of a more accurate diagnosis. However, these studies are more difficult to perform in children younger than 6 years of age.

Other roentgenographic studies may be necessary to document the presence of complications of PUD. Abdominal films in the upright or lateral decubitus position may demonstrate free air in the abdomen if perforation has occurred. Celiac axis

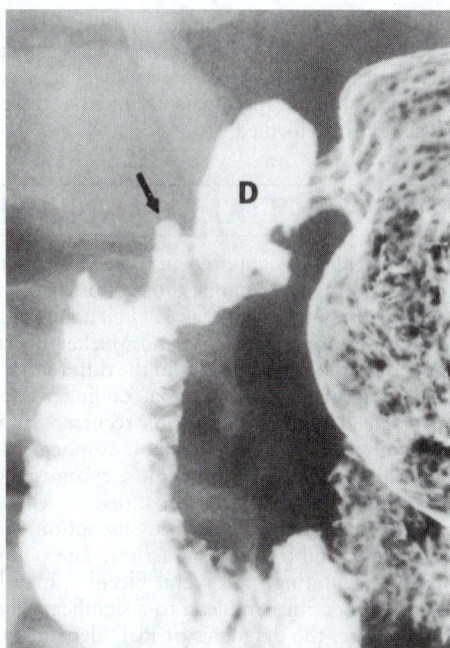

FIGURE 347.1. Peptic ulcer disease. Note the postapical ulcer crate (*arrow*). There are edematous folds radiating from its base and marked spasm of the postapical portion of the duodenum. D, duodenal bulb. (Used with permission from Swischuk LE. *Emergency imaging of the acutely ill or injured child,* 4th ed. Philadelphia: Lippincott Williams & Wilkins, 2000:218.)

angiography may be helpful to identify the source of persistent upper gastrointestinal bleeding caused by PUD if upper endoscopy is unavailable.

COMPLICATIONS

Hospitalization for PUD usually is unnecessary unless the complications of intractable pain, obstruction, active bleeding, or perforation are present. If signs of gastric outlet obstruction are found, food should be withheld and nasogastric suction applied. Surgical intervention should be considered if the obstruction does not resolve within 72 hours of nasogastric drainage. If upper gastrointestinal bleeding is present, a large-bore nasogastric tube should be inserted and the stomach lavaged repeatedly with normal saline. Vital signs and hematocrit values should be monitored carefully to determine whether blood transfusions are necessary. During severe hemorrhage, upper endoscopy may be necessary to identify the site of bleeding. Intravenous octreotide or endoscopic cautery may control active bleeding. Surgical intervention should be considered when the requirement for blood transfusion approaches one-third to one-half of total blood volume.

ENDOSCOPY

Fiber-optic endoscopy is the diagnostic procedure of choice for the detection of PUD in children. Gastroesophagoduodenoscopy is indicated to determine the source of upper gastrointestinal bleeding and to make the initial diagnosis of PUD, particularly when roentgenographic findings are absent in symptomatic patients. Endoscopy confirms the diagnosis of PUD in 97% of the patients examined for this purpose. A nodular appearance of the gastric antrum may be evident in 50% of children with infection with *H. pylori*. Confirmation of the presence of *H. pylori* requires cultures, measurement of urease activity (CLO [*Campylobacter*-like organisms] test, Delta West, Australia), or Warthin-Starry silver stains of antral or duodenal biopsy tissue specimens obtained at the time that upper endoscopy is performed.

DIFFERENTIAL DIAGNOSIS

The diagnosis of PUD in children may be difficult to make because the symptoms often mimic those of other diseases. Errors in diagnosis may be as high as 12%. The most common incorrect diagnoses are appendicitis and Meckel diverticulum. The principal conditions to consider in the differential diagnosis are nonspecific functional dyspepsia, Zollinger-Ellison syndrome, antral G-cell hyperplasia, chronic recurrent (functional) abdominal pain, gastroesophageal reflux, esophagitis, pancreatitis, eosinophilic gastritis or duodenitis, cytomegalic gastritis (Menetrier disease), graft-versus-host disease, cholecystitis, appendicitis, Meckel diverticulum, intussusception, inflammatory bowel disease, and infectious diarrhea. The symptoms of abdominal pain, vomiting, and rectal bleeding may be common to all of these entities and lead to a significant diagnostic dilemma. Therefore, the diagnosis of PUD depends primarily on the physician's clinical acumen and should be considered early in the differential diagnosis of abdominal pain.

Nonspecific functional dyspepsia may present with the classic manifestations of PUD or with atypical features characterized by poorly localized, periodic abdominal pain and tenderness, abdominal discomfort, nausea, vomiting, belching, bloating, flatus, early satiety, and anorexia. When symptoms occur in the absence of demonstrable disease, the term *nonspecific functional dyspepsia* is used. This condition is indistinguishable clinically from PUD, and the diagnosis must be made by exclusion after upper endoscopy and biopsies are performed.

Zollinger-Ellison syndrome, a rare diagnosis in children, is characterized by hypersecretion of gastric acid, intractable ulcer disease, and intestinal malabsorption caused by a gastrin-secreting tumor (gastrinoma) of the pancreas. Fasting serum gastrin levels usually are increased and may assist in the differential diagnosis. In some instances, secretin stimulation studies and computed tomography (CT) scanning of the abdomen are necessary to differentiate between PUD and this entity. Antral G-cell hyperplasia, or pseudo–Zollinger-Ellison syndrome, is characterized by hyperchlorhydria, peptic ulceration, and an exaggerated postprandial gastrin response. Other conditions associated with acid hypersecretion include systemic mastocytosis, short bowel syndrome, hyperparathyroidism, and cystic fibrosis.

Chronic recurrent abdominal pain occurs in approximately 10% of school-aged children and may be difficult to distinguish from PUD. The precipitating factors associated with chronic recurrent abdominal pain often are vague or have a psychosocial overlay in an otherwise well child. The diagnosis of functional abdominal pain usually is determined by excluding other organic illnesses using appropriate diagnostic studies, including endoscopy, if necessary.

Gastroesophageal reflux, esophagitis, pancreatitis, eosinophilic gastritis or duodenitis, cytomegalovirus gastritis (Menetrier disease), graft-versus-host disease, cholecystitis, Crohn disease, and appendicitis may be confused with primary PUD because these illnesses have similar clinical features, including epigastric or periumbilical abdominal pain, nausea, and vomiting. Similarly, Meckel diverticulum, intussusception, ulcerative colitis, and infectious diarrhea may manifest with rectal bleeding and can mimic the pattern of secondary peptic ulcers. Multiple diagnostic studies, including serum amylase and lipase determinations, liver function studies, stool cultures for pathogenic bacteria and smears for parasites, ultrasonography, roentgenographic studies, radionuclide imaging, and upper or lower endoscopy, may need to be performed to delineate the cause of the illness and eliminate the possibility of PUD.

THERAPY

The goal of medical therapy is to relieve ulcer pain, promote healing, and prevent complications. The control of gastric acid production by drugs and diet and the avoidance of factors that stimulate acid secretion are essential (Box 347.2). The eradication of *H. pylori* from infected patients is imperative to prevent ulcer recurrence.

The mainstay of medical management for PUD includes proton pump inhibitors and histamine-2 (H_2)-receptor antagonists. Proton pump inhibitors inhibit the hydrogen ion pump in the parietal cell, thereby blocking the final common pathway for acid formation. They demonstrate consistent gastric pH control and are not associated with the development of tachyphylaxis with repeated dosing. These drugs are indicated for the treatment of recalcitrant ulcers unresponsive to H_2-blocker therapy, healing and prevention of ulcers caused by nonsteroidal antiinflammatory drugs, hypersecretory states such as Zollinger-Ellison syndrome, and *H. pylori* antritis and duodenal ulcer disease. Dosages required for symptomatic relief and healing of ulcers may be greater than those for adults because of differences in the pharmacokinetics of proton pump inhibitors in children. Proton pump inhibitors generally are well tolerated. Reported side effects may include headache, nausea, abdominal pain, and diarrhea. Elevated gastrin levels and an increased number of antral G cells may occur, but the clinical significance of these findings is unclear.

H_2-receptor antagonists are potent inhibitors of basal and food-stimulated acid production. Their use is associated with a healing rate of 90% in children with PUD. H_2-receptor therapy also is effective in the prophylaxis of gastrointestinal bleeding after critical illness, brain injury, or surgery. Side effects associated with this drug are uncommon occurrences; rebound hypersecretion of hydrochloric acid may occur after discontinuation of the medication. Therapy with H_2-receptor antagonists beyond 1 year is not recommended, although serious long-term side effects have not been documented.

BOX 347.2 | **Treatment of Peptic Ulcer Disease in Children**

Medical
Hospitalization
Nasogastric suction and lavage
Blood transfusion
Medications (proton pump inhibitors, histamine-2-receptor antagonists, cytoprotective drugs, anticholinergics, antibiotics)
Diet (selected food avoidance)
Abstinence (cigarette smoking, alcohol, selected drugs)

Surgical
Truncal or selective vagotomy
Pyloroplasty
Antrectomy

Other medications such as antacids, anticholinergic drugs, and sucralfate may be added to the therapeutic regimen. Antacids promote the healing of ulcers and provide relief of symptoms by neutralizing gastric acid. The side effects of antacid therapy, either diarrhea or constipation, can be ameliorated by adjusting the proportion of magnesium and aluminum in the dosing regimen. Calcium antacids and sodium bicarbonate are unsuitable for chronic use because of the potential for increased acid secretion after buffering capacity ceases or systemic alkaline and sodium loading, respectively. Anticholinergics such as propantheline bromide decrease acid secretion, but the effective dose often produces side effects such as blurred vision and dry mouth. Sucralfate binds to the erosive surface of the ulcer and protects the mucosa from further damage. This drug is indicated for the short-term management of ulcer disease because of its ability to provide pain relief. However, it has the potential to alter the bioavailability of other drugs and must be administered separately from other drugs. Other cytoprotective drugs (e.g., misoprostol) have not been studied adequately in children to warrant their use. Medications such as octreotide may be helpful in reducing active bleeding from ulcers.

The most commonly used treatment regimen for *H. pylori*-associated PUD in children is triple-drug therapy. The multidrug regimens that are effective in adults have not been tested with the same rigor in children. The treatment regimen currently recommended includes a proton pump inhibitor in combination with two antibiotics, one being clarithromycin and the other being either amoxicillin or metronidazole, all given in therapeutic doses for 2 weeks. Combination therapy results in the successful eradication of *H. pylori* in more than 80% of compliant patients. Although proton pump inhibitors have anti-*H. pylori* activity *in vitro*, they are not effective in eradicating the organism *in vivo* when used alone as monotherapy.

Dietary intervention in conjunction with medical management promotes healing of ulcers. Milk feedings raise the gastric pH and prevent gastrointestinal bleeding in children. The factors responsible for the reduction of gastric acidity are unknown, although several peptides and hormones found in bovine and human milk have been implicated. Food may ameliorate symptoms, although acidic foods or beverages such as soft drinks, juices, pickles, tomatoes, and spices exacerbate gastric ulcer pain. Alcoholic beverages, cigarette smoking, aspirin, and other drugs that damage the gastric mucosal barrier are contraindicated.

The surgical management of PUD is reserved for patients with complications of ulcers, including intractable pain, perforation, hemorrhage, and obstruction. Truncal or selective vagotomy with pyloroplasty and antrectomy is the procedure performed in children with PUD. However, with highly effective acid-suppression medications and the aggressive treatment of *H. pylori* ulcer disease, these operations have become virtually obsolete in children.

PROGNOSIS

Prognostic reports of primary PUD in children and adolescents may be invalid because of recent information about the role of *H. pylori* in ulcer disease. Previous reports stated that ulcer disease recurred within 1 year in 35% to 50% of all patients, and at least two-thirds had repeated relapses over the course of years. More recent reports indicate that the annual ulcer relapse rate in children is 5% after successful eradication of *H. pylori* infection. With current advances in our understanding about the role of *H. pylori* infection in ulcer disease, the prognosis of PUD in children will be altered radically in the future.

The prognosis of secondary stress ulcers is affected by the precipitating illness or injury. The outcome in the neonate with gastric hemorrhage and perforation is poor. Healing generally occurs in infants and children who develop an acute ulcer, although emergency surgery may be necessary for hemorrhage or perforation. Recurrences of stress ulcers are unlikely with resolution of the underlying illness.

Acknowledgments

This work is a publication of the USDA/ARS Children's Nutrition Research Center, Department of Pediatrics, Baylor College of Medicine, and Texas Children's Hospital, Houston, Texas. This project has been funded in part with federal funds from the U.S. Department of Agriculture, Agricultural Research Service, under Cooperative Agreement number 58-7-MN1-6-100. The contents of this publication do not necessarily reflect the views or policies of the U.S. Department of Agriculture, nor does mention of trade names, commercial products, or organizations imply endorsement by the U.S. government.

Suggested Readings

Andersson T, Hassall E, Lundborg P, et al. Pharmacokinetics of orally administered omeprazole in children. *Am J Clin Gastroenterol* 2000;95:3101.

Go MF. Review article: natural history and epidemiology of *Helicobacter pylori* infection. *Aliment Pharmacol Ther* 2002;16:3.

Gold BD. Current therapy for *Helicobacter pylori* infection in children and adolescents. *Can J Gastroenterol* 1999;13:571.

Hassall E. Guidelines for approaching suspected peptic ulcer disease or *Helicobacter pylori* infection: where we are in pediatrics, and how we got there. *J Pediatr Gastroenterol Nutr* 2001;32:405.

Hyams JS, Davis P, Sylvester FA, et al. Dyspepsia in children and adolescents: a prospective study. *J Pediatr Gastroenterol Nutr* 2000;30:413.

Kuusela A-L, Maki M, Tuuska T, et al. Stress-induced gastric findings in critically ill newborn infants: frequency and risk factors. *Intensive Care Med* 2000;26:1501.

Lacy BE, Rosemore J. *Helicobacter pylori*: ulcers and more: the beginning of an era. *J Nutr* 2001;131:2789S.

Malaty HM. *Helicobacter pylori* infection and eradication in paediatric patients. *Paediatr Drugs* 2000;2:357.

Matysiak-Budnik T, Heyman M. Food allergy and *Helicobacter pylori*. *J Pediatr Gastroenterol Nutr* 2002;34:5.

Roma E, Kafritsa Y, Panayiotou J, et al. Is peptic ulcer a common cause of upper gastrointestinal symptoms? *Eur J Pediatr* 2001;160:497.

Sherman P, Czinn S, Drumm B, et al. *Helicobacter pylori* infection in children and adolescents: working group report of the first world congress of pediatric gastroenterology, hepatology, and nutrition. *J Pediatr Gastroenterol Nutr* 2002;35:S128.

Sherman P, Hassall E, Hunt RH, et al. Canadian *Helicobacter* study group consensus conference on the approach to *Helicobacter pylori* infection in children and adolescents. *Can J Gastroenterol* 1999;13:553.

Stringer MD, Veysi VT, Puntis JW, et al. Gastroduodenal ulcers in the *Helicobacter pylori* era. *Acta Paediatr* 2000;89:1181.

Uc A, Chong SF. Treatment of *Helicobacter pylori* gastritis improves dyspeptic symptoms in children. *J Pediatr Gastroenterol Nutr* 2002;34:281.

CHAPTER 348 ■ INTUSSUSCEPTION

MARY L. BRANDT

Intussusception is the most common cause of intestinal obstruction in infants aged 3 months to 3 years. Intussusception rarely occurs in the first month of life and has a peak occurrence in infants between the ages of 5 and 9 months. The incidence of intussusception has considerable regional variation, from less than 0.5 to 4 per 1,000 live births. The highest incidences worldwide are found in northern New York, southern Quebec, and China.

PATHOPHYSIOLOGY

Intussusception is the result of invagination or telescoping of a portion of the bowel into the more distal bowel (Fig. 348.1). The portion of the bowel that invaginates into the more distal bowel, the intussusceptum, is pulled along with its mesentery by peristaltic waves. As the proximal bowel is pulled into the lumen of the intussuscipiens, or distal bowel, the mesentery is compressed and angled, resulting initially in lymphatic obstruction and subsequently in venous obstruction. The intussuscepted mass quickly obstructs the intestinal lumen, resulting in distention and peristaltic rushes proximal to the obstructing mass. With each peristaltic rush, the patient experiences colicky pain. As the edema from lymphatic obstruction and venous engorgement increases, the hydrostatic pressure within the intussusception increases until it equals the arterial pressure, at which time arterial inflow ceases. The intestinal mucosa becomes ischemic, with an outpouring of mucus into the intestinal lumen. Venous engorgement results in leakage of blood into the intestinal lumen, and the blood and mucus form the classic "currant jelly" stools. Although currant jelly stools are

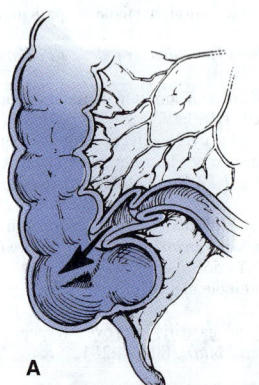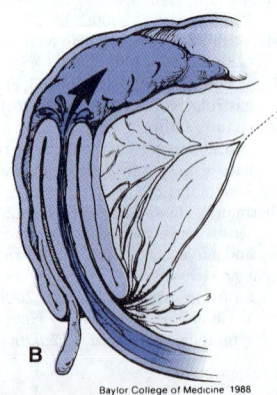

Baylor College of Medicine 1988

FIGURE 348.1. The development of an ileocolic intussusception. **A:** The invagination typically begins several centimeters proximal to the ileocecal valve. As the ileum is drawn into the more distal bowel, the lumen is obstructed and the mesenteric vessels become compressed. **B:** Edema and venous engorgement develop, with accumulation of blood and mucus ("currant jelly") in the lumen of the colon. If not reduced, infarction of the intussusceptum occurs.

relatively diagnostic, they occur in only a small percentage of patients and are a fairly late sign of intussusception.

ETIOLOGY

Most infants who develop intussusception are healthy and well nourished. Approximately 10% of patients have a previous history of diarrhea, and many have signs and symptoms of respiratory tract infections. Approximately 65% of intussusceptions occur before the patient's first birthday, and in almost all of these patients, no clear cause of the intussusception can be identified. Enlarged lymphoid tissue in the wall of the terminal ileum (Peyer patches) is a common finding in children with intussusception and probably acts as the lead point for the intussusception. An inexperienced surgeon may confuse this tissue with tumor and request a biopsy or resect the bowel unnecessarily. The association of intussusception with viral syndromes and the presence of this enlarged lymphoid tissue support a viral cause for the majority of the "idiopathic" intussusceptions. Adenovirus and rotavirus, in particular, have been implicated in the pathophysiology of intussusception.

Approximately 2% to 3% of older children with intussusception have a lesion such as polyps, Meckel diverticulum, ectopic pancreas, small enterogenous cysts, lymphomas, and benign tumors of the ileal wall that serves as a lead point. Localized edema or hemorrhage of the bowel wall such as that seen in patients with Henoch-Schönlein purpura, abdominal trauma, hemophilia, and leukemia also may act as a lead point. Altered intestinal motility or uncoordinated peristalsis (such as that seen after head injuries, use of anticholinergic medication, or enteritis associated with acquired immunodeficiency syndrome) also has been associated with the development of intussusception. Postoperative intussusception occurs most often after retroperitoneal dissections, particularly for tumors, and after fundoplication, presumably as a result of vagal manipulation. Nearly all intussusceptions associated with altered motility are located in the small bowel. Patients with cystic fibrosis may develop intussusception as a result of mucus-laden hypertrophied mucosal glands, which act as lead points, and as a result of the thick, tenacious fecal material associated with enzymatic insufficiency (Box 348.1). The average age for patients with cystic fibrosis who develop an intussusception is 9 years. Chronic indwelling tubes may be associated with intussusception; edema of the bowel wall caused by the tube serves as the intussuscepting point.

CLINICAL PRESENTATION

Nearly all affected infants present with vomiting and colicky pain. Because these two symptoms are nonspecific and common, infants typically are seen later in the course of illness, at which time they are more likely to have bloody stools and high fever. The classic triad of colicky abdominal pain, vomiting, and bloody stools occurs in as few as 10% of children diagnosed with an intussusception. Early in the course of illness, because of the acute distention of the small bowel, the affected infant evacuates the distal colon and passes several partially formed stools. In fact, this finding is so universal that the presence of a large amount of stool in the rectum by examination or radiography renders the presence of an intussusception mass less likely. The same reflex is responsible for the vomiting. Initially, the vomitus is clear, but as the intestinal obstruction progresses, the vomitus becomes bile-stained and eventually fecaloid. The peristaltic rushes and colicky pain first occur at intervals of several minutes and last only a few seconds. During the intervals between peristaltic rushes, the infant appears to be in no discomfort, and the abdomen is soft and scaphoid. Children with intussusception may develop a profound lethargy, mimicking a true coma. In fact, in some children this condition may be the presenting symptom.

At the time of presentation, a mass usually is palpable. Because 95% of the cases of intussusception are ileocolic, with the invaginating bowel beginning just proximal to the ileocecal valve, the sausage-shaped mass can be found in the distribution of the colon, commonly in the area of the hepatic flexure but occasionally more distally. At times, the intussusception mass is located medial to the lateral edge of the rectus abdominis muscle and below the edge of the liver, rendering palpation difficult. In 3% of the cases, the intussuscepting intestine prolapses through the rectum. The right lower quadrant may feel empty to palpation, a finding known as *Dance sign*.

If complete intestinal obstruction ensues, the child may develop abdominal distention, fluid loss from vomiting and sequestration of intraluminal fluid, and continuous abdominal pain. If further delay in establishing the diagnosis and initiating treatment occurs, infarction of the intussusceptum occurs. In most cases, infarction of the intussusceptum is associated with generalized peritonitis; if untreated, the patient dies within 2 to 5 days.

DIFFERENTIAL DIAGNOSIS

Intussusception should be included in the differential diagnosis of any condition characterized by abdominal pain, blood in the stool, or an intraabdominal mass. Intussusception often is confused with gastroenteritis. Although intermittent colicky abdominal pain is typical of both, the pain associated with intussusception is more consistently episodic. Early in the illness, the infant with intussusception appears well between paroxysms of pain. Intussusception, particularly cecal-colic intussusception, occasionally results in partial, rather than complete, intestinal obstruction and presents with liquid, blood-streaked,

loose stools similar to those seen with infectious enterocolitis. The bloody mucoid or currant jelly stools seen in patients with intussusception also may be seen in other processes that result in bowel ischemia, such as volvulus and incarcerated internal hernia.

DIAGNOSIS

The diagnosis of intussusception is made from a clinical history of intermittent, colicky pain lasting only a few seconds and extending over the course of several hours, after which the patient becomes lethargic, vomits, and shows signs and symptoms of intestinal obstruction. On physical examination, a palpable sausage-shaped mass in the distribution of the colon, typically in the area of the transverse colon, confirms the diagnosis. If bloody stools are noted in association with a sausage-shaped mass and intermittent colicky pain, the diagnosis is virtually assured.

Plain radiography of the abdomen may be diagnostic of the small bowel obstruction, but it also may show more specific findings of an intussusception. Signs that are suggestive of an intussusception include reduced gas in the jejunum, lateralization of the ileum, inability to see the cecum, absence of stool in the rectum, and ability to visualize the intussusceptum as it is outlined by air in the lumen. A true lateral abdominal radiograph may be helpful in seeing the intussusceptum. Ultrasound may be useful in establishing the diagnosis of intussusception and is used in many institutions instead of a contrast enema, particularly as a screening study. In some institutions, ultrasound is used not only to diagnose the intussusception, but also to document reduction with an air or water contrast enema. Ultrasound often is the most useful test in diagnosing a postoperative small bowel intussusception, which is difficult to diagnose by contrast study. Because it also is therapeutic in many cases, the contrast enema remains the standard method of establishing the diagnosis in most institutions.

Any infant or young child with signs and symptoms typical of an intussusception should undergo a contrast enema. Other patients with less classic presentations can be screened with diagnostic ultrasound before undergoing a contrast enema.

TREATMENT

The treatment of suspected intussusception begins with a diagnostic, and often therapeutic, contrast enema. Before proceeding with the enema, the child must be resuscitated adequately and plans should be made for surgery, should the reduction attempt be unsuccessful or result in a perforation. A large intravenous catheter should be placed for intravenous administration of isotonic fluids and, if necessary, blood products, and appropriate boluses (10 to 20 mL/kg) should be given until the child's volume status is normalized. Blood samples should be sent for serum electrolytes and hemoglobin and hematocrit. If the patient's hemoglobin is low, blood should be typed and cross-matched. Gastric aspiration through a nasogastric tube prevents further vomiting and enteric accumulation of fluid. Before performing the enema reduction, some surgeons give a single dose of an appropriate antibiotic as prophylaxis for any possible perforation of compromised bowel. Antibiotics to cover enteric bacteria are mandatory for patients before surgery.

Only after resuscitation has been initiated should the patient be taken to the radiology suite for a diagnostic contrast enema examination with fluoroscopy. Once the diagnosis is confirmed by contrast enema, a decision must be made regarding whether to attempt hydrostatic reduction (Fig. 348.2). Although the reduction is less likely to be successful in very young children,

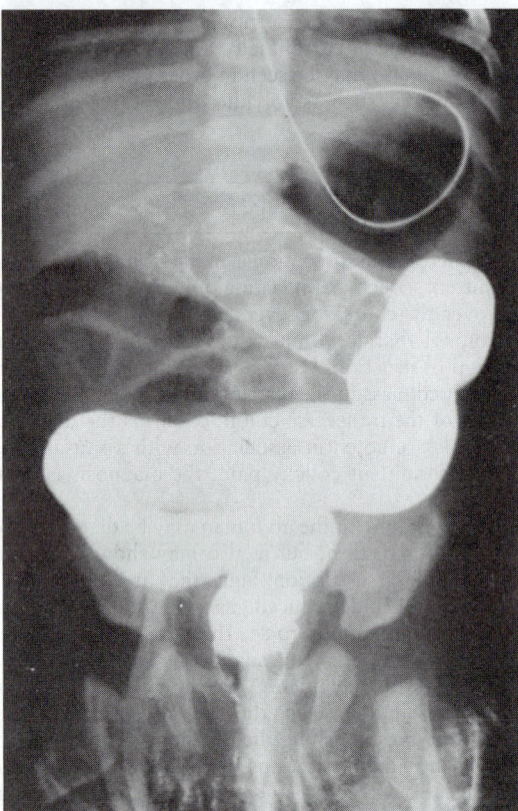

FIGURE 348.2. Barium enema study showing the coiled-spring pattern of barium around the intussusceptum in the transverse colon.

Principles of Contrast Enema Reduction of Intussusception

1. Arrange for immediate laparotomy if reduction is not successful by obtaining a surgical consult prior to attempting reduction.
2. Initiate resuscitation with intravenous fluids and nasogastric suction.
3. Insert ungreased Foley catheter in rectum, distend balloon, and pull down against levators. Tape catheter in place and hold buttocks tightly together. Wrap legs.
4. Let contrast run from a height of 3 feet, 6 inches above the table while intermittently fluoroscoping the patient.
5. Abandon procedure if contrast column is stationary and its outline is unchanged for 10 minutes.
6. Reduction is marked by free flow of contrast well into the ileum, expulsion of feces and flatus with the contrast, disappearance of the mass on physical examination, and clinical improvement of the child.
7. Failure to reduce the intussusception requires prompt operative intervention.

Adapted from Ravitch MM. Intussusception. In: Welch KJ, Randolph JG, Ravitch MM, et al., eds. *Pediatric surgery.* Chicago: Year Book, 1987:868.

children with a prolonged history, or children with a complete bowel obstruction, the only absolute contraindications to hydrostatic reduction are free intraperitoneal air, signs of peritonitis on physical examination, or systemic signs of compromised intestine. The current treatment protocol and guidelines for the contrast enema are described in Box 348.2. A Foley catheter is placed in the rectum, and the buttocks are held or taped together to prevent leakage. At present, contrast materials for reduction include air, water, water-soluble contrast, and barium. If the risk of perforation is high, air, water, or water-soluble contrast is a better choice than is barium. Three efforts at reduction are attempted, under fluoroscopic guidance, by raising the bag of barium 3 feet above the patient. If water-soluble contrast is used, the column of contrast can be raised to 5 feet instead of 3 feet. If air is used, the air is insufflated to a pressure not to exceed 100 to 120 mm Hg. These protocols can be used as guidelines, but some patients may benefit from more aggressive maneuvers in an attempt to avoid laparotomy. If perforation occurs, complications can be minimized if the patient has received antibiotics, a safe contrast medium such as air is being used, and no delay occurs in taking the patient to the operating room. Although most radiologists use fluoroscopy to monitor the reduction attempt, ultrasound also can be used to determine if the intussusception is reduced.

Hydrostatic and pneumatic reduction is successful in 30% to 80% of the patients with intussusception. To be sure that complete reduction has occurred, contrast or air must be seen in the terminal ileum. If the intussusceptum is reduced but the terminal ileum is not visualized, a second attempt at reduction several hours later may be successful. A second attempt is more likely to be successful if good movement of the intussusceptum occurred with the first attempt and if some relief of the patient's symptoms was achieved. Patients with free air or peritoneal signs and patients in whom reduction clearly is

unsuccessful should be taken directly to the operating room for operative reduction. Because the intussusceptum causes vascular compromise, these incidents are true surgical emergencies. Successful operative reduction can be accomplished in most patients; however, nearly 25% of infants requiring surgery require resection because reduction is impossible or the intestine is nonviable. The compromised bowel may be excised and a primary anastomosis performed. In rare cases, when the patient is unstable or the contamination is extreme, the surgeon may choose to create an ileostomy instead. A temperature spike after radiologic or surgical reduction of an intussusception is an extremely common occurrence. It most likely is mediated by endotoxin as blood culture results are almost universally negative in these patients. The recurrence rate after both hydrostatic reduction and surgical reduction is close to 5%; recurrences usually occur in the first 24 hours after a successful reduction has been achieved.

Suggested Readings

Bhisitkul DM, Listernick R, Shkolnik A, et al. Clinical application of ultrasonography in the diagnosis of intussusception. *J Pediatr* 1996;121:182

Connolly B, Alton D, Ein S, Daneman A. Partially reduced intussusception: when are repeated delayed reduction attempts appropriate? *Pediatr Radiol* 1995;25:104.

Conway E. Central nervous system findings and intussusception: how are they related? *Pediatr Emerg Care* 1993;9:15.

Daneman A, Alton D, Win S, et al. Perforation during attempted intussusception reduction in children—a comparison of perforation with barium and air. *Pediatr Radiol* 1995;25:81.

Den Hollander D, Burge D. Exclusion criteria and outcome in pressure reduction of intussusception. *Arch Dis Child* 1993;68:79.

Guo J, Ma X, Zhou Q. Results of air pressure enema reduction of intussusception: 6396 cases in 13 years. *J Pediatr Surg* 1986;21:1201.

Kirks D. Diagnosis and treatment of pediatric intussusception: how far should we push our radiologic techniques? *Radiology* 1994;191:622.

Luks F, Yazbeck S, Brandt M, Desjardins J. Transient fever associated with a reduction of intestinal invagination. *Chir Pediatr* 1990;31:157.

Meradji M, Hussain S, Robben S, Hop W. Plain film diagnosis in intussusception. *Br J Radiol* 1994;67:147.

Meyer J, Dangman B, Buonomo C, Berlin J. Air and liquid contrast agents in the management of intussusception: a controlled, randomized trial. *Pediatr Radiol* 1993;188:507.

Paler S, Ein S, Stringer D, Alton D. Intussusception: barium or air? *J Pediatr Surg* 1991;26:271.

Peh W, Khong P, Chan K, et al. Sonographically guided hydrostatic reduction of childhood intussusception using Hartmann's solution. *AJR Am J Roentgenol* 1996;167:1237.

Shanbhogue R, Hussain S, Meradji M, et al. Ultrasonography is accurate enough for the diagnosis of intussusception. *J Pediatr Surg* 1994;29:324.

Stringer M, Pablot S, Brereton R. Paediatric intussusception. *Br J Surg* 1992;79:867.

CHAPTER 349 ■ MOTILITY DISORDERS

ELLEN L. BLANK

Movement of nutrients through the gut results from coordinated contractions of the intestinal smooth muscles. Gastrointestinal motility is regulated by myogenic, neural, and neuroendocrine input during fasting and digestion. Development of uncoordinated human gastric contractions occurs as early as 26 weeks' gestation, although gastric emptying is slow and feeding intolerance occurs commonly. Increasing strength and coordination of gastric and small intestinal muscle contractions develop at approximately 30 weeks' gestation, allowing for enteral feedings by tube. By 36 weeks' gestation, motility patterns similar to those of term infants and the appearance of coordinated sucking and swallowing allow preterm infants to feed orally.

Motility disorders may arise from abnormalities of any of the regulatory inputs anywhere in the digestive tract. Recurrent signs and symptoms of intestinal dysfunction without any demonstrable obstructing lesion present a diagnostic dilemma. Common complaints include dysphagia, anorexia, heartburn, nausea, vomiting, chest pain, abdominal bloating, abdominal pain, diarrhea, and constipation. These symptoms may occur acutely as a reversible ileus with infection. Postsurgical syndromes such as ileus, duodenogastric (bile) reflux, and rapid gastric emptying seen in dumping syndrome and postvagotomy also are regarded commonly as disorders of gastrointestinal motility.

Chronic intestinal pseudoobstruction is a heterogeneous group of disorders presenting with signs and symptoms of mechanical bowel obstruction without any demonstrable obstruction. Primary pseudoobstruction occurs more commonly in children and may occur sporadically or as part of a familial syndrome. Approximately 20% of cases are familial. Neural or myopathic abnormalities may be responsible. Dysfunction also may occur in other organs containing smooth muscle, such as the urinary bladder, gallbladder, and eyes. The onset of symptoms may occur in infancy or in a previously healthy child.

Secondary pseudoobstruction has a similar presentation but can be explained by another disease process or drug effect. Diseases affecting gastrointestinal smooth muscle include scleroderma, dermatomyositis, systemic lupus erythematosus, amyloidosis, myotonic and muscular dystrophy, and ceroidosis. Hormonal disorders impairing gastrointestinal function include hypothyroidism, multiple endocrine neoplasia type IIB, hypoparathyroidism, and pheochromocytoma. Neurologic abnormalities causing neural gastrointestinal dysfunction include diabetic autonomic gastropathy, Hirschsprung disease, and familial dysautonomia. Miscellaneous disorders that can impair gastrointestinal motility include severe inflammatory bowel disease, small bowel transplantation, Chagas disease, and radiation enteritis. Drugs such as opiates, phenothiazines, tricyclic antidepressants, anticholinergic agents, clonidine, and calcium channel blockers also may impair gut motor function.

Barium radiographic studies are helpful in locating areas of intestinal dilatation (Fig. 349.1). Contrast or ultrasound

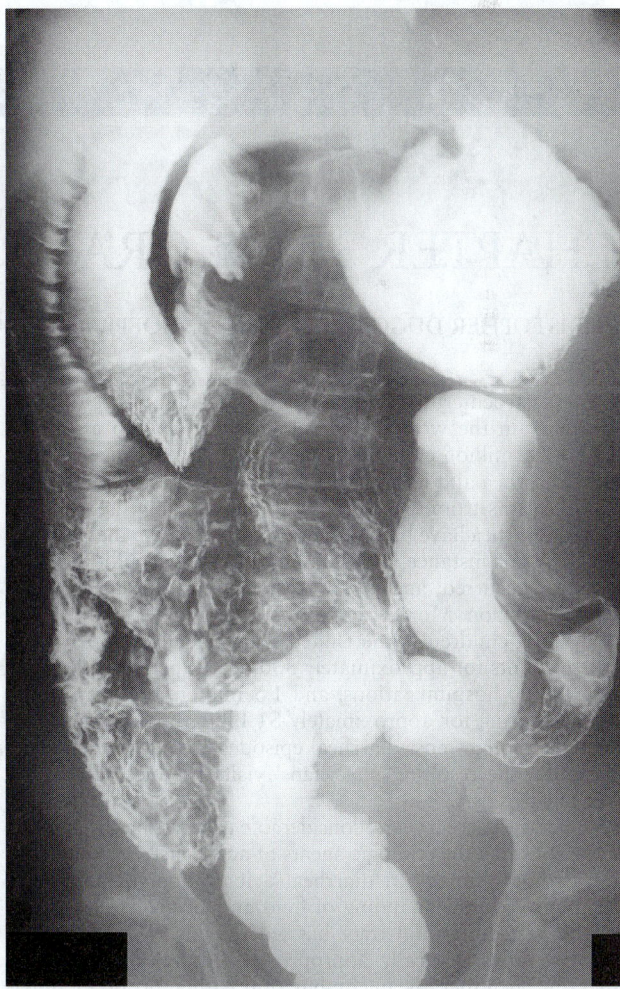

FIGURE 349.1. Barium contrast study of a child with pseudoobstruction syndrome. Delayed gastric emptying, dilated air- and fluid-filled loops of small bowel, and a dilated rectum, all suggestive of obstruction, are seen without any identifiable anatomic obstruction. Courtesy of Children's Hospital of Wisconsin, Milwaukee, WI.

studies of the gallbladder and urinary bladder demonstrate any associated anomalies. If full-thickness intestinal biopsy specimens are available, enteric nervous system abnormalities may be identified using the Smith method of silver staining, and smooth muscle abnormalities can be seen with hematoxylin-eosin or Masson trichrome stains.

Manometric studies have shown abnormalities in the esophagus and small intestine of patients with chronic intestinal pseudoobstruction. Esophageal motility studies have demonstrated decreased resting lower esophageal sphincter pressure, failure of lower esophageal sphincter relaxation normally seen with swallowing, and disordered muscle contractile patterns through the esophagus. Antroduodenal motility studies have demonstrated at least three types of abnormalities: absent migrating myoelectric complexes, usually found during fasting; abnormal postprandial motility; and lower than normal amplitude of intestinal smooth muscle contractions.

Most children with untreated pseudoobstruction syndromes have failure to thrive. Vigorous nutritional support has decreased the morbidity and mortality rates of affected children. When dysphagia or unpalatability of nutrient supplements occurs, bolus intragastric feedings may be useful. For children who have delayed gastric emptying, continuous intragastric feedings may be required. Long-term tube feedings usually are easier to administer, are more comfortable for the child, and allow decompression of gastric distension by a percutaneous or surgically placed gastrostomy. Patients with gastroparesis may benefit more by having continuous jejunal feedings. Total parenteral nutrition also may be necessary to achieve optimal growth. Prokinetic agents, such as bethanechol, metoclopramide, erythromycin, and domperidone, largely have been unsuccessful in improving gastrointestinal motility in pseudoobstruction syndromes. Cisapride has had limited success in relieving gastrointestinal complaints. Antibiotics are helpful in treating bacterial overgrowth. Cathartics may be helpful in treating constipation. Conservative management of obstructive symptoms should be used as much as possible to avoid repeated laparotomies.

Suggested Readings

Berseth C. Gastrointestinal motility in the neonate. *Clin Perinatol* 1996;23:179.

Milla PJ. Intestinal motility during ontogeny and intestinal pseudo-obstruction in children. *Pediatr Clin North Am* 1996;43:511.

Navarro J, Sonsino E, Boige N, et al. Visceral neuropathies responsible for pseudo intestinal pseudo-obstruction syndrome in pediatric practice: analysis of 26 cases. *J Pediatr Gastroenterol Nutr* 1990;11:179.

CHAPTER 350 ■ ORAL REHYDRATION THERAPY

CHRISTOPHER DUGGAN, JULIUS G. K. GOEPP, AND MATHURAM SANTOSHAM

Acute gastroenteritis continues to be a leading cause of child mortality in the world. In developing nations, an estimated 1.5 to 2.5 million children younger than 5 years die annually from diarrhea and its complications. Although the total number of deaths from diarrhea is still unacceptably high, deaths due to diarrhea have been reduced dramatically in the past two decades. For instance, in 1982, an estimated 5 million deaths per year occurred, and in 1992, the estimated annual deaths fell to 3 million. More recent estimates are lower still.

Among children in the United States, acute gastroenteritis still accounts for approximately 300 deaths per year, 160,000 to 200,000 hospitalizations, and 1.5 million physician visits, all accounting for approximately $1 billion in direct medical costs. Although most diarrheal episodes among U.S. children are mild, the resulting physicians' visits produce substantial health care costs.

Over the past 30 years, considerable progress has been made in establishing the etiologic agents of acute gastroenteritis and the pathophysiology of diarrheal dehydration. In particular, an improved understanding of fluid and electrolyte transport in the gastrointestinal tract has led directly to the development of physiologically appropriate solutions for oral fluid therapy. Such therapy, in combination with appropriate nutritional management of the child with gastroenteritis, has come to be known as *oral rehydration therapy* (ORT).

Early attempts at treating dehydration resulting from diarrhea were described in the medical literature in the 1830s during epidemics of *Vibrio cholerae* infections. These attempts at parenteral fluid therapy were largely unsuccessful because of inadequate aseptic technique and poor equipment and because the physiologic effects of diarrhea and volume depletion in humans were poorly understood. Even those patients who improved with this therapy worsened when therapy was discontinued, and more than 75% still died. By 1926, awareness of treating acidosis in dehydration led Powers to administer solutions of glucose, saline, and bicarbonate, along with blood; fasting also was recommended. He reported a reduction in the mortality rate among hospitalized patients to 33%. During the ensuing 2 decades, the use of saline solutions with dextrose, accompanied by enforced fasting, was ineffective at further reducing the hospital mortality rate below 30%. In 1946, Darrow and Harrison, following careful balance studies of salt and water losses, added potassium to rehydration fluids and reported a mortality rate as low as 6%, still in fasting children.

Oral electrolyte solutions were pioneered in the 1940s by Harrison. The first commercially available solution (Lytren, Mead, Johnson Co.) was developed in the 1950s. Simultaneous reports of hypernatremic dehydration and increased rates of mortality led to a widespread distrust of ORT among pediatricians in the United States. In fact, the epidemic of hypernatremia was attributable to the inappropriate management of diarrhea and to the packaging of Lytren itself, not to intrinsic ORT problems: (a) Boiled skimmed milk was recommended frequently for use in diarrhea, and its high osmolality contributed to high serum sodium values; (b) Lytren was sold in bulk to be mixed at home, and parents often mixed the solution improperly; and (c) Lytren contained 8% glucose, which made it excessively osmotic (see following discussion of the osmolarity of oral rehydration solutions). A valuable lesson learned from the 1950s experience is that ORT use must be appropriately taught to caregivers and that proper feeding practices should be followed during diarrhea, not that ORT itself is a dangerous treatment.

In the 1950s and 1960s, laboratory models of fluid and electrolyte transport in mammalian intestines, combined with improved measurements of stool electrolyte losses in cholera, led to the development of the first oral solutions truly tailored to the needs of patients with gastroenteritis, specifically cholera. Subsequently, numerous studies have documented the effectiveness of ORT among children and adults with dehydration from gastroenteritis caused by a variety of infectious agents.

The critical role of nutrition during diarrhea episodes has only been relatively recently appreciated. Although Park in 1924 and Chung in 1948 were among the first to challenge the notion that feedings should be withheld during diarrhea, their views were not accepted until studies in the 1980s demonstrated improved outcomes with continued feeding during diarrhea episodes.

Management of gastroenteritis and dehydration has moved to the forefront of pediatric medicine over several decades. Practice guidelines emphasizing ORT as a cornerstone of therapy were released by the Centers for Disease Control and Prevention (CDC) in 1992 and 2003. The American Academy of Pediatrics (AAP) Practice Parameter for the Management of Acute Gastroenteritis in Young Children identifies ORT as the preferred treatment of children with mild to moderate dehydration caused by diarrhea. Paradoxically, ORT is used least in the industrialized countries where much of the original basic scientific research was done. Like any therapy, ORT relies on appropriate teaching and implementation for its ultimate effectiveness. In the balance of this chapter, we describe the pathophysiology of gastroenteritis, the mechanisms of action of ORT, and practical aspects of ORT delivery, particularly in an industrialized world setting.

PATHOPHYSIOLOGY AND ETIOLOGY OF ACUTE DEHYDRATING GASTROENTERITIS

Although the terms dehydration and rehydration strictly refer to loss and replacement of water alone, they are used commonly to reflect overall fluid and electrolyte status. More accurately, a patient with diarrhea usually has sustained volume depletion, reflecting losses not only of water but of sodium and other electrolytes as well. Initial losses of sodium during gastroenteritis are from the extracellular fluid compartment (ECF). With progressive loss of circulating volume and total body potassium depletion, sodium is also shifted from the ECF into the intracellular fluid compartment. Thus, regardless of the measured serum sodium or potassium concentration, total body sodium and potassium content is invariably diminished during dehydration from gastroenteritis.

Pathophysiologic Considerations

Intestinal Absorption

A grasp of basic intestinal physiology is vital to understanding the concepts underlying fluid therapy of the volume-depleted patient. Here, we consider absorption of various substances from the bowel and their physiologic roles in homeostasis.

Fluids and electrolytes are secreted at a tremendous rate in the healthy bowel (approximately 9 L daily in adults). Therefore, powerful mechanisms for reabsorption must be present; otherwise, rapid volume depletion would ensue. The normal flow of fluid into and out of the bowel lumen creates a circulatory pattern: Secretions from salivary glands, the pancreas, and the gallbladder are added to the intrinsic bowel secretions to digest nutrients, and the vast bulk of fluid, as well as sodium and other electrolytes, is rapidly reabsorbed by mechanisms residing in the epithelial cells of the small and large bowel. This complex system is modulated by the interactions of hormonal and intracellular mediators common to most tissues: the adenosine and guanosine nucleotide messenger systems, intracellular calcium, and metabolites of arachidonic acid (leukotrienes and prostaglandins).

The immediate driving force for active water absorption in the bowel is the movement of sodium. Uptake of sodium occurs by means of a two-step process, the first involving active pumping of the ion out of intestinal epithelial cells at the basolateral membrane, followed by sodium entry down the resulting gradient from the bowel lumen into the cell (Fig. 350.1). Sodium entry also occurs passively by several ion-coupled mechanisms: sodium–hydrogen exchange and coupled sodium chloride absorption. Sodium cotransport with small organic molecules such as glucose and amino acids also occurs. Although various mechanisms and ratios of sodium to organic substrate have been proposed, the clinical relevance resides in the fact that uptake of sodium and therefore water is dramatically increased when organic substrate is present with sodium at a molecular ratio of approximately 1:1 in the intact intestine. This observation is exploited in the design of oral rehydration solutions (ORSs).

Modulation of sodium uptake and water absorption occurs in part by the effects of aldosterone on sodium channels in enterocyte membranes. Elevated aldosterone levels result in increased sodium absorption. Antidiuretic hormone and glucocorticoids also affect water and salt uptake from bowel. Catecholamines have profound acute stimulatory effects on sodium absorption.

Absorption of other electrolytes is also important, but these substances play a smaller direct role in the movement of fluid, except as modulators of sodium uptake. Luminal potassium rapidly equilibrates with serum levels; even a severely potassium-depleted patient may continue to lose potassium in the stool. Additionally, elevated aldosterone in dehydration

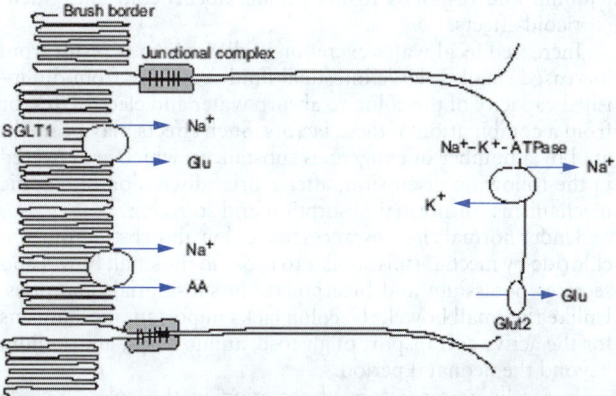

FIGURE 350.1. Solute-coupled sodium transport into the intestinal epithelial cell. SGLT1, sodium glucose cotransport protein 1; GLUT2, glucose transport protein 2. (From King CK, Glass RI, Bresee JS, Duggan C. Managing acute gastroenteritis among children: oral rehydration, maintenance and nutritional therapy. *MMWR Morb Mortal Wkly Rep* 2003;52:1.)

contributes to urinary potassium losses. Bicarbonate is secreted in substantial quantities by the pancreas and must be reabsorbed to maintain systemic pH. Luminal bicarbonate stimulates absorption of sodium as well.

Features of Intestinal Secretion

As with water and electrolyte absorption, secretory processes in the mammalian intestine occur by various mechanisms that are responsive to a host of intrinsic and extrinsic modulators. Rates of secretion between the small and large intestine vary greatly; therefore, we discuss each portion of the bowel individually and then describe the action of various substances on secretion in the intestine as a whole.

In the healthy gastrointestinal tract, net fluid absorption exceeds secretion, whereas in dehydrating diarrheal illness, net intestinal losses exceed absorption. Such net loss may result from increased secretion in the proximal gut or from diminished absorption distally, or both. Each of the substances considered here may act on one or more of the secretory or absorptive processes to affect this balance. Their mechanisms of action are briefly discussed here.

Secretion in the Small Intestine. Most absorptive processes in the small intestine occur in cells at the villous tip, whereas secretion takes place chiefly in crypt cells. The secretion of chloride ion is a major determinant of fluid movement into the gut lumen. Chloride secretion occurs by energy-requiring, pump-mediated entry at the basal cell membrane, with subsequent conductive, channel-mediated exit at the apical membrane.

Control and modulation of chloride secretion in the small bowel depend on the interrelationship of several intracellular messenger systems, which appear to be fundamental signaling processes in most enterocytes. Known mediators of chloride secretion include free calcium ion (Ca^{2+}), cyclic adenosine monophosphate (cAMP), cyclic guanosine monophosphate (cGMP), and intracellular pH. Various endocrine and paracrine substances exert their ultimate effects on intestinal secretion by affecting one or more of these messenger systems.

Regulation of Absorption and Secretion in the Colon. The mammalian colon shares certain features of fluid and electrolyte transport with the small intestine but differs in a number of significant aspects. The rate and volume of electrolyte and water absorption are segmentally heterogeneous in the colon and may depend on volume, composition, and rate of flow of the luminal contents. Colonic sodium recovery occurs across a gradient three to four times greater than that found in the jejunum and responds to both mineralocorticoid and glucocorticoid effects.

Increased fecal water excretion in diarrhea may result from increased small or large intestinal fluid secretion, from diminished capacity of the colon to absorb water and electrolytes, or from a combination of these factors. Such effects may be mediated by a number of exogenous substances, which are covered in the following discussion, after a brief discussion of colonic mechanisms for normal absorption and secretion.

Under normal circumstances, the colon absorbs sodium and chloride by mechanisms similar to those in the small bowel and secretes potassium and bicarbonate in substantial quantities. Unlike the small bowel, the colon lacks important mechanisms for the active cotransport of glucose, amino acids, and sodium beyond the neonatal period.

Intracellular mediators of secretion in the colon include those discussed previously for the small intestine: calcium, cAMP, and cGMP. cAMP appears to increase colonic secretion of chloride and potassium, probably by increasing apical membrane conductances. Additionally, cAMP reduces net sodium chloride absorption. The effects of increased intracellular cal-

cium are similar to those in the small intestine, and evidence exists that increased cAMP may result in elevation of intracellular concentrations of Ca^{2+}. cGMP may also play a role in colonic electrolyte modulation, but its effects are less well understood than those of calcium or cAMP.

As in the small bowel, the metabolites of arachidonic acid, prostaglandin (PG) E and leukotrienes, play a role in the regulation of colonic fluid and electrolyte movement. These arachidonic acid metabolites serve as intermediaries that increase cAMP levels and exert a direct effect by some as yet unspecified intracellular mechanism independent of adenylate cyclase.

Etiologic Agents of Diarrhea: Mechanisms of Action

A variety of intrinsic and extrinsic agents pathologically stimulate secretion in the small or large intestine. These substances may be conveniently divided into three categories: (a) a single group of intrinsic biochemical signals (hormones, neurotransmitters, and mediators of inflammation), (b) extrinsic biologic pathogens (bacteria, viruses, and enterotoxins), and (c) extrinsic chemical secretagogues (laxatives). Each of the clinically important members of these categories appears to have its ultimate effect on one of the final common intracellular mediators discussed previously—calcium, cAMP, or cGMP.

The effects of enterotoxins on secretory processes are most prominent in the small bowel. Many of these agents act by raising intracellular levels of cAMP; they are all heat-labile multiunit toxins that bind and activate cellular adenylate cyclase. The ultimate effect of these intracellular changes is that secretion in crypt cells is switched on, whereas absorption in villous cells is switched off. Toxins that act by this mechanism include the heat-labile *V. cholerae* and *Escherichia coli* toxins, as well as those produced by certain strains of *Salmonella*, *Campylobacter*, and possibly *Shigella*.

A second group of toxins appears to function by stimulation of the guanylate cyclase pathway. This group comprises the heat-stable toxins of *E. coli*, *Yersinia enterocolitica*, and *Klebsiella pneumoniae*. Evidence suggests that the effect of the toxins is mediated in part by calcium and PGE, which in turn stimulate cGMP production.

Effects of enterotoxin on fluid and electrolyte transport in the colon are less well understood and may be less important clinically in water loss from diarrhea. Nonetheless, reduced sodium chloride absorption in cholera has been suggested. In addition to the enterotoxin effects, bacterial pathogens stimulate a host inflammatory response, resulting in release of mediators such as PGE and leukotrienes. These act directly as stimulators of secretion and indirectly as modulators of intracellular second messengers.

Viral agents such as rotavirus appear to exert their pathologic effects by inducing sloughing of intestinal villous (i.e., absorptive) cells in excess of crypt (i.e., secretory) cells. Because the damage to villous cells is patchy and absorption in the surviving cells is intact, oral fluid replacement in such cases is usually still effective.

ORAL REHYDRATION SOLUTIONS

ORT is based on glucose–sodium cotransport in the intestinal epithelial cell.

Water passively follows the osmotic gradient generated by the transcellular transport of electrolytes and nutrients. While three principle mechanisms of sodium absorption have been described, the mechanism essential to the efficacy of ORSs was shown to result from the coupled transport of sodium and glucose molecules at the intestinal brush border (Fig. 350.1). Cotransport across the luminal membrane is facilitated by the protein SGLT1 (sodium glucose cotransporter 1). Once in the enterocyte, the transport of glucose into the blood is facilitated by GLUT2 (glucose transporter type 2) in the basolateral membrane. The Na^+-K^+-ATPase provides the gradient that drives the process. Clinical studies have demonstrated that this mechanism remains intact even in patients with severe diarrhea.

Composition of Standard Oral Rehydration Solutions

In 1975, the World Health Organization (WHO) and the United Nations Children's Fund (UNICEF) agreed to promote a single ORS (WHO-ORS) containing (in mmol/L) sodium 90, potassium 20, chloride 80, citrate 30, and glucose 111 (2%) for use among diverse populations in different countries. This composition was selected to allow for a single solution to be used for treatment of diarrhea caused by a variety of infectious agents and associated with varying degrees of electrolyte loss. WHO-ORS has been proven for over 30 years to be safe and effective at rehydration and maintenance for children and adults with all types of infectious diarrhea.

A review of the separate components of ORS is helpful in understanding the rationale behind a new and possibly improved version of ORS. The inclusion of sodium and glucose are of course necessary for the cotransport mechanism noted previously, which drives water into the cell. Promotion of sodium cotransport can occur over a range of glucose concentrations (from 10 to 25 g/L, or 56 to 140 mmol/L). However, when glucose concentrations exceed 30 g/L (3%), as is the case with most fruit juices and sodas, osmotic forces may counteract the cotransport phenomenon and draw water back into the gastrointestinal lumen.

The sodium component of ORSs has engendered much research and debate. Since early experience with ORSs originated in areas of the world where cholera was an important cause of diarrhea, early oral solutions contained 100 to 120 mEq/L of sodium to mimic the electrolyte losses of an actively purging cholera patient. Since sodium losses in noncholera diarrhea are lower, the utility of these original solutions for viral and other gastrointestinal infections was questioned by some. Controlled clinical trials later confirmed that solutions with 90 or 75 mEq/L (or even lower amounts) of sodium worked well as a rehydration solution for noncholera diarrhea, as long as adequate replacement fluid was given. However, the unique programmatic advantage of being able to prescribe a single solution for all causes of diarrhea (cholera and noncholera) led the WHO and other policy-making bodies to argue for the deployment and use of a solution with a single composition. Recently, a solution with a sodium concentration of 75 mEq/L has been recommended for global use (see below).

Potassium is needed since stool losses of this electrolyte can be compounded by urinary losses in the setting of increased aldosterone levels, and hypokalemia is a well-recognized complication of diarrhea. With severe hypokalemia, a paralytic ileus can ensue and reduced intestinal fluid absorption can follow. Most ORSs contain 20 mmol/L of potassium, which is an amount that can only begin to replace potassium losses of the child with diarrhea. Additional sources of potassium from diet are needed.

The importance of additional alkali to rehydration solutions was noted in the early twentieth century when mortality rates due to diarrhea fell with the addition of base. Trisodium citrate provides three bicarbonate ions per molecule, is stabler than sodium bicarbonate, and is currently the source of base in many ORSs. Bicarbonate also stimulates intestinal sodium absorption independently of other organic substrates.

Newer Oral Rehydration Solutions

Since the 1975 WHO UNICEF solution was agreed upon, many efforts have been made to improve upon its rehydration capabilities. Studies in the 1980s and 1990s emphasized the use of additional or alternative cotransport molecules such as amino acids and starches. To date, the amino acid preparations do not appear more effective than traditional ORSs and are more costly. Rice-based ORSs may be recommended where training is adequate and home preparation is preferable, and it appears particularly effective in treating diarrhea from cholera. Nevertheless, given the simplicity and safety of ORS packets in developing countries and of commercially available ORSs in developed countries, these remain the first choice for most clinicians.

Other potential additives to ORSs include substances capable of liberating short-chain fatty acids such as amylase-resistant starch derived from corn and partially hydrolyzed guar gum. The presumed mechanism of action is the enlistment of increased colonic sodium uptake coupled to short-chain fatty acid transport. Other possible future ORS composition changes include the addition of probiotics, prebiotics, or zinc. The addition of zinc to the therapeutic armamentarium might be especially notable given the extensive literature that has developed concerning the importance of zinc supplementation in preventing or reducing the severity of diarrheal diseases in areas of the world with poor zinc dietary intake.

More recent clinical trials have documented that a reduced osmolarity ORS is better designed for the management of children with acute noncholera diarrhea. Specifically, use of a reduced osmolarity ORS was associated with less vomiting, less stool output, and a reduced need for unscheduled intravenous infusions when compared with standard ORSs in these patients. In cholera infection, a trial in adults showed no clinical difference between subjects treated with the lower osmolarity solution and those treated with the standard solution, apart from some increased incidence of asymptomatic hyponatremia. On the basis of those findings, UNICEF and WHO now recommend a reduced osmolarity solution for global use. In May 2002, WHO announced a new ORS formulation consistent with these recommendations, with 75 mEq/L sodium, 75 mmol/L glucose, and a total osmolarity of 245 mosm/L. The newer hypotonic WHO ORS is also recommended for use in treating adults and children with cholera, although postmarketing surveillance is under way to confirm the safety of this indication.

The composition of several commonly available oral rehydration solutions is quite distinct from other beverages frequently used inappropriately for rehydration (Table 350.1).

Limitations of Oral Rehydration Therapy

Although ORT provides simple, safe, and effective therapy for the majority of children with dehydration, certain limitations exist. As indicated in the preceding section, ORSs are limited in the quantities of solute they can contain without becoming physiologically hyperosmolar and exacerbating fluid losses. Glucose-based ORSs (G-ORSs), therefore, provide good rehydration but have no effect by themselves on stool output or duration of illness. Solutions that contain complex carbohydrate molecules (see following discussion) may overcome this barrier and may provide sufficient substrate to reverse fluid losses and decrease diarrhea.

TABLE 350.1

COMPOSITION OF COMMERCIAL ORAL REHYDRATION SOLUTIONS AND COMMONLY CONSUMED BEVERAGES (WHICH ARE NOT APPROPRIATE FOR DIARRHEA TREATMENT)

Solution	CHO (gm/L)	Na (mmol/L)	K (mmol/L)	Cl (mmol/L)	Base* (mmol/L)	Osmolarity (mosm/L)
Oral rehydration solutions						
WHO-ORS (2002)	13.5	75	20	65	30	245
WHO-ORS (1975)	20	90	20	80	30	311
ESPGHAN ORS	16	60	20	60	30	240
Enfalyte†	30	50	25	45	34	200
Pedialyte‡	25	45	20	35	30	250
Rehydralyte‡	25	75	20	65	30	305
Ceralyte§	40	50–90	20	40–80	30	220
Commonly used beverages						
Apple juice‖	120	0.4	44	45	—	730
Coca Cola¹	112	1.6	—	—	13.4	650
Gatorade²	46	23.5	2.5	17	3	330
Chicken broth‖	8	260	0.5	260	—	450
Tea‖	—	6	—	—	6	

*Actual or potential bicarbonate, such as lactate, citrate, or acetate.
†Mead-Johnson Laboratories, Princeton, NJ.
‡Ross Laboratories, Columbus, OH (data for flavored and freezer pop Pedialyte are identical).
§http://www.ceralyte.com/index.htm. Accessed December 8, 2003.
‖U.S. Department of Agriculture.
¹Coca-Cola Corporation, Atlanta, GA (figures do not include electrolytes, which may be present in local water used for bottling; base = phosphate).
²The Gatorade Company, Chicago, IL.
From King CK, Glass RI, Bresee JS, Duggan C. Managing acute gastroenteritis among children: oral rehydration, maintenance and nutritional therapy. *MMWR Morb Mortal Wkly Rep* 2003;52:1.

Another limitation concerns children presenting with shock and severe dehydration. Children with shock constitute a medical emergency and should be managed initially with intravenous or intraosseous solutions until their level of consciousness allows for the safe administration of oral solutions.

Children with very high rates of stool output (more than 10 mL/kg/hour) may be unable to maintain positive fluid balance orally. Although theoretically a concern, practical experience confirms that most children in fact do retain sufficient fluid for repletion to occur. Careful intake and output measurements should be kept, and parenteral fluids should be provided for the occasional child who is unable to be rehydrated with ORT.

A small proportion (approximately 1%) of children with acute gastroenteritis experience carbohydrate malabsorption, heralded by a dramatic increase in stool volume and reducing substances when ORS is given. In infants with carbohydrate malabsorption, if ORS is discontinued and parenteral fluids are provided, a dramatic reduction in stool output occurs.

Vomiting is often and inaccurately cited as a contraindication to ORT. Most children with vomiting can be rehydrated successfully if fluids are provided in small, frequent quantities. To prevent the thirsty child from rapidly consuming a large volume of fluid with subsequent vomiting related to gastric distention, we recommend that ORSs be given in small volumes using a 5-mL syringe or teaspoon. Persistent gentle encouragement of parents is critical in this setting; administration of large volumes of ORS may aggravate vomiting. As tissue acidosis is corrected, vomiting generally ceases, although an occasional child may benefit from an initial few hours of parenteral fluid therapy. The majority of children who present with vomiting can be adequately hydrated with ORS when it is properly administered.

Limitations of ORT use in the clinical setting are related predominantly to misperceptions by physicians and nurses that lead to management decisions that undermine the use of ORT. Some of these misperceptions include the notions that ORT is excessively time consuming, that it is labor intensive to staff, and that parents in the developed world are resistant to its use. We have found that each of these perceived barriers can be overcome. They are discussed more fully below.

DIETARY CONSIDERATIONS

Although Chung and Viscorova in 1948 reported good results among children who were fed during diarrhea, many pediatricians have historically recommended delayed feeding until improvement or cessation of the diarrhea. By contrast, the AAP and CDC guidelines for management of children with diarrhea and dehydration recommend early feeding of appropriate foods to children with diarrhea once rehydration has been achieved. The nutritional consequences of fasting are profound. Children in the developing world may experience two to ten episodes of diarrhea annually, each of 3 to 5 days' duration. Serious energy deprivation and ultimately growth retardation may ensue; these findings have been noted in industrialized countries as well. Fasting also has been demonstrated to inhibit enterocyte renewal, which, along with increased susceptibility to new infection, places the child at risk for prolonged or renewed diarrheal losses.

Enteral feeding, on the other hand, has been shown to increase cell renewal in the gut and to diminish intestinal permeability. In a careful balance study by Brown et al., the calories provided during feeding were shown to result in improved nutritional parameters among children with diarrhea. We have also demonstrated reductions in both duration and volume of diarrhea among inpatient Apache infants fed a soy-based, lactose-free formula compared with those receiving G-ORS only for the first 24 hours.

Role of Lactose-Containing Feedings

Although the use of feedings early in the course of diarrheal illness is now widely recommended, the role of lactose-containing formulas or nonhuman milks remains controversial. A large number of studies have tried to identify the best formula for children with acute gastroenteritis by comparing lactose-containing to lactose-reduced or lactose-free diets. A review of these studies identified the following issues. Studies suggesting that lactose-containing feedings resulted in worse outcomes generally included children whose illness was more severe at enrollment. A single study of known lactose malabsorbers found differences between lactose and nonlactose regimens, whereas studies that excluded such patients did not. The studies in which control patients were given truly lactose-free feedings tended to show differences between groups, whereas those providing reduced lactose feedings to controls were less likely to demonstrate differences. A formal meta-analysis of 29 randomized controlled trials of 2,215 patients concluded that virtually all children with acute diarrhea can be managed successfully with continued feeding of undiluted nonhuman, lactose-containing milk.

Breast-Feeding during Diarrhea

Human breast milk contains more lactose than does cow's milk or milk-based formulas, and breast-feeding has in the past been discouraged during diarrhea. At least one trial of continued breast-feeding during diarrhea in hospitalized children demonstrated reduced stool output among breast-fed children compared with those whose feedings were interrupted.

Although no completely satisfactory explanation has been articulated, a number of reasons have been proposed for the improved outcomes among breast-fed infants. Breast milk has lower osmolality and contains secretory antibodies, enzymes, and growth factors that may reduce the severity of infections. Also, continued feedings may be superior to intermittent feedings, and breast-feeding may more closely resemble continuous feedings. Mothers whose nursing patterns are interrupted may experience reduction or cessation of subsequent milk flow. Such mothers may then abandon breast-feeding entirely, to the nutritional detriment of the infant. For all of the previously mentioned reasons, breast-feeding should not be interrupted during diarrheal episodes.

DELIVERY OF ORAL REHYDRATION THERAPY

General Recommendations

Like any other form of treatment, ORT must be delivered in a controlled and reliable fashion to be effective. When delivered in this manner, failure rates (i.e., the need for intravenous fluid therapy) should be less than 5%, as found in a meta-analysis of ORT efficacy trials in developed nations. Because of its simplicity, many health care providers tend to offer ORSs to patients without properly instructing them in its use and without adequate monitoring of its effects. The results are often discouraging both for parents and providers. We have found that when the following recommendations are observed, therapy is most likely to be successful.

Clinical Assessment and Management

Patients presenting for therapy of acute gastroenteritis initially should be examined in light of their relevant history to rule out clinical conditions such as appendicitis, volvulus, intussusception, or other serious systemic illnesses. In patients with uncomplicated diarrhea, the physical examination should be directed at the assessment of dehydration. Table 350.2 shows the clinical classification of dehydration that we have used for many years. In children and infants with uncomplicated acute watery diarrhea, we discourage the routine use of laboratory diagnostic studies. Urine specific gravity, however, may provide a useful parameter for monitoring the progress of rehydration therapy.

The management of the dehydrated child is divided into two phases: rehydration and maintenance (Table 350.3). Replacement of ongoing fluid losses as well as maintenance fluids and diet should be provided throughout the treatment period.

TABLE 350.2

SIGNS OF DEHYDRATION

Sign	Minimal or no Dehydration	Mild to Moderate Dehydration	Severe Dehydration
Percent loss of body weight	<3%	3–9%	>9%
Mental status	Well, alert	Normal, fatigued or restless, irritable	Apathetic, lethargic, unconscious
Thirst	Drinks normally, may refuse	Thirsty, eager to drink	Drinks poorly, unable to drink
Heart rate	Normal	Normal to increased	Tachycardia, with bradycardia in most severe cases
Quality of pulses	Normal	Normal to decreased	Weak, thready, or impalpable
Breathing	Normal	Normal, fast	Deep
Eyes	Normal	Slightly sunken	Deeply sunken
Tears	Present	Decreased	Absent
Mouth and tongue	Moist	Dry	Parched
Skin fold	Instant recoil	<2 seconds	>2 seconds
Capillary refill	Normal	Prolonged	Prolonged, minimal
Extremities	Warm	Cool	Cold, mottled, cyanotic
Urine output	Normal to decreased	Decreased	Minimal

From King CK, Glass RI, Bresee JS, Duggan C. Managing acute gastroenteritis among children: oral rehydration, maintenance and nutritional therapy. *MMWR Morb Mortal Wkly Rep* 2003;52:1; and World Health Organization. *The treatment of diarrhoea: a manual for physicians and other senior health workers.* Geneva: WHO CDR, 1995:95.3.

TABLE 350.3

SUMMARY OF TREATMENT BASED ON DEGREE OF DEHYDRATION

Degree of Dehydration	Rehydration Therapy	Replacement of Losses	Nutrition
Minimal or no dehydration	N/A	<10 kg: 60–120 mL ORS for each diarrheal stool or vomiting episode >10 kg: 120–240 mL oral rehydration solutions for each diarrheal stool or vomiting episode	Continue breast-feeding. Resume age-appropriate normal diet after initial hydration, including adequate caloric intake for maintenance*
Mild to moderate dehydration	ORS, 50–100 mL/kg over 3–4 hours	Same as above	Same as above
Severe dehydration	LR or NS in 20 mL/kg IV boluses until perfusion and mental status improve. Then give 100 mL/kg ORS over 4 hours or 100 mL/kg D5 ½ NS IV over 8 hours	Same as above; if unable to drink, give via nasogastric tube or give IV D5 ¼ NS with 20 mEq/L KCl	Same as above

*Overly restricted diets should be avoided during acute diarrhea. Breast-fed infants should continue to nurse *ad libitum* even during acute rehydration. Infants too weak to eat may be given breast milk or formula via nasogastric tube. Lactose-containing formulas are generally well tolerated. If lactose malabsorption appears clinically significant, lactose-free formulas may be used. Complex carbohydrates, fresh fruits, lean meats, yogurt, and vegetables are all recommended. Carbonated drinks and/or commercial juices with a high concentration of simple carbohydrates should be avoided.
D5, 5% dextrose; KCl, potassium chloride; LR, lactated Ringer solution; NS, normal saline.
From King CK, Glass RI, Bresee JS, Duggan C. Managing acute gastroenteritis among children: oral rehydration, maintenance and nutritional therapy. *MMWR Morb Mortal Wkly Rep* 2003;52:1.

Rehydration Phase

In the rehydration phase, the total fluid deficit is intended to be replaced over a 4-hour period. This rapid restoration of circulating volume reverses systemic acidosis and improves tissue perfusion more efficiently than does the traditionally recommended repletion over 24 hours. Children with mild to moderate dehydration should be given 50 to 100 mL/kg of ORS over 4 hours. Patients with severe dehydration (frank or impending shock) should receive an initial bolus of normal saline or Ringer lactate by the intravenous or intraosseous routes at 40 mL/kg/hour, until signs of shock resolve. The degree of dehydration should then be recalculated, and the ORS should be continued as outlined previously. While parenteral access is being sought, nasogastric infusion of fluid using a small (5 to 7 Fr.) soft catheter may be initiated at a rate of 40 mL/kg/hour, as long as the patient's airway protective reflexes remain intact.

At the end of each hour of rehydration, ongoing losses (stool and emesis) should be calculated and replaced. This fluid should consist of ORS (or isotonic intravenous fluid in children receiving initial parenteral therapy). Alternatively, parents may be instructed to provide 10 mL/kg (i.e., approximately 4 oz for a 12-kg child) of ORS for each diarrheal stool.

As soon as rehydration is complete, clinical assessment should be repeated. If signs of dehydration persist, the rehydration phase should be repeated until fluid repletion has occurred. When rehydration is complete, the maintenance phase is begun (see Table 350.3).

Older Child. Toddlers and school-aged children may present a special challenge for ORT because they often refuse to drink physiologically appropriate solutions because of the salty taste. Fortunately, such children are at lower risk for severe dehydration compared to infants because of their smaller body surface area–to-volume ratio. Fruit-flavored ORS freezer pops have become commercially available (Pedialyte Freezer Pops, Ross Laboratories, Columbus, OH), which may be more palatable to older children. The child's usual diet should be continued; however, fluids that are high in simple sugars such as undiluted commercial fruit juices and colas should be avoided. Ongoing stool losses should be replaced with appropriate ORSs as is recommended for infants.

Vomiting Child. Infants and children with acute gastroenteritis often vomit. Vomiting is exacerbated by systemic acidosis, hypokalemia, and gastric distention. Most vomiting children can be rehydrated successfully orally, and vomiting generally resolves as systemic fluid repletion occurs. Parents should be instructed to provide ORS in small quantities (1 tsp or 5 mL) frequently (every minute) and to persevere in spite of the vomiting, which may continue in the initial phases. As gastric distention is minimized and acidosis is corrected, the frequency of vomiting generally is diminished and the rate of fluid administration can be increased. Children with truly intractable vomiting (as defined by an increasing or persisting negative fluid balance 4 hours after beginning therapy) should receive parenteral fluid therapy. Oral treatment usually can begin once vomiting ceases.

Antiemetic medications may have adverse effects and are usually unnecessary in acute diarrhea management. The use of phenothiazines, for example, may interfere with oral rehydration by causing sleepiness. Recent trials have shown that ondansetron, a serotonin antagonist, either by the oral or IV route, was effective in decreasing vomiting and limiting hospital admission, but cost-effective analyses should be done before this class of agents is routinely prescribed for diarrhea.

Maintenance Phase

The goals during the maintenance phase are twofold: to replace ongoing losses and to meet baseline metabolic fluid and nutritional needs.

Replacing Ongoing Losses. Ongoing stool losses should be replaced with ORS on a 1:1 basis. In hospitals and clinics, this can be accomplished using diaper weights. At home, 10 mL/kg or approximately 4 to 8 oz of ORS should be given for each watery stool (2 to 4 oz in infants weighing less than 10 kg). Parents should be instructed about the gastrocolic reflex that often results in a bowel movement immediately after a feeding and may result in poor compliance with ORT at home. Parents should be reassured that the fluid given by mouth is absorbed and is likely to exceed in quantity the amount lost in stool. Because of their high osmotic load and low sodium content, fluids such as full-strength juices, punches, and soft drinks should be actively discouraged during diarrhea.

Nutritional and Baseline Fluid Needs. Once the rehydration phase has been completed and vomiting has diminished, infants and children should be started back on regular feedings. In breast-fed infants, maintenance fluid and nutritional requirements should be met with breast milk on demand. Formula-fed infants should continue their usual formula immediately upon rehydration in amounts sufficient to satisfy energy and nutrient requirements. Lactose-free or lactose-reduced formulas usually are not necessary. A meta-analysis of clinical trials shows no advantage of lactose-free formulas over lactose-containing formulas for most infants, although some infants with malnutrition or severe dehydration recover more quickly when given lactose-free formula. Patients with true lactose intolerance will have exacerbation of diarrhea when a lactose-containing formula is introduced.

For toddlers and children, a regular diet also should be reinstated once the rehydration phase is completed. We have found that the standard BRAT (banana, rice, applesauce, toast) diet is unnecessarily restrictive and may provide inadequate dietary energy and fat for the recovering child. Foods high in complex carbohydrates and low in fats and simple sugars are usually well tolerated. Families then may make sensible choices from a wide variety of appropriate foods that are culturally acceptable (e.g., rice, bread, cereal, potatoes, vegetables, yogurt, lean meat, and fruit).

Perceived Obstacles to Implementation of Oral Rehydration Therapy

Barriers to the successful use of ORT in the industrialized world generally involve perceptions on the part of health care providers that are inaccurate or wholly mistaken. The following are examples of such misperceptions along with recommended responses:

- Myth: Parental involvement in the medical care of children is impractical. Parents often demand high-technology care of their children by the health care system. However, parents can be incorporated into the system so that they become active partners. Parents who have successfully provided ORSs to their child and watched the child improve in their own hands often prefer the use of ORT to intravenous therapy. A randomized trial of ORS versus IV rehydration for dehydrated children demonstrated shorter stays in emergency departments and improved parental satisfaction with oral rehydration.
- Myth: ORT takes too long. Parenteral fluid delivery usually is seen as a more rapid, direct, and assured means of fluid repletion, whereas time spent teaching parents to provide ORSs may be perceived as wasted. Several studies have favorably compared the timeliness of ORT with intravenous solutions. When 5 mL (1 tsp) of ORS is taken per minute, 300 mL (10 oz) is delivered hourly, representing a rate of fluid administration sufficient to meet the needs of most children during the rehydration phase without inducing gastric distention.
- Myth: ORT can only be used in mild dehydration. Providers are often concerned that moderately or severely ill children will not tolerate ORS or that electrolyte abnormalities or acidosis mandate intravenous therapy. In fact, standard ORSs contain more base and potassium than do standard intravenous solutions and are rapidly absorbed. As indicated previously, ORSs can be delivered

rapidly to the infant. Finally, a nasogastric tube may be used to deliver ORSs to a child who is unable to drink (provided airway protective reflexes remain intact). One study showed that rapid nasogastric rehydration was well tolerated, more cost effective, and associated with fewer complications than IV rehydration.

- Myth: ORT cannot be used if a child is vomiting. Although children with truly intractable vomiting require parenteral fluids for a time, most can be rehydrated enterally when small volumes are presented to the stomach. The use of a 5-mL syringe or medicine cup can facilitate fluid delivery. The volume of emesis usually is overestimated by parents and staff. Generally, when careful measurements are made, children are found to maintain a net positive fluid balance.

Real Obstacles to Implementation of Oral Rehydration Therapy

Certain genuine obstacles remain to the proper widespread use of ORT. One of these is cost: Although ORT is cheaper than is intravenous therapy, the cost of the former is often borne by the parent because many third-party insurers do not pay for ORT in hospitals or clinics. Currently, commercially available solutions cost from $3 to $7 per liter, a prohibitive expense for many families. Public assistance programs such as WIC provide solutions in only approximately one-half of the United States. One approach to the cost issue is to use packaged dry salts as is done by WHO. These packets (Oral Rehydration Salts, Jianis Bros., Kansas City, MO) provide salts for 1 L of ORS at less than $0.75 per packet. Generic brands of premixed ORS are also widely available. A safety and effectiveness study of homemade and reconstituted packet cereal-based ORSs found that errors in mixing occurred in 1% to 3% of cases, highlighting the risks of these methods over ready-to-use ORT. A cereal-based packet form of ORT is also available (Cera-lyte, Cera Products, LLC, 8265-I Patuxent Range Road, Jessup, MD). The AAP recommends the use of dry ORT packets when provided with an appropriately sized container for mixing to reduce the potential for misuse.

SUMMARY AND CONCLUSIONS

Acute gastroenteritis and dehydration continue to be a leading cause of infant mortality globally. Proper use of any therapy is critical to its success and depends on a thorough understanding of the pathophysiology of the disease process in question, the physiology of the therapeutic intervention itself, and the available systems for delivery of the treatment. In this chapter, we have endeavored to provide the clear physiologic basis for the use of ORT, as well as a practical framework to ensure its appropriate use and delivery. Although the last three decades have seen enormous progress in development and implementation of ORT programs, a large gap still remains between scientific knowledge of ORT and the practical use of this therapy. Only through the continued process of research, development, and education in this area will further progress be made. Technology and knowledge must be transferred not only from the research centers to the field, but also from providers to parents, incorporating parents into the health care team. We also must continue efforts to effect the transfer of experience and skills from the less-developed to the more-developed nations. Efforts to adapt ORT technology to the industrialized world represent the beginning of such an effort.

Suggested Readings

American Academy of Pediatrics PC, Subcommittee on Acute Gastroenteritis. Practice parameter: the management of acute gastroenteritis in young children. *Pediatrics* 1996;97:424.

Atherly-John Y, Cunningham S, Crain E. A randomized trial of oral vs intravenous rehydration in a pediatric emergency department. *Arch Pediatr Adolesc Med* 2002;156:1240.

Brown KH, Peerson JM, Fontaine O. Use of nonhuman milks in the dietary management of young children with acute diarrhea: a meta-analysis of clinical trials. *Pediatrics* 1994;93:17.

Darrow DC, Pratt EL, Flett JJ, et al. Disturbances of water and electrolytes in infantile diarrhea. *Pediatrics* 1949;3:129.

Duggan C, Nurko S. "Feeding the gut": the scientific basis for continued enteral nutrition during acute diarrhea. *J Pediatr* 1997;131:801.

Field M. Intestinal ion transport and the pathophysiology of diarrhea. *J Clin Invest* 2003;111:931.

Gore SM, Fontaine O, Pierce NF. Efficacy of rice-based oral rehydration. *Lancet* 1996;348:193.

Gore SM, Fontaine O, Pierce NF. Impact of rice-based oral rehydration solution on stool output and duration of diarrhoea: meta-analysis of 13 clinical trials. *BMJ* 1992;304:287.

Hirschhorn N. The treatment of acute diarrhea in children. An historical and physiological perspective. *Am J Clin Nutr* 1980;33:637.

Hirschhorn N, Greenough WB. Progress in oral rehydration therapy. *Sci Am* 1991; 264:50.

Kilgore PE, Holman RC, Clarke MJ, Glass RI. Trends of diarrheal disease-associated mortality in U.S. children, 1968 through 1991. *JAMA* 1995;274:1143.

King CK, Glass RI, Bresee JS, Duggan C. Managing acute gastroenteritis among children: oral rehydration, maintenance and nutritional therapy. *MMWR Morb Mortal Wkly Rep* 2003;52:1.

Kosek M, Bern C, Guerrant RL. The global burden of diarrhoeal disease, as estimated from studies published between 1992 and 2000. *Bull World Health Organ* 2003;81:197.

Nager, AL, Wang VJ. Comparison of nasogastric and intravenous methods of rehydration in pediatric patients with acute dehydration. *Pediatrics* 2002; 109:566.

Parashar U, Hummelman E, Bresee J, et al. Global illness and deaths caused by rotavirus disease in children. *Emerg Infect Dis* 2003;9:565.

Pizarro D, Posada G, Villavicencio N. Oral rehydration in hypernatremic and hyponatremic diarrheal dehydration: treatment with oral glucose/electrolyte solution. *Am J Dis Child* 1983;137:730.

Ramakrishna BS, Venkataraman S, Srinivasan P, et al. Amylase-resistant starch plus oral rehydration solution for cholera. *N Engl J Med* 2000;342:308.

Santosham M, Daum RS, Dillman L, et al. Oral rehydration therapy of infantile diarrhea: a controlled study of well-nourished children hospitalized in the United States and Panama. *N Engl J Med* 1982;306:1070.

Santosham M, Fayad I, Zikri MA, et al. A double-blind clinical trial comparing World Health Organization oral rehydration solution with reduced osmolarity solution containing equal amounts of sodium and glucose. *J Pediatr* 1996;128:45.

Santosham M, Keenan EM, Tulloch J, et al. Oral rehydration therapy for diarrhea: an example of reverse transfer of technology. *Pediatrics* 1997;100:E10.

CHAPTER 351 ■ ANORECTAL MALFORMATIONS

DAVID E. WESSON

Formation of the anus and rectum and separation from the urogenital tract occur primarily between the 4-mm (fourth week) and 16-mm (sixth week) stage of embryonic development but continue to the 56-mm stage. Major anorectal malformations occur in 1 per 1,500 live births. Imperforate anus does not follow a simple mendelian pattern of inheritance, although it has been reported in siblings and in members of one family over three generations.

and Rice, largely has been replaced by a lateral radiograph of the pelvis taken with a marker on the anal dimple and the infant in the prone position with the pelvis elevated off the bed. This study should be done more than 12 hours after birth to allow sufficient time for air to reach the rectum. If the end of the rectal air column is within 1 cm of the perineal skin, a fistula indicating a low lesion is likely to be present.

ETIOLOGY AND CLASSIFICATION

The Hedgehog family of cell signals plays a key role in the development of the anorectal region in all vertebrate and invertebrate species. Sonic Hedgehog, an endoderm-derived signaling molecule, induces mesodermal gene expression in the hindgut of the chick embryo. Defective Hedgehog signaling in mice leads to a constellation of anomalies strikingly similar to the VACTERL (described later) association seen in humans. Mutations in *Gli* genes, which participate in the transduction of Hedgehog signaling, cause Palliser-Hall syndrome in humans, a prominent feature of which is imperforate anus.

Table 351.1 lists types of anorectal malformations according to gender, the level of rectal descent, and the presence or absence of a fistula. The level of rectal descent may be determined by perineal inspection or with the aid of plain radiographs, perineal ultrasound, voiding cystourethrography (VCUG), computed tomographic scanning, and magnetic resonance imaging. The traditional invertography, as described by Wangensteen

TABLE 351.1

CLASSIFICATION OF ANORECTAL MALFORMATIONS

Female	Male
High	**High**
Rectal atresia and stenosis	Rectal atresia and stenosis
Cloaca	Rectovesical (bladder neck) fistula
Rectovaginal fistula (rare)	Rectourethral prostatic fistula
Rectovestibular fistula*	Rectourethral bulbar fistula
Imperforate anus with no fistula	Imperforate anus with no fistula
Low	**Low**
Anovestibular fistula*	Perineal fistula
Perineal fistula	Anal stenosis
Anal stenosis	

*Rectovestibular fistulas differ from anovestibular fistulas in that they have a long tract and share a long common wall with the vagina.

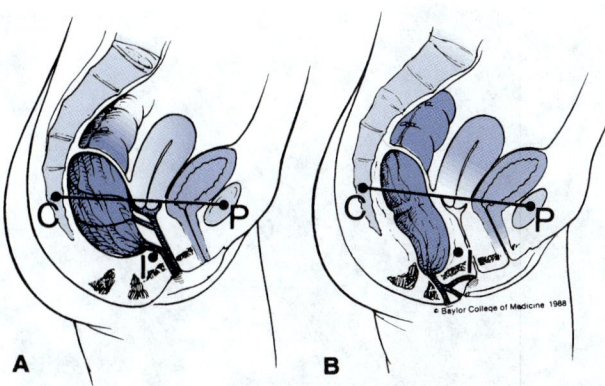

FIGURE 351.1. Anorectal anomalies in the female infant. **A:** High lesions usually have a cloaca, fistula to the vagina (rare), or a fistula to the vestibule. **B:** Low lesions also may have a fistula to the vestibule without a long shared wall with the vagina or a fistula to the fourchette or perineum.

Lesions close to the anus occur more commonly than do high lesions in girls; high lesions are seen more often in boys. Nearly 80% of the boys with a high lesion have a fistula to the urinary tract, and nearly all girls with a high lesion have a cloacal anomaly (Figs. 351.1 and 351.2).

DIAGNOSIS

The basic steps in management of neonates with anorectal malformations are as follows:

> Determine whether the level is high or low.
> Check for associated defects, especially cardiac and renal.
> Ensure free drainage of urine and stool.

A full assessment may require 24 to 48 hours because this length of time often is required for meconium to appear in the urine (high lesion) or perineum (low lesion). To defer any decision regarding primary repair or creation of a colostomy for at least 24 hours is wise. All patients require ultrasound screening for hydronephrosis and hydrocolpos before an operation is performed.

Several findings on physical examination suggest the level of an imperforate anus. A flat bottom with no crease or anal dimple and no evidence of an external sphincter predicts a high

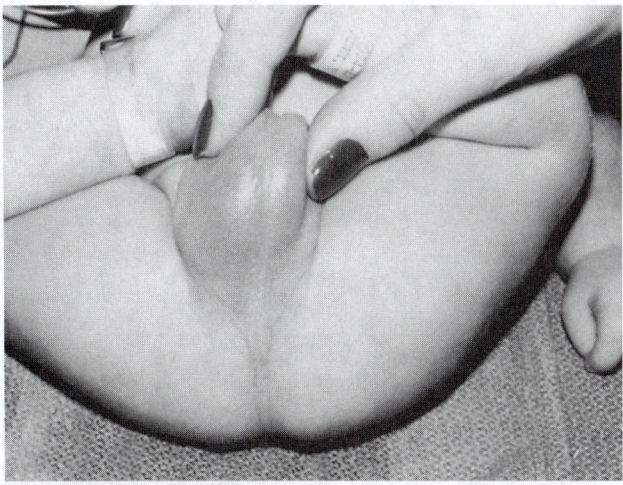

FIGURE 351.3. Perineum of a male infant with a high lesion and a rectourethral fistula. After 24 hours, there was no evidence of a fistula to the perineum or raphe. A colostomy was done on the second day of life, and reconstruction of the anus and rectum was performed when the child was 1 year old. Today, it would be done much earlier.

imperforate anus (Fig. 351.3). A prominent anal dimple not always is associated with a low anomaly. Nonetheless, a well-developed raphe, an anal dimple, and a bucket-handle deformity usually suggest a low lesion. Ninety percent of boys with a low lesion have a fistula to the perineum. Whitish inspissated mucus (perineal pearls) or meconium-stained material may be expressed from the fistula in the subcutaneous tract along the raphe of the perineum, scrotum, or even ventral surface of the penis (Fig. 351.4). Often the perineal fistula is not obvious at

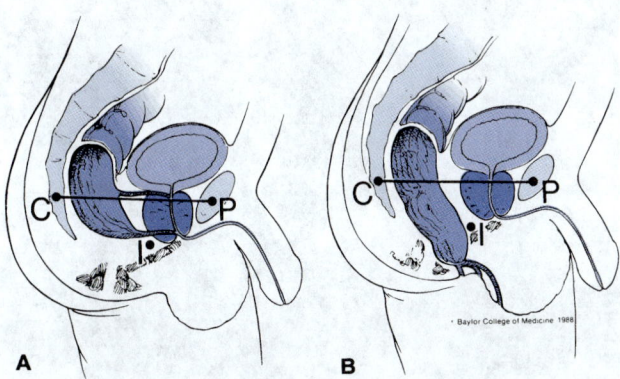

FIGURE 351.2. Anorectal anomalies in the male infant. **A:** Eighty percent of high lesions have fistulas to the bulbar or membranous urethra. **B:** Ninety percent of male infants with low lesions have a fistula to the perineum or median raphe.

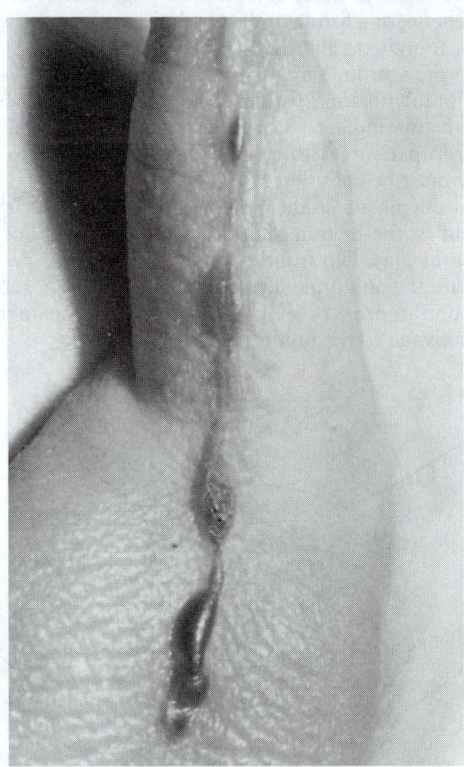

FIGURE 351.4. Male infant with a low lesion and a fistula to the median raphe. Note meconium along the median raphe. A perineal anoplasty was done shortly after birth.

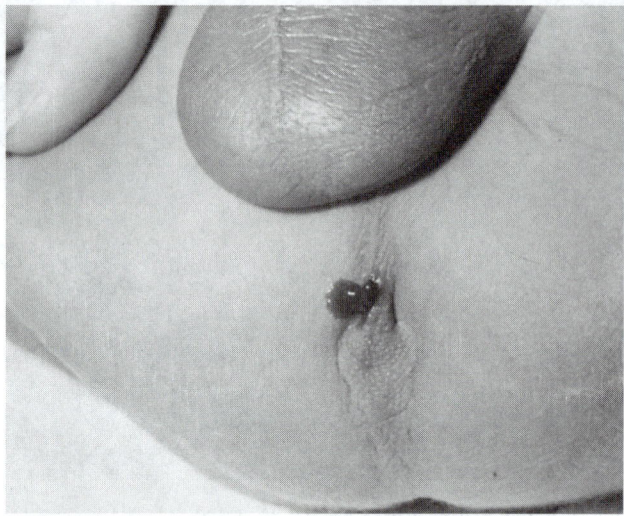

FIGURE 351.5. Male infant with a perineal fistula. Meconium did not appear until 18 hours after birth. A perineal anoplasty was done on the child's second day of life.

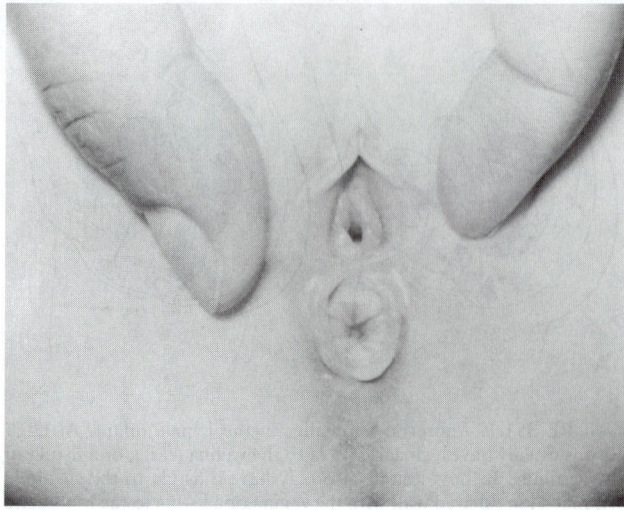

FIGURE 351.7. Ectopic perineal anus located posterior to the fourchette but anterior to the external sphincter. The patient did well with dilations until 6 months of age, when the anus was moved to the normal location.

birth but becomes evident with the passage of a small fleck of meconium during the first 24 hours of life (Fig. 351.5). Not all lesions with a perinela fistula are low. Boys with a flat bottom and a fistula from the rectum to the perineum greater than 1.0 cm in length may have a high lesion requiring treatment as such. The passage of flatus or meconium in the urine is diagnostic of a high anomaly with a fistula to the urethra or bladder.

Low lesions are found more frequently in girls (Fig. 351.6). Nearly all girls with a low lesion have a fistula to the perineum in the form of an anterior ectopic anus (Fig. 351.7), a fistula to the fourchette, or a fistula to the vestibule, which is between the posterior fourchette and the hymenal ring (Fig. 351.8). Openings into the vestibule may be associated with low lesions or high lesions with long fistulas. The complete absence of an external fistula indicates a high lesion. Fistulas to the vagina are rare. In patients with a single perineal opening, a cloacal anomaly must be considered.

Initial diagnostic studies are designed to identify the level of descent of the rectum and to detect associated anomalies, including fistulas. Ultrasound and VCUG must be performed to evaluate the anatomic integrity of the urinary tract. A retrograde urethrogram or VCUG may further delineate the presence of a fistula to the urethra or bladder.

The urine should be examined for meconium or squamous epithelial cells. Chest radiography may be performed with a nasogastric tube in place to rule out esophageal, cardiac, and vertebral anomalies. Echocardiography also should be performed to diagnose the presence of cardiac anomalies. Plain radiographs may reveal anomalies of the lumbosacral spine. An ultrasound scan or a magnetic resonance imaging scan of the spinal cord also should be obtained to screen for a tethered cord and other spinal anomalies.

ASSOCIATED MALFORMATIONS

Associated anomalies are reported in 40% to 50% of patients with imperforate anus and must be sought in infants with all forms of anorectal malformations. The genitourinary,

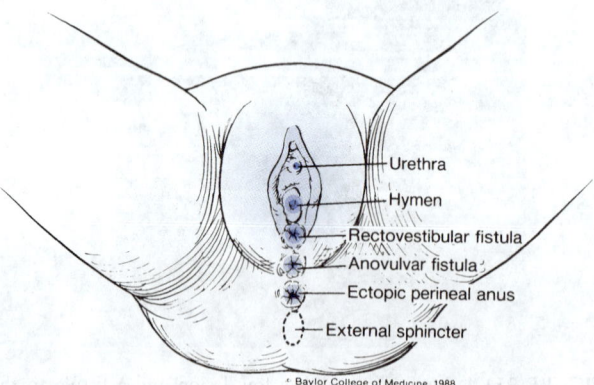

FIGURE 351.6. Appearance of fistulas on the female perineum.

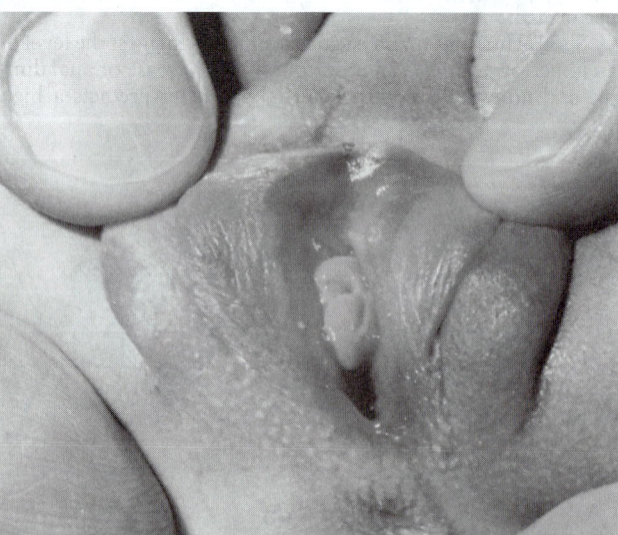

FIGURE 351.8. Rectovestibular fistula located between the hymen and fourchette in the fossa navicularis. A colostomy was performed on the child's second day of life, and anorectal reconstruction was performed at 1 year. Now it would be done much earlier.

gastrointestinal, skeletal, and cardiovascular systems may be affected. In addition to imperforate anus, esophageal atresia, vertebral anomalies, and radial and renal anomalies make up the VATER association. This association has been expanded to VACTERL, in which C represents cardiac lesions and L represents limb deformities. When any one of these anomalies is seen, the others should be sought.

Nearly 40% of the infants with imperforate anus have genitourinary anomalies ranging from minor genital anomalies, such as hypospadias, to renal agenesis. Unilateral renal agenesis is the most common defect, occurring in 8% to 25% of patients with imperforate anus.

Gastrointestinal anomalies occur in 10% to 15% of the children with imperforate anus. Esophageal atresia is the most common anomaly and often is associated with maternal polyhydramnios. Duodenal atresia also may accompany imperforate anus and also is associated with maternal polyhydramnios. Although an uncommon occurrence, Hirschsprung disease occasionally is seen in patients with imperforate anus and may complicate the postoperative course. This association has been reported in Pallister-Hall syndrome.

Cardiovascular anomalies are reported in 7% to 12% of the patients with imperforate anus. Ventricular septal defect and tetralogy of Fallot are two of the more common anomalies.

Skeletal anomalies are found in 6% to 20% of patients with anorectal malformations. Vertebral anomalies, usually sacral, are the most common. As many as 50% of the patients with high lesions have sacral vertebral anomalies. The development of the sacrum, levator musculature, and sacral nerves is integrated closely. Neurologic control of both the rectum and bladder is provided by nerves arising from the second, third, and fourth sacral segments. Normal innervation and sphincter muscle development may occur in patients with deficiencies of the fourth and fifth sacral vertebrae. Loss of the second through fifth sacral segments usually results in uncorrectable fecal and urinary incontinence.

In addition to the absence of the sacral vertebrae, other spinal abnormalities that result from improper midline fusion of bony, mesenchymal, and neural structures have been reported in patients with anorectal malformations. These abnormalities, referred to as *spinal dysraphism*, include intraspinal masses, lipomyelomeningoceles, tethered cord, and occult meningocele. They may cause a progressive neurologic deficit and impaired continence. Once neurologic function is lost, it often does not return to normal despite neurosurgical intervention.

TREATMENT

The treatment of imperforate anus depends on the level of descent of the rectum and on the presence or absence of a fistula to the urinary tract, vagina, or perineum. Children with an ectopic or anterior anus usually are asymptomatic during infancy but may develop refractory constipation when their diet changes and their stools become more formed and solid. In such patients, the anus should be surgically moved posteriorly to its normal location.

Infants with low lesions and perineal fistulas can undergo surgical repair in the newborn period. They may require only dilation of the tract to allow defecation. If the tract is small, a perineal anoplasty (a Y-V anoplasty or a minimal posterior sagittal anorectoplasty [PSARP]) may be performed to enlarge the anal opening and to prevent rectal and colonic dilation. Girls with perineal (cutaneous) fistulas have a very good plane of separation between the rectum and the vagina. They may be managed with dilations or a minimal PSARP, with no need for a protective colostomy. In girls with a fistula to the fourchette, the opening is between the mucosa of the vestibule and the perineal

skin. At 3 to 6 months of age, these patients should undergo surgical translocation of the anus to its normal location on the perineum (anal transposition) or PSARP with or without a protective colostomy.

Openings into the vestibule in girls may be either high with long fistulas (rectovestibular) or low (anovestibular). Low openings also may be treated initially by dilation and, when the child is 3 to 6 months of age, by anal transposition or PSARP with a protective colostomy. High lesions with a long fistula require that the child undergo a diverting colostomy in the neonatal period. Repeated dilations usually are inadequate to prevent chronic constipation with rectal dilation, and dilations may injure the septum between the rectal fistula and vagina, resulting in a rectovaginal fistula.

A child with a high lesion should undergo a diverting colostomy as soon as the diagnosis is confirmed and the patient has been screened for other anomalies. Colostomies are prone to complications such as prolapse, obstruction, and skin breakdown. They must be created and cared for meticulously. In most cases, the stoma should be constructed near the junction between the descending and sigmoid colon. A colostomy is particularly important in patients with fistulas to the urinary tract. Most authorities recommend a divided colostomy with a proximal end stoma and distal mucus fistula because failure to divert the fecal stream from the fistula completely may result in recurrent urinary tract infections.

Hyperchloremic acidosis may result from the passage of urine through the rectourinary fistula, where it is absorbed from the colon. Closure of the fistula eliminates this problem. Occasionally, one encounters a girl with a cloacal anomaly in whom the urine empties into a dilated, poorly emptying vagina, which leads to recurrent urinary tract infections. In these patients, the urinary tract must be decompressed to divert the urine, and the vagina must be drained adequately. Patients with high lesions undergo PSARP or abdominosacral-perineal pull-through when they are 3 to 6 months of age. A distal colostogram through the mucus fistula is extremley useful in planning the definitive operation. Although laparoscopic repair of a high imperforate anus has been reported, most pediatric surgeons continue to perform the open transperineal operation popularized by Pena. Girls with cloacal malformations require that special attention be given to associated vaginal and uterine anomalies, which should be addressed at the time of the PSARP.

After the anal anastomosis has healed, usually 3 weeks after the PSARP is performed, daily anal dilations are started. Once the anus reaches an adequate size (12 to 14 mm), the colostomy may be closed.

PROGNOSIS

The outcome for children with anorectal malformations depends on anatomic development or maldevelopment, operative technique, and the patient's cooperation. Nearly all patients with low malformations have normal anorectal function. Significant proportions of children born with high lesions suffer long-term problems with defecation (fecal incontinence and constipation), micturition (incontinence), and sexual dysfunction. Only 75% have voluntary bowel movements, and half of these experience fecal incontinence. At least 33% are totally incontinent of stool.

In the early postoperative period, constipation may be caused by stenosis and, rarely, by Hirschsprung disease, but more often it is caused by a lack of rectal sensation for fecal material, which leads to fecal impaction. Attention must be given to regular evacuations to prevent impaction. Once impaction develops, the rectum and distal colon become overdistended and lose their muscular tone and peristaltic function. This condition must be prevented. In some instances, daily laxatives or enemas are required. In a few selected cases, excision of a dilated, atonic rectosigmoid pouch is beneficial.

Significant numbers (up to 50%) of the patients with high anomalies have sacral vertebral defects. Patients with anomalies of S3 have varying degrees of neurologic deficit to the perineum, including the rectal and bladder sphincters. Patients with an absence of S2 to S5 lack all innervation to the perineum. These patients usually develop fecal or urinary incontinence.

Finally, rarely does a child with a high anomaly have perfect rectal function. Toilet training may be difficult until the child is older, often 5 or 6 years of age. The rectal function and fecal continence continue to improve into early adolescence. If the patient and his or her family can be supported through the early postoperative years, rectal function nearly always improves to an acceptable level.

Patients who remain totally incontinent may be helped by daily colonic irrigations using an enema continence catheter, appendicostomy, or cecostomy. A skin-level stoma or an indwelling tube may be used for this purpose. This procedure usually allows the patient with inadequate sphincters to stay clean. A combination of meticulous surgical repair and persis-tent bowel management will ensure an excellent quality of life for most children with anorectal anomalies.

Acknowledgments

I wish to acknowledge the late William J. Pokorny, M.D., whose chapter on anorectal malformations from an earlier edition of this textbook was used extensively in writing this chapter.

Suggested Readings

Kim J, Kim P, Hui CC. The VACTERL association: lessons from the Sonic hedgehog pathway. *Clin Genet* 2001;59:306.

Pena A. *Atlas of surgical management of anorectal malformations*. New York: Springer-Verlag, 1990.

Pena A, Hong A. Advances in the management of anorectal malformations. *Am J Surg* 2000;180:795.

Pena A, Hong AR, Midulla P Levitt, M. Reoperative surgery for anorectal anomalies. *Semin Pediatr Surg* 2003;12:118.

CHAPTER 352 ■ ULCERATIVE COLITIS

W. DANIEL JACKSON, STEPHEN L. GUTHERY, AND RICHARD J. GRAND

Ulcerative colitis (UC) is a chronic relapsing inflammatory disease of the colon and rectum of unknown origin. It was described first by Wilks and Moxon in 1875 as a chronic inflammatory bowel disease (IBD) distinct from infectious colitis. After the recognition that the colon could be involved in patients with the regional enteritis described by Crohn and associates in 1932, criteria differentiating UC from Crohn colitis were established by 1960. Nonetheless, as many as 15% of cases of noninfectious chronic inflammatory colitis remain indeterminant. Therefore, this chapter should be read in conjunction with Chapter 353.

PATHOLOGY

The inflammation in UC is limited to the colon and rectum. Table 352.1 contrasts the patterns of pathologic involvement in UC and Crohn disease (CD). On the basis of these patterns, a distinction between the two entities usually can be made. The distal colon is affected most severely, and the rectum is involved in most patients with UC. Although 60% to 70% of these patients may present with universal or pancolitis, ultimately as many as 90% of children presenting by age 10 years may have inflammation of the entire colon. Inflammation is limited primarily to the mucosa and consists of continuous involvement along the length of the bowel, with varying degrees of ulceration, hemorrhage, edema, and regenerating epithelium. A recent study suggests that focal inflammatory changes may occur in early-onset UC. Although considered to be limited to the colon, inflammation may extend uninterrupted to the cecum and up to 25 cm into the terminal ileum as *backwash ileitis* without stenosis or distortion. In severe disease in which the mucosal epithelium has been destroyed, inflammation may extend beyond the muscularis mucosae into the submucosa. Intervening areas of granulation tissue and regenerating epithelium may form islands of tissue, termed *pseudopolyps*. Thickening of the bowel wall with fibrosis is a rare finding, although shortening of the colon and focal colonic strictures may occur in long-standing disease. Fistulas and perianal disease do not occur.

The histology of UC lesions demonstrates continuous acute and chronic inflammation with mucosal and submucosal infiltration by polymorphonuclear leukocytes and mononuclear cells rarely extending beyond the muscularis (Fig. 352.1). The colonic crypts show the most characteristic changes. Cryptitis and crypt abscesses characterize acute inflammation, which may lead to chronic changes of crypt distortion with branching and dropout, diminished goblet mucous cells, and Paneth cell metaplasia. No granulomas and little fibrosis occur.

ETIOLOGY

The origin of UC is unknown, but it involves a perpetuated dysregulated immune response that injures colonic epithelial elements. No convincing infective agent has been found, although the lesions resemble changes seen with infectious colitis, and luminal bacteria or their products may be implicated

TABLE 352.1

COMPARATIVE FEATURES OF ULCERATIVE COLITIS AND CROHN'S DISEASE

	Ulcerative Colitis	Crohn Disease
Site of Disease		
Upper gastrointestinal tract	0%	20%
Ileum alone	0%	19%
Ileum and colon	Backwash ileitis	52%
Colon alone	85%–90% (distal colon predominant)	15% (proximal colon predominant)
Rectum	Approximately 100%	Relative sparing
Rectum alone	10%–15%	Rare
Perianal disease	Rare	25% (tags, fissures, abscesses)
Fistulas	0%	14% (enteroenteral, enterovesical, enterovaginal, enterocutaneous)
Gross Pathology/Histology	Hemorrhagic mucosa, diffuse continuous inflammation, pseudopolyps, loss of haustra, no perianal disease	Segmental involvement, skip regions, aphthae, thickened bowel wall, serosal fat, narrow separate bowel loops, anal tags, fistulas
Histology	Mucosal and submucosal inflammation, cryptitis, crypt abscess and distortion, depletion of goblet cells	Transmural inflammation, noncaseating granulomas, prominent lymphoid tissue, preserved goblet cells, fibrosis

in inducing and perpetuating the inflammatory response. Although no specific heritable patterns exist, 15% to 40% of patients may have other family members with IBD, with an incidence approximately ten times greater when a positive family history exists. However, concordance between monozygotic twins is only 20%, and human leukocyte antigen (HLA) markers (e.g., DR2) and linkages to other genetic syndromes (e.g., Hirschsprung, Down, and Turner) indicate that other factors, environmental and genetic, may determine susceptibility given a familial predisposition. Mutations in *CARD15*, an IBD susceptibility gene on chromosome 16, have been associated with CD but not UC. Other susceptibility loci for UC are being sought.

Evidence exists of autoimmunity in terms of serum antibodies, immune complex complement activation, and lymphocytes directed against colonic epithelium and activated to release cytokine mediators of inflammation. The efficacy of glucocorticoids and other immunosuppressants in controlling the activity of UC certainly is related to attenuation of the immune response. Rodent models of colitis, especially the interleukin-2–deficient mouse, support a hypothesized derangement of T-lymphocyte immunoregulation, specifically loss of suppression of the inflammatory response to luminal antigens, including bacterial and food-related antigens.

The association of UC with a high familial prevalence of atopic diseases and with extraintestinal manifestations of ery-

thema nodosum, arthritis, uveitis, and vasculitis supports the presence of genetic immunologic factors in the pathogenesis. However, data are insufficient at present to determine whether immune mechanisms have a primary causal or secondary perpetuating role. Allergic colitis rarely is seen after infancy and usually is transient. Evidence is insufficient for establishing an allergic origin for UC. No specific dietary practices have been implicated unequivocally in the cause or as risk factors.

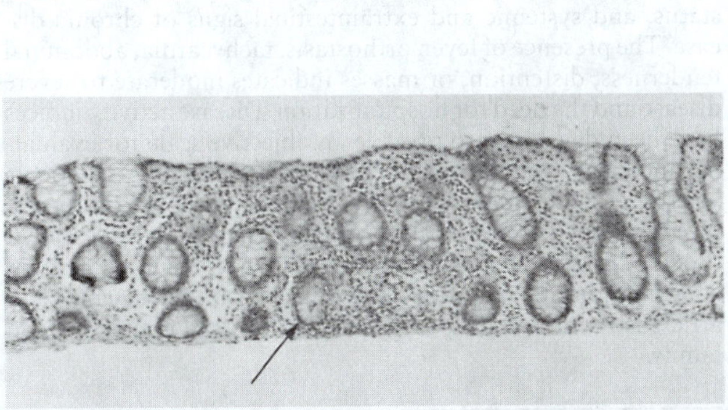

Early gastroenteritis and lack of breast-feeding have been proposed as risk factors. Nonsmokers are overrepresented relative to CD, with nicotine proposed to have a therapeutic role only in UC. No data support a psychosomatic origin in terms of stress, personality type, or psychiatric illness, although emotional and other psychosocial factors may affect the presentation and course of the disease.

EPIDEMIOLOGY

The incidence of UC in children appears to have reached a plateau after 1978. The incidence in the general population ranges from 4.1 to 7.3 cases per 100,000, with a prevalence ranging from 41.1 to 79.9 cases per 100,000 population. The disease is more prevalent in whites, with increased representation among those of Jewish backgrounds. UC occurs more commonly in northern Europe and North America, with an urban predominance. A recent review of cases in Wisconsin revealed that the incidence of UC in children may be as low as 2.14 cases per 100,000, and these investigators detected no ethnic, racial, familial, or urban predominance. Affected female patients outnumber affected male patients by approximately 50%. The distribution of age at onset is bimodal, with the major peak occurring in the second and third decades and a second peak in the fifth and sixth decades. Between 15% and 40% of all patients with UC present for evaluation before they reach age 20 years, with a peak onset occurring in adolescence. The incidence of UC in the 10- to 19-year-old age group has been estimated at 2 to 4 cases per 100,000 population. Approximately 20% of pediatric cases may present for evaluation by the time the children are age 10 years, with a mean age of approximately 6 years. The disease rarely occurs in children younger than 2 years old, although cases in infants have been reported. Most cases of noninfectious infantile colitis are caused by cow's milk or soy protein allergy and are transient, with no proved relationship to later IBD.

FIGURE 352.1. Rectal biopsy specimen of an adolescent girl with ulcerative colitis. Note the increased acute and chronic inflammatory cells in the lamina propria with invasion of the crypts, producing cryptitis and a crypt abscess (*arrow*). There is mild distortion of the crypt architecture consistent with chronic disease.

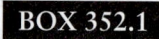

BOX 352.1   Patterns of Presentation of Ulcerative Colitis

Extraintestinal (<5%)
Growth failure, arthropathy, erythema nodosum, pyoderma gangrenosum, occult fecal blood, elevated sedimentation rate, nonspecific abdominal pain, altered bowel pattern, cholangitis

Mild Disease (50%–60%)
Diarrhea, mild rectal bleeding, abdominal pain
No systemic disturbance

Moderate Disease (30%)
Bloody diarrhea, cramps, urgency, abdominal tenderness
Systemic disturbance: anorexia, weight loss, mild fever, mild anemia

Severe Disease (10%)
More than six bloody stools per day, abdominal tenderness with or without distention, tachycardia, fever, weight loss, significant anemia, leukocytosis, hypoalbuminemia

CLINICAL PRESENTATION

UC presents in at least four patterns that differ in the extent of mucosal inflammation and systemic disturbance (Box 352.1). The most common presentation is the insidious onset of diarrhea and hematochezia (overt rectal bleeding), usually without systemic signs of fever, weight loss, or hypoalbuminemia. In these patients, the disease often is confined to the distal colon and rectum; the physical examination is normal, without abdominal tenderness; and the course remains mild, with intermittent exacerbations.

Approximately 30% of patients have signs of moderate systemic disturbance and present with bloody diarrhea, cramps, urgency, anorexia and weight loss, malaise, mild anemia, and low-grade or intermittent fever. Physical examination may reveal abdominal tenderness, and stool shows varying amounts of blood and leukocytes.

The inflammation may progress to severe colitis in approximately 10% of cases, characterized by the following: more than six bloody stools per day, significant anemia often requiring transfusion, hypoalbuminemia caused by intestinal mucosal exudation, fever, tachycardia, and weight loss. The abdomen may be diffusely tender or distended. A subgroup of patients with severe colitis may not respond to medical therapy and may require early colectomy. Criteria for recognizing which patients may require surgery are presented in the later discussion on therapy.

Finally, extraintestinal manifestations of disease, including growth disturbance, may be presenting features and may precede as well as accompany overt gastrointestinal manifestations of colitis. The first sign of disease may be growth disturbance characterized by decreased linear growth velocity caused by subtle chronic dietary caloric deficits attributed to relative anorexia or to the increased metabolic demands of inflammation. Thyroid abnormalities have been discerned in patients with IBD. Nondestructive arthritis involving peripheral large joints may occur before and may not be correlated with intestinal symptoms. The skin lesions of erythema nodosum may be seen on the extensor surfaces of the arms and legs before colitis is recognized. Pyoderma gangrenosum, a severe necrotizing ulceration of skin, may evolve in areas of trauma, of surgical incisions, or around an ileostomy. The erythrocyte sedimentation rate may be elevated, suggesting a systemic inflammatory process, or stool examination may reveal occult blood and leukocytes because of the underlying colitis. Biochemical signs of liver involvement are uncommon. Approximately 4% of patients, predominantly those who have serology positive for perinuclear staining antineutrophil cytoplasmic antibody (pANCA), either develop or present with primary sclerosing cholangitis, characterized by fatigue, pruritus, and the gradual appearance of jaundice.

COMPLICATIONS

The most serious complication of UC, toxic megacolon, occurs in fewer than 5% of patients and is a medical and surgical emergency. In this entity, dilatation of the diseased colon is accompanied by fever, tachycardia, hypokalemia, hypomagnesemia, hypoalbuminemia, and dehydration. Leukocytosis with a predominance of immature neutrophils may be present. Some of these signs, particularly fever and tenderness, may be attenuated by high-dose corticosteroid treatment. The patient with toxic megacolon is at risk for development of colonic perforation, gram-negative sepsis, and massive hemorrhage. Effective monitoring requires supine and upright radiography to assess colonic caliber and to exclude the presence of intraabdominal free air, which would indicate perforation. Management should include stool bacterial culture, assay for *Clostridium difficile* toxins, and treatment with broad-spectrum antibiotics and high-dose corticosteroids. Because most distention occurs in the anteriorly located transverse colon, positioning the patient in the prone position may be helpful. Patients who fail to respond promptly to aggressive medical measures require colectomy.

In patients with long-standing disease, colonic stricture may occur. In adults, it may be caused by carcinoma; in children, benign postinflammatory fibrotic stricture is more likely to be present. Intraabdominal and hepatic abscesses occur less often than in CD, except after perforation or colectomy.

DIAGNOSIS

The diagnosis of UC is based on clinical presentation, radiologic findings, mucosal appearance, and histologic features, as well as on the exclusion of other known causes of colitis. A complete history should be obtained, with attention given to family history, exposure to infectious agents or antibiotic treatment, retardation in growth or sexual development, and extraintestinal manifestations. The physical examination should include assessment of hydration, nutritional status, and systemic and extraintestinal signs of chronic disease. The presence of fever, orthostasis, tachycardia, abdominal tenderness, distention, or masses indicates moderate to severe disease and the need for hospitalization. Disease activity indices have been developed to provide an objective scale for evaluating and measuring the severity or intensity of disease in patients with UC. These indices are based on frequency of stools, rectal bleeding, mucosal appearance, and physician global assessment (Box 352.2). Optimal evaluation and management will require coordination of care among the primary care physician, pediatric gastroenterologist, surgeon, psychosocial counselor, and family.

Laboratory Evaluation

A complete blood cell count discloses leukocytosis or anemia. The erythrocyte sedimentation rate is elevated in 60% to 70% of patients and is a marker of inflammatory activity. Electrolyte

BOX 352.2	Ulcerative Colitis Disease Activity Index

1. Stool frequency (number = points)
   - 0 = normal
   - 1 = one to two stools/day more than normal
   - 2 = three to four stools/day more than normal
   - 3 = more than four stools/day more than normal
2. Rectal bleeding
   - 0 = none
   - 1 = streaks of blood
   - 2 = obvious blood
   - 3 = mostly blood
3. Mucosal appearance on sigmoidoscopy
   - 0 = normal
   - 1 = mild friability
   - 2 = moderate friability
   - 3 = spontaneous bleeding
4. Physician assessment of symptoms
   - 0 = no symptoms
   - 1 = mild symptoms
   - 2 = moderate symptoms
   - 3 = severe symptoms

Sum for total score: range, 0 to 12

Reprinted from Sutherland LR, Martin F, Greer S, et al. 5-Aminosalicylic acid enema in the treatment of distal ulcerative colitis, proctosigmoiditis, and proctitis. *Gastroenterology* 1987;92:1894.

disturbances are uncommon findings except in patients with dehydration, but serum protein and albumin levels may be low, indicating significant exudation. Because of either poor intake or losses from colonic inflammation and bleeding, levels of serum iron, zinc, and magnesium may be low. The low level of iron may be caused by elevated acute-phase proteins (transferrin) or may represent true deficiency or effects of chronic disease. Hypomagnesemia may prevent correction of hypocalcemia. Low alkaline phosphatase and cholesterol are indicators of depletion in zinc. Elevated serum transaminases, gammaglutamyl transferase, and alkaline phosphatase may signify sclerosing cholangitis. Stool should be examined for blood, leukocytes, and ova and parasites. Culture of fresh stool should allow exclusion of *Salmonella, Shigella, Campylobacter,* toxigenic or hemorrhagic *Escherichia coli, Aeromonas hydrophila,* and *Yersinia.* Serologic titers may help to exclude *Entamoeba histolytica.* The colitis caused by the toxins of *C. difficile* may resemble the lesions in UC or CD or may complicate underlying IBD. An assay for *C. difficile* toxins should be obtained on all patients, regardless of prior antibiotic treatment. False-positive tests for *C. difficile* toxin A may be more common in severe colitis; if available, the cytotoxin B assay also should be requested. Finding a pathogen does not exclude underlying IBD in which the prevalence of secondary infections is increased.

pANCA is found in 50% to 80% of patients with UC and in 10% to 25% with CD, especially those patients with colitis. Enzyme-linked immunosorbent assays for pANCA antibodies have a sensitivity of approximately 90% and a specificity of 70% for detection of UC. At the cost of sensitivity, the specificity can be increased to 92% by applying a cutoff level and confirming perinuclear staining, thus yielding a positive predictive value of 54% and a negative predictive value of 93%.

The serologic marker anti-*Saccharomyces cerevisiae* antibody (ASCA) is found in approximately 50% to 70% of patients with CD and in only approximately 5% of patients with UC. Some investigators and commercial laboratories have advocated the use of combinations of these serologic tests to differentiate IBD from other causes of gastrointestinal symptoms, specifically functional abdominal pain, as well as to help distinguish UC from CD. Reliance on serologic diagnostic strategies must be deferred until diagnostic and methodologic standards are validated for the relatively low prevalence of IBD in general pediatric practice.

Radiology

In the clinically ill patient, chest and abdominal radiography, both upright and supine, shows the extent of colonic dilatation and helps to exclude obstruction caused by stricture and pneumoperitoneum from perforation. These films form a baseline for later comparisons. Barium enema examination no longer is recommended as a screening procedure because colonoscopy has greater diagnostic value. If colonoscopy is not available, patients with mild to moderate disease can be evaluated using a cautiously performed barium enema, avoiding excessive distention of the colon. Barium enema never should be performed in patients with severe active colitis because of the risk of causing perforation or precipitating toxic megacolon. A barium enema may reveal the chronic changes of foreshortening, loss of haustrations, continuous involvement, pseudopolyps, and strictures as well as spasm (Fig. 352.2). However, direct inspection by flexible sigmoidoscopy may be safer and is more informative, allowing tissue biopsy to be performed. An upper gastrointestinal barium series and small bowel follow-through with fluoroscopic study of the terminal ileum are necessary to exclude small bowel involvement. The most sensitive and specific study of the small intestine is obtained with a barium enteroclysis, requiring nasojejunal intubation. In Crohn colitis, the ileum may be stiffened, nodular, and contracted, whereas in the backwash ileitis of UC, mucosal detail is effaced and the ileum is dilated but remains pliable. In UC, no other signs of small bowel involvement should be present. In moderately to severely ill patients with dilated bowel, extensive bleeding, persistent fever, or an abdominal mass, abdominal ultrasound or computed tomographic scanning may demonstrate abscesses and may assist in evaluating the ileum. Radionuclide-labeled leukocyte studies may be helpful indicators of the pattern of involvement if barium studies cannot be done safely. A newer image modality, wireless capsule endoscopy, may be validated and adapted to pediatrics in the future.

Endoscopy

Flexible sigmoidoscopic or colonoscopic inspection of the colon and ileum, in conjunction with mucosal biopsies, is the most sensitive and specific means of evaluating intestinal inflammation and is preferred over barium enema. Active disease is characterized by diffuse continuous involvement of the mucosa with edema, erythema, and friability. Erosions may occur in the acute stages, followed by mucosal regeneration forming pseudopolyps in the atrophic mucosa of chronic disease. In UC, rectal inflammation or proctitis usually is present, and, although the entire colon may be involved, the distal colon usually is affected more severely. Focal, segmental, or right-sided colonic inflammation with rectal sparing suggests CD, and small bowel involvement should be excluded. Biopsy specimens should be obtained from multiple colonic levels, including the rectum.

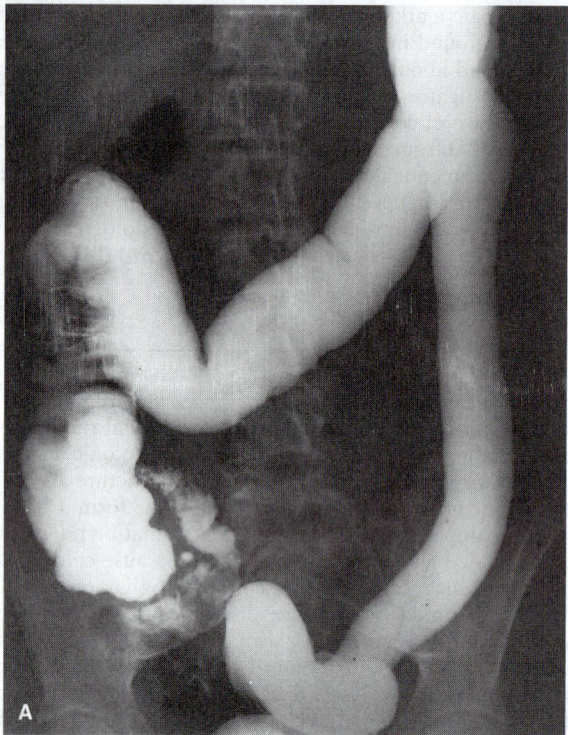
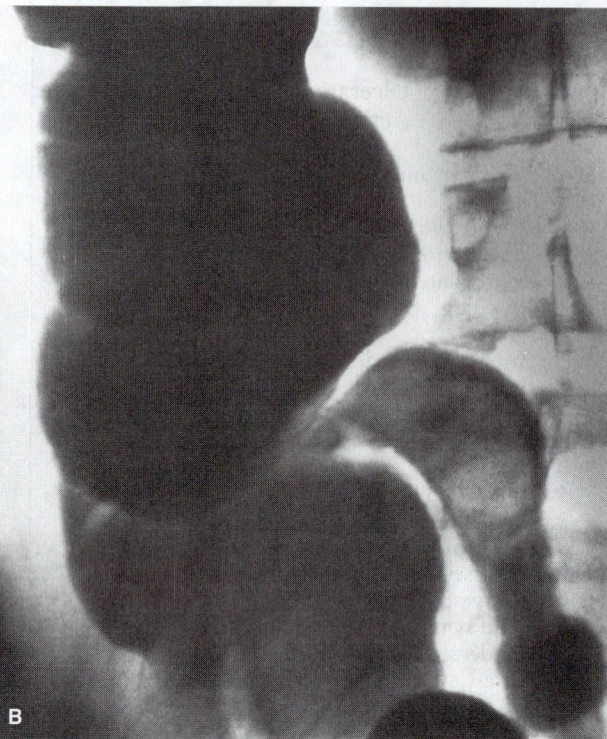

FIGURE 352.2. Single-contrast barium enema study in a 16-year-old girl with ulcerative colitis. **A:** Continuous involvement of the distal colon exists, with reflux of barium into the terminal ileum through a normal ileocecal valve. The small caliber and loss of haustra of the featureless transverse and descending colon indicate long-standing disease. The ascending colon and cecum appear normal. **B:** Spot film of the ileocecal region shows a distensible, pliable, nondisplaced terminal ileum. No strictures or signs of obstruction exist.

DIFFERENTIAL DIAGNOSIS

Gastrointestinal complaints are prevalent in children: as many as 10% of children, particularly those aged 7 to 11 years, may seek medical attention for the complaint of recurrent abdominal pain, usually periumbilical in location. In most of these cases, extensive evaluation for IBD is contraindicated unless associated features of fever, diarrhea, growth disturbance, or other extraintestinal manifestations are present. Conversely, the periumbilical location of the pain is nonspecific and should not be considered pathognomonic for functional abdominal pain because it also is a common occurrence in IBD. In cases of uncomplicated recurrent abdominal pain, constipation or stool retention, giardiasis, lactose intolerance, urinary tract infection, peptic disease, or functional motility, related causes should be considered.

Rectal bleeding may be caused by Meckel diverticulum, hemolytic-uremic syndrome, polyposis, hemorrhoids, or anal fissures. The hematochezia from Meckel diverticulum usually is painless, copious, maroon, and without fecal leukocytes. Hemolytic-uremic syndrome often can be excluded by urinalysis, inspection of the blood smear, and measuring the blood urea nitrogen. Henoch-Schönlein purpura may present with severe cramping abdominal pain or hematochezia before emergence of the characteristic vasculitic rash on dependent areas. Polyps may be detected by sigmoidoscopy or barium enema. Fissures may be secondary to constipation or may be the perianal manifestations of CD, particularly if they are off the sagittal plane or if inflammation is prominent.

Colitis, characterized by fecal leukocytes accompanying the bleeding and sigmoidoscopic evidence of inflammation, may be caused by infection or allergy. Infection with *Salmonella,* *Shigella, Campylobacter, Yersinia, Aeromonas,* certain strains of *E. coli,* and the protozoa *E. histolytica* or *Blastocystis hominis* may resemble UC and should be excluded. *C. difficile* pseudomembranous colitis may be present even in the absence of a history of antibiotic treatment and seems to be more prevalent in patients with IBD. Food proteins, usually cow's milk or soy protein in infancy, may produce allergic colitis difficult to distinguish from UC unless histologic examination reveals a predominant eosinophilic infiltration of the mucosa. Except for rare eosinophilic gastroenteritis, such a response occurs only in infants and responds promptly to exclusion of the allergenic protein.

Before experiencing the onset of overt gastrointestinal manifestations of UC, the patient may be followed for prodromal growth retardation or extraintestinal disease, in which case Crohn colitis should be considered. Extraintestinal signs of UC or CD may be mistaken for primary endocrine disorders, rheumatologic diseases, or anorexia nervosa.

THERAPY

Because UC is confined to the colon, total proctocolectomy is curative. However, because of the potential complications of surgery and the challenges in a patient's adjustment to an ileostomy and life without a colon, medical management is attempted initially. In addition, always some residual diagnostic uncertainty exists about the exclusion of Crohn colitis. Therefore, surgery is reserved for failure to respond to medical management, severe hemorrhage or complications, chronic corticosteroid dependence, or finding of mucosal dysplasia or adenomas in colonoscopic surveillance of long-standing disease.

BOX 352.3   **Pharmacologic Therapy for Ulcerative Colitis**

Mild or Localized Distal Colitis
Sulfasalazine: 50–75 mg/kg/day in two to three divided doses
5-Aminosalicylates: 30–80 mg/kg/day oral, enema, or suppository (proctitis)
Folate supplement: 1 mg/day (with sulfasalazine)

Moderate to Severe Colitis
Methylprednisolone or prednisone: 1–2 mg/kg/day in two divided doses for 2 weeks; taper to 1 mg/kg/day once daily over 4–6 weeks, depending on clinical response. When clinical remission is achieved, taper to once every other day and discontinue over another 4 weeks
Sulfasalazine: 40–50 mg/kg/day in two to three divided doses initiated gradually during steroid taper in daily 250-mg increments until full dose is achieved (maximum, 3–4 g/day)

5-Aminosalicylates: 30–80 mg/kg/day, oral and/or nightly enema
Folate: 1 mg/kg/day (with sulfasalazine)
Hydrocortisone enemas

Refractory or Steroid-Dependent Disease
Azathioprine: 2–2.5 mg/kg/day
6-Mercaptopurine: 1–1.5 mg/kg/day
Cyclosporine: 2–4 mg/kg/day intravenously (trough level <300 ng/mL)

Maintenance
Sulfasalazine: 50–75 mg/kg/day in two to three divided doses
5-Aminosalicylates: 30–80 mg/kg/day
Folate: 1 mg/day (with sulfasalazine)

Medical Therapy

The goals of medical therapy in children with UC are to control inflammation and symptoms and to sustain remission and prevent relapses. The choice of therapy depends on the severity of the inflammation (Box 352.3).

Mild to moderate cases of colitis unaccompanied by systemic signs can be managed on an outpatient basis with the gradual introduction of sulfasalazine or a nonsulfa aminosalicylate (5-ASA) alternative. Mesalamine or balsalazide increasingly are replacing sulfasalazine as first-line agents to allow administration of higher dosages without incurring dose-related side effects. Response to treatment, with reduction in stool frequency, bleeding, and cramps, is expected to be achieved within 2 to 4 weeks. Subsequently, activity and diet may be liberalized as tolerated.

Moderate to severe disease, when colitis is accompanied by systemic signs, occasionally requires hospitalization for proper evaluation, observation for complications, and management. For patients with moderate disease, high-dose (up to 4.8 g/day for adults) oral mesalamine or balsalazide may be sufficient, with remission expected to occur within 30 days. Corticosteroids are reserved for those who fail to respond to high-dose mesalamine or for those with severe disease requiring hospitalization. Hypoalbuminemia and anemia may require infusion of albumin or blood transfusion to optimize recovery. The immunomodulator azathioprine and its active metabolite 6-mercaptopurine are useful in approximately 75% of patients with refractory disease who are dependent on long-term corticosteroid therapy.

Severe disease with copious bloody diarrhea, weight loss, fever, abdominal tenderness or distention, leukocytosis, anemia, and hypoalbuminemia indicates loss of homeostasis and should be treated as an emergency, with hospitalization and surgical consultation. Some of these patients eventually require colectomy for failure to respond to medical therapy or because of the emergence of life-threatening complications such as toxic megacolon, hemorrhage, or perforation. Anemia and hypoalbuminemia should be corrected with transfusions of blood and albumin. Dehydration and electrolyte disturbances should be anticipated and reversed. Magnesium is essential to colonic

function and often is depleted, a finding reflected in low urinary magnesium excretion after a parenteral challenge dose of magnesium sulfate, even in the presence of normal serum magnesium levels. After blood has been drawn for culture and stool obtained for bacterial culture, parasite examination, and *C. difficile* toxin assay, broad-spectrum intravenous antibiotic coverage should be instituted. High-dose intravenous corticosteroid treatment is essential. Serial abdominal radiography should be obtained for surveillance of complications, which may be masked by corticosteroid treatment. Computed tomography, radionuclide-labeled leukocyte scans, or ultrasound examination to search for abscesses is indicated in patients who fail to respond to treatment. Traditional teaching has maintained that most patients who fail to respond to a maximal medical regimen within 2 weeks ultimately require colectomy. Prolonging medical treatment and postponing surgery in these cases increase the risk of development of complications caused by immunosuppression, corticosteroid therapy, central venous catheters, transfusions, and hospitalization. Despite concerns regarding the advisability of their use in a disease that is surgically curable, new options for immunomodulation are being explored. Cyclosporine is an immunosuppressive agent that may be effective in controlling severe or fulminant steroid-resistant colitis until the slow-onset long-term immunomodulating agents (azathioprine or 6-mercaptopurine) can exert their corticosteroid-sparing effects. At this time, evidence is insufficient to support the addition of infliximab to the treatment arsenal for UC, although an argument can be made for its use in indeterminate colitis before colectomy.

Rates of relapse or ongoing active disease are estimated at 45% to 70% per year, with the rate increasing with severity of disease and relapse correlating with presence of pANCA. Maintenance of remission or prevention of relapse is a major goal of long-term therapy. Sulfasalazine and nonsulfa 5-ASA compounds have been shown to be roughly equivalent in efficacy for maintaining remission compared with placebo. 5-ASA compounds that do not contain sulfa, such as mesalamine and balsalazide, have increasing efficacy at increasing doses without a significant increase in adverse effects. Increasing the dose of sulfasalazine, conversely, significantly increases the risk of development of adverse effects, mainly resulting from the sulfapyridine moiety.

Specific Pharmacologic Agents

ASA agents and corticosteroids are the principal therapeutic agents for UC. Sulfasalazine, the oldest of the ASA-based medications, has proved efficacious in controlling mild disease and in reducing the frequency of relapses once remission of disease has been obtained. Sulfasalazine is an azo-bonded combination of a 5-ASA and sulfapyridine. The parent compound is split by colonic flora into the two constituents. The 5-ASA is poorly absorbed and is considered to be the active antiinflammatory moiety, presumably through inhibition of prostaglandin synthesis. The following are among the effects attributed to 5-ASA: inhibition of lipoxygenase activity, which mediates migration of polymorphonuclear leukocytes; inhibition of prostaglandin E_2 synthesis; reduction in the levels of thromboxane B_2 and 6-keto-prostaglandin F_1; and antisecretory effects. The sulfapyridine is absorbed and excreted in the urine. Sulfapyridine is responsible for the side effects of allergy, hemolytic anemia, rash, headaches, and nausea. These effects are relatively common, often dose-dependent, and may be transient. Oligospermia has been reported and is considered reversible. The principal role of the azo-bonded sulfapyridine seems to be to prevent small intestinal absorption of the salicylate because little of the parent compound is transported across the intestinal mucosa. Children at risk for glucose-6-phosphate dehydrogenase deficiency should be screened before receiving treatment with sulfasalazine. Because of the potential for intolerance, the sulfasalazine dosage should be increased gradually from 10 mg/kg/day over the course of 1 week to a maximum dosage of 50 to 75 mg/kg in two to three divided doses. Symptoms and blood cell counts should be monitored closely. Because sulfasalazine impairs absorption of folate, folate supplements, 1 mg/day, are given.

Alternative poorly absorbed nonsulfa 5-ASA preparations have been formulated to avoid the complications associated with sulfapyridine. These agents include 5-ASA or mesalamine incorporated into a pH-sensitive resin (Asacol), releasing drug in the relatively alkaline ileum and colon or into a time-release resin (Pentasa), allowing mesalamine delivery to more proximal small bowel, or a diazo-bonded dimers of 5-ASA (balsalazide [Colazal] or olsalazine sodium [Dipentum]) cleaved by colonic bacteria with little small bowel availability. These medications do not appear to inhibit absorption of folate. Sulfasalazine may be formulated in suspension, and balsalazide capsules may be opened, facilitating treatment in younger children. Mesalamine has been implicated in renal papillary necrosis and tubulointerstitial nephritis, and renal function and urinalysis should be monitored periodically.

Corticosteroids are effective in initial control of moderate to severe acute UC but are not to be continued for long-term maintenance therapy. In the acute context, corticosteroids do not seem to affect surgical outcome adversely should surgery become necessary. Treatment is begun with a relatively high dosage of prednisone or methylprednisolone (1 to 2 mg/kg/day) in divided doses and is sustained until disease is controlled, usually within 2 weeks, and then is maintained in a single daily dose of at least 1 mg/kg/day for another 2 to 4 weeks. Subsequently, with adjunctive use of sulfasalazine or nonsulfa ASAs, the dose is tapered gradually by 5-mg decrements weekly and discontinued. If exacerbation of disease activity prevents the withdrawal of corticosteroids, the addition of immunomodulator therapy with azathioprine or 6-mercaptopurine (its metabolite) may be necessary. Effects of short-term glucocorticoid treatment on growth are equivocal because the activity of disease itself may cause growth retardation. Some patients resume normal growth velocity only after corticosteroid suppression of their disease activity occurs. Other patients whose disease remains in remission may show catch-up growth velocity only after withdrawal of corticosteroids. Of importance for compliance, documentation, and patient safety is to have a printed steroid dosing and tapering schedule in managing an exacerbation of disease. Nonetheless, long-term steroid therapy is not recommended for long-term treatment of UC.

Studies have confirmed the efficacy of 5-ASA enemas in the control of left-sided or distal colitis and in maintenance of remission. Patients with proctocolitis may respond to mesalamine suppositories. Hydrocortisone enemas and foam have been used in an attempt to reduce the dose of systemic corticosteroids necessary to control distal disease. Poorly absorbed topical corticosteroid enemas and oral delayed-release preparations (e.g., budesonide) are other options.

Immunomodulators such as azathioprine and its active metabolite 6-mercaptopurine have proved useful in the control of corticosteroid-dependent IBD in children. These agents have a mean 3-month lag until full corticosteroid-sparing efficacy is obtained but may be useful in acute disease, with adult data showing that intravenous loading of azathioprine may accelerate time to efficacy. Treatment may be optimized and toxicity minimized by monitoring active metabolite 6-thioguanine and hepatotoxic metabolite 6-methylmercaptopurine levels after 2 to 4 weeks of therapy and at 6-month intervals. Rare cases of severe bone marrow depression may occur in patients with low thiopurine methyltransferase (TPMT) activity. Prospective TPMT genotyping has been promoted to identify patients at risk. Complete blood counts and liver and pancreatic enzymes should be monitored after initiation of treatment and every 3 months. Cyclosporine and tacrolimus (FK-506) have shown short-term efficacy in arresting fulminant colitis and in allowing transition to maintenance therapy with azathioprine or 6-mercaptopurine. The major risks are the consequences of immunosuppression and bone marrow suppression, including leukopenia and opportunistic infection. Lymphoproliferative malignant disease, a potential complication of these agents, is considered rare. One estimate of risk of lymphoma with 6-mercaptopurine and azathioprine treatment was 1 case per every 300 patient-years. As with prolonged corticosteroid treatment, the potential benefits and risks of these agents must be weighed against the curative benefits and surgical risks of colectomy.

New agents targeted on cytokines or their receptors, including anti-tumor necrosis factor antibodies, are under study and currently are indicated for steroid-dependent or fistulizing CD. Enemas of short-chain fatty acids, a preferred substrate of colonic epithelium that can prevent or heal diversion colitis, are being studied for an expanded role. Probiotic manipulation of intestinal flora, hypothesized to alter intestinal permeability and to modulate the inflammatory response, may find a therapeutic role in IBD.

Nutritional Therapy

The goals of nutritional therapy are to restore metabolic homeostasis by correcting nutrient deficits and replacing ongoing losses, to provide sufficient energy and protein for positive nitrogen balance or net protein synthesis, and to promote catch-up growth toward premorbid percentiles. The provision of adequate nutrients is essential for optimal healing. In UC, in which malabsorption is unlikely to occur and increased metabolic requirements are small or unproved, the undernutrition is caused by a reduced voluntary intake of calories and protein with a variable contribution of protein losses by inflammatory exudation. On the basis of diet diary analysis of current intake, oral protein and calorie supplements are prescribed to make up calorie and protein deficits. Guidelines for supplementation are to provide at least 140% of the recommended daily allowance for height and age for both energy and protein. Continuous nocturnal nasogastric infusions of enteral formula through a soft Silastic catheter may be necessary for patients who cannot voluntarily increase their intake. Nutritional support is less likely to help establish a remission in patients with UC than in patients with CD. Nonetheless, correcting nutrient deficiencies and maintaining adequate nutritional status are valuable in preventing deterioration of the patient's medical condition and in preparing patients for surgery. Common mineral deficiencies include magnesium and zinc, which should be treated. Calcium intake and vitamin D status should be optimized in patients treated with corticosteroids and with disease of long duration because of an increased risk for development of osteopenia.

Surgery

Surgery is indicated when medical and nutritional therapies fail to control the disease or prevent significant morbidity caused by either disease or treatment. Although in most cases medical management is successful in controlling UC and prolonged remissions are possible, a cure can be obtained only by surgical excision.

Indications for colectomy in acute UC include uncontrolled hemorrhage, severe colitis that fails to respond within 2 weeks to intensive treatment (including corticosteroids, cyclosporine, and nutritional support), and complications of toxic megacolon, stricture, or perforation. Elective colectomy is indicated in patients with prolonged corticosteroid dependence or corticosteroid-induced complications caused by treatment of chronic active disease, in patients with retardation of growth and sexual maturation despite nutritional support, and in those with long-standing disease or epithelial dysplasia of rectal or colonic mucosa, which increases the risk of development of carcinoma. The risk of morbidity and mortality of elective colectomy in a patient whose disease activity is controlled and whose nutritional status has been optimized are less than in the acutely ill patient.

Several surgical options exist. Partial or subtotal colectomy usually is performed, leaving a rectal stump as a blind or Hartmann pouch and creating a terminal ileostomy. If the rectal disease cannot be controlled or if permanent ileostomy ultimately is necessary, proctectomy should be performed. The risks of development of extraintestinal complications and carcinoma remain as long as residual diseased rectal mucosa is present. If the disease in the rectal segment can be controlled with a combination of topical and systemic corticosteroids, performing a careful and complete rectal mucosectomy, with preservation of the pelvic nerves and the rectal musculature and sphincters, through which the ileum may be pulled and anastomosed to the anus, is possible. Some surgeons prefer to leave a short segment of transitional anorectal mucosa (potentially diseased) at the anorectal junction to reduce risks of injury to the complex nerves of this area. A variety of ileal pouches may be constructed to create a reservoir, aiding continence. Postoperative inflammation of the neorectum or ileal pouch, termed *pouchitis,* suggests stasis, possible CD (which must be excluded by biopsy), or failure of complete dissection of the rectal mucosa before ileal pull-through. Metronidazole and ciprofloxacin have been the most effective agents in treating pouchitis. Mesalamine suppositories may be useful for any residual proctitis. Recent small but well-designed studies indicate that a probiotic mixture of nonpathogenic bacterial species is effective in the prevention and maintenance of remission of pouchitis after colectomy and ileoanal pull-through. With the ileoanal pull-through and the use of antimotility agents such as loperamide, the patient often can achieve complete continence, with an average of five bowel movements per day. Perianal irritation is treated topically with sitz baths, careful hygiene, and cholestyramine ointment, which may absorb irritating bile acids. Before surgery, psychological preparation and consulta-

tion with an enterostomal specialist can ease the child's transition to life with an ileostomy.

PROSPECTIVE MANAGEMENT AND PROGNOSIS

UC is a chronic disease requiring careful surveillance, patient education, and expert management by a team consisting of a pediatrician, gastroenterologist, nutritionist, psychiatrist or psychologist, social worker, and nurse. An alliance with a pediatric surgeon familiar with IBD is essential for the management of potential complications. The success of management depends on the degree to which the patient and family understand and participate in the treatment. Interest is increasing in developing patient self-management protocols to allow early intervention in exacerbations as well as appropriate adjustments of medication with changes in activity of the disease. Nutrition and growth, sexual maturation, psychosocial adjustment to disease, and compliance with therapy all should be monitored as carefully as one monitors the clinical signs and symptoms of disease activity outlined previously. Several internet web sites can be recommended as valid sources of information; they include the sites of the Crohns and Colitis Foundation of America (www.ccfa.org) and the North American Society for Pediatric Gastroenterology, Hepatology and Nutrition (NASPGHAN www.naspghan.org). A patient handbook has been developed to assist children and adolescents in participating in the management of their disease and is available through NASPGHAN.

The frequency of follow-up depends on the course of disease activity, but intervals should be no longer than 6 months. Most children have the potential for a full, active life with good general health. Ten percent of patients experience only the presenting episode of colitis but still must be followed long term because of the risk of development of cancer in later life. Approximately 20% of patients have intermittent symptoms, 50% have chronic disease, and the remaining 20% have chronic, active, incapacitating disease.

The risk of colonic carcinoma in pediatric-onset UC increases by an estimated 0.5% to 1% per year after the first 10 years of disease, depending on the extent of involvement and family history. Because the risk is cumulative, patients with persistent symptoms and pancolitis of early onset in youth are at greatest risk. The risk of colorectal cancer in patients with pancolitis diagnosed before they reach age 15 years may be as high as 40% after 35 years. The risk of development of carcinoma appears to be less in patients with left-sided colitis or proctitis. Carcinoma in the context of colitis may not follow a typical adenoma-to-adenocarcinoma sequence and may arise from flat mucosa, thus increasing the challenge of surveillance. Histologic evidence of any degree of dysplasia may be associated with extant adenocarcinoma and warrants considering proctocolectomy. Annual colonoscopy with multiple biopsies at 5- to 10-cm intervals circumferentially (approximately 35 samples) to detect dysplasia or polyps has been recommended for patients with disease of more than 10 years' duration. However, such surveillance is costly, fallible, and not without morbidity, and the efficacy of surveillance in preventing development of lethal cancer is unproved. These considerations have led some physicians to advocate performing prophylactic colectomy in patients with long-standing disease that began in childhood or adolescence. Evidence indicates a reduction of risk by long-term treatment with 5-ASA agents, with putative preventive efficacy of ursodeoxycholic acid and folate. More study is needed to determine the optimal management of risk of development of carcinoma.

The advent of corticosteroids and potent immunosuppressants has altered the prognosis for medical management of UC significantly; fewer patients require surgery to control the disease. Most patients can resume full activities, including school attendance and athletics. UC has no specific effect on fertility and poses no risk to the fetus. The 5-ASA products appear to be safe during pregnancy. However, poor nutritional status increases the risks for pregnant women, and sulfasalazine may produce reversible oligospermia. Azathioprine and 6-mercaptopurine may increase the risk of spontaneous abortion and prematurity, based on current data. UC that manifests during pregnancy may be more severe, and approximately 30% to 50% of patients with preexisting disease may experience exacerbations during pregnancy.

Despite the successes achieved with medical management, no medical cure exists for UC. The medications used to control the disease have potential morbidity, and the risk of development of colonic carcinoma is significant and cumulative, warranting careful surveillance. Confronting a chronic disease that entails frequent medical visits and frustrating relapses or the prospects of surgery in childhood and adolescence is a tremendous emotional burden for both the patient and family and requires ongoing psychosocial support. Colectomy both cures the disease and eliminates the risk of colorectal carcinoma but adds variables of surgical morbidity, inconvenience, and discomfort. All these factors must be considered and reconciled by the patient, family, and medical team in the long-term management of children with UC.

Suggested Readings

Chong SKF, Blackshaw AJ, Morson BC, et al. Prospective study of colitis in infancy and early childhood. *J Pediatr Gastroenterol Nutr* 1986;5:352.

Ekbom A, Helmick C, Zack M, Adami H. Ulcerative colitis and colorectal cancer: a population-based study. *N Engl J Med* 1990;323:1228.

Escher JC, Taminiau JA, Niewenhuis EE, et al. Treatment of inflammatory bowel disease in childhood: best available evidence. *Inflamm Bowel Dis* 2003; 9:34.

Fonkalsrud EW. Surgery for pediatric ulcerative colitis. *Curr Opin Pediatr* 1995; 7:323.

Garrelds IM, van Meeteren ME, Meijssen MA, Zijlstra FJ. Interleukin-2–deficient mice: effect on cytokines and inflammatory cells in chronic colonic disease. *Dig Dis Sci* 2002;47:503.

Gionchetti P, Rizzello F, Habal F, et al. Standard treatment of ulcerative colitis. *Dig Dis* 2003;21:157.

Gionchetti P, Rizzello F, Helwig U. Prophylaxis of pouchitis onset with probiotic therapy: a double blind, placebo-controlled Trial. *Gastroenterology* 2003;124:1202.

Gryboski JD. *Clostridium difficile* in inflammatory bowel disease relapse. *J Pediatr Gastroenterol Nutr* 1991;13:39.

Gryboski JD. Ulcerative colitis in children 10 years old or younger. *J Pediatr Gastroenterol Nutr* 1993;17:24.

Hyams JS, Davis P, Grancher K, et al. Clinical outcome of ulcerative colitis in children. *J Pediatr* 1996;129:81.

Kelly DG, Fleming CR. Nutritional considerations in inflammatory bowel diseases. *Gastroenterol Clin North Am* 1995;24:597.

Kugathasan S, Judd R, Hoffmann R, et al. Epidemiologic and clinical characteristics of children with newly diagnosed inflammatory bowel disease in Wisconsin: a statewide population-based study. *J Pediatr* 2003;143:525.

Lichtiger S, Present DH, Kornbluth A, et al. Cyclosporine in severe ulcerative colitis refractory to steroid therapy. *N Engl J Med* 1994;330:1841.

Lindsley CB, Schaller JG. Arthritis associated with inflammatory bowel disease. *J Pediatr* 1974;84:6.

Odze R. Diagnostic problems and advances in inflammatory bowel disease. *Mod Pathol* 2003;16:347.

Podolsky DK. Inflammatory bowel disease. *N Engl J Med* 2002;347:417.

Price AB, Morson BC. Inflammatory bowel disease: the surgical pathology of Crohn's disease and UC. *Hum Pathol* 1975;6:7.

Roberts EA. Primary sclerosing cholangitis in children. *J Gastroenterol Hepatol* 1999;14:588.

Rubin D, Hanauer S. Screening and surveillance for individuals with inflammatory bowel disease. *Semin Colon Rectal Surg* 2000;11:34.

Rubin D, Hanauer SB, Kornbluth A, et al. Use of 5-ASA is associated with decreased risk of dysplasia and colorectal cancer in ulcerative colitis. *Gastrointest Endosc News* 2003;10:1.

Ruemmele FM, SR Targan, G Levy, et al. Diagnostic accuracy of serologic assays in pediatric inflammatory bowel disease. *Gastroenterology* 1998;115:822.

Sands B. Therapy of inflammatory bowel disease. *Gastroenterology* 2000;118: S68.

Sutherland LR, Martin F, Greer S, et al. 5-Aminosalicylic acid enema in the treatment of distal ulcerative colitis, proctosigmoiditis, and proctitis. *Gastroenterology* 1987;92:1894.

CHAPTER 353 ■ CROHN DISEASE

W. DANIEL JACKSON, STEPHEN L. GUTHERY, AND RICHARD J. GRAND

Crohn disease (CD) is a transmural inflammatory process that may affect any segment of the gastrointestinal (GI) tract from mouth to anus in a discontinuous fashion. The small bowel is involved in 90% of cases, predominantly the distal ileum (70%), usually in combination with colitis as ileocolitis (more than 50%). Isolated colonic disease without clinical or radiologic evidence of small bowel involvement occurs in approximately 10% of patients. The small bowel involvement is responsible for many of the specific nutritional complications of CD, whereas the colonic involvement poses the greatest challenge for differentiation from other infectious and inflammatory bowel diseases. Although CD shares many features with ulcerative colitis (UC), several features allow differentiation of the two disorders (Table 352.1). This chapter, therefore, complements Chapter 352.

PATHOLOGY

Unlike the findings in UC, the inflammation in CD usually does not involve a continuous segment of bowel and often appears as *discrete focal ulcerations* (e.g., aphthae) with relatively intact intervening mucosa. As the disease progresses, in the 60% of cases involving the colon, right-sided or proximal colonic inflammation predominates, with relative sparing of the rectum. *Anal involvement*, in the form of skin tags, anal fissures, abscesses, and fistulas, occurs in approximately 25% of patients, often preceding intestinal symptoms. The inflammation of CD usually is *transmural* and can be recognized as mesenteric inflammation; fat encroachment on the serosal surface of the intestine; stiffening of the small bowel loops caused by

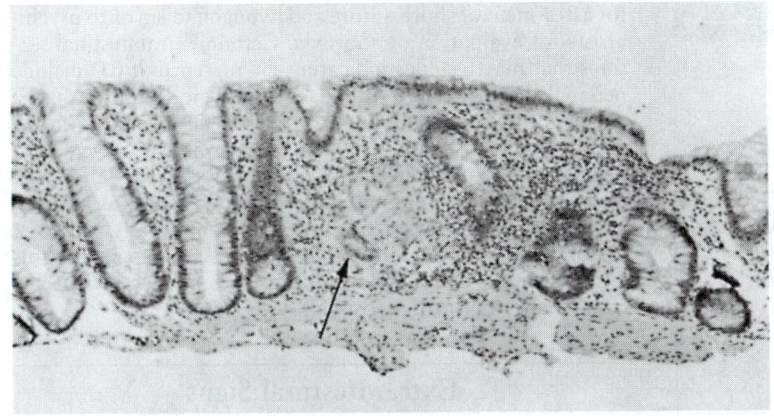

FIGURE 353.1. Colonic biopsy of an adolescent girl with active Crohn disease. Note the distortion of the crypt architecture with a prominent noncaseating granuloma and giant cells (*arrow*) amid increased acute and chronic inflammation of the lamina propria.

fibrosis; and adhesions, stricture formation, and fistulas to other loops of bowel, bladder, vagina, or skin.

The histology of the lesions in CD reveals the transmural nature of the acute and chronic inflammation, often showing edema, lymphoid aggregates, and significant fibrosis. Mucosal changes may resemble those of ulcerative or infectious colitis characterized by acute polymorphonuclear leukocyte invasion of crypt epithelium to cause cryptitis or crypt abscesses, as well as chronic features of crypt branching and dropout distorting normal crypt architecture. Some areas of the bowel may be normal or may show only mild chronic inflammation. Noncaseating granulomas may be found in as many as 50% of the patients, and coupled with the transmural inflammation, disease distribution, and clinical presentation, their presence provides strong support for the diagnosis of CD (Fig. 353.1).

ETIOLOGY

As in UC, the cause of CD is unknown, with evidence existing for the collusion of multiple factors, including genetics, luminal agents, altered mucosal integrity, and immunologic response, in the pathogenesis. A current hypothesis suggests that CD is caused by an inappropriate cellular immune response to enteral bacterial products in a genetically susceptible host. The pathogenesis of the chronic inflammation may involve abnormalities in the regulation of the immune response to infectious, toxic, or dietary-derived intestinal antigens or an inappropriate immune response to an unusual antigen or infectious agent. No consistent pathogen has been identified. Altered colonic flora or bacterial products may play a role in the pathogenesis, given the attenuation or absence of disease in germ-free animal models and the therapeutic usefulness of antibiotics. Impaired intestinal mucosal exclusion of luminal antigens may be a causal factor or simply a consequence of inflammation. Inappropriately regulated immune or cytokine responses have been implicated on the basis of the favorable response to corticosteroids, other immunosuppressive agents, and cytokine antagonists. Although evidence for an activated T-lymphocyte population and cytokine production exists, no specific markers of autoimmunity have been demonstrated.

A genetic basis of CD is supported by several observations. First, the prevalence of CD is higher among some subpopulations (e.g., Ashkenazi Jews). Second, concordance of disease among monozygotic twins is approximately 67%. Third, multiple independent genome-wide scans have revealed susceptibility loci in families with several affected members. Finally, mutations in the *CARD15/NOD2* gene on chromosome 16 confer an increased risk among both heterozygotes (two- to fourfold) and homozygotes (40-fold). The normal pro-

tein product of *CARD15/NOD2* is responsible for binding intracellular bacterial products and transducing intracellular inflammatory signals involved in bacterial recognition by monocytes. Not all individuals with CD have mutations in *CARD15/NOD2*; conversely, not all those with mutations in *CARD15/NOD2* develop CD. These features, as well as the several other identified susceptibility loci (e.g., on chromosomes 5 and 7), suggest that CD has a non-Mendelian complex genetic basis.

EPIDEMIOLOGY

A recent epidemiologic study of children diagnosed by pediatric gastroenterologists in Wisconsin revealed an incidence of inflammatory bowel disease (IBD) of 7.05 cases per 100,000 per year. The majority of cases, 4.56 per 100,000 population, were CD, more than twice the incidence of UC. In most cases, no family history existed. Unlike previous studies indicating an increased prevalence among whites (especially in the Jewish population) in the developed world, the incidence was not affected by racial or urbanization factors. Male and female representation is approximately equal, as is bimodal age at onset, with peaks occurring in the second and third and again in the sixth decades of life. Approximately 2% of cases, including rare cases in infancy presenting as intractable diarrhea, occur before the patient reaches 10 years of age.

CLINICAL PRESENTATION

The presentation of CD in children depends on the location and extent of inflammation. In many cases, the onset is insidious with nonspecific features of GI involvement or extraintestinal manifestations leading to delayed or incorrect diagnosis. Diarrhea, abdominal pain (most frequently postprandial periumbilical cramping), fever, and weight loss are the most common presenting features. Rectal bleeding, seen in 30% of CD cases, is seen much less commonly than in UC and signifies colonic involvement. The three general patterns of clinical presentation based on anatomic involvement show considerable overlap: (1) diarrhea and lower abdominal cramping representing colonic inflammation; (2) nausea, vomiting, anorexia, and/or early satiety due to upper gastrointestinal or small intestinal disease; and (3) extraintestinal symptoms and signs, including delayed maturation and growth impairment (Box 353.1).

Colonic involvement may present as diarrhea, often associated with cramps and urgency to defecate after any distention of the inflamed colon by the fecal stream. Other signs of colitis may be indistinguishable from those seen in UC and consist

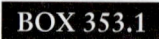

BOX 353.1   Crohn Disease: Patterns of Involvement

Extraintestinal signs and growth retardation
Anorexia, malaise, fatigue
Perianal disease, oral aphthae
Erythema nodosum, pyoderma gangrenosum
Anemia, hepatitis, nephrolithiasis, arthritis, clubbing

Small bowel involvement
Nausea, early satiety
Abdominal mass, postprandial cramps
Diarrhea, malabsorption
Mineral and vitamin deficiencies (iron, zinc, magnesium, folate, vitamin B$_{12}$)

Colonic features
Diarrhea, urgency
Rectal bleeding, fecal leukocytes
Perianal fistula, abscess

of an inflammatory exudate of neutrophils into the lumen and occult or overt rectal bleeding. Perianal disease and relative sparing of the rectum occur more frequently in Crohn colitis than in ulcerative colitis and may be the only differentiating features. Perianal skin tags and fissures may be the first physical sign of disease, especially if they are off the sagittal plane. Perianal abscesses and perineal fistulas also should suggest the diagnosis of Crohn colitis. A rare complication, toxic dilation with risk of perforation and sepsis known as *toxic megacolon*, has been reported in Crohn colitis, though less often than in UC; treatment is the same as that outlined for toxic megacolon complicating severe ulcerative colitis (see Chapter 352).

Another pattern of presentation is produced by upper gastrointestinal inflammation, which probably accounts for much of the postprandial cramping, early satiety, nausea, and anorexia that patients report. Rare involvement of the esophagus or gastroduodenal segments may mimic peptic disease and respond partially to acid control therapy. Gastritis or duodenal ulceration in the absence of *Helicobacter pylori* infection or use of nonsteroidal antiinflammatory agents should suggest possible CD. Diarrhea may occur in 90% of patients with small bowel involvement and, in the absence of colitis, most likely signifies malabsorption of bile acids by the terminal ileum or nutrients. Estimates of the prevalence of malabsorption in children with CD depend on the nutrient that is malabsorbed but range from 17% for lactose and 29% for fat to 70% for protein. The frequency of lactose malabsorption is normal when adjusted for that expected for the ethnic distribution of patients with CD but in some patients may be a consequence of small bowel inflammation. Deficiencies of iron, zinc, magnesium, folate, and vitamin B$_{12}$ may be more pronounced in patients with small bowel disease, particularly those with terminal ileum involvement.

Patients may present with nonspecific extraintestinal manifestations and growth retardation (see Box 353.1). Overt clinical signs of involvement of the GI tract may not appear for years, although this inflammation may be extensive enough to cause early satiety, nausea, anorexia, and distention as signs of malabsorption or impaired transit and partial obstruction. Over the course of time, net energy and protein deficits are reflected in decreased weight velocity followed by decreased height velocity and delayed skeletal and sexual maturation. As a consequence of nutritional, growth, and maturational problems, patients may be referred to specialists in endocrinology

for assessment of short stature and hypogonadism or to psychiatrists for evaluation of anorexia. Certain extraintestinal features that may be clues indicating the presence of CD include perianal disease, oral aphthae, erythema nodosum, arthritis, uveitis, and digital clubbing. A microcytic anemia with reduced total iron-binding capacity, an elevated leukocyte and platelet count, and an elevated erythrocyte sedimentation rate may be present. Abdominal radiography may show an unusual gas pattern with some small bowel dilation; usually, however, radiography does not establish a diagnosis. Recognizing this insidious mode of presentation leads to timely use of specific tests to confirm the diagnosis.

Extraintestinal Signs

The systemic nature of CD is apparent in the range of potential involvement of extraintestinal organs. Arthritis and arthralgias may occur in as many as 11% of cases and usually present as a seronegative monoarticular arthritis of large joints such as a knee or ankle or as a migratory polyarthritis. Arthritis occurs more commonly in patients with colonic involvement (e.g., colitis, ileocolitis) and seems to parallel the activity of disease, although occasionally it precedes overt gastrointestinal signs. Sacroiliitis and ankylosing spondylitis rarely occur, predominantly in patients with histocompatibility gene *HLA-B27*.

Fewer than 5% of patients develop cutaneous lesions of erythema nodosum or pyoderma gangrenosum. The latter condition is a severe deep ulceration of the skin, often preceded by minor trauma or associated with surgical incisions or stoma sites. Management requires control of the underlying bowel disease, often with the addition of metronidazole, topical tacrolimus, dapsone, local corticosteroid injection, and occasional skin grafting.

Signs of liver disease occur in fewer than 4% of patients with CD. Mild histologic abnormalities of steatosis may be more common findings. Involvement of the liver correlates with the activity of bowel disease but rarely progresses to cirrhosis or chronic active hepatitis. Sclerosing cholangitis has been reported in two adolescents with Crohn colitis and is not associated exclusively with UC. Cholelithiasis, usually asymptomatic, may occur after ileal dysfunction or resection that interrupts the enterohepatic circulation of bile acids, leading to the decreased cholesterol solubility characteristic of lithogenic bile. Prolonged periods of bowel rest without meal-stimulated contraction of the gallbladder allows stasis of bile in the gallbladder, which contributes to sludge and formation of stones.

Urologic manifestations include calcium oxalate renal calculi caused by increased intestinal oxalate absorption accompanying steatorrhea and subsequent increased renal excretion. Ureteral inflammation may develop from adjacent transmural bowel inflammation and leads to pyuria, obstruction, and infection. Hydroureter or hydronephrosis may result from renal stones, inflammation, or external compression from adjacent intestinal masses. Recurrent urinary tract infections and pneumaturia may herald enterovesical fistulas.

Other signs include uveitis, acutely symptomatic in fewer than 3% and asymptomatic in as many as 30% of patients; aphthous stomatitis; osteoporosis; anemias of chronic disease; iron, vitamin B$_{12}$, and folate deficiencies; zinc deficiency, implicated when there is taste dysfunction, acrodermatitis, and poor healing; thyroid dysfunction and enlargement; and growth failure.

Undernutrition and Growth Failure

Weight loss occurs in as many as 87% of children presenting with CD. Often accompanying the weight loss are impaired

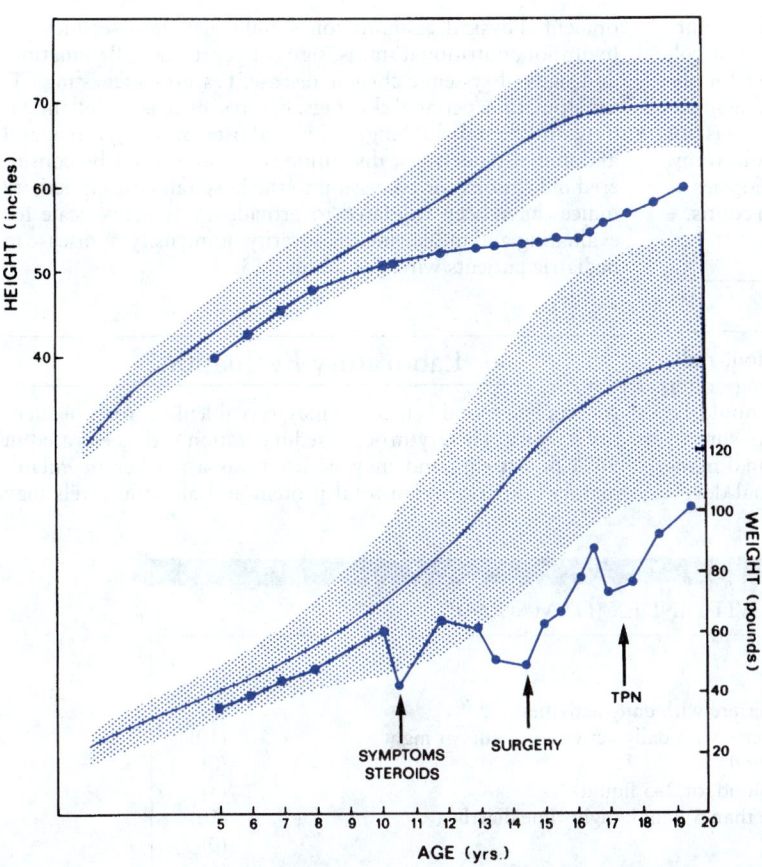

FIGURE 353.2. Growth curve of an adolescent with Crohn disease. The reduction in linear growth preceded the acute weight loss and onset of symptoms. Although growth accelerated after corticosteroid treatment, limited surgical resection, and total parenteral nutrition (TPN), premorbid percentiles were not achieved.

linear growth, retarded bone development and mineralization, and delayed sexual maturation. These changes may be subtle initially and often precede development of overt bowel disease by months or years. Most of these effects seem to be caused by undernutrition because they can be reversed by nutritional supplementation.

The cause of undernutrition in IBD is multifactorial. In most patients with growth failure, dietary energy intake is less than the average requirement for age and may be the result of anorexia from altered taste, early satiety, or meal-related cramps or diarrhea. Some cases are complicated by steatorrhea (29%) and increased enteric protein excretion (70%). Hypoalbuminemia (50%), hypomagnesemia, hypocalcemia, fat-soluble vitamin losses, and deficiencies in iron, folate, vitamin B_{12}, and zinc may be present. Nutrient requirements are increased by the metabolic demands of chronic inflammation, losses through fistulas, and demands for repletion of lean body mass and fat deficits beyond those normally imposed by growth, especially in adolescents.

Most endocrine test results are normal in patients with growth retardation and short stature associated with CD. Although bone age may be delayed and serum insulinlike growth factor-1 levels depressed, both respond to nutritional therapy, and pituitary, thyroid, adrenal, and growth hormone studies typically are normal. One study revealed a high prevalence of thyroidomegaly and hypothyroidism in adults with CD. Sexual maturation, arrested by disease and nutrient deficits leading to delayed puberty and menarche, resumes after nutritional therapy is initiated and inflammation is controlled.

Growth failure may occur with or without corticosteroid therapy. Despite evidence that corticosteroids may suppress linear growth, their use in controlling the inflammation of CD often permits growth to resume at normal rates. Whether accelerated or catch-up growth sufficient to reach the premorbid growth percentiles can be achieved during high-dose cortico-

steroid treatment is unclear. The patient with long-standing disease may adapt to a state of chronic undernutrition, characterized by height stunted below expected percentiles, appropriate weight for height, and normal to subnormal linear growth velocity. The consequences of untreated chronic undernutrition in a child with CD are poor disease control, increased complications, delayed puberty, and permanent short stature (Fig. 353.2).

COMPLICATIONS

The major intestinal complications of CD are related to the transmural nature of the inflammation that extends from mucosa to serosa. Contiguous loops of bowel or other organs may become enveloped in inflammation. Adhesions, strictures, and abscesses may develop, with a risk of development of an obstruction or bacterial overgrowth. Fistulas may form to any abdominal or pelvic structure and should be suspected to underlie any chronic draining ulcer or sinus. Enterocutaneous, enteroenteric, perirectal, labial, enterovaginal, and enterovesical fistulas may pose a nutritional hazard because they are conduits for major losses of protein and other nutrients. Perianal disease occurs in 25% of patients with CD, most often in the context of colonic inflammation and fistula formation. Skin tags, anal fissures, and perianal or perirectal abscesses may precede other signs of intestinal CD or develop during an exacerbation of colitis. Although often minor in appearance, these lesions can create severe discomfort and be quite refractory to treatment. Massive hemorrhage and toxic megacolon, which are potential complications of UC, occur only rarely in CD.

The risk of malignancy of all types appears to be increased in patients with CD and is estimated to be 20 times greater than normal for patients with CD diagnosed before the patient is 21 years of age. Nonetheless, the incidence of small bowel carcinoma is low, and the rates of colonic adenocarcinoma are lower than those in patients with UC. However, rates of colorectal cancer approach those of UC when adjusted for the extent of colonic involvement in Crohn colitis. The association of colonic mucosal dysplasia with carcinoma in CD is not established sufficiently to recommend prophylactic colectomy, although performing surveillance colonoscopy and biopsies as in UC is prudent in patients with long-standing Crohn colitis.

DIAGNOSIS

The diagnosis of CD is based on clinical presentation, radiologic findings, and mucosal appearance and histology after exclusion of alternative causes. A complete history should be obtained, with attention given to family history, exposure to infectious agents or antibiotic treatment, extraintestinal manifestations, and retardation in growth rate or in sexual devel-opment. Physical examination should include assessment of hydration, nutritional status, signs of peritoneal inflammation, and signs of systemic chronic disease. Features suggesting CD are stomatitis; perianal skin tags, fissures, fistulas, or inflammation; and digital clubbing. Fever, orthostasis, tachycardia, and abdominal tenderness, distention, or mass should be considered indications for admission to the hospital. Disease activity indices have been validated to provide an objective scale for evaluating and measuring the severity or intensity of disease in pediatric patients with CD (Table 353.1).

Laboratory Evaluation

A complete blood cell count may reveal leukocytosis or identify anemia. The erythrocyte sedimentation rate is elevated in 90% of patients and may be useful as a marker of inflammatory activity. Serum total protein and albumin levels may

---

TABLE 353.1

PEDIATRIC CROHN DISEASE ACTIVITY INDEX (ITEM SCORE)

History

Abdominal pain:	None	(0)
	Mild, does not interfere with daily activities	(5)
	Mod/severe, interferes with daily activities, occurs at night	(10)
Stools per day:	0–1 formed, no blood	(0)
	2 or fewer, small blood, or 2–5 liquid	(5)
	Large blood, more than 5 liquid, night-time diarrhea	(10)
General well-being:	Normal	(0)
	Occasional limitation	(5)
	Frequent difficulty	(10)

Laboratory

Hematocrit (age based): scale 0, 2.5, 5 depending on severity of anemia

Erythrocyte sedimentation rate:		
	<20	(0)
	20–50	(2.5)
	>50	(5)
Albumin:		
	>3.4	(0)
	3.1–3.4	(2.5)
	<3.1	(5)

Examination

Weight:	
Gain or stable	(0)
Involuntary weight loss of 1–9%	(5)
Weight loss exceeding 10%	(10)
Height:	
Height velocity 0 to −1 standard deviations (SDs) below mean	(0)
Height velocity −1.1 to −2.0 SDs	(5)
Height velocity less than −2.0 SDs	(10)
Abdomen:	
No tenderness; no mass	(0)
Tenderness or mass without tenderness	(5)
Tenderness, involuntary guarding, definite mass	(10)
Perirectal disease:	
None, asymptomatic tags	(0)
1–2 indolent fistulas with minimal drainage, nontender	(5)
Active fistula, drainage, tenderness, or abscess	(10)
Extraintestinal manifestations:	
fever >38.4°C for ≥3 days the previous week; arthritis, uveitis, erythema nodosum, pyoderma gangrenosum	
None	(0)
1	(5)
2 or more	(10)

From Hyams JS, Ferry GD, Mandel FS, et al. Development and validation of a pediatric Crohn disease activity index. *J Pediatr Gastroenterol Nutr* 1991;12:439.

be low as a consequence of undernutrition and enteric protein losses. Serum magnesium, iron, and plasma zinc levels may be low because of poor intake coupled with cumulative losses from sloughed intestinal epithelial cells or bleeding. Ileal dysfunction may be revealed by low levels of vitamin B_{12} and fat-soluble vitamins. Urinalysis may reveal pyuria. Fresh stool should be obtained for visual inspection and laboratory examination for blood, leukocytes, and parasites; cultured for infectious pathogens, including pathogenic *Escherichia coli* and *Yersinia enterocolitica*; and assayed for *Clostridium difficile* toxins A and B. Serologic titers may help exclude *Y. enterocolitica* and *Entamoeba histolytica*. Detection of pathogens may not exclude the existence of underlying CD, but the infections must be treated first.

The serologic marker anti-*Saccharomyces cerevisiae* antibody (ASCA) is found in approximately 60% of patients with CD and only approximately 10% of patients with UC. The perinuclear staining antineutrophil cytoplasmic antibody (pANCA) is another marker, found in approximately 70% of patients with UC and 20% with CD, especially those patients with colitis. Detectable ASCA antibodies have sensitivities ranging between 41% and 76% and specificities between 88% and 94% for the identification of CD. Positive predictive values have been reported between 70% and 85%, with negative predictive values ranging between 82% and 91%. The low sensitivity of the ASCA assay limits its utility as a screening marker for CD, although its high specificity may be useful in discriminating between UC and CD. Some investigators and commercial laboratories have advocated the use of combinations of these serologic tests to differentiate IBD from other causes of similar symptoms—specifically functional abdominal pain.

Radiology

Although the extent of radiographic involvement has not correlated with activity of clinical disease, radiologic studies often are helpful in establishing the diagnosis and providing treatment. In the acutely ill patient, upright and supine radiographs of the abdomen and a chest radiograph demonstrate the extent of bowel dilatation and help exclude ileus, intestinal obstruction, or pneumoperitoneum, signifying perforation. Although contraindicated in severe colitis, if mild to moderate clinical colitis is present and colonoscopy is unavailable, a barium enema study with air contrast may demonstrate characteristic aphthous lesions and show cecal or segmental involvement or right-sided predominance (Fig. 353.3). Because the ileum may not be defined adequately by barium enema, an upper GI series with small bowel follow-through or the more definitive nasojejunal enteroclysis study, combined with careful fluoroscopic study of the terminal ileum, is essential to define the small bowel involvement, which affects as many as 90% of patients with CD (Fig. 353.4). The small bowel enteroclysis study, although uncomfortable, provides the best definition of small bowel lesions, stenosis, and fistulas. The terminal ileum or other loops may be relatively rigid, constricted, and nodular, with fixed deformities despite fluoroscopic manipulation, features caused by the transmural inflammation in CD. This appearance may be contrasted with that of the "backwash" ileitis seen in UC, in which mucosal detail is effaced and dilation occurs without signs of thickening of the bowel wall. An abdominal mass, persistent focal tenderness, fever, or obstruction should be evaluated by ultrasound or computed tomography (CT) to exclude abscess. If CD is suspected but difficult to demonstrate, or if complications are suspected, CT often can demonstrate the bowel wall thickening, fat wrapping, or abscesses (Fig. 353.5). Radionuclide-labeled leukocyte scans may be useful as adjuncts to these standard techniques to detect and

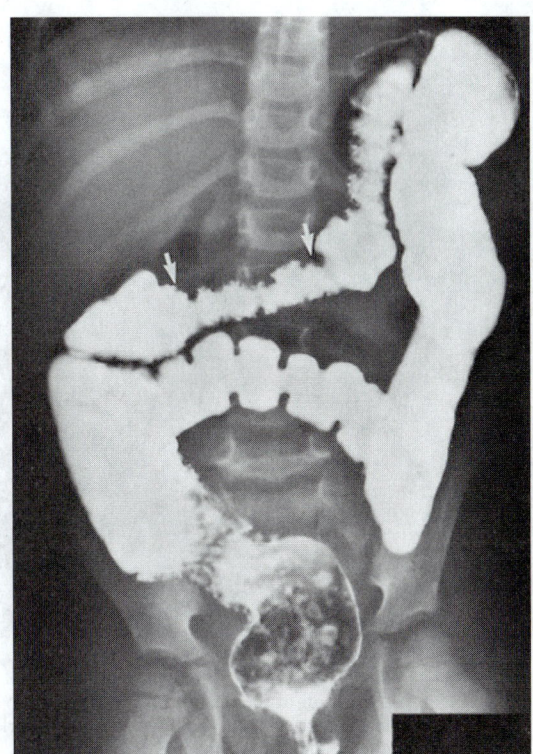

FIGURE 353.3. Barium enema study in an 8-year-old girl with Crohn disease reveals segmental colitis involving discrete regions of the transverse colon (*between arrows*). Notice the irregular mucosal margins consistent with active ulceration and edema. The rectum, shown with residual stool, was spared.

monitor patterns of inflammation, but they may lack the resolution and specificity required for establishing the diagnosis and, like other imaging modalities, may not correlate with clinical status. Wireless capsule endoscopy may identify otherwise unrecognized lesions in nonstrictured cases.

Endoscopy

Colonoscopy with biopsy of the colon and terminal ileum is the most sensitive and specific test for evaluating Crohn ileocolitis. As reflected in its pathology, the lesions of CD may appear as discrete ulcerations or aphthae of the mucosa, often with a central exudate and corona of erythema. Severe or chronic disease may present with a cobblestone mucosal pattern caused by linear or stellate ulcerations and nodularity or with strictures or stenosis. Intervening areas may be normal in appearance and histologic characteristics. In the more than 60% of patients with colonic involvement, disease is more active in the proximal colon and cecum. Although perianal disease may be present, the rectum often is relatively spared. Because the histology of regions that appear grossly normal may show signs of nonspecific chronic inflammation, biopsies must be obtained from multiple sites, regardless of gross endoscopic appearance. Endoscopy to explore the esophagus, stomach, and duodenum is indicated when involvement is suspected on clinical or radiologic grounds.

DIFFERENTIAL DIAGNOSIS

GI disorders are common occurrences in pediatric patients, with as many as 10% of children between the ages of 7 and

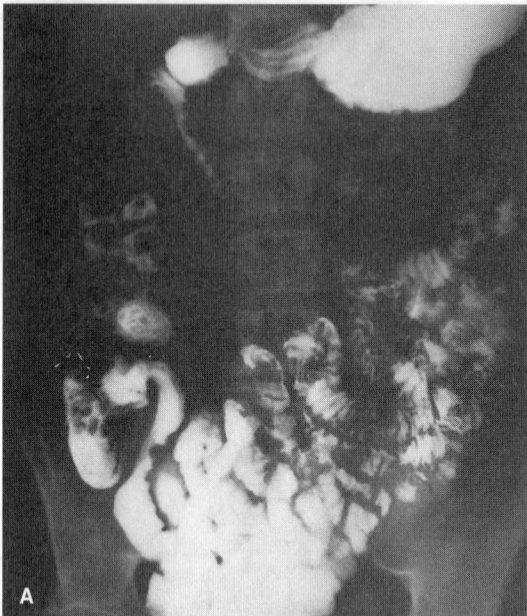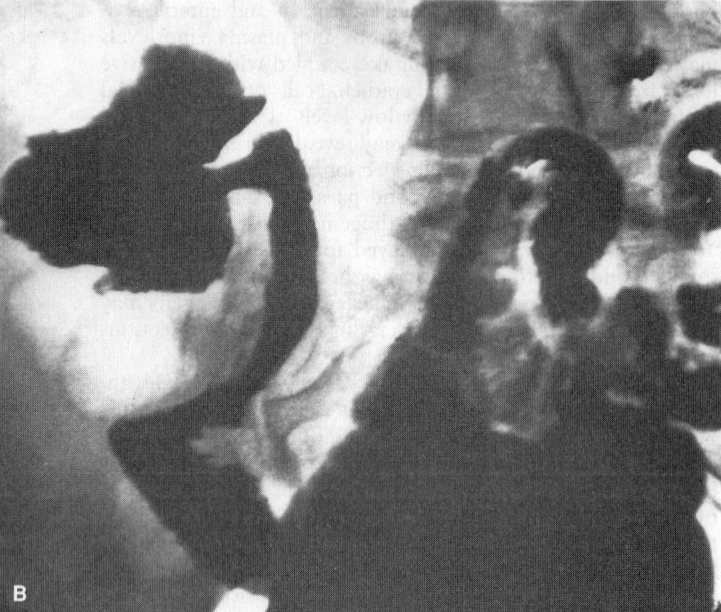

FIGURE 353.4. A: Enteroclysis small bowel study of a 15-year-old girl shows some distortion but no obstruction of the distal ileum and irregular cecal mucosa. **B:** Spot film of the terminal ileum reveals a long, constricted, and rigid segment with marked distortion at the ileocecal valve. The separation of loops indicates markedly thickened bowel walls.

11 years seeking medical attention for the complaint of recurrent abdominal pain, usually periumbilical in location. Because the location and character of pain in children with either functional abdominal pain or IBD are quite similar, differentiating between the two disorders based on pain alone is difficult. In uncomplicated recurrent abdominal pain, discomfort caused by stool retention, lactose intolerance, peptic disease, urinary tract infection, pelvic inflammatory disease, or irritable bowel syndrome should be considered and eliminated. Unless signs of inflammation or growth disturbance are present, extensive evaluation for IBD is not indicated in the patient with recurrent abdominal pain. Variability in the presentation of CD renders establishing the diagnosis and differentiating from other entities challenging. Signs of inflammation (e.g., fever, tenderness), extraintestinal lesions, or an elevated sedimentation rate often can differentiate inflammatory causes of growth failure

from endocrine or psychogenic syndromes such as growth hormone deficiency, hypopituitarism, and anorexia nervosa. This last condition may be especially difficult to differentiate from CD, as both have features in common, such as inability to maintain ideal body weight, inadequate caloric intake, and amenorrhea. Signs of colitis on stool examination, barium study, or colonoscopy with biopsy or the presence of oral aphthae or perianal disease can localize the inflammation to the GI tract. The presence of extracolonic disease or granulomas on biopsy favors CD over UD, although in the absence of such features, CD cannot be excluded. Specific criteria may be met favoring the diagnosis of Behçet syndrome, especially with conjunctival and genital involvement. In at least 5% of cases, often fulminant colitis, Crohn colitis may be indistinguishable clinically and histologically from UC until characteristic extracolonic or new histologic features appear. Early UC may show focal inflammation with the typical skip lesions associated with CD. These cases are represented by the term *indeterminate colitis*. Occasionally, evidence of CD does not appear until inflammation develops in the ileostomy or ileoanal pouch of a patient who has had a colectomy for what was presumed to be UC.

Rectal bleeding occurs more commonly in UC than in CD and has many causes in addition to colitis, such as Meckel diverticulum, hemolytic-uremic syndrome, Henoch-Schönlein purpura, intestinal polyps, or hemorrhoids. Anal fissures secondary to constipation usually present without signs of colitis or chronic perianal inflammation and skin tags.

Pathogens such as *C. difficile*, *Y. enterocolitica*, enteropathogenic *E. coli*, *Aeromonas hydrophila*, *Giardia lamblia*, and *E. histolytica* must be excluded, along with the customary *Salmonella*, *Shigella*, and *Campylobacter* cultured in the setting of enterocolitis. These agents often are overlooked in the initial evaluation and may produce a chronic inflammatory picture resembling Crohn ileocolitis. Tuberculosis, *Yersinia*, and lymphoma may involve the small bowel, predominantly the terminal ileum, which is rich in lymphoid tissue, and may resemble CD clinically and radiographically.

The patient with acquired immunodeficiency syndrome (AIDS) may present with enterocolitis caused by a variety of

FIGURE 353.5. Computed tomographic scan of the lower abdomen of a 12-year-old girl with Crohn ileocolitis. Notice the thickened bowel wall of terminal ileum (*solid arrow*) and cecum (*open arrow*) and the thickened mesentery. No abscesses or fistulas were demonstrated.

pathogens, including cytomegalovirus, cryptosporidium, Isospora, and mycobacteria, as well as anorectal involvement with condylomata acuminata, chlamydia, or herpes simplex virus. Esophageal or gastric ulceration, especially esophageal candidiasis, may occur. AIDS should be considered if these signs are accompanied by splenomegaly and lymphadenopathy or high-risk factors.

Unlike most other rheumatologic diseases of childhood, the arthritis of IBD, including colitis caused by *C. difficile* or *Yersinia*, usually is asymmetric, involving large joints of the lower extremities without deformity.

THERAPY

Because no pharmacologic regimen has been shown to alter the long-term outcome of CD, the goals of treatment are to minimize the morbidity of disease exacerbations without introducing iatrogenic morbidity. Optimal management mandates consultation with a pediatric gastroenterologist and may require the perspective of a pediatric surgeon. The pharmacotherapy of CD has been based on a therapeutic triangle in which the base represents maximized use of 5-aminosalicylic acid (ASA) preparations and the apex new or investigational biologic agents (Fig. 353.6). Future approaches directed at arresting the activity of disease with an agent specifically targeting a critical pathway of inflammation followed by a potent maintenance medication may indeed alter the natural history of CD.

Pharmacologic Therapy (Box 353.2)

Sulfasalazine and other 5-aminosalicylate agents have been used for the induction and maintenance of remission of mild to moderate CD. The response rates to these agents have been mixed, with some trials reporting equivalent response rates to corticosteroids, whereas others have demonstrated no difference compared to placebo. Results of meta-analyses and larger clinical trials also are inconsistent, although mesalamine appears to be effective in the prevention of postoperative relapse. Heterogeneity in distribution of disease (ileitis versus ileocolitis versus colitis) and variable strategies for dosing are possible explanations for these disparate results. Although it is being supplanted in the therapy of CD, sulfasalazine has been useful in the management of Crohn colitis. In conjunction with corticosteroid treatment, sulfasalazine is better than is placebo in treating ileocolitis. Although it has not been proved effective in

---

| BOX 353.2 | Pharmacologic Therapy of Crohn Disease |

Acute exacerbation
Mesalamine: 30–60 mg/kg/day in three to four divided doses
Mesalamine enema qhs (for distal colitis)
Methylprednisolone or prednisone: 1–2 mg/kg/day in two divided doses, taper to 1 mg/kg/day qam and then to qod over 4–6 weeks, depending on clinical response
When remission is achieved, taper and discontinue

Remission
Sulfasalazine: 50–75 mg/kg/day in three to four divided doses (maximum, 4 g/day)
Nonsulfa 5-aminosalicylates: 30–60 mg/kg/day in three to four divided doses
Folate supplement: 1 mg/day (with sulfasalazine)

Perianal disease or fistula
Metronidazole: 15 mg/kg/day in divided doses q8h
Ciprofloxacin: 250–500 mg twice per day

Refractory disease
Azathioprine: 2–3 mg/kg/day in two divided doses
6-Mercaptopurine: 1–2 mg/kg/day in two divided doses
Methotrexate 15 mg subcutaneous or IM q week.
Infliximab (anti-tumor necrosis factor receptor): 5 mg/kg intravenous infusion over 2 hours

---

preventing relapse or in treating small bowel disease, it often is continued in a chronic regimen. Sulfasalazine optimally is introduced gradually, depending on the patient's tolerance. It often can be reintroduced in small tolerance-inducing increments after discontinuation because of side effects of headache, nausea, vomiting, or bloody diarrhea. Neutropenia and oligospermia are reversible side effects. Folate malabsorption caused by competitive inhibition of absorption is treated with 1-mg/day supplements. Because the side effects of sulfasalazine are caused primarily by the sulfapyridine moiety and the antiinflammatory effects are caused by the topical activity of the relatively poorly absorbed 5-aminosalicylate moiety, alternative oral nonsulfa preparations of 5-ASA have been created to prevent proximal GI absorption. Evidence exists that these agents are effective in the colitis of CD as well as UC although a recent meta-analysis of studies yielded only a small sub-clinical improvement in disease activity. Some forms of 5-ASA or mesalamine allow drug release as early as the proximal small intestine and distal ileum with efficacy in Crohn enteritis and ileitis. Adverse effects of mesalamine are uncommon developments, but severe tubulointerstitial nephritis and pancreatitis have been reported, prompting recommendations to monitor renal function as frequently as monthly. Colitis distal to the splenic flexure may be managed with nightly 5-ASA retention enemas, and proctitis may respond to 5-ASA suppositories.

Metronidazole and ciprofloxacin both have been used to induce remission in mild to moderate disease, although the latter is not approved for use in children. Both of these agents are likely to be more helpful in patients with ileocolitis or colitis than in those with isolated small intestinal disease. The use of metronidazole or ciprofloxacin is supported primarily by small randomized trials or uncontrolled studies in adults. Metronidazole has been shown to be superior to placebo in prevention of postoperative recurrence, although this benefit declines over the course of time, such that by 3 years, no difference exists between the results achieved with metronidazole and those with

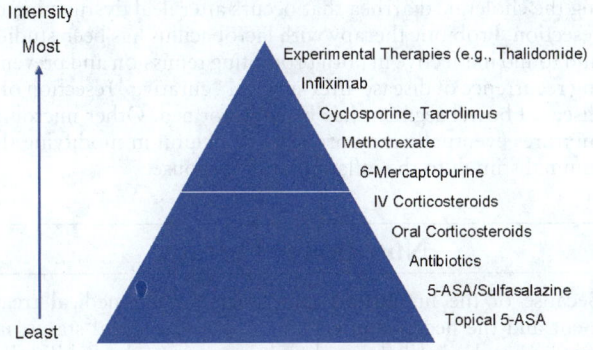

Therapeutic Triangle for IBD

Intensity

Most

- Experimental Therapies (e.g., Thalidomide)
- Infliximab
- Cyclosporine, Tacrolimus
- Methotrexate
- 6-Mercaptopurine
- IV Corticosteroids
- Oral Corticosteroids
- Antibiotics
- 5-ASA/Sulfasalazine
- Topical 5-ASA

Least

IV=intravenous; 5-ASA =5-aminosalicylic acid

FIGURE 353.6. Therapeutic triangle for Crohn disease.

placebo. Antimicrobial agents may have a role in reducing any bacterial antigen-stimulated inflammatory response. Metronidazole is an antimicrobial agent effective against anaerobic bacteria, including *C. difficile* and the protozoa *E. histolytica* and *G. lamblia,* that is indicated in patients with Crohn colitis that is unresponsive to 5-ASA agents or with complications of perianal disease or small intestinal bacterial overgrowth. Clinical series support its role in healing perineal fistulas, with up to a 70% response rate for children with perianal disease. Potential morbidity includes reversible peripheral neuropathy with chronic use and a potential increased risk of development of malignancy. Ciprofloxacin has proved efficacious in treating perianal disease, including fistulas and abscesses, with minimal toxicity in adults with CD. Despite some concerns regarding effects on cartilage development in youth, ciprofloxacin has been used increasingly in pediatrics (e.g., in cystic fibrosis) and may be prescribed for children with CD that is unresponsive to antiinflammatory agents and metronidazole. Clarithromycin, initially proposed within a model of mycobacterial pathogenesis of CD, may be helpful in treating children with mild to moderate CD, regardless of mycobacterium studies.

Corticosteroids are effective for induction of remission in 70% of patients with moderate to severe CD. Although corticosteroids clearly are beneficial, their use is limited by their adverse effects and the individual variation in therapeutic response. Corticosteroid therapy is indicated for symptoms refractory to other agents, extensive small bowel disease, severe or persistent systemic and extraintestinal complications, and postoperative recurrences.

In active disease, induction of remission is achieved with a dosage of 1 to 2 mg/kg/day of prednisone or methylprednisolone (up to 60 mg/day), tapered after 3 to 4 weeks by 5-mg weekly decrements over 4 to 6 weeks. The corticosteroid then may be tapered to an alternate-day regimen and discontinued as allowed by the patient's symptoms. Continuous low-dose treatment does not seem to prevent relapse. Higher-dose, alternate-day corticosteroids have been shown to control symptoms with a minimum of side effects and a lower risk of growth retardation. However, the availability of immunosuppressive therapy has led to reduced reliance on a chronic or alternate-day regimen of steroids, which are not recommended for maintenance treatment.

Potential morbidity of high-dose corticosteroid therapy includes adrenal suppression, hypertension, osteoporosis, glaucoma, cataracts, masking of symptoms, pseudotumor cerebri, hirsutism, cutaneous striae, altered body composition, and psychosis. An alternate-day regimen may minimize these effects once the activity of the disease has been controlled. The effects on growth are equivocal because active disease itself may cause growth retardation, and some patients resume normal growth velocity during corticosteroid suppression of activity of disease. Other patients, whose disease is quiescent, may show catch-up growth velocity only after withdrawal of corticosteroids. A general principle is to use the least amount of corticosteroid necessary to control disease activity and allow growth and full function. Budesonide is a glucocorticoid with low systemic bioavailability that is active topically when administered as enema. The controlled ileal release preparation appears to be as effective as prednisone and more effective than mesalamine for the treatment of mild to moderate ileocolitis, with significantly fewer adverse effects occurring than with prednisone. Nonetheless, budesonide does not appear to be effective in sustaining a steroid- or surgically induced remission in adults, and chronic use has been associated with growth retardation in children.

Immunomodulating agents such as azathioprine and 6-mercaptopurine are useful in establishing or maintaining remission and in allowing reduction in corticosteroid dosage. Although bone marrow suppression and opportunistic infection are potential risks, current evidence from clinical trials suggests that these complications are rare and can be weighed against the known morbidity of chronic corticosteroid treatment. Lymphoid malignancy is a rare complication of immunosuppressive therapy. These agents seem to be useful in acute management, although several months of treatment may be required before full clinical efficacy is achieved in terms of corticosteroid-sparing or healing perianal disease and fistulas. A recent multicenter, randomized, placebo-controlled trial indicates that 6-mercaptopurine plus corticosteroids is more effective in achieving remission than are corticosteroids alone in children with moderate to severe CD. Treatment may be optimized and toxicity minimized by monitoring active metabolite 6-thioguanine and hepatotoxic metabolite 6-methyl-mercaptopurine levels after 2 to 4 weeks and at 6-month intervals. Complete blood counts and liver and pancreatic enzymes should be monitored after initiation of treatment and every 3 months.

Methotrexate given subcutaneously once weekly is effective in maintaining remission and as a steroid-sparing agent. Adverse effects of methotrexate include nausea, stomatitis (prevented by supplementing with folic acid), and pain at the injection site. Methotrexate has been associated rarely with interstitial pneumonitis and hepatic fibrosis. Widespread use in children with rheumatoid arthritis has provided evidence for a low risk of side effects.

Infliximab, a humanized mouse monoclonal anti-tumor necrosis factor-alpha (TNF-α) antibody, has been shown to be beneficial in treating patients with CD for the induction of remission, the maintenance of remission, and the treatment of fistulous disease. It is contraindicated in the setting of strictures that may progress with treatment. Infliximab is administered as an intravenous infusion at 5 mg/kg/dose, with three doses given in a 6-week period for induction of remission and every 6 to 8 weeks to maintain remission. Infusion reactions can occur and appear to be higher in patients who have developed antibodies to infliximab. Patients receiving immunosuppressive agents concurrently (such as azathioprine, 6-mercaptopurine, or methotrexate) appear to have less of a risk of generating antibodies to infliximab. The concurrent use of immunosuppressive agents in patients receiving maintenance infliximab is advocated. Other adverse effects include a serum sickness-like illness and reactivation of tuberculosis. A full assessment of risk of developing tuberculosis is mandatory prior to administering infliximab. As with any immunoglobulin infusion, anaphylaxis precautions should be in place.

Antimotility agents such as loperamide may be used to prolong intestinal transit time and facilitate fluid absorption, providing relief from diarrhea at night and at social functions. These agents should be used with caution and discontinued if symptoms of cramping, distention, or fever occur. Agents that bind bile acids, such as cholestyramine, may be useful in reducing the choleraic diarrhea that occurs after ileal dysfunction or resection. Probiotic therapy with lactobacillus has been studied and found ineffective in both promoting remission and preventing recurrence of disease after surgical "curative" resection of a diseased bowel segment has been performed. Other microbial mixtures eventually may prove to be helpful in modifying the luminal stimuli to the inflammatory response.

Nutritional Therapy

Because of the limitations and morbidity of medical treatment and the negative effect of CD on nutritional status, increased emphasis has been placed on nutritional rehabilitation and therapy. Optimal prospective management in patients with IBD should include regular assessment of growth and nutritional status. Data of value are height, weight, triceps skin fold, midarm muscle circumference, and serum levels of protein, albumin, and transferrin. A reduction in growth velocity over an interval of time may presage or contribute to an exacerbation of CD activity. Maintenance of optimal nutritional status with aggressive support of intake of energy and protein may prolong remission or allow corticosteroid treatment to be reduced. The goals of nutritional therapy in CD must include recovery of metabolic homeostasis by correcting specific nutrient deficits and replacing ongoing losses, provision of sufficient energy and protein for positive nitrogen balance (i.e., protein synthesis) and healing, and promotion of catch-up growth toward premorbid percentiles.

Deficiencies in iron, folate, or vitamin B_{12} should be corrected with appropriate supplements. Urinary methylmalonic aciduria or elevated serum homocysteine is a more sensitive indicator of vitamin B_{12} deficiency in patients with ileitis than are blood levels or macrocytosis. Magnesium depletion, better reflected in low urinary excretion after a challenge dose than in plasma concentration, should be corrected by parenteral magnesium sulfate. Low plasma zinc levels, low cholesterol, or low alkaline phosphatase suggests a zinc deficit caused by low dietary intake, redistribution to circulating hepatic pools as a consequence of chronic inflammation, or depletion caused by active mucosal inflammation and enteric losses. Treatment consists of supplements of zinc sulfate (1 to 2 mg/kg/day of elemental zinc). Oral protein and calorie supplements are prescribed to make up deficits revealed by dietary analysis of voluntary intake. The guidelines for supplementation suggest providing at least 140% of the recommended daily allowance for height and age for energy and protein intake. Continuous nocturnal nasogastric infusions given through a soft Silastic catheter may be necessary in patients who cannot voluntarily increase their intake. An elemental formula may need to be given if significant malabsorption, symptoms from partial obstruction, or a goal of reducing the antigen load to an inflamed colon are present, although nonelemental diets appear to have equal efficacy in achieving remission. A gastrostomy tube is an option for those without gastric involvement who cannot tolerate a nasogastric tube yet need chronic supplementation. In severe or complicated CD, when enteral feeding is not possible or bowel rest is desired, parenteral nutrition provided through a central venous catheter is necessary to achieve nutritional goals.

The optimal nutritional therapy serves as an adjunct to medical therapy in controlling symptoms and inducing remission. Short-term remissions have been achieved by aggressive enteral or parenteral nutritional support alone. Polymeric, elemental or semielemental formula diets all have been advocated as primary initial therapy to induce remission until immunosuppressive agents become effective. A meta-analysis of nine adult and pediatric studies revealed no difference in remission rates between polymeric diets and elemental formulas, with analysis of four trials showing a lower remission rate than that with steroids. Nutritional therapy alone has been variably effective in closing fistulas, but most eventually require surgery. After nutritional rehabilitation and remission of disease have been achieved, efforts should continue to ensure catch-up growth rates toward premorbid percentiles occur.

Surgery

Unlike UC, in which disease is limited to the colon and can be cured by total colectomy, no definitive surgical cure for CD exists. For these reasons and because of the high incidence of complications requiring repeat operation, surgery is reserved for the acute and chronic complications of CD refractory to medical or nutritional therapy (Box 353.3). Although failure of medical therapy to control symptoms or allow appropriate growth is the most common indication, remissions seem to be shorter in these cases than after resection for a specific complication presenting early in the course of the disease. Such indications include intestinal obstruction or stricture, abscess or perforation, fistula, uncontrolled hemorrhage, appendectomy, or rare toxic megacolon. Local resection is more successful for isolated small bowel and ileocecal disease than for colitis. Intractable colitis is managed by total proctocolectomy with ileostomy or segmental colectomy with anastomosis. The endorectal pull-through operation used for intractable UC never should be used for CD because of the risk of perirectal or pelvic abscess or perianal disease. Perianal abscesses often need draining with probing or injection of contrast to exclude underlying fistulas; proctectomy rarely is required to control perianal disease; and anal tags should not be excised. One series reported prolonged remission in 56% of pediatric patients with CD after resection. The remainder relapsed after 0.4 to 18.1 years of remission (median, 1.8 years).

BOX 353.3	Surgical Indications for Crohn Disease (N = 204)	
Failed medical therapy	22%	(44)
Intraabdominal abscess or perforation	7.5%	(15)
Obstruction	7.4%	(15)
Fistula	6.4%	(13)
Hemorrhage	2%	(4)
Appendectomy	1.5%	(3)
Total requiring surgery	46%	(94)

Reprinted with permission from Patel HI, Leichtner AM, Colodny AH, Shamburger RC. Surgery for Crohn disease in infants and children. *J Pediatr Surg* 1997;32:1063.

PROSPECTIVE MANAGEMENT AND PROGNOSIS

CD is a chronic incurable disease requiring careful surveillance, patient education, and expert management by a team consisting of a pediatrician, gastroenterologist, nutritionist, psychiatrist or psychologist, social worker, and nurse. An alliance with a pediatric surgeon familiar with IBD is essential for management of potential complications. The success of long-term management is determined in part by the degree to which the patient and family understand and participate in the treatment.

Nutritional status, growth, sexual maturation, psychosocial adjustment to disease, and compliance with therapy should be monitored as carefully as one monitors the clinical signs and symptoms of activity of disease. The frequency of follow-up depends on the course of disease activity, but intervals should be no longer than 6 months. Most children with CD can expect to live full, productive lives with good general health. The mortality rate is low, but the morbidity rate is high, especially in patients with colonic involvement. Fertility is unaffected in CD unless malnutrition or inflammatory damage to reproductive organs occurs. Activity of the disease often remains stable or improves during pregnancy, although an exacerbation may occur after delivery. The fetus seems to have no increased risk. The incidence of colorectal carcinoma is increased in Crohn colitis. Surveillance colonoscopy is mandatory in patients with duration of disease exceeding 10 years. Because adenocarcinoma may arise in strictured bowel, patients with persistent strictures must be observed closely in order to plan timely resection. The management of CD in children is complex, and the patient must adapt to the lifelong unpredictable nature of this disease, the morbidity associated with chronic medication and hospital visits, and the demands of adolescent development. A willingness to become active in the management of his or her condition and to work with the team involved in each case probably is the patient's best prognostic feature. The motivated patient and family will want to avail themselves of resources of the Crohns and Colitis Foundation of America and the North American Society for Gastroenterology, Hepatology, and Nutrition (see Chapter 352).

Suggested Readings

Baldassano R, Braegger CP, Escher JC, et al. Infliximab (REMICADE) therapy in the treatment of pediatric Crohn disease. *Am J Gastroenterol* 2003;98:833.

Bernstein L. Complications of inflammatory bowel disease. *Pract Gastroenterol* 1987;11:35.

Dady IM, Thomas AG, Miller V, Kelsey AJ. Inflammatory bowel disease in infancy: an increasing problem? *J Pediatr Gastroenteral Nutr* 1996;23:569.

D'Agata ID, Vanounou T, Seidman E. Mesalamine in pediatric inflammatory bowel disease: a 10-year experience. *Inflamm Bowel Dis* 1996;2:229.

Escher JC, Taminiau JA, Niewenhuis EE, et al. Treatment of inflammatory bowel disease in childhood: best available evidence. *Inflamm Bowel Dis* 2003;9:34.

Ferry GD, Buller HA, eds. Mechanisms of growth retardation, drug therapy, and nutritional support in pediatric inflammatory bowel disease: a workshop sponsored by the North American and European societies for pediatric gastroenterology and nutrition. *Inflamm Bowel Dis* 1995;1:313.

Hanauer SB, Sandborn W. Management of Crohn disease in adults. *Am J Gastroenterol* 2001;96:635.

Hyams, JS, Ferry GD, Mandel FS, et al. Development and validation of a pediatric Crohn disease activity index. *J Pediatr Gastroenterol Nutr* 1991;12:439.

Kelly DG, Fleming CR. Nutritional considerations in inflammatory bowel diseases. *Gastroenterol Clin North Am* 1995;24:597.

Kugathasan S, Judd R, Hoffmann R, et al. Epidemiologic and clinical characteristics of children with newly diagnosed inflammatory bowel disease in Wisconsin: a statewide population-based study. *J Pediatr* 2003;143:525.

Markowitz J, Daum F, Aiges M, et al. Perianal disease in children and adolescents with Crohn's disease. *Gastroenterology* 1984;86:829.

Markowitz J, Grancher K, Kohn N, et al. A multicenter trial of 6-mercaptopurine and prednisone in children with newly diagnosed Crohn disease. *Gastroenterology* 2000;119:895.

Odze R. Diagnostic problems and advances in inflammatory bowel disease. *Mod Pathol* 2003;16:347.

Patel HI, Leichtner AM, Colodny AH, Shamburger RC. Surgery for Crohn disease in infants and children. *J Pediatr Surg* 1997;32:1063.

Podolsky DK. Inflammatory bowel disease. *N Engl J Med* 2002;347:417.

Prantera C, Scribano M, Falasco G, et al. Ineffectiveness of probiotics in preventing recurrence after curative resection for Crohn disease: a randomized controlled trial with *Lactobacillus* GG. *Gut* 2002;51:405.

Price AB, Morson BC. Inflammatory bowel disease: the surgical pathology of Crohn disease and ulcerative colitis. *Hum Pathol* 1975;6:7.

Ruemmele FM, Targan SR, Levy G, et al. Diagnostic accuracy of serologic assays in pediatric inflammatory bowel disease. *Gastroenterology* 1998;115:822.

Seidman E, LeLeiko N, Ament M, et al. Nutritional issues in pediatric inflammatory bowel disease. *J Pediatr Gastroenterol Nutr* 1991;12:424.

Stein RB, Lichtenstein GR. Medical therapy for Crohn disease: the state of the art. *Surg Clin North Am* 2001;81:71.

Vermeire S, Joosens S, Peeters M, et al. Comparative study of ASCA (anti-*Saccharomyces cerevisiae* antibody) assays in inflammatory bowel disease. *Gastroenterology* 2001;120:827.

Zachos M, Tondeur M, Griffiths A. Enteral nutritional therapy for inducing remission of Crohn disease. *Cochrane Database Syst Rev* 2001;3:CD000542.

CHAPTER 354 ■ ANTIBIOTIC-ASSOCIATED DIARRHEA AND COLITIS

W. DANIEL JACKSON AND RICHARD J. GRAND

A spectrum of gastrointestinal disturbances ranging from transient diarrhea to frank pseudomembranous colitis has been associated with antibiotic treatment in adults and children. Diarrhea has been reported in 10% to 15% of patients treated with amoxicillin, amoxicillin/clavulanate and cefixime, and, less frequently, other antibiotics. Usually the diarrhea is uncomplicated and self-limited, resolving after discontinuation of the antibiotics. In some cases, the diarrhea may become fulminant, accompanied by signs of systemic illness, or progress to hemorrhage and protein-losing enteropathy, associated with the evolution of pseudomembranous colitis. Diarrhea or colitis may be associated with parenteral as well as enteral routes of antibiotic administration.

Studies have identified cytopathic toxins elaborated by *Clostridium difficile* as the cause of most cases of antibiotic-associated pseudomembranous colitis and most nosocomial cases of antibiotic-associated diarrhea. Other pathogens include *Salmonella, Clostridium perfringens, Staphylococcus aureus*, and *Candida albicans*, among organisms resistant to antibiotics used in treating another illness. Reduced fecal flora counts may alter fermentation rates for malabsorbed carbohydrates, fiber, and bile acids, causing osmotic and secretory stimulation of the colon. Antibiotics also may cause diarrhea via

motility effects such as erythromycin stimulation of motilin receptor-mediated, antroduodenal, migrating motor complexes, or clavulanate stimulation of small bowel motility.

EPIDEMIOLOGY

C. difficile is considered part of the normal flora of infants younger than 1 year and has been isolated from 25% to 50% of neonates and 45% of infants younger than the age of 12 months. Significant toxin B titers may be measured in 25% to 50% of asymptomatic infants. The reasons for asymptomatic carriage in infancy are unknown but may include the absence of toxin receptors, maternal antitoxin, or immature inflammatory responses. *C. difficile* colonization occurs in only 4% to 18% of older children and is isolated rarely from the stools of healthy adults, although it is a common vaginal species. In one study of self-limited mild diarrhea associated with antibiotic treatment in a group of very young children, most of whom were infants younger than 1 year of age, no correlation of symptoms with *C. difficile* colonization or toxin was found. Nonetheless, numerous cases of protracted diarrhea occur in infants in whom *C. difficile* is the only identified pathogen.

C. difficile is implicated most frequently in chronic or colitic diarrhea. In a study of adults with antibiotic-associated diarrheal states, 27% had demonstrable *C. difficile* toxin. In both adults and children, *C. difficile* colonization with toxin production is responsible for at least 95% of antibiotic-associated pseudomembranous colitis. Pseudomembranous colitis caused by *C. difficile* has been reported in settings in which antibiotics have not been used. In addition, rare reports exist of pseudomembranous enterocolitis attributed to other organisms, such as *C. perfringens* and *S. aureus*.

MICROBIOLOGY

C. difficile is a gram-positive, spore-forming obligate anaerobic bacillus resistant to most antibiotics. *C. difficile* is present in soil and can be cultured from hospital surfaces. Spores may be acquired directly from the environment or by fecal–oral transmission from colonized contacts. It may be isolated from blood agar culture and inoculated into chopped meat broth media made selective by the addition of cycloserine and cefoxitin, followed by subtyping for toxigenic strains. *C. difficile* produces two exotoxins implicated in the secretory and inflammatory features of enterocolitis. Toxin A is a potent enterotoxin and chemotactic agent causing inflammation and secretion of a hemorrhagic exudate in ligated rabbit ileal loops but having little effect on cultured fibroblast cells used for cytopathic assay. Conversely, toxin B is one of the most potent cytotoxins in cultured fibroblast assays, leading to its diagnostic utility. Although toxin B has been the traditional diagnostic marker, toxin A, usually elaborated in much greater amounts, has been considered the principal agent in the pathogenesis of *C. difficile*-related diarrhea and colitis. However, the clinical importance of toxin B is supported by the discovery of pathogenic strains of *C. difficile* in both animal and human hosts that produce toxin B without producing toxin A and by some evidence that the two toxins may act synergistically.

PATHOGENESIS

The indigenous, mixed bowel flora form an important host defense mechanism, limiting proliferation and colonization of potential bacterial pathogens. The composition of the bowel flora is kept remarkably constant with a thousandfold predominance of anaerobic bacteria, despite a great variety of dietary and physiologic changes. The ability of the indigenous flora to limit proliferation or exclude colonization of pathogenic bacteria is called *colonization resistance* and is important in protecting the host at the gut interface with the environment.

Oral or intravenous antibiotic agents that produce fecal levels sufficient to alter the bowel flora, particularly antibiotics active against the indigenous anaerobic population, reduce the colonization resistance of the intestinal lumen to *C. difficile*. *C. difficile* may be harbored normally in limited numbers or may be introduced from environmental reservoirs, vaginal sources, other colonized contacts, or environmental surfaces. The relative resistance of *C. difficile* to most conventional antibiotics allows it to proliferate and elaborate its cytopathic enterotoxins associated with invasiveness, inflammation, and secretion. The superficial inflammation may progress to mucosal necrosis and exudation of protein and leukocytes, continuing until the conditions are poor for *C. difficile* proliferation because of competition with other bowel flora or the introduction of specific antibiotic therapy. Because the toxins A and B are responsible for the inflammation, agents that bind or eliminate toxins, such as cholestyramine or other resins, may have some efficacy. Gastric acid suppression, especially by potent proton

pump inhibitors, has been implicated as a risk factor for *C. difficile*-related diarrhea in adults. The elderly and neonates may have attenuated gut flora and lower colonization resistance, leading to increased susceptibility to colonization.

The mechanism of toxin A-mediated inflammation begins with receptor binding and internalization by colonocytes, followed promptly by localization in mitochondria causing cessation of production of adenosine 5′-triphosphate (ATP) and generation of reactive oxygen species. Cytoskeletal damage related to Rho protein glucosylation, observed for both toxins A and B, includes disruption of intercellular tight junctions in colonic epithelium, increasing permeability and leading to cell injury. The severe inflammatory response is mediated by toxin A-induced cytokine release, stimulation of enteric sensory neurons to release substance P, calcitonin gene–related peptide, and neurotensin, amplifying mast cell and macrophage activity. A similar mechanism is suspected for the cytopathic effects of the structurally similar toxin B. These processes account for the intense secretory response, inflammation, and necrosis of colonic epithelium exposed to *C. difficile* toxins.

CLINICAL PRESENTATION

Diarrhea is a common, often expected, side effect of antibiotic treatment in children and usually is a self-limited, dose-related, and mild consequence, resolving after the course of treatment is completed. These uncomplicated sporadic cases are unlikely to be caused by *C. difficile* proliferation. In a subset of patients, however, a severe chronic enterocolitis may develop, with profuse watery diarrhea beginning 4 to 10 days after initiation or as late as 4 weeks after discontinuation of antibiotic treatment. The diarrhea may be associated with dehydration, electrolyte depletion, vomiting, and abdominal distention. Hypokalemia, hypoalbuminemia, and metabolic acidosis may occur. The onset of fever, crampy abdominal pain, tenesmus or urgency, and neutrophilic leukocytosis, with or without hematochezia, suggests inflammation of the colon. Significant hypoproteinemia, edema, ascites, and pleural effusion complicate the most severe cases of pseudomembranous colitis and are ominous signs. Dilation of the colon may herald toxic megacolon. The risks of perforation, peritonitis, and sepsis render this outcome a medical and surgical emergency.

Another pattern of antibiotic-associated enterocolitis is diarrhea of variable severity without evolution of signs of frank colitis. The diagnosis in this situation may be delayed for months until colitis develops or *C. difficile* is considered and the toxin assay is performed. Despite lack of clinical signs of overt pseudomembranous colitis, focal colitis may be found on colonoscopy. Chronic *C. difficile* diarrhea may resemble other malabsorptive syndromes such as celiac disease or Crohn disease and contribute to growth failure in children.

Rarely, patients have presented with massive stool retention and abdominal distention apparently related to colonic dysmotility in the presence of proliferation of *C. difficile* and production of toxin and responding to treatment directed against *C. difficile*.

Most cases of antibiotic-associated enterocolitis occur in patients without underlying gastrointestinal disorders who are treated with antibiotics for other conditions (e.g., respiratory illness, often with questionable indication) or receive short-term preoperative antibiotics. Almost all classes of antibiotics have been implicated in the cause of *C. difficile* enterocolitis, but the most commonly cited ones are ampicillin and amoxicillin, clindamycin, and cephalosporins, all potent in suppressing normal bowel anaerobic flora but with relatively little activity against *C. difficile*. The prevalence of ampicillin- and cephalosporin-associated enterocolitis in children reflects the prevalence of administration of these drugs by pediatricians.

Clindamycin, administered relatively infrequently to children, is associated with diarrhea and enterocolitis in children less frequently than it is in adults. Other antibiotics implicated include penicillins, sulfonamides, trimethoprim-sulfamethoxazole, and quinolones. The incidence of antibiotic-associated enterocolitis has not been correlated with specific antibiotic combinations or dosage, although an animal model suggests that duration of therapy is most important.

DIAGNOSIS

C. difficile-associated enterocolitis should be suspected in any patient with the acute onset of severe diarrhea or colitis with concomitant or prior oral or intravenous antibiotic treatment; diarrhea beginning after the third hospital day; chronic diarrhea of unknown cause, with or without a history of prior antibiotic treatment; or an exacerbation of suspected or previously documented inflammatory bowel disease (Box 354.1).

In addition to delineating antibiotic treatment, the history should elicit details regarding fever, vomiting, pain, tenesmus, urgency, and rectal bleeding. Physical examination should assess hydration status, hemodynamic stability, and abdominal tenderness or distention, the last suggesting toxic dilation. Laboratory findings typically show a neutrophilic leukocytosis, which can be impressive (greater than 30,000/μL) in pseudomembranous colitis or minimal in mild, chronic *C. difficile*–induced diarrhea. Hypoproteinemia is a common finding in pseudomembranous enterocolitis but rare in chronic diarrhea. Examination of stool for occult blood and leukocytes may confirm the presence of colitis. Routine stool cultures for *Salmonella, Shigella, Campylobacter,* toxigenic *Escherichia coli,* and *Yersinia* spp., as well as examination for parasites, should exclude other pathogens. Serology for *Entamoeba histolytica* or *Yersinia enterocolitica* may be considered. Few microbiological laboratories will isolate *C. difficile.*

The most sensitive and specific test for *C. difficile* disease is the cytotoxic assay for toxin B in serially diluted stool samples, measuring cytopathic effects in cultured fibroblasts. The cytopathic activity is specifically neutralized by an antitoxin derived from another *Clostridium* species, *C. sordellii.* After infancy, the presence of toxin B usually is associated with clinical disease, although cytotoxic titers do not correlate with severity. Unfortunately, the assay requires 18 to 24 hours and laboratory tissue culture technology. Most efforts have been directed toward the development of a rapid, sensitive, and specific assay for toxin A. Latex agglutination assays have proved to be too low in specificity and sensitivity for clinical reliability. A highly sensitive and specific enzyme-linked immunoassay to toxin A has become standard in most laboratories and can produce results within several hours. Newer immunoassays for both toxins A and B are available. Because many hospital laboratories no longer provide the more specific and sensitive yet cumbersome cytotoxin B assay, and some strains of *C. difficile* do not elaborate toxin A, some false-negative assays will occur. In addition, false-positive toxin A determinations, with negative cytotoxin assays and cultures, have occurred in several patients with exacerbations of inflammatory bowel disease. The predictive value of cytotoxin assays in infants appears to be quite low given the frequency with which *C. difficile* colonization and cytotoxin can be identified in asymptomatic neonates and infants. Hypogammaglobulinemia may increase risks of pathogenicity in these infants. Flat and upright abdominal radiography may show signs of ileus with small bowel dilatation and air-fluid levels but are nonspecific. Barium enema examination may show edema, ulcerations, and "thumb printing" or nodular contour defects caused by edema and pseudomembranes, but this study is unnecessary for establishing the diagnosis and increases the risk of bowel perforation occurring. Sigmoidoscopy or colonoscopy may reveal characteristic findings of discrete or confluent pseudomembranous inflammation of the rectum and colon and confirm the diagnosis (Figs. 354.1 and 354.2). Disease may occur more proximally in the presence of an unimpressive sigmoidoscopic examination. Colonoscopy usually is negative in cases of chronic diarrhea that show no other signs of colitis, although biopsies may show signs of focal inflammation. The availability of rapid *C. difficile* toxin assays renders establishing a diagnosis by sigmoidoscopy unnecessary except in severe or equivocal cases in which immediate treatment is necessary.

| **BOX 354.1** | Diagnostic Strategy for Antibiotic Associated Diarrhea in Children |

1. Test patients at risk for *Clostridium difficile* enterocolitis:
   Persistent, fulminant, or secretory diarrhea
   Evidence of colitis: hematochezia, fecal leukocytes, hypoalbuminemia
   Antibiotic exposure regardless of duration, timing, or agents
   Onset after third day of hospitalization
   Inflammatory bowel disease, immunosuppression, cystic fibrosis
2. Exclude non-*C. difficile* pathogens if <u>third</u> hospital day or earlier.
3. Enzyme immunoassays for both toxins A and B on diarrheal stool.
4. Cytotoxin assay for toxin B.
5. Abdominal radiographs for abdominal tenderness or distention.
6. Treatment trial of metronidazole.
7. Sigmoidoscopy and biopsy for atypical or unresponsive cases.

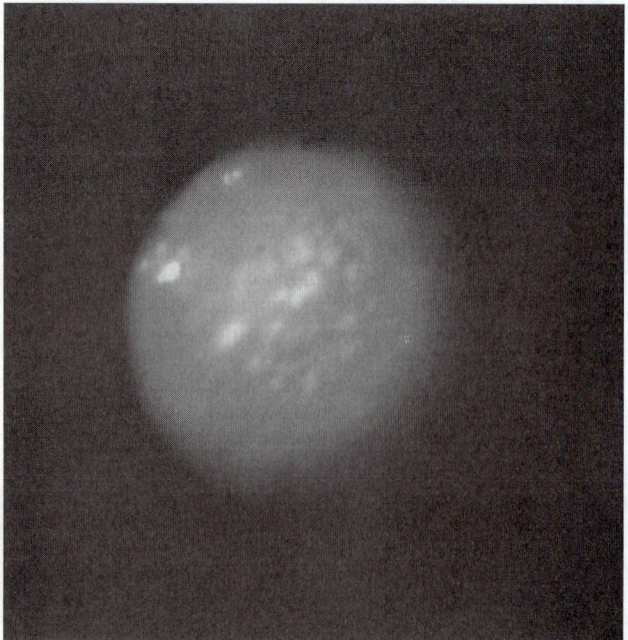

FIGURE 354.1. Colonoscopic photograph of an array of early purulent eruptions in *Clostridium difficile* colitis.

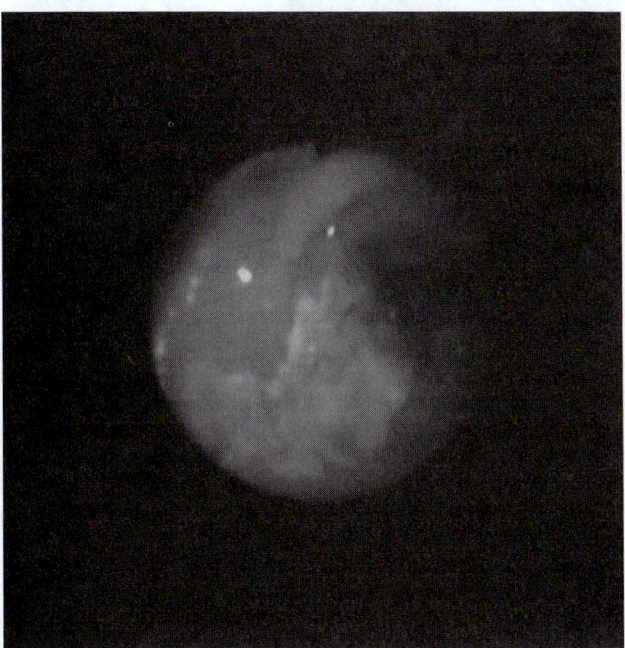

FIGURE 354.2. Colonoscopic photograph of a confluent pseudomembrane in *Clostridium difficile* colitis.

DIFFERENTIAL DIAGNOSIS

Chronic diarrhea may be caused by a variety of viral and bacterial pathogens. Susceptibility to the more common enteric bacterial pathogens, *Shigella, Salmonella, Campylobacter, E. coli,* and *Yersinia,* also is increased in the host whose intestinal flora have been altered or eradicated by broad-spectrum antibiotic treatment. Cytomegalovirus, *Entamoeba histolytica, Blastocystis hominis,* and other pathogens may cause chronic diarrheal states and focal colitis. Lactose intolerance, giardiasis, celiac disease, cystic fibrosis, acquired immunodeficiency, and other disorders associated with malabsorption should be entertained in the differential diagnosis of chronic diarrhea. Patients with cystic fibrosis who routinely receive prolonged courses of broad-spectrum antibiotics in the hospital, in conjunction with maldigestion providing substrate for colonic bacterial fermentation, are at greater risk for having colonization with *C. difficile.*

Pseudomembranous colitis unassociated with antibiotic treatment has been observed in association with necrotizing enterocolitis of neonates, diversion colitis developing after bowel surgery, Hirschsprung enterocolitis, uremic colitis, hemolytic-uremic syndrome, congenital heart disease with bowel ischemia related to congestive heart failure, and inflammatory bowel disease. Inflammatory bowel disease may present similarly or may be complicated by *C. difficile* enterocolitis. Patients with IBD appear to be more susceptible to colonization by *C. difficile* than are healthy hosts. The sigmoidoscopic appearance may resemble either Crohn disease or ulcerative colitis. *C. difficile* infection also has been suggested but not proved to be a potentiating factor in the pathogenesis of inflammatory bowel disease.

PATHOLOGY

Pseudomembranous colitis is a term denoting the characteristic endoscopic and pathologic features found in antibiotic-associated colitis. The rectal mucosa is erythematous and friable with small (less than 5 mm), raised, yellowish plaques that may be discrete or confluent. Histologically, these lesions are superficial mucosal erosions surmounted by a tenacious pseudomembrane consisting of fibrin, mucus, polymorphonuclear leukocytes, and necrotic epithelium. The submucosa is edematous with acute and chronic inflammatory infiltrates and mucus-congested glands and goblet cells. Cryptitis and crypt abscesses may be present. However, chronic features of crypt architectural distortion, including branching, and fibrosis are atypical and raise concern for the presence of underlying chronic inflammatory bowel disease. Although typically involved in pseudomembranous colitis, the rectum may be spared. Rare cases in which significant disease was recognized only on small bowel biopsy or colonoscopy to the proximal colon have been reported.

THERAPY

Hemodynamic homeostasis should be established using vigorous rehydration, correction of electrolyte disturbances, and albumin infusions as indicated by clinical findings, such as orthostasis, dehydration, and edema (Box 354.2). If possible, antibiotics should be discontinued or changed to an intravenous preparation known to be associated less frequently with anaerobic bacterial suppression and pseudomembranous colitis. Antimotility agents such as diphenoxylate hydrochloride with atropine sulfate (Lomotil), paregoric, or loperamide should be discontinued because of the risk of stasis and the induction of toxic megacolon. Enteric hygienic precautions should be instituted to prevent the spread of *C. difficile* to other patients or family members at risk, especially those being treated with antibiotics.

After the diagnosis is supported sufficiently by clinical and sigmoidoscopy findings or confirmed by demonstration of *C. difficile* toxin, oral metronidazole, administered as 30 mg/kg/day in four divided doses, up to 500 mg per dose, should be administered for 7 to 10 days. An alternative for patients intolerant of metronidazole or with refractory disease or apparent bacterial resistance is oral vancomycin, administered as 40 mg/kg/day in four divided doses, up to 250 mg per dose, for 7 to 10 days. Metronidazole and vancomycin are equally

---

BOX 354.2	**Therapeutic Strategy for Suspected *Clostridium difficile* Enterocolitis in Children**

1. Ensure hemodynamic homeostasis.
2. Discontinue antibiotics or substitute more selective or intravenous alternative.
3. Discontinue antimotility agents.
4. Institute enteric precautions.
5. Administer pharmacologic agents:
   Metronidazole: 30 mg/kg/day in four divided doses for 7–10 days
   Vancomycin: 40 mg/kg/day in four divided doses for 7–10 days
   Intravenous (if unable to tolerate oral): metronidazole, 30 mg/kg/day in divided doses q6h
6. Monitor clinical response. Immediate posttreatment testing is not advised.
7. Management of relapse:
   Repeat course of antibiotic.
   Investigate and eliminate sources of reinfection.
   Give prolonged course of antibiotic and/or addition of probiotics.
   Exclude chronic inflammatory bowel disease.

efficacious against *C. difficile*, with clinical response expected to be achieved in 2 to 10 days. The advantages of metronidazole include its minimal suppression of normal aerobic fecal flora, avoidance of selection for vancomycin-resistant *Enterococcus* and other organisms, and low cost. The rate of relapse also may be lower, based on its limited suppression of aerobic fecal flora, allowing recovery of colonization resistance. Because biliary excretion and mucosal exudation lead to bactericidal fecal drug levels, intravenous metronidazole also is effective in patients who cannot receive oral medication because of ileus or surgery. Parenteral vancomycin does not produce effective intraluminal levels and is not recommended. Bacitracin, miconazole, and tetracycline have been used successfully to eradicate *C. difficile* but have no advantages over metronidazole in efficacy or cost. Strategies to alter the colonic flora by introducing probiotics to restore colonization resistance have been proposed. Several randomized, double-blind controlled trials have shown some efficacy of *Saccharomyces boulardii* yeast and several *Lactobacillus* species in reducing the incidence of antibiotic-associated diarrhea, including *C. difficile*-related diarrhea.

Relapses associated with the reappearance of symptoms and production of toxins are relatively common occurrences and may occur after apparent eradication of *C. difficile* toxin in as many as 14% of patients within 21 days after receiving vancomycin treatment of pseudomembranous colitis and in as many as 67% of children with chronic diarrhea. *C. difficile* may be cultured from the stools of some patients who are toxin-free and asymptomatic after receiving treatment. Toxin B may be detectable in a subset of patients after clinical resolution has been achieved but does not imply or predict relapse. Although some patients suffer recurrent relapses with any antibiotic treatment, others may harbor the organism without disease during subsequent antibiotic treatment. Multiple relapses warrant performing evaluation for underlying chronic IBD. The reasons for variable resistance to antibiotic-associated enterocolitis undoubtedly are complex but probably are related to host factors such as the composition of the indigenous bowel flora, transit time, presence of receptors for toxins, and immunologic defenses. Bacterial spores may survive therapy and repopulate the colon, or organisms may be acquired from environmental exposures. Clusters of occurrence in hospital settings have been reported directly from patient contact and indirectly from environmental surfaces. Family and day-care contacts, including adults, frequently harbor the organism and may be sources of reinfection. *C. difficile* also is part of the normal vaginal flora, which may account for the high rates of colonization in neonates.

Mild diarrheal relapses may resolve spontaneously and do not warrant initiating treatment. Although metronidazole-resistant *C. difficile* strains have been isolated, development of resistance usually is not the cause of relapse. Most relapses respond to a second course of metronidazole or vancomycin. Multiple relapses may require strategies of extending the course of treatment to 3 weeks, gradually tapering the frequency of doses over additional weeks to allow reestablishment of normal colonic flora, or intermittent dosing every other day to eliminate newly active spores. Rifampin, bacitracin, oral intravenous immune globulin, cholestyramine, *S. boulardii*, or *Lactobacillus* spp. each has been reported to be effective in some refractory cases.

PREVENTION

Prophylactic administration of broad-spectrum antibiotics, particularly antibiotics such as ampicillin or amoxicillin com-

monly implicated in *C. difficile*–associated enterocolitis, should be done only when strictly indicated. The risk of suppression of bowel flora and increased susceptibility to *C. difficile* enterocolitis should be weighed in the selection of antibiotic treatment. The prevalence of nosocomial contamination and infection within the hospital mandates enforcement of scrupulous hand washing and universal enteric hygiene for all patients. Hospitalized patients with documented disease should be isolated on a strict basis from other susceptible antibiotic-treated patients, and hospital rooms should be disinfected thoroughly. Asymptomatic family contacts may be screened and treated in cases of recurrent relapses, but no evidence suggests that vancomycin or metronidazole can eliminate the carrier state. Altering bowel flora with probiotics such as the yeast *S. boulardii* or *Lactobacillus* spp. may serve as an adjunct to therapy for relapses or for prevention. A prophylactic role of prebiotics such as dietary supplementation with soluble fiber or oligopolysaccharides has not been established.

PROGNOSIS

Before pseudomembranous colitis or chronic antibiotic-associated diarrhea was recognized as being associated with the toxins of *C. difficile*, the mortality rate from pseudomembranous colitis in children was as high as 28%. The availability of safe and efficacious treatment, coupled with the recognition of the spectrum of presentation of antibiotic-associated enterocolitis and its propensity for relapse, has improved the prognosis dramatically, and severe complications and death are now rare occurrences.

Suggested Readings

Bartlett JG. Antibiotic-associated diarrhea. *N Engl J Med* 2002;346:334.

Bolton RP, Tait SK, Dear PR, Losowsky MS. Asymptomatic neonatal colonisation by Clostridium difficile. *Arch Dis Child* 1984;59:466.

Borriello SP. Pathogenesis of *Clostridium difficile* infection. *J Antimicrob Chemotherapy* 1998;41:13.

Chang T, Gorbach SL. Rapid identification of *Clostridium difficile* by toxin detection. *J Clin Microbiol* 1982;15:465.

Cremonini F, Di Caro S, Santarelli L, et al. Probiotics in antibiotic-associated diarrhoea. *Dig Liver Dis* 2002;34:S78.

Farrell RJ, LaMont JT. Pathogenesis and clinical manifestations of *Clostridium difficile* diarrhea and colitis. *Curr Top Microbiol Immunol* 2000;250:109.

Gryboski JD. *Clostridium difficile* in inflammatory bowel disease relapse. *J Pediatr Gastroenterol Nutr* 1991;13:39.

Hentges DJ. The protective function of the indigenous intestinal flora. *Pediatr Infect Dis* 1986;5:S17.

Kader HA, Piccoli DA, Jawad AF, et al. Single toxin detection is inadequate to diagnose *Clostridium difficile* diarrhea in pediatric patients. *Gastroenterology* 1998;115:1329.

Kelly CP, Pothoulakis C, LaMont JT. *Clostridium difficile* colitis. *N Engl J Med* 1994;330:257.

Kim K, Dupont HL, Pickering LK. Outbreak of diarrhea associated with *Clostridium difficile* and its toxin in day-care centers: evidence of person-to-person spread. *J Pediatr* 1983;102:376.

Pothoulakis C, Lamont JT. Microbes and microbial toxins: paradigms for microbial-mucosal interactions; II. The integrated response of the intestine to *Clostridium difficile* toxins. *Am J Physiol Gastrointest Liver Physiol* 2001;280:G178.

Savidge TC, Pan WH, Newman P, et al. *Clostridium difficile* toxin B is an inflammatory enterotoxin in human intestine. *Gastroenterology* 2003;125:413.

Sutphen JL, Grand RJ, Flores A, et al. Chronic diarrhea associated with *Clostridium difficile* in children. *Am J Dis Child* 1983;137:275.

Tedesco FJ. Antibiotic-associated pseudomembranous colitis with negative proctosigmoidoscopy examination. *Gastroenterology* 1979;77:295.

Thompson CM, Gilligan PH, Fisher MC, Long SS. *Clostridium difficile* cytotoxin in the pediatric population. *Am J Dis Child* 1983;137:271.

Tucker KD, Carrig PE, Wilkins TD. Toxin A of *Clostridium difficile* is a potent cytotoxin. *J Clin Microbiol* 1990;28:869.

CHAPTER 355 ■ CHRONIC RECURRENT ABDOMINAL PAIN

WILLIAM J. KLISH

Chronic recurrent abdominal pain undoubtedly is the most frustrating problem a pediatrician must manage. It also is a common occurrence. Unless the diagnosis is dealt with in a positive manner and the patient's parents develop confidence in that diagnosis, they will seek medical advice constantly and will frequently shop for answers.

The symptom of abdominal pain is frightening to the average parent. It conjures up images of life-threatening problems such as appendicitis or obstruction. Many children who experience chronic recurrent abdominal pain of any cause obviously are in great discomfort. They grip their stomachs, frequently become pale, and are not interested in engaging in play. If the physician casually writes off the symptom as functional or psychological, he or she will lose the confidence of the parents, who observe their child in pain and know that the symptom is not "in the child's head." Physicians themselves frequently worry about missing a diagnosis in these cases, and this self-doubt may be conveyed subtly to the parents.

The physician must approach the diagnosis of chronic recurrent abdominal pain with confidence. The pediatrician must never doubt that the child is in actual pain and must build a trusting relationship with the parents. He or she should discuss the differential diagnosis with the parents at the beginning and should rule out potential diagnoses in a logical manner. If the diagnosis of functional pain is made, the pediatrician should discuss it at length, emphasizing that the pain is not life-threatening. These measures usually allay the fears of the parents sufficiently that they can deal with the symptom effectively. Occasionally, the child's fear of going to school or some other phobia may be so deep-seated that removal of the pain as a defense mechanism may lead to its replacement with something else. These children should be referred for psychological therapy.

PATHOGENESIS OF VISCERAL PAIN

When Aristotle described the five senses, he omitted the sensation of pain. The ancient Greeks considered pain to be an emotion or something unpleasant, the opposite of pleasure. For centuries, arguments have raged over whether pain is a separate, distinct sensation or a psychological reaction to a complex feeling. Even though perception of pain now is assigned to a specific sensory faculty, the chronic recurrent abdominal pain of childhood, more than any other form of pain, exemplifies this historical uncertainty.

Receptors for transmitting pain are described morphologically as undifferentiated nerve endings. They can be stimulated by mechanical, chemical, or thermal stimuli. In the case of the viscera, these receptors are most sensitive to mechanical stimuli. Receptor substance is contained within vesicles at the nerve ending and is released on stimulation, thus causing depolarization of the nerve when it combines with receptors on the external surface. This action is terminated by a specific hydrolytic enzyme surrounding the nerve terminal. If severe trauma to tissue occurs, this hydrolytic enzyme may be destroyed, resulting in prolonged depolarization of the nerve cells by the receptor substance and persistent pain. One of the receptor substances thought to be active in pain fibers is substance P, an 11-amino acid peptide, but other substances also have been identified.

The afferent nerve fibers involved in the transmission of pain follow a course through the sympathetic ganglion chain and enter the dorsal horn of the spinal cord, where they synapse. Afferents from the viscera enter the dorsal horn along with afferents from cutaneous structures of the corresponding dermatome. These two sources of nerve impulses overlap at the synaptic junctions and give rise to the phenomenon of referred pain. As the input from visceral structures increases, more impulses are received by the fibers, which share their input between visceral and cutaneous structures. This input eventually is perceived by the brain as arising from cutaneous structures.

Another mechanism that may play a role in the cutaneous localization of visceral pain is the peritoneocutaneous reflex of Morley. Certain somatic nerve endings in the parietal peritoneum may extend into the roots of the mesentery and posterior portion of the diaphragm. When these nerves are stimulated, pain is referred to the corresponding skin area. This reflex usually is the result of inflammation from peritonitis.

Neurons that synapse with afferents from the viscera in the dorsal horn of the spinal cord cross to the opposite side and ascend through the lateral spinothalamic tract to the thalamus. A third neuron then carries the sensation by means of the internal capsule to the cerebral cortex.

A satisfactory theory of pain must account for the evidence that local factors in the spinal cord, and events occurring in the cerebral cortex (e.g., anxiety) may influence the perception or threshold of pain. The gate theory is an attempt to explain this phenomenon. It proposes that pain fibers are subject to the influence of larger-diameter afferents that originate in the substantia gelatinosa of the spinal cord. These neurons interact through an axoaxonic synapse that, under normal conditions, is dominant, and the gate is closed. As excitation from the viscera increases, this modulating effect is overcome, and pain is felt. Feedback from the brain may alter the transmission from this interneuron. In functional abdominal pain, anxiety may decrease the modulating effect to the point that normal intestinal sensations are perceived as pain. The interneuronal receptors in the system are opiate receptors that normally are activated by the endogenously produced opiates, enkephalins, and endorphins.

Under normal circumstances, the only stimulus that is adequate to initiate pure visceral pain is increased intravisceral pressure caused by stretching, distention, or contraction of the viscus. Inflammation decreases the visceral threshold for pain so sensations from temperature or chemical irritants may be felt. With the exception of colonic pain, true visceral pain is felt at or near the midline of the body; colonic pain tends to be referred to the area directly above the point of stimulation.

Pain referred away from the midline suggests several possibilities: inflammation of a viscus rather than a simple disturbance of motor function, which lowers the pain threshold and gives rise to referred pain; a stimulus of extreme severity, such as the passage of a calculus, which refers pain because of its high-intensity stimulus; or extension of the disease process to the peritoneum, which stimulates somatic nerve endings.

DIFFERENTIAL DIAGNOSIS

Most children who have chronic recurrent abdominal pain unassociated with other significant symptoms have functional pain. However, because no specific diagnostic test is available, this diagnosis is one of exclusion. Discussing this diagnosis with the parents before making an evaluation is important, so if other potential diagnoses are excluded, the parents do not attribute the diagnosis of functional pain to the physician's inability to diagnose something more serious.

The common entities that cause chronic recurrent abdominal pain of childhood are listed in Box 355.1 in their approximate order of frequency. Most of these diagnoses can be screened for without having to perform a multitude of laboratory and radiographic examinations.

Lactose intolerance probably is the second most common cause of abdominal pain in children. If a child is programmed genetically to become lactase-deficient, the activity of this enzyme gradually begins to decrease when that child is approximately 4 to 6 years of age. If drinking milk continues at a constant rate, the enzyme activity eventually will not be sufficient to hydrolyze the entire amount of lactose ingested; as a result, some lactose spills into the distal small bowel and colon, where it is fermented by bacteria, and gases such as hydrogen and carbon dioxide are produced. This gas production, if great enough, may cause intestinal dilatation and pain. As the syndrome progresses, diarrhea results from the osmotic effect of the unabsorbed sugar and its fermentative products. Early in the development of lactose intolerance, pain may be the sole symptom.

Diagnosing lactose intolerance as a cause of abdominal pain sometimes is difficult because the laboratory tests (e.g., breath hydrogen production, lactose tolerance test) tend to be too sensitive, and the condition is overdiagnosed as a result. Establishing cause and effect from these tests is difficult. Dietary restriction may be the easiest way to establish lactose intolerance as a cause of abdominal pain. The child should be given a lactose-free diet for approximately 2 weeks. If the abdominal pain disappears, the diagnosis can be suspected. However,

it should be confirmed by giving the child lactose again and observing for exacerbation of symptoms. This cycle should be completed twice to ensure that lactose intolerance is present. After the diagnosis is established, the parents can be counseled intelligently. Because lactose intolerance is a dose-related phenomenon, most children can tolerate some lactose-containing foods. Low-lactose dairy products (e.g., cheese) should be reintroduced as tolerated, which would preclude the need for supplementation of calcium.

Children with simple constipation frequently complain of abdominal pain. Parents and children do not make the association between the number of bowel movements and the pain. Unless the physician asks specifically about the frequency of bowel movements, the diagnosis may go unrecognized for a long time. Rectal examination is helpful in establishing this diagnosis, but a trial of a mild stimulant may be necessary to establish the cause.

Musculoskeletal pain arising from the abdominal muscles is a diagnosis that can be overlooked easily. School-aged children frequently are engaged in competitive sports and are subjected to intensive exercise training programs. These exercises result in strained muscles and chronic myositis of specific muscle bundles. The pain usually is described as sharp or knifelike and may be triggered by various activities or body positions. It usually is located at or near the insertion of the rectus or oblique muscles into the costal margin or iliac crest. Palpating along these insertions with a fair degree of pressure may locate a trigger point that reproduces the pain and establishes the diagnosis. If the abdominal muscles are tightened during the physical examination and the pain still is reproduced by palpation, the origin undoubtedly is musculoskeletal.

Occasionally, intestinal parasites (e.g., *Giardia*, pinworms) may cause only abdominal pain. Stool should be examined for ova and parasites as part of the evaluation of all children with this problem.

Inflammatory bowel disease, *Helicobacter pylori* gastritis, and peptic ulcers usually cause symptoms sufficient to make their diagnosis apparent. However, an occasional patient may complain initially of nonspecific abdominal pain and nothing else. A complete blood count, reticulocyte count, sedimentation rate, *H. pylori* antibody test, and stool guaiac test are helpful for screening for these diagnoses. If the child is anemic, has an elevated reticulocyte count or positive results on the stool guaiac test, or has an elevated sedimentation rate or *H. pylori* antibody, additional studies (e.g., endoscopy, radiographic examinations) should be obtained.

Many other diseases can cause abdominal pain in children, but most of the other diagnoses are associated with other symptoms. If the child complains only of abdominal pain and the results of all the tests suggested earlier are negative, the physician should feel comfortable in making the diagnosis of functional abdominal pain.

BOX 355.1	**Common Entities that Cause Chronic Recurrent Abdominal Pain**

Functional abdominal pain
Lactose intolerance
Simple constipation
Musculoskeletal pain
Parasitic infection
Reflux esophagitis
Helicobacter pylori gastritis
Peptic ulcer disease
Mesenteric lymphadenopathy
Inflammatory bowel disease

TREATMENT

The treatments for most of the diagnoses previously discussed are obvious. Lactose intolerance requires restriction of dairy products in the diet, and simple constipation is treated best by a bulk agent (e.g., psyllium) or a mild stimulant (e.g., senna). Salicylate used for 1 week as an antiinflammatory agent frequently is enough to allow musculoskeletal pain to subside.

If the diagnosis of functional abdominal pain is made, discussing this diagnosis with the parents in the same manner as organic disease is helpful. The physician must convey the message that the pain is real but is not caused by a process that will become progressively worse and threaten the life of the child. The analogy of a headache in an adult is useful. The pain of a headache is real, but it is treated only as pain and, under normal circumstances, it is not allowed to interfere with daily responsibilities. A child's responsibility is to go to school, and pain should not prevent him or her doing so. If the pain is severe, it could be treated with medications, such as acetaminophen. Antimotility agents usually are ineffective. Using a hot pad or hot water bottle as a counterirritant sometimes is helpful. Above all, the physician should instill confidence in parents that the pain is not threatening to their child's well-being and will disappear as the child matures.

Suggested Readings

Alfven G. One hundred cases of recurrent abdominal pain in children: diagnostic procedures and criteria for a psychosomatic diagnosis. *Acta Paediatr* 2003;92:43.

Bishop B. Pain: its physiology and rationale for management. *Phys Ther* 1980; 60:13.

Bowsher D. Pain pathways and mechanisms. *Anesthesia* 1978;30:935.

Klish WJ. Visceral pain. In: Chey WY, ed. *Functional disorders of the digestive tract.* New York: Raven, 1983:237.

Moir CR. Abdominal pain in infants and children. *Mayo Clin Proc* 1996;71:984.

Ness TJ, Gebhart GF. Visceral pain: a review of experimental studies. *Pain* 1990;41:167.

Perquin CW, Hazebroek-Kampschreur AA, Hunfeld JA, et al. Pain in children and adolescents: a common experience. *Pain* 2000;87:51.

Vayner N, Coret A, Polliack G, et al. Mesenteric lymphadenopathy in children examined by US for chronic and/or recurrent abdominal pain. *Pediatr Radiol* 2003;33:864.

Walker LS, Garber J, Greene JW. Somatic complaints in pediatric patients: a prospective study of the role of negative life events, child social and academic competence, and parental somatic symptoms. *J Consult Clin Psychol* 1994;62:1213.

Zeiter DK, Hyams JS. Clinical aspects of recurrent abdominal pain. *Pediatr Ann* 2001;30:17.

CHAPTER 356 ■ PROTEIN-LOSING ENTEROPATHY

DAN W. THOMAS AND FRANK R. SINATRA

Numerous disorders result in excessive loss of serum proteins from the gastrointestinal (GI) tract. This form of intestinal dysfunction is called *protein-losing enteropathy* (PLE). The presence of PLE indicates an underlying GI disturbance, but it is not pathognomonic of a specific disorder. The maladies frequently associated with PLE in children are listed in Box 356.1.

On a collective basis, the occurrence of PLE is relatively common.

PATHOPHYSIOLOGY

The exact mechanism of serum protein exudation is not known in all instances of PLE. Three basic causes have been proposed: mucosal ulceration, epithelial alteration, and impaired lymphatic flow. A combination of these mechanisms often is responsible for the PLE that occurs in many disorders.

BOX 356.1

Pathophysiologic Classification of Disorders Associated with Protein-Losing Enteropathy in Children

Epithelial Alteration
Ménétrier disease
Celiac disease
Gastrointestinal allergy
Graft-versus-host disease
Infectious gastroenteritis/bacterial overgrowth syndrome
Pneumonia/systemic infections
Parasitic infestations
Carbohydrate-deficient glycoprotein syndrome
Segmental mesenteric thrombosis/ischemia

Mucosal Ulceration
Crohn disease
Ulcerative colitis
Enterocolitis (e.g., necrotizing, allergic, vasculitic, segmental mesenteric thrombosis/ischemia, infectious, radiation, toxic, bacterial overgrowth syndrome)

Alteration in Lymphatic Flow
Primary lymphangiectasia
   Isolated intestinal lymphangiectasia
   Generalized lymphangiectasia

   Noonan syndrome
   Klippel-Trenaunay-Weber syndrome
   Hennekam syndrome
   Familial lymphangiectasia
Secondary lymphangiectasia
   Lymphoma/posttransplant lymphoproliferative disease
   Graft-versus-host disease
   Radiation enteritis
   Crohn disease
   Parasitic infestations
   Scleroderma
   Abdominal tuberculosis
   Cardiovascular diseases
      Congestive heart failure
      Constrictive pericarditis
      Cardiomyopathy
      Fontan procedure sequela
Hepatic/mesenteric venous obstruction
Congenital intestinal lymphatic hypoplasia

Examples include Crohn disease, posttransplant lymphoproliferative disease, and messenteric venous thrombosis or ischemia. Impaired lymphatic flow probably is the most frequent cause of protracted PLE. Reduced systemic venous return, such as that found in cardiac failure or constrictive pericarditis, can lead indirectly to PLE by compromising lymph flow through the thoracic duct into the systemic circulation. In addition to compromised mesenteric lymphatic flow, bowel wall edema and damage also are likely contributing factors when hepatic or splanchnic venous blood flow or both are hindered (e.g., hepatic, portal, and mesenteric venous thrombosis; intermittment, segmental intestinal volvulus). These factors are thought to be responsible for the devastating PLE that occurs in children who have undergone Fontan operations for congenital heart disease.

In affected children, Ménétrier disease, also termed *hypertrophic gastritis*, appears to follow a self-limited clinical course, as opposed to the progressive form of this disorder that afflicts adults, probably because childhood Ménétrier disease often is caused by viral gastritis. Similarly, other GI infections are transient causes of PLE; intestinal bacterial overgrowth syndrome also is a cause. Pneumonia or systemic infections can result in PLE. The mechanism is unknown at present but could involve alteration of gut permeability secondary to systemic cytokine release.

A growing group of recognized inherited diseases that result in defective glycosylation of serum proteins, termed the carbohydrate-deficient glycoprotein syndromes, also now is a recognized cause of PLE. These disorders are thought to result in a defective epithelial basement membrane barrier or extracellular mucosal matrix in the gut that are the putative mechanisms for PLE.

PLE appears to be a nonselective process. Cellular elements, usually lymphocytes, also may be lost from the bowel, especially in patients with impaired intestinal lymphatic drainage. Levels of serum proteins with short half-lives, such as fibrinogen, are less affected than are those with long turnover times, such as albumin. Hypoproteinemia does not occur in every case of PLE because increased hepatic synthesis of serum proteins can compensate for ongoing losses. This synthesis is possible both because of the efficiency of intraluminal digestion and reabsorption of protein exuded from the bowel and because of the capacity of the liver to increase its rate of protein synthesis if nutritional intake is adequate. Disproportionate protein loss occurs in patients with GI bleeding from generalized intestinal mucosal diseases, such as chronic inflammatory bowel disease or posttransplant lymphoproliferative disease.

Many other primary GI disturbances can be associated with PLE. Frequently, generalized malabsorption occurs with PLE if the bowel wall lymphatics or mucosal surfaces are severely involved (e.g., lymphangiectasia, celiac disease). Children with severe fat malabsorption, as manifested by steatorrhea or low serum levels of fat-soluble vitamins but without concomitant PLE, are likely to have a primary disorder of intraluminal digestion (e.g., pancreatic insufficiency resulting from cystic fibrosis). The finding of gross or occult blood in the stool also may help to localize the site of dysfunction or damage to the intestinal mucosal surface.

CLINICAL FINDINGS

In most cases of PLE, the clinical findings of the primary underlying disorder dominate the picture. The associated PLE is suggested by edema or hypoproteinemia. Occasionally, these findings are the presenting manifestations of the underlying disease. PLE should be considered in all cases of unexplained edema or hypoproteinemia. Anemia and lymphocytopenia can occur concomitantly with PLE.

Intestinal lymphangiectasia is a focal segmental or generalized dilatation of the intestinal lymphatic system. It may occur as a primary anomaly (primary lymphangiectasia) or may be secondary to lymphatic obstruction (secondary lymphangiectasia). Primary lymphangiectasia may be limited to the enteric lymphatic system or may be part of a generalized lymphatic disorder. Dilated lymphatics in the mucosal or submucosal layers can become disrupted, with loss of lymphocytes and protein into the intraluminal or intraperitoneal space. Generalized edema caused by hypoproteinemia is the most common clinical finding. GI symptoms include diarrhea, vomiting, and abdominal pain. When intestinal lymphangiectasia occurs as part of a generalized lymphatic disorder, asymmetric nonpitting edema can occur in a single extremity as a result of local lymphatic abnormalities. Chylous ascites or chylothorax also may occur as a consequence of abnormal lymphatics.

In several syndromes, intestinal lymphangiectasia is present. Hennekam syndrome is an autosomal recessive disorder in which intestinal lymphangiectasia occurs in association with facial anomalies and mild mental retardation. A consanguineous Arab family demonstrated a familial form of lymphangiectasia in which edema, growth retardation, diarrhea, abdominal pain, clubbing, and hepatic vein stenosis were present. Children with Noonan syndrome and Klippel-Trenaunay-Weber syndrome can have intestinal lymphangiectasia. Congenital intestinal lymphatic hypoplasia also has been reported.

DIAGNOSIS

Methods for detecting PLE were unavailable until the 1960s, when radiolabeled protein excretion tests were developed. Before that time, a large percentage of patients whose disorder was diagnosed as "idiopathic hypercatabolic hypoproteinemia" probably had unrecognized PLE. The technique used most frequently was the fecal quantitation of excreted radioactivity after the intravenous injection of chromium-51–labeled albumin. Physiologically normal subjects excrete less than 1% of the administered radioactive dose over a 2- to 4-day collection period. These studies contributed to our understanding of normal GI protein catabolism and demonstrated the frequent association of PLE with a wide variety of GI disorders. Studies involving the use of iodine-131–labeled albumin indicated that as much as 10% of daily protein catabolism occurs in the GI tract of healthy persons. Widespread use of these techniques was not possible in pediatric patients. Performing these studies was difficult; they required a 3- to 4-day hospitalization, used radioactive agents, and were relatively expensive. Generally, the radiolabeled proteins used for these studies are not available for clinical purposes in the United States.

Attempts to measure protein loss in stool were unsuccessful because of intraluminal protein digestion. Losses were underestimated consistently because of the efficiency of protein digestion and reabsorption. Fecal nitrogen quantitation is an inaccurate method of diagnosing PLE. Malabsorption of dietary nitrogen may alter the results of these studies significantly. Typically, children with cystic fibrosis have azotorrhea and steatorrhea without PLE, and patients with Crohn disease may have PLE and normal fecal nitrogen excretion.

A practical technique for screening for PLE now exists. The screening test is the measurement of fecal alpha-1-antitrypsin (AAT) excretion. The properties of this protein render it uniquely suited as a natural marker of PLE. Normally, AAT is a major serum protein component that accounts for approximately 4% of the total serum protein content and has a molecular weight similar to that of albumin. It is relatively resistant to intestinal and bacterial proteolytic enzymes and, therefore is excreted relatively intact in stool. These properties allow for the quantitation of fecal AAT to serve as a marker for excessive serum protein loss from the bowel. Clinical studies have shown that determination of fecal AAT is a simple and reliable screening test for PLE. Disorders known to result in PLE are associated with increased fecal AAT excretion. An exception appears to be PLE associated with the loss of serum protein from the gastric mucosa. In these cases of gastritis, AAT appears to be degraded in the acid environment of the stomach.

Fecal AAT excretion may be expressed as stool concentration, intestinal clearance, or total daily output. Normal intestinal clearance is considered to be 13 to 40 mL/day and is calculated by the following formula:

$$\text{Clearance} = \text{Fecal AAT} \times \text{Daily stool output} / \text{Serum AAT}$$

In most clinical situations, a single AAT determination on a random specimen appears adequate. Healthy persons excrete approximately 1 to 2 mg of AAT/1 g of dry stool. Young, exclusively breast-fed or formula-fed infants appear to have higher fecal AAT concentrations, but total daily excretion is not increased because of the decreased total stool volume in breast-fed and formula-fed infants.

Human technetium-99m–labeled albumin and other labeled scintigraphy imaging agents have been used to detect PLE. This technique has proven to be very helpful in localizing the site of bowel protein loss in difficult cases and can aid in directing further evaluation of selected refractory cases of PLE by endoscopy or surgical exploration. These cases usually are in children with segmental intestinal volvulus or forms of lymphangectasia. Conventional imaging tests, such as an upper GI series with small bowel follow-through or a computed tomography scan with contrast, are indicated before exploratory laparotomy in such cases. Lymphoscintigraphy also is useful in some children in whom intestinal lymphangiectasia is likely to be present. Lymphatic defects present on scintigraphy support the diagnosis of generalized lymphangiectasia with probable involvement of the GI tract if associated PLE is present.

Screening for PLE by determining fecal AAT can be used to identify and follow the clinical course of various GI disorders associated with PLE. In children with Crohn disease, PLE is the most common functional abnormality. Screening for PLE, therefore, can be used to aid in the diagnosis of Crohn disease and to follow disease activity.

Usually, evaluations of children with suspected PLE are prompted by the finding of hypoproteinemia. An approach to the evaluation of a hypoproteinemic child is given in Box 356.2.

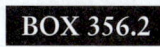

BOX 356.2 — **Evaluation for Hypoproteinemia**

Estimate Dietary Intake
Evaluate for Hypercatabolic Stress
Signs of infection, systemic vasculitis, neoplasm

Initial Laboratory Tests
Total serum protein
Liver chemistry panel
Prothrombin time
Urinalysis, quantitative urinary protein excretion
Complete blood cell count
Erythrocyte sedimentation rate

Screening Tests for Digestive Dysfunction
72-hour fecal fat
Fecal alpha-1-antitrypsin
Test for fecal occult blood

TREATMENT

Management of children with PLE depends on the successful treatment of the primary underlying condition. Reversal of the PLE that occurs in some children after they undergo the Fontan procedure has been observed with treatment with corticosteroids and also with low-dose heparin therapy. The primary mechanism of action of either the corticosteroids or heparin in these cases is not understood. However, these therapeutic responses may lead to further research to provide a better understanding of the pathogenesis of PLE. The treatment of specific GI and non-GI disorders associated with PLE is discussed elsewhere in this book.

Suggested Readings

Bhan MK, Khoshoo V, Chowdhary D, et al. Increased fecal alpha-1-antitrypsin excretion in children with persistent diarrhea associated with enteric pathogens. *Acta Paediatr Scand* 1989;78:265.

Donnelly JP, Rosenthal A, Castle VP, et al. Reversal of protein-losing enteropathy with heparin therapy in three patients with univentricular hearts and Fontan palliation. *J Pediatr* 1997;130:474.

Gabrielli O, Catassi C, Carlucci A, et al. Intestinal lymphangiectasia, lymphedema, mental retardation and typical face: confirmation of the Hennekam syndrome. *Am J Med Genet* 1991;40:244.

Halaby H, Bakheet SM, Shabib S, et al. 99m Tc-human serum albumin scans in children with protein-losing enteropathy. *J Nucl Med* 2000;40:215.

Hilliard RI, McKendrym JBJ, Phillips MJ. Congenital abnormalities of the lymphatic system: a new clinical classification. *Pediatrics* 1990;86:988.

Klar A, Shoseyov D, Berkun Y, et al. Intestinal protein loss and hypoalbuminemia in children with pneumonia. *J Pediatr Gastroenterol Nutr* 2003;37:120.

Lee WS, John P, McKiernan P, et al. Inferior vena cava occlusion and protein-losing enteropathy after liver transplantation in children. *J Pediatr Gastroenterol Nutr* 2002;34:413.

Marks MP, Lanza MV, Kahlstrom EJ, et al. Pediatric hypertrophic gastropathy. *AJR Am J Roentgenol* 1986;147:1031.

Mertens L, Hagler D, Sauer U, et al. Protein-losing enteropathy after the Fontain operation: an international multicenter study. *J Thorac Cadiovasc Surg.* 1998;115:1063.

Niehues R, Hasilik M, Alton G, et al. Carbohydrate-deficient glycoprotein syndrome type Ib: phosphomannose isomerase deficiency and mannose therapy. *J Clin Invest* 1998;101:1414.

Shields E, Tucker T, Meyers W, Chung C. Visualization of protein-losing enteropathy in infantile systemic hyalinosis with Tc-99m HSA after albumin challenge. *Clin Nucl Med* 1996;21:415.

Stormon MO, Mitchell JD, Smoleniec JS, et al. Congenital intestinal lymphatic lymphatic hypoplasia presenting as non-immune hydrops *in utero*, and subsequent neonatal protein-losing enteropathy. *J Pediatr Gastroenterol Nutr* 2002;35:691.

Su J, Smith MB, Rerknimitr R, Marrow D. Small intestine bacterial overgrowth presenting as protein-losing enteropathy. *Dig Dis Sci* 1998;43:679.

Thomas DW, McGilligan KM, Carlson M, et al. Fecal alpha-1-antitrypsin and hemoglobin excretion in healthy human milk-, formula-, or cow's milk-fed infants. *Pediatrics* 1986;78:305.

Thomas DW, Sinatra FR, Merritt RJ. Random fecal alpha-1-antitrypsin concentration in children with gastrointestinal disease. *Gastroenterology* 1981;80:776.

Vallet HL, Holtzapple PG, Eberlein WR, et al. Noonan syndrome with intestinal lymphangiectasia. *J Pediatr* 1972;80:269.

Waldman TA. Protein-losing enteropathy. *Gastroenterology* 1966;50:422.

Younes BS, Ament ME, McDiarmid SV, et al. The involvement of the gastrointestinal tract in posttransplant lymphoproliferative disease in pediatric liver transplantation. *J Pediatr Gastroenterol Nutr* 1999;28:380.

CHAPTER 357 ■ PROTEIN INTOLERANCE

JONATHAN E. TEITELBAUM AND W. ALLAN WALKER

Allergy is derived from the Greek word for "other." Food allergy or protein intolerance is an immunologic reaction to a dietary protein component considered foreign, or "other than oneself." The manifestations of this immune reaction are complex and varied. The development of food intolerance depends on many variables and reflects the interaction between genetic factors and environmental exposure. Because the pathophysiologic mechanisms are incompletely understood, food allergies have been suspected in numerous clinical situations ranging from altered behavior to anaphylaxis. This chapter focuses on those reactions with a suspected immune basis that are reproducible with food challenge. Particular attention is paid to the gastrointestinal manifestations of food allergy seen in infants and likely to come to the attention of pediatricians.

COMMON FOOD ANTIGENS

Typically, antigens responsible for food allergies are 10- to 40-kd glycoproteins or acid proteins resistant to enzyme and heat denaturation. Allergic reactions to cow's milk protein are the most significant in infancy. Whether these reactions occur because cow's milk protein is the first foreign antigen introduced into the diet of an inappropriately reacting neonate or because of its antigenic nature is not certain. The whey protein beta-lactoglobulin, a dimer of 24 kd, which is part of the calycine family, was thought to be the prime allergen. However, now recognized are more than 30 antigenic proteins, including caseins, bovine serum albumin, gamma globulin, and alpha-lactalbumin, all of which can trigger immune-mediated responses.

Soy proteins can induce allergic disease with clinical symptoms and intestinal biopsies resembling those of cow's milk allergy. Soy allergy is an especially common occurrence in Japan, where soy constitutes a major dietary source of protein. In Scandinavian countries, allergy to fish protein is a common occurrence. Eggs, peanuts, and other legumes, nuts, citrus fruits, and yeast also have highly antigenic proteins. The enteropathy associated with gluten sensitivity (e.g., celiac disease) is a special type of food intolerance and is discussed in Chapter 361.

ANTIGEN PROCESSING IN THE GASTROINTESTINAL TRACT

The relationship between the movement of antigens through the intestine and the development of symptoms is complex. After migration, dietary antigens may be expelled in the feces or can cross the mucosal barrier and encounter the local or systemic immune system. Proposed mechanisms of antigenic transfer include passage through M cells, enterocytes (via endocytosis and exocytosis), or intercellular gaps.

Several physical barriers limit the number of foreign antigens that gain access to the immune system. Nonspecific barriers to this process include proteolytic enzymes of the stomach and pancreas and lysosomal enzymes of the intestinal epithelial cells, which degrade complex proteins into smaller peptides and amino acids. Gastrointestinal (GI) peristalsis leads to presentation to the local immune system of fewer antigens per unit of time. Mucous secretions overlying the enterocyte provide a physical barrier.

Specific immunologic components of antigen handling include the gut-associated lymphoid tissue (GALT): the large number of phagocytes, eosinophils, mast cells, and T and B lymphocytes found in the lamina propria, Peyer patches, and among the epithelial cells (intraepithelial lymphocytes) throughout the GI tract. Immunoglobulin A (IgA) is made and secreted in response to certain food antigens and plays a crucial role in the host defense.

An important aspect of this complex system is its alteration with age and illness. Developmental aspects of the immune system may be important in its formation. Infants younger than 1 year old have lower levels of intestinal IgA, fewer intraepithelial lymphocytes, and higher permeability to antigens than do older children. *In vitro* studies suggest that in states of tolerance, protein-specific IgA antibodies prevent the triggering of a local or systemic reaction by a given antigen. However, when the immune system is regulated improperly, a nonspecific IgA response to numerous antigens occurs. In addition, mononuclear cells, perhaps responding to antigens presented on the class II major histocompatibility complex of the enterocyte, release such cytokines as tumor necrosis factor–alpha (TNF-α). *In vitro* studies suggest that TNF-α enhances eosinophil cytotoxicity and perturbs epithelial barrier function by opening the tight junction, thus rendering it more permeable to macromolecules. The immune dysregulation and increase in intestinal permeability to antigens likely contribute to an allergic response.

Recently, researchers have appreciated that gut microflora play an important role in regulating the intestinal and systemic immune system and in inducing tolerance. This role is related to the hygiene hypothesis that was born out of epidemiologic data that showed an inverse correlation between family size and allergic rhinitis. The concept then was generalized to other atopic diseases. Thus, reduced contact with microbes and a diminished burden of infectious disease at an early age may lead to weakened immunologic drive in the Th1 direction and result in overactivity of Th2 responsiveness. This is relevant because Th1 cells generally secrete cytokines which activate other T cells (i.e., interleukin 2, interferon gamma) or other inflammatory cells (i.e., TNF) and thus initiate and augment inflammatory reactions and enhance MHC expression. On the other hand, Th2 cells secrete cytokines that activate B cells (i.e., interleukin 4 and 5) or induce T cells and other hematopoietic cells (i.e., interleukin 6) to grow and differentiate, thus leading to enhanced B cell antibody production and inhibition of Th1 cytokine production. Indeed, the fetal immune response is thought to be Th2- predominant, and the acquisition of certain bacteria, more commonly found in the colon of breast-fed infants, is thought to dampen this Th2 response. However, one should realize that this paradigm is overly simplified, and ongoing research is devoted to defining what are likely novel regulatory T cell classes that are essential in the acquisition and maintenance of mucosal and systemic tolerance.

COW'S MILK–PROTEIN INTOLERANCE

Allergic reactions to foods have been described since ancient times. Hippocrates noted that some infants developed prolonged diarrhea, vomiting, and urticaria, which resolved with elimination of cow's milk from the diet. Cow's milk allergy still was considered to be a rare occurrence before 1950. However, since 1960, when food technology advanced the development and acceptance of cow's milk-based artificial formulas, the incidence of cow's milk-protein intolerance has increased.

Based on an increased understanding of the underlying immunopathophysiology, children with cow's milk allergy can be classified into one of two groups. The first are immediate reactions, those occurring within 2 hours after exposure, and likely represent a type I or IgE-dependent mechanism. This group of reactions is discussed more completely in Chapter 422, Food Allergies. The second group with delayed reactions, occurring more than 2 hours after ingestion, likely represent a type II, III, or IV non–IgE-dependent, T cell–mediated reaction. Most gastrointestinal reactions are of this latter group.

Several prospective studies with a variety of clinical and laboratory definitions of milk allergy placed the prevalence of cow's milk-protein intolerance at 0.5% to 7.5% among Europeans and North American infants. Infants have presented within 28 hours of birth with cow's milk allergy, suggesting intrauterine sensitization. Most children develop symptoms by the time they are 3 months old; however, if affected children are not exposed to cow's milk formula early in infancy, the reaction can be delayed. Retrospective studies indicate that 50% of affected patients have a reaction within the first week after exposure and 75% do by 4 weeks after exposure. Risk factors include a family history of atopy and early dietary exposure to cow's milk. Exclusively breast-fed infants can develop symptoms of protein intolerance to those proteins that pass through the mother's milk.

Gastrointestinal Manifestations

Symptoms referable to the GI tract (including diarrhea, vomiting, and weight loss) are among the most common ones associated with cow's milk allergy, occurring in 50% to 80% of allergic patients. Several clinical entities have been described (Box 357.1).

Colitis

The presentation of milk-induced colitis ranges from asymptomatic occult GI blood loss to explosive, grossly bloody diarrhea and hypovolemic shock. The typical child generally is healthy, with specks or streaks of blood and mucus in his stool. The stool often is noted to be somewhat looser and more frequent, and some colicky pain may be associated with the passage of the stool. Because the blood loss often is minimal, anemia rarely occurs. The differential diagnosis includes infectious colitis (e.g., *Salmonella, Shigella, Yersinia, Campylobacter, Escherichia coli* O157:H7, and *Clostridium difficile*), anal fissure, necrotizing enterocolitis, arteriovenous malformations, inflammatory bowel disease, intussusception, volvulus, Meckel diverticulitis, polyps, Hirschsprung enterocolitis, and bowel infarction (Box 357.2).

Because the rectosigmoid area commonly is abnormal, the diagnosis can be confirmed by flexible sigmoidoscopy. Endoscopic findings include a friable mucosa and increased nodu-

---

BOX 357.1   **Signs and Symptoms of Milk Protein Allergy**

Gastrointestinal
  Colitis (e.g., Bloody diarrhea)
  Vomiting
  Diarrhea with poor weight velocity
  Vomiting
  *Irritable bowel syndrome
  *Abdominal migraine
  *Constipation
  *Chronic aphthous ulcerations
  *Colic
Nongastrointestinal Manifestations
  Shock caused by anaphylactic reaction
  Urticarial rashes
  Lip swelling
  Laryngeal edema
  Atopic dermatitis
  Respiratory symptoms, including wheezing
  †Rhinorrhea
  †Nasal obstruction
  †Conjunctivitis
  †Otitis media
  Heiner syndrome
  *Neonatal thrombocytopenia
  *Iron-losing enteropathy

*Insufficient evidence to prove a causal relationship.
†Rarely seen as the only manifestation of cow milk protein allergy.

---

larity suggestive of lymphonodular hyperplasia. More severe cases may have multiple superficial erosions or, rarely, frank ulcerations with exudate. Microscopically, the presence of focal infiltrates of eosinophils in all mucosal compartments, particularly the lamina propria, often is striking. Histologic analysis shows maintenance of the mucosa without features of chronicity. Crypt abscesses with neutrophils and eosinophils can occur. A retrospective study of affected patients noted that the presence of no fewer than 60 eosinophils per high-powered field in the lamina propria and of degranulated eosinophils correlates with allergic colitis rather than with infectious colitis.

BOX 357.2   **Differential Diagnosis of Colitis**

Infectious colitis (e.g., *Salmonella, Shigella, Yersinia, Campylobacter, Escherichia coli* O157:H7, and *Clostridium difficile*)
Anal fissure
Necrotizing enterocolitis
Arteriovenous malformations
Inflammatory bowel disease
Intussusception
Volvulus
Meckel diverticulitis
Polyps
Hirschsprung enterocolitis
Bowel infarction

Although dietary manipulation that removes antigen (see Treatment below) often results in resolution of gross blood within 3 to 7 days, the presence of microscopic blood loss in the stool may be ongoing for weeks. Testing for the presence of occult blood in the stool of an otherwise healthy child is, therefore, discouraged. The long-term effects of enduring small amounts of gross blood in the stool of a thriving child have not been studied, but anecdotally it appears to be well-tolerated and ultimately self-limited, without any obvious sequelae.

Malabsorption Syndrome

In infants experiencing poor growth and chronic diarrhea, a small bowel enteropathy secondary to milk allergy should be suspected. In addition to celiac disease (in children who have been exposed to gluten), other causes of enteropathy or malabsorption in infancy that should be considered include immunodeficiency (e.g., acquired immunodeficiency syndrome), autoimmune enteropathy, chronic infectious enteritis (e.g., Giardia), chronic protein malnutrition, bacterial overgrowth, primary or secondary lactase deficiency, pancreatic insufficiency (e.g., cystic fibrosis, Shwachman syndrome), and chronic liver disease. An examination of stool from affected patients may show evidence of carbohydrate and fat malabsorption, and accompanying symptoms of allergic processes (e.g., eczema or wheezing) may be present. A separate entity of protein-losing enteropathy secondary to cow's milk allergy also has been described. Small-bowel biopsies of allergic patients reveal villous atrophy with a patchy distribution; severe enteropathy can resemble the total villous atrophy of celiac disease. Biopsies of the gastric antrum in affected patients almost always are abnormal, demonstrating dense infiltration of eosinophils.

Vomiting

Between 40% and 50% of patients with cow's milk allergy have emesis as a symptom, creating an obvious diagnostic problem because gastroesophageal reflux (GER) disease in infancy is a relatively common finding. Some studies suggest that as many as 42% of patients who have GER are allergic to cow's milk. These studies use a double-blind, placebo-controlled food challenge, endoscopy, and pH probe monitoring to confirm the diagnosis. The differential diagnosis of vomiting in children would include physiologic GER, pyloric stenosis, intestinal malrotation with volvulus, and intestinal duplication. A pH probe in allergic patients may identify a distinct pattern, in which a progressive reduction in pH begins at the end of a feeding and continues until the initiation of the next feeding, when the pH steeply rises. The debate as to how many of such patients truly are allergic is heightened because GER, like allergy-related diseases, often resolves with time.

Other Gastrointestinal Symptoms

Symptoms and syndromes, including irritable bowel syndrome, abdominal migraine, constipation, and chronic aphthous ulcerations, have been ascribed to protein intolerance but usually without convincing proof of an immunologic basis. Colic has been considered an allergic process and often is treated by dietary manipulation, although its relation to true protein intolerance rarely is documented. Food intolerance or allergy may cause colic in 10% to 12% of otherwise healthy infants who have reproducible symptoms during a double-blind, placebo-controlled food challenge. Of these, as many as 33% will develop other manifestations of allergy by the time they are 6 months of age. The resolution of colic coincident with a change in formula is necessary, but not sufficient, to prove an allergic cause for these symptoms. Because frequent changes in formula during infancy can convince involved parents that affected children are susceptible to allergies, any treatment of colic with dietary manipulation should be done with the reassurance that food allergy in infants usually is a short-lived phenomenon and that many factors likely contribute to colic.

Nongastrointestinal Manifestations

In addition to being a target organ of immune reactions related to protein allergy, the intestinal tract acts as a conduit for various antigens, allowing immune responses to occur in other organ systems. Shock caused by anaphylactic reactions to food represents a true type I hypersensitivity reaction, although it is the least common form of food allergy. Other immediate reactions include urticarial rashes, lip swelling, and laryngeal edema. A study of 13 fatal or near-fatal anaphylactic reactions to food (most often peanuts) found that two-thirds of the fatal (but none of the nonfatal) reactions occurred at school, heightening the need for public awareness of and preparedness for such emergencies. Patients with prior severe reactions or respiratory sequelae to foods should be encouraged to carry epinephrine at all times.

Atopic dermatitis has been associated with food allergy. Sampson et al. (1985) found evidence of food hypersensitivity in 63 of 113 patients with severe eczema; egg, peanut, and milk proteins accounted for 72% of the reactions. However, only those children who fail standard medical therapy (e.g., topical steroids and emollients) have a sufficiently high incidence of food allergy to warrant evaluation. In addition, care should be taken in the treatment of patients with eczema to avoid emollients that contain common sensitizing proteins (e.g., peanut oil), because anecdotal reports have cited cases in which such patients subsequently developed allergy to those proteins.

Respiratory symptoms, including wheezing, have been attributed to food protein allergy, and many infants who exhibit dermatologic findings also have acute bronchospasm. In older children, reactive airway disease can be a manifestation of protein allergy, although symptoms often take hours to days to occur; hence, establishing the diagnosis is difficult. Rhinorrhea, nasal obstruction, conjunctivitis, and otitis media rarely are secondary to cow's milk–protein allergy, particularly when they are the sole complaints. Heiner syndrome, a symptom complex of pulmonary hemosiderosis, wheezing, chronic rhinitis, otitis media, and anemia, resolves with the dietary elimination of cow's milk proteins.

Other conditions with a possible link to cow's milk intolerance include neonatal thrombocytopenia and an iron-losing enteropathy. Methemoglobinemia in patients with severe allergy-related diarrhea also has been reported.

DIAGNOSIS

The multiplicity of symptoms and overlapping mechanisms of food-allergy disorders creates difficulties in establishing an appropriate diagnosis. The use of double-blind, placebo-controlled food challenges has aided the scientific study of food intolerance greatly and has become the gold standard for diagnosis. Clinicians rely on history, but studies using double-blind, placebo-controlled food challenge determined that only one-third of patients with a history identifying a specific antigen develop a significant reaction to the antigen on challenge. Children who have been asymptomatic while being exposed to a given antigen for longer than 6 months rarely are allergic to that protein. A family history of allergy or atopy appears to increase children's risk of having this allergy. If one parent is allergic, the child's risk is twice that of the general population. This risk appears to be more significant if a mother is the affected parent. If both parents are allergic, the risk for the child is five times that of the general population.

A peripheral eosinophilia is seen in 16% to 19% of patients with colitis. Some patients affected with colitis have eosinophils in their stool, a low serum albumin, or both. Newborn cord blood with an elevated IgE level or IgE antibodies against bovine proteins has been shown to correlate with a predisposed state. One study reported such elevation in 76% of patients who later developed cow's milk allergy. This finding contrasts to the elevation of total IgE in infancy, when no clinical significance seems to exist.

Radioactive immunosorbent tests (RASTs) to detect food allergy are limited by the technique's measurement of IgE antibodies, which are the immunologic mediators in only a small group of patients with gastrointestinal allergy. In patients with acute-onset dermatologic or respiratory manifestations of cow's milk allergy, the sensitivity of a RAST may be as high as 80%, although even higher numbers have been reported in those instances in which the specific IgE level was very high. For these patients with immediate reactions, the negative predictive value of RAST testing is thought to be 95%. In patients with only GI symptoms, usually a RAST is much less helpful because these reactions are less dependent on IgE-mediated inflammation.

Alternative and complimentary medicine approaches to allergic disorders commonly are utilized by patients. Very few studies support the validity of these tests. The testing of specific serum immunoglobulins (e.g., IgG or IgA) directed towards certain food antigens appears to be unhelpful because they are found in healthy controls and merely represent exposure, not a pathologic reaction, to food proteins. Studies have refuted the use of applied kinesiology and provocation-neutralization testing in diagnosis.

Skin tests in the assessment of food allergy can provide a clue to affected patients' physiologic response to an antigen and usually are less expensive than is a RAST. Performing skin testing on infants can be difficult and is more reliable in children older than 3 years, when a more specific IgE response has developed. Again, such testing is less reliable when searching for the offending antigen in a non-IgE-mediated reaction. Indeed, positive results are seen in only 40% of individuals with cow's milk allergy. Research is ongoing on the usefulness of patch testing, in which the antigen is applied to a patch and exposure to the skin is hours to days, in identifying food antigens causing delayed-type reactions.

Intestinal biopsy offers a means of documenting the inflammatory reaction. The presence of a primarily eosinophilic infiltration of the mucosa may be helpful. However, the mucosal lesion may be focal, and thus sampling error can result in negative biopsies. Furthermore, the presence of allergic inflammation does not identify the causative antigen. Finally, even tissue eosinophilia is not diagnostic of allergy because it can be present in other conditions such as inflammatory bowel disease, GER, collagen vascular disease, and eosinophilic gastroenteropathies, including eosinophilic esophagitis.

In approximately 10% of affected patients, the symptoms of protein intolerance are vague, and even double-blind, placebo-controlled food challenge is inconclusive. Typically, patients demonstrate a particular class of reaction to a given antigen. For example, a type I immediate anaphylactoid reaction rarely is seen in a patient who previously had a delayed GI reaction. Occasionally, a subgroup of patients with severe atopy appears to be an exception to this rule. Nonetheless, all challenges should be performed under close medical supervision. Bock et al. (1988) produced guidelines for office-based food challenges.

THERAPY

The treatment of protein intolerance is strict dietary avoidance of the offending antigen. If parents or affected patients suspect food allergy, often they perform some type of dietary elimination before seeking medical advice. These diets may not eliminate the proposed antigen completely unless all food labels are scrutinized. A milk-avoidance diet, for instance, must exclude cow's milk and all dairy products. At the other extreme, self-imposed elimination diets can be so strict as to endanger the intake of calories and nutrients necessary for normal growth and development. Care must be taken in the design of exclusionary diets so that they remain palatable and nutritionally adequate. The input of a skilled nutritionist is crucial.

In the case of cow's milk-protein allergy resulting in colitis or enteritis, the use of soy-based formula is not recommended by the American Academy of Pediatrics (AAP) because as many as 25% to 60% of these infants are intolerant to soy protein. Similarly, goat's milk and sheep's milk, which may pose additional problems secondary to inadequate vitamin supply (e.g., folic acid, vitamin B_{12}, and vitamin B_6), also have shared antigenicity with cow's milk proteins. For this reason, casein hydrolysate formulas are recommended by the AAP's Committee on Nutrition for the treatment of protein intolerance. Casein hydrolysate formulas undergo the *in vitro* breakdown of casein to small peptides with molecular weights of less than 1,500 daltons, which has been demonstrated to reduce their antigenicity significantly. Indeed, the AAP allows a formula to be designated as hypoallergenic only if modification of the protein results in 90% of allergic subjects tolerating the formula with 95% confidence. However, these formulas (e.g., Pregestimil, Alimentum, and Nutramigen), in which 97% of the proteins are less than 1,000 daltons, are expensive and often unpalatable. Whey hydrolysate formulas (e.g., Carnation Good Start) contain larger peptides (greater than 1,500 daltons) and may be less suitable for the dietary management of food allergy; thus, they are not recommended by the AAP for use in allergic individuals. Laboratory analysis of hydrolysate formulas reveals that they contain small amounts of intact antigenic proteins, as supported by case reports of highly sensitive children who continue to have allergic reactions while on these formulas. This situation has led to the availability of amino acid-based formulas (e.g., Neocate, EleCare) that are significantly less antigenic. Some studies suggest that supplementation of vitamins A and D and of calcium may be beneficial in patients on hydrolysate formulas.

Children who are breast-fed exclusively can develop cow's milk allergy. Indeed, an analysis of breast milk shows that intact protein can be detected in a significant number of cases, and as many as 70% of breast-fed children will have antibodies to cow's milk protein, indicating that they were exposed to the proteins. In some instances, allergic symptoms may resolve if involved mothers adhere to a strict milk-free diet, although doing so often is difficult in practice.

In rare instances, low-dose systemic steroids are used for allergic colitis, if an elemental diet has yielded no effect. An investigation of other immune therapies continues in the laboratory setting. Interferon-gamma can increase the expression of major histocompatibility complex and adhesion molecules on epithelial cells, which may confer an increased IgA response, IgA receptor expression, and decreased intestinal permeability. Animal studies with IgE-mediated reactions suggest that anti-IL-1 antibodies can prevent sensitization and subsequent allergic reactions. Given the recent interest in the hygiene hypothesis, the study of probiotic bacteria has been the focus of much allergy-related research. The ingestion of bacteria such as *Lactobacillus* GG has been shown to hydrolyze cow's milk proteins and possibly decrease the antigenicity of these proteins, suppress lymphocyte proliferation, increase the expression of IgA, affect levels of interferon gamma, and decrease levels of TNF-α. Clinical studies suggest this use may decrease the incidence of atopy in high-risk infants and aid in the treatment of atopic dermatitis. Although this use generally is considered safe, rare instances of bacteremia have been described, although typically not in normal hosts.

Other approaches that are undergoing investigation include the use of pancreatic enzymes for the treatment of atopic dermatitis associated with cow's milk allergy, oral desensitization, the infusion of IgE antibodies, and vaccination with plasmid DNA. The food industry also has begun to investigate the tolerability of crops in which the immunogenic antigens are removed while preserving the food's nutritional quality.

The natural history of cow's milk allergy reveals that fewer than 1% of affected individuals will have a life-long allergy, with affected children demonstrating immediate reactions being at greatest risk for nonresolution. As many as 85% of children with delayed reactions will have tolerance after 1 year. However, overall studies, including all categories of allergic patients, suggest that tolerance by 1 year occurs in only 45% to 56%. Protein tolerance by 2 years and 3 years is 60% to 77% and 71% to 87%, respectively.

PREVENTION

Human colostrum and breast milk are thought to facilitate GI tract maturation and to provide passive protection against bacteria, viruses, and other antigens. Because many of the symptoms of cow's milk-protein intolerance occur in the first year of life, exclusive breast-feeding during this time, with delayed introduction of solid foods until the child reaches the age of 5 to 6 months, may be beneficial in preventing the onset of food allergy. Indeed, the incidence of allergy among breast-fed infants is 0.5% as compared to 2.0% to 7.5% in bottle-fed infants. Breast-feeding should be encouraged in parents of infants with a strong family history of atopy and is in keeping with the AAP recommendations for infant nutrition. Most studies suggest that breast feeding seems to protect against the development of allergic disease, especially among children at high risk due to a family history of atopy. These studies suggest a protective effect during the first decade of life; however, long-term outcome data are not available. Studies also suggest that the use of extensively hydrolyzed cow's milk-based formulas reduces the risk of developing cow's milk allergy.

Few existing data support the restriction of the mothers' diets to various antigens while they are breast-feeding as a means of preventing the formation of a food allergy. Similarly, studies have been undertaken to assess whether altering mothers' diets during the third trimester of pregnancy would change the incidence of allergies in their infants. Two controlled, prospective studies of Swedish women with a family history of atopy failed to show any effect.

Suggested Readings

Baehler P, Chad Z, Seidman EG, et al. Distinct patterns of cow's milk allergy in infancy defined by prolonged, two-stage double-blind, placebo-controlled food challenges. *Clin Exp Allergy* 1996;26:254.

Bock SA, Sampson HA, Atkins FM, et al. Double-blind, placebo-controlled food challenge (DBPCFC) as an office procedure: a manual. *J Allergy Clin Immunol* 1988;82:986.

Cavataio F, Iacono G, Corroccio A, et al. Clinical and pH-metric characteristics of gastro-oesophageal reflux secondary to cows' milk protein allergy. *Arch Dis Child* 1996;75:51.

Goldman H, Proujansky R. Allergic proctitis and gastroenteritis in children: clinical and mucosal biopsy features in 53 cases. *Am J Surg Pathol* 1986;10:75.

Heyman M, Darmon N, Desjeux JF, et al. Mononuclear cells from infants allergic to cow's milk secrete tumor necrosis factor α, altering intestinal function. *Gastroenterology* 1994;106:1514.

Host A, Jacobsen HP, Halken S, et al. The natural history of cow's milk protein allergy/intolerance. *Eur J Clin Nutr* 1995;49(Suppl 1):S13.

Insoft RM, Sanderson IS, Walker WA. The development of immune function within the human intestine and its role in neonatal diseases. *Pediatr Clin North Am* 1996;43:551.

Jenkins HR, Pincott JR, Soothill JF, et al. Food allergy: the major cause of infantile colitis. *Arch Dis Child* 1984;59:326.

Lake AM, Whitington PF, Hamilton SR. Dietary protein-induced colitis in breast-fed infants. *J Pediatr* 1982;101:906.

Rautava S, Ruuskanen O, Ouwehand A, et al. The hygiene hypothesis of atopic disease-an extended version. *J Pediatr Gastroenterol Nutr* 2004;38:378.

Sampson HA. Food allergies. *Curr Opin Gastroenterol* 1995;11:548.

Sampson HA, McCaskill CC. Food hypersensitivity and atopic dermatitis: evaluation of 113 patients. *J Pediatr* 1985;107:669.

Sampson HA, Mendelson L, Rosen JP. Fatal and near-fatal anaphylactic reactions to food in children and adolescents. *N Engl J Med* 1992;327:380.

Stern M, Walker WA. Food allergy and intolerance. *Pediatr Clin North Am* 1985;32:471.

Zeiger RS. Food allergen avoidance in the prevention of food allergy in infants and children. *Pediatrics* 2003;111:1662.

CHAPTER 358 ■ EOSINOPHILIC GASTROINTESTINAL DISEASES

GLENN T. FURUTA AND PETER NGO

Eosinophilic gastrointestinal diseases are clinicopathologic entities requiring a mucosal biopsy for diagnosis. Eosinophilic gastroenteritis, the classical eosinophilic gastrointestinal disease, presents with a broad range of symptoms, with mucosal biopsies revealing eosinophilic inflammation of the stomach and small bowel. Clinical manifestations vary depending on the location of eosinophilic infiltration but can include abdominal pain, vomiting, bloody diarrhea, and failure to thrive. Exclusion of other causes of gastrointestinal eosinophilia such as drug reactions, parasitic infections, gastroesophageal reflux disease (GERD), and inflammatory bowel disease is required to make the diagnosis. The cause of eosinophilic gastrointestinal disorders is unclear, but several lines of evidence implicate allergy as a primary cause. The last decade has witnessed a dramatic rise in the recognition and incidence of eosinophilic esophagitis (EE). EE occurs more commonly than does eosinophilic gastroenteritis and has better defined features.

EOSINOPHILIC ESOPHAGITIS

Pathogenesis

Increasing evidence supports the concept that EE is related to an allergic response. Between 33% and 100% of affected patients have atopic disease or peripheral eosinophilia. The affected esophageal mucosa demonstrates increased expression of interleukin (IL)-5, an eosinophiliotropic cytokine. Specific antigens initiating the inflammatory cascade are likely unique to the individual, but food and aeroallergens are suspected. Mechanisms of the allergic response are not certain; some patients have elevated IgE, whereas others do not. Dysphagia and predisposition for food impaction are thought to be due to either esophageal dysmotility or proximal esophageal strictures. Esophageal motility studies document increased ineffective contractions. Endoscopic ultrasonic evaluation revealed thickening of mucosal, submucosal, and muscularis layers of the esophagus, suggesting muscular involvement.

Clinical Manifestations

Symptoms associated with EE can be very similar to those observed in GERD and include vomiting, dysphagia, regurgitation, chest pain, epigastric pain, nausea, aversive feeding behavior, failure to thrive, or respiratory symptoms such as coughing and wheezing. In contrast to children with GERD, patients with EE do not have a clinical response to acid blockade. The most characteristic symptom of EE is dysphagia, which often is accompanied by food impaction. Not all children with EE will report these symptoms, thus mandating a high level of suspicion.

Diagnosis

Histologic evaluation of esophageal tissue is the cornerstone of diagnosis. When symptoms are unresponsive to acid blockade, upper endoscopy with mucosal biopsy is indicated. The healthy esophageal mucosa is devoid of eosinophils, whereas in patients with EE, greater than 15 to 20 eosinophils per high power field are seen on light microscopy. The proximal as well as the distal esophagus can be involved, and eosinophilic aggregates or microabscesses often are present. A speckled pattern of pinpoint white papules, which appears similar to *Candida* infection, actually represents these superficial eosinophilic microabscesses (Fig. 358.1). Other gross endoscopic findings include mucosal furrowing (linear folds along the esophageal mucosa), concentric rings in the esophageal wall, and proximal strictures (Fig. 358.2). pH monitoring of the distal esophagus typically is normal.

Therapy

Consistent with the hypothesis that food allergens provide antigenic stimuli for eosinophilic inflammation, studies have shown convincingly that elemental diets and targeted dietary elimination can result in clinical and histologic resolution. Consultation with an allergist is recommended and may identify a specific allergen via skin prick, radioallergosorbent (RAST),

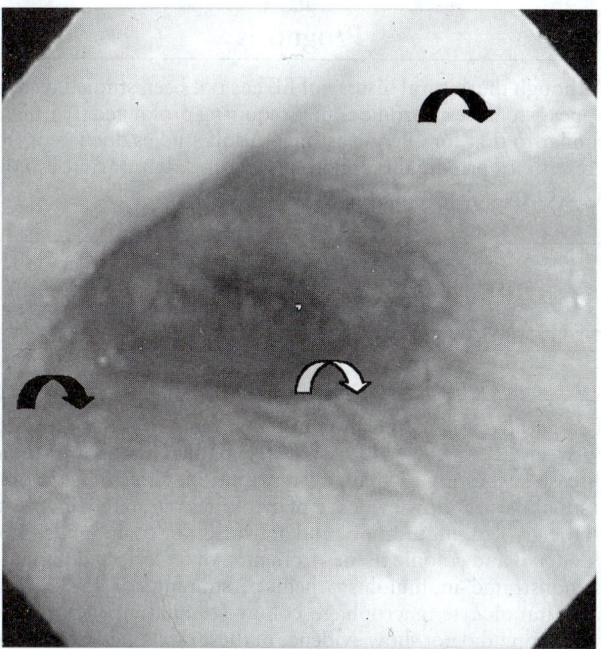

FIGURE 358.1. Whitish exudate on esophageal mucosa of patient with eosinophilic esophagitis.

or skin patch testing. If dietary elimination does not produce satisfactory results, immunosuppression with corticosteroids should be considered. Although systemic corticosteroids can produce clinical and histologic improvement, they are associated with undesirable side effects. To decrease these effects, topical application of corticosteroids have been used and shown to be effective in several studies. Aerosolized corticosteroids such as fluticasone propionate delivered via a metered-dose canister can provide a topical coating of corticosteroid if the medication is swallowed instead of inhaled.

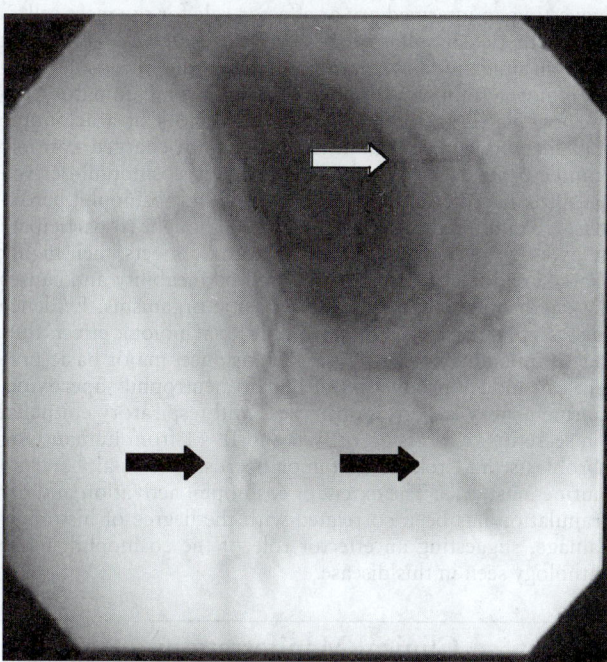

FIGURE 358.2. Longitudinal furrows on esophageal mucosa of patient with eosinophilic esophagitis.

Prognosis

Although the natural history of EE has not been studied well, it appears to have a chronic course requiring prolonged treatment similar to that for allergic asthma. Adult studies document the presence of proximal esophageal strictures, but Barrett esophagus or metaplasia has not been reported.

EOSINOPHILIC GASTROENTERITIS

Pathogenesis

The pathogenesis of eosinophilic gastroenteritis is unknown. Between 20% and 70% of affected patients have an atopic disease suggesting an allergic contribution. Affected gastrointestinal tissues show evidence of cytokines intimately involved in the growth, maturation, and activation of eosinophils. The duodenal and colonic tissues from nine of ten affected patients demonstrated immunohistochemical staining for IL-3, IL-5, and granulocyte-macrophage colony-stimulating factor. The tissues that did not show evidence of these cytokines came from a patient who had undergone treatment with corticosteroids. Interestingly, the serum level of IL-5 was undetectable in all patients examined, suggesting that the intestinal immunologic milieu provides a compartment that is separate from the systemic and is conducive to eosinophil growth and proliferation.

Other evidence suggesting an allergic participation is the patient's response to such immunologically active treatments as corticosteroids and mast-cell stabilizing agents. Corticosteroid treatment induces the prompt resolution of symptoms and histologic abnormalities in most patients with eosinophilic gastroenteritis. The reasons for this response remain unknown, but inhibition of the cytokine production that can stimulate eosinophil proliferation and activation, such as IL-3, IL-5, and granulocyte-macrophage colony-stimulating factor, has been proposed. In addition, case series have shown that the mast cell stabilizing agents cromolyn and ketotifen improve symptoms and, in some patients, reduce the eosinophilic infiltrate, suggesting an intermediary or effector role for the mast cell.

Whether eosinophils are protective cells defending the host from an unidentified toxin, microbe, or other antigenic stimuli is not certain. Eosinophils produce proinflammatory cytokines, platelet-activating factors, mediators of arachidonic acid metabolism, and at least four highly charged cationic granule proteins (i.e., major basic protein, eosinophil-derived neurotoxin, eosinophil cationic protein, and eosinophil peroxidase). Traditionally, these proteins are thought to participate in disease processes through their cytotoxic effects; their highly charged cationic nature increases cell permeability and causes the death of resident cells and parasitic organisms. Evidence suggests that these proteins have additional biologic effects during an inflammatory response. For instance, major basic protein can induce production of human neutrophil superoxide, murine airway hyperresponsiveness and respiratory epithelial ion secretion, expression of IL-6 and IL-11 from human lung fibroblasts, and release of tumor necrosis factor-alpha from murine mast cells. The extent of eosinophil activation and degranulation has been correlated with the degree of histologic damage, suggesting an effector role of the eosinophil in the pathology seen in this disease.

Clinical Manifestations

The clinical presentations are varied and depend on the part of the intestinal tissue that is affected. The mucosa of the gastric antrum or small intestine is the site most commonly affected in the pediatric form of eosinophilic gastroenteritis, and these patients can present with symptoms seen in Crohn disease: failure to thrive, diarrhea, hematochezia, vomiting, or protein-losing enteropathy.

When muscular involvement is predominant, obstructive symptoms are common findings. Eosinophilic infiltration of the muscular layer of the antrum can cause gastric outlet obstruction. When it occurs during the neonatal period, eosinophilic gastroenteritis can be confused with pyloric stenosis. Older patients can present with symptoms of appendicitis or intussusception.

Patients with serosal infiltration may present with increasing abdominal girth caused by exudative eosinophilic ascites. Those patients do not have associated hepatic disease, and the ascitic fluid appears to develop as a result of the interruption of the normal lymph flow.

Eosinophilic colitis is characterized by isolated eosinophilic infiltration of the colon on biopsy. It may be seen as a form of primary eosinophilic gastrointestinal disease but more commonly is seen in parasitic disease, drug reactions, vasculitis such as Churg-Strauss syndrome, or with a diagnosis of allergic colitis of infancy, also known as dietary protein-induced colitis of infancy. Allergic colitis of infancy is the most common cause of bloody stools in the first year of life. Cow's milk protein and soy protein are implicated most frequently, and the vast majority of these patients can tolerate these proteins without sequelae by the time they reach 1 to 3 years of age.

Diagnosis

Physical findings are nonspecific and include abdominal tenderness and blood in the stool of affected patients. Long-standing disease may produce evidence of malnutrition. Periorbital and peripheral edema occur as a result of hypoalbuminemia. Peripheral eosinophilia is an inconsistent finding, occurring in 13% to 85% of patients. Hypoalbuminemia occurs in 33% to 100% of patients and usually is a result of protein-losing enteropathy. Usually, results of intestinal tests of malabsorption are normal. IgE levels can be elevated in severe disease. Charcot-Leyden crystal proteins, a marker of eosinophil degranulation, can be found in the stool. When ascitic fluid is present, it appears turbid and is rich in eosinophils.

Radiographic bowel abnormalities are nonspecific. The small bowel may appear normal or can demonstrate narrowing with proximal dilation, flocculation, or mucosal thickening with nodularity. In mucosal disease, air contrast studies of the antrum may reveal an irregular lacy antral pattern instead of the normal smooth surface. If the colon is involved, a cobblestone pattern similar to that of granulomatous colitis may be seen.

Gastrointestinal biopsies are the cornerstone for establishing the diagnosis. Affected tissue can appear erythematous, nodular, or ulcerated, but, in some patients, it can appear normal. Because lesions may appear normal and involvement often is patchy, multiple biopsy samples should be obtained. When serosal disease presents with an acute abdomen or muscular disease causes complete obstruction, the diagnosis is made during exploratory laparotomy. If biopsies are suggestive of eosinophilic gastroenteritis, confirmation of diagnosis rests on the exclusion of the other possible causes.

Differential Diagnosis

The nonspecific symptoms seen in cases of eosinophilic gastroenteritis render diagnosis difficult to establish unless a high index of suspicion is maintained. The finding of peripheral eosinophilia may be helpful, but, when it is present, conditions such as lymphoma, collagen-vascular diseases (especially polyarteritis nodosa), and enteroinvasive parasitic infestation should be excluded.

The radiographic abnormalities may be seen in other types of gastritis, such as aspirin-induced gastritis, peptic ulcer disease, or chronic granulomatous disease, and in such infections as histoplasmosis and tuberculosis. Gastric tumors (e.g., carcinoma, lymphoma, leiomyoma, leiomyosarcoma) and *Helicobacter pylori* infection can exhibit nodular radiographic abnormalities. Hypertrophic gastric folds can be seen in Zollinger-Ellison syndrome and Ménétrier disease.

The combination of gastric lesions and small bowel radiographic abnormalities suggests the diagnosis of eosinophilic gastroenteritis, but Crohn disease and granulomatous infections should be excluded.

Tissue eosinophilia can be seen in inflammatory bowel disease, peptic disease, amebiasis, or other parasitic infections. Usually, eosinophilic granulomatous disease, tropical sprue, and inflammatory bowel disease have different clinical signs and symptoms.

Therapy

No specific treatment or consistently effective diet is available. Elimination diets should be attempted if the clinical symptoms are mild and a specific allergen can be identified. The use of elimination diets in patients without clear identification of an offending food has not been particularly useful and, in fact, can be deleterious if growing pediatric patients are deprived of adequate nutrition. If elimination diets are used for prolonged periods, care should be taken to ensure that the child has appropriate caloric, mineral, and micronutrient intake.

Corticosteroids should be used if symptoms are significant or the response to an elimination diet is not satisfactory. Oral corticosteroids have improved both symptoms and the associated histologic abnormalities. Generally, clinical improvement occurs promptly, and often patients tolerate reduction in corticosteroid doses. Some patients may need intermittent low-dose or alternate-day corticosteroids for long-term control. Other therapies, including sodium cromolyn and ketotifen, have been used with varying success. Although surgery often is needed for lesions producing complete obstruction, corticosteroid therapy often can relieve this mechanical symptom.

Prognosis

Eosinophilic gastroenteritis is a chronic disease with a large variation in clinical expression. The prognosis varies according to the type and extent of eosinophilic infiltration. Patients with muscle layer disease have an excellent prognosis, particularly if surgical intervention alleviates the symptoms. Those with diffuse mucosal disease have a less clear prognosis. Some patients have long-term remissions, whereas others develop chronic disease requiring prolonged, intermittent steroid therapy. Complications include small bowel bacterial overgrowth, hemorrhage, and perforation, but no malignant transformation has been reported.

Suggested Readings

Caldwell JH, Mekhjian HS, Hurtubise PE, Beman FM. Eosinophilic gastroenteritis with obstruction. Immunological studies of seven patients. *Gastroenterology* 1978;74:825.

Chen MJ, Chu CH, Lin SC, et al. Eosinophilic gastroenteritis: clinical experience with 15 patients. *World J Gastroenterol* 2003;9:2813.

Desreumaux P, Bloget F, Seguy D, et al. Interleukin 3, granulocyte-macrophage colony-stimulating factor, and interleukin 5 in eosinophilic gastroenteritis. *Gastroenterology* 1996;110:768.

Faubion WA Jr, Perrault J, Burgart LJ, et al. Treatment of eosinophilic esophagitis with inhaled corticosteroids. *J Pediatr Gastroenterol Nutr* 1998;27:90.

Fox VL, Nurko S, Furuta GT. Eosinophilic esophagitis: it's not just kid's stuff. *Gastrointest Endosc* 2002;56:260.

Fox VL, Nurko S, Teitelbaum JE, et al. High-resolution EUS in children with eosinophilic "allergic" esophagitis. *Gastrointest Endosc* 2003;57:30.

Goldman H, Proujansky R. Allergic proctitis and gastroenteritis in children. Clinical and mucosal biopsy features in 53 cases. *Am J Surg Pathol* 1986;10:75.

Katz AJ, Goldman H, Grand RJ. Gastric mucosal biopsy in eosinophilic (allergic) gastroenteritis. *Gastroenterology* 1977;73:705.

Kelly KJ, Lazenby AJ, Rowe PC, et al. Eosinophilic esophagitis attributed to gastroesophageal reflux: improvement with an amino acid-based formula. *Gastroenterology* 1995;109:1503.

Keshavarzian A, Saverymuttu SH, Tai PC, et al. Activated eosinophils in familial eosinophilic gastroenteritis. *Gastroenterology* 1985;88:1041.

Liacouras CA, Wenner WJ, Brown K, Ruchelli E. Primary eosinophilic esophagitis in children: successful treatment with oral corticosteroids. *J Pediatr Gastroenterol Nutr* 1998;26:380.

Lim JR, Gupta SK, Croffie JM, et al. White specks in the esophageal mucosa: an endoscopic manifestation of non-reflux eosinophilic esophagitis in children. *Gastrointest Endosc* 2004;59:835.

Orenstein SR, Shalaby TM, Di Lorenzo C, et al. The spectrum of pediatric eosinophilic esophagitis beyond infancy: a clinical series of 30 children. *Am J Gastroenterol* 2000;95:1422.

Rothenberg ME. Eosinophilic gastrointestinal disorders (EGID). *J Allergy Clin Immunol* 2004;113:11.

Spergel JM, Beausoleil JL, Mascarenhas M, Liacouras CA. The use of skin prick tests and patch tests to identify causative foods in eosinophilic esophagitis. *J Allergy Clin Immunol* 2002;109:363.

Straumann A, Spichtin HP, Grize L, et al. Natural history of primary eosinophilic esophagitis: a follow-up of 30 adult patients for up to 11.5 years. *Gastroenterology* 2003;125:1660.

Talley NJ, Shorter RG, Phillips SF, Zinsmeister AR. Eosinophilic gastroenteritis: a clinicopathological study of patients with disease of the mucosa, muscle layer, and subserosal tissues. *Gut* 1990;31:54.

Teitelbaum JE, Fox VL, Twarog FJ, et al. Eosinophilic esophagitis in children: immunopathological analysis and response to fluticasone propionate. *Gastroenterology* 2002;122:1216.

CHAPTER 359 ■ SHORT BOWEL SYNDROME

CARLOS H. LIFSCHITZ

Short bowel syndrome can be caused by prenatal events, such as volvulus, small bowel atresia, gastroschisis or malformation. Acquired causes of the syndrome include necrotizing enterocolitis, volvulus, meconium ileus, massive trauma to the abdomen and, although rarely in children, Crohn disease (Box 359.1).

Because most cases occur in the perinatal period, the remaining bowel must be capable of adapting to provide sufficient absorption of water and electrolytes to maintain homeostasis and nutrients sufficient to sustain growth. Compensatory intestinal growth dominated by villous hyperplasia usually occurs within

---

BOX 359.1   Etiology of Short Bowel Syndrome

Congenital
  Intestinal atresia
  Gastroschisis
  Apple peel/Christmas tree deformity
  Hirschsprung disease involving ileum and colon
Acquired
  Necrotizing enterocolitis
  Volvulus
  Meconium ileus
  Trauma
  Crohns disease (rare in children)
  Tumors (rare in children)
  Radiation enteritis (rare in children)
  Mesenteric vascular occlusion (rare in children)

---

3 years after resection. In the more severe cases, various degrees of nutrient malabsorption may persist, rendering it impossible for affected patients to sustain life or growth without additional intravenous nutrition. In addition, poor peristalsis as a result of damaged bowel from the initial insult or from narrowing of intestinal surgical anastomosis or peritoneal fibrosis or both may impair enteral nutrition.

Ultimately, total oral or enteral nutrition may be feasible if at least 20 to 30 cm of small bowel remains and the ileocecal valve is intact. During the adaptation period, and sometimes during periods of accelerated growth, the administration of intravenous nutrition may be mandatory. Some patients may tolerate enteral feedings only when they are administered as a constant infusion through a gastrostomy. The degree of nutrient malabsorption that results from a short bowel is related to the extent of the resection, the topography of the segment of bowel resected, and the existence of the ileocecal valve. Removal of the ileocecal valve complicates the clinical condition because it facilitates bacterial overgrowth. In some cases, however, intestinal peristalsis may be affected, and nutrient absorption can be impaired, even when a reasonable length of bowel remains functional.

CLINICAL MANIFESTATIONS AND COMPLICATIONS

Although disaccharidases are more abundant in the jejunum, they occur also in the ileum, and carbohydrate malabsorption may not be severe if the jejunum is resected. Carbohydrate malabsorption can be secondary to decreased surface absorptive area and diminished disaccharidase activity as a result of diminished bowel length, mucosal irritation resulting from gastric hypersecretion (frequently observed in the early phase of extensive small bowel resections), accelerated transit time, and/or small bowel bacterial overgrowth. In the last situation, bacteria may use the carbohydrate before it is absorbed, causing the formation of gas and diarrhea.

Protein is malabsorbed to an extent less than that evinced by other nutrients. The decreased absorption of protein is proportional to the amount of intestine resected but, in addition, bacterial overgrowth in the small bowel may lead to enteric protein losses.

The degree of fat absorption impairment is related to the segment and length of bowel resected. Because fat cannot be absorbed in the jejunum, severe malabsorption of fat occurs in cases of extensive ileal resection. The ileum is the site for reab-

sorption of bile salt; removal of this segment of bowel causes malabsorption of the bile salts and a decrease in the bile acid pool, which impairs the formation of micelles and causes the malabsorption of fat and fat-soluble vitamins. Malabsorption of vitamin B_{12} occurs also with ileal resection and may need to be replaced for life.

After proximal small bowel resection, iron, zinc, and folate deficiency may occur in addition to a decreased absorption of calcium, magnesium, and phosphorus. Resection of the colon may result in water and sodium losses. The small bowel may compensate for the absence of the colon through an increased capacity to reabsorb water and electrolytes. Calcium and magnesium soaps may form in the lumen of the bowel in cases of fat malabsorption and can lead to hypocalcemia and hypomagnesemia. Pancreatic secretions may be decreased after the patient undergoes a proximal resection because of the loss of stimulation by cholecystokinin.

THERAPY

The treatment of short bowel syndrome (Box 359.2) includes the use of lactose-free, semi–lactose-free, or elemental diets with low osmolality. Resins to bind bile acids (e.g., cholestyramine) may be helpful in treating bile acid–induced diarrhea, which usually occurs after shorter resections. A low-fat diet is indicated after extensive resections, particularly those that include the distal ileum. The use of medium-chain triglycerides may be advantageous because the formation of micelles is not necessary for their absorption. However, essential fatty acid deficiency may occur with the use of low-fat diets that contain predominantly medium-chain triglycerides. If gastric hypersecretion develops, it may be controlled by therapy with H_2 receptor blockers or proton pump inhibitors. If small bowel bacterial overgrowth occurs, it must be treated (see Chapter 360, Small Bowel Bacterial Overgrowth). Such surgical intervention as bowel lengthening (Bianchi procedure and serial transverse enteroplasty) may improve nutrient absorption in certain patients. These procedures consist of utilizing the existing hyperplastic and dilated bowel by dividing it into two and joining the pieces lengthwise. A minimum amount of remaining bowel of at least 5 cm in diameter is required for these operations. The cycling of total intravenous nutrition, limited parenteral administration of protein, and enteral nutrition may decrease cholestasis and slow the process of liver fibrosis. Intestinal transplantation is a new option for selected patients

---

BOX 359.2   Management Alternatives for Short Bowel Syndrome

Nutritional
  Enteral nutrition through a gastrostomy button
  Intravenous nutrition
  Menhaden oil (experimental)
  Glutamine (experimental)
Surgical
  Creation of an antiperistaltic segment (no longer performed)
  Creation of a valve (no longer performed)
  Lengthening (Bianchi and STENT procedures)
Hormonal
  Human growth hormone (experimental)
  Glucagon-like peptide-2 (experimental)
Other
  Short-chain fatty acids (experimental)

---

with short bowel syndrome, in whom intravenous access becomes unavailable and or liver failure is imminent. Intestinal transplantation is the last resort for many patients.

Suggested Readings

Bianchi A. Experience with longitudinal intestinal lengthening and tailoring. *Eur J Pediatr Surg* 1999;9:256.

Buchman AL, Scolapio J, Fryer J. AGA technical review on short bowel syndrome and intestinal transplantation. *Gastroenterology* 2003;124:1111.

Thompson JS, Langnas AN, Pinch LW, et al. Surgical approach to short-bowel syndrome. Experience in a population of 160 patients. *Ann Surg* 1995;222:600.

Vanderhoof JA., Young RJ. Short bowel syndrome. In: Lifschitz C, ed. *Pediatric gastroenterology and nutrition in clinical practice.* New York, M. Dekker 2002:701.

Kim HB, Fauza D, Garza J, et al. Serial transverse enteroplasty for short bowel syndrome (STEP): a novel bowel lengthening procedure. *J Pediatr Surg* 2003; 38:425.

CHAPTER 360 ■ SMALL BOWEL BACTERIAL OVERGROWTH

CARLOS H. LIFSCHITZ

In healthy persons, the stomach, duodenum, and upper small bowel are sterile, or the number of organisms never surpasses 10^5 colony-forming units per milliliter. The organisms commonly found are lactobacilli, streptococci, *Haemophilus influenzae, Haemophilus parainfluenzae, Veillonella,* and *Propionibacterium acnes.* Such mechanisms as gastric acidity, secretions of the intestine and pancreas, immunoglobulins, and, especially, intestinal peristalsis, aid in maintaining a low bacterial count. The distal ileum contains as many as 10^9 colony-forming units per milliliter, including gram-negative bacilli and anaerobes. The ileocecal valve is important in preventing the growth of an anaerobic, colonic-type flora in the distal small bowel. The impairment of any of these mechanisms may result in bacterial overgrowth in the small bowel (Box 360.1).

Frequently, bacterial overgrowth in the small bowel leads to malabsorption of carbohydrates because of intraluminal use by bacteria. Presenting symptoms are abdominal distention as a result of formation of gas, excessive eructation, halitosis, vomiting, and diarrhea. Diarrhea can result from bacterial degradation of brush border disaccharidases and from a decrease in small-bowel villous height and a consequent decrease in the transport of monosaccharides.

Hypoproteinemia, which usually occurs in patients with bacterial overgrowth in the small bowel, can be the result of protein loss due to mucosal injury caused by the bacteria or of altered dietary protein absorption due to luminal bacterial degradation.

Bile acids, on which anaerobic bacteria act in the upper portion of the small bowel, are deconjugated, become unabsorbable, and cause diarrhea when they reach the colon. The lack of reabsorption of bile acids results in a diminished bile acid pool and impaired fat absorption. Bacterial overgrowth in the small bowel also can produce intestinal mucosal changes that interfere with the formation of chylomicrons. Colonic bacteria act on malabsorbed fat and transform it into hydroxylated fatty acids, which also cause diarrhea.

The absorption of fat-soluble vitamins can be impaired by a similar mechanism. Patients with bacterial overgrowth in the small bowel are at risk for developing bleeding disorders that result from vitamin K deficiency, night blindness caused by vitamin A malabsorption, and rickets caused by vitamin D

BOX 360.1   **Causes of Small Bowel Bacterial Overgrowth**

Congenital Bowel Abnormalities
Gastroschisis
Small bowel atresia
Meconium ileus
Malrotation
Duodenal webs

Abdominal Surgery
Postoperative adhesions
Intestinal bypass
Roux-en-Y procedures
Short bowel syndrome
Absence (by surgical removal) of ileocecal valve
Vagotomy

Acquired Bowel Abnormalities
Crohn disease
Fistulas
Tumors

Changes in Peristalsis
Parasites
Chronic diarrhea
Pseudo-obstruction
Scleroderma
Diabetes

Nutritional Factors
Celiac disease
Severe malnutrition
Hypokalemia

Other
Hypochlorhydria
Nasojejunal tubes
H_2 receptor blockers
Proton pump inhibitors
Cystic fibrosis
Immunodeficiency

deficiency. Vitamin B_{12} deficiency also occurs in patients with bacterial overgrowth in the small bowel, and the deficiency appears to result from bacterial use of vitamin B_{12}.

The diagnosis of bacterial overgrowth in the small bowel is made by intestinal intubation, aspiration, culture, and colony count of intestinal fluid. High fasting-breath hydrogen levels (15 to 20 ppm or higher) may herald bacterial overgrowth.

Treatment includes the correction of the underlying abnormality through the resection of intestinal strictures or adhesions or the use of sulfonamides or oral antibiotics, such as kanamycin, neomycin, or gentamicin. In older children, metronidazole or tetracyclines may be used. An ion exchange resin, such as cholestyramine, may help to bind such bacterial products as bile acids.

Suggested Readings

Sherman PM, Lichtman SN. Bacterial overgrowth. In: Walker W, Durie PR, Hamilton JR, et al., eds. *Pediatric gastrointestinal disease: pathophysiology, diagnosis, management.* St. Louis: Mosby, 1996:816.

Thompson JS. Surgical management of short bowel syndrome. *Surgery* 1993; 113:4.

Toskes PP. The changing nature of small intestine bacterial overgrowth. *Curr Gastroenterol Rep* 1999;1:267.

CHAPTER 361 ■ CELIAC DISEASE

CARLOS H. LIFSCHITZ

Celiac disease (CD) is an immune-mediated disease, characterized by villous atrophy of the proximal small bowel, that responds to the withdrawal of gluten from the diet. The fraction of gluten called *gliadin* has been identified as the agent responsible for the disease. The relationship between CD and intolerance to dietary wheat and rye was recognized by Dicke in 1950. The highest rate of CD occurs in Ireland, where 1 in 300 persons is affected.

EPIDEMIOLOGY

A sensitivity to gluten is the precipitating factor leading to the changes found in the intestinal mucosa in patients with CD. These proteins are found in all forms of wheat (including durum, semolina, spelt, kamut, einkorn, and faro) and related grains such as rye and barley. The disease is closely associated with genes that code for human leukocyte antigens (HLA) DQ2 and DQ8. Transglutaminase 2 appears to be an important component of the disease, both as a deamidating enzyme that can enhance the immunostimulatory effect of gluten and as a target autoantigen in the immune response. The prevalence of CD in children between 2.5 and 15 years of age in the general population is 3 to 13 per 1,000 children, or approximately 1:300 to 1:80 children. The female to male ratio is of 2:1.

CLINICAL MANIFESTATIONS AND COMPLICATIONS

The age at which cereal is introduced into the diet and the amount and type of cereal ingested may affect the presentation of the disease. Breast-feeding also may provide temporary protection. Precocious presentation may occur in children between 10 and 18 months of age and includes frothy, liquid, foul-smelling stools. Affected children acquire the celiac aspect, characterized by wasting and severe abdominal distention, at approximately 1 year of age. The other form of presentation occurs in children between ages 2 to 3 years old and includes poor feeding, lack of weight gain for several months or actual weight loss, irritability, and diarrhea consisting of foul-smelling, bulky stools (Box 361.1). Monosymptomatic forms may present with constipation or severe, recurrent abdominal pain. The disease has been diagnosed in adolescents who had no major gastrointestinal complaints but consulted a physician because of short stature. Less common forms of presentation include anemia and, in adults, CD may be associated with a wide spectrum of neurologic manifestations including cerebellar ataxia, epileptic seizures, dementia, neuropathy, myopathy, and multifocal leukoencephalopathy (Box 361.2).

DIAGNOSIS

Laboratory analyses are nonspecific. Serum abnormalities such as low hemoglobin, iron, albumin, cholesterol, calcium, phosphate, vitamin A, or carotene levels are related to the malabsorption but are nonspecific for the disease. Fat globules may be identified in a stool smear, and the malabsorption of fat can be quantified by means of a 72-hour stool collection (i.e., normal absorption, 95% of ingested fat), but this test rarely is needed. The test to measure absorption of D-xylose no longer is used. Antigliadin antibodies no longer should be ordered as a screening test because they have low sensitivity and poor specificity. Although elevated serum levels of tissue transglutaminase are highly indicative of the disease, the diagnosis requires a peroral small bowel biopsy. In cases of immunoglobulin A deficiency,

BOX 361.1	Common Manifestations of Celiac Disease

Diarrhea
Abdominal distention
Malnutrition
Failure to thrive

BOX 361.2   Nongastrointestinal Manifestations of Celiac Disease

Dermatitis herpetiforms
Dental enamel hypoplasia
Osteopenia/osteoporosis
Short stature
Delayed puberty
Anemia (nonresponsive to iron therapy, seen in adults only)
Hepatitis
Arthritis
Brain calcifications
Neurologic symptoms

BOX 361.3   Associations with Celiac Disease

Type 1 diabetes
Autoimmune thyroiditis
IgA deficiency
Down syndrome
Turner syndrome
Williams syndrome
First-degree relatives of patients with CD

---

which sometimes is associated with CD, the test could provide a false-negative answer. Therefore, in individual cases, the assessment of serum Ig A may be helpful. A small-bowel biopsy can demonstrate moderate to severe villous atrophy and a chronic inflammatory infiltrate of the lamina propria. If the biopsy results support the clinical and laboratory findings, affected patients are placed on a gluten-free diet for 6 to 12 months. Small-bowel biopsy repeated at the end of this period should demonstrate a normalization of the villous architecture. The third, confirmatory biopsy, after the patient has been reexposed to gluten, is needed only in certain situations, one of which is if the diagnosis was done prior to the patient reaching 2 years of age. Determination of HLA-DQ2 may have a role in excluding the diagnosis in equivocal cases, but its utility is limited because of its high frequency of occurrence in the normal population.

Although small-bowel villous atrophy in conjunction with the clinical picture described is characteristic of CD, such other abnormalities as dietary protein intolerance can present in a similar manner.

THERAPY

Treatment with a gluten-free diet (GFD) is recommended for all symptomatic children with intestinal histopathologic abnormalities that are characteristic of CD. Clinical experience has demonstrated that children with persistent diarrhea and poor weight gain resulting from CD have complete resolution of symptoms on treatment with a GFD.

The transient malabsorption of lactose can be observed in some patients with CD as a result of decreased lactase activity, but this is rare. For such patients, lactose-free or lactose-hydrolyzed milk is recommended. Malabsorption of fat and fat-soluble vitamins also is seen in patients with CD. The inability to absorb fat probably is not related solely to a mucosal defect because fat is absorbed primarily in the distal ileum, a part of the small bowel that is less affected in CD. A decreased contraction of the gallbladder, probably caused by a lack of secretion of cholecystokinin by the damaged enterocytes of the proximal small bowel, may explain the lack of bile acid secretion and consequent malabsorption of fat. In patients with pro-

longed malnutrition, potassium deficiency may result in muscle dysfunction, which may lead to bowel distention, stasis, and bacterial overgrowth in the small bowel.

Treatment entails the complete removal of gluten from the diet and supplementation of calories during the period of catch-up growth; vitamin and mineral supplements are recommended during this time. The recommendation that affected patients remain on a GFD for life is questioned by some investigators.

Celiac Crisis

The celiac crisis is a medical emergency that can occur in patients in whom exposure to gluten has been prolonged or who are intentionally or inadvertently reexposed to gluten. Patients present in shock, with diarrhea, abdominal distension, and severe hypokalemia. Intercurrent illnesses may precipitate a celiac crisis.

Investigation of Family Members and in Associated Conditions

The prevalence of CD among first-degree relatives is much higher than in the general population. Most of these patients have an atypical form of presentation. Serologic testing is recommended for all first-degree relatives of CD patients; these individuals also should undergo HLA typing to detect those whose HLA phenotype is consistent with CD.

Serologic testing also may be indicated in patients with hypothyroidism, Down syndrome, and Type I diabetes, in whom the incidence of the disease is higher than in the normal population (Box 361.3).

Suggested Readings

Fabiani E, Catassi C; International Working Group. The serum IgA class antitissue transglutaminase antibodies in the diagnosis and follow up of coeliac disease. Results of an international multi-centre study. International Working Group on Eu-tTG. *Eur J Gastroenterol Hepatol* 2001;13:659.

Hill ID, Dirks MH, Liptak GS, et al. Guideline for the diagnosis and treatment of celiac disease in children: recommendations of the North American Society for Pediatric Gastroenterology, Hepatology, and Nutrition. *J Pediatr Gastroenterol Nutrit* 2005;40:1.

Polanco I. Celiac disease. In: Lifschitz C, ed. *Pediatric gastroenterology and nutrition in clinical practice.* New York: M. Dekker, 2002:517.

CHAPTER 362 ■ IMMUNODEFICIENCY STATES

CARLOS H. LIFSCHITZ

ACQUIRED IMMUNODEFICIENCY SYNDROME

The acquired immunodeficiency syndrome (AIDS) has been reported in children since 1983 and may be found among hemophiliacs, transfusion recipients, infants born to high-risk parents, and adolescents. The gastrointestinal (GI) manifestations observed in patients with AIDS include esophagitis and diarrhea with or without parasitic, viral, or bacterial infections. Nutrient malabsorption is not always a factor in the illness, although children may have nutrient malabsorption even if they do not have overt symptoms. Esophagitis caused by *Candida albicans* can be the presenting symptom in patients with AIDS and may or may not be associated with oral thrush.

Organisms commonly associated with the diarrhea that occurs in patients with AIDS are *C. albicans*, *Cryptosporidium*, cytomegalovirus, atypical mycobacteria, and *Salmonella typhimurium*. Even in the absence of systemic or enteric infections or malignancy, many adult and pediatric patients with AIDS suffer from chronic diarrhea, anorexia, and weight loss. *Mycobacterium avium-intracellulare* has been found in the small bowel of patients with AIDS and has been associated with diarrhea. The organism is an acid-fast bacillus that has been found in macrophages of the lamina propria of the small bowel. Patients with cytomegalovirus infections may have diarrhea, and viral inclusions can be found at different levels of the GI tract. Ileitis or colitis, together with esophageal and colonic ulcers from which the virus can be cultured, has been reported.

The GI symptoms of AIDS can mimic those of other diseases. The symptoms of patients with AIDS who suffer from chronic diarrhea and have marked abdominal distention and malnutrition have been compared with the symptoms of celiac disease. The histologic picture of the small-bowel mucosa is compatible with partially treated celiac disease in that it has patchy atrophy alternating with more normal segments of mucosa. In other patients, the clinical symptoms are similar to those of inflammatory bowel disease. These patients complain of abdominal pain, weight loss, diarrhea, and fever. AIDS in children may manifest also as pseudomembranous necrotizing jejunitis.

AIDS may be expressed as a failure to thrive, with or without diarrhea. Diarrhea and malabsorption are more prevalent occurrences in patients with documented GI infections. Frequently, increased fecal fat, diminished appetite, and weight loss are observed in these patients. A small-bowel biopsy can identify infiltration of the lamina propria with chronic inflammatory cells and occasional subtle villous atrophy. Nonspecific inflammatory cell infiltrate also can be seen in the colon. These histologic and functional abnormalities have been called *AIDS enteropathy*. The evaluation of patients who have AIDS and present with GI symptoms should include a careful search for bowel pathogens. However, in many patients in whom pathogens can be identified, often diarrhea persists despite a variety of therapeutic interventions, including systemic treatment for fungal or mycobacterial disease and the intravenous administration of antibiotics for other infections. Feedings can be administered through a nasogastric tube if affected children are too debilitated to take food orally. This technique also may facilitate gastric emptying and tolerance of formula.

IMMUNOGLOBULIN A DEFICIENCY

Selective immunoglobulin A (IgA) deficiency is the most common of the primary immunodeficiency states, affecting approximately 1 in 700 of the population. Because other immunoglobulins, such as IgM, may compensate for the deficiency, only 13% of the patients have significant GI symptoms. The GI manifestations of IgA deficiency are chronic diarrhea, steatorrhea, lactose malabsorption, milk-protein intolerance, and those secondary to infestation by *Giardia lamblia*. The relationship between serum or secretory IgA deficiencies and GI symptoms has not been clarified completely, but a secretory IgA deficiency appears to be the form associated with malabsorption. Celiac disease, lymphonodular hyperplasia, ulcerative colitis, Crohn disease, and disaccharidase deficiencies have been associated with IgA deficiency. Moreover, small-bowel villous atrophy has been observed in patients with IgA deficiency and giardiasis. Usually, diarrhea and malabsorption improve after treatment for *G. lamblia*.

PANHYPOGAMMAGLOBULINEMIA

Approximately 60% of patients with the common variable form of immunoglobulin deficiency have chronic or recurrent diarrhea; most of these patients also have malabsorption. Infestation by *G. lamblia* is a common occurrence, and secondary disaccharidase deficiencies and clinical carbohydrate intolerance may occur. However, malabsorption can occur also in patients in whom *Giardia* cannot be found. The intestinal mucosa may reveal that altered villous architecture, despite malabsorption, is present, although the small-bowel histology is normal. Small-bowel bacterial overgrowth can complicate the clinical picture in some patients, but treatment of this condition does not necessarily resolve the symptoms. Malabsorption also can result from the development of gastric achlorhydria and deficiency of intrinsic factor leading to vitamin B_{12} malabsorption and myeloblastic anemia. In rare cases, the syndrome can include neutropenia and pancreatic exocrine insufficiency. A rare condition, ulcerative jejunoileitis, may complicate common variable hypogammaglobulinemia and can result in severe nutrient malabsorption.

X-LINKED HYPOGAMMAGLOBULINEMIA

Patients with X-linked hypogammaglobulinemia suffer from diarrhea and malabsorption less often than do those with common variable hypogammaglobulinemia. Usually, diarrhea

TABLE 362.1

ORGANISMS ASSOCIATED WITH IMMUNODEFICIENCIES

Secretory IgA deficiency	*Giardia lamblia*
AIDS	*Candida albicans*
	Cryptosporidium
	Cytomegalovirus
	Atypical mycobacteria
	Salmonella typhimurium
	Mycobacterium avium-intracellulare
Panhypogammaglobulinemia	*Giardia lamblia*
T-cell deficiency	*Candida albicans*

resolves after the child reaches 2 years of age. Giardiasis occurs frequently and can lead to malabsorption.

COMBINED IMMUNODEFICIENCIES

Usually, patients with such rare conditions as Wiskott-Aldrich syndrome have a history of chronic, blood-tinged diarrhea early in infancy. The second most common primary immunodeficiency syndrome is severe combined immunodeficiency. Diarrhea and malabsorption are common findings in infants who have deficient humoral and cellular immune mechanisms. Few studies have traced the pathogenesis of the malabsorption state. The villi of the jejunal mucosa are stunted, and marked mucosal edema and a large number of vacuolated macrophages can be seen. Malabsorption may be limited initially to lactose, but eventually it encompasses other nutrients. Treatment by bone marrow grafting may cause a graft-versus-host reaction and can result in marked villous shortening, diarrhea, enteral

protein loss, and nutrient malabsorption. Small-bowel bacterial overgrowth may aggravate malabsorption.

T-CELL DEFICIENCY

Frequently, patients with DiGeorge syndrome have oral and esophageal candidiasis and prolonged diarrhea.

THERAPY

Organisms commonly associated with GI symptoms in immunosuppressed patients are listed in Table 362.1. Metronidazole or quinacrine hydrochloride (Atabrine) can be used to eradicate *Giardia*. Treatment for *Cryptosporidium* can be attempted with albendazole, and multiple antibiotics can be administered for *M. avium-intracellulare*, but generally such treatment is not successful. Nutritional support should include a lactose-free diet and preferably the use of hydrolyzed proteins. The elimination of fresh vegetables and fruits may reduce the risk of introducing pathogenic bacteria into immunosuppressed persons.

Suggested Readings

Barton LL, Moussa SL, Villar RG, Hulett RL. Gastrointestinal complications of chronic granulomatous disease: case report and literature review. *Clin Pediatr* (Phila) 1998;37:231.

Gurbindo C, Seidman EG. Gastrointestinal manifestations of primary immunodeficiency diseases. In: Walker W, Durie PR, Hamilton JR, et al., eds. *Pediatric gastrointestinal disease: pathophysiology, diagnosis, management*. St. Louis: Mosby, 1996:585.

Kahn E. Gastrointestinal manifestations in pediatric AIDS. *Pediatr Pathol Lab Med* 1997;17:171.

Winter HS, Madden J. Nutritional support of the chronically ill child. In: Lifschitz C, ed. *Pediatric gastroenterology and nutrition in clinical practice*. New York: M. Dekker, 2002:399.

CHAPTER 363 ■ ENZYME AND TRANSPORT DEFECTS

SANDY T. HWANG AND ROBERT J. SHULMAN

CARBOHYDRATE MALABSORPTION

Pathophysiology and Clinical Findings

Disorders of carbohydrate absorption are linked integrally with dysfunction of the small-intestinal mucosal carbohydrate-digesting enzymes: lactase, sucrase, alpha-dextrinase, trehalase, and glucoamylase. Lactase activity increases substantially between 35 weeks' gestation and birth. Lactase is the only enzyme capable of hydrolyzing lactose. Sucrase and alpha-

dextrinase are two enzymes that are linked covalently in the intestinal brush border and develop full activity in early fetal life. Sucrase can hydrolyze sucrose, maltose, and the 1,4 bonds in glucose polymers and starches. Alpha-dextrinase can hydrolyze maltose but not sucrose, and it is the only enzyme that can hydrolyze the 1,6 bonds found in starches. Trehalose, a carbohydrate found in mushrooms and insects, is hydrolyzed by trehalase. Glucoamylase activity also is developed early in gestation and can hydrolyze maltose and the 1,4 linkages from the nonreducing ends of starches (i.e., glucose polymers, complex starches). If lactose, sucrose, trehalose, and maltose are not hydrolyzed and absorbed, they remain as osmotically active molecules in the lumen of the bowel. Unabsorbed glucose polymers and starches have a similar but smaller effect inversely proportional to molecular size. All disorders associated with significant carbohydrate malabsorption can induce a net secretion of water that increases the rate of intestinal transit and can decrease the absorptive capacity for other nutrients. The result is watery diarrhea and cramping that cease if patients are not fed.

Malabsorbed carbohydrate passes into the colon, where it is converted by bacterial fermentation to fatty acids, which also are osmotically active, and to hydrogen gas. These conversion products are absorbed partially; some of the hydrogen gas is excreted in breath. When carbohydrate is malabsorbed beyond the capacity of bacterial fermentation, the result is acid stools (pH less than 6) and fecal carbohydrate loss (i.e., stools positive for reducing substances, such as glucose).

Disorders of carbohydrate digestion or absorption may or may not be associated with failure to thrive in infancy, depending on the degree of exposure to the offending carbohydrate. Nutritional or growth abnormalities do not result if the diet is nutritionally adequate and contains little or no offending carbohydrate.

Primary Disorders

Infants with the rare condition of congenital lactase deficiency are symptomatic at birth if a lactose-containing diet (e.g., breast milk, formula) is fed. Lactose tolerance appears to increase during childhood for reasons that are not understood entirely. Late-onset lactase deficiency, an autosomal recessive trait, develops between ages 3 and 5 years. It occurs in 5% to 20% of white children and 70% to 75% of black children in North America, in 74% of Hispanic children, and in 55% of Filipino children. Evidence suggests that the decline in lactase activity can be due to changes in gene transcriptional regulation or posttranslational processing. Although lactose malabsorption also occurs in late-onset deficiency, lactose intolerance—characterized by watery diarrhea, abdominal pain, and/or cramping—may not be present, because symptoms depend in part on patients' subjective response to gas and pain, the lactose load, the rate of gastric emptying, and, in some cases, the residual lactase activity.

In North America, the incidence of sucrase and alpha-dextrinase deficiency is 0.2%. In this autosomal recessive disorder, patients have a defect in the posttranslational processing of the enzymes; sucrase activity is absent, and dextrinase activity is partially or completely absent. Usually, patients become symptomatic in infancy when a sucrose-containing diet is introduced. As with congenital lactase deficiency, patients appear to develop tolerance to sucrose with age.

Trehalase deficiency is a rare autosomal recessive condition particularly prevalent in the Greenland Inuit population (10% to 15%). Symptoms have been reported after the ingestion of large amounts of mushrooms.

A recently identified condition, glucoamylase deficiency, is included in the differential diagnosis of chronic diarrhea in children. Usually, the activity levels of sucrase, dextrinase, maltase, and lactase are normal. Significant growth failure is not a common feature.

In glucose and galactose malabsorption (an autosomal recessive disease), hydrolysis of carbohydrates proceeds normally, but patients lack the ability to absorb glucose or galactose (carbohydrates that appear to have a common transport mechanism). The defect appears to be a mutation in the sodium glucose cotransporter gene. Often, the disorder is associated with abnormal renal tubular glucose transport, which results in a decreased threshold for glucose reabsorption. Symptoms occur if the diet contains lactose, sucrose, maltose, or starches.

Isolated fructose malabsorption has been described. Often, symptoms of abdominal pain, bloating, and diarrhea follow the malabsorption of such fructose-containing foods as fruits and fruit juices. Symptoms do not develop after the ingestion of sucrose. Clinical evidence suggests this condition can coexist with glucose–galactose malabsorption.

Secondary Disorders

All the entities described must be differentiated from secondary carbohydrate intolerance, which results from damage to the enzyme-containing villous epithelial cells. Usually, lactase is the enzyme affected most severely because of its normally low activity and the slow rate of recovery, compared with that of the other enzymes. In contrast to sucrose and maltose, the rate-limiting step in lactose absorption is hydrolysis, not absorption. Lactase deficiency in infancy results commonly from enteric virus infections (e.g., rotavirus) or small-intestinal bacterial pathogens. A clinically significant deficiency may last from 3 to 4 weeks after an episode of acute gastroenteritis. Celiac disease and iron deficiency are other disorders that may be associated with lactase deficiency in older infants and children. If mucosal injury is severe, sucrase, alpha-dextrinase, and glucoamylase can be affected. In the worst cases, glucose absorption is impaired as a consequence of the reduced surface area available for absorption resulting from blunted and damaged villi.

Diagnosis and Treatment

An accurate diet history is critical in the diagnosis of carbohydrate intolerance. Often, the diagnosis can be confirmed by exclusion of the suspected carbohydrate from the diet, followed by rapid abatement of the symptoms (Fig. 363.1). Confirmatory evidence of carbohydrate malabsorption includes acid stools (i.e., pH less than 6, measured with Nitrazine paper on a fresh stool sample) and, in severe cases, stools positive for glucose. Stools are glucose positive because of bacterial breakdown of the disaccharides to their component sugars.

The diagnosis of carbohydrate malabsorption can be confirmed with an oral tolerance test, but this is neither sensitive nor specific. The hydrogen breath test is a more useful diagnostic tool. In the oral tolerance and the breath hydrogen tests, a 2-g load of the carbohydrate per 1 kg of body weight is administered as a 20% solution. In response to the oral tolerance test, a rise in blood glucose of less than 25 mg/dL is presumptive evidence of carbohydrate malabsorption, as is a rise in breath hydrogen greater than 10 parts per million over baseline. A definitive diagnosis is achieved when normal histology (in the primary disorders) or abnormal histology (in the secondary deficiencies) is found and enzyme activity is absent in a small-intestinal biopsy specimen obtained perorally.

The treatment of choice for the primary disorders is exclusion of the offending carbohydrate from the diet, presumably for life. However, tolerance generally improves with age, and small amounts of the carbohydrate can be consumed without clinical symptoms. Lactose intolerance can be overcome when meals are supplemented with the lactase enzyme obtained from the fungus *Aspergillus oryzae* (Lactrase, Lactaid). Sucrase and alpha-dextrinase intolerance can be improved by adding fresh bakers' yeast (*Saccharomyces cerevisiae*) to meals. A more palatable alternative is liquid yeast sucrase (Sucraid). The exclusion of starches from the diet improves symptoms in glucoamylase deficiency. Glucose and galactose malabsorption requires the use of fructose as the dietary carbohydrate, because fructose transport by facilitated diffusion is unaffected in this disorder. Fructose malabsorption requires the removal of free fructose from the diet.

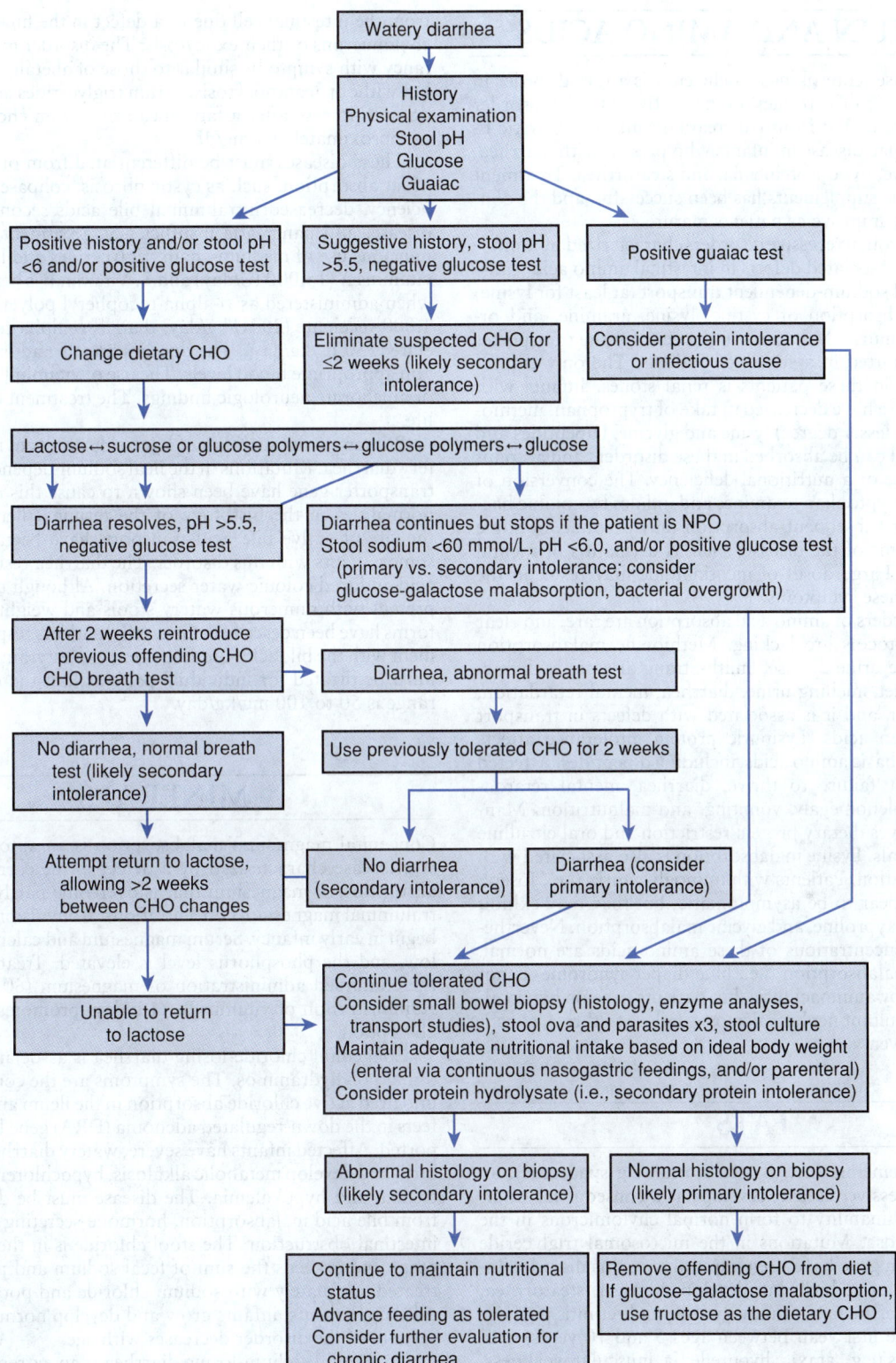

FIGURE 363.1. Scheme for diagnosing and treating primary and secondary carbohydrate malabsorption. This general outline may have to be individualized. It is important that only one change at a time be made in the feeding regimen (e.g., carbohydrate concentration, volume of the feeding) and adequate time is allowed between changes to assess the results. CHO, carbohydrate; NPO, nothing by mouth.

PROTEIN AND AMINO ACIDS

Enteropeptidase (enterokinase) deficiency is a rare disorder in which pancreatic proenzymes are not activated. The disorder must be differentiated from pancreatic insufficiency, cystic fibrosis, and celiac disease in infants who present with diarrhea, failure to thrive, hypoproteinemia, and steatorrhea. Treatment with pancreatic supplements has been successful, and the condition tends to improve as patients mature.

Many autosomal recessive disorders characterized by aminoaciduria have associated defects in intestinal amino acid transport. A lack of sodium-dependent transport (at least for lysine) leads to malabsorption of cystine, lysine, arginine, and ornithine in cystinuria. Mutations in the gene for the transporter have been reported in a subset of patients. The only clinical manifestation in these patients is renal stones. Infants with Hartnup disease have decreased uptake of tryptophan, methionine, and (to a lesser degree) lysine and glycine. Dipeptides and tripeptides still can be absorbed in these disorders and account for the absence of a nutritional deficiency. The conversion of malabsorbed tryptophan to amines and indoles by colonic bacteria and their subsequent absorption may account for some of the symptoms of the disease, such as dermatitis or mental deterioration. Large doses of nicotinamide may result in the remission of these symptoms.

Other disorders of amino acid absorption are rare, and clear treatment protocols are lacking. Methionine malabsorption (i.e., oasthouse urine disease, Smith-Strang disease) is characterized by sweet-smelling urine, diarrhea, mental retardation, and white hair, and it is associated with defects in transport of other amino acids. Lysinuric protein intolerance affects transport of dibasic amino acids, including dipeptides. Affected infants exhibit failure to thrive, diarrhea, mental retardation, hepatosplenomegaly, vomiting, and malnutrition. Management involves dietary protein restriction and oral citrulline taken with meals. Lysine malabsorption is also associated with mental retardation. Patients with iminoglycinuria (i.e., Joseph syndrome) appear to be asymptomatic, but they may exhibit proline, hydroxyproline, and glycine malabsorption. Nevertheless, serum concentrations of these amino acids are normal. Tryptophan malabsorption (i.e., blue diaper syndrome) is not accompanied by aminoaciduria, but patients develop hypercalcemia with resultant nephrocalcinosis, failure to thrive, constipation, and fever.

FATS

Abetalipoproteinemia (i.e., Bassen-Kornzweig syndrome), an autosomal recessive disease, develops as a consequence of affected infants' inability to form normal chylomicrons in the intestinal mucosa. Mutations in the microsomal triglyceride transfer protein gene have been implicated in this disorder. Infants are normal at birth but develop diarrhea, steatorrhea, failure to thrive, anemia, acanthocytosis, and retinitis pigmentosa during the first year. Between ages 5 and 10 years, neurologic findings (e.g., ataxia, hyporeflexia, muscular weakness, and athetoid movements, probably due to vitamin E deficiency) characteristically develop. Serum triglyceride levels are lower than 10 mg/dL, and the cholesterol level is less than 50 mg/dL.

Hypobetalipoproteinemia is an autosomal dominant disorder that, in the homozygous form, is indistinguishable from abetalipoproteinemia. Abnormalities in the apolipoprotein B protein have been identified in these patients. Heterozygotes have milder hypolipemia (triglycerides, 50 to 100 mg/dL; cholesterol, less than 100 mg/dL) and neurologic symptoms.

Chylomicron retention disease, an autosomal recessive disorder, is characterized by inability to transport chylomicrons from the intestinal cell due to a defect in the final assembly of chylomicrons or their exocytosis. The disorder manifests in infancy with symptoms similar to those of abetalipoproteinemia but without acanthocytosis. Serum triglycerides are normal but do not increase after a fatty meal; the serum cholesterol level is approximately 65 mg/dL.

These diseases must be differentiated from other disorders of fat absorption, such as cystic fibrosis, colipase or lipase deficiency, decreased intraluminal bile acids secondary to liver disease, and pancreatic insufficiency. Treatment includes the judicious use of medium-chain triglycerides and large doses of vitamins A (15,000 IU/day) and E. Vitamin E is better absorbed when administered as D-alpha-tocopheryl polyethylene glycol 1,000 succinate (20 IU/kg/day) than as D-alpha-tocopheryl acetate (150 IU/kg/day). The dosages must be adjusted to maintain appropriate blood levels. The use of vitamin E may prevent or ameliorate neurologic findings. The treatment continues for life.

Primary malabsorption of bile acids results in nonfatty, watery diarrhea. Mutations in the ileal sodium-dependent bile acid transporter gene have been shown to cause this disorder. Abnormalities in the histology of the terminal ileum, which is the site of active bile acid transport, have been observed in some patients with this disorder. The diarrhea results from bile acid–induced colonic water secretion. Although most patients present with numerous watery stools and weight loss, milder forms have been described. Generally, patients respond to treatment with the bile acid–binding agent cholestyramine. The dose must be titrated for individual patients, but the usual dosage range is 50 to 100 mg/kg/day.

MINERALS

Congenital magnesium malabsorption is an autosomal recessive disease characterized by a defect in the carrier-mediated absorption of magnesium that is overcome partly by high intraluminal magnesium concentrations. Convulsions and tetany begin in early infancy. Serum magnesium and calcium levels are low, and the phosphorus level is elevated. Treatment entails the continued administration of magnesium (60 mg/kg/day). Administration of vitamin B_6 (1 g/day) promotes magnesium absorption.

Congenital chloride-losing diarrhea is associated with maternal polyhydramnios. The symptoms are the consequence of impaired active chloride absorption in the ileum and colon. Defects in the down-regulated adenoma (DRA) gene have been reported. Affected infants have severe, watery diarrhea soon after birth and develop metabolic alkalosis, hypochloremia, hyponatremia, and hypokalemia. The disease must be differentiated from bile acid malabsorption, hormone-secreting tumors, and intestinal obstruction. The stool chloride is in the 150 mEq/L range and exceeds the sum of fecal sodium and potassium. If treated adequately with sodium chloride and potassium chloride supplements, infants grow and develop normally, and the severity of the disorder decreases with age.

Congenital sodium-losing diarrhea is an extremely rare autosomal recessive disorder that also manifests with polyhydramnios. Although thought to be related to genes encoding for sodium/proton exchangers, it is not related to mutations in the genes encoding for currently known sodium/proton exchangers NHE1, NHE2, NHE3, and NHE5. Patients develop acidosis and hypokalemia because of a defect in intestinal sodium and hydrogen ion exchange. Stool sodium is in the range of 100 mEq/L. Patients are treated for the disorder with sodium and potassium citrate solutions. Reported patients have succumbed primarily to complications related to their management (e.g., central venous catheter infections).

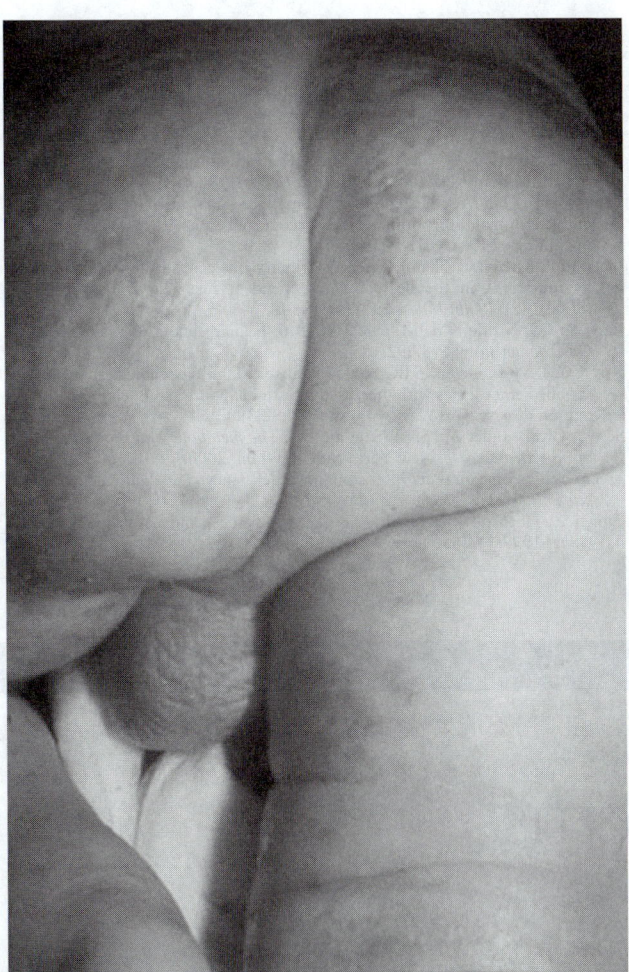

FIGURE 363.2. Perianal rash seen in a patient with acrodermatitis enteropathica.

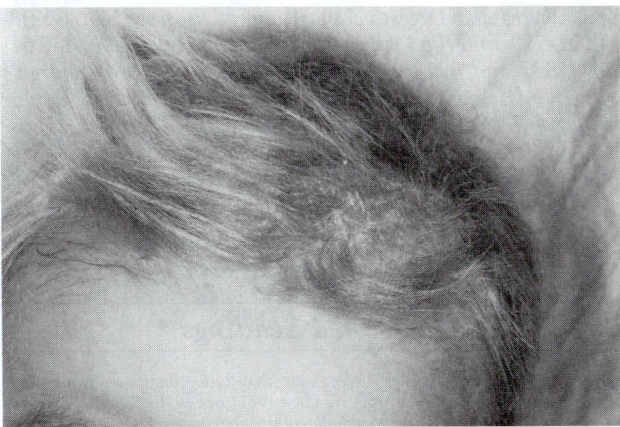

FIGURE 363.3. Hair changes seen in a patient with Menkes disease.

Acrodermatitis enteropathica is an autosomal recessive disorder that leads to zinc deficiency due to zinc malabsorption. Mutations in the recently identified intestinal zinc transporter have been reported in some patients. A ligand in human milk facilitates zinc absorption, and symptoms appear at weaning. Affected infants develop diarrhea and a red, excoriated rash that begins in the perioral and perianal areas and then spreads (Fig. 363.2). Other symptoms include alopecia, recurrent infections, and neurologic disturbances. Usually, patients have low plasma levels of zinc. However, the diagnosis is confirmed most easily by a rapid response to zinc therapy. The recommended initial dose of elemental zinc is 10 mg/kg/day until there is complete healing and then a lower maintenance dose of 1 to 2 mg/kg/day. Higher initial doses may be required for some patients. There is usually a rapid improvement in symptoms within 48 hours after the onset of therapy. Treatment is continued indefinitely for complete and continued resolution of the symptoms.

A widespread defect in copper transport that also involves the duodenum and jejunum causes Menkes disease, a recessive X-linked disorder. The defective gene involved in this disease encodes for an intracellular copper-binding adenotriphosphatase and results in the accumulation of copper within affected tissues. It is characterized by broken, stubby hair (Fig. 363.3), hypopigmentation, osteoporosis, flared metaphyses, pudgy facies with drooping jowls, low serum copper and ceruloplasmin levels, and progressive cerebral degeneration. Treatment with subcutaneous injections of copper-histidine may prevent the progression of neurologic symptoms if given early, but it has no effect on the connective tissue disorder.

Hemochromatosis is an autosomal recessive disorder characterized by an abnormally increased rate of iron absorption by the gastrointestinal tract. Thus far, mutations in three genes involved in intestinal iron absorption have been identified in patients. The increased iron absorption and the reduced iron storage by the reticuloendothelial system lead to systemic iron overload with resulting cirrhosis, diabetes, heart failure, and skin pigmentation. Because iron accumulation takes many years, the disease is rare in children. The amount of iron in the diet probably determines the onset of the disease. The treatment of choice is routine phlebotomy.

VITAMINS

Cobalamin (vitamin B_{12}) malabsorption (i.e., Imerslund-Grasbeck syndrome) is an autosomal recessive disorder that may be caused by a decrease in the number or function of ileal receptors for cobalamin or by a defect in cobalamin intracellular transport. Mutations in the gene for cubilin, the ileal receptor for the cobalamin-intrinsic factor complex, have been reported in these patients. Usually, patients present in the first 2 years of life (but sometimes later) with megaloblastic anemia, poor feeding, ataxia, paresthesia, and low serum levels of cobalamin. This disorder must be differentiated from others of cobalamin metabolism: lack of intrinsic factor, inactive or rapidly degraded intrinsic factor, ineffective splitting of R binders from cobalamin due to pancreatic insufficiency, or binding of cobalamin by intestinal bacteria in bacterial overgrowth syndromes. Except for the associated proteinuria, other symptoms resolve with cobalamin administration (200 to 1,000 μg/month, given intramuscularly).

Congenital folate malabsorption occurs almost exclusively in girls and manifests with a megaloblastic anemia and anorexia between ages 2 and 3 months in association with mental impairment. Whether treatment completely prevents the central nervous system disease is unclear, because patients appear to have impaired uptake of folate into cerebrospinal fluid. Treatment with folinic acid (1.5 mg/day given intramuscularly) probably is necessary throughout life.

Acknowledgments

This study was supported by the U.S. Department of Agriculture/Agricultural Research Service (USDA/ARS) under Cooperative Agreement No. 6250-51000-043; the National Institute of Diabetes and Digestive and Kidney Diseases, No. 1-K08-DK02-550; and the National Institutes of Health No. 1-R01-NR05337 and is a publication of the USDA/ARS Children's Nutrition Research Center, Department of Pediatrics, Baylor College of Medicine, and Texas Children's Hospital, Houston, Texas. The contents of this publication do not necessarily reflect the views or policies of the USDA, nor does mention of trade names, commercial products, or organizations imply endorsement by the U.S. government.

Suggested Readings

Barr RG, Perman JA, Schoeller DA, et al. Breath tests in pediatric gastrointestinal disorders: new diagnostic opportunities. *Pediatrics* 1978;62:393.

Bondy PK, Rosenberg LE, eds. *Metabolic control and disease.* Philadelphia: Saunders, 1980.

Cooper BA, Rosenblatt DS. Inherited defects of vitamin B$_{12}$ metabolism. *Ann Rev Nutr* 1987;7:291.

Danks DM. Inborn errors of trace mineral metabolism. *Clin Endocrinol Metab* 1985;14:591.

Davis RE. Clinical chemistry of folic acid. *Adv Clin Chem* 1985;25:233.

Gishan FK, Lee PC, Lebenthal E, et al. Isolated congenital enterokinase deficiency: recent findings and review of the literature. *Gastroenterology* 1983;85:727.

Gitomer WL, Pak CYC. Recent advances in the biochemical and molecular biological basis of cystinuria. *J Urol* 1996;156:1907.

Holmberg C. Congenital chloride diarrhoea. *Clin Gastroenterol* 1986;15:583.

Iacono G, Carroccio A, Cavataio F, et al. Congenital fructose-glucose-galactose malabsorption. *J Pediatr Gastroenterol Nutr* 1995;21:95.

Lebenthal E, Khin MU, Zheng BY, et al. Small intestinal glucoamylase deficiency and starch malabsorption: a newly recognized alpha-glucosidase deficiency in children. *J Pediatr* 1994;124:541.

Oelkers P, Kirby LC, Heubi JE, et al. Primary bile acid malabsorption caused by mutations in the ileal sodium-dependent bile acid transporter gene (SLC10A2). *J Clin Invest* 1997;99:1880.

Popovic OS, Kostic KM, Milovic VB, et al. Primary bile acid malabsorption. *Gastroenterology* 1987;92:1851.

Roy CC, Levy E, Green PHR, et al. Malabsorption, hypocholesterolemia, and fat-filled enterocytes with increased intestinal apoprotein B: chylomicron retention disease. *Gastroenterology* 1987;92:390.

Scriver CR, Beaudet AL, Sly WS, et al., eds. *The metabolic and molecular bases of inherited disease.* New York: McGraw-Hill, 2000.

Treem WR. Congenital sucrase-isomaltase deficiency. *J Pediatr Gastroenterol Nutr* 1995;21:1.

Tümer Z, Horn N. Menkes disease: recent advances and new aspects. *J Med Genet* 1997;34:265.

CHAPTER 364 ■ APPENDICITIS

WALTER PEGOLI, JR.

Appendicitis is the most common clinical entity leading to emergency abdominal operations in children. Pathologist Reginald Fitz initially described the condition in 1886. T. G. Morton performed the first successful appendectomy in 1887. Despite recognition of appendicitis as a surgically significant clinical entity more than 100 years ago, appendicitis remains a condition that can be difficult to diagnose. It is the responsibility of pediatricians and surgeons to make an early, accurate diagnosis to permit prompt intervention.

EPIDEMIOLOGY

Understanding the embryologic development of the appendix can aid clinicians in making the diagnosis of appendicitis. The appendix arises from the cecum during the eighth week of fetal development. It rotates from its initial position along the lateral aspect of the cecum to a more medial position near the ileocecal valve. Rotational arrest can occur at any point, resulting in variations in the final position of the appendix within the abdominal cavity. Variability in appendiceal position, especially the tip, can lead to alterations in the point of maximal tenderness on physical examination when inflammation is present.

The risk of developing appendicitis during an average lifetime has been estimated to range from 6% to 20%. The risk is lowest during infancy and greatest during adolescence. Approximately 1% of all children age 15 years or younger will develop appendicitis, with a peak incidence between 10 and 12 years. The incidence of perforation present at the time of surgery ranges between 10% and 50%.

PATHOPHYSIOLOGY

Luminal obstruction is the most common etiology of acute appendicitis. Most often, obstruction is the result of inspissated fecal material (appendicolith). However, appendicoliths are present in only 30% to 50% of patients at the time of appendectomy.

Bacterial or viral infections can lead to periappendiceal lymphoid hyperplasia. Lymphoid hyperplasia located near the base of the appendix can result in extrinsic compression. Obstruction, either intrinsic or extrinsic, is followed by an increase in intraluminal pressure distal to the point of obstruction, secondary to increased mucus production and venous engorgement. Unabated, the inflammatory process leads to thrombosis of the vascular strictures within the wall of the appendix. Thrombosis, with progressive ischemia, results in full thickness necrosis, which ultimately leads to perforation.

CLINICAL MANIFESTATIONS AND COMPLICATIONS

Early diagnosis and treatment are essential to the successful management of patients with appendicitis. Usually, patients present with the triad of nausea (with or without vomiting), fever, and abdominal pain. The pain associated with appendicitis exhibits a classic migratory pattern, which is a result of the particular neural pathways associated with the perception of abdominal pain. Obstruction of the appendiceal lumen leads to distention of the organ; impulses via wall-stretch receptors then are relayed through visceral nerve fibers to the tenth

Differential Diagnosis of Right Lower Quadrant Pain

Medical Conditions
Constipation
Diabetic ketoacidosis
Gastroenteritis (viral or bacteria)
Hemolytic-uremic syndrome
Henoch-Schönlein purpura
Inflammatory bowel disease
Pneumonia
Primary peritonitis
Sickle cell crisis
Urinary tract infection

Gynecologic Conditions
Ectopic pregnancy
Mittelschmerz
Ovarian torsion
Pelvic inflammatory disease
Ruptured ovarian cyst

Surgical Conditions
Intussusception
Meckel diverticulitis

thoracic ganglion. Pain initially is perceived in the periumbilical region. As the inflammatory process progresses and becomes full-thickness, parietal peritonitis results. Pain localizes in the right lower quadrant (RLQ) at McBurney's point (two-thirds of the way between the umbilicus and the anterior superior iliac spine).

Anorexia, nausea, and vomiting are important symptoms in patients with acute appendicitis. One or more of these symptoms occur subsequent to the onset of abdominal pain. The differential diagnosis of RLQ pain is extensive (Box 364.1). A detailed history and physical examination are of utmost importance and may effectively rule out a number of other conditions. Laboratory data and radiographic findings may offer additional important information.

The cardinal physical finding is pain that localizes in the RLQ of the abdomen. The point of maximal tenderness varies with the location of the appendiceal tip. For example, the distal appendix may lie across the psoas muscle or in the depths of the pelvis. In such situations, pain is not perceived at McBurney's point, but rather as back or suprapubic discomfort. However, one may elicit tenderness by extending the hip (psoas sign) or flexing and internally rotating the thigh (obturator sign). Rebound tenderness denotes peritoneal inflammation and occurs late in the disease process. The diagnostic value of the rectal examination in patients who may have appendicitis should not be underestimated. Induration or focal tenderness in the right hemipelvis can be suggestive of acute appendicitis. In cases of long-standing perforated appendicitis with a periappendiceal abscess, a fluctuant mass can be palpated.

DIAGNOSIS

Although many different laboratory studies have been used by clinicians to aid in the diagnosis of appendicitis, none has been consistently reliable. The white blood cell (WBC) count and differential blood cell count offers the most valuable information. An elevated leukocyte count, with a predominance of polymor-

phonuclear cells (a so-called left shift), is consistent with an intraabdominal inflammatory process. However, nonsurgical illnesses such as enterocolitis (bacterial versus inflammatory), Meckel diverticulitis, or ruptured ovarian cysts can be associated with an elevated WBC count and an abnormal differential blood cell count.

Other tests, such as C-reactive protein and erythrocyte sedimentation rate, may be beneficial in diagnosing patients with appendicitis but are nonspecific. In adolescent females with abdominal pain, a urinary beta–human chorionic gonadotropin should be obtained to rule out intrauterine or ectopic pregnancy. A urinalysis can offer important information in patients evaluated for abdominal pain. The presence of WBCs or red blood cells (or both) in the urine should raise the question of a urinary tract infection. However, red or white blood cells in the urine does not rule out the diagnosis of appendicitis. An inflamed appendix can lie over the ureter or bladder, which can result in transmural inflammation with subsequent hematuria or pyuria.

Radiographic examination may be helpful if the diagnosis is in doubt or if abscess formation is suspected. On plain-film abdominal radiography, an appendicolith can be visualized in the RLQ in 10% to 20% of cases. Other plain-film findings are abnormal bowel gas patterns (dilated loops) in the RLQ, focal lower thoracolumbar scoliosis, and obliteration of the psoas shadow.

Ultrasound can aid in the diagnosis of appendicitis, especially in female adolescents. Sonography can determine the thickness of the appendical wall, luminal character, and appendiceal compressibility. An edematous, distended (greater than 6 mm), noncompressible appendix accurately predicts acute appendicitis, especially when its location corresponds to the point of maximal tenderness. The diagnosis of other conditions, such as ovarian cysts, tumors, and intra- or extrauterine pregnancies, may prevent unnecessary negative laparotomies. Most recent studies report sensitivities and specificities of 80% to 95% for the ultrasonographic diagnosis of acute appendicitis.

Computed axial tomography (CT) of the abdomen is of great value in the diagnosis and management of patients with complicated appendicitis. CT may be helpful in establishing the diagnosis in those who are neurologically impaired, immunologically suppressed, or obese. In addition, a CT scan may aid in the differentiation of abdominal masses, in distinguishing inflammation (phlegmon) from abscess, and in demonstrating bowel-wall thickening in patients with inflammatory bowel disease. The study can be used to guide subsequent drainage of a periappendiceal abscess. For patients who are immunologically suppressed, a CT scan may be helpful in differentiating bacterial enteritis (typhlitis) involving the ileocecal area from acute appendicitis.

THERAPY

Once the diagnosis of appendicitis has been made, all efforts should be made to prepare the patient for definitive treatment: appendectomy. In uncomplicated cases, an intravenous line should be established, and physiologic saline solution should be administered. In cases of complicated appendicitis (gangrene, rupture, and diffuse peritonitis), affected individuals may exhibit significant dehydration and will require volume resuscitation prior to surgery. The most expedient method of resuscitation involves the administration of repeated boluses of lactated Ringer's solution (or normal saline), 20 mL/kg over a 20-minute period. During resuscitation, vital signs and urine output should be monitored closely. When the patient achieves a urine output of 1 to 2 mL/kg/hour and vital signs normalize, adequate circulating blood volume has been achieved. Very rarely, myocardial contractility is impaired, and cardiotropic agents, such as dopamine, may be required. In patients who manifest signs and symptoms consistent with septic shock, adequate resuscitation may take up to 4 and 6 hours.

Preoperative antibiotic therapy is empiric, and based on the extent of perceived intraabdominal contamination. Enteric bacteria (*Escherichia coli*, enterococci, pseudomonads, and bacteroids) are the organisms isolated most frequently from the luminal and the periappendiceal fluid in patients with appendicitis. The antibiotic regimen chosen should be bacteriocidal for enteric organisms. In patients with uncomplicated appendicitis, a broad-spectrum second-generation cephalosporin, such as cefoxitin or cefotetan, is adequate. However, if perforation is suspected, triple antibiotic therapy using ampicillin, gentamicin, and metronidazole or clindamycin is recommended.

Studies have shown that surgical risks, postoperative complications, and overall hospital costs incurred do not depend on the operative technique used to remove the appendix. The technique utilized—conventional versus minimally invasive—is based on the surgeons' familiarity with laparoscopic procedures and the patient's body habitus.

The open, conventional technique requires a RLQ muscle-splitting incision. The appendix is then mobilized and its blood supply is ligated and divided. The base of the appendix is ligated and amputated. The abdomen is irrigated with saline solution, and the incision is closed in layers.

For patients undergoing laparoscopic appendectomy, general anesthesia is required. A nasogastric tube and Foley catheter are placed in the operating room. Two or three 1-cm incisions usually are made: one below the umbilicus for insertion of the camera and the other in the RLQ overlying the appendix. The appendix is grasped using laparoscopic forceps and is delivered through the RLQ incision. In some cases, a third port is required to perform the procedure intracorporeally. The mesentery and appendiceal base are treated as in the open technique, using stapling devices. Laparoscopy offers the advantage of a more complete examination of the abdominal cavity, which is beneficial in those patients with abdominal pain of uncertain etiology. Most pediatric surgeons prefer the laparoscopic approach in the adolescent females, when the diagnosis is in question, or in the morbidly obese patient in whom access to the peritoneal cavity using open techniques would require an excessively large incision.

Patients with uncomplicated acute appendicitis require minimal postoperative care. Maintenance intravenous fluids should be continued until gastrointestinal function returns. Usually, this occurs within the first 12 to 24 hours after surgery. A single dose of perioperative antibiotics has been shown to be sufficient in uncomplicated cases. However, in patients with appendicitis complicated by perforation, defuse peritonitis, or abscess formation, a nasogastric tube may be necessary. In most complicated cases, bowel function returns in 3 to 5 days. Broad-spectrum antibiotics (ampicillin, gentamicin, and clindamycin or metronidazole) should continue until such patients are afebrile, exhibit a normal leukocyte and differential blood cell count, and return to normal bowel function.

The most common complications in patients with appendicitis are infections. Wound infections are heralded by increasing pain, induration, and erythema. Infected draining wounds should be opened and treated with wet to dry dressings. If patients exhibit a persistently draining wound, spiking fever, and an elevated WBC count, an intraabdominal abscess must be presumed. CT of the abdomen and pelvis may identify an intraabdominal or pelvic abscess. If the abscess is monolocular and favorably positioned, percutaneous drainage may be performed. However, if the location of the abscess is unfavorable, open surgical drainage often is necessary. Late complications include adhesive postoperative bowel obstructions (2% to 5% of patients with uncomplicated appendicitis) and infertility (women with pelvic abscess who develop adhesions about the fallopian tubes).

Suggested Readings

Angel CA, Rao BN, Wren E, et al. Acute appendicitis in children with leukemia and other malignancies: still a diagnostic dilemma. *J Pediatr Surg* 1992;27:476.

El Ghoneiml A, Valla JS, Limonne B, et al. Laparoscopic appendectomy in children: report of 1,379 cases. *J Pediatr Surg* 1994;29:786.

Gardner, MWL. When to operate immediately and when to observe. *Seminars in Pediatric Surgery* 1997;6:74.

Lund DP, Murphy EP. Management of perforated appendicitis in children: a decade of aggressive treatment. *J Pediatr Surg* 1994;29:1130.

Peal RH, Hale DA, Molloy M, et al. Pediatric appendectomy. *J Pediatr Surg* 1995;30:173.

Sherlock DJ. Acute appendicitis in the over 60 age group. *Br J Surg* 1985;72:245.

CHAPTER 365 ■ ASCITES

WILLIAM J. COCHRAN

Ascites is derived from the Greek word "askos," which means bladder or bag. Ascites is the accumulation of fluid in the peritoneal cavity; it is a manifestation of an underlying disorder, such as cirrhosis, congestive heart failure, nephrotic syndrome, protein-losing enteropathy, or malnutrition associated with hypoalbuminemia. Hippocrates stated, "When the liver is full of fluid and this overflows into the peritoneal cavity so that the belly becomes full of water, death follows." Indeed, this was the case for Beethoven, who, in 1827, died 2 days after having a paracentesis performed. Although the predicted outcome is less bleak today, ascites resulting from cirrhosis still is associated with significant morbidity and mortality. In adults having cirrhosis and ascites, the 1-year survival is about 50%, compared with over 90% for those having cirrhosis without ascites.

PATHOGENESIS

The presumed initiating factor in the development of ascites in cases of congestive heart failure is increased hydrostatic pressure. In patients with the nephrotic syndrome, protein-losing enteropathy, or malnutrition, the associated hypoalbuminemia results in a decreased oncotic pressure. These alterations in Starling forces cause fluid to move from the intravascular space to the extravascular space. When the rate of extravascular fluid production exceeds the ability of the lymphatic system to reabsorb this fluid and transport it back to the vascular system, fluid accumulates in the peritoneal cavity, resulting in ascites.

The exact role of hypoalbuminemia in the development and maintenance of ascites is controversial, because many patients with hypoalbuminemia or analbuminemia do not have ascites. Approximately 50% of patients with serum albumin concentrations of less than 2.5 g/dL develop ascites. The pathogenesis of ascites in cirrhosis is less well defined and remains an area of active research.

In the past, two major theories had been proposed to explain the formation of ascites associated with cirrhosis: the underfill theory and the overflow theory. According to the underfill theory, ascitic fluid accumulates in the peritoneal cavity secondary to the alterations in Starling forces. Intrahepatic venous obstruction, caused by hepatic inflammation, scarring, and regenerative nodules, increases hydrostatic pressure in the hepatosplanchnic venous system. Increased hydrostatic pressure, in conjunction with a low oncotic pressure due to decreased hepatic protein synthesis, forces fluid out of the hepatosplanchnic vascular space and into the interstitial space. As the fluid in the interstitial space increases, eventually it exceeds the ability of the lymphatic system to reabsorb it, resulting in the accumulation of fluid in the peritoneal cavity as ascites. The intravascular volume is decreased, which stimulates the renin-angiotensin-aldosterone system to retain renal sodium to replenish the intravascular volume. Sodium retention increases the hydrostatic pressure in the hepatosplanchnic circulation, which promotes the accumulation of more ascitic fluid, establishing a vicious cycle.

Current evidence does not support this theory. If this theory were correct, vascular resistance should be increased along with a decrease in the cardiac index and plasma volume, which is not the case in patients with cirrhosis and ascites. More important, sodium retention has been well documented to precede the formation of ascites, rather than being the consequence of ascites.

The overflow theory proposes that the primary cause of ascitic fluid accumulation is renal sodium retention and subsequent plasma volume expansion. The sodium retention causes an expansion of the intravascular space, which increases the hydrostatic pressure in the hepatosplanchnic circulation and results in fluid extravasation into the peritoneal cavity. Several theories have been proposed to account for this increased sodium reabsorption, including decreased hepatic clearance of sodium-retaining substances or a reduced synthesis of a natriuretic substance. The major problem with this theory is that, instead of having an arterial vascular space that is overfilled, patients with cirrhosis and ascites actually have an arterial vascular system that is underfilled, even though the overall plasma volume and cardiac index are increased.

The most commonly accepted theory at this time is the arterial vasodilatation theory. This theory proposes that the initiating event is the development of peripheral arterial vasodilation resulting from an overproduction of vasodilators, primarily nitric oxide. The source of increased nitric oxide production is the endothelial cells of the splanchnic bed. In addition to overproduction, theoretically, diminished hepatic function results in the decreased inactivation of endogenous vasodilators, such as glucagon, vasoactive intestinal polypeptide, or substance P. The accumulation of endogenous vasodilators decreases the systemic vascular resistance, which decreases effective blood volume. This decrease in effective arterial blood volume is detected by arterial receptors, which in turn results in the stimulation of the renin-angiotensin-aldosterone system and the sympathetic nervous system, prompting renal sodium and water retention. The activation of the renin-angiotensin-aldosterone system increases renal vascular resistance and promotes the proximal and distal tubular reabsorption of sodium. In addition to increasing renal vascular resistance, activation of the sympathetic nervous system also promotes the proximal tubular reabsorption of sodium directly and increases renin secretion. This outcome increases the total blood volume, increasing the hepatosplanchnic circulation and its hydrostatic pressure, and resulting in fluid extravasation. Splanchnic arterial vasodilation occurs relatively early in the course of chronic liver disease. This finding is manifested clinically by a resting tachycardia and a wide pulse pressure found in persons with cirrhosis without ascites.

Several lines of evidence support this proposed mechanism of ascites formation. First, increased levels of multiple vasodilators have been noted in patients with cirrhosis and ascites. In addition, it has been determined that an increased production of nitric oxide occurs in patients with cirrhosis and ascites, as compared with normal individuals. Also supportive of this theory is the fact that the activity of the renin-angiotensin-aldosterone system and the sympathetic nervous system is increased in patients with cirrhosis and ascites. These patients have elevated levels of renin, antidiuretic hormone, and aldosterone.

Although the arterial vasodilation theory does not account for all the complex cardiovascular and renal changes in patients with cirrhosis and ascites, it is the explanation accepted most commonly. Additional research is needed to elucidate the pathogenesis of ascites in these patients.

DIAGNOSIS

The causes of ascites are subdivided into eight major categories: portal hypertension, hypoalbuminemia, infectious ascites, chylous ascites, urinary ascites, gastrointestinal ascites, miscellaneous causes, and pseudoascites (Box 365.1). Portal hypertension, the most common cause of ascites in North Americans, can have a prehepatic, hepatic, or posthepatic origin. The major cause of prehepatic portal hypertension is portal vein thrombosis or occlusion, which can result in the development of esophageal varices but rarely causes ascites. Often, hepatic-origin portal hypertension is secondary to hepatic fibrosis or cirrhosis. These disorders can result from congenital hepatic fibrosis, neonatal hepatitis, biliary atresia, alpha-1-antitrypsin deficiency, cystic fibrosis, chronic active hepatitis, or one of several storage diseases (see Chapter 370, Cirrhosis). Primary and metastatic hepatic tumors rarely may cause portal hypertension and ascites. Hepatic cysts, which may result in ascites, occur with polycystic kidney disease. Posthepatic causes of portal hypertension include the Budd-Chiari syndrome (i.e., hepatic vein thrombosis), constrictive pericarditis, or congestive heart failure. These latter two emphasize the importance of a thorough cardiac examination in the evaluation of a patient with ascites.

Hypoalbuminemia may be associated with ascites. The disorder associated most commonly with hypoalbuminemia and ascites is the nephrotic syndrome, although protein-losing enteropathy, malnutrition, and hydrops fetalis also can be responsible.

BOX 365.1   Categories in the Differential Diagnosis of Ascites

Portal hypertension
Prehepatic
    Portal vein thrombosis or occlusion
Hepatic
    Fibrosis
    Cirrhosis
    Tumors
    Cysts
Posthepatic
    Budd-Chiari syndrome
    Constrictive pericarditis
    Congestive heart failure
Hypoalbuminemia
Nephrotic syndrome
Protein-losing enteropathy
Malnutrition
Hydrops fetalis
Infectious causes
Bacterial peritonitis
Fungal peritonitis
Tuberculous peritonitis
Cytomegalovirus
Toxoplasmosis
Syphilis
Chylous causes
Traumatic
Lymphatic obstruction
Lymphatic abnormalities
Urinary causes
Posterior urethral valves
Bladder perforation
Ureteral stenosis
Urethral stenosis
Neurogenic bladder
Gastrointestinal causes
Pancreatic causes
Intestinal atresia
Meconium peritonitis
Bile peritonitis
Miscellaneous causes
Gynecologic disorders
Ventriculoperitoneal shunts
Eosinophilic peritonitis
Hypothyroidism
Pseudoascites
Omental cysts
Mesenteric cysts
Enteric duplication

Ascites caused by infectious agents requires prompt diagnosis and treatment. Primary infections that may be associated with ascites include bacterial, fungal, or tuberculosis infections. Congenital cytomegalovirus, toxoplasmosis, or syphilis infections may be associated with significant ascites. Spontaneous bacterial peritonitis occurs in patients who have preexisting ascites and subsequent peritoneal infection by the hematogenous route. Patients with ascites may develop secondary bacterial peritonitis when a bowel perforation leads to peritoneal infection.

Chylous ascites can be associated with trauma, lymphatic obstruction, or lymphatic abnormalities. Traumatic chylous as-

cites can result from a surgical procedure, an accidental blunt or penetrating injury, or child abuse. The most common cause of lymphatic obstruction that produces chylous ascites is lymphadenopathy. Neoplasms are a rare cause of chylous ascites in children, although they are the cause of chylous ascites found most commonly in adults. The major lymphatic abnormalities associated with chylous ascites are lymphangiectasia, lymphangiomatosis, and congenital "leaky lymphatics." The latter disorder occurs in infants who are younger than 2 months and have chylous ascites of unknown cause. The disorder is thought to result from delayed maturation of the lacteals, allowing chyle to leak into the peritoneal cavity.

Urinary ascites results from leakage of urine into the peritoneal cavity. This process is responsible for approximately 50% of the cases of neonatal ascites. Posterior urethral valves cause approximately 60% of cases, and spontaneous congenital bladder perforation is responsible for 20%. Less common causes of urinary ascites are ureteral stenosis, urethral stenosis, and neurogenic bladder. Renal scintigraphy can be useful for localizing the area of leakage in these disorders.

Gastrointestinal disorders are an uncommon cause of ascites. Pancreatic ascites can be associated with pancreatitis or pancreatic pseudocysts. Pancreatic ascites is due to the contiguous spread of the pancreatic inflammation to the peritoneum, with extravasation of pancreatic secretions into the peritoneal cavity resulting in peritonitis. Rarely, neonatal ascites has a pancreatic origin. Other potential gastrointestinal causes of neonatal ascites are intestinal atresia, meconium peritonitis, and bile peritonitis.

Ascites rarely results from gynecologic disorders, such as ovarian cysts or pelvic inflammatory disease. Infrequently, ventriculoperitoneal shunts are associated with ascites. Eosinophilic peritonitis is a rare cause of ascites in children but is diagnosed readily from a markedly elevated eosinophil count in the ascitic fluid. Hypothyroidism may be associated with ascites, which resolves with thyroid replacement therapy.

Disorders that can mimic ascites, or pseudoascites, include omental cysts, mesenteric cysts, and enteric duplication. Failure to differentiate pseudoascites from true ascites before performing a paracentesis may be detrimental to the patient.

Physical Examination

The clinical hallmark of ascites is abdominal distention (Fig. 365.1). Other potential physical findings include bulging flanks, protrusion of the umbilicus, and labial and scrotal swelling. Patients with portal hypertension may have a prominent abdominal venous pattern (Fig. 365.2).

Massive ascites (see Fig. 365.1) renders affected patients' condition obvious. In less dramatic presentations, three physical signs can help to detect ascites: flank dullness, shifting dullness, and fluid wave. Flank dullness is verified with the patient in the supine position. In patients with ascites, the gas-filled loops of bowel float to the center of the abdomen, on top of the ascitic fluid. When the physician percusses the abdomen, it is tympanitic at the umbilicus and dull below the level of fluid into the flanks. Shifting dullness can be assessed by percussing the abdomen with the patient in the supine position and then in the right and left lateral decubitus positions. Ascites is suggested if the point of dullness shifts with changes in position. A fluid wave is elicited by having affected patients place the lateral aspect of their hands longitudinally on the abdomen. The examiner taps the lateral abdominal wall lightly while feeling the opposite wall for a fluid wave. Flank dullness and shifting dullness have the greatest sensitivity, and the fluid wave has the greatest specificity.

Previously, the puddle sign was advocated to test for ascites. After having been prone for 5 minutes, affected patients

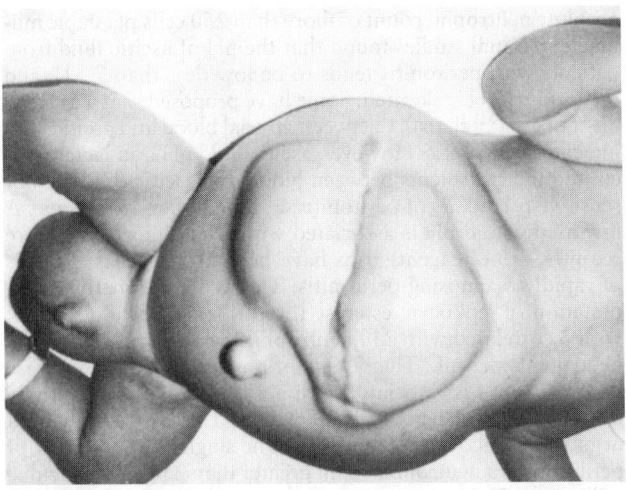

FIGURE 365.1. A 6-month-old infant with severe neonatal hepatitis. Note the marked abdominal distention, bulging of the flanks, wound and umbilical herniation, and scrotal swelling.

rise on their hands and knees while the examiner lightly taps the flanks, auscultating the most dependent portion of the abdomen. The test is positive for ascites if a sloshing sound or change in the percussive sound occurs with lateral movement of the stethoscope.

The physical examination alone is not sufficiently specific or sensitive to detect ascites. In one study of patients with equivocal ascites, the physical examination alone had an accuracy of approximately 50%.

Patients in whom ascites is secondary to cirrhosis may have physical signs of chronic liver disease, such as large hemorrhoids, peripheral edema, scleral icterus, dilated abdominal vessels, spider telangiectasia, and splenomegaly. Other aspects of a physical examination that require particular attention in ascites patients are the cardiac and chest examinations. As discussed, several potential cardiac causes of ascites have been identified, including constrictive pericarditis and right ventricular failure. A thorough cardiac examination is required in all patients with ascites. The examination should include a search

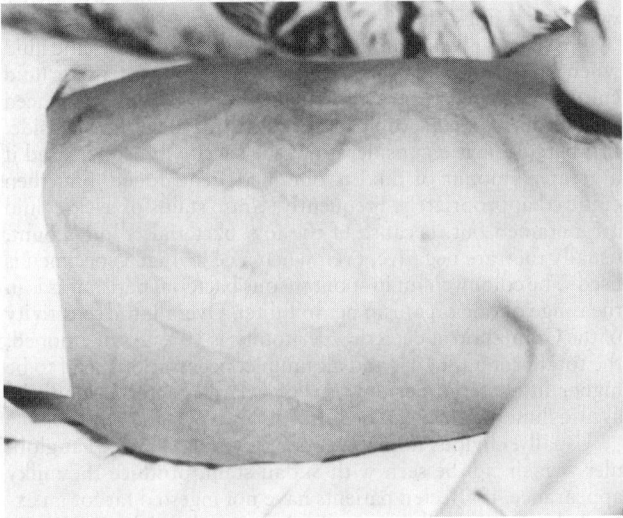

FIGURE 365.2. An 11-year-old child with portal vein obstruction. Note the prominent abdominal vasculature.

for jugular venous distention that suggests right ventricular failure. Some patients with right ventricular failure notice a pulsatile sensation on palpation of the liver. Patients with massive ascites may be tachypneic, owing to compromised intrathoracic volume. Some patients may develop sympathetic pleural effusions. The thyroid gland also should be palpated to evaluate for enlargement, which would suggest hypothyroidism.

Blood pressure also should be obtained; if it is elevated, a nephrogenic cause for the ascites should be considered. The presence of facial edema also suggests a nephrogenic cause for the ascites, although it is uncommon in those with ascites of liver or cardiac origin.

A physical assessment of nutritional status should be performed. Patients with ascites may be compromised nutritionally because of the underlying disorder. Patients with massive ascites may experience early satiety, resulting in inadequate intake, or they may have malabsorption secondary to an edematous intestinal tract; both these conditions can affect nutritional status adversely. Patients with cirrhosis also may develop deficiencies of fat-soluble vitamins or essential fatty acids, nutritional signs for which physicians must be alert.

Radiologic Evaluation

Because physical examination is not sensitive enough to detect small and moderate ascites, other means are required. Plain radiography of the abdomen may be helpful. The classic radiographic findings of ascites include separated and floating bowel loops, abdominal haziness, indistinct psoas muscle shadows, and increased pelvic density in the upright position. These nonspecific signs are not sufficiently sensitive to detect ascites. More reliable signs include an increased distance (greater than 2 mm) between the properitoneal fat stripe and the right colon (i.e., McCort or flank stripe sign), a radiolucent shadow between the lateral wall of the liver and the abdominal wall (i.e., Hellmen sign), radiodensity superior and lateral to the bladder (i.e., dog's-ear sign), and obliteration of the lower lateral hepatic angle. Of these four signs, the flank stripe sign and obliteration of the lower hepatic angle are the most sensitive indicators of ascites, being present in 55% and 85% of patients, respectively.

Ultrasonography, unlike plain film radiography, is sensitive and specific for ascites. Ultrasonography can demonstrate as little as 100 mL of fluid, and can differentiate free from loculated fluid or detect causes of pseudoascites, such as an omental cyst. Before performing paracentesis, abdominal ultrasonography should be obtained during the initial evaluation of every patient with ascites, to differentiate true ascites from pseudoascites, for which paracentesis may be detrimental. Ultrasonography is the diagnostic procedure of choice because of its sensitivity, specificity, and noninvasive nature.

Computed tomography (CT) is extremely sensitive in the detection of ascites, but it should be performed only in special circumstances, because of its expense and risk of patient exposure to radiation.

Analysis of Ascitic Fluid

Ascitic fluid for diagnostic evaluation is obtained by abdominal paracentesis after abdominal ultrasonography is performed. Paracentesis is indicated in the assessment of patients who present with new onset of ascites, those with suspected peritonitis, patients who have cirrhosis and ascites and deteriorate suddenly, and possibly of patients with blunt abdominal trauma. Paracentesis also can be used therapeutically in certain situations.

Paracentesis is performed with affected patients in a supine position. The preferred sites of needle insertion are the avascular linea alba midway between the umbilicus and the pubic symphysis or either lower quadrant lateral to the abdominal rectus muscle. To minimize leakage, the latter site may be preferable in patients with tense ascites. In those with prominent hepatosplenomegaly, an abdominal ultrasound examination may be helpful in determining an appropriate site. Patients should void or be catheterized before paracentesis to avoid puncture of a distended bladder. The needle should not be placed through a scar because of the increased possibility of bowel perforation. Care should be taken to avoid any distended abdominal vessels. Local anesthesia can be obtained with the use of topical 2.5% lidocaine and 2.5% prilocaine cream or by infiltrating the site with 1% lidocaine. One can utilize either a 16- or 18-guage intravenous catheter or a formal 15-guage paracentesis needle. The paracentesis needle has fenestrations on the side. Use of a paracentesis needle in those who have a large-volume paracentesis has been associated with increased speed and efficiency of resolution, compared with an intravenous catheter. After the site is prepared aseptically and local anesthesia is administered, the needle is inserted at an angle until ascitic fluid is obtained. Insertion of the needle in a Z-track fashion minimizes fluid leakage. Approximately 20 to 50 mL of fluid should be removed for diagnostic evaluation.

Paracentesis is a safe procedure, with a complication rate of 1% to 3%. Potential complications include persistent leakage, bladder or intestinal perforation, scrotal swelling, pneumoperitoneum, and bleeding. Paracentesis is not contraindicated for patients with coagulopathies or thrombocytopenia. Studies in adult patients with coagulopathy or thrombocytopenia show no benefit of correction of these disorders prior to paracentesis. Data are limited regarding this in children. Some experts recommend that platelets be provided to children with a platelet count of less than 50,000. In addition, for children whose prothrombin time is prolonged by more than 5 seconds, fresh frozen plasma should be administered.

Various tests can be performed to classify the ascitic fluid further and to determine its cause. Traditionally, peritoneal fluid has been separated into transudative and exudative categories. Most often, ascitic fluid is a transudate and is associated with an increased hydrostatic pressure in the portal system or with decreased serum oncotic pressure. Typically, transudative ascitic fluid is clear or straw colored, with total protein concentrations of less than 2.5 to 3.0 g/dL or less than one-half the plasma total protein concentration. The concentrations of electrolytes, urea, creatinine, glucose, triglycerides, cholesterol, and hydrogen ions in ascitic fluid are almost identical to those plasma levels. Trace elements, such as zinc, tend to be present in lower concentrations in ascitic fluid than in plasma. The level of fibrin split products may be increased in ascitic fluid relative to plasma. The leukocyte count is fewer than 250 to 500 cells per cubic millimeter; less than one-third of the cells are neutrophils. Gram stain and cultures reveal no organisms.

Exudative ascitic fluid is secondary to inflammation of the peritoneum or abdominal viscera (i.e., peritonitis, pancreatitis) or is caused by leakage of lymph or chyle into the peritoneal cavity. Usually, exudative peritoneal fluid is turbid or cloudy. Characteristically, the protein content is elevated, with the total protein concentration typically in excess of 3 g/dL. The protein content may be less in patients with hypoproteinemia. The ratio of ascitic protein to plasma protein can be determined in such patients, and tends to be greater than 0.5 in exudative ascites. Lactate dehydrogenase (LDH) is elevated relative to plasma; the ratio of ascitic fluid LDH to plasma LDH is greater than 0.6. An elevated leukocyte count is common in patients with peritonitis; the count is greater than 500 leukocytes per cubic millimeter, and more than 50% of the cells are neutrophils (i.e.,

absolute neutrophil count of more than 250 cells per cubic millimeter). Initial studies found that the pH of ascitic fluid from patients with peritonitis tends to be low (less than 7.31), and the lactate level is elevated. Some have proposed that a pH gradient of greater than 0.1 between arterial blood and ascitic fluid indicates peritonitis. However, ascitic fluid pH and lactate levels and their gradients between blood and ascitic fluid are not sensitive predictors of peritonitis, although they are specific. A low ascitic fluid pH is associated with a high mortality. More recently, urine reagent strips have been proposed as a means of rapidly diagnosing peritonitis. This is a colorimetric determination of leukocyte esterase that utilizes a scale of 0 to 4, with 3 correlated with 250 neutrophils per mL and 4 with 500 neutrophils per mL. The finding of positive leukocyte esterase of grade 3 or 4 is associated with peritonitis, with a sensitivity of 89% and specificity of 99%. A 0 or 1 is associated with a negative predictive value of 99%. The single best predictor of peritonitis is a neutrophil count greater than 250 cells per cubic millimeter. The leukocyte count in ascites can increase during diuretic treatment, but the neutrophil count does not. Peripheral leukocytosis does not affect the leukocyte or neutrophil count of ascites.

The classification of ascites into transudative and exudative categories on the basis of total protein and LDH levels is inaccurate. Many patients with cirrhosis and ascites have elevated protein concentrations in their ascitic fluid. The protein concentration can be increased in the ascitic fluid through diuretic therapy. Some have proposed that the serum-ascites albumin gradient is superior in differentiating transudative and exudative ascites. If the serum-ascites albumin concentration gradient [serum albumin (in grams per deciliter) minus ascites albumin (in grams per deciliter)] is greater than 1.1 g/dL, the ascites can be designated as transudative. Typically, exudative ascites has a serum-ascites albumin concentration gradient of less than 1.1 g/dL. The serum and ascites albumin concentration must be measured simultaneously. The serum-ascites albumin ratio is not a valid test if the ascitic fluid albumin is less than 1 g/dL. The serum-ascites albumin ratio is based on the rationale that, if the ascites is secondary to portal hypertension, a high oncotic gradient should be evident between the serum and ascitic fluid. Because albumin is the greatest contributor protein to oncotic pressure, the ratio is high. In such states as peritonitis, the albumin level in the ascitic fluid increases, and the ratio decreases. Using only the total ascitic fluid protein for classifying the fluid as a transudate or exudate will differentiate them correctly only 50% to 60% of the time. The serum-ascitic albumin ratio predicts transudative ascites and exudative ascites with sensitivities of 90% and 95%, respectively.

Physicians always should obtain a culture of the ascitic fluid when a paracentesis is performed. The sensitivity of ascitic fluid cultures is increased greatly if 10 to 20 mL of fluid is placed into aerobic and anaerobic blood culture bottles at the bedside. If tuberculosis is a consideration, the sensitivity is increased if a greater amount of fluid is obtained, centrifuged, and then cultured appropriately. Frequently, Gram stains of ascitic fluid are obtained but, because of the low bacterial colony count, usually they are negative, even when a centrifuged specimen is used. The colony count in spontaneous bacterial peritonitis is in the range of one organism per milliliter. Overall, the sensitivity of the Gram stain at detecting peritonitis is 10%. As mentioned, the total protein, LDH, and albumin concentrations tend to be higher in bacterial peritonitis. For a large bacterial load, the ascitic fluid glucose may be low.

Usually, chylous fluid appears milky (Fig. 365.3). Fat globules, which can be seen with Sudan stain, produce the milky appearance. If affected patients have not ingested fat for an extended period, the fluid may be clear or yellowish, and lymph ascites may be a more appropriate term. The leukocyte count

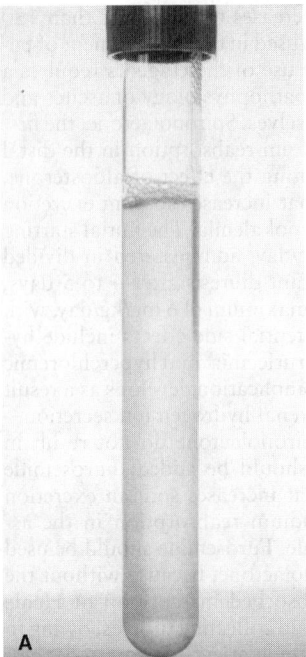
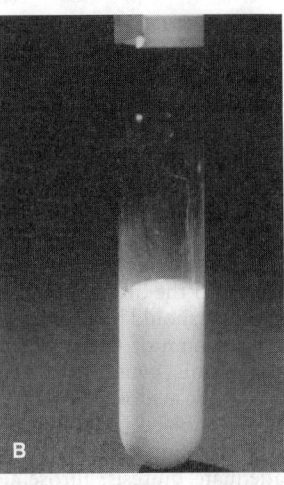

FIGURE 365.3. A: Ascitic fluid from a patient with cirrhosis, with its typical yellowish appearance. B: Ascitic fluid from a patient with chylous ascites, with its characteristic milky appearance. See Figure 365.3 in color section.

is higher in chylous ascites than in ascites of other causes, with the exception of infectious peritonitis. The average leukocyte count is 1,000 to 5,000 cells per cubic millimeter, with lymphocytes constituting the majority of cells. The concentration of triglycerides in chylous fluid is much greater than that in serum. The cholesterol concentration, however, is similar to serum levels.

Pancreatic ascitic fluid has exudative characteristics, with an elevated protein level and leukocyte count. Pancreatic ascites can develop in cases of acute pancreatitis, chronic pancreatitis, or pancreatic pseudocyst. Usually, the gross appearance of pancreatic ascitic fluid is turbid, but it may be tea colored or bloody in hemorrhagic pancreatitis. The hallmark of pancreatic ascites is peritoneal amylase and lipase levels that are greater than those in serum. Infants younger than 4 to 6 months are relatively amylase deficient; in infants with pancreatic ascites, the amylase level in the ascitic fluid may be low, rendering determination of the lipase level imperative.

Urinary ascites is typified by increased creatinine and urea levels in the peritoneal fluid—higher than serum levels. Sodium and chloride levels tend to be lower than those in serum, and potassium levels tend to be higher.

Bile ascites is a rare disorder that occurs in neonates secondary to spontaneous perforation of the bile ducts. The ascitic fluid is bile stained, just as it is in a patient with ascites and cholestasis; unlike the latter condition, bile ascites is associated with levels of total and direct bilirubin that are greater in the peritoneal fluid than in serum.

Malignant ascites, rare in children, is characterized by elevated protein and LDH levels. The serum-ascites albumin concentration gradient is less than 1.1 g/dL in 93% of affected patients.

The glucose level may be low, and the fluid may be bloody. Ascitic fluid secondary to the nephrotic syndrome has the characteristics of ascitic fluid associated with cirrhosis. It is straw colored, with a total protein concentration of less than 2.5 g/dL and an albumin gradient of greater than 1.1 g/dL.

Complications

Complications associated with ascites can be secondary to the presence of ascites itself or to the therapeutic modalities used to treat the ascites. Massive ascites can impair respiratory function by pushing up the diaphragm, thereby decreasing intrathoracic volume, or by the presence of pleural effusions. Ascites can increase intraabdominal pressure, resulting in gastroesophageal reflux or early satiety. Massive ascites can cause patient discomfort and can reduce mobility.

Spontaneous bacterial peritonitis (SBP) is a complication that occurs when the ascitic fluid becomes infected (i.e., peritonitis) in the absence of a local source of infection, such as a perforation. The incidence of SBP is approximately 15%, but it occurs most commonly in patients with cirrhosis and ascites, and occurs much less frequently when the ascites is caused by the nephrotic syndrome or by congestive heart failure. The mechanism of infection is believed to be the result of a translocation of enteric bacteria through the gastrointestinal tract wall to the lymphatics and then to the bloodstream before seeding the ascitic fluid. The reticuloendothelial system phagocytic activity is decreased in cirrhosis, accounting for the increased incidence of SBP. The ascitic fluid of affected persons has lower total protein and complement levels, which predispose such patients to developing SBP. Aerobic gram-negative organisms are recovered most commonly, and these are responsible for approximately 70% of cases. *Escherichia coli* is the most common aerobic gram-negative organism, followed by *Klebsiella*. Aerobic gram-positive organisms are the next most frequently detected organisms, with streptococcal species accounting for 20% and enterococcal species being the cause in approximately 5% of these infections. Anaerobes are rarely responsible for SBP. If multiple organisms are recovered from the ascitic fluid, a secondary cause for the infection, such as perforation, should be sought. The organisms responsible for SBP in patients with ascites secondary to the nephrotic syndrome are the same as those associated with cirrhosis. The overall incidence of SBP, however, is much lower in nephrotic syndrome than in cirrhosis.

Most commonly, patients with SBP present with fever and abdominal pain but with no other source of infection. They may present also with hypotension, diarrhea, portosystemic encephalopathy, or unexplained deterioration in liver function despite previously stable cirrhosis. Ten percent of patients with SBP are totally asymptomatic at the time of presentation. The key to making the correct diagnosis is to be alert to the possibility and to perform paracentesis if affected patients have any symptoms compatible with SBP. Due to the presence of SBP in asymptomatic individuals, it has been recommended that all hospitalized patients with ascites have a diagnostic paracentesis at the time of admission.

Therapy should be instituted for any patient if the neutrophil count of the ascitic fluid is greater than 250 cells per cubic millimeter. Treatment should not wait until cultures are positive, because patients with SBP deteriorate rapidly if appropriate treatment is not instituted promptly. Ampicillin and an aminoglycoside provide good coverage, but administering a nephrotoxic drug to patients with cirrhosis and diminished renal function may not be advisable. Cefotaxime is considered the drug of choice for presumed SBP. A repeat paracentesis can be considered after 48 hours of therapy to assess response. Therapy should be continued for 5 to 10 days. Blood and urine cultures should be obtained before starting therapy, because 50% and 40%, respectively, are positive. An important adjuvant therapy for SBP is intravascular volume expansion. An important complication of SBP is renal impairment. It has been shown in adults that treatment of SBP with cefotaxime and intravenous albumin was associated with lower rates of renal impairment, hospital mortality, and 3-month mortality, compared with those who were treated with cefotaxime alone.

SBP is associated with a mortality of 20%. Even in those who survive the first episode of SBP, the 1-year survival rate is only 30% to 40%. A high SBP recurrence rate is seen in those who survive the initial episode, with a probability of recurrence of 70% within 1 year. Because of the high mortality and frequent recurrence of SBP, cirrhosis patients who recover from the initial episode of SBP should be considered for liver transplantation after the infection has resolved. In anticipation of liver transplantation, such prophylactic antibiotics as trimethoprim-sulfamethoxazole or norfloxacin should be administered. The prognosis of SBP in patients with nephrotic syndrome is not so bleak, with SBP not adversely affecting their overall prognosis.

THERAPY

Several medical and surgical therapeutic modalities can be used to treat ascites. Treatment of ascites is not associated with improved survival, but it does improve the quality of life. The initial therapy must be directed at the underlying disorder and at promoting growth. The mere presence of ascites does not mandate therapy. Therapy should be instituted on development of secondary complications, such as patient discomfort, reduced mobility, or impaired respiratory, cardiovascular, or gastrointestinal function. The treatment of patients should focus on reducing symptoms, with a minimum of complications induced by the treatment.

Medical treatment consists primarily of nutritional and diuretic therapies. Frequently, bed rest is recommended for adults with ascites, because of the theoretic possibility that an upright position activates the renin-angiotensin-aldosterone and sympathetic nervous systems, which increases tubular reabsorption of sodium. Prolonged bed rest for pediatric patients is not a practical therapeutic modality; the goal of normalizing the lives of pediatric patients to promote sound psychological development is served poorly by enforced bed rest.

In the treatment of ascites, salt restriction is the mainstay of nutritional therapy and should be instituted immediately. Sodium retention, whether primary or secondary, is responsible for maintaining ascites. Moderate to marked salt restriction alone can result in significant diuresis in 10% to 15% of patients. Sodium intake should be restricted to 1 or 2 mEq/kg/day, even if diuretics are prescribed; sodium restriction may reduce diuretic requirements. Indeed, inadequate sodium restriction is a relatively common cause of diuretic-resistant ascites. More severe sodium restriction can result in a large negative sodium balance; then ascites is decreased at the expense of growth.

Therapy must be directed at the normalization and maintenance of nutritional status. Patients with massive ascites may have early satiety because of gastric compression, or they may have gastroesophageal reflux, which can limit intake, ultimately producing malnutrition. Patients with ascites and hypoalbuminemia may have an edematous intestinal tract, which causes malabsorption and deterioration in their nutritional status. In patients with ascites caused by liver disease, fat and fat-soluble vitamins might be malabsorbed, a condition that might require specific therapy. Such patients may benefit from an elemental formula containing medium-chain triglycerides that are absorbed more readily than are long-chain triglycerides, from tube feedings for inadequate intake, and from supplemental vitamins.

Although water intake may have to be restricted in some patients with cirrhosis, water intake need not be a concern for most of those who can excrete the amount of fluid normally consumed. Excessive fluid intake should be discouraged. Fluid restriction of 50% to 70% of maintenance should be in-

stituted if the serum sodium decreases to much less than 130 mEq/L. Frequently, diuretics are used in the management of patients with ascites. The rational use of these agents requires a thorough understanding of the pathophysiology of ascites and knowledge of the diuretics themselves. Spironolactone, the first diuretic to be used, inhibits sodium reabsorption in the distal and collecting tubules by inhibiting the effect of aldosterone. It is a weak natriuretic agent that increases sodium excretion by only 2%; it does not cause hypokalemia. The initial starting dose is between 2 and 3 mg/kg/day, administered in divided doses. In the absence of significant diuresis after 4 to 5 days, the dose should be doubled to a maximum of 6 mg/kg/day, with a maximum of 400 mg/day. Potential side effects include hyperkalemia, gynecomastia, hyperuricemia, and hyperchloremic metabolic acidosis. The latter complication develops as a result of spironolactone inhibition of renal hydrogen ion secretion.

If sodium restriction and spironolactone do not result in adequate diuresis, furosemide should be added. Furosemide is a potent natriuretic agent that increases sodium excretion 20% to 25%, by inhibiting sodium reabsorption in the ascending limb of the loop of Henle. Furosemide should be used only in conjunction with spironolactone, because without the latter agent, the sodium not absorbed in the loop of Henle would be absorbed in the distal and collecting tubules, owing to the hyperaldosteronemia of affected patients. Furosemide therapy can be started at 1 to 2 mg/kg/day in divided doses, with a maximum of 6 mg/kg/day (maximum dose, 240 mg). The major complication associated with furosemide is a marked kaluresis, which can cause hypokalemia and metabolic alkalosis. Hypokalemia may result in arrhythmias and growth failure. Hypokalemia may precipitate hepatic encephalopathy, because hypokalemia causes an increased renal production of ammonium. Other potential complications of furosemide use include hyponatremia, hypochloremia, ototoxicity (especially when used in conjunction with aminoglycosides), nephrocalcinosis, and azotemia. Other newer loop diuretics, such as bumetanide, have been used successfully. The dose of bumetanide is 0.015 to 0.1 mg/kg once a day with a maximum daily dose of 10 mg.

Diuresis should be induced gradually. After diuretic therapy is begun, fluid comes initially from the intravascular space and then from edema or ascitic fluid. Edema fluid is mobilized more readily than is ascitic fluid. Patients with ascites and edema can be diuresed more aggressively than those without edema, at a maximal rate of 1 kg per day for adults. Patients without edema probably should not be diuresed more than 0.5 kg/day. Recommended maximum weight loss for pediatric patients is 10 grams per kg of body weight per day. Aggressive diuresis should be avoided in patients with decreased renal function because of the possible development of hypovolemia, further reduction in renal function, and development of the hepatorenal syndrome. All patients who receive diuretic therapy should have electrolyte, urea, and creatinine levels monitored closely.

Albumin can be infused intravenously in conjunction with furosemide to achieve a more rapid diuresis in patients who are acutely symptomatic. Albumin is administered in a dose of 1.0 g/kg over 1 to 2 hours, and furosemide, 1 mg/kg, is given intravenously halfway through the infusion. Because albumin enters the peritoneal fluid, the effect is transient. This therapy is expensive, may result in increased portal pressure, and may cause variceal bleeding.

Nonsteroidal antiinflammatory agents should be used with caution in patients with cirrhosis and ascites. These agents inhibit renal prostaglandin synthesis, which causes a marked reduction in renal blood flow, glomerular filtration rate, and free-water clearance. These agents also reduce the natriuretic activity of furosemide.

Many patients do not respond to nutritional and diuretic therapy; these patients are said to have diuretic-resistant ascites. Their physicians must consider surgical therapy for these patients. Surgical therapy consists of large-volume paracentesis, insertion of a peritoneovenous shunt, transjugular intrahepatic portosystemic shunt, or liver transplantation. In the past, the removal of a large amount of ascitic fluid was discouraged strongly because of potential electrolyte abnormalities, renal impairment, and hypovolemia. However, multiple studies of adult patients have documented that large-volume paracentesis (5 L/day) can be performed safely and without adversely affecting hemodynamic or renal functions, if it is accomplished in conjunction with the intravenous administration of albumin. Albumin is replaced at a dose of 6 to 8 g/L of ascitic fluid removed, administered over 1 to 2 hours. The mobilization of ascitic fluid by therapeutic paracentesis with albumin infusion is more effective and safer than is conventional diuretic therapy and is considered the treatment of choice by many for the management of tense ascites. Chronic paracentesis without albumin infusion is associated with the loss of a large amount of protein, which can reduce serum protein levels further and can affect the patient's nutritional status adversely. Large volume paracentesis (greater than 50 mL/kg) with albumin infusion has been shown to be effective and safe in children in the management of tense ascites. Use of a paracentesis needle results in more rapid paracentesis than an IV catheter. Albumin at a dose of 1 g/kg of body weight should be infused over 1 to 2 hours as the paracentesis is being performed.

Two peritoneovenous shunts have been used in the treatment of refractory ascites: the LeVeen and the Denver. The LeVeen shunt consists of a perforated tube connected to another tube with a one-way, pressure-sensitive valve. The perforated portion is placed in the abdominal cavity; the other end is tunneled subcutaneously over the chest and inserted into the superior vena cava. When abdominal pressure exceeds superior vena caval pressure, ascitic fluid is drawn into the circulatory system. The Denver shunt is similar, except that it also contains a bulb that can be pumped to transfer ascitic fluid to the circulatory system. Although experience with these shunts in children has been limited, the results have been successful in controlling the ascites. However, their use has not improved survival.

Both types of shunts are associated with a high rate of complications. Patients with peritoneovenous shunts may develop persistent infections, most commonly staphylococcal, which require shunt removal. The incidence of bacterial infections can be decreased by giving prophylactic antibiotics before procedures. Intravascular coagulation occurs in approximately 25% of persons with shunts, probably because of the large amount of fibrin split products and other clotting factors in the ascitic fluid transported to the vascular system. This high incidence of intravascular coagulation can be decreased by removing the ascites completely at the time of shunt surgery. Frequently, the shunts also become occluded: mean length of patency is 6 months. Other potential complications include pulmonary embolism, congestive heart failure, bleeding varices, and small-bowel obstruction. The high incidence of complications and occlusion, along with the advent of transjugular intrahepatic portosystemic shunts, limits the usefulness of the peritoneovenous shunts.

Transjugular intrahepatic portosystemic shunt (TIPS) was developed during the 1980s, for the treatment of complications of portal hypertension in adult patients with cirrhosis including refractory ascites (see Chapter 371, Portal Hypertension). TIPS is performed by an interventional radiologist placing a stent that bridges the hepatic vein and the branches of the portal vein. TIPS is effective in the treatment of refractory ascites; however, these shunts frequently become occluded (70% at 1 year), and a significant risk of hepatic encephalopathy (30% in adult studies) is present. This limits the usefulness of TIPS in the treatment of refractory ascites, and it is considered a second-line option. Pediatric experience using TIPS is limited, but the data indicate that it is as effective in pediatric patients as in adults, with success rates in the range of 75% to 90%.

In pediatric patients with cirrhosis and ascites, the optimal long-term treatment is liver transplantation. Liver transplantation is the only treatment of ascites associated with cirrhosis that has been shown to improve survival. The 1-year survival rate of pediatric liver transplantation is approximately 90%.

Suggested Readings

Athow AC, Wilkinson ML, Saunders AJ, et al. Pancreatic ascites presenting in infancy, with review of the literature. *Dig Dis Sci* 1991;36:245.

Boyer TD. Transjugular intrahepatic portosystemic shunt: current status. *Gastroenterology* 2003;124:1700.

Castellote J, Lopez C, Gornals J, et al. Rapid diagnosis of spontaneous bacterial peritonitis by use of reagent strips. *Hepatology* 2003;37:893.

Churchill RJ. CT of intra-abdominal fluid collections. *Radiol Clin North Am* 1989;27:653.

Cochran WJ, Klish WJ, Brown MR, et al. Chylous ascites in infants and children: a case report and literature review. *J Pediatr Gastroenterol Nutr* 1985;4:668.

Fiedorek SC, Casteel HB, Reddy G, et al. The etiology and clinical significance of pseudoascites. *J Gen Intern Med* 1991;6:77.

Garcia-Tsao G. Current management of the complications of cirrhosis and portal hypertension: variceal hemorrhage, ascites, and spontaneous bacterial peritonitis. *Gastroenterology* 2001;120:726.

Heyman MB, LaBerge JM. Role of transjugular intrahepatic portosystemic shunt in the treatment of portal hypertension in pediatric patients. *J Pediatr Gastroenterology Nutr* 1999;29:240.

Inadomi J, Cello JP, Koch J. Ultrasonographic determination of ascitic fluid. *Hepatology* 1996;24:549.

Kramer RE, Sokol RJ, Yerushalmi B, et al. Large-volume paracentesis in the management of ascites in children. *J Pediatr Gastroenterol Nutrition* 2001;33:245.

Machin GA. Diseases causing fetal and neonatal ascites. *Pediatr Pathol* 1985;4:195.

McHutchison J. Differential diagnosis of ascites. *Semin Liver Dis* 1997;17:191.

Moore KP, Wong F, Gines P, et al. The management of ascites in cirrhosis: report on the consensus conference of the international ascites club. *Hepatology* 2003;38:258.

Rimola A, Garcia-Tsao G, Navasa M, et al. Diagnosis, treatment and prophylaxis of spontaneous bacterial peritonitis: a consensus document. *J Hepatol* 2000;32:142.

Runyon B. Historical aspects of treatment of patients with cirrhosis and ascites. *Semin Liver Dis* 1997;17:163.

Sabri M, Saps M, Peters JM. Pathophysiology and management of pediatric ascites. *Curr Gastroenterol Rep* 2003;5:240.

Williams JW, Simel DL. Does this patient have ascites? How to divine fluid in the abdomen. *JAMA* 1992;267:2645.

Zervos EE, Rosemurgy AS. Management of medically refractory ascites. *Am J Surg* 2001;181:256.

CHAPTER 366 ■ PANCREATITIS

STEVEN L. WERLIN

ACUTE PANCREATITIS

Acute pancreatitis is most common pancreatic disorder in children, second only to cystic fibrosis in prevalence. Blunt abdominal trauma, viral infections (especially mumps), and multisystem disease account for the majority of cases of known etiology. Other causes are much less common (Box 366.1). Child abuse is recognized as a major cause of traumatic pancreatitis in young children. More recently defined causes of pancreatitis include organic acidemias and protease inhibitors used in the treatment of acquired immunodeficiency syndrome (AIDS). Improved techniques have led to increased recognition of congenital abnormalities.

Acute pancreatitis is believed to occur after the activation of proteolytic pancreatic proenzymes, which follows colocalization with lysosomal hydrolases within the acinar cell. This process then leads to autodigestion and further activation and release of active proteases. In the lysosome, trypsinogen is activated to trypsin by lysosomal hydrolases. Then trypsin activates other proteases, elastase, and phospholipase A_2. Lecithin is activated by phospholipase A_2 into the toxic lysolecithin. These activated enzymes then spill into the cytoplasm and interstitium, initiating the inflammatory process. The healthy pancreas is protected by three factors: (a) pancreatic proteases synthesized as inactive proenzymes, (b) digestive enzymes segregated into secretory granules, and (c) the presence of protease inhibitors.

The histopathologic findings of acute pancreatitis are related to the release of activated proteolytic and lipolytic enzymes. Interstitial edema appears early. Later, as the episode of pancreatitis progresses, localized and confluent necrosis, blood vessel disruption leading to hemorrhage, and an inflammatory response in the peritoneum may develop.

The definition of acute pancreatitis and its differentiation from chronic pancreatitis have been the subject of much dispute. The definition accepted most widely holds that acute pancreatitis is an isolated episode, with complete morphologic and histologic resolution. Acute pancreatitis may recur but, unless structural damage occurs, it rarely becomes chronic.

Clinical Manifestations and Complications

Clinically, children with acute pancreatitis have continuous, midepigastric, and periumbilical abdominal pain often radiating to the back; vomiting; and frequently fever. They appear acutely ill and are both restless and uncomfortable. They may lie on their side. The pain increases in severity for 24 to 48 hours. During this interval, vomiting may increase, and affected patients may require hospitalization for fluid and electrolyte therapy. Usually, acute cases are self-limited, and the prognosis is excellent.

In more severe cases, jaundice, ascites, and pleural effusions may occur. Acute hemorrhagic pancreatitis, the most severe form of acute pancreatitis, is rare in children. In this life-threatening condition, affected children are severely ill with intractable nausea, vomiting, and abdominal pain. The pancreas may become necrotic and may be transformed into an infected, inflammatory, hemorrhagic mass or phlegmon. Mortality from shock, renal failure, infection, massive gastrointestinal bleeding, and other complications approaches 50%. A number of classification systems have been devised to predict

---

| BOX 366.1 | Etiology of Acute Pancreatitis in Children |

Drugs and Toxins
Alcohol
L-Asparaginase
Azathioprine
Cimetidine
Corticosteroids
Dideoxycytidine
Didanosine
Enalapril
Erythromycin
Estrogen
Furosemide
6-Mercaptopurine
Mesalamine
Methyldopa
Pentamidine
Scorpion bites
Sulfonamides
Sulindac
Tetracycline
Thiazides
Valproic acid

Hereditary Pancreatitis
Infections
Coxsackie B virus
Epstein-Barr virus
Hepatitis A, B
Influenza A, B
Leptospirosis
Malaria
Measles
Mumps
Mycoplasma
Reye syndrome
   (varicella, influenza B)
Rubella
Rubeola

Obstructive Causes
Ampullary disease
Ascariasis

Biliary tract malformations
Cholelithiasis and
   choledocholithiasis
Clonorchis
Duplication cyst
Endoscopic retrograde
   cholangiopancreatography
   complication
Pancreas divisum
Pancreatic ductal
   abnormalities
Postoperative conditions
Sphincter of Oddi dysfunction
Tumor

Systemic Disease
Brain tumor
Collagen-vascular diseases
Cystic fibrosis
Diabetes mellitus
Head trauma
Hemochromatosis
Hemolytic uremic syndrome
Hyperlipidemia types I, IV, V
Hyperparathyroidism
Kawasaki disease
Malnutrition
Organic acidemia
Peptic ulcer
Periarteritis nodosa
Renal failure
Systemic lupus
   erythematosus
Transplantation (bone
   marrow, heart,
   liver, kidney, pancreas)

Trauma
Blunt injury
Child abuse
Surgical trauma
Total body cast

the outcome of a case of pancreatitis. None of these systems are relevant to pediatric patients.

Diagnosis

Because no test is accepted as a reference standard for the diagnosis of pancreatitis, many individual tests have been recommended. The tests used most widely are those that determine serum amylase and lipase activities. Typically, the serum amylase level is elevated for 4 to 5 days, whereas the lipase is increased for 8 to 14 days. Both false-positive and false-negative results occur. A large number of nonpancreatic conditions have been associated with hyperamylasemia. False-positive results may occur in diabetic ketoacidosis, renal failure, burn patients, and in the presence of an elevation of salivary amylase, as may occur in mumps. The fractionation of serum amylase into the salivary and pancreatic components can be performed readily in most clinical laboratories. We prefer to determine the serum lipase, which may be more specific than is amylase for acute pancreatitis. Once the diagnosis of acute pancreatitis is made, we follow only the amylase, because normalization of the lipase lags the amylase by several days. Newer tests, such as those that determine the levels of serum pancreatic elastase 1 and phospholipase A_2 and urinary trypsin activation peptide, still are under study.

Commonly found laboratory abnormalities include leukocytosis, hyperglycemia, glucosuria, hypocalcemia, and hyperbilirubinemia. Usually, radiologic findings are nonspecific. A sentinel loop of small bowel or a segmental ileus may be seen. Although imaging studies are not useful in the management of uncomplicated pancreatitis, ultrasonography (US) and computed tomography (CT) currently are cornerstones in the diagnosis and management of the complications of pancreatitis. These studies may demonstrate diffuse pancreatic enlargement, indeterminate pancreatic masses, pancreatic and extrapancreatic fluid collections, and peripancreatic abscesses. Importantly, 20% or more of patients with acute pancreatitis will have a normal CT examination.

Therapy

The treatment of mild and moderate episodes of acute pancreatitis is supportive and expectant. The aims of therapy are to relieve pain and to restore homeostasis. Meperidine is given as necessary for pain control. Fluid and electrolyte balance is maintained. Nasogastric suction is useful to control vomiting, but does not speed the resolution of the underlying pancreatitis. Antibiotics are used only for the treatment of specific infection. Usually, improvement occurs in 2 to 4 days. Patients with acute pancreatitis may be fed when clinical symptoms have resolved and the serum amylase has returned to near normal. A low-fat diet is given for several weeks. Surgery is rarely required. Often, the treatment of severe acute pancreatitis is prolonged and may require total parenteral nutrition and surgical drainage.

PANCREATIC PSEUDOCYST

Pancreatic pseudocyst formation is an uncommon sequela of pancreatitis. Pseudocysts are delineated by a fibrous wall in the lesser peritoneal sac, which may enlarge or extend in almost any direction, thus producing a wide variety of symptoms. A pseudocyst is suggested when an episode of pancreatitis fails to resolve, when an abdominal mass develops after an episode of pancreatitis, or when pancreatitis relapses shortly after resolution. Clinical features may include pain, nausea, vomiting, and jaundice. The most useful diagnostic techniques are US

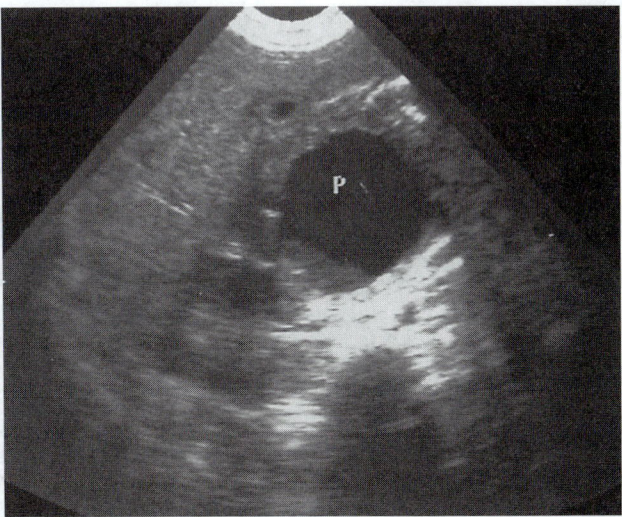

FIGURE 366.1. Pancreatic pseudocyst (*P*). This pseudocyst, 5 cm in diameter, developed in a 16-year-old boy 2 weeks after recovery from an episode of acute pancreatitis. (Courtesy of Dr. John Sty.)

(Fig. 366.1), CT scanning, and endoscopic retrograde cholangiopancreatography (ERCP). Because of its ease of use, availability, and low cost, US is the test of first choice. Sequential studies of patients with pancreatitis have demonstrated that pancreatic pseudocysts frequently are asymptomatic and resolve spontaneously. Most gastroenterologists recommend that US be performed routinely 2 to 4 weeks after an episode of pancreatitis for the evaluation of possible pseudocyst formation.

Almost always, pseudocysts smaller than 4 cm resolve spontaneously. Until recently, the treatment of nonresolving and large pseudocysts was surgical. Percutaneous and endoscopic drainage of pancreatic pseudocysts are accepted nonsurgical forms of treatment. If surgery is required, the pseudocyst must be allowed to mature for 4 to 6 weeks before surgical drainage is performed. A delay is not required before percutaneous or endoscopic drainage.

CHRONIC PANCREATITIS

Usually, chronic or recurrent pancreatitis in children is due to hereditary pancreatitis, traumatic damage, cystic fibrosis, or anomalies of the pancreatic or biliary ductal systems. Descriptions of many kindreds have described the transmission of pancreatitis as an autosomal dominant trait with incomplete penetrance. Frequently, symptoms begin in the first decade but usually are mild at onset. Although spontaneous recovery from each attack occurs in 4 to 7 days, episodes become progressively more severe. Hereditary pancreatitis is diagnosed when the disease is present in successive generations of a family. The gene for hereditary pancreatitis has been localized to the short arm of chromosome 7, and has been cloned. Mutations on the cationic trypsinogen gene that have been identified allow autoactivation of trypsinogen to trypsin. Evaluation during symptom-free intervals may be unrewarding until calcifications, pseudocysts, or pancreatic insufficiency develops mutations of cystic fibrosis (CFTR) and SPINK1 genes may also lead to pancreatitis. Other conditions associated with chronic relapsing pancreatitis are hyperlipoproteinemia (types I and V), hyperparathyroidism, and ascariasis. The majority of cases of recurrent pancreatitis in childhood are due to anatomic abnormalities.

All children who have experienced more than one episode of pancreatitis must be evaluated thoroughly. Serum lipid, calcium, and phosphorus levels are determined. In the appropriate

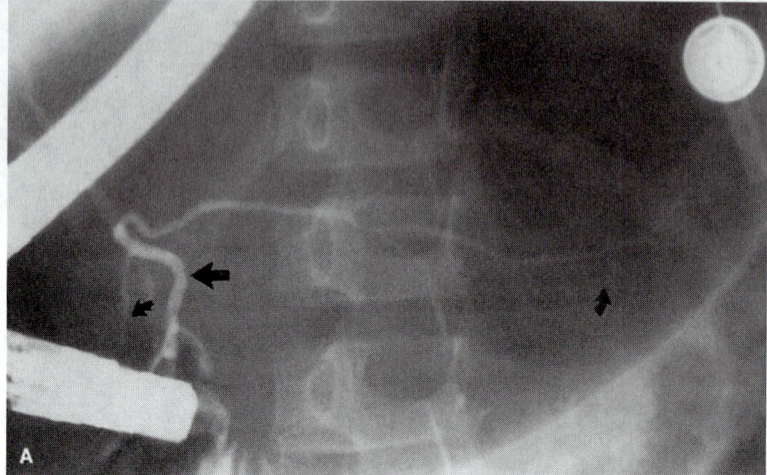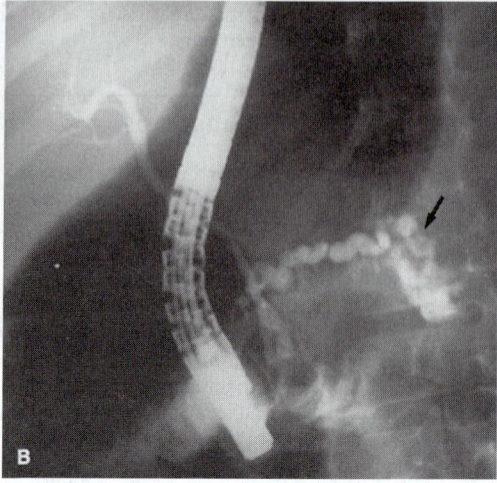

FIGURE 366.2. A: Normal pancreatogram. Note the excellent visualization of the side branches. Main pancreatic duct (*large arrow*); side branches (*small arrows*). (Courtesy of Dr. Anthony Bohorfoush.) **B:** Chronic pancreatitis. Note dilatation and tortuosity of the main pancreatic duct. Filling defects represent intraductal stones (*arrow*).

clinical setting, stools are evaluated for ascaris. A sweat test is performed. Plain-film abdominal radiographs are evaluated for the presence of pancreatic calcifications. US or CT is performed to detect the presence of a pseudocyst or biliary lithiasis.

ERCP, which defines the anatomy of the gland, should be considered in the evaluation of children with nonresolving pancreatitis, recurrent acute pancreatitis or chronic pancreatitis, and before operation in patients with pseudocyst. In such cases, ERCP may detect unsuspected anatomic defects amenable to surgical therapy (Fig. 366.2). This technique is useful and safe (even in very young children) if performed by experienced investigators. Pancreatograms from a normal child and from a child with chronic pancreatitis are found in Figure 366.2.

DISORDERS OF THE DUCTS AND SPHINCTER

Although a wide variety of anatomic defects leading to pancreatitis have been described in case reports, only two—choledochal cysts and pancreas divisum—are seen commonly in practice.

Choledochal Cysts

A choledochal cyst is a congenital dilatation of the extrahepatic biliary tract and usually causes symptoms of biliary tract obstruction (such as the classic triad of pain, jaundice, and abdominal mass) and nausea, vomiting, and fever. These symptoms are thought to be due to an anomalous, long, common channel of the pancreatic and common bile ducts. At times, the presentation may be that of pancreatitis. Usually, the diagnosis is made easily by US or CT.

A choledochocele (an intraduodenal choledochal cyst) at times can be diagnosed only by ERCP. The symptoms of choledochocele may be those of pancreatitis or biliary tract obstruction. The treatment of all forms of choledochal cyst is surgical resection.

Pancreas Divisum

In normal embryologic development, the dorsal and ventral pancreatic anlage fuse by the end of the sixth week of gestation. Incomplete fusion may lead to pancreas divisum, a condition in which the dorsal and ventral portions of the pancreas drain into the duodenum independently. A large body of literature developed over recent years debates whether these anomalies predispose to pancreatitis. Various anomalies of the ductal system are present in 30% to 40% of normal individuals, and pancreas divisum is seen in 5% to 15%. Although the controversy is not settled yet, the present consensus is that pancreas divisum predisposes to pancreatitis when it is associated with an anomaly (e.g., stenosis) of the accessory sphincter. A number of surgical and therapeutic endoscopic procedures have been recommended, with only mixed success.

Suggested Readings

Bettinger JR, Grendell JH. Intracellular events in the pathogenesis of acute pancreatitis. *Pancreas* 1991;6:S2.

Brown CW, Werlin SL, Geenen JE, et al. The diagnostic and therapeutic role of endoscopic retrograde cholangiopancreatography in children. *J Pediatr Gastroenterol Nutr* 1993;17:19.

Jaffe RB, Arata JA, Matlak ME. Percutaneous drainage of traumatic pancreatic pseudocysts in children. *AJR Am J Roentgenol* 1989;152:591.

Haddock G, Coupar G, Youngson GG, et al. Acute pancreatitis in children: a 15-year review. *J Pediatr Surg* 1994;29:719.

Kahler SG, Sherwood WG, Woolf D, et al. Pancreatitis in patients with organic acidemias. *J Pediatr* 1994;124:239.

McArthur KE. Drug-induced pancreatitis [review]. *Aliment Pharmacol Ther* 1996;10:23.

Orebaugh SL. Normal amylase levels in the presentation of acute pancreatitis. *Am J Emerg Med* 1994;12:21.

Parenti DM, Steinberg W, Kang P. Infectious causes of acute pancreatitis. *Pancreas* 1996;13:356.

Sternby B, O'Brien JF, Zinsmeister AR, et al. What is the best biochemical test to diagnose acute pancreatitis? A prospective clinical study. *Mayo Clin Proc* 1996;71:1138.

Weizman Z, Durie PR. Acute pancreatitis in childhood. *J Pediatr* 1988;113:24.

Werlin SL, Kugathasan S, Fruitrchy BC. Pancreatitis in children. *J Pediatr Gastroenterol Nutr* 2003;143:525.

Whitcomb DC, Gorry MC, Preston RA, et al. Hereditary pancreatitis is caused by a mutation in the cationic trypsinogen gene. *Nat Genet* 1996;14:141.

CHAPTER 367 ■ DISORDERS OF THE LIVER AND BILIARY SYSTEM

DONALD A. NOVAK, FREDERICK J. SUCHY, AND WILLIAM F. BALISTRERI

Significant changes in hepatic anatomy and physiology occur in neonates. These rapid maturational alterations are required for infants to cope with their changing environment.

THE LIVER AND GALLBLADDER IN EARLY LIFE

Postnatally, the liver grows in proportion to infants' height, weight, and age; in addition, the proportions of the liver change. The liver may account for as much as 10% of the total body volume in fetuses, but constitutes approximately 5% of body weight at birth and only 2% of adult weight.

Clinical Assessment of Liver Size

The standard clinical indices of liver size are the degree of projection of the liver edge below the right costal margin, the span of dullness on percussion, and the length of the vertical axis of the liver, estimated radiographically. Several studies have provided a baseline of age-related values. In 1957, McNicholl's study of 317 healthy infants and children established values for the projection of the liver edge below the costal margin and emphasized that a projection of greater than 3.5 cm in the midclavicular line (MCL) in the newborn indicated hepatic enlargement. The measurement of liver span may be subject to less variability than is the degree of projection. Younoszai and Mueller measured liver span (vertical height) in older patients by percussing the upper margin and palpating the lower edge in the right MCL. A linear increase in the span, similar in both genders, correlated with body weight and age. Lawson et al. determined the liver span in the MCL in 350 infants and children by percussion of the upper and lower borders. The mean liver span was found to be curvilinearly related to age; by extrapolation, the range was estimated to be 1.9 cm at 1 week of life, to 7.7 cm (for men) and 6.3 cm (for women) at age 20. Age and gender were the major factors correlating liver size in children with normal growth patterns. The expected span of liver dullness in the MCL in children ages 12 to 20 can be obtained by the following equations:

$$\text{Boys: span (cm)} = [0.032 \times \text{weight (lb)}] + [0.18 \times \text{height (in.)}] - 7.86$$

$$\text{Girls: span (cm)} = [0.027 \times \text{weight (lb)}] + [0.22 \times \text{height (in.)}] - 10.75$$

Reiff and Osborn determined that the mean liver span in 100 healthy newborns was 5.9 ± 0.8 cm by percussion; this value, much larger than the one cited earlier, suggests that extrapolation of the curve by Lawson et al. may not be accurate for the neonatal age range. It exhibited a poor correlation of span with measurement of liver projection below the costal margin. Reiff and Osborn emphasized the clinical utility of the assessment of liver span.

Liver volume may reflect liver size more accurately because a change in shape may not necessarily be distributed equally. Liver volume, as assessed by ultrasonography, a reproducible and noninvasive method, correlated inversely ($r = -0.79$) with age. The relative volume (expressed per unit of body weight) in the first year of life (approximately 48 mL/kg) was almost twice the volume at age 15 (approximately 25 mL/kg).

Clinical Assessment of Gallbladder Size

The gallbladder is visualized readily in children, even in neonates, using high-frequency real-time ultrasonographic imaging. A gallbladder that may be distended in sick infants, often in conjunction with sepsis, mandates essential definitions of those criteria useful in differentiating a normal gallbladder in a newborn from a gallbladder or biliary tract that is pathologically enlarged or atretic. In a study of children between ages 1 month and 16 years, ultrasonography scans showed a gradual age-related increase in the size of the gallbladder. Wall thickness never was more than 3 mm; the lumen of the common hepatic duct increased with age but never was greater than 4 mm.

Functional Alterations during Development

Specific deficiencies in hepatic function have been observed repeatedly in normal, healthy newborn infants. This finding has led to an extensive investigation of the alterations in the quantitative pattern of various enzymes during embryonic development. Despite marked intraspecies differences, several general concepts can be stated.

During late fetal and early postnatal development, the differentiation of tissue function depends on *de novo* synthesis of enzymes, not on activation of enzymes already present in the embryonic tissue. Greengard documented the quantitative pattern of enzymatic differentiation in early life and observed that the increase in their concentrations (i.e., emergence) occurs in clusters that correlate with the changing functional requirements of the developing organism. Substrate and hormonal flow across the placenta and dietary and hormonal input in the postnatal period modulate the emergence of these enzymatic processes. The lipid composition of various cell and organelle membranes changes rapidly in response to alterations in the composition of dietary lipids. The role of genetic preprogramming (i.e., effect of the biologic clock) also must be considered in understanding the ontogeny of metabolic activities.

Age-Related Differences in Standard Biochemical Assays

Well-defined, age-related changes are seen in the biochemical parameters of hepatic function. Normal reference values are cited in Appendix A. For example, serum ceruloplasmin and alpha$_1$-antitrypsin values do not vary significantly with age after the immediate perinatal period. Kattwinkel et al. determined that serum levels of aspartate aminotransferase, gamma-glutamyltransferase, 5′-nucleotidase, and total alkaline phosphatase and its bone isoenzymes exhibit significant age dependency in normal children. Throughout early life, cholesterol concentrations increase rapidly. Importantly, clinicians at each institution must establish a working range using their instrumentation.

Alkaline Phosphatase

The total activity of alkaline phosphatase in human serum varies considerably with age and, to some degree, with gender. The largest proportion of these age-dependent differences is caused by an increased isoenzyme originating in bone; these fluctuations are therefore most significant during periods of accelerated bone growth. Values must be interpreted in the context of these known physiologic changes. In newborns, the reference normal values may be as much as four times the values of adults; throughout the remainder of childhood, alkaline phosphatase activity may be three times the adult value, with a decline after puberty.

Ammonia

Except for a transient increase in the ammonia content of peripheral blood in normal neonates, ammonia nitrogen values during early life are similar to adult values. Transient hyperammonemia is seen in early life, possibly due to the shunting of blood through the ductus venosus and immaturity of metabolic processes.

Alpha-Fetoprotein

The concentrations of alpha-fetoprotein (αFP), a glycoprotein synthesized by embryonic tissues (e.g., liver, yolk sac), are highest in serum during the tenth to fourteenth weeks of fetal life. Concentrations decrease rapidly, especially in the perinatal period.

Gamma-Glutamyltransferase (γ-GTP)

Gamma-glutamyltransferase (gamma-glutamyl transpeptidase) is a multifunctional, membrane-bound glycoprotein that serves catalytic and detoxification functions. Because of the difficulty in interpreting alkaline phosphatase values, the measurement of gamma-glutamyl transpeptidase may be beneficial in the pediatric population; activity is normally high at birth and declines rapidly with maturation.

5′-Nucleotidase

Usually, serum 5′-nucleotidase activity is elevated in hepatobiliary diseases. However, unlike serum alkaline phosphatase, its activity is not increased in infancy, childhood, skeletal disorders, or pregnancy.

CONGENITAL ANOMALIES AND ABERRATIONS OF HEPATIC PHYSIOLOGY IN EARLY LIFE

Hepatic structural and functional abnormalities due to congenital or acquired defects can manifest in the perinatal period. The response of the neonatal liver to injury from a variety of insults may be stereotypic: the formation of giant cells, inflammation, and cell necrosis.

Anomalies

Reductions or increases in the external lobation of the liver are rare. More frequent are abnormalities of the hepatic ducts and gallbladder, such as partial or complete duplication or congenital absence of the gallbladder. Riedel's lobe, a tongue-shaped mass of normal liver tissue that projects downward from the right lobe, is a common anatomic variation.

Hepatomegaly

In the evaluation of unexplained hepatomegaly (Box 367.1), ultrasonography can demonstrate hepatic size and consistency. A hyperechogenic (bright) appearance of the hepatic parenchyma is common in children and can be caused by metabolic disease (e.g., glycogen storage disease) or a fatty liver (e.g., obesity, malnutrition, hyperalimentation, steroid therapy). This ultrasonographic finding in children can guide further evaluation, such as liver biopsy with quantitative and qualitative assays for fat or specific enzyme assays.

Chronic Cholestasis

Infants and children with hepatobiliary dysfunction, regardless of the cause, are at risk for the sequelae of prolonged cholestasis. These sequelae include malabsorption of fats and fat-soluble vitamins, secondary to diminished intestinal bile acid concentrations, and retention of endogenous compounds, such as bilirubin and bile acids, usually excreted by the liver. Chronic liver disease, with resultant impairment of hepatic function, may alter nutrient metabolism. Growth failure may result from aberrations in hormonal balance. Hepatic disease may progress, with the eventual development of hepatic cirrhosis, portal hypertension, and liver failure. Therapy is largely symptomatic; in most cases, progression of the underlying hepatic disease cannot be halted. General recommendations for therapy are given in Table 367.1.

Patients with chronic cholestasis may develop intense pruritus, manifest in early life. The cause of pruritus remains obscure; xanthomas also may develop. Xanthoma formation may be related to the elevated serum lipid values found in chronic cholestasis. Therapy for both complications is aimed at inducing more efficient excretion of these endogenous compounds. Ursodeoxycholic acid (10 to 30 mg/kg/day in divided doses) is the agent of choice. Cholestyramine resin (8 to 16 g/day) also may be given to stimulate bile excretion. The usefulness of this agent is limited by the extent of residual bile flow. In addition, cholestyramine is unpalatable, its administration is difficult, and it may cause constipation and fat-soluble vitamin deficiency. Rifampin (10 mg/kg/day; maximum, 300 mg/day) has been evaluated in a few pediatric patients with pruritus and has been found efficacious, as has partial biliary diversion. Therapy with ultraviolet B (UVB) light has proven useful in the control of pruritus in adults. Plasma perfusion and therapy using carbamazepine or hydroxyzine have been used in adults, but their usefulness in children must be evaluated. Newer therapies have focused on the central causes of pruritus. Specifically, naltrexone, an opiate receptor antagonist, and ondansetron, acting via 5-hydroxytryptamine receptors, have been shown to be efficacious in relieving the pruritus associated with cholestasis in adults.

Often, nutritional inadequacies are a problem in children with chronic cholestasis. Fat malabsorption is common, because of diminished intestinal bile acid concentrations. It is

---

BOX 367.1 Pathophysiology and Differential Diagnosis of Liver Enlargement

Increased Number of Cells in the Liver
Inflammation (hepatocyte or Kupffer cell enlargement, inflammatory cells)
  Viral, acute or chronic
  Bacterial (sepsis, abscess, cholangitis)
  Toxic
  Autoimmune
Storage
  Fat
    Nonalcoholic fatty liver disease
    Reye syndrome/mitochondrial disease
    Malnutrition
    Lipid infusion
    Cystic fibrosis
    Diabetes
  Glycogen (multiple forms of glycogen storage disease)
Specific lipid storage disease
    Gaucher disease
    Niemann-Pick disease
    Wolman disease
  Miscellaneous
    Alpha one antitrypsin deficiency
    Wilson disease
    Hypervitaminosis A
Infiltration
  Primary tumors
    Hepatoblastoma
    Hepatocellular carcinoma
    Hemangioma
    Focal nodular hyperplasia
  Secondary or metastatic tumors
    Lymphoma
    Leukemia
    Neuroblastoma
    Wilms tumor
    Hemophagocytic lymphohistiocytosis

Increased Size of Vascular Space
Intrahepatic obstruction to hepatic vein outflow
  Venoocclusive disease
  Hepatic vein thrombosis (Budd-Chiari)
  Hepatic vein web
Suprahepatic
  Congestive heart failure
  Pericardial disease
    Tamponade
    Constrictive pericarditis

Increased Size of Biliary Space
Congenital hepatic fibrosis
Caroli disease

Idiopathic (benign?)

---

essential to provide adequate calories and supplements containing medium-chain triglycerides (which are absorbed more readily) as orally administered formula or through nasogastric drip. Fat-soluble vitamin (e.g., A, D, E, K) deficiency is common in children with chronic cholestasis. Vitamin D deficiency may cause rickets; vitamin K deficiency may be responsible for intracranial hemorrhage; vitamin E deficiency may be responsible for a progressive neuromuscular syndrome once thought to be an inherent feature of multiple cholestatic diseases. A deficiency (i.e., malabsorption) of vitamin E causes a neuropathy

characterized by progressive loss of the myelinated axons of peripheral nerves and a degeneration of spinal cord posterior columns; the neuronal tocopherol content may be low. Clinically, areflexia, cerebellar ataxia, ophthalmoplegia, and peripheral neuropathies are seen. Because these lesions appear to be partly reversible in young children, careful monitoring of fat-soluble vitamin levels is necessary. Vitamin E levels may be elevated falsely because of elevated serum lipid levels, and the ratio of serum vitamin E to total serum lipids (normal ratio, less than 0.6 mg/g in children younger than 12 years) should be followed. Oral supplementation should be given as necessary, but intramuscular administration has been required in some patients. D-Alpha-tocopheryl polyethylene glycol-1,000 succinate (TPGS) is a water-soluble form of vitamin E that is adsorbed well after oral administration and is safe and effective for the prevention and correction of the vitamin E deficiency of chronic cholestasis.

Despite careful attention to caloric intake, mineral balance, and vitamin status, poor hepatic synthetic function may limit growth. At this point, affected patients may become candidates for orthotopic liver transplantation (OLT). Survival rates up to 90% are reported following OLT. The success rates and degree of organ availability increase significantly as infants attain adequate size (larger than 10 kg), although hepatic size–reduction techniques have made transplantation more available to smaller children, as has the use of living related donors.

Total Parenteral Nutrition–Related Cholestasis

Parenteral nutrition is a life-saving form of therapy in neonates, children, or adults who are unable to receive enteral nutrition. However, serious complications are frequent, among which is cholestasis related to total parenteral nutrition (TPN), second in incidence only to catheter-related sepsis.

Cholestasis associated with TPN occurs primarily in premature infants, although hepatobiliary lesions, including triaditis and steatosis, have been described in older children and adults. In an early report, the incidence of cholestasis in children receiving TPN was 50% in infants with birth weights of less than 1,000 g and 18% in infants with birth weights of 1,000 to 1,500 g. Other investigators have confirmed the inverse relation between gestational age and the incidence of TPN-related cholestasis. The onset of cholestasis appears to be related to the duration of infusion, usually occurring after at least 2 weeks of therapy. Frequently, TPN-related hepatic disease occurs in sick, premature infants, typically those undergoing episodes of sepsis, shock, abdominal surgery, and necrotizing enterocolitis.

TPN-related cholestasis has an insidious onset. Jaundice may be observed, but it is attributed to "physiologic" hyperbilirubinemia. Often, the diagnosis of TPN-related cholestasis is entertained first when routine parenteral nutrition–related surveillance laboratory tests reveal elevated serum levels of conjugated bilirubin. Usually, serum bile acid levels are elevated; often, an increase in serum bile acid levels is the earliest biochemical abnormality associated with TPN-related cholestasis. Later in the disease course, serum aminotransferase and serum alkaline phosphatase levels may become abnormal. Typically, hepatic synthetic function remains normal until late in the disease course.

The differential diagnosis of TPN-related cholestasis includes the many causes of neonatal cholestasis and is a diagnosis of exclusion. The evaluation should concentrate on identifying other potentially treatable causes of cholestasis, including infectious, metabolic, or anatomic disorders that may be detected in as many as 10% of infants evaluated for possible TPN-related liver dysfunction. This exercise is imperative, because alternative therapy may be available.

TABLE 367.1

SUGGESTED MEDICAL MANAGEMENT OF THE CONSEQUENCES OF PERSISTENT CHOLESTASIS

Effect	Management
Malnutrition	
Malabsorption of dietary long-chain triglyceride	Replace with dietary formula or supplement containing medium-chain triglyceride: adequate protein (vegetable sources), adequate calories (complex starch)
Fat-soluble vitamin deficiency	Supplement and monitor
Vitamin A (e.g., night blindness, thick skin)	Replace with 5,000–25,000 IU/d as Aquasol A
Vitamin E (e.g., neuromuscular degeneration)	Replace with 50–400 IU/kg/d as alphatocopherol
Vitamin D (e.g., metabolic bone disease)	Replace with 5,000–8,000 IU/d of D_2 or 3–5 μg/kg/d of 25-hydroxycholecalciferol
Vitamin K (e.g., hypoprothrombinemia)	Replace with 2.5–5.0 mg/d as water-soluble derivative of menadione
Micronutrient deficiency	Calcium, phosphate, and zinc supplementation
Deficiency of water-soluble vitamins	Supplement with twice the recommended daily allowance
Retention of biliary constituents	
Bile acids and cholesterol (itch or xanthomas)	Remove or chelate
	Bile acid binders (cholestyramine, 8–16 g/d)
	Ursodeoxycholic acid (15 mg/kg/d)
	Rifampin (10 mg/kg/d)
	Hydroxyzine (2mg/kg/d)
	Potential therapies (UV-B light, carbamazepine, naloxone, ondansetron)
Trace elements, such as copper (e.g., hepatotoxicity)	Possible role of avoidance of food enriched in copper; potential role of chelating agents
Progressive liver disease	
Variceal hemorrhage	Management of variceal bleeding
	Acute: lavage, endoscopic sclerotherapy, octreotide or vasopressin, balloon tamponade
	Chronic: sclerotherapy or banding, beta-blockade, surgical (i.e., shunt versus variceal ligation)
Ascites	Ascites management
	Sodium restriction (1–2 mEq/kg/d)
	Spironolactone (2–3 mg/kg/d in divided doses); if diuresis is inadequate after 2–4 days, double dose; follow urine and serum electrolyte concentrations
	Further diuretic therapy (i.e., furosemide or thiazides) with albumin
End-stage liver disease	Transplantation

The hepatic pathology of TPN-related cholestasis is nonspecific. Early changes include hepatocyte and canalicular cholestasis, extramedullary hematopoiesis, giant cell transformation, and pseudoacinar formation. Later changes reflect worsening disease, with inflammatory infiltrates, ductular proliferation, and fibrosis. Although hepatic fibrosis, cirrhosis, and hepatic failure have been documented in patients receiving long-term TPN, milder changes, including ductular proliferation and inflammation, can reverse upon discontinuation of TPN and resumption of oral feedings.

The cause of TPN-related cholestasis is unknown. In early life, affected infants have a period during which hepatic uptake and (presumably) the excretion of bile acids and other organic anions is diminished. Premature infants may be unusually susceptible to cholestasis. Elevated serum concentrations of the potentially toxic bile acid lithocholate occur during prolonged TPN administration and may potentiate cholestasis. Fasting alone may predispose affected infants to cholestasis through lack of the hormonal stimulation of bile secretion. Sepsis, common in the infant receiving TPN, is known to cause cholestasis. Repeated episodes of intravascular catheter infection seem to be associated with worsening disease, especially in patients with short bowel syndrome. Amino acids have been implicated in the cause of TPN-associated cholestasis, and indirect evidence suggests that amino acid infusions may influence the development of cholestasis. Certain amino acids have been shown to inhibit hepatic bile acid uptake. The amino acid composition of TPN infusates is capable of altering bile flow rates in animals. Unfortunately, a specific amino acid deficiency or toxicity syndrome resulting in cholestasis has not been identified

in the human. Choline deficiency is common in patients on long-term TPN, and may result in hepatic steatosis, as may excessive rates of glucose infusion. Little evidence is available to suggest that intravenous fat or glucose infusions are associated with cholestasis. Other possible factors in the genesis of TPN-related cholestasis include deficiencies or excesses of various minerals or trace elements.

The management of patients with TPN-related cholestasis is difficult. Continuation of TPN may result in worsening hepatic disease. Conversely, complete withdrawal of TPN may result in a catabolic state and poor growth. A prudent approach is to attempt the slow introduction of enteral feeding, to stimulate gastrointestinal hormone release and bile flow. The protein infusion should be limited to the lowest amount required for growth. Avoiding episodes of sepsis, through scrupulous care of indwelling catheters, as well as of bacterial translocation, through the use of enteral feedings, with resultant improvement in mucosal integrity may be beneficial. The use of intermittent courses of oral antibiotics also has been advocated, especially in those patients with short bowel syndrome who suffer from bacterial overgrowth. The use of minimal enteral feedings through the oral administration of approximately 10% of the daily caloric needs may prevent or ameliorate TPN-related cholestasis.

Generally, the prognosis for infants who develop TPN-related cholestasis is good. However, long-term follow-up studies are not available.

TPN-related cholelithiasis occurs primarily in preterm infants. Patients may be asymptomatic or may present with signs and symptoms of acute cholecystitis, including vomiting, rapid rise of serum bilirubin, fever, and sepsis. Diagnosis depends on clinical suspicion and ultrasonography. Factors important in the genesis of TPN-related cholestasis also may play a role in the causation of cholelithiasis; in particular, fasting may be associated with gallbladder stasis. Continued fasting and TPN administration may cause biliary sludge, composed of thick bile intermixed with pigment granules, calcium bilirubinate, and cholesterol crystals. Sludge, identifiable by ultrasonography, appears to be the precursor of stone formation, and prolonged gallbladder stasis may predispose to stone formation. The administration of furosemide and of TPN solutions may increase calcium secretion into bile, increasing its lithogenicity. Gallbladder sludge resolves spontaneously with the resumption of enteral feedings. Rarely, gallstones have been reported to clear with feeding. Cycling of TPN administration does not appear to be helpful.

Total Parenteral Nutrition–Associated Hepatobiliary Dysfunction in Older Patients

Although hepatic dysfunction with TPN is reported most often in infants, some reports describe the development of cholestasis—associated with bile ductular proliferation, periportal inflammation, and fibrosis—in older patients who have undergone massive intestinal resection, requiring prolonged parenteral nutrition. Less severe abnormalities, including steatosis without cholestasis, have been observed in adults with GI dysfunction requiring TPN. It is unclear whether these cases share a pathogenesis similar to that of TPN-related cholestasis of infancy.

METABOLIC DISEASE OF THE LIVER

The liver plays a central role in carbohydrate, lipid, and amino acid synthesis and degradation. Not surprisingly, the liver is involved primarily or secondarily in many states of metabolic derangement. For example, the absence of a crucial enzyme may cause a build-up of toxic metabolites; this condition is found in patients with tyrosinemia. Conversely, the sequestration of a synthesized product within the liver may lead to hepatic and systemic damage, as is seen in alpha$_1$-antitrypsin deficiency.

Hepatic metabolic disease may be suggested by a family history or by the pattern of symptom onset. For example, liver injury after the initiation of fructose ingestion should suggest the diagnosis of fructosemia. Clinical features of liver-based metabolic diseases are nonspecific but include jaundice, hepatosplenomegaly, failure to thrive, dysmorphism, developmental delay, hypotonia, seizures, and progressive neuromuscular dysfunction. Screening laboratory data may reveal hypoglycemia, hyperammonemia, increased serum aminotransaminase levels, acidosis, or hypoprothrombinemia. The metabolic disease can be confirmed in a variety of ways. Percutaneous hepatic biopsy allows histologic examination and measurement of specific enzyme activities or substrate accumulation. Accurate diagnosis is important in that it may allow effective therapy and genetic counseling. Therefore, physicians must remain alert to the possibility of metabolic disease.

Disorders of Tyrosine Metabolism

Tyrosine is an amino acid important in the synthesis of melanin, thyroid hormones, and catecholamines. Metabolism of tyrosine to fumaric acid and acetoacetic acid proceeds down a pathway with several intermediates. Deficiency or immaturity of any of the enzymes catalyzing these steps may lead to hypertyrosinemia. Transient neonatal tyrosinemia is a self-limiting condition of premature neonates, presumably caused by an immaturity of tyrosine aminotransferase activity. Vitamin C may be effective in enhancing enzyme activity in these patients. Hypertyrosinemia may occur also in any form of severe hepatic injury, typically in concert with high serum methionine levels.

Hereditary Tyrosinemia

Type 1 hereditary tyrosinemia is an autosomal recessive disorder. The acute form manifests in infancy with symptoms of jaundice, failure to thrive, anorexia, hepatosplenomegaly, ascites, hypoprothrombinemia, clinical bleeding, rickets, and hepatic failure or cirrhosis. Usually, the chronic form is seen later in life, accompanying cirrhosis or hepatocellular carcinoma. Episodic, severe, acute peripheral neuropathy is common in patients surviving infancy and is an important cause of morbidity and mortality.

Laboratory features include diminished hepatic synthetic function, including decreased vitamin K–dependent clotting factors and hypoalbuminemia. Serum aminotransferase levels are mildly to moderately elevated, as is serum bilirubin. Hemolytic anemia or hypoglycemia may occur. Fanconi syndrome, with attendant hyperphosphaturia, glycosuria, proteinuria, and aminoaciduria, often is evident. Rickets, presumably secondary to hypophosphatemia, may complicate the picture. Serum tyrosine values are extraordinarily high, as may be serum methionine levels. The phenolic acid by-products of tyrosine metabolism (i.e., *p*-hydroxyphenyl lactic, *p*-hydroxyphenyl pyruvic, and *p*-hydroxyphenyl acetic acids) are excreted in the urine, as are succinyl acetone and succinyl acetoacetate.

Pathogenesis

The enzymatic defect in type 1 tyrosinemia appears to be at the level of fumarylacetoacetate (FAH). The gene responsible for this activity has been mapped to human chromosome 15, and multiple mutations have been associated with the phenotype of type 1 tyrosinemia. This deficiency causes a build-up of potentially toxic metabolites, including succinyl acetone (SA) and succinyl acetoacetate (SAA). These intermediates are toxic reactive metabolites that may cause renal and hepatic damage as a result of binding to sulfhydryl groups of proteins.

Hepatic Pathology

The hepatic injury in tyrosinemia presumably begins *in utero*, as illustrated by elevated cord blood αFP levels with normal serum tyrosine levels. The liver exhibits nodular cirrhosis and extensive fibrosis. Pseudoacinar formation, fatty infiltration, and iron deposition may occur. Hepatocellular carcinoma may be found in older patients with cirrhosis.

Therapy

The acute form of type 1 tyrosinemia, without therapy, typically is fatal in the first year of life. Dietary modifications to limit the intake of phenylalanine, tyrosine, and methionine appear to improve renal dysfunction, but the effects on the hepatic disease are unclear. Proper diagnosis is important for genetic counseling, and prenatal diagnosis is available. The treatment of choice for infants with type 1 tyrosinemia is 2-(2-nitro-4-trifluoromethylbenzoyl)-cyclohexane-1,3-dione, an inhibitor of 4-hydroxyphenylpyruvate dioxygenase. Further study is required to determine the role of this agent in preventing both ongoing hepatic damage and subsequent malignant transformation; however, current evidence suggest that this agent, when begun early in life, may significantly diminish the severity of hepatic disease as well as the incidence of hepatocellular carcinoma in those afflicted with tyrosinemia. Liver transplantation can correct most of the biochemical abnormalities of hereditary tyrosinemia and, therefore, has been recommended for all tyrosinemic children with cirrhotic nodules demonstrated on computed tomography (CT) or ultrasonographic examinations, because of the great risk of developing hepatocellular carcinoma. Neurologic crises provide an additional reason to consider early liver transplantation.

(Disorders of carbohydrate and lipoprotein metabolism and their effect on the liver are discussed in Chapters 387 and 388.)

DISORDERS OF PROTEIN METABOLISM: UREA CYCLE ENZYME DEFECTS

Hyperammonemia

The differential diagnosis of childhood hyperammonemia includes disorders of the urea cycle, mitochondrial disorders, organic acidemias, disorders of fatty acid oxidation, transient hyperammonemia of the neonate, Reye syndrome, drug toxicity (e.g., secondary to valproate), and hepatic failure. Differentiation of these situations is important because specific therapy is available for certain disorders.

Ammonia is eliminated from the body through the formation of urea in the liver (Fig. 367.1). An accumulation of this potentially toxic substrate can be ascribed to primary or acquired alterations in any of the enzymatic steps in this cycle. Episodes of hyperammonemia may depress consciousness and eventually may produce permanent impairment of neurologic function, or death. Symptoms in newborns may be more subtle.

Most often, hyperammonemia in newborns is secondary to inherited defects in urea cycle enzymes. If untreated, deficiency in ornithine transcarbamylase, a sex-linked recessive disorder, is fatal in the neonatal period. Affected heterozygous girls also may have episodic hyperammonemia, with subsequent mental retardation or death. Citrullinemia and argininosuccinic acidemia may manifest in the neonatal period with hyperammonemic coma or, in a subacute form with mental retardation; those with argininosuccinate lyase deficiency may undergo progressive hepatic fibrosis. Type II citrullinemia has been associated with idiopathic neonatal hepatitis. Patients with argininemia have hyperammonemia and spastic diplegia. Affected newborns may have a clinical picture resembling that caused by sepsis. A high index of suspicion is required. An algorithm for the workup of infants with hyperammonemia is shown in Figure 367.2.

Hyperammonemia may be reduced through the use of peritoneal dialysis, hemodialysis, or venovenous hemofiltration. Efforts should be made to induce ammonia excretion through alternative pathways. Therapy should be tailored to individual disorders. In addition to the administration of low-protein diets, sodium benzoate often is given to allow the excretion of ammonia in the form of hippurate. Arginine or citrulline may be given to enhance the excretion of nitrogen. Sodium phenylacetate or phenylbutyrate may be given in argininosuccinase deficiency; glutamine may be conjugated with phenylacetate, resulting in the renal excretion of phenylacetylglutamine and the accompanying excretion of nitrogen. These steps have allowed the successful management of many episodes of hyperammonemia, with longer survival of affected patients. However, catastrophic episodes still may occur despite adequate therapy. Efforts at identifying carriers and prenatal diagnosis are critical. Specific prenatal diagnosis of ornithine transcarbamylase deficiency has been described. Early, prospective treatment of at-risk infants results in more favorable outcomes. Liver transplantation may be curative if performed before irreversible neurologic injury.

Such organic acidemias as propionic acidemia, isovaleric acidemia, methylmalonic acidemia, glutaric acidemia, and multiple carboxylase deficiencies also may manifest with neonatal hyperammonemia. Typically, serum ammonia levels are elevated to a degree less than that observed in urea cycle defects, and usually acidosis and ketosis are evident. Evaluation includes a careful analysis of the pattern of urinary organic acid excretion. Therapy focuses on correcting specific defects, including acidosis and removal of ammonia through the use of dialysis. Subsequent medical or dietary therapy (or a combination) is tailored to individual disorders; hepatic transplantation

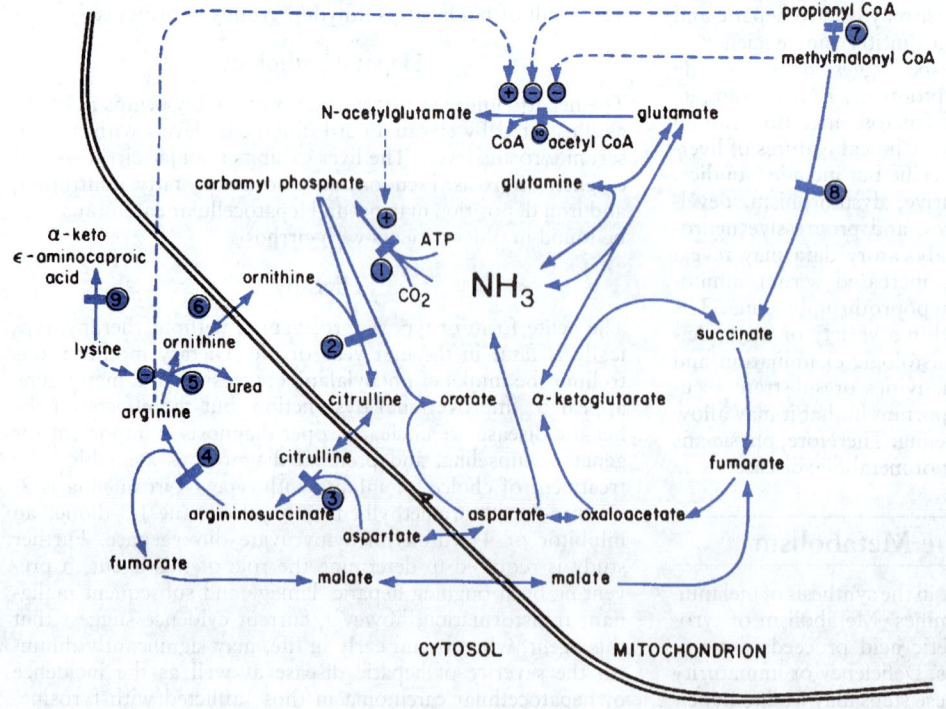

FIGURE 367.1. Urea cycle. Major metabolic pathways for the use of ammonia. Solid bars indicate sites of primary enzyme defects (or suspected sites of primary enzyme defects) in various inherited metabolic disorders associated with hyperammonemia. 1, carbamyl phosphate synthetase I; 2, ornithine transcarbamylase; 3, argininosuccinate synthetase; 4, argininosuccinate lyase; 5, arginase; 6, mitochondrial ornithine transport 7, propionyl coenzyme A (CoA) carboxylase; 8, methylmalonyl CoA mutase; 9, 4-L-lysine dehydrogenase; 10, N-acetylglutamate synthetase. Dotted lines indicate sites of pathway activation (+) or inhibition (−). ATP, adenosine triphosphate. (Reprinted with permission from Flannery DB, Hsia YE, Wolf B. Current status of hyperammonemic syndromes. *Hepatology* 1982;2:495.)

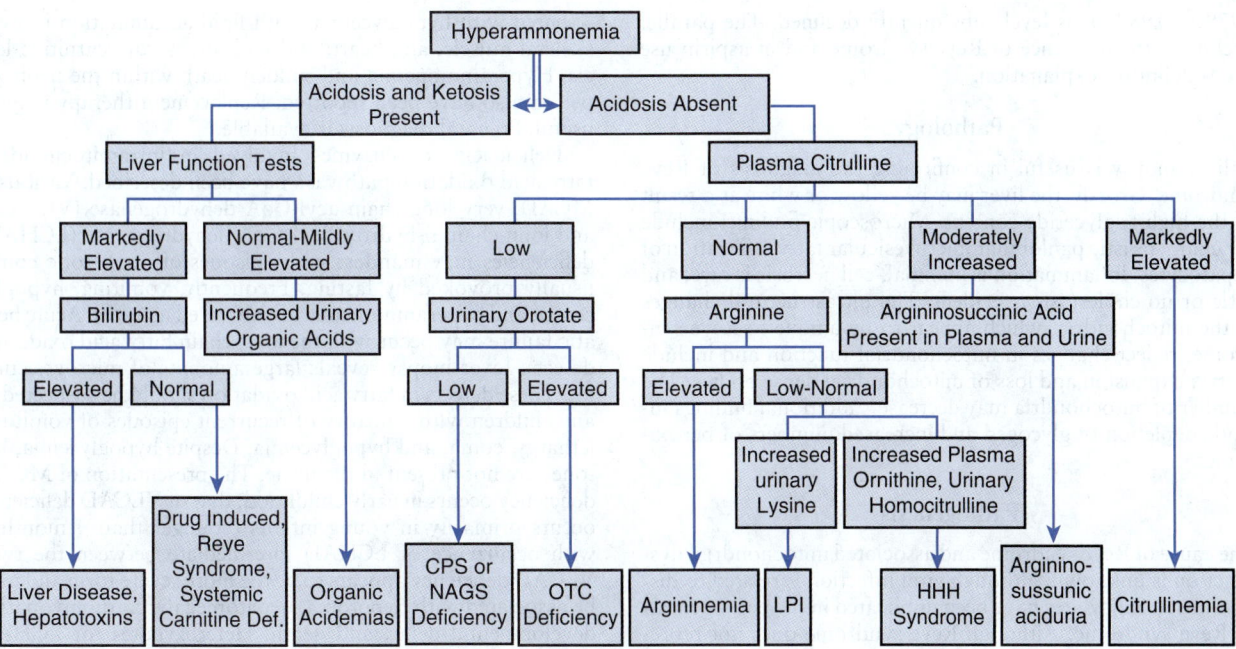

FIGURE 367.2. Differential diagnosis of hyperammonemia. CPS, carbamyl phosphate synthetase; Def., deficiency; HHH, hyperornithinemia-hyperammonemia-homocitrullinemia; LPI, lysinuric protein intolerance; NAGS, N-acetyl glutamate synthetase; OTC, ornithine transcarbamylase. (Reprinted with permission from Batshaw ML. Hyperammonemia. *Curr Probl Pediatr* 1984;14:1.)

has been performed for selected disorders, however neurologic outcome may not be altered by this therapy.

The liver is a major target organ of inherited disorders of oxidative phosphorylation. Liver disease of varying severity may occur at different ages, in association with deficiencies of the respiratory chain complexes. Neonatal liver failure has been described with deficiency of complexes III and IV. Mitochondrial DNA depletion, with a general reduction in activity of respiratory chain complexes encoded by the mitochondrial genome (complexes I, III, and IV), also has been described. These infants present within the first months of life with hypoglycemia, coagulopathy, hyperbilirubinemia, and hyperammonemia. A significant lactic acidemia and elevated lactate-to-pyruvate ratio is present. Liver biopsy specimens show microvesicular and macrovesicular steatosis. Death from liver failure is common. Liver transplantation should not be done in the presence of progressive neuromuscular disease, which occurs frequently in these patients and is not reversed through this treatment modality.

Transient hyperammonemia of infancy is a disorder found primarily in premature infants, often in conjunction with respiratory distress. Typically, ammonia levels rise rapidly during the first days of life, producing central nervous system (CNS) depression and coma in the second and third days of life. Family history is negative, unlike that often found for infants with urea cycle defects or organic acidemias. The cause of this disorder is unknown, although diminished hepatic blood flow in the neonatal period has been postulated. Therapy is aimed at reducing serum ammonia levels, and dialysis has been used. Prognosis appears to be good for patients whose disease is treated aggressively and who survive the neonatal period.

Reye Syndrome

Reye syndrome became a topic of widespread interest in the mid-1970s, when a dramatic increase in incidence was observed. Although the ensuing years have brought a better under-

standing of the epidemiology and therapy of Reye syndrome, its cause remains unclear. Clearer, however, is that most cases presenting as "Reye syndrome" are due to defects in mitochondrial metabolism. Despite its declining incidence, therefore, the disease continues to attract interest as a paradigm for other mitochondrial disorders.

Clinical and Laboratory Features

Classic Reye syndrome, or acute encephalopathy and fatty degeneration of the viscera, follows a biphasic course. Within a week after recovery from a generally mild prodromal viral illness, pernicious vomiting occurs, usually without fever. Irritability and lethargy may be present initially. Most patients do not progress further; however, some may display delirium and stupor followed by progression to seizure, coma, or death due to brainstem herniation. Focal neurologic findings are absent. Mild hepatic enlargement occurs, although jaundice does not. The cerebrospinal fluid is normal. The encephalopathy may continue for 24 to 96 hours, by which time gradual improvement in neurologic function begins to occur in patients who eventually recover, or deterioration in those for whom progression is obvious.

The laboratory features of this syndrome include an elevation of serum aminotransferase levels to at least threefold above normal. Serum ammonia may be normal or elevated at presentation, as may the prothrombin time; however, serum ammonia levels above 100 mg/dL and a corrected prothrombin time of 3 seconds or longer than control levels on admission are harbingers of progression to deeper coma grades. Hypoglycemia may affect primarily infants and younger children. The differential diagnosis of children presenting with a Reye syndrome–like picture includes CNS infections, salicylate toxicity, valproate and other drug toxicity, urea cycle disorders, disorders of fatty acid oxidation, and organic acidemias.

Epidemiology

The incidence of Reye syndrome rose dramatically in the early mid-1970s, to a peak of 555 cases reported nationally from

1979 to 1980. This level subsequently declined. The parallel decline in the incidence of Reye syndrome and in aspirin use needs definitive explanation.

Pathology

A liver biopsy is useful in confirming the diagnosis of Reye syndrome. Grossly, the liver may be yellow or white as a result of the high triglyceride content. Microscopic findings include the characteristic panlobular microvesicular fatty infiltration of hepatocytes. Inflammation is minimal, cell necrosis is rare, and little or no cholestasis is evident. The ultrastructural changes in the mitochondria, which appear to be unique to Reye syndrome, reflect changes in mitochondrial function and include matrix expansion and loss of mitochondrial dense bodies. The number of mitochondria may decrease. Additional findings include depletion of glycogen and increased numbers of peroxisomes.

Pathogenesis

The cause of Reye syndrome and associated mitochondrial dysfunction is unknown, although viral infection is related to disease onset. Salicylates have been implicated in the pathogenesis of Reye syndrome. Although Reye syndrome does not represent acute salicylate toxicity, multiple studies have suggested a higher incidence of aspirin use in patients developing Reye syndrome. Therefore, current recommendations are to withhold aspirin use in children, especially during periods of increased varicella and influenza activity.

Therapy

The treatment of Reye syndrome involves careful monitoring for progression in the early, less severe stages and intensive supportive care addressing increased intracranial pressure and the other consequences of mitochondrial dysfunction in the more severe stages. Specific therapy is unavailable.

Prognosis

The prognosis for patients with grade I disease is excellent, with rapid recovery expected. Prognostic indices include the degree of elevation of serum ammonia and prolongation of prothrombin time on admission. Neurologic deficits may occur after recovery from more severe disease; they include deficits in measured intelligence, achievement, visuomotor integration, and concept formation.

Diseases Resembling Reye Syndrome

Many diseases, including urea cycle defects and organic acidemias, may present with episodes of hyperammonemia. Although most of these disorders present primarily in infancy, some, such as the heterozygous form of ornithine transcarbamylase deficiency, may appear later in childhood with Reye syndrome–like illnesses. Other entities that may appear in infancy or childhood include medium-chain acyl-CoA dehydrogenase (MCAD) deficiency, long-chain acyl-CoA dehydrogenase deficiency, and short-chain acyl-CoA dehydrogenase deficiency; carnitine-acylcarnitine translocase deficiency; and 3-hydroxy-3-methyl glutaric acidemia. Common features shared by these defects include acute metabolic decompensation associated with fasting, chronic involvement of fatty acid–dependent tissues (e.g., cardiac and skeletal muscle), episodes of hypoketotic hypoglycemia, and an alteration in the esterification of plasma or tissue carnitine.

Carnitine aids in the transfer of long-chain fatty acids across the inner mitochondrial membrane, where they undergo beta-oxidation. Carnitine-acylcarnitine translocase deficiency is associated with hypoglycemia; with lipid accumulation in liver, skeletal muscle, and heart; and with low serum carnitine levels. Hyperammonemia and sudden death within the neonatal period also have been reported. Replacement therapy may be useful. Prenatal diagnosis is available.

Deficiencies of enzymes involved in intramitochondrial fatty acid oxidation pathways have been described. Variously, MCAD, very long-chain acyl-CoA dehydrogenase (VLCAD), and long-chain 3-hydroxyacyl-CoA dehydrogenase (LCHAD) deficiencies may manifest with episodes of nonketotic coma, usually provoked by fasting. Frequently, vomiting, hypoglycemia, and hyperammonemia are observed features. Acute hepatic failure may occur with the long-chain fatty acid oxidation defects. Liver biopsy reveals large amounts of microvesicular fat. These defects in fatty acid oxidation should be suspected in any children with a history of recurrent episodes of vomiting, lethargy, coma, and hypoglycemia. Despite hypoglycemia, ketones are not present in the urine. The presentation of MCAD deficiency occurs in early childhood; that of VLCAD deficiency occurs primarily in young infants (younger than 4 months), with occurrence of LCHAD intermediate between the two. VLCAD deficiency appears to be the more severe form and may be associated with hypotonia, hepatomegaly, cardiomyopathy, developmental delay, and death. Heterozygotes for LCHAD deficiency may present as adults with acute fatty liver of pregnancy. MCAD deficiency has been associated with sudden infant death syndrome. Although this disorder previously was thought to be relatively benign, prospective studies have identified a moderate incidence of neurologic deficits in children with the disease.

Diagnostic efforts should include a search for characteristic patterns of urine dicarboxylic acid excretion during acute episodes of illness or after fasts. A total plasma carnitine concentration of less than 30 μmol/L suggests a fatty-acid oxidation disorder. Other diagnostic measures may include measurement of acyl-CoA dehydrogenase activity in liver or in fibroblasts. Postnatal DNA screening for MCAD deficiency has been advocated. Mutations responsible for VLCAD and LCHAD also have been identified. Treatment modalities are unproven and therefore remain speculative, but they have included high-carbohydrate, low-fat diets, carnitine supplementation, and use of dietary medium-chain triglyceride oil in patients with VLCAD. Avoidance of fasting is recommended. In acutely ill children, glucose should be administered at rates sufficient to prevent fatty-acid mobilization (approximately 10 mg/kg/minute) until oral feeding can be resumed. (For further discussion of disorders of fatty acid oxidation, see Chapter 386.)

Nonalcoholic Steatohepatitis (NASH)

Fatty infiltration of the liver may be seen in a wide variety of conditions, including malnutrition/malabsorption, cystic fibrosis, Wilson disease, the use of specific drugs, hypercortisolism, Reye syndrome, abetalipoproteinemia, peroxisomal and mitochondrial disease, and alcohol abuse, among others. Excluding those patients with significant concurrent alcohol use, children with fatty infiltration of the liver are said to have nonalcoholic fatty liver disease (NAFLD). Obese patients, as well as those with type II diabetes, also are at risk of NAFLD. In fact, 10% to 20% of obese children have elevated serum aminotransferases, and approximately 20% of obese children with normal aminotransferases have ultrasonographic findings that suggest fatty infiltration of the liver. The prevalence of this problem in pediatrics is underlined by the finding that 60% of adolescents found to have elevated serum aminotransferases are overweight. In a series of 24 children in whom ultrasound examination suggested fatty infiltration (the majority of whom were obese), all had hepatic steatosis on biopsy. The mechanisms by which fat infiltration of the liver occurs presumably vary according to underlying etiology. In general, however, steatosis implies either enhanced hepatic free fatty acid delivery or synthesis, or diminished excretion/degradation, either through diminished β-oxidation or diminished VLDL synthesis or excretion. Hyperinsulinemia favors hepatic steatosis through the stimulation of fatty acid synthesis in combination with both diminished oxidation and VLDL excretion.

Nonalcoholic steatohepatitis (NASH) represents a form of NAFLD in which hepatic steatosis is noted in combination with hepatic inflammation. Patients with NASH are generally asymptomatic, although right upper quadrant pain may occur, as may symptoms associated with portal hypertension (ascites, variceal hemorrhage, etc.) in advanced cases. Hepatomegaly may be noted in as many as 25% of adult patients. Serum ALT values are generally elevated two- to threefold. Unfortunately, these findings are not specific to NASH, and do not allow it to be distinguished clinically from NAFLD. Pathologic findings range from Grade 1 (steatosis, mild inflammation in the hepatic lobule) to Grade 3 (severe steatosis, lobular and portal inflammation, ballooning degeneration of hepatocytes). Severe disease also may be associated with fibrosis, which may progress to cirrhosis. Of 24 children with biopsy-proved steatosis, 88% had inflammation on biopsy, and 75% had fibrosis. Of these, seven children had fibrosis classified as moderately severe, and one child had cirrhosis. Progression to cirrhosis may be rapid—in one reported child, it occurred within a 2-year period.

The pathophysiology of NASH, especially as distinguished from NAFLD, is uncertain. Possible inciting factors include enhanced oxidant stress and direct hepatocyte toxicity from elevated serum free fatty acid levels. The latter is supported by studies in which animals deficient in peroxisome proliferator-activated receptor alpha (PPAR-α) and peroxisomal fatty acyl-CoA oxidase (AOX) develop steatohepatitis, suggesting that endogenously produced fatty acids, usually oxidized by AOX, may act as nuclear transcription factors, important in the pathogenesis of NASH. Steatohepatitis also develops in animals deficient in methionine adenosyltransferase 1A, important in the formation of S-adenosylmethionine (AdoMet). Animals depleted in AdoMet demonstrate enhanced oxidative stress and lipid peroxidation.

The mainstay of the therapy of NASH in the obese child is weight loss and exercise. In a series of 38 obese children with NAFLD inferred from ultrasound, 79% of those who lost weight demonstrated improvement or clearing of previous ultrasound findings. Similar findings have been documented in adults. Supplementation with vitamins E and C may also be beneficial, presumably because of their antioxidant properties. Betaine (a methyl-group donor) also has shown promise in preliminary studies. Hepatic transplantation may be required in severe cases.

DISORDERS OF METAL METABOLISM

Wilson Disease

Wilson disease (i.e., hepatolenticular degeneration) is an autosomal recessive disorder of copper metabolism. The clinical presentation is highly variable, but symptoms rarely are evident before age 5. Patients younger than age 20 tend to present with predominantly hepatic manifestations, such as asymptomatic hepatomegaly, an illness mimicking acute hepatitis, and with a picture similar to other forms of chronic active hepatitis. Hepatic insufficiency associated with cirrhosis may develop slowly

and may manifest with signs of portal hypertension, including ascites, edema, and variceal hemorrhage. Conversely, patients may present with acute liver failure (ALF) associated with a brisk hemolytic anemia; this specific presentation is almost uniformly fatal if orthotopic liver transplantation is not performed. Older patients present with predominantly neurologic and psychiatric disturbances. Often, these disorders initially are subtle and include deterioration in school or job performance, behavioral changes, slurred speech, and tremors. If untreated, severe dysarthria and dystonia result, often leading to psychiatric hospitalization or institutionalization. Kayser-Fleischer rings (i.e., copper deposits on the inner surface of Descemet's membrane) invariably are found if neurologic disease exists, but they may be absent in younger patients having liver disease only. Hemolysis, presumably secondary to the release of copper from the liver, may be present, as may calcified, pigmented gallstones. Other clinical features may include Fanconi syndrome, with progressive renal disease and arthritis.

Pathogenesis

The clinical manifestations of Wilson disease are thought to result from an excessive accumulation of copper in the liver, eyes, CNS, and kidneys. The reason for copper accumulation is unknown, but the most likely explanation may be the defective excretion of copper from hepatocytes into the bile, presumably secondary to an undefined lysosomal defect. A gene linked to Wilson disease has been mapped to the long arm of chromosome 13; the product of this gene is a P-type copper-transporting adenosine triphosphatase (ATPase; ATB7B; Wilson disease protein (WNDP)). Multiple mutations in this gene, resulting in the Wilson disease phenotype, have been identified; distinct mutations may be associated with distinct phenotypes. The inheritance pattern is autosomal recessive. WNDP is found primarily in the trans-Golgi apparatus of cells, where it is thought to transfer copper to copper-dependent enzymes and proteins, including ceruloplasmin. When intracellular concentrations of copper are increased, WNDP also is found in vesicles into which copper is thought to be sequestered, thus protecting the cell from toxicity. Data also indicate defective synthesis of the copper-binding protein ceruloplasmin in patients with WD. The defect appears to reside at the level of messenger RNA production. The precise cause of copper hepatotoxicity is unclear, but a postulated mechanism is the oxidation of sulfhydryl groups, which depletes stores of reduced glutathione. Copper also may inhibit a variety of enzymatic processes.

The natural history of Wilson disease begins with the asymptomatic storage of copper in hepatocytes. As saturation occurs, hepatocyte necrosis occurs, with the stored copper released into the circulation. This process may result in hemolysis and copper deposition in the eye, kidney, and CNS. Hepatic fibrosis and cirrhosis occur in conjunction with the progressive deposition of copper in other tissues.

Laboratory features of Wilson disease may include a low serum ceruloplasmin level. Serum copper may be elevated, particularly during episodes of hemolysis, and urinary copper excretion is markedly increased. The examination of urine copper excretion after a dose of D-penicillamine may be particularly valuable. Hepatic copper content is increased to more than 250 μg/g dry weight, although sampling error may be an issue with percutaneous needle biopsy specimens. Liver tissue may contain fatty infiltration, glycogen granules, and enlarged Kupffer cells. A lesion indistinguishable from that observed in autoimmune hepatitis may be observed in some patients. Advanced cases may demonstrate hepatic fibrosis and cirrhosis.

Diagnosis

The diagnosis of Wilson disease should be considered in all children with unexplained hepatic disease. A high level of clinical suspicion must be maintained. Signs of chronic liver disease must be sought. Kayser-Fleischer rings should be sought through a careful slit-lamp examination. Neurologic signs, especially in older patients, may be found. CNS lesions may be demonstrated with CT or magnetic resonance imaging (MRI) scans. Helpful laboratory features include decreased serum ceruloplasmin levels and an elevated serum copper level; the 24-hour urinary copper excretion rate, normally less than 40 μg/24 hours, may be more than 100 μg/24 hours in Wilson disease. However, this finding may be present in other forms of chronic liver disease. To discriminate, a dose of oral D-penicillamine increases urinary copper excretion in Wilson disease to levels of 1,200 to 2,000 μg/day. Hepatic biopsy, when assessed for histologic change and hepatic copper content, is the single best method for the diagnosis of Wilson disease. In patients exhibiting the fulminant presentation of Wilson disease, serum alkaline phosphatase and serum aminotransferase levels often are disproportionately low, but the serum and urine copper content is elevated markedly. Genetic testing currently is unavailable.

Therapy

Untreated, Wilson disease is uniformly fatal. Adequate therapy is available in the form of triethylene tetramine dihydrochloride (Triene), a copper chelating agent. D-Penicillamine (beta, beta-dimethyl-cysteine) may be used alternatively, and is given orally in initially low doses, increasing to 1 g/day for adults and 0.50 to 0.75 g/day for younger children. Urinary copper excretion increases initially during chelating therapy, leading to the "decoppering" of affected patients. Urinary copper levels later stabilize, reflecting the maintenance of copper balance. In conjunction with this therapy, a diet low in copper must be instituted; foods with a high copper content, such as liver, chocolate, nuts, and shellfish, should be avoided. These restrictions should maintain the daily copper intake below 1 mg/day. Water sources should be analyzed for copper content. With the institution of therapy, usually an improvement in hepatic and neurologic function is found, and the Kayser-Fleischer rings regress. This therapeutic program must be followed for life. One study found that patients who discontinue therapy often die within 3 years. Zinc acetate, administered orally, may maintain a negative copper balance in some patients with Wilson disease, and it can be a useful form of maintenance therapy, particularly in patients unable to tolerate other chelator therapy, or in combination with chelator therapy. At present, its sole use as initial therapy in symptomatic patients cannot be recommended. Zinc appears to exert its effect primarily by decreasing the intestinal absorption of copper. Tetrathiomolybdate shows promise in the therapy of patients with preexisting neurologic disease, in whom the institution of D-penicillamine may be associated with worsening of symptoms, although data are limited at present.

For Wilson disease patients who present with ALF associated with hemolysis, intensive support is indicated; plasma perfusion, hemodialysis, and peritoneal dialysis may be efficacious in lowering the serum copper and in decreasing the copper burden. However, the hepatic injury apparently is irreversible; after stabilization, efforts should be directed toward rapid diagnosis and referral of affected patients for liver transplantation, which is curative.

Prognosis

Untreated Wilson disease is uniformly fatal; death may occur from hepatic, neurologic, renal, or hematologic complications. The prognosis for patients presenting with ALF and hemolysis is uniformly poor without liver transplantation. With proper therapy, usually the prognosis for most patients with Wilson

disease is good, although individual differences in response to chelation therapy exist. Siblings of patients with Wilson disease should be screened carefully for the disease, and therapy should be instituted in asymptomatic patients.

Indian Childhood Cirrhosis

Indian childhood cirrhosis is a form of familial childhood cirrhosis that occurs primarily in Indian Hindu families, but has been described also in Central American, Middle Eastern, and West African children. Studies suggest the presence of a similar disorder in children in the United States. Typically, onset of the disease occurs in children younger than 3 years. Affected patients present with hepatomegaly, pale stools, fever, and behavioral changes. Jaundice may be evident. Typically, the hepatic disease progresses rapidly. Hepatic biopsy confirms the progression from a nonspecific early stage to one with progressive fibrosis and, subsequently, to widespread necrosis and cirrhosis. Usually, the disease is fatal within the first 5 years of life. Suggested causes include excessive dietary intake of copper, perhaps through the use of copper and brass cooking and storage vessels. A genetic defect in the North American form of this disorder, specifically, an arginine to tryptophan mutation in the protein cirhin, expressed predominately in fetal liver, has been localized to chromosome 16q22. Therapy using D-penicillamine may allow complete recovery, especially if started early in the disease course.

Neonatal Iron Storage Disease

Neonatal iron storage disease (NISD) is a poorly characterized disorder in which hepatic insufficiency develops within the first 4 to 7 days of life. Typically, affected infants are born prematurely, and an increased familial incidence appears possible. Often, a hemorrhagic diathesis is prominent. Affected patients may die within the first week of life. Pathologic examination reveals increased iron deposition in multiple organs, including the liver, pancreas, heart, and thyroid glands. The patients have no evidence of hemolytic disease. Although the respective roles of extrinsic iron, infection, and genetic predisposition remain obscure, NISD does not appear to be related genetically to hereditary hemochromatosis. Diagnosis may be made by finding hemosiderosis in minor salivary glands on biopsy of oral mucosa, or MRI demonstrating nonparenchymal iron (pancreas, heart, etc.). Effective treatment may necessitate liver transplantation. The use of an antioxidant "cocktail" including desferrioxamine, prostaglandin E_1, alpha-tocopherol, N-acetylcysteine, and selenium has been reported, however no definitive evidence exists to support efficacy.

MISCELLANEOUS ERRORS OF METABOLISM AFFECTING THE LIVER

Cystic Fibrosis

Given the presence of the cystic fibrosis transmembrane regulator protein (CFTR) within the biliary epithelium, it is not surprising that the hepatobiliary system is involved in 20% to 50% of patients with CF. In most cases, this involvement is clinically insignificant but, with improved life expectancies in this disorder, more hepatobiliary complications are being reported. Scott-Jupp et al. observed among 1,100 CF patients a progressive rise in the prevalence of clinically apparent liver disease from 0.3% in a 0- to 5-year-old group to a peak of 8.7% among those between ages 16 and 20. An increased risk of hepatic disease has been associated with specific polymorphisms of the glutathione S-transferase P1 gene.

Infants with CF may present with persistent neonatal cholestasis, often in association with meconium ileus. Infants with this syndrome may appear to have a hypoplastic extrahepatic biliary tract at operative cholangiography, and hepatoportoenterostomy occasionally has been performed because of misdiagnosis. In nonoperated patients, bile flow spontaneously resumes in time. CF should be considered in all infants with neonatal cholestasis.

The liver pathology of affected infants reflects biliary ductal obstruction, presumably by inspissated secretions. Excessive biliary mucus is associated with periportal inflammation and mild intrahepatic bile ductular hyperplasia. Older patients with CF may develop steatosis of the liver. Tender hepatomegaly may occur with right ventricular heart failure. Focal biliary cirrhosis may occur in early childhood, but it becomes more prominent in adulthood. Approximately 24% of patients who die of CF have changes consistent with focal biliary cirrhosis found during autopsy. A small percentage of patients with focal biliary cirrhosis subsequently develop multilobular biliary cirrhosis associated with jaundice, portal hypertension, and hepatic failure. Variceal hemorrhage may occur in this condition.

The management of patients with CF and significant hepatic disease focuses on the management of portal hypertension; liver cell failure is uncommon. Options include sclerotherapy, shunting, and orthotopic liver transplantation. The administration of ursodeoxycholic acid (20 mg/kg/day; higher doses may be required in infants) often results in biochemical and functional improvement in the hepatic disease associated with CF. Long-term effects and prognosis remain uncertain.

The biliary complications of CF include microgallbladder in 15% to 20% of patients and gallstones in as many as 15% of patients. Gallstone formation may involve abnormal gallbladder size and motility, excessive amount and viscosity of gallbladder and biliary mucus, and diminished bile acid output, lithogenic bile, and probable cholesterol supersaturation of bile. Stenosis of the common bile duct also may occur.

Alpha₁-Antitrypsin Deficiency

Alpha₁-antitrypsin, a 50-kd glycoprotein synthesized in the liver, functions as a protease inhibitor to neutralize a broad spectrum of proteolytic enzymes, although its major target protease is leukocyte elastase. Alpha₁-antitrypsin accounts for approximately 80% of the serum alpha₁-globulin fraction. Homozygous deficiency of alpha₁-antitrypsin is associated with neonatal cholestasis and with childhood and adulthood cirrhosis; an increased incidence of primary liver cancer has been proposed. Homozygous- and heterozygous-deficient persons are at risk for pulmonary disease.

Alpha₁-antitrypsin occurs in more than 75 variant forms, designated as *Pi phenotypes*, each inherited in a codominant fashion. The normal phenotype is MM; the type associated most often with hepatic disease is ZZ. Patients with ZZ phenotypes have low serum alpha₁-antitrypsin levels, usually 10% to 15% of normal. A Pi null-null phenotype has been described in which no alpha₁-antitrypsin is present in the serum. Adults with cirrhosis also have been described in conjunction with MZ, M Malton, and M Duarte phenotypes.

The incidence of the PiZZ (homozygous-deficient) phenotype is estimated to be 1 in 2,000 to 4,000. The clinical manifestations of the PiZZ phenotype in children vary. Approximately 10% of these patients present with clinical evidence of neonatal hepatic disease. Another 40% to 50%, although asymptomatic, have hepatic biochemical abnormalities when tested at age 3 months. Patients presenting with neonatal cholestasis may be jaundiced in the first week of life, and acholic stools and hepatomegaly may be observed. Often, jaundice clears by the fourth month of life. Approximately equal proportions of these infants continue to have abnormal liver function and, if untreated, die by age 10 of complications related to hepatic cirrhosis; persistently abnormal hepatic function with slow progression to cirrhosis; continued mild hepatic dysfunction and fibrosis, with survival into adulthood; or resolving hepatic disease with a return to normal function.

Pathologic findings in the liver may correlate with any of the previously described clinical conditions. In the neonatal period, the hepatic lesion may be indistinguishable from that usually found in neonatal hepatitis. Cirrhosis has been reported in neonates and in preterm infants. Variable degrees of bile-duct proliferation may occur early in the disease; this specific histologic feature portends a more severe course. The characteristic hepatic lesion in alpha₁-antitrypsin deficiency is the presence of diastase-resistant hepatocyte inclusions that stain positively for periodic acid–Schiff. These globules, antigenically related to alpha₁-antitrypsin, occur predominantly in periportal hepatocytes. These inclusions may not be visible before age 4 months, but their size increases with age. In more advanced disease, biopsy findings may reveal extensive fibrosis, and few intrahepatic bile ducts may be found.

The pathophysiology of the hepatic disease observed in alpha₁-antitrypsin deficiency is unclear. Patients with the PiZZ phenotype produce, because of a point mutation, an abnormal alpha₁-antitrypsin protein characterized by the substitution of lysine for glutamate at position 342. The abnormal alpha₁-antitrypsin protein is polymerized within the endoplasmic reticulum; therefore, entrance into the Golgi apparatus does not occur, resulting in accumulations of abnormal proteins within the hepatocyte. These deposits occur also in the absence of hepatic disease; toxicity of retained alpha₁-antitrypsin probably relates to its rate of degradation within the hepatocyte. Breast-feeding does not appear to influence prognosis favorably.

Diagnosis involves ascertaining the patient's alpha₁-antitrypsin phenotype; measurement of alpha₁-antitrypsin levels is less reliable. Characteristic hepatic biopsy findings are confirmatory. Family members of affected patients should be screened.

The treatment of hepatic disease associated with alpha₁-antitrypsin deficiency is supportive. Hepatic transplantation, if required, is curative. The utility of alpha₁-antitrypsin replacement therapy in hepatic disease is unknown but may be detrimental. Future therapy may involve a modulation of gene expression to turn off protein production.

VIRAL HEPATITIS

Viral hepatitis in children is a major health concern throughout the world. Multiple hepatotropic viruses that cause disease in humans have been identified. These include hepatitis A, hepatitis B, the delta agent (i.e., hepatitis D), hepatitis C and, rarely, the more recently described hepatitis E. Hepatitis G virus is a recently recognized cause of chronic viremia, but no link between this virus and acute or chronic hepatitis has been established. Other viruses capable of causing hepatitis include Epstein-Barr virus, cytomegalovirus, varicella virus, rubella, parvovirus B19, human herpesviruses (including 6, 7, and 8), and coxsackievirus B; typically, these organisms cause hepatitis as part of a multisystem presentation, and they are discussed in other chapters.

Hepatitis A

Hepatitis A virus (HAV), a member of the picornavirus family, is an RNA virus. Hepatitis A accounts for as many as 25% of cases of hepatitis in the developing world. Usually, transmission is through the fecal–oral route, although parenteral transmission has been recorded. Usually, the consumption of contaminated food or water is implicated. No carrier state is known, and transmission is by person-to-person spread during the preicteric stage of disease. Fecal viral shedding is maximal during the late incubation period (28 days), immediately before or after symptom onset. As a result of this method of spread, infants may be ideal vectors of HAV infection, with spread to other family members or to other children at day-care centers. Institutionalized children also are at high risk for disease acquisition.

The clinical symptoms of HAV infection may be absent or (especially in children younger than age 2) may consist of nausea, vomiting, and diarrhea. Young patients with HAV are often anicteric. In older children, symptoms of acute hepatitis predominate. Approximately two-thirds of those with symptoms become jaundiced. Prodromal symptoms of fever, headache, and anorexia may occur. In most patients, HAV infection has a mild course, and clinical improvement occurs rapidly. Aminotransferase levels, which peak within 1 week of disease onset, usually normalize within several weeks but may remain elevated for several months (Fig. 367.3). The diagnosis may be confirmed through the demonstration of anti-HAV IgM in serum; anti-HAV IgG develops later and persists for life. No evidence suggests that chronic hepatitis is due to HAV. A small percentage of patients may develop fulminant hepatitis due to HAV, accounting for a fatality rate of less than 1% for those infected with HAV.

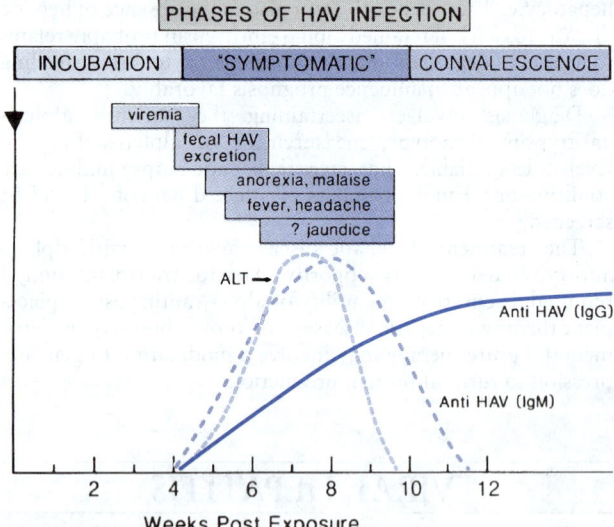

FIGURE 367.3. Typical course of hepatitis A infection. The period of viremia, which occurs during the incubation phase, is brief. The duration of fecal excretion overlaps this prodromal phase and is present early in the symptomatic phase. Jaundice may occur up to 6 weeks after exposure but is not present in all cases. The alanine aminotransferase (ALT, or serum glutamate pyruvate transaminase) elevation also precedes the development of clinical symptoms; usually, values remain abnormal after serum bilirubin returns to normal. Anti-hepatitis A virus (HAV) is detectable early in the acute "symptomatic" phase of the illness; the initial response is anti-HAV IgM, which peaks shortly after the onset of symptoms and progressively declines. This is succeeded by a gradual rise in anti-HAV of the IgG class, which peaks after the symptomatic phase and remains detectable indefinitely. Arrow indicates exposure.

The treatment of HAV infection is symptomatic, and hospitalization rarely is required. Dietary therapy has no proven role. Prevention of disease spread is a major goal of therapy. Infected infants should not return to their day-care center until 2 weeks after onset of symptoms to minimize the exposure of others to fecal shedding. If HAV is documented in a day-care center employee or attendee (or in a parent of an attendee), 0.02 mL/kg of immune globulin should be given to all employees and children. Standard immune globulin is effective in modifying the clinical manifestations of HAV infection, but must be given within 2 weeks of exposure. Immune globulin prophylaxis is not required for casual contacts of patients with HAV infection outside the day-care center. Inactivated hepatitis A vaccines have been approved for children older than age 2 years. In general, these vaccines are well tolerated and effective. Children living in areas with a high incidence of hepatitis A should be immunized, as should other at-risk individuals. Vaccination more than 1 month before exposure obviates the need for postexposure immune globulin prophylaxis.

Hepatitis B

The hepatitis B virus (HBV) is a DNA virus of the hepadnavirus family. HBV-related viral particles can be found in the serum and tissues of infected persons. Contained within the virion is the core protein (HB_cAg), within which is the viral DNA. Other components of the HBV virion are the surface antigen (HB_sAg), DNA polymerase, and the e antigen (HB_eAg). Diagnostic efforts focus on identification of antigens HB_sAg or HB_eAg, antibodies generated in response to them (e.g., anti-HB_s, anti-HB_e, anti-HB_c), or viral DNA in serum.

Usually, the transmission of HBV occurs by the parenteral route, through exchange of blood or body secretions. The virus has been demonstrated in blood, semen, saliva, and breast milk. Transmission may occur through intimate contact of any type and through vertical (i.e., mother-to-infant) transmission. Persons at high risk include those with frequent exposure to blood or blood products. Children at greatest risk in the United States include those born to mothers who had acute hepatitis B in the third trimester or are chronic HB_sAg carriers. Institutionalized children, hemophiliacs, hemodialysis patients, and intravenous drug abusers are at risk for disease. The prevalence of the HB_sAg carrier state in the United States is approximately 0.1%.

The incubation period of HBV is estimated at 60 to 180 days, and often the subsequent infection is subclinical, but symptoms occur in 25% to 30% of patients (Fig. 367.4). Early symptoms may be systemic and include fever, symmetric arthropathy, skin eruptions, and urticarial or (in some children) a papular acrodermatitis known as *Gianotti-Crosti syndrome*. Often the disease is anicteric. Malaise, right upper quadrant pain, and a variety of nonspecific GI complaints may occur. The diagnosis of acute hepatitis B is made in the proper clinical setting through the demonstration of HB_sAg and anti-HB_c IgM in serum. HB_sAg positivity in the absence of anti-HB_c IgM suggests chronic infection.

The outcome of HBV infection varies. Typically, adults and older children infected with HBV have a benign course with complete resolution. Approximately 1% of patients may have fulminant hepatitis. A chronic carrier state may ensue after HBV infection in fewer than 1% to 10% of older patients. At least 20% of preschool-aged children with acute HBV infection become chronic carriers. Virtually all infants born to HB_sAg-positive mothers contract HBV unless intervention is initiated; of these, approximately 90% become chronic carriers. Transmission in the neonatal period may occur at delivery when infants are in contact with large amounts of maternal blood. Infants may become infected postnatally from the mother or from infected siblings. In each case, development of the chronic

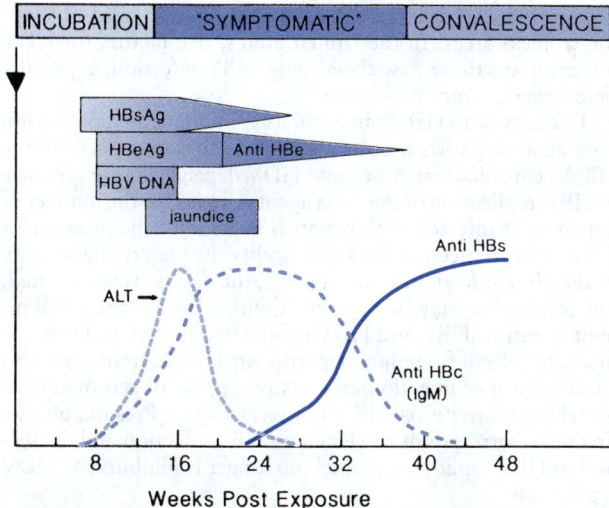

FIGURE 367.4. Typical course of hepatitis B infection. After exposure to hepatitis B virus (HBV; *arrow*), the earliest detectable serum marker is a rise in HB$_s$Ag, which may appear at any time (weeks 1 to 10) post-exposure; HBV DNA and HBAg follow closely. HB$_e$Ag is detectable 2 to 8 weeks before the onset of the symptomatic phase, which is heralded by an increase in alanine aminotransferase (ALT) levels, serum bilirubin concentrations, and constitutional signs. Clearance of HB$_s$Ag by immune aggregation with anti-hepatitis B core antigen (HB$_c$) occurs by 6 to 8 months postinfection; those who fail to clear are termed HB$_s$Ag carriers. Anti-HB$_c$, which appears just before the symptomatic phase, is the first detectable, host-induced immunologic marker of hepatitis B infection. Anti-HB$_c$ of the IgM class may be the only marker of HBV infection in serum after clearance of HB$_s$Ag and before a rise in anti-HB$_s$. Anti-HB$_c$ is not a neutralizing antibody and therefore, in contrast to anti-HB, is not protective.

carrier state is common. Typically, infection acquired during the neonatal period is asymptomatic. Less commonly, a mild icteric hepatitis may occur. In rare cases, ALF may occur, particularly after infection with a precore defective variant of HBV.

Children who are chronic HB$_s$Ag carriers are usually asymptomatic and seldom have a history of previous hepatitis. Problems inherent in the chronic carrier state include risk of disease transmission to others and increased risk for the development of cirrhosis and hepatocellular carcinoma. Chronic infection may be associated with asymptomatic infection or chronic hepatitis. The diagnosis of chronic HBV hepatitis rests on the demonstration of elevated aminotransferases and HB$_s$Ag positivity, often accompanied by HBV DNA or HB$_e$Ag seropositivity. Patients with HB$_e$Ag positivity are in the "replicative" phase of disease, during which active viral replication and hepatic inflammation occur. Eventually, the viral genome is inserted into the hepatocyte genome of affected patients; integration of the viral genome may form the basis of future malignant transformation. Subsequently, such patients may become anti-HB$_e$ positive, indicating a low level or absence of viral replication. Usually, seroconversion to anti-HB$_e$ positivity is associated with a remission of chronic liver disease. This seroconversion, however, frequently is preceded by a period in which viral replication increases, often accompanied by a flare of hepatic disease. The transformation from HB$_e$Ag positivity to anti-HBe positivity occurs spontaneously at a rate of 5% to 15% annually in infected children. Inactivation is not permanent in all cases, and reactivation of disease with resumption of HB$_e$Ag positivity may occur. Approximately 30% of patients who lose HB$_e$Ag revert to HB$_e$Ag positivity. These reversions are associated also with exacerbations of hepatic disease. As

many as 15% of patients with HB$_s$Ag positivity spontaneously may become HB$_s$Ag-negative.

Studies of adults and children suggest a role for interferon-alpha in the treatment of chronic HBV infection. Specifically, 30% to 40% of adults with chronic, replicative hepatitis B infection given 5 million units of interferon daily for 16 weeks had a sustained loss of hepatitis B viral replication, defined as a loss of HB$_e$Ag and HBV DNA. Patients most likely to respond include those with HBV DNA levels of less than 100 pg/mL and those with pretreatment alanine aminotransferase values exceeding 100 U/L. The results of treating groups of children have been promising, with meta-analysis highlighting the clearance of HBV DNA in approximately 30% (20% to 58%) of treated patients, as compared with 8% to 17% of controls. Although standard doses have not been established, the loss of viral replication has been suggested in 30% to 50% of Hispanic children treated with 5 to 10 million U/m^2 given three times per week. Response rates may be lower in perinatally infected patients, who generally have high HBV DNA levels in association with normal serum aminotransferase levels. Likely, the poor response in these children was the result of the profound immunologic tolerance to HBV induced by exposure to the virus early in life. Usually, the duration of interferon therapy is 6 months; side effects include fever (predominantly in the first month of therapy), malaise, autoimmune phenomena, and bone marrow suppression. Patients with decompensated HB$_s$Ag-positive liver disease may develop hepatic failure during treatment. Patients who respond to interferon-alpha are less likely to develop hepatocellular carcinoma on long-term follow-up. Lamivudine (2′,3′-dideoxycytosine) has been shown to suppress HBV DNA production. In HB$_s$Ag-positive children (HB$_e$Ag, HBV DNA positive; ALT greater than 1.3 times normal), 23% of those treated with lamivudine for one year responded with clearance of HBV DNA and HB$_e$Ag, as compared with 13% of controls. A longer duration of therapy may result in increased rates of clearance. Lamivudine was well tolerated. As in adult studies, use was associated with the development of lamivudine-resistant mutant virus in approximately 20% of treated children.

Despite the promise of pharmacologic therapy, attention must remain focused on disease prevention. Infants born to infected mothers should be given hepatitis B immune globulin and hepatitis B vaccine at birth. Universal vaccination of children against HBV is recommended. Despite current uncertainty concerning optimal immunization schedules and the duration of protection, universal immunization in Taiwan has dramatically decreased new cases of HBV infection and its complications, including hepatocellular carcinoma. The effectiveness of early screening programs for hepatocellular carcinoma in patients with chronic HBV infection, including serial αFP determinations and high-resolution ultrasonography, must be verified.

Hepatitis C

Hepatitis C virus (HCV) is the major cause of post-transfusion and community-acquired NANB hepatitis. The HCV consists of a single-stranded RNA genome and shares with the flavivirus family some similarities in nonstructural proteins. Cloning of the agent and ongoing refinement of HCV-specific serologic assays have led to rapid advances in our understanding of the clinical course of acute and chronic infection and in the seroepidemiology of the virus. The overall prevalence in the United States of antibody against HCV is approximately 0.6%. Transmission has occurred primarily by blood or blood products. Serologic screening of blood donors, as well as heat treatment of coagulation factors, has led to a dramatic decrease in cases associated with these therapies, but transmission by intravenous drug use and sexual contact remain important. Vertical transmission from mother to infant may occur, particularly in the setting of maternal human immunodeficiency virus (HIV) infection. The overall risk of transmission is approximately 5% and is related to the level of maternal viremia. The breast milk of infected mothers may contain HCV RNA but, in a small group of breast-fed infants of infected mothers, transmission was not detected at 1 year follow-up. Household spread is not frequent.

Usually, the clinical manifestations of acute HCV infection are mild and may be missed unless tests of liver injury are evaluated serially after a possible exposure. The virus does not appear to be an important cause of fulminant hepatitis, but chronic infection develops in more than 50% of the patients. Often, the illness in affected patients is characterized by a fluctuating pattern of aminotransferase elevations and few symptoms, but as many as 25% of these patients ultimately develop cirrhosis. A strong association also exists between HCV infection and the development of hepatocellular carcinoma. In children, hepatic disease is generally mild, although cirrhosis requiring hepatic transplantation during childhood has been reported. The long-term outlook for infected children as they age is uncertain. Several studies have documented recovery or a chronic, mild disease. Progression to end-stage disease is uncommon. However, given the prevalence and persistence of this infection, a proportion of patients may develop significant liver disease as adults.

The diagnosis of HCV infection relies on the detection of antibodies (anti-HCV) against recombinant viral antigens by enzyme immunoassay. Confirmation, if necessary, may be obtained through the detection of viral RNA (HCV-RNA) via polymerase chain reaction (PCR) or branched DNA reactions. In patients with acute transfusion-associated or sporadic hepatitis, serologic assays may detect antibody within 8 weeks; most affected patients test positive by 20 weeks after exposure. Serial measurement of anti-HCV antibodies may be required to exclude infection. Infants born to HCV-positive mothers may have a persistence of maternal antibody until the age of 18 months, in the absence of infection. Screening of antibody-positive infants includes HCV PCR at 6 weeks and 6 months of age. PCR-positive (6 months) infants are presumed to be infected, whereas PCR-negative children should be followed to document the clearance of HCV antibodies.

The pathologic findings in the liver of infected children include steatosis (fat), portal lymphoid aggregates, and sinusoidal lymphocytosis. Bile duct damage and fibrosis also may occur.

The treatment of chronic hepatitis C infection with interferon-alpha for 6 to 12 months improves liver test results and histopathologic abnormalities in approximately 50% of adults. At least one-half of affected patients can be expected to relapse after discontinuation of therapy, but usually they respond to retreatment. Longer treatment periods produce a further improvement in rates of sustained response, as does cotreatment with ribavirin and the use of pegylated interferon. Several studies of children treated with interferon-alpha have suggested response rates that are similar or superior to those obtained in adults. Response rates of patients infected with viral genotype 1 are significantly lower than those of patients infected with other genotypes. Limited data suggest that the combination of ribavirin and interferon is safe and effective in children; pegylated interferon has yet to be studied in children. Currently, no recommended postexposure prophylaxis against hepatitis C is available.

Hepatitis Delta Infection

The hepatitis delta virus (HDV) is a defective RNA virus that requires HBV coinfection to cause infection. The virion, a 36-nm particle enclosing HDV RNA, is encased within an HB_sAg coat. The modes of transmission of the delta agent ap-

pear to be similar to those discussed for hepatitis B. Endemic areas include the Amazon Basin (i.e., Labrea hepatitis), the Mediterranean basin, areas of European Russia, and developing tropical areas. In the United States, risk factors for HDV infection are those associated with HBV infection, especially percutaneous transmissions.

Infection with HDV can occur as a simultaneous coinfection with acute hepatitis B or as a superinfection with HDV in the HB_sAg chronic carrier. Because HDV depends on the presence of HBV, replication of the delta agent is limited to the number of hepatocytes infected with hepatitis B. Usually, the presence of delta virus coinfection does not modify the underlying severity of the HBV infection. In most cases, the disease is self-limited, but coinfection may be associated with a higher rate of fulminant hepatitis. HBV and HDV coinfection is responsible for as much as 30% of fulminant hepatitis worldwide; frequently, this specific form of infection exhibits two peaks of serum aminotransferase activity, usually a few weeks apart. Presumably, the first peak corresponds to HDV and HBV infection and the second to HBV replication, which no longer is inhibited by HDV replication.

Superinfection with HDV occurs in chronic carriers of HBV subsequently exposed to HDV. In these patients, the presence of HBV-colonized hepatocytes allows the rapid establishment of HDV infection, with a resultant increase in disease severity. Frequently, fulminant hepatitis occurs in HBV-infected persons who then are superinfected with HDV. Chronic active hepatitis occurs in as many as 60%. The outcome varies. A chronic HDV carrier state may develop, usually associated with severe progressive chronic liver disease. Conversely, HDV or HBV infection may resolve.

The diagnosis of HDV infection rests on a high level of clinical suspicion; all patients with ALF and patients known to be carriers of HB_sAg and having acute exacerbation of disease activity must be studied serologically. The presence of delta antigen or of IgM antibodies to HDV (anti-HDV) is evidence of infection. No specific treatment for HDV is available. Preventive measures are aimed at the prevention of HBV infection.

Hepatitis E

The E form of hepatitis appears to be transmitted enterically, probably through fecally contaminated water supplies. Epidemics may involve large numbers of cases. Outbreaks have occurred in Asia, Africa, and Russia. The incubation period appears to range between 35 and 45 days, with a peak point of incidence between 15 and 40 days. The disease may be mild to severe in intensity, with an approximately 20% incidence of fatality in pregnant women. No evidence suggests that hepatitis E causes chronic infection. The responsible agent appears to be a 32- to 34-nm viruslike particle that also is transmissible to animals. The viral genome of these particles, designated *hepatitis E*, has been cloned. While unclassified, the viral genome resembles that of the calicivirus and togavirus families. Serologic assays for this agent are available, although no pharmacologic therapies currently are available. A recombinant vaccine currently is undergoing clinical evaluation.

CHRONIC HEPATITIS

Chronic hepatitis may occur as a result of persistent hepatic viral infection, as seen in conjunction with hepatitis B, D, and C. Drugs also may precipitate or induce hepatitis. Chronic lupoid or autoimmune hepatitis (AIH), first described by Waldenström, may be responsible for chronic hepatitis with rapid progression to cirrhosis. Metabolic disorders, such as Wilson disease and alpha$_1$-antitrypsin deficiency, may present with clinical and histologic features similar to those found in chronic hepatitis. Biliary tract disease, particularly primary sclerosing cholangitis, must be considered in the differential diagnosis. The clinical manifestations have an insidious onset, usually heralded by the finding of abnormally elevated serum aminotransferase levels. Between 30% and 50% of pediatric patients with AIH present with acute illness. The onset of ascites, encephalopathy, hypoalbuminemia, hypergammaglobulinemia, and hypoprothrombinemia may be sudden.

Regardless of the mode of onset, a liver biopsy is required to establish the diagnosis of chronic hepatitis and the severity of the underlying histopathologic process, both essential in the determination of appropriate treatment. Characteristic pathologic findings of specific disease entities may be found. In chronic hepatitis B, hepatocytes have a "ground glass" appearance, exhibiting orcein-positive inclusions. Biopsies from patients with chronic hepatitis C may exhibit fatty infiltration, acidophilic bodies, bile duct damage, and lymphoid aggregates. Hepatitis due to drug toxicity histologically resembles viral disease. Biopsy specimen in AIH contains an infiltrate of plasma cells. In addition, the severity of the histologic lesion may provide significant information regarding the stage of the underlying pathologic process. Current systems of nomenclature have used an etiologic designation (i.e., chronic hepatitis B) in conjunction with a description of the degree or grade of inflammation (both portal and lobular) present. In addition, the degree of fibrosis (ranging from none to cirrhosis) is documented. These schemes allow more a precise description of pathologic findings. Noteworthy is that histologic features may vary throughout the course of a disease process and that, therefore, biopsy findings represent only a brief "snapshot."

Autoimmune Hepatitis

As many as 20% of chronic hepatitis cases are ascribed to AIH, a disorder diagnosed most frequently in young women aged 15 to 25 years. The disease may be associated with other disorders of presumably immunologic origin, including thyroiditis, inflammatory bowel disease, arthritis, rash, and Coombs-positive hemolytic anemia. Commonly, presenting features resemble those of acute viral hepatitis and may include weakness, nausea, vomiting, behavioral changes, malaise, and jaundice. Less commonly, patients may be asymptomatic, and the disease may be discovered when liver function abnormalities are uncovered in the course of routine evaluations. Laboratory features include elevated serum aminotransferases, often in the range of 500 to 1,000 IU. Usually, coagulation defects and hypergammaglobulinemia exist. Serologic abnormalities include positive lupus erythematosus cell tests in approximately 15% of cases, and antinuclear and anti–smooth-muscle antibodies in 70% (type I autoimmune hepatitis). In addition, some cases of AIH in children and adults are associated with the presence of anti–liver-kidney microsome antibodies (anti-LKM), directed against cytochrome P-450 2D6. These patients may form a distinct subset of patients with AIH, characterized by early age at onset (type II autoimmune hepatitis). HLA-B8 and HLA-DR3 and DR4 appear to be associated with the development of AIH. Often, findings on physical examination include jaundice, mild hepatomegaly, and splenomegaly. Signs of chronic liver disease, including spider telangiectasia and palmar erythema, may be present. In advanced cases, findings may reflect underlying hepatic cirrhosis and may include edema, ascites, variceal hemorrhage, and hepatic encephalopathy.

Pathologic findings include the characteristic plasma-cell infiltrate and interface hepatitis. In more severe disease, bands of necrosis may spread from portal area to portal area, central area to portal area, or central area to central area (bridging necrosis). Fibrosis extends into the lobule, eventually causing cirrhosis. Usually, bridging or multilobular necrosis denotes severe, progressive disease. Cirrhosis may be present at the time of diagnosis.

Pathophysiology

In AIH, a generalized increase in immune system activity is observed. Serum gamma-globulin levels are elevated, and autoantibodies often are present, although in young children AIH may be present in the absence of serum autoimmune markers. Interestingly, IgA deficiency is common. Autoimmune hepatitis is associated with non–T-cell-mediated, antibody-dependent, and cell-mediated cytotoxic reactions against hepatocytes. Decreased suppressor T-cell function has been found. Corticosteroids appear to improve suppressor T-cell function in AIH.

Clinical Manifestations, Prognosis, and Therapy

Controlled studies of the therapy of AIH and the natural history of the untreated condition have been performed only in adults; typically, untreated patients had a 5-year mortality of 30% to 50%. Children and adults respond to immunosuppressive therapy. Corticosteroid therapy, with or without the addition of azathioprine, improves the clinical, biochemical, and histologic features of AIH and prolongs life in most patients, but progression to cirrhosis may not be prevented.

The decision to treat depends on affected patients' clinical status and on histologic findings. Patients with extreme elevations of serum aminotransferase values and gamma-globulin levels and those with bridging or multilobular necrosis on hepatic biopsy carry a high risk of rapid progression to cirrhosis and deserve therapy. Usually, prednisone is begun with a dosage of 1 to 2 mg/kg/day; this dosage is continued until clinical and biochemical remission (i.e., aminotransferase values less than twice normal) is achieved, usually within the first 3 months of therapy. Subsequently, the dosage is lowered in decrements of 5 mg every 4 to 6 weeks until a maintenance dosage of 10 to 20 mg/day (in adults and older children) is achieved. Evidence of biochemical or clinical relapse necessitates a return to the starting dose. The use of azathioprine (1 to 2 mg/kg/day) should be considered in all patients, especially in those who cannot be maintained on low-dose steroids or who develop serious side effects. Monitoring for bone marrow suppression is essential. Because daily steroid use may suppress linear growth in children, anecdotal reports suggest the use of alternate-day steroids in the long-term management of AIH. This form of therapy, although capable of normalizing aminotransferase values, has not produced sustained histologic remission in adults. Despite the reported salutary effect of an alternate-day steroid regimen on the growth of children with AIH, this form of therapy should be used only with caution.

Therapy should be assessed at 6 to 12 months after initiation, with a repeat percutaneous liver biopsy to ensure histologic resolution. Disappearance of symptoms, normalization of biochemical abnormalities, and regression of histologic findings justify attempts at slow withdrawal of the medication.

Generally, response to steroid therapy is good. Approximately 70% of treated patients respond initially to therapy, but many of these patients relapse shortly (within 6 months) after discontinuation of medication and again require immunosuppressive therapy. Patients who relapse do not appear to have a morbidity or mortality from hepatic disease higher than those in whom remission is sustained. However, the incidence of medication-related side effects may limit future therapy. Cyclosporin A, tacrolimus, and/or mycophenolate mofetil have been used in an increasing number of children with refractory disease. Generally, good results have been obtained; however, relapse often occurs after withdrawal of these medications. Orthotopic liver transplantation is a therapeutic option for patients who progress to end-stage liver disease; however, the disease may recur within the transplanted organ. In addition, episodes of rejection in transplanted AIH patients are often particularly severe and require aggressive therapy.

DRUG-INDUCED LIVER DISEASES

Drug-related hepatotoxicity occurs in children less often than in adults, presumably because children receive fewer drugs than do adults. Probably, age-related differences in hepatic metabolism also play a role. For example, halothane hepatotoxicity rarely occurs in children, but sodium valproate hepatotoxicity has been described almost exclusively in children. In the former instance, immaturity of hepatic metabolic processes may limit the production of toxic metabolites; in the latter situation, degradation of toxic compounds may be limited by immaturity, thus resulting in hepatotoxicity.

Many agents are capable of producing hepatotoxicity. They include environmental and "natural" hepatotoxins (i.e., *Amanita*) and medicinal agents. Most drug reactions affecting the liver in children are the result of exposure to analgesics (acetaminophen), steroids, or antiinflammatory, antiinfective, or antineoplastic drugs. The liver is uniquely sensitive to toxic agents, presumably because of its central role in the metabolism and detoxification of xenobiotics. Phase 1 enzymes activate drugs to reactive intermediates consisting of a carboxyl, phenol, epoxide, or hydroxyl group. The cytochrome P-450 enzymes are central to this process. The reactive metabolites often are toxic and are enzymatically conjugated in phase 2 reactions with glucuronic acid, sulfate, or glutathione, allowing excretion into urine or bile. Genetic polymorphisms underlie the variable expression and function of drug metabolizing enzymes and transporters. Gender, age, use of multiple drugs, nutritional status, and other systemic illnesses also can influence the hepatotoxic potential of a given substance.

Pathogenesis

Agents that produce hepatic disease may do so in several ways. Direct hepatotoxins injure the hepatocyte through peroxidation of membrane lipids, with subsequent cell necrosis. Carbon tetrachloride is a direct hepatotoxin. Indirect hepatotoxins interfere with specific cellular metabolic pathways. These agents may be cytotoxic (e.g., galactosamine, tetracycline, 6-mercaptopurine) or cholestatic (e.g., estrogenic steroids). Direct and indirect hepatotoxins cause predictable liver injury, with effects that generally are dose-dependent. Idiosyncratic hepatotoxins cause hepatic disease in an unpredictable fashion that generally is not dose-related. In some cases, drug-related hypersensitivity may play a role. Typically, these cases are accompanied by rash, fever, and eosinophilia, and they require prior exposure to the offending agent, usually 1 to 5 weeks before reaction onset. Other idiosyncratic reactions include those that depend on the presence of specific metabolic defects. Affected patients may produce and be unable to metabolize specific toxic intermediates of drug metabolism. In these instances, the systemic features of hypersensitivity are not present, and hepatotoxicity may occur after various periods of drug exposure. Phenytoin, sodium valproate, and some isoniazid toxicity may be secondary to this mechanism.

Pathology

The pathologic findings of drug-related hepatotoxicity vary, and may mimic virtually every form of acute and chronic liver disease. In general, predictable reactions are associated with characteristic patterns of hepatic damage; e.g. carbon tetrachloride and acetaminophen cause centrilobular hepatocyte damage. Often, idiosyncratic toxins cause diffuse changes of necrosis or cholestasis. Inflammation may be prominent, and

the hepatic lesion produced may be similar to that seen in acute viral hepatitis. Steatosis is observed with tetracycline (microvesicular) toxicity and with ethanol (macrovesicular) toxicity. Cholestatic changes with inflammatory infiltrates may be found with the injury associated with erythromycin estolate and chlorpromazine. Usually, cholestasis without inflammation is seen with estrogenic and androgenic steroids. Androgenic steroids also affect the development of peliosis hepatis. Hepatic vein thrombosis has been linked to oral contraceptive use, and hepatic venoocclusive disease may be observed after the use of antineoplastic drugs. Hepatic tumors have been associated with anabolic steroid and oral contraceptive use. Autoimmune hepatitis may be triggered by drug administration (e.g. minocycline).

Clinical Manifestations and Diagnosis

Often, the clinical manifestations of drug-related toxicity are mild and nonspecific. In the case of hypersensitivity, fever, rash, and arthralgia may be present. Because many cases of drug-related hepatotoxicity occur in ill, hospitalized patients, separating the symptoms of underlying illness from those related to drug toxicity may be difficult. Similarly, elevated hepatic enzyme levels may be attributed to the underlying illness. Other causes of hepatic dysfunction must be considered, including (in the appropriate clinical setting) viral hepatitis, biliary tract disease, inborn errors of metabolism, sepsis, and hypoxia.

The laboratory features of drug-related hepatotoxicity are variable and nonspecific. Hepatocellular necrosis leads to marked increases in serum aminotransferase levels. Serum alkaline phosphatase and 5'-nucleotidase values also may increase, although usually to a lesser degree. The prothrombin time may be prolonged in the presence of extensive hepatic necrosis, serum albumin values may be depressed, and jaundice may develop. Hyperammonemia may be found in sodium valproate hepatotoxicity or in acute hepatic failure. A milder elevation of serum aminotransferase levels may occur in microvesicular steatosis or with the use of drugs that stimulate the cytochrome P-450 enzyme system. The diagnosis of drug hepatotoxicity syndromes depends on a high level of clinical suspicion and an appropriate clinical history. In some cases, such as in acute acetaminophen overdose, serum drug levels may be useful in predicting hepatotoxicity. A hepatic biopsy may help to identify characteristic patterns of hepatic injury attributable to specific drugs.

Therapy

Usually, the treatment of drug-related hepatotoxicity rests on the withdrawal of the offending agent. In some cases, specific therapy is available. Examples include the use of N-acetylcysteine in acetaminophen overdose and chelation therapy in toxicity due to iron overload. Generally, therapy is supportive. The prognosis of drug-related hepatotoxicity is good after the involved drug is withdrawn. The prognosis of ALF is poor, with survival rates of less than 50%. Recovery, if it occurs, usually is complete. Continued use or rechallenge with the hepatotoxic drug may be associated with fatal liver injury.

For drug-associated chronic hepatitis, removal of the offending drug usually results in arrest of hepatic inflammation and, in most cases, complete recovery. Corticosteroids have a limited utility, but may be of value in treating the hepatotoxicity associated with a generalized hypersensitivity reaction. Hepatic failure may ensue if the involved agent is not identified and discontinued rapidly. Rechallenge a drug suspected of causing this form of liver injury is not justified because fulminant liver failure may occur. Liver transplantation may be required in patients suffering massive hepatic necrosis.

ACUTE HEPATIC FAILURE

ALF results from acute, massive hepatocellular necrosis or from sudden, severe impairment of hepatocellular function. Typically, patients have no evidence of prior hepatic dysfunction. Hepatic encephalopathy is a prerequisite for the diagnosis of ALF in older patients; this may not be evident in infants with ALF. In cases of viral hepatitis, encephalopathy must occur within 8 weeks of onset. Hepatic failure complicating chronic liver disease may present with similar clinical and laboratory features. In ALF, usually all hepatic functions are impaired, including hepatic synthetic, excretory, and detoxifying functions.

Epidemiology

ALF may be caused by acute viral hepatitis. Variously, hepatitis A, B, D, and E may cause ALF, as may Epstein-Barr virus, herpes viruses, and enteroviral infections. Fulminant hepatitis C is rare. The most common cause of ALF in children, accounting for 40% to 50% of cases, is an undefined (probably viral nonA, nonB, nonC) agent. Other unusual infectious agents include cytomegalovirus, varicella, rubeola, yellow fever, Lassa, Ebola, Marburg, dengue, and togaviruses. Rarely, leptospirosis and malaria also have been associated with ALF. Hepatotoxic drugs may be responsible for 25% of ALF cases. Acetaminophen toxicity is a common cause. Less commonly associated agents include intravenous tetracycline, halothane, sodium valproate, ethanol, carbon tetrachloride, methyldopa, and isoniazid. Poisoning due to the ingestion of the mushroom *Amanita phalloides* may be responsible. Rarely, autoimmune hepatitis may present as ALF. Hepatic ischemia due to endotoxic shock, vascular occlusion, or congenital heart disease may result in massive necrosis. In childhood, metabolic disorders, including galactosemia, tyrosinemia, mitochondrial disorders, NISD, hereditary fructose intolerance, and Wilson disease, may cause ALF. Finally, infiltrative processes, including hemophagocytic lymphohistiocytosis and leukemia, should be considered.

Pathogenesis

The pathogenesis of ALF is understood poorly. Anoxia or hypoxia of the liver may lead to hepatocellular necrosis, and multiple drugs may cause hepatocyte necrosis through direct hepatocellular membrane damage, through the formation of toxic intermediate products of metabolism, or through interference with cell metabolic pathways. Not as well understood is the mechanism through which viral hepatitis produces ALF in some patients and mild self-limiting infection in others. The direct effects of viral infection and individual systemic immune responses to that infection presumably play a role. The final common pathway is hepatic necrosis, with effects on hepatic synthetic, excretory, and detoxifying functions. Other factors that may contribute to ALF include infection, endotoxemia, tissue hypoxia, and individual differences in hepatocyte regenerative capabilities.

The cause of hepatic encephalopathy probably is multifactorial. Several theories have attempted to correlate observed biochemical abnormalities with hepatic encephalopathy. These theories include the ammonia theory, the synergism theory, the false neurotransmitter theory, and the gamma-aminobutyric acid (GABA)-ergic neurotransmission theory.

The ammonia theory proposes that hepatic encephalopathy is caused by elevated serum ammonia levels due to colonic production of free ammonia ion and failure of the liver to convert ammonia to urea. Contradicting this theory is the finding that hepatic encephalopathy may occur before an elevation of serum ammonia levels. Moreover, elevated serum ammonia levels in animals do not produce changes consistent with those of hepatic encephalopathy on electroencephalograms or visual evoked potential testing. In contrast to the seizures frequently observed with isolated hyperammonemia, seizures usually are not seen with hepatic encephalopathy unless a complication such as hypoglycemia, intracranial bleeding, or meningitis occurs.

The synergism theory proposes that hyperammonemia, in conjunction with methionine derivatives (i.e., mercaptans produced by intestinal bacteria) and short-chain fatty acids, is capable of causing hepatic encephalopathy.

The false neurotransmitter theory proposes that intestinal bacteria produce compounds such as octopamine during episodes of hepatic encephalopathy. These false neurotransmitter substances may reach the brain because of disordered blood–brain barrier function and may cause cerebral dysfunction. The plasma levels of amino acids are increased in hepatic encephalopathy. These substances may enter the CNS and become false neurotransmitters through beta-hydroxylation. It is not clear whether these substances are capable of producing the behavioral and neurologic changes consistent with hepatic encephalopathy.

GABA-like compound, also produced by colonic bacteria, may play a role in the production of hepatic encephalopathy. GABA receptors possess binding sites for benzodiazepines and barbiturates, which appear to enhance the inhibitory response to GABA. Specific benzodiazepine antagonists partially and temporarily may reverse the effects of hepatic encephalopathy.

Cerebral edema, observed in many cases of ALF, may occur because of a disruption of the blood–brain barrier, expansion of the interstitial space, or failure of cellular autoregulatory (e.g., osmotic regulation) mechanisms. Attempts to control cerebral edema have included steroid and mannitol administration. Steroids do not appear to help, but mannitol may be effective in diminishing intracranial pressure. The use of intracranial pressure monitors in children with ALF remains controversial. (The therapy for ALF is discussed in Chapter 455, Acute Hepatic Failure.)

Clinical Manifestations and Complications

Affected patients may have had a recent episode of acute viral hepatitis or recent drug and toxin ingestion. Patients or their parents may report the onset of lethargy, nausea, vomiting, fever, lack of appetite, and abdominal pain. Jaundice may have developed. Initially, hepatic encephalopathy may manifest with minor behavioral or motor disturbances. Infants may become irritable, eat poorly, and exhibit disturbed sleep patterns; older children may be confused and might exhibit slurred speech. Asterixis, elicited through dorsiflexion of the hand at the wrist, may be demonstrable. Hepatic encephalopathy may progress to deep coma. Often, fetor hepaticus is present. Ascites may develop, as may frequent episodes of bleeding. Hyperventilation may be an early sign, with hypoventilation becoming a problem in more advanced stages of disease. Often, cardiac arrhythmias (e.g., tachycardia, bradycardia) and hypotension occur. Hepatomegaly may occur, and a rapidly decreasing hepatic size is an ominous sign.

Diagnosis

Laboratory features include elevation of conjugated and unconjugated serum bilirubin. Initially, serum aminotransferases may be markedly elevated, although a subsequent decrease after massive hepatocyte necrosis may occur as the patient's condition worsens. Commonly, indices of hepatic synthetic function are altered. Serum albumin concentrations may be normal at presentation but decrease with time. The prothrombin time is elevated markedly and usually does not improve with vitamin K administration; values in excess of 50 seconds or an international normalized ratio (INR) greater than 4 (or both) have been associated with poor outcome. The serum concentrations of clotting factors synthesized in the liver (i.e., factors I, II, V, VII, IX, and X) usually are low, and factor VIII levels are normal or increased. Levels of factor VII, which has a short plasma half-life, of less than 8% of normal have been associated with a very poor outcome. Platelet concentrations may be diminished secondary to bone marrow suppression, disseminated intravascular coagulation, or hypersplenism. Platelet function also may be abnormal. Serum ammonia usually is elevated, but the onset of encephalopathy may precede this rise or may occur with a normal or only a slightly elevated serum ammonia concentration. Frequently, serum sodium values are diminished in the setting of the renal resorption of sodium and elevated total-body sodium values. Hypokalemia may result from an increased renal excretion of potassium. Hypoglycemia may occur, particularly in children, presumably because of the depletion of hepatic glycogen, inadequacy of gluconeogenesis, and hormonal dysfunction. Azotemia may occur; serum creatinine values rise, and blood urea nitrogen values may remain stable or fall because of deficient urea synthesis. Hypophosphatemia, hypocalcemia, and hypomagnesemia may occur. Hyperventilation may cause systemic alkalosis, but cell necrosis may result in systemic acidosis. Hepatic biopsy, which seldom is possible in patients with ALF because of marked coagulopathy, reveals massive hepatocellular necrosis, which may be patchy or zonal. Bridging necrosis and sparse inflammation also may be seen. In cases of tetracycline toxicity or acute fatty liver of pregnancy, microvesicular fatty infiltration of hepatocytes occurs. Hepatic failure in these cases presumably is secondary to hepatocyte organelle dysfunction. Evidence of preexisting liver disease also may be present, as observed in Wilson disease or in some cases of autoimmune hepatitis.

Prognosis

Recovery from ALF, if it occurs, usually is complete, with no residual hepatic dysfunction. Patients with ALF due to HBV and especially those (45%) with HBV and HDV coinfection may have chronic active hepatitis after recovery.

The survival rate is best for patients with ALF due to HAV (60% to 70%) and acetaminophen intoxication (50%). Lowest survival rates are found for those with ALF secondary to nonA, nonB, nonC hepatitis and idiosyncratic reactions to halothane (10% to 20%). Aplastic anemia occurs in about 10% of patients after recovery from or transplantation for ALF caused by the undefined agent. Multiple prognostic indicators have been proposed. The following factors are associated with a poor prognosis:

- Acetaminophen toxicity associated with a pH of less than 7.3 (95% mortality), prothrombin time of more than 100 seconds, and a creatinine level of more than 300 μmol/L with grade 3 encephalopathy (77% mortality)
- Viral hepatitis and drug reactions associated with ages of up to 11 years or older than 40, jaundice more than 7 days before onset of encephalopathy, bilirubin levels higher than 300 μmol/L, and a prothrombin time greater than 50 seconds

Other proposed variables have included factor V levels of less than 20% or factor VII levels of less than 8% of controls. Grade 4 coma, renal failure, and major episodes of GI bleeding have been identified as poor prognostic signs in the pediatric population. The decision to transplant is difficult and must be based on the relative outcomes of ALF and transplantation. Death prior to orthotopic liver transplantation (while awaiting an organ) is not uncommon. For those who receive organs, the survival rate is approximately 60%. Although patients with transplantation secondary to fulminant hepatitis B infection may remain serologically positive, they rarely have clinical disease, unlike those receiving transplantations for chronic HBV. Others have suggested that the need for transplantation be determined by grade 4 encephalopathy and the need for continued fresh-frozen plasma infusions to keep the prothrombin time within 10 seconds of control values.

Hepatocellular failure is the cause of death in 20% of the patients with ALF. Eighty percent of these deaths are caused by complications, including cerebral edema, GI hemorrhage, and sepsis.

PORTAL HYPERTENSION

Portal hypertension occurs in children because of obstruction to the flow of portal blood at extrahepatic (presinusoidal) and intrahepatic (sinusoidal and postsinusoidal) sites. Regardless of the underlying etiology, clinical manifestations of portal hypertension are similar, but complications, management, and outcome may differ if hepatic insufficiency is present.

Extrahepatic Portal Hypertension

Etiology

An extrahepatic or presinusoidal block may occur in children as a result of obstruction to blood flow in the portal vein or one of its branches. In approximately 40% of children with this lesion, a history of portal vein injury may be elicited. Causes of injury include thrombogenic tendencies, umbilical vein catheterization, neonatal omphalitis, or surgical trauma. Older children may have a history of abdominal trauma or pancreatitis. Clinical signs at presentation may include abdominal pain, diarrhea, and abdominal distention. Usually, splenomegaly is found, although the liver size is normal. Ascites and GI hemorrhage, usually from esophageal varices, may occur. Laboratory findings are consistent with hypersplenism: thrombocytopenia, neutropenia, or anemia. Secondary abnormalities of coagulation factors may be detected; in some cases hypercoagulability may be primary and presumably causative.

Diagnosis

Diagnosis is by ultrasonography, angiography of the portal venous system, and MRI, all of which are useful in demonstrating the anatomy of the portal venous system. A key feature of extrahepatic portal vein obstruction on imaging is the cavernous transformation of the portal vein, in which an extensive complex of tortuous collateral vessels form to bypass the obstruction. Because intrinsic liver disease must be excluded, hepatic biopsy may be required.

Prognosis

Frequently, hemorrhage from esophageal varices occurs in cases of extrahepatic portal hypertension. Presumably because of relatively intact hepatocellular function, most of these bleeding episodes are tolerated well and may be treated conservatively with endoscopic sclerotherapy or ligation. Portosystemic shunt procedures also have been used, but shunt surgery in young children carries a high risk of failure because of shunt thrombosis. In addition, the long-term risk of encephalopathy exists. In affected children, bleeding episodes usually decrease in frequency with age, often ceasing entirely in the third decade of life, presumably because of the development of effective collateral circulation. However, significant bleeding still may occur during adolescence and may eventually lead to a shunting procedure.

Intrahepatic Portal Hypertension

Other forms of portal hypertension include those caused by intrahepatic sinusoidal lesions and those secondary to postsinusoidal defects. Examples of the former are the most common causes of portal hypertension and include hepatic cirrhosis due to biliary atresia, alpha$_1$-antitrypsin deficiency, congenital hepatic fibrosis, or Wilson disease. Examples of the latter include Budd-Chiari-like syndromes, due to obstruction of the inferior vena cava at the level of the diaphragm, hepatic venous occlusion due to vasculitis; tumor; masses; or polycythemia. Other causes of postsinusoidal block include hepatic venoocclusive disease, typically associated with bone marrow transplantation, and constrictive pericarditis with resultant relative obstruction to vena caval flow.

Clinical Manifestations

The clinical manifestations of portal hypertension include splenomegaly and, in some cases, hepatomegaly. Caput medusae (i.e., dilated abdominal wall veins) may develop. Hepatopulmonary syndrome, caused by intrapulmonary vascular dilation with subsequent hypoxemia, may occur. Anastomoses between the systemic and splanchnic venous circulations may occur throughout the abdomen. These anastomoses include connections between the spleen and kidneys and between the mesenteric and gonadal veins. Other connections are found in the areas of the rectum and, most important clinically, in the region of the gastroesophageal junction. Esophageal varices are submucosal veins that connect the azygos and hemiazygos veins to the portal circulation. When portal hypertension occurs, flow develops from the high-pressure portal venous system through these vessels, with resultant vessel dilation. Factors predisposing to variceal hemorrhage include portal venous pressure gradients of at least 12 mm Hg, decreasing thickness of varix walls, increasing variceal transmural pressure, and increasing varix radii. Large, thin-walled vessels are more likely to bleed than are small varices. Not all patients with these varices have episodes of hemorrhage. Other risk factors for variceal hemorrhage include the ingestion of salicylate- and ethanol-containing products. Typically, variceal hemorrhage manifests as painless, massive hematemesis. Blood may be passed rectally as hematochezia or as melena. Affected patients may be known through prior studies—including barium swallow or upper endoscopy—to have esophageal varices. The precise diagnosis in patients who present with acute upper GI tract bleeding must await hemodynamic stabilization. After stabilization, the site of bleeding should be ascertained through endoscopy of the esophagus, stomach, and duodenum. Endoscopy should be performed on an emergency basis, but only in a well-controlled environment, such as an intensive care unit or an operating room. Airway protection may be necessary. The differential diagnosis includes gastritis, Mallory-Weiss tears, and peptic ulcer disease.

Therapy of Variceal Hemorrhage

Gastric lavage is performed before and after endoscopy, usually with saline to remove large blood clots. No clear advantage accrues from lavage with chilled fluids, and this procedure may result in significant hypothermia in pediatric patients. Intravascular volume replacement is administered as needed, with care taken to avoid the overadministration of sodium or of volume, which can worsen the variceal hemorrhage. Monitoring the central venous pressure may be useful in this regard. Replacement of erythrocytes, clotting factors, and platelets may be required. Vital signs must be monitored frequently.

These measures are sufficient to control variceal hemorrhage in most children. If hemorrhage continues, sclerotherapy may be performed on an emergent basis. This technique, in which a sclerosing agent, such as ethanol or sodium tetradecyl sulfate, is injected into or around esophageal varices through an endoscope, is performed most often after an affected patient's medical condition has stabilized. Variceal hemorrhage is controlled in 80% to 95% of patients treated. Subsequent injections are required to obliterate varices. Rebleeding may occur in as many as one-third of patients during the course of sclerotherapy. Studies comparing sclerotherapy with shunt surgery in adults suggest that the two modalities are similar in terms of patient survival; those receiving shunts appear more likely to develop hepatic encephalopathy, and those receiving sclerotherapy are more likely to have repeated episodes of variceal hemorrhage, some requiring shunt procedures. Studies suggest that sclerotherapy is safe and effective in children; the sclerosant volumes used are lower than those used in adults. Prophylactic sclerotherapy has been used also in adults before the first episode of variceal hemorrhage, but this procedure is not recommended. Although generally safe, sclerotherapy may cause esophageal perforation and stricture. Long-term control of bleeding from gastric varices may not be achieved through this technique.

In older children, the control of variceal hemorrhage, particularly in nonurgent situations, may be attained through the use of variceal banding or ligation. This technique, performed through an endoscope, ligates varices by constricting them with rubber bands. Efficacy is similar to that obtained with sclerotherapy, and complications are reduced significantly. Because of this reduced complication rate, the use of prophylactic ligation seems merited in adults; however, the prophylactic therapy of significant varices utilizing this technique has not been studied in children. Performance of esophageal banding in younger children is limited by the size of required instrumentation.

If control of variceal hemorrhage is not attained through use of the foregoing techniques, octreotide may be administered intravenously. Although not well studied in infants, octreotide, which may reduce splanchnic blood flow in humans and has minimal systemic side effects, has become the pharmacologic agent of choice for the control of acute variceal hemorrhage. Doses for use in younger children have not been elucidated. Vasopressin, a nonspecific vasoconstrictor that reduces blood flow through splenic, gastric, and intestinal arterioles to reduce portal venous pressure, also may be of use. Side effects, more common in adults than in children, include myocardial infarction and ischemic bowel disease.

Another pharmacologic agent that has been proposed in the management of variceal hemorrhage is nitroglycerin; given in concert with vasopressin, it may decrease portal pressure further and may ameliorate the side effects of vasopressin therapy. Few data address this combination in pediatric patients.

Propranolol has been used to prevent initial and recurrent variceal hemorrhage in adults, with a corresponding prolongation of survival. Limited data suggest that this agent may be effective in decreasing portal pressure in children with portal hypertension. However, during acute hemorrhage, propranolol decreases cardiac output and heart rate and is contraindicated.

Continuing hemorrhage after the use of the aforementioned techniques is an indication for balloon tamponade of varices using the Sengstaken-Blakemore tube. This form of therapy controls hemorrhage in 40% to 80% of patients. In some cases, hemorrhage is controlled with inflation of only the gastric balloon in conjunction with traction on the tube. Balloon tamponade is associated with a relatively high incidence of re-bleeding (as high as 60% in some series). Potential side effects of therapy include pulmonary aspiration if the airway is left unprotected, esophageal rupture, and suffocation.

Other methods of controlling variceal hemorrhage include the surgical creation of a portosystemic shunt and transthoracic ligation of esophageal varices. Although portosystemic shunts occasionally have been used successfully in children, performing them in young children is technically difficult. Splenorenal shunts are preferred. Success rates are limited by the small vessel size, and shunt surgery carries a high death rate, especially when performed as an emergency procedure. Hepatic encephalopathy may occur in the postoperative period, even with a technically successful shunt. Shunt surgery may render future attempts at hepatic transplantation more difficult. A transjugular intrahepatic portosystemic shunt (TIPS), in which a catheter is placed by an interventional radiologist between the right hepatic vein and the right or left portal vein branch, has been used in children as young as 2 years, although the need for periodic revision and dilation makes them most useful as a bridge to future hepatic transplantation.

Good results have been reported using the Sugiura and modified Sugiura procedures, consisting of esophageal transection with devascularization. Rebleeding episodes appear to be rare (approximately 2%), and encephalopathy does not occur. This procedure may be an option for children with variceal bleeding, but large series in the United States have not been reported.

Portal hypertension caused by intrahepatic disease has a poor prognosis, particularly if associated with poor liver function. Patients with portal hypertension and progressive liver disease ultimately require liver transplantation.

ASCITES

Ascites, a collection of free fluid within the peritoneal cavity, complicates cirrhosis and portal hypertension. (See also Chapter 365, Ascites.) Physical examination findings consistent with ascites include recent enlargement of abdominal girth, protuberance of the umbilicus, and shifting dullness on physical examination; a "fluid wave" may be detected.

Pathophysiology

Multiple factors interplay in the cause of ascites in patients with portal hypertension. Although the mechanisms by which ascites accumulate remain uncertain and probably are multifactorial, patients with cirrhosis and portal hypertension demonstrate an impaired renal excretion of sodium. Although at first related to direct hepatorenal interaction, later, this defect is exacerbated by the development of peripheral arterial vasodilation, caused in part by nitric oxide, with a subsequent release of aldosterone and vasopressin. These factors, in association with increased sympathetic nervous system activity and abnormalities in atrial natriuretic factor excretion or metabolism, lead to water and sodium retention, with the eventual formation of edema or ascites.

Diagnosis

Ascites may be diagnosed from historic evidence of chronic liver disease associated with compatible physical examination findings. The radiographic signs of ascites may include diffuse haziness of the abdomen, displacement of bowel loops medially, indistinct hepatic margins, and displacement of the lateral liver border medially. Abdominal ultrasonography or CT scans may confirm the presence of ascites. Diagnostic paracen-

tesis should be performed in all patients with new-onset ascites to rule out acute peritonitis. Useful studies include peritoneal fluid polymorphonuclear cell count (i.e., more than 500 cells per unit suggest peritonitis), Gram stain, culture, total protein, glucose, and lactate dehydrogenase levels.

Therapy

Treating ascites in children with liver disease is difficult. A marked accumulation of ascites may be associated with discomfort, dyspnea, anorexia, and gastroesophageal reflux. The control of ascites, although not shown to prolong life, may result in improved patient comfort. Effective therapy must be aimed at the altered renal handling of salt and water in liver disease. Usually, dietary sodium intake is limited to 1 to 2 mEq/kg/day as a first step, but the restriction of dietary sodium must be tempered by the necessity of maintaining adequate caloric intake. Typically, fluid restriction is not required in patients with adequate urine output and no hyponatremia.

If sodium restriction is insufficient to produce diuresis, pharmacologic therapy may be required. The goal of diuretic therapy is to inhibit renal sodium retention and to produce a gradual diuresis without simultaneously decreasing circulating plasma volume. In adults, the maximal rate of peritoneal ascitic fluid absorption is 700 to 900 mL/day. Diuresis of more than 900 mL/day results in volume contraction, with the attendant risks of renal insufficiency and hyperkalemia. Accompanying edema may allow more rapid diuresis. Similar data are unavailable in children. Usually, therapy is initiated with spironolactone, an inhibitor of aldosterone, which is begun in a dosage of 2 to 3 mg/kg/day. Spironolactone acts on the distal tubule and is potassium-sparing. Usually, diuresis occurs within 3 to 5 days of therapy initiation; adequate response may be confirmed by the achievement of an elevation of the urine sodium-to-potassium ratio above 1. If the response is inadequate, the dose may be doubled or an additional diuretic agent with a proximal tubular site of action, such as a thiazide, furosemide, or ethacrynic acid, may be added. Complications of diuretic agents include hypokalemia and hyponatremia and, if circulating vascular volume is decreased, renal insufficiency and encephalopathy. Urine and serum electrolyte concentrations must be followed carefully.

Large-volume paracentesis, often followed by intravenous colloid (i.e., albumin) infusion is a safe and effective method of removing ascites in adults. Recent studies indicate that the technique may be safely employed in children and may be particularly useful in patients becoming refractory to diuretic therapy or with respiratory compromise from tense ascites.

HEPATORENAL SYNDROME

The hepatorenal syndrome denotes the occurrence of unexplained progressive renal disease in patients with hepatic disease. The kidneys in these patients are structurally normal. Several factors appear to be involved in its etiology, including a decreased renal perfusion pressure, activation of the renal sympathetic nervous system and increased synthesis of several vasoactive mediators.

The hepatorenal syndrome occurs in patients with ascites and portal hypertension after a precipitating event, most often one producing a decrease in circulating plasma volume. Laboratory features include low urine sodium in conjunction with azotemia. The differential diagnosis of oliguria in cirrhotic patients also includes prerenal causes and acute tubular necrosis; if acute tubular necrosis is present, support with dialysis is necessary until renal function returns.

No specific therapy for hepatorenal syndrome exists, but sodium and fluid intake should be limited. Dialysis may be useful for patients who have acute hepatic dysfunction and in whom adequate hepatic function is expected to return. The prognosis for patients with hepatorenal syndrome and chronic liver disease is poor, and transplantation should be considered.

HEPATIC TRANSPLANTATION

With the availability of the immunosuppressive agent cyclosporine, liver transplantation has become a viable option for many patients with acute liver failure and chronic hepatic disease. (See also Chapter 459, Care of Children with Solid-Organ Transplants.) Potential candidates for liver transplantation include those with the conditions listed in Box 367.2.

Contraindications to liver transplantation include unresectable extrahepatic primary malignancy, malignancy metastatic to the liver, or terminal disease uncorrectable by liver transplantation. In children, those disorders for which liver transplantation is commonly required include biliary atresia, alpha$_1$-antitrypsin deficiency, ALF, hepatic tumors, and Wilson disease with ALF. The Pediatric End-Stage Liver Disease (PELD) scoring system is used to prioritize patients waiting for liver transplantation based on the severity of liver disease. The PELD score—based on the objective findings of the serum albumin, bilirubin, INR, age less than 1 year, and growth failure—is used to predict death or movement to an intensive care unit over time.

Survival rates at 1 year after liver transplantation approach 90% or better in many centers. Slightly lower rates of survival are reported for infants younger than 1 year and weighing 5 to 10 kg. Size is a major limiting factor in transplantation because of technical difficulties and because of the lack of donors weighing less than 10 kg. Split liver transplants and the use of living related donors have partially ameliorated this problem. The potential complications of liver transplantation include hepatic artery thrombosis, graft necrosis, biliary anastomotic leakage, GI bleeding, and GI perforation. Viral and bacterial sepsis may occur. Despite immunosuppression with cyclosporine or tacrolimus, episodes of rejection may occur. The treatment of these episodes includes bolus administration of corticosteroids and, if needed, additional immunosuppressive agents, including monoclonal antilymphocyte antibody preparations. Intensive immunosuppression may result in EBV-related posttransplantation lymphoproliferative disease (PTLD).

Despite these limitations, liver transplantation is a life-saving and potentially curative procedure for many patients with hepatic disease. A 20-year survival of 64% has been reported in one large series. This improved to a 10-year survival of 83% with use of tacrolimus-based immunosuppression. The follow-up of children who have undergone liver transplantation entails careful monitoring of immunosuppressant levels and hypertension, which often occurs after liver transplantation. Episodes of rejection must be differentiated quickly from episodes of viral hepatitis, ordinarily by percutaneous hepatic biopsy. Additional psychosocial issues arise as affected patients and their families return to their social environment.

BILIARY TRACT DISEASE: PRIMARY SCLEROSING CHOLANGITIS

Primary sclerosing cholangitis (PSC) is a disorder characterized by the inflammation and subsequent fibrosis of the hepatobiliary system. The term implies the absence of other biliary lesions, including postsurgical abnormalities, ischemic injury, drug toxicity, biliary infection associated with immunodeficiency, choledocholithiasis, and bile duct carcinoma. Reports suggest that PSC is much more common in both children and adults than has been previously recognized.

Thirty to eighty percent of children with PSC have idiopathic inflammatory bowel disease, usually chronic ulcerative colitis, and approximately 4% to 5% of patients with inflammatory bowel disease have PSC. Young men are affected most commonly. A distinct form, with onset in the neonate, has been described. An autoimmune hepatitis/PSC overlap syndrome also may occur.

Pathogenesis

Theories proposing a role for bacterial or viral infections or for specific bile duct toxins are not supported by the evidence. However, an immunologic cause is suggested strongly by the elevated serum IgG levels and autoantibody positivity in childhood PSC. Supportive evidence includes a positive association with HLA-B8 and HLA-DR3, the presence of circulating immune complexes, and the apparent T-lymphocyte–mediated destruction of bile ducts observed in PSC. The precise mechanism of pathogenicity is unknown.

Clinical Manifestations and Complications

The clinical features of PSC at presentation vary widely. In adults, the insidious onset of fatigue and pruritus is followed by jaundice. In children, abdominal pain, fever, jaundice, and pruritus variously have been reported as presenting features. Acute bacterial cholangitis may occur. PSC has been diagnosed before the onset of symptoms through abnormal hepatic function tests in the setting of inflammatory bowel disease. Patients may present with hepatomegaly or hepatosplenomegaly, with or without jaundice. Usually, one or more of these findings is seen in 50% to 75% of patients at presentation. The course and severity of PSC is independent of the activity of inflammatory bowel disease.

BOX 367.2   **Conditions Found in Potential Candidates for Liver Transplantation**

- Diseases that demonstrate a progressive, irreversible, downhill course, such as biliary atresia after a failed Kasai procedure
- Decompensated hepatic disease, especially if accompanied by life-threatening complications, such as ascites with spontaneous bacterial peritonitis and variceal hemorrhage
- Intractable pruritus or severe metabolic bone disease with resultant social invalidism
- Diseases for which no alternative therapy is available, such as the type I Crigler-Najjar syndrome in which intense phototherapy has failed

---

Diagnosis

Usually, children and adults with PSC have elevated serum alkaline phosphatase or gamma-glutamyl transpeptidase levels;

both are markers of cholestasis. The serum bilirubin level may or may not be elevated. Often, serum aminotransferase levels are increased only moderately. In children, serum immunoglobulin levels may be elevated, and serum antinuclear antibodies and anti–smooth-muscle antibodies are found more commonly in children with PSC than in adults. Antineutrophil cytoplasmic antibodies (ANCA) with a perinuclear distribution are found in about 40% of children with PSC.

Radiologic Features

The radiologic features of PSC reflect its characteristic progressive injury of bile ducts. Usually, endoscopic retrograde cholangiography is performed to visualize the biliary tree. Other potentially useful techniques include magnetic resonance cholangiography, percutaneous transhepatic cholangiography and, in rare cases, operative cholangiography. Typical radiographic features of PSC include diffuse, 1- to 2-cm strictures of the intrahepatic and extrahepatic biliary systems, often with intervening, slightly dilated segments that produce a beaded appearance. Narrow, bandlike strictures may be seen, as may diverticulum-like outpouchings. Similar changes may be found in immunodeficient patients and in those with histiocytosis.

Hepatic Pathology

Histologic abnormalities in PSC include bile duct lesions— periductal fibrosis and inflammation with subsequent ductal obliteration. The course of PSC can be divided into four stages: enlargement of portal tracts with edema, increased connective-tissue, and bile duct proliferation with inflammation; growth of fibrous tissue into the periportal parenchyma; formation of fibrotic septa; and biliary cirrhosis. The hepatic biopsy finding of "pericholangitis" in patients with inflammatory bowel disease is thought to represent PSC of the small bile ducts. Pathologically, the livers of children with PSC may exhibit inflammation and piecemeal necrosis, and the condition may be mistaken for autoimmune hepatitis.

Therapy

No effective therapy is available for PSC. In patients with associated chronic ulcerative colitis, proctocolectomy does not appear to influence the course of PSC favorably, and peristomal varices may form in patients so treated. Ursodeoxycholic acid may produce a transient improvement in biochemical abnormalities, but controlled studies have not demonstrated improvements in clinical course or long-term outcomes. The usefulness of other immunosuppressive agents (e.g., corticosteroids, azathioprine, cyclosporine) and of antifibrogenic agents (e.g., colchicine) has not been proven, even in patients with the autoimmune hepatitis/PSC overlap syndrome. Episodes of cholangitis may occur and should be treated vigorously. Dominant stricture formation may occur, accompanied by increases in serum bilirubin levels and episodes of cholangitis. The conservative management of these strictures in adult patients has included transhepatic or endoscopic balloon dilation. Cholangiocarcinoma may occur. Orthotopic liver transplantation is required in patients progressing to end-stage liver disease, although PSC may recur in the allograft.

The prognosis for patients with PSC is highly variable. Several studies in children have shown a median survival (50%) from onset of disease without liver transplantation of 10 to 12 years.

Other hepatobiliary disorders associated with inflammatory bowel disease include steatosis, chronic hepatitis, hepatic granulomas, cholelithiasis, and occlusion of the portal or hepatic veins.

SPONTANEOUS PERFORATION OF THE COMMON BILE DUCT

Spontaneous perforation of the common bile duct typically occurs at the junction of the cystic and common bile ducts, which suggests an area of developmental weakness at this site. The disorder commonly is detected in the first 3 months of life. Symptoms of infants at and before diagnosis include failure to thrive, irritability, vomiting, and acholic stools. Physical examination may reveal jaundice and occasionally abdominal distention, often with bile-stained hydrocele and hernia sacs secondary to the bile-stained ascites. Laboratory features may include leukocytosis and conjugated hyperbilirubinemia. Serum aminotransferase values may be elevated mildly. The diagnosis may be suggested by hepatobiliary scintigraphy, which demonstrates tracer activity outside the biliary tract. Paracentesis may yield bile-stained ascitic fluid.

The diagnosis depends on a demonstration of a bile duct perforation at the time of operative cholangiography. Hepatic pathology is nonspecific in this condition: Cholestasis may be present, portal tracts may be edematous, and bile duct proliferation occasionally is found.

Surgical therapy is required; drainage with or without suture closure of the perforation has been recommended. Alternatively, internal drainage through a Roux-en-Y loop anastomosis to the gallbladder has been performed in some cases.

CYSTIC DISEASES OF THE LIVER

Cystic diseases of the liver include choledochal cysts, autosomal recessive and dominant forms of polycystic kidney disease, congenital hepatic fibrosis, and Caroli disease. Although similar pathologic features may occur in several of these disorders, differences in the manner of inheritance and distinct morphometric and clinical features suggest that the disorders have separate causes.

Choledochal Cysts

Choledochal cysts occur in as many as 2% of infants with obstructive jaundice. This potentially correctable lesion must be sought in all infants with cholestasis.

Clinical Manifestations and Complications

Choledochal cysts may manifest at any age. A 3:1 female predominance is evident. Usually, the infantile form presents in the first few months of age with jaundice and acholic stools; hepatomegaly may develop. A palpable abdominal mass may be found in as many as 60% of these patients. Approximately 50% of infants experience vomiting and failure to thrive. Infants with choledochal cysts have various degrees of hepatic impairment at diagnosis. Usually, those with cirrhosis and portal hypertension have a poor prognosis despite cyst resection.

Children older than 2 years may present with the classic signs of abdominal pain (often secondary to pancreatitis), jaundice, and an abdominal mass, but all three findings are present in fewer than 25% of affected patients. Episodes of recurrent cholangitis also may occur. Usually, hepatic injury due to obstruction caused by the cyst is less severe in patients who are seen first at an older age; their prognosis is better. Abnormalities of the pancreatic duct are common in patients with late-onset choledochal cysts, as are coexisting hepatic and biliary anomalies, including double common duct, double gallbladder, and accessory hepatic ducts. Biliary and pancreatic calculi may be detected.

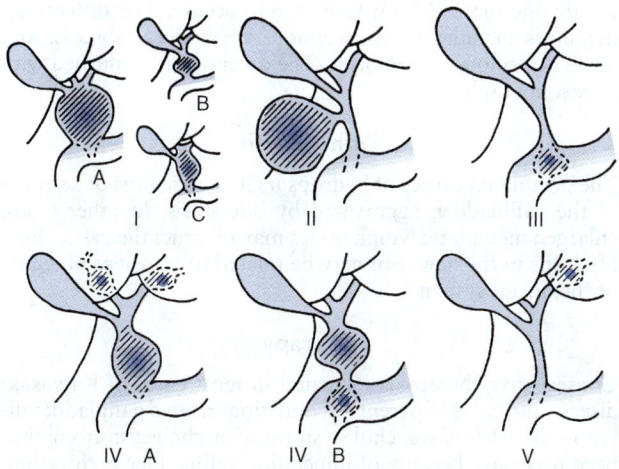

FIGURE 367.5. Classification of choledochal cysts. Please see text for description.

Pathology

Five types of choledochal cysts have been described (Fig. 367.5). Type I cysts (93%) represent fusiform dilation of the extrahepatic bile ducts. Type II cysts (6%) are diverticula of any portion of the extrahepatic bile duct. Type III cysts (2%) are choledochoceles of the distal common duct. Type IV cysts are similar to type I cysts but, in addition to fusiform dilation of the extrahepatic duct, intrahepatic and extrahepatic duct cysts or extrahepatic cysts are present. Type V cysts may contain one or more cystic dilatations of the intrahepatic bile ducts. Hepatic pathology depends in part on age at diagnosis. In infants, the hepatic pathology resembles that seen in biliary atresia. Prolonged obstruction may result in cirrhosis with portal hypertension or recurrent pancreatitis.

Pathogenesis

The pathogenesis of choledochal cysts is unknown. Theories formulated to explain the features of this disorder include the possibility that the cysts are congenital malformations or that they are acquired as a result of injury to bile duct walls from infection or pancreatic enzymes.

Diagnosis

Usually, the diagnosis of choledochal cysts is made with ultrasonography, which has demonstrated choledochal cysts *in utero*. Other potentially useful techniques include radionuclide scintigraphy, CT scans, endoscopic retrograde cholangiopancreatography, and percutaneous transhepatic cholangiography.

Therapy

Usually, therapy involves surgical excision of the cyst. A Roux-en-Y loop of jejunum is used to drain the proximal duct system. Cholangitis may occur postoperatively, and the development of malignancy in retained cystic tissue is an ongoing risk.

Polycystic Kidney Disease

Autosomal Dominant Polycystic Disease

Autosomal dominant polycystic disease (ADPKD) is one of the most common inherited diseases, affecting 1 in 1,000 live births. It is characterized by progressive renal cyst development and enlargement and by an array of extrarenal manifestations. A high degree of intrafamilial and interfamilial variability is seen in the clinical expression of the disease. At least three genetic loci underlie the cases of ADPKD. The *PKD1* gene encoding a novel protein of 460 kd called *polycystin* has been localized to chromosome 16p13.3 and accounts for 85% of the cases. *PKD2* is on chromosome 4q13–23 and accounts for approximately 15%. A third locus remains unmapped but has been demonstrated in some reported families. The *PKD2* protein, polycystin-2, a nonspecific calcium permeable channel, is thought to interact in some fashion with polycystin-1.

Multiple hepatic lesions have been associated with ADPKD and include the ductal plate malformation with cystic communicating duct elements, dilated and apparently noncommunicating cysts, biliary microhamartomas (the so-called von Meyenburg complexes), segmental dilatation of the intrahepatic ducts or so-called Caroli disease, and congenital hepatic fibrosis. Approximately 50% of patients with renal failure have demonstrable hepatic cysts that are not in continuity with the biliary tract. Often, these cysts are asymptomatic, but they may cause pain and occasionally are complicated by hemorrhage or infection. The prevalence of hepatic cysts increases with age; they are extremely uncommon before the age of 16. Although the frequency of cysts is similar in men and women, the development of large hepatic cysts is largely a complication of women. Selected patients with severe symptomatic polycystic liver disease and favorable anatomy benefit from liver resection and fenestration with acceptable morbidity and mortality.

Autosomal Recessive Polycystic Disease

Autosomal recessive polycystic kidney disease (ARPKD) is characterized by bilateral enlargement of the kidneys, caused by a generalized dilatation of the collecting tubules. Invariably, the disorder is associated with congenital hepatic fibrosis and a varying degree of biliary ductal ectasia. The gene responsible for ARPKD (polycystic kidney and hepatic disease 1, PKHD1), is located on chromosome 6p21 and has been cloned. It encodes a 450kDa protein called fibrocystin, which may function as a receptor involved in renal collecting duct and biliary differentiation. Normally, ARPKD presents in early life, often shortly after birth, and generally is more severe than is ADPKD. Patients with ARPKD may die in the perinatal period due to renal failure or lung dysgenesis. Such patients demonstrate varying degrees of periportal fibrosis, bile ductular hyperplasia, and biliary dysgenesis. Often, the hyperplastic bile ductules are arranged in a disordered pattern consistent with the findings of congenital hepatic fibrosis. Liver disease and complications from hepatic fibrosis are most likely to be clinically significant in patients whose kidney disease allows prolonged survival. The most prominent clinical problem in older patients with ARPKD and congenital hepatic fibrosis is portal hypertension. In 30% to 70% of such patients, hematemesis or melena may be the presenting sign. Although portal hypertensive bleeding may occur during the first year of life, it presents more commonly in older children. In such cases, usually firm or hard hepatomegaly is present. Splenomegaly also is a frequent finding accompanied by hypersplenism. Because of dilatation of the intrahepatic bile ducts, affected patients are at increased risk of bacterial cholangitis. Caroli disease, or a congenital, segmental, saccular dilatation of the intrahepatic bile ducts, may coexist with congenital hepatic fibrosis and ARPKD.

Congenital Hepatic Fibrosis

Congenital hepatic fibrosis appears to be inherited in an autosomal recessive fashion, although sporadic cases occur. The hepatic lesion is characterized by broad bands of periportal or perilobular fibrous tissue surrounding irregularly shaped islands of normal hepatocytes. These bands of fibrous tissue may contain clusters of distorted biliary duct elements, sometimes described as *bile duct hamartomas,* which appear to communicate with the biliary tree. Portal venous anomalies may exist. Frequently, renal anomalies occur in this disorder. The lesion most commonly associated is renal tubular ectasia. Another associated lesion resembles that seen in adult polycystic kidney disease. Nephronophthisis may be associated with hepatic findings of congenital hepatic fibrosis; affected patients have severe, progressive renal disease.

Usually, the signs and symptoms of congenital hepatic fibrosis begin in childhood and include hepatomegaly and splenomegaly. Indices of hepatic function, including serum albumin levels and prothrombin time, are normal, as are serum bilirubin and aminotransferase values. Portal hypertension is common, and hemorrhage from esophageal varices may occur. A subset of patients with congenital hepatic fibrosis and associated bile duct dilation may experience repeated episodes of cholangitis and microabscess formation. Biliary calculi may form.

The medical management of patients with congenital hepatic fibrosis is directed toward the consequences of portal hypertension. For example, endoscopic sclerotherapy or banding is used in those with variceal hemorrhage. The vigorous treatment of episodes of cholangitis is necessary. Syndromes associated with hepatic lesions similar to those in congenital hepatic fibrosis include the Meckel (i.e., encephalocele, polydactyly, cystic renal disease), Jeune, Ellis–van Creveld, and Ivemark syndromes, tuberous sclerosis, as well as congenital disorders of glycosylation.

Caroli Disease

Caroli disease is characterized by a saccular dilation of the intrahepatic bile ducts, an absence of portal hypertension or cirrhosis, and a high incidence of cholangitis and lithiasis. Renal cystic disease may be associated with the liver disease. Overlap exists between Caroli disease and congenital hepatic fibrosis with intrahepatic biliary duct dilation. Type IV and V choledochal cysts also may share certain features.

Often, patients with Caroli disease present in childhood with episodes of abdominal pain, fever, jaundice, and tender hepatomegaly, all attributable to episodes of cholangitis. Laboratory features include elevated serum alkaline phosphatase and conjugated bilirubin levels. Ultrasonography or CT scans may suggest the diagnosis. Percutaneous transhepatic cholangiography is useful in determining the extent of disease.

Episodes of cholangitis require antibiotic therapy. Biliary calculi may necessitate surgery. Disease localized to a single lobe of the liver may be treated by partial hepatectomy. Other surgical drainage procedures have been used, with variable results. Cholangiocarcinoma has been reported in patients with Caroli disease.

GALLBLADDER DISEASE

Hydrops

Hydrops of the gallbladder denotes noninflammatory, noncalculous distention of the gallbladder, often associated with illnesses such as scarlet fever, familial Mediterranean fever, polyarteritis nodosa, leptospirosis, and Kawasaki disease. Patients receiving long-term parenteral nutrition may have acute distention of the gallbladder, presumably secondary to prolonged fasting. Affected children present with abdominal pain (100%), vomiting (75%), right upper quadrant tenderness (93%), and

a palpable mass (55%); fever rarely occurs. The differential diagnosis includes intussusception, appendiceal abscess, and acute acalculous cholecystitis. The diagnosis is confirmed with ultrasonography.

Pathogenesis

The postulated causes of hydrops include vasculitis or serositis of the gallbladder, aggravated by bile stasis. In other cases, enlarged mesenteric lymph nodes may obstruct the cystic duct. Hydrops in the newborn may be related to transient plugging of the ductal system.

Therapy

Conservative therapy is indicated in most cases of Kawasaki disease and cases of parenteral nutrition–related gallbladder dilation. In other cases, cholecystotomy or cholecystectomy has been necessary because of impending gallbladder perforation. Typically, green, black, or white bile is drained from the acutely dilated gallbladder; no stones are found, and bile cultures are sterile. The lack of inflammation in the gallbladder wall differentiates this disorder from acute acalculous cholecystitis.

Acute Acalculous Cholecystitis

Acute acalculous cholecystitis accounts for 5% to 15% of cases of cholecystitis in adults and 5% to 30% of cases in children. Clinical features include jaundice (approximately 30%), abdominal pain (95%), fever, anorexia, nausea, and vomiting. The acute onset of right-sided abdominal tenderness suggests this diagnosis. The differential diagnosis includes appendicitis, intussusception, calculous cholecystitis, and peritonitis. Laboratory features include hyperbilirubinemia, leukocytosis, and elevated serum alkaline phosphatase levels.

Acute acalculous cholecystitis has been associated with severe trauma and has been seen in postoperative patients. Associated autoimmune disorders include systemic lupus erythematosus, diabetes mellitus, and rheumatoid arthritis, which suggests that vasculitis underlies the lesion. Anatomic anomalies of the cystic duct also may be associated with hydrops. Acalculous cholecystitis has been related also to TPN, but most cases appear to be associated with infection. Specific organisms include *Salmonella,* group A and B streptococci, such parasites as *Giardia lamblia* and *Ascaris,* and tuberculosis.

Ultrasonographic scans can suggest the diagnosis of acute acalculous cholecystitis, although findings such as gallbladder wall edema and the presence of pericholecystic fluid are nonspecific, particularly in critically ill patients and those with hypoalbuminemia. Radionuclide scintigraphy and CT scans also may be useful.

The treatment of this disorder involves cholecystectomy and the treatment of any systemic infection. The gallbladder mucosa is edematous and demonstrates an inflammatory infiltrate. Usually, the gallbladder bile is sterile on culture.

Cholelithiasis

Cholelithiasis is less common in children than in adults; in many affected children, a specific cause can be identified. The clinical presentation varies, and often gallstones are discovered in asymptomatic patients undergoing abdominal examination for other reasons. Symptoms of gallstone disease include abdominal pain, nausea, vomiting and, in older patients, fatty food intolerance. The abdominal pain may resemble colic and may radiate to the right scapula or (in older patients) may localize to the right upper quadrant. Dark urine or jaundice, perhaps secondary to hemolytic anemia, may be noticed; fever rarely occurs.

Pigment stones, composed primarily of calcium bilirubinate in polymeric or monomeric forms, or cholesterol stones may be identified. Several factors may contribute to pigment stone formation, including increased secretion of unconjugated bilirubin into bile or deconjugation of conjugated bilirubin in bile, probably by bacterial beta-glucuronidase.

Hemolytic anemias are associated with pigment-stone formation in children. Sickle cell disease is associated with an incidence of gallstone formation of approximately 42% by age 18 years. Wilson disease may be associated with stone formation, as may other erythrocyte hemoglobinopathies and enzymopathies. Children receiving long-term TPN may develop pigment stones.

Cholesterol gallstones form in three stages. In stage I, bile becomes supersaturated with cholesterol because of the increased biliary secretion of cholesterol or diminished biliary bile acid secretion, perhaps because of increased fecal bile acid losses. The cholesterol-saturated bile then must undergo nucleation or cholesterol crystallization from a saturated solution. Factors that probably add to the risk of cholesterol stone formation include gallbladder stasis or dysmotility; absence of putative inhibitors of gallstone nucleation, including apolipoprotein AI and AII; and the presence of promoters of gallstone nucleation, including mucous glycoproteins and congenital disorders of canalicular phospholipid transport.

Usually, cholesterol gallstones in the pediatric population occur in adolescent girls; obesity and parity correlate with the incidence of cholelithiasis in these patients. Children with CF, ileal Crohn disease, and ileal resections have excessive fecal bile acid loss and may form gallstones. Chronic cholestasis also increases the risk of gallstone formation.

Diagnosis

Plain-film abdominal roentgenography may reveal pigment (i.e., radiopaque) stones. Cholesterol stones are radiolucent. Ultrasonography is the method of choice for detecting gallstones, but radionuclide scintigraphy may aid in assessing gallbladder function.

Therapy

Laparoscopic cholecystectomy is the method of choice for treating symptomatic gallstone disease in children. Endoscopic retrograde cholangiopancreatography and sphincterotomy (if necessary) may be performed preoperatively in children in whom the presence of common duct stones is suspected. Operative cholecystectomy with operative cholangiography may be required for suspected choledocholithiasis in children or infants too small for endoscopic retrograde cholangiopancreatography and sphincterotomy. The role of surgery in children with asymptomatic cholelithiasis is controversial. The course of children with asymptomatic gallstones has not yet been defined, and no alternative therapeutic methods for children are available. Nonoperative gallstone dissolution using oral ursodeoxycholic acid, fragmentation of stones with extracorporeal shock waves, and biliary tract perfusion with solvents are methods untried in children. The prognosis after gallstone removal is excellent.

LIVER DYSFUNCTION IN HEART DISEASE

Children and adults with congenital or acquired cardiac disease may have secondary hepatic dysfunction. Congestive heart failure may cause diminished hepatic blood flow and elevated hepatic venous pressure. Midzonal distention, atrophy, and necrosis then may result. Cirrhosis may occur in advanced cases, especially in children with chronic elevations of right-sided pressures. Left-sided heart failure leads to diminished cardiac output, with resultant decreases in hepatic blood flow. Central zonal hypoxia and necrosis then may follow. Clinical findings include tender hepatomegaly, especially in cases of venous congestion. Laboratory features include prolongation of the prothrombin time, unresponsiveness to vitamin K, and markedly increased aminotransferase and serum bilirubin levels. Hypoglycemia may be severe. Autopsy studies of children with hypoplastic left-sided heart syndrome and coarctation of the aorta have shown a high incidence of hepatic necrosis, compared with other forms of congenital heart disease.

SICKLE CELL DISEASE

Patients with sickle cell disease are at high risk for hepatic abnormalities. Autopsy studies reveal cirrhosis in 10% of patients with sickle cell disease. The postulated causes of injury include hypoxic injury from sickling, viral hepatitis, gallstones, right ventricular failure, iron overload, and alcohol and drug abuse. Hepatic sickle cell crisis may occur in as many as 10% of patients admitted to the hospital with sickle cell disease. Manifestations include jaundice, nausea, abdominal pain, and fever. Often, tender hepatomegaly is found. Serum aminotransferase and bilirubin values are elevated. Viral hepatitis, ALF, and gallbladder disease also may occur in patients with sickle cell disease. Children with sickle cell disease may develop extreme hyperbilirubinemia, with total serum bilirubin values of 20 mg/dL, presumably owing to intrahepatic sickling. These markedly increased levels are not associated with extreme pain, fever, or hemolytic or venoocclusive crisis. Usually, the clinical course of disease in affected patients is benign, with gradual resolution of bilirubin values. Rarely, hepatic failure may occur; in these cases exchange transfusion may be helpful, although hepatic transplantation may sometimes be required.

Suggested Readings

Alpha₁-Antitrypsin Deficiency

Garver RI, Mornex J, Nukiwa T, et al. Alpha₁-antitrypsin deficiency and emphysema caused by homozygous inheritance of nonexpressing alpha₁-antitrypsin genes. *N Engl J Med* 1986;314:762.

Norman MR, Mowat AP, Hutchison DC. Molecular basis, clinical consequences and diagnosis of alpha₁-antitrypsin deficiency. *Ann Clin Biochem* 1997;34:230.

Qu D, Teckman JH, Perlmutter DH. Review: alpha₁-antitrypsin deficiency–associated liver disease. *J Gastroenterol Hepatol* 1997;12:404.

Sveger T. Liver disease in alpha₁-antitrypsin deficiency detected by screening of 200,000 infants. *N Engl J Med* 1976;294:1316.

Sveger T, Eriksson S. The liver in adolescents with alpha₁-antitrypsin deficiency. *Hepatology* 1995;22:514.

Wu Y, Whitman I, Molmenti E, et al. A lag in intracellular degradation of mutant alpha₁-antitrypsin correlates with the liver disease phenotype in homozygous PiZZ alpha₁-antitrypsin deficiency. *Proc Natl Acad Sci USA* 1994;91:9014.

Ascites

Kramer RE, Sokol RJ, Yerushalmi B, et al. Large-volume paracentesis in the management of ascites in children. *J Pediatr Gastroenterol Nutr* 2001;33:245.

Martin PY, Schrier RW. Pathogenesis of water and sodium retention in cirrhosis. *Kidney Int Suppl* 1997;59:S43.

Sabri M, Saps M, Peters JM. Pathophysiology and management of pediatric ascites. *Curr Gastroenterol Rep* 2003;5:240.

Aspects of Hepatic Development

Arey LB. *Developmental anatomy*, 2nd ed. Philadelphia: Saunders, 1965.

Castell DO, O'Brien KD, Muench H, et al. Estimation of liver size by percussion in normal individuals. *Ann Intern Med* 1969;70:1183.

Coppoletta JM, Wolbach SB. Body length and organ weights of infants and children: a study of the body length and normal weights of the more important vital organs of the body between birth and 12 years of age. *Am J Pathol* 1933;9:55.

Greengard O. Enzymic differentiation of human liver: comparison with the rat model. *Pediatr Res* 1977;11:669.

Henning SJ. Postnatal development: coordination of feeding, digestion and metabolism. *Am J Physiol* 1981;241:G199.

McGahan JP, Phillips HE, Cox KL. Sonography of the normal pediatric gallbladder and biliary tract. *Radiology* 1982;144:873.

Younoszai MK, Mueller S. Clinical assessment of liver size in normal children. *Clin Pediatr* 1975;14:378.

Choledochal Cysts

de Vries JS, de Vries S, Aronson DC, et al. Choledochal cysts: age of presentation, symptoms, and late complications related to Todani's classification. *J Pediatr Surg* 2002; 37:156.

Mackenzie TC, et al. The management of prenatally diagnosed choledochal cysts. *J Pediatr Surg* 2001;36:1241.

Metcalfe MS, Wemyss-Holden SA, Maddern GJ. Management dilemmas with choledochal cysts. *Arch Surg* 2003;138:333.

Cholelithiasis

Apstein MD, Carey MC. Pathogenesis of cholesterol gallstones: a parsimonious hypothesis. *Eur J Clin Invest* 1996;26:343.

Gamba PG, Zancan L, Midrio P, et al. Is there a place for medical treatment in children with gallstones?. *J Pediatr Surg* 1997;32:476.

Holcomb GW Jr., Holcomb GW III. Cholelithiasis in infants, children and adolescents. *Pediatr Rev* 1990;11:26B.

Lucena JF, Herrero JI, Quiroga J, et al. A multidrug resistance 3 gene mutation causing cholelithiasis, cholestasis of pregnancy, and adulthood biliary cirrhosis. *Gastroenterology* 2003;124:1037.

Newman KD, Powell DM, Holcomb GW. The management of choledocholithiasis in children in the era of laparoscopic cholecystectomy. *J Pediatr Surg* 1997;32:1116.

Rescorla FJ. Cholelithiasis, cholecystitis, and common bile duct stones. *Curr Opin Pediatr* 1997;9:276.

Chronic Cholestasis

Bergasa NV. The pruritus of cholestasis. *Semin Dermatol* 1995;14:302.

Cynamon HA, Andres JM, Iafrate RP. Rifampin relieves pruritus in children with cholestatic liver disease. *Gastroenterology* 1990;98:1013.

Whitington PF, Whitington GL. Partial external diversion of bile for the treatment of pruritus associated with intrahepatic cholestasis. *Gastroenterology* 1988;95:130.

Wolfhagen FH, Sternieri E, Hop WC, et al. Oral naltrexone treatment for cholestatic pruritus: a double-blind, placebo-controlled study. *Gastroenterology* 1997;113:1264.

Chronic Hepatitis

Alvarez F, Schwarz K. Immune diseases of the liver and biliary tract. *J Pediatr Gastroenterol Nutr* 2002;35(Suppl 1):S39.

Czaja AJ. Treatment of autoimmune hepatitis. *Semin Liver Dis* 2002;22(4):365.

Czaja AJ. Diagnosis and therapy of autoimmune liver disease. *Med Clin North Am* 1996;80:973.

Fitzgerald JF. Chronic hepatitis. *J Pediatr* 1984;104:893.

Gregorio GV, Portmann B, Karani J, et al. Autoimmune hepatitis/sclerosing cholangitis overlap syndrome in childhood: a 16-year prospective study. *Hepatology* 2001;33(3):544.

Gregorio GV, Portmann B, Reid F, et al. Autoimmune hepatitis in childhood: a 20-year experience. *Hepatology* 1997;25:541.

Ishak KG. Chronic hepatitis: morphology and nomenclature. *Mod Pathol* 1994;7:690.

Johnson PJ, McFarlane IG, Williams R. Azathioprine for long-term maintenance of remission in autoimmune hepatitis. *N Engl J Med* 1995;333:958.

Ludwig J. The nomenclature of chronic active hepatitis: an obituary. *Gastroenterology* 1993;105:274.

Cystic Fibrosis

Balistreri WF. The Liver-the next frontier in the treatment of patients with cystic fibrosis. In: Reyes HB, Leuschner U, Arias I, eds. *Pregnancy, sex hormones, and the liver.* Proceedings of the 89th Falk Symposium. Lancaster, UK: Kluwer Academic Publishers, 1996:114.

Colombo C, Battezzati PM, Podda M, et al. Ursodeoxycholic acid for liver disease associated with cystic fibrosis: a double-blind multicenter trial. The Italian Group for the Study of Ursodeoxycholic Acid in Cystic Fibrosis. *Hepatology* 1996;23:1484.

Colombo C, Castellani MR, Balistreri WF, et al. Scintigraphic documentation of an improvement in hepatobiliary excretory function after treatment with ursodeoxycholic acid in patients with cystic fibrosis and associated liver disease. *Hepatology* 1992;15:677.

Ferenchak AP, Sokol RJ. Cholangiocyte biology and cystic fibrosis liver disease. *Semin Liver Dis* 2001;21:471.

Nousia-Arvanitakis S, Fotoulaki M, Economou H, et al. Long-term prospective study of the effect of ursodeoxycholic acid on cystic fibrosis-related liver disease. *J Clin Gastroenterol* 2001;32:324.

Park RW, Grand RJ. Gastrointestinal manifestations of cystic fibrosis: a review. *Gastroenterology* 1981;81:1143.

Riordan JR, Rommens JM, Kerem B, et al. Identification of cystic fibrosis gene: cloning and characterization of complementary DNA. *Science* 1989;245:1066.

Rommens JM, Iannuzzi MC, Kerem BS, et al. Identification of the cystic fibrosis gene: chromosome walking and jumping. *Science* 1989;245:1059.

Scott-Jupp R, Lama M, Tanner MS. Prevalence of liver disease in cystic fibrosis. *Arch Dis Child* 1991;66:698.

Sokol RJ, Durie PR. Recommendations for management of liver and biliary tract disease in cystic fibrosis. *J Pediatr Gastroen Nutr* 1999;28(1):S1.

van de Meeberg PC, Houwen RH, Sinaasappel M, et al. Low-dose versus high-dose ursodeoxycholic acid in cystic fibrosis–related cholestatic liver disease. Results of a randomized study with 1-year follow-up. *Scand J Gastroenterol* 1997;32:369.

Drug-Induced Liver Disease

Buratti S, Lavine JE. Drugs and the liver: advances in metabolism, toxicity, and therapeutics. *Curr Opin Pediatr* 2002;14:601.

Lee WM. Medical Progress: Drug-induced liver disease. *N Engl J Med* 2003;349:474.

Fibrocystic Diseases

Calvet JP, Grantham JJ. The genetics and physiology of polycystic kidney disease. *Semin Nephrol* 2001;21:107.

Birnbaum A, Suchy FJ. The intrahepatic cholangiopathies. *Semin Liver Dis* 1998;18:263.

D'Agata ID, Jonas MM, Perez-Atayde AR, et al. Combined cystic disease of the liver and kidney. *Semin Liver Dis* 1994;14:215.

Desmet VJ. Ludwig symposium on biliary disorders—part I. Pathogenesis of ductal plate abnormalities. *Mayo Clin Proc* 1998;73:80.

Guay-Woodford LM, Desmond RA. Autosomal recessive polycystic kidney disease: the clinical experience in North America. *Pediatrics* 2003;111:1072.

Johnson CA, Gissen P, Sergi C. Molecular pathology and genetics of congenital hepatorenal fibrocystic syndromes. *J Med Genet* 2003;40:311.

Sutters M, Germino GG. Autosomal dominant polycystic kidney disease: molecular genetics and pathophysiology. *J Lab Clin Med* 2003;141:91.

Zerres K, Rudnik-Schoneborn S, Senderek J, et al. Autosomal recessive polycystic kidney disease (ARPKD). *J Nephrol* 2003;16:453.

Fulminant Hepatic Failure

Bhaduri BR, Mieli-Vergani G. Fulminant hepatic failure: pediatric aspects. *Semin Liver Dis* 1996;16:349.

Emre S, Schwartz ME, Shneider B, et al. Living related liver transplantation for acute liver failure in children. *Liver Transpl Surg* 1999;5:161.

Lee WM. Management of acute liver failure. *Semin Liver Dis* 1996;16:369.

Schiodt FV, Atillasoy E, Shakil AO, et al. Etiology and outcome for 295 patients with acute liver failure in the United States. *Liver Transpl Surg* 1999;5:29.

Hepatic Transplantation

Heffron TG. Living related liver transplantation. *Semin Liver Dis* 1995;15:165.

Jain A, Mazariegos G, Kashyap R, et al. Pediatric liver transplantation. A single center experience spanning 20 years. *Transplantation* 2002;73:941.

McDiarmid SV, Anand R, Lindblad AS. Development of a pediatric end-stage liver disease score to predict poor outcome in children awaiting liver transplantation. *Transplantation* 2002;74:173.

Hepatitis (General)

Bader TF. Hepatitis A vaccine. *Am J Gastroenterol* 1996;91:217.

Balistreri WF, Chang MH, Ciocca M, et al. Acute and chronic hepatitis: Working Group Report of the First World Congress of Pediatric Gastroenterology, Hepatology, and Nutrition. *J Pediatr Gastroenterol Nutr* 2002;35(Suppl 2): S62.

Bortolotti F, Giacchino R, Vajro P, et al. Recombinant interferon-alfa therapy in children with chronic hepatitis C. *Hepatology* 1995;22:1623.

Broderick AL, Jonas MM. Hepatitis B in children. *Semin Liver Dis* 2003; 23(1):59.

Di MV, Lo IO, Almasio P, et al. Long-term efficacy of alpha-interferon in beta-thalassemics with chronic hepatitis C. *Blood* 1997;90:2207.

Dienstag JL, Perrillo RP, Schiff ER, et al. A preliminary trial of lamivudine for chronic hepatitis B infection. *N Engl J Med* 1995;333:1657.

Dusheiko G, Main J, Thomas H, et al. Ribavirin treatment for patients with chronic hepatitis C: results of a placebo-controlled study. *J Hepatol* 1996;25:591.

Gonzalez-Peralta RP. Hepatitis C virus infection in pediatric patients. *Clin Liver Dis* 1997;1:691.

Hoofnagle JH, Di Bisceglie AM. Serologic diagnosis of acute and chronic viral hepatitis. *Semin Liver Dis* 1991;11:73.

Hupertz VF, Wyllie R. Perinatal hepatitis C infection. *Pediatr Infect Dis J* 2003;22(4):369.

Jonas MM. Children with hepatitis C. *Hepatology* 2002;36(5 Suppl 1):S173.

Kesson AM. Diagnosis and management of paediatric hepatitis C virus infection. *J Paediatr Child Health* 2002;38(3):213.

Koff RS. Natural history of acute hepatitis B in adults reexamined. *Gastroenterology* 1987;92:2035.

Lemon SM. Type A viral hepatitis. *N Engl J Med* 1985;313:1059.

National Institutes of Health. Consensus Development Conference Panel statement: management of hepatitis C. *Hepatology* 1997;26:2S.

Schwarz KB, Balistreri W. Viral hepatitis. *J Pediatr Gastroenterol Nutr* 2002; 35(Suppl 1):S29.

Schwimmer J, Balistreri, WF. The transmission, natural history and treatment of hepatitis C virus infection in the pediatric age population. *Semin Liver Dis* 2000;20:37.

Smedile A, Rizzetto M. The hepatitis delta virus and its disease. *Viewpoints Dig Dis* 1987;19:1.

Stevens CE, Taylor PE, Tong MJ, et al. Yeast-recombinant hepatitis B vaccine: efficacy with hepatitis B immune globulin in prevention of perinatal hepatitis B virus transmission. *JAMA* 1987;257:2612.

Torre D, Tambini R. Interferon-alpha therapy for chronic hepatitis B in children: a meta-analysis. *Clin Infect Dis* 1996;23:131.

Hepatorenal Syndrome

Van Roey G, Moore K. The hepatorenal syndrome. *Pediatr Nephrol* 1996;10:100.

Arroyo V, Guevara M, Gines P. Hepatorenal syndrome in cirrhosis: pathogenesis and treatment. *Gastroenterology* 2002;122:1658.

Hyperammonemia

Brusilow SW, Batshaw ML, Waber L. Neonatal hyperammonemic coma. *Adv Pediatr* 1982;29:69.

Brusilow SW, Maestri NE. Urea cycle disorders: diagnosis, pathophysiology, and therapy. *Adv Pediatr* 1996;43:127.

Jan D, Poggi F, Jouvet P, et al. Definitive cure of hyperammonemia by liver transplantation in urea cycle defects: report of three cases. *Transplant Proc* 1994;26:188.

Kiwaki K, Matsuda I. Gene therapy for ornithine transcarbamylase deficiency. *Acta Paediatr Jpn* 1996;38:189.

Metabolic Disease

Dhawan A, Mieli-Vergani G. Liver transplantation for mitochondrial respiratory chain disorders: to be or not to be? *Transplantation* 2001;71(5):596.

Dubern B, Broue P, Dubuisson C, et al. Orthotopic liver transplantation for mitochondrial respiratory chain disorders: a study of 5 children. *Transplantation* 2001;71(5):633.

Holme E, Lindstedt S. Diagnosis and management of tyrosinemia type I. *Curr Opin Pediatr* 1995;7:726.

Hostetter MK, Levy HL, Winter HS, et al. Evidence for liver disease preceding amino acid abnormalities in hereditary tyrosinemia. *N Engl J Med* 1983;308:1265.

Koiwai O, Nishizawa M, Hasada K, et al. Gilbert's syndrome is caused by a heterozygous missense mutation in the gene for bilirubin UDP-glucuronosyltransferase. *Hum Mol Genet* 1995;4:1183.

Levy HL. Nutritional therapy for selected inborn errors of metabolism. *J Am Coll Nutr* 1989;8:549.

Murcia FJ, Vazquez J, Gamez M, et al. Liver transplantation in type I tyrosinemia. *Transplant Proc* 1995;27:2301.

Odievre M. Clinical presentation of metabolic liver disease. *J Inherit Metab Dis* 1991;14:256.

Paradis K. Tyrosinemia: the Quebec experience. *Clin Invest Med* 1996;19:311.

Rootwelt H, Chou J, Gahl WA, et al. Two missense mutations causing tyrosinemia type 1 with presence and absence of immunoreactive fumarylacetoacetase. *Hum Genet* 1994;93:615.

Saheki T, Kobayashi K. Mitochondrial aspartate glutamate carrier (citrin) deficiency as the cause of adult-onset type II citrullinemia (CTLN2) and idiopathic neonatal hepatitis (NICCD). *J Hum Genet* 2002;47(7):333.

St-Louis M, Tanguay RM. Mutations in the fumarylacetoacetate hydrolase gene causing hereditary tyrosinemia type I: overview. *Hum Mutat* 1997;9:291.

Nonalcoholic Steatohepatitis

Green RM. NASH-hepatic metabolism and not simply the metabolic syndrome. *Hepatology* 2003;38(1):14.

Harrison SA, Kadakia S, Lang KA, et al. Nonalcoholic steatohepatitis: what we know in the new millennium. *Am J Gastroenterol* 2002;97(11):2714.

Molleston JP, White F, Teckman J, Fitzgerald JF. Obese children with steatohepatitis can develop cirrhosis in childhood. *Am J Gastroenterol* 2002;97(9):2460.

Nadeau K, Klingensmith G, Sokol RJ. Case report: nonalcoholic steatohepatitis in a teenage girl with type 2 diabetes. *Curr Opin Pediatr* 2003;15(1):127.

Neuschwander-Tetri BA, Caldwell SH. Nonalcoholic steatohepatitis: summary of an AASLD Single Topic Conference. *Hepatology* 2003;37(5):1202.

Rashid M, Roberts EA. Nonalcoholic steatohepatitis in children. *J Pediatr Gastroenterol Nutr* 2000;30(1):48.

Parenteral Nutrition-Related Cholestasis

Btaiche IF, Khalidi N. Parenteral nutrition-associated liver complications in children. *Pharmacotherapy* 2002;22(2):188.

Briones ER, Iber FL. Liver and biliary tract changes and injury associated with total parenteral nutrition: pathogenesis and prevention. *J Am Coll Nutr* 1995; 14:219.

Buchman A. Total parenteral nutrition-associated liver disease. *J Parenter Enteral Nutr* 2002;26(5 Suppl):S43.

Fleming CR. Hepatobiliary complications in adults receiving nutrition support. *Dig Dis* 1994;12:191.

Misra S, Ament ME, Vargas JH, et al. Chronic liver disease in children on long-term parenteral nutrition. *J Gastroenterol Hepatol* 1996;11:S4.

Portal Hypertension

Lykavieris P, Gauthier F, Hadchouel P, et al. Risk of gastrointestinal bleeding during adolescence and early adulthood in children with portal vein obstruction. *J Pediatr* 2000;136:805.

Miga D, Sokol RJ, Mackenzie T, et al. Survival after first esophageal variceal hemorrhage in patients with biliary atresia. *J Pediatr* 2001;139:291.

Ryckman FC, Alonso MH. Causes and management of portal hypertension in the pediatric population. *Clin Liver Dis* 2001;5:789.

Sarin SK, Agarwal SR. Extrahepatic portal vein obstruction. *Semin Liver Dis* 2002;22:43.

Sclerosing Cholangitis

Feldstein AE, Perrault J, El-Youssif M, et al. Primary sclerosing cholangitis in children: a long-term follow-up study. *Hepatology* 2003;38:210.

Gregorio GV, Portmann B, Karani J, et al. Autoimmune hepatitis/sclerosing cholangitis overlap syndrome in childhood: a 16-year prospective study. *Hepatology* 2001;33:544.

Mieli-Vergani G, Vergani D. Sclerosing cholangitis in the paediatric patient. *Best Pract Res Clin Gastroenterol* 2001;15:681.

Mitchell SA, Chapman RW. Review article: the management of primary sclerosing cholangitis. *Aliment Pharmacol Ther* 1997;11:33.

Reye Syndrome and Mimickers

Bennett MJ, Powell S. Metabolic disease and sudden, unexpected death in infancy. *Hum Pathol* 1994;25:742.

Bhala A, Willi SM, Rinaldo P, et al. Clinical and biochemical characterization of short-chain acyl-coenzyme A dehydrogenase deficiency. *J Pediatr* 1995;126:910.

Brown-Harrison MC, Nada MA, Sprecher H, et al. Very long chain acyl-CoA dehydrogenase deficiency: successful treatment of acute cardiomyopathy. *Biochem Mol Med* 1996;58:59.

Hale DE, Bennett MJ. Fatty acid oxidation disorders: a new class of metabolic diseases. *J Pediatr* 1992;121:1.

Hardie RM, Newton LH, Bruce JC, et al. The changing clinical pattern of Reye's syndrome 1982–1990. *Arch Dis Child* 1996;74:400.

Ibdah JA, Yang Z, Bennett MJ. Liver disease in pregnancy and fetal fatty acid oxidation defects. *Mol Genet Metab* 2000;71:182.

Nada MA, Vianey-Saban C, Roe CR, et al. Prenatal diagnosis of mitochondrial fatty acid oxidation defects. *Prenat Diagn* 1996;16:117.

Sims HF, Brackett JC, Powell CK, et al. The molecular basis of pediatric long chain 3-hydroxyacyl-CoA dehydrogenase deficiency associated with maternal acute fatty liver of pregnancy. *Proc Natl Acad Sci USA* 1995;92:841.

Strauss AW, Powell CK, Hale DE, et al. Molecular basis of human mitochondrial very-long-chain acyl-CoA dehydrogenase deficiency causing cardiomyopathy and sudden death in childhood. *Proc Natl Acad Sci USA* 1995;92:10496.

Treem WR. Inherited and acquired syndromes of hyperammonemia and encephalopathy in children. *Semin Liver Dis* 1994;14:236.

Ziadeh R, Hoffman EP, Finegold DN, et al. Medium chain acyl-CoA dehydrogenase deficiency in Pennsylvania: neonatal screening shows high incidence and unexpected mutation frequencies. *Pediatr Res* 1995;37:675.

Wilson Disease and Presumed Defects of Metal Metabolism

Bavdekar AR, Bhave SA, Pradhan AM, et al. Long-term survival in Indian childhood cirrhosis treated with D-penicillamine. *Arch Dis Child* 1996;74:32.

Bull PC, Thomas GR, Rommens JM, et al. The Wilson disease gene is a putative copper transporting P-type ATPase similar to the Menkes gene. *Nat Genet* 1993;5:327.

Dufour JF, Kaplan MM. Muddying the water: Wilson's disease challenges will not soon disappear [editorial, comment]. *Gastroenterology* 1997;113:348.

Gollan JL. Treatment of Wilson's disease: in D-penicillamine we trust–what about zinc? *Hepatology* 1987;7:593.

Lutsenko S, Efremov RG, Tsivkovskii R, et al. Human copper-transporting ATPase ATP7B (the Wilson's disease protein): biochemical properties and regulation. *J Bioenerg Biomembr* 2002;34(5):351.

Prasad R, Kaur G, Nath R, et al. Molecular basis of pathophysiology of Indian childhood cirrhosis: role of nuclear copper accumulation in liver. *Mol Cell Biochem* 1996;156:25.

Roberts EA, Schilsky ML. A practice guideline on Wilson disease. *Hepatology* 2003;37(6):1475.

Scheinberg IH, Jaffe ME, Sternlieb I. The use of trientine in preventing the effects of interrupting penicillamine therapy in Wilson's disease. *N Engl J Med* 1987;317:209.

Schilsky ML, Scheinberg IH, Sternlieb I. Prognosis of Wilsonian chronic active hepatitis. *Gastroenterology* 1991;100:762.

Shneider BL. Neonatal liver failure. *Curr Opin Pediatr* 1996;8:495.

Tanzi RE, Petrukhin K, Chernov I, et al. The Wilson disease gene is a copper transporting ATPase with homology to the Menkes disease gene. *Nat Genet* 1993;5:344.

Vulpe C, Levinson B, Whitney S, et al. Isolation of a candidate gene for Menkes disease and evidence that it encodes a copper-transporting ATPase. *Nat Genet* 1993;3:7.

CHAPTER 368 ■ LIVER ABSCESS

PRATHIBA NANJUNDIAH AND WILLIAM J. KLISH

Because the liver has systemic and portal circulations, the infrequency of liver abscess in infants and children is surprising. The low incidence is partly attributable to the extensive network of reticuloendothelial cells that line the sinusoids and are capable of clearing bacteria. Early use of antibiotics and improved medical and surgical care have reduced the liver's exposure to bacteria and account for the infrequency of this disorder.

The exact incidence of hepatic abscess in children is unknown. Dehner and Kissane reported a 0.38% incidence at autopsy in patients younger than 15 years. In this large series studied from 1917 to 1967, 41% of the patients were younger than 2 years and 67% were 2 to 5 years of age. The incidence was estimated to be 3 per 100,000 admissions to a large pediatric hospital. In another review, the incidence was 25 per 100,000 pediatric hospital admissions. These findings suggest an increase in the incidence of this disorder, which may be related to the use of advanced diagnostic techniques. The prolonged lifespan of patients with primary and secondary immune defects could also account for the number of older children with pyogenic liver abscess.

Pyogenic liver abscess does occur in neonates and accounts for 0.026% of admissions to a neonatal intensive care unit in one study. No definite sex predilection is seen except that patients with chronic granulomatous disease, which is more frequently seen in boys, have an increased risk of developing liver abscess.

PATHOGENESIS

Infectious agents may reach the liver by direct invasion from contiguous structures, through the portal vein, by systemic (hematogenous) bacteremia, or by direct inoculation during surgery or through traumatic events. Cases in which the mode of transmission is obscure are described as cryptogenic.

Systemic bacteremia with hematogenous spread to the liver through the hepatic artery appears to be the most common source of liver abscess in children. In the series of Dehner and Kissane, the hematogenous route was responsible for 78% of the cases.

The portal system is the second most common route by which bacteria may reach the liver, and this route accounts for most cases of hepatic abscess in neonates. Among newborns, solitary liver abscess (usually due to gram-negative organisms) has been reported as a complication of umbilical venous catheterization or omphalitis. Prematurity and necrotizing enterocolitis are other important predisposing factors in neonates.

Portal vein inflammation and bacteremia can be associated with infections of the abdominal cavity. Appendicitis, perirectal abscess, Crohn disease, ulcerative colitis, and omphalitis are possible sources of portal vein sepsis. Liver abscess in Crohn disease may be secondary to seeding of the mesenteric vessels with portal bacteremia from the inflamed loops of bowel.

Direct extension of infection from contiguous structures accounts for 11% of the liver abscesses in children. Ascending cholangitis is a frequent complication of hepatic portoenterostomy in patients with biliary atresia and may lead to abscesses of the liver in these patients. Liver abscesses also may develop after liver transplantation, especially if technical problems with vascular supply or biliary drainage occur. Hepatic artery thrombosis can be a significant risk factor.

Penetrating and nonpenetrating trauma to the liver may lead to liver abscesses, presumably from the proliferation of bacteria within the localized hematomas or biliary collection that may result from trauma. This mode of infection is rare in children.

Cryptogenic hepatic abscesses have been reported in children with fever of unknown origin and account for a small percentage of patients. Hepatic abscesses also have been reported in patients with cat-scratch disease.

An increased incidence of hepatic abscess is found in immunocompromised children. Children with chronic granulomatous disease and acute leukemia are at increased risk. The pathophysiology may be related to chronic, low-grade intestinal infection or the small number of viable granulocytes and monocytes. Patients being treated with corticosteroids are at risk because of suppression of the natural host defenses.

Pyogenic liver abscess has been reported as a complication of anaerobic bacterial invasion of hepatic infarcts in patients with sickle cell anemia. These patients have other abnormalities that may contribute to their increased risk, such as splenic dysfunction and increased gut permeability to certain bacteria from microinfarcts.

Liver abscesses can result from infection of central parenteral nutrition catheters or ventriculoperitoneal shunts. Biliary tract disease predisposes the patient to the development of multiple liver abscesses, and portal vein inflammation usually results in a single abscess. Solitary abscess is most common in the right lobe of the liver.

ETIOLOGY

Staphylococcus aureus was the most common pathogen seen in 44%, enteric organisms in 25%, and anaerobes in 10% of the cases in a review of 96 children with pyogenic liver abscess. Gram-negative organisms such as *Escherichia coli, Aerobacter, Pseudomonas, Proteus,* and *Klebsiella* species have been isolated frequently from liver abscesses in neonates. With improvement in culture techniques, anaerobes (e.g., *Actinomyces, Fusobacterium,* and *Bacteroides* species) and mycobacteria (i.e., typical and atypical species in patients infected with human immunodeficiency virus) have been identified in children. Fungi, especially *Candida albicans,* have been isolated from liver abscesses in neonates and leukemic patients on total parenteral nutrition. *Entamoeba histolytica* is a well-known cause of liver abscess. Liver abscess due to *Mycobacterium tuberculosis* and *M. avium intracellulare* can be the presenting infection in patients with acquired immunodeficiency syndrome.

PATHOLOGY

Microscopically, liver abscesses are characterized by an area of necrosis surrounded by polymorphonuclear leukocytes, large mononuclear cells, and lymphocytes. Adjacent to the inflammatory cell infiltrate, fibrous tissue intermingled with hepatocytes may be seen. Microorganisms may be seen in the necrotic center or at the periphery of the abscess cavity.

CLINICAL MANIFESTATIONS

The signs and symptoms of hepatic abscess are nonspecific and frequently are related to the underlying disease, especially in the neonate. A history of recent travel to areas where amebiasis is endemic, previous abdominal surgery, trauma, immunodeficiency, or inflammatory bowel disease may be elicited. Fever, abdominal pain, nausea, vomiting, loss of appetite, weakness, and malaise are the most constant and prominent symptoms. Weight loss, diarrhea, and pleuritic pain occur less frequently. A history of fever of unknown cause, with or without abdominal pain, in an otherwise healthy child should suggest the diagnosis of liver abscess. Patients with multiple abscesses generally experience a more acute illness, and patients with solitary abscesses usually show a subacute or chronic disease course.

Hepatomegaly occurs in 40% to 80% of patients. Tenderness is usually elicited on percussion of the right upper quadrant of the abdomen but may not be appreciated unless the physician specifically examines this region. Jaundice is not a clinical feature of liver abscess unless associated biliary tract disease is present. Other physical findings include abdominal distention and decreased breath sounds or crackles from pulmonary involvement due to pleural effusion or fixed hemidiaphragm.

DIAGNOSIS

Initial laboratory studies may show some degree of anemia and leukocytosis. The erythrocyte sedimentation rate may be elevated. Nonspecific elevations in the levels of transaminases, glutamine peptidase, and alkaline phosphatase may be seen in some patients. If the abscesses are secondary to biliary tract disease, bilirubin and alkaline phosphatase levels may be elevated.

Blood cultures are frequently positive in patients with multiple liver abscesses. Chest radiographs may reveal a pleural effusion or a fixed hemidiaphragm. Ileus and air in the liver abscess may be seen on abdominal radiographs.

Abdominal imaging techniques are particularly useful in younger children, who are unable to localize pain. Ultrasonography is a sensitive technique that does not require exposure to radiation and is recommended as the first imaging modality in children. However, imaging techniques such as magnetic resonance imaging and computed tomography (CT) are considerably more sensitive and have improved the diagnosis of these infections (Fig. 368.1). Although both of these techniques are expensive, they provide accurate information about the number, size, and location of abscesses within the liver parenchyma. Lesions of approximately 1 cm in diameter can be detected. With intravenous contrast studies, hypodense abscesses are demonstrated readily and can be differentiated from vascular lesions and tumors of the liver.

DIFFERENTIAL DIAGNOSIS

The differential diagnosis of fever, abdominal pain, vomiting, and malaise in young children often includes hepatitis, appen-

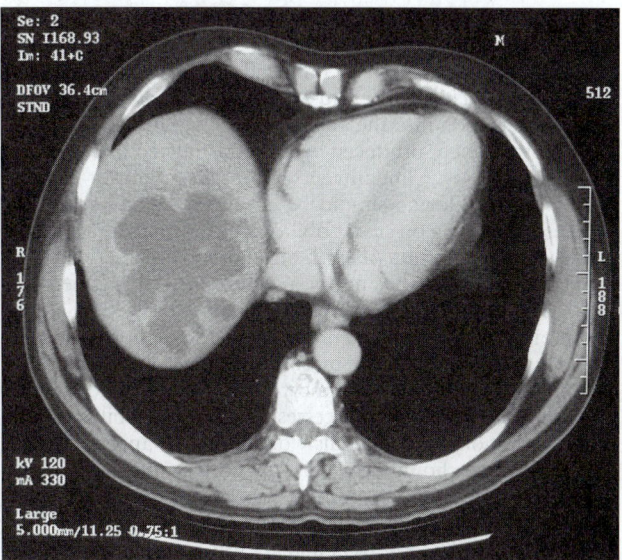

FIGURE 368.1. Computed tomography scan of the liver shows lobulated pyogenic liver abscess. Cultures from the abscess revealed *Klebsiella*. (Pictures courtesy of Gary W. Radner, MD, pediatric radiologist.)

dicitis, tuberculosis, pyelonephritis, bowel obstruction, occult trauma, and liver tumors. In adolescents, choledochal disease is possible, and gonorrheal or chlamydial perihepatitis or Fitz-Hugh–Curtis syndrome should be considered in girls.

The differentiation of amebic abscess from pyogenic liver abscess is difficult. In one large pediatric series, many patients with amebic abscesses had traveled to an area where amebiasis is endemic. The most common presenting symptoms included fever, cough or difficulty breathing, abdominal pain, loss of appetite, and weight loss. Diarrhea was not a constant symptom. Seventy-seven percent of the patients had an isolated mass in the right hepatic lobe, and 81% had hepatomegaly on physical examination.

Examination of stool specimens for cysts and trophozoites of *E. histolytica* is positive in only 10% to 30% of the patients with amebic abscess. The presence of *E. histolytica* trophozoites in the abscess is diagnostic, but they are usually found only in the wall of an abscess cavity. Counterimmunoelectrophoresis of serum for the detection of antibody to *E. histolytica* is a rapid test and establishes a presumptive diagnosis. A positive titer (more than 1:128) on the indirect hemagglutination assay of serum is confirmatory and has an accuracy of 85% to 95%.

THERAPY

Untreated and undiagnosed liver abscess is fatal. Although surgical intervention of a solitary pyogenic abscess is mandatory, antibiotic therapy with a percutaneous drainage is the main treatment. A catheter is placed into the abscess cavity under CT or ultrasound guidance, the contents are aspirated, and a draining catheter is placed. Surgical support is essential for this procedure, because spillage of abscess material into the peritoneal or pleural cavity, hemorrhage, or other complications may occur.

Percutaneous aspiration is useful in all cases of liver abscess except amebic abscess as a guide to proper antibiotic therapy. Antibiotic therapy should be based on information gained from Gram stain of the abscess material, culture, and antibiotic susceptibility testing. However, empiric antibiotic therapy should not be delayed pending the abscess drainage procedure. A combination of a semisynthetic penicillin or cephalosporin and an aminoglycoside has been recommended for initial therapy of liver abscess in children. Third-generation cephalosporins have better penetration into the abscess cavity and may work in the acidic environment produced by bacteria and necrotic debris in the abscess cavity. Clindamycin, cefoxitin sodium, or metronidazole hydrochloride should be administered for anaerobic isolates, depending on susceptibility. The optimal duration and route of administration of antibiotics for children with drained solitary liver abscess has not been determined. A regimen of 2 to 4 weeks of parenteral antibiotic therapy followed by a minimum of 4 to 6 weeks of oral therapy with an appropriate antibiotic is recommended by most physicians. The combination of amphotericin B and 5-fluorocytosine is recommended in the treatment of fungal liver abscesses unless susceptibility testing suggests that other antifungals would be more appropriate.

The aspirate should be evaluated cytologically, particularly in patients who fail to respond to treatment or who have negative ameba titers, to exclude malignant lesions. Multiple liver abscesses are difficult to treat and are not amenable to surgical therapy. Prolonged antibiotic treatment may be required for immunocompromised children. Serial imaging studies may be required to document appropriate response and shrinkage of the abscess cavity.

COMPLICATIONS AND PROGNOSIS

Complications of hepatic abscess include pleural and pulmonary inflammation, peritonitis, subphrenic or subhepatic abscesses, hemobilia, septicemia, and shock. Mortality associated with liver abscess was 27% before 1997. However, a review of 109 cases in children, excluding neonates, from 1977 to 1988 reported a decrease in mortality to 15%. A recent series from India reported an 11% mortality rate in children with pyogenic liver abscess. Increased vigilance and early diagnosis, in conjunction with better imaging modalities, advanced microbial isolation techniques, and newer antimicrobials, has significantly reduced the mortality of this disease.

Suggested Readings

Chusid MJ. Pyogenic hepatic abscess in infancy and childhood. *Pediatrics* 1978;62:554.
Dehner LP, Kissane JM. Pyogenic hepatic abscess in infancy and childhood. *J Pediatr* 1969;74:763.
Doerr CA, Demmler GJ, Garcia-Prats JA, Brandt ML. Solitary pyogenic liver abscess in neonates, report of three cases and review of the literature. *Pedeatr Infect Dis J* 1994;13:64.
Donovan AJ, Yellin AE, Ralls PW. Hepatic abscess. *World J Surg* 1991;15:162.
Haffer A, Boland F, Edwards MS. Amebic liver abscess in children. *Pediatr Infect Dis* 1982;1:5.
Kaplan SL. Pyogenic liver abscess. In: Feigin RD, Cherry JD, eds. *Textbook of pediatric infectious diseases,* 4th ed. Philadelphia: Saunders, 1998;1:655.
Kumar A, Srinivasan S, Sharma AK. Pyogenic liver abscess in children—South Indian experience. *J Pediatr Surg* 1998;33:417.
Kusne S, Dummer JS, Singh N, et al. Infections after liver transplantation: an analysis of 101 consecutive cases. *Medicine* 1988;67:132.
Laurin S, Kaude JV. Diagnosis of liver-spleen abscesses in children with emphasis on ultrasound for the initial and follow-up examination. *Pediatr Radiol* 1984;14:198.
MacDonald GA, Greenson JK, DelBuono EA, et al. Mini-microabscess syndrome in liver transplant recipients. *Hepatology* 1997;26:192.
Moss TJ, Pysher JT. Hepatic abscess in neonates. *Am J Dis Child* 1981;135:726.
Nolan JP. Bacteria and the liver. *N Engl J Med* 1978;299:1069.
Pineiro-Carrero VM, Andres JM. Morbidity and mortality in children with pyogenic liver abscess. *Am J Dis Child* 1989;143:1424.
Rabkin JM, Orloff SL, Corless CL, et al. Hepatic allograft abscess with hepatic artery thrombosis. *Am J Surgery* 1998;175:354.
Vachon L, Diament MJ, Stanley P. Percutaneous drainage of hepatic abscesses in children. *J Pediatr Surg* 1986;21:366.
Weinberg RJ, Klish WJ, Brown MR, et al. Hepatic abscess as a complication of Crohn's disease. *J Pediatr Gastroenterol Nutr* 1983;2:174.

CHAPTER 369 ■ CHOLECYSTITIS

KATHLEEN J. MOTIL

Cholecystitis is an inflammatory disease of the gallbladder that may be acute or chronic. In some instances, acute cholecystitis may be superimposed on the preexisting chronic form of the disease. Acute and chronic cholecystitis may be classified further as calculous or acalculous, based on the presence or absence of gallstones. In developed countries, gallstones are present in 50% to 70% of children who have cholecystitis, but in developing countries, acalculous cholecystitis may predominate. Chronic cholecystitis with cholelithiasis is the most common pattern, occurring in almost two-thirds of children with this diagnosis (Table 369.1).

ETIOLOGY AND PATHOGENESIS

Acute cholecystitis may result from any of three primary events in the gallbladder: bile stasis, an inflammatory response, or ischemia. Stasis usually results from obstruction of the cystic duct due to gallstones but may occur secondary to the edema produced by stones, hyperplastic lymph nodes, or a neoplasm. Starvation, dehydration, and immobilization are associated with stasis due to interruption of gallbladder contraction and

TABLE 369.1

PATTERNS OF CHOLECYSTITIS AND THEIR FREQUENCY

Type	Frequency (%)
Acute Cholecystitis	
Calculous	19
Acalculous	5
Chronic Cholecystitis	
Calculous	64
Acalculous	12

emptying. Bile salts, lysolecithin, pancreatic juice, and bacteria have been implicated as agents responsible for inciting the inflammatory response. Torsion of the gallbladder or systemic vascular disease may lead to ischemic changes of the biliary tract. Empyema or gangrene may lead to perforation. After the initial attack subsides, the mucosal surface of the biliary tract heals, and the wall becomes scarred. If the inflammation subsides but the cystic duct remains obstructed, the gallbladder may become distended (i.e., hydrops). Recurrent attacks of obstruction and inflammation lead to progressive scarring of the gallbladder with loss of function and additional gallstone formation. Rarely, adenomatous hyperplasia with polyp formation may portend cholecystitis.

PATHOLOGY

The pathologic features of acute cholecystitis include an enlarged gallbladder that is filled with turbid bile, fine sandy gravel, or gallstones. The gallbladder wall is thickened and may be ulcerated or perforated. The inflammatory response is characterized by edema, polymorphonuclear cell infiltration, vascular congestion, and necrosis.

The pathologic features of chronic cholecystitis vary. The gallbladder may be contracted or enlarged. The gallbladder wall is thickened, and the mucosal folds may be flattened. The lumen contains clear, mucoid bile; formed stones usually are present. Ninety percent of all gallstones are made of calcium bilirubinate and calcium carbonate. Rarely, gallstones consist primarily of cholesterol. Microscopic features of chronic cholecystitis include increased subepithelial fibrosis and an infiltrate of lymphocytes, plasma cells, macrophages, and mononuclear cells. Cholesterolosis occurs when crystals of cholesterol are deposited in the submucosal macrophages of the gallbladder.

EPIDEMIOLOGY

The incidence of cholecystitis in children ranges from less than 1% to 4%. Although this disorder is less common in children than in adults, its frequency in childhood appears to be increasing. Girls are affected more commonly than are boys after adolescence. Both sexes are affected equally before this age. The occurrence of cholecystitis in the white population is almost twice that in the black population. Acute and chronic cholecystitis, with or without gallstones, has been reported in all age ranges and may even occur in the fetus. Approximately 40% of all pediatric cases occur in children less than 11 years of age and 60% occur in children 11 to 20 years of age. Acalculous cholecystitis affects younger children more commonly, and calculous cholecystitis occurs more frequently in adolescents.

PREDISPOSING FACTORS

Several entities have been implicated as predisposing factors for cholecystitis in children (Table 369.2). Hemolytic disease, including congenital spherocytosis, sickle cell anemia, and thalassemia, has been found in more than one-third of children with cholecystitis and gallstones. Children who receive cyclosporine in conjunction with heart transplantation are known to be at risk for cholecystitis, possibly because of hepatotoxicity and bile stasis. Children who are maintained on total parenteral nutrition for more than 4 weeks are at risk of developing biliary tract disease due to bile stasis. Ileal abnormalities, particularly ileal resection and the loss of the ileocecal valve associated with necrotizing enterocolitis, intestinal atresia, short gut syndrome, cystic fibrosis, cirrhosis, or Crohn disease, potentiate the development of biliary tract disease and

TABLE 369.2

FACTORS ASSOCIATED WITH CHOLECYSTITIS IN CHILDHOOD

Factors	Frequency (% of Cases)
Hemolytic disease	37
Ileal abnormalities	37
Pregnancy	31
Obesity	27
Total parenteral nutrition	19
Infection	12
Family history of biliary disease	12
Previous abdominal surgery	9
Cystic fibrosis	7
Biliary tract anomalies	6
Cirrhosis	4
Trauma	1
Other (congenital anomalies, drugs, ventilatory support)	<1

gallstone formation. Pregnancy, with its attendant hormonal alterations, and obesity each are associated with approximately 30% of the cases of cholecystitis and cholelithiasis.

Bacterial (e.g., *Salmonella, Shigella, Yersinia, Aerobacter, Brucella, Pseudomonas, Staphylococcus*, group B streptococci, *Leptospira, Listeria, Escherichia coli, Clostridium, Vibrio cholerae*), fungal (*Candida albicans*), parasitic (*Giardia, Ascaris, Leishmania donovani*), and protozoan (*Cryptosporidium, Plasmodium falciparum*) infections, viral gastroenteritis, infectious hepatitis (type A), urinary tract infections, sepsis, Kawasaki disease, measles, scarlet fever, endocarditis, and pneumonia have been implicated as causes of acalculous cholecystitis.

A family history of biliary or hepatic disease may be identified in 12% of the children with cholecystitis. Abdominal, cardiac, and scoliosis surgery, bone marrow transplantation, burn injury, blunt abdominal trauma, and shock have been associated with cholecystitis. Congenital or acquired malformations of the biliary tract (e.g., septate gallbladder, choledochal cyst, stenosis of the cystic duct, biliary dyskinesia) and anomalies of other organs (e.g., exstrophy of the bladder, rectal atresia, hypospadias, tracheoesophageal fistula, pulmonary stenosis, skeletal anomalies) have been noted in children with cholecystitis. Other factors such as drugs (e.g., furosemide, narcotics) and ventilatory support have been associated with cholecystitis.

CLINICAL FEATURES

The clinical presentation of cholecystitis varies from total absence of symptoms to florid illness. The symptoms of cholecystitis in children are similar to those in adults (Table 369.3). Episodic abdominal pain localized to the right upper quadrant and epigastrium or radiating to the back or shoulder is the most common complaint and occurs in two-thirds of the children with cholecystitis. Abdominal tenderness, generalized or localized to the right upper quadrant, is found on examination in at least two-thirds of the children with cholecystitis. Vomiting and dietary fat intolerance affect 30% to 40% of patients. Jaundice develops in at least one-third of the patients and is more common in children than in adults. Jaundice usually is attributed to inflammation around the common duct rather than to obstruction secondary to choledocholithiasis. Fever occurs in at least one-fourth of the patients. Infrequently, a mass (hydrops) may be palpated and may be associated with acute acalculous cholecystitis. Symptoms may be noticed for only a

TABLE 369.3

CLINICAL FEATURES OF CHOLECYSTITIS IN CHILDHOOD

Finding	Frequency (% of Cases)
Symptom	
Abdominal pain	67
Right upper quadrant	79
Epigastrium	19
Radiation to back, shoulder	38
Vomiting	41
Dietary fat intolerance	33
Sign	
Abdominal tenderness	68
Jaundice	35
Fever	27
Mass	17

few days, but they may be present as long as 10 years before the correct diagnosis of cholecystitis is made.

LABORATORY AND RADIOGRAPHIC STUDIES

Although leukocytosis and elevated serum bilirubin and alkaline phosphatase levels may be found in many patients, laboratory studies, including liver function tests, are of limited diagnostic value. A complete blood cell count and hemoglobin electrophoresis may be indicated to determine the presence of an underlying hemolytic disorder.

Abdominal ultrasonography is the most effective, noninvasive method of delineating gallbladder dilation, thickened walls, and the presence of stones in the gallbladder or common bile and hepatic ducts (Fig. 369.1). Oral cholecystography is not performed any longer because of the accuracy of ultrasonography. Computed tomography (CT) scans may be obtained for more global diagnostic purposes. Sonography and CT scans are reported to be highly sensitive (92%) and highly specific (96%).

Hepatobiliary imaging with a ^{99m}Tc-labeled iminodiacetic acid derivative may be useful to demonstrate a nonfunctioning gallbladder in acute cholecystitis. Cholecystokinin-stimulated hepatobiliary scans may be useful to detect gallbladder dyskinesia associated with chronic cholecystitis. Endoscopic retrograde cholangiopancreatography (ERCP) may be indicated in the presence of obstructive jaundice and recurrent pancreatitis, both of which may be found in the presence of cholelithiasis.

An abdominal flat plate serendipitously may show asymptomatic calcified gallstones. Because gallstones are not calcified in at least 50% of children, they will not be seen on a plain roentgenogram of the abdomen. Moreover, calcifications constitute a nonspecific finding that is consistent with other diagnoses, including tuberculosis, bacterial or amebic abscesses, intrahepatic calculi, hemangioma, echinococcal cysts, neuroblastoma, or hepatic neoplasms.

DIFFERENTIAL DIAGNOSIS

Cholecystitis may mimic other diseases and cause a significant delay in the correct diagnosis. In various studies, 13% of the children with cholecystitis were given the preoperative diagnosis of appendicitis, and 21% with sickle cell disease were diagnosed initially as having a sickle cell crisis. Cholecystitis should be considered early in the differential diagnosis of abdominal pain, especially in high-risk children who have a family history of gallbladder or sickle cell disease.

The principal conditions to consider in the differential diagnosis of cholecystitis are appendicitis, pancreatitis, gastroesophageal reflux, esophagitis, peptic ulcer disease, hepatitis, hepatic abscess or tumor, intussusception, pyelonephritis or nephrolithiasis, and pneumonitis. Acute appendicitis is the disease most often confused with acute cholecystitis. Colicky abdominal pain, fever, and leukocytosis are the clinical features more typical of cholecystitis. A preoperative diagnosis of cholecystitis and cholelithiasis should be made by ultrasonography. Laparoscopy or laparotomy can resolve the diagnostic dilemma.

Cholecystitis may be difficult to differentiate from acute pancreatitis because these illnesses have similar clinical features and because serum amylase levels may be elevated in acute cholecystitis although the pancreas is normal. Pancreatitis may occur in conjunction with acute cholecystitis. Cholelithiasis may cause acute pancreatitis as stones traverse the common bile duct and ampulla of Vater. Abdominal ultrasound scans may aid in the differential diagnosis of pancreatitis and cholecystitis. Gastroesophageal reflux, esophagitis, or peptic ulcer

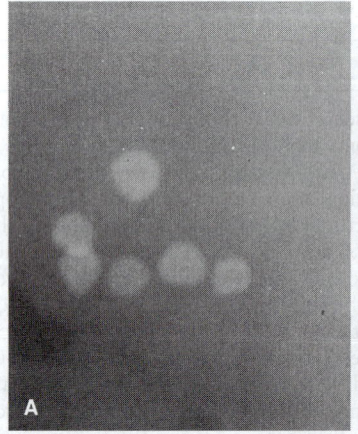
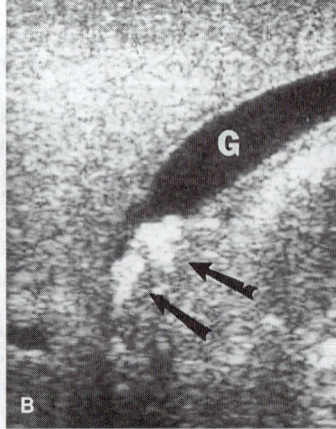
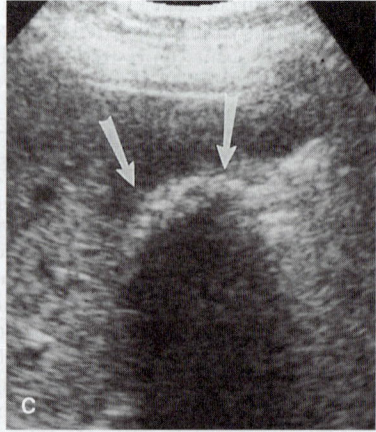

FIGURE 369.1. Gallstones. **A:** Note the calcified gallstones in a patient with sickle cell disease. **B:** A conglomeration of gallstones (*arrows*) located in the neck of the gallbladder (*G*). **C:** Sonogram of the gallbladder demonstrates an echogenic arc (*arrows*) characteristic of a gallbladder completely filled with gallstones. (Used with permission from Swischuk LE. *Imaging of the newborn, infant, and young child,* 5th ed. Philadelphia: Lippincott Williams & Wilkins, 2004:499.)

disease may be confused with cholecystitis. Gastroesophageal endoscopy with biopsies is an appropriate test to differentiate among these entities.

The spectrum of diseases that may affect the liver (e.g., hepatitis, abscess, tumor) is broad. Multiple diagnostic modalities such as liver function tests, abdominal ultrasound, computerized tomography, or liver biopsy may be necessary to delineate the cause of the illness and eliminate the possibility of cholecystitis. Intussusception should be considered in the child with acute abdominal pain. Ultrasonography or contrast roentgenography may be necessary to rule out gastrointestinal obstruction. Renal and pulmonary disease may also be associated with abdominal pain. Abnormalities on auscultation of the lungs, urinalysis, and appropriate radiographic studies should clarify these issues.

TREATMENT

The treatment of acute cholecystitis includes hospitalization, hydration with intravenous fluids, correction of electrolyte abnormalities, and discontinuation of oral feedings. Medications (e.g., meperidine) should be administered for pain relief. Antibiotics, such as ampicillin and gentamicin, are used to treat acute cholecystitis because they are excreted in bile or provide adequate coverage for enteric organisms. Second- or third-generation cephalosporins (e.g., cefoperazone, cefoxitin, cefotaxime) may be an alternate choice, particularly in protracted biliary disease. Antimicrobial therapy alone may be curative in selected cases of acalculous cholecystitis. Antihelminthic and antispasmodic drugs should be used to treat helminthic causes of cholecystitis. ERCP may be required to treat the obstructive complications associated with helminthic infestations.

Laparoscopic cholecystectomy is the treatment of choice for the management of uncomplicated acute cholecystitis. The current recommendation is to proceed with surgery 3 to 7 days after bowel rest and antibiotics have been initiated. Nearly all children respond to medical management, thereby allowing surgery to be performed safely. If the child does not respond to bowel rest and antibiotics, or complications of cholecystitis are apparent, surgery must be performed immediately. If the child's condition is precarious, cholecystostomy may be the preferred temporary procedure. Urgent cholecystectomy under these circumstances has been associated with a high rate of surgical complications. Lithotripsy with oral bile acid therapy is not a satisfactory alternative to cholecystectomy and has limited use in children.

Laparoscopic cholecystectomy is considered to be the treatment of choice for chronic cholecystitis, particularly in the case of symptomatic cholelithiasis. Controversy exists about the treatment of asymptomatic cholelithiasis in children. Because spontaneous disappearance of gallstones in infancy has been reported, a period of observation for 9 to 12 months of the asymptomatic patient who has sludge or noncalcified stones in the gallbladder may be warranted. However, elective cholecystectomy is advised for all symptomatic patients, those with calcified stones, and those asymptomatic patients with or without underlying medical disorders, in whom sludge or noncalcified stones do not resolve after 9 to 12 months. The operative mortality rate for open or laparoscopic cholecystectomy is less than 1% for children. Operative cholangiography and exploration of the common duct are indicated for choledochal stones, recurrent pancreatitis, a history of jaundice, serum bilirubin levels greater than 6 mg/dL, or dilation of the common bile duct. However, ductular stones have been identified in only 6% of the children who have undergone cholecystectomy. ERCP may be a valuable prelaparoscopic adjunct to identify the patient who may require a choledochal exploration. ERCP may identify ductal stones in patients who present with jaundice and ultrasound findings of either choledocholithiasis or a dilated common bile duct. ERCP with sphincterotomy may be the initial procedure for extraction of ductular stones if they do not pass spontaneously.

COMPLICATIONS

The major complications of acute cholecystitis are gangrene, empyema, and perforation, the latter of which may manifest initially as a localized pericholecystic abscess, with subsequent extension into the peritoneal cavity and generalized peritonitis or the formation of a cholecystenteric fistula, primarily with the duodenum or the hepatic flexure of the colon. Surgical intervention is indicated for these complications. Less frequently, ascending cholangitis, liver abscess, or sepsis may complicate the clinical course of acute cholecystitis.

The complications of chronic cholecystitis in the absence of cholelithiasis are minimal. Patients with gallstones are at risk for recurrent bouts of acute cholecystitis, pancreatitis, perforation, bile peritonitis, biliary obstruction, biliary cirrhosis, and cancer of the gallbladder.

PROGNOSIS

The prognosis after surgery for children with cholecystitis but without underlying hemolytic disease is excellent. The overall mortality rate for acute and chronic cholecystitis is less than 2% for children. Ten-year follow-up of children with gallbladder disease detected no further illness after cholecystectomy in 97% of patients. In children with hemolytic disorders, 82% had resolution of their episodes of abdominal pain and jaundice for as long as 6 years after cholecystectomy.

Acknowledgments

This work is a publication of the U. S. Department of Agriculture (USDA)/Agricultural Research Service (ARS) Children's Nutrition Research Center, Department of Pediatrics, Baylor College of Medicine, and Texas Children's Hospital in Houston, Texas. This project has been funded in part with federal funds from the ARS of the USDA under Cooperative Agreement number 58-7MN1-6-100. The contents of this publication do not necessarily reflect the views or policies of the USDA, nor does mention of trade names, commercial products, or organizations imply endorsement by the U.S. government.

Suggested Readings

Bahu Mda G, Baldisseroto M, Custodio CM, et al. Hepatobiliary and pancreatic complications of ascariasis in children: a study of seven cases. *J Pediatr Gastroenterol Nutr* 2001;33:271.

Bailey PV, Connors RH, Tracy TF, et al. Changing spectrum of cholelithiasis and cholecystitis in infants and children. *Am J Surg* 1989;158:585.

Chirdan LB, Iya D, Ramyil VM, et al. Acalculous cholecystitis in Nigerian children. *Pediatr Surg Int* 2003;19:65.

Clements RH, Holcombe GW III. Laparoscopic cholecystectomy. *Curr Opin Pediatr* 1998;10:310.

Debray D, Pariente D, Gautier F, et al. Cholelithiasis in infancy: a study of 40 cases. *J Pediatr* 1993;122:385.

Holcombe GW III, Morgan WM III, Neblett WW III, et al. Laparoscopic cholecystectomy in children: lessons learned from the first 100 patients. *J Pediatr Surg* 1999;34:1236.

Kikiros C, Arunachalam P, Lam MH. Adenomatous hyperplastic polyp of the gallbladder associated with cholelithiasis in a child. *Pediatr Surg Int* 2003; 19:118.

Lobe TE. Cholelithiasis and cholecystitis in children. *Semin Pediatr Surg* 2000; 9:170.

Safford SD, Safford KM, Martin P, et al. Management of cholelithiasis in pediatric patients who undergo bone marrow transplantation. *J Pediatr Surg* 2001;36:86.

Sakopoulos AG, Gundry S, Razzouk AJ, et al. Cholelithiasis in infant and pediatric heart transplant patients. *Pediatr Transplant* 2002;6:231.

CHAPTER 370 ■ CIRRHOSIS

WILLIAM J. COCHRAN

Cirrhosis is a chronic liver disease characterized by a marked increase in connective tissue and by diffuse destruction and regeneration of hepatic parenchymal cells. Fibrosis results from the accumulation of excess extracellular matrix and is potentially reversible. Conversely, cirrhosis is an irreversible state in which portal areas are bridged by fibrous connective tissue, which results in the formation of regenerative nodules. The word *cirrhosis* comes from the Greek word *kirrhos*, which means tawny. This term was used because the liver was a tawny color in the first recognized type of cirrhosis, alcoholic cirrhosis. Cirrhosis is the final or end stage of chronic liver disease and is secondary to many causes. Pediatricians should have a basic knowledge of the disorder and its inevitable complications. This chapter reviews the classification, causes, complications, and treatment of cirrhosis.

CLASSIFICATION

Cirrhosis has been classified according to morphologic, histologic, and etiologic findings. Little correlation is found between the cause and the pathology, because the liver reacts to insults in a limited number of ways, and cirrhosis is the final stage of response. The etiologic classification is probably the most practical for clinicians, although others are discussed briefly because they are mentioned frequently in the literature. The exact mechanism of the development of cirrhosis is unknown but is an area of active research. The major etiologic categories of pediatric cirrhosis include biliary tract disorders; genetic and metabolic disorders; infectious, cardiac, immune, nutritional, drug-related, and toxin-related disorders; and miscellaneous diseases (Box 370.1). Because many cases represent inherited diseases, determining the cause and providing appropriate genetic counseling is important. In most cases, determination of the cause of cirrhosis does not alter the therapeutic plan for the affected child.

The morphologic classification characterizes the gross appearance of the liver according to the size of the nodule. It identifies three major groups: micronodular, macronodular, and mixed micronodular and macronodular (Box 370.2). Micronodular cirrhosis consists of diffuse, small nodules less than 3 mm in diameter. It is commonly found in alcohol-induced cirrhosis. Patients with biliary atresia, Indian childhood cirrhosis, and hemochromatosis may have micronodular cirrhosis.

Macronodular cirrhosis consists of different-sized nodules, most greater than 3 mm in diameter, some several centimeters

---

BOX 370.1   Etiologic Classification of Cirrhosis

Biliary tract disorders
  Biliary atresia
  Choledochal cysts
  Caroli disease
  Intrahepatic bile duct paucity
    Alagille syndrome
    Nonsyndromic
  Congenital hepatic fibrosis
  Cystic fibrosis
  Primary sclerosing cholangitis
Genetic and metabolic disorders
  Alpha-1-antitrypsin deficiency
  Disorders associated with copper
    Wilson disease
    Indian childhood cirrhosis
  Disorders associated with iron
    Hemochromatosis
    Juvenile hemochromatosis
    Neonatal iron storage disease
    Iron overload
  Progressive familial intrahepatic cholestasis
  Galactosemia
  Hereditary fructose intolerance
  Hereditary tyrosinemia
  Glycogen storage disease

Lipid storage disorders
  Wolman disease
  Niemann-Pick disease
  Gaucher disease
Peroxisomal disease
  Zellweger syndrome
  Refsum disease
  Neonatal adrenoleukodystrophy
Mitochondrial disorders
  Complexes I, III, and IV deficiencies
  Alpers disease
  Pearson syndrome
  Mitochondrial DNA depletion syndrome
Infection
  Hepatitis B
  Hepatitis C
  Cytomegalovirus
  Syphilis
Cardiac cirrhosis
  Autoimmune disease
  Nutritional disorders
  Drugs and toxins
  Miscellaneous
    Neonatal hepatitis

in diameter. Wilson disease (i.e., hepatolenticular degeneration) and alpha-1-antitrypsin deficiency are examples of macronodular cirrhosis. Other disorders that initially appear micronodular may progress to macronodular cirrhosis if the patient lives long enough.

In mixed micronodular and macronodular cirrhosis, both types of nodules (less than and greater than 3 mm in diameter) occur in equal numbers. The cirrhosis that results from autoimmune hepatitis is characterized by this mixed type of morphology.

The histologic classification divides cirrhosis into biliary cirrhosis, postnecrotic cirrhosis, posthepatic (cardiac) cirrhosis, and unique liver disease (Box 370.3). Biliary cirrhosis is characterized clinically by cholestasis and histologically by bile stasis and increased fibrosus tissue extending from the portal areas. Examples of pediatric biliary cirrhosis include biliary atresia, progressive familial intrahepatic cholestasis, and cystic fibrosis. Postnecrotic cirrhosis is the result of chronic liver cell injury and is characterized histologically by piecemeal necrosis at the junction of the hepatocytes and the portal area. Children with neonatal hepatitis, chronic hepatitis B, and chronic hepatitis C may develop postnecrotic cirrhosis. Cardiac cirrhosis develops secondary to elevated right heart pressure, which leads to increased hepatic vein pressure and, finally, to centrilobular hemorrhagic necrosis with cirrhosis. Unlike the morphologic classification, which is nonspecific, the histologic classification may enable precise determination of the cause of the disease, such

as Wilson disease with increased copper deposition; hemochromatosis with excessive iron deposition; and alpha-1-antitrypsin deficiency with periodic acid-Schiff positive, diastase-resistant granules.

SPECIFIC DISEASES THAT CAUSE CIRRHOSIS

Biliary Tract Disorders

Biliary Atresia

Biliary tract disorders are responsible for the greatest number of cases of cirrhosis in the pediatric population; extrahepatic biliary atresia is most common (see also Chapter 367, Disorders of the Liver and Biliary System). Biliary atresia is a progressive inflammatory cholangiopathy that results in fibrosis and complete obstruction of the extrahepatic biliary tree.

Biliary atresia is the most common cause of cholestasis in nonpremature infants 0 to 3 months of age and is the single most common pediatric etiology requiring liver transplantation. The incidence of biliary atresia is 1 in 8,000 to 12,000 live births with a female-to-male ratio of 1.2:1.0. Approximately 10% of patients with biliary atresia have associated anomalies such as malrotation and polysplenia. Biliary atresia is the result of progressive obliteration of the extrahepatic biliary tree; it appears to be an acquired disorder rather than a consequence of abnormal development, as evidenced by the rare occurrence of biliary atresia in autopsied fetuses and premature newborns. Many theories regarding the etiology of biliary atresia have been proposed. For additional details about these theories, see Box 370.4.

Clinical Manifestations. Biliary atresia presents clinically as cholestasis in the first several months of life. Some have divided this disorder into two major types, classic or perinatal and embryonic or fetal type. The classic type accounts for the greatest number of cases and is characterized by patent ducts at birth that subsequently become obliterated secondary to inflammation. This type of biliary atresia is uncommonly associated with other congenital anomalies. The second type, embryonic or fetal, has an earlier onset of cholestasis and is more commonly associated with other congenital anomalies such as polysplenia.

Diagnosis. Unfortunately, no laboratory tests or radiographic studies exist that accurately differentiate biliary atresia from other cholestatic disorders of the newborn such as neonatal hepatitis. Total and direct bilirubin are elevated as are liver enzymes, in particular gamma-glutamyltransferase (GGT). Indeed, some authors feel that if an infant with cholestasis has a GGT in excess of 500 the diagnosis is biliary atresia until proven otherwise. A hepatobiliary scan can be helpful in ruling out the diagnosis of biliary atresia by demonstrating excretion of the tracer by the liver into the intestinal tract. Lack of excretion, however, is a nonspecific finding. The best diagnostic test, other than exploratory laparotomy, is percutaneous needle biopsy of the liver. The histologic hallmark of biliary atresia is bile duct proliferation and a widened portal area. The liver biopsy is a sensitive diagnostic test; if the described findings are present, exploratory laparotomy and intraoperative cholangiography are indicated. More recently, endoscopic retrograde cholangiopancreatography has been used to evaluate the extrahepatic biliary system in infants with cholestasis, although this procedure can be difficult to perform in infants.

Treatment. If biliary atresia is found during laparotomy, a Kasai procedure (i.e., portoenterostomy) should be performed.

BOX 370.4   Etiology of Biliary Atresia

The three most prominent theories are (a) viral infection, (b) an immune-mediated process, and (c) a defect in morphogenesis. The two viruses that have received the most attention are reovirus type 3 and group C rotavirus. One study noted that 62% of infants with biliary atresia had antibodies to reovirus type 3, whereas 52% of infants with neonatal hepatitis and 12% of normal infants had such antibodies. Another study documented that mice injected intraperitoneally with reovirus type 3 develop a lesion similar to biliary atresia. A more recent study demonstrated reovirus RNA in the liver and bile ducts of infants with biliary atresia as well as those with choledochal cyst at a greater rate than infants with neonatal hepatitis. Rotavirus has also been implicated in the development of biliary atresia. A multicenter study demonstrated that 10 of 20 patients with biliary atresia had group C rotavirus (detected by polymerase chain reaction), whereas none of the control patients tested positive. Rotavirus, like reovirus, when provided to mice has been noted to result in a lesion similar to biliary atresia.

An immune-mediated process has also been implicated in the pathogenesis of biliary atresia. This theory was first proposed because the inflammatory infiltrate present in the bile ducts of biliary atresia is similar to that seen in primary sclerosing cholangitis, an immune disorder. The increased frequency of HLA-B12 and of haplotypes A9-B5 and A28-B35 in infants with biliary atresia compared to healthy children supports this premise.

Defects in morphogenesis have also been postulated as a cause of biliary atresia. There is remodeling of the primitive bile ducts that results in the final development of the biliary tree. Defects in this process secondary to genes or a defective protein could result in biliary atresia. The term that has been used to describe this process is *ductal plate malformation*.

Controversy surrounds the use of the Kasai procedure when the infant is older than 3 months and shows advanced fibrosis because patients with biliary atresia who undergo surgery after the age of 3 months have a poor prognosis. These infants have a 10-year survival rate of approximately 13% without liver transplantation, compared with 57% for infants in whom surgery is performed before the age of 2 months. Moreover, if liver transplantation is required, the surgical procedure may be more difficult if abdominal surgery has been performed previously. Unfortunately, 80% of patients, even if operated on before 3 months of age, develop cirrhosis and require a liver transplant.

Choledochal Cysts

Choledochal cysts are a relatively uncommon cause of cirrhosis; the incidence is 1 in 13,000 to 15,000 live births (see also Chapter 367). Females are affected four times more frequently than are males. Five major types of choledochal cysts are found. Type I is a congenital cystic dilation of the common bile duct and is the most common type of choledochal cyst. Type II choledochal cyst is a diverticular outpouching of the common bile duct. Type III is a choledochocele with an ampullary obstruction. Type IV has both extrahepatic and intrahepatic bile duct

cystic dilations. Type V, or Caroli disease, consists of intrahepatic bile duct cysts. Although patients may present with a choledochal cyst at any age, approximately one-third of patients present in the first year of life and more than two-thirds in the first 6 years of life. The classic triad of abdominal pain, right upper quadrant mass, and jaundice is present in only 10% to 20% of patients. More commonly, patients with a choledochal cyst present with jaundice, abdominal pain, vomiting, acholic stools, or hepatomegaly. A choledochal cyst can be diagnosed with abdominal ultrasonography, which may reveal cystic dilations of the intrahepatic and extrahepatic biliary trees. A hepatobiliary scan can aid in the diagnosis by showing a rounded extrahepatic structure that retains the tracer and is distinguishable from the gallbladder. More recently, endoscopic retrograde cholangiopancreatography (ERCP) and magnetic retrograde cholangiopancreatography (MRCP) have been utilized to more specifically look at the biliary anatomy. If untreated, patients develop cirrhosis. A high incidence of cholangiocarcinoma is seen in this patient population. The incidence varies from 2% to 26% in patients who remain untreated and is up to 50% in those who had an enteric drainage procedure with the cyst still present. A higher incidence of cancer in the gallbladder also appears to exist. Treatment consists of excision of the cyst and performance of a choledochojejunostomy and a cholecystectomy.

Congenital segmental dilation of the intrahepatic biliary tree may progress to cirrhosis. Caroli disease, an autosomal recessive disorder, is characterized by hepatomegaly and dilated intrahepatic ducts that contain bile. A significant potential exists for the formation of stones within these dilated ducts and for the development of cholangitis. Although affected patients tend not to develop cirrhosis, a subset of patients has severe periportal fibrosis and do develop cirrhosis.

Intrahepatic Bile Duct Paucity

Intrahepatic bile duct paucity refers to a group of disorders characterized by a reduction or absence of bile ductules in the portal triads of the liver. Rather than the one to two bile ductules usually found per portal triad, the paucity syndromes are characterized by less than one-half bile duct per triad. This group of disorders can be subdivided into two major categories: syndromic and nonsyndromic. The syndromic form comprises Alagille syndrome (i.e., arteriohepatic dysplasia). The incidence of Alagille syndrome is 1:2,500 live births. In addition to the paucity of intrahepatic bile ducts, Alagille syndrome is associated with at least two of the four major associated abnormalities: abnormal facies (see Chapter 462), congenital heart disease, ocular abnormalities, and vertebral arch defects. The typical facial pattern is characterized by a broad forehead, mild hypertelorism, a straight nose, and a small, pointed chin. The most common congenital heart defect is pulmonary valve stenosis while peripheral pulmonic stenosis is the most common vascular disorder. Posterior embryotoxin in the anterior chamber of the eye is the most frequently noted ocular abnormality. Other potential associated anomalies include growth retardation, pancreatic insufficiency, mental retardation, hypogonadism, and renal abnormalities. Alagille syndrome is inherited in an autosomal dominant fashion, although a spontaneous mutation rate of 15% to 50% is seen. The gene responsible for this disorder, *Jagged I*, was identified in 1997. The clinical spectrum of this disorder is large. Some individuals will have mild liver disease while others will develop liver failure and require liver transplantation in the first year of life. Treatment is primarily supportive. Prognosis for patients with Alagille syndrome is variable. Survival in patients with their native liver is 51% and 38% at 10 and 20 years, respectively. Most patients die of liver disease, heart disease, or infections. Ten to twenty percent of these patients develop cirrhosis. It has been estimated that 30% to 50% of patients require liver transplantation by 19 years of age due to cirrhosis, pruritus, or osteodystrophy. Patients with Alagille syndrome and cirrhosis are at increased risk for developing hepatic malignancy.

The nonsyndromic form comprises intrahepatic bile duct paucity that is not due to Alagille syndrome. This form includes bile duct paucity with and without an associated primary disorder. Disorders that may be associated with a decreased number of bile ducts include cystic fibrosis, alpha-1-antitrypsin deficiency, Down syndrome, hypopituitarism, inborn errors of bile acid metabolism, and graft-versus-host disease. The prognosis for these patients depends on the underlying disorder. Those with intrahepatic bile duct paucity but no associated disorder typically do not progress to severe liver disease; however, isolated reports have noted a rate of cirrhosis of up to 50% in such patients.

Congenital Hepatic Fibrosis

Congenital hepatic fibrosis is a rare autosomal recessive disorder characterized by the formation of multiple bands of fibrous tissue running throughout the liver and dysmorphic bile ducts within the fibrous tissue. The exact cause is unknown, but the condition is thought to be secondary to abnormal development of the bile ducts. Most patients have associated renal disease in the form of renal tubular ectasia or autosomal recessive polycystic kidney disease. The clinical manifestations are variable and age dependent; infants present primarily with renal disease and older patients present primarily with liver disease. Those with liver disease tend to show hepatosplenomegaly, especially of the left lobe, and portal hypertension. They may also develop cholangitis, biliary calculi, and intrahepatic abscesses. Therapy is supportive.

Cystic Fibrosis

Cystic fibrosis is the most common lethal genetic disease affecting whites (see also Chapter 236). It is inherited in an autosomal recessive pattern and is found in approximately 1 in 2,000 live births. The lungs and pancreas are the primary organs affected, although multiple organ systems are involved. Hepatobiliary disorders occur in 20% to 60% of patients with cystic fibrosis, and the incidence increases with age. Ten to thirty-five percent of patients with cystic fibrosis will have asymptomatic elevation of their liver function tests. Hepatic steatosis is the most common liver abnormality, occurring in at least one-third of patients with cystic fibrosis. This complication is in part secondary to malnutrition, which is prevalent in these patients. Thirty percent of patients have microgallbladders, and 5% to 10% have cholelithiasis. Some infants with cystic fibrosis present with neonatal cholestasis secondary to sludge in the biliary tree. Patients with cystic fibrosis may develop focal biliary cirrhosis or multilobular cirrhosis, although cirrhosis rarely is the presenting manifestation of cystic fibrosis. Focal biliary cirrhosis occurs in 10% to 60% of patients with cystic fibrosis. Histologically, this lesion is characterized by inspissation of eosinophilic microprotein in the bile ducts, bile duct proliferation, chronic inflammation, and portal fibrosis. Focal biliary cirrhosis is of little clinical consequence. Multilobular cirrhosis, on the other hand, is very significant clinically and can lead to end-stage liver disease requiring liver transplantation. As with other liver diseases associated with cystic fibrosis, the incidence of multilobular cirrhosis increases with age; it is present in approximately 5% of patients older than 12 years and 10% to 15% of those older than 25 years. Due to the frequency of liver disease in patients with cystic fibrosis, it is recommended that all patients have liver blood tests performed on an annual basis.

Medical management is primarily supportive with nutritional therapy being the mainstay. Administration of ursodeoxycholic acid, 20 mg per kg per day in two divided doses, to patients with cystic fibrosis and liver disease has led to improvements in liver enzyme levels, but the long-term effect on the course of liver disease is still unknown.

Primary Sclerosing Cholangitis

Primary sclerosing cholangitis is a chronic inflammatory disease of unknown cause that rarely occurs in children. It is characterized by progressive fibrosis of the intrahepatic and extrahepatic biliary ducts. These ducts are best visualized by ERCP, which reveals multiple focal areas of stricture and irregularities. Three categories are identified, based on age of onset and the presence of associated disease states: primary sclerosing cholangitis of neonatal onset (27% of cases), that of postneonatal onset associated with a disease (55%), and that of postneonatal onset not associated with another disease (18%). Sclerosing cholangitis in the pediatric population is most commonly associated with inflammatory bowel disease (80%). Other disorders associated with primary sclerosing cholangitis include autoimmune thyroiditis, histiocytosis X, or immunodeficiency states. Patients commonly present with abdominal pain, fatigue, jaundice, and hepatosplenomegaly. Liver enzyme levels, in particular GGT, are almost always elevated. Two-thirds of individuals have hypergammaglobulinemia and in 70% antinuclear antibody (ANA) and anti-smooth muscle antibodies are present. Liver biopsy reveals portal fibrosis, ductular proliferation, and pericholangitis. The progression to frank cirrhosis is inevitable, although it tends to occur 5 to 10 years after diagnosis. Multiple medications have been used in an attempt to halt the progression of this disease; some, such as ursodeoxycholic acid, may result in improvement of liver enzyme levels, but they do not appear to alter the progression of the disease. Liver transplantation is the only life-extending therapeutic option for end-stage liver disease.

Genetic and Metabolic Disorders

Alpha-1-Antitrypsin Deficiency

Alpha-1-antitrypsin deficiency (described in more detail in Chapter 367) is the prototypic genetic and metabolic disorder resulting in cirrhosis in pediatric patients. It is the most common genetic cause of liver disease in the pediatric population. In addition, this disorder is the most common inherited disorder for which liver transplantation is required. Alpha-1-antitrypsin is an acute-phase reactant that is synthesized in the liver and is the major antiproteolytic agent in the body. Alpha-1-antitrypsin deficiency is a disorder of glycoprotein metabolism with a prevalence of 1 in 1,600 to 1,800 persons. The gene responsible for the deficiency state resides on chromosome 14 and is associated with a single amino acid substitution resulting in the production of an abnormal protein. The liver disease associated with alpha-1-antitrypsin deficiency is believed to be the result of the accumulation of this abnormal protein, which undergoes polymerization that is concentration and temperature dependent. The diagnosis is made by determining the phenotype or Pi (protease inhibitor) type (Box 370.5).

The disorder can manifest in infancy, childhood, or adulthood. In infancy, patients present with cholestasis, bleeding (in the gastrointestinal tract or central nervous system, or from the umbilical stump), or transaminase elevation. In childhood or adulthood, patients present with chronic hepatitis, cirrhosis, or portal hypertension. A strong association also is seen between alpha-1-antitrypsin deficiency and the development of emphysema in young adults.

Genetics of Alpha-1-Antitrypsin Deficiency

Normal individuals are protease inhibitor (Pi) MM, and individuals homozygotic for the deficiency are PiZZ. PiZZ persons have 15% to 20% of the normal alpha-1-antitrypsin levels; PiMZ and PiSS persons have levels 60% and 65% of normal, respectively. Interestingly, most individuals with the PiZZ phenotype are normal; only 10% to 15% of these individuals have demonstrable liver disease. Although rare, liver disease has been reported in patients with the PiMZ and PiSZ phenotypes. PiNull is associated with no detectable level of alpha-1-antitrypsin and these individuals do not develop liver disease, supporting the premise that it is the accumulation of the abnormal protein that results in the liver disease rather than a low level of the normal protein. Because alpha-1-antitrypsin is an acute-phase reactant, PiZZ individuals may have a low-normal level of alpha-1-antitrypsin when an acute infection is present. Liver biopsy can also be useful in making the diagnosis. PiZZ individuals have an accumulation of periodic acid-Schiff–positive, diastase-resistant eosinophilic granules in the hepatocytes located primarily in the periportal area. These eosinophilic granules may be difficult to find in the first several months of life.

Treatment is primarily supportive unless severe liver disease ensues, in which case liver transplantation is curative. Intermittent intravenous infusion of purified alpha-1-antitrypsin from plasma has normalized serum alpha-1-antitrypsin levels and halted the progression of lung disease in adults. This therapy offers little benefit to those with liver disease because the liver pathology is secondary to the retained abnormal protein and is not due to the low serum levels of alpha-1-antitrypsin. The prognosis for pediatric patients with liver disease is more favorable than believed previously when the studies were hospital based. In a long-term study, Swedish children with alpha-1-antitrypsin deficiency and liver disease in infancy were followed from infancy to 18 years of age. Eleven percent died in infancy of liver disease; another 11% died as young children of other causes but at autopsy showed cirrhosis or fibrosis. The other 78% had no clinically demonstrable liver disease at 18 years of age; 13% of these had minimally elevated liver enzymes with normal procollagen, a marker of fibrogenesis in liver disease.

Disorders Associated with Copper

Wilson Disease

Wilson disease (i.e., hepatolenticular degeneration) is an inherited disorder of copper metabolism (see also Chapter 367). The prevalence of Wilson disease is approximately 1 in 30,000 to 100,000. Wilson disease is an autosomal recessive disorder; the gene responsible for the defect in copper metabolism is *ATP7B* located on chromosome 13. The defect in copper metabolism appears to result from decreased incorporation of copper into ceruloplasmin, thus limiting excretion of copper out of the hepatocyte as well as other cells. As a result, there is accumulation of copper in the cells of most organs, especially the liver, brain, and kidneys.

Wilson disease is usually detected in patients after 5 years of age; however, case reports are found of patients as young as 2 years. Many presentations are possible, although younger patients usually present with liver disease and older patients with neurologic symptoms. The liver disease can manifest as acute or chronic hepatitis, steatohepatitis, cholestasis, portal hypertension, cirrhosis, or liver failure. The neurologic symptoms range from deterioration in handwriting and personality changes to athetoid movements, Parkinson-like state, and psychosis. Patients with Wilson disease may have other extrahepatic manifestations, including hemolytic anemia, arrhythmias, arthropathy, osteomalacia and skeletal fractures, renal tubular acidosis, or Fanconi syndrome.

The diagnosis of Wilson disease is based on the physical examination (presence of Kayser-Fleischer rings), increased level of urinary copper excretion, and decreased serum copper and ceruloplasmin levels. The copper content of the liver is significantly elevated. Kayser-Fleischer rings result from the deposition of copper in Descemet membrane of the cornea. These rings increase in size with the duration of the disease and resolve over time with appropriate therapy. The finding of Kayser-Fleischer rings is essentially diagnostic. Genetic testing is also available for research purposes.

Therapy is directed toward achieving and maintaining a negative copper balance for life. Penicillamine, which chelates copper, is used when significant copper overload exists. It is not typically used in those with neurologic symptoms since it is associated with worsening of neurologic symptoms in 10% to 50% of cases. Triethylene tetramine (trientine hydrochloride) also chelates copper and is used in those who do not tolerate penicillamine. Maintenance therapy consists of a reduction in dietary copper and the use of zinc acetate to decrease absorption of dietary copper. A newer therapeutic alternative is ammonium tetrathiomolybdate, which has two anticopper mechanisms. Ammonium tetrathiomolybdate binds with dietary copper, limiting its absorption. In addition, it also complexes with copper and albumin, rendering copper unavailable for uptake by cells. Liver transplantation can be performed for end-stage liver disease and results in correction of the metabolic defect. Although the prognosis for untreated patients is dismal (i.e., early death is essentially universal), patients who are diagnosed early enough and treated appropriately have a normal life expectancy. If the diagnosis and appropriate therapy are delayed, permanent neurologic or hepatic damage can take place. In addition, siblings and offspring of patients with Wilson disease should be screened for this disorder with a complete physical examination, including slit lamp examination and measurement of liver enzymes, serum copper, and ceruloplasmin levels, and a 24-hour urine collection for copper.

Indian Childhood Cirrhosis

Indian childhood cirrhosis (copper-associated liver disease in childhood), a rare disorder of copper metabolism once thought to be confined to India, has now been detected in other regions, including North America and Europe. The cause of the disorder is uncertain, but it is most likely due to increased dietary copper from water or cooking utensils. Some authors believe the condition is due to an inborn error of copper metabolism because an increased incidence is seen in families with an affected child. A family history of affected siblings is present in 30% of cases. The disorder affects children 1 month to 10 years of age, with a peak incidence between 1 and 3 years. Affected patients typically present with hepatosplenomegaly and hepatitis of unknown cause.

Early in the course of the disease, the liver histology is characterized by a diffuse inflammatory process with ballooning degeneration, Mallory bodies, and fibrosis. A large amount of copper is deposited in the liver, as in Wilson disease; however, patients with Indian childhood cirrhosis do not have low ceruloplasmin levels.

Therapy with penicillamine prior to the establishment of severe liver disease has been shown to improve clinical symptoms, reduce hepatic copper content, and improve liver histology. The use of penicillamine after the establishment of cirrhosis, however, has no beneficial effect, and liver transplant is necessary for long-term survival. Death frequently occurs within 8 months of onset of symptoms if no treatment is provided. Initiation of public health measures to reduce the copper consumption of infants and young children in India has resulted in a decreased incidence of this disorder.

Disorders Associated with Iron

Hemochromatosis

Hemosiderosis, a condition characterized by increased iron stores, is associated with disorders such as hemochromatosis, juvenile hemochromatosis, neonatal iron overload syndrome (neonatal hemochromatosis), secondary iron overload (which can occur with multiple blood transfusions), alcoholic liver disease, and excessive dietary iron intake (see also Chapter 367).

Primary Hemochromatosis (Hemochromatosis Type I). Primary hemochromatosis is an autosomal recessive disorder associated with increased iron absorption leading to an increase in total body iron of 10 to 50 times that normally present. Hereditary hemochromatosis is the most common recessively inherited disease in North America, with an incidence of 3 to 6 per 1,000 persons; 10% of the population is heterozygous for this disorder. The gene is located on the short arm of chromosome 6, with more than 80% of the mutations being C282Y. This condition presents most commonly in adulthood. More pediatric patients are likely to be diagnosed with this disorder as a result of screening after the parents have been diagnosed. The iron is deposited in all organs of the body, particularly in the liver, pancreas, skin, endocrine glands, and heart.

Symptoms of hemochromatosis can be very nonspecific (i.e., fatigue and abdominal pain), and the physician must maintain a high index of suspicion to make the correct diagnosis early and prevent some of the irreversible complications. Clinical manifestations of hemochromatosis include metallic gray or bronze skin pigmentation, diabetes, hypogonadism, amenorrhea, arthropathy, cardiomyopathy, and arrhythmias. Hepatic manifestations include hepatomegaly, hepatitis, cirrhosis, and portal hypertension.

Several laboratory studies can be used in making the diagnosis of hemochromatosis. Plasma iron and transferrin saturation are elevated, although the transferrin level itself is low because of the severity of the liver disease. Transferrin saturation ([iron]/[total iron-binding capacity or transferrin level] × 100%) normally is less than 40%; those with hemochromatosis typically have values above 50%. Levels greater than 70% are almost diagnostic of hemochromatosis. Ferritin level, which reflects iron stores, is elevated and may be in the thousands. The amount of iron excreted in the urine after administration of deferoxamine is significantly increased and correlates relatively well with the quantity of excess iron stores. False-negative and false-positive results may be obtained from these tests, and additional testing may be required to confirm the diagnosis. A liver biopsy is extremely important in the evaluation of a patient with hemochromatosis. Special iron stains reveal increased iron deposition, which is greatest in zone I early in the disease and becomes panlobular with time. The liver should also be analyzed for total iron content, which is normally 200 to 2,400 μg/g of dry weight liver. Because the amount of iron increases with age, another parameter that has been proposed is the hepatic iron index (HII). The HII is the hepatic iron content in micromoles per gram divided by the patient's age in years. Normally the HII is less than 2; a value greater than 2 is typical in hemochromatosis. The liver biopsy also provides information regarding the degree of fibrosis, if any, and allows other liver pathologies to be ruled out. Further confirmation can be obtained with molecular testing to document the presence of the mutation (C282Y) in the HLA-linked iron-loading gene (HFE).

Treatment of hemochromatosis requires removal of iron from the body. Iron removal can be achieved with repeated phlebotomy or with chelation therapy. Because each pint of blood contains approximately 200 mg of iron, repeated phlebotomy for prolonged periods can remove significant quantities of iron. Phlebotomy is initially performed on a weekly basis; 7 to 10 mL/kg to a maximum of 500 mL is removed at a time. Once the ferritin level has normalized, the frequency is reduced to once every 1 to 4 months to maintain ferritin and transferrin saturation in the low normal range. Hemoglobin levels need to be monitored during this process. Chelation therapy with deferoxamine is used much less frequently because of the ease, safety, and efficacy of phlebotomy. Untreated patients die of cirrhosis or heart failure.

Screening for hereditary hemochromatosis is somewhat controversial. Clinicians generally agree that all first-degree relatives of patients with hemochromatosis should be screened; the most effective screening test is measurement of transferrin saturation. Some have advocated screening the entire population using transferrin saturation testing or genetic screening because of the frequency and potential severity of this disorder.

Juvenile Hemochromatosis (Type II Hemochromatosis). Juvenile hemochromatosis is an autosomal recessive disorder that, like type I hemochromatosis, is associated with increased iron absorption resulting in excessive iron accumulation in different organs (Table 370.1). Iron absorption is greater in type II compared to type I hemochromatosis. Juvenile hemochromatosis differs from type I hemochromatosis in multiple ways. First, this disorder is uncommon, unlike type I hemochromatosis, the most common inherited disease in North America. Juvenile hemochromatosis presents early in life with heart disease and/or hypogonadism. Type I hemochromatosis typically presents in middle-aged adults with liver disease or diabetes. The earlier onset of disease in type II is felt to be secondary to the more rapid accumulation of iron in tissues due to the greater rate of absorption. In addition, the genetic defect associated with type II hemochromatosis is located on the long arm of chromosome 1 while type I hemochromatosis is due to mutations in the HFE gene. The laboratory evaluation and liver biopsy in type II are similar to that for type I.

Treatment of type II hemochromatosis is as noted for type I.

Neonatal Iron Storage Disease

Another disorder of iron metabolism is neonatal hemochromatosis or neonatal iron storage disease (see also Chapter 367).

TABLE 370.1

COMPARISON BETWEEN TYPES I AND II HEMOCHROMATOSIS

Characteristic	Type I	Type II
Inheritance	Autosomal recessive	Autosomal recessive
Frequency	Common	Uncommon
Clinical presentation	Middle age as liver disease or diabetes mellitus	Early in life as heart disease or hypogonadism

This disorder, which is felt to be autosomal recessive, is distinct from hemochromatosis. Unlike patients with hemochromatosis, in whom the hepatic injury occurs after years of excessive iron accumulation, patients with neonatal hemochromatosis present in the first week of life with fulminant liver failure. Frequently a history of prematurity, intrauterine growth retardation, and oligohydramnios is noted. Neonatal hemochromatosis differs from most other causes of neonatal liver disease except congenital infections in that the liver disease begins *in utero* and fulminant liver disease is present in the first several days of life. These infants present with signs of liver failure including hypoalbuminemia, hyperbilirubinemia, coagulopathy, ascites, and hypoglycemia, but unlike many neonatal liver disorders, serum transaminase levels are relatively low. The pathogenesis of neonatal hemochromatosis is unknown. Many theories have been proposed, including a defect in divalent metal transporter 1 (DMT1) that transports iron across the endosomal membrane into the cytoplasm.

Diagnosis of neonatal hemochromatosis is made after other causes of neonatal liver failure have been ruled out and by having the typical laboratory and pathologic findings noted in neonatal hemochromatosis. Laboratory evaluation reveals an elevated ferritin level, low transferrin level, increased transferrin saturation, coagulopathy, cholestasis, and hyperammonemia. The low transaminase levels probably reflect a decreased amount of viable hepatocytes. Liver biopsy reveals diffuse fibrosis, bile duct proliferation, giant cells, and increased iron. Cirrhosis is universally present. As in hemochromatosis, excessive iron is found in other visceral organs, including the heart, pancreas, and thyroid. Excess iron, however, is not noted in the reticuloendothelial cells. Magnetic resonance imaging also may demonstrate increased iron stores.

Treatment is primarily supportive until a liver transplantation can be performed. Survival without liver transplantation is extremely rare. Use of an antioxidant cocktail containing selenium, prostaglandin E, vitamin E, and *N*-acetylcysteine along with deferoxamine has met with limited success. Removal of iron by itself has little or no effect, unlike in hemochromatosis.

Secondary Iron Overload

In addition to the previously mentioned disorders of iron metabolism, excess iron can accumulate in the liver and result in chronic liver disease and cirrhosis because of excess iron administration. This happens most commonly in those who require frequent and repeated transfusions of red blood cells. Examples of these types of disorders include thalassemia, as well as those with certain types of malignancies such as acute lymphocytic leukemia. Due to repeated blood transfusions, iron accumulates and is deposited in the liver. The excess iron, as in hemochromatosis, results in liver injury that can progress to chronic hepatitis and cirrhosis. Patients who require frequent transfusions should be monitored for secondary iron overload by periodically measuring ferritin levels.

Treatment of secondary iron overload consists of removal of excess iron from the liver. Unlike hemochromatosis where this is most commonly accomplished by phlebotomy, individuals with secondary iron overload suffer from anemia; therefore, phlebotomy is not a viable option. These individuals require chelation therapy that is most commonly performed with deferoxamine. This can be accomplished by administering deferoxamine IV at a dose of 15 mg/kg/hour to a maximum of 12 g/day or via a subcutaneous infusion at a dose of 20 to 50 mg/kg/day to a maximum of 2 g/day over 8 to 12 hours. Supplemental vitamin C should be avoided during this treatment as this can increase iron absorption in the gastrointestinal tract. In addition, the combination of vitamin C and deferoxamine has been associated with impaired cardiac function. Ferritin levels

---

> **BOX 370.6** **Major Categories of Progressive Familial Intrahepatic Cholestasis**
>
> Progressive familial intrahepatic cholestasis (PFIC) I, which had previously been referred to as Byler disease, was first observed in an Amish kindred but has now been reported throughout the world, especially in those groups that practice consanguineous marriage. It is believed to result from impaired canalicular secretion of chenodeoxycholic acid; the acid accumulates and exerts a direct hepatotoxic effect. PFIC II is secondary to bile salt export protein deficiency, resulting in impaired bile acid transport into the bile canaliculus. This disorder is more common in people of Middle Eastern and European decent. Patients with PFIC I and II clinically present with cholestasis, pruritus, hepatomegaly, and growth failure. Some also have diarrhea and pancreatic insufficiency. A feature that distinguishes these disorders from other cholestatic disorders of infancy is the fact that levels of gamma-glutamyltransferase (GGT) and cholesterol tend to be normal or minimally elevated. Liver biopsy is nonspecific and can reveal intrahepatic bile duct paucity or neonatal hepatitis with giant cells with varying degrees of fibrosis to frank cirrhosis. PFIC III is felt to be secondary to a deficiency in multidrug resistance protein 3 that appears to result in a defect in phospholipid secretion. PFIC III presents in a similar fashion to PFIC I and II, but differs in that the GGT is elevated and the liver biopsy reveals bile duct proliferation.

should be monitored during treatment, and once normalized, maintenance therapy can be instituted.

Progressive Familial Intrahepatic Cholestasis

Progressive familial intrahepatic cholestasis (PFIC) is a group of disorders that appear to be inherited in an autosomal recessive pattern and that are characterized by progressive chronic cholestasis. These disorders appear to be secondary to defects in bile canalicular transport. There are three major categories of PFIC (Box 370.6).

For all three types of PFIC, cirrhosis and hepatic failure almost universally develop if the patient remains untreated. Numerous medical therapies—including administration of choleretic agents such as ursodeoxycholic acid, bile acid sequestrants (cholestyramine), and others—have been used with limited success. Surgical therapy consisting of partial biliary diversion has been shown to be an effective therapeutic modality. In this procedure, a segment of jejunum is anastomosed between the gallbladder and the skin, resulting in external diversion of bile. If the surgery is performed before the development of cirrhosis, it may resolve the symptoms and prevent the development of cirrhosis. If cirrhosis is already established, liver transplantation is required.

Storage Diseases Causing Cirrhosis

Galactosemia

Galactosemia is an inherited disorder of galactose metabolism that results in severe liver disease in infancy, which progresses

TABLE 370.2

STORAGE DISEASES CAUSING CIRRHOSIS

Disorder	Enzymatic Defect	Clinical Manifestations	Treatment
Galactosemia	Galactose 1-phosphate uridyltransferase	Vomiting, diarrhea, cholestasis Failure to thrive, developmental delay	Dietary restriction of galactose
Fructose	Intolerance Fructose-1,6 biphosphotate aldolase	Vomiting, irritability, diarrhea Cholestasis, hypoglycemia, Seizure, hepatomegaly	Dietary restriction of fructose
Tyrosinemia	Fumarylacetoacetate hydrolase	Liver failure, renal tubular dysfunction Vitamin D resistant rickets	Dietary restriction of tyrosine, methionine & phenylalanine Treatment with NTBC
GSD I	Glucose-6-phosphatase	Hepatomegaly, hyopglycemia metabolic acidosis, short stature	High carbohyrate meals Nocturnal feedings
GSD III	Amylo-1, 6-glucosidase	Growth failure, hepatomegaly	High carboydrate meals Nocturnal feedings
GSDIV	1,4 glucan-6-glycosly transferase	Hepatosplenomegaly, FTT	Nocturnal feedings
Cholesterol ester storage disease	Lysosomal acid lipase def	Hepatomegaly, +/− splenomegaly Hypercholesterolemia	HMG-Co A reductase inhibitor
Wolman disease	Lysosomal acid lipase deficiency	Diarrhea, failure to thrive Hepatosplenomegaly	No treatment
Niemann Pick	Lysosomal sphingomyelinase deficiency	Hepatosplenomealy, failure to thrive Neurological deterioration	No treatment
Gaucher disease	Glucocerebrosidase	Type I: hepatosplenomegaly osteopenia delayed Puberly poor growth thrombocytopenia	Intravenous Glucocerebrosidase
		Type II: Rapid neurologic deterioration hepatosplenomegaly	No treatment
		Type III: Hepatosplenomegaly, slower Neurologic deterioration	Intravenous Glucocerebrosidase

to cirrhosis if left untreated (see also Chapter 387, Disorders of Carbohydrate Metabolism) (Table 370.2). It is an autosomal recessive disorder that occurs with a frequency of 1 in 10,000 to 30,000 live births. A deficiency of galactose 1-phosphate uridyltransferase causes an accumulation of galactose 1-phosphate in the liver, brain, lenses, kidneys, and adrenal glands. These infants, if fed lactose, a disaccharide of glucose and galactose, present in infancy with vomiting, diarrhea, failure to thrive, developmental delay or retardation, cataracts, cholestasis, or cirrhosis. Liver biopsy is nonspecific and reveals hepatic steatosis, fibrosis, necrosis, and pseudoacinar formation. The latter is a nonspecific finding in several metabolic disorders. A preliminary diagnosis is made when reducing substances other than glucose are found in the urine. Diagnosis is confirmed by a finding of low levels of galactose 1-phosphate uridyltransferase in erythrocytes. Treatment consists of excluding galactose from the diet; if treatment is instituted early enough, symptoms resolve, and the patient has a normal life expectancy.

Hereditary Fructose Intolerance

Hereditary fructose intolerance is an autosomal recessive disorder with a prevalence of 1 in 40,000 (see also Chapter 387). Affected patients have a deficiency in the enzyme fructose-1,6 biphosphate aldolase (aldolase B), which results in the hepatic accumulation of fructose 1-phosphate. This latter compound is a competitive inhibitor of phosphorylase and interferes with the breakdown of glycogen to glucose. The reduction in glycolysis results in hypoglycemia and lactic acidosis. Intracellular

phosphate and adenosine triphosphate levels are also reduced because phosphate is sequestered as fructose 1-phosphate. Patients with this disorder usually present in infancy with vomiting, irritability, diarrhea, cholestasis, hepatomegaly, and seizures from hypoglycemia after ingesting the disaccharide sucrose, which is composed of glucose and fructose.

Laboratory evaluation reveals fructose in the urine and elevated levels of liver enzymes and bilirubin. The liver biopsy is nondiagnostic but reveals hepatic steatosis, necrosis, cholestasis, and pseudoacinar formation. Eventually, fibrosis and cirrhosis develop. The definitive diagnosis is based on low levels of aldolase B in a liver biopsy specimen. In addition, one can perform DNA analysis to determine if one of the several mutations known to cause this disorder is present. The confirmatory study is a fructose tolerance test. This test consists of administering intravenous fructose and then serially measuring blood glucose, phosphorus, lactate, and uric acid levels. In patients with hereditary fructose intolerance, blood glucose and phosphorus levels fall, whereas uric acid and lactate levels rise. Fructose tolerance tests should be performed in a controlled setting, since hypoglycemia and shock may occur. Treatment consists of eliminating fructose from the diet. If treatment is instituted early, symptoms resolve, and the patient has a normal life expectancy.

Hereditary Tyrosinemia

Hereditary tyrosinemia type I is a rare disorder of tyrosine metabolism that shows an autosomal recessive mode of inheritance (see also Chapter 385). Several areas of the world have relatively high frequency of this disorder including the Lac-St. Jean region of Quebec, Canada, and in Scandinavia. In the former region, the frequency of heterozygotes has been estimated at 7%. The gene for hereditary tyrosinemia type I has been mapped to chromosome 15q. This disorder is the result of a deficiency of fumarylacetoacetate hydrolase (i.e., fumarylhydrolase), the last enzyme in the degradation of tyrosine. As a result, the serum levels of tyrosine and other intermediates, such as succinylacetone, rise; these substances appear to be responsible for the tissue injury. These patients develop severe liver disease and frequently die of liver failure in the first year of life. They may present also with cirrhosis, renal tubular dysfunction (including Fanconi syndrome), or vitamin D–resistant rickets. Tyrosinemia is diagnosed if elevated blood levels of tyrosine and methionine are found and if succinylacetone is detected. The level of fumarylacetoacetate can be measured in red blood cells, cultured fibroblasts, or liver. Prenatal evaluation can be performed by measuring the level of this enzyme in cells from amniotic fluid or by measuring succinylacetone in the amniotic fluid after 15 weeks' gestation. It is now also possible to utilize amniotic cells to do DNA analysis to assess for the gene responsible for hereditary tyrosinemia. Patients with tyrosinemia are at very high risk for developing hepatocellular carcinoma; the disease is seen in up to 37% of patients with tyrosinemia and can occur as early as 2 years of age. Therapy is directed at reducing dietary tyrosine, phenylalanine, and methionine, which may help normalize the serum amino acid pattern and improve the renal tubular disease. The liver disease typically progresses, however, and the risk of hepatocellular carcinoma is not reduced. Liver transplantation has been performed successfully in patients with tyrosinemia and had been the only hope for survival in patients with severe progressive liver disease. An investigational therapeutic option is 2-(2-nitro-4-trifluoro-methylbenzyol)-1,3 cyclohexanedione (NTBC). This compound inhibits phenylpyruvate dioxygenase, the enzyme involved in the second step of tyrosine metabolism, thereby decreasing the generation of toxic metabolites of tyrosine catabolism. Treatment with NTBC has been associated with improved liver function in 95% of treated cases as well as significant improvement in kidney function. This treatment does not appear to alter the risk for hepatocellular carcinoma, however, and liver transplantation may be considered in an attempt to prevent this complication.

Glycogen Storage Diseases

Glycogen storage diseases (GSDs) are rare inherited disorders of glycogen metabolism; each type is the result of a specific enzyme deficiency (see also Chapter 387). Many types of glycogen storage diseases are associated with glycogen accumulation and subsequently with some degree of hepatomegaly; the exceptions are those that involve only skeletal muscle. Types I, III, and IV are those in which the untreated patient can develop significant liver disease.

Type I glycogen storage disease (von Gierke) is the most common form and is subdivided into two subtypes, GSD Ia and GSD Ib. GSD type Ia is due to a deficiency in glucose-6-phosphatase. Type Ib is secondary to glucose-6-phosphatase transporter deficiency. Children with GSD I most commonly present with hepatomegaly, hypoglycemia, and metabolic acidosis. Short stature in association with excess adipose tissue is frequently present. Xanthomas may also be noted. Laboratory abnormalities are most marked in the fasting state and include hypoglycemia, metabolic acidosis with elevated lactic acid, hyperuricemia, hypophosphatemia, and hyperlipidemia. Those with GSD type Ia may also have thrombocytopenia while GSD type Ib can be associated with neutropenia. Fever and recurrent infections can occur in those with GSD Ib secondary to the neutropenia. Hepatic transaminases are mildly elevated but

normalize with maintenance of euglycemia. GSD type I does not progress to cirrhosis; however, there is an increased risk of hepatic adenomas. Patients with GSD type I may also have renal enlargement secondary to glycogen deposition. Over time, this can progress to nephropathy.

Type III GSD (Forbes disease) is secondary to amylo-1, 6-glucosidase deficiency (debranching enzyme). Patients with this form of GSD most commonly present with growth failure and hepatomegaly. Unlike GSD type I, untreated patients with GSD type III frequently develop fibrosis, but infrequently does it progress to cirrhosis. Splenomegaly is noted later on in childhood secondary to hepatic fibrosis and portal hypertension.

Type IV glycogen storage disease (Andersen disease) is the type most frequently associated with cirrhosis. This is secondary to a deficiency in 1,4-glucan-6-glycosyl transferase deficiency (brancher enzyme). Those with this disorder most commonly present between 3 and 15 months of age with hepatosplenomegaly and growth failure. Approximately one-half will experience abnormal neuromuscular development.

Liver biopsy can be extremely useful in making the diagnosis of glycogen storage disease. Excess glycogen is the most common abnormality noted. This is demonstrated with periodic acid-Schiff (PAS) staining in which the glycogen is pink and disappears with diastase, an enzyme that metabolizes glycogen. The histology of the glycogen in the various types can often be differentiated by electron microscopy. Type I GSD is associated with significant hepatic steatosis and nuclear hyperglycogenosis. Type III, debranching enzyme deficiency, has nuclear glycogenosis similar to that found in type I but less steatosis. Fibrosis may be prominent in type III but typically does not occur in type I. Type IV, brancher enzyme deficiency, is the glycogen storage disease associated with the most rapid development of cirrhosis, which typically occurs in the first 2 years of life. Broad bands of fibrous tissue form, and hepatocytes have eccentric nuclei and glycogen-filled lysosomes. The definitive diagnosis can be made by direct measurement of these enzymes in liver tissue.

Treatment is directed toward avoidance of hypoglycemia and its associated hormonal disruption, which is thought to contribute to the complications of glycogen storage disease. Type I and type III are treated with frequent high-carbohydrate meals. Uncooked cornstarch in doses of 2 g/kg every 6 hours has been utilized to help maintain glucose levels. The ingested cornstarch is gradually metabolized by amylase, resulting in a prolonged generation of glucose. In addition, patients with type III may benefit from higher protein intake. Continuous nocturnal nasogastric or gastrostomy feedings are utilized for all types of glycogen storage diseases to avoid hypoglycemia. This regimen has resulted in a reduction in liver size, improved liver function, normalization of liver enzymes, and decreased levels of liver glycogen in those with types I and III. For patients with type IV disease and cirrhosis, the only treatment option is liver transplantation.

Lipid Storage Disorders

Several lipid storage disorders associated with hepatic fibrosis or cirrhosis include cholesterol ester storage disease, Wolman disease, Niemann-Pick disease, and Gaucher disease (see also Chapter 389). Cholesterol ester storage disease and Wolman disease are both autosomal recessive disorders caused by lysosomal acid lipase deficiency but represent allelic variants. Lysosomal acid lipase is the enzyme responsible for the hydrolysis of triglyceride and cholesterol esters in lysosomes. Patients with cholesterol ester storage disease present with hepatomegaly and hypercholesterolemia any time from several weeks of age to adulthood. Splenomegaly is present in 50% of cases, and hypertriglyceridemia is present in one-half of the cases as well. Liver biopsy reveals intralysosomal lipid primarily in the form of cholesterol esters, although an excess of triglyceride also is seen. Varying degrees of fibrosis are found, with some cases developing frank cirrhosis. Definitive diagnosis for this and Wolman disease is based on the measurement of lysosomal acid lipase in white blood cells or skin fibroblasts. Prenatal testing is available. No specific therapy exists, although use of HMG-CoA reductase inhibitors, such as lovastatin, has been noted to reduce serum lipid levels as well as hepatocellular lysosomal lipid content. Efforts are under way to develop enzyme replacement therapy for this disorder and initial studies in mice have been promising. Liver transplantation may be required. The mortality rate of individuals with cholesterol ester storage disease is approximately 6%.

Wolman disease is the more severe variant of lysosomal acid lipase deficiency. Cholesterol esters and triglycerides are deposited in the liver, small intestine, bone marrow, lymph nodes, kidneys, thymus, brain, and adrenal glands. These patients can present in infancy with diarrhea, vomiting, malabsorption, failure to thrive, icterus, and hepatosplenomegaly. Unlike patients with cholesterol ester storage disease, cholesterol and triglyceride levels tend to be normal. A flat plate of the abdomen almost universally reveals calcification of the adrenal glands. Results of liver biopsy in Wolman disease are similar to those in cholesterol ester storage disease, with increased intralysosomal lipid consisting of cholesterol esters and triglycerides and varying degrees of fibrosis. No effective treatment exists, and patients usually die during the first year of life.

Niemann-Pick disease is an autosomal recessive disorder secondary to lysosomal sphingomyelinase deficiency. As a result of this enzymatic deficiency, sphingomyelin and cholesterol accumulate in the reticuloendothelial cells, especially in the liver, spleen, brain, and bone marrow. Hepatocytes are vacuolated, and Niemann-Pick foam cells are seen in liver biopsy specimens. Periportal fibrosis can be evident; however, progression to cirrhosis is uncommon. Electron micrographs of the liver reveal intracytoplasmic whorls of sphingomyelin. Of the two major types, the most common is the acute neuronopathic infantile form (type IA), manifesting in infancy with hepatosplenomegaly, failure to thrive, and neurologic deterioration. No effective therapy exists, and the prognosis for patients with infantile-type Niemann-Pick disease is poor.

Gaucher disease is the most common lysosomal storage disease. It is an autosomal recessive disorder that results from a deficiency in glucocerebrosidase (beta-glucosidase), resulting in accumulation of glucocerebroside in the lysosomes of macrophages. There are three phenotypes of Gaucher disease based on the presence and rate of progression of neurologic symptoms. Type I is the most common, accounting for approximately 90% of cases, and occurs most frequently in the Ashkenazi Jewish population. Patients with this type present at any time from infancy to adulthood with splenomegaly, hepatomegaly, osteopenia, bone pain, and/or bleeding secondary to thrombocytopenia. Hepatic involvement is a major component of type I Gaucher disease consisting of hepatomegaly and hepatic fibrosis. Although fibrosis occurs, patients rarely develop cirrhosis and portal hypertension. Type I Gaucher disease does not have the neurologic symptoms that dominate the other two types. Type II, acute neuronopathic Gaucher disease, is the rarest form and presents in infancy with rapidly progressive neurologic deterioration. Type III, subacute neuronopathic Gaucher disease, presents with anemia, osteopenia, and neurologic abnormalities in childhood and is more slowly progressive than is type II.

Laboratory evaluation reveals thrombocytopenia, mildly elevated liver enzymes, and an elevated acid phosphatase. Liver biopsy reveals lipid-filled Gaucher cells with a typical "wrinkled tissue paper" appearance. These histiocytic cells are located around the central vein and the sinusoids. The diagnosis of Gaucher disease is confirmed by measurement of glucocere-

brosidase in white blood cells. Prenatal testing is also available. Gaucher disease is one of only a few metabolic diseases where enzyme replacement therapy is available. Treatment consists of the intravenous administration of glucocerebrosidase (alglucerase, imiglucerase). Studies indicate that macrophage-targeted glucocerebrosidase may be helpful in improving thrombocytopenia and reducing hepatosplenomegaly.

Peroxisomal Disease

Several disorders of peroxisomal metabolism are associated with liver disease and the potential to develop cirrhosis, including Zellweger syndrome, infantile Refsum disease, and neonatal adrenoleukodystrophy (see also Chapter 390). Peroxisomes are subcellular organelles involved in multiple metabolic pathways, including beta oxidation of very long-chain fatty acids (VLSFAs), oxidase-mediated metabolism of amino acids, cholesterol and bile acid synthesis, and metabolism of hydrogen peroxide. Zellweger syndrome (i.e., cerebrohepatorenal syndrome) is a rare autosomal recessive disorder that most commonly presents in infancy with hypotonia, absent reflexes, facial dysmorphism, and liver disease. The characteristic facial features include midfacial hypoplasia, hypertelorism, micrognathia, high narrow forehead, large fontanelles, and inner epicanthal folds. Other associated anomalies include cortical cysts of the kidney, abnormal calcification of the patella, clinodactyly, cryptorchidism, hypospadias, pigmentary retinopathy, central nervous system malformations, and cardiac lesions such as patent ductus arteriosus and septal defects. Neurologic involvement is frequent and severe, consisting of hypotonia, areflexia, mental retardation, and seizures. Liver disease is often mild early on, with patients showing hepatomegaly and cholestasis. Later, if these patients survive the neonatal period, the development of severe liver disease is essentially a universal phenomenon; cortical cysts of the kidney and cirrhosis are present as early as 6 months of age. The cause of the cirrhosis is unknown, but appears to be related to the accumulation of metabolic products normally catabolized by the peroxisome—especially intermediate bile acids. Support for this is derived from one case in which an infant with Zellweger syndrome received primary bile acids (cholic acid and chenodeoxycholic acid) in an attempt to decrease the amount of the toxic bile acid intermediates. This resulted in improvement in liver function and histology. Liver biopsy reveals foamy, lipid-filled hepatocytes, giant cells, and varying degrees of necrosis and fibrosis. Evaluation by electron microscope reveals absence of hepatic peroxisomes, abnormal mitochondria, and lipid-filled macrophages. The diagnosis is made in an individual with the typical clinical findings, a liver biopsy with absent peroxisomes, and the typical electron-micrographic findings noted previously. In addition, levels of VLCFAs, phytanic acid, and pipecolic acid are elevated, while that of docosahexaenoic acid (DHA) is low. No definitive therapy exists at this time. Dietary restriction of VLCFAs, pipecolic acid, and phytanic acid has shown little to no effectiveness. As noted above, administration of primary bile acids may be of benefit. In addition, one study determined that administration of DHA normalized serum DHA levels, decreased VLCFAs, and improved liver enzymes. Due to the involvement of multiple organ systems and their severe neurologic problems, these patients are not candidates for liver transplantation. Median survival time of patients with Zellweger syndrome is 5 months.

Infantile Refsum disease and neonatal adrenoleukodystrophy also are autosomal recessive disorders of peroxisomal metabolism that appear clinically as milder forms of Zellweger syndrome. These disorders are associated with reduced levels of peroxisomes but not their absence. Although milder than

Zellweger syndrome, these disorders have a very bad prognosis, with only a few surviving into the second decade of life.

In addition to these disorders associated with absence or marked reduction in the number of peroxisomes, rare disorders of isolated peroxisomal enzyme deficiency have been noted. Two such deficiencies have been associated with hepatic fibrosis and cirrhosis, bifunctional enzyme deficiency and acyl-CoA oxidase deficiency.

Mitochondrial Disorders

There has been increasing information regarding mitochondrial disorders and liver disease over the last decade. Deficiencies in complexes I, III, and IV of the electron transport chain have been associated with neonatal liver failure. Infants present with poor feeding, lethargy, and hypotonia. Laboratory evaluation reveals hypoalbuminemia, hyperammonemia, coagulopathy, and hypoglycemia. A metabolic acidosis with elevation of lactate and pyruvate is present with the molar ratio of lactate to pyruvate being elevated (normal less than 20:1). Liver biopsy reveals hepatic steatosis with both microvesicular and macrovesicular steatosis. Hepatic mitochondria exhibit increased density. Periportal fibrosis of varying degrees is noted and cirrhosis may be present. There is no specific therapy for these disorders. Liver transplantation is a consideration in the absence of severe impairment of another organ system.

Alpers disease (progressive neuronal degeneration of childhood) is another defect in electron transport. This is an autosomal recessive disorder secondary to a deficiency in complex I and can be a rare cause of cirrhosis (see also Chapter 386, Disorders of Mitochondrial Fatty Acid Oxidation). Patients present with progressive neuromuscular degeneration, seizures, and liver disease; death often occurs by 5 years of age.

Pearson bone marrow pancreas syndrome is secondary to mitochondrial DNA rearrangements resulting in electron transport defects. Hematologic characteristics of Pearson include macrocytic anemia, thrombocytopenia, and neutropenia with vacuolization of the erythroid and myeloid precursors in the bone marrow. Exocrine pancreatic insufficiency accounts for the diarrhea noted in those with this syndrome. Hepatomegaly, which can be marked, is a common feature. Liver histology reveals hepatic steatosis, fibrosis, and potentially cirrhosis.

Mitochondrial DNA depletion syndrome is due to a generalized reduction in mitochondrial DNA, which in turn results in reduced activity of the respiratory chain complexes I, III, and IV. Affected individuals present in infancy or childhood with myopathy, lactic acidosis, hypoglycemia, and liver failure.

Infection

Many organisms can infect the liver and cause hepatitis, including the hepatitis A, hepatitis B, hepatitis C, hepatitis D, hepatitis E, and hepatitis G viruses; Epstein-Barr virus; cytomegalovirus; rubella virus; and *Treponema pallidum* (see also Chapter 367). Chronic hepatitis tends to occur only after infections with hepatitis B, hepatitis D, and hepatitis C viruses; *T. pallidum*; cytomegalovirus; and possibly hepatitis G virus. In the absence of neonatal immunization the risk of the newborn contracting hepatitis B from a mother who is HBsAg and HBe AG positive is 85% to 90%. Risk of neonatal acquisition is greater when the mother contracts acute hepatitis B in the third trimester compared to the first or second trimester. Neonates who acquire hepatitis B from their mother typically are asymptomatic; however, approximately 6% will develop acute or fulminant hepatitis around 2 to 3 months of age. Chronic hepatitis B infection occurs in 90% to 95% of infants who become infected in the neonatal period, compared with 1% to 5% who develop

this infection as an adult. These infants have the ability to transmit the disease to others. Liver disease in these individuals may progress to cirrhosis, and there is an increased risk of developing hepatocellular carcinoma, rarely in childhood. It may be prudent to annually monitor those with hepatitis B and cirrhosis with alpha-fetoprotein levels and ultrasound examination to screen for this complication. The optimal therapeutic approach to chronic hepatitis is its prevention by universal use of hepatitis B vaccine, which has been shown to be 95% effective in preventing acquisition of hepatitis B by infants born to infected mothers. There are two medications approved by the U.S. Food and Drug Administration (FDA) for treatment of hepatitis B in children: interferon-alpha and lamivudine. Interferon-alpha, administered at a dose of 6 million U/m^2 (maximum 10 MU) three times a week subcutaneously for 6 months, has resulted in clearance of hepatitis B virus DNA and/or HBeAg seroconversion to negative in 20% to 58% of cases, compared with 8% to 17% of controls. Higher doses have not been associated with higher clearance rates. Side effects are common with interferon, although they resolved with discontinuation of the medication. Transient influenza-like symptoms occur in most treated individuals early in the therapy. Neutropenia occurs in up to 40% but severe neutropenia and infection are uncommon. Significant psychological problems can also occur, and interferon should be used with caution in those with significant depression. Interferon should not be used in children less than 2 years of age due to the risk of developing diplegia. Treated individuals who demonstrate a virologic response also show improvement in liver histology, and this may be associated with decreased risk of cirrhosis and hepatocellular carcinoma. Lamivudine is a nucleoside analogue that blocks viral replication by inhibition of hepatitis B polymerase. It is administered at a dose of 3 mg/kg/day (maximum 100 mg) orally for 1 year. The rate of seroconversion (loss of hepatitis B DNA and or HBe AB development) with lamivudine is similar to that of interferon-alpha, but the rate of loss of HBsAg is only 5% with lamivudine versus 3% to 33% with interferon-alpha. Lamivudine is well tolerated even by those with severe liver disease.

Hepatitis C is the most common cause of chronic liver disease in the United States and is the most common reason for liver transplantation in adults. Since the implementation of screening for hepatitis C by blood banks in 1990, the incidence of new cases of hepatitis C has decreased. After acute hepatitis C infection, 85% of patients develop chronic hepatitis and 20% to 30% develop cirrhosis. Patients with chronic hepatitis C are at increased risk of developing hepatocellular carcinoma. The combination of pegylated (PEG)-interferon and ribavirin is now the accepted treatment for hepatitis C in adults. At present, there is no FDA-approved treatment of hepatitis C in children. Interferon-alpha, 3 to 6 million U/m^2 three times a week subcutaneously for 1 year, has been shown to be effective in the treatment of hepatitis C in children. Five to forty-five percent of children treated with interferon-alpha have a sustained viral response (absence of hepatitis C virus RNA by PCR 6 months after cessation of therapy). Several genotypes of hepatitis C exist, with genotype I being the most common in the United States. Sustained viral response is related to the genotype of hepatitis C, with lower rates noted in genotype I (27%) than in non-I genotypes (70%). As in adults, combination of interferon with ribavirin is more effective in children than interferon-alpha alone, with sustained viral response of 47% to 70%. The dose of ribavirin has ranged from 8 to 15 mg/kg/day. Ribavirin is a teratogen and should be used with caution in those of childbearing age. Ribavirin is also associated with hemolytic anemia, requiring frequent monitoring of hemoglobin.

Cirrhosis is a rare complication of congenital syphilis and cytomegalovirus infection. With appropriate therapy, the hepatitis resolves, and cirrhosis does not develop.

Cardiac Cirrhosis

Cirrhosis may develop secondary to congenital heart disease or congestive heart failure as a result of passive congestion and ischemia of long duration. The signs and symptoms of the heart disease are prominent, with few or none referable to the liver disease other than hepatosplenomegaly. The initial lesion consists of dilation of the central vein and the sinusoids. As time passes, centrilobular hemorrhage, necrosis, and fibrosis are seen. Liver enzymes are elevated; bilirubin levels show minimal elevation except in severe cases. As cardiac failure persists, the centrilobular fibrosis extends into the lobule, and if the patient survives long enough, cirrhosis develops. If cardiac function is normalized before cirrhosis develops, liver disease can stabilize or resolve, depending on its stage.

Budd-Chiari syndrome (i.e., obstruction or thrombosis of the hepatic vein) and constrictive pericarditis result in similar hepatic lesions, which improve after appropriate treatment of the underlying disorder.

Autoimmune Disease

Autoimmune chronic active hepatitis is an uncommon disorder in the pediatric population, but it has potentially severe consequences (see Chapter 367). Approximately 75% of patients are female. The exact cause of autoimmune hepatitis is unknown, but there appears to be a genetic predisposition, with affected patients frequently having a family history of autoimmune disease. In addition to the genetic predisposition, environmental factors are involved. Viral infections appear to be one such factor, and it is now recognized that autoimmune hepatitis can develop after hepatitis A infection. Autoimmune hepatitis can also develop *de novo* in children who underwent liver transplantation for nonautoimmune liver disease. Autoimmune hepatitis has been classified as type I or type II based on the pattern of autoantibodies. Type I autoimmune hepatitis is characterized by the presence of ANA and or antismooth muscle antibody (ASMA). Type II autoimmune hepatitis is associated with the presence of antiliver kidney microsomal antibody (anti-LKM). There is some overlap, with 25% of type I patients having anti-LKM in addition to being positive for ANA and/or ASMA. Patients with type I more commonly have IgA deficiency (45%) compared to type II patients (10%). Cirrhosis is more common in patients with type I than type II autoimmune hepatitis, 69% versus 38%. Patients with autoimmune hepatitis may initially presents as any other hepatitis with nonspecific symptoms, hepatomegaly, and jaundice. Others will present with acute or chronic liver failure. Evaluation fails to produce evidence of infectious causes of hepatitis or evidence of other causes of liver disease, such as Wilson disease or alpha-1-antitrypsin deficiency. Laboratory evaluation of autoimmune hepatitis reveals the erythrocyte sedimentation rate and immunoglobulin levels to be elevated. In addition to ANA, ASMA, and anti-LKM, autoantibodies, such as anti–soluble-liver antigen antibodies, or antiactin antibodies may be found in as many as 80% of patients. The liver biopsy is nonspecific and reveals chronic hepatitis with portal tract inflammation. Special stains for copper and iron should be performed to further rule out Wilson disease and hemochromatosis. Reports indicate that many patients with autoimmune chronic hepatitis have cirrhosis at the time of presentation.

Treatment of this disorder consists of immunosuppression. Physicians generally agree on initial therapy with prednisone 2 mg/kg/day. Some physicians also recommend use of azathioprine (0.5 to 2 mg/kg/day) at the onset, but others use such therapy only when prednisone alone has proven unsuccessful. Most children with autoimmune hepatitis will require lifelong immunosuppression. Cyclosporine has been tried in patients who do not respond to the other therapies. Inadequate response to therapy results in progression of the liver disease and the development of liver failure; liver transplantation is required in 25% to 50% of such patients. Studies of adult patients indicate that approximately 15% to 25% of those transplanted for autoimmune hepatitis have a recurrence of the disease in the transplanted liver.

Nutritional Disorders

Malnutrition in the form of undernutrition and overnutrition is a worldwide problem. The most common hepatic abnormality in infants and children with malnutrition is hepatic steatosis. This disorder occurs in children with severe protein-calorie malnutrition as well as in obese patients. The frequency of hepatic steatosis in obese patients ranges from 25% to 50%. Evidence is accumulating that hepatic steatosis can progress to cirrhosis, although this claim remains controversial (see Chapter 372).

Total parenteral nutrition is a commonly used therapeutic modality. Cholestasis is often encountered when total parenteral nutrition is used, especially in premature infants. Hepatic fibrosis and cirrhosis can occur after prolonged administration of total parenteral nutrition.

Jejunoileal bypass surgery was performed relatively frequently to treat the morbidly obese in the 1960s and 1970s. Unfortunately, approximately one-third of these patients develop liver disease, including fibrosis, hepatitis, and micronodular cirrhosis. Approximately 10% of these patients develop cirrhosis over a period of many years. Many theories exist regarding the cause of cirrhosis in these patients, although the exact mechanism is unknown.

Vitamin A, a fat-soluble vitamin, is an essential nutrient required for many metabolic processes. Hypervitaminosis A, however, can result in pseudotumor cerebri and liver disease. Ingestion of more than 40,000 IU of vitamin A for prolonged periods can result in cirrhosis.

Drugs and Toxins

Although many drugs are hepatotoxic, relatively few contribute to the development of cirrhosis. Alcohol ingestion is the primary cause of drug-induced cirrhosis. Alcohol abuse results in micronodular cirrhosis. Approximately 75% of patients who consume 1 pint of alcohol per day for 15 years have significant liver disease. Use of methotrexate sodium can cause portal cirrhosis, and the potential for development of cirrhosis is increased by alcohol intake, daily use of methotrexate sodium, prior liver disease, and obesity. Patients on long-term methotrexate sodium therapy probably should undergo a liver biopsy after administration of each 1.0 to 1.5 g of the drug. One to two percent of patients taking chlorpromazine become jaundiced after 1 to 2 months of therapy. In most of these patients, the liver disease resolves over 1 year. A small percentage of these patients develop biliary cirrhosis. Other drugs that can potentially result in cirrhosis are amiodarone hydrochloride and perhexiline maleate.

Toxins that can cause cirrhosis include carbon tetrachloride, dimethylnitrosamine, vinyl chloride, arsenic, and aflatoxin.

Neonatal Hepatitis

Neonatal hepatitis is a relatively common disorder of unknown cause that initially presents as cholestasis in the newborn period. Other causes for cholestasis, such as infections, metabolic disorders, and biliary atresia, should be excluded. As knowledge of metabolic disorders causing neonatal cholestasis has increased, the frequency of idiopathic neonatal hepatitis has decreased. Histologically, cholestasis, lobular disarray, inflammation, necrosis, and multinucleated giant cells are seen. Unlike in biliary atresia, no bile duct proliferation is seen. Ten percent of cases have a family history of a previously affected infant. The prognosis for idiopathic neonatal hepatitis has improved, primarily because multiple metabolic disorders that previously went unrecognized and were diagnosed as neonatal hepatitis are now no longer classified in this idiopathic group, and many of these metabolic disorders have bad prognoses, as discussed previously. Currently, most infants with idiopathic neonatal hepatitis do well, but a small percentage still develops cirrhosis.

CLINICAL MANIFESTATIONS OF CIRRHOSIS

Clinical manifestations of this hepatic condition are the same regardless of the cause of the disease. Children with cirrhosis fail to thrive and become malnourished unless aggressive nutritional support is provided. The cause of the malnutrition is multifactorial and includes decreased hepatic protein synthesis, malabsorption of fat and fat-soluble vitamins due to a reduction in enteric bile salts, anorexia secondary to chronic disease, and early satiety as a result of ascites. The fat malabsorption and edema of the intestinal tract can result in chronic diarrhea.

Portal hypertension develops as a result of cirrhosis, and these children have hepatosplenomegaly. Late in the course of cirrhosis, liver size can decrease secondary to a loss of hepatocytes. The spleen can become significantly enlarged and cause hypersplenism with its associated thrombocytopenia and possible leukopenia and anemia. Patients with portal hypertension may also have prominent abdominal vessels, varices, and hemorrhoids.

Patients with cirrhosis frequently are edematous because of decreased serum albumin and increased total body water, which is caused primarily by increased extracellular fluid volume. Cirrhotic patients have various degrees of jaundice. If jaundice occurs during the time when the teeth are forming, the teeth can develop a greenish color. Because of the decreased ability to excrete bile salts, the serum bile acid level is elevated and can result in pruritus. When severe, excoriations and lichenification are noticed. Other potential physical findings in cirrhosis include palmar erythema, spider angiomas, digital clubbing, and delayed sexual maturation.

COMPLICATIONS OF CIRRHOSIS

Many potentially serious complications of cirrhosis may occur. Failure to thrive, delayed sexual development, and hypersplenism have been discussed briefly. Ascites and peritonitis, portal hypertension, and gastrointestinal hemorrhage frequently accompany cirrhosis and are discussed in Chapters 365, 371, and 346, respectively. Hepatorenal syndrome and hepatopulmonary syndrome are discussed in Chapter 372. Other potential complications of cirrhosis are hematologic abnormalities, coagulation disorders, hepatic encephalopathy, malnutrition, fat-soluble vitamin deficiencies, liver failure, pruritus, and cholelithiasis.

Hematologic abnormalities include thrombocytopenia, leukopenia, and anemia. Thrombocytopenia and leukopenia are secondary to hypersplenism. Hypersplenism results in platelet counts in the range of 50,000 to 100,000 cells/μL. If the platelet

count is less than 20,000 cells/mm^2, another cause for thrombocytopenia should be sought. Essential fatty acid deficiency also can contribute to thrombocytopenia. Several factors lead to anemia in patients with cirrhosis, including hypersplenism, iron deficiency due to gastrointestinal bleeding, and hemolytic anemia, which can be associated with chronic active hepatitis. Anemia also can be caused by vitamin E deficiency or alterations in erythrocyte membrane lipid component. Malabsorption of fats and fat-soluble vitamins can lead to alterations in the fatty acid component and the cholesterol-phospholipid ratio in the erythrocyte membrane and can cause decreased erythrocyte survival. Elevated serum lithocholic acid levels, which can occur in patients with cirrhosis, can induce spur cell anemia.

Coagulation disorders are common in patients with cirrhosis. These patients may be deficient in vitamin K and have a reduction in the vitamin K–dependent clotting factors II, VII, IX, and X. Factor VII has the shortest half-life and is the first to become reduced when vitamin K levels are deficient. The prothrombin time is the most sensitive coagulation indicator of vitamin K deficiency. The potential exists for reduction in all hepatic clotting factors in advanced stages of cirrhosis because hepatocyte mass and its synthetic capabilities are reduced.

Patients with severe liver disease may have findings consistent with disseminated intravascular coagulation. These findings consist of thrombocytopenia, elevated prothrombin and partial thromboplastin times, decreased fibrinogen levels, and elevated levels of fibrin split products. The cause of the thrombocytopenia and reduced clotting factors has been discussed. Fibrin split products are normally cleared by the liver; if the clearance is impaired by severe liver disease, the result is increased levels of fibrin split products, which are typically greater than 10 and less than 40 μg/mL. Finding these abnormalities in a patient with severe liver disease does not necessarily indicate true disseminated intravascular coagulation.

Hepatic encephalopathy is a complex neuropsychiatric disorder thought to be caused by the metabolic alterations associated with hepatocellular failure. The elevation in serum ammonia that occurs with liver failure had long been thought to cause hepatic encephalopathy. It is now known that hyperammonemia is not solely responsible and that the cause of hepatic encephalopathy is multifactorial. Other contributory factors include alterations in the permeability of the blood–brain barrier, the presence of other neurotoxins (e.g., mercaptans, short-chain fatty acids) and false neurotransmitters (e.g., octopamine and gamma-aminobutyric acid), and alterations in serum amino acid patterns (e.g., decreased ratio of branched-chain amino acids to aromatic amino acids). Patients initially have impaired intellectual functioning, followed by lethargy, coma, and seizures. They manifest asterixis, hyperreflexia, and decerebrate posturing.

Controversy exists regarding the treatment of hepatic encephalopathy. Therapy generally is directed toward improving hepatocellular function and decreasing potential aggravating factors. Unfortunately, except for liver transplantation, little can be done to improve hepatocellular function other than to discontinue administration of any potentially hepatotoxic drug. Attempts should be made to reduce production and absorption of ammonia. Neomycin therapy has long been used for this disorder to decrease bacterial formation of ammonia. Administration of lactulose helps prevent the absorption of ammonia by decreasing intraluminal pH and retaining the ammonium ion in the gut, from which it is subsequently excreted. Whether these agents should be used alone or together remains a subject for debate. Another potential therapeutic modality includes reducing protein intake in an attempt to decrease endogenous ammonia production. Protein intake should not be curtailed totally, because the result is increased catabolism of endogenous protein and subsequent ammonia production. The use of branched-chain amino acid and total parenteral nutrition formulas has been somewhat successful at temporarily improving central nervous system function, but this treatment does not alter the course of the disease. Patients with portosystemic encephalopathy should be checked for *Helicobacter pylori* and, if it is found, should be treated to decrease gastric ammonia production.

Other neurologic problems can develop in children with chronic cholestasis secondary to vitamin E deficiency. Vitamin E deficiency is encountered almost universally in children with chronic cholestasis. The first neurologic deficit to develop is areflexia, followed by ataxia, peripheral neuropathy, and ophthalmoplegia. If the deficiency is not corrected early enough, severe neurologic impairment may become permanent; therefore, vitamin E deficiency should be aggressively sought and treated in patients with chronic liver disease. Vitamin E status is best determined by comparing the level of vitamin E to the level of total serum lipids (cholesterol, triglyceride, and phospholipid). Normally, vitamin E levels are related to serum lipid levels. In patients with cholestasis in whom total serum lipids are increased, a normal vitamin E level may actually represent a deficiency. Normally, the relation of vitamin E to total lipids should be greater than 0.6 mg of vitamin E per gram of lipid. Vitamin E replacement is best done with D-alpha-tocopheryl polyethylene glycol (TPGS). In this preparation, vitamin E is linked to polyethylene glycol, which is readily absorbed via the intestinal tract. Absorption of vitamin E is significantly better with this form than with the typical water-soluble vitamin E. TPGS is initially given at a dosage of 25 IU/kg/day and adjusted as needed to maintain a normal ratio of vitamin E to total lipids.

Acute hepatic failure can occur after viral hepatitis, Reye syndrome, or drug exposure, or it can result from progressive cirrhosis. Acute hepatic failure is associated with a mortality of approximately 70%, and hepatic failure secondary to end-stage cirrhosis is uniformly fatal unless a liver transplant is performed.

The biochemical hallmark of hepatic failure in cirrhotic patients is reduced levels of the transaminases with a progressive increase in bilirubin levels, prothrombin and partial thromboplastin times, and ammonia levels. The blood urea nitrogen may decrease secondary to inability of the liver to manufacture urea, or it may increase in response to the development of the hepatorenal syndrome. Treatment is primarily supportive and directed at maintaining cerebral, renal, cardiac, and hepatic function. The complications of hepatic failure, such as encephalopathy, hepatorenal syndrome, and bleeding disorder, should be anticipated, and attempts made to prevent their occurrence. Nutritional support for these patients is complicated because of the need to restrict protein intake and because of the potential for fluid and electrolyte problems.

Pruritus is a frequent complication of chronic liver disease and can dramatically interfere with the child's life. Pruritus was originally thought to be secondary to elevated levels of bile salts, but there may also be a central neurogenic component.

An increased incidence of cholelithiasis is found in patients with cirrhosis. Gallstones occur more frequently in patients with decompensated cirrhosis (35% of cases) than in those with compensated cirrhosis (7% of cases). Cholelithiasis should be considered in the differential diagnosis of increasing jaundice in cirrhotic patients.

TREATMENT

Prevention of cirrhosis is the ultimate goal. After cirrhosis is established, no specific therapy exists other than liver transplantation. The disorders in which cirrhosis is potentially preventable and the specific preventive steps were discussed previously. Supportive therapy for patients with cirrhosis is directed toward the improvement and maintenance of nutritional status. The aim is to support growth, prevent gastrointestinal bleeding, avoid hepatotoxic drugs and toxins, and aggressively treat any of the potential complications encountered.

Nutritional support is the major therapy, especially because most patients with cirrhosis are malnourished. The cause of malnutrition in these patients is multifactorial; contributing factors include anorexia secondary to chronic disease, early satiety due to ascites, and malabsorption of nutrients, especially fats and fat-soluble vitamins, due to a decrease in intraluminal bile acids. In addition to fat-soluble vitamins, other nutrients in which patients may potentially be deficient include folic acid, riboflavin, and iron.

A nutritional assessment should be performed at the initial visit, and various anthropometric measurements and laboratory tests should be administered periodically. Anthropometric measurements that are readily obtainable include weight, height, weight for height, body mass index, and skinfold thickness; of these, weight is the most variable and is not necessarily a good index of nutritional status. Without any significant change in nutritional status, the patient's weight can increase or decrease significantly as a result of alterations in the amount of ascitic fluid present. Measurement of the triceps skinfold thickness (TSF) can yield some information about fat stores, which usually are depleted in these patients. Determination of midarm muscle circumference (i.e., midarm circumference [in centimeters] – 3.14 × TSF [in centimeters]) can provide information about the patient's muscle mass. In addition to measurements of liver function and liver enzyme levels, other laboratory tests that provide information about the patient's nutritional status should be performed periodically; these include determination of the levels of serum albumin, prealbumin, calcium, phosphorous, iron, vitamin A, and 25-dihydroxyvitamin D; determination of the ratio of vitamin E to total serum lipids; and measurement of prothrombin time. The blood urea nitrogen is normally low in these patients due to malnutrition unless the patient has significant renal failure. Creatinine level, too, is typically low because of the decreased muscle mass in patients with end-stage liver disease. Therefore, patients with cirrhosis may have normal renal function tests even in the face of renal impairment.

Patients in the early stage of cirrhosis should consume high-protein, high-calorie diets. Protein intake may range from 2.5 to 3.0 g/kg/day. Care must be taken to avoid precipitation of hepatic encephalopathy. Administration of a formula with medium-chain triglycerides (e.g., Pregestimil, Alimentum) may help improve fat absorption; medium-chain triglyceride absorption has a low requirement for bile salts compared to absorption of long-chain triglycerides. Formulas with extremely high levels of medium-chain triglycerides (e.g., Portagen) and, therefore, low levels of long-chain triglycerides may be deleterious and result in essential fatty acid deficiency and thus should be avoided. Because of the anorexia and early satiety frequently reported in cirrhotic patients, nighttime nasogastric feedings may be required to ensure adequate intake.

Fat-soluble vitamins should be supplemented and their levels monitored because of the potential for malabsorption in cirrhotic patients. Supplementation should include vitamin A (Aquasol A), 5,000 to 25,000 IU/day; Mephyton (AquaMephyton); 25-hydroxyvitamin D, 3 to 5 μg/kg/day; and vitamin E as TPGS, 25 IU/kg/day. The absorption of the fat-soluble vitamins is improved if they are administered simultaneously with TPGS. These patients may reasonably be supplemented with a daily multiple vitamin. Calcium supplements also may be necessary because of the loss of calcium from saponification with malabsorbed fats.

Patients with cirrhosis frequently have pruritus, which can be treated by the administration of choleretic agents such as phenobarbital, ursodeoxycholic acid, or cholestyramine. Antipruritic agents (e.g., diphenhydramine, hydroxyzine) can provide significant relief. Studies have shown rifampin, naloxone hydrochloride, and propofol to be effective. The patient's nails should be trimmed to avoid excoriation and possible infection.

Other potential complications of cirrhosis, such as ascites, peritonitis, gastrointestinal bleeding, hepatic encephalopathy, and the hepatorenal syndrome, are discussed elsewhere in this book. Liver transplantation has been a major advance in the treatment of cirrhosis. The procedure is performed successfully in infants and children. The use of tacrolimus has significantly improved the survival rate of transplant patients. The current 1-year survival rate is approximately 90%. The transplantation procedure is difficult and expensive, however; postoperative complications, including rejection, infection, and posttransplant lymphoproliferative disease, are frequent. Transplantation also is extremely stressful for the patient and family. Nevertheless, for a patient with end-stage cirrhosis of the liver, transplantation is the only hope for survival and one that potentially offers a good quality of life.

Suggested Readings

Andrews NC. Disorders of iron metabolism. *New Engl J Med* 1999;341:1986.
Balistreri WF. Intrahepatic cholestasis. *J Pediatr Gastroenterol Nutr* 2002;35: S17.
Birnbaum A, Suchy FJ. The intrahepatic cholangiopathies. *Seminar Liver Dis* 1998;18:263.
Broderick AL, Jonas MM. Hepatitis B in children. *Semin Liver Dis* 2003;23:59.
Camaschella C, Roetto A, De Gobbi M. Juvenile hemochromatosis. *Semin Hematol* 2002;39:242.
Feldstein AE, Perrault J, El-Youssif M, et al. Primary sclerosing cholangitis in children: a long-term follow-up study. *Hepatology* 2003;38:210.
Grompe M. The pathophysiology and treatment of hereditary tyrosinemia type 1. *Semin Liver Dis* 2001;21:563.
Kurbegov AC, Setchell KDR, Haas JE, et al. Biliary diversion for progressive familial intrahepatic cholestasis: improved liver morphology and bile acid profile. *Gastroenterology* 2003;125:1227.
Lykavieris P, Hadchouel M, Chardot C, Bernard O. Outcome of liver disease in children with Alagille syndrome: a study of 163 patients. *Gut* 2001;49: 431.
Martinez M, Vazquez E, Garcia-Silva MT, et al. Therapeutic effects of docosahexaenoic acid ethyl ester in patients with generalized peroxisomal disorders. *Am J Clin Nutr* 2000;71:376S.
Miyano T, Yamataka A. Choledochal cysts. *Curr Opin Pediatr* 1997;9:283.
Murray KF, Kowdley KV. Neonatal hemochromatosis. *Pediatrics* 2001;108:960.
Perlmutter DH. Liver injury in alpha-1-antitrypsin deficiency. *Clin Liv Dis* 2000;4:387.
Piccoli DA, Spinner NB. Alagille syndrome and the Jagged I gene. *Semin Liver Dis* 2001;21:525.
Roberts EA, Schilskky ML. A practice guideline on Wilson's disease. *Hepatology* 2003;37:1475.
Singh I, Johnson GH, Brown FR III. Peroxisomal disorders. Biochemical and clinical diagnostic considerations. *Am J Dis Child* 1988;142:1297.
Sokol RJ, Durie PR. Recommendations for management of liver and biliary tract disease in cystic fibrosis. *J Pediatr Gastroenterol Nutr* 1999;28:S1.
Sokol RJ, Mack C, Narkewicz MR, Karrer FM. Pathogenesis and outcome of biliary atresia: current concepts. *J Pediatr Gastroenterol Nutr* 2003;37:4.
Sokol RJ, Treem WR. Mitochondria and childhood liver diseases. *J Pediatr Gastroenterol Nutr* 1999;28:4.
Wirth S, Lang T, Gehring S, Gerner P. Recombinant alfa-interferon plus ribavirin therapy in children and adolescents with chronic hepatitis C. *Hepatology* 2002;36:1280.

CHAPTER 371 ■ PORTAL HYPERTENSION

WILLIAM J. COCHRAN

The portal vein is formed at the junction of the superior mesenteric vein and the splenic vein. The inferior mesenteric vein joins with either the splenic or superior mesenteric vein. The portal vein goes to the hilum of the liver, where it bifurcates into right and left branches. These vessels continue to bifurcate until forming the hepatic sinusoids. The hepatic sinusoids then coalesce to form the hepatic vein, which ultimately joins the inferior vena cava.

Portal hypertension is an abnormal condition of sustained elevated pressure in the portal venous system. Normal portal vein pressure is between 5 and 10 mm Hg. Portal vein measurements rarely are made in clinical practice, because the methods for obtaining them are difficult and invasive. Several studies have documented that the complications of portal hypertension do not occur until the portal pressure gradient (i.e., the pressure gradient between the portal vein and the hepatic vein on the inferior vena cava) exceeds 10 to 12 mm Hg. Normal is less than 5 mm Hg. Above this threshold value, the absolute portal pressure correlates poorly with the complications associated with portal hypertension. The portal and hepatic veins do not have valves; therefore, the increased portal pressure results in increased blood flow and simultaneously increased pressure in the splanchnic system. This condition prompts the formation of portosystemic collaterals, which divert portal blood to the systemic circulation. In severe cases of cirrhosis, as much as 90% of the portal blood enters the systemic circulation through these collaterals and bypasses the liver.

Portal hypertension occurs more frequently in adult patients than in pediatric patients. Because adults are more frequently affected and clinical studies are more difficult to perform in the pediatric population, most of our knowledge regarding the etiology and treatment of portal hypertension comes from adult studies and from animal experiments.

ETIOLOGY

The two major factors that contribute to the development and maintenance of portal hypertension are increased vascular resistance and increased splanchnic blood flow. Increased vascular resistance to portal blood flow is the initiating factor responsible for the development of portal hypertension.

Three major sites of increased vascular resistance are seen: prehepatic, intrahepatic, and posthepatic (Box 371.1). Prehepatic portal hypertension is secondary to obstruction of portal venous flow. Within the prehepatic category, portal vein

> **BOX 371.1** **Causes of Portal Hypertension**
>
> *Prehepatic origin*
> Portal vein thrombosis
> *Intrahepatic origin*
> Presinusoidal
>   Schistosomiasis
>   Neoplasms
>   Hepatic cysts
> Sinusoidal
>   Cirrhosis
> Postsinusoidal
>   Venoocclusive disease
> *Posthepatic origin*
> Thrombosis
>   Budd-Chiari syndrome
> Cardiac disease
>   Right-sided heart failure
>   Constrictive pericarditis

thrombosis is the most common cause of portal hypertension in the pediatric population. Portal vein thrombosis can develop as a result of sepsis, pancreatitis, dehydration, shock, hypercoagulable states, umbilical vein catheterization, or omphalitis. Over half of the cases, however, are idiopathic. Other congenital anomalies are noted in 40% of the idiopathic cases compared with 12% of those with an identified postnatal cause. When this condition evolves, many small collateral veins develop to transport portal blood around the thrombosed portal vein to the liver. This condition is known as *cavernomatous transformation of the portal vein*, in which the normal portal vein is replaced by many small tortuous veins. Despite the presence of portal hypertension in these patients, their liver function studies and liver enzymes are normal. Patients with cavernomatous transformation of the portal vein can present at any age with splenomegaly or variceal bleeding or both. Classically, the frequency of variceal bleeding in this disorder was considered to decrease after adolescence, but more recent studies indicate that this is not the case. Variceal bleeding secondary to portal vein thrombosis can occur at any age and can result in massive, life-threatening bleeding.

Increased vascular resistance in intrahepatic portal hypertension is secondary to increased intrahepatic and portocollateral resistance. Two major components of this increased intrahepatic vascular resistance are an irreversible component due to anatomic alterations and a reversible component that results from an increase in vascular tone.

The sites of anatomic abnormalities in intrahepatic portal hypertension can be divided into three major groups: presinusoidal, sinusoidal, and postsinusoidal. Hepatic schistosomiasis is the most common cause of presinusoidal portal hypertension worldwide, although it is exceedingly rare in North America. Patients with hepatic schistosomiasis develop portal hypertension as a result of ova deposition in the portal venules and the subsequent periportal granulomatous reaction. Overall, hepatic schistosomiasis is second only to cirrhosis as the most common cause of portal hypertension. Neoplasms and hepatic cysts, as seen in polycystic disease or Caroli disease, may compress the portal venules and result in presinusoidal portal hypertension.

The primary cause of sinusoidal portal hypertension in pediatric and adult patients is cirrhosis. As noted previously,

cirrhosis is the most common cause of portal hypertension in adult and pediatric patients. Numerous pediatric disorders can lead to cirrhosis, in part because the liver responds to injury in a limited manner and cirrhosis is the final common pathway. The most common cause of cirrhosis in the pediatric population is biliary atresia, but many other disorders are associated with cirrhosis. These include alpha-1-antitrypsin deficiency, cystic fibrosis, infectious hepatitis, autoimmune hepatitis, and other metabolic disorders (see Chapter 370).

Venoocclusive disease is an example of a disorder causing intrahepatic postsinusoidal portal hypertension. Histologically, venoocclusive disease is characterized by sclerosis of the terminal hepatic veins, which results in increased resistance and the subsequent development of portal hypertension. This condition is relatively uncommon in children but occurs most frequently after bone marrow transplantation or in patients with immune deficiency. The risk that bone marrow transplant patients will develop venoocclusive disease is increased when leukemia is the reason for transplantation, when preexisting hepatic dysfunction is present, and when the procedure is the second bone marrow transplantation.

The classic cause of posthepatic portal hypertension is the Budd-Chiari syndrome, which is a thrombus in the hepatic vein at the entry to the inferior vena cava. Posthepatic portal hypertension also can develop as a result of severe right heart disease or constrictive pericarditis.

Anatomic changes are the most important component (the irreversible component) of increased intrahepatic resistance. The reversible component of increased hepatic resistance, increased intrahepatic vascular tone, has been shown to be present in patients with chronic liver disease and portal hypertension. Two cell types are involved: stellate cells and sinusoidal endothelial cells. Stellate cells (also called *Ito cells*) surround the sinusoidal endothelial cells. When injured, these cells produce collagen as well as smooth-muscle–like protein; the latter can contract when exposed to a number of substances, such as endothelin, angiotensin II, substance P, thrombin, and thromboxane. Current evidence supports the theory that, with injury, these stellate cells produce smooth-muscle actin, which results in perisinusoidal contraction and thereby alters sinusoidal blood flow.

The sinusoidal endothelial cells also respond to various vasoactive substances. Alterations in vasoactive compounds contribute to the reversible component of this increased intrahepatic vascular resistance. Evidence indicates that several vasoconstrictors including endothelin, angiotensin, norepinephrine, and vasopressin are increased in those with cirrhosis. Simultaneously, there is a reduction in several vasodilators including nitric oxide. These changes then result in increased vascular tone of the sinusoidal endothelial cells, thus contributing to the increased intrahepatic resistance.

CLINICAL MANIFESTATIONS

Portal hypertension can present as gastrointestinal (GI) bleeding, splenomegaly, ascites, or prominent abdominal vasculature. GI bleeding is frequently the presenting manifestation of portal hypertension and can occur as early as infancy. The bleeding is most frequently from esophageal varices but can occur from gastric, duodenal, or colonic varices. Rectal hemorrhoids are very uncommon in infants and young children; the presence of rectal hemorrhoids in this population should suggest portal hypertension. Portal gastropathy and portal colopathy are other sources of GI bleeding in patients with portal hypertension.

Splenomegaly is the second most frequent mode of presentation. These patients may present with splenomegaly or with hypersplenism. Most patients with portal hypertension eventually

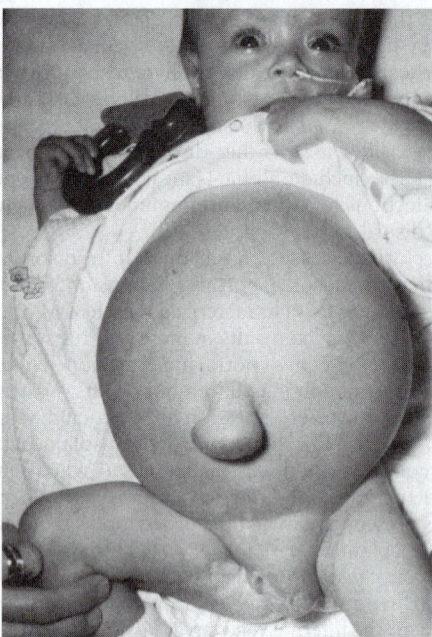

FIGURE 371.1. Female infant with cirrhosis due to biliary atresia. Note abdominal distension, umbilical hernia, and labial swelling due to massive ascites.

develop splenomegaly, although no direct correlation is found between spleen size and the portal pressure gradient. The presence of upper GI bleeding in a patient with splenomegaly should be considered due to portal hypertension until proven otherwise.

Ascites is frequently a problem in patients with sinusoidal and postsinusoidal portal hypertension but is uncommon in patients with presinusoidal hypertension. Ascites may be minimal, detected only incidentally on ultrasound examination of the abdomen, or it may be massive and be associated with an umbilical hernia, labial or scrotal enlargement, or respiratory insufficiency (Fig. 371.1).

Much less commonly, portal hypertension presents with prominent abdominal vasculature. The prominence of abdominal vasculature is the result of diversion of portal blood, as in the case of varices. When these vessels radiate from the umbilicus, the condition is known as *caput medusa*.

DIAGNOSIS

The existence of portal hypertension can be determined by several modalities (Box 371.2), but the condition is diagnosed most frequently by physical examination. The most common physical manifestations of portal hypertension are splenomegaly, ascites, prominent abdominal vasculature, and hemorrhoids or rectal varices. When portal hypertension is secondary to chronic liver disease, other physical manifestations may be present, including icterus, a firm to hard liver, asterixis, spider hemangiomas, palmar erythema, encephalopathy, and malnutrition.

Several invasive and noninvasive techniques can be used to document portal hypertension. The two major noninvasive techniques are the barium swallow test and ultrasonography. Before the advent of flexible endoscopy, the barium swallow was the test performed most commonly to detect portal hypertension and its major complication, esophageal varices. The majority of patients with long-standing portal hypertension have esophageal varices, which can be identified by barium

---

BOX 371.2   Diagnosis of Portal Hypertension

Physical examination
Splenomegaly
Ascites
Prominent abdominal vessels
Esophageal varices
Hemorrhoids/rectal varices
Evidence of chronic liver disease

Noninvasive techniques
Barium swallow
Ultrasonography

Invasive techniques
Endoscopy
Direct measurement of portal pressure
Measurement of hepatic venous pressure gradient
Angiography
Splenoportography

---

swallow as worm-like structures in the esophagus (Fig. 371.2). Ultrasonography is extremely useful in evaluating children with portal hypertension. In addition to predicting the presence of portal hypertension, ultrasonography is helpful in evaluating causes such as cirrhosis, hepatic cysts, or portal vein thrombosis. Ultrasonography also can assess spleen size, detect the presence of ascites, and determine if any associated renal abnormalities exist, such as are noted in congenital hepatic fibrosis. A classic ultrasonographic finding of portal hypertension in adult patients is an enlarged portal vein diameter. The portal vein also should be assessed in relation to respiration. In normal patients, the portal vein increases in diameter with inspiration. This increase with inspiration does not occur in patients with portal hypertension, and its absence may be a more reliable indicator of portal hypertension than is the actual diameter of the portal vein. A more reliable marker of portal hypertension in pediatric patients is the ratio of portal vein diameter (in millimeters) to body surface area (in square meters). If this ratio

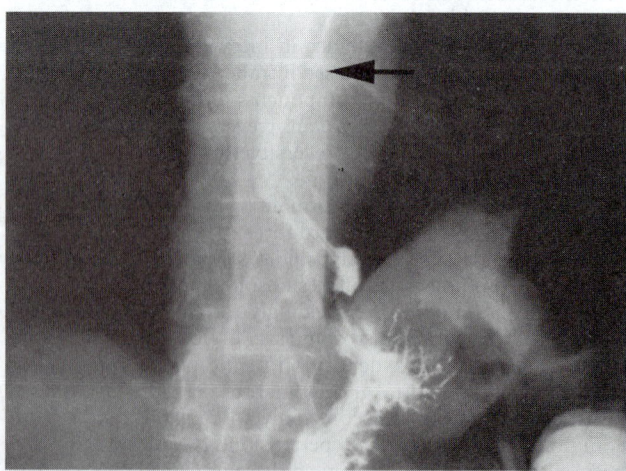

FIGURE 371.2. Barium swallow test in a patient with portal hypertension and esophageal varices. The linear structures (*arrow*) in the esophagus indicate esophageal varices. (Courtesy of Dr. Thomas Colley, Geisinger Clinic, Danville, PA.)

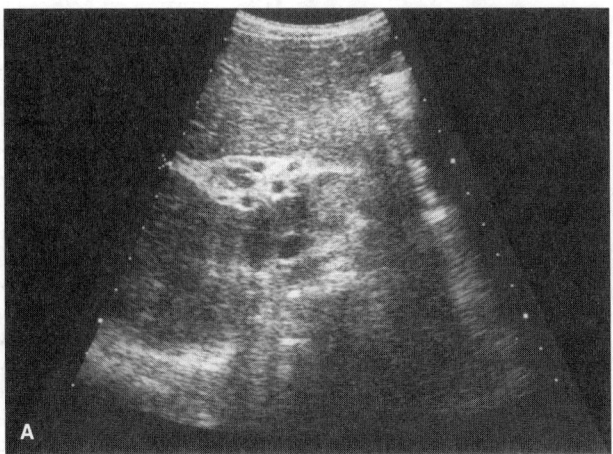

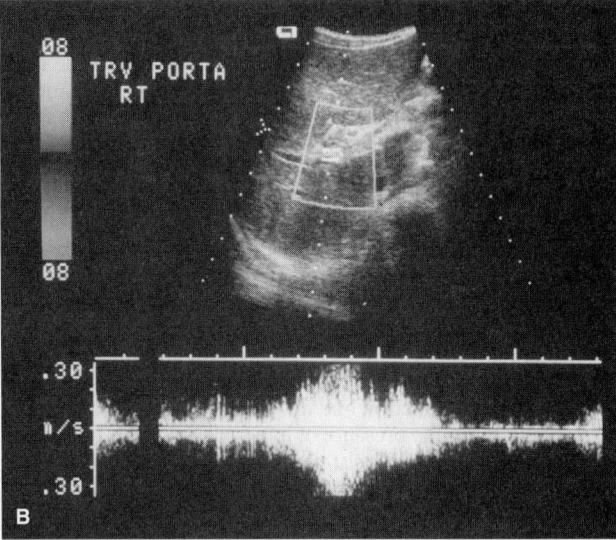

FIGURE 371.3. **A:** Ultrasonic examination of patient with cavernomatous transformation of the portal vein demonstrating the small collateral veins. **B:** Doppler ultrasonographic study of the same patient; the collateral veins are enclosed in the rectangle. See Color Figure 371.3B in color section; the collateral veins appear blue in that image.

exceeds 12, esophageal varices are likely. Another parameter is the ratio of the lesser omentum thickness to aortic diameter. In patients with portal hypertension, blood flow through the lesser omentum rises, increasing its thickness and thus increasing this ratio. A ratio of greater than 1.9 is a good predictor of the presence of esophageal varices.

Doppler ultrasonography can be used to assess blood flow within the portal vein, which normally is 10 to 30 mL/second and hepatopetal in direction. Because of increasing vascular resistance, blood flow decreases as portal hypertension increases and, in severe cases, the direction of the blood flow may be reversed (hepatofugal flow). In cases of cavernomatous transformation of the portal vein, color Doppler ultrasonography can help to determine the presence of small collaterals around the obstructed portal vein (Fig. 371.3).

Other studies using Doppler ultrasonography in children suggest that portal vein pulsatility is a sensitive and specific finding indicative of portal hypertension in children. Another potentially useful parameter is maximal velocity of the main portal vein. This value decreases as the severity of liver disease increases.

Invasive techniques to determine the presence of portal hypertension include endoscopy, direct measurement of portal pressure, measurement of hepatic venous pressure gradient, angiography, contrast-enhanced computed topography, magnetic resonance angiography, and splenoportography. Endoscopy can be performed safely in pediatric patients and is more sensitive in detecting esophageal varices than is the barium swallow test or ultrasonography. Endoscopy allows visual inspection of the varices to determine size and color, which is helpful in predicting the risk of bleeding (Fig. 371.4). Endoscopy can also determine the presence of portal gastropathy and gastric and duodenal varices.

Portal pressure can be measured directly by percutaneously puncturing an intrahepatic branch of the portal vein or during abdominal surgery by inserting a needle directly into the portal vein. The former procedure is difficult to perform in pediatric patients, and the latter procedure is unacceptable for the sole purpose of diagnosing portal hypertension. Direct measurements are most commonly performed in a research setting.

The hepatic venous pressure gradient is measured by placing a catheter in the hepatic vein under fluoroscopic control.

The free hepatic venous pressure is obtained, and the catheter is advanced until the catheter occludes a small hepatic vein. The pressure is obtained in this position and is known as the *wedged hepatic venous pressure*. The hepatic venous pressure gradient is the difference between the wedged hepatic venous pressure and the free hepatic venous pressure. This gradient is normally less than 5 mm Hg; a value greater than 10 mm Hg is indicative of portal hypertension. Complications of portal hypertension typically do not occur until the hepatic venous pressure gradient exceeds 12 mm Hg. Patients with prehepatic portal hypertension, as in portal vein thrombosis, have a normal hepatic venous pressure gradient. Pressure gradient measurement is also invasive and is most commonly used in adult studies assessing the efficacy of pharmacologic agents to reduce portal pressure.

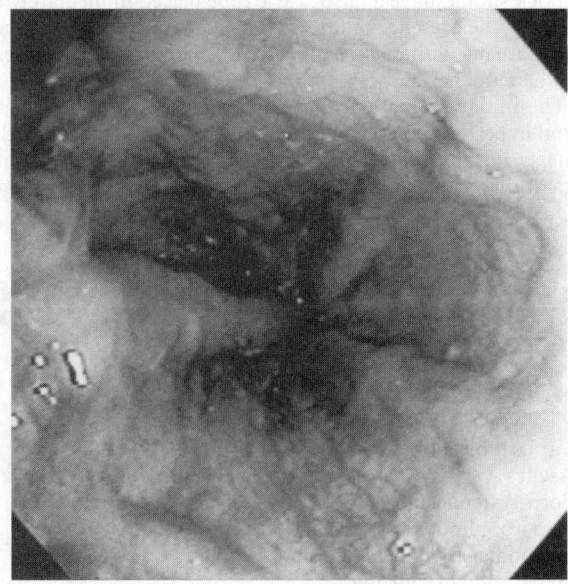

FIGURE 371.4. Endoscopic view of esophageal varices.

The major role of angiography in patients with portal hypertension is to rule out vascular thrombosis, as in the Budd-Chiari syndrome or portal vein thrombosis, and to define the vascular anatomy if surgery is contemplated. Recent advances in contrast-enhanced computed topography and magnetic resonance angiography have limited the use of mesenteric angiography.

Splenoportography is performed by the direct puncture of the spleen percutaneously. Because of the high risk associated with this procedure and because the portal system can be visualized with less invasive techniques, it is rarely performed. The procedure should not be used unless surgery can be performed immediately should complications occur.

Various laboratory studies are important in patients with portal hypertension—not to diagnose the condition but to further assess hepatic function and the patient's nutritional status and to evaluate for the presence of hypersplenism. This laboratory evaluation should consist of a complete blood count and measurement of serum electrolytes, coagulation studies, and liver and renal profiles.

COMPLICATIONS AND TREATMENT

Six major potential complications of portal hypertension are variceal bleeding, ascites, portosystemic encephalopathy, hepatopulmonary syndrome, hepatorenal syndrome, and splenomegaly with associated hypersplenism (Box 371.3). Variceal bleeding is the most frequent and potentially life-threatening complication of portal hypertension. Varices are present in 50% of patients with cirrhosis, and 10% to 30% experience an episode of variceal hemorrhage per year. After an initial episode of variceal hemorrhage, the risk of recurrent bleeding is high—40% at 6 weeks and 70% at 1 year. The mortality rate among adults with variceal bleeding is 30% to 50%. The mortality rate is lower among children but remains significant at 3% to 8%. Bleeding occurs most commonly from esophageal varices but may occur secondary to gastric, duodenal, or colonic varices as well as from ulcers, portal gastropathy, or portal colopathy.

Patients with upper GI hemorrhage most commonly present with hematemesis. Other presenting manifestations include melena, abdominal pain, syncope, and shock. Therefore, any patient with portal hypertension who presents with syncope or in shock should have a nasogastric tube placed immediately to assess for the presence of upper GI bleeding. Although uncommon, patients with massive upper GI hemorrhage may present with hematochezia.

The initial evaluation and management of a patient with portal hypertension and an acute upper GI hemorrhage are the same as for any other patient with upper GI bleeding. Rapid evaluation of the patient's circulatory status is imperative, and

if it is compromised, aggressive therapy is required. The patient's vital signs must be checked to determine whether the patient is hypotensive or whether orthostatic changes are present. If less than 10% of the blood volume has been lost, few signs or symptoms are present other than tachycardia. Patients receiving beta blockers may not develop tachycardia despite being hypovolemic. Not until more than 10% of blood volume has been lost are orthostatic changes noted. A loss of 20% or more of blood volume is associated with shock, tachycardia, hypotension, and decreased perfusion. Patients with GI bleeding require adequate IV access to allow rapid restoration of blood volume. The largest IV tube possible should be placed to allow high rates of infusion because the flow through an IV tube is proportional to the fourth power of the radius. If IV access cannot rapidly be obtained, an intraosseous line can be placed or a venous cutdown performed. Once IV access is obtained, normal intravascular volume must be established and maintained. A 20-mL/kg bolus of normal saline or Ringer lactate should be administered rapidly and repeated as needed until normal intravascular volume is obtained. These patients should not be overhydrated because this increases portal pressure and worsens the variceal bleeding. Placement of a central venous line may be helpful in monitoring central venous pressure to ensure normal intravascular volume and avoid overhydration. Packed red blood cells or whole blood should be administered as needed. In the event that a blood transfusion is required before blood has been typed and cross-matched, type O Rh-negative blood should be administered.

Laboratory studies to be obtained as soon as possible include a complete blood count, type, and cross-match; liver function studies including coagulation studies; serum electrolyte levels; and renal function tests. Platelets should be administered if the platelet count is less than 50,000 per deciliter. Prolonged coagulation should be corrected with 10 mL/kg of fresh-frozen plasma and vitamin K.

A nasogastric tube should be placed and gastric lavage performed as part of the initial evaluation. This procedure documents the presence of an upper GI bleed, assesses the degree of bleeding, prepares the patient for endoscopy, and allows the removal of protein load (i.e., blood) that could precipitate encephalopathy. No evidence exists that placement of a nasogastric tube precipitates variceal bleeding. If large clots that prevent lavage are present, a large-bore oral gastric tube such as an Ewald or Edlich tube can be used. These large tubes may compromise the airway, so elective intubation may be considered before their passage. Intubation may also prevent aspiration, which can occur with massive bleeding. Classically, iced saline has been used for lavage; however, no evidence exists to support its use over that of saline at room temperature. In addition, use of iced saline in infants may result in hypothermia.

The use of prophylactic antibiotics in adult patients with cirrhosis and variceal hemorrhage is now considered standard of care. The use of antibiotics in this situation has been shown to not only decrease the incidence of infection but also to increase survival. The antibiotic of choice in this situation is norfloxacin for 7 days. There is no pediatric data available to substantiate the use of prophylactic antibiotics but it is advocated. Cefotaxime or ceftriaxone are the antibiotics used for the pediatric population.

After initial stabilization of the patient, an upper endoscopy should be performed both for diagnostic and therapeutic purposes. When patients with known portal hypertension and esophageal varices present with an acute upper GI hemorrhage, one cannot assume that the bleeding is from the varices. In 40% to 50% of adult patients, the bleeding is from a source other than esophageal varices. In one study of cirrhotic pediatric patients with GI bleeding, the source was other than variceal in 36% of cases. Appropriate therapy depends on the cause of the

---

BOX 371.3 **Complications of Portal Hypertension**

Variceal bleeding
Ascites
Portosystemic encephalopathy
Hepatopulmonary syndrome
Splenomegaly/hypersplenism
Hepatorenal syndrome

BOX 371.4   **Therapy of Acute Variceal Hemorrhage**

Endoscopic techniques
  Sclerotherapy
  Band ligation
Pharmacologic therapy
  Vasopressin
  Terlipressin
  Somatostatin
  Octreotide
Balloon tamponade
  Sengstaken-Blakemore tube
  Minnesota tube
Surgical techniques
  Transjugular intrahepatic portosystemic shunts
  Surgically created portosystemic shunts
    Portocaval
    Splenorenal
    Distal splenorenal
  Devascularization
  Liver transplantation

---

bleeding, so it is imperative to determine the source of bleeding. Patients with portal hypertension may bleed from ulcers or gastritis, in which case therapy with an acid-suppressing agent should be instituted. These agents, however, exert no beneficial effect on bleeding esophageal varices. Patients with an upper GI hemorrhage should not have a barium swallow test in an attempt to diagnose the cause of the bleeding. Although this study may detect esophageal varices, it does not prove that the bleeding is from the varices. Gastric blood and clots make interpretation of the gastric component of an upper GI series challenging. Ingested barium makes it difficult to adequately perform an upper endoscopy, the most sensitive diagnostic test in the evaluation of an upper GI hemorrhage.

Therapeutic endoscopy, sclerotherapy, and band ligation form the mainstay of treatment for esophageal variceal hemorrhage (Box 371.4). Sclerotherapy had been the primary therapeutic modality used in pediatric patients; however, band ligation is now felt by many to be the procedure of choice. Sclerotherapy can be performed with conscious sedation or under general anesthesia. After the flexible endoscope is passed, a varix is visualized and then injected with a sclerosing agent. Injections are best placed several centimeters above the lower esophageal sphincter and can be intravariceal or paravariceal because these are equally effective. Various sclerosing agents can be used; the most common are morrhuate sodium, ethanolamine oleate, and absolute alcohol used in volumes of 1 to 3 mL per varix and at a maximum of 10 to 15 mL per session. In pediatric patients, as in adults, sclerotherapy is effective in controlling bleeding in 70% to 90% of the cases. Unfortunately, rebleeding occurs in 10% to 30% of these patients. Complications from sclerotherapy occur in 10% to 30% of patients, with a mortality rate of 1%. The most common complications are fever, retrosternal chest pain, esophageal ulceration, bleeding, perforation, and stricture formation. If all the varices are not obliterated during the initial session, a repeat elective session should be performed in 2 to 4 weeks.

Esophageal variceal ligation is accomplished by passing the endoscope with a banding device on the end that holds multiple bands. Once the varix to be banded is isolated, suction is applied via the endoscope to bring the varix into the de-

vice, and the band is then released over the varix, occluding it. Esophageal band ligation is as effective as sclerotherapy in the control of acute variceal bleeding and is associated with fewer complications and reduced mortality.

A newer endoscopic therapeutic modality is endoscopically placed hemoclips. These jaw-like clips mechanically clamp the varix to control the bleeding. These have been used successfully to control bleeding varices in adults and to a limited degree in pediatric patients.

Pharmacologic therapy is an important modality for treating esophageal variceal hemorrhage. Pharmacologic therapy can be instituted as soon as variceal hemorrhage is suspected, even prior to endoscopy. Several drugs are available that can be used in the therapy of acute variceal bleeding: vasopressin, terlipressin, somatostatin, and octreotide. Vasopressin has been the mainstay of pharmacologic therapy for variceal bleeding. Vasopressin is a short-acting vasoconstrictor that increases splanchnic vascular resistance, thereby decreasing splanchnic blood flow and portal pressure. In addition, vasopressin increases the lower esophageal sphincter pressure, which may compress the submucosal blood vessels and decrease variceal blood flow. Vasopressin is administered intravenously because no benefit is derived from selective administration, and the latter is associated with a high frequency of complications. Because of its short half-life, vasopressin is administered via a continuous infusion at a dosage of 0.3 to 0.4 U/kg/hour. Some investigators recommend administration of a bolus (0.3 U/kg over 20 minutes) before starting the continuous infusion. Therapy should be started at a lower dose and increased as needed to control bleeding to a maximal dosage of 48 U/hour. Above this level, a high incidence of side effects occurs with little further reduction in portal pressure. The major side effects of vasopressin are related to its vasoconstrictive effects and include bowel ischemia, myocardial ischemia, decreased cardiac output, bradycardia, cerebrovascular accidents, and diarrhea. It may exert an antidiuretic effect, resulting in hyponatremia. After bleeding ceases, the vasopressin is continued for several hours and then tapered by 20% every 4 hours until it is discontinued. Overall, the success rate of using vasopressin alone to control variceal hemorrhage is in the range of 75% to 80%.

Nitroglycerin, a vasodilator, is recommended in conjunction with vasopressin. The systemic vasodilation caused by nitroglycerin results in reflex splanchnic vasoconstriction, which decreases portal pressure. The major side effects of vasopressin are from its systemic vasoconstrictive effects; these are reduced by the systemic vasodilatory effects of nitroglycerin. Multiple adult studies have documented that use of a combination of vasopressin and nitroglycerin is more effective and is associated with fewer side effects than is use of vasopressin alone. Pediatric experience with this combination is limited. Nitroglycerin is started at a dose of 0.25 to 0.5 μg/kg/minute and is increased by 0.5 μg/kg/minute every 5 minutes to a total of 1 to 2 μg/kg/minute. Even when used in combination with nitroglycerin, vasopressin is associated with significant side effects, which limits its usefulness.

Terlipressin is a synthetic vasopressin analogue that was developed in an attempt to decrease the side effects associated with vasopressin. The half-life of terlipressin is longer than that of vasopressin, allowing for bolus administration instead of continuous infusion. The adult dosage is 2 mg intravenously every 4 hours for the first 24 hours of therapy; the dosage is then decreased to 1 mg every 4 hours. Multiple adult studies have documented its efficacy at controlling variceal hemorrhage in more than 70% of cases. The complication rate associated with terlipressin is less than that of vasopressin, even when the latter is combined with nitroglycerin. Its use is not yet approved in the United States, however.

Newer pharmacologic therapies for bleeding esophageal varices include somatostatin and octreotide. Somatostatin appears to cause splanchnic vasoconstriction by inhibiting the release of several vasodilatory substances, including glucagon, substance P, and vasoactive intestinal peptide. In addition, octreotide appears to have a direct splanchnic vasoconstrictor effect. Its net effect is to reduce splanchnic and hepatic blood flow, which results in a decrease in portal pressure. The vasoconstrictor effect is limited to the splanchnic system without the systemic vasoconstriction associated with vasopressin. Complication rates are very low, with the most common complication being hyperglycemia. Meta-analytic studies comparing somatostatin to vasopressin noted somatostatin to be more effective in controlling variceal bleeding, and it is associated with fewer side effects than is vasopressin. The adult dosage of somatostatin is a 250-μg bolus given intravenously, followed by a continuous infusion of 250 μg/hour. Somatostatin is not currently available in the United States.

Octreotide, a synthetic analogue of somatostatin, exhibits the same effect on the portal circulation and is as efficacious in controlling acute variceal hemorrhage as somatostatin. The half-life of octreotide is longer than that of somatostatin but is still short enough to require continuous intravenous infusion. In adults, octreotide is administered as a bolus of 50 μg, followed by a constant infusion of 50 μg/hour. Pediatric experience with octreotide in gastrointestinal bleeding associated with portal hypertension is limited. The largest pediatric series to date noted bleeding to cease in 70% of cases. Recommended pediatric dose is a bolus of 1 to 2 μg/kg to a maximum of 50 μg, followed by a constant infusion of 1 to 3 μg/kg/hour to a maximum of 50 μg/hour. Several studies have noted octreotide to be safer and more effective than vasopressin, making octreotide the drug of choice in the treatment of variceal hemorrhage.

Another therapeutic modality that has been used in patients with resistant bleeding esophageal varices is balloon tamponade. The most commonly used tubes are the Sengstaken-Blakemore tube and the Minnesota tube. The Sengstaken-Blakemore tube has a gastric and an esophageal balloon with a gastric lumen. The Minnesota tube is similar but has a gastric and an esophageal lumen in addition to the two balloons. The ability to suction esophageal contents makes the Minnesota tube preferable. Use of these tubes should be restricted to intensive care units, and the patient should be intubated to prevent aspiration. The tube is inserted, and the gastric balloon is inflated and then pulled back, applying pressure on the gastroesophageal junction. A radiograph of the abdomen should be obtained to confirm the balloon's position. If bleeding does not stop, the esophageal balloon is inflated. The gastric and esophageal lumens should be suctioned continuously to monitor bleeding and help prevent aspiration. Esophageal balloon inflation should not exceed 24 hours. Different sizes of tubes are available for pediatric use. Balloon tamponade may control variceal bleeding in 80% of cases, but its use is limited because it is associated with a high rate of complications, including esophageal rupture and aspiration. Early rebleeding is a frequent problem with balloon tamponade even when the initial bleeding event is controlled, with rebleeding rates in the range of 50%. As a result, balloon tamponade should be reserved for those patients in whom endoscopic and pharmacologic therapy has failed, as a temporary means before surgical intervention.

Transjugular intrahepatic portosystemic shunt (TIPS) placement is a relatively new therapeutic modality available for the management of portal hypertension. This shunt functions on the same principle as other surgically created portosystemic shunts to decrease portal pressure. The shunting is accomplished by passing a catheter through the internal jugular vein into the hepatic vein under fluoroscopic control. The hepatic vein is punctured, and the catheter advanced into a branch of the portal vein. A metallic mesh stent is then placed between the portal vein and the hepatic vein. The result is a decrease in absolute portal pressure and an increase in vena cava pressure. The combined effect is a reduction in the portal pressure gradient. TIPS is also associated with an increase in cardiac output, an increase in right atrial pressure, and a decrease in systemic vascular resistance. TIPS is contraindicated in patients with portal vein thrombosis.

TIPS can be performed successfully in 90% of adult patients; the mortality rate is approximately 1%. Complications include peritoneal bleeding (1% to 2%); variceal rebleeding (10% to 20%); and transient deterioration in liver function. Worsening of liver function is secondary to decreased hepatic blood flow. The liver capsule is punctured in 30% of cases. With correction of coagulopathy prior to the procedure, this complication corrects itself and does not typically require surgical intervention. Hemolysis occurs in 10% to 15% of patients and typically resolves spontaneously in 3 to 4 weeks. As with surgically created portosystemic shunts, TIPS is associated with portosystemic encephalopathy, which occurs in 20% to 30% of cases. Unfortunately, TIPS frequently becomes partially or totally occluded. Thrombosis of the catheter occurs in 10% to 15%. Stenosis occurs in 18% to 78% of patients after 1 year. Doppler ultrasound can be used to monitor for this complication but if suspected, angiography is required.

TIPS has been used successfully to treat acute variceal bleeding and to prevent recurrent variceal bleeding. Patients with refractory ascites have also responded to TIPS treatment. The frequency of occlusion and the development of portosystemic encephalopathy limit its use in long-term management of portal hypertension. Current indications for TIPS placement include acute variceal bleeding not controlled by conventional medical therapy and recurrent variceal bleeding before performance of a liver transplantation. Evidence exists that TIPS may also be beneficial in treatment of the hepatorenal syndrome. TIPS has been used successfully in the pediatric population; however, its availability is limited to major institutions.

If aggressive medical management fails to control acute variceal bleeding, several surgical procedures can be considered, such as devascularization of the stomach and esophagus, portosystemic shunt surgery, and liver transplantation. Devascularization surgery, although effective for controlling acute variceal bleeding, is rarely performed because of the high rate of associated rebleeding (40% to 50%) and the availability of newer therapeutic modalities. Portosystemic shunt surgery, too, is effective but is performed less frequently than before 1990. Several portosystemic shunt procedures are used. Portosystemic shunts can be nonselective or selective. The nonselective shunts are the portocaval and splenorenal shunts. Because of the diversion of blood flow away from the liver, these shunts are associated with a high rate of postoperative encephalopathy, which occurs in 15% to 30% of patients. Selective shunts, such as the distal splenorenal shunt, attempt to decompress the gastric and esophageal venous component of the portal system while maintaining hepatic blood flow. Because hepatic blood flow is maintained, these shunts are associated with a lower incidence of portosystemic encephalopathy (10%) and are therefore generally preferred to the nonselective shunts. Long-term survival also appears to be better in patients with the distal splenorenal shunt than in patients with nonselective shunts. Mortality rates associated with emergency shunt surgery are high and are greatest in those with more severe bleeding and with the most hepatic dysfunction. Portosystemic shunts are more difficult to perform in young children and are more likely to become occluded, which minimizes their usefulness in this population. In pediatric patients with hepatic portal hypertension and variceal hemorrhage, liver transplantation is preferable to shunt surgery for long-term management.

Shunt surgery can be considered for patients with extrahepatic portal hypertension accompanied by variceal bleeding unresponsive to medical therapy. In the past, one of the portosystemic shunts would be performed. More recently, however, a shunt bypassing the thrombosed portal vein has been used with success. This shunt grafts the jugular vein between the superior mesenteric vein and the distal portion of the left portal vein (Rex shunt).

Liver transplantation is an accepted therapeutic modality for the treatment of pediatric patients with end-stage liver disease; the survival rate is approximately 90%. Liver transplantation is commonly performed in patients for significant complications of portal hypertension, including acute variceal hemorrhage. Variceal hemorrhage should first be managed medically; however, if the patient is unresponsive to this treatment, liver transplantation should be considered even before emergent portosystemic shunt surgery for those with end-stage liver disease.

Ascites (see Chapter 365) is a frequent problem in patients with sinusoidal and postsinusoidal portal hypertension. It is uncommon in patients with presinusoidal portal hypertension. The pathogenesis of ascites in patients with portal hypertension is multifactorial. The portal hypertension results in increased hydrostatic pressure and, in patients with associated liver disease accompanied by hypoalbuminemia, decreased oncotic pressure is seen. These alterations in Starling forces cause fluid to move from the intravascular space to the extravascular space. When the rate of extravascular fluid production exceeds the ability of the lymphatic system to reabsorb this fluid and transport it back to the vascular system, the fluid accumulates in the peritoneal cavity; the result is ascites. Another factor contributing to the development of ascites in patients with cirrhosis is renal sodium retention and subsequent plasma volume expansion. This increase in intravascular volume increases the hydrostatic pressure in the hepatosplanchnic circulation, resulting in fluid extravasation into the peritoneal space.

Ascites can be minimal, detected only incidentally on ultrasonic examination, or it can be massive, resulting in early satiety and malnutrition or respiratory distress. Medical therapy for ascites consists of normalization of the patient's nutritional status, salt restriction, and use of diuretics such as spironolactone. If the patient is having acute symptoms such as respiratory distress, a large-volume therapeutic paracentesis can be performed or albumin can be administered intravenously at a rate of 1 g/kg over 1 to 2 hours, with furosemide, 1 mg/kg, given intravenously halfway through the infusion. In cases of refractory ascites, the patient can undergo peritoneovenous shunt placement (LeVeen or Denver shunt) or TIPS procedure. The high incidence of complications and occlusion along with the advent of TIPS limits the usefulness of the peritoneovenous shunts.

Another potential complication of ascites with portal hypertension is spontaneous bacterial peritonitis (SBP). The organisms most commonly involved are *Escherichia coli*, *Klebsiella*, *Streptococcus*, and *Enterococcus*. Cefotaxime sodium is considered the drug of choice for SBP; therapy should be continued for 5 to 10 days. SBP is associated with a mortality rate of 20%. SBP also has a high recurrence rate in those who survive, with a probability of recurrence of 70% in 1 year. Due to the high mortality rate and rate of recurrence, patients with cirrhosis who recover from the initial episode of SBP should be considered for liver transplantation. Administration of trimethoprim and sulfamethoxazole or norfloxacin appears to be effective prophylaxis for the prevention of SBP in patients with cirrhosis and ascites.

Portosystemic encephalopathy is a neuropsychiatric disorder characterized by alterations in consciousness, impaired intellectual abilities, and several neuromuscular signs such as asterixis. Laboratory evaluation of affected patients reveals elevated ammonia levels, and an electroencephalogram demonstrates diffuse slowing. This condition develops most often in patients with severe liver disease who have portosystemic shunts. These shunts can develop spontaneously or can be the result of TIPS surgery or surgically created portosystemic shunts. Although multiple theories have been put forward to explain the pathogenesis of portosystemic encephalopathy, its exact cause is unknown. Precipitating factors include dehydration, use of diuretics, GI bleeding, infection, and use of sedatives. Therapy is directed toward reducing serum ammonia levels by decreasing dietary protein to decrease endogenous ammonia production, controlling any ongoing GI hemorrhaging, and removing blood from the GI tract. Neomycin can be administered to decrease enteric bacterial ammonia production, and lactulose is given to trap ammonia in the gut. Protein intake should not be curtailed totally, because the result is increased catabolism of endogenous protein and subsequent ammonia production. The use of branched-chain amino acid and total parenteral nutrition formulas has been somewhat successful at temporarily improving central nervous system function, but this treatment does not alter the course of the disease. Any precipitating cause of portosystemic encephalopathy, such as bacterial infection, should be treated. Patients with portosystemic encephalopathy should be checked for *Helicobacter pylori* and, if it is found, should be treated to decrease gastric ammonia production.

Splenomegaly and associated hypersplenism is a frequent problem in patients with portal hypertension. Patients may have massive splenomegaly, predisposing them to splenic rupture after blunt abdominal trauma. Symptoms vary from moderate left upper quadrant pain or left shoulder pain to overt shock. Patients with hypersplenism have a reduction in one or more hematologic components. Thrombocytopenia (platelet counts of 50,000 to 150,000/mm^3) is typical. If the condition is severe, treatment consists of splenectomy, liver transplantation, or the creation of a portosystemic shunt. The major risk of splenectomy is overwhelming sepsis. If splenectomy is to be performed, pneumococcal vaccine and meningococcal vaccine should be administered to children older than 2 years, and penicillin should be administered prophylactically after splenectomy.

Hepatopulmonary syndrome (HPS) is an uncommonly recognized complication of liver disease or portal hypertension. It is estimated that 40% of patients with cirrhosis and portal hypertension will have pulmonary vasodilation and 10% to 25% will have HPS. It is uncertain if the frequency and severity of HPS correlates with the degree of hepatic synthetic dysfunction or portal hypertension. This syndrome is the result of a pulmonary vasculopathy leading to intrapulmonary vasodilation and a widened alveolar–arterial gradient and the development of hypoxemia. The mechanism responsible for the intrapulmonary vasodilation is unknown, but it is theorized to be due to altered metabolism or clearance of vasoactive substances such as nitric oxide. Patients with HPS present clinically with shortness of breath, dyspnea on exertion, clubbing, cyanosis, and cutaneous spider angiomas. An arterial blood gas measurement should be obtained in a patient with possible HPS. Normal arterial oxygenation and alveolar–arterial gradient exclude HPS. An abnormality requires further evaluation, consisting of a chest radiograph to rule out other pulmonary disorders and contrast echocardiography to document intrapulmonary vasodilation. Radionuclide lung perfusion scanning with technetium-labeled macroaggregated albumin particles can be used to quantify intrapulmonary vasodilation. Unfortunately, no effective medical therapy exists for HPS. Supplemental oxygen may be of benefit. TIPS surgery can temporarily improve gas exchange, but the only effective long-term therapy is liver transplantation. There is a significant increased mortality rate in those with HPS. Even after successful transplantation, weeks to months can be required for resolution of pulmonary abnormalities.

Hepatorenal syndrome is a severe complication associated with cirrhosis and portal hypertension. The incidence of hepatorenal syndrome in adult patients hospitalized with ascites is 7% to 15%. The mortality rate associated with this disorder is exceedingly high, 80% at 4 weeks and 90% at 10 weeks. Hepatorenal syndrome is characterized by a low glomerular filtration rate (GFR) with an elevated serum creatinine greater than 1.5 mg/dL and/or 24-hour creatinine clearance of less than 40 mL/minute without any other obvious cause such as hypovolemia. Laboratory findings with this disorder include a low urine sodium (less than 10 mEq/L), urine osmolality greater than plasma osmolality, urine red blood cells less than 50 per high power field, and a serum sodium less than 130 mEq/L. Hepatorenal syndrome has been divided into two subtypes. Type I is acute (less than 2 weeks) renal impairment with a doubling of serum creatinine level to greater than 2.5 mg/dL or by a 50% reduction of the initial creatinine clearance to a level lower than 20 mL/minute. Type II is the slower onset of renal impairment. The prognosis of type I is much worse than is type II. Precipitating factors are identified in approximately two-thirds of patients who develop hepatorenal syndrome. These factors contribute to the development of hypovolemia and hypotension and include gastrointestinal bleeding; infection such as peritonitis; diarrhea or vomiting; and aggressive diuresis. Use of nephrotoxic drugs can contribute to renal impairment and care should be taken to avoid their use in individuals with cirrhosis and portal hypertension. The pathophysiologic hallmark of hepatorenal syndrome is peripheral vasodilation and renal vasoconstriction. Studies have documented an overproduction of intestinal nitric oxide, a potent systemic vasodilator, in these patients. As a consequence of this systemic vasodilation and decrease in effective arteriolar blood volume, there is a compensatory activation of vasoconstrictor systems including the sympathetic nervous system and renin–angiotensin–aldosterone system and a release of vasopressin. In addition, a reduction in renal vasodilators, prostaglandins E_2 and I_2, in patients with hepatorenal syndrome have been noted. The net effect is a reduction in renal blood flow resulting in renal impairment. Endotoxins play a role in the development of hepatorenal syndrome in those with infections. Endotoxin is known to induce thromboxane A2 and leukotrienes, which cause renal vasoconstriction. Due to the potential for infection, any patient with cirrhosis and portal hypertension who develops renal impairment should have cultures of blood, urine, and ascites obtained. Because it is difficult to differentiate between hypovolemia and hepatorenal syndrome, all patients should receive a fluid bolus and renal function should be reassessed prior to making a diagnosis of hepatorenal syndrome. Medical therapy was initially directed at the use of renal vasodilators. A number of studies have now documented that dopamine in renal doses is of no benefit in the management of hepatorenal syndrome. One study noted improvement in renal function with the use of N-acetylcysteine. N-acetylcysteine has renal medullar vasodilator properties as well as being an antioxidant. More studies are needed, however, prior to recommending its routine use. Vasopressin's potent splanchnic vasoconstrictor effect reduces portal blood flow and pressure, leading to a reduction in renal vasoconstrictors. Use of vasopressin has been of some temporary benefit in treating those with hepatorenal syndrome. Other means of reducing portal pressure such as TIPS can improve renal function. The only definitive long-term treatment of hepatorenal syndrome is liver transplantation. Vasopressin and TIPS are used to improve renal function until liver transplantation can be performed.

PREVENTION

Preventive measures in patients with portal hypertension are directed at reducing the incidence of initial or recurrent variceal bleeding. The risk of initial variceal hemorrhage for patients with small esophageal varices is 5% per year and 15% per year for those with large varices. Due to the frequency of variceal hemorrhage and the high morbidity and mortality rates associated with variceal bleeding, one should attempt to prevent the initial hemorrhage. Therapeutic modalities available for primary prevention of variceal bleeding include medical and surgical approaches. These same therapeutic modalities can be used in an attempt to prevent recurrent variceal bleeding. All patients with portal hypertension should wear a bracelet or chain stating that they have portal hypertension and indicating their blood type and any medications they are taking.

Products that can precipitate or worsen variceal bleeding should be avoided in children with portal hypertension. Aspirin use is a potentially aggravating factor in variceal bleeding. Because aspirin is a component of several medications, patients and parents should be taught to read the labels of medications to avoid inadvertent consumption of aspirin. Prophylaxis with acid-suppressing agents, histamine-2 (H_2) blockers, and proton pump inhibitors offers no benefit in the prevention of variceal bleeding and should be used only if the patient has acid peptic disease or gastroesophageal reflux. Theoretically, agents that increase lower esophageal sphincter pressure may be beneficial by decreasing blood flow in esophageal varices; however, no benefit of these agents has been documented.

Pharmacologic therapy for prevention of variceal hemorrhage is directed at reducing portal pressure. This reduction can be accomplished by decreasing blood flow into the portal system or by decreasing vascular resistance in the vessels at the site of origin of the portal hypertension and their collaterals. Propranolol hydrochloride, a nonselective beta blocker, is the agent most commonly used in the prevention of primary and secondary variceal hemorrhage. Propranolol hydrochloride reduces splanchnic blood flow and portal pressure by blocking vasodilatory splanchnic beta-adrenergic receptors and by decreasing cardiac output. The result is a reduction in gastroesophageal collateral blood flow, which decreases the risk of variceal bleeding. Propranolol hydrochloride has been shown to be more effective at reducing portal pressure than is atenolol, a cardioselective $beta_1$ blocker. The dose administered is that required to decrease the heart rate by 25% or to a resting heart rate of 55. Some evidence exists that abrupt cessation of propranolol hydrochloride therapy can result in a relatively rapid onset of variceal bleeding. Patients treated with propranolol hydrochloride should be cautioned not to discontinue use abruptly so that rebound bleeding can be avoided.

Adult studies have provided ample documentation that administration of propranolol hydrochloride significantly reduces the incidence of initial variceal bleeding and the frequency of fatal hemorrhage compared to administration of a placebo. For this reason, adults with portal hypertension should be screened for esophageal varices. Endoscopy is the gold standard for the detection and quantitation of esophageal varices. If large esophageal varices are present and the use of beta blockers is not contraindicated, therapy with propranolol hydrochloride should be instituted.

Use of pharmacologic therapy in pediatric patients is controversial. No controlled study has assessed the use of propranolol hydrochloride in children with portal hypertension, although it has been used in selected pediatric patients with an apparent beneficial response. In the vast majority of pediatric patients with esophageal varices, cirrhosis is the cause of the portal hypertension. These patients eventually require liver transplantation to survive. Therefore, most authorities advocate liver transplantation in pediatric patients with cirrhosis and esophageal varices as the optimal and permanent means of preventing initial variceal hemorrhage instead of a temporary measure such as administration of propranolol hydrochloride.

Another pharmacologic agent to be considered for prevention of initial variceal bleeding is isosorbide mononitrate. This agent is a vasodilator that acts by increasing nitric oxide formation in vascular smooth-muscle cells, resulting in a decrease in venous return and possibly a reduction in arterial pressure, leading to splanchnic vasoconstriction and decreased portal blood flow. Isosorbide mononitrate has been shown to be somewhat less effective than propranolol hydrochloride in the prevention of initial variceal hemorrhage. Isosorbide mononitrate also has been associated with a higher mortality rate than that associated with propranolol use. At this time it is recommended not to use isosorbide mononitrate as a single agent to prevent initial variceal bleeding. Several trials assessing the efficacy of combining propranolol hydrochloride and isosorbide mononitrate found it to be no more effective than propranolol alone in decreasing the risk of variceal bleeding. Pediatric use of isosorbide mononitrate is extremely limited.

Administration of spironolactone has been shown to reduce the hepatoportal venous gradient in cirrhotic patients with ascites. No studies exist evaluating the use of spironolactone as a single agent in the prevention of variceal hemorrhage; however, its use should be considered in those patients with ascites. Low-sodium diets exert no beneficial effect on portal pressure, but high sodium intake should be avoided.

Use of sclerotherapy or band ligation in the prevention of initial variceal hemorrhage is not recommended because it may not be as effective as therapy with propranolol hydrochloride and it has potential complications. Endoscopic band ligation can be considered for primary prevention in those with large varices who have contraindications to the use of propranolol. Portosystemic shunt surgery should not be used to prevent initial variceal hemorrhage. Studies assessing the efficacy of portosystemic shunt surgery revealed that the incidence of initial variceal hemorrhage was reduced. However, shunt surgery was associated with a high incidence of portosystemic encephalopathy, and survival was not as good as for medically treated patients.

The risk of recurrent variceal hemorrhage in patients who survive their initial hemorrhage is high; the recurrence rate is greater than 60% within 1 year of the initial bleed. The highest risk of rebleeding occurs in the first 2 weeks after the index bleed. Administration of propranolol hydrochloride, sclerotherapy, variceal band ligation, portosystemic shunt surgery, and TIPS have all been shown to be effective in reducing the risk of recurrent variceal hemorrhage. Unfortunately, no improvement in survival rate has been consistently demonstrated with any of these therapeutic modalities. Adult studies indicate that propranolol is safer and more effective than are endoscopic procedures. TIPS is more effective than propranolol but it is associated with a high rate of hepatic encephalopathy. Studies assessing the combination of propranolol and isosorbide mononitrate have revealed conflicting data, as has the combination of propranolol and band ligation.

Because of the high rate of rebleeding and the fact that the highest risk of rebleeding is within the first 2 weeks after the initial bleed, pediatric patients with cirrhosis who experience a variceal hemorrhage should be transferred to a liver transplant center and should undergo liver transplantation as soon as possible. Pediatric patients who experience an episode of variceal bleeding should undergo sclerotherapy or variceal band ligation. If they continue to experience rebleeding, portosystemic shunt surgery should be considered if liver transplantation is unavailable or inappropriate.

Suggested Readings

Bosch J, D'Amico G, Garcia-Pagan JC. Portal hypertension. In: *Schiff's diseases of the liver.* Philadelphia: Lippincott Williams & Wilkins, 2003:429.

Boyer TD. Transjugular intrahepatic portosystemic shunt: current status. *Gastroenterology* 2003;124:1700.

De Ville de Goyet J, Alberti D, Falchetti, et al. Treatment of extrahepatic portal hypertension in children by mesenteric-to-left portal vein bypass: a new physiological procedure. *Eur J Surg* 1999;165:777.

Eroglu Y, Emerick KM, Whitington PF, Alonso EM. Octreotide therapy for control of acute gastrointestinal bleeding in children. *J Pediatr Gastroenterol Nutr* 2004;38:41.

Fox VL, Carr-Locke DL, Conners PJ, Leichtner AM. Endoscopic ligation of esophageal varices in children. *J Pediatr Gastroenterol Nutr* 1995;20:202.

Garcia-Tsao G. Current management of the complications of cirrhosis and portal hypertension: variceal hemorrhage, ascites, and spontaneous bacterial peritonitis. *Gastroenterology* 2001;120:726.

Heaton ND, Davenport M, Howard ER. Symptomatic hemorrhoids and anorectal varices in children with portal hypertension. *J Pediatr Surg* 1992;27:833.

Heyman MB, LaBerge JM. Role of transjugular intrahepatic portosystemic shunt in the treatment of portal hypertension in pediatric patients. *J Pediatr Gastroenterol Nutr* 1999;29:240.

Hyams JS, Treem WR. Portal hypertensive gastropathy in children. *J Pediatr Gastroenterol Nutr* 1993;17:13.

Iannitti DA, Henderson JM. The role of surgery in the treatment of portal hypertension. *Clin Liver Dis* 1997;1:99.

Karrer FM, Narkewicz MR. Esophageal varies: current management in children. *Semin Pediatr Surg* 1999;8:193.

Kramer L, Horl WH. Hepatorenal syndrome. *Semin Nephrol* 2002;22:290.

McKiernan PJ. Treatment of variceal bleeding. *Gastrointest Endosc Clin North Am* 2001;11:789.

Peters JM. Management of gastrointestinal bleeding in children. *Curr Treatment Opt Gastroenterol* 2002;5:399.

Rabinowitz SS, Norton KI, Benkov KJ, et al. Sonographic evaluation of portal hypertension in children. *J Pediatr Gastroenterol Nutr* 1990;10:395.

Ryckman FC, Alonso MH. Causes and management of portal hypertension in the pediatric population. *Clin Liver Dis* 2001;5:789.

Schenk P, Schoniger-Hekele M, Fuhrmann V, et al. Prognostic significance of the hepatopulmonary syndrome in patients with cirrhosis. *Gastroenterology* 2003;125:1042.

Schenker S, Bay MK. Portal systemic encephalopathy. *Clin Liver Dis* 1997;1:157.

Shun A, Delaney DP, Martin HCO, et al. Portosystemic shunting for paediatric portal hypertension. *J Pediatr Surg* 1997;32:489.

Sudan DL, Shaw BW Jr. The role of liver transplantation in the management of portal hypertension. *Clin Liver Dis* 1997;1:115.

CHAPTER 372 ■ HEPATIC STEATOSIS

WILLIAM J. COCHRAN

Hepatic steatosis is a common entity that frequently goes unrecognized in the pediatric population. The term *hepatic steatosis* is used to describe excessive fat in the liver. Normally, fat accounts for less than 5% of the weight of the liver. Hepatic steatosis is not a primary disease process and can occur in many situations. Steatohepatitis is the presence of excessive hepatic fat in conjunction with inflammation. Ludwig in 1980 first used the expression nonalcoholic hepatic steatohepatitis (NASH) to

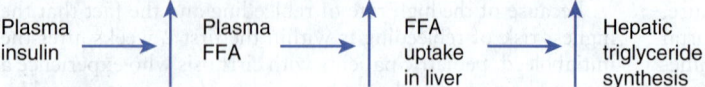

FIGURE 372.1. Increases in plasma free fatty acids (FFAs) leads to increased uptake of FFAs by the liver and subsequently increased hepatic triglyceride synthesis. This is an issue in obese children who tend to have hyperinsulinemia, which increases plasma FFA.

describe steatohepatitis not associated with excessive alcohol consumption. Subsequently this term has been dropped in favor of nonalcoholic fatty liver disease (NAFLD) to describe the spectrum of liver disease associated with excessive hepatic fat. NAFLD associated with obesity in adults has been recognized for almost 50 years. Moran was the first to report this entity in pediatric patients in 1983.

PATHOPHYSIOLOGY

Fat accumulates in the liver in a complex and, in certain situations, unknown manner. Although a complete discussion of hepatic lipid metabolism is beyond the scope of this chapter, several excellent reviews exist. Fat accumulation usually results from increased uptake, increased synthesis, decreased oxidation, or decreased secretion of fat by the liver.

Uptake of free fatty acids by the liver is proportional to the amount of free fatty acids to which the liver is exposed (Fig. 372.1). Ingestion of carbohydrates, especially glucose and fructose, as well as increased uptake of free fatty acids promotes hepatic triglyceride synthesis (Fig. 372.2). If triglyceride release in the form of lipoproteins does not increase proportionally, fat accumulates in the liver. Several factors are associated with increased plasma free fatty acid levels: acute starvation, elevation of several hormones (e.g., adrenocorticotropic hormone, thyrotropin, thyroid hormone, growth hormone, insulin), obesity, and use of certain drugs (e.g., corticosteroids, epinephrine).

A reduction in the oxidation of fatty acids may also result in development of hepatic steatosis. This can occur secondary to ingestion of chemicals such as hypoglycin A or amanitotoxin as well as to defects in fatty acid metabolism such as long-chain fatty acyl dehydrogenase deficiency (Fig. 372.3). Obesity is now the most common entity associated with NAFLD; therefore, its pathogenesis deserves further elaboration. The pathogenesis of NAFLD is felt to result from two metabolic alterations—hyperinsulinemia (Fig. 372.1) and increased oxidative stress, which is thought to be a cause of the inflammation in NAFLD and may be caused by increased fatty acids, which are hepatotoxic in their own right and also adversely affect intracellular membranes.

Many obese children have hyperinsulinemia. Elevated insulin levels promote an increase in plasma free fatty acids, which, as noted above, leads to increased uptake of free fatty acids by the liver and subsequently increased hepatic triglyceride synthesis. One means by which the liver can reduce its fat content is by re-esterification of fatty acids and subsequent secretion of triglycerides from the hepatocytes into the blood.

There is some evidence that obese individuals may have a decreased ability to accomplish this. Together, increased fatty acid uptake by the liver due to hyperinsulinemia and decreased ability to remove fat from the liver would result in increased hepatic fat. Support for the importance of oxidative stress in this process is derived from a study documenting improvement in children with NAFLD treated with the antioxidant vitamin E.

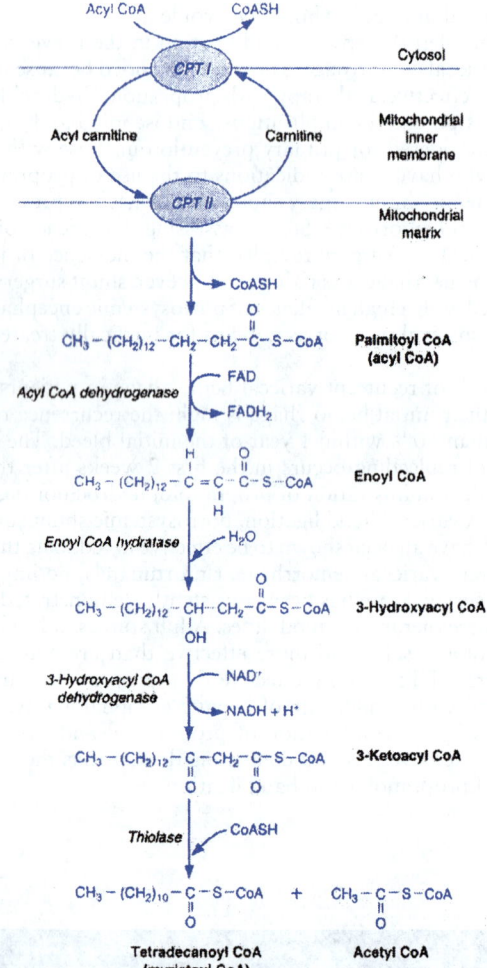

FIGURE 372.3. Fatty acids (acyl CoA in this example) are transported into the mitochondria in a carnitine-dependent process. Carnitine deficiency can thus be associated with hepatic steatosis secondary to decreased fatty acid oxidation. Within the mitochondria, fatty acids undergo beta oxidation as shown in this diagram. Ingestion of chemicals such as hypoglycin A or amanitotoxin as well as defects in fatty acid metabolism such as long-chain fatty acyl dehydrogenase deficiency (see fourth reaction within mitochondria) can result in decreased fatty acid oxidation, and thus hepatic steatosis. Reduction of mitochondrial fatty acid oxidation also may contribute to the hepatic steatosis in patients with Reye syndrome. (Reprinted with permission from Davidson, Sittman. *Biochemistry*, 4th ed. Philadelphia: Lippincott Williams & Wilkins, 1999.)

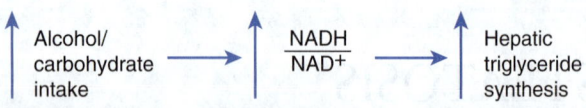

FIGURE 372.2. Hepatic triglyceride synthesis is increased in several disorders, but the condition secondary to alcoholism is best known. Metabolism of alcohol by the liver increases the ratio of the reduced form of nicotinamide adenine dinucleotide (NADH) to the nonreduced form (NAD^+), which promotes hepatic triglyceride synthesis. Ingestion of carbohydrates, especially glucose and fructose, also promotes hepatic triglyceride synthesis.

Disorders Associated with Hepatic Steatosis

The various disorders often associated with hepatic steatosis can be divided into several broad categories: nutritional, toxin- or drug-induced, metabolic, endocrine, infectious, and idiopathic (Box 372.1).

Hepatic steatosis is associated with several nutritional disorders, the first of which—protein-calorie malnutrition—was noticed by Williams in 1933. Hepatic steatosis is uncommon in patients with marasmus (i.e., protein and calorie deprivation) but common in patients with kwashiorkor (i.e., protein deprivation), in whom fat can account for 50% of the weight of the liver. The exact mechanism of hepatitic steatosis is unknown but is probably multifactorial, including elevation in the level of free fatty acids, reduction in peroxisomes associated with decreased oxidation of fat, decrease in apolipoprotein synthesis, and decrease in lipoprotein secretion. These patients frequently develop hepatomegaly, and their liver enzyme levels may be mildly elevated. Fat deposition begins first in the periportal area and progresses out to the central vein. With appropriate nutritional therapy, the fat disappears, first from the central area and last from the periportal area. Other isolated nutritional deficiencies, such as pyridoxine or riboflavin deficiency, may be associated with hepatic steatosis, although this is uncommon.

NAFLD is common among patients with overnutrition. Due to the current epidemic in pediatric obesity, obesity is now felt to be the most common cause of hepatic steatosis in the pediatric population in developed countries. Ten to twenty percent of obese children have elevated liver enzyme levels attributed to NAFLD. Studies using ultrasound have noted hepatic steatosis in 25% to 50% of obese children. There also appears to be a good correlation between the severity of obesity and the degree of hepatic steatosis. Liver biopsies in these obese children reveal varying degrees of macrovesicular and microvesicular hepatic steatosis, inflammation, and fibrosis. Several studies have documented fibrosis in 60% to 70% of obese children at the time of their initial evaluation. Some of these patients have bridging fibrosis, which, if uncorrected, could progress to cirrhosis. Indeed, there are several reports of cirrhosis in obese children secondary to NAFLD. Fifteen percent of adults with nonalcoholic steatohepatitis have cirrhosis. If patients lose weight, the inflammation and fatty changes can resolve. Thus, because of the potential seriousness of this disorder, obese patients should be screened for NAFLD by determining liver enzyme levels; if they are elevated, an ultrasound examination should be performed and other causes of hepatitis ruled out. These individuals should then be placed on a weight-reduction program. If liver enzymes do not return to normal levels, a liver biopsy should be performed and consideration be given to pharmacologic therapy such as vitamin E or metformin. Some individuals recommend more complete evaluation of NAFLD in all obese patients since adult studies have noted that significant steatohepatitis and fibrosis can be present even with normal alanine aminotransferase (ALT) levels.

Hepatic steatosis can be caused by many toxins and drugs, the most common of which is alcohol. As many as one-third of alcoholics without symptoms of liver disease have hepatic steatosis. Acute deposition of hepatic fat actually can occur after just one alcoholic binge. Other drugs associated with hepatic steatosis include tetracycline, valproic acid, steroids, zidovudine, tamoxifen, amiodarone, diltiazem, and, in excessive doses, vitamin A. Antineoplastic agents associated with the development of hepatic steatosis include methotrexate sodium, l-asparaginase, actinomycin D, mitomycin C, and bleomycin sulfate.

Although the exact mechanism is uncertain, total parenteral nutrition (TPN) can be associated with hepatic steatosis. The cause of hepatic steatosis associated with TPN is probably multifactorial. This disorder may develop secondary to the delivery of excessive glucose or fat. Excessive glucose increases fatty acid synthetase, increasing hepatic fatty acid production. Infusion of excessive lipids also results in increased serum fatty acid levels. Carnitine is not routinely supplemented in TPN, but it can be synthesized from lysine and methionine. Carnitine supplementation has not been shown to be effective in preventing TPN-induced fatty liver. Choline, too, is not typically added to TPN. Because choline is required in apolipoprotein synthesis, its absence may contribute to TPN-associated hepatic steatosis. Choline supplementation resulted in resolution of this disorder in one study. In children, it appears that a toxic reaction to the TPN also may occur.

Food contaminated with *Aspergillus flavus* can result in the development of hepatic steatosis. This fungus produces aflatoxin, which inhibits the incorporation of thymidine into DNA and RNA polymerase, resulting in hepatic steatosis. Consumption of the mushroom *Amanita phalloides*, which produces amanitotoxin, also is associated with acute fatty liver and with

---

BOX 372.1 Disorders Associated with Hepatic Steatosis

Nutritional
Undernutrition (kwashiorkor)
Obesity
Carnitine deficiency
Choline deficiency

Toxin or drug induced
Aflatoxin
Amanitotoxin
Hypoglycin A
Carbon tetrachloride
Dimethylformamide
Total parenteral nutrition
Vitamin A
Corticosteroids
Alcohol
Tetracycline
Valproic acid
Zidovudine
Tamoxifen
Methotrexate
L-Asparaginase
Actinomycin D
Amiodarone
Diltiazem
Mitomycin C
Bleomycin sulfate

Metabolic
Disorders of carbohydrate metabolism
Glycogen storage disease
Galactosemia
Congenital lactic acidosis
Fructose 1,6-diphosphatase deficiency

Disorders of protein metabolism
Methylmalonic acidemia
Urea cycle defects

Tyrosinemia
Homocystinuria

Disorders of fat metabolism
Hyperlipidemia
Abetalipoproteinemia
Wolman disease
Cholesterol ester storage disease
Niemann-Pick disease
Fatty acyl CoA dehydrogenase deficiency
Gangliosidoses
Tangier disease

Other metabolic disorders
Wilson disease
Sialidosis
Refsum disease
Fucosidosis

Endocrine
Cushing disease
Diabetes mellitus

Disorders associated with insulin resistance
Dysmetabolic syndrome
Mauriac syndrome
Lipoatrophy

Infectious
Hepatitis C

Idiopathic
Reye syndrome
Fatty liver of pregnancy
Jejunoileal bypass
Inflammatory bowel disease
Celiac disease
Cystic fibrosis
Nephrotic syndrome
Shwachman syndrome

other gastrointestinal, renal, and central nervous system disturbances. Jamaican vomiting sickness, once common in the Caribbean, is now rare. The illness resulted from the consumption of unripe akee fruit, which contains hypoglycin A. In addition to other severe disturbances, hypoglycin A can cause hepatic steatosis.

Inborn errors of carbohydrate, protein, and lipid metabolism may have hepatic steatosis as a morphologic component of the disease. Disorders of carbohydrate metabolism associated with hepatic steatosis include glycogen storage disease, galactosemia, fructose 1,6-diphosphatase deficiency, and congenital lactic acidosis. Methylmalonic acidemia, urea cycle defects, and tyrosinemia are disorders of protein metabolism that may involve increased amounts of hepatic fat, although this is a relatively minor histologic component of the latter disorder. Defects in lipid metabolism that can be associated with increased hepatic fat include hyperlipidemia, abetalipoproteinemia, medium-chain fatty acyl CoA dehydrogenase deficiency, long-chain fatty acyl CoA dehydrogenase deficiency, carnitine deficiency, choline deficiency, the gangliosidoses, fucosidosis, Wolman disease, cholesterol ester storage disease, and Niemann-Pick disease. In most disorders that result in hepatic steatosis, the excess fat occurs as triglycerides. Although this is true for patients with hyperlipoproteinemia, the excess fat occurs as cholesterol esters in those with Wolman disease and cholesterol ester storage disease. Glycolipids accumulate in patients with gangliosidoses, and glycosphingolipids in those with fucosidosis. Both cholesterol and glycosphingolipids accumulate in those with Niemann-Pick disease. Abnormalities in copper metabolism as in Wilson disease also can be associated with excessive hepatic fat.

The endocrine disorders that result in excessive hepatic fat are Cushing disease and diabetes mellitus. The frequency of fatty liver is 50% in adults with type 2 diabetes and less than 5% in those with juvenile-onset diabetes. The reason for this difference is most likely related to the hyperinsulinemia that occurs with type II diabetes.

Most infections of the liver result in inflammation with little accumulation of fat. The single infection that can result in a fatty liver is hepatitis C.

Idiopathic disorders associated with hepatic steatosis include Reye syndrome (see Chapter 405), fatty liver of pregnancy, jejunoileal bypass, and inflammatory bowel disease. Fatty liver of pregnancy usually occurs during the third trimester of the patient's first pregnancy. The patient has a sudden onset of nausea, vomiting, and abdominal pain, after which jaundice, encephalopathy, and hematemesis, along with premature labor, may develop. Laboratory evaluation reveals hyperbilirubinemia, elevated liver enzyme levels, and leukocytosis. This disorder is not readily differentiated from viral hepatitis unless a liver biopsy is performed; the biopsy reveals a centrilobular microvesicular hepatic steatosis with little or no inflammation. Subtle signs of necrosis are present, but no diffuse hepatic necrosis is seen. Evaluation by electron microscope reveals abnormal mitochondria, but they are different from those in patients with Reye syndrome. Fatty liver of pregnancy has a mortality rate greater than 20% and is treated with supportive therapy and rapid delivery of the infant. Infant mortality is also high, in excess of 40%. The hepatic lesion resolves spontaneously with the delivery of the infant. Acute fatty liver of pregnancy is unlikely to occur in subsequent pregnancies.

Jejunoileal bypass has been performed to treat morbid obesity in adults and may be associated with hepatic steatosis. This condition is believed to develop secondary to malnutrition, bacterial overgrowth, or various nutritional deficiencies.

Hepatic steatosis occurs in up to one-third of patients with inflammatory bowel disease, making it the most common hepatobiliary disorder associated with inflammatory bowel disease. The cause of hepatic steatosis in inflammatory bowel disease

is unknown, but it is most likely multifactorial. Malnutrition, corticosteroid use, and bacterial toxins have been implicated in the pathogenesis.

DIAGNOSIS

Liver biopsy is the definitive means for identifying hepatic steatosis. Percutaneous liver biopsies can be performed easily and safely in children. The major potential complications associated with liver biopsy are bleeding, pneumothorax, and perforation of the gallbladder. An ultrasonographic examination of the liver should be obtained before a liver biopsy is performed to rule out liver pathology, such as a hemangioma of the liver, that may be a contraindication to performing this procedure.

Two general histologic patterns of hepatic steatosis are seen: macrovesicular and microvesicular. Macrovesicular hepatic steatosis is the term applied if large lipid vacuoles fill the hepatocyte, displacing the nucleus to the cell's periphery (Fig. 372.4A). Macrovesicular steatosis is associated with alcohol abuse, corticosteroid use, nutritional and metabolic disorders, and obesity. Liver function is relatively well preserved in

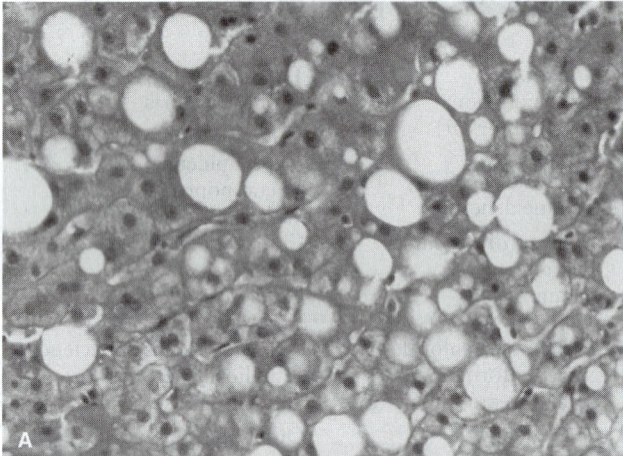

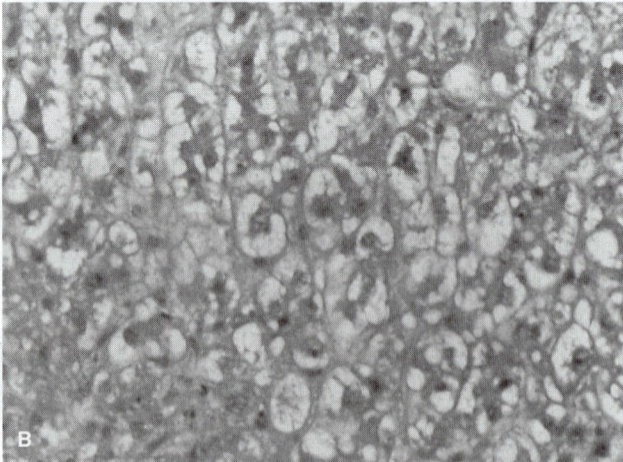

FIGURE 372.4. A: Macrovesicular hepatic steatosis in alcoholic liver disease. Large lipid vacuoles are evident and, in some hepatocytes, the nucleus is displaced to the cell's periphery. (Original magnification ×312.5.) B: Microvesicular hepatic steatosis in a fatal case of fatty liver of pregnancy. Coalescing lipid vacuoles within the hepatocytes distort the cell outlines and give a foamy appearance. The nucleus remains in the center of the cell. (Original magnification ×312.5.) (Courtesy of Dr. P. Cera, Geisinger Clinic, Danville, PA.)

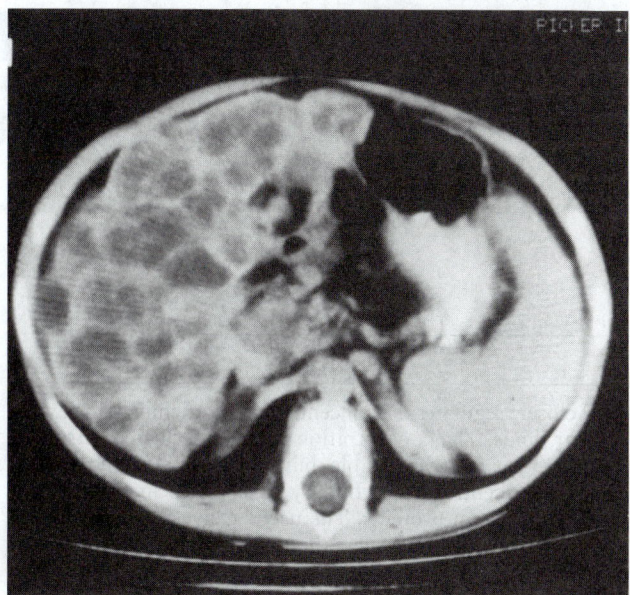

FIGURE 372.5. Computed tomographic scan of patient with cystic fibrosis and focal hepatic steatosis. Note the low attenuation filling defects throughout the liver. (Courtesy of Dr. M. Maksimak, Geisinger Clinic, Danville, PA.)

this type of steatosis. Microvesicular hepatic steatosis is characterized by small lipid vacuoles that are dispersed throughout the cytoplasm, with the nucleus remaining in the center of the hepatocyte (Fig. 372.4B). This pattern of fatty deposition is associated with the ingestion of toxins or drugs such as hypoglycin A and tetracycline, with fatty liver of pregnancy, and with Reye syndrome. Unlike entities associated with macrovesicular steatosis, disorders associated with microvesicular steatosis are characterized by clinical and laboratory evidence of significant liver dysfunction.

Noninvasive means of detecting hepatic steatosis include ultrasonography, computed tomography (CT), and magnetic resonance imaging (MRI). Hepatic steatosis results in a brightly reflective ultrasound echo pattern, a pattern fairly specific for hepatic steatosis. Hepatic steatosis is more readily identified by CT examination, which demonstrates the liver parenchyma to be of lower density (lower attenuation) than the spleen. CT can help in differentiating focal fatty infiltrates from tumor (Fig. 372.5). Focal hepatic infiltration is more difficult to evaluate by means of ultrasonography. MRI accurately detects both diffuse and focal hepatitic steatosis; however, it is more expensive than CT is and offers no significant advantages.

TREATMENT AND PROGNOSIS

Hepatic steatosis is a nonspecific finding in many disorders. Treatment should address the underlying disorder (i.e., weight loss for obese individuals). There is no established specific therapy for NAFLD. A number of pharmacologic agents have been utilized in the treatment of NAFLD secondary to obesity. These have focused on two major categories: drugs that improve insulin resistance, such as metformin, and those that are cytoprotective. Metformin has been noted in several uncontrolled studies of adults to have lowered liver enzymes levels. Currently, there are no pediatric studies that have assessed the effectiveness and safety of metformin. Cytoprotective drugs used in the treatment of NAFLD include ursodeoxycholic acid and vitamin E. Uncontrolled trials in adults have noted improvement in liver enzyme levels with ursodeoxycholic acid. One pediatric study found no benefit to the use of ursodeoxycholic acid. High-dose vitamin E (400 to 1,200 IU/day) was associated with significant improvement in liver enzymes in obese children with NAFLD. Another study of children noted radiologic improvement with the use of taurine supplements. Further research is required prior to recommending any pharmacologic therapy for NAFLD in obese children.

The prognosis for patients with hepatic steatosis depends on the primary disease process responsible. Although some investigators believe that hepatic steatosis itself is not detrimental, accumulating evidence supports the theory that NAFLD may progress to cirrhosis. While cirrhosis secondary to NAFLD may be more common in adults, it has been reported in obese children as young as 9 years of age.

Suggested Readings

American Gastroenterological Association. Medical position statement: nonalcoholic fatty liver disease. *Gastroenterology* 2002;123:1702.
American Gastroenterological Association. Technical review on nonalcoholic fatty liver disease. *Gastroenterology* 2002;123:1705.
Bradfury MW, Berk PD. Lipid metabolism in hepatic steatosis. *Clin Liver Dis* 2004;8:639.
Bugianesi E, Leone N, Vanni E, et al. Expanding the natural history of nonalcoholic steatohepatitis: from cryptogenic cirrhosis to hepatocellular carcinoma. *Gastroenterology* 2002;123:134.
Fishbein MH, Miner M, Mogren C, Chalekson, J. The spectrum of fatty liver in obese children and the relationship of serum aminotransferases to severity of steatosis. *J Pediatr Gastroenterol Nutr* 2003;36:54.
Lavine JE. Vitamin E treatment of nonalcoholic steatohepatitis in children: a pilot study. *J Pediatr* 2000;136:734.
Mehta K, Van Thiel DH, Shah N, Mobarhan S. Nonalcoholic fatty liver disease: pathogenesis and the role of antioxidants. *Nutr Rev* 2002;60:289.
Mofrad P, Contos MJ, Haque M, et al. Clinical and histologic spectrum of nonalcoholic fatty liver disease associated with normal ALT values. *Hepatology* 2003;37:1286.
Neuschwander-Tetri BA, Caldwell SH. Nonalcoholic steatohepatitis: summary of an AASLD single topic conference. *Hepatology* 2003;37:1202.
Obinata K, Maruyama T, Hayashi M, et al. Effect of taurine on the fatty liver of children with simple obesity. *Adv Exp Med Biol* 1996;403:607.
Roberts EA. Steatohepatitis in children. *Best Practice Res Clin Gastroenterol* 2002;16:749.
Sathya P, Martin S, Alverez F. Nonalcoholic fatty liver disease (NAFLD) in children. *Curr Opin Pediat* 2002;14:593.
Vajro P, Franzese A, Valerio G, et al. Lack of efficacy of ursodeoxycholic acid for the treatment of liver abnormalities in obese children. *J Pediatr* 2000;136:739.

SECTION VIII ▪ DISEASES OF THE ENDOCRINE SYSTEM

CHAPTER 373 ▪ PARATHYROID GLANDS

JOHN L. KIRKLAND

INTRODUCTION

The parathyroid glands promote calcium homeostasis through a sensitive and complex self-regulating system. The intricacy and stability of this system are remarkable. Nonetheless, defects in vitamin D synthesis; mutations in the calcium-sensing receptor gene; insensitivity of the target organ; disturbances in the dietary intake of calcium, phosphorus, and vitamin D; and diseases of the parathyroid gland, liver, and kidney may cause significant disorders in calcium homeostasis.

PHYSIOLOGY

Parathyroid Hormone

Parathyroid hormone (PTH) is secreted as an 84-amino acid peptide with a half-life of less than 4 minutes. PTH secretion is stimulated physiologically by changes in calcium levels. A 2% change in ionized calcium levels produces a significant release of PTH. Changes in ionized calcium levels are detected by a calcium-sensing receptor located on the membranes of parathyroid gland cells. This receptor is a member of the G protein–coupled receptor superfamily consisting of seven membrane-spanning domains.

Circulating immunoreactive PTH includes less than 30% of the intact hormone due to proteolytic modifications. Inactive fragments constitute the remaining amounts. The first 34-amino acid residues contain high-affinity binding domains to PTH/PTH-related protein (PTHrP) receptors located on bone and kidney cells. C-terminal portions of PTH have a longer half-life than does the intact PTH and constitute the major fragments in the circulation. The C-terminal fragments are biologically inactive and may complicate laboratory measurements of PTH. Exogenous manipulation of the calcium levels in experimental animals alters the ratio of intact to fragmented PTH hormone components, suggesting an active intragland conversion system. Kupffer cells and hepatocytes degrade PTH in the liver, and the kidney tubular cells excrete PTH fragments in the urine. PTH exerts its major actions by binding to receptors located on osteoblastic and renal tubular cells. These target cells are activated through the adenylate cyclase or the phospholipase C and D signaling cascades. PTH indirectly activates the osteoclasts in bone to increase resorption of mineralized bone, resulting in mobilization of calcium and phosphorus. However, small amounts of PTH delivered intermittently may stimulate bone growth in specific clinical situations, probably through the production of local growth factors. PTH activates the proximal and distal tubular cells in the kidney to promote resorption of calcium and to inhibit resorption of phosphorus. In addition, PTH stimulates the production of 1-alpha,25-dihydroxyvitamin D in the kidney.

Calcium

PTH closely regulates the concentration of calcium in the extracellular fluids. The concentration of ionized calcium throughout the day is relatively stable, but variations exist in the total calcium concentration secondary to changes in the concentrations of serum proteins. The usual daily variation of total calcium concentrations is less than 2%. The extracellular concentration of calcium is 10^{-3} mol, contained in three major components. The unbound component, or free calcium, accounts for approximately 50% of the total amount of calcium and is the most important regulator of physiologic processes. The bound components account for the other 50%, with protein binding accounting for approximately 40% and anion binding for approximately 10%. Albumin is the most abundant protein-binding calcium, with each albumin molecule capable of binding as many as 12 calcium molecules, depending on the extracellular pH. Acidosis decreases the binding capacity and increases the free extracellular concentration of calcium, whereas alkalosis increases the binding capacity and decreases the free extracellular concentrations of calcium. These alterations in binding capacity explain the variations in clinical signs that occur with disturbances in acid-base regulation. Bicarbonate, citrate, and phosphate complexes compose the anion-binding system. The intracellular concentration of calcium is approximately 10^{-6} mol and is maintained by cellular transport systems. Numerous critical metabolic processes require a rigid control of calcium concentration. These processes include the permeability of plasma membranes in neural tissue, the mineralization of developing bone, the promotion of coagulation, and cardiac contractility, as well as calcium's intracellular role as a modulator for multiple processes.

Low levels of serum calcium stimulate the immediate release of preformed PTH, followed by increased production of prepro-PTH mRNA. The calcium-selective transmembrane channels and calcium sensors play a significant role in this process. High levels of serum calcium inhibit the previously mentioned process. The increased levels of PTH stimulate other important compensatory mechanisms, as previously mentioned.

Vitamin D

An understanding of calcium homeostasis must include an explanation of vitamin D. Vitamin D has two entry points into the body. The first is from the skin, and the second is from dietary supplementation. The skin contains the pre-vitamin D compound 7-dehydrocholesterol. Ultraviolet B waves from the sun or other sources convert this substance to a pre-vitamin D compound, which is converted by heat-sensitive reactions to vitamin D_3. A serum-binding protein transfers vitamin D_3 to the liver. The second entry point for vitamin D is from dietary supplementation, either by irradiated ergosterol, vitamin D_2, or vitamin D_3. Vitamins D_2 and D_3 differ slightly in their structure, but they have similar functions physiologically. Vitamins D_2

and D$_3$ are hydroxylated in the liver at the 25 position by a cytochrome P-450-vitamin D-25-hydroxylase enzyme. Diseases of the liver, as well as pharmacologic agents such as phenytoin and phenobarbital, interfere with this important hydroxylation step. Interference in this step may result in functional vitamin D deficiency. 25-hydroxyvitamin D is transported to the kidney, where the cytochrome P-450-monooxygenase 25-hydroxy-1-alpha-hydroxylase converts 25-hydroxyvitamin D to 1-alpha,25-dihydroxyvitamin D and 24,25-dihydroxyvitamin D. 1-alpha,25-dihydroxyvitamin D is the most active metabolite and is responsible for many actions of vitamin D. PTH, estrogen, growth hormone, prolactin, and insulin stimulate 1-alpha-hydroxylation. 1-alpha,25-dihydroxyvitamin D exerts its effects by binding to intracellular receptors that contain a DNA-binding region. Mutations within the vitamin D receptor gene are responsible for end-organ resistance to 1-alpha,25-dihydroxyvitamin D. The vitamin D nuclear receptor complex joins the retinoic acid X receptor to form a heterodimer. This heterodimer binds to the vitamin D-responsive element of target genes promoting or inhibiting transcription of other genes. For example, gene expression of calbindin, a calcium-binding protein, which facilitates the transport of calcium from the intraluminal space of the intestines to the extracellular compartment, is stimulated positively. However, the heterodimer-receptor complex affects PTH gene expression negatively.

Another role of vitamin D is the stimulation of osteoclasts from progenitor cells. Osteoclasts enhance the release of calcium from bone, thereby providing the body with a method to compensate for acute hypocalcemia. 1-alpha,25-dihydroxyvitamin D also has cell proliferative and differentiation effects in some biologic systems.

Parathyroid Hormone-Related Protein

PTHrP produces effects similar to those of PTH. The role of PTHrP in calcium homeostasis remains poorly understood, but the hypercalcemia and hypophosphatemia of malignancy are related to its production. Islet cell tumors and pheochromocytomas are two examples of malignancies producing PTHrP. PTHrP exists in three isoforms, with initial sequences in all three similar to those of PTH. PTHrP binds to common receptors with an affinity similar to that of PTH. Fetal tissues such as placenta and parathyroid glands, as well as breast milk, contain large amounts of PTHrP. PTHrP also regulates cell and organ growth, differentiation, and migration. Loss of the PTHrP gene in experimental animals is lethal in the embryonic stage.

Calcitonin

Calcitonin, a 32-amino acid protein secreted by the C cells of the thyroid gland, binds a G-protein coupled cell surface receptor. Calcitonin's physiologic role remains obscure. An acute increase in serum calcium levels increases secretion of calcitonin, but a chronic increase in serum calcium levels does not always increase secretion of calcitonin. Normal gastrointestinal proteins such as gastrin and cholecystokinin are calcitonin secretagogues. Biologic effects include inhibition of osteoclastic resorption, producing hypocalcemia and hypophosphatemia. Calcitonin receptors are present also in the central nervous system, testes, lymphocytes, placenta, and skeletal muscle. Elevated levels of calcitonin are observed in medullary thyroid carcinomas (multiple endocrine neoplasia type 2), but hypocalcemia does not occur. Treatment of hypercalcemic pediatric patients with calcitonin is beneficial in some cases, such as the hypercalcemia of immobilization and neonatal hypophosphatasia.

Phosphorus

The intracellular concentration of phosphorus is approximately 10^{-4} mol, whereas that of the extracellular fraction is approximately 2×10^{-4} mol. The serum concentration of phosphorus is less regulated than is calcium. Eighty-five percent of the phosphorus is contained in the skeleton and, with calcium, provides structural support for the body. The phosphate esters and other phosphorylated compounds provide the generation and transfer of cellular energy.

HYPOPARATHYROIDISM

Hypoparathyroidism in children is a rare finding, excluding transient hypoparathyroidism in neonates. Hypoparathyroidism is recognized biochemically by hypocalcemia usually associated with hyperphosphatemia. The clinical manifestations of hypocalcemia are secondary to neuromuscular instability. The most common presentation is a seizure. Numbness and tingling sensations in the extremities may occur before the seizure. Chvostek sign (stimulation of the ipsilateral facial muscle by tapping the facial nerve in front of the ear), Trousseau sign (carpopedal spasm produced by inflation of the blood pressure cuff to greater than the systolic blood pressure for 2 minutes), laryngospasm, bronchospasm, and prolonged QT intervals on electrocardiographs can occur. The cause of hypoparathyroidism and treatment of hypocalcemia are discussed in the following sections.

Autoimmune Hypoparathyroidism

Hypoparathyroidism may occur alone or as part of the autoimmune polyendocrinopathy-candidiasis-ectodermal dystrophy (APECED) syndrome. APECED is an autosomal recessive disease caused by a mutation in the autoimmune regulating (AIRE) gene. AIRE is a transcription factor with an unknown target(s). A consistent component of APECED is immunologic destruction of the hormone-producing cells. Approximately 30% to 40% of patients have antibodies against the parathyroid gland, but the role of antibodies as a causative factor is uncertain. Lymphocytic infiltration of the parathyroid glands is a common pathologic finding. Mucocutaneous candidiasis may precede the development of hypoparathyroidism. Other endocrinopathies include hypoadrenalism, hypogonadism, hypothyroidism, and diabetes mellitus. Frequent clinical, physical, and laboratory assessments are required to detect the subtle onset of these disorders.

Neonatal Hypocalcemia

Neonatal hypocalcemia occurring within the first 3 days of life is defined as early, whereas hypocalcemia occurring after the fifth day of life is defined as late. Early neonatal hypocalcemia may develop from agenesis or hypoplasia of the parathyroid gland, either as an isolated finding or as part of a recognizable group of clinical findings. DiGeorge syndrome was described originally in infants with congenital absence of the thymus and the parathyroid glands, as well as deficient cell-mediated immunity. Later descriptions included cardiovascular malformations involving the aortic arch. They included truncus arteriosus and aortic arch syndromes. Additional findings include dysmorphic features of the face, such as low-set ears, short philtrum, micrognathia, and a small "fish-like" mouth. The velocardiofacial syndrome includes facial dysmorphisms, palatal abnormalities, congenital heart disease, and other clinical findings consistent with DiGeorge syndrome. Genetic analysis of both conditions reveals deletions of chromosome 22q11, suggesting a common origin with a broad clinical spectrum. An autosomal dominant trait has been documented in some cases. The natural history is quite variable, with the hypoparathyroidism resolving in some affected children during the first year, whereas others may have latent hypoparathyroidism.

Other causes of early neonatal hypocalcemia include preterm delivery with low birth weight, birth asphyxia, and presence of diabetes in the mother. The causes of these disorders are understood poorly. Possible reasons for the hypocalcemia include increased calcitonin levels, target-organ resistance to 1-alpha,25-dihydroxyvitamin D, delayed feeding, decreased excretion of PTH, and diminished biologic effects of PTH.

Late neonatal hypocalcemia may occur secondary to hypoparathyroidism of any cause, either as an isolated entity or as part of a syndrome. Examples of the latter include Kearns-Sayre syndrome and Kenny-Caffey syndrome. Maternal hyperparathyroidism may produce neonatal hypocalcemia by suppression of neonatal PTH. Increased phosphorus intake of any cause, including cow's milk-based formulas, may lower serum calcium. Why only a small percentage of neonates fed a high phosphate-containing formula develop hypocalcemia is unclear. The increased phosphorus levels may antagonize PTH actions or secretion of PTH or produce increased calcium and phosphorus deposition in bones, leading to hypocalcemia.

Illnesses

Acute illnesses, including gram-negative sepsis, toxic shock syndrome, acquired immunodeficiency syndrome, and severe acute respiratory syndrome (SARS) often are associated with hypocalcemia secondary to hypoparathyroidism. The cause of the hypoparathyroidism in ill children is unknown, but it may be related to macrophage-generated interleukins that mimic calcium ionophores. A critically ill child admitted to an intensive care unit is a prime candidate for hypocalcemia. Recognition of hypocalcemia may be delayed because of concurrent resuscitation or diagnostic procedures. However, correction of the hypocalcemia is mandatory because many cardiovascular agents require normal concentrations of calcium for biologic effects. Levels of ionized calcium, as opposed to levels of total serum calcium, reflect the child's true calcium status because disturbances in total serum calcium determination from hypoalbuminemia, fluctuations in the pH, and the presence of radiographic contrast media may influence measurements of total serum calcium.

Isolated Hypoparathyroidism

Isolated hypoparathyroidism not associated with other endocrine diseases, or as a result of thyroid surgery, can occur. The cause of isolated hypoparathyroidism is known is some cases, but unknown in others. Known causes include mutations in the mammalian glial cells missing homolog, GCMb; mutations in the signal peptide of the preproparathyroid hormone gene; and mutations of the transcription factor family of GATA. The clinical and laboratory findings, as well as treatment, are identical to those of other forms of hypoparathyroidism. The familial forms may be caused by gene mutations near the PTH gene located on the short arm of chromosome 2. Hypoparathyroidism also occurs as a consequence of deposition of iron in the parathyroid gland from frequent transfusions, such as in thalassemia major, or as a result of deposition of copper, such as occurs in Wilson disease.

Autosomal Dominant Hypoparathyroidism

Autosomal dominant hypoparathyroidism is a rare form of hypocalcemia caused by a gain of function mutation in the calcium-sensing receptor. Affected individuals also may have hypomagnesemia, hyperphosphatemia, and hypercalcuria. Treatment with vitamin D may produce eucalcemia but also promote hypercalciuria, leading to nephrogenic diabetes insipidus and nephrocalcinosis. Thiazide diuretics have proven beneficial in several patients by increasing serum calcium and reducing levels of urinary calcium, but most patients do not require treatment.

Hypomagnesemia

Chronic magnesium deficiency, either congenital or acquired, produces hypocalcemia secondary to diminished production and effectiveness of PTH. Interestingly, acute-onset hypomagnesemia increases production of PTH. Chronic hypomagnesemia caused by urinary or gastrointestinal losses develops from unknown cellular defects, most likely defects in calcium and magnesium-permeable cation channels. Affected individuals have other metabolic disturbances, such as hypokalemia. Acquired hypomagnesemia usually is secondary to another disease, such as intestinal malabsorption. Clinical manifestations include tetany, carpopedal spasms, or seizures. Laboratory findings include serum levels of magnesium less than 1.5 mEq/L. Treatment consists of magnesium administered intravenously, intramuscularly, or orally. Magnesium levels should be measured frequently. Diarrhea may result from oral administration of magnesium. If diarrhea develops, the oral replacement dosage should be decreased accordingly, then slowly increased.

Laboratory Findings

The characteristic laboratory findings of hypoparathyroidism include hypocalcemia and hyperphosphatemia. Levels of PTH are low in most situations discussed previously. Radiographs of bones usually do not show any diagnostic features. The differential diagnosis includes hypocalcemia for other reasons, such as phosphate-induced hypocalcemia; renal failure; and hypocalcemic rickets. Clinical history, laboratory assessment, and radiographs can facilitate the evaluation. Children with pseudohypoparathyroidism (end-organ resistance to PTH action) present with hypocalcemia and hyperphosphatemia, but levels of PTH are elevated.

TREATMENT OF HYPOCALCEMIC DISORDERS

The acute treatment of symptomatic hypocalcemia in the disorders previously mentioned can be generalized if modifications are made for each cause. Intravenous calcium usually is required. Numerous intravenous preparations exist. Pediatricians frequently use 10% calcium gluconate initially as an intravenous solution. One milliliter of this solution supplies 9 mg of elemental calcium. Infants with seizures and laryngospasm may require an initial dose of 1 to 2 mL/kg. The infusion of calcium should be slow, 1 mL or less per minute, with strict attention paid to the heart rate or an electrocardiographic monitor. Bradycardia is an indication to decrease the rate of infusion of calcium. Subsequent intravenous calcium is administered at a rate of 25 to 100 mg of elemental calcium per kilogram of body weight per day, depending on the severity of the hypocalcemia. Extravasation of intravenous calcium may result in necrosis of tissue. This complication may develop despite the continuous monitoring of intravenous sites, prompting some physicians to administer intravenous calcium only as an intermittent bolus. However, intermittent dosages of intravenous calcium may decrease serum pH, rapidly increase tonicity, and produce an intermittent "overshoot" hypercalcemia. A solution of 10% solution of calcium chloride also can be used for intravenous treatment, but it is more irritating to the veins than is calcium gluconate. One milliliter of this solution contains 27.3 mg of elemental calcium. Both 10% calcium chloride and 10% calcium gluconate can be diluted with glucose solutions for intravenous administration. Oral treatment with calcium supplementation may be initiated immediately. Calcium glubionate (Neo-Calglucon) contains 23 mg of elemental calcium per milliliter. Other commercial preparations have varying amounts of elemental calcium. The amount of elemental calcium administered to maintain eucalcemia varies from 50 to 150 mg/kg/day. Because calcium administered through the gastrointestinal system is dependent on the presence of 1-alpha, 25-dihydroxyvitamin D or its analogues, it is not surprising that treatment of moderate or severe hypoparathyroidism with oral calcium alone rarely is successful.

Treatment with vitamin D or its analogues usually is required to treat most chronic hypocalcemic states such as hypoparathyroidism. Most vitamin D supplementation is undertaken with dihydrotachysterol, 25-hydroxyvitamin D, or 1-alpha, 25-dihydroxyvitamin D. Vitamin D was used previously in large amounts, but its long half-life rendered adjustments in dosage difficult to make. Dihydrotachysterol is administered in a dose of 0.05 to 0.50 mg/day. A liquid solution facilitates small changes in the dosage required to maintain eucalcemia. 25-hydroxyvitamin D is begun at 20 μg on a daily or every-other-day basis, and the dosage is increased slowly. Experience in infants and children is limited. 1-alpha,25-dihydroxyvitamin D is initiated in infants at .04 to .08 μg/kg/day and at a dose of 0.25 μg/day in older children. The dosage is changed according to the level of serum calcium. This preparation has a more rapid onset of action than does dihydrotachysterol, and therapeutic manipulation is easier to achieve. 1-alpha,25-dihydroxyvitamin D may be administered intravenously, but its use in children is limited.

Synthetic PTH administered twice daily controls hypocalcemia in patients with hypoparathyroidism, but neither it nor its analogues are readily available. The goal of long-term management is to maintain eucalcemia and eucalciuria. Children may require monthly tests for calcium levels and 24-hour urine collections twice yearly for calcium and creatinine ratios. The optimal level of serum calcium is in the low range of normal. For children older than 8 years of age, the level of urinary calcium should be less than 0.3 mg of calcium per milligram of creatinine. For children younger than 8 years of age, levels of urinary calcium should be less than 0.8 mg of calcium per milligram of creatinine, depending on the child's age. Older patients may require levels of serum calcium slightly below the normal range to avoid development of hypercalciuria. Changing the dosage of exogenous calcium and vitamin D may be required to titrate the levels of serum calcium to the desired range.

HYPERPARATHYROIDISM

Hyperparathyroidism is an uncommon occurrence in pediatric patients, but it is extremely important because an aggressive therapeutic approach may prevent development of chronic renal diseases from nephrocalcinosis. The clinical manifestations of hypercalcemia from any cause are similar. The neuromuscular and gastrointestinal systems are affected initially. Muscle weakness, paralysis, or hyporeflexia may be observed in the former, whereas constipation, anorexia, and nausea may be observed in the latter. Antidiuretic hormone action on the kidney may be affected adversely, with resulting development of polyuria and polydipsia suggesting diabetes insipidus. Nephrocalcinosis may occur later. The cardiovascular symptoms may reveal bradycardia and a reduced QT interval. The causes of hyperparathyroidism are discussed in the following sections. Non–parathyroid gland hypercalcemia in children is mentioned briefly.

Neonatal Severe Hyperparathyroidism

A rare form of hypercalcemia in neonates is neonatal severe hyperparathyroidism secondary to a homozygous loss of function of the calcium sensing receptor on chromosome 3q21-24. Loss of function mutations disable the normal negative feedback mechanisms that control the secretion and production of PTH. Genetic analysis suggests that neonatal severe hyperparathyroidism is a homozygous form of familial hypocalciuric hypercalcemia. Thus, neonates inherit mutated calcium-sensing receptor genes from both parents and, as a result, have severe hypercalcemia. However, *de novo* mutations in the calcium-sensing receptor are reported. The increased levels of PTH promote resorption of bones producing hypercalcemia, as well as increased renal tubular loss of phosphate. Attempts to control hypercalcemia with dietary restrictions of calcium may result in rickets. Failure to thrive occurs frequently. Medical treatment as outlined below usually is inadequate to manage the hypercalcemia, and total parathyroidectomy is required. Parathyroid gland autoimplants are successful in some cases. Ectopically transplanted parathyroid tissue can be removed selectively to treat hypercalcemia.

Parathyroid Adenoma and Parathyroid Gland Hyperplasia

Hypercalcemia in older children may be secondary to hyperparathyroidism from parathyroid adenomas and chief cell hyperplasia. Parathyroid carcinomas in children are rare findings. Other causes of hyperparathyroidism include chronic renal disease and sex-linked hypophosphatemic rickets. Presenting clinical signs may include paralytic ileus, osseous deformities, and personality changes, or the child may be asymptomatic. Unfortunately, many cases are undiagnosed until hypercalcemic complications develop. The diagnosis is confirmed biochemically by hypercalcemia, hypophosphatemia, and elevated levels of PTH for the degree of hypercalcemia. Hypercalciuria may be present also. Radiographic findings include osteitis fibrosa cystica and genu valgum. Advances in sonographic techniques and the use of delayed technetium 99m sestamibi single photon emission computed tomography may assist in presurgical localization and differentiate between parathyroid gland hyperplasia and adenoma. Transient hypocalcemia may occur after surgery as remaining parathyroid tissues recover from suppression and calcium deficits in bone are replaced.

Multiple Endocrine Neoplasia Types 1 and 2

Multiple endocrine neoplasia (MEN) 1 is characterized by neoplasia of the pancreas, anterior pituitary gland, and parathyroid gland. MEN 1 is an autosomal dominant inherited disease with high penetrance and variable expression. Hyperparathyroidism occurs in almost all of the patients. Pancreatic tumors and pituitary adenomas occur less frequently. Almost all patients with hyperparathyroidism have hyperplastic parathyroid tissue. Genetic analysis reveals a loss of heterozygosity at chromosome 11q13 loci, producing inactivation of menin, a tumor-suppressor gene. Some cases have an onset in neonates. Hypercalcemia, elevated levels of PTH, and the familial occurrence confirm the diagnosis. Treatment consists of subtotal parathyroidectomy with implants of a small amount of parathyroid tissue to the muscles of one extremity.

MEN 2A consists of medullary carcinoma of the thyroid gland, pheochromocytoma, and hyperparathyroidism. The hyperparathyroidism has been related to mutations in the *RET* gene. Treatment of the hyperparathyroidism is surgical.

Familial Hypocalciuric Hypercalcemia

Familial hypocalciuric hypercalcemia is an autosomal dominant form of hypercalcemia secondary to a heterozygous loss of function of the calcium-sensing receptor gene localized in some families to the long arm of chromosome 3. The diagnosis is unsuspected in most children unless other family members have hypercalcemia. The cardinal findings are mild to moderate hypercalcemia and relative hypocalciuria. Serum calcium levels rarely are greater than 14 mg/dL. Urinary calcium expressed in terms of milligram of calcium per milligram of creatinine for age is normal or elevated slightly, but it is less than would be expected from the degree of hypercalcemia. Nephrocalcinosis does not occur. Levels of PTH may be normal but are elevated for the degree of hypercalcemia. Phosphorus levels are variable. Serum magnesium levels are elevated in some children. Other biochemical studies related to calcium and vitamin D metabolism, such as 1-alpha,25-dihydroxyvitamin D, calcitonin, urinary cAMP levels, and radiographic examination of the skeleton, do not reveal consistent abnormalities or have normal results. The asymptomatic nature of this disorder, as opposed to the signs and symptoms of hypercalcemia secondary to hyperparathyroidism, can corroborate the diagnosis.

The inactivation of the calcium-sensing receptor results in mild to moderate resistance to the inhibitory effects of hypercalcemia on secretion of PTH. Surgical removal of all parathyroid tissue results in hypoparathyroidism. Removal of only parts of the parathyroid gland does not improve the hypercalcemia. No treatment is recommended currently.

NON–PARATHYROID GLAND HYPERCALCEMIC DISORDERS

Profound hypercalcemia may occur in illnesses unrelated to abnormalities of the parathyroid gland. The causes are diverse, but treatment is similar to that for the hypercalcemia of hyperparathyroidism.

Williams Syndrome

Individuals with Williams syndrome usually are small for gestational age with facial abnormalities, hypotonia, developmental and motor retardation, supravalvular aortic stenosis, and a gregarious and friendly character ("cocktail party" personality). The hypercalcemia usually resolves by the end of the first year of life. The gene responsible for this disorder has been localized to the long arm of chromosome 7. Deletions of the entire elastin gene result in Williams syndrome, whereas partial deletions result in isolated supravalvular aortic stenosis. Treatment for symptomatic hypercalcemia may require hydration, furosemide, glucocorticoids, and low-calcium diets.

Idiopathic Infantile Hypercalcemia

The inheritance and pathogenesis of idiopathic infantile hypercalcemia remain largely unknown. In some cases, excessive maternal supplementation of vitamin D during pregnancy can result in birth defects similar to those seen in Williams syndrome. The infants may have supravalvular aortic stenosis and musculoskeletal abnormalities as observed in Williams syndrome. The hypercalcemia may persist for longer than 1 year. Elevated levels of PTHrP may occur with hypercalcemia.

Immobilization Hypercalcemia

Immobilization of patients for any reason infrequently may produce hypercalcemia and hypercalciuria. The cause is unknown, but it may be related to the normally fast turnover of calcium in the skeletal system of children. The best treatment is ambulation, but bisphonates are reported to lower serum calcium levels.

Hypophosphatasia

Severe infantile hypophosphatasia is an autosomal recessive disorder resulting from a large spectrum of mutations in the tissue-nonspecific alkaline phosphatase gene with a highly variable clinical expression. These mutations result in deficient mineralization and rickets. Hypercalcemia results from an imbalance in absorption of calcium and deposition of calcium in bones. Urinary phosphoethanolamine levels may be elevated, but the test is not pathognomonic. No effective treatment exists for this disorder, but hypercalcemia may improve with calcitonin.

Hypercalcemic Granulomatous Disorders

Numerous granulomatous diseases (including sarcoidosis, tuberculosis, and neonatal subcutaneous fat necrosis) have been associated with hypercalcemia. The macrophages involved in the granuloma produce increased amounts of 1-alpha,25-dihydroxyvitamin D. Treatment with glucocorticoids has been effective in producing eucalcemia.

Laboratory Findings

Elevated levels of PTH concomitant with hypercalcemia and hypophosphatemia usually distinguish hyperparathyroidism from other causes. The negative feedback system between calcium and PTH permits differentiation from other causes of hypercalcemia. For example, low levels of PTH accompany the hypercalcemia of hypervitaminosis D. Ultrasound and radiopharmaceutical evaluation of parathyroid gland size permit differentiation of hyperplasia and adenomas. The diagnosis of familial hypercalcemic hypocalciuria usually is based on a normal level of PTH, relative hypocalciuria, modest hypercalcemia, and the similar biochemical findings in other family members.

TREATMENT OF HYPERCALCEMIC DISORDERS

Treatment of hypercalcemia secondary to hyperparathyroidism must include treatment of the underlying disorder. The acute treatment requires hydration, which can be performed orally in cooperative children or by intravenous methods in uncooperative ones. Twice the maintenance fluid rates or more are used.

Dehydration secondary to nausea, vomiting, and polyuria can occur with hypercalcemia. The total volume of fluid replacement should include deficits as well as the increased maintenance amounts. The administration of intravenous saline after rehydration is achieved offers an added benefit because excretion of calcium is enhanced by sodium excretion. Furosemide, 2 mg/kg/day, or other loop diuretics may be used because they increase excretion of sodium as well as excretion of calcium. Glucocorticoids such as prednisone, 2 mg/kg/day, are useful because they decrease intestinal absorption of calcium. Sunlight, any form of vitamin D, and dairy products should be avoided during courses of hypercalcemia. The treatments previously mentioned usually suffice in children, but further treatment can be undertaken with phosphorus, mithramycin, and peritoneal dialysis. Calcitonin, 5 U/kg administered subcutaneously every

12 hours over the course of 36 hours, and pamidronate, 1 mg/kg administered intravenously over the course of 24 hours, have been used in children, but their use is limited. The potential side effects of bisphonates on growing bone is unknown.

Suggested Readings

Favus MJ. *Primer on the metabolic bone diseases and disorders of mineral metabolism*, 5th ed. Philadelphia: Lippincott-Raven, 2003.

Harrison HE, Harrison HC. *Disorders of calcium and phosphorus metabolism in childhood and adolescence*. Philadelphia: Saunders, 1979.

Langman CB. New developments in calcium and vitamin D metabolism. *Curr Opin Pediatr* 2000;12:135.

Pearce SH. Clinical disorders of extracellular calcium-sensing and molecular biology of the calcium sensing receptor. *Ann Med* 2002;34:201.

CHAPTER 374 ■ PUBERTY AND GONADAL DISORDERS

LESLIE P. PLOTNICK AND DOMINIQUE N. LONG

Because the range of normal onset and progression of puberty is broad and is different in boys and girls, pediatricians must have a solid grasp of normal pubertal events to assess when a child falls outside the normal range and needs evaluation or treatment.

Puberty is initiated by changes in the sensitive negative feedback system that exists among the gonads, hypothalamus, and pituitary in the prepubertal child. Puberty involves an increase in gonadal steroid production (i.e., gonadarche) and an increase in adrenal steroid production (i.e., adrenarche).

In most girls, puberty begins between 8 and 13 years of age and is completed, on average, in 4.2 years (range, 1.5 to 6.0 years). In 90% of girls, breast development (thelarche) is the first sign of puberty. The time from onset of breast buds to menarche is 2.3 ± 1.0 years.

A 1997 cross-sectional study conducted by Herman-Giddens et al. showed that a substantial portion of girls have pubertal changes at age 7 years. The changes occurred earlier in black than in white girls. In 2002, Wu et al. reported data from the Third National Health and Nutrition Examination Survey (NHANES III), conducted between 1988 and 1994, showing that, on average, black girls enter puberty first, followed by Mexican American and then white girls. Including current body mass index (BMI) did not modify the relationship between race/ethnicity and pubertal status, with the exception of attainment of menarche. Higher BMI led to earlier age at the onset of menarche. Sun et al. also reported data from NHANES III in 2002 finding little statistical difference between sexual development in non-Hispanic white girls and Mexican American girls. Using NHANES III, Sun et al. and Wu et al. both found the median age for onset of breast development was 9.48, 10.38, and 9.80 in non-Hispanic black girls, non-Hispanic white girls, and Mexican American girls, respectively. Similarly, the median age for onset of pubic hair in girls was 9.5, 10.5, and 10.3, respectively.

Chumlea et al. used NHANES III data in 2003 to show that the median age for attainment of menarche is 12.43 years, which is not significantly different from that reported for U.S.

girls in 1973. Again, non-Hispanic black girls had a significantly earlier age of onset of menarche than did non-Hispanic white and Mexican American girls (12.06 years, 12.55 years, and 12.25 years, respectively).

In the vast majority of boys, puberty begins between 9 and 14 years of age and is completed, on average, in 3.5 years (range 2.0 to 4.5 years). In most boys, testicular enlargement (length greater than 2.5 cm) is the first sign of puberty. Sun et al. reported data from NHANES III showing the median age of genital development in boys to be 9.2 years, 10 years, and 10.3 years for non-Hispanic black boys, non-Hispanic white boys, and Mexican-American boys, respectively.

Classically, if a girl shows signs of pubertal maturation before she is 8 years of age or a boy shows signs of puberty before he is 9 years of age, the child should be evaluated for precocious puberty. The 1997 data by Herman-Giddens et al. were interpreted as lowering the age for evaluation to 6 years for black girls and 7 years for white girls. These recommendations are controversial, although detailed etiologic evaluations in 6- to 8-year-old girls usually are not revealing of pathology. Each child must be considered individually, including past medical history, tempo of puberty, and physical examination. Conversely, if no signs of pubertal development occur by 13 years of age in girls or by 14 years of age in boys, the child should be evaluated for pubertal delay. Timing and progression of puberty is important. Pubertal changes that progress too rapidly or arrest in progression require evaluation.

HYPOTHALAMIC–PITUITARY–GONADAL PHYSIOLOGY

Pituitary release of luteinizing hormone (LH) and follicle-stimulating hormone (FSH) is regulated by the hypothalamic factor gonadotropin-releasing hormone (GnRH; also called LH-releasing hormone or factor). The hypothalamic secretion of this peptide is controlled by various neurotransmitters, which can be influenced by higher signals such as visual and olfactory stimuli and stress. GnRH is secreted in pulses, the frequency of which is important for pituitary secretion of LH and FSH. At the onset of puberty, an increase in GnRH, LH, and FSH pulsatile secretion occurs. LH and FSH become more responsive to GnRH, and an increase in GnRH receptors occurs in the pituitary.

LH and FSH stimulate the testes to produce testosterone and the ovaries to produce estrogen and stimulate ovulation. The gonadal sex steroids feed back centrally. The feedback usually is negative, except that positive feedback of estrogens is needed to produce the LH surge required for ovulation.

PRECOCIOUS SEXUAL DEVELOPMENT

Causes of precocious or inappropriate sexual development are listed in Box 374.1. Evaluating a child for sexual precocity requires obtaining a careful medical and family history. Does

---

| **BOX 374.1** | **Precocious or Inappropriate Sexual Development** |

True or central precocious puberty (central gonadotropin secretion)
Idiopathic
Central nervous system tumors: hamartomas, gliomas (with neurofibromatosis), and others
Other central nervous system disorders: trauma, postinfectious, hydrocephalus, radiation, surgery
Severe primary hypothyroidism

Precocious puberty independent of pituitary gonadotropins
Girls
    Exogenous estrogen exposure
    Estrogen-secreting tumors (adrenals or ovaries)
    Ovarian cysts
    McCune-Albright syndrome
Boys
    Exogenous androgen exposure
    Adrenal androgen secretion
        Congenital adrenal hyperplasia
    Adrenal tumors
    Testicular androgen secretion
    Tumors
    Familial Leydig cell hyperplasia
    Gonadotropin-secreting tumors
    McCune-Albright syndrome

Heterosexual development
Virilization in girls
    Exogenous androgen exposure
    Congenital adrenal hyperplasia
    Adrenal tumors
    Ovarian tumors
Feminization in boys
    Exogenous estrogen exposure
    Adrenal tumor
    Testicular tumor
    Increased peripheral conversion of androgens to estrogens

Variations of normal puberty
Premature thelarche
Premature adrenarche
Pubertal gynecomastia

---

the child have any history of central nervous system (CNS) disorder? Previous growth measurements are valuable. What is the child's growth pattern? Is there evidence of acceleration of linear growth? When did the various pubertal changes begin? How fast have these changes progressed? When did the parents and sibling have pubertal changes? Is there a family history of early sexual development? Questions regarding exposure to any exogenous source of sex steroids must be asked. Creams and pills can contain sex steroids, especially estrogens, and oral contraceptives are found readily in many homes. Are any athletes in the home taking anabolic steroids or is anyone in the family using topical androgen preparations?

The physical examination should include a careful examination of the fundi (looking for papilledema). The child's skin should be inspected for signs of oiliness or acne (androgen effect) and café au lait spots (McCune-Albright). The thyroid should be palpated. The presence of axillary hair and odor, the amount of breast tissue, and whether the nipples and areolae are enlarging should be evaluated. The abdomen should be palpated for masses. The amount, location, and character of pubic hair should be noted.

In girls, the clitoris, labia, and vaginal orifice should be examined carefully. Is there evidence of maturation of the labia minora? Does the vaginal mucosa look red and shiny (prepubertal) or pink and dull (estrogenized)? Is the clitoris of normal size? Are vaginal secretions evident on the genitalia or on the child's underwear?

In boys, the stretched length and width of the penis should be evaluated (this may require pushing down on a suprapubic fat pad). Careful palpation and measurement of the testes are key. Are the testes prepubertal in length (less than 2.5 cm), or are they enlarging? Is there a difference in size and consistency of the two testes, suggesting a unilateral mass? Transillumination of the testes may be helpful, especially if discrepancies in size exist. Is the scrotum thinning, or does is look thick and nonvascular (i.e., prepubertal)? Are the results of the neurologic examination normal?

TRUE OR CENTRAL PRECOCIOUS PUBERTY

True or central precocious puberty is caused by early maturation of hypothalamic GnRH secretion. In many cases, no definable CNS abnormality can be found, and the problem falls into the idiopathic category, which occurs more frequently in girls than in boys. In idiopathic precocious puberty, although the onset is at an early age, the pattern and timing of progression of pubertal events are normal.

A search for an underlying CNS abnormality should be made by imaging of the CNS with computed tomography (CT) or magnetic resonance imaging (MRI). CNS tumors, especially hypothalamic hamartomas, are known causes of central precocious puberty. Hypothalamic hamartomas contain GnRH neurons that function independently of CNS inhibition. Neurofibromas, gliomas, and other tumors have been found with some frequency. Other CNS lesions also are associated with precocious puberty, such as hydrocephalus, posttrauma, and postinfectious encephalitis or meningitis.

Children with central precocious puberty have accelerated linear growth, advanced bone ages, and pubertal levels of LH, FSH, and the sex steroids estradiol and testosterone. Because levels of LH and FSH fluctuate, single samples may be inadequate to make the diagnosis but are most helpful if drawn at 8 AM. An alternative includes drawing multiple samples taken at 20-minute intervals for 1 or more hours. Most reliable is a GnRH stimulation test with levels of LH and FSH determined at regular intervals, which often can help clarify the diagnosis. Newer, highly sensitive gonadotropin assays may allow establishing the diagnosis of central puberty by a single basal LH measurement or by a single LH measurement 40 minutes after a subcutaneous GnRH injection. In boys, the finding of bilateral pubertal-sized testes almost always indicates central precocious puberty. This point is extremely important in the physical examination because it determines the diagnostic workup.

The discovery that the pulse frequency of endogenous GnRH is important for pituitary secretion of LH and FSH has had a major effect on designing treatments for blocking release of LH and FSH. GnRH agonists that provide consistent, not fluctuating, GnRH levels lower LH and FSH levels. Long-acting GnRH analogues have been successful in inhibiting pituitary release of LH and FSH and in stopping the progression of puberty. In many cases, secondary sex characteristics have regressed.

Treatment with GnRH analogues produces a prepubertal hormonal state, and growth acceleration, bone age advancement, and the progression of secondary sex characteristics cease. The first GnRH analogue to treat precocious puberty was approved by the Food and Drug Administration in the early 1990s, with others following. Most GnRH analogues are given as monthly intramuscular injections. Other preparations may be given as a depot intramuscular injection every 3 months, as well as daily subcutaneous injections.

The decision to treat should depend on several factors. First, the age of the child and his or her adjustment to the pubertal changes must be considered. A 2-year-old child is in need of treatment, but a 7-year-old child psychologically may handle the changes well. The rapidity of pubertal progression, as well as chronologic age, must be considered. In the older child with precocious puberty, the major issues in deciding whether to treat are the magnitude of bone age advancement and the rapidity of its progression, the degree of compromise of adult stature, and the decrease in predicted adult height.

Any form of pituitary gonadotropin-independent precocious sex hormone exposure causes accelerated linear growth and advanced bone age. If the bone age is advanced enough after the pathologic cause is removed, the child may experience spontaneous gonadotropin-dependent puberty. This puberty, although precocious for the chronologic age, is not precocious for bone age. This situation typically is seen in a boy in whom the diagnosis of congenital adrenal hyperplasia was made late and treatment with glucocorticoids was begun at an advanced bone age. In this situation, treatment with a GnRH analogue may be indicated.

In some patients with severe prolonged untreated primary hypothyroidism, precocious sexual development may be seen and is associated with pubertal levels of LH and FSH. These patients exhibit poor linear growth and usually delayed bone age. When overproduction of the thyroid-stimulating hormone is suppressed by exogenous thyroxine, the concentrations of LH and FSH decrease to prepubertal levels, and the pubertal changes regress.

PRECOCIOUS PUBERTY INDEPENDENT OF PITUITARY GONADOTROPINS

Girls

Girls with precocious puberty independent of pituitary gonadotropins have a nongonadotropin-stimulated or independent source of estrogens producing their pubertal changes. An exogenous source of estrogens must be sought. The use of skin creams and medications must be pursued and the labels read to see whether they contain estrogen. Birth control pills are used widely, and, although they may not be in the child's home,

grandparents, friends, and baby-sitters may keep them in unprotected locations. A positive association was found between consumption of various meat products and an outbreak of premature thelarche in girls younger than 2 years of age in Puerto Rico between 1978 and 1981. However, more than 50% of the cases examined had no exposure to this risk factor. No other associations between meat products and precocious puberty have been reported.

Estrogen-producing tumors of the ovary and adrenal gland must be considered. Adrenal estrogen-producing tumors are rare findings and are associated with high estradiol levels and increased levels of other adrenal sex hormones. They should be visible with abdominal CT or MRI scans. Estrogen-producing ovarian tumors are found more commonly and may be palpable during careful bimanual examination. As with adrenal tumors, estradiol levels usually are high. Ultrasound and CT scans usually demonstrate the ovarian mass. Ovarian cysts, associated with high levels of estradiol, are another cause of gonadotropin-independent precocious puberty and are demonstrable with imaging. Girls with estradiol-secreting ovarian cysts often present with premature breast development, with or without an isolated episode of vaginal bleeding. In some cases, the cyst has resolved by the time the pelvic ultrasound is obtained.

Treatment entails removal of the source of estrogen if exogenous exposure is the cause. If an adrenal or ovarian tumor is found, surgical excision and, if the tumor is malignant, additional treatment are indicated. Ovarian cysts are difficult to treat because they may recur, and surgical excision may make no difference in the patient's long-term clinical course.

McCune-Albright syndrome is an unusual syndrome of irregular café au lait spots, polyostotic fibrous dysplasia, and precocious puberty. McCune-Albright syndrome is seen in both sexes and is caused by a mutation in the gene that codes for the alpha subunit of Gs, the G protein that stimulates formation of adenyl cyclase. This mutation produces constitutive activation. It is a somatic mutation and can produce constitutive activation in various glands, including the thyroid, parathyroid, and adrenal. Treatments with ketoconazole (see following discussion) and aromatase inhibitors have been tried with variable success. A recent multicenter trial showed that tamoxifen treatment reduced vaginal bleeding and slowed growth velocity and the rate of skeletal maturation.

Boys

Boys with gonadotropin-independent precocious puberty have a source of androgens independent of central gonadotropin secretion. Exogenous androgen exposure must be considered. With the widespread abuse of androgens (i.e., anabolic steroids) by athletes, young children are at risk of being exposed. Also, recent availability of topical androgens may contribute to the risk of being exposed.

An adrenal source of androgens, including an adrenal tumor or an adrenal biosynthetic defect (e.g., 21-hydroxylase deficiency), causes precocious puberty in boys. Those with an adrenal or exogenous androgen source show clinical virilization, including acceleration of linear growth and advancement of bone age, but have prepubertal testes on examination.

Adrenal tumors are associated with high levels of adrenal androgens that are not suppressed with glucocorticoid administration. Performing CT or MRI is important in establishing the diagnosis. Adrenal enzyme deficiencies show characteristic precursor and androgen patterns, and the elevated androgen levels are suppressible with exogenous glucocorticoids.

Testicular tumors may produce elevated androgens and cause precocious puberty. On examination, the testes show a discrepancy in size: the testis with the tumor is larger and often has an irregular consistency.

Familial Leydig cell hyperplasia, or testotoxicosis, is another gonadotropin-independent cause of precocious puberty in boys. It is a sex-limited autosomal recessive disorder that causes pubertal levels of testosterone despite prepubertal LH patterns. This disorder is caused by activating mutations in the LH receptor. These patients are fertile as maturation of spermatogenesis occurs.

Treatment of gonadotropin-independent precocious puberty in boys entails removal of the androgen source in exogenous exposure. Excision of adrenal or testicular tumors is indicated, with additional treatment given if the lesions are malignant. Deficiencies in adrenal enzymes require appropriate glucocorticoid replacement.

GnRH analogue treatment is ineffective in familial Leydig cell hyperplasia. Some reports indicate that ketoconazole, which inhibits enzymes in the testosterone biosynthetic pathway, may be a useful treatment. Spironolactone, an antiandrogen, combined with testolactone, an inhibitor of p450 aromatase (the key enzyme in the conversion of testosterone to estrogen) also may be used to treat gonadotropin-independent precocious puberty.

An additional cause of precocious puberty in boys is human chorionic gonadotropin (hCG)-producing tumors. These tumors may be in the CNS (i.e., germinoma) or elsewhere in the body (e.g., hepatoma, hepatoblastoma, teratoma, chorioepithelioma). Because some LH assay antibodies cross-react with hCG, laboratory test results may show factitiously elevated levels of LH and prepubertal levels of FSH. Specific assays document that the gonadotropin is hCG. Because a gonadotropin is being secreted, the testes may be enlarged, and boys with this problem clinically may resemble those with central precocious puberty.

Heterosexual Development

Heterosexual development is defined as virilization in girls and feminization in boys. When it occurs before the normal age of puberty, it can be called *heterosexual precocity*. But whether it occurs at a prepubertal age or later, the diagnostic causes, evaluation, and treatment are the same.

Virilization in girls can be caused by exogenous androgen exposure and adrenal and ovarian lesions. Adrenal enzyme deficiencies (e.g., 21-hydroxylase, 11-hydroxylase, and 3 beta-hydroxysteroid dehydrogenase deficiencies) produce virilization. Typically, girls with these enzyme deficiencies have genital ambiguity as neonates, but other manifestations may occur later, sometimes as subtle as hirsutism or acne in a teenager or adult. Adrenal or ovarian androgen-producing tumors must be sought in any female patient with virilization by measuring plasma levels of sex steroids and by diagnostic imaging with ultrasound, CT, or MRI.

Boys with signs of feminization may have an exogenous estrogen exposure, an adrenal estrogen-producing tumor, a testicular tumor, or increased peripheral conversion of androgens to estrogens, as with a familial increase in aromatase activity or certain tumors such as hepatomas.

Measurement of sex hormone levels, diagnostic imaging, tests of suppression with glucocorticoids, and adrenocorticotropin (ACTH) stimulation tests are helpful in defining the cause.

VARIATIONS OF NORMAL PUBERTY

Three variations of normal pubertal development, premature thelarche (in girls), premature adrenarche (in girls and boys), and pubertal gynecomastia (in boys), occur frequently and must be differentiated from progressive and pathologic processes.

Premature Thelarche

Premature thelarche is a common entity, with clinical evidence of mild estrogenization in girls, typically when they are between 1 and 4 years of age. Breast enlargement, which may be unilateral, occurs, often without development of nipples and areolae. No sexual hair develops, and no linear growth acceleration occurs. It is an isolated phenomenon, and lack of progression is the hallmark. Evaluation shows incomplete estrogenization of the vaginal mucosa, a normal bone age, and prepubertal gonadotropin patterns. Estradiol levels usually are prepubertal, but they may be slightly increased.

Postulated causes include ovarian cysts and transient pituitary gonadotropin secretion. No treatment is necessary. Close follow-up is important because the early stages of precocious puberty may be clinically indistinguishable from those of premature thelarche.

Premature Adrenarche

Premature adrenarche is caused by early activation of adrenal androgens, producing development of pubic and axillary hair and axillary odor. In girls, the pubic hair often begins on the labia. No other signs of pubertal changes and no signs of abnormal virilization exist. If signs of gonadarche are observed, an evaluation for precocious puberty is indicated. If virilization occurs, a workup for virilizing lesions is necessary. Some children with premature adrenarche may have mild neurologic problems. Height and bone age often are slightly greater than the mean but fall within two standard deviations. Plasma adrenal androgens and urinary androgen metabolites (17-ketosteroids) are increased to the early pubertal range.

Typically, premature adrenarche occurs in 6- to 8-year-old children, but it may be seen in much younger children. The sexual hair gradually increases. Evidence suggests that a substantial percentage of children with this diagnosis may have mild 21-hydroxylase deficiency, and an ACTH stimulation test is useful for making this diagnosis. In some girls, premature adrenarche may be a marker for future polycystic ovarian syndrome.

Pubertal Gynecomastia

Pubertal gynecomastia is a common occurrence in teenage boys (greater than or equal to 40%), typically beginning in Tanner stage 2 or 3 and lasting for approximately 2 years. In some boys, the ratio of estradiol to testosterone may be elevated. Severely affected boys may require surgical reduction. Tamoxifen and testolactone may be effective for treating gynecomastia in moderate cases.

Pathologic causes of gynecomastia must be considered. Hypogonadism (e.g., Klinefelter syndrome [47XXY]); partial androgen insensitivity; partial blocks in testosterone biosynthesis; hyperthyroidism; adrenal, testicular, or LH- and hCG-producing tumors; liver tumors or disease; and chronic debilitating illness causing malnutrition all have been associated with gynecomastia. A variety of drugs can cause gynecomastia: androgens, estrogens, hCG, psychoactive drugs (e.g., phenothiazines), marijuana and other street drugs and alcohol, testosterone antagonists (e.g., ketoconazole, cimetidine, spironolactone), and antituberculosis and cytotoxic agents.

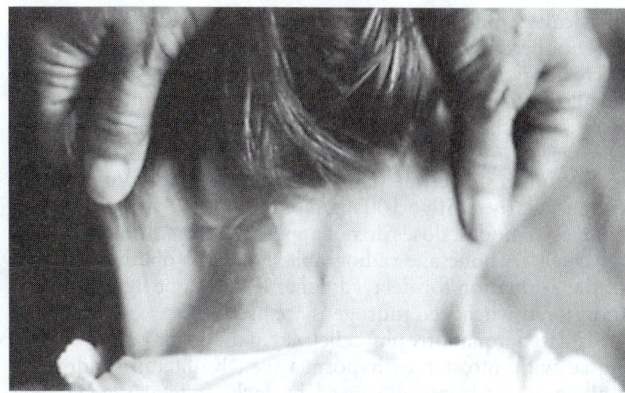

FIGURE 374.1. Turner syndrome. (Used with permission from Avery GB, Fletcher MA, MacDonald MG. *Neonatology: pathophysiology and management of the newborn*, 5th ed. Philadelphia: Lippincott Williams & Wilkins, 1999:851.)

Obese teenage boys may present with large breasts that are only adipose tissue and of no pathologic consequence. However, determining whether glandular breast tissue exists in an extremely obese boy may be difficult.

DELAYED PUBERTY

The causes of delayed puberty are listed in Box 374.2. An evaluation for pubertal delay is indicated if no signs of puberty are observed in a girl by the time she reaches 13 years of age or in a boy by 14 years of age. Evaluation also is indicated if an arrest in pubertal maturation occurs.

The differential diagnosis of delayed or absent puberty rests on the initial levels of gonadotropin. If LH and FSH levels are high, a primary gonadal abnormality exists. If LH and FSH levels are normal or low, a search for central hormonal abnormalities or chronic disease must be undertaken.

Elevated Gonadotropin Level

Patients with elevated LH and FSH levels have evidence of bilateral gonadal failure and lack of appropriate sex steroid levels to feed back centrally. After LH and FSH levels are found to be elevated, a karyotype should be determined. Common causes of gonadal failure are chemotherapy, radiation therapy, and autoimmune glandular failure.

Girls with an XY karyotype who have complete androgen insensitivity develop breasts at the appropriate age, but no sexual hair develops, and no menses occur. Girls with an XY karyotype and complete 17-alpha-hydroxylase deficiency (i.e., no sex steroids can be formed) have no secondary sex characteristics. If these syndromes are partial, enough androgen is present to cause genital ambiguity in the neonate or virilization during puberty.

Turner syndrome is a common cause of absent breast development and elevated gonadotropin levels (Fig. 374.1). Turner syndrome invariably is associated with short stature and often with other anomalies, including webbed neck, increased nevi, high-arched palate, shield chest, coarctation of the aorta, renal anomalies, an increased arm-carrying angle, and edema of the hands and feet. Most girls with this syndrome have a 45X karyotype, but many have a mosaic pattern (45X/46XX) or an X-chromosomal structural abnormality (e.g., ring or isochrome). Buccal smears are not adequate for establishing this diagnosis. Sexual hair develops in girls with Turner syndrome because adrenal androgens are not affected.

Boys with Klinefelter syndrome (47XXY) usually come to attention because of gynecomastia and small testes (i.e., inadequate masculinization). They usually are clinically normal at birth, and throughout childhood they are tall with slim builds and long limbs. They also may have mosaic chromosome patterns (e.g., 46XY/47XXY) or multiple X chromosomes.

Treatment of patients with gonadal failure involves replacing sex steroids. Depending on the age of the patient and whether height is an issue, replacement can be done gradually over the course of several years or more abruptly.

In young teenage boys, injectable testosterone can be used. A typical regimen is testosterone enanthate administered intramuscularly in a dose of 50 mg/month initially and gradually increased to full adult doses of 300 mg every 3 weeks or 200 mg every 2 weeks. Long-term replacement therapy with oral testosterone preparations is not recommended because of the hepatotoxicity of 17-alpha-alkylated steroids. Testosterone patches and topical gel preparations are available and can be used to induce and maintain puberty.

In girls, conjugated estrogens can be started at 0.3 mg/day, with doses increased gradually until satisfactory breast development is achieved. After 1 to 2 years of estrogen treatment or if vaginal spotting occurs, treatment with estrogens in cycles of approximately 25 days per month, with a progestational agent overlapping for approximately the last 10 to 14 days of each cycle, should be started. Estradiol also can be given in gradually increasing doses. Depot estrogen preparations given monthly have been used. New transdermal estrogen patches may be useful in long-term treatment. After adequate estrogenization has occurred, long-term treatment can be achieved with a combination oral contraceptive pill. Bone age should be monitored.

Normal or Low Gonadotropin Levels

The most common cause of pubertal delay is constitutional delay, which is discussed in Chapter 375. Usually, a careful physical examination in a midteenaged boy reveals signs of early puberty, and signs of the appropriate progression of puberty are noted on follow-up examinations. Reassurance may be all that is necessary. However, more severely affected boys may be psychologically disabled by this problem, and serious consideration should be given to providing a short course of exogenous testosterone (e.g., testosterone enanthate given intramuscularly as 50 to 100 mg/month for 4 to 6 months). Short courses of modest doses do not appear to affect ultimate stature adversely. A bone age radiograph should be obtained as part of the evaluation for delayed puberty, and bone age should be monitored whenever androgens are used.

Isolated gonadotropin deficiency may or may not be associated with anosmia or hyposmia (i.e., Kallmann syndrome). Kallmann syndrome is caused by lack of fetal GnRH neuron migration caused by lack of adhesion molecule production (coded by the KAL gene). Hypogonadotropic hypogonadism may be difficult to differentiate from constitutional delay in certain cases, and using GnRH stimulation testing may be helpful. Baseline LH and FSH levels may not differentiate prepubertal or hypogonadotropic from early pubertal levels. Search for an organic cause requires imaging of the CNS. Prolactin-secreting pituitary adenomas may produce gonadotropin deficiency. LH and FSH deficiency is associated more commonly with other pituitary hormone deficiencies, especially growth hormone deficiency. The differential diagnosis of hypopituitarism is discussed in Chapter 375. Induction and maintenance of puberty in these patients must be coordinated with other hormonal replacement therapy. Traditionally, puberty has been induced and maintained with exogenous sex steroids, as discussed earlier in this chapter. Gonadotropin injections can be used to induce fertility in patients with central gonadotropin deficiency. GnRH has been given in pulsatile fashion to induce puberty and to produce fertility.

Some adolescent girls may develop normally, but because they lack normal central cyclic hormonal function, they do not have normal menses. Any chronic disease during childhood and adolescence may delay puberty and growth. Particular attention must be paid to the possibility of subtle gastrointestinal disease, especially inflammatory bowel disease and celiac disease, and to the patient's nutritional status. Inadequate caloric intake or excessive exercise can delay puberty and cause amenorrhea.

Certain syndromes are associated with central gonadotropin deficiency, particularly the Prader-Willi and Laurence-Moon-Biedl syndromes. Hypothyroidism can cause delayed puberty or precocious puberty.

Blind children may have pubertal delay, and associated pituitary-hypothalamic dysfunction must be considered in these children.

In virtually all patients with primary gonadal failure or central gonadotropin deficiency, treatment with sex steroids can induce and maintain satisfactory sexual maturation and satisfactory sexual functioning. With the use of gonadotropins or GnRH preparations, patients with central gonadotropin deficiency have hope for fertility.

Suggested Readings

Chumlea WC, Schubert CM, Roche AF, et al. Age at menarche and racial comparison in US girls. Pediatrics 2003;111:110.

Eugster EA, Rubin SD, Reiter EO, et al. Tamoxifen treatment for precocious puberty in McCune-Albright syndrome: a multicenter trial. J Pediatr 2003; 143:60.

Grumbach MM, Styne DM. Puberty: ontogeny, neuroendocrinology, physiology and disorders. In: Wilson JD, Foster DW, eds. William's textbook of endocrinology. Philadelphia: Saunders, 1994:1139.

Herman-Giddens ME, Slora EJ, Wasserman SC, et al. Secondary sexual characteristics and menses in young girls seen in office practice: a study from the pediatric research in office settings network. Pediatrics 1997;99:505.

Kaplan SL, Grumbach MM. Pathophysiology and treatment of sexual precocity. J Clin Endocrinol Metab 1990;71:785.

Lee PA, O'Dea L. Primary and secondary testicular insufficiency. Pediatr Clin North Am 1990;37:1359.

Mahoney CP. Adolescent gynecomastia: differential diagnosis and management. Pediatr Clin North Am 1990;37:1389.

Miller WL. Pathophysiology, genetics and treatment of hyperandrogenism. Pediatr Clin North Am 1997;44:375.

Pescovitz OH. Precocious puberty. Pediatr Rev 1990;11:229.

Plotnick LP. Precocious puberty. In: Carpenter S, Rock J, eds. Pediatric and adolescent gynecology. New York: Raven, 1992:153.

Plotnick LP, Kritzler RK. Sexual development alterations. In: Hoekelman RA, ed. Primary pediatric care. St. Louis: Mosby–Year Book, 1997:1105.

Rosenfield RL. Diagnosis and management of delayed puberty. J Clin Endocrinol Metab 1990;70:559.

Rosenfield RL. The ovary and female sexual maturation. In: Kaplan SA, ed. Clinical pediatric endocrinology. Philadelphia: Saunders, 1990:259.

Styne DM. The testes: disorders of sexual differentiation and puberty. In: Kaplan SA, ed. Clinical pediatric endocrinology. Philadelphia: Saunders, 1990:367.

Styne DM. New aspects in the diagnosis and treatment of pubertal disorders. Pediatr Clin North Am 1997;44:505.

Sun SS, Schubert CM, Chumlea WC, et al. National estimates of the timing of sexual maturation and racial differences among US children. Pediatrics 2002; 110:911.

Wheeler MD, Styne DM. Diagnosis and management of precocious puberty. Pediatr Clin North Am 1990;37:1255.

Wilson DM, Rosenfeld RG. Treatment of short stature and delayed adolescence. Pediatr Clin North Am 1987;34:865.

Wu T, Mendola P, Buck GM, et al. Ethnic differences in the presence of secondary sex characteristics and menarche among us girls: the third national health and nutrition examination survey, 1988–1994. Pediatrics 2002;110:752.

CHAPTER 375 ■ GROWTH, GROWTH HORMONE, AND PITUITARY DISORDERS

LESLIE P. PLOTNICK AND RYAN S. MILLER

Problems related to growth are commonly observed in pediatric practice. Short stature can be defined as height more than two standard deviations (SDs) below the mean and tall stature as height more than two SDs above the mean. By definition, 3% of children have short stature and 3% have tall stature. On the

other hand, growth is dynamic, and growth velocity is defined as the increase in length or height over time.

Measurement of growth velocity over a period of time in addition to determination of stature at any given point in time both are essential in deciding whether a child may have a problem with growth. A child may have normal height and weight but a subnormal rate of growth, indicating the need for an evaluation. The growth of an individual can be assessed adequately only through obtaining regular height and weight measurements and accurately plotting these measurements on growth curves to detect deviations from normal velocities (see Chapter 5, Pediatric History and Physical Examination, for height and weight curves for girls and boys, birth to 36 months and 2 to 18 years).

Because the timing of puberty affects growth rate, Tanner has modified the growth curves to include curves for early and late developers. These curves are especially useful in evaluating adolescents with early-normal and late-normal onset of puberty and should be used to assess the normality of growth in these children (Fig. 375.1).

Growth velocity curves are important to use when evaluating children for disorders of growth. These curves are shown in Fig. 375.2. Velocities for children with early-normal and late-normal puberty are superimposed on the curves.

Bone age also is important in evaluating a child for a growth problem. A child with normal bone age is unlikely to have a systemic chronic disease or a hormonal abnormality as the cause of the growth problem. Significantly delayed or advanced bone ages (i.e., greater than two SDs from the mean) may indicate pathology and require evaluation.

SHORT STATURE OR POOR LINEAR GROWTH

A child with a height below the third percentile or whose growth curve has been crossing percentiles downward should be examined carefully for a pathologic cause of poor growth (Box 375.1). However, for children who are born smaller or larger than their genetic growth potential to gradually shift percentiles, up or down, for height and weight is not unusual. For example, a child who at birth is in the 90th percentile for length and weight but whose parents are in the tenth percentile for height may decelerate gradually to the tenth percentile over the course of the first 2 years of life. Sometimes differentiating this pattern from pathologic growth is difficult. The key points are a gradual deceleration of height and weight proportionally, deceleration not below the genetically anticipated percentile, and once the percentile is reached, velocities normalizing and height and weight remaining at that percentile. If the deceleration is abrupt and falls to less than the third percentile or to a percentile below the parents' percentile, further evaluation is needed.

A large percentage of children with poor growth have major organ system disease that is responsible for their growth failure. Most patients in this category have a disorder that is not subtle, and the history and physical examination disclose the problem without extensive laboratory testing. However, some disorders may not be evident from history and physical examination and, therefore, require laboratory studies for diagnosis.

Renal disorders, particularly renal tubular acidosis, require evaluation by electrolytes, chemistries, and urinalysis. Particularly difficult to define are patients with gastrointestinal (GI) abnormalities. Patients with inflammatory bowel disease, especially Crohn disease, may have growth failure for several years before GI symptoms become evident. A complete blood cell count with an erythrocyte sedimentation rate and/or C-reactive protein may be helpful, but GI contrast studies and endoscopy are required to make the diagnosis. Patients with celiac disease may not have the classic history of malabsorption and hyperphagia. These children may have poor appetites or may have no symptoms other than poor growth. Laboratory tests (tissue transglutaminase and antiendomysial antibodies)

may help with this diagnosis, but the definitive diagnostic test is a small-bowel biopsy. The decision as to when to do more extensive GI studies (e.g., radiologic, endoscopic) rests on the persistence of a poor growth rate over time, with other laboratory tests remaining normal and no other diagnosis being made, especially if the child's weight is affected more than is height. Malnutrition of any cause, including malabsorption or inadequate caloric intake, is associated with poor growth.

Poor growth also may be due to inborn metabolic errors, chromosomal abnormalities, and a variety of dysmorphic syndromes including Turner syndrome, Prader-Willi syndrome (PWS), Russell-Silver syndrome, and Noonan syndrome. Turner syndrome and its variants (i.e., absence or structural abnormalities of one X chromosome or a mosaic pattern) may manifest with classic phenotypic features or may have only minor clinical features. Girls with non-45X karyotypes (i.e., mosaics, rings, isochromes, or partial X deletions) are more likely to lack the classic phenotypic features. All short girls with subnormal growth rates should have banded karyotyping as part of the laboratory evaluation. Turner syndrome may be as common as growth hormone (GH) deficiency and should be considered in all short girls. Growth curves for girls with Turner syndrome are available.

Children born small for gestational age (SGA), which is defined as weight or length greater than or equal to two SDs below the mean for gestational age, may have poor postnatal growth and resultant short stature. These children may have dysmorphic features, indicating a specific syndrome associated with intrauterine growth retardation. They may be nondysmorphic but thin, especially with very thin extremities, minimal body fat, and thin, narrow faces. Bone ages may be delayed or normal. Approximately 15% fail to catch up by 2 years of age, and approximately half of these children will remain short as adults.

Skeletal dysplasias resulting in poor growth occasionally may be subtle. The skeletal abnormalities usually are evident on physical examination. Careful measurement of upper and lower segment ratios may aid in establishing the diagnosis. Radiologic studies can help identify the specific abnormalities.

Nutritional deficiencies are an important cause of growth retardation throughout the world. In the developed countries, it may be caused by GI pathology, familial psychosocial problems, or self-imposed caloric deprivation. The last one is an important problem in the United States. Anorexia nervosa is associated with both inadequate weight gain and linear growth retardation. Normal GH levels and low insulinlike growth factor (IGF-1) have been observed. Linear growth and lab markers typically normalize with refeeding.

Psychological factors also have been associated with poor growth. Children in disturbed families may have psychosocial dwarfism, with disturbed eating and sleeping behaviors and transient pituitary hormone deficiencies, especially of GH and adrenocorticotropic hormone. When the child is removed from the adverse home environment, catch-up growth occurs and the hormonal levels normalize.

Various medications may produce poor growth. Glucocorticoids will be discussed later in this chapter. Stimulants such as amphetamines and methylphenidate and similar medications, especially in high doses, have been associated with short-term impairment of weight and height. However, longer-term studies have shown no evidence of height deficits in late adolescence and no difference in adult stature.

Familial or genetic short stature is characterized by height below the third percentile, normal growth rate, and skeletal age appropriate for chronologic age. It is a common cause of short stature in children. Usually the parents' heights are in the lower normal percentiles for adults. Children with familial short stature are entirely normal. Their heights usually are at or slightly below the third percentile but not at or more than

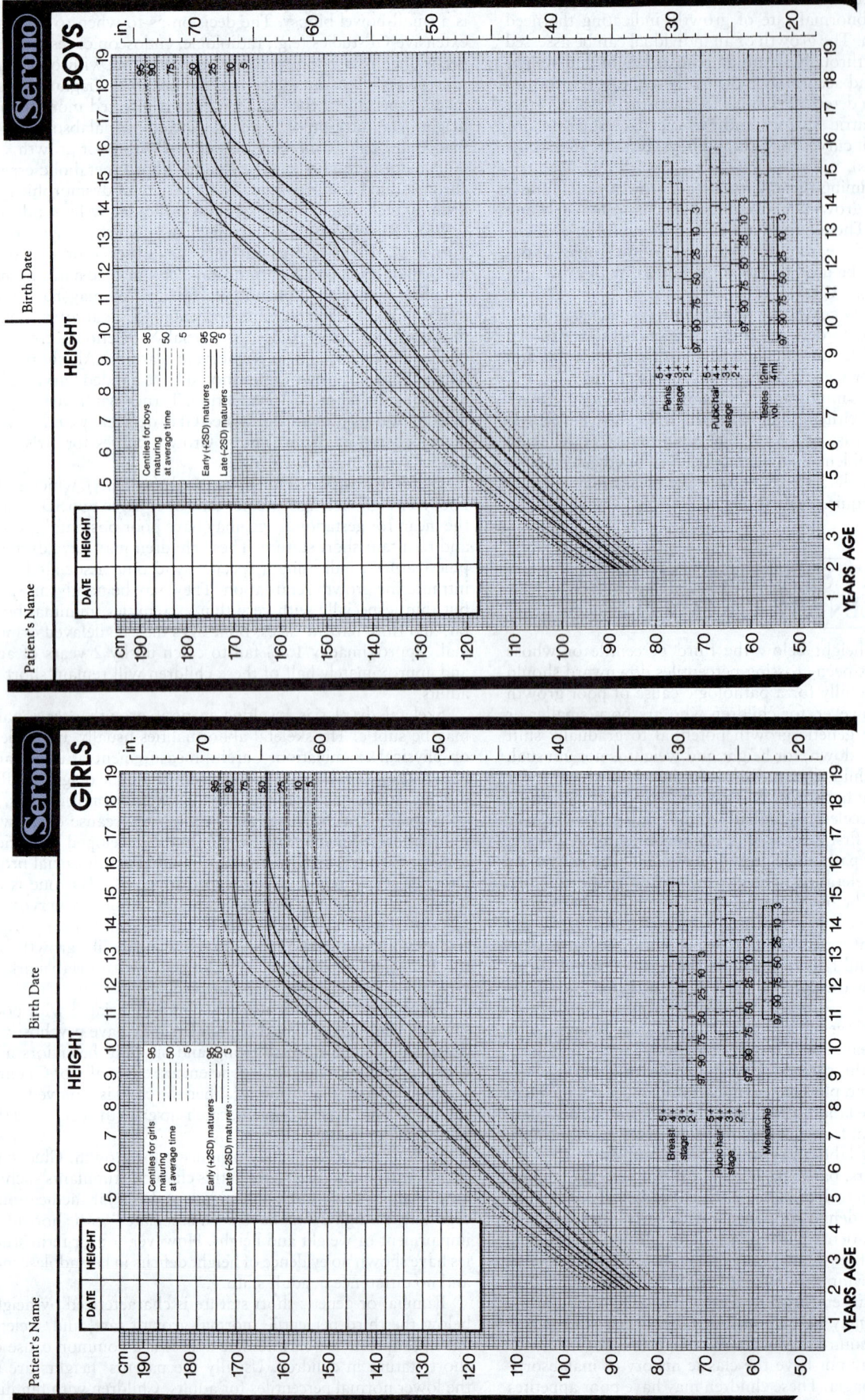

FIGURE 375.1. Early and late puberty curves for girls and boys, superimposed on the average curve. (Reprinted with permission from Tanner JM. North American growth and development longitudinal standards. Height: distance and velocity for girls and boys. *J Pediatr* 1985;107. Distributed by Serono Laboratories, Randolph, MA.)

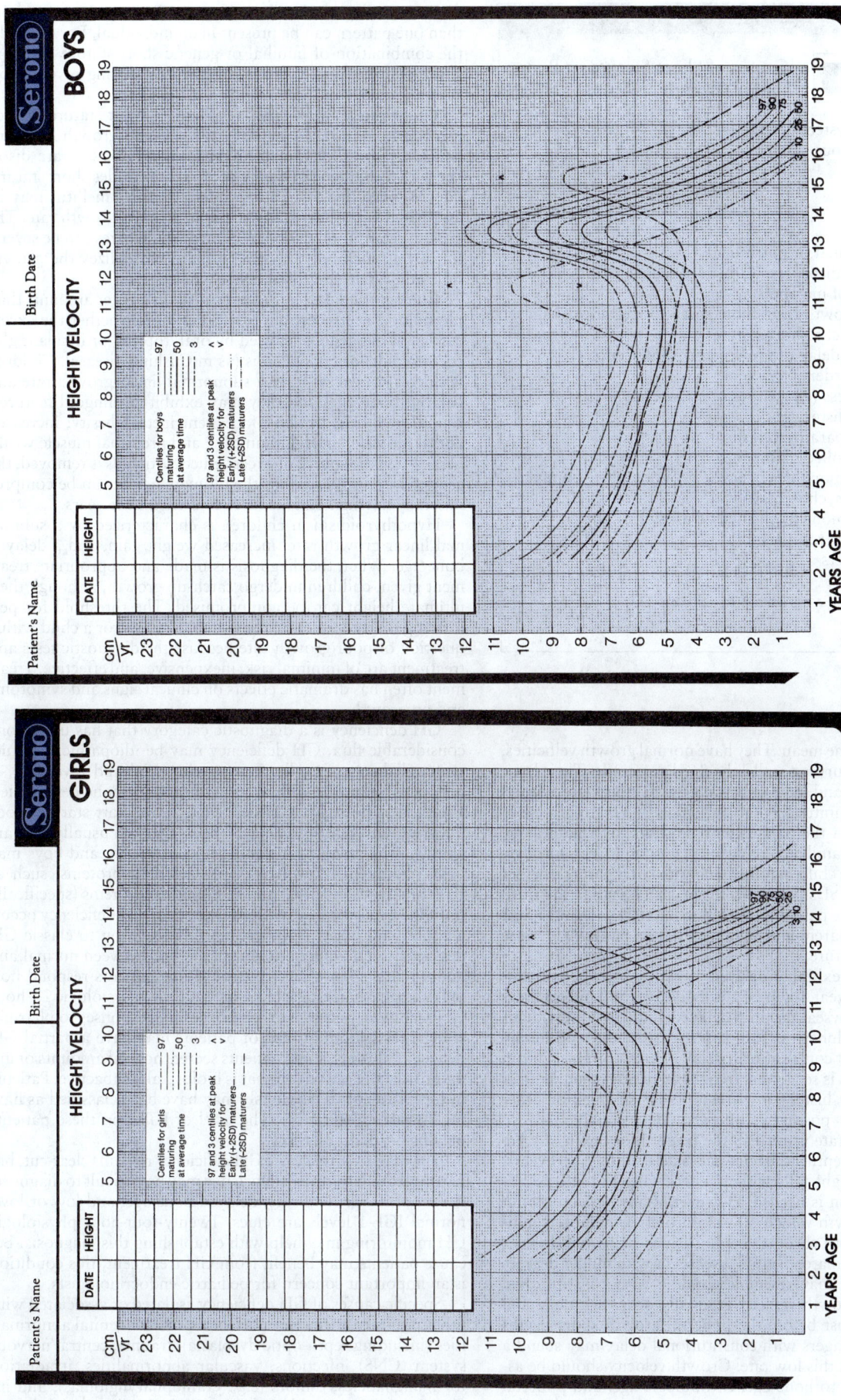

FIGURE 375.2. Growth velocity curves for girls and boys, including early and late pubertal patterns. (Reprinted with permission from Tanner JM. North American growth and development longitudinal standards. Height: distance and velocity for girls and boys. *J Pediatr* 1985;107. Distributed by Serono Laboratories, Randolph, MA.)

BOX 375.1 — Causes of Short Stature or Poor Linear Growth

Major organ system disease
  Central nervous system
  Cardiac
  Pulmonary
  Hematologic
  Renal
  Gastrointestinal or nutritional
Chromosomal disorders: Turner syndrome, others
Inborn errors of metabolism
Intrauterine growth restriction (small for gestational age)
Familial or genetic short stature
Constitutional delay of growth and adolescence
Endocrine disorders
  Cortisol excess (exogenous or endogenous)
  Hypothyroidism
  Pseudohypoparathyroidism
  Poorly controlled diabetes
  Growth hormone deficiency (e.g., idiopathic, organic,
    familial, psychosocial)
  Growth hormone insensitivity (resistance)
Shifting linear percentiles
Skeletal disorders
Nutritional
Deprivation or psychosocial dwarfism
Medications

---

three SDs below the mean. They have normal growth velocities, and their height curves parallel the third percentile. Their bone ages are normal, and their pubertal growth spurts are normal in timing and magnitude.

One or both of the parents may be short for a pathologic reason, such as familial GH deficiency or mild chondrodysplasias, which the child may have inherited. If a parent's height is more than two SDs below the mean (i.e., less than the third percentile) or if the parent is disproportionately short for his or her family, both parent and child may have a pathologic cause for their short stature.

Children may exhibit a delayed growth pattern, characterized by a 2- to 4-year lag in height, bone age, and pubertal development. Epiphyseal fusion is delayed, and most individuals reach normal adult height. This pattern of growth is commonly a manifestation of constitutional delay of growth. This variant of normal growth is seen more frequently in boys than in girls. Often, the family history in parents, older siblings, or other family members is positive for this growth pattern.

If the growth rate is normal, the height is at or slightly below the third percentile, the bone age is delayed by 2 to 4 years, and predicted height falls within genetic target range, no additional evaluation is needed. However, if any concern about a subnormal growth velocity exists, further evaluation is indicated. Patients with chronic illness, such as sickle cell disease, asthma, or inflammatory bowel disease, or with milder degrees of GH deficiency may resemble children with constitutional delay. Because growth velocity gradually drops with age and is at its lowest just before the pubertal growth spurt begins (Fig. 375.2), teenagers with constitutional delay may spend a prolonged time at this low rate. Growth velocity should be assessed in relation to bone age, chronologic age, and pubertal stage.

Patterns of growth failure often are distinct. However, more than one pattern can be present in an individual. For example, the combination of familial or genetic short stature and constitutional delay may occur together, producing severe short stature.

Endocrine abnormalities resulting in short stature include glucocorticoid excess, hypothyroidism, and growth hormone deficiency. Pseudohypoparathyroidism (PHP) is a rare disorder with a characteristic phenotype that includes short stature. Poorly controlled insulin-dependent diabetes mellitus may be associated with short stature and poor linear growth rate. The growth retardation in poorly controlled diabetes can be severe. Improving metabolic control usually normalizes the growth rate, and catch-up growth can occur.

Glucocorticoid excess (i.e., cortisol in greater amounts than physiologic needs) produces short stature, whether the excess cortisol is exogenous (caused by oral, topical, or inhalant glucocorticoids) or endogenous (as in Cushing disease). Children with cortisol excess have a subnormal linear growth rate and delayed bone age, and they may exhibit cushingoid features: round, plethoric "moon" face; centripetal obesity; increased dorsal fat pad ("buffalo hump"); and proximal muscle weakness. When the source of excess glucocorticoids is removed, the growth rate increases, but the ultimate height can be compromised by having had glucocorticoid excess for years.

Hypothyroidism in children is characterized by a subnormal linear growth rate, increased weight gain, and a delayed bone age. When the diagnosis is made and appropriate treatment given, children undergo catch-up growth, although their ultimate height can be compromised. The threshold for performing thyroid function tests should be low for a child with a question of poor growth rate because the diagnostic tests and treatment are of minimal risk, inexpensive, and effective. Treatment often has dramatic effects on clinical signs and symptoms and on growth.

GH deficiency is a diagnostic category that has undergone considerable flux. GH deficiency may be idiopathic, organic, or familial; occasionally, it is psychosocial and reversible. It may occur alone or with other pituitary hormone deficiencies. Children with classic GH deficiency have short stature, poor linear growth rate, and delayed bone age, and usually they are chubby. They may have fasting hypoglycemia, and boys may have micropenis. Levels of GH-dependent proteins, such as IGF-1 (somatomedin-C) and IGF-binding proteins (specifically IGFBP-3), may be low. Various degrees of GH deficiency occur; a continuum exists from normal GH secretion to classic GH deficiency, and where one draws the line between normal and abnormal is somewhat arbitrary. Some patients respond normally to pharmacologic tests but have low physiologic 24-hour GH secretion, and some have borderline responses to pharmacologic tests; both groups of patients may have a partial GH deficiency. Rarely, some patients secrete normal amounts of immunologically active GH that is biologically subactive. Patients in these categories previously may have been classified as having constitutional delay. The level of IGF-1 in these patients may be borderline or low.

The diagnosis of classic GH deficiency remains clear-cut, but partial growth hormone deficiency may be difficult to diagnose. A subnormal growth rate, delayed bone age, and low or low-normal IGF-1 levels are clues. Twenty-four-hour physiologic GH monitoring may help with establishing this diagnosis. Because patients may benefit from GH treatment, this condition is an important concern for pediatric endocrinologists.

Specific causes of GH deficiency, isolated or associated with other pituitary hormone deficiencies, are congenital abnormalities (including septo-optic dysplasia), trauma, central nervous system (CNS) infections, vascular abnormalities, irradiation for malignancies, tumors (e.g., craniopharyngiomas), and infiltrative processes such as histiocytosis. Midline facial defects such as cleft palate or single central incisor often can be associated with pituitary abnormalities.

Craniopharyngiomas are the most common tumors associated with pituitary and hypothalamic deficiencies. They are tumors of the Rathke pouch and usually are suprasellar, but they may be entirely intrasellar. Patients with craniopharyngiomas usually present with headache, visual abnormalities, and neurologic symptoms. They also may have growth failure and symptoms of diabetes insipidus. On physical examination, they may have visual defects (e.g., field defects, optic atrophy, papilledema) and signs of pituitary hormone deficiencies. Imaging of the CNS identifies the tumors. Treatment is surgical excision, often followed by radiation therapy, and appropriate hormonal replacement therapy.

Syndromes of primary GH insensitivity or resistance occur because of defects in the GH receptor or its signal transduction or IGF-1 synthesis. Secondary causes of GH insensitivity include inhibiting GH antibodies, malnutrition, liver disease, and renal failure.

TALL STATURE AND EXCESSIVE LINEAR GROWTH

Most children with tall stature (i.e., height more than two SDs above the mean) have familial or genetic tall stature; their parents or other family members are tall. This, like familial short stature, is not pathologic. These children grow above the 95th percentile, but their growth curves are parallel to it. Their linear growth velocities are normal, and their bone ages are normal. Their pubertal growth spurt is normal in timing and magnitude, although they tend to grow in the upper normal velocity percentiles.

Certain syndromes are associated with tall stature and should be sought on examination. Marfan syndrome, cerebral gigantism, homocystinuria, Klinefelter syndrome (XXY), and XYY karyotypes are associated with tall stature.

Nutritional obesity often is associated with tall stature. Obese children typically show linear growth in the upper normal percentiles and also may have bone ages at the upper limits of normal (i.e., approximately one to two SDs above the mean). This growth is in contrast to the weight gain associated with endocrine abnormalities such as hypothyroidism, Cushing disease, and GH deficiency, in which linear growth rate is subnormal and bone age is delayed. Endocrine abnormalities also can cause tall stature. Children with hyperthyroidism may have an excessive linear growth rate during the hyperthyroid period, but this finding usually is not a presenting complaint.

GH excess (i.e., pituitary gigantism) causes excessive linear growth rates. GH excess is a rare occurrence in childhood and adolescence and usually is caused by a pituitary GH-producing tumor or sometimes by excess production of GH-releasing factor from a hypothalamic or peripheral tumor, such as a pancreatic tumor. Some children with tall stature and excessive linear growth rates have precocious secretion of sex hormone caused by central precocious puberty or a variety of gonadal or adrenal abnormalities (see Chapter 374). Children with precocious secretion of sex hormone have excessive linear growth rates initially. However, the hormones also cause rapid advancement of bone age and early epiphyseal fusion, which compromise adult stature.

High doses of sex steroids have been used occasionally to treat tall stature if the predicted adult height is excessive. A modest effect on adult stature may be seen. Patients have been reported with aromatase deficiency who cannot convert androgen to estrogen, and one patient was reported to have an estrogen-receptor defect. All have tall stature, lack of epiphyseal fusion, and osteopenia, despite normal or elevated andro-

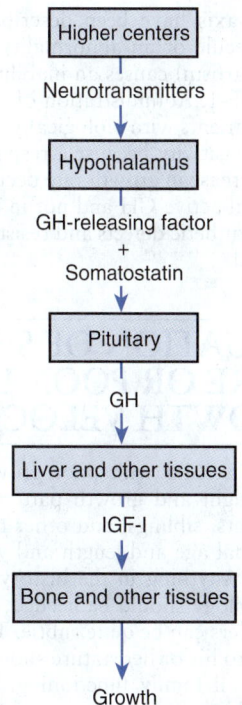

FIGURE 375.3. Regulation of growth hormone (*GH*) secretion. IGF-1, insulinlike growth factor-1.

gen levels. These patients indicate the crucial role of estrogen in stopping linear growth by causing epiphyseal fusion.

HYPOTHALAMIC–PITUITARY–GROWTH HORMONE PHYSIOLOGY

The regulation of GH secretion is shown in outline form in Fig. 375.3. Pituitary release of GH is controlled by two hypothalamic factors, a GH-releasing factor and an inhibiting factor (somatostatin). Hypothalamic release of these factors is controlled by neurotransmitters secreted by higher neurons that respond to factors such as sleep, exercise, and physical and emotional stress. GH is released in bursts, and the levels fluctuate markedly during the day and night, with higher values usually occurring during the early hours of sleep. Most of the effects of GH on linear growth are mediated by another class of hormones called the *somatomedins* or *insulin-like growth factors*, of which IGF-1 is the predominant growth-promoting factor. IGF-1 is thought to be generated mostly in the liver. IGF-1 generation in other tissues (e.g., the growth plate) may be more important than circulating IGF-1 for linear growth.

For GH to generate IGF-1, the GH must be normally biologically active and able to bind to its receptor. The receptor and all postreceptor steps must be intact. IGF-1 acts through its receptors on target tissues to produce linear growth. IGF-1 and GH also exert negative feedback at the pituitary and hypothalamic levels, affecting secretion of GH.

A defect anywhere in the GH–IGF-1 axis can produce short stature and a clinical picture identical to that of GH deficiency. Various defects along the axis can be distinguished from each other only by laboratory testing.

Some cases of GH deficiency may be caused by mutations in genes coding for GH, the GH-releasing hormone receptor, or transcription factors (e.g., Pit-1). Patients with other disorders of the GH–IGF-1 axis have been described. A biologically subactive GH molecule or an abnormality in the GH receptor (i.e., Laron dwarfism) causes an inability to generate normal amounts of IGF-1. Administration of exogenous GH can help differentiate patients with biologically subactive GH from those with GH insensitivity because a response of an increase in IGF-1 and an increase in growth rate occurs in only patients with biologically subactive GH and not in those with GH insensitivity. IGF-1 synthetic defects and resistance to IGF-1 also have been described.

EVALUATION OF SHORT STATURE OR POOR LINEAR GROWTH VELOCITY

The evaluation of a child with poor growth begins with a careful history. Height and growth patterns and the timing of puberty in parents, siblings, and other relatives should be obtained. Gestational age and length and weight at birth are important factors. Anything in the history to suggest major organ system pathology should be heeded, remembering that renal and GI disorders can be quite subtle. The child's psychological adjustment to his or her stature should be investigated, as should the overall family functioning. Nutritional issues should be discussed.

The child's growth curve should be evaluated carefully. If no previous growth data are available, questions about changes in shoe and clothing sizes and about how the child's growth compares with that of siblings and peers can be helpful. For example, "He used to be a head taller than his sister, who's 3 years younger, but now they're the same height," is revealing information. Every effort should be made to obtain previous height and weight data.

The complete physical examination is important. Any features of chronic disease should be noted. Obtaining accurate height and weight measurements is mandatory. Careful funduscopic examination looking for evidence of optic nerve abnormalities and confrontation visual fields should be performed. Because dentition reflects bone age, the age appropriateness of primary and secondary teeth should be assessed. Are there any dysmorphic features of the face or body habitus or extremities? The thyroid should be palpated carefully. Are there signs of sexual maturation? If the patient is a boy, is the penis abnormally small? Are there any clinical features of cortisol excess or of Turner syndrome? Is the child's appearance proportionate or disproportionate for arm span and for upper and lower segment ratios? If clues to a specific diagnosis are found, a complete laboratory workup is unnecessary. For example, if the child appears normal on examination and the history and growth curve strongly suggest familial short stature, no workup is necessary. Perhaps only a bone age evaluation to assess predicted height should be performed. If the child is clearly cushingoid, the specific cause should be pursued.

In many children, no clear cause is evident after the history has been obtained and a physical examination has been performed. In these children, a screening evaluation can include bone age radiograph, complete blood count, erythrocyte sedimentation rate and/or C-reactive protein, chemistry panel including electrolytes, thyroid hormone levels (i.e., T_4, TSH), banded karyotyping for girls, IGF-1, IGFBP-3, and a screen for celiac disease (antiendomysial antibodies or tissue transglutaminase and IgA). In addition, urinalysis and urine culture can be considered.

Any specific abnormalities should be investigated further, but if nothing abnormal is seen other than perhaps a significant bone age delay, the next step depends on the clinical impression and on the child's growth curve and current growth rate.

BOX 375.2   **Tests for Growth Hormone Deficiency**

Screening tests
  Exercise: before and after 20 minutes of jogging on a level surface or up and down stairs
  Sleep: useful for inpatients; measure growth hormone approximately 45 minutes after onset of nighttime sleep
Pharmacologic tests (arginine through glucagon in the following list measure ability of the hypothalamic-pituitary unit to secrete growth hormone)
  Arginine
  L-Dopa
  Insulin hypoglycemia
  Clonidine
  Glucagon
  Growth hormone-releasing factor (i.e., measures only pituitary growth hormone function)
Physiologic tests: sampling every 20 to 30 minutes, intermittently or with a continuous blood withdrawal pump

---

Growth is an ongoing dynamic process, and evaluation over the course of time reveals a pattern that may lead to the diagnosis. If a child's growth rate is persistently subnormal such that he or she gradually or abruptly falls away from a normal curve, formal GH testing is indicated.

Tests for GH deficiency are summarized in Box 375.2. Random GH measurements are not useful to screen for deficiency because secretion is pulsatile. IGF-1 levels are low in GH deficiency and also are low with poor nutritional status. The level of IGF-binding proteins, particularly IGFBP-3, correlates with GH production and along with IGF-1 also may be a useful screening tool for GH deficiency. Physiologic screening tests (exercise, sleep; see Box 375.2) may be helpful. An inadequate response to a screening test indicates the need for formal GH testing.

For classic GH deficiency to be diagnosed, a patient must fail two definitive pharmacologic tests. Most laboratories use a level of 7 to 10 ng/mL peak value as the cutoff point between normal and subnormal. Different assays have different normal ranges. Some investigators contend that formal GH testing is not more reliable than are low IGF-1 and IGFBP-3 levels in properly selected patients.

Despite the sophisticated diagnostic testing available, some children have clearly negative workup results, do not fit the diagnosis of constitutional delay, and are left with a diagnosis of idiopathic short stature. Children in this category need careful follow-up because a specific cause may become evident with time.

TREATMENT OF SHORT STATURE

If a specific diagnosis is made, the condition is treated appropriately. For example, if primary hypothyroidism is found, thyroid replacement therapy is indicated. This section discusses primarily treatment with exogenous GH for children with GH deficiency and other disorders resulting in short stature.

From 1958 to 1985, GH in the United States and elsewhere was obtained exclusively from cadaver pituitaries. In 1985, pituitary GH was withdrawn because a few young men treated with pituitary GH in the 1960s and 1970s died of Creutzfeldt-Jakob disease, thought to be related to infected pituitary tissue.

In October 1985, the first recombinant DNA-produced biosynthetic GH was approved for use in GH-deficient children. Several other preparations have been approved since then. Pituitary GH and biosynthetic GH have identical effects.

Until recombinant GH became widely available, GH therapy was limited strictly to patients with GH deficiency. A GH-deficient child usually grows 3 to 4 inches in the first year of treatment and 2 to 3 inches in each successive year. Catch-up growth to the normal range may be gradual. Recommended doses depend on the type of preparation and the diagnosis. Daily treatment for GH deficiency using approximately 0.20 to 0.30 mg/kg/week divided into six or seven subcutaneous injections has supplanted thrice-weekly therapy for many patients because of data documenting that better growth rates were achieved on daily treatment regimens.

GH also has been approved for use in growth failure associated with chronic renal insufficiency, Turner syndrome, Prader-Willi syndrome, children born small for gestational age, and idiopathic short stature. Use for other diagnostic categories is investigational.

Women with Turner syndrome are approximately 20 cm shorter than are normal women within respective populations. One randomized, controlled trial of GH in girls with Turner syndrome reported a final height difference of 4.8 cm in treated versus untreated girls.

Growth failure related to GH deficiency is a principal feature of PWS. Treatment with GH has been shown to increase linear growth, increase lean body mass, and decrease fat mass. However, deaths have been reported with use of GH in patients with PWS and severe obesity or respiratory impairment (including sleep apnea and respiratory infection), and it is contraindicated in these patients.

Children born small for gestational age who fail to manifest catch-up growth by age 2 years may benefit from GH therapy, but other causes of growth failure should be excluded before initiating treatment. With long-term treatment, as many as 85% of patients can reach adult stature within their targeted genetic potential.

Some children with mild deficiencies in GH secretion may resemble clinically patients with constitutional delay. Because these patients may benefit from GH treatment, a trial of GH may be considered for patients with subnormal growth velocities and low-normal IGF-1 levels.

Idiopathic short stature is a diagnostic label for short children who do not fall into any specific diagnostic category. A child who may be small for the family; who has a negative history, normal physical examination, and negative laboratory evaluation; and who does not fit the category of constitutional delay is considered to have idiopathic short stature. The use of growth hormone therapy in otherwise healthy children with short stature has been very controversial. In 2003, the Food and Drug Administration (FDA) approved the use of GH for this indication in children who are more than 2.25 SDs below the mean height for age and have predicted heights below 63 inches for boys and 59 inches for girls. In children enrolled in randomized, controlled studies and treated for an average duration of 6 years, final height exceeded that of the control groups by an average of 1.5 to 3 inches. However, 20% of patients studied failed to improve on their predicted height, indicating that care must be taken not to foster unrealistic expectations.

Boys with constitutional delay clearly may benefit from treatment with androgens during their teenage years. Low-dose testosterone given by monthly injection for 4 to 6 months can gently accelerate growth, bone age, and spontaneous puberty. Anabolic steroids may be helpful for younger children with constitutional delay, although these steroids are not used routinely.

Children with familial short stature grow at normal velocities and do not need any treatment to help them achieve a ge-netically appropriate height. Often, parents exert tremendous pressure to intervene in some way and put the child on GH treatment. In some families, the focus on being taller as a cure for all ills suggests the need for psychiatric intervention.

The use of GH treatment in children with constitutional delay has been studied by several investigators. In some published studies, as many as 50% of treated children had significant increases in their growth rates. After GH treatment is stopped, the growth rate in many patients decelerates, sometimes to or below the pretreatment growth rate. The data are conflicting on whether GH treatment can increase the adult height of children with constitutional delay, and this issue remains controversial.

The side effects of biosynthetic GH treatment include development of various degrees of insulin resistance (although hyperglycemia is rare), mild sodium and water retention that is not clinically significant, development of anti-GH antibodies that is not clinically significant, and transient lowering of thyroxine levels. Occasionally, slipped capital femoral epiphyses, worsening of scoliosis, pseudotumor cerebri, and gynecomastia have been reported. Deaths in patients with PWS are discussed previously.

The issue of most concern regarding GH therapy is the possibility that it could increase the development of malignancies, especially leukemia. Studies in GH recipients do not show an increase in leukemia in those without risk factors (i.e., prior tumors). GH therapy does not increase the risk of recurrence of CNS tumors. One study showed an increase in colon cancer in adults who had been treated with cadaver GH before 1985. The authors of this study state that no evidence is available as to whether growth hormone in modern dosage regimens is associated with an increased risk of developing colon cancer.

DISORDERS OF ANTIDIURETIC HORMONE

Antidiuretic hormone (ADH) (vasopressin) is released from the posterior pituitary by neurons originating in the hypothalamic supraoptic and periventricular nuclei. Release of ADH is mediated through osmoreceptors and baroreceptors, and secretion increases in response to hypovolemia and hyperosmolality. ADH acts by means of the kidney to reabsorb water, which decreases urine volume and increases urine osmolality.

Diabetes Insipidus

Diabetes insipidus is a disorder of subnormal secretion of ADH or reduced kidney responsiveness to ADH. Renal responsiveness can be established by monitoring the response to exogenous vasopressin. ADH deficiency may be genetic, but more often it is caused by lesions in the hypothalamic area, commonly tumors and infiltrative disorders such as histiocytosis. Trauma, inflammatory processes, and vascular abnormalities also are causes of ADH deficiency.

ADH deficiency manifests with symptoms of polyuria and polydipsia with large volumes of dilute urine. Symptoms often are dramatic and may be abrupt in onset. The search for an organic cause requires brain magnetic resonance imaging, a search for histiocytosis, and an evaluation for dysfunction of other hormones of the hypothalamic-pituitary axis.

The best diagnostic test is water deprivation. This test should be performed under careful observation in a well-hydrated child. Body weight, urine volumes and osmolality, and serum sodium and osmolality should be measured at baseline, frequently during the test, and at the end of the test. Levels of ADH can be measured at the onset and conclusion of the test, but the ADH level is not essential for the diagnosis. If serum osmolality and serum sodium values increase above normal in the context of poor urine concentration, the diagnosis of diabetes insipidus is made. A weight loss of a maximum of 5% is allowed. At the end of the water deprivation test, exogenous ADH (injection of aqueous vasopressin or deamino-8-D-arginine vasopressin [DDAVP] or intranasal DDAVP) is given to assess renal responsiveness.

Children with psychogenic or neurogenic polydipsia as the primary problem must be differentiated from those with diabetes insipidus. These children usually have low serum sodium and osmolality.

Diabetes insipidus caused by ADH deficiency is treated with exogenous ADH. The best mode of treatment is with intranasal or oral DDAVP, a long-acting analogue of arginine vasopressin. To eliminate nighttime awakening to urinate and drink, treatment begins with low doses that are increased gradually. DDAVP also can be given parenterally. In many patients, DDAVP can be given every 12 hours.

Because infants' diets have a low solute load, their urine should remain dilute, and long-acting ADH preparations may more readily produce hyponatremia. Low-dose vasopressin injections have been successful in managing diabetes insipidus in infants without producing significant hyponatremia.

An intact thirst mechanism allows patients on ADH preparations to regulate their fluid balance easily on their own as long as they have free access to water. In the unusual patient with abnormal thirst, regulation becomes difficult, and strict prescriptions of fluid intake may be required.

Syndrome of Inappropriate Antidiuretic Hormone Secretion

Excess endogenous or exogenous ADH without fluid restriction leads to water intoxication: water retention and weight gain, hyponatremia, and production of small amounts of concentrated urine. The typical symptoms are lethargy, weakness, nausea, vomiting, headaches, and seizures.

In children, the most likely causes of the syndrome of inappropriate antidiuretic hormone secretion are intracranial disease (e.g., meningitis), neurosurgery, head trauma, and pulmonary disease. Malignancies producing excess ADH are uncommon occurrences in children.

The treatment is fluid restriction. In severe cases, use of hypertonic saline with diuretic therapy (e.g., furosemide) may be indicated. Slow and steady correction is required.

PROLACTIN

Prolactin is the one pituitary hormone for which the major physiologic control is an inhibiting factor, dopamine. Pathologic processes occur when prolactin is secreted in excess amounts because of a prolactin-secreting pituitary adenoma or when loss of hypothalamic dopamine inhibition occurs because of interruption of normal pathways, especially by trauma, tumors, or infiltrative processes in the hypothalamus. Certain drugs (e.g., phenothiazines, cimetidine, opiates) can cause

hyperprolactinemia. Excess prolactin suppresses pituitary secretion of LH and follicle-stimulating hormone (FSH) and is associated with galactorrhea. The decrease in LH and FSH leads to impotence, oligomenorrhea, amenorrhea, infertility, and delayed puberty.

The diagnosis of excess secretion of prolactin is made by finding an elevated prolactin level in a euthyroid, nonpregnant patient. CNS imaging with magnetic resonance imaging and a workup for evidence of dysfunction of other hypothalamic–pituitary hormones is necessary. Very high prolactin levels usually are associated with large tumors.

Treatment options include careful observation, medical therapy with dopamine agonists, and surgery. Dopamine agonists (bromocriptine or cabergoline) are the major therapeutic options, and the response to treatment is rapid. In some cases, bromocriptine therapy has been associated with regression in tumor size. Surgery may be useful in addition to medical therapy. For patients who do not respond well to medical therapy or surgery, radiation therapy may be indicated.

Suggested Readings

Allen DB, Fost N, Blizzard RM, eds. Access to treatment with human growth hormone: medical, ethical and social issues. *Growth Genet Horm* 1992;8:1.

Blethen SL. Safety of recombinant deoxyribonucleic acid-derived growth hormone: The National Cooperative Growth Study experience. *J Clin Endocrinol Metab* 1996;81:1704.

Cuttler L, Silver JB, Singh J, et al. Short stature and growth hormone therapy. A national study of physician recommendation patterns. *JAMA* 1996;276:531.

Haqq AM, Stadler DD, Jackson RH, et al. Effects of growth hormone on pulmonary function, sleep quality, behavior, cognition, growth velocity, body composition, and resting energy expenditure in Prader-Willi syndrome. *J Clin Endocrinol Metab* 2003;88:2206.

Hintz RL, Attie KM, Baptista J, Roche A. Effect of growth hormone treatment on adult height of children with idiopathic short stature. *N Engl J Med* 1999; 340:502.

Root AW, Bercu BB, Diamond FB. Growth hormone secretagogues: physiology and function. *Growth Genet Horm* 1997;13:33.

Rosenbloom AL, Rosenfeld RG, Guevara-Aguirre J. Growth hormone insensitivity. *Pediatr Clin North Am* 1997;44:423.

Rosenfeld RG. Consultation with the specialist: growth hormone. *Pediatr Rev* 1996;17:143.

Rosenfeld RG. Is growth hormone just a tall story? *J Pediatr* 1997;130:172.

Rosenfeld RG, Albertsson-Wikland K, Cassorla F, et al. Diagnostic controversy: the diagnosis of childhood growth hormone deficiency revisited. *J Clin Endocrinol Metab* 1995;80:1532.

Rosenfeld R, Allen DB, MacGillivray MH, et al. Growth hormone use in pediatric growth hormone deficiency and other pediatric growth disorders. *Am J Manag Care* 2000;6:S805.

Rosenfeld RG, Frane J, Attie KM, et al. Six-year results of a randomized, prospective trial of human growth hormone and oxandrolone in Turner syndrome. *J Pediatr* 1992;121:49.

Saenger P. The case in support of GH therapy. *J Pediatr* 2000;136:103.

Swerdlow AJ, Higgins CD, Adlard P, Preece MA. Risk of cancer in patients treated with human pituitary growth hormone in the UK, 1959–1985: a cohort study. *Lancet* 2002;360:273.

Vimalachandra D, Craig JC, Cowell CT, Knight JF. Growth hormone treatment in children with chronic renal failure: a meta-analysis of randomized controlled trials. *J Pediatr* 2001;139:560.

Van Pareren Y, Mulder P, Houdijk M, et al. Adult height after long-term, continuous growth hormone treatment in short children born small for gestational age: results of a randomized, double-blind, dose-response GH trial. *J Clin Endocrinol Metab* 2003;88:3584.

Wilson DM, Rosenfeld RG. Treatment of short stature and delayed adolescence. *Pediatr Clin North Am* 1987;34:865.

Zitelli B. Sneetches and growth hormone. *J Pediatr* 2002;140:493.

CHAPTER 376 ■ CHILDHOOD OBESITY

WILLIAM H. DIETZ

Childhood obesity has now become the most prevalent nutritional disease of children and adolescents in the United States. Estimates from the 1999–2000 National Health and Nutrition Examination Survey (NHANES) indicate that approximately 15% of children in the United States are overweight. Furthermore, comparison of the prevalence of overweight in NHANES 1999–2000 with data from NHANES II completed in 1980 indicates that the prevalence of overweight doubled in 6- to 11-year old children and tripled in 12- to 17-year old adolescents. The prevalence of overweight, and its association with a variety of morbidities in childhood and adolescence, indicates that the prevention of overweight and the treatment of overweight among children and adolescents must become a high priority for pediatricians.

IDENTIFICATION

Childhood and adolescent overweight should be identified through the use of the body mass index (BMI) (weight in kg/height in m^2). The BMI appears to be a reasonable index of adiposity, because it correlates reasonably well with the percentage of body weight attributable to fat among those with a BMI greater than or equal to the ninety-fifth percentile, it does not covary with height like the weight for height index, and an increased BMI predicts persistence and cardiovascular disease risk factors. The appropriate cutoff points for the identification of those at risk of being overweight and those who are overweight are the eighty-fifth and ninety-fifth percentiles, respectively, using the Centers for Disease Control and Prevention growth charts (www.cdc.gov/growthcharts and Chapter 5). The ninety-fifth percentile is the percentile identified by a BMI of greater than or equal to 30 in young adults, which corresponds to class I obesity in adults. Therefore, this approach makes the identification of childhood and adolescent obesity congruent with the criteria used to identify adult obesity.

Because of the concern about spuriously labeling a child as overweight who may have an increased BMI because of an increase in muscle or bone mass, the approach indicated in Figure 376.1 should be followed in the assessment of a child with an increased BMI. One approach to distinguish children with an increased BMI attributable to fat from those whose BMI reflects an increase in fat-free mass or bone is the measurement of the triceps skinfold thickness (TSF). The TSF provides a relative but direct measure of body fat. If a child has an increased BMI, but normal TSF, the child is likely overweight, but not overfat. Both the child and the family should be reassured that the child's increased BMI represents a growth variant, but that continued monitoring will be essential. If the child has an increased TSF, the additional screening tests noted in Figure 376.1 should be performed to assess whether an associated morbidity exists. Children whose BMI is at the eighty-fifth percentile or children who have had rapid weight gain of more than two BMI units annually should be considered at risk and followed carefully.

PERIODS OF RISK

Identification of the periods of risk for the development of childhood and adolescent obesity will help identify the times and populations that represent reasonable targets for counseling efforts. Young children at greatest risk for the development of adult obesity are children of two obese parents, regardless of the weight status of the child. Therefore, counseling with respect to diet and activity for children of two obese parents should begin early.

The first important period of risk for persistent obesity independent of the risk of parental obesity is the prenatal period. Children with birth weights greater than or equal to 4 kg have an increased risk of subsequent overweight. Maternal weight

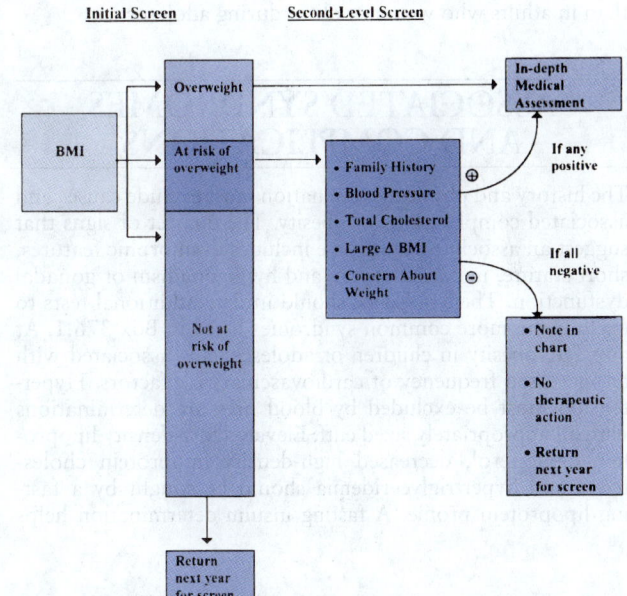

FIGURE 376.1. Algorithm for the assessment of children with an increased body mass index (BMI). Children with a BMI greater than the 95th percentile should receive in-depth assessment including measurement of the triceps skinfold thickness (TSF) to confirm that the increase in BMI is attributable to an increase in fat. If both the BMI and TSF are increased, a complete history and physical are required to exclude the syndromes and complications associated with obesity. Children whose BMI is between the 85th and 95th percentiles require a more detailed history, and a close follow-up to ensure that their weight does not progress. Children with a BMI between the 85th and 95th percentile who have a family history of obesity, have elevated blood pressure or cholesterol, have a large change in BMI, or are concerned about their weight should have an in-depth assessment like that for children or adolescents whose weight exceeds the 95th percentile. (Reproduced with permission form Himes JH, Dietz WH. Guidelines for overweight in adolescent preventive services: recommendations from an expert committee. *Am J Clin Nutr* 1994;59:307.)

gain during pregnancy is an important determinant of birth weight. The mechanisms that account for the effect of birth weight on subsequent growth include increases in cell number or alterations in brain growth or satiety centers.

A second potential period is the period of BMI rebound. After an initial increase in the BMI in the first year of life, the BMI begins to decline and reaches a nadir at 6 to 8 years of age. Thereafter, the BMI begins to increase again. Although it has been suggested that children in whom BMI rebound begins early are at increased risk for persistently increased BMI, this effect may be mediated by the BMI in early childhood rather than the time of BMI rebound. Inspection of the BMI growth charts indicates that children in the upper BMI percentiles have an earlier BMI rebound than do children in lower percentiles. The factors that affect fatness during this period remain uncertain. Factors in early childhood that affect food preference or alter regulation of food intake, or exposure of the child to environments that affect food or activity outside the home may alter energy balance to promote gains in body fat.

The third period of risk for the development of obesity or its complications is adolescence. Body fat increases in girls during adolescence, whereas body fat decreases in boys. In girls, however, body fat is deposited gluteally, whereas body fat in boys is deposited centrally. Visceral fat deposition increases the risk of a variety of cardiovascular morbidities such as hyperlipidemia, glucose intolerance, and hypertension. The risk of persistent obesity in adolescent girls is therefore greater than in boys, but the risk of subsequent mortality associated with obesity is greater in boys than in girls. Morbidity in adulthood associated with adolescent obesity is greater in both genders than in adults who were not obese during adolescence.

ASSOCIATED SYNDROMES AND COMPLICATIONS

The history and physical examination must exclude causes and associated complications of obesity. The quartet of signs that suggest an associated syndrome includes dysmorphic features, short stature, impaired vision, and hypogonadism or gonadal dysfunction. Their presence should initiate additional tests to exclude the more common syndromes listed in Box 376.1. At any age, obesity in children or adolescents is associated with an increased frequency of cardiovascular risk factors. Hypertension must be excluded by blood pressure determinations with an appropriately sized cuff. Elevated low-density lipoprotein cholesterol, decreased high-density lipoprotein cholesterol, and hypertriglyceridemia should be sought by a fasting lipoprotein profile. A fasting insulin determination helps

exclude glucose intolerance. Although children or adolescents with acanthosis nigricans have been thought to be at particular risk for glucose intolerance, glucose intolerance and acanthosis nigricans appear more strongly related to the severity of obesity.

The most urgent complications of obesity include sleep apnea, pseudotumor cerebri, Blount disease, and imminent slipped capital femoral epiphysis. Sleep apnea is characteristically associated with snoring and daytime somnolence. Tonsillar enlargement may contribute to sleep apnea, and a tonsillectomy may be curative. However, obese children should receive careful postoperative monitoring after a tonsillectomy, because postoperative peripharyngeal edema may cause a fatal respiratory obstruction. Headaches and papilledema require a careful workup to confirm pseudotumor and exclude malignancies. Blount disease or bowing of the lower extremities associated with overgrowth of the medial aspect of the proximal metaphysis requires weight reduction to halt the progression of the disease or to prevent recurrence after surgical correction. Slipped capital femoral epiphysis usually presents with hip pain and a limp. The morbidities associated with these complications merit aggressive weight reduction.

A final concern is the impact of childhood or adolescent overweight on the severity or complications of obesity in adulthood. Overweight that begins before 8 years of age is associated with a mean BMI of over 40 (approximately 100 lb overweight) in adulthood. In addition, overweight present in adolescence is associated with an increased mortality in males and an increased risk of comorbidities, such as diabetes and cardiovascular disease, in adulthood. These sequelae appear independent of the effect of adolescent weight on weight at age 55 years.

ETIOLOGY

Obesity can only result from an energy intake in excess of energy expenditure. However, whether energy intake is a more important factor than energy expenditure remains unclear. Limitations in the measurement of energy intake and energy expenditure, and the lack of longitudinal measures of each, contribute to our lack of knowledge about these critical features of obesity. Therefore, although the discussion in Box 376.2 considers logical causal factors, only a limited number of studies link these behaviors to the onset or persistence of obesity.

PREVENTION

The natural history of overweight suggests that several periods in childhood and adolescence should be targeted for prevention. In infancy and early childhood, as indicated previously, the highest risk of obesity occurs in the child whose parents are both overweight, regardless of the weight status of the child. Therefore, families with two obese parents should be targeted for preventive efforts. Although the focus of prevention has not been clearly determined, several logical targets exist. Infants who are breast-fed appear to have a lower prevalence of subsequent overweight, even after control for socioeconomic class. Breast-fed infants also accept the introduction of new foods more readily than infants who are fed formula. Although not carefully studied, acceptance of a variety of foods by infants may enhance the likelihood that when they are older, children will accept foods such as fruits and vegetables that are likely to reduce the caloric density of the diet. In addition, mothers who are restrained eaters or who try to control the quantity of food that their child consumes have children who

---

BOX 376.1   **Syndromes Associated with Childhood Obesity**

Alstrom-Hallgren syndrome
Carpenter syndrome
Cohen syndrome
Laurence Moon Biedl syndrome
Polycystic ovary disease
Prader-Labhart-Willi syndrome
Pseudohypoparathyroidism
Turner syndrome

BOX 376.2   Energy Relationships in Obesity

Studies of dietary intake have focused on the role of dietary fat in the genesis of obesity. Dietary fat is calorically more dense than carbohydrate, and, in contrast to carbohydrate, increased fat intake is not associated with increased fat oxidation. Therefore, excessive fat intake may predispose to fat deposition. However, recent increases in the prevalence of obesity in the U.S. population have occurred despite a reduction in the proportion of dietary energy derived from fat. Furthermore, restriction of dietary fat alone in children whose caloric intake was not limited produced no differences in the change in BMI over a 1-year period. Nonetheless, the conclusion that fat plays no role in the genesis or persistence of obesity must be tempered by several limitations of the dietary methodologies.

Patterns of food intake may offer a more targeted approach to weight control. Almost half of an average family's income spent on food is spent on food consumed outside the home. Furthermore, almost 70% of children consume lunch away from home, and almost 20% of children consume breakfast or dinner outside the home. The foods consumed on these occasions, especially if they constitute fast food or take-out foods, tend to be higher in fat and calories, and are often consumed in larger portions than comparable foods that are prepared and consumed at home. Soft drink consumption, which includes both soda and 10% juice, now accounts for over 10% of an average adolescent's daily caloric intake. Although children who consume a greater quantity of fruits and vegetables should be less likely to become overweight, no data yet link increased fruit and vegetable intake to a reduced risk for the development of overweight. Likewise, no data yet link snack frequency or snack choice to the development of obesity. Family interactions around food constitute a final area of interest and concern. Parental control of the quantity of food intake may impair the ability of the child to regulate energy balance. No population-based studies have examined this variable to determine whether the prevalence of obesity is increased in families in which parents attempt to regulate food intake.

Few definitive studies have examined the link between either resting metabolic rate, the energy spent on activity, or total daily energy expenditure and the development of overweight. The few short-term studies that have examined this problem have failed to demonstrate that reductions in any one of these components of energy expenditure place children or adolescents at increased risk for the development of increased adiposity. Activity constitutes the second variable in the energy balance equation. At the outset of high school, 50% of boys but less than 30% of girls participate in regular vigorous activity. By the end of high school, participation among boys declines slightly, whereas among girls the rates decline to approximately 15%. Although no data yet link the decline in vigorous activity in girls to the development of overweight during adolescence, the coincidence of the decline in vigorous activity with the period at which the prevalence of obesity increases in girls should not be dismissed.

Inactivity or sedentary behavior appears to represent a domain independent of activity. Television viewing represents the most important form of inactivity for children and adolescents in the United States. The average child spends over 4 hours per day watching television. Furthermore, cross-sectional and prospective population studies in children and adults have linked the amount of time spent viewing television with the development of obesity in children and adolescents. Although children who are watching television are sedentary, television viewing also affects food consumption. Advertisements for food constitute the most frequent commercials on children's television programs. Consumption of the foods advertised on television and food consumption while watching television are directly related to the prevalence of obesity. Therefore, the effects of television viewing on the prevalence of obesity may reflect both inactivity and increased food consumption.

---

are less capable of controlling their own caloric intake. This observation suggests that parents should be in charge of what their children are offered and when, and children can decide whether to eat what is offered or not. Implicit in this division of responsibility is that if children do not decide to eat what is offered, parents are not obligated to offer alternative choices. After children learn that they will be hungry if they do not eat what is offered, it is much more likely that they will consume that food when it is next offered. However, negotiations about food must be conducted in a neutral manner. Failure to accept what is offered should not be met with a punitive response. Otherwise, attitudes about food will likely develop an emotional overlay. Finally, children should not be encouraged to eat, because encouragement may make it less likely that the child will consume the food he or she is encouraged to eat. In each of these areas, parents may need assistance in building the skills necessary to negotiate these developmental steps successfully.

After early childhood, the overweight status of the child or adolescent has a greater effect than does parental obesity status on the risk of persistence. The two groups at greatest risk for persistent obesity are children with early onset of overweight and girls during adolescence. At any age, the more severely overweight have an increased risk of persistent obesity.

TREATMENT

The first goal of therapy should be weight maintenance. In children with a BMI between the eighty-fifth and ninety-fifth percentiles, weight maintenance may be the only therapy required for the child to return to the normal BMI range. The goal of weight maintenance may be easiest for the male preadolescent, in whom adolescence is accompanied by a loss of fat and an increase in fat-free mass.

Because the child's dietary choices and exercise patterns occur in a family context, the family must be included in decisions about what modifications are necessary and how they should be implemented. How primary care providers approach families of overweight children is critical. Questions to the family such as "How concerned are you about your child's weight?" will help establish whether the family views the child's weight as a serious problem and may help establish their readiness for change. A family that does not view their child's weight as a serious problem should be counseled regarding the potential adverse physical and psychosocial effects of obesity and told that the primary care provider will be happy to help them if they become more concerned. A question such as "What do you think has made your child overweight" addresses what the family views as the cause of their child's obesity and moves the discussion toward therapy. A question such as "What changes do you have to make in order to control your child's weight?" allows the family to begin to define the changes necessary to achieve weight maintenance and, subsequently, weight loss. In families where adolescents are in conflict with their parents about what and when they should eat, the neutrality of the primary care provider often provides the successful arbitration that allows the provider to build an alliance with the adolescent and support the adolescent's role in self-care.

The same rules that govern the division of responsibility outlined above apply to the overweight child and adolescent. Careful dietary histories to establish caloric intake are not helpful, because they underestimate food intake. However, dietary histories that focus on the pattern of food intake or the consumption of high caloric density snacks may offer more specific targets for reduction or elimination. Consumption of foods outside the home at day-care, school, or after-school programs may represent an important source of excess calories in families that carefully control the foods offered at home.

Activity also plays a crucial role in weight maintenance and reduction. Increased activity increases energy expenditure. Although several studies suggest that increases in activity play a modest role in weight reduction, at least one study of adults demonstrated a significant effect of increased activity on weight maintenance.

Several clinical and school-based studies have indicated that reductions in inactivity may be a more effective approach to weight loss in children than efforts to increase activity. For more details about this approach, see Box 376.3.

How to achieve increases in activity in primary care settings has not been carefully investigated. Parents should be encouraged to limit television time, not only because of the positive effect such limitations have on obesity, but also because of the effect it has on a wide variety of other behaviors. Furthermore, children must be given opportunities to play. Time with parents walking or playing outdoors represent times valued by both participants. One important hazard is the guilt that working parents feel when their schedules offer few opportunities for their children to play. In many neighborhoods, safe environments for children do not exist. In these cases, alliances with other groups committed to neighborhood safety and community improvement may help to make schools or other facilities available for children to play after school or on weekends.

Children or adolescents with morbid complications of their obesity, such as sleep apnea, Blount disease, slipped femoral capital epiphysis, or pseudotumor cerebri are candidates for rapid weight loss. A consensus on the treatment of the morbidly obese child or adolescent, defined as a body weight 200% of ideal, does not yet exist. In cases where either a morbid complication of obesity or morbid obesity exists, referral to a specialist in the treatment of obese children and adolescents is warranted. In such cases, aggressive family therapy used in conjunction with a low-calorie diet such as the protein-modified fast may be helpful.

At present, drug therapy must be reserved for those adolescents with a morbid complication of obesity who have failed more conservative approaches to weight reduction. Trials of sibutramine and orlistat in adolescents have indicated more weight loss than can be achieved with a placebo, but the results are still quite modest. Furthermore, these drugs cost approximately $1,100 per year, few insurance companies pay for their use, and weight gain will likely recur when drug therapy is discontinued. Finally, neither has yet been approved for use in the pediatric age group. Therefore, if pharmacotherapy is used to treat obesity, a study protocol and informed consent should be required. As with more restrictive dietary therapy, the use of medications to treat obesity should be referred to an obesity treatment specialist.

The frequency of bariatric surgery for adult obesity has gained increasing acceptance in the management of severe obesity in adults, and may also be considered under selected conditions for adolescents with severe obesity. An expert committee has recently recommended that bariatric surgery only be considered when more conservative therapy by comprehensive pediatric obesity programs have failed, and then only for adolescents whose growth has been completed. Surgery should be reserved for adolescents with a BMI of greater than or equal to 40 with a comorbid condition. Surgical approaches also should be considered an unproven approach for which informed consent is warranted. Because only limited experience exists, such patients should agree to lifelong follow-up after surgery.

| BOX 376.3 | Decreased Inactivity as an Approach of Weight Loss in Children |

In a study including parents and children and comparable control of caloric intake by the elimination or reduction of specific high caloric density foods, a program with decreased inactivity in the form of less television time produced greater short-term and 1-year weight losses than did a program with increased activity. In most cases, the reduction in inactivity was achieved by a reduction in television viewing. Furthermore, the attitudes of children toward vigorous activity were more positive among children reinforced for reductions in inactivity than among children reinforced for increased activity. The lack of improvement in attitudes among children reinforced for increased activity may reflect a forced choice. Children who were reinforced for increased activity may have felt pressured to increase their activity and were therefore less positive about their choices than were children who were reinforced to decrease their inactivity and who chose freely what to do in place of inactivity.

Suggested Readings

Barlow SE, Dietz WH. Obesity evaluation and treatment: Expert committee recommendations. *Pediatrics*. Available at: www.pediatrics.org/cgi/content/full/102/3/e29. Accessed December 20, 2005.

Dier WH, Robinson TN. Overweight children and adolescents. *New Engl J Med* 2005;352:2100.

Dietz WH. Critical periods in childhood for the development of obesity. *Am J Clin Nutr* 1994;59:955.

Epstein LH, Valoski AM, Vara LS, et al. Effects of decreasing sedentary behavior and increasing activity on weight change in obese children. *Health Psychol* 1995;14:109.

Freedman DS, Dietz WH, Srinivasan SR, Berenson GS. The relation of overweight to cardiovascular risk factors among children and adolescents: the Bogalusa Heart Study. *Pediatrics* 1999;103:1175.

Himes JH, Dietz WH. Guidelines for overweight in adolescent preventive services: recommendations from an expert committee. *Am J Clin Nutr* 1994;59:307.

Inge T, Krebs N, Garcia V, et al. Bariatric surgery for severely overweight adolescents: concerns and recommendations. *Pediatrics* 2004;114:217–223.

Whitaker RC, Wright JA, Pepe MS, et al. Predicting obesity in young adulthood from childhood and parental obesity. *New Engl J Med* 1997;337:869.

CHAPTER 377 ■ NEUROENDOCRINE DISORDERS

THOMAS MOSHANG JR. AND ADDA GRIMBERG

Neuroendocrinology, the study of the body's homeostatic control mechanisms, examines the interactions between the nervous and endocrine systems. Both neurons and endocrine cells exert their actions through release of chemical messengers that bind to specific cell receptors, although the former classically release messengers across synapses and the latter into the circulation. Both systems seem to converge in the hypothalamic–pituitary unit, sometimes referred to as the body's *master gland*. Neuroendocrine disorders in children disturb growth, sexual maturation and function, water balance, and adrenal and thyroid functions. The rising number of childhood cancer survivors constitutes an increasingly important subgroup of children with neuroendocrine disorders due to the sequelae of radiotherapy and chemotherapy.

NORMAL CONTROL MECHANISMS: ANATOMY AND PHYSIOLOGY

The hypothalamic–pituitary unit is located at the base of the third ventricle where the hypothalamus receives multiple afferent neural connections from higher brain centers. Also, chemical agents from the cerebrospinal fluid are transmitted from the third ventricle to hypothalamic axon terminals and capillaries via tanycytes, bipolar ependymal cells. The hypothalamus communicates with the anterior pituitary gland through a special portal circulation that not only is fenestrated (the exception to the blood–brain barrier) but that also transmits information bidirectionally. The link to the posterior pituitary is a direct physical connection; the axons of the posterior pituitary actually have their cell bodies in the hypothalamic nuclei (Fig. 377.1).

Afferent signals from the brain and hypothalamus stimulate pituitary hormone secretion, which in turn activates hormone synthesis and release by other endocrine glands in the body. These hormones provide quantitative data to the hypothalamic–pituitary unit to determine the need for ongoing activity (positive feedback) or termination of signal (negative feedback). An extra step of modulation occurs in the anterior pituitary, as the hypothalamus secretes releasing and inhibitory factors (e.g., growth hormone–releasing hormone [GHRH] and somatostatin) into the portal network to control activity of the anterior pituitary hormones: growth hormone (GH), thyroid-stimulating hormone (TSH), the gonadotropins (luteinizing hormone [LH] and follicle-stimulating hormone [FSH]), adrenocorticotropin hormone (ACTH), and prolactin. Vasopressin (antidiuretic hormone [ADH]) and oxytocin, the two hormones secreted by the posterior pituitary, are synthesized by cell bodies within the hypothalamic nuclei and transferred in secretory granules via axonal transport down the pituitary stalk (Table 377.1; see Fig. 377.1).

NEUROENDOCRINE DISORDERS

Neuroendocrine disorders may present at any age with variable clinical manifestations dependent on the cause and the hormones that are produced or deficient (Table 377.2). Growth failure is the most common presentation of neuroendocrine disturbances in children. It may arise from deficiencies of several pituitary hormones, either in combination or singly, or from loss of growth signals from the hypothalamus and higher brain centers. Thus, accurate and consistent plotting of a child's growth curve is often the pediatrician's first clue to an underlying neuroendocrine problem.

Congenital or Genetic Forms of Neuroendocrine Disease

Congenital or genetic forms of neuroendocrine disorders may present in the newborn period or later in life. The genetic causes

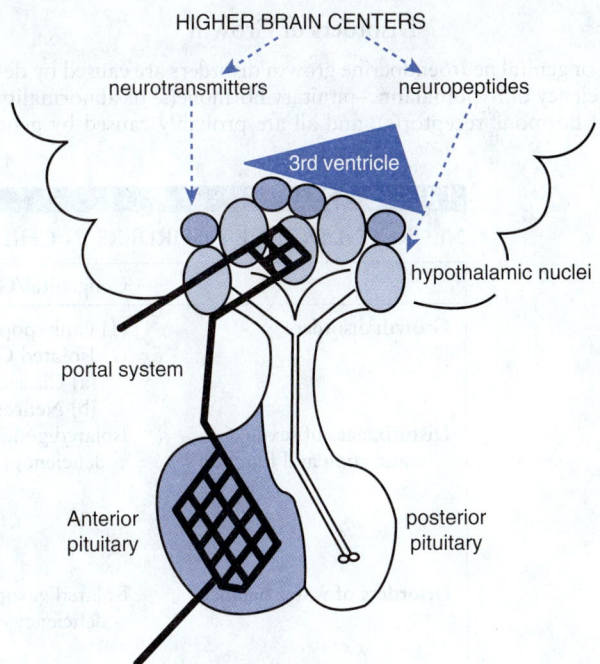

FIGURE 377.1. Anatomy of communication within the hypothalamic–pituitary unit. Input to the hypothalamic nuclei originates from higher brain centers, the cerebrospinal fluid in the third ventricle, and the anterior pituitary through a special bidirectional fenestrated portal circulatory network. The hypothalamic nuclei affect anterior pituitary functioning through releasing and inhibitory factors transmitted by the portal capillaries and posterior pituitary functioning by axonal transport.

TABLE 377.1

OVERVIEW OF THE NEUROENDOCRINE AXES AND THEIR FEEDBACK LOOPS*

	Pituitary Hormone	Target Organ	Feedback
Anterior pituitary			
Hypothalamic-Releasing Factor			
GHRH (stim); somatostatin (inhib)	GH	Liver; skeleton, cartilage, muscle	Insulinlike growth factor-1 (IGF-1)
TRH	TSH	Thyroid	Thyroxine (T_4), triiodothyronine (T_3)
GnRH	LH, FSH	Ovaries, testes	Estrogen, testosterone
CRH	ACTH	Adrenals	Cortisol
Dopamine (inhib)	PRL	Mammary gland	Auto feedback
Posterior pituitary			
Hormone: Made in Hypothalamic Nuclei, Secreted by Posterior Pituitary			
Vasopressin (ADH)		Renal collecting ducts; vascular smooth muscle	Plasma osmolality; blood pressure and volume
Oxytocin		Myoepithelial cells surrounding the mammary acini	Relaxin (inhib); mammary suckling and vaginal distension (stim)

*The hypothalamic modulators of anterior pituitary function are growth hormone–releasing hormone (GHRH), thyrotropin-releasing hormone (TRH), gonadotropin-releasing hormone (GnRH), and corticotropin-releasing hormone (CRH). GH, growth hormone; LH, luteinizing hormone; PRL, prolactin; TSH, thyroid-stimulating hormone.

of a number of these disorders are known, including mutations in the GHRH receptor, GH gene, *Pit1* gene, *Prop1* gene, Kallmann syndrome (hypogonadotropism with anosmia), and others. It is beyond the scope of this section to discuss the details of these gene mutations, but the clinical aspects are presented here. Parks et al. recently reviewed the heritable disorders of pituitary development.

Disorders of Growth

Congenital neuroendocrine growth disorders are caused by deficiency of hypothalamic–pituitary hormone(s) or abnormality of hormone receptor(s), and all are probably caused by gene mutations, although some of the genetic defects have not yet been elucidated.

Panhypopituitarism. Congenital panhypopituitarism, or the deficiency of more than one pituitary hormone, is caused by gross malformation and histologic or molecular abnormalities of the hypothalamic–pituitary unit. Gross hypothalamic–pituitary malformation may be associated with other midline brain malformations, including holoprosencephaly and anencephaly. Holoprosencephaly, characterized by ventral midline fusion of forebrain structures, is the most frequent brain malformation in humans. Because induction of hypothalamic development is intimately involved in forebrain midline signaling

TABLE 377.2

NEUROENDOCRINE DISORDERS IN CHILDREN*

	Congenital/Genetic	Acquired
Growth disorders	(1) Panhypopituitarism (2) Isolated GH deficiency 　(a) Classical 　(b) Neurosecretory	(1) Panhypopituitarism (2) Isolated GH deficiency (3) Psychosocial dwarfing (4) Accelerated growth
Disturbances of sexual maturation and function	Isolated gonadotropin deficiency	(1) Sexual precocity 　(a) Central 　(b) Primary hypothyroidism 　(c) Radiation-induced (2) Sexual infantilism (3) Amenorrhea
Disorders of water balance	Isolated vasopressin (ADH) deficiency	(1) Diabetes insipidus (2) Syndrome of inappropriate ADH (3) Cerebral salt wasting
Disturbances of the ACTH-adrenal axis	Isolated ACTH deficiency	(1) Cushing disease (2) ACTH deficiency
Disorders of thyroid function	(1) Isolated TRH deficiency (2) Familial thyroid resistance	TRH or TSH deficiency

*Pediatric neuroendocrine disorders are most readily classified as congenital/genetic or acquired, and by the specific hormonal axis affected. This listing, though not exhaustive, summarizes the disorders discussed in this chapter. ACTH, adrenocorticotropin hormone; GH, growth hormone; TRH, thyrotropin-releasing hormone; TSH, thyroid-stimulating factor.

during embryogenesis, mild cases of holoprosencephaly may present clinically with only hypothalamic/pituitary dysfunction. Four genes have been shown to cause holoprosencephaly in humans when mutated, including sonic hedgehog (*SHH*). Septooptic dysplasia, or de Morsier syndrome, describes the association of optic nerve hypoplasia with septum pellucidum agenesis; additional associations may be schizencephaly or callosal absence, and a case of septooptic dysplasia with cerebrocortical dysplasia has been reported. Septooptic dysplasia occurs with variable degrees of neuroendocrine dysfunction, primarily hypothalamic involvement and GH deficiency. Septooptic dysplasia has been associated with mutations of the *HESX1* homeobox gene. Thus, mutations in transcription factors active during early hypothalamic–pituitary development frequently result in gross abnormalities that may be visualized with brain imaging. Mutations in factors active later during cellular differentiation and function (such as *Pit1* or *PROP1*) may result in histologic and functional changes, but not radiologically apparent abnormalities. Nonetheless, the clinical characteristics are similar.

Common clinical findings in the newborn with panhypopituitarism include hypoglycemia and jaundice and, in boys, micropenis. Newborn screening for hypothyroidism may detect a low thyroxine level (T_4) with a normal TSH level. In infants with gross malformations, there may be midline defects (such as cleft palate), neurologic signs, and visual defects (especially nystagmus). In the older child, there may be a single central incisor or, most commonly, growth failure. Treatment consists of replacing the identified deficient hormones and addressing the underlying cause.

Isolated Growth Hormone Deficiency. Isolated GH deficiency (GHD) occurs as a spectrum of clinical diseases, all sharing growth failure as the main phenotypic trait. The familial forms

include autosomal recessive and autosomal dominant patterns of inheritance. Complete or classic GHD is not difficult to diagnose. However, partial GHD or insufficiency is often more difficult to confirm biochemically because of the hormone's circadian rhythm. Indirect means of measuring GH function have therefore been devised, including random growth factor (insulinlike growth factor-1 [IGF-1] and IGF-binding protein [IGFBP]-3) levels, provocative GH testing, and overnight serum GH sampling. Because all of these tests have questionable specificity, interassay differences, or, in the case of GH, paucity of published age-, gender-, or pubertal-specific normal ranges, diagnosis of GHD cannot rely on any single parameter. The combination of subnormal growth velocity, delayed bone age, and two provocative stimulation tests with failing results is accepted as adequate indication of GHD. Provocative GH testing falsely passes children with neurosecretory GHD; the pharmacologic stimulus bypasses the defect and prompts release of normal levels of GH by the unaffected pituitary gland, whereas spontaneous GH secretion in these children is blunted because of the defect in the hypothalamic or higher brain centers' triggering of GH release. Clinical concern based upon the knowledge that neurosecretory GHD exists, especially after cranial irradiation, can be diagnosed by overnight GH sampling. The various neuromodulators of GH secretion are listed in Table 377.3. Children with GH insufficiency, including neurosecretory GHD, achieve improvements in final height with GH therapy, as do children with classic GHD but not children with non-GHD short stature.

Disorders of Sexual Maturation and Function

Isolated Gonadotropin Deficiency. Isolated gonadotropin deficiency actually may be more common than GHD. However, most patients present to reproductive endocrinologists with

TABLE 377.3

NEUROMODULATORS OF GH SECRETION[a]

Class of Neuromodulator	Example	Second Messenger or Mechanism	Effect on GH Secretion
Growth hormone–releasing hormone (GHRH)	GHRH	Calcium influx	Stimulatory[b]
Somatostatin	SRIH	G proteins	Inhibitory
Alpha-2-adrenergic agonist	Clonidine, norepinephrine, epinephrine	G proteins; stimulate GHRH	Stimulatory[b]
Beta-2-adrenergic agonist	Epinephrine	G proteins; increase SRIH	Inhibitory[b]
Dopaminergic agonist	Dopamine	Adenyl cyclase (pituitary receptors); increase SRIH	Inhibitory[b]
Serotonergic agonist	Serotonin	G proteins, K channel	Stimulatory
Cholinergic agonists	Acetylcholine	G proteins (muscarinic receptors); inhib SRIH	Stimulatory
Histaminergic agonists	Histamine	H_1 receptors	Stimulatory
Gamma-aminobutyric acid (GABA)	GABA	Chloride influx	Stimulatory
Amino acids	Arginine	Depress SRIH	Stimulatory[b]
Hypoglycemia	Insulin		Stimulatory[b]
Hyperglycemia	Diabetes mellitus	Suppress GHRH	Inhibitory
Free fatty acids		Inhibit GHRH	Inhibitory
Calcitonin	Calcitonin	Block GHRH	Inhibitory
Prostaglandins	E series	Adenyl cyclase (Pit); increase GHRH	Stimulatory
Insulinlike growth factors (IGFs)	IGF-1, IGF-2	Negative feedback: stimulate SRIH, inhibit GHRH	Inhibitory
Exercise, stress		Catecholamines	Stimulatory[b]

SRIH, Somatostatin.

[a]The many neuromodulators of growth hormone (GH) secretion include the hypothalamic peptides, GHRH and SRIH, the negative feedback of the insulinlike growth factors, and several neurotransmitters, neuropeptides, amino acids, and other molecules.

[b]Class utilized for GH provocative testing (GHRH, alpha-2-adrenergic agonist clonidine, beta-2-adrenergic antagonist propranolol, dopaminergic l-DOPA, amino acid arginine, hypoglycemia induced by insulin, and exercise).

the chief complaint of infertility. More complete deficiency of gonadotropins presents as inadequate adolescent sexual development. Distinguishing idiopathic hypogonadotropic hypogonadism from constitutional delay of growth and development as well as from psychological dysfunction (depression or anorexia nervosa) can be difficult. Gonadotropin-releasing hormone (GnRH) testing, evaluating the gonadotropin response to an administered GnRH bolus, may be misleading, because the latter conditions also do not demonstrate a gonadotropin response to GnRH. Partial gonadotropin deficiency, conversely, may proceed slowly through puberty and a GnRH bolus testing will cause release of gonadotropins. Patients with Kallmann syndrome (clinically manifested by delayed puberty associated with anosmia) are often easier to diagnose because of the anosmia. This is a familial syndrome, and genetic analysis often detects a mutation in the X chromosome KAL locus that encodes a developmental chemoattractant for both GnRH-secreting and olfactory neuron migration.

Disorders of Water Balance

Isolated Vasopressin (Antidiuretic Hormone) Deficiency. Idiopathic diabetes insipidus (DI), or isolated ADH deficiency, may be familial or sporadic. The familial cases of DI result from autosomal dominant point mutations in the preprohormone synthesis; the gene for the X-linked recessive form has not yet been cloned. A familial DI syndrome linked with diabetes mellitus, optic atrophy, and deafness (DIDMOAD) also exists. Idiopathic DI must be distinguished from other causes of polyuria and polydipsia, including diabetes mellitus, hypercalcemia, renal disease, and primary (psychogenic) polydipsia. Additionally, the evaluation of isolated ADH deficiency must include biochemical studies to eliminate the possible association with anterior pituitary deficiency as well as a magnetic resonance imaging (MRI) scan to rule out anatomic abnormalities such as histiocytosis and germinoma; when the posterior pituitary is deficient, its hyperintense signal is absent on MRI.

Disturbances of the Adrenocorticotropin Hormone–Adrenal Axis

Isolated Adrenocorticotropin Hormone Deficiency. Isolated ACTH deficiency is also extremely rare, but well-documented families with ACTH deficiency, presenting with neonatal or infantile hypoglycemia, have been reported. Isolated ACTH deficiency does not lead to sodium loss or hyperkalemia because the angiotensin-renin regulation of aldosterone production remains intact. However, the ACTH and glucocorticoid deficiency can result in hypoglycemia as well as shock and vascular collapse.

Disorders of Thyroid Function

Isolated Thyroid-Stimulating Hormone Deficiency. In patients with multiple pituitary deficiencies, thyrotropin-releasing hormone (TRH) testing can detect secondary or tertiary hypothyroidism. However, isolated TSH deficiency is believed to be extremely rare. There are reports of poor growth attributed to central hypothyroidism, as determined by frequent nocturnal sampling of TSH but not by TRH testing, but these studies must be confirmed. Measurement of the circulating concentration of free T_4 is another useful screen. Measurement of total T_4 and TSH are not helpful, as in primary hypothyroidism, because their values may be low-normal in central disease.

Familial Thyroid Hormone Resistance. Familial thyroid hormone resistance is an autosomal dominant disorder caused by insensitivity of the hypothalamic–pituitary and peripheral thyroid hormone receptors and is manifested by elevated serum levels of thyroid hormones with normal or high-normal levels of TSH. The patient may manifest clinical symptoms of hyperthyroidism, hypothyroidism, or euthyroidism, depending on whether the peripheral thyroid receptors are also insensitive. The initial studies reported a family with clinical signs of hypothyroidism and deaf-mutism, now referred to as *Refetoff syndrome*. However, familial thyroid hormone resistance is associated clinically most often with only hypothalamic–pituitary resistance but not peripheral resistance and thus findings of mild hyperthyroidism (i.e., poor weight gain, poor concentration with evidence of attention deficits, and mild tachycardia). A small goiter is generally palpable. No treatment exists, but beta-adrenergic blockade is occasionally useful.

Acquired Neuroendocrine Disorders

Pediatric acquired neuroendocrine disorders result from numerous causes. Trauma leading to glandular infarction or hemorrhage may occur at any age, including perinatal distress. Destruction of the pituitary stalk by head trauma or neurosurgical transection results in pituitary isolation syndrome, characterized by DI and variable anterior pituitary failure caused by both loss of hypothalamic connections and pituitary infarction. Although hypopituitarism also can arise from infections or masses, the most common cause is iatrogenic after the treatment of brain tumors and childhood cancer.

Surgical resection of brain tumors near the hypothalamus and pituitary often results in multiple pituitary deficiencies, including DI. Although multiple factors, including nutritional insufficiency, psychosocial dysfunction, and the malignant disease process itself, contribute to the neuroendocrine failure in pediatric cancer patients, numerous studies now indicate that radiotherapy and chemotherapy both play a role in the development of long-term neuroendocrine disturbances.

Disturbances of Growth

Although seasonal variations in growth rates occur, a prolonged period (6 months or more) of accelerated or decelerated growth that deviates from the norm should be regarded by the clinician as inappropriate.

Accelerated Growth. A sudden growth acceleration is more often caused by a return to good health (catch-up growth) and less likely to be secondary to an acquired neuroendocrine disturbance. GH-producing adenomas are exceedingly rare in childhood. The most sensitive test for the possibility of pituitary gigantism is a measurement of somatomedin-C (IGF-1), which will be clearly elevated for age. Rapid growth together with precocious puberty, on the other hand, can be associated with brain tumors, especially hypothalamic glioma. Exogenous obesity is an increasingly common cause of growth acceleration in childhood.

Growth Failure. Growth failure is the single most sensitive sign that something is amiss with a child. Child abuse, neglect, and deprivation can cause growth failure through emotional and nutritional disturbances that translate into functional GHD and GH insensitivity. Known as *psychosocial dwarfing*, this syndrome is unique in its reversibility. Correction of GH functioning and catch-up growth are achieved by removing the child from the socially harmful environment and placing him or her into a nurturing home or hospital; return to the original family setting prompts relapse. Furthermore, treatment with exogenous GH while the child remains in the neglectful or abusive environment fails to restore normal growth.

GH is also the most common hormonal deficiency in children with acquired organic neuroendocrine disease. Intrasellar tumors may present with growth failure alone, although generally associated neurologic symptoms occur, such as visual field deficits and headache. Hypothalamic tumors may lead to GHD,

DI, and sexual precocity. GHD also may result from surgery in the pituitary area, and it is the most frequent neuroendocrine disturbance after cranial irradiation. In children treated with radiotherapy for brain tumors, 40% to 75% developed growth deceleration and subnormal physiologic GH secretion. Similar outcomes occurred with cranial radiotherapy for the treatment of systemic malignancies such as acute lymphoblastic leukemia or with total body irradiation as part of bone marrow transplantation protocols.

Several factors determining the growth-stunting effects of radiotherapy have been characterized, including total dose, fraction size, patient age, and time interval to testing. The total dose of radiation reaching the hypothalamic–pituitary axis, especially doses beyond 1,800 to 2,000 cGy, correlates with the incidence, severity, and speed of onset of GHD. Doses of 1,800 cGy diminish and alter the pubertal increase in spontaneous GH secretion, doses of 2,400 cGy decrease all spontaneous GH secretion yet may maintain normal provocative secretion, and doses of 2,700 cGy or more blunt both spontaneous and provocative secretion. However, fraction size may be as important as total radiation dose in causing GH aberrations. A larger fraction size administered over a shorter treatment period increases the risk of GHD for a given total radiation dose. Furthermore, younger children are more likely than older children to develop GHD with the same radiation treatment. Finally, the time interval between radiation treatment and endocrine testing also affects the frequency of GHD, with the incidence increasing over time. Most studies have revealed GHD within 1 to 2 years after radiotherapy.

Many of the treatment protocols involve a combination of radiotherapy with chemotherapy, and it has become clear that chemotherapy also plays a part in the growth failure of childhood cancer survivors. In fact, the two modalities are synergistic. When chemotherapy is used in conjunction with cranial or craniospinal irradiation, the growth failure is more profound, the incidence of GHD is increased, and the development of GHD is earlier. More recent information is suggestive that chemotherapy can cause GHD, even without irradiation.

Disturbances of Sexual Maturation

Precocious puberty was defined as breast development in a girl before the age of 8 years and testicular enlargement in a boy younger than 9 years. This definition has been brought into question by a 1997 survey of primary care practices in the United States that found breast changes in over 5% of Caucasian girls at age 7 years and over 5% of African American girls at age 6 years; the average age of menarche has remained unchanged at 12.5 years. Delayed adolescence is lack of breast development in a girl older than 12.5 years and lack of testicular enlargement in a boy older than 14 years. Within a given clinical context, however, such as after cranial irradiation, the clinician should be aware that earlier than anticipated sexual development, even if not by definition precocious, may limit the child's growth potential. Similarly, poor progression of adolescent changes, even if not delayed, may reflect neuroendocrine failure in oncologic patients.

Sexual Precocity. Central precocious puberty is caused by premature activation of the hypothalamic–pituitary-gonadal axis. Whereas the majority of cases in girls are idiopathic, some girls and most boys develop central precocious puberty because of an organic brain lesion or after cranial irradiation. Most lesions, including hydrocephalus, meningoencephalitis, severe head trauma, neurofibromas, tuberous sclerosis, optic gliomas, and other tumors in the sella turcica, are believed to cause sexual precocity by disrupting the normal hypothalamic prepubertal gonadotropin suppression. In contrast, hypothalamic hamartomas can induce puberty by secreting LH-releasing hormone, and pineal germinomas by secreting human chori-

onic gonadotropin. Thus, once the diagnosis of central precocious puberty is confirmed with an advanced bone age and pubertal level of LH (best done with an ultrasensitive assay), neuroimaging with computed tomography or preferably MRI should be obtained to exclude a central nervous system lesion. Aside from addressing the underlying cause, central precocious puberty can be halted with long-acting GnRH agonists that suppress gonadotropin secretion.

Another form of central precocious puberty is found with prolonged untreated severe hypothyroidism. The strikingly elevated levels of TSH may cause sexual development despite the drastically delayed bone age. Because TSH, FSH, and LH are all glycoproteins secreted by basophilic cells and sharing the same alpha-subunit, nonspecific stimulation of gonadotropins results from the excessively high TRH levels. This form of sexual precocity is readily corrected by restoring euthyroid status with thyroxine replacement.

Gonadotropins are second to GH in radiation sensitivity, and radiation treatment frequently leads to pubertal aberrations. Earlier puberty and even true precocious puberty have been found to occur following cranial radiation of 1,800 cGy or greater. Age at pubarche also is correlated positively with age at radiotherapy, with the youngest children radiated having a higher frequency of early puberty. Although more common in girls, precocious puberty following cranial irradiation also occurs in boys.

Sexual Infantilism. Brain tumors and cancer therapy also can cause delayed puberty. Primary gonadotropin deficiency may result from pituitary tumors, including craniopharyngioma, prolactinoma, and nonfunctioning pituitary adenoma, and from secondary gonadotropin deficiency from hypothalamic tumors (germinoma). Except for prolactinomas or nonfunctioning pituitary adenomas, evidence of other pituitary hormone deficiencies usually occurs.

Cranial radiation treatment in very high doses causes hypogonadotropic hypogonadism. In a large series of children with hypothalamic glioma, one-third of the teenaged children developed hypogonadotropic hypogonadism and all had significant cranial irradiation (greater than 2,500 cGy) at an early age. Furthermore, 70% of postpubertal women experienced oligomenorrhea and 30% of adult men had low serum testosterone concentrations after cranial radiation for brain tumors, with both genders demonstrating GnRH deficiency on endocrine testing.

Radiation directed at the gonads causes primary testicular and ovarian failure. Even relatively low doses of irradiation decrease spermatogenesis and follicular development. Significant dosages (greater than 1,000 cGy) directed at the gonads lead to hormonal failure as well. The testis is more sensitive to radiation effects than is the ovary, and the postpubertal gonad is more radiosensitive than is the prepubertal gonad. Chemotherapy, notably the alkylating agents, can cause gonadal failure, especially when administered postpubertally.

Amenorrhea. Several types of amenorrhea demonstrate the profound influence the nervous system can exert on endocrine functioning. Functional amenorrhea, the single most common cause of secondary amenorrhea except pregnancy, results from psychic stress and is therefore transient and self-resolving. It likely is mediated by functional abnormalities in the hypothalamic gonadotropin-regulating areas. Pseudocyesis, false or phantom pregnancy, describes the emotionally driven condition in which a nonpregnant woman develops amenorrhea, increasing weight, expanding abdominal girth, and morning sickness. Amenorrhea from prolonged, intense exercise and from anorexia nervosa may have a psychogenic component in addition to gonadotropin disturbances caused by diminished body fat.

Disorders of Water Balance

ADH, the main neuroendocrine hormone regulating water balance and hence blood volume and tonicity, is also a potent vasoconstrictor and neurotransmitter. ADH deficiency results in free water loss, volume depletion, and serum hyperosmolality (DI). Inappropriate regulation of ADH (i.e., unresponsiveness to stretch receptors indicating volume expansion) causes fluid retention and hyponatremia (syndrome of inappropriate ADH [SIADH]).

Diabetes Insipidus. Acquired central DI is most commonly caused by hypothalamic injury and disease. Head trauma, intraoperative manipulation, and resection of the pituitary stalk frequently precipitate DI. A triphasic pattern, in which initial ADH insufficiency causes polyuria, followed by improved urinary concentrating ability caused by the release of ADH by dying neurons and ending in permanent polyuria when the neurons are irreversibly lost, can span up to 2 weeks after injury. Other central causes of DI include craniopharyngiomas and dysgerminomas, histiocytosis X, intraventricular hemorrhage, asphyxia, and severe intracranial infections. Cranial irradiation does not cause DI.

Regardless of the cause, central DI is treated with ADH analogues, most often DDAVP. DDAVP should not be used, however, in the immediate postoperative fluid management after surgical craniopharyngioma resection because its long half-life may overlap with the onset of the middle triphasic period in which the potential sudden release of endogenous ADH may lead to water overload with hyponatremic seizure. As well, a number of patients have developed cerebral salt wasting (discussed below) after surgery and/or radiation. This sudden onset of polyuria associated with dehydration but either normal or low levels of serum sodium must be judiciously managed by fluid and electrolytes alone. In all cases of DI secondary to surgical treatment, fluid balance must therefore be monitored carefully and, if necessary, intravenous vasopressin must be administered judiciously (except in the cases of salt wasting).

Syndrome of Inappropriate Antidiuretic Hormone. SIADH in children occurs because of brain or lung disease. SIADH often complicates bacterial meningitis, but also can be seen with encephalitis, Guillain-Barré syndrome, and head trauma. Pulmonary infections, status asthmaticus, and mechanical ventilation of very low-birth-weight premature infants also can be associated with SIADH. The treatment of SIADH is water restriction. Administration of hypertonic saline prolongs what is generally a transient condition and should not be used.

Cerebral Salt Wasting. Cerebral salt wasting is caused by production of central nervous system (CNS) factors related to atrial natriuretic hormone after brain injury, often during or after cranial radiation treatment. The CNS peptide can now be measured as *brain natriuretic peptide* (BNP). BNP and perhaps other CNS factors prompt both sodium and water loss, characterized by polyuria, volume depletion, and hyponatremia, thereby distinguishing this clinical condition from DI and SIADH. During radiation treatment for a primary CNS lesion, cerebral salt wasting can occur superimposed on DI and cause a confusing clinical situation. The polyuria suggests inadequate vasopressin treatment, but increasing the dose of vasopressin leads to worsening hyponatremia. Restriction of fluid (because of the possibility of SIADH) causes further volume depletion. The management of cerebral salt wasting, which is generally transient, is to withhold vasopressin therapy and replace fluid loss with salt and water, possibly requiring hypertonic (3%) saline and significant quantities of fluid.

Disturbances of the Adrenocorticotropin Hormone–Adrenal Axis

Cortisol negatively inhibits corticotropin-releasing hormone (CRH)-ACTH release, but the mechanisms causing upregulation of CRH and ACTH, as during stress, are still not clear. ACTH excess (Cushing disease) and deficiency may be encountered.

Cushing Disease. Hyperadrenocorticism caused by an ACTH-producing pituitary adenoma or dysregulated CRH-ACTH production is far more common in the adult than pediatric age range. Tumors producing ACTH-like peptides are not seen in children. Nonetheless, Cushing disease should be suspected in a child with linear growth deceleration and exaggerated weight gain that is accompanied by hypertension, hyperpigmentation, pigmented striae, truncal obesity, acne, and virilization. Midnight or bedtime collection of saliva for cortisol concentration has been demonstrated to be specific and sensitive as a diagnostic test for excess cortisol production. Collection of saliva is a good way to screen for Cushing disease in children since urinary collections are occasionally difficult. However, repeated 24-hour urinary free cortisol determinations are the best diagnostic test for Cushing syndrome. Cushing disease is distinguished from Cushing syndrome, or primary hypercortisolism, by the unsuppressed ACTH level and by imaging studies of the adrenal and pituitary glands. Unfortunately, Cushing disease is difficult to treat and recurrence is common. Treatment modalities include transsphenoidal surgery, total adrenalectomy, and pituitary irradiation. A recent study suggests that pituitary Cushing disease may be cured in most cases following transsphenoidal surgery, by pituitary irradiation for recurrent disease. The use of medical therapies such as ketoconazole or mitotane to temporize excessive adrenal cortisol production until radiation ablation is complete is important.

Adrenocorticotropin Hormone Deficiency. Acquired ACTH deficiency is almost always secondary to brain tumor or its treatment, especially surgical resection. Cranial irradiation, *per se*, is unlikely to cause ACTH or CRH deficiency. Prolonged high-dose glucocorticoid treatment can also cause a reversible suppression of ACTH; although transient, it may last for 6 to 12 months depending on the degree of prior glucocorticoid exposure. Clinical signs and symptoms include lethargy, weakness, nausea, anorexia, hypotension, hypoglycemia, and acidosis (but without hyperkalemia or hyponatremia because of maintenance of normal mineralocorticoid activity by the intact renin-angiotensin system). Laboratory studies suggestive of ACTH insufficiency include low morning cortisol levels with low normal ACTH levels; the diagnosis should be confirmed by intravenous low-dose ($1-\mu$g) synthetic ACTH stimulation testing or by CRH testing. These patients require physiologic glucocorticoid replacement as well as pharmacologic dose administration during periods of illness and severe stress such as surgery. Cortisol replacement dose, although based on production rates in healthy children, should be titrated to symptomatic relief and restoration of blood pressure. The absence of pituitary ACTH as a marker of cortisol sufficiency makes glucocorticoid replacement difficult because no good biochemical parameters exist that can be followed. Excessive cortisol replacement results in poor growth, osteopenia, and other manifestations of Cushing syndrome. Inadequate cortisol replacement results in poor weight gain, growth, and potential shock.

Disturbances of Thyroid Function

Acquired hypothalamic or pituitary TRH or TSH deficiency is most often caused by tumor or tumor treatment and almost never occurs without other pituitary disturbances. The most common causes in childhood are craniopharyngioma and surgical resection of hypothalamic or other pituitary tumors. Cranial irradiation rarely causes TSH deficiency. Clinically, secondary or tertiary hypothyroidism is not as severe as primary hypothyroidism and certainly does not cause myxedema, but it can compound the growth failure of the concurrent GHD; GH treatment without thyroxine replacement in these cases cannot normalize the growth pattern. Therefore, pediatricians must check serum-free thyroxine concentrations in any child with GHD. Total T_4 levels may be low or low-normal, and the usual compensatory elevation in TSH level in primary hypothyroidism is absent because of the impaired hypothalamus and pituitary.

ENDOCRINE MANAGEMENT OF CHILDHOOD CANCER SURVIVORS

Radiation- and chemotherapy-induced neuroendocrine dysfunction presents several acute and long-term management issues for the pediatrician caring for children with cancer. Perhaps most critical in the immediate phase of oncologic treatment is obtaining accurate baseline growth measurements: height (standing and sitting), weight, and bone age. Also during treatment, evaluation for hypothyroidism and thyroxine replacement, as indicated, should be pursued. Although growth deceleration may arise because of the toxicity of oncologic treatment, even in patients with documented GHD, GH therapy should be delayed until the child has been disease-free usually for 1 year after completion of any oncologic treatment. Some children experience spontaneous catch-up growth, and the GHD does not need to be corrected immediately. Furthermore, the incidence of relapse is highest in the first few years after cancer diagnosis and treatment, although no evidence exists of GH therapy stimulating cancer recurrence.

Pediatricians and internists caring for survivors of childhood cancer must vigilantly monitor for signs of long-term neuroendocrine sequelae from radiotherapy, chemotherapy, or both. Growth should be assessed via measurements every 6 months and annual bone ages; growth failure should prompt provocative GH stimulation testing. The use of growth factors (IGF-1 or IGFBP-3) for screening of GHD is less reliable in children with brain tumors or after cranial irradiation. GH therapy for GHD is indicated for both growth in children and maintenance of body composition and cardiovascular integrity in adults. Recent long-term studies have demonstrated the safety of GH therapy in children surviving brain tumor in terms of both tumor recurrence or new second tumors. Outcome studies indicate that the dose of growth hormone should be 0.043 mg/kg/day, which provides better adult height outcomes as compared to studies from European centers that tend to use 0.02 mg/kg/day. Continued screening for hypothyroidism, secondary adrenal insufficiency, and gonadal axis disturbances also must be conducted because impairments may become manifest years after radiation and chemotherapy.

Suggested Readings

Constine LS, Woolf PD, Cann D, et al. Hypothalamic-pituitary dysfunction after radiation for brain tumors. *N Engl J Med* 1993;328:87.
Kaplowitz PB, Oberfield SE, the Drug and Therapeutics and Executive Committees of the Lawson Wilkins Pediatric Endocrine Society. Reexamination of the age limit for defining when puberty is precocious in girls in the United States: implications for evaluation and treatment. *Pediatrics* 1999;104:936.
Moshang T Jr. Pediatric brain tumors: outcomes as regards growth and sexual development. *Curr Opin Endocrinol Diabetes* 1997;4:80.
Moshang T Jr, Grimberg A. The effects of irradiation and chemotherapy on growth. *Endocrinol Metab Clin North Am* 1996;25:731.
Packer RJ, Boyett J, Janss A, et al. Growth hormone replacement therapy in children with medulloblastoma: use and effect on tumor control. *J Clin Oncol* 2001;19:480.
Parks JS, Brown MR, Hurley DL, et al. Heritable disorders of the pituitary. *J Clin Endocrin Metab* 1999;84:4362.
Oberfield SE, Allen JC, Pollack J, et al. Long-term endocrine sequelae after treatment of medulloblastoma: prospective study of growth and thyroid function. *J Pediatr* 1986;108:219.
Ogilvy-Stuart AL, Clayton PE, Shalet SM. Cranial irradiation and early puberty. *J Clin Endocrinol Metab* 1994;78:1282.
Sklar CA, Mertens AC, Mitby P, et al. Risk of disease recurrence and second neoplasms in survivors of childhood cancer treated with growth hormone: a report from the Childhood Cancer Survivor Study. *J Clin Endocrinol Metab* 2002;87:3136.

CHAPTER 378 ■ TYPE 1 (INSULIN-DEPENDENT) DIABETES MELLITUS

LESLIE P. PLOTNICK

Type 1 (insulin-dependent) diabetes mellitus is a common, serious disease of children and adolescents. The diagnosis usually is straightforward, but long-term management is a major challenge for the child, family, and health care team. Developments since the 1980s have rendered the attainment of metabolic control a technical possibility. However, achievement of true metabolic normalcy remains an elusive goal. In addition, diabetes management is stressful to the family, and psychological and behavioral issues often interfere with the goal of metabolic control. Few other diseases require the extensive self-care management needed to care for type 1 diabetes.

DEFINITION AND DIAGNOSTIC CRITERIA

In 1997, an expert committee reclassified and updated diagnostic criteria for diabetes. Type 1 diabetes is the type most frequently found in children and adolescents. It has been called *juvenile-onset, ketosis-prone, brittle diabetes,* and, until most recently, *type 1 or insulin-dependent diabetes mellitus* (IDDM). Patients with type 1 diabetes are insulinopenic and need exogenous insulin to prevent development of ketosis and to preserve life.

Type 2 diabetes is found more commonly in adults and obese persons. This type also has been called *adult-onset, maternity-onset, ketosis-resistant, stable diabetes,* and, until most recently, *type 2 or non–insulin-dependent diabetes mellitus* (NIDDM). As obesity increases in the pediatric and adolescent populations, type 2 diabetes is becoming increasingly common in this age group. Type 2 diabetes is discussed in detail in Chapter 379. It is caused primarily by insulin resistance without adequate compensatory insulin secretion. Thus, a relative, not absolute, insulin deficiency occurs. Affected patients are not dependent on insulin for survival and are less ketosis-prone, but they may need exogenous insulin for metabolic control, and they can develop ketosis and ketoacidosis in certain situations. Sometimes distinguishing between type 1 and type 2 is difficult at presentation.

Other specific types of diabetes occur due to causes such as genetic defects in beta-cell function (maturity-onset diabetes in youth [MODY]) and insulin action, and others are caused by diseases of the exocrine pancreas.

To be diagnosed with diabetes, a child or adolescent must have classic symptoms with a random plasma glucose level at or above 200 mg/dL (11.1 mmol/L). If the patient is asymptomatic, fasting plasma glucose must be at or above 126 mg/dL (7.0 mmol/L) or the 2-hour plasma glucose levels on an oral glucose tolerance test must be at or above 200 mg/dL. The asymptomatic criteria require confirmation by repeat testing (on another day). The diagnosis of diabetes in a child rarely is subtle. Most children present with the classic symptoms of polyuria, polydipsia, polyphagia, weight loss, and lethargy. Glucose tolerance testing rarely is necessary for establishing the diagnosis.

EPIDEMIOLOGY

The prevalence of type 1 diabetes in the United States in children and adolescents varies somewhat according to different sources, with most studies reporting a rate of 1.2 to 1.9 cases per 1,000 members of the population of this age group. This incidence is age-dependent with a range of fewer than 1 per 1,000 at age 5 years to approximately 3 per 1,000 at age 16 years. The U.S. incidence is about 12 to 15 new cases per year per 100,000 of the pediatric population.

Major worldwide variations in incidence exist, with the United States having an intermediate incidence. Incidence increases with age and peaks in early to middle puberty. A seasonal distribution of newly diagnosed cases exists: for unknown reasons, more cases are diagnosed in the cooler months. Male and female subjects are approximately equally affected.

GENETICS, ETIOLOGY, AND PATHOGENESIS

Our understanding of the genetics, cause, and pathogenesis of type 1 diabetes has increased greatly. No one diabetes gene exists. Instead, certain genetic alterations raise or lower the risk of beta-cell damage. Inheritance of HLA antigens DR3 and DR4 is associated with an increased risk of developing type 1 diabetes. Inheritance of one of these HLA antigens confers a three- to fivefold risk of developing type 1 diabetes; inheritance of both confers an approximately tenfold risk. DR3 or DR4 occurs in

---

BOX 378.1	**Risk of Developing Type 1 Diabetes if One Sibling is Affected**

Identical twins: <50%
HLA identical: 1 in 5
HLA haploidentical: 1 in 20
HLA nonidentical: 1 in 100

---

approximately 95% of persons with type 1 diabetes. Variations on the DQ antigens also account for changes in the risk of developing type 1 diabetes. An amino acid variation at position 57 of the DQ beta chain (nonaspartic acid) is associated with a marked increase in risk. In addition, a higher risk is conferred by an arginine at position 52 of the DQ alpha chain.

The chance of type 1 diabetes developing in a second sibling is summarized in Box 378.1 and is related directly to the shared HLA haplotypes. Approximately 5% of a diabetic patient's siblings develop type 1 diabetes.

Less than 50% of identical twins are concordant for type 1 diabetes, indicating that a susceptibility to type 1 diabetes, rather than the disease itself, is inherited. This inherited susceptibility appears to place the beta cell at unusual risk for immunologic, inflammatory damage. The less than 50% concordance in identical twins and the marked geographic variation in incidence of type 1 diabetes support the significance of external factors in the process of beta-cell damage.

Beta-cell destruction occurs in genetically susceptible people. Researchers suggest that at least 80% of the functional beta-cell mass must be destroyed before overt glucose intolerance occurs. The process of beta-cell destruction in most cases is immune-mediated, probably takes months or years, and may be initiated by environmental factors. Whether the process is relentless and progressive, inevitably producing type 1 diabetes, or may wax and wane over the course of time and sometimes enters remission remains controversial. One hypothesis is that the exposure to the environmental factors may be recurrent and intermittent or continuous (e.g., viral infections, dietary factors, environmental toxins, stress) rather than a single triggering event. Viruses or other environmental factors may precipitate beta-cell destruction by direct damage (exposing antigens for future immunologic attack) or by molecular mimicry caused by similar protein sequences in beta-cell antigens and the offending agent (e.g., virus, bovine serum albumin). The damaged beta cell presents antigens recognized as nonself to the immune system. The ability of macrophages to present these antigens to helper T cells depends on the class II (D) HLA molecules and their three-dimensional structure, which is determined by the amino acid sequence of the HLA molecules' alpha and beta chains. Another hypothesis suggests that certain HLA types may bind the antigens intracellularly, preventing their exposure to the immune system and protecting against the development of type 1 diabetes.

The autoimmune processes release cytokines that are destructive in the beta cells directly or that destroy tissue by generating free radicals. The process of beta-cell destruction probably occurs in two phases: an early cytokine-dependent initiation phase and a later phase with antigen-specific T-lymphocyte proliferation, which amplifies and perpetuates beta-cell destruction. Beta-cell protective mechanisms may help beta cells resist immunologic damage.

Type 1 diabetes susceptibility probably is conferred by unfavorable combinations of common gene alleles for HLA and beta-cell destructive and beta-cell protective mechanisms.

Specific HLA types appear to be necessary for development of type 1 diabetes, but they are not sufficient.

Most patients with newly diagnosed type 1 diabetes have measurable immunologic markers: islet cell antibodies (ICAs) and insulin autoantibodies (IAAs). ICAs may be cytoplasmic or surface antibodies. High-titer ICAs confer a greater risk of subsequently developing type 1 diabetes than do low titers. ICAs probably are more predictive in children, as is the persistence of positivity.

Another important immunologic marker is IAAs. IAAs in combination with ICAs and high-titer IAAs are associated with an increased risk of developing type 1 diabetes. Other beta-cell autoantigens, including glutamic acid decarboxylase (GAD65), also are important markers.

PATHOPHYSIOLOGY

Insulin is the body's major anabolic hormone. In the fed state, it stimulates energy storage in the forms of glycogen, protein, and adipose tissue. When insulin levels are low or deficient, mobilization of stored substrate occurs (i.e., glycogenolysis, proteolysis, lipolysis) and tissue uptake of glucose is inhibited. Because insulin is a potent antilipolytic hormone, a greater degree of insulin deficiency is required for lipolysis than for glucose intolerance to occur. In the early stages of insulin deficiency, hyperglycemia predominates, and a more severe degree of insulin deficiency is necessary for ketonuria, ketonemia, and acidosis to develop.

In addition to insulin deficiency, a relative excess of counterregulatory hormones (e.g., growth hormone, cortisol, glucagon, catecholamines) must exist to produce the picture of diabetic ketoacidosis (DKA). Hyperglycemia produces an osmotic diuresis, causing the symptoms of polyuria and polydipsia. Passive electrolyte loss occurs along with the osmotic diuresis. Weight loss is caused by the general catabolic state and the osmotic diuresis. Eventually, dehydration results and is especially severe if the child cannot drink enough fluid to compensate for the diuresis, as in the case of vomiting or a decreased level of consciousness. Lipolysis results in production of ketones, causing metabolic acidosis.

CLINICAL PRESENTATION

Most children with type 1 diabetes present with the classic symptoms of polyuria, polydipsia, polyphagia, and weight loss; many also complain of lethargy. If the diagnosis is not made and treatment is not begun, further metabolic decompensation occurs, with worsening DKA.

In young children and infants, the diagnosis is more likely to be missed in its early stages because of difficulty in recognizing early symptoms, and children of these ages are more likely to present with severe ketoacidosis. If pediatricians inquire specifically about the classic symptoms in patients with nonspecific signs of illness and weight loss, this diagnosis is more likely to be made quickly. Establishing the diagnosis early avoids further metabolic decompensation and the risks of DKA and its treatment.

Most children with new-onset type 1 diabetes have symptoms of less than 1 month's duration, but some have had mild to moderate symptoms for several months. Questions about bedwetting, nocturia, number of diapers used, or leaving class to use the bathroom may help uncover the presence of polyuria.

Type 1 diabetes must be considered in any child with clinical dehydration who continues to urinate regularly. Too often, frequent urination leads the parent or physician to conclude incorrectly that the child is not dehydrated. Routine dipstick testing for urine glucose and ketones in patients with non-

specific symptoms such as lethargy, weight loss, nausea, and vomiting and in those with specific type 1 diabetes symptoms could enhance greatly the early establishment of diagnosis of this disease before severe metabolic decompensation has occurred.

New-onset type 1 diabetes may be managed in an inpatient or outpatient setting, depending on the severity of the patient's metabolic abnormalities and the health care resources available.

CLINICAL COURSE

After the initial presentation, many children with newly diagnosed type 1 diabetes undergo a honeymoon period or remission phase. During this period, the remaining functional beta cells regain the ability to produce insulin, possibly as a result of elimination of hyperglycemia. Measurement of C-peptide levels has demonstrated that improved secretion of insulin occurs during this phase. Because endogenous insulin secretion increases, requirements for exogenous insulin decrease, usually dropping to less than 0.5 U/kg per day. Hypoglycemia becomes a potential problem. This phase usually begins within 1 to 3 months after diagnosis is made and lasts for several months, sometimes as long as 12 to 24 months. The honeymoon period is a period of relative well-being, with metabolic near normalcy as indicated by normal glycosylated hemoglobin levels. Information about the honeymoon period must be included in the education of the newly diagnosed patient because denial of having the disease and subsequent failure to monitor it are likely to occur unless patients and families learn about this phase and expect its occurrence and its end.

As this phase ends, the remaining beta cells lose their capacity to secrete insulin, and requirements for exogenous insulin increase. This phase usually occurs gradually, but, as in cases of acute infection, it may be abrupt. Careful monitoring and frequent adjustments of doses are extremely important during the end of the remission phase, and close contact between the patient and physician is necessary.

GOALS OF TREATMENT

The overall goals of treatment of type 1 diabetes center around the (currently unattainable) goal of true metabolic normalcy, which in day-to-day life means avoiding short-term complications (hypoglycemia, hyperglycemia, ketosis, and DKA) and minimizing risks of developing long-term complications. In addition, helping the child and family achieve normal psychological maturation and independence is an ongoing and lifelong goal. Certain specific goals are discussed below.

Normal Growth

Normal growth in height and weight and normal timing of adolescent pubertal development are important goals of long-term management. Chronically undertreated children with poorly controlled type 1 diabetes often fail to grow and gain weight normally and have delayed skeletal maturation (i.e., bone age) and delayed sexual maturation. The growth retardation can be severe. Growth is an important factor to follow, and height, weight, and pubertal development should be monitored carefully. The causes for deviations from normal velocities should be sought.

Children receiving excessive doses of insulin may gain weight too rapidly. Excessive doses of insulin, which can cause rebound hyperglycemia and ketosis, can produce on occasion a similar degree of growth retardation, as can chronically inadequate doses. Mauriac syndrome (diabetes with growth retardation and hepatomegaly) is caused by poor diabetic control, and, although patients with this syndrome usually are receiving inadequate insulin doses, excessive doses on occasion have been associated with this clinical picture.

Effective Management Choices

Education of the patient and family with the goal of independent management of type 1 diabetes at home is important. Some families achieve independence quickly. Others require intensive and repeated education on a one-to-one basis or in group programs. Independent decision making by patients and families who are well educated about diabetes and its management enhances independence, feelings of control, and self-esteem and is important for long-term psychological success. Most day-to-day decisions regarding hyperglycemia, hypoglycemia, illness, ketonuria, and unusual activities or eating schedules can be handled appropriately by knowledgeable families. Frequent blood glucose monitoring, which is discussed later in this chapter, is mandatory.

Children and adolescents with type 1 diabetes should be encouraged to participate in any activities that are appropriate for their ages and interests. An adolescent with sports practice three times a week after school can learn how to increase calories or decrease insulin doses and keep blood glucose levels in an acceptable range during the activity. Certain precautions must be taken. For example, a source of sugar must be readily available during a physical activity. When adolescents drive, a readily available glucose source must be in easy and rapid reach. Medic-Alert bracelets or necklaces should be worn.

The choice of insulin regimen, including lifestyle choices, education level, and motivation to do the work needed for diabetes management, should meet the needs of the individual child and family.

The diet should be designed around the child's and family's food preferences and habits, using sound nutritional principles. Families should participate in the planning of the diet, and the amount of food must be adequate for satiety to maximize adherence. With basal/bolus insulin regimens, discussed below, dietary flexibility is the norm.

Avoiding Metabolic Abnormalities

Avoidance of metabolic abnormalities is another important goal. Monitoring blood glucose levels several times a day along with urinary ketone checks is mandatory for successful management. Significant hyperglycemia and hypoglycemia should be avoided. In young children, especially preschoolers, blood glucose levels often vary widely. To avoid development of serious hypoglycemia in this age group, compromises may have to be made in tolerating hyperglycemia. Glycosylated hemoglobin levels should be monitored regularly, usually every 3 months, with a goal of achieving a level as close to the normal range as possible. Normal values vary depending on the laboratory method used. Blood lipids should be monitored and dietary modifications made if hyperlipidemia occurs.

Ketonuria should be treated early. In most patients who monitor regularly, DKA can be avoided by responding to hyperglycemia, ketosis, and periods of illness with adjustments in insulin doses. The demands of the diabetes management regimen are high and require care and understanding on the part of the families and the health care team to maximize the child's chances for successful emotional development.

MANAGEMENT

Insulin

Many insulin preparations, including standard insulin and new "designer" insulin analogues, are available. Animal (beef and pork) insulin no longer is available; all insulin now is human, made by recombinant DNA methods.

Three rapid-acting insulin analogues are available. The first, lispro (Humalog, Eli Lilly), was approved for use in 1996. Aspart (NovoLog, Novo-Nordisk), and glulisine (Apidra Snofi-Aventis) were approved more recently. These are biosynthetic analogues of regular insulin and are absorbed and cleared more rapidly than is regular insulin and, therefore, more closely mimic pancreatic insulin secretion. They can be used effectively even after a meal in children with unpredictable eating habits.

Regular insulin is short-acting and is the standard insulin used in intravenous infusion to treat DKA. Neutral protamine hagedorn (NPH) or Lente is intermediate in peak and duration of action. Ultralente is a longer-acting insulin than is NPH, with a duration of approximately 18 to 22 hours, and has a significant peak. Glargine (Lantus, Aventis) is an insulin analogue that is the first peakless long-acting insulin, with a duration of action of approximately 20 to 24+ hours (Table 378.1). Levemir (Detemir, Novo Nordisk) is a long acting insulin given 1 to 2 times per day.

With the advent of insulin analogues, many options for insulin regimens now are possible.

Split/Mixed Regimens

These regimens are the basic two or three injections using an intermediate insulin (e.g., NPH) or a longer-acting one (e.g., Ultralente). Most children and adolescents require at least two injections per day of short- and intermediate-acting insulin to achieve satisfactory metabolic control; the injections are administered shortly before breakfast and dinner. During the honeymoon period, when insulin requirements are at a minimum, one injection per day may be satisfactory for control. Except for this period, achieving control with a single daily injection is nearly impossible. Absorption may vary from different injection sites and is more rapid in exercised sites and at higher temperatures. Injection into hypertrophied sites may slow absorption.

These regimens use, for example, NPH and regular insulin at breakfast and again at dinner. The total dose is split into two shots, and each shot is a mix of NPH and regular insulin. A rapid-acting analogue can be used instead of regular insulin.

TABLE 378.1

TIMING OF ACTION OF AVAILABLE INSULIN (TIMES ARE APPROXIMATE)

	Onset	Peak	Duration (Hour)
Rapid acting analogues			
Lispro	0.25	0.5–1.0	3
Aspart	0.25	0.7–1.0	3+
Regular	0.5–1.0	2–3	4–6
NPH/Lente	1–4	4–10	10–16
Ultralente	1–4	8–16	18–20
Long-acting analogue			
Glargine	1–2	No peak	20–24

Several different mixes that combine different percents of short- or rapid-acting insulin with intermediate acting insulin are available.

BOX 378.2	**Example of Split/Mixed Insulin Regimen for a 30-kg Child on a Diet with a Fixed Number of Carbohydrates per Meal**

Morning (before breakfast): 12 NPH
Before dinner or at bedtime: 6 NPH
Sliding scale regular, lispro or aspart dose

Blood	glucose
<50	3
50–100	4
100–150	5
150–200	6
200–250	7
250–300	8
>300	9

BOX 378.3	**Example of a Basal Bolus Regimen for a 40-kg Child on a Diet with no Fixed Number of Carbohydrates**

Total daily insulin dose = 32 units
50% basal = 16 units for basal insulin given as either 16 units glargine per day OR 0.6 units per hour of lispro or aspart as pump basal rate
Bolus doses: Insulin-to-carbohydrate ratio for meals and snacks: 450 divided by total insulin dose (450/32 = 14). Use 1 unit per 15 carbohydrate grams.
Correction factor: 1,800 rule = 1,800 divided by total insulin dose (1,800/32 = 56). Use 1 unit per 60 blood glucose points (or 0.5 unit per 30 blood glucose points) above target. Target might be 120 in the daytime and 150 at night.

A variation of this schedule is to split the evening dose further into regular insulin or a rapid-acting analogue taken with dinner and move the time for taking the NPH to bedtime. The peak actions of the insulin used in split/mixed regimens do not correlate well with usual mealtimes, and excess of between-meal insulin levels causes a need for snacks to avoid development of hypoglycemia. There is an increased risk of development of nocturnal hypoglycemia. Use of a rapid-acting insulin instead of regular insulin helps somewhat with this problem, but the peaks of NPH and Ultralente remain nonphysiologic (Box 378.2).

Basal/Bolus Regimens

These regimens are attempts to achieve more physiologic insulin levels. One insulin type is given to provide basal (or fasting) insulin needs, and another insulin type is used to cover "bolus" needs (food requirements). Bolus doses are determined based on the amount and type of food ingested (mainly carbohydrates) and on the blood glucose level at the time the meal is eaten. Basal insulin can be provided either with the basal rate on an insulin pump or with glargine. Bolus doses are provided by use of rapid-acting analogues. Basal requirements usually are approximately 50% of total daily insulin needs.

No matter which regimen is used, frequent blood glucose monitoring is necessary so that patients can respond to the levels by adjusting their insulin doses. For example, with a split/mixed regimen, if an occasional fasting blood glucose level falls above the target range, the morning short-acting insulin dose should be increased. If the fasting blood glucose level is increased for several consecutive days, the evening NPH dose should be increased.

During the honeymoon period, dose requirements may drop to less than 0.5 U/kg/day. Except during this period, most preadolescent children need approximately 0.75 to 1.0 U/kg/day. Teenagers usually require approximately 1.0 to 1.2 U/kg/day.

Patients on a *split/mixed* regimen typically need approximately two-thirds of the total dose in the morning and one-third before eating dinner. The doses usually are split between one-third short- or rapid-acting (regular, lispro, or aspart) and two-thirds NPH to one-half short- or rapid-acting and one-half NPH. More short- or rapid-acting insulin usually is required in the morning because of the dawn phenomenon, which is caused by normal nocturnal increases in some counterregulatory hormones, producing less insulin sensitivity in the early morning.

Use of a *basal/bolus* regimen requires either an insulin pump or use of daily glargine (given once or sometimes twice per day) and doses of lispro or aspart before meals and snacks. Glargine cannot be mixed with any diluent nor with any other insulin, which means that use of this regimen requires multiple daily injections. Lispro and aspart can be given with use of an insulin pen device, which simplifies administration. Starting dose calculations are shown in Box 378.3. These doses are based on empiric formulas, and modifications can be made once responses to starting doses are assessed. Bolus doses with rapid-acting insulin have two parts to the dose: the amount of insulin needed to cover the carbohydrates in the meal (the insulin-to-carbohydrate ratio) and the amount of insulin needed to correct for a blood glucose level outside the target range (the correction or sensitivity factor). Thus, the bolus dose for a meal is calculated based on the insulin-to-carbohydrate ratio and the amount of carbohydrates the child plans to eat, and then the calculated dose is increased or decreased based on the amount that the blood glucose is above or below the target range. Target ranges may be set at 80 to 120 for daytime and 100 to 150 at bedtime, for example. When converting a child from a two- or three-shot regimen with NPH to a basal/bolus regimen, the total daily dose usually is lower and recommendations are to use 50% to 80% of the NPH dose for the initial basal insulin dose, with the lower percentages used for younger children.

Insulin pumps offer the ability to have different basal rates at different times of the day. Basal/bolus regimens offer near complete flexibility in timing and amount and content of meals and snacks.

When insulin doses are more than 1.5 U/kg/day and especially when they are at or more than 2 U/kg/day, overtreatment must be considered. Excess doses of insulin can worsen control and produce a clinical picture of widely variable blood glucose values. The Somogyi phenomenon is rebound hyperglycemia after hypoglycemia, which may be asymptomatic. It is caused by release of counterregulatory hormones (e.g., catecholamines, cortisol, glucagon, growth hormone) in response to hypoglycemia.

Improvements in the purity of insulin preparations have decreased local and systemic allergic reactions markedly. Lipoatrophy, the loss of subcutaneous adipose tissue, is a rare finding. Lipohypertrophy, increased deposits of adipose tissue, still occurs and may be related to poor injection technique. Proper site rotation is important in preventing lipohypertrophy.

Medical Nutrition Management

Children and adolescents with type 1 diabetes require a nutritionally balanced diet with adequate calories and nutrients for normal growth. The recommended diet usually contains 50% to 55% carbohydrate calories, 20% protein, and approximately 30% fat. Most carbohydrate calories are complex carbohydrates, and the fat portion should emphasize low levels of cholesterol and saturated fats. For patients using split/mixed insulin regimens, timing of meals is important in minimizing blood glucose variability. In addition to the usual three meals, midafternoon snacks are necessary, particularly because they are timed to coincide with the typical peak of the morning NPH insulin dose and with most after-school sports activities. Bedtime snacks are important for most children receiving evening NPH doses. Midmorning snacks are useful in preschool-aged children, but most school-aged children find them disruptive to their school routine. This snack usually is not recommended after a child begins elementary school. Occasional treats should be allowed by the diet plan, and patients and families should learn how to adjust insulin doses for times of increased caloric intake, such as holidays and birthdays. For patients using basal/bolus regimens, nearly total flexibility in timing and amount and content of meals is possible. The ability to achieve it requires understanding and execution of accurate counting of carbohydrates and calculation of insulin doses based on an insulin-to-carbohydrate ratio and a correction factor based on blood glucose level (Box 378.3).

Control of calories with avoidance of obesity is necessary for certain patients. A sense of satiety and a diet that fits with the family's food preferences are necessary for maximum and realistic adherence to dietary recommendations. The diet should be individualized for each child and family.

Some centers have reported an increased frequency of eating disorders, particularly in adolescent girls with type 1 diabetes. When a disorder occurs, its metabolic consequences can be devastating, and aggressive intervention (e.g., admission to an eating disorders unit) is indicated.

Nutritional management is complex, especially in sophisticated regimens when carbohydrate counting and insulin-to-carbohydrate ratios are used to determine insulin doses. This regimen is prescribed best by a nutritionist with expertise in management of diabetes.

Exercise

Physical fitness and regular exercise are important for all patients with type 1 diabetes. Insulin requirements may be lower, metabolic control improved, and self-esteem and body image improved in the physically fit child. During periods of exercise, extra calories or lower insulin doses may be needed to prevent development of hypoglycemia. Monitoring blood glucose to assess the effects of exercise on blood glucose levels and the response to therapeutic maneuvers should be performed to arrive at an effective regimen for the individual patient. Regular exercise is to be encouraged at any age because it then can become part of the child's health care regimen.

When metabolic control is poor (e.g., the child has hyperglycemia, especially with ketosis), the stress of exercise may worsen metabolic control. Some patients have a delayed hypoglycemic response to exercise, and if this response occurs, adjustments must be made in insulin dose and in calories.

Monitoring

One of the major advances since the late 1970s has been the technique of self-monitoring blood glucose. Numerous reagent strips, glucose meters, and finger-lancing devices are available. Glucose meters are small, portable, and accurate. Improvements and advances include memory storage of several hundred readings, with the date and time of the reading; the ability to add carbohydrate amounts and insulin doses to the meter memory; the ability to download the information to computers with specialized software programs; and communication of the level from the meter to an insulin pump. Development of a noninvasive blood glucose meter remains elusive.

Blood glucose traditionally is monitored before meals, before snacks (e.g., midmorning, midafternoon, bedtime), and in the middle of the night (e.g. at approximately 3:00 AM, the anticipated lowest nighttime point) if evening NPH is used. Basal/bolus regimens require a blood glucose level each time one ingests any calories to decide on what insulin dose to take. Postprandial levels are very helpful in assessing whether the selected dose was satisfactory. Many people monitor at least eight to ten times per day, more often with sports, when ill, or during periods of metabolic instability. Fasting and preprandial blood glucose readings in the 100 to180 range for preschool-aged children, 90 to 180 for school-aged children, and 90 to 130 for teenagers are reasonable goals. Bedtime or overnight levels of 110 to 200 in preschoolers, 100 to 180 in school-aged children, and 90 to 150 in teenagers also are reasonable.

Glycated hemoglobin (HbA1c) is an objective level that measures average blood glucose concentration over approximately the previous 2 months. Various assay methods are available, and normal ranges may vary. The method used in the Diabetes Control and Complications Trial (DCCT) had a normal HbA1c range of less than 6.05%.

Some patients can achieve values in the normal or near-normal range with relative ease. These children may have some residual endogenous insulin secretion. Diabetes management teams can be successful in helping patients achieve improved HbA1c levels, but some patients may not achieve levels in the goal range. HbA1c goals vary with age. For preschoolers, 7.5% to 8.5%, for school-aged children less than 8%, for adolescents <7.5% and for adults <7.0% may serve as goals. However, the occurrence of hypoglycemia will limit one's ability to achieve these goals. And, with limitations of current insulins and their methods of administration, often these target levels cannot be reached.

Urinary ketones also should be monitored. Even patients who monitor blood glucose accurately and regularly need to check urinary ketones, particularly when the blood glucose levels are above 250 mg/dL, when they have a fever, when they feel nauseous or are vomiting, or when they are just not feeling well. This monitoring is important in achieving the goal of avoiding DKA episodes by treating early ketosis.

Blood lipids should be monitored periodically. Because type 1 diabetes is associated with other autoimmune diseases, especially thyroid disease celiac disease, periodic monitoring should be performed (e.g., thyroid antibodies, thyroid-stimulating hormone, thyroxine). Patients should be seen by the health care team approximately every 3 months. Regular monitoring for ophthalmologic complications and for nephropathy is discussed later in this chapter.

Education

Education is fundamental to management and control of diabetes. Patients and families need to understand all aspects of diabetes, including acute and long-term complications. They must understand details of insulin action, including duration and timing; injection techniques; mechanics of insulin pumps; dietary information; blood glucose monitoring; and urinary ketone checks. They must gain skills in integrating the demanding clinical regimen into their schedules so that they can achieve emotional stability and ongoing psychological growth.

Education must be appropriate to the child's age and the family's educational background, and it must be ongoing. Shifting responsibility from parent to child for diabetes self-care skills (e.g., insulin injections) should be done gradually and when the child shows interest and readiness to do so. Premature shifting of responsibility may be a cause of deterioration in metabolic control. Management of diabetes is a family affair.

The life of the entire family is affected by having a child with type 1 diabetes. Sharing responsibilities and attending support groups and camps for type 1 diabetes children can help with psychological adjustment.

Teaching about diabetes management is best handled by a diabetes management team, including a physician, nurse educator, dietitian, and mental health professional. Excellent comprehensive educational manuals for children and families are available, and several comprehensive Web sites are exceptional (see end of chapter for a list of these Web sites).

PREDICTION AND PREVENTION

Knowledge concerning persistent insulin secretion after the onset of hyperglycemia and the prodrome of positive immune markers that exists prior to the onset of hyperglycemia has led to the hope that intervention to arrest or alter immune destruction could preserve beta-cell function. Unfortunately, no intervention tried to date has been successful in realizing this hope. Recent trials with insulin (Diabetes Prevention Trial [DPT1]) and a European trial with nicotinamide have not altered the natural history. Prediction models used in DPT1, though, were accurate. New national studies (Diabetes TrialNet) are being planned for the future.

Pharmacologic intervention in newly diagnosed type 1 diabetes or as a preventive measure in genetically susceptible people with positive immune markers should be done only in carefully controlled trials by qualified investigators. Treatment of individual patients with these new methods outside clinical trials should not be done. One goal of these studies may be cure. However, another important goal is maintaining some beta-cell function to produce a less severe and easier-to-manage diabetes, which should allow a significant reduction in acute and chronic diabetic complications.

TRANSPLANTATION

Whole or partial pancreas transplants have been successful in patients with type 1 diabetes, but they require lifelong immunosuppression. These transplants usually are performed only in patients with type 1 diabetes who already are receiving or will need immunosuppressive treatment for a kidney transplant. Patients with severe diabetic complications have received solo pancreatic transplants if the risk of immunosuppressive treatment was deemed to be outweighed by the risk of the diabetic complications.

Newer immunosuppressive agents and improvement in surgical approaches may broaden the criteria for pancreatic transplantation in the future.

Another approach to transplantation has been to use isolated beta cells. Some success has been achieved, with the Edmonton protocol, and additional studies in the United States are being conducted. An additional problem that remains is the source of islets. The number of brain-dead cadaver donors in the United States is insufficient to provide pancreas tissue for all the established and newly diagnosed patients with type 1 diabetes. The risk-to-benefit ratio of chronic immunosuppressive therapy does not warrant pancreatic transplantation in chil-

dren and adolescents with type 1 diabetes at this time. Studies with stem cells and novel immunologic approaches continue to be performed, with great hopes for the future.

CONTROL TO PREVENT COMPLICATIONS

The DCCT was a national study designed to assess the relation between metabolic control and microvascular complications. The primary prevention group addressed the question of whether good metabolic control can prevent the onset of diabetic complications. The secondary intervention group addressed whether improved metabolic control can prevent progression or cause regression of early complications. Released in 1993, study results showed a significant improvement in the time of onset and the rate of progression of microvascular complications in patients with intensive control compared with those with standard diabetes control. One worrisome complication of intensive control in this study was a threefold greater incidence of development of severe hypoglycemia (requiring assistance from another person).

Several other studies have shown that diabetic complications, background retinopathy, proliferative retinopathy, and nephropathy occur more frequently in patients with poorer diabetic control. The duration of type 1 diabetes correlates with the incidence of complications. The physician should aim for the best possible level of metabolic control possible for that particular child in his or her family at that specific point in time and should strive for ongoing improvement. Episodes of severe hypoglycemia may cause temporary relaxation of goals.

Blood glucose targets have been discussed previously. Even with these targets, grouped data generally show HbA1c levels 1.5 to 2.0 times that of the nondiabetic mean, and even with this level of control, the frequency of hypoglycemia may be high. Use of basal/bolus regimens including insulin infusion pumps has been successful in lowering and maintaining improved HbA1c. Possibly, the attention and motivation given to achieve good metabolic control may be more important than the actual insulin regimen. The prudent approach is to try to achieve the best possible metabolic control for each patient, tempered by the frequency and severity of hypoglycemia, concerns about excessive weight gain, and the degree of metabolic vigilance tolerable to that particular child and family.

COMPLICATIONS

Acute Complications

Hypoglycemia

Hypoglycemia (i.e., blood glucose less than 50 to 60 mg/dL) occurs in patients on insulin whether or not they are in tight metabolic control. It can occur more frequently when blood glucose levels are kept close to normal, depending on the insulin regimen used. Hypoglycemic symptoms may be mild (i.e., adrenergic symptoms of tremors, sweating, hunger, palpitations), moderate (i.e., adrenergic plus neuroglycopenic symptoms of headache, irritability or other mood change, sleepiness, confusion, inattentiveness, impaired judgment, weakness), or severe (i.e., unresponsiveness, coma, convulsions). Mild and moderate reactions can be treated by ingesting simple sugars (i.e., 10 to 15 g of glucose). Moderate reactions may require assistance by another person and additional carbohydrates. Severe reactions require treatment with intravenous glucose or parenteral glucagon (0.1 mg/kg to a maximum of 1.0 mg intramuscularly or subcutaneously). All patients' families, day-care providers, teachers, coaches, and others should learn the signs and symptoms of hypoglycemia, have a readily available source of glucose to treat it (e.g., a tube of cake frosting), and ideally have and know how to use glucagon injections to treat severe reactions. Evidence suggests that a longer duration of disease and tight metabolic control and more hypoglycemic episodes are associated with a diminished counterregulatory hormone response to hypoglycemia, and some patients develop hypoglycemic unawareness. These factors increase the risk of developing severe hypoglycemia. Young children often cannot notify their parents of hypoglycemic symptoms, and goals for metabolic control may need to be loosened. Concern exists that hypoglycemia may have deleterious effects on learning. Fear of hypoglycemia, particularly after a severe reaction, may cause long-lasting acceptance by patients and families of unacceptably high blood glucose levels (e.g., greater than 200 mg/dL).

Hyperglycemia and Ketosis

Patients with type 1 diabetes and their families must learn how to adjust insulin doses to treat the inevitable hyperglycemia that occurs with type 1 diabetes or when to call their health care provider for assistance. When ketosis occurs, they must know how to respond. Use of additional insulin doses to respond to hyperglycemia and ketosis is important in preventing progression to DKA.

Diabetic Ketoacidosis (DKA)

DKA is a common and potentially life-threatening acute complication of type 1 diabetes. DKA is the most common cause of death in patients with type 1 diabetes who are younger than mid-20s. In the United States, overall mortality from DKA is 1% to 3%. Severe DKA has a higher risk for morbidity and death. DKA can be defined as a blood glucose level usually greater than 250 mg/dL, pH less than 7.2 or 7.3, and plasma bicarbonate level of 15 or less. Severe DKA is defined as a pH of 7.1 or less and a bicarbonate level of 5 or less. Milder forms may be seen. Careful monitoring of blood glucose and urinary ketones and appropriate treatment responses to early metabolic abnormalities can prevent a significant number of DKA episodes in patients with established type 1 diabetes. In new-onset type 1 diabetes, attention given to early signs and symptoms of diabetes by the primary health care providers and families may help lower the number of newly diagnosed patients presenting with severe DKA.

The basic cause of DKA is absolute or relative insulin deficiency. Elevated levels of counterregulatory or stress hormones (e.g., glucagon, cortisol, growth hormone, catecholamines) are present. These hormonal abnormalities produce hyperglycemia (by increased glucose production and decreased utilization), which leads to an osmotic diuresis and dehydration, lipolysis and hyperlipidemia, acidosis caused by the production of ketones (i.e., acetoacetate, beta-hydroxybutyrate) from fatty acids, and electrolyte abnormalities caused by intracellular–extracellular shifts and urinary losses. Box 378.4 lists the common errors made in establishing the diagnosis of and managing DKA.

Presentation and Definition. The usual manifestations of DKA include a history of classic signs and symptoms of polyuria, polydipsia, and weight loss. After patients are sufficiently ketotic and acidotic, they have the fruity breath odor of ketosis. Many also exhibit nausea, vomiting, and lethargy. State of consciousness may vary from awake and alert (with mild DKA) to drowsiness or coma. Hyperventilation and dehydration also occur. Abdominal pain and an elevation in leukocytes may be caused solely by DKA and may be confused with an acute ab-

---

| BOX 378.4 | Common Errors in Diagnosis and Management of Diabetic Ketoacidosis |

Taking good urine output to mean the patient is not significantly dehydrated (usually occurs with new-onset type 1 diabetes)

Delaying initiation of insulin: waiting for all laboratory values to be done or waiting for infusion pump

Letting the blood glucose drop too low by not adding enough glucose to the intravenous fluids

Fluid intake that is too aggressive (too rapid or too much)

Feeding patient too early, causing nausea and vomiting before gastric peristalsis normalizes

Decreasing the intravenous insulin rate or discontinuing intravenous insulin when the blood glucose has decreased but the patient is still acidotic

Not anticipating cerebral edema

Not heeding and treating symptoms of cerebral edema (e.g., worsened sensorium, severe headache)

Not carefully reviewing clinical and laboratory data and adjusting the treatment plan as needed (i.e., rigidly adhering to a predetermined treatment regimen)

Stopping the intravenous insulin before starting subcutaneous insulin

Not giving subcutaneous insulin before a meal or snack

---

domen. These clinical findings usually resolve with therapy of DKA, but if not, an underlying cause (e.g., appendicitis) must be sought. DKA must be considered in children who are vomiting and appear dehydrated but continue to urinate excessively.

In a known diabetic patient, DKA may be precipitated by an acute infection, but it usually is caused by omission of insulin that may be deliberate or based on a misconception that insulin doses should be eliminated or significantly decreased because of anorexia or vomiting. Disconnection from insulin infusion without proper monitoring in patients on insulin pumps also is a cause. Careful monitoring of blood glucose levels and urinary ketones and appropriate therapeutic response can help avoid many DKA episodes.

Recurrent DKA in most cases now is thought to be caused by deliberate omission of insulin, sometimes by a child without the parents' knowledge and sometimes by the child and parents in collusion. Putting a responsible adult in charge of the insulin injections and using a simplified regimen may be successful in lowering the number of or in eliminating the DKA episodes.

The degree of hyperglycemia does not correlate necessarily with the degree of acidosis, and patients may be severely acidotic but only minimally hyperglycemic. The diagnosis of DKA can be established rapidly at the bedside with a meter glucose reading and a urinary or serum ketone determination using strips or tablets.

Treatment. The basic components of DKA treatment are fluid and electrolyte replacement (with careful attention to potassium) and insulin, which must be performed with frequent monitoring of clinical and laboratory factors, using a flow sheet (Table 378.2) and paying careful attention to details and trends.

Fluid Replacement. Dehydration affects virtually all patients with DKA. Water and electrolyte losses occur because of polyuria caused by the osmotic diuresis produced by glycosuria, hyperventilation, vomiting, and diarrhea. The best measure of dehydration is the patient's current weight compared

TABLE 378.2

DIABETIC KETOACIDOSIS FLOW SHEET

Feature	Monitoring Schedule
Clinical data	
Weight	Onset of treatment
Vital signs	Onset of treatment and every 1–2 hours initially
State of consciousness	Onset of treatment and every 1–2 hours initially
Laboratory data	
Electrolytes (Na, K, Cl, and HCO$_3$), venous pH	Every 1–2 hours for the first 4–8 hours, then every 2–4 hours until diabetic ketoacidosis is cleared
Glucose	Hourly
Blood urea nitrogen, creatinine, calcium, phosphate levels	Every 4–8 hours depending on initial levels and type of fluids used
Urinary ketone level	Every void
Fluids	Type and rate; record hourly input
Urine output	Record every void
Potassium, phosphate, bicarbonate	Record amounts added to fluid
Insulin	Dose, rate, and route

with a recent, healthy weight. Dry mucous membranes, poor skin turgor, and orthostatic hypotension are clinical indications of dehydration. Most patients with DKA are 5% to 10% dehydrated. Patients in shock may have greater degrees of dehydration.

Adequate intravenous replacement of fluids is extremely important and should begin as soon as the diagnosis of DKA is established. Normal saline (NS) or Ringer lactate, an isotonic solution, is recommended initially because it helps to restore the intravascular volume and, thereby, maintain blood pressure and kidney perfusion, which enhances glucose loss through the kidney, resulting in a lower blood glucose level.

A variety of published recommendations exist for the amount and rate of fluid replacement. The recommendations discussed in this section are the ones most generally accepted. For initial rehydration or resuscitation, 10 to 20 mL/kg of NS is given in the first hour. Some clinicians prefer Ringer lactate. Rarely, colloid (i.e., albumin) may be needed for patients in shock. After the first hour, the patient's state of hydration should be reassessed. If evidence of poor perfusion (e.g., hypotension, delayed capillary refill) still is present, another infusion of NS (10 to 20 mL/kg) may be needed in the second hour.

After this initial reexpansion, half isotonic saline (0.45 NS) should be used unless the patient is significantly hyperosmolar, when NS should continue. This phase of replacement and rehydration takes into account maintenance requirements, replacement of the fluid deficit, and, if excessive, ongoing losses. Maintenance requirements plus the deficit can be given evenly over the course of 48 hours. Slower replacement (over the course of 48 hours or longer) may be needed when marked hyperosmolality or high calculated serum sodium levels are present. Recommendations for a maximum of 4 L/m^2/day of fluid also have been made (see paragraph on cerebral edema in Complications, later). Urinary catheters rarely are needed. Nasogastric tubes may be needed in obtunded, vomiting patients; for patients in shock, monitoring central venous pressure may be needed.

Insulin. Continuous low-dose insulin infusion is the method of choice. Short-acting (regular) insulin is used. The advantages of a continuous intravenous insulin infusion are the elimination of the problem of poor absorption from subcutaneous and intramuscular sites in a dehydrated patient and rapid clearance, allowing easy dose adjustment, which renders management more controllable. The usual recommended dose is 0.1 U/kg/hour. Sometimes a bolus of the same dose is given before starting the insulin infusion. Running the infusate (30 to 50 mL) through the tubing to saturate binding sites on the tubing is recommended. The insulin infusion is given best separately from the replacement fluids so that the rates can be adjusted independently, and it is best to use an infusion pump.

If no improvement in acidosis is seen within approximately 2 hours, the intravenous insulin rate should be increased to 0.15 or 0.20 U/kg/hour.

Glucose. A decrease in glucose should occur at a rate of approximately 75 to 100 mg/dL/hour. In the first hour or two of treatment, a decrease in glucose level from the initial rehydration fluids occurs as intravascular volume expands.

The blood glucose level corrects to normal levels more quickly than does the acidosis, and intravenous insulin must be continued until the acidosis is cleared. Continuing the intravenous insulin infusion until urinary ketones are cleared may enable easier management after the infusion is discontinued and subcutaneous insulin is started. If the blood glucose level decreases to 250 mg/dL and acidosis is still present, glucose should be added to intravenous fluids, starting with 5% dextrose and increasing as needed to 7.5% or 10% dextrose to keep the blood glucose at approximately 250 mg/dL. If the blood glucose level is less than 300 at the onset of treatment, adding 5% dextrose at the onset of therapy is useful. In some patients, despite the use of 10% dextrose, the blood glucose may fall too low (perhaps less than 100 mg/dL), and decreasing (not discontinuing) the intravenous insulin infusion rate may be necessary.

Potassium. Patients with DKA have total-body potassium depletion, but the measured serum potassium may be high, normal, or low. An exchange of intracellular potassium ions for extracellular hydrogen ions occurs. Treatment with insulin causes potassium to move intracellularly, causing a decrease in serum potassium. Both hypokalemia and hyperkalemia are potential causes of death, and, therefore, the serum potassium must be monitored every 1 to 2 hours; potassium should not be added to the intravenous fluids until the serum potassium level is known and the patient is voiding. Electrocardiography performed while awaiting the potassium level can help assess whether hypokalemia or hyperkalemia is present.

If serum potassium is elevated at the onset of treatment, adding potassium to the intravenous fluids should not be done until the serum potassium has fallen into the normal range. If the potassium is normal or low, potassium should be added to the intravenous fluids unless renal failure exists. Generally, 40 mEq/L is used. If the serum potassium is low, more than 40 mEq/L may be needed and careful monitoring (e.g., electrocardiography, frequent blood determinations) is required. Potassium chloride, potassium phosphate, or potassium acetate may be used.

Sodium. Patients with DKA have lost sodium through the urine and have a total-body sodium loss. Most have low serum sodium levels, probably caused by hyperglycemia, which has osmotic pressure and causes dilution of the extracellular sodium. Lipemic serum falsely lowers the sodium level. During DKA treatment, serum sodium levels should be monitored closely to ensure that the sodium concentration is not decreasing. A failure of serum sodium to increase as glucose levels decrease may be a marker for excess free water (see paragraph on cerebral edema in Complications, later). An increase in serum sodium as the glucose level falls helps prevent rapid osmolality changes. The osmolality should be calculated (2 [Na] + [glucose]/18) to ensure that it remains in the normal (not low) range. Sodium replacement involves intravenous NS, 10 to 20 mL/kg during the first hour and 10 to 20 mL/kg during the second hour, if indicated. After this initial volume reexpansion, 0.45 NS is recommended. If serum osmolality drops, NS (instead of 0.45 NS) is needed.

Phosphate. Phosphate depletion occurs in DKA because of poor food intake, the catabolic state, and urinary losses. Insulin treatment causes phosphate to move intracellularly, lowering serum phosphate levels. In clinical studies, routine administration of phosphate has not been demonstrated to have any advantage in treatment of DKA. Potential theoretic benefits for use of phosphate exist; phosphate depletion can impair the central nervous system and myocardial function, cause insulin resistance, and shift the hemoglobin–oxygen dissociation curve to impair oxygen delivery to the tissues.

Phosphate replacement is indicated when the serum phosphate is very low, less than 2 mEq/L. Many clinicians recommend some phosphate replacement (not more than 1.5 mEq/kg/day) for approximately 8 to 12 hours after the initial fluid reexpansion, with potassium added as half potassium chloride and half potassium phosphate. One advantage of using part potassium phosphate instead of all potassium chloride is that less chloride is given. When phosphate is given, a risk of hypocalcemia exists, and calcium levels must be monitored.

Bicarbonate. Treatment of DKA with bicarbonate to help correct acidosis has been controversial. The treatment of DKA with insulin generates bicarbonate as ketones are metabolized, and bicarbonate is not needed in mild or moderate DKA. These patients gradually correct their acidosis as insulin and fluid treatment proceed. Potential risks of bicarbonate include overtreatment producing a metabolic alkalosis, greater risks of hypokalemia, and paradoxic cerebrospinal fluid acidosis. Clinical trials of bicarbonate in severe DKA have not shown improvement in outcome of DKA whether or not bicarbonate was used. Bicarbonate use should be reserved for patients who are severely acidotic when the acidosis may threaten respiratory or cardiac function (e.g., pH less than 7.0 and bicarbonate less than 5) and only for a small partial correction (e.g., to raise the pH to 7.2, maximum). Generally, 1 to 2 mEq/kg of bicarbonate given over the course of approximately 2 hours and added to the first bottle of half-NS (0.45 NS) can be given. The pH should be rechecked approximately 30 minutes after the infusion is given. Bicarbonate should not be given to hypokalemic patients until treatment with potassium is ongoing.

Converting to Subcutaneous Insulin. Patients should be continued on intravenous fluids and an intravenous insulin infusion until they are clinically stable with normal sensorium and normal vital signs, until the acidosis is cleared (i.e., normal venous pH and bicarbonate), and until they can take fluids and food orally without vomiting. Any identified precipitating factor (e.g., infection) should have been treated. Subcutaneous insulin requires time to take effect, and the intravenous insulin infusion must be continued for approximately 30 minutes after the first subcutaneous dose of insulin is given to prevent insulin levels from becoming too low, which would allow recurrence of lipolysis and ketogenesis. A dose of short- or rapid-acting insulin is given before a meal, and then the insulin drip is discontinued approximately 30 minutes later.

The switch from intravenous to subcutaneous insulin is done best during the daytime.

The choice of which insulin regimen, a split/mixed regimen or a basal/bolus regimen, to start the treatment can be discussed with the family and then begun as DKA clears. Frequent blood glucose measurements and urinary ketone checks are important. Adjustment of the dose depends on the patient's blood glucose responses to previous subcutaneous doses. When the patient's usual insulin requirement is known and the precipitating factor of the DKA is cleared, the patient may be able to resume his or her usual dose of insulin as soon as normal caloric intake is reestablished. For example, a well-controlled child who had an episode of moderate DKA because an insulin dose was skipped while the child had a viral gastroenteritis probably could resume the usual insulin schedule fairly soon after the DKA has cleared and he or she can eat normally. For example, DKA is cleared at approximately 1 AM, the intravenous fluids and intravenous insulin have been continued through the night, vomiting has ceased, and the child can eat and drink without nausea. The usual morning dose may be satisfactory before breakfast. Some patients may need lower insulin doses after a DKA episode because of decreased caloric intake, but some may need more. Frequent monitoring of blood glucose and urinary ketones is imperative. Newly diagnosed patients need to have their current insulin requirements established, after discussion about which type of regimen to use.

Two common errors occur during this transition period. First, the intravenous insulin infusion is discontinued without giving subcutaneous insulin, and the patient becomes hyperglycemic, ketotic, and even acidotic within several hours. This decision is made because the blood glucose is normal or low and the acidosis may or may not have cleared. If this condition occurs during the night, 4 to 8 hours may transpire before the deterioration of the patient's metabolic control is appreciated. The second common error is to withhold insulin before a meal because the blood glucose is normal or low. When this is done, the blood glucose increases to high levels after eating, and the general response is to give insulin to lower the blood glucose level, which may fluctuate over a wide range during the remainder of the day. The best approach is to give short- or rapid-acting insulin before eating to prevent a postprandial glucose rise.

DKA Prevention. Many episodes of DKA can be prevented by vigilance and careful monitoring of blood glucose and urinary ketones. Urinary ketones should be checked whenever blood glucose is elevated to approximately 250 mg/dL or higher and if the patient is feeling ill. This requirement cannot be overemphasized. When ketone test results become positive (moderate to large), extra short- or rapid-acting insulin can be given until the ketones are clear. Failure to monitor, failure to recognize or pay attention to symptoms of illness, and failure to contact the health care team early may lead to episodes of DKA that could have been prevented. Proper sick day management can prevent DKA. Recurrent DKA is caused uniformly by deliberate insulin omission, often in dysfunctional families, but it also may be caused by putting too much responsibility for management of the diabetes on a child or adolescent without providing adequate parental supervision.

Sick Day Management. Deterioration of metabolic control during infections in children is caused in part by the increase in stress or counterregulatory hormones, which have hyperglycemic and lipolytic effects and which produce relative insulin deficiency and requirements for increased insulin. Alternatively, because decreases in caloric intake occur with illness in children, especially with nausea and vomiting, insulin requirements may drop, and hypoglycemia may occur. The goals of sick day management are the prevention and treatment of hypoglycemia and significant hyperglycemia and ketosis, and the prevention of DKA. The physician's advice is essential, as is parental supervision. Sick day management should not be left to a child or teenager. The underlying illness (e.g., infection) needs to be diagnosed and treated. The basis of management includes frequent blood glucose and urinary ketone checks (at least every 4 hours for blood glucose and every void for urinary ketones); insulin adjustment (using short- or rapid-acting insulin) based on blood glucose levels and urinary ketones; and substitution of equivalent calories of sugar-containing fluids (e.g., soda, fruit juice, Jell-O, popsicles) if the child cannot or will not eat solids. Depending on the type of illness, the insulin dose may be the usual daily dose, with short- or rapid-acting insulin doses adjusted up or down for blood glucose levels; a decrease in the usual daily dose with short- or rapid-acting insulin adjusted for blood glucose levels; or only short- or rapid-acting insulin given approximately every 3 to 4 hours. Persistent vomiting (i.e., several times in a row so that no calories are retained) or refusal to take fluids or food orally requires an emergency department or clinic visit. Glucagon must be available in the home. Supplemental short- or rapid-acting insulin at doses of 10% to 20% of the 24-hour requirement given every 3 to 4 hours often is effective in preventing significant hyperglycemia and in clearing or preventing ketosis.

Other Management Topics. Ketones (e.g., acetoacetate) interfere with creatinine measurements. A child with DKA may have an elevated creatinine, suggesting he or she is in renal failure when it is a spurious measurement. Creatinine should be rechecked as the ketoacidosis clears. Use of Acetest tablets to determine the presence of serum ketones helps to establish a diagnosis of DKA rapidly. However, serum dilutions (titers) on Acetest tablets are not useful in establishing the severity of the acidosis. Acetest tablets (i.e., nitroprusside reaction) do not measure beta-hydroxybutyrate, which is the major ketone in DKA. Because treatment of DKA causes a shift toward acetoacetate from beta-hydroxybutyrate, using this qualitative ketone method may suggest that the patient's condition is worsening, although total ketones and acidosis are improving. Thus, this method is not useful in following the course of DKA treatment. It is not necessary to wait for an infusion pump to arrive to start insulin. One hour's worth of insulin can be put in an intravenous solution and infused over the course of 1 hour. If the timing is not exact, no harm occurs. Delay in starting fluids and insulin leads to worsening of the patient's clinical status.

The diagnosis of DKA can be established rapidly at the bedside by a meter blood glucose reading and a rapid assessment of serum ketones (i.e., Acetest method). Usually, a venous pH measure will be available rapidly. The initial fluid reexpansion then can be started. Insulin can be started immediately or delayed by 1 to 2 hours. Treatment should be started if the diagnosis of DKA is evident, without waiting for all the laboratory results. However, potassium should not be added to the intravenous fluids until the serum potassium level is known. Electrocardiography can help establish rapidly whether the serum potassium level is low, normal, or high.

Cerebral Edema

Cerebral edema is an unpredictable, often fatal, and uniformly feared complication of treating DKA. It usually occurs when biochemical abnormalities are improving. Cerebral edema probably accounts for one-half or more of DKA-associated deaths. Subclinical brain swelling occurs often during treatment of DKA. Factors implicated but not pinpointed as possible causes of cerebral edema are a decrease in blood glucose that is too rapid, decreasing the blood glucose to an excessively low level, excessive administration of fluids, tonicity of intravenous fluids, failure of the serum sodium to increase during treatment, and the use of bicarbonate.

Rosenbloom's comprehensive review of 69 cases of intracerebral complications in DKA found that infants and children younger than 5 years old and patients with new-onset diabetes made up an excessive proportion of cases. In this review, rate or tonicity of hydration fluids, rate of decrease of blood glucose, amount of sodium given, degree of decrease in serum sodium concentration, or the use of bicarbonate could not be implicated as causes of cerebral edema. One-half of the patients had histories suggesting that dramatic changes in neurologic status occurred before respiratory arrest occurred, and patients receiving treatment before respiratory arrest had a better outcome. This review indicated that close neurologic monitoring and providing treatment to decrease raised intracranial pressure (ICP), when definite signs of neurologic deterioration occur, could improve outcome. Rosenbloom concluded, "Treatment appears to be successful in only 50 percent of patients who give sufficient warning for such intervention, and they comprised half of the study population."

Prevention of DKA is essential. Other studies have shown that fluid intakes above 4.0 L/m^2/day are associated with more cases of cerebral edema. Failure of serum sodium to increase in the face of decreasing glucose levels, which may indicate excess administration of free water, occurs more frequently in patients with complications attributable to brain edema. Use of bicarbonate also has been associated with cerebral edema. Until the causes of cerebral edema are better defined, paying attention to all of these factors in the treatment of DKA seems to be prudent, but anticipating cerebral edema, knowing it occurs more commonly in infants and young children and with new-onset diabetes, is important. The physician should be prepared to recognize the signs and symptoms of increased ICP, such as severe headache, changes in arousal and sensorium or behavior, changes in blood pressure, dilated pupils, problems with temperature regulation, slow pulse, and onset of incontinence. Careful clinical monitoring is essential. Treatment involves providing intravenous mannitol 1 g/kg. Mannitol should be located by the bedside or nearby for the first 24 hours of treatment. However, even early treatment did not prevent severe or fatal central nervous system damage in almost one-half of the patients in one study.

Chronic Complications and Comorbidities

Autoimmune Disease

Associated autoimmune disease, particularly thyroid dysfunction, occurs with greater frequency with type 1 diabetes. Thyroid function should be monitored periodically (every 1 to 2 years in patients with type 1 diabetes). Thyroid-stimulating hormone, T_4, and thyroid antibodies may be monitored. Although rare, autoimmune adrenal hypofunction can occur, and symptoms to suggest its presence should prompt appropriate testing.

Celiac disease also occurs more frequently in children with type 1 diabetes, and all patients should be screened for it at least once. Tissue transglutaminase and antiendomysial antibodies are more sensitive and specific than are antigliadin antibodies. Also, because these are IgA antibodies, ensuring that the individual patient is not IgA-deficient by obtaining an IgA level is important.

Joint Dysfunction

Limited joint mobility, perhaps caused by glycosylation of tissue proteins, is a marker for long-term poor control and is associated with other complications (e.g., retinopathy, nephropathy, and neuropathy). The hands and other joints should be examined.

Growth Disturbance

Linear growth is affected negatively by poor diabetic control. Decreased growth velocity, crossing percentiles downward for height and weight, eventual short stature, and delayed skeletal and sexual maturation are associated with chronic undertreatment with insulin. An extreme form of this—the Mauriac syndrome, or diabetic dwarfism—occurs rarely and usually is associated with hepatomegaly. Careful height and weight measurements should be obtained at every appointment and plotted on growth curves so that deviations from normal velocities can be detected early. Alternatively, treatment with excessive insulin doses often leads to excessive weight gain, causing the weight curve to cross percentiles upward. The maintenance of normal growth curves for height and weight is an important goal of diabetes management.

Retinopathy

Most patients with type 1 diabetes develop background retinopathy after 15 to 20 years of having the disease. The percentage of patients developing proliferative retinopathy is less, with studies reporting incidences of 20% to 50%. Approximately 5% to 10% of patients with type 1 diabetes become blind. Early treatment with laser photocoagulation can reduce significantly the rate of progression to blindness. All patients with type 1 diabetes should be evaluated annually by an ophthalmologist, with regular-interval eye examinations performed by the child's pediatrician and diabetes physician. These yearly examinations should begin 3 to 5 years after the diagnosis of diabetes is established, once the child is 10 years old or older. Factors increasing the risk of development of retinopathy are hypertension, poor metabolic control, elevated blood lipids, smoking, and pregnancy. Increased diabetes duration also is associated with increased risk of developing retinopathy. The DCCT clearly showed that intensive blood glucose control delayed onset and slowed progression of retinopathy.

Nephropathy

Approximately 30% to 40% of patients with type 1 diabetes eventually develop end-stage renal disease and need dialysis or transplantation. End-stage renal disease is an important cause of morbidity and mortality. Diabetic nephropathy is characterized by proteinuria, which may be severe, producing a nephrotic syndrome, hypertension, initial hyperfiltration (i.e., increased glomerular filtrate rate), and progressive renal insufficiency (i.e., increasing serum creatinine and urea nitrogen, decreasing glomerular filtrate rate). Glomerular damage, especially mesangial expansion and basement membrane thickening, is the most characteristic histologic finding. The importance of tight metabolic control to prevent nephropathy or slow its progression has been shown by the DCCT.

A genetic predisposition may be an important underlying factor. All patients with type 1 diabetes should be monitored by urine microalbumin at least annually after the first few years of having the disease, but perhaps starting in the first year after the diagnosis is made. Blood pressure should be monitored accurately several times a year. If hypertension, overt proteinuria, or elevation in serum creatinine or urea nitrogen is found, monitoring of renal function several times each year and consultation with a nephrologist is warranted. Microalbuminuria (less than 200 to 250 mg/day) is a marker for the early stages of nephropathy. Low-protein diets have been successful in slowing or preventing progression of renal insufficiency in type 1 diabetes, but concerns exist about their use in growing children.

Hypertension is an extremely important factor that is known to accelerate the progression of nephropathy. It should be treated aggressively. Angiotensin-converting enzyme inhibitors are recommended. Whether using angiotensin-converting enzyme inhibitors to lower blood pressures already in the normal range is useful in preventing or retarding nephropathy is not known. Patients should avoid other risk factors, such as smoking.

Neuropathy

Symptomatic diabetic neuropathy, peripheral or autonomic, is an uncommon occurrence in children and adolescents with type 1 diabetes, although changes in nerve conduction may be measured after they have had the disease for 4 to 5 years. Overall, neuropathy is a common type 1 diabetes complication, and its frequency increases with the duration of disease and degree of hyperglycemia. Improvements in glycemic control may help neuropathic symptoms.

Macrovascular Complications/Lipids

Patients with type 1 diabetes tend to have coronary artery, cerebrovascular, and peripheral vascular disease more often, at an earlier age, and more extensively than does the nondiabetic population. Hypertension, elevated blood lipid levels, and cigarette smoking are other risk factors for developing macrovascular complications. Risk factor assessment, including lipid panels, blood pressure measurements, and determination of smoking status, should be done, and treatment should be instituted as indicated. A strong admonition against smoking and referral to an appropriate program for patients who already are smokers is indicated. Studies continue to show that lower and lower low-density lipoprotein (LDL) levels are beneficial in lowering the risk of development of vascular disease, and recommendations continue to evolve. Recommendations at the current time are to treat children with LDL cholesterol at or above 160 and to consider treatment if LDL is at or above 130 if life style and dietary changes are not successful and if other risk factors are present. Treatment goals are to achieve an LDL below 100. Although bile acid sequestrants usually are recommended as the first line in children, they are tolerated poorly and effective therapeutic data is lacking. Thus, statins should be considered with appropriate monitoring. Of course, dietary counseling and blood glucose control are important parts of management.

Web Sites

International Society for Pediatric and Adolescent Diabetes diabetes guidelines: www.ispad.org
American Diabetes Association: www.diabetes.org
Children with Diabetes: www.childrenwithdiabetes.com

Suggested Readings

American Academy of Pediatrics. Screening for retinopathy in the pediatric patient with type 1 diabetes mellitus. *Pediatrics* 1998;101:313.

American Diabetes Association. Management of dyslipidemia in children and adolescents with diabetes. *Diabetes Care* 2003;26:2194.

American Diabetes Association. Nephropathy in diabetes. *Diabetes Care* 2004; 27:S79.

American Diabetes Association. Standards of medical care for patients with diabetes mellitus. *Diabetes Care* 2004: 27:S15.

Brink SJ, Moltz K. The message of the DCCT for children and adolescents. *Diabetes Spectrum* 1997;10:259.

Chase HP. *Understanding insulin dependent diabetes (Pink Panther)*, 10th ed. Denver: Barbara Davis Center for Childhood Diabetes, Children's Diabetes Foundation, 2002.

Chase HP, Dixon B, Pearson J, et al. Reduced hypoglycemic episodes and improved glycemic control in children with type 1 diabetes using insulin glargine and NPH. *J Pediatr* 2003;143:737.

DCCT Research Group. The effect of intensive diabetes treatment on long-term complications in adolescents with IDDM: the DCCT. *J Pediatr* 1994; 125:177.

DCCT Research Group. The effect of intensive diabetes treatment on the development and progression of long-term complications in IDDM: the DCCT. *N Engl J Med* 1993;329:977.

Diabetes Prevention Trial-Type 1 Diabetes Study Group. Effect of insulin in relatives of patients with type 1 diabetes mellitus. *N Engl J Med* 2002;346:1685.

Duck SC, Wyatt DT. Factors associated with brain herniation in the treatment of DKA. *J Pediatr* 1988;113:10.

Ellis EN. Concepts of fluid restriction in DKA and HHNC. *Pediatr Clin North Am* 1990;37:313.

Expert Committee. Report of the Expert Committee on the diagnosis and classification of diabetes mellitus. *Diabetes Care* 1997;20:1183.

Glaser N, Barnett P, McCaslin I, et al. Risk factors for cerebral edema in children with diabetic ketoacidosis. The Pediatric Emergency Medicine Collaborative Research Committee of the American Academy of Pediatrics. *N Engl J Med* 2002;344:264.

Harris GD, Fiordalisi I, Harris WL, et al. Minimizing the risk of brain herniation during treatment of DKA: a retrospective and prospective study. *J Pediatr* 1990;117:22.

Marcin JP, Glaser N, Barnett P, et al. Factors associated with adverse outcomes in children with diabetic ketoacidosis-related cerebral edema. *J Pediatr* 2002;141:793.

Plotnick LP, Clark LM, Brancati FL, Erlinger T. Safety and effectiveness of insulin pump therapy in children and adolescents with type 1 diabetes. *Diabetes Care* 2003;26:1142.

Plotnick LP, Henderson R. *Clinical management of the child and adolescent with diabetes.* Baltimore: Johns Hopkins University Press, 1998.

Rewers M, Klingensmith GJ. Prevention of type 1 diabetes. *Diabetes Spectrum* 1997;10:282.

Rosenbloom AL. Intracerebral crises during treatment of DKA. *Diabetes Care* 1990;13:22.

Ryan CM, Becker DJ. Hypoglycemia in children with type 1 diabetes-risk factors, cognitive function and management. *Endocrinol Metab Clin North Am* 1999; 28:883.

Silverstein J, Klinginsmith G, Copeland K, et al. Care of children and adolescents with type 1 diabetes. A statement of the American Diabetes Association *Diabetes Care* 2005;28:186.

Tamberlane WV, Ahern J. Implications and results of the DCCT. *Pediatr Clin North Am* 1997;44:285.

White NH, Cleary PA, Dahma W, et al. Beneficial effects of intensive therapy of diabetes during adolescence: outcomes after the conclusion of the DCCT. *J Pediatr* 2001;139:804.

CHAPTER 379 ■ TYPE 2 DIABETES MELLITUS

DAVID W. COOKE

Type 2 diabetes mellitus is a disorder of glucose and lipid regulation caused by a combination of decreased insulin effectiveness at the cellular level and impaired insulin secretion. Because untreated type 2 diabetes does not generally deteriorate to ketoacidosis, it is a form of non–insulin-dependent diabetes mellitus (NIDDM). Until recently, type 2 diabetes was considered a disease of adulthood, being rarely diagnosed in children. In fact, it is a disease whose prevalence increases with age so that it was also uncommon in young adults. In recent decades, however, the prevalence of type 2 diabetes has been increasing in adults, and it has been identified in larger numbers of younger adults. This "epidemic" of type 2 diabetes has extended into childhood so that now significant numbers of children diagnosed with diabetes have type 2 diabetes, in contrast to the recent past, when type 1 diabetes would have been the only likely diagnosis.

EPIDEMIOLOGY

The recent diabetes epidemic has resulted in a 40% increase in the prevalence of diabetes in U.S. adults during the 1990s, with more than 6.5% of the U.S. population now having diabetes. Type 2 diabetes is the most common form of diabetes, accounting for 90% or more of these cases. Both genetic and environmental factors contribute to the risk of developing type 2 diabetes. Genetic factors explain the increased risk in individuals with a positive family history, as well as the variation in the prevalence of the disease across different racial and ethnic groups, with increased risk in African American, Hispanic, Asian, and Native American populations compared to Caucasians. The most significant environmental factor is the association of type 2 diabetes with obesity: whereas type 2 diabetes can occur in nonobese individuals, more than 90% of those who develop diabetes are obese. Criteria for screening children for type 2 diabetes are listed in Box 379.1.

Before the 1990s, fewer than 2% of children with diabetes were thought to have type 2 diabetes. During the 1990s, however, reports began to document a rising prevalence of type 2 diabetes in pediatric patients. The percentage of cases of diabetes in children and adolescents that are type 2 diabetes depends on the proportion that are adolescents, the prevalence and degree of obesity, and the racial and ethnic composition of the population, but now it may be as high as one-half of

---

BOX 379.1 | **Criteria for Screening Children for Type 2 Diabetes**

Age ≥10 years or children <10 years of age in whom puberty has begun

   Plus

Overweight (body mass index [BMI] >85th percentile for age and sex, weight for height >85th percentile, or weight >120 percentile of ideal for height)

   Plus

Any two of the following risk factors:

- Family history of type 2 diabetes in first- or second-degree relatives
- Of the following race/ethnicity: American Indian, African American, Hispanic, Asian/Pacific Islander
- Signs of insulin resistance or conditions associated with insulin resistance (acanthosis nigricans, hypertension, dyslipidemia, polycystic ovary syndrome)

Adapted from American Diabetes Association. Type 2 diabetes in children and adolescents. *Pediatrics* 2000;105:671.

newly diagnosed cases. Although there are not yet accurate population-wide prevalence estimates for type 2 diabetes in children and adolescents, the data indicate a rising prevalence that has yet to plateau. There has been a female predominance in diagnosed cases of type 2 diabetes, with a female-to-male ratio of approximately 2:1.

The majority of children presenting with type 2 diabetes are obese (body mass index [BMI] above the 95th percentile for age), with many being extremely obese. As in adults, however, a small percentage of children with type 2 diabetes are not obese. Most children will present with type 2 diabetes during puberty. The explanation for this is that in all children, puberty is associated with an approximately 30% decrease in insulin sensitivity; in the predisposed individual this additional challenge to glucose homeostasis may not be met, resulting in type 2 diabetes. Thus far, it remains relatively uncommon for children to present with type 2 diabetes before puberty, although that does occur.

Hypertension and a specific form of dyslipidemia (hypertriglyceridemia and decreased high-density lipoprotein [HDL] cholesterol level) associate together in obese adults in a syndrome referred to as the metabolic syndrome or syndrome X. Insulin resistance, one of the main defects leading to type 2 diabetes, is also a part of this syndrome, and adults with the metabolic syndrome are at increased risk of type 2 diabetes, so that hypertension and dyslipidemia may also indicate an increased risk of type 2 diabetes in children.

Adults who have blood glucose levels that fall within a "prediabetes" range of impaired glucose regulation are at very high risk of developing type 2 diabetes within several years—up to 40% in 5 to 10 years. However, there are not yet data available to demonstrate that impaired fasting glucose (IFG) or impaired glucose tolerance (IGT; see later) in children or adolescents indicates the same increased risk for the development of type 2 diabetes as in adults. One possible confounder that could alter this relationship of glucose levels with later risk of diabetes is the insulin resistance of puberty that resolves at the end of puberty.

There is a strong genetic component to the risk of type 2 diabetes (Box 379.2).

PATHOGENESIS

Because the emergence of type 2 diabetes as a significant pediatric disease has been a recent development, there may be aspects of the disease specific to pediatric patients that are not yet known. Current knowledge, however, has indicated that

---

BOX 379.2   Genetic Factors as a Cause of Type 2 Diabetes

Virtually all children identified with type 2 diabetes will have a family history of type 2 diabetes, and most will have a parent with type 2 diabetes. Type 2 diabetes is felt to be a multigenic disorder; that is, it is caused by the combined effects of a number of genes (and the effects of environmental factors) rather than being the result of a mutation of a single gene. Although a number of genes have now been implicated as potential contributors to the genetic risk of type 2 diabetes (including the genes for the peroxisome proliferator-activated receptor-gamma [PPAR-gamma]; the beta-3-adrenergic receptor; calpain-10; and insulin receptor substrate 1 [IRS-1]), current knowledge of the identity of type 2 diabetes genes is very incomplete. Notably, many genes in the glucose metabolism, insulin secretion, and insulin signaling pathways have been investigated and excluded as significant type 2 diabetes genes. Individuals with homozygous or compound heterozygous mutations of the insulin receptor do have syndromes with extreme insulin resistance, but these are distinct from type 2 diabetes. The phenotype associated with these mutations varies from relatively normal glucose control (rarely) or diabetes identified in adolescence (type A insulin resistance) to more severe phenotypes evident in infancy (Rabson-Mendenhall syndrome and leprechaunism, which is usually fatal in infancy).

There is a type of non–insulin-dependent diabetes for which the genetic cause is known. These are the single gene mutations that lead to maturity-onset diabetes in youth (MODY), inherited in an autosomal dominant manner and resulting in diabetes that usually has its onset before age 25 years. Six separate MODY types have been identified. These are due to mutations in the genes for glucokinase (MODY2) and for transcription factors: hepatocyte nuclear factor (HNF)-4-alpha (MODY1); HNF-1-alpha (MODY3); insulin promoter factor-1 (IPF1; MODY4); HNF-1-beta (MODY5); and neurogenic differentiation 1/beta-cell E-box transactivator 2 (NeuroD1/BETA2; MODY6). These genes are all expressed in the pancreatic beta cell, and heterozygous mutations cause a deficiency in insulin secretion. Because insulin resistance is not part of the pathophysiology, obesity is not a feature of MODY. The severity of the insulin deficiency varies for the different MODY types, and consequently the severity of the untreated diabetes can vary from mild, sometimes unrecognized hyperglycemia with little risk of long-term microvascular diabetic complications to severe hyperglycemia with a very high risk of microvascular complications. However, in contrast to the ultimately total insulin deficiency of type 1 diabetes, there is generally sufficient insulin secretion in MODY to prevent ketosis. It is necessary to emphasize that the recent increased prevalence of non–insulin-dependent diabetes in children is not due to children with MODY. MODY is a relatively uncommon cause of diabetes, responsible for less than 5% of adult cases of diabetes. As in adults, the vast majority of children and adolescents with non–insulin-dependent diabetes have type 2 diabetes.

Genetic and environmental factors affecting fetal growth may also alter the risk for the development of type 2 diabetes. Intrauterine growth restriction (IUGR) is associated with an increased risk of type 2 diabetes in adulthood, and children with a history of IUGR have decreased insulin sensitivity. As other environmental factors increase the risk of diabetes, the increased insulin resistance in these children is likely to further increase their risk of developing type 2 diabetes during childhood. At the opposite extreme, overnutrition of the fetus, as occurs in infants born to diabetic mothers, also increases the risk of type 2 diabetes for the offspring. From a public health perspective, this is very concerning, given the increasing prevalence of diabetes in younger individuals, the result of which potentially will lead to more pregnancies in women with diabetes, setting the stage for an explosion of the type 2 diabetes epidemic.

the pathophysiology of type 2 diabetes in children mirrors that of the adult disease, although physiologic changes of puberty contribute a unique aspect to the pathophysiology.

Two defects are present in patients with type 2 diabetes: insulin resistance and defective insulin secretion. Insulin resistance refers to a decreased effectiveness of insulin in activating signals distal to binding of insulin to the insulin receptor. Insulin resistance itself, except in the most extreme situation, will not lead to diabetes, as normal metabolic control can be maintained by a compensatory increase in insulin secretion. When a second defect results in an inability to respond to the requirement for increased insulin secretion imposed by insulin resistance, type 2 diabetes mellitus occurs. There is evidence, however, that at least in some of the at-risk ethnic populations, the increased risk of diabetes is related to increased insulin resistance. The data supporting this are strongest for African Americans and Native Americans, and the increased insulin resistance in these populations is almost certainly genetically based. Additional information about the role of insulin resistance and insulin secretion in the pathogenesis of type 2 diabetes is presented in Box 379.3.

CLINICAL MANIFESTATIONS AND COMPLICATIONS

Many children with type 2 diabetes present with the same classic symptoms of diabetes mellitus as children with type 1 diabetes: polyuria, polydipsia, and polyphagia (in contrast to type 1 diabetes, significant weight loss is less likely to have occurred with type 2 diabetes). However, in contrast to children presenting with type 1 diabetes, where the symptoms are typically present for only a few weeks, children with type 2 diabetes may have had these symptoms for many months. Many children with type 2 diabetes will not have any specific symptoms, and diabetes will be diagnosed based on screening tests obtained due to the presence of risk factors for type 2 diabetes or because a urinalysis obtained for other reasons indicates glucosuria. Finally, although diabetic ketoacidosis (DKA) is much less common in patients with type 2 diabetes than in patients with type 1 diabetes, a significant number of children with type 2 diabetes will present in DKA. (See Chapter 378 for discussion of the presenting features of DKA.)

Patients with diabetes mellitus are at risk for both acute and chronic complications. The acute complications (hypoglycemia, DKA, and nonketotic hyperosmolar coma) can occur at any time after the diagnosis of diabetes, while the chronic complications, including macrovascular and microvascular complications, develop over many years. A more detailed discussion of these complications is presented in Chapter 378.

Diabetic ketoacidosis

In established type 1 diabetes, without treatment with insulin, the patient will quickly develop DKA. In contrast, patients with type 2 diabetes generally have sufficient insulin action to restrain lipolysis, limiting free fatty acid delivery to the liver and subsequent ketoacid production. Because of this, patients with type 2 diabetes are at much lower risk of developing DKA, even without treatment for their diabetes. However, significant numbers of children who have ultimately been determined to have type 2 diabetes have presented with DKA. While these children require initial treatment with insulin, many can ultimately be managed with oral medications. It is likely that in these children, hyperglycemia has induced sufficient *glucotoxicity* on the beta cell to diminish insulin secretion to such a degree that DKA can occur. Once this toxicity is relieved by

appropriate glycemic control, sufficient endogenous insulin secretion is restored to allow the discontinuation of exogenous insulin treatment. It is not yet clear why children with type 2 diabetes appear to have a greater risk of DKA than is seen in adults. Nonetheless, although DKA is uncommon in children with type 2 diabetes, the child and family should be taught the skills necessary to detect developing ketosis and prevent deterioration into DKA, just as is done for the child with type 1 diabetes. The child with type 2 diabetes who presents in DKA (or has an episode of DKA subsequent to the diagnosis of type 2 diabetes) should be considered at higher risk for subsequent episodes of DKA.

Nonketotic Hyperosmolar Coma

The classic hyperglycemic crisis in patients with type 2 diabetes is nonketotic hyperosmolar coma. This is similar to DKA, in that stress hormones (epinephrine, cortisol, growth hormone) are increased due to an intercurrent illness and antagonize insulin action, inducing an acute worsening of hyperglycemia. The hyperglycemia induces an osmotic diuresis, and if not compensated for with increased fluid intake, the dehydration compounds the hyperglycemia by impairing glucose clearance by the kidneys. Marked hyperglycemia, hyperosmolarity, and dehydration result. In contrast to DKA, at most only moderate levels of ketones are present in the blood. Because nonketotic hyperosmolar coma is due to an inability to maintain hydration in the face of ongoing fluid loss from the osmotic diuresis and develops insidiously over a period of a number of days, it typically only develops in debilitated patients with type 2 diabetes. It therefore is not a common feature in type 2 diabetes in children.

Hypoglycemia

Treatment of diabetes with insulin seeks to match the dose of insulin given to the current insulin requirement. If more insulin is given than is needed, there is a risk of producing hypoglycemia. This is true whether insulin is used to treat type 1 or type 2 diabetes, although hypoglycemia is generally less common in insulin-treated patients with type 2 diabetes than in patients with type 1 diabetes.

The insulin secretagogues, which include the sulfonylureas and the newer meglitinide analogues, act by stimulating endogenous insulin secretion. Treatment with these medications carries the risk that they will stimulate more insulin secretion than is needed to meet the current insulin requirement and induce hypoglycemia. This risk in the typical child with type 2 diabetes is quite low. The meglitinide analogue secretagogues are very short acting, intended to be given at mealtime. As such, they have an even lower risk of hypoglycemia than the longer-acting sulfonylureas, where there is some risk of hypoglycemia if meals are missed. The signs, symptoms, and treatment of hypoglycemia in type 2 diabetes, whether induced by insulin or insulin secretagogue treatment, is the same as in type 1 diabetes; see Chapter 378 for a further discussion of hypoglycemia in diabetes.

Microvascular Complications

The hyperglycemia from diabetes of any type leads to damage to the microvascular circulation, resulting in tissue and organ damage, most notably in the retina, kidneys, and nerves. Due to these microvascular complications, diabetes mellitus is a leading cause of blindness, end-stage renal disease, and neuropathy. Increasing degrees of hyperglycemia are the main risk factor for microvascular complications. Genetic factors are also likely to

| BOX 379.3 | The Role of Insulin Resistance and Insulin Secretion in the Pathogenesis of Type 2 Diabetes |

Insulin Resistance

Obesity and low levels of physical activity both lead to insulin resistance, explaining their very high association with type 2 diabetes. It is the marked increase in the rates and severity of obesity and sedentary behavior in both adults and children that has led to the marked increased prevalence of type 2 diabetes over the past decade. The mechanisms through which obesity and poor physical conditioning lead to insulin resistance remain incompletely understood. However, a number of factors that are secreted by adipocytes can alter insulin sensitivity. Increased secretion of some of these factors due to the increased mass of adipose tissue present in obesity, or unknown effects of obesity leading to either increased or decreased secretion of these factors, may lead to the insulin resistance of obesity. For example, free fatty acid concentrations are increased in the serum of obese individuals, and free fatty acids impair insulin sensitivity in both liver and muscle. Notably, excess intraabdominal adiposity has a much higher association with insulin resistance than obesity with a more peripheral (subcutaneous) distribution, and intraabdominal fat tissue has a higher lipolytic rate compared to subcutaneous adipose tissue, lending support for the role of free fatty acids in the insulin resistance of obesity. Abnormal secretion by the adipocyte of a number of other factors, referred to as adipokines and including tumor necrosis factor-alpha (TNF-alpha), resistin, adiponectin, and leptin, has also been implicated in the pathophysiology of the insulin resistance of obesity. Even less is understood about how decreased physical activity leads to insulin resistance. However, its effect is clearly demonstrated by the finding that increased physical activity with regular exercise, even in the absence of weight loss, can significantly increase insulin sensitivity–sufficient in some cases to correct the hyperglycemia of type 2 diabetes without the need for other treatments.

Insulin sensitivity declines by approximately 30% in all children at the beginning of puberty, resolving as puberty ends. The cause of this decreased insulin sensitivity is due to the insulin antagonizing action of the increased growth hormone secretion that occurs during puberty. The increased insulin resistance of puberty explains why most children do not present with type 2 diabetes until after puberty has begun: most obese children are able to increase insulin secretion sufficient to compensate for the insulin resistance of their obesity, but in some of these children, the addition of the insulin resistance of puberty results in insulin requirements that exceed the child's insulin secretory capacity.

A final cause of insulin resistance is hyperglycemia itself. While this cannot explain the prediabetic development of insulin resistance, hyperglycemia can exacerbate insulin resistance in uncontrolled diabetes, further impairing metabolic control.

Insulin Secretory Defect

In the nondiabetic individual, glucose homeostasis is maintained by the ability of the pancreatic beta cells to match insulin secretion to insulin requirements. Thus, in the presence of insulin resistance such as that due to obesity, there is a compensatory increase in insulin secretion, leading to elevated fasting and meal-stimulated insulin levels. In the majority of individuals this compensation persists and glucose homeostasis is maintained. In genetically predisposed individuals, however, the beta cell is unable to continue to meet the increased insulin requirements. Environmental factors may also contribute to insulin secretion becoming inadequate, as for example, if insulin resistance rises further due to increasing obesity, or to the additional burden of pubertal insulin resistance. The inability to maintain normal fasting or postprandial glucose levels indicates the presence of impaired insulin secretion. Although appropriate information about children is not yet established, data in adults indicate that once impaired insulin secretion is present, there is a high risk that the insulin secretory defect will worsen. As the beta-cell dysfunction worsens, metabolic control will further deteriorate from mildly abnormal (glucose levels above normal but below criteria for a diagnosis of diabetes) to diabetes. Insulin levels early in this progression are still elevated compared to individuals with normal insulin sensitivity, but are not elevated sufficient to maintain normal glucose control. With time (again based on data from adults) the insulin secretory defect continues to worsen, including loss of beta cells, requiring increasing use of medications to maintain control of blood glucose levels.

The direct cause of the beta-cell dysfunction in type 2 diabetes is not known, although both genetic and environmental factors are likely involved. A number of mechanisms related either directly or indirectly to insulin resistance have been implicated. The persistent stimulus imposed by insulin resistance on the beta cell to oversecrete insulin appears to be a key contributor to the loss of beta-cell function. The increased metabolic activity of the hyperstimulated beta cell may lead to oxidative damage, to which the beta cell is particularly sensitive. In addition, the increased stimulation of the beta cell in insulin resistance leads to an increased secretion of islet amyloid polypeptide (IAPP), which is cosecreted with insulin from the beta cell. In the majority of patients with type 2 diabetes, IAPP accumulates in the islets as amyloid, potentially impairing beta-cell function. The increased free fatty acid levels present in insulin resistance likely contribute to defective insulin secretion, just as they can contribute to insulin resistance because long-term exposure to increased free fatty acids impairs beta-cell function, and may be responsible for beta-cell death by apoptosis. Similarly, just as hyperglycemia can further impair insulin sensitivity, prolonged exposure to increased glucose levels imposes a *glucotoxicity* on the beta cell. Clinically this can be significant, in that if glucose levels are normalized in a patient with type 2 diabetes, endogenous insulin secretion may be significantly improved, at least temporarily.

As is true in adults, a significant percentage of children with characteristics that otherwise indicate they have type 2 diabetes (including a lack of requirement for insulin treatment for prolonged periods of time) have diabetes-specific autoantibodies. Therefore, autoimmune destruction of beta cells may contribute to the loss of beta-cell function in at least a subset of children with type 2 diabetes. Based on studies in adults with type 2 diabetes, it is likely that these children with evidence of diabetes-specific autoimmunity will have an earlier requirement for treatment with insulin to maintain metabolic control.

play a role. The risk of microvascular complications increases with time, with the earliest evidence uncommon prior to a duration of hyperglycemia of 5 years. It is extremely unlikely that pediatric patients with type 2 diabetes will demonstrate significant microvascular disease until after they reach adulthood. However, the fact that these children have a lifetime with diabetes ahead of them puts them at very high risk of accumulating microvascular complications. It is therefore important to begin to establish glycemic control as soon as possible to minimize the risk of these complications.

Macrovascular Complications

Atherosclerotic vascular disease (ASVD) occurs at a higher frequency and develops at a younger age in patients with diabetes than in the general population. This risk is likely even higher in patients with type 2 diabetes compared to those with type 1 diabetes. Even in the absence of diabetes, insulin resistance itself is associated with an increased risk for ASVD. Thus, over half of patients with type 2 diabetes die from cardiovascular disease, including coronary artery and cerebrovascular disease, and peripheral vascular disease is a major factor in the necessity for lower limb amputations in significant numbers of adults with long-standing diabetes. As for microvascular complications, children with type 2 diabetes will not develop evidence of these macrovascular complications until they are adults, but the pathologic changes leading to vessel occlusion begin accumulating in childhood, so that efforts to decrease the risk of developing ASVD should be started early.

DIAGNOSIS

The diagnosis of diabetes in a child requires documentation of significant hyperglycemia. Once a diagnosis of diabetes is made, the type of diabetes is determined based on clinical and laboratory information. For a child with classic symptoms of diabetes (principally polydipsia and polyuria), a random plasma glucose level of 200 mg/dL or more is sufficient to make the diagnosis of diabetes. For children with type 1 diabetes, this will be how the diagnosis is established in the vast majority of children, as type 1 diabetes rarely has a significant asymptomatic period.

In contrast to the case for type 1 diabetes, patients with type 2 diabetes may be asymptomatic for many years (this is based on data from adults with type 2 diabetes; similar information is not yet known for children with type 2 diabetes). Because microvascular and macrovascular damage accumulates even in asymptomatic diabetes, it is appropriate to screen for this disease. However, while the rising prevalence of type 2 diabetes is alarming, screening the entire child population cannot be justified, so only children at higher risk should be screened

for type 2 diabetes. Box 379.1 lists the recommendations for screening.

If screening for type 2 diabetes is performed, the diagnosis of diabetes is based on an elevated plasma glucose measured either in the fasting state or 2 hours after oral glucose ingestion (1.75 g/kg up to a maximum of 75 g, performed in the fasting state). The criteria were developed based on data in adults; levels indicating diabetes were defined based on glucose concentrations that predict an increased risk for the development of microvascular complications; levels indicating impaired glucose regulation were defined to identify individuals at risk of developing diabetes in the near future. The diagnostic criteria have been extended for use in the diagnosis of diabetes and impaired glucose regulation in children, although rigorous validation of these diagnostic criteria in children has not been performed. Table 379.1 presents the diagnostic glucose levels. The fasting glucose level has been recommended as the preferred screening test due to the greater ease in obtaining this test and better reproducibility than the 2-hour plasma glucose level. The hemoglobin A1$_c$ level (HbA1$_c$) is not currently recommended as a screen for diabetes. However, if an elevated HbA1$_c$ level is documented, that should be considered evidence of diabetes.

There are tests that can be performed to quantitate insulin sensitivity in an individual (and thereby identify those with insulin resistance). The fasting insulin level and other computed measures of insulin sensitivity that include the fasting insulin and glucose levels are useful for research in type 2 diabetes. However, insulin resistance itself is not a diagnosis that requires specific treatment, and therefore quantifying insulin resistance is not useful in a clinical setting.

Classification

Once a diagnosis of diabetes mellitus is made in a child, it is necessary to classify the disorder as type 1 or type 2. Diagnosing a child with type 1 diabetes indicates an absolute requirement for treatment with insulin, while there are additional options for treatment of children with type 2 diabetes.

In many cases, the classification of diabetes type is straightforward. The diabetes is classified as type 2 if it is diagnosed based on screening blood tests obtained on a child at increased risk of type 2 diabetes. The diabetes is classified as type 1 if a child with no risk factors for type 2 diabetes presents with DKA. In addition, because type 2 diabetes remains uncommon prior to the onset of puberty, prepubertal children should generally be diagnosed with type 1 diabetes, although unusual circumstances may justify a cautious and tentative diagnosis of type 2 diabetes.

The classification of diabetes in symptomatic adolescents is based on an assessment of the presence and absence of features suggestive of type 1 versus type 2 diabetes, as outlined in

---

TABLE 379.1

DIAGNOSTIC CRITERIA FOR DIABETES MELLITUS AND IMPAIRED GLUCOSE REGULATION

	Normal	Impaired	Diabetes
Fasting plasma glucose	<100 mg/dL	100–125 mg/dL (IFG)	≥126 mg/dL
2-hour plasma glucose	<140 mg/dL	140–199 mg/dL (IGT)	≥200 mg/dL

IFG, impaired fasting glucose; IGT, impaired glucose tolerance. Two-hour plasma glucose is obtained after 1.75 g/kg of glucose (maximum of 75 g) is ingested orally in the fasting state. Results indicative of diabetes should be confirmed by repeat testing on a different day. Glucose levels in mmol/L are obtained by dividing the above levels by 18.
Adapted from The Expert Committee on the Diagnosis and Classification of Diabetes Mellitus. Follow-up report on the diagnosis of diabetes mellitus. *Diabetes Care* 2003;26:3160.

TABLE 379.2

CHARACTERISTICS SUGGESTIVE OF TYPE 1 VERSUS TYPE 2 DIABETES AT PRESENTATION

	Type 1	Type 2
Polydipsia and polyuria	Present for days to weeks	Absent, or present for weeks to months
Ethnicity	Caucasian	African American, Hispanic, Native American, Asian
Weight	Weight loss more common	Obese
Other findings		Acanthosis nigricans
Family history	Negative	Positive
Insulin or C-peptide level	Low	High
Ketoacidosis	More common	Less common
Autoantibodies	Positive	Less common

Table 379.2. However, no factor is absolutely diagnostic of type 1 or type 2 diabetes:

- While it is not necessary to measure beta-cell autoantibodies in all adolescents with diabetes to classify their diabetes, in some cases it may be helpful. An absence of these antibodies makes type 1 diabetes unlikely. However, as many as 15% of children with type 1 diabetes will not have detectable autoantibodies to a given beta-cell autoantigen, and 5% will not have any detectable beta-cell autoantibodies. In addition, just as in adults, a significant fraction of children with type 2 diabetes will have measurable beta-cell autoantibodies.
- Type 2 diabetes is very unlikely in a nonobese child, but obesity does not protect against type 1 diabetes, and with the high and rising prevalence of obesity, the occurrence of type 1 diabetes in an obese adolescent will not be uncommon.
- The high prevalence of type 2 diabetes will also result in the occurrence of type 1 diabetes in children with a family history of type 2 diabetes.
- While insulin and C-peptide levels are lower in children presenting with type 1 diabetes than those presenting with type 2 diabetes, the overlap is large, so that these levels are often not helpful in differentiating early type 1 from type 2 diabetes. This is particularly true if levels are measured at the time of presentation, when glucotoxicity may be having a significant effect on insulin secretion.
- Acanthosis nigricans is velvety soft, hyperpigmented, thickened skin that can be found around the neck and in the axilla, groin, and other intertriginous areas. Acanthosis nigricans is an indicator of insulin resistance and hyperinsulinism. It is much more common in African Americans and Hispanics than in Caucasians, even with similar degrees of insulin resistance.
- Insulin resistance is a significant component of the pathophysiology of polycystic ovary syndrome (PCOS).
- The presence of DKA does not exclude a diagnosis of type 2 diabetes, as DKA is not uncommon in adolescents with type 2 diabetes and can be just as severe as that which occurs in type 1 diabetes.

In some cases definite classification is difficult and a tentative classification is made but can be reconsidered after observation of the clinical course of the disease. Recurrences of ketosis, especially if resulting in DKA, should prompt a consideration for reclassification in a patient initially designated as having type 2 diabetes. Conversely, significant C-peptide levels more than 2 years after diagnosis is uncommon in type 1 diabetes, so that such a finding should prompt reevaluation in a patient classified as having type 1 diabetes.

THERAPY

The goal of therapy in type 2 diabetes is to minimize the risk of long term microvascular and macrovascular complications while avoiding short-term complications. Long-term studies in adults, notably the United Kingdom Prospective Diabetes Study (UKPDS), have demonstrated that the risk of microvascular complications in type 2 diabetes can be lowered by maintaining lower blood sugar levels. Therefore, one goal of treatment is to return blood glucose levels to as close to normal as possible. It is not yet clear that lower blood sugar levels will decrease the risk of ASVD. However, reduction of other risk factors for ASVD can decrease this risk and is an important aspect of the treatment of type 2 diabetes. Treatment of type 2 diabetes is best accomplished by cooperative efforts between the patient, his or her family, and a medical team that may include physicians, nurses, and nutritionists. The natural history of type 2 diabetes includes declining beta-cell function over time. Therefore, escalation of therapy is generally required to maintain the desired level of glycemic control.

Approach to Treatment

The overall goal of treatment of type 2 diabetes is to achieve normal or near-normal glucose levels. The $HbA1_c$ level should be measured up to every 3 months, with a goal of achieving a value less than 7%. A minority of patients will be able to achieve this with lifestyle changes that lead to weight loss and an increase in exercise levels. A much larger percentage of patients will require treatment with a single antidiabetes medication, either insulin injections or one of the oral agents. Some patients will require a combination of medications to achieve the desired level of glycemic control.

For many patients, it is reasonable to recommend lifestyle changes as the initial treatment for type 2 diabetes. However, if this has not resulted in achieving the desired degree of glycemic control within 3 to 6 months, treatment with medication should be started. In addition, if the patient presents with evidence of marked hyperglycemia, such as an $HbA1_c$ of over 9%, a period of treatment with medication to correct the hyperglycemia and remove the glucotoxic effect on insulin secretion and insulin sensitivity may be needed before lifestyle changes could be effective, even if the patient is successful in fully implementing the lifestyle changes.

Ketoacidosis is an indication of severe insulin deficiency and must always be treated with insulin, whether the child has type 1 or type 2 diabetes. In addition, patients whose fasting blood glucose level is above 200 to 250 mg/dL (or with an $HbA1_c$ above 9%) will often have difficulty achieving adequate glycemic control if they are begun on an oral medication alone. Patients with either of these presentations should be treated initially with insulin. However, because improvement in their glycemic control will relieve the glucotoxic effect of hyperglycemia on the beta cell, in some of these patients insulin treatment may later be discontinued with adequate control and then maintained with oral medications.

In most children with type 2 diabetes, the initial treatment of choice will be metformin. Unlike insulin treatment or insulin secretagogues, treatment with metformin does not have any significant risk of hypoglycemia. In addition, treatment with insulin or the secretagogues may lead to weight gain, which is clearly undesirable. For patients in whom metformin cannot be used, either because of specific contraindications or because the patient is unable to tolerate it due to gastrointestinal (GI) side effects, an insulin secretagogue may be a reasonable initial treatment option. Insulin treatment may also be used, although its requirement for injections often makes this alternative less desirable. The alpha-glucosidase inhibitors are rarely used as first-line treatment, although if they are tolerated, they may be effective in patients with only mild hyperglycemia.

Each of the oral antidiabetes medications lowers the $HbA1_c$ by 1% to 2% in adults with diabetes (comparable data in children are only available for metformin, where the efficacy was similar to that in adults). Therefore, it can be anticipated that a patient with an $HbA1_c$ greater than 9% will require more than one medication to achieve the desired degree of glycemic control. As noted previously, one option would be treatment with insulin until the $HbA1_c$ is significantly lowered, followed by transition to an oral agent (again, generally metformin).

Most adult patients with type 2 diabetes will have declining beta-cell function over time, requiring the use of additional medications to maintain glycemic control. While data are not yet available to determine how quickly beta-cell function will decline in children with type 2 diabetes, the approach to maintaining glycemic control should be the same as in adults. If glycemic control cannot be maintained with the maximal dose of a single medication (e.g., as demonstrated by an $HbA1_c$ above 7%), another medication should be added to the treatment regimen. For the patient taking metformin, this could be the addition of an insulin secretagogue or an alpha-glucosidase inhibitor. In some patients it may be appropriate to add a thiazolidinedione.

Unlike the oral antidiabetes medications, there is no maximal effective dose for insulin; doses can always be increased to give a greater glucose-lowering effect. The only factor limiting insulin doses is hypoglycemia. Therefore, treatment with insulin should be considered for patients who cannot achieve glycemic control on oral agents. It may be worthwhile to continue treatment with metformin to maintain some improved insulin sensitivity to help minimize insulin requirements.

Just as in type 1 diabetes, aggressive treatment of hypertension, dyslipidemia, and microalbuminuria (with angiotensin-converting enzyme inhibitors) is appropriate to minimize the risk of long-term microvascular and/or macrovascular complications. In addition, the additive effect of smoking on ASVD risk should be presented to adolescents to emphatically discourage smoking.

Lifestyle Management

The ideal treatment for type 2 diabetes would reverse the pathophysiologic changes that resulted in the development of diabetes. In this regard, the best treatment is to increase insulin sensitivity through weight loss and increased exercise. Even modest weight loss can result in sufficient improvement in insulin sensitivity to result in normalization of blood glucose levels in patients with diabetes with modest hyperglycemia without the need for medication. In addition, exercise has a weight-loss–independent effect on improving insulin sensitivity. The direct and immediate benefit of successful efforts at making these lifestyle changes can be used to help motivate adolescents with diabetes and their families. Unfortunately, although weight loss and increased exercise can effectively treat type 2 diabetes, less than 10% of children and adolescents can be expected to be successful in achieving and maintaining sufficient changes in dietary and exercise habits to maintain adequate levels of glycemic control without medications. However, weight loss and exercise are beneficial in reducing ASVD risk, so even if medication is required, these lifestyle changes should be encouraged.

Medications

Only limited studies have investigated treatments for type 2 diabetes in pediatric patients, and only insulin and metformin are currently approved by the Food and Drug Administration for the treatment of diabetes in children. However, adequate treatment will often require the use of alternative or additional medications.

Insulin

The main underlying abnormality in type 2 diabetes is an imbalance between insulin requirements and endogenous insulin production. This can be overcome by treatment with insulin injections. The use of insulin to treat type 2 diabetes is, for the most part, no different than that used to treat type 1 diabetes, and further information on insulin treatment can be found in Chapter 378. One aspect specific to type 2 diabetes, however, is that if the patient has sufficient preservation of endogenous insulin secretion, treatment with just an intermediate- or long-acting insulin, such as NPH insulin or insulin glargine, may be all that is necessary to achieve normal or near-normal glycemia.

Metformin

Metformin is a biguanide, which is one of the two classes of insulin-sensitizing agents used in the treatment of type 2 diabetes. Its primary effect is to increase the insulin sensitivity of the liver, suppressing the inappropriately elevated hepatic glucose production in type 2 diabetes. Because metformin does not directly increase insulin levels, it rarely causes hypoglycemia. Metformin has an anorectic effect in some patients, which can lead to a modest decrease in weight.

Initiation of treatment with metformin is frequently associated with GI symptoms, including diarrhea and abdominal cramps. This can be minimized by taking metformin with meals and starting with a low dose that is then increased to an effective dose. These effects generally resolve with time; patients should be informed of the transient nature of these GI side effects to discourage discontinuation of the metformin.

Metformin can cause lactic acidosis. While this is extremely rare, it can be fatal. The lactic acidosis occurs with excessive accumulation of metformin. Metformin is cleared by the kidneys, so that its use is contraindicated in patients with renal impairment. In addition, metformin should be temporarily discontinued at times that renal function may be compromised, such as with the use of intravenous radiographic contrast agents, or when there is a risk of dehydration, such as with significant vomiting and dehydration. (Urine ketones should be measured if there is significant vomiting to determine if ketoacidosis is the cause of the vomiting.) Metformin is also contraindicated in patients with liver dysfunction, as this can impair lactate clearance. Mild elevations of serum transaminase levels (up to two to three times the upper limit of normal) can occur due to accumulation of triglyceride in hepatocytes in obese individuals and is not a contraindication to treatment with metformin; in fact, metformin treatment may normalize the transaminase levels in patients with fatty liver disease.

Insulin Secretagogues

Insulin secretagogues include the sulfonylureas (such as glimepiride, glipizide, and glyburide) and the newer meglitinide analogues (nateglinide and repaglinide). These agents stimulate insulin secretion by the beta cell. As with insulin treatment, insulin secretagogues have a risk of hypoglycemia and may promote weight gain. The risk of hypoglycemia is low unless there is a significant decrease in food intake. Therefore, as with patients treated with insulin, patients treated with sulfonylureas should be cautioned not to skip meals, and blood sugar levels must be monitored during illnesses that decrease food intake. The short-acting meglitinide analogues are taken with each meal; the risk of hypoglycemia with these medications is then very low if the medication is skipped if a meal is skipped. However, the need to take the meglitinide analogues with every meal is likely to make compliance difficult, particularly for the adolescent who may eat many meals away from home. The long-acting sulfonylureas can be taken once a day.

Alpha-Glucosidase Inhibitors

Acarbose and miglitol inhibit the intestinal enzyme alpha-glucosidase. They are taken with meals, which delays carbohydrate absorption and allows endogenous insulin secretion to better meet prandial insulin requirements, helping to control postprandial glucose levels. GI side effects are common, but can be minimized if a low dose is begun.

Thiazolidinediones

Pioglitazone and rosiglitazone are insulin sensitizers that act mainly to increase peripheral insulin sensitivity (the stimulation of glucose uptake into muscle and adipose tissue). Like metformin, they do not cause hypoglycemia. These drugs are quite new, so only limited long-term safety data are available, particularly in children. The initial drug in this class, troglitazone, was removed from the market because it caused liver dysfunction and in rare cases lead to fulminant liver failure. Although pioglitazone and rosiglitazone do not appear to have the same risk of liver injury as troglitazone, liver enzymes must be monitored in patients treated with thiazolidinediones. There is some evidence suggesting that thiazolidinediones may have unique advantages in the treatment of type 2 diabetes, including improvement in serum lipid abnormalities, direct antiatherogenic effects, and perhaps preservation of endogenous insulin secretion. However, until further safety data are available, they should rarely be used in children as first-line treatment, and then used only with caution.

PREVENTION

The best approach for prevention of a disease is to address modifiable risk factors. For diabetes, insulin resistance is the one risk factor that can be corrected. From a public health standpoint, the prevention of diabetes will require societal changes that decrease the prevalence of obesity and increase physical activity on a population-wide basis. Similarly, healthy eating habits that avoid excess weight gain and lifestyles that incorporate regular physical activity can be recommended for all children.

Children who are at high risk of developing diabetes can be identified. These are the children that fulfill the criteria for screening for type 2 diabetes outlined in Box 379.1. An even higher risk subgroup would be those children who have either impaired fasting glucose or impaired glucose tolerance (although the risk of progression from the impaired categories to diabetes is not yet as well defined for children as it is in adults). Because of the enormous negative impact of diabetes on the long-term health of patients, it would be highly desirable to intervene in a specific way in these high-risk children to prevent the development of diabetes.

A number of studies have demonstrated that intensive lifestyle interventions can decrease the percentage of high-risk adults who develop type 2 diabetes. In two large studies, the Diabetes Prevention Program and the Finnish Diabetes Prevention Study, the development of diabetes was reduced by 58% in obese adults with impaired glucose tolerance by interventions that sought to increase exercise and lose weight. These studies had goals for weight loss of 5% to 7%, and goals for exercise of 20 to 30 minutes per day. While similar studies have not yet been completed in children at high risk of developing type 2 diabetes, these same goals for lifestyle modification should be recommended for children at risk of developing diabetes.

The ability of medications to prevent the development of diabetes in high-risk adults has also been investigated in a number of studies. Acarbose, troglitazone, and metformin have all been demonstrated to decrease the percentage of high-risk adults who develop type 2 diabetes. Except for troglitazone, the medications were less effective than were the intensive lifestyle interventions. However, until more data are available, including longer-term studies and studies in children, the use of medications to prevent type 2 diabetes in high-risk children cannot be routinely recommended.

Suggested Readings

American Diabetes Association. Type 2 diabetes in children and adolescents. *Pediatrics* 2000;105:671.

Arslanian S. Childhood obesity and type 2 diabetes. *Pediatrics* 2005;116:473.

Arslanian S. Type 2 diabetes in children: clinical aspects and risk factors. *Hormone Res* 2002;57:19.

Fagot-Campagna AF, Pettit DJ, Engelgau MM, et al. Type 2 diabetes among North American children and adolescents: an epidemiologic review and a public health perspective. *J Pediatr* 2000;136:664.

Kaufman FR. Type 2 diabetes in children and youth. *Rev Endocr Metabol Disord* 2003;4:33.

Ludwig DS, Ebbeling CB. Type 2 diabetes mellitus in children: primary care and public health considerations. *JAMA* 2001;286:1427.

CHAPTER 380 ■ THYROID GLAND

RUBINA A. HEPTULLA

NORMAL THYROID DEVELOPMENT AND THYROID HORMONE SYNTHESIS

The thyroid gland first appears in the fourth week of gestation as an epithelial proliferation and invagination of the endoderm of the foregut, and the synthesis of thyroglobulin begins at this time. The thyroid then penetrates the mesoderm and migrates downward but remains connected to the floor of the foregut by means of the thyroglossal duct. This duct eventually becomes solid and, in normal individuals, involutes completely. By the seventh week of development, the now bilobed gland reaches its normal position anterior to the trachea. By the tenth to eleventh week, the fetal thyroid begins to trap and oxidize iodide, and by the twelfth week, colloid formation is detectable. By the eleventh week of gestation, the thyroid gland secretes thyroxine (T_4) and triiodothyronine (T_3). By the thirteenth week, thyroxine-binding globulin (TBG) and thyroid-stimulating hormone (TSH) are detectable in serum. Maturation of the fetal hypothalamic-pituitary-thyroid axis usually occurs by the twentieth week of gestation.

The synthesis of thyroid hormone is regulated through a central biologic feedback system. Under the stimulatory influence of the hypothalamic tripeptide thyrotropin-releasing hormone (TRH), also known as *thyrotropin-releasing factor*, the pituitary thyrotrophs secrete TSH. TSH enters the circulation and binds to specific receptors on the thyroid gland to stimulate production of T_4. This stimulation occurs within the cell through a second messenger system, guanine nucleotide-coupled cyclic adenosine monophosphate production, a mechanism common to many peptide hormones. The circulating levels of T_4 and T_3 feed back at the level of the pituitary and the hypothalamus to regulate the release of TSH.

Thyroid hormone synthesis is a multistep procedure that begins when circulating iodide is trapped by the iodine pump and undergoes organification by thyroperoxidase. Organic iodide binds to the tyrosine residues of thyroglobulin, resulting in the formation of monoiodotyrosine and diiodotyrosine. Monoiodotyrosine and diiodotyrosine condense to form T_3 and T_4, the major thyroid hormones produced. T_3 and T_4 are stored on the thyroglobulin molecule in the form of colloid or are released from the thyroglobulin molecule into the circulation. Thyroglobulin itself normally is not released into the plasma and, if detected, may indicate a thyroid cell abnormality such as thyroiditis or carcinoma. Although the major thyroid hormone produced in and secreted by the thyroid gland is T_4, its effects are exerted in peripheral tissues through its deiodination to the much more potent T_3. The amount of T_3 secreted by the thyroid gland itself adds a minimal fraction to the total circulating T_3 under physiologic conditions. Inborn errors in thyroid hormone metabolism have been described for all of these steps.

The thyroid gland produces a third thyroid hormone, reverse T_3 (rT_3), which is synthesized from T_4 by a deiodinase different from that which produces T_3. Its physiologic role is unknown. The rT_3 levels are high during fetal life, when T_3 levels normally are lower than those in postnatal life. After birth, rT_3 levels decrease markedly, and T_3 levels increase into the normal range. In certain conditions, such as the euthyroid sick syndrome, the levels of circulating rT_3 may be elevated.

T_4 and T_3 are transported in the plasma bound to the thyroid hormone-binding proteins TBG, the major binding protein, and thyroxine-binding prealbumin. Albumin also binds thyroid hormone with low affinity. The protein-bound fractions of circulating T_4 and T_3 account for more than 99% of the total hormone, and more than 70% of the total is bound to TBG. Even minor changes in the levels of the thyroid hormone-binding proteins can result in a significant change in the level of total circulating hormone, although the free (i.e., metabolically available, not protein-bound) hormone remains the same. For the same reason, TBG acts as a buffer to protect the tissues from fluctuations in T_4 levels. As with inborn errors of thyroid hormone synthesis, many disorders of thyroid hormone-binding proteins, the most common of which is the X-linked recessive condition of TBG deficiency, have been described.

The physiologic effects of thyroid hormone are protean, accounting for the myriad symptoms that occur in thyroid disorders. These effects include protein synthesis, cell growth and differentiation, critical effects on the maturation of the central nervous system (CNS) and skeleton, maintenance of oxidative metabolism and heat production, and maintenance of cardiovascular function. The circulating levels of thyroid hormone also affect muscle tone, deep tendon reflexes, and maturation of the epidermis.

The thyroid gland also is the source of calcitonin, produced by the so-called C cells. These cells are embryologically derived from the neural crest and, thus, are not truly thyroid in origin. The physiologic effects of calcitonin oppose those of parathyroid hormone.

THYROID FUNCTION TESTS

Static Tests

The static tests of thyroid function include measurement of plasma levels of the various components of the thyroid system. Normal values for many of these components are given in Table 380.1.

Total T_4 and free T_4 concentration is determined by an immunometric assay that is the most widely used test of thyroid function and reflects the total of the protein-bound and free hormone. Total T_4 is not a direct measurement of T_4. Changes in serum-binding protein levels produce corresponding changes in total T_4, although physiologically active free T_4 is unchanged. This change results in abnormal serum total T_4 levels in a physiologically normal patient. To overcome this obstacle, free T_4 by equilibrium dialysis is used and is a direct measurement of free T_4. Because the direct measurement of the active hormone accurately measures the free hormone level, it is

TABLE 380.1

THYROID FUNCTION TESTS IN INFANCY, CHILDHOOD, AND ADULTHOOD[a]

Age	Thyroxine (μg/dL)	Free Thyroxine (ng/dL)	Triiodo-Thyronine (ng/mL)	Thyroxine-Binding Globulin (mg/dL)	Thyroid-Stimulating Hormone[b] (μU/mL)
Cord blood	7.5–16.8 (11.2)	1.5–3.7 (2.1)	10–90 (58)	2.5–5.1 (3.9)	—
Premature (26–30 weeks) 3–4 days	2.6–14.0 (6.4)	0.4–2.8 (1.5)	24–132 (65)	1.2–3.8 (2.4)	<32 weeks: 0.8–4.1
Full term					
1–3 days	8.2–19.9 (14.6)	2.0–4.9 (3.5)	89–405 (273)	1–24 months: 2.1–6.0 (4.6)	4 days: 1.3–16.0
1 week	6.0–15.9 (12.0)	—	91–300 (190)		
1–12 months	6.1–14.9 (9.8)	0.9–2.6 (1.6)	85–250 (175)		0.97–7.70
Prepubertal children	1–3 years: 6.8–13.5 (9.3); 3–10 years: 5.5–12.8 (8.6)	0.8–2.2 (1.6)	119–218 (168) 80–185 (116)	2–10 years: 2.0–5.3 (3.5)	0.6–5.5
Pubertal children and adults	4.2–13.0 (8.0)	0.8–2.3 (1.5)	55–170 (105)	1.8–4.2 (2.8)	0.5–4.8 (1.6)

[a]Values represent normal range with mean shown in parentheses.
[b]Thyroid-stimulating hormone levels surge in the postpartum period and peak at 25 to 160 μU/mL by 30 minutes, then decline to cord blood levels by the third day.
Data are from Esoterix, Calabasas Hills, CA, and were used with permission. Other laboratories may have different reference ranges.

unaffected by serum-binding protein abnormalities or thyroid-binding protein excess or deficiency. However, this assay is expensive, time-consuming, and technically demanding, limiting its widespread commercial use. Total and free T_3 concentrations are determined using the methods described for T_4. In normal individuals, two-thirds of the T_3 measured in plasma arises from peripheral deiodination of T_4, and only one-third arises from direct secretion from the thyroid gland.

The T_3 resin uptake (T_3RU) once was used routinely to estimate the number of thyroid hormone-binding protein sites, reflecting the circulating level of free T_4. T_3RU is not a measure of plasma T_3 concentration. Radiolabeled T_3 is added to an aliquot of the patient's serum and binds to all available (i.e., unoccupied) TBG binding sites. Because TBG has a greater affinity for T_4 than for T_3, the radioactive T_3 does not displace the patient's T_4 from the TBG molecule. A resin that binds T_3 is added, and the unbound radioactive T_3 is taken up by the resin. This percentage increases as the number of available TBG binding sites decreases. The T_3RU test is useful only if the total T_4 concentration is known. The free thyroxine index, an estimation of the free T_4 concentration, is calculated from the total T_4 concentration and the T_3RU using the following formula:

$$\text{Free } T_4 \text{ index} = T_4 \times \frac{T_3\text{RU (patient)}}{T_3\text{RU (average for laboratory)}}$$

The T_3RU and free thyroxine index have been replaced largely by direct measurement of free T_4 concentration.

TSH levels are determined by an ultrasensitive immunometric assay and are helpful in the interpretation of thyroid hormone levels. The pituitary gland is exquisitely sensitive to changes in thyroid hormone levels, and elevated levels may indicate early thyroid gland failure or inadequate thyroid hormone replacement therapy before plasma thyroxine concentrations decrease below the normal range.

Measurement of TBG levels now is widely available, and this information is useful for interpreting abnormal thyroid hormone levels. TBG levels may be altered by a variety of conditions and medications (Box 380.1).

Many drugs may affect thyroid function test results because of interactions at various levels of thyroid hormone synthesis, release, and metabolism (Table 380.2). Obtaining a thorough

history of medications is essential in the evaluation of a patient with an abnormality of thyroid function.

Immunoglobulin measurements helpful in the diagnosis of thyroid disorders include antithyroglobulin and antimicrosomal antibodies, which may be present in autoimmune disorders of the gland, and thyroid-stimulating immunoglobulin (TSI), which is important in the pathogenesis of hyperthyroidism. TSH-blocking antibodies can be measured at some centers and have been implicated in the pathogenesis of hypothyroidism.

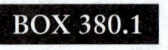
BOX 380.1   **Factors that Influence Thyroid-Binding Globulin Levels**

Increased thyroid-binding globulin
Congenital (X-linked)
Hepatitis
Porphyria
Heroin, methadone
Estrogens, pregnancy
Oral contraceptives
Tamoxifen
5-Fluorouracil
Perphenazine (Trilafon)

Decreased thyroid-binding globulin
Congenital (X-linked)
Hepatic cirrhosis
Nephrotic syndrome
Androgens
Antiestrogens
Glucocorticoids
Nicotinic acid
Acromegaly
Protein-losing enteropathy
Protein-calorie malnutrition
Hyperthyroidism

TABLE 380.2

DRUGS THAT INFLUENCE THYROID HORMONE LEVELS

Characteristic	Drug	Effect
Drugs that have a transient CNS effect to alter thyroid hormone levels	Octreotide, dopamine, L-dopa, glucocorticoids	Decreased TSH secretion
	Metoclopramide	Increased TSH
Drugs that directly decrease thyroid hormone synthesis, most often by decreasing iodide organification; exceptions are nitroprusside, which inhibits iodide trapping, and lithium, which inhibits release of T_4 and T_3 from thyroglobulin	p-Aminosalicylate, phenylbutazone, sulfonamides, aminoglutethimide, nitroprusside, lithium, inorganic iodide*	Decreased T_4 and free T_4; increased TSH
Compounds that decrease the gut absorption of orally administered thyroxine	Cholestyramine, soybean flour, aluminum hydroxide, ferrous sulfate, sucralfate	Decreased T_4 and free T_4 and thus increased TSH
Drugs that inhibit the binding of T_4 and T_3 to TBG; phenytoin also acts to increase cellular uptake of T_4, which decreases the free T_4 concentration	Salicylates, phenylbutazone	Decreased T_4; normal free T_4 and TSH
	Phenytoin	Decreased T_4 and freeT_4; normal T_3 and TSH
Drugs that change uptake or metabolism of thyroid hormones, including decreased conversion of T_4 to T_3	Heparin	Normal T_4; increased free T_4; normal T_3 and TSH
	Phenytoin	Decreased T_4 and free T_4; normal T_3 and TSH
	Glucocorticoids	Decreased T_4, free T_4, and T_3; normal TSH
	Propanolol	Decreased T_3 (only in hyperthyroidism)
	Amiodarone	Complex effects may cause hypothyroidism or hyperthyroidism, but most patients are euthyroid with slightly high TSH levels early in treatment
	PTU, methimazole	Decreased T_4 and T_3; increased TSH; PTU: levels decreased peripheral T_4 to T_3 conversion
Drugs that induce hepatic mixed function oxidases and enhance clearance of thyroxine; effect may be accompanied by increased T_4 to T_3 conversion	Diphenylhydantoin, phenobarbital, carbamazepine, rifampin	Decreased T_4 and free T_4 with normal T_3 and TSH because of combined effects
Drugs that enhance T_4 to T_3 conversion	Exogenous growth hormone	Decreased T_4 and free T_4; normal T_3 and TSH
Drugs that induce autoimmune thyroiditis	Interferon-alpha	Induction of antithyroid antibodies with transient hypothyroidism or hyperthyroidism
	Interleukin-2	Transient painless thyroiditis

CNS, central nervous system; PTU, propylthiouracil; T_3, triiodothyronine; T_4, thyroxine; TBG, thyroxine-binding hormone; TSH, thyroid-stimulating hormone.

*Many commonly used compounds contain iodide, including expectorants, amiodarone, topical antiseptics, radiographic contrast dyes, and antiasthmatic drugs.

Adapted from Kaplan MM. Interactions between drugs and thyroid hormones. Thyroid Today 1981;4:5; Burger AG. Effects of certain pharmacologic agents on the peripheral metabolism of thyroxine. In: Ingbar SH, Braverman LE, ed. Werner's the thyroid: a fundamental and clinical text. Philadelphia: Lippincott–Raven, 1986:351; Surks MI, Sievert R. Drugs and thyroid function. N Engl J Med 1995;333:1688.

Dynamic Tests

The TRH stimulation test of TSH release is a helpful tool in the evaluation of patients whose thyroid hormone and TSH levels do not establish a diagnosis. In response to an intravenous infusion of TRH, the normal person has a brisk increase in serum TSH, followed by a slower return to the normal range. This pattern is accompanied by a similar increase and decrease in the serum prolactin concentration. The magnitude and timing of the TSH response to TRH help to differentiate normal from abnormal thyroid function. This test is useful in infants as well as older patients. An exaggerated TSH response occurs in pri-

mary hypothyroidism, whereas a blunted response occurs in hyperthyroidism. In addition, the TSH response to TRH may allow differentiation of central hypothyroidism caused by hypothalamic or pituitary dysfunction.

The T_3 suppression test is helpful in differentiating hyperthyroidism caused by autonomous gland hyperfunction (i.e., TSI stimulation) from other causes. After a baseline of early radioactive iodine uptake has been determined, the patient is treated with exogenous T_3 for 1 week, at which time the radioactive iodine uptake test is repeated. An autonomously hyperfunctioning gland does not show the normal decrease in radioiodine uptake.

Radiologic Studies

Radiologic studies of the thyroid gland involve the administration of radioactive isotopes, which are taken up by the thyroid gland and, to a lesser extent, by certain other tissues. Because the percentage of administered radioactive isotopes taken up by the thyroid gland is higher in infants and children than in adults and because the radiation risk to the thyroid gland is cumulative, the use of these studies for infants and children should be minimized. The commonly accepted indications for performing these studies in children include the evaluation of thyroid nodules, as an adjunctive test for elucidation of the cause of hyperthyroidism; localization of ectopic thyroid tissue; evaluation of dyshormonogenesis; and assistance in establishing the diagnosis when the combination of other static and dynamic tests of thyroid function is inconclusive.

Three radioactive isotopes are used commonly for thyroid studies. Iodine-131 results in the highest absorbed dose of radioactivity and has the longest half-life; its use generally is reserved for thyroid ablative therapy and for imaging studies in patients with thyroid cancer. Iodine-123 emits much less beta-radiation and is the isotope usually used for iodine uptake studies. Technetium (Tc)-99m pertechnetate results in the lowest dose of radioactivity, but once taken up by the thyroid gland, it is not further metabolized and, therefore, is not useful in studies of thyroid hormone metabolism and release. However, it can be used in the evaluation of thyroid nodules (i.e., hot versus cold) and goiters (e.g., homogeneous versus nonhomogeneous uptake; increased versus decreased uptake).

The 24-hour uptake of radioactive iodine (^{123}I or ^{131}I, depending on the clinical situation) is a common method for assessing the presence of thyroid tissue and for determining the daily iodine turnover of the thyroid gland. The daily turnover reflects the cumulative effect of thyroid clearance, renal clearance, thyroid retention, and dietary intake, and it is reported as the percentage of the total dose given.

In the early or 20-minute uptake test, the percentage of uptake for 20 minutes after administration of the intravenous dose of isotope is measured cumulatively. This uptake reflects thyroid uptake and organification of the circulating iodine load and is less affected by factors that modify the 24-hour uptake. Some patients, particularly patients with cancer preparing for a total body uptake study, are advised to consume a diet low in iodine before the test so that uptake of the iodine isotope is maximal.

The perchlorate or thiocyanate discharge test, which is performed after the 20-minute uptake, measures the amount of radioactive iodine that can be released from the gland after uptake. This test is useful for evaluating suspected dyshormonogenesis.

The T$_3$ suppression test described earlier is helpful in establishing the diagnosis of hyperthyroidism. It also can be used as a method to detect relapses in Graves disease without interrupting the patient's medical therapy.

Ultrasound of the thyroid gland can be used to differentiate solid from the more rare cystic nodules and may be as useful as is a low-risk screening procedure for this purpose. Ultrasound also is useful in differentiating thyroidal from nonthyroidal masses.

ABNORMAL THYROID CONDITIONS

Abnormalities of the thyroid gland may result from altered function (e.g., hypothyroidism, hyperthyroidism), altered structure (e.g., enlargement, nodule), or nonthyroidal causes (e.g., drugs, other illnesses).

Hypothyroidism

Hypothyroidism is defined as a state in which the thyroid gland fails to secrete sufficient quantities of thyroid hormone. Primary hypothyroidism results from a problem inherent to the gland itself, and secondary or central hypothyroidism results from the failure of pituitary stimulation of the thyroid gland. Primary and central hypothyroidism can be either congenital or acquired.

Congenital Hypothyroidism

Congenital hypothyroidism is a disease with an overall prevalence of approximately 1 in 4,000 live births, including 1 of 2,000 persons of Far Eastern or Hispanic descent, 1 of 5,500 persons of European descent, and 1 of 32,000 persons of African descent. Ninety-five percent of all cases are sporadic, and 5% are genetic, most often reflecting a dyshormonogenesis. It has a 2:1 female-to-male predominance, and associations with specific HLA types have been reported in certain populations. Newborn screening for congenital hypothyroidism is performed in all 50 states in the United States, but the methods of screening vary. Healthy, premature infants have lower T$_4$ concentrations than do term infants of the same chronologic age, which must be considered when evaluating the results of the newborn screen. If the newborn screen blood sample is obtained within the first day of life, the TSH level may be falsely elevated because of the peripartum TSH surge.

Etiology. The causes of congenital hypothyroidism are considered here according to the types of hypothyroidism they produce.

Permanent primary hypothyroidism denotes irreversible failure of the thyroid gland to produce sufficient thyroid hormone. The most common cause is an ectopic thyroid gland, which results from improper migration during fetal development. It accounts for more than two-thirds of all cases detected by newborn screening worldwide. The ectopic thyroid tissue often can be demonstrated by Tc-99m scanning, and it is found most commonly at the base of the tongue (i.e., lingual thyroid). These aberrantly located glands do not function properly and do not produce an adequate amount of thyroid hormone.

The next most common cause of congenital primary hypothyroidism is hypoplasia, or aplasia of the gland, and this thyroid dysgenesis may result from the same pathophysiologic process, as does ectopy of the gland. In some cases, immunoglobulins have been implicated in the pathogenesis. A TSH-binding inhibitor immunoglobulin (TBII) has been described in sibling cases of nongoitrous neonatal hypothyroidism and in association with maternal chronic lymphocytic thyroiditis. TBII may be associated with a transient form of hypothyroidism in the newborn. TBII is detectable in both maternal and infant sera. Another antibody, known as *thyroid growth-blocking immunoglobulin*, has been associated with thyroid dysgenesis. It can block the growth of thyroid cells *in vitro*. Antithyroglobulin and antimicrosomal antibodies are not known to play direct roles in the pathogenesis of congenital hypothyroidism.

The third most common cause of congenital primary hypothyroidism is dyshormonogenesis, an inborn error of thyroid hormone synthesis, secretion, or metabolism. Dyshormonogenesis is responsible for most of the familial cases of congenital hypothyroidism. The most common form is a defect in the organification of iodide. Other causes of familial congenital hypothyroidism include deiodination defects, abnormal thyroglobulin, iodide trapping defects, abnormalities of the TSH receptor (e.g., familial unresponsiveness to TSH), and failure of thyroid hormone secretion. A rare peripheral resistance to thyroid hormone in which affected patients have clinical hypothyroidism but elevated T_4 levels and normal TSH levels that prevent neonatal recognition of the disease has been described.

Congenital hypothyroidism may result from maternal radioactive iodine treatment if it has been given after the eighth week of gestation, when fetal iodide trapping has begun.

Transient primary hypothyroidism is a self-limited process, and the cause is determined by a careful history. The causes include maternal iodine deficiency (e.g., endemic goiter), fetal or neonatal exposure to iodine (e.g., maternal medications, amniofetography, painting of the cervix, painting of the umbilical stump), maternal antithyroid drugs, maternal antibodies (e.g., TBII), and, rarely, association with the nephrotic syndrome (i.e., urinary loss of iodine). Transient hypothyroidism is more likely to occur in premature than in full-term infants. Although transient, some of these conditions may require temporary treatment with thyroid hormone. Hypothyroxinemia of prematurity (low T_4 with normal TSH) is not understood clearly, but treatment with thyroxine generally is not recommended.

Permanent central hypothyroidism generally is associated with congenital hypopituitarism and may account for as many as 5% of cases of congenital hypothyroidism. Hypopituitarism may be associated with midline craniofacial defects (e.g., septooptic dysplasia, cleft lip, cleft palate), pituitary aplasia, idiopathic hypopituitarism, and malformations of the central nervous system (CNS).

Low T_4 levels without hypothyroidism are caused most commonly by TBG deficiency, an X-linked recessive disorder with a frequency similar to that of central hypothyroidism. TBG deficiency is differentiated easily from true hypothyroidism because the level of free T_4 is normal, the T_3RU level is high, and the TBG level is low. This condition does not require treatment. Low T_4 levels may occur in ill neonates as a manifestation of the euthyroid sick syndrome (i.e., nonthyroidal illness), which is discussed later.

Diagnosis. Congenital hypothyroidism is diagnosed only rarely from clinical abnormalities. These children have normal birth weight and length and a slightly larger than average head circumference at birth, and one-third have longer than average gestation. Most cases are detected as a result of newborn screening tests, which must be confirmed by thyroid function tests using a venous blood sample. The dried blood filter-paper test is not a satisfactory confirmatory test.

Certain clinical features of hypothyroidism, listed in Box 380.2, may suggest the diagnosis before the results of the newborn screening tests are available. Features that suggest the possibility of hypopituitarism (e.g., midline defects, hypoglycemia, micropenis) should lead to an evaluation for central hypothyroidism. Goiters rarely are present in patients with congenital hypothyroidism, even in cases of dyshormonogenesis. They

---

BOX 380.2	Signs and Symptoms of Congenital Hypothyroidism

Large fontanelles	Prolonged jaundice
Umbilical hernia	Constipation
Macroglossia	Lethargy
Mottled, dry skin	Difficulty feeding
Hypotonia	Cool skin (hypothermia)
Abdominal distention	Sleeps through the night (newborn Hoarse cry period)
Respiratory distress	Goiter (rare)

---

may occur in cases of placental transmission of a goitrogen, and they may be large enough to produce upper airway obstruction.

The hormonal patterns found in congenital hypothyroxinemia are summarized in Table 380.3. In true hypothyroidism, other tests may be helpful in determining the cause of the disease. They include thyroid scanning; urinary iodine if iodine toxicity or deficiency is suspected; bone age, which may be quite delayed in long-standing hypothyroidism; thyroglobulin level, which may help differentiate ectopic from dysplastic glands; and alpha-fetoprotein levels, which may be elevated in long-standing disease.

Treatment. The treatment of congenital hypothyroidism consists of prompt, early replacement of thyroid hormone with oral levothyroxine in a single daily dose of 10 to 15 μg/kg/day. The tablet can be given crushed in a small amount of breast milk or formula and fed using a spoon to ensure adequate delivery to the neonate. Soy products sometimes interfere with thyroid hormone absorption and, hence, using soy formula should be avoided for children with congenital hypothyroidism. The total replacement dose may be used at the outset of therapy unless evidence of cardiac disease is present, in which case a stepwise increase in dosage is recommended. Breast-feeding is not a substitute for replacement therapy because thyroid hormones, although measurable in breast milk, do not provide adequate serum levels in the hypothyroid infant. The goals of treatment include maintenance of the T_4 level in the upper half of the normal range for the age- and weight-dependent titration of dose. Recent data suggest that developmental outcomes have improved with administration of early and high-dose treatment with thyroid hormones.

With prompt and adequate treatment, children with congenital hypothyroidism have the potential to have normal somatic and intellectual growth and development. If left untreated,

---

TABLE 380.3

HORMONAL PATTERNS IN CONGENITAL HYPOTHYROXINEMIA

Cause	First Newborn Screen			Follow-up Confirmation		
	T_4[a]	TSH	T_4	T_3RU	TSH	Free T_4
Primary hypothyroidism	Low	High	Low	Low/normal	High	Low
Central hypothyroidism	Low	Normal[b]	Low	Low/normal	Normal[b]	Low
Transient hypothyroidism	Low	High	Normal	normal	Normal	Normal
Thyroid-binding globulin deficiency[c]	Low	Normal	Low	High	Normal	Normal

T_3RU, triiodothyronine resin uptake; T_4, thyroxine; TSH, thyroid-stimulating hormone.
[a] Many state newborn screening programs do not measure T_4, but only thyroid-stimulating hormone levels.
[b] The normal level of thyroid-stimulating hormone seen in central hypothyroidism is inappropriately low for the decreased level of free T_4.
[c] The diagnosis of thyroid-binding globulin deficiency is made most accurately by demonstration of a low thyroid-binding globulin level.

severe mental retardation and neurologic dysfunction ensue and are more severe in children with primary than with central hypothyroidism. Patients in whom treatment is begun before they reach 6 weeks of age have an average IQ of 100. If treatment is begun when they are 6 weeks to 3 months of age, the average IQ decreases to 95; if begun at 3 to 6 months, the average IQ is 75; and after 6 months, the average IQ is 55 or less.

A variety of other neurologic and learning disorders, including hearing loss, ataxia, attention deficit disorder, abnormalities of muscle tone, and speech defects, have been associated with untreated congenital hypothyroidism. Somatic growth and skeletal development also are impaired, and other clinical manifestations become apparent (see Box 380.2). With severe hypothyroidism, cardiac failure may develop. The sequelae of untreated congenital hypothyroidism are devastating. If an infant has evidence of congenital hypothyroidism on the basis of the newborn screen result and a speedy diagnosis cannot be made after the confirmatory test results have been obtained, therapy should be initiated before establishing the diagnosis. In infants with a possible central hypothyroidism, adrenocorticotropic hormone deficiency must be ruled out before starting thyroid hormone replacement. Levothyroxine treatment is inexpensive and has a low risk if thyroid hormone levels are measured frequently. In uncertain cases, the child should be treated until 2.5 to 3 years of age, when the medication can be discontinued for 1 to 2 months without risk while a diagnosis is established.

Acquired Hypothyroidism

Acquired hypothyroidism appears after the newborn period in a child who did not have congenital hypothyroidism. The estimated prevalence is 1 in 500 to 1,000 school-aged children, with a female-to-male preponderance of 4:1. Certain types of acquired hypothyroidism are familial.

Etiology. As with congenital hypothyroidism, the causes of acquired hypothyroidism can be divided into those that produce primary or those that produce central hypothyroidism. Patients who are critically ill with a nonthyroidal illness may appear to have chemical hypothyroidism, a condition known as the *euthyroid sick syndrome.*

Primary acquired hypothyroidism in childhood is characterized by low T$_4$ levels, elevated TSH, and a variety of clinical manifestations (Box 380.3). It most often results from immunologic destruction of the thyroid gland, but many nonimmunologic causes are known.

The most common cause is chronic lymphocytic thyroiditis (CLT), also known as *Hashimoto thyroiditis.* A defect in cell-mediated immunity results in lymphocytic infiltration and enlargement of the thyroid gland. Titers of antithyroglobulin and antimicrosomal antibodies are elevated in more than 80% of patients. Patients with CLT present with nontender enlargement of the gland, which may be asymmetric or even nodular. The patients often are euthyroid, but some may present with transient hyperthyroidism or have signs and symptoms of hypothyroidism.

CLT may occur alone or in association with other autoimmune endocrine diseases known as the *autoimmune polyglandular syndromes types I and II* (Table 380.4). Because of this association, patients with CLT should be observed for signs of other autoimmune processes, some of which may result in severe illnesses such as Addison disease and diabetes mellitus. An increased incidence of CLT exists among patients with chromosomal abnormalities, including Down syndrome, Turner syndrome, and Klinefelter syndrome. This factor is particularly important for patients with Down syndrome because many of the clinical manifestations of hypothyroidism are seen also in

patients with Down syndrome and may cause a delay in diagnosing hypothyroidism.

Several nonimmune-mediated causes of acquired hypothyroidism exist. Subacute thyroiditis may produce hypothyroidism in some patients. Environmental causes of primary hypothyroidism include goitrogen ingestion (e.g., iodides, antithyroid drugs, other medications; see Table 380.2), thyroidectomy, and radioactive iodine ablative therapy. Infiltrative diseases that can cause hypothyroidism include Langerhans histiocytosis and nephropathic cystinosis.

Some of the causes of congenital hypothyroidism (e.g., ectopic gland, dyshormonogenesis) may not result in thyroid decompensation and the inability to meet metabolic demands until after infancy.

Central acquired hypothyroidism is caused by pituitary or hypothalamic dysfunction. This central process itself may be primary (i.e., idiopathic) or the result of another disease

---

BOX 380.3	Signs and Symptoms of Acquired Hypothyroidism

Short stature, decreased growth velocity
Obesity, myxedema
Goiter (primary hypothyroidism)
Delayed skeletal and dental age
Cold intolerance
Constipation
Dry, cool skin
Thinning of hair
Lethargy
Delayed reflex return
Bradycardia
Delayed puberty
Abnormal menses
Precocious puberty (rare)
Muscular pseudohypertrophy (rare)
Galactorrhea (rare)*

---

*Hypothalamic thyroid-releasing hormone stimulates prolactin release from the posterior pituitary. In primary hypothyroidism, increased thyroid-releasing hormone may produce hyperprolactinemia and galactorrhea.

TABLE 380.4

CLINICAL FEATURES OF AUTOIMMUNE POLYGLANDULAR SYNDROMES

Type I	Type II
Primary hypothyroidism	Primary hypothyroidism
Primary hypogonadism	Primary hypogonadism
Vitiligo	Vitiligo
Pernicious anemia	Pernicious anemia
Alopecia	Alopecia
Malabsorption	Malabsorption
Adrenal insufficiency	Adrenal insufficiency
Mucocutaneous candidiasis	Myasthenia gravis
Chronic active hepatitis	Type I diabetes mellitus
Hypoparathyroidism	Hyperthyroidism
Onset in infancy or childhood	Onset in adulthood
Probably autosomal recessive	Autosomal dominant
No HLA association	HLA-B8, -DR3 associated

process. Idiopathic hypopituitarism is manifested by deficiencies of some or all of the anterior pituitary hormones, including TSH, growth hormone, adrenocorticotropic hormone, luteinizing hormone, and follicle-stimulating hormone. Hypopituitarism can be secondary to infiltrative disease (e.g., histiocytosis), tumor (e.g., craniopharyngioma), head trauma, surgery, and radiation therapy. A greater chance of posterior pituitary involvement occurs in secondary hypopituitarism than in idiopathic hypopituitarism. Posterior pituitary involvement most often is manifested by the presence of diabetes insipidus (i.e., vasopressin deficiency).

TSH deficiency usually is associated with generalized pituitary or hypothalamic dysfunction. Isolated TSH deficiency is a rare occurrence and may be caused by a lack of TRH stimulation (e.g., receptor defects in the pituitary, tumor invasion of the critical hypothalamic nuclei), or it may be idiopathic.

Diagnosis. The diagnosis of hypothyroidism usually is straightforward. The clinical features are listed in Box 380.3. The earliest sign of hypothyroidism in a child often is a slowing of the linear growth rate, as skeletal growth is sensitive to thyroid hormone levels, which is reflected in a delayed bone age and often in delayed puberty. In rare cases of primary hypothyroidism, precocious puberty occurs as a result of secretion of luteinizing hormone and follicle-stimulating hormone, accompanying the increased TSH release. These children may have normal or relatively advanced bone ages caused by the effects of sex steroids, but they do not have the associated pubertal growth spurt. A severe loss of height potential may occur.

Except in the rare cases of peripheral resistance to thyroid hormone, circulating levels of T_4 and T_3 are low in hypothyroidism. Tests that assess concentrations of thyroid hormone–binding proteins (e.g., T_3RU, TBG level) or free T_4 levels must be performed before therapy is initiated. TSH levels help differentiate primary from secondary hypothyroidism. The cause of primary hypothyroidism often can be determined by obtaining a careful history of goitrogen exposure, surgery, or radiation exposure or by assessing antithyroid antibody levels. Determination of the cause of secondary hypothyroidism must involve an assessment of other aspects of the hypothalamic-pituitary system, and performing radiologic studies of the brain may be necessary to rule out tumor or infiltrative disease.

Treatment. The treatment of acquired hypothyroidism is thyroid hormone replacement with a single daily dose of oral levothyroxine (5 to 6 μg/kg/day for 1- to 5-year-olds, 4 to 5 μg/kg/day for 6- to 12-year-olds, 2 to 3 μg/kg/day for adolescents, and 1.7 μg/kg/day for adults). The dose of levothyroxine needs to be titrated based on laboratory (T_4 and TSH values) and growth parameters. Long-standing hypothyroidism affects final height, and early detection and treatment are necessary to prevent this complication. Many children who commence treatment after having long-standing hypothyroidism may experience school and behavioral problems, which may be related to a decrease in attention span and an increase in energy level as they become euthyroid. In cases of hypothyroidism caused by exposure to goitrogen, treating the hypothyroidism by eliminating the exposure may be possible.

The euthyroid sick syndrome, also known as the *low T_3 syndrome*, is a condition present in patients with nonthyroidal illness in whom the total T_3 level is lower than normal, the total T_4 level often is low, and the TSH level is in the normal range. The rT_3 levels may be elevated or normal. Impaired conversion of T_4 to T_3 results in low T_3 levels. The patient's illness may cause increased metabolic clearance of T_4 and a decreased ability of the pituitary to secrete TSH. As a result, total concentration of T_4 may decrease, but free T_4 may remain normal because of the presence of a circulating inhibitor of T_4 binding to TBG. Cytokines such as interleukin (IL)-1, IL-6, and tumor necrosis factor-alpha are thought to play a role as well. In cases of a low level of free T_4, tissue hypothyroidism may exist in this syndrome, but it may be adaptive and even beneficial in severe illness. If the patient recovers from the underlying illness, serum TSH levels increase and may become elevated before the T_3 and T_4 levels return to normal. Replacement therapy with T_4 is not recommended.

Hyperthyroidism

Hyperthyroidism occurs when excessive amounts of circulating thyroid hormone are present. The clinical manifestation is called *thyrotoxicosis*. Like hypothyroidism, hyperthyroidism may be congenital or acquired. Hyperthyroidism in childhood is rare and accounts for less than 5% of all cases of hyperthyroidism.

Congenital Hyperthyroidism

Congenital hyperthyroidism, more often called *neonatal thyrotoxicosis*, occurs almost exclusively in infants of mothers with Graves disease (GD). Neonatal thyrotoxicosis may be transient, lasting up to several weeks, or prolonged, lasting more than 6 months. Neonatal thyrotoxicosis is a serious illness requiring prompt and aggressive management. This disease occurs in as many as 1 of 70 infants of mothers with GD. It has an equal gender distribution, unlike the later-onset form of thyrotoxicosis, which has a female preponderance. If maternal TSI titers are more than five times the normal values, regardless of whether the mother has had ablative thyroid therapy, the risk of neonatal thyrotoxicosis is greatly increased. Neonatal thyrotoxicosis accounts for approximately 1% of all cases of pediatric thyrotoxicosis.

Etiology. The cause of the transient form of neonatal thyrotoxicosis usually is transplacental passage of TSI (i.e., maternal immunoglobulin G) from a mother with GD or, more rarely, Hashimoto thyroiditis. TSIs may continue to be produced even after thyroid ablation (surgery or radioactive iodine). Neonatal thyrotoxicosis secondary to the passage of TSIs is a transient disorder and resolves upon clearance of maternal antibodies from the baby's circulation. However, a rare form of persistent neonatal hyperthyroidism may occur due to activating mutations in the TSH receptor. This disorder should be suspected if the child has a family history of other members with thyrotoxicosis and/or the neonatal form is inherited in an autosomal dominant fashion. Another inherited form may be associated with McCune-Albright syndrome. The prolonged form of the disease also may be caused by endogenously produced TSI from the infant's own lymphocytes or from transplacentally acquired maternal lymphocytes. The incidence of intrauterine death is increased (5% to 7%) in offspring of mothers receiving medical or surgical treatment for thyrotoxicosis and in 24% of offspring of untreated, hyperthyroid mothers. Preterm delivery commonly occurs with this condition and is higher in mothers who are untreated.

Diagnosis. In a neonate, symptoms may be apparent at birth or may be delayed for many days. Affected patients often have low birth weight and microcephaly. They also exhibit marked irritability and hyperactivity, tachycardia, tachypnea, prominent eyes, thyroid enlargement, and a failure to gain weight despite marked hyperphagia. The glandular enlargement may be so marked that it causes respiratory distress requiring endotracheal intubation. Other features include vomiting, severe diarrhea, hepatosplenomegaly, jaundice, thrombocytopenia, and cardiac failure. Eye signs such as periorbital edema, lid retraction, and exophthalmos may be present even in the absence of maternal eye signs. The mortality rate of untreated cases is 15% to 25%, and death usually is caused by cardiac failure.

Fetal tachycardia and intrauterine growth restriction may suggest the diagnosis. The severity of the disease does not correlate with the size of the goiter, but it may be related to maternal TSI levels. The diagnosis is made on the basis of clinical findings combined with elevated levels of T_4, free T_4, and T_3. The diagnosis occasionally may be available prenatally through cordocentesis for fetal thyroid hormone levels, or, alternatively, *in utero* serial ultrasounds have proved to be a useful noninvasive tool in the diagnosis of neonatal thyrotoxicosis.

Treatment. The treatment of neonatal thyrotoxicosis is directed toward immediate management of the symptoms and reduction in the amount of thyroid hormone produced. This treatment may need to be initiated in the intensive care nursery, with adequate cardiopulmonary monitoring and venous access.

Therapy consists of a combination of propylthiouracil, administered as 5 to 10 mg/kg/day, and propranolol, given at a dosage of 2 mg/kg/day. Iodine solutions such as Lugol solution (5% iodine and 10% potassium iodide), given as one drop every 8 hours may be used in conjunction to suppress thyroid hormone synthesis. Treatment with dexamethasone is helpful in some cases. If no improvement occurs within 24 hours, the doses of Lugol solution and propylthiouracil should be increased by at least 50%. If evidence of cardiac failure arises, the infant should be given digoxin or diuretics or both promptly. Adequate caloric intake is vital in these hypermetabolic infants. Serum levels of thyroid hormone must be monitored carefully to ensure adequate therapy and to avoid hypothyroidism. In milder cases, Lugol solution and propranolol may not be needed.

Breast-feeding is not contraindicated for mothers on thioamides; propylthiouracil (PTU) is preferred for maternal treatment and is excreted in much lower concentrations than is methimazole.

Long-term complications of neonatal thyrotoxicosis can occur even in patients who receive prompt and adequate treatment. These complications include premature craniosynostosis and neurodevelopmental defects, particularly intellectual impairment; both may be caused by intrauterine thyrotoxicosis. The intellectual impairment usually correlates with premature craniosynostosis, but a direct effect of thyrotoxicosis on the developing brain cannot be ruled out.

Acquired Hyperthyroidism

Acquired hyperthyroidism most often is caused by GD (i.e., autoimmune thyrotoxicosis). GD has a strong female predominance, with the female-to-male ratio ranging from 3:1 to 5:1. It has a familial tendency, and many genes have been implicated in GD susceptibility. They include MHC-HLA, CTLA-4 gene, and IL-1. The mechanisms by which they confer susceptibility to autoimmune thyroid disease remain unknown. It may occur in the autoimmune polyglandular syndrome. Emotional stress as a precipitating factor of thyrotoxicosis has been described frequently.

Etiology. The cause of GD is autonomous hyperfunction of the thyroid gland, stimulated by TSI. TSI levels are elevated in most patients. TSI binds to the TSH receptors on the thyroid cells, producing the stimulatory effect. GD is serologically related to chronic lymphocytic thyroiditis (CLT) in that antithyroid antibodies may be elevated in patients with GD and in their unaffected family members. The events that stimulate the production of TSI and their relation to antithyroid antibodies are unknown.

BOX 380.4	Signs and Symptoms of Hyperthyroidism

Goiter
Anxiousness, nervousness
Tachycardia
Widened pulse pressure
Increased appetite
Weight loss or gain
Tremor
Proptosis
Heat intolerance
Increased growth velocity
Diarrhea
Sleep disturbances
Fatigue

Diagnosis. The diagnosis of GD is based on the combination of clinical findings (Box 380.4) and the characteristic elevations of thyroid hormone levels. The thyroid gland almost invariably is enlarged, and tachycardia, nervousness, and widened pulse pressure occur in more than 80% of patients. Most patients experience weight loss, although weight gain may occur because of a significantly increased appetite. Proptosis or exophthalmos is a common finding, but the Graves ophthalmopathy in children usually is less severe than that in adults. Pretibial myxedema seen in 1% to 2% of adults rarely is seen in children. Other autoimmune diseases associated with GD are type 1 diabetes, systemic lupus erythematosus, rheumatoid arthritis, Addison disease, and pernicious anemia.

The thyroid hormone profile characteristically shows elevated total T_4, free T_4, and T_3 levels, accompanied by very low or undetectable levels of TSH. In some cases, the T_3 level is elevated with a normal level of T_4 (i.e., T_3 toxicosis). The source of T_3 in patients with T_3 toxicosis is direct secretion by the gland. In these patients, the contribution of T_3 secreted by the gland may equal or exceed that of peripheral T_4 deiodination to the total circulating T_3.

In patients with hyperthyroidism without exophthalmos, differentiating among early CLT, subacute thyroiditis, and GD may be difficult. If TSI levels are not elevated, a radioactive iodine uptake scan aids in establishing the diagnosis. Characteristically, patients with GD have elevated uptake that is not suppressed with administration of T_3. Patients with CLT or subacute thyroiditis generally have normal or decreased uptake of [123]I.

Treatment. The three forms of treatment for GD are medical treatment, radioactive iodine ablation, and surgical treatment. Depending on the clinical circumstances, any of these methods may be used as the initial therapy.

The mainstay of medical management is antithyroid medication with methimazole (Tapazole) or PTU. Both agents are equally effective in decreasing the production of T_4 and T_3 by the thyroid gland, but PTU also blocks the peripheral deiodination of T_4 to T_3. PTU is not known to decrease significantly thyroid gland secretion of T_3 and, therefore, may not provide a significant advantage over methimazole in patients with T_3 toxicosis. The dosage of PTU is 5 to 10 mg/kg/day, divided into three equal doses. The daily dose of methimazole is approximately one-tenth that of PTU, and it has the advantage of having a longer serum half-life, allowing twice-daily or even once-daily doses. If the symptoms of thyrotoxicosis are particularly bothersome to the patient, they may be alleviated by treatment with propranolol (10 to 20 mg every 6 to 8 hours) concomitantly with antithyroid medication until the symptoms improve. With successful treatment, the patient should become euthyroid within 6 weeks.

The medical therapy of thyrotoxicosis is somewhat controversial. In some centers, the dosage of antithyroid medication is increased until the patient becomes hypothyroid, at which time thyroid hormone replacement is added to the regimen. This increase gives the theoretic advantage of maximal suppression of the gland, minimizing the likelihood that relapse will occur. This theory has been supported by clinical trials. In other centers, the dose of antithyroid medication is titrated to maintain the patient in a euthyroid state. After the patient becomes euthyroid using either method, treatment is continued for usually not less than 1 year before the child is assessed for remission by a T_3 suppression test or by discontinuing antithyroid medication. If relapse occurs, the antithyroid medication can be restarted or alternative treatment can be instituted.

Approximately 5% to 10% of patients treated with antithyroid medication experience side effects from the medication. Most of these side effects are minor and include erythematous skin rashes, urticaria, and arthralgias. Granulocytopenia is the most frequent serious side effect and generally is heralded by a fever or sore throat. Vasculitis, at times severe enough to cause pulmonary hemorrhage, is another serious side effect. If side effects occur, discontinuation of the drug generally reverses the problem. The patient then may be treated with a different antithyroid preparation; however, the same reaction may occur.

If medical treatment is not successful because of side effects, frequent relapses, or inability to comply with the treatment schedule, or if the patient or physician prefers an immediate cure, thyroid ablative therapy should be implemented. [131]I ablation has been used widely to treat thyrotoxicosis in adults. Its use in children has increased during the last two decades. With increasing long-term experience, in the future it may be more widely used in the pediatric population. The limitation in its use has been a theoretic risk of the later development of thyroid cancer or other malignancies. However, the data currently available suggest that ^{131}I treatment in childhood or adolescence does not affect the risk of developing thyroidal or nonthyroidal cancers or leukemia and does not increase the risk of birth defects occurring in the patients' offspring. Remission from thyrotoxicosis should occur within several weeks, and remission most often is followed by permanent hypothyroidism after several months.

Surgical subtotal thyroidectomy is effective and has low morbidity when performed by an experienced surgeon. The patient must be euthyroid for surgery, and preoperative treatment with iodides such as Lugol solution often is recommended to decrease vascularity of the gland. The risks include those associated with general anesthesia as well as hypothyroidism (up to 50%); transient hypocalcemia (10% to 20%) and, rarely, hypoparathyroidism; recurrent laryngeal nerve damage; or recurrence of thyrotoxicosis.

Prognosis. The prognosis for children with GD generally is good. Evidence suggests that with antithyroid medication alone, remission of GD, defined as being euthyroid for 1 year after stopping medication, occurs at a rate of approximately 25% every 2 years. In some cases, relapse of hyperthyroidism or spontaneous hypothyroidism may occur after remission.

Thyroid Storm and Thyrotoxic Periodic Paralysis

Although rare, thyroid storm and thyrotoxic periodic paralysis (TPP) are two endocrine emergencies reported with hyperthyroidism. Thyroid storm, also called *thyrotoxic crisis*, is a life-threatening manifestation of thyrotoxicosis, which is a

clinical diagnosis based on the manifestations of exaggerated and uncontrolled hyperthyroidism. Patients generally present with marked hyperthermia and tachycardia and may develop cardiac failure, vomiting, diarrhea, and CNS abnormalities, including confusion, apathy, and coma. Thyroid storm can be precipitated by many events but most often is associated with infection, surgery, or trauma. The therapy includes aggressive antithyroid treatment, including PTU or methimazole, Lugol solution, or lithium carbonate; prevention of thyroid hormone action with beta-blockade; antipyretics; support of life-threatening conditions using intravenous hydration, oxygen, and digitalis; and treatment of any underlying infection.

TPP is a reversible cause of sudden-onset weakness that most commonly affects hyperthyroid patients of Asian descent. However, it has been observed in other persons as well. At presentation, signs and symptoms of thyrotoxicosis may be subtle and may be overlooked. Proximal muscle limb weakness commonly occurs. Mental, sensory, or respiratory muscles are spared. Rhythm and electrocardiographic abnormalities have been noted. The exact mechanism of this disorder is unknown. Altered plasma membrane permeability to sodium and potassium, a function of Na^+-K^+, has been theorized. Treatment includes hospital observation of cardiac rhythm, potassium correction if indicated, and antithyroid medications. Treatment of hyperthyroidism causes a resolution of paralysis. Precipitating factors such as strenuous exercise and high carbohydrate intake should be avoided.

Other causes of hyperthyroxinemia are rare. They include subacute thyroiditis, pituitary resistance to thyroid hormone, activating mutations of TSH receptor, generalized resistance to thyroid hormone, familial dysalbuminemias, excess TBG, factitious hyperthyroidism from excessive intake of exogenous thyroid hormone, and TSH-secreting pituitary tumors. In generalized resistance to thyroid hormone, mutant thyroid hormone receptors result in high thyroxine and TSH levels, but the patients are clinically euthyroid. They have a high incidence (46%) of attention-deficit hyperactivity disorder. However, patients with this disorder do not have a higher than expected incidence of generalized resistance to thyroid hormone, and they have only a slightly higher incidence of thyroid function abnormalities than that of the general population.

Thyromegaly

Thyromegaly, or enlargement of the thyroid gland or goiter, is an uncommon finding in children. Causes include neoplasm, infiltration, inflammation, or stimulation of the gland. The enlargement may be diffuse or nodular (Box 380.5). Enlargement of certain nonthyroidal structures may mimic thyromegaly.

Diffuse Thyromegaly

Diffuse thyromegaly most often is caused by autoimmune thyroid diseases, including Hashimoto thyroiditis (i.e., CLT) and GD. Autoimmune thyroid disease accounts for more than 90% of the patients with diffuse thyromegaly. A female preponderance exists among children with diffuse thyromegaly. The cause, diagnosis, and treatment of these two diseases were discussed previously.

Two rarer forms of thyroiditis also may produce diffuse thyromegaly. Subacute thyroiditis, presumably caused by a viral infection, occurs much less frequently in children than in adults. It usually presents with firm, tender enlargement of the gland during or immediately after a viral syndrome involving pharyngitis, fever, myalgia, and fatigue. A painless enlargement of the thyroid gland also has been described in this disease. At the time of presentation, thyroid function test results often

---

BOX 380.5   **Causes of Thyromegaly**

Diffuse
Hashimoto thyroiditis
Thyrotoxicosis
    Graves disease
Thyroiditis
    Thyroid–stimulating hormone–secreting adenoma
    Pituitary resistance to thyroid hormone
Goitrogen exposure
Dyshormonogenesis
Iodine deficiency (endemic)
Idiopathic (simple) goiter
Acute, subacute thyroiditis

Nodular
Hashimoto thyroiditis
Thyroid cyst
Thyroid adenoma
Hyperfunctional (hot)
Hypofunctional (cold)
Thyroid carcinoma
    Papillary
    Follicular
    Mixed papillary or follicular
    Anaplastic
    Medullary
Nonthyroidal masses
    Lymphadenopathy
    Branchial cleft cyst
    Thyroglossal duct cyst

---

suggest thyrotoxicosis, with elevated thyroid hormone levels and undetectable TSH levels caused by inflammatory destruction of the gland and release of stored T_4 and T_3 into the circulation. However, in contrast to GD, the 24-hour uptake of radioactive iodine is very low.

After the hyperthyroid phase of several weeks to months, a recovery phase that may last several months occurs. During this phase, the thyroid function test results reveal chemical hypothyroidism, with decreased serum T_4 and elevated TSH levels and an abnormally high radioactive iodine uptake. After the hypothyroid phase, the patient usually recovers completely, with normal thyroid function test results and a gland of normal size and consistency. In rare cases, permanent hypothyroidism has been described. Antithyroid antibodies may be measurable during the acute and hypothyroid phases, but generally they disappear after recovery.

Treatment includes antiinflammatory therapy, including aspirin and possibly glucocorticoids, during the acute phase. If the patient is disturbed by the symptoms of hyperthyroidism, propranolol may be added, but treatment with antithyroid medication generally is not indicated. During the recovery phase, hypothyroidism should be treated with thyroxine replacement for several months, at which time the dose is tapered and serum T_4 and TSH levels are remeasured.

Acute (suppurative) thyroiditis is a rare cause of diffuse thyromegaly, especially in the United States. Acute thyroiditis is caused by a bacterial infection of the gland and may be unilateral or bilateral. Most cases occur during or after an upper respiratory tract infection. The most common organisms cultured from an acutely infected thyroid gland are *Staphylococcus aureus* and *Streptococcus hemolyticus* or *Streptococcus pneumoniae*.

The patient presents with acute onset of fever, chills, sore throat, and dysphagia and with an extremely tender and enlarged gland. Thyroid function test results, including radioactive iodine uptake, usually are normal, and antithyroid antibodies are undetectable. Early treatment with parenteral antibiotics, after aspiration for culture, is necessary to avoid formation and rupture of an abscess. With prompt and aggressive treatment, full recovery is expected. In some children, acute thyroiditis has been associated with a fistula of the piriform sinus. In these patients, the left lobe of the gland is involved more often.

In certain parts of the world, diffuse thyromegaly caused by iodine deficiency (i.e., endemic goiter) still is a common occurrence, but supplementation of dietary salt with iodine has rendered iodine deficiency a rare problem in North America.

In some cases of diffuse thyromegaly, particularly in adolescent girls, no cause can be determined, and the diagnosis of idiopathic (simple) goiter is made. Other causes of enlargement of the thyroid gland (see Box 380.5) are ingestion of a goitrogen (including antithyroid medication), other drugs, and certain foods; familial dyshormonogenesis; and rare pituitary abnormalities, such as pituitary resistance to thyroid hormone or a TSH-secreting pituitary adenoma.

Nodular Thyromegaly

Nodular thyromegaly, an enlargement of one or more areas of the thyroid gland, may be unilateral or bilateral and usually is nontender. Some causes of nodular thyromegaly are listed in Box 380.5. Certain nonthyroidal tissues may present with an enlargement in the area of the thyroid gland, including lymph nodes, cysts (e.g., thyroglossal duct, branchial cleft), neurofibromas, hemangiomas, and lymphangiomas.

Thyroid nodules are rare findings in children. The most common cause of asymmetric enlargement of the thyroid gland is Hashimoto thyroiditis. However, the incidence of malignant neoplasms is higher in children's nodules than in adults' nodules. Performing a comprehensive and rapid diagnostic evaluation of solitary or multiple thyroid nodules is imperative.

The history should include questions about previous irradiation to the head, neck, or thorax for any reason (including repeated fluoroscopy) because such irradiation has been shown to increase the risk for later development of thyroid neoplasia. This risk is proportional to the dosage of irradiation, and the neoplasm may appear anywhere between 3 and 35 years later. Rapid and painless enlargement of the nodule may suggest neoplasia. If the nodule is tender or intermittently painful, more likely it is caused by acute or subacute thyroiditis or a hemorrhagic cyst. The risk of malignancy is higher in solitary than in multiple nodules. Symptoms that suggest hypothyroidism or hyperthyroidism are less likely to occur with malignant than with benign lesions.

Family history is especially important in the case of multiple endocrine neoplasia (MEN) syndromes, which are associated with medullary carcinoma of the thyroid gland. This carcinoma is derived from the C cells that secrete calcitonin. Depending on the particular type of MEN syndrome within the family, other neoplasms, such as multiple mucosal neuromas, pheochromocytoma, and parathyroid adenoma, may occur (see Chapter 382).

Physical examination of the neck must include careful palpation of the gland and its surrounding structures, including local lymph nodes. Consistency, mobility, and tenderness of the nodule must be evaluated.

The diagnostic evaluation of thyroid nodularity includes blood and radiologic tests of thyroid function. Blood tests that are indicated include thyroid hormone and TSH levels (often normal in malignant lesions), antithyroid antibodies (in CLT), and calcitonin levels before and after pentagastrin stimulation if medullary carcinoma of the thyroid is suspected. In individuals at risk for development of MEN syndromes, genetic testing often is helpful in identifying affected individuals before neoplasms are clinically obvious. Thyroglobulin levels, although helpful in the follow-up of treated thyroid carcinoma as a marker for recurrence, are not always helpful in the initial evaluation.

Radiologic studies are of great importance in the evaluation of thyroid nodules. Radiography may show calcification of the gland or local lymph nodes or demonstrate pulmonary metastases. Ultrasound can differentiate solid from cystic nodules. Radioisotope scanning can assess the functional activity of the nodule. A hyperfunctional (hot) nodule is more likely to be caused by an adenoma, thyroiditis, or thyrotoxicosis than by a carcinoma. A hypofunctional (cold) nodule is more likely to be malignant or nonthyroidal, whereas a solitary isofunctional (warm) nodule is more likely to be benign.

In most pediatric centers, a definite tissue diagnosis made by needle biopsy or surgical excision is recommended for all thyroid nodules. In the case of warm nodules, a trial of thyroid hormone suppression may be undertaken in an attempt to shrink the nodule. If the nodule enlarges or fails to decrease, a tissue diagnosis is necessary.

Thyroid Tumors in Children

Thyroid cancer is rare in children. Papillary carcinoma is the most common form, and the tumor usually is well-differentiated. Medullary thyroid carcinoma may occur in association with MEN syndromes. Radiation exposure such as occurred with the Chernobyl disaster resulted in a 100-fold increase in the incidence of pediatric thyroid cancer. Radiation and chemotherapy associated with other childhood malignancies also has been implicated in the occurrence of thyroid malignancy.

Diagnosis

Thyroid function with thyroglobulin levels and genetic testing of the *RET* gene in at-risk children for MEN 2 should be included. Imaging studies using thyroid scans, ultrasonography, computed tomography, or magnetic resonance imaging scans are helpful in delineating the size and extent of disease. Histopathologic confirmation requires ultrasound-guided fine-needle aspiration biopsy and/or biopsy of the mass.

Treatment

Surgical removal of the tumor and involved lymph nodes is the mainstay of therapy with radioactive iodine ^{131}I for residual disease.

Suggested Readings

Ballabio M, Nicolini U, Jowett T, et al. Maturation of thyroid function in normal human fetuses. *Clin Endocrinol* 1989;31:565.

Burger AG. Effects of certain pharmacologic agents on the peripheral metabolism of thyroxine. In: Ingbar SH, Braverman LE, eds. *Werner's the thyroid: a fundamental and clinical text*. Philadelphia: Lippincott-Raven, 1986:351.

Delange F, Dalhem A, Bourdoux P, et al. Increased risk of primary hypothyroidism in preterm infants. *J Pediatr* 1984;105:462.

Fisher DA. The hypothyroxinemia of prematurity [editorial]. *J Clin Endocrinol Metab* 1997;82:1701.

Fisher DA. The thyroid. In: Kaplan SA, ed. *Clinical pediatric endocrinology*. Philadelphia: Saunders, 1990:95.

Fisher DA. The thyroid. In: Rudolph AM, ed. *Pediatrics*. Norwalk, CT: Appleton & Lange, 1987:1504.

Fisher DA, Vanderschueran-Lodeweyckx M. Laboratory tests for thyroid diagnosis in infants and children. In: Delange F, Fisher DA, Malvaux P, eds. *Pediatric thyroidology*. Basel: S Karger, 1985:127.

Foley T, Malvaux P, Blizzard R. Thyroid disease. In: Kappy MS, Blizzard RM, Migeon CJ, eds. *Wilkins' the diagnosis and treatment of endocrine disorders in childhood and adolescence*, 4th ed. Springfield, IL: Charles C Thomas, 1994: 457.

Hashizume K, Ichikawa K, Sakurai A, et al. Administration of thyroxine in treated Graves disease: effects on the level of antibodies to thyroid-stimulating hormone receptors and on the risk of recurrence of hyperthyroidism. *N Engl J Med* 1991;324:947.

Hung W. Thyroid nodules and thyroid cancer. In: Delange F, Fisher DA, Malvaux P, eds. *Pediatric thyroidology*. Basel: S Karger, 1985:271.

Kaplan MM. Interactions between drugs and thyroid hormones. *Thyroid Today* 1981;4:5.

Koch CA, Sarlis NJ. The spectrum of thyroid diseases in childhood and its evolution during transition to adulthood: natural history, diagnosis, differential diagnosis and management. *J Endocrinol Invest* 2001;24:659.

Linder N, Davidovitch N, Reichman B, et al. Topical iodine-containing antiseptics and subclinical hypothyroidism in preterm infants. *J Pediatr* 1997; 131:434.

Lippe BM, Landaw EM, Kaplan SA. Hyperthyroidism in children treated with long-term medical therapy: twenty-five percent remission every two years. *J Clin Endocrinol Metab* 1987;64:1241.

Rivkees SA, Sklar C, Freemark M. Clinical review 99: the management of Graves' disease in children, with special emphasis on radioiodine treatment. *J Clin Endocrinol Metab* 1998;83:3767.

Thorpe-Beeston JG, Nicolaides KH, Felton CV, et al. Maturation of the secretion of thyroid hormone and thyroid stimulating hormone in the fetus. *N Engl J Med* 1991;324:532.

Van Vliet G. Treatment of congenital hypothyroidism. *Lancet* 2001;358:86.

Weiss RE, Stein MA, Trommer B, Refetoff S. Attention-deficit hyperactivity disorder and thyroid function. *J Pediatr* 1993;123:539.

CHAPTER 381 ■ ADRENAL CORTEX

PATRICIA A. DONOHOUE

NORMAL ADRENAL DEVELOPMENT AND STEROID HORMONE SYNTHESIS

The fetal adrenal cortex develops from coelomic mesothelium in proximity to the developing bipotential gonads. The cortex then separates from the gonads, which eventually migrate to their adult positions. For this reason, rests of adrenocortical tissue may appear along the paths of migration or near or within the gonads in adults. By the sixth week of gestation, steroid-producing cells appear in the adrenal cortex, and by the tenth week, the fetal zone (comprising 80% of the total volume) and the adult (definitive) zone are producing steroid hormones under the stimulatory control of adrenocorticotropic hormone (ACTH) stimulation. The fetal zone, whose major products are estrogen and androgen precursors, begins to degenerate by the eighth month of gestation. At that time, the adult zone begins to develop and then differentiate into a mature adult cortex that secretes the three families of steroid hormones: mineralocorticoids, glucocorticoids, and androgens. This differentiation is not completed until the child is approximately 3 years of age.

The adult adrenal cortex constitutes approximately 90% of the mature gland and is composed of three zones. The outermost zone, the zona glomerulosa, accounts for 15% of the cortical volume and is the site of mineralocorticoid synthesis. The zona fasciculata constitutes 75% of the cortex, and the reticularis (the innermost zone) constitutes 10%. The zona fasciculata and zona reticularis are one functional unit, involved in glucocorticoid and androgen biosynthesis. The zona reticu-

laris is thought to secrete steroids under basal conditions, and the zona fasciculata stores lipids for stress steroidogenesis.

All three groups of steroid hormones are produced from cholesterol, which is supplied by the circulation or produced endogenously. Under the stimulation of the anterior pituitary hormone ACTH, cholesterol is converted to pregnenolone. This conversion is the rate-limiting step in steroid hormone biosynthesis. Pregnenolone serves as the precursor for all three families of adrenal steroid hormones (Fig. 381.1).

Pituitary ACTH release is controlled by the hypothalamic peptide, corticotropin-releasing hormone (CRH). ACTH secretion also may be under the influence of the immune system. Normal ACTH secretion occurs in a diurnal pattern, which results in the normal diurnal fluctuation in serum cortisol levels: highest in the early morning and lowest in the evening. The serum cortisol level completes the feedback loop by stimulating (low cortisol levels) or suppressing (high cortisol levels)

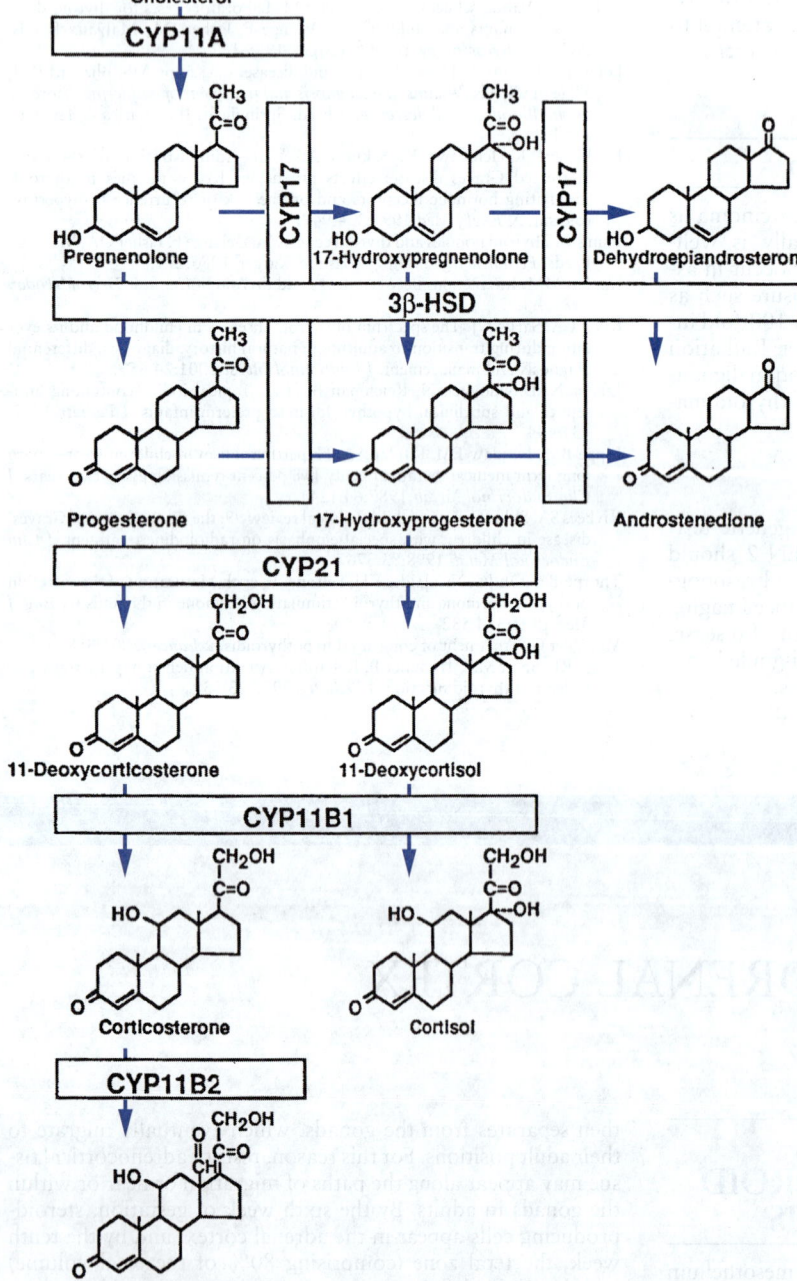

FIGURE 381.1. Adrenal steroid biosynthetic pathways. The 20-hydroxylase, 22-hydroxylase, and 20,22-desmolase are activities of the same CYP11A enzyme. Both 17-alpha-hydroxylase and 17,20-desmolase activities are properties of the same CYP17 enzyme. However, 11-beta-hydroxylase and CMO activities are properties of two different isozymes, CYP11B1 and CYP11B2, encoded by different adjacent genes. The single enzyme that has CMOI and CMOII activities is termed aldosterone synthase (CYP11B2). In addition, several isoforms of 3-beta-HSD exist, some of which are expressed in extraadrenal sites. 3β-HSD, 3-beta-hydroxysteroid dehydrogenase, Δ^5,Δ^4-isomerase; CMO, corticosterone methyl oxidase; CYP11B1, 11-beta-hydroxylase; CYP11B2, 18-hydroxylase (CMOI) and 18-dehydrogenase (oxidase) (CMOII); CYP17, 17-alpha-hydroxylase and 17,20-desmolase (lyase); CYP21, 21-hydroxylase; CYP11A, 20-hydroxylase, 22-hydroxylase, 20,22-desmolase. (From Donohoue PA, Parker KL, Migeon CJ. Congenital adrenal hyperplasia. In: Scriver CR, Beaudet AL, Sly WS, Valle D, eds. *The metabolic and molecular bases of inherited disease,* 8th ed. New York: McGraw-Hill, 2001:4077, with permission from McGraw-Hill Publishers.)

TABLE 381.1

GLUCOCORTICOID DOSAGES

Preparation	Physiologic Replacement Dose*
Hydrocortisone	12.5 mg/m^2/day IM or IV 15–25.0 mg/m^2/day PO
Cortisone acetate	16 mg/m^2/day IM or IV 25–32 mg/m^2/day PO
Prednisolone	3–5 mg/m^2/day PO

IM, intramuscularly; IV, intravenously; PO, *per os* (by mouth).
*Recommended doses for daily physiologic replacement of glucocorticoid. The actual optimal dose must be titrated for each patient.

hypothalamic CRH secretion and pituitary ACTH secretion. Serotonin stimulates and norepinephrine inhibits hypothalamic CRH secretion. The daily cortisol secretion rate initially was determined to be 12.1 ± 3 mg/m^2 of body surface area (the total daily cortisol production increasing with growth), and this value still is widely accepted. More recent studies, employing different techniques, suggest a lower but more variable secretion rate. Based on the average daily production of cortisol and the potencies of various pharmacologic glucocorticoid preparations, recommendations can be made about the average daily dose of each that would be required for physiologic replacement (Table 381.1). Many preparations also have a mineralocorticoid effect (Table 381.2). In times of physiologic stress (fever or other illnesses), the recommendation is that the oral cortisol replacement doses be increased by threefold.

Most cortisol circulates in the blood bound to cortisol-binding globulin (CBG), also known as *transcortin*, an alpha-globulin secreted by the liver. The free fraction of cortisol is the biologically active hormone. Estrogens increase levels of CBG, and liver disease and the nephrotic syndrome are associated with decreased levels of CBG. However, levels of free cortisol are unaffected by these conditions.

The major physiologic metabolic effects of cortisol are glycogen synthesis, gluconeogenesis, fat catabolism, and protein catabolism. At high levels, glucocorticoids induce a wide variety of metabolic changes, including immunosuppression, osteoporosis, glucose intolerance, increased gastric acid secretion, and altered central nervous system (CNS) function, resulting in psychiatric symptoms.

Mineralocorticoid (e.g., aldosterone) secretion is controlled mainly by the renin-angiotensin system and also by serum

TABLE 381.2

RELATIVE POTENCIES OF CORTICOSTEROIDS

Steroid Preparation	Effect* Glucocorticoid	Mineralocorticoid (mg)
Cortisone	100	100
Hydrocortisone	80	80
Prednisone	20	100
Prednisolone	20	100
Methylprednisolone	16	No effect
9-alpha-Fluorocortisol	5	0.2
Dexamethasone	2	No effect

*Relative glucocorticoid and mineralocorticoid potencies. The doses given for each preparation represent approximately equivalent clinical effects. For example, the mineralocorticoid effect of 0.2 mg 9-alpha-fluorocortisol (Florinef) is equivalent to the mineralocorticoid effect of 100 mg cortisone. Prednisone and prednisolone are potent glucocorticoids and weak mineralocorticoids.

potassium levels. The cells of the zona glomerulosa, which have specific membrane receptors for angiotensin II, secrete aldosterone and its precursors. Stimulation of the adrenal cortex with ACTH produces only a transient increase in levels of aldosterone. The average daily aldosterone secretion rate is not related to body surface area and is similar for infants and adults (approximately 100 μg/day). The major physiologic effect of mineralocorticoids is exerted at the level of the distal convoluted tubule, where they promote retention of sodium and excretion of potassium.

The factors that control secretion of adrenal androgen are not understood as well. In prepubertal children, the production of adrenal androgens is very low. At puberty, their production increases and normal adrenarche occurs. The most potent adrenal androgen is androstenedione, which is converted outside the adrenal gland to the more potent androgen testosterone. At very high levels, dehydroepiandrosterone, a weak androgen, may exert androgenic effects. In pubertal and adult males, the adrenal gland contributes little to the total production of androgen. However, in pubertal and adult females, at least 50% of the circulating testosterone is derived from adrenal androstenedione.

TESTS OF ADRENOCORTICAL FUNCTION

Static Tests

The static tests of adrenocortical function provide important but limited information and often must be accompanied by dynamic testing in the diagnostic evaluation of adrenal disorders. Normal values for some levels of adrenal steroids and responses to dynamic tests are given in Table 381.3.

The level of serum cortisol is measured by immunoassay and is interpretable only if the time of day that the sample was obtained is known. If the cortisol level is subnormal at 8 AM, the time of a normal peak, hypocortisolism is suspected. However, this test does not discriminate among primary adrenal failure, ACTH deficiency, or an enzymatic defect in the biosynthesis of cortisol. A low level of cortisol late in the day is normal and has little value in the assessment of adrenal failure. However, if the level is elevated in a nonstressed patient, it may indicate absence of the normal pattern of diurnal variation often seen in Cushing syndrome. Because the level of serum cortisol rises briskly in response to such stresses as fever, trauma, surgery, fear, or anxiety, single determinations of levels of cortisol cannot be used reliably to diagnose hypercortisolism.

Determination of the level of serum ACTH is useful only if it is accompanied by other tests of adrenal function. The diurnal variation in levels of cortisol is preceded by similar fluctuations in levels of ACTH. An extremely elevated level of ACTH in the setting of subnormal levels of serum cortisol suggests primary adrenal failure. However, because ACTH mediates the rise in serum cortisol in response to stress, its levels vary widely.

Mineralocorticoid status is assessed by measuring concentrations of serum electrolytes and plasma renin activity (PRA), which is elevated in mineralocorticoid deficiency. PRA is a measure of the rate of conversion of angiotensinogen to angiotensin I. Such factors as blood pressure, posture, intake of sodium, and renal function affect PRA and must be considered in the interpretation of the test result. The PRA assay may be useful in monitoring the adequacy of mineralocorticoid replacement therapy. A direct renin assay also is now available. Levels of plasma or urinary excretion of aldosterone and deoxycorticosterone also are useful for assessing secretion of mineralocorticoids.

TABLE 381.3

NORMAL PLASMA AND URINARY STEROID HORMONE LEVELS WITH STATIC AND DYNAMIC TESTS

Test	Values[a]		
Static tests			
Plasma cortisol[b]	*μg/dL*		
Premature infants (day 4)			
26–28 weeks	1–11 (6.0)		
31–35 weeks	2.5–9.1 (6.4)		
Full-term infants			
3 days	1.7–14 (6.2)		
7 days	2–11 (4.4)		
31 days–11 months	2.8–23 (9.4)		
Children			
12 months–15 years (0800)	3–21 (9.8)		
Adults			
0800	8–19 (11.0)		
1600	4–11 (5.9)		
	mg/g creatinine	*mg/24 hours*	
Urinary 17-hydroxy corticosteroids (17-OHCS)	Prepubertal children		
1–4 years	1.7–6.4 (4.1)	0.2–2.5 (0.8)	
5–9 years	2.2–6.0 (3.5)	0.5–2.5 (1.2)	
Pubertal children and adults			
Male	2.4–4.3 (3.2)	3–10 (6.4)	
Female	1.6–3.6 (2.3)	2–6 (2.8)	
	μg/g creatinine	*μg/24 hours*	
Urinary free cortisol	Prepubertal children	7–25 (15)	3–9 (5.2)
	Adult men	7–45 (21)	11–84 (40)
	Adult women	9–32 (19)	10–34 (20)
	Pregnancy	14–59 (38)	16–60 (47)
	(μg/dL)		
Salivary cortisol	Prepubertal children		
0800	0.17–1.2		
1600	0.10–0.33		
2300	0.03–0.19		
Adults			
0800	0.18–0.95		
1600	0.10–0.28		
2300	0.05–0.17		
Postdexamethasone (after 1 mg @ 2300)			
0800	<0.1		
Dynamic tests			
Adrenal capacity	Plasma cortisol at 1 hour is double baseline level and >18 μg/dL		
Rapid IV test: 0.25 mg Cortrosyn over 1 minute:			
Prolonged test: 20 U/m²Acthar gel IM every 12 hours for 3 days, or 0.25 mg Cortrosyn IV over 8–12 hours beginning at 0800 for 3 days:	Urinary 17-OHCS: three- to fivefold increase over baseline		
ACTH capacity[c]			
Oral metyrapone 15 mg/kg every 4 hours six times from 0800 to 1600:	Urinary 17-OHCS increase two- to fourfold or serum 11-deoxy-cortisol increase to >10 ng/dL		
Oral metyrapone: 30–40 mg/kg (up to 3.0 g) at midnight:	8 AM: Increase in serum 11-deoxycortisol to >7 μg/dL, with a decrease in serum cortisol to <5 μg/dL		
Regular insulin 0.05–0.10 U/kg IV or glucagon 0.1 mg/kg IM:	Rise in serum cortisol by 10 μg/dL or to >20 μg/dL		
Pituitary suppression tests:			

Overnight test

20 μg/kg dexamethasone PO (up to 1.0 mg*) at 2300, with serum cortisol level at 0800 the following morning.
  Normal response: 0800 cortisol <5 μg/dl rules against Cushing syndrome[†,‡]

Low-dose test

48 hour, 2 mg/day (0.5 mg PO q6h)
  Normal response: 0800 cortisol level obtained 2 hours after the last dose of dexamethasone ≤1.8 μg/dL rules against Cushing syndrome[§]

48 hour, 2 mg/day test combined with CRH stimulation test at 0800, 2 hours after the last dose of dexamethasone
    Normal response: serum cortisol <1.4 μg/dl, 15 minutes after CRH 1 μg/kg IV (or 100 μg IV in adults) rules against Cushing syndrome

(Continued)

TABLE 381.3

(CONTINUED)

Test	Values[a]

High-dose test for differential diagnosis of ACTH-dependent Cushing syndrome[ǁ]
48 hour, 8 mg/day (2 mg dexamethasone PO q6h)
    Suppression of urinary 17-OHCS by >50% consistent with pituitary source of ACTH
Overnight test (8 mg dexamethasone PO at 2300)
    Serum cortisol at 0800 the mornings before and after show suppression of serum cortisol by >50% suggests pituitary source of ACTH	

ACTH, adrenocorticotropic hormone; CRH, corticotropin-releasing hormone; IM, intramuscularly; IV, intravenously.
*The use of a 1.5- or 2.0-mg dose offers no better discrimination between the presence and absence of Cushing syndrome.
†There are some patients with Cushing syndrome whose serum cortisol will suppress to <5 μg/dL. A cutoff of ≤1.8 μg/dL effectively excludes all cases of Cushing syndrome.
‡Some suggest simultaneous measurement of a dexamethasone level to ensure compliance if the testing is performed as an outpatient.
§The original report of Liddle (Tests of pituitary-adrenal suppressibility in the diagnosis of Cushing syndrome. *J Clin Endocrinol Metab* 1960;20:1539) described suppression of urinary 17-hydroxycorticosteroid excretion as the expected outcome.
ǁThis test is utilized *after* excess ACTH has been demonstrated. It has been largely replaced by high-resolution radiologic studies, bilateral inferior petrosal sampling, and CRH stimulation testing.
[a]Normal ranges and means (in parentheses) for static test values are based on reference ranges from Esoterix Laboratories, Calabasas Hills, California, and are used with permission.
[b]Stress or anxiety may cause elevation of cortisol levels far above the stated normal range.
[c]In many centers, metyrapone no longer is available for diagnostic testing. Insulin-induced hypoglycemia or glucagon stimulation will be the tests of choice for ACTH capacity. The specific details of the glucagon stimulation test are described in Vanderschueren-Lodeweyckx M, Wolter R, Malvaux P, et al. The glucagon stimulation test: effect on plasma growth hormone and on immunoreactive insulin, cortisol, and glucose in children. *J Pediatr* 1974;85:182.

Levels of plasma adrenal androgen are affected less by physiologic conditions, such as stress and state of hydration, than are other static tests of adrenocortical function. They are useful in evaluating hyperandrogenic states caused by a variety of factors, such as adrenal tumors and adrenal enzyme deficiencies. However, elevated levels must be investigated further with the appropriate stimulation or suppression tests.

Plasma levels of numerous of steroid precursors and adrenal androgens are helpful in establishing the diagnosis and providing therapeutic management of the inherited steroidogenic enzyme deficiencies (e.g., congenital adrenal hyperplasia). Normal values for these levels depend on the reference laboratory, but age and gender differences are reflected in the representative set of normal values provided in Table 381.4.

Measurement of urinary steroids and their metabolites may be a helpful adjunct to determination of levels of plasma steroids. The 24-hour excretion of urinary 17-hydroxycorticosteroids is a measure of daily glucocorticoid production. The 24-hour urinary-free cortisol is used widely in screening for Cushing syndrome. The 24-hour excretion of urinary 17-ketosteroids reflects the total daily production of adrenal androgen (androstenedione) and is useful in the diagnostic evaluation and assessment of treatment adequacy in hyperandrogenic states.

Dynamic Tests

Adrenocorticotropic Hormone Stimulation Test

The ACTH stimulation test is used to evaluate the response of the adrenal cortex to pharmacologic levels of ACTH. The short intravenous ACTH test is used for assessing production (ACTH responsiveness) of cortisol in a patient with failing adrenal glands or ACTH deficiency. Levels of serum cortisol are measured 60 minutes after the patient receives rapid intravenous infusion of synthetic ACTH (cosyntropin [Cortrosyn]) or during and after an 8- to 12-hour infusion. A subnormal response in a patient who has not received glucocorticoid therapy may indicate primary adrenal failure (i.e., Addison disease). If the failed response is accompanied by high PRA or by hyponatremia and hyperkalemia, primary adrenal failure is diagnosed. If electrolytes are normal, measurement of PRA and levels of

aldosterone may reveal evidence of failing but compensated mineralocorticoid production. If the mineralocorticoid status is normal and the patient has a failed cortisol response to IV ACTH, then a prolonged test (2 weeks of IM ACTH as Acthar gel) may be indicated. If the levels of cortisol rise with prolonged stimulation of ACTH, then central ACTH deficiency is suspected.

The intravenous ACTH test can be used also to assess the adrenal gland's recovery after a prolonged course (more than 1 month) of pharmacologic doses of glucocorticoids. A subnormal response reflects the loss of ability to respond to stimulation of ACTH after prolonged suppression of ACTH secretion. Unlike patients with Addison disease, these patients should have normal production of mineralocorticoids, and they should have a normal cortisol response to a 2-week course of Acthar gel. Patients with ACTH suppression caused by prolonged corticosteroid therapy will have responses to ACTH testing similar to those seen in patients with ACTH deficiency caused by partial or panhypopituitarism.

The short intravenous ACTH test is useful also in assessing adrenal enzyme deficiencies, especially 21-hydroxylase deficiency. The cortisol precursors progesterone and 17-hydroxyprogesterone are measured before and 30 minutes (and sometimes 60 minutes) after the patient is given a rapid infusion of ACTH. The rate of rise is calculated and compared with normal ranges according to age, gender, and stage of the menstrual cycle. Results can be used to identify both heterozygous carriers and affected individuals. This test should be performed during the follicular phase of the cycle in menstruating females.

Adrenocorticotropic Hormone Secretion Tests

Several dynamic tests are available for assessing ACTH secretion in patients with suspected hypopituitarism. Perhaps the most sensitive test of ACTH release is insulin-induced hypoglycemia. After the patient has been given an intravenous bolus of regular insulin, serial measurements of levels of blood glucose, cortisol, and growth hormone are made. Symptomatic hypoglycemia is the desired end-point, but changes in levels of consciousness must be treated with prompt administration of intravenous dextrose. The test is not recommended for young infants because of the risk of damage to the central nervous system resulting from hypoglycemia.

TABLE 381.4

NORMAL VALUES FOR ADRENAL ANDROGENS AND COMMONLY MEASURED CORTISOL PRECURSORS

	Androstenedione (ng/dL)	DHEA (ng/dL)	17-Hydroxyprogesterone (ng/dL)
Cord blood	30–150 (90)	200–1,590 (600)	900–5,000 (1,900)
Premature infants (day 4)			
26–28 wk	92–892 (254)	236–3,640 (941)	124–841 (471)
31–35 wk	80–446 (207)	80–3,150 (811)	26–568 (248)
Full-term infants	1–7 d: 20–290 (150)	3 d: 65–1,250 (570)	3 d: 7–77 (36)
	1–11 mo: 6–68 (23)	8–30 d: 50–760 (285)	1–11 mo Boys*Girls: 13–106 (31)
		31d–5 mo: 26–385 (113)	
		6–11 mo: 20–100 (40)	
Prepubertal	1–10 yr: 8–50 (24)	12 m–5 yr: 20–130 (29)	1–10 yr: 3–90 (38)
		6–7 yr: 20–275 (93)	
Puberty		8–10 yr: 31–345 (156)	
Tanner 1			
Male (<9.8 y)	8–50 (24)	31–345 (156)	3–90 (38)
Female (<9.2 y)	8–50 (24)	31–345 (156)	3–82 (31)
Tanner 2			
Male (9.8–14.5 y)	31–65 (45)	110–495 (300)	5–115 (51)
Female (9.2–13.7y)	42–100 (65)	150–570 (330)	11–98 (49)
Tanner 3			
Male (10.7–15.4 y)	50–100 (67)	170–585 (390)	10–138 (57)
Female (10.0–14.4 y)	80–190 (123)	200–600 (385)	11–155 (70)
Tanner 4			
Male (11.8–16.2 y)	48–140 (82)	160–640 (395)	29–180 (80)
Female (10.7–15.6y)	77–225 (131)	200–780 (430)	10–230 (91)
Tanner 5			
Male (12.8–17.3 y)	65–210 (105)	250–900 (505)	24–175 (97)
Female (11.8–18.6 y)	80–240 (160)	215–850 (540)	20–265 (108)
Adults (18–40 y)	Men: 75–205 (115)	160–800 (455)	Men: 27–199 (103)
	(20–50 y)		
	Women: 60–245†		Women
			Postmenopausal: 30–120
			Follicular: 15–70 (46)
			Luteal: 35–290 (165)

DHEA, dehydroepiandrosterone.
*Levels increase after the first week to 40–200 between 1 and 2 months, then decline to the prepubertal range by 1 year.
†Entire menstrual cycle.
Normal ranges and means (in parentheses) are based on reference ranges from Esoterix Laboratories, Calabasas Hills, California, and are used with permission.

The use of the glucagon stimulation test is more appropriate in the younger age group. After the patient receives an intramuscular injection of glucagon, the blood glucose level rises initially and then drops rapidly because of the release of endogenous insulin. Levels of serum cortisol and growth hormone should increase in response to this fall in blood glucose.

The metyrapone test may be used in the assessment of ACTH secretory ability. Metyrapone blocks the activity of the enzyme 11-hydroxylase, which is needed to convert 11-deoxycortisol to cortisol (see Fig. 381.1). When levels of cortisol drop, ACTH secretion is stimulated, increasing the production of cortisol precursors. It can be measured by a rise in serum levels of ACTH and 11-deoxycortisol and in urinary 17-hydroxycorticosteroids. The ACTH-stimulated gland eventually overrides the enzymatic block, allowing production of cortisol to occur. However, patients must be observed closely while this test is being performed because acute adrenal insufficiency may be precipitated if the patient has marked ACTH deficiency.

In patients who have overproduction of glucocorticoids or adrenal androgens, determining whether the hypersecretion is autonomous or suppressible is important. The dexamethasone suppression test is useful in these cases and can be administered as a low- or high-dose test. After oral administration of dexamethasone, a potent glucocorticoid, pituitary ACTH secretion should be inhibited. Patients with elevated adrenal androgen

levels secondary to biosynthetic block have decreased production of androgen while ACTH stimulation is suppressed. In patients with Cushing syndrome caused by an autonomous ACTH-producing tumor, such as a pulmonary carcinoma, hypercortisolism does not respond to dexamethasone.

ADRENOCORTICAL ABNORMALITIES

Congenital Adrenal Hyperplasia

Congenital adrenal hyperplasia (CAH) is a family of diseases caused by an inherited deficiency of any of the enzyme activities necessary for the biosynthesis of cortisol (see Fig. 381.1). These enzymes, with the exception of 3-beta-hydroxysteroid dehydrogenase, are members of the cytochrome P-450 family. These cytochromes are microsomal or mitochondrial terminal oxidases involved in electron transport, and they require NAD and flavoproteins as cofactors. Deficient activity of any one of these enzymes results in decreased production of cortisol and increased secretion of ACTH. With ACTH stimulation, the adrenal cortex becomes hyperplastic and steroid precursors preceding the specific enzymatic block accumulate. These accumulated precursors are shunted, if possible, to a steroidogenic

TABLE 381.5

CLINICAL FEATURES OF THE DIFFERENT FORMS OF CONGENITAL ADRENAL HYPERPLASIA AT DIAGNOSIS

Deficient Enzyme	Clinical Form	Elevated Levels	Abnormal Sexual Development
21-Hydroxylase:			
Complete deficiency	Salt-losing	Urinary 17-ketosteroids, plasma 17-hydroxy-progesterone, plasma androstenedione, PRA, ACTH	Girls: ambiguous genitalia
Partial deficiency	Simple virilizing	Same as in complete deficiency	Girls: ambiguous genitalia Boys and girls: postnatal virilization
Mild deficiency	Attenuated, late-onset	Same as in complete deficiency, but milder elevations	Female adults or adolescents: menstrual irregularities, hirsutism
11-beta-Hydroxylase*	Hypertensive	Urinary 17-hydroxycorticosteroids, urinary 17-ketosteroids, plasma DOC, plasma 11-deoxycortisol, plasma androstenedione	Girls: ambiguous genitalia Boys and girls: postnatal virilization
17-alpha-Hydroxylase	Hypertensive	Plasma DOC, plasma corticosterone	Boys: incomplete or no virilization
3-beta-Hydroxysteroid dehydrogenase			
Complete deficiency	Salt-losing	Plasma DHEA, 17-hydroxypregnenolone, PRA, ACTH	Boys and girls: ambiguous genitalia
Partial deficiency	Mild	Plasma DHEA, 17-hydroxypregnenolone	Female adolescents: hirsutism, premature pubarche
Cholesterol side-chain cleavage	Salt-losing, "lipoid"	No steroids produced	Boys: absent virilization

ACTH, adrenocorticotropic hormone; DHEA, dehydroepiandrosterone; DOC, 11-deoxycorticosterone; PRA, plasma renin activity.
*A late-onset form of 11-beta-hydroxylase deficiency has been reported.

pathway that is unaffected by the enzymatic block. Each form of CAH is manifested by the clinical features produced by deficient end products (e.g., glucocorticoid, mineralocorticoid, or androgen) and by accumulated or shunted precursors (e.g., mineralocorticoid or androgen excess). CAH is inherited as an autosomal recessive disorder and has an equal sex distribution. A summary of these diseases and their clinical features is given in Table 381.5. The severity of the clinical features varies among families, representing very severe to mild or even asymptomatic forms.

The most common form of CAH is caused by 21-hydroxylase (21-OH) deficiency, which accounts for more than 90%

of the cases. The most severe form, the salt-losing form, is caused by complete absence of 21-OH activity and results in cortisol and mineralocorticoid deficiencies. Affected girls have ambiguous genitalia at birth caused by excessive secretion of adrenal androgens, which are converted to testosterone (Fig. 381.2). Usually, affected and untreated girls and boys present with symptoms of acute adrenal insufficiency, known as a *salt-losing crisis*, at ages 1 to 3 weeks.

The simple virilizing form is caused by a partial 21-OH deficiency. Patients with this disease produce adequate amounts of cortisol and aldosterone under the stimulation of excess ACTH and elevated PRA levels but at the expense of excess

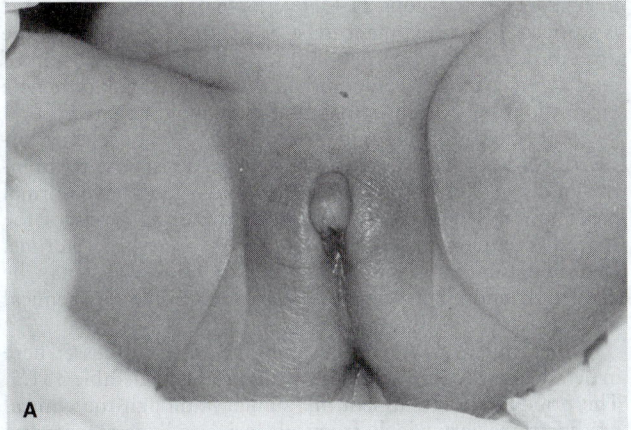
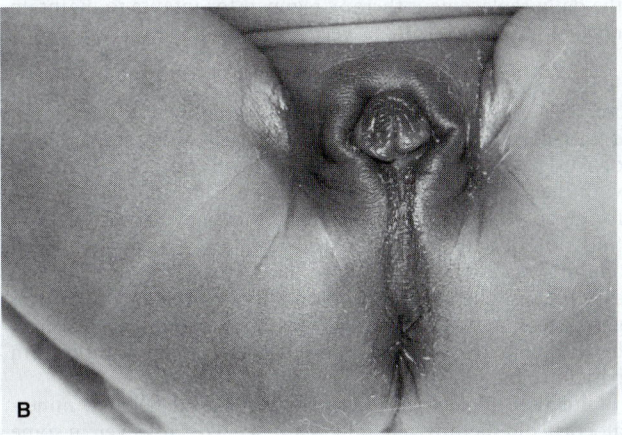

FIGURE 381.2. Ambiguous genitalia in female pseudohermaphrodites with congenital adrenal hyperplasia. Both cases exhibit enlargement of the clitoris, posterior fusion of the vaginal orifice, and development of rugae of the labia majora. **A:** Female infant with salt-losing 21-hydroxylase deficiency, whose ambiguous genitalia were not detected at the time of her newborn physical examination. **B:** Female infant with 11-beta-hydroxylase deficiency.

production of androgen. Girls may present with ambiguous genitalia or postnatal virilization, and boys may present with suspected isosexual precocious puberty, although the testes remain prepubertal in size. The combined frequencies of the salt-losing and simple virilizing forms approximate 1 in 10,000 to 13,000 births among Caucasians. The incidence among populations of Asian and African descent is somewhat lower.

A mild degree of 21-OH deficiency, the attenuated, late-onset or nonclassical form, manifests as hirsutism or menstrual irregularities in adolescent or adult females. In the asymptomatic or cryptic form, biochemical abnormalities consistent with 21-OH deficiency are present, but no clinical features are evident.

Diagnosis

The diagnosis of CAH caused by 21-OH deficiency is made when elevated levels of hormones preceding the enzymatic block (see Fig. 381.1) are demonstrated in a child with the typical clinical findings. A female infant with virilization of the external genitalia or a male infant with a salt-losing crisis (dehydration with hyponatremia, hyperkalemia, and acidosis) has elevated plasma 17-hydroxyprogesterone, progesterone, and androstenedione levels; increased urinary 17-ketosteroids; elevated levels of PRA and ACTH; and normal or low serum cortisol concentrations. Older children who present with inappropriate virilization (i.e., simple virilizing form) have normal cortisol and electrolyte levels but the same elevated hormone levels as those described for the younger group. Such children also have growth acceleration and advanced skeletal age caused by the effects of excess androgen.

In the salt-losing form, treatment is directed first at correcting the life-threatening metabolic abnormalities of adrenal crisis by correcting dehydration with intravenous saline and dextrose; by correcting hyperkalemia with insulin and glucose if necessary; and, after a blood sample is obtained for measurements of steroid hormones, by replacing glucocorticoid with the rapidly acting intravenous glucocorticoid, hydrocortisone (Solu-Cortef), at a "stress" dosage, which is three times the calculated dose for daily physiologic replacement. In general, this dose is 25 mg/day for children younger than 3 years of age. Because parenteral mineralocorticoid preparations no longer are available, prolonged treatment with high-dose glucocorticoids is necessary until oral mineralocorticoids can be tolerated. This treatment allows sufficient mineralocorticoid effect from the glucocorticoid preparation to achieve a lowered concentration of serum potassium and adequate retention of urinary sodium. In many cases, supplemental sodium chloride must be added to the daily replacement therapy regimen for infants to maintain normal serum electrolyte levels.

Treatment

Treatment with glucocorticoids promptly decreases the level of ACTH and the excess production of androgen. Children with the salt-losing form of CAH have a lifelong requirement for glucocorticoid replacement, but they may tolerate discontinuation of daily mineralocorticoid therapy when they reach adulthood. Careful titration of glucocorticoid therapy is necessary because the balance between undertreatment (i.e., androgen excess) and overtreatment (i.e., cushingoid features) may be within a narrow dosage range and varies significantly from patient to patient.

For the simple virilizing form of 21-OH deficiency, mineralocorticoid therapy generally is not needed. However, in some patients, mineralocorticoid supplementation has been used successfully to decrease the required glucocorticoid dose for adequate suppression of adrenal androgen levels. The mechanism of this effect is thought to be through suppression of secretion of vasopressin, a stimulator of CRH secretion. Glucocorticoid therapy must be titrated for optimal results, as in the salt-losing form. Treatment of the late-onset form of 21-OH deficiency is with glucocorticoid replacement as well.

In treating patients with all forms of this disease (as for all children receiving glucocorticoid therapy), the dosage must be increased during times of stress; parents must be trained to administer intramuscular hydrocortisone during times when children cannot take the medication orally.

Prognosis

The prognosis for children with 21-OH deficiency is good with careful follow-up and titration of hormonal replacement therapy. Some degree of morbidity is associated with surgical treatment of the external genitalia in girls, and it may be significant if multiple surgical procedures are needed. Fertility usually is normal in adequately treated males with the salt-losing form, but females with this form may have decreased fertility. In the simple virilizing form and late-onset forms, generally fertility is unaffected in males and in females who receive adequate treatment.

Prenatal Diagnosis

The prenatal diagnosis of 21-OH deficiency is available for families at risk using one of several methods. The diagnosis can be made in the presence of elevated amniotic fluid levels of 17-hydroxyprogesterone and androstenedione. The genes for 21-OH lie within the HLA complex on chromosome 6 and are inherited with the HLA complex. If the HLA haplotypes of a previously affected sibling are known and no HLA recombination has occurred, the 21-OH status of the fetus can be determined by the HLA type of amniotic cells. More commonly, chorionic villus biopsy specimens are analyzed directly for 21-OH gene mutations if the genotype of a previously affected sibling is known.

Prenatal Treatment

Prenatal treatment is effective in preventing or reducing the ambiguity of the genitalia in female infants, but only if it is instituted early in the first trimester, before the ninth week of gestation. A mother at risk is treated with dexamethasone until chorionic villus sampling or amniocentesis can provide information about the genetic sex and 21-OH genotype and/or HLA type of a fetus. If the fetus has an XY karyotype or if it has a normal or heterozygous 21-OH genotype, the dexamethasone is stopped. If the treatment must be continued until term, the dose of dexamethasone required for adequate suppression of fetal adrenal steroid secretion (and thus reduced risk of female virilization) may produce maternal cushingoid features.

Unaffected siblings can be tested for 21-OH deficiency carrier status to provide genetic counseling. In response to an intravenous ACTH stimulation test, heterozygotes have normal baseline levels with an exaggerated increase in levels of the steroid precursors progesterone and 17-hydroxyprogesterone. Determination of 21-OH genotypes or HLA types may be used to diagnose heterozygotes or to confirm the biochemical findings.

Other causes of CAH occur rarely and are not discussed here in detail. Some features of these forms are listed in Table 381.5. The principles of treatment are similar, although the clinical presentations vary widely from salt-losing to hypertensive and from abnormal virilization in females to inadequate virilization in males. Although prenatal diagnosis based on biochemical and genetic testing is available for other forms of CAH, 21-OH deficiency is the only HLA-linked form.

Hypofunction of the Adrenal Cortex

Hypofunction of the adrenal cortex is a rare finding in children and may be either primary or secondary to ACTH deficiency. Enzymatic defects in cortisol biosynthesis that are caused by adrenal insufficiency have been discussed already in the section on congenital adrenal hyperplasia.

Primary Adrenal Insufficiency

Primary adrenal insufficiency or failure usually is caused by Addison disease. The most common cause of Addison disease in developed countries is autoimmune destruction of the adrenal cortex, as occurs in the autoimmune polyglandular syndromes (APSs) (Table 381.6). Approximately 45% of patients with autoimmune Addison disease (i.e., caused by antiadrenal antibodies) develop one or more other autoimmune endocrinopathies, most often thyroid disease. APS type 1 is due to a mutation in the *AIRE* (**A**uto **i**mmune **Re**gulator) gene, the product of which apparently is required to prevent autoimmunity. Other, rarer causes of primary adrenal failure are congenital adrenal hypoplasia, bilateral adrenal hemorrhage (as in the Waterhouse-Friderichsen syndrome), trauma, thrombosis, infection (e.g., tuberculosis), destruction caused by tumor metastases, or degeneration (as seen in adrenoleukodystrophy).

In primary adrenal failure, decreased or absent production of all three groups of adrenal steroid hormones occurs. In most cases, the signs and symptoms of adrenal insufficiency, particularly the hyperpigmentation associated with increased ACTH, develop slowly. ACTH is a proteolytic cleavage product of the anterior pituitary prohormone proopiomelanocortin. Other cleavage products produced in equimolar amounts to ACTH are beta-endorphin and melanocyte-stimulating hormones, and activity of the latter hormone produces hyperpigmentation. The clinical features of adrenal insufficiency are listed in Box 381.1.

The diagnosis of primary adrenal failure is based on demonstration of elevated levels of ACTH levels with decreased or absent cortisol and mineralocorticoid production. The fasting 8 AM cortisol level is low and fails to rise with ACTH stimulation. The fasting glucose value may be low, and hyponatremia with hyperkalemia may be present. Usually, PRA is elevated. Levels of adrenal androgen may be below normal in adolescent patients. Levels of antiadrenal antibody should be measured, as should antibodies to other endocrine glands.

Treatment includes physiologic replacement with glucocorticoid and mineralocorticoid. Glucocorticoid dosage must be increased during times of stress.

TABLE 381.6

AUTOIMMUNE POLYGLANDULAR SYNDROMES (APSs) ASSOCIATED WITH CHRONIC HYPOADRENOCORTICISM (ADDISON DISEASE)

General	Type I	Type II*
Prevalence	Rare	Not as rare as type 1
Age at onset	Infancy/young childhood	Adolescence/adulthood
Inheritance	Autosomal recessive	Dominant
Gender predominance	None	Female
Cause	AIRE gene mutations	Polygenic/multifactorial
HLA association	None	HLA DR/DQ association
Hormonal Abnormalities		
Hypoparathyroidism	>80%	Rare
Addison disease	>60%	Common but Variable†
Hypogonadism	>30%	<10%
Autoimmune thyroid disease	<10%	>70%
Type 1 diabetes	<20%	40–50%
Hypopituitarism	Uncommon	Rare
Other Clinical Features		
Mucocutaneous candidiasis	80–100%	Not seen
Ectodermal dysplasia	>75%	Not seen
Alopecia	25–30%	<10%
Pernicious anemia	10–15%	Variable
Autoimmune hepatitis	10–15%	Rare
Intestinal malabsorption	10–25%	Rare
Vitiligo	10%	<10%
Asplenism	Uncommon	Not seen
Keratoconjunctivitis	Uncommon	Rare

*APS types II, III, and IV also have been described. APS type III consists of autoimmune thyroid disease associated with one or more autoimmune diseases *other than Addison disease*. Its prevalence is increased in Down syndrome, Turner syndrome, and Klinefelter syndrome. APS type IV consists of any two autoimmune-affected organ diseases in a combination not included in types I, II, or III, or associated with non–organ-specific autoimmune disease.
†The association of Addison disease with autoimmune thyroid disease is known as Schmidt syndrome. When type 1 diabetes is added, the triad is known as Carpenter syndrome.
Data adapted from the following references: Brown RS. The autoimmune polyglandular syndromes: a pediatric perspective. In: A current review of pediatric endocrinology. Rockland, MA: Serono Symposia International, Inc., 2003:51; Neufeld M, Maclaren NK, Blizzard RM. Two types of autoimmune Addison syndrome associated with different polyglandular autoimmune (PGA) syndromes. *Medicine* 1981;60:355; and Schatz DA, Winter WE. Autoimmune polyglandular syndrome II: clinical syndrome and treatment. *Endocrinol Metab Clin North Am* 2002;31:338.

| BOX 381.1 | Signs and Symptoms of Adrenal Insufficiency |

Glucocorticoid deficiency
  Fasting hypoglycemia
  Increased insulin sensitivity
  Decreased gastric acidity
  Gastrointestinal symptoms (e.g., nausea, vomiting)
  Fatigue
  Headaches
Mineralocorticoid deficiency
  Muscle weakness
  Weight loss
  Fatigue
  Nausea, vomiting, anorexia
  Salt craving
  Hypotension
  Hyperkalemia, hyponatremia, acidosis
Androgen deficiency (in older children and adults)
  Decreased pubic and axillary hair
  Decreased libido
  Increased proopiomelanocortin cleavage products
  Hyperpigmentation due to melanocyte stimulation

Secondary Adrenocortical Insufficiency

Secondary adrenocortical insufficiency usually is caused by ACTH deficiency. Rarely, resistance to ACTH may occur.

ACTH deficiency may be caused by idiopathic hypopituitarism (congenital), congenital malformations of the pituitary or hypothalamus, destruction of the pituitary or hypothalamus (infection, hemorrhage, tumor, irradiation, infiltrative disease), or iatrogenic causes (prenatal glucocorticoid treatment of the mother, or postnatal pharmacologic glucocorticoid treatment).

In the absence of primary adrenal disease, ACTH deficiency does not result in mineralocorticoid deficiency. Therefore, hyponatremia, hyperkalemia, and dehydration are not seen as manifestations of ACTH deficiency. In fact, cortisol deficiency may result in decreased renal clearance of free water, resulting in retention of fluids. Often, it is apparent in patients with diabetes insipidus, who may appear to have improvement of their disease if ACTH deficiency develops.

The diagnosis of ACTH deficiency is based on absence of the 8 AM peak in serum cortisol and on lack of response to tests of ACTH secretion (insulin-induced hypoglycemia, glucagon stimulation, metyrapone). In cases of partial ACTH deficiency, affected patients may produce enough ACTH for normal daily physiologic needs (normal 8 AM cortisol, normal 24-hour urinary 17-hydroxycorticosteroids) but may be unable to respond to stress and will fail the tests of stimulated ACTH secretion. In any child with ACTH deficiency, the secretion of other anterior and posterior pituitary hormones must be assessed carefully.

ACTH deficiency is treated with glucocorticoid at physiologic replacement doses. The dosage must be titrated carefully to prevent overtreatment, which seems to occur at lower doses in children with ACTH deficiency than in those with primary adrenal failure. Mineralocorticoid treatment is unnecessary.

Adrenocortical Hyperfunction

Adrenocortical hyperfunction is manifested most often by the effects of glucocorticoid excess, called *Cushing syndrome*.

| BOX 381.2 | Causes of Cushing Syndrome |

ACTH-independent
Iatrogenic (e.g., glucocorticoid therapy)
Adrenocortical tumors (e.g., adenoma, carcinoma, micronodular disease)

ACTH-dependent
Hypothalamic CRH-producing tumor
Pituitary ACTH-producing tumor
Ectopic CRH-producing tumor (e.g., pancreas, lung)
Ectopic ACTH-producing tumor (e.g., lung, bronchus, gut)
Iatrogenic (e.g., ACTH therapy)
Increased serotonin levels (e.g., idiopathic)

ACTH, adrenocorticotropic hormone; CRH, corticotropin-releasing hormone.

Etiology

The most common cause of Cushing syndrome is iatrogenic administration of pharmacologic doses of a glucocorticoid as an antiinflammatory or immunosuppressive agent. Other causes of Cushing syndrome are rare findings in children (Box 381.2). These causes include ACTH-dependent hypercortisolism (Cushing disease) and primary adrenal hypercortisolism. Among children who have hypercortisolism and are not receiving exogenous glucocorticoids, those younger than 7 years old are more likely to have a primary adrenal cause. Those older than age 7 are more likely to have ACTH-dependent hypercortisolism. The clinical features of hypercortisolism are listed in Box 381.3.

Diagnosis

The diagnosis of Cushing syndrome is based on demonstration of hypercortisolism and the determination of its source in patients not receiving glucocorticoid treatment. Measurement of levels of serum cortisol at 8 AM and in late afternoon may fail to show the normal diurnal variation. However, the diurnal pattern may not mature in normal children until after they are 3 years old. The value of serum ACTH levels is limited. Low

---

| BOX 381.3 | Clinical Features of Hypercortisolism |

Obesity with violaceous striae (generalized in infants, truncal in older children with moon facies or buffalo hump)
Decreased height velocity (short stature, delayed bone age)
Plethora, increased hematocrit
Easy bruising
Hypertension
Osteoporosis
Glucose intolerance
Poor wound healing
Increased frequency of infections
Renal stones, hypercalciuria
Weakness, muscle wasting (unusual in infants)
Depression or other psychiatric symptoms

levels do not rule out the possibility of an ACTH-producing tumor, but high levels usually rule out a primary adrenal cause. Usually, the 24-hour urinary 17-hydroxycorticosteroid levels and levels of free cortisol are elevated, as are 17-ketosteroid levels in some cases. Midnight salivary cortisol levels also are elevated.

In children with equivocal clinical features and baseline static test results, an overnight dexamethasone suppression test may be the most advantageous dynamic screening test. After a single dose of dexamethasone (20 μg/kg up to maximum of 1 mg, given orally at 11 PM), the 8 AM serum cortisol should be less than 5 μg/dL in a normal child. If the child fails the overnight test, a low-dose and then a high-dose dexamethasone suppression test should be performed (see Table 381.3). Failure to respond to the low-dose test in conjunction with appropriate suppression on the high-dose test suggests an ACTH-producing pituitary adenoma. Failure to respond to the high-dose dexamethasone test suggests an ectopic ACTH-producing tumor or an adrenal tumor.

If a pituitary, adrenal, or ectopic ACTH-producing tumor is suspected, radiologic imaging studies must be performed to visualize the tumor. Bilateral inferior petrosal sinus sampling may help lateralize a suspected but radiologically undetectable pituitary tumor secreting ACTH. Some ACTH-producing pituitary tumors are microadenomas, visible only at the time of transsphenoidal pituitary exploration.

Treatment

The treatment of Cushing syndrome is removal of the cause of hypercortisolism. In cases of iatrogenic disease, that removal is not always possible because the nature of the disorder requires glucocorticoid treatment.

In cases of ACTH-dependent disease, the source of production of ACTH usually must be removed surgically. In cases of pituitary Cushing disease, such medications as cyproheptadine and bromocriptine have been more effective in lowering levels of ACTH in adults than in children. Bilateral adrenalectomy once was the only treatment for ACTH-dependent disease, but most patients then developed Nelson disease (i.e., pituitary enlargement caused by hyperplasia of ACTH-producing cells). In primary adrenal disease, adrenalectomy (unilateral in the case of a tumor and bilateral in micronodular disease) is the treatment of choice.

The side effect of these treatments most commonly encountered is adrenal insufficiency, caused by ACTH deficiency or adrenalectomy. In the case of unilateral adrenalectomy, the contralateral adrenal gland will need time to recover from prolonged lack of ACTH stimulation. Patients who undergo pituitary exploration have a small risk of developing panhypopituitarism.

Prognosis

The prognosis for patients with Cushing syndrome is based on the underlying cause. Patients with adrenal or pituitary adenomas have a good prognosis after adequate surgical resection is performed. Those who have adrenal or ectopic ACTH-producing carcinomas have a poorer prognosis.

Hypersecretion of adrenal androgens may be caused by CAH or by an adrenal tumor. In addition, feminizing adrenocortical tumors have been described. Adrenal tumors, including adenomas and carcinomas, are rare findings in children; they are treated by surgical resection and, in some cases, by adjunctive therapies.

Hypersecretion of mineralocorticoids may be caused by the hypertensive form of CAH (see Table 381.5) or by primary hyperaldosteronism. In CAH caused by 11-OH or 17-OH deficiency, glucocorticoid replacement therapy results in lowering of mineralocorticoid levels and lowering of the blood pressure from the hypertensive range. Hyperaldosteronism is an exceedingly rare occurrence in children and is treated with the aldosterone inhibitor spironolactone.

Rare causes of apparent mineralocorticoid excess include an inherited defect in the conversion of cortisol to cortisone due to deficiency of 11-beta-hydroxysteroid dehydrogenase type 1 (11BHSD1). Apparent mineralocorticoid excess may be associated with ingestion of licorice. Licorice root contains glycyrrhetinic acid, which inhibits 11BHSD1.

Suggested Readings

Brown RS. The autoimmune polyglandular syndromes: a pediatric perspective. In: *A current review of pediatric endocrinology*. Rockland, MA: Serono Symposia International, 2003:51.

Donohoue PA. The adrenal gland and its disorders. In: Kappy MS, Allen OB, Geffner ME, eds. *Principles and Practice of Pediatric Endocrinology*. Springfield, IL: Charles C. Thomas, 2005:357.

Donohoue PA, Parker KL, Migeon CJ. Congenital adrenal hyperplasia. In: Scriver CR, Beaudet AL, Sly WS, Valle D, eds. *The metabolic and molecular bases of inherited disease*, 8th ed. New York: McGraw-Hill, 2001:4077.

Donohoue PA, Saenger PH. Ambiguous genitalia. In: Finberg L, Kleinman R, eds. *Saunders manual of pediatric practice*, 2nd ed. Philadelphia: Harcourt Health Sciences Companies, 2002:872.

Joint LWPES/ESPE CAH Working Group. Consensus statement on 21-hydroxylase deficiency from the Lawson Wilkins Pediatric Endocrine Society and the European Society for Paediatric Endocrinology. *J Clin Endocrinol Metab* 2002;87:4048.

CHAPTER 382 ■ ADRENAL MEDULLA

PATRICIA A. DONOHOUE

NORMAL ADRENAL MEDULLARY DEVELOPMENT AND SECRETIONS

Early in embryogenesis, primitive sympathetic nervous system ganglion cells migrate from neural ectoderm, differentiate into pheochromoblasts, and penetrate the adrenal cortex. These pheochromoblasts develop into the chromaffin cells of the adrenal medulla.

The adrenal medulla is innervated by sympathetic nerves that originate in the splanchnic system. This sympathoadrenal system is controlled by a complex set of central neural connections and is involved in the production, storage, and secretion of catecholamines. The adrenal medulla is exposed to

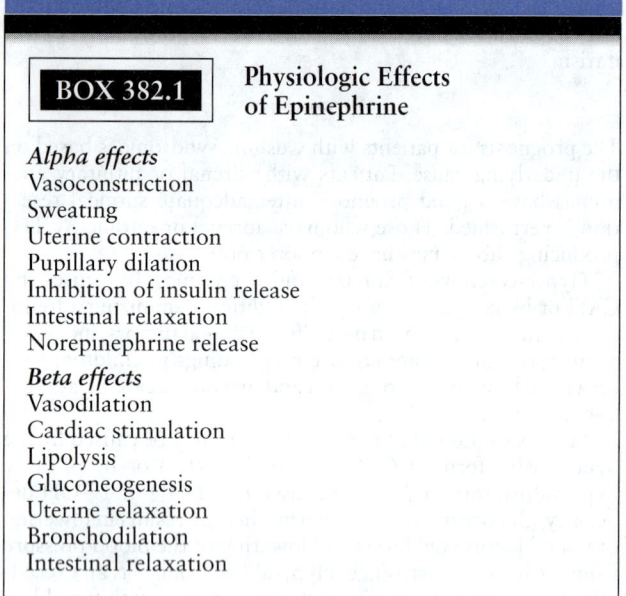

BOX 382.1   Physiologic Effects of Epinephrine

Alpha effects
Vasoconstriction
Sweating
Uterine contraction
Pupillary dilation
Inhibition of insulin release
Intestinal relaxation
Norepinephrine release

Beta effects
Vasodilation
Cardiac stimulation
Lipolysis
Gluconeogenesis
Uterine relaxation
Bronchodilation
Intestinal relaxation

TABLE 382.1

FEATURES OF THE MULTIPLE ENDOCRINE NEOPLASIA (MEN) SYNDROMES

Neoplasia	MEN1	MEN2A	MEN2B
Pheochromocytoma	−	+	+
Medullary thyroid carcinoma	−	+	+
Multiple neural tumors	−	−	+
Parathyroid tumors/ hyperplasia	+	+	−
Pancreatic tumors	+	−	−
Anterior pituitary tumors	+	−	−
Gastrinoma	+	−	−
Carcinoid	+	−	−
Other features:			
Marfanoid habitus	−	−	+
Cutaneous lichen amyloidosis	−	+	−
Hirschsprung disease	−	+	−

the relatively high concentration of cortisol found in the venous drainage of the adrenal cortex.

The major catecholamines in humans are dopamine, norepinephrine, and epinephrine, all of which are synthesized in nerve endings. Epinephrine is the major product of the adrenal medulla. In its biosynthesis, tyrosine is hydroxylated to form dopa, which then is converted to dopamine, a neurotransmitter within the central nervous system (CNS). Dopamine also acts as the precursor for synthesis of norepinephrine, the principal neurotransmitter of the sympathetic nervous system. Then norepinephrine is converted to epinephrine in the adrenal medulla, in an enzymatic step controlled by cortisol. Epinephrine exerts its physiologic effects by interaction with alpha- and beta-adrenergic receptors. The physiologic effects of epinephrine are widespread and are separated into the alpha- and beta-receptor effects (Box 382.1).

TESTS OF ADRENAL MEDULLARY PRODUCTS

Measurements of single catecholamine levels, such as norepinephrine and epinephrine, generally are not helpful because patients who produce excessive amounts of these catecholamines may have periods of low blood levels, and persons with normal production have high levels in response to stress. Persons with symptoms of excess of catecholamines are evaluated best by measuring their catecholamines and their metabolites. The most helpful tests include 24-hour urinary normetanephrine, metanephrine, homovanillic acid, vanillylmandelic acid (VMA), and plasma-free metanephrine. Serial measurements of these compounds in blood and urine after paroxysmal attacks of catecholamine release also may be informative.

ABNORMALITIES OF THE ADRENAL MEDULLA

Abnormalities of the adrenal medulla are caused by benign or malignant tumors that secrete catecholamines. Adrenal medullary deficiency, which occurs after adrenalectomy or in

patients with congenital adrenal hyperplasia caused by 21-hydroxylase deficiency, is not known to pose a significant health risk.

Pheochromocytoma

Pheochromocytoma is a rare occurrence in children but must be considered in children with hypertension or other symptoms of catecholamine excess. This tumor may arise from any chromaffin tissue, but it is found most often in the adrenal medulla. Bilateral adrenal or extraadrenal tumors are seen more commonly in pediatric than in adult pheochromocytomas, and often they are associated with the familial multiple endocrine neoplasia (MEN) syndromes. The neoplasias associated with the various MEN syndromes are listed in Table 382.1. Features consistent with these associated tumors (e.g., medullary carcinoma of the thyroid) should be sought in any patient with pheochromocytoma. The MEN syndromes are inherited and are expressed variably. The MEN type I syndrome is caused by germline mutations of a gene termed *MEN1*. The MEN type II syndromes (i.e., IIA and IIB) and familial medullary carcinoma of the thyroid are caused by germline-activating mutations of the *RET* protooncogene. Tumor cells from sporadic pheochromocytomas may contain mutations of this gene as well. Pheochromocytomas also are associated with neuroectodermal dysplasias (e.g., neurofibromatosis) and with the Von Hippel-Lindau syndrome.

Pheochromocytoma is benign in more than 90% of pediatric patients. A male preponderance exists among children with this tumor, but the sex ratio is reversed in adults. The peak incidence in the pediatric group occurs in children between 9 and 12 years of age. The signs and symptoms of pheochromocytoma are those of catecholamine excess (Box 382.2). These features vary greatly and are likely to be paroxysmal, but the hypertension may be sustained. Hypertensive crisis may occur while the patient is receiving anesthesia without proper adrenergic blockade.

Diagnosis

The diagnosis of pheochromocytoma is based on demonstration of increased catecholamines and their metabolites in a 24-hour urine collection and in blood, or plasma-free metanephrine. These substances are urinary-free epinephrine and norepinephrine, metanephrine, and VMA. Urinary VMA levels may be elevated falsely with certain drugs, such as aspirin, penicillin, acetaminophen, and sulfa preparations. If these test results are inconclusive, performing a clonidine suppression test may be useful.

Clonidine causes a decrease in blood catecholamine levels only if they are not elevated owing to secretion from an autonomous source. If suspected as being present from the biochemical tests, the tumor usually can be localized by ultrasonography, computed tomography, magnetic resonance imaging, or intravenous pyelography. Venography to demonstrate elevated levels of catecholamines should be performed only after administration of adequate alpha-blockade with phentolamine mesylate (Regitine) to prevent occurrence of a hypertensive crisis. Scintigraphic imaging with ^{131}I-metaiodobenzylguanidine (MIBG scan) has been used to demonstrate the presence of a pheochromocytoma. MIBG is similar in structure to norepinephrine and is concentrated in tissues that are synthesizing catecholamines by means of norepinephrine in storage granules.

Treatment

The treatment of pheochromocytoma is surgical excision and requires extensive preoperative treatment with alpha- and beta-blockade and with alpha-methyltyrosine if needed. If performing a bilateral adrenalectomy is necessary, treatment for primary adrenal insufficiency must be instituted promptly. Postoperative recordings of blood pressure and catecholamine levels are needed to monitor for recurrence of the tumor. Malignant tumors are diagnosed on the basis of functional tumor in nonchromaffin tissue areas. Benign tumors may cause blood vessel or capsular invasion, but they do not spread beyond chromaffin tissue areas. Malignant tumors grow slowly and are resistant to irradiation and chemotherapy. Symptoms are treated medically, with various degrees of success.

Neuroblastoma

Neuroblastoma is one of the most common solid tumors of childhood and may arise from the adrenal medulla. It can be sporadic or familial. The diagnosis is based on demonstration of elevated homovanillic acid or VMA levels in the urine and on radiologic localization. The treatment and prognosis of neuroblastoma are discussed elsewhere.

Other Tumors

Other tumors of the adrenal medulla include ganglioneuroblastoma and ganglioneuroma. These tumors may manifest with chronic watery diarrhea owing to tumor secretion of vasoactive intestinal peptide. The diarrhea resolves after excision of the tumor.

Suggested Readings

Brandi ML, Gagel RF, Angeli A, et al. Guidelines for diagnosis and therapy of MEN type 1 and type 2. *J Clin Endocrinol Metab* 2001;86:5658.

Bravo EL, Gifford RW Jr. Pheochromocytoma: diagnosis, localization and management. *N Engl J Med* 1984;311:1298.

Donohoue PA. The adrenal gland and its disorders. In: Kappy MS, Allen OB, Geffner ME, eds. *Principles and Practice of Pediatric Endocrinology*. Springfield, IL: Charles C. Thomas, 2005:357.

Reckler JM, Vaughan ED Jr, Tjeuw M, Carey RM. Pheochromocytoma. In: Vaughan ED Jr, Carey RM, eds. *Adrenal disorders*. New York: Thieme Medical Publishers, 1989:259.

Sawka AM, Jaeschke R, Singh RJ, Young WF Jr. A comparison of biochemical tests for pheochromocytoma: measurement of fractionated plasma metanephrines compared with the combination of 24-hour urinary metanephrines and catecholamines. *J Clin Endocrinol Metab* 2003;88:553.

SECTION IX ■ INBORN ERRORS OF METABOLISM

CHAPTER 383 ■ INTRODUCTION TO INBORN ERRORS OF METABOLISM

REBECCA S. WAPPNER AND BRYAN E. HAINLINE

The concept of inherited biochemical genetic disorders was described first by Garrod in his 1908 published lecture, "Inborn Errors of Metabolism." His original description of four disorders has been expanded greatly since then. This expansion has occurred mainly since the late 1970s, through the development of improved diagnostic testing and advances in the molecular understanding of the bases for the disorders.

Inborn errors of metabolism are genetically determined abnormalities in the biochemical processes of the body. Most often, a single defective protein disrupts a metabolic pathway at a specific step, leading to an excessive accumulation of immediate or precursor substrates and a deficiency of immediate and subsequent products of the reaction. The clinical manifestations of the disorders are related to the abnormal metabolism that occurs.

Individual disorders result from point mutations, deletions, or other alterations of DNA or RNA processing. Defects may occur in nuclear-encoded genes located on the autosomes or X chromosome or in genes located in mitochondrial DNA. Most disorders produce abnormalities in a single enzyme protein, but a regulatory, protective, or activator protein for the enzyme can be involved. Other inborn errors may be due to the faulty transport of molecules. Occasionally, several enzymes may be affected, giving a composite clinical picture incorporating features of several enzyme deficiencies. Multiple sulfatase deficiency and combined methylmalonic acidemia and homocystinuria are typical examples. Conversely, identical clinical phenotypes may be seen with mutations in different proteins. An example of the latter is Sanfilippo syndrome, which may be caused by the deficient activity of any one of four different enzymes.

Most of the disorders are inherited as autosomal recessive traits. Some are inherited as X-linked conditions, whereas others show maternal, or mitochondrial, inheritance. An accurate diagnosis should be established so that appropriate information and genetic counseling can be given to family members and affected individuals concerning prognosis, treatment options, recurrence risks, carrier detection, and prenatal diagnosis.

CLINICAL MANIFESTATIONS AND COMPLICATIONS

The inborn errors of metabolism vary widely in clinical presentation and age of onset. Those that affect essential pathways in the body are more severe and present at early ages with acute metabolic disease (i.e., urea cycle defects or organic acidemias). Others are indolent and associated with the gradual onset of organomegaly (i.e., Gaucher disease) or neurologic impairment (i.e., phenylketonuria). Still others are benign and result in no significant clinical problems (i.e., iminoglycinuria or pentosuria). Although inborn errors of metabolism classically have been considered disorders of childhood, they may present at any age. Mild variants of all types have been reported with increasing frequency in adolescents and adults.

Often, the pattern of clinical findings points to a specific inborn error and usually is related directly to the pathway affected. Those involving amino acid or organic acid metabolism may have an acute metabolic presentation with decreased intake and lethargy, followed by encephalopathy, coma, or death if not recognized and treated. Laboratory testing will reveal profound acidosis (often with hyperammonemia) that is refractory to standard therapy. Unusual odors may be noted. Frequently, patients with urea cycle disorders develop acute neurologic deterioration in the neonatal period. Often, disorders of fatty acid oxidation and carbohydrate metabolism present with lethargy, encephalopathy, and hypoglycemia at times of decreased carbohydrate intake or fasting. Hepatomegaly and hypotonia frequently are noted. Lactic acidosis, cardiomyopathies, myopathies, and other neurologic symptoms commonly are seen with mitochondrial disorders. Lysosomal storage disorders are characterized by progressive hepatomegaly, splenomegaly, neurologic regression, short stature, and coarse facies. Frequently, patients with peroxisomal disorders have dysmorphic features and neurologic problems. Other inborn errors present with only psychomotor handicaps. Rarely, inborn errors result in urinary tract stones, immunodeficiencies, and self-mutilation.

A history of cyclic vomiting and lethargy, especially if related to the intake of protein or specific carbohydrates, should arouse suspicions, as should repeated episodes of acute, life-threatening events. A family history possibly may reveal similarly affected individuals or unexplained early infant deaths.

Table 383.1 lists the patterns of clinical findings associated with certain groups of the disorders. Table 383.2 lists the findings in specific inborn errors. Table 383.3 lists the abnormal

TABLE 383.1

CLINICAL MANIFESTATIONS OF INBORN ERRORS OF METABOLISM

Clinical Manifestation	General Type of Disorder								
	AA	OA	UREA	FAO	MIT	CARB	PER	MPS	SL
Episodic nature	++	++	++	++	+	+	−	−	−
Poor feeding	+	+	++	+	+	+	+	−	−
Abnormal odor	+	+	−	+	−	−	+	−	−
Lethargy, coma	+	++	++	++	+	+	+	−	−
ALTE	+	+	+	+	+	+	−	−	−
Seizures	+	+	+	−	+	+	+	+	+
Developmental regression	+	+	+	−	+	−	+	++	+
Hepatomegaly	+	+	+	+	+	+	+	+	+
Hepatosplenomegaly	−	−	−	−	−	−	−	+	+
Splenomegaly	−	−	−	−	−	−	−	−	+
Hypotonia	+	+	+	+	+	+	+	+	+
Cardiomyopathy	−	+	−	+	+	+	+	+	+
Coarse facies	−	−	−	−	−	−	−	++	+
Birth defects	−	+	−	+	+	−	+	−	+
Hypoglycemia	+	+	−	+	+	+	−	−	−
Acidosis	+	++	−	+	+	+	−	−	−
Hyperammonemia	+	+	++	+	+	−	−	−	−
Ketosis	+	+	−	+	−	+	−	−	−
Hypoketosis	−	−	−	+	−	−	−	−	−

++, usually present; +, may be present; −, usually not present; AA, amino acidopatheis; ALTE, acute life-threatening event; CARB, disorders of carbohydrate; FAO, mitochondrial fatty acid oxidation defects; MIT, mito-chondrial disordes of oxidative phosphorylation; MPS, mucopolysaccharidoses; OA, organic acidopathies PER, peroxisomal disorders; SL, sphingolipidoses; UREA, disorders of the urea cycle.
Adapted from Wappner RS. Biochemical diagnosis of genetic diseases. *Pediatr Ann* 1993;22;283.

TABLE 383.2

PHYSICAL FINDINGS OF INBORN ERRORS OF METABOLISM

Finding	Related Disorder
Skin	
Absent or reduced pigment	Albinism, cystinosis, Menkes s., PKU, sialidosis
Alopecia	Acrodermatitis enteropathica, hereditary generalized resistance to 1,25-dihydroxyvitamin D
Angiokeratoma	Fabry d., fucosidosis, galactosialidosis, beta-mannosidoses, Schindler d., sialidosis
Dermatitis	Acrodermatitis enteropathica, biotinidase deficiency, Hartnup d., PKU, prolidase deficiency
Edema	GM_1 gangliosidosis, prolidase deficiency
Fat pads	CDG
Hair, sparse	Biotinidase deficiency, Menkes s.
Hair, kinky	Argininosuccinic aciduria, Menkes s.
Hirsutism	GP, ML, MPS
Ichthyosis	Multiple sulfatase deficiency, steroid sulfatase deficiency
Inverted nipples	CDG
Keratosis palmoplantaris	Tyrosine aminotransferase deficiency
Masses	Farber d.
Photosensitization	Porphyrias
Xanthomas	Hyperlipoproteinemias and other disorders of lipoproteins
Head	
Coarse facies	GP, ML, MPS
Macrocephaly	Canavan, glutaric acidemia I, GP, ML, MPS
Microcephaly	CDG, leukodystrophies, PKU, maternal PKU syndrome, tyrosine aminotransferase deficiency
Eyes	
Arcus juvenilis	Hyperlipoproteinemias
Cataracts	Aspartylglucosaminuria, cerebrotendinous xanthomatosis, Fabry d., Farber d., lysinuric protein intolerance, alpha-mannosidase deficiency, mitochondrial ox/phos, Niemann-Pick d., sialidosis, SLO, steroid sulfatase deficiency, Zellweger and other peroxisomal disorders
Cherry-red macular spots	Farber d., galactosialidosis, GM_1 and GM_2 gangliosidoses, Krabbe d., Niermann-Pick d., sialidosis
Corneal clouding	GP, ML, MPS, Tangier d., sialidosis
Corneal opacities	Farber d., fish eye d., alpha-mannosidosis, mitochondrial ox/phos, steroid sulfatase deficiency, Tangier d.
Dislocated lens	Homocystinuria, sulfite oxidase deficiency
Gyrate atrophy of retina	Ornithine aminotransferase deficiency
Kayser-Fleischer rings	Wilson d.
Keratitis	Tyrosine aminotransferase deficiency
Retinitis pigmentosa	Abetalipoproteinemia, CDG, cystinosis, mitochondrial ox/phos, peroxisomal disorders
Ears	
Deafness	Biotinidase deficiency, Hunter s. and other MPS, PPRP-S overactivity, mitochondrial ox/phos, SL
Mouth	
Gingival hyperplasia	GP, ML, MPS
Heart	
Cardiomyopathy	CDG, Fabry d., galactosialidosis, GSD, GM_1 gangliosidosis, hepatorenal tyrosinemia, 3-methylglutaconic acidemia, ML, mitochondrial fatty acid oxidation defects, mitochondrial ox/phos, MPS, myoadenylate deaminase deficiency, Pompe d.
Abdomen	
Acute visceral attacks	Fabry d., hepatic porphyrias
Musculoskeletal system	
Arthritis	Farber d., gout and other purine disorders
Dorsal kyphosis (gibbus)	GM_1 gangliosidosis, GP, ML, MPS, multiple sulfatase deficiency
Marfanoid appearance	Homocystinuria
Rickets	Familial hypophosphatemic rickets, disorders of vitamin D metabolism, disorders with renal tubular dysfunction
Neurologic system	
Dystonia	Glutaric acidemia I, organic acidemias, Wilson d.
Muscle cramping after exercise	Mitochondrial fatty acid oxidation defects, muscle glycogenoses and other GSD, myoadenylate deaminase deficiency
Myopathy	Mitochondrial fatty acid oxidation defects, mitochondrial ox/phos, muscle glycogenoses and other GSD, Pompe d.

(Continued)

TABLE 383.2

(CONTINUED)

Finding	Related Disorder
Paresthesia	Fabry d., sialidosis
Peripheral neuropathy	CDG, leukodystrophies, peroxisomal disorders, Tangier d.
Psychoses	Adult Tay-Sachs d., homocystinuria, porphyrias, purine disorders
Self-mutilation	Adenylosuccinase deficiency, Lesch-Nyhan s., tyrosine aminotransferase deficiency
Renal system	
Renal cysts	CDG, CPT II deficiency, glutaric acidemia II, peroxisomal disorders
Renal failure	Fabry d., GSD I, methylmalonic acidemia, disorders with urinary tract stones
Renal tubular dysfunction	Cystinosis, galactosemia, GSD I, hereditary fructose intolerance, hepatorenal tyrosinemia
Stones	Cystinuria, gout, and other purine disorders; hyperoxaluria, orotic acidemia
Other findings	
Adrenal insufficiency	Adrenoleukodystrophy, adrenomyeloneuropathy, glycerol kinase deficiency
Amenorrhea	Galactosemia (females)
Hypogonadism	Adrenoleukodystrophy, adrenomyeloneuropathy, mitochondrial ox/phos, SLO
Immunodeficiency	Adenosine deaminase deficiency, purine nucleoside phosphorylase deficiency
Urine and diaper color	
Black	Homogentisic aciduria
Blue	Tryptophan malabsorption
Pink	Disorders with hematuria, stone formation
Port wine	Porphyrias
Yellow-orange	Disorders with increased uric acid
Urine odor	
Acrid	Glutaric acidemia II
Cabbage	Tyrosinemia
Fishy	Trimethylaminuria
Maple syrup	Maple syrup urine disease
Mousy	PKU
Sweaty feet	Isovaleric acidemia
Sweet	2-Methylacetoacetyl-CoA 3-oxothiolase deficiency
Swimming pool	Hawkinsinuria

CDG, carbohydrate-deficient glycoprotein syndrome; CPT, carnitine palmitoyl transferase; d., disease; GP, glycoproteinoses; GSD, glycogen storage disease; ML, mucolipidoses; MPS, mucopolysaccharidoses; ox/phos, oxidative phosphorylation; PKU, phenylketonuria; PPRP-S, phosphoribosylpyrophosphate synthetase; s., syndrome; SL, sphingolipidoses; SLO, Smith-Lemli-Opitz syndrome.

common laboratory testing results that may suggest an inborn error of metabolism. Table 383.4 lists specific specialty testing for inborn errors of metabolism. These tables and lists may aid physicians in determining which disorder to consider and which tests to perform. Although clinical features of disorders of mitochondrial oxidative phosphorylation, disorders of copper metabolism, and the porphyrias are listed in the tables for comprehensive coverage, these disorders are discussed in Chapters 386 and 412.

In the United States, all state-mandated newborn screening programs test for phenylketonuria; other disorders for which testing is done vary from state to state. Supplemental screening, employing testing with tandem mass spectrometry, may detect additional disorders of fatty acid oxidation and amino acid and organic acid metabolism. This type of testing is being added to screening panels in many states and also is available commercially. Clinicians should be aware of the disorders that are included in their state newborn screening program. Biologic false-positive and false-negative results may occur with screening testing. Thus, even if a patient has been screened for a specific disorder and the results are negative, if the patient has features of the disorder, then the patient should be tested again, because cases can be missed.

Acute Metabolic Disease

The initial therapy for treatment of an acute metabolic crisis should include all usual measures needed for support of a critically ill patient. Acidosis and hypoglycemia should be corrected; vasopressors may be used. Affected patients should be monitored for signs of increased intracranial pressure. All sources of protein should be stopped, and the patient given only glucose as the carbohydrate source. Intravenous solutions containing lactate or fructose should be avoided. Vitamins or cofactors for the suspected disorder may be given after diagnostic specimens are obtained. Occasionally, acidosis or hyperammonemia will require hemodialysis or hemofiltration. Consultation with a specialist in metabolic disorders should be considered to aid in the diagnosis and management of the patient.

Samples for diagnostic testing should be obtained when the patient is most symptomatic. Urine metabolic screening profiles that are available include spot testing for ketoacids (oxoacids) and sulfhydryl groups; amino acid, mucopolysaccharide, oligosaccharide, and carbohydrate qualitative or quantitative chromatography may be included. Definitive amino acid testing should be done by quantitation. Organic acid analysis should be done by gas chromatography combined with mass spectrometry. Acyl-carnitine profiles require tandem mass spectrometry. Enzymatic testing or other bioassays should be performed to confirm an exact diagnosis. Molecular genetic techniques, such as mutation analysis, may be helpful in establishing a diagnosis and are important for family and prenatal genetic counseling and testing.

Often, physicians are faced with a patient who is in extremis and for whom a diagnosis of an inborn error is being considered. If time permits, consultation with a metabolic

TABLE 383.3

ABNORMAL COMMON LABORATORY TESTING RESULTS THAT SUGGEST AN INBORN ERROR OF METABOLISM

Finding	Disorders
Hematologic	
Pancytopenia	Organic acidemias, Gaucher disease, Pearson syndrome (mitochondrial disorder)
Thrombocytopenia	Gaucher disease, other lysosomal storage disorders with splenomegaly
Neutropenia	Barth syndrome (3-methylglutaconic acidemia type II)
Hemolytic anemia	Disorders of pyrimidines
Defective T- and B-cell function	Adenine deaminase deficiency
Defective T-cell function	Purine-nucleoside phosphorylase deficiency
General Chemistry	
Acidosis	Organic acidemias, amino acidemias, mitochondrial disorders of energy production
Lactic acidosis	Mitochondrial disorders, organic acidemias, glycogen storage disease type I (GSD I)
Elevated ammonia	Urea cycle defects, organic acidemias, amino acidemias, mitochondrial fatty acid oxidation disorders
Increased anion gap	Organic acidemias, amino acidemias
Hypoglycemia	Mitochondrial fatty acid oxidation disorders, glycogen storage diseases, pyruvate carboxylase deficiency, 3-hydroxy-3-methyl-glutaric acidemia, hereditary fructose intolerance, fructose-1,6-diphosphatase deficiency.
Lowered blood calcium	Disorders of vitamin D activation or utilization, long-chain hydroxy acyl-CoA dehydrogenase (LCHAD) deficiency
Lowered blood phosphorus	Familial hypophosphatemic rickets
Elevated uric acid	GSD I, purine disorders
Lowered uric acid	Purine disorders
Elevated alkaline phosphatase	Hyperphosphatasia
Lowered alkaline phosphatase	Hypophosphatasia
Elevated creatine kinase	Mitochondrial fatty acid oxidation defects, mitochondrial myopathies
Urinalysis	
Hematuria	Disorders with renal stones, methylmalonic acidemia, vitamin B_{12} activation defects
Ketonuria	Organic acidemias, amino acidemias, mitochondrial fatty acid oxidation defects, glycogen storage disorders
Myoglobinuria	Mitochondrial fatty acid oxidation defects, mitochondrial myopathies
Positive reducing substance	Galactosemia, hereditary fructose intolerance

TABLE 383.4

SPECIALTY TESTING FOR INBORN ERRORS OF METABOLISM*

Name of Test	Indications
Acyl-carnitine profile	Disorders of mitochondrial fatty acid oxidation, organic acidemias, mitochondrial disorders of energy production
Amino acids, quantitative	Disorders of amino acids
Ammonia	Disorders of the urea cycle, amino acidopathies, organic acidemias, or mitochondrial fatty acid oxidation defects
Biotinidase	Biotinidase deficiency
L-Carnitine	Organic acidemias and disorders of mitochondrial fatty acid oxidation
Cholestanol	Cerebrotendinous xanthomatosis
7-Dehydrocholesterol	Smith-Lemli-Opitz syndrome
Lactate, pyruvate	Disorders of mitochondrial energy production
Lysosomal acid hydrolases	Lysosomal storage disorders
Organic acids, urine	Organic acidemias, amino acidopathies, mitochondrial fatty acid oxidation disorders, mitochondrial disorders of energy production
Orotic acid, urine	Urea cycle defects
Total homocystine	Homocystinuria, hyperhomocysteinemia
Transferrin, carbohydrate deficient	Carbohydrate deficient glycoprotein disorders
Very long chain fatty acids and plasmalogens	Disorders of peroxisomes

*See specific disorder for additional testing.

specialist will assist in determining the specific studies that are indicated. If time does not allow consultation, samples of frozen plasma or serum (2 mL or more) and frozen urine (10 mL or more), along with dried blood filter-paper dots (as used for newborn screening), should be collected. If the affected patient dies, quick-frozen samples of muscle and liver also should be obtained (preferably within 1 hour of death) and stored without preservative at −70°C. In addition, a skin biopsy for cultured fibroblasts should be performed, and the sample placed in a sterile container without preservative or in tissue culture media. The samples then may be used for diagnostic testing after consultation with the metabolic specialist.

Acknowledgments

This work was supported in part by a grant from the Indiana State Department of Health, Indianapolis, IN.

Suggested Readings

Blau N, Duran M, Blaskovics ME, et al. *Physician's guide to the laboratory diagnosis of metabolic disorders*, 2nd ed. Berlin, Heidelberg: Springer-Verlag, 2003.

Bove KE. The metabolic crisis: a diagnostic challenge. *J Pediatr* 1997;131:181.

Burton BK. Inborn errors of metabolism in infancy: a guide to diagnosis. *Pediatrics* 1998;102:E69.

Clarke JTR. *A clinical guide to inherited metabolic diseases*. Cambridge, UK: Cambridge University Press, 1996.

Fearing MK, Marsden D. Expanded newborn screening. *Pediatr Ann* 2003; 32:509.

GeneReviews at GeneTests: Medical Genetics Information Resource (database online). Copyright, University of Washington, Seattle. 1997–2003. Available at http://www.genetests.org.

Goodwin G, Msall ME, Vohr BR, et al. Newborn screening: an overview with an update on recent advances. *Curr Prob Pediatr Adolesc Health Care* 2002; 32:144.

Online Mendelian Inheritance in Man, OMIM™. McKusick-Nathans Institute for Genetic Medicine, Johns Hopkins University (Baltimore, MD) and National Center for Biotechnology Information, National Library of Medicine (Bethesda, MD), 2000. World Wide Web URL: http//80-www.ncbi.nlm.nih.gov.

Morris AA, Leonard JV. Adults with inherited disorders of intermediary metabolism. *Br J Hosp Med* 1997;57:246.

Saudubray JM, Nassogne MC, de Lonlay P, et al. Clinical approach to inherited metabolic disorders in neonates: an overview. *Semin Neonat* 2002;7:3.

Saudubray JM, Sharpentier C. Clinical phenotypes: diagnosis/algorithms. In: Scriver CR, Beaudet AL, Sly WS, et al., eds. *The metabolic and molecular bases of inherited disease*, 8th ed. New York: McGraw-Hill, 2001:1327.

Schulze A, Lindner M, Kohlmuller D, et al. Expanded newborn screening for inborn errors of metabolism by electrospray ionization-tandem mass spectrometry: results, outcome, and implications. *Pediatrics* 2003;111:1399.

Wilken B, Wiley V, Hammond J, et al. Screening newborns for inborn errors of metabolism by tandem mass spectrometry. *N Engl J Med* 2003;348: 2304.

CHAPTER 384 ■ DISORDERS OF TRANSPORT

REBECCA S. WAPPNER

An increasing number of inborn errors of metabolism are being recognized to result from defects in the transport of various types of metabolites or compounds across cell or organelle membranes. Most often the defect involves a specific carrier mechanism, often protein-based, which is subject to genetic mutation. This chapter discusses the classic defects involving the renal transport of amino acids and that of phosphate. Examples of other defects in transport, discussed elsewhere in this section, include lysinuria protein intolerance and hyperammonemia–hyperornithinemia–homocitrullinuria, discussed with disorders of the urea cycle; microsomal glucose transporter defects associated with glycogen storage diseases types Ib and Ic; and defective lysosomal transport of free sialic acid in Salla disease and infantile free sialic acid storage disease, cystine in cystinosis, and vitamin B_{12} in combined homocystinuria and methylmalonic acidemia.

DISORDERS OF RENAL AMINO ACID TRANSPORT

Cystinuria

Cystinuria is named after the extremely elevated urinary cystine concentration found in affected persons. The very low solubility of cystine leads to its precipitation and recurrent stone formation in the genitourinary tract. Affected patients may present at any age with acute abdominal or flank pain (colic), hematuria, urinary tract infection, renal failure, or hydronephrosis or other obstruction of the urinary tract. The disorder may be accompanied by a history of passing small stones known as "gravel" or crystals in diapers. Occasionally, presymptomatic patients will be diagnosed by the finding of characteristic hexagonal cystine crystals on routine urinalysis.

The disorder results from defects in the low-specificity, high-capacity renal tubular reabsorption transport system for the dibasic amino acids (ornithine, arginine, and lysine) and cystine. Fig. 384.1 shows the similar structure of four amino acids involved; the amino groups are approximately the same distance apart. Lysine is excreted in much larger amounts than is cystine but, because it is fairly soluble, it does not form stones. Intestinal transport of dibasic amino acids also is affected but is not of clinical significance.

Cystinuria occurs in approximately 1 in 7,000 persons. The disorder results from mutations at two separate genetic loci, SLC3A1 on chromosome 2 and SLC7A9 on chromosome 19, which code for the heavy and light chains, respectively, of the renal cystine/dibasic amino acid transport system. Clinically, two types of the disorder are recognized, which are distinguished by the urine cystine excretion pattern in carriers and by the mode of inheritance. Carriers for type I cystinuria have normal urinary excretion of cystine. Type I cystinuria, inherited on an autosomal recessive basis, is most often associated with mutations at the *SLC3A1* locus, but can be seen with *SLC7A9* mutations. Carriers for nontype I cystinuria (previously termed type II and type III) have moderately increased urinary cystine levels, even to the extent that occasionally they form stones. This pattern of inheritance is most consistent with an autosomal dominant mode with incomplete penetrance. Nontype I

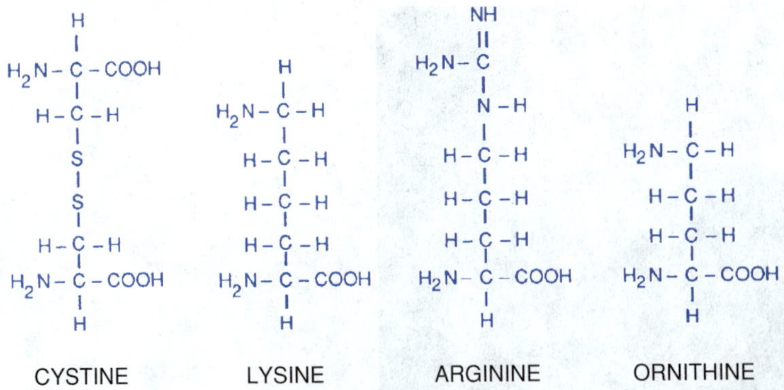

CYSTINE   LYSINE   ARGININE   ORNITHINE

FIGURE 384.1. The four amino acids excreted in excess in cystinuria.

cystinuria most often results from mutations at the *SLC7A9* locus. Affected persons with type I, nontype I, or heterozygous combined type I/nontype I cystinuria cannot be distinguished by clinical findings or urine cystine levels. Type I cystinuria and nontype I cystinuria are of approximately equal incidence.

The diagnosis may be suggested by analysis of excreted stones. Quantitative measurement of amino acids in a timed urine sample will document the disorder in patients older than 6 months. Before that time, immaturity of renal tubular transport frequently interferes with the ability to distinguish homozygotes from heterozygotes for nontype I cystinuria. Usually, urinary cystine excretion of more than 250 mg/g of creatinine is diagnostic of cystinuria.

Management is directed at preventing stone formation. Oral intake of liquids is increased to keep the urinary cystine concentration to less than 300 mg/L. Alkalinization of the urine to a pH of more than 7.5 will increase the solubility of cystine. If recurrent stones form, the use of D-penicillamine or one of its homologues, 2-mercaptopropionylglycine, may be indicated. These compounds form a mixed disulfide with the cysteinyl residues of cystine that are soluble and excreted readily. Renal transplantation may be needed for advanced renal disease.

Iminoglycinuria

Iminoglycinuria, a benign disorder, results from defects in another low-specificity, high-capacity transport system of the renal tubule that is shared by the two imino acids—proline and hydroxyproline—and glycine. The diagnosis is confirmed by quantitative urine amino acid measurements. Plasma concentrations of all three acids will be normal or low.

Other disorders resulting in increased plasma proline or hydroxyproline concentrations also may cause iminoglycinuria in that the specific imino acid involved will so overload the renal tubular reabsorption system as to interfere with reabsorption of the other imino acid and that of glycine. Transient iminoglycinuria may be seen also in normal neonates.

Hartnup Disease

Hartnup disease involves the third low-specificity, high-capacity transport system of the renal tubule and of the gastrointestinal tract. This "neutral" amino acid system transports all the amino acids except those transported by the dibasic and iminoglycine systems and the dicarboxylic amino acids, which have yet another system of their own. Clinical manifestations result from the intestinal malabsorption of tryptophan, which is a precursor for nicotinic acid (niacin) and nicotinamide. Affected persons have findings resembling that of pellagra, or niacin deficiency. Symptoms include a photosensitive dermatitis in exposed areas that may become depigmented or desquamated; such neuropsychiatric problems as cerebellar ataxia,

tremors, behavioral problems, and mild psychomotor handicaps; and diarrhea. The urinary amino acid pattern is diagnostic, demonstrating increased excretion of all the neutral amino acids except proline, hydroxyproline, and glycine. Bacterial degradation of unabsorbed fecal tryptophan results in increased formation of indican and indolic acids, which can be absorbed and excreted in the urine of affected patients. Symptomatic patients respond to nicotinamide supplementation at twice the recommended dietary intake for age. Neurologic complications, however, may not be reversible.

This autosomal recessive disorder has an incidence of approximately 1 in 30,000; this figure is based on results from newborn screening programs. Affected patients rarely present with clinical manifestations, however. The relatively high nicotinic acid dietary intake in developed countries, from an adequate daily protein intake and fortified cereals and grains, usually is enough to meet the increased requirements of affected persons. Carriers cannot be identified. The disorder results from mutations at the *ASCT1* gene locus on chromosome 19, which codes for a neutral amino acid transporter.

HYPOPHOSPHATEMIC RICKETS

Familial hypophosphatemic rickets, also known as vitamin D–resistant rickets, is an X-linked dominant disorder that results from defective proximal renal tubular reabsorption of phosphate and abnormal regulation of renal 25-hydroxyvitamin D-1-alpha-hydroxylase activity. The normal increase in activity of 1-alpha-hydroxylase and subsequent synthesis of 1,25-dihydroxyvitamin D in response to the lowered blood phosphate levels does not occur. Evidence also corroborates that intestinal absorption of phosphorus is reduced. Mutations in the *PHEX* gene, a phosphate-regulating gene with homologies to the endopeptidases located at chromosome Xp22.1, are associated with the disorder and result in parathyroid hormone dysregulation.

Affected hemizygous boys will have renal loss of phosphate and lowered blood phosphate levels from birth. Alkaline phosphatase becomes elevated by age 1 month. Most present between ages 1 and 2 years with short stature and bowed legs. Often, the head is enlarged or dolichocephalic. Enlargement at the wrists and ankles and a "rachitic rosary" at the growing ends of ribs from overgrowth of uncalcified cartilage may be noted. Blood levels of phosphorus vary with age and should be compared to age-matched normals. Blood calcium levels are normal or low-normal; urine calcium levels are low. Parathyroid levels are normal or slightly elevated. The hypocalcemia, seizures, and hypotonia seen with nutritional rickets do not occur. Renal loss of bicarbonate and electrolytes, as seen in renal Fanconi syndrome, is not present. Serum levels of 25-hydroxyvitamin D are normal; levels of 1,25-dihydroxyvitamin D are normal or slightly low. Radiographs show fraying, widening, and

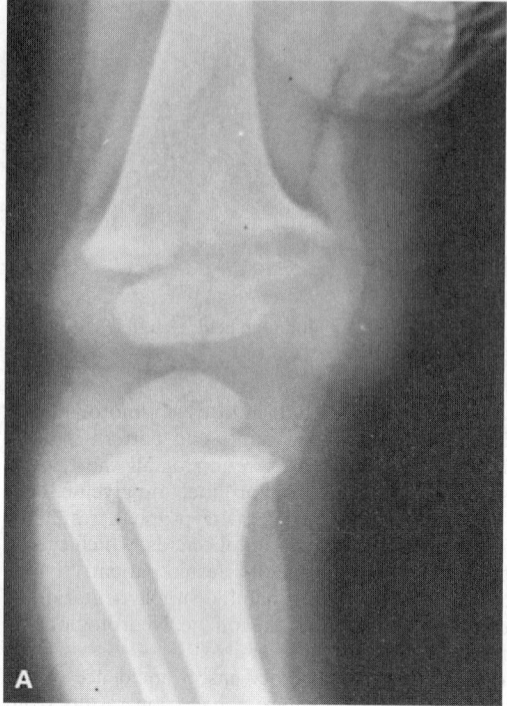

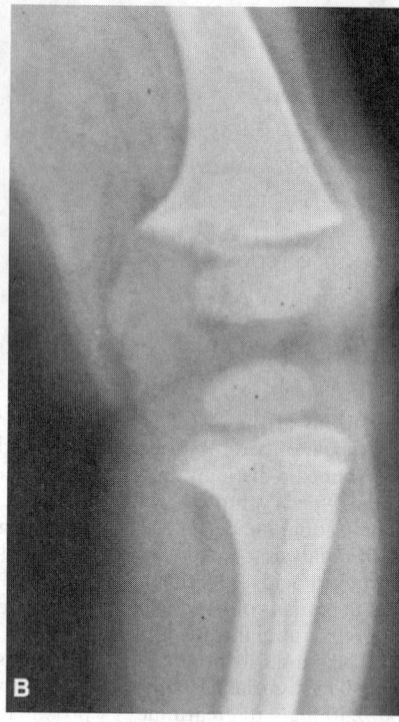

FIGURE 384.2. Familial hypophosphatemic rickets. **A:** Right knee radiogram. **B:** Left knee radiogram. Note the moth-eaten appearance of the epiphyses, particularly medially, and the various deformities of the diaphyses of the tibias and femurs.

cupping of the metaphyseal areas of the long bones that are most pronounced in the distal medial femoral areas (Fig. 384.2).

Usually, treatment with titrated doses of neutral phosphorus salts (up to 2 g/day in four to five divided doses) and 1,25-dihydroxyvitamin D (0.01 to 0.05 μg/kg/day, divided into twice-daily doses; maximum 3 μg daily) results in clinical improvement. The dosage of phosphate must be started low and slowly increased to avoid loose stooling. Blood and urine laboratory values must be carefully monitored to determine exact dosages and to avoid hypercalcemia, hypercalciuria, nephrocalcinosis, decreased renal function, and secondary and tertiary hyperparathyroidism. Most affected male subjects require surgical correction of bowing deformities of the legs.

Heterozygous affected female subjects show varying degrees of involvement. Almost all have lowered blood phosphorus levels. However, only approximately one-half will show clinical signs of rickets and will need treatment with oral medications. Occasionally, they require osteotomies to correct bowing deformities (Fig. 384.3).

Children with the disorder need dental intervention for an increased risk of caries and abscesses due to abnormal dental enamel formation and delayed dental eruption. Untreated older children and adults develop thick cortical bones and coarse,

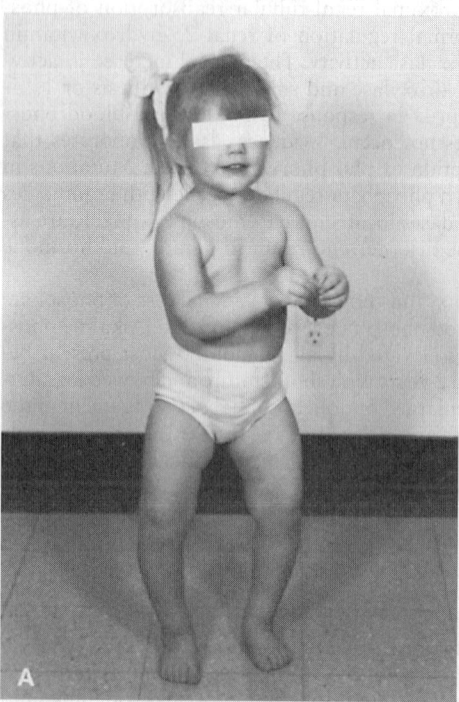

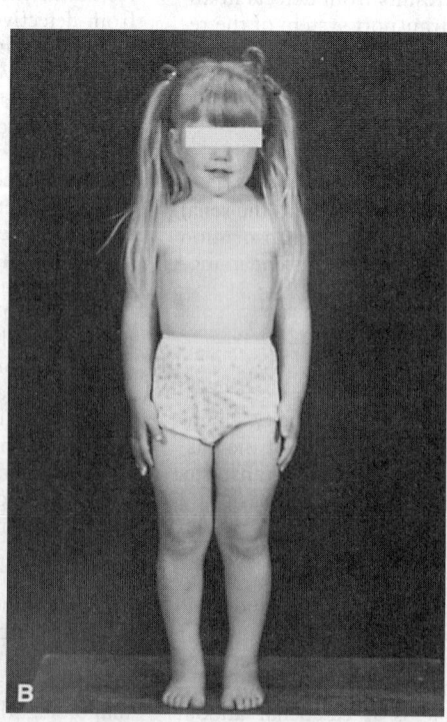

FIGURE 384.3. Familial hypophosphatemic rickets in a patient before (A) and after medical therapy and surgical osteotomies (B).

dense trabecular bones. Although osteomalacia is present, the increased total mass of incompletely calcified osteoid may give increased values for bone density. Occasionally, spinal stenosis with compression of the spinal cord requires decompressive laminectomy. Untreated adults frequently develop a progressing ankylosis of the spine and major joints. Sensorineural hearing loss has been reported.

Because the disorder is inherited as an X-linked dominant trait, all daughters of affected men will be heterozygous, with a variable risk for severity of the disorder. Children of affected women will have a 50% risk of being affected; of the children who inherit the disorder, sons clinically will show the disorder and daughters will be affected variably. Prenatal diagnosis may become available in the future with molecular genetic techniques.

Other, very rare genetic forms of familial hypophosphatemia are inherited as autosomal dominant (hypophosphatemic bone disease) or autosomal codominant (hereditary hypophosphatemic rickets with hypercalciuria) traits. Oncogenic hypophosphatemic osteomalacia may occur with small mesenchymal tumors that have osteoclast-like multinucleated giant cells.

Suggested Readings

Barbey F, Joly D, Rien P, et al. Medical treatment of cystinuria: critical reappraisal of long-term results. *J Urol* 2000;163:1419.

Botzenhart E, Vester U, Schmidt C. Cystinuria in children: distribution and frequencies of mutations in the SLC3A1 and SLC7A9 genes. *Kidney Int* 2002; 62:1136.

Carpender TO, Keller M, Schwartz D, et al. Dihydroxyvitamin D supplementation corrects hyperparathyroidism and improves skeletal abnormalities in X-linked hypophosphatemic rickets—a clinical research center study. *J Clin Endocrinol Metab* 1994;78:1378.

Grieff M. New insights into X-linked hypophosphatemia. *Curr Opin Nephrol Hypertens* 1997;6:15.

Jan de Beur SM, Levine MA. Molecular pathogenesis of hypophosphatemic rickets. *J Clin Endorinol Metab* 2002;87:2467.

Makitie O, Doria A, Kooh SW, et al. Early treatment improves growth and biochemical and radiographic outcome in X-linked hypophosphatemic rickets. *J Clin Endocrinol Metab* 2003;88:3591.

Nozaki J, Dakeishi M, Ohura T, et al. Homozygosity mapping to chromosome 5p15 of a gene responsible for Hartnup disorder. *Biochem Biophys Res Comm* 2001;284:255.

Pietrow PK, Auge BK, Weizer AZ, et al. Durability of the medical management of cystinuria. *J Urol* 2003;169:68.

Quarles LD. FGF23, PHEX, and MEPE regulation of phosphate homeostasis and skeletal mineralization. *Am J Physiol Endocrinol Metab* 2003;285:E1.

Rowe PS, Oudet CL, Sinding FF, et al. Distributions of mutations in the *PEX* gene in families with X-linked hypophosphatemic rickets (HYP). *Hum Mol Genet* 1997;6:539.

Rutchik SD, Resnick MI. Cystine calculi. Diagnosis and management. *Urol Clin North Am* 1997;24:163.

Scriver CR, Beaudet AL, Sly WS, et al., eds. *The metabolic and molecular bases of inherited disease*, 8th ed. Part 21: Membrane transport systems. New York: McGraw-Hill, 2001:4891.

Strologo LD, Pras E, Pontesilli C, et al. Comparison between SLC3A1 and SLC7A9 cystinuria patients and carriers: a need for a new classification. *J Am Soc Nephrol* 2002;13:2547.

CHAPTER 385 ■ DISORDERS OF AMINO ACID AND ORGANIC ACID METABOLISM

REBECCA S. WAPPNER

DISORDERS OF PHENYLALANINE AND TYROSINE METABOLISM

Phenylalanine is an essential amino acid in that it cannot be synthesized in the body. Tyrosine is considered nonessential in normal individuals because it may be synthesized from phenylalanine. Both phenylalanine and tyrosine are present in natural foods; the amount varies with the protein content of the food source. Phenylalanine and tyrosine are precursor amino acids for such important compounds as thyroid hormone, neurotransmitters, and melanin. The metabolism of phenylalanine and tyrosine is shown in Figure 385.1.

Phenylketonuria

Phenylketonuria (PKU), perhaps the most recognized inborn error of metabolism, results from deficient activity of phenylalanine hydroxylase (PAH). It occurs in 1 in 12,000 births and is seen most frequently among persons of white and Asian backgrounds. Affected patients appear normal at birth. Untreated, they gradually develop severe psychomotor retardation, microcephaly, hyperreflexia, seizures, autistic-appearing

behaviors, eczematoid-appearing rashes, and pigment dilution over the first few years of life. Intelligence quotients that are normal at birth fall to an average of approximately 60 by age 1 year and to an average of approximately 40 by age 4. Before newborn screening, most patients with PKU were diagnosed during an evaluation for delayed psychomotor development.

Untreated patients have markedly elevated blood and urine levels of phenylalanine and phenylalanine metabolites, such as phenylacetic acid and phenylpyruvic acid, which are known also as *phenylketones*. Levels of tyrosine are normal or low-normal. The elevated levels of phenylalanine are thought to interfere with brain growth and myelination. Increased levels of phenylacetic acid will result in a distinctive "mousy" body and urine odor. A positive blue-green color with ferric chloride urine testing indicates the presence of elevated levels of phenylpyruvic acid. Usually, enzymatic testing for PAH activity is not performed to confirm the disorder, because enzymatic activity is expressed only in liver. Mutations at the *PAH* genetic locus may be shown with peripheral blood leukocytes.

Newborn screening for PKU occurs throughout the United States. At birth, the infant's blood phenylalanine level reflects that of the mother. As protein-containing feedings of breast milk or infant formula are introduced, the affected infant's blood phenylalanine rises. Samples for newborn screening are

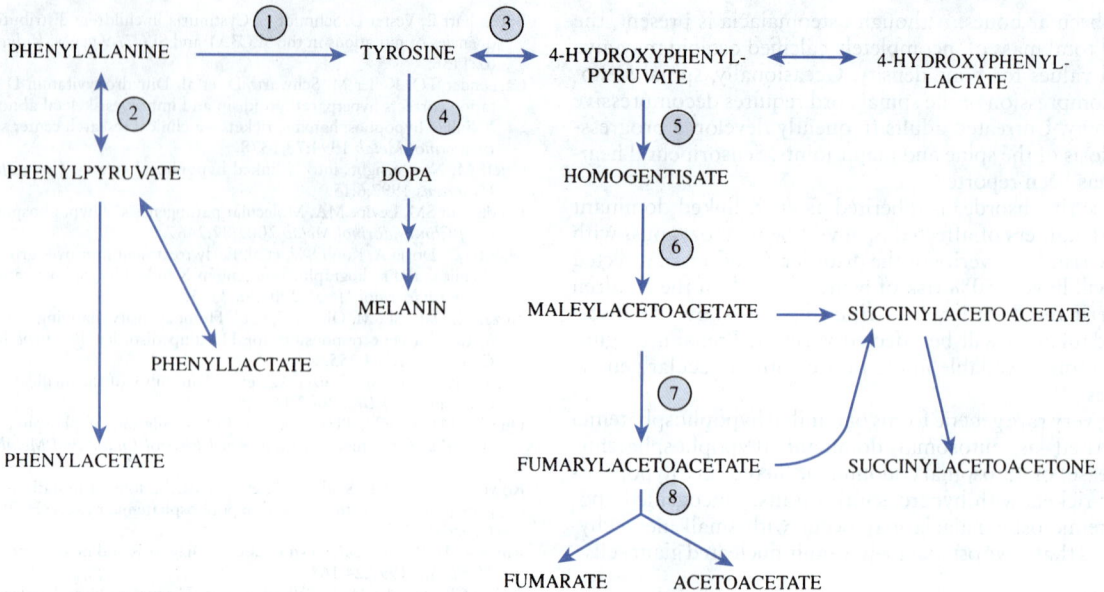

FIGURE 385.1. Metabolism of phenylalanine and tyrosine. 1, phenylalanine hydroxylase; 2, phenylalanine aminotransferase; 3, tyrosine aminotransferase; 4, tyrosine hydroxylase; 5, 4-hydroxyphenylpyruvate dioxygenase; 6, homogentisic acid oxidase; 7, maleylacetoacetate isomerase; 8, fumarylacetoacetate hydrolase. DOPA, 3,4-dihydroxyphenylalanine.

usually taken after 24 hours of feedings. The exact requirement, based on the age of the infant or the duration of feedings, will vary from state to state, depending upon the testing laboratory's method and upper limits of normal (cutoff). Infants screened earlier than recommended should have repeat testing done prior to 1 week of age. Ill neonates should have testing obtained no later than 1 week of age, regardless of feeding status. Mobilization of body stores for caloric needs and intravenous feedings containing routine amino acid mixtures usually will sufficiently load the phenylalanine pathway to give a valid result. Neonates with positive screening should be referred promptly to a program or clinic that specializes in PKU care for confirmation and treatment of their disorder. The best outcomes occur in those patients in whom control of blood phenylalanine levels occurs before 2 weeks of age and in those whose blood phenylalanine levels are kept continuously within recommended treatment ranges. With treatment, all symptoms of the disorder are reversible except for loss of intellectual potential, which usually is not reversible once it has occurred. Special medical foods, low in or devoid of phenylalanine and containing tyrosine, are used. Small, measured amounts of natural foods also are given to supply the amount of phenylalanine necessary for growth. Blood phenylalanine levels are monitored frequently and dietary adjustments made to keep the phenylalanine level within the recommended control range for age. Dietary prescriptions are individualized for affected persons and their tolerance of phenylalanine. The degree of control of blood phenylalanine levels, especially during early childhood, correlates with intellectual outcome. To achieve and maintain phenylalanine control requires continuing education and support of affected patients and their families.

Dietary control of blood phenylalanine levels, including the use of special medical foods, is needed indefinitely. Children and adolescents who discontinue the special diet have increasing problems with "executive" planning skills, school performance, and behavior. Adults not in dietary control have problems retaining employment, unusual personalities, panic attack–like episodes, and other neuropsychiatric problems. Actual (not just performance) intelligence may decrease. A few patients have had an acute demyelinating encephalopathy.

Magnetic resonance imaging reveals "dysmyelination," which may improve with dietary control. Other patients with PKU discontinue their special medical foods and continue to take a very low natural protein diet. These patients are at additional risk of developing multiple nutritional deficiencies, especially of cobalamin, folate, and calcium.

PKU is inherited as an autosomal recessive trait. Multiple mutations have been found at the *PAH* gene locus at chromosome 12q24.1. Certain mutations are more common with specific ethnic backgrounds. However, no single mutation is most common among white populations, as in cystic fibrosis. Many individuals with PKU are, in fact, compound heterozygotes for two different mutations. Carrier detection and prenatal diagnosis are available by using molecular genetic techniques in families in whom the exact mutation or polymorphisms at the *PAH* locus are known.

Certain mild variants of PKU allow a nearly normal dietary phenylalanine intake and do not require the use of special medical foods. Blood phenylalanine levels are elevated persistently (greater than 2 mg/dL) but are lower than the levels seen with classic PKU. Affected patients have at the *PAH* locus different mutations that allow for some residual activity of PAH. Importantly, girls and women with milder variants of PKU should be followed for the long term because they may have a risk of having offspring with maternal PKU syndrome (discussed in the next section) if their blood levels are elevated to more than 5 mg/dL during pregnancy.

Maternal Phenylketonuria Syndrome

The offspring of women with uncontrolled PKU during pregnancy have a significantly increased risk for cardiac malformations, microcephaly, psychomotor retardation, poor prenatal and postnatal growth, and an unusual facies, similar to that seen with fetal alcohol exposure. An increased risk for miscarriage also is present. During pregnancy, phenylalanine concentrations in the fetus are approximately 1.5 times that of the mother. Thus, if the mother's phenylalanine levels are more than the currently recommended range of between 1 mg/dL and 3 to 5 mg/dL during pregnancy, those of the fetus will be

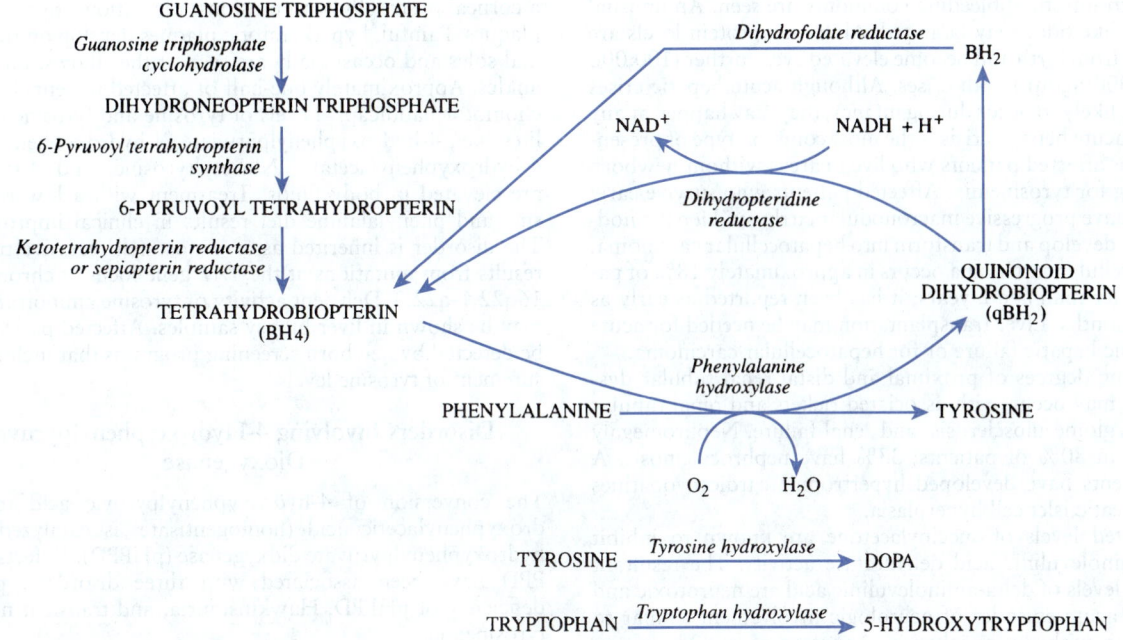

FIGURE 385.2. Biopterin synthesis and recycling. DOPA, 3,4-dihydroxyphenylalanine; NAD$^+$, oxidized form of nicotinamide adenine dinucleotide; NADH, reduced form of nicotinamide adenine dinucleotide.

even higher and may reach a level that is known to be teratogenic and affect brain growth and development in the fetus. The psychomotor development of the offspring has been shown to be inversely related to the mother's blood phenylalanine level during pregnancy. This risk occurs because of the mother's metabolic disorder, regardless of the PAH status of the fetus. All offspring of PKU mothers will be carriers for PKU; approximately 1 in 150 offspring also will have PKU, depending on the carrier status of the father.

Improved outcomes can be seen with control of the mother's phenylalanine level, optimally before and throughout the pregnancy. A great deal of commitment and effort is needed, however, to achieve this degree of control of phenylalanine levels during pregnancy. Women with mild forms of PKU also may be at risk (as discussed in Phenylketonuria, earlier). Women with all forms of PKU should receive counseling concerning their risks for maternal PKU syndrome, optimally before planning a pregnancy or becoming pregnant.

Tetrahydrobiopterin Synthesis and Recycling Defects

Tetrahydrobiopterin is a cofactor for PAH and for tyrosine hydroxylase and tryptophan hydroxylase. The synthesis and recycling of tetrahydrobiopterin is shown in Figure 385.2. Approximately 1% to 2% of patients with elevated phenylalanine levels will have defects in the synthesis or recycling of tetrahydrobiopterin. Deficient activities of guanosine triphosphate cyclohydrolase or of 6-pyruvoyl tetrahydropterin synthase are synthetic defects that result in tetrahydrobiopterin deficiency. Deficient activity of dihydropteridine reductase results in failure of recycling of tetrahydrobiopterin. In addition to having PKU, affected patients develop progressive neurologic deterioration during infancy as a result of decreased production of the neurotransmitters dopamine (3,4-dihydroxyphenylalanine) and 5-hydroxytryptophan. All infants with persistent hyperphenylalaninemia should be tested for biopterin defects, a procedure easily performed on filter-paper samples of blood and urine. Untreated, most affected infants die by age 1 year. Treat-

ment with lowered phenylalanine diets will improve the elevated phenylalanine levels but will not improve the neurologic status. The use of tetrahydrobiopterin, folinic acid, and neurotransmitter replacement has resulted in varied outcomes. The disorders are inherited as autosomal recessive traits.

Tyrosinemia

Elevated levels of tyrosine, or hypertyrosinemia, may occur with inherited disorders of tyrosine metabolism, severe liver dysfunction, scurvy (ascorbic acid deficiency), hyperthyroidism, or malnutrition.

Hepatorenal or Hereditary Tyrosinemia

Hepatorenal tyrosinemia, also known as *hereditary tyrosinemia* or *tyrosinemia type I*, results from deficient activity of fumarylacetoacetate hydrolase (FAH). The disorder is inherited as an autosomal recessive trait and is seen most commonly in Scandinavia and in the Saguenay-Lac St. Jean region of Quebec, where the incidence is 1 in 1,846 births. In the general population, it occurs in 1 in 100,000 to 120,000 births. Originally, the disorder was named after the markedly elevated levels of tyrosine and tyrosine metabolites found in body fluids of affected patients. Clinical manifestations seen in affected patients, however, now are thought to result from elevated levels of succinylacetone and succinylacetoacetone, which accumulate as a result of the deficient activity of FAH.

Hepatorenal tyrosinosis is a progressive multisystem disorder affecting the liver, kidneys, and peripheral nervous system. Progressive hepatic dysfunction with marked impairment of synthetic function starts in infancy. Transaminase levels may be normal or elevated only slightly. Jaundice rarely is seen early in the disease. Some patients have a rapidly progressing course and develop hepatic failure by 1 year of age. Others have acute hepatic crises that often are preceded by intercurrent illness. Markedly abnormal liver enzymes, jaundice, ascites, and gastrointestinal bleeding commonly are seen. An unusual cabbage-like odor may be noted. Alpha-fetoprotein levels are elevated from birth and become elevated even further (100,000 to 400,000 ng/mL) with crises. Although acute hepatic crises are most likely to occur during infancy, they may happen at any age. An acute hepatic crisis is the most common type of presentation for affected patients who live in areas without newborn screening for tyrosinemia. Affected patients who survive early infancy have progressive macronodular cirrhosis. Hepatic nodules may develop and transform into hepatocellular carcinoma. Hepatocellular carcinoma occurs in approximately 18% of patients older than age 2 years; it has been reported as early as age 33 months. Liver transplantation may be needed for acute or chronic hepatic failure or for hepatocellular carcinoma.

Varying degrees of proximal and distal renal tubular dysfunction may occur, with associated rickets and renal tubular acidosis, glomerulosclerosis, and renal failure. Nephromegaly is noted in 80% of patients; 33% have nephrocalcinosis. A few patients have developed hypertrophic cardiomyopathies or pancreatic islet cell hyperplasia.

Elevated levels of succinylacetone are known to inhibit delta-aminolevulinic acid dehydratase activity. The resultant elevated levels of delta-aminolevulinic acid are neurotoxic and produce acute episodes of neurologic involvement similar to those seen with the porphyrias. Approximately 42% of patients develop acute episodes of neurologic crisis that most often begin as painful paresthesias. Autonomic involvement with hypertension, tachycardia, and ileus may occur. One-third of patients with neurologic crises develop a progressive paralysis that may require assisted ventilation. Peripheral nerves show axonal degeneration and secondary demyelination. Repeated neurologic crises may lead to chronic weakness. Most affected children are developmentally normal. Psychomotor regression is rare unless an acute hepatic encephalopathy develops from hepatic failure.

Dietary therapy with special medical foods devoid of or low in phenylalanine, tyrosine, and methionine along with limited amounts of natural protein from formulas or foods results in improved tyrosine levels. However, diet therapy alone will not stop the production of succinylacetone, prevent the progression of liver and kidney disease, or reduce the risk for neurologic crises or hepatocellular carcinoma. Treatment with 2-(2-nitro-4-trifluoromethylbenzoyl)-1,3-cyclohexanedione (NTBC), an inhibitor of 4-hydroxyphenylpyruvate dioxygenase, reduces succinylacetone production and should be started, along with dietary therapy, once the disorder is confirmed. NTBC therapy has been shown to improve hepatic and renal function and to eliminate neurologic crises. Even with NTBC therapy, affected patients still may go on to develop hepatocellular carcinoma and require liver transplantation.

Elevated levels of urinary succinylacetone and succinylacetoacetone may be demonstrated with special gas chromatography–mass spectroscopy techniques. Deficient activity of FAH may be documented in erythrocytes, peripheral blood lymphocytes, or liver biopsy samples. Newborn screening for tyrosinemia type I may be accomplished by measurement of tyrosine or succinylacetone levels in dried blood filter-paper cards. Mutations in the FAH gene locus, at chromosome 15q23-q25, have been shown in affected patients. Carrier testing may be done if the mutation or polymorphisms at the FAH locus are known. Prenatal diagnosis is available.

Oculocutaneous Tyrosinemia

Oculocutaneous tyrosinemia, also known as *type II tyrosinemia* or the *Richner-Hanhart syndrome*, is associated with deficient activity of tyrosine aminotransferase. Symptoms most often start during the first year of life; however, presentation has been reported as late as age 38. Affected patients develop a corneal dystrophy with erosions, ulcerations, opacities, and plaques. Painful, hyperkeratotic plaques develop on the palms and soles and occasionally are seen at the elbows, knees, and ankles. Approximately one-half of affected patients have psychomotor handicaps. Levels of tyrosine and tyrosine metabolites (i.e., 4-hydroxyphenylpyruvate, 4-hydroxyphenyllactate, 4-hydroxyphenylacetate, N-acetyltyrosine, and 4-tyramine) are elevated in body fluids. Treatment with a lowered tyrosine and phenylalanine diet results in clinical improvement. The disorder is inherited as an autosomal recessive trait and results from mutations at the TAT gene locus at chromosome 16q22.1-q22.3. Deficient activity of tyrosine aminotransferase may be shown in liver biopsy samples. Affected patients may be detected by newborn screening programs that include measurement of tyrosine levels.

Disorders Involving 4-Hydroxyphenylpyruvate Dioxygenase

The conversion of 4-hydroxyphenylpyruvic acid to dihydroxyphenylacetic acid (homogentisate) is catalyzed by 4-hydroxyphenylpyruvate dioxygenase (pHPPD). Defects in pHPPD have been associated with three disorders: primary deficiency of pHPPD, Hawkinsinuria, and transient neonatal tyrosinemia.

Deficient Activity of 4-Hydroxyphenylpyruvate Dioxygenase. Primary deficiency of pHPPD is a rare disorder characterized by seizures, psychomotor retardation, and episodes of acute ataxia and lethargy. Hepatic and oculocutaneous problems do not occur. Elevated levels of 4-hydroxyphenyllactate, 4-hydroxyphenylacetate, and 4-hydroxyphenylpyruvate are noted on urine organic acid profiles. Deficient activity of pHPPD may be shown in biopsy samples of liver or kidney.

Hawkinsinuria. The pHPPD reaction is complex and involves the formation of epoxy intermediates. This rare disorder is associated with the accumulation of epoxy intermediates, which may combine with glutathione to produce (2-L-cystein-S-yl-1,4-dihydroxycyclohex-5-en-1-yl)-acetic acid. This compound was named *hawkinsin* after the first family in whom the disorder was reported. Depletion of glutathione results in increased production of 5-oxoproline, which may be responsible for the acidosis and hemolysis noted in affected infants. Affected patients may be asymptomatic or present during infancy with failure to thrive and metabolic acidosis. One reported patient had hemolytic anemia. A chlorine-like, or "swimming pool," odor may be noted. Plasma tyrosine is normal or elevated mildly. Most symptomatic patients respond to a lowered protein diet and supplemental ascorbic acid, a cofactor for pHPPD.

Transient Neonatal Tyrosinemia. As many as 10% of premature infants and some full-term neonates have transient immaturity of pHPPD. The relatively higher protein intake with infant formula as compared to human breast milk and a lowered intake of dietary ascorbic acid at this age also may contribute to the pathogenesis of the disorder. Many affected infants are asymptomatic, although lethargy, feeding problems, prolonged jaundice, and metabolic acidosis may occur. Elevated blood and urine levels of phenylalanine, tyrosine, and tyrosine metabolites are noted. Frequently, patients respond to supplemental ascorbic acid, a cofactor for pHPPD, and a lowered protein diet. Most affected infants are detected during newborn screening for PKU or tyrosinemia.

Alcaptonuria

Alcaptonuria, an autosomal recessive disorder, is associated with deficient activity of homogentisic acid oxidase and elevated levels of homogentisic acid. Homogentisic acid polymerizes to form a pigment deposited in connective tissues throughout the body (ochronosis). Usually, pigment deposition is evident first in ear cartilage and sclera between ages 20 and 30 years. Later, deposition in the large joints and lumbosacral spine may lead to decreased range of motion and ankylosis. Acute inflammatory "ochronotic arthritis" may occur. Urine from affected patients may appear dark brown or may turn dark brown if left standing (i.e., autooxidize) or with alkalinization. If washed with alkaline solutions, cloth diapers will show dark-brown staining. A brownish discoloration may be noted in the axillary and inguinal areas of affected individuals. Perspiration will stain clothes. Elevated levels of homogentisic acid are noted in blood, urine, or tissue samples. Supplemental ascorbic acid may delay the onset of the disorder and reduce the severity of clinical symptoms.

DISORDERS OF HISTIDINE METABOLISM

Histidine, an essential amino acid in infants and children, is needed for nitrogen retention and growth. Histidine is metabolized through urocanic acid to formiminoglutamic acid and, ultimately, to glutamic acid.

Histidinemia

Histidinemia is associated with deficient activity of histidase (histidine ammonia lyase), which normally catalyzes the conversion of histidine to urocanic acid. This autosomal recessive condition occurs in approximately 1 in 12,000 births and results from mutations at the *HAL* gene locus at chromosome 12q22-q23. Affected patients have elevated plasma and urine levels of histidine. Increased urinary levels of histidine metabolites (i.e., imidazolepyruvic acid, imidazolelactic acid, and imi-

dazoleacetic acid) produce a green color with the ferric chloride reagent, which can be confused with the blue-green color noted with phenylpyruvic acid in PKU. The majority of affected patients have no clinical effects from the elevated histidine levels. Approximately 1%, however, have psychomotor retardation and speech problems that suggest that the elevated histidine levels may play a role in the development of neurologic problems by enhancing the effects of other adverse clinical problems (i.e., perinatal hypoxia) at an early age. Special low-histidine diets will lower blood histidine levels and may be indicated in symptomatic patients. Deficient activity of histidase can be shown in liver or uncultured skin biopsies.

Urocanic Aciduria

Urocanic aciduria results from deficient activity of urocanase, which normally catalyzes the conversion of urocanic acid to imidazole propionic acid. Elevated levels of urocanic acid are found in the urine of affected patients. It remains unclear whether this finding has any clinical significance or is related to the psychomotor or growth retardation noted in some affected patients.

DISORDERS OF TRANSSULFURATION

The transsulfuration pathway is shown in Figure 385.3. Methionine, an essential amino acid, is converted to homocystine and subsequently is metabolized through cystathionine and cystine to inorganic sulfur, which is excreted from the body. Homocystine also may be remethylated to methionine by two pathways, which use either 5-methyltetrahydrofolate or betaine as methyl donors for the reaction. *S*-adenosylmethionine,

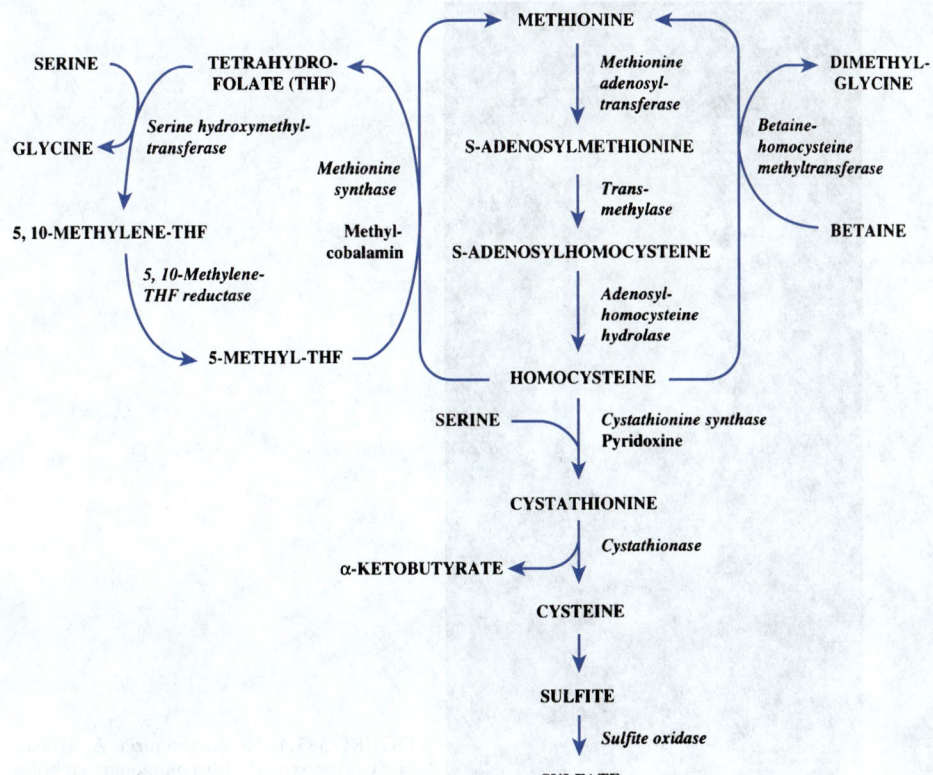

FIGURE 385.3. The transsulfuration pathway.

an intermediate in the conversion of methionine to homocystine, is an important donor for methyl groups needed for DNA and RNA modification and for reactions that involve neurotransmitter, myelin, and phospholipid metabolism. Because the demand for methyl groups often is greater than the amount that dietary methionine can supply, at least one-half of the homocystine produced from methionine is remethylated to methionine to meet this need.

Hypermethioninemia

Hypermethioninemia that occurs without elevation of other amino acids of the transsulfuration pathway results from deficient activity of methionine S-adenosyltransferase. No associated clinical manifestations are apparent. Most affected infants are detected by newborn screening programs that use measurement of blood methionine levels to detect homocystinuria. No specific treatment is needed. Elevated methionine levels may be seen also with severe liver dysfunction, hepatorenal tyrosinemia, and treatment with 6-azauridine or isoniazid.

Homocystinuria

Homocystinuria may occur as a result of cystathionine synthase deficiency. It may be the result also of defects in the remethylation pathway catalyzed by methionine synthase, which converts homocystine to methionine.

Cystathionine Synthase Deficiency

Classic homocystinuria is associated with deficient activity of cystathionine synthase. The disorder is inherited as an autosomal recessive trait and has an incidence of approximately 1 in 344,000 births. Elevated levels of methionine and homo-

cystine are found in the body fluids of affected patients. Cystine levels are low. Affected patients appear normal at birth, then slowly develop clinical features of the disease during early childhood. As in hypermethioninemia, the elevated methionine levels appear to be benign. The major clinical manifestations are related to the elevated homocystine levels. Interference in the cross-linkage of collagen leads to dislocated lens, osteoporosis, scoliosis, and a marfanoid body habitus. Most patients are tall, with long, thin extremities. In contrast to Marfan syndrome, often they have decreased range of motion at the elbows and knees and develop pes cavus foot deformities (Fig. 385.4). Elevated homocystine levels also disrupt the vascular endothelium, and thrombus formation can occur in any vessel at any age. Hypertension, pulmonary emboli, myocardial infarctions, and cerebrovascular accidents occur. Approximately 25% of patients have a major thromboembolic event by age 20 years; 50% have a major event by age 28. Psychomotor retardation develops; the average intelligence quotient is 64. Unusual personalities, behavioral problems, and other neuropsychiatric problems are common.

Plasma and urine quantitative amino acid determinations will show elevated levels of methionine and homocystine and lowered levels of cystine. Other sulfur-containing amino acids may be noted (i.e., the mixed disulfide of cysteine and homocysteine, homolanthionine, and S-adenosyl homocysteine). Protein-bound homocystine levels will be elevated. Deficient activity of cystathionine synthase may be shown in phytohemagglutinin-stimulated lymphocytes or in cultured skin fibroblasts.

Treatment is aimed at reducing homocystine levels to as nearly undetectable as possible and at normalizing cystine levels. Limited amounts of natural foods and special methionine-free medical foods with added cystine are given. Betaine, which serves as a methyl donor in the remethylation of homocystine to methionine, is used in addition to dietary therapy. Supplemental vitamins may be needed to ensure adequate intake of

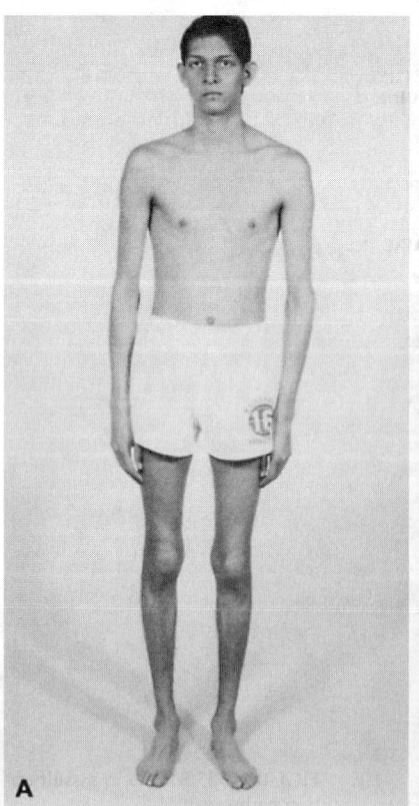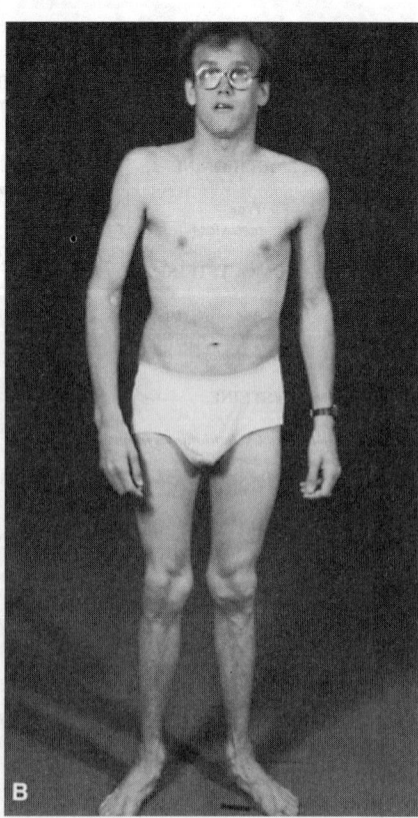

FIGURE 385.4. Homocystinuria. **A:** Teenage boy who presented with a pulmonary embolus. **B:** Young adult.

pyridoxine, vitamin B_{12}, and folate. Although treatment is indicated for life, achieving compliance with dietary therapy in adolescents and adults may be difficult.

Approximately 50% of patients with homocystinuria have some residual cystathionine synthase activity and are responsive to high-dose pyridoxine therapy. Usually, these patients have less severe clinical manifestations of the disorder. Many have normal intelligence. Doses of 300 to 900 mg/day of pyridoxine may be given in adults. Doses in children should be proportionately lower and not exceed 900 mg/1.73 m^2/day. Special medical foods and betaine therapy may be needed in some patients for control of the disorder. Others require only a relatively lowered natural protein diet.

The gene that encodes for cystathionine synthase (*CBS*) is located at chromosome 21q22.3. At least 92 mutations in the *CBS* gene have been reported in affected patients, some of which are associated with pyridoxine responsiveness. Carrier detection may be performed if the mutation or polymorphisms at the *CBS* locus are known. Prenatal diagnosis is available.

Newborn screening for homocystinuria occurs in some states and in Europe by testing blood methionine levels in dried blood filter-paper samples. In many affected infants the disorder has not been detected, however, mainly owing to the slow rise in blood methionine levels during the first few days of life when screening samples are customarily obtained in the United States. In those infants with homocystinuria who were detected by newborn screening and who were started on dietary therapy in early infancy, the natural course of the disease has been modified. Psychomotor handicaps and dislocated lenses have been prevented or delayed in onset. With the use of more sensitive newborn screening methods such as tandem mass spectrometry, which many states are now adopting, it is anticipated that improved early detection of homocystinuria patients will occur.

Homocystinuria Due to Remethylation Defects

Homocystinuria may result from defects in the remethylation pathway. Affected patients have deficient activity of methionine synthase or inherited disorders in folate or cobalamin metabolism that affect methionine synthase activity. Homocystine levels are elevated but to a degree less than that seen with cystathionine synthase deficiency. Methionine levels are low or normal. Cystathionine levels may be elevated. Usually, progressive central nervous system involvement occurs in addition to features of classic homocystinuria. All the disorders are inherited as autosomal recessive traits. Prenatal diagnosis is available. Carrier detection may be performed if the mutation or polymorphisms at the genetic loci involved are known. Nutritional deficiencies of folate or cobalamin may result in similar biochemical and clinical abnormalities.

Deficient Activity of Methionine Synthase. Methionine synthase (5-methyltetrahydrofolate homocysteine S-methyltransferase) catalyzes the remethylation of homocystine to methionine. Patients with the disorder present most often as infants with poor feeding, lethargy, hypotonia, delayed development, and megaloblastic anemias. One adult patient presented with neurologic problems and macrocytic anemia. Serum vitamin B_{12} and folate levels are normal. Some patients respond to treatment with intramuscular hydroxocobalamin, betaine, and folic acid. The disorder results from mutations in the gene *MTF,* located at chromosome 1q43, which encodes for methionine synthase. Previously, patients with methionine synthase deficiency were designated as having type cblG (cobalamin G) defects (named after the complementation groups noted in studies with cell lines of patients with various defects of cobalamin metabolism).

Defects in Tetrahydrofolate Metabolism. Deficient activity of 5,10-methylenetetrahydrofolate reductase (MTHFR) results in lowered levels of 5-methyltetrahydrofolate, the major transport form of folate, and the methyl donor for the methionine synthase reaction. The disorder may present at any age; clinical severity is related to the amount of residual enzyme activity present. The patients most severely affected are neonates who present with apnea, seizures, and a progressive demyelinating encephalopathy. Most do not survive beyond age 1 year. Other patients less severely affected have developmental delay, incoordination, gait abnormalities, paresthesias, seizures, recurrent strokes, or psychiatric problems. Some have a marfanoid body habitus. Megaloblastic anemias do not occur. Serum folate levels are normal or low; vitamin B_{12} levels are normal. Perivascular changes, demyelination, macrophage infiltration, and astrogliosis of the central nervous system occur in addition to thrombus formation as seen with cystathionine synthase deficiency. Patients with milder forms may respond to treatment with betaine, folic acid, pyridoxine, and hydroxocobalamin. Methionine supplementation also may be needed. Residual neurologic impairments may improve slowly with treatment and rehabilitation.

Deficient activity of MTHFR may be shown in peripheral blood leukocytes or cultured skin fibroblasts. A number of mutations have been reported in the gene *MTHFR* located at chromosome 1p36.3, which encodes for the enzyme. The disorder is inherited as an autosomal recessive trait. Carrier detection is available for families in whom the mutation or polymorphisms are known. Prenatal diagnosis is available.

A specific allele at the *MTHFR* locus (C677T) encodes for a thermolabile enzyme. Homozygosity for this allele, if combined with low tissue folate levels, may result in elevated plasma homocystine (hyperhomocystinemia) and an increased risk for atherosclerotic vascular disease. The allele also may play a role in the prevention of neural tube birth defects by folic acid.

Defects in Cobalamin Metabolism. Dietary cobalamin (vitamin B_{12}) is taken up into the cells as hydroxocobalamin, is processed in lysosomes, and then is further metabolized to either methylcobalamin, a cofactor for methionine synthase, or adenosylcobalamin, a cofactor for methylmalonyl-CoA mutase. Depending on the site of the metabolic block, patients with defects in cobalamin metabolism may have only homocystinuria, only methylmalonic acidemia, or combined homocystinuria and methylmalonic acidemia. Table 385.1 lists the biochemical genetic features of the disorders of cobalamin metabolism along with classic homocystinuria and methylmalonic acidemia. The disorders have been classified into seven complementation groups, cblA to cblG, according to studies in cell lines from affected patients.

Deficient activity of methionine synthase reductase. Functional deficiency of methionine synthase results from defects in the formation of its cofactor methylcobalamin. Patients with type cblE complementation group have methionine synthase reductase deficiency as a result of mutations in the *MTRR* gene located at chromosome 5p15.3-p15.2. This defect in the formation of methylcobalamin occurs intracellularly after lysosomal processing of hydroxocobalamin. Affected patients present in infancy with clinical findings similar to those seen in methionine synthetase deficiency, including poor feeding, lethargy, hypotonia, and delayed development. They have megaloblastic anemias but do not have methylmalonic acidemia. Serum folate and vitamin B_{12} levels are normal. Most respond to treatment with large doses of intramuscular hydroxocobalamin. Betaine and folic acid also may be needed. One patient with cblE disease was detected and treated prenatally by maternal intramuscular hydroxocobalamin injections. This patient continues to do well on hydroxocobalamin therapy.

Abnormalities in cobalamin metabolism and activation that affect the formation of both methylcobalamin and adenosylcobalamin result in *combined homocystinuria and methylmalonic*

TABLE 385.1

BIOCHEMICAL GENETIC FEATURES OF METHYLMALONIC ACIDEMIA AND HOMOCYSTINURIA

Disorder	Enzymatic or Other Defect	Gene Location	Classification
Methylmalonic acidemia	Methylmalonyl-CoA mutase deficiency	MUT 6p21	Type mut⁰: essentially no enzyme activity
			Type mut⁻: structurally abnormal enzyme with some residual activity
	Defects in the formation of adenosylcobalamin, cofactor for methylmalonyl-CoA mutase	MMAA 4q31.1-q31.2	Type cblA: defect in mitochondrial hydroxocobalamin reduction and adenosylation
		MMAB 12q24	Type cblB: deficient activity of mitochondrial hydroxocobalamin adenosyltransferase
Combined methylmalonic acidemia and homocystinuria	Defects in the formation of both adenosylcobalamin and methylcobalamin	Unknown	Type cblC: unknown defect in hydroxocobalamin metabolism
			Type cblD: unknown defect in hydroxocobalamin metabolism
			Type cblF: defect in the exit of hydroxocobalamin from lysosomes
Homocystinuria	Methionine synthase reductase deficiency	MTRR 5p15.3-p15.2	Type cblE: defect in the remethylation of homocystine to methionine
	Methionine synthase deficiency	MTR 1q43	Defect in the remethylation of homocystine to methionine (prior type cblG)
	5,10-Methylenetetrahydrofolate reductase deficiency	MTHRF 1p36.3	Failure to form 5-methyltetrahydrofolate, methyl donor for methionine synthase reaction
	Cystathionine synthase deficiency	CBS 21q22.3	Mutations without pyridoxine responsiveness
			Mutations with pyridoxine responsiveness

cbl, cobalamin complementation group, based on studies with cell lines from patients with various types of methylmalonic acidemia; mut, mutase.

$acidemia$. Patients have reduced activities of methionine synthase and methylmalonyl-CoA mutase and clinical features of both associated disorders. Three complementation groups—cblC, cblD, and cblF—are associated with these abnormalities. Type cblF results from a defect in the transfer of hydroxocobalamin from lysosomes to the cytosol. The exact intracellular metabolic defects in types cblC and cblD are unknown. Most affected patients present in infancy with failure to thrive, poor feeding, lethargy, hypertonicity, and progressive neurologic dysfunction. Cortical atrophy and myelopathies may be seen, especially in those patients with later onset of their disease. Pigmentary retinopathies and abnormal maculae have been reported with types cblC and cblD. Type cblC may present with hemolytic-uremic syndrome. One case of sudden death was reported with type cblF. Some older patients have a marfanoid habitus. Megaloblastic or megalocytic anemias and, occasionally, pancytopenia occur. Serum cobalamin and folate levels are normal. Moderately elevated homocystine and normal or lowered methionine levels are noted on quantitative amino acid determinations. Urine organic acid analysis will show moderate to marked elevation of methylmalonate but less than that seen in classic methylmalonic acidemia. Usually, severe metabolic acidosis does not occur. Some patients respond to treatment with large doses of intramuscular hydroxocobalamin, betaine, and diets lower in natural protein. Psychomotor handicaps, however, may not be reversible. Others do not respond to therapy and die in infancy. Prenatal diagnosis is available.

Cobalamin metabolism abnormalities that affect only the formation of adenosylcobalamin, complementation groups cblA and cblB, result in methylmalonic acidemia. They are discussed with that disorder.

Cystathioninuria

Elevated levels of cystathionine and related sulfur-containing compounds, from cystathioninase (cystathionase) deficiency, are benign and not associated with any significant clinical manifestations. The elevated levels of cystathionine may normalize with pyridoxine treatment.

Increased levels of cystathionine may be seen also transiently in normal neonates. They also may occur with nutritional pyridoxine deficiency, thyrotoxicosis, hepatic dysfunction, and certain tumors (i.e., neuroblastomas, ganglioblastomas, and hepatomas).

Sulfite Oxidase Deficiency

Sulfite oxidase deficiency is a rare autosomal recessive disorder that results in the accumulation and increased urinary excretion of sulfite, thiosulfate, and S-sulfocysteine. Affected patients present as neonates with severe, generalized, intractable seizures. Dislocated lens and a demyelinating central nervous system deterioration occur in those who survive the neonatal period.

Deficiency of the molybdenum cofactor for sulfite oxidase deficiency is more common than is isolated sulfite oxidase deficiency and presents with similar clinical findings. Molybdenum is a cofactor also for xanthine dehydrogenase and aldehyde oxidase. Affected patients have low levels of uric acid; elevated levels of urinary xanthine, hypoxanthine, and taurine; and accumulation of sulfite, thiosulfate, and S-sulfocysteine. Milder variants have been reported. Deficient activity of sulfite oxidase

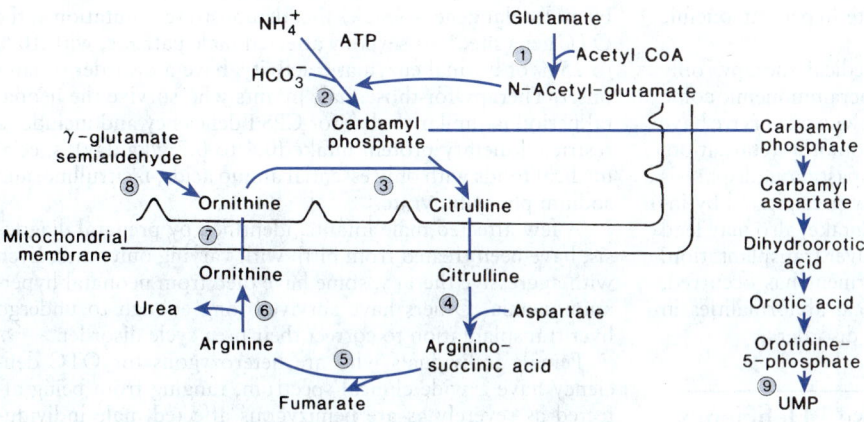

FIGURE 385.5. Urea cycle. 1, N-acetyl-glutamate synthetase; 2, carbamyl phosphate synthetase I; 3, ornithine transcarbamylase; 4, argininosuccinate synthetase; 5, argininosuccinate lyase; 6, arginase; 7, mitochondrial ornithine transport defect (hyperammonemia–hyperornithinemia–homocitrullinuria); 8, ornithine aminotransferase; 9, decarboxylase, site of allopurinol block in pyrimidine pathway. ATP, adenosine triphosphate; CoA, coenzyme A; UMP, uridine monophosphate.

or xanthine dehydrogenase may be demonstrated in cultured skin fibroblasts or liver biopsy samples. No specific treatment is available. Prenatal diagnosis is available.

DISORDERS OF AMMONIA METABOLISM

Excess dietary or waste nitrogen (remaining after what is needed for protein synthesis and tissue maintenance is used) normally is not stored in the body but is converted into urea by a series of reactions known as the *urea cycle* (Fig. 385.5). Disorders of the urea cycle are associated with the accumulation of ammonia and its precursors (i.e., glutamine, glutamic acid, aspartic acid, and glycine). Elevated plasma ammonia levels that exceed three times the upper limits of normal are toxic and associated with cytotoxic changes in the brain and liver. With rising ammonia levels, affected patients develop poor feeding, anorexia, behavioral changes, irritability, vomiting, lethargy, ataxia, and seizures. As the hyperammonemia progresses, affected patients become comatose, and ventilatory support may be needed. Circulatory collapse and cerebral edema may occur. The classic cases are neonates who appear asymptomatic for 24 to 48 hours and then develop progressive neurologic deterioration. Milder forms of the disorders may present later in infancy, may produce intermittent symptoms over a period of years, or may be detected in older children or adults with neurologic problems or psychomotor retardation. As a group, the disorders are estimated to occur in approximately 1 in 30,000 live births. All the disorders of ammonia metabolism are inherited as autosomal recessive traits, except for ornithine transcarbamylase (OTC) deficiency, which is inherited as an X-linked trait, and transient hyperammonemia of the newborn, which is not genetic in origin.

The diagnosis of a specific urea cycle disorder is made on the basis of the pattern of plasma and urine amino acid abnormalities and the presence or absence of orotic aciduria. Confirmation of specific enzymatic deficiencies requires only erythrocytes or cultured skin fibroblasts for some of the disorders but necessitates liver biopsy for others. Molecular genetic studies may be used also with many of the disorders to confirm the diagnosis and for carrier and prenatal testing.

Secondary hyperammonemia, associated with other amino acidemias or organic acidurias, usually can be excluded by the absence of acidosis. Urinary organic acid determination, however, should be obtained to rule out the rare case that might present initially with hyperammonemia (i.e., with maple syrup urine disease [MSUD], methylmalonic acidemia, or propionic acidemia). Secondary hyperammonemia may occur also with disorders of mitochondrial fatty acid oxidation or oxidative phosphorylation and with severe liver dysfunction or liver failure.

Treatment of acute hyperammonemia, either at the initial presenting episode or at a subsequent intercurrent episode, is a medical emergency. With the initial episode, blood and urine samples should be collected for diagnostic testing, but treatment should be started immediately, before a specific diagnosis is established. Therapy should include the removal of all exogenous protein sources and the administration of intravenous glucose to prevent protein catabolism. Reduction of markedly elevated plasma ammonia and ammonia precursors is carried out most effectively by hemodialysis. Alternatively, hemofiltration may be used. For a temporary delay in hemodialysis or hemofiltration, peritoneal dialysis may be performed but is less effective. Because the duration of time in coma is inversely related to outcome, prompt referral to a tertiary medical center is indicated if hemodialysis or hemofiltration are not readily available.

Drugs that use alternate pathways for waste nitrogen excretion, such as sodium benzoate and sodium phenylacetate, may be used intravenously to control acute mild to moderate hyperammonemia (less than 350 μmol). One must be prepared to start hemodialysis or hemofiltration immediately in the absence of significant improvement in ammonia levels within a short period after this therapy is instituted, however. These drugs are used enterally also to maintain plasma ammonia levels within the normal range between intercurrent episodes in patients with the more severe forms of the disorders. Sodium benzoate combines with glycine to form hippurate. Sodium phenylacetate combines with glutamine to form phenylacetylglutamine. Both hippurate and phenylacetylglutamine are excreted rapidly by the kidneys and remove a significant amount of nitrogen, the ammonia precursor. A combination preparation of sodium benzoate and sodium phenylacetate is commercially available (previously investigational new drug) for intravenous use. Sodium phenylbutyrate, which is converted into sodium phenylacetate in the body and is less odorous than phenylacetate, also is commercially available in tablet or powder form for enteral use. Before these drugs were developed, many patients with severe forms of the disorders did not survive past age 1 year.

Once plasma ammonia levels fall to less than 100 μmol, the patient may be started on enteral therapy. Special medical foods, free of protein or with protein content composed of only essential amino acids, may be necessary to meet basic caloric and other nutrient needs. Depending on the type of disorder and its severity, a fairly limited protein intake with or without essential amino acid supplementation will be needed. Specific amino acid supplementation with L-citrulline or L-arginine also is given for relative insufficiencies of these amino acids and to "prime" the urea cycle. Intravenous L-arginine hydrochloride is used for the same purpose during acute hyperammonemic episodes.

Even with prompt and aggressive medical therapy, only 30% to 50% of neonates who develop hyperammonemic coma survive the neonatal period. Most of those who do survive have significant neurologic deficits and psychomotor retardation. Seizure disorders, cortical atrophy, and spastic quadriparesis are common. Later acute episodes, usually precipitated by intercurrent infections or excessive protein intake, also may lead to further neurologic sequelae or death. Liver transplantation, done before significant neurologic impairment has occurred, has been shown to correct the biochemical abnormalities in children affected with severe forms of the disorders.

Carbamyl Phosphate Synthetase I Deficiency

Carbamyl phosphate synthetase I (CPS I) is a mitochondrial enzyme that catalyzes the formation of carbamyl phosphate from ammonia, adenosine triphosphate, and bicarbonate in the presence of N-acetylglutamate. N-Acetylglutamate, a critical cofactor for this reaction, is formed from acetyl CoA and glutamate in the presence of N-acetylglutamate synthetase. Inhibition of N-acetylglutamate synthetase by organic acids, especially propionic acid, is thought to be the reason for the secondary hyperammonemia seen with organic acidurias.

Most patients with CPS I deficiency present with neonatal hyperammonemic coma. Near-zero levels of citrulline and lowered arginine and elevated levels of glutamine, alanine, and glycine are noted on quantitative plasma amino acid determinations. No elevation of urinary orotic acid occurs. Less than 10% of normal CPS I activity is noted on liver, rectal, or duodenal biopsy. Partial deficiencies, with 10% to 25% of normal enzyme activity, have been reported with later onset of symptoms. Treatment includes a fairly restrictive dietary protein intake (0.5 to 0.7 g/kg/day), special medical foods with only essential amino acids, L-citrulline, and sodium phenylbutyrate. Liver transplantation may be needed in the severe form of the disorder. The disorder is inherited as an autosomal recessive trait. The gene that encodes for CPS I, CPS I, is located at chromosome 2q35. Carrier detection is available only in families with known mutations or polymorphisms at the CPS I locus. Prenatal diagnosis is possible using molecular genetic techniques or by fetal liver biopsy for enzymatic analysis.

N-Acetylglutamate Synthetase Deficiency

N-Acetylglutamate synthetase deficiency is a very rare disorder with neonatal presentation. Plasma citrulline and arginine levels and urinary orotic acid levels are normal. Therapy is similar to that for CPS I deficiency, except that arginine, an activator of N-acetylglutamate synthetase, and N-carbamylglutamate, a congener of N-acetylglutamate, are given.

Ornithine Transcarbamylase Deficiency

OTC deficiency, the most common of the urea cycle disorders, is inherited as an X-linked trait. Usually, affected male individuals present as neonates with massive hyperammonemia. Plasma ammonia levels often exceed 1,000 µmol. Citrulline levels are reduced markedly. Levels of glutamine, glycine, and alanine are elevated, along with other nonspecific elevations associated with massive hyperammonemia (i.e., lysine and proline). Urinary orotic acid is elevated markedly. Even with aggressive management, many patients do not survive the neonatal period. The enzymatic deficiency may be confirmed with liver biopsy or

by molecular genetic studies that demonstrate a mutation at the OTC gene site. Less severely affected male patients, with 10% to 25% of normal enzymatic activity, have a disorder of later onset. Therapy for those male infants who survive the neonatal period is similar to that for CPS I deficiency and includes a restricted dietary protein intake (0.4 to 0.7 g/kg/day), special medical foods with only essential amino acids, L-citrulline, and sodium phenylbutyrate.

A few affected male infants, identified by prenatal diagnosis, have been treated from birth with varying outcomes. Even with aggressive therapy, some have died from neonatal hyperammonemia. Others have survived long enough to undergo liver transplantation to correct their urea cycle disorder.

Female individuals who are heterozygous for OTC deficiency have a wide clinical spectrum, ranging from being affected as severely as are hemizygous affected male individuals to being asymptomatic. The degree of relative lyonization (random X chromosome inactivation) in hepatocytes of normal and abnormal OTC genes in female individuals determines the clinical severity of their disease. Approximately 20% of female heterozygotes for OTC are symptomatic. At least three severely affected female infants have not survived the neonatal period. More often, symptomatic carrier female individuals have 10% to 20% of normal OTC activity and, during childhood, a diagnosis is made on the basis of symptoms of intermittent hyperammonemia (i.e., cyclic vomiting, lethargy, and coma) or protein intolerance or avoidance. Neurologic problems (i.e., strokes, cerebral atrophy, dementia, or other encephalopathic processes) may be seen. Acute hyperammonemia in the postpartum period also has been reported. Therapy for symptomatic heterozygous female individuals depends on the degree of severity of their disease.

Importantly, female relatives of affected patients should be evaluated to determine whether they are carriers for OTC deficiency. Approximately two-thirds of mothers of affected male infants will be carriers for the disorder. Carrier detection will allow early identification of women at risk for hyperammonemic episodes and may be helpful also in reproductive planning. Measurement of urinary orotic acid or orotidine while taking allopurinol, which inhibits the pyrimidine pathway beyond orotic acid, will detect most (but not all) OTC carriers. Over 100 mutations at the OTC locus, at chromosome Xp21.1, have been identified. Molecular genetic techniques are available for both carrier detection and prenatal diagnosis in families with known mutations or polymorphisms at the OTC locus.

Citrullinemia

Citrullinemia is associated with deficient activity of argininosuccinate synthetase. Most patients present in the neonatal period with massive hyperammonemia. Plasma and urine citrulline levels are elevated markedly. Plasma argininosuccinic acid is absent; plasma glutamine and alanine are elevated. Urinary orotic acid may be increased but to a lesser degree than with OTC deficiency. Milder forms with partial argininosuccinate synthetase deficiency have been reported with presentation in early childhood.

Because citrulline is excreted fairly rapidly in the urine (a means for waste nitrogen excretion), usually this disorder is managed more easily than is OTC or CPS I deficiency after the neonatal period. Patients still require a protein-restricted diet (0.8 to 1.5 g/kg/day), special medical foods, and sodium phenylbutyrate. L-Arginine supplementation is given. The disorder is inherited as an autosomal recessive trait. The diagnosis may be confirmed by measurement of argininosuccinate synthetase in cultured skin fibroblasts or liver biopsy specimens. At least 18 mutations have been identified in the gene ASS, located at chromosome 9q34, which encodes for argininosuccinate synthase. Carrier detection and prenatal diagnosis are available.

Citrin Deficiency

Citrin is a mitochondrial carrier protein responsible for catalyzing an efflux of aspartate into the cytosol in exchange for the entry of glutamate into the mitochondria. The aspartate in the cytosol combines with citrulline to form argininosuccinic acid. Deficiency of citrin leads to decreased concentrations of cytosolic aspartate available for argininosuccinic acid formation, secondary argininosuccinate synthetase deficiency, and the elevated citrulline levels and hyperammonemia seen in affected patients. Decreased levels of citrin also result in decreased production of NAD$^+$ by the malate-aspartate NADH shuttle. Elevated NADH is thought to inhibit UDP galactose-4-epimerase activity, which results in the elevated galactose levels seen in citrin-deficient patients.

Citrin deficiency occurs as two forms. Both forms are most common in Japan. The *adult onset form*, or citrullinemia type 2 (CTLN2), presents over age 10 years with elevated levels of citrulline and hyperammonemia. Affected patients often die within a few years of the onset of their disorder, usually from hyperammonemia-associated cerebral edema. Some have been treated with liver transplantation.

The *neonatal intrahepatic cholestasis form of citrin deficiency* (NICCD) presents between 1 and 4 months of age with direct hyperbilirubinemia, impaired coagulation, hypoalbuminemia, mildly elevated liver transaminases, and mild hyperammonemia. Bile acid and alpha-fetoprotein levels are elevated. Liver biopsies show fatty changes and variable fibrosis. Blood and urine amino acid determinations show markedly elevated levels of citrulline and methionine and moderate elevation of threonine, tyrosine, lysine, and arginine. Mild elevation of phenylalanine and ornithine also may occur. Disturbed galactose metabolism leads to elevated levels of blood and urine galactose and positive urine testing for reducing substances. Treatment with a lowered protein and/or galactose-free diet often improves the hepatic dysfunction and aminoacidopathy. Supplements of fat-soluble vitamins may be required. The hepatic dysfunction frequently spontaneously resolves during the first year of life, but it may persist and require liver transplantation. Some infants have recovered only to relapse into the adult form in late puberty or adolescence.

Affected infants often have positive newborn screening testing as a result of the elevated galactose and amino acid levels. With expanded newborn screening programs being instituted in many locations, it is anticipated that additional cases in countries other than Japan will be identified. Citrin is encoded by the gene *SLC25A13*, located at chromosome 7q21.3. There is no genotype-phenotype correlation. The same mutation may be found in patients with either one of the two forms of the disorder.

Argininosuccinic Aciduria

Argininosuccinic aciduria results from argininosuccinase (argininosuccinate lyase) deficiency. Plasma and urine argininosuccinic acid levels are elevated markedly. Plasma arginine is reduced markedly; plasma glutamine and alanine are elevated. No marked increase occurs in urinary orotic acid.

The disorder presents in the neonatal period but as late as age 1 to 2 weeks. Milder forms have presented in childhood or have been detected by urinary newborn screening. Many patients have chronic hepatomegaly with fatty infiltration and fibrosis on biopsy. Arginine deficiency may lead to trichorrhexis nodosa with friable hair and erythematous maculopapular rashes, both of which respond to arginine therapy. The rapid excretion of argininosuccinic acid in the urine serves as a means for waste nitrogen excretion as in citrullinemia. Usually, patients respond well to intravenous and oral L-arginine therapy. Protein restriction may be needed. Intercurrent hyperammonemic episodes also may require the use of intravenous sodium benzoate and sodium phenylacetate, but usually they are not required otherwise. The disorder is inherited as an autosomal recessive trait and may be confirmed by demonstrating deficient activity of argininosuccinate lyase in erythrocytes, cultured skin fibroblasts, or liver biopsy specimens. At least 12 mutations have been identified in the gene *ASL*, located at chromosome 7cen–q11.2, which encodes for argininosuccinase. Carrier detection and prenatal diagnosis are available.

Argininemia

Argininemia is a rare disorder associated with deficient activity of arginase and modest hyperammonemia (100 to 300 μmol). Usually, patients do not have neonatal hyperammonemia. More often, they reveal a history of episodic vomiting, headache, irritability, seizures, cerebral atrophy, psychomotor retardation, and progressive spastic quadriparesis. Hepatomegaly may be present along with abnormal liver function tests. Multifocal hydropic changes are noted on liver biopsy. Plasma arginine (greater than 500 μmol) and urinary arginine levels are elevated. Urinary lysine, cystine, and ornithine may be increased as a result of competition with the large amounts of arginine for a shared renal tubular reabsorption system. Urinary orotic acid is increased. Because of arginine stimulation of N-acetylglutamate synthetase, the amount of carbamyl phosphate produced is greater than the urea cycle can use, and the excess is channeled into the pyrimidine pathway. Therapy includes protein restriction, special medical foods, sodium phenylbutyrate, and supplementation of lysine and ornithine. Deficient activity of arginase may be demonstrated in erythrocytes, leukocytes, or liver biopsy samples. The disorder is inherited as an autosomal recessive trait. The disorder results from mutations in the gene *ARG1*, located at chromosome 6q23, which encodes for arginase. Carrier detection and prenatal diagnosis may be accomplished by molecular genetic techniques in families in whom mutations or polymorphisms at the *ARG1* locus are known. Otherwise, fetal liver biopsy or fetal blood sampling is required for prenatal diagnosis because the enzyme is not expressed in cultured fibroblasts.

Lysinuric Protein Intolerance

Two disorders involved with the transport of dibasic amino acids, lysinuric protein intolerance, and the hyperammonemia–hyperornithinemia–homocitrullinuria (HHH) syndrome are associated with hyperammonemia and faulty urea synthesis.

Lysinuric protein intolerance results from faulty renal tubular, intestinal, and hepatic transport of dibasic amino acids. Urinary levels of lysine, arginine, and ornithine are elevated. Urinary levels of cystine, another dibasic amino acid, are not elevated, which distinguishes the urinary findings from those noted in cystinuria. Plasma levels of lysine, arginine, and ornithine are low. Plasma citrulline may be elevated. As a result of the low levels of ornithine, urea synthesis is impaired. Modest hyperammonemia (100 to 300 μmol) and orotic aciduria occur. Patients may have signs of intermittent or acute hyperammonemia. They are noted also to have short stature, osteoporosis, hypotonia, lens opacities, hyperelastic skin, hyperextensible joints, friable hair, psychomotor retardation, and hepatosplenomegaly. Pancytopenia may be present. Treatment includes dietary protein restriction and L-citrulline supplementation. The disorder is inherited as an autosomal recessive trait and is most common in persons of Finnish background. The disorder results from mutations at the *LPT* locus at chromosome 11q11.2.

Hyperammonemia–Hyperornithinemia–Homocitrullinuria Syndrome

HHH syndrome is a rare, autosomal recessive disorder. Defective ornithine transport into the mitochondria leads to decreased urea synthesis. Plasma ornithine levels are elevated moderately (200 to 1,100 μmol), and lysine levels may be decreased. Urinary orotic acid is increased in one-half of affected patients. Intermittent increases in urine levels of cystine, ornithine, arginine, and lysine may occur with episodes of hyperammonemia. Also, urinary excretion of homocitrulline, a metabolite of lysine, is increased. Plasma ammonia levels are elevated only mildly except during intercurrent episodes. Most patients present during the first year of life with symptoms of intermittent hyperammonemia. Treatment includes protein restriction and supplemental ornithine or citrulline administration. The disorder results from mutations at the *ORNT1* locus at chromosome 13q14.

Gyrate Atrophy of the Retina

Ornithine aminotransferase (OAT) is a mitochondrial, pyridoxal phosphate–dependent enzyme involved in ornithine synthesis and degradation. Deficient activity of OAT is associated with hyperornithinemia (400 to 1,400 μmol) without hyperammonemia. Patients may have a dibasic aminoaciduria. No increased urinary homocitrulline occurs, as is seen with HHH. The major clinical feature of the disorder is a characteristic gyrate atrophy of the choroid and retina with progressive loss of vision. Myopia and decreased peripheral and night vision start in childhood. Posterior subcapsular cataracts develop. Complete loss of vision commonly occurs between ages 20 and 50 years. Treatment includes supplementation with L-lysine or alpha-aminoisobutyric acid in an attempt to increase renal excretion of ornithine; administration of pyridoxine (to which some patients are responsive); supplementation with proline and creatine; and dietary protein restriction, especially of arginine. The disorder is inherited as an autosomal recessive trait. Approximately one-third of reported cases have occurred in Finnish individuals. More than 60 mutations have been found at the *OAT* locus on chromosome 10q26. Carrier detection and prenatal diagnosis are available.

Transient Hyperammonemia of the Newborn

In contrast to primary disorders of the urea cycle, which often are characterized by a 1- to 2-day period or longer before the onset of symptoms, patients with transient hyperammonemia of the newborn present with symptomatic hyperammonemia during the first 2 days of life. Often, they are premature infants who rapidly develop respiratory distress, lethargy, and coma. Frequently, plasma ammonia levels are massively elevated (2,000 to 4,000 μmol). Plasma citrulline levels may be normal or elevated mildly. Urinary orotic acid levels usually are normal but may be elevated mildly for a brief period. The hyperammonemia should be treated aggressively; the associated mortality and morbidity rates are similar to those for primary urea cycle defects that present with neonatal hyperammonemic coma. For individuals who survive, recurrent hyperammonemia is rare, even with a normal protein intake. The cause for the disorder is unknown but may be related to a transient immaturity of the urea cycle.

Infants who weigh less than 2,500 g at birth may have plasma ammonia levels approximately twice the upper limits of normal for the first 6 to 8 weeks of life. This usually asymptomatic mild hyperammonemia also is thought to result from transient immaturity of the urea cycle.

DISORDERS OF LYSINE METABOLISM

Familial Hyperlysinemia

Familial hyperlysinemia is a benign disorder associated with elevated blood and urine levels of lysine and, occasionally, saccharopine. Reduced activity of the bifunctional enzyme alpha-aminoadipic semialdehyde synthase, which consists of the activities of lysine ketoglutarate reductase and saccharopine dehydrogenase, may be shown in cultured skin fibroblasts. The disorder is associated with mutations at the *AASS* locus at chromosome 7q31.3.

Saccharopinuria

Saccharopinuria is a very rare variant of familial hyperlysinemia. Affected patients have markedly elevated urine levels of saccharopine, deficient activity of saccharopine dehydrogenase, and partial reduction in the activity of lysine ketoglutarate reductase. Although two reported patients had psychomotor retardation, whether the biochemical abnormalities were related is unclear.

Glutaric Acidemia Type I

Glutaric acidemia type I is an autosomal recessive disorder most common in persons with Swedish background, the Saulteaux-Ojibway Indians in Canada, and the Old-Order Amish of Lancaster County, Pennsylvania. The disorder is associated with deficient activity of glutaryl-CoA dehydrogenase and elevated levels of glutaric acid, a derivative of lysine and tryptophan. Progressive macrocephaly starts from birth. During the first 2 years of life, functional hypotonia, dystonia, dyskinesia, and increased motor tone may develop slowly or may occur acutely with an episode of metabolic decompensation. Episodes are characterized by ketoacidosis, hypoglycemia, hyperammonemia, hepatomegaly, coma, and seizures. Computed tomography and magnetic resonance imaging show neuronal degeneration of the caudate and putamen and cortical atrophy with compensatory dilation of the lateral ventricles and widening of the sulci. Urine organic acid profiles show elevated glutaric and 3-hydroxyglutaric acids. Elevated levels of glutaconic acid and dicarboxylic acids will occur also with acute episodes. A few affected patients have had normal urine organic acid profiles. Plasma total and free carnitine levels will be low; esterified carnitine levels will be elevated. Acyl-carnitine profiles are usually abnormal and diagnostic. Deficient activity of glutaryl-CoA dehydrogenase may be shown in cultured skin fibroblasts.

Acute episodes should be treated vigorously with intravenous hydration with glucose and electrolytes and correction of the acidosis with bicarbonate to prevent additional neurologic sequelae. Treatment includes a lowered natural protein diet; occasionally special medical foods devoid of lysine and tryptophan are needed. Riboflavin, a cofactor for glutaryl-CoA dehydrogenase, and L-carnitine should be given. Baclofen may be helpful in controlling the dystonia. Some patients have improved motor tone in response to oral creatine. The best outcomes occur in patients who are started on therapy before they develop acute episodes or neurologic involvement.

Over 60 mutations have been identified in the gene *GCD* that encodes for glutaryl-CoA dehydrogenase at chromosomal location 19p13.2. Carrier detection and prenatal diagnosis are available. The disorder may be detected by newborn screening programs that employ tandem mass spectrometry.

Elevated levels of glutaric acid are seen also with glutaric acidemia type II (which is discussed with disorders of mitochondrial fatty acid oxidation in Chapter 386) and with glutaric acidemia type III (which is discussed with the peroxisomal disorders in Chapter 390).

2-Ketoadipic Acidemia

2-Ketoadipic acid is an intermediate in the metabolism of lysine, hydroxylysine, and tryptophan. Increased excretion of 2-ketoadipic, 2-aminoadipic, and 2-hydroxyadipic acids occurs. The disorder results from decreased activity of 2-ketoadipic dehydrogenase and appears to be benign.

Lysinuric protein intolerance is discussed with the disorders of ammonia metabolism.

DISORDERS OF GLYCINE METABOLISM

Nonketotic Hyperglycinemia

Glycine is a neurotransmitter that is mainly inhibitory in the spinal cord and brain stem and excitatory in the cerebral cortex and other forebrain areas. Nonketotic hyperglycinemia is an autosomal recessive disorder associated with increased body fluid levels of glycine as a result of deficient activity of the mitochondrial glycine-cleaving enzyme complex. Most affected infants present at birth or in the early neonatal period with severe hypotonia, central nervous system depression, and generalized or myoclonic seizures. Often, they are apneic and require assisted ventilation. Psychomotor development does not progress. Affected patients who survive the neonatal period are profoundly handicapped. Prolonged survival, even into adolescence, has occurred. Electroencephalography shows independent multifocal spike discharges or hypsarhythmia patterns. Often, controlling seizures is difficult. Valproate should be avoided because it potentiates the hyperglycinemia and has resulted in clinical deterioration in some affected patients. Although no treatment is effective, sodium benzoate and/or dextromethorphan may improve seizure control in some patients.

Less severely affected patients present at later ages with varying degrees of seizures and psychomotor handicaps. An infantile type has the onset of seizures and delayed development after 6 months of age. The childhood form is characterized by mild mental handicaps with episodes of delirium, chorea, and vertical gaze palsy with febrile illnesses. A late-onset form consists of progressive spastic paraparesis and optic atrophy without mental handicap. Rarely, transient hyperglycinemia may occur in neonates, with variable outcome.

Glycine levels are elevated markedly, especially in the cerebrospinal fluid (CSF). The diagnosis may be established by comparing the simultaneous level of glycine in the CSF to that in plasma. A ratio of CSF to plasma glycine of more than 0.08 is diagnostic. Decreased activity of the glycine-cleaving enzyme complex may be demonstrated in liver biopsy samples.

The glycine-cleaving enzyme complex is composed of four distinct proteins, termed *P*, *H*, *T*, and *L*. The P protein, encoded by the gene *GCSP (GLDC)* at chromosomal location 9p22, is a pyridoxal phosphate–dependent glycine decarboxylase. The H protein, encoded by the gene *GCSH* at chromosome location 16p24, is a lipoic acid–containing protein. The T protein, encoded by the gene *GCST (AMT)* at chromosome location 3p21.2–p21.1, is a tetrahydrofolate-requiring aminomethyltransferase. The L protein, with genetic site unknown, is a lipoamide dehydrogenase. Mutations in the P protein usually are seen in affected neonates. Defects in the H and T proteins have been reported in patients with later-onset disease. Carrier detection and prenatal diagnosis may be accomplished if the mutation or polymorphisms at the genetic locus involved are known. Prenatal diagnosis also may be done by measuring activity of the glycine-cleaving enzyme complex in chorionic villus samples.

Elevated glycine levels may occur also with organic acidemias (i.e., propionic acidemia and methylmalonic acidemia), with valproate anticonvulsant therapy, and in children with a high dietary intake of gelatin.

DISORDERS OF PROLINE AND HYDROXYPROLINE

The imino acids proline and hydroxyproline are nonessential amino acids. Proline may be synthesized from ornithine or glutamate and, along with its metabolite pyrroline-5-carboxylate, is important in the regulation of protein synthesis and the production of phosphoribosyl pyrophosphate and purine nucleotides. Hydroxyproline is formed by the hydroxylation of proline in procollagen and exists mainly bound to peptides in collagen (iminopeptides). The disorders of proline and hydroxyproline metabolism are inherited as autosomal recessive traits.

Hyperprolinemia and Hyperhydroxyprolinemia

Type I hyperprolinemia results from deficient activity of proline oxidase, which is encoded by the gene *PRODH* at chromosomal location 22q11.2. Affected patients have elevated plasma and urine levels of proline. Urine levels of hydroxyproline and glycine are elevated also, owing to overload of the renal tubular transport system shared by the three amino acids. The disorder appears to be a benign condition.

In *type II hyperprolinemia*, elevated blood and urine levels of pyrroline-5-carboxylate and elevated urine levels of pyrroline-3-hydroxy-5 carboxylate are noted in addition to the biochemical abnormalities noted with type I hyperprolinemia. The disorder results from deficient activity of delta-1-pyrroline-5-carboxylate dehydrogenase, encoded by the gene *ALDH4A1* at chromosomal location 1p36. The majority of affected patients have seizure disorders, and some have psychomotor handicaps. Otherwise, asymptomatic patients also have been reported. Deficient activity of delta-1-pyrroline-5-carboxylate dehydrogenase may be shown in peripheral blood leukocytes and cultured skin fibroblasts.

Hyperhydroxyprolinemia is associated with deficient activity of 4-hydroxyproline oxidase. Elevated blood levels of hydroxyproline and urine levels of hydroxyproline, proline, and glycine are thought to be of no clinical significance.

Elevated urine levels of proline, hydroxyproline, and glycine also occur in iminoglycinuria, which is discussed with the disorders of transport in Chapter 384.

Prolidase Deficiency

Deficient activity of prolidase, also known as *peptidase D*, is associated with increased urinary levels of iminopeptides that contain proline and hydroxyproline (i.e., glycylproline). Affected patients have a chronic erythematous dermatitis on the face, palms, and soles. Severe, progressive ulcerations may develop on the lower legs. Many affected patients have psychomotor retardation and recurrent infections. Occasionally, splenomegaly, prominent sutures, abnormally shaped skulls, ptosis, or ocular proptosis occur. Other patients detected by newborn screening programs have been asymptomatic. There is no specific effective treatment. Deficient activity of prolidase may be demonstrated in peripheral blood leukocytes, erythrocytes, or cultured skin fibroblasts. Mutations have been reported in affected patients in the *PEPD* gene, located at chromosome 19q, which encodes for prolidase.

DISORDERS OF GLUTATHIONE

Glutathione (L-gamma-glutamyl-L-cysteinyl-glycine) is an important component of many metabolic processes. It is involved with the formation and maintenance of sulfhydryl groups of proteins and enzymes (i.e., CoA), facilitates the transport of amino acids across cell membranes, provides reducing capacity for several reactions (i.e., the formation of deoxyribonucleotides), and functions in the detoxification of peroxides, free radicals, and other compounds, including some medications. All the disorders of glutathione metabolism are rare autosomal recessive diseases.

5-Oxoprolinuria

5-Oxoprolinuria, or pyroglutamic aciduria, results from generalized deficiency of glutathione synthetase. Glutathione synthetase normally catalyzes the conversion of gamma-glutamylcysteine to glutathione, the second step in the synthesis of glutathione. In affected patients, the low intracellular levels of glutathione and lack of normal feedback inhibition to the first step in its synthesis lead to overproduction of gamma-glutamylcysteine, which is converted to 5-oxoproline. Affected patients present as infants with chronic metabolic acidosis, mild hemolytic anemia, progressive psychomotor retardation, and cerebellar dysfunction. They also may have neutropenia, defective granulocyte function, and an increased susceptibility to bacterial infections. Treatment for an acute episode of acidosis should include intravenous hydration and bicarbonate. Often, maintenance therapy with bicarbonate or other buffers is needed. Affected patients also should avoid medications that require glutathione in their metabolism (i.e., acetaminophen) and situations that may result in the formation of free radicals (i.e., therapeutic oxygen). Supplements of vitamin E may improve erythrocyte survival and granulocyte function. Blood levels of glutathione will be decreased. Markedly elevated urine levels of 5-oxoproline may be shown with organic acid determinations that use gas chromatography–mass spectrometry. Reduced activity of glutathione synthetase may be shown in erythrocytes and cultured skin fibroblasts.

Deficient activity of glutathione synthetase, limited to erythrocytes, results in lowered erythrocyte levels of glutathione and a compensated hemolytic anemia. Central nervous system involvement, acidosis, and elevated 5-oxoproline do not occur. Occasionally, patients require splenectomy.

The gene *GSS* that encodes for glutathione synthetase is located at chromosome 20q11.2. Patients with the form of the disorder limited to erythrocytes have mutations that differ from those encountered in the generalized form of the disorder.

Gamma-Glutamylcysteine Synthase Deficiency

Deficient activity of gamma-glutamylcysteine synthase, the second step in the synthesis of glutathione, results in generalized glutathione deficiency and low levels of gamma-

glutamylcysteine. Levels of 5-oxoproline are normal. Affected patients have mild hemolytic anemias, spinocerebellar degeneration, peripheral neuropathies, myopathies, and a generalized aminoaciduria. Reduced levels of glutathione and decreased activity of gamma-glutamylcysteine synthase may be shown in erythrocytes. The disorder results from mutations in the gene *GCLC*, at chromosome 6p12, which encodes for gamma-glutamylcysteine synthase.

Gamma-Glutamyl Transpeptidase Deficiency

Deficient activity of gamma-glutamyl transpeptidase, involved with the transport of amino acids across cell membranes, has been reported in young adults with psychomotor handicaps. Elevated blood and urine levels of glutathione, gamma-glutamylcysteine, and cysteine occur. Hemolytic anemia does not occur. Deficient activity of gamma-glutamyl transpeptidase may be shown in cultured skin fibroblasts. The disorder results from mutations in the gene *GGTI*, at chromosome 22q11.1-q11.2, which encodes for gamma-glutamyl transpeptidase.

5-Oxoprolinase Deficiency

Deficient activity of 5-oxoprolinase, which normally converts 5-oxoproline to glutamic acid, is associated with moderately elevated blood and urine levels of 5-oxoproline. Affected patients do not have any significant clinical findings, however, and the disorder is considered to be benign.

Elevated levels of 5-oxoproline have been seen also with severe burns, with Stevens-Johnson syndrome, with homocystinuria, and in patients on artificial diets.

DISORDERS OF BRANCHED-CHAIN AMINO ACID METABOLISM

The branched-chain amino acids (BCAAs) leucine, isoleucine, and valine are essential amino acids needed for protein synthesis and growth. They are metabolized to compounds important in fatty acid and cholesterol synthesis, gluconeogenesis, and the production of energy. The metabolism of the BCAA is illustrated in Figure 385.6. The majority of the disorders of BCAAs result in the accumulation of organic acids, which may cause significant metabolic acidosis. Secondary inhibition of the urea cycle, from inhibition of N-acetylglutamate synthetase, often results in hyperammonemia that may be as severe as that seen with primary disorders of the urea cycle. Hyperglycinemia may occur from inhibition of the glycine-cleaving enzyme complex. Bone marrow depression may result in neutropenia, thrombocytopenia, or pancytopenia. Often, the severe forms of the disorders present in the newborn period or early infancy with life-threatening illness. Less severe forms present at later ages with psychomotor handicaps, seizures, episodic lethargy or vomiting, or acute metabolic decompensation with intercurrent illness.

With acute episodes, affected patients accumulate abnormal patterns of organic acids that often suggest a specific disorder. Those who are severely ill also accumulate lactic acid and ketones from dehydration, poor perfusion, and mobilization of tissue stores. Urine dipsticks for ketones and spot testing for ketoacids with dinitrophenylhydrazine may be positive. The abnormal pattern of metabolites may be shown by organic acid analysis, which should be performed by methods that use gas chromatography combined with mass spectrometry. Because of rapid excretion of organic acids, determinations are best

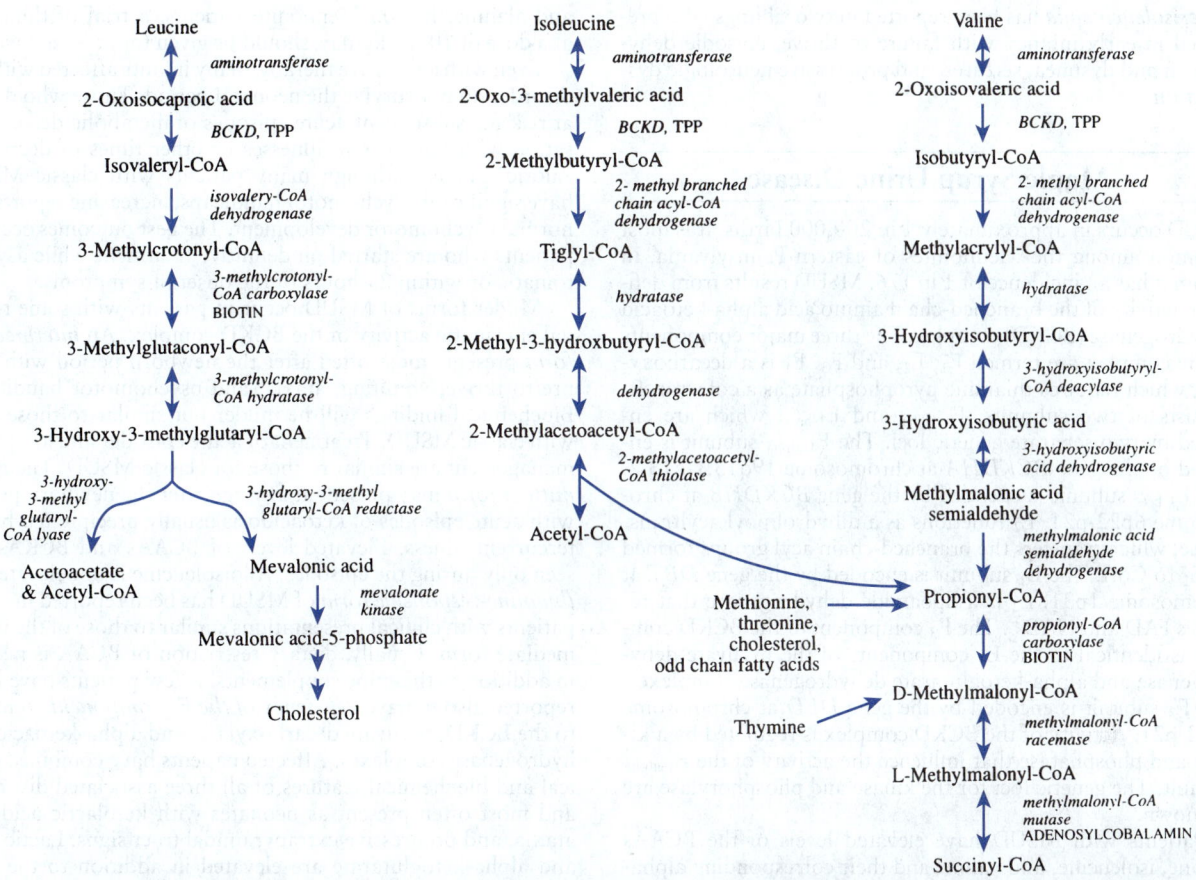

FIGURE 385.6. Metabolism of the branched-chain amino acids. BCKD, branched-chain alpha-ketoacid (2-oxoacid) dehydrogenase complex; CoA, coenzyme A; TPP, thiamine pyrophosphate.

performed on urine samples. Blood organic acid determinations can be performed on those who are anuric or oliguric. Acyl-carnitine profiles, determined by tandem mass spectrometry on plasma or dried blood filter-paper specimens, will detect abnormal compounds that form CoA esters with carnitine (i.e., isovaleryl-carnitine, propionyl-carnitine). Acyl-glycine profiles will show abnormal compounds that conjugate with glycine (i.e., isovaleryl-glycine). Blood and urine quantitative amino acid profiles show accumulation of the BCAA with MSUD and the branched-chain aminotransferase deficiencies. Because the pathways are not reversible at the alpha-ketoacid dehydrogenase complex step, accumulation of branched-chain amino acids will not occur with disorders after that step (i.e., isovaleric acidemia, propionic acidemia, and methylmalonic acidemia).

Acute episodes of metabolic decompensation require aggressive management to minimize residual neurologic dysfunction. Hemodialysis or hemofiltration may be needed for persistent acidosis or hyperammonemia. Cofactors for suspected specific enzymatic deficiencies may be given once diagnostic specimens are obtained. Special medical foods devoid of the offending amino acids are important in suppressing catabolism with acute illnesses and usually are needed for long-term management. Affected patients are at risk to develop acute episodes of metabolic decompensation with times of stress, infection, or catabolism for the remainder of their lives. Plans for "sick day" management should be formulated and started by patients' families once symptoms appear, as in the care of diabetics. The patients are managed best by metabolism specialists experienced with the disorders.

All the disorders of branched-chain amino acid metabolism are inherited as autosomal recessive traits except for the cardiac-neutropenia form of 3-methylglutaconic acidemia, which is inherited as an X-linked trait. Frequently, carrier testing is available only by molecular genetic techniques. Depending on the specific disorder involved, molecular genetic analysis, measurement of metabolite levels in amniotic fluid, or enzymatic testing may be used for prenatal diagnosis. Many of the disorders can be detected through newborn screening programs, especially those programs that include tandem mass spectrometry.

Branched-Chain Aminotransferase Deficiencies

The branched-chain amino acids are converted into their corresponding alpha-ketoacids (2-oxoacids) by either cytosolic or mitochondrial aminotransferases before oxidative decarboxylation. Although the aminotransferases are equally active toward all three amino acids, reports of patients with isolated hypervalinemia and combined hyperleucinemia and hyperisoleucinemia suggest that different mutations in the aminotransferases may alter substrate specificity. *Hypervalinemia* has been reported in three patients. One presented with neonatal failure to thrive, vomiting, delayed development, and neurologic problems. The others were siblings with psychomotor retardation. *Combined hyperleucinemia and hyperisoleucinemia* has been reported in two siblings who presented in early infancy with failure to thrive, episodic dehydration and dyspnea, seizures, and progressive neurologic dysfunction.

Maple Syrup Urine Disease

MSUD occurs in approximately 1 in 200,000 births. It is most common among the Mennonites of eastern Pennsylvania, in whom it has an incidence of 1 in 176. MSUD results from deficient activity of the branched-chain amino acid alpha-ketoacid dehydrogenase (BCKD) complex. The three major components of the complex are termed E_1, E_2, and E_3. E_1 is a decarboxylase, which requires thiamine pyrophosphate as a cofactor. E_1 consists of two subunits, $E_{1-alpha}$ and E_{1-beta}, which are encoded by two separate genetic loci. The $E_{1-alpha}$ subunit is encoded by the gene *BCKDHA* at chromosome 19q13.1-q13.2. The E_{1-beta} subunit is encoded by the gene *BCKDHB* at chromosome 6p22-p21. E_2 functions as a dihydrolipoyl acyltransferase, which transfers the branched-chain acyl groups formed by E_1 to CoA. The E_2 subunit is encoded by the gene *DBT* at chromosome 1p31. E_3 is a lipoamide dehydrogenase that requires FAD and NAD^+. The E_3 component of the BCKD complex is identical to the E_3 components of the pyruvate dehydrogenase and alpha-ketoglutarate dehydrogenase complexes. The E_3 subunit is encoded by the gene *DLD* at chromosome 6p22-p21. Activity of the BCKD complex is regulated by a kinase and phosphatase that influence the activity of the $E_{1-alpha}$ subunit. The genetic loci for the kinase and phosphorylase are unknown.

Patients with MSUD have elevated levels of the BCAAs leucine, isoleucine, and valine, and their corresponding alpha-ketoacids (BCKAs), 2-oxoisocaproic acid, 2-oxo-3-methylvaleric acid, and 2-oxoisovaleric acid, respectively. The disorder derives its name from the 2-oxo-3-methylvaleric acid, which has an odor similar to maple syrup or burnt sugar. Alloisoleucine, a metabolite of leucine and 2-oxo-3-methylvaleric acid, also is elevated and unique to MSUD. Plasma quantitative amino acid determinations show elevated BCAAs and alloisoleucine. Elevated BCKAs are seen with urine organic acid profiles. Spot testing for ketoacids can be performed with dinitrophenylhydrazine and is useful for home monitoring.

MSUD exists in five clinical forms. The most common, *classic form*, presents in the first 2 weeks of life with poor feeding, irritability, lethargy, alternating hypotonia and hypertonia, abnormal movements, and seizures, which progress to cerebral edema and coma. Severe metabolic acidosis and ketosis may occur, often with hyperammonemia and hypoglycemia. Intravenous hydration with glucose and electrolytes along with correction of the acidosis with bicarbonate is indicated. Patients should be monitored carefully for cerebral edema; serum osmolality should be kept in the normal range. Hypertonic saline, mannitol, and furosemide may be needed. Hemofiltration or hemodialysis may be required to correct the acidosis or hyperammonemia. Suppression of catabolism is highly important in controlling the disorder and may be accomplished by enteral feedings with special medical foods or intravenous hyperalimentation with special amino mixtures devoid of the BCAA. The additional use of insulin and propranolol has been successful in controlling severe episodes.

Maintenance therapy includes the use of special medical foods devoid of the BCAA. Although all three BCAAs are elevated, it is now thought that the elevated leucine levels are primarily responsible for the pathologic features of the disorder. Limited amounts of natural protein to supply leucine requirements, along with small amounts of valine, and occasionally isoleucine are given to maintain plasma BCAAs within the recommended treatment range. Severely affected patients may benefit also from additional supplements of glutamine and alanine. In non-Mennonite patients, a trial of thiamine, at a dose of 10 mg/kg/day, should be given for at least 3 weeks.

Even with aggressive therapy, many infants affected with the disorder do not survive the neonatal period. Those who do are at risk for subsequent acute episodes of metabolic decompensation with intercurrent illnesses or other times of decreased caloric intake. Although many patients with classic MSUD have significant psychomotor handicaps, increasing reports cite normal psychomotor development. The best outcomes occur in patients who are started on definitive treatment while asymptomatic or within 24 hours of the onset of symptoms.

Milder forms of MSUD occur in patients with some residual enzymatic activity of the BCKD complex. An *intermediate form* presents most often after the newborn period with failure to thrive, vomiting, ataxia, and psychomotor handicaps. Biochemical findings will be milder but similar to those seen with classic MSUD. Treatment of acute episodes and long-term management are similar to those for classic MSUD. The *intermittent form* may present at any age after the newborn period with acute episodes of ketoacidosis usually precipitated by intercurrent illness. Elevated levels of BCAAs and BCKAs are seen only during the episodes. Alloisoleucine is not elevated. A *thiamine-responsive form* of MSUD has been reported in a few patients with clinical presentations similar to those of the intermediate form. Usually, dietary restriction of BCAA is needed in addition to thiamine supplements. A few patients have been reported also to have *deficiency of the E_3 component* common to the BCKD, pyruvate decarboxylase, and alpha-ketoacid dehydrogenase complexes. Affected patients have combined clinical and biochemical features of all three associated disorders and most often present as neonates with ketolactic acidosis, ataxia, and progressive extrapyramidal tract signs. Lactic acid and alpha-ketoglutarate are elevated in addition to the biochemical findings of MSUD.

Newborn screening for MSUD is available in some areas of the United States. Most programs test for leucine levels in dried blood filter-paper samples. Many infants affected with the classic form of the disease will be symptomatic by the time the results of newborn screening are available. Others will be asymptomatic and should be evaluated immediately. Milder forms of the disorder probably will not be detected by newborn screening.

Mutations in genes that encode for the components of the BCKD complex have been demonstrated in patients with MSUD. $E_{1-alpha}$ mutations have been reported with the classic and the intermediate forms of the disorder. A specific $E_{1-alpha}$ mutation (Y393N) is found in Mennonite families; it may occur also in non-Mennonite patients in the United States. Two E_2 mutations have been reported in thiamin-responsive patients. Carrier detection is available for those families in whom the genetic mutation or polymorphisms are known. Prenatal diagnosis may be performed by molecular genetic techniques or by enzymatic assay.

Disorders of Leucine Metabolism

Isovaleric Acidemia

Isovaleric acidemia results from deficient activity of isovaleryl-CoA dehydrogenase. The most severe form of the disorder presents in the first 2 weeks of life with poor feeding, vomiting, lethargy, seizures, and hypothermia, which progress to lethargy and coma. Marked metabolic acidosis and secondary hyperammonemia occur. Bone marrow depression may be seen. Approximately one-half of affected neonates do not survive the newborn period. Other affected infants present later, during the first year of life, with acute episodes of ketoacidosis, vomiting, lethargy, and coma. Affected patients are at risk to develop subsequent episodes of metabolic decompensation at times of increased protein intake or decreased caloric intake (i.e., with intercurrent illness).

With episodes, patients accumulate isovaleric acid, which has a characteristic offensive odor described as "sweaty feet." Urine organic acid profiles show elevated levels of isovaleryl-glycine, 3-hydroxisovalerate, 4-hydroxyisovalerate, and other oxidation and conjugation products of isovaleric acid. Plasma or serum levels of isovaleric acid may be detected by short-chain volatile organic acid profiles. Such determinations, however, are not readily available in most areas. Blood and urine quantitative amino acid determinations will not show elevated BCAAs. Because isovaleryl-CoA may conjugate with carnitine or glycine, acyl-carnitine or acyl-glycine profiles will be abnormal. Affected patients also have lowered levels of total and free carnitine and elevation of carnitine esters.

Initial treatment should include intravenous hydration with glucose and electrolytes and correction of the acidosis with bicarbonate. Hemodialysis or hemofiltration may be needed for persistent acidosis or hyperammonemia. L-Carnitine may be given initially intravenously and later in enteral form. Special medical foods devoid of leucine are given along with limited amounts of natural protein. Glycine supplements may be used in addition to or in place of L-carnitine. Many patients with neonatal onset of the disorder have psychomotor handicaps. Normal psychomotor development is possible and frequently is noted in those with later onset of their disease.

Deficient activity of isovaleryl-CoA dehydrogenase may be shown in peripheral blood leukocytes or cultured skin fibroblasts. Mutations have been shown in affected patients at the IVD gene locus, at chromosome 15q14-q15, which encodes for isovaleryl-CoA dehydrogenase. Carrier detection is available by molecular genetic techniques in families with known mutations or polymorphisms at the gene site. Prenatal diagnosis may be done with molecular genetic techniques, by measuring isovaleryl-glycine levels in amniotic fluid with stable isotope dilution analysis, or by enzymatic assay in cultured amniocytes. The disorder may be detected by newborn screening programs that include testing by tandem mass spectrometry.

Elevation of isovaleryl compounds and the "sweaty feet" odor occur along with other metabolic abnormalities in glutaric acidemia type II (multiple acyl-CoA dehydrogenase deficiency), which is discussed with the disorders of mitochondrial fatty acid oxidation in Chapter 386.

3-Methylcrotonyl-CoA Carboxylase Deficiency

Patients with deficient activity of 3-methylcrotonyl-CoA carboxylase present in infancy with poor feeding, vomiting, irritability, lethargy, seizures, and hypotonia, which may progress to coma. Hypoglycemia, hyperammonemia, ketosis, and mild metabolic acidosis occur. Asymptomatic affected individuals also have been identified by family studies and expanded newborn screening. Urine organic acid profiles show elevated levels of 3-methylcrotonylglycine and 3-hydroxyisovalerate. Acyl-carnitine profiles are abnormal. Plasma levels of free carnitine are low; esterified carnitine fractions are elevated. Treatment includes a lowered protein and leucine diet, along with supplements of L-carnitine. The disorder may occur also as part of multiple carboxylase deficiency, which results from deficient activity of holocarboxylase synthetase or biotinidase (see Multiple Carboxylase Deficiency, later). For this reason, affected patients also should receive biotin until the exact diagnosis is established. Deficient activity of 3-methylcrotonyl-CoA carboxylase may be determined in peripheral blood leukocytes or cultured skin fibroblasts. Prenatal diagnosis is available. The disorder may be detected by newborn screening programs that include testing by tandem mass spectrometry.

3-Methylcrotonyl-CoA carboxylase is composed of two subunits, alpha and beta. The alpha subunit is encoded by the gene MCC1 at chromosome location 3q15-q27; the beta sub-unit is encoded by MCC2 at 5q12-q13. Mutations at both gene locations have been shown in affected patients.

3-Methylglutaconic Acidemia

3-Methylglutaconic acidemia exists in at least four forms. Type I is associated with deficient activity of 3-methylglutaconyl-CoA hydratase. The basis for the elevated levels of 3-methylglutaconate in the other forms presently is unknown.

Patients with type I 3-methylglutaconic acidemia present in infancy or childhood with delayed language development and variable degrees of psychomotor handicaps. Mild metabolic acidosis, hepatomegaly, and macrocephaly may occur. Urine organic acid profiles show elevated levels of 3-methylglutaconate, 3-methylglutarate, and 3-hydroxyisovalerate. Acyl-carnitine profiles are abnormal. Lowered free and elevated esterified carnitine fractions are noted. Treatment includes a relatively lowered dietary intake of protein and L-carnitine supplements. Occasionally, special medical foods devoid of leucine are needed for metabolic control during infancy. Bicarbonate or citrate buffers may be needed for treatment of the acidosis. This form of the disorder is inherited as an autosomal recessive trait. Deficient activity of 3-methylglutaconyl-CoA hydratase may be shown in cultured skin fibroblasts. Prenatal diagnosis is available. The gene AUH, on chromosome 9, encodes for the hydratase. The disorder may be detected by newborn screening programs that include testing by tandem mass spectrometry.

Type II 3-methylglutaconic acidemia, or the cardiac-neutropenic form, also known as Barth syndrome, is inherited as an X-linked trait. Affected patients have dilated cardiomyopathies, myopathies, neutropenia, and growth retardation. Mild lactic acidosis, hypocholesterolemia, and hypoglycemia may occur. Mildly elevated urine levels of 2-ethylhydracrylic acid are noted in addition to mild elevations of 3-methylglutaconate and 3-methylglutarate. Elevation of 3-hydroxyisovalerate does not occur. Plasma carnitine values usually are normal. Specific activity of 3-methylglutaconyl-CoA hydratase is normal. There is no specific treatment. Some patients respond to pantothenic acid and/or L-carnitine supplements. The disorder has been linked by molecular genetic studies to the TAZ gene locus at chromosome Xq28. The gene encodes for a protein, tafazzin, that is highly expressed in cardiac and skeletal muscle, but for which no function is currently known.

Type III 3-methylglutaconic acidemia, or Costeff optic atrophy syndrome, presents in infancy with bilateral optic atrophy, choreiform movements, ataxia, mild spasticity, and variable developmental handicaps. Urine organic acids show elevated 3-methylglutaconate and 3-methylglutarate. Elevation of 3-hydroxyisovalerate does not occur. Plasma carnitine values usually are normal. Specific activity of 3-methylglutaconyl-CoA hydratase is normal. There is no specific treatment. The disorder is most common in Iraqi Jewish individuals and has been linked to the gene OPA3 at chromosome 19q13.2-q13.3.

Type IV 3-methylglutaconic acidemia, the idiopathic or unclassified form, presents with a variety of neurologic problems, including severe progressive encephalopathy, movement disorders, hypotonia, spastic quadriparesis, optic atrophy, and psychomotor regression. The disorder has been reported in both male and female patients. Mild to moderate elevation of 3-methylglutaconate and 3-methylglutarate is noted. Elevation of 3-hydroxyisovalerate does not occur. Specific activity of 3-methylglutaconyl-CoA hydratase is normal. Some patients have had abnormal mitochondrial electron transport chain studies or Pearson syndrome. The basis for this form of the disorder is unknown; there is no specific therapy.

3-Hydroxy-3-Methylglutaric Acidemia

3-Hydroxy-3-methylglutaric acidemia results from deficient activity of 3-hydroxy-3-methylglutaryl-CoA lyase. Most affected patients present before 1 year of age with vomiting, lethargy, hypotonia, and seizures. Severe hypoglycemia, metabolic acidosis, and, occasionally, hyperammonemia occur. Owing to the site of the metabolic block, few if any ketones can be formed. Urine organic acid profiles show increased levels of 3-hydroxy-3-methylglutarate, 3-hydroxyisovalerate, 3-methylglutaconate, and 3-methylglutarate. Acyl-carnitine profiles are abnormal. Plasma carnitine levels will show relatively elevated esterified fractions. Treatment of acute episodes should include intravenous hydration with glucose and electrolytes and bicarbonate to correct the acidosis. Diets high in carbohydrates and lower in protein and fat are recommended, along with L-carnitine supplements. Fasting should be avoided as it may precipitate hypoglycemia. Approximately 20% of affected patients die with an acute episode. Some affected patients have psychomotor handicaps; most have normal development. Deficient activity of 3-hydroxy-3-methylglutaryl (HMG)-CoA lyase may be shown in peripheral blood leukocytes or cultured skin fibroblasts. The disorder may be detected by newborn screening programs that include testing by tandem mass spectrometry. The lyase is encoded by the gene *HMGCL* at chromosome 1pter-p33.

Mevalonic Acidemia

Mevalonic acidemia is a rare disorder that results from deficient activity of mevalonate kinase, the first step in the synthesis of cholesterol and related compounds. Affected patients present in early infancy with severe failure to thrive, psychomotor retardation, hypotonia, and episodes of fever, rash, vomiting, or diarrhea. Hepatosplenomegaly, anemia, cataracts, ataxia, and dysmorphic features may occur. Less severely affected patients present at later ages with hypotonia, ataxia, and elevated creatine kinase levels. Urinary organic acid profiles show markedly elevated levels of mevalonic acid. Plasma cholesterol levels are normal or slightly low. Metabolic acidosis does not occur. No treatment is effective. Severely affected patients have died in infancy. Deficient activity of mevalonate kinase may be determined in peripheral blood leukocytes or cultured skin fibroblasts. Prenatal diagnosis is available. Mevalonate kinase is encoded by the gene *MVK* at chromosome 12q24.

Disorders of Isoleucine Metabolism

2-Methylacetoacetyl-CoA 3-Oxothiolase Deficiency

The clinical severity of deficient activity of mitochondrial 2-methylacetoacetyl-CoA 3-oxothiolase (also known as *beta-ketothiolase deficiency*) varies widely. Most severely affected patients present between ages 1 and 2 years with failure to thrive and recurrent episodes of severe metabolic ketoacidosis. Some present in the newborn period. Hypoglycemia may occur. A "sweet" odor is noticed. Urine organic acid determinations show elevated levels of 2-methyl-3-hydroxybutyrate. Elevated levels of 2-methylacetoacetate, 2-butanone, and tiglylglycine also may be noted. Acyl-carnitine profiles are abnormal. Acute episodes should be treated with intravenous hydration with glucose and electrolytes and bicarbonate to correct acidosis. Long-term management includes a lowered protein diet and avoidance of fasting. Normal psychomotor development is possible. Deficient activity of 2-methylacetoacetyl-CoA thiolase may be demonstrated in peripheral blood leukocytes and cultured skin fibroblasts. Prenatal diagnosis is possible. The disorder may be detected by newborn screening programs that include testing by tandem mass spectrometry. The disorder is associated with mutations at the gene *ACAT1* located at chromosome 11q22.3-q23.1.

Disorders of Valine Metabolism

3-Hydroxyisobutyryl-CoA Deacylase Deficiency

The one reported patient with 3-hydroxyisobutyryl-CoA deacylase deficiency presented at birth with multiple congenital anomalies, poor feeding, hypotonia, and profound developmental delay. The patient died at age 3 months. Acidosis did not occur. Routine organic acid profiles were normal. S-(2-carboxypropyl)-cysteine and S-(2-carboxypropyl)-cysteamine were noted in urine by high-voltage electrophoresis. The compounds are formed by 3-methylacrylyl-CoA reacting with cysteine and cysteine derivatives.

3-Hydroxyisobutyric Acidemia

Patients with 3-hydroxyisobutyric acidemia present as infants with dysmorphic features, brain dysgenesis, hypotonia, failure to thrive, seizures, and episodic ketoacidosis or lactic acidosis. Urine organic acid profiles reveal large amounts of 3-hydroxyisobutyric acid, along with increased levels of 3-hydroxypropionate, 2-ethyl-3-hydroxypropionate, and 3-hydroxyisovalerate. The exact metabolic defect has not been established, but deficient activity of 3-hydroxybutyric acid dehydrogenase or methylmalonic semialdehyde dehydrogenase may be involved. Treatment with a lowered protein diet and L-carnitine is indicated. Prenatal diagnosis is possible.

Disorders of Propionate Metabolism

Normally, propionyl-CoA is metabolized by propionyl-CoA carboxylase to methylmalonyl-CoA. Methylmalonyl-CoA is metabolized to succinyl-CoA, which enters the Krebs cycle. Isolated propionic acidemia results from deficient activity of propionyl-CoA carboxylase. Biotin is a cofactor for propionyl-CoA carboxylase and three additional carboxylases. Propionic acidemia may occur also with multiple carboxylase deficiency, which results from either biotinidase deficiency or holocarboxylase synthase deficiency.

Propionyl-CoA Carboxylase Deficiency

Most affected patients present in the newborn period with poor feeding, vomiting, hypotonia, and lethargy that progresses to coma. Hepatomegaly, seizures, and other neurologic problems may occur. Other patients with less severe forms of the disorder may present as late as adulthood with episodic vomiting and lethargy, failure to thrive, psychomotor handicaps, seizures, dystonia, or protein intolerance or avoidance. Acute episodes of metabolic decompensation result in severe metabolic acidosis and ketosis. Hyperammonemia of varying degrees, from inhibition of the urea cycle by abnormal organic acids, is common. Secondary depression of the bone marrow may lead to neutropenia, thrombocytopenia, or pancytopenia. Urine organic acid profiles show markedly elevated levels of propionyl-CoA metabolites, such as 3-hydroxypropionic acid, methylcitrate, and tiglylglycine. Plasma short-chain volatile organic acid profiles reveal elevated propionate levels. Elevated levels of glycine, from inhibition of the glycine-cleaving enzyme complex, will be noted on blood or urine quantitative amino acid determinations. Plasma levels of total and free carnitine are low; esterified carnitine levels will be elevated. Acyl-carnitine or acyl-glycine profiles will be abnormal and reveal propionyl conjugates. The disorder may be detected by newborn screening programs that employ tandem mass spectrometry.

Initial treatment of an acute episode should include intravenous hydration with electrolytes and glucose. Hypoglycemia (if present) and acidosis should be corrected. Hemodialysis or hemofiltration may be needed for persistent or massive hyperammonemia or acidosis. All sources of natural protein should be stopped. Once diagnostic specimens are obtained, biotin should be given enterally until clarification of whether the patient has propionyl-CoA carboxylase deficiency or a disorder of biotin metabolism. Patients with isolated propionyl-CoA carboxylase deficiency usually do not respond to biotin, whereas those with defects in biotin metabolism will. Intravenous, and later oral, L-carnitine is indicated. Special medical foods devoid of precursor amino acids for propionyl-CoA (i.e., methionine, threonine, valine, and isoleucine) usually are needed to control the disorder. Small amounts of natural protein needed for growth also are given. Intermittent use of metronidazole, which reduces gastrointestinal tract bacterial formation of propionyl-CoA, may improve appetite and metabolic control.

Some severely affected patients will not survive the initial episode. Others occasionally die with a subsequent acute episode of metabolic decompensation. Although long-term survival and normal intellectual development are possible, many affected patients have significant psychomotor handicaps.

The diagnosis is established by demonstrating deficient activity of propionyl-CoA carboxylase in peripheral blood leukocytes or cultured skin fibroblasts. Prenatal diagnosis may be obtained by measurement of methylcitrate levels in amniotic fluid or by measurement of propionyl-CoA carboxylase activity or radiolabeled propionate studies in cultured amniotic fluid cells.

Propionyl-CoA carboxylase is comprised of two subunits, alpha and beta, encoded by two separate genes. The alpha subunit is encoded by *PCCA* at chromosome 13q32; the beta subunit is encoded by *PCCB* at chromosome 3q21-p22. Mutations in affected patients have been found in both subunits and are clinically indistinguishable.

Multiple Carboxylase Deficiency

Biotin is an essential, water-soluble vitamin found in many dietary sources. Biotin may be synthesized also by intestinal flora. Although nutritional deficiency of biotin is rare, it can occur with chronic total parenteral nutrition that does not contain biotin. Biotin deficiency has been reported also in some patients on chronic anticonvulsant therapy with phenytoin, primidone, or carbamazepine. Biotin deficiency results in cutaneous and neurologic manifestations, including alopecia, erythematous perioral rashes, dry skin, superficial *Candida* infections, depression, apathy, myalgias, hyperesthesias, and paresthesias. Most symptoms rapidly respond to biotin replacement.

Biotin serves as a cofactor for four carboxylases: cytosolic acetyl-CoA carboxylase, which is involved in the biosynthesis of long-chain fatty acids; mitochondrial 3-methylcrotonyl-CoA carboxylase, involved with leucine metabolism; mitochondrial pyruvate carboxylase, involved in pathways of gluconeogenesis; and mitochondrial propionyl-CoA carboxylase, involved with the metabolism of four amino acids, odd-chain fatty acids, and cholesterol. The carboxylases are synthesized as inactive apoenzymes. Biotin is attached covalently to the carboxylases by the action of holocarboxylase synthase. The resulting holocarboxylase, consisting of a biotin-apoenzyme complex, is enzymatically active. After the holocarboxylase activity is completed, biotin is released from the complex by the action of biotinidase. The free biotin then may be recycled and used again for the formation of holocarboxylase complexes.

Multiple carboxylase deficiency may occur from deficient activity of holocarboxylase synthase or biotinidase. The clinical manifestations are a composite of those findings seen with the four individual carboxylase disorders. Affected patients respond to biotin therapy.

Holocarboxylase Synthase Deficiency. Holocarboxylase synthase deficiency is less common than is biotinidase deficiency. Most affected patients present in the neonatal period or early infancy with symptoms similar to isolated propionic acidemia and 3-methylcrotonyl-CoA carboxylase deficiency (i.e., poor feeding, vomiting, lethargy, hypotonia, seizures, and occasionally coma). Those with a later onset may have alopecia, perioral rashes, dermatitis, delayed development, ataxia, deafness, and optic atrophy. Metabolic ketolactic acidosis with secondary hyperammonemia and bone marrow depression is common. Urine organic acid determinations show elevated levels of 3-hydroxyisovaleric acid, 3-methylcrotonylglycine, 3-hydroxypropionate, methylcitrate, tiglylglycine, and lactate. Acyl-carnitine profiles are abnormal. Initial management is similar to that for propionic acidemia, with intravenous hydration and correction of hypoglycemia and acidosis, if present. Oral free biotin therapy (10 mg daily) should be started once diagnostic specimens are obtained. Although biotin therapy will correct the metabolic disorder, residual neurologic dysfunction, including optic atrophy and hearing loss, may remain.

Reduced activity of three of the four affected carboxylases (pyruvate carboxylase, propionyl-CoA carboxylase, and 3-methylcrotonyl-CoA carboxylase) may be shown in peripheral blood leukocytes or cultured skin fibroblasts. Leukocyte studies should be drawn before starting biotin therapy. Biotinidase activity also should be determined and will be normal. Direct measurement of holocarboxylase synthase activity may be done in lymphocytes, cultured skin fibroblasts, or cultured lymphoblasts. Prenatal diagnosis is available by measurement of 3-hydroxyisovaleric acid and methylcitrate levels in amniotic fluid or by determination of enzymatic activity for the carboxylases in cultured amniotic fluid cells. The disorder may be detected by newborn screening programs that include testing by tandem mass spectrometry. Holocarboxylase synthase is encoded by the gene *HLCS* at chromosome 21q22.1.

Biotinidase Deficiency. Biotinidase deficiency occurs in approximately 1 in 112,000 births and is most common among French Canadians. Although an acute presentation in the neonatal period can occur, most affected patients present between ages 3 months and 3 years with chronic dermatologic and neurologic problems. Symptoms are similar to those seen with late-onset holocarboxylase synthase deficiency. Neurologic problems include psychomotor delay, ataxia, myoclonic seizures, hypotonia, deafness, visual problems, and optic atrophy. Dermatologic problems include partial or complete alopecia, perioral rashes, and conjunctivitis. Urine organic acid profiles will be abnormal and similar to those seen with holocarboxylase synthase deficiency. Treatment with free biotin, starting at 5 to 10 mg daily, will result in a fairly prompt clinical response. Residual neurologic dysfunction, including optic atrophy and deafness, may occur.

Deficient activity of biotinidase may be shown in serum, leukocytes, or cultured skin fibroblasts. Newborn screening occurs in some states; most methods use measurement of biotinidase in dried blood filter-paper specimens. Activity of the carboxylases will be normal in cultured skin fibroblasts but may be lowered in leukocytes if they are obtained before starting biotin replacement therapy. Prenatal diagnosis is available. Biotinidase is encoded by the gene *BTD* at chromosome 3p25.

Partial Biotinidase Deficiency. Partial biotinidase deficiency occurs in approximately 1 in 129,000 births and is usually detected by newborn screening for biotinidase deficiency. Affected patients may become symptomatic with intercurrent gastroenteritis, which interrupts the uptake of exogenous biotin. Most often they only have dermatologic problems such as alopecia or dermatitis. Treatment with free biotin at doses of 1 to 5 mg daily is recommended. Mutations at the *BTD* locus allow for residual activity. Patients with partial deficiency usually have 10 to 30% of normal mean biotinidase activity, compared to the less than 10% activity seen in the classic disease.

Biotin Uptake Deficiency. Patients with a defect in the uptake and transport of biotin will present with clinical features similar to those of biotinidase deficiency. They respond to free biotin supplementation. Specific activity of biotinidase and of the carboxylases is normal. The uptake defect can be shown in cultured skin fibroblasts or transformed lymphoblasts.

Methylmalonic Acidemia

Normally, methylmalonyl-CoA is metabolized to succinyl-CoA by methylmalonyl-CoA racemase and methylmalonyl-CoA mutase. Methylmalonyl-CoA mutase requires adenosylcobalamin, an active form of cobalamin (vitamin B_{12}), as its cofactor. Defects in either the mutase or its cofactor adenosylcobalamin may cause methylmalonic acidemia.

Methylmalonyl-CoA Mutase Deficiency

Methylmalonyl-CoA mutase deficiency occurs in at least 1 in 50,000 births. The disorder exists in two forms. Patients with the mut° (mutase) form have essentially no mutase activity, whereas those with the mut⁻ form translate a structurally abnormal mutase that has some residual enzymatic activity. Most patients present in the first week of life with poor feeding, lethargy, vomiting, hypotonia, and respiratory distress that rapidly progresses to coma. Hepatomegaly may occur. Less severely affected patients may present at older ages with failure to thrive, psychomotor difficulties, dystonia, and other neurologic problems, or with an acute episode of metabolic decompensation during an intercurrent illness. Severe metabolic ketoacidosis and hyperammonemia are common findings. Secondary bone marrow depression may lead to neutropenia, thrombocytopenia, or pancytopenia. Megaloblastic anemias are not seen, and levels of cobalamin and folate are normal. Urine organic acid profiles show massive elevation of methylmalonate in addition to metabolites of propionyl-CoA (i.e., 3-hydroxypropionate and methylcitrate). Increased levels of beta-hydroxybutyrate, lactate, and pyruvate, from dehydration and poor perfusion, also occur. Acyl-carnitine profiles are abnormal. On quantitative amino acid determinations, glycine will be elevated, owing to secondary inhibition of the glycine-cleaving enzyme complex. Plasma levels of free and total carnitine are usually low; esterified carnitine levels are markedly high. The disorder may be detected by newborn screening programs that employ tandem mass spectrometry.

Initial treatment should include intravenous hydration with electrolytes and glucose and correction of the metabolic acidosis. Hypoglycemia should be corrected if present. All sources of natural protein should be stopped. Hemodialysis or hemofiltration may be needed for persistent or massive acidosis or hyperammonemia. Intravenous (and later enteral) L-carnitine should be given. Large doses of intramuscular hydroxocobalamin (preferred) or cobalamin should be given daily until the type of the disorder is known. Usually, patients with mutase defects do not respond to hydroxocobalamin, whereas those with defects in the synthesis of adenosylcobalamin frequently do.

Some severely affected patients do not survive their initial episode. Others die later from an acute episode of metabolic decompensation. Although long-term survival and normal intellectual development are possible, many affected patients have significant psychomotor handicaps. Older patients may develop interstitial nephritis and chronic renal failure.

Special medical foods devoid of methionine, threonine, valine, and isoleucine, along with small amounts of natural protein limited to that required for growth, usually are needed for control of this disorder. Supplements of L-carnitine are given. Intermittent use of metronidazole to reduce gastrointestinal tract bacterial formation of propionyl-CoA, a precursor of methylmalonyl-CoA, may increase appetite and improve metabolic control.

Table 385.1 lists the biochemical genetic features of methylmalonic acidemia and homocystinuria, including the cobalamin defects.

Defects in Adenosylcobalamin Metabolism

Cobalamin (vitamin B_{12}) is taken up in cells as hydroxocobalamin, processed in lysosomes, and then metabolized to either adenosylcobalamin, a cofactor for methylmalonyl-CoA mutase, or methylcobalamin, a cofactor involved with homocystine remethylation. Using studies in cell lines from affected patients, seven complementation groups, designated *cbl* (cobalamin) *types A to G*, have been noted with defects in cobalamin metabolism. Of these, types cblA and cblB are associated with defects in the formation of adenosylcobalamin and methylmalonic acidemia. The other types, associated with either homocystinuria or combined methylmalonic acidemia and homocystinuria, are discussed with homocystinuria in Disorders of Transsulfuration, earlier.

In general, type cblA and cblB patients are clinically indistinguishable from patients with methylmalonyl-CoA mutase deficiency. However, their disorder tends to have a later onset and may present up to age 1 year. Approximately 90% of type cblA patients and 40% of type cblB patients respond to treatment with large doses of intramuscular hydroxocobalamin. Two patients with type cblA have been detected and treated prenatally with maternal injections of cobalamin. Special medical foods, L-carnitine supplementation, and intermittent metronidazole also may be needed for control of the disorder.

Of patients with methylmalonic acidemia, approximately 33% will have the mut° form, 11% will have the mut° form, 31% will have the type cblA form, and 25% will have the type cblB form of the disorder. All types of the disorder are inherited as autosomal recessive traits. Carrier detection is available. Prenatal diagnosis has been accomplished by measurement of methylmalonic acid levels in amniotic fluid for all types of the disorder and by radiolabeled propionate studies in cultured amniotic fluid cells for the mutase deficiency.

DISORDERS OF BETA–AMINO ACID AND GAMMA–AMINO ACID METABOLISM

Beta-alanine, R-beta-aminoisobutyric acid, S-beta-aminoisobutyric acid, beta-leucine, and gamma-aminobutyric acid (GABA) occur as free amino acids. Beta-alanine and GABA are also components of the imidazole dipeptides carnosine (beta-alanyl-L-histidine), anserine (beta-alanyl-1-methyl-L-histidine), and homocarnosine (gamma-aminoisobutyryl-L-histidine). GABA, beta-alanine, and carnosine function as neurotransmitters. Anserine and carnosine appear to act as intracellular buffers and antioxidants in skeletal muscle during anaerobic glycolysis. The disorders of beta– and gamma–amino acid metabolism are rare, autosomal recessive diseases. Some are benign, whereas others are associated with neurologic problems.

Disorders of Beta-Alanine and Beta-Aminoisobutyric Acid

Hyper–Beta-Alaninemia

Hyper–beta-alaninemia is associated with markedly elevated levels of beta-alanine and GABA in plasma and CSF and increased urinary excretion of beta-alanine, GABA, beta-aminoisobutyric acid, and taurine. The increased excretion of beta-aminoisobutyric acid and taurine occurs due to competition with the markedly elevated levels of beta-alanine for a shared renal transport system for these amino acids. The exact metabolic defect is unknown, but deficient activity of an aminotransferase involved with the catabolism of beta-alanine is proposed. Of two reported patients, one who presented as a lethargic neonate developed intractable seizures at 7 weeks and died at age 5 months. The other patient, a 4-year-old with intermittent lethargy and seizures, was treated with pyridoxine, a known cofactor for aminotransferases, with response.

Hyper–Beta-Aminoisobutyric Acidemia

Hyper–beta-aminoisobutyric acidemia is a benign disorder associated with deficient activity of R-beta-aminoisobutyric-pyruvate transaminase. Elevated levels of beta-aminoisobutyric acid (R-isomer) are noted on urine organic acid profiles. The disorder occurs in 5% to 10% of whites and in 40% to 95% of Asian populations.

Abnormal metabolism of beta-alanine and beta-aminoisobutyric acid occurs also in combined uraciluria-thyminuria, which is discussed with the disorders of pyrimidine metabolism in Chapter 391.

Disorders of Gamma-Aminobutyric Acid

GABA is a major inhibitory neurotransmitter in the central nervous system. GABA is produced mainly from glutamic acid by the action of glutamic acid decarboxylase and is metabolized to succinic semialdehyde and subsequently to succinic acid, which enters the tricarboxylic acid cycle. The disorders of GABA metabolism are associated with neurologic dysfunction. Measurement of total and free GABA and GABA metabolites in quick-frozen samples of CSF often is needed for confirmation of the disorders.

Pyridoxine Dependency

Pyridoxal-5′-phosphate is a cofactor for glutamic acid decarboxylase, which catalyzes the formation of GABA from glutamic acid. Deficient activity of glutamic acid decarboxylase is associated with generalized seizures that present most often before or shortly after birth. The seizures are relatively unresponsive to conventional anticonvulsant therapy but are responsive to intravenous or oral pyridoxine. *In utero* treatment has been reported. Some affected patients have a later onset of their disorder and develop seizures after age 5 months. Levels of GABA in the brain and CSF are low and increase with pyridoxine therapy. Treatment with pyridoxine is needed indefinitely. Dosage requirements may be as low as 10 mg/day and should not exceed 900 mg/1.73 m²/day.

Gamma-Aminobutyric Acid Transaminase Deficiency

4-Aminobutyrate-alpha-ketoglutarate aminotransferase, specific for GABA (GABA transaminase), catalyzes the conversion of GABA to succinic semialdehyde. Deficient activity of GABA transaminase is a rare disorder associated with severe psychomotor retardation, hypotonia, hyperreflexia, seizures, accelerated linear growth, and death by age 3 years. A leukodystrophy of the brain was noted at autopsy in one patient. Levels of beta-alanine are elevated in plasma and CSF. Free and total GABA, homocarnosine, and other GABA conjugates are elevated in CSF. Increased urinary excretion of GABA, beta-alanine, beta-aminoisobutyric acid, and taurine occurs. The increased excretion of beta-aminoisobutyric acid and taurine results from competition for a shared renal transport system, as in hyper–beta-alaninemia. Elevated fasting plasma growth hormone levels occur presumably from the growth hormone–releasing effect of GABA. Deficient activity of GABA

transaminase may be shown in peripheral blood leukocytes. GABA transaminase is encoded by the gene *GABAT* at chromosome 16p13.3.

4-Hydroxybutyric Acidemia

4-Hydroxybutyric acidemia results from deficient activity of succinic semialdehyde (SSA) dehydrogenase, which normally catalyzes the conversion of SSA to succinic acid. SSA accumulates and is reduced to 4-hydroxybutyric acid by 4-hydroxybutyrate dehydrogenase, resulting in elevated body fluid levels of 4-hydroxybutyric acid. Affected patients present with variable degrees of global psychomotor retardation. Hypotonia, hyporeflexia, ataxia, oculomotor apraxia, seizures, and myopathy may occur. Bilateral globus pallidus abnormalities may be noted with magnetic resonance imaging. Elevated levels of 4-hydroxybutyric acid are found in urine, plasma, and CSF, which decrease with age. Detecting 4-hydroxybutyric acid, however, is difficult by routine gas chromatography–mass spectrometry analysis, owing to its volatility. Analysis in experienced laboratories may be needed. Affected patients also will have elevated urine levels of 4-hydroxybutyric acid metabolites (i.e., 3,4-dihydroxybutyrate; 3-oxo-4-hydroxybutyrate; glycolic acid; 2,4-dihydroxybutyrate; and 3-hydroxypropionate). Plasma and urine glycine levels may be elevated. Treatment with vigabatrin (gamma-vinyl-GABA) may improve attention span and cerebellar dysfunction in some patients. Deficient activity of succinic semialdehyde dehydrogenase may be shown in peripheral blood lymphocytes or cultured lymphoblasts. Prenatal diagnosis is available. The disorder results from mutations in the gene *ALDH5A1* at chromosome 6p22.

Serum Carnosinase Deficiency

Most beta-alanine exists as the dipeptide carnosine (beta-alanyl-L-histidine), which is present in skeletal muscle and brain. Skeletal muscles of birds, rabbits, rats, and whales also contain anserine (beta-alanyl-1-methyl-L-histidine). Normally, anserine is absent in human tissues. Significant amounts of carnosine and anserine are detected only in plasma after the ingestion of large amounts of fowl, rabbit, or other dietary sources of the dipeptides. Normal persons excrete beta-alanine and 1-methylhistidine, carnosine, and anserine after consuming foods containing the dipeptides. Homocarnosine (GABA-L-histidine) is present in human brain and CSF; levels in infants are higher than those in adults. Homocarnosine is not present in plasma, and only insignificant amounts are found in urine.

Carnosinase exists in two forms in humans: a tissue (cytosolic) isoenzyme and a serum isoenzyme. Only the serum carnosinase isoenzyme hydrolyzes carnosine, anserine, and homocarnosine. The tissue isoenzyme, also known as *prolinase*, is involved with proline metabolism.

Deficient activity of serum carnosinase is a benign trait associated with persistently elevated blood and urine levels of carnosine. Anserine is excreted in the urine also after taking foods with high anserine content; little or no urinary 1-methylhistidine is produced. Although many patients with serum carnosinase deficiency (including a family reported with "homocarsinosis") have neurologic abnormalities, the neurologic problems appear to be unrelated to the biochemical abnormalities.

OTHER DISORDERS OF AMINO ACID METABOLISM

Sarcosinemia

Sarcosinemia is a rare, autosomal recessive disorder associated with deficient activity of sarcosine dehydrogenase, which normally catalyzes the conversion of sarcosine (*N*-methylglycine) to glycine. Elevated blood and urine levels of sarcosine occur. The disorder is benign and is not associated with any significant clinical abnormalities. Sarcosinemia is also seen in patients with severe folate deficiency.

Trimethylaminuria

Trimethylamine (TMA), a malodorous compound, is produced from food substances high in choline, trimethylamine-*N*-oxide, or carnitine by the action of intestinal bacteria. TMA is absorbed into the circulation and normally is oxidized in the liver to trimethylamine oxide, a nonodorous compound. In affected patients, lack of hepatic TMA *N*-oxidation results in high levels of TMA in the urine, sweat, and breath and the unpleasant body odor of "rotting fish." Treatment consists of dietary avoidance of foods high in choline (egg yolks, liver, kidney, legumes, soy beans, peas), trimethylamine-*N*-oxide (saltwater fish), and carnitine (meats, milk). Also beneficial may be special deodorant preparations made with resins that absorb TMA and short courses of neomycin or metronidazole to alter intestinal microflora and to suppress TMA production. The disorder is inherited as an autosomal recessive trait and most probably results from deficient activity of the flavin-containing monooxygenase FMO_2.

Aspartoacylase Deficiency (Canavan Disease)

Spongy degeneration of the brain, or Canavan disease, is an autosomal recessive disorder most common in individuals of Eastern European Jewish ancestry. A leukodystrophy with optic atrophy, macrocephaly, hyperreflexia, rigidity, and neurologic deterioration starts in early infancy and results in death by age 3 years. Increased levels of *N*-acetylaspartic acid (NAA) are noted in the blood and urine of affected patients. Deficient activity of aspartoacylase may be demonstrated in cultured skin fibroblasts. Mutations in the gene that encodes for aspartoacylase (*ASPA*), located at chromosome 17pter–p13, have been shown in affected patients. Three of the mutations are seen commonly in patients with Eastern European Jewish ancestry. Carrier detection is available if the genetic mutation or polymorphisms are known. Prenatal diagnosis is available. There is no specific effective therapy.

Guanidinoacetate Methyltransferase Deficiency

Creatine plays an important role in the storage and transmission of phosphate-bound energy in brain and muscle. Creatine is synthesized in the liver and pancreas from glycine and arginine, which combine to form guanidinoacetate. The guanidinoacetate then is methylated to form creatine by the action of guanidinoacetate methyltransferase (GAMT). Creatine and creatine-phosphate may be converted by nonenzymatic cyclization to creatinine. Deficient activity of GAMT results in the accumulation of guanidinoacetate in the brain and the systemic depletion of creatine and creatine-phosphate. Affected patients present in early infancy with progressive extrapyramidal signs, ataxia, hypotonia, seizures, autistic-like behaviors, and delayed development.

Electroencephalograms show abnormally low background activity and multifocal spike patterns. Magnetic resonance imaging shows abnormal signal intensities in the globus pallidus. Low blood levels of creatinine, creatine, and creatine-phosphate and decreased urinary excretion of creatinine are

noted. Guanidinoacetate levels are elevated in body fluids. Patients respond to treatment with oral creatine monohydrate. Decreased activity of GAMT may be shown in cultured fibroblasts or lymphocytes. Prenatal diagnosis is available. The disorder is inherited as an autosomal recessive trait and results from mutations in the gene *GAMT* at chromosome location 19p13.3.

Suggested Readings

Azen C, Koch R, Friedman E, et al. Summary of findings from the United States Collaborative Study of children treated for phenylketonuria. *Eur J Pediatr* 1996;155:S29.

Bachmann C. Outcome and survival of 88 patients with urea cycle disorders: a retrospective evaluation. *Eur J Pediatr* 2003;162:410.

Barth PG, Wanders RJ, Vreken P, et al. X-linked cardioskeletal myopathy and neutropenia (Barth syndrome). *J Inherit Metab Dis* 1999;22:555.

Beasley MG, Costello PM, Smith I. Outcome of treatment in young adults with phenylketonuria detected by routine neonatal screening between 1964 and 1971. *Q J Med* 1994;87:155.

Blau N, Duran M, Blaskovics ME, Gibson KM. *Physician's guide to the laboratory diagnosis of metabolic diseases*, 2nd ed. Berlin: Springer-Verlag, 2002.

Cederbaum S. Phenylketonuria: an update. *Curr Opin Pediatr* 2002;14:702.

Cleary MA, Walter JH, Wraith JE, et al. Magnetic resonance imaging in phenylketonuria: reversal of cerebral white matter change. *J Pediatr* 1995;127:251.

Cockburn F, Barwell BE, Brenton DP, et al. Report of Medical Research Council Working Party on Phenylketonuria. Phenylketonuria due to phenylalanine hydroxylase deficiency: an unfolding story. *BMJ* 1993;306:115.

Cockburn F, Barwell BE, Brenton DP, et al. Report of Medical Research Council Working Party on Phenylketonuria. Recommendations on the dietary management of phenylketonuria. *Arch Dis Child* 1993;68:426.

Costeff H, Gadoth N, Apter N, et al. A familial syndrome of infantile optic atrophy, movement disorder, and spastic paraplegia. *Neurology* 1989;39:595.

Dasouki M, Buchanan D, Mercer N, et al. 3-Hydroxy-3-methylglutaric aciduria: response to carnitine therapy and fat and leucine restriction. *J Inherit Metab Dis* 1987;10:142.

Efrat BS, Kobayashi K, Shaag A, et al. Infantile citrullinemia caused by citrin deficiency with increased dibasic amino acids. *Mol Genet Metab* 2002;77:202.

Elpeleg ON, Costeff H, Joseph A, et al. 3-Methylglutaconic aciduria in the Iraqi-Jewish "optic atrophy plus" (Costeff) syndrome. *Dev Med Child Neurol* 1994;36:167.

Fries MH, Rinaldo P, Schmidt-Sommerfeld E, et al. Isovaleric acidemia: response to a leucine load after three weeks of supplementation with glycine, L-carnitine, and combined glycine-carnitine therapy. *J Pediatr* 1996;129:449.

Gibson KM, Bennett MJ, Naylor EW, et al. 3-Methylcrotonyl-coenzyme A carboxylase deficiency in Amish/Mennonite adults identified by detection of increased acylcarnitines in blood spots of their children. *J Pediatr* 1998;132:519.

Gibson KM, Breuer J, Nyhan WL. 3-Hydroxy-3-methylglutaryl-coenzyme A lyase deficiency. Review of 18 reported patients. *Eur J Pediatr* 1998;148:180.

Gordon N. Ornithine transcarbamylase deficiency: a urea cycle defect. *Eur J Paediatr Neurol* 2003;7:115.

Guttormsen AB, Ueland PM, Nesthus I, et al. Determinants and vitamin responsiveness of intermediate hyperhomocysteinemia (equal to or greater than 40 micromoles/liter): the Hordaland homocysteine study. *J Clin Invest* 1996;98:2174.

Hamosh A, McDonald LW, Valle D, et al. Dextromethorphan and high-dose benzoate therapy for nonketotic hyperglycinemia in an infant. *J Pediatr* 1992;121:131.

Hanley WB, Koch R, Levy HL, et al. The North American Maternal Phenylketonuria Collaborative Study, developmental assessment of the offspring: preliminary report. *Eur J Pediatr* 1996;155:S169.

Holme E, Lindstedt S. Diagnosis and management of tyrosinemia type I. *Curr Opin Pediatr* 1995;7:726.

Jakobs C, Jaeken J, Gibson KM. Inherited disorders of GABA metabolism. *J Inherit Metab Dis* 1993;16:704.

Jouvet P, Jugie M, Rabier D, et al. Combined nutritional support and continuous extracorporeal removal therapy in the severe acute phase of maple syrup urine disease. *Intensive Care Med* 2001;27:1798.

Kang SS, Wong PWK, Susmano A, et al. Thermolabile methylenetetrahydrofolate reductase: an inherited risk factor for coronary artery disease. *Am J Hum Genet* 1991;48:536.

Kaplan P, Mazur A, Field M, et al. Intellectual outcome in children with maple syrup urine disease. *J Pediatr* 1991;119:46.

Kind T, Levy J, Lee M, et al. Cobalamin C disease presenting as hemolytic-uremic syndrome in the neonatal period. *J Pediatr Hematol Oncol* 2002;24:327.

Leonard JV, Morris AAM. Urea cycle disorders. *Semin Neonatol* 2002;7:27.

Mardach R, Zempleni J, Wolf B, et al. Biotin dependency due to a defect in biotin transport. *J Clin Invest* 2002;109:1617.

Mazzocco MMM, Nord AM, Van Doorninck W, et al. Cognitive development among children with early-treated phenylketonuria. *Dev Neuropsychol* 1994;10:133.

Morton DH, Strauss KA, Robinson DL, et al. Diagnosis and treatment of maple syrup disease: a study of 36 patients. *Pediatrics* 2002;109:999.

Ogier de Baulny H, Saudubray JM. Branched-chain organic acidurias. *Semin Neonatal* 2002;7:65.

Ohura T, Kobayashi K, Abukawa D, et al. A novel inborn error of metabolism detected by elevated methionine and/or galactose in newborn screening: neonatal intrahepatic cholestasis caused by citrin deficiency. *Eur J Pediatr* 2003;162:317.

Ostman-Smith I, Brown G, Johnson A, et al. Dilated cardiomyopathy due to type II X-linked 3-methylglutaconic aciduria: successful treatment with pantothenic acid. *Br Heart J* 1994;72:349.

Pietz J, Fatkenheuer B, Burgard P, et al. Psychiatric disorders in adult patients with early-treated phenylketonuria. *Pediatrics* 1997;99:345.

Scriver CR, Beaudet AL, Sly WS, Valle D, eds. *The metabolic and molecular bases of inherited disease,* 8th ed. New York: McGraw-Hill, 2001.

Stockler S, Isbrandt D, Hanefeld F, et al. Guanidinoacetate methyltransferase deficiency: the first inborn error of creatine metabolism in man. *Am J Hum Genet* 1996;58:914.

Strauss KA, Morton DH. Branched-chain ketoacyl dehydrogenase deficiency: maple syrup disease. *Curr Treat Options Neurol* 2003;5:329.

Thompson GN, Chalmers RA, Halliday D. The contribution of protein catabolism to metabolic decompensation in 3-hydroxy-3-methylglutaric aciduria. *Eur J Pediatr* 1990;149:346.

Weglage J, Funders B, Wilken B, et al. School performance and intellectual outcome in adolescents with phenylketonuria. *Acta Paediatr* 1993;81:582.

Wilcken B, Wiley V, Hammond J, et al. Screening newborns for inborn errors of metabolism by tandem mass spectrometry. *N Engl J Med* 2003;348:2304.

CHAPTER 386 ■ DISORDERS OF MITOCHONDRIAL FATTY ACID OXIDATION

BRYAN E. HAINLINE AND REBECCA S. WAPPNER

FATTY ACID METABOLISM

One of the primary functions of mitochondria, the aerobic production of energy from fatty acids, is discussed in this chapter. Other biochemical reactions taking place within these organelles are discussed in Chapters 384 to 388 and 409. Mitochondria assume a wide variety of sizes and shapes that depend on the metabolic and physiologic needs of the tissue in which they are located. A prototypic mitochondrion is 1 to 2 μm long, is roughly cylindric, and has rounded ends. The outer surface is bounded by the outer membrane, which is permeable to low-molecular-weight compounds. The inner membrane is much more restrictive to biomolecules, however, and most substances cannot enter or leave the mitochondrial matrix unless a specific transport system is available. The inner membrane is folded narrowly into cristae at somewhat regular intervals, which project more or less deeply into the matrix. The narrow space between the outer and inner membranes (the intermembrane space) is continuous with the narrow space within the crista. In general, the areas at which the inner membrane is contiguous with the outer membrane primarily have transport functions, whereas those inner membrane areas that form the cristae have primarily electron transport–oxidative phosphorylation functions. The matrix has its own complement of enzymes that are involved with various metabolic functions and contains the mitochondrial DNA, whose genes encode RNA and additional molecules needed for protein synthesis and mitochondrial oxidative phosphorylation.

Mitochondrial beta-oxidation of fatty acids is an important source of energy for metabolic processes including normal fasting, muscular activity, illness with stress (e.g., infection), and nonshivering thermogenesis. After long-chain fatty acids are mobilized from adipose tissue, they are transported, bound to albumin, to the liver and other tissues, where plasma membrane uptake is mediated by fatty acid–binding proteins. Long-chain fatty acids are "activated" to their coenzyme A (CoA) esters by long-chain acyl-CoA synthase, are transported across the mitochondrial membrane by a carnitine-mediated system, and are oxidized to ketone bodies in the mitochondrial matrix. Medium-chain fatty acids are transported across the mitochondrial membranes in a noncarnitine-dependent process, activated by a corresponding matrix medium-chain acyl-CoA synthase, and they are then oxidized in a manner similar to the long-chain molecules. Disorders involving mitochondrial beta-oxidation of fatty acids are characterized by faulty ketone body formation, impaired energy production, and the accumulation of partially oxidized fatty acid metabolites during periods of stress and fasting. All are inherited as autosomal recessive traits. Biochemical aspects of these disorders, including the importance of carnitine, are described in Box 386.1. The disorders have widely varying clinical manifestations.

Dietary sources of carnitine include meats and dairy products. Endogenous carnitine may be synthesized from methylated lysine, which can be derived from such muscle proteins as myosin. Usually, secondary carnitine deficiency states are associated with organic acidemias or faulty beta-oxidation. Deficiencies may be seen also in patients with renal tubular disorders, vitamin C and pyridoxine deficiencies, strict vegetarian diets, total parenteral nutrition, hemodialysis, and valproate anticonvulsant therapy.

Systemic carnitine deficiency, regardless of its cause, results in faulty fatty acid oxidation and has been associated with poor tolerance of fasting, hypoketotic hypoglycemia, liver dysfunction, hypotonia, myopathies, cardiomyopathies, and recurrent myoglobinuria and myalgias.

DISORDERS OF FATTY ACID OXIDATION

The clinical features of disorders of fatty acid oxidation are summarized in Table 386.1. Additional details are provided in the following sections. It should be noted that the introduction of expanded newborn screening using tandem mass spectrometry will affect the identification and management of

---

BOX 386.1   Biochemical Aspects of Fatty Acid Metabolism

As shown in Figure 386.1, long-chain (C10 to C25) fatty acids are activated by long-chain acyl-CoA synthase (located in the outer mitochondrial membrane) to form long-chain acyl-CoA esters. Then the esters are transesterified with carnitine by carnitine palmitoyl transferase (CPT) I, which resides on the inner aspect of the outer mitochondrial membrane. The long-chain acyl-carnitines (and nonesterified carnitine) cross the inner mitochondrial membrane by a process mediated by carnitine-acyl-carnitine translocase. On the matrix side of the inner mitochondrial membrane, the long-chain acyl-carnitines are reesterified to long-chain acyl-CoA esters by a separate transferase, CPT II. The "activated" long-chain acyl-CoA esters then enter the beta-oxidation pathway. Medium-chain (C6 to C12) and short-chain (C4 and C6) fatty acids do not need carnitine-mediated transport to transverse the membranes. They are "activated" to their respective acyl-CoA esters by medium- or short-chain acyl-CoA synthases (synthetases) located in the mitochondrial matrix before entering the beta-oxidation pathway. With each cycle through the beta-oxidation pathway, the fatty acid–CoA ester is reduced in length by two carbons to form an acetyl-CoA group that can be metabolized further to ketone bodies in the liver and kidneys or can enter the tricarboxylic acid cycle in heart and skeletal muscle.

The beta-oxidation pathway includes a series of chain length–specific acyl-CoA dehydrogenases, enoyl-CoA hydratases, 3-hydroxyacyl-CoA dehydrogenases, and 3-oxoacyl-CoA thiolases. The four acyl-CoA dehydrogenases are flavoproteins (derived from riboflavin) that transfer electrons from acyl-CoA esters to electron transfer flavoprotein (ETF) and subsequently to the mitochondrial electron transport chain to form adenosine triphosphate. Very long-chain acyl-CoA dehydrogenase (VLCAD) is a membrane-bound protein that catalyzes the oxidation of fatty acids with chain lengths of 16 to 24 carbons; long-chain acyl-CoA dehydrogenase (LCAD) catalyzes the reaction for 12- to 18-carbon fatty acid esters; medium-chain acyl-CoA dehydrogenase (MCAD) catalyzes the reaction for chain lengths of 4 to 14 carbons; and short-chain acyl-CoA dehydrogenase (SCAD) catalyzes the reaction for chain lengths of 4 or 6 carbons. Fatty acid acyl-CoA esters with odd chain lengths are oxidized similarly until a three-carbon propionyl-CoA is formed. Unsaturated fatty acids require additional enzymes, long- and short-chain 3-*cis*, 2-*trans*-enoyl-CoA iso-

merase and 2,4-dienoyl-CoA reductase, for complete beta-oxidation of these compounds. An enzyme related to SCAD may be responsible for oxidation of branched-chain substrates. The long-chain activities for enoyl-CoA hydratase, 3-hydroxyacyl-CoA dehydrogenase, and 3-oxoacyl-CoA thiolase exist together in a trifunctional protein (TFP) complex. Individual soluble enzymes with short-chain enoyl-CoA hydratase, short-chain 3-hydroxyacyl-CoA dehydrogenase, and 3-oxoacyl-CoA thiolase activities have been found in the mitochondrial matrix.

The acetyl-CoA and acyl-CoA esters formed as a result of beta-oxidation exit the mitochondrial matrix by carnitine-mediated transport similar to that for the entrance of long-chain acyl-CoA esters. Acetyl-carnitine is formed by carnitine acetyltransferase and is transported by the translocase to the cytosol.

ETF and ETF:ubiquinone oxidoreductase (ETF:QO) are proteins that mediate the transfer of electrons from flavin-containing acyl-CoA dehydrogenases (i.e., VLCAD, LCAD, MCAD, SCAD, and others) to the main respiratory chain at the level of ubiquinone (coenzyme Q). The energy of these electrons is used for the formation of adenosine triphosphate and the ultimate reduction of molecular oxygen to form water.

L-Carnitine (gamma-trimethyl-beta-hydroxy-butyrobetaine) is needed for transport of long-chain fatty acid acyl-CoA esters into the mitochondrial matrix and for the return of acyl-CoA intermediates to the cytosol. L-Carnitine also functions to remove the metabolites of faulty beta-oxidation and certain other abnormal organic acids from the mitochondrial matrix by forming carnitine esters with these compounds. The abnormal acyl-carnitine compounds then are transported to the cytosol, from which they exit the cell, enter the circulation, and are excreted in the urine. Usually, plasma carnitine measurements are reported as total, free, and esterified in micromolar concentrations. In some patients with disorders of beta-oxidation or organic acidemias, both the total and free carnitine levels are low. In other patients, the total plasma carnitine level is normal, but the esterified fraction is abnormally high (greater than 40% of total carnitine). This condition results in a relative deficiency of free carnitine, which is needed for appropriate fatty acid transport.

---

these disorders. Although screening of asymptomatic newborns will identify most individuals with severe disorders, especially medium-chain acyl-CoA dehydrogenase (MCAD) deficiency, the remaining disorders may not be recognized early. Clinical suspicion should remain high when children or older patients present with symptoms described below, despite a history of a negative newborn acyl-carnitine screening test.

Medium-Chain Acyl-CoA Dehydrogenase Deficiency

MCAD deficiency, the most common of the disorders of fatty acid oxidation, occurs in approximately 1 in 15,000 births, varying from 1 in 6,500 to 1 in 17,000 in different populations.

This disorder is seen almost exclusively in whites, especially those with Northwestern European heritage, among whom the carrier rate may be as frequent as 1 in 40 for the most common mutation, K304E. Most patients present between ages 5 and 24 months with vomiting, lethargy, and hypotonia that occur after a decreased carbohydrate intake associated with an intercurrent illness or fasting. Mild hepatomegaly and seizures may occur. Hypoglycemia, mildly elevated blood ammonia, and increased liver enzyme levels usually are noted. Any acidosis usually is mild. Urine and plasma ketones may be either absent or present in trace amounts, which has led to the term *hypoketotic hypoglycemia* for this group of disorders. However, some patients may make ketone bodies when severely stressed. The amount of ketones produced in these patients, as determined by plasma beta-hydroxybutyrate levels, is inappropriately low for the degree of hypoglycemia and the marked elevation of

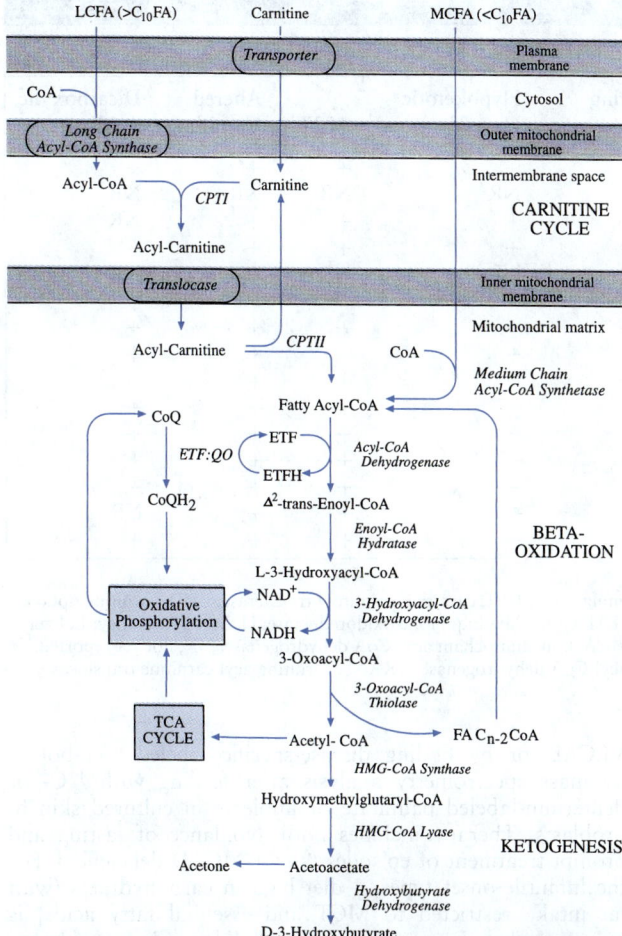

FIGURE 386.1. Mitochondrial metabolism of fatty acids. In the beta-oxidation section, a series of chain-length specific enzymes occurs at each of the four steps involved: VLCAD (very long-chain acyl-CoA dehydrogenase), LCAD (long-chain), MCAD (medium-chain), and SCAD (short-chain) at the acyl-CoA dehydrogenase step (see also text). C, carbon length; CoA, coenzyme A; CoQ, coenzyme Q; $CoQH_2$, reduced coenzyme Q; CPT, carnitine palmitoyl transferase; ETF, electron transport flavoprotein; ETF:QO, ETF:ubiquinone oxidoreductase; FA, fatty acid; LCFA, long-chain fatty acids; MCFA, medium-chain fatty acids; NAD^+, oxidized form of nicotinamide adenine dinucleotide; NADH, reduced form of nicotinamide adenine dinucleotide; TCA, tricarboxylic acid (citric acid).

plasma free fatty acids. The pathophysiologic reason for the hypoglycemia is understood incompletely but is believed to result from failure of the normal increase in gluconeogenesis with fasting, which usually occurs in response to increased acetyl-CoA and ketone body production.

Clinical presentation varies widely. Some patients have been identified in the newborn period due to a history of early hypoglycemia, whereas others were asymptomatic and were detected only by family studies or state-mandated newborn screening. Ill, affected patients may have a rapidly deteriorating course with an episode that progresses to coma and death from cardiorespiratory collapse or cerebral edema. The accumulation of acyl-CoA compounds, especially those with chain lengths of three carbons or more, frequently is associated with encephalopathy and may result in cerebral edema. Mortality has been reported to be highest (59%) at between ages 15 and 26 months. Approximately 25% of patients die with their first episode, which frequently is unrecognized as being a result of a disorder of fatty acid oxidation until the disorder is diagnosed in a second child in the family. Many of the deaths have been attributed to Reye syndrome or to sudden infant death syndrome. Autopsy findings include fatty infiltration of the liver, the pattern of which may be macrovesicular or microvesicular. Mitochondrial changes in the liver on electron microscopy differ from those seen in Reye syndrome. Condensed mitochondria, with increased matrix density and intracristal widening, or enlarged and abnormally shaped mitochondria, with an increase in the number of cristae and crystalloids in the matrix, may be seen.

With episodes, affected individuals accumulate metabolites of medium-chain length (C6 to C12), especially octanoic acid and 4-decanoic acid. Owing to the excessive accumulation of fatty acyl-CoA intermediates of medium-chain length in the mitochondria, alternative pathways of microsomal (omega and omega$_1$) oxidation and peroxisomal beta-oxidation become involved and lead to excessive production of (omega$_1$)-hydroxy acids and medium-chain dicarboxylic acids, such as adipic, suberic, and sebacic acids. Organic acid analysis using gas or liquid chromatography–mass spectrometry may detect these metabolites in the blood or urine of patients during episodes. Acyl-CoA compounds may be conjugated with glycine or with carnitine. Abnormal metabolites of medium-chain length may be detected as urinary acyl-glycine conjugates (stable isotope dilution gas chromatography–mass spectrometry) or by plasma or dried blood filter-paper sample acyl-carnitine profiles (fast atom bombardment with tandem mass spectrometry). The latter two tests are more sophisticated and sensitive than are routine organic acid measurements. Their use is indicated particularly in the evaluation of all patients suspected of having a defect in fatty acid oxidation. Between episodes, asymptomatic affected patients may have normal routine organic acid studies. However, urine acyl-glycine or dried blood filter-paper or plasma acyl-carnitine profiles usually are abnormal. Frequently, affected patients have abnormal plasma and urinary carnitine levels, with lowered total and elevated esterified fractions. Such patients should not be subjected to a provocative fast because of the possibility of inducing a fatal acute episode. The use of acyl-carnitine profiles from dried blood filter-paper samples has not only allowed identification of asymptomatic affected children, but also has led to retrospective diagnosis in children who have died, including several affected newborns. Those infants identified by newborn screening tests should have the diagnosis confirmed by repeat testing at a separate standard laboratory. Confirmation of deficient activity of MCAD may be shown in cultured skin fibroblasts by finding disease-specific labeled metabolites using tandem or electrospray mass spectrometry assay after feeding with carbon 14– or deuterium-labeled palmitate or linoleate.

Molecular genetic analysis of the *MCAD* gene has led to localization of the gene on chromosome 1p31. A common point mutation at position 985 of the MCAD cDNA (K304E) is present in approximately 90% of patients with the disorder. Twenty-one less common mutations account for the remaining alleles. A new mutation, 199T-C, has been found in population screening at a frequency of 1 in 500. It has, however, not yet been associated with symptomatic disease. Confirmation of the disease and determination of carrier status for the common K304E mutation may be performed using DNA extracted from dried blood filter-paper samples. Prenatal diagnosis may be done by molecular genetic techniques or by using the labeled-metabolite assay.

The basis for treatment is the avoidance of fasting and lipolysis. Frequent meals or feedings with a high carbohydrate and relatively lowered fat intake is recommended. Medium-chain triglyceride (MCT) oil in any form should be avoided. Premature infant formulas often contain MCT oil and should not be used. Treatment should be started as soon as the diagnosis is considered, even if test results are not yet available. L-Carnitine supplementation is indicated in symptomatic patients. Only the

TABLE 386.1

CLINICAL FEATURES OF DISORDERS OF MITOCHONDRIAL FATTY ACID OXIDATION

Enzyme Defect	Gene Location	Common Mutation	Tissue Involved	Fasting Intolerance	Hypoketotic Hypoglycemia	ALTE	Altered Carnitine	Dicarboxylic Acids
CPT IA	11q13	No	K, L	+	+	+	+*	−
CPT1B	22pter	No	H, M, A	NR	NR	NR	NR	NR
CPT II	1p32	Yes	H, L, M	+	+	+	+	NR
CUD	5q33.1		H, M	+	+	+	+	−
DCR	8q21.3		L, M	NR	NR	NR	+	NR
ETF	15q23–q25 (ETFA)		H, K, L, M					
	19q13.3 (ETFB)			+	+	+	+	+
ETF:QO	4q32qter		H, K, L, M		+		+	+
LCHAD	2p23 (alpha)	Yes	H, L, M	+	+	+	+	+
TFP	2p23 (alpha/beta)	No	H, L, M	+	+	+	+	+
MCAD	1p31	Yes	L	+	+	+	+	+
SCAD	12q22qter		L, M	−	−	+	+	+
SCHAD	4q22–q26		L, M	+	−	+	+	+
TRANS	3p21.31		H, M	+	+	+	+	NR
VLCAD	17p11.2–p11.13	No	H, M	+	+	+	+	+

*Elevated.

+, Usually present; −, usually not present; A, adipose; ALTE, acute life-threatening event; CPT, carnitine palmitoyl transferase; CUD, carnitine uptake defect; DCR, 2,4-dienoyl-CoA reductase; ETF, electron transport flavoprotein; ETF:QO, ETF:ubiquinone oxidoreductase; H, heart; K, kidney; L, liver; LCHAD, long-chain 3-hydroxyacyl-CoA dehydrogenase; M, skeletal muscle; MCAD, medium-chain acyl-CoA dehydrogenase; NR, not yet reported; SCAD, short-chain acyl-CoA dehydrogenase; SCHAD, short-chain 3-hydroxyacyl-CoA dehydrogenase; TRANS, carnitine-acyl-carnitine translocase; VLCAD, very long-chain acyl-CoA dehydrogenase.

prescription form of L-carnitine should be used, not the D,L-form available in health food stores. Episodes should be treated promptly with intravenous glucose and hydration, to which most patients respond. Intravenous L-carnitine may be needed for severe episodes or in situations where enteral intake is not feasible. Once the disorder is recognized and treated, many patients do well. However, residual neurologic dysfunction from severe episodes will persist.

Very Long-Chain Acyl-CoA Dehydrogenase Deficiency

Very long-chain acyl-CoA dehydrogenase (VLCAD) deficiency is less common than is MCAD. Originally, the disorder was attributed to a deficiency of long-chain acyl-CoA dehydrogenase (LCAD). However, the discovery of a separate very long-chain enzyme, along with the reassessment of fibroblast cell lines from originally reported LCAD patients, has shown that virtually all have a deficiency in VLCAD. VLCAD deficiency has clinical features similar to those in MCAD deficiency, including nonketotic hypoglycemia, hyperammonemia, carnitine deficiency, and hepatomegaly. The disorder may be distinguished from MCAD deficiency by earlier onset (usually before age 6 months), more severe acute episodes, and higher mortality. Often, a dilated cardiomyopathy is present. Hypotonia, muscle weakness, and developmental delay may occur, especially in those patients who have become ill from their disorder. Milder variants have been reported with initial symptoms similar to those of MCAD deficiency. Other patients have developed symptoms later in life, with recurrent episodes of stress-related myalgias and rhabdomyolysis. Liver biopsies in the more severe types may reveal portal fibrosis in addition to steatosis. During episodes, urinary organic acid (gas chromatography–mass spectroscopy) profiles show elevated long-chain (C12 and C14) and medium-chain dicarboxylic acids. Because long-chain acyl-carnitines are not excreted readily in the urine, urinary acyl-carnitine profiles frequently are normal. Urinary acyl-glycine profiles and plasma or dried blood filter-paper sample acyl-carnitine profiles often are abnormal. Lowered total and elevated esterified plasma carnitine levels are noted. The disorder is confirmed by demonstrating reduced activity of

VLCAD or by finding disease-specific labeled metabolites by mass spectrometry analysis after feeding with [14]C- or deuterium-labeled palmitate or linoleate in cultured skin fibroblasts. Therapy includes both avoidance of fasting and prompt treatment of episodes (as for MCAD deficiency). For the infantile-onset types, a diet high in carbohydrates (with fat intake restricted to MCT and essential fatty acids) is recommended. For patients with rhabdomyolysis, carbohydrate loading is recommended before exercise. L-Carnitine supplementation may be beneficial to patients with all types of the disorder. The VLCAD gene has been cloned and localized to chromosome 17p11.2–17p11.13. At least 14 mutations or deletions have been demonstrated for the disorder. Prenatal diagnosis may be performed using the deuterium-labeled mass spectrometry technique and enzymatic testing.

Short-Chain Acyl-CoA Dehydrogenase Deficiency

Short-chain acyl-CoA dehydrogenase (SCAD) deficiency is a rare disorder. In contrast to patients with MCAD and VLCAD deficiencies, patients with SCAD deficiency are able to tolerate fasting and are capable of ketone body production, because their metabolic block allows the normal beta-oxidation of medium- and long-chain fatty acids. Some patients are asymptomatic while others have died in episodes thought to be related to their disorders. Two forms of the disorder have been identified. Patients with the "infantile form" of the disorder present with poor feeding, metabolic acidosis, failure to thrive, developmental delay, hepatomegaly, and progressive hypotonia. Lipid deposition occurs in the liver and muscle. Usually, abnormal organic acid profiles with elevated butyric acid and ethylmalonic acid are noted. Carnitine deficiency is often not a feature. The "adult form" of SCAD deficiency presumably is limited to skeletal muscle. Affected patients have episodic weakness and lipid deposits in type I fibers on muscle biopsy. Mitochondria may have osmiophilic inclusions or may be normal. Usually, the dried blood filter-paper acyl-carnitine profile is abnormal, but it can be intermittently normal in asymptomatic patients. The infantile type of SCAD deficiency can be confirmed by using cultured skin fibroblasts or skeletal muscle to demonstrate reduced activity of SCAD or by finding disease-specific labeled metabolites by mass spectrometry analysis after feeding with ^{14}C- or deuterium-labeled palmitate or linoleate. DNA sequencing to determine mutations is frequently utilized to confirm the diagnosis. Testing for alterations in oxidative phosphorylation is often undertaken to ensure that a mitochondrial myopathy is not the underlying disorder for those patients with myopathic symptoms. Treatment includes L-carnitine and riboflavin (may enhance any residual SCAD activity) therapy in addition to the avoidance of prolonged fasting.

The *SCAD* gene has been cloned and localized to chromosome 12q22qter. The disorder is biochemically heterogeneous; two mutations have been identified to date. Prenatal diagnosis should be feasible using the ^{14}C- or deuterium-labeled palmitate–mass spectrometric assay. However, the finding of asymptomatic patients has called into question the usefulness of such testing.

Long-Chain Hydroxyacyl-CoA Dehydrogenase and Trifunctional Protein Deficiency

Isolated long-chain hydroxyacyl-CoA dehydrogenase (LCHAD) deficiency is a disorder with clinical features similar to those seen with infantile VLCAD deficiency. Patients with LCHAD deficiency may also have deficiencies of long-chain 2-enoyl-CoA hydratase and 3-ketoacyl-CoA thiolase activities that result in the trifunctional protein (TFP) complex deficiency. Isolated deficiency of the LCHAD, however, is the most common form of the disorder. Symptoms of nonketotic hypoglycemia, carnitine deficiency, cardiomyopathy, acute or chronic progressive liver dysfunction, pigmentary retinopathy, muscle weakness, and peripheral neuropathy have been noted. Hypocalcemia, suggestive of hypoparathyroidism, has been reported. In contrast to VLCAD deficiency, the cardiomyopathy is usually hypertrophic, sometimes associated with pericardial effusion, and the hepatic dysfunction is more severe, owing to extensive lipid infiltration that may extend to cirrhosis. Affected patients may present with sudden and rapid collapse of circulatory function that often is fatal. Three clinical phenotypes for TFP deficiency have been suggested including a severe neonatal presentation with cardiomyopathy, Reye-like symptoms, and early death; a hepatic form with recurrent, hypoketotic hypoglycemia; and a milder, childhood-onset neuromyopathic type with episodic myoglobinuria. The last group of patients experience a later onset of symptoms in childhood, with clinical features similar to those of VLCAD deficiency, including muscle weakness, rhabdomyolysis, progressive hypotonia, and fatty infiltration of the liver. Adults with recurrent rhabdomyolysis, exercise intolerance, and muscle weakness also are known. Patients with late-onset TFP deficiency rarely have symptoms of liver disease as a presenting feature.

During pregnancy, mothers carrying children affected with LCHAD or trifunctional protein deficiency may develop acute fatty liver of pregnancy (AFLP) syndrome or HELLP (*h*emolysis, *e*levated *l*iver enzymes, *l*ow *p*latelets) syndrome. AFLP syndrome is associated with anorexia, nausea or vomiting, abdominal pain, and jaundice in the third trimester of pregnancy. The more common HELLP syndrome may occur as a severe form of preeclampsia. Microvesicular fatty infiltration of the liver in the mother resolves with delivery of the affected child. All children born of mothers with either AFLP or HELLP syndrome during pregnancy should be evaluated for LCHAD and the trifunctional protein deficiency.

With episodes, affected patients excrete 3-hydroxydicarboxylic acids and 3-hydroxymonocarboxylic acids. Plasma or dried blood filter-paper acyl-carnitine profiles are abnormal.

Some patients may show abnormal profiles only when ill. Plasma carnitine levels reveal elevated esterified fractions. The defective enzyme activity and abnormal metabolites can be demonstrated in cultured skin fibroblasts in a manner similar to those discussed for the foregoing disorders. Treatment is similar to that for VLCAD deficiency with a low-fat diet, L-carnitine, and MCT supplementation.

The trifunctional protein complex is composed of four alpha and four beta subunits. The genes that encode for both the alpha and beta subunits have been localized to chromosome 2p23. A frequent mutation in the alpha subunit (G1528C) has been described for 60% to 90% of patients with isolated LCHAD deficiency. A number of other mutations have been found in each of the two subunits that are associated with trifunctional protein deficiency. Prenatal diagnosis should be possible with the use of either the labeled substrate assay or DNA techniques for families of patients with known mutations.

Medium- and Short-Chain Hydroxyacyl-CoA Dehydrogenase Deficiency

Medium- and short-chain hydroxyacyl-CoA dehydrogenase (M/SCHAD) deficiency was previously thought to be a disorder deficient in short-chain 3-hydroxyacyl-CoA dehydrogenase activity. Recent characterization of the encoding gene has suggested broader substrate specificity than previously thought. Deficiency has been associated with three presentations. The infantile form presents as a recurrent Reye-like illness with fasting intolerance, ketosis, and hypoglycemia suggestive of ketotic hypoglycemia. Nonhydroxylated and 3-hydroxy dicarboxylic acids with C6 to C14 chain lengths and abnormal carnitine esters have been noted. An older-onset variant was reported with recurrent myoglobinuria, hypoketotic hypoglycemic encephalopathy, and hypertrophic cardiomyopathy. The enzymatic defect was found in skeletal muscle but not in cultured skin fibroblasts. A third set of patients has been identified with symptoms of severe liver dysfunction without muscle abnormalities. Treatment with a high-carbohydrate, low-fat diet and the avoidance of fasting has limited symptoms to some degree in these patients. The gene for SCHAD has been cloned.

Dienoyl-CoA Reductase Deficiency

Mitochondrial 2,4-dienoyl-CoA reductase deficiency is unique in that it is the first enzymatic defect reported to involve only unsaturated fatty acid oxidation. The only reported case to date presented in the neonatal period with hypotonia, hyperlysinemia, and lowered total and free carnitine levels. Failure to thrive, microcephaly, and shortened trunk, arms, and fingers also were noted; the patient died at age 4 months of respiratory acidosis. An unusual acyl-carnitine, 2-*trans*, 4-*cis*-decadienoylcarnitine, was noted in the plasma and urine. The level of reductase activity was reduced to 40% of controls in the liver and 17% of controls in muscle. Management is similar to that for VLCAD. The cDNA for the enzyme has been cloned.

Carnitine Plasma Membrane Transporter Deficiency

Carnitine plasma membrane transporter deficiency is due to a defective carrier protein responsible for sodium-dependent transport of carnitine across plasma membranes. This is the only known defect to be considered a cause of primary carnitine deficiency. The defect is present in cultured skin fibroblasts, in cardiac and skeletal muscle, and in kidneys but not in liver. The majority of patients have been identified between ages 2 and 7 years with a progressive cardiomyopathy and skeletal muscle weakness. Other patients present at between ages 3 months and 2 years with symptoms similar to those of MCAD deficiency, including fasting-induced hypoglycemia, hyperammonemia, and decreased ketone body production. Symptomatic cardiac involvement may develop later. Plasma and tissue total carnitine levels are markedly low, often less than 10 μM. Carriers (heterozygotes) have levels intermediate between normal controls and homozygous affected patients. Urine organic acid profiles are normal. Most patients respond well to high-dose L-carnitine supplementation. The diagnosis is confirmed by measurement of carnitine transport into fibroblasts. The gene has been cloned. The incidence of the disorder in Japan has been estimated at 1 in 40,000.

Carnitine-Acyl-Carnitine Translocase Deficiency

Carnitine-acyl-carnitine translocase deficiency is very rare and has been associated with fasting hypoketotic hypoglycemia, coma, chronic hyperammonemia and liver dysfunction, hypotonia, muscle weakness, cardiac arrhythmias, and cardiomyopathy in early infancy. Often, the plasma carnitine level is low with an increased esterified fraction. Plasma acyl-carnitine profiles will be abnormal and show both medium- and long-chain acyl-carnitines. Urine organic acid analysis shows medium- and long-chain dicarboxylic acids. Treatment includes avoidance of long-chain fat and supplementation with MCT. The gene has been cloned and several mutations have been identified.

Carnitine Palmitoyl Transferase I and Carnitine Palmitoyl Transferase II Deficiencies

Two immunologically distinct isoforms of CPT I are known. Two separate genes, located on chromosomes 11q and 22pter, respectively, encode the hepatic isoform (*CPT1A*) and an isoform found in skeletal muscle, heart, and adipose tissue (*CPT1B*). The hepatic isoform has been shown to be expressed developmentally in rat heart muscle and accounts for 25% of CPT I activity in the newborn heart and 2% to 3% in adult heart.

CPT I deficiency is very rare. The infantile "hepatic" form occurs in young infants who have clinical symptoms similar to those of MCAD deficiency, including fasting hypoglycemia and hypoketonemia, lethargy or coma, hyperammonemia, hepatomegaly, and seizures. Renal tubular acidosis has been reported in one patient. Usually, cardiac and muscle involvement do not occur. Laboratory studies show liver dysfunction and elevated free fatty acids and triglycerides without ketonuria or ketonemia. Free and total carnitine levels are markedly elevated with reported levels as high as 140 μM. Acyl-carnitine metabolites show no specific abnormalities. The diagnosis has been made by measuring CPT I activity in cultured skin fibroblasts, leukocytes, or liver. The level of activity in muscle is not affected. Dried blood filter-paper acyl-carnitine profiles and deuterated palmitate or linoleate labeling of fibroblasts show nonspecific results. Treatment includes frequent feedings and MCT supplementation. The *CPT1A* gene has been cloned and several mutations have been identified.

CPT II deficiency is more common than is CPT I deficiency. The majority of patients have a "muscular" form of the disorder that presents in adolescents and young adults with recurrent attacks of rhabdomyolysis. Fasting, exercise, cold, or infection may precipitate episodes. Hepatic and cardiac involvement rarely is seen. Although the disorder is inherited as an autosomal recessive trait, almost all patients have been males. The incidence of anesthetic-related malignant hyperthermia also is higher. Deficient activity of CPT II may be shown in muscle, liver, cultured skin fibroblasts, or leukocytes. Usually, patients with the "muscular" form of the disorder have 20% to 25% residual specific activity.

A more severe, sometimes lethal "infantile" form of CPT II deficiency, with 0% to 10% residual activity, has been described. Most affected infants present before age 6 months with hypoketotic hypoglycemia, metabolic acidosis, hyperammonemia, hypotonia, cardiomyopathy, and occasionally cardiac arrhythmias, renal cortical cysts, and brain malformations. Liver involvement has varied. As these individuals approach puberty, they may develop symptoms of the more common "muscle" form such as muscle weakness, and exercise-induced muscle pain and/or rhabdomyolysis. Often, reduced concentrations of total and free carnitine are seen. Dried blood filter-paper and plasma acyl-carnitine profiles frequently are abnormal and show accumulation of long-chain acyl-carnitines. Treatment is similar to that for VLCAD deficiency.

The gene for CPT II has been localized to chromosome 1p32. The two forms of the disorder have been shown to result from different mutations. Prenatal diagnosis should be possible for CPT II using the labeled metabolite assay.

Multiple Acyl-CoA Dehydrogenase Deficiency

Multiple acyl-CoA dehydrogenase deficiency, or glutaric acidemia type II, is a complex disorder due to deficient function of either electron transfer flavoprotein (ETF) or ETF: ubiquinone oxidoreductase (ETF:QO) dehydrogenase. ETF and ETF:QO mediate the transfer of electrons from flavin-containing acyl-CoA dehydrogenases to CoQ in the respiratory chain. The flavin-containing acyl-CoA dehydrogenases include those involved with mitochondrial beta-oxidation of fatty acids (i.e., VLCAD, MCAD, or SCAD) and several involved with amino acid metabolism (i.e., dimethylglycine, sarcosine, isovaleryl-CoA, 2-methylbutyryl-CoA, and glutaryl-CoA dehydrogenases).

The disorder exists in four distinct clinical forms. Two "severe" forms of ETF and ETF:QO deficiency present in the neonatal period and are distinguished by the presence or absence of congenital anomalies. Often, the patients are premature and by age 2 days develop hypotonia, hepatomegaly, hypoglycemia, metabolic acidosis, hyperammonemia, and an acrid odor (similar to that of sweaty feet) derived from isovaleric acid. In the severe dysmorphic form, patients exhibit features resembling those found in Zellweger syndrome, with a high forehead, hypoplastic midface, hypertelorism, and low-set ears. Rocker-bottom feet, muscular defects of the abdominal wall, anomalies of the external genitalia, enlarged cystic kidneys, and brain malformations also have been noted. Most patients with the severe forms die by age 1 week. A few who have lived longer have developed cardiomyopathies. Serum and urine organic acid profiles show marked elevations of metabolites of varying chain length, including glutaric, ethylmalonic, 3-hydroxyisovaleric, 2-hydroxyglutaric, 5-hydroxyhexanoic, adipic, suberic, sebacic, and dodecanedioic acids. Abnormal levels of short-chain volatile acids, such as isovaleric, isobutyric, and 2-methylbutyric, have been noted, as have isovaleryl-, isobutyryl-, and 2-methylbutyryl-glycine conjugates. A generalized aminoaciduria along with elevations of proline and hydroxyproline is common. Usually, ketonuria is not present. Treatment with riboflavin, carnitine, and a diet low in fat and protein may be attempted but usually is not effective.

In the infantile or "childhood" form, usually patients do not have physical anomalies. This mild form, also known as *ethylmalonic-adipic aciduria*, varies in onset from infancy to adulthood. It is accompanied by episodic vomiting, hypoglycemia, acidosis, and hypotonia similar to that in Reye syndrome. Some patients have hepatomegaly and myopathies. With episodes, urinary organic acid profiles will show a pattern similar to, but less elevated than, that of the severe form. Sometimes, the only finding will be an elevation in urine ethylmalonic acid. Plasma acyl-carnitine profiles may be abnormal with metabolites typical of more than one enzymatic defect, especially when the affected patients are acutely ill. Elevated blood and urine sarcosine levels may be noted. Plasma carnitine levels may be low or show an elevated esterified fraction. Treatment with riboflavin, carnitine, and a diet low in protein and fat is indicated. Episodes should be treated vigorously with intravenous glucose and hydration.

A fourth form of the disorder was reported in adults with progressive lipid storage myopathies and episodic ketosis. Most patients respond to riboflavin treatment.

ETF and ETF:QO deficiencies have been reported with both forms of the disorder. The severe neonatal form with congenital anomalies is more likely to be associated with ETF:QO deficiency. ETF is composed of two subunits, alpha and beta. Several mutations and deletions have been reported for the alpha subunit and the beta subunit genes, at chromosomal locations 15q23-q25 and 19q13.3, respectively. Mutations have been found also in the gene that encodes for ETF:QO (ETF dehydrogenase, ETFDH), which is located at chromosome 4q32qter. Prenatal diagnosis is available for the severe forms.

Suggested Readings

Andresen BS, Bross P, Vianey-Saban C, et al. Cloning and characterization of human very-long-chain acyl-CoA dehydrogenase cDNA, chromosomal assignment of the gene and identification in four patients of nine different mutations within the VLCAD gene. *Hum Mol Genet* 1996;5:461.

Bennett M, Weinberger MJ, Kobori JA, et al. Mitochondrial short-chain L-3-hydroxyacyl-coenzyme A dehydrogenase deficiency: a new defect of fatty acid oxidation. *Pediatr Res* 1996;39:185.

Brown-Harrison MC, Nada MA, Sprecher H, et al. Very long chain acyl-CoA dehydrogenase deficiency: successful treatment of acute cardiomyopathy. *Biochem Mol Med* 1996;58:59.

Eaton S, Bartlett K, Pourfarzam M. Mammalian mitochondrial beta-oxidation. *Biochem J* 1996;320:345.

Frerman FE, Goodman SI. Defects of electron transfer flavoprotein and electron transfer flavoprotein-ubiquinone oxidoreductase: glutaric acidemia type II. In: Scriver CR, Beaudet AL, Sly WS, Valle D, eds. *The metabolic and molecular bases of inherited disease*, 8th ed. New York: McGraw-Hill, 2001;2357.

Gobin S, Bonnefont JP, Prip-Buus C, et al. Organization of the human liver carnitine palmitoyltransferase 1 gene (CPT1A) and identification of novel mutations in hypoketotic hypoglycaemia. *Hum Genet* 2002;111:179.

Iafolla AK, Thompson RJ, Roe CR. Medium-chain acyl coenzyme A dehydrogenase deficiency: clinical course in 120 affected children. *J Pediatr* 1994;124:409.

Largilliere C, Vianey-Saban C, Fontaine M, et al. Mitochondrial very long chain acyl-CoA dehydrogenase deficiency—a new disorder of fatty acid oxidation. *Arch Dis Child* 1995;73:F103.

Nada MA, Vianey-Saban C, Roe CR, et al. Prenatal diagnosis of mitochondrial fatty acid oxidation defects. *Prenat Diagn* 1996;16:117.

Rinaldo P, Matern D, Bennett MJ. Fatty acid oxidation disorders. *Annu Rev Physiol* 2002;64:477.

Roe CR. Clinical experience with carnitine deficiency. *J Rare Dis* 1997;3:5.

Roe CR, Ding J. Mitochondrial fatty acid oxidation disorders. In: Scriver CR, Beaudet AL, Sly WS, Valle D, eds. *The metabolic and molecular bases of inherited disease*, 8th ed. New York: McGraw-Hill, 2001:2297.

Spiekerkoetter U, Sun B, Khuchua Z, et al. Molecular and phenotypic heterogeneity in mitochondrial trifunctional protein deficiency due to beta-subunit mutations. *Hum Mutat* 2003;21:598.

Stanley CA, DeLeeuw S, Coates PM, et al. Chronic cardiomyopathy and weakness or acute coma in children with a defect in carnitine uptake. *Ann Neurol* 1991;30:706.

Stanley CA, Hale DE, Berry GT, et al. A deficiency of carnitine-acylcarnitine translocase in the inner mitochondrial membrane. *N Engl J Med* 1992;327:19.

Strauss AW, Powell CK, Hale DE, et al. Molecular basis of human mitochondrial very-long-chain acyl-CoA dehydrogenase deficiency causing cardiomyopathy and sudden death in childhood. *Proc Natl Acad Sci USA* 1995;92:10496.

Turnbull DM, Bartlett K, Stevens DL, et al. Short-chain acyl-CoA dehydrogenase deficiency associated with a lipid storage myopathy and secondary carnitine deficiency. *N Engl J Med* 1984;311:1230.

Tyni T, Pihko H. Long-chain 3-hydroxyacyl-CoA dehydrogenase deficiency. *Acta Pediatr* 1999;88:237.

Yamaguchi S, Indo Y, Coates PM, et al. Identification of very-long-chain acyl-CoA dehydrogenase deficiency in three patients previously diagnosed with long-chain acyl-CoA dehydrogenase deficiency. *Pediatr Res* 1993;34:111.

CHAPTER 387 ■ DISORDERS OF CARBOHYDRATE METABOLISM

REBECCA S. WAPPNER

CARBOHYDRATE METABOLISM

Dietary carbohydrates include polymeric starch from plant sources, glycogen from animal sources, disaccharides in the form of lactose from milk sources and sucrose from fruit and vegetable sources, and, to a lesser extent, such monosaccharides as glucose, galactose, and fructose. The polymers and disaccharides are hydrolyzed to monosaccharides by enzymes present in the brush border of intestinal villi. The free monosaccharides—glucose, galactose, and fructose—are absorbed and transported to the liver, where they are used rapidly. Carbohydrate metabolism in the liver is concerned primarily with maintenance of blood glucose concentration. Glucose may be formed by the metabolism of dietary carbohydrates, from degradation of glycogen, or by gluconeogenesis from amino acids, glycerol, and lactate. Glucose-6-phosphate occupies a central position in the pathways in that all sources for free glucose first must be converted to glucose-6-phosphate except for that resulting from the action of debrancher enzyme on glycogen. In addition to being used for free glucose, glucose-6-phosphate also may be used for glycogen synthesis; for glycolysis and the production of lactate and CO_2 by the Embden-Meyerhof pathway; for the production of the reduced form of nicotinamide adenine dinucleotide and CO_2 by entering the pentose cycle; and for glucuronate formation. The major disorders of carbohydrate metabolism involve the intermediary metabolism of glycogen, galactose, and fructose.

DISORDERS OF GLYCOGEN SYNTHESIS AND DEGRADATION

Glycogen Metabolism

Glycogen, the principal storage form of carbohydrate in humans, is found primarily in liver and muscle. It is a high-molecular-weight, highly branched, spherical structure composed of up to 60,000 glucosyl residues attached to a single glycogenin protein molecule. The glucosyl residues are joined in alpha-1,4-linkage to form linear chains. Branch points occur at intervals of four to ten residues where the connecting glucosyl residues are attached in alpha-1,6-linkage. Ten percent of the glucosyl residues are at the nonreducing end of the molecules; 60% of them are on outer branches, making them readily accessible for glycogenolysis. The usual concentration of glycogen in liver is less than 5 g per 100 g of wet weight. Additional information about glycogen metabolism is presented in Box 387.1.

Classification of Glycogen Storage Disorders

The disorders associated with abnormal synthesis and degradation of glycogen vary widely in their clinical spectrum. Overall they occur in one in 20,000 to 25,000 live births. Table 387.1 lists the disorders according to their currently accepted type and specific enzymatic or other metabolic defect. The disorders may have primarily hepatic or muscle involvement.

Hepatic Glycogen Storage Disorders

The hepatic glycogen storage disorders are estimated to occur in at least 1 in 60,000 births. Often, the pathogenesis of the various disorders may be predicted by the site of their associated enzymatic defects. All cause some degree of hepatomegaly and (usually) hypoglycemia. Functional testing may help to distinguish between the disorders. The presence of fasting hypoglycemia, the response to glucagon in the fasting and fed state, the response of blood glucose to the administration of such other carbohydrates as galactose, and the type of glucose response noted with a glucose tolerance test may be used to help differentiate between the disorders. All fasting and tolerance testing should be done with caution and close observation of the patient. For the severe disorders, the presence of lactic acidosis and hypoglycemia may be considered a relative contraindication to proceeding with fasting, glucagon stimulation,

---

BOX 387.1   Glycogen Metabolism

Glycogen is synthesized from glucose-1-phosphate by the actions of three enzymes (Fig. 387.1). Uridine diphosphate (UDP)-glucose pyrophosphorylase converts glucose-1-phosphate to UDP-glucose. Glycogen synthetase catalyzes the transfer of glucosyl residues from the UDP-glucose to a glycogenin protein molecule to form a glycogen primer. Glycogen synthetase also catalyzes the attachment of additional glucosyl residues in alpha-1,4-linkage to lengthen the chains. And, the brancher enzyme, amylo-1,4-1,6-transglucosylase, creates the branch points by attaching glucosyl residues in alpha-1,6-linkage to the linear chains.

Glycogen degradation involves sequential removal of nonreducing terminal glucosyl residues by a phosphorylase system and the debrancher enzyme. Phosphorylase exists in both inactive (b) and active (a) forms. Conversion of the phosphorylase to the active form requires the presence of adenosine triphosphate (ATP) and active phosphorylase kinase. Phosphorylase kinase also exists in inactive (b) and active (a) forms and is activated in the presence of ATP by a protein kinase generated in response to increased cyclic adenosine monophosphate (cAMP) formation from hormonal and chemical influences on the hepatic parenchymal cell plasma membrane. The activated phosphorylase a cleaves the alpha-1,4-linkages of the outer chains to within four glucosyl residues of the branch points and liberates glucose-1-phosphate. Then debrancher enzyme is needed for further degradation to proceed. Debrancher functions both as a transferase, which moves the three outermost glucosyl residues to another linear chain, and as an amylo-1,6-glucosidase, which then removes the final glucosyl residue in branched alpha-1,6-linkage with liberation of free glucose. In this manner, approximately 10% free glucose and 90%

glucose-1-phosphate is released. The glucose-1-phosphate is converted to glucose-6-phosphate by phosphoglucomutase. Then, glucose-6-phosphate is converted to free glucose and inorganic phosphate by the glucose-6-phosphatase system.

The active site of microsomal glucose-6-phosphatase is located within the lumen of the endoplasmic reticulum. Substrates and products of its activity thus must cross the endoplasmic reticulum membrane. Five different proteins are now recognized to be necessary for normal hepatic glucose-6-phosphatase activity. The catalytic subunit of glucose-6-phosphatase hydrolyzes glucose-6-phosphate. At least four microsomal transport proteins also are involved. Microsomal transport protein T1 transports glucose-6-phosphate, the substrate for the reaction, into the lumen of the endoplasmic reticulum. Two microsomal transport proteins transport inorganic phosphate, pyrophosphate, and carbamyl phosphate across the microsomal membrane and out of the lumen where they would inhibit glucose-6-phosphatase activity. And, microsomal transport protein GLUT2, one of a family of proteins that facilitate transport of glucose across plasma membranes, transports free glucose from the microsomal lumen to the cytosol.

The synthesis and degradation of hepatic glycogen are regulated primarily by cAMP, glucose, and glycogen. An increased demand for blood glucose results in increased activation of phosphorylase and suppression of glycogen synthetase activity. Hepatic glycogen functions as a reserve for blood glucose. In contrast, muscle glycogen functions mainly as a fuel reserve for ATP generation, which is needed during exercise and usually does not contribute to blood glucose levels. Under anaerobic conditions, muscle glycogen can be degraded also to lactate by glycolysis.

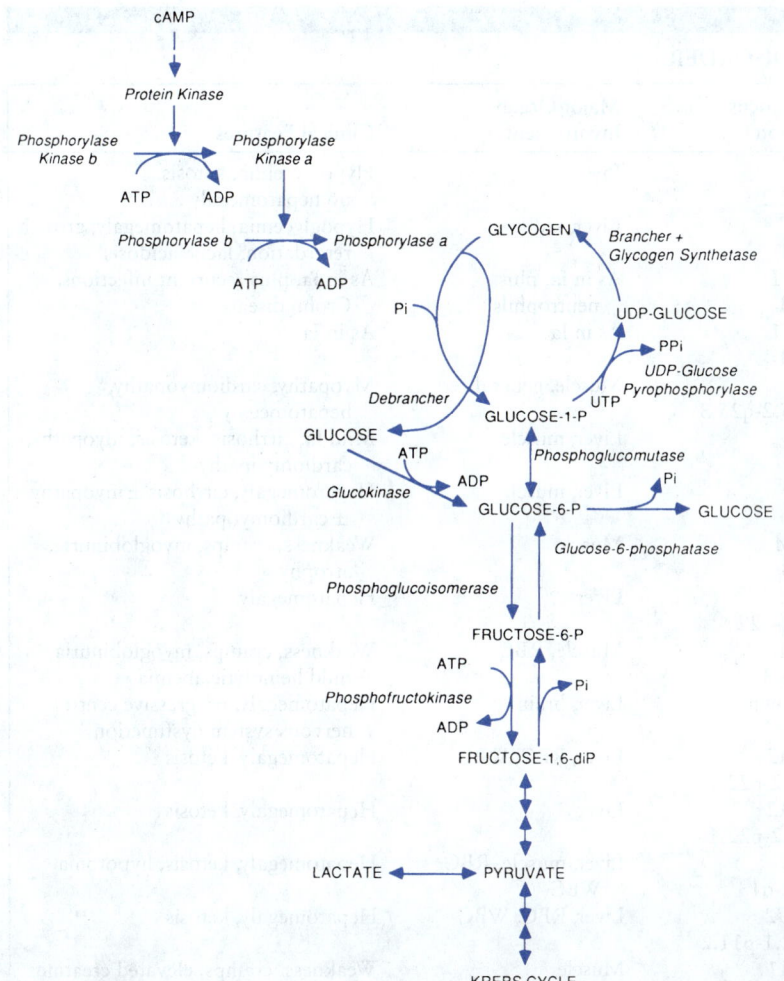

FIGURE 387.1. Glycogen synthesis and degradation. ADP, adenosine diphosphate; ATP, adenosine triphosphate; cAMP, cyclic adenosine monophosphate; diP, diphosphatase; P, phosphatase; Pi, inorganic phosphate; PPi, inorganic pyrophosphate; UDP, uridine diphosphate; UTP, uridine triphosphate.

and other tests in the classic fashion. Liver and muscle biopsies may be performed to assess the total content of glycogen and the type of glycogen structure present and to document deficient activity of specific enzymes. Open liver biopsies and muscle biopsies, rather than punch biopsies, are preferred because of the sample size needed for these analyses. Muscle biopsy should be performed simultaneously with open liver biopsy, regardless of the suspected clinical type of glycogen storage. Most important is that an experienced laboratory be contacted before obtaining the samples to ensure appropriate handling. Because many of the disorders may be documented by enzymatic analysis or by molecular genetic techniques in leukocytes, erythrocytes, or cultured skin fibroblasts, these less invasive procedures should be performed first, if possible.

All the disorders are inherited as autosomal recessive traits except for three forms of type IX glycogen storage disease (GSD), which are inherited as X-linked traits. Carrier detection and prenatal diagnosis vary, depending on the tissue distribution of the enzyme involved and whether molecular genetic testing is available for the specific disorder.

Type Ia (von Gierke Disease). Type Ia GSD, also known as *hepatorenal GSD*, is associated with deficient activity of glucose-6-phosphatase in the liver, kidney, and intestine. Patients have a defective catalytic subunit of the enzyme. Affected individuals experience marked hepatomegaly, lactic acidosis, and hypoglycemia. The disorder is diagnosed most often between ages 3 and 4 months but may be recognized in the neonatal period.

Milder forms may present at later ages with hepatomegaly and short stature. Other clinical features include a doll-like appearance, decreased muscle mass, renal enlargement, vomiting, diarrhea, and failure of maturation in puberty. Many affected infants are obese as a result of demanding frequent feedings, including nocturnal feedings beyond the time this behavior usually disappears (Fig. 387.2).

Fasting hypoglycemia may be profound and often results in no clinical symptoms in untreated patients. This tolerance of hypoglycemia is thought to be the result of the ability of these patients to use alternative substrates for glucose in the brain. Glucose-6-phosphatase is essential for the normal release of hepatic free-glucose, whether it is the product of glycogenolysis or gluconeogenesis. Dietary carbohydrates other than glucose also cannot be converted to glucose because the conversion involves glucose-6-phosphatase as the final step. The fasting hypoglycemia results in activation of phosphorylase and hepatic glycogenolysis, which leads to the formation of glucose-6-phosphate. The glucose-6-phosphate then is metabolized to lactate by glycolysis. Gluconeogenesis also is stimulated, and a recycling between lactate and glycogen occurs, resulting in a net increase in lactate. Stimulation of the glycolytic and gluconeogenic pathways also results in elevated triglyceride, cholesterol, very low-density lipoprotein, free fatty acid, and uric acid levels. Xanthomas, lipemia retinalis, gout, and uric acid nephropathy may occur. Biotinidase activity, frequently measured as part of newborn screening panels, is elevated in Type Ia, but not Type Ib GSD.

TABLE 387.1

CLASSIFICATION OF GLYCOGEN STORAGE DISORDERS

Type	Enzyme or Metabolic Process Affected	Gene Locus Location	Major Organ Involvement	Clinical Features
0	Glycogen synthetase	GYS2 12p12.2	Liver	Hypoglycemia, ketosis, no hepatomegaly
Ia	Glucose-6-phosphatase	G6PT 17q21	Liver, kidney	Hypoglycemia, hepatomegaly, growth retardation, lactic acidosis
Ib	Microsomal transport of glucose-6-phosphate	G6PT1 11q23	As in Ia, plus neutrophils	As in Ia, plus recurrent infections, Crohn disease
Ic	Microsomal transport of phosphate	G6PT1 11q23	As in Ia	As in Ia
II	Lysosomal alpha-glucosidase	GAA 12q25.2-q25.3	Muscle, generalized	Myopathy, cardiomyopathy, hepatomegaly
III	Debrancher	AGL 1p21	Liver, muscle	Mild Ia, cirrhosis, ketosis, myopathy, cardiomyopathy
IV	Brancher	GBE1 3p12	Liver, muscle	Hepatomegaly, cirrhosis $\pm$ myopathy $\pm$ cardiomyopathy
V	Muscle phosphorylase	PYGM 11q13	Muscle	Weakness, cramps, myoglobinuria, atrophy
VI	Hepatic phosphorylase	PYGL 14q21-q22	Liver	Hepatomegaly
VII	Muscle phosphofructokinase	PFKM 12q13.3	Muscle, RBC	Weakness, cramps, myoglobinuria $\pm$ mild hemolytic anemia
VIII	Loss of activation of phosphorylase	Unknown	Liver, brain	Hepatomegaly, progressive central nervous system dysfunction
IXa-1	Phosphorylase kinase (PK), alpha-liver subunit	PHKA2 Xp22.2-p22.1	Liver, RBC, WBC	Hepatomegaly, ketosis
IXa-2	PK, alpha-liver subunit	PHKA2 Xp22.2-p22.1	Liver	Hepatomegaly, ketosis
IXb	PK, beta subunit	PHKB 16q12-q13	Liver, muscle, RBC, WBC	Hepatomegaly, ketosis, hypotonia
IXc	PK, gamma-testis/liver subunit	PHKG2 16p12.1-p11.2	Liver, RBC, WBC	Hepatomegaly, ketosis
IXd	PK, alpha-muscle subunit	PHKA1 Xq12-q13	Muscle	Weakness, cramps, elevated creatine kinase
IXe	PK, subunit defect unknown	Unknown	Muscle	Myopathy
IXf	PK, subunit defect unknown	Unknown	Heart	Neonatal cardiomyopathy $\pm$ hypoglycemia
X	cAMP-dependent kinase	Unknown	Liver, muscle	Hepatomegaly $\pm$ mild hypotonia
XI	Microsomal transport of glucose	GLUT2 3q26.1-q26.3	Liver, kidney	Hepatomegaly, renal tubular dysfunction

The types are numbered according to chronologic order of recognition.
cAMP, cyclic adenosine monophosphate; RBC, red blood cell; WBC, white blood cell.

Liver transaminases are normal or elevated only slightly. Within the liver parenchyma, adenomatous nodules may develop, which before current dietary therapy occasionally were reported to transform into hepatic carcinoma. Abnormal bleeding tendencies that occur are thought to result from decreased platelet adhesiveness associated with the hypoglycemia. Hypercalcuria and, occasionally, renal tubular dysfunction may be present during childhood. Frequently, adults develop progressive renal disease, including focal segmental glomerulosclerosis and interstitial fibrosis.

Because patients with type I GSD frequently become hypoglycemic after 2 to 3 hours of fasting, any tolerance or stimulation test should be done cautiously and with intravenous glucose at hand. Glucose tolerance testing gives a diabetic-type early response. Fasting insulin levels are low. No glycemic response to galactose occurs (1 to 2 g/kg of 20% solution, orally or intravenously). Glucagon stimulation (20 to 30 μg/kg intramuscularly or intravenously; maximum dose, 1 mg) occasionally will produce a response, which is defined as a rise in blood glucose of 50% more than baseline. Lactic acid levels will rise with fasting and with glucagon or galactose administration. Glycogen content is elevated in the liver, kidney, and intestine. Glycogen structure is normal. On liver biopsy, the hepatocytes are noted to have glycogen in the nuclei and lipid droplets of varying size in the cytoplasm. Cirrhosis is not evident. The diagnosis may be confirmed by demonstrating a recognized mutation at the glucose-6-phosphatase gene locus in peripheral leukocytes or by measurement of glucose-6-phosphatase in liver or intestinal biopsy samples. Prenatal diagnosis and carrier detection are available only in families in whom the molecular defects are known.

Treatment is directed at supplying continuous exogenous glucose. Infants are given a formula with glucose or glucose polymers as the only carbohydrate source. Older children are given similar enteral supplements and are restricted in their intake of natural sources of galactose and fructose. Frequent daily feedings every 2 to 3 hours are supplemented with nocturnal nasogastric or gastrostomy drip feeding. Uncooked cornstarch

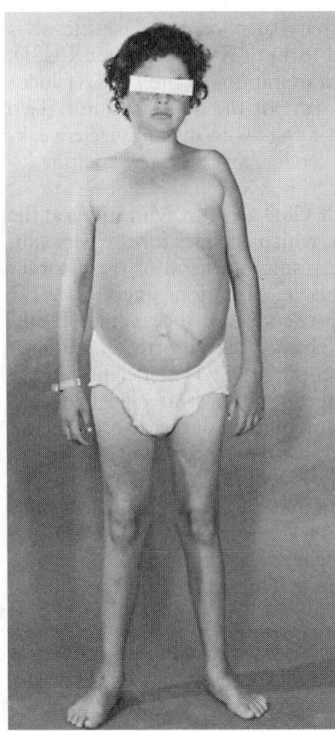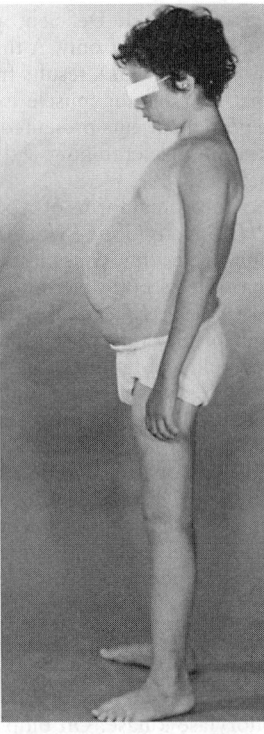

FIGURE 387.2. Glycogen storage disease Ia in a 13-year-old patient.

slurries may be used with older children and adults. Clinical and laboratory improvement is remarkable with dietary therapy. Usually, hepatic adenomas regress. Long-term survival is possible. However, affected patients continue to be at risk for significant acidosis and hypoglycemia with intercurrent illnesses or if enteral feedings are interrupted. Renal transplantation has been performed for renal failure. Liver transplantation has been shown to correct attendant biochemical abnormalities and should be considered if malignant transformation of adenomas occurs.

Type Ib. Type Ib GSD is similar in clinical and laboratory findings to type Ia GSD. Patients also have abnormalities of neutrophil mobility and neutropenia, recurrent infections, and Crohn disease. The disorder is caused by defective transport of glucose-6-phosphate across the microsomal membrane of hepatocytes and leukocytes, owing to a defective microsomal transport protein, T1. Decreased levels of the T1 transport protein in liver biopsy samples will confirm the diagnosis. Treatment is similar to that for type Ia GSD. In addition, the neutropenia usually is responsive to recombinant human granulocyte-monocyte colony-stimulating factor or granulocyte colony-stimulating factor. Patients also will need the care of a pediatric hematologist and gastroenterologist.

Type Ic. Type Ic GSD has been reported in a few patients with deficient microsomal transport of inorganic phosphate and pyrophosphate. The clinical features are similar to that for type Ia GSD.

Type II (Pompe Disease). Pompe disease is associated with deficient activity of lysosomal alpha-glucosidase (acid maltase) and generalized storage of glycogen. Major clinical findings include progressive myopathy, cardiomyopathy, and hepatomegaly. The disorder is discussed with the lysosomal storage disorders in Chapter 389.

Type III (Cori Disease). Type III GSD is associated with deficient activity of the debrancher enzyme amylo-1,6-glucosidase.

The disorder also is known as *limit dextrinosis* because glycogen of abnormal structure, similar to limit dextrin with short outer chains, is stored in liver and muscle. Most affected patients have both hepatic and muscle involvement. During early childhood, hepatic involvement predominates, and patients present in the first year of life with fasting hypoglycemia, hepatomegaly, and growth retardation. Occasionally, myopathy or cardiomyopathy occurs. No renal enlargement is noted, but renal tubular dysfunction may be seen. Mild inflammatory disease of the liver and cirrhosis may occur.

As adults, the patients often develop a progressive myopathy with abnormal electromyographs and nerve conduction velocities. Cardiomyopathy may occur. Some patients with debrancher deficiency, however, have only hepatic involvement and do not develop progressive muscle involvement.

Functional studies with glucose tolerance testing will reveal a diabetic-type early response. The response to glucagon varies but usually is normal in the fed state; no response is seen in the fasted state. Fasting lactate levels are normal but become elevated after a glucose load. Fasting ketonuria and elevated liver transaminations are seen commonly, which help to distinguish type III from type I GSD. Blood levels of cholesterol and uric acid may be elevated. Glycogen content is elevated in liver, muscle, and erythrocytes. The glycogen structure is abnormal. Liver biopsy samples have more nuclear glycogen and fewer lipid droplets than are seen with type Ia GSD. Often, fibrous septa are present. Treatment includes frequent feedings that are high in protein. Carbohydrate intake is not restricted because gluconeogenesis is intact. Galactose and fructose are converted readily to glucose. During childhood, however, nocturnal drip feedings may be required for fasting hypoglycemia. Usually, hepatic symptoms improve with age.

The diagnosis may be established by showing deficient activity of debrancher in many tissues, including leukocytes, erythrocytes, and cultured skin fibroblasts, and in liver and muscle biopsies. DNA-based diagnosis also is available. Confirmation of the risk for significant muscle involvement before clinical symptoms are present, however, can be made only by demonstrating debrancher deficiency in muscle biopsies in addition to other tissues.

Type IV (Andersen Disease). Type IV GSD is associated with deficiency of the brancher enzyme amylo-1,4-1,6-transglucosylase. The disorder also is known as *amylopectinosis* because the glycogen stored has fewer than the normal number of branch points and long outer chains similar to what is seen in amylopectin. The decreased branching makes the glycogen less soluble. The cirrhosis seen in this disease is thought to result from a foreign-body reaction to the abnormal glycogen. Usually, affected infants are normal at birth but develop hepatomegaly and failure to thrive within a few months of age. Often, progressive fibrosis of the liver leads to cirrhosis, splenomegaly, and liver failure. Liver transplantation has been performed with variable outcomes. Some patients present with poor motor development, hypotonia, muscle atrophy, and absent reflexes as major clinical manifestations. Cardiac involvement may occur and can be severe. Many severely affected patients die by age 4 years. Patients with milder cases have a longer lifespan and, in some, the condition even improves with age. Usually, liver, muscle, and erythrocyte glycogen concentrations are normal, but the glycogen has an abnormal structure. The enzymatic defect may be demonstrated in leukocytes, cultured skin fibroblasts, and liver. Carrier detection and prenatal diagnosis are available.

Type VI (Hers Disease). Type VI GSD is a rare disorder associated with deficient activity of hepatic phosphorylase and hepatomegaly. Hypoglycemia is rare, and hepatomegaly may recede with age. Occasionally, patients have hepatic fibrosis and elevated serum lipids and transaminases. Glucagon usually produces no glycemic response. Elevation of liver glycogen content of normal structure occurs. Deficient activity of hepatic phosphorylase may be demonstrated in liver. The disorder may be indistinguishable clinically from the hepatic forms of type IX GSD and type X GSD.

Type VIII. Type VIII GSD is a very rare disorder characterized by the onset of hepatomegaly and progressive central nervous system degeneration shortly after birth. No clinical problems are found with glucose homeostasis. Glycogen concentration is increased in the liver and on cerebral biopsy. The particulate matter in the brain appears larger than usual on electron microscopy. Liver phosphorylase activity is low and is thought to result from impaired regulation of phosphorylase activation. The exact biochemical defect is not known.

Type IX. Type IX GSD is associated with deficient activity of phosphorylase kinase. Varying clinical and genetic forms of the disorder exist that correlate with the molecular findings. Four different subunits of the enzyme are termed *alpha*, *beta*, *gamma*, and *delta* on the basis of descending order of molecular weight. The subunits have tissue-specific isoforms that account for the clinical variability of the disease. Genetic loci for the subunits are located on both autosomes and the X chromosome, which explains the genetic variability. Additional information about the genes that code for the different subunits is presented in Box 387.2.

Type IXa-1 GSD, a common form accounting for approximately 25% of cases, results from mutations at the *PHKA2* locus on the X chromosome that encodes for the liver isoform of the alpha subunit. Affected boys present during early childhood with massive hepatomegaly, growth retardation, and mild delays in motor development. Any fasting hypoglycemia is mild. Fasting lactate levels may be normal or slightly elevated, fasting ketonuria is common, and response to glucagon is normal. Elevated triglycerides, cholesterol, and liver function tests are noted. In most patients, the hepatomegaly and other clinical findings resolve by adult life. A few patients have developed nodular cirrhosis with portal hypertension in late childhood. Glycogen of normal structure is elevated. Deficient activity of phosphorylase kinase may be demonstrated in the liver, leukocytes, erythrocytes, and cultured skin fibroblasts. *Type IXa-2 GSD*, a rare X-linked disorder, results from mutations at the *PHKA2* locus, allelic to but different from those associated with type IXa-1 GSD. Clinical presentation is similar to that

for type IXa-1. Deficient activity of phosphorylase kinase is confined to liver only. A third form of X-linked type IX GSD, termed *IXd GSD*, results from mutations in the *PHKA1* locus that encodes for muscle isoforms of the alpha subunit. Two reported patients presented as adults with distal muscle weakness, muscle cramping with exercise, and elevated creatine kinase levels.

Autosomal forms of type IX GSD are rare. Mutations at the *PHKB* locus (*Type IXb GSD*), which encodes for the beta subunit of phosphorylase kinase, result in a form of the disorder that affects both liver and muscle. Mutations at the *PHKG2* locus (*Type IXc GSD*), which encodes for the gamma-T subunit of phosphorylase kinase, have been reported in patients with clinical findings similar to type IXa-1. Deficient activity of phosphorylase kinase has been demonstrated in liver and blood cells. And, a third autosomal form of the disorder (*Type IXf GSD*) is characterized by a severe progressive neonatal cardiomyopathy. One patient was reported also to have neonatal hypoglycemia. The molecular basis for the disorder is unknown. Deficiency of phosphorylase kinase is confined to cardiac muscle. The inheritance pattern is unclear for *Type IXe GSD*, which affects muscle only. The subunit defect and genetic locus are likewise unknown.

Type X. Type X GSD is associated with failure of activation of hepatic and muscle phosphorylase caused by deficiency of a cAMP-dependent protein kinase needed for activation of phosphorylase kinase. On biopsy, phosphorylase is found only in the b or inactive form. The disorder is similar to types VI and IX GSD. One reported patient also had minimal muscle symptoms.

Type XI (Fanconi-Bickel Syndrome). Type XI GSD is characterized by marked hepatomegaly, growth retardation, and proximal renal tubular dysfunction of the Fanconi type during childhood. Renal bicarbonate and phosphate wasting may lead to acidosis and rickets. Affected patients also have galactose intolerance from decreased galactose utilization and may have mild fasting hypoglycemia. Liver transaminases and lactic acid levels are normal. Glycogen accumulation is noted in hepatocytes and proximal renal tubular cells. Treatment includes a galactose-restricted diet along with replacement of electrolytes, bicarbonate, phosphorus, and vitamin D for the renal tubular dysfunction. The disorder results from deficiency of the GLUT2 microsomal transport protein that transports free glucose in hepatocytes, pancreatic beta cells, and the basolateral membranes of intestinal and renal epithelial cells.

Type O. Type O GSD is associated with deficient activity of hepatic glycogen synthetase. Patients present during the first year of life with fasting hypoglycemia and ketosis. Hepatomegaly is not present. Often, clinically distinguishing the disorder from ketotic hypoglycemia is difficult. Lactate may increase after a glucose load or after 12 hours of fasting. The glucose tolerance test is diabetic type. Hypoglycemia is not responsive to glucagon. The diagnosis is made by confirmation of the enzymatic defect on liver biopsy. The hepatic glycogen concentration is reduced markedly but is not absent. Treatment consists of frequent high-protein feedings.

Muscle Glycogen Storage Disorders

Two disorders of glycogen metabolism, types V and VII GSD, affect only muscle. They have a similar clinical presentation and often can be distinguished only by demonstration of the specific enzymatic defect on muscle biopsy. Resting muscle derives its energy from the oxidation of glucose and fatty acids. With exercise, the requirement for adenosine triphosphate (ATP) may increase several hundredfold, and the demand for substrates for aerobic metabolism may exceed that supplied from the blood. The additional ATP required must come from glycogenolysis. In both disorders, the enzymatic defects occur in the glycolytic

---

| BOX 387.2 | **Genetic Variability in Type IX Glycogen Storage Disease** |

Two genes—*PHKA1* (alpha-muscle) and *PHKA2* (alpha-liver)—encode alpha subunit isoforms and are located at two separate sites, Xq12-q13 and Xp22.2-p22.1, respectively, on the X chromosome. The beta subunit is encoded by only one gene (*PHKB*) at autosomal location chromosome 16q12-q13. Isoforms of the beta subunit exist, but as a result of alternative mRNA splicing rather than of being encoded by different genetic loci. The gamma subunit isoforms are encoded by genes *PHKG1* (gamma-muscle) and *PHKG2* (gamma-T, or testis-liver-other not muscle) at separate chromosomal sites 7q21 and 16p12.1-p11.2, respectively. Also, the delta subunit is encoded by the gene *PHKD1* (also termed *CALM1*) at chromosomal location 14q24-q31. The gamma subunit is the catalytic subunit; the other subunits are regulatory. The delta subunit is one of a family of calmodulins, or calcium-binding regulatory proteins.

pathway, and no increase in muscle or blood lactate occurs with exercise. During childhood and adolescence, affected patients are noted to have increased fatigability. Between ages 20 and 40 years, severe muscle cramps, myoglobinuria, and elevated blood levels of lactate dehydrogenase, aldolase, and creatine kinase are noted with exercise. After age 40, the cramps and myoglobinuria are less evident, but muscle wasting and weakness appear with increasing severity. Reduced exercise tolerance may be demonstrated by having the patient perform an ischemic exercise test. With a blood pressure cuff on the arm inflated to more than systolic pressure, repeated pressure on a rubber ball by the hand usually will produce severe muscle cramping. Measurement of venous lactate levels in the same arm before and after exercise will fail to show the normal rise. Skeletal muscle biopsy reveals increased glycogen deposits in the cytoplasm beneath the sarcolemma. Treatment involves avoidance of strenuous exercise, which may result in myoglobinuria and acute renal failure.

Type V (McArdle Disease). Type V GSD is associated with deficient activity of muscle phosphorylase. Elevated muscle glycogen content and the enzymatic defect may be demonstrated on muscle biopsy. Severe early-onset variants, presenting in a neonate and a 4-year-old, have been reported.

Type VII (Tarui Disease). Type VII GSD is associated with deficient activity of muscle phosphofructokinase, which catalyzes the conversion of fructose-6-phosphate to fructose-1,6-diphosphate. Phosphofructokinase is important in the regulation of glycolysis in muscle and affects the use of both glycogen and glucose in muscle. Glycogen content of muscles is increased secondary to increased stimulation of glycogen synthetase and uridine diphosphate (UDP)-glucose pyrophosphorylase. An abnormal polysaccharide, with a fine fibrillar appearance resembling amylopectin, is present. Usually, the disorder is more severe than is type V GSD. Erythrocyte phosphofructokinase activity also is decreased to approximately 50% of normal, and patients may have a mild hemolytic anemia. A severe variant of the disorder has been described in a child who died at age 6 months from respiratory failure. The enzymatic defect may be demonstrated on muscle biopsy.

DISORDERS OF GALACTOSE METABOLISM

Galactose Metabolism

Galactose, the major dietary carbohydrate in infants, must be converted to glucose to be used as an energy source. This conversion occurs primarily in hepatocytes by the Leloir pathway (Fig. 387.3). Galactose first is phosphorylated to galactose-1-phosphate by a specific galactokinase. The galactose-1-phosphate then reacts with UDP-glucose to form UDP-galactose and glucose-1-phosphate in the presence of galactose-1-phosphate uridyl transferase. UDP-galactose is converted to UDP-glucose by UDP-galactose-4-epimerase.

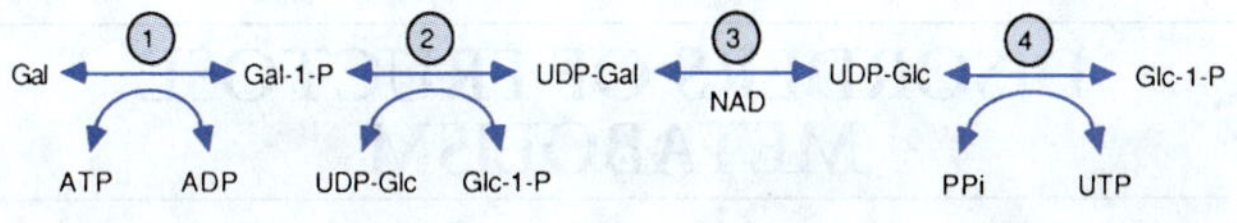

FIGURE 387.3. Disorders of galactose metabolism. 1, galactokinase; 2, galactose-1-phosphate uridyltransferase; 3, UDP-galactose-4-epimerase; 4, UDP-glucose phosphorylase; ADP, adenosine diphosphate; ATP, adenosine triphosphate; Gal, galactose; Glc, glucose; NAD, nicotinamide adenine dinucleotide; P, phosphate; PPi, inorganic pyrophosphate; UDP, uridine diphosphate; UTP, uridine triphosphate.

The UDP-glucose formed may reenter the Leloir pathway at the transferase step and react with pyrophosphate to form glucose-1-phosphate, or it may be used to form glycogen in the presence of glycogen synthetase.

Galactose may be reduced also by a nonspecific aldose reductase in the presence of the reduced form of nicotinamide adenine dinucleotide to form galactitol. In patients with kinase and transferase deficiencies, elevated galactitol levels lead to osmotic swelling and disruption of lenticular fibers, resulting in cataract formation.

UDP-galactose also may be synthesized in the body from glucose-1-phosphate by reversing the Leloir pathway. In this manner, UDP-galactosyl residues needed for biosynthesis of macromolecules, such as gangliosides, may be generated even in the absence of dietary galactose. The UDP-galactose may be converted also to galactose-1-phosphate by pyrophosphorylase, which is thought to be the source of the galactose-1-phosphate seen in patients with well-controlled transferase deficiency.

Galactokinase Deficiency

Galactokinase deficiency, an autosomal recessive trait that occurs in approximately 1 in 150,000 births, is associated with increased galactose in body fluids. The disorder results from mutations in the *GALK1* gene at chromosome location 17p24. The major clinical manifestation is nuclear cataracts, which begin to form after birth and usually are apparent clinically by early infancy if a lactose-containing diet is taken. Frequently, the cataracts are not completely reversible and require surgery. Occasionally, patients develop pseudotumor cerebri. No natural aversion to milk or milk products is seen, nor is the generalized multisystem involvement that occurs in the other types of galactose metabolic defects.

Urinary galactose levels are elevated and may be detected by spot-testing for non–glucose-reducing sugars. Tests for reducing sugars (i.e., Clinitest) will be positive, whereas simultaneous testing specific for glucose (i.e., with Combistix, Glucostix) will be negative or only slightly positive. False negatives may occur in patients on galactose-restricted diets and in those with poor intake. False positives may occur in neonates (especially those who are premature), in patients with intestinal lactase deficiency, and in those with severe liver dysfunction. Galactokinase deficiency may be detected by newborn screening programs that measure blood galactose elevation but not by those programs that measure only galactose-1-phosphate elevation or that screen only for the transferase deficiency. The disorder may be confirmed by demonstrating deficient activity of galactokinase in erythrocytes or cultured skin fibroblasts. Treatment consists of strict dietary elimination of all lactose and galactose sources. Milk and milk products must be avoided strictly, as must other sources of lactose, such as medications (vehicles) and prepared foods. Infants should be given a lactose-free formula. Older children may be given lactose-free calcium supplements. Therapy will arrest further cataract formation but, even with improvement, some visual impairment may remain. Carrier testing and prenatal diagnosis are available.

Galactose-1-Phosphate Uridyl Transferase Deficiency (Classic Galactosemia)

Galactose-1-phosphate uridyl transferase deficiency is the most common disorder of galactose metabolism. It is inherited as an autosomal recessive trait and, in its classic form, occurs in approximately 1 in 62,000 births. Affected infants appear normal at birth. With the ingestion of dietary galactose, symptoms of failure to thrive, vomiting, diarrhea, and lethargy usually are evident by age 1 week. Prolonged physiologic jaundice or the appearance of hepatotoxic jaundice may be evident after age 1 week with increased direct bilirubin. Exchange transfusion and phototherapy may be indicated. Hepatomegaly and abnormal liver function tests are common. Ascites and cirrhosis may occur. Extrahepatic biliary atresia may have been considered. Nuclear cataracts appear within days or weeks and may become irreversible. Often, the cataracts are evident only on slit lamp examination. Renal tubular dysfunction with generalized aminoaciduria, proteinuria, and galactosuria develops. Marasmus and an encephalopathy follow. The symptoms are rapidly progressive, and most untreated infants do not survive past age 6 weeks. Deaths are due most commonly to liver failure and septicemia, especially with *Escherichia coli*. The cataracts are thought to be the result of lenticular accumulation of galactitol, as with the kinase deficiency. Galactose-1-phosphate levels are elevated markedly in the tissues and are thought to be responsible for the hepatic, renal, and central nervous system manifestations of the disorder.

The presence of non–glucose-reducing substances in the urine may be demonstrated, as in galactokinase deficiency. Care should be taken because false-negative results may be obtained in those infants with poor intake, vomiting, or marasmus or in those receiving a galactose-free diet. Galactose tolerance testing is dangerous and should be avoided. The disorder may be confirmed by demonstrating deficient activity of galactose-1-phosphate uridyl transferase in erythrocytes. If an affected child has received a transfusion or an exchange transfusion, a falsely elevated level of erythrocyte enzymatic activity may be obtained. The disorder may be detected also by newborn screening programs that test for elevated blood galactose or galactose-1-phosphate or screen for the transferase by spot enzyme assay (Beutler test). All screening tests should be confirmed with quantitative enzymatic testing and electrophoresis, which can be performed with erythrocytes or cultured skin fibroblasts. Because of the seriousness of the disorder, patients who are presumed to be affected on the basis of newborn screening or on clinical grounds should be changed promptly to a galactose-free diet while awaiting the results of confirmatory testing.

Galactosemia results from mutations at the *GALT* gene locus on chromosome 9p13. Over 300 mutations have been identified. The Q188R mutation is the most common in North American and European patients who have the classic form of the disease. Carrier testing and prenatal diagnosis are available.

Treatment includes strict dietary restriction of all galactose and lactose sources, as for galactokinase deficiency. Affected children improve gradually and dramatically when placed on the diet. Markedly elevated galactose-1-phosphate intracellular levels decrease slowly and may remain elevated for 10 to 15 days. Some persistent mild elevation of erythrocyte galactose-1-phosphate may be seen in patients compliant with galactose restriction and is thought to occur as a result of *in vivo* formation from UDP-galactose. The hepatic and renal manifestations improve slowly and may be reversed entirely. The cataracts improve significantly, but residua may remain, which usually do not interfere with vision. Effects on the central nervous system and ovaries, however, are not reversible. Approximately 60% of patients who are treated early have later psychomotor difficulties and learning disabilities, especially in expressive language, mathematics, and spatial relationships. Behavioral problems with attention deficits and other psychological problems may occur. At least 70% of women have hypergonadotropic hypogonadism with ovarian atrophy. Amenorrhea can be primary or secondary. Men have normal gonadal function. Because of lack of improvement in galactose tolerance with age, the dietary restriction must continue indefinitely. Intermittent erythrocyte galactose-1-phosphate determinations may help to guide clinical management.

Milder forms of classic galactosemia may present with a less severe clinical picture during infancy. Some children present even later in childhood with a history of intermittent milk aversion or partial treatment. The findings of cataracts, hepatic involvement, and psychomotor difficulties should raise the possibility of this diagnosis.

Variants of Transferase Deficiency. A number of other mutant alleles at the transferase locus are known to be associated with varying enzyme activity (0% to 140%) and starch-gel electrophoretic patterns. Some are associated with clinical manifestations when present in the homozygous state, and others are symptomatic only when present in compound heterozygosity with the classic galactosemia (G) gene. The Duarte (D) allele is the most common variant and is associated with an N314D mutation at the *GALT* gene locus. Between 8% and 13% of the population are carriers for the Duarte allele, which produces 50% of normal transferase activity. The compound heterozygote (D/G) for Duarte and classic galactosemia is the most frequent form of transferase abnormality and usually will be detected by newborn screening programs. D/G galactosemia is estimated to occur in approximately 1 in 4,000 births. Affected infants have an average 25% transferase activity; most have elevated erythrocyte galactose-1-phosphate levels in infancy. Some have clinical signs of galactose toxicity. Dietary galactose restriction is recommended for at least the first 6 months of life, at which time a controlled oral galactose tolerance test with measurement of plasma and erythrocyte galactose and galactose-1-phosphate levels may be performed. Approximately 90% of patients will have normal galactose tolerance by this age. Usually, the remainder have normal galactose tolerance by age 1 year. D/G galactosemia may be confirmed by quantitative determination of enzymatic activity and a distinctive banding pattern with starch-gel electrophoresis of erythrocyte hydrolysates.

Uridine Diphosphate Galactose-4-Epimerase Deficiency

Two forms of the autosomal recessive disorder uridine diphosphate galactose-4-epimerase deficiency have been documented. The more common form occurs in approximately 1 in 46,000 births. Deficient enzymatic activity occurs only in leukocytes, lymphocytes, and erythrocytes. The overall ability to metabolize galactose is normal, and no significant clinical abnormalities are seen. Erythrocyte galactose-1-phosphate is elevated; usually, galactosemia and galactosuria do not occur. The disorder may be detected in newborn screening programs that use measurement of erythrocyte galactose-1-phosphate in screening.

The second, very rare form of epimerase deficiency is characterized by a generalized deficiency of epimerase activity in all tissues. The clinical manifestations are similar to those seen with classic galactosemia. Elevation of blood galactose and erythrocyte galactose-1-phosphate occurs. The disorder should be considered in neonates who have symptoms of classic galactosemia, yet have normal transferase levels. Therapy is similar to that for classic galactosemia except that small amounts of dietary galactose must be given to supply the UDP-galactose needed for formation of gangliosides during growth periods. Careful monitoring of erythrocyte galactose-1-phosphate and UDP-galactose levels is indicated. Epimerase deficiency is associated with mutations in the *GALE* gene at chromosome 1p36-p35. Deficient activity of epimerase may be shown in erythrocytes, cultured skin fibroblasts, and the liver.

DISORDERS OF FRUCTOSE METABOLISM

Fructose Metabolism

Sucrose and small amounts of fructose and sorbitol are distributed widely in fruits, vegetables, and other natural and

BOX 387.3   Fructose Metabolism

Fructose is converted to intermediates of the gluco-neogenic and glycolytic pathways and is metabolized primarily to glucose and lactate (Fig. 387.4). Fructokinase catalyzes the phosphorylation of fructose to fructose-1-phosphate. In normal individuals, this process is associated with a decrease in intracellular inorganic phosphate and ATP concentration and with secondary transient mild hyperuricemia, hypermagnesemia, hyperkalemia, hypophosphatemia, and hypoglycemia. An exaggeration of this response is thought to be the basis for the clinical symptoms seen in hereditary fructose intolerance. Fructose-1-phosphate is cleaved to D-glyceraldehyde and dihydroxyacetone phosphate in the presence of aldolase. Aldolase also catalyzes the cleaving of fructose-1,6-diphosphate to D-glyceraldehyde-3-phosphate and dihydroxyacetone phosphate. Three forms of aldolase exhibit different tissue distributions: Aldolase A is the major form in muscle, aldolase B is the major form in the liver, and aldolase C is the major form in the brain. Triokinase catalyzes the phosphorylation of D-glyceraldehyde to D-glyceraldehyde-3-phosphate. Other pathways exist for the conversion of D-glyceraldehyde to triosephosphate intermediates, such as D-glyceraldehyde-3-phosphate and phosphoglycerate. Glyceraldehyde-3-phosphate then may be metabolized to pyruvate or it may be condensed with dihydroxyacetone phosphate to form fructose-1,6-diphosphate, which ultimately is converted to glucose and glycogen. Fructose-1,6-diphosphatase, which irreversibly catalyzes the formation of fructose-6-phosphate from fructose-1,6-diphosphate, plays a key role in gluconeogenesis. In glycolysis, phosphofructokinase irreversibly catalyzes this step in reverse order. The products of fructose metabolism may be diverted to gluconeogenesis and glycogen synthesis or to glycolysis and the Krebs cycle, depending on the metabolic need at the time.

---

sweetened foods and comprise a major portion of the daily dietary carbohydrate consumption in Western societies. After hydrolysis of sucrose, a large portion of ingested fructose is absorbed unchanged in the small intestine and is transported to the liver, the main site of fructose metabolism. Some of the fructose is converted to glucose in the small intestine, and some is metabolized in muscle, adipose tissue, and the kidneys. Ingested sorbitol is converted to fructose by sorbitol dehydrogenase. Additional information concerning fructose metabolism is presented in Box 387.3.

Hepatic Fructokinase Deficiency (Essential Fructosuria)

Hepatic fructokinase deficiency, a benign autosomal recessive disorder associated with mutations in the *KHK* gene at chromosome 2p23.3-p23.2, occurs in approximately 1 in 130,000 individuals. Fructosuria may be detected on routine urinalysis if the procedure includes testing for reducing substances.

Fructose-1-Phosphate Aldolase B Deficiency (Hereditary Fructose Intolerance)

Fructose-1-phosphate aldolase B deficiency, an autosomal recessive disorder, is associated with reduced activity of aldolase B in the liver, renal cortex, and small intestine. Considerable heterogeneity is seen in residual activity among affected pa-

tients, who usually have less than 15% of normal hepatic aldolase B activity. The true incidence of the disorder is unknown; it is estimated to occur in 1 in 20,000 individuals in Switzerland and Great Britain. The disorder results from mutations in the *ALDOB* gene at chromosome 9q22.3.

The symptoms of this disorder, which occur only after the ingestion of dietary fructose, are related to acute hypoglycemia and chronic hepatic and renal dysfunction. In young infants, usually the symptoms do not start until weaning or the introduction of fruits, vegetables, and juices. Symptoms may occur before this time if the infant is taking a formula with fructose or sucrose as the carbohydrate source. The symptoms of an acute ingestion, which are more severe in young infants than in older children and adults, are associated with hypoglycemia and include sweating, trembling, emesis, lethargy, coma, seizures, and even shock and death. Acute fructose ingestion results in depletion of intracellular inorganic phosphate and ATP and in secondary inhibition of gluconeogenesis and glycolysis. More chronic symptoms include poor feeding, failure to thrive, vomiting, diarrhea, irritability, tremors, hepatomegaly, hepatic dysfunction leading to cirrhosis and hepatic failure, and proximal renal tubular dysfunction of the Fanconi type. The accumulation of fructose-1-phosphate in the liver, kidney, and small intestine is thought to be responsible for these manifestations. The pattern of these chronic symptoms, with intermittent acute episodes associated with the ingestion of fructose-containing foods, points to the disorder clinically. Older children and adults will have a nutritional history of avoidance of fruits and sweets and may be referred for bizarre eating patterns.

Laboratory findings associated with acute episodes will include hypoglycemia, hypophosphatemia, hypermagnesemia, hyperuricemia, hyperkalemia, lactic acidosis, and fructosemia and fructosuria. The presence of a non–glucose-reducing substance in the urine should be confirmed as fructose by sugar chromatography. Fructosuria will not be present in those patients with intake of foods or fluids with other carbohydrate sources and may not be seen in patients with poor intake or those without recent exposure to fructose. Laboratory findings from chronic exposure are those associated with hepatic dysfunction and proximal renal tubular dysfunction. Liver biopsy samples reveal diffuse steatosis, scattered hepatic necrosis, periportal and intralobular fibrosis, and cirrhosis in later stages. Renal biopsy reveals granulation and vacuolization of epithelial cells with dilated proximal tubules. Small intestinal biopsy samples may exhibit submucosal or serosal hemorrhages.

Treatment with avoidance of all dietary sources of sucrose and fructose, including that in foods and medications, should be instituted once the disorder is suspected. Sorbitol is metabolized to fructose and thus also must be avoided. Acute episodes respond to intravenous glucose infusion. Once a fructose-restricted diet is started, usually clinical improvement is evident within days. Small children may have persistent hepatomegaly, and some progress to liver failure requiring transplantation. After several weeks of treatment, an intravenous fructose tolerance test with a maximum dose of 200 mg/kg may be administered with caution. An oral fructose tolerance test may lead to a severe acute episode and should be avoided. The disorder can be documented also by demonstrating a known mutation at the aldolase B gene locus in peripheral leukocytes or by enzymatic assay of aldolase B in biopsy samples from the liver or small intestine. Because aldolase B is not expressed in cultured skin fibroblasts or amniocytes, carrier and prenatal testing is available only for families in whom the molecular genetic defect is known.

Fructose-1,6-Diphosphatase Deficiency

Fructose-1,6-diphosphatase deficiency is a rare, autosomal recessive disorder associated with deficient activity of fructose-1,

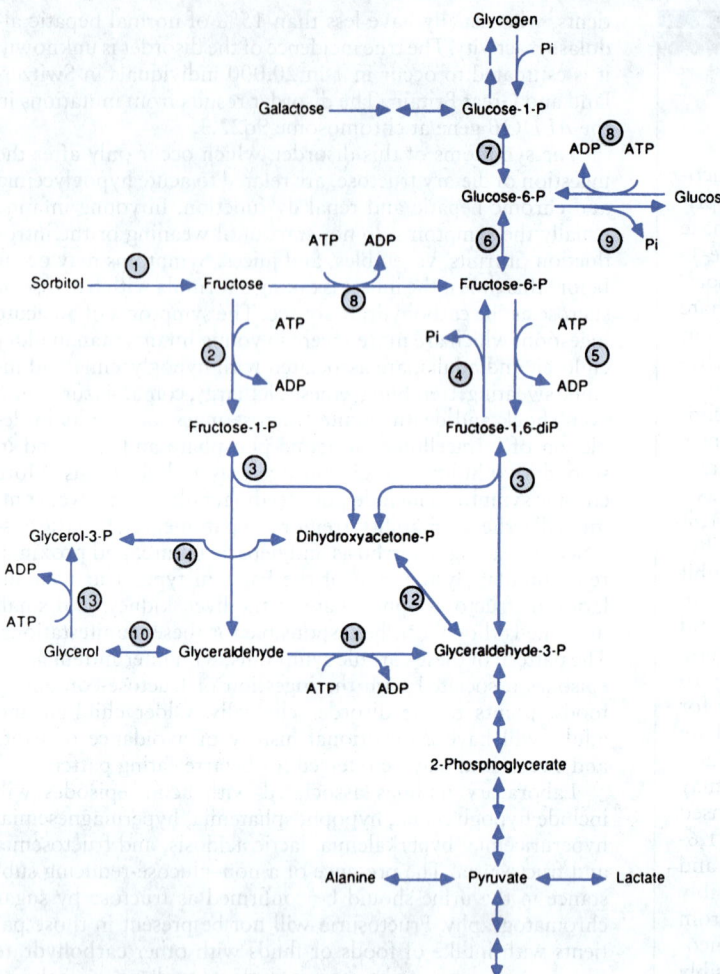

FIGURE 387.4. Pathways of fructose metabolism. 1, sorbitol dehydrogenase; 2, fructokinase; 3, fructoaldolase; 4, fructose-1,6-diphosphatase; 5, phosphofructokinase; 6, phosphohexose isomerase; 7, phosphoglucomutase; 8, hexokinase; 9, glucose-6-phosphatase; 10, alcohol dehydrogenase; 11, triokinase; 12, triose phosphate isomerase; 13, glycerol kinase; 14, glycerophosphate dehydrogenase; ADP, adenosine diphosphate; ATP, adenosine triphosphate; P, phosphate; Pi, inorganic phosphate.

6-diphosphatase in the liver, jejunum, and kidney. It is a severe disorder of gluconeogenesis associated with life-threatening episodes of hypoglycemia, lactic acidosis, and ketosis, which are triggered by fasting. Approximately one-half of affected patients present in the first 4 days of life with hypoglycemia and ketoacidosis. Moderate hepatomegaly and hypotonia may be present. Seizures, apnea, and cardiac arrest may occur. Usually, the episodes respond to intravenous glucose and bicarbonate. Later episodes may be triggered by intercurrent infections and other states that increase the metabolic need for glucose or when the patients are fasted or have repeated vomiting. Laboratory testing at the time of an episode will reveal hypoglycemia, ketosis, and elevated lactate, pyruvate, alanine, and uric acid levels. Usually, fructosuria is not present, nor is there an aversion to dietary fructose.

Treatment includes dietary restriction of fructose sources and the avoidance of fasting. Tolerance of fasting improves with age. Most patients respond well with regression of hepatomegaly. An intravenous (never oral) fructose tolerance test with a maximum dosage of 200 mg/kg may be cautiously performed, but the results will not be as striking as those seen with hereditary fructose intolerance. A fasting test, with close monitoring of the patient, may reveal an increase in lactic acid and ketosis as blood glucose decreases. Usually, glucagon produces a glycemic response in the fasting state. Also noted is a glycemic response to glucose or galactose but not to fructose, glycerol, alanine, or dihydroxyacetone. Deficient activity of fructose-1,6-diphosphatase may be demonstrated in peripheral leukocytes and in liver and jejunal biopsy samples. The

disorder results from mutations in the *FBP1* gene at chromosome 9q22.2-q22.3. Carrier testing and prenatal diagnosis are available using molecular genetic techniques.

OTHER DISORDERS OF CARBOHYDRATE METABOLISM

Pentosuria

Essential pentosuria is a benign, autosomal recessive disorder associated with excessive urinary excretion of 1 to 4 g of L-xylulose daily. It is most common in persons of Jewish heritage and results in the presence of a non–glucose-reducing substance on urinalysis. Essential pentosuria is caused by deficient activity of NADP-linked L-xylitol dehydrogenase, which catalyzes the conversion of L-xylulose to xylitol in the glucuronic acid pathway. The L-xylulose may be demonstrated by sugar chromatography.

Glycerol Kinase Deficiency

Glycerol kinase deficiency, inherited as an X-linked trait, is associated with elevated serum and urine glycerol levels. It may be suspected in individuals found to have a very high triglyceride blood level when the laboratory uses methods that measure the amount of glycerol released with the hydrolysis of triglyceride (pseudohypertriglyceridemia). The disorder exists in three clinical forms. Isolated glycerol kinase deficiency, or the juvenile form, presents during early childhood with episodic vomiting, lethargy that may progress to coma, and often significant metabolic acidosis that requires intravenous hydration and bicarbonate. Markedly elevated glycerol levels are noted on urinary organic acid testing by gas chromatography–mass spectroscopy; marked pseudohypertriglyceridemia is present. Treatment includes a low-glycerol (low-fat) diet and prompt treatment of episodes, which may occur with intercurrent illnesses or times of fasting.

Usually, the benign, or adult, form of isolated glycerol kinase deficiency is asymptomatic, does not require dietary therapy, and is recognized by finding pseudohypertriglyceridemia as part of an evaluation for hyperlipidemia.

The microdeletion, or complex form, of glycerol kinase deficiency results from deletions in the p21 region of the X chromosome, which involve the glycerol kinase gene (*GK*) locus and one or both of the closely linked, contiguous, Xp21 loci for congenital adrenal hypoplasia (*AHC*) and Duchenne muscular dystrophy (*DMD*). Boys with one of these disorders should be evaluated for the others. Treatment includes glycerol dietary restriction in addition to any therapy, such as adrenal hormone replacement therapy, that is indicated for the associated disorders. Deficient activity of glycerol kinase may be noted in peripheral blood leukocytes, fibroblasts, or transformed lymphoblast cell lines. Molecular genetic studies also should be performed to rule out the microdeletion forms.

Ketotic Hypoglycemia

With fasting, blood glucose levels are maintained initially by breakdown of hepatic glycogen. Adults are able to continue glycogenolysis for as long as 6 to 12 hours, whereas children—who have smaller glycogen stores and a proportionately greater demand for glucose for the central nervous system—may be able to sustain glycogenolysis for only 4 to 6 hours. Glycogenolysis is stimulated by epinephrine and glucagon, which activate the hepatic phosphorylase system. Once hepatic glycogen stores are depleted, gluconeogenesis ensues and is stimulated by growth hormone and cortisol. In adults, approximately 50% of glucose is derived from amino acid precursors (especially alanine) through breakdown of skeletal muscle, 30% is derived from lactate, and 10% is formed from glycerol from adipose tissue stores. Gluconeogenesis occurs mainly in the liver but also may occur in the kidney with prolonged fasting. Also, with prolonged fasting, adipose tissue is metabolized with the release of free fatty acids and glycerol from triglyceride stores. Free fatty acids may be used directly or oxidized in the liver for energy with the resultant formation of ketone bodies. Abnormalities in any of the pathways involved, in the hormonal influences, or in availability of substrates for gluconeogenesis may result in fasting hypoglycemia.

Ketotic hypoglycemia is a common disorder that presents with fasting hypoglycemia and ketosis in patients between ages 1 and 5 years. Most patients present between ages 18 and 24 months. The disorder also has been termed *accelerated starvation, idiopathic hypoglycemia,* or *substrate-limited hypoglycemia.* Many patients are not able to fast longer than 8 to 16 hours before symptoms develop. Affected patients often exhibit a history of transient hypoglycemia and being small for gestational age in the neonatal period. As young infants, such patients feed frequently; as toddlers, usually they are observed to want to eat immediately on arising or after fasting for what commonly would be considered a short time for their age. They often are thin, rather than obese, and have a relatively smaller muscle mass than that expected for their age. Episodic hypoglycemia occurs with situations that lead to caloric deprivation, such as intercurrent illnesses with associated decreased intake, missing meals, or sleeping longer than usual. Acute hypoglycemia is associated with the usual signs of lethargy, coma, and seizures. Although the exact biochemical basis for the disorder is unknown, it is thought to be the result of decreased availability or impaired mobilization of muscle amino acids for gluconeogenesis. Usually, plasma alanine levels are lowered in fasting states in these patients. Excretion of epinephrine is blunted in response to hypoglycemia induced by insulin or a ketogenic diet. Maturation of the adrenal response to hypoglycemia may be delayed. Because of accelerated starvation, free fatty acid oxidation leads to markedly elevated levels of plasma and urine ketone bodies, for which the disorder is named. The ability to fast improves with age, and most children "outgrow" the disorder by puberty. This disorder is not inherited and affects males more commonly than females.

Treatment during acute episodes requires prompt normalization of blood glucose levels, usually with intravenous glucose administration. Clinical symptoms subside rapidly. Between episodes, a high-protein, high-carbohydrate, frequent feeding diet is given. Parents of affected patients should be instructed in the measurement of urinary ketones and should be directed to increase carbohydrate sources at those times when ketones are detected or carbohydrate intake decreases. Situations that require fasting, such as surgery or persistent vomiting with intercurrent illness, often will necessitate the use of intravenous glucose administration to maintain normal glucose levels.

Diagnosis of the disorder is established by exclusion of the many other disorders involving hormonal deficiencies and metabolic defects that also present with fasting hypoglycemia with ketosis. Diagnostic testing may be performed during an acute episode before glucose therapy or with a carefully monitored provocative fast. Because even normal children become ketotic and hypoglycemic after 24 to 36 hours of fasting, children suspected of having ketotic hypoglycemia must be monitored carefully, and the fast must not extend beyond 16 to 24 hours. An intravenous line without glucose (but with electrolytes) should be placed in children who have a history of significant hypoglycemia occurring frequently or after only a short period of fasting. Blood glucose levels should be monitored at least every 4 hours for the first 8 hours of fasting, then every 2 hours for the remainder of the test, unless the glucose level is dropping or symptoms occur, in which case it should be monitored more frequently. Glucose oxidase test strips may be used, but all low values should be confirmed with immediate laboratory blood glucose measurements. Monitoring urine ketones during the fast is helpful because usually they will become positive before hypoglycemia develops. When the glucose drops to 40 mg/dL or less, or at 16 to 24 hours of fasting with ketone-positive urine, or at 24 hours, blood and urine sampling should be obtained. Blood testing (with expected results) should include measurements of glucose (less than or equal to 40 mg/dL), insulin (low or less than 0.25 to 0.50 of glucose level), growth hormone (elevated), cortisol (elevated), quantitative amino acids (decreased alanine), carnitine (normal total, esterified fraction less than 40% of total), and an acyl-carnitine profile (normal ketones, no abnormal fatty acid oxidation metabolites). Blood testing for free fatty acids, ketones, and beta-hydroxybutyrate levels is optional. Liver function testing, electrolytes, pH, and lactate levels also should be obtained if one suspects a glycogenosis or if hypoglycemia occurs before 8 hours of fasting. Urine should be tested for reducing substances (negative), ketones (markedly positive), and organic acids (elevated ketones only). Additional samples of frozen heparinized plasma (1 mL) and urine (20 mL) and a dried blood filter-paper card (as used for newborn screening) should be held in case further studies are needed.

Children should be fed or given intravenous glucose after samples are obtained at the termination of the provocative testing, especially if they are symptomatic. In patients with ketotic hypoglycemia, glucagon produces no response in the fasted state, but a response is present in the fed state. Glucagon stimulation testing is not absolutely necessary unless a glycogenosis is suspected and should not be performed if symptomatic hypoglycemia has occurred. If the studies are obtained during an acute episode before treatment by an astute physician, provocative fasting may not be necessary. Abnormalities that differ from those mentioned (i.e., failure to note elevated cortisol levels) should prompt additional diagnostic testing.

Other metabolic diseases that present with fasting hypoglycemia and ketosis include disorders of mitochondrial fatty acid oxidation (except for medium-chain acyl-CoA dehydrogenase deficiency), intermittent maple syrup urine disease, glycogen synthetase deficiency (Type O GSD), and fructose-1,6-diphosphatase deficiency.

Suggested Readings

Ali M, Ellos P, Cox TM. Hereditary fructose intolerance. *J Med Genet* 1998; 35:353.

Arn PH. Galactosemia. *Curr Treat Options Neurol* 2003;5:343.

Bodamer OA, Feillet F, Lane RE, et al. Utilization of cornstarch in glycogen storage disease type Ia. *Eur J Gastroenterol Hepatol* 2002;14:1251.

Bosch AM, Bakker HD, van Gennip AH, et al. Clinical features of galactokinase deficiency: a review of the literature. *J Inherit Metab Dis* 2002;25:629.

Chou JY, Matern D, Mansfield BC, Chen YT. Type I glycogen storage diseases: disorders of the glucose-6-phosphatase complex. *Curr Mol Med* 2002;2:121.

Cleary MA, Heptinstall LE, Wraith JE, Walter JH. Galactosaemia: relationship of IQ to biochemical control and genotype. *J Inherit Metab Dis* 1995;18:151.

Dieckgraefe BK, Korzenik JR, Hussain A, Dieruf L. Association of glycogen storage disease 1b and Crohn disease: results of a North American survey. *Eur J Pediatr* 2002;161:S88.

Garty BZ, Douglas SD, Danon YL. Immune deficiency in glycogen storage disease type 1B. *Isr J Med Sci* 1996;32:1276.

Gordon N. Glycogenosis type V or McArdle's disease. *Dev Med Child Neurol* 2003;45:640.

Hansen TW, Henrichsen B, Rasmussen RK, et al. Neuropsychological and linguistic follow-up studies of children with galactosaemia from an unscreened population. *Acta Paediatr* 1996;85:1197.

Kaufman FT, Xu YK, Ng WG, et al. Gonadal function and ovarian galactose metabolism in classic galactosemia. *Acta Endocrinol* 1989;120:129.

Leslie ND. Insights into the pathogenesis of galactosemia. *Annu Rev Nutr* 2003; 23:59.

Rake JP, Visser G, Labrune P, et al. Guidelines for management of glycogen storage disease type I-European Study on Glycogen Storage Disease Type I (ESGSDI). *Eur J Pediatr* 2002:161:S112.

Scriver CR, Beaudet AL, Sly WS, et al., eds. *The metabolic and molecular bases of inherited disease*, 8th ed. New York: McGraw-Hill, 2001.

Shen JJ, Chen YT. Molecular characterization of glycogen storage disease type III. *Cur Mol Med* 2002;2:145.

Tolan DR. Molecular basis of hereditary fructose intolerance: mutations and polymorphisms in the human aldolase B gene. *Hum Mutat* 1995;6:210.

Walter JH, Roberts REP, Besley GTN, et al. Generalised uridine diphosphate galactose-4-epimerase deficiency. *Arch Dis Child* 1999;80:374.

Webb AL, Singh RH, Kennedy MJ, Elsas LJ. Verbal dyspraxia and galactosemia. *Pediatr Res* 2003;53:396.

Widhalm K, Miranda da Cruz BD, Koch M. Diet does not ensure normal development in galactosemia. *J Am Coll Nutr* 1997;16:204.

Wolfsdorf JI, Weinstein DA. Glycogen storage diseases. *Rev Endocr Metab Disord* 2003;4:95.

CHAPTER 388 ■ DISORDERS OF LIPOPROTEINS

REBECCA S. WAPPNER

LIPOPROTEIN METABOLISM

Lipids are a primary source of energy. They also function as the structural components of cell membranes and are precursors of biologically important compounds, including bile acids, vitamin D, and steroid hormones. Plasma lipoproteins vary widely in their composition and consist of spherical particles that have a central core of nonpolar lipids (i.e., triglycerides and cholesterol), surrounded by a surface monolayer of polar lipids (i.e., phospholipids) and apolipoproteins. The plasma lipoproteins are classified according to size, density, and electrophoretic charge.

By ultracentrifugation, plasma lipoproteins are separated by density into chylomicrons, very low-density lipoproteins (VLDL), low-density lipoproteins (LDL), intermediate-density lipoproteins (IDL), and high-density lipoproteins (HDL). Chylomicrons are the largest, least dense, and have the lowest protein content, whereas HDL are the smallest, contain the most protein, and are the most dense. Lipoprotein electrophoresis separates the lipoproteins on the basis of charge into chylomicrons, beta-lipoproteins (LDL), pre–beta-lipoproteins (VLDL), and alpha-lipoproteins (HDL). The chylomicrons have the lowest charge and remain near the origin, whereas HDLs have the highest charge and greatest mobility. The electrophoretic findings are the basis for the Fredrickson classification of hyperlipoproteinemias, as shown in Table 388.1.

Apolipoproteins are an integral part of lipoproteins and function as ligands for lipoprotein receptors and as cofactors for many of the enzymes involved with lipoprotein metabolism. Table 388.2 lists the major apolipoproteins with their associated lipoproteins and specific functions.

Several enzymes are involved with lipoprotein metabolism. *Lipoprotein lipase* (LPL), produced in adipose tissue and striated muscle and present on the endothelial surface of capillaries, hydrolyzes the triglycerides of plasma chylomicrons, VLDL, and IDL to free fatty acids and glycerols. LPL requires activation by apolipoprotein C-II (apoC-II). *Hepatic lipase*, produced by hepatocytes and present on hepatic endothelial cells, hydrolyzes the triglycerides of VLDL and IDL in the formation of LDL and hydrolyzes the phospholipids and triglycerides of HDL. The free fatty acids and glycerols released by the actions of the lipases may be oxidized as fuel or used for the resynthesis of lipoproteins, depending on the metabolic need at the time. *Lecithin-cholesterol acyltransferase* (LCAT) catalyzes the transfer of fatty acids from lecithin to cholesterol to create cholesterol esters. ApoA-I is the major cofactor for LCAT. *Cholesterol ester transfer protein* (CETP) transfers cholesterol esters formed by the action of LCAT to acceptor lipoproteins (i.e., LDL, VLDL, and HDL). A specific species of HDL, with

TABLE 388.1

CLASSIFICATION OF HYPERLIPOPROTEINEMIA

Electrophoretic Phenotype	Increased Lipoproteins	Plasma Elevations	Atherosclerotic Risk	Incidence	Associated Defects	Associated Genetic Disorders
Ia	Chylomicrons	Triglycerides	Not increased	Rare	LPL deficiency, LPL inhibitor	LPL deficiency
Ib	Chylomicrons	Triglycerides	Not increased	Rare	ApoC-II deficiency	ApoC-II deficiency
IIa	LDL	Cholesterol	High	1 in 500 (FH); 5 in 100 (PH)	LDL receptor, apoB-100 binding site defects (FH); multifactorial (PH)	FH; PH; familial combined hyper-lipoproteinemia
IIb	LDL + VLDL	Cholesterol and triglycerides	High	1 in 200	Overproduction of apoB and VLDL	Familial combined hyperlipo-proteinemia
III	beta-VLDL	Cholesterol and triglycerides	High	1 in 5,000	ApoE-2/E-2 genotype	Familial dysbetalipo-proteinemia
IV	VLDL	Triglycerides	May be increased	Genetic uncommon, secondary common	Overproduction and decreased clearance of VLDL	Familial hypertriglyc-eridemia (mild forms); familial combined hyper-lipoproteinemia
V	Chylomicrons + VLDL	Triglycerides and cholesterol	May be increased	Uncommon	ApoE mutations	Familial hypertri-glyceridemia (severe forms)

Apo, apolipoprotein; FH, familial hypercholesterolemia; LDL, low-density lipoprotein; LPL, lipoprotein lipase; PH, polygenic hypercholesterolemia; VLDL, very low-density lipoprotein.

associated apoD, functions with LCAT and CETP to take up cholesterol esters from peripheral tissues and transfer them to VLDL, IDL, and LDL. IDL and LDL transport the cholesterol esters back to the liver, thereby effecting reverse cholesterol transport and decreasing atherosclerotic risk.

Chylomicrons and VLDL are the major transport forms of triglycerides. Chylomicrons, formed from dietary long-chain triglycerides, are considered exogenous triglycerides, whereas VLDLs, formed in the liver, are considered endogenous. Cir-

culating chylomicrons, with associated apoB-48 and apoA-I, acquire apoC-II and apoE and are metabolized to chylomicron remnants with the release of triglycerides by LPL. The chylomicron remnants, now richer in cholesterol ester, are taken up by hepatocytes through receptor-mediated endocytosis and further hydrolyzed to free fatty acids, glycerol, and cholesterol. In the hepatocytes, endogenous triglycerides are formed, which are then secreted into the circulation as VLDL, with associated apoB-100 and small amounts of apoE. After acquiring

TABLE 388.2

APOLIPOPROTEINS

Apolipoproteins	Associated Lipoproteins	Function
A-I	Chylomicrons, HDL	Cofactor for LCAT
A-II	Chylomicrons, HDL	Transport of HDL
A-IV	Chylomicrons, HDL	Cofactor for LCAT; promotes cholesterol efflux from cells
B-48	Chylomicrons and chylomicron remnants, VLDL, IDL	Chylomicron transport
B-100	Chylomicrons and chylomicron remnants, VLDL, IDL	Ligand for LDL receptor; transport of VLDL, IDL, LDL
C-I	Chylomicrons, VLDL, IDL, HDL	Cofactor for LCAT; inhibits binding of apoE-containing lipoproteins to LRP and LDL receptor
C-II	Chylomicrons, VLDL, IDL, HDL	Cofactor for LPL
C-III	Chylomicrons, VLDL, IDL, HDL	Inhibits binding of apoE-containing lipoproteins to LDL receptor
D	HDL	Transport of cholesterol esters between lipoproteins
E	Chylomicrons and chylomicron remnants, VLDL, IDL, HDL	Ligand for remnant receptor and LDL receptor
F	HDL	Possibly involved with cholesterol transport or esterification
G	HDL	Unknown
H	Chylomicrons, VLDL, HDL	Cofactor for LPL with apoC-II

HDL, high-density lipoprotein; IDL, intermediate-density lipoprotein; LCAT, lecithin-cholesterol acyltransferase; LDL, low-density lipoprotein; LPL, lipoprotein lipase; LRP, low-density lipoprotein receptor-related protein; VLDL, very low-density lipoprotein.

apoC-II, the VLDL undergoes hydrolysis of its triglycerides by LPL, with the formation of more cholesterol ester-rich IDL; further hydrolysis of IDL results in LDL. IDL and LDL, with associated apoB-100, are taken up by hepatocytes or adrenal cells through receptor-mediated endocytosis, and the molecules are hydrolyzed further to release free fatty acids, glycerol, and cholesterol. The resultant increase in hepatocyte intracellular concentration of cholesterol, whether from the endocytosis of chylomicron remnants, IDL, or LDL, results in feedback inhibition of *de novo* synthesis of cholesterol from acetoacetate. This rate-limiting step is catalyzed by 3-hydroxy-3-methylglutaryl–coenzyme A (HMG-CoA) reductase. In addition, other feedback effects include down-regulation of receptor synthesis and esterification of cholesterol by acyl-CoA cholesterol acyl transferase.

HYPERLIPOPROTEINEMIA

Diagnosis

In children, the diagnosis of a hyperlipoproteinemia is established by a 12- to 18-hour fasting lipid profile that includes total cholesterol, LDL (calculated), HDL, and triglyceride levels. Adults and older adolescents should fast for 18 to 24 hours before blood sampling. Younger children, who are less tolerant of fasting, may fast for only 8 to 12 hours. Plasma lipid levels vary with age. Tables of normal values for children and adults are available (see the section, Suggested Readings). In general, total cholesterol levels of less than 170 mg/dL are desirable; levels greater than 200 mg/dL are elevated. LDL levels of less than 110 mg/dL are desirable; levels greater than 130 are elevated. Triglyceride levels greater than 200 mg/dL and HDL levels of less than 35 mg/dL are considered abnormal. Elevated LDL levels and reduced HDL levels correlate positively with an increased risk for premature atherosclerosis. Lipoprotein electrophoresis helps establish the pattern of elevation and also demonstrates chylomicrons, if present.

Family history is frequently helpful in determining which children are at high risk for hyperlipoproteinemia. Questions should be asked concerning the presence of xanthomas, arcus cornea, angina, peripheral vascular disease, strokes, or coronary artery disease before the age of 55 years, and the lipid levels of both parents should be ascertained. Children with a positive family history for hyperlipoproteinemia should have a fasting lipid profile done starting at age 2 years. Most of the familial disorders are inherited as autosomal dominant traits, and each child of an affected parent has a 50% chance to inherit the disorder. Children found to be affected should be started on therapy appropriate for age and the degree and pattern of hyperlipoproteinemia. At-risk children with normal results should have the testing repeated at 5-year intervals. Children with borderline results should have repeat testing done in 1 year. An exception occurs in families in which both parents have a known genetic hyperlipoproteinemia. When both parents have hyperlipoproteinemias, the children have a 50% chance to also have the disorder and inherit it from one of the parents. But, in addition, they have a 25% chance to inherit a gene for the disorder from each parent and have a severe homozygous form of hyperlipoproteinemia. Such children should be tested in infancy so that appropriate therapy may be started before clinical symptoms appear. Any child at any age with symptoms of severe hyperlipoproteinemia (i.e., pancreatitis, angina, arcus cornea, or xanthomas) should have testing done.

Because testing children for hyperlipoproteinemia on the basis of family history alone may miss a significant number of children with hyperlipoproteinemia, screening for hypercholes-

terolemia in a wider population may be considered. As many as 20% to 25% of children have elevated lipid levels. Only the minority have genetic hyperlipoproteinemias. Most lipid elevations result from a dietary intake high in total and saturated fats, sedentary lifestyle, reduced exercise, and obesity. Other children have increased lipid levels from diabetes, hypothyroidism, nephrosis, liver dysfunction, and medications (i.e., corticosteroids and contraceptives). Hypertension, chronic alcoholism, and smoking also increase the risk for premature atherosclerosis. Children with other risk factors should be considered for cholesterol screening starting at 5 years of age. Children with elevated cholesterol levels on repeated testing should have a fasting lipid profile performed.

Therapy

The American Heart Association Step One and Step Two diets are used for the nutritional therapy of hyperlipoproteinemia. The Step One diet limits total fat intake to 30% of calories, with equal amounts from saturated, monounsaturated, and polyunsaturated fats. Total cholesterol intake is limited to 300 mg/day. An increased intake of complex carbohydrate and fiber also is recommended. The Step One diet is prudent and applicable to the general population, as well as children older than 5 years with hyperlipoproteinemia. It may be used cautiously in children with hyperlipoproteinemia between ages 2 and 5 years. In children, total fat intake should not be lower than 20% of total caloric intake. Dietary modification is indicated if the total cholesterol levels remain persistently higher than 200 mg/dL or LDL levels remain higher than 130 mg/dL. The Step Two diet further reduces the saturated fat intake to 7% of total calories and cholesterol intake to less than 200 mg/day. The Step Two diet should not be implemented in children unless hyperlipoproteinemia persists while on a Step One diet.

In addition to the Step One and Step Two diets, persons with hypertriglyceridemia also should reduce free carbohydrate intake. An American Diabetes Association–type diet, with reduced free sugar intake, reduced total fat and cholesterol intake, and caloric intake to maintain a normal weight-for-height ratio is recommended. In obese individuals, hypertriglyceridemia may resolve with normalization of weight for height. The avoidance of ethanol, a significant source of carbohydrates, is important in adults. Response to dietary therapy may take as long as 3 to 6 months to be appreciated.

An over-restriction of dietary lipid intake may result in failure to thrive and essential fatty acid nutrient deficiencies. Parents should be cautioned that the dietary restrictions used for the treatment of hyperlipoproteinemias in adults are not recommended for use in very young children, especially those younger than 2 years. Once the diagnosis of a hyperlipoproteinemia is established in children, dietary plans and instructions should be given by an experienced pediatric nutritionist. Growth parameters should be monitored frequently.

Resins that bind bile salts, such as cholestyramine and colestipol, may be used in those children with hyperlipoproteinemias who have persistently elevated lipid levels after an adequate trial of dietary therapy. Resins are added to diet therapy and do not replace it. Most children who require resin therapy have total cholesterol levels greater than 300 mg/dL and LDL levels of more than 190 mg/dL before starting dietary therapy. Slurries of the resin, wetted in cold juice or skim milk, may be used with younger children. Tablets also are available for older children and adults. Resins should be taken twice daily, before morning and evening meals. Doses of 1 to 4 g/day may be used in children; adolescents may require up to 8 g/day. Side effects of bloating and constipation can be lessened by cautiously increasing doses. Supplemental multivitamins and folate, given at least 30 minutes before or 4 hours after the resin, lessen the risk for those deficiencies of fat-soluble vitamins and folate reported with the use of resins. Response to therapy with resins also may take some time to occur; follow-up laboratory testing and monitoring growth parameters should be done at 2- or 3-month intervals.

Inhibitors of HMG-CoA reductase should not be used before age 11 years or mid-puberty and then only in those children with homozygous or other severe forms of the hypercholesterolemias. Although recent short-term studies have shown statins to be effective in lowering LDL cholesterol levels in children, long-term benefits and safety have not been established. Relatively recently developed cholesterol absorption inhibitors (i.e., ezetimibe) may be used alone or in combination with HMG-CoA reductase inhibitors in older children with severe forms of the disorders. Nicotinic acid therapy also may be of benefit in some children, especially those with hypertriglyceridemia. Nicotinic acid may be used with diet and resins, but it should not be used with HMG-CoA reductase inhibitors because of an increased risk for rhabdomyolysis and hepatic toxicity with this combination of drugs. Fibric acid derivatives, often used in adults with hypertriglyceridemias, usually are not given to children. For severe forms of the disorders, unresponsive to other therapeutic approaches, LDL apheresis may be indicated. Liver transplantation also has been performed in very severely affected patients.

The treatment of hyperlipoproteinemias during childhood also should include other measures known to improve lipid levels or decrease the risk for premature atherosclerosis. A routine exercise plan should be maintained throughout the year and not just on a seasonal basis, a normal weight-for-height ratio should be maintained, smoking should be avoided, and stress minimized or alleviated if possible.

GENETIC HYPERLIPOPROTEINEMIAS

Familial Hypercholesterolemia (Type IIa Hyperlipoproteinemia)

Familial, or type IIa, hyperlipoproteinemia is characterized by elevated plasma total cholesterol and LDL and an increased risk for premature atherosclerosis. More than 420 different mutations have been documented in the LDL receptor gene (*LDLR*) at chromosome location 19p13.2. The mutations lead to a reduced number or reduced function of LDL receptors, reduced clearance of LDL and IDL from plasma, and deposition of LDL-derived cholesterol in tissues. With decreased intracellular cholesterol concentration, the feedback inhibition of HMG-CoA reductase does not occur, and endogenous cholesterol is synthesized continuously. The disorder is inherited as an autosomal dominant trait. Approximately 1 in 500 persons are heterozygotes for the disorder and have approximately one-half the normal number of functioning LDL receptors. In heterozygotes, total cholesterol levels range from 270 to 500 mg/dL, with an average level of 350 mg/dL. Mean plasma LDL is two to three times normal. Occasionally, elevated VLDL and triglycerides occur, especially if the person has obesity or another factor associated with secondary hyperlipoproteinemia. Lipoprotein electrophoresis shows a type IIa pattern. Although elevated cholesterol and LDL are present from birth, clinical symptoms usually do not occur before late adolescence. Tendinous xanthomas may occur in the fingers or Achilles tendons. Tuberous and subperiosteal xanthomas may be noted at the elbows and knees. Arcus cornea and palpebral xanthomas develop. The mean age of onset of severe coronary artery disease is 43 years in men and 53 years in women. Compared with the general population, heterozygotes for familial hyperlipoproteinemia have three to six times the incidence of coronary artery disease and a 20-fold increase in the incidence of cerebral vascular accidents.

A dietary reduction of total and saturated fat intake and an increased intake of complex carbohydrates and fiber, in addition to the administration of resins that bind bile salts and, occasionally, nicotinic acid usually is needed to lower the levels of cholesterol and LDL to acceptable ranges during childhood. Use of HMG-CoA reductase and cholesterol absorption inhibitors, in addition to diet and resin therapy, frequently is indicated in postpubertal adolescents and adults.

A severe homozygous form of the disorder occurs in approximately 1 in 1 million persons. These patients have essentially no LDL receptor activity. Total cholesterol levels range from 600 to 1,200 mg/dL, and LDL levels are four to six times normal. Generalized atherosclerosis, xanthomas, and arcus cornea usually are present by mid-childhood (Fig. 388.1). Deaths have been reported as early as 18 months of age; most untreated patients do not survive beyond 30 years of age. Treatment with diet, resins, cholesterol absorption inhibitors, and HMG-CoA reductase inhibitors may not be successful, and LDL apheresis may be required. Liver transplantation has been performed. Gene vector therapy may become available in the future. Prenatal diagnosis is possible.

In addition, 1 in 800 persons has a mutation at the apoB-100 genetic locus that affects LDL receptor binding and results in clinical findings similar to those seen with familial hyperlipoproteinemia. These mutations also are inherited as autosomal dominant traits.

Polygenic Hypercholesterolemia

Polygenic hypercholesterolemia is of multifactorial etiology. Cholesterol and LDL are moderately elevated. Lipoprotein electrophoretic patterns usually show a type IIa pattern, but type IIb also may be seen. Both environmental influences and genetic factors play a role in the development of atherosclerosis in affected individuals. An underlying genetic disorder may be present and may result in increased synthesis of apoB or cholesterol, or increased susceptibility to dietary cholesterol. Environmental and life-style influences (i.e., obesity, diabetes, or lack of exercise) enhance the risk. Polygenic hypercholesterolemia occurs in 5% of the adult population and is noted in 85% to 90% of persons with moderate elevations of cholesterol and LDL. Treatment is similar to that for familial hypercholesterolemia.

Familial Combined Hypercholesterolemia

Familial combined hypercholesterolemia, an autosomal dominant disorder that occurs in 0.5% to 1.0% of the population, is the most common genetic disorder associated with an increased risk for atherosclerosis. The disorder results from the increased synthesis of apoB and VLDL. Many affected patients have combined elevations of both cholesterol and triglycerides, whereas others have only elevated cholesterol or only elevated triglycerides. Lipoprotein electrophoresis patterns vary, even among members of the same family; types IIa, IIb, IV, and occasionally type V are seen. Affected children often have elevation of only triglycerides and go on to develop the combined phenotype at later ages. Xanthomas are uncommon. Pancreatitis may occur because of markedly elevated triglyceride levels. Ten percent of affected patients develop significant coronary artery disease by 60 years of age. Familial combined hypercholesterolemia is inherited as an autosomal dominant trait. Family studies may be needed to establish this diagnosis, given the widely varying

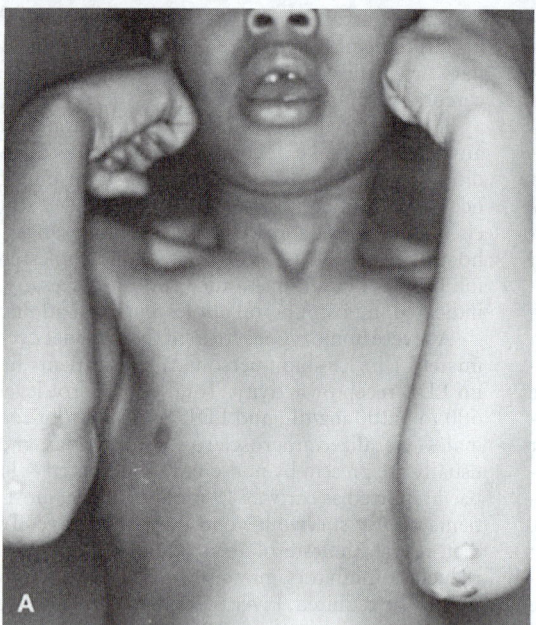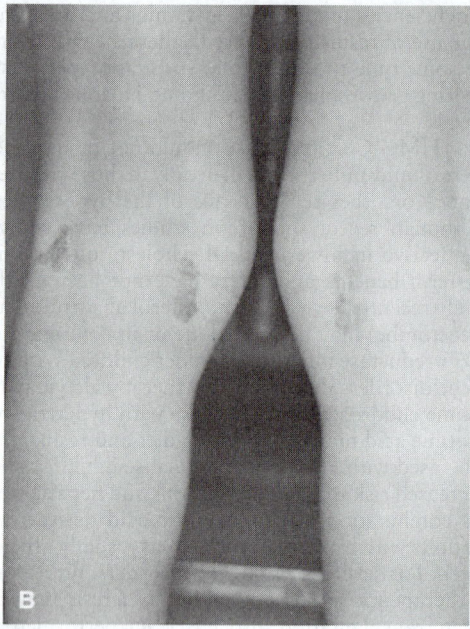

FIGURE 388.1. Homozygous hypercholesterolemia in a 7-year-old boy. Cutaneous xanthomas had been present since the age of 4 years. A: Elbows. B: Popliteal fossa.

clinical phenotype. Treatment consists of normal weight maintenance, dietary reduction of total fat and cholesterol, and avoidance of dietary free sugars and ethanol. HMG-CoA reductase inhibitors, cholesterol absorption inhibitors, or nicotinic acid may be needed. Fibric acid derivatives are usually not effective.

Familial Hypertriglyceridemia

Familial hypertriglyceridemia, an autosomal dominant disorder that affects 0.2% to 0.3% of the population, is associated with mutations in the *HTGS* gene on chromosome 15q11.2–q13.1. Plasma triglyceride levels are elevated moderately at 250 to 500 mg/dL. VLDL is elevated, but cholesterol is not. Lipoprotein electrophoretic patterns of type IV or, on occasion, type V are seen. Symptoms usually are not evident during childhood. Environmental factors (i.e., diabetes, obesity, alcoholism, estrogen or corticosteroid therapy) that increase VLDL and triglyceride levels may potentiate symptoms in affected adults. The exact metabolic defect is unknown. An overproduction of endogenous triglycerides or delayed catabolism of VLDL may underlie this disorder. As with familial combined hypercholesterolemia, family studies may be needed to establish the exact diagnosis. Treatment is similar to that for familial combined hypercholesterolemia. Correction of any environmental or other medical problems often corrects the hypertriglyceridemia. A very low fat intake may be needed to prevent secondary pancreatitis.

The severe form of familial hypertriglyceridemia is an autosomal dominant disorder of adults characterized by elevated triglycerides (600 to 3,000 mg/dL), fasting chylomicronemia, eruptive xanthomas, recurrent abdominal pain and pancreatitis, and a type V lipoprotein electrophoretic pattern. Many symptomatic adults have additional environmental and lifestyle factors that increase the risk for hyperlipoproteinemia and premature atherosclerosis. The disorder results from mutations at the apoE gene locus that lead to defective binding with the LDL receptor and other LDL receptor–related proteins.

DISORDERS OF APOLIPOPROTEINS

Apolipoprotein A Disorders

Familial apoA-I deficiency is a rare autosomal recessive disorder that results in markedly low levels of HDL, severe coronary atherosclerosis, cutaneous and tendinous xanthomas, and corneal clouding. Because apoA-I is a cofactor for LCAT, LCAT activity is decreased to approximately one-half of normal. Plasma cholesterol and LDL are normal; triglycerides may be normal or increased. The apoA-I, apoC-III, and apoA-IV genes are adjacent to each other and form a gene cluster at chromosomal location 11q23. Deletions involving apoA-I and apoC-III or all three contiguous genes have been reported in patients with clinical features similar to isolated apoA-I deficiency. No specific treatment is available.

Apolipoprotein B Disorders

ApoB-48 and apoB-100 are encoded by the same gene locus, *APOB*, located at chromosome 2p24. ApoB-100 is a full-length translation of the gene that is formed in the liver. ApoB-48, formed in the intestine, is a truncated product of the same gene that contains only 2,152 amino acid residues, in comparison with the 4,563 of apoB-100.

The absence of both apoB-48 and apoB-100 in plasma characterizes the autosomal recessive disorder *abetalipoproteinemia*. The disorder is associated with the absence of a microsomal triglyceride transfer protein (MTP) that is involved in the assembly, processing, or secretion of apoB-containing lipoproteins. Affected patients have absent postprandial plasma chylomicrons, VLDL, and LDL. Cholesterol and triglyceride levels are very low. Severe fat malabsorption is present from birth. The abnormal lipid status affects the membranes of erythrocytes, causing spiny projections (acanthocytosis) to develop. An associated defect occurs in the intestinal absorption and transport of tocopherol (vitamin E) that leads to spinocerebellar ataxia, peripheral neuropathy, ceroid myopathy, and pigmentary retinopathy. Treatment includes a lower-fat diet to prevent steatorrhea, along with supplemental fat-soluble vitamins, especially vitamin E, to improve neurologic status. Supplements of essential fatty acids may also be needed.

Hypobetalipoproteinemia results from the reduced production of apoB or from mutations at the apoB locus that encode truncated (shortened) forms of apoB. The disorder is inherited as an autosomal dominant trait. Homozygous affected patients have clinical symptoms similar to abetalipoproteinemia; treatment also is similar. Heterozygotes have partially reduced levels of LDL and cholesterol; most are asymptomatic, but occasionally neurologic symptoms or acanthocytosis occur. Treatment is similar to that for abetalipoproteinemia.

Chylomicron retention disease is a rare autosomal recessive disorder characterized by fat malabsorption and the absence of postprandial plasma chylomicrons. Ataxia, neuropathy, and acanthocytosis occasionally occur. A defect occurs in the formation and secretion of chylomicrons. ApoB-48 is synthesized and present in enterocytes, but not in plasma. ApoB-100 is not affected. Treatment is similar to that for abetalipoproteinemia.

Mutations at the apoB-100 locus that affect LDL receptor binding are associated with familial hypercholesterolemia and are discussed in that section.

Apolipoprotein C Disorders

Patients with *deficiency of apoC-II*, an activator for LPL, have markedly elevated chylomicron and triglyceride levels, and these patients experience repeated attacks of abdominal pain and pancreatitis that may start during childhood. HDL and LDL are low. A type I lipoprotein electrophoretic pattern is seen. Atherosclerotic risk is not increased. The disorder is inherited as an autosomal recessive trait and results from mutations in the *APOC2* gene at chromosome location 19q13.2. Treatment includes significantly lowering dietary fat intake. Transfusions of normal plasma may be needed with severe pancreatitis.

Apolipoprotein E Disorders

ApoE facilitates the binding of chylomicron remnants and VLDL to the LDL receptor. Three major isoforms of apoE, termed *apoE-2*, *apoE-3*, and *apoE-4*, are encoded by three different alleles at the apoE locus, *APOE*, at chromosome location 19q13.2. Sixty percent of the population has the normal homozygous apoE-3/E-3 genotype. Compound heterozygotes for apoE-3/E-2 and apoE-3/E-4 make up approximately 37% of the population.

The apoE-2/E-2 genotype occurs in approximately 1% of the population. These persons have a latent defect that may lead to type III hyperlipoproteinemia (dysbetalipoproteinemia) if another condition occurs that is associated with secondary hyperlipoproteinemia (i.e., diabetes, obesity, hypothyroidism). ApoE-2 has a greatly decreased binding affinity for the LDL receptor, when compared with apoE-3. Reduced clearance and the accumulation of cholesterol-rich chylomicron remnants and partially degraded VLDL gives an abnormal "broad beta" band on lipoprotein electrophoresis. Plasma cholesterol and triglyceride levels are increased. Fifty percent of affected adults have a distinctive xanthoma striata palmaris; tuberoeruptive and periosteal xanthomas may be seen. Most patients respond to diet therapy. Nicotinic acid, fibric acid derivatives, and HMG-CoA reductase inhibitors also may be used.

The apoE-4/E-4 genotype also occurs in approximately 1% of the population and is associated with elevated LDL levels that may contribute to an increased risk for atherosclerosis in patients with various forms of hypercholesterolemia.

Mutations at the apoE locus that result in defective binding to the LDL receptor and other LDL receptor–related proteins may lead to type V hyperlipoproteinemia, a severe form of familial hypertriglyceridemia.

Lp(a)

Lp(a), a variant of LDL, consists of an LDL-like molecule that has one or two copies of the glycoprotein Lp(a) attached to its apoB-100. Multiple isoforms of Lp(a) exist; at least 20 common alleles have been found at the Lp(a) genetic locus *LPA*. Approximately 20% of the general population have high levels of Lp(a) that double the risk for premature atherosclerosis. A fivefold risk exists if both Lp(a) and LDL are elevated. Lp(a) is present in atherosclerotic plaques; it is thought that the Lp(a) may in some way interfere with the dissolution of fibrin clots. Treatment is similar to that for familial hypercholesterolemia.

OTHER DISORDERS OF LIPOPROTEIN METABOLISM

Tangier Disease

Tangier disease is a rare, autosomal recessive disorder named after the isolated island off of the Virginia coast where it was first recognized. The nonlysosomal accumulation of cholesterol esters in the reticuloendothelial system and other tissues leads to enlarged, orange-yellow tonsils and adenoids, splenomegaly, and peripheral neuropathies. Occasionally, corneal infiltration is noted on slit-lamp examination. HDL, total cholesterol, apoA-I, and apoA-II levels are markedly decreased. Plasma triglycerides are normal or increased. Fasting chylomicronemia is common. Lipoprotein electrophoresis shows the absence of alpha lipoproteins. HDL and other lipoproteins have altered apolipoprotein content. The risk for premature atherosclerosis, however, is not increased. Heterozygotes for the disorder have partially reduced HDL, total cholesterol, apoA-I, and apoA-II levels. The disorder results from mutations in the *HDLDT1* gene at chromosome 9q31. The gene codes for ATP-binding cassette transporter 1 (ABC1), suggesting that defective lipid transport and efflux of lipids may be involved. No specific treatment exists.

Lipoprotein Lipase Deficiency

LPL hydrolyzes triglycerides in chylomicrons and VLDL and is encoded by the *LPL* gene at chromosome 8p22. *Deficient activity of LPL*, an autosomal recessive disorder, results in eruptive xanthomas, hepatosplenomegaly, and repeated attacks of abdominal pain and pancreatitis starting in childhood. Chylomicrons and triglyceride levels are markedly elevated; HDL and LDL are low. A type I pattern is noted on lipoprotein electrophoresis. The presence of a *familial inhibitor to LPL* is an autosomal dominant disorder that presents during childhood with fasting hyperchylomicronemia, pancreatitis, and eruptive xanthomas. Laboratory findings are similar to that for LPL deficiency. The risk for atherosclerosis is not increased with either disease. Treatment includes significant dietary fat restriction. Nicotinic acid and fibric acid derivatives may be needed.

Hepatic Lipase Deficiency

Hepatic lipase (hepatic triglyceride lipase) hydrolyzes triglycerides of HDL and surface phospholipids. Patients with deficient activity of hepatic lipase have eruptive and plantar xanthomas and increased risk for premature atherosclerosis. Elevated cholesterol, triglycerides, and a species of HDL with a high triglyceride content are noted. The disorder results from mutations in the *LIPC* gene at chromosome 15q21–q23. Treatment consists of a lowered-fat diet along with fibric acid derivatives, nicotinic acid, or HMG-CoA reductase inhibitors.

Lecithin-Cholesterol Acyltransferase Deficiency

LCAT facilitates the transfer of fatty acids from lecithin to cholesterol in the synthesis of cholesterol esters. Two disorders, inherited as autosomal recessive traits, result from mutations at the *LCAT* gene locus at chromosome 6q22.1. *Familial deficiency of LCAT* is a rare disorder associated with a markedly reduced activity of LCAT that results in the deposition of unesterified cholesterol and phospholipids in tissues. Affected patients have juvenile corneal opacities, anemia, target cells, proteinuria, and occasionally renal failure. Xanthomas and an increased risk for premature atherosclerosis may occur. *Fish-eye disease* is characterized by corneal opacities in young adults. The other clinical features associated with familial deficiency of LCAT do not occur. In fish-eye disease, LCAT fails to esterify HDL, but retains its ability to esterify other lipoproteins. No specific treatment is available.

Cholesterol Ester Transfer Protein Deficiency

Cholesterol ester transfer protein (CETP) transfers cholesterol esters formed by the action of LCAT to acceptor lipoproteins (i.e., LDL, VLDL) and facilitates the exchange of HDL cholesterol esters with other lipoproteins. A deficiency of CETP results in elevated levels of HDL; no significant clinical disease appears to be associated with this finding, however.

OTHER DISORDERS OF LIPID AND CHOLESTEROL METABOLISM

Cerebrotendinous Xanthomatosis

Cerebrotendinous xanthomatosis is a rare, autosomal recessive disorder associated with the deficient activity of hepatic mitochondrial 27-hydroxylase and the deficient biosynthesis of bile salts. Intermediates of bile salt biosynthesis (i.e., cholestanol and other bile alcohols) and cholesterol accumulate in most tissues, including the brain, and are excreted in urine, bile, and feces. Plasma cholesterol levels, however, usually are normal or only slightly elevated. Affected patients have a progressive dementia, cerebellar ataxia, spinal cord paresis, tuberous and tendinous xanthomas, cataracts, and early atherosclerosis. The onset and clinical spectrum are variable. Psychomotor retardation, xanthomas, and cataracts may occur during childhood. Spasticity and ataxia usually develop in young affected adults. Most patients respond to treatment with chenodeoxycholic acid and HMG-CoA reductase inhibitors.

Phytosterolemia (beta-Sitosterolemia)

Patients with phytosterolemia develop subcutaneous and tendinous xanthomas before 10 years of age and premature atherosclerosis by age 20 years. Plasma, erythrocyte, and tissue levels of sitosterol and other sterols of plant and shellfish origin are elevated, presumably as a result of increased intestinal absorption or decreased biliary excretion of the compounds. Plasma cholesterol is normal or moderately elevated. Treatment includes avoidance of dietary sources of the compounds and cholestyramine. The disorder is inherited as an autosomal recessive trait.

Both cerebrotendinous xanthomatosis and phytosterolemia should be considered in children with xanthomas who have normal or only slightly elevated plasma cholesterol levels. Cerebrotendinous xanthomatosis should be considered in any child with juvenile cataracts.

Smith-Lemli-Opitz Syndrome

Smith-Lemli-Opitz syndrome is a well-recognized dysmorphic syndrome that occurs in 1 in 30,000 births in the United States. Affected patients have an unusual facies with a narrow, sloping anterior forehead. Ptosis of the eyelids, anteverted nares, epicanthal folds with wide nasal bridge, micrognathia, and low-set slanted or posteriorly rotated ears may be noted (Fig. 388.2). Congenital cataracts, cleft palate, postaxial polydactyly, transverse palmar creases, valgus deformities of the feet, and dislocated hips often occur. Hypoplasia of the labia, hypospadias, and cryptorchidism are frequently noted. Defects in brain morphogenesis and neuronal organization result in hypoplasia of the frontal lobes, cerebellum, and brainstem. Microcephaly, seizures, and moderate to severe psychomotor retardation occur.

The disorder results from the deficient activity of a 3β-hydroxysterol Δ^7-reductase, which is responsible for the reduction of the double bonds of 7-dehydrocholesterol (7DHC) during cholesterol synthesis. Affected patients have markedly elevated plasma and tissue levels of 7DHC and other cholesterol precursors that are thought to interfere with normal embryonic development. Blood cholesterol levels are reduced, but this is not apparent by usual laboratory methods that use colorimetric methods to measure cholesterol. Measurement of

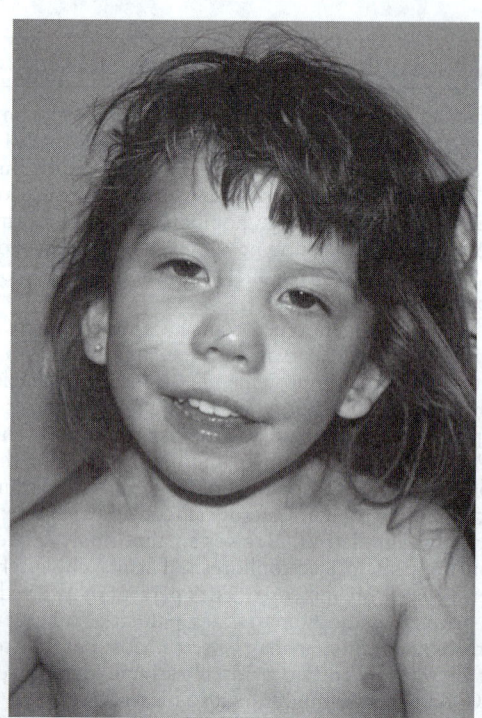

FIGURE 388.2. Three-year-old girl with Smith-Lemli-Opitz syndrome. Note the abnormal facies with low-set, posteriorly rotated ears.

7DHC requires special laboratory techniques that combine gas chromatography with mass spectrometry. Using this method, an abnormal pattern of elevated cholesterol precursors and lowered cholesterol can be shown in the plasma, erythrocytes, or cultured skin fibroblasts from affected patients. Most patients respond to treatment with cholesterol supplements. Sun-blocking creams are used to prevent the photosensitivity reactions that occur as a result storage of 7DHC in the skin. The disorder is inherited as an autosomal recessive trait and is associated with mutations in the DHCR7 gene at chromosome location 11q12–q13. Prenatal diagnosis is available.

Suggested Readings

Coletti RB, Neufeld EJ, Roff NK, et al. Niacin treatment of hypercholesterolemia in children. *Pediatrics* 1993;92:78.

de Jongh S, Kerckhoffs MC, Grootenhuis MA, et al. Quality of life, anxiety and concerns among statin-treated children with familial hypercholesterolaemia and their parents. *Acta Paediatr* 2003;92:1096.

Dennison BA, Jenkins PL, Pearson TA. Challenges to implementing the current pediatric cholesterol screening guidelines into practice. *Pediatrics* 1994; 94:296.

Diller PM, Huster GA, Leach PL, et al. Definition and application of the discretionary screening indicators according to the National Cholesterol Education Program for Children and Adolescents. *J Pediatr* 1995;126:345.

Dirisamer A, Hachemian N, Bucek RA, et al. The effect of low-dose simvastatin in children with familial hypercholesterolaemia: a 1-year observation. *Eur J Pediatr* 2003;162:421.

Gagne C, Gaudet D, Ruckert E. Efficacy and safety of ezetimibe coadministered with atorvastatin or simvastatin in patients with homozygous familial hypercholesterolemia. *Circulation* 2002;105:101.

Irons M, Elias ER, Abuelo D, et al. Treatment of Smith-Lemli-Opitz syndrome: results of a multicenter trial. *Am J Med Genet* 1997;68:311.

Kelley RI. Editorial: A new face for an old syndrome. *Am J Med Genet* 1997; 65:251.

Klish W, for the Committee on Nutrition, American Academy of Pediatrics. Committee statement: cholesterol in childhood. *Pediatrics* 1998;101:141.

Lauer RM. National Cholesterol Educational Program. Report of the expert panel on blood cholesterol levels in children and adolescents. *Pediatrics* 1992; 89(Suppl):525.

Robins SJ. *Management of lipid disorders. A basis and guide for therapeutic intervention.* Baltimore: Williams & Wilkins, 1997.

Scriver CR, Beaudet AL, Sly WS, et al., eds.Lipids, part 12. In: *The metabolic and molecular bases of inherited disease,* 8th ed. New York: McGraw-Hill, 2001:2705.

Tonstad S. Children and statins. *Acta Paediatr* 2003;92:1001.

Tonstad S, Knudtzon J, Sivertsen M, et al. Efficacy and safety of cholestyramine therapy in peripubertal and prepubertal children with familial hypercholesterolemia. *J Pediatr* 1996;129:42.

Valente AM, Newburger JW, Lauer RM. Hyperlipidemia in children and adolescents. *Am Heart J* 2001;142:433.

CHAPTER 389 ■ LYSOSOMAL STORAGE DISORDERS

REBECCA S. WAPPNER

Lysosomes are cytoplasmic, single membrane–bound organelles that contain hydrolytic enzymes responsible for the degradation of a variety of compounds, including mucopolysaccharides, sphingolipids, and glycoproteins. The substances to be degraded are either exogenous material that has been taken into the cell by endocytosis, or endogenous material contained in cytoplasm, which has been segregated into autophagosomes. Deficient activity of a specific lysosomal acid hydrolase leads to progressive accumulation of partially degraded material, which distends the cells and disrupts cellular function. The reduced activity of an acid hydrolase may be the result of a genetic mutation at the enzyme locus that results in lowered specific activity or reduced stability of the enzyme, failure of formation of a protective protein or activator for the enzyme, or failure of formation of a recognition marker on the enzyme, which targets it for lysosomal location. Lysosomal storage of material also may result from failure of active transport of small molecules from the lysosome.

The pattern of clinical findings seen with the various disorders is related to the type of compound stored and its natural distribution in the body. All the disorders are inherited as either autosomal recessive or X-linked traits. Carrier testing and prenatal diagnosis are available for most of the disorders, but only in a limited number of experienced laboratories. An exact enzymatic and, often, molecular diagnosis is essential for accurate carrier and prenatal studies.

Current therapy mainly consists of symptomatic and supportive therapy for the patient and family. Enzyme replacement therapy (ERT) with intravenous infusions of human recombinant enzyme is presently available for Gaucher disease, Fabry disease, mucopolysaccharidosis type I (Hurler, Hurler-Scheie, and Scheie syndromes), and mucopolysaccharidosis type VI (Maroteaux-Lamy syndrome). Clinical trials with human recombinant enzymes are currently underway for ERT for mucopolysaccharidosis type II (Hunter syndrome) and alpha-glucosidase deficiency (Pompe disease). It is anticipated that ERT for additional lysosomal storage disorders will be developed in the future. Enzyme replacement therapy decreases lysosomal storage of abnormal compounds and improves visceral and skeletal involvement, but the infused enzyme usually will not cross the blood–brain barrier to correct central nervous system involvement. Bone marrow or stem cell transplantation has also been successful in correcting many of the findings of the disorders and may be considered prior to significant central nervous system involvement. Although donor macrophages may cross the blood–brain barrier and replace brain microglial cells, it may take months or years to do so. Animal models are available that may be used for the investigation of new therapies.

For most of the disorders, the associated genes have been mapped and cloned. Heterogeneity has been noted in the molecular basis for many of the disorders and often correlates with the varying clinical presentations.

MUCOPOLYSACCHARIDOSES

The mucopolysaccharidoses are associated with lysosomal accumulation of partially degraded acid mucopolysaccharides (MPSs). MPSs, also termed *glycosaminoglycans,* are large molecules composed of linear repeating sulfated hexuronate or hexosamine disaccharide units attached to a protein core. MPSs normally are degraded by a series of acid hydrolases that remove the sulfate and carbohydrate residues in a stepwise manner. Deficiency of a specific hydrolase results in partial degradation of the molecules and lysosomal storage of the residual fragments.

The degradation of heparan sulfate, dermatan sulfate, keratan sulfate, or chondroitin sulfate, alone or in combination, may be involved, depending on the specific hydrolase affected. Disorders associated with heparan sulfate storage usually have central nervous system involvement and progressive mental retardation, those associated with dermatan sulfate storage have visceral and bone involvement, and those associated with keratan sulfate storage have bone involvement as their major clinical feature.

Radiography shows a distinct pattern of abnormalities termed *dysostosis multiplex.* The skull is enlarged and elongated (dolichocephaly) and the calvarium thickened. The sella may be J-, wooden shoe–, or boot-shaped (Fig. 389.1). The vertebral bodies in the lower thoracic and upper lumbar areas have a beaking of the anterior inferior surface caused by hypoplasia of their anterosuperior areas (Fig. 389.2). A dorsal kyphosis, or gibbus deformity, develops. The ribs are thickened, except where they join the spine, and they have an oar-shaped appearance (Fig. 389.3). The metacarpals have a proximal narrowing with distal widening, giving them a baby-bottle appearance. The distal humerus and ulna show an abnormal angulation termed a *Madelung deformity* (Fig. 389.4). The pelvis shows flaring of the iliac bones, shallow acetabular areas, and progressive coxa valga. The long bones become shortened, thickened, and may have signs of expansion of the medullary cavity. Hypoplasia of the odontoid process may occur. Radiography in Morquio syndrome, which is associated with keratan sulfate and chondroitin-6-sulfate storage, shows a different pattern,

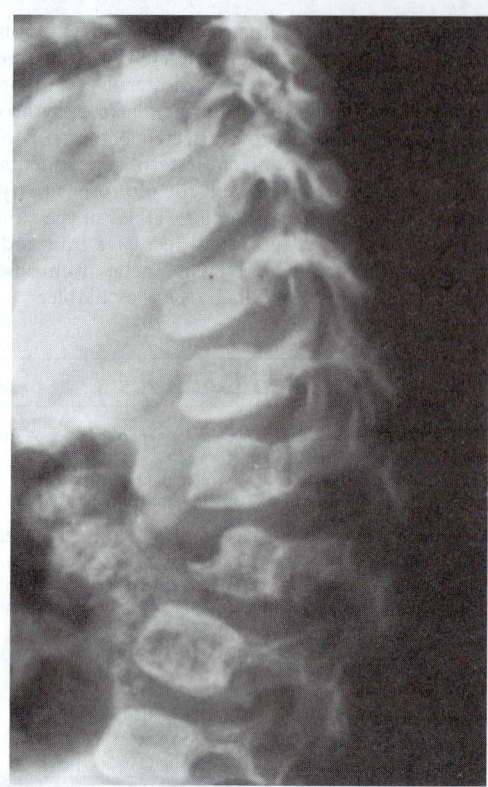

FIGURE 389.2. Lateral spine radiogram in Hurler syndrome. "Beaking" (anterior inferior projection) occurs in the lower thoracic and upper lumbar vertebral bodies from hypoplasia of the anterior superior surfaces. This results in an anterior kyphosis or "gibbus" formation.

with a platyspondyly that resembles that seen with the spondyloepiphyseal dysplasias (Fig. 389.5).

The age of onset, severity, and pattern of clinical and radiographic findings help to distinguish between the various types of mucopolysaccharidoses. Although urinary MPS testing may be helpful in some cases, the diagnosis is made on the basis of enzymatic testing. Demonstration of deficient activity of a specific lysosomal hydrolase may be done with serum or peripheral leukocytes for most of the disorders. Cultured skin fibroblasts may be required for others. DNA mutation analysis can confirm the disorder and may be helpful in establishing

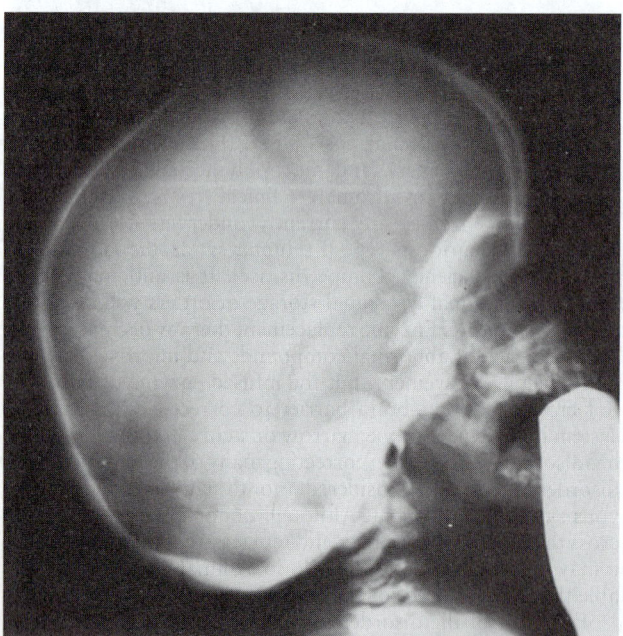

FIGURE 389.1. Lateral skull radiogram in Hurler syndrome. The skull is enlarged and elongated (dolichocephaly), with a "J" shape to the sella and thickened calvarium.

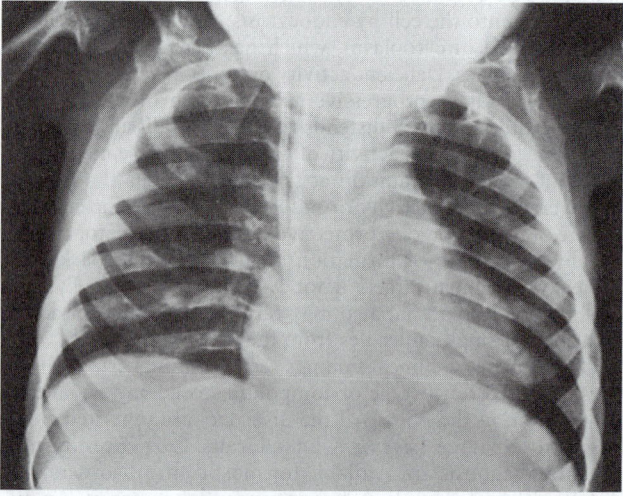

FIGURE 389.3. Anteroposterior chest radiogram in Hurler syndrome. The ribs are thickened, except where they join the spine, and they obscure more of the lung fields than usual.

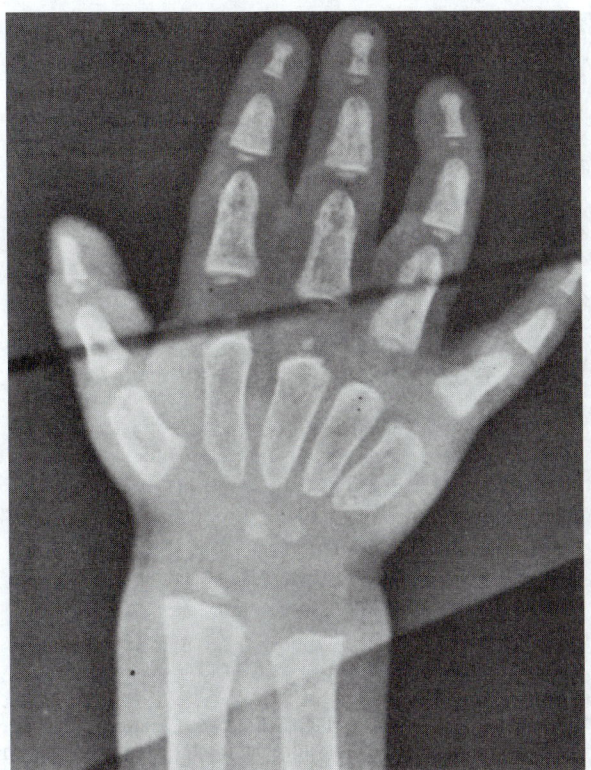

FIGURE 389.4. Anteroposterior hand and wrist radiogram in Hurler syndrome. There is abnormal angulation of the distal ends of the radius and ulna and proximal narrowing of the metacarpals (baby-bottle appearance). The hands have a claw-like appearance from joint contractures and connective tissue involvement.

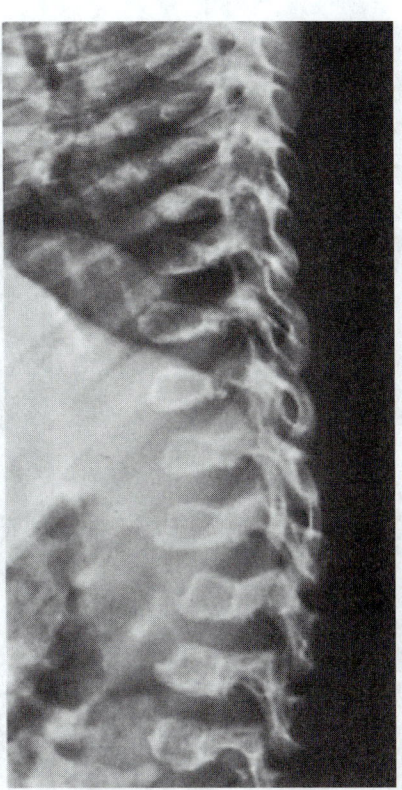

FIGURE 389.5. Lateral spine radiogram in Morquio syndrome. The vertebral bodies are flattened (platyspondyly). "Beaking" occurs in the lower thoracic and upper lumbar areas.

prognosis if different forms of the disorder occur. DNA mutation analysis may also be needed for accurate carrier testing. Table 389.1 gives molecular genetic information for the MPS storage disorders.

Hurler Syndrome (Mucopolysaccharidosis I-H)

Hurler syndrome, the prototype for the mucopolysaccharidoses, is associated with deficient activity of alpha-L-iduronidase and excessive storage of heparan and dermatan sulfate.

Hurler syndrome is inherited as an autosomal recessive trait and occurs in approximately 1 in 100,000 births.

Children with Hurler syndrome appear normal at birth. Between 6 and 12 months of age, they have the onset of gradual coarsening and prominence of facial features, with flattening of the midfacial areas and widening of the nasal bridge. Clouding of the corneas, gingival hyperplasia, and thickening of the alveolar ridge develop. Dental eruption is delayed. Deafness may occur and often is helped transiently by amplification. Respiratory involvement results from thickening of the soft tissues in the nasal and pharyngeal areas. Initially, the child may have persistent rhinorrhea or noisy breathing. Gradual upper airway obstruction results in sleep apnea and cor pulmonale. Cardiac involvement usually develops between 2 and 5 years of age and

---

TABLE 389.1

MUCOPOLYSACCHARIDOSES

Type	Name	Gene	Chromosome Location	Enzyme Affected
MPS IH	Hurler	*IDUA*	4p16.3	alpha-L-Iduronidase
MPS IS	Scheie	*IDUA*	4p16.3	alpha-L-Iduronidase
MPS IH/IS	Hurler/Scheie	*IDUA*	4p16.3	alpha-L-Iduronidase
MPS II	Hunter	*IDS*	Xq28	Iduronate sulfatase
MPS IIIA	Sanfilippo A	*SGSH*	17q25.3	Heparan *N*-sulfatase
MPS IIIB	Sanfilippo B	*NAGLU*	17q21	alpha-*N*-Acetylglucosaminidase
MPS IIIC	Sanfilippo C	*MPS3C*	14	Acetyl-CoA:alpha-glucosaminide acetyltransferase
MPS IIID	Sanfilippo D	*GNS*	12q14	*N*-Acetylglucosamine-6-sulfatase
MPS IVA	Morquio A	*GALNS*	16q24.3	*N*-Acetylgalactosamine-6-sulfate sulfatase
MPS IVB	Morquio B	*GLB1*	3p21.33	beta-Galactosidase, specific for keratan sulfate
MPS VI	Maroteaux-Lamy	*ARSB*	5q11–q13	Arylsulfatase B
MPS VII	Sly	*GUSB*	7q21.11	beta-Glucuronidase
MPS IX	Hyaluronidase deficiency	*HYAL1*	3p21.3–p21.2	Hyaluronidase

MPS V and MPS VIII are vacant.

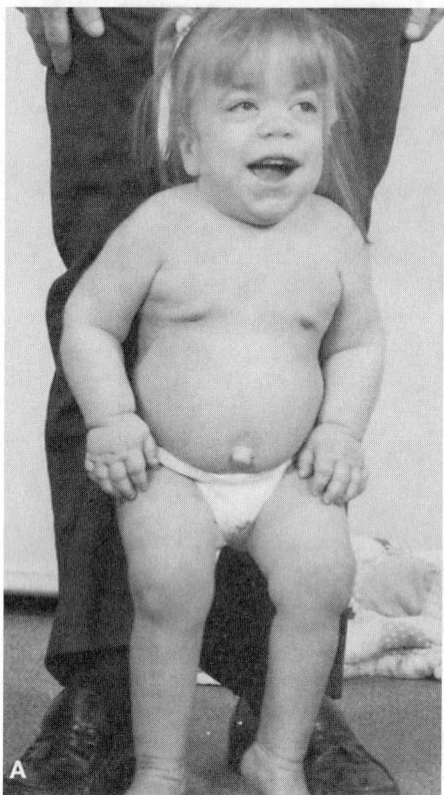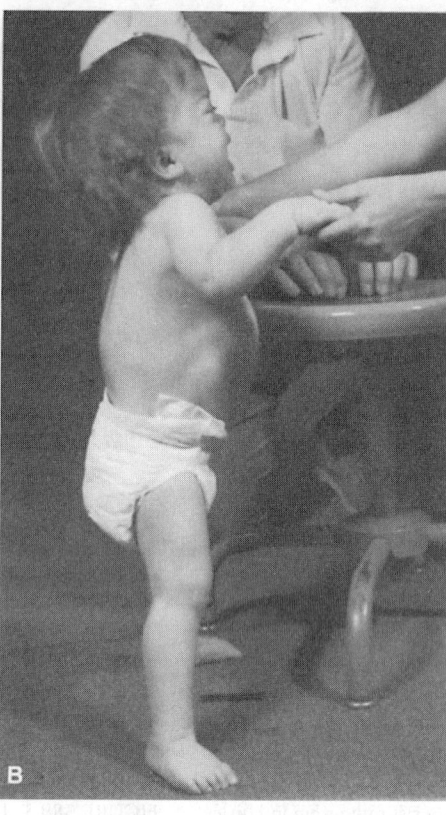

FIGURE 389.6. Children with Hurler syndrome at ages 37 months (**A**) and 27 months (**B**). Note the dolichomacrocephaly and dorsal kyphosis.

may result in thickened valve leaflets, pseudoatheromatosis of the coronary arteries, cardiomyopathy, and congestive heart failure. Hepatosplenomegaly develops during the first year. Infrequently hypersplenism results in thrombocytopenia or pancytopenia. Umbilical and inguinal hernias often require surgical correction (Figs. 389.6 and 389.7).

Bone growth is delayed and there usually is minimal linear growth after 2 to 3 years of age. The gibbus deformity, a dorsolumbar kyphosis, develops during the first year and may progress. The head becomes enlarged and dolichocephalic, with prominence of the frontal areas and suture lines. Radiography shows a progression of the dysostosis multiplex. Overproduction of collagen and elastin may accompany the MPS storage and result in joint stiffness, carpal tunnel syndrome, thickening of the meninges with hydrocephalus, and decreased compliance of the thoracic cage.

Psychomotor development appears normal for the first year, remains on a plateau for 1 to 2 years, and then gradually regresses. Physical limitations are noted as a result of the joint stiffness and bone involvement. Contractures in the lower extremities lead to a "jockey stance," and the hands become stiff and claw-like in appearance, with limited manual dexterity. Physical therapy may be prescribed, with the restriction that flexion and extension of the neck should not be done because of possible hypoplasia of the odontoid process. Adaptive equipment may be of benefit. Most children eventually become wheelchair-bound and do not live past their early teenage years. Death may occur earlier from cardiopulmonary involvement. Enzyme replacement therapy with human recombinant enzyme is currently available for patients with alpha-L-iduronidase deficiency and has shown clinical and biochemical improvement in nonneurologic manifestations of the disorder.

Hurler syndrome may be confirmed by demonstrating deficient activity of alpha-L-iduronidase in peripheral leukocytes or cultured skin fibroblasts. At least 46 mutations have been identified at the alpha-L-iduronidase locus (*IDUA*) that are associated with Hurler syndrome. Two common mutations, W402X

and Q70X, along with one minor allele, P533R are found in over one-half of the alleles in patients from Caucasian populations. Carrier detection is available, but considerable overlap exists between carriers and noncarriers with enzymatic testing. More accurate carrier detection may be done in families of patients in whom the exact genetic mutation is known. Prenatal diagnosis is available with both chorionic villi sampling and cultured amniotic fluid cells.

Scheie Syndrome (Mucopolysaccharidosis I-S)

Scheie syndrome, formerly called *MPS V*, is an autosomal recessive disorder that also results from deficient activity of alpha-L-iduronidase. Most patients have mutations at the *IDUA* locus that allow the enzyme to retain the ability to degrade heparan sulfate. Thus, mainly dermatan sulfate is stored.

Scheie syndrome is one of the mildest forms of the mucopolysaccharidoses. Patients have normal intelligence and usually are of normal stature. Clinical symptoms begin after 5 years of age and include mild coarsening of facial features, severe clouding of the corneas, and pronounced joint involvement in the hands and feet. Aortic valvular problems are common. Carpal tunnel syndrome, degeneration of the retina, glaucoma, and deafness may occur. The disorder usually is associated with a normal or near-normal lifespan. Enzyme replacement therapy with human recombinant alpha-L-iduronidase is available.

Hurler-Scheie Syndrome (Mucopolysaccharidosis I-H/I-S)

Hurler-Scheie syndrome is a rare disorder associated with deficient activity of alpha-L-iduronidase. The clinical features are intermediate between those of Hurler and Scheie syndromes. The onset usually is during the first 2 years of life; survival has

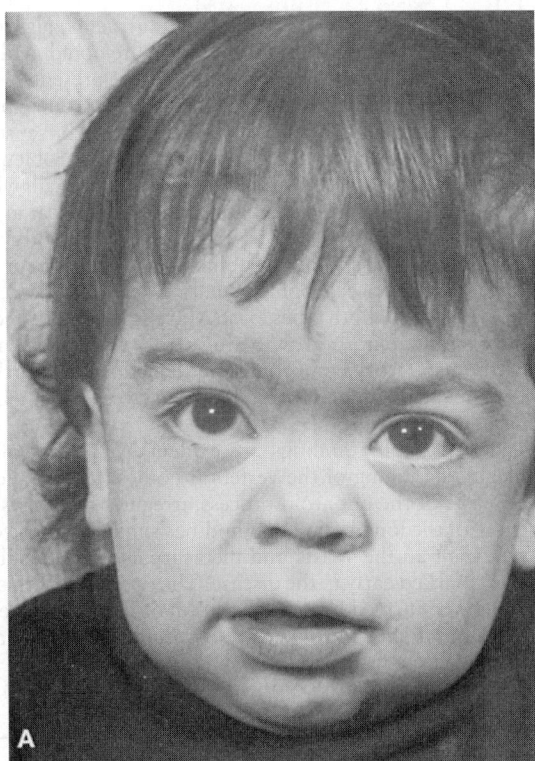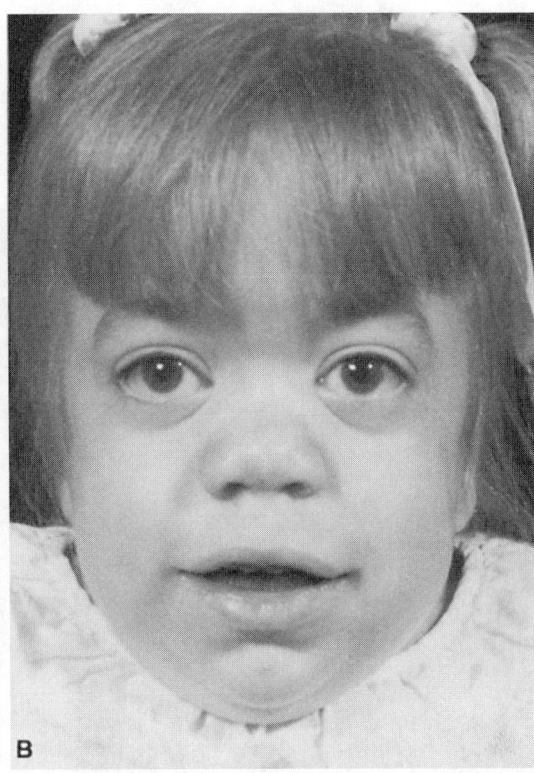

FIGURE 389.7. Face in Hurler syndrome. **A:** Aged 27 months. **B:** Aged 37 months. Prominence of facial features, increased facial hair, flat nasal bridge, and corneal clouding increase with age.

been reported into the third decade of life. By molecular genetic analysis, some affected patients are compound heterozygotes (i.e., they have one gene for Hurler syndrome and another that allows some residual activity) or they may have other allelic mutations at the alpha-L-iduronidase locus specific for Hurler-Scheie syndrome. Enzyme replacement therapy with human recombinant alpha-L-iduronidase is available.

Hunter Syndrome (Mucopolysaccharidosis II)

Hunter syndrome is an X-linked disorder associated with deficient activity of iduronate sulfatase and storage of heparan and dermatan sulfate. Both severe (type A) and mild (type B) forms exist. The clinical features of the severe form are similar to those of Hurler syndrome except that the onset is between 1 and 2 years of age, the course of the disease is somewhat slower, and no corneal clouding occurs (Fig. 389.8). Deafness is common. Skin lesions, consisting of ivory raised papules, often are noted on the upper back and on the lateral upper arms and thighs. Patients commonly survive until the second or third decades. The milder type of this disorder is comparable with Scheie syndrome, usually with normal intelligence and survival into the sixth or seventh decade. Deficient activity of iduronate sulfatase may be noted in serum, peripheral leukocytes, and cultured skin fibroblasts. Accurate carrier detection may be done only with molecular genetic techniques. Prenatal diagnosis is available using chorionic villi sampling and cultured amniotic fluid cells. Enzyme replacement therapy with human recombinant iduronate sulfatase is presently in clinical trials.

Sanfilippo Syndrome (Mucopolysaccharidosis III)

Four forms of Sanfilippo syndrome exist that are clinically indistinguishable. All are inherited as autosomal recessive

traits and are associated with the storage of heparan sulfate. Type A (MPS IIIA) is associated with deficient activity of heparan N-sulfatase (sulfamidase), type B (MPS IIIB) with alpha-N-acetylglucosaminidase, type C (MPS IIIC) with acetyl CoA:alpha-glucosaminide acetyltransferase, and type D

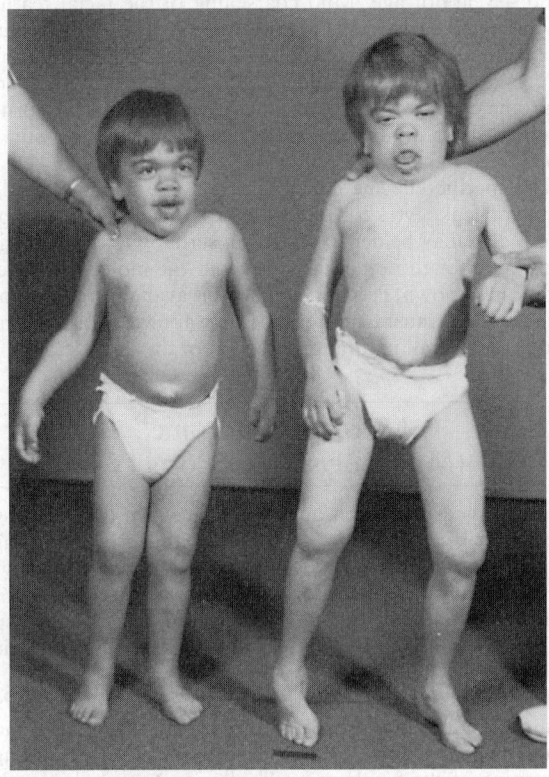

FIGURE 389.8. Brothers, ages 5 and 15 years, with Hunter syndrome.

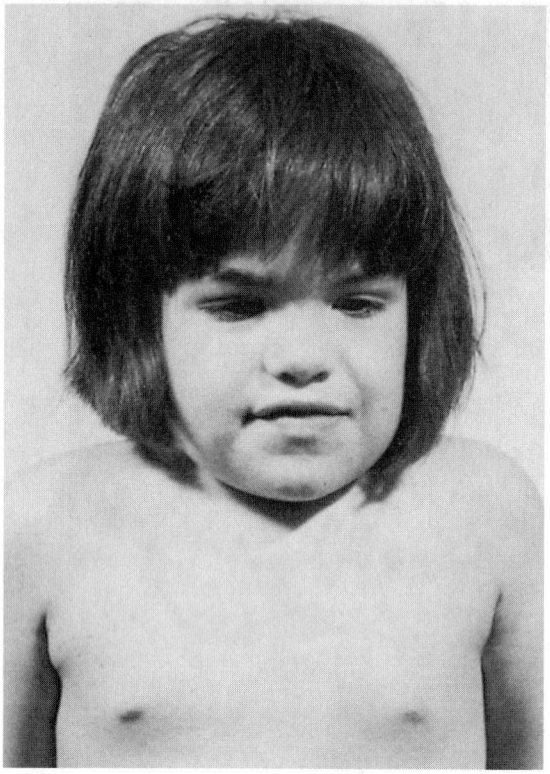

FIGURE 389.9. Patient with Sanfilippo syndrome, age 6 years. Note the minimal coarsening of facial features compared with the other mucopolysaccharidoses.

(MPS IIID) with deficient activity of N-acetylglucosamine-6-sulfatase.

The major clinical findings are related to progressive debilitation from central nervous system involvement. Developmental delay and behavior problems usually are first noted between 2 and 4 years of age. Mild coarsening of the facial features may be noted early in the disease process (Fig. 389.9). Later, joint stiffness, hepatosplenomegaly, hernias, and radiographic findings similar to, but milder than, those seen with Hurler syndrome occur. Affected patients usually do not have corneal clouding, short stature, or cardiac involvement. Most survive into their teenage years.

The specific enzyme deficiencies may be demonstrated in peripheral leukocytes and cultured skin fibroblasts for all types. Type B also may be demonstrated in serum. Carrier detection is available for those families in whom the molecular genetic mutation is known. Prenatal diagnosis is available for all types. Bone marrow transplantation does not appear to significantly change the overall natural progression of the disorder.

Morquio Syndrome (Mucopolysaccharidosis IV)

Morquio syndrome is an autosomal recessive disorder associated with keratan sulfate and chondroitin-6-sulfate storage. Two forms of this disorder exist. Type A is associated with deficient activity of N-acetylgalactosamine-6-sulfate sulfatase (galactose-6-sulfatase) and type B with beta-galactosidase, specific for keratan sulfate. The two forms are similar in clinical findings.

The major clinical feature is skeletal involvement. Psychomotor retardation usually is not present. The onset of short stature and joint laxity occurs at approximately 1 year of age. Shortening of the trunk and neck, flaring of the ribs, promi-

nence of the sternum (pectus carinatum), genu valgum, and enlargement and instability of the joints are noted. Mild corneal clouding and hepatosplenomegaly may be present. Enamel hypoplasia is noted in type A Morquio syndrome, but not in type B. Progressive hearing loss, either mixed or sensorineural, may require hearing aids. Cardiorespiratory problems usually are secondary to the skeletal involvement; valvular heart disease also may be present. Acute or chronic cervical myelopathy is associated with the severe hypoplasia of the odontoid process and with atlantoaxial subluxation. Posterior spinal fusion of the upper cervical spine usually is required. Both mild and severe forms of both types exist. More severely affected patients have minimal linear growth after 6 to 7 years of age and die of cardiorespiratory compromise in their third or fourth decade. Patients with milder forms have survived into their seventh decade.

Radiographic findings are evident by 2 years of age and include flattening of the vertebral bodies (platyspondyly), hypoplasia of the odontoid process, irregular metaphyses, shortening of the long bones, and findings similar to those of Hurler syndrome in the wrists and metacarpals. Keratansulfaturia is most marked early in the disease. The two types of this disorder may be confirmed by demonstration of the enzyme deficiencies in cultured skin fibroblasts. No specific therapy is available. Bone marrow transplantation has not been successful in changing the natural course of the disorder.

Maroteaux-Lamy Syndrome (Mucopolysaccharidosis VI)

Maroteaux-Lamy syndrome is an autosomal recessive disorder associated with dermatan sulfate storage and deficient activity of arylsulfatase B (N-acetylgalactosamine-4-sulfatase). Three forms of the disorder—mild, intermediate, and severe—vary in severity and age of onset. Clinical features of the severe form are similar to those of Hurler syndrome. Psychomotor retardation, however, usually is not present. Survival is possible into the third decade of life. Hydrocephalus and increased intracranial pressure may occur. Mitral and aortic insufficiency may be present. The mild form resembles Scheie syndrome except that patients are short. An intermediate type also has been reported (Figs. 389.10 and 389.11). Deficient activity of arylsulfatase B may be shown in peripheral leukocytes or cultured skin fibroblasts. Carrier detection and prenatal diagnosis are available. Bone marrow or stem cell transplantation may be considered before significant cardiac involvement. Enzyme replacement therapy is available.

Beta-Glucuronidase Deficiency (Mucopolysaccharidosis VII)

Beta-glucuronidase deficiency, also known as *Sly syndrome*, is an autosomal recessive disorder associated with the storage of heparan sulfate, dermatan sulfate, chondroitin-4-sulfate, and chondroitin-6-sulfate. Clinical features may be similar to Hurler syndrome in some patients and milder, without mental retardation, in others. The disorder also may present in the neonatal period with hydrops fetalis and features of a storage disorder. The enzyme deficiency may be demonstrated in peripheral leukocytes and cultured skin fibroblasts.

Hyaluronidase Deficiency (Mucopolysaccharidosis IX)

Hyaluronidase deficiency has been reported in a 14-year-old girl with short stature, periarticular soft tissue masses, and

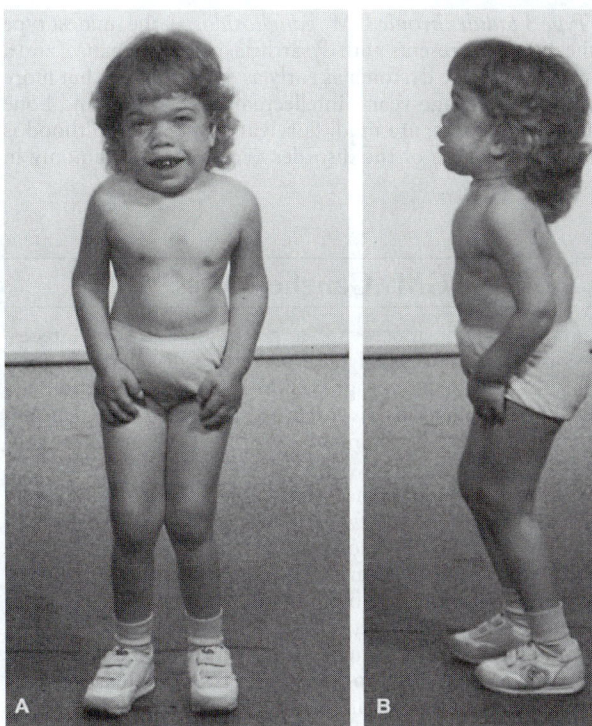

FIGURE 389.10. Patient with Maroteaux-Lamy syndrome, severe form, age 10 years. Note the coarse facial appearance, shortened thorax, hand and joint contractures, and "gibbus" formation of the thoracic spine.

a mildly dysmorphic facies with flattened nasal bridge. Psychomotor development and neurologic and ophthalmologic examinations were normal. Radiography of the pelvis showed nodular intraarticular soft tissue masses and acetabular erosions. Histologic studies of the masses and skin fibroblasts revealed membrane-bound storage of MPS-like material in histocytes. Plasma hyaluronidase activity was absent and plasma hyaluronan levels elevated. The disorder is inherited as an autosomal recessive trait.

SPHINGOLIPIDOSES

The sphingolipidoses are associated with lysosomal accumulation of glycosphingolipids, gangliosides, and sphingomyelin. Faulty degradation of the molecules results from deficient activity of a lysosomal acid hydrolase or a missing sphingolipid activator protein needed for enzyme-lipid stabilization and interaction.

Ceramide, the basic structure for these molecules, is composed of sphingosine, to which a long-chain fatty acid, usually C16, has been attached at the amino group (Fig. 389.12). Attachment of neutral carbohydrate groups in an oligosaccharide chain occurs at the hydroxyl group of the sphingosine. The attachment of a glucosyl residue in beta linkage as the first

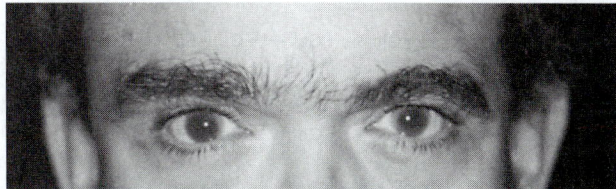

FIGURE 389.11. Eyes in adult-onset Maroteaux-Lamy syndrome. Note the corneal clouding.

neutral sugar leads to a glucosylceramide (glucocerebroside) series of glycosphingolipids. Attachment of a galactosyl residue leads to a galactosylceramide (galactocerebroside) series. The neutral sugars of the oligosaccharide side chain may be in alpha or beta linkage and are derived from glucose, galactose, N-acetyl-galactosamine, or N-acetyl-glucosamine. If the first neutral sugar is a sulfated galactosyl, the compound is called a *sulfatide*. If sialic acid, or N-acetyl-neuraminic acid, is attached to the neutral sugars, the structure is termed a *ganglioside*.

Current nomenclature of the gangliosides, according to the Svennerholm classification, is determined by the number of sialic acid residues that are attached to the oligosaccharide chain (M = mono, D = di, T = tri) and by the number (5 minus *n*) of neutral sugars in the chain. For example, GM_1 ganglioside would have one sialic acid residue and four (5 minus 1) neutral sugars in the oligosaccharide chain attached to the ceramide. Degradation of glycosphingolipids involves stepwise removal of the neutral sugars, sulfate, and sialic acid by a series of lysosomal hydrolases (Fig. 389.13). Table 389.2 gives molecular genetic information for the sphingolipidoses.

GM_1 Gangliosidosis

GM_1 gangliosidosis is inherited as an autosomal recessive trait and associated with acid beta-galactosidase deficiency. Storage of GM_1 ganglioside, GA_1 ganglioside, keratan sulfate, and other glycoproteins and oligosaccharides that contain beta-galactoside residues occurs in the brain, viscera, bones, and other tissues of affected patients. Three major types of the disorder vary in clinical severity and age of onset, corresponding to different mutations at the beta-galactosidase gene locus.

Type 1 (infantile form or generalized gangliosidosis) is associated with a complete lack of acid beta-galactosidase activity (Fig. 389.14). Symptoms begin at or shortly after birth and include severe progressive central nervous system degeneration, coarse facial features, corneal clouding, macroglossia, gingival hyperplasia, hepatosplenomegaly, hernias, joint stiffness, dorsal kyphosis, and edema of the extremities. Cherry-red macular spots may be seen in one-half of the patients. Radiography shows dysostosis multiplex. Foamy histiocytes may be noted in bone marrow and visceral organs. Death usually occurs by 2 years of age. Carrier detection and prenatal diagnosis are available.

Type 2 (late infantile or juvenile GM_1 gangliosidosis) is a milder disorder with less severe symptoms of MPS storage. The

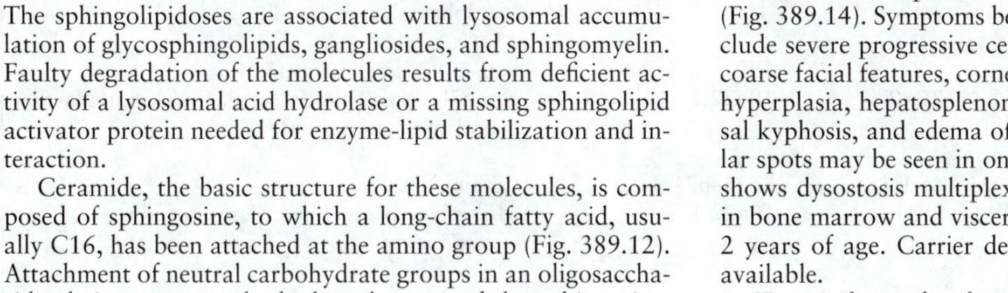

A. $CH_3(CH_2)_{12} - CH = CH - \underset{\underset{OH}{|}}{CH} - \underset{\underset{NH}{|}}{CH} - CH_2 - O - \underset{\underset{OH}{\overset{O}{\|}}}{P} - O - CH_2 - CH_2 - \underset{\underset{CH_3}{\overset{CH_3}{|}}}{N^+} - CH_3$

B. $CH_3(CH_2)_{16} - C = O$

D.

C.

FIGURE 389.12. Structure of sphingomyelin. A, sphingoid (sphingosine); B, fatty acid (stearoyl); C, ceramide; D, phosphoryl choline.

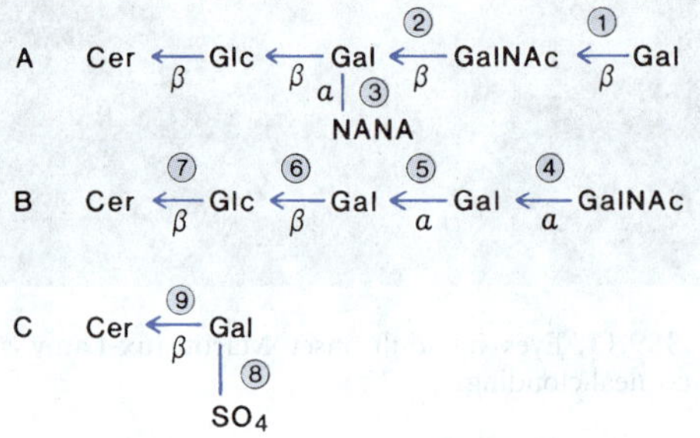

FIGURE 389.13. Examples of sphingolipid degradation. A, GM$_1$ ganglioside; B, asialoganglioside; C, sulfatide; 1, GM$_1$-beta-galactosidase (GM$_1$ gangliosidosis); 2, beta-N-acetylgalactosaminidase, beta-hexosaminidase A and B (GM$_2$ gangliosidoses); 3, GM$_3$-alpha-neuraminidase; 4, alpha-N-acetylgalactosaminidase, alpha-galactosidase B (Schindler disease); 5, alpha-galactosidase A (Fabry disease); 6, ceramide-lactoside beta-galactosidase; 7, beta-glucosidase (Gaucher disease); 8, arylsulfatase A (metachromatic leukodystrophy); 9, beta-galactosidase (Krabbe disease); Cer, ceramide; Gal, galactose; GalNAc, N-acetylgalactosamine; Glc, glucose; NANA, N-acetylneuraminic acid, sialic acid.

onset of ataxia between 1 and 2 years of age is followed by progressive mental and motor deterioration, spasticity, seizures, and blindness. Death occurs between 3 and 10 years of age. There usually is no coarsening of the facial features, hepatosplenomegaly, corneal clouding, or macular changes. Radiography may show mild changes of dysostosis multiplex.

Type 3 (adult chronic GM$_1$ gangliosidosis), the mildest type of the disorder, presents with dysarthria, gait disturbance, and a slowly progressive dystonia as early as 4 years of age, but more often in the teenage years. Intellectual involvement and bone changes, if present, are mild. Survival into early adulthood is possible. This type of the disorder occurs most commonly in Japan.

GM$_2$ Gangliosidoses

The GM$_2$ gangliosidoses are a group of autosomal recessive disorders associated with cerebral degeneration secondary to lysosomal storage of GM$_2$ ganglioside and related glycosphingolipids. The disorders are associated with deficient activity of the beta-hexoaminidases or the GM$_2$ activator protein.

Beta-hexosaminidase has two subunits, alpha and beta, which are the products of two separate genetic loci, HEXA and HEXB, located on chromosomes 15 and 5, respectively. The isoenzymes of beta-hexosaminidase are composed of different combinations of these subunits. Hexosaminidase A is composed of an alpha and a beta subunit, whereas hexosaminidase B contains two beta subunits. Hexosaminidase A usually accounts for 55% to 70% of the total hexosaminidase-specific activity, whereas hexosaminidase B accounts for 30% to 45%. Genetic mutations at the alpha subunit gene locus lead to hexosaminidase A deficiency and Tay-Sachs disease. Mutations at the beta subunit gene locus lead to deficiency of both hexosaminidase A and B and result in Sandhoff disease. A GM$_2$

TABLE 389.2

SPHINGOLIPIDOSES

Name	Gene	Chromosome Location	Enzyme or Process Affected
GM$_1$ gangliosidosis	GLB1	3p21.33	beta-Galactosidase
GM$_2$ gangliosidoses			
Tay-Sachs disease	HEXA	15q23–q24	Hexosaminidase A
Sandhoff disease	HEXB	5q13	Hexosaminidase B
GM$_2$ ganglioside activator protein deficiency	GM2A	5q31.3–q33.1	Hexosaminidase A
Fabry	GLA	Xq22.1	alpha-Galactosidase (alpha-galactosidase A)
Schindler	NAGA	22q11	alpha-N-Acetylgalactosaminidase (alpha-galactosidase B)
Glucocerebrosidoses			
Gaucher	GBA	1q21	beta-Glucocerebrosidase
Sphingolipid activator protein 2 (saposin C) deficiency	PSAP	10q22.1	beta-Glucocerebrosidase, galactosylceramidase, and sphingomyelinase
Ceramidoses			
Farber	ASAH	8p22–p21.3	Ceramidase
Prosaposin (saposin precursor) deficiency	PSAP	10q22.1	Multiple lysosomal hydrolases including ceramidase
Sphingomyelin-cholesterol lipidoses			
Niemann-Pick types A and B	SMPD1	11p15.4–p15.1	Sphingomyelinase
Niemann Pick type C1	NPC1	18q11–q12	Defect in cholesterol transport and esterification
Niemann Pick type C2	NPC2	14q24.3	Defect in cholesterol transport and esterification
Krabbe	GALC	14q31	beta-Galactosidase specific for galactosylceramide (galactosylceramidase)
Sulfatide lipidoses			
Metachromatic leukodystrophy	ARSA	22q13.31-qter	Arylsulfatase A (cerebroside sulfatase)
Sphingolipid activator protein 1 (saposin B) deficiency	PSAP	10q22.1	Arylsulfatase A plus 19 other glycolipid hydrolases
Multiple sulfatase deficiency	SUMF1	3p26	Sulfatase-modifying factor 1

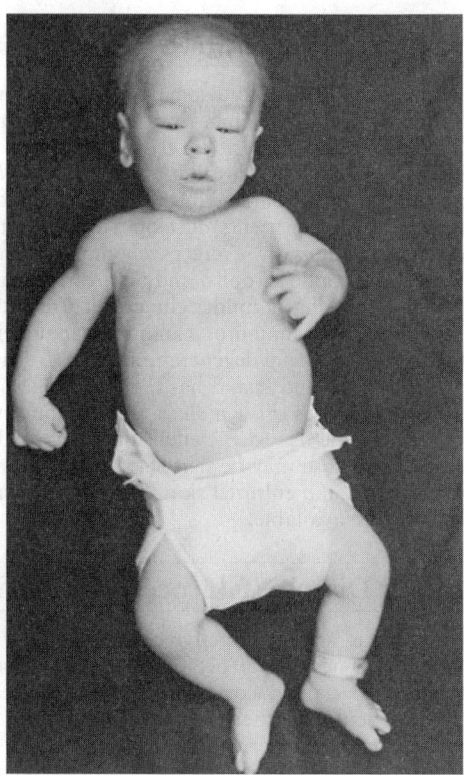

FIGURE 389.14. Patient with GM$_1$ gangliosidosis. This child has a mildly coarse facial appearance, facial edema, and an enlarged abdomen from hepatosplenomegaly. An early "gibbus" formation was noted in the thoracic spine.

activator protein, encoded by the *GM2A* locus on chromosome 5, is needed for stabilization of the GM$_2$ ganglioside-hexosaminidase A complex. At least 93 mutations at the *HEXA* locus, 26 at the *HEXB* locus, and 4 at the *GM2A* locus have been characterized to date.

Tay-Sachs Disease (GM$_2$ Gangliosidosis, Type 1)

Tay-Sachs disease is associated with the storage of GM$_2$ ganglioside and progressive central nervous system degeneration. Affected children are usually normal at birth. Between 6 and 12 months of age, hypotonia and psychomotor retardation become evident. An exaggerated startle response to stimuli, termed *hyperacusis*, may be noted. Starting at approximately 1 year of age, spasticity, loss of vision, seizures, and macrocephaly develop. Cherry-red spots in the macular area may be seen as early as 3 months of age and represent a normal red macular area surrounded by a white area of storage. Later in the disorder, the spots appear dark brown as macular degeneration advances. Affected children usually require nasogastric or gastrostomy feedings and have problems with oral secretions after 18 to 24 months of age. Intercurrent respiratory problems frequently occur. Most affected children die between 3 and 4 years of age. The diagnosis is confirmed by measurement of hexosaminidase A in serum, plasma, peripheral leukocytes, or cultured skin fibroblasts. Severe deficiency of hexosaminidase A exists, which may be expressed in specific activity units or as a percentage of the total enzyme. Because hexosaminidase B is not affected and may be increased, the total amount of beta-hexosaminidase is normal.

The disorder is most common in individuals of Eastern European Jewish ancestry, among whom the carrier rate is 1 in 31. Since the 1970s, community education and carrier testing programs have identified at-risk couples, in which both individuals are carriers for Tay-Sachs disease, before the birth of an affected child. The current recommendation is that all persons of Eastern European Jewish ancestry have carrier testing performed before conception so that timely and appropriate genetic counseling can be given. Because the carrier rate among individuals of other backgrounds is approximately 1 in 256, the possibility of Tay-Sachs disease should not be excluded in non-Jewish children if the disorder is suspected on clinical grounds. Prenatal diagnosis is available using chorionic villi sampling or amniocentesis.

Sandhoff Disease (GM$_2$ Gangliosidosis, Type 2)

Sandhoff disease is associated with total deficiency of beta-hexosaminidase and storage in the brain and viscera of GM$_2$ ganglioside, as well as other glycolipids, glycoproteins, and oligosaccharides that contain beta-hexosaminide residues. Clinical features are similar to those in Tay-Sachs disease. Hepatosplenomegaly and renal storage may be noted. Sandhoff disease occurs in children of all backgrounds. Carrier detection and prenatal diagnosis are available.

GM$_2$ Gangliosidosis Variants

Juvenile forms of both Tay-Sachs disease and Sandhoff disease present between 2 and 6 years of age with ataxia or developmental regression, followed by loss of speech, spasticity, athetosis, and minor motor seizures. Macular changes may not be present; optic atrophy and retinitis pigmentosa are seen occasionally. Death occurs between 5 and 15 years of age. Mutations at the *HEXA* or *HEXB* locus in these patients usually allow some residual enzymatic activity.

An *adult form* of Tay-Sachs disease has been reported in patients with atypical spinocerebellar degeneration and occasionally psychoses. The onset has varied widely from between 2 and 4 years of age to as late as 16 years of age. These patients have been shown to have a specific mutation at the *HEXA* locus that results in an unstable alpha subunit protein.

Affected patients of all types have been found to have normal enzyme activity when tested with standard methods that use artificial substrates. Deficient activity may be demonstrated by testing with natural substrates. Some of these patients have a *GM$_2$ activator protein deficiency*, whereas others have mutations that affect substrate specificity.

Conversely, otherwise normal adults have been noted to have absent hexosaminidase A when tested with artificial substrates, but only partially reduced activity when tested with natural substrates. These individuals are usually compound heterozygotes who have one gene for classic Tay-Sachs disease and the other for a pseudodeficiency allele that does not allow measurement of enzyme activity with artificial substrates. Approximately 35% of enzymatically determined non-Jewish heterozygotes and 2% of Jewish heterozygotes are carriers for one of the two pseudodeficiency alleles at the *HEXA* locus. Individuals found to be heterozygotes by enzymatic testing should have mutational analysis done to determine whether they are carriers for the pseudodeficiency allele or carriers for Tay-Sachs disease, so that accurate genetic counseling may be given concerning disease risks for their children.

Fabry Disease (alpha-Galactosyl-Lactosyl Ceramidosis)

Fabry disease is an X-linked disorder associated with deficient activity of alpha-galactosidase (formerly termed *alpha-galactosidase A*). Storage of glycosphingolipids with terminal

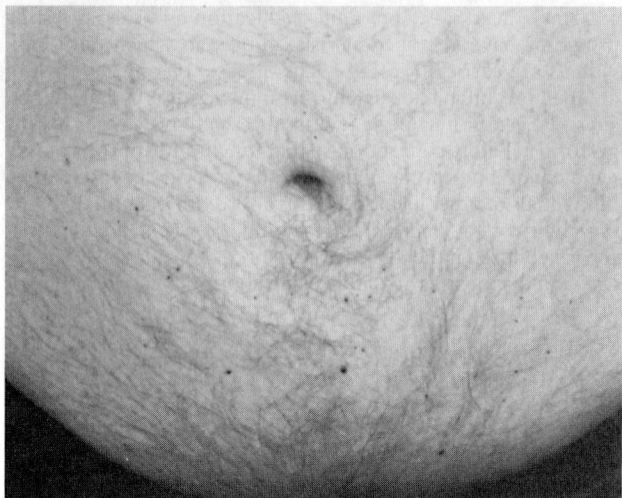

FIGURE 389.15. Angiokeratomas in a patient with Fabry disease.

galactosyl residues in alpha linkage, such as globotriaosylceramide, galabiosylceramide, and blood group B substances, occurs in the eyes, kidneys, skeletal and cardiac muscle, the central and autonomic nervous systems, and the vascular endothelium and smooth muscle throughout the body.

Clinical symptoms usually are evident by 10 years of age. Acroparesthesia often is the presenting symptom. Intermittent painful crises, lasting minutes to days, may involve the extremities or the abdomen. Because episodes often are accompanied by a low-grade fever and an elevated erythrocyte sedimentation rate, they may be mistaken for other causes of an acute abdominal crisis. A characteristic whorl-like corneal dystrophy with spoke-like or propeller-like cataracts may be seen. Angiokeratoma corporis diffusa, consisting of punctate, flat to slightly raised, dark red to blue-black papules, usually appear in clusters in areas between the umbilicus and knees (bathing suit area) (Fig. 389.15). Angiokeratoma also may be found on the conjunctiva or mucosal surfaces. Hypohidrosis is common.

With advancing age, affected patients complain of fatigue, weakness, and poor vision. Cardiac involvement may lead to myocardial infarction, cardiomyopathies, or conduction defects. Vascular involvement of the central nervous system may lead to aneurysms, vascular occlusion, or hemorrhage. Patients frequently become hypertensive. Renal dysfunction, initially evident as proteinuria, usually progresses to renal failure by 30 to 40 years of age. Renal dialysis or transplantation may be indicated.

Deficient activity of alpha-galactosidase may be shown in peripheral leukocytes or cultured skin fibroblasts. Low-dose diphenylhydantoin or carbamazepine may improve the acroparesthesia and painful crises. Enzyme replacement therapy employing human recombinant alpha-galactosidase is currently available and has been shown to reduce the tissue level of stored glycosphingolipid and improve clinical status. Accurate carrier detection may be done with molecular genetic techniques. Prenatal diagnosis is available.

Female carriers for Fabry disease often have milder, but similar, clinical findings. The most frequent of these is corneal dystrophy. With advancing age, many become symptomatic, and deaths have occurred from vascular, renal, or cardiac involvement, as in male subjects. Enzyme replacement therapy is also indicated for symptomatic female carriers for Fabry disease.

Schindler Disease

Schindler disease is a rare, autosomal recessive disorder associated with deficiency of alpha-N-acetylgalactosaminidase (formerly called *alpha-galactosidase B*) and the storage of glycoproteins and oligosaccharides that contain alpha-N-acetylgalactosaminyl residues. Three clinical forms of the disorder are recognized. *Type I* patients develop a neuroaxonal dystrophy during infancy with severe psychomotor retardation, myoclonic seizures, optic atrophy, and progressive neurologic deterioration. *Type II* has a milder clinical picture and occurs in adults with mild psychomotor handicaps, angiokeratoma, and peripheral neuroaxonal degeneration. *Type III* is intermediate between types I and II and has a variable age of onset. Urinary oligosaccharides show a characteristic abnormal pattern in all types of the disorder. Deficient activity of alpha-N-acetylgalactosaminidase may be demonstrated in plasma, peripheral leukocytes, and cultured skin fibroblasts. Carrier and prenatal testing are available.

Gaucher Disease (Glucocerebrosidosis)

Gaucher disease is an autosomal recessive disorder associated with deficient activity of beta-glucocerebrosidase (beta-glucosidase). Storage of glucocerebroside (glucosylceramide) occurs in the reticuloendothelial system. Three forms of the disorder vary in clinical severity.

Type 1, the chronic nonneuronopathic form of Gaucher disease, is the most common sphingolipid storage disorder. Its highest incidence is among persons of Eastern European Jewish ancestry. Affected patients may present at any age with asymptomatic splenomegaly. More severely affected patients present during childhood with massive splenomegaly and pancytopenia. Hepatomegaly with mildly elevated liver function test results also occurs. Cirrhosis and liver failure occasionally develop. Infiltration of the bone marrow interferes with bone growth and mineralization and compounds the pancytopenia. Pulmonary storage may lead to abnormal pulmonary function and cor pulmonale. Bone marrow and other tissues from the reticuloendothelial system have large, lipid-laden, fusiform histiocytes with dense eccentric nuclei that resemble wrinkled tissue paper or crumpled silk (Gaucher cells). Radiography shows an expanded cortex of the distal femur termed an *Erlenmeyer-flask deformity;* bone erosion with cyst-like changes of varying sizes is noted. Painful avascular crises in long bones and vertebral bodies, pseudoosteomyelitis, and avascular necrosis of the femoral or humeral heads may occur. Serum acid phosphatase levels are elevated from bone involvement. Older patients may have yellow or brown discoloration of the exposed skin or pingueculae on the conjunctiva. Primary central nervous system disease does not occur. The disorder is slowly progressive, and many patients who present in childhood live well into adult life. Other patients have a relatively mild disease and are identified by splenomegaly when they are adults.

Enzyme replacement therapy with intravenous infusions of macrophage-targeted modified human recombinant glucocerebrosidase results in significant clinical improvement in symptomatic patients. Responses in hematologic parameters and reduction in the size of the liver and spleen occur more rapidly than skeletal changes. Although extremely expensive, enzyme replacement therapy should be considered for any symptomatic patient with type 1 or 3 Gaucher disease. Bone marrow transplantation also may be considered, but it is associated with considerable risks when compared with enzyme replacement therapy. Gene transfer therapy is being investigated.

Before enzyme replacement therapy was available, many patients required splenectomy for persistent thrombocytopenia and bleeding diatheses. Postsplenectomy management should include prophylactic antibiotics and immunization, as for other asplenic individuals. Orthopedic problems are often difficult to treat and should be referred to specialists who are experienced with Gaucher patients.

Type 2, the acute neuronopathic form of Gaucher disease, has its onset between birth and 18 months of age. Massive hepatosplenomegaly is accompanied by a rapidly progressing central nervous system deterioration. Trismus, strabismus, and retroflexion of the head are pathognomonic. Spasticity, hyperreflexia, and seizures occur. Feeding and respiratory problems are common. Death usually occurs by 2 years of age. Treatment is symptomatic and supportive. Enzyme replacement therapy has been shown to improve organomegaly and hematologic status, but does not prevent central nervous system deterioration.

Type 3, the subacute neuronopathic form of Gaucher disease, has features of both types 1 and 2. Most cases occur in individuals with northern Swedish (Norrbottnian) ancestry. The onset of hepatosplenomegaly in childhood usually precedes the progressive neurologic symptoms. Behavioral changes, oculomotor apraxia, extrapyramidal and cerebellar signs, seizures, and developmental regression occur. Many patients live into early adulthood. Enzyme replacement therapy improves organomegaly and hematologic status and appears to stabilize, and in some cases has improved, central nervous system involvement.

The diagnosis for all three types of Gaucher disease is established by the demonstration of deficient activity of beta-glucosidase in peripheral leukocytes or cultured skin fibroblasts in experienced laboratories. Molecular genetic studies help differentiate between type 1 and type 3 disease in young patients. Atypical juvenile cases have been associated with *deficiency of sphingolipid activator protein 2* (saposin C). Carrier detection and prenatal diagnosis are available.

Farber Disease (Ceramidosis, Lipogranulomatosis)

Farber disease, an autosomal recessive disorder, is associated with deficient activity of acid ceramidase (acylsphingosine deacylase). Ceramide and other gangliosides are stored in the skin, lymph nodes, viscera, and brain. Connective tissue granuloma forms in response to the storage. *Type 1*, the *classic* and most common form of the disorder, presents between 2 weeks and 4 months of age. A hoarse cry, swollen painful joints, periarticular nodules, and pulmonary infiltration are noted. Older patients have more widely distributed skin nodules over pressure points and in the periorbital and perioral regions. Joint contractions develop. Granulomatous lesions of the conjunctiva occur. Occasionally, macular changes and corneal or lens opacities are noted. Swallowing and respiration are hindered by granulomas in the pharynx and upper respiratory tract. Valvular cardiac lesions, hepatosplenomegaly, and a generalized lymphadenopathy may occur. Psychomotor deterioration, seizures, hypotonia, hyporeflexia, and failure to thrive are noted. Death usually occurs within a few years of onset, but some patients have survived to the late teenage years. Other forms of this rare disorder differ in the age of onset, clinical severity, and degree of visceral involvement. They are named as follows: *type 2*, or the *intermediate* form; *type 3*, or the *mild* form; *type 4*, or the *neonatal visceral* form; *type 5*, or the *progressive neurologic* form; *type 6*, which consists of type 1 in combination with Sandhoff disease; and *type 7*, which is associated with *deficiency of prosaposin*, the precursor protein for the sphingolipid activator proteins (SAPs). Current therapy is supportive only.

Deficient activity of ceramidase may be shown in peripheral leukocytes or cultured skin fibroblasts. Carrier detection and prenatal diagnosis are available.

Niemann-Pick Disease (Sphingomyelin-Cholesterol Lipidosis)

Niemann-Pick disease consists of a group of disorders that are associated with the storage of sphingomyelin, unesterified cholesterol, bis(monoacylglyceryl)phosphate, and other related glycosphingolipids in the reticuloendothelial system, viscera, and brain. All are inherited as autosomal recessive traits. The disorders are divided into two groups on the basis of cause. Types A and B are associated with deficient activity of sphingomyelinase. Both type A and B result from mutations at the sphingomyelinase genetic locus; patients with type B have some residual activity that spares significant central nervous system involvement. Type C is associated with defects in intracellular transport and esterification of cholesterol that lead to secondary reduction in activity of sphingomyelinase. Lipid-filled foam cells may be noted in the bone marrow, brain, and viscera of affected patients. Sea-blue histiocytes may be demonstrated with Romanovsky staining.

Type A Niemann-Pick disease, the most common form of the disorder, is seen more frequently in persons of Eastern European Jewish ancestry in whom the carrier rate is estimated to be 1 in 80. Hepatosplenomegaly develops between birth and 6 months of age and is followed by a rapidly progressing central nervous system deterioration. Lymphadenopathy and pulmonary infiltration occur. A yellow-brown discoloration of the skin and seizures may be noted. One-half of patients have cherry-red spots in the macular areas. Failure to thrive and respiratory problems are common. Most affected children die by 2 to 3 years of age.

Type B Niemann-Pick disease is less severe than is type A. Like type A, type B is most often observed in patients of Eastern European Jewish heritage. Hepatosplenomegaly begins during early childhood. Progressive pulmonary infiltration may lead to chronic lung disease and cor pulmonale. Lymphadenopathy is noted frequently. Little or no central nervous system involvement occurs. Many patients survive into adulthood. Enzyme replacement therapy is being developed for type B disease.

Deficient activity of sphingomyelinase may be demonstrated in peripheral leukocytes or cultured skin fibroblasts for types A and B Niemann-Pick disease. Carrier detection and prenatal diagnosis are available.

Type C Niemann-Pick disease has a spectrum of clinical presentation. The disorder most often presents during childhood with variable hepatosplenomegaly and a slowly progressive central nervous system deterioration. Behavioral changes, psychomotor delay and regression, incoordination, and ataxia develop. Hyperreflexia, spasticity, dysarthria, dystonia, and seizures occur. Vertical supranuclear ophthalmoplegia is a common and pathognomonic finding. Survival to late teenage years is possible. Other affected patients present with neonatal hepatic failure or the onset of progressive neurologic involvement, with or without hepatic involvement, during early infancy. Still other patients present as adults with psychosis or progressive dementia. Genetic isolates, with an increased incidence of the disorder, occur among the French Arcadians in Nova Scotia and Hispanic-Americans in southern Colorado. Current therapy is mainly supportive. The benefit of a lowered cholesterol intake and the use of inhibitors of endogenous cholesterol synthesis are being investigated. Defects in cholesterol transport and esterification may be shown in cultured skin fibroblasts. Carrier detection and prenatal diagnosis may be done with molecular genetic techniques. Two forms of type C Niemann-Pick disease exist, type C1 and type C2, which result from mutations at two separate genetic loci, *NPC1* and *NPC2*, respectively. Both forms have variable clinical findings. Some patients with type C2 have a severe and rapid disease course or severe pulmonary involvement.

Krabbe Disease (Globoid Cell Leukodystrophy, Galactosylceramidosis)

Krabbe disease is associated with deficient activity of the beta-galactosidase specific for removing the terminal beta-galactosyl residue from galactosylceramide (galactosylceramidase). Storage of galactosylceramide (galactocerebroside) occurs in the white matter of the central nervous system and in the peripheral nervous system. Globoid cells (globoid bodies) are large, distended, multinucleated, modified macrophages that are found in clusters in the perivascular areas of the white matter of affected patients.

The *infantile type* of Krabbe disease usually presents before 6 months of age with increased motor tone, irritability, hypersensitivity to external stimuli, episodic hypothermia, optic atrophy, and developmental regression. Thereafter follows a rapidly progressing degeneration of the central and peripheral nervous systems, with hypotonia and loss of vision and hearing. Cherry-red spots may be seen. Seizures and peripheral neuropathy are common. Cerebrospinal fluid protein concentration may be elevated markedly (100 to 500 mg/dL); nerve conduction velocity is decreased. Severe brain atrophy with demyelination and gliosis occurs. Most patients die by 2 years of age.

The *late-onset variants* of Krabbe disease (late infantile, juvenile, and adult forms) become clinically symptomatic between 6 months and 35 years of age. Decreased vision with optic atrophy, spastic quadriparesis with pyramidal signs, acute polyneuropathy, ataxia, spinocerebellar degeneration, and psychomotor regression may be seen. Elevated cerebrospinal fluid protein concentrations and decreased nerve conduction velocities are variable.

Krabbe disease, inherited as an autosomal recessive trait, is most common in persons of Scandinavian ancestry. Deficient activity of galactosylceramidase (galactocerebroside beta-galactosidase) may be demonstrated in peripheral leukocytes and cultured skin fibroblasts. Carrier detection and prenatal diagnosis are available.

Metachromatic Leukodystrophy (Sulfatide Lipidosis)

Metachromatic leukodystrophy is associated with the accumulation of galactosyl sulfatide (cerebroside sulfatide) in the white matter of the central nervous system and in the peripheral nervous system. In addition, galactosyl sulfatide and sulfated galactoglycerolipids accumulate in the kidney, gallbladder, and other visceral organs. Along with the storage of sulfatides, demyelination, gliosis, spongy degeneration, and atrophy of the brain occur. The storage of the acidic sulfatides gives rise to the metachromatic staining noted with acetic acid–cresyl violet stain for which the disorder is named.

Three clinical types of metachromatic leukodystrophy exist, which are classified according to age of onset. All types are inherited as autosomal recessive traits.

The *late-infantile type* of metachromatic leukodystrophy has its onset between 1 and 2 years of age. Delayed development, ataxia, gait disturbances, weakness, or peripheral neuropathy may be presenting signs. Thereafter follows a progressive psychomotor regression and central and peripheral nervous system deterioration. Weakness, hypotonia, and hyporeflexia progress to dysarthria and loss of speech, optic atrophy and blindness, nystagmus, loss of truncal and limb control, and spasticity. Respiratory and feeding problems are common as a result of bulbar and pseudobulbar palsies. Seizures may occur. A gray discoloration of the macular areas

may be present. The cerebrospinal fluid protein concentration is elevated. Nerve conduction velocities are slowed. Computed tomographic scanning of the head reveals atrophy of the white matter with enlargement of the ventricles and widening of the sulci. Metachromatic granules may be demonstrated in urine sediment. Bone marrow examination usually does not provide specific findings. Most children die between 2 and 4 years after the onset of their disease.

The *juvenile type* of metachromatic leukodystrophy usually becomes apparent between 5 and 7 years of age but may have its onset as late as 16 to 20 years of age. Changes in personality or school performance, gait disturbances, ataxia, speech problems, or incontinence often are presenting symptoms. The disorder progresses in a manner similar to, but slower than, the late infantile type. Seizures are more common. Most affected individuals do not live past their teenage years or for more than 4 to 6 years after the onset of the disease.

The *adult type* of metachromatic leukodystrophy has its onset after puberty. Initial symptoms may be emotional lability, apathy, personality change, weakness, incontinence, dementia, or psychosis. Thereafter follows progressive dementia, ataxia, dystonia, optic atrophy, and spasticity. Most patients live 5 to 10 years after the onset of the disease, but some have a slower course, with survival for several decades.

Deficient activity of galactosyl-3-sulfate-ceramide sulfatase (cerebroside sulfatase), also termed *arylsulfatase A*, is associated with all three types of clinical presentation. The variation is the result of different allelic mutations at the genetic locus for the enzyme, with preservation of some residual activity in the milder forms. *Deficiency of a cerebroside sulfatase activator protein* (sphingolipid activator protein 1, or saposin B) has been found in some patients with the juvenile form of the disorder.

Carrier detection and prenatal diagnosis are available, but may require radiolabeled sulfatide accumulation studies or molecular genetic techniques. Healthy adults have been reported who have absent or reduced arylsulfatase A activity when tested using artificial substrates but normal radiolabeled sulfatide accumulation studies. This pseudodeficiency is not rare and can be problematic if parents of affected children are not tested before prenatal diagnosis.

Multiple Sulfatase Deficiency (Mucosulfatidosis, Austin Disease)

Multiple sulfatase deficiency is a rare disorder that results from impaired activation of multiple lysosomal and nonlysosomal sulfatases. The lysosomal enzymes known to be involved and the disorders associated with the isolated deficiency of each include arylsulfatase A (metachromatic leukodystrophy), arylsulfatase B (Maroteaux-Lamy syndrome), iduronate sulfatase (Hunter syndrome), heparan sulfamidase (Sanfilippo syndrome A), N-acetylglucosamine-6-sulfate sulfatase (Sanfilippo syndrome D), and N-acetylgalactosamine-6-sulfate sulfatase (Morquio syndrome A). All are discussed elsewhere in this chapter. Other enzymes involved include glucuronate-2-sulfatase, glucosamine-3-sulfatase, and arylsulfatases C, D, E, and F. Deficiency of arylsulfatase C is associated with X-linked ichthyosis, corneal opacities, and elevated blood cholesterol sulfate levels. Deficiency of arylsulfatase E results in X-linked chondrodysplasia punctata. The function of the other enzymes is unknown.

Multiple sulfatase deficiency, an autosomal recessive disorder, is associated with clinical manifestations that are a combination of those features seen with late-infantile metachromatic leukodystrophy, the mucopolysaccharidoses, and steroid

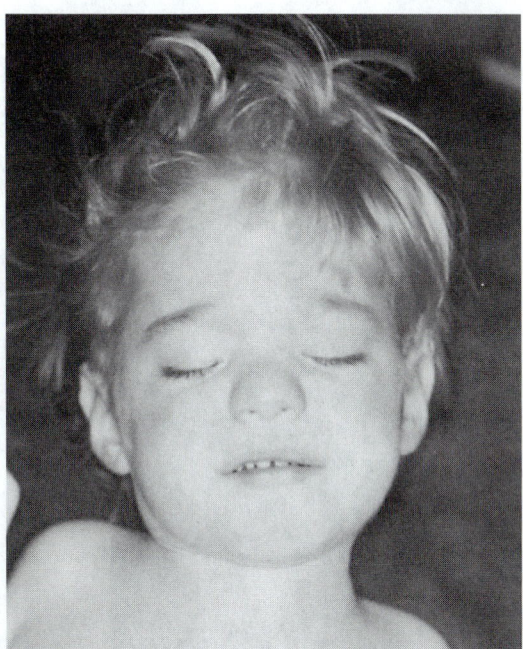

FIGURE 389.16. Patient with multiple sulfatase deficiency. Note the mildly coarse facial appearance. The patient also had a "gibbus" formation in the lower thoracic spine and mild joint contractions.

sulfatase deficiency. Patients usually present by 2 years of age with coarse facial features, dysostosis multiplex, hepatosplenomegaly, weakness, deafness, ichthyosis, and psychomotor delay. An early-onset, more severe form of the disorder has been noted at birth. Elevated urinary excretion of dermatan and heparan sulfates, slowed nerve conduction velocities, and increased cerebrospinal fluid protein concentrations occur. The progression of this disorder is similar to that of late-infantile metachromatic leukodystrophy. Most children do not live past 10 years of age (Fig. 389.16).

DISORDERS OF LYSOSOMAL ENZYME TRANSPORT (MUCOLIPIDOSES)

Before we reached our current biochemical understanding of this group of disorders, it was recognized that affected patients had features of both the mucopolysaccharidoses and the sphingolipidoses; hence, the disorders were called *mucolipidoses*. Of the previously classified subgroups of mucolipidoses, type I (sialidosis) now is known to result from alpha-neuraminidase deficiency and is described with the glycoproteinoses. Types II and III still retain the name *mucolipidosis* and are associated with faulty synthesis of the recognition marker needed for transport of the acid hydrolases into lysosomes. Deficient activity of multiple acid hydrolases occurs.

Lysosomal acid hydrolases are glycoproteins that require posttranslational processing. After leaving the membrane-bound polysomes, they enter the endoplasmic reticulum, where mannose-rich oligosaccharide side chains are attached. The enzymes then enter the Golgi apparatus, where the mannose groups are phosphorylated by a series of steps in which N-acetylglucosamine-1-phosphate is attached to the 6-hydroxyl groups of terminal mannose residues by N-acetylglucosamine-1-phosphotransferase. The N-acetylglucosamine then is removed by a phosphodiesterase to expose the mannosyl-6-phosphate. This mannosyl-6-phosphate is the signal for receptor sites in the Golgi cisternae that transport the enzymes into the lysosomes. Without the mannosyl-6-phosphate signal, the enzymes do not become localized in the lysosomes and are excreted from cells. The enzymes also do not undergo the usual final processing in the lysosome to mature enzymes and have additional sialic residues attached, which alters their biochemical properties.

The defect in most patients with mucolipidoses II and III is failure to phosphorylate the terminal mannose residues because of deficient activity of N-acetylglucosamine-1-phosphotransferase. Patients with mucolipidosis III have some residual activity and, thus, milder disease than do those with mucolipidosis II. In addition, some patients with mucolipidosis III have been found to have normal levels of the phosphotransferase but defective recognition function.

In both mucolipidosis II and mucolipidosis III, the specific activity of many lysosomal hydrolases is markedly increased (10 to 20 times normal) in plasma and serum and is lowered or absent in cultured skin fibroblasts. Peripheral leukocytes have normal or decreased activity. Arylsulfatase A, beta-galactosidase, beta-hexosaminidase, and alpha-L-iduronidase may be measured to show this effect. Acid phosphatase and beta-glucosidase are not affected. Deficient activity of the phosphotransferase may be demonstrated in cultured skin fibroblasts. Both disorders are inherited as autosomal recessive traits. Carrier detection and prenatal diagnosis are available.

Mucolipidosis II (I-Cell Disease)

Most patients with mucolipidosis II present shortly after birth with features similar to those associated with Hurler syndrome and GM_1 gangliosidosis. Prominent gingival hypertrophy occurs. Severe dysostosis is present from birth. Most patients do not live past 5 years of age. The disorder is named after the numerous dense inclusions that are seen with phase-contrast microscopy in cultured skin fibroblasts from affected patients. Urinary MPS excretion is normal, but sialooligosaccharide concentrations may be increased (Figs. 389.17 and 389.18).

Mucolipidosis III (Pseudo-Hurler Polydystrophy)

Patients with mucolipidosis III have a milder clinical course than do those with mucolipidosis II. The onset of stiffness of the large and small joints occurs between 2 and 4 years of age. The disorder is similar to the intermediate form of Maroteaux-Lamy syndrome (MPS VI). Affected patients may have mild psychomotor handicaps. Cardiac valvular lesions are common. Carpal tunnel syndrome and atlantoaxial subluxation may require surgical correction. Many patients have lived to be young adults.

Table 389.3 gives molecular genetic information for the disorders of lysosomal enzyme transport, glycoproteinoses, lysosomal membrane transport defects, and other disorders of lysosomal storage.

GLYCOPROTEINOSES

Glycoproteins structurally are oligosaccharide chains attached to a peptide core. Two major classes of glycoproteins differ in structure because of variations in synthetic pathways. The protein portions of glycoproteins are synthesized on membrane-bound polysomes and then pass to the smooth endoplasmic

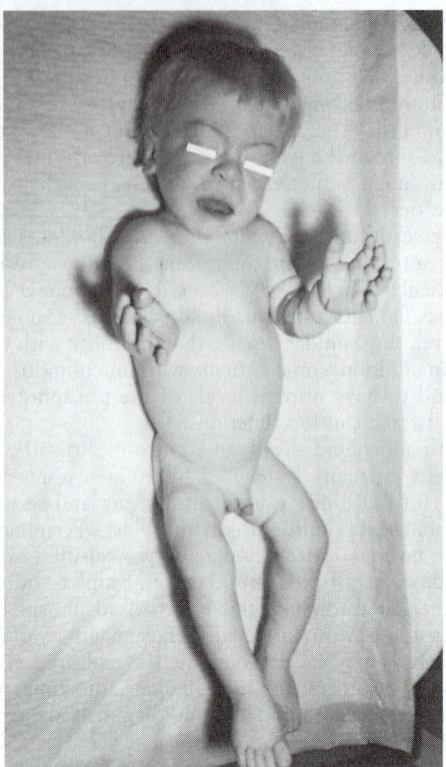

FIGURE 389.17. Patient with I-cell disease (mucolipidosis II). Note the macrocephaly with coarse facial features, thickened gingiva, foreshortened thorax and proximal extremities, hand and joint contractures, and enlarged abdomen from hepatosplenomegaly.

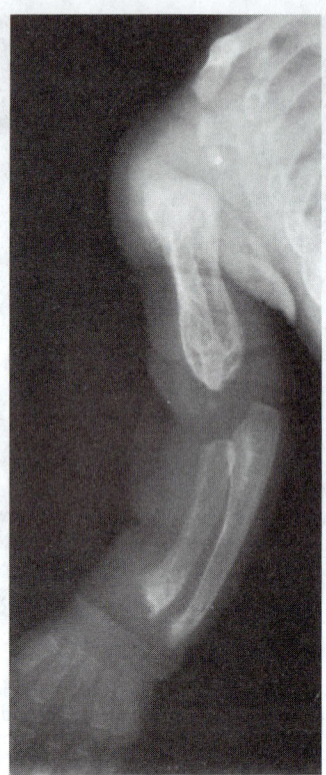

FIGURE 389.18. Radiogram in a patient with I-cell disease (mucolipidosis II). Note the severe dysostosis multiplex and the "bone within bone" appearance.

reticulum and Golgi apparatus, where the carbohydrate side chains are added. In one major class, the glycoprotein oligosaccharide side chains are synthesized by a sugar-nucleotide pathway, which involves the stepwise addition of single sugars from sugar-nucleotides catalyzed by a series of specific glyco-

syltransferases (O-glycosylation). The oligosaccharide chains are attached to the protein core by N-acetylgalactosaminyl residues, which bind with the hydroxyl groups of serine or threonine. Examples of this group include blood group substances, immunoglobulin A (IgA), and submaxillary mucins.

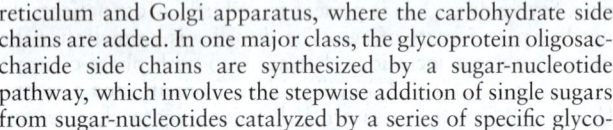

TABLE 389.3

OTHER LYSOSOMAL STORAGE DISORDERS

Name	Gene	Chromosomal Location	Enzyme or Process Affected
I. Disorders of lysosomal enzyme transport (mucolipidoses)			
Mucolipidosis II	*GNPTA*	4q21–q23	N-Acetylglucosamine-1-phosphotransferase
Mucolipidosis III	*GNPTA*	4q21–q23	N-Acetylglucosamine-1-phosphotransferase
II. Glycoproteinoses			
Fucosidosis	*FUCA1*	1p34	alpha-Fucosidase
alpha-Mannosidosis	*MAN2B1*	19cen–q12	alpha-Mannosidase
beta-Mannosidosis	*MANBA*	4q22–q25	beta-Mannosidase
Sialidosis	*NEU1*	6p21.3	alpha-Neuraminidase
Galactosialidosis	*PPCA*	20q13.1	Protective protein for beta-galactosidase and alpha-neuraminidase (cathepsin A)
Aspartylglucosaminuria	*AGA*	4q32–q33	Aspartylglucosaminidase
III. Lysosomal membrane transport defects			
Free sialic acid storage disorders (infantile free sialic acid storage disease, Salla disease)	*SLC17A5*	6q14–q15	Solute carrier family 17 (sodium phosphate) member 5
Cystinosis	*CTNS*	17p13	Cystinosin (lysylcystine transport protein)
IV. Other disorders of lysosomes			
Glycogen storage disease II (Pompe disease)	*GAA*	17q25.2–q25.3	Acid alpha-glucosidase (acid maltase)
Acid lipase deficiency (Wolman disease, cholesteryl ester storage disease)	*LIPA*	10q24–q25	Lysosomal acid lipase

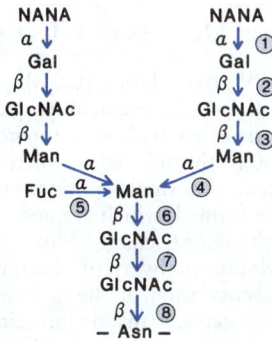

FIGURE 389.19. Degradation of glycoproteins. 1, alpha-neuraminidase; 2, beta-galactosidase; 3, beta-N-acetylglucosaminidase, beta-hexosaminidase A and B; 4, alpha-mannosidase; 5, alpha-fucosidase; 6, beta-mannosidase; 7, endo-beta-N-acetylglucosaminidase or beta-hexosaminidase A and B; 8, beta-aspartylglucosaminidase; Asn, asparagine; Fuc, fucose; Gal, galactose; GlcNAc, N-acetylglucosamine; Man, mannose; NANA, N-acetylneuraminic acid, sialic acid.

Alternatively, the glycoproteins may be synthesized by a dolichol pathway (N-glycosylation) that uses phosphorylated sugar-dolichol intermediates in addition to the sugar-nucleotides. In this synthetic pathway, the oligosaccharide chains are attached to the protein core by N-acetylglucosaminyl residues, which bind with the amino group of asparagine. In addition, as the oligosaccharide chains are formed, they receive a large number of mannosyl residues, which subsequently are trimmed, and then glucosyl, glucosaminyl, galactosyl, fucosyl, and sialic acid (N-acetyl neuraminic acid) residues are added to form the final complex branched structure (Fig. 389.19). Examples of glycoproteins formed by the dolichol pathway include ovalbumin, thyroglobulin, and IgM.

The degradative enzymatic defects in the glycoproteinoses involve failure of sequential removal of specific carbohydrate residues from the oligosaccharide chains as a result of deficient activity of specific lysosomal acid hydrolases. Because oligosaccharide linkages also appear in sphingolipids and MPS, more than one type of partially degraded material may be stored in the individual disorders. Many of the clinical features of these disorders resemble those described for the mucopolysaccharidoses, mucolipidoses, and sphingolipidoses. Usually, vacuolization of peripheral lymphocytes and abnormal patterns of urinary oligosaccharide excretion are found.

An expanding group of disorders involving the synthesis or processing of glycoproteins, known as congenital defects in glycosylation, affect central nervous system functioning and may involve other systems or organs. The disorders are discussed at the end of this section.

Fucosidosis

Fucosidosis is an autosomal recessive disorder associated with alpha-fucosidase deficiency and the storage of fucose-containing sphingolipids, glycoproteins, and oligosaccharides. Many affected individuals are of Italian and Hispanic-American origin. *Type I* fucosidosis has its onset between 3 and 18 months of age and is characterized by short stature, coarse facial features, macroglossia, hepatosplenomegaly, cardiac involvement, dysostosis multiplex, seizures, and psychomotor retardation. Many patients have elevated sweat chloride levels. Most die before 10 years of age. *Type II* fucosidosis is a milder disorder with onset between 1 and 2 years of age and survival to young adulthood. Patients with this variant usually do not have hepatosplenomegaly or elevated sweat chloride levels, but they may have angiokeratomas. Deficient activity of alpha-fucosidase may be demonstrated in peripheral leukocytes or cultured skin fibroblasts. Carrier detection and prenatal diagnosis are available.

Mannosidosis (alpha-Mannosidase Deficiency)

Mannosidosis is an autosomal recessive disease associated with deficient activity of alpha-mannosidase and storage of mannose-containing glycoproteins. *Type I* mannosidosis has its onset between 3 and 12 months of age. Clinical findings include coarse facial features, hepatosplenomegaly, psychomotor retardation, mild dysostosis multiplex, posterior spoke-like cataracts, corneal opacities, frequent infections, hearing loss, and hypotonia. Most patients die between 3 and 12 years of age. *Type II* mannosidosis is a milder disorder with onset between 1 and 4 years of age and survival to young adult life. Deficient activity of alpha-mannosidase may be shown in peripheral leukocytes and cultured skin fibroblasts. Carrier detection and prenatal diagnosis are available.

beta-Mannosidase Deficiency

Deficient activity of beta-mannosidase is a rare autosomal recessive disorder that presents with psychomotor retardation and mild facial dysmorphism during childhood. Other reported clinical features are variable and have included angiokeratomas, behavioral problems, cerebral atrophy, increased motor tone, hearing loss, seizures, and status epilepticus. Deaths have occurred as early as 15 months of age. Other affected patients have lived to be adults. The urine from affected patients contains mannosyl-beta-N-acetylglucosamine. Deficient activity of beta-mannosidase may be shown in peripheral leukocytes and cultured skin fibroblasts.

Sialidosis

Sialidosis is an autosomal recessive disorder associated with deficient activity of alpha-neuraminidase, which cleaves the terminal alpha-N-acetyl-neuraminic acid (sialic acid) residues from glycoproteins and oligosaccharides. The disorder previously was classified as type I mucolipidosis. Two forms of the disorder are known.

Type I sialidosis, or the *normosomatic type*, also has been called the cherry-red spot–myoclonus syndrome. Symptoms begin between 8 and 25 years of age. Progressive visual impairment occurs, along with cherry-red macular spots and, occasionally, punctate lenticular opacities. The myoclonus is generalized and debilitating, and it may be difficult to control with medication. A painful neuropathy (as in Fabry disease), delayed nerve conduction velocities, hyperreflexia, ataxia, nystagmus, and major motor seizures may occur. Most patients die as young adults. The disorder is seen most often in patients of Italian background.

Type II sialidosis, the more *severe dysmorphic form*, has three subgroups, which vary in age of onset and clinical severity. In addition to the features of type I sialidosis, affected patients also have coarse facial features and dysostosis multiplex. The *juvenile form* has its onset between 2 and 20 years of age. There usually is no hepatosplenomegaly or renal involvement. Angiokeratomas may be present. Many patients have survived to the fourth or fifth decade of life. This form is most common in Japan, and many reported patients may actually have galactosialidosis, rather than sialidosis. The *infantile form* has its onset between birth and 12 months of age. Hepatosplenomegaly and renal involvement occur. Most patients die by 10 to 20 years of age. The *congenital form* may result in stillbirth of an infant with an appearance similar to that of hydrops fetalis. Other infants survive for a few months. Facial edema, ascites, hepatosplenomegaly, inguinal hernias, renal involvement, stippling of the epiphyses, and corneal clouding may be seen.

Deficient activity of alpha-neuraminidase may be noted in cultured skin fibroblasts. Carrier detection and prenatal diagnosis are available.

Galactosialidosis

Galactosialidosis, an autosomal recessive disorder, is associated with deficiency of both alpha-neuraminidase and beta-galactosidase, as a result of deficiency of a protective protein (cathepsin A) that complexes with both enzymes. The clinical findings are similar to those seen with sialidosis and generalized gangliosidosis. Foam cells may be seen in bone marrow and vacuolated lymphocytes noted on peripheral smears. Three major forms of the disorder exist that vary in clinical severity and age of onset.

The *early infantile form* of the disorder has its onset between birth and 3 months of age. Fetal hydrops, neonatal edema, coarse facies, hepatosplenomegaly, cardiomegaly, renal failure, telangiectasias, and psychomotor delay are common. Cherry-red macular spots and corneal clouding may occur. Dysostosis multiplex is noted on radiography. Most patients die by 20 months of age.

The *late infantile form* presents between 1 and 3 years of age with coarse facial features, hepatosplenomegaly, growth retardation, deafness, and cardiac valvular disease. Radiography shows dysostosis multiplex. Cherry-red macular spots and corneal clouding may be seen. Although mild psychomotor delay may be present, central nervous system deterioration and seizures usually do not occur.

The *juvenile/adult form* of the disorder is seen most often in patients with Japanese heritage. Approximately 70% of patients with galactosialidosis have this form of the disorder. The mean age of onset is 15 years, but symptoms may start as early as 1 year or as late as 40 years of age. Coarse facial features, platyspondyly, cardiac involvement, hernias, corneal clouding, and cherry-red macular spots are commonly seen. A progressive neurologic course with myoclonus, generalized seizures, and ataxia occurs. One-half of patients have angiokeratomas. Hepatosplenomegaly is occasionally seen. Deaths have occurred as early as 13 years and as late as 45 years.

Deficient activity of alpha-neuraminidase and beta-galactosidase may be shown in peripheral leukocytes or cultured skin fibroblasts. Carrier and prenatal testing are available.

Aspartylglucosaminuria

Aspartylglucosaminuria, an autosomal recessive disorder that is most common in Finland, is associated with deficient activity of aspartylglucosaminidase. Gradual coarsening of the facial features, sagging skin, and psychomotor deterioration start to develop between 1 and 5 years of age. Mild dysostosis multiplex, lenticular opacities, acne, and photosensitivity usually occur. Some patients also have joint laxity, macroglossia, short stature, hypotonia, and spasticity. Many live into the fourth decade of life. Deficient activity of aspartylglucosaminidase may be shown in peripheral leukocytes and cultured skin fibroblasts.

Congenital Defects of Glycosylation

Congenital defects of glycosylation (CDG), previously known as carbohydrate-deficient glycoprotein syndromes, are rare autosomal recessive disorders with an estimated incidence of 1 in 40,000 to 60,000 births in Sweden, where the disorders are most commonly seen. Abnormal isoforms of glycoproteins and glycoconjugates are formed, which are underglycosylated and have shortened carbohydrate chains. Most of the disorders affect the N-glycosylation pathway of glycoprotein formation. Others affect O-glycosylation or the glycosylation of glycolipids. Serum glycoproteins, transport proteins, lysosomal hydrolases, and coagulation factors and inhibitors are affected.

Modification of the terminal carbohydrate residues of serum transferrin, a glycoprotein, results in an abnormal isoform pattern on isoelectric focusing (IEF). Determination of the serum transferrin IEF pattern will detect most patients with CDG. Some patients, especially those with types IIb and IIc and defects of O-glycosylation, however, will be missed by this technique. Confirmation of the associated enzyme deficiencies can be done in leukocytes for types Ia and Ib; the other types will need cultured skin fibroblast lines for testing. Because the serum IEF transferrin pattern is normal *in utero* and for the first few weeks of life, testing by this method should be deferred until after 3 weeks of age. Lowered levels of thyroxine-binding globulin, one of the affected glycoproteins, may cause false-positive results with newborn screening for hypothyroidism; many affected infants have been identified in this manner.

Two major forms of the disorders exist. Type I disorders involve defects in the *synthesis* of glycoproteins that are formed by the N-glycosylation pathway. Type II disorders mainly affect *processing and posttranslational modification* of the glycoproteins. A few type II defects involve the O-glycosylation synthetic pathway. Table 389.4 lists the currently recognized defects and associated enzymatic deficiencies and molecular findings. The majority of the disorders affect the central nervous system. Some have multisystemic involvement, whereas others only affect a single organ or system. Carrier testing and prenatal diagnosis vary with the specific form involved. For additional information about the various forms of CDG, see Box 389.1.

Two disorders involving O-glycosylation are recognized. Patients with *muscle–eye–brain disease* have congenital glaucoma and myopia, retinal and optic disc hypoplasia, congenital muscular dystrophy with severe hypotonia, myoclonic jerks, electroencephalogram (EEG) abnormalities, hydrocephalus, and delayed development. Pachygyria/microgyria, cerebellar hypoplasia, and normal or thin corpus callosum are noted on magnetic resonance imaging of the brain. The more severe *Walker-Warburg syndrome* is characterized by agyria, hydrocephalus, absent corpus callosum, retinal dysplasia, and microphthalmia. Congenital muscular dystrophy, congenital glaucoma, cataracts, and encephaloceles may occur. Most patients do not survive infancy.

An increasing number of disorders are being reported as associated with defects in glycosylation as our knowledge of molecular genetics expands. Patients with the *progeria variant of Ehlers-Danlos syndrome* have been found to have a defect in glycosylation leading to defective biosynthesis of precursors of dermatan sulfate. *Hereditary multiple exostoses* has been associated with two genes, *EXT1* and *EXT2*, which code for proteins involved with glycosyltransferase activity needed for the formation of heparan sulfate. *Congenital dyserythropoietic anemia type II* (CDAII), also known as hereditary erythroblastic multinuclearity with positive acidified-serum test (HEMPAS), has been associated with a defect in glycosylation limited to erythrocyte membrane proteins. Affected patients have hemolytic anemia, splenomegaly, and bi- and multinucleated erythroblasts.

TABLE 389.4

CONGENITAL DEFECTS OF GLYCOSYLATION (CDG)

Type	Gene	Chromosomal Location	Enzyme or Process Affected
I. Defects in *N*-linked glycan synthesis			
CDG type Ia	*PMM2*	16p13.3–p13.2	Phosphomannomutase 2
CDG type Ib	*PMI*	15q22–qter	Phosphomannose isomerase
CDG type Ic	*hALG6*	1p22.3	Dol-P-Glc:Man$_9$GlcNAc$_2$-PP-Dol alpha-1,3-glucosyltransferase
CDG type Id	*hALG3*	3q27	Dol-P-Man:Man$_5$GlcNAc$_2$-PP-Dol mannosyltransferase
CDG type Ie	*DPM1*	20q13	Dol-P-Man synthase 1
CDG type If	*MPDU1*	17p13.1–p12	Man-P-Dol utilization defect 1
CDG type Ig	*hALG12*	22	Dol-P-Man:Man$_7$GlcNAc$_2$-PP-Dol alpha-6-mannosyltransferase
CDG type Ih	*hALG8*	Unknown	Dol-P-Glc:Glc-1-Man$_9$GlcNAc$_2$-PP-Dol alpha-3-glucosyltransferase
CDG type Ii	*hALG2*	9q22	GDP-Man:ManGlcNAc$_2$-PP-Dol mannosyltransferase
CDG type Ij	*DPAGT1*	11q23.3	UDP-GlcNAc:Dol-P-GlcNAc phosphotransferase
II. Defects in *N*-linked glycan processing			
CDG type IIa	*MGAT2*	14q21	GlcNAc-transferase II
CDG type IIb	*GCS1*	2p12–p13	alpha-Glucosidase I
CDG type IIc	*FUCT1*	11	GDP-fucose transporter 1
CDG type IId	*B4GALT1*	9p13	UDP-galactose:GlcNAc-beta-1,4-galactosyltransferase I
III. Defects in *O*-glycosylation			
Walker-Warburg Syndrome	*POMT1*	9q34.1	O-Mannosyltransferase
Muscle-eye-brain disease	*POMGNT1*	1p34–p33	O-Mannose beta-1,2-GlcNAc transferase
IV. Other			
Progeria variant of Ehlers-Danlos syndrome	*XGPT1*	5q35.2–q35.3	Xylosylprotein 4-beta-galactosyltransferase I
Hereditary multiple exostosis type I	*EXT1*	8q24.11–q24.13	Exostosin-1 (Glucosyltransferase)
Hereditary multiple exostosis type II	*EXT2*	11p12–p11	Exostosin-2 (Glucosyltransferase)
Congenital dyserythropoietic anemia type II	*CDAN2*	20q11.2	Exact defect unknown

Dol, dolichol; GDP, guanosine diphosphate; Glc, glucose; GlcNAc, *N*-acetylglucosamine; *h*, human analogue of yeast gene (*Saccharomyces cerevisiae*); Man, mannose; P, phosphate; UDP, uridine diphosphate.

LYSOSOMAL MEMBRANE TRANSPORT DEFECTS

Carrier-mediated transport systems are needed for small molecules to pass from the lysosomal space into the cytosol. Systems have been described for monosaccharides and amino acids. Defective transport also has been associated with lysosomal storage of free sialic acid and cystine.

Free Sialic Acid Storage Disease

Two major forms of free sialic acid storage disease exist: Salla disease and the more severe infantile free sialic acid storage disease. Both are inherited as autosomal recessive traits. Patients with intermediate forms have been described, as well as patients with a mild clinical presentation but markedly increased urinary excretion of sialic acid comparable with that seen in the severe forms.

Salla disease is most common in the Salla region of Finland. Patients present with hypotonia, ataxia, psychomotor retardation, and coarse facies between 3 and 12 months of age. Progressive central nervous system involvement leads to impaired coordination, dysarthrias, dyspraxias, dystonias, seizures, muscle rigidity, and dementia. Affected individuals may live to be adults.

Infantile free sialic acid storage disease, the more generalized sialic acid storage disease, presents within the first 2 months of life with coarse facies, hepatosplenomegaly, psychomotor retardation, hypopigmentation, anemia, and diarrhea. Ascites may be present. Dysostosis multiplex may be noted on radiography. The disorder is rapidly progressive, and most patients do not live past the first few years of life.

Lysosomal levels of free sialic acid, or *N*-acetylneuraminic acid, are 10 to 30 times higher than normal in patients with Salla disease and up to 200 times higher than normal in those with infantile free sialic acid storage disease. Urinary excretion of free sialic acid is increased with both disorders, more so in the severe form. Activity of neuraminidase is normal. The disorders may be documented by elevated levels of free sialic acid in cultured skin fibroblasts and peripheral leukocytes. Prenatal diagnosis is possible. Carrier detection is not.

Cystinosis

Cystinosis, an autosomal recessive disorder, is associated with the lysosomal accumulation of free cystine in many tissues throughout the body. Most patients have the infantile nephropathic type, which presents between 3 and 18 months of age with renal Fanconi syndrome. Poor linear growth and hypothyroidism are common. The patients have a fair complexion and relatively light hair because of poor melanin production;

BOX 389.1   Specific Congenital Defects of Glycosylation

Type Ia congenital defects of glycosylation (CDG), the most common, is a multisystem disorder that has been documented in over 500 patients. Hypotonia, restricted movement of large joints, and severe to profound psychomotor handicaps are present from birth. Nonimmune fetal hydrops may occur. Poor feeding, lethargy, and hypothermia are common in affected neonates. Failure to thrive, growth retardation, hyporeflexia, and ataxia are seen during early infancy. Cerebellar, and often cerebral, atrophy is noted with radioimaging. Pericardial effusions, ventricular hypertrophy, cardiac failure, and hepatic dysfunction or failure may occur. Proteinuria, large renal simple cysts, or microcysts may be noted. Liver biopsy shows unusual lysosomal vacuoles, with concentric membrane-like inclusions, as well as steatosis with slight to moderate fibrosis. The skin and subcutaneous tissues, especially over the thighs and buttocks, are uneven in consistency and may feel tough. Fat pads may be present over the buttocks. Lipoatrophic streaks or patches may be noted on the lower legs. Inverted, often laterally displaced, nipples may be present.

Coagulopathies may develop from reduced levels of factors IX and XI or reduced levels of coagulation inhibitors (i.e., antithrombin II, protein C, protein S, and heparin cofactor II). Approximately 20% of patients die during early infancy from severe infection, cardiomyopathy, or hepatic failure.

A slowly progressive peripheral neuropathy and retinitis pigmentosa occur in older infants and children. Affected patients have stroke-like episodes of stupor, coma, loss of vision, seizures, and hemiplegia that may be precipitated by intercurrent illnesses. Older teenagers and young adults frequently develop severe scoliosis and kyphosis.

In contrast to type Ia, *type Ib CDG* mainly affects the gastrointestinal system and is one of two forms of the disorders for which specific treatment is available. Psychomotor development is normal. Chronic diarrhea starts during the first year of life. A protein-losing enteropathy may occur; partial villus atrophy may be noted on duodenal biopsy. Cyclic vomiting may lead to failure to thrive; hypoglycemia is common. Occasionally, hepatic fibrosis with abnormal liver function is seen. The defect results in decreased endogenous production of mannose-6-phosphate. Although treatment with oral mannose results in rather prompt clinical improvement, it may take several months to see improvement in the transferrin isoform pattern.

The remainder of the type I CDG disorders are rare and have been reported only in a small number of patients. *Types Ic through Ii CDG* have central nervous system involvement as their major clinical finding. Seizures, hypotonia, and psychomotor handicaps predominate. Types Id, Ie, Ig, and Ih CDG patients are reported to have dysmorphic features including hypertelorism, short philtrum, abnormal uvula, high-arched palate, coloboma of the iris, and dysplastic ears or nails. Retinitis pigmentosa and ichthyosis were noted in type If CDG patients. Supragluteal fat pads were noted in Type Ig CDG patients. Hepatomegaly and coagulopathies were noted in type Ih CDG patients. *Type Ij CDG* resembles type Ib CDG in that the prominent findings are hepatomegaly and protein-losing enteropathy. Psychomotor development is normal and there are no dysmorphic features.

Type IIa CDG presents with profound psychomotor retardation, hypotonia, and stereotypic behaviors. Brain magnetic resonance imaging shows cortical atrophy, focal white matter lesions, and delayed myelination. In contrast to type Ia CDG, peripheral neuropathy does not occur and deep tendon reflexes are normal. Dysmorphic features include a coarse facies, large low-set ears, and widely spaced nipples.

Type IIb CDG has been reported in one patient, who had a broad nose, high-arched palate, small chin, and overlapping fingers. Hypotonia, abnormal nerve conduction, and seizures were noted. Hepatic fibrosis occurred. The patient required assisted ventilation for apnea and died at age 2.5 months.

Type IIc CDG is also known as leukocyte adhesion deficiency type II (LAD II). Affected patients have dysmorphic features including short stature, short limbs, flat facies with a broad depressed nasal bridge, broad palms, and long eyelashes. They also have moderate to severe psychomotor handicaps. Decreased fucose content of glycoconjugates causes decreased adhesion of the leukocytes to endothelial cells and failure of migration of neutrophils to infection focuses, resulting in increased peripheral leukocyte counts and immune deficiency. Patients also lack detectable ABO blood group markers on their erythrocytes (Bombay blood type). Some patients will respond to oral fucose supplementation.

Type IId CDG has been reported in one patient with hypotonia, coagulopathy, and a Dandy-Walker malformation with congenital macrocephaly and progressive hydrocephalus. Elevated serum creatine kinase levels were noted.

---

hypohidrosis is common. Extreme photophobia is caused by cystine deposition in the corneas, which may be evident with slit lamp examination. Affected patients may have a peripheral pigmentary retinopathy and other ophthalmologic problems. Cystine crystals may be noted by electron microscopy in renal interstitial tissues, bone marrow, lymph nodes, and conjunctivae. Before therapy with cysteamine was available, most patients developed renal failure by 10 years of age. An intermediate, adolescent type of cystinosis, with onset between 10 and 20 years of age and slower progression of the disease, and an adult type without significant renal involvement also exist.

The disorder may be documented by showing elevated levels of free cystine in peripheral leukocytes or cultured skin fibroblasts. Carrier detection and prenatal diagnosis are available. Treatment includes the use of the free thiol cysteamine (beta-

mercaptoethylamine) in enteral and eyedrop forms. This depletes intracellular cystine by forming a mixed disulfide with the cysteinyl residues of cystine. The disulfide is transported across the lysosomal membrane by a different, unaffected carrier system. Cysteamine treatment results in improved growth and may preserve renal function if started within the first 2 years of life. Corneal crystals dissolve. Symptomatic therapy for the renal tubular dysfunction is similar to that for primary Fanconi syndrome. Thyroid and other hormone replacement therapy should be given. Renal dialysis and transplantation may be indicated if renal failure develops. Although cystine storage does not occur in the donor kidney, extrarenal progressive storage of cystine may lead to loss of vision, corneal erosions, diabetes mellitus, pancreatic insufficiency, hypogonadism, and progressive neurologic involvement in transplanted patients.

OTHER DISORDERS OF LYSOSOMES

Lysosomal alpha-Glucosidase Deficiency

Glycogenosis (glycogen storage disease) type II is associated with deficient activity of lysosomal acid alpha-glucosidase (acid maltase), which catalyzes the hydrolysis of glucose residues from lysosomal glycogen. The disorder may occur at any age. Three groups have been identified based on clinical severity and age of onset of symptoms.

The *classic infantile form* of the disorder, also known as *Pompe disease* or *generalized glycogenosis*, presents shortly after birth with a rapidly progressive generalized myopathy and hypertrophic cardiomyopathy. The appearance of a prominent tongue may be the result of macroglossia or the fact that the mouth is held open because of the hypotonia. Hepatomegaly may be present and often is associated with cardiac failure. Intellect usually is not impaired. Death occurs by 1 year of age from cardiac or respiratory failure. Electrocardiography shows gigantic QRS complexes in all leads and a shortened PR interval. Echocardiography reveals biventricular hypertrophy with left outflow tract obstruction. Electromyography shows pseudomyotonic discharges, high-frequency discharges, and fibrillations. Hypoglycemia and other biochemical abnormalities noted with defects in cytosolic glycogen metabolism do not occur. Lysosomal accumulation of glycogen occurs in the muscle, heart, liver, and most other tissues of the body.

Less severe forms occur at later ages, with skeletal muscle wasting and weakness and little or no cardiac involvement. The *juvenile form* has its onset in early childhood; most patients die of respiratory failure by 20 years of age. The *adult form* is characterized by a chronic proximal myopathy with onset between the second and fourth decades of life. Electromyopathic findings in the milder forms are variable, but can be similar to those in the infantile form. Elevated levels of creatine kinase and hepatic enzymes occur.

Increased lysosomal glycogen content may be found in muscle biopsy samples. Deficient activity of alpha-glucosidase may be shown in muscle or cultured skin fibroblasts. Care should be taken if the enzyme is measured in peripheral leukocytes because of the presence of an unaffected renal isoenzyme. The disorder is inherited as an autosomal recessive trait. Carrier testing and prenatal diagnosis are available. Enzyme replacement therapy with human recombinant alpha-glucosidase is being developed and is presently in clinical trials.

Lysosomal Acid Lipase Deficiency

Lysosomal acid lipase is needed for hydrolysis of cholesteryl esters and triglycerides. Two allelic autosomal recessive disorders, Wolman disease and cholesteryl ester storage disease, are associated with deficient activity of lysosomal acid lipase. These disorders may be confirmed by demonstrating deficient activity of acid lipase in peripheral leukocytes or cultured skin fibroblasts. Carrier detection and prenatal diagnosis are available.

Wolman disease presents in the first few weeks of life with vomiting, diarrhea, steatorrhea, abdominal distention, hepatosplenomegaly, and calcification of the adrenal glands. Liver function test results are abnormal. Total plasma cholesterol and triglyceride levels usually are normal; elevated very low-density lipoprotein levels have been noted in a few cases. Severe failure to thrive leads to death by 6 months of age. Storage of cholesteryl esters and triglycerides occurs in the liver, spleen, adrenals, intestines, lymph nodes, bone marrow, and interstitial tissues throughout the body. Lymphocytes may be vacuolated. Foam cells and sea-blue histiocytes may be noted in bone marrow. The liver also may show portal fibrosis.

Cholesteryl ester storage disease is a milder disorder. Hepatomegaly may not be present until adult life. Splenomegaly, hepatic fibrosis or micronodular cirrhosis, esophageal varices, and intestinal involvement occur in some patients. Hypercholesterolemia with variable hypertriglyceridemia usually is present, and atherosclerosis may develop. Adrenal calcification does not occur, and foam cells are not prominent. Treatment with dietary reduction of total and saturated fats and free carbohydrates, resins that bind bile salts, and inhibitors of endogenous cholesterol synthesis may result in clinical improvement in some patients.

Suggested Readings

Amalfitano A, Bengur AR, Morse RP, et al. Recombinant human acid alpha-glucosidase enzyme therapy for infantile glycogen storage disease type II: results of a phase I/II clinical trial. *Genet Med* 2001;3:132.

Aula P, Gahl WA. Disorders of free sialic acid storage. In: Scriver CR, Beaudet AL, Sly WS, Valle D, eds. *The metabolic and molecular bases of inherited disease*, 8th ed. New York: McGraw-Hill, 2001:5109.

Bosman DK, Hollak CE, Aerts JM, et al. The effect of enzyme therapy in a patient with Gaucher disease type III. *J Inherit Metab Dis* 1996;19:703.

Brady RO, Barton NW. Enzyme replacement and gene therapy for Gaucher's disease. *Lipids* 1996;31:S137.

Breunig F, Knoll A, Wanner C. Enzyme replacement therapy in Fabry disease: clinical implications. *Curr Opin Nephrol Hypertens* 2003;12:491.

Brooks DA. Alpha-L-iduronidase and enzyme replacement therapy for mucopolysacchridosis I. *Expert Opin Biol Ther* 2002;2:967.

Desnick RJ, Brady R, Barranger J, et al. Fabry disease, an under-recognized multisystemic disorder: expert recommendations for diagnosis, management, and enzyme replacement therapy. *Ann Intern Med* 2003;138:338.

Erikson A, Astrom M, Mansson JE. Enzyme infusion therapy of the Norrbottnian (type 3) Gaucher disease. *Neuropediatrics* 1995;26:203.

Gahl WA, Thoene JG, Schneider JA. Cystinosis: a disorder of lysosomal membrane transport. In: Scriver CR, Beaudet AL, Sly WS, Valle D, eds. *The metabolic and molecular bases of inherited disease*, 8th ed. New York: McGraw-Hill, 2001:5085.

Grabowski GA, Hopkin RJ. Enzyme therapy for lysosomal storage disease: principles, practice, and prospects. *Annu Rev Genomics Hum Genet* 2003;4:403.

Grunewald S, Matthijs G, Jaeken J. Congenital disorders of glycosylation: a review. *Pediatr Res* 2002;52:618.

Harms HK, Zimmer KP, Kurnik K, et al. Oral mannose therapy persistently corrects the severe clinical symptoms and biochemical abnormalities of phosphomannose isomerase deficiency. *Acta Paediatr* 2002;91:1065.

Kakkis ED, Muenzer J, Tiller GE, et al. Enzyme-replacement therapy in mucopolysaccharidosis I. *N Eng J Med* 2001;344:182.

Kaplan P, Mazur A, Manor O, et al. Acceleration of retarded growth in children with Gaucher disease after treatment with alglucerase. *J Pediatr* 1996;129:149.

Marquardt T, Denecke J. Congenital disorders of glycosylation: review of their molecular bases, clinical presentations and specific therapies. *Eur J Pediatr* 2003;162:359.

Marquardt T, Luhn K, Srikrishna G, et al. Correction of leukocyte adhesion deficiency type II with oral fucose. *Blood* 1999;94:3976.

Mehta AB, Lewis S, Laverey C. Treatment of lysosomal storage disorders. *BMJ* 2003;327:462.

Muenzer J, Lamsa JC, Garcia A, et al. Enzyme replacement therapy in mucopolysaccharidosis type II (Hunter syndrome): a preliminary report. *Acta Paediatr Suppl* 2002;91:98.

Natowicz MR, Short MP, Wang Y, et al. Clinical and biochemical manifestations of hyaluronidase deficiency. *N Engl J Med* 1996;335:1029.

Prows CA, Sanchez N, Daugherty C, et al. Gaucher disease: enzyme therapy in the acute neuronopathic variant. *Am J Med Genet* 1997;71:16.

Raben N, Plotz P, Byrne BJ. Acid alpha-glucosidase deficiency (glycogenosis type II, Pompe disease). *Curr Mol Med* 2002;2:145.

Ries M, Ramaswami U, Parini R, et al. The early clinical phenotype of Fabry disease: a study on 35 European children and adolescents. *Eur J Pediatr* 2003;162:767.

Scriver CR, Beaudet AL, Sly WS, Valle D, eds. *Lysosomal disorders, part 16. The metabolic and molecular bases of inherited disease*, 8th ed. New York: McGraw-Hill, 2001:3371.

Vincent I, Bu B, Erickson RP. Understanding Niemann-Pick type C disease: a fat problem. *Curr Opin Neurol* 2003;16:155.

Wasserstein MP, Larkin AE, Glass RB, et al. Growth restriction in children with type B Niemann-Pick disease. *J Pediatr* 2003;142:424.

Wenger DA, Coppola S, Liu SL. Insights into the diagnosis and treatment of lysosomal storage diseases. *Arch Neurol* 2003;60:322.

CHAPTER 390 ■ PEROXISOMAL DISORDERS

REBECCA S. WAPPNER

Peroxisomes are small, single membrane–bound, electron-dense, subcellular organelles associated with a growing number of recognized biochemical functions and related disorders. Initially termed *microbodies,* the name later was changed to *peroxisomes* when catalase, which reduces hydrogen peroxide to water, and a series of oxidases were found to be localized to this organelle. Peroxisomes are formed by division or budding of preexisting peroxisomes. They then are enlarged and become functional by acquiring newly synthesized membrane and matrix proteins, which contain peroxisomal targeting signals that allow them to be imported into the peroxisomes through receptor-mediated processes.

At least 50 enzymatic reactions are known to occur in peroxisomes. Abnormalities noted in patients with peroxisomal disorders have included catalase deficiency; reduced beta-oxidation of very long-chain fatty acids (VLCFA; carbon chain length greater than 22); reduced biosynthesis of isoprenoids, cholesterol, bile salts, and ether lipids such as plasmalogens; reduced oxidation of phytanic acid, pipecolic acid, and 2-methyl branched-chain fatty acids; and abnormalities in glyoxylate metabolism.

Peroxisomal beta-oxidation of fatty acids differs from that in mitochondria in that the process is not linked to oxidative phosphorylation. Also, the energy produced is not conserved but is dissipated as heat (Fig. 390.1). The peroxisome appears to be the exclusive site for the beta-oxidation of unsaturated VLCFA and plays a major role in the beta-oxidation of monounsaturated long-chain fatty acids (C22:1). Faulty beta-oxidation of VLCFA leads to elevated plasma levels and tissue storage of VLCFA, especially tetracosanoic acid (lignoceric acid; C24:0) and hexacosanoic acid (cerotic acid; C26:0).

Plasmalogens are ether phospholipids that are major constituents of cell membranes, myelin, and platelet-activating factor. Dihydroxyacetone phosphate (DHAP) acyltransferase and alkyl DHAP synthase, peroxisomal enzymes involved with the first two steps of plasmalogen synthesis, have been shown to be deficient in patients with certain peroxisomal disorders.

Peroxisomal mevalonate kinase catalyzes the early steps in the biosynthesis of cholesterol and isoprenoids. Biosynthesis of bile acids (chenodeoxycholic and cholic acids) from cholesterol involves a series of peroxisomal reactions similar to those for beta-oxidation of VLCFA. Faulty biosynthesis leads to the accumulation of bile acid precursors such as dihydroxycholestanoic and trihydroxycholestanoic acids in the serum, urine, and bile.

Phytanic acid, an unusual 20-carbon branched-chain fatty acid mainly of dietary origin, has been noted to be elevated in certain types of the peroxisomal disorders as a result of faulty phytanic acid alpha-oxidation caused by deficient activity of phytanoyl-CoA hydroxylase. Pristanic acid, a metabolite of phytanic acid, accumulates, along with bile salt precursors, in 2-methylacyl-CoA racemase deficiency. Pipecolic acid, an intermediary in the degradation of lysine, also has been noted to be elevated in certain disorders as a result of the deficient activity of pipecolic acid oxidase. Alanine-glyoxylate aminotransferase, which is deficient in hyperoxaluria type 1, is peroxisomal in location.

CLASSIFICATION OF PEROXISOMAL DISORDERS

The peroxisomal disorders presently are classified into two groups. Group 1 includes disorders of peroxisomal biogenesis. Peroxisomal membrane and matrix proteins are not imported into peroxisomes, resulting in generalized peroxisomal dysfunction and the deficient activity of multiple peroxisomal enzymes. The peroxisomal enzymes are transcribed, but remain in the cytosol, where they are degraded. Membranous structures, termed *peroxisomal ghosts,* may be seen on electron microscopy in tissues from affected patients. These structures may contain some membrane proteins, but they are missing catalase and most other matrix enzymes. Mutations have been shown in *PEX* (peroxin) genes that encode for peroxisomal membrane proteins, proteins involved with peroxisomal membrane and matrix protein import, and peroxisomal receptors for peroxisomal targeting signals. Considerable variability of

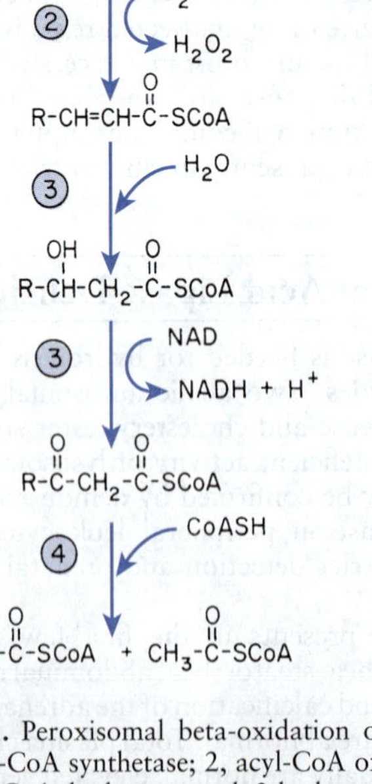

FIGURE 390.1. Peroxisomal beta-oxidation of fatty acids. 1, very long-chain acyl-CoA synthetase; 2, acyl-CoA oxidase; 3, bifunctional enzyme: enoyl-CoA hydratase and 3-hydroxyacyl-CoA dehydrogenase; 4, 3-oxoacyl-CoA thiolase; AMP, adenosine monophosphate; ATP, adenosine triphosphate; CoASH, uncombined coenzyme A; NAD, nicotinamide adenine dinucleotide; NADH, reduced nicotinamide adenine dinucleotide; PPi, inorganic pyrophosphate.

TABLE 390.1

BIOCHEMICAL ABNORMALITIES IN PEROXISOMAL DISORDERS

	Elevated VLCFA	Faulty Plasmalogen Synthesis	Faulty Bile Acid Synthesis	Elevated Phytanic Acid	Elevated Pipecolic Acid	Other, Not Lipid
Group 1: Disorders of peroxisomal biogenesis						
Zellweger syndrome	+	+	+	+/−	+	−
Neonatal ALD	+	+	+	+/−	+	−
Infantile Refsum disease	+	+	+	+	+	−
Hyperpipecolic acidemia	+	+	+	+/−	+	−
Rhizomelic chondrodysplasia punctata	+	+	−	+	−	−
Group 2: Deficient activity of a single peroxisomal enzyme						
Pseudo-Zellweger syndrome	+	−	+	−	−	−
Pseudoneonatal ALD	+	−	−	−	−	−
Bifunctional enzyme deficiency	+	−	+	+*	−	−
DHAP acyltransferase deficiency	−	+	−	−	−	−
Alkyl DHAP synthase deficiency	−	+	−	−	−	−
X-linked ALD/AMN	+	−	−	−	−	−
Adult Refsum disease	−	−	−	+	−	−
2-Methylacyl-CoA racemase deficiency	−	−	+	+/−*	−	−
Mevalonate kinase deficiency	−	−	−	−	−	+
Hyperoxaluria type I	−	−	−	−	−	+
Acatalasemia	−	−	−	−	−	+
Glutaryl-CoA oxidase deficiency	−	−	−	−	−	+

+, abnormal; −, normal; ALD, adrenoleukodystrophy; AMN, adrenomyeloneuropathy; DHAP, dihydroxyacetone phosphate; VLCFA, very-long-chain fatty acids; *, also elevated pristanic acid.

clinical phenotype exists within the same genotype. Some patients have severe forms of the disorders that present in the neonatal period, whereas other forms are milder and present at older ages. Group 1 includes classic and mild Zellweger syndrome, classic and severe neonatal adrenoleukodystrophy (ALD), infantile Refsum disease, hyperpipecolic acidemia, and the rhizomelic form of chondrodysplasia punctata (RCDP).

Group 2 is comprised of disorders associated with the deficient activity of a single peroxisomal enzyme. These disorders result from single gene mutations and include a group of three Zellweger-like conditions termed *pseudo-Zellweger syndrome* (3-oxoacyl-CoA thiolase deficiency), *pseudoneonatal ALD* (acyl-CoA oxidase deficiency), and the *bifunctional enzyme deficiency* (functions as both enoyl-CoA hydratase and 3-hydroxyacyl-CoA dehydrogenase). Other disorders in Group 2 include two RCDP-like conditions associated with the isolated deficient activity of DHAP acyltransferase or alkyl DHAP synthase; X-linked ALD and adrenomyeloneuropathy (AMN); adult Refsum disease; mevalonate kinase deficiency; 2-methylacyl-CoA racemase deficiency; hyperoxaluria type I; acatalasemia; and peroxisomal glutaryl-CoA oxidase deficiency. Table 390.1 summarizes the biochemical findings in the disorders presently recognized as involving peroxisomal function.

DISORDERS ASSOCIATED WITH DEFECTS IN PEROXISOMAL BIOGENESIS

Zellweger Syndrome

Zellweger syndrome (cerebrohepatorenal syndrome) previously was classified as a dysmorphic syndrome affecting almost every organ system. Major dysmorphic features include a flat midfacial area with shallow orbital ridges and epicanthal folding; large fontanelle; flat occiput; high, prominent forehead; dolichocephaly; Brushfield spots; mild micrognathia; external ear anomalies; and transverse palmar creases. Retinitis pigmentosa, with impaired vision; hearing problems; hepatomegaly, with impaired function and cirrhosis; albuminuria; renal cortical cysts; and impaired cortisol response to adrenocorticotropic hormone or adrenal atrophy usually are noted. Marked generalized hypotonia, present from birth, often is associated with feeding and respiratory problems. Some patients also have congenital cataracts, glaucoma, punctate mineralization of joints, cardiac defects, and elevated serum iron levels. Abnormal fetal brain development with macrogyria and polymicrogyria, and failure of myelination and white-matter development lead to severe progressive psychomotor retardation and seizures. Most children have marked failure to thrive and do not live past 6 months of age (Fig. 390.2).

Zellweger syndrome is associated with generalized peroxisomal dysfunction. Elevated plasma and tissue levels of VLCFA, phytanic acid, pipecolic acid, and bile salt precursors, as well as decreased plasmalogen synthesis, are noted. Deficient enzyme activities associated with these findings have been shown. Current therapy is symptomatic and supportive, including correction of coagulopathies using vitamin K and adrenal corticosteroid hormone replacement therapy, if indicated. Attempts to improve the clinical status of affected patients using supplements of bile salts and dietary restriction of VLCFA and phytate precursors are being investigated. The disorder is inherited as an autosomal recessive trait. The molecular basis for the disorder and its mild variants (discussed in the next paragraph) is heterogeneous and can involve any one of 11 gene loci. Most commonly, a molecular defect occurs in *PEX1*, located at chromosome 7q21-q22. Prenatal diagnosis is available. Carrier detection is available in families in which the molecular defect is known.

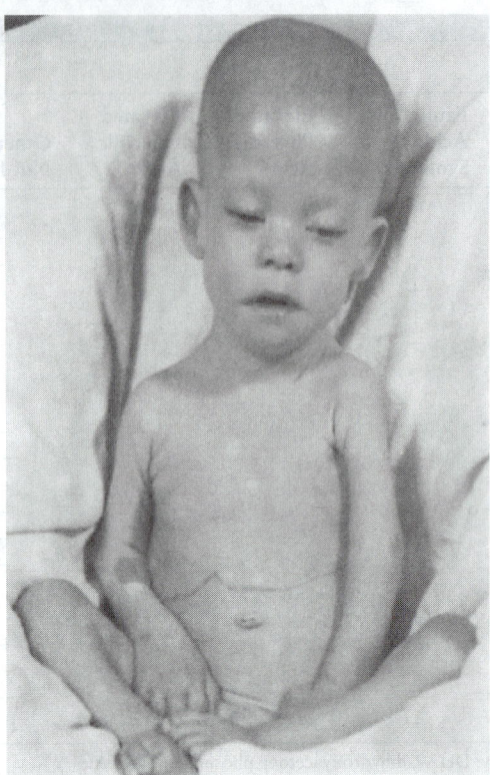

FIGURE 390.2. Child with Zellweger syndrome at age 8.5 months. (The spots are from film processing and are not caused by hypopigmentation.)

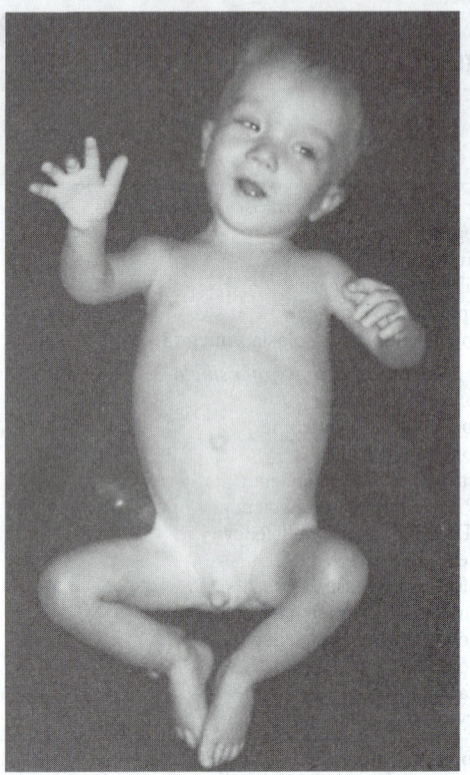

FIGURE 390.3. Child with mild Zellweger syndrome at age 15 months.

Neonatal Adrenoleukodystrophy, Infantile Refsum Disease, Hyperpipecolic Acidemia, and "Mild" Zellweger Syndrome

Neonatal ALD, infantile Refsum disease, hyperpipecolic acidemia, and mild Zellweger syndrome are similar in clinical and biochemical features. It has been proposed that they be termed *peroxisomal polydystrophy syndromes*. All are associated with generalized peroxisomal dysfunction, but the biochemical defects are often less severe than those seen in classic Zellweger syndrome. Likewise, the clinical features may be milder and later in onset, the dysmorphic features may be variable, and usually no renal cysts or chondrodysplasia punctata are present (Fig. 390.3).

Rhizomelic Form of Chondrodysplasia Punctata

RCDP, an autosomal recessive disorder, is associated with elevated plasma phytanic acid levels and faulty plasmalogen biosynthesis as a result of deficient activities of phytanoyl-CoA hydroxylase and DHAP acyltransferase, respectively. Affected patients also have an unprocessed form of 3-oxoacyl-CoA thiolase. Clinical features, present from birth, include disproportionate short stature affecting the proximal part of the extremities (rhizomelia); abnormal facies, with frontal bossing and flat nasal bridge; congenital cataracts; joint contractures; microcephaly; mental retardation; and failure to thrive. Most affected patients die in infancy. Radiographic findings include severe, symmetric epiphyseal and extraepiphyseal calcifications that spare the vertebral column. Splaying and metaphyseal cupping occur, as well as shortening of the humeri

or femora (Fig. 390.4). The disorder most commonly results from mutations in the *PEX7* gene, which encodes a cytosolic peroxisomal receptor for peroxisomal targeting signal 2.

DISORDERS ASSOCIATED WITH DEFICIENT ACTIVITY OF A SINGLE PEROXISOMAL ENZYME

Pseudo-Zellweger Syndrome, Pseudoneonatal Adrenoleukodystrophy, and Bifunctional Enzyme Deficiency

Patients with clinical features similar to those seen with disorders of peroxisomal biogenesis have been reported with single-enzyme deficiencies. These disorders include pseudo-Zellweger syndrome (3-oxoacyl-CoA thiolase deficiency), pseudoneonatal ALD (acyl-CoA oxidase deficiency), and the bifunctional enzyme deficiency. Dysmorphic features are noted with pseudo-Zellweger syndrome but are only minimal in those with pseudoneonatal ALD and usually absent with the bifunctional enzyme deficiency. All three disorders have disturbances in peroxisomal beta-oxidation of VLCFA. In addition, patients with pseudo-Zellweger syndrome and those with the bifunctional enzyme deficiency have abnormal bile acid synthesis. Patients with the bifunctional enzyme deficiency also have increased phytate and pristanic acid levels.

Variants of the Rhizomelic Form of Chondrodysplasia Punctata

Variants of RCDP may result from isolated deficiencies of either DHAP acyltransferase or alkyl DHAP synthetase. These

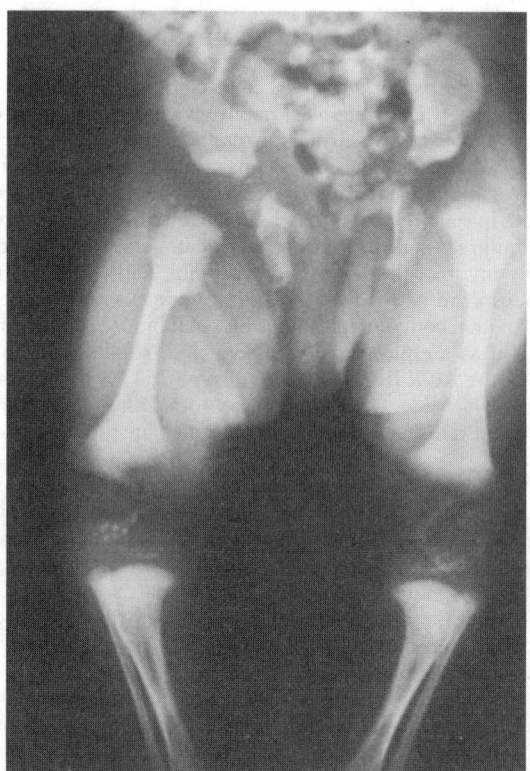

FIGURE 390.4. Radiograph of a patient with the rhizomelic form of chondrodysplasia punctata. Note the extraepiphyseal calcifications.

patients only have abnormal plasmalogen synthesis, in contrast to patients with classical RCDP, who have abnormalities in both plasmalogen synthesis and phytate oxidation.

X-Linked or Childhood Adrenoleukodystrophy and Adrenomyeloneuropathy

X-linked or childhood ALD is characterized by the onset, between 4 and 8 years of age, of changes in behavior or school performance, disturbances in vision or hearing, abnormalities in gait and coordination, dysarthrias, and dysphagias. Thereafter follows a progressive central and peripheral nervous system inflammatory demyelination with gradual loss of vision, hearing, mental and motor abilities, and the development of seizures. Most boys die within 3 to 5 years after the onset of symptoms. Adrenocortical atrophy or insufficiency and a suppressed response to adrenocorticotropic hormone occurs in more than 90% of affected boys. Occasionally, a patient will exhibit Addison disease before the neurologic symptoms are noted. Some affected male subjects, ascertained through family studies, do not develop progressive neurologic disease.

AMN, an adult variant of ALD that usually occurs in men in their twenties, is characterized by progressive spastic paraparesis, sensory deficits, and polyneuropathy. Adrenal insufficiency occurs in two-thirds of affected men. Primary hypogonadism, with low testosterone and elevated follicle-stimulating hormone levels, is common. Because both ALD and AMN are inherited as X-linked traits and have occurred in the same sibship, AMN is considered to be a milder phenotypic variant of ALD. Approximately 20% of female carriers for ALD/AMN also develop progressive neurologic disorders with spastic paraparesis; 50% will have mild neurologic findings.

ALD and AMN result from the defective degradation of VLCFA. A reduced activity of peroxisomal very long-chain acyl-CoA synthetase (also known as *lignoceroyl-CoA synthetase*), the first step in beta-oxidation of VLCFA, has been shown in cultured fibroblasts from affected patients. Patients with ALD and AMN, as well as most female carriers of these disorders, have elevated plasma levels of VLCFA. Affected male subjects accumulate saturated VLCFA in the ganglioside of cerebral white matter and in the cholesteryl ester fraction of the adrenal cortex and cerebral white matter (Fig. 390.5).

Hormone replacement therapy is indicated for adrenal and testosterone insufficiency. Investigational studies have shown that dietary restriction of C26:0, in addition to glycerol trierucate (C22:1) and glycerol trioleate (C18:1) supplementation, results in lowered plasma levels of VLCFA. Some affected male patients with ALD appear to respond to this therapy if it is started before the onset of neurologic symptoms. Whether the therapy prevented neurologic progression in these patients or whether these patients were those fortunate enough to be destined not to have progressive neurologic disease was unclear. The therapy is not effective in patients with AMN. Agents that modify inflammatory response are being investigated. Bone marrow transplantation may be considered for male patients

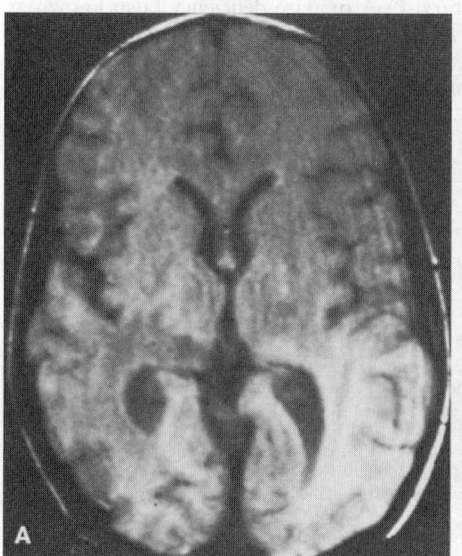
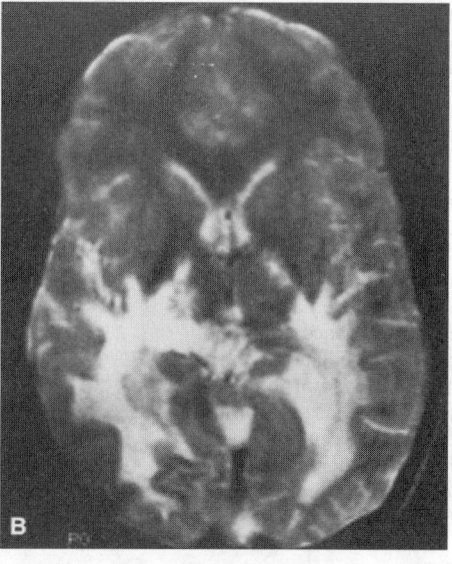

FIGURE 390.5. Adrenoleukodystrophy. **A:** T1-weighted magnetic resonance image. **B:** T2-weighted magnetic resonance image. Note the increased periventricular signal in the posterior areas.

with ALD early in their disease and before significant neurologic involvement.

The gene *ALD*, located at chromosome Xq28, encodes the ALD protein, which is thought to be a peroxisomal transport protein involved with the import or anchoring of very long-chain acyl-CoA synthetase at the peroxisomal membrane. Multiple different mutations at the *ALD* locus have been reported in affected male patients. Because approximately 10% to 15% of obligate female carriers for ALD/AMN have false-negative results when tested by plasma VLCFA levels alone, molecular genetic techniques using mutation analysis must be used for accurate carrier detection. This testing is especially important if a sister is being considered as a bone marrow transplant donor. Prenatal diagnosis is available.

Adult Refsum Disease

Adult Refsum disease, a rare autosomal recessive disorder, is associated with the deficient activity of phytanoyl-CoA hydroxylase and elevated plasma, serum, and tissue levels of phytanic acid. The age of onset is variable, but cerebellar ataxia, peripheral polyneuropathy, retinitis pigmentosa, and elevated spinal fluid protein concentrations are noted in most patients before 20 years of age. They also may have ichthyosis, anosmia, skeletal abnormalities, sensorineural hearing loss, and cardiac conduction defects. Treatment through the strict reduction of dietary phytanic acid sources (meats, diary products, fish) may result in clinical improvement. Occasionally, plasmapheresis combined with dietary therapy may be needed to reduce phytanic acid stores during initial therapy. The disorder results from mutations in the *PAHX* gene at chromosome 10pter–p11.2.

2-Methylacyl-CoA Racemase Deficiency

Peroxisomal 2-methylacyl-CoA racemase, encoded by the AMACR gene at chromosome 5p13.2–q11.1, is involved in the oxidation of long branched-chain fatty acids and bile salts. A deficient activity of the racemase results in elevated body fluid levels of pristanic acid, a product of phytanic acid metabolism, and of bile salt precursors, di-, and trihydroxycholestanoic acids. Minimal elevation of phytanic acid is noted. Levels of very long-chain fatty acids are normal. Two of three reported patients presented with an adult-onset peripheral sensory and motor neuropathy. One patient additionally had retinitis pigmentosa, seizures, and hypogonadism. The other had long-tract neurologic findings, as seen with AMN. The third patient was a child with coexisting Niemann-Pick Type C disease, who was identified during biochemical investigations for the other condition.

Mevalonate Kinase Deficiency

Mevalonate kinase is involved in the early steps of the biosynthesis of isoprenoids and cholesterol. Affected patients have variable clinical features. Severe forms of the disorder result in failure to thrive, psychomotor handicaps, hypotonia, and recurrent crises, which are characterized by fevers accompanied by rashes, vomiting, or diarrhea. Ataxia, cerebellar atrophy, hepatosplenomegaly, cataracts, anemia, and dysmorphic features may occur. Urine organic acids will disclose large amounts of mevalonolactone. Most patients expire between 6 months and 4 years of age. Milder forms of the disorder have some residual activity. The clinical and biochemical findings are not as severe and longer survival is possible. No specific treatment is available.

Primary Hyperoxaluria Type I

Primary hyperoxaluria type I is characterized by recurrent calcium oxalate nephrolithiasis, nephrocalcinosis, chronic renal failure, and excessive urinary excretion of oxalic, glyoxylic, and glycolic acids. The age of onset and clinical severity are variable, but most patients are symptomatic by the age of 5 years. Initial symptoms may be related to uremia and chronic renal failure. Oxalosis (extrarenal calcium oxalate deposition) usually involves the bones, myocardium, and testes but may be widespread with advanced disease. Crystals may be seen in the proximal convoluted tubules on renal biopsy. The disorder, inherited as an autosomal recessive trait, results from mutations in the *AGXT* gene at chromosome 2q37.3 and is associated with deficient activity of peroxisomal alanine-glyoxylate aminotransferase. Glyoxylate is the immediate precursor of oxalate.

Treatment includes the use of pyridoxine in an attempt to reduce oxalate synthesis by stimulating an alternate pathway, the avoidance of dietary sources high in oxalate and ascorbic acid (an oxalate precursor), and the administration of magnesium or phosphate to increase urinary oxalate solubility. Renal transplantation is successful only temporarily, because it does not correct the basic disorder. However, combined liver and kidney transplants have been successful.

Hyperoxaluria type II, which is not classified as a peroxisomal disorder, has a milder clinical presentation, without renal insufficiency. Hyperoxaluria type II is associated with excessive urinary excretion of oxalate and L-glyceric acid and deficient activity of cytosolic D-glycerate dehydrogenase and glyoxylate reductase. Secondary hyperoxaluria may result from pyridoxine deficiency, ascorbic acid ingestion, ethylene glycol poisoning, increased intake of oxalate or oxalate precursors, and increased oxalate absorption with small bowel disorders and steatorrhea.

Acatalasemia

Acatalasemia (catalase deficiency), inherited as an autosomal recessive trait, may be associated with varying degrees of ulcerating gangrenous lesions of the oral cavity during childhood. Most homozygous persons are asymptomatic, however.

Peroxisomal Glutaryl-CoA Oxidase Deficiency

Peroxisomal glutaryl-CoA oxidase deficiency (also known as *glutaric aciduria type III*) has been reported in one patient with failure to thrive, vomiting, and elevated urinary glutaric acid levels. Riboflavin supplements lowered the levels of glutaric acid.

Suggested Readings

Baumgartner MR, Saudubray JM. Peroxisomal disorders. *Semin Neonatol* 2002; 7:85.

Berger J, Moser HW, Forss-Petter S. Leukodystrophies: recent developments in genetics, molecular biology, pathogenesis and treatment. *Curr Opin Neurol* 2001;14:305.

Bezman L, Moser AB, Raymond, et al. Adrenoleukodystrophy: incidence, new mutation rate, and results of extended family screening. *Ann Neurol* 2001; 49:512.

Ferdinandusse S, Denis S, Clayton PT, et al. Mutations in the gene encoding peroxisomal alpha-methylacyl-CoA racemase cause adult-onset sensory motor neuropathy. *Nat Genet* 2000;24:188.

Fitzpatrick DR. Zellweger syndrome and associated phenotypes. *J Med Genet* 1996;33:863.

Gartner J. Organelle disease: peroxisomal disorders. *Eur J Pediatr* 2000;159S3: S236.

Loes DJ, Fatemi A, Melhem ER, et al. Analysis of MRI patterns aids prediction of progression in X-linked adrenoleukodystrophy. *Neurology* 2003;61:369.

McLean BN, Allen J, Ferdinandusse S, et al. A new defect of peroxisomal function involving pristanic acid: a case report. *J Neurol Neurosurg Psychiatry* 2002;72:396.

Moser HW, Powers JM, Smith KD. Adrenoleukodystrophy: molecular genetics, pathology and Lorenzo's oil. *Brain Pathol* 1995;5:259.

Percy AK, Rutledge SL. Adrenoleukodystrophy and related disorders. *Ment Retard Dev Disabil Res Rev* 2001;7:179.

Ramond GV. Peroxisomal disorders. *Curr Opin Neurol* 2001;14:783.

Ronghe MD, Barton J, Jardine PE, et al. The importance of testing for adrenoleukodystrophy in males with idiopathic Addison's disease. *Arch Dis Child* 2002;86:185.

Scriver CR, Beaudet AL, Sly WS, et al., eds. Peroxisomes, part 11. *The metabolic and molecular bases of inherited disease,* 8th ed. New York: McGraw-Hill, 2001;3181.

Zhang LX, Bakshi R, Fine E, et al. Clinical and electrophysiological improvement of adrenomyeloneuropathy with steroid treatment. *J Neurol Neurosurg Psychiatry* 2003;74:822.

CHAPTER 391 ■ DISORDERS OF PURINE AND PYRIMIDINE METABOLISM

REBECCA S. WAPPNER

PURINE AND PYRIMIDINE METABOLISM

Purine and pyrimidine nucleotides are important constituents of RNA, DNA, nucleotide sugars, and other high-energy compounds and of cofactors such as adenosine triphosphate and nicotinamide-adenine dinucleotide. Both purines and pyrimidines may be synthesized *de novo* from ribose-5-phosphate and carbamyl phosphate, respectively, as shown in Figs. 391.1 and 391.2. The nucleosides guanosine, adenosine, cytidine, uridine, and thymidine are formed by the addition of ribose-1-phosphate to their respective purine bases (guanine and adenine) and pyrimidine bases (cytosine, uracil, and thymine). Phosphorylation of the nucleosides results in monophosphate, diphosphate, and triphosphate nucleotides. Recycling and interconversion of the compounds occur (salvage pathways); these processes, in turn, conserve the nucleotides and nucleosides and exert a negative feedback on *de novo* synthesis.

The disorders of purine and pyrimidine metabolism exhibit a wide array of clinical symptoms, which include renal calculi, neurologic problems, delayed physical and mental development, self-mutilation, hemolytic anemias, and immunodeficiencies. Table 391.1 gives a summary of the findings, diagnostic testing, and treatment for the disorders.

DISORDERS OF PURINE METABOLISM

Gout

Gout is characterized by hyperuricemia, uric acid nephrolithiasis, and inflammatory arthritis. The disorder may present at any age, but most often it is seen in adults, with an increasing incidence with age. The prevalence is estimated to be 1 in 167 men and 1 in 1,000 women. Primary gout is associated with the overproduction or decreased renal excretion of uric acid. The biochemical basis of the disorder is unknown in most patients, and the disorder is considered to be a polygenic trait. Primary gout also can be seen with the overproduction of uric acid associated with increased activity of phosphoribosylpyrophosphate synthetase (PPRP-S) and deficiency of hypoxanthine guanine phosphoribosyltransferase (HGPRT), inherited disorders that are discussed in the following sections. In addition, familial juvenile gout appears to include a group of rare, inherited disorders that occur at younger ages than primary polygenic gout. Secondary gout may be seen with other conditions or disorders associated with increased production or decreased excretion of uric acid (i.e., starvation, dehydration, prolonged exercise, lactic acidosis, ketoacidosis, hypertension, renal dysfunction, myeloproliferative disorders, and glycogen storage disease type I). Secondary gout also may be seen during treatment with diuretics, low-dose salicylates, pyrazinamide, ethambutol, and niacin or during the treatment of malignant diseases. Environmental factors may play a role in the pathogenesis of gout in that excessive purine, ethanol, or carbohydrate ingestion appears to be related to increased production of uric acid.

Gouty arthritis results from monosodium urate crystal deposition in joints and surrounding tissues. The presentation usually is monoarticular and peripheral, and the most commonly affected site is the metatarsophalangeal joint of the great toe. Untreated, an acute arthritic attack resolves spontaneously within a few days to a few weeks. During acute attacks, colchicine, corticosteroids, and nonsteroidal antiinflammatory agents may be used. Chronic arthritis may lead to joint damage and deformity. Monosodium urate crystals may be noted in joint fluid. Tophi, which are monosodium urate crystal deposits, may occur over the helix of the ears and over points of insertion of tendons at the elbows, knees, and feet. Urolithiasis may occur before or after the onset of the arthritis. Calcium oxalate and urate stones are seen. Uric acid stones are yellow-orange, smooth, hard, and radiolucent, and they crush with difficulty. Renal dysfunction is thought to be related to underlying hypertension and renal vascular disease, rather than to hyperuricosuria.

Most patients with elevated uric acid levels are asymptomatic, never develop gout, and do not require long-term treatment. Symptomatic gout is more likely to develop in patients with serum uric acid levels greater than 10 mg/dL. Patients with frequent attacks of gouty arthritis, chronic gout, tophi, or uric acid nephrolithiasis may benefit from treatment

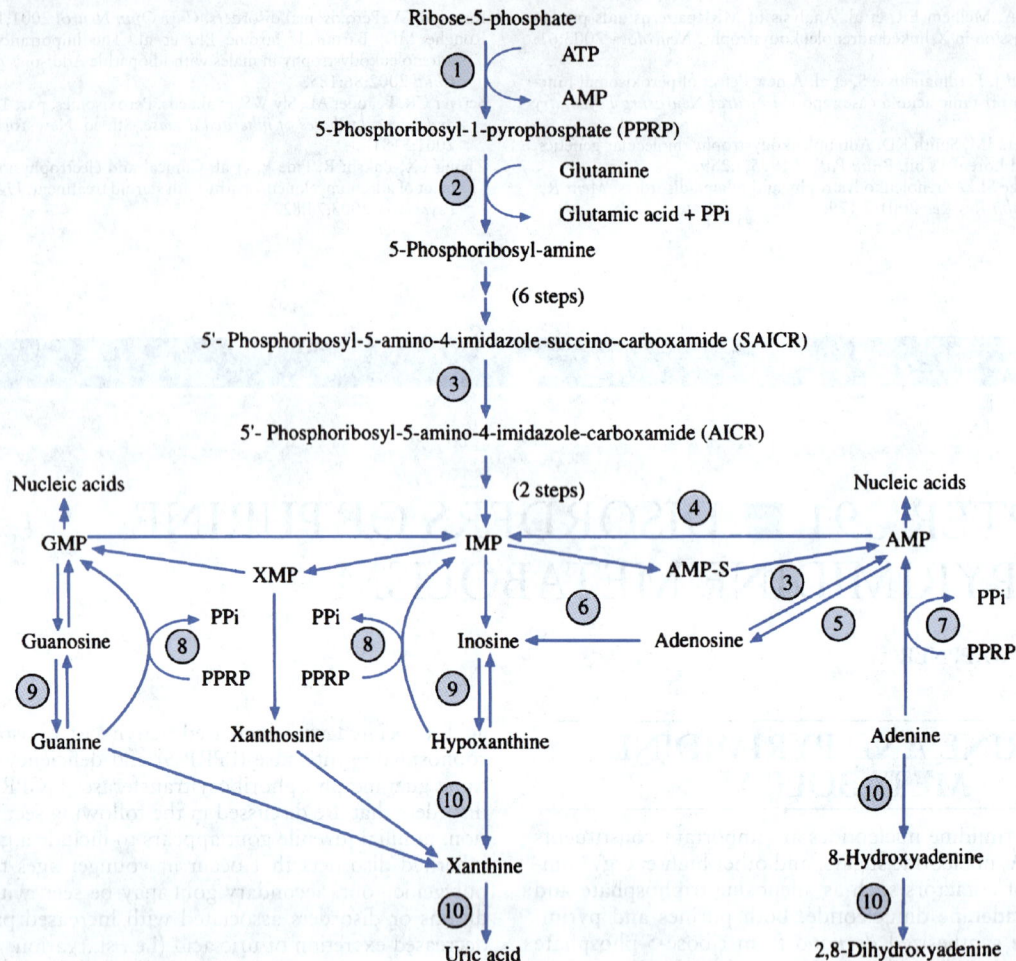

FIGURE 391.1. Purine metabolism. *1*, phosphoribosylpyrophosphate synthetase; *2*, amido-phosphoribosyltransferase; *3*, adenylosuccinate lyase (catalyzes AMP-S to AMP); *4*, adenylate deaminase; *5*, purine-5′-nucleotidase; *6*, adenosine deaminase; *7*, adenine phosphoribosyltransferase; *8*, hypoxanthine guanine phosphoribosyltransferase; *9*, purine-nucleoside phosphorylase; *10*, xanthine oxidoreductase. Only the ribose forms of the nucleosides and nucleotides are illustrated. The deoxyribose forms follow similar pathways. AMP, adenosine monophosphate; AMP-S, adenylosuccinic acid; ATP, adenosine triphosphate; GMP, guanosine monophosphate; IMP, inosine monophosphate; PPi, inorganic pyrophosphate; XMP, xanthosine monophosphate.

of hyperuricemia. Allopurinol, which inhibits xanthine oxidase (oxidoreductase) activity and results in reduced purine biosynthesis and reduced excretion of uric acid, is the treatment of choice for those with urate nephropathy. Probenecid and sulfinpyrazone, which increase uric acid clearance, may be used with patients with normal renal function and no uric acid renal stones. Alkalinization of the urine, which increases uric acid solubility, and increased fluid intake, which decreases the concentration of urinary uric acid, may help to prevent renal stone formation. Dietary reduction of purine-containing foods, correction of obesity, and cessation of ethanol ingestion help to lessen environmentally related causes of hyperuricemia.

Phosphoribosylpyrophosphate Synthetase Overactivity

PPRP-S catalyzes the transfer of the pyrophosphate group of adenosine triphosphate to ribose-5-phosphate to form PPRP. PPRP-S is induced by lowered purine nucleotide levels under normal circumstances. The resulting PPRP acts as an in-

ducer of amidophosphoribosyl transferase, the next step in the purine biosynthetic pathway. The increased levels of purine nucleotides that result then act by means of negative feedback to inhibit purine biosynthesis. This X-linked recessive disorder is associated with reduced sensitivity of PPRP-S to nucleotide inhibition and increased specific activity of PPRP-S *in vitro*. The result is a continuous overproduction of purines by *de novo* biosynthesis. Patients have hyperuricemia and hyperuricosuria and present during the teenage or young adult years with severe gout or renal calculi. A more severe form of the disorder exists in which severe psychomotor retardation, autistic features, hypotonia, and nerve deafness also occur. Female carriers of the severe form may have deafness and gout.

Elevated PPRP levels may be detected in erythrocytes, lymphocytes, and cultured skin fibroblasts. Treatment includes allopurinol, high fluid intake, and alkalinization of the urine.

Adenylosuccinate Lyase Deficiency

Adenylosuccinate lyase (ADSL) is associated with two steps in purine metabolism. In the *de novo* synthetic pathway, it

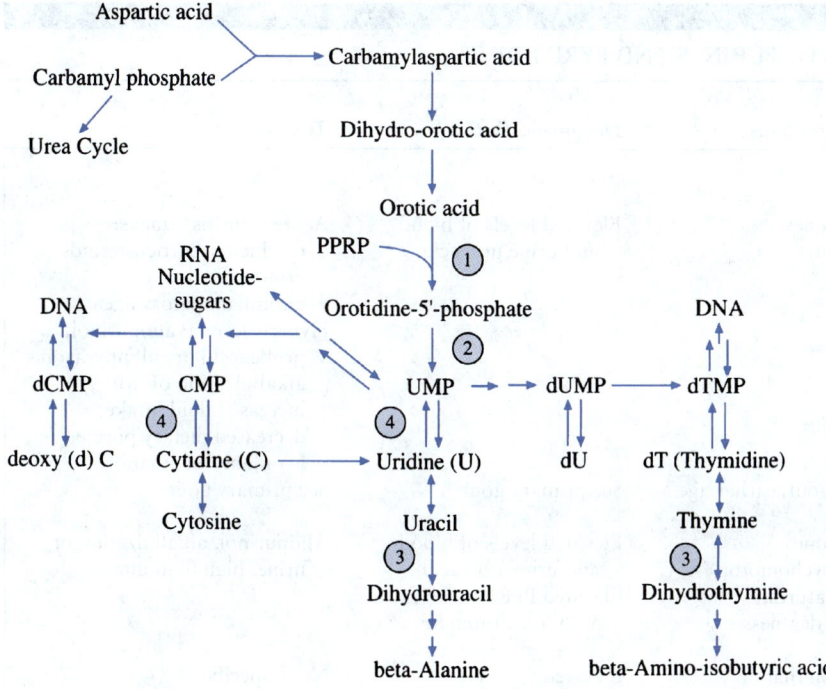

FIGURE 391.2. Pyrimidine metabolism. *1,* orotic acid phosphoribosyltransferase; *2,* orotidine phosphate decarboxylase; *3,* dihydropyrimidine dehydrogenase; *4,* pyrimidine-5′-nucleotidase, MP, monophosphate; PPRP, phosphoribosylpyrophosphate.

catalyzes the conversion of succinyl aminoimidazole carboxamide ribotide to aminoimidazole carboxamide ribotide with release of fumarate. In the second reaction, adenylosuccinic acid is converted to adenosine monophosphate, also with release of fumarate. Deficient activity of ADSL is associated with the accumulation of both substrates for the enzyme in their nucleoside-derivative forms, succinyl aminoimidazole carboxamide riboside and succinyl adenosine. ADSL deficiency is a rare autosomal recessive disorder, associated with mutations in the *ADSL* gene located at chromosome 22q. Elevated succinyl purine levels are neurotoxic and result in varying degrees of psychomotor handicaps and neurologic involvement, which are usually evident by 2 years of age. More severely affected patients present with neonatal seizures. Hypotonia, autistic features, and growth retardation may occur. Computed tomography of the brain may show cerebellar hypoplasia, mainly of the vermis, and cortical and subcortical hypotrophy. Magnetic resonance imaging of the brain often shows a disturbed myelin or leukodystrophy pattern. The diagnosis is established by the finding of elevated levels of succinyl aminoimidazole carboxamide ribotide and succinyl adenosine in the plasma, urine, and cerebrospinal fluid. No effective therapy is currently available.

Myoadenylate Deaminase Deficiency

Adenylate deaminase catalyzes the deamination of adenosine monophosphate to inosine monophosphate and is composed of multiple isoenzymes that are tissue specific. Deficient activity of muscle adenylate deaminase (myoadenylate deaminase) is an autosomal recessive disorder associated with muscle cramping and myalgia after exercise. Exercise does not lead to ammonia production, which normally would stimulate glycolysis. Muscle adenosine triphosphate and total purine content decrease to a greater extent than normally occurs with exercise. The exact metabolic abnormalities in muscle energy metabolism are not known fully. Increased creatine kinase has been noted in 60% of patients. Some patients also have hypotonia, and a few have been reported to have hyperuricemia and gout. A single mutant allele at the myoadenylate deaminase locus *AMPD1*, resulting in a truncated peptide, has been found in all cases

evaluated to date. Myoadenylate deaminase deficiency may be shown in muscle biopsy samples by histochemical staining or measurement of specific enzymatic activity.

Secondary muscle adenylate deaminase deficiency has been reported in association with other neuromuscular disorders (i.e., hypokalemic paralysis, muscular dystrophy, motor neuron disorders, polymyositis, and other collagen-vascular diseases). Molecular genetic evaluations in these patients have shown reduced transcription of myoadenylate deaminase. Patients with muscle adenylate deaminase deficiency also appear to be at higher risk for malignant hyperthermia. In general, no specific therapy exists. Ribose administration has resulted in varying responses.

Adenosine Deaminase Deficiency

Adenosine deaminase (ADA) catalyzes the deamination of deoxyadenosine to deoxyinosine and, to a lesser extent, the deamination of adenosine to inosine. Under normal circumstances, adenosine usually is converted to adenosine monophosphate by adenylate kinase. Deficiency of ADA is associated with elevated levels of deoxyadenosine and deoxyadenosine nucleotides, especially deoxyadenosine triphosphate. These elevations lead to activation of adenosine monophosphate deaminase and cytoplasmic 5′-nucleotidase, which results in depletion of adenosine triphosphate and other adenosine nucleotides. Elevated levels of deoxyadenosine nucleotides and decreased levels of adenosine nucleotides are noted in plasma, erythrocytes, and platelets of patients. Plasma and urine levels of deoxyadenosine are markedly elevated, as are plasma levels of adenosine. The elevated levels of deoxyadenosine bind with *S*-adenosylhomocysteine hydrolase and decrease its specific activity, which results in reduced methylation reactions. The elevated levels of deoxyadenosine also inhibit ribonucleoside diphosphate reductase and DNA synthesis in T-cell and B-cell precursors and are thought to be responsible for the severe combined immunodeficiency that is associated with ADA deficiency.

Most patients have symptoms of repeated infections and failure to thrive by 2 years of age. T-cell function usually is completely impaired, whereas B-cell function is variable. Mild

TABLE 391.1

CLINICAL FINDINGS IN THE DISORDERS OF PURINES AND PYRIMIDINES

Disorder (Inheritance Pattern)	Major Signs and Symptoms	Diagnostic Testing	Treatment
Disorders of Purine Metabolism			
Primary gout (Polygenic trait)	Uric acid urinary stones Inflammatory arthritis	Elevated levels of blood and urine uric acid	Acute arthritis attacks: colchicine, corticosteroids, nonsteroidal antiinflammatory agents Hyperuricemia: allopurinol, probenecid or sulfinpyrazone, alkalinization of urine, increased fluid intake, decreased dietary purine, avoidance of ethanol
Familial juvenile gout (AD)	Similar to primary gout, earlier age of onset	See primary gout	See primary gout
Phosphoribosyl pyrophosphate synthetase (PPRP-S) overactivity (X-linked)	Uric acid urinary stones Severe form with psychomotor delays, autistic features, hypotonia, nerve deafness	Elevated levels of blood and urine uric acid Elevated PPRP in RBCs, WBCs, cultured SFs	Allopurinol, alkalinization of urine, high fluid intake
Adenylosuccinate lyase (ADSL) deficiency (AR)	Variable presentation that may include neonatal seizures, hypotonia, psychomotor delays, autistic features, growth retardation Cerebellar hypoplasia and disturbed myelin pattern on radioimaging	Elevated succinyl aminoimidazole carboxamide ribotide (SAICR) and succinyl adenosine in plasma, urine, cerebrospinal fluid	None specific
Myoadenylate deaminase deficiency (AR)	Muscle cramps and myalgia with exercise Occasional hypotonia, gout, hyperuricemia	Elevated serum creatine kinase with exercise Deficient activity of adenylate deaminase in muscle biopsy	Ribose, with variable response At risk for malignant hyperthermia
Adenosine deaminase (ADA) deficiency (AR)	Severe combined immunodeficiency (SCID)	Deficient activity of ADA in plasma, RBCs, WBCs, cultured SFs	Polyethylene glycol (PEG)-modified bovine ADA BMT/SCT
Purine-nucleoside phosphorylase (PNP) deficiency (AR)	Defective T-cell-mediated immunity Psychomotor handicaps; familial autoimmune hemolytic anemia	Decreased body fluid levels of uric acid. Deficient activity of PNP in lysed RBCs	Intermittent transfusions of irradiated normal RBCs BMT/SCT
Adenine phosphoribosyl transferase (APRT) deficiency (AR)	2,8-Dihydroxyadenine urinary stones Only 15% of patients become symptomatic	Elevated levels of urine adenine, 8-hydroxyadenine, and 2,8-dihydroxyadenine Deficient activity of APRT in RBCs, WBCs, cultured SFs	Allopurinol, decreased dietary intake of purine, large fluid intake
Hypoxanthine guanine phosphoribosyl transferase (HGPRT) deficiency (X-linked)	Severe form known as Lesch-Nyhan syndrome Uric acid urinary stones Choreoathetosis, dystonia, self-mutilation Milder variants without self-mutilation	Elevated urine uric acid at all ages Elevated blood uric acid after puberty Deficient activity of HGPRT in RBCs or cultured SFs	Allopurinol, in carefully titrated doses
Hereditary xanthinuria (AR)	Isolated deficiency of xanthine oxidoreductase (XOR) Uric acid urinary stones Molybdenum cofactor deficiency variants with urinary stones (deficiency of XOR and aldehyde oxidase) or neonatal intractable seizures, microcephaly, dislocated lens (deficiency of XOR, aldehyde oxidase, and sulfite oxidase)	Low serum and urine uric acid. Elevated urine xanthine and hypoxanthine Deficient activity of XOR in liver or intestinal mucosa biopsy	Lowered purine diet High fluid intake Lowered sulfur-containing amino acid (methionine, cystine) diet with sulfite oxidase deficiency

(Continued)

TABLE 391.1

(CONTINUED)

Disorder (Inheritance Pattern)	Major Signs and Symptoms	Diagnostic Testing	Treatment
Disorders of Pyrimidine Metabolism			
Hereditary orotic aciduria (AR)	Severe macrocytic, hypochromic anemia Psychomotor handicaps Occasionally birth defects, immune deficiencies, or urinary tract obstruction	Increased urine orotic acid Deficient activity of the uridine monophosphate synthetase complex in RBCs, WBCs, cultured SFs, and liver biopsy	Uridine
Hereditary combined uraciluria-thyminuria (AR)	Complete deficiency with variable, early-onset neurologic problems Inability to detoxify 5FU Partial deficiency (pharmacokinetic form), later onset, with symptoms only after exposure to 5FU	Elevated body fluids levels of uracil, thymine, and 5-hydroxymethyluracil Decreased beta-alanine and beta-aminoisobutyrate Decreased activity of dihydropyrimidine dehydrogenase in WBCs or cultured SFs	Avoidance of treatment with 5FU
Dihydropyrimidinase (DPH) deficiency (AR)	May have neurologic symptoms, seizures, microcephaly Inability to detoxify 5FU Inability to activate IRCF-187	Elevated body fluids levels of dihydrouracil and dihydrothymine Decreased beta-alanine Deficient activity of DPH in liver biopsy	Avoidance of treatment with 5FU Avoidance of combined treatment of doxorubicin (Adriamycin) with IRCF-187
Pyrimidine-5′-nucleotidase (P5N) deficiency (AR)	Nonspherocytic hemolytic anemia	Elevated erythrocyte uridine triphosphate and cytidine triphosphate Deficient activity of P5N in RBCs	Usually none Occasionally need transfusions and splenectomy
Pyrimidine-5′-nucleotidase (P5N) superactivity (AR)	Delayed development, seizures, ataxia Multiple infections	Low urine uric acid Increased activity of P5N in cultured SFs	Uridine

AD, autosomal dominant; AR, autosomal recessive; BMT, bone marrow transplant; 5FU, f-fluorouracil; ICRF-187, [1,2-bis(3,5-dioxopiperazinyl-1-yl)propane]; RBC, erythrocyte; SCT, stem cell transplant; SF; skin fibroblast; WBC, leukocyte/lymphocyte.

forms have been reported. This autosomal recessive disorder may be confirmed by the finding of deficient activity of ADA in erythrocytes, plasma, lymphocytes, and cultured skin fibroblasts. Most obligate carriers have approximately one-half normal erythrocyte ADA activity, but overlap with physiologically normal individuals occurs. Mutation analysis of the *ADA* gene locus, located at chromosome 20q13.11, may be used for carrier testing. Prenatal diagnosis is available.

General treatment is similar to that for other forms of severe combined immunodeficiency. Bone marrow transplantation is the treatment of choice and is indicated if an appropriate donor exists. Treatment with injections of polyethylene glycol (PEG)–modified bovine ADA has resulted in clinical improvement in all patients treated to date. Gene therapy with *ex vivo* retrovirus-mediated gene transfer into stem and myeloid cells and T-lymphocytes is being investigated. All patients with severe combined immunodeficiency should be tested for ADA deficiency because this disorder may account for 20% to 25% of all cases of severe combined immunodeficiency.

Purine-Nucleoside Phosphorylase Deficiency

Purine-nucleoside phosphorylase catalyzes the conversion of inosine, deoxyinosine, guanosine, and deoxyguanosine to their corresponding bases. The enzyme has a wide tissue distribution and plays a major role in purine salvage. Deficiency of purine-nucleoside phosphorylase results in elevated levels of the nucleosides and deoxynucleosides in body fluids and leads to markedly elevated levels of deoxyguanosine triphosphate.

This disorder is associated with defective T-cell–mediated immunity. Most patients have failure to thrive and repeated infections during infancy. B-cell function usually is normal; serum immunoglobulin levels are normal or elevated. The elevated deoxyguanosine triphosphate levels are thought to lead to inhibition of ribonucleoside diphosphate reductase, which results in decreased synthesis of deoxyribonucleotides and DNA in T-cell precursors. Many patients also have neurologic findings including psychomotor retardation, hypotonia, and spastic quadriparesis, which may preceed the onset of the immunodeficiency. Others have had a milder disease with familial autoimmune hemolytic anemia.

Patients have elevated plasma and urinary levels of inosine, deoxyinosine, guanosine, and deoxyguanosine. Hypoxanthine and guanine, which have been produced by gut bacterial action, may be found in the urine of severely affected individuals. Reduced plasma and urine uric acid levels occur. Deficiency of purine-nucleoside phosphorylase may be shown in lysed erythrocytes. The disorder, inherited as an autosomal recessive trait, results from mutations at the *PNP* locus at chromosome 14q13. Carrier detection and prenatal diagnosis are available. Intermittent transfusions of irradiated normal erythrocytes, to supply patients with exogenous enzyme, results in clinical improvement in only one-half of patients who receive it. PEG-modified PNP is being developed. Bone marrow transplantation should be considered if a suitable donor exists.

Adenine Phosphoribosyl Transferase Deficiency

Adenine phosphoribosyl transferase (APRT) catalyzes the conversion of adenine to adenine monophosphate. With APRT deficiency, adenine is not salvaged and is converted to 8-hydroxyadenine and the extremely insoluble 2,8-dihydroxyadenine by xanthine oxidase. The disorder, inherited as an autosomal recessive trait, results from mutations at the APRT gene locus at chromosome 16q24.3. Great clinical heterogeneity exists among patients. Only 15% of patients become symptomatic. The disorder may appear as early as 2 years of age and as late as the fourth decade. The major clinical findings are related to urinary stone formation, with urinary tract infections, hematuria, crystalluria, renal colic, and renal failure. The renal calculi are soft, creamy gray, and radiolucent, and they crush with ease. Urinary levels of adenine, 8-hydroxyadenine, and 2,8-dihydroxyadenine are elevated. Plasma uric acid levels are normal. The enzymatic defect may be noted in erythrocytes, lymphocytes, and cultured skin fibroblasts. A variant with partial APRT deficiency has been reported in Japan. Treatment includes a high fluid intake, dietary purine restriction, and allopurinol, which inhibits the conversion of adenine to its metabolites.

Hypoxanthine Guanine Phosphoribosyl Transferase Deficiency

HGPRT catalyzes the conversion and salvage of the purine bases guanine and hypoxanthine to their corresponding nucleotides, guanosine monophosphate and inosine monophosphate. Under normal circumstances, the nucleotides so formed exert a strong negative feedback inhibition on de novo purine biosynthesis. In addition, the salvage of these purines restricts the renal loss of purines in the form of uric acid. Deficiency of HGPRT is associated with loss of inhibition of purine biosynthesis and subsequent overproduction and overexcretion of purines in the form of uric acid.

Complete HGPRT deficiency (Lesch-Nyhan syndrome) may present as early as the first week of life with yellow-orange crystalluria. Renal failure and gout may develop. Hyperuricemia may not be present in young children but usually is present after puberty. Hyperuricosuria occurs at all ages. Affected patients also have elevated plasma and urinary hypoxanthine levels. Neurologic manifestations usually begin between 6 and 8 months of age and are noted first as athetosis and loss of motor abilities. A movement disorder with choreoathetosis and dystonia develops. Spasticity may be severe and often leads to dislocated hips. Deep tendon reflexes are brisk, and Babinski signs often are present. The patients usually are not ambulatory. Although mental handicaps are prominent and most patients have an estimated intelligence quotient of less than 50, their motor handicaps may limit their performance during testing, and innate intelligence actually may be higher. Patients have a compulsive-aggressive behavior disorder, which includes self-mutilation. Most commonly, they bite their lips and fingers and experience pain while doing so. Tooth extraction and physical restraints may be required. They also may be aggressive toward caretakers. With age, they become verbally abusive and aggressive. There may be recurrent emesis and failure to thrive.

The disorder is inherited as an X-linked recessive trait. Some female carriers have hyperuricemia and gout. HGPRT deficiency may be noted in erythrocytes or cultured skin fibroblasts. Mutations at the HGPRT locus at chromosome Xq26-q27 are heterogenous; almost every patient evaluated has had a different mutation. DNA mutation analysis may be used for carrier detection. Prenatal diagnosis is available. Treatment consists of careful administration of allopurinol, because these patients are very sensitive to this drug. Monitoring of urinary xanthine and oxypurinol levels must be done to prevent urolithiasis from the purines. No successful treatment for the neurologic manifestations exists.

Partial deficiency of HGPRT presents with hyperuricemia, gout, renal dysfunction, and urolithiasis during adolescence or early adulthood. The severe neurologic manifestations of Lesch-Nyhan syndrome usually are not present. The disorder is inherited as an X-linked recessive disorder; female carriers occasionally have clinical manifestations. Partial deficiency of HGPRT may be noted in lysed erythrocytes and cultured skin fibroblasts. Treatment is similar to that for primary gout.

An intermediate form of HGPRT deficiency presents during childhood with hyperuricemia, gout, choreoathetosis, and spasticity. The abnormal behaviors and mental retardation seen with classic HGPRT deficiency do not occur.

Hereditary Xanthinuria

Xanthine oxidoreductase (XOR) catalyzes the degradation of hypoxanthine and xanthine to uric acid. Deficiency of activity of XOR, an autosomal recessive disorder known as hereditary xanthinuria, is associated with increased excretion of xanthine and, to a lesser extent, hypoxanthine. Patients also have low serum and urine uric acid levels. Approximately 50% of patients are asymptomatic. The disorder is usually detected by blood screening panels, which reveal a low level of uric acid. Others have symptoms related to the elevated levels of the relatively insoluble xanthine in the urine. Renal colic and calculi, repeated urinary tract infections, hydronephrosis, and renal failure may occur at any age. Xanthine stones are brownish orange, smooth, oval, and radiolucent. No specific therapy exists other than high fluid intake and treatment of the calculi and infections. The enzymatic deficiency may be noted in liver and intestinal mucosal biopsies.

Two variants of hereditary xanthinuria result from defects in the molybdenum cofactor needed for activity of XOR and for activity of aldehyde oxidase and sulfite oxidase. One variant, a result of a defect in the sulfide ligand of the cofactor, results in combined deficiencies of XOR and aldehyde oxidase. Affected patients have clinical and biochemical findings similar to those seen with isolated XOR deficiency. In addition, these patients are unable to oxidize allopurinol, pyrazinamide, and N-methylnicotinamide. The second variant is associated with the inability to synthesize the pteridyl moiety of the molybdenum cofactor. These patients have combined XOR, aldehyde oxidase, and sulfite oxidase deficiencies and present in the neonatal period with intractable seizures, microcephaly, and dislocated lens. Milder forms also have been reported.

DISORDERS OF PYRIMIDINE METABOLISM

Hereditary Orotic Aciduria

Hereditary orotic aciduria is a rare, autosomal recessive disorder associated with deficient activity of both orotate phosphoribosyltransferase and orotidine 5'-monophosphate decarboxylase. The enzymes exist as a complex, are associated with a multifunctional protein carrier, and catalyze the conversion of orotic acid to uridine monophosphate. The bifunctional enzyme complex is termed uridine monophosphate (UMP) synthetase. Deficient activity of the enzyme complex, associated with mutations in the UMPS gene at chromosome 3q13, results in interruption of the biosynthesis of pyrimidines and markedly elevated urinary excretion of orotic acid. The disorder becomes apparent during the first year of life with severe macrocytic, hypochromic anemia with megaloblastic changes in the bone marrow. Psychomotor handicaps are common. Occasionally, congenital malformations or immune deficiencies are noted. Crystalluria and urinary tract obstruction may occur with the massive orotic aciduria. Uric acid clearance also is elevated, most probably as a result of a uricosuric effect of orotic acid. The enzymatic defect may be shown in liver, cultured skin fibroblasts, lymphoblasts, erythrocytes, and leukocytes. Treatment with uridine results in clinical improvement and a reduction in orotic acid excretion. Heterozygotes may have a mild orotic aciduria. Prenatal diagnosis is possible. Orotic aciduria also can result from defects in the urea cycle, discussed in Chapter 385.

Hereditary Combined Uraciluria-Thyminuria

Hereditary combined uraciluria-thyminuria results from deficient activity of dihydropyrimidine dehydrogenase (DPD), which catalyzes the degradation of the pyrimidine bases, uracil and thymine, to dihydrouracil and dihydrothymine, respectively. Dihydrouracil and dihydrothymine are further degraded by dihydropyrimidinase (DPH) and ureidopropionase to beta-alanine and beta-aminoisobutyric acid, respectively. Affected patients have increased urinary excretion of uracil, thymine, and 5-hydroxymethyluracil, a metabolite of thymine. Increased levels of these compounds also may be noted in plasma and cerebrospinal fluids. Decreased levels of beta-alanine and beta-aminoisobutyric acid occur. The neurologic symptoms seen with the disorder are thought to result from the decreased beta-alanine levels and resultant disruption in neurotransmitter function. Deficiency of DPD also results in impaired clearance and catabolism of 5-fluorouracil, which can lead to severe toxicity of the drug, including encephalopathy, when it is given. Two forms of the disorder exist, which are associated with different mutations at the *DPD* gene locus at chromosome 1p22. The early-onset form of the disorder presents during childhood with varying degrees of delayed development, seizures, hypertonia, hyperreflexia, microcephaly, and dysmyelination. Patients with the later-onset, pharmacokinetic form have a partial DPD deficiency and develop symptoms only after exposure to 5-fluorouracil. Deficient activity of DPD may be shown in peripheral blood leukocytes, lymphocytes, or cultured skin fibroblasts.

Dihydropyrimidinase Deficiency

DPH catalyzes the conversion of dihydrouracil and dihydrothymine to beta-ureidopropionic and beta-ureidobutyric acid, respectively. Deficiency of DPH results in elevated body fluid levels of dihydrouracil and dihydrothymine. Most affected patients have varying degrees of psychomotor hand-

icaps, seizures, and microcephaly. Others are asymptomatic. Decreased beta-alanine levels are thought to be responsible for the neurologic problems as occurs with DPD deficiency. Moreover, as with DPD deficiency, affected patients are unable to detoxify 5-fluorouracil. In addition, they are also unable to activate IRCF-187 [1,2-bis(3,5-dioxopiperazinyl-1-yl)propane], a compound given with doxorubicin (Adriamycin) to reduce doxorubicin toxicity. Deficient activity of DPH can be shown only in liver biopsy samples.

Pyrimidine-5′-Nucleotidase Deficiency

Pyrimidine-5′-nucleotidase (P5N) is a major enzyme in the pyrimidine salvage pathway that catalyzes the conversion of monophosphated nucleotides to their respective nucleosides. Deficiency of erythrocyte P5N, an autosomal recessive disorder, is associated with elevated levels of the erythrocyte pyrimidine nucleotides uridine triphosphate and cytidine triphosphate. Patients present either in childhood or as adults with nonspherocytic hemolytic anemia. The disorder usually is relatively benign, and transfusions and splenectomy are seldom required. Deficient activity of P5N may be shown in erythrocytes.

Pyrimidine-5′-Nucleotidase Superactivity

P5N superactivity is a very rare disorder characterized by developmental delay, seizures, ataxia, recurrent infections, hyperactivity, and poor social interaction. The only biochemical abnormal finding is persistent hypouricosuria. Most patients respond to treatment with uridine. Increased specific activity of P5N may be shown in cultured skin fibroblasts.

Suggested Readings

Aiuti A. Advances in gene therapy for ADA-deficient SCID. *Curr Opin Mol Ther* 2002;4:515.

Brewerton LJ, Fung, E, Synder FF. Polyethlene glycol-conjugated adenosine phosphorylase: development of alternative enzyme therapy for adenosine deaminase deficiency. *Biochim Biophys Acta* 2003;1637:171.

Hershfield MS. PEG-ADA replacement therapy for adenosine deaminase deficiency: an update after 8.5 years. *Clin Immunol Immunopathol* 1995;76:S228.

Howe S, Thrasher AJ. Gene therapy for inherited immunodeficiencies. *Curr Hematol Rep* 2003;2:328.

Nyhan WL, Wong DF. New approaches to understanding Lesch-Nyhan disease. *N Engl J Med* 1996;334:1602.

Rott KT, Agudelo CA. Gout. *JAMA* 2003;289:2857.

Scriver CR, Beaudet AL, Sly WS, et al., eds. Purines and pyrimidines. In: Scriver CR, Beaudet AL, Sly WS, Valle D, eds. *The metabolic and molecular bases of inherited disease,* 8th ed. New York: McGraw-Hill, 2001:2513.

Simmonds HA, Duley JA, Fairbanks LD, McBride MB. When to investigate for purine and pyrimidine disorders: introduction and review of clinical and laboratory indications. *J Inherit Metab Dis* 1997;20:214.

Vidotto C, Fouser D, Akkermann M, et al. Purine and pyrimidine metabolites in children's urine. *Clin Chim Acta* 2003;335:27.

CHAPTER 392 ■ HERITABLE DISORDERS OF CONNECTIVE TISSUE

BART L. LOEYS, MICHAEL J. WRIGHT, AND HARRY C. DIETZ III

The diversity of clinical features in connective tissue diseases pays witness to the ubiquitous nature of connective tissue itself. Therefore, determining what is and is not a connective tissue disease can be difficult and subject to individual interpretation. We have chosen to follow the lead set in *McKusick's Heritable Disorders of Connective Tissue* and *Connective Tissue and Its Heritable Disorders* in this matter. We recommend both these texts as excellent sources of detailed reviews regarding the normal physiology of connective tissue and the molecular basis of heritable disorders. In this chapter, we do not cover the chondrodysplasias. For further discussion of skeletal dysplasias, we refer the reader to Chapter 433 and to the excellent review by Kornak and Mundlos.

MARFAN SYNDROME AND RELATED PHENOTYPES

Marfan Syndrome

Marfan syndrome is one of the best studied and most fully understood of the connective tissue diseases. It is a dominantly inherited disorder with a birth incidence estimated at 1 in 5,000. This may be an underestimation because of the high degree of clinical variability and the lack of a fully sensitive diagnostic test.

Clinical Features

Although the genetic defect that underlies Marfan syndrome is known, the diagnosis still largely depends on the identification of specific clinical features. Those features are found mainly in the skeleton, the cardiovascular system, the eyes, the lungs, and the integument. Abnormalities of the skeleton, along with a degree of muscle hypoplasia, give rise to the distinctive appearance of individuals with Marfan syndrome (Fig. 392.1). The increased total height that may be present from birth is caused by expansion of the lower segment, measured from the symphysis pubis to the floor in an individual standing in bare feet. Consequently, the ratio of the upper segment to the lower segment is decreased as compared with controls. Usually, the ratio in individuals with Marfan syndrome is more than 2 standard deviations below the mean for age and, in general terms, is less than 1.0 at 0 to 5 years, less than 0.95 at 6 to 7 years, less than 0.90 at 8 to 9 years, and less than 0.85 in those older than 10 years. Upper extremity involvement is reflected in an increased span-to-height ratio, with greatest diagnostic significance given to values greater than 1.05. Arachnodactyly is a subjective finding that can be assessed clinically by eliciting the thumb sign (positive if the entire distal phalanx of the thumb projects beyond the ulnar border of the palm when the thumb is opposed maximally) and the wrist sign (positive if the distal phalanges of the thumb and little finger completely overlap when wrapped around the contralateral wrist). Joint laxity affects both large and small joints and may give rise to recurrent dislocation. It is particularly problematic in the feet, where pes planus and instability of the ankle can cause difficulties with ambulation. Paradoxically, limitation of movement or even joint contracture, especially of the elbow and fingers, may be present. Later in life, arthritis may develop in previously hypermobile joints. Protrusio acetabuli (deep protrusion of the femoral head into the pelvis) occurs in up to 50% of cases but rarely causes clinical manifestations.

The axial skeleton is prominently involved: scoliosis with or without kyphosis of the thoracic spine occurs in approximately 60% of cases. Spondylolisthesis may be found in the lumbosacral spine. Physiologic thoracic kyphosis can be replaced by a "straight back" or even by thoracic lordosis; in association with the pectus excavatum, this condition may give rise to significant reduction in anteroposterior diameter of the chest. Pectus excavatum and pectus carinatum arise as a result of rib overgrowth.

Abnormalities of the bones of the skull and face manifest as dolichocephaly, a long, thin face, malar hypoplasia, a high, arched palate (giving rise to dental crowding and malocclusion), and micrognathia. Other facial findings include deeply set eyes and downward slant of the palpebral fissures.

The increased mortality associated with Marfan syndrome at all ages is explained almost exclusively by cardiovascular complications. The most common cardiovascular complications are mitral valve prolapse and aortic root dilatation. Mitral valve prolapse may give rise to mitral regurgitation with the concomitant risks of congestive heart failure and dysrhythmia secondary to left atrial enlargement. Mitral valve disease is the most common indication for cardiovascular surgery and the most common source of early mortality in the pediatric population. Aortic root dilatation predisposes an affected individual not only to aortic regurgitation but to the most feared of all complications of Marfan syndrome: aortic dissection and rupture. Usually, dilatation is limited to the ascending aorta, but it can involve to the abdominal aorta and the pulmonary artery. Commonly, echocardiography is used to monitor cardiovascular involvement and for planning appropriate intervention (see the later discussion of management). Importantly, subsets of individuals show primary involvement of the descending thoracic and abdominal aorta. This may increase in incidence as people with Marfan syndrome are living longer as a result of therapeutic interventions. Computed tomographic or magnetic resonance imaging modalities should be used to monitor the descending aorta.

Subluxation or complete dislocation of the lens is the classic ocular sign in Marfan syndrome. This condition may be present at birth but can present or progress throughout childhood. Formal slit-lamp examination is essential to confirm this feature, but the presence of iridodonesis (a shimmering of the iris on accommodation) is indicative. In addition to myopia and retinal detachment secondary to increased length of the eyeball, glaucoma and cataracts occur at greater than expected frequency and earlier in life than in the general population.

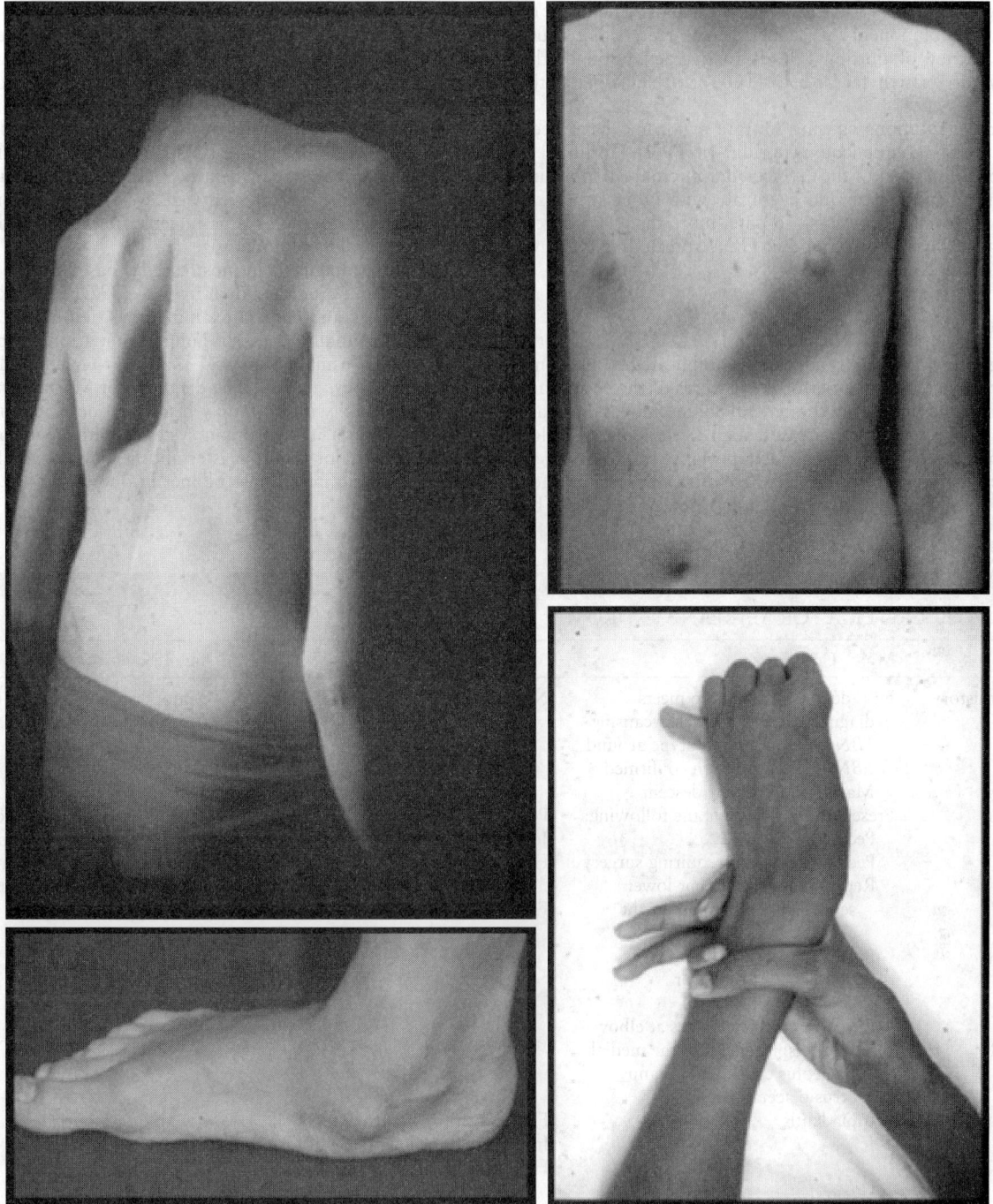

FIGURE 392.1. Major skeletal manifestations of Marfan syndrome such as scoliosis, pectus carinatum, pes planum, and positive wrist and thumb signs.

Dural ectasia has become recognized as a feature of both diagnostic and clinical importance. In this defect, the dural sac gradually expands with erosion of sacral bone. Usually, this condition remains asymptomatic but should be considered in the differential diagnosis of back or leg pain in individuals with Marfan syndrome. Rarely, dural ectasia produces a meningocele presenting as a pelvic mass.

Despite a reported association between Marfan syndrome and attention-deficit/hyperactivity disorder, it remains unclear whether attention-deficit disorder occurs at an increased frequency in this patient population.

Striae distensae may occur, particularly after puberty, affecting the shoulders, thighs, and, often and most impressively, the lumbar region. Recurrent inguinal or incisional hernias also are common. Otherwise, the skin is involved minimally.

Often, spontaneous pneumothorax is perceived as a common complication of Marfan syndrome; in reality, it is relatively rare. Pulmonary function may be compromised by severe scoliosis and chest wall deformity.

Pathology

Aortic dilatation begins at the sinuses of Valsalva and extends into the ascending aorta and (in some cases) beyond. Commonly, dissection begins at the site of maximal dilatation. Histologically, the medial layer of the aorta is disorganized, with fragmentation of the elastic matrix and accumulation of other matrix components. Recent evidence suggests that structural deficiency of fibrillin-1 leads to overactivation of the transforming growth factor-beta (TGF-beta) signaling pathway.

To date, mutations causing Marfan syndrome have been found only in the gene encoding fibrillin-1 (*FBN1*). Fibrillin-1 is the major component of the extracellular microfibril. Fibrillin-1 molecules multimerize and aggregate with other structural proteins to form microfibrils. To date, more than 560 different mutations have been found in *FBN1*, precluding effective population screening.

Diagnosis

The diagnosis of Marfan syndrome is complicated by the common occurrence of a number of the features of the condition, both as isolated findings in the general community and as part of other connective tissue diseases, such as the Ehlers-Danlos syndromes and familial mitral valve prolapse syndromes (see later). In an attempt to overcome these difficulties, criteria for diagnosing Marfan syndrome were established, as reported by Beighton and associates and more recently were revised, as noted by De Paepe and colleagues. The discovery of the molecular basis of Marfan syndrome, as reported by Dietz and colleagues, has not allowed for the creation of a definitive and universally applicable diagnostic test, because of the large number of separate causative mutations and the finding that related but distinct conditions can be caused by mutations in the same gene. Linkage analysis can identify at-risk individuals and pregnancies in families of sufficient size even if a mutation is not known, but discovery of a pathogenic mutation renders this possible regardless of family size.

Therefore, diagnosis in most cases is based on the clinical assessment and criteria shown in Table 392.1. In addition to careful history and clinical examination, the only specialized investigations required are slit-lamp examination, echocardiography, and plasma amino acid analysis (to exclude the diagnosis of homocystinuria). The diagnosis of Marfan syndrome in an individual with no family history requires identification of major criteria in two organ systems, with involvement of a third. If a major criterion is established by virtue of family history, major criteria must be met in one organ system and another must be involved.

TABLE 392.1

DIAGNOSTIC CRITERIA FOR MARFAN SYNDROME*

	Major Criteria	Minor Criteria	Involvement
Family history	First-degree relative who meets diagnostic criteria Marfan-causing *FBN1* mutation Haplotype around *FBN1* associated with confirmed Marfan inherited by descent	None	Major criterion must be met or family history is noncontributory
Skeletal	Presence of any four of the following: Pectus carinatum Pectus excavatum requiring surgery Reduced upper segment-lower segment ratio or span/height >1.05 Positive wrist and thumb signs Scoliosis >20 degrees or spondylolisthesis Extensiom <170 degrees at elbow Medial displacement of the medial melleolus causing pes planus Protrusio acetabulae	Pectus excavatum Joint hypermobility High arched palate with dental crowding Facial appearance	Two of the components of the major criteria or one of the components of the major criteria and two minor criteria
Ocular	Ectopia lentis	Flat cornea (by keratometry) Increased globe length (by ultrasound) Hypoplastic iris or hypoplastic ciliary muscle causing decreased miosis	Two minor criteria
Cardiovascular	Dilation of the ascending aorta with or without aortic regurgitation involving at least the sinuses of Valsalva Dissection of the ascending aorta	Mitral valve prolapse with or without mitral regurgitation Dilation of main pulmonary artery without other cause at age 40 years or younger Calcification of the mitral annulus at age 40 years or younger Dilation or dissection of the descending thoracic or abdominal aorta at age 50 years or younger	One major or one minor criterion
Pulmonary	None	Spontaneous pneumothorax Apical blebs (radiographically)	One minor criterion
Skin and central nervous system	Lumbosacral dural ectasia	Striae atrophicae not associated with marked weight changes, pregnancy, or repetitive stress Recurrent or incisional herniae	One major or one minor criterion

*To make a diagnosis of Marfan syndrome in an individual with no family history requires major criteria in two organ systems and involvement of a third. If there is a family history, major criteria must be met in one organ system and another must be involved.

Management

Management of aortic root dilatation or dissection, aortic regurgitation, and mitral valve abnormalities is important because appropriate treatment can have significant effects on morbidity and mortality. Echocardiographic measurement of aortic root diameter at the sinuses of Valsalva and assessment of aortic and mitral valve function should be carried out at least yearly. More frequent evaluations may be necessary with severe regurgitation or aortic dilatation, or with rapid rate of growth of the aorta. Charts of aortic root diameter plotted against body surface area are available for normalization, as reported by Roman and associates. Surgical intervention should proceed at any age when the maximal aortic root diameter reaches 5.0 cm. This guideline is based on the observation of aortic dissection in older children or adults that cross this threshold. Given the extreme rarity of aortic complications in young children, it has been difficult to establish rules with similar predictive value and conviction. Current consensus suggests that surgery should be considered in young children who develop severe aortic regurgitation or aortic root growth that exceeds 1 cm/year. Indications based on aortic size have been impossible to validate, and the recent trend has been to tolerate aortic dimensions up to 5.0 cm irrespective of age. It is anticipated that these guidelines will be refined with further experience.

Various surgical techniques have been developed, but recently the results of valve-sparing procedures have been quite encouraging. This procedure avoids lifelong anticoagulation and is particularly appealing for young woman who anticipate pregnancy. Use of a homograft remains an alternative for very young children who require surgery. Given the primary involvement of the pulmonary artery, the Ross procedure, which involves replacing the aortic root with a pulmonary autograft, is contraindicated in Marfan syndrome and in other connective tissue disorders. Severe left ventricle enlargement or dysfunction and valve insufficiency are indications for surgical repair or replacement of the aortic or mitral valves.

Beta blockade has been shown to slow the rate of aortic root dilatation and to reduce the incidence of aortic dissection in Marfan syndrome. Our policy has been to treat all individuals, including children with a confirmed diagnosis of Marfan syndrome, with atenolol in sufficient doses to maintain the heart rate after submaximal exercise at less than 110 beats/minute. This treatment is generally well tolerated in children and adults with Marfan syndrome. Treatment with verapamil should be considered in individuals who do not tolerate beta blockade.

Individuals with Marfan syndrome should remain active with aerobic activities performed in moderation. Contact sports, competitive sports, exercise to the point of exhaustion, and isometric exercises (e.g., weight lifting) should be avoided because of the increased risk of aortic dilatation, dissection, or rupture. Antibiotic prophylaxis should be liberally prescribed, because the inherent abnormality of the valve tissue (e.g., myxomatous mitral valve changes) can predispose patients to bacterial endocarditis.

The development and progression of scoliosis should be monitored by clinical and radiographic assessment. Rapid progression is particularly likely at times of maximal growth. Bracing should be considered when the curve progresses beyond 20 degrees. If bracing is unsuccessful or if the curve is between 40 and 50 degrees, surgical correction is likely to be necessary. Management of hypermobile joints may require physical therapy to increase strength of surrounding muscle groups and may call for splinting to allow for adequate function. Importantly, chest wall deformity is largely a cosmetic concern, with documented cardiopulmonary dysfunction only at extreme severity. Although pectus excavatum can contribute to restrictive pulmonary abnormalities, current evidence suggests that operative repair after early childhood fails to reverse this situation. Give

the high rate of recurrence, intervention is rarely performed before early adolescence. In adolescence and adulthood, the development of arthritis and back pain can become a major and difficult management issue.

Yearly review by an ophthalmologist is recommended, with particular attention paid to the maximal correction of myopia and screening for the development of glaucoma, cataracts, and retinal detachment. Management of ectopia lentis in individuals with Marfan syndrome requires the expertise of an ophthalmologist with considerable experience.

Often, individuals with Marfan syndrome have significant problems with psychosocial adjustment. Contact with other affected families and individuals of similar age through such organizations as the National Marfan Foundation can be very helpful in this regard.

Related Phenotypes

Table 392.2 describes the phenotypes, their clinical features, and the molecular defect (when known) that most commonly enter the differential diagnosis of Marfan syndrome. Comparison of Tables 392.1 and 392.2 should allow these conditions to be differentiated from Marfan syndrome.

Related Disorders

Recently, a new syndrome (Loeys-Dietz syndrome) characterized by the triad of hypertelorism, cleft palate/bifid uvula, and aortic aneurysm with arterial tortuosity, was identified. This syndrome has variable clinical expression with alterations in the skeletal, craniofacial, cardiovascular, and neurocognitive development. This autosomal dominant disease is caused by mutations in genes encoding for TGF receptor 1 or 2 (*TGFBR1* or *TGFBR2*), localized on chromosome 9q and 3p, respectively. These findings identify the crucial contribution of TGF-beta signaling to diverse developmental and homeostatic processes and provide definitive proof of its role in the pathogenesis of many common human phenotypes, such as cleft palate and craniosynostosis. Importantly, aortic dissections in the Loeys-Dietz syndrome seem to occur at smaller aortic root diameters than in Marfan syndrome.

In addition, the gene responsible for the recessive form of Weill-Marchesani syndrome has been identified. This disorder is characterized by short stature, brachydactyly, joint stiffness, and lens abnormalities and caused by mutations in the *ADAMTS10* gene. At present, it is unclear whether the autosomal dominant form of this disease with mutations in the *FBN1* gene is a truly different disease or whether patients with this disorder have atypical Marfan syndrome.

EHLERS-DANLOS SYNDROMES

The Ehlers-Danlos syndromes (EDSs) comprise a heterogeneous group of disorders having as their cardinal features hyperextensible skin with a velvety texture, dystrophic scarring, easy bruising, joint hypermobility (Fig. 392.2), and connective tissue fragility. The spectrum of severity of these cardinal features and additional specific abnormalities have produced a number of classification systems. The foregoing numbered classification of EDS is currently still in use. However, it is relatively impenetrable to those who do not use it frequently. In an attempt to rationalize the classification of these disorders (especially in light of molecular genetic advances), a new nomenclature based on the cause of each type shown has been proposed. The two nosologies are compared in Box 392.1. A brief description of the different types of EDS is given in the following sections, and information about their inheritance patterns is presented in Box 392.1.

TABLE 392.2

DIFFERENTIAL DIAGNOSIS OF MARFAN SYNDROME

	Clinical Features	Basic Defect	Inheritance
MASS phenotype (*mitral*, *aortic*, *skin*, *skeletal*)	Mitral valve prolapse, mild aortic dilatation without progression to dissection, skin involvement, skeletal involvement	Some resulting from *FBN1* (low mutant transcript)	AD
Loeys-Dietz syndrome	Hypertelorism, cleft palate/bifid uvula, aortic aneurysm with arterial tortuosity	*TGFBR1* or *TGFBR2*	AD
Mitral valve prolapse syndrome	Familial mitral valve prolapse with or without skeletal involvement	Loci on 11p15.4, 16p11.2–12.1, and Xq28	AD, XL
Homocystinuria	Ocular: ectopia lentis (dislocated downward), glaucoma, retinal detachment, optic atrophy Musculoskeletal: osteoporosis, dolichostenomelia, scoliosis, joint contractures Cardiovascular: intravascular thrombosis, atherosclerosis Skin: thin skin, malar flushing, cutis marmorata Neurologic: variable mental retardation, stroke, seizures, dystonia, psychiatric disturbance	Deficiency of cystathionine beta-synthase; 5-methyltetrahydrofolate homocysteine methyltransferase (methionine synthase); 5,10-methylenetetrahydrofolate reductase	AR
Congenital contractural arachnodactyly	Arachnodactyly, contractures, crumpled ears, dolichostenomelia, scoliosis; no lens or aortic involvement	*FBN2*	AD
Annuloaortic ectasia	Familial thoracic aortic aneurysm, familial cystic medial necrosis without associated systemic features	*FBN1*, loci on 3p24.2–25, 5q13–15, and 11q23.2–24	AD
Isolated skeletal features	Familial tall stature with or without other skeletal features	*FBN1*, likely genetic heterogeneity	AD
Isolated ectopia lentis	Ectopia lentis, usually associated with mild skeletal findings	*FBN1*, possible genetic heterogeneity	AD
Klinefelter syndrome	Marfanoid habitus, small testes and genitalia, gynecomastia, learning difficulty	Supernumerary X chromosome(s)	AD
Stickler syndrome	Marfanoid habitus, progressive myopia, chorioretinal and vitreal degeneration, cleft palate, midface hypoplasia, sensorineural hearing loss, articular hypermobility, degenerative arthropathy	*COL2A1, COL11A1, COL11A2*	AD
Shprintzen-Goldberg syndrome	Features of Marfan syndrome, craniosynostosis, mental retardation, hypertelorism, proptosis, camptodactyly, recurrent hernias	*FBN1*, likely genetic heterogeneity	AD
Fragile X syndrome	Marfanoid habitus, mental retardation, prominent jaw, large ears, macroorchidism, joint hypermobility, mitral valve prolapse	*FMR1*	XL
Weill-Marchesani syndrome	Short stature, spherophakia, stiff joints, short digits	*FBN1, ADAMTS10*	AD, AR
Bicuspid aortic valve	Ascending aortic aneurysm, coarctation of the aorta		AD

AD, autosomal dominant; AR, autosomal recessive; XL, X-linked.

Classic or Type I/II Ehlers-Danlos Syndrome

Classic EDS predominantly involves the skin. Dystrophic scarring is marked, with the formation of cigarette-paper scars. Scars are often seen on the shins, on the forehead, and under the chin when affected children begin to walk. Joint hypermobility gives rise to early degenerative arthritis. Pes planus and scoliosis are common and are thought to result from ligamentous laxity, which is also responsible for delayed motor development. Easy bruising is a hallmark feature. Mitral valve prolapse has been described in up to 50% of cases. Aortic dilatation is rare, mild if present, and generally nonprogressive.

Hypermobile or Type III Ehlers-Danlos Syndrome

The skin manifestations in the hypermobile type of EDS are mild. Joint laxity can be severe. Associated findings include recurrent dislocations, joint pain, and early arthritis. Pain can be out of proportion to the objective findings but is debilitating and should not be trivialized. Patients can also have severe postural orthostatic tachycardia syndrome, presumably resulting from venous pooling, and chronic fatigue. These problems can require aggressive management.

Vascular or Type IV Ehlers-Danlos Syndrome

The major clinical features are thinning of the skin (over the anterior chest in particular), marked bruising, and a characteristic facial appearance with "tight" skin, a thin nose, and a staring expression. Hypermobility is limited mainly to small joints of the hand. The major complications are related to rupture of arteries or hollow organs and are responsible for a reduced life expectancy, with the mean age at death in one survey being in the fourth decade. Major bleeding and hollow-organ rupture are unusual before the age of 20 years, but, ultimately, arterial rupture causes more than 90% of deaths in men. The

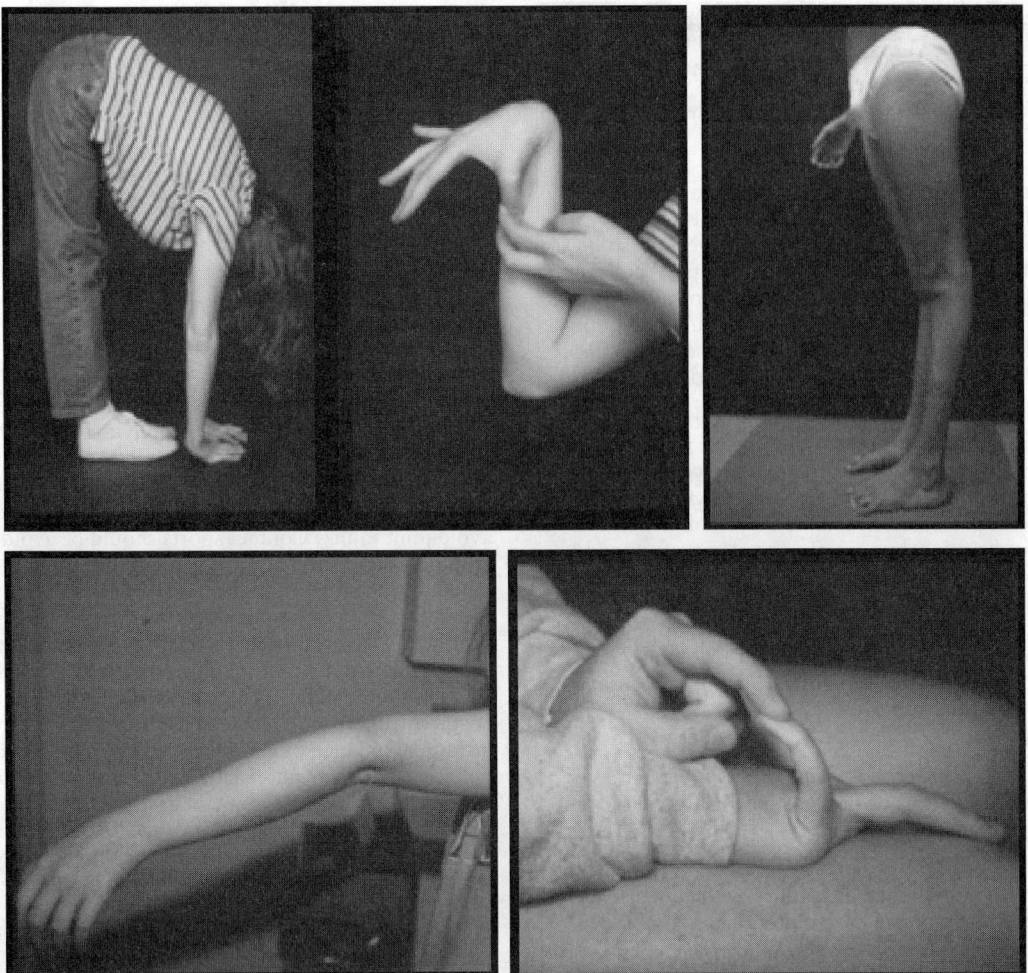

FIGURE 392.2. Joint hypermobility as seen in Ehlers-Danlos syndrome: ability to put hands flat on the ground, thumb abduction sign, and hyperextension of fingers, elbows, and knees.

percentage is slightly lower in women, with some female deaths caused by rupture of the gravid uterus. Unlike the experience with Marfan syndrome, successful treatment protocols have not yet been found for EDS type IV, and the prognosis for affected individuals remains poor.

Ocular-Scoliotic or Type VI Ehlers-Danlos Syndrome

Cardinal findings include early-onset scoliosis and eye involvement, principally microcornea, fragility of the globe, and retinal detachment. Patients also present with soft, velvety hyperextensible skin and joint hypermobility. Arterial rupture has been described in a number of patients with this type of EDS.

Arthrochalasia or Types VIIA and VIIB Ehlers-Danlos Syndrome

The EDS type VII phenotype is a group of related disorders featuring prominent joint hypermobility. EDS types VIIA and VIIB are clinically similar conditions showing joint dislocation (especially congenital dislocation of the hip), short stature, micrognathia, wormian bones, and long bone fractures, but relatively normal skin.

Dermatosparaxis or Type VIIC Ehlers-Danlos Syndrome

Dermatosparaxis or type VIIC EDS is a rare recessively inherited condition that features congenital and recurrent joint dislocations, extremely fragile and easily bruised skin, hernia formation, and blue sclerae. Electron microscopic studies of skin have shown a characteristic ribbon-like appearance of collagen fibrils.

Periodontal or Type VIII Ehlers-Danlos Syndrome

The most prominent feature of EDS type VIII is periodontal disease leading to loss of teeth by early adulthood. The skin is fragile, with scars over bony prominences reminiscent of necrobiosis diabeticorum. Skin elasticity and joint mobility are relatively normal. Periodontitis has been described in patients with EDS type IV.

Miscellaneous Types

The features of EDS type V are similar to those found in type II, with less severe bruising and joint hypermobility. The differentiating factor is the pattern of inheritance, which is believed

---

| BOX 392.1 | Inheritance Patterns in Ehlers-Danlos Syndrome |

Type I/II

Classic Ehlers-Danlos syndrome (EDS) is inherited in an autosomal dominant manner. Intrafamilial and interfamilial variability is common. Molecular genetic studies of classic EDS have shown mutations in type V collagen in less than 50% of patients. Moreover, not all families show linkage to this locus, but linked and unlinked families appear clinically indistinguishable. In some families, mutations in the *COL1A1* gene have been described.

Type III

In most cases, the pattern of inheritance is dominant. However, small subsets of patients show recessive inheritance owing to mutations in the tenascin X-gene (*TNXB*). These patients presented with joint hypermobility and extensive skin bruising but no abnormal scar formation. It was subsequently shown that heterozygous carriers of tenascin X mutations also present with joint hypermobility. A mutation in type III collagen has been found in one family. However, it is not clear whether this family has a mild form of the vascular form of EDS with later onset of arterial or intestinal rupture.

Type IV

The pattern of inheritance is dominant. Abnormalities of synthesis and secretion of procollagen III are caused by mutations in the *COL3A1* gene.

Type VI

The pattern of inheritance in families with this disorder is recessive. Most patients have mutations in the *PLOD1* gene that encodes the enzyme lysyl hydroxylase 1. This enzyme is essential for normal intermolecular cross-linking of type I and type III collagens. Deficient activity can be detected by elevation of the urinary lysyl pyridinoline–hydroxylpyridinoline ratio.

Type VIIA and VIIB

Both conditions are the result of mutations in the splice sites around exon 6 of the *COL1A1* gene in EDS type VIIA and the *COL1A2* gene in EDS type VIIB, resulting in skipping of the exon during messenger RNA processing.

Type VIIC

Type VIIC is the result of deficiency of procollagen N-protease that acts at a cleavage site encoded by exon 6 of *COL1A1* and *COL1A2* to produce mature alpha$_1$ and alpha$_2$ collagen chains.

Type VIII

Phenotypic overlap with type VIII exists. However, type III collagen abnormalities have not been consistently demonstrated in families with type VIII EDS. Recently, a locus for this type of EDS has been mapped to chromosome 12p13 in a large Swedish pedigree. However, genetic study of other pedigrees revealed locus heterogeneity.

---

to be X-linked in type V, although some researchers have suggested that reported families actually may be consistent with dominant inheritance with variable expression.

EDS type IX is known also as *occipital horn syndrome*. It has been reclassified as *X-linked cutis laxa* (see the later section on cutis laxa).

EDS type X or *fibronectin defect* is an autosomal recessive disorder, so far described in a single family, in which features resembling EDS type II and type III were associated with petechiae caused by a platelet aggregation defect correctable by the addition of fibronectin. Platelet aggregation defects are not unique to EDS type X, however, and some researchers have suggested that type X may not represent a unique phenotype.

Finally, EDS type XI or *familial joint hypermobility syndrome* has been removed from the EDS nosology.

Management

Because definite treatment is not available, medical intervention is focused on prophylaxis, symptomatic treatment, and psychosocial support. For the prophylaxis of scarring, children should wear protective pads or bandages. In case of trauma, numerous fine stitches should be used and left in place for twice as long as usual. The goal of orthopedic management should be to avoid joint injury. Contact sports should be avoided, but regular non–weight-bearing exercises (e.g., swimming) will stabilize joints, diminish pain, and improve psychosocial status. Bracing, splinting, and pain medication may be necessary. Surgery should be a last resort. The vascular form of EDS is even more challenging from a treatment perspective. Patients with vascular EDS should carry a medical identification paper with diagnostic information. General recommendations for this group include avoidance of central catheters and arterial lines, conservative management of arterial dissection or internal bleeding (if possible), total colectomy in case of colon perforation, very close monitoring of pregnancy (up to 15% mortality rate), and avoidance of medications that interfere with platelet function or coagulation. Finally, behavorial and psychological counseling therapy can be beneficial.

OSTEOGENESIS IMPERFECTA

The osteogenesis imperfecta (OI) syndromes are a group of disorders characterized by decreased bone density leading to increased frequency of fractures and a number of associated features that allow classification on a clinical basis. At a molecular level, defects in type I collagen have been found in patients with each subtype.

Type I

The most common of OI, type I, is associated with blue sclerae, hearing impairment in approximately 50% of affected adults, hypermobility of the joints of the hands and feet, bowing of the lower limb bones, and, in some cases, wormian bones in the skull. Usually, deformity is limited to the sites of fractures that may rarely be present at birth but ordinarily occur after the first year of life with the onset of walking. Most fractures occur in the first 2 decades of life, with improvement in the clinical course at the onset of adolescence. A recrudescence of fractures may occur after menopause. Dentinogenesis imperfecta, which is recognized by opalescence of the teeth, identifies a subgroup of individuals who are likely to have a more severe prognosis, with an increased number of fractures and more significant deformity.

Mutations leading to decreased production of the proalpha subunits of type I collagen are thought to be responsible for most cases of OI type I. Inheritance is autosomal dominant, and approximately 90% of obligate heterozygotes experience fractures.

Type II

OI type II is characterized by severe bone fragility, with consequent multiple fractures and intrauterine or early neonatal death. The severe undermineralization, particularly of the skull, leads to multiple wormian bones. Ribs can show a beaded appearance. Shortening of long bones gives raise to an accordion-like appearance of the femurs. The sclerae are dark blue, the nose is small, and micrognathia is evident. Type II is a dominant disorder, with sibling recurrence usually the result of gonadal mosaicism. Overall, autosomal recessive inheritance in type II OI seems exceedingly rare.

In general, type II OI is also heterogeneous at the molecular level, although most of the cases studied have been shown to result from mutations in *COL1A1* or *COL1A2*. These mutations result in the production of abnormal type I collagen molecules that have the capacity to interfere globally with type I collagen fibrillogenesis via a dominant-negative mechanism. In contrast, the milder OI type I phenotype is generally associated with mutations that decrease production of type I collagen from the mutant allele but do not interfere with the function of the protein derived from the wild-type allele (haploinsufficiency).

Type III

OI type III is the so-called progressively deforming subgroup of this disorder. Usually, children are born with multiple fractures that continue to occur throughout life. The long bones may be overmodeled at birth, with widened metaphyses and marked angulation, but later they show undermodeling, which produces a broad bone appearance. The membranous skull is deossified severely, with multiple wormian bones. Progressive kyphoscoliosis is a major complication that develops throughout childhood and adolescence and, if left untreated, results in cardiopulmonary compromise. The sclerae may be blue at birth but become white. Usually, the teeth are normal, and hearing is unaffected.

In most cases, OI type III is a dominant disorder, but recessive inheritance has been documented in a well-recognized subgroup. Mutations in both *COL1A1* and *COL1A2* have been found in some individuals with OI type III. However, both genes have been excluded as the site of causative mutations in others.

Type IV

OI type IV is a dominant disorder with a phenotype similar to that of type I. However, the sclerae are white in patients with type IV OI, and deafness is not a feature. Fractures are present at birth in approximately 25% of patients and are common in childhood; however, as in type I, they improve in adolescence. Long bone deformity and kyphoscoliosis are more severe than in type I and overlap with the mild end of the type III spectrum. As in type I, subgroups with and without dentinogenesis imperfecta exist. Mutations in both *COL1A1* and *COL1A2* have been found in patients with OI type IV.

Type V

Recently, a subgroup of patients with a clinical picture like that of OI type IV has been separated based on the presence of hypertrophic callus formation after fractures. One of the major clinical features distinguishing this group from type IV is limitation of pronation and supination of the forearms as a result of calcification of the intraosseous membrane. Neither blue sclera nor dentinogenesis imperfecta is part of the phenotype. The biochemical or genetic cause of this autosomal dominant form has not yet been identified.

Management

The management of patients with OI has focused on maximizing mobility and minimizing deformity. Instruction for parents in handling techniques and environmental adaptations aimed at minimizing fractures is necessary. Physical therapy to increase mobility and strength must be provided. Recently, promising medical strategies such as the use of bisphosphonates and bone marrow transplantation as a source of osteoblastic stem cells have emerged. Clinics catering specifically to these needs are available in a number of centers, and active self-help groups exist.

OTHER CONNECTIVE TISSUE DISEASES

Cutis Laxa

Hereditary cutis laxa refers to a heterogeneous group of disorders characterized by cutaneous abnormalities and variable systemic manifestations. The most constant clinical feature is loose skin, sagging over the face and trunk. An autosomal dominant and two autosomal recessive forms of cutis laxa have been described. A previously defined X-linked form, caused by mutations in the *ATP7A* gene, is now classified within the group of copper deficiency syndromes and has been shown to be allelic with Menkes disease. All forms are very rare, and no precise data about their prevalence are available. The autosomal dominant form, a relatively mild condition without systemic abnormalities, can be caused by mutations in the elastin gene, but molecular heterogeneity cannot be excluded. Type I autosomal recessive cutis laxa is characterized by pulmonary emphysema, umbilical and inguinal hernias, and gastrointestinal and vesicourinary tract diverticuli; this type has the poorest prognosis. The type II recessive form is called cutis laxa with joint laxity and developmental delay. Recessive type I is believed to be less frequent than type II. Histopathologic examination of skin in patients with cutis laxa reveals loss and/or fragmentation of elastic fibers. Homozygosity for a mutation in the fibulin-5 gene was recently demonstrated in a family segregating a severe form of recessive type I cutis laxa. It was subsequently shown that a heterozygous mutation in the fibulin-5 gene can also result in cutis laxa.

In a number of families, additional features of recessive variants with mental retardation and corneal clouding (De Barsy syndrome) and joint laxity, wormian bones, and osteoporosis (geroderma osteodysplastica) have been described. A recessive deficiency of lysyl oxidase was suggested in other affected individuals, but the primary defect has not yet been discovered. The nomenclature of these disorders remains confusing and will be resolved only by elucidation of their molecular basis.

Pseudoxanthoma Elasticum

Pseudoxanthoma elasticum is a rare disorder involving the skin, the eyes, and the cardiovascular system. Skin changes affect the face, neck, axillae, cubital fossa, inguinal region, and periumbilical area. Initially, the skin is thickened and grooved, with a yellowish discoloration that has been described as *peau citrine* (orange peel) and, less elegantly, as a plucked-chicken appearance. Later, affected skin becomes lax and redundant.

Mottling of the retinal pigment progresses to salmon spots, and angioid streaks develop, owing to disruption of Bruch membrane. Neovascular membranes form, with consequent retinal detachment and retinal hemorrhage, causing severe visual impairment.

Premature medial arterial calcification leads to reduced or absent peripheral pulses and claudication affecting mainly the lower limbs. The coronary arteries also are involved, with angina and myocardial infarction as frequent complications. The vasculature of the gastrointestinal tract is involved, giving rise to frequent gastrointestinal hemorrhage, although the exact pathogenesis of these events is not yet resolved. The cardiovascular complications are responsible for increased mortality, even though survival to old age is well documented. Genetic linkage analysis using positional cloning strategies resulted in mapping of the *PXE* gene to chromosome 16p13.1 and subsequent identification of causal mutations in the *MRP6* or *ABCC6* gene. The biologic function of this gene product remains unknown. It has been suggested that *PXE* could be inherited either in autosomal recessive or dominant pattern, but clinical and molecular analysis has proven only recessive inheritance and showed pseudodominance or mild manifestations in heterozygotes in the so-called dominant families.

Acknowledgments

The preparation of this chapter was supported by the Greenberg Center for Skeletal Dysplasias, the Smilow Family Foundation, the National Marfan Foundation, the National Institutes of Health, and the Howard Hughes Medical Institute.

Suggested Readings

Beighton PE, ed. *McKusick's heritable disorders of connective tissue,* 5th ed. Baltimore: Mosby, 1993.

Beighton PE, De Paepe A, Danks D, et al. International nosology of heritable disorders of connective tissue, Berlin 1986. *Am J Med Genet* 1988;29:581.

Beighton PE, De Paepe A, Steinmann B, et al. Ehlers-Danlos syndromes: revised nosology, Villefranche 1997. *Am J Med Genet* 1998;77:31.

De Paepe A, Dietz HC, Devereux RB, et al. Revised diagnostic criteria for the Marfan syndrome and related conditions. *Am J Med Genet* 1996;62:417.

Dietz HC, Cutting GR, Pyeritz RE. Marfan syndrome caused by a recurrent missense mutation in the fibrillin gene. *Nature* 1991;352:337.

Gray JR, Davies SJ. Marfan syndrome. *J Med Genet* 1996;33:403.

Kornak U, Mundlos S. Genetic disorders of the skeleton: a developmental approach. *Am J Hum Genet* 2003;73:447.

Kucher MS, Shapiro F. Osteogenesis imperfecta. *J Am Acad Orthop Surg* 1998; 6:225.

Online Mendelian Inheritance in Man (OMIM) Center for Medical Genetics, Johns Hopkins University, Baltimore; National Center for Biotechnology Information, National Library of Medicine, Bethesda, MD: http://www.ncbi. nlm.nih.gov/omim.

Pope FM, Burrows NP. Ehlers-Danlos syndrome has varied molecular mechanisms. *J Med Genet* 1997;34:400.

Pyeritz RE, Fishman EK, Bernhardt A, Siegelman S. Dural ectasia is a common pleiotropic feature of the Marfan syndrome. *Am J Hum Genet* 1988;43:726.

Rimoin DL, Connor JM, Pyeritz RE, Korf BR eds. *Emery and Rimoin's principles and practice of medical genetics,* 4th ed. Edinburgh: Churchill Livingstone, 2002.

Roman MJ, Devereux RB, Kramer-Fox R, O'Loughlin J. Two-dimensional echocardiographic root dimensions in normal children and adults. *Am J Cardiol* 1989;64:507.

Royce PM, Steinmann B, eds. *Connective tissue and its heritable disorders. Molecular, genetic, and medical aspects,* 2nd ed. New York: Wiley-Liss, 2002.

Silverman DI, Burton KJ, Gray J, et al. Life expectancy in the Marfan syndrome. *Am J Cardiol* 1995;75:157.

Taybi H, Lachman RS. *Radiology of syndromes, metabolic disorders, and skeletal dysplasias,* 4th ed. St. Louis: Mosby, 1996.

Wynne-Davis R, Hall CM, Apley AG. *Atlas of skeletal dysplasias.* Edinburgh: Churchill Livingstone, 1985.

CHAPTER 393 ■ INBORN ERRORS ASSOCIATED WITH FAULTY BONE MINERALIZATION

REBECCA S. WAPPNER

DISORDERS OF ALKALINE PHOSPHATASE

Hypophosphatasia

Alkaline phosphatase is contained in membrane-enclosed vesicles located at the sites of mineral deposition in bone matrix and cartilage. Alkaline phosphatase appears to act as a pyrophosphatase, which releases phosphate ions needed for calcification. Usually, serum levels of alkaline phosphatase in children are approximately three times those in adults because of an increase in the bone fraction that is associated with active bone growth.

Deficiency of alkaline phosphatase, termed *hypophosphatasia,* is characterized by faulty bone mineralization. Four currently recognized forms of the disorder vary in age of onset and clinical severity. All are associated with reduced serum levels of alkaline phosphatase and elevated levels of plasma and urinary pyridoxal-5′-phosphate, inorganic pyrophosphate, and phosphoethanolamine, which are natural substrates for the enzyme. Varying degrees of hypercalcemia and hypercalciuria occur. Mutations in the tissue-nonspecific alkaline phosphatase (*TNSALP* or *ALPL*) gene, located at chromosome 1p36.1-p34, show genotype-phenotype correlation with the differing forms of the disorder. Prenatal diagnosis is available for the severe forms.

The *perinatal* or *lethal* form of hypophosphatasia is the most severe and is expressed *in utero.* Polyhydramnios may occur. Almost complete lack of skeletal mineralization, shortened extremities, and severe craniotabes occur. Serum alkaline phosphatase levels are extremely low and often are less than 10% of the lower limit of normal for infants. Many affected individuals are stillborn, whereas others live a few days and then die in the immediate neonatal period of respiratory insufficiency.

Radiography will help to differentiate this disorder from other severe forms of bone dysplasia. This form of the disorder is inherited as an autosomal recessive trait.

The *infantile* form of hypophosphatasia is a severe, autosomal recessive disorder that presents within the first year of life with generalized skeletal demineralization. Shortened extremities, fractures, failure to thrive, hypercalcemia, hypercalciuria, nephrocalcinosis, premature synostosis of the skull, and respiratory infections are common. Serum alkaline phosphatase levels are moderately reduced, with levels usually less than 25% of the lower limit of normal for children. Initial treatment with calcitonin may correct elevated calcium levels. Long-term therapy with chlorothiazide has resulted in decreased hypercalciuria and may improve bone mineralization. Dietary reduction of vitamin D and calcium may be needed to control the hypercalcemia. Reduced exposure to sunlight and use of sunscreens also may be required. Importantly, however, children should receive between 200 and 400 IU of vitamin D daily to prevent secondary rickets from developing. Serial measurement of 25-hydroxyvitamin D levels will help to monitor intake. Premature synostosis may not be appreciated on routine radiography or computed tomography, owing to the demineralization. Increased intracranial pressure may require surgical correction. Although many children with the infantile form die during childhood, long-term survival is possible. Bone marrow transplantation resulted in clinical improvement in one reported patient.

The *childhood* form of hypophosphatasia is characterized by premature loss of deciduous teeth, short stature, and clinical features of rickets. Joint swelling and discomfort and a nonprogressive myopathy often occur. Affected patients have an increased incidence of scoliosis and fractures. Radiography shows demineralization and rachitic changes. Focal areas of radiolucency project from growth plates into the metaphyseal areas. Craniosynostosis has been reported. Serum alkaline phosphatase levels are variably reduced and range between 20% and 75% of the lower limit of normal for children. Hypercalcemia and hypercalciuria may occur. Treatment is similar to that for the infantile form of the disorder. This form may be inherited as an autosomal dominant or an autosomal recessive trait.

Patients with the relatively mild *adult* form of hypophosphatasia may have a history of early loss of deciduous teeth, repeated fractures, or "rickets" in infancy. Stress fractures, pseudofractures, and arthritis may occur. Serum alkaline phosphatase levels are low, but not as reduced as in the more severe forms, and they may be just under the lower limit of normal for age. Usually, significant hypercalcemia and hypercalciuria are not noted. In some patients, the disorder is detected on screening blood panels. This form of the disorder may be inherited as an autosomal dominant or an autosomal recessive trait.

Pseudohypophosphatasia

Pseudohypophosphatasia has clinical and radiographic findings similar to those of the infantile form of hypophosphatasia, including elevated urinary phosphoethanolamine levels. However, serum alkaline phosphatase levels are normal.

Hyperphosphatasemia

Hyperphosphatasemia, or elevation of alkaline phosphatase levels, may be seen in children with rickets, fractures, liver dysfunction, growth spurts, or inherited genetic disorders.

Transient hyperphosphatasemia of infancy has its onset between ages 2 months and 3 years, although occurrences as late as 6 years have been reported. The disorder is detected most often when screening panels are carried out for some illness, usually an acute infection. Alkaline phosphatase fractionation studies indicate that both bone and liver isoenzymes are elevated. Usually, alkaline phosphatase activity normalizes within 4 months. Occasionally, resolution may take as long as 18 months or more. Nonspecific effects of infection or medication have been cited as possible causes. The condition is sporadic and benign and requires no therapy.

Familial hyperphosphatasemia also is a benign condition that may be differentiated from transient hyperphosphatasemia of infancy by the finding that it will not resolve. Because it is inherited as an autosomal dominant trait, one of the parents also will have hyperphosphatasemia.

Hyperphosphatasemia *with osteoectasia* (juvenile Paget disease) is a rare, autosomal recessive disorder associated with elevated bone alkaline phosphatase levels, abnormal bone remodeling, severe osteoporosis, and bone fragility leading to progressive skeletal deformities. Most patients come from a Puerto Rican or Native American background. The onset occurs between ages 1 and 3 years. Arterial complications of the disease frequently lead to death in adulthood. Radiographic findings are characteristic, with the long bones having a cylindric appearance, pseudocysts, irregular trabeculation, and dilated shafts (osteoectasia). Calcitonin and bisphosphonate therapy may improve clinical and radiographic findings. The disorder results from mutations in the *TNFRSF* (tumor necrosis factor receptor superfamily) *11B* gene, at chromosome 8q24.2, which encodes for osteoprotegerin, a glycoprotein involved with regulation of bone resorption.

DISORDERS OF VITAMIN D METABOLISM

Vitamin D exists as ergocalciferol (vitamin D_2) and cholecalciferol (vitamin D_3). In humans, exposure to ultraviolet light results in the photoconversion of 7-dehydrocholesterol to vitamin D_3 in the skin and usually is sufficient to supply the daily recommended need. Ergocalciferol is added routinely to commercial milk and infant formulas to prevent dietary vitamin D deficiency as a result of inadequate exposure to sunlight. Both vitamin D_2 and vitamin D_3 are stored in plasma, muscle, and adipose tissue and are converted to their active metabolites by hydroxylation. Vitamin D (D_2 or D_3) is converted to 25-hydroxycalciferol (calcidiol, calcifediol; 25-OH-D) in the liver by microsomal 25-cholecalciferol hydroxylase. Then the 25-OH-D is transported to the kidney, where it undergoes a second hydroxylation step by mitochondrial 1-alpha-hydroxylase to form 1,25-dihydroxycholecalciferol (calcitriol; 1,25-diOH-D). The 1,25-diOH-D binds to receptor sites in target organs. The resultant activated vitamin D–receptor complex is transported to the nucleus of the cell; there it induces translation, with resulting production of specific proteins (e.g., calcium-binding protein) that are related to the physiologic actions of activated vitamin D. Defects in hydroxylation, receptor binding, nuclear uptake, and postreceptor processing have been demonstrated in patients and are associated with autosomal recessive patterns of inheritance.

Clinical manifestations are similar to those seen with dietary vitamin D deficiency. Patients appear well at birth, but physical and biochemical findings of rickets develop during the first year of life. Many have hypocalcemic seizures (tetany) by age 4 months. Hypotonia, repeated respiratory infections, failure to thrive, and delayed motor milestones are common. Radiography shows classic florid rickets with decreased mineralization, fraying and cupping of epiphyseal areas, and fractures and pseudofractures. Widening of the wrists and knees, enlargement of costochondral junctions (rachitic rosary), craniotabes of the skull, frontal bossing, and bowing of long bones may be seen. Occasionally, pseudotumor cerebri develops. The serum calcium concentration is low, the phosphorus concentration may be low, and alkaline phosphatase and parathyroid hormone levels are elevated.

Hereditary deficiency of 25-OH-D has been reported in two siblings, presumably a result of deficient activity of hepatic microsomal 25-cholecalciferol hydroxylase. Treatment with high-dose vitamin D_2 or 25-OH-D_3 will correct the associated rickets.

Hereditary deficiency of 1,25-diOH-D (vitamin D–dependent rickets, type I) is associated with deficient activity of renal 1-alpha-hydroxylase and reduced serum levels of 1,25-diOH-D. Serum 25-OH-D levels are normal or elevated. Treatment includes 1,25-diOH-D (calcitriol) in doses that usually range from 0.3 to 2 μg/day. The disorder results from mutations in the gene *PDDR* (pseudovitamin D deficiency rickets), at chromosome 12q14, which encodes for 1-alpha-hydroxylase.

Hereditary generalized resistance of 1,25-diOH-D (vitamin D–dependent rickets, type II) results from abnormalities in the 1,25-diOH-D–receptor sites in cell membranes in most patients. Other, very rare forms have been associated with defects in postreceptor processing. Serum 25-OH-D levels are normal, and 1,25-diOH-D levels are usually elevated. Patients are affected more severely than are those with 1-alpha-hydroxylase deficiency. Many patients are presented for evaluation at birth, and 50% have alopecia totalis. Very large doses of 1,25-diOH-D are given, which may need to be as high as 5 to 60 μg/day for severly affected individuals. Large doses of enteral (and occasionally intravenous) calcium are also needed for the treatment of hypocalcemia in severely affected infants. Mutations in the VDR (vitamin D receptor) gene, at chromosome 12q12-q14, have been reported in affected patients.

Suggested Readings

Barcia JP, Strife F, Langman C. Infantile hypophosphatasia: treatment options to control hypercalcemia, hypercalciuria, and chronic bone demineralization. *J Pediatr* 1997;130:825.

Casella SJ, Reiner BJ, Chen TC, et al. A possible genetic defect in 25-hydroxylation as a cause of rickets. *J Pediatr* 1994;124:929.

Cockerill FJ, Hawa NS, Yousof N, et al. Mutations in the vitamin D receptor gene in three kindreds associated with hereditary vitamin D–resistant rickets. *J Clin Endocrinol Metab* 1997;82:3156.

Demir E, Bereket A, Ozkan B, et al. Effect of alendronate treatment on the clinical picture and bone turnover markers in chronic idiopathic hyperphosphatasia. *J Pediatr Endocrinol Metab* 2000;13:217.

Liberman UA, Marx SJ. Vitamin D and other calciferols. In: Scriver CR, Beaudet AL, Sly WS, Valle D, eds. *The metabolic and molecular bases of inherited disease,* 8th ed. New York: McGraw-Hill, 2001:4223.

Mornet E. Hypophosphatasia: the mutations in the tissue-nonspecific alklaine phosphatase gene. *Hum Mutat* 2000;15:309.

Tuysuz B, Mercimek S, Ungur S, et al. Calcitonin treatment in osteoectasia with hyperphosphatasia (juvenile Paget's disease): radiographic changes after treatment. *Pediatr Radiol* 1999;29:838.

Wang JT, Liu CJ, Burridge SM, et al. Genetics of vitamin D 1-alpha-hydroxylase deficiency in 17 families. *Am J Hum Genet* 1998;63:1694.

Whyte MP. Hypophosphatasia. In: Scriver CR, Beaudet AL, Sly WS, Valle D, eds. *The metabolic and molecular bases of inherited disease,* 8th ed. New York: McGraw-Hill, 2001:5313.

Whyte MP, Kurtzberg J, McAlister WH, et al. Marrow cell transplantation for infantile hypophosphatasia. *J Bone Miner Res* 2003;18:624.

Whyte MP, Obrecht SE, Finnegan PM, et al. Osteoprotegerin deficiency and juvenile Paget's disease. *N Engl J Med* 2002;347:175.

Zurutuza L, Muller F, Gibrat JF, et al. Correlations of genotype and phenotype in hypophosphatasia. *Hum Mol Genet* 1999;8:1039.

SECTION X ■ DISEASES OF THE NERVOUS SYSTEM

CHAPTER 394 ■ EVALUATION OF THE CHILD WITH NEUROLOGIC DISEASE

MARVIN A. FISHMAN

PATIENT HISTORY AND NEUROLOGIC EXAMINATION

The most important parts of the evaluation of a child with neurologic symptoms are the history and physical examination. Principles used during the general evaluation are applicable to the child with a neurologic problem. Slight modification of the approach can increase the amount of information obtained. The purpose of taking the history is to elicit information that enables a tentative diagnosis to be made. With a tentative diagnosis in mind, the physician performs the neurologic examination to see whether the findings are consistent with the postulated diagnosis. For example, if a patient is thought to have idiopathic epilepsy but has an abnormal neurologic examination, the possibility that a structural lesion is causing the seizures should be considered. In the case of a child with a complaint of weakness, cerebellar dysfunction should be considered, as well as disease of nerve or muscle, because unsteadiness may be interpreted as weakness by the family. Tests of coordination, power of individual muscle groups, reflexes, and sensation can help to differentiate the cause of the symptom.

Information obtained from the history should allow the tempo of the illness to be assessed and the findings to be interpreted in accord with neuroanatomic and neurophysiologic principles. The physician should determine whether the disease process is acute or chronic and whether the onset was abrupt or insidious. Occasionally, an event such as intercurrent illness or trauma results in closer than usual observation of a child and discovery of a preexisting problem; a history dating the beginning of neurologic symptoms may not always be accurate. A decrease in the rate of acquisition of new developmental skills or loss of previously acquired skills suggests a degenerative process. Specific questions should be asked to help clarify the meaning of terms used by the historian. *Dizziness* may indicate vertigo or light-headedness. *Weakness* may refer to loss of muscle power, fatigue, or unsteadiness. *Blurred vision* may indicate diplopia, decreased acuity, a visual field defect, or scotomata. Each of these conditions has different importance in terms of localizing the area of dysfunction. The physician must decide whether the symptoms can be explained by dysfunction of one part of the nervous system or whether the process is diffuse or multifocal. Different physical findings correlate with each of these possibilities.

Information obtained during history taking should include details of the mother's pregnancy, labor, and delivery. Occasionally, insults may affect the nervous system of the fetus or neonate and can produce immediate or subsequent neurologic problems. Particular attention given to the schedule of acquisition of motor and language developmental milestones yields information about when the disorder began and whether the problem involves specific areas of function. A summary of normal developmental milestones is given in Box 394.1.

Many neurologic illnesses are familial, and important clues to the child's illness may be obtained from careful review of the family history. Family members may not know the specific name of the disease being considered but may be familiar with symptoms and signs, particularly in cases of familial diseases involving the cerebellum, peripheral nerves, or muscle. Subtle manifestations of neurocutaneous syndromes may not have been appreciated previously, and the finding of tuberous sclerosis or neurofibromatosis in the child can result in identification of other affected relatives. Occasionally, diseases are diagnosed erroneously by family members. Any severe headache may be referred to mistakenly as migraine. Eliciting a detailed history in family members to see whether the symptoms do suggest migraine is important.

The physical examination begins when the child enters the examining room; observations continue during the history taking. Significant information about cranial nerves and cerebellar and motor function can be obtained by watching an infant crawl, walk, or play with toys. The general physical examination should include measurement of head size. The presence of dysmorphic features or cutaneous abnormalities may help to establish a diagnosis. Performing a Wood light examination may be necessary to detect the depigmented ash-leaf lesions seen in tuberous sclerosis. Metabolic disorders resulting in the accumulation of excessive amounts of lipids or other materials may result in enlargement of the liver and spleen. Cardiac murmurs may signify abnormalities that predispose to neurologic complications such as embolic strokes and cerebral abscesses. A cranial bruit may suggest a large intracranial vascular malformation. Cutaneous abnormalities, dimples, vascular malformations, and tufts of hair over the lower back may be associated with occult spinal dysraphism. Limb growth asymmetry suggests chronic hemiparesis.

The formal neurologic examination is used to confirm the information obtained by observation and to corroborate the diagnosis suspected from the history. Examination often is easier to perform with the infant seated in the mother's lap rather than with the infant seated or lying on an examining table. Beginning the examination with the child's legs and working upward results in better cooperation than if more unpleasant aspects of the examination, such as funduscopy, are performed first.

Cranial nerve testing is easy to perform. Cranial nerve I, the olfactory nerve, often is not tested unless there is a specific indication for doing so. Cranial nerve II, the optic nerve, can be inspected and tested. Vision can be assessed by several methods in children who are too young to cooperate in formal testing with visual acuity charts. Various revolving drums or tapes can be used to elicit optokinetic nystagmus in young infants. With infants older than 6 months of age, various small objects, even a fleck of paper, can be placed in front of them, and their attempts to pick it up can be observed. Each eye can be tested separately. Cranial nerves III, IV, and VI are responsible for eye movements, pupillary responses, and lid opening. They can be tested by observing spontaneous eye movements and by having the child watch toys such as puppets. Facial sensation is supplied by cranial nerve V and can be tested with a wisp of cotton. The motor branch of cranial nerve V supplies the muscles of mastication. These muscles can be tested by having the child open the jaw against resistance and by palpating the masseter muscles as the teeth are clenched. Facial movements, a function of cranial nerve VII, can be assessed when the child smiles and laughs and with volitional movements. Asking the child to smile allows observation of the symmetry of the nasolabial folds; the symmetry of burying the eyelashes can be observed as the eyes are closed. The symmetry of the strength of the eyelid closure can be tested by attempting to open the upper lids while the child tries to keep the eyes tightly closed. Auditory acuity, controlled by cranial nerve VIII, can be tested by using a tuning fork or watch or by giving whispered instructions out of sight of the child. Lower cranial nerves IX, X, XI, and XII can be tested by eliciting a gag reflex, watching the palate contract, and observing movements of the tongue, shoulders, and neck.

In preschool-aged children, motor function is assessed by watching the child play, crawl, climb, or walk. Activities can be designed to test functions of upper or lower extremities. Lifting a child with the examiner's hands placed in the patient's axillae tests shoulder girdle function. Lifting a child off the ground while the child holds the examiner's thumbs tests hand strength. Tone is tested by passively moving the child's limbs.

Deep tendon reflexes are elicited in children by techniques similar to those used with adults. Infants have developmental reflexes in the newborn period that disappear with normal development. The more common developmental reflexes are listed in Table 394.1. The abnormal persistence of these reflexes usually is accompanied by other abnormalities in the neurologic examination or a lack of appropriate developmental skills. The isolated persistence of one of these reflexes should be interpreted cautiously because of the significant variation in the age at which they normally disappear.

Cerebellar function can be assessed in young infants and preschool children by watching them play; this method is particularly useful for observing upper extremity function as well as balance. The skill with which young children perform fine motor tasks is age-dependent, and the assessment of normal function must take this fact into consideration. Infants often can be coaxed into reaching for small objects, and during these maneuvers, fine motor coordination and hand function are observed. The presence of adventitial or associated movements can be evaluated at this time. Watching a child walk or run is helpful in determining cerebellar function and motor strength, peripheral nerve function, and abnormalities of tone.

The sensory examination often is difficult to perform and interpret accurately in infants and preschool children. When it is performed near the end of a history-taking and examination session, attention and cooperation may be lacking. Under these circumstances, completing the sensory examination at a later time may yield more useful information. Engaging the child in "play games" often enhances effort and interest. Testing of cortical or sensory modalities, such as double simultaneous stimulation, stereognosis, or graphesthesia, requires accurate reporting by the examinee. Reliable information often is difficult to obtain until the child is of school age.

LABORATORY INVESTIGATIONS

The laboratory tests frequently used in the evaluation of children with neurologic problems are discussed briefly. A few indications are given for each test, but the discussion is neither complete nor comprehensive. Readers can refer to other sections of this book that discuss the use of laboratory tests in the context of specific diseases or problems.

BOX 394.1   Normal Developmental Milestones

Newborn
In ventral suspension, hangs head down
When prone, has pelvis raised and knees under abdomen
Shows complete head lag on traction
Shows walking reflex
Shows grasp reflex

8 weeks
In ventral suspension, holds head in same plane as
    rest of body
When prone, lifts chin off couch
Holds hands open part of the time
Fixes and follows object through an arc of more than
    90 degrees
Smiles and makes sounds

12 weeks
In ventral suspension, holds head above rest of body
Bobs head when supported sitting
Shows no grasp reflex
Turns head to sound, notices hands, follows object through a
    180-degree arc
Recognizes mother

20 weeks
When prone, holds chest off couch and weight on forearms
Shows no head lag on traction
Can grasp objects and bring them to mouth
Smiles at mirror
Excites with feeding
Laughs aloud

28 weeks
When prone, can support upper trunk with weight
    on hands and arms extended
Rolls prone to supine
Sits on floor with support of hands
Bears weight on legs in standing position
Transfers objects
Imitates sounds
Responds to name
Drinks from cup
States syllables

40 weeks
Creeps on abdomen
Achieves sitting position independently
Shows pincer grasp
Waves bye-bye

52 weeks
Walks like bear
May walk independently
Releases toys
Plays simple games
Shows interest in picture books
Uses two to three words with meaning
Understands simple phrases

15 months
Creeps upstairs
Can sit in chair

Achieves standing position independently
Stacks two to three cubes
Uses cup, rotates spoon
Knows some body parts

18 months
Pulls toys when walking
Takes off shoes and socks
Uses jargon and normal language
Imitates mother
Follows simple request
Turns pages in groups

2 years
Walks up stairs placing both feet on each step
Kicks ball
Stacks more than five cubes
Puts on socks
Shows some dressing skills
Uses phrases
Names common objects
Turns pages singly
Places objects in form board puzzles

2½ years
Jumps with both feet
Holds crayon in hand
Is toilet trained
Knows name and sex
Follows instructions
Identifies objects
May name a color

3 years
Rides tricycle
Draws circles and tries to imitate cross
Dresses self independently except for buttons
Shows normal speech
Goes upstairs one foot at a time
May know nursery rhymes
Begins to understand prepositions

4 years
Walks down stairs with one foot on each step
Copies cross
Asks numerous questions
Engages in imaginative play

5 years
Skips on both feet
Can tie shoelace
Copies square
Knows age
Distinguishes morning from afternoon
Begins to draw a person

6 years
Copies a diamond
Repeats digits
Counts
Knows number of fingers

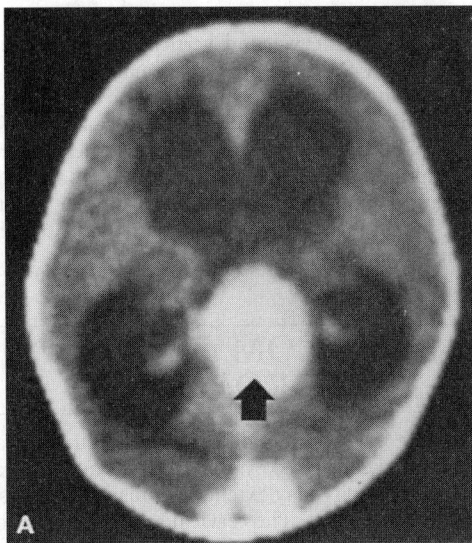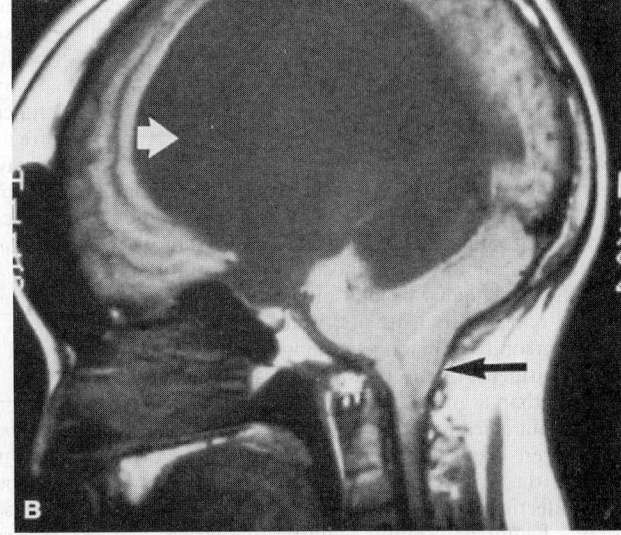

FIGURE 395.1. A: Computed tomographic scan with contrast enhancement demonstrates hydrocephalus secondary to an aneurysm of the vein of Galen (*arrow*). **B:** A magnetic resonance image in the sagittal plane demonstrates hydrocephalus (*white arrow*) and a Chiari type II malformation (*black arrow*) with downward displacement of the brainstem into the cervical canal. (Courtesy of Dr. Clark Carrol, Texas Children's Hospital, Houston, TX.)

brain tumors, and arachnoiditis caused by bleeding into the subarachnoid space from a ruptured arteriovenous malformation, aneurysm, or trauma. Premature infants may develop hydrocephalus secondary to intraventricular hemorrhage.

Symptoms and Signs

The primary process (e.g., tumor, infection, bleeding) and the symptom and signs caused by increased ICP secondary to the hydrocephalus may contribute to the clinical picture. The severity of the findings is influenced by the rate at which the hydrocephalus develops and the development of alternate pathways of absorption of CSF. Nonspecific symptoms include headaches that are variable in location and intensity; they occasionally occur early in the morning and are associated with vomiting. Personality and behavior changes, including irritability or indifference, sometimes occur. Lethargy and drowsiness are relatively late symptoms. Nausea and vomiting are secondary to increased ICP, particularly with posterior fossa lesions. Nonspecific signs include third and sixth cranial nerve deficits, which result in paresis of extraocular muscles and may lead to diplopia. Papilledema may be a late finding if the ICP is not markedly elevated and the process is slow and chronic. Changes in vital signs occur relatively late and indicate distortion of the brainstem. In young children, the anterior fontanelle may become full or distended; this condition is accompanied by excessive head growth and dilatation of scalp veins. The "setting-sun sign" is produced by paralysis of upward gaze so the sclera above the iris is visible. Spasticity develops first in the lower extremities and then in the arms and results from stretching of motor fibers around the bodies of the lateral ventricles. Dilatation of the third ventricle may cause pressure on the hypothalamus, resulting in disturbances in sexual development and in fluid and electrolyte imbalances. Specific deficits produced by focal lesions include hemiparesis, ataxia, tremor, speech and language disorders, gaze disorders, facial weakness, and difficulty in swallowing. Seizures are unusual isolated presenting symptoms of hydrocephalus and often are caused by the underlying associated condition.

Diagnosis and Therapy

Neuroimaging techniques such as CT or MRI have made the diagnosis of hydrocephalus relatively straightforward. The pattern of ventricular dilatation, the presence of interstitial edema (i.e., CSF in the white matter surrounding the ventricles), and an underlying cause for obstruction of CSF flow usually are readily apparent (Fig. 395.1). The CSF should be examined if a relatively recent infection is suspected or if subarachnoid bleeding is suspected but no evidence of such is found on neuroimaging studies. In infancy, chronic subdural hematomas may present in a similar fashion and can be detected by neuroimaging procedures.

Treatment includes specific therapy for any underlying condition associated with the hydrocephalus, such as brain tumor, abscess, and chronic meningitis. Surgery is the most effective means of treating progressive hydrocephalus; a shunt system is placed between the cerebral ventricles and the peritoneal cavity. Shunt placement is a palliative measure and not a cure. The complication rate is relatively high. Problems encountered include mechanical obstruction of the shunt system. The failure rate may be as high as 40% in the first year. Infections within the shunt system may produce meningitis or ventriculitis. Shunt infections may be indolent and often are caused by organisms that usually are not considered pathogens, such as *Staphylococcus epidermidis*. Other surgical procedures include third ventriculotomies in certain conditions. Shunt infections occur in approximately 5% to 10% of procedures. Most occur within the first 6 months of placement of the shunt. Medical therapy designed to decrease production of CSF may be used when the hydrocephalus is slowly progressive and perhaps transitory. Such conditions include the ventricular enlargement sometimes seen after subarachnoid hemorrhage or meningitis. The therapeutic agents used include acetazolamide, furosemide, and glycerol. Diuretic therapy in newborns with posthemorrhage ventricular dilatation does not appear to be effective in reducing the need for placement of a shunt system. These agents also may be used in the interim between the removal of an infected shunt system and insertion of a new system. Serial lumbar punctures in preterm infants with posthemorrhagic ventriculomegaly do not appear to be effective in reducing the risk for shunt placement, death, or disability.

Prognosis

Intellectual function and motor function in hydrocephalic children are determined by the problem causing the hydrocephalus rather than by the ventricular dilatation itself. The natural history of intrauterine infections, meningitis, brain tumors, or other disorders determines the prognosis. The disabilities produced by the hydrocephalus include motor problems related to spasticity or coordination deficits, visual impairment secondary to optic atrophy from long-standing increased ICP, and intellectual impairment. Intellectual ability usually is affected less significantly than is motor performance because the gray matter of the brain is less affected by the hydrocephalus than is the white matter. The incidence of seizures varies according to the origin of the hydrocephalus. The rate is estimated to be 50% with infections, 30% with cerebral malformations or intraventricular hemorrhage, and 7% with spina bifida.

CHIARI MALFORMATION

The Chiari malformation involves the brainstem and the lower portion of the cerebellum. These structures are displaced downward into the cervical canal. Various degrees of the malformation occur. In type I, caudal cerebellar tonsillar ectopia is present, and the cerebellar tonsils extend into the foramen magnum for more than 5 mm. In type II, the cerebellar vermis, medulla, and fourth ventricle are elongated and extend into the spinal canal. The downward displacement may be such that the cervical spinal cord is kinked on itself, and the foramen magnum and upper cervical canal may be packed tightly with the displaced tissue. A strong association exists with hydrocephalus and myelodysplasia. Children with meningomyeloceles and hydrocephalus usually have an associated Chiari malformation. Hydromyelia and syringomyelia may be present in as many as 50% of children younger than age 6 years. Other minor malformations include breaking of the tectal plate and large massa intermedia. In the rare type III malformation, associated cervical spina bifida, with herniation of brain tissue through the defect, is present.

The symptoms related to Chiari malformation type I include neck pain, back pain, scoliosis, torticollis, motor dysfunction, and apnea. Children younger than 3 years of age often present with oropharyngeal dysfunction (i.e., aspiration, regurgitation, choking, dysphagia). Older children often present with scoliosis and headache. The pain may be occipital to suboccipital in location. The headaches may be associated with activities that increase ICP (e.g., coughing and straining). Some patients with Chiari I malformations are asymptomatic and are thought to have "incidental" malformations. These patients may be followed with periodic neurologic examinations and managed conservatively. The incidence of asymptomatic Chiari I lesions depends on the definition (i.e., the degree of tonsillar descent), but even patients whose tonsils are 5 mm or more below the foramen magnum may be asymptomatic. Some children have associated syringomyelia and present with scoliosis. The downward displacement of the hindbrain can be detected by neuroimaging procedures (see Fig. 395.1). In addition to MRI of the posterior fossa, MRI of the spinal cord may be necessary to detect the associated malformations.

Type II Chiari malformations usually occur in children with spina bifida and hydrocephalus. The symptoms and signs are those caused by the malformations. With significant downward displacement of the hindbrain, stretching of the lower cranial nerves may occur, which can produce facial paralysis, hoarseness or stridor, or difficulty in swallowing. If the upper segments of the spinal cord are involved, motor deficits in the arms may be seen. Cerebellar ataxia and vertical nystagmus also have been described in patients with Chiari malformation.

Symptoms attributable to hindbrain or cervical cord dysfunction in patients with Chiari I malformations often are treated with occipital decompression, and cervical laminectomy should be considered. Shunting of an associated hydrocephalus and repair of the meningomyelocele are the first procedures attempted in treating patients with Chiari II malformations.

SYRINGOMYELIA AND HYDROMYELIA

Syringomyelia is a rare condition in children. It is a cavity within the spinal cord lined by glial elements and is paracentral in location. The cavity may extend over many segments or may be isolated to just a few. The cervical area often is involved. If the syrinx extends into the brainstem, the condition is known as *syringobulbia*. Syringomyelia may be associated with abnormalities of the cervicomedullary junction, including Chiari malformation, intramedullary spinal cord tumors, spinal cord trauma, and arterial insufficiency to the spinal cord. The signs and symptoms depend on the location of the syrinx and any associated condition. Often, wasting of the small muscles of the hands and sensory deficits involving the arms are present. Deep tendon reflexes may be absent. Involvement of the descending tracts may cause spasticity in the lower extremities. A dissociated sensory disturbance with loss of temperature sensation but preservation of touch may occur; it may show a segmental distribution and results from destruction of the commissural

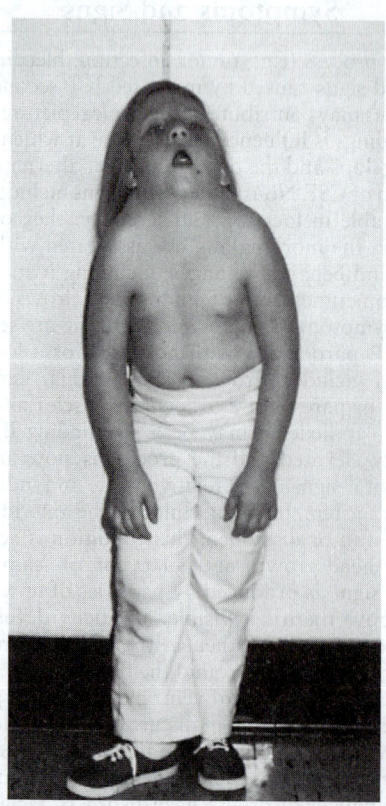

FIGURE 395.2. Girl with Klippel-Feil syndrome has a short neck and retrocollis resulting from limited neck flexion. Her lateral neck rotation is also limited. Her low occipital hairline is not visible in this photograph.

fibers of the spinal cord by the cavity. Recently, some children presenting with scoliosis were studied by MRI, and approximately 20% were found to have syringomyelia. The diagnosis may be made by MRI of the spinal cord. Treatment consists of therapy for the primary lesion, such as associated tumor or cervical medullary junction abnormality, and decompression of the syrinx itself in some patients.

Hydromyelia involves symmetric dilatation of the central canal of the spinal cord. The enlarged canal is lined by ependymal and often communicates with the fourth ventricle. The enlargement may extend over many segments and may include the entire length of the spinal cord. It often is associated with other malformations, including communicating hydrocephalus, Chiari malformation, and aqueductal stenosis. The signs and symptoms often are related to the associated malformations, and therapy is directed toward them. Whether any findings are related to the dilatation of the central canal itself is unclear.

KLIPPEL-FEIL SYNDROME

The three characteristic clinical findings of Klippel-Feil syndrome are short neck, limited neck motion, and low occipital hairline (Fig. 395.2). The type I form of the syndrome consists of fusions involving the cervical and upper thoracic vertebrae.

In type II, only the cervical vertebrae are involved, and fusion of several segments may be present. In type III, lesions similar to those found in types I and II occur, but lower thoracic and lumbar vertebrae are involved. Various forms of the syndrome have been transmitted as autosomal dominant and autosomal recessive traits. Mutations in *PAX3* gene have been implicated as possibly associated with this syndrome. Malformations in other organ systems are common findings. They include extraocular muscle palsies, deafness, macrocephaly, hydrocephalus, and meningoceles. Neurologic abnormalities include mirror movements, nystagmus, and mental retardation. Musculoskeletal anomalies include thoracic scoliosis, spina bifida occulta, abnormalities of ribs, and Sprengel deformity. Webbing of the neck and facial asymmetry may be evident. Less commonly, congenital heart disease and genitourinary anomalies are found. Cleft lip and palate and abnormalities of the gastrointestinal tract, lungs, and skin also have been reported.

MACROCEPHALY

Macrocephaly refers to a head size 2 standard deviations (SDs) above the mean. The condition can have many causes. Box 395.1 lists the more common conditions associated with large head size. In some children, a large brain (i.e., megalencephaly) may be the underlying condition. It may be familial and may

---

BOX 395.1   Large Head Syndromes

Hydrocephaly
Congenital
    Aqueductal stenosis: with or without meningomyelocele and Chiari malformation
    Communicating: with or without meningomyelocele and Chiari malformation
Dandy-Walker syndrome
Hydranencephaly
Porencephaly
Holoprosencephaly
Genetic
    Chromosomal malformation
    Sex-linked transmission
Cysts
Infectious
    Postinflammatory disease (meningitis)
    Viral (cytomegalovirus, mumps, other)
    Parasitic (toxoplasmosis)
Vascular
    Postsubarachnoid hemorrhage
    Arteriovenous malformation
    Vein of Galen aneurysm
Tumor
    Choroid plexus papilloma
    Posterior fossa neoplasm
    Other

Subdural
Effusion
Hematoma
Hygroma
Empyema

Neurocutaneous Disorders
Neurofibromatosis
Tuberous sclerosis
Multiple hemangiomatosis

Incontinentia pigmenti
Basal cell nevus syndrome
Neurocutaneous melanosis

Toxic-Metabolic Causes
Benign increased intracranial hypertension associated with antibiotics, vitamin A, endocrine disorders, catch-up growth after malnutrition, galactosemia, anemias

Cranioskeletal Dysplasias
Anemias
Achondroplasia
Osteogenesis imperfecta
Osteopetrosis
Metaphyseal dysplasia
Platybasia
Fibrous dysplasia (Albright syndrome)

Storage and Degenerative Diseases
Leukodystrophies
    Canavan spongy degenerative disease
    Alexander disease
Lysosomal disease
    Tay-Sachs disease
    Generalized gangliosidosis
    Mucopolysaccharidosis
    Metachromatic leukodystrophy
Peroxisomal disorders
    Neonatal adrenoleukodystrophy
Amino acid disorders
    Maple syrup urine disease

Unknown Causes
Cerebral gigantism
Megalencephaly
    Familial disorder
    Dominant transmission
Beckwith-Wiedemann syndrome

not be accompanied by any additional symptoms and signs or may include an associated mental deficiency and other neurologic abnormalities such as hypotonia. Infantile macrocephaly is a risk factor for developing autistic spectrum disorders. An error in neuroepithelial proliferations is thought to be responsible for some cases of macrocephaly.

Infants who are macrocephalic and whose head growth parallels a normal growth pattern but is higher than the ninety-fifth percentile have been described. Imaging demonstrates slight ventricular dilatation and increased width of the subarachnoid space over the convexities of the hemispheres. The development of most of these children is normal or only slightly delayed. If head growth continues parallel to the ninety-fifth percentile, no intervention is necessary. The exact cause of this condition is uncertain. It has been called *extraventricular obstructive hydrocephalus, benign communicating hydrocephalus,* and *external hydrocephalus.* Another possibility is that the fluid over the convexities represents small subdural hematomas with secondary hydrocephalus. The diagnosis can be established by CT or MRI, and the children can be followed with serial head circumference measurements. Any deviation from the anticipated growth pattern warrants performing repeat neuroimaging studies. Usually, by the preschool years, the head size deviates less from the ninety-fifth percentile, and the fluid collections remain stable or decrease.

MICROCEPHALY

Microcephaly indicates a head size smaller than 2 SDs below the mean. The condition results from a small brain (i.e., microencephaly), the causes of which are many. In primary microcephaly, no identifiable insult occurs to the developing brain that subsequently inhibits its growth. The primary microcephalies include familial forms and cases that seem to occur in isolation. Newborn infants with primary microcephaly often do not exhibit striking deficits, unlike the infants who have sustained a major insult *in utero.* Eventually, intellectual impairment becomes apparent, and some children develop motor deficits and epilepsy. Other anomalies sometimes associated with microcephaly include agyria, lissencephaly, micropolygyria, schizencephaly, macrogyria, and heterotopia. These infants usually have severe deficits that are apparent in the neonatal period. Microcephaly can result from a variety of disorders resulting from chromosomal anomalies, intrauterine infections, inherited metabolic disorders, intrauterine anoxia or vascular events, and teratogenic insults in the perinatal period.

Suggested Readings

Barnett HJM, Foster JB, Hudgson P. Syringomyelia. In: Walton JH, ed. *Major problems in neurology.* Philadelphia: WB Saunders, 1973.

Bolton PF, Roobol M, Allsopp L, Pickles A. Association between idiopathic infantile macrocephaly and autism spectrum disorders. *Lancet* 2001;358: 726.

Bourgeois M, Sainte-Rose C, Cinalli G, Maixner W. Epilepsy in children with shunted hydrocephalus. *J Neurosurg* 1999;90:274.

Casey AT, Kimmings EJ, Kleinlugtebeld AD, Taylor WA. The long-term outlook for hydrocephalus in childhood: a ten year cohort study of 155 patients. *Pediatr Neurosurg* 1997;27:63.

Chumas P, Tyagi A, Livingston J. Hydrocephalus: what's new? *Arch Dis Child Fetal Neonatal Ed* 2001;85:F149.

Clark, GD. Brain development and the genetics of brain development. *Neurol Clin* 2002;20:4.

DeMyer W. Megalencephaly in children: clinical syndromes, genetic patterns and differential diagnosis from hydrocephalus. *Neurology* 1972;22:634.

Dure LS, Percy AK, Check WR, Laurent JP. Chiari type I malformation in children. *J Pediatr* 1989;115:573.

Fishman MA. Hydrocephalus. In: Eliasson SG, Prensky AL, Hardin WB, eds. *Neurological pathophysiology.* New York: Oxford University Press, 1978.

Foster JB, Hudgson P, Pearce GW. The association of syringomyelia and congenital cervicomedullary anomalies: pathological evidence. *Brain* 1969;92: 25.

Fransen E, Van Camp G, Vits L, Willems PJ. L1-associated diseases: clinical geneticists divide, molecular geneticists unite. *Hum Mol Genet* 1997;6: 1625.

Greenlee JDW, Donovan KA, Hasen DM, et al. Chiari I malformation in the very young child: the spectrum of presentations and experience in 31 children under 6 years of age. *Pediatrics* 2002;110:6.

Gunderson CH, Greenspan RH, Glaser GH, Lubs HA. The Klippel-Feil syndrome: genetic and clinical re-evaluation of cervical fusion. *Medicine (Baltimore)* 1967;46:491.

Hanieh A, Autherland A, Foster B, Cundy P. Syringomyelia in children with primary scoliosis. *Childs Nerv Syst* 2000;16:200.

Hoppe-Hirsch E, Laroussinie F, Brunet L, Sainte-Rose C. Late outcome of the surgical treatment of hydrocephalus. *Childs Nerv Syst* 1998;14:97.

International PHVD Drug Trial Group. International randomized controlled trial of acetazolamide and furosemide in posthaemorrhagic ventricular dilatation in infancy. *Lancet* 1998;352:433.

Javadpour M, Mallucci C, Broadbelt A, Golash A. The impact of endoscopic third ventriculostomy on the management of newly diagnosed hydrocephalus in infants. *Pediatr Neurosurg* 2001;35:131.

Lorber J, Priestley BL. Children with large heads: a practical approach to diagnosis in 557 children, with special reference to 109 children with megalencephaly. *Dev Med Child Neurol* 1981;23:531.

McGaughran JM, Oates A, Donnai D, Tassabehji M. Mutations in *PAX1* may be associated with Klippel-Feil syndrome. *Eur J Hum Genet* 2003;11:468.

McLone DG, ed. *Pediatric neurosurgery, surgery of the developing nervous system,* 4th ed. Philadelphia: WB Saunders, 2001.

Portnoy HD, Croissant PD. Megalencephaly in infants and children. *Arch Neurol* 1978;35:306.

Pryor H, Thelander H. Abnormally small head size and intellect in children. *J Pediatr* 1968;73:593.

Schrander-Stumpel C, Fryns JP. Congenital hydrocephalus: nosology and guidelines for clinical approach and genetic counselling. *Eur J Pediatr* 1998;157: 355.

Shapiro S, Boaz J, Kleiman M, Kalsbeck J. Origin of organisms infecting ventricular shunts. *Neurosurgery* 1988;22:868.

Whitelaw A, Kennedy CR, Brion LP. Diuretic therapy for newborn infants with posthemorrhagic ventricular dilatation. *Cochrane Database Sys Rev* 2001;2:CD002270.

Whitelaw A. Repeated lumbar or ventricular punctures for preventing disability or shunt dependence in newborn infants with intraventricular hemorrhage. *Cochrane Database Sys Rev* 2000;1:CD000216.

Yasuda T, Tomita T, McLone DG, Donovan M. Measurement of cerebrospinal fluid output through external ventricular drainage in one hundred infants and children: correlation with cerebrospinal fluid production. *Pediatr Neurosurg* 2002;36:22.

CHAPTER 396 ■ CEREBRAL PALSY

BRUCE K. SHAPIRO AND ARNOLD J. CAPUTE

Cerebral palsy is a disorder of movement and posture that results from an insult to or anomaly of the immature central nervous system (CNS). This definition recognizes the central origin of the dysfunction and differentiates cerebral palsy from neuropathies and myopathies. The definition implies that the cause is static and excludes progressive neurologic disorders. The simplicity of the definition belies the diversity of the dysfunctions that result from diffuse neurologic damage.

Although a static encephalopathy, cerebral palsy is not unchanging. As the CNS matures, peripheral manifestations of the central lesions change. Some children improve, some require bracing and surgery, and others reach a plateau.

HISTORICAL PERSPECTIVE

Just as the disorder changes with time, so has the approach to cerebral palsy. Although known from ancient and biblical times, cerebral palsy was not differentiated from other crippling disorders until William John Little described spastic diplegia and related it to birth injury. Little treated the handicap that resulted from cerebral palsy, and others, including Sigmund Freud and William Osler, focused on classification and clinicopathologic associations.

At the turn of the twentieth century, the emphasis had shifted to the prevention of handicaps. Bronson Crothers and his coworkers are credited with initiating the first programs of physical therapy for cerebral palsy. Winthrop Phelps, an orthopedic surgeon, expanded the treatment for children with cerebral palsy using a comprehensive method of treatment that addressed nonmotor and motor dysfunctions. As scientific capabilities have increased, two major trends have emerged: reevaluation of clinicopathologic correlations with noninvasive techniques to define anatomy and physiology and, objective quantification of movement to define therapy more reliably. Early identification and intervention are mandated.

EPIDEMIOLOGY

Cerebral palsy is the most common movement disorder of childhood. Estimates of its frequency vary from 1 to 6 per 1,000, but most recent studies report a prevalence of 1 to 2 per 1,000. The lower rate should be regarded as a minimum estimate because milder cases are not included; more severe cases may be obscured by other developmental disabilities, such as seizure disorders or mental retardation, and patients with the most severe cases may die.

Traditionally, spastic cerebral palsy has been the most frequent type, accounting for approximately 50% of cases. It is followed by athetosis (approximately 20% of cases), rigidity, ataxia tremor, and mixed forms (approximately 25% of cases). However, obtaining good estimates of the frequency of cerebral palsy is difficult. Time trends have not been consistent, with some researchers reporting an increase and others a decrease. Disagreement ensues about whether to include children

with acquired cerebral palsy (e.g., owing to neurotrauma or infection) and at what age cerebral palsy should be diagnosed because the diagnosis is less stable in infants.

The causes of cerebral palsy have changed. Acute infantile hemiplegia, which was a common occurrence during the late nineteenth century, has become rare. Modern obstetric techniques have diminished major birth trauma markedly. The understanding and successful prevention of hemolytic disease of the newborn have changed the spectrum of extrapyramidal cerebral palsy of the choreoathetoid type.

Most cerebral palsy is found in children who do not possess identifiable risk factors. Traditional risk factors associated with cerebral palsy are birth asphyxia, prematurity, and intrauterine growth retardation. When risk factors are analyzed in a multivariate fashion, the strongest determinants of cerebral palsy are found not to be related to events of labor or delivery. Data from the perinatal collaborative study more strongly support the hypothesis that abnormal antenatal events yield difficult pregnancies, labors, and deliveries and that perinatal difficulties are associated with, not the cause of, cerebral palsy.

The impact of prematurity on the incidence of cerebral palsy is not clear. As neonatal care has improved, the incidence of cerebral palsy in heavier-birth-weight groups has decreased. Very low-birth-weight infants (less than 1,500 g) may have a higher incidence of cerebral palsy, but the lower number of children at this birth weight should modify the contribution that these children make to the total pool of cerebral palsy cases.

Some studies have reaffirmed the relationship between maternal infection and cerebral palsy. Multiple gestation markedly increases the incidence of cerebral palsy. Some researchers have suggested that cytokines are the mediators that tie together infection, asphyxia, multiple births, and prematurity.

CLASSIFICATION

The classification of cerebral palsy is multiaxial and includes the type of dysfunction (e.g., physiologic), the site of dysfunction (e.g., topographic), associated dysfunctions (e.g., supplemental), and etiologic, neuroanatomic, functional, and therapeutic axes. Only the first three axes are used and discussed here. The neuroanatomic axis awaits definition, and the etiologic, functional, and therapeutic axes have been abandoned. The current classification is most useful for older infants and children. All patients with cerebral palsy pass through a hypotonic phase, and attempts at early classification must be viewed as tentative until the evolution of the neurologic syndrome stabilizes. The changing peripheral manifestations also limit prognostication.

Physiologic Classification

Cerebral palsy can be divided into two major types, the pyramidal (spastic) and the extrapyramidal (nonspastic). Extrapyramidal cerebral palsy can be subdivided into choreoathetoid, ataxic, dystonic, and rigid forms. These groups are clinically useful but are not well correlated with neuropathologic findings.

The neurologic findings of the pyramidal type are consistent and persistent, varying little with movement, tension, emotion, or sleep. Variability is the main feature of extrapyramidal types; findings are increased with activity, tension, and emotions and are decreased with sleep or relaxation.

The characteristic type of hypertonus seen in spasticity is clasp knife, similar to the opening and closing of a penknife with a consistent hitch. The tone in extrapyramidal types varies from hypotonic to hypertonic. Extrapyramidal hypertonus is of the lead pipe or candle-wax type, but it is variable and can be diminished by repetitive movement (i.e., "shaking it out"). The persistence of spastic hypertonus may be a factor in the development of contractures. The variability of extrapyramidal tone may protect against such development.

Pathologic reflexes, such as Babinski or Chaddock, are elicited readily in patients with spastic forms. A true Babinski reflex must be differentiated from the extensor plantar response that is seen as part of athetotic posturing. Sustained ankle clonus usually is associated with spasticity. Primitive reflexes are more evident in the extrapyramidal forms.

Topographic Classification

The topographic classification is limited to the spastic types. Generally, it is not used with extrapyramidal types because these types show four-limb involvement and are classified by the nature of the movement disorder. The topographic axis includes hemiplegia, diplegia, quadriplegia, and bilateral hemiplegia.

Hemiplegia (i.e., hemiparesis) describes involvement of either lateral side of the body. The upper extremities are more severely impaired than are lower ones, and upper extremity dysfunction usually brings the child to attention.

Diplegia refers to four-limb involvement, with the upper limbs involved only minimally, although significant lower extremity impairment is present. The good upper extremity function seen in diplegia is of major assistance to habilitative efforts. The designation *paraplegia* is reserved for spinal and lower motor neuron dysfunctions, such as myelodysplasia.

Spastic quadriplegia is four-limb involvement with significant impairment of all extremities. Upper limbs may be less severely impaired than are lower ones, but substantial functional limitations exist. Some researchers consider quadriplegia a furtherance of diplegia.

Bilateral hemiplegia designates significant spasticity of both sides of the body, with upper extremities significantly more severely impaired. Monoplegia and triplegia are *formes frustes* or combinations of hemiplegia and quadriplegia.

The value of physiologic or topographic classification is that syndromes emerge that are related to patterns of neurologic deficit. For example, hemiplegia may be associated with growth arrest, a visual field defect (e.g., homonymous hemianopia), sensory impairment (e.g., astereognosis, deficiencies in two-point discrimination, position sense), and seizures. Cerebral palsy resulting from bilirubin encephalopathy has been associated with choreoathetoid movements that evolve into dystonia during adolescence, brown-green discoloration and dentin dysplasia of the deciduous teeth, upward-gaze apraxia, and high-frequency hearing loss, often associated with central auditory processing dysfunction.

Supplemental Classification

The child with cerebral palsy has an abnormally functioning CNS. The problem is expressed in many ways, all of which are associated with the primary problem. Cognitive, communicative, and behavioral disturbances are common. Seizures, sensory loss, and visual and auditory occurrences influence treatment programs.

Cerebral palsy rarely occurs without associated deficits. The diagnosis of cerebral palsy alone is not sufficient. In some cases, the cerebral palsy is not the most limiting condition. Associated dysfunctions alter treatment and affect long-term outcomes. An understanding of the interaction of the motor components and associated deficits is necessary for setting realistic goals. Evaluation and delineation of the associated deficits comprise part of the evaluation of cerebral palsy.

The presence of associated deficits, each with its own spectrum of severity, renders each case of cerebral palsy unique. A complete description of the child's areas of strength and weakness must be obtained because no "garden variety" of cerebral palsy exists. Failure to define a developmental profile usually results in incomplete habilitation, unrealistic goals, and therapeutic frustration.

Mental retardation coexists with cerebral palsy in approximately 60% of patients. In spastic forms of cerebral palsy, mental retardation occurs more frequently and more severely in proportion to the number of limbs involved. However, motor impairment does not always mean that the child also has mental retardation.

Children who escape mental retardation are nonetheless brain damaged and have processing impairments that may present as communicative disorders in the preschool child or as learning disabilities in the older child. The communicative disorders are of central origin and must be differentiated from the speech disorders that result from oral motor dysfunction.

Deafness has been reported in approximately 10% of people with cerebral palsy, with the athetoid type having the highest incidence. Strabismus occurs in 50%, although it is seen less commonly in children with hemiplegia. However, visual field cuts occur in 25% of children with hemiplegia. Refractive errors also occur more commonly in cerebral palsy.

Abnormal neural control of oral motor mechanisms may result in speech and articulation problems, swallowing abnormalities, and repeated episodes of aspiration. Drooling, poor articulation, and difficulties in breath control are more evident in nonspastic forms of cerebral palsy. Most children can be managed successfully with oral motor treatment techniques and appropriate positioning. Swallowing abnormalities and aspiration are seen in children who have severe rigidity or dystonia. Severe oral motor dysfunction may be complicated by gastroesophageal reflux and may cause growth failure. In treating the child with severe oral motor dysfunction, the nutritional and motor aspects should be assessed separately. If the child is failing to grow appropriately, has repeated episodes of dehydration, or has gastroesophageal reflux, a feeding gastrostomy with or without an antireflux procedure should be considered.

Sensory impairments associated with hemiplegia are thought to be caused by parietal lobe dysfunction. A limb with sensory impairment (i.e., a blind limb) is functionally useless. Fine testing of cortical sensory function is not possible in children younger than 7 years of age, and sensory impairment should be suspected in the child who uses the more motor-involved limb for function.

Seizures occur in one-third of children with cerebral palsy. Most seizures are controlled easily with standard approaches. Recalcitrant seizure disorders, such as infantile spasms or Lennox-Gastaut syndrome, are associated more commonly with increased motor dysfunction. Hemiplegia is associated most commonly with seizures.

Behavioral disturbances occur in many children with cerebral palsy. Neurobehavioral disturbances, such as short attention span, impulsivity, distractibility, perseveration, and self-stimulation, may be seen. Emotional disturbances may intensify as the child nears adolescence, when issues of independence and peer-group interactions cannot be resolved successfully.

Expanded Classification

The traditional definition of cerebral palsy does not specify that motor impairment is present to a handicapping degree, nor does it allow for temporal changes. If the physician concentrates only on the children with obvious motor handicap, a larger, more mildly dysfunctioning group of children will be overlooked. This oversight is unfortunate because many of these children have lasting developmental problems outside the motor area and require surveillance and tailoring of treatment programs.

Children who have subclinical forms of cerebral palsy require neither motor therapy nor orthopedic surgical procedures for their motor dysfunctions. These children demonstrate clumsiness, awkwardness, transitory abnormalities of tone or postural responses, and other minor neuromotor signs. These signs are markers of central processing dysfunction and place the child at risk for having a preschool learning disorder or a specific learning disability. The term *cerebral palsy* should not be used with the parents because it does not assist in counseling and may cause the focus to be placed on the basis of the motor disturbance rather than on the processing dysfunction.

The current definition of cerebral palsy is incomplete because it does not address the entire spectrum of motor dysfunction in children. Although the motor dysfunction may not be handicapping, deviations in motor development are markers for other developmental dysfunctions in cognitive and behavioral domains. Table 396.1 is a classification scheme that expands the definition of cerebral palsy to include the entire spectrum of motor dysfunction of childhood.

DIAGNOSIS

Some physicians have challenged the classification of cerebral palsy as a static encephalopathy. Brains that have suffered an insult continue to develop in deviant fashion, even if the insult is not ongoing. The results of the insult may continue to unfold as the child ages. A person could appropriately ask, "What is static about cerebral palsy?" Two related clinical findings lend support to this dynamic view of cerebral palsy. The clinical picture changes in the first several years of life, and contractures and postural deformity may occur later in life.

The changing clinical picture in the first year of life has been noticed since the initial clinical descriptions of cerebral palsy. The younger the child, the less secure the diagnosis of cerebral palsy. The inability to appreciate the manifestations of brain injury until late in a child's first year led physicians to link cerebral palsy to teething. In the absence of signs of severe brain dysfunction, motor failure, or associated dysfunctions that interfere with physiologic homeostasis, establishing the diagnosis of cerebral palsy is difficult. The early abundance of primitive reflexes, the lack of inhibition of deep tendon reflexes until substantial myelination has taken place, and the inability to predict the development of tone confound an early diagnosis. Overidentification and underidentification are not uncommon in the first year of life, but the mandates for early intervention services have increased attempts at earlier diagnosis. Evaluation of children with suspected cerebral palsy is described in Box 396.1.

Neonatal Period

In the neonatal period, cerebral palsy cannot be diagnosed by clinical methods. The relative immaturity of the full-term newborn limits the prognostic ability of the neonatal examination. Although a normal neurologic examination may be reassuring,

TABLE 396.1

EXPANDED CLASSIFICATION OF CEREBRAL PALSY

Rates of Motor Development	Motor Signs	Associated Dysfunction
Minimal normal: MQ 75–100 Qualitative abnormalities only	Subtle, transient abnormalities of tone Persistence, exaggeration of some primitive reflexes to a mild degree Soft signs reflected as clumsy or awkward motor performance	Communicative disorders Specific learning disabilities ADHD
Mild: MQ 50–74	Transient abnormalities of tone Occasional "hard" signs Persistent primitive reflexes; delayed postural responses Soft signs may be present to functionally important degree (i.e., tremor, synkinesis, poor coordination)	Communicative disorders Specific learning disabilities ADHD

Moderate: MQ 40–50
    Assisted ambulation
    May need bracing
    Usually does not require assistive devices
    Pharmacotherapy or nerve blocks may be used
	Traditional neurologic findings
	Many exaggerated obligatory primitive reflexes, some obligatory
	Postural responses delayed or absent
		Mental retardation
		Communicative disorders
		Specific learning disabilities
		Seizures
		ADHD+
		Stereotypic behaviors

Severe, profound: MQ <35
    Wheelchair mobility
    Usually requires bracing, assistive devices, and surgery
	Traditional neurologic signs predominate
	Obligatory primitive reflexes
	Absent postural reponses
		Mental retardation
		Seizures
		ADHD++
		Stereotypic behaviors

ADHD, attention-deficit hyperactivity disorder; MQ, motor quotient.
Modified from Shapiro BK, Palmer FB, Capute AJ. Cerebral palsy: history and state of the art. In: Gottlieb M, Wilhams J, eds. *Textbook of developmental pediatrics*. New York: Plenum Publishing, 1987.

BOX 396.1   Evaluation of the Child with Suspected Cerebral Palsy

Evaluation seeks to determine the cause of the disorder and to delineate associated dysfunctions. The basis for the evaluation of the child with cerebral palsy is the same as that for a child with any other condition—history, physical examination, and appropriate confirmatory tests. The main justifications for attempts to determine the cause of cerebral palsy are prevention of subsequently affected children and alleviation of parental guilt. As part of the process of accepting the diagnosis, parents frequently express a desire to know the cause of the cerebral palsy. Establishing the cause can reassure parents that they were not responsible for their child's cerebral palsy.

Determining the cause of the cerebral palsy often is difficult. Many potentially damaging events may occur to the same child, or no risk factors may be present. The clinician must decide whether to go on a "fishing expedition" or follow the patient until signs are manifested. Taking an aggressive approach means many negative evaluations, but a less aggressive attitude may mean an affected sibling.

For children with substantial motor dysfunction, a magnetic resonance imaging (MRI) scan permits the establishment of a diagnosis of gross brain anomalies and allows an assessment of myelination. If the MRI scan suggests a stroke, evaluation for coagulopathy is warranted. If a developmental malformation is present, genetic evaluation should be considered. In the absence of an MRI abnormality, the presence of atypical findings, a positive family history of cerebral palsy, or evidence of degeneration, evaluation of possible metabolic disorders is warranted. Although no uniformity exists in such an evaluation, we recommend obtaining a complete blood count and measurement of the levels of electrolytes, glucose, uric acid, pyruvate and lactate, ammonia, plasma amino acids, and very-long-chain fatty acids, as well as assessment of kidney (including uric acid) and liver functions. Quantification of urinary organic acids by gas chromatography may be warranted, although the yield is low and indications are not clarified. Chromosomal analysis, when positive, rarely yields classic syndromes but more often shows deletions, insertions, or transpositions.

Evaluation of associated deficits is important for proper habilitation. To focus solely on the motor deficit and to miss significant cognitive dysfunction may be harmful to the child and family. Specialists in audiology, dentistry, education, nursing, nutrition, neurology, occupational therapy, ophthalmology, orthopedics, otolaryngology, physical therapy, psychology, social work, and speech and language commonly have roles to play in assisting in the management of the child with cerebral palsy. Evaluations are necessary to define associated deficits, but overdoing it is possible. The primary care provider must direct the evaluation of the associated deficits.

---

abnormal findings in the neonatal period usually do not prognosticate cerebral palsy.

Advances in noninvasive techniques of neuroimaging, particularly in ultrasonography, have provided an alternative means of assessment that may better predict cerebral palsy than does the clinical examination. Periventricular cysts, although uncommon findings, are specific for cerebral palsy. As the natural history of ultrasonic lesions is better appreciated and as techniques for assessing metabolism and blood flows (e.g., emission tomography) are applied increasingly to neonates, the ability to diagnose cerebral palsy in the neonatal period will improve.

Birth to 6 Months

Attempts to identify cerebral palsy at an early age were hindered by a reticence to diagnose cerebral palsy until a handicap was clearly evident. This practice was based in part on the observation that some children evidenced early aberrations in motor development that were associated with transitory abnormalities of tone. These abnormalities frequently did not result in a long-term motor handicap, and establishing a diagnosis was delayed to prevent misclassification. In recent years, the desire to ameliorate the effects of cerebral palsy has outweighed the fear of potential adverse effects occuring from misclassification.

The earliest presentations of cerebral palsy are subtle because the infant has not yet developed a wide range of volitional movement. Feeding difficulties related to hypotonia or uncoordinated sucking and swallowing, difficulty with diapering because of adductor tightness, and behavioral disturbance, such as impaired periodicity, excessive colic, or cerebral irritability, are common manifestations of cerebral palsy.

The motor examination of the young infant is made difficult by the differential maturation of the underlying precursors of volitional movement. Flexor hypertonus occurs in full-term newborns and normalizes during the infant's first half-year. Primitive reflexes appear during the last trimester of pregnancy, are displayed at birth, and are suppressed during the first 6 months of life. Movement is undifferentiated and reciprocating initially, but it becomes more specific as the infant ages. Although rolling usually is considered the first motor milestone, predictable motor sequences that may assist in making early diagnosis occur before rolling.

Observing spontaneous movement is the most important aspect of the motor examination. Decreased amounts of the movement may be generalized or confined to specific limbs. The baby may not kick equally, may exhibit fisting in one hand but not the other, may transfer in only one direction, or may show hand preference at too early an age. Such asymmetries are not normal.

Eliciting movements may yield information about axial abilities. In the prone position, the baby may clear the face at birth, lift the head by 1 month of age, lift the chest by 2 months, get up on the forearms by 3 months, and push up on the wrists by 4 months. By 5 months, the infant should be able to shift weight in a prone position while attempting to obtain a toy. In prone suspension, many infants are able to move their faces perpendicularly to the plane of their bodies, with vertebral extension (i.e., Landau reflex) by 3 months. The full-term baby has only minimal overshoot when being pulled into the sitting position, and the 2-month-old infant can maintain the head in line with the body if gently displaced laterally from supported sitting. The 4-month-old infant flexes the neck from a supine position. The newborn can step and momentarily support his or her weight when held in vertical suspension (i.e., neonatal positive support). By 2 to 3 months, the infant loses this stepping response and is able to support his or her weight (i.e., mature positive support response). Neuromotor signs indicating increased lower extremity tone, such as "scissoring" or assumption of an equinus position, are not normal.

The components of early movement may assist in delineating the nature of the dysfunction, but they are distant from the motor action and are not directly related. Passive tone assessment or measurement of deep tendon reflex activity yields little in infants of this age. Primitive reflexes are difficult to interpret except when they are abnormally absent or in obligatory forms or when the most immature of the primitive reflexes exist (e.g., a Moro reflex beyond 6 months or stepping beyond 2 months).

If the pediatrician sees generalized decreases in movement, notices asymmetric findings, or elicits a neurodevelopmental examination that approximates that of an infant of one-half the child's chronologic age, the examination is abnormal. The examination has limited prognostic value because the situation is likely to change with maturation. However, early identification permits early intervention and monitoring. An abnormal motor examination requires delineation of other areas of neural functioning because dysfunction usually is diffuse.

6 to 18 Months

Motor delay is the basis for the diagnosis of cerebral palsy. However, lesser motor delays may not be significant and may resolve with maturation. One technique for qualifying the amount of motor delay is to compare the child's motor age with the chronologic age to develop a motor quotient. Motor quotients of less than 50% are associated with significant motor dysfunction and should be investigated further.

The examination of the infant who has delay in acquisition of motor skills consists of assessing the degree and duration of primitive reflexes, evaluating the child for postural responses that should be developing, noticing reactions that are never normal (e.g., asymmetry), and searching for neurologic dysfunction in other areas, such as language.

As is true of the younger infant, direct observation of spontaneous movement is a sensitive method for detecting movement disorders. Watching the child's sitting, the child's locomotion in prone posture, standing, and walking, and the child's transitions between postures reveals important information about gross movement. Assessment of transferring, reaching, raking, finger isolation (e.g., pincer use), and voluntary release reveals the status of the upper extremities.

The interweaving of the suppression of the primitive reflexes and the onset of postural responses serves as the basis for volitional movement. Persistence of significant primitive reflex activity beyond the first half-year is abnormal. The Moro reflex (Fig. 396.1), or embrace response, is elicited by sudden neck extension or by slapping the side of the pillow; extension, adduction, and abduction of the upper extremities occur, followed

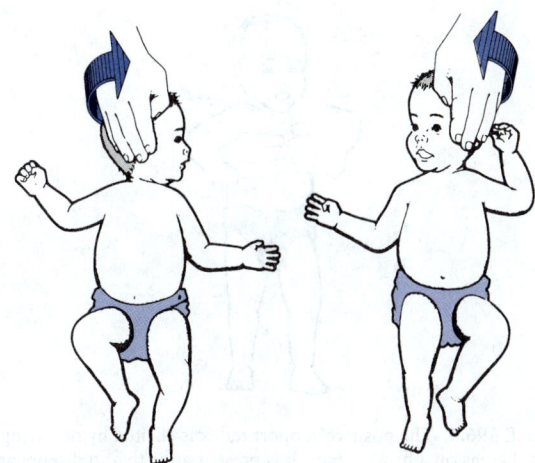

FIGURE 396.2. In the asymmetric tonic neck reflex, or "fencer" response, limbs extend on the side to which the chin is turned, and limbs on the opposite side are flexed. The reflex is present at birth and disappears at 3 to 6 months.

by semiflexion of fingers, wrists, and elbows. The asymmetric tonic neck reflex (Fig. 396.2), or "fencer" response, is elicited by turning the child's head laterally with relative extension of the limbs on the chin side and relative flexion on the occiput side. The tonic labyrinthine reflex (Fig. 396.3) is elicited by extending or flexing the neck, which alters the relation of the labyrinths and is associated with shoulder retraction and hip extension or shoulder protraction and hip flexion. If present to a substantial degree, these three reflexes interfere with midline activities, inhibit rolling, and preclude sitting.

A fourth reflex is the positive support reflex of the neonatal type (Fig. 396.4), which gives some indication of neurologic integrity of the lower extremities. It is elicited by stimulating (i.e., bouncing) the hallucal areas on a firm surface; the result is momentary lower extremity extension followed by flexion

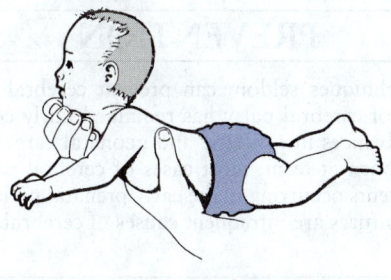

extension

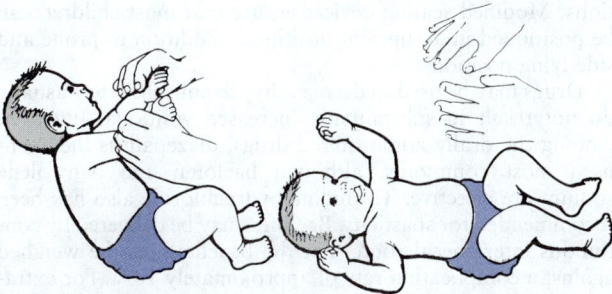

FIGURE 396.1. The Moro, or embrace, reflex is elicited by sudden neck extension or by slapping the side of the baby's pillow. The reflex is present at birth and disappears at 3 to 6 months.

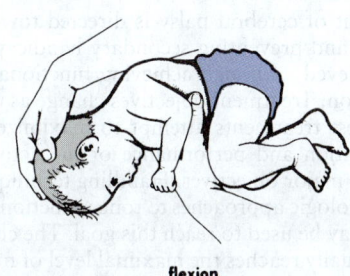

flexion

FIGURE 396.3. The tonic labyrinthine reflex is elicited by extending or flexing the neck. The reflex is present at birth and disappears at 3 to 6 months.

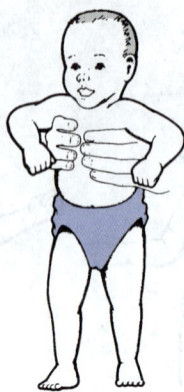

FIGURE 396.4. The positive support reflex is elicited by bouncing the hallucal areas on a firm surface. It is present at birth and disappears at 2 to 3 months.

caused by cocontractions of the hip flexors and extensors. This neonatal or immature response is followed at 2 to 3 months of age by the more mature one in which the extremities support the body weight for a longer period.

Just as important as the delineation of movement-inhibiting primitive reflexes is the evaluation of postural responses (e.g., righting, equilibrium). Postural responses appear in the second half of the first year of life and coincide with volitional movement. Postural responses keep the head and neck in vertical alignment with the body. The 5-month derotative responses are defined as the body's following the turning of the head in a derotative fashion or the head's following the axial displacement of the body. Resistance to anterior displacement by extension of the arms (i.e., anterior propping) occurs at 5 months, lateral propping is seen at 7 months, and posterior propping is noted at 9 months. Anterior propping is associated with the ability to sit in a tripod fashion, lateral propping correlates with independent sitting, and posterior propping permits pivoting in sitting. Propping responses without primitive reflex activity portend a good prognosis in the motor-delayed child.

PREVENTION

Current techniques seldom can prevent cerebral palsy. The prevalence of cerebral palsy has remained fairly constant despite the advances in obstetric and neonatal care. In children who were born at term, most cases of cerebral palsy can be traced to events occurring in the early prenatal period. Obstetric misadventures are infrequent causes of cerebral palsy.

TREATMENT

The treatment of cerebral palsy is directed toward maximizing function and preventing secondary handicaps. Normality rarely is achieved, although achieving functional outcomes is not uncommon. Treatment objectives change as the child ages.

The earliest treatments attempt to maximize motor function. Ambulation and performance of the activities of daily living are the major objectives. Handling techniques, positioning, pharmacologic approaches to tone reduction, bracing, and surgery all may be used to reach this goal. The child with cerebral palsy usually reaches the maximal level of motor function by the time he or she reaches early years of school.

In the preschool years, enhancing communication becomes increasingly important. Communicative abilities are related more closely to long-term outcome than is motor function.

The most efficient means of communication is oral. However, oral communication may not be possible for some children, and alternative methods may be used to circumvent oral motor dysfunction. Children whose motor dysfunction is sufficiently severe to render intelligible speech an unlikely goal, but who possess the necessary cognition, may be treated with augmentative methods of communication that circumvent oral communication. These methods may range from boards that require looking at the proper answer, to scanning systems, to pointing, to computer-synthesized speech.

As the child ages, concerns about communication evolve into concerns about school performance. Cognitive deficits, peer acceptance, and environmental issues are areas that commonly require intervention. Management of motor deficits focuses on the prevention of postural deformity and seeks to maintain gross motor function.

Focusing on the motor impairment alone may meet with early therapeutic success, but it ultimately fails. Long-term outcomes are related more to associated deficits and motivation than to motor ability. Communication, ability to perform activities of daily living, and circumvention of transportation barriers are related more to societal integration than to gross motor status.

Motor Therapy

The motor deficit in cerebral palsy results from the combination of abnormal tone and abnormal control of movement. Normalizing tone may permit the expression of more functional abilities. Although conceptually simple, the application of specific techniques is complex because of the different patterns of tone that may be encountered. Hypertonus, hypotonus, mixed patterns of hypertonus and hypotonus, and shifting tone occur. Most techniques are designed to decrease hypertonus and its effects. Low tone in extreme forms is treated by positioning and support. Shifting tone is the most difficult to treat. No techniques have been consistently effective in achieving control of disordered movement.

Specific techniques of handling are the mainstays of physical therapy. The physical therapy of cerebral palsy is a diverse set of approaches. Table 396.2 lists the various objectives of physical therapy. Neurodevelopmental physical therapy is the type most commonly used in the United States, but most therapists take an eclectic approach and modify their programs by using other techniques to augment standard approaches. Motor therapy is tailored to the child and is determined empirically.

In young infants and in children with severe motor deficits, handling techniques are supplemented by positioning. Positioning seeks to diminish asymmetries and tonic influences of primitive reflexes and to normalize tone. Proper positioning enhances the child's opportunity to interact with the environment. Benefits for oral motor function may be seen in improved feeding abilities and in diminished difficulty in handling secretions. Modified seating devices ensure that most children can be positioned in an upright position in addition to prone and side-lying positions.

Drugs may be used to decrease hypertonus, but they usually do not result in substantially increased volitional function. Among the orally administered drugs, diazepam is the agent used most commonly, although baclofen and dantrolene sodium are effective. Tizanidine hydrochloride also has been recommended for spasticity. Baclofen may be delivered by continuous interathecal route, but the benefits must be weighed against a complication rate of approximately 10%. For extrapyramidal dysfunction, L-dopa/carbidopa or trihexyphenidyl hydrochloride has been used. Most of the experience with these agents is not derived from their use in children with cerebral palsy, and only limited data exist regarding their effects in

TABLE 396.2

PHYSICAL THERAPY OBJECTIVES AND OUTCOMES

Objective	Outcome	Length of Therapy	Intensity	Efficacy
1. Recover function acquired previously (e.g., postsurgical)	Attain previous level of function	Short term	High	Yes
2. Acquire new skill for which readiness is demonstrated	Attain targeted skill	Short term	High	Yes
3. Improve quality of a skill	Efficiency, speed, distance	Variable	Variable	?
4. Maintain current level of function	No loss of skills	Long term	Moderate/intermittent	Possibly
5. Develop the prerequisite skills for a functional boost	Skills present to move to level 2	Long term	Moderate	?
6. Prevent postural deformity, contractures	Range of motion	Long term	Low	Not provable
7. Circumvent functional limitation	Achieve function using technology	Short term	High	Yes

Modified from Shapiro BK, Capute AJ. Cerebral palsy. In: McMillan JA, DeAngelis CA, Feigin RD, et al., eds. *Oski's pediatrics: principles and practice,* 3rd ed. Philadelphia: Lippincott-Raven, 1999.

motor and nonmotor areas (e.g., effects on learning with long-term use). Pharmacologic approaches must be coupled with targeted, measurable goals.

Nerve blocks with agents such as alcohol or phenol have been used to treat localized motor dysfunction caused by spasticity (e.g., heel cord tightness or adductor overactivity). Botulinum toxin now is the agent used most commonly for nerve block. These agents are more specific than are other forms of pharmacotherapy, but the effects are not permanent. Whether nerve blocks can prevent surgical interventions is not clear.

Bracing may be used to assist function, to prevent deformity, or to normalize tone. For example, in children who have spastic diplegia and obligatory positive supporting responses, such as marked equinus, bracing of the ankle and foot may be used to stretch tight muscles and to prevent contracture or provide a more stable base for walking. By providing a fixed point to work against, bracing may improve the function of children with choreoathetosis. Bracing is used most commonly for foot and ankle problems, but splinting of the upper extremity may improve hand function.

Although surgery is the oldest intervention used in cerebral palsy, it is the approach in the greatest state of change. Surgical goals are similar to those of other motor therapies: improvement of function and prevention of deformity. Surgery may correct deformity. It clearly changes the nature of the motor deficit, although the timing and appropriate procedure frequently are debated. Surgical approaches have moved away from consideration of static, single-joint function to more dynamic, multilevel approaches. This move has been facilitated by techniques such as gait analysis that objectively quantify movement in great detail and permit the delineation of individual muscle action during the course of a movement. As a result, surgery performed on the lower extremity is becoming more specific to the physiologic disturbance. Long-term study of these techniques is necessary to validate their efficacy.

Hand function is essential to the ultimate outcome in cerebral palsy. Good hand function may permit the person with cerebral palsy to circumvent other motor deficits. Surgical approaches to aid upper extremity function traditionally have been deferred until the child reaches late adolescence to allow for full growth and maximal cooperation from the patient. Techniques for the surgical management of the upper extremity are evolving.

Neurosurgical approaches to cerebral palsy primarily seek to alter the abnormal control of movement. Some techniques also normalize tone. Selective posterior rhizotomy is the neurosurgical technique applied most commonly. Ventrolateral thalamotomy, cerebellar pacing, and electronic stimulation also have been used. Systematic study of these approaches is difficult to achieve, and criteria for their use are still being defined.

Needs of Parents and Family

The parents of a child with cerebral palsy are expected to perform many tasks. In addition to performing normal parenting roles, they act as therapists, case managers, and advocates. They are charged with selecting the best options from seemingly contradictory recommendations, coordinating evaluations and treatment, and ensuring that their child receives the services guaranteed by federal and state laws. They are required to provide skilled nursing care. At times, the amount of effort the child requires seems endless. Sometimes, this care is accomplished to the detriment of spouses and other children.

The continuing relationship with the family affords the pediatrician the opportunity to take the long-term view. Pediatricians can assist parents by providing health care to the child, reviewing treatment goals to ensure that they are attainable and prioritized, periodically updating evaluations and imparting new information, and providing a listening ear. The pediatrician's interactions with the family place him or her in a position to consider the needs of the entire family and to see that those needs are taken into account in the development of a treatment program.

Suggested Readings

Capute AJ, Shapiro BK. The motor quotient: a method for the early detection of motor delay. *Am J Dis Child* 1985;139:940.

Capute AJ, Shapiro BK, Palmer FB. Spectrum of developmental disabilities: continuum of motor dysfunction. *Orthop Clin North Am* 1981;12:3.

Cheney PD, Palmer FB. Cerebral palsy. *Ment Retard Dev Disab Res Rev* 1997; 3:1.

Clark SL, Hankins GD. Temporal and demographic trends in cerebral palsy: fact and fiction. *Am J Obstet Gyenecol* 2003;188:628.

Crothers BS, Paine RS. *The natural history of cerebral palsy.* Cambridge, MA: Harvard University Press, 1959.

Guzzetta F, Shackelford GD, Volpe S, et al. Periventricular intraparenchymal echodensities in the premature newborn: critical determinant of neurologic outcome. *Pediatrics* 1986;78:996.

Murphy N, Such-Neibar T. Cerebral palsy diagnosis and management: the state of the art. *Curr Probl Adolesc Health Care* 2003;33:146.

Nelson KB, Ellenberg JH. Antecedents of cerebral palsy: multivariate analysis of risk. *N Engl J Med* 1986;315:81.

Park TS, Owen JH. Current concepts: surgical management of spastic diplegia. *N Engl J Med* 1992;326:745.

Penney JB Jr, Young AB. Movement disorders. In: Johnston MV, Macdonald RL, Young AB, eds. *Principles of drug therapy in neurology*. Philadelphia: FA Davis, 1992:50.

Scrutton D, ed. *Management of the motor disorders of children with cerebral palsy*. Philadelphia: JB Lippincott, 1984.

Shapiro BK, Palmer FB, Capute AJ. Cerebral palsy: history and state of the art. In: Gottlieb M, Wilhams J, eds. *Textbook of developmental pediatrics*. New York: Plenum Publishing, 1987.

Stanley F, Alberman E, eds. *The epidemiology of the cerebral palsies*. Philadelphia: JB Lippincott, 1984.

CHAPTER 397 ■ ACUTE ENCEPHALOPATHIES

JULIE THORNE PARKE

The term *encephalopathy* refers to a diffuse disturbance of brain function resulting in behavioral changes, altered consciousness, or seizures. The term usually is reserved for noninfective causes of brain dysfunction. The term *encephalitis* refers to brain dysfunction resulting from an infectious process. Clinically, it may be difficult to differentiate the two, and an infectious process must always be considered in a patient with evidence of an acute disturbance of brain function.

Many conditions can cause acute brain dysfunction in children that results in progressive alterations of consciousness (Box 397.1). Many of these conditions are treatable and may have a favorable outcome if an accurate diagnosis is made and appropriate therapy is instituted.

BOX 397.1   Causes of Acute Encephalopathy in Childhood

Oxygen or Substrate Deprivation
Hypoxia-Ischemia
  Cardiorespiratory arrest
  Cardiac dysrhythmia
  Congestive heart failure
  Hypotension
  Diffuse intravascular coagulation
  Near drowning
  Suffocation
  Pulmonary disease
  Carbon monoxide poisoning
Hypoglycemia
  Ketotic hypoglycemia
  Defects in gluconeogenesis
  Insulin-secreting pancreatic tumors
  Hepatitis
  Reye syndrome
  Alcohol intoxication

Metabolic and Endocrinologic Disturbance
Fluid and electrolyte imbalance
  Water intoxication
  Hyponatremia or hypernatremia
  Hypomagnesemia or hypermagnesemia
  Hypocalcemia or hypercalcemia
  Hypophosphatemia or hyperphosphatemia
  Acidosis or alkalosis
  Burn encephalopathy
Endocrinologic disturbance
  Diabetes mellitus
  Hypothyroidism or hyperthyroidism

Hypoparathyroidism or hyperparathyroidism
  Hypopituitarism
Organ failure
  Hepatic
  Renal
  Pancreatic
  Intussusception or volvulus
  Hypertensive encephalopathy
Inborn errors of metabolism
  Aminoacidurias (branched-chain ketoacidosis)
  Organic acidurias (propionic, methylmalonic, isovaleric acidemias, beta-ketothiolase deficiency)
  Urea cycle defects
  Disorders of fatty acid oxidation
  Disorders of pyruvate metabolism
  Mitochondrial respiratory chain disorders
  Carnitine deficiency syndromes

Postinfectious Disorders
  Acute disseminated encephalomyelitis
  Reye syndrome

Exogenous Toxins
  Drugs (sedatives, anticholinergics, psychotropics, salicylates)
  Insecticides/pesticides
  Heavy metals, lead

Modified from Plum F, Posner JB, eds. *The diagnosis of stupor and coma*, 3rd ed. Philadelphia: FA Davis, 1982.

PATHOPHYSIOLOGY

To function normally, the brain must be supplied adequately with substrates and cofactors for production of energy and for synthesis of structural components. Adequate blood flow to deliver the substrates and to remove waste products must be present. Many encephalopathies are caused by cytotoxic injury, which occurs if production of energy is disrupted by a lack of oxygen or glucose or by inadequate cerebral blood flow. Cytotoxic injury also may occur with direct poisoning of the neuron by exogenous toxins or drugs or by endogenous toxins arising from an error of metabolism or from inadequate removal of toxic wastes by the kidneys or liver. Cytotoxic injury frequently is accompanied by cerebral edema and increased intracranial pressure (ICP), which amplifies cerebral ischemia.

Other encephalopathies may be caused by interference with neurotransmission rather than actual cytotoxic injury. Severe electrolyte disturbances may alter the electrical properties of cellular membranes. Various toxins and drugs may produce similar interference with polarization of membranes or may alter neurotransmitters, thus interfering with neuronal activity.

CLINICAL PRESENTATION

The earliest signs of acute encephalopathy may be subtle and may include personality disturbances, a shortened attention span, and changes in mentation. Cognitive deficits, such as difficulty in processing new information and perceptual and memory deficits, occur commonly in the initial stages. Abnormal movements, particularly fine tremors, asterixis, or myoclonus, may be present. Primitive reflexes, such as the grasp, snout, sucking, and rooting responses, may be elicited on examination. With increasing severity of brain dysfunction, alteration in the level of consciousness occurs, progressing from lethargy and obtundation to stupor and coma. Some patients retain an alert appearance but become increasingly disoriented and agitated. Other patients have alternating periods of hyperalertness and drowsiness, gradually progressing to longer periods of unresponsiveness. Seizures occur frequently and may be generalized or focal.

Diffuse symmetric abnormalities in motor tone and strength are common findings. Focal motor abnormalities are seen uncommonly and, if present, tend to fluctuate in severity or change in location. The pupillary examination may be helpful in determining the cause of the encephalopathy. Preservation of the pupillary light reflexes in the presence of respiratory depression and deep coma suggests a metabolic coma. The absence of pupillary light reflexes suggests asphyxia, ingestion of an anticholinergic drug or glutethimide, or structural disease as the cause of coma.

ETIOLOGY

Hypoxic-Ischemic Encephalopathy

Oxygen and glucose are the two major substrates needed for production of energy in the brain. The supply of these two substrates and the cofactors necessary to allow their usage depend on an adequate cerebral blood flow. The brain is particularly vulnerable to even brief interruptions of blood flow or oxygen supply because it possesses almost no reserves of nutrients and metabolizes at one of the highest rates of any organ in the body. If the brain's oxygen supply is insufficient, whether because of decreased availability or decreased delivery, consciousness is lost rapidly. If oxygenation is restored immediately, consciousness returns without sequelae. However, if oxygen deprivation lasts longer than 1 or 2 minutes, signs of encephalopathy may persist for hours or permanently. Total ischemic anoxia lasting longer than approximately 4 minutes usually results in severe, irreversible brain damage. In rare instances, especially near-drowning events, recovery of brain function occurs despite more prolonged periods of anoxia.

Major causes leading to hypoxic-ischemic encephalopathy include obstruction of the airway, as in drowning, choking, or suffocation, and sudden decrease in cardiac output, as in cardiorespiratory arrest, severe dysrhythmias, severe hypotension, or massive systemic hemorrhage. Carbon monoxide poisoning may produce hypoxic encephalopathy because carbon monoxide binds tightly to hemoglobin and diminishes its oxygen-carrying capacity. Subacute chronic hypoxia, such as occurs in congestive heart failure, severe anemia, or pulmonary disease, also may cause encephalopathy. However, severe neurologic changes usually occur only after a prolonged period of chronic hypoxia, and the cause of hypoxia generally is evident. Cerebral edema is a consistent feature in patients who have had an acute anoxic-ischemic event and may be quite severe. Some patients may show a "lucent" interval of 12 to 24 hours before lapsing into coma with signs of cerebral edema. Occasionally, patients who have had oxygen deprivation or carbon monoxide intoxication develop delayed postanoxic encephalopathy characterized by rapid neurologic deterioration several weeks after the initial insult.

The treatment of hypoxic-ischemic encephalopathy includes adequate oxygenation, rapid restoration of perfusion, management of cerebral edema, and maintenance of good fluid and electrolyte balance. Anticonvulsant therapy also may be necessary. The prognosis is difficult to determine early in the course because patients may remain comatose for days and may eventually recover with few sequelae. Early evidence of brainstem dysfunction is a poor prognostic sign.

Metabolic and Endocrinologic Disturbances

Hypoglycemia

Hypoglycemia is a serious, correctable cause of metabolic encephalopathy. The tolerance to hypoglycemia varies, but symptoms usually occur when blood glucose levels fall to less than 40 mg/dL. The severity of symptoms is determined by the availability of alternative substrates for cerebral metabolism. Patients with hypoglycemic encephalopathy may present with a variety of neurologic symptoms, including simple confusion, delirium, abrupt focal neurologic signs resembling a stroke, focal or generalized seizures, or coma. Because the spectrum of clinical presentations is so wide, hypoglycemia should be suspected in every patient with acute neurologic dysfunction. Blood should be drawn immediately for a glucose determination, and glucose should be administered. If treated promptly, neurologic symptoms are reversible. Persistent deficits may occur with prolonged or recurrent hypoglycemic attacks. The most common symptomatic form of hypoglycemia in children is ketotic hypoglycemia (Box 397.2).

Diabetic Ketoacidosis

Diabetes mellitus is the most common endocrine disease presenting as acute encephalopathy, although pituitary, adrenal, parathyroid, and thyroid disorders occasionally present with similar symptoms. Diabetic ketoacidosis typically occurs in patients with relatively severe diabetes who neglect to take their insulin or who have an associated acute infection. Polyuria, polydipsia, and fatigue lead to a dehydrated state with metabolic acidosis. Nausea, vomiting, and acute abdominal pain

---

BOX 397.2   Ketotic Hypoglycemia

Ketotic hypoglycemia is seen most frequently in thin, young children who have a mild infectious illness that precipitates vomiting, altered mental status, and seizures, accompanied by hypoglycemia and ketosis. The cause of this disorder is not clear, but it may be the result of limited liver glycogen stores and an inability to mobilize gluconeogenic precursors. Patients with this disorder should be treated immediately with glucose and then should be maintained on dietary therapy consisting of frequent feedings during the day and bedtime snacks. Another common cause of hypoglycemia is insulin overdose. Less common causes of hypoglycemia include hereditary defects in gluconeogenesis, insulin-secreting pancreatic tumors, deficiency of growth hormone or cortisol, hepatitis, and Reye syndrome. Excessive ingestion of alcohol also may produce hypoglycemia.

---

may be prominent early in the course. Hyperventilation occurs commonly and reflects the body's attempt to compensate for the metabolic acidosis. The neurologic examination is nonfocal, and brainstem function usually is intact.

The treatment of diabetic ketoacidosis may have serious neurologic consequences. Sudden lowering of serum osmolality may produce a shift of water into the brain, thus causing marked cerebral edema. This condition should be suspected when patients recovering from diabetic ketoacidosis complain of headache or become increasingly lethargic. Profound hypophosphatemia may occur as dehydration is corrected and the serum glucose level is lowered, causing further neurologic dysfunction. In addition to ketoacidosis, hypoglycemia, uremia, hypertension, and cerebral infarction should be considered in the diabetic patient presenting with acute encephalopathy.

Disorders of Fluid and Electrolyte Balance

Disturbances in water and sodium metabolism can cause a spectrum of neurologic signs and symptoms, ranging from confusion and seizures to deep coma with increased ICP. Neuronal function depends on a correct ionic environment and can be altered by any changes in composition or volume of body fluids. Electrolyte disturbances occur fairly frequently in young children because their cutaneous water losses are relatively higher than those of adults and renal conservation of water is less efficient than that in adults. Young children have a reduced tolerance for water deprivation or abnormal water loss. Disorders of electrolytes and serum osmolality are common causes of acute encephalopathy in children. Consciousness is altered if serum osmolality is less than 260 mOsm/kg or greater than 330 mOsm/kg. The total concentration of osmotically active materials in the interstitial and intracellular fluids is equal because water diffuses freely across the cell membranes. A decrease in extracellular osmolality leads to cellular overhydration, whereas an increase in extracellular osmolality leads to cellular dehydration.

Hyponatremia. Hyponatremia or water intoxication may be caused by a sudden hypotonic water load, a disproportionate loss of sodium, or inappropriate retention of water. Numerous neurologic disorders stimulate release of antidiuretic hormones in excess of the amount required to maintain a normal concentration of serum sodium. Meningitis, head trauma, brain neoplasms, and acute or subacute peripheral neuropathy have been associated with the syndrome of inappropriate levels of antidiuretic hormone. Various endocrine disorders, pulmonary disorders, and drug ingestions increase secretion of antidiuretic hormones and predispose the patient to development of hyponatremia. Chronic hyponatremia, which may occur in chronic renal disease, is better tolerated than are acute changes in sodium balance. Moderately severe hyponatremia may cause confusion, delirium, and multifocal myoclonus. Seizures and coma usually are associated with severe hyponatremia and may be life-threatening. Seizures may be multifocal or generalized and typically occur with serum sodium concentrations between 95 and 110 mEq/L.

The treatment of hyponatremia depends on the cause. Infants with hyponatremic dehydration are rehydrated with isotonic solutions. Patients with water intoxication resulting from excess antidiuretic hormones or a free water load often can be treated with fluid restriction. Hypertonic saline solutions should be reserved for patients with severe hyponatremia manifested by seizures or coma.

Hypernatremia. Acute hypernatremia usually is caused by severe water depletion in children with diarrhea. It also may occur in patients receiving excessively concentrated solutions by tube feeding or in patients with diabetes insipidus. Symptoms of encephalopathy usually occur with serum sodium levels in excess of 160 mEq/L or total osmolalities of 340 mOsm/kg or more. Most of the dehydration in hypertonic states is intracellular. Because circulatory volume is relatively well maintained, clinical signs of dehydration, such as tachycardia and poor skin turgor, are less prominent than in hyponatremic or isotonic dehydration. Brain shrinkage predisposes the child to petechial brain hemorrhages and to extraaxial hemorrhage. Venous sinus thrombosis and cerebral infarctions also may occur. The mortality rate is high, and many survivors have permanent neurologic sequelae, including hemiparesis, seizure disorders, and mental retardation.

The treatment of hypernatremic dehydration involves the slow replacement of fluids. Rapid rehydration predisposes to cerebral edema with seizures and other manifestations of water intoxication.

Hypocalcemia. Hypocalcemia produces hyperexcitability of the peripheral and central nervous systems. Headaches and muscular cramping and twitching are early signs. Positive Chvostek and Trousseau signs are elicited easily, and carpopedal spasm may be prominent. Seizures commonly occur and may be generalized, focal, or multifocal. Management consists of correction of the metabolic disturbance with intravenous administration of calcium gluconate. Long-term oral administration of calcium and vitamin D may be necessary, depending on the underlying cause.

Hypercalcemia. Neurologic manifestations of hypercalcemia include headaches, hallucinations, rigidity, tremor, and psychotic behavior. Some patients present with slowly progressive dementia. Treatment depends on the cause. Severe hypercalcemia may require the use of a chelating agent.

Hypomagnesemia. Symptoms of hypomagnesemia, which occur when serum magnesium drops to less than 1 mEq/L, include confusion, irritability, hallucinations, and coma. Muscle twitching, myoclonic jerks, and tremors are common occurrences. Generalized seizures may occur. Examination shows increased muscle tone, carpopedal spasm, and positive Chvostek and Trousseau signs. Treatment consists of slow intravenous administration of magnesium sulfate.

Hypermagnesemia. Severe hypermagnesemia causes somnolence, lethargy, coma, and respiratory failure. Peripheral neuromuscular paralysis with loss of the deep tendon reflexes occurs. Treatment, which is difficult to provide, may include the administration of calcium and neostigmine, and hemodialysis may be necessary in severe cases.

Organ Failure

Hepatic Encephalopathy. Acute hepatic failure during childhood has numerous causes, including inborn errors of metabolism, acute viral hepatitis, Reye syndrome, and ingestion of hepatotoxic substances. Other disorders, including hepatolenticular degeneration (Wilson disease), chronic heart failure, and biliary atresia, are more likely to cause symptoms of chronic hepatic failure. Acute hepatic encephalopathy may be precipitated in these patients by intercurrent infection, excessive protein intake, or gastrointestinal hemorrhage. Numerous metabolic disturbances, many of which may contribute to the encephalopathic state, occur in hepatic failure. Hyperammonemia, hypokalemia, hypomagnesemia, and alkalosis are common findings. Short- and medium-chain fatty acids and beta-hydroxylated phenylethylamines accumulate and may act as toxins or false neurotransmitters. Alterations in the pattern of serum amino acids also occur.

Patients may show initial apathy, confusion, or lethargy. Some patients have visual hallucinations and become extremely agitated. Coarse, flapping tremor of the hands (asterixis) frequently occurs. Grimacing, jerking, and other motor disturbances are also common. Seizures can occur at any time during the encephalopathy. The level of consciousness may fluctuate dramatically from confusion to reversible decerebrate or decorticate posturing. The laboratory examination is helpful in making the diagnosis of hepatic coma because many of the liver function test results are abnormal and the arterial blood ammonia level usually is markedly elevated. A bleeding diathesis may predispose the patient to development of an intracranial hemorrhage. The electroencephalogram shows diffuse slowing in the early stages and progresses to an unusual pattern of triphasic waves as the patient becomes stuporous.

Treatment of acute hepatic encephalopathy focuses on correcting multiple metabolic abnormalities, reducing ammonia generation, and managing cerebral edema. Intake of protein should be severely limited, and broad-spectrum antibiotics and lactulose may help to reduce the accumulation of ammonia. Exchange blood transfusions or hemodialysis can be used to correct the metabolic abnormalities and to improve clotting functions. Liver transplantation should be considered in cases of severe encephalopathy. Although hepatic coma may be reversible, the mortality rate is high.

Uremic Encephalopathy. Both acute renal failure and chronic renal failure are associated with numerous neurologic complications, including uremic encephalopathy, peripheral neuropathy, hypertensive encephalopathy, hemorrhagic complications, and dialysis dysequilibrium syndrome. Common systemic diseases with renal manifestations in childhood include poststreptococcal glomerulonephritis, Henoch Schönlein purpura, systemic lupus erythematosus, and hemolytic-uremic syndrome. The precise cause of the encephalopathy associated with uremia has not been determined, and the severity of neurologic symptoms does not correlate well with the level of azotemia. Encephalopathic features have been reported in patients with blood urea nitrogen values as low as 48 mg/100 mL, but such features have been absent in other patients with blood urea nitrogen values exceeding 200 mg/100 mL. Some investigators have suggested that increased permeability of cell membranes allows access to the brain by neurotoxic compounds such as organic acids that normally are excluded. The clinical picture of uremic encephalopathy is nonspecific. Early symptoms include lethargy or agitation, tremulousness, asterixis, and myoclonic jerks. Tetany that is unresponsive to administration of calcium may occur. Muscle tone usually is increased. Generalized or focal seizures may occur, and meningeal irritation with nuchal rigidity has been described. Myokymic twitching of muscles, cramps, and intractable hiccups are possible.

Treatment of uremia by dialysis may lead to a form of encephalopathy known as the *dialysis dysequilibrium syndrome*. This syndrome is characterized by the abrupt onset of lethargy, visual hallucinations, and generalized seizures progressing to a comatose state; it can occur at the end of dialysis or up to 24 hours later. Papilledema and other signs of increased ICP may be observed. These symptoms are secondary to cellular overhydration, which occurs when urea is removed from the circulation and extracellular space but remains high in the intracellular space. The dialysis dysequilibrium syndrome can be prevented by avoiding overly aggressive dialysis. Symptoms may be treated with mannitol or saline.

Hypertensive Encephalopathy. Acute encephalopathy with seizures or coma may be the initial symptom of hypertensive disease. Neurologic symptoms may begin abruptly with severe headache, vomiting, and seizures, which tend to be focal, progressing to obtundation and coma. Patients frequently have focal weakness or focal neurologic signs on examination. Visual obscurations may occur. Most patients with hypertensive encephalopathy have abnormal funduscopic examinations with retinal artery spasm, retinal exudates, or papilledema, although the fundi may be normal. Hypertensive encephalopathy usually is associated with a sustained diastolic pressure of 120 mm Hg or greater, but it may occur at lower pressures that are higher than age-dependent normal baseline values. Initially, neurologic signs tend to be focal and fleeting in duration because they are caused by vasoconstriction. In the later stages, the patient experiences focal increases in vascular permeability, focal edema, and necrosis. Neurologic signs become more persistent, typically lasting a few minutes to several days but then disappearing, leaving little residual deficit. Spinal fluid pressure usually is elevated, as is cerebrospinal fluid protein. Magnetic resonance imaging (MRI) may show a posterior cerebral edema syndrome. Prognosis is good if hypertension is controlled aggressively.

Pancreatic Encephalopathy. Acute pancreatitis may cause encephalopathy, and chronic relapsing pancreatitis may cause episodic stupor or coma. The encephalopathy usually begins several days after the onset of pancreatitis and is characterized by agitation or stupor, focal or generalized convulsions, and signs of bilateral corticospinal tract dysfunction. The pathogenesis is not understood, although postmortem evidence of patchy demyelination of white matter in the brain has led to the hypothesis that enzymes liberated from the pancreas play a role. Biochemical complications of acute pancreatitis, such as hyperosmolality, acidosis, and hypocalcemia, also may contribute to the encephalopathy.

Reye Syndrome

Reye syndrome, an encephalopathy with fatty degeneration of the viscera, may occur after numerous viral infections, but it most commonly follows influenza B viral infections and varicella. However, no virus has been recovered from brain tissue, and the disease is not caused by active viral invasion. This syndrome may occur in persons of all ages but usually does so among children and adolescents. The mortality rate is high, and many survivors have significant neurologic sequelae.

The origin of Reye syndrome is unknown. Several environmental toxins and drugs, particularly salicylates, have been implicated as possible causative agents. Reye syndrome probably is not a specific disease but is a common presentation of multiple different conditions. Characteristically, profuse vomiting and confusion occur several days after an upper respiratory tract infection or varicella. A phase of hyperexcitability with restlessness, disorientation, and combativeness follows. More severely affected children become comatose with decorticate or decerebrate posturing. Classic signs of rostrocaudal deterioration with progressive loss of brainstem reflexes may occur. Numerous laboratory abnormalities are seen, the most significant of which are elevated serum transaminase levels, hyperammonemia, and hypoprothrombinemia. The bilirubin level is normal. Hypoglycemia occurs in 40% of patients, most often in children younger than 2 years old. The serum cholesterol concentration is decreased, as are levels of several serum proteins, including lipoproteins, clotting factors, and components of the complement system. The histopathologic features in the liver are characteristic, showing microvesicular steatosis, glycogen depletion, and abnormal mitochondria. Mitochondrial abnormalities have been seen in neurons, renal tubular cells, and other organs. The most prominent neuropathologic feature is marked cytotoxic cerebral edema.

The treatment of Reye syndrome is directed at supportive care to correct metabolic abnormalities and to manage cerebral edema, which may be massive. Administration of hypertonic solutions of glucose and mannitol, early elective intubation, hyperventilation, and monitoring of ICP have roles in the standard treatment of Reye syndrome. Other treatment modalities that may be helpful include use of neomycin and lactulose, if serum ammonia concentrations are high, and intravenous administration of L-carnitine. Controversial treatment modalities include corticosteroid therapy, induction of coma with pentobarbital sodium, induction of deep hypothermia, and exchange transfusions. The incidence and severity of Reye syndrome have declined dramatically in recent years, possibly because of a reduced use of salicylates, earlier recognition of inborn errors of metabolism, or changes in the characteristics of the viral agents responsible for Reye syndrome. Current opinion is that salicylates add additional metabolic insult to a patient already experiencing a primary mitochondrial injury. Aspirin should not be given to children at risk of developing Reye syndrome.

Inborn Errors of Metabolism

Many inborn errors of metabolism may cause acute, often recurrent, encephalopathic symptoms. In many patients, the enzyme deficiency is incomplete. Children with inborn metabolic errors, particularly those with disorders of fatty acid oxidation, may be completely well for years until a minor illness or prolonged fasting triggers a metabolic crisis that results in acute encephalopathy. In addition to disorders of fatty acid oxidation, defects in pyruvate metabolism, mitochondrial respiratory chain disorders, urea cycle defects, carnitine deficiency syndromes, glycogen storage disorders, and numerous amino acidopathies and organic acidurias may cause recurrent episodes of vomiting, ataxia, and altered sensorium.

A history of similar episodes, a family history of consanguinity, or a previously affected sibling strongly suggests an inherited defect in metabolism. Collection of laboratory samples at the time of presentation is important because laboratory abnormalities may correct rapidly with administration of intravenous fluids. Diagnostic studies should measure levels of blood ammonia, lactate, glucose, serum amino acids, a carnitine and acylcarnitine profile, and urine organic acids and acylglycines.

Intoxications

Drug-induced encephalopathy always must be considered in the child presenting with unexplained seizures or an alteration in mental status, particularly if evidence of involvement of other organ systems is present. Drug-induced encephalopathy may be caused by accidental ingestion, therapeutic overdosage,

---

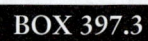

BOX 397.3   Exogenous Toxins Causing Acute Encephalopathy

Pharmacotherapeutic Agents
Sedative/hypnotics (barbiturates, glutethimide, benzodiazepines)
Narcotic analgesics
Antihistamines
Anticholinergics
Anticonvulsants
Phenothiazines
Tricyclic antidepressants
Salicylates
Iron
Penicillin
Cimetidine
Steroids

Drugs of Abuse
Alcohol
Amphetamines
Narcotics
Cannabis
Lysergic acid diethylamide (LSD)
Mescaline
Psilocybin
Phencyclidine
Solvents

Environmental Toxins
Carbon monoxide
Lead and heavy metals
Organophosphates
Dichlorodiphenyltrichloroethane (DDT)
Hydrocarbons
Solvents

---

or deliberate abuse. Many drugs in common use are capable of producing agitation, delirium, stupor, and coma when they are taken in large amounts (Box 397.3).

Sedatives

Sedatives such as barbiturates, benzodiazepines, glutethimide (Doriden), and alcohol produce coma if taken in large enough amounts. Nystagmus, ataxia, and dysarthria frequently precede signs of impaired consciousness in sedative overdosage. In larger amounts, most sedatives selectively depress the level of consciousness and respiratory function but spare pupillary light reflexes. The pupils may remain small and reactive even with large ingestions that produce coma, hypotension, respiratory failure, and flaccid paralysis with areflexia. A notable exception is glutethimide, which characteristically produces midposition or moderately dilated pupils that are unequal and fixed to light. Glutethimide tends to cause prolonged coma with marked fluctuations in the level of consciousness. Treatment is primarily supportive, but dialysis may be useful in patients with severe cases.

Anticholinergics

Intoxication with antihistamines and anticholinergic agents such as tricyclic antidepressants and scopolamine causes central nervous system excitation with confusion, anxiety, hallucinations, and delirium. Other symptoms may include flushing, dry skin, dilated pupils, tachycardia, and urinary retention. Hyperpyrexia, seizures, and coma may occur. Anticholinergic intoxication may be reversed by repetitive intravenous administration of physostigmine salicylate. Cardiac dysrhythmias frequently occur with overdosage of tricyclic antidepressants and may require aggressive therapy.

Salicylates

Encephalopathic symptoms may occur with acute or chronic salicylate intoxication. Initial symptoms include hyperpnea, vomiting, tinnitus, restlessness, and delirium. Lethargy, convulsions, and coma with respiratory failure and cardiovascular collapse may follow. Salicylate ingestion must be differentiated from Reye syndrome and organic acidurias that cause metabolic acidosis. Treatment consists of intravenous fluid replacement with correction of acidosis. Acetazolamide administration increases the excretion of salicylates. Exchange transfusion, peritoneal dialysis, or hemodialysis may be necessary in patients with severe cases. The neurologic symptoms are potentially reversible, although severe poisoning may be fatal.

Environmental Toxins

Numerous environmental toxins can cause acute encephalopathic symptoms. Chlorinated insecticides may cause a period of excitability with disorientation, tremor, muscle twitching, and headache, which is followed by seizures and respiratory failure.

Inorganic lead poisoning occurs with long-term ingestion of the metal from lead-containing paint or putty or from exposure to smelters. Nonspecific symptoms of systemic involvement precede the development of encephalopathy. Initial symptoms may include irritability, anorexia, failure to gain weight, constipation, vomiting, and anemia. The onset of the encephalopathy often is abrupt, with a brief period of ataxia and persistent vomiting followed by intractable seizures and signs of massive cerebral edema. Papilledema and cranial nerve VI palsies are common occurrences. Focal motor signs and focal or multifocal seizures may suggest a mass lesion rather than diffuse encephalopathy. Lumbar puncture generally is contraindicated because of the likelihood of herniation. However, if performed to rule out infection, it may show an elevated protein concentration and mild mononuclear pleocytosis.

Initial management involves treatment of cerebral edema and control of seizure activity. Chelation therapy is indicated in severe cases. The prognosis for patients with acute lead encephalopathy is poor. The mortality rate is high, and patients who recover have a high incidence of permanent neurologic deficits, including mental retardation, behavioral disorders, motor disabilities, and persistent seizure disorders.

Acute Disseminated Encephalomyelitis

Symptoms of acute encephalopathy occasionally occur after or in conjunction with a systemic illness. In some cases, the encephalopathy is caused by direct viral invasion of the nervous system. However, other instances appear to be caused by an indirect, immune-mediated reaction to the infection. Acute disseminated encephalomyelitis (ADEM) is an acute demyelinating disease that occurs after administration of some immunizations or after infections including rubella, rubeola, varicella, herpes zoster, mumps, mycoplasma pneumoniae, Epstein-Barr virus, and other viruses. The demyelination is thought to occur as a result of an acquired, delayed hypersensitivity to myelin and a direct attack on the myelin sheath by sensitized lymphocytes. Alternatively, one suggestion is that damage to small vessels may be the primary event in the pathogenesis of the illness with a secondary loss of myelin.

Clinical evidence of neurologic deterioration appears in a few days to 3 weeks after a vaccination or a viral illness. Initial symptoms include nonspecific signs such as fever, headache, vomiting, anorexia, and meningismus. The nonspecific symptoms may be followed by the acute onset of seizures, with rapid progression to confusion, lethargy, and coma. Other patients develop motor deficits, visual field defects, optic neuritis, aphasia, ataxia, movement disorders, myelopathy, or cranial nerve abnormalities. Younger patients may have generalized seizures and evidence of cerebral edema rather than multifocal signs. The disease usually is acute, progressing to maximal severity within 1 week. The duration varies; some patients show a rapid improvement within days, and others improve slowly over the course of several weeks. No pathognomonic laboratory findings occur in ADEM. The cerebrospinal fluid protein level may be mildly elevated, and lymphocytic pleocytosis may be present. The electroencephalogram usually is abnormal, showing diffuse, nonspecific slowing. MRI is helpful diagnostically, revealing disseminated multifocal lesions in white matter, basal ganglia, and brainstem consistent with edema, inflammation, and demyelination. Hemorrhagic white matter lesions may occur.

Treatment focuses on reduction of cerebral edema and aggressive management of seizures. Corticosteroids and immunoglobulin therapy may be helpful. The mortality rate is high, with death occurring in 10% to 30% of patients. Approximately one-third of the survivors have neurologic sequelae.

Suggested Readings

Andreoli S. Renal manifestations of systemic diseases. *Semin Nephrol* 1998; 18:270.

DeVivo D. Reye syndrome and associated metabolic encephalopathies. In: Fishman M, ed. *Pediatric neurology*. Orlando, FL: Grune & Stratton, 1986:203.

Green A, Hall M. Investigation of metabolic disorders resembling Reye's syndrome. *Arch Dis Child* 1992;67:1313.

Jackson M, Schaefer J, Johnson M, et al. Presentation and clinical investigation of mitochondrial respiratory chain disease. *Brain* 1995;118:339.

Jones B, Egelhoff J, Patterson R. Hypertensive encephalopathy in children. *AJNR Am J Neuroradiol* 1997;18:101.

Longo N. Mitochondrial encephalopathy. *Neurol Clin* 2003;21:817.

Marks N, Bodensteiner J, Bobele G, et al. Parainflammatory leukoencephalomyelitis: clinical and magnetic resonance imaging findings. *J Child Neurol* 1988;3:205.

Parke J. Para-infectious neurologic syndromes. In: Fishman M, ed. *Pediatric neurology*. Orlando, FL: Grune & Stratton, 1986:219.

Pavlakis S, Phillips P, DiMauro S, et al: Mitochondrial myopathy, encephalopathy, lactic acidosis, and strokelike episodes: a distinctive clinical syndrome. *Ann Neurol* 1984;16:481.

Piomelli S, Rosen J, Chisolm J, Graif J. Management of childhood lead poisoning. *J Pediatr* 1984;105:523.

Plum F, Posner J. Multifocal, diffuse, and metabolic brain diseases causing stupor and coma. In: Plum F, Posner J. *The diagnosis of stupor and coma*, 3rd ed. Philadelphia: FA Davis, 1982:177.

Polinsky M. Neurologic manifestations of renal disease. In: Berg B, ed. *Principles of child neurology*. New York: McGraw-Hill, 1996:1327.

Roberts M, Slover R, Chase H. Diabetic ketoacidosis with intracerebral complications. *Pediatr Diabetes* 2001;2:109.

Signorini E, Lucchi S, Mastrangelo M, et al. Central nervous system involvement in a child with hemolytic uremic syndrome. *Pediatr Nephrol* 2000;14:990.

Trauner D. Neurologic complications of gastrointestinal and liver disease. In: Berg B, ed. *Principles of child neurology*. New York: McGraw-Hill, 1996: 1317.

Treem W. Inherited and acquired syndromes of hyperammonemia and encephalopathy in children. *Semin Liver Dis* 1994;14:236.

Vaquero J, Chung C, Cahill M, Blei A. Pathogenesis of hepatic encephalopathy in acute liver failure. *Semin Liver Dis* 2003;23:259.

Wright R, Mathews K. Hypertensive encephalopathy in childhood. *J Child Neurol* 1996;11:193.

CHAPTER 398 ■ STATIC ENCEPHALOPATHY

TIMOTHY E. LOTZE

Static encephalopathy is a syndrome of abnormal motor functions and postural mechanisms caused by nonprogressive abnormalities of the developing brain. The term encompasses a heterogenous group of disorders whose causes are diverse, and it often is used synonymously with the term *cerebral palsy* (see Chapter 396). In addition to the motor dysfunction, which may range from mild to severe, associated neurologic difficulties, including mental retardation, seizures, communication dysfunction, and visual and hearing deficits, may be present. Furthermore, a variety of musculoskeletal problems may result. In the United States, as many as 500,000 children and adults may be affected. Thus, they represent an important public health responsibility.

The classification of static encephalopathy has changed little from Freud's description of more than a century ago. These categories reflect the involvement, individually or in combination, of the following structures: the cerebral hemispheres, leading to upper motor neuron signs including hypertonia and spasticity; the basal ganglia, leading to extrapyramidal signs; and the cerebellum, leading to hypotonia and ataxia. The resulting classification includes spastic forms (hemiplegia, diplegia, or tetraplegia), extrapyramidal forms (choreoathetosis or dystonia), and a cerebellar form (ataxia). Frequently, the clinical picture is not pure, and mixed forms often are described. The comparative frequency of each form of static encephalopathy as determined from Swedish studies is shown in Table 398.1. The preponderance of spastic forms is evident. In general, male subjects outnumber female subjects at a ratio of 1.2:1.0. The increasing prominence of diplegic forms (symmetric lower extremity involvement greater than that in the upper extremities) is the result of increased survival of low-birth-weight infants (Table 398.2).

The prevalence of static encephalopathy has changed substantially since 1960. During the 1960s, a decline in the prevalence of static encephalopathy to 1.5 per 1,000 live births was attributed to improved prenatal and perinatal care. In particular, better treatment of Rh incompatibility, with resulting decrease in damage to basal ganglia from kernicterus, has led to a reduction of the extrapyramidal form. Conversely, through the 1970s, the prevalence steadily increased, related to better perinatal care, especially of very low-birth-weight infants. The current overall prevalence of static encephalopathy is 2.1 per 1,000 live births, and this rate has not changed significantly during the past 3 decades. For the most recent reporting period from the Swedish population-based studies, gestation-related prevalences were 86 per 1,000 live births for extremely premature infants of less than 28 weeks' gestation, 60 per 1,000 for infants of 29 to 31 weeks' gestation, 6 per 1,000 for those of 32 to 36 weeks' gestation, and 1.3 per 1,000 for infants of more than 36 weeks' gestation. Overall, nearly 50% of affected children were low-birth-weight infants (i.e., less than 2,500 grams). A slight increase in the prevalence for static encephalopathy among infants of less than 31 weeks' gestation occurred for this period. This increase has been attributed in part to the rise in multiple births owing to more frequent use of assisted fertilization.

RISK FACTORS

Risk factors for static encephalopathy vary with the period or timing of the insult. More than a century ago, Little described static encephalopathy and related it causally to difficulties in the birth process. However, data from several large population-based studies confirmed the subsequent theory, first advanced by Freud, that static encephalopathy in most children cannot be attributed to birth asphyxia and that "difficult birth in itself is merely a symptom of deeper effects that influenced the development of the fetus." Intrapartum asphyxia is thought to be causely related in only 20% of cases of static encephalopathy. Congenital disorders may account for 30% to 40% of the total, and infections of the central nervous system account for another 5% to 10%. In fact, no specific cause can be identified for as many as 50% of infants in whom the condition develops. In infants born at term, neonatal events that previously have been attributed to asphyxia are at least *as likely to occur* in association with underlying congenital disease. These events include meconium in the amniotic fluid, low 10-minute Apgar scores, neonatal seizures, apnea, newborn neurologic abnormalities, and slow head growth. The term infant with low Apgar scores from a late asphyxial event who does not show signs of newborn encephalopathy will not develop static encephalopathy. Furthermore, epilepsy and mental retardation alone do not follow birth asphyxia as the sole cause. Prematurity, low birth weight, and placental dysfunction are increasingly important factors in the genesis of static encephalopathy. Risk factors in the very low-birth-weight infant include hypotension, acidosis, sepsis, seizures, pneumothorax, and prolonged ventilation.

Spastic diplegia most commonly is the result of prematurity and postnatal complications of premature birth, including periventricular leukomalacia and intraventricular hemorrhage. When it occurs in the full-term infant, spastic diplegia usually is the result of a complicated pregnancy and delivery. Spastic diplegia does not occur in the term infant whose only insult at birth is late asphyxia (i.e., antenatal risk factors must be considered).

Since 1960, infant mortality has decreased dramatically in the developed countries of the world. This decrease has been attributed to improved prenatal and perinatal care. That these improvements have not had a favorable effect on the frequency of static encephalopathy provides further support for causative factors other than the birth process itself in this disorder.

TABLE 398.1

COMPARATIVE PERCENTAGE DISTRIBUTION OF STATIC ENCEPHALOPATHY (SWEDISH SERIES, 1991 TO 1994)

Hemiplegia	33%
Tetraplegia	6%
Diplegia	44%
Ataxia	4%
Dyskinesia	12%

TABLE 398.2

COMPARATIVE GESTATIONAL PERCENTAGE DISTRIBUTION OF STATIC ENCEPHALOPATHY (SWEDEN, 1991 TO 1994)

Type	<28 Weeks	29–31 Weeks	32–36 Weeks	>36 Weeks
Hemiplegia	9%	10%	32%	44%
Diplegia	83%	76%	56%	25%

Extensive evaluation of electronic fetal monitoring revealed that this technique did not improve the outcome in terms of neurologic development in either term or preterm infants.

To define a causal relationship between intrapartum events and cerebral palsy more clearly, the International Cerebral Palsy Task Force developed a set of specific criteria that were refined further in 2003. These criteria are described in Box 398.1. Additionally, the investigators concluded that only cerebral palsy involving spastic quadriplegia is associated with significant intrapartum events and that purely dyskinetic or ataxic forms generally are genetic in origin. Infants injured during the prenatal period may have had time to recover before parturition and thus may not have perinatal encephalopathy. Their static problems can be assigned clearly to insults occurring at a time other than birth.

Static encephalopathy also may result from postnatal events such as infection, trauma, or cardiac disease, although only 10% to 20% have this origin. Less commonly, systemic disease (hematologic, immunologic, or metabolic), neoplasm, vascular malformation, or dysmyelinating disease is responsible. Postnatal events leading to static encephalopathy may occur throughout infancy and childhood. Of these, infection and trauma are the most significant.

PATHOPHYSIOLOGY OF MOTOR DYSFUNCTION

The developing brain has specific areas of greater vulnerability to insult based on cellular and vascular factors. These areas of vulnerabilty change as the brain matures. In the preterm infant, the periventricular region is a watershed area particularly sensitive to oxidative stress. Damage to this region results in spastic diplegia as the cortical fibers projecting to the lower extremities are more medially placed. By term, the basal ganglia and parasagittal structures are more prone to damage.

The abnormalities of motor function that accompany static encephalopathy represent disorders of tone, posture, balance, and involuntary movement. When static encephalopathy occurs in premature infants, as many as 80% have a diplegic form. Disorders of balance reflect cerebellar involvement and are characterized by ataxia and, to some extent, hypotonia. Disorders of involuntary movement are accompanied by dystonia and choreoathetosis and indicate an insult to the basal ganglia.

Neuropathologic evaluation of static encephalopathy demonstrates a fixed, nonprogressive lesion. The motor dysfunction hardly is static, however. The spastic disorders, particularly the diplegic form, commonly present with hypotonia, and only over the course of weeks or months does the pattern of spasticity develop. Similarly, the movements of choreoathetosis that signify extrapyramidal involvement seldom are present in early infancy and often begin to emerge after the child's first birthday. The evolution of motor involvement reflects the interplay of maturing normal neural elements and impaired or abnormal neural elements.

The pathophysiology of these motor disorders may be divided into six major categories. The categories may overlap in some children, and not every individual displays the full array of abnormalities, except possibly those who are impaired most severely. This classification provides a useful framework, however, for understanding the pathophysiology of motor difficulties in persons with static encephalopathy (Box 398.2).

BOX 398.1

Criteria that Define an Acute Intrapartum Hypoxic Event as Sufficient to Cause Cerebral Palsy

All four essential criteria must be met to support an association.

Essential Criteria
1. Metabolic acidosis (pH <7 and base deficit of 12 mmol/L)
2. Early onset of severe or moderate neonatal encephalopathy in infants born at 34 or more weeks of gestation
3. Spastic quadriplegic or dyskinetic type of static encephalopathy
4. Exclusion of other identifiable causes such as trauma, coagulation disorders, infectious conditions, or genetic disorders

Suggestive But Not Specific Criteria
- A recognized sentinel event
- Sudden and sustained fetal bradycardia or the absence of heart rate variability in the presence of persistent, late, or variable decelerations, usually after a hypoxic sentinel event when the pattern previously was normal
- Apgar scores of 0 to 3 beyond 5 minutes
- Onset of multisystem involvement within 72 hours of birth
- Early imaging study showing evidence of acute nonfocal cerebral abnormality

Adapted from: Haukins GD, Speer M. Defining the pathogenisis and pathophysiology of neonatal encephalopathy and cerebral palsy. *Obstet Gynecol* 2003;102:628.

ASSOCIATED ABNORMALITIES

Associated neurologic abnormalities may be seen in patients with each form of static encephalopathy. Approximately 65% of the total population with static encephalopathy has some degree of mental retardation. Other common associations include visual deficits (approximately 20%) and seizures (approximately 30%). Nearly 50% of affected children have strabismus. Approximately 60% are able to ambulate. Among the spastic forms of the disorder, children with tetraplegia generally have profound retardation, cortical blindness, and seizures. In addition, they are likely to have swallowing difficulties as a

BOX 398.2

Classification of Pathophysiology of Motor Difficulties in Persons with Static Encephalopathy

- Disorders of postural fixation result in an inability to orient the trunk and extremities to attain a vertical posture and are caused by spasticity in the limbs and hypotonia of the trunk.
- Failure to suppress brainstem postural reflexes similarly disrupts proper orientation to the environment. These reflex centers rely on labyrinthine (vestibular) input to modulate extensor tone, thus increasing extensor tone in the supine position and flexor tone in the prone position. In neither position can the child interact effectively with his or her external surroundings.
- Disorders of tone are associated with spasticity (increased velocity dependent reistance) in the antigravity muscles, which are the flexor muscles of the upper extremities and the extensor muscles of the lower extremities. The end result consists of flexed upper extremities and extended lower extremities, which prevent the performance of both individual and integrated motor activities and can ultimately lead to fixed postural deformities.
- Disorders of voluntary movement are characterized by a lack of motor planning and integrated motor activities, which can be noted most easily in walking, running, or hand dexterity.
- Disorders of involuntary movement encompass dystonia and choreoathetosis. Such movements often are exacerbated by attempts to initiate voluntary motor acts and may be heightened by anxiety or tension. In some children, these involuntary movements may progress over the course of time to rigidity, in effect reducing involuntary movements and virtually prohibiting voluntary acts.
- Failure of development of cortical reactions results in the inability of a child to generate appropriate self-protection mechanisms or to suppress certain primitive reflexes such as the palmar and plantar grasps.

manifestation of pseudobulbar palsy, to be at greater risk for poor nutrition and for aspiration and its attendant problems, and to be nonambulatory. The hemiplegic and diplegic forms of static encephalopathy are accompanied by retardation and seizures in one-third of affected children. Hemianopia (a visual field deficit) may occur in one-third of all patients with hemiplegia. Children with choreoathetosis may have normal intellect and rarely have seizures. Their severe motor disorder can limit functional mobility severely, and these children frequently are assumed to be more cognitively impaired than they may be.

DIFFERENTIAL DIAGNOSIS

Static encephalopathy is a diagnosis of exclusion and one that should not be based on a single examination. Repeat examinations are necessary to distinguish static encephalopathy from progressive disorders and from familial disorders of similar appearance. Progressive static encephalopathy is a contradiction in terms and should prompt careful review of the diagnosis. As an acquired disorder, static encephalopathy does not exhibit a familial pattern. It often presents with hypotonia and must be distinguished from other causes of hypotonia. In patients

with static encephalopathy, the degree of hypotonia exceeds the degree of weakness, and the deep tendon reflexes usually are brisk. Injury to the spinal cord may produce weakness and hypotonia initially. Spinal muscular atrophy or anterior horn cell disease (Werdnig-Hoffmann disease) is characterized by weakness, hypotonia, and areflexia. Disorders of peripheral nerves and muscles cause weakness and hypotonia that are proportional, and, in the case of peripheral nerve disease, hyporeflexia also is present.

The spastic forms of static encephalopathy must be differentiated from other neurologic disorders that are associated with upper motor neuron signs, including the following: intracranial mass lesions such as a neoplasm, brain abscess, or subdural fluid collection; hydrocephalus; cerebrovascular disease, such as vasculitis or arteriovenous malformation; metabolic disorders such as arginase deficiency; and disorders of white matter, to include various types of leukodystrophies or multiple sclerosis. The clinical presentation of these disorders should be distinguishable readily from that of static encephalopathy. The extrapyramidal forms of static encephalopathy must be differentiated from other extrapyramidal disorders of childhood, including the different forms of dystonia, benign familial chorea, and Huntington disease.

TREATMENT AND PROGNOSIS

A multidisciplinary team approach is required for adequate management of patients with static encephalopathy. Team members include the child's primary care provider, therapists, teachers, social workers, and consultants from neurology and physical medicine and rehabilitation, among others. Treatment goals for patients with static encephalopathy include optimizing the motor and intellectual capabilities of each child and providing for realistic social interaction. Motor dysfunction requires an individualized physical and occupational therapy program and an appropriate educational curriculum. Physical therapy is essential to minimize contractures and orthopedic deformities from muscle imbalance. In some instances, surgical intervention may be required; in others, orthotic devices may be sufficient to treat these problems. Pharmacologic interventions for spasticity include centrally acting benzodiazepines or baclofen. Baclofen also can be administered intrathecally by a surgically implanted pump. Alternatively, botulinum A toxin has proved effective in reducing spasticity after injection in selected muscles or muscle groups. Efficacy is time-limited, necessitating repeated treatments every 3 to 6 months. Phenol injections and dorsal rhizotomy sometimes are performed in selected populations to reduce spasticity, although improvement in functional mobility may be variable and may reflect other impairments, including difficulties with motor planning and interference from involuntary movements.

Regular reassessment of the child with static encephalopathy is essential to evaluate the status of the therapeutic and educational regimen and to provide for appropriate modifications. In some instances, deterioration or apparent deterioration occurs and must be assessed carefully. Possible explanations for apparent deterioration are as follows: inaccurate initial assessment; inappropriate expectations of parents and therapists; an inadequate or inappropriate treatment program; depression; medication side effects; progressive musculoskeletal deformity secondary to growth or limited mobility from pain or weight gain; or unrecognized, slowly progressive disorders such as muscular dystrophy, spinal muscular atrophy, leukodystrophy, neuronal storage disease, a neoplasm, or a chronic infection such as human immunodeficiency disease, acquired immunodeficiency syndrome, or subacute sclerosing panencephalitis.

The possible role of depression deserves emphasis. Children with static encephalopathy can be identified readily by their motor dysfunction. By preschool age, these children are capable of recognizing that they are different, and appropriate attention must be given to their mental health as well.

The prognosis for a child with static encephalopathy depends on numerous factors, including the extent of the motor dysfunction, the extent of associated abnormalities, and the availability of appropriate educational and therapeutic programs. A child with spastic tetraplegia is least likely to demonstrate significant progress, whereas a child with mild spastic hemiplegia or diplegia has a very favorable prognosis. In either case, the roles of the family and society will be major determinants. As predictors for ambulation, independent sitting by 24 months and crawling by 30 months are useful indicators. Virtually all children with hemiplegic static encephalopathy will walk and, as a group, have the best prognosis.

As many as 90% of patients with static encephalopathy will survive into adulthood, thus reinforcing the need for long-term planning and preparation.

FUTURE CONSIDERATIONS

The prevention of static encephalopathy should be a long-term research goal. Improved prenatal and perinatal care is responsible for previously improved incidence rates, and advances in the treatment of Rh incompatibility states have reduced the occurrence of extrapyramidal forms of the disorder. Improved perinatal care also has led to increased survival, however, especially of preterm infants, thereby enlarging the group that is at risk. Effective strategies, including neuroprotective therapies, are required to minimize this possibility. Similarly effective strategies must be developed to promote the treatment and education of these children and to integrate them into their families and society. Advances in brain imaging and spectroscopy (nuclear magnetic resonance imaging, near-infrared and single photon emission computed tomography) may provide fundamental information regarding the functional capabilities of the brain in neonates who are at risk for having static encephalopathy. This information can serve as a guide to treatment strategies for such children during their later years.

Suggested Readings

American College of Obstetricians and Gynecologists, Kudrjavcev T, Schoenberg BS, Kurland LT, et al. Cerebral palsy (CP)—trends in incidence and changes in concurrent neonatal mortality: Rochester, Minnesota, 1950–1976. *Neurology* 1983;33:1433.

Bax M. Terminology and classification of cerebral palsy. *Dev Med Child Neurol* 1964;6:295.

Davies PA, Drillien CM, Foley J, et al. Cerebral palsy. In: Drillien CM, Drummond MB, eds. *Neurodevelopmental problems in early childhood.* Oxford: Blackwell, 1977:259.

Dormans JP, Pellegrino L. *Caring for children with cerebral palsy: a team approach.* Baltimore, MD: Paul H. Brookes Publishing Co., 1998.

Grant A, Joy MT, O'Brien N, et al. Cerebral palsy among children born during the Dublin: randomised trial of intrapartum monitoring. *Lancet* 1989;2:1233.

Hagberg B, Hagberg G, Olow I, et al. The changing panorama of cerebral palsy in Sweden VII. Prevalance and origin in the birth year period 1987–1990. *Acta Paediatr* 1996;85:954.

Hagberg B, Hagberg G, Beckung E, et al. Changing panorama of cerebral palsy in Sweden VIII. Prevalance and origin in birth year 1991–1994. *Acta Paediatr* 2000;90:271.

Haukins GD, Speer M. Defining the pathogenisis and pathophysiology of neonatal encephalopathy and cerebral palsy. *Obstet Gynecol* 2003;102:628.

Miller G, Clark GD, eds. *The cerebral palsies: causes consequences, and management.* Butterworth-Heinemann; 1998.

Murphy DJ, Hope PL, Johnson A. Neonatal risk factors for cerebral palsy in very preterm babies: case-controlled study. *BMJ* 1997;314:404.

Nelson KB. What proportion of cerebral palsy is related to birth asphyxia? *J Pediatr* 1988;112:572.

Percy AK. Neonatal asphyxia and static encephalopathies. In: Fishman MA, ed. *Pediatric neurology.* Orlando, FL: Grune & Stratton, 1986:57.

Swaiman KF, Russman BS. Cerebral palsy. In: Swaiman KF, Ashwal S, eds. *Pediatric neurology: principles and practice,* 3rd ed. St. Louis: CV Mosby, 1999:312.

Teplin SW, Howard JA, O'Connor MJ. Self-concept of young children with cerebral palsy. *Dev Med Child Neurol* 1981;23:730.

Torfs CP, van den Berg BJ, Oechsli FW, Cummins S. Prenatal and perinatal factors in the etiology of cerebral palsy. *J Pediatr* 1990;116:615.

Williams K, Hennessy E, Alberman E. Cerebral palsy: effects of twinning, birthweight, and gestational age. *Arch Dis Child* 1996;75:F178.

CHAPTER 399 ■ IDIOPATHIC INTRACRANIAL HYPERTENSION

MARVIN A. FISHMAN

Idiopathic intracranial hypertension is a syndrome in which increased intracranial pressure (ICP) occurs in patients who have no history of an acute insult to the nervous system such as hypoxic-ischemic disease or trauma, no acute encephalopathy such as Reye syndrome, no focal or lateralizing neurologic signs, no evidence of intracranial tumor or obstruction to cerebrospinal fluid (CSF) flow, and normal results of CSF analyses except for increased pressure. This syndrome occurs in children of all ages. No gender predilection exists as it does in adults, in whom a significant preponderance is noted in women. The syndrome has been recognized for more than 80 years. Most of the earlier reported cases were associated with otitis media, mastoiditis, and lateral sinus thrombosis. The condition then was described as *otitic hydrocephalus*. Complications of otitis media have become less frequent precipitating factors, presumably related to the more aggressive use of antibiotics in the treatment of middle-ear infections. Various conditions have been associated with this syndrome (Box 399.1). A common cause now is catch-up growth, which occurs in pediatric patients after the successful treatment of an underlying illness. It may be associated with numerous conditions such as cystic fibrosis and nutritional deprivation syndromes, correction of chronic conditions such as patent ductus arteriosus, and complications of prematurity. Rarely, a familial form of the syndrome has been reported.

Recently, diagnostic criteria for idiopathic intracranial hypertension have been proposed, as reported by Friedman and Jacobson. These criteria include the following: (a) if symptoms

> ### BOX 399.1   Causes of Idiopathic Intracranial Hypertension
>
> **Circulatory-Hematologic Conditions**
> Gastrointestinal hemorrhage
> Polycythemia
> Iron deficiency anemia
> Hemophilia
> Dural sinus thrombosis
> Hypercoagulable state
> Pernicious anemia
> Obstruction of superior vena cava
> Sickle cell anemia
> Cryofibrinogenemia
>
> **Drugs**
> Tetracycline
> Nalidixic acid
> Corticosteroid administration
> Corticosteroid withdrawal
> Progestational agents
> Indomethacin
> Sulfamethoxazole
> Oral contraceptives
> Lithium carbonate
> Thyroid hormone
> Penicillin
> Minocycline
> Gentamicin
>
> **Endocrine Conditions**
> Hyperparathyroidism
> Hypoparathyroidism
>
> Adrenal insufficiency
> Hyperadrenalism
> Menarche
> Obesity
> Menstrual abnormalities
> Pregnancy
> Hyperthyroidism
>
> **Infections**
> Infectious mononucleosis
> Mastoiditis
> Lyme disease
> Postinfectious states
>
> **Neurologic Conditions**
> Guillain-Barré syndrome
> Recurrent polyneuritis
> Head trauma
>
> **Systemic Conditions**
> Lupus erythematosus
> Sarcoidosis
> Paget disease
> Chronic hypoxia
> Pulmonary hypoventilation
> Serum sickness
> Cryoglobulinemia
> Catch-up growth
> Nephrotic syndrome
> Allergies
> Connective tissue syndromes
> Wiskott-Aldrich syndrome
> Galactosemia
> Renal insufficiency

are present, they may reflect only those of generalized intracranial hypertension or papilledema; (b) if signs are present, they may reflect only those of generalized intracranial hypertension or papilledema; (c) elevated ICP measured in the lateral decubitus position is documented; (d) CSF composition is normal; (e) no evidence of hydrocephalus, mass, structural or vascular lesion is seen on magnetic resonance imaging (MRI) and magnetic resonance (MR) venography; and (f) no other cause of intracranial hypertension is identified. Thus, increased ICP associated with many of the conditions listed in Box 399.1 would be excluded from the idiopathic intracranial hypertension syndrome using this definition.

PATHOGENESIS

The exact pathogenesis of the increased ICP is not known. Different mechanisms may be operative depending on the origin. Obstruction of the dural venous sinus system by thromboses resulting in increased intracranial venous pressure may cause decreased CSF absorption and intracranial hypertension. Alternatively, the increase in intracranial venous pressure may be transmitted directly to the CSF compartment. When the intracranial venous sinus pressure is elevated in the absence of anatomic obstructions, the pressure is thought to be secondary to the ICP. Immediate reduction in the venous pressure is noted

when the CSF pressure is lowered. The elevated venous pressure is thought to be caused by reversible compression of the sinuses.

In other situations, the mechanism is less clear. Additional possibilities include an increased rate of CSF formation, an increase in brain volume secondary to an increase in interstitial fluid volume or cerebral blood volume, or a decreased rate of CSF absorption by arachnoid villi. Increased production of CSF in the absence of a choroid plexus papilloma is highly unlikely. Studies using positron emission tomography have demonstrated that the intracerebral blood volume is not increased sufficiently to account for the increase in ICP. In addition, no evidence exists to support the presence of either vasogenic or cytotoxic brain edema to account for an increase in brain volume that could produce intracranial hypertension. The most attractive hypothesis is that of altered absorption of CSF. Supporting evidence for this hypothesis has been derived from CSF perfusion studies in patients with idiopathic intracranial hypertension that have demonstrated reduced conductance to CSF outflow. Studies of the transport of intrathecal iodine-131 human serum albumin have revealed decreased plasma absorption of intrathecally injected isotope and abnormal transport of the material within the CSF pathways, thus indicating stasis and decreased absorption.

SYMPTOMS AND SIGNS

The onset of symptoms in patients with idiopathic intracranial hypertension may be insidious or abrupt. The most common complaint is headache. Nausea, vomiting, and visual disturbances also are noted frequently. The visual complaints have included double vision, blurred vision, soreness of the eyes, and transient obscurations. Occasional complaints have included dizziness, vertiginous sensations, tinnitus, neck pain, paresthesias, radicular pain, and facial pain. The level of consciousness is relatively unimpaired.

The neurologic examination reveals no focal deficits. Occasionally, minor tremors and alterations in tone and reflexes have been noted. Abnormalities have been related primarily to the eyes and visual system. Papilledema has been noted in most cases. Young infants whose fontanelles and cranial sutures are open may not have disc edema. Occasional cases have been reported in adults without papilledema, but they have met the diagnostic criteria and had documented increased ICP by lumbar puncture. The papilledema almost always is bilateral. Sometimes, unilateral or asymmetric involvement has been reported. In children old enough to cooperate for examination, visual field defects may be noted. The most common finding is an enlarged blind spot. Other findings include generally constricted visual fields, altitudinal defects, and nasal defects, often in the inferior quadrant. Decreased visual acuity is a late finding.

DIAGNOSIS

The diagnosis of idiopathic intracranial hypertension has been facilitated by the development of noninvasive neuroimaging techniques, mainly computed tomography (CT) and MRI. The diagnosis is one of exclusion. Clinically, the patient has a relatively normal neurologic examination, normal CSF except for increased ICP, and an imaging study (CT or MRI) that shows no evidence of a mass lesion or obstruction to CSF flow. Conditions listed in Box 399.1 should be considered. Conditions that may mimic idiopathic intracranial hypertension include carcinomatous meningitis, fungal meningitis, and diffuse gliomatosis cerebri. Recently, using newer methods of MR venography, sinovenous stenoses have been identified in most patients with idiopathic intracranial hypertension. However, these findings may be secondary to the increased ICP.

TREATMENT

Approaches to lowering ICP are applicable to all patients. In children in whom a specific cause is identified (e.g., iron deficiency anemia), treatment of the underlying disorder may result in resolution of the intracranial hypertension. Similarly, discontinuation of an antibiotic thought to precipitate the syndrome often results in improvement. In patients in whom no precipitating event or other identifying condition can be treated, symptomatic therapy is instituted. No controlled studies are available regarding the effectiveness of any proposed method of therapy; in approximately 25% of patients, the problem resolves after the initial diagnostic lumbar puncture is performed.

Suggested treatment includes performing a lumbar puncture after obtaining a normal neuroimaging study. The lumbar puncture confirms the diagnosis of idiopathic intracranial hypertension and is the first therapeutic intervention. Many patients experience relief of symptoms after removal of CSF. A second lumbar puncture should be done several days later, even in an asymptomatic patient, to measure CSF pressure again. If the pressure remains elevated after several additional examinations, pharmacologic intervention is indicated. Treatment with acetazolamide may help to decrease formation of CSF and thus lower ICP. Fairly large doses, approximately 50 mg/kg/day in children, are needed to achieve a concentration sufficient to inhibit CSF-forming enzymes in the choroid plexus. Other agents, such as furosemide, 1 mg/kg/day, or glycerol, 1 to 2 g/kg every 6 hours, have been used. Raising the serum osmolality has been shown to decrease production of CSF, and this approach may be the mechanism whereby these agents reduce increased ICP when they are administered on a long-term basis. If this approach does not result in resolution of the increased ICP, a course of corticosteroids can be attempted. The goal of therapy is to relieve symptoms and to avoid development of permanent visual disabilities. Therefore, whenever possible, visual fields and the blind spot should be assessed in patients who do not respond promptly to treatment. Deterioration in the results of this examination is an indication for providing more aggressive therapy. In children in whom visual changes are present and the pressure remains elevated despite administration of pharmacologic therapy, surgical intervention should be considered. CSF diversion procedures, optic nerve sheath decompression, and lumbar thecoperitoneal shunts have been used effectively.

PROGNOSIS

The resolution of symptoms, particularly headache, after the initiation of therapy does not necessarily indicate that the pressure has been relieved. Papilledema may take weeks to months to resolve and therefore is not a good parameter by which to judge the immediate effectiveness of therapy. Direct measurement of CSF pressure is necessary to monitor treatment.

The main purpose of treatment is the prevention of persistent visual disabilities. The clinical findings early in the course of the disease do not differentiate those patients who are likely to have sequelae. The papilledema usually resolves within 3 to 6 months. Symptoms in patients who have been treated effectively usually disappear before this time. Rarely, papilledema may persist for longer than 12 months. Some patients have spontaneous resolution of the syndrome, and, in many others, the increased ICP remits as soon as any type of therapy is initiated.

Persistent impaired visual acuity is not related to the presence of transient visual obscurations or the degree of papilledema. Fortunately, only a few patients have persistent visual defects or diminished acuity. Loss of visual acuity and visual fields may be reversed with rapid, vigorous therapy, and patients may have good functional recovery. Therefore, close observation is extremely important.

A rare complication of idiopathic intracranial hypertension is the development of the empty sella syndrome. This development is thought to occur in patients with congenital absence of the diaphragmatic sella. Continued pressure on the pituitary is thought to compress the gland and to result in the eventual appearance of the sella being empty. Usually, no associated endocrine symptoms are present, but growth hormone deficiency may occur.

Recurrent episodes of idiopathic intracranial hypertension have been noted. They are unusual and are thought to occur in approximately 10% of all patients.

Suggested Readings

Amacher AL, Spence JD. Spectrum of idiopathic intracranial hypertension in children and adolescents. *Childs Nerv Syst* 1985;1:81.

Babikian P, Corbett J, Bell W. Idiopathic intracranial hypertension in children: the Iowa experience. *J Child Neurol* 1994;9:144.

Baker RS, Baumann RJ, Buncie JR. Idiopathic intracranial hypertension (pseudotumor cerebri) in pediatric patients. *Pediatr Neurol* 1989;5:5.

Baker RS, Carter D, Hendrick EB, Buncie JR. Visual loss in pseudotumor cerebri of childhood. *Arch Ophthalmol* 1985;103:1681.

Brooks DJ, Beaney RP, Leenders KL, et al. Regional cerebral oxygen utilization, blood flow, and blood volume in idiopathic intracranial hypertension studied by positron emission tomography. *Neurology* 1985;35:1030.

Corbett JJ, Degre K. Idiopathic intracranial hypertension. *Neurology* 2002;58:5.

Corbett JJ, Savino PJ, Thompson S, et al. Visual loss in pseudotumor cerebri. *Arch Neurol* 1982;39:461.

Corbett JJ, Thompson HS. The rational management of idiopathic intracranial hypertension. *Arch Neurol* 1989;46:1049.

Couch R, Camfield PR, Tibbles JAR. The changing picture of pseudotumor cerebri in children. *Can J Neurol Sci* 1985;12:48.

Farb RI, et al. Idiopathic intracranial hypertension: the prevalence and morphology of sinovenous stenosis. *Neurology* 2003;60:1418.

Fishman RA. The pathophysiology of pseudotumor cerebri. *Arch Neurol* 1984;41:257.

Friedman DI, Jacobson DM. Diagnostic criteria for idiopathic intracranial hypertension. *Neurology* 2002;59:1492.

King JO, Mitchell PJ, Thomson KR, et al. Manometry combined with cervical puncture in idiopathic intracranial hypertension. *Neurology* 2002;58:26.

Raichle ME, Grubb RL, Phelps ME, et al. Cerebral hemodynamics and metabolism in pseudotumor cerebri. *Ann Neurol* 1978;4:104.

Silberstein SD, McKinstry EC. The death of idiopathic intracranial hypertension? *Neurology* 2003;60:1406.

CHAPTER 400 ■ CEREBROVASCULAR DISEASE IN CHILDHOOD

BRADLEY L. SCHLAGGAR, ANDREW J. KORNBERG, AND ARTHUR L. PRENSKY

Cerebrovascular disease can be divided broadly into two primary pathophysiologic processes: occlusion and hemorrhage. In occlusive vascular disease, cerebral blood vessels are blocked by the formation of a clot (thrombosis) or by the migration of clotted material (emboli) from the heart, vessels, or other organs. In hemorrhagic vascular disease, rupture of blood vessels occurs with bleeding into cerebral parenchyma, subarachnoid, subdural, or epidural spaces.

These processes reduce blood flow (i.e., ischemia) to brain parenchyma. When severe ischemia leads to death of neurons and the surrounding neuropil, the process is termed *infarction*. With hemorrhage, in addition to physical disruption of nerve tissue, pressure on parenchyma can further obstruct blood flow locally, leading to ischemia and infarction.

PATHOPHYSIOLOGY

Two important factors, the blood supply and the metabolic needs of the brain region supplied, govern the extent of damage to nervous tissue produced by cerebrovascular disease. Blood is supplied to the brain by two essentially separate circulations, the carotid (anterior) and vertebrobasilar (posterior) systems, and to a lesser extent by small perforating blood vessels from the meninges. Anastomoses between the carotid and vertebrobasilar systems exist at the circle of Willis and in the meninges. These anastomoses are important because they may prevent hypoperfusion when circulation is reduced in the territory of a single vessel. The efficiency of these anastomoses in preventing ischemia and infarction is dependent on how quickly flow is interrupted. With slower occlusion, the region of brain supplied by the vessel more likely will remain adequately perfused by collateral vessels, and the area of ischemia and subsequent infarction will be minimized. When end arteries, which are smaller vessels that have few or ineffective anastomoses, become occluded, the likelihood of infarction is relatively higher. Brain parenchyma situated between the most distal portions of the two circulations or major arteries within a circulation (e.g., those from the anterior and middle cerebral arteries in the anterior circulation) is termed a *watershed zone* or *area*. These "zones" have some blood supply from both circulations and, consequently, have some protection from occlusion of one or other circulation. However, watershed areas are especially vulnerable to damage from a general decrease in the cerebral perfusion pressure that can occur with severe systemic hypotension or with very high intracranial pressure (ICP) that produces decreased cerebral perfusion.

Two fundamental mechanisms protect the brain in the setting of decreased perfusion and oxygenation: autoregulation and elevation of the oxygen extraction fraction. Autoregulation is an important physiologic mechanism that supports maintained normal cerebral perfusion (the difference between mean arterial pressure and ICP or central venous pressure) in the setting of decreased and increased systemic pressures by altering the resistance of blood vessels in the brain. To what extent the developing cerebral vasculature can autoregulate or modulate oxygen extraction and at what age the capacity for these mechanisms reaches maturity remain unclear.

Recent research has improved the understanding of the pathophysiologic processes involved in stroke and has suggested some therapeutic strategies. Experimental data suggest that ischemic brain injury is an evolving process, with the amount of injury related to the degree of diminution of local cerebral blood flow (CBF). The *ischemic penumbra* in stroke refers to a region of tissue that is electrically silent as a result of absent or decreased perfusion. Ultimately, the central core of this ischemic penumbra will be damaged irreversibly, and a surrounding ischemic zone will, with return of perfusion, survive with normal or near-normal function. If blood flow falls further in these surrounding regions, more extensive infarction will occurs, and "progression" of the stroke will be seen. When flow to these ischemic regions is restored, then clinical improvement occurs. In adults, CBF is roughly 50 mL/100g/minute. Clinical manifestations of cerebral ischemia manifest when CBF falls to less than 20 mL/100g/minute. When CBF is less than 15 mg/mL/minute, recipient tissue becomes electrically silent. CBF of less than 8 to 10 mg/mL/minute leads to the failure of ion conductance. The corresponding parameters are not well understood in the developing brain. The concept of a penumbra has suggested strategies for decreasing the ultimate size of infarcted tissue by effectively restoring blood flow to ischemic regions. Therapeutic strategies include reperfusion of ischemic areas by thrombolytic drugs or angioplasty, neuroprotection using drugs that may ameliorate the neurotoxicity of released chemicals, and anticoagulation to prevent further embolic phenomena. Prompt diagnosis and treatment may decrease the extent of infarction and may thereby reduce the ultimate morbidity in stroke.

A stroke also can be caused by obstructing the outflow of blood from the brain, which can be seen if cerebral veins or the venous sinuses are occluded. The pathophysiology of this entity is related to "backpressure," which results in stasis and subsequent ischemia, as well as raising ICP and decreasing the perfusion of the brain. This type of backpressure also may result in the rupture of smaller vessels that feed the venous sinuses.

A transient ischemic attack (TIA) is defined as loss of neurologic function lasting less than 24 hours with subsequent complete return of normal function. By definition, TIA is caused by ischemia, but not infarction, of brain tissue.

Classically, the clinical presentation of cerebrovascular disease is thought to depend on the specific brain regions and/or white matter pathways damaged and the functions subserved by these regions. Indeed, a great deal of what is known about the localization of function in the human brain stems from the consequence of cerebrovascular disease and stroke. Strokes in the anterior (internal carotid) system usually present with hemiplegia, hemisensory loss, aphasia, or hemianopsia, whereas events in the posterior (vertebrobasilar) circulation typically present with brainstem dysfunction such as bilateral motor, sensory, and visual disturbances, vertigo, abnormal eye movements, and problems with balance and coordination. Specific stroke syndromes have been well characterized but are beyond the scope of this chapter. The reader is referred to standard neurology textbooks for detailed accounts.

Stroke is a relatively rare occurrence in children. In population-based studies from Minnesota and California, the annual incidence rate was roughly 2.5 cases per 100,000 population, or approximately one-half the incidence for primary intracranial neoplasm. Of these, 0.6 to1.2 per 100,000 were ischemic strokes and 1.1 to 1.9 per 100,000 were hemorrhages, depending on whether patients with sickle cell anemia were included in the analysis (absent for Minnesota, present for California). Adult series report between 90 and 110 cerebrovascular accidents per 100,000 adults/year. Of these, most are thrombotic strokes related to occlusive vascular disease. African American children are more likely to develop ischemic strokes and hemorrhagic strokes, even when those with sickle cell disease are excluded. Their risk of death also is greater. Male patients, in general, are more likely to die of stroke in childhood.

Many strokes in children are without a known origin or are a complication of a disease originating outside the central nervous system (CNS). Congenital heart disease, sickle cell disease, vasculitis, infection, hypercoagulable states, vascular dissection, and trauma are the usual causes of childhood stroke. Although these diseases usually are evident before the stroke occurs, sometimes stroke is the presenting problem. Atherosclerosis and hypertension, the major systemic disorders associated with occlusive vascular disease in adults, are rare causes of stroke in the pediatric population.

DIFFERENTIAL DIAGNOSIS

Cerebrovascular disorders usually present as an acute alteration in neurologic function, but changes occasionally occur in a gradual or stepwise fashion. Other disorders may present with similar symptoms and need to be considered in the differential diagnosis of acute neurologic dysfunction. Brain tumors may mimic cerebrovascular disorder because of the rapid onset of surrounding edema or hemorrhage into the tumor. Unwitnessed focal seizures may present as hemiparesis, but, in contrast to hemiparesis caused by a vascular event, the signs usually begin to resolve at around 6 hours and are resolved completely within 24 to 48 hours (e.g., Todd paresis). In embolic stroke or stroke associated with an arteriovenous malformation (AVM), a focal seizure may herald the event. In these cases, the hemiparesis usually will persist for more than 24 hours. Intracranial infections, such as meningitis, may be associated with cerebrovascular events because they can involve vessel walls leading to spasm or local thrombotic occlusion. Tuberculous meningitis, a chronic form of meningitis, may present with gradual neurologic dysfunction and/or may be associated with stroke. Cerebral abscess may mimic a cerebrovascular event, but other symptoms such as fever or a source of infected emboli should help to differentiate an abscess from a vascular occlusion.

OCCLUSIVE CEREBROVASCULAR DISEASE

Mechanisms for thrombotic and embolic occlusive cerebrovascular disease in children are listed in Box 400.1.

Thrombosis

More than three-fourths of thrombotic and thromboembolic events occur in the territory of the carotid artery or branches of the middle cerebral artery. A specific cause can be identified in approximately 50% to 60% of patients, and an arterial occlusion without a specific cause can be identified in a further 20%. A cause should aggressively be sought because treatment of the primary disorder may possibly prevent recurrent episodes of stroke.

Atherosclerosis

When atherosclerosis occurs in children, generally it is because they have an inherited disorder of lipid or lipoprotein metabolism. Types 1, 2, and 4 of the hyperlipoproteinemias are associated with premature atherosclerosis, including plaques in the major cerebral vessels, in children. The same problem can be found in children with hypercholesterolemia with low levels of high-density lipoproteins and in hyperlipidemia associated with juvenile diabetes. Disorders predisposing to accelerated atherosclerosis such as juvenile diabetes, Down syndrome, and progeria also may predispose to stroke. A history of cerebrovascular disorders or coronary artery disease occurring before the age of 40 years in other family members is an indication for an evaluation of serum lipids and lipoproteins in a child with a suspected vascular accident. The management of these children involves lowering blood lipids with dietary manipulation or medication.

Arteritis

Arteritis refers to inflammatory changes in the arterial wall, which narrows or occludes the vessel, thus producing tissue ischemia. The arteritides affect a variety of different vessel sizes, with certain disorders, such as systemic lupus erythematosus (SLE), often affecting smaller vessels. The arteritides usually are associated with systemic symptoms such as fever, myalgia, arthralgia, and weight loss. Multiple organ systems, particularly the kidneys or lungs, often are involved. Significant laboratory findings include an elevated sedimentation rate, decreased serum complement, and elevated antinuclear antibody titers. However, if the arteritis is limited to the CNS, these laboratory abnormalities usually are absent, and frequently no systemic symptoms are present.

SLE is one of the most common collagen-vascular diseases in childhood. Between 13% and 30% of children with SLE have neurologic complications from their disease. In some series, 3% of children with SLE develop cerebrovascular occlusive disease. Most of them have significant multisystem disease at the onset of their neurologic complications.

Takayasu disease is an arteritis of unknown origin that primarily involves the aorta and its branches. The disorder occurs most commonly in female patients between the second and fifth decade of life, but it has been reported in infancy. Claudication in the upper extremities and loss of pulses with bruits commonly are seen. When left untreated, the disorder is progressive and may lead to death. Stroke is uncommon, occurring in approximately 10% of cases.

Other causes of arteritis such as polyarteritis nodosa and Henoch-Schönlein purpura are unusual events in children. Varicella infection has been described, with the presumed pathophysiology of arteritis involving large vessels. Stroke also should be considered in children with acquired immunodeficiency syndrome who develop focal neurologic signs because that infection also may produce an arteritis of large vessels.

Delayed-onset hemiparesis after primary spasm or thrombosis of the arteries at the base of the brain occurs with severe meningitis. This type of occlusive vascular disease is seen more commonly with chronic fungal and tuberculous meningitides, but it also can be seen with acute bacterial meningitis in children, particularly if treatment is delayed. The chances of full

BOX 400.1	Occlusive Cerebrovascular Diseases in Children and Adolescents

Thrombosis
Abnormalities of the arterial wall
    Atherosclerosis
        Lipid abnormalities
        Down syndrome
        Progeria
    Arteritis
        Isolated central nervous system vasculitis
        Systemic lupus erythematosus
        Polyarteritis nodosa
        Takayasu disease
        Henoch-Schönlein purpura
        Radiation
        Infection
            Meningitis
            Mastoiditis
            Varicella
            Human immunodeficiency virus infection
        Other
Trauma
    External and internal trauma
    Dissection
Congenital and hereditary disorders
    Sickle cell disease
    Kinking and tortuosity of vessels
    Fibromuscular dysplasia
    Williams syndrome
    Neuroectodermal disorders
        Sturge-Weber syndrome
        Neurofibromatosis 1
        Tuberous sclerosis
    Metabolic disorders
        Homocystinuria
        MELAS syndrome (mitochondrial myopathy, encephalopathy, lactic acidosis, and stroke-like episodes)
        Menke disease

    Fabry disease
    Other
Moyamoya syndrome
    Moyamoya disease
    Migraine
Acute infantile hemiplegia
Hypercoagulable states
    Dehydration
    Hemolytic-uremic syndrome
    Nephrotic syndrome
    Cryoglobulinemia
    Polycythemia
    Leukemia and its treatment
    Thrombocytosis
    Fibrinogen
    Plasminogen
    Antithrombin III deficiency
    Protein C deficiency
    Protein S deficiency
    Factor V G1691A (Leiden) mutation (activated protein C resistance)
    Lipoprotein (a)
    Prothrombin G20210A mutation
    MTHFR 677TT (hyperhomocysteinemia)
    Antiphospholipid antibodies
        Anticardiolipin
        Anti-beta-2-glycoprotein 1
        Lupus anticoagulant

Embolism
Cardiac disease
    Cyanotic heart disease
    Valvular disease
    Bacterial endocarditis
    Arrhythmias
    Tumor
Peripheral thrombosis and embolism

recovery are poor. Major strokes rarely occur when bacterial meningitis is treated early. Radiation therapy for brain tumors may predispose to arteritis of both small and larger vessels (see later).

Magnetic resonance angiography (MRA) may allow ready evaluation without the risk of formal angiography if the pathologic process is suspected to be in major vessels that supply the brain or their larger branches. Because MRA is based on flow, it is very susceptible to producing radiologic "overcalls" of vessel disease. Smaller vessels likely are best visualized by conventional percutaneous angiography, which also affords an opportunity to visualize the great vessels. The presence of multiple areas of narrowing or occlusion suggests, but is not pathognomonic of, arteritis.

The treatment of arteritis depends in part on its cause. If the inflammation is a result of an underlying infectious disorder, the infection must be treated appropriately. Antiplatelet medications may be used transiently, depending on the blood count. Arteritis seen with hypersensitivity reactions or autoimmune disorders usually is treated with immunosuppressants, including steroids, cyclophosphamide, prostacyclin, plasma exchange, and high-dose gammaglobulin, depending on the cause of the disease, the rate of progression, and other organs in-

volved. An important point is that no data exist regarding optimal treatment of childhood arteritis.

Trauma

Trauma probably is the single most common cause of occlusion of the extracranial portions of the carotid system in children. The pathophysiology associated with trauma initially is an intimal tear, then formation of a dissecting aneurysm of the involved vessel, and subsequent occlusion of the vessel by thrombosis. The thrombus may then extend distally, or an embolus can arise from the thrombus and occlude more distal vessels. The pathophysiologic events involved agree well with the clinical features. The neurologic deficit may be acute or associated with a delay in onset of symptoms with a subsequent progressive, stuttering course, often with headache and/or neck pain. Occasionally, the initial symptom is recurrent headache alone. Trauma may occur to the carotid artery in the neck as a result of intraoral trauma such as falling onto a pencil or a stick. Vertebral artery dissections associated with twisting or traction of the neck, such as in chiropractic manipulations, have been described in adults and children. Traumatic dissection should be considered in any patient presenting with neurologic complaint whose activity increases the risk of injury to the head and neck. Blunt, nonpenetrating injuries to the neck or head rarely cause thrombotic occlusion of major intracerebral vessels with or without dissection.

Congenital and Hereditary Disorders

Extracranial vessels, in particular the carotid arteries, sometimes are extremely tortuous. They may form kinks and interrupt blood flow. These vessel irregularities have been associated with transient ischemic episodes and stroke.

Fibromuscular dysplasia (FMD) is a nonatherosclerotic, noninflammatory angiopathy of unknown origin affecting medium-sized and small arteries. It usually affects female patients in their second to fifth decades of life but is a well-recognized cause of cerebral arterial obstruction causing ischemic stroke in children. Pathologically, segmental hyperplasia with intervening saccular dilatation is present. The diagnosis is made by angiography, with affected vessels showing evidence of luminal narrowing alternating with areas of mural dilatation, producing the so-called "string of beads" appearance. Finding these abnormalities in the arterial system at more than one site renders the diagnosis of FMD highly likely. Diagnosis previously was made using conventional angiography, but more recent advances in MRA have allowed FMD to be diagnosed using this less invasive technique. Ischemic stroke secondary to intracranial multifocal cerebral stenoses has been described in Williams syndrome (see Appendix B), a multisystem disorder also associated with cardiovascular and renal vascular disease.

Several neuroectodermal disorders have been associated with stroke in children. The Sturge-Weber syndrome is a congenital malformation of venous vasculature that is manifested by a facial angioma (port-wine stain) involving the first or second division of the trigeminal nerve and an associated leptomeningeal angioma on the ipsilateral side to the port-wine stain. The disorder commonly is manifest by glaucoma, progressive hemiparesis, focal seizures, mental retardation, and occasionally cerebral hemorrhage. The pathophysiologic process primarily consists of abnormal venous return through the vessels of the angioma, stagnation of blood, and local hypoxemia with subsequent damage to neurons. Diagnosis is based on identification of the clinical features and the typical calcifications on computed tomography (CT) scan that resemble a railroad track. However, only a few children with facial port wine lesions have this syndrome. Neurofibromatosis 1 has been associated with moyamoya syndrome (see later), particularly after cranial irradiation has been performed for an optic glioma or other intracranial tumors early in life. Tuberous sclerosis has been associated with embolic stroke, possibly related to emboli from cardiac rhabdomyomas. The CNS white matter changes in incontinentia pigmenti have been postulated to be secondary to vascular events *in utero*.

Sickle Cell Disease. Sickle cell disease refers to a recessively inherited hemoglobinopathy in which hemoglobin S comprises more than 50% of the hemoglobin in red cells. It is the most common hemoglobinopathy in the United States, and approximately 8% of the African American population have the trait. The prevalence of stroke in individuals with sickle cell anemia ranges from 5% to 17% in different series. Most of these patients will develop the complications before reaching age 15 years. Ischemic strokes tend to occur in younger individuals, whereas intracranial hemorrhage typically occurs in young adults. Cognitive deficits correlate with the location and volume of presumed "silent strokes" evident on MR imaging (MRI). Approximately 22% of children with sickle cell disease have these lesions. Most occur before the child reaches age 10 years. A large multicenter study is under way to investigate whether transfusion therapy prevents or ameliorates the cognitive burden caused by the cerebrovascular disease in sickle cell disease. Such treatment certainly reduces the number of clinically overt strokes.

Hemoglobin S forms intracellular aggregates, especially under conditions of low oxygen tension. This event leads to a rigid, deformed red blood cell membrane (the sickle cell). Initially, the sickling is reversible on restoration of normal oxygenation, but with repeated episodes of sickling, the membrane is damaged and remains sickled. The abnormal shape of the red cell may impede movement though the microvasculature and cause regional hypoperfusion. Although this mechanism long has been presumed to be the cause of stroke, radiologic and pathologic studies have provided evidence that the mechanism of stroke is a large-vessel occlusive vasculopathy. The vessels primarily involved include the supraclinoid internal carotid artery and the proximal areas of the middle and anterior cerebral arteries. The stenosis or occlusion of large intracranial vessels at the base of the skull can lead to the angiographic appearance of moyamoya syndrome (see later); and emboli from proximal vessels may result in distal hypoxia and further exacerbation of sickling and ischemia, especially in watershed areas. The clinical features are similar to those of other cerebrovascular events, but focal or generalized seizures commonly herald the onset of the stroke. The prognosis of an acute stroke in a patient with sickle cell disease is poor. Approximately 75% have permanent deficits, and 50% to 60% develop seizures. Management involves providing adequate oxygenation, hydration, and hypertransfusion therapy to maintain Hemoglobin S levels lower than 20%. The use of anticoagulation during thrombotic events may be indicated. Recurrent events occur commonly, but studies have shown the predictive value of transcranial ultrasonography in patients with sickle cell anemia, a technique that may allow hypertransfusion therapy to be used in high-risk individuals to prevent these events.

Metabolic Disorders. The prototype metabolic disorder associated with stroke in childhood is homocystinuria. In this recessively inherited disorder, patients have an accumulation of the amino acid homocysteine and of its derivative homocystine. Homocystine has been thought to increase platelet stickiness and possibly damage the intima of vessels. Both events predispose to development of intravascular thrombosis. Thrombi and emboli can be seen in all types and sizes of vessels of the CNS, including venous thrombosis (see later). The disorder is characterized by marfanoid habitus, mild to moderate retardation, and ectopic lenses. Homocystinuria is diagnosed by the finding of homocystine in blood or excessive amounts of the amino acid in the urine. The phenotype can be produced by different enzymatic abnormalities, with the most common type responsive to pyridoxine (vitamin B_6) because of activation of cystathionine synthase.

Other metabolic disorders associated with stroke include the mitochondrial disorders, particularly mitochondrial myopathy, encephalopathy, lactic acidosis, and stroke-like episodes (MELAS syndrome), but strokes are also seen in the following: Leigh disease and Menke syndrome; organic acidurias such as methylmalonic, propionic, and isovaleric acidemias and glutaric aciduria type 1; Fabry disease; sulfite oxidase deficiency; and ornithine transcarbamylase deficiency. These conditions are very rare causes of vascular occlusion. When present, the event usually occurs in infancy or early childhood. Laboratory diagnosis of these conditions in a child presenting with a stroke includes evaluation of blood and urine for amino acids, urine for sulfite, serum ammonia, serum copper, and both arterial and cerebrospinal fluid (CSF) lactate and pyruvate (increased in mitochondrial disorders). Specific tests for common mitochondrial gene mutations now are available commercially. Treatment of the underlying disorder may prevent recurrence.

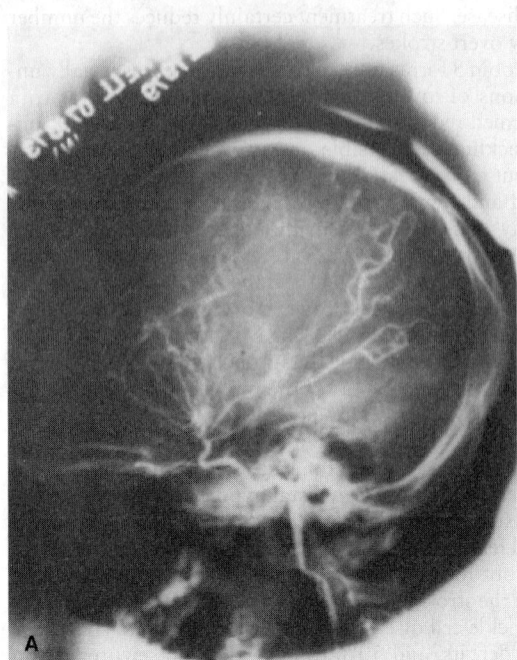

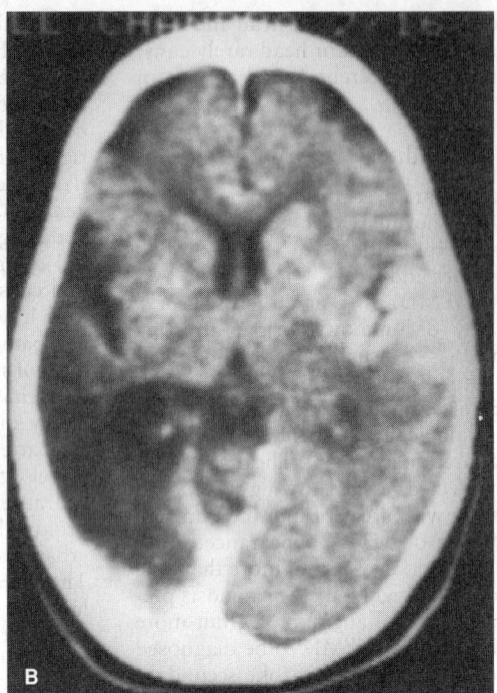

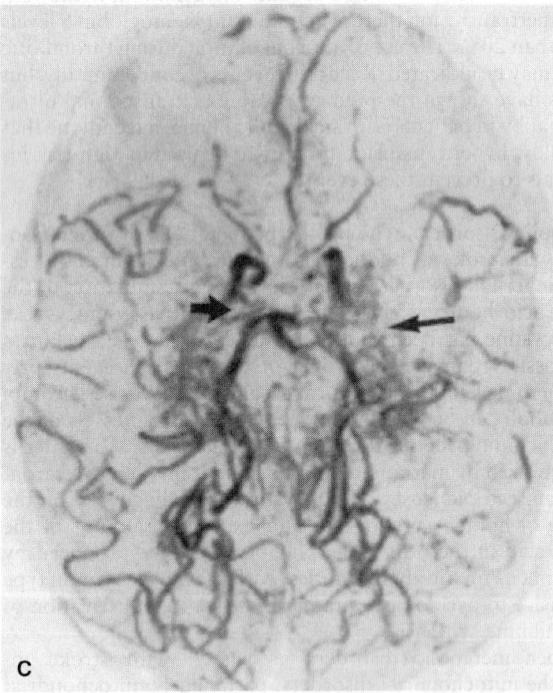

FIGURE 400.1. Moyamoya disease. **A:** A network of fine collateral vessels is seen deep in the cerebrum lateral to the sella turcica. The vessels originate, for the most part, from the branches of the external carotid artery and help to supply the internal circulation. A tortuous leptomeningeal anastomosis also helps to supply the brain. **B:** Multiple strokes of different ages are seen in both cerebral hemispheres. **C:** Magnetic resonance angiography demonstrates the fine collateral vessels deep in the cerebrum (*arrow*) and the cutoff of intracranial vessels around the circle of Willis (*arrowhead*).

Moyamoya Syndrome. Moyamoya syndrome is a chronic progressive arterial disease of unknown origin, characterized by progressive stenosis and occlusion of the intracranial portion of the internal carotid arteries and other vessels that comprise the circle of Willis. The posterior circulation is involved less often. The slow progression of the disorder allows collateral vessels to form from the external carotid circulation as well as the vertebrobasilar system. Other collateral vessels from transdural and leptomeningeal vessels occur and predispose patients to subdural bleeding. The disease is named after the appearance on angiography of the collateral vessels that supply the distal internal carotid and the middle and anterior cerebral arteries from the external carotid circulation. The Japanese term *moyamoya*, "something hazy, like a puff of smoke drifting in the air," describes the distinctive angiographic appearance (Fig. 400.1A). Most Japanese cases have no known cause, and approximately 10% are familial. However, a variety of disorders can give a similar appearance on angiography, and, therefore, this appearance should be considered a syndrome rather than a specific disease entity. Examples of these disorders include sickle cell anemia, neurofibromatosis type 1, cranial irradiation, FMD, Down syndrome, tuberculous meningitis, and Fanconi anemia. Very few cases of moyamoya disease in Western nations are familial unless the underlying cause is identified and is an inherited disorder.

Symptoms occur in childhood and affect girls more frequently than boys. Various clinical patterns have been identified, with the most common that of multiple transient ischemic events in which some of the transient episodes are followed by permanent residual neurologic abnormalities (Fig. 400.1B). Less common presentations include an acute stroke, TIAs without permanent abnormalities, and acute intracranial hemorrhage related to rupture of thin-walled collateral vessels. The disorder is progressive and is associated with declining intelligence and focal seizures. The diagnosis is based on the clinical presentation and the characteristic findings on angiography. MRI and MRA also have been shown to demonstrate the abnormalities (Fig. 400.1C). The availability of a noninvasive technique such as MRA is particularly important in children, because considerable technical difficulties are associated with formal conventional angiography (see the later discussion of new methods of investigation). However, MRA may not be as sensitive for depicting moyamoya findings as conventional angiography, so clinical judgment will dictate which test is used.

Treatment of moyamoya syndrome includes the use of antiplatelet agents, such as aspirin, and surgical procedures. Unfortunately, various medical therapies, including steroids, have failed to retard the progression of this disorder. In some studies, surgical techniques directed at improving the perfusion to partially ischemic areas of brain have improved the long-term prognosis. These procedures include arterial anastomoses between extracranial vessels such as superficial temporal or occipital arteries and dural or other cerebral arteries or by revascularization using muscle or omental grafts (encephalomyo or omental-dural anastomoses). These synangiosis procedures appear to facilitate the natural tendency to form transdural anastomoses, which are thought to sustain cerebral perfusion after completion of occlusion of the circle of Willis. Results appear to be best in those children whose disease is progressing slowly and when the surgical procedure is done before intellectual deterioration occurs.

Migraine. Migraine headaches occur in 10% to 25% of the population, with a significant percentage beginning in childhood or young adulthood. Complicated migraine, that is, migraine complicated by significant neurologic deficits such as hemiplegia lasting well into or beyond the headache, has been estimated to occur in 1% of the population. Most migraine-related neurologic events are brief, last less than 1 hour, and are associated with a full recovery. However, occasionally longer-lasting events or permanent deficits are seen. In a review of 34 years of the literature, Featherstone defined persons at risk of developing a stroke associated with migraine. Such individuals more commonly are female, have a prior history of classic or complicated migraine, and usually are younger than 40 years of age. Only approximately 15% of individuals who develop stroke after migraine are children. Adolescents and young women who take birth control pills regularly also are at greater risk. The prognosis for migraine-related stroke may be slightly better than that of other causes. The diagnosis is based on exclusion of other causes of stroke, a past history that is diagnostic for migraine headaches, and the association of the event with a migraine attack. Treatment is supportive, and use of vasodilators or anticoagulation at the onset of a neurologic abnormality has not been shown to be of definite benefit. Prophylactic treatment of migraine can reduce the frequency and severity of headache and possibly may decrease the risk for having a stroke. Ergotamines and triptans, vasoconstrictive agents used as migraine abortives, are contraindicated in patients with history of cerebrovascular disease or a history of hemiplegic or vertebrobasilar migraine.

Acute Infantile Hemiplegia

This term has been used in a variety of ways. It has been used to describe the sudden onset of a stroke with hemiplegia when no specific cause is found and also to describe a particular syndrome of fever and partial seizures of acute onset with subsequent hemiparesis. The seizures are difficult to control, and consciousness may or may not be impaired. Typically, the convulsions last for many hours, and on their resolution, the child is left with flaccid hemiparesis. The hemiparesis may improve, but 80% of the children are left with significant disabilities, including mental retardation. Epilepsy usually occurs within the following year. CT or MRI scans show evidence of an acute infarction, but no occlusion can be demonstrated with angiography in many patients. No cause of this syndrome has been defined. Because many of these catastrophes occur with acute throat infections, researchers have postulated that the cause in these cases may be inflammation of the wall of the carotid artery, but this theory never has been proven.

Perinatal Stroke

The prevalence of perinatal stroke likely is higher than previously recognized and may be on the order of 1 in 5,000 to 10,000 term births. One theory of the origin of perinatal stroke is that it is the consequence of a transient thrombophilia of pregnancy. Further, the presence of a patent foramen ovale or ductus arteriosus renders the brain more susceptible to emboli from clots in the venous system and the placenta. This scheme fits with the clinical experience that infants with perinatal stroke have a very low risk of subsequent childhood stroke. Recent studies suggest the risk to be roughly 1% to 4%. A recent case-control study demonstrated that in nearly 70% of neonates identified with perinatal stroke, at least one genetic or acquired risk for thrombophilia could be identified. Importantly, in the control population, 24% of subjects had at least one prothrombotic risk.

Hypercoagulable States

Hypercoagulability, or the tendency for circulating blood to form a thrombus spontaneously, is a potential cause of stroke in the pediatric patient. The site for formation of a clot can be in either the arterial or the venous circulation, including the dural sinuses draining the brain. Hypercoagulable states may be divided into primary and secondary causes. The primary causes include states having an absence or dysfunction of a substance or substances usually present to prevent thrombus formation. These disorders usually are inherited and present early in life. Usually, the patient has a history of recurrent thrombosis or a family history of thrombosis. These causes include protein C, protein S, antithrombin III deficiencies; plasminogen, lipoprotein (a), and fibrinogen pathway abnormalities, as well as mutations in the prothrombin gene (*G20210A*), factor V (the factor V Leiden mutation [*G1691A*], typically detected through measuring activated protein C resistance), and the methylene tetrahydrofolate reductase gene (*677TT*) causing elevated serum homocysteine. The secondary (acquired) causes are a group of diseases or drugs causing a high frequency of intravascular thrombosis, by depleting substances preventing thrombosis, increasing the propensity of blood to clot, or damaging the endothelium of blood vessels. Antiphospholipid antibodies (including antibodies to cardiolipin and beta-2-glycoprotein 1 and the lupus anticoagulant) may play a role in cases of stroke in childhood. Some other causes are found in Box 400.1. Treatment involves treating the underlying cause. In principle, if a stroke is thought to be caused by an antiphospholipid syndrome, then warfarin (Coumadin) should be considered for treatment. However, anticoagulating a hemiparetic toddler, for example, may introduce more risk than benefit. Furthermore, no specific data exist to guide management of stroke caused by antiphospholipid antibody syndrome in childhood. What is becoming clear is that these genetic and acquired risk factors for thrombophilia modulate the risk for having a recurrent arterial ischemic stroke (at least for nonperinatal stroke).

Results from a recent international (United Kingdom, Canada, Germany) collaborative effort presented at the thirty-second annual Child Neurology Society meeting demonstrated that recurrent arterial ischemic stroke occurred in roughly 10% of the nearly 700 children studied, with roughly 60% of recurrences occurring within the first 6 months after stroke. Investigators also found that the presence of a prothrombotic risk independently increases the risk of recurrence, and the risk increase is higher when multiple prothrombotic risks are present. This particular analysis found that elevated fibrinogen, lipoprotein (a), and homocysteine were the thrombophilic risk factors most likely to be linked to recurrence, but regional and population differences in prothrombotic risk and recurrence may exist. These findings eventually may have implications for treatment decisions such as dietary folate to lower serum homocysteine or limited antiplatelet/anticoagulation therapy in recognition that most recurrence takes place in the first 6 months after a stroke. Whether these risk factors conspire to modulate recurrent risk in patient populations with better-characterized risks, such as structural heart defects or sickle cell disease, is not clear. Likely, as in adults, multiple risk factors (e.g., hypertension, hypercholesterolemia, diabetes mellitus) can appear to conspire to increase the risk of cerebrovascular disease.

The adult literature suggests that thrombophilic risk factors appear to increase the risk of venous thrombosis, not arterial thrombosis. Clearly, much work remains to be done to characterize risks of stroke in the pediatric population.

Venous Thromboses

Dehydration, infection, and hypercoagulable states are the major known causes of occlusion of cerebral veins. Clinically, venous thrombosis presents with partial seizures or focal neurologic findings such as hemiparesis. Signs or symptoms of raised ICP, such as headache, vomiting, lethargy, visual disturbances, and papilledema, may be seen. Diagnosis can be difficult to establish. Particular patterns seen on CT scan such as filling defects in the occluded sinus with displacement of contrast media by thrombus (negative delta sign), angiography (particularly the venous phase), radionucleotide studies, and most recently MR venography may be helpful in establishing a diagnosis. Banker pointed out the difficulty of establishing a diagnosis in life when, in a study of autopsied cases for occlusive cerebrovascular disease, she demonstrated pathologic features that affected primarily the venous system in more than 50% of strokes in infants and children. However, many of her patients died of intracranial infections. MRI is the best initial investigation because it readily identifies the infarct, if any, whereas MR venography, which can be done at the same time, can identify thrombosed vessels (including cortical veins). Dural sinus thrombosis in children usually is treated by trying to relieve elevated ICP by lumbar puncture and removal of CSF or medication to reduce CSF production. The optic nerves must be protected and their function evaluated repeatedly over short time intervals. As of yet, no study proves that anticoagulants or thrombotic agents improve the outcome of dural sinus thrombosis in children.

Embolism

Embolic occlusive vascular disease in children has several sources, including paradoxical emboli from the venous system, phlebitis of pulmonary veins resulting from lung infections, cardiac disease, and lesions of the aorta and great vessels in the neck. For practical purposes, almost all embolic occlusions that occur in children beyond the perinatal period are the result of congenital or acquired heart disease. Most of these emboli are associated with cyanotic congenital heart disease, particularly tetralogy of Fallot and truncus arteriosus. Clinical studies suggest that embolic occlusions may occur in 5% to 10% of children with these two disorders. Approximately three-fourths of these strokes occur within the first 2 years of life. Pathology studies of children who die of congenital heart disease before or after surgical correction of these disorders suggest that the incidence of emboli may be as high as 15% to 20% and that many emboli occur after catheterization and surgical attempts have been made to correct the cardiac deformity.

Other cardiac lesions also can be a source of emboli. Disease of the mitral or aortic valves can result in cerebral emboli. Since the decline in the incidence of rheumatic fever, this cause of embolization is relatively unusual. Prolapsed mitral valves have been associated with an increased risk of embolization, particularly in the first or second decade of life. Brain emboli also may result from subendocardial fibroelastosis, cardiomyopathies, tumors of the heart such as atrial myxomas and rhabdomyomas, bacterial endocarditis, and cardiac dysrhythmias. On rare occasions, cerebral emboli also can arise from lesions in the walls of the great vessels of the thorax and neck. Coarctation of the aorta may be a source of emboli to the brain. Paradoxical embolus via a patent foramen ovale or atrial septal defect also should be considered.

Distinguishing an embolic from a thrombotic cerebrovascular event is not always possible. Strokes caused by emboli are said to be more sudden in onset, often accompanied by focal seizures or headache, and to cause of more limited deficit. At times, the deficit may be complete but improves rapidly as the clot breaks up and the area is reperfused. Unfortunately, no combination of these clinical parameters successfully distinguishes between embolization and thrombosis. If a child has a disorder in which the incidence of embolization is high, that fact becomes extremely important in establishing the diagnosis. The patient may benefit from treatment with anticoagulants or, less often, antiplatelet agents such as aspirin until the cause of the embolus can be corrected.

INTRACRANIAL HEMORRHAGE

Common causes of intracranial hemorrhage are shown in Box 400.2.

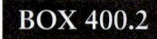

BOX 400.2   Causes of Hemorrhagic Vascular Disease

Abnormalities of the Clotting Mechanism
Decreased clotting factors
Thrombocytopenia
Disseminated intravascular coagulation

Vascular Malformations
Arteriovenous malformation
Cerebral aneurysm
  Congenital
  Acquired: mycotic, traumatic, embolic

Hypertensive Cerebrovascular Disease

Intracranial Neoplasm

Trauma

Infection
Hemorrhagic meningoencephalitis (e.g., herpes simplex virus)

Abnormalities of the Clotting Mechanism

Deficiency of clotting factors such as in hemophilia (factor VIII deficiency), factor IX deficiency (Christmas disease), von Willebrand disease, and thrombocytopenia (particularly idiopathic thrombocytopenic purpura and disseminated intravascular coagulation) can be associated with spontaneous or posttraumatic intracerebral hemorrhage. The presenting symptoms and signs of intracranial hemorrhage are seizures, focal neurologic signs, or evidence of increased ICP. The underlying diseases responsible for abnormalities in the clotting mechanism need to be corrected to ensure recovery and to prevent recurrence. On occasion, the clot may need to be evacuated surgically if control of the raised ICP cannot be achieved medically.

Vascular Malformations

Congenital abnormalities of cerebral blood vessels are a common cause of intracranial bleeding. These malformations include AVMs, angiomas, and aneurysms.

Arteriovenous Malformations

AVM is the most common malformation and pathologically consists of normal and abnormal veins and arteries. AVMs usually are found in the distribution of the internal carotid and middle cerebral arteries, but they also can occur in the posterior circulation and posterior fossa. They may present clinically as an intracranial mass, as a focal or generalized seizure disorder, or as an acute hemorrhage. Between 50% and 70% of children with AVMs present with intracranial hemorrhage, and approximately 25% to 40% present with seizures. Of those who do present with hemorrhage, most have blood in the subarachnoid space. Some have blood within the brain substance that produces acute focal neurologic signs. Presentation as a mass lesion is unusual, but the patient may have symptoms of raised ICP and slowly progressive neurologic symptoms or signs.

At the time of acute rupture, blood mixed in the CSF may result in nuchal rigidity, severe headache, nausea, and vomiting. Excessive numbers of red blood cells or xanthochromia in the CSF may lead one to suspect that a hemorrhage has occurred. Bruits can be heard over the cranial vault in approximately 25% of symptomatic AVMs. The larger the malformation, the more likely one is to hear a bruit. Most AVMs are large enough to be identified by the radiographic scanning techniques now in use, but improvement in imaging techniques may improve diagnosis further. Occasionally, a small malformation is not demonstrated by scan if no surrounding hemorrhage is present or if the AVM is obliterated by the bleeding. If an AVM is suspected, arteriography is the most useful diagnostic procedure available. MRA, based on blood flow, may fail to detect flow through a vascular malformation. Conventional angiography also is needed to determine which vessels feed and drain the malformation and to decide whether the lesion is surgically treatable. If the lesion is too extensive to be treated surgically, it may be reduced in size by introducing artificial emboli to obstruct the arteries that feed the lesion.

Telangiectasias are the second most common vascular malformations in children. They are essentially capillary angiomas. The vessels that make up the lesion look like widely dilated capillaries. These lesions occur anywhere in the brain but frequently are seen in the posterior fossa, particularly in the basis pontis. Such malformations often are asymptomatic throughout life and can be inherited (Osler-Weber-Rendu syndrome, also known as hereditary hemorrhagic telangiectasia). When symptoms are produced, they are almost always the result of intracerebral hemorrhage. Occasionally, these hemorrhages are large enough to produce elevated ICP, either by acting as a

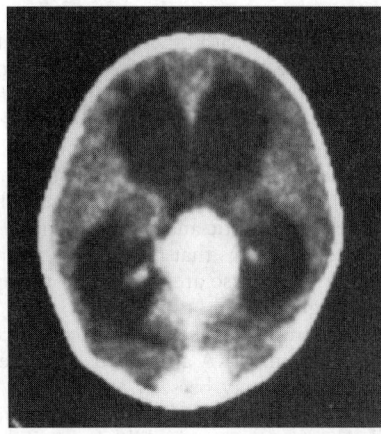

FIGURE 400.2. Aneurysm of the vein of Galen. A large aneurysm of the vein of Galen in a 6-week-old infant is shown. The aneurysm compromises the aqueduct of Sylvius and results in severe hydrocephalus.

mass or by obstructing the flow of CSF and producing hydrocephalus. The most common presentation, however, is the acute onset of focal symptoms and signs without elevated ICP. The hemorrhage often can be seen on CT scan. Usually, these hemorrhages are not large enough to require surgical evacuation. In many instances, the bleeding obliterates the associated malformation.

An aneurysm of the vein of Galen (Fig. 400.2) is, in reality, a vascular malformation involving both arteries and veins. It lies above the tectum of the midbrain and can obstruct the aqueduct of Sylvius and produce hydrocephalus. Like any other very large vascular malformation, an aneurysm of the vein of Galen may present with marked shunting of blood between arteries and veins, causing high-output congestive heart failure. This presentation is a common finding in the neonate. Infants with less severe involvement may present with increased heart size and macrocephaly because of hydrocephalus. A cranial bruit usually can be auscultated. The accepted treatment of this malformation is to occlude the feeding vessels, if possible, either by clipping of the arteries or by therapeutic embolization with metal coils. The prognosis is poor for patients presenting with a massive aneurysm or congestive cardiac failure.

Venous angiomas are common incidental findings on MRI and rarely are symptomatic. Hemorrhage is rare. Diagnosis is based on the characteristic enhanced CT or MRI findings. These lesions usually are not visualized on MRA.

Arterial Aneurysms

Aneurysms are rare findings in children. Fewer than 2% of all aneurysms become symptomatic in patients younger than age 19 years. Approximately 90% of aneurysms that become symptomatic during childhood are located in the anterior or middle cranial fossa. Most aneurysms are congenital. Arterial aneurysms have a defect in the arterial wall, and the internal elastic lamina and the media are missing. However, increased proportions of symptomatic aneurysms in children are caused by infection (particularly emboli from bacterial endocarditis), trauma, and, in rare instances, tumor. Congenital aneurysms in children occur most frequently at the distal portion of the internal carotid and the proximal middle cerebral arteries, as well as at the anterior and posterior communicating vessels. Although most aneurysms in children do present with subarachnoid and, less frequently, intracerebral hemorrhage, some act as masses and present primarily with compression of the oculomotor or other cranial nerves. A higher incidence exists of congenital aneurysms with FMD, kinking and coiling of carotid vessels, coarctation of the aorta, and autosomal dominant polycystic kidney disease, as well as with other diseases affecting elastin. Autosomal inheritance of aneurysms has been reported.

Mycotic aneurysms can result from embolization from the heart as well as from bacterial and fungal disorders affecting the meninges. Mycotic and traumatic aneurysms are present less often at the bifurcation of the major intracranial vessels and are more commonly seen distally in the middle and anterior cerebral arteries. Mycotic aneurysms are more likely to be multiple than are aneurysms that result from trauma or those that are congenital. They also are more likely to rupture, especially with anticoagulation.

Cerebral arteriography is the procedure of choice for the diagnosis of an aneurysm. MRA also has been refined to such a degree that aneurysms may be seen, particularly if they are located in larger vessels at the base of the brain. Approximately two-thirds of symptomatic children have abnormalities on CT scan, including evidence of intracerebral or subarachnoid hemorrhage or a focal enhancing lesion. Because congenital aneurysms in children frequently are larger than those seen in adults, these lesions are more apt to be found by conventional scanning techniques before rupture. The treatment of aneurysms in children is surgical and does not differ appreciably from that for the adult population. Treatment involves either clipping the aneurysm or using interventional radiographic techniques. Vasospasm occurs in the presence of subarachnoid bleeding in children, and treatment with volume expansion to produce mild hypertension and with calcium channel blockers may be useful.

Other Causes of Intracranial Hemorrhage

A cerebral hemorrhage can be a manifestation of both leukemia and the drugs used to treat it. Asparaginase has been linked to hemorrhagic and thrombotic cerebrovascular complications, but, in particular, it has been associated with cerebral venous and dural sinus thrombosis. High-dose methotrexate therapy also has been linked to stroke-like syndromes.

Hypertension is a much less frequent cause of hemorrhage in children than in adults, but such catastrophes can occur because of elevated blood pressures in conjunction with renal, cardiovascular, or endocrine disorders. Trauma certainly is the most common cause of subarachnoid hemorrhage in infants and young children and is associated with both accidental and nonaccidental injury. Child abuse should be considered strongly in an infant or toddler presenting with intracranial and retinal hemorrhages.

Bleeding into a preexisting tumor may be responsible for an intracerebral hemorrhage. An area of severe cerebral edema surrounding the lesion may be a pointer to this diagnosis.

NEW TECHNIQUES IN THE DIAGNOSIS OF CEREBROVASCULAR DISEASE

Various imaging techniques have evolved over recent years and are especially important in the diagnostic evaluation of pediatric patients with cerebrovascular disease. MRI has become the imaging modality of choice. It provides superb images with the advantages of little or no artifact related to bone. It demonstrates abnormalities before they are visible on CT, provides excellent images of the venous sinuses, and allows the diagnosis of venous sinus thrombosis to be made readily (Fig. 400.3). It has the advantage of not using radiation, as conventional CT does. The disadvantage is primarily that acquisition of data takes a considerable amount of time (although it is becoming shorter)

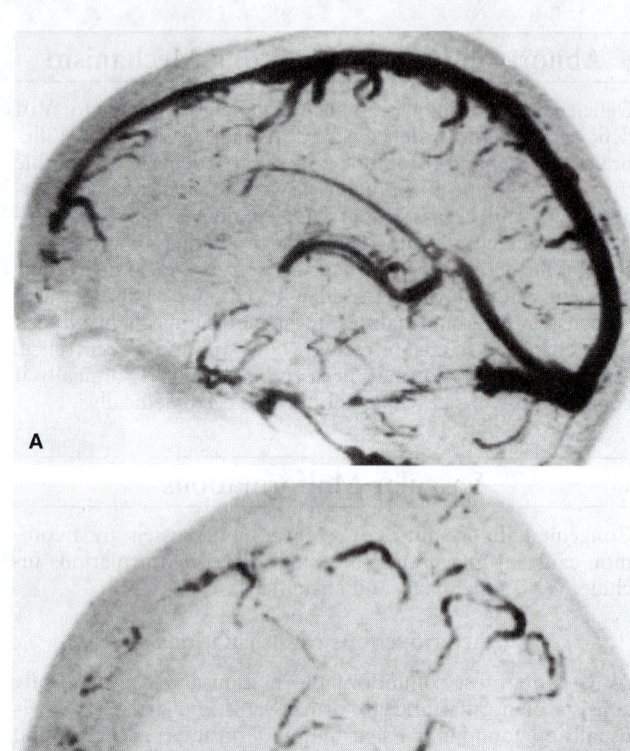

FIGURE 400.3. Sinus vein thrombosis. **A:** A magnetic resonance (MR) venogram demonstrates patent sinus veins. **B:** Sagittal sinus vein thrombosis is readily demonstrated by MR venography with a void in the signal in the sagittal sinus.

and that the images are degraded by movement. For this reason, many pediatric patients require sedation or anesthesia to provide optimal images. Conventional angiography is associated with a greater risk of morbidity and mortality. In addition to the risks of the procedure itself are the additional risks of general anesthesia and allergy to contrast medium. The procedure has an increased degree of technical difficulty in young children compared with older children and adults. MRA is a rapid, safe, and technically simpler procedure compared with conventional angiography, especially in children. At present, whether MRA will supersede conventional angiography completely is unknown, but new-generation scanners combined with more sensitive and reproducible imaging sequences may render MRA comparable to conventional angiography for some conditions such as FMD and dissection. MRA provides information on both the arterial side (Fig. 400.4) and the venous side (MR venography) (see Fig. 400.3) of the cerebrovascular system. However, until studies can show that MRA is as sensitive as conventional angiography, particularly in defining pathologic features in smaller vessels, the latter will remain the "gold standard" for the diagnosis of cerebrovascular disease.

Diffusion-weighted MRI has made a substantial impact on the evaluation of acute stroke. MRI can image the extent of water diffusion in a given volume of tissue. Infarcted tissue has greater cytotoxic edema and less water diffusion than normal tissue. Certain MRI sequences are particularly sensitive to detecting blood product, thus rendering the technique a

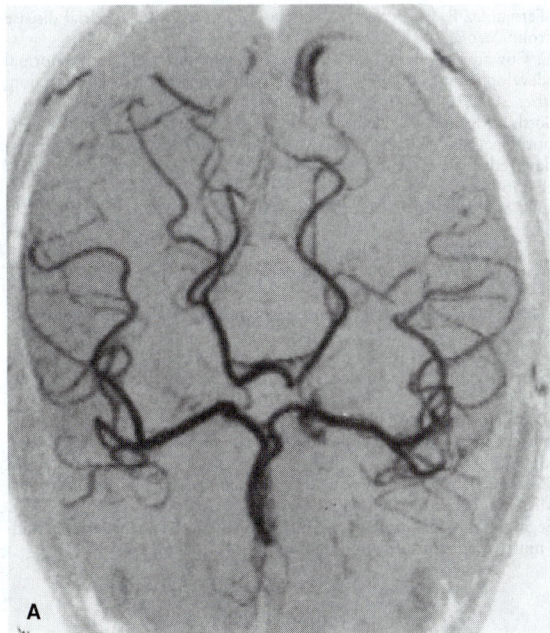
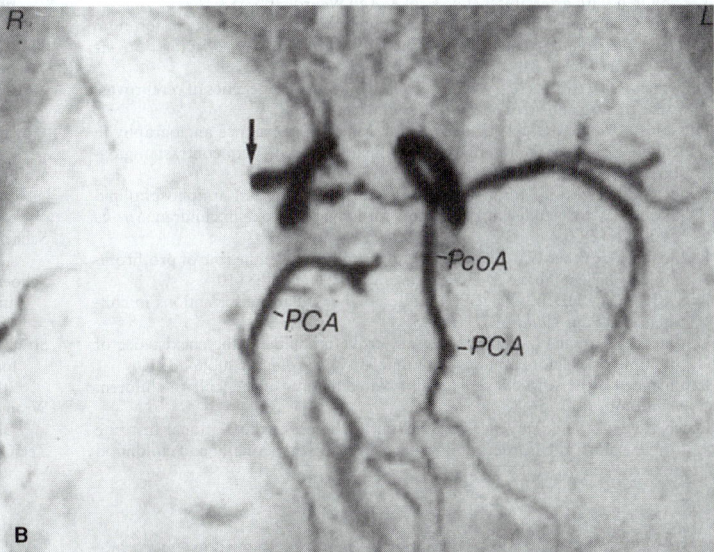

FIGURE 400.4. Magnetic resonance (MR) angiography. **A:** A normal MR angiogram. Clear, accurate images of cerebral vessels are readily obtained. **B:** An occlusion of the right middle cerebral artery is readily demonstrated (*arrow*). PCA, posterior cerebral artery; PcoA, posterior communicating artery.

useful approach to diagnosing hemorrhage. Further, the age of a hemorrhage can be delineated through MRI. Current work is directed at correlating MRI changes with discerning the time of hypoxic-ischemic injury in the neonatal period.

APPROACH TO THE PATIENT

A detailed approach to a patient with acute stroke is beyond the scope of this chapter. In general, however, the approach to a patient with cerebrovascular disease is twofold. First, providing general support and specific treatment of the event is necessary. An excellent review by Oppenheimer and associates of the complications of acute stroke is recommended reading. Second, obtaining prompt and directed diagnostic evaluation is mandatory. The diagnostic evaluation in a child presenting with a presumed cerebrovascular disorder should be geared toward identifying a cerebrovascular lesion, eliminating other causes of acute neurologic dysfunction, and identifying a cause. The importance of making an etiologic diagnosis cannot be overstated because it may enable prognostic information to be given to the family and may have potential immediate and long-term therapeutic implications in attempting to reduce the risk of recurrence. Diagnostic evaluation should be performed in an efficient manner with the diagnostic workup influenced by the most likely cause in that patient. Evaluation typically includes detailed hematologic, immunologic, cardiologic, and radiologic investigations, which are discussed in greater detail in earlier sections of this chapter. The articles by Fisher and Caplan are excellent reviews of current and potential therapies in cerebrovascular disease.

The U.S. Food and Drug Administration (FDA) has approved the use of tissue plasminogen activator (t-PA) for the treatment of acute stroke in adults. t-PA can be administered in adults within 3 hours of known onset of ischemic stroke so long as no specific contraindications are present. Currently, no study has looked at the role of this or any other thrombolytic agent in the treatment of acute stroke in children, although case reports have been published. Since the mid-1990s, several

dozen clinical trials involving putative neuroprotective agents have been performed in adults with acute stroke. At present, no agent has demonstrated the safety or efficacy to warrant approval by the FDA.

Controversies persist in the use of anticoagulant therapy in the treatment of acute stroke. At present, no evidence-based guidelines exist for the use of anticoagulation in the treatment of acute stroke in children.

In the acute setting, the general approach to a patient with stroke should include maintaining reasonable oxygen saturation and normoglycemia. Avoiding hyperthermia (maintaining temperature around 37°C) is thought to be beneficial. Intravenous fluids should be isotonic to avoid delivering excessive free water and thus potentiating cerebral edema. Seizures and elevated ICP should be treated. Immobile patients are at risk for development of deep venous thrombosis; measures such as low-dose subcutaneous heparin and compression stockings may be beneficial, particularly in a patient with known thrombophilia.

Certain acute stroke types warrant transfer of a patient to a center with neurosurgical capabilities. These include hemorrhagic stroke, posterior fossa (hemorrhagic or ischemic) stroke, and large hemispheric strokes.

Suggested Readings

Adams RJ. Stroke prevention and treatment in sickle cell disease. *Arch Neurol* 2001;58:565.

Banker BQ. Cerebral vascular disease in infancy and childhood. I. Occlusive vascular disease. *J Neuropathol Exp Neurol* 1961;20:127.

Caplan LR. New therapies for stroke. *Arch Neurol* 1997;54:1222.

Chabrier S, Lasjaunias P, Husson B, et al. Ischaemic stroke from dissection of the craniocervical arteries in childhood: report of 12 patients. *Eur J Paediatr Neurol* 2003;7:39.

Chiu D, Shedden P, Bratina P, Gortta JC. Clinical features of moyamoya disease in the United States. *Stroke* 1998;29:1347.

deVeber G, Andrew M, Canadian Pediatric Ischemic Stroke Study Group. Cerebral sinovenous thrombosis in children. *N Engl J Med* 2001;345:417.

Featherstone HJ. Clinical features of stroke in migraine: a review. *Headache* 1986;26:128.

Fisher M. Characterizing the target of acute stroke therapy. *Stroke* 1997;28:866.

Fullerton HJ, Wu YW, Zhao S, Johnston SC. Risk of stroke in children: ethnic and gender disparities. *Neurology* 2003;61:189.

Ganesan V, Prengler M, McShane MA, et al. Investigation of risk factors in children with arterial ischemic stroke. *Ann Neurol* 2003;53:167.

Günther G, Junker R, Strater R, et al. Symptomatic ischemic stroke in full-term neonates: role of acquired and genetic prothrombotic risk factors. *Stroke* 2000;31:2437.

Hademenos GJ, Alberts MJ, Awad I, et al. Advances in the genetics of cerebrovascular disease and stroke. *Neurology* 2001;56:997.

Husson B, Rodesch G, Lasjaunias P, et al. Magnetic resonance angiography in childhood arterial brain infarcts: a comparative study with contrast angiography. *Stroke* 2002;33:1280.

Kenet G, Sadetzki S, Murad H, et al. Factor V Leiden and antiphospholipid antibodies are significant risk factors for ischemic stroke in children. *Stroke* 2000;31:1283.

Kirkham FJ, deVeber GA, Chan A, et al. Recurrent stroke: the role of prothrombotic disorders (abstract). *Ann Neurol* 2003;54(suppl):S110.

Lagos JC, Riley HD Jr. Congenital intracranial vascular malformations in children. *Arch Dis Child* 1971;46:285.

Lanthier S, Carmant L, David M, et al. Stroke in children: the coexistence of multiple risk factors predicts poor outcome. *Neurology* 2000;54:371.

Lanthier S, Lortie A, Michaud J, et al. Isolated angiitis of the CNS in children. *Neurology* 2001;56:837.

Lynch JK, Hirtz DG, DeVeber GA, Nelson K. Report of the National Institute of Neurological Disorders and Stroke workshop on perinatal and childhood stroke. *Pediatrics* 2002;109:116.

Martinez-Fernandez E, Gil-Peralta A, Garcia-Lozano R. Mitochondrial disease and stroke. *Stroke* 2001;32:2507.

Mercuri E, Cowan F, Gupte G, et al. Prothrombotic disorders and abnormal neurodevelopmental outcome in infants with neonatal cerebral infarction. *Pediatrics* 2001;107:1400.

Nowak-Göttl U, Sträter R, Heinecke A, et al. Lipoprotein (a) and genetic polymorphisms of clotting factor V, prothrombin and methylenetetrahydrofolate reductase are risk factors of ischemic stroke in childhood. *Blood* 1999;94:3678.

Oppenheimer S, Hachinski V. Complications of acute stroke. *Lancet* 1992;339:721.

Rothman SM, Fulling KH, Nelson JS. Sickle cell anemia and central nervous system infarction: a neuropathological study. *Ann Neurol* 1986;20:684.

Schatz J, Brown RT, Pascual JM. Poor school and cognitive functioning with silent cerebral infarcts and sickle cell disease. *Neurology* 2001;54:1109.

Schoenberg BS, Mellinger JF, Schoenberg DG. Cerebrovascular disease in infants and children: a study of incidence, clinical features, and survival. *Neurology* 1978;28:763.

Sträter R, Becker S, von Eckardstein A, et al. Prospective evaluation of risk factors for recurrent stroke during childhood: results of the 5-year follow-up. *Lancet* 2002;360:1540.

Wraige E, Hajat C, Jan W, et al. Ischaemic stroke subtypes in children and adults. *Dev Med Child Neurol* 2003;45:229.

Zee C-S, Segall HD, McComb JG, et al. Intracranial arterial aneurysms in childhood: more recent considerations. *J Child Neurol* 1986;1:99.

CHAPTER 401 ■ EPILEPSY

KEVIN CHAPMAN AND DANIEL G. GLAZE

Epilepsy is the symptomatic expression of an underlying brain disease or disordered brain function, not a disease in the usual sense. The incidence of epilepsy has been reported to range from 0.8% to 1.1%. Epilepsy is the most common neurologic disorder seen in children, and approximately 50% of all cases of epilepsy start in childhood. Epilepsy is defined as a randomly recurring stereotyped symptom complex resulting from an unprovoked episodic disturbance of central nervous system (CNS) function, associated with an excessive, self-limited, neuronal discharge. Variation in clinical manifestations results from variation in the portion of the brain involved.

Epilepsy can have many causes; in general, any event having the potential to produce insult to the brain can result in epilepsy. In many children, the cause is static or nonprogressive encephalopathy secondary to historical antecedents such as hypoxia, hemorrhage, CNS infection, head trauma, and developmental defects of the brain. Cerebral insult as a consequence of labor and delivery complications is a much less common cause than previously thought. Although specific entities such as tuberous sclerosis, neurofibromatosis, brain tumors, some degenerative diseases, and certain inborn errors of metabolism can present initially with recurrent seizures, these diagnoses are suggested by other signs and symptoms revealed by the history and physical examination. For certain seizure disorders, historical evidence of a genetic predisposition may be present. Several gene mutations affecting membrane channels have been identified as the cause of an increasing number of epileptic syndromes. Mutations in the sodium channel genes have been linked to the syndrome of generalized epilepsy with febrile seizures plus, severe myoclonic epilepsy of infancy, and benign neonatal infantile seizure. gamma-Aminobutyric acid (GABA) receptor mutations have been associated with autosomal dominant juvenile myoclonic epilepsy. Most of these gene tests currently are available for research purposes only, but they highlight the increasing recognition that genetic factors have an integral role in the evaluation of epilepsy. Seizures can occur in certain autosomal recessive disorders (e.g., phenylketonuria), X-linked disorders (e.g., fragile X syndrome), chromosomal abnormalities (e.g., Angelman syndrome, Down syndrome), and mitochondrial disorders (e.g., mitochondrial myopathies). In approximately one-half of all children with recurrent seizures, the diagnostic workup does not disclose a specific cause.

Isolated seizures can occur as a consequence of hypoglycemia or other acute metabolic derangements. Such seizures do not constitute epilepsy because specific therapy for the primary disorder obviates the necessity of maintenance therapy with antiepileptic drugs (AEDs). The risk of experiencing unprovoked seizures by age 5 years in children with developmental disability is 3%, which is approximately fourfold greater than that of the general population. Selected subgroups with major impairments account for most of this increased risk. The risk is only 1%, similar to the general population, in those without cerebral palsy or mental retardation.

CLASSIFICATION AND DESCRIPTION OF SEIZURE TYPES

Diagnostic accuracy and treatment options have improved greatly since the 1980s as a consequence of advances made in many areas. These areas include the adoption of a universally accepted descriptive classification system, the increased availability of serum drug monitoring, the development of new AEDs, advances in video-electroencephalographic (EEG) monitoring and neuroimaging techniques, and improved knowledge of drug interactions. Nonetheless, a carefully detailed history and physical examination remain of prime importance to diagnosis.

Epilepsy is a clinical, not a laboratory, diagnosis, and errors in diagnosis, seizure classification, and subsequent treatment are most often the consequence of an inadequate history and physical examination. Numerous relatively benign, episodic spells often are misdiagnosed and even treated as seizures. They include breath-holding spells, benign paroxysmal vertigo, syncope, tics, and even masturbation. The physician rarely has the opportunity actually to witness a clinical seizure and usually must rely on a description provided by the parents. A seizure often is a frightening experience for parents, and their ability to recall details, time relationships, and the sequence of events understandably can be limited. Frequently, the parents may not have witnessed the event and can report only what they were told by a teacher or other witness. Often, obtaining a description by telephone from the actual witness is worthwhile. When the available clinical description is vague and unconvincing, an appropriate approach may be to delay definitive diagnosis and treatment and to instruct parents about what to look for should attacks recur. Asking the parents to videotape an event may provide useful information for the clinician.

The classification system for epileptic seizures currently in use is based on both clinical and EEG features (Box 401.1). It divides seizures into two major categories, generalized and partial. Generalized seizures are those in which the clinical features indicate the involvement of both cerebral hemispheres from the start. Consciousness usually is impaired, and, when motor involvement is present, it is bilateral and relatively symmet-

ric from the beginning. Conversely, partial seizures are characterized by clinical features suggesting that only a limited functional area of one cerebral hemisphere is involved. These seizures begin focally, although they may become generalized. Partial seizures are divided further into those with elementary or simple symptoms and those with complex symptoms. In children, elementary partial seizures most commonly are focal motor or focal sensory phenomena, and consciousness is preserved unless secondary generalization occurs. Complex partial seizures usually have their origin in temporal or frontal lobe structures, and the clinical features encompass a spectrum of complex phenomena, including behavioral automatisms, alterations of perception, hallucinations, changes in affect and memory, and ideational distortions.

Generalized Seizures

Generalized tonic-clonic seizures are characterized clinically by an abrupt arrest of activity and an immediate loss of consciousness. The tonic phase, consisting of sustained, generalized contraction of flexor or extensor muscles, usually lasts only a few seconds. The clonic phase that follows is characterized by symmetric, rhythmic, clonic activity consisting of alternating contraction and relaxation of major appendicular or axial muscle groups. The clonic phase lasts longer than the tonic phase, but often it terminates spontaneously in less than 5 minutes. Respiration may be irregular and stridulous, and sphincter incontinence may or may not be present. The clonic phase usually is followed by a variable period of confusion and lethargy, which may persist from minutes to hours, and sleep is common.

Clonic seizures are identical to the clonic phase of tonic-clonic seizures. Generalized tonic seizures are characterized by sustained contraction of flexor or extensor muscle groups, thus giving the child a stiff or rigid appearance. A coarse tremor may be superimposed, but it should not be confused with the rhythmic, alternating muscle contraction and relaxation of clonic activity. A distinction often can be made by asking the parents to supplement their verbal description with a demonstration of what they observed. Both clonic and tonic seizures are followed by postictal signs and symptoms similar to those seen with generalized tonic-clonic seizures.

Myoclonic seizures are characterized by brief, random contractions of a muscle or group of muscles occurring unilaterally or bilaterally, either singly or in clusters. Consciousness usually is preserved. Myoclonic seizures are seen most often with progressive or degenerative types of encephalopathy accompanied by intellectual deficits, as well as other overt abnormalities, on neurologic examination. Atonic or "drop" attacks are a subclass of myoclonic seizures and are characterized by a precipitous loss of postural tone. The child abruptly becomes limp and drops to the floor. With nonambulatory infants, precipitous loss of tone resulting in head nodding or slumping forward may occur. The duration of myoclonic seizures is only a few seconds, and immediate resumption of normal activity with no postictal lethargy or confusion occurs.

Absence seizures are characterized clinically by brief episodes of altered awareness during which transient arrest of activity occurs and the child appears to stare blankly. The duration of these episodes seldom is longer than 5 to 10 seconds, but they can recur many times a day. They rarely are seen in children younger than 3 years old, and most have their onset before 10 years of age. The child commonly is not aware that a seizure has occurred and frequently is assumed to be daydreaming. A child who is daydreaming, however, is aware of doing so and usually responds when his or her name is called or he or she is touched. In contrast, a child with absence seizures usually denies awareness of any lapse and does not respond to verbal

---

BOX 401.1 **Classification of Epileptic Seizures**

Generalized Seizures
Tonic-clonic
Clonic
Tonic
Atonic
Myoclonic
Absence

Partial Seizures
Elementary symptomatology
    With motor symptoms
    With sensory symptoms
Complex symptomatology
    With impairment of consciousness only
    With cognitive symptoms
    With affective symptoms
    With psychosensory symptoms
    Compound forms
Secondarily generalized

Reprinted from Commission on Classification and Terminology of the International League Against Epilepsy. Proposal for revised clinical and electroencephalographic classification of epileptic seizures. *Epilepsia* 1981;22:489.

or physical stimuli. Subtle motor activity such as rhythmic eye blinking, drooping of the head, or slight movements of the arms may accompany the staring episodes. The seizure is terminated by the immediate return of environmental awareness, and the child may resume an activity at the point at which it was interrupted. A generalized, symmetric three/second spike-and-wave pattern, which may be induced with hyperventilation, is the EEG hallmark of absence seizures.

Partial Seizures

Partial seizures are classified based on the loss or preservation of consciousness. During complex partial seizures, awareness is lost, compared with simple partial seizures, in which the patient remembers the event. The initial semiologic features of a partial seizure are especially important. Tonic deviation of the head and eyes to one side, or some other localized motor or sensory feature preceding a secondarily generalized tonic-clonic seizure, may be a clue to focal cortical origin of the attack. In children, elementary partial seizures usually are focal motor or sensory. The initial feature may be focal twitching involving the distal portion of an extremity, which may remain localized or spread to become a hemiconvulsion. Similarly, focal sensory seizures may be initiated by the appearance of a sensation of numbness or tingling in an extremity, which may remain confined to that area or spread to involve the entire side of the body. Consciousness often is preserved but is lost if secondary generalization occurs.

Various types of auras may precede and herald the onset of a complex partial seizure. These subjective cognitive symptoms may be characterized clinically by an abrupt alteration in mental state that involves disruption of time relationships and memory. Older children sometimes describe feelings of unreality, remoteness, detachment, or depersonalization. Forced thinking, a deluge of thoughts, or perseveration of a thought also have been described. *Déjà vu* or *jamais vu*, the impression of an inappropriate familiarity or unfamiliarity with a place or situation, occasionally may be reported. Attacks characterized by *affective symptoms* may be described as inexplicable feelings of fear or dread or other emotional experiences that intrude abruptly on the patient's prevailing affective state. Attacks characterized by *somatosensory disturbances* are notable for distortions of perception or hallucinations. Some children report transient distortions of perception concerning the size of objects (micropsia or macropsia), and others describe hallucinations involving taste or smell, as well as formed visual hallucinations.

Complex partial seizures have a variety of clinical expressions and are subclassified on this basis. One form that causes impairment of consciousness only is characterized by transient, blank staring or confusion. These episodes can be mistaken for absence seizures, but the attacks usually last 30 seconds or longer, whereas absence episodes commonly last less than 10 seconds. An EEG can be helpful in distinguishing between the two forms because a three/second generalized spike-and-wave pattern is the hallmark of absence seizures, whereas focal discharge from temporal or frontal areas is seen in complex partial seizures.

Probably the most familiar complex partial seizure is the psychomotor attack that is characterized by semipurposeful motor automatisms. The stereotyped automatisms may be persistent, and the child exhibits continuing repetition of the activity in which he or she was engaged before the onset of the seizure. For example, if the child were walking, he or she may continue to walk, but without purposeful direction. If the child was writing, he or she may continue to move the pencil across the page without producing decipherable script. The simplest types of automatisms are masticatory, sucking, and lip-pursing movements. Patting, scratching, or picking at clothing also may be seen. More complex behaviors such as fumbling with clothing as if to undress or turning about as if searching for something are less common. Finally, *compound forms* that incorporate various elements of the several varieties just described may be seen. In an individual child, the form taken usually is stereotyped from one attack to another.

Epileptic Syndromes

The international classification of epileptic seizures is confined to a description of individual seizure types. Increasing numbers of distinct epileptic syndromes are recognized, and the terminology used in daily communication consists of descriptions of syndromes. The Commission on Classification and Terminology of the International League Against Epilepsy has proposed a classification system for the epileptic syndromes. This system initially divides all epileptic syndromes according to whether the epilepsy is partial, generalized, or uncertain and then subdivides these categories according to the presence or absence of presumed cause. The epilepsy is considered to be secondary (or symptomatic) if obvious disease is demonstrable, if the patient has a history of or demonstrates neurologic or mental impairment, or if the causes are presumed on the basis of studies of previous patients with the same seizure type and location. A modified classification of the epileptic syndromes is shown in Box 401.2.

Several epileptic syndromes are unique to childhood and contain certain features that distinguish them from the more typical primary or secondary types of epilepsy. Infantile spasms or infantile massive spasms are peculiar to infancy and early childhood, with a peak incidence of onset occurring in children between 2 and 7 months of age. They have been described as occurring in three clinical forms. Flexor spasms consist of sudden flexion of the neck, trunk, and extremities, which may be so violent that the torso will jackknife at the waist. Extensor spasms consist of abrupt extension of the neck and trunk with adduction or abduction of the extremities. The predominant form is a mixed flexor-extensor spasm most commonly consisting of flexion of the neck, trunk, and arms with extension of the legs and, less commonly, flexion of the legs and extension of the arms. Infantile spasms tend to occur in clusters, with each cluster consisting of 2 to 125 individual spasms. Each individual spasm lasts only for a few seconds, although a cluster may extend over several minutes. Spasms rarely occur during actual sleep but frequently occur on arousal. In most instances, the EEG shows the distinctive pattern of hypsarrhythmia.

Infantile spasms must be distinguished from benign myoclonus of early infancy and benign neonatal sleep myoclonus, which are characterized by normal EEG results, normal development, and occurrence during sleep. Massive spasms frequently are misinterpreted as startle responses or attacks of colic. A careful history usually elicits the absence of a preceding startle stimulus or the information that the episodes are too precipitous in onset and offset and too short in duration to fit the usual clinical picture of colic. Although crying may follow an infantile spasm, it is not the inconsolable crying that is encountered in infants with cramping abdominal pain.

Infantile spasms have occurred in association with numerous and seemingly unrelated pathologic states, and no one specific factor or circumscribed group of factors has been identified as a common etiologic abnormality. Etiologic associations provide the basis for division of these spasms into two broad groups. In the idiopathic or cryptogenic group, no demonstrable cause is present, the child's development usually has been normal until the onset of spasms, and the results of magnetic resonance imaging (MRI) scans of the brain are normal. In the symptomatic group, a specific etiologic factor can be identified,

---

BOX 401.2   **Modified Classification of Epileptic Syndromes**

1. Localization-related (focal, local, partial) epilepsies and syndrome
   Idiopathic with age-related onset
     Benign childhood epilepsy with centrotemporal spikes
     Childhood epilepsy with occipital paroxysms
     Primary reading epilepsy
   Symptomatic, all other partial epilepsies consequent to a known or suspected disorder of the central nervous system
2. Generalized epilepsies and syndromes
   Idiopathic with age-related onset
     Benign neonatal familial convulsions
     Benign neonatal convulsions
     Benign myoclonic epilepsy in infancy
     Childhood absence epilepsy
     Juvenile absence epilepsy
     Juvenile myoclonic epilepsy
   Cryptogenic or symptomatic
     West syndrome (infantile spasms)
     Lennox-Gastaut syndrome
   Symptomatic
     Nonspecific origin
       Early myoclonic encephalopathy
     Specific syndromes such as those associated with inborn—errors of metabolism, malformations
3. Epilepsies and syndromes undetermined, whether focal or generalized
   With both generalized and focal seizures
     Neonatal seizures
     Severe myoclonic epilepsy in infancy
     Acquired epileptic aphasia (Landau-Kleffner syndrome)
   Without unequivocal generalized or focal features
4. Special syndromes
   Situation-related seizures
     Febrile convulsions
     Isolated seizures
     Seizures occurring only when there is an acute metabolic or toxic event

---

Reprinted from Commission on Classification and Terminology of the International League Against Epilepsy. Proposal for revised classification of epilepsies and epileptic syndromes. *Epilepsia* 1989;30:389.

---

developmental or neurologic abnormalities have preceded the onset of spasms, and the results of MRI scans of the brain often are abnormal. The cryptogenic group represents no more than 10% to 15% of the total, and it has a better prognosis than the symptomatic group.

Causes associated with the symptomatic group of infantile spasms include cerebral dysgenesis, intrauterine infections, and genetic disorders. Two syndromes of cerebral dysgenesis that have been associated with infantile spasms are the Miller-Dieker syndrome (lissencephaly with or without a deletion in the *LIS-1* gene on chromosome 17) and the Aicardi syndrome (girls with agenesis of the corpus callosum, distinctive chorioretinopathy, and mental retardation).

The relationship of pertussis immunization to the onset of infantile spasms has generated interest and concern for many years. The Child Neurology Society and the American Academy of Neurology have reviewed this subject, reached similar conclusions, and issued position papers based on the scientific data available. These organizations concluded that no specific clinical or neuropathologic syndrome is associated with diphtheria-tetanus-pertussis (DTP) vaccine and no means exist by which a diagnosis of brain damage resulting from DTP immunization can be established in an individual case. Well-designed, controlled epidemiologic studies have failed to prove an association between DTP immunization and infantile spasms. Children receive their initial DTP immunizations at an age when infantile spasms have their onset. The administration of pertussis vaccine is associated with a short-term increase in the risk of seizures (mostly febrile seizures), and complete recovery is expected. Children whose neurologic problems begin soon after immunization warrant a full diagnostic workup.

The Lennox-Gastaut syndrome is one type of symptomatic or cryptogenic generalized epilepsy, that is age-dependent. The Lennox-Gastaut syndrome is characterized by the onset in early childhood of mixed seizures (including tonic, tonic-clonic, atonic, akinetic or myoclonic, and absence), refractoriness to common AEDs, an abnormal EEG pattern (generalized, slow-spike and slow-wave activity), and a high incidence of developmental and mental retardation. This syndrome frequently is preceded by infantile spasms. Etiologic factors are similar to those outlined with infantile spasms. In 30% of the cases, the Lennox-Gastaut syndrome appears in children who have no antecedents, previous epilepsy, or clinical or neurologic evidence of brain damage and who have had previously normal development.

Benign focal epilepsy of childhood (also called *benign epilepsy of childhood with rolandic or centrotemporal spikes*) is a form of partial epilepsy that is characterized by an onset between the ages of 4 and 10 years. The seizures typically occur during sleep, although daytime seizures also may be seen. The seizures most frequently begin with clonic twitching of one side of the face. Involvement of the tongue or an upper extremity, and secondary generalization may occur. If the child is awake, he or she may experience paresthesias involving the mouth and throat. The child usually appears well immediately after the seizure. The occurrence of seizures during sleep may cause uncertainty regarding whether the child has had a nightmare or a seizure. The children are otherwise well and have a history of normal development. Neuroimaging studies in these children have been unremarkable. The EEG is characterized by independent spike discharges occurring focally in one or both central (rolandic) regions. Focal spike activity is enhanced during sleep and may occur only at this time. EEG background activity is otherwise normal. Both the seizures and the spike focus typically have a short natural history and usually are resolved by puberty or soon afterward. This natural history, in addition to normal development of the child and normal results of neuroimaging studies, suggests the terminology of benign focal epilepsy. The EEG trait (the central spike with a normal background) may be inherited as an autosomal dominant gene with a particular age penetrance. The inheritance pattern of the seizures is familial, but it appears to be multifactorial. Similar varieties of benign focal epilepsy have been identified in association with temporal, parietal, and occipital spike foci.

Childhood epilepsy with occipital paroxysms is associated with an EEG pattern that is characterized by unilateral or bilateral occipital spike or sharp waves and seizures that are hemiclonic or consist of automatisms and that typically are preceded by visual symptoms (amaurosis, phosphenes, illusions, or hallucinations). In 25% of the cases, the seizures are followed immediately by migraine-like headaches.

ANCILLARY LABORATORY STUDIES

In approaching the laboratory evaluation, the physician must recall that epilepsy is primarily a clinical diagnosis. Some laboratory studies are necessary to establish a baseline for future comparison, and others can help with formulating medical treatment and prognosis. Indications for laboratory studies should be based on information extracted from the history and physical examination. If specific disease entities such as hypocalcemia, hypoglycemia, or other metabolic, toxic, or degenerative disorders are valid considerations, additional studies relevant to the particular entity are, of course, appropriate.

Electroencephalography

An EEG has value only when it is interpreted in the context of the child's age, history, and physical findings. The quality of information gained from an EEG is related directly to the standards of the laboratory and the training and experience of the personnel. A routine EEG always should be recorded during wakefulness and sleep and, in older children, during hyperventilation and photic stimulation. Because normal organizational and frequency characteristics change rapidly with advancing age and cerebral maturation, it is of particular importance that the interpretation of EEGs in infants and young children be done by an electroencephalographer who has had specific training and experience with this age group. EEGs in many laboratories are interpreted by neurologists with little or no experience with infants and young children. Additional information about the use of EEGs in epilepsy is presented in Box 401.3.

Normal EEG results should not necessarily dissuade a physician from making a diagnosis of epilepsy in the presence of a convincing clinical description. The initial EEG often does not contain epileptiform discharges. Investigators have found that the initial EEG in 25% to 58% of affected children may be normal or borderline without epileptiform abnormalities. Similarly, abnormal EEG results do not necessarily confirm a clinical suspicion of epilepsy. The type and location of an abnormality are expected to correlate with the clinical data. When the available clinical and EEG data do not provide a basis for confident classification regarding seizure type, or in cases in which pseudoseizures are suspected, video-EEG monitoring may be justified. Medically refractory patients may undergo video-EEG monitoring to assess their candidacy for epilepsy surgery. Patients with daily episodes may need only short-term monitoring, whereas those with infrequent seizures may need longer monitoring with tapering or discontinuation of medication to encourage seizures.

Neuroimaging

Routine skull radiography seldom is indicated or helpful except when overt bony disease is detected by physical examination. Neuroimaging studies may be indicated in cases of partial seizures or if the history and physical examination suggest structural lesions, degenerative diseases, or a congenital structural abnormality. High-resolution ultrasound is a useful technique in the investigation of premature infants and term neonates with seizures. MRI has virtually replaced computed tomography in the evaluation of patients with epilepsy. MRI allows for the clear imaging of intraparenchymal structures, without bony artifacts and exposure to ionizing radiation; it allows acquisition of multiplanar anatomic data and the ability to reconfigure the data for enhanced visualization; and it visualizes important substrates of epilepsy such as malformations of cortical development, abnormal neuronal and glial proliferation, abnormal neuronal migration, tumors, vascular malformations, encephalomalacia, and mesial temporal sclerosis. The development of the fast fluid-attenuated inversion-recovery imaging (FLAIR) technique provides superior detection of small cortical-based epileptogenic lesions and improved ability to identify gliosis. MRI should be customized to answer the appropriate clinical question, and discussion regarding the region of interest with the neuroradiologist may improve detection of smaller lesions.

Hematologic and Hepatic Tests

Because most of the AEDs in use have the potential to produce hematologic or hepatic side effects, a baseline complete blood count, platelet count, and liver enzyme analysis should be obtained, dependent on the known toxic effects of the drug to be used.

MEDICAL TREATMENT

Successful treatment of a child with epilepsy demands more than just preventing recurrent seizures. The sensitive physician must adopt both an educational and an advocacy position, thus ensuring acceptance of the child's epilepsy by the family, teachers, classmates, and the community. Misconceptions about epilepsy still abound and often have an adverse effect on a child's self-esteem and psychosocial development. Time invested in providing a clear explanation, in lay language, of the nature of epilepsy, the objectives of treatment, and the simple fundamentals of pharmacokinetics can allay apprehensions, dispel misconceptions, and promote compliance with the prescribed drug regimen.

Population studies suggest that approximately 70% of patients in whom epilepsy is diagnosed ultimately become free of seizures and that most can expect to discontinue anticonvulsant

---

BOX 401.3 — **Electroencephalography in Epilepsy**

The duration of a routine electroencephalogram (EEG) in most laboratories is approximately 1 hour. This 1-hour sample is taken to be representative of the patient's cerebral electrical activity during any average 24-hour period. An obvious potential exists for sampling to take place at a time when no epileptiform activity is present. A sleep-deprived EEG or a routine EEG obtained at a subsequent date may demonstrate abnormalities that were not evident in the initial sample. The yield of useful information is enhanced when the EEG can be scheduled in particular relation to a clinical seizure. The EEG should be recorded as soon as possible after any seizures that occur in neonates and infants up to 6 months of age. If an EEG is recorded in children with febrile seizures who are 6 to 36 months of age, the test should be delayed until 5 to 10 days after the seizure because the child's postictal brain wave activity may be transiently and diffusely slow for several days, and its significance could be misinterpreted. For patients with nonfebrile seizures, the EEG should be recorded as soon as possible after the event.

medication. Nearly 50% of patients become seizure free with the first AED prescribed at moderate doses. A higher likelihood of remission has been reported in children than in adults. Children with epilepsy in association with mental retardation or cerebral palsy, however, have low rates of remission. The literature does not reflect universal agreement on the optimal duration of anticonvulsant therapy. In most instances, a seizure-free period of at least 2 to 3 consecutive years is a conservative objective before the gradual withdrawal of medication should be considered. Monitoring serum drug levels at reasonable intervals can provide a guideline for adjusting drug dosages as the child grows. Complete seizure control is not possible in some children, and, in those instances, the occurrence of an occasional seizure is preferable to an increase in the dosage of anticonvulsants to levels that produce sedation and dysequilibrium, thereby compromising both cognitive function and social interaction.

Treatment after the Nonfebrile First Seizure

The initiation of AED therapy after an initial, nonfebrile seizure in otherwise well children continues to be controversial. The decision to treat should be individualized and should take into consideration the risk of seizure recurrence, the consequences of having another seizure, and the risks of AED therapy. The observation that many children, possibly as many as one-half, who present with a single unprovoked seizure do not experience a second seizure has caused many clinicians to elect not to begin AED therapy after the first seizure. Some children may have a benign developmental disorder of seizure threshold that they outgrow. These include children whose generalized tonic-clonic seizures begin between 1 and 10 years of age and who have normal neurologic examinations and normal or nonspecific abnormal EEG results and children with benign epilepsy with rolandic spikes.

The importance of identifying epileptic syndromes has been recognized. For example, children with West syndrome (infantile spasms), childhood absence epilepsy, and juvenile myoclonic epilepsy have high recurrence risks, whereas children with benign epilepsy with rolandic spikes appear to have good outcomes without AED therapy. Some physicians believe that the stigma attached to the diagnosis of epilepsy and the potential adverse side effects of AEDs, especially on behavior and cognitive function, outweigh the risk of recurrent seizures.

The risk for recurrence in children with a first, nonfebrile seizure has been addressed in only a few studies and has been reported to vary from 52% to 61%. Past studies indicated that recurrence rates are much higher after a second seizure (79% to 90%), and most seizures recur within 6 months of the first (70% to 74%). Recurrence rates are highest in patients with abnormal results on neurologic examination, focal spikes in the EEG, and complex partial seizures. Recurrence rates in otherwise normal children, who have normal EEG results after the first, nonfebrile, generalized tonic-clonic seizure, range from 10% to 30%. The diagnosis of epilepsy is conventionally made after two unprovoked seizures.

Whether prevention of further seizures alters the tendency of many children to outgrow epilepsy is not clear. One study suggests that the number of seizures before AED treatment has little influence on ease of seizure control unless that number is ten or greater. At that point, the chance of seizure control appears to be decreased, but if control is achieved, the chance of success of discontinuation is unchanged. This study did not include children with epileptic syndromes with high recurrence risks, as indicated previously. In other cases, however, some delay in initiating AED therapy may have no significant effect on seizure control and subsequent remission.

In children, the consequences of seizure recurrences are primarily social, unless a prolonged episode of status epilepticus occurs. Even in the latter case, if no acute cause is present and the episode is unprovoked, the outcome usually is favorable. The social consequences are not to be minimized. Many patients with epilepsy beginning in childhood may have persistent and significant social adjustment and competence problems as adults. As yet, no universally accepted consensus exists regarding withholding treatment after the occurrence of a first such seizure during childhood. A clinician who sees a child after a single seizure, especially a child who is neurologically and mentally normal and who has normal EEG results, may consider, after discussion with the patient and parents, withholding therapy pending the occurrence of a second seizure. If a decision is made to delay initiation of AED therapy, it should be done after a full discussion with the child's caretaker of potential risks and benefits, practical restrictions to avoid potentially harmful situations if the child does have another seizure (e.g., not bathing alone), and what to do if the child does have another brief or prolonged seizure.

Antiepileptic Drugs

Optimal response to drug therapy and control of seizures can be obtained in approximately 70% of children if a few general principles are observed carefully:

- Initiate therapy with a drug that is known to be effective for the specific type of seizure disorder treated. If several drugs are equally effective, start with the one that is least toxic, least expensive, and available in appropriate dosage forms and that requires the least amount of laboratory monitoring.
- Always initiate therapy with a single drug. The introduction of more than one variable complicates the assessment of side effects and therapeutic efficacy.
- Start with a dosage that falls near the lower end of the known therapeutic range (Table 401.1).
- Dosage intervals should be based on the half-life of the drug being used (see Table 401.1). It may be necessary to administer drugs with relatively short half-lives two to three times a day. Even though drugs with long half-lives, such as phenobarbital (PBS), can be delivered in a single daily dose, transient sedation may be noted at peak levels, or sluggishness may be seen during the early morning hours when the total dose is delivered at bedtime.
- Maintain the initial dosage for an interval that is sufficient to achieve a steady state before assessing therapeutic efficacy or checking blood levels. Drug metabolism and excretion begin almost immediately after absorption, and the drug continues to accumulate in the body until the elimination rate is in equilibrium with the daily intake. As a general rule, long-term oral administration for approximately five times the half-life of the drug is required to achieve a steady state.
- If the initial dosage does not produce satisfactory seizure control, advance it incrementally until seizure control is obtained or the patient exhibits dose-related side effects (e.g., sedation, ataxia). Serum concentrations of anticonvulsants can be measured as a guideline for adjusting the administered dosage and compliance (see Table 401.1).
- If the addition of a second drug becomes necessary, add only one drug at a time. If little or no improvement was seen with the initial drug, consideration should be given to withdrawing it gradually after the second drug has reached therapeutic blood levels and seizures are improved significantly or are controlled.

TABLE 401.1

ANTIEPILEPTIC DRUG DOSING GUIDELINES

Medication	Adults	Children	Level	Formulation
Carbamazepine				
Starting dose	200 mg twice daily	5–10 mg/kg/day divided bid	8–12	Tablet (chewable): 100 mg Tablet: 200 mg Extended-release tablet: 100, 200, 400 mg Suspension: 100 mg/ 5 mL Carbatrol: 200, 300 mg
Increase by	200 mg/day weekly	5–10 mg/kg/day divided weekly		
Typical maintenance	800–1,200 mg/day divided tid (or bid if extended release)	15–45 mg/kg/day divided bid to qid		
Ethosuximide				
Starting dose	500 mg/day divided bid	10 mg/kg/day divided bid	40–100	Syrup: 250 Capsule: 250 mg
Increase by	250 mg/day weekly	5–10 mg/kg/day weekly		
Typical maintenance	1,000–2,000 mg/day divided bid to tid	15–40 mg/kg/day divided bid to tid		
Felbamate				
Starting dose	400 mg tid	15 mg/kg/day divided tid	40–100	Tablet: 400, 600 mg Syrup: 600 mg/5 mL
Increase by	1,200 mg/day weekly	15 mg/kg/day weekly		
Typical maintenance	1,200 mg tid	45–60 mg/kg/day divided tid		
Gabapentin				
Starting dose	300 mg qid	10 mg/kg/day divided bid	4–16	Tablet: 100, 300, 400 mg Capsules: 600, 800 mg Syrup: 1,000 mg/5 mL
Increase by	300 mg/day (going to tid)	10 mg/kg/day (going to tid)		
Typical maintenance	900–3,600 mg/day divided tid	30–100 mg/kg/day divided tid		
Lamotrigine (without valproic acid)				
Starting dose	>12 years old 50 mg qd for 2 weeks	<12 years old 0.6 mg/kg/day divided bid for 2 weeks	2–10 (total) 1–9 (free)	Tablets: 25, 100, 150, 200 mg Chewable dispersable: 2, 5, 25 mg
Increase by	50 mg bid for 2 weeks	1.2 mg/kg/day divided bid for 2 weeks		
Subsequent increments	100 mg/day divided bid every 1–2 weeks	1.2 mg/kg/day divided bid every 1–2 weeks		
Typical maintenance	300–500 mg/day divided bid	5–15 mg/kg/day divided bid		
Lamotrigine (with valproic acid)				
Starting dose	>12 years old 25 mg qod for 2 weeks	<12 years old 0.15 mg/kg/day qd for 2 weeks	2–20 (total) 1–9 (free)	Tablet: 25, 100, 150, 200 mg Chewable dispersable: 2, 5, 25 mg
Increase by	25 mg qd for 2 weeks	0.3 mg/kg/day qd or bid every 2 weeks		
Subsequent increments	25–50 mg divided bid every 1–2 weeks	0.3 mg/kg/day divided bid every 1–2 weeks		
Typical maintenance	100–400 mg/day divided bid	1–5 mg/kg/day divided bid		
Levetiracetam				
Starting dose	500 mg divided bid	10 mg/kg/day divided bid	5–45	Tablets: 250, 500, 750 mg
Increase by	1,000 mg/day weekly	10–20 mg/kg/day weekly		
Typical maintenance	1,500 mg bid	40–60 mg/kg/day divided bid		

(Continued)

TABLE 401.1

(CONTINUED)

Medication	Adults	Children	Level	Formulation
Oxcarbazepine			10–35	Tablets: 150, 300, 600 mg
Starting dose	300 mg bid	8–10 mg/kg/day divided bid		Suspension: 300 mg/5 mL
Increase by	600 mg/day weekly	10 mg/kg/day weekly		
Typical maintenance	1,200 mg bid	20–45 mg/kg/day divided bid		
Phenytoin			10–20	Capsules: 100 mg
Starting dose	100 mg/day weekly	1–2 mg/kg/day weekly		Extended-release
Increase by				capsules: 30, 100 mg
Typical maintenance	200–600 mg/day qd or bid	4–8 mg/kg/day divided bid		Chewable capsule: 50 mg
				Suspension: 125 mg/5 mL
Phenobarbital			20–40	Solution: 20 mg/5 mL
Starting dose	60–90 mg at night	2–6 mg/kg/day qd or divided bid		Tablets: 15, 30, 60, 100 mg
Increased by	30 mg monthly	1–2 mg/kg/day biweekly		
Typical maintenance	60–120 mg divided qd or bid	2–6 mg/kg/day divided bid		
Primidone			5–10	Tablets: 50, 250 mg
Starting dose	62.5 mg qhs	1–2 mg/kg/day for 4–5 days		Suspension: 250 mg/5 mL
Increase by	62.5 mg every 3 days	1–2 mg/kg/day every 3 days		
Typical maintenance	10–20 mg/kg/day divided tid	5–20 mg/kg/day divided tid or qid		
Tiagabine			5–200	Tablets: 2, 4, 12, 16, 20 mg
Starting dose	4 mg/day	0.1 mg/kg/day		
Increase by	4 mg/day every 1–2 weeks divided bid, tid	0.1 mg/kg/day every 1–2 weeks divided tid		
Typical maintenance	32–56 mg/day divided bid or tid	0.6–1 mg/day divided tid		
Topiramate			2–25	Tablets: 25, 100, 200 mg
Starting dose	25–50 mg/day divided bid	0.5–1 mg/kg/day divided qhs or bid		Capsules: 15, 25 mg (sprinkles)
Increase by	25–50 mg/day every 1–2 weeks	0.5–1 mg/kg/day divided bid every 1–2 weeks		
Typical maintenance	200–400 mg/day divided bid	5–9 mg/kg/day divided bid		
Valproic acid			50–100	Depakene capsule: 250 mg
Starting dose	500–1,000 mg/day divided bid	10–15 mg/kg/day divided bid		Syrup: 250 mg/5 mL
Increase by	250 mg/day weekly	10–15 mg/kg/day weekly		Depakote tablets: 125, 250, 500 mg
Typical maintenance	1,000–3,000 mg/day divided bid, tid (extended-release formulation may be given qd)	30–60 mg/kg/day divided bid, tid		Sprinkles: 125 mg
				Extended release: 250, 500 mg
Zonisamide			15–30	Capsules: 25, 100 mg
Starting dose	100–200 mg/day qd or bid	1–2 mg/kg/day qd or bid		
Increase by	100 mg/day every 1–2 weeks	1–2 mg/kg/day every 1–2 weeks		
Typical maintenance	200–600 mg/day qd or bid	4–8 mg/kg/day qd or bid		

bid, twice daily; qd, once daily; qhs, at bedtime; qod, every other day; tid, three times daily.
Adapted from Holland KD. Efficacy, pharmacology, and adverse effects of antiepileptic drugs. *Neurol Clin* 2001;19:313.

BOX 401.4   **Pharmacokinetics of Antiepileptic Drugs**

Most antiepileptic drugs (AEDs) are weak acids and are absorbed slowly from the small intestine. Absorption can be influenced by antacids, rapid gut transit time, malabsorption syndromes, and variations in solubility characteristics among generic preparations. By the time most AEDs reach the bloodstream, they are bound (to varying degrees) to plasma proteins. The protein-bound fraction of the drug does not cross the blood-brain barrier and thus does not reach the site of intended biologic action. Both therapeutic effectiveness and clinical symptoms of dose-related toxicity are accounted for by the *free* or unbound fraction. The routine blood levels that are used as a guide in clinical practice reflect the total drug concentration, including both the free and the protein-bound fractions. In most instances, the extent of protein binding of a given drug is relatively stable from patient to patient.

The following clinical situations may raise the suspicion of altered protein binding. The child who exhibits clinical signs and symptoms of drug intoxication in the context of a blood level that is within the therapeutic range may have an elevated concentration of free drug as a result of some drug interaction. This situation also may be seen in the rare child who has an inherently low protein-binding capacity. Conversely, the child who seems to require large doses and "supertherapeutic" levels to achieve seizure control but who exhibits no clinical symptoms of toxicity may have a higher than average binding capacity. In both these clinical situations, the determination of free levels may serve as a better guideline for dosage adjustment. Most laboratories are capable of measuring free drug in plasma ultrafiltrate.

- No logic supports the simultaneous administration of two drugs in the same chemical group.
- Periodic laboratory monitoring is indicated when drugs that are known to have a significant incidence of hematologic or hepatic side effects are used.
- The withdrawal of AEDs always should be gradual to avoid the precipitation of status epilepticus.

Pharmacokinetics

A basic understanding of pharmacokinetics is required if AEDs are to be used successfully. Familiarity with the absorption and distribution characteristics of the drug, the degree to which it is bound to plasma proteins, and the way in which it is metabolized and excreted is essential if blood concentrations are to be maintained at therapeutic levels with minimal fluctuation between doses. Additional information about the pharmacokinetics of AEDs is presented in Box 401.4.

Blood Level Monitoring

Blood level monitoring permits the dosage requirement of anticonvulsant medications to be tailored to the individual needs of a given patient. Ideally, dosage adjustment should be made on the basis of *trough* drug levels. Doing so may not always be practical, however, because families have difficulty coming in to have blood specimens drawn before the child takes the morning dose of medication. In actual practice, most blood levels prob-

ably are obtained during return office visits at varying times of the day. However, making note of the interval between collection of the blood specimen and ingestion of the most recent dose can be useful in determining whether the measurement more nearly approximates a peak or a trough level based on the known half-life and peak time of the drug used.

The blood levels of AEDs that define a therapeutic range (see Table 401.1) are intended to be used as general guidelines, always in the context of the clinical state of the child. The lower limit of the range identifies the minimal level required to produce seizure control in the average patient. The upper limit identifies the level at which the average patient exhibits clinical symptoms of dose-related toxicity. Seizures can be controlled in a few children with blood levels somewhat lower than the minimum range, but others require and tolerate levels somewhat above the maximum. The circumstances in which blood levels can be useful in clinical decision making are as follows: 5 to 14 days (five times the drug half-life) after treatment has been initiated at a given dosage, or after a change is made in the dosage (levels drawn before a steady state is achieved will not reflect accurately the optimal concentrations that can be achieved with the dose being used); when previously controlled seizures begin to recur (the most common explanation for this circumstance is noncompliance, but occasionally a child will have been allowed to outgrow a dosage); when clinical symptoms of toxicity become evident or when suspected drug interactions need assessment; and every 6 to 8 months in a rapidly growing child, especially one whose seizures have been controlled easily at low therapeutic levels.

Specific Medications

Since 1993, nine new drugs have been approved for use in the treatment of epilepsy by the U.S. Food and Drug Administration (FDA). In some instances, these drugs have advantages over the traditional drugs (e.g., phenobarbital [PBS], phenytoin [PHT], carbamazepine [CBZ], valproic acid [VPA]), with fewer side effects, less drug interaction, and different routes of metabolism. The newer agents often cost more per dose than do the traditional drugs, although their cost can be mitigated by the decreased need for routine laboratory monitoring for toxicity. Table 401.2 provides some guidelines for the treatment of different seizure types with antiepileptic medications. Suggested first-line therapy is provided, while alternative second-line therapies are listed alphabetically. Guidelines have been proposed regarding the safety and efficacy of the newer AEDs medications, but data pertaining to the pediatric population are lacking. Table 401.2 attempts to provide a brief synopsis for treatment options, but other medications may be recommended under the supervision of a pediatric neurologist. Table 401.1 provides an overview of the doses, levels, and available formulations of some of the common AEDs. The AEDs are discussed in further detail in the following sections.

Benzodiazepines. Benzodiazepines (BZDs) exert their effect by binding to the GABAa receptor and thus causing an increase in the frequency of inhibitory chloride channel opening. BZDs are effective in multiple seizure types, including myoclonic, absence, and atonic seizures. They are considered first-line therapy in the acute treatment of status epilepticus. Side effects include sedation and ataxia, and the development of tolerance limits their use on a long-term basis. Lorazepam, diazepam, and midazolam are the BZDs most frequently used for status epilepticus. Clonazepam has been used mostly as adjunctive treatment for epilepsy.

Carbamazepine (Tegretol). CBZ works through the blockade of voltage-dependent sodium channels and is effective in the treatment of complex partial, simple partial, and generalized

TABLE 401.2

PRACTICAL ANTIEPILEPTIC TREATMENTS BASED ON SEIZURE TYPE

Seizure Type	First-Line Antiepileptic Drug	Other Treatment Options (Listed Alphabetically, Not in Order of Preference)
Partial seizure with or without secondary generalization	Oxcarbazepine	Carbamazepine, lamotrigine, levetiracetam, phenobarbital, phenytoin, topiramate, valproic acid, zonisamide
Tonic-clonic	Valproic acid	Lamotrigine, levetiracetam, topiramate, zonisamide
Atonic	Valproic acid	Lamotrigine, levetiracetam, topiramate, zonisamide
Myoclonic	Valproic acid	Benzodiazepines, lamotrigine, levetiracetam, topiramate, zonisamide
Absence	Ethosuximide	Lamotrigine, valproic acid
Infantile spasm	Adrenocorticotropic hormone	Vigabatrin*
Neonatal seizure	Phenobarbital	Phenytoin

*Vigabatrin is possibly effective in the treatment of infantile spasm. Data are insufficient to determine whether valproic acid, benzodiazepines, pyridoxine, zonisamide, topiramate, or combination therapy is effective in the treatment of infantile spasms.
Adapted from Jarrar RG, Buchhalter JR. Therapeutics in pediatric epilepsy. Part 1: the new antiepileptic drugs and the ketogenic diet. *Mayo Clin Proc* 2003;78:359.

tonic-clonic seizures. CBZ is metabolized by the cytochrome P-450 system, and its half-life may be affected by drugs that affect this pathway, such as the coadministration of macrolide antibiotics. Dose-related side effects include dysequilibrium, drowsiness, and diplopia. Hepatic, dermatologic, and hematologic side effects may occur and have been estimated to be fatal in 1 in 50,000 to 200,000 treated patients. Liver function tests and complete blood counts are followed regularly when initiating the medication.

Ethosuximide (Zarontin). The mechanism of action of ethosuximide is through modulation of low-threshold (T-type) calcium currents in the thalamus. Ethosuximide has a narrow spectrum of action, but it is the drug of choice for the treatment of childhood absence epilepsy. The main side effects associated with ethosuximide are nausea and vomiting, which can be limited with administration after meals.

Gabapentin (Neurontin). Gabapentin has no significant interactions with other drugs and is not metabolized in the liver. Side effects can include weight gain and involuntary movements. Drawbacks include a short half-life (5 to 7 hours), necessitating multiple daily doses, and that it is dependent on renal function, has a limited spectrum of effectiveness, is ineffective against primary generalized seizures such as absence and myoclonic seizures, and has limited effectiveness as monotherapy in children.

Lamotrigine (Lamictal). Lamotrigine (LTG) has a demonstrated effect of blockade of sodium channel. In addition to effectiveness for partial seizures, LTG appears especially effective in the treatment of generalized epilepsy in children, including generalized absence seizures and Lennox-Gastaut syndrome, although it is less effective for treatment of myoclonic seizures. Side effects include increase in seizure frequency and rash. A higher incidence (in comparison with adults) of rash, typically maculopapular but including Stevens-Johnson syndrome, has been reported in children. Rash typically occurs within 2 to 8 weeks, but it has been reported on the first day and as late as the fifth month after LTG initiation. The occurrence of rash, in some reports, has been related to rapid escalation of the dose of LTG and to concurrent use of VPA. After discontinuance of VPA, LTG has been reintroduced without recurrence of rash. As monotherapy, its half-life is 24 hours; used with VPA, it is 59 hours; and used with enzyme-inducing AEDs (CBZ, PHT, PBS), it is 15 hours.

Levetiracetam (Keppra). The mechanism of action of Levetiracetam (LEV) is unclear. LEV has been FDA-approved for adjunctive treatment of partial seizures in adults. Some reports have noted its effectiveness in generalized seizures. LEV has been associated with somnolence, dizziness, and behavioral problems. Psychosis has been noted in some patients, which resolved after discontinuation of LEV.

Oxcarbazepine (Trileptal). Oxcarbazepine (OXC) is chemically related to CBZ and has a similar blockade of voltage-sensitive sodium channels. OXC is approved for the treatment of partial seizures in adults and children aged 4 years and older. Side effects associated with OXC include somnolence and ataxia and rarely hyponatremia but the toxic hematologic and hepatic side effects seen with CBZ have not been reported.

Phenytoin. PHT is similar to CBZ in its ability to block voltage-dependent sodium channels. It also has the ability to block voltage-dependent calcium channels at higher doses. PHT is effective in the treatment of complex partial, simple partial, and generalized tonic-clonic seizures. PHT metabolism is through the cytochrome P-450 enzyme system, and the drug is excreted in bile and urine. PHT is highly protein-bound (90%), and the free fraction may be increased in patients with hypoalbuminemia or by drugs that compete with its binding sites. Side effects often are dose-related and include nystagmus, ataxia, and somnolence. Movement disorders including chorea and dystonia have been associated with its use, and long-term exposure may cause cosmetic side effects, including gingival hyperplasia and hirsutism. A rash may develop in 5% to 10% of patients and rarely may cause Stevens-Johnson syndrome. A parenteral formulation of 50 mg/mL is available and can be infused no faster than 50 mg/minute.

Fosphenytoin was introduced in 1996 as an alternative to the parenteral form of PHT. It has fewer cutaneous side effects and can be administered more quickly than can PHT. The common loading dose is 18 to 20 mg PHT equivalents (PE)/kg, and it can be administered at a rate of 3 mg PE/kg/minute or 150 mg PE/kg/minute in adults.

Phenobarbital. PBS exerts its anticonvulsant effects through augmenting the effect of GABA-mediated chloride channel inhibition and by inhibiting the effect of glutamate, thus diminishing excitatory neurotransmission. PBS has been used for treatment of simple or complex partial seizures, as well as primary or secondarily generalized seizures. Some of the properties of PBS render it especially attractive in the treatment of neonatal seizures. PBS is metabolized through the cytochrome P-450 enzyme system, and the dose may need to be adjusted in patients with hepatic disease. A parenteral formulation is available. Primidone (Mysoline) is similar to PBS in structure and efficacy, but side effects tend to limit its usefulness.

Tiagabine (Gabitril). Tiagabine (TGB) inhibits the uptake of GABA into neurons and glia, which increases inhibition. TGB appears to be an effective AED for partial seizures, but it may exacerbate primary generalized seizures. Its short half-life (8 hours monotherapy; 2 to 3 hours when used with CBZ or PHT), decreased rate of absorption with food, and diurnal variation (lower levels in evening than morning) may complicate the use of TGB. Side effects include generalized weakness (dose dependent), abnormal thinking, and depression.

Topiramate (Topamax). Topiramate (TPM) has multiple mechanisms of action *in vitro*. TPM is FDA approved for adjunctive treatment of partial and generalized seizure in patients older than 2 years. TPM has demonstrated usefulness in the treatment of Lennox-Gastaut syndrome and infantile spasms. Increases in the PHT serum levels reportedly occur occasionally with the addition of TPM. Side effects include psychomotor slowing, difficulty with concentration and language problems. Rarely, renal stones and acute myopia have been reported. Therefore, attention to hydration is emphasized, because TPM is a weak carbonic anhydrase.

Valproic Acid (Depakene) and Divalproex Sodium (Depakote). The mechanism of action of VPA is not understood entirely, but it appears to increase GABA levels and to block voltage-sensitive sodium channels. VPA has a wide range of clinical efficacy, and it has been used in the treatment of partial-onset seizures, absence seizures, generalized tonic-clonic seizures, myoclonic seizures, and Lennox-Gastaut syndrome. Its effectiveness in treating epilepsy is tempered by its varied side effects. It may induce fatal hepatotoxicity, pancreatitis, and hematopoietic dysfunction. Tremor occurs in about 10% of patients and is dose-related. Other side effects include polycystic ovarian disease, weight gain, and hair loss, thus necessitating its use cautiously in adolescent patients. Routine blood screening of hepatic function and blood counts are recommended. A parenteral form is available, and loading with intravenous VPA, with doses of 15 to 25 mg/kg, has been used in the treatment of status epilepticus.

Zonisamide (Zonegran). Zonisamide exerts its antiepileptic effects through sodium channel blockade, blocking of T-type calcium current, and inhibition of carbonic anhydrase. It has been approved for the use of treatment of partial seizures in adults. Zonisamide has been used for the treatment of a broad spectrum of seizure types, including primary generalized seizures, absence seizures, infantile spasms, and myoclonic seizures. A half-life of 24 to 60 hours allows for once-daily dosing. Side effects include somnolence, cognitive problems, and anhidrosis.

Other Agents. Felbamate (Felbatol) was approved for use in 1993, but its use has been limited by an increased incidence of aplastic anemia and hepatotoxicity. Felbamate currently is used mainly in patients with refractory Lennox-Gastaut syndrome. Adrenocorticotropic hormone (ACTH) is used specifically in the treatment of infantile spasms, although its mechanism of action remains unknown. ACTH has multiple side effects including cushingoid features, weight gain, hypertension, immunosuppression, and irritability. An alternative treatment to ACTH for infantile spasms may involve oral steroids. Vigabatrin (Sabril) is not approved for use in the United States owing to concentric visual field loss, but it is available in many other countries. Vigabatrin is used for the treatment of partial seizures and infantile spasms, but it may exacerbate idiopathic generalized epilepsy. Pregabalin (Lyrica) was approved in 2005 as adjunctive therapy for adults with partial onset seizures. Its use in pediatric populations has not been adequately studied to make recommendations regarding applications and dosing.

Ketogenic Diet

Interest in the ketogenic diet has had a resurgence. However, the diet has a long history as an effective and safe method for treatment of intractable childhood epilepsy. Its use predates almost all AEDs, except PBS and bromides. Many clinical reports indicate that at least one-third to two-thirds of patients benefit from the use of the diet. Whether the effect of the diet is caused by the direct anticonvulsant effect of high levels of ketones or to a ketone-induced secondary change in cerebral metabolism is unclear. Current practice has been to initiate the diet in children whose conditions are intractable to medical therapy. The diet appears to be most effective for patients with symptomatic forms of epilepsy that are hard to control, especially epileptic encephalopathies associated with atypical absence seizures, myoclonic seizures, and atonic seizures. The diet, to a lesser degree, may have efficacy for partial seizures. Although the diet is most successful in children aged 2 to 5 years, it also has been used in infants and in older children. Infants must have adequate nutrition to support growth and development. A highly motivated family and an experienced dietitian are key to the successful use of the diet.

The ketogenic diet produces a state of chronic ketosis by manipulation of protein, fat, and carbohydrates. To achieve the required amount of daily calories for daily activity, fat is added to achieve a fat-to-carbohydrate ratio of 4:1 or 3:1 and thereby leads to the accumulation of ketone bodies. A daily intake of protein of 0.75 g/1.2 kg is maintained to meet requirements for growth.

The diet should be given at least a 4- to 6-week trial, with ketosis well maintained. If the frequency of seizures has not changed significantly, a return to standard therapy should be considered. If a significant decrease in the number of seizures occurs, the diet should be maintained for 2 years, an attempt to reduce and stop AEDs should be made, and, at the end of 2 years, the diet should be discontinued gradually. Potential side effects include reduction in bone mass, renal calculi, thinning of hair, and, rarely, alopecia. The long-term cardiovascular effects need further study. Sugar-free supplements of multivitamins and calcium need to be provided. The use of medium-chain triglyceride oil is an alternative to the traditional diet. Evidence suggests that medium-chain triglycerides can reduce the likelihood of hypoglycemia and high cholesterol levels, which have been reported with the 4:1 diet. Control of sugar intake while patients are on the diet is strict, and commonly used medications such as antibiotics, as well as daily used substances such as toothpaste, must be monitored closely for their carbohydrate content.

Vagus Nerve Stimulation

Vagus nerve stimulation (VNS) was approved for the treatment of medically refractory, partial-onset seizures in children 12 years old and older by the FDA in 1997. VNS has been used in many children and has been proven to be effective in reducing the number of seizures in patients with medically intractable epilepsy. VNS involves the implantation of a pulse stimulator under the skin of the anterior chest attached to bipolar leads, which wrap around the left vagus nerve in the neck. The stimulator provides intermittent electrical pulses, and a magnet can be used by the family or patient to activate the stimulator to attempt to terminate or shorten a seizure. Studies have demonstrated that as many as 60% of patients may experience a 50% decrease in seizure frequency, although other studies have shown less benefit. Side effects of the stimulator include voice alteration (57%), coughing (37%), and rarely sleep apnea. Although the cost of VNS is expensive, some patients may derive a clear benefit from the device, thus allowing for a reduction of AEDs, which may decrease some of the side effects of medical therapy.

EPILEPSY SURGERY

Although a thorough discussion of epilepsy surgery is beyond the scope of this chapter, it has proven effective in selected patients with intractable focal epilepsy. Candidates with focal lesions on neuroimaging, focal electrographic patterns, and involvement of noneloquent cortex are best suited for resective surgery. Seizure freedom rates may be as high as 91% in patients with hippocampal sclerosis, whereas patients with malformations of cortical development, which are more common in the pediatric age group, have seizure freedom rates of about 50% after undergoing resection. When treatment is effective, some patients may not require AEDs; therefore, all patients who have partial-onset epilepsy in whom medical therapy has failed should be evaluated for epilepsy surgery.

DISCONTINUING ANTIEPILEPTIC DRUGS

The use of AEDs in children involves at least three major decisions. Two of these, whether to start AEDs and which AED to use, have been discussed. The third concerns when to discontinue AED therapy. To reduce further exposure to AEDs, a growing tendency is to remove children from AED therapy after shorter seizure-free periods. The decision to discontinue AEDs should take into consideration the likelihood of when remission may occur for an individual patient, the benefits versus potential adverse effects of continuing AED therapy, and the risks associated with medication discontinuation. The risks of seizure relapse after discontinuation of AEDs in children have varied between 6% and 40%, depending on the population studied, the types of epilepsy and their causes, and the follow-up period.

Adverse effects of AEDs are reported to occur in as many as 50% of individuals receiving AEDs; however, in only 7% were the side effects so significant that the AED needed to be stopped. Although currently used AEDs appear to be relatively safe when used by children, the concern is that they may be associated with adverse behavioral and cognitive side effects. Cognitive impairment secondary to AED therapy in children may be overstated. Long-term treatment with PBS or BZDs may be associated with behavioral disturbances and cognitive impairment in selective patients. In general, children and adults maintained on nontoxic doses of AEDs usually have little, if any, cognitive impairment. Even if most children tolerate AEDs well, other factors should be considered. They include the psychological consequences and expense of taking daily medications, including the cost of the drugs and the monitoring of laboratory studies. Discontinuing AED therapy after 2 seizure-free years has been reported to be associated with a relapse risk similar to that of longer treatment periods up to 5 years.

Regardless of treatment duration from the last seizure, an estimated 30% to 40% of children experience a recurrence after AED withdrawal. However, the risks of status epilepticus and physical injury after withdrawal, although present, are low. Most children are likely to regain seizure control after reestablishment of AED therapy. Continued AED therapy is not a guarantee against recurrent seizures. As many as 22% of those who remain on medication may have a seizure recurrence during the first 2 years. One study reported the outcome for children withdrawn from AED therapy at 1 year after their last seizure. In this series, 61% continued to be free of seizures after 24 months. This figure is similar to those in studies requiring longer seizure-free treatment periods.

Multivariate analysis revealed four factors predicting recurrent seizures after withdrawal at 1 year, namely female gender, age greater than 10 years at onset of seizure, partial seizures (other than those associated with benign epilepsy of childhood with rolandic spikes), and clinical evidence of neurologic abnormality. When three or four of these factors were present, fewer than 50% of the children remained free of seizures; for children with one, two, or none of these factors, more than 80% remained free of seizures. In addition, younger children with more severe forms of epilepsy (e.g., Lennox-Gastaut syndrome) are unlikely to experience a year without seizures. However, a significant portion of children with cerebral palsy with significant motor problems may remain free of seizures after AED withdrawal. In selected children, no advantage has been noted in prolonging AED therapy beyond 1 year of the last seizure.

The American Academy of Neurology, recognizing that withdrawal of AEDs is a common problem in the management of patients with epilepsy and that the decision often is made in the absence of data, developed practice parameters to serve as a guideline for making this decision (Box 401.5).

In summary, numerous studies have attempted to address the question of when to terminate AED therapy. Many children who have remained free of seizures for 2 to 5 consecutive years do not experience a recurrence after medication is withdrawn. Other children may need to continue medication indefinitely, particularly if they have fixed, major neurologic deficits in addition to seizures or certain epileptic syndromes such as juvenile myoclonic epilepsy. In general, children in whom seizures came under prompt control and who have no other significant

---

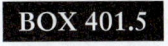

BOX 401.5 American Academy of Neurology Recommendations Concerning Withdrawal of Antiepileptic Drugs

Children or adults who meet the following profile have the greatest chance for successful drug withdrawal:

- Seizure-free interval of 2 to 5 years while taking antiepileptic drugs
- Single type of partial or generalized seizure
- Normal neurologic examination and normal intelligence quotient
- Electroencephalogram normalized with treatment

The recommendation is that drug withdrawal be offered to patients who meet this profile and who have complied with treatment. Children meeting this profile are expected to have at least a 69% chance for successful withdrawal. However, discontinuation of antiepileptic drugs may be appropriate in patients not meeting this profile, even though the risk of recurrence may be higher than 31% for these children.

neurologic deficits tend to remain free of seizures when medication is discontinued. No agreement has been reached regarding whether age at seizure onset or particular EEG characteristics are significant risk factors for recurrence. Some clinicians obtain an EEG at the initiation or conclusion of drug withdrawal and prolong treatment in the presence of markedly abnormal EEG results, including active epileptiform abnormalities. Seizures in children are most likely to recur during the period of drug withdrawal.

We believe that children who have been maintained free of seizures for 2 consecutive years should be considered for drug withdrawal. AEDs should be discontinued gradually, usually over a period of 4 to 6 weeks. Only one drug should be withdrawn at a time if the child has been taking multiple drugs. In the case of adolescents, it seems reasonable to exercise extra caution regarding driving during the period of drug withdrawal or to attempt AED withdrawal before the patient reaches driving age.

COGNITIVE AND BEHAVIORAL EFFECTS OF DRUGS

Many factors may have adverse effects on cognitive function and behavior in children with epilepsy. They include seizure type and frequency, cause, accompanying neurologic deficits, basic intellectual endowment, and the psychosocial milieu. Learning difficulties appear to be more frequent in children with epilepsy than in the general population. Many studies have attempted to assess the adverse effects of AEDs on cognitive function. Cross-study comparison has been difficult for numerous reasons, including variability in patient age, drug regimens, drug levels, seizure type and frequency, psychological and educational test instruments used, and bias inherent in data obtained from parent and teacher questionnaires. Certainly, PBS can produce paradoxical hyperkinesis in some children, and common sense suggests that drug doses that are sufficient to produce lethargy or sedation will affect learning and social interaction.

Although evidence suggests that many, if not all, AEDs have adverse effects on behavior or cognition in certain children, more well-controlled studies are required to resolve this issue. Physicians should heed the reports of parents and teachers in assessing the potential effects of AEDs on the cognitive skills and behavior of individual children. If the high probability is that a given drug is producing adverse effects, the physician should consider altering the dose or substituting another drug.

COUNSELING PATIENTS AND PARENTS

Diagnosing the condition and initiating appropriate drug therapy are only the initial steps in caring for a child with a seizure disorder. Parents and children often have many questions, misconceptions, and fears. They always want to know if the child will outgrow seizures, what to do during a seizure, and how seizures may influence participation in school and sports. Dispelling misconceptions and providing guidance are just as important as dispensing medication. Anxious and overprotective parents or overly solicitous teachers and peers can affect the child's psychosocial development adversely. Parents and older children should have a clear understanding that epilepsy is not a disease entity *per se,* but rather is the symptomatic expression of disordered cerebral function, and that the prognosis for seizure control depends on underlying etiologic factors and may vary significantly from one child to another. On the basis of specific etiologic factors, or the absence thereof, the physician

can provide the family with an individualized understanding and prognosis.

Frequently, parents are concerned that their child may die during a seizure. One should emphasize that the objective of maintenance drug therapy is to prevent seizure recurrence and that a period of observation is required to optimize the medication dosage. If further seizures occur, they most likely will be brief. Most seizures terminate spontaneously within 5 minutes, and death as a result of seizures is exceedingly rare. Indeed, fatalities usually are the consequence of the patient's being engaged in a potentially hazardous activity when a seizure occurs (swimming unattended, operating a motorized vehicle, or climbing to some high place).

Parents should be reassured that the brevity of most seizures obviates the necessity of rushing to the emergency department. If a seizure persists beyond 10 to 15 minutes, seeking medical assistance is appropriate. Teachers and school nurses also should be advised that sending a child home after a brief, uncomplicated seizure is not necessary. Excessive zeal in this regard can only diminish self-esteem, raise anxiety levels, and alter social interaction with classmates. The family should be fully informed of the rationale for drug choice and use and of the potential dose-related and non-dose-related side effects. Compliance can be enhanced by advising the patient to use an inexpensive pillbox that is compartmentalized to hold daily medications.

Precautions

In general, the child with epilepsy should be treated as a neurologically normal child, with a few notable precautions. As with all children, swimming always should be supervised. Until seizures are well-controlled, bicycle riding with a helmet should be restricted to low-traffic residential areas, and climbing onto rooftops should be discouraged. Sports and athletic activities often are extremely important to young people, and decisions regarding participation should involve the parents, patient, and physician in an open discussion. In most instances, epilepsy should not exclude a child from participation in sports activities. Situations in which a seizure could cause a dangerous fall, such as rope climbing, activities on parallel bars, and high diving, should be avoided, as should competitive underwater swimming. Participation in contact collision sports should be given individual consideration. Common sense suggests, however, that contact or collision sports could pose significant risks to a patient who is continuing to have several seizures per month.

Immunizations

Current recommendations state that pertussis immunization may affect seizure risk adversely and should be deferred in children with a personal history of seizures and in those with certain neurologic conditions such as tuberous sclerosis, certain inherited metabolic disorders, or other conditions predisposing them to seizures. The pertussis component of the DTP vaccine should be eliminated from subsequent immunizations in the child who has had a seizure within 48 hours of receiving a prior DTP immunization.

Puberty

Puberty traditionally has been considered to have an adverse effect on the course of epilepsy, especially in girls. An increase, a decrease, and no change in seizure frequency during puberty have been reported. Physicians have been cautioned against withdrawing AEDs during this period, even when the patient has met currently accepted criteria for discontinuing therapy. This attitude is not supported by the evidence, however.

Teratogenesis

Physicians have a special obligation to adolescents and potentially sexually active girls and their parents in making them aware of the potential teratogenic effects of AEDs. No woman should receive AEDs unnecessarily, and, in the girl who has been free of seizures for several years, consideration should be given to gradual withdrawal of medication before a pregnancy is planned. The discontinuation of AEDs in pregnant women who have required medication to control seizures is not recommended because prolonged seizures could cause serious harm to both the woman and the fetus.

The traditional AEDs have been reported to produce congenital malformations, ranging from minimal defects such as cleft lip (amenable to satisfactory cosmetic repair) to major cardiac defects and spinal dysraphism. Few human data on the newer AEDs are available, although LTG was noted to be associated with a lower incidence of major malformations in one study. In general, however, the pregnant woman with epilepsy who requires drugs for seizure control has approximately a 90% chance of delivering a normal child. Daily folate supplementation (suggested dose, 4 to 6 mg/day) for women of childbearing age who are receiving AEDs is recommended, especially for those receiving VPA.

Driver's Licensure

The restriction imposed by epilepsy on eligibility for a driver's license is a major concern for teenagers. In some instances, the aspiration for licensure can be a potent motivation for compliance with medication regimens. Legal requirements and the duration of restrictions vary from state to state, and physicians must be acquainted with the regulations of the state in which they practice. In general, the recommendation is that patients be free of seizures for at least 6 to 12 consecutive months before they are licensed to drive. The physician may be required to attest to the seizure-free interval and to the patient's compliance with the prescribed drug regimen. For medicolegal purposes, it may be useful for the physician to document by an entry in the clinical record that the patient and the parents have been advised of the relevant regulations.

Suggested Readings

Ad Hoc Committee for the Child Neurology Society Consensus Statement on Pertussis Immunization and the Central Nervous System. Pertussis immunization and the central nervous system. *Ann Neurol* 1991;29:458.

American Academy of Neurology and the Child Neurology Society. Practice parameter: medical treatment of infantile spasms. *Neurology* 2004;62: 1668.

Bird TD. Major patterns of human inheritance: relevance to the epilepsies. *Epilepsia* 1994;35(suppl 1):S2.

Bourgeois BF. New antiepileptic drugs in children: which ones for which seizures? *Clin Neuropharmacol* 2000;23:119.

Camfield C, Camfield P, Gordon K, et al. Does the number of seizures before treatment influence ease of control or remission of childhood epilepsy? Not if the number is 10 or less. *Neurology* 1996;46:41.

Commission on Classification and Terminology of the International League against Epilepsy. Proposal for revised clinical and electroencephalographic classification of epileptic seizures. *Epilepsia* 1981;22:489.

Commission on Classification and Terminology of the International League against Epilepsy. Proposal for revised classification of epilepsies and epileptic syndromes. *Epilepsia* 1989;30:389.

Dalessio DJ. Seizure disorders and pregnancy. *N Engl J Med* 1985;312:559.

Delgado MR, Riela AR, Mills J, et al. Discontinuation of antiepileptic drug treatment after two seizure-free years in children with cerebral palsy. *Pediatrics* 1996;97:192.

Dooley J, Gordon K, Camfield P, et al. Discontinuation of anticonvulsant therapy in children free of seizures for 1 year: a prospective study. *Neurology* 1996;46:969.

Farrell K, Connolly MB, Munn R, et al. Prospective open-label, add-on study of lamotrigine in 56 children with intractable generalized epilepsy. *Pediatr Neurol* 1997;16:201.

Glauser TA. Topiramate. *Semin Pediatr Neurol* 1997;4:34.

Hauser E, Freilinger M, Seidl R, et al. Prognosis of childhood epilepsy in newly referred patients. *J Child Neurol* 1996;11:201.

Holland KD. Efficacy, pharmacology, and adverse effects of antiepileptic drugs. *Neurol Clin* 2001;19:313.

Jarrar RG, Buchhalter JR. Therapeutics in pediatric epilepsy. Part 1: the new antiepileptic drugs and the kerogenic diet. *Mayo Clin Proc* 2003;78: 359.

Kuzniecky RI. Neuroimaging in pediatric epilepsy. *Epilepsia* 1996;37(suppl 1): S10.

Kwan P, Brodie M. Effectiveness of first antiepileptic drug. *Epilepsia* 2001; 42:1255.

Marson AG, Kadir ZA, Hutton JL, et al. The new antiepileptic drugs: a systematic review of their efficacy and tolerability. *Epilepsia* 1997;38:859.

Nordli DR Jr, De Vivo DC. The ketogenic diet revisited: back to the future. *Epilepsia* 1997;38:743.

Ottman R, Annegers JF, Risch N, et al. Relations of genetic and environmental factors in the etiology of epilepsy. *Ann Neurol* 1996;39:442.

Pellock JM, Willmore LJ. A rational guide to routine blood monitoring in patients receiving antiepileptic drugs. *Neurology* 1991;41:961.

Quality Standards Subcommittee of the American Academy of Neurology. Practice parameters: a guideline for discontinuing antiepileptic drugs in seizure-free patients-summary statement. *Neurology* 1996;47:600.

Quality Standards Subcommittee of the American Academy of Neurology and the Practice Committee of the Child Neurology Society. Practice parameters: treatment of the child with a first unprovoked seizure. *Neurology* 2003; 60:166.

Shinnar S, Berg AT, Moshe SL, et al. The risk of seizure recurrence after a first unprovoked afebrile seizure in childhood: an extended follow-up. *Pediatrics* 1996;98:216.

Therapeutics and Technology Assessment Subcommittee and Quality Standards Subcommittee of the American Academy of Neurology and American Epilepsy Society. Efficacy and tolerability of the new antiepileptic drugs. Part 1: treatment of new onset epilepsy. *Neurology* 2004;62:1252.

Wheless JW, Maggio V. Vagus nerve stimulation therapy in patients younger than 18 years. *Neurology* 2002;59:S21.

Zupanc ML. Neuroimaging in the evaluation of children and adolescents with intractable epilepsy. Part 1: magnetic resonance imaging and the substrates of epilepsy. *Pediatr Neurol* 1997;17:19.

CHAPTER 402 ■ STATUS EPILEPTICUS

KEVIN CHAPMAN AND DANIEL G. GLAZE

Status epilepticus (SE) may be defined classically as seizure activity that lasts longer than 30 minutes or repeated seizures between which the child does not return to the baseline level of consciousness. Some studies have challenged the duration of a seizure before it can be called SE, and progressively shorter times are being used in the definition. In convulsive SE, the child has a prolonged, generalized tonic-clonic seizure or the repetition of such seizures without a return to full consciousness between episodes. In nonconvulsive SE, such as absence status and complex partial status, the clinical presentation is a change in mental state that often manifests as prolonged *twilight* or semicoma. In epilepsia partialis continua, consciousness is preserved in the presence of continuous, focal motor activity. Most SE episodes in children appear to be generalized convulsive in character. Of those SE episodes beginning with partial seizures, most secondarily generalize. Careful history taking and observation suggest that most (64% of adults and children) SE episodes begin as partial seizures that generalize so the final character is generalized.

The burden of SE is significant. The overall (in adults and children) incidence of SE appears to be 41 to 61 per 100,000, and SE results in an estimated 42,000 deaths (in children and adults) per year in the United States. The age distribution of SE suggests two age peaks: during the first year of life (the time of the highest frequency of SE) and in individuals 60 years old or older. In children, 21% of all cases of SE occur in the first year of life, and 64% occur in the first 5 years. Approximately 12% of patients with newly diagnosed epilepsy have a seizure lasting 30 minutes or longer. Most cases of SE occur in children, and fewer than 25% occur as idiopathic events. The occurrence of SE should prompt a full diagnostic workup. Previously, overall short-term mortality figures as high as 30% were reported, but investigators have reported more recently a mortality rate of 3% to 6% in children. The long-term mortality rate in children has been found to be 7% over the subsequent 10 years. This decrease in mortality rates is the result of faster diagnosis and support, combined with better medical treatment and improved intensive care. Death usually is attributable to the underlying cause of SE rather than to a prolonged seizure. When this information is considered, mortality related to prolonged seizures *per se* has been reported to occur in as few as 1% to 2% of cases. SE can be associated with significant mortality rates and morbidity that can include epileptic brain damage, neurologic cognitive defects, and continuing recurrent seizures.

Three factors appear to be related to mortality and morbidity: duration of SE, age, and cause. Greater incidence of mortality is observed if SE lasts longer than 1 hour. Prolonged seizures can lead to a series of metabolic derangements that potentially can cause neuronal damage. Tonic-clonic SE that progresses beyond 60 minutes may be associated with severe, permanent brain damage or death. The significance of prolonged or refractory SE, frequently defined as seizures having a duration of longer than 1 hour, has been observed in humans and experimental animals. In animals with experimentally induced seizures lasting less than 1 hour, reversible neuronal injuries are produced. However, if the duration of seizure is greater than 1 hour, neuronal death involving susceptible regions, including the hippocampus, amygdala, thalamus, and middle cerebral cortical layers, is observed. This neuronal death occurs even if a patient is well ventilated and irrespective of metabolic derangements. Neuron-specific enolase, a marker for brain injury, is significantly elevated after prolonged SE. Initial increases in cerebral blood flow and glucose consumption are followed after 60 to 120 minutes of seizure activity by decreased cerebral blood flow but continuing glucose consumption. Excessive enhancement of local metabolic rates may result in selective cell death. Animal studies in adult rats have demonstrated that the hippocampus is particularly susceptible and may undergo reorganization that leads to a reduction of seizure threshold. One longitudinal quantitative magnetic resonance imaging study in adults demonstrated progressive loss of hippocampal volume in patients with temporal lobe epilepsy, whereas other studies have demonstrated decreases in the ratio of N-acetylaspartic acid (NAA) to choline on magnetic resonance spectroscopy following SE, findings suggesting neuronal loss after seizures has occurred. The initial systemic effects of SE include an increase in plasma catecholamines, an increase in blood pressure, tachycardia, and hyperpyrexia. These effects are self-correcting with the cessation of SE. Late effects that may be less amenable to correction include hypotension, hypoglycemia, acidosis, pulmonary edema, hyperpyrexia, and rhabdomyolysis. They may contribute to significant mortality rates and morbidity. These findings in humans and animal models emphasize the importance of ensuring prompt cessation of SE and of managing and correcting the systemic effects of SE.

In most series, mortality rates are significantly lower in children. One study found that the overall mortality rate was less than 5% in children versus 26% in adults and more than 50% in adults older than 80 years of age. Differences in origin in children versus adults contribute to this observation. SE may occur in the setting of an acute illness, in patients with established epilepsy, or as a first unprovoked seizure. Causes can be classified as idiopathic, remote symptomatic, febrile, acute symptomatic, or associated with progressive encephalopathy. Although 6% to 12% of SE episodes in children represent a first unprovoked seizure, a cause should be investigated.

Infectious processes, toxic or metabolic disorders, and chronic forms of encephalopathy, as well as the sudden withdrawal of antiepileptic drugs, may underlie or precipitate this condition in children. In patients with known epilepsy, antiepileptic drug noncompliance or low levels should be considered. If a child has a known preexistent neurologic or other medical abnormality, complications such as shunt malfunction, central nervous system (CNS) hemorrhage or infection should be considered. In adults, anoxic/hypoxic-ischemic insults account for a significant incidence of mortality; these causes are uncommon in children. Etiologic factors observed more frequently in children include infections of the CNS (meningoencephalitis), metabolic aberrations, febrile seizures, and "idiopathic" epilepsy. These conditions have a lower incidence of associated mortality and morbidity. In children, most

TABLE 402.1

GUIDELINE FOR EMERGENCY MANAGEMENT OF STATUS EPILEPTICUS
IN CHILDREN

Duration of Seizure	Action
0–5 minutes	Monitor airway, breathing, circulation (ABCs)
	Administer high-flow oxygen
	Obtain history and perform physical examination
	Place intravenous access
5–10 minutes	Give lorazepam 0.1 mg/kg IV (maximum dose 4 mg)
	Or diazepam 0.2–0.5 mg/kg IV (maximum dose 10 mg)
	If no IV access, give diazepam rectally: 2–5 years old, 0.5 mg/kg; 6–11 years old, 0.3 mg/kg; >12 years old, 0.2 mg/kg
	Obtain laboratory studies, including bedside glucose testing
10–25 minutes	Give fosphenytoin 20 mg/kg PE IV at 3 mg/kg/min
	Or alternatively in neonates: phenobarbital 20 mg/kg
	May administer second dose of lorazepam or diazepam
25–40 minutes	Give phenobarbital 20 mg/kg IV
	Or alternatively rebolus with fosphenytoin 10 mg/kg PE IV
	Transfer to intensive care setting and monitor closely for respiratory depression
40–60 minutes	Administer anesthetic doses of pentobarbital or midazolam
	Start bedside electroencephalographic monitoring

IV, intravenously; PE, phenytoin equivalents.
Adapted from Working Group on Status Epilepticus. Treatment of convulsive status epilepticus: recommendations of the Epilepsy Foundation of America's working group on status epilepticus. *JAMA* 1993;270:854.

fatalities are associated with acute insult to the CNS or progressive neurologic disorders.

Neurologic sequelae in children with idiopathic or febrile SE are rare developments (1.5% versus 9.1% for all causes). In addition, the incidence of recurrent seizures after SE in children is low. The risk of recurrent episodes of convulsive SE is 58% in neurologically abnormal children but is very low in neurologically normal children (3%). After SE as the first unprovoked seizure in a neurologically normal child, no increased risk of recurrence of seizures is observed. However, if the patient has recurrence of a seizure, it is more likely to be prolonged. Some authors suggest that initiating long-term therapy for a neurologically normal child whose first seizure is an episode of SE is not necessary. Factors influencing a favorable outcome of SE in children may be related to advances in therapy, prompt and aggressive management of seizure and systemic abnormalities, and the resistance of the immature brain to damage from seizures.

TREATMENT

Tonic-clonic SE is a life-threatening situation and represents a neurologic emergency. The longer the seizure lasts, the more difficult it will be to stop. Animal studies have demonstrated that antiepileptic drugs have a time-dependent decreased effectiveness in SE. The therapeutic measures outlined here are appropriate in cases in which a seizure or repeated seizures continue unabated for 10 to 30 minutes. Any patient with persistent clonic seizures on arrival to the emergency room should be treated as having SE because of the time of transportation. Some clinicians consider almost any tonic-clonic seizure to be an episode of SE and intervene with both supportive and drug therapy.

Therapy must address the immediate problem of stopping the seizure, providing supportive measures (e.g., supplemental oxygen, a clear airway, an intravenous glucose source), detecting and correcting any predisposing or precipitating factors, and incorporating a drug with a long half-life to prevent the recurrence of seizures once they have been arrested. Table 402.1 provides a guideline for treatment of SE in children. Supportive measures are listed in Box 402.1.

BOX 402.1   Supportive Measures

The preservation of vital functions takes precedence:

- Blood pressure, respiration, and cardiac function are maintained to avoid hypoxic-ischemic damage to the brain. Resuscitation equipment should be available.
- Blood samples are obtained for electrolyte, glucose, blood urea nitrogen, calcium, and magnesium measurements and, if the patient has been treated previously for seizures, for antiepileptic drug level determinations. Bedside blood glucose testing should be performed to evaluate quickly for hypoglycemia, which needs immediate correction.
- An intravenous line is inserted for the infusion of a glucose solution to maintain the blood glucose level at approximately 150 mg/dL. Fluids should be limited initially to 1,000 to 1,200 mL/m^2.
- Increased intracranial pressure is treated if evident.
- A detailed history should be obtained focusing on recent illness, trauma, and history of seizures and medications. A thorough physical and neurologic examination should be performed evaluating for evidence of head trauma or central nervous system infection.

Drug Therapy

Initial treatment with a benzodiazepine is considered first-line therapy for the control of SE. Lorazepam is the benzodiazepine most widely used. In a comparison study, it was found to terminate SE in 65% of patients and was significantly better than was phenytoin alone. Lorazepam has a rapid onset and a more prolonged duration of anticonvulsant action than does diazepam. Although its half-life of 10 to 15 hours is less than that of diazepam, lorazepam continues to achieve effective brain levels for 8 to 24 hours. The suggested dose in children is 0.05 to 0.10 mg/kg (maximum dose, 4 mg) given intravenously and repeated one or two times as needed. Diazepam may be used alternatively and is administered in an intravenous dose of 0.25 to 0.30 mg/kg, excluding infants younger than 2 to 3 months old (maximum dose, 5 mg in children younger than 5 years and 10 mg in children 5 to 10 years old). In children who are 5 to 10 years old, an alternative method of calculating the dose is 1 mg/year of age to a maximum of 10 mg. In patients without intravenous access or in the prehospital setting, diazepam is available and may be administred as a rectal gel formulation, with rapid absorption and onset. The dosage varies based on age and weight of the patient: 2 to 5 years old, 0.5 mg/kg; 6 to 11 years old, 0.3 mg/kg; and older than 12 years of age, 0.2 mg/kg. Intramuscular midazolam, at a suggested dose of 0.2 mg/kg, may be as effective as is intravenous diazepam. The intramuscular route may be particularly useful in the physician's office, in the prehospital setting, and for children with difficult intravenous access.

Patients who have seizures that continue despite receiving an adequate trial of benzodiazepines should be treated with a medication with a longer half-life. Fosphenytoin has replaced phenytoin as a drug of choice in the treatment of SE. Fosphenytoin is a prodrug of phenytoin with equal efficacy. It has a more neutral pH than does phenytoin, is water soluble and rapidly converted to phenytoin, and has a low rate of reactions at the injection site. Fosphenytoin is given as phenytoin equivalents (PE), and the dose is 10 to 20 mg PE/kg given intravenously for the treatment of SE. Fosphenytoin can be given in normal saline or dextrose at a rate of 3 mg/kg/minute. A maximum dose of 150 mg/minute has been suggested, although levels are available rapidly after slower (50 to 100 mg/minute) administration. Side effects may include vomiting, somnolence, ataxia, nystagmus, and pruritus (typically perineal) and paresthesias. Although fosphenytoin is not reported to have significant cardiovascular side effects in children and infants, monitoring of cardiac rhythm and vital signs is suggested. Intramuscular administration of fosphenytoin can give rapid, adequate levels of phenytoin, but it is not recommended for the treatment of SE. In children younger than 1 year of age, close monitoring of phenytoin levels is suggested based on reports of difficulties achieving and maintaining adequate serum levels with fosphenytoin in this age group. An advantage associated with the use of fosphenytoin is the general absence of sedation and of respiratory depression. If seizures persist after the initial doses of lorazepam and fosphenytoin are given, an additional bolus of lorazepam may be given with an addition 10 mg/kg of fosphenytoin. Phenobarbital, at a dose of 10 to 20 mg/kg at a rate of 1–2 mg/kg/minute or 30 mg/min, may be used. Respiratory depression and excessive sedation should be monitored closely. If this regimen is unsuccessful, neurologic consultation is appropriate.

In neonates and very young infants, administration of intravenous phenobarbital at a dose of approximately 20 mg/kg is advised. The dose may be repeated up to a maximum of 40 mg/kg. If necessary, it may be followed by fosphenytoin given intravenously in doses starting at 10 mg PE/kg at rates of 1 mg/kg/minute. A dose of 10 mg PE/kg may be repeated if seizures continue.

Suggested Readings

Appleton R, Choonara I, Martland T, et al. The treatment of convulsive status epilepticus in children: the Status Epilepticus Working Party. *Arch Dis Child* 2000;83:415.

Crawford TO, Mitchell WG, Fishman LS, et al. Very high dose phenobarbital for refractory status epilepticus in children. *Neurology* 1988;38:1035.

Crawford TO, Mitchell WG, Snodgrass SR. Lorazepam in childhood status epilepticus and serial seizures. *Neurology* 1987;37:190.

Delgado-Escueta AV, Bajorek JG. Status epilepticus: mechanisms of brain damage and rational management. *Epilepsia* 1982;23(suppl 1):529.

DeLorenzo RJ, Hauser WA, Towne AR, et al. A prospective, population-based epidemiologic study of status epilepticus in Richmond, Virginia. *Neurology* 1996;46:1029.

Giang DW, McBride MC. Lorazepam versus diazepam for the treatment of status epilepticus. *Pediatr Neurol* 1988;4:358.

Gross-Tsur V, Shinnar S. Convulsive status epilepticus in children. *Epilepsia* 1993;34(suppl 1):512.

Hauser WA. Status epilepticus: epidemiological considerations. *Neurology* 1990;5(suppl 2):9.

Holmes GL. Do seizures cause brain damage? *Int Pediatr* 1988;3:158.

Holmes GL. Seizure-induced neuronal injury: animal data. *Neurology* 2002;59(suppl 5):S3.

Lockman LA. Treatment of status epilepticus in children. *Neurology* 1990;5(suppl 2):43.

Logroscine G, Hesdorffer DC, Cascino GD, et al. Long-term mortality after a first episode of status epilepticus. *Neurology* 2002;58:537.

Mitchell WG. Status epilepticus and acute repetitive seizures in children, adolescents, and young adults: etiology, outcome, and treatment. *Epilepsia* 1996;37(suppl 1):574.

Pellock JM. Recent advances concerning status epilepticus. *Int Pediatr* 1990;5:189.

Pellock JM. Fosphenytoin use in children. *Neurology* 1996;46(suppl 1):S14.

Phillips SA, Shanahan RJ. Etiology and mortality of status epilepticus in children: a recent update. *Arch Neurol* 1989;46:74.

Shinnar S, Maytal J, Krasnoff L, Moshe SL. Recurrent status epilepticus in children. *Ann Neurol* 1992;31:598.

Treiman DM, Meyers PD, Walton NY, et al. A comparison of four treatments for generalized convulsive status epilepticus. *N Engl J Med* 1998;339:792.

Working Group on Status Epilepticus. Treatment of convulsive status epilepticus. Recommendations of the Epilepsy Foundation of America's working group on status epilepticus. *JAMA* 1993;270:854.

CHAPTER 403 ■ FEBRILE SEIZURES

MARVIN A. FISHMAN

Febrile seizures are a worldwide problem and occur in 2% to 4% of children younger than 5 years of age. In some populations, the incidence is as high as 15%, which may be the result of closer living arrangements among family members, thereby making detection more likely, as well as racial or geographic differences. A febrile seizure is defined as a convulsion that is associated with an elevated temperature greater than 38°C occurring in a child who is younger than 6 years of age. Exclusions to the diagnosis include a history of a previous afebrile seizure, infection or inflammation of the central nervous system, or acute systemic metabolic abnormalities that may produce convulsions. Febrile seizures are classified into two groups based on their clinical features. *Simple* (benign) febrile seizures are those that last less than 15 minutes, do not have focal features, and, if they occur in a series, have a total duration of less than 30 minutes. *Complex* febrile seizures include those that last longer than 15 minutes, have focal features, or postictal paresis, and occur in series with a total duration greater than 30 minutes.

PATHOGENESIS

Febrile seizures are an age-related phenomenon and occur in children between the ages of 6 months and 6 years. The reason that febrile seizures occur only in infants and young children is unclear, as are the mechanism whereby fever induces the seizure.

Febrile seizures occur during both bacterial and viral infections and may occur more frequently in patients with illnesses that are accompanied by severe constitutional symptoms. One study found that infection with human herpesvirus 6 accounted for approximately one-third of the first-time febrile seizures in children 2 years old or younger. These children are more likely to have clusters of seizures and long-lasting partial seizures with postictal paralysis. Attempts have been made to link susceptibility to febrile seizures with abnormalities of neurotransmitters. The concentration of gamma-aminobutyric acid (GABA), an inhibitory transmitter, was found to be reduced in the cerebrospinal fluid (CSF) of children who were studied after their first or second febrile seizure. No correlation was found between the duration of the seizure and the concentration of GABA; however, because the samples were obtained after the convulsion occurred, the abnormality possibly was a secondary phenomenon rather than a primary event.

Genetic factors appear to be important in the expression of the condition. An increased incidence of febrile seizures exists among first-degree relatives—10% to 20% of parents and siblings—of children with febrile seizures. The concordance rate for febrile seizures in monozygotic twins is much higher than that in dizygotic twins, in whom the rate is similar to that of other siblings. A complex segregation analysis of febrile seizures occurring in more than 450 families during a 30-year period was completed. Different models explained the rate of occurrence based on the frequency of febrile convulsions in the proband. In children who had a single febrile convulsion, a polygenic (common familial environment) model was most appropriate. If the proband had experienced multiple febrile convulsions, however, the most consistent model was that of a single major locus with nearly dominant seizure susceptibility.

A relationship between febrile seizures and an increased incidence of epilepsy in families of the proband appears to exist. Siblings and parents of patients with febrile seizures have a 4% to 10% incidence of epilepsy. Moreover, siblings of patients with epilepsy are at increased risk for having febrile seizures.

Recently, several autosomal dominant genetic syndromes that increase the susceptability to febrile seizures have been identified. The loci are found on 8q13-21, 19p, 19q, 2q23-24, and 5q14-15.

Generalized epilepsy with febrile seizures plus (GEPS+) is a newly identified autosomal dominant syndrome. The phenotype in families consists of children who have febrile seizures that persist beyond 6 years of age and may have afebrile tonic-clonic as well as other seizure types. Some families have had an association between myoclonic epilepsy, as well as partial seizures, and atonic seizures beginning between 1 and 4 years of age. Several genes have been identified, and they all involve sodium channel mutations. Families with the GEFS+ phenotype who have evidence of GABA receptor dysfunction also have been described. Mutations in the same receptor have been found in families with childhood absence epilepsy and febrile seizures. This finding suggests that the mutation has age-dependent effects and involves different neuronal networks because the ages of onset and the physiologic features of the seizure types are different.

SIGNS AND SYMPTOMS

Most febrile seizures are simple. Prolonged convulsions occur in fewer than 10% of children with febrile seizures, and focal features are seen in fewer than 5%. Generalized seizures mainly are clonic, but both atonic and tonic episodes have been noted. Involvement of the facial and respiratory muscles is noted frequently. Complex febrile seizures occur as the initial convulsion in most children who experience them. An initial simple febrile seizure can be followed by a subsequent complex febrile seizure, however, and vice versa. Children usually have significantly elevated body temperatures, but approximately 25% of febrile convulsions occur in children whose temperatures are between 38° and 39°C. Children who have repeated febrile seizures do not always experience them with the same degree of fever. In addition, these seizures do not occur every time the child has a temperature elevation similar to the one associated with the preceding febrile seizure. Most febrile seizures occur on the first day of illness, and, in some children, they are the first sign of the accompanying infection.

DIFFERENTIAL DIAGNOSIS

The main concern in evaluating an infant or child with a febrile convulsion is the possible presence of underlying meningitis or encephalitis. A thorough evaluation by an experienced clinician almost always detects the child with meningitis. If the only indication for performing a lumbar puncture is a febrile seizure, meningitis is found in fewer than 1% of patients. Fewer than one-half of these patients have bacterial meningitis. In children who have meningitis presenting with seizures, as many as 40% (particularly younger infants) may not have meningeal signs. They may have other symptoms and findings, however, that strongly suggest the presence of meningitis. Thus, a diagnosis of bacterial meningitis based solely on a routine evaluation of CSF after a febrile seizure is exceedingly rare.

Seizures usually are distinguished easily from other types of involuntary movements occurring in sick infants. Chills usually consist of fine, rhythmic oscillatory movements about a joint and are not clonic in nature. They rarely involve facial or respiratory muscles. Moreover, chills are not accompanied by loss of consciousness, which does occur during a generalized seizure.

An underlying metabolic disorder presenting as a seizure in a febrile child rarely is detected. A careful review of the history usually provides other clues suggesting the likelihood of an underlying problem.

DIAGNOSTIC TESTS

The routine performance of lumbar punctures in all children with febrile seizures does not seem warranted. Children who may be considered candidates for examination of the CSF include young infants, children whose febrile seizures occur after the second day of illness, cases in which the clinician is unsure of his or her judgment regarding the presence or absence of meningitis, and situations in which the patient cannot be observed. The American Academy of Pediatrics recommends that after the first seizure with fever in infants younger than 12 months of age, performing a lumbar puncture should be considered strongly. The routine performance of skull radiography in children with febrile seizures is useless. If imaging of the brain is indicated by abnormal head size, by an abnormal neurologic examination (especially with focal features), or by signs or symptoms of increased intracranial pressure, computed tomography or magnetic resonance imaging should be performed. Measurement of serum electrolytes, blood sugar, calcium, and urea nitrogen concentrations are of very low yield and need not be performed routinely. These tests should be done when indicated by the results of the history or physical examination. Patients with significant vomiting, diarrhea, and abnormal fluid intake may be suspected of having acute metabolic disturbances, and routine serum chemistry testing should be performed in these children. The routine use of electroencephalography in all children with febrile seizures is not warranted. A tracing obtained within 1 week of the seizure is abnormal in at least one-third of these children. Febrile convulsions of long duration or with focal features increase the likelihood that abnormalities will be found. Abnormal electroencephalographic results do not identify children in whom epilepsy subsequently will develop and should not be used as the basis for deciding which children need anticonvulsant therapy.

TREATMENT

Short-Term Treatment

A child who is convulsing actively needs to be treated urgently, especially if the seizure has been present for 5 minutes or longer and shows no signs of abating. Immediate attention should be directed toward ensuring that the patient has an adequate airway, is breathing well, and has satisfactory perfusion and circulatory status. A blood sample should be obtained for the determination of electrolyte and glucose levels, if indicated. At this point, antiepileptic drugs should be administered, intravenously if possible. One strategy is to give a short-acting anticonvulsant such as lorazepam (0.05 to 0.10 mg/kg). If seizures persist, an additional dose can be given. The clinician should be ready to intubate the child if respirations become inadequate. Rarely, additional treatment with fosphenytoin (15 to 20 mg/kg) may need to be given if seizures persist. It should be administered slowly to avoid the development of cardiac dysrhythmias and hypotension. For persistent status epilepticus, phenobarbital may need to be administered (20 mg/kg).

Rectally administered diazepam, at a dosage of 0.5 mg/kg (maximum, 5 mg), has been used for the control of febrile seizures. Rectally administered diazepam is effective in approximately 80% of patients. After the seizures are under control, the fever should be treated with antipyretic agents such as acetaminophen or aspirin and with physical methods such as sponging with tepid water and using a cooling mattress, if necessary.

Prophylactic Treatment

The Committee on Quality Improvement, Subcommittee on Febrile Seizures of the American Academy of Pediatrics has issued a practice parameter regarding the long-term treatment of the child with simple febrile seizures. The Committee concluded the following:

> Based on the risk and benefits of effective therapies, neither continuous nor intermittent anticonvulsive therapy is recommended for children with one or more simple febrile seizures. The American Academy of Pediatrics recognizes that recurrent episodes of febrile seizures can create anxiety in some parents and their children and as such appropriate educational and emotional support should be provided.

After reviewing the appropriate literature, the Committee concluded that, although anticonvulsive therapy with phenobarbital or valproic acid is effective in decreasing recurrent febrile seizures, the risks and potential side effects of these medications outweigh the benefit.

The effectiveness of these two anticonvulsants was confirmed in a metaanalytic review of studies for the prevention of recurrent febrile seizures (odds ratio for recurrence 0.54 and 0.09, respectively); in comparison, no difference in the risk for recurrence between children receiving intermittent diazepam and a placebo was found. The latter finding is in contrast to a controlled trial in which oral diazepam (0.33 mg/kg every 8 hours during the first few days of a febrile illness) was as effective as was the continuous administration of phenobarbital in reducing episodes of recurrent febrile seizures.

In summary, children with febrile seizures are at increased risk for developing afebrile seizures, but no available data suggest that the prevention of recurrent febrile seizures reduces the risk of developing afebrile seizures. For children who have had febrile seizures, treatment with antipyretics at the time of a febrile illness is helpful in overall management but does not appear to affect the recurrence rate of febrile seizures.

PROGNOSIS

The prognosis for children with febrile seizures can be divided into three categories: recurrence rate for febrile seizures, development of neurologic sequelae, and development of epilepsy. The major factor influencing the recurrence of febrile seizures is the age of the infant at the time of the first seizure. The younger the child, the more likely it is that febrile convulsions will recur. If the first seizure occurs when the child is younger than 1 year of age, the recurrence rate is approximately 50% to 65%, in contrast to a rate of 28% if the first seizure occurs after that point. If the first seizure does not occur until the child is at least 2.5 years of age, the recurrence rate is reduced to approximately 20%. Other factors that have been shown in some studies to influence the recurrence rate have been abnormal development before the first febrile seizure occurs, a history of afebrile seizures in parents and siblings, and the number of subsequent febrile illnesses. Approximately 50% to 75% of recurrences take place within 1 year of the initial seizure, and approximately 90% occur within 2.5 years. This recurrence rate can be influenced by the intermittent use of rapidly acting antiepileptic drugs.

Neurologic sequelae reported as a result of febrile seizures include death, status epilepticus, motor coordination deficits, mental retardation, and learning and behavioral problems. The exact incidence of these complications is uncertain, but it appears to be exceedingly low. They occur only in children who have experienced complex febrile seizures. Many of the reports documenting these complications have been anecdotal and derived from biased populations consisting of children who were evaluated at hospitals or clinics. In population-based studies, the incidence of these complications is very low. In the National Collaborative Perinatal Project, approximately 5% of children who had febrile seizures had episodes lasting longer than 30 minutes. No children in that study sustained permanent motor deficits, and none of the patients had impaired mental development unless afebrile seizures developed subsequently. Another study also has confirmed that status epilepticus as a result of febrile seizures does not cause new neurologic deficits. Children with prior neurologic abnormalities do have a higher risk of subsequently having febrile as well as afebrile seizures than do neurologically normal children after an episode of status epilepticus. A trend for recurrent febrile status epilepticus in these children exists. Neurologically normal children, however, do not have significantly increased risk for subseqent development of febrile seizures (prolonged or brief) or afebrile seizures after febrile status epilepticus.

Children who have febrile seizures are at increased risk for the development of epilepsy. In a neurologically normal child who has a simple febrile seizure, this risk may be twice that of the general population, or 1.0% versus 0.5%. Abnormal neurologic development in the presence of complex febrile seizures, particularly focal seizures, greatly increases the risk, by as much as 30- to 50-fold. In the National Collaborative Perinatal Project, children who were neurologically abnormal and who had a focal seizure had a 15.4% incidence of afebrile seizures by the time they reached 7 years of age. In a population-based study in Rochester, Minnesota, in which patients were observed into adulthood, the risk ranged from 2.4% among children with simple febrile convulsions to as high as 49% among children with focal, prolonged, and repeated episodes within 24 hours. These risk factors often were associated with partial unprovoked seizures, whereas subsequent unprovoked generalized seizures were more likely to be associated with the number of febrile convulsions experienced and a family history of unprovoked seizures. In the National Collaborative Perinatal Project, one-half of the children who had nonfebrile seizures never had recurrent febrile seizures. Thus, recurrence does not appear to be a prerequisite for the development of epilepsy.

Whether temporal lobe epilepsy develops after prolonged febrile seizures occur remains controversial. Patients considered for temporal lobe surgery often have histories of prolonged febrile seizures. Moreover, studies measuring hippocampal volume in adults with epilepsy have found a link between a history of febrile seizures and smaller hippocampi. However, in some studies of familial febrile seizures, asymmetry in the size of the hippocampi was found in some members who had febrile seizures and did not develop epilepsy, as well as in some unaffected members. Therefore, preexisting lesions may predispose patients to the development of epilepsy rather than being a consequence of the febrile seizures. In other studies, infants with very prolonged febrile status epilepticus had acute edema of the hippocampus demonstrated by magnetic resonance imaging. Some had developed hippocampal atrophy on follow-up studies. The possibility of preexisting lesions could not be excluded. Community-based epidemiologic studies have not been able to confirm the association between febrile seizures and temporal lobe epilepsy. In summary, febrile seizures have not clearly and consistently been demonstrated to be a cause of temporal lobe epilepsy.

Suggested Readings

Abou-Khalil B, Ge Q, Desai R, et al. Partial and generalized epilepsy with febrile seizures plus and a novel SCN1A mutation. *Neurology* 2001;57:2265.

American Academy of Pediatrics Provisional Committee on Quality Improvement, Subcommittee on Febrile Seizures. Practice parameter: the neurodiagnostic evaluation of the child with a first simple febrile seizure. *Pediatrics* 1996;97:769.

Annegers JF, Hauser WA, Shirts SB, Kurland CT. Factors prognostic of unprovoked seizures after febrile convulsions. *N Engl J Med* 1987;316:493.

Barum TZ, Shinnar S, eds. *Febrile seizures*. San Diego: Academic Press, 2002.

Baulac S, Huberfeld G, Gourfinkel-An I, et al. First genetic evidence of GABA$_A$ receptor dysfunction in epilepsy: a mutation in the γ2-subunit gene. *Nat Genet* 2001;28:46.

Berg AT, Shinnar S, Hauser SW, et al. A prospective study of recurrent febrile seizures. *N Engl J Med* 1992;327:1122.

Berg AT, Shinnar S, Levy SR, Testa FM. Childhood-onset epilepsy with and without preceding febrile seizures. *Neurology* 1999;53:1742.

Camfield PR, Camfield CS, Shapiro SH, Cummings C. The first febrile seizure: antipyretic instruction plus either phenobarbital or placebo to prevent recurrence. *J Pediatr* 1980;97:16.

Ellenberg JH, Nelson KB. Febrile seizures and later intellectual performance. *Arch Neurol* 1978;35:17.

Escayg A, MacDonald BT, Meisler MH, et al. Mutations of SCN1A, encoding a neuronal sodium channel, in two families with GEFS+2. *Nat Genet* 2000;24:343.

Fernandez G, Effenberger O, Vinz B, et al. Hippocampal malformation as a cause of familial febrile convulsions and subsequent hippocampal sclerosis. *Neurology* 1998;50:909.

Fishman MA. Febrile seizures. In: Fishman MA, ed. *Pediatric neurology*. Orlando, FL: Grune & Stratton, 1986.

Gerber MA, Berliner BC. The child with a "simple" febrile seizure: appropriate diagnostic evaluation. *Am J Dis Child* 1981;135:431.

Hall CB, Long CE, Schnabel KC, et al. Human herpesvirus-6 infection in children: a prospective study of complications and reactivation. *N Engl J Med* 1994;331:432.

Knudsen FU. Febrile seizures: treatment and outcome. *Brain Dev* 1996;18:438.

Lerche H, Weber YG, Baier H, et al. Generalized epilepsy with febrile seizures plus: further heterogeneity in a large family. *Neurology* 2001;57:1191.

Maytal J, Shinnar S. Febrile status epilepticus. *Pediatrics* 1990;86:611.

Nakayama J, Hamano K, Iwasaki N, et al. Significant evidence for linkage of febrile seizures to chromosome 5q14-q15. *Hum Mol Genet* 2000;9:87.

Nelson KB, Ellenberg JH. Predictors of epilepsy in children who have experienced febrile seizures. *N Engl J Med* 1976;295:1029.

Nelson KB, Ellenberg JH. Prognosis in children with febrile seizures. *Pediatrics* 1978;61:720.

Rantala H, Tarkka R, Uhari M. A meta-analytic review of the preventive treatment of recurrences of febrile seizures. *J Pediatr* 1997;131:922.

Rosman NP, Colton T, Labazzo J, et al. A controlled trial of diazepam administered during febrile illnesses to prevent recurrence of febrile seizures. *N Engl J Med* 1993;329:79.

Scheffer IE, Berkovic SF. Generalized epilepsy with febrile seizures plus: a genetic disorder with heterogeneous clinical phenotypes. *Brain* 1997;120:479.

Singh SR, Andermann E, Whitehouse WP, et al. Severe myoclonic epilepsy of infancy: extended spectrum of GFES+? *Epilepsia* 2001;42:837.

Suga S, Suzuki K, Ihira M, et al. Clinical characteristics of febrile convulsions during primary HHV-6 infection. *Arch Dis Child* 2000;82:62.

Sugawara T, Mazaki-Miyazaki E, Ito M, et al. Na$_v$1.1 mutations cause febrile seizures associated with afebrile partial seizures. *Neurology* 2001;57:703.

VanLandingham KE, Heinz ER, Cavazos JE, Lewis DV. Magnetic resonance imaging evidence of hippocampal injury after prolonged focal febrile convulsions. *Ann Neurol* 1998;43:413.

Wallace RH, Marini C, Petrou S, et al. Mutant GABAa receptor γ2-subunit in childhood absence epilepsy and febrile seizures. *Nat Genet* 2001;28:49.

CHAPTER 404 ■ THE COMATOSE CHILD

JAMES OWENS AND DANIEL G. GLAZE

DEFINITION AND PATHOPHYSIOLOGY

Coma is not a specific disorder, but a sign of central nervous system (CNS) dysfunction. It may be caused by either a primary or a systemic condition affecting the CNS. A patient in a coma is unresponsive to any environmental stimuli. Coma is a medical emergency and represents a life-threatening situation; it requires prompt supportive therapy to prevent hypoxia and rapid etiologic diagnosis to ensure that proper specific therapy is initiated.

The term *coma* often is used inappropriately to describe virtually any state of altered consciousness. The terms used in this chapter to describe altered states of consciousness are defined here. The correct use of these terms in clinical practice and in publications is recommended (Box 404.1).

BOX 404.1   **Terms and Definitions**

Coma: A state of altered consciousness in which the patient is unresponsive to any environmental stimuli.

Stupor or obtundation: A state in which the patient appears to be awake or in light sleep, can be aroused by mild external stimulation, and will respond to questions or commands, but lapses into an immobile or sleeplike state when the stimulus is removed.

Vegetative state: A clinical condition of complete unawareness of the self and the environment. Vegetative state is accompanied by sleep-wake cycles, with either complete or partial preservation of hypothalamic and brainstem autonomic functions. Patients in a vegetative state show no evidence of sustained, reproducible, purposeful, or voluntary behavioral responses to visual, auditory, tactile, or noxious stimuli; show no evidence of language comprehension or expression; have bowel and bladder incontinence; and have variably preserved cranial-nerve and spinal reflexes. Response is limited to primitive postural and reflex movements. Persistent vegetative state has been defined as a vegetative state present 1 month after acute traumatic or nontraumatic injury or lasting for at least 1 month in patients with degenerative or metabolic disorders or developmental malformations.

Locked-in syndrome: Quadriplegia and mutism with preserved consciousness demonstrated by communication by intact vertical eye movements.

Brain death: Irreversible cessation of all brain functions, including the brainstem, a state characterized by no CNS function above the level of the spinal cord.

The standardized Glasgow Coma Scale (GCS) is used widely in evaluating a patient's responsiveness after traumatic coma and, more recently, nontraumatic coma (Table 404.1). This scale, which depends only on a clinical examination performed at the bedside, allows staging by serial examinations of the patient and has permitted comparative study of patients in different centers. Its usefulness in young children is limited somewhat, however, because some of the parameters depend on the patient's understanding and responding to language.

In general, the underlying pathophysiology of coma is accounted for by two types of lesions or processes: those that affect the reticular formation of the brainstem (which also may involve centers maintaining respiratory and circulatory integrity) and those that affect the brain diffusely (bilateral hemispheric dysfunction). The latter category includes CNS lesions, systemic infections, and toxic or metabolic disturbances. These disturbances also may be associated with brain edema and prolonged seizures, which in themselves may cause brain damage.

EVALUATION AND TREATMENT

Short-Term Treatment

The evaluation and treatment of the comatose child fall into two phases. During the immediate phase, treatment precedes establishment of a diagnosis, and its most important aspects include stabilizing the child and protecting him or her from sustaining further brain damage. An evaluation of etiologic possibilities for the coma follows. After providing immediate treatment to the comatose child, the physician must be prepared to manage the potential complications of a prolonged altered state of consciousness. Knowledge of the probable prognosis for recovery or long-term impairment will facilitate provision of patient care and will improve communication with the child's parents.

During the initial phase of treatment, the physician must ensure that the patient's brain is receiving adequate substrate for energy production. The airway must be maintained, and sufficient oxygen and ventilation must be provided; a child with inadequate respiratory effort needs intubation and respirator assistance. The patient's cardiac output must be evaluated, and cardiac dysrhythmias and hypotension must be treated appropriately. Treatment also should include control of body temperature, especially in children with hyperthermia (greater than 42°C), to prevent irreversible damage to the CNS. The possibility of reversible hypoglycemic encephalopathy being present should be considered, and immediate treatment of the patient (after blood is obtained for determination of the serum glucose level) should include the administration of 1 mg/kg of concentrated glucose solution (50% dextrose).

Recurrent or prolonged seizures can produce brain damage; iatrogenic paralysis and ventilation do not protect against this damage. Therefore, status epilepticus requires emergency treatment (see Chapter 402).

TABLE 404.1

MODIFIED GLASGOW COMA SCALE

Response	Older than 5 Years Old	Younger than 5 Years Old	Score
Eye opening	Spontaneous	Spontaneous	4
	To speech	To speech	3
	To pain	To pain	2
	None	None	1
Verbal	Oriented	Alert, normal sounds	5
	Confused	Less than normal, irritable	4
	Inappropriate words	Cries to pain	3
	Incomprehensible sounds	Moans to pain	2
	None	No response	1
Best motor	Obeys commands	Normal spontaneous movements	6
	Localizes pain	Localizes pain (>9 months)	5
	Withdraws	Withdraws	4
	Abnormal flexion	Abnormal flexion	3
	Extension response	Extension response	2
	None	None	1

Modified from Kirkham, F. Non-traumatic coma in children. *Arch Dis Child* 2001;85:303.

During the initial treatment period, a rapid physical examination should be performed to search for signs of trauma that could necessitate performing immediate laboratory testing and surgical or neurosurgical intervention. The child should be evaluated for signs of increased intracranial pressure (ICP), keeping in mind that papilledema may not be apparent for hours after the onset of ICP. Loss of venous pulsations may be helpful in the early identification of ICP. If intracranial hypertension is present, immediate therapy, including hyperventilation to reduce the partial pressure of carbon dioxide to 25 to 30 mm Hg and elevation of the head, should be initiated. (For further therapeutic measures for intracranial hypertension, see Chapter 399.)

After immediate assessment and treatment have been performed, further historical information should be obtained. The diagnostic workup should include measurement of serum electrolyte, arterial blood gas, and serum calcium levels, along with liver and renal function tests and a complete white blood cell count. Lumbar puncture should be considered in the presence of signs of meningeal irritation, such as nuchal rigidity, to evaluate for such possibilities as meningitis or subarachnoid hemorrhage. Signs of meningeal irritation may be absent in young children or infants. When the history is suggestive or the cause of coma is not clear, blood and urine evaluations for toxicologic studies should be performed.

Physical Examination

The general physical examination can provide clues to the cause of coma. Of particular importance are signs of trauma and vital signs, including respiratory pattern, heart rate and rhythm, and blood pressure. The neurologic examination must include particular attention given to pupillary size and reactivity, ocular motility, respiratory rate and pattern, and motor response to pain.

Pupils

Metabolic coma or early-stage rostral-caudal herniation with interruption of descending sympathetic pathways is associated with small but reactive pupils; involvement of the midbrain is associated with nonreactive, midposition, or mildly dilated (5 to 7 mm) pupils; intoxication or poisoning by organophosphates, phenothiazines, or opiates is associated with miosis

(pupils less than 2 mm in diameter). Less frequently, small pupils may be seen with pontine lesions.

Extraocular Motility

In a comatose child, intact brainstem function is suggested by full-reflex eye movements in response to the doll's eye maneuver, which is performed by holding the patient's eyes open and rocking the head from side to side multiple times. If the eyes remain in the primary position or straight ahead during this maneuver, function of the brainstem is compromised. Caloric stimulation is a more sensitive test that may be performed after the tympanic membrane is determined to be intact. The head is positioned in the midline and is raised 30% from the horizontal. Then, 50 mL of ice water is instilled into the external auditory canal against the intact tympanic membrane. Tonic deviation of the eyes to the side in which the ice water was instilled indicates an intact brainstem; any asymmetry or absence of eye deviation implies a structural or metabolic brainstem lesion.

Respiration

Bilateral cortical damage may result in Cheyne-Stokes respiration, which is characterized by periodically alternating episodes of hyperventilation and apnea. Metabolic disturbances, such as respiratory alkalosis or metabolic acidosis, or a midbrain lesion may cause central neurogenic hyperventilation characterized by rapid regular breathing.

True neurogenic hyperventilation is a rare finding; the tachypneic hypocapnia that is observed commonly in unconscious individuals probably is the result of stimulation by pulmonary congestion of afferent peripheral reflexes arising in the lung and chest wall. Pontomedullary damage may be associated with an atactic or irregular respiratory pattern.

Motor Response

The quality of the patient's motor response may be assessed after the administration of a painful stimulus such as supraorbital ridge compression. Purposeful movement with localization of the stimulus by the patient suggests a high level of intact brain function. Lesions compressing the brain at the thalamic level may be associated with decorticate posturing, which is characterized by flexion of the upper extremities at the elbow and extension with internal rotation of the lower extremities.

Midbrain lesions may be associated with decerebrate posturing, which is characterized by extension and internal rotation of both the upper and lower extremities. Pontomedullary lesions frequently are associated with no response to pain.

Etiologic Factors

Once the child's condition has been stabilized, a more exhaustive search for a cause of the coma may be necessary. In general, the causes of coma can be divided into two major categories: traumatic and nontraumatic.

Blunt trauma to the head is a common occurrence in childhood. Alteration of consciousness that lasts less than 24 hours after blunt trauma is termed *concussion*. The neuropathologic implication of concussion is that no microscopic or gross change in the brain has resulted. If the period of unresponsiveness lasts longer than 24 hours, the clinical diagnosis is *contusion* of the brain. The neuropathologic changes associated with contusion include focal hemorrhage and necrosis of brain tissue. The magnitude of alteration caused in brain function after blunt trauma depends on several variables, including the amount of force exerted on the skull, the area of the skull involved, the direction of force against the skull, the relative mobility of the skull, and the angular velocity of the brain after the trauma. The frontal, temporal, and occipital lobes are especially prone to injury caused by rotational acceleration forces when rotation and flexion of the skull on the neck have occurred. Flexion and rotational acceleration may cause brainstem injury.

Radiologic evaluation of pediatric head trauma should begin with a noncontrast computed tomography (CT) scan, followed by a magnetic resonance imaging (MRI) scan if significant neurologic deficits are found on examination. Even in children with only mild alteration in consciousness (GCS score of 13 to 14), the incidence of intracerebral hemorrhage was shown in one study to be approximately 19% (30 of 135 patients). Depressed skull fractures may be associated with laceration of the brain and dura, and they should be identified and evaluated quickly. Fractures across the middle meningeal artery groove may be associated with tearing of the meningeal artery and subsequent epidural hemorrhage. Epidural hematoma frequently is associated with a biphasic clinical presentation: an initial episode of coma occurring immediately after the injury, followed by a lucid interval, after which loss of consciousness ensues as the hematoma enlarges. Periorbital ecchymosis, cerebrospinal fluid (CSF) rhinorrhea, and hemorrhage behind the tympanic membrane are signs of basilar skull fracture. Acute subdural hematoma may develop after laceration of the dura associated with depressed skull fracture occurs.

Chronic subdural hematoma may develop after closed head injury, which causes tearing of the bridging veins. Subarachnoid hemorrhage in children most commonly is the result of head trauma or ruptured arteriovenous malformations. Subarachnoid hemorrhage may be suggested by an abnormal funduscopic examination showing subhyaloid (preretinal) hemorrhages, signs of meningeal irritation (which may be absent in comatose children), and xanthochromic CSF. A history of trauma dictates a search for injury to visceral organs or long bones. These injuries may be associated with hemorrhage and hypovolemic shock or with fat embolism from fractures of the long bones.

The nontraumatic causes of coma in children fall into four categories: toxic and metabolic disorders, mass lesions, infections, and seizures.

Toxic and metabolic abnormalities affect the CNS diffusely and are characterized by a history of progressive CNS dysfunction leading to coma. Neurologic findings usually are symmetric, although motor signs that vary from one side to the other may be present at times. Typically, the pupillary light reflex is preserved; however, in cases of glutethimide intoxication, anoxia, profound hypothermia, atropine intoxication, or barbiturate intoxication leading to apnea, the pupillary light reflex may be absent. More typically, drug ingestion is associated with miotic pupils. In cases of narcotic overdose, administration of the narcotic antagonist naloxone hydrochloride (initial dose, 0.1 mg/kg intravenously) is diagnostic and is associated with arousal of the patient and pupillary dilatation. Coma may occur if the serum osmolality is less than 260 mOsm/kg or greater than 330 to 350 mOsm/kg. Levels of blood sodium less than 120 mEq/L, and especially levels less than 100 mEq/L, may be associated with coma. Arterial blood gas and acid-base abnormalities may occur in comatose children and may provide clues to the underlying etiologic factors. For example, diabetic ketoacidosis, uremic encephalopathy, and lactic acidosis are associated with metabolic acidosis; hepatic encephalopathy and salicylate intoxication are associated with respiratory alkalosis; and respiratory depressant drugs or acute or chronic pulmonary failure may be associated with respiratory acidosis.

Although they are infrequent occurrences, arterial thrombosis and intracranial hemorrhages may occur in association with inborn errors of metabolism such as homocystinuria, with collagen-vascular diseases, with deficiencies of plasma-clotting factors such as factor VIII, with disorders giving rise to thrombocytopenia such as leukemia, and with types of hemoglobinopathy such as sickle cell disease. Venous thrombosis occurs more commonly than does arterial thrombosis and may follow severe dehydration and pyogenic infection of the middle ear or mastoid or paranasal sinuses.

Although less common at present, a history of severe vomiting, rapidly developing coma, and laboratory signs of hepatic dysfunction after a minor illness should suggest the possibility of Reye syndrome. This disorder likely is associated with hepatic and CNS dysfunction caused by acute mitochondrial failure. Coma may occur in children with diabetes mellitus, either secondary to osmotic diuresis with glycosuria, dehydration, ketoacidosis, and depletion of salt or as a result of an overdose of insulin and associated hypoglycemia because of either miscalculation or failure to consume sufficient carbohydrates in relation to the insulin administered. Other endocrine disorders, including thyrotoxicosis, myxedema, adrenal insufficiency, and Cushing disease, may lead to coma, although systemic signs of endocrine dysfunction usually are evident in these cases before coma supervenes.

In evaluating the comatose child, determining whether the condition has been caused by an intracranial mass lesion is critical. Such lesions may require neurosurgical intervention, in contrast to toxic and metabolic disorders, infections, or seizures, for which medical treatment is indicated. Intracranial mass lesions that may be associated with coma include intracerebral hemorrhage, subdural and epidural hematomas, brain abscesses, brain tumors, and cerebral infarction with edema. Usually, supratentorial mass lesions initially are associated with focal or lateralizing signs and symptoms, such as hemiparesis or hemispheric sensory deficits, before they produce coma. With progressive involvement, coma may occur, and deterioration proceeds in a rostral-caudal manner, beginning with hemispheric dysfunction and followed by impaired function of the thalamus, the midbrain pons, and then the medulla. This progressive deterioration usually is reflected by changes in reflex eye movements, pupillary size and reactivity, motor response to pain, and respiratory pattern. Recognition of these signs of transtentorial herniation is important because immediate neurosurgical intervention may be indicated. Other supratentorial lesions may be so placed as to cause herniation of the medial portion of the temporal lobe (the uncus) and to produce midbrain compression and signs of midbrain compromise, including ipsilateral pupillary dilatation, before coma supervenes.

Infratentorial lesions that involve the brainstem may alter consciousness early, and the typical rostral-caudal progression of signs may not occur. Impairment in eye movements and pupillary function may be early localizing signs. Midbrain lesions usually are associated with midpositional pupils that are nonreactive to light stimulus; pontine lesions may be associated with pinpoint pupils. Dysconjugate eye movements or conjugate deviation of the eyes away from the side of the lesion and the side of the hemiparesis are suggestive of an infratentorial lesion involving the brainstem.

Infections of the CNS and the meninges must be suspected in every comatose child, and a lumbar puncture for CSF analysis should be performed in all cases except those with strong evidence of an intracranial mass lesion that could be associated with herniation. Signs of meningeal irritation may not be present in infants and young children. The differential diagnosis of infections involving the CNS should include not only acute bacterial meningitis but also tuberculous meningitis, viral encephalitis, and fungal and rickettsial diseases. Any severe systemic infection may lead to coma, and common childhood illnesses may be followed by symptoms similar to those of encephalomyelitis. Acute hemorrhagic leukoencephalopathy may follow a course much like that of parainfectious encephalomyelitis and may be associated with abnormal CSF findings, including elevated pressure, pleocytosis of mononuclear cells and red blood cells, and elevated levels of protein.

Seizures may be associated with impaired consciousness. Usually, the duration of postictal unresponsiveness is brief, but prolonged postictal coma may occur after status epilepticus or in some children with underlying head trauma, CNS infections, or severe forms of metabolic encephalopathy.

Laboratory Evaluation

In addition to blood tests and CSF examination, two other tests may be particularly helpful in evaluating the comatose child. CT of the head is indicated in certain cases of head injury, including those associated with coma, and when an intracranial mass is suspected. An MRI scan may be performed to evaluate parenchymal injury more definitively. Magnetic resonance spectroscopy, a noninvasive method of assaying cerebral metabolites such as lactate, has not proven useful in isolation but may help to predict outcome when combined with other clinical criteria. An electroencephalogram (EEG) performed at the time of presentation may provide information on the underlying pathophysiologic process responsible for coma: bilateral hemispheric involvement versus brainstem lesion, diffuse versus lateralized lesions or processes, and the occurrence of seizures. Characteristics of the EEG may suggest a specific category of disorders, such as metabolic aberrations or drug intoxications. Serial EEG examinations may be helpful in monitoring the patient's recovery. Although more useful in adults, somatosensory evoked potentials (SEPs) provide prognostic data with the probability of recovery significantly diminished when, combined with other clinical criteria, SEPs are absent. In particular, after 24 hours of coma, bilateral absence of the N20 SEP wave, combined with a GCS score of less than 5, absent respiratory drive, absent pupillary responses, and a discontinuous or epileptiform EEG has a positive predictive value of 100% for an unfavorable outcome (severe disability, presistent vegetative state, or death) in comatose children.

Long-Term Treatment and Complications

The physician must be aware that, after the initial immediate treatment of the comatose child, numerous late complications may occur, including seizures. In the case of head injury, most children who have seizures show evidence of them soon after the injury.

Of children who are hospitalized after incurring a head injury, approximately 5% have seizures within the first week after the traumatic event. Among children surviving severe head injury, 20% to 25% have unprovoked seizures. In adults with severe traumatic brain injury, prophylactic treatment with phenytoin decreases the risk of early, but not late, posttraumatic seizures. The efficacy of seizure prophylaxis in pediatric traumatic brain injury has not been established. During a study of children younger than 16 years who had experienced moderate to severe blunt head injury, phenytoin did not substantially reduce the rate of early posttraumatic seizures. Some children may relapse into an encephalopathic state during the first few days after apparent partial or complete recovery from anoxic or hypoglycemic insults. The prognosis in these instances is variable, and some patients may not recover or may die.

Numerous systemic problems may complicate a patient's course after sustaining a brain injury associated with coma. Inappropriate secretion of antidiuretic hormone may complicate the initial phase of treatment. Central diabetes insipidus may occur as a late sequela of brain injury and may require treatment with antidiuretic hormone analogues. Elevated blood pressure occurs frequently in the acute phase of injury and may persist as a difficult treatment problem. Propranolol has been suggested as the most effective drug if therapy is required. Significant numbers of children with severe brain injury require prolonged intubation or tracheostomy because of aspiration, apnea, or hypoventilation. These patients may have difficulty handling secretions and be at risk for development of atelectasis and pneumonia. These children also are at increased risk for acquisition of various infections (including ventriculitis if ICP monitoring or ventriculoperitoneal shunt devices have been required), aspiration pneumonia, or urinary tract infections. In addition, they are at risk for development of decubitus ulcers. An increased incidence of sinusitis and otitis media has been observed in children with nasogastric or nasotracheal tubes. These infections usually are caused by nosocomial flora, which may be resistant to commonly used antimicrobial agents.

PROGNOSIS AND OUTCOME

Predicting the outcome of a comatose child frequently is difficult. In comatose children, the mortality rate resulting from nontraumatic causes is 46%, but it varies significantly by the underlying cause. Indeed, of all the factors that may bear on prognosis, the cause of the coma probably is the most important. For example, the prognoses for children whose comas are consequent to drug overdose or a toxic or metabolic disorder appear to be much more favorable, with a mortality rate of approximately 3%, than the prognoses for those with coma resulting from most other causes. Coma caused by hypoxic-ischemic insult has a very poor prognosis in most cases. After coma caused by head trauma, infants and children appear to have better outcomes than do adults.

The relationship of the GCS score to the outcome in children with traumatic brain injury has been examined. Except for patients who have had prolonged hypoxemia, all children, including those with GCS scores of 3 to 5, apparently can have a satisfactory outcome. The mortality rate is higher among those with GCS scores of 3 to 5 than among those with scores of 6 or greater. Death occurs predominantly in children with GCS scores of 3. Nonsurvivors have an increased incidence of shock, a need for cardiopulmonary resuscitation, and higher ICP. Most deaths occur in patients who have no heart rate at the scene. Survivors with GCS scores of 3 to 5 have longer stays in the intensive care unit and longer intervals before recovery of cognition than do those with scores of 6 or greater. Of all survivors, 17% to 37% may have deficits in either memory or speech and language, as well as a motor function deficit, attention-deficit disorder, or both. A hypoxic-ischemic insult at the time of the accident appears to be a devastating and confounding variable in patients with head injury. GCS scores alone have been reported to have limited predictive value in the absence of factors that included presence of hypoxia on admission and features on CT scans of subarachnoid hemorrhage, diffuse axonal injury, and brain swelling. In the absence of hypoxic-ischemic injury, children with traumatic brain injury and GCS scores of 3 to 5 may recover independent function. Aggressive treatment is warranted for children with severe head injury, even if the GCS scores are low. Conversely, even mild head injuries may be associated with a detectable drop in cognitive function. The duration of the coma may have prognostic significance.

Numerous studies have attempted to evaluate the effectiveness of laboratory tests, such as the EEG and evoked potentials, in formulating a prognosis. EEGs showing no evidence of brain activity may be recorded in patients with drug overdoses who experience complete recovery. Repeatedly abnormal EEG results (e.g., no detectable brain activity or burst suppression pattern) during coma that is not associated with an uncomplicated drug overdose or a reversible toxic or metabolic disorder indicate an extremely poor prognosis for significant recovery.

A few studies on the outcome and prognosis for children whose coma is secondary to nontraumatic disorders have noted numerous influential or predictive factors. Coma caused by hypoxia-ischemia appears to have a poorer outcome than does coma resulting from other factors. Moreover, the need for assisted ventilation, increased ICP for longer than 2 days, and the duration of the coma (especially if it is more than 2 weeks) appear to be associated with a very poor prognosis. Poor outcomes for children following near drowning in warm or nonicy waters have been reported when purposeful movements remain absent 24 hours after near drowning or when a combination of absent pupillary light reflexes, increased initial blood glucose, and male gender is present. In children with coma secondary to trauma, certain features of the examination, including absence of the pupillary light reflex, absent or impaired spontaneous eye movements, and absent motor responses or posturing, have been associated with a poor prognosis for recovery or with death. These observations have not been confirmed in a study of children whose comas resulted from nontraumatic disorders.

Persistent Vegetative State

The term *persistent vegetative state* is used to describe a clinical syndrome that is present after brain damage in which, after the initial period of coma, patients seem to be in a state of wakefulness without awareness. As many as 12% of patients who survive coma remain in a persistent vegetative state. Patients who make a reasonable recovery after sustaining brain damage associated with coma usually do not pass through this state. Although the suggestion has been made that this term be applied to any patient who fails to regain functional awareness of his or her environment after at least 1 month in a coma, more recent observations suggest that patients may enter this state very early and that certain features (including decerebrate or decorticate responses, roving eye movements, and spontaneous blinking) may be early clues to its occurrence.

Although a persistent vegetative state may occur after a coma resulting from any one of many causes, it appears to follow hypoxia and ischemia most commonly. The pathologic features of a persistent vegetative state vary with the underlying etiologic factors, but findings usually include diffuse neuronal damage in the cerebral hemispheres. The few studies that have been performed on persistent vegetative states in children indicate that such children have extremely poor prognoses for recovery. In a consensus statement, the Multi-Society Task Force reported that recovery of consciousness from a posttraumatic persistent vegetative state is unlikely after 12 months in adults and children. Recovery from a nontraumatic persistent vegetative state after 3 months is exceedingly rare in both adults and children. Patients with degenerative or metabolic disorders or congenital malformations who remain in a persistent vegetative state for several months are unlikely to recover consciousness. The survival rate for children 3 years of age or older in a persistent vegetative state is 63% at 8 years. Factors that suggest more rapid mortality include a degenerative cause and the need for gastrostomy tube feedings.

Locked-In Syndrome

The term *locked-in syndrome* is used to denote the clinical state of quadriplegia and mutism with preserved consciousness, which usually is demonstrated by communication by intact vertical eye movements. These patients are entirely awake and responsive, although their repertoire of responses is limited to blinking and sometimes to jaw and eye movement. The locked-in syndrome commonly results from bilateral ventral pontine infarction after basilar artery occlusion, but it has been reported with other conditions, such as tumors, drug overdose, trauma, brainstem encephalitis, and hemorrhage. EEG results that indicate reactivity to external stimuli may be useful in confirming the diagnosis. In most adults and children, the prognosis for recovery is poor, but recognition of the locked-in syndrome is important for humane patient care.

Brain Death

Brain death is the term used for the irreversible cessation of all functions of the entire brain, including the brainstem. Medical standards for the determination of brain death in children have been reported. The report emphasizes the need to determine and ensure the absence of remediable or reversible factors, including toxic and metabolic disorders, sedative-hypnotic drugs, paralytic agents, hypothermia, hypotension, and surgically remediable conditions, and it sets forth the physical examination criteria found in Box 404.2.

Hysterical Nonorganic Coma

Hysterical coma, although rare in young children, may be seen in adolescents. Episodes of feigned or hysterical coma may be precipitated by some stressful, emotional situation and usually begin with observers present. The neurologic examination is normal. Lateral eye movements after oculocephalic testing may be absent because visual fixation can suppress this reflex. Other maneuvers, however, such as placing the patient on his or her side and then turning the patient to the opposite side may demonstrate lateral eye movements. The eyes usually are closed tightly and, if opened by force, will close again rapidly. Cold caloric testing that demonstrates nystagmus virtually proves that the coma is feigned or hysterical.

| **BOX 404.2** | Physical Examination Criteria for Brain Death |

Coma and apnea must coexist. The patient must exhibit complete loss of consciousness, vocalization, and volitional activity.

The absence of brainstem function must be indicated by the following: midposition or fully dilated pupils that do not respond to light; the absence of spontaneous eye movements and those induced by oculocephalic and caloric (oculovestibular) testing; and the absence of movement of bulbar musculature, including facial and oropharyngeal muscles. The corneal, gag, cough, sucking, and rooting reflexes are absent; respiratory movements are absent with the patient off the respirator. Protocols for apnea testing in children have been suggested. The absence of spontaneous respiratory effort at a partial pressure of arterial carbon dioxide of 60 mm Hg or higher traditionally has been accepted as the respiratory criteria for the determination of brain death. Preoxygenation with 100% oxygen has been suggested. Continuous cardiovascular monitoring is important, and the test may need to be terminated if significant changes in heart rate or blood pressure develop.

The patient must not be significantly hypothermic or hypotensive for his or her age.

The tone should be flaccid and spontaneous, or induced movements should be absent, excluding spinal cord events such as reflex withdrawal or spinal myoclonus.

The examination should remain consistent with brain death throughout the observation and testing. The required duration of these clinical criteria varies with the age of the patient and the laboratory tests used. In patients between 7 days and 2 months of age, the Task Force for the Determination of Brain Death in Children recommends that two examinations and EEGs be performed at least 48 hours apart. In patients between 2 months and 1 year of age, the recommendation is for two examinations and EEGs to be performed at least 24 hours apart, although a second examination and EEG are not necessary if a concomitant radionuclide angiographic study demonstrates no perfusion of the intracerebral arteries (absence of brain parenchymal uptake of intravenously injected isotope after 30 to 60 minutes). In patients older than 1 year of age, laboratory testing is not required; the Task Force recommends an observation period of at least 12 hours. The Task Force also suggests that if assessing the extent and irreversibility of brain damage is difficult, a more prolonged period of observation lasting at least 24 hours should be undertaken; however, this observation can be reduced if the EEG demonstrates cerebral electrical silence or the concomitant radionuclide angiographic study does not reveal perfusion of the intracerebral arteries.

Suggested Readings

Antony JH. Relapsing encephalopathy after hypoxia. *J Pediatr* 1978;72:433.

Banaskiak K, Lister G. Brain death in children. *Curr Opin Pediatr* 2003;15:288.

Barlow KM, Spowart JJ, Minns RA. Early posttraumatic seizures in nonaccidental head injury: relation to outcome. *Dev Med Child Neuro* 2000;42:591.

Bernardi B, Zimmerman R, Bilaniuk L. Neuroradiologic evaluation of pediatric craniocerebral trauma *Top Magn Reson Imaging* 1993;5:161.

Bratton SL, Jardine DS, Morray JP. Serial neurologic examinations after near drowning and outcome. *Arch Pediatr Adolesc Med* 1994;148:167.

Chang BS, Lowenstein DH. Practice parameter: antiepileptic drug prophylaxis in severe traumatic brain injury: report of the Quality Standards Subcomitee of the American Academy of Neurology. *Neurology* 2003;60:10.

Facco E, Zuccarello M, Pittoni G, et al. Early outcome prediction in severe head injury: comparison between children and adults. *Childs Nerv Syst* 1986;2:67.

Feinberg WM, Ferry PC. A fate worse than death: the persistent vegetative state in childhood. *Am J Dis Child* 1984;138:128.

Gillies JD, Seshia SS. Vegetative state following coma in childhood: evolution and outcome. *Dev Med Child Neurol* 1980;22:642.

Golden GS, Leeds N, Kremenitzer MW, et al. The "locked-in" syndrome in children. *J Pediatr* 1976;89:596.

Graf WD, Cummings P, Quan L, et al. Predicting outcome in pediatric submersion victims. *Ann Emerg Med* 1995;26:312.

Grmec S, Gasparovic V. Comparison of APACHEII, MEES, and Glasgow Coma Scale in patients with nontraumatic coma for predictions of mortality. *Crit Care* 2001;5:19.

Hawley C, Ward A, Magnay A, Long J. Outcomes following childhood head injury: a population study. *J Neurol Neurosurg Psychiatry* 2004;75:737.

James HE. Emergency management of acute coma in children. *Am Fam Physician* 1993;48:473.

Jennett B, Teasdale G, Braakman R, et al. Predicting outcome in individual patients after severe head injury. *Lancet* 1976;1:1031.

Johnston RB, Mellits ED. Pediatric coma: prognosis and outcome. *Dev Med Child Neurol* 1980;22:3.

Kirkham, F. Non-traumatic coma in children. *Arch Dis Child* 2001;85:303.

Lieh-Lai MW, Theodorou AA, Sarnaik AP, et al. Limitations of the Glasgow Coma Scale in predicting outcome in children with traumatic brain injury. *J Pediatr* 1992;120:195.

Mahoney WJ, D'Souza BJ, Haller JA, et al. Long-term outcome of children with severe head trauma and prolonged coma. *Pediatrics* 1983;71:756.

Margolis HK, Shaywitz BA. The outcome of prolonged coma in childhood. *Pediatrics* 1980;65:477.

Multi-Society Task Force on PVS. Medical aspects of the persistent vegetative state. *N Engl J Med* 1994;330:1499.

Ong L, Selladurai BM, Dhillon MK, et al. The prognostic value of the Glasgow Coma Scale, hypoxia and computerized tomography in outcome prediction of pediatric head injury. *Pediatr Neurosurg* 1996;24:285.

Paret G, Barzilay Z. Apnea testing in suspected brain dead children: physiological and mathematical modeling. *Intensive Care Med* 1995;21:247.

Perry HE, Shannon MW. Diagnosis and management of opoid- and benzodiazepine-induced comatose overdose in children. *Curr Opin Pediatr* 1996;8:243.

Plum F, Posner JB. *The diagnosis of stupor and coma*, 3rd ed. Philadelphia: FA Davis, 1982.

Strauss DJ, Ashwal S, Day SM, Shavelle RM. Life expectancy of children in vegetative and minimally conscious states. *Pediatr Neurol* 2000;23:312.

Strauss DJ, Shavelle RM, Anderson TW. Long-term survival of children and adolescents after traumatic brain injury. *Arch Phys Med Rehabil* 1998;79:1095.

Task Force for the Determination of Brain Death in Children. Guidelines for the determination of brain death in children. *Ann Neurol* 1987;22:616.

Trubel HK, Novotny E, Lister G. Outcome of coma in children. *Curr Opin Pediatr* 2003;15:283.

Wang MY, Griffith P, Sterling J, et al. A prospective study of pediatric trauma patients with mild alterations in consciousness (Glasgow Coma Scale score of 13–14). *Neurosurgery* 2000;46:1093.

Young KD, Okada PJ, Sokolove PE, et al. A randomized, double-blinded, placebo-controlled trial of phenytoin for the prevention of early posttraumatic seizures in children with moderate to severe blunt head injury. *Ann Emerg Med* 2004;43:435.

CHAPTER 405 ■ REYE SYNDROME

PENELOPE TERHUNE LOUIS

Reye syndrome, first described in 1963, is an acute, life-threatening, postinfectious, metabolic encephalopathy that affects predominantly school-aged children, occasionally infants, and rarely adults. Over the years, the disease and its clinical manifestations have received widespread recognition.

Characteristically, a prodromal illness, most often influenza or varicella infection, is followed in 3 to 5 days by the onset of persistent and intractable vomiting. Initially, patients are well oriented but irritable and lethargic. Some patients have no change in consciousness and remain only lethargic, with no progression to unconsciousness. The alanine aminotransferase (ALT) and aspartate aminotransferase (AST) levels are 3 to 30 times normal. The serum bilirubin level rarely exceeds 1 mg/dL. Serum ammonia concentrations are variable at presentation. As the encephalopathy worsens to a hyperexcitable state, the patient is intermittently out of contact with the environment. Further progression to a deeper comatose state is characterized by decerebrate and decorticate posturing, hyperventilation, and, finally, flaccid paralysis with loss of involuntary ventilatory control. The comatose patient uniformly has an elevated ammonia concentration ranging from 3 to 20 times normal. The encephalopathy typically persists for 24 to 96 hours, with gradual improvement occurring in survivors. Recovery of consciousness in patients with permanent neurologic impairment may require weeks.

Criteria for the case definition of Reye syndrome include the following: an acute, noninflammatory encephalopathy documented clinically by an alteration in consciousness and, if available, cerebrospinal fluid containing fewer than eight leukocytes per microliter; hepatopathy documented by liver biopsy on autopsy or a threefold or greater increase in the ALT, AST, or serum ammonia level; and no more reasonable explanation for the cerebral or hepatic abnormalities.

Accurately assessing the severity of the illness is important because the therapies for severely affected children are aggressive, invasive, and dangerous. Several staging systems have been developed, culminating in the National Institutes of Health Staging System (Box 405.1). The peak incidence of this disorder occurred in the 1960s and 1970s, and only rare cases have been reported since 1985.

PATHOGENESIS

Despite intensive study, the pathogenesis of Reye syndrome remains incompletely defined. Whether the pathogenesis can be explained by a primary injury to the mitochondria of multiple organs, including the brain, liver, and muscle, with its metabolic consequences, or by a primary hepatic injury that leads to metabolic consequences producing the biochemical abnormalities and encephalopathy remains unclear. Morphologic and biochemical studies have confirmed the presence of a characteristic injury. Pleomorphic, enlarged mitochondria with disrupted cristae, electron-lucent matrices, and reduced numbers of dense bodies are characteristic of the hepatic pathologic features of Reye syndrome. Associated reductions in mitochon-

drial enzymes involved in ureagenesis and gluconeogenesis and in enzymes associated with the citric acid cycle have been observed. Further evidence of mitochondrial injury is suggested by the finding of dicarboxylic acids in the urine and serum.

Morphologic and biochemical studies of the brain in patients with Reye syndrome have revealed swollen astrocytes and myelin blebs. Alterations in the morphologic features of the mitochondria have been identified only in neurons. Despite these morphologic changes, mitochondrial enzyme activities in the brain are not reduced as they are in the liver. This finding is somewhat surprising because it suggests that brain mitochondrial injury may play an unimportant role in the observed encephalopathy of Reye syndrome.

The role of salicylates in the pathogenesis of Reye syndrome remains unclear, although salicylate use commonly precedes the onset of the syndrome. Serum salicylate concentrations are increased in patients with the disorder compared with those in control patients; however, no correlation has been found between coma grade and serum concentration. Salicylates are known to stimulate macrophages that are activated by a viral infection, endotoxin, and phagocytosis. The stimulation of macrophages results in the release of tumor necrosis factor and interleukin-1, which are mediators of the toxic and metabolic effects that are similar to those observed in Reye syndrome.

In 1982, the Committee on Infectious Disease of the American Academy of Pediatrics issued a statement warning against the use of salicylates in children with possible varicella or influenza infection, and a program of public education was initiated. Some authors have cited the reduction in use of aspirin and the decrease in the occurrence of Reye syndrome as an argument to support the association between administration of aspirin and development of this disorder. Other authors

---

BOX 405.1   **National Institutes of Health Staging System**

Stage I: Lethargy; follows verbal commands; normal posture; purposeful response to pain; brisk pupillary light reflex; and normal oculocephalic reflex

Stage II: Combative or stuporous; inappropriate verbalizing; normal posture; purposeful or nonpurposeful response to pain; sluggish pupillary reflexes; and conjugate deviation on doll's eye maneuver

Stage III: Comatose; decorticate posture; decorticate response to pain; sluggish pupillary reaction; and conjugate deviation on doll's eye maneuver

Stage IV: Comatose; decerebrate posture and decerebrate response to pain; sluggish pupillary reflexes; and inconsistent or absent oculocephalic reflex

Stage V: Comatose; flaccid; no response to pain; no pupillary response; no oculocephalic reflex

dispute these conclusions and state that even the prospective, controlled, epidemiologic study performed by the U.S. Public Health Service showed histologic support for the diagnosis of Reye syndrome in only 27% of the patients, and no electron microscopic evidence was presented. This decline in the incidence of Reye syndrome was seen at the same time as knowledge of metabolic diseases was expanding rapidly, and an alternative explanation may be that fewer patients with an underlying genetic metabolic disease were being incorrectly diagnosed as having Reye syndrome.

Based on available evidence, apparently a primary mitochondrial injury stimulates multiple metabolic disturbances, resulting in hyperammonemia, free fatty acidemia, lactic acidosis, and dicarboxylic acidemia. The metabolic abnormalities and the underlying mitochondrial injury synergistically lead to the observed pathophysiologic findings through mechanisms that remain incompletely understood. Fatty acids, dicarboxylic acids, salicylates, and other factors may inhibit mitochondrial ureagenesis and may potentiate their individual metabolic effects. Alternatively, they may inhibit adenosine triphosphate synthesis and may lead to profound reductions in high-energy phosphate, which is required to catalyze an array of enzymatic reactions.

TREATMENT

The treatment of children with Reye syndrome ranges from relatively simple provision of glucose to children with stage I findings to extremely complex neurologic intensive care for children with more severe stages of the disease. Therapy is significantly dependent on the stage of the disease in patients with Reye syndrome.

Children who are in stage I require close neurologic evaluation, frequent determinations of glucose levels, and daily measurements of ammonia, liver enzymes, and electrolyte levels.

Hypoglycemia is avoided by the provision of intravenous glucose, coupled with close monitoring of the glucose level. Children with stage I Reye syndrome have an excellent prognosis if they undergo observation in the hospital and receive glucose and electrolyte intravenous therapy.

Children who have disease of stage II or higher Reye syndrome require significantly more care and must be treated in the hospital's intensive care facility. In all patients with stage III disease or with stage II disease progressing toward stage III, aggressive therapy should consist of intubation, hemodynamic monitoring, monitoring and control of intracranial pressure, and therapies to reduce ammonia.

Suggested Readings

Casteels-VanDael M, VanGeet C, Wouters C, et al. Reye syndrome revisited: a descriptive term covering a group of heterogenous disorders. *Eur J Pediatr* 2000;159:641.

Centers for Disease Control and Prevention. Reye's syndrome surveillance: United States, 1989. *MMWR Morb Mortal Wkly Rep* 1991;40:88.

Forsyth BW, Horwitz RI, Acampora D, et al. New epidemiologic evidence confirming that bias does not explain the aspirin/Reye's syndrome association. *JAMA* 1989;261:2517.

Glascow JF, Middleton B. Reye syndrome: insights on causation and prognosis. *Arch Dis Child* 2001;85:351.

Hall SM, Lynn R. Reye's syndrome. *N Engl J Med* 1999;341:345.

Hardie RM, Newton LH, Bruce JC, et al. The changing clinical pattern of Reye's syndrome, 1982–1990. *Arch Dis Child* 1996;74:400.

Hurwitz ES, Barret MJ, Bergman D, et al. Public health study of Reye's syndrome and medications. *JAMA* 1987;257:1905.

Orlowski JP, Gillis J, Kilham HA. A catch in the rye. *Pediatrics* 1987;80:638.

Reye RDK, Morgan G, Baral J. Encephalopathy and fatty degeneration of the viscera: a disease entity in childhood. *Lancet* 1963;2:749.

Stumpf DA. Reye syndrome: an international perspective. *Brain Dev* 1995; 17(suppl):77.

Trauner DA. What is the best treatment for Reye's syndrome? *Arch Neurol* 1986; 43:729.

Treem WR. Inherited and acquired syndromes of hyperammonemia and encephalopathy in children. *Semin Liver Dis* 1994;14:236.

CHAPTER 406 ■ DISORDERS OF THE ANTERIOR HORN CELL

JULIE THORNE PARKE

The anterior horn cells may be involved selectively in a number of acquired and inherited diseases. Certain viruses, particularly poliomyelitis, demonstrate a specific affinity for these nerve cells. Herpes zoster and coxsackievirus also occasionally affect anterior horn cells. Inherited conditions influencing the anterior horn cells include the spinal muscular atrophies (SMAs) and numerous metabolic disorders. Damage to the anterior horn cells is characterized clinically by weakness, atrophy, and hyporeflexia. Fasciculations are common findings. Because the dorsal sensory root is not involved in these disorders, sensory abnormalities are not present. Motor nuclei in the brainstem are involved commonly, so bulbar dysfunction is seen frequently.

SPINAL MUSCULAR ATROPHIES

The SMAs are hereditary degenerative diseases affecting the motor neurons of the brain stem and spinal cord. Several distinct clinical presentations exist (Table 406.1), differing by age at onset of symptoms, severity of symptoms, and length of survival. SMA I, SMA II, and SMA III are autosomal recessive disorders, all caused by a mutation of the survival motor neuron gene (*SMN*) on chromosome 5q13. A large, 500-kilobase duplication is present on 5q, containing two *SMN* genes. The pathogenic gene *SMN1* is in the telomeric copy of the duplication. The homozygous absence of *SMN1* is the primary cause of SMA. A centromeric copy of the gene *SMN2* differs slightly

TABLE 406.1

PROGRESSIVE SPINAL MUSCULAR ATROPHIES

Disorder	Inheritance	Age of Onset	Clinical Features
Acute infantile SMA (acute Werdnig-Hoffmann disease, SMA type I)	Autosomal recessive	*In utero* to 6 mo	Frog-leg posture; severe weakness with some movements of fingers and toes; most are unable to sit; areflexia; tongue atrophy and fasciculations; progressive swallowing and respiratory problems; survival <3 years
Intermediate SMA (chronic Werdnig-Hoffmann disease, SMA type II)	Autosomal recessive; rarely autosomal dominant	3 mo to 15 yr	Proximal weakness; most sit, some walk until teens; decreased or absent reflexes; long periods of apparent arrest; high incidence of scoliosis, contractures; unusual tremor (minipolymyoclonus); survival varies several years to third decade
Juvenile SMA (Kugelberg-Welander disease)	Autosomal recessive; rarely autosomal dominant	5–15 yr	May be part of continuous disease spectrum of SMA type II; proximal weakness with hip and shoulder atrophy; calf hypertrophy; decreased or absent reflexes; may remain ambulatory into fourth decade

SMA, spinal muscular atrophy.

and encodes an unstable, truncated protein. The severity of the disease is determined mainly by the number of *SMN2* copies present. Most infants with SMA I have one or two copies of *SMN2*. Most individuals with SMA II or SMA III have three or more copies, thus producing more SMN protein. The SMN protein is an essential factor in the cytoplasmic assembly of spliceosomes. It also may play a role in the renewal or regeneration of spliceosomes in the nucleus. The clinical categories of SMA continue to be useful in describing the severity of disease, although they now are recognized as variants of the same disease (Box 406.1).

Acute Infantile Spinal Muscular Atrophy (Werdnig-Hoffmann Disease, Spinal Muscular Atrophy Type I)

Patients with the most severe form of SMA present a stereotypic picture, with the onset of symptoms occurring within the first 6 months of life. In one-third of cases, the onset occurs *in utero,* with a notable decrease in fetal movements during the last months of pregnancy. These infants are hypotonic and weak in the neonatal period, and they have significant feeding difficulties and respiratory distress. Other children may appear

physiologically normal for the first few weeks of life while generalized weakness of the extremities, trunk, and bulbar muscles gradually develops. A typical *frog-leg* posture, characterized by abduction of the arms with flexion at the elbows and abduction of the legs with flexion at the knees, is seen in the early stages of the disease.

Physical examination reveals marked hypotonia and generalized and symmetric weakness. Movements may be limited to flickering of the fingers and toes. The tendon reflexes almost invariably are absent. The child is unable to support the head and cannot straighten the trunk when held in ventral suspension. Respirations are shallow, and chest movements may be paradoxic. Feeding difficulties occur early, and secretions pool in the mouth as swallowing becomes further impaired. Visible atrophy and fasciculations of the tongue may be present. The extraocular muscles are not affected. The child appears alert and attentive, and development is normal with the exception of motor skills. Contractures are not seen commonly in the early stages of the disease, although a few patients have congenital contractures or dislocation of the hip. The natural course is one of gradually increasing weakness, with development of feeding difficulties and respiratory compromise. In most cases, death occurs from a pulmonary infection with respiratory failure before the patient reaches 3 years of age.

Electromyographic examination shows fibrillation potentials suggesting active denervation and a marked reduction in number of voluntary motor unit potentials. Nerve conduction velocities are normal, thus distinguishing SMA from peripheral neuropathy. Histologically, striking differences in the muscle occur between SMA I and other neurogenic atrophies. Large groups of small round or oval fibers with well-preserved architecture are present, a finding suggesting an arrest in maturation rather than atrophy of mature muscle fibers (Fig. 406.1). Molecular genetic diagnosis is available both for establishing a definitive diagnosis and for prenatal testing.

The treatment of acute infantile SMA is limited to supportive care. Respiratory insufficiency frequently becomes a problem before the child reaches 1 year of age, and survival beyond 2 or 3 years is rare. Life can be prolonged with mechanical respiratory support, but the patient's quality of life may be very poor.

BOX 406.1   **Types of Spinal Muscular Atrophy**

Acute infantile spinal muscular atrophy (spinal muscular atrophy type I)
    Werdnig-Hoffmann disease
Intermediate spinal muscular atrophy (spinal muscular atrophy type II)
Juvenile spinal muscular atrophy (spinal muscular atrophy type III)
    Kugelberg-Welander disease

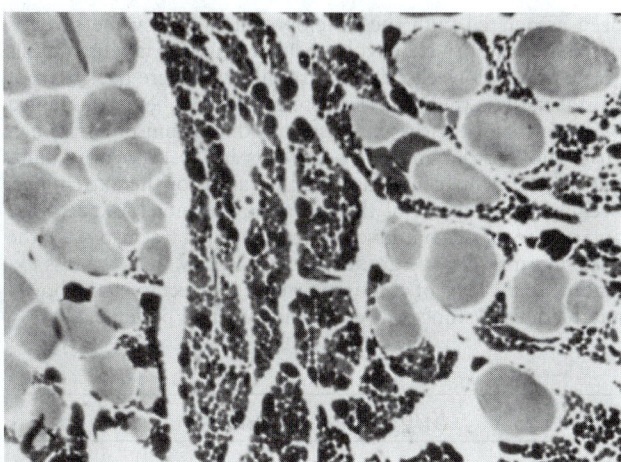

FIGURE 406.1. Muscle biopsy sample of a patient with Werdnig-Hoffmann disease showing characteristic groups of rounded, atrophic type II (dark) muscle fibers adjacent to groups of normal sized or hypertrophic type I (light) muscle fibers.

Intermediate Spinal Muscular Atrophy (Spinal Muscular Atrophy Type II)

SMA II usually presents after the child reaches 6 months of age. The child may learn to sit independently and to stand, but independent walking usually is not achieved. Weakness is symmetric, and proximal muscles and trunk tend to be involved more severely than distal muscles. A characteristic fine tremor is noted with hands outstretched. Tongue fasciculations and atrophy are noted in approximately one-half of the patients, but chewing and swallowing difficulties are rare. The deep tendon reflexes are absent or diminished. As in patients with the acute form of the disease, intelligence is normal. Many patients have a stable course after the initial months of progressive weakness and may survive until adulthood.

No specific treatment is available for this disorder. Therapy should be directed toward preventing contractures by a combination of physical therapy, bracing, and orthopedic procedures. Attention should be paid to maintaining correct posture of the spine because scoliosis may be rapidly progressive and can cause severe thoracic distortion, thereby adding to the respiratory impairment.

Juvenile Spinal Muscular Atrophy (Kugelberg-Welander Disease, Spinal Muscular Atrophy Type III)

Typically, juvenile SMA begins when children are between 5 and 15 years of age, although earlier and later times of onset have been described. Weakness frequently starts in the hip girdle and causes difficulty in walking, climbing stairs, and rising from a seated position. As pelvic girdle weakness progresses, the child may use the hands to push off the knee when rising from the floor (Gower maneuver). The calf muscles may appear hypertrophied in comparison with the atrophic thigh muscles, leading to the erroneous diagnosis of Duchenne or Becker muscular dystrophy. Involvement of the shoulder and arm muscles becomes apparent in the later stages of the illness. Facial weakness and bulbar symptoms are rare developments. Most patients remain ambulatory until their third or fourth decade, at which time severe hip weakness necessitates the use of a wheelchair. Skeletal deformities are not common developments early in the course of the disease, but scoliosis and contractures may occur when the patient becomes nonambulatory.

OTHER HEREDITARY DISORDERS

Numerous less common diseases can affect the anterior horn cell. Some of these diseases have distinctive clinical features, but, for many, their genetic nature is not established yet. A rare disorder, progressive juvenile bulbar palsy (Fazio-Londe disease), causes progressive weakness of the facial, ocular, and bulbar muscles, starting when the child is in the first decade of life. As the disease advances, the trunk and limb muscles also become involved, and death occurs within several years. Pathologically, loss of motor nuclei occurs throughout the brainstem and in anterior horn cells in the spinal cord. A form of infantile-onset pontocerebellar hypoplasia has been associated with anterior horn cell disease resembling SMA I, but with a normal *SMN* gene. A rare infantile form of anterior horn cell disease associated with respiratory distress (SMARD 1) is characterized by marked, early diaphragmatic involvement and relentlessly progressive respiratory insufficiency, with death occurring within weeks or months. The specific gene pathogenic for SMARD 1 has been identified as immunoglobulin mu-binding protein 2 *(IGHMBP2)*. The function of the gene is unknown. Numerous descriptions of children with progressive weakness and atrophy of the shoulder girdle and peroneal muscles have been reported. Some of these cases of scapuloperoneal or facioscapulohumeral muscular atrophy appear to be caused by anterior horn cell disease, although others seem to have a myopathic basis.

Arthrogryposis multiplex congenita is a syndrome consisting of multiple contractures of the joints of the arms and legs that are present at birth. This syndrome may be caused by a pathologic process in the anterior horn cell, peripheral nerve, neuromuscular junction, muscle, or joints and joint capsules. The anterior horn cell type is the most common and results from a marked decrease in the number of anterior horn cells in the cervical and lumbar spinal cord. The patients are profoundly weak and have decreased range of motion of the joints, with multiple contractures. Deep tendon reflexes are absent. The typical posture is one of extension of the arms with internal rotation of the forearms and finger flexion. The thighs usually are flexed at the hips and are rotated externally, and the feet have a talipes equinovarus deformity. Weakness generally is not progressive in these patients, and orthopedic procedures may improve function of the joints.

Numerous metabolic conditions have been associated with anterior horn cell involvement. Several patients have been described who have progressive proximal muscle weakness, fasciculations, cramps, and hyperreflexia suggestive of motor neuron disease but are found to have hexosaminidase deficiency. In patients with classic Tay-Sachs disease, the anterior horn cells may be involved by the storage of ganglioside, producing hypotonia and weakness. Anterior horn cell disease has been noted in patients with Pompe disease, infantile neuroaxonal dystrophy, and ceroid lipofuscinosis. Hyperglycinemia, beta-hydroxyisovaleric aciduria, and beta-methylcrotonylglycinuria have been associated with clinical conditions similar to those of SMA. More recently, mitochondrial disorders have been associated with the clinical phenotype of SMA. In many of these disorders, the disease picture is dominated by pathologic features in other parts of the nervous system.

INFECTIOUS DISEASES

Poliomyelitis is an acute viral disease that exhibits a specific predilection for the anterior horn cells. The illness begins with fever, malaise, and, frequently, gastrointestinal symptoms. These symptoms are followed by a meningitic illness, with stiffness and pain in the neck and pain in the back muscles. In a small percentage of infections, paralysis develops during the acute meningeal illness. Occasionally, paralysis may be delayed for 1 to 2 weeks after the onset of meningeal symptoms. The legs usually are more severely involved than are the arms, but weakness may occur in any muscle group. The muscular weakness may be associated with fasciculations and pain initially and then may progress to a flaccid paralysis. Muscular involvement may be asymmetric and restricted to muscles in one extremity, or it may involve the trunk and all the extremities. Bulbar involvement occurs in 10% to 30% of children with paralytic poliomyelitis and causes difficulty in swallowing or breathing. Examination of the cerebrospinal fluid reveals lymphocytosis, with a normal glucose level and a normal or slightly elevated protein level. The virus cannot be isolated from the cerebrospinal fluid, but it may be recovered from stool suspensions or throat washings. Electromyography reveals evidence of denervation (fibrillation potentials) after a period of approximately 3 weeks. As recovery progresses, polyphasic motor unit action potentials of increasingly large amplitude are recorded, indicating reinnervation.

The prognosis of patients with paralytic poliomyelitis varies depending on the site and severity of the paralysis. The mortality rate in bulbar disease is approximately 10%, with death usually resulting from respiratory failure. The mortality rate associated with spinal poliomyelitis is approximately 1%. Gradual improvement occurs in most cases, but many patients are left with residual weakness. Poliomyelitis has become a rare disease since the advent of widespread immunization, but sporadic cases still occur.

Coxsackievirus infections occasionally show an affinity for anterior horn cells and cause a paralytic illness similar to poliomyelitis. Numerous other viruses and immunizations have been associated with the development of transverse myelitis with anterior horn cell involvement. Transverse myelitis begins abruptly 1 to 3 weeks after a viral illness. Severe back or root pain usually is the initial symptom and may be accompanied by fever, malaise, neck stiffness, and diffuse muscular aching. Disruption of the anterior horn cells in the cervical or lumbar enlargements causes a flaccid paralysis of the extremities. Because involvement of the spinal cord is not limited to the anterior horn cells but involves corticospinal tracts as well, the flaccidity may change gradually to spasticity. Sensory loss extending to the level of cord impairment is detectable, and bowel and bladder dysfunctions occur in almost all patients.

Suggested Readings

Crawford T. Spinal muscular atrophies. In: Jones H, DeVivo D, Darras B, eds. *Neuromuscular disorders of infancy, childhood and adolescence*. Philadelphia: Butterworth Heinemann, 2003:145.

Di Donato C, Ingraham S, Mendell J, et al. Deletions and conversion in spinal muscular atrophy patients: is there a relationship to severity? *Ann Neurol* 1997;41:230.

Dubowitz V. Disorders of the lower motor neurone: the spinal muscular atrophies In: Dubowitz V, ed. *Muscle disorders in childhood*. Philadelphia: WB Saunders, 1995:325.

Fidzianska A. Spinal muscular atrophy in childhood. *Semin Pediatr Neurol* 1996;3:53.

LeFebvre S, Burglen L, Reboullet S, et al. Identification and characterization of a spinal muscular atrophy-determining gene. *Cell* 1995;80:155.

Parano E, Pavone L, Falsaperla R, et al. Molecular basis of phenotypic heterogeneity in siblings with spinal muscular atrophy. *Ann Neurol* 1996;40:247.

Pons R, Andreetta F, Wang C, et al. Mitochondrial myopathy simulating spinal muscular atrophy. *Pediatr Neurol* 1996;15:153.

Russman B, Iannacone S, Buncher C, et al. Spinal muscular atrophy: new thoughts on the pathogenesis and classification schema. *J Child Neurol* 1992;7:347.

CHAPTER 407 ■ PERIPHERAL NEUROPATHIES

JULIE THORNE PARKE

Involvement of the peripheral nerves may occur in a variety of different disorders, including systemic diseases, infections, and poisonings. In addition, degeneration of the peripheral nerves is a major feature in numerous diseases. Diseases of the peripheral nerve have been classified in several ways. They may be categorized according to type of functional impairment (motor, sensory, autonomic, or mixed), site of pathologic involvement (primary involvement of axon or myelin), clinical course and tempo (acute, subacute, or chronic), presumed etiology, or, in an increasing number of instances, molecular genetics. None of these systems of classification is entirely satisfactory, and combinations of clinical, electrophysiologic, and pathologic features usually are used to determine the etiology. Despite a thorough diagnostic search, the cause of polyneuropathy remains obscure in more than one-half of all cases.

CLINICAL MANIFESTATIONS AND COMPLICATIONS

The term *polyneuropathy* signifies a generalized disorder of nerve function that usually is symmetric; *mononeuropathy* implies a disorder of a single peripheral nerve; and *mononeuropathy multiplex* refers to the dysfunction of multiple single nerves. The clinical signs of a neuropathy reflect the function of the peripheral nerves involved.

The characteristic symptoms of a polyneuropathy are weakness and sensory impairment. The weakness usually is more pronounced distally and often is more severe in the lower extremities than in the upper extremities. A gait disturbance may be an early feature of the disorder. Patients with primarily motor involvement commonly have a *high stepping gait* that is used to overcome their bilateral foot drop. The distal tendon reflexes usually are absent. In long-standing diseases, such as the hereditary types of neuropathy, wasting of the affected distal musculature may occur, producing an *inverted champagne bottle* or *stork leg* appearance of the legs. In a few forms of polyneuropathy, notably Guillain-Barré syndrome (GBS), weakness tends to be proximal and may be attributed mistakenly to a myopathic process. The sensory abnormalities in most neuropathies, similar to the weakness, tend to be distal, becoming gradually less severe in more proximal parts of the limbs. Thus, sensory loss appears to be in a glove-and-stocking distribution on examination. In infants and young children, profound sensory loss may lead to self-mutilation, involving injury to the insensitive areas. The involvement of motor and sensory neurons may be found in association with various spinocerebellar degenerations, such as Friedreich ataxia, which shows a selective involvement of the posterior column of the spinal cord and results in a marked impairment of proprioceptive and vibratory sensation and less impairment of pain and temperature sensations.

Pure motor or sensory forms of neuropathy occur, but most disorders cause a combination of motor and sensory symptoms. Predominantly motor polyneuropathies include GBS and the neuropathy of porphyria. Types of neuropathy with severe sensory disturbances but little motor disability include the hereditary sensory neuropathies and some drug-induced neuropathies. If autonomic nerves are affected, abnormalities of pupillary reaction, impaired sweating, impaired bladder and bowel control, and postural hypotension may be noted. Autonomic involvement is a constant feature of the polyneuropathy that is associated with diabetes mellitus and of one form of hereditary sensory neuropathy, the Riley-Day syndrome.

DIAGNOSIS

Several physical signs are helpful in establishing the diagnosis of polyneuropathy. Skeletal deformities, such as pes cavus and hammertoe, are suggestive of long-standing disorders beginning in infancy and usually are caused by hereditary neuropathies (Fig. 407.1). If scoliosis is present, it also is suggestive of a long-standing hereditary neuropathy. Associated retinitis pigmentosa, sensorineural deafness, cerebellar ataxia, or cardiomyopathy suggests a hereditary rather than an acquired disorder. The peripheral nerves usually are normal to palpation, but they may be enlarged in patients with some forms of hypertrophic neuropathy. Enlargement of the peripheral nerves occurs predominantly in patients with demyelinating neuropathies and may be found in those with chronic inflammatory neuropathies and some hereditary neuropathies, such as Charcot-Marie-Tooth disease and Refsum disease.

Electrodiagnostic studies are particularly helpful in diagnosing peripheral neuropathy. Motor and sensory conduction velocities are slowed to varying degrees in patients with most forms of polyneuropathy. In contrast, nerve conduction velocities in patients with anterior horn cell disease or myopathy usually are normal. Nerve conduction velocities may be normal or slowed only slightly in patients with primarily axonal neuropathies, but the amplitude of the compound motor action potential is reduced markedly in these patients. Specialized studies of proximal nerve conduction velocity may be necessary to demonstrate proximal lesions, such as those that occur

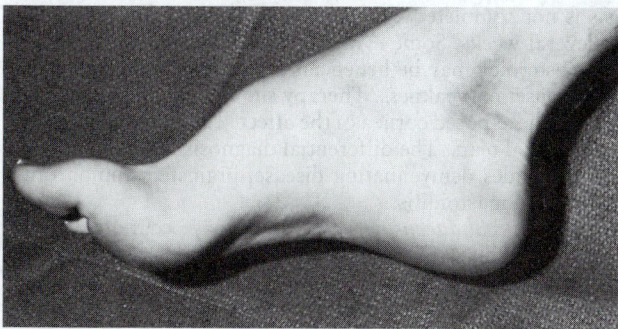

FIGURE 407.1. Pes cavus in a child with a hereditary hypertrophic neuropathy.

in GBS. A biopsy of the sural nerve may be useful in making the diagnosis by revealing evidence of either an axonal or a demyelinating process. The specific cause of the neuropathy, however, rarely is established by biopsy alone.

SPECIFIC ETIOLOGIES

Inflammatory Polyradiculoneuropathy (Guillain-Barré Syndrome)

GBS is the most common cause of acute weakness from peripheral nerve involvement. This syndrome is characterized by the acute or subacute development of a polyradiculoneuropathy, usually after an upper respiratory tract infection or an episode of gastroenteritis. Numerous infectious agents, including Epstein-Barr virus, coxsackievirus, influenza viruses, echoviruses, cytomegalovirus, and *Mycoplasma pneumoniae*, have been associated with the illness. *Campylobacter jejuni* infection has been associated with GBS, particularly the axonal form. GBS may occur after immunization against rabies. Pathologically, the disorder is characterized by the presence of inflammatory lesions, with segmental demyelination scattered throughout the peripheral nervous system. The most severely involved segments are the rootlets and the proximal portions of the peripheral nerves.

Much evidence supports an immunologic basis for this disease. The neuropathologic and clinical features are similar to those of an experimental condition known as *experimental allergic neuritis*, which is induced in animals through the injection of Freund adjuvant into peripheral nerve tissue. Experimental allergic neuritis can be transferred passively between animals by sensitized lymphocytes but not by serum, thus suggesting that experimental allergic neuritis is mediated by a delayed hypersensitivity mechanism. The prevailing opinion is that demyelination in GBS is secondary to a cell-mediated immune response that is directed against a component of peripheral myelin. Humoral immunity also has been found to be altered in patients with GBS, and it may contribute to the pathogenesis of the disorder.

Clinical symptoms typically manifest after an antecedent infection, following a latent period that varies in length from several days to several weeks. The most common initial symptoms are numbness and paresthesias of the hands and feet, followed by progressive weakness involving all four extremities. Motor impairment usually begins in the lower extremities and progresses in an ascending pattern to involve the upper extremities, trunk, and cranial nerves. A descending pattern of weakness also has been observed. Occasionally, the onset is abrupt, with simultaneous involvement of all extremities. The weakness usually is symmetric, although minor differences between the sides may occur.

A spectrum of motor involvement, varying from mild weakness to a complete flaccid quadriplegia, occurs. Muscle stretch reflexes are markedly reduced or absent. Involvement of the cranial nerves is seen commonly, with facial diplegia occurring in 50% of patients. Lower cranial nerve dysfunction may give rise to dysarthria and difficulty in swallowing and coughing. Significant respiratory muscle weakness occurs in 20% of patients and may necessitate artificial ventilation. Sensory symptoms are much less prominent than is weakness, but a distal sensory loss, particularly involving proprioception and vibratory sensation, may be present.

The autonomic nervous system is involved frequently, with episodes of paroxysmal hypertension or hypotension, tachycardia or bradycardia, facial flushing, and sweating abnormalities. Bowel and bladder functions may be impaired early in the course of the disease, but sphincter dysfunction usually is short-lived. The neurologic symptoms evolve fairly rapidly over the

TABLE 407.1

CRITERIA FOR DIAGNOSIS OF GUILLAIN-BARRÉ SYNDROME

Required
Progressive motor weakness in more than one extremity
Areflexia (or distal areflexia with hyporeflexia of biceps and knee jerks)

Strongly supportive
Clinical features (in order of importance):
    Progression up to 4 weeks into illness
    Relative symmetry
    Mild sensory symptoms or signs
    Cranial nerve involvement (facial weakness in 50%)
    Recovery beginning 2–4 weeks after progression ceases
    Autonomic dysfunction
    Absence of fever at onset of symptoms
Cerebrospinal fluid features:
    Protein level elevated after first week of symptoms
    Ten or fewer mononuclear leukocytes per microliter
Electrodiagnostic features:
    Nerve conduction slowing or block (80%)
    Prolongation of F wave latencies

Casting doubt
Marked, persistent asymmetry of weakness
Persistent bowel or bladder dysfunction
Bowel or bladder dysfunction at onset
More than 50 mononuclear leukocytes per microliter in cerebrospinal fluid
Presence of polymorphonuclear leukocytes in cerebrospinal fluid
Sharp sensory level

Rule out the diagnosis
Current history of hexacarbon abuse
Abnormal porphyrin metabolism
Recent diphtheritic infection
Evidence of lead neuropathy or intoxication
Purely sensory syndrome
Definite diagnosis of poliomyelitis, botulism, hysterical paralysis, or toxic neuropathy

Adapted from Asbury AK. Diagnostic considerations in Guillain-Barré syndrome. *Ann Neurol* 1981;9(suppl):1.

course of the first few days, with maximum disability reached within 1 week in most cases. A stable period of 1 to 3 weeks occurs, after which recovery begins. The recovery may be rapid, taking place in 6 to 8 weeks, or it may be slow, lasting many months.

Many patients with GBS have some variation in clinical presentation or laboratory test results. The currently accepted criteria for the diagnosis of this syndrome are listed in Table 407.1. Several variants of GBS are recognized; the most common one occurring in childhood is a syndrome of acute external ophthalmoplegia, ataxia, and areflexia known as the *Miller-Fisher syndrome*. The ophthalmoplegia often is bilateral and may be complete, with pupillary involvement. The course usually is benign, with recovery taking place within 3 to 6 months. More recently, a severe acute sensory variant has been described.

The most important laboratory finding in patients with GBS is an elevated cerebrospinal fluid (CSF) protein content without a pleocytosis (albuminocytologic disproportion). The total CSF protein level may be normal in the early stages of the illness, but it is elevated in almost all patients after an interval of several days. The protein content continues to increase after the disease

stabilizes, reaching a peak 2 to 4 weeks after the onset of the disease and ranging from 45 to 800 mg/dL.

Electrophysiologic studies are helpful in diagnosing GBS, with abnormalities of motor and sensory conduction occurring in 90% of patients. Characteristic electrodiagnostic features include marked slowing of conduction velocities, prolonged distal latencies, and dispersion of the evoked responses. Proximal nerve conduction, which characteristically is slow and can be measured by studying the latency of the F response, may be the only abnormal electrophysiologic finding in the early stages of the disease. In later stages of the disease, electromyographic studies may show denervation potentials indicating axonal damage, which is associated with a poor prognosis for complete recovery.

The treatment of GBS is largely supportive. Careful monitoring of respiratory function is important during the early stages of the illness to prevent death as a result of respiratory failure. Elective intubation and mechanical ventilation should be used aggressively in patients with any evidence of respiratory compromise because respiratory failure may occur abruptly if they become fatigued. Good nursing care and physiotherapy are important in severely affected patients. Most children with GBS recover completely, although the convalescence may be prolonged. Plasmapheresis and intravenous immunoglobulin have been shown to be beneficial both in shortening the length of the illness and in lessening the severity of the associated long-term disability.

Numerous entities may produce a clinical picture similar to that of GBS. The ascending form of acute transverse myelitis and early cord compression may be difficult to distinguish from GBS initially. The presence of pyramidal tract signs, a clear sensory level, and persistent sphincter disturbances support involvement of the spinal cord rather than the root and peripheral nerve. Acute paralytic poliomyelitis may present with weakness simulating GBS, but generally more systemic symptoms, more marked meningeal signs, and a cellular response in the CSF are present. Uncommon conditions that may cause acute symmetric weakness include porphyria, diphtheritic polyneuropathy, heavy-metal intoxication, systemic lupus erythematosus, periodic paralysis, tick paralysis, rabies, and botulism.

Postinfectious Neuropathies

Bell palsy, an acute paralysis of the face, is the most common postinfectious neuropathy. It frequently occurs after mild upper respiratory tract infections or episodes of otitis media. Patients often complain of pain localized in the ear, which is followed by the rapid development of weakness of the entire side of the face. The nasolabial fold on the affected side is flattened, and the child may be unable to close the eye. Taste sensation may be altered, and hyperacusis may occur as a result of involvement of the nerve to the stapedius muscle.

The prognosis for recovery is good, particularly if the paralysis is not complete. Convalescence begins within a few days to several weeks. Some evidence suggests that treatment with corticosteroids may be beneficial if started within 2 to 3 days of the onset of weakness. Therapy should include measures to protect the exposed cornea of the affected eye by taping and using artificial tears. The differential diagnosis of an acute facial palsy includes demyelinating disease, brainstem tumor, otitis media, and mastoiditis.

A painless *abducens nerve paralysis* may occur after a nonspecific viral illness. The prognosis for this type of cranial nerve VI palsy is excellent, with improvement beginning in 3 to 6 weeks and total recovery seen in most children by 3 months. Isolated oculomotor, glossopharyngeal, and hypoglossal nerve palsies occur much less commonly.

Brachial Plexopathy

An acute brachial plexopathy may occur in children after acute febrile illnesses or immunizations. The disorder is characterized by the sudden onset of pain in the shoulder and upper arm, followed by the rapid development of flaccid weakness involving primarily those muscles that are innervated by the upper roots of the brachial plexus. The paralysis may be severe, and atrophy of the affected muscles occurs. Sensory loss is minimal or absent. Electrophysiologic studies reveal a slowing of nerve conduction velocities, low-amplitude evoked responses, and evidence of denervation. Physiotherapy is required to prevent contractures, because recovery tends to be very slow, occurring over the course of many months.

Genetically Determined Neuropathies

The genetically determined neuropathies tend to be slowly progressive, symmetric disorders that may be inherited as autosomal dominant, autosomal recessive, or X-linked traits (Table 407.2). These forms of neuropathy are predominantly motor and usually are associated with deformities of the feet, such as pes cavus and hammertoe. The foot deformities may precede the development of weakness by many years and, in some cases, may be the only manifestation of the disease. The hereditary neuropathies are classified on the basis of clinical, electrophysiologic, genetic, and pathologic features. The specific metabolic defects are known in only a minority of the disorders (Table 407.3).

Hereditary Motor and Sensory Neuropathy Type I (Hypertrophic Peroneal Muscular Atrophy, Charcot-Marie-Tooth Disease 1)

Hereditary motor and sensory neuropathy type I (HMSN I), or Charcot-Marie-Tooth Disease 1 (CMT1), is the most common of the hereditary neuropathies. This type of peroneal muscular atrophy usually is inherited in an autosomal dominant manner. The most common form of the disease (CMT1A) is associated with a large, tandem DNA duplication on chromosome 17p11.2–12, containing the gene encoding peripheral myelin protein (PMP22). Sixty to ninety percent of patients with CMT1 have this duplication. The duplication mutation arises *de novo* at a fairly high frequency and may be responsible for some of the presumed autosomal recessive cases of CMT disease. Other cases of CMT1 are caused by missense mutations in the myelin protein zero (MPZ) gene on chromosome 1 (CMT1B) and in the early growth response 2 (EGR2) gene on chromosome 10 (CMT1D). Marked variability occurs in the clinical features among different family members. The onset occurs in childhood, and the disorder is characterized by progressive weakness and atrophy beginning in the intrinsic foot muscles and the peroneal muscles. A history of foot abnormalities, such as pes cavus or hammertoe, is found commonly, and some family members with foot deformities do not have apparent weakness. The progressive footdrop causes the child to become progressively more clumsy and to trip frequently. The small muscles of the feet and the distal leg become atrophic, giving a stork leg or inverted champagne bottle appearance to the legs. As the disease progresses, intrinsic hand muscles and muscles of the proximal legs may become involved. Stretch reflexes are decreased or absent. Sensory function is normal or impaired only slightly. Peripheral nerves may be hypertrophic on palpation.

Reduced motor nerve conduction velocities are a hallmark of HMSN I. Conduction velocities usually are less than one-half of normal in the upper extremities and may be slowed profoundly in the lower extremities. Pathologically, a predominant loss of myelinated fibers in the peripheral nerves, with evidence of attempted remyelinization, is present. Whorls of Schwann cells and multiple layers of poorly formed regenerating myelin cause a characteristic onion-bulb appearance (Fig. 407.2).

No specific treatment exists for HMSN I, although ankle orthoses may help to alleviate the footdrop and improve the gait. Life expectancy is not reduced significantly, and patients usually remain ambulatory throughout life.

Hereditary Neuropathy with Liability to Pressure Palsies (Tomaculous Neuropathy)

Hereditary neuropathy with liability to pressure palsies (HNPP) is an autosomal dominant disorder caused by a deletion of the same region of chromosome 17 containing the PMP22 gene that is duplicated in CMT1A. It is characterized by recurrent mononeuropathies, sometimes triggered by minor trauma. Patients have intermittent sensory or motor symptoms in the distribution of individual nerves, suggesting compression or entrapment. Symptoms may be brief, lasting for only minutes, or may persist up to several months. Mononeuropathies are extremely rare in children, and, when present, should raise suspicion of an underlying neuropathy.

X-Linked Charcot-Marie-Tooth Disease

The second most common form of CMT, X-linked Charcot-Marie-Tooth disease (CMTX), is caused by mutations in the gap junction beta-1 (GJβ1) gene located on the X chromosome, encoding for the protein connexin. Symptoms usually begin in late teenage years or young adulthood. Weakness is slowly progressive and is limited to distal musculature. Female patients occasionally develop symptoms in adulthood.

Hereditary Motor and Sensory Neuropathy Type II (Axonal Form of Peroneal Muscular Atrophy, Charcot-Marie-Tooth Disease 2)

HMSN II (CMT2) refers to dominantly inherited axonal neuropathy. Clinically, this disorder is similar to HMSN I, although the onset may be later and have less involvement of the hand muscles. Distinguishing clinically between HMSN I and HMSN II requires electrodiagnostic testing. The hallmarks of HMSN II are reduced amplitude of compound muscle action potentials with normal or mildly slowed conduction velocities and evidence of denervation on needle electromyography. Molecular genetic studies show HMSN II to be heterogeneous, with the identification of multiple gene loci.

Hereditary Motor and Sensory Neuropathy Type III (Déjérine-Sottas Disease, Hypertrophic Neuropathy of Infancy)

Déjérine-Sottas disease initially was classified as a severe hypomyelinating neuropathy with onset in infancy and recessive inheritance. However, advances in molecular biology suggest that Déjérine-Sottas disease is a heterogeneous group that does not constitute an entity. Many patients presumed to have Déjérine-Sottas have been found to have autosomal dominant

TABLE 407.2

CURRENT CLASSIFICATION OF HEREDITARY MOTOR AND SENSORY NEUROPATHIES

Designation	Type/Description
HMSN I	**Autosomal Dominant**
CMT1A	HMSN type Ia Duplication 17p11.2–12 or point mutation *PMP22*
CMT1B	1b Deletion or point mutation *MPZ*
CMT1C	Ic Mutation unknown
HNPP	Deletion 17p11.2–12 or point mutation *PMP22*
HMSN I	**Autosomal Recessive**
CMT4A	With linkage to 8q
CMT4B	With focally folded myelin; some due to *myotubularin* (*MTMR2*) mutations (11q22)
CMT4C	With linkage to 5q23–33
CMT4D	HMSNL (Lom); *N-myc downstream regulated gene 1* (*NDRG1*) mutations (8q24)
CMT4E	Due to *early growth response 2 (EGR2)* mutations
CMT4F	Due to *periaxin (PRX)* mutations (19q13.1–13.3)
?	With basal lamina onion bulbs
HMSNX	**X-linked**
CMTX	1 *dominant* mutation or deletion Xq13.1 (*connexin* [cX32] mutations)
	2 *recessive* linked to Xp22.2
	3 *recessive* linked to Xq26–q27
HMSN II	**Autosomal Dominant**
CMT2A	HMSN Type IIa Linkage to 1p35–p36
CMT2B	IIb Linkage to 3q13–q22
CMT2C	IIc Unknown
CMT2D	IId Linkage to 7p14
CMT2E	IIe Linkage to 8p21 *Neurofilament-light chain (NF-L)* mutations
?	IIf Linkage to 3p14.1–q13
HMSN II	**Autosomal Recessive**
	Infantile form with respiratory failure (often fatal) (SMARD) *IGHMBP2* mutations
	Axonal type with onset in early childhood
HMSN III*	**Variable Inheritance**
	Point mutation *PMP22* or *MPZ* (hetero- or homozygous)
	Compound heterozygous
	Other myelin protein mutations (*EGR2, periaxin*)
HMSN IV and CMT4†	
HMSN V	With spastic paraparesis
HMSN VI	With optic atrophy
HMSN VII	With retinitis pigmentosa
Other rare and complex forms	

HNPP, hereditary neuropathy with liability to pressure palsies; HMSN, hereditary motor and sensory neuropathy; IGHMBP2, immunoglobulin mu-binding protein 2; SMARD, spinal muscular atrophy with respiratory distress.

*The term HMSN III should be restricted to hereditary neuropathies in which hypomyelination is the dominant feature. This would include congenital hypomyelinating neuropathy and Déjérine-Sottas disease.
†HMSN type IV originally was proposed to indicate Refsum disease, whereas CMT4 describes recessive forms of HMSN.

Reprinted with permission from Ouvrier R, Wilmshurst J. Overview of the Neuropathies. In: Jones H, DeVivo D, Darras B, ed. *Neuromuscular disorders of infancy, childhood and adolescence*. Philadelphia: Butterworth Heinemann, 2003:344.

mutations caused by mutations in *PMP22*, *MPZ*, and *EGR2*. Pathologically, severe disruption of the myelin occurs in many different nerves, with marked onion-bulb formation and nerve hypertrophy. The onset of clinical features occurs in infancy, with delayed motor development and severe generalized weakness. Walking is delayed, and patients may be unable to run. Weakness increases in severity during the second decade. Skeletal deformities, such as pes cavus and scoliosis, are common

findings. Nerves are hypertrophic to palpation. Pupillary responses and lower cranial nerve function also may be affected. Motor nerve conduction velocities are reduced markedly, consistent with a severe demyelinating disorder. CSF protein values may be elevated significantly. Because the onset occurs in infancy, other infantile demyelinating neuropathies, including metachromatic leukodystrophy and Krabbe disease, must be excluded.

TABLE 407.3

HEREDITARY NEUROPATHIES WITH KNOWN BIOCHEMICAL ABNORMALITY

Disorder	Inheritance	Biochemical Defect	Associated Clinical Features
Acute intermittent porphyria	Autosomal dominant	Uroporphyrinogen 1 synthetase deficiency	Abdominal pain; acute psychosis; progressive weakness; tachycardia; hypertension.
Krabbe disease	Autosomal recessive	Galactocerebroside betagalactosidase deficiency	Irritability; spasticity; loss of milestones in early infancy; elevated cerebrospinal fluid protein level. Death within 1–2 years.
Metachromatic leukodystrophy	Autosomal recessive	Arylsulfatase A deficiency	Ataxia; spasticity; intellectual regression; loss of reflexes at age 2–3 years; elevated cerebrospinal fluid protein level. Slower juvenile form.
Adrenoleukodystrophy	X-linked recessive	Peroxisomal defect in fatty acid oxidation (very long-chain fatty acid accumulation)	Behavior changes; gait disturbance; vision loss; adrenal insufficiency between ages 5 and 10 years. Later onset forms occur.
Refsum disease	Autosomal recessive	Peroxisomal defect (alpha-oxidation of long-chain fatty acids, phytanic acid accumulation)	Ataxia; ichthyosis; deafness; retinitis pigmentosa; progressive sensorimotor neuropathy.
Fabry disease	X-linked recessive	alpha-Galactosidase A deficiency	Painful sensory neuropathy (burning feet); angiokeratomas in bathing-suit distribution; renal failure; stroke.
Bassen-Kornzweig disease (abetalipoproteinemia)	Autosomal recessive	beta-Lipoprotein deficiency	Fat malabsorption; vitamin A, E, and K deficiencies; progressive ataxia; retinitis pigmentosa; developmental retardation; acanthocytosis; low cholesterol level.
Tangier disease	Autosomal recessive	alpha-Lipoprotein deficiency	Yellow tonsils; hepatosplenomegaly; sensory neuropathy.

Refsum Disease

Refsum disease is a recessively inherited disorder characterized by a diffuse polyneuropathy, ataxia, and retinitis pigmentosa. Additional features include progressive deafness, cardiomyopathy, ichthyosis, and night blindness. Skeletal malformations occur frequently and include pes cavus and shortened metacarpal bones. The onset varies from early childhood to the second decade. The peripheral neuropathy is progressive and symmetric. Episodes of acute exacerbation of weakness, from which the patient may recover, may occur. These exacerbations may resemble closely inflammatory polyradiculoneuropathy. Sensory deficits are present. The cardiomyopathy may be clinically important, with the development of left ventricular failure or cardiac dysrhythmias.

Numerous laboratory test abnormalities are detected in patients with Refsum disease. The CSF protein level may be elevated significantly. The electroretinogram results may be severely altered. Both motor and sensory nerve conduction velocities are prolonged. Sural nerve biopsy reveals demyelination, showing onion-bulb formation. The Schwann cells often contain sudanophilic and metachromatic droplets, which may represent phytanic acid deposition. The diagnosis of this disorder can be confirmed by measuring the serum phytanic acid level. Patients with Refsum disease are unable to metabolize phytanic acid through alpha-oxidation, so the substance accumulates in the tissues. Studies in recent years have characterized Refsum disease as a peroxisomal disorder.

The treatment of Refsum disease focuses on the exclusion of dietary phytanic acid, which is found in dairy products,

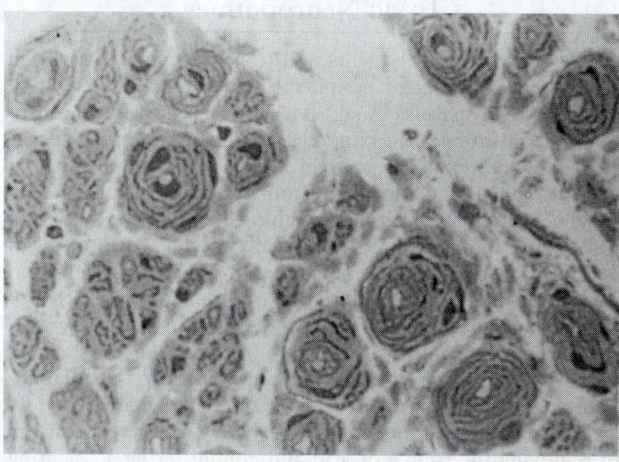

FIGURE 407.2. Sural nerve biopsy sample in a patient with hereditary motor and sensory neuropathy type I (Charcot-Marie-Tooth disease 1) shows multiple laminations of Schwann cells producing a characteristic onion-bulb formation.

vegetables, fatty meats, fish, chocolate, and nuts. Improvement in muscular strength and nerve conduction velocities has been seen to occur after adherence to a strict diet. Plasmapheresis has been helpful in patients with severe, life-threatening episodes.

Hereditary Sensory Autonomic Neuropathies

Hereditary sensory neuropathies occur much less frequently than do sensorimotor neuropathies. The major feature of type I and type II forms is distal sensory loss to pain and temperature. Type I is inherited dominantly and is characterized by neuropathic pain and ulceration of the feet, with onset between the second and fourth decades. It has been shown to be caused by mutations in the serine palmitoyltransferase subunit-1 gene (*SPTLC1*) on 9q22. Type II is a recessive trait, presenting in infancy or early childhood with severe sensory loss of the hands and trunk as well as the feet. Traumatic injuries leading to severe infections of skin and bone and self-mutilation occur commonly. Autonomic dysfunction is present to a variable degree. Pathologically, the number of myelinated fibers is decreased or the fibers are totally absent.

Familial dysautonomia (FD, Riley-Day syndrome) is a sensory neuropathy noted for its involvement of the autonomic nervous system. Familial dysautonomia is a rare familial disorder that is inherited in an autosomal recessive manner, primarily in individuals of Jewish ancestry, with onset occurring in infancy. It is caused by mutations in the gene encoding for IκB kinase complex-associated protein (IKAP) on chromosome 9q31–33. Familial dysautonomia is characterized by poor feeding, vomiting, irritability, and recurrent pulmonary infections. Signs of autonomic dysfunction include abnormal temperature regulation with profuse sweating, decreased or absent tearing, blotching of the skin, cyclical vomiting, breath-holding spells, and episodes of hypotension or hypertension. The tongue is smooth and lacks fungiform papillae. Generalized insensitivity to pain, involving the cornea as well as the skin, is present. Muscle stretch reflexes are decreased or absent. Mental retardation has been reported. Death usually occurs in young children as a result of chronic pulmonary failure or aspiration. Morphologic studies show a loss of neurons in cervical and thoracic sympathetic ganglia. Several metabolic abnormalities have been reported and include increased amounts of homovanillic acid and decreased amounts of vanillylmandelic acid in the urine, as well as reduced levels of plasma dopamine beta-hydroxylase, the enzyme that converts dopamine to norepinephrine.

Toxic Neuropathies

Many pharmaceutical agents and toxic chemicals have been implicated as causes of peripheral neuropathy. The onset of these polyneuropathies usually is insidious, occurring after prolonged exposure to the toxin. A careful history of drug use and environmental exposure to toxins is of utmost importance in making a diagnosis. Some of the more common agents causing toxic neuropathies are listed in Table 407.4.

Lead poisoning in children typically produces symptoms of encephalopathy. On occasion, however, a peripheral neuropathy may precede the development of encephalopathic symptoms. Lead usually causes a motor neuropathy with only mild sensory impairment. The distribution of weakness is distal, with patients having either footdrop or wristdrop. The diagnosis is suggested by a history of pica and may be confirmed by an elevated lead concentration in the blood. Treatment consists of removing the source of lead and administering a chelating agent. Long-term arsenic intoxication may cause paresthesias and symmetric distal weakness, primarily in the feet and legs. Sensation is decreased in a glove-and-stocking distribution, and the tendon reflexes are depressed. Transverse white striae (Mees

TABLE 407.4

TOXIC NEUROPATHIES

Industrial chemicals and insecticides
Acrylamide
Carbon disulfide
Cyanide
n-Hexane
Organophosphates (cholinergic symptoms with delayed-onset neuropathy)
Trichloroethylene (facial numbness)
Tri-orthocresylphosphate

Metals
Lead (especially neuropathy of radial nerve, causing wristdrop)
Arsenic (Mees lines, sensory deficit)
Mercury
Thallium (ataxia, alopecia, seizures)

Pharmaceutical agents
Chloramphenicol
Cisplatin
Diphenylhydantoin
Disulfiram
Gold (may be acute)
Hydralazine
Isoniazid
Metronidazole
Vincristine

lines) are seen in the fingernails 6 weeks after exposure. Cranial nerve involvement is an unusual finding, and the CSF protein concentration is normal, helping to differentiate arsenic poisoning from GBS.

Suggested Readings

Arnason B, Soliven B. Acute inflammatory demyelinating polyradiculo-neuropathy. In: Dyck P, Thomas P, Griffin J, et al., eds. *Peripheral neuropathy*, 3rd ed. Philadelphia: Saunders, 1993:1437.

Asbury A. Diagnostic considerations in Guillain-Barré syndrome. *Ann Neurol* 1981;9(Suppl):1.

Axelrod F, Pearson J. Congenital sensory neuropathies. Diagnostic distinction from familial dysautonomia. *Am J Dis Child* 1984;138:947.

Brune P, McKusick V. Familial dysautonomia. Report of genetic and clinical studies with a review of the literature. *Medicine (Baltimore)* 1970;49:343.

Dubowitz V. Disorders of the lower motor neurone, hereditary motor neuropathies. In: Dubowitz V, ed. *Muscle disorders in childhood*. Philadelphia: Saunders, 1995:370.

Epstein M, Sladky J. The role of plasmapheresis in childhood Guillain-Barré syndrome. *Ann Neurol* 1990;28:65.

Gabreels-Festen A, Joosten E, Gabreels F, et al. Hereditary and sensory neuropathy of neuronal type with onset in early childhood. *Brain* 1991;114:1855.

Guillain-Barré Syndrome Study Group. Plasmapheresis and acute Guillain-Barré syndrome. *Neurology* 1985;35:1096.

Kamholz J, Menichella D, Jani A, et al. Charcot-Marie-Tooth disease type 1: molecular pathogenesis to gene therapy. *Brain* 2000;123:222.

Lupski J, de Oca-Luna R, Slaughenhaupt S, et al. DNA duplication associated with Charcot-Marie-Tooth disease type 1A. *Cell* 1991;66:219.

Murakami T, Garcia C, Reiter L, et al. Charcot-Marie-Tooth disease and related inherited neuropathies. *Medicine* 1996;75:233.

Oh S, LaGanke C, Claussen G. Sensory Guillain-Barré syndrome. *Neurology* 2001;56:82.

Ouvrier R, Wilmshurst J. Overview of the Neuropathies. In: Jones H, DeVivo D, Darras B, ed. *Neuromuscular disorders of infancy, childhood and adolescence*. Philadelphia: Butterworth Heinemann, 2003:339.

Ropper A. *Campylobacter* diarrhea and Guillain-Barré syndrome. *Arch Neurol* 1988;45:655.

Tyson J, Ellis D, Fairbrother U, et al. Hereditary demyelinating neuropathy of infancy. A genetically complex syndrome. *Brain* 1997;120:47.

Vedanaryanan V, Kandt R, Lewis D, et al. Chronic inflammatory demyelinating polyradiculoneuropathy of childhood: treatment with high dose intravenous immunoglobulin. *Neurology* 1991;41:828.

CHAPTER 408 ■ DISEASES OF THE NEUROMUSCULAR JUNCTION

JULIE THORNE PARKE

Numerous conditions may interfere with the transmission of the electrical impulse across the neuromuscular junctions, which consist of the terminal portion of a motor nerve, the synaptic cleft, and the end-plate region of a muscle. The nerve impulse originates in the anterior horn cell and is propagated down the axon of the motor nerve into the motor nerve terminals. Depolarization of the nerve terminals opens calcium channels, causing the release of acetylcholine into the synaptic cleft. Acetylcholine binds to receptors on the muscle end plate, altering its permeability to ions and causing localized depolarization of the end plate (the end-plate potential). If the amplitude of the end-plate potential reaches threshold, a muscle fiber action potential is generated. The muscle action potential is propagated along the muscle fiber and into the interior of the muscle fiber by the T tubules, thus initiating muscle fiber contraction. Acetylcholine acts at the postsynaptic membrane for only a brief period before it is broken down by an enzyme, cholinesterase, into two inactive components, choline and acetic acid. The choline is taken up by the presynaptic nerve terminal, where choline acetyltransferase catalyzes the resynthesis of acetylcholine.

Neuromuscular transmission can fail if insufficient acetylcholine is released (presynaptic process) or if the number of acetylcholine receptors is insufficient to interact with the acetylcholine (postsynaptic disorder). Conditions interfering with the presynaptic events include some forms of congenital myasthenia gravis, botulism, hypocalcemia, hypermagnesemia, and neuromuscular blockade from antibiotics. Disorders affecting the postsynaptic events include autoimmune myasthenia gravis, some types of congenital myasthenia gravis, organophosphate poisoning, and iatrogenic neuromuscular blockade with curare (Table 408.1). Neuromuscular transmission failure also may occur when inhibition of or a deficiency in acetylcholinesterase occurs, causing a depolarization block.

Disorders of neuromuscular transmission are manifested clinically by muscle weakness, which is exacerbated by exercise and improved by rest. Defects in neuromuscular transmission can be documented by pharmacologic tests and by electrophysiologic studies, including repetitive nerve stimulation and single-fiber electromyography.

JUVENILE MYASTHENIA GRAVIS

Pathophysiology

The juvenile and adult forms of myasthenia gravis are autoimmune disorders characterized by an autoimmune attack on the acetylcholine receptor. Circulating antibodies to the acetylcholine receptor bind to the receptor on the muscle end plate, blocking its function. Morphologic studies show a simplified postsynaptic membrane with poorly developed folds and clefts and a loss of functional acetylcholine receptor sites. Antibody can be demonstrated on the postsynaptic membrane, further implicating an immunologic process in its destruction. Circulating acetylcholine receptor antibodies can be measured, but the titer does not correlate well with the clinical condition of affected patients. A lymphocyte-mediated immune response to acetylcholine receptors also has been identified. The thymus plays a role in the disease, possibly by sensitizing specific lymphocytes to produce acetylcholine receptor antibodies.

Clinical Manifestations and Complications

Usually, the onset of juvenile myasthenia gravis occurs after age 10, although it can appear much earlier. Girls are affected more commonly than are boys. The cardinal feature of the disease is easy fatigability. Usually, the onset is gradual, with symptoms most apparent in the afternoon or evening, when the patient is tired. Occasionally, the onset is fairly sudden and may appear to have been precipitated by an infectious illness. Characteristically, the weakness abates with rest and worsens with sustained effort. In approximately one-half of patients, weakness first appears in the ocular muscles, causing ptosis or diplopia (Fig. 408.1). Frequently, ptosis is asymmetric and may be unilateral. It tends to fluctuate during the day and to vary from day to day. Involvement of the ocular muscles is variable, but it may be severe, causing a total ophthalmoplegia. Approximately one-fourth of affected patients have weakness of the bulbar musculature, resulting in difficulties in speaking, swallowing, or chewing. The facial muscles are involved in most affected patients. Weakness of the palate and

TABLE 408.1

DISORDERS OF NEUROMUSCULAR TRANSMISSION

Presynaptic
Botulism
Eaton-Lambert syndrome
Hypermagnesemia
Hypocalcemia
Snake bite
Antibiotics
Congenital myasthenia gravis
? Tick paralysis

Inhibition or Deficiency of Acetylcholinesterase
Organophosphates
Congenital myasthenia gravis

Postsynaptic
Autoimmune myasthenia gravis
Curare (D-tubocurarine)
alpha-Bungarotoxin
Congenital myasthenia gravis

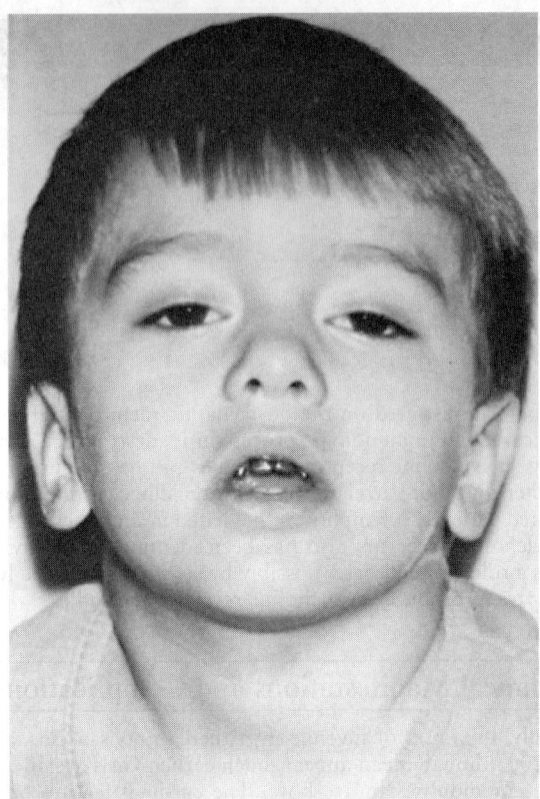

FIGURE 408.1. Four-year-old child with juvenile myasthenia gravis, exhibiting fluctuating ptosis and bilateral facial weakness.

tongue may render speech unintelligible. Affected children's voices may be strong initially, becoming softer and less distinct during continued conversation. Difficulty chewing food is a common problem, and many patients support their jaw in one hand to assist with chewing. Swallowing difficulties and choking spells may occur. Weakness of the muscles of the neck, particularly the neck extensors, causes the head to fall forward. Patients with predominantly bulbar symptoms are at risk of developing respiratory failure, particularly during an intercurrent infection.

A smaller number of children (approximately 20%) have generalized weakness of the extremities. Fatigability may be demonstrated in younger children by having them climb stairs or hold their arms outstretched for an interval. In older children, repetitive testing of deltoid strength or performance of multiple deep knee bends may help to disclose the weakness. Regardless of the distribution of weakness, the principal features are a fluctuating quality in the weakness and a susceptibility to fatigue. These features differ from those of other neuromuscular disorders, which produce relatively constant symptoms.

Diagnosis

Usually, the diagnosis of myasthenia gravis can be made on the basis of the history and physical examination, and it may be confirmed by pharmacologic tests. A small dose of an anticholinesterase drug produces a dramatic improvement in strength. Edrophonium chloride (Tensilon) is preferred because of its rapid onset and short duration of action. The availability of acetylcholine is increased by inhibiting the enzyme cholinesterase, thereby improving neuromuscular transmission. A placebo injection of normal saline should be given

before the edrophonium. A test dose of one-tenth of the total dose is given initially. If no complications occur with the test dose, the remainder of the full dosage of 0.1 mg/kg (maximum dosage, 10 mg) is given intravenously. The affected patient's heart rate and blood pressure must be monitored throughout the test, and atropine sulfate should be immediately available because a cholinergic crisis occasionally occurs, manifest by extreme bradycardia or transient respiratory weakness requiring ventilatory support. Usually, a marked but short-lived improvement in weakness is seen in patients with myasthenia. A more prolonged effect can be achieved with intramuscular or subcutaneous Neostigmine if a longer observation period is necessary to evaluate limb strength. Neostigmine is especially useful in infants and younger children.

Electrophysiologic studies are helpful in documenting transmission failure at the neuromuscular junctions. Repetitive nerve stimulation produces a characteristic fall in amplitude between the first and the fourth or fifth responses (decremental response). Testing several muscles may be necessary because the abnormality may not be present in all muscles. Selective single-fiber electromyography is possible in some older patients and may confirm the variability in synaptic transmission time in patients with rather mild disease. Antibodies to the human muscle acetylcholine receptor are found in the serum of as many as 90% of patients. However, patients with negative antibody test results are those who typically present with a purely ocular weakness or mild generalized weakness and in whom the diagnosis is uncertain. A negative test result does not exclude the diagnosis.

Therapy and Prognosis

Numerous different therapeutic modalities are available for treating myasthenia gravis. The selected approach should consider the age of the affected patient, the severity of the disease, and the potential benefits and risks of each form of therapy. Cholinesterase inhibitors improve neuromuscular transmission by inhibiting the enzymatic degradation of acetylcholine and thereby prolonging its effect on muscle end plates. These agents result in symptomatic improvement in strength in most patients with myasthenia gravis and may be sufficient to produce normal or near-normal strength in some. Pyridostigmine bromide (Mestinon) and neostigmine bromide (Prostigmin) are the agents used most commonly. Pyridostigmine is preferred because of its longer half-life and more favorable side-effect profile. An initial dosage of 1.0 mg/kg/day in divided dosages is typical in pediatric patients. Adolescents and adults typically are started at dosages of 30 to 60 mg every 4 to 6 hours. The dosage and the dosing interval must be adjusted carefully on the basis of close clinical observation. The dosage required by given individuals may vary during the day and from one day to the next. A cholinergic crisis may result from excessive anticholinesterase dosing, as a result of the accumulation of acetylcholine at neuromuscular junctions. Both nicotinic symptoms, such as increased muscle weakness and fasciculations, and muscarinic symptoms, such as diarrhea, pallor, sweating, increased salivation, cardiovascular disturbances, and visual blurring, may occur (Table 408.2). Clinicians may have difficulty in distinguishing between an overdose of anticholinesterase medications (producing weakness in respiratory muscles) and respiratory distress from myasthenic crisis (causing respiratory insufficiency). Close monitoring of the affected patient's muscle strength, pulmonary function, and ability to cough adequately is critical during these periods. Elective intubation and ventilatory support should be instituted before respiratory insufficiency occurs.

Other treatment modalities, including thymectomy, corticosteroid therapy, and immunosuppressive agents, are aimed

TABLE 408.2

SIDE EFFECTS OF CHOLINESTERASE INHIBITORS

Muscarinic
Abdominal cramps
Diarrhea
Nausea
Vomiting
Increased salivation
Increased bronchial secretions
Irritability
Anxiety
Sleep disturbances
Coma
Seizures

Nicotinic
Muscle fasciculations
Muscle weakness

more directly at the basic immunologic mechanism of the disease. Corticosteroid therapy, given on an alternate-day schedule, is effective in many patients who have an incomplete response to anticholinesterase drugs. However, the complications of corticosteroid therapy in young children may make its long-term use unsatisfactory. The importance of the thymus gland in myasthenia gravis long has been recognized, and thymectomy has been accepted as a successful method of treatment. The beneficial effects of thymectomy are not understood fully, but likely the thymus sensitizes lymphocytes to form antibodies directed at the acetylcholine receptors in the postsynaptic membrane. Total removal of the thymus gland is essential for maximal benefit. Often, the postoperative care of affected children is complex, and careful monitoring and observation in an intensive care setting is required. The efficacy of thymectomy appears to be greatest in patients with primarily bulbar symptoms. It is less effective and generally not recommended for patients with solely ocular symptoms. Plasmapheresis has been used as an intensive, short-term intervention in patients with myasthenia. It is helpful in patients who have had a short-term exacerbation of weakness during myasthenic crisis or after a thymectomy. It is used also to produce a rapid improvement in strength in preparation for thymectomy. Intravenous immunoglobulin (IVIG) also has been shown to be effective for the short-term management of myasthenia gravis, in myasthenic crises, and in preparing patients for surgery.

The prognosis for patients with juvenile myasthenia gravis is relatively good, in that complete or partial remissions occur in 25% within 2 years of disease onset. Often, however, the disease is characterized by a fluctuating course of remissions and exacerbations. The severity of symptoms varies, and some children have severe disease that necessitates frequent hospitalizations and mechanical ventilatory support. Approximately 80% of children improve after undergoing thymectomy.

TRANSIENT NEONATAL MYASTHENIA GRAVIS

The syndrome of transient neonatal myasthenia gravis is found in infants born of mothers with myasthenia gravis. The disease is caused by the transplacental passage of the IgG acetylcholine receptor antibodies and occurs in approximately 15% of the newborn children of affected mothers. Usually, symptoms appear in the first few hours after birth, although the onset may be delayed for several days. Initial symptoms include hypoto-

nia, diffuse muscle weakness, respiratory distress, and feeding difficulties. Ptosis or ocular motility problems may occur. Usually, symptoms last for several weeks, but they may persist for several months. The affected children recover fully and have an incidence of the later onset of myasthenia gravis no greater than that of the general population. The severity of an affected mother's illness is not correlated with the occurrence or severity of her infant's myasthenia. The diagnosis of neonatal myasthenia may be made by performing repetitive nerve stimulation studies, documenting the presence of circulating antibody to acetylcholine receptors, and evaluating the response to short-acting anticholinesterase medication. Supportive care and anticholinesterase agents are necessary in approximately 80% of patients.

CONGENITAL MYASTHENIA GRAVIS

Several rare varieties of congenital myasthenia gravis exist, exhibiting onset at birth or in early childhood and producing persistent symptoms. Usually, the disorders are familial, and most are inherited through an autosomal recessive mechanism, with the exception of the dominantly inherited slow-channel syndrome. Congenital myasthenia gravis differs from acquired myasthenia gravis by lack of evidence of an autoimmune etiology. Detailed physiologic and morphologic studies have identified specific abnormalities in neuromuscular junctions in patients with several of the syndromes. A number of mutations in different genes have been found that cause presynaptic, synaptic, or postsynaptic defects of neuromuscular transmission. Similar to other disorders of neuromuscular transmission, the syndromes are characterized by fluctuating weakness. Because of their heterogenous pathophysiology, the clinical manifestations of these syndromes vary. Recurrent episodes of apnea may occur. Severe ocular muscle weakness is characteristic of several of the syndromes. Bulbar or respiratory involvement may be accentuated by crying or prolonged activity. Motor milestones may be delayed. A progression of symptoms may occur during adolescence; in some cases, presentation may not occur until adolescence or early adult life. Patients with these disorders do not respond to immunosuppressive therapy or to thymectomy. The response to acetylcholinesterase inhibitors varies. The slow-channel syndrome and acetylcholinesterase deficiency syndrome may be worsened by acetylcholinesterase inhibitors.

BOTULISM

Pathophysiology

The exotoxin of *Clostridium botulinum* is one of the most potent neurotoxins known. It is absorbed from the intestine or an infected wound and is distributed in a hematogenous manner to peripheral cholinergic nerve synapses, such as neuromuscular junctions. The toxin irreversibly blocks acetylcholine release from the presynaptic nerve terminals. Recovery occurs through the sprouting of terminal motor neurons and the formation of new motor end plates.

In children and adults, poisoning may occur after ingestion of the toxin in inadequately cooked or improperly canned food. The anaerobic bacillus and the exotoxin it produces are destroyed by heat, so proper cooking of food should eliminate outbreaks. At high altitudes, where water boils at a lower temperature, the exotoxin is not destroyed during boiling, accounting for the greater frequency of botulism in mountain locales. The majority of outbreaks of botulism can be traced to home-canned foods, particularly vegetables, fruits, fish, and condiments. Wound botulism results from the infection of traumatized tissue by the organism, with subsequent toxin production. Most cases occur subsequent to wounds sustained in open fields or on farms, particularly in compound extremity fractures.

A third type of botulism, infant botulism, differs from foodborne and wound botulism because it is caused by the ingestion of the spores of *C. botulinum* rather than by the exotoxin. It occurs almost exclusively in children in the first year of life, usually in those between ages 5 and 12 weeks. The ingested spores colonize the intestinal tract and produce the *C. botulinum* toxin. Frequently, the source of the spores is not found. Honey has been implicated as the source in approximately 20% of patients, and environmental sources, such as yard soil, have been implicated in other cases.

Seven antigenically distinct types of *C. botulinum* toxin have been identified. Disease in humans is caused primarily by toxin types A, B, E, and F. Almost always, type E botulism can be traced to fish and fish products. Almost all cases of infant botulism have been caused by toxin types A or B.

Clinical Manifestations and Complications

Clinical symptoms appear within 1 to 2 days after the consumption of contaminated food or within 1 to 2 weeks after wound inoculation. The initial symptoms of food-borne infection may resemble those of food poisoning: vomiting, diarrhea, and abdominal pain. Commonly, similar symptoms develop in several members of a family. Weakness of the extraocular muscles occurs, causing blurred vision and diplopia. Failure of convergence may be the first symptom. Often, vision problems are accompanied by other bulbar symptoms, including dizziness, dysarthria, and dysphagia. Some patients have only bulbar symptoms; others have varying degrees of extremity weakness. Weakness may occur fairly rapidly after the ingestion of large amounts of toxin, causing a flaccid paralysis and respiratory failure. In wound botulism, the toxin is released slowly into the circulation, so that the onset of symptoms and the progression of weakness are slower. Examination reveals involvement of the extraocular muscles. Pupillary responses may or may not be affected. Typically, tendon reflexes are absent, but they may be present. Sensory abnormalities are not seen. In patients with milder disease, fatigability is not as prominent as in patients with myasthenia gravis.

The clinical appearance of infant botulism is different from that of food-borne or wound botulism. Constipation is the first sign of illness, although frequently this symptom may be overlooked. Infants gradually become listless and weak over a period of days to weeks. As the bulbar muscles become involved, difficulty in feeding occurs, and the cry becomes weaker. Drooling and pooling of food and secretions in the posterior pharynx may occur. Ptosis, ophthalmoplegia, and diminished facial expression are present. Most often, hypotonia and generalized muscle weakness are manifest initially as a loss of head control. Respiratory arrest may occur abruptly in patients with severe disease. Botulism may be responsible for some cases of unexpected sudden death in infancy.

Diagnosis

Electrophysiologic studies are helpful in demonstrating a disturbance in neuromuscular transmission in patients with botulism. The compound muscle action potential elicited by a single stimulus to the nerve is small, and the amplitude declines with repetitive stimulation at a slow rate. Repetitive stimulation at fast rates produces an increase in the amplitude of muscle action potentials. Needle examination demonstrates a distinctive pattern of brief, small, abundant motor unit potentials that may be diagnostic of botulism in the context of the clinical syndrome. Confirmation of the diagnosis of botulism depends on detecting the toxin or the organism in affected patients or in the implicated food. In infant botulism, the organism may be isolated from stool culture.

Differential Diagnosis

Botulism in children must be distinguished from myasthenia gravis, Guillain-Barré syndrome, tick paralysis, and chemical intoxications. Typically, patients with myasthenia gravis have preserved pupillary reactions and usually do not have areflexia. Fatigability is much more prominent in myasthenia gravis, and the edrophonium chloride (Tensilon) test result is dramatically positive. Clinical differentiation from Guillain-Barré syndrome may be difficult. Usually, patients with Guillain-Barré syndrome have ascending weakness, with a later onset of cranial nerve involvement. Frequent paresthesias and elevated cerebrospinal fluid protein content also help to distinguish this disorder. Electromyography is helpful in differentiating both Guillain-Barré syndrome and myasthenia gravis from botulism.

In addition to these disorders, the differential diagnosis of infant botulism includes Werdnig-Hoffmann disease, poliomyelitis, and diphtheria. The early extraocular muscle and pupillary involvement, the symmetry of weakness, and the absence of fever or pharyngitis, in addition to the characteristic electrophysiologic findings, should increase the suspicion of botulism.

Therapy and Prognosis

The treatment of all forms of botulism is directed toward aggressive supportive care, with particular attention paid to respiratory support. Generally, the prognosis is good if the patient is supported adequately, although recovery may be very slow, taking weeks to many months in severely affected individuals. In cases of food-borne botulism, if affected patients are seen early, emetics and gastric lavage should be used to reduce the amount of unabsorbed toxin. Antitoxin may be given, although evidence of its efficacy once neurologic manifestations have occurred is lacking. If food-borne botulism is suspected, state and federal health officials should be notified immediately. The treatment of wound botulism includes exploration and débridement of the site, in conjunction with antitoxin and antibiotic therapy. Guanidine may be of some value in improving muscle strength in mild or moderately severe cases of food-borne or wound botulism. Infant botulism is a self-limiting disease, generally lasting 2 to 6 weeks. The use of antitoxin and antibiotics has not been shown to influence its course. Antibiotics may exacerbate symptoms because bacterial death may liberate *C. botulinum* toxin, thus increasing the amount of toxin in the gastrointestinal tract. Aggressive supportive care is required throughout the period of hypotonia and weakness, and many infants require prolonged ventilator support. Constipation may persist for months and may improve with the use of stool softeners and adequate hydration. The mortality from botulism is 20% to 25% in cases of food-borne or wound botulism. The mortality of recognized cases of infant botulism is approximately 3%. A relapse of infant botulism after apparent resolution of clinical symptoms may occur, making close follow-up necessary.

TICK PARALYSIS

Pathophysiology

A progressive, ascending flaccid paralysis may be caused by the attachment of certain species of ticks. In North America, the disease is caused most commonly by *Dermacentor andersoni* (wood tick) or *Dermacentor variabilis* (dog tick). *Ixodes holocyclus* (scrub tick) is the cause of the disease in Australia. Most cases of tick paralysis occur in the spring or summer and involve young children, especially girls with long hair. Frequently, the tick attaches near the hairline, where it remains unnoticed. Clinical symptoms begin within several days after the tick attaches. Tick paralysis is thought to be caused by a toxin released by the ticks, but the exact mechanism and site of the toxin's action are not known. The toxin may prevent depolarization in the terminal portions of the motor neurons.

Clinical Manifestations and Complications

Tick paralysis may begin with such general symptoms as irritability and diarrhea. Initial neurologic signs include gait ataxia and areflexia. Weakness of the legs then becomes apparent and advances in an ascending, symmetric pattern to involve the trunk and upper extremities. If the tick remains attached, the weakness may progress to involve the bulbar musculature, producing dysarthria, dysphagia, blurred vision, and facial weakness. Respiratory compromise may occur. Patients may complain of numbness and tingling of the extremities, but objective sensory abnormalities are rare.

Diagnosis

Routine laboratory studies are not helpful in establishing the diagnosis of tick paralysis. The cerebrospinal fluid protein level is normal, which helps to distinguish tick paralysis from Guillain-Barré syndrome. Usually, electrophysiologic studies reveal a reduced amplitude of the compound muscle action potential, with no significant incremental or decremental response on repetitive stimulation. Motor and sensory nerve conduction velocities are decreased slightly in the distal segments.

Therapy and Prognosis

Recovery occurs within 1 to 5 days after removal of the tick. Intensive supportive care, with assisted ventilation for respiratory failure, may be required during this period. The tick must be removed for recovery to occur. Removal is achieved best by covering the tick with petrolatum to cause it to withdraw before removing it with forceps. Care should be taken to remove the entire tick so that secondary infection does not occur.

NEUROMUSCULAR TOXINS

Numerous pharmacologic and environmental agents may interfere with neuromuscular transmission (Table 408.3). Organophosphates, such as parathion, cause the irreversible inhibition of acetylcholinesterase, resulting in an accumulation of acetylcholine in the synaptic cleft. These insecticides cause muscle paralysis with prominent autonomic symptoms. Common

TABLE 408.3

DRUGS AFFECTING NEUROMUSCULAR TRANSMISSION

Antibiotics (tetracyclines, trimethoprim, polymyxins, aminoglycosides, lincomycin, clindamycin, tobramycin, streptomycin, erythromycin, colistin, ciprofloxacin, norfloxacin, ofloxacin, pefloxacin)
D-Penicillamine
beta-Adrenergic blockers (propranolol)
Phenytoin
Amitriptyline
Procainamide
Quinidine
Chloroquine
Lithium
Phenothiazines
Neuromuscular blocking agents (succinylcholine, pancuronium bromide, D-tubocurarine, vecuronium, others)
Anticholinesterases
Calcium channel blockers
Iodinated contrast agents
Magnesium (milk of magnesia, Maalox)
Adrenocorticotropic hormone
Corticosteroids
Many others

neuromuscular-blocking agents used in anesthesia, such as succinylcholine, may cause prolonged paralysis in patients with clinical or subclinical myasthenia gravis. Numerous antibiotics interfere with the release of acetylcholine and aggravate preexisting neuromuscular-transmission problems. Several other drugs, including propranolol, phenytoin, calcium channel blockers, and corticosteroids, may have a similar effect on neuromuscular transmission. The treatment of drug-induced neuromuscular blockade consists of supportive care and the substitution of a different drug.

Suggested Readings

Andrews P, Sanders D. Juvenile myasthenia gravis. In: Jones H, DeVivo D, Darras B, eds. *Neuromuscular disorders of infancy, childhood and adolescence.* Philadelphia: Butterworth Heinemann, 2003:575.

Crawford T. Infantile botulism. In: Jones H, DeVivo D, Darras B, eds. *Neuromuscular disorders of infancy, childhood and adolescence.* Philadelphia: Butterworth Heinemann, 2003:547.

Dubowitz V. Myasthenia. In: Dubowitz V. *Muscle disorders in childhood,* 2nd ed. Philadelphia: Saunders, 1995:398.

Engel A. Myasthenia gravis and myasthenic syndromes. *Ann Neurol* 1984;16:519.

Engel A, Ohno K, Sine S. Congenital myasthenic syndromes: progress over the past decade. *Muscle Nerve* 2003;27:4.

Lefvert A, Osterman P. Newborn infants to myasthenic mothers: a clinical study and an investigation of acetylcholine receptor antibodies in 17 children. *Neurology* 1983;33:133.

Long S. Botulism in infancy. *Pediatr Infect Dis J* 1984;3:266.

Papazian O. Transient neonatal myasthenia gravis. *J Child Neurol* 1992;7:135.

Rodriquez M, Gomez M, Howard F, et al. Myasthenia gravis in children: long-term follow-up. *Ann Neurol* 1983;13:504.

Sanders D, Scoppetta C. The treatment of patients with myasthenia gravis. *Neurol Clin* 1994;12:343.

Venkataraman V, Evans O, Subramony S. Tick paralysis in children. *Neurology* 2002;59:1088.

Wolfe G. Treatment review and update for myasthenia gravis. *J Clin Neuromusc Dis* 2004;6:54.

CHAPTER 409 ■ HEREDITARY AND ACQUIRED TYPES OF MYOPATHY

DARRYL C. DE VIVO AND SALVATORE DIMAURO

Molecular genetics has revolutionized our current understanding of neuromuscular diseases. The inherited conditions embrace all patterns of heredity, both mendelian and non-mendelian. The term *muscular dystrophy* is used to describe a group of conditions that are inherited, progressive, and characterized by myodegeneration. Other conditions are designated as types of myopathy, such as congenital myopathy (e.g., central core disease) or metabolic myopathy. In general, forms of metabolic myopathy are classified according to the involved pathway (e.g., types of glycogenoses, forms of mitochondrial myopathy), and often the specific biochemical defect is known. Whenever possible, these diseases are classified according to the molecular, genetic, or biochemical defect because the phenotypic expression of one molecular defect may be fairly heterogeneous. Thus, Duchenne-type muscular dystrophy (DMD) and Becker muscular dystrophy (BMD) are allelic diseases, whereas McLeod syndrome and the dystrophy associated with glycerol kinase deficiency are due to contiguous genes involvement. We know now that the heterogeneous phenotypes associated with a specific genetic defect may result from the variable involvement of contiguous genes, depending on the size of the deleted genetic segment.

The acquired muscle disorders are classified according to etiologic factors whenever possible or by the characteristics of the tissue reaction. Hence, we use the terms *inflammatory*, *toxic*, *nutritional*, and *endocrinologic* to describe these diverse conditions.

HEREDITARY TYPES OF DYSTROPHY

X-Linked Diseases

Duchenne Muscular Dystrophy

DMD is the most severe form of progressive primary muscular degeneration. It affects approximately one in 3,000 live-born male infants, with one-third of all cases representing new mutations. DMD is associated with mutations in a gene located in band 1 of region 2 of the short (p) arm of the X chromosome (Xp21), which encodes for a large protein called dystrophin. DMD is manifest at birth, becomes clinically evident when children are between 3 and 5 years of age, and progresses inexorably over the course of the next 2 decades before culminating in death. Most patients become wheelchair-dependent when they are between 10 and 12 years of age.

Pathogenesis. DMD is associated with mutations in a gene located in band 1 of region 2 of the short (p) arm of the X chromosome (Xp21), which encodes for a large protein called dystrophin. The genetic cause of DMD is known, but the pathophysiology remains obscure. The dystrophin gene—the

largest identified thus far—encompasses 80 exons, with multiple spliced isoforms and many tissue-specific promoters. The typical DMD phenotype is due to lack of the full-length muscle dystrophin transcript that encodes a dystrophin isoform of 427 kd. The most common gene defects associated with DMD are deletions involving one or more exons. The severity of the clinical phenotype depends largely on how a deletion affects the reading frame. If the "residual" gene still can be spliced together into an abnormal but still "readable" mRNA, then an abnormal dystrophin is made and the clinical presentation is milder, usually BMD (see section, Becker Muscular Dystrophy). If, however, the deletion causes a frame shift and generates an unreadable mRNA, then no dystrophin is made and clinical presentation is severe DMD.

Dystrophin, with a molecular weight of 440 kd, is a central component of the membrane cytoskeleton, in close association with other proteins, including sarcoglycans, dystroglycans, and laminin (Fig. 409.1). This complex confers structural integrity to the muscle plasma membrane, which is subject to the mechanical stress of contraction. Thus, a simple—perhaps simplistic—pathogenic hypothesis is that "tears" in the plasma membrane lead to cell death. However, this mechanism does not explain the presymptomatic period or the progressive nature of the disease. Other hypotheses consider the partial compensatory roles of other cytoskeletal proteins (such as utrophin), the limited regenerating potential of continually damaged myofibers, and the potential contribution of inflammation and fibrosis. The histopathologic abnormalities seen in the various types of DMD are distinctive but are not specific for any entity (Box 409.1).

Clinical Manifestations and Complications. Infant macroglossia has been noted occasionally, and motor milestones may be delayed. One-third of patients with DMD are late walkers (i.e., they do not walk independently until they are between 15 and 18 months of age). Parents retrospectively report developmental clumsiness and motor sluggishness in running, climbing stairs, rising from the ground after falling, and pedaling a tricycle. Abnormalities of gait and posture appear in middle childhood, with the emergence of increasing lumbar lordosis, pelvic waddling, frequent falling, and Gowers sign. Although Gowers sign is distinctive in DMD, it may be seen in patients with any condition that causes pelvic girdle weakness. Enlargement of the musculature becomes evident, with characteristic involvement of calf, gluteal, lateral vastus, deltoid, and infraspinatus groups. Weakness is more evident in the proximal muscles, and tendon reflexes are diminished at the knees, biceps, and triceps. Only in the preterminal phase are the distal tendon reflexes affected noticeably. Before ambulation is lost, contractures of the iliotibial bands, hip flexors, and heel cords develop. After ambulation is lost, the muscles decrease in size, contractures progress with loss of joint mobility, and kyphoscoliosis develops with further compromise of respiratory function.

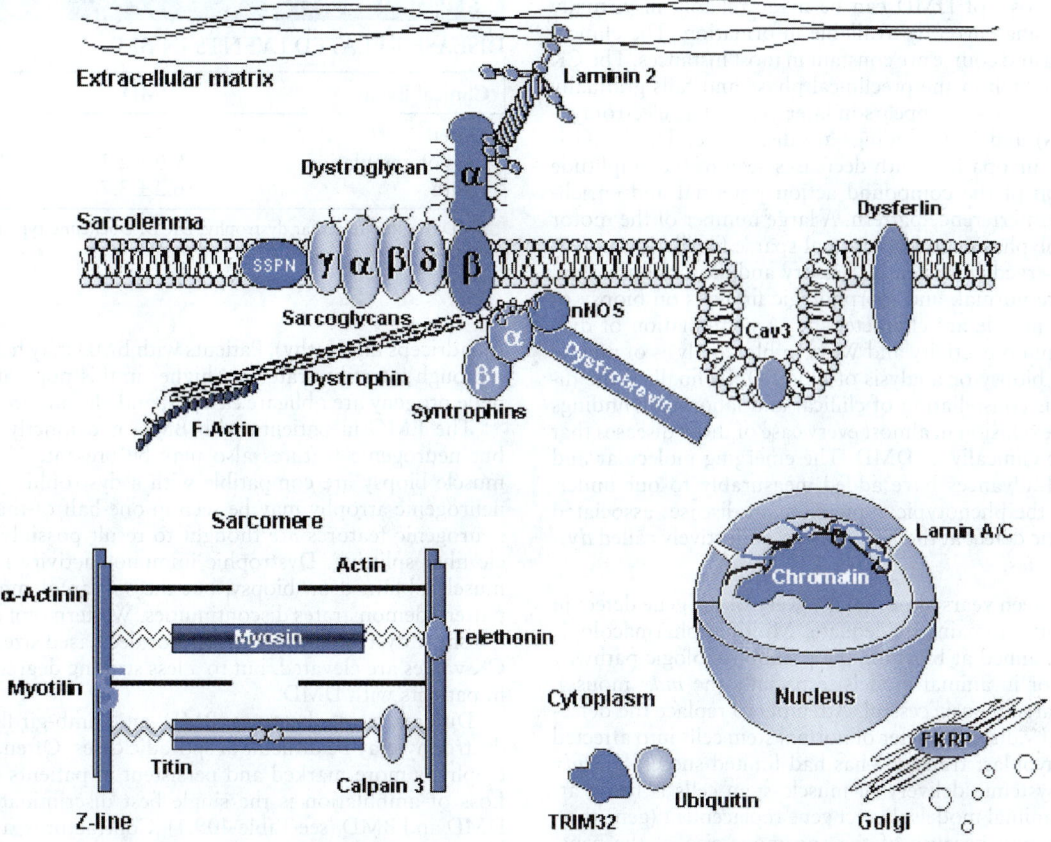

FIGURE 409.1. Schematic representation of the proteins involved in the muscular dystrophies. (Reproduced with permission from Barresi R, Campbell KP. Limb-girdle muscular dystrophies. In: Rosenberg RN, Prusiner SB, DiMauro S, et al, eds. *The molecular and genetic basis of neurologic and psychiatric disease*, 3rd ed. Boston: Butterworth-Heinemann, 2003:479.)

Complications may result from the following:

■ Cardiac involvement is evident in all patients with DMD but rarely is the cause of death. Similarly, cardiac abnormalities may be noted in female carriers of DMD, even when the serum creatine kinase (CK) values are normal. Degenerating muscle fibers and small foci of fibrosis are scattered throughout the myocardium and conduction systems. The posterobasal region and adjacent lateral wall of the left ventricle are involved commonly and prominently. The changes in electrocardiogram (ECG) are distinctive: tall right precordial R waves and deep Q waves in the left precordial and limb leads.

■ Nervous system involvement has been recognized since the earliest descriptions of DMD. It is a nonprogressive process and may be associated with the "atrophy" of the brain seen on computed tomography (CT). Some patients also have macrocephaly. The mean IQ is approximately 80, and individual IQ values correspond to a gaussian, bell-shaped distribution curve.

Diagnosis. The differential diagnosis of DMD includes BMD, autosomal recessive forms of congenital muscular dystrophy or limb-girdle dystrophy (see later discussion), muscle carnitine deficiency, the childhood form of acid maltase deficiency, and juvenile spinal muscular atrophy (Kugelberg-Welander syndrome). Female patients with clinical features of DMD must undergo genetic and cardiologic examination. Such patients may represent sporadic cases of autosomal recessive limb-girdle dystrophy, manifesting carriers of DMD, or genuine examples of DMD resulting from selective chromosomal aberrations. These aberrations include Turner syndrome (XO karyotype), mosaic states (X/XX or X/XX/XXX), a structurally abnormal X chromosome, an X autosomal translocation, and, perhaps more important, a skewed inactivation of the X chromosome favoring the one carrying the mutant gene.

BOX 409.1   Histopathology of Duchenne Muscular Dystrophy

Necrosis and regeneration dominate the histopathologic findings in biopsy samples from young patients with DMD, and end-stage biopsy samples obtained from patients with preterminal disease reveal the replacement of muscle cells with fat cells and fibrous tissue. Groups of necrotic degenerating fibers are the most prominent early features in DMD. These clusters of necrotic cells are invaded by phagocytes, and the infiltration is followed by active regeneration. A variation in fiber size becomes evident, with small atrophic fibers located adjacent to hypertrophied elements. Some of the large fibers are hypercontracted or have undergone hyalinization. Endomysial and perimysial connective tissue gradually increases with progression of disease. Plasma membrane defects have been seen by electron microscopy in non-necrotic muscle fibers and are thought to represent an early or possibly basic change in DMD. The basal lamina overlying the plasma membrane defect is normal.

The diagnosis of DMD can be made reliably in virtually every case using currently available information. The clinical presentation and course are constant in most instances. The CK value is very high in the preclinical phase and falls gradually as the muscle mass disappears in later years. The electromyogram (EMG) and ECG findings are distinctive. The EMG is distinctively myopathic, with decreases seen in the amplitude and duration of the compound action potential and enrichment of the interference pattern. A large number of the motor units are polyphasic, and occasional sparse fibrillation potentials are observed consistently. Sensory and motor conduction velocities are normal, and morphologic findings on biopsy of the skeletal muscle are characteristic. A combination of dystrophin immunoreactivity and Western blot analysis of muscle obtained at biopsy or analysis of blood DNA finalizes the diagnosis. This constellation of clinical and laboratory findings permits the exclusion in almost every case of those diseases that masquerade clinically as DMD. The emerging molecular and biochemical advances have added measurably to our understanding of the phenotypic expressions of diseases associated with a genetic defect at the Xp2.1 locus, collectively called *dystrophinopathies*.

Therapy. Fifteen years after the discovery of the gene defect in DMD, therapy remains inadequate. Multiple pharmacologic approaches, aimed at blocking the pathophysiologic pathway in humans or in animal models (especially the *mdx* mouse), have been largely unsuccessful. Attempts to replace the defective protein by direct transfer of normal stem cells into affected muscles—myoblast transfer—has had limited success in *mdx* mice. The systemic delivery of muscle stem cells is being attempted in animal models. Direct gene replacement (gene therapy) is daunting because of the enormous size of the gene, the need for appropriate vectors, and the risks of immunologic reaction occurring. However, the use of truncated genes (minigenes) carried by adeno-associated virus (AAV) has shown some success in animals. Thus, for now, traditional methods of care remain important. Family counseling, physical therapy, proper use of orthotic devices, selective surgical interventions to treat joint contractures and spinal deformities, and dietary management are important ways to improve the quality and length of life for patients with DMD.

Clinical trials of promising therapeutic regimens have been conducted by the Collaborative Investigation of Duchenne Dystrophy (CIDD) group sponsored by the Muscular Dystrophy Association. The CIDD has documented the clinical course of DMD carefully and has developed rigorous protocols to assess the efficacy of various drugs and hormones used in its treatment. Treatment with prednisone, 0.75 mg/Kg/day, has been shown in double-blind, placebo-controlled trials to slow the decline of muscle strength and to increase muscle mass.

Becker Muscular Dystrophy

Two other disorders share a genetic defect at or near the Xp2.1 locus: BMD and the McLeod syndrome. BMD represents a more benign version of DMD, most commonly due to a deletion in the dystrophin gene that does not alter the reading frame of the transcript (as described earlier, in the section Duchenne Muscular Dystrophy). Current information indicates that BMD and DMD are allelic gene abnormalities. BMD is similar to DMD, but the age of onset is later and the progression is slower (Table 409.1).

Pseudohypertrophy is striking, and frequently pes cavus deformities are present in patients with BMD. Unlike in DMD, cardiac or nervous system involvement is an unusual finding, but "pure" dilated cardiomyopathy can occur in patients with BMD in the absence of muscle weakness. Other unusual clinical phenotypes include recurrent myoglobinuria or idiopathic hyper-CKemia, and weakness confined to the quadriceps

TABLE 409.1

DISEASE-RELATED EVENTS IN BMD AND DMD

Clinical Event	DMD	BMD
Onset	3–5	12
Loss of ambulation	9.0 ± 2.3	30.5 ± 12.0
Death	16.2 ± 3.7	42.0 ± 15.9

BMD, Becker muscular dystrophy; DMD, Duchenne-type muscular dystrophy.

(quadriceps myopathy). Patients with BMD may have children, although infertility rates are higher in this population. All female progeny are obligate carriers, and all sons are unaffected.

The EMG in patients with BMD is distinctly myopathic, but neurogenic features also may be present. The results of muscle biopsy are compatible with a dystrophic process, but neurogenic atrophy may be seen in one-half of the cases. The neurogenic features are thought to result possibly from muscle fiber splitting. Dystrophic immunoreactivity is present in muscle obtained on biopsy, but the subsarcolemmal staining pattern demonstrates discontinuities. Western blot analyses often show dystrophin of increased or decreased size. The serum CK values are elevated, but to a less striking degree than those in patients with DMD.

Differentiating between BMD and limb-girdle muscular dystrophy may be difficult in sporadic cases. Often, calf hypertrophy is more marked and persistent in patients with BMD. Loss of ambulation is the single best discriminator between DMD and BMD (see Table 409.1). Contractures, a rigid spine, and the absence of pseudohypertrophy help to distinguish Emery-Dreifuss muscular dystrophy from BMD. The treatment approaches and genetic counseling are similar to those for DMD.

McLeod Syndrome

The McLeod syndrome has been viewed by some physicians as the minimal expression of the Xp2.1 gene abnormality. The gene encoding the Kx antigens in the Kell red blood cell antigen system is contiguous to the DMD locus. McLeod syndrome is manifested by absence of the Kx antigens, hemolytic anemia, acanthocytosis, elevated serum CK activity, and a benign nonprogressive myopathy. The skeletal muscle biopsy reveals muscle fiber necrosis and regeneration. One classic patient had the genetic misfortune of having chronic granulomatous disease, McLeod red cell phenotype, DMD, retinitis pigmentosa, idiopathic intestinal pseudo-obstruction, and mental retardation. The McLeod syndrome may be confused with polymyositis.

Emery-Dreifuss Syndrome

Emery-Dreifuss syndrome also is inherited as an X-linked recessive condition, but autosomal dominant or recessive inheritance also is seen in a minority of patients. This disease begins in early childhood and progresses very slowly. Weakness is evident first in the legs, with later involvement of the pectoral girdle. Contractures of the elbows and heel cords are prominent, and early features and rigidity of the spine also may be present. Distal muscles are spared, and no pseudohypertrophy ensues. Atrial conduction abnormalities may occur and, ultimately, the cardiac involvement may result in sudden death. Serum CK values are elevated moderately. Scoliosis and hyperextension of the cervical vertebrae are conspicuous features in the rigid spine syndrome, a form of congenital muscular dystrophy. The gene responsible for Emery-Dreifuss syndrome at Xq28 contains only six exons and five introns. It encodes a 254-amino acid serine-rich protein called emerin, which is localized to the inner nuclear membrane. Patients with autosomal dominant or autosomal recessive forms of Emery-Dreifuss syndrome harbor mutations in the lamin A/C gene (*LMNA*), which encodes lamins A and C: like emerin, both lamin A and lamin C are components of the nuclear lamina.

Autosomal Types of Dystrophy

The generalized types of dystrophy that are inherited in an autosomal manner include the various forms of myotonia, periodic paralyses, limb-girdle dystrophies, and congenital dystrophies.

Myotonia

Myotonia is divided into two categories: progressive and nonprogressive. Myotonic dystrophy is the only progressive disorder. The nonprogressive disorders include myotonia congenita, paramyotonia, and numerous atypical myotonic disorders.

Myotonic dystrophy type 1 follows a pattern of autosomal dominant inheritance and has been subdivided into a "classical form" (Steinert disease) or dystrophia myotonica type 1 (DM-1) and two proximal myotonic dystrophy syndromes (PROMM), DM-2/PROMM and DM3/PROMM. In DM-1, gene mapping studies have localized the defect to the long arm of chromosome 19 and characterized it as an unstable CTG repeat expansion in the noncoding region of a serine-threonine protein kinase (*DMPK*) gene. This trinucleotide amplification correlates with the clinical phenomenon of anticipation. The clinical manifestations of myotonic dystrophy are protean, and this disorder is viewed more properly as a systemic disorder with muscle involvement. Virtually all systems are involved. Severe brain involvement may occur in the congenital form, and adults have mental deterioration. Smooth, striated, and cardiac muscle tissues are affected. Myotonia involves striated muscle and anal sphincter; smooth-muscle involvement has been seen in the gastrointestinal tract, gallbladder, uterus, ureter, and ciliary body of the eye. Endocrine disturbances include testicular tubular atrophy, pituitary dysfunction, and diabetes mellitus associated with peripheral insulin resistance. Baldness and cataracts are common manifestations, as is hypogammaglobulinemia. Cataracts are represented as multicolored subcapsular opacities visualized best by slit-lamp examination.

In virtually all affected infants with congenital myotonic dystrophy, the mother is the affected parent, despite the fact that the gene is transmitted as an autosomal dominant trait. Numerous complications of pregnancy have been recognized, including an increased rate of spontaneous abortion, reduced fetal movements, polyhydramnios, uterine inertia during labor, and postpartum hemorrhage (often associated with retained placental fragments). The neonatal mortality rate is increased, and affected infants display numerous abnormal features. Neonatal respiratory distress, paralyzed diaphragm, hypotonia, bilateral facial weakness, talipes, and delayed motor and mental retardation are common clinical features. Myotonia is conspicuously absent and is not clinically evident until later in the patient's first decade of life. Congenital hip dislocation and hernias are the result of muscular laxity. Mild mental retardation is evident in most, if not all, affected children, and hydrocephalus has been reported in some instances. The correlation between maternal myotonic dystrophy and the congenital form of the disease is overwhelming but unexplained.

The muscle histopathology of myotonic dystrophy is distinctive. Type I fiber atrophy and centrally placed nuclei are characteristic, even in the congenital form. These and other findings suggest an arrest in muscle development: hypoplasia rather than active degeneration. Other common features include ringed fibers, sarcoplasmic masses, and nuclear chains.

Myotonic dystrophy type 2 (DM-2/PROMM) typically starts in adults and is characterized by myotonic stiffness or weakness of proximal leg muscles or finger flexors. Myalgia is a common finding; it is unrelated to exercise or to the severity of myotonia and typically fluctuates in intensity. Unlike patients with DM-1, patients with DM-2/PROMM do not show facial muscle weakness and wasting or distal limb muscle wasting. Myotonia is elicited best by percussion of forearm or thenar muscles. Cataracts are common findings. The gene defect on chromosome 3q21 is an unstable quadruplet (CCTG) repeat expansion in the gene for the zinc finger 9 protein (*ZNF9*). Some families with autosomal dominant inheritance of very similar symptoms and signs do not show linkage to the DM-1 or the DM-2 loci, and their gene defect is unknown: this form of myotonic dystrophy is called DM-3/PROMM.

Treatment of the various types of myotonia is directed toward their symptoms and toward the debilitating features of myotonic dystrophy specifically. The myotonia may be relieved with quinine sulfate, procainamide, or phenytoin. Patients with myotonic dystrophy need general medical supervision and support. Cardiac conduction disturbances and sensitivity to various anesthetics may be life-threatening. Medical and rehabilitative intervention, insertion of cardiac pacemakers, treatment of respiratory problems, and the use of various orthotic devices are helpful.

Periodic Paralyses, Cardiac Arrhythmias, Congenital Myotonia, and Malignant Hyperthermia

These clinically diverse conditions all are caused by mutations in genes encoding subunits of ion channels (sodium, calcium, or potassium) and, therefore, often are labeled collectively as channelopathies.

Periodic Paralyses. Often, the periodic paralyses are associated with high or low serum potassium values. The primary periodic paralyses are inherited as an autosomal dominant trait, whereas the secondary disorders result from acquired conditions that perturb body water and electrolyte status or thyroid function. The genetically determined conditions are associated with modest disturbances of potassium homeostasis, in contrast to the nongenetic conditions. Thyrotoxic periodic paralysis resembles hypokalemic periodic paralysis. It occurs remarkably more commonly in men (6:1) and Asians (3:1). The condition is sporadic and resolves with effective treatment of the hyperthyroidism.

Traditionally, the primary periodic paralyses have been divided into hypokalemic, hyperkalemic, and normokalemic. A fourth (rarer) form of periodic paralysis is associated with a bidirectional ventricular tachycardic dysrhythmia.

Hypokalemic periodic paralysis presents in middle to late childhood. Attacks are accompanied by a modest fall in the level of serum potassium and in the urinary retention of sodium, potassium, chloride, and water. These electrolyte changes can produce a characteristic change on the ECG. The attacks, which affect limb and trunk muscles but typically spare bulbar, respiratory, and cardiac muscles, may be provoked by the ingestion of carbohydrate or sodium or by excitement. Initially, the attacks occur infrequently, but daily attacks may occur during early adulthood. The episodes decrease in frequency in late adulthood, but older patients may have a fixed limb weakness. Glucose-insulin infusion may provoke an attack, and oral potassium salts attenuate the episode. These findings are diagnostic of the condition. Two common mutations have been identified in the L-type calcium channel subunit gene (*CACNA1S*) located on chromosome 1q31.

Hyperkalemic periodic paralysis also is inherited as an autosomal dominant trait, with initial presentation occurring during the patient's first or second decade of life. The serum potassium value rises modestly during the attack, accompanied by a kaliuresis. Between paralytic episodes, some patients have myotonia involving facial, lingual, thenar, or finger extensor muscles. Primary hyperkalemic periodic paralysis can be provoked by the oral administration of potassium chloride. Mutations in the sodium channel gene (SCN4A) have been identified in patients with hyperkalemic periodic paralysis.

Long QT syndrome and idiopathic ventricular fibrillation is a channelopathy affecting cardiac muscle and characterized by delayed repolarization, showing in surface ECGs as a prolonged QT interval. This important and not uncommon disorder (1 in 7,000 persons) causes ventricular arrhythmias with syncope or sudden death occurring in young asymptomatic individuals, often during exercise. Long QT syndrome is transmitted as an autosomal dominant (rarely recessive) trait and is caused by mutations in the various genes encoding subunits of the potassium channel. Muscle biopsy often reveals few or an absence of abnormalities in patients, with the periodic paralyses manifesting during the early symptomatic years, even during a paralytic episode. Later, a distinctive vacuolar myopathy develops. Often, these biopsy results correlate with fixed limb weakness.

Lack of electrical excitability of muscle fiber surface membranes is common to the various forms of primary periodic paralysis, and an abnormality of the sodium channel that characterizes the electrophysiologic study results in patients with paramyotonia congenita and those with hyperkalemic periodic paralysis (in agreement with molecular genetic data). The resting membrane potential, studied *in vitro*, is reduced in patients with primary hypokalemic periodic paralysis and in those with the acquired form associated with thyrotoxicosis. Both insulin and thyroid hormone are known to increase the activity of the sodium-potassium pump, but this information does not facilitate an understanding of the clinical symptomatology associated with modest decreases in serum potassium values.

Treatment begins with accurately establishing the diagnosis of the syndrome. Aggravating environmental factors must be avoided to minimize the frequency and intensity of the attacks. Acetazolamide is the preferred drug for both the hypokalemic and hyperkalemic forms of primary periodic paralysis; it may be useful also in the paralysis associated with cardiac dysrhythmias. However, treatment of the paralysis may worsen the cardiac disturbance. Imipramine has been useful in one patient in controlling the dysrhythmia. Acetazolamide is ineffective in treating the paralysis associated with hyperthyroidism. Propranolol is helpful, but control of the thyroid disease is more important.

Congenital Myotonia. The nonprogressive types of myotonia as a group are rare, and the symptomatology is limited to skeletal muscle, unlike that of myotonic muscular dystrophy. *Myotonia congenita* is an autosomal dominant trait that appears in infants. Muscular hypertrophy is evident. Becker later distinguished the autosomal dominant (Thomsen) form of nonprogressive myotonia from the recessive form, in which generalized myotonia first appears in early to middle childhood. Muscular hypertrophy is even more striking in the recessive form of the disease. Subtle weakness also may be present. Both the dominant and the recessive forms of myotonia congenita result from mutations in the skeletal muscle chloride channel CLCN1 gene. Disturbances of chloride conductance, a crucial factor in the repolarization and electrical stability of the sarcolemma, explain the myotonic runs observed on EMG.

Potassium-aggravated myotonia refers to a childhood-onset syndrome resembling myotonia congenita, without associated weakness or periodic paralysis. The myotonia is alleviated by repeated contractions ("warm-up" phenomenon) and worsened by potassium intake. Some patients have hypertrophy of neck and shoulder muscles. In children, potassium-rich meals

may cause hypoventilation due to stiffness of thoracic muscles. This condition has been associated with mutations in the sodium channel gene (SCN4A).

Paramyotonia congenita has two clinical signatures: (a) it is paradoxically worsened by repetitive exercise (the reverse of the "warm-up" phenomenon) and (b) it is triggered by exposure to cold. Onset is during infancy, and inheritance is autosomal dominant. Episodes of paralysis may be induced by intake of potassium, similar to hyperkalemic periodic paralysis. As in hyperkalemic periodic paralysis, mutations affect the sodium channel gene (SCN4A).

Malignant Hyperthermia. Malignant hyperthermia has occurred in association with several of the forms of myopathy discussed, especially central core disease (discussed more fully in the section, Congenital Myopathies). However, most patients with malignant hyperthermia have no obvious clinical symptoms of muscle disease, and the EMG and muscle histology results are normal or nonspecifically abnormal. These latter patients do have an underlying myopathy that may be manifested by increased serum CK values or *in vitro* studies that document sensitivity to caffeine or anesthetic agents. Malignant hyperthermia is inherited in most patients in an autosomal dominant pattern. However, this condition may not be recognized until the patient is exposed to such anesthetic agents as halothane or succinylcholine, and such exposure may be catastrophic. A family history of an untoward anesthetic experience, recurrent myoglobinuria, or sudden death should suggest the possible presence of this muscle condition.

The molecular basis of malignant hyperthermia has been clarified, at least partially. More than 50% of autosomal dominant families harbor mutations in the gene (RYR1) that encodes the sarcoplasmic reticulum calcium release channel or ryanodine receptor. Mutations in RYR1 may cause malignant hyperthermia or central core disease, which are allelic diseases for this locus and can occur together in the same family. A smaller number of families with malignant hyperthermia harbor mutations in genes for calcium channel subunits: CACNA1S, encoding the alpha-1-subunit of the voltage-dependent L-type calcium channel (malignant hyperthermia linked to this locus is allelic to hypokalemic periodic paralysis), or CACNL2A, encoding the alpha-2-subunit of the same channel.

The symptom complex is characterized by rapidly rising body temperature, tachycardia, tachypnea, cyanosis, and respiratory and metabolic acidosis. Usually, affected patients experience rigidity and myoglobinuria. Unexplained fevers, muscle cramps, and increased serum CK values may represent clinical clues to the presence of malignant hyperthermia. The clinical syndrome can be aborted by the intravenous administration of dantrolene.

Congenital Muscular Dystrophies

Many primary muscle diseases may present in early infancy, but only a few are known as congenital types of muscular dystrophy. This distinction, therefore, is arbitrary and, to some degree, confusing. The conditions discussed here are two syndromes that cause dystrophic changes in skeletal muscle, as noted by biopsy. These syndromes are distinguished by the presence or absence of nervous system pathology.

Congenital muscular dystrophy without nervous system involvement (also called classical, occidental, or pure CMD) appears to be inherited as an autosomal recessive trait, although many cases are sporadic. Affected infants are weak at birth, and often hypotonia is present, although not invariably. Similarly, joint contractures frequently accompany the weakness (arthrogryposis multiplex congenita). Respiratory difficulties may be present and largely determine the outcome. The "dystrophic" process itself is rather stationary, in part controverting the use of the term. Affected infants do reasonably well if they survive past infancy. Weakness does not progress in any measurable way, but orthopedic complications may supervene and require therapeutic intervention.

The laboratory abnormalities are variable. CK values are elevated, but tend to decrease with time. The EMG is distinctly myopathic, and fibrillations are scarce. The muscle tissue is abnormal, with fiber diameter variability and an abundance of endomysial and perimysial connective tissue. Necrosis of single muscle fibers is a fairly unusual occurrence.

The clinical course of affected patients is influenced largely by the respiratory complications that develop. The muscle disease appears to be primarily nonprogressive in most patients, and many of these children are very bright. Aggressive support and orthopedic corrective surgery are warranted in any children who have survived past infancy.

Approximately one-half of patients with typical congenital muscular dystrophy show deficiency of *laminin-2*, also known as *merosin*, a protein that links the dystroglycan complex of the sarcolemma with the extracellular matrix (see Fig. 409.1). The dystroglycans, together with dystrophin and with the sarcoglycans, are essential in maintaining the integrity of muscle membranes during the harsh mechanical stress imposed by muscle contraction. For additional information about merosin in CMD, see Box 409.2.

Congenital muscular dystrophy with nervous system pathology has a less favorable prognosis. In Japan, the birth incidence of *Fukuyama syndrome* is approximately one-half that of DMD. Mothers of affected infants report decreased fetal movements, and the newborn is weak and hypotonic. Sucking efforts and crying are weak, and facial expression is decreased. The calves may be enlarged, and contractures of the knee joints and elbows are common findings; tendon reflexes are decreased or absent. Generalized convulsions may occur in one-half of affected patients, and motor retardation is evident during later development. Eventually, many children sit or crawl, but few are able to walk. Atrophy of limb muscles is increasingly evident, and most affected children die within their first decade.

The association of Fukuyama muscular dystrophy and xeroderma pigmentosum led to the identification of the locus for Fukuyama muscular dystrophy on chromosome 9q31–33. The gene has been identified, and at least two independent point mutations have been identified in affected individuals. The gene encodes a novel protein called *fukutin*, which is expressed in various tissues in normal individuals but not in patients in whom the mutated gene contains a retrotransposal insertion of sequences repeated in tandem.

The serum CK values are elevated ten- to 50-fold in most instances, and the EMG is distinctly myopathic. The skeletal muscle examined at biopsy is abnormal, with variation of fiber-type diameter, necrosis of fibers, scattered foci of inflammation, and increased endomysial and perimysial connective tissue. The neuropathology is equally remarkable and descriptive of altered neuronal migration and cortical sulcation. The cortex is thick and smooth, particularly in the temporal and occipital regions. These findings are indicative of lissencephaly or polymicrogyria. Reduction in central white matter and associated cerebral ventricular enlargement are evident.

Another condition combining congenital muscular dystrophy and congenital brain abnormalities is the *Muscle-Eye-Brain disease (MEB)*, first described in Finland, where the disease is encountered most frequently. Patients have congenital hypotonia, mental retardation, and visual failure, including severe progressive myopia, retinal degeneration, and optic atrophy. Seizures are common manifestations. Dystrophic changes occur in muscle, with normal immunohistochemistry for dystrophin but often secondary partial defect of laminin alpha-2. Brain abnormalities include cobblestone lissencephaly, frontal pachygyria, and occipital micropolygyria. White matter is affected minimally. After the locus for MEB was assigned to chromosome 1p32–34 by linkage analysis and homozygosity mapping, mutations were identified in a gene (POMGnT1) that encodes a glycosyltransferase. A third condition, clinically similar to MEB, is Walker-Warburg Syndrome (WWS; MIM 236670). WWS is inherited as an autosomal recessive trait and characterized clinically by ocular abnormalities, muscular dystrophy, and severe neuronal migration defects. The condition results from mutations in the o-mannosyltransferase gene POMT1. These recent studies suggest that glycosylation defects are important causes of congenital muscular dystrophies and that overexpression of the gene *LARGE*, which encodes a glycosyltransferase, can circumvent the defective glycosylation of alpha-dystroglycan in cells from patients. This observation opens new vistas on therapeutic approaches.

BOX 409.2 — Merosin and Congenital Myotonic Dystrophy

The gene for the protein merosin is located on chromosome 6q2, and several mutations have been identified. Several children with merosin-deficient CMD have white matter abnormalities on cerebral magnetic resonance imaging (MRI), typically, white matter hypodensity on T2-weighted images. Otherwise, the brain usually is structurally normal. Immunohistochemistry of muscle shows more or less severe deficiency of laminin alpha-2 (for an accurate diagnosis, it is important to use antibodies to different portions of the laminin alpha-2 chain). Identification of mutations in the *LAMA2* gene confirms the diagnosis.

Merosin-positive patients with CMD are a heterogeneous group, but certain clinical features allow division into distinctive subgroups that are associated increasingly with specific gene defects. Thus, linkage analysis in some families with CMD and rigid spine syndrome (caused by axial muscle contractures) has identified a locus on chromosome 1 (*RSMD1*), and the sequence of candidate genes has revealed pathogenic mutations in a gene encoding a selenoprotein (*SEPN1*). Another form of merosin-positive CMD, Ullrich muscular dystrophy, is characterized by distal hyperextensibility contrasting with proximal joint contractures: the gene responsible for Ullrich disease (*COL6A3*) encodes subunits of type VI collagen.

Localized Types of Dystrophy

Many forms of muscular dystrophy are characterized by localized muscular involvement. These syndromes may involve the limb-girdle musculature preferentially, facioscapulohumeral (FSH) groups, scapular and peroneal groups, distal limb musculature, extraocular muscles, or oropharyngeal muscles. Most of these categories are fairly heterogeneous, and phenotypic features are varied.

Limb-Girdle Syndromes

In 1954, Walton and Nattrass introduced the term *limb-girdle muscular dystrophy* to describe, in a number of patients, a disorder that did not fulfill the clinical criteria for DMD or FSH dystrophy. Affected patients were of both genders, often were in middle to late childhood, and had serum enzyme, EMG, and skeletal muscle biopsy abnormalities of the type commonly encountered in patients with a muscular dystrophy.

TABLE 409.2

CLASSIFICATION OF THE LIMB-GIRDLE MUSCULAR DYSTROPHIES (LGMD)

Form	Chromosome	Gene Product	Characteristics
Autosomal Dominant			
LGMD1A	5q31	Myotilin	
LGMD1B	1q11–21	Lamin A/C	
LGMD1C	3p25	Caveolin 3	Usual normal early development, with a proximal myopathy in childhood, often accompanied by calf hypertrophy
			Caveolin is localized at the sarcolemma and is not part of the dystrophin-glycoprotein complex (DGC, see Fig. 409.1); interacts with the dystrophin-binding site of β-dystroglycan
LGMD1D	6q23	Unknown	
LGMD1E	7q	Unknown	
Autosomal Recessive			
LGMD2A	15q15–21	Calpain-3	Usually slowly progressive proximal weakness in adolescence, although onset varies widely in different families
LGMD2B	2p13	Dysferlin	Onset occurs in childhood or adolescence, and the course is slowly progressive.
			Allelic to Miyoshi distal myopathy
			Recent data suggest that dysferlin has an important role in muscle repair
LGMD2C (SCARMD)	13q12	γ-Sarcoglycan	Severe proximal myopathy involving primarily the lower limbs, confining patients to a wheelchair by the time they are in their teens and causing respiratory insufficiency soon thereafter
			Before the molecular defect was identified, this disorder, observed initially in consanguineous North African families and simulating Duchenne dystrophy, was called SCARMD
LGMD2D	17q12–21	α-Sarcoglycan	Proximal myopathy that varies in severity from a Duchenne dystrophy-like presentation to late-onset and relatively mild weakness
			Severity of the phenotype appears to be proportional to the residual amount of α-sarcoglycan
LGMD2E	4q12	β-Sarcoglycan	Proximal weakness and calf hypertrophy can mimic Duchenne dystrophy in boys, but onset can be late and ambulation preserved into adulthood
			Initially identified in inbred Indiana Amish families
LGMD2F	5q33–34	δ-Sarcoglycan	Onset occurs in childhood, progression is rapid, and death usually occurs before the patient reaches 20 years of age
			Dominant gene mutations can manifest as dilated cardiomyopathy without myopathy
LGMD2G	17q11–12	Telethonin	Onset of weakness occurs in early adolescence, and progression to wheelchair dependence takes one or two decades
			Cardiomyopathy may coexist.
LGMD2H	9q31–34	TRIM32	
LGMD2I	19q13.4	Fukutin-related protein	Weakness and wasting of shoulder girdle muscles, calf hypertrophy, and sometimes macroglossia
			Secondary reduction of laminin α2 and impaired glycosylation of α-dystroglycan (see Fig. 409.1)
LGMD2J	2q31	Titin	

SCARMD, severe congenital autosomal recessive muscular dystrophy.
Note: This classification is still expanding.

This large and ill-defined group of patients has been subdivided into 15 entities associated with specific gene defects. The conventional nomenclature assigns the number 1 (LGMD1) to the forms transmitted by autosomal dominant inheritance and the number 2 (LGMD2) to the autosomal recessive forms. The capital letters that follow (LGMD1A-E and LMGD2A-J) identify specific gene defects (Table 409.2). Figure 409.1 shows the proteins involved in these and other muscular dystrophies. Although LGMDs traditionally are considered diseases of adults, many of them can start in childhood and are outlined in Table 409.2.

Facioscapulohumeral Dystrophy

The syndrome of FSH dystrophy and its variants are inherited as autosomal dominant traits, and their expression may be fairly variable, even among family members. As the term implies, facial, periscapular, and humeral muscle groups are affected. Unlike that in most forms of dystrophy, involvement may be asymmetric, and an isolated congenital absence of a muscle may occur. Generally, the condition is benign, presenting in adolescence and progressing slowly over the course of decades, often with periods of clinical arrest. A few cases have started in infants, with a more malignant course. Initial presentation as Möbius syndrome, with congenital facial weakness, also has been described. Early childhood onset may be associated with a sensorineural hearing loss or an exudative telangiectasia of the retina (Coats disease). The clinical presentation in children, however, usually is more subtle. Patients may sleep with their eyes partially open and have difficulty in whistling or sipping through a straw. One variant is known as the *scapuloperoneal syndrome*; scapular winging and foot-drop are common signs. Subtle weakness of the facial muscles may coexist or may develop later.

The pathogeneses of these syndromes are obscure. Some cases seem to have myopathic elements, and others are distinctly neurogenic. The biopsy samples also may have some prominent inflammatory features, raising the question of an inflammatory myopathy and justifying a clinical trial with corticosteroids. In some patients, surgical fixation of the scapulae to the posterior thoracic wall improves shoulder-girdle function.

Molecular genetic studies have localized the gene responsible for FSH muscular dystrophy distal to 4q35, where deletions of an integral number of copies of a 3.3 kb DNA repeat labeled D4Z4 were identified. Normal individuals have 15 or more copies of the 3.3 kb repeats, whereas patients with FSH dystrophy have 12 or fewer repeats. The pathogenetic significance of these findings is difficult to interpret because the deletions do not disrupt an expressed gene. However, the deletions bring the FSH gene closer to heterochromatic telomeric DNA, and this could interfere with gene expression, a phenomenon known as *position effect variegation*. In practical terms, establishing a molecular diagnosis is feasible in more than 95% of cases.

Distal Limb Syndromes

Distal muscle syndromes are distinctly rare events at all ages and particularly so in children. Progress in our understanding of the molecular bases of several distal myopathies is providing a rational classification, which is shown in Box 409.3.

Ocular Syndromes

Eye involvement may be isolated (ocular myopathy) or combined with pharyngeal dysfunction (oculopharyngeal nbsp;dystrophy). Many other conditions, such as thyroid disease, inflammatory disorders, myasthenia gravis, and mitochondrial disorders, also cause ocular muscle dysfunction. Usually, the two genetic forms of ocular dystrophy are transmitted as autosomal dominant traits. Typically, the onset occurs in middle adulthood, and progression of the disease is slow. Serum CK values are normal. *Ocular dystrophy* is manifested by ptosis and weakness of facial and proximal limb musculature. Early manifestations may be evident in late childhood. *Oculopharyngeal muscular dystrophy (OPMD)* develops much later, with ptosis and dysphagia. Eye, facial, and limb-girdle muscles are less involved. OPMD is caused by expansions of the GCG trinucleotide repeat. These conditions are distinctly rare and should not be confused with congenital ptosis, which is benign, nonprogressive, and often unilateral.

HEREDITARY TYPES OF MYOPATHY

Congenital Myopathies

A group of neuromuscular diseases present in young infants are inherited as mendelian traits and are recognized by distinctive histochemical abnormalities. Often, these disorders are designated as benign, nonprogressive forms of myopathy. They are not invariably nonprogressive, however, and whether the defect is intrinsic to the muscle fiber is not certain. As a group of disorders, they exhibit considerable overlap in phenotypic expression. Congenital hip dislocation, kyphoscoliosis, infantile hypotonia, and decreased responsiveness of tendon reflexes are common clinical features. The distinctive histochemical abnormality involves the type I muscle fiber exclusively or preferentially. CK values and nerve conduction velocities are normal, and the EMG shows brief, abundant, polyphasic potentials of short duration and low amplitude.

Central core disease was the first entity to be described in this group of disorders. In 1956, Shy and Magee studied five family members who had been slow in learning to walk and continued to have mild weakness throughout life. Several members had congenital dislocation of the hips. The genetic pattern was consistent with an autosomal dominant trait. The

---

BOX 409.3   Types of Distal Myopathy

Welander distal myopathy was described first in several generations of a Swedish family who showed a distal weakness that was transmitted as an autosomal dominant trait. Symptoms become manifest in adulthood; effects primarily occur in the hands and forearms. The progression of the disorder is slow, and serum enzyme values are normal. Linkage analysis has localized the locus to chromosome 2p13, very close to, and possibly coinciding with, the dysferlin gene, mutations of which cause either a limb-girdle muscular dystrophy (LGMD2B) or a distal myopathy (Miyoshi myopathy).

Tibial muscular dystrophy (Markesbery-Griggs-Udd distal myopathy) is another form of adult-onset, slowly progressing myopathy, affecting muscles of the anterior leg compartment first, then wrists and finger extensors. Muscle biopsy shows rimmed vacuoles in addition to dystrophic features. The disease has been linked to chromosome 2q31, but the gene responsible is not known.

Nonaka distal myopathy is an autosomal recessive condition of young adults affecting initially ankle dorsiflexors and foot extensors and causing foot-drop and steppage gait. Proximal weakness may develop later, but the quadriceps typically are spared. Muscle biopsy shows, in addition to dystrophic features, characteristic rimmed vacuoles that are virtually indistinguishable from those seen in patients with hereditary inclusion body myopathy (hIBM). In agreement with this observation, Nonaka distal myopathy has been linked to the same locus as has hIBM on chromosome 9p12–13. Mutations in the gene for UDP-N-acetyl-glucosamine 2 epimerase/N-acetyl mannosamine-kinase (GNE) have been documented in hIBM and may be associated with Nonaka myopathy.

Miyoshi distal myopathy often starts in adolescence and affects first the gastrocnemii muscles, causing difficulty walking on toes and climbing stairs. Relative early onset, posterior leg muscle involvement, and high serum CK values distinguish Miyoshi myopathy from other distal myopathies. The condition is autosomal recessive, and the responsible gene encodes dysferlin (i.e., Miyoshi myopathy is allelic to LGMD2B). Dysferlin has an important role in plasma membrane repair.

Another distal myopathy that also can present as an autosomal dominant limb-girdle syndrome (*LGMD1C*) is caused by mutations in the gene encoding caveolin 3 (*CAV3*).

muscle biopsy in all five individuals revealed a unique alteration. The central cores of most myofibers were compacted and amorphous and failed to stain with oxidative enzyme histochemical reactions. Electron microscopy demonstrated relatively normal-appearing myofibrils, with no mitochondria in the central core region. This disorder increases the risk of developing malignant hyperthermia. In fact, central core disease and malignant hyperthermia have been established to be allelic disorders caused by mutations in a gene on chromosome 19q12–13.2 (*RYR1*) that encodes the *ryanodine receptor*, an important regulator of calcium concentration in the cytoplasm. In this sense, central core disease could be classified as a channelopathy (see earlier sections).

Multicore (mini-core) disease also has been described in a few cases, with variable clinical presentations. Some patients resemble those with central core diseases, others have congenital myopathy with rigid spine syndrome, and still others have partial or complete ophthalmoplegia. Fibers of both types contain the multicore pattern. This histologic entity is genetically heterogeneous. In agreement with the variable clinical presentation, some cases have been associated with mutations in the selenoprotein N (*SEPN1*) gene, which also causes congenital muscular dystrophy with rigid spine (see earlier discussion). In other cases, mutations occurred in the ryanodine receptor gene (*RYR1*), stressing the similarity with central core disease. However, these two mutations do not explain all cases of multicore myopathy.

Nemaline myopathy was the second entity to be described in this group of diseases. In 1963, Shy, Engel, Somers, and Wanko reported a clinical syndrome of infantile hypotonia, muscular hypoplasia, mild weakness, reduced or absent tendon reflexes, and relative sparing of intelligence. Subsarcolemmal accumulations of rodlike structures were present and were seen more commonly in the type I fibers. The rods were similar to Z disk material, from which they presumably are derived. Female individuals are affected more often, but the genetic pattern is autosomal dominant or recessive. The weakness is relatively nonprogressive, but death may result from respiratory failure. Dysmorphic features, which are more characteristic in nemaline myopathy, include elongated facial features, high-arched palate, kyphoscoliosis, pectus excavatum, and pes cavus. Mutations in as many as five genes have been associated with nemaline myopathy, explaining in part the different types of inheritance. The gene most commonly affected in the autosomal recessive congenital form is *NEB*, encoding the giant structural protein nebulin. Most autosomal dominant cases harbor mutations in the *ACTA1* gene, which encodes skeletal muscle alpha-actinin. Rarer genetic defects involve the genes for alphatropomyosin (*TPM3*), beta-tropomyosin (*TPM2*), or troponin T (*TNNT1*).

Myotubular (centronuclear) myopathy was the third of these diseases to be described. Several investigators have suggested that this disorder may represent an arrest in embryonic muscle development. Rows of centrally placed nuclei are characteristic, predominantly in type I fibers. Type I fiber predominance and hypotrophy also may coexist.

The clinical syndrome is more varied in myotubular myopathy and can be life-threatening. Prenatal onset of the disorder is suggested by diminished fetal movements. The postnatal presentation may vary, with one group of patients being weak at birth. Motor development is slow, respiratory effort may be compromised, and death may occur before affected children reach 3 years of age. Generalized weakness is evident, with preferential involvement of eye, facial, and neck muscles. A second group of patients is detected in early childhood with a gait abnormality and difficulty in climbing stairs. Focal or generalized seizures may coexist in this group. Other patients may not have symptoms until their second or third decade of life.

The combination of ophthalmoparesis and facial diplegia is distinctive in children with myotubular myopathy. Genetic transmission is variable from one family to another, including autosomal dominant or X-linked recessive patterns. Some researchers have segregated type I muscle fiber hypotrophy with central nuclei from myotubular myopathy as a separate entity, but the distinctions may be only apparent. Most affected males with the X-linked form harbor mutations in the myotubularin gene (*MTM1*) on Xq27–q28. Deletions in this area or skewed X-chromosome inactivation can explain how some girls can be affected as severely as boys. Myotubularin is a dual-specific phosphatase involved in the control of muscle growth and differentiation, thus explaining the "immature" muscle phenotype. The genetic bases of the autosomal forms of myotubular myopathy remain to be clarified.

A heterogeneous group of structurally defined myopathies, usually manifesting in young adults and often affecting respiratory muscles and the heart, goes under the label of *myofibrillar myopathies*. These myopathies are characterized by the accumulation of different abnormal proteins, most commonly desmin. *Desmin myopathy* is characterized morphologically by an accumulation of material staining bluish with the Gomori trichrome and immunoreactive to antibodies against desmin. Ultrastructurally, myofibrillar disruption, streaming of the Z band, and accumulation of dense, amorphous material occur. Numerous mutations in the desmin gene have been identified in families with an autosomal dominant transmission of myopathy with or without cardiomyopathy.

Rehabilitative efforts should be undertaken, and respiratory function should be protected, particularly during intercurrent illnesses. A cuirass may be helpful in compromised patients during pulmonary infection. Affected patients may use the cuirass at night to obtain adequate rest. Some patients may have difficulty with negative pressure units because of laxity of pharyngeal muscles and resulting obstructive apnea. Oximetry used in conjunction with the cuirass is an effective way to monitor airway patency under these circumstances. Annual vaccination for the influenza viruses is an important preventive measure.

Metabolic Myopathies

Glycogenoses

Thirteen distinct enzyme defects are known to affect glycogen metabolism (Fig. 409.2). Eleven of these defects affect muscle directly: type II, acid maltase deficiency (Pompe disease); type III, debrancher deficiency (Cori-Forbes disease); type IV, brancher deficiency (Andersen disease); type V, myophosphorylase deficiency (McArdle disease); type VII, muscle phosphofructokinase (PFK) deficiency (Tarui disease); type VIII, phosphorylase kinase deficiency; type IX, phosphoglycerate kinase (PGK) deficiency; type X, phosphoglycerate mutase deficiency; type XI, lactic dehydrogenase (LDH) deficiency; type XII, aldolase A deficiency; and type XIII, beta-enolase deficiency.

Type II: Acid Maltase Deficiency. Two major clinical syndromes are associated with acid maltase deficiency. The first syndrome (Pompe disease) presents in early infancy and is associated with death before the infant reaches 1 year of age. The clinical picture is distinctive, with infantile hypotonia, weakness, areflexia, macroglossia, massive cardiomegaly, and moderate hepatomegaly. Affected infants are alert and exhibit little clinical measure of central nervous system dysfunction. Death results from cardiac and pulmonary failure. The peripheral lymphocytes contain vacuoles that are positive on periodic acid-Schiff staining, and acid maltase activity is virtually absent in all tissues. The condition is transmitted as an autosomal recessive trait. The glycogen content is increased in all

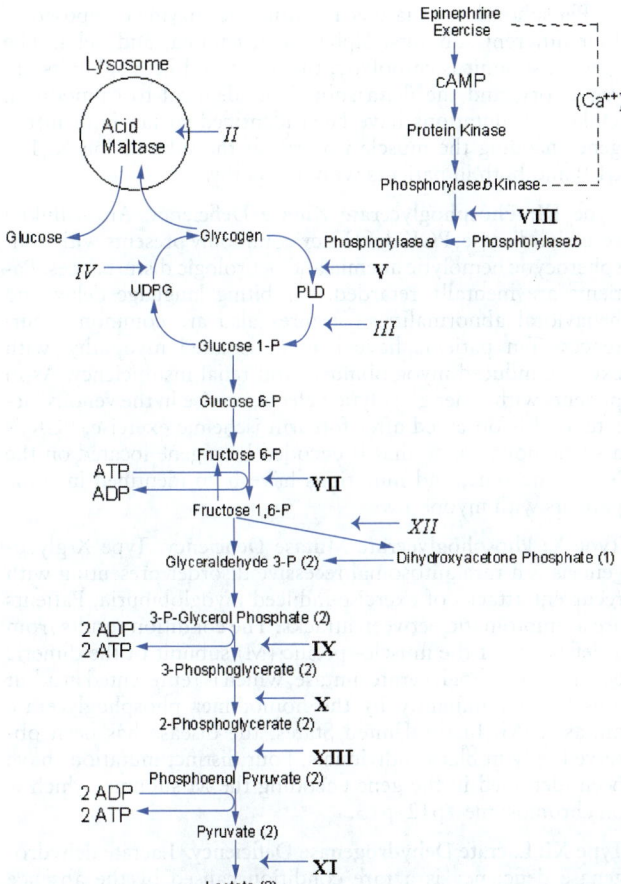

FIGURE 409.2. Glycogen metabolism and glycolysis. Sites of documented enzyme defects: I, glucose-6-phosphatase; II, acid maltase; III, debranching; IV, branching; V, muscle phosphorylase kinase; VII, muscle phosphofructokinase; VIII, phosphorylase b kinase; IX, phosphoglycerate kinase; X, phosphoglycerate mutase; XI, lactate dehydrogenase; XII, aldolase; XIII, beta-enolase. ADP, adenosine diphosphate; AMP, adenosine monophosphate; ATP, adenosine triphosphate; PLD, phosphorylase-limit dextrin; UDPG, uridine diphosphate glucose.

tissues, with the predominant accumulation occurring within lysosomes. The presence of much free glycogen in tissues also has been noted, however.

The serum CK values are elevated moderately, and the EMG is myopathic, with bizarre high-frequency pseudomyotonic discharges. The potentials are polyphasic, and the interference pattern is reduced. Chest radiography reveals massive cardiomegaly. The ECG demonstrates a shortened PR interval, depressed ST segments, and inverted T waves. Muscle biopsy reveals a severe vacuolar myopathy with material that is positive on periodic acid-Schiff staining stored in lysosomes and increased free glycogen particles present in the cytoplasm. In the nervous system, glycogen accumulates in glial and neuronal cell bodies. The anterior horn cells are engorged with glycogen. Severe involvement of brainstem and spinal motor neurons contributes to the clinical appearance of spinal muscular atrophy with weakness, hypotonia, and areflexia. Impressive improvement has been described in some infants treated with genetically engineered human alpha-glucosidase expressed in rabbit milk.

The second syndrome associated with acid maltase deficiency is a more benign neuromuscular disorder that presents in children or young adults. Usually, this syndrome is limited to skeletal muscle, with progressive weakness and respi-

ratory insufficiency developing. The condition in young children simulates DMD, with calf enlargement and Gowers sign. The serum CK values may range from 200 to 2,000 IU/L, and the EMG results are distinctly abnormal. In the adult form, the clinical appearance may be confused with that of limb-girdle dystrophy or chronic polymyositis. Cardiac function is normal in patients with the childhood and adult versions of acid maltase deficiency. Although a therapeutic approach based on high-protein diet and aerobic exercise has been advocated, enzyme replacement therapy—when more easily available—should benefit myopathic patients even more than generalized (Pompe disease) patients.

Nearly 90 distinct mutations have been identified in the gene on chromosome 17q23–q28 that encodes acid maltase. Establishing the genotype-phenotype correlation is difficult because of the frequency of compound heterozygotes, but, in general, good correspondence is found between the severity of the mutation and the severity of the clinical phenotype. Thus, deletions or missense mutations usually are associated with the infantile variant (Pompe disease), whereas "leaky" mutations are associated with the childhood and adult variants.

Type III: Debrancher Deficiency. Type III glycogenosis results from a deficiency of amylo-1,6-glucosidase. The classic presentation in infancy is one of fasting hypoglycemia, ketonuria, growth retardation, and hepatomegaly. Patients are weak and hypotonic and have poor head control. Usually, these signs remit gradually near the time of puberty, although a few patients exhibit slowly progressive weakness into adult life. The muscle biopsy sample reveals a severe vacuolar myopathy with storage of glycogen. Commonly, weakness is more evident in the proximal groups, but distal wasting may be fairly noticeable and can suggest a motor neuron disease or chronic neuropathy. Motor nerve conduction velocities actually may be decreased, and the EMG may contain a mixed pattern, including fibrillations, positive sharp waves, and myotonic discharges. No effective treatment is available for this autosomal recessive condition, but infants and young children should be protected from fasting hypoglycemia with frequent feedings and nocturnal gastric infusions of glucose and uncooked corn starches. The gene encoding the human debranching enzyme has been cloned and sequenced; it has been assigned to chromosome 1p21. More than 15 mutations have been reported.

Type IV: Brancher Deficiency. Type IV deficiency is the result of a deficiency of the enzyme amylo-1,4-1,6-transglucosidase. Typically, it is a rapidly progressive, fatal condition manifested by hepatosplenomegaly, progressive cirrhosis, and chronic liver failure. Death occurs in late infancy or early childhood. However, it has become apparent that branching enzyme deficiency can cause a wide spectrum of clinical phenotypes, variably affecting liver, heart, muscle, and brain. Myopathy was reported in numerous patients, either alone or in association with hepatopathy or cardiopathy. Onset can be intrauterine (with fetal hydrops) or congenital (often associated with cardiopathy) or can occur in childhood or in adult life. No effective therapy is available for this autosomal recessive condition, but liver transplantation is an option in children with liver cirrhosis and portal hypertension. The gene encoding the human branching enzyme has been assigned to chromosome 3, and numerous mutations have been identified. Knowledge of the molecular defects in infants or children with severe presentation renders genetic counseling and prenatal establishment of diagnosis possible.

Type V: Myophosphorylase Deficiency. Myophosphorylase deficiency was the first glycogenosis to be described. In 1951, McArdle reported a syndrome associated with weakness, fatigue, and muscle cramping with pain after exercising. He also observed a lack of lactic acid production by the exercising muscle and proposed a defect in glycolysis. Intense exercise may lead to muscle necrosis and myoglobinuria in patients with myophosphorylase deficiency. Irreversible renal failure may ensue. Most patients recover muscle function between attacks, but approximately 25% have some fixed weakness. Serum CK values are elevated at rest and may increase dramatically during an attack of myoglobinuria. Rarely, the condition may present as a fatal, infantile myopathy. Heart function is normal in patients with McArdle disease. The nervous system is not involved, although seizures occur more commonly than would be expected. Hypoglycemia and hyperventilation may be factors that contribute to convulsions in patients with this disorder. The diagnosis is suspected when a flat lactate response to ischemic exercise is obtained, and it is confirmed by examination of tissue from skeletal muscle obtained at biopsy.

Dietary manipulations (high-protein diet) and aerobic exercise may be beneficial in attenuating the symptoms of myophosphorylase deficiency. Myoglobinuria can be minimized by avoiding strenuous, prolonged physical exercise. Moderate sustained exercise leads to a "second-wind" phenomenon that presumably represents a metabolic conversion from carbohydrate to fatty acids as a fuel source for skeletal muscle. This condition is transmitted as an autosomal recessive trait.

The gene encoding human myophosphorylase has been assigned to chromosome 11q13, and more than 30 mutations have been identified in patients with McArdle disease. In white patients, by far the most common molecular defect is an Arg49Stop mutation in exon 1. The frequency of this mutation is such that the diagnosis often can be established through a molecular analysis of genomic DNA in blood, thus avoiding the need for a muscle biopsy. The genotype-phenotype correlation in McArdle disease remains fuzzy: the most common genetic defect in typical adult patients (homozygous Arg49Stop) was found also in two infants who had died of the fatal variant.

Type VII: Muscle Phosphofructokinase Deficiency.
Type VII deficiency was described by Tarui in 1965, and it resembles McArdle disease clinically. Typically, symptoms begin in the patient's second decade of life and include intolerance for exercise, cramps, and myoglobinuria. A more severe and possibly heterogeneous clinical presentation of PFK deficiency affects infants or young children, who may present with arthrogryposis congenita and generalized weakness, but who also have signs of multisystem involvement, including seizures, cortical blindness, corneal opacifications, and cardiopathy.

Erythrocyte PFK activities are reduced by 50% in this syndrome, and it is transmitted as an autosomal recessive trait. The partial PFK deficiency that occurs in red cells may cause erythrocytosis and mild hemolytic anemia. In patients with typical presentation, numerous mutations have been identified in the gene encoding the muscle subunit of PFK, which is on chromosome 1. In contrast, no mutations have been found in patients with the fatal infantile presentation.

Type VIII: Myophosphorylase Kinase Deficiency.
Type VIII syndrome is a rare condition resulting from a deficiency of the kinase that converts the inactive "b" form of myophosphorylase to the active "a" form. Total phosphorylase activity is normal, but the active form represents less than 10% of the total enzyme activity.

Phosphorylase kinase deficiency causes four main clinical syndromes: (a) an X-linked, benign liver disease of infancy, with hepatomegaly, growth retardation, delayed motor development, and fasting hypoglycemia; (b) an apparently autosomal recessive liver and muscle disease, with hepatomegaly and nonprogressive myopathy; (c) myopathy, intolerance for exercise, and, rarely, myoglobinuria, inherited as an autosomal recessive or X-linked recessive trait; and (d) probably autosomal recessive fatal infantile cardiomyopathy.

Phosphorylase kinase is a multimeric enzyme composed of four different subunits: alpha, beta, gamma, and delta. The gamma subunit is catholytic, the alpha and beta subunits are regulatory, and the delta subunit is identical to calmodulin. Only two mutations have been identified so far, both in the gene encoding the muscle isoform of the subunit (on Xq12–q13) and both in patients with myopathy.

Type IX: Phosphoglycerate Kinase Deficiency.
An X-linked recessive disease, PGK deficiency commonly presents with nonspherocytic hemolytic anemia and neurologic disturbances. Patients are mentally retarded, exhibiting language delay and behavioral abnormalities. Seizures also are common occurrences. Ten patients have had an isolated myopathy, with exercise-induced myoglobinuria and renal insufficiency. As in patients with other glycolytic defects, no rise in the venous lactate level is observed after forearm ischemic exercise. PGK is a single polypeptide that is encoded by a gene located on the X chromosome, and mutations have been identified in some patients with myopathy.

Type X: Phosphoglycerate Mutase Deficiency.
Type X glycogenosis is a rare autosomal recessive disorder presenting with recurrent attacks of exercise-induced myoglobinuria. Patients are asymptomatic between attacks. The condition results from a deficiency of the muscle-specific (M) subunit of the dimeric enzyme phosphoglycerate mutase, which is represented in adult muscle predominantly by the homodimer phosphoglycerate mutase-MM. In the United States, the disease has been observed only in black individuals. Four distinct mutations have been identified in the gene encoding the M subunit, which is on chromosome 7p12–p13.

Type XI: Lactate Dehydrogenase Deficiency.
Lactate dehydrogenase deficiency is a rare condition caused by the absence of the M subunit and associated with exercise-induced myoglobinuria. One Japanese family has been studied in detail, and the findings are compatible with an autosomal recessive pattern. Forearm ischemic exercise produces a marked rise in the pyruvate level, with little or no rise in the lactate level. The lactate dehydrogenase M subunit has been assigned to a gene on chromosome 11, and several mutations have been identified both in Japanese and in white patients.

Type XII: Aldolase A Deficiency.
A new form of muscle glycogenosis was identified in 1995, and it was attributed to a deficiency of aldolase A, the isoform that predominates in skeletal muscle and erythrocytes. The clinical picture in a 4-year-old boy was dominated by episodes of intolerance for exercise and weakness after febrile illnesses, with markedly increased levels of serum CK but without pigmenturia. The molecular defect in this child was identified as a missense mutation (Glu206Lys) in the aldolase A gene on chromosome 16q22–q24.

Type XIII: Beta-Enolase Deficiency.
One patient with this enzyme defect was identified in 2001, a 47-year-old man with adult-onset but rapidly progressive intolerance for exercise, exercise-related myalgia, and chronically increased serum CK. Enolase is a dimeric enzyme, which, in adult human muscle is represented predominantly by the beta homodimer. The patient was compound heterozygous for two mutations in the gene encoding the beta subunit (ENO3).

Mitochondrial Diseases

Defects of mitochondrial metabolism are recognized with increasing frequency. The most common morphologic abnormality of muscle mitochondria can be shown at the light-microscopical level with the modified Gomori trichrome stain. Excessive accumulations of mitochondria give these fibers a *ragged-red* appearance. Ragged-red fibers (RRFs) are distinctive and usually represent the morphologic counterpart of

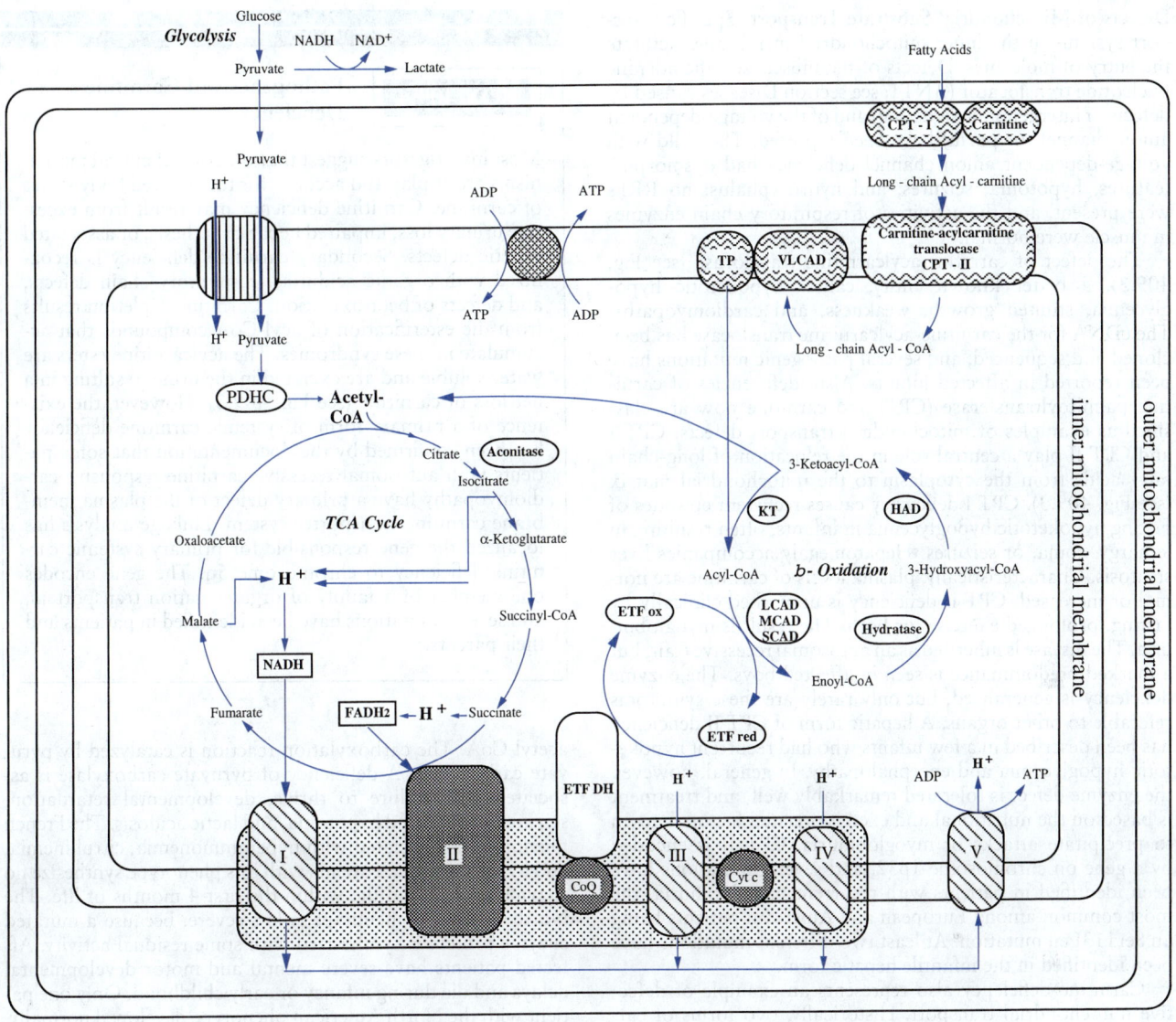

FIGURE 409.3. Schematic representation of mitochondrial metabolism. Respiratory chain components or complexes encoded exclusively by the nuclear DNA are solid; complexes containing some subunits encoded by the nuclear genome and others encoded by mtDNA are cross-hatched. PDHC, pyruvate dehydrogenase complex; CPT, carnitine palmitoyltransferase; VLCAD, very long-chain acyl-CoA dehydrogenase; TP, trifunctional protein; LCAD, long-chain acyl-CoA dehydrogenase; MCAD, medium-chain acyl-CoA dehydrogenase; SCAD, short-chain acyl-CoA dehydrogenase; HAD, 3-hydroxyacyl-CoA dehydrogenase; KT, 3-ketothiolase; ETFox, oxidized form of electron transfer flavoprotein; ETFred, reduced form of electron transfer flavoprotein; ETF-DH, ETF-coenzyme Q oxidoreductase. (Reproduced with permission from DiMauro S, Bonilla E, Mitochondrial encephalomyopathies. In: Engel AG, Franzini-Armstrong C, eds. *Myology*. New York: McGraw-Hill, 1623.)

suspected or proven biochemical defects of the mitochondrial respiratory chain. Although the presence of RRFs is a useful diagnostic clue, their absence does not rule out mitochondrial dysfunction, thus emphasizing the need for a classification scheme predicated on biochemical and molecular genetic criteria.

The current classification of mitochondrial diseases is based on the principal metabolic pathways located in this organelle and on the dual genetic control of the respiratory chain (Fig. 409.3). Carbohydrates (converted to pyruvate in the cytoplasm by the glycolytic pathway) and fatty acids (transported into mitochondria and converted to acetyl-CoA by the intramitochondrial beta-oxidation spiral), are the principal sources of fuel, and each substrate is metabolized to acetyl-CoA. Acetyl-

CoA condenses with oxaloacetate to form citric acid. Citric acid is oxidized in the Krebs cycle. The reducing equivalents generated during oxidation enter the electron transport chain (which includes complexes I, II, III, and IV, plus coenzyme Q and cytochrome *c*) and are reoxidized. The energy of oxidation is coupled to the phosphorylation of adenosine diphosphate by complex V (ATP synthetase), ultimately yielding adenosine triphosphate (ATP). Together, the electron transport chain and ATP synthetase form the *respiratory chain*.

The mitochondrial diseases of muscle or brain can be subdivided into four major groups, according to the site of the biochemical lesion: defects of mitochondrial transport, defects of substrate use, defects of the Krebs cycle, and defects of the respiratory chain.

Defects of Mitochondrial Substrate Transport. Specific transport systems in the inner mitochondrial membrane facilitate the entry of molecules. Defects of the muscle-specific adenine nucleotide translocator (ANT1; see section Diseases caused by defects of intergenomic signaling) and of the voltage-dependent anion channel (or porin) have been reported. The child with voltage-dependent anion channel deficiency had dysmorphic features, hypotonia, seizures, and hydrocephalus; no RRFs were present, and the activities of respiratory chain enzymes in muscle were normal.

The defect of carnitine-acylcarnitine translocase (see Fig. 409.3), a better known entity, causes hypoketotic hypoglycemia, stunted growth, weakness, and cardiomyopathy. The cDNA for the carnitine-acylcarnitine translocase has been cloned and sequenced, and several pathogenic mutations have been reported in affected infants. Also, deficiencies of carnitine palmitoyltransferase (CPT) and carnitine now are classified as examples of mitochondrial transport defects. CPT I and CPT II play a central role in the relocation of long-chain fatty acids from the cytoplasm to the mitochondrial matrix (see Fig. 409.3). CPT I deficiency causes recurrent episodes of fasting hypoketotic hypoglycemia in infants, often resulting in lethargy, coma, or seizures. Hepatomegaly accompanies liver steatosis. Characteristically, plasma levels of carnitine are normal or increased. CPT II deficiency is unmasked clinically by fasting, prolonged exercise, or both. The result is myoglobinuria. The disease is inherited as an autosomal recessive trait, but a marked predominance is seen in affected boys. The enzyme deficiency is generalized, but only rarely are these symptoms referable to other organs. A hepatic form of CPT II deficiency has been described in a few infants who had recurrent hypoketotic hypoglycemia and encephalopathy. In general, however, the enzyme defect is tolerated remarkably well, and treatment is based on the nutritional and exercise-related factors known to precipitate attacks of myoglobinuria. CPT II is encoded by a gene on chromosome 1p32, and several mutations have been identified in patients with recurrent myoglobinuria, the most common among European and American patients being an Ser113Leu mutation. At least two different mutations have been identified in the infantile hepatic form.

Carnitine deficiency also represents an example of defective mitochondrial transport. Historically, two forms of carnitine deficiency have been discussed: one confined to muscle (myopathic) and the second involving a generalized defect in carnitine (systemic). The myopathic form involves a defect in the uptake of carnitine by muscle. Consequently, the transport of long-chain fatty acids across the inner mitochondrial membrane is blocked, producing a resulting accumulation of neutral lipids in the cytoplasm. This lipid storage is associated with a progressive weakness that begins in childhood. The carnitine concentrations are decreased in muscle but are normal in blood and liver. A defect in the active transport of carnitine into muscle has been suspected but never proved. Some patients respond to carnitine supplementation or to prednisone. The mechanism of action of prednisone is unknown.

Systemic carnitine deficiency is manifested by recurrent encephalopathy that often is triggered by an intercurrent infection. This presentation is very similar to that of Reye syndrome. Concentrations of carnitine are decreased in the serum and tissues, and excessive urinary excretion of carnitine ensues. The legitimacy of systemic carnitine deficiency has been questioned since its first description in 1975. Box 409.4 presents additional information about the pathogenesis of carnitine deficiency. Carnitine supplementation is life-saving in affected patients, and supplementation is recommended whenever carnitine deficiency is documented.

Defects of Substrate Use. Pyruvate has two major metabolic fates: carboxylation to oxaloacetate or decarboxylation to

---

| BOX 409.4 | **Pathogenesis of Carnitine Deficiency** |

Most investigators suggest that other biochemical mechanisms are at play and account for the reduced body stores of carnitine. Carnitine deficiency may result from excessive urinary loss, impaired hepatic synthesis, or associated genetic defects. Secondary carnitine deficiency is recognized with organic acidurias, respiratory chain defects, and defects of beta-oxidation. Carnitine depletion results from the esterification of acyl-CoA compounds that accumulate in these syndromes. The acylcarnitine esters are water-soluble and are excreted in the urine, resulting in a net loss of carnitine (see Fig. 409.3). However, the existence of a primary form of systemic carnitine deficiency has been confirmed by the documentation that some patients with autosomal recessive carnitine-responsive cardiomyopathy have a primary defect of the plasma membrane carnitine transporter system. Linkage analysis has localized the gene responsible for primary systemic carnitine deficiency to chromosome 5q. The gene encodes one member of a family of organic cation transporters, and several mutations have been identified in patients and their parents.

---

acetyl-CoA. The carboxylation reaction is catalyzed by pyruvate carboxylase. A deficiency of pyruvate carboxylase is associated with failure to thrive, developmental retardation, seizures, generalized hypotonia, and lactic acidosis. The French phenotype is associated with hyperammonemia, citrullinemia, and hyperlysinemia. Patients with this phenotype synthesize no enzyme protein and die within the first 4 months of life. The North American phenotype is less severe, because a mutated enzyme protein is synthesized with some residual activity. Affected patients have severe mental and motor developmental delays and die during infancy or early childhood. Only one patient with the North American phenotype developed normally, although experiencing intermittent metabolic crises. Pyruvate carboxylase activity also may be impaired secondarily by a deficiency of holocarboxylase synthetase or biotinidase. Deficiency of biotinidase is treated easily with large doses of biotin.

The pyruvate dehydrogenase complex (PDHC; see Fig. 409.3) is composed of five enzymes, two of which—a kinase and a phosphatase—regulate the activity of the complex by phosphorylation (deactivation) and dephosphorylation (activation) of the first enzyme component (E1). The E1 component is composed of an alpha subunit and a beta subunit. The genes for these two subunits have been cloned, and their sequence has been determined. The alpha subunit is the site of phosphorylation involving three serine residues. Currently, the alpha subunit appears to be the most vulnerable genetic locus of the PDHC, and the gene for this subunit is located on the proximal portion of the short arm of the X chromosome. Syndromes of varying severity are associated with deficiency of PDHC. These syndromes vary from a benign condition of intermittent ataxia to a devastating condition of congenital lactic acidosis, failure to thrive, developmental delay, generalized hypotonia, and death in early infancy. These children have the neuropathologic and neuroradiologic features of Leigh syndrome (LS). Most patients with LS have mutations in the gene encoding the E1 alpha-subunit of PDH, but the first patients with LS and mutations in the gene for the E1 beta-subunit have been reported. Male infants are affected predominantly with the fatal congenital form, whereas female patients exhibit primarily the chronic progressive form. These female patients represent manifesting carriers of an X-linked trait.

A distinctive facial dysmorphism has been described in some infants with PDHC deficiency. The dysmorphic features are similar to those described in patients with the fetal alcohol syndrome, and elevated acid aldehyde levels have been suggested as a possible common pathogenetic mechanism linking these two disorders.

More than 20 defects of fatty acid and ketone-body metabolism have been described. Some of the defects involving the carnitine cycle were discussed earlier in this section and include the membrane carnitine transporter defect, the defect of carnitine-acylcarnitine translocase, and CPT II deficiency. A deficiency of CPT I has been described in approximately 30 patients. These patients have an illness similar to Reye syndrome in infancy and may have associated renal tubular acidosis. This symptom responds to treatment with medium-chain triglycerides. Patients with CPT II deficiency have normal tissue and plasma carnitine concentrations. Patients with CPT I deficiency may have normal or high carnitine concentrations. Patients with defects involving the carnitine cycle demonstrate little, if any, dicarboxylic aciduria.

In contrast, patients with defects involving beta-oxidation have remarkable dicarboxylic aciduria and carnitine deficiency. Five of these defects involve the first step in beta-oxidation, which is the conversion of acyl-CoA to a,b-unsaturated acyl-CoA. In addition to the four classic beta-oxidation reactions in the mitochondrial matrix (flavin adenine dinucleotide [FAD]-dependent dehydrogenation of acyl-CoAs; hydration of 2-enoyl-CoAs; nicotinamide adenine dinucleotide-dependent oxidation of 3-hydroxyacyl-CoAs; and CoA-hydrogen sulfide-dependent thiolysis of 3-hydroxy-acyl-CoAs), two additional enzymes bound to the inner mitochondrial membrane, very long-chain acyl-CoA dehydrogenase (VLCAD) and the trifunctional protein (TFP), prepare fatty acids for β-oxidation in the matrix (see Fig. 409.3). Jointly, VLCAD and TFP act on long-chain fatty acyl-CoAs, whereas the matrix enzymes act on medium- and short-chain acyl-CoAs. Reoxidation of FAD is accomplished by two FAD-dependent electron carriers: electron transfer factor (ETF) and ETF-dehydrogenase. Ultimately, the electrons are transferred to coenzyme Q10, which is located centrally within the respiratory chain. Acetyl-CoA, resulting from the beta-oxidation of fatty acids, enters the Krebs cycle or the HMG-CoA cycle that is important in the biosynthesis of ketone bodies.

Severe hypoglycemic hypoketotic crises developing during prolonged fasting, physical exercise, or intercurrent infections characterize the clinical presentation of most patients with defects of beta-oxidation. Both VLCAD and TFP deficiencies are associated with devastating infantile syndromes characterized by hypoglycemia with Reye syndrome episodes, cardiomyopathy, and sudden infant death syndrome (SIDS). However, milder manifestations of VLCAD or TFP deficiency cause recurrent episodes of myoglobinuria in children or adults, simulating CPT II deficiency. The genes for VLCAD and for both alpha and beta subunits of TFP have been isolated, and increasing numbers of mutations are reported in patients. Medium-chain acyl-CoA dehydrogenase deficiency is the most common of these defects. Hundreds of cases of medium-chain acyl-CoA dehydrogenase deficiency have been described since 1983. The clinical presentation is reasonably uniform, with a history of recurrent metabolic crises in infancy or childhood, often triggered by infectious episodes and poor feeding. Hypoglycemia, with or without hyperammonemia, and inappropriately low urinary ketone-body excretion are highly suggestive of a fatty acid oxidation defect. Liver biopsy may reveal fatty metamorphosis. The accumulation of lipids in skeletal muscle is evident in long-chain acyl-CoA dehydrogenase deficiency. Cardiac involvement also is prominent in the latter disorder.

Medium-chain acyl-CoA dehydrogenase is encoded by a gene on chromosome 1p31, and numerous mutations have been identified, the most common being an A-to-G transition at nucleotide 985 of the coding region, resulting in the substitution of a highly conserved lysine at position 304 by a glutamate (Lys304Glu).

Short-chain acyl-CoA dehydrogenase (SCAD) deficiency has been described in more than 20 cases, with different clinical presentations. One patient suffered muscle weakness and lactic acidosis after exercising, suggesting a muscle-specific defect. She benefited from supplementation of oral carnitine. Another patient had an infantile multisystem disorder characterized by failure to thrive, progressive muscle weakness, microcephaly, and psychomotor retardation. Two common SCAD gene variants (625G → A and 511C → T) confer disease susceptibility. Proving SCAD deficiency remains difficult.

Usually, glutaric aciduria type II (multiple acyl-CoA dehydrogenase deficiency) is associated with respiratory distress, hypoglycemia, hyperammonemia, generalized carnitine deficiency, and hypoketotic metabolic acidosis in the neonatal period, with death following within the first several weeks. However, a few affected patients have become symptomatic in childhood or adulthood, with findings of a lipid storage myopathy, weakness, or premature fatigue. The biochemical lesion of glutaric aciduria type II appears to affect the ETF or the ETF-dehydrogenase systems. As a result, all acyl-CoA dehydrogenases are affected indirectly, presenting with a characteristic urinary organic acid pattern. ETF is composed of two subunits, a and b; the genes encoding both subunits have been cloned and sequenced, and several mutations have been identified in each gene. Similarly, a few molecular defects have been identified in the gene encoding ETF-dehydrogenase. A defect of ETF is responsible also for a milder disorder known as *ethylmalonic-adipic aciduria*. This disorder develops in older children and is characterized by recurrent episodes of vomiting, acidosis, and hypoglycemia. A few patients with the milder form of multiple acyl-CoA dehydrogenase deficiency have responded to riboflavin supplementation.

The two remaining syndromes associated with the first step in beta-oxidation include glutaric aciduria type I, which results from a specific defect of glutaryl-CoA dehydrogenase, and isovaleric acidemia, which results from a defect of isovaleryl-CoA dehydrogenase. Both conditions are transmitted as autosomal recessive disorders. Glutaric aciduria type I presents in young infants as a pyramidal tract disorder. Later, affected patients have a movement disorder, implicating involvement of the extrapyramidal system. Young patients with isovaleric acidemia have acute attacks of vomiting, lethargy, and coma. Fifty percent of affected patients die during the first episode. Isovaleric acidemia can be treated with a glycine-rich, low-protein diet. The excretion of short-chain fatty acids produces a distinctive odor of sweaty feet in patients with isovaleric acidemia.

Defects of the Krebs Cycle. In general, biochemical defects involving the Krebs cycle have been assumed to result in fetal wastage, and such may be the case in most instances. Four defects involving the Krebs cycle have been described (Box 409.5).

Defects of the Respiratory Chain. Defects of the respiratory chain must be subclassified further, because this metabolic pathway is controlled by both the nuclear genome and the mitochondrial genome. The primary molecular defect is located in the nuclear DNA (nDNA) in some instances and in the mitochondrial DNA (mtDNA) in other instances. A subgroup of the nDNA defects involves a secondary disturbance of mitochondrial DNA. These conditions have been called *defects of intergenomic signaling*.

BOX 409.5   Defects of the Krebs Cycle

Defect of Dihydrolipoyl Dehydrogenase

This enzyme is shared by the PDHC (E3), the alpha-ketoglutarate dehydrogenase complex, and the branched-chain alpha-keto acid dehydrogenase complex. As a result, affected patients may have a distinctive organic acid profile, including elevated lactate, pyruvate, alpha-ketoglutarate, and branched-chain alpha-keto acid levels. Dihydrolipoyl dehydrogenase is encoded by a gene on chromosome 7. An occasional affected patient may respond to lipoic acid supplementation.

Defect in Mitochondrial and Cytosolic Isoforms of Fumarase

This enzyme is encoded by the same gene located on chromosome 1. Fumarase deficiency has been documented in cultured skin fibroblasts, skeletal muscle, and liver. Affected children have mental delay, microcephaly, hypotonia, and cerebral atrophy. The primary laboratory finding in this disorder is the excretion of large amounts of fumaric acid in the urine.

Defect of Succinate Dehydrogenase (Complex II of the Mitochondrial Respiratory Chain)

A few patients have had a myopathy or encephalomyelopathy resulting from a defect of succinate dehydrogenase. One patient had a muscle tissue—specific syndrome of limb weakness and myoglobinuria associated with combined deficiencies of aconitase and succinate dehydrogenase.

Defect of the Alpha-Ketoglutarate Dehydrogenase Complex

Patients with this disorder in infancy exhibit a severe encephalopathy and associated lactic acidosis.

Diseases caused by mutations in mtDNA. Primary mtDNA defects occur sporadically or are inherited as maternal, non-mendelian traits. Maternal inheritance resembles X-linked and autosomal dominant inheritance patterns in that the maternally transmitted trait is passed from affected mothers to their children, and the disease appears in consecutive generations. The maternally inherited trait differs from the X-linked inherited trait because both male and female progeny inherit the condition from their mothers. Similarly, the maternally inherited trait differs from the autosomal dominant trait because a higher percentage (theoretically, 100%) of the progeny are affected. The phenotypic expression of a maternally inherited trait is modulated by replicative segregation and the threshold effect. These two concepts are predicated on the facts that multiple mtDNA copies are found in each mitochondrion and that hundreds or thousands of mitochondria are found in each cell (*polyplasmy*). As a result, the distribution of wild-type mtDNA and mutated mtDNA (i.e., the degree of *heteroplasmy*) drifts randomly in each successive cell division. As the percentage of mutated mtDNA copies reaches a threshold, the cellular phenotype reflects the genotype and displays energy failure.

Kearns-Sayre syndrome (KSS) is characterized by three fundamental features: pigmentary degeneration of the retina, ophthalmoplegia, and clinical onset before age 20. Often, other signs, including heart block, cerebellar syndrome, and cerebrospinal fluid (CSF) protein concentration in excess of 100 mg/dL, occur. Endocrine disturbances are associated with this syndrome, and short stature is a common problem. Diabetes mellitus and hypoparathyroidism may develop and may contribute to fatal episodes of coma or to seizures, respectively. RRFs are present in skeletal muscle obtained at biopsy, and they are do not stain with the cytochrome c oxidase (COX) histochemical reaction (COX-negative RRF). A spongy degeneration is seen in the brain of all patients examined at autopsy. Levels of folic acid are reduced in the CSF. Therapy with folic acid and coenzyme Q10 (CoQ10) often is employed, but it has limited effect. A cardiac pacemaker is necessary as therapy for heart block.

Virtually all reported cases of KSS have been sporadic, and patients have major, single deletions of the mitochondrial genome. Sporadic cases of progressive external ophthalmoplegia (PEO) also have been associated with these deletions, suggesting that this abnormality of ocular motility is the minimal clinical expression of KSS. Large mitochondrial DNA deletions have been observed also in infants with Pearson syndrome, a usually fatal sporadic disease of infancy manifested by pancytopenia and pancreatic exocrine dysfunction. In addition, large mitochondrial DNA deletions were described recently in a family with maternally inherited diabetes mellitus and deafness, but later this family was found also to have harbored an mtDNA duplication, which can explain both the origin of the deletion and the maternal inheritance.

Myoclonus epilepsy and RRFs (MERRF) is dominated by myoclonus, ataxia, limb weakness, and generalized seizures. Most patients have symptoms in childhood or early adolescence. Associated signs often include dementia, optic atrophy, short stature, hearing loss, peripheral neuropathy, and multiple lipomas.

Although spongy degeneration of the brain is a common occurrence, frequently neuronal loss also is seen in MERRF, and it affects preferentially the cerebellum, brainstem, and spinal cord. CT scans and magnetic resonance imaging (MRI) reveal brain atrophy. Characteristically, electroencephalography shows paroxysmal epileptiform discharges that are either focal or generalized. As a rule, the blood and CSF lactate values are increased. The CSF protein level also is increased, but rarely above 100 mg/dL. Magnetic resonance spectroscopy (MRS) of the brain shows abnormal lactate peaks, both in the CSF of the ventricles and in the brain parenchyma. MERRF is inherited as a maternal trait. Muscle biopsy shows RRFs, which are COX-negative. The mutation associated most commonly with MERRF is in the tRNA^{Lys} gene (*A83344G*). No effective treatment is available for patients with MERRF, aside from seizure control.

MELAS (*m*itochondrial myopathy, *e*ncephalopathy, *l*actic *a*cidosis, and *s*trokelike episodes) probably is the most common maternally inherited mitochondrial disorder. The original criteria included normal early development, short stature, seizures, and sudden onset of hemiparesis, hemianopsia, or cortical blindness. Dementia was prominent in several cases, as was episodic vomiting, headache, and hearing loss. CT scan revealed focal stroke-like lucencies in several cases and basal ganglia calcifications in some. Diffuse spongy degeneration of the brain and focal encephalomalacia were seen at autopsy. Muscle biopsy shows RRFs, but, unlike those found in other mtDNA-related disorders, most RRFs in MELAS are COX-positive; another morphologic peculiarity of MELAS is the mitochondrial proliferation in the walls of blood vessels (strongly

SDH-reactive vessels, SSVs). MELAS is inherited as a maternal trait, and approximately 80% of patients fulfilling the clinical criteria for this condition have a mutation in the tRNA$^{Leu(UUR)}$ gene of mtDNA (*A3243G*). Numerous other mutations, both in tRNA genes and in protein-encoding genes (especially in the ND5 gene of complex I), have been associated with MELAS. Coenzyme Q10 is somewhat beneficial in treatment, and vigorous attempts should be made to control seizure activity.

A third maternally inherited condition of pediatric importance is NARP/MILS (*neuropathy, ataxia, and retinitis pigmentosa/maternally inherited Leigh syndrome*). As the acronym implies, this multisystem disorder includes peripheral neuropathy, ataxia, and retinitis pigmentosa, plus dementia, seizures, and proximal weakness. In some family members, the clinical presentation started in infancy and was more severe, fulfilling the clinical and neuropathologic criteria of Leigh syndrome. NARP/MILS has been linked with a mtDNA point mutation—T8993G—affecting subunit 6 of ATP synthetase (ATPase, complex V). In fact, NARP/MILS is an excellent example of the pathogenic role of the mutation load: at high mutation loads, the clinical phenotype changes from NARP to Leigh syndrome. Other mutations in the ATPase 6 have been associated with Leigh syndrome or bilateral striatal necrosis.

Yet another important maternally inherited disease caused by mutations in mtDNA protein-coding genes is Leber hereditary optic neuropathy (LHON), associated with three "primary" mutations, all of them in genes encoding complex I subunits: G3460A in ND1; G11778A in ND4; and T14484C in ND6. Approximately ten additional point mutations in complex I genes ("secondary mutations") put affected patients at increased risk of developing optic neuropathy. By 2004, more than 100 pathogenic point mutations in mtDNA have been reported, reflecting the explosive pace of discoveries in this area.

Diseases caused by defects of intergenomic signaling. Two conditions transmitted by mendelian inheritance but affecting mtDNA integrity or abundance define the group of disorders known as *defects of intergenomic signaling*. The first is characterized by multiple mtDNA deletions and can be transmitted by autosomal dominant or recessive inheritance. The clinical hallmark of multiple mtDNA deletions is PEO, usually associated with a variety of other symptoms and signs, including progressive limb weakness, peripheral neuropathy, ataxia, parkinsonism, and psychiatric problems. Mutations in the gene encoding one isoform of the adenine nucleotide translocator 1 (*ANT1*) have been identified in some, but not all, patients with autosomal dominant PEO. Mutations in a gene called *Twinkle*, a helicase, also are associated with autosomal dominant PEO, whereas mutations in the gene encoding polymerase γ (*POLG*) may cause either autosomal dominant or autosomal recessive PEO. A special form is the *mitochondrial neurogastrointestinal encephalomyelopathy* (MNGIE) syndrome, an autosomal recessive multisystem disorder caused by mutations in the gene (*TP*), encoding the enzyme thymidine phosphorylase. As the acronym indicates, mitochondrial neurogastrointestinal encephalomyopathy is characterized by PEO, peripheral neuropathy, and gastrointestinal symptoms, including chronic diarrhea and intestinal pseudoobstruction. MRI of the brain shows leukodystrophy. Usually, onset occurs in individuals in their teens, and death occurs in their fourth or fifth decade of life. Interestingly, two of the proteins affected in patients with PEO and multiple mtDNA deletions (ANT1 and TP) are involved in the regulation of the mitochondrial nucleotide pool.

The second example of a mtDNA abnormality caused by a nDNA defect is the mitochondrial DNA depletion syndrome. This condition is inherited as an autosomal recessive trait and presents as a fatal congenital condition or as an infantile-onset myopathy. Limb weakness and hypotonia are distinctive in the setting of lactic acidosis and RRFs. Some affected patients have

a fatal hepatopathy, and others have an associated nephropathy. The congenital cases were associated with an 83% to 98% depletion of mitochondrial DNA in skeletal muscle; affected patients with infantile-onset disease had a 66% to 83% depletion of mitochondrial DNA. Mutations in two genes, both involved in mitochondrial nucleotide homeostasis, have been associated with mtDNA depletion, although they do not explain all cases. Mutations in the gene encoding thymidine kinase (*TK2*) are found commonly in patients with depletion of myopathic mtDNA, whereas mutations in the gene encoding deoxyguanosine kinase (*dGK*) predominate in patients with hepatic or multisystemic mtDNA depletion syndromes.

Diseases caused by mutations in nDNA. Most respiratory chain subunits are encoded by nDNA genes, and many more nuclear genes are needed for the correct assembly and functioning of the respiratory chain. Thus, it is not surprising that mendelian disorders of the respiratory chain are numerous, although their description has lagged behind the avalanche of reports on mtDNA mutations that took place during the past 15 years. This group of disorders can be subdivided further into five subgroups based on the type of molecular defect: (a) mutations in genes encoding subunits of respiratory chain complexes; (b) mutations of genes encoding "ancillary proteins" (i.e., factors needed for the correct assembly and function of respiratory chain complexes); (c) mutations in genes controlling the importation and correct localization of nDNA-encoded protein from the cytoplasm into mitochondria; (d) mutations affecting the lipid composition of the inner mitochondrial membrane; and (e) mutations affecting mitochondrial motility, fusion, or fission.

Mutations in genes encoding respiratory chain subunits. These mutations are "direct hits," that is to say, they alter components of the respiratory chain directly. Thus far, this pathogenic mechanism is known only for complex I and complex II. These complexes have been associated mostly with autosomal recessive forms of LS (Table 409.3). LS probably is the most important clinical and pathologic entity associated with mitochondrial dysfunction during brain development. This encephalopathy of infancy or childhood is defined by the characteristic neuropathology first described by Leigh in 1951: focal symmetrical areas of necrosis in the basal ganglia, brainstem, and posterior columns of the brainstem. Microscopically, these spongiform lesions show cystic cavitation, vascular proliferation, neuronal loss, and demyelination. Correspondingly, T_2-weighted MRI scans of the brain typically show bilateral

---

TABLE 409.3

BIOCHEMICAL AND GENETIC CAUSES OF LEIGH SYNDROME (LS) IN APPROXIMATE ORDER OF FREQUENCY

Biochemical or Molecular Defect	Transmission
Pyruvate dehydrogenase (PDH)	E1 XR
Cytochrome *c* oxidase (COX)	AR
Complex I (NDUF genes)	AR
ATPase 6 (T8993G)	Maternal
Complex II	AR
Complex I (ND5 gene)	Maternal
A8344G (MERRF)	Maternal
ATPase 6 (T8993C)	Maternal
Other ATPase 6 mutations	Maternal
Single mtDNA deletion	Sporadic
mtDNA depletion	AR

XR, X-linked recessive; AR, autosomal recessive; MERRF, myoclonus epilepsy with ragged-red fibers.

| BOX 409.6 | Disorders Caused by Mutations in Genes That Encode Ancillary Proteins |

Mutations in the assembly protein BCSIL cause complex III deficiency and are responsible for Leigh syndrome (LS) and for a fatal infantile disorder prevalent in Finland and dubbed GRACILE (*g*rowth *r*etardation, *a*minoaciduria, *c*holestasis, *i*ron overload, *l*actic acidosis, and *e*arly death).

Mutations in the *SURF1* gene, which encodes a COX-assembly protein, are the most important causes of LS with complex IV deficiency and should be looked for in all children with autosomal recessive LS and COX deficiency. Mutations in other COX-assembly proteins characteristically cause LS brain involvement but also involvement of another target tissue. Thus, mutations in *SCO2* cause a rapidly fatal "encephalocardiomyopathy," as do mutations in *COX15*, whereas mutations in *SCO1* cause an "encephalohepatopathy," and mutations in *COX10* cause an "encephalonephropathy." Application of the new technology of integrative genomics led to the identification of the gene (*LRPPRC*, encoding an mRNA-binding protein), responsible for COX deficiency in the French-Canadian form of LS.

Finally, mutations in *ATP12*, an assembly gene for complex V (ATP synthetase), have been described in a rapidly fatal multisystem disease of infancy.

basal ganglia hyperintensities. Clinically, the patient has psychomotor retardation or, more commonly, regression, nystagmus, recurrent vomiting, optic atrophy, dystonia, and abnormal respiration. Some clinical features suggest specific etiologies. Thus, normal early development is a common occurrence in COX deficiency, whereas retinitis pigmentosa is virtually pathognomonic of NARP/MILS.

Mutations in several highly conserved complex I genes have been associated with autosomal recessive LS or leukodystrophy. Mutations in the *SDHA* gene of complex II were identified in a few families with autosomal recessive LS.

Mutations in genes encoding ancillary proteins. These mutations are "indirect hits," in that the mutant proteins are not components of respiratory chain complexes but are indispensable for their correct assembly. This pathogenic mechanism has been documented in patients with defects of complex III, complex IV, and complex V. Box 409.6 contains more information about these mutations. These remarkable advances in our molecular genetic understanding of LS have important practical applications because we can now offer sound genetic counseling and prenatal diagnosis to young families who have lost a first child to LS.

Some respiratory chain disorders, including various forms of apparently primary coenzyme Q10 deficiency, two myopathies with COX deficiency, and a rare defect in oxidative phosphorylation known as Luft syndrome, have not yet been elucidated at the molecular level.

At least three different clinical presentations have been associated with *muscle deficiency of coenzyme Q10 (CoQ10)*, a component of the respiratory chain that carries electrons from complexes I and II to complex III. These defects of CoQ10 presumably are primary and are transmitted as autosomal recessive traits. The *myopathic form* of CoQ10 deficiency was described in five patients with a characteristic triad of myopathy with recurrent myoglobinuria, RRF with lipid storage in muscle

biopsies, and brain dysfunction with seizures, ataxia, or mental retardation. The *ataxic form* of CoQ10 deficiency was reported in approximately 20 patients with childhood-onset of cerebellar ataxia, cerebellar atrophy, variably associated with central and peripheral nervous system signs, including seizures, mental retardation, weakness, or peripheral neuropathy. Muscle biopsies do not show RRFs. The third presentation of CoQ10 deficiency is a mitochondrial encephalomyopathy of infancy associated with renal disease. It is important to keep this entity in mind because patients with all three forms—but especially those with the myopathic and the generalized infantile forms—benefit remarkably from oral supplementation of high-dose CoQ10. Presumably, the different presentations are due to different defects of CoQ10 biosynthesis, but no specific biochemical or molecular defects are known.

Two forms of myopathy are caused by COX deficiency presumably due to nuclear mutations in which the molecular defects remain obscure. The first form is a fatal infantile myopathy associated with generalized weakness, respiratory insufficiency, and death before the patient reaches 1 year of age. Lactic acidosis is prominent, and renal dysfunction is manifested by glycosuria, phosphaturia, and aminoaciduria. Simultaneous involvement of the heart or liver has been described, but the nervous system has been spared. The second phenotype is a remarkable syndrome of muscle involvement, termed *benign infantile mitochondrial myopathy* because the metabolic and biochemical abnormalities disappear during late infancy. Affected children have a severe neonatal myopathy and lactic acidosis. The clinical condition improves spontaneously and disappears by early childhood. The cytochrome oxidase deficiency is severe in skeletal muscle obtained at biopsy shortly after birth, but the enzyme activity increases to normal values by the time the patient is 1 or 2 years of age.

Defects of mitochondrial protein importation. Mitochondrial proteins synthesized in the cytoplasm have mitochondrial targeting signals that direct them to the appropriate organellar compartment. Transport across outer and inner membranes requires a battery of factors, including docking proteins, chaperonins, and proteases. Several mutations in targeting sequences have been documented, preventing individual proteins from reaching their final destination. For example, one rare defect of PDH E1 alpha-subunit causing LS was not caused by a mutation in the protein itself but by a mutation in its targeting sequence.

In contrast, few genetic defects are known to impair the general transport machinery, presumably because the resulting impairment in mitochondrial function would not be compatible with life. However, one X-linked disease, the deafness-dystonia syndrome (Mohr-Tranebjaerg syndrome), characterized by neurosensory hearing loss, dystonia, cortical blindness, and psychiatric symptoms, is caused by mutations in the *TIMM8* gene, which encodes the deafness-dystonia protein (DDP1), a component of the protein transport machinery.

Alterations of the lipid milieu of the inner mitochondrial membrane. This situation is exemplified by *Barth syndrome*, an X-linked recessive disorder characterized by mitochondrial myopathy, cardiopathy, growth retardation, and leucopenia. The tafazzin gene (*TAZ*) responsible for this disorder encodes a family of proteins ("tafazzins") that are homologous to phospholipids acyltransferases. Analysis of phospholipids in target tissues from patients with Barth syndrome showed decreased concentration (and altered composition) of cardiolipin, the main lipid component of the mitochondrial inner membrane and an important cofactor of respiratory chain complexes.

Alterations of mitochondrial motility, fusion, or fission. Mitochondria are dynamic organelles that move around the cell along microtubular "rails" propelled by energy-requiring dynamins. Also, in most cells, mitochondria exist as a dynamic tubular network, requiring tubules to fuse and fragment in a coordinated fashion. We already know of two human diseases caused by impaired mitochondrial fusion. The first is autosomal dominant optic atrophy, an important cause of blindness in young adults (the mendelian counterpart of LHON), caused by mutations in the *OPA-1* gene. The second is Charcot-Marie-Tooth (CMT) type 2A, a severe axonal neuropathy, which is inherited as an autosomal dominant trait and has been associated with mutations in the gene (MFN2) encoding mitofusin 2.

Myoadenylate Deaminase Deficiency

Myoadenylate deaminase deficiency has failed to establish a firm basis in muscle nosology because the clinical manifestations are both protean and vague. Some affected patients, in fact, are asymptomatic; others demonstrate varying signs of weakness, hyporeflexia, periodic paralysis, paresthesias, and recurrent infections in childhood. The most common symptoms are muscle cramping and stiffness or pain after exercise. Myoglobinuria never has been reported, but serum CK values may be elevated slightly. Muscle specimens obtained at biopsy may appear normal or can demonstrate nonspecific minor changes. The specific histochemical stain for myoadenylate deaminase has revealed that the enzyme deficiency is a common occurrence, a concept confirmed by molecular genetic studies showing that a nonsense mutation (C-to-T at codon 12) in the gene encoding the muscle isozyme of adenylate deaminase (*AMPD1*) occurs in 2% of the population. Given the high frequency of this mutation, not surprisingly a few cases of genetic "double trouble" already have been reported. These entities consist of the association in the same patient of two homozygous mutations, the *AMPD1* mutation and a second mutation in a gene encoding another enzyme, such as myophosphorylase or phosphofructokinase. Affected patients appear to have more severe clinical manifestations than expected, as though the *per se* rather benign myoadenylate deaminase deficiency worsened the clinical presentation of the accompanying enzyme defect, a disease susceptibility mutation, of sorts, similar to the SCAD variant.

ACQUIRED DISORDERS

Muscle symptoms or frank weakness may be associated with numerous acquired illnesses in infancy or childhood, but, in the aggregate, these conditions are rare events when compared to the hereditary disorders. The acquired disorders may be associated with three primary processes: inflammatory changes, toxic or nutritional insults to muscle, or various endocrinologic disturbances.

Inflammatory Myopathy

Pathogenesis

Inflammatory forms of myopathy are classified according to their diverse etiologic factors. Known infectious agents include viruses, bacteria, fungi, and parasites. Those disorders that result from viral processes may be subdivided into three groups: acute benign myositis (caused by influenza viruses A and B, parainfluenza virus, and adenovirus II), acute myoglobinuria (caused by influenza viruses A and B, coxsackievirus B5, echovirus 9, adenovirus 21, herpes simplex virus, and Epstein-Barr virus), and epidemic pleurodynia (caused by group B coxsackieviruses). Bacterial infections are less common occurrences and are more localized. *Staphylococcus aureus* is the organism encountered most frequently in the subtropical

and tropical regions of the world. Clostridial, tuberculous, syphilitic, and leprous infections of muscle are distinctly rare events but have been described in children. Fungal infections are rarer still, but parasitic infections may be encountered occasionally. Toxoplasmosis, cysticercosis, and trichinosis are the likely agents in this category of infections.

The pathogenesis of dermatomyositis-polymyositis remains unknown. An immunogenetic predisposition to a viral infection is suspected because 72% of affected patients have the HLA-B8 haplotype.

Clinical Manifestations and Complications

The childhood inflammatory myopathic conditions encountered most commonly are idiopathic and include the dermatomyositis-polymyositis complex. Children with dermatomyositis exhibit a rather stereotyped syndrome in most cases. Muscle tenderness, joint discomfort, and tissue edema are associated with the weakness. Such children are extremely irritable and unhappy and frequently cry when examined. *Misery* is the term often used to describe the clinical picture. Occasionally, the cutaneous features are subtle or absent, in which case the term *polymyositis* is appropriate. Pure polymyositis in children is an exceedingly rare event. The annual incidence of dermatomyositis-polymyositis is approximately three to five cases per 1 million children. Girls are affected more frequently, with a 3:2 female-to-male ratio. Usually, the onset is insidious, but fulminant presentations with severe weakness do occur.

Spontaneous exacerbations and remissions also occur, and death may result from gastrointestinal ulceration, perforation, or hemorrhage; cardiac dysrhythmias or myocarditis; respiratory failure; overwhelming sepsis; or suicide. Dystrophic calcification of soft tissues is a serious complication, often developing 2 or 3 years after the initial onset of clinical symptoms. Characteristically, the rash involves the upper eyelids, the malar region of the face, the ears, the extensor regions of the limbs, and lateral aspects of the rib cage. Increased tortuosity of capillaries is evident in these regions and beneath the nail beds. These observations indicate that the target cell in this idiopathic condition is the endothelium, with prominent involvement of the intramuscular blood vessels. Immune complexes have been shown in venules within the skeletal muscle of affected children.

The clinical course of patients with dermatomyositis is variable. Some follow a monocyclic course, with full recovery occurring in 6 to 24 months. Others experience a chronic polycyclic course, and a third group has a chronic continuous course. The prognosis for complete recovery was decidedly poor before the availability of corticosteroids and other therapeutic agents. Before 1960, approximately one-third of patients died, one-third survived with severe residual disability, and one-third experienced a satisfactory recovery. However, some patients have severe residual weakness, joint contractures, evidence of smoldering disease, and soft-tissue nbsp;calcifications despite receiving optimal therapeutic intervention. Calcinosis occurs more commonly in children than in adults, ranging in incidence from 40% to 75%. Factors that correlate with the eventual development of calcinosis include severe disease at the outset, poor response to corticosteroids, persistent weakness, and severe generalized cutaneous vasculitis.

Diagnosis

The clinical picture is sufficiently distinctive to permit establishing a precise diagnosis in most cases. The laboratory findings, on the other hand, vary. A leukocytosis and an elevated erythrocyte sedimentation rate may be detected in acutely ill children, and serum enzyme levels, specifically those of CK and the transaminases, may be increased. Some patients have a positive antinuclear antibody test result, with the speckled pattern being the most common. The results of these blood studies may be normal in the presence of active muscle inflammation, however, and the degree to which the results are abnormal does not correlate very well with affected patients' conditions. The principal factors correlating with response to treatment, therefore, are the patient's clinical condition and perception of weakness.

The EMG is helpful in making the diagnosis. EMG findings include a mixture of neurogenic and myopathic features. Increased insertional activity indicates muscular irritability, fibrillations reflect the denervation of individual muscle fibers and fiber splitting, and decreased amplitude and duration of the compound action potential reflect direct injury to the muscle fiber. Some investigators have used the term *neuromyositis* to describe this mixed picture of muscle-tissue involvement.

Often, the results of muscle biopsy are distinctive, with inflammatory infiltration, necrosis, phagocytosis, and a gradual increase of endoneural connective tissue noted. An atrophy of muscle fibers at the periphery of the fascicle is the morphologic hallmark of this disease process. This distinctive finding has been termed *perifascicular atrophy*, and it suggests an ischemic mechanism as the explanation. Banker and Victor proposed the term *systemic angiopathy* instead of *dermatomyositis*, considering it to be a more accurate description of the disease process.

Therapy

The mainstay of therapy in dermatomyositis is a corticosteroid. Prednisone is used commonly, and recommendations call for a high-dose regimen to be started immediately and for treatment to be projected over a long period, often 18 to 36 months. The recommended dosage is 60 to 100 mg/m^2/day, the equivalent of 2 to 3 mg/kg/day. Initially, the daily amount of medication should be divided into three or four doses to effect maximal suppression of the disease as quickly as possible. Within 2 to 6 weeks, an attempt should be made to adjust the regimen to a single dose each morning and then to an alternate-day schedule if the drug continues to be effective. Approximately two-thirds of affected children respond to this regimen and recover satisfactorily. Treatment should be continued for 2 or 3 years in most patients. Therefore, it is essential that the side effects of prednisone be reviewed in detail with affected children and their parents at the outset. Potassium supplementation, antacids, and proper dietary instruction are most important in this regard. A diet low in salt and carbohydrates and relatively high in protein appears to be beneficial and seems to be associated with less severe cushingoid features. Most series of patients described since the early 1960s indicate a significant reduction in mortality rates (5% to 10%) and a considerable improvement in satisfactory outcome (65% to 75%). Other treatment regimens, including intravenous infusions of gamma globulins (IVIG) using various protocols, have been employed.

However, a remaining subgroup of patients does not do well. Often, they respond poorly to corticosteroids at the outset and exhibit prominent cutaneous manifestations of the disorder. A small number of affected patients may not absorb the orally administered steroids satisfactorily, but parenteral administration may be successful. More likely, however, is that an alternative treatment regimen will be necessary using an antimetabolite, plasmapheresis, or cyclosporine. No statement can be made regarding the efficacy of these alternative therapies because the total reported experience is limited and no controlled studies have been performed. Anecdotal experience with cyclosporine, limited as it is, is encouraging. The consensus is that chemotherapy should be considered early in those children who are at risk for the development of calcinosis, particularly because no known therapy can eradicate this complication once it has occurred.

Physical therapy and rehabilitation are critical elements of treatment throughout the illness. Passive and active range-of-motion exercises and the proper use of assistive devices to facilitate ambulation are important for physical and psychological well-being and for the restoration of good muscle function after the inflammatory process subsides.

Toxic and Nutritional Myopathy

Toxic and nutritional forms of myopathy are distinctly rare occurrences in children and often are publishable as case reports when they are recognized. Muscle necrosis and fibrosis associated with contractures may result from intramuscular injections of certain drugs.

Vincristine causes weakness affecting mainly the type 2 muscle fibers. This complaint is reversible when the drug is discontinued. Chloroquine and emetine also cause reversible types of myopathy.

Muscle necrosis and myoglobinuria may follow exposure to numerous drugs and toxins. Exogenous toxins include sea snake poisons, hornet poisons, and an unidentified myotoxic factor that has caused epidemic myoglobinuria in small fishing villages of northern Europe (Haff disease).

Hypokalemia from any cause may lead to muscle necrosis. Myoglobinuria has been reported after the administration of various kaliuretic agents, including amphotericin B and licorice. Succinylcholine may cause myoglobinuria in normal children. This phenomenon is to be distinguished from the myoglobinuria that follows the administration of anesthetic agents in children with the genetic trait for malignant hyperthermia (as discussed).

Malnutrition causes severe muscle wasting and weakness. Hypotonia may accompany rickets caused by vitamin D deficiency, and muscle weakness may result (rarely) from vitamin E deficiency.

Endocrine Causes of Myopathy

Muscle weakness and atrophy may accompany several endocrine disorders. Perhaps seen most commonly is the weakness that accompanies corticosteroid therapy. This complication may contribute to an affected patient's disability when steroids are being used to treat a primary muscle disease, such as dermatomyositis. Potassium wasting may compound this insult to muscle. Characteristically, the muscle biopsy sample reveals nonspecific atrophy of the type 2 fibers. This finding, however, is nondiagnostic and may be seen in nutritional and toxic states, disease atrophy, and infantile hypotonia resulting from cerebral factors. Proximal weakness is seen commonly in Cushing syndrome.

Frequently, weakness and wasting of the pelvic girdle muscles are seen with hyperparathyroidism, and the clinical syndrome may simulate a motor neuron syndrome. Serum CK values are normal. Muscle irritability and tetany may be the result of hypoparathyroidism and hypocalcemia.

Hyperthyroidism may cause several muscle disorders, but these conditions seldom are seen in children. Thyrotoxic periodic paralysis is similar to the familial hypokalemic form of this disorder (as discussed) and often is seen in adult male Asians. Thyrotoxic myopathy causes a slowly progressive weakness, and exophthalmic ophthalmoplegia may occur in the absence of clinically apparent hyperthyroidism. Congenital cretinism and childhood hypothyroidism can cause generalized muscular hypertrophy (Kocher-Debré-Sémélaigne syndrome). Hypothyroidism is associated with delayed contraction and relaxation of muscle fibers, increased CK values, and distinctive EMG abnormalities. These abnormalities have been termed *pseudomyotonic* and include bizarre, high-frequency, polyphasic discharges. Generally, the muscle symptoms in patients with these diverse forms of endocrinopathy revert to normal when the hormonal excess or deficiency is corrected.

Suggested Readings

Barresi R, Michele DE, Kanagawa M, et al. LARGE can functionally bypass α-dystroglycan glycosylation defects in distinct congenital muscular dystrophies. *Nature Med* 2004;10:696.

Dalakas MC, Park K-Y, Semino-Mora C, et al. Desmin myopathy, a skeletal myopathy with cardiomyopathy caused by mutations in the desmin gene. *N Engl J Med* 2000;342:770.

DiMauro S, Schon EA. Mitochondrial respiratory-chain diseases. *N Engl J Med* 2003;348:2656.

Engel AG, Franzini-Armstrong C. *Myology.* New York: McGraw-Hill, 2004.

Jones HR, De Vivo DC, Darras DT. *Neuromuscular disorders of infancy, childhood, and adolescence.* Boston: Butterworth-Heinemann, 2003.

Karpati G. *Structural and molecular basis of skeletal muscle diseases.* Basel: ISN Neuropath Press, 2002.

Laval SH, Bushby KMD. Limb-girdle muscular dystrophies—from genetics to molecular pathology. *Neuropath Appl Neurobiol* 2004;30:91.

Ozawa E, Nishino I, Nonaka I. Sarcolemmopathy: muscular dystrophies with cell membrane defects. *Brain Path* 2001;11:218.

Rosenberg RN, Prusiner SB, DiMauro S, et al. *The molecular and genetic basis of neurological and psychiatric disease.* Boston: Butterworth-Heinemann, 2003.

Schuelke M, Wagner KR, Stoltz LE, et al. Myostatin mutation associated with gross muscle hypertrophy in a child. *N Engl J Med* 2004;350:2682.

Toda T, Kobayashi K, Kondo-Iida E, et al. The Fukuyama congenital muscular dystrophy story. *Neuromusc Disord* 2000;10:153.

Vervoort VS, Holden KR, Ukadike KC, et al. POMGnT1 gene alterations in a family with neurological abnormalities. *Ann Neurol* 2004;56:143.

CHAPTER 410 ■ SLOW VIRUS INFECTIONS AND TRANSMISSIBLE SPONGIFORM ENCEPHALOPATHIES OF THE CENTRAL NERVOUS SYSTEM

WILLIAM J. BRITT

Transmissible central nervous system (CNS) diseases with unusually long incubation periods and prolonged clinical syndromes have been recognized in domestic animals for several hundred years. Only in the latter half of the twentieth century have physicians appreciated similar diseases in humans. The term *slow virus diseases* was coined in 1954 by Danish veterinary pathologist Bjorn Sigurdsson to unify the descriptions of these unique diseases. Characteristically, slow virus diseases exhibited a long period of latency, often measured in months to years, followed by a protracted but progressive clinical course that usually was confined to a single organ system. Initially, only diseases of domestic animals, such as scrapie and maedi of sheep, were included in this group of transmissible diseases. Subsequently, Gadjusek's natural history studies of kuru and Hadlow's description of similar histopathologic features of kuru and scrapie suggested that such neurodegenerative diseases as Creutzfeldt-Jakob disease (CJD) could be transmissible. During the same period, other investigators described a slowly progressive CNS degeneration associated with persistent measles virus infection. Thus, progressive and protracted human CNS diseases caused by either conventional or unconventional viral agents were grouped into the category of slow virus diseases.

A common feature of slow virus diseases in humans is the involvement of the CNS. Although in most cases, many of the pathogenetic details of these infectious processes are not understood completely, several unique characteristics of the CNS appear to predispose this organ system to chronic, destructive infections. The immune-mediated clearance of infectious agents from the CNS is limited because of the paucity of lymphoid structures in the CNS, as compared with other organs. The tight junctions of the endothelium of the CNS vasculature limit the passage of soluble immune effector molecules and cells of the systemic immune system. In addition, resident cells of the CNS express reduced levels of class I and II major histocompatibility complex molecules, thus limiting their ability to present foreign antigens or to regulate immune responses. Thus, the CNS offers an ideal compartment for chronic virus infection, especially for those agents that fail to evoke a strong systemic immune response, thereby limiting infiltration of the CNS by cells of the systemic immune system. Finally, the limited self-renewal capacity of cells within the CNS and the requisite bidirectional interactions among cells of the CNS often result in significant neurologic abnormalities in the absence of cytopathology. Perhaps this condition can be illustrated best by the fulminant clinical course of rabies, which often is associated with minimal CNS inflammation.

Although many infectious agents can induce latent CNS infections, the progressive and stereotypic clinical course of human slow virus diseases is unique to a limited number of diseases. This discussion is restricted to four diseases (Table 410.1), with the understanding that human retroviral infection of the CNS also could be included but is covered in Chapter 139, Pediatric Human Immunodeficiency Virus Infection.

SLOW VIRUS DISEASES ASSOCIATED WITH CONVENTIONAL AGENTS

Within the category of slow virus diseases associated with conventional agents are two relatively uncommon diseases—subacute sclerosing panencephalitis (SSPE) and progressive

TABLE 410.1

CONVENTIONAL AND UNCONVENTIONAL AGENTS ASSOCIATED WITH SLOW VIRUS DISEASE

Agent	Disease
Conventional	
Measles virus	Subacute sclerosing panencephalitis (SSPE)
Rubella virus	Progressive multifocal leukoencephalopathy (PML)
Polyoma virus (JC Virus)	Progressive rubella panencephalitis (PRP)
Unconventional	**Human Diseases**
Transmissible spongiform encephalopathies (prion diseases)	Creutzfeldt-Jakob disease (CJD)
	Gerstmann-Straussler-Scheinker syndrome
	Fatal familial insomnia
Sporadic	Familial Creutzfeldt-Jakob disease
Familial	Creutzfeldt-Jakob disease (iatrogenic)
Infectious	Variant Creutzfeldt-Jakob disease (vCJD)
	Kuru
	Animal Diseases
Infectious	Bovine spongiform encephalopathy (BSE)
	Scrapie (sheep)
	Chronic wasting disease (deer, elk)
	Transmissible mink encephalopathy (mink)

multifocal leukoencephalopathy (PML)—and an extremely rare degenerative disease, progressive rubella panencephalitis (PRP). Each of these diseases has been shown to follow infection of the CNS by a well-characterized virus, yet the pathogenesis of each disease is unique. SSPE can be explained most readily by the immunologic selection of viral mutants, whereas PML likely represents an extension of viral tropism secondary to a failure of normally protective immune responses. The pathogenesis of PRP remains unknown, and, because so few cases have been reported, one can only speculate on possible pathways that lead to disease.

Subacute Sclerosing Panencephalitis

SSPE is an infrequent but almost always fatal progressive panencephalitis. The clinical and histopathologic descriptions of this disease can be found in the medical literature dating from early in this century; however, not until 1950 was the term *subacute sclerosing panencephalitis* used to describe a progressive encephalitis with characteristic histologic findings of perivascular infiltrates of CD4$^+$ lymphocytes and plasma cells in both the gray and white matter and CD8$^+$ lymphocytes in the brain parenchyma. In the 1960s, measles virus was identified as the causative agent of SSPE, a finding that has been validated by the dramatic drop in the number of cases of SSPE after the institution of universal measles immunization in the United States and northern Europe. Several pathogenic mechanisms for the development of SSPE have been proposed, but most experimental data have been consistent with persistence of the measles virus in the CNS. The persistence of measles virus is associated with unique mutational events of the measles matrix protein and possibly positive immune selection of those genes encoding

the viral fusion and hemagglutinin proteins. The mechanisms leading to persistence of measles virus in the CNS in the face of host immune responses likely is secondary to extended viral tropism resulting from an immunologic selection of variants and evasion of protective host responses. Alternatively, persistence could be a direct result of extended viral tropism without a requirement of immune selection.

Natural history studies have demonstrated that the incidence of disease is approximately one in 10 million in the developed world, whereas in some Asian countries, such as Pakistan, the incidence may be 100-fold higher. A recent report from New Guinea documented an incidence of nearly 10 cases per 100,000 population, nearly 1,000-fold higher than that observed in North America and northern Europe. In the United States, SSPE previously has been reported to occur more frequently in white children from rural areas and, in particular, those in the southeastern United States. Risk factors for the development of SSPE within a population include a high incidence of wild-type measles virus infection and the acquisition of measles before the second year of life. Interestingly, both these risk factors have been modified by measles vaccination. Studies from the Netherlands demonstrated a tenfold drop in the incidence of SSPE after the incorporation of measles virus into routine immunization schedules. No genetic markers have been associated with the development of SSPE, although the disease occurs approximately two to three times more commonly in men than in women. Cases of SSPE have been reported after measles vaccination, with an estimated incidence of 1.0 to 2.5 cases per 1 million doses of vaccine. However, these studies failed to determine whether subclinical, wild-type measles virus infection occurred in these cases before administration of vaccine. In fact, no direct evidence exists that the vaccine strains of measles virus can cause SSPE, and vaccine strains of measles virus have not been isolated from the brains of patients with SSPE.

The clinical signs and symptoms of SSPE present in patients between the ages of 6 and 10 years (range, ages 2 to 49 years). Two cases of SSPE have been reported in infants younger than 2 years of age and have been thought to be associated with the congenital or perinatal acquisition of measles virus. In most cases, the onset of SSPE occurs 4 and 8 years after having wild-type measles virus infection. The clinical course of SSPE has been described by various staging systems, the most widely used being that suggested by Jabbour. Usually, clinical presentation or stage I includes such progressive psychointellectual disturbances as mood changes, poor school performance, depression, or hyperactivity. Often, this stage lasts for less than 6 months. Physical findings in stage I are nonspecific, although a pigmented retinopathy has been reported in a small percentage of patients. Stage II can include a variety of motor disorders, including seizures, myoclonic jerks, and akinetic drop attacks. Intellectual function continues to deteriorate during this stage. In contrast to the relatively brief duration of stage I, patients may exhibit findings consistent with stage II for 6 months to more than 1 year. Progression to stage III is heralded by the increased frequency of myoclonic jerks, spasticity, rigidity, and decorticate posturing. Often, hypothalamic dysfunction is manifest by hyperpyrexia, pallor, and flushing. Similar to stage I, stage III often is brief, lasting less than 6 months. Stage IV often is associated with a vegetative state. Although most patients follow a clinical course consistent with this staging system, approximately 5% to 10% of patients may survive for several years, remaining static in stage II or stage III. Alternatively, a similar number of patients may have a fulminant and progressive course lasting less than 3 months.

Laboratory findings consistent with the diagnosis of SSPE include a characteristic electroencephalogram (EEG), the presence of oligoclonal IgG in the cerebrospinal fluid (CSF), and an elevated titer of antimeasles antibody in the CSF. Both computed tomography (CT) and magnetic resonance imaging (MRI) have been used to demonstrate focal lesions in the brain. The imaging findings usually begin in the cortical-subcortical white matter and progress to periventricular white matter; however, these findings do not reflect the clinical stages of the disease. The EEG finding of periodic, synchronous bilateral discharges on a background of suppressed electrical activity (burst-suppression pattern) has been suggested to be characteristic of SSPE. However, the EEG is not diagnostic, and the absence of this finding does not exclude the diagnosis of SSPE. A more consistent finding is CSF pleocytosis consisting of lymphocytes and elevated protein, presumably secondary to the presence of increased levels of IgG. The increased CSF IgG results from oligoclonal antimeasles IgG, which can represent as many as 20% to 40% of the total CSF IgG. The finding of measles-specific oligoclonal IgG in the CSF, together with a compatible clinical course, is diagnostic of SSPE.

The treatment of SSPE has been unsuccessful. Early trials with the antiviral compound isoprinosine suggested a possible clinical benefit; however, subsequent trials and questions surrounding the study design of the original trial have led to the conclusion that this compound does not alter the natural history of SSPE in most patients. Other compounds used to treat SSPE include interferon-alpha, ribavirin, and immune-response modifiers. To date, significant efficacy has not been reported for any of these agents. Therefore, the most effective therapeutic strategy appears to be aggressive implementation of universal measles vaccine programs.

Progressive Multifocal Leukoencephalopathy

PML is a demyelinating, degenerative CNS disease that is caused by persistent infection with the human polyoma virus, JC virus. Initially, the disease was described in patients with underlying immunodeficiencies associated with lymphoproliferative disorders and congenital immunodeficiencies. Subsequently, it was associated with immunosuppressive therapy in allograft recipients. Although the number of organ allotransplantations increased dramatically during the early 1980s, PML remained a very rare disease, with fewer than 200 cases reported in the literature. When the incidence of human immunodeficiency virus 1 (HIV-1) infection increased exponentially during the 1980s, acquired immunodeficiency syndrome (AIDS) rapidly became the most common underlying disease associated with the development of PML. Between 1981 and 1990, 971 documented cases of PML were reported to the Centers for Disease Control and Prevention (CDC). Estimates have suggested that as many as 5% of patients with untreated AIDS will develop PML. PML is a disease primarily of adults; however, well-documented cases have been described in pediatric patients with congenital immunodeficiencies, those undergoing immunosuppressive therapy after receiving allografts, and children with AIDS.

The etiology of PML was discovered in 1971, after the isolation of a novel human polyoma virus of the papovavirus family—JC virus—from a patient with PML. Subsequent studies have shown that JC virus infection can be found in the vast majority of cases of PML. The pathogenesis of this disease is described in Box 410.1.

However, JC virus has been isolated also from the brain of individuals without PML. Thus, whether PML represents dissemination of virus from distant sites or local reactivation after immune suppression remains unclear. Interestingly, different genotypes of JC virus have been documented in different regions of the brain, suggesting that spread to the brain can be asynchronous. Either mechanism is consistent with the

---

| BOX 410.1 | Pathogenesis of Progressive Multifocal Leukoencephalopathy (PML) |

The pathogenesis of PML is explained most readily by persistent lytic replication of the JC virus in oligodendrocytes. More recently, oligodendrocytes infected with JC virus have been shown to undergo apoptosis. Both processes can lead to demyelination. The nucleotide sequencing of JC viral genomes from PML lesions has demonstrated differences in the genetic structure of PML-associated virus, as compared to the sequence of JC virus from normal individuals without evidence of PML. This result has suggested a possible link between genetic variants and development of disease. The multifocal distribution and relatively synchronous development of lesions has suggested hematogenous spread of the virus to the CNS. Genotyping of JC virus from the blood and brain of patients with PML infections has revealed nearly identical sequences in the transcriptional control regions of the viral genome, consistent with virus spread from blood to brain.

---

finding that more than 50% of children have antibody to JC virus by the time they reach age 6 years, and 80% to 90% of adults are seropositive. Viral DNA has been detected in the urine of approximately 20% of normal volunteers. Thus, infection with JC virus is nearly universal in the adult population. Other human polyomaviruses, most notably BK virus, have been isolated from the urine of immunocompromised patients but have not been associated with PML.

The clinical course of PML is characterized best by an insidious onset of a variety of neurologic abnormalities in patients with significant underlying immunodeficiency. Abnormalities in motor, sensory, and intellectual functions may present simultaneously. Weakness is a common complaint. Cognitive disturbances and disorders in speech also have been reported. Fever is not a component of PML. Usually, death follows the development of coma and occurs approximately 3 to 6 months after onset of symptoms, although the rate of progression can vary considerably. In patients with AIDS, the course of PML can be altered dramatically with successful antiretroviral therapy (ART). Similar to inflammatory eye disease (immune recovery uveitis) seen in patients with AIDS and CMV retinitis after immune reconstitution in those patients receiving ART, an accelerated symptomology presumably associated with inflammatory cell infiltrates in the brain can develop in patients with AIDS and PML successfully treated with ART.

Laboratory and imaging studies can be used to confirm the diagnosis of PML in an immunocompromised patient with a slowly evolving neurologic syndrome. MRI has been shown to be a very useful noninvasive technique for evaluating patients with suspected PML and has demonstrated lesions in such noncortical areas of the brain as the basal ganglia and brainstem. In contrast to the appearance of PML in allograft recipients or patients with congenital immunodeficiencies, lesions in ART-treated patients with AIDS may enhance with contrast agents secondary to surrounding inflammation. Usually, the EEG reveals only nonspecific changes that are nondiagnostic of PML. The use of polymerase chain reaction to demonstrate JC virus DNA in CSF has been reported to have a sensitivity of approximately 85%. Quantitation of JC virus genome copy in CSF of patients with PML has revealed a correlation between high copy number (more than 4 logs) and poor outcome, but a correlation between copy number and extent of disease has not been demonstrated. Brain biopsy using CT-guided stereotaxic techniques can provide a definitive diagnosis but often cannot be accomplished because of the location of the lesion. Detection of JC-specific antibody responses are of no value because of the near-universal seropositivity of the population and the possibility of deficient antibody responses in immunocompromised patients at risk for developing disease.

The treatment of PML in the face of ongoing immunosuppression has yielded only disappointing results. Several antiviral agents have been used with little, if any, effect, although case reports have suggested that treatment with the nucleoside analogy cidofovir may provide some benefit. The discontinuation of immunosuppression in transplant recipients can limit the progression of the disease, but often patients are left with significant neurologic deficits. In patients with AIDS, successful ART can stabilize the disease. In these cases, reconstitution of CD4+ lymphocytes responses and CD8+ cytotoxic T-lymphocyte activity have been shown to correlate with stabilization of disease and a more favorable clinical outcome.

Progressive Rubella Panencephalitis

PRP, an extremely rare degenerative disease of the CNS, has been associated with persistent infection by rubella virus. To date, fewer than ten cases have been documented in the medical literature. Isolation of rubella virus from the brain of children with PRP and elevated levels of serum and CSF antirubella antibody in other cases have provided evidence for the role of rubella virus in this disease. The development of PRP in children with congenital rubella syndrome is consistent with the proposed etiology of PRP. The lack of additional cases of PRP has limited the understanding of its pathogenesis. Several histopathologic findings of specimens from patients with PRP have suggested that persistent viral replication within the CNS leads to lymphocytic infiltration and local immune-mediated damage. Mineralization of vessels within the CNS suggests that vasculitis may be a component of the disease, yet histopathologic studies of autopsy specimens have failed to provide evidence of active vasculitis. Two possible explanations have been proposed, both of which require persistence of rubella virus replication for years. The first one suggests that viral mutants that favor persistence in the CNS arise and are responsible for the slowly progressive CNS damage seen in PRP. Rubella virus has been isolated from only one case, but this finding could argue for the presence of a defective virus that cannot be propagated *in vitro*. The second mechanism involves the production of immune complexes secondary to the persistence of rubella virus and the host antibody response. Immune complexes could be associated with a subacute vasculitis in the host CNS, leading to the observed damage to the CNS. Similar changes in other organs that often are targets of immune complex–mediated damage, such as the kidney, have not been reported in children with PRP.

The clinical features of PRP include progressive neurologic deterioration, with the onset of the disease often heralded by nonspecific intellectual dysfunction and behavioral changes. More specific clinical findings have included ataxia, seizures, and dementia. Evidence of CNS inflammation, such as meningismus, headache, or fever, have not been described. Although the disease is progressive, continued survival with significant CNS damage can exceed 2 years. No effective treatment for this extremely rare infection is known. Laboratory diagnosis of PRP is made most readily by examination of the CSF. Pleocytosis consisting of mononuclear cells and normal CSF glucose values are present in patients with PRP. The CSF protein is elevated secondary to the presence of oligoclonal IgG specific for rubella virus. Often, imaging studies demonstrate

cortical atrophy, but they are nonspecific and thus provide little specific diagnostic information.

TRANSMISSIBLE SPONGIFORM ENCEPHALOPATHIES

The group of neurodegenerative diseases (CJD, Gerstmann-Straussler-Scheinker disease, fatal familial insomnia, bovine spongiform encephalopathy [BSE] variant of CJD [vCJD], and kuru) that have been designated as *transmissible spongiform encephalopathies* (TSEs) represents a subset of amyloid diseases that also includes Alzheimer disease and multiple myeloma (see Table 410.1). Together, these diseases have in common the accumulation of polymeric protein fibrillary material (amyloid) in involved organs. In contrast to other known amyloid diseases, the spongiform encephalopathies are transmissible, perhaps by an abnormal protein that accumulates in the amyloid plaques that are characteristic of TSEs, or perhaps by an as yet unidentified conventional infectious agent that triggers the production of the TSE amyloid.

Although the TSE of sheep—scrapie—has been appreciated for more than 200 years and prompted Sigurdsson's original description of slow virus diseases, only recently have the TSEs of humans become the focus of laboratory investigation. In 1997, Prusiner received the Nobel Prize for his hypothesis that a transmissible protein, termed the *prion*, can elicit disease with a reproducible phenotype. Intense interest in this group of diseases has followed the identification of a vCJD in Great Britain. This TSE appears to be similar (if not phenotypically identical) to BSE, or mad-cow disease, which has been shown to be transmissible to other ungulates as well as to large cats in zoos and possibly to domestic cats. Although direct evidence that the BSE agent also is causative of vCJD has not been reported, experimental transmission of BSE to primates, similar phenotypic characteristics of BSE and vCJD in small animal models of TSE, and similar biochemical characteristics of prions derived from these two diseases strongly argue for a link between the two diseases. These findings suggest that the agent responsible for the BSE likely was transmitted from cattle to humans. The outbreak of BSE in the 1980s, coupled with the more recent increase in the incidence of CJD in young adults in Great Britain and the identification of vCJD, contributed to a decision by members of the European Common Market to ban the importation of British beef. The estimated economic impact of this outbreak on the cattle industry in England was in excess of 4 billion U.S. dollars. Similarly, the recent discoveries of BSE in U.S. and Canadian cattle herds have been estimated to have resulted in more than 1 billion U.S. dollars in lost revenues. More recently, a TSE of deer and elk (chronic wasting disease, CWD) has been reported with increasing frequency in the United States. How and where this disease arose is unclear, but one possibility is that it was introduced into wild deer herds by animals that had escaped from game farms and subsequently joined resident herds. The pathogenesis of TSEs remains controversial (Box 410.2).

TSEs, specifically CJD, generally are not considered pediatric diseases because the mean age of onset is between 60 and 65 years, with an incubation period of 10 to 15 years. CJD is an uncommon disease, with a worldwide incidence of 0.5 to 1.0 in 1 million population, except in populations with specific mutations within the cellular gene that encodes the prion protein (PRP) that can be associated with an increase in the misfolding of the normal PRP. In these latter cases, the variant disease behaves as an autosomal dominant, inherited neurodegenerative disease. Approximately 20 pediatric cases of CJD in the United States resulted from the use of cadaveric growth hormone. The pediatric cases had a typical clinical

BOX 410.2   Pathogenesis of Transmissible Spongiform Encephalopathy (TSE)

Prusiner's infectious protein hypothesis suggests that a mutant isoform of a normal cellular protein (PrP) can initiate amyloid formation within the CNS, similar to that observed during crystallization of proteins *in vitro*. The finding that the infectious scrapie agent had a protein counterpart in normal, unaffected cells provided support for this mechanism of disease transmission. Furthermore, transgenic mice in which this cellular gene had been deleted were resistant to the mouse-adapted scrapie agent, a finding that demonstrated that the cellular protein was necessary for the development of scrapie. Yet, even this elegant experiment failed to demonstrate directly that the etiologic agent of this group of diseases was an infectious protein. Perhaps the most exciting observation made in the recent past has been that a mutant form of the protein could cause conversion of the normal cellular isoform into the amyloid-forming isoform *in vitro*. This finding was consistent with the infectious protein hypothesis and suggested that an abnormal isoform of a normal cellular protein could act as a seed to promote misfolding of the cellular protein and eventual amyloid formation. The unique feature of this pathogenic mechanism is that the phenotypic expression of the disease is reproduced when protein only is inoculated into an experimental animal. Thus, no genetic information in the form of a conventional nucleic acid is required.

As noted, the infectious protein for the experimental models of TSE has been termed a *prion*. These small proteinaceous particles have been shown to be resistant to treatments such as the ionizing radiation that inactivates infectious agents (including small viruses) that contain nucleic acids, but they are sensitive to enzymes (proteases), chemical agents that degrade proteins. Interestingly, this infectious material is resistant to standard methods of sterilization, including heat and pressure, a finding that explained the etiology of iatrogenic cases of CJD, which have occurred after stereotaxic neurosurgical procedures and the use of dural grafts. These published findings, together with observations in experimental models of TSE, have suggested the possibility that the agent could be present in blood. As a result, the American Red Cross placed restrictions on donors who have resided in Great Britain because of concern about the possibility of blood-borne transmission.

Although numerous observations have been consistent with the infectious protein hypothesis, none has addressed the hypothesis directly, thus leading other investigators to question the evidence supporting the prion hypothesis and to suggest that the hypothesis has not been tested rigorously. Experimental findings that have argued against an infectious protein etiology of this group of diseases include the inability to transmit disease using recombinant-derived, *in vitro*-generated prions; observations that suggest the existence of prion strains, thus indicating the possibility of genetically determined phenotypes of disease; and the lack of transmissibility of other amyloid diseases that also are associated with misfolded proteins. Although a careful review of the experimental data supporting the protein-only hypothesis has revealed several alternative interpretations, and definitive evidence for the protein-only hypothesis has not been presented, one must appreciate that the inoculation of highly purified material obtained from the CNS (and devoid of any detectable infectious agent that contains nucleic acid) can transmit disease reliably to experimental animals. Most recently, investigators have demonstrated that RNA can increase greatly the efficiency of *in vitro* prion generation, thus suggesting that strains of prions could arise, depending on their interactions with specific RNAs. The controversy surrounding the etiology of TSEs remains; however, investigators appear to agree that the nature of the agent(s) responsible for this group of diseases is far from understood.

---

course after an incubation period of 12 to 13 years. The use of recombinant growth hormone eliminated this route of transmission. More recently, cases of CJD (possibly vCJD) have occurred in young adults in Great Britain. Because these cases occurred in young adults without risk factors for iatrogenic CJD, these cases have been proposed to arise from consumption of BSE-contaminated meat. Consistent with this explanation has been a mean age of 27 years in the approximately 130 cases of vCJD reported in Great Britain. The young age of patients with vCJD is in marked contrast to the mean age of patients with sporadic CJD.

The initial clinical findings of TSE include both motor and sensory dysfunction. Memory loss and either anxiety or depression are common presenting symptoms. Objective findings include gait and visual disturbances, paresthesias, and speech disturbances. Late in the course of disease, neuroendocrine disorders may develop, as may disturbances in circadian rhythms followed by insomnia. Progressive disease is a hallmark of TSE, and most patients enter a vegetative state within 1 year of onset of the disease. In the early descriptions of juvenile cases of kuru, death usually occurred within 6 months after the appearance of clinical symptoms. Currently, no treatment is available for this group of diseases.

Laboratory diagnosis is accomplished best by brain biopsy. The findings of neuronal loss, status spongiosis, proliferation of astrocytes, and microgliosis are characteristic histologic findings. These findings are focal, and areas of normal brain can be found within the same biopsy specimen. *Status spongiosis* is a term used to describe the vacuolation of the neuropil caused by neuronal loss and collapse of the normal architecture of the brain. Amyloid plaques may be present, although their presence is not required for establishing the diagnosis. In different forms of the diseases, the amyloid plaques may take on a different morphology that is characteristic of each disease. Such is the case of the florid plaques observed in biopsy specimens from patients with vCJD. Lesions may be distributed throughout the brain, and often their distribution is unique to each clinical variant of TSE and, in some cases, it can be related to the clinical presentation. Monoclonal antibody reagents have been shown to be useful in the detection of the mutant isoform of PRP in biopsy specimens, including biopsy specimens from non-CNS tissue such as the tonsils. Noninvasive imaging techniques are helpful in providing an accurate diagnosis. MRI and CT have documented cortical atrophy late in the course of the disease. Serial EEG also can point to the diagnosis, if characteristic tracings are observed, but it does not provide a definitive diagnosis. Routine examination of CSF is of little or no value. Currently, no treatment is available for this group of diseases. Some early *in vitro* studies have suggested that some polyanions such as Congo Red could inhibit amyloid formation, but studies to date have not identified a compound that could be expected to stabilize disease in patients with TSE.

Suggested Readings

Progressive Multifocal Leukoencephalopathy

Antinori A, Cingolani A, Lorenzini P, et al. Clinical epidemiology and survival of progressive multifocal leukoencephalopathy in the era of highly active antiretroviral therapy: data from the Italian Registry Investigative Neuro AIDS (IRINA). *J Neurovirol* 2003;9(Suppl 1):47.

Cinque P, Bossolasco S, Brambilla AM, et al. The effect of highly active antiretroviral therapy-induced immune reconstitution on development and outcome of progressive multifocal leukoencephalopathy: study of 43 cases with review of the literature. *J Neurovirol* 2003;9(Suppl 1):73.

Du Pasquier RA, Clark KW, Smith PS, et al. JCV-specific cellular immune response correlates with a favorable clinical outcome in HIV-infected individuals with progressive multifocal leukoencephalopathy. *J Neurovirol* 2001;7:318.

Gasnault J, Kahraman M, de Goer de Herve MG, et al. Critical role of JC virus-specific CD4 T-cell responses in preventing progressive multifocal leukoencephalopathy [see comment]. *AIDS* 2003;17:1443.

Gasnault J, Kousignian P, Kahraman M, et al. Cidofovir in AIDS-associated progressive multifocal leukoencephalopathy: a monocenter observational study with clinical and JC virus load monitoring. *J Neurovirol* 2001;7:375.

Hammarin AL, Bogdanovic G, Svedhem V, et al. Analysis of PCR as a tool for detection of JC virus DNA in cerebrospinal fluid for diagnosis of progressive multifocal leukoencephalopathy. *J Clin Microbiol* 1996;34:2929.

Koralnik IJ. Overview of the cellular immunity against JC virus in progressive multifocal leukoencephalopathy. *J Neurovirol* 2002;8(Suppl 2):59.

Mader I, Herrlinger U, Klose U, et al. Progressive multifocal leukoencephalopathy: analysis of lesion development with diffusion-weighted MRI. *Neuroradiology* 2003;45:717.

Marra CM, Rajicic N, Barker DE, et al. A pilot study of cidofovir for progressive multifocal leukoencephalopathy in AIDS. [erratum appears in *AIDS* 2003;17:281.]. *AIDS* 2002;16:1791.

Miralles P, Berenguer J, Lacruz C, et al. Inflammatory reactions in progressive multifocal leukoencephalopathy after highly active antiretroviral therapy. *AIDS* 2001; 15:1900.

Thurnher MM, Thurnher SA, Muhlbauer B, et al. Progressive multifocal leukoencephalopathy in AIDS: initial and follow-up CT and MRI. *Neuroradiology* 1997;39:611.

Progressive Rubella Panencephalitis

Weil ML, Itabashi HH, Cremer NE, et al. Chronic progressive panencephalitis due to rubella virus simulating subacute sclerosing panencephalitis. *N Engl J Med* 1975;292:994.

Subacute Sclerosing Panencephalitis

Gascon GG. Subacute sclerosing panencephalitis. *Semin Pediatric Neurology* 1996;3:260.

Gurses C, Ozturk A, Baykan B, et al. Correlation between clinical stages and EEG findings of subacute sclerosing panencephalitis. *Clin Electroencephalogr* 2000;31:201.

Hara S, Kimura H, Hoshino Y, et al. Combination therapy with intraventricular interferon-alpha and ribavirin for subacute sclerosing panencephalitis and monitoring measles virus RNA by quantitative PCR assay. *Brain Dev* 2003; 25:367.

Ozturk A, Gurses C, Baykan B, et al. Subacute sclerosing panencephalitis: clinical and magnetic resonance imaging evaluation of 36 patients. *J Child Neurol* 2002;17:25.

Schneider-Schaulies J, Meulen V, Schneider-Schaulies S, et al. Measles infection of the central nervous system. *J Neurovirol* 2003;9:247.

Schneider-Schaulies S, ter Meulen V. Pathogenic aspects of measles virus infections. *Arch Virol* 1999;15(Suppl):139.

Takasu T, Mgone JM, Mgone CS, et al. A continuing high incidence of subacute sclerosing panencephalitis (SSPE) in the Eastern Highlands of Papua New Guinea. *Epidemiol Infect* 2003;131:887.

Transmissible Spongiform Encephalopathies

Bessen RA, Kocisko DA, Raymond GJ, et al. Non-genetic propagation of strain-specific properties of scrapie prion protein. *Nature* 1995;375:698.

Chesebro B. Introduction to the transmissible spongiform encephalopathies or prion diseases. *Br Med Bull* 2003;66:1.

Chesebro B. Prion protein and the transmissible spongiform encephalopathy diseases. *Neuron* 1999;24:503.

Collinge J. Prion diseases of humans and animals: their causes and molecular basis. *Annu Rev Neurosci* 2001;24:519.

Cousens SN, Zeidler M, Esmonde TF, et al. Sporadic Creutzfeldt-Jakob disease in the United Kingdom: analysis of epidemiological surveillance data for 1970–96. *Br Med J* 1997;315:389.

Hill AF, Collinge J. Subclinical prion infection. *Trends Microbiol* 2003;11:578.

Prusiner SB. Molecular biology and pathogenesis of prion diseases. *Trends Biochem Sci* 1996;21:482.

Prusiner SB. Prions and neurodegenerative disease. *N Engl J Med* 1987;317:1571.

Woolhouse ME, Anderson RM. Understanding the epidemiology of BSE. *Trends Microbiol* 1997;5:421.

CHAPTER 411 ■ LEUKODYSTROPHIES

ALAN K. PERCY

The leukodystrophies are a group of progressive inherited neurodegenerative disorders affecting myelin formation in the central and (in some instances) peripheral nervous systems. As such, they should be distinguished from disorders characterized by demyelination, such as multiple sclerosis, inflammatory disorders, or toxic processes. The leukodystrophies can be categorized as dysmyelinating (abnormal myelin formation), hypomyelinating (failure of myelin formation), or vacuolating (dissolution of myelin). The leukodystrophies are associated mainly with infants and children, but adult variants are recognized with increasing frequency. These disorders are recessive conditions involving both autosomal and X-linked inheritance. Typically, the clinical pattern of the leukodystrophies is characterized by the loss of previously acquired capabilities, whether motor or cognitive, signifying a degenerative disease. In in-

fants, this condition reflects loss of acquired developmental milestones, whereas during childhood or adolescence, changes in behavior or school performance are more typical.

When the degenerative process occurs in infancy or early childhood, often white matter or myelin dysfunction can be distinguished from gray matter or neuronal dysfunction on the basis of the clinical appearance of the disorder. Children with disorders of white matter display a loss of acquired motor capabilities (e.g., ambulation or hand use), hypotonia, or ataxia or signs of corticospinal tract involvement, such as spasticity, hyperreflexia, or extensor plantar responses. Children with disorders of gray matter demonstrate intellectual or cognitive deficits, such as loss of language or communication skills, seizures, and blindness. This formulation may be an effective guide to conducting clinical and laboratory assessments early in the disease process. Global nervous system involvement limits the effectiveness of this approach during later stages.

During infancy, the various types of leukodystrophy must be differentiated from an emerging static encephalopathy. In the presence of rapid, clear-cut regression, making this determination is straightforward. Subtle regression or a plateau in development, however, presents a greater diagnostic challenge. In older children, consideration must be given to such demyelinating processes as multiple sclerosis, acute disseminated encephalomyelitis, or polyneuropathy (e.g., Guillain-Barré syndrome). In addition, other conditions must be excluded, including nutritional deficiency, a toxic encephalopathy (from heavy-metal or drug intoxication with such drugs as neuroleptics, hypnotics, or anticonvulsants), a neoplasm of the central nervous system (CNS), an immunopathologic condition (systemic lupus erythematosus), or a chronic infectious process (human immunodeficiency virus, acquired immunodeficiency syndrome, or subacute sclerosing panencephalitis).

As a group, the leukodystrophies have an incidence of one in 50,000, based on recent data from Germany. This incidence figure should be regarded as a minimum number because underdiagnosis is likely. Efforts to provide useful screening tools have focused on cranial magnetic resonance imaging (MRI) and cerebrospinal fluid (CSF) analyses. In particular, cranial MRI has increased the recognition and elucidation of an emerging group of leukodystrophies, such as vanishing white matter disease (see Section, Vanishing White Matter Disease). Cranial MRI also is an effective mechanism for monitoring the progression of disease and assessing the efficacy of treatment during the conduct of clinical trials. Effective treatment presently is limited for those entities described in the following sections.

Metachromatic leukodystrophy and globoid cell leukodystrophy (Krabbe disease) are autosomal recessive disorders of sphingolipid metabolism. The sphingolipids are a group of unique lipid compounds that are important constituents of biologic membranes. The tissue distribution of the individual sphingolipids differs dramatically. Some sphingolipids are prominent within neural elements, and others are present in nonneural tissues. The sphingolipids sulfatide and galactosylceramide are critical components of myelin in both the central and peripheral nervous systems, whereas the group of sphingolipids called *gangliosides* are associated particularly with neurons and their axons and dendrites. (Disorders of ganglioside metabolism are described in Chapter 389, Lysosomal Storage Disorders.)

Adrenoleukodystrophy is an X-linked disorder of very long-chain fatty acid (VLCFA) metabolism. Canavan disease, an autosomal recessive disorder, is caused by abnormal acetylaspartate metabolism. Pelizaeus-Merzbacher disease, an X-linked disorder, is caused by duplications or point mutations of the proteolipid protein (PLP) gene. Alexander disease, an autosomal recessive disorder, results from mutations in the gene for glial fibrillary acidic protein. Vanishing white matter disease is caused by mutations in genes encoding the eIF2B translation factor.

Effective therapy for these disorders is limited. Bone marrow transplantation has been performed with variable success. Gene therapy strategies are being investigated. Dietary therapy with erucic acid (Lorenzo oil) has been employed without clear benefit in clinically affected children, but it may be beneficial in delaying onset in the presymptomatic stage. Symptomatic therapy should be used as indicated to treat infections, seizures, and other medical problems. Affected families should be provided with appropriate support, as the stress associated with caring for such children can be overwhelming.

The prenatal diagnosis of many of these disorders is feasible. Analysis of amniotic fluid cells or chorionic villus samples can provide an accurate assessment of the fetus. Population-based screening currently is not realistic. As such, prenatal diagno-

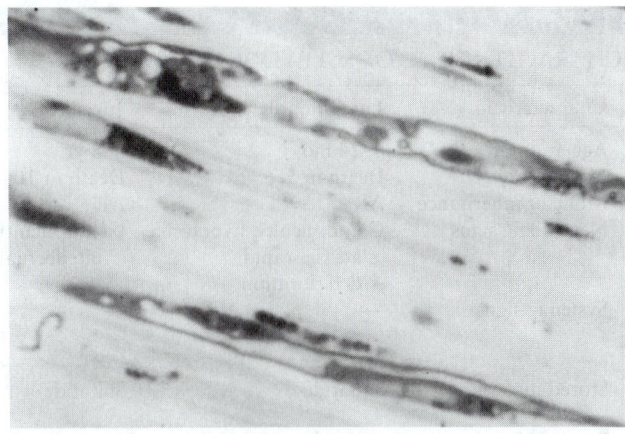

FIGURE 411.1. Light micrograph of peripheral nerve in longitudinal section from a patient with metachromatic leukodystrophy, showing lipid inclusion material within the Schwann cell cytoplasm and in the interstitial space.

sis is practical only in families with a known risk for having affected offspring. Despite the identification of specific mutations in these disorders, in many instances, a determination of the relevant enzyme or metabolite remains the preferred diagnostic modality.

METACHROMATIC LEUKODYSTROPHY (SULFATIDE LIPIDOSIS)

Metachromatic leukodystrophy is an autosomal recessive disorder with an incidence of one per 40,000 people. The biochemical basis is the inability to degrade the sphingolipid, sulfatide, or galactosylceramide-3 sulfate (Figs. 411.1 and 411.2). Sulfatide, along with galactosylceramide, is an important constituent of central and peripheral nervous system myelin. Metachromatic leukodystrophy results from a deficiency of sulfatide sulfatase (arylsulfatase A), the lysosomal enzyme responsible for the degradation of sulfatide. This deficiency causes an accumulation of sulfatide in both neural and non-neural (especially kidney and gallbladder) tissues, where it can be detected as metachromatic granules. Both central and peripheral myelin

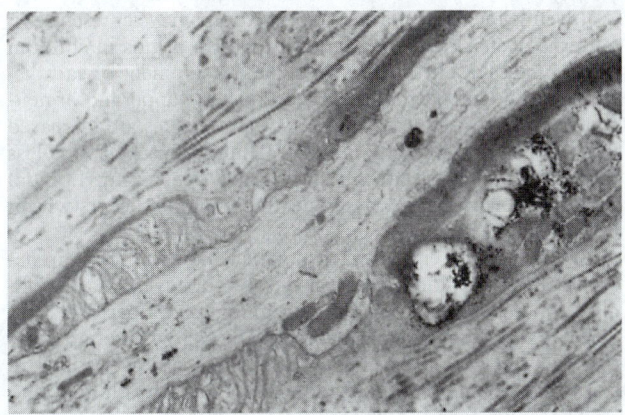

FIGURE 411.2. Electron micrograph of peripheral nerve in longitudinal section from a patient with metachromatic leukodystrophy, showing densely staining inclusion material within the Schwann cell cytoplasm.

TABLE 411.1

CHARACTERISTICS OF SULFATIDE LIPIDOSES

Characteristic	Late Infantile	Juvenile	Adult	Multiple Sulfatase Deficiency
Age at onset	6–24 mo	4–8 yr	15 yr or older	6–18 mo
Prognosis	Death in 5–6 yr	Death in 10–15 yr	Slow progression	Death by age 10–12 yr
Mode of inheritance	AR	AR	AR	AR
Neurologic signs	Gait difficulty, hypotonia, ataxia, rapid deterioration	Gait difficulty, ataxia, intellectual decline	Dementia, depression, psychosis, motor difficulty	Gait difficulty, hypotonia, ataxia, rapid deterioration
Systemic signs	—	—	—	Coarse features, hepatosplenomegaly, skeletal deformity, ichthyosis
Stored material	Sulfatide	Sulfatide	Sulfatide	Sulfatide, cholesterol sulfate, mucopolysaccharide sulfate
Enzyme defect	Sulfatide sulfatase (arylsulfatase A)	Sulfatide sulfatase (arylsulfatase A)	Sulfatide sulfatase (arylsulfatase A)	Multiple sulfatases
Feasibility of prenatal diagnosis	Yes	Yes	Yes	Yes

AR, autosomal recessive.

are abnormal. Neuropathology consists of the widespread loss of myelin and oligodendroglia in the brain and segmental demyelination of the peripheral nerves.

Forms of the Disease

Metachromatic leukodystrophy occurs in three principal forms: late infantile (the most common), juvenile, and adult (Table 411.1). The distinction of separate phenotypes is arbitrary, however, as this variability reflects the continuum of phenotypes rather than separate entities. As specific mutations are identified, the genotype-phenotype correlations become clearer and the continuum of clinical involvement becomes more evident. The late infantile form appears in affected children between ages 1 and 2 years, after they have experienced normal early development, often including ambulation. Early signs are regression of motor skills, gait difficulties, ataxia, hypotonia, and extensor plantar responses. Muscle stretch reflexes are diminished or absent as a result of peripheral nerve involvement. Optic atrophy is prominent early. The disorder progresses fairly rapidly, with loss of motor and mental capabilities and ultimately loss of meaningful contact with the environment. Death usually occurs by the time the child is age 6 years.

Juvenile metachromatic leukodystrophy may represent two patterns of disease. An early juvenile form begins in children between ages 4 and 8 years, with the development of gait disturbance and intellectual decline. Ataxia and upper motor neuron signs are prominent. Muscle stretch reflexes are increased initially but subsequently are lost. Clinical progression is less rapid than that in the late infantile form. Often, extrapyramidal signs and seizures appear, and death commonly occurs within 6 years of onset.

Alternately, juvenile metachromatic leukodystrophy can begin in affected children between ages 6 and 16 years as personality and behavior changes and declining school performance. Seizures are common occurrences, and motor dysfunction eventually ensues. The progression of this form is slower still, and survival is possible into late adolescence or early adulthood. The adult form of metachromatic dystrophy presents as dementia or psychosis as early as age 16 years or as late as age 60 years. Often, declining school or work performance is the first sign of the disease. Motor dysfunction is an inevitable development, but its progression may be very slow.

Multiple sulfatase deficiency combines features of the late infantile form of metachromatic leukodystrophy, steroid sulfatase deficiency, and the mucopolysaccharidoses (see Table 411.1). Mucopolysaccharide storage is suggested by the presence of coarse facial features, ichthyosis, hepatosplenomegaly, and skeletal abnormalities. Tissue accumulation of sulfatides, sulfated steroids, and mucopolysaccharides reflects the pervasive deficiency of multiple sulfatase activities.

Diagnosis and Therapy

The diagnosis of metachromatic leukodystrophy is accomplished by careful clinical assessment and the performance of appropriate laboratory studies. The diagnosis is suggested by a history of regression and progressive deterioration of motor function, and signs of gait difficulties with weakness, hypotonia, hyporeflexia, and extensor plantar responses in the early forms, or behavioral and motor disability in older children or adolescents. Nerve conduction velocities are reduced as a reflection of peripheral nerve involvement. The CSF protein level is increased. Cranial computed tomography (CT) or MRI scans reveal symmetric white matter lesions in the early forms of the disease and may demonstrate cortical atrophy in the later forms. Decreased activity of the enzyme arylsulfatase A, preferably in leukocytes or skin fibroblast cultures, establishes the diagnosis. The availability of biochemical analysis has eliminated the role of peripheral nerve biopsy, which typically will reveal metachromatic granules.

A determination of arylsulfatase A activity in affected individuals is an ineffective means of differentiating the various clinical forms. Fibroblast cultures may be useful, however, on the basis of their ability to degrade exogenous sulfatide. Little sulfatide is metabolized in the late infantile form, whereas greater residual metabolic activity is present in the adult form. This differentiation may not be straightforward in some cases. Some individuals with the juvenile-onset pattern have normal levels of arylsulfatase A. Instead, such patients lack an activator protein necessary for sulfatide degradation. This deficiency also can be demonstrated by the abnormal catabolism of exogenous sulfatide in cultured fibroblasts and by the absence of the activator protein in leukocytes or fibroblast cultures using specific antibodies.

Arylsulfatase A maps to chromosome 22q. Advances in molecular genetics revealed two major arylsulfatase alleles associated with metachromatic leukodystrophy: one was detected exclusively in the late infantile form and the other in the juvenile and adult forms, thus providing a molecular basis for understanding the phenotypic heterogeneity of the disease. Additional mutant alleles also have been identified. This multiplicity of allelic variants requires continued reliance on arylsulfatase determinations for definitive diagnosis.

Carrier detection and prenatal diagnosis may be accomplished by measuring the activity of arylsulfatase A. In families with known mutations, molecular analysis for the specific mutation should be performed. Some normal individuals exhibit a pseudodeficient arylsulfatase A state by biochemical assay; in such cases, prenatal diagnosis could yield ambiguous results. In these circumstances, evaluating the ability of the amniotic or trophoblastic cells to catabolize exogenous sulfatide in culture is necessary before deciding on the status of the fetus.

No effective treatment is available for metachromatic leukodystrophy. Enzyme replacement through bone marrow transplantation has possible benefit in terms of improving the activity of arylsulfatase A and slowing the progression of disease, but convincing evidence of long-term efficacy within the CNS is lacking. Careful consideration should be given to therapies that may modify the natural history in a way that would produce greater chronicity without affecting resolution. Supportive therapy is indicated to ensure proper nutrition and to treat medical problems, including seizures, as they occur.

GLOBOID CELL LEUKODYSTROPHY (GALACTOSYLCERAMIDE LIPIDOSIS, KRABBE DISEASE)

Globoid cell leukodystrophy is an autosomal recessive disorder that has an incidence in Sweden of approximately one per 50,000 people but is seen less commonly outside Scandinavia. The inability to degrade the sphingolipid galactosylceramide represents the biochemical abnormality. Galactosylceramide also is an important component of central and peripheral nervous system myelin. Hence, both are affected in this disorder. Globoid cell leukodystrophy reflects a fundamental failure in myelinogenesis. The small amount of myelin that is formed (less than 1% of normal) has a normal composition. Also, unlike metachromatic leukodystrophy, with its marked storage of

sulfatide, galactosylceramide levels in brain actually are deficient.

Globoid cells, multinucleate giant cells that occur in clusters throughout brain and brainstem white matter, especially around venules, are elicited by galactosylceramide, levels of which actually are increased. In addition, white matter is marked by a reduction or loss of oligodendroglia and by the presence of diffuse gliosis. Segmental demyelination is noted in peripheral nerves. Failure to synthesize myelin may be attributed to the cytotoxic effect on oligodendrocytes of galactosylsphingosine, which is formed by removing the fatty acid from galactosylceramide. Levels of this compound in the brains of affected children are as much as 100 times normal.

Forms of the Disease

Globoid cell leukodystrophy occurs in two principal forms: infantile (the more common) and late-onset (Table 411.2). Infantile globoid cell leukodystrophy presents early in the first year of life, usually by the time the infant is age 6 months, and it is characterized by extreme irritability, hypertonia, and developmental stagnation and then regression, followed quickly by extensor posturing, rigidity, exaggerated startle response, optic atrophy, and cortical blindness. Initially, muscle stretch reflexes are prominent but gradually are lost, and hypotonia replaces hypertonia. Both hypotonia and hyporeflexia are signs of peripheral nerve involvement. Death from intercurrent illness usually occurs by the time the child is age 12 months, although survival to ages 18 to 24 months has occurred.

Late-onset globoid cell leukodystrophy appears in children between ages 1.5 and 5.0 years, after a period of normal development. Typical features are gait abnormalities and ataxia, spasticity, loss of vision with optic atrophy and cortical blindness, and mild to profound psychomotor retardation, with slow but relentless progression. Adult onset also has been reported, with clinical features predominantly those of spastic paraparesis and preserved mentation.

Diagnosis and Therapy

The definitive diagnosis of globoid cell leukodystrophy can be made by enzymatic assay. Galactosylceramide beta-galactosidase activity, mapped to chromosome 14, is deficient and can be assayed in leukocytes and fibroblast cultures. As in metachromatic leukodystrophy, numerous mutant alleles have

TABLE 411.2
GLOBOID CELL LEUKODYSTROPHY

Characteristic	Infantile	Late Infantile
Age at onset	Infancy	1–5 yr
Prognosis	Death by age 2 yr	Death by age 10–12 yr
Mode of inheritance	Autosomal recessive	Autosomal recessive
Neurologic signs	Irritability, extensor rigidity, optic atrophy, cortical blindness, rapid deterioration	Ataxia, gait difficulty, vision loss, psychomotor decline
Stored material	Galactosylceramide, galactosylsphingosine (psychosine)	Galactosylceramide, galactosylsphingosine (psychosine)
Enzyme defect	Galactosylceramide beta-galactosidase	Galactosylceramide beta-galactosidase
Feasibility of prenatal diagnosis	Yes	Yes

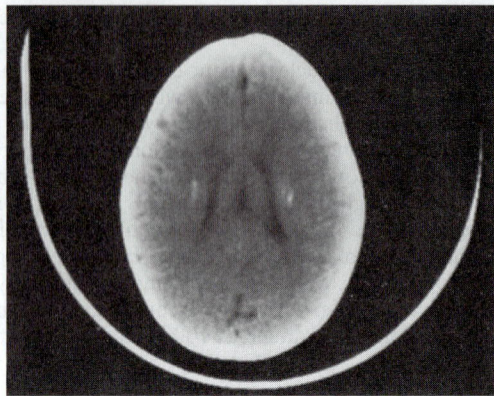

FIGURE 411.3. Nonenhanced brain computed tomographic scan of an infant with galactosylceramide lipidosis (Krabbe disease), demonstrating lesions of increased density adjacent to the lateral ventricles.

been identified, thus providing phenotype-genotype correlations for the variant forms. The need to assess galactosylceramide beta-galactosidase activity will be suggested by a careful history and physical assessment and by the demonstration of reduced nerve conduction velocities and marked elevation of the CSF protein level (usually in excess of 3 g/L). Cranial CT scans will show decreased white matter and increased density of the internal capsule, thalamus, and basal ganglia (Fig. 411.3). Cranial MRI scans will demonstrate the failure of myelination through a reversal of the usual gray-white appearance.

Genetic counseling and prenatal diagnosis may be provided for potential carriers. However, the existence of a pseudodeficiency state in carriers may cloud the picture and could necessitate an assessment of the ability of amniotic cell or trophoblast cultures to degrade exogenous galactoceramide. Caution must be exercised in interpreting such studies. Effective therapy for globoid cell leukodystrophy is lacking. Nonetheless, supportive care is important to assist the family during this difficult period.

ADRENOLEUKODYSTROPHY

Adrenoleukodystrophy is a multifaceted disease complex that includes X-linked adrenoleukodystrophy (ALD) and adrenomyeloneuropathy (AMN) and an autosomal recessive form, neonatal ALD, that appears in infancy (Table 411.3). Each form is characterized by excessive levels of VLCFA in plasma and tissues.

Forms of the Disease

X-linked adrenoleukodystrophy, the most common of the three disease forms, is a progressive disorder of young boys aged 3 to 16 years (mean age, 8 years) that generally begins with personality changes or altered school performance and motor deficit. Seizures occur in 20% of affected children and occasionally signal the onset of the disorder. Motor involvement may be unilateral at first. Although expression of disease is highly variable, generally, progression is relentless and results in profound psychomotor retardation, spasticity, and extensor posturing. Death occurs within 10 years of diagnosis. Adrenal insufficiency is important clinically in approximately 40% of children, although an equal number may have inadequate cortisol response to adrenocorticotropic hormone challenge. An "Addison disease only" phenotype of ALD is recognized, and may account for 40% of cases of Addison disease in men.

X-linked AMN has its onset in the third decade of life as a slowly progressive spastic paraparesis and a distal sensorimotor neuropathy. Bowel and bladder dysfunction accompany the motor disability. Adrenal insufficiency is noted frequently. X-linked ALD and AMN may occur in the same family.

Neonatal ALD is the least common of the three conditions. Beginning in early infancy, this autosomal recessive disorder represents a fundamental abnormality of the subcellular organelle known as the *peroxisome* and is related thereby to Zellweger syndrome and to neonatal Refsum disease. Neonatal

TABLE 411.3

ADRENOLEUKODYSTROPHY COMPLEX

Characteristic	Adrenoleukodystrophy	Adrenomyeloneuropathy	Neonatal Adrenoleukodystrophy
Age at onset	3–16 yr (mean, 8 yr)	20–40 yr	Infancy
Prognosis	Death in 1–10 yr	Prolonged survival	Death in 1–4 yr
Mode of inheritance	XLR	XLR	AR
Neurologic signs	Behavior problems, poor school performance, quadriparesis, blindness	Spastic paraparesis, distal neuropathy, urinary retention, impotence	Hypotonia, seizures, rapid deterioration, mild dysmorphism, hepatomegaly
Systemic signs	Hypoadrenalism in 50%, diminished response to ACTH, skin hyper-pigmentation	Hypoadrenalism, hypogonadism	Normal adrenal function, hypoplastic adrenal glands
Stored material	Very long-chain fatty acids	Very long-chain fatty acids	Very long-chain fatty acids, phytanic acid, bile acid precursors, reduced plasmalogens
Enzyme defect	Peroxisomal fatty acyl-CoA synthetase import	Peroxisomal fatty acyl-CoA synthetase	Absent or deficient peroxisomes
Feasibility of prenatal diagnosis	Yes	Yes	Yes

ACTH, adrenocorticotropic hormone; AR, autosomal recessive; XLR, X-linked recessive.

ALD is characterized by neonatal seizures, profound hypotonia, mild dysmorphic features, hepatomegaly with impaired function, and pigmentary abnormalities of the retina. Its progression is rapid, and often death occurs by the child's first birthday.

Neuropathologic evaluation of X-linked ALD/AMN demonstrates a demyelinating process with a vigorous perivascular inflammatory response corresponding to the areas of clinical involvement. Adrenal atrophy is prominent. Adrenal cortical cells are swollen, but medullary cells are spared. In addition, adrenal cortical cells contain birefringent laminar inclusions (due to VLCFA cholesterol esters) in the X-linked disorders and the neonatal form. The characteristic pathologic feature of neonatal leukodystrophy is the absence or marked reduction and morphologic alteration of peroxisomes. In addition to prominent hypomyelination, the neuropathology of the neonatal form includes heterotopias and polymicrogyria, both features common to the peroxisomal deficiency disorders (e.g., Zellweger syndrome).

A definitive diagnosis of each of these disorders depends on the demonstration of elevated levels of VLCFAs (26-carbon chain) or an elevated ratio of C26:0/C22:0 fatty acids. Thus, the metabolic defect is a failure of VLCFA beta-oxidation, a function located in the peroxisome and distinct from mitochondrial fatty-acid beta-oxidation. The specific enzymatic abnormality in X-linked ALD/AMN is the defective activation of LCFA by the peroxisomal enzyme fatty acyl coenzyme A synthetase. The molecular abnormality, however, involves a gene at Xq28 encoding a protein (ALDP) that is essential for the transport of fatty acyl-CoA synthetase into peroxisomes. Multiple mutations have been identified in this gene. This molecular heterogeneity may explain the variability in clinical expression, although it does not explain the occurrence of both X-linked forms in the same family. A separate ALDP-like protein isoform may be partially protective. The pathogenesis of demyelination, however, remains unexplained.

Neonatal ALD is marked by generalized peroxisomal dysfunction. It is accompanied by elevated phytanic acid and deficient plasmalogen and bile acid synthesis, in addition to abnormal VLCFA oxidation.

Diagnosis and Therapy

The clinical diagnosis of X-linked ALD is based on careful history and physical examination, characteristic changes seen on cranial CT (confluent hypodensities in parietooccipital white matter, with contrast enhancement at the margins suggesting active demyelination; Fig. 411.4) or cranial MRI (symmetric periventricular signal increase) examination, normal nerve conduction velocities, abnormal brainstem auditory-evoked responses (prolonged interpeak latency between waves I and V), and elevated CSF protein levels. In contrast, X-linked AMN is characterized by normal CSF protein levels and normal results on neuroimaging of the brain (mild cerebral atrophy is a possible late finding) but abnormal nerve conduction velocities and brainstem auditory-evoked responses. In addition to having elevated VLCFA levels and altered peroxisomes, children with neonatal ALD demonstrate reduced plasmalogens and elevated phytanic acid and pipecolic acid levels in plasma. Marked abnormalities of brainstem auditory-evoked responses, visual-evoked responses, and electroretinography also may assist in the clinical diagnosis.

Heterozygote detection may be accomplished reliably for X-linked ALD by combining the measurement of levels of VLCFA in plasma and cultured skin fibroblasts with that of levels of ALDP in leukocytes and cultured skin fibroblasts. As many as 5% of possible heterozygotes for X-linked ALD still may es-

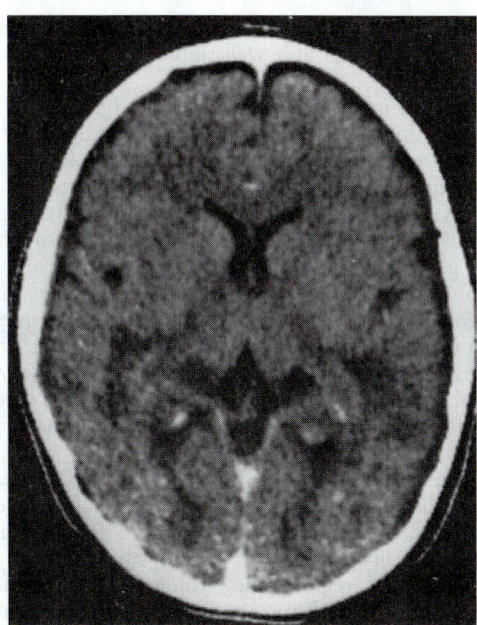

FIGURE 411.4. Enhanced brain computed tomographic scan of a child with adrenoleukodystrophy, indicating symmetric low-density lesions located posteriorly in the parietooccipital regions, with areas of contrast enhancement.

cape detection, however. Heterozygote detection is not possible for neonatal ALD. Nonetheless, prenatal diagnosis is feasible for each disorder in families known to be at risk.

Fifteen percent or more of female heterozygotes for X-linked ALD may have a relatively mild form of the disease. Such cases are characterized by a progressive spastic paraparesis, mild peripheral neuropathy, normal adrenal function, and elevated VLCFA levels in plasma or fibroblasts.

Effective therapy for the various forms of ALD is under active study. Bone marrow transplantation has not been helpful in neurologically impaired children with the X-linked ALD, but it may retard disease onset in normal or mildly affected children. Dietary therapy aimed at restricting the intake of LCFAs and at modifying their endogenous formation seems to function similarly by restricting disease onset in presymptomatic individuals. This treatment strategy appears ineffective for progressive disease.

ALEXANDER DISEASE

Alexander disease, a rare disorder of white matter caused by astrocyte dysfunction, recently was associated with mutations in glial fibrillary acidic protein (GFAP) gene, *GFAP*. Infantile, juvenile, and adult forms have been described. The infantile form appears in children from birth to age 2 years and is characterized by psychomotor retardation, spastic quadriparesis, seizures, and megalencephaly. Progression to death is rapid. Juvenile- and adult-onset forms occur much less commonly. In these forms, neurologic involvement appears to be confined to the brainstem and spinal cord, and mentation is less affected or may remain intact. In the juvenile form, onset occurs in affected children between ages 5 and 10 years and features spastic paraparesis, dysphagia, and cognitive decline, all of which are slowly progressive. Death may occur within a few years, secondary to bulbar dysfunction, or the disease course may extend to middle life. The adult form is a quite uncommon occurrence and generally presents in a way similar to multiple sclerosis (MS).

Eosinophilic inclusions, called *Rosenthal fibers,* and severe hypomyelination that vary in severity depending on the age at onset represent the characteristic neuropathologic findings. Rosenthal fibers are found near astrocyte filaments and consist largely of GFAP, alpha-beta–crystallin, and heat shock protein 27. Although these fibers are seen in individuals with other disorders (e.g., glial tumors, MS, syringomyelia), their abundance in Alexander disease is the diagnostic key. Demyelination is prominent in frontal white matter and in the brainstem. Elevated alpha-beta-crystallin and heat shock protein 27 levels in CSF have been reported. Recently, mutations in *GFAP,* including phenotype-genotype correlations, have been described. Prior to this discovery, diagnosis was based on the neuropathologic findings.

The clinical diagnosis of Alexander disease in the presence of psychomotor retardation, megalencephaly, and seizures may be aided by brain imaging (CT or MRI) that demonstrates low-density lesions in cerebral white matter, particularly the frontal region, and symmetric enhancement of caudate nuclei, the thalamus, and periventricular white matter after the administration of a contrast agent. The identification of mutations in *GFAP* will confirm the diagnosis. As such, histopathologic examination of brain tissue is no longer necessary.

Treatment is supportive, with emphasis placed on the administration of appropriate anticonvulsant agents.

CANAVAN DISEASE

Canavan disease is an autosomal recessive leukodystrophy that is noted frequently in Ashkenazi Jews and is associated neuropathologically with spongy degeneration of the brain. Onset occurs most frequently in early infancy, usually leading to death within the first decade of life. Characteristic clinical features include psychomotor retardation, spasticity, blindness with optic atrophy, and megalencephaly. Seizures may occur in 25% to 50% of patients, but generally they are not problematic. Milder forms have been described, reflecting the heterogeneity of molecular abnormalities. Brain imaging (CT or MRI) reveals diffuse white matter changes without ventriculomegaly. The finding of markedly elevated *N*-acetyl aspartic acid levels in the blood, urine, and CSF of affected children led to the identification of aspartoacylase deficiency as the biochemical abnormality and to the subsequent capability of prenatal diagnosis. The gene defect has been mapped to chromosome 17p. Multiple mutant alleles have been identified, three of which account for almost all affected Ashkenazi Jews; other mutant alleles predominate in non-Jewish individuals. The precise role of *N*-acetyl aspartic acid in the pathogenesis of this disorder is unclear, but it may involve excitatory neurotransmitter systems. No effective therapy is available.

PELIZAEUS-MERZBACHER DISEASE

Pelizaeus-Merzbacher disease (PMD) is an X-linked disorder due to duplication or point mutations in the gene, *PLP,* located at chromosome Xq22. *PLP* encodes the proteolipid protein, the major CNS myelin protein. PMD presents most commonly in infancy, with impaired motor developmental, ataxia, nystagmus (often rotatory), and cognitive impairment. Spastic

paraparesis, ataxia, and athetotic upper extremity movements dominate motor signs. Optic atrophy may be seen. Although deterioration is inevitable, developmental progress continues through childhood before a slow-paced regression becomes evident. As such, PMD occasionally is misdiagnosed as static encephalopathy. Survival into middle age is expected. A so-called connatal form may be seen shortly after birth. This form is more rapidly progressive, with death occurring by the time the affected child reaches the age of 10 years. In addition to the above features, feeding difficulties are prominent, as are seizures, optic atrophy, and stridor. Treatment is supportive in both forms.

Spastic paraparesis type 2 (SPG2) is allelic with PMD. Onset typically occurs in childhood and features spastic paraparesis and hyperreflexia without evidence of intracranial involvement. An intermediate form also may be seen, again dominated by the spastic paraparesis but with earlier onset (2 to 5 years) and the variable appearance of optic atrophy, nystagmus, and mild cognitive impairment.

In both PMD and SPG2 forms, cranial MRI reveals symmetrical white matter abnormalities indicative of hypomyelination with reversal of the typical gray-white appearance. In SPG2, the abnormalities tend to be more scattered. In PMD, cerebral white matter may have a "tigroid" pattern indicative of alternating areas with or without myelin, whereas the connatal form displays total absence of myelin. Peripheral nerve myelin appears normal. In addition, markedly abnormal visual-, auditory-, and somatosensory-evoked responses may aid in the clinical assessment.

Numerous duplications and point mutations have been identified in *PLP* and clear phenotype-genotype correlations developed. DM20, an isoform of PLP, is a closely related myelin protein. *PLP* mutations that do not alter the DM20 isoform result in the milder phenotype associated with SPG2. Establishing prenatal diagnosis is feasible.

The precise molecular defect varies among individuals, however, indicating marked molecular heterogeneity. A further complication is that fewer than 50% of individuals with clinical features of PMD have mutations in the coding region of the PLP gene. The involvement of alternative genes has been described in some individuals with similar phenotypes.

VANISHING WHITE MATTER DISEASE

Vanishing white matter (VWM) disease, also called childhood ataxia with diffuse hypomyelination (CACH) syndrome, is a rare, autosomal recessive disorder involving hypomyelination. VWM disease was mapped recently to chromosome 3q27. Onset begins in late infancy or early childhood, following initially normal development. Neurologic involvement features progressive spasticity and ataxia. Seizures, dysarthria, and optic atrophy also may be noted. Onset often occurs after acute infections or head injury followed by a relapsing and remitting pattern, again in association with infections or head injury. Survival is variable: relatively brief or extending to middle life. Cranial MRI demonstrates diffuse, symmetrical hypomyelination, a feature confirmed at pathologic examination without evidence of an inflammatory process. Mutations in the elF2B translation initiation factor have been identified in VWM disease. This protein has five subunits. Mutations have been found in each subunit. This translation initiation factor appears to be sensitive to fever, which may explain the role of infection (or trauma) in the relapsing-remitting course of this disorder.

Suggested Readings

Berger J, Löschl B, Bernheimer H, et al. Occurrence, distribution, and phenotype of arylsulfatase A mutations in patients with metachromatic leukodystrophy. *Am J Med Genet* 1997;69:335.

Bezman L, Moser AB, Raymond GV, et al. Adrenoleukodystrophy: incidence, new mutation rate, and results of extended family screening. *Ann Neurol* 2001;49:512.

Cailloux F, Gauthier-Barichard F, Mimault C, et al. Genotype-phenotype correlation in inherited brain myelination defects due to proteolipid protein gene mutations. Clinical European Network on Brain Dysmyelinating Disease. *Eur J Hum Genet* 2000;8:837.

Hodes ME, Pratt VM, Dlouhy SR. Genetics of Pelizaeus-Merzbacher disease. *Dev Neurosci* 1993;15:383.

Kaul R, Gao GP, Aloya M, et al. Canavan disease: mutations among Jewish and non-Jewish patients. *Am J Hum Genet* 1994;55:34.

Moser HW. Adrenoleukodystrophy: phenotype, genetics, pathogenesis, and therapy. *Brain* 1997;120:1485.

Percy AK. The inherited neurodegenerative disorders of childhood: clinical assessment. *J Child Neurol* 1987;2:82.

Rodriguez D, Gauthier F, Bertini E, et al. Infantile Alexander disease: spectrum of GFAP mutations and genotype-phenotype correlation. *Am J Hum Genet* 2001;69:1134.

Scriver CR, Beaudet AL, Sly WS, et al. *The metabolic and molecular bases of inherited disease*, 8th ed. New York: McGraw-Hill, 1995.

Traeger EC, Rapin I. The clinical course of Canavan disease. *Ped Neurol* 1998; 18:207.

van der Knaap MS, Leegwater PA, Konst AA, et al. Mutations in each of the five subunits of translation initiation factor eIF2B can cause leukoencephalopathy with vanishing white matter. *Ann Neurol* 2002;51:264.

Wenger DA, Rafi MA, Luzi P. Molecular genetics of Krabbe disease (globoid cell leukodystrophy): diagnostic and clinical implications. *Hum Mutat* 1997;10: 268.

CHAPTER 412 ■ METABOLIC ENCEPHALOPATHIES

EDWARD R. B. McCABE

Many of the metabolic disorders include among their clinical features abnormalities of the central nervous system (CNS). A significant portion of these disorders can be treated to prevent progression of the encephalopathy. Because of the potential for treatment, arriving quickly at a definitive diagnosis is extremely important so that appropriate treatment may be instituted promptly. Rapid and definitive diagnosis also allows the family to plan realistically for their child's future, even if a specific treatment is not available. Genetic counseling is much more accurate and informative when the diagnosis is known, and ensuring that family members have this information while they still are in their childbearing years is important. A delay in the diagnosis until a subsequent pregnancy or birth of an affected sibling occurs is particularly unfortunate.

DISORDERS OF CARBOHYDRATE METABOLISM

Hypoglycemia is a common, treatable, and often preventable cause of encephalopathy in children. Glucose is a critical substrate for energy production in the brain; when its availability is interrupted, significant CNS dysfunction results. The signs and symptoms of CNS dysfunction include convulsions and coma, but they may be less severe, involving confusion, irritability, listlessness, headache, eye rolling, and agitation. Night terrors also may accompany hypoglycemia in some patients. In addition, affected children may evidence hunger, tachycardia, or sweating, the last being especially noticeable on the brow and hands, which may be cold and clammy to the touch. Although the heart depends on fatty acids for its primary energy supply, glucose represents an important substrate; therefore, cardiomegaly with or without overt cardiac failure may be associated with hypoglycemia. Symptoms in neonates and young infants may include poor feeding, a weak or high-pitched cry, limpness, cyanosis, and vomiting. Signs and symptoms should resolve rapidly with normalization of the blood glucose level, unless the episode has been sufficiently profound or prolonged to result in dysfunction extending beyond the hypoglycemic episode. In such cases, the possibility of developing long-term sequelae is significant.

Hypoglycemia has been defined classically as a whole-blood glucose level of less than 20 mg/dL or a serum or plasma glucose level of less than 25 mg/dL in preterm or low-birth-weight infants during the first week of life; a blood glucose level of less than 30 mg/dL or a serum glucose level of less than 35 mg/dL in full-sized or term neonates from birth to 72 hours; and a blood glucose level of less than 40 mg/dL or a serum glucose level of less than 46 mg/dL thereafter. Other physicians suggest that these definitions represent population norms rather than physiologically acceptable glucose concentrations and that a blood glucose level of less than 40 mg/dL or a serum glucose level of less than 45 to 50 mg/dL should be considered hypoglycemia regardless of the age of the individual. The differential diagnosis of hypoglycemia is extensive, but the history and clinical assessment can be helpful in narrowing the possibilities (Table 412.1). Specific diagnostic testing is recommended for these disorders to tailor management, prevent recurrences, and treat the hypoglycemia effectively.

The primary complication of hypoglycemia is irreversible CNS damage. The goal of diagnosis and treatment is to prevent acute and chronic hypoglycemia, with its attendant CNS compromise. A severe acute insult may result in respiratory compromise and death from status epilepticus or coma. The clinician must carry out the diagnostic evaluation with care and discretion so as to prevent hypoglycemia. For example, medium-chain acyl-CoA dehydrogenase (MCAD) deficiency may be diagnosed by the measurement of octanoylglycine and other organic acids using tandem mass spectrometry (MS/MS) (e.g., as part of the newborn screen) without risk to the patient, whereas a fast or a fat challenge may lead to significant hypoglycemia and the risk of developing sequelae.

TABLE 412.1

METABOLIC DISORDERS ASSOCIATED WITH HYPOGLYCEMIA

Metabolic Disorders	Diagnostic Comments
Primary disorders of carbohydrate metabolism	
Glycogen storage disease	Hepatomegaly and fasting hypoglycemia with:
IA. Glucose-6-phosphate deficiency	Prominent short stature, lactic acidemia
IB. Glucose-6-phosphate translocase deficiency	Neutropenia
III. Debrancher deficiency	Elevated red blood cell glycogen
VI. Hepatic phosphorylase deficiency	Frequently a milder course
IXA. X-linked hepatic phosphorylase kinase deficiency	Mild course
IXB. Autosomal hepatic and muscle phosphorylase kinase deficiency	Mild course
IXC. Autosomal hepatic phosphorylase kinase deficiency	More severe than IXA and B, and may include hepatic cirrhosis
Fructose-1,6-diphosphatase deficiency	Profound hypoglycemia and acidemia
Hereditary fructose intolerance	
Fructose-1-phosphate aldolase deficiency	Jaundice and hepatomegaly develop after child begins sucrose-fructose intake; hypoglycemia and hypophosphatemia with fructose load
Galactosemia (galactose-1-phosphate uridylyl transferase deficiency)	Hypoglycemia rare, except with significant galactose load, and more frequently a consequence of liver disease
Glycerol intolerance	Hypoglycemia associated with fat ingestion or glycerol challenge; includes patients with fructose-1,6-diphosphate deficiency
Disorders of amino acid and organic acid metabolism	
Organic acidemias, including maple syrup urine disease, methylmalonic acidemia, propionic acidemia, isovaleric acidemia, glutaric acidemia, acetoacetyl-CoA thiolase deficiency, and others	Hypoglycemia associated with acidemia and, in some cases, with a "Reye-like" syndrome with hyperammonemia, and cerebral edema
Congenital lactic acidoses	Lactic acidemia with disturbance of gluconeogenesis or energy metabolism
Biotinidase deficiency	Hypoglycemia associated with complex organic acidemia, ataxia progressing to seizures and coma, alopecia, and rash
Disorders of fat metabolism	
MCAD, LCAD, VLCAD, LCHAD deficiency	Fasting, hypoketotic hypoglycemia associated with dicarboxylic acidemia; seen among patients with sudden infant death syndrome and acute life-threatening episodes
Endocrine disorders	
Hyperinsulinism	Postprandial and post-glucose infusion hypoglycemia; may be caused by increased islet-cell mass (as with islet cell adenoma and nesidioblastosis) or functional hyperresponsiveness (as with leucine hypersensitivity); may be exogenous, as in diabetics who receive too much insulin or individuals with Münchhausen or Münchhausen-by-proxy syndrome
Infant of a diabetic mother	A specific form of hyperinsulinism found in large-for-gestational-age neonates with a history of maternal diabetes mellitus
Hypopituitarism	Hypothalamic or pituitary hormonal deficiencies resulting in the inability to mount a normal glycemic response to stress or to tolerate starvation; may include deficiencies of growth hormone, adrenocorticotropic hormone, or thyroid hormone
Adrenal insufficiency	Seen with the congenital adrenal hyperplasias and congenital adrenal hypoplasias and with adrenal medullary unresponsiveness
Limited substrate availability	
Malnutrition	History of limited intake of protein or calories; signs and symptoms of kwashiorkor or marasmus
Ketotic hypoglycemia	Fasting, ketotic hypoglycemia; frequently preceded by intercurrent illness; also known as *accelerated starvation*; typically seen between ages 1 and 7 years
Infectious and postinfectious	
Sepsis	Hypoglycemia in all age groups; particular vigilance essential in neonatal period, when signs and symptoms of hypoglycemia may be subtle
Reye syndrome	History of chickenpox or flu-like illness; aspirin is an important risk factor; inherited metabolic diseases represent an increasing proportion of cases
Neonatal	Must seek underlying etiology, especially sepsis, maternal diabetes; limited substrate availability renders neonates particularly vulnerable
Shock	Must consider hypoglycemia as possibly contributory in any individual with shock until glycemic status is determined
Liver disease	Must consider metabolic and nonmetabolic disorders as underlying etiologies
Toxic	Includes exogenous insulin, sulfonylureas, salicylates, propranolol, L-asparaginase, and others

LCAD, long-chain acyl-CoA deficiency; LCHAD, long-chain hydroxy acyl-CoA deficiency; MCAD, medium-chain acyl-CoA dehydrogenase; VLCAD, very long-chain hydroxy acyl-CoA deficiency.

To avoid repeated hypoglycemic episodes, if a definitive diagnosis has not been made, and the risk of spontaneous or challenge-induced hypoglycemia exists, the diagnostic plan should be worked out well ahead of time so that the necessary information may be obtained if the child becomes symptomatic. A secure intravenous line should be in place in any hospitalized patient who is at risk for developing iatrogenic or spontaneous hypoglycemia, and the blood glucose should be measured at an appropriate frequency to attempt to anticipate and prevent symptomatic episodes and their sequelae.

The treatment of an acute hypoglycemic episode involves the rapid restoration of normoglycemia to supply this substrate to the CNS. If venous access is readily available, the most rapid and effective therapy is the administration of intravenous glucose delivered at a rate of 0.5 to 1.0 g/kg, or 2 to 4 mL/kg of a 25-g/dL (25%) dextrose solution given at a rate of 1 mL/minute. The glucose infusion should continue at a rate of 8 to 10 mg/kg/minute, with frequent measurement taken of the blood glucose concentration and necessary adjustments made in the infusion rate to maintain a normal blood glucose level. If hypoglycemia persists despite increasing glucose infusion rates, hyperinsulinism should be considered. After the blood glucose level has stabilized and feeding has been reinitiated, the infusion rate may be decreased slowly but never discontinued abruptly. Even in the absence of pathologic hyperinsulinemia, the insulin level will rise physiologically in response to the administration of glucose; therefore, the glucose infusion must be tapered slowly (by decrements of 4 to 6 mg/kg/minute at 4- to 6-hour intervals) to prevent rebound hypoglycemia.

Hypoglycemia is a medical emergency and, if percutaneous venous access is not achieved rapidly, a cutdown should be performed by someone who is skilled in this technique; alternatively, in the young child, interosseous access should be considered. Additional supportive measures, including endotracheal intubation, may be necessary.

For the child with milder hypoglycemia, oral glucose may be beneficial, but care must be taken to protect against aspiration if the child is becoming obtunded. Glucagon (0.03 to 0.30 mg/kg, up to a maximum total dose of 1 mg intramuscularly) may be given, but with the knowledge that if it is effective, the benefit may be only transient. For patients with certain glycogen storage diseases, ketotic hypoglycemia, and other disorders in which glycogen has been depleted or is unavailable, it may have a minimal effect or none at all. Diazoxide, an antihypertensive agent that also suppresses insulin release, may be useful in certain patients with hyperinsulinemia. The usual starting dosage of diazoxide is 8 to 12 mg/kg/day, given orally in divided doses every 8 to 12 hours, but the dose may range between 5 and 20 mg/kg/day. Marked hypertrichosis is a prominent side effect that should be discussed with the parents at the time the drug is started because it may become objectionable enough to them to interfere with compliance. The hypertrichosis is reversible when the drug is discontinued. Hemoglobin A_1c may be used to monitor the magnitude of hyperglycemic excursions. Small, frequent feedings are useful for many patients with hypoglycemia, although the composition of the feedings differs according to the underlying disorder. Feedings may be supplemented with a slow-release glucose in the form of uncooked cornstarch, starting at 1.6 g/kg every 4 hours for children younger than 2 years of age and 1.75 to 2.50 g/kg every 6 hours in older children. Water or diet drinks are the preferred vehicles for suspension of the uncooked cornstarch (weight-to-volume ratio, 1:2) because these liquids avoid other sugars, which is important for certain hypoglycemic disorders, and do not contain natural amylases, such as may be present in some natural juices.

Home glucose monitoring may be valuable for many patients because of the variable course and response of any individual. With proper education and oversight, home monitoring will provide reassurance to patients and families and can reduce the risk of developing hypoglycemia.

With severe and prolonged hypoglycemia, permanent encephalopathy is not an unusual event, particularly in young children. Learning disability, attention deficit disorder, developmental delay, ataxia, spasticity, or seizures may be seen. Seizures associated with normal blood glucose concentrations should be treated with the usual anticonvulsant medications. The family of a child with sequelae should be counseled regarding infant stimulation and special education. Most families have concerns regarding the genetic risk of recurrence, although they may not voice their concerns to the physician; therefore, this topic should be addressed with all families.

DISEASES OF COPPER METABOLISM

Menkes Syndrome

Menkes syndrome, also known as *kinky-hair disease* or *steely hair disease*, is an X-linked disorder characterized by progressive neurologic deterioration beginning in the first 4 to 8 weeks of life, with apathy, somnolence, feeding difficulties, and myoclonic seizures. Many of these patients are born prematurely, fail to thrive, and have hypothermia. Patients also can be seen with sepsis. Their muscle tone varies from hypotonia and flaccidity to hypertonia and spasticity. The descriptive names for this disorder derive from the dull, hypopigmented, sparse, and kinky appearance of the hair (resembling steel wool). Microscopically, pili torti and monilethrix with friable, short hair are present. The child's face typically is pale, with pudgy cheeks, a prominent vermilion border (described as a "cupid's bow" mouth), and microcephaly. The arteries are tortuous, with defective, fragmented elastic fibers. Generalized or focal cerebral and cerebellar degeneration may be present and may result from the vascular abnormalities. Low serum copper concentrations, low circulating ceruloplasmin levels, and decreased hepatic and brain copper content are observed.

Copper absorption from the intestine is deficient in Menkes syndrome, and elevated copper content in the intestinal mucosa, kidney, spleen, lung, muscle, pancreas, and placenta has suggested defective copper transport. The copper level is increased in cultured fibroblasts. The gene responsible for Menkes syndrome maps to Xq12–q13 and codes for the adenosine triphosphatase (ATPase), Cu^{2+}-transporting, alpha polypeptide (ATP7A). ATP7A is a copper-binding P-type ATPase that is involved in the transport of copper and homeostasis.

Although progression followed by death in infancy or during the toddler years is a typical occurrence, individuals with milder forms of this disorder have been described. Patients with the occipital horn syndrome have allelic mutations in ATP7A and also have cutis laxa, bladder diverticula with occasional rupture, skeletal abnormalities, and mild mental retardation.

Treatment with copper in the form of copper histidinate has been reported to prevent progression of the neurodegeneration, but this treatment remains experimental, with considerable question existing with regard to its general efficacy in patients with this disease. If it has any possibility of being effective, treatment with copper must be initiated as early as possible in patients with Menkes syndrome.

Wilson Disease

Wilson disease, or hepatolenticular degeneration, is a disorder with a variable clinical presentation, but typical features

TABLE 412.2

THE HUMAN PORPHYRIAS

Disease	Deficient Enzyme	Genetics	Porphyria Classification	Major Symptoms		
				Neuro-Psychiatric	Visceral	Photo-Sensitivity
ALAD porphyria	(2*) ALAD	AR	Acute hepatic	+	+	−
Acute intermittent porphyria	(3) HMB synthase	AD	Acute hepatic	+	+	−
Congenital erythropoietic porphyria	(4) Urogen III cosynthase	AR	Erythropoietic	−	−	+
Porphyria cutanea tarda	(5) Urogen decarboxylase	AD	Hepatic	−	−	+
Hepatoerythropoietic porphyria	(5) Urogen decarboxylase	AR	Hepatoerythropoietic	−	±	+
Hereditary coproporphyria	(6) Coprogen oxidase	AD	Acute hepatic	+	+	±
Variegate porphyria	(7) Protogen oxidase	AD	Acute hepatic	+	+	±
Erythropoietic protoporphyria	(8) Ferrochelatase	AD	Erythropoietic	−	±	+

−, not elevated; ±, may or may not be elevated; +, elevated; AD, autosomal dominant; ALA, delta-aminolevulinic acid; ALAD, delta-aminolevulinic acid dehydratase; AR, autosomal recessive; Copro, coproporphyrinogen (coprogen); 7-CP, 7-carboxylic porphyrins; HMB, hydroxymethylbilane; IsoCP, isocoproporphyrins; Proto, protoporphyrinogen (protogen); RBCs, red blood cells; Uro, uroporphyrinogen (urogen).
*Number in parentheses is enzyme sequence in the heme synthetic pathway.

include neurologic manifestations, hepatocellular disease, Kayser-Fleischer rings of the cornea, a low serum ceruloplasmin level, and increased concentrations of copper in the serum, urine, and liver. Two neurologic forms are recognized, although their signs and symptoms overlap. Commonly, the dystonic form is associated with liver disease in children, and symptoms include rigidity progressing to contractures. Choreiform or athetoid movements are manifestations of the lenticular degeneration. The pseudosclerotic form is typified by tremors and adult onset, with a longer-term progression than that of the dystonic form. The neurologic dysfunction associated with Wilson disease primarily is motor, with no sensory component. Psychiatric manifestations may be seen, may be the primary complaint, and may be diagnosed as schizophrenia. Frequently, deterioration in school performance, alterations of mood, and acting out are not recognized as manifestations of organic disease in these patients and are attributed to problems of preadolescent and adolescent socialization. Even if neurologic features are subtle or absent, the presence of Kayser-Fleischer rings by gross visual or slit-lamp examination provides valuable clinical information. The corneal rings are present in virtually all patients with neurologic or psychiatric symptoms but only in two-thirds or fewer of those with hepatic abnormalities.

Additional features of Wilson disease include acute or chronic hepatocellular disease, renal dysfunction, hemolytic anemia, neutropenia, thrombocytopenia, osteoporosis, osteomalacia, pathologic fractures, arthritis, cardiomyopathy, and hypoparathyroidism. Renal manifestations may range from generalized aminoaciduria to full renal Fanconi syndrome, uricosuria with hypouricemia, renal lithiasis, nephrocalcinosis, and renal failure. In affected patients, generally the serum ceruloplasmin level is less than 20 mg/dL. Normal ceruloplasmin values are low in young infants (younger than 3 months), however, and ceruloplasmin levels may be normal in as many as 5% of patients with Wilson disease. An elevated copper content, detected on liver biopsy, is a particularly valuable measure. Although normal values vary among laboratories, the hepatic copper content of affected patients generally is at least two- to fivefold above the upper limit of normal and frequently is elevated tenfold or more. The serum copper concentration may

be low, but overlap with the normal range renders it a less useful diagnostic test. Urinary copper excretion is increased from less than 40 μg/24 hours in normal individuals to 100 to 1,000 μg/24 hours in affected patients. A test dose of penicillamine at 10 mg/kg results in an increase in copper excretion to 1,200 to 3,000 μg/24 hours in patients with Wilson disease. Ensuring that all containers, solutions, and equipment (including biopsy needles) used to collect tissue and fluids for copper determination are free of contaminating copper is important because its presence could interfere with accurate measurement. The incorporation of intravenously administered radioactive copper into ceruloplasmin also has been used in diagnosing this condition.

Wilson disease is an autosomal recessive disorder involving a gene that maps to 13q14.3, is designated *ATYP7B*, and has striking similarity to the P-type ATPase ATP7A responsible for Menkes syndrome.

Because the clinical features and age at onset of Wilson disorder are so variable, physicians should subject siblings of affected patients to clinical and laboratory examination. Mildly symptomatic or presymptomatic individuals can be detected in this manner. Because of the variability in clinical expression of Wilson disease, the differential diagnosis can be very broad, including acute viral hepatitis, chronic active hepatitis, alpha$_1$-antitrypsin deficiency, and other causes of liver disease associated with progressive neurologic deterioration or dementia, including the porphyrias. Kayser-Fleischer rings, when present, however, are definitive.

The treatment of Wilson disease using D-penicillamine (Cuprimine) or triethylene tetramine (TETA or trientine) for copper chelation, or zinc sulfate or acetate to block copper absorption, should be instituted as early as possible in the course of the disease, with the best results obtained in patients in whom treatment has been started before symptoms arise. The usual dosage of penicillamine is 20 mg/kg/day up to 500 to 750 mg/day in children younger than 10 years and 1,000 mg/day in older individuals, although dosages as high as 3,000 mg/day have been used. D-Penicillamine is given in two to four divided doses. It is an agent with a significant incidence of side effects, including allergic reactions, bone marrow suppression, and a variety of rashes. These effects may be prevented or

TABLE 412.2

(CONTINUED)

Tissue for Enzyme Diagnosis[†]	Increased Intermediates in RBC			Increased Intermediates in Urine					Increased Intermediates in Stool		
	Uro	Copro	Proto	ALA	PBG	Uro	Copro	7-CP	Copro	Proto	IsoCP
RBCs	−	−	+	+	−	−	+	−	−	−	−
RBCs, fibroblasts, liver, lymphocytes, amniotic fluid cells	−	−	−	+	+	−	−	−	−	−	−
RBCs, fibroblasts, aminocytes	+	±	−	−	−	+	+	−	+	−	−
RBCs, liver	−	−	−	−	−	+	±	+	±	−	+
RBCs, fibroblasts	−	−	+	−	−	+	−	+	−	−	+
Fibroblasts, leukocytes	−	−	−	+	+	+	+	−	+	±	−
Fibroblasts, lymphocytes	−	−	−	+	+	−	+	−	+	+	−
Erythrocytes, fibroblasts	−	−	+	−	−	−	−	−	±	+	−

[†]Enzymatic diagnosis may be possible using other tissues but has been well documented in those tissues listed. Prenatal diagnosis at an enzymatic level theoretically is possible in all, but data are limited. In autosomal dominant disorders, family studies may be necessary in an attempt to evaluate heterozygous levels of activity.

minimized by starting the drug at a dosage of 200 to 250 mg/day and increasing the dosage at weekly intervals by increments of 200 to 250 mg/day to achieve urinary copper excretions of greater than 2 mg/day early in treatment. TETA is given before meals, three times a day, as 400- to 800-mg doses to achieve a 24-hour urinary copper excretion similar to that for penicillamine, and it apparently has minimal side effects, as compared with penicillamine. Zinc sulfate or acetate is given in three to four doses per day at least 1 hour before meals at 100 to 150 mg zinc per day. The restriction of copper intake should be considered, although strict restriction may be impractical. Supplementation of zinc not only induces metallothionein but prevents zinc deficiency from chelation and decreases copper absorption by competition for uptake. Vitamin B_6 should be supplemented in patients receiving penicillamine because this drug (particularly the L-isomer, but perhaps the D-isomer to a lesser extent) inhibits pyridoxine-dependent enzymes and can produce signs of pyridoxine deficiency.

The prognosis for patients with Wilson disease and acute fulminant hepatitis is poor, but treatment should include peritoneal dialysis and possibly plasmapheresis. The aggressive and effective extraction of copper may not be successful in saving the lives of such individuals. Liver transplantation has been effective in treating patients with Wilson disease, even those with acute disease, and should be considered in patients who do not respond to chelation, including those with acute, fulminant disease.

PORPHYRIAS

The porphyrias are inborn errors of the heme biosynthetic pathway. Not all the porphyrias are associated with encephalopathy, but all are described here for the purposes of differential diagnosis and completeness. Those porphyrias with neuropsychiatric features are the acute hepatic porphyrias (Table 412.2).

Heme biosynthesis is diagrammed in Figure 412.1 and explained in Box 412.1. Table 412.2 details the clinical features of the porphyrias, listing them according to the enzyme sequence from step 2 through step 8. The disorders are discussed in the same sequence in the text.

Aminolevulinic acid (ALA) synthase is the initial and rate-limiting enzyme of heme biosynthesis, and it is regulated by negative feedback from the end product of the pathway, heme.

Two genes are recognized for this enzyme: *ALAS1* encodes the housekeeping gene and maps to 3p21, and *ALAS2* is the erythroid-specific gene and maps to Xp11.21. A defect in *ALAS2* results in X-linked sideroblastic anemia, which is characterized by hypochromic microcytic anemia that frequently is detected in childhood, hemochromatosis that leads to death at a relatively young age, hyperferricemia, increased peripheral siderocytes after splenectomy, and reduced protoporphyrin levels in the microcytes.

Delta-Aminolevulinic Acid Dehydratase Porphyria

ALA dehydratase deficiency is an extremely rare autosomal recessive porphyria. Affected patients have varied from an infant with severe involvement and failure to thrive to a man in his seventh decade with minimal involvement. Hypotonia and paralysis may result in respiratory failure. Other features include vomiting and pain involving the extremities and abdomen. Remissions and exacerbations are typical occurrences, with exacerbations associated with inanition, stress, or ethanol intake. ALA dehydratase activity is decreased in erythrocytes to approximately 2% of normal levels. Intermediate ALA dehydratase activity to approximately 50% has been documented in parents and other relatives of affected individuals, without associated symptomatology. The ALA dehydratase gene has been mapped to 9q34, and mutation analysis has been performed. The treatment of acute episodes using intravenous glucose may be helpful in some patients. Clinical similarities with acute intermittent porphyria (AIP) suggest consideration of a treatment regimen modeled on that for the more common AIP.

Acute Intermittent Porphyria

AIP is an autosomal dominant deficiency of hydroxymethyl-bilane (HMB) synthase, formerly known as porphobilinogen (PBG) deaminase, which maps to the long arm of chromosome 11 (11q23.3). It is considered to be the most common of the inborn errors of porphyrin metabolism, with an estimated incidence of five to 10 per 100,000 in the United States, although as many as 90% of individuals with PBG deaminase deficiency are asymptomatic.

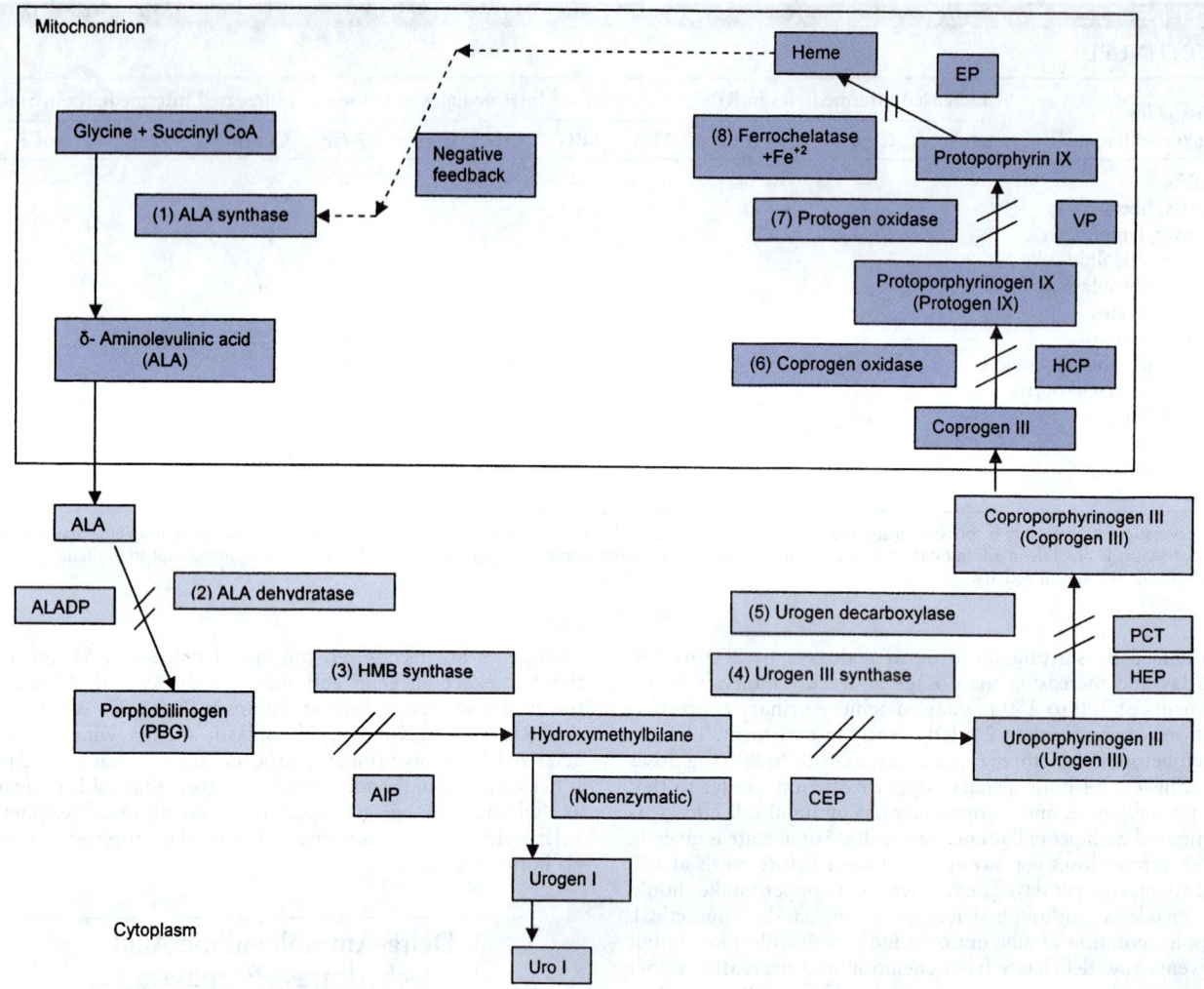

FIGURE 412.1. Heme biosynthesis, showing the eight enzymatic steps. AIP, acute intermittent porphyria; ALADP, delta-aminolevulinic acid dehydratase porphyria; CEP, congenital erythropoietic porphyria; EP, erythropoietic protoporphyria; HCP, hereditary coproporphyria; HEP, hepatoerythropoietic porphyria; PCT, porphyria cutanea tarda; Uro, urogen decarboxylase; VP, variegate porphyria.

The characteristic features of acute episodes are severe abdominal pain and port wine urine. Associated vomiting, constipation, abdominal distention, and ileus may lead to the diagnosis of surgical abdomen, but surgery should be avoided whenever possible during these attacks. Diarrhea and urinary retention or incontinence may be seen. Tachycardia, hypertension or hypotension, fever, leukocytosis, and seizures may accompany attacks, as may psychiatric disturbances, including disorientation, hallucinations, paranoia, anxiety, and depression. Motor neuropathy is seen more commonly than is sensory neuropathy and is of extreme concern because bulbar paralysis and respiratory insufficiency can occur and may be fatal.

Symptomatic AIP is a rare occurrence before puberty but has been reported. Acute attacks are precipitated by a variety of drugs, most of which induce ALA synthase. Prominent among these agents are barbiturates, phenytoin (Dilantin), oral contraceptives, sulfonamides, and valproic acid. AIP attacks also may occur with menstrual periods, decreased food intake, and stress. Stress factors include infections, ethanol intoxication, and surgery.

Frequently, PBG and ALA levels are elevated in the urine, but they may be normal or minimally increased, especially in asymptomatic individuals with HMB synthase deficiency. HMB synthase activity in erythrocytes is reduced to approximately 50% of normal; however, because the wide variation in normal values can lead to an overlap of enzyme activity between patients with AIP and normal control individuals, enzyme activity should be measured in the parents of affected children and in other family members. Occasionally, patients have normal red cell HMB synthase levels, and cultured fibroblasts may be used to measure enzyme activity. The enzyme deficiency also is expressed in amniotic fluid cells, liver, and lymphocytes. The HMB synthase mutations have been analyzed.

The mainstay of treatment is to prevent attacks by avoiding precipitating influences, including known exacerbating medications and stresses. An increased oral intake of carbohydrates should be attempted early in an attack; if the patient does not respond to this treatment, intravenous dextrose infusions should be used. These patients should be monitored for inappropriate antidiuretic hormone secretion. Propranolol has been used to control tachycardia and hypertension. The pain of an acute attack is severe, but it may be treated with a narcotic analgesic (e.g., morphine) and a phenothiazine (e.g., chlorpromazine), although the narcotic analgesic increases the

---

BOX 412.1   Steps in Heme Biosynthesis

- Of the eight enzymatic steps in this pathway, four are mitochondrial: delta-aminolevulinic acid (ALA) synthase (step 1), coproporphyrinogen (coprogen) oxidase (step 6), protoporphyrinogen (protogen) oxidase (step 7), and ferrochelatase (step 8).
- Four enzymes are cytoplasmic: ALA dehydratase (step 2), porphobilinogen (PBG) deaminase (step 3), uroporphyrinogen III (urogen III) synthase (UROS, step 4), and urogen decarboxylase (UROD, step 5).
- Clinical disorders are associated with all eight steps: step 1 with X-linked sideroblastic anemia and steps 2 through 8 with porphyrias. ALA and coprogen III move between the mitochondrial and cytoplasmic compartments, but no defects in the transport of these intermediates have been noted.
- Eight clinically distinct porphyrias are associated with seven enzymes (steps 2 to 8): Porphyria cutanea tarda (PCT) is caused by the heterozygous deficiency of step 5 (urogen decarboxylase), and hepatoerythropoietic porphyria is caused by the homozygous deficiency of this same enzyme.

tendency toward constipation and urinary retention. Intravenous hematin is used for acute attacks and for prophylaxis. The intravenous preparation may be given in a dosage of up to 3 to 4 mg/kg over the course of at least 30 minutes, as often as every 12 hours. Administration of hematin has been associated with reversible renal shutdown after excessive doses and with a coagulopathy. Frequently, phlebitis and thrombophlebitis are seen with the administration of intravenous hematin in as many as 50% of patients treated at the higher dose. For prophylaxis against recurrent perimenstrual attacks, the dose is 200 mg weekly.

Congenital Erythropoietic Porphyria

Congenital erythropoietic porphyria (CEP) is a rare autosomal recessive porphyria resulting from homozygous deficiency for urogen III synthase (UROS), which maps to 10q25.2–q26.3. Although usually its onset occurs in infancy, some patients are asymptomatic until adulthood. Frequently, CEP is suspected first on the basis of reddish to brown staining in a neonate's or infant's diapers. Photosensitivity is noted in an infant or young child, with the presence of vesicles and bullae that become crusted and superinfected in exposed areas of the skin. Scarring associated with hyperpigmentation and deformity, with particular involvement of the phalanges, ears, and nose, is seen in some patients. Hypertrichosis in the form of fine, downy hair over the face and extremities is a common finding. Porphyrin deposits in the teeth cause a reddish or brownish discoloration. The teeth and the serous vesicular fluid exhibit a red fluorescence under ultraviolet light because of the elevated content of porphyrin. Other features include hemolytic anemia, splenomegaly, gallstones, and pathologic fractures.

UROS activity can be measured in erythrocytes, fibroblasts, and amniocytes, and mutation analysis has been performed. Treatment involves protection from sunlight by limiting exposure and using sunscreen, administration of beta-carotene, protection from trauma, and aggressive treatment of cutaneous

infections to prevent scarring and deformity. Hypersplenism is an indication for performing total or subtotal splenectomy, and some patients respond with reduced photosensitivity. Infusions of hematin have been used successfully in patients with this disorder. Charcoal, which binds porphyrins, has been used orally with beneficial results: plasma and cutaneous porphyrin levels were reduced and symptoms were abated. Bone marrow transplantation is effective in some patients.

Porphyria Cutanea Tarda

PCT is a common porphyria, and two types represent the majority of patients: type I, or "sporadic," and type II, or familial. Levels of urogen decarboxylase (UROD) are decreased to 50% in both types, with the reduction typically found only in the liver in type I but generalized, including the liver and erythrocytes, in type II. The sporadic form occurs in association with ethanol abuse, estrogen intake, or iron ingestion, as well as with other toxins or disorders. Type I PCT may occur in more than one individual in a family and may be genetically heterogeneous. Type I PCT is seen more commonly in adults, whereas type II typically has its onset in childhood. Vesicles and bullae of the exposed skin, with crusting, scarring, and hyperpigmentation, occur in both types, as does increased fragility of the skin. Hypertrichosis of the face may develop. Hepatic cirrhosis and siderosis are common findings, and an increased incidence of hepatocellular carcinoma is present.

The urinary concentration of uroporphyrin exceeds that of coproporphyrin. The UROD locus maps to 1p34. UROD mutation analysis has been performed in familial PCT.

Treatment includes the avoidance of precipitating exposures and protection from sunlight. Phlebotomy has been used and is presumed to work by decreasing total body iron levels. Chloroquine may be effective by forming a complex with porphyrins and improving their clearance, but its use has been associated with retinopathy.

Hepatoerythropoietic Porphyria

Hepatoerythropoietic porphyria is a rare porphyria caused by a homozygous deficiency of urogen decarboxylase. Patients may be seen at any age, from infancy through adulthood. The porphyrins in this disorder have their origins in the liver and bone marrow. Clinical features include cutaneous photosensitivity, hypertrichosis, pigmentation of the urine and teeth, hemolytic anemia, and hepatosplenomegaly. The severity of the photosensitivity is similar to that seen in patients with CEP and more severe than that noted in individuals with erythropoietic protoporphyria (EP). Red cells and fibroblasts may be used for enzymatic diagnosis, and mutation analysis has been carried out. Current therapy relies on protection from sun exposure, although oral charcoal might prove beneficial, as it has for CEP.

Hereditary Coproporphyria

Hereditary coproporphyria (HCP) is an autosomal dominant disorder that is characterized by approximately 50% activity of coprogen oxidase that maps to 3q12, although several cases of homozygous HCP also have been seen. The clinical features of HCP are similar to those of AIP and include abdominal pain, gastrointestinal disturbances, and neuropsychiatric complaints, but approximately 30% of affected patients have photosensitivity as well. Paralysis, respiratory failure, and death have been reported. The disease has presented in the second decade of life and beyond. Precipitating features are similar to those of other acute hepatic porphyrias, with barbiturates being a common offender. Excessive urinary excretion of coproporphyrin is typical, with elevated excretion of ALA, PBG, and uroporphyrin during acute episodes. Coprogen oxidase can be assayed in the fibroblasts and leukocytes of patients with the disease, and mutation analysis is available. A homozygous HCP with an earlier onset also has been described. Treatment is similar to that for AIP.

Variegate Porphyria

Typically, variegate porphyria (VP) is the autosomal dominant heterozygous deficiency of protoporphyrinogen (protogen) oxidase. A relatively common disorder in South African whites, elsewhere it is somewhat less common than is AIP. This acute hepatic porphyria may present with neuropsychiatric and visceral features similar to those of AIP and HCP or with cutaneous photosensitivity. The skin findings are identical to those in patients with PCT, and the diagnosis of PCT may be made erroneously when the presentation is solely cutaneous. Precipitating factors are those of AIP and HCP. Homozygous VP is a rare occurrence and presents clinically in childhood with more severe manifestations of the usual symptoms; it also may include mental retardation, prominent neurologic features, and growth delay.

"Pseudoporphyria" has been described, with porphyrin excretion resembling that in VP after the consumption of excessive quantities of porphyrin-containing brewers' yeast tablets. The plasma of patients with VP has a characteristic fluorescence emission at 626 nm. Protogen oxidase can be measured in lymphocytes and fibroblasts. The gene for protogen oxidase maps to 1q22, and mutations have been determined. Treatment involves the avoidance of factors associated with acute episodes, protection from the sun, and other measures described for AIP.

Erythropoietic Protoporphyria

EP is the autosomal dominant heterozygous deficiency of ferrochelatase (18q21.3), the final step in heme synthesis that involves the insertion of iron into protoporphyrin. EP is the most common of the erythropoietic porphyrias. Cutaneous photosensitivity is relatively mild and is noted first in childhood, usually before the child reaches 10 years of age, with exposure to the sun or other bright light causing burning, edema, itching, and erythema. Generally, lesions resolve after a few hours, although petechiae, purpura, vesicles, and crusting may develop and may last several days before clearing. Scarring and disfigurement are not typical features of this porphyria, although mild scarring and hyperkeratosis may be seen after chronic eczematoid lesions have resolved. Anemia is a rare occurrence and, when present, is nonhemolytic. Gallstones are relatively common findings. Hepatocellular disease is a rare occurrence but may be severe, progressing rapidly to cirrhosis and death. The presence of protoporphyrin in the red cells, plasma, and stool is characteristic of patients with EP. Ferrochelatase activity varies between 15% and 50% of normal in affected individuals, and mutation analysis is available.

The primary cause of clinical problems in patients with EP is sunlight or strong artificial light. If exposure cannot be avoided, topical sunscreens may be of some help if they have a high sun protection factor (SPF 26 or greater). Oral high-dose beta carotene (usually 120 to 180 mg/day to reach the recommended serum concentration of 600 to 800 μg/dL) is considered useful but requires several weeks or months before tolerance to

sunlight improves. In addition, the dosages necessary may lead to carotene discoloration of the skin. In the past, drugs and chemicals were not considered precipitating factors; with a recognition of the potential severity of the associated liver disease, however, more attention is being paid to protecting patients from these agents. Iron, vitamin E, and cholestyramine have been recommended to prevent progression once hepatocellular disease is noted, but data on their efficacy are limited. Hypertransfusion therapy may be beneficial through the suppression of hematopoiesis. Liver transplantation for patients with hepatic failure has produced only transient benefit because of the accumulation of protoporphyrin by the transplanted liver.

DISORDERS OF AMINO AND ORGANIC ACID METABOLISM

Hypoglycemia with or without Hyperammonemia

Hypoglycemic disorders, including maple syrup urine disease, methylmalonic acidemia, propionic acidemia, isovaleric acidemia, glutaric acidemia, and acetoacetyl-CoA thiolase deficiency, generally present with acidemia that may be associated with a condition similar to Reye syndrome, and these disorders should be considered in any patient with Reye syndrome, especially in those with a family history or a history of recurrence. Quantitative serum amino acid levels are diagnostic in patients with maple syrup urine disease and may be helpful, but they are not diagnostic in patients with those other organic acidemias that are characterized as ketotic hyperglycinemias. Urine organic acid analysis is diagnostic in the latter and is indicated by the metabolic acidemia, odor (in patients with maple syrup urine disease and isovaleric acidemia, or "sweaty feet" disease), and neurologic symptoms. Acetoacetyl-CoA thiolase deficiency should be considered in the differential diagnosis of "idiopathic ketotic hypoglycemia." These patients have metabolic acidemia during hypoglycemic episodes. The urine organic acid analysis may reveal only beta-hydroxybutyrate, and measurement of enzyme activity may be required for diagnosis.

MCAD deficiency is characterized by nonketotic or hypoketotic fasting hypoglycemia. The urine organic acid analysis may show dicarboxylic aciduria, with adipic, suberic, and sebacic acids. Octanoylglycine is diagnostic of MCAD deficiency. Frequently, affected patients show evidence of a reduced serum free-carnitine concentration, with an increased proportion of acyl carnitines. Additional disorders of fatty-acid metabolism that present typically with hypoketotic hypoglycemia are long-chain acyl-CoA dehydrogenase deficiency, very long-chain acyl-CoA dehydrogenase deficiency, and long-chain hydroxy acyl-CoA deficiency.

Hyperammonemias

Hyperammonemia is characteristic of the urea cycle disorders, but it also may be seen in patients with lysinuric protein intolerance, the hyperornithinemia-hyperammonemia-homocitrullinuria syndrome, transient hyperammonemia, and organic acidemias, as mentioned earlier. Neonates exhibit poor feeding, vomiting, and lethargy, which progresses to seizures, coma, and death. Patients with milder disease, who are seen later in infancy or childhood, may have episodic problems, including ataxia. Respiratory alkalosis from central stimulation, along with vomiting, are typical features of hyperammonemia.

The determination of blood ammonia, quantitative serum amino acids (with particular attention to citrulline), and urine organic acid levels is important diagnostic testing that should be followed by specific enzymatic assays.

Intractable Seizures

Hypsarrhythmia and myoclonus beginning early in life are typical of nonketotic hyperglycinemia. This autosomal recessive deficiency of cleavage enzyme can be diagnosed by the detection of elevated cerebrospinal fluid glycine levels; generally, serum and urine glycine concentrations are increased as well. Beta-alaninemia is an extremely rare disorder with a similar clinical presentation.

Developmental Delay

Phenylketonuria (PKU) is the prototype among these amino acid disorders. Others, however, including variants of maple syrup urine disease and the organic acidemias, may have mental retardation as the main characteristic. Quantitative serum amino acid measurements, including MS/MS, urine homocys-tine detection, and urine organic acid analyses, are used to screen for these disorders.

Autistic Behavior and Psychiatric Disturbances

Older children with untreated PKU may evidence autistic behavior and schizophrenic symptoms. Schizophrenic behavior also has been described in some older patients with homocystinuria.

OTHER DISORDERS

Other disorders that should be included in the differential diagnosis of the metabolic encephalopathies, and that can be investigated by specific laboratory tests, include many of the lysosomal storage diseases, certain of the peroxisomal disorders (especially Zellweger cerebrohepatorenal syndrome with elevated very long-chain fatty acid levels), Lesch-Nyhan syndrome (hypoxanthine-guanine phosphoribosyltransferase deficiency), and primary or secondary hypophosphatemia.

CHAPTER 413 ■ RETT SYNDROME

ALAN K. PERCY

Rett syndrome is a pervasive developmental disorder affecting predominantly females. After a period of apparently normal development, affected children experience a plateau in development and then a rapid decline in motor and cognitive function, usually between the ages of 6 to 18 months. The principal clinical features are loss of purposeful hand use; development of stereotypic hand movements, such as hand washing, hand wringing, and hand tapping (Fig. 413.1); and loss of communication and socialization skills. Generally, these children say a few words initially, but meaningful verbal communication is lost with onset of the disorder. In addition, eye contact is very poor, leading to interpretation of their behavior as being autistic. Acquired deceleration of head growth is noted as early as 3 months of life; other features include periodic breathing, including breath holding or hyperventilation or both, while awake. Seizures occur in many of these children and may consist of staring spells, complex partial, and generalized tonic-clonic events. Pervasive growth failure, including poor weight gain, short stature, and small hand and foot size, is evident. In addition, the hands and feet tend to be markedly cooler and discolored (bluish) when compared to the remainder of the extremities. Diminished response to pain often is noted. Gastrointestinal dysfunction manifested as gastroesophageal (GE) reflux and constipation may be prominent. In later childhood and early adolescence, scoliosis is a common finding.

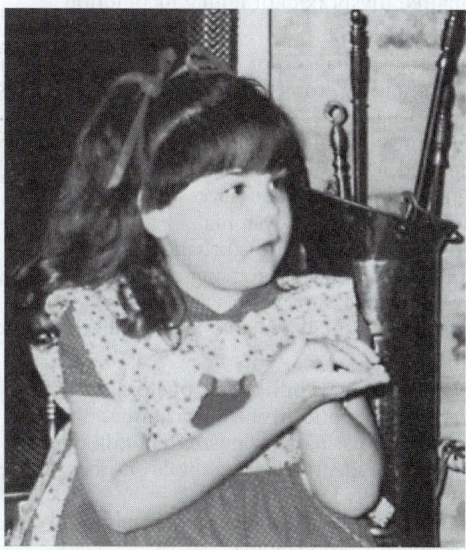

FIGURE 413.1. Photograph of a 5-year-old girl with Rett syndrome, demonstrating the typical hand position associated with the disorder.

Although the behavioral mannerisms (hand stereotypies and periodic breathing) seen in Rett syndrome are confined to wakefulness, sleep often is interrupted, and uncontrollable screaming is a common occurrence, especially during the first few years of life. A lengthy, relatively stable phase, during which the episodes of screaming and the behavioral mannerisms may become milder, follows the early period of decline. Attentiveness and eye contact improve such that communication may occur through gaze or eye pointing or augmentative communication. Survival into adulthood is typical. Because Rett syndrome has been recognized for only 40 years, and accurate clinical diagnosis only since the 1980s, the natural history including survival of Rett syndrome has not been elucidated fully.

In 1999, our understanding of Rett syndrome advanced dramatically, with the identification of mutations in the gene *MECP2*, which encodes methyl-CpG-binding protein 2. Mutations in *MECP2* have been identified in up to 95% of females fulfilling the clinical criteria for Rett syndrome (Box 413.1). As such, the diagnosis of Rett syndrome still is based on well-established clinical criteria. Further, the spectrum of clinical expression in females has widened considerably, with descriptions of several variant forms being based on different patterns of expression. With the identification of mutations in *MECP2*,

affected males also have been detected. However, they generally present a quite different clinical picture, ranging from severe, fatal encephalopathy both sporadically and in the male siblings of affected females to typical Rett syndrome in males with Klinefelter syndrome or somatic mosaicism. Familial X-linked mental retardation has been noted in males with *MECP2* mutations, but lacking other features of Rett syndrome.

Neuroimaging reveals no parenchymal abnormalities except for mild to moderate cerebral atrophy. Volumetric studies indicate specific reductions in frontal cortex and caudate nuclei. The electroencephalogram (EEG) typically is abnormal, featuring slowing, loss of occipital dominant rhythm, and the appearance of multifocal spike-and-wave epileptiform activity. Previous reports of biogenic amine metabolite reduction in the cerebrospinal fluid (CSF) have not been found consistently. Elevated CSF beta-endorphin levels have been noted in most instances, but this finding is not specific to Rett syndrome. Abnormalities have been described also in glutamate and nerve growth factor levels in CSF and in acetylcholine, dopamine, and glutamate neurotransmitter systems in the brain. Neuropathologic assessment has revealed intriguing abnormalities in addition to reduced brain weight. The principal findings have been reduced pigmentation within neurons of the substantia nigra, reduced neuronal size, and reduced synaptic connections. These findings suggest a fundamental abnormality in brain development, most likely occurring near the time of birth. The exact role of *MECP2* in this process is unknown at present. The availability of mouse models should provide insight into the pathobiologic mechanism.

The prevalence rate for Rett syndrome is one per 10,000 to 15,000, exceeding that of phenylketonuria in females. Most affected individuals are the result of new mutations, the majority of which appear to occur in the paternal germline. The recurrence of Rett syndrome within individual families has been reported in fewer than 1% of cases. When recurrence has been described in more than one generation, transmission has occurred through the mother. The association of *MECP2* mutations and Rett syndrome has allowed the development of phenotype-genotype correlations. Indeed, some mutations do produce milder clinical involvement. However, variations in X-inactivation patterns are likely to modify the effect of specific mutations. The predominance of Rett syndrome in females is explained partly by the modifying influence of the normal X chromosome, whereas similar mutations in males likely will produce a more severe phenotype. In addition, the occurrence of new mutations in the father will yield only affected females.

The differential diagnosis of Rett syndrome includes infantile autism, with which it has been confused most frequently. If the clinical criteria for autism and Rett syndrome are applied carefully, however, one should have no difficulty in making the distinction. In addition, all children with acquired deceleration of head growth and a diagnosis of progressive cerebral palsy should be evaluated carefully for Rett syndrome. Angelman syndrome, often associated with a 15q deletion, may resemble Rett syndrome during early stages and should be excluded with appropriate molecular testing. Finally, other neurodegenerative disorders, such as infantile neuronal ceroid lipofuscinosis, should be considered. Periodic breathing also occurs in children with Joubert syndrome. Children with Joubert syndrome have structural abnormalities of the cerebellum on neuroimaging, differentiating them from those of Rett syndrome.

No specific therapy is available. Most affected children achieve independent walking. Some will lose this capability in later stages and thus become susceptible to the complications of relative immobility, including orthopedic deformities, particularly progressive scoliosis. Antiepileptic agents are indicated if seizures occur. Carbamazepine has been particularly

---

BOX 413.1 — Diagnostic Criteria for Rett Syndrome

Necessary Criteria

1. Apparently normal prenatal and perinatal history
2. Psychomotor development largely normal through the first 6 months or may be delayed from birth
3. Normal head circumference at birth
4. Postnatal deceleration of head growth in the majority
5. Loss of achieved purposeful hand skill between ages of 6 months to 2.5 years
6. Stereotypic hand movements such as hand wringing/squeezing, clapping/tapping, mouthing and washing/rubbing automatisms
7. Emerging social withdrawal, communication dysfunction, loss of learned words, and cognitive impairment
8. Impaired (dyspraxic) or failing locomotion

Supportive Criteria

1. Awake disturbances of breathing (hyperventilation, breath-holding, forced expulsion of air or saliva, air swallowing)
2. Bruxism
3. Impaired sleep pattern from early infancy
4. Abnormal muscle tone successively associated with muscle wasting and dystonia
5. Peripheral vasomotor disturbances
6. Scoliosis/kyphosis progressing through childhood
7. Growth retardation
8. Hypotrophic small and cold feet; small, thin hands

Exclusion Criteria

1. Organomegaly or other signs of storage disease
2. Retinopathy, optic atrophy, or cataract
3. Evidence of perinatal or postnatal brain damage
4. Existence of identifiable metabolic or other progressive neurologic disorder
5. Acquired neurological disorders resulting from severe infections or head trauma

effective; lamotrigine and valproate are suitable alternatives. Nutritional supplementation, including gastrostomy feeding to promote adequate dietary intake, may be required. Constipation is a common occurrence and requires careful attention. Early childhood education and programs involving physical and occupational therapy should be tailored to individual children. Prolonged survival requires appropriate prospective care to minimize the development of future medical and orthopedic complications.

Suggested Readings

Amir RE, Van den Veyver IB, Schultz R, et al. Influence of Mutation Type and X Chromosome Inactivation on Rett Syndrome Phenotypes. *Ann Neurol* 2000;47:670.

Amir RE, Van den Veyver IB, Wan M, et al. Rett syndrome is caused by mutations in X-linked *MECP2*, encoding methyl-CpG-binding protein 2. *Nature Genet* 1999;23:185.

Armstrong DD. Review of Rett syndrome. *J Neuropathol Exp Neurol* 1997;56: 843.

Hagberg B, Aicardi J, Dias K, et al. A progressive syndrome of autism, dementia, ataxia, and loss of purposeful hand use in girls: Rett's syndrome—report of 35 cases. *Ann Neurol* 1983;14:471.

Hagberg B, Hanefeld F, Percy A, Skjeldal O. An update on clinically applicable diagnostic criteria in Rett syndrome. *Europ J Paediatr Neurol* 2002;6:293.

Percy A, Gillberg C, Hagberg B, et al. Rett syndrome and the autistic disorders. *Neurol Clin* 1990;8:659.

Percy AK, Lane JB. Rett syndrome: clinical and molecular update. *Curr Opin Pediatr* 2004;16:670.

Rett A. Uber ein eigenartiges hirnatrophisches syndrome bei hyperammonämie im kindesalter. *Wien Med Wochenschr* 1966;116:723.

Schanen C, Houwink EJF, Dorrani N, et al. Phenotypic manifestations of *MECP2* mutations in classical and atypical Rett syndrome. *Am J Med Genet* 2004;126:129.

Shahbazian MD, Young JI, Yuva-Paylor LA, et al. Mice with truncated MeCP2 recapitulate many Rett syndrome features and display hyperacetylation of histone H3. *Neuron* 2002;35:243.

CHAPTER 414 ■ BASAL GANGLIA AND NEUROTRANSMITTER DISORDERS

JOSEPH JANKOVIC

Biochemical or structural pathology in the basal ganglia may be manifested by movement disorders, groups of neurologic diseases, or syndromes that are characterized either by slowness, paucity, and "freezing" of voluntary movement (bradykinesia, akinesia) or by excess abnormal involuntary movement (hyperkinesia, dyskinesia). The basal ganglia seem to be important in the initiation, scaling, and controlling of the amplitude and direction of movement. This complex of deep nuclei is divided anatomically into the corpus striatum, the globus pallidus, and the substantia nigra (Fig. 414.1). The corpus striatum, which includes the caudate nucleus and the putamen, receives input from the cerebral cortex and the thalamus and, in turn, projects to the globus pallidus. The substantia nigra is divided into the dopamine-rich pars compacta, which

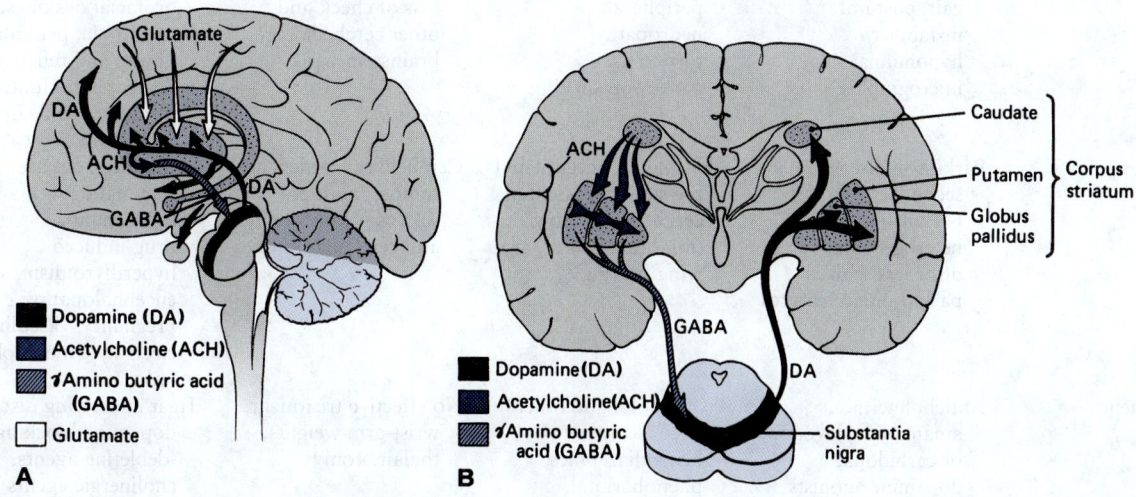

FIGURE 414.1. Brain diagram showing some important neurotransmitter pathways involved in disorders of the basal ganglia. **A:** Sagittal section. **B:** Coronal section.

is darkly pigmented because of a high content of neuromelanin, and the less dense pars reticularis. The pars reticularis is similar histologically and chemically to the medial segment of the globus pallidus, and both project by way of the thalamus to the premotor and motor cortex. The pars compacta gives rise to the nigral-striatal pathway, which is the main dopaminergic tract. The output of the basal ganglia, which once was thought to be in parallel with the pyramidal system (hence the term *extrapyramidal*), projects by way of the thalamus to the cerebral cortex and then to the pyramidal system. Integration of the basal ganglia with the cortex facilitates motor control.

The diagnosis of a particular movement disorder depends primarily on careful observation of the clinical phenomena. Often, the bradykinetic movement disorders are accompanied by rigidity, postural instability, and loss of automatic associated movements. The hyperkinetic involuntary movements are differentiated phenomenologically according to their characteristic clinical features: rapidity and duration of contractions, rhythmicity, pattern, and suppressibility (Table 414.1). In general, abnormal involuntary movements are exaggerated with stress and disappear during sleep; however, certain forms of myoclonus and tics may persist during all stages of sleep. In a clinic devoted to movement disorders, tics are the hyperkinetic movements observed most commonly in children, followed in lessening frequency by dystonia, stereotypies, choreoathetosis, tremors, and myoclonus.

PARKINSONISM

Parkinson Disease

Parkinson disease (PD) usually is a condition of middle and late life, but the early-onset parkinsonism (before age 40) and juvenile parkinsonism (before age 20) seems to be recognized with increasing frequency. Although the rigid, akinetic form of parkinsonism appears to occur more commonly in the juvenile cases, the typical resting tremor is present in many affected patients. Dystonia (often involving the legs), levodopa-induced dyskinesias, and clinical fluctuations seem to be particularly common occurrences in the juvenile cases. Some patients with familial juvenile parkinsonism belong to group with the "hereditary dystonia-parkinsonism syndrome." The pathogenesis of PD is further described in Box 414.1. Many other types of parkinsonism, some of which have their onset in childhood (Box 414.1), have been identified.

Wilson Disease

Wilson disease (WD) is one of the most important causes of juvenile parkinsonism and other movement disorders. Failure to

---

TABLE 414.1

DIFFERENTIAL DIAGNOSIS OF HYPERKINETIC MOVEMENT DISORDERS

| Clinical Features | Tremor | | | Chorea |
	At Rest	Postural	Kinetic	
Characteristics	3- to 7-Hz supination-pronation oscillatory ("pill rolling"): hands, legs, lips, jaw (alternating contractions of antagonists)	4- to 12-Hz flexion-extension oscillatory movement with arms outstretched: hands, arms, head, voice, legs (simultaneous contractions of antagonists)	3- to 5-Hz intention tremor on finger-to-nose and heel-to-shin test	Rapid, abrupt, flowing, unsustained, random, semipurposeful, nonpatterned; athetosis is a slow chorea (writhing movement)
Associated features	Bradykinesia, rigidity (cog-wheel), shuffling gait, postural instability, hypomimia, micrographia	Dystonia, parkinsonism, and hereditary peripheral neuropathy, torticollis, parkinsonism	Ataxia, titubation, dysdiadochokinesia, loss of check and other cerebellar or brainstem signs	"Milkmaid's grip," darting tongue, orofacial dyskinesia, hypotonia, pendular or "hung-up" reflexes, dementia in Huntington disease, carditis in Sydenham chorea
Etiology	Parkinson disease, secondary parkinsonism, heterogeneous disorders with parkinsonian features	Physiologic, accentuated physiologic, essential cerebellar outflow (midbrain rubral, wing beating)	Cerebellar disorders and tumors, multiple sclerosis, brainstem and cerebellar strokes	Huntington disease, rheumatic fever (Sydenham), drug-induced hyperthyroidism, static encephalopathy, pregnancy, vasculitis, electrolyte metabolic imbalance
Treatment	Anticholinergics, amantadine, levodopa or carbidopa, dopamine agonists	Propranolol and other beta-blockers, benzodiazepines, phenobarbital, pyrimidine, clonazepam, amantadine, alcohol	No effective treatment, wrist-arm weights, thalamotomy	Treat underlying disorder, dopamine-blocking or -depleting agents, cholinergic agents

diagnose this condition may have tragic consequences, including death, as a result of irreversible liver cirrhosis and profound neurologic deficit. The gene for this autosomal recessive hepatolenticular degenerative disease has been linked to the esterase D locus on the long arm of chromosome 13. Numerous mutations have been identified in the WD gene, which encodes copper-transporting P-type adenosine triphosphatase (ATPase) and has been termed *ATP7B*. The prevalence of the gene in the overall population is approximately 1%, although symptomatic WD is a relatively rare event (estimated prevalence, 30 per 1 million). The hepatic and neurologic dysfunction associated with WD is caused by a defect in copper metabolism, resulting from a reduction in the rate at which copper is incorporated into ceruloplasmin and a decrease in the rate at which it is excreted from the liver. Usually, low ceruloplasmin levels are found in patients with WD, but they do not seem to

be the primary defect because some patients with the disease and some heterozygotes have normal levels. Furthermore, the ceruloplasmin gene has been mapped to chromosome 3, not to chromosome 13. The excess copper not only accumulates in the liver and brain but also can cause renal tubule damage, osteoporosis, and arthropathy. Kayser-Fleischer rings, the best-recognized ophthalmologic sign of WD, are caused by the deposition of copper in the cornea.

Usually, the onset of WD occurs between adolescence and age 40, and its presentation seems to be age-dependent, with hepatic failure being more common in children and neurologic or psychiatric symptoms occurring frequently in adults. In a nonselected population of 31 patients with WD, the mean age at onset was 21 ± 5 years; 61% had neurologic symptoms, 13% had liver symptoms, and 10% had a combination of neurologic and liver problems. Approximately one-third of patients

TABLE 414.1

DIFFERENTIAL DIAGNOSIS OF HYPERKINETIC MOVEMENT DISORDERS (CONTINUED)

| | | | Myoclonus | | |
Stereotypy	Dystonia	Ballism	Generalized	Segmental	Tics
Repetitive, purposeless movements resembling normal voluntary movements	Sustained, twisting, usually low but may be rapid and may progress to fixed contractures (dystonic postures)	Abrupt, random, forceful, violent, flinging, usually proximal and unilateral, often spontaneously remits	Abrupt, irregular, brief, jerklike contractions of one or more muscles occurring synchronously or asynchronously, may be stimulus-sensitive	Rhythmic contraction of agonists, not stimulus-sensitive, may persist during sleep	Rapid, sudden, unpredictable, coordinated jerks preceded by inner urge, waxing and waning, temporarily suppressible
Often associated with akathisia (sensory and motor restlessness)	Torticollis, writer's cramp, blepharospasm, spasmodic dysphonia, essential tremor, hypertrophy of contracted muscles	Initial hemiparesis, later choreoathetosis	Encephalopathy, seizures, dementia, periodic electroencephalogram, enhanced somatosensory evoked potentials	Palatal myoclonus may be associated with bulbar palsy; spinal myoclonus may be associated with myelopathy	Vocalizations, coprolalia, echolalia, copropraxia, echopraxia, obsessive-compulsive behavior, attention deficit disorder, sleep disturbance
Usually drug-induced (tardive dyskinesia) schizophrenia, autism, mental retardation, Rett syndrome	Dystonia musculorum deformans, adult-onset torsion dystonia, drug-induced	Lesion of contra-lateral subthalamic nucleus (hemorrhage, infarction, rarely tumor)	Postanoxic, uremic, and other encephalopathies, Creutzfeldt-Jakob disease, subacute sclerosing panencephalitis, myoclonic epilepsy, Ramsay Hunt syndrome	Brainstem or spinal cord infarction, hemorrhage, myelitis, demyelinating disease	Gilles de la Tourette syndrome, transient tic of childhood
May improve with dopamine blockers or depleters, beta-blockers, opioid agonists or antagonists	Muscle relaxants, anti-cholinergics, tetra-benazine, baclofen, dopamine agonists, levodopa for diurnal dystonia, C botu-linum toxin injections, thalamotomy	Dopamine-blocking or -depleting agents, thalamotomy	Clonazepam, 5-hydroxy-tryptophan, sodium valproate, piracetam, lisuride	Tetrabenzine, 5-hydroxytryptophan, clonazepam, anti-cholinergics	Dopamine-blocking or -depleting agents

BOX 414.1   Classification of Parkinsonism

Primary Parkinson Disease
Idiopathic, dominated by:
  Tremor
  Postural instability, gait difficulty
  Akinesia (freezing)
  Dementia
  Depression
  Sensory disturbance
  Autonomic dysfunction
Inherited, associated with essential tremor, dystonia, or
  peripheral neuropathy
Young-onset, associated with dystonia or essential tremor

Secondary Parkinsonism
Drugs (dopamine-blocking and -depleting drugs,
  alpha-methyldopa, lithium, diazoxide, flunarizine,
  cinnarizine)
Toxins (manganese, mercury, carbon monoxide, cyanide,
  carbon disulfide, methanol, ethanol, MPTP)
Metabolic (parathyroid, acquired hepatocerebral degen-
  eration, GM$_1$ gangliosidosis, Gaucher disease)
Encephalitis and postencephalitic syndrome
Slow virus (Creutzfeldt-Jakob disease)
Vascular (multiinfarct, Binswanger disease)
Brain tumor
Trauma and pugilistic encephalopathy
Hydrocephalus (normal and high-pressure)
Syringomesencephalia

Multiple System Degenerations (Parkinsonism Plus)
Sporadic
  Progressive supranuclear palsy (ophthalmoparesis)
  Shy-Drager syndrome (dysautonomia)
  Olivopontocerebellar atrophy (ataxia)
  Parkinsonism-dementia-amyotrophic lateral sclerosis
    complex
  Striatonigral degeneration
  Corticodentonigra degeneration with neuronal
    achromasia
  Alzheimer disease
Inherited
  Huntington disease
  Wilson disease
  Hallervorden-Spatz disease
  Familial parkinsonism-dementia syndrome
  Familial basal ganglia calcification
  Neuroacanthocytosis
  Spinocerebellar-nigral degeneration and Joseph disease
  Glutamate dehydrogenase deficiency

MPTP, 1-methyl-4-phenyl-1,2,3,6-tetrahydropyridine.
Modified with permission from Jankovic J. Parkinson's disease
and related disorders of movements. In: Calne DB, ed. *Handbook
of experimental pharmacology*. Berlin: Springer-Verlag, 1989:
227.

findings at first evaluation were dysarthria (97%), dystonia (65%), dysdiadochokinesia (58%), rigidity (52%), gait and postural abnormalities (42%), tremor (32%), abnormal eye movements (32%), hyperreflexia (29%), drooling (23%), and bradykinesia (19%).

Because of its variable clinical expression, establishing the diagnosis of WD often is delayed. Almost all patients with neurologic disease have Kayser-Fleischer rings, but this yellow-brown deposit at the limbus of the cornea may be noted also in patients with primary biliary cirrhosis and active hepatitis with cirrhosis. Occasionally, a "sunflower cataract" may be seen as a result of copper deposition in the lens.

Usually, the diagnosis of WD is confirmed by the demonstration of low serum copper and ceruloplasmin levels, increased urine copper concentrations after a dose of penicillamine, and a rise in the level of copper in the liver (Table 414.2). The ratio of radioactivity in the plasma at 24 hours to that at 2 hours after the administration of an oral or intravenous dose of copper[64] is less than 0.5 in patients with WD (the equivalent value being greater than 0.8 in normal individuals). Other laboratory abnormalities often detected in patients with WD include aminoaciduria, hypercalciuria, glycosuria, leukopenia, hemolytic anemia, thrombocytopenia, and renal tubal deficit. In approximately one-half of affected patients, computed tomographic (CT) scanning of the brain reveals characteristic hypodense areas in the region of the basal ganglia, and often magnetic resonance imaging (MRI) reveals on T2-weighted images hypointensity that extends from the globus pallidum into the putamen. Extensive degeneration of the corpus striatum, particularly the putamen, is seen at autopsy. Also, the cerebellum, brainstem, and subcortical white matter may be involved.

The goals of treating patients with WD are to reduce copper intake and to create a negative copper balance by increasing copper output in the urine. D-Penicillamine at dosages of 0.5 to 2.0 g/day has been used successfully to chelate copper. However, penicillamine often produces considerable toxicity, including fever, urticaria, leukopenia, nephritis, thrombocytopenia, systemic lupus erythematosus, hemolytic anemia, Goodpasture syndrome, pyridoxine deficiency, and a syndrome resembling myasthenia gravis. Trientine hydrochloride (Syprine) in dosages of 400 to 800 mg three times daily before meals has been approved for the treatment of penicillamine-sensitive patients with WD. In addition to the chelating agents, zinc sulfate at a dosage of 300 to 1,200 mg/day between meals may reduce the absorption of copper. When early diagnosis is made and dietary and chelating therapies are instituted, the progression of liver and neurologic dysfunction can be halted and even reversed. At least 2,000 μg of copper should be excreted during the first 24 hours of penicillamine therapy. Approximately one-third of patients with WD experience deterioration despite receiving penicillamine therapy, but most improve, sometimes after a latent period lasting several weeks or months. In patients with parkinsonian symptoms, levodopa and anticholinergic therapy may provide symptomatic relief.

Besides the treatment of patients with symptomatic WD, of paramount importance is screening all their relatives and instituting therapy immediately if the disease is diagnosed in any of them. Patients who fail to improve with chelating or other pharmacologic therapy may experience marked relief of neurologic symptoms several months after undergoing liver transplantation.

Huntington Disease

The usual onset of Huntington disease (HD) occurs in the fourth and fifth decades of life, but it is seen in approximately

had psychiatric symptoms, including depression, emotional lability, personality change, and slow mentation, at onset of disease. Another one-third had neurologic symptoms, particularly parkinsonism, pseudobulbar palsy, tremor, and dystonia; 14% had symptoms of liver disease; and 17% had their condition diagnosed by family screening. The most common neurologic

TABLE 414.2

LABORATORY TESTS IN WILSON DISEASE

Laboratory Tests (Units)	Normal	Wilson Disease
Serum copper (μg/dL)	90–140	<60 (10–100)
Serum ceruloplasmin (mg/dL)	24–45	<15 (0–30)
Urine copper (μg/24 hr)	<40	>200 (100–1,000)
Urine copper after penicillamine (μg/6 hr)	<400	>800
Liver copper (μg/g wet weight)	<10	>30
Liver uptake (^{64}Cu at 24 hr)	>60%	<50%
Plasma (^{64}Cu 24:2 hr ratio)	>0.8	<0.5

10% of affected patients during childhood or adolescence. Both juvenile and adult-onset HD are autosomal dominant traits, with a defective gene mapped to a terminal band of the short arm of chromosome 4. The gene mutation was found to consist of an unstable enlargement of the CAG repeat sequence at 4p16.3. Most patients with juvenile HD have the akinetic-rigid syndrome termed the *Westphal variant*. Other features of juvenile HD include dementia, seizures, and ataxia. In addition, patients with juvenile HD are more likely to have inherited the abnormal gene from their father than from their mother, and they tend to segregate within families. Although the medium-sized spiny neurons (type I cells) usually are affected first in the adult form of HD, the large spiny cells have been suggested to degenerate first in the juvenile form. In contrast to the caudate nucleus, which typically is involved in the adult form of HD, the putamen seems to be most damaged in the juvenile form of the disease.

The diagnosis of HD can be established with 100% accuracy with the demonstration of the presence of more than 40 CAG repeats in one of the alleles in the HD gene. The psychological and social impact of such testing, however, must be considered carefully before presymptomatic individuals are tested.

The most remarkable biochemical change observed in the brains of adults with HD is a reduction in the activity of glutamic acid decarboxylase, particularly in the corpus striatum, substantia nigra, and other basal ganglia. In contrast, thyrotropin-releasing hormone, neurotensin, somatostatin, and neuropeptide Y are increased in the corpus striatum. The depletion of gamma-aminobutyric acid in the corpus striatum may result in disinhibition of the nigral-striatal pathway. Coupled with the accumulation of somatostatin, the net result may be the release of striatal dopamine, which results in chorea. Dopamine-blocking drugs, such as haloperidol, and dopamine-depleting agents, including tetrabenazine, often are useful in controlling chorea. In patients with childhood HD, which usually is manifested by parkinsonian features, levodopa may provide symptomatic relief.

Hallervorden-Spatz Disease

In contrast to WD, which is characterized by the abnormal deposition of copper, the hallmark of neurodegeneration with brain iron accumulation (NBIA), previously referred to as Hallervorden-Spatz disease, is the deposition of iron, particularly in the globus pallidus and substantia nigra. Usually, NBIA starts in patients between the ages of 4 and 12 years, but occasionally it presents as parkinsonian dementia in adult life. Children with NBIA have posture and gait abnormalities, bradykinesia, rigidity, and other parkinsonian features, including tremor. In addition, other hyperkinetic movement disorders,

particularly dystonia and choreoathetosis, may be seen. Further symptoms include progressive dysarthria, dementia, ataxia, spasticity, seizure disorder, optic atrophy, and retinitis pigmentosa.

Most cases are inherited in an autosomal recessive pattern, but many occur sporadically, and some phenotypically similar cases seem to be inherited by autosomal dominant transmission. Mutations in the gene *PANK2*, localized to 20p12.3–p13, have been identified in a subset of patients with NBIA, referred to as pantothenate kinase-associated neurodegeneration (PKAN). Testing for the most frequent mutations has been used to confirm the diagnosis of PKAN. The disease also may be suspected when a MRI scan shows a central focus of increased T2-signal intensity surrounded by a zone of decreased signal in the region of the globus pallidus (eye-of-the-tiger sign) (Fig. 414.2).

Furthermore, increased iron uptake in the basal ganglia may be demonstrated by scintillation counting after the infusion of radioactive iron (^{59}Fe). Increased iron uptake is confirmed also by postmortem examination, which reveals pigmentary degeneration of the basal ganglia, particularly the internal segment of the globus pallidus and the zona reticularis of the substantia nigra. These pigmentary changes are caused by a threefold to fourfold accumulation of iron in these areas. Another distinctive pathologic feature of NBIA is marked neuroaxonal degeneration, with the formation of spheroids. These glycoprotein-containing axonal swellings have been attributed to abnormal peroxidation. The abnormal accumulation of cysteine was demonstrated in one of our patients with NBIA. This increased cysteine may chelate ferrous iron, which in turn promotes the generation of free radicals, causing the characteristic neuropathologic changes of the disease. Iron chelation with desferrioxamine and antioxidant therapy has been tried in patients with NBIA, but no benefit has been demonstrated.

Levodopa and anticholinergic drugs may provide modest symptomatic relief of parkinsonian symptoms. In addition, botulinum toxin injections usually are effective in the treatment of focal dystonia (see the section, Dystonia).

HYPERKINETIC MOVEMENT DISORDERS

Tremor

Essential tremor (ET) is the most common cause of an oscillatory involuntary movement during childhood (Box 414.2). ET may start at any age, including infancy. One form of infantile ET is the hereditary chin tremor, which consists of rhythmic,

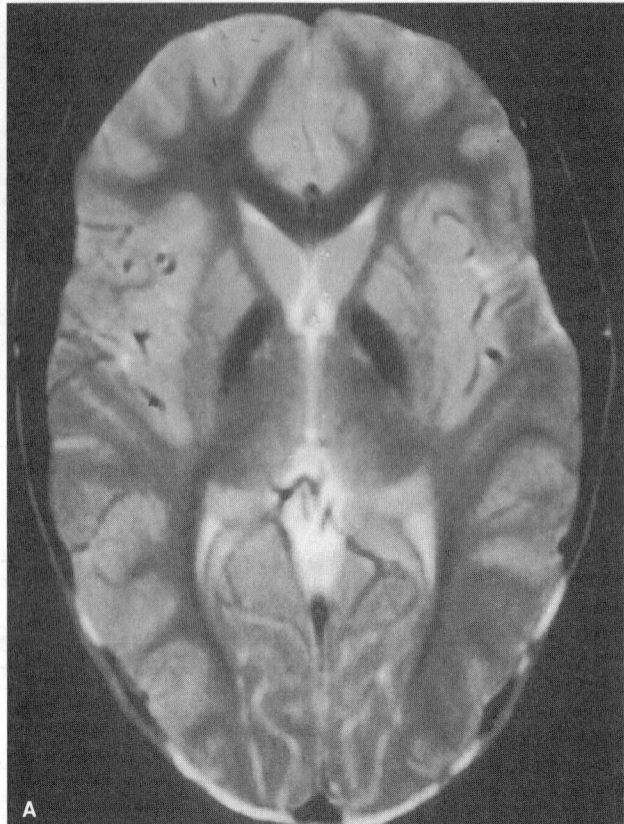

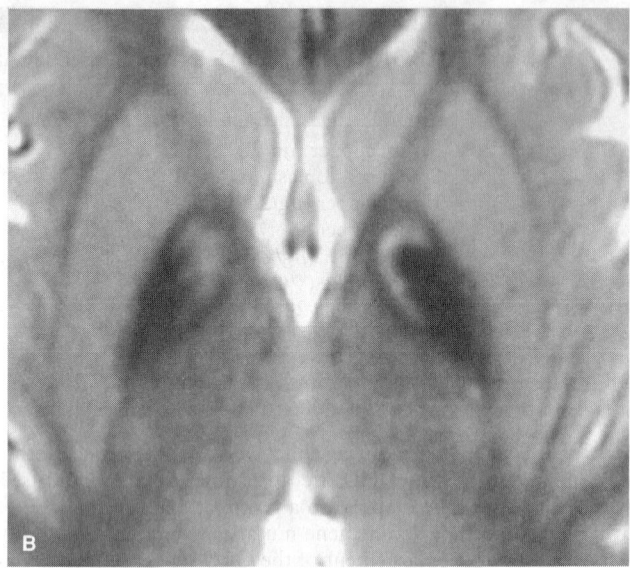

FIGURE 414.2. MRI of a patient with NBIA showing hypointensity with relative hyperintensity in the anteromedial globus pallidus on T_2-weighted MRI, the so-called "eye-of-the-tiger" sign.

three-per-second contractions of the chin that often are associated with deafness and are inherited in an autosomal dominant pattern. Another form of ET that begins during infancy or early childhood is so-called shuddering attacks. Affected children may have more than 100 attacks a day, but symptom-free intervals may last as long as 2 weeks. The attacks are characterized by bursts of rapid trembling of the entire body, occasionally associated with head turning, involuntary sniffing, and throat clearing. During the attacks, affected children usually sink to the floor; the attacks may persist during sleep.

In addition to these forms of ET, the characteristic action-postural tremor also may be seen in children. Often, the slower tremor (approximately 6.5 Hz) involves the head and neck, whereas the more rapid tremor (8 to 12 Hz) tends to involve the hands. Many other variants of ET have been recognized, however. Although ET usually is "benign," it occasionally can progress to a very disabling movement disorder, interfering with writing, feeding, speaking, and other activities of daily living.

Usually, ET is inherited in an autosomal dominant manner, and a locus has been found on chromosome 2p22–p25. Although abnormalities of neurotransmitters in the basal ganglia are suspected to underlie ET, no pathologic changes have been documented in the few brains that have been examined at autopsy. Besides the beta blockers, primidone, gabapentin, topiramate, lorazepam, alprazolam, clonazepam, amantadine, clonidine, and ethanol may improve ET.

Other oscillatory involuntary movements occasionally seen in infants and children are "head nodding," which often is associated with congenital nystagmus, including spasmus nutans, and the "bobble-headed doll's syndrome," which is seen with diencephalic lesions, including third-ventricle cysts or tumors, craniopharyngioma, hydrocephalus, and hypothalamic lesions.

Chorea, Athetosis, and Ballism

Chorea consists of continuous, unsustained, rapid, abrupt, and random contractions, whereas athetosis consists of nonpatterned, writhing movements that represent a form of "slow chorea." In contrast, ballism is a form of severe, coarse chorea; usually, it is unilateral (hemiballism) and often is the result of a lesion in the contralateral subthalamic nucleus and adjacent structures. Many acquired and hereditary types of chorea can become manifest during childhood (Box 414.3). Almost all normal infants make movements that resemble chorea, but usually this physiologic chorea resolves by the time they reach the age of 8 months. Children with attention deficit disorder and hyperactivity have distal chorea called *chorea minima*.

Cerebral Palsy

Of the various causes of chorea that occur in childhood, static encephalopathy (cerebral palsy) probably is the most common (see Chapter 396). Approximately one-third of patients with cerebral palsy have chorea or athetosis (choreoathetosis) as the predominant motor disturbance, but dystonia also was seen in 70% of such patients in one study of dyskinetic cerebral palsy. The involuntary movements are notable in one-half of affected patients during the first year, and athetosis develops in the remainder over the subsequent 4 or 5 years. In one study, 82% of

---

BOX 414.2   Classification of Tremors

Rest tremors
Parkinson tremor
Parkinson disease
Secondary parkinsonism
  Postencephalic
  Toxic disorder (phenothiazines, butyrophenones,
    metoclopramide, reserpine, tetrabenazine, carbon
    monoxide, manganese, MPTP, carbon disulfide)
  Tumor
  Trauma
  Vascular disorder
  Metabolic tremor: hypoparathyroidism, chronic
    hepatocerebral degeneration
Parkinsonism plus (heterogeneous system
  degenerations)
Olivopontocerebellar atrophy
Progressive supranuclear palsy
Wilson disease
Huntington disease
Spasmus nutans
Hereditary chin quivering
Other
Midbrain (rubral) tremor
Severe essential tremor
Roussy-Lévy syndrome

Action tremors
Postural tremors
Physiologic tremor
  Normal physiologic tremor
  Accentuated physiologic tremor
    Stress-induced (anxiety, fight, fatigue, fever)
    Endocrine (thyrotoxicosis, hypoglycemia,
      pheochromocytoma)
    Drugs, toxins (epinephrine, isoproterenol, caffeine,
      theophylline and other sympathomimetic agents,
      levodopa, amphetamines, lithium, tricyclic
      antidepressant, phenothiazines, butyrophenones,
      thyroxine, hypoglycemic agents,
      adrenocorticosteroids, alcohol withdrawal, mercury,
      lead, arsenic, bismuth, carbon monoxide,
      methylbromide, monosodium glutamate, sodium
      valproate, metrizamide, meperidine)
Essential tremor
  Autosomal dominant
  With peripheral neuropathy: Charcot-Marie-Tooth
    disease (Roussy-Lévy syndrome)

With other movement disorders (parkinsonism, torsion
  dystonia, spasmodic torticollis, myoclonus)
Factors that accentuate physiologic tremor and also
  enhance or unmask essential tremor
Vitamin E deficiency
Action tremor of parkinsonism
Neuropathic tremor
  Peripheral neuropathies
  Motor neuron disease
Cerebellar postural hypotonic tremor (titubation)
Midbrain ("rubral") tremor
Dystonic (axial) tremor
Kinetic (intention) tremor
Cerebellar outflow tremor (superior cerebellar peduncle
  lesion)
  Multiple sclerosis
  Posterior circulation strokes
  Cerebellar degenerations
  Wilson disease
  Drugs, toxins (phenytoin, barbiturates, lithium,
    meperidine, alcohol, mercury, 5-fluorouracil,
    vidarabine, amiodarone, cimetidine, tocainide)
Midbrain ("rubral") tremor
Primary handwriting tremor
Dystonic (distal) tremor
Familial benign chorea and tremor
Miscellaneous tremors and other rhythmic movements
Idiopathic
Hysterical
Involuntary rhythmic movements not classified as tremors
  Cardiac and respiratory movements
  Convulsions
  Nystagmus
  Segmental myoclonus
  Oscillatory myoclonus
  Asterixis
  Fasciculations
  Clonus
  Minipolymyoclonus
  Shivering
  Shuddering
  Head flopping or nodding movements

MTP, 1-methyl-4-phenyl-1,2,3,6-tetrahydropyridine.
Modified from Jankovic J. *Neurologic consultant.* New York:
Lawrence Della Corte, 1984:1.

---

patients with athetotic cerebral palsy had jaundice, asphyxia, or both during the postnatal period, and approximately 60% had a history of premature birth.

Although the neurologic impairment in cerebral palsy usually is nonprogressive, patients have been described as having had delayed-onset progressive choreoathetosis and dystonia. These cases have been attributed to sprouting and denervation supersensitivity of receptors in the basal ganglia.

Kernicterus, a syndrome that usually is seen in premature infants having total serum bilirubin concentrations exceeding 10 mg/dL, may be manifested by choreoathetosis, tremor, dystonia, rigidity, dysarthria, deafness, and limitation of upward gaze. Another cause of chorea that occurs in premature infants is severe bronchopulmonary aplasia. The rate of mortality in these infants is approximately 30%, and evidence of neuronal loss in the basal ganglia has been noted at autopsy. Generally, surviving infants have a good prognosis, and the chorea usually resolves.

Hereditary Chorea

Although most children with HD have a parkinsonian syndrome, approximately one-fourth have chorea. Another form

---

BOX 414.3   Classification of Choreas

Developmental choreas
Physiologic chorea of infancy
Kernicterus, cerebral palsy, "minimal cerebral dysfuntion"
  (the choreiform syndrome)

Hereditary choreas
Amino acid disorders
Glutaric acidemia, cystinuria, homocystinuria,
  phenylketonuria, Hartnup disease,
  argininosuccinicaciduria
Carbohydrate disorders
Mucopolysaccharidoses, mucolipidoses, galactosemia,
  pyruvate dehydrogenase deficiency
Lipid disorders
Sphingolipidosis (Krabbe), globoid cell leukodystrophy,
  metachromatic leukodystrophy, Gaucher, GM_1 and GM_2
  gangliosidosis, ceroid lipofuscinosis
Other metabolic disorders
Lesch-Nyhan syndrome, leigh disease, sulfite-oxidase
  deficiency, porphyria
Heredodegenerative disorders
Hallervorden-Spatz, ataxia-telangiectasia, tuberous
  sclerosis, Sturge-Weber, Wilson disease, myoclonus
  epilepsy, familial inverted choreoathetosis, hemoglobin SC
  disease, xeroderma pigmentosum, Pelizaeus-Merzbacher,
  familial striatal necrosis, Huntington disease, benign
  familial chorea (hereditary chorea without dementia),
  choreoacanthocytosis (amyotrophic chorea),
  paroxysmal kinesigenic choreoathetosis, paroxysmal
  dystonic choreoathetosis (Mount-Reback), familial
  calcification of the basal ganglia, joseph disease,
  olivopontocerebellar atrophies (hereditary ataxia)

Drug-induced and toxic choreas
Antipsychotic neuroleptics
Tardive dyskinesia
Antiparkinsonian drugs
Dopaminergic (levodopa, bromocriptine, pergolide,
  lisuride), amantadine, anticholinergics
Anticonvulsants
Phenytoin, carbamazepine
Noradrenergic stimulants
Amphetamines, methylphenidate, aminophylline,
  theophylline, caffeine, pemoline
Steroids
Oral contraceptives, anabolic steroids

Opiates
Methadone
Miscellaneous drugs
Amoxapine, antihistamines, cimetidine, cyclizine, diazoxide,
  digoxin, isoniazid, lithium, methyldopa, metoclopramide,
  reserpine, triazolam, tricyclic antidepressants
Toxins
Alcohol intoxication and witdrawal, carbon monoxide,
  manganese, mercury, thallium, toluene, glue sniffing
Metabolic disorders
Hyponatremia and hypernatremia, hypocalcemia,
  hypoglycemia and hyperglycemia, hypomagnesemia,
  hepatic encephalopathy (acquired hepatocerebral
  degeneration), renal encephalopathy
Endocrine disorders
Hyperthyroidism, hypoparathyroidism,
  pseudohypoparathyroidism, hyperparathyroidism,
  chorea gravidarum (pregnancy), Addison disease
Nutritional disorders
Beriberi, pellagra, vitamin B_{12} deficiency in infants
Infectious disorders
Sydenham chorea (poststreptococcal), scarlet fever
  (streptococcal erythrogenic toxin), diphtheria, pertussis,
  typhoid fever, viral encephalitis (mumps, measles,
  varicella, echovirus, influenza), postvaccinal,
  neurosyphilis, mononucleosis, legionnaires disease,
  bacterial endocarditis, sarcoidosis, mycobacterium
  tuberculosis, bacterial meningitis
Immunologically mediated chorea
Systemic lupus erythematosus, periarteritis nodosa, Behçet
  syndrome, Henoch-Schönlein purpura, multiple sclerosis

Cerebrovascular choreas
Basal ganglia infarction, basal ganglia hemorrhage,
  arteriovenous malformation, polycythemia vera,
  migraine, transient cerebral ischemia

Miscellaneous choreas
Posttraumatic, epidural hematoma, subdural hematoma,
  electrical injury to the nervous system, brain tumor,
  degeneration of nucleus centrum medianum of thalamus,
  hydrocephalus

Modified from Kurlan R, Shoulson I. Facial choreas. In: Jankovic
J, Tolosa E, eds. *Advanced neurology*, vol 49. New York: Raven,
1988.

---

of hereditary chorea is benign hereditary chorea, an autosomal dominant disorder that may present during infancy, childhood, or adolescence. Although it is benign, it may persist as a lifelong condition and rarely may be associated with intellectual impairment. Usually, caudate atrophy is not seen, but ^{18}F-2-fluorodeoxyglucose positron emission tomography (PET) may indicate decreased cerebral glucose metabolism in the caudate nucleus.

Another cause of genetic childhood chorea is the Lesch-Nyhan syndrome. This complex motor-behavioral syndrome is inherited as an X-linked recessive trait and is a result of defective activity of the enzyme hypoxanthine-guanine phosphoribosyltransferase. The diagnosis is suspected when a young boy with delayed developmental milestones, spasticity, and

choreoathetosis develops self-mutilating behavior and is found to have sandlike deposits in his urine. Often, affected patients have complications of hyperuricemia, including gouty arthritis, tophus formation, and obstructive nephropathy. Cerebrospinal fluid (CSF) studies of monoamine metabolites and postmortem biochemical assays have provided evidence of reduced dopamine and norepinephrine turnover in patients with this disorder.

Sydenham Chorea

The high frequency of complications of chronic rheumatic heart disease in patients with Sydenham chorea (SC) suggests an association between rheumatic fever and this neurologic disorder. Unlike arthritis and carditis, which occur soon after such infection, chorea and various neurobehavioral symptoms may be delayed for 6 months or longer and may be the sole manifestation of rheumatic fever. Coincident with a dramatic decline in cases of acute rheumatic fever, the incidence of SC also is decreasing rapidly. Irritability, emotional lability, and other behavioral problems usually accompany the involuntary movements of this disorder. In approximately 20% of cases, the chorea is strictly unilateral (hemichorea). Besides chorea, other clinical features of SC include the "milkmaid's grip," "spooning," and "hung-up" reflexes.

In most cases, the chorea subsides within 5 to 15 weeks, but it may recur in as many as 30% of patients within 2 years. Recurrence is particularly likely to occur during pregnancy (chorea gravidarum). Usually, although the motor symptoms resolve completely, mental changes (particularly emotional lability) and cardiac problems may persist indefinitely. Persistent dopaminergic supersensitivity in affected individuals has been suggested by the high frequency of adverse reactions to central stimulants and to neuroleptics, together with psychotic features.

In addition to elevated titers of antistreptolysin, IgG antibodies reacting with neurons in the caudate and subthalamic nuclei have been found in most patients. Because a latency period of approximately 1 to 6 months may occur after the streptococcal infection develops and before the onset of chorea occurs, patients with SC may have normal erythrocyte sedimentation rates and normal antistreptolysin and antistreptococcic antibody levels. The pathology of SC has not been studied well, but some brains have had vasculitis, chiefly involving the basal ganglia, cortex, and cerebellum. Besides SC, many other infectious causes of chorea, including meningitis, exist.

Although cephalosporins are equally effective, penicillin G, 500 to 1,000 mg four times per day, or one intramuscular injection of 600,000 to 1.2 million units of benzathine penicillin, is considered the drug of choice for pharyngitis caused by beta-hemolytic streptococcal infection. Despite administration of an adequate (10-day) course, the bacteriologic failure rate is as high as 15%, and some patients develop rheumatic fever. Therefore, oral rifampin, 20 mg/kg every 24 hours in four doses, is recommended during the last 4 days of the 10-day course of penicillin therapy. Alternately, oral rifampin, 10 mg/kg, can be given every 12 hours for 8 doses, with one dose of intramuscular benzathine penicillin G. Another alternative is oral clindamycin, 20 mg/kg/day in three doses for 10 days. The best ways to prevent rheumatic fever are establishing an accurate diagnosis and providing adequate treatment of the initial acute pharyngitis. Penicillin prophylaxis is advisable in all patients for at least 10 years. In addition to an initial course of penicillin followed by the administration of prophylactic oral penicillin until the patient reaches 20 years of age, a trial of corticosteroids, haloperidol, pimozide, reserpine, or tetrabenazine may be needed in severe cases.

Dystonia

Dystonia consists of repetitive, patterned, twisting, and sustained movements that may be either slow or rapid. The distribution of dystonia seems to be age-dependent: in children, often the disorder starts distally, whereas in adults, a cranial-cervical distribution is found more commonly. Approximately 30% of all patients with dystonia have onset of the involuntary movements before they attain age 20. Childhood dystonia tends to progress to generalized dystonia, but usually adult dys-

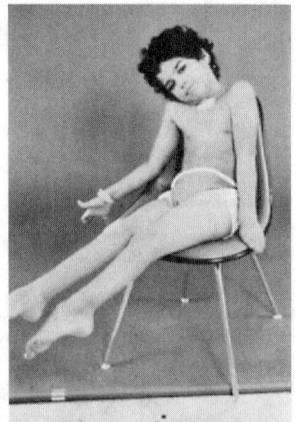
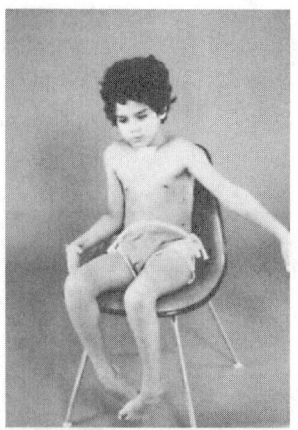
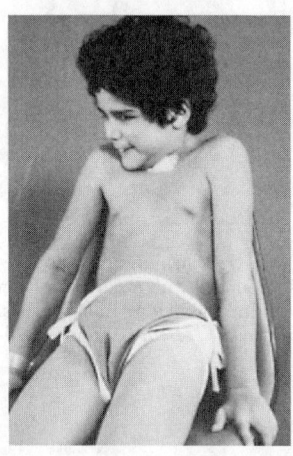
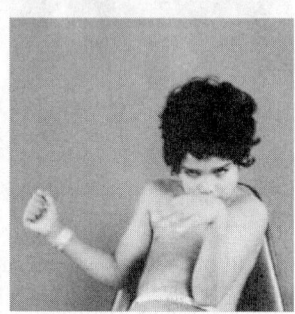

FIGURE 414.3. An 8-year-old boy with autosomal dominant, generalized torsion dystonia. As result of severe dystonic contractions, he had muscle breakdown, myoglobinuria, and renal failure requiring a temporary curarization and tracheostomy. (Reproduced with permission from Jankovic J, Fahn S. Dystonic disorders. In: Jankovic J, Tolosa E, eds. *Parkinson's disease and movement disorders*, 3rd ed. Baltimore: Williams & Wilkins, 1998:513.)

tonia remains focal or segmental (Fig. 414.3). Hemidystonia (unilateral dystonia) involving one-half of the body seems to be a particularly common finding among children and young adults (Fig. 414.4). Approximately three-fourths of patients with hemidystonia have evidence of a structural lesion in the contralateral basal ganglia, particularly the putamen. The causes include infarction or hemorrhage in one-third and perinatal trauma in one-fifth of cases. In many patients with secondary dystonia, particularly children, a delay of several years after the acute event often may occur before the contralateral hemidystonia becomes manifest.

The severity of dystonia varies from one individual to another, and often it depends on a particular circumstance. For example, in some patients, it occurs only on participating in certain activities, the so-called task-specific dystonias, such as cramping during writing or typing or "musician's hands." As the dystonia progresses, often it "overflows" to adjacent muscles and eventually becomes apparent even at rest. Rarely, the spasms become so severe as to cause cervical disk, nerve, or root problems and muscle breakdown with myoglobinuria.

Dystonic states may be classified (according to cause) into primary dystonia, secondary dystonia, or psychogenic dystonia (Box 414.4). The term *primary dystonia* has replaced the old terminology of *dystonia musculorum deformans* or *idiopathic torsion dystonia*. By definition, primary dystonia, whether

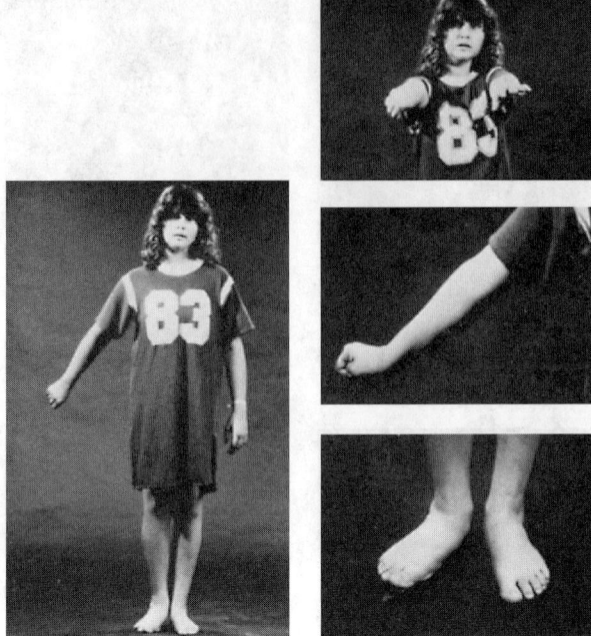

FIGURE 414.4. A 14-year old girl with right hemidystonia as a result of left striatal injury at age 2. (Reproduced with permission from Jankovic J, Fahn S. Dystonic disorders. In: Jankovic J, Tolosa E, eds. *Parkinson's disease and movement disorders*, 3rd ed. Baltimore: Wiliams & Wilkins, 1998:513.)

sporadic or inherited, is not associated with any other neurologic impairment, such as intellectual, pyramidal, cerebellar, or sensory deficits. Approximately 20% of patients with primary dystonia, however, have associated tremor that is phenomenologically identical to ET; in some families, dystonia and ET can coexist. Cerebral palsy probably is the most common cause of secondary dystonia seen in children, but many other causes of secondary dystonia exist (see Box 414.4).

Most cases of primary childhood-onset dystonia are inherited as an autosomal dominant disorder. Additional information about the genetics of dystonia is presented in Box 414.2. A specific gene mutation also has been identified in dopa-responsive dystonia (DRD), and many affected patients have a diurnal variation in the severity of their dystonia in that they are asymptomatic in the morning or after a daytime nap, but, as the day progresses, they experience fatigability and dystonic movements, usually starting in the legs and later progressing to a more generalized dystonia. Some patients also have associated hyperreflexia, rigidity, tremor, and other parkinsonian features. Although the homovanillic acid level in the CSF often is low, usually the fluorodopa PET scan is normal. The most characteristic feature of DRD is the marked sensitivity to dopaminergic therapy. Besides experiencing marked improvement with levodopa or dopamine agonists, affected patients also respond favorably to anticholinergic therapy.

No specific morphologic changes have been noted at postmortem examination of the brains of patients with primary dystonia. A marked reduction in the concentrations of norepinephrine in the posterior and lateral hypothalamus and an increase in the red nucleus have been reported in the few brains of patients with primary dystonia examined at autopsy. Further studies, however, are needed before consistent abnormalities of neurotransmitters can be confirmed.

Certain orthopedic and musculoskeletal problems peculiar to the pediatric population may produce postural deformities that resemble dystonia. Congenital torticollis, caused by contracture of the sternocleidomastoid muscle, may produce a palpable mass and neck deformity in the child's first 6 to 8 months of life. Such congenital torticollis may be the result of local trauma that occurred during a breech or difficult forceps delivery, spondylosis, asymmetric facet joint, basal impression, atlantoaxial dislocation, or other cervical-cranial anomaly. The number of cases of infantile or juvenile scoliosis that actually represent axial dystonia is not known.

Usually, dystonia consists of continual muscle contractions, although they may be modified by a specific action or position (e.g., sensory tricks). In some patients, dystonia fluctuates markedly in a paroxysmal or diurnal manner, such as is seen in DRD paroxysmal kinesigenic and nonkinesigenic dystonia (Table 414.3). The chief difference is that the kinesigenic dystonia is precipitated by a sudden movement, such as arising rapidly from a chair or turning suddenly, whereas the nonkinesigenic dystonia occurs spontaneously. The kinesigenic form of paroxysmal dystonia is seen predominantly in boys and has its onset when they are between the ages of 5 and 15 years. Usually, the attacks last a few seconds and recur as many as 100 times a day; the dystonia often is asymmetric and associated with choreoathetosis and epilepsy. Most patients with kinesigenic dystonia improve with anticonvulsant therapy, including phenytoin, carbamazepine, and barbiturates. The nonkinesigenic form of paroxysmal dystonia may begin in infancy, with the attacks lasting minutes to hours and recurring two or three times a month. The attacks may be precipitated by alcohol, coffee, fatigue, stress, exercise, or excitement. Besides dystonia, many patients with nonkinesigenic dystonia have choreoathetosis and ataxia, particularly during the attacks. This form of dystonia is resistant to pharmacologic therapy, but some patients improve with the administration of clonazepam, oxazepam, acetazolamide, valproate, carbamazepine, and haloperidol. Gastroesophageal reflux (Sandifer syndrome) is another cause of paroxysmal dystonic postures occurring in infants and children, including torticollis and opisthotonos. Multiple sclerosis, thyrotoxicosis, such metabolic disorders as Hartnup disease, paroxysmal dystonia in sleep (hypnogenic dystonia), and "infectious torticollis" also produce paroxysmal or fluctuating dystonia.

Establishing an accurate diagnosis is the first step in treating patients with torsion dystonia. Usually, more extensive diagnostic investigation is prompted by the presence of atypical features, such as impaired intellect, seizures, neuroophthalmologic abnormalities, ataxia, corticospinal tract signs, sensory deficits, severe speech disturbance, and unilateral distribution of the dystonia (Box 414.5). WD is one of the most important causes of dystonia because it is curable. Another treatable, and possibly preventable, type of childhood dystonia is the drug-induced form. Dystonic movements may be caused by levodopa, bromocriptine, anticonvulsants, and ergots, but only the dopamine receptor-blocking drugs, such as the antipsychotics and antiemetics, produce persistent tardive dystonia. Although acute transient dystonic reaction is a well-recognized complication of therapy with these drugs, a small percentage of patients treated with the neuroleptics have persistent and often disabling dystonia. In such cases of tardive dystonia, the offending drug should be stopped and, if no spontaneous improvement occurs, the patient should be given trials of muscle relaxants, anticholinergic drugs, and tetrabenazine. Approximately two-thirds of children with idiopathic torsion dystonia obtain some benefit from high-dose anticholinergic therapy (30 to 60 mg/day of trihexyphenidyl). When trihexyphenidyl is used, it must be introduced in small doses and increased gradually over a period of several weeks or months

BOX 414.4	Classification of Dystonic States

Primary idiopathic dystonia
Inherited (hereditary torsion dystonia, dystonia musculorum deformans)
Autosomal dominant
Autosomal recessive (pseudodominant)
X-linked recessive
Dystonia with marked diurnal variation*
Paroxysmal kinesigenic and nonkinesigenic dystonia*
Parkinsonism-dystonia*
Sporadic (idiopathic torsion dystonia)
Generalized
Segmental (usually secondary dystonias)
Hemidystonia
Multifocal
Focal (torticollis, occupational cramps, oromandibular dystonia, blepharospasm, spasmodic dysphonia)
Secondary Dystonia
Associated with other neurodegenerative disorders
Wilson disease
Huntington disease
Parkinsonism
Progressive supranuclear palsy
Progressive pallidal degeneration
Hallervorden-Spatz disease
Joseph disease
Ataxia-telangiectasia
Multiple sclerosis
Neuroacanthocytosis
Rett syndrome
Intraneuronal inclusion disease
Infantile bilateral striatal necrosis
Familial basal ganglia calcifications
Associated with metabolic disorders
Amino acid disorders
    Glutaric aciduria type I
    Methylmalonic acidemia
    Homocystinuria
    Hartnup disease
    Tyrosinosis
Lipid disorders
    Metachromatic leukodystrophy

Ceroid lipofuscinosis
Juvenile dystonic lipidosis ("sea-blue" histiocytosis; GM_1- and GM_2-variant gangliosidoses: neurovisceral storage disease with supranuclear ophthalmoplegia)
Miscellaneous metabolic disorders
  Leigh disease
  Leber disease and mitochondrial encephalopathies
  Lesch-Nyhan syndrome
  Triosephosphate isomerase deficiency
  Vitamin E deficiency
Result of known specific cause
Perinatal cerebral injury and kernicterus (possibly be delayed in onset)
Infection: viral encephalitis, encephalitis lethargica, tuberculosis, Reye syndrome, subacute sclerosing panencephalitis, Creutzfeldt-Jakob disease, acquired immunodeficiency syndrome; syphilis; acute infectious torticollis
Paraneoplastic brainstem encephalitis
Head trauma
Peripheral trauma
Atlantoaxial dislocation, subluxation, plagiocephaly
Gastroesophageal reflux (Sandifer syndrome)
Cerebrovascular injury
Brain tumor
Arteriovenous malformation
Central pontine myelinolysis
Cerebral ectopia and syringomyelia
Torticollar tilt
Toxins (manganese, carbon monoxide, carbon disulfide, methane, wasp sting)
Drugs (levodopa, bromocriptine, antipsychotics, metoclopramide, fenfluramine, ergots, anticonvulsants)

Psychogenic Dystonia

---

*Also may occur sporadically.
Modified with permission from Jankovic J, Fahn S. Dystonic syndromes. In: Jankovic J, Tolosa E, eds. *Parkinson's disease and movement disorders*. Baltimore: Urban and Schwarzenberg, 1988:283.

---

until symptomatic improvement is noted or such side effects as mental dullness, blurring of vision, and other anticholinergic adverse reactions prevent further increase in the dosage. In addition to anticholinergic drugs, tetrabenazine, a monoamine-depleting agent, is effective in some patients with dystonia; occasionally, we combine it with pimozide, a postsynaptic dopamine receptor–blocking drug. Other drugs that occasionally prove useful in the treatment of dystonia include oral and intrathecal baclofen, carbamazepine, valproate, primidone, and lithium. All patients with childhood-onset dystonia, particularly that combined with parkinsonism, should be treated with levodopa, because they may have DRD. When pharmacologic therapy fails, *Clostridium botulinum* toxin injections may be tried, particularly for patients with focal dystonia. Usually, stereotactic thalamotomy, cervical rhizotomy, and other surgical therapies are reserved for patients who have

disabling dystonia and whose disease does not respond to pharmacologic therapy or chemodenervation using botulinum toxin.

Tics

Approximately 25% of normal children have transient tics, rendering this the childhood-onset involuntary movement seen most frequently in a movement disorders clinic. One of the most common causes of pathologic tics in childhood is the Gilles de la Tourette syndrome (TS). This motor-behavioral disorder is the expression of a genetic disturbance affecting the central nervous system (CNS). Usually, the onset occurs when the child is between ages 2 and 15 years, although, in some

TABLE 414.3

IDIOPATHIC FLUCTUATING OR PAROXYSMAL DYSTONIAS

| Characteristic | Diurnal | Paroxysmal | |
		Kinesigenic	Nonkinesigenic
Male-to-female ratio	1:1	4:1	3:2
Age at onset (years)	<10	5–15 (1–35)	<5 (0–25)
Inheritance	AD, AR, sporadic	AD, sporadic	AD, sporadic
Duration of attacks	Hours	<5 minutes	Minutes to hours
Frequency of attacks	1 per day	100 per day	3 per month
Associated features	Postural tremor, parkinsonism, hyperreflexia	Choreoathetosis, epilepsy	Choreoathetosis, ataxia
Asymmetry	+++	++	+
Ability to suppress attacks	0	+++	+++
Induced or precipitating factors	Afternoon and evening fatigue	Sudden movement, startle	Alcohol, coffee, fatigue, stress, exercise, excitement
Medical therapy	Levodopa, anticholinergics	Phenytoin, carbamazepine, barbiturates	Clonazepam, oxazepam, acetazolamide, valproate, carbamazepine, haloperidol

+, occasionally; ++, usually; +++, almost always; AD, autosomal dominant; AR, autosomal recessive.
Modified with permission from Jankovic J, Fahn S. Dystonic syndrome. In: Jankovic J, Tolosa Ed, eds. *Parkinson's disease and movement disorders.* Baltimore: Urban and Schwarzenberg, 1988:283.

cases, the initial manifestation may not be appreciated until he or she reaches the age of 21 years. The clinical expression of TS is gender-influenced: in boys, motor and vocal manifestations seem to dominate, whereas in girls, such behavioral problems as obsessive-compulsive disorder (OCD) seem to occur more commonly. In addition to OCD, other comorbidities, particularly attention deficit disorder (ADD) with or without hyperactivity (ADHD), occur sometime during the course of the illness in most patients with TS.

In addition to such simple tics as blinking, facial grimacing, shoulder shrugging, and head jerking, many patients with TS have complex sequences of coordinated movements,

---

BOX 414.5   **Investigation of Patients with Atypical Dystonia**

Blood Studies
Ceruloplasmin, copper, creatine phosphokinase, myoglobin, glucose, lactate, pyruvate, uric acid, creatinine, workup for autoimmune disease
Examination of red blood cells for acanthocytosis or sickle cell disease; lymphocytes for vacuolation (light microscopy) or inclusions (electron microscopy)
Leukocytes (lysosomal enzymes, hypoxanthine guanine phosphoribosyltransferase)

Urine Studies
Screening tests (amino acids, 24-hour copper, column chromatography for oligosaccharides and mucopolysaccharides)

Cerebrospinal Fluid Studies
Lactate, pyruvate

Biopsies
Liver (morphology, copper)
Bone marrow ("sea-blue" histiocytes, vacuolation)
Skin (fibroblasts for lysosomal enzymes)
Conjunctivae (neuronal inclusions)
Rectal mucosa (neuronal inclusions)
Muscle (mitochondrial abnormalities)
Brain (neuronal inclusions or deposits)

Other Studies
Slit-lamp examination for Kayser-Fleischer ring, cataracts, etc.
CT or MRI (basal ganglia calcifications or necrosis and other abnormalities)
PET scan (glucose metabolism, blood flow, ^{18}F-L-dopa, receptor ligand studies)
Spine radiographs or myelogram (atlantoaxial subluxation, Klippel-Feil deformity)
Upper gastrointestinal study (hiatal hernia in Sandifer-Kinsbourne syndrome)
Videotape (quantitative rating scale and polyelectromyograph for documentation)
Electrophysiologic studies (electroencephalogram; electroretinogram; visual-brainstem, somatosensory, and cortical evoked responses; polysomnography; electromyography; nerve conduction tests) (particularly useful in evaluation of paroxysmal and posttraumatic dystonia)

CT, computed tomography; MRI, magnetic resonance imaging; PET, positron emission tomography.
Modified with permission from Jankovic J, Fahn S. Dystonic syndromes. In: Jankovic J, Tolosa Ed, eds. *Parkinson's disease and movement disorders.* Baltimore: Urban and Schwarzenberg, 1988: 283.

including bizarre gait, kicking, jumping, body gyrations, scratching, and seductive or obscene gestures. The waxing and waning nature of tics, the irresistible urge before a tic and relief after a tic, the temporary suppressibility of the tics, and the recurrence of tics during sleep often result in the misdiagnosis of the disorder as having a psychogenic origin. The psychogenic nature of the condition also is suggested erroneously by the involuntary vocalizations that occur, which range from simple noises to coprolalia (obscene words), echolalia (repetition of words), and palilalia (repetition of a phrase or word with increasing rapidity). Coprolalia, although it is one of the most recognizable symptoms of TS, has been seen in only 40% of our patients thus far. Many patients also experience copropraxia, echopraxia, bizarre thoughts and ideas, thought fixation, compulsive ruminations, and perverse sexual fantasies. Sleep complaints, including restlessness, insomnia, enuresis, somnambulism, nightmares, and bruxism, have been noted in approximately one-half of our patients, and approximately two-thirds had evidence of motor tics recorded by polysomnography. If a broad spectrum of behavioral problems is included, approximately 1% of all individuals manifest one or more aspects of the TS gene.

Disturbance in the mesencephalic-mesolimbic system, which results in disinhibition of the limbic system, has been suggested as the pathogenetic mechanism underlying TS. Neither imaging nor postmortem studies of the brains of patients with TS have shown any abnormalities consistently.

Although haloperidol and pimozide are recommended most frequently in the treatment of TS, we find risperidone, fluphenazine, and tetrabenazine to be more effective and better tolerated. Patients with predominant behavioral symptoms, particularly impulse control problems and rage attacks, may benefit from clonidine and the selective serotonin uptake inhibitors (SSRIs). The SSRIs also are fairly effective in treating associated OCD. When TS is associated with ADD or ADHD, such CNS stimulants as methylphenidate, dextroamphetamine (Dexedrine), and guanfacine may be needed. These agents, however, should be used cautiously because they may precipitate or exacerbate tics. Atomoxetine, a norepinephrine uptake inhibitor, also has been found to be effective in treating some patients with ADHD.

Myoclonus

In contrast to tics, myoclonus is a simple, jerk-like movement that is not coordinated or suppressible and often is activated by volitional movement (Box 414.6). Benign neonatal sleep myoclonus, which occurs in the first month of life, usually is stimulus-sensitive and occurs in the early stages of sleep. It should be differentiated from neonatal seizures and infantile spasms. Usually, essential myoclonus begins before the person reaches 20 years of age, is inherited in an autosomal dominant pattern, and may be associated with ET.

Cortical myoclonus may be manifested as a continuous, repetitive, focal jerking. It can be triggered by external stimuli or can be evoked by muscle stretch reflex or by quick, passive, movement of distal phalanx (cortical reflex myoclonus) or by movement (cortical action myoclonus). Cortical reflex myoclonus is characterized by a time-locked electroencephalographic (EEG) event preceding the myoclonic movement and by enhanced amplitude of the somatosensory evoked potential. The most common causes of epilepsia partialis continua include cortical stroke and Rasmussen encephalitis, a disorder of childhood or adolescence caused by focal cortical lesion or inflammation, possibly caused by viral infection. In contrast to the hyperexcitable sensorimotor cortex that underlies cortical myoclonus, presumably, reticular reflex myoclonus is the result of hyperexcitable brainstem reticular formation, particularly the nucleus reticularis gigantocellularis.

Progressive myoclonus epilepsy consists of myoclonus, seizures, and a progressive clinical course. One form of progressive myoclonus epilepsy, Unverricht-Lundborg disease (also known as *Baltic myoclonus* or *EPM1*), is characterized by stimulus-sensitive myoclonus that usually begins when affected patients are between 6 and 15 years of age. Such patients also have dysarthria, ataxia, intention tremor, and mild intellectual decline, and most become bedridden within 5 years after onset of the disease. Epileptiform EEG findings may be seen as long as 3 years before the onset of clinical symptoms. The disease is inherited in an autosomal recessive pattern, and at least some cases may be associated with mitochondrial myopathy and encephalopathy. The gene responsible for EPM1, localized to 21q22.3, encodes cystatin B, a cysteine protease inhibitor. Several different mutations have been identified in this gene in patients with EPM1, but the most common is an unstable expansion of a dodecamer mini-satellite repeat unit in the promoter region of the cystatin B gene.

Another form of progressive myoclonus, Lafora body disease, usually begins in patients between 11 and 18 years of age and is characterized by progressive dementia, apraxia, and cortical blindness, with total disability resulting within 5 to 8 years after onset. Biopsy of the skin (particularly the axillary skin), liver, muscle, or brain reveals typical inclusions (Lafora bodies) that are positive on periodic acid-Schiff staining.

Ramsay Hunt syndrome is a group of heterogeneous disorders dominated by a combination of progressive myoclonus and cerebellar ataxia. Myoclonus also may be a manifestation of viral encephalitis and typically is seen in patients with subacute sclerosing panencephalitis. In this subacute disorder, progressive dementia and "slow" myoclonus that occur approximately every second are associated with periodic complexes on the EEG. Another form of myoclonic encephalopathy that occurs in young children is the opsoclonus-myoclonus syndrome or the "dancing eyes–dancing feet" syndrome. Usually, it is seen after a febrile illness or in association with a neuroblastoma, and marked improvement may be achieved with steroid therapy. Stimulus-sensitive myoclonus resembles another jerk-like movement disorder called *the startle disease* or *hyperexplexia*. Hereditary hyperexplexia, an autosomal dominant disorder of childhood, has been found to be caused by a point mutation in the gene coding for the alpha-1 subunit of the glycine receptor on chromosome 5, but not all forms of hereditary hyperexplexia are caused by the same genetic and physiologic abnormality. Small myoclonic jerks (minipolymyoclonus) also have been reported in children with chronic spinal muscular atrophy. The idiopathic, generalized, or segmental forms of myoclonus may improve with treatment using clonazepam, sodium valproate, 5-hydroxytryptophan, tetrabenazine, reserpine, levodopa, trihexyphenidyl, lisuride, and piracetam.

Stereotypies

Stereotypies are such repetitive, purposeless, and seemingly voluntary movements as chewing, rocking, twirling, or touching. These movements usually are seen in the setting of infantile autism or mental retardation. Attention increasingly has been directed toward another disorder characterized by marked stereotypy: Rett syndrome. This condition occurs only in girls who have normal prenatal and perinatal growth and development. At the age of 6 to 18 months, they regress in their verbal and motor skills, lose purposeful use of their hands, and have jerky ataxia and typical stereotyped movements of

---

BOX 414.6   Classification of Myoclonus

Physiologic myoclonus (normal individuals)
Sleep jerks (hypnic jerks)
Anxiety-induced
Exercise-induced
Hiccough (singultus)
Benign infantile myoclonus with feeding

Essential myoclonus (no known cause and no other gross neurologic deficits)
Hereditary (autosomal dominant)
Sporadic
  Ballistic movement overflow myoclonus
  Oscillatory myoclonus
  Segmental myoclonus (rhythmic and nonrhythmic)
  Nocturnal myoclonus
  Restless legs syndrome

Epileptic myoclonus (seizures dominant and no encephalopathy, at least initially)
Isolated epileptic myoclonic jerks
Cortical reflex myoclonus
Reticular reflex myoclonus
Primary generalized epileptic myoclonus
Epilepsia partialis continua
Photoconvulsive response
Infantile spasms
Childhood epileptic encephalopathy with slow spike and slow waves (Lennox-Gastaut syndrome, myoclonic-ataxic epilepsy, cryptogenic myoclonic epilepsy)
Familial myoclonic epilepsy (janz)
Familial myoclonic epilepsy (Rabot)
Progressive myoclonus epilepsy (Baltic myoclonus, or Unverricht-Lundborg)

Symptomatic myoclonus (progressive or static encephalopathy dominates)
Progressive myoclonus epilepsy
  Lafora body disease
  Neuronal ceroid lipofuscinosis
  Sialidosis (types I, II)
  Mitochondrial encephalopathy
  Noninfantile neuronopathic Gaucher disease
  Biotin-responsive encephalopathy
  Lipidoses (GM_2 gangliosidosis, Tay-Sachs, Krabbe)
Spinocerebellar degeneration
  Ramsay Hunt syndrome
  Friedreich ataxia
  Ataxia-telangiectasia

Basal ganglia degenerations
  Wilson disease
  Torsion dystonia
  Hallervorden-Spatz disease
  Progressive supranuclear palsy
  Huntington disease
  Parkinson disease
Dementias
  Creutzfeldt-Jakob disease
  Alzheimer disease
Viral types of encephalopathy
  Subacute sclerosing panencephalitis
  Encephalitis lethargica
  Arbovirus encephalitis
  Herpes simplex encephalitis
  Postinfection encephalitis
Metabolic types
  Hypoxic-ischemic encephalopathy
  Hepatic failure
  Renal failure
  Dialysis syndrome
  Hyponatremia
  Hypoglycemia
  Infantile myoclonic encephalopathy (polymyoclonus with or without neuroblastoma)
  Nonketotic hyperglycemia
Toxic types of encephalopathy
  Bismuth
  Heavy metal poisons
  Methyl bromide dichlorodiphenyltrichloroethane
  Drugs, including levodopa
Physical types of encephalopathy
  Posttraumatic encephalopathy
  Heat stroke
  Electric shock
  Decompression injury
Focal central nervous system damage
  Poststroke disorder
  Postthalamotomy disorder
  Tumor
  Trauma
  Segmental myoclonus (branchial, spinal)

Modified from Patel V, Jankovic J. Myoclonus. In: Appel SH, ed. *Current neurology*, vol 8. St. Louis: Mosby, 1988:77.

---

the hands resembling hand washing and kneading. In addition to the motor manifestations, girls with Rett syndrome often have breath-holding spells, hyperventilation, loss of facial expression, poor eye contact, bruxism, dystonia, occasional seizures, apparent insensitivity to pain, and a variety of self-injurious and aggressive behaviors. The pathogenesis of Rett syndrome is unknown, and the vast majority of the cases occur sporadically, although some are familial. Mutations in the X-linked gene encoding methyl-CpG binding protein 2 (MECP2) have been found to be responsible for most Rett cases. A broad range of mutations in the *MECP2* gene as well as other genes (e.g., *NLGN-3*, *NLGN-4*) have been described involving not only girls and women, but also males, and in a variety of autistic spectrum disorders, such as Asperger syndrome, Angelman syndrome, learning disability, and mental retardation.

Suggested Readings

Higgins JJ, Loveless JM, Jankovic J, Patel P. Evidence that a gene for essential tremor maps to chromosome 2p in four families. *Mov Disord* 1998; 13:972.

Jankovic J. Botulinum toxin in clinical practice. *J Neurol Neurosurg Psychiatry* 2004;75:951.

Jankovic J. Tourette's syndrome. *N Engl J Med* 2001;345:1184.

Jankovic J, Fahn S. Dystonic disorders. In: Jankovic J, Tolosa E, eds. *Parkinson's disease and movement disorders*, 4th edition. Philadelphia: Lippincott Williams and Wilkins, 2002:331.

Jankovic J, Madisetty J, Vuong KD. Essential tremor in children. *Pediatrics* 2004; 114:1203-1205.

Lotze T, Jankovic J. Paroxysmal kinesigenic dyskinesias. *Semin Pediatr Neurol* 2003;10:68.

Manji H, Howard RS, Miller DH, et al. Status dystonicus: the syndrome and its management. *Brain* 1998;121:243.

Neul JL, Zoghbi HY. Rett syndrome: a prototypical neurodevelopmental disorder. *Neuroscientist* 2004;10:118.

Pranzatelli MR, Travelstead AL, Tate ED, et al. B- and T-cell markers in opsoclonus-myoclonus syndrome: immunophenotyping of CSF lymphocytes. *Neurology* 2004;62:1526.

Prashanth LK, Taly AB, Sinha S, et al. Wilson's disease: diagnostic errors and clinical implications. *J Neurol Neurosurg Psychiatry* 2004;75:907.

Singer HS, Loiselle CR, Lee O, et al. Anti-basal ganglia antibodies in PANDAS. *Mov Disord* 2004;19:406.

Thomas M, Hayflick SJ, Jankovic J. Clinical heterogeneity of neurodegeneration with iron accumulation–1 (Hallervorden-Spatz Syndrome) and pantothenate kinase associated neurodegeneration (PKAN). *Mov Disord* 2004;19:36.

Tijssen MAJ, Voorkamp LA, Padgberg GW, et al. Startle responses in hereditary hyperexplexia. *Arch Neurol* 1997;54:388.

CHAPTER 415 ■ DISEASES WITH ASTROCYTE ABNORMALITIES

MARVIN A. FISHMAN

ALEXANDER DISEASE

Alexander disease is a degenerative disorder of the nervous system caused by a mutation in the gene encoding glial fibrillary acidic protein (GFAP). The disease usually presents in infancy, but later-onset forms have been described.

Pathology and Pathogenesis

GFAP is the main intermediate filament protein in astrocytes. Mutations appear to exert a dominant toxic gain of function. The vast majority of mutations are found in exons 1, 4, 6, and 8. They involve changes in a single nucleotide. The altered protein presumably affects the interaction between astrocytes and oligodendrocytes. The histologic correlate is a finding of Rosenthal fibers in the brains of affected children. The fibers are the result of a conglutination of altered glial filaments, which form eosinophilic hyalin spheres in the cytoplasm of astrocytes. The spheres are particularly prevalent beneath the pia mater and around blood vessels. Several stress proteins plus glial fibrillary protein have been identified as major constituents of Rosenthal fibers. Hypomyelination or demyelination occurs, but it is thought to be a secondary event and not to represent a feature of the primary pathogenesis of the disease. Abnormally enlarged mitochondria have been noted, but whether this finding is indicative of an abnormality of mitochondria metabolism is unclear.

The common feature of all the variants of Alexander disease is the presence of refractile eosinophilic bodies in relation to astrocytes. These bodies are most abundant in the subpial, subependymal, and perivascular areas, but they may be found throughout the nervous system in both the white and gray matter and may be seen in the spinal cord. The eosinophilic bodies are found in large, hypertrophied astrocytes, which have a perpendicular orientation to the surface of the brain in the subpial area and form a radial array around blood vessels. In the juvenile form of the disease, the brainstem may be involved predominantly, and the medulla has been noted to be hypertrophied. Electron microscopy demonstrates filaments of granular osmophilic material that form the Rosenthal fibers in the astrocytes. Alpha B-crystallin, a stress protein, is a major protein component of Rosenthal fibers, but its gene structure is normal. A variable loss of myelin occurs in patients with Alexander disease and results in a soft and retracted appearance of the white matter. In infantile cases, the myelin loss may be marked and present in a diffuse pattern. In patients with the juvenile- and adult-onset forms of the disease, demyelination is more limited and patchy. Rosenthal fibers are not specific for Alexander disease and have been noted in patients with a variety of disorders, including syringomyelia, astrocytic glioma, optic nerve glioma, multiple sclerosis, central pontine myelinolysis, disseminated cerebral gliomatosis, and neurofibromatosis.

Clinical Manifestations and Complications

Three variants of Alexander disease have been described and are distinguished by their age of onset: infantile, juvenile, and adult. Recently, a neonatal form of the disease that begins within the first month of life has been suggested. These variants are grouped together under the term *Alexander disease* because they result in similar pathologic changes in various portions of the central nervous system (CNS), and mutations in the GFAP gene have been found in the first three forms.

The infantile form affects children between birth and 2 years of age, but the average age of onset of the illness is at 6 months. The course usually is 2 to 3 years, but the duration of the disease varies from months to more than 5 years. Psychomotor retardation, megalencephaly (with or without hydrocephalus), spasticity, and seizures are prominent features. The head may not be large at birth, but it increases progressively in size during infancy. Increased intracranial pressure (ICP) may be present, even without hydrocephalus. When hydrocephalus is present, it often is the result of a partial obstruction of the aqueduct by proliferating astrocytes in the ependymal lining. Clinical examination does not disclose any abnormality of peripheral nervous system function.

The juvenile-onset form of the disease is much less common than is the infantile form. This type is seen in patients between 7 and 14 years of age. Its course is longer, varying between 1 and more than 10 years (average, 8 years). The intellect remains intact, unlike in the infantile form. Findings are related to dysfunction of the brainstem and include ptosis, nystagmus, facial diplegia, difficulty in swallowing, nasal speech, and tongue atrophy. Other features include generalized spasticity, weakness, and ataxia.

The adult-onset type of Alexander disease is rarest and occurs in young adults. The clinical syndrome resembles that of multiple sclerosis and includes blurred vision, spasticity, nystagmus, dysarthria, and dysphagia.

The neonatal form has onset within the first month of life and is characterized by refractory seizures, hydrocephalus, and severe motor and mental retardation. The course is rapidly progressive, leading to severe disability or death within the first 2 years of life.

Diagnosis and Therapy

Molecular genetic testing of the gene encoding GFAP is available. The diagnosis also can be confirmed by the detection of astrocytic bodies on examination of brain tissue. The syndrome occurs in a sporadic fashion, and familial cases rarely are noted.

The diagnosis can be suspected on the basis of characteristic findings on magnetic resonance imaging (MRI). Abnormality of the white matter, predominantly involving the frontal regions, can be seen, as can abnormalities in the periventricular regions. Abnormal signals also are noted in the basal ganglia and thalamus. Abnormalities in the brainstem may be present. Contrast enhancement may occur in the involved areas. The imaging findings may suggest the diagnosis even when the clinical picture is nonspecific.

Supportive therapy is helpful for patients with Alexander disease. Antiepileptic drugs are used to treat the associated seizures. Attention to nutrition and control of infections with antibiotics are indicated. Psychosocial support of the family should be undertaken.

CANAVAN DISEASE

Canavan disease is a spongy degeneration of the CNS caused by a deficiency of the enzyme aspartoacylase. It is an autosomal recessive disorder. Several clinical variants have been described and are categorized by age of onset into neonatal, infantile, and juvenile forms. The vast majority of cases are of the infantile type. The other two variants have not been studied thoroughly at the biochemical and molecular levels. Thus, the mutations leading to the various phenotypes are not well-delineated.

Pathology and Pathogenesis

The pathogenesis of Canavan disease is unknown. The absence of the enzyme aspartoacylase leads to excess urinary excretion of its substrate, N-acetylaspartic acid (NAA), as well as an increase in its concentration in the blood. High levels of NAA occur in brain tissue, but its role in brain metabolism is unclear. The enzyme has been localized to the white matter, but the synthesis of NAA occurs primarily in the gray matter. Hydrolysis of NAA appears to be important to the maintenance of white matter. Proton-nuclear magnetic resonance spectroscopy of brain tissue demonstrates increased levels of NAA. In many other neurologic diseases, NAA levels are decreased, and this finding is thought to be a general marker for neuronal loss. The

human gene for aspartoacylase (ASPA) has been cloned and localized to the terminal end of the short arm of chromosome 17.

Astrocytes in affected individuals have been noted to have abnormal mitochondria and reduced levels of adenosine triphosphatase. The possible metabolic disturbance has been thought to result in excessive fluid accumulation, which produces vacuoles and gives the brain the spongy appearance that is the pathologic hallmark of the disease. The excessive fluid appears to occur within the cytoplasm of the astrocytes and also within myelin lamellae. Whether the changes noted in the mitochondria are primary or represent secondary effects of the disease is unclear.

In the infantile form of Canavan disease, the weight of the brain is increased. If the child survives more than 2 years, however, the weight tends to decline and return to the normal range. This weight loss often is accompanied by enlargement of the ventricular system secondary to the loss of brain substance rather than to the obstruction of flow of the cerebrospinal fluid (CSF). Vacuoles appear in the deep cortical layers and in the subcortical white matter. With long-standing disease, myelin, axons, and neurons are lost. Changes in the cerebellum are characterized by decreased numbers of Purkinje cells and granular cells. Vacuoles also have been noted in the spinal cord.

Electron microscopy shows that the vacuoles are related to astrocytes swollen with watery cytoplasm and to split myelin lamellae at the intraperiod line. The mitochondria of the astrocytes are abnormal in appearance and elongated. The matrix and cristae are distended and distorted.

Clinical Manifestations and Complications

The neonatal form of Canavan disease is seen extremely rarely. It is characterized by lethargy, crying, decreased spontaneous movement, and difficulty swallowing and sucking. Affected neonates are hypotonic and remain so. They have Cheyne-Stokes respiration and often die within a few weeks. This form of disease appears to occur in sporadic fashion; it is not clearly autosomal recessive or dominant, and no familial inheritance pattern has been reported.

The infantile form is autosomal recessive and is the most common type of Canavan disease. It occurs predominantly in Ashkenazi Jews, although patients from a variety of ethnic backgrounds have been described. Onset occurs within the first 6 months of life. Most children die within the first decade, but survival beyond that time is recognized more frequently than in the past as older patients are identified through biochemical and molecular studies. At onset, the infant appears sluggish and hypotonic and has poor head control. Macrocephaly is present in most affected infants. Development ceases, and in the second 6 months of life, the hypotonia changes to spasticity. When this event occurs, auditory, visual, or tactile stimuli may precipitate decorticate or decerebrate posturing. Vision deteriorates with the development of optic atrophy and nystagmus. Occasionally, increased ICP is noted, and it is not caused by hydrocephalus. Focal and myoclonic seizures, as well as other types of seizure activities, may develop. Occasionally, choreoathetosis is present. In the end stages of the disease, paroxysmal episodes of sweating, hyperthermia, vomiting, and hypotension may occur.

The juvenile form of Canavan disease may have a long course, with onset occurring after the child is 5 years of age. It is characterized by a progressive cerebellar syndrome, in addition to dysarthria, dementia, and spasticity. Ataxia and tremor may be noted early in the course of the disease. Eventually, visual disturbances occur that are characterized by loss of vision, optic atrophy, and abnormal retinal pigmentation. Unlike in the infantile form of the disease, the size of the child's head is not increased. Other features rarely noted have included partial deafness, hyporeflexia, and muscle wasting. Possible involvement of other organ systems has been suggested because of the presence of diabetes mellitus, probable hyperaldosteronism, and heart block. Many of these patients were described before biochemical diagnostic testing was available.

Diagnosis and Therapy

Patients with Canavan disease have a deficiency of aspartoacylase in fibroblasts, accompanied by an increased concentration of NAA in the urine and blood. Computed tomography of the brain has demonstrated diffuse attenuation of the white matter. MRI demonstrates changes consistent with a leukodystrophy. Two predominant mutations in the aspartoacylase gene, Glu285Ala, a missense mutation in exon 6, and Tyr231Xaa, a nonsense mutation in exon 5, account for 97% of the cases in Ashkenazi Jewish patients. Molecular diagnosis of carriers among Ashkenazi Jews can be determined in approximately 98% of cases. Mutation analysis using cells obtained from chorionic villus sampling or amniocentesis is helpful in identifying of an affected conceptus. Prevention programs through carrier testing in Jewish individuals is recommended by the American College of Medical Genetics and the American College of Obstetrics and Gynecology. Many different mutations occur in non-Jewish patients, thus diminishing the utility of screening programs.

No specific therapy is available for patients with Canavan disease. Symptomatic support includes nutritional therapy and administration of antiepileptic drugs and antibiotics as indicated. Providing psychosocial support for the family is important.

Suggested Readings

Adachi M, Schneck L, Cara J, et al. Spongy degeneration of the central nervous system (Van Bogaert and Bertrand type; Canavan's disease). *Hum Pathol* 1973;4:331.

Alexander WS. Progressive fibrinoid degeneration of fibrillary astrocytes associated with mental retardation in a hydrocephalic infant. *Brain* 1949;72:373.

Aoki Y, Haginoya K, Munahata M, et al. A novel mutation in glial fibrillary acidic protein gene in a patient with Alexander disease. *Neurosci Lett* 2001;312:71.

Brenner M, Johnson AB, Boespflug-Tanguy O, et al. Mutations in GFAP, encoding glial fibrillary acidic protein, are associated with Alexander disease. *Nature Genet* 2001;27:117.

Goodhue WW Jr., Couch RD, Namiki H. Spongy degeneration of the CNS. *Arch Neurol* 1979;36:481.

Gorospe JR, Naidu S, Johnson AB, et al. Molecular findings in symptomatic and pre-symptomatic Alexander disease patients. *Neurology* 2002;58:1494.

Head MW, Corbin E, Goldman JE. Overexpression and abnormal modification of the stress proteins alpha B-crystallin and HSP27 in Alexander disease. *Am J Pathol* 1993;143:1743.

Jellinger K, Seitelberger F. Juvenile form of spongy degeneration of the CNS. *Acta Neuropathol* (Berl) 1969;13:276.

Kaul R, Gao GP, Matalon R, et al. Identification and expression of eight novel mutations among non-Jewish patients with Canavan disease. *Am J Hum Genet* 1996;59:95.

Matalon R, Kaul R, Casanova J, et al. Aspartoacylase deficiency: the enzyme defect in Canavan disease. *J Inherit Metab Dis* 1989;12:329.

Matalon R, Matalon KM. Canavan disease: Prenatal diagnosis and genetic counseling. *Obstet Gynecol Clin* 2002:29:2.

Matalon R, Michals K, Kaul R. Canavan disease: from spongy degeneration to molecular analysis. *J Pediatr* 1995;127:511.

Namekawa M, Takiyama Y, Aoki Y, et al. Identification of GFAP gene mutation in hereditary adult-onset Alexander's disease. *Ann Neurol* 2002;52:779.

Rodriguez D, Gauthier F, Bertini E, et al. Infantile Alexander disease: spectrum of GFAP mutations and genotype-phenotype correlation. *Am J Hum Genet* 2001;69:1140.

Sistermans ES, de Coo RF, van Beuendonk HM, et al. Mutation detection in the aspartoacylase gene in 17 patients with Canavan disease: four new mutations in the non-Jewish population. *Eur J Hum Genet* 2000;8:557.

CHAPTER 416 ■ PHAKOMATOSES AND OTHER NEUROCUTANEOUS SYNDROMES

SHARON E. PLON

NEUROFIBROMATOSIS

Neurofibromatosis (NF) is the term used for a set of distinct disorders that share some clinical characteristics, with NF types 1 and 2 being described most clearly. NF type 1 (NF-1) previously called Von Recklinghausen disease, accounts for at least 85% of all patients with NF and is one of the most common dominant genetic disorders.

Neurofibromatosis Type 1 (Von Recklinghausen Disease)

NF-1 occurs with a frequency of approximately 1 in 2,500 to 4,000 persons. It is inherited as an autosomal dominant trait, with an affected parent having a 50% risk of transmitting the disease to each child. However, approximately one-half of the

index cases represent new mutations, so that a negative family history is a common finding in the pediatric setting, and children with features of NF-1 should be evaluated regardless of family history. The disorder is essentially the same whether it is inherited from an affected parent or results from a new mutation. The likelihood that a person with an NF-1 mutation will have clinical features of the disease (termed the penetrance) is close to 100%. However, the severity of NF-1 is highly variable in its expression from one family to another, from one person to another within a given family, and from one body part to another within a given person. Additional information concerning the genetics and molecular biology of NF-1 is presented in Box 416.1.

Clinical Manifestations and Complications

Because of the difficulty of performing molecular analysis, most patients are diagnosed on clinical grounds. A checklist of the

BOX 416.1 — Genetics and Molecular Biology of Neurofibromatosis Type 1

The gene mutated in NF-1 (*NF1*) resides on the proximal long arm of chromosome 17, specifically in band 17q11.2. However, it is a very large gene, with no major hotspots of mutations, which has limited clinical testing for *NF1* mutation. One exception is the finding that approximately 5% of patients have deletion of the entire gene, which is associated with significant developmental delay, early development of neurofibromas, and dysmorphic features.

DNA genetic linkage analysis of large numbers of families with NF-1, along with molecular analysis of translocations involving chromosome band 17q11.2, has resulted in the rapid identification and cloning of the *NF1* gene. The *NF1* gene product, neurofibromin, is expressed in virtually all tissues studied, from both normal individuals and those with NF-1. Neurofibromin functions to regulate the activity of the ras-mediated signaling pathways, which implies, in turn, that loss of neurofibromin at key times in a cell's life may lead to abnormal growth promotion. Loss of the remaining normal copy of the *NF1* gene (termed loss of heterozygosity) has been documented in MPNST, myeloid malignancies associated with NF-1, and some neurofibromas. Thus, *NF1* appears to function as a tumor-suppressor gene. However, mouse models containing mutations in the paralogous gene have demonstrated that the development of tumors results both from the neoplastic cell losing the second copy of the *NF1* gene and supporting cells (including mast cells) containing the inherited *NF1* mutation. Thus, new treatment research is focusing on inhibiting the function of these supporting cells to decrease tumor burden.

BOX 416.2 — Anatomic-Structural and Functional Features in Neurofibromatosis Type 1

Anatomic-Structural Features

Skin pigmentation
  Café au lait spots; freckling: axillary, elsewhere; hyperpigmentation over a plexiform neurofibroma; other hyperpigmentation; hypopigmentation

Discrete neurofibromas
  Cutaneous: general, areola, nipple; subcutaneous; oral-pharynx-larynx; deep

Plexiform neurofibromas
  Craniofacial: orbital, other; chest wall; paraspinal: cervical, thoracic, lumbosacral; abdominal, retroperitoneal; limb; visceral

Central nervous system (CNS)
  Orbit: glioma, other; intracranial: chiasm, other; astrocytoma, schwannoma, meningioma, other; spinal

Other tumors
  Schwannoma (non-CNS); malignant peripheral nerve sheath tumor; pheochromocytoma; carcinoid; other benign; malignancy

Ocular
  Lisch nodules; hypertrophied corneal nerves; choroidal hamartomas; congenital glaucoma; eyelid ptosis; cataracts

Skeletal
  Short stature; macrocephaly; craniofacial dysplasia; vertebral dysplasia; kyphoscoliosis/scoliosis; lumbar scalloping; pseudoarthrosis: tibial, other; genu valgum/varum; pectus excavatum; other skeletal

Miscellaneous
  Colon ganglioneuromatosis; xanthogranulomas (skin); vascular: angiomas, renal, cerebral, other; pulmonary fibrosis; cerebrospinal fluid: ventricle dilation, hydrocephalus, other abnormality; excess dental caries; electroencephalographic abnormality; other anatomic features

Functionl Features
  Cosmetic disfigurement; hypertrophic impairment; weakness/paralysis; incoordination; pain; seizures; other neurologic features; strabismus; visual impairment; hearing impairment; speech impediment; developmental delay; learning disability; school performance problems; mental retardation; psychosocial burden; psychiatric symptoms; headache; puberty disturbance; pruritus; constipation; gastrointestinal bleeding; hypertension; surgery; other functional features

---

features that are characteristic of all types of NF, with an emphasis on NF-1, is provided in Box 416.2. Café au lait spots (CALS) (hyperpigmented macules) are the hallmark of NF-1. Segmental NF refers to the rare patients who have clinical features of NF in only one segment of the body, and CALS are limited to that area. CALS are seen variably in patients with NF-2 but typically are much fewer in number compared with patients with NF-1. Small numbers of CALS also are seen in other cancer-predisposing syndromes and thus are not specific to the neurofibromatoses.

In patients with NF-1, CALS are larger than 15 mm in diameter and have sharply defined edges and a uniform intensity of coloration (Fig. 416.1). CALS often develop during the child's first year of life and increase in number during the first few years. The pattern of CALS then stabilizes. CALS are different from freckling, which in NF-1 is most likely to occur in regions of skin apposition, particularly the axilla. Multiple (six or greater) CALS may be the only feature of NF-1 in a 1-year-old child and are sufficient to merit a full diagnostic evaluation for NF-1.

Neurofibromas are of four types: cutaneous, subcutaneous, nodular plexiform, and diffuse plexiform. Cutaneous neurofibromas are the most common variety, eventually occurring in virtually all patients with NF-1. Often, they do not appear until just before the patient enters puberty or coincident with it. They are present in highest density over the trunk (Fig. 416.2). Subcutaneous neurofibromas usually become apparent toward the end of the first decade of life or in early adulthood, and

they may be painful or tender. Nodular plexiform neurofibromas are complex clusters of subcutaneous-like neurofibromas along proximal nerve roots and major nerves. With continued growth along the spinal column, they lead to spinal erosion and, eventually, spinal cord compression. Diffuse plexiform neurofibromas, with or without overlying hyperpigmentation, are congenital lesions that tend to enlarge steadily with age (Fig. 416.3). Both diffuse and nodular plexiform lesions can result in significant morbidity and deformity.

Lisch nodules (lesions of the iris) are relatively specific for NF-1. They develop over the course of time and are present in

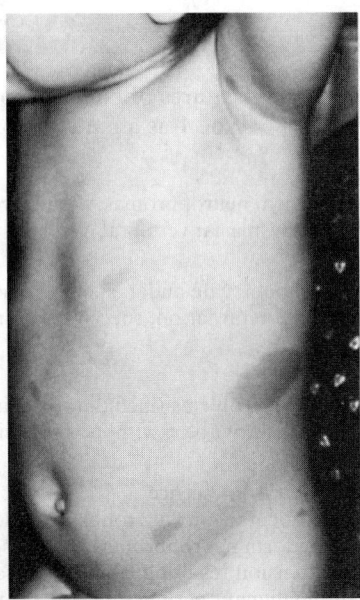

FIGURE 416.1. In patients with neurofibromatosis type 1, café au lait spots usually are larger than 15 mm in diameter, the edges usually are defined sharply, and the intensity of the coloration is uniform.

fewer than 10% of patients with NF-1 who are younger than 6 years old. Ninety to 100% of NF-1 patients who are older than 10 years old have Lisch nodules, and thus they are a very helpful diagnostic finding. If large in size or number, Lisch nodules may be easy to see with an ordinary ophthalmoscope, but ruling out their presence requires careful slit-lamp examination by an ophthalmologist who is familiar with these lesions. The examination of parents for the presence of Lisch nodules (coupled with a skin examination) can be very useful in determining whether an affected child carries a new mutation or inherited

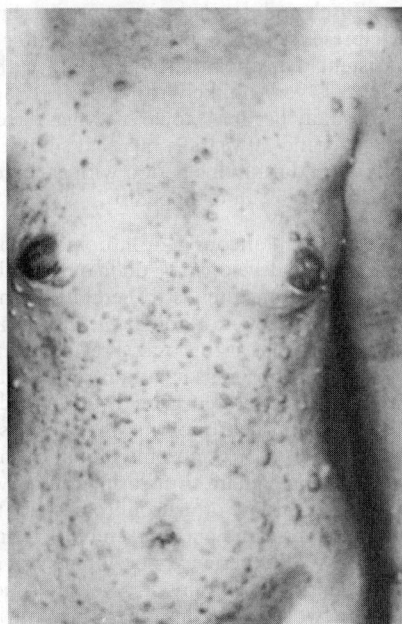

FIGURE 416.2. Cutaneous neurofibromas often are not apparent until puberty and are present in highest density over the trunk.

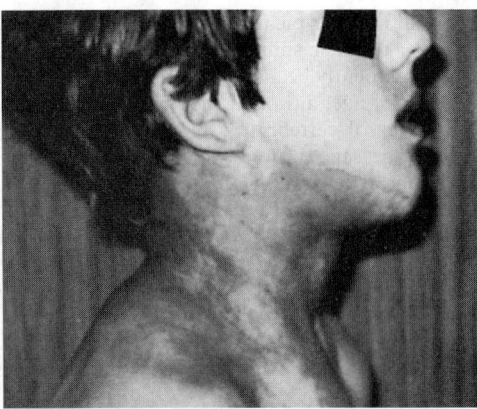

FIGURE 416.3. Plexiform neurofibromas, with or without overlying hyperpigmentation, are congenital lesions that have variable growth patterns during childhood and adolescence.

it from an affected parent. It is important to reassure parents that the development of Lisch nodules does not impact vision.

Optic pathway tumors (OPT) are characteristic of NF-1, occurring in 15% of patients with this disorder. In approximately 5% of children with NF, these lesions result in morbidity, including blindness, thus necessitating a careful ophthalmic examinations of all young children with NF-1. However, given the variable natural history of these lesions and the controversy concerning appropriate treatment, no consensus with regard to recommendations for routine neuroimaging to detect these lesions presymptomatically has been established. In addition to having optic gliomas, children with NF-1 are at increased risk for developing other central nervous system (CNS) neoplasms. Neuroimaging of children with NF-1 utilizing T2-weighted magnetic resonance imaging (MRI) revealed the frequent occurrence of areas that were unusually bright. These lesions have been referred to by many names, including unidentified bright objects, NF-1 bright spots, and, more recently, vacuolation changes. These lesions wax and wane and often disappear later in childhood. Whether the number of lesions correlates with any cognitive dysfunction is unclear. Although suggestive of NF-1, their presence is not a diagnostic criterion.

Learning disabilities, distinct from mental retardation, are present in 40% to 60% of children with NF-1. These disabilities may be foreshadowed by a delay in attaining developmental milestones, but in any event, they usually are apparent by the time the child begins the first grade of school. Mental retardation occurs in approximately 8% of patients with NF-1, but its presence should not be presumed to be the result of NF-1 until an investigation for other causes has been completed and found to be negative or unrevealing. Mental retardation and dysmorphic features are found with children who have a large deletion encompassing the whole NF-1 gene. Speech impediments may involve articulation or language elements and usually are obvious by the time the child is 3 years of age.

Pseudoarthrosis, or bowing of the tibia, may occur as an independent lesion, but it often is one of the characteristic congenital lesions of NF-1. The congenital nature of the pseudoarthrosis may be masked by a delay in diagnosis until weight bearing or walking is attempted. Any child with tibial pseudoarthrosis should be evaluated thoroughly for other clinical features of NF-1. Sphenoid wing dysplasia is another congenital skeletal feature of NF-1. Similar to pseudoarthrosis, it is a congenital primary bony dysplasia, although sometimes an associated orbital or periorbital diffuse plexiform neurofibroma may occur.

The scoliosis that is typical of NF-1 usually involves the cervical and upper thoracic spine and has an anterior angulation (kyphosis). It frequently becomes apparent in children between 6 and 10 years of age, although the presence of a hair whorl overlying an area of vertebral dysplasia (Riccardi sign) at an earlier age may presage future problems.

Renovascular hypertension is one of the clinical problems of NF-1 that can be anticipated and treated effectively. All individuals who have NF-1 are at risk for developing the disorder and must receive regular blood pressure monitoring, regardless of their age, although adolescents and pregnant women are most likely to be affected. Pheochromocytoma is another source of systemic hypertension, both intermittent and sustained. NF-1 patients with hypertension should be evaluated for these two causes of hypertension.

Malignant peripheral nerve sheath tumor (MPNST), previously referred to as neurofibrosarcoma, has an overall lifetime incidence of 3% to 5% among patients with NF-1. Although the magnitude of this risk may be small, the relative risk is at least two orders of magnitude above that of the general population, and NF-1 patients diagnosed with MPNST have a very poor prognosis. These malignancies usually are found in an area of a preexisting plexiform neurofibroma. Thus, a MPNST must be ruled out in a child with a history suggestive of such a lesion (i.e., pain, acceleration in growth of a plexiform lesion, a rapidly enlarging tumor, or an otherwise unexplained neurologic deficit).

Several other common medical conditions show an increased frequency in NF-1, one of which is puberty disturbance. More important, premature or delayed puberty may indicate the presence of a chiasmal or hypothalamic glioma. Short stature is seen in at least 16% of patients with NF-1, and growth curves for children with NF-1 are available. Macrocephaly also is present in 16% or more of affected patients. This finding not always is apparent in infancy and is not correlated with any known functional compromise.

Natural History

The timing of onset of the features of NF-1 is well established (Box 416.3).

Congenital Features. Congenital glaucoma may occur in approximately 1% of infants with NF-1, and screening for glaucoma should be included in the ophthalmic evaluation of infants with NF-1. Tibial pseudoarthrosis may be obvious by congenital bowing of the distal leg, or it may not become apparent until weight bearing or ambulation is attempted. Diffuse plexiform neurofibromas almost always are present at birth, but they may be subtle (i.e., apparent only from associated overlying hyperpigmentation or large CALS) or internal (e.g., apparent only on radiographic studies). Sphenoid wing dysplasia sometimes is associated with an orbital or periorbital diffuse plexiform neurofibroma. Similarly, vertebral dysplasia occasionally is associated with a diffuse plexiform neurofibroma, but it is unlikely to be a source of concern until later in childhood.

Infantile Features. Optic-pathway gliomas often are detected first on MRI neuroimaging during the child's second year of life. They usually are not apparent clinically until visual compromise can be appreciated by a parent or clinician and, in some cases, not until the tumor mass causes proptosis. Thus, significant visual compromise may occur in children with OPT if the diagnosis of NF-1 is not made and ophthalmic evaluation not initiated. In most cases, children who have no evidence of optic pathway involvement on neuroimaging by the time they are age 3 years are very unlikely to develop symptomatic OPT later in life. Also, as noted previously, CALS become apparent when the child is between 6 and 18 months of age.

> ### BOX 416.3   Features of Neurofibromatosis Type 1 as a Function of Age
>
> **Congenital**
> Glaucoma; plexiform neurofibromas; pseudoarthrosis; sphenoid wing dysplasia; vertebral dysplasia
>
> **Infancy to 6 Years**
> Optic-pathway glioma; café au lait spots; learning disability; mental retardation; speech impediment; seizures
>
> **6 to 10 Years**
> School performance problems (including learning disability); scoliosis, with or without kyphosis; iris Lisch nodules
>
> **Preadolescence and Adolescence**
> Cutaneous and subcutaneous neurofibromas; accelerated growth of plexiform neurofibromas; psychosocial burden; hypertension resulting from renovascular involvement; malignant peripheral nerve sheath tumor
>
> **Adulthood**
> Variable increase in number and size of cutaneous and subcutaneous neurofibromas; hypertension resulting from renovascular involvement; malignant peripheral nerve sheath tumor; pheochromocytoma

---

Often, the parents of a young child with NF-1 are concerned that he or she will have diffuse plexiform neurofibromas and, as a result, be seriously disfigured. In general, these lesions develop early in childhood and if not evident (on careful examination) by middle childhood are unlikely to develop. Moreover, even in children with a diffuse plexiform neurofibroma, the prediction of growth is difficult and extreme disfigurement is unusual.

Later Childhood Features. School performance problems resulting from learning disabilities usually become important in patients with NF-1 in the middle to later years of childhood (8 to 14 years). Lisch nodules in the iris cause no clinical problems, but their presence in patients with NF-1 after 6 years of age is so consistent that after that age a child without Lisch nodules or CALS is very unlikely to have NF-1. Scoliosis or kyphoscoliosis usually becomes apparent when the child is between the ages of 5 and 10 years, a fact that supports particularly close follow-up during this period with early recognition and prompt treatment by an orthopedist.

Adolescent Features. Cutaneous neurofibromas, subcutaneous neurofibromas, or both develop most often during adolescence, and their initial appearance tends to herald the onset of puberty rather than to follow it. Nodular plexiform neurofibromas may become apparent at this time. Previously appreciated diffuse plexiform neurofibromas have an irregular growth pattern and may show accelerated growth during adolescence. However, any plexiform neurofibroma that has a substantial change in growth pattern or symptoms should be investigated for the possibility of malignant transformation to MPNST. In view of the increased activity of neurofibromas and the associated social stigmatization and personal emotional turmoil that children with NF-1 may experience, development of significant psychosocial difficulties during this stage of life is not surprising. Renovascular hypertension becomes apparent in this age group.

Adult Features. Cutaneous and subcutaneous neurofibromas almost always increase significantly in number and size during all phases of adulthood, but the absolute number of lesions is highly variable. Pregnancy may initiate or aggravate the appearance and growth of neurofibromas. Pruritus associated with the accelerated growth of neurofibromas may be a prominent and distressing symptom. Renovascular hypertension also continues to appear in young adulthood, particularly in women during pregnancy. MPNST may develop in adult life and may occur in patients with NF-1 whose disease otherwise has been relatively mild. Pheochromocytomas associated with NF-1 almost always occur in adults, and pregnancy also may contribute to their development. Chronic pain caused by the development of spinal neurofibromas is a common occurrence in adults with NF-1.

Diagnosis

According to the guidelines developed by the original 1987 National Institutes of Health Consensus Development Conference on Neurofibromatosis and the review of those guidelines in 1997, the diagnostic criteria for NF-1 are met in an individual if two or more of the following are found: six or more CALS larger than 5 mm in greatest diameter in prepubertal individuals and larger than 15 mm in greatest diameter in postpubertal individuals; two or more neurofibromas of any type, or one plexiform neurofibroma; freckling in the axillary or inguinal regions; optic-pathway glioma; two or more iris Lisch nodules; a distinctive osseous lesion, such as sphenoid wing dysplasia or thinning of long-bone cortex, with or without pseudoarthrosis; and a first-degree relative (parent, sibling, or offspring) with NF-1 diagnosed by the above criteria.

Establishing the diagnosis of NF-1 rarely is a problem in a child who is 1 year or older and has a positive family history for the disease because the requisite number of CALS usually are obvious by that age. Establishing such diagnosis is more problematic in a young child without a family history of the disease because one or more additional features may or may not be present at an early age. In addition to NF-1, much rarer inherited syndromes, including Russell-Silver syndrome and McCune-Albright syndrome, are associated with CALS. Excluding the diagnosis of NF-1 in a young child with CALS is difficult. Molecular testing looking for mutations in the NF-1 gene has been difficult, but more sensitive sequence-based tests are now available and may aid in establishing the diagnosis. Testing may be particularly helpful if parents are uncomfortable with the uncertainty in the diagnosis. Approximately 50% of infants with CALS will develop other diagnostic features of NF-1. If the diagnosis is suspected but cannot be established after the patient reaches 2 or 3 years, she should be evaluated for an alternative form of NF, including NF-2.

Genetic Counseling

Because 50% of the index cases of NF-1 represent new mutations, many parents will be unaffected. However, because the clinical expression of NF-1 is highly variable, careful examination of the parents (including skin and eye examinations) should be undertaken before they are counseled about their risk of having more children with NF-1. If they clearly are unaffected, this risk is less than 1%, with families only rarely having a second affected child due to germline mosaicism in a parent. If a parent is affected with NF-1, then the recurrence risk for each subsequent pregnancy is 50%. The severity of NF-1 in the offspring is unrelated to the severity of the disorder in the affected parent, and we have no means of predicting the clinical severity of the disease. Prenatal diagnosis is now available as better mutation-detection methods have been developed. If an NF-1 mutation has been detected through the molecular analysis of DNA from an affected family member, then the prenatal diagnosis of subsequent pregnancies is possible.

Screening and Follow-Up

The current recommendation is that children suspected of having NF-1 be evaluated in a multidisciplinary NF clinic. Such a clinic normally includes specialists from the disciplines of genetics, neurology, dermatology, neurosurgery, and plastic surgery. The first purpose of a screening evaluation is to confirm the diagnosis of NF-1 by identifying features of the disease that are not apparent from the history and general physical examination. The second goal of clinic care is to detect potentially compromising lesions before they become symptomatic, thereby minimizing the ultimate severity of the symptoms (e.g., identifying an optic-pathway glioma before it causes irreversible blindness). At the initial visit, a full family history is taken and the genetics of NF, including the potential recurrence risk in other offspring, are explained to the parents.

In addition to a full physical, dermatologic, and neurologic examination, additional evaluation includes a slit-lamp ocular examination to identify Lisch nodules, choroidal hamartomas, hypertrophied corneal nerves, and perhaps signs of an optic-pathway glioma. As mentioned previously, the use of neuroimaging for asymptomatic children with NF-1 is controversial. A panel convened by the National Neurofibromatosis Foundation did not recommend presymptomatic screening. However, many clinicians who follow children with NF-1 continue to perform neuroimaging on patients younger than 3 years to look for optic-pathway tumors, given the difficulty of detecting visual loss in very young children. Developmental evaluation is useful to identify learning disabilities so that special efforts can be initiated on behalf of the youngster in school.

If the results of a detailed history, physical examination, and presymptomatic screening fail to reveal any potentially serious problems, annual routine follow-up visits are recommended. In the absence of new problems, follow-up efforts can be restricted to history taking and physical examination; repeated routine screening is unnecessary. If new, evolving, or established clinical problems are present, the appropriate follow-up interval and the extent of evaluation are determined by the nature and severity of the clinical concerns. Referral of the patient or family to a local chapter of the National Neurofibromatosis Foundation for further information about the disorder and general support usually is helpful.

Therapy

Medical therapy for problems arising from NF-1 is similar to that used for the same conditions when they occur in the absence of NF-1; these conditions include seizures, headaches, hyperactivity, learning disabilities, anxiety, and renovascular hypertension. Antineoplastic chemotherapy and radiotherapy have no role in the treatment of benign neurofibromas, although carboplatin-based treatment is used to treat enlarging optic-pathway gliomas. Treatment regimens for MPNST can include surgery, chemotherapy, and radiation therapy, although these lesions often are resistant to all three modalities. Children with NF-1 who receive radiotherapy for CNS lesions appear to have an increased incidence of toxicity.

Surgery is the mainstay of therapy for patients with NF-1, particularly for removing or debulking tumors (e.g., neurofibromas, neurofibrosarcomas, pheochromocytomas), for treating skeletal dysplasia (e.g., tibial pseudoarthrosis, sphenoid wing dysplasia), for correcting scoliosis or kyphoscoliosis, and for treating at least some individuals with renovascular or other types of vascular compromise. In general, the surgical removal of neurofibromas is associated with suboptimal results; the tumors tend to recur, and the possibility of a consequent neuropathy developing is significant. Surgical removal of a neurofibroma should be undertaken only if a specific clinical goal (e.g. decompression of a vital structure) can be established beforehand.

Neurofibromatosis Type 2 (Bilateral Acoustic Neurofibromatosis)

NF-2 is distinct from NF-1 both in clinical terms and in terms of the gene locus. The *NF2* gene resides on the middle long arm of chromosome 22, specifically in band 22q11.2. Information about the molecular biology of NF-2 is presented in Box 416.4. NF-2 is a much less common disorder than is NF-1, and more of the serious manifestations develop in adolescence and young adulthood.

Clinical Manifestations and Complications

The definitive feature of NF-2 is the presence of bilateral acoustic neuromas, which actually are vestibular schwannomas. Intracranial and spinal cord meningiomas also occur frequently, as do spinal cord astrocytomas. Paraspinal schwannomas and neurofibromas are common occurrences at all levels, but particularly in the cervical and lumbar regions. Cutaneous and subcutaneous neurofibromas generally are fewer in number. Cutaneous schwannomas are relatively common findings, even in young children; they may have the same coloration as the skin or be slightly hyperpigmented with or without associated hypertrichosis. Their size ranges from 3 to 8 mm. CALS are few in number and relatively pale in color, and they tend to be somewhat less clearly demarcated and larger in size than those that are typical of NF-1. Posterior subcapsular cataracts are present consistently, even in children of a young age. Retinal hamartomas are another feature of NF-2. Both the cataracts and the retinal hamartomas may be particularly useful features for delineating the diagnosis of NF-2 in a child. This disease is clinically distinct from NF-1; in particular, optic-pathway gliomas, Lisch nodules, and plexiform neurofibromas are not features of NF-2.

Diagnosis

In contrast to the diagnosis of NF-1, that of NF-2 may be difficult to establish in children. The inclusive diagnostic criteria for NF-2 are the bilateral eighth cranial nerve masses seen with neuroimaging studies (computed tomography [CT] or, MRI) or a first-degree relative with NF-2 and either a unilateral eighth cranial nerve mass or two of the following: neurofibroma, meningioma, spinal astrocytoma, schwannoma, and posterior subcapsular cataracts. Children with NF-2 may be asymptomatic through the first 15 years of life, although the cutaneous schwannomas, cataracts, and retinal hamartomas may be detectable during this period. The most frequent symptoms include headaches, hearing loss, and tinnitus, which most often are unilateral in the earliest stages of the disease. Once symptoms appear, however, progression generally is constant and relatively gradual, although rapid deterioration occurs occasionally. Early mortality is apparent approximately 10 years after diagnosis, with earlier presentation being associated with a more severe clinical course. The progression of symptoms results from the appearance and growth of the various CNS tumors. Women have more meningiomas than do men with NF-2, and whether pregnancy worsens the clinical course is unclear. Recognition of the disorder usually results from the development of symptoms from a CNS tumor, a characteristic eye finding, or the presence of an affected first-degree relative.

Genetic Counseling

NF-2 is an autosomal dominant disorder; each offspring of an affected patient carries approximately a 50% risk for bearing the mutant gene and ultimately manifesting the disorder. A larger proportion of index cases of NF-2 than of NF-1 appear to represent new mutations, with some of the index cases being mosaic for the *NF2* mutation. Mosaicism refers to the finding that only some cells in the body may carry the mutation. The finding of mutations in only about 40% to 60% of patients with NF-2 has been attributed at least partly to mosaicism. Mosaic individuals also have a slightly lower risk of having an affected child. Thus, in a two-generation pedigree, it is preferable to do genetic testing on the affected child, who will not be mosaic. Genetic evaluation is recommended as for NF-1, although with some differences: (a) excluding the diagnosis in children who are at risk for NF-2 on clinical grounds is much more difficult and (b) testing for mutations in the *NF2* gene is simpler. For families with a detected mutation, prenatal diagnosis is available. For some additional families with multiple living affected members, linkage analysis also can be used for prenatal diagnosis. Patients who carry a missense mutation (encoding the exchange of one amino acid for another) have a milder course than do patients with mutations that disrupt the production of the NF2 protein.

Therapy

Surgery for the removal or debulking of intracranial, spinal, or paraspinal tumors is the mainstay of therapy for patients with NF-2. The most appropriate treatment for acoustic neuromas is controversial. The consequences of surgical removal of an acoustic neuroma may include further hearing loss and ipsilateral facial nerve palsy. However, microsurgical techniques, radiosurgery, and conformal radiation therapy often are used for very small lesions (within the internal auditory canal) and may preserve hearing and facial nerve function. For this reason, patients with positive findings on imaging should be referred to an experienced ear, nose, and throat (ENT) surgeon and radiation oncologist to discuss treatment options before hearing loss develops. For patients with more advanced lesions, for whom hearing preservation is not possible, brainstem implants to restore some degree of hearing have been approved by the U.S. Food and Drug Administration (FDA) for patients with NF-2 who have large lesions accompanied by loss of hearing. Studies from the United Kingdom suggest that patients have better prognoses when treated at centers with significant experience

BOX 416.5

Molecular Biology of Tuberous Sclerosis

Because tuberous sclerosis (TS) is caused by mutations in one of two specific genes, the identification of these genes allows the determination of whether certain genotypes are more likely to result in specific manifestations of the disease than are others. Overall, children with a mutation in *TSC2* versus *TSC1* are more likely to have cognitive deficits (67% versus 31%) and generally have a more severe phenotype. The function of these genes is not understood clearly, but tuberin encodes a protein that regulates the ras/gap pathway of signal transduction. Somatic mutations in the normal allele in TS-associated tumors suggest that these genes act as tumor suppressors. As described for NF-2, individuals who appear to be the first member of the family with TS may be mosaic for the mutation, which complicates genetic testing. Children with clinical features of TS and polycystic kidney disease harbor a deletion that encompasses the *TSC2* and neighboring *PKD1* genes. These children need careful surveillance by a nephrologist to monitor renal function.

in NF-2. Severe disorientation may occur when patients are diving or swimming underwater, and drowning may result. All individuals who have or are at risk for developing NF-2 should be advised of this risk and should be cautioned never to swim alone. Families affected with NF-2 should consider learning sign language, given the significant risk of hearing loss occurring.

Tuberous Sclerosis

Tuberous sclerosis (TS) is characterized by hypoepigmented lesions of the skin, tumors of the CNS, seizures, and ocular hamartomas; it shows an autosomal dominant pattern of inheritance. Because it combines developmental abnormalities of the skin, nervous system, and eyes, this disorder traditionally has been grouped with the neurofibromatoses and von Hippel–Lindau disease (VHL) in the category known as the phakomatoses. TS is caused by mutations in one of two genes: *TSC1* (encoding hamartin) on 9q34 and *TSC2* (encoding tuberin) on 16p13. Information about the molecular biology of TS is presented in Box 416.5.

Natural History

TS is a complex disorder, with some problems apparent from infancy and other lesions developing throughout childhood and early adulthood. Marked variation occurs in the expression of the disorder; patients can have very mild to very severe symptoms. Although several patient series have found most patients to have mental retardation and seizures, some bias in how the patients in these series were identified exists. More recently, population-based studies confirm that approximately 30% have profound disability, 15% mild to severe impairment, and 55% have IQs in the normal range. In addition, recent studies document that children with TS have a high rate of autistic spectrum disorders that can further complicate their social adjustment and developmental progress.

One exception to the general rule of progressivity may be seen for cardiac rhabdomyomas; these congenital cardiac tumors tend to regress, at least to some degree, with age. In any

event, once the diagnosis of TS is made, the patient must be observed closely, and the appropriate clinical, laboratory, and imaging techniques must be used to identify new lesions and to monitor the progression of those already identified. The malignant degeneration of benign tumors (e.g., astrocytomas, fibromas) is not a common feature of TS.

Although the use of vaccines with a pertussis component was thought to be contraindicated in patients with TS, more recent studies do not demonstrate any association between vaccination and seizure pattern or outcome in children with TS.

Diagnosis

When multiple features of TS are present, the diagnosis is relatively easy to establish. When only one feature is present, the diagnosis is likely to be considered only tentatively, if not overlooked entirely.

- Skin. Hypopigmented macules, usually elliptic in shape (ash-leaf spots); fibroadenomas (adenoma sebaceum, shown in Fig. 416.4), typically involving the malar regions of the face; periungual fibromas; shagreen patches, seen most commonly over the lower trunk; and a distinctive brown patch on the forehead. The last lesion is especially important because it may be the first and most readily recognizable feature of TS to be appreciated on the physical examination of neonates and infants with the disorder.
- Teeth. Characteristic pits of the enamel
- Eyes. Choroidal hamartomas; hypopigmented defects of the iris
- CNS. Periventricular tubers; cerebral astrocytomas; sacrococcygeal chordomas seen on CT examination; nonspecific electroencephalographic abnormalities, including hypsarrhythmia
- Cardiovascular system. Cardiac rhabdomyomas; aortic and major artery constrictions
- Kidneys. Renal angiomyolipomas
- Lungs. Diffuse interstitial fibrosis

Seizures are not listed as a diagnostic feature because they are nonspecific, but that does not minimize their frequency in TS. Seizures of all types, but particularly myoclonic jerks associated with hypsarrhythmia, and mental retardation are the most common symptoms leading to the consideration of the diagnosis of TS. MRI scans of the brain in patients with TS are virtually diagnostic and should be obtained for all individuals suspected of having the disorder. Heart failure or a cardiac

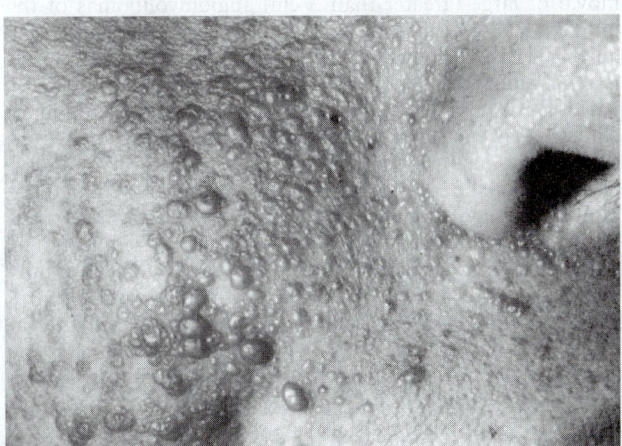

FIGURE 416.4. Fibroadenomas (adenoma sebaceum) in a child with tuberous sclerosis at age 7.

murmur may indicate the presence of a cardiac rhabdomyoma, and deficient circulation or decreased pulses may indicate the presence of arterial tree involvement. Renal failure or an abdominal mass may lead to the recognition of angiomyolipomatous kidney involvement during adolescence or early adulthood. A subset of children with TS have concurrent polycystic kidney disease. Dyspnea may indicate the presence of pulmonary involvement, particularly in adult women with TS.

The diagnosis of TS is made on clinical grounds. A recent revision of these guidelines recommends the diagnosis of definite TS when three major criteria are present and of probable TS when two major and one minor criteria are present. Major criteria include forehead plaque, shagreen patch, three or more hypomelanotic macules, periungual fibromas, lymphangiomatosis, renal angiomyolipomas, cardiac rhabdomyoma, multiple retinal nodular hamartomas, cortical tuber, subependymal nodule, and subependymal giant cell astrocytoma.

Genetic Counseling

TS is the result of a mutation in one of two autosomal dominant genes. Precisely because new mutations are relatively common, a negative family history does not exclude the diagnosis. Moreover, once the diagnosis of TS has been established in the proband, all first-degree relatives must be evaluated carefully for subtle signs of the disorder before one can assume that the child represents a new mutation. Thus, counseling of parents regarding the risk of having another child affected with TS should be undertaken by geneticists familiar with TS who have examined the parents. Anyone who meets the clinical criteria for TS or is documented to carry a TS mutation carries a 50% risk that each of his or her offspring will have the disorder. Genetic testing for mutations in both *TSC1* and *TSC2* is clinically available. Once a mutation is identified, this information can be used to test at-risk family members and to make a prenatal diagnosis. Ultrasound evaluation of a potentially affected pregnancy normally is unrevealing except for the possible identification of cardiac rhabdomyomas. A negative ultrasound study clearly does not rule out the presence of TS in the fetus.

Therapy

No specific medical treatment is available for TS itself. The medical treatment used for seizures and other complications (e.g., heart failure, renal failure) is the same as if TS were not present, unless surgery on the primary lesions is indicated. For example, surgical removal of a cardiac rhabdomyoma may rarely be warranted. Some clinicians recommend surgical removal of large (greater than 3 cm) angiomyolipomas of the kidney because of the risk of hemorrhage into the lesion. Very advanced cases of renal disease (primarily in adults) can result in renal failure.

Children with TS benefit from care in a multidisciplinary clinic that offers services including genetics, neurology, ophthalmology, nephrology, dermatology, neurosurgery, and plastic surgery. The Tuberous Sclerosis Consensus Conference published a set of guidelines for the initial evaluation and management of children with TS, which is summarized here. The initial screening evaluation should include a detailed family history, medical history, developmental history, and physical examination focused on the dermatologic and neurologic features of TS. Ophthalmic evaluation to identify characteristic lesions is helpful in making the diagnosis. The routine monitoring of a child with TS is recommended and should include annual physical examination, ophthalmic examination, developmental assessment, and review of school progress. The increased risk of autistic spectrum disorders also should be considered. Routine imaging studies are recommended for all

---

BOX 416.6 | **Molecular Biology of Von Hippel-Landau Disease**

The loss of heterozygosity of 3q markers in renal cell carcinomas, both from patients with VHL and from those with isolated tumors, pointed to the locus for VHL. Identification of the gene revealed constitutional mutations in patients with VHL and somatic mutations in sporadic renal-cell carcinomas. Families with renal-cell carcinoma are likely to carry mutations that disrupt the production of the VHL protein, including nonsense mutations, frameshifts, and deletions. Specific missense mutations in the VHL gene increase the risk that a patient with VHL will develop pheochromocytomas. The function of the VHL protein has been elucidated recently; it regulates the stability of the hypoxia-sensing transcription factor, HIF1α. Cells lacking VHL function mimic hypoxic cells, even in a normal oxygen environment, thus explaining the high vascularity of VHL-associated tumors. Anti-angiogenesis agents are being used in clinical trials of patients with VHL to determine if they will block or reverse tumor formation.

---

children with TS, including renal ultrasonography every 1 to 3 years, cranial CT every 1 to 3 years, or cranial MRI every 1 to 3 years.

Von Hippel-Lindau (VHL) Disease

VHL traditionally is grouped with the neurofibromatoses and TS as a phakomatosis because of the direct involvement of the CNS, vascular abnormalities, diffuse cystic changes in multiple organs, and malignant tumors of the kidney that characterize the disease. It, too, is an autosomal dominant, heritable condition and is caused by mutations in the *VHL* gene on chromosome 3q. Information about the molecular biology of VHL is presented in Box 416.6.

Natural History

VHL is progressive. Regardless of the mode of presentation, patients with VHL must have life-long surveillance for the progression of prior lesions and the development of new ones. The most likely tumors to be diagnosed during early childhood are retinal angiomas and pheochromocytomas. Both require surgical treatment. CNS hemangioblastomas may cause serious problems during adolescence, requiring surgery. Renal cysts may be apparent on imaging in childhood, but frank renal-cell carcinomas typically develop in young adulthood. More recently, researchers have recognized that individuals with VHL also have an increased risk of developing endolymphatic sac tumors (ELST) that can result in hearing loss. Before the use of surveillance regimens, a shortened life span was typical of this disorder. The goal of careful screening is to detect the complications of VHL at a more curable stage to prolong life span.

Diagnosis

The clinical diagnosis of VHL is based on identifying two of the characteristic features or one feature and a positive family history. Because lesions associated with VHL may not cause symptoms, one cannot exclude the diagnosis based solely on physical examination and medical history. A thorough imaging evaluation, including evaluation of the brain, spine, and kidneys, is required. Also, unlike in the other phakomatoses, molecular testing for mutations in the *VHL* gene has a near 99% sensitivity; thus, genetic testing is used as a key part of the diagnostic work-up. Clinical presentations can include visual disturbances and glaucoma associated with retinal vascular hamartomas, headache, cerebellar dysfunction, and signs of increased ICP associated with CNS hemangioblastomas or tachycardia, hypertension, and headache associated with pheochromocytoma. The renal lesions often are clinically silent, but diffuse cystic lesions throughout the kidneys and solid renal lesions may be detected on imaging.

Genetic Counseling

VHL is an autosomal dominant disorder. Approximately 15% of patients present as the first affected member of the family, which is lower than the nearly 50% seen in the other phakomatoses. Individuals diagnosed with VHL have a 50% risk of having an affected child. Again, the parents of any child diagnosed with VHL should be screened carefully for evidence of the disease because they may be asymptomatic but have unsuspected tumors. The isolation of the *VHL* gene has allowed for the development of clinical mutation testing with a very high level of sensitivity and specificity. Similar to other disorders, the *VHL* gene may have unique mutations in a given family, so testing of an affected member of the family is done first to identify the specific mutation in that family. Once a mutation is identified, other at-risk individuals in the family can be tested to determine which children require surveillance and which do not. Genetic testing performed in specialized laboratories is considered part of routine medical care for VHL families. For families with VHL without an identified mutation, linkage analysis is available if a sufficient number of living affected relatives can be found. Either direct mutation testing or linkage can be used for prenatal diagnosis.

Therapy

The hallmark of treatment is careful life-long surveillance, following a program of imaging of the brain and abdomen, as well as yearly ophthalmologic and screening for pheochromocytoma. All patients with VHL should be followed carefully in a center familiar with the multiple complications of this disorder (Box 416.7). The medical treatment of VHL is tailored by the physician based on the knowledge that the patient is at increased risk for developing recurrent or ipsilateral

---

BOX 416.7	Screening Protocols for Individuals with the Clinical Diagnosis of von Hippel–Lindau Disease or a Known VHL Mutation

Clinical assessment annually
Retinal examination annually from infancy
Testing of urinary vanillylmandelic acid and catecholamine or plasma metanephrine levels annually from age 2
Magnetic resonance imaging of brain and spine every 2 years for those older than age 11; every 5 years for those older than age 60
Ultrasound scan of upper abdomen annually from age 11 to age 20; computed tomographic examination of abdomen every 1–2 years from age 20
Directed imaging of the inner ear for endolymphatic sac tumors if hearing loss or tinnitus develop.

---

tumors. For example, in the case of renal-cell carcinoma, surgeons will wait until a lesion is approximately 3 cm in size and use nephron-sparing procedures in contrast to a total nephrectomy. Cerebellar hemangioblastomas that have an enlarging cystic component are most likely to become symptomatic and require surgical removal at the first sign of symptoms. Laser technology to treat early retinal angiomas is used commonly in patients with VHL.

Sturge-Weber Disease

Sturge-Weber disease (SWD) also is called encephalofacial angiomatosis and sometimes is considered the "fourth phakomatosis." It differs from the neurofibromatoses, TS, and VHL by virtue of the absence of three features: cutaneous pigmentation defects, a clear excess of tumors, and heritability. To date, no clear mutational mechanism has been found that underlies SWD, although researchers have proposed it to be secondary to a somatic mutation.

Clinical Manifestations and Complications

In addition to a facial port wine stain and intracranial angiomatosis, primary involvement of the anterior chamber of the eye, specifically the trabecular network, and Schlemm canal may lead to glaucoma (in either eye) in as many as 30% of patients with SWD. Macrocephaly and cutaneous xanthogranulomas also may be seen. No one feature is associated uniformly with any other, and histopathologic features cannot establish a diagnosis beyond confirming the type of lesion.

Natural History

The anatomic features of SWD may be associated with mental retardation, seizures, hemiparesis, and visual deficits, including homonymous hemianopsia. A recent study of adults with SWD reveals that patients with seizures have a significantly increased incidence of developmental delay and special educational placement. Forty percent of adults were financially independent.

Diagnosis

The diagnosis of SWD depends on the presence of a port wine stain (nevus flammeus) on the face, primarily in the first division of the trigeminal nerve; leptomeningeal angiomatosis (including angiomatous involvement of the choroid plexus or choroid of the eye); or both.

Genetic Counseling

No clear evidence exists for assigning an inherited cause for SWD. Recurrence among siblings to the proband is unlikely. One study of 20 children born to adults with SWD revealed one case of TS and no children with SWD. Only a few cases of an affected person having a child with SWD have been reported in the literature.

Therapy

No medical treatment is available for SWD, and the role of surgical treatment has yet to be defined. The use of lasers to treat the facial and ocular angioma lesions has been at least partially successful.

McCune-Albright Syndrome

McCune-Albright syndrome is referred to by many names including Albright syndrome (AS) or polyostotic fibrous dysplasia, but it is distinct from Albright hereditary osteodystrophy.

The cardinal features of the disorder are fibrous dysplasia of one or more bones, precocious puberty, and general autonomous activation of the endocrine system and CALS. Although some features of McCune-Albright syndrome overlap with those of one or more of the neurofibromatoses (e.g., CALS), the diseases rarely present a diagnostic dilemma. McCune-Albright syndrome is caused by mutations to GNAS1, which encodes a specific G-protein subunit that regulates signal transduction from membrane receptors.

Although heritability has not been an element of McCune-Albright syndrome, researchers have reasoned that a mutation of the alpha subunit of the G protein (Gs alpha) might be present in a mosaic form. Indeed, such a mutation has been found. This finding is important for two reasons. First, it documents a somatic mutation as a mechanism to account for human disease. Thus, the disorder has a genetic basis but not a germ cell or heritable basis. Second, the role of the G protein in determining the nature and availability of a nucleoside phosphate moiety (cyclic adenosine monophosphate) is similar to one of the functions of neurofibromin, the *NF1* gene product. The result of the mutation is the autonomous stimulation of signal transduction pathways in the absence of hormone, resulting in the hyperactive endocrine disorders so commonly seen in this condition.

Clinical Manifestations and Complications

The fibrous dysplasia of AS may involve any bone, but the most frequent sites are the femur, tibia, pelvis, phalanges, ribs, and humerus. Radiography reveals a combination of radiolucent and radiopaque elements, except at the base of the skull, where diffuse sclerosis usually is seen. Precocious puberty or sexual precocity, as it relates to this disorder, more accurately is termed pseudoprecocious puberty; that is, blood levels of sex steroids are elevated, but levels of gonadotrophic hormones are normal and are reported to occur in more than 50% of affected girls. Early spermatogenesis and fertility can accompany these endocrine changes. CALS, when they are present, usually are fewer in number, larger in size and have a rougher contour than are those seen in patients with NF (particularly NF-1). Hyperthyroidism may be seen in approximately 30% of patients with AS. Other features, including acromegaly and elevated levels of growth hormone in the blood, intramuscular myxomas, hyperplastic reticuloendothelial tissues, and lymphoid or myeloid metaplasia, also have been reported, although much less frequently.

Natural History

Progressive worsening of the osseous lesions in patients with McCune-Albright syndrome commonly occurs, although they rarely become quiescent. Fractures may result, as may shortening and deformity of the involved bones. Malignant degeneration apparently does occur, but in fewer than 1% of patients with AS. The sexual precocity usually develops in the last half of the first decade of life, although it has been noted as early as 3 months of age. As mentioned, fertility may be part of the sexual precocity, although pregnancies are unusual. Adult fertility apparently is not affected. Hyperthyroidism may occur at any time in childhood and beyond.

Genetic Counseling

McCune-Albright syndrome is caused by missense mutations in the GNAS1 gene at 20q13.2, which encodes a G-protein subunit. The lack of familial cases is explained by the finding that the patients are mosaic for the mutation, with the individual having a combination of normal cells and mutant cells due to a somatic mutation. Thus, recurrence risk for the parents of an affected child is very low.

Therapy

The treatment of the premature puberty is performed best under the auspices of a specialized pediatric endocrinology center. Bone grafting and subsequent surgical procedures to correct deformities may be indicated, depending on the extent and complications of the lesions. Close observation of the fibrous dysplasia lesions for malignant degeneration is warranted.

Suggested Readings

Gutinan DH, Aylsworth A, Carey JC, et al. The diagnostic evaluation and multidisciplinary management of neurofibromatosis 1 and neurofibromatosis 2. *JAMA* 1997;278:51.

Korf BR. Clinical features and pathobiology of neurofibromatosis 1. *J Child Neurol* 2002;17:573.

Lonser PL, Glenn GM, Walther M, et al. Von Hippel-Lindau disease. *Lancet* 2003;361:2059.

Roach, ES, DiMario, FJ, Kandt, RS, et al. Tuberous Sclerosis Consensus Conference: recommendations for diagnostic evaluation. National Tuberous Sclerosis Association. *J Child Neurol* 1999;14:401.

CHAPTER 417 ■ HEADACHE

ARTHUR L. PRENSKY

Headache is one of the most common neurologic complaints of children. Bille found that 2.5% of schoolchildren frequently had headaches at age 7 and that 15.7% had similar complaints at age 15. More recent surveys indicate an even higher prevalence. In several Scandinavian countries, as many as 7% of all schoolchildren aged 7 to 8 years have more than one headache each month. Ten to twenty percent of the adolescent population has chronic headache symptoms. Despite the many treatments available to reduce or relieve headaches in children, cephalgia remains a frequent complaint, and it impairs the schooling of many pediatric patients.

Whereas the brain is insensitive to pain, pain-sensitive fibers are found in the walls of intracranial arteries and veins, the dural sinuses, the periosteum of bone, extracranial vessels, the muscle and skin of the scalp, the mucosal surfaces of the nasal sinuses, the teeth and gums, and the temporomandibular joint.

Inflammation, stretching, torsion, or contraction of these innervated structures can activate these fibers and produce pain. This pain may be felt at the site of the irritation, but as elsewhere in the body, pain can be projected to other areas of the head or neck. For example, irritation or stretching of the undersurface of the tentorium cerebelli can project to the occipital region, whereas the superior surface of the tentorium may project frontally because it is innervated by fibers of the first division of the fifth cranial nerve. Inflammation of the ethmoid sinuses may produce pain that projects frontally or temporally, whereas pain from inflammation of the maxillary or frontal sinuses is felt at the site of the infection.

Headache syndromes can be classified as acute, subacute, or chronic, depending on the length of time the child has been bothered by the symptoms. This distinction is valuable because differentiating headaches that are due to intracranial disease from those of an extracranial origin is essential. Considerable overlap exists in the symptoms of both groups of headaches, but most intracranial disorders that produce headaches do so acutely or produce increasingly severe episodes of pain over the course of days to weeks, causing the child to be evaluated after a relatively short period of time. The vast majority of children who present to a physician complaining of headache have chronic symptoms that have occurred over the course of months to years. They are brought to see a physician because their headaches are becoming more severe or occurring more frequently. The physician is responsible for deciding the source of the pain, its cause, and the appropriate treatment.

The diagnosis of the most common headache syndromes of children—migraine, tension headache, and chronic daily headache—are not associated with visible pathology. Therefore, the diagnosis is established entirely by the history and the absence of physical findings. Recurrent headaches presenting over the course of several months caused by intracranial pathology usually are associated with physical findings. Physical findings need not be present if the history of pain is brief. Some extracranial headaches also have physical findings such as limitation of neck motion, tight cervical muscles, sinus tenderness, or a mandibular joint click when chewing. Searching for these findings is part of the routine examination. Laboratory tests, including scans, usually are not helpful unless the headaches started recently, have unusual complications, or are associated with physical findings.

CHRONIC HEADACHE SYNDROMES

Although children get chronic, frequent headaches for many reasons, the most common cause of this symptom is migraine. A survey of Scots schoolchildren from Aberdeen indicated that migraine was a far more common occurrence than was tension headache in the 5- to 15-year-old age group. Children who had chronic headaches, particularly migraine, had significantly reduced school attendance.

Migraine Headaches

In 1962, the Committee on Classification of Headache described migraines as "recurrent attacks of headache widely varied in intensity, frequency, and duration." Migraine headaches come in four forms. *Common migraine* accounts for approximately three-fourths of the migraine headaches seen in children. These headaches do not have a prodrome and are less likely to be well-localized or unilateral. *Classic migraine* is that form of the disorder in which an aura exists; usually it is visual, but it can involve other sensory or motor changes. The headache often is unilateral and limited to one area of the cranium. *Complicated migraine* is a syndrome in which the aura is prolonged and the neurologic symptoms may last hours or even days, persisting through and beyond the headache at times. The disorder often is defined by the neurologic symptoms. For example, if confusion and delirium predominate, the child is said to have acute confusional migraine; if the child is paralyzed on one side of the body for a lengthy period of time, the child is said to have hemiplegic migraine; if the neurologic symptoms are predominantly in the territory of the basilar artery and involve ataxia, dizziness, bilateral sensory motor findings, diplopia, or bilateral vision loss, the disorder is defined as basilar migraine. The familial form of hemiplegic migraine, an autosomal dominant disorder, has been localized to chromosome 19. *Cluster headaches* are a fourth subdivision of migraine. In this disorder, headaches occur in groups. The pain usually is unilateral and often around or above the eye. Associated autonomic changes, such as profuse tearing or nasal discharge, are present. It occurs rarely in children.

In 1988, the Classification Committee of the International Society for Headache redefined migraine headache. The diagnosis of common migraine would require at least five attacks of headache, each lasting longer than 4 hours and accompanied by either nausea or vomiting or photophobia and phonophobia, as well as two of the following: unilateral location, pulsating quality, an intensity that inhibits daily activities, or aggravation by routine physical activity. Common migraine is defined as "migraine without aura." The diagnosis presumes that neither the history nor the physical examination suggests other diseases that would produce repeated headaches. The Committee then defined migraine with aura. The aura can be brief, as in classic migraine, or prolonged, as in complicated migraine. The Committee separated ophthalmoplegic migraine, a rare disorder most commonly seen in infants, in which repeated attacks of headache are associated with paresis of one or more ocular cranial nerves in the absence of demonstrable intracranial lesion, and retinal migraine, in which repeated attacks of headache occur that are associated with scotoma or blindness in one eye.

The suitability of these criteria for the diagnosis of migraine headache in children has been questioned repeatedly. Children are less able to describe the specific characteristics of a headache, particularly the type of pain. They often report the onset inaccurately, and they do not complain until pain is severe. Thus, many headaches that otherwise could be classified as migraine may not be reported as lasting 4 or more hours. Recurrent headaches lasting at least 2 hours would seem a more reasonable criteria for the usual childhood migraine. In addition, too great a reliance is put on gastrointestinal symptoms, which may be lacking in children. Also, because few children report both photophobia and phonophobia, a more inclusive and accurate classification would demand that only one of these two symptoms be present.

Another generally accepted group of criteria for the diagnosis of both common and classic migraine in children includes repeated episodes of headache accompanied by at least three of the following symptoms: (a) recurrent abdominal pain (with or without headache) or nausea or vomiting; (b) an aura, which usually is visual but may be sensory, motor, or vertiginous; (c) throbbing or pounding pain; (d) pain restricted to one side of the head (although it may shift sides from one headache to the next); (e) relief of pain obtained by brief periods of sleep; and (f) family history of migraine in one or more immediate relatives.

Children with common migraine usually have nausea or some type of abdominal distress, are helped by sleep, and have a family history of migraine. Localized, throbbing pain and an aura are seen more frequently during and after puberty. These criteria have been criticized for placing excessive emphasis on a family history of similar headaches.

Migraines in children differ from those in adults in that males account for approximately 60% of patients affected before reaching age 12 years compared with approximately 33% in the adult population; unilateral headaches occur less commonly in prepubertal children; and a visual aura is seen much less frequently. The incidence of epilepsy with migraine ranges from 5.4% to 12.3% in children in various series, but in adults it is less than 3%. Nausea and vomiting occur in approximately the same percentage of cases for both adults and children, and approximately 70% of children and adults have a strong family history of migraine. Childhood migraine is more likely to vary in frequency than in severity. Children who otherwise fit the criteria for the diagnosis of migraine may have one headache a month and then gradually, or sometimes abruptly, begin to have five or more headaches a week. Approximately 2% to 3% of adolescents and adults have these daily headaches. Occasionally, these exacerbations can be related to changes in mood, particularly depression, or to stress or a prior infection or head injury. Matthews has suggested that overuse of analgesics may lead to "transformed migraine" and produce daily headaches, the most severe of which have the characteristics of migraine. However, frequently, no predisposing factor can be found to explain the variation in frequency or severity of headache.

Studies indicate that approximately 15% to 20% of adolescents with migraine experience remission in their second decade of life; a small number of headaches persist, but the symptoms associated with migraine disappear, and the headaches can be reclassified as tension headaches.

The pathophysiology of migraine still is uncertain. The previously held view that the aura was a loss of neurologic function caused by vasoconstriction of vessels supplying specific areas of the brain and that the cephalgia that followed was due to extracerebral vasodilatation no longer is tenable. Olesen et al. have noted no correlation between the locus and severity of pain in common migraine and regional cerebral blood flow. Nor have they found a correlation with neurologic symptoms and the area of cerebral blood flow reduction in patients with migraine. The genesis of migraine headache appears to lie within the central nervous system, and vascular changes could be secondary phenomena. However, no doubt exists that severe vasoconstriction can occur later in the headache and, in some patients, may lead to a permanent loss of function as a result of a stroke. The hypotheses most commonly accepted concerning the cause of migraine pain is that, initially, cortical changes in current flow lead to neuronal inactivation (spreading depression). This spreading depression activates reticular neurons that, in turn and for unknown reasons, activate efferent fibers of the trigeminal nerve. This results in the dilatation of meningeal vessels outside the brain and the release of inflammatory and pain-mediating peptides. Trigeminal sensory fibers then transmit the sensation of pain back to the brain, where it is processed through the thalamus and cortex.

Serotonin has been suggested as an important chemical mediator for pain within both the nervous system and the vascular wall. The evidence for this suggestion is that serotonin levels fall in both platelets and sera during a migraine attack, whereas the level of a metabolite of serotonin, 5-hydroxy-indoleacetic acid, increases in the urine. The drug reserpine, which lowers levels of serotonin, induces migraine, whereas injections of 5-hydroxytryptamine (5-HT) relieve migrainous pain. A series of new drugs, the triptans, act as agonists for 5-HT (ib, id) receptors in the brain and meningeal vessels. The fact that they effectively treat migraine in 70% to 80% of patients further supports the relation of migraine to serotonin.

The diagnosis of migraine is made by history. The physical examination generally is normal. Laboratory studies usually are not needed for confirmation unless physical signs or a doubtful history is present. Aspects of the clinical history that should alert the physician to study the child further include (a) a strong family history of occlusive cerebrovascular disease early in life or of intracranial hemorrhage, (b) persistent localization of headaches to one side of the cranium with no shift to the other hemisphere, (c) onset of motor or sensory symptoms well after the headache has started rather than before the headache occurs, (d) failure of motor or sensory symptoms to clear within 24 hours after the headache has ceased, and (e) association of focal headaches with partial seizures involving the same hemisphere. Focal physical findings or evidence of increased intracranial pressure (ICP) on examination also indicate the need for further evaluation or even hospitalization. Neuroimaging usually clarifies whether these symptoms or signs are associated with an underlying structural disorder of the brain. At the present time, magnetic resonance imaging (MRI) scans of the brain and the arterial system are the most satisfactory studies to rule out an underlying disorder. Unless seizures are suspected, the electroencephalogram (EEG) has little place in the evaluation of a child suspected of having migraine. The EEG frequently is abnormal in children who have migraine, and as many as 10% of them may be paroxysmal. However, unless the abnormality on the EEG is focal, the tracing does not have any prognostic significance. Focal tracings do suggest the possible presence of an underlying lesion and mandate further study by neuroimaging. Children with complicated migraine almost always are evaluated by neuroimaging. Children with basilar migraine often are evaluated by EEG because distinguishing between the symptoms of basilar migraine and those of occipital lobe epilepsy sometimes is difficult. In addition, some patients with basilar migraine have extremely abnormal, epileptiform EEGs. Their symptoms may be treated best with anticonvulsants. This small group forms a borderland between migraine and epilepsy. Recurrent headaches that are clinically indistinguishable from migraine have been described in association with metabolic diseases affecting the mitochondria and CNS vascular disease, such as moyamoya disease, sickle cell disease, and cerebral autosomal dominant arteriopathy with subcortical infarcts and leukoencephalopathy (CADASIL) attributed to the Notch 3 mutation on chromosome 19. However, without other symptoms or signs leading the physician to suspect such disorders, further laboratory studies are not indicated.

Many children have symptoms that are said to be "migraine variants." Children who have migraine variants may not have a headache with each attack. The syndrome is related to migraine on the basis of one of two pieces of information: (a) a strong family history of migraine or (b) the known tendency of children with these disorders to develop more typical forms of migraine later in life. Patients who have or later develop migraine may have isolated attacks of confusion or loss of memory. They may have recurrent attacks of delirium. These patients may not complain of headaches, although a strong family history may suggest migraine. Motion sickness is a very common symptom in patients who have or will develop migraine. Recurrent attacks of paroxysmal vertigo in younger children (benign paroxysmal vertigo) are considered a migraine variant, although not all of these children later develop migraine. Children with benign paroxysmal vertigo have a normal neurologic examination and a normal EEG, as do those with benign paroxysmal torticollis. Infants who have attacks of hemiplegia that alternately affect the left and right sides of the body have been considered to have a migraine variant because a strong family history of migraine often exists and many of these children later go on to complain of migraine. However, these children often have other paroxysmal phenomena, such as tonic spells and movement disorders, and many do not develop normal physical or mental function as they grow older. Although some investigators have claimed success in modifying this disorder by treating these infants or children with calcium channel blockers, the relationship between migraine and alternating infantile hemiplegia remains unclear.

Many children with recurrent episodes of abdominal pain develop typical migraine headaches later in life. Paroxysmal abdominal pain is more likely to be a migrainous than an epileptic syndrome, although paroxysmal EEGs are seen commonly with the disorder. Most children with recurrent abdominal pain have neither migraine nor epilepsy when they are followed into adult life, but they may continue to have bouts of unexplained abdominal pain. Cyclical vomiting also sometimes is considered a migraine variant, although it usually does not respond to antimigraine medications.

Patients who have a genetic predisposition to migraine seem to react more severely to relatively minor head injuries. Sometimes a minor episode of trauma is followed by the onset of common or classic migraine or parts of the syndrome, such as isolated vomiting or loss of vision. Transient blindness or motor and sensory loss can occur without significant headache. These episodes are short-lived, and this fact, as well as the absence of any evidence of intracranial injury on neuroimaging, suggests that the symptoms and signs are caused by migraine and are not the result of a contusion.

The treatment of migraine can be divided into two parts: (a) the treatment of the acute attack and (b) prevention of numerous future attacks by the use of daily medication (Box 417.1).

The current recommendation is to give acetaminophen, 20 mg/kg, at the onset of the headache and to give 10 to 20 mg/kg in 2 or more hours if needed, up to four times per day. Repeated use of high doses day after day can cause liver damage. Ibuprofen should be given initially in a dose of 20 mg/kg, up to 800 mg/kg in one dose, to be repeated in 2 to 4 hours, but no more than three doses should be given in a 24-hour period. Furthermore, the drug should not be used if the patient begins to complain of abdominal pain, dizziness, or tinnitus. Naproxen sodium can be given to children older than 12 years of age. One tablet should be taken at the onset of the headache, and the dose may be repeated up to three times a day at 8- to 12-hour intervals. Again, nausea that worsens or epigas-

tric pain is a contraindication to continued use of the drug. If these mild analgesics fail, prescription preparations such as acetaminophen/caffeine/butalbital (Fioricet) or isomethepten/acetaminophen/dichlorphenazone (Midrin) may be used in older children. One to two tablets of Midrin can be taken at the onset of the headache, and the dose can be repeated in 60 minutes. Adolescents should take two tablets at the onset of the headache, a third tablet at 60 minutes from onset, and hourly thereafter, up to 6 tablets daily. Stronger, addicting medications, such as oxycodone or butorphanol nasal spray, should be reserved for extremely severe, relatively infrequent headaches.

Ergotamine preparations still have a limited place in the treatment of infrequent migraine attacks, although they potentiate nausea and vomiting. They largely have been replaced by the use of triptans. Children aged 6 to 12 years should take 1 mg at the onset of a headache and 0.5 mg every 30 to 60 minutes thereafter, until a total of 4 mg is ingested or the vomiting or headache subsides. Children aged 12 to 18 years may take 1 to 2 mg at the onset of a headache and 1 mg every 30 minutes thereafter until a total of 6 mg is reached. Some of these preparations come as suppositories. If suppositories are used, 2 mg should be taken at the onset of the headache; the drug can be given again in 1 hour if needed. The same dosage is used for sublingual preparations. Dihydroergotamine mesylate still is used widely and often is effective in the treatment of migraine. It is used most commonly for intractable headaches, for which it is given intravenously, but it can be given at home either by intramuscular injection or by nasal spray. When injected, one milligram is given at the onset of the headache; the dose can be repeated twice at 1-hour intervals, but no more than 3 mg should be given to a patient in a 24-hour period. Use in children is restricted to those older than age 12 years. The nasal spray delivers 0.5 mg. per spray. One spray should be given in each nostril. It should be repeated in 15 minutes.

The triptans are a new class of drugs specifically designed to treat migraine. They are not pain relievers, although they do relieve migraine headache, as well as nausea and photophobia. These 5HT agonists affect central transmission and inhibit peripheral trigeminal effects on meningeal vessels, thus reducing the dilatation of these blood vessels and the formation of nociceptive peptides. At least seven different triptans are available. All can be taken orally as a tablet or capsule. Some come in forms that dissolve sublingually (rizatriptan and zomatriptan), whereas sumatriptan also is formulated as a nasal spray and for subcutaneous injection. Approximately 70% of patients have moderate to total relief of their headaches usually within 2 to 4 hours. In a significant percentage, headaches recur within the next 24 hours, and the dose usually can be repeated once during that time. The rapidity of the onset of pain relief depends on the individual, the method of administration (being most rapid when injected or given as a spray), and the product formulation. Rizatriptan, for example, produces relief more rapidly in a susceptible population than does frovatriptan. These remarkable drugs have made life tolerable for many people incapacitated by migraine attacks; however, they are not universally effective, and they are extremely expensive. They are not approved for patients younger than age 12 years and usually not for those younger than 18 years of age. They, like over-the-counter medications, work best when given at the onset of the headache. They, too, cannot be used on a daily basis over a long period.

Migraine often is treated prophylactically when disabling headaches occur more frequently than four times per month. These medicines have no direct effect on pain but are taken daily to reduce the number and severity of headaches. The medications were designed to treat other disorders such as depression, hypertension, cardiac disease, or epilepsy, but their effect on neuronal circuitry often helps migraineurs. Dosages of these

---

BOX 417.1 | **Principles in the Treatment of an Acute Migraine Headache**

- Drug therapy is more likely to be effective if it is used before the headache becomes severe, which may necessitate taking medication to school. Oral medication, unless sublingual, does not work once the patient has started to vomit.
- Unless they are specifically contraindicated, over-the-counter preparations should be used initially.
- The more frequent the headaches, the more reluctant the physician should be to prescribe powerful but addicting analgesics. These drugs should not be given to patients who experience more than six headaches per month. When patients have frequent headaches that occur three or four times per week, the use of even simple analgesics (e.g., ibuprofen or acetaminophen) or caffeine can potentiate the recurrence of headaches as patients strive to withdraw from the drug.
- If headaches occur relatively infrequently, but the pain is severe and disabling and interrupts activities, the initial dose of an analgesic should be a large one if it does not have a sedative added to it. Aspirin generally is not used for the treatment of headaches in children because of its past association with Reye syndrome.

drugs often are increased slowly, and the effects are not immediate. Usually, the patient must keep an accurate headache diary for weeks or months to be sure that an effect is being achieved. The drug best studied is the tricyclic antidepressant amitriptyline hydrochloride (1 to 2 mg/kg/day). Although they are more effective as antidepressants, serotonin reuptake inhibitors seem less effective in relieving chronic headaches in children who are not depressed. Other prophylactic medications include beta-blocking agents such as propanolol (1 to 2 mg/kg/day), calcium channel blockers, cyproheptadine hydrochloride (0.3 mg/kg/day in divided doses), and antiepileptics. Dilantin and phenobarbital have been used for decades to treat migraine headaches, but newer antiepileptics have proven to be more effective. Divalproex sodium (increase slowly from 10 to 40 mg/kg/day) and topiramate (from 25 to 200 mg/day raised over 8 to 12 weeks) seem to be the most effective medications in this group. Gabapentin (from 400 to 2,600 mg/day raised slowly) is less effective, but it has fewer drug interactions and serious side effects. Adjunctive medications include riboflavin and magnesium and, for more chronic cases, the alpha-adrenergic agonist, tizanidine.

During the past decade, the most common forms of headache in children have been treated by biofeedback and relaxation therapy. Initial studies were poorly controlled, but increasing evidence indicates that pediatric, as well as adult, patients with common migraine and tension headaches do respond to this type of treatment. Of children who can complete a course of biofeedback or relaxation technique training successfully, 60% to 80% have a positive response that consists of a reduction in the severity or frequency of the headaches; this rate compares favorably with the rate of response to medication. Follow-up studies suggest that the benefits of this training last for at least 1 year. Problems associated with undertaking these forms of behavioral therapy include (a) limited availability of the facilities, which often are restricted to large medical centers; (b) the cost of the therapy, which often is not covered by insurance; and (c) the failure of children to practice these learned techniques regularly. The most likely cause of failure of behavioral therapy, however, is an unstable and unhappy home life.

The use of special diets to treat headaches generally is not successful, nor is desensitization to common allergens. No substantial evidence has established that migraine headache is an allergic disorder. However, some children do get headaches after eating specific foods that contain amines such as tyramine. Chocolate, cheese and other milk products, and wine are major offenders. Some children also seem to have an increased number of headaches if they drink a great deal of soda containing caffeine or diet soda containing aspartame. Such children usually ingest one to two cans of soda a day, or more. If the relationship of a headache to a specific food is well established, withdrawal of the particular food from the diet can be helpful.

Teenage girls who have migraine with aura have a somewhat higher incidence of stroke. This risk is increased if they take birth control pills, and, hence, this form of birth control should be avoided by such patients.

Tension Headaches

Differentiating common migraine from tension headaches solely by the description of the headache often is difficult. No single factor in the history separates them, and people who have either type of headache tend to have a normal physical examination. The Classification Committee of the International Headache Society indicates that tension headaches may last from 30 minutes to 7 days. The headache is subdivided as chronic or episodic, depending on how frequently the headaches bother the child. The pain is a pressing or tightening type of pain that is mild to moderate in intensity, is bi-

lateral, and does not worsen with routine physical activity. Nausea and vomiting are absent, but either phonophobia or photophobia may be present. These criteria are used to differentiate tension headache from migraine headache. However, in children at least, the differentiation using these criteria is not sharp. Children who appear to have tension and not migraine headaches by other criteria do have nausea and vomiting when the headache is extremely severe. Other factors in the history help the physician establish a diagnosis. Tension headaches tend to occur and to be more severe during periods of obvious stress. This association is seen with migraine, but it is not as clear-cut. Migraine headaches tend to involve the frontal and, to a lesser degree, the temporal regions of the head or to be localized to one side of the head; tension headaches tend to involve the occipital or temporal regions bilaterally and often extend to the neck. They also tend to be diffuse. Tension headaches tend to be continuous; they fluctuate throughout the day, but often they last for days. Patients who have tension headaches are less likely to have immediate family members who have typical migraine headaches.

The pathophysiology of tension headaches once was considered to be the result of contracting scalp muscles caused by anxiety or stress. Electrophysiologic studies indicate that many patients with tension headaches do not have contraction of scalp muscles while they are in pain, and, hence, another etiology—as yet undefined—must explain the pain for this subgroup of patients. Some patients with both tension and migraine headaches have overt depression and a history of clear-cut changes in mood, self-image, interest in their usual day-to-day activities, appetite, and sleep habits. They often have other somatic complaints. The headaches in these children do not disappear until the underlying mood disorder is recognized and treated. The subgroup with EMG changes or tender scalp muscles now are called chronic tension-type headache with a disorder of the pericranial muscles.

The pain resulting from tension headaches usually can be treated by analgesics such as those recommended for the treatment of pain in children with migraine. When tension headaches occur frequently, biofeedback and relaxation therapy are useful. Recently, muscle relaxation using botulinum toxin has been used. Antidepressants occasionally may help patients who have chronic tension headaches without depression. However, that population of children whose headaches are related to depression, an anxiety neurosis, or a conversion reaction requires a psychiatric referral.

Many adolescents and a few children younger than age 12 years have chronic daily headache. These patients have tight, pressing, generally nonthrobbing headaches lasting part or all of the day, virtually every day. The headaches are diffuse or bilateral, are not associated with gastrointestinal symptoms, and frequently do not inhibit daily activities. However, many children with this type of headache are unable to go to school. Yet, a careful search fails to reveal that they are stressed at school in any way. In our experience, most children with chronic daily headache have had headaches in the past that meet the criteria for the diagnosis of migraine and have headaches that are migrainous in quality when their chronic headaches are severe (i.e., they frequently vomit, their headaches become worse with activity, and they have photophobia or phonophobia or both). Children who have these headaches often have a family history of migraine headaches. However, their headaches are not unilateral, they do not throb, they have no aura, and they are not relieved by sleep. Chronic daily headaches are the most difficult form of cephalgia to treat. Fortunately, they tend to subside over the course of several years, even if therapy is unsuccessful. In this type of headache, the excessive use of analgesic agents may compound the recurrence of pain when drug use is decreased. The use of increasingly powerful analgesics leads to addiction. Patients must try to live with their headaches and limit taking analgesics to three days a week. The headaches sometimes respond to tricyclics or other types of antidepressants, even if no history of frank depression exists. However, the response is not as gratifying as that seen with simple migraine. Prophylactic treatment using valproate has produced partial relief in more than half the patients tested. Biofeedback and relaxation therapy also may help, but, again, the results are not as satisfactory as those achieved in simple migraine or episodic tension headaches. Constant, intractable headaches also can be associated with infection, such as a low-grade viral meningitis. These headaches may persist for months following an infection, usually viral but sometimes bacterial. The most notable example is continuous headache that occurs after a recent contact with the EB virus.

Sinus Headaches

Chronic or recurrent headaches occur in approximately 15% of children with chronic sinusitis. Sinus disease also may exacerbate the symptoms of migraine in children who are subject to that disorder. Frequently, no increase in temperature occurs. The most common accompanying symptoms are rhinorrhea, postnasal drip, coughing, sneezing, wheezing, and headache. However, none of these symptoms predicts sinus infection. Pain or pressure over the frontal or maxillary sinuses may be present, and these cavities can fail to transilluminate. (The frontal sinuses form later in childhood and are not fully developed in most children until they reach the end of puberty.) Most sinus headaches in children result from infection of the sphenoid or ethmoid sinuses, which cannot be palpated or visualized by transillumination in the office. Pain from these sinuses usually is referred to the frontotemporal region, but it can occur over any part of the cranial vault. Sinus headaches often occur at the same time each day, build slowly, often are throbbing, and vary quite markedly with change in position because positional change may promote sinus drainage. The only certain way to diagnose sinus headaches is by radiography. The sinuses should be clouded, exhibit a fluid level, or have a thickened mucosa, or the diagnosis should not be made. However, the degree of abnormality on computed tomography (CT) scan does not correlate well with the severity of the pain. Although simple analgesics may help decrease the pain of sinus headaches, sustained relief usually depends on long-term therapy using appropriate antibiotics and nasal decongestants for the underlying disease. Sinus infections rarely clear after 10 days of antibiotic treatment. A broad-spectrum antibiotic should be given for 21 days and the CT scan repeated. In less tractable disorders, the sinuses may have to be drained surgically and passages may have to be opened to prevent them from becoming infected once again.

A related syndrome, called the *middle turbinate syndrome*, that produces headache usually behind the eye or frontal sinus on one side of the head has been described. The middle turbinate enlarges and presses on either the nasal septum or the lateral nasal wall, resulting in pain. The diagnosis usually can be confirmed by endoscopy or CT. The treatment is surgery to eliminate the point of contact.

Cervicogenic Headaches

Although not recognized by the International Headache Society, pathology in the upper neck, particularly the C_2-C_3 dermatomes apparently can produce pain in the neck and the posterior head that may radiate to the temporal areas and sometimes to the shoulders. The symptoms may mimic migraine or tension headaches, but the patient may have tightness of cervical muscles and occasionally some limitation of the neck motion. In children, it can occur after trauma or rarely be an isolated symptom of a Chiari I malformation. If no anatomic pathology is found, treatment usually is massage, muscle relaxants, and over-the-counter anti-inflammatory drugs.

Ocular Headaches

Pain in or around the eye usually is caused by local diseases of the eye. The sclera often is red. Light, movement of the eye, or pressure on the eyeball may make the pain worse. Severe eye pain caused by glaucoma, uveitis, inflammation of tissues of the orbit, or masses within the orbit rarely are confused with headache from other sources. Errors of refraction and strabismus are not associated with an increased incidence of headache, other than perhaps in hypermetropia or astigmatism; the latter usually produces a dull, aching sensation in and about the eye or, at worst, a mild frontal headache when the eyes are used in close work, such as reading, for a long period.

Temporomandibular Joint Disease

The most common symptoms of temporomandibular joint disease are pain in the face and jaws, stiffness of the jaws in the morning, sounds of clicking or movement of the joint when chewing, and fatigue when chewing. Patients with temporomandibular joint disease often clench their jaws and have bruxism. Patients who have these symptoms, including older children and adolescents, often complain of chronic headache. The pain predominantly is in the temporal or frontotemporal region and may be unilateral or bilateral. At other times, patients complain of throat, occipital, neck, and back pain. The physical examination is helpful if limited movement of the temporomandibular joint occurs or a click is palpated when the patient makes chewing movements. Pain also may occur when the lateral mandibular muscles are pressed. Evaluations of children who have malocclusion and require orthodontic treatment do not indicate that they have more symptoms related to temporomandibular joint disease than do other children of the same age. Whether temporomandibular joint disease contributes to chronic headache in children remains uncertain. Many children exhibit bruxism but have little else in the way of symptoms or signs to suggest joint disease. If sufficient findings exist to suspect that the joint is the cause of chronic cephalgia, the patient should be referred to a dental surgeon for occlusal splint therapy.

Epilepsy

Lateralized or generalized headaches frequently occur after epileptic seizures and occasionally precede partial seizures as an aura. No consensus exists as to whether headache can be the sole manifestation of an epileptic seizure. Headaches, often diagnosed as migraine, do occur more frequently in children who have epilepsy than in the general pediatric population. Children who have complex-partial seizures tend to have headaches of brief duration and abrupt onset and termination at times when they are not having an epileptic seizure. These headaches usually are relieved by anticonvulsant therapy; however, the headaches do not necessarily represent a seizure because anticonvulsants are effective in relieving migraine in children who have no history or signs of epilepsy.

Trauma

A traumatic injury to the head may produce intracranial lesions that are associated with headaches. Some patients with acute traumatic lesions, particularly intracerebral hemorrhage or acute subdural bleeding, may be alert enough to complain of headache. If so, the pain usually is severe and nonthrobbing. It often is localized on the same side as the site of the lesion, but it sometimes is diffuse. Intracranial injuries also can be associated with more chronic, increasingly severe headaches, which again may be localized or diffuse and may have no other special characteristics. This type of headache is seen with enlarging subdural hematomas. Regardless of the severity or location of the headache, severe or persistent cephalgia that occurs after cranial trauma should be investigated by neuroimaging, even if the patient does not have neurologic signs.

Chronic or recurrent headaches may occur after head trauma when no focal lesion is revealed by cerebral imaging. As noted, trauma can be a triggering stimulus for the onset or worsening of migraine. Headache also is an integral part of the postconcussive syndrome, which also includes dizziness and personality changes. Fortunately, the syndrome is seen less commonly in children than in adults. When the headache does occur, it can persist for months. Standard criteria for the diagnosis of a postconcussive headache require that the concussion be severe enough to have caused a transient loss of consciousness or posttraumatic amnesia lasting longer than 10 minutes. The headaches should occur within 14 days of regaining consciousness. The postconcussion syndrome often is accompanied by anxiety, irritability, and, at times, frank depression. These emotional changes may help to prolong the headache and make it more intense.

The treatment of posttraumatic headaches depends on their causes. The therapy for posttraumatic migraine headaches does not differ from that of migraine headaches in children who have not been traumatized. Analgesics are used to treat postconcussive headaches; however, as in other syndromes featuring chronic daily headaches, these agents may be abused and may be difficult to withdraw, so that they become a part of the continuing problem. If these headaches persist for months and no associated structural lesion is discovered, the child may need behavioral treatment or psychiatric evaluation.

SUBACUTE HEADACHE SYNDROMES

Children with subacute headache syndromes have had no headaches or rare headaches until 2 to 3 months before they come for evaluation. They are brought to a physician because their headaches have become increasingly frequent and severe during this brief period. Distinguishing the intracranial from extracranial causes of such headaches by history alone may not be possible. However, certain features of the headache do suggest the possibility that the cause could be an intracranial lesion. These features include (a) severe occipital headache; (b) headache made worse by straining, sneezing, or coughing; (c) headache that awakens the patient from a deep sleep; (d) headache that is exacerbated or improved markedly by a change in position; (e) headache associated with projectile vomiting or vomiting without nausea; and (f) headache with a history of focal seizures. Headaches that occur day after day in the same area with increasing intensity also are worrisome. Even if one or more of these symptoms are present, statistically, most children do not have an intracranial lesion. As noted, patients who have had headaches caused by intracranial mass lesions almost always have physical findings if the headaches have been present for several months. These findings include papilledema, unilateral or bilateral sixth-nerve palsies, ataxia, and spasticity (particularly in the lower extremities), as well as more localized indications of brain dysfunction involving movement, vision, or language, depending on the site of the lesion. Although physical findings are much more suggestive of an intracranial lesion,

all children with a history of headaches of recent onset whose pain is becoming progressively worse or more frequent should be investigated by neuroimaging.

Headaches result from intracranial lesions for one of two reasons: (a) a localized or generalized increased pressure occurs within the skull, which stretches and distorts vessels at the surface of the brain or distorts the meninges, which also contain pain-sensitive fibers, or (b) the pain-sensitive fibers in these brain coverings become irritated by infection or bleeding. Tumors or other masses, such as an abscess or hemorrhage, usually are responsible for local distortion of brain vessels or meninges. However, nearly 80% of tumors in children occur either in the posterior fossa or near the midline. Thus, they frequently can obstruct the circulation of cerebrospinal fluid and result in hydrocephalus. When this occurs, the elevation of ICP is more diffuse, and the headache frequently is bifrontal or generalized rather than localized over one part of the hemicranium.

Pseudotumor cerebri produces the same type of headache that is found when ICP is elevated from other causes, such as a mass lesion or hydrocephalus. Frequently, vomiting or blurred vision are accompanying complaints, and papilledema, sixth-nerve palsies, ataxia, and, less frequently, spasticity may be found on physical examination. As the name implies, no mass is found on neuroimaging. Because it is possible to visualize the dural venous sinuses using MRI techniques, an increasingly large proportion of patients with pseudotumor are found to have occlusion of one of these sinuses. However, in most cases, the cause remains unknown. Pseudotumor cerebri occurs more frequently in adult obese females, but this finding is not true of children. It has been associated with both high and low levels of serum vitamin A, the use of drugs such as lithium or antibiotics, and disorders of endocrine function.

The treatment of headaches resulting from tumor or hemorrhage is not within the scope of this chapter. If the diagnosis of pseudotumor cerebri is made, the patient often may be relieved by a single lumbar puncture performed for diagnostic reasons. If, as is often the case, symptoms recur and the ICP returns to high levels within 3 to 4 days, dexamethasone (2 to 4 mg every 6 hours) may be used for 3 to 5 days and then withdrawn rapidly. Alternatively, acetazolamide (20 mg/kg/day) can be given in three divided doses. If this treatment fails to relieve the patient's symptoms, repeated lumbar punctures may need to be performed whenever the symptoms recur. Oral glycerol still is used rarely as an osmotic agent to lower ICP. The dosage is increased gradually from 0.5 to 2.0 mg/kg/day, in three divided doses, as tolerated. Obesity and chronic diarrhea are complications of this form of therapy. The major danger of chronic elevation of ICP caused by pseudotumor is damage to the visual system, and vision should be followed on a regular basis by an ophthalmologist. In patients with intractable pseudotumor that cannot be treated by drugs or repeated lumbar puncture, the optic nerve must be protected. This protection can be accomplished in one of two ways: fenestration of the optic nerve sheath, which protects the nerve against high pressures, or, alternatively, placement of a lumbar peritoneal shunt that reduces ICP. Anticoagulants and thrombolytic agents have been used to treat sinus thrombosis, when found, but its benefit to children has yet to be proven.

ACUTE HEADACHE SYNDROMES

A headache may be so severe that it brings a child to a doctor's office or to the emergency department seeking both a diagnosis and immediate relief of pain. Under these circumstances, distinguishing between an intracranial and extracranial source for the headache, deciding if hospital admission is necessary, and providing a plan that relieves the child's pain as quickly as possible are extremely important. The basis of any diagnosis remains the history and physical examination, but in the face of an acute cephalgia, deciding if the child requires an immediate CT scan of the head or lumbar puncture to assist in the diagnosis and planning of care often is crucial.

Common intracranial causes of acute, severe headache are a mass lesion, infection, and intracranial hemorrhage. Extracranial causes include migraine, tension headaches, and, rarely, sinusitis. The most decisive factor in the child's history is whether this is the first such headache the child has experienced or another headache in an already established pattern that has been evaluated in the past. Determining whether this particular headache has been associated with an unusual antecedent event such as head injury, seizure, fever, or changes in sensory or motor function also is important. Critical physical findings include meningismus; focal neurologic signs; papilledema or split sutures; evidence of cranial trauma, including blood in or behind the ear; and a depressed level of consciousness.

If this attack is the first of severe cephalgia without a significant prior headache history, immediate neuroimaging is recommended if any of the following is present: history of recent trauma, recent onset of seizures, unusual behaviors predating the headache, fever, meningismus, papilledema, focal neurologic signs, or a depressed level of consciousness. Early neuroimaging is indicated if the physician considers that drugs that significantly depress consciousness are needed to relieve the child's pain. Meningeal irritation usually results in an acute, diffuse, rapidly progressive headache that becomes so intense that it may be unbearable. If the cause of the irritation is bleeding, the onset may be explosive (a "thunderclap" headache), and the headache may become excruciating within a matter of a minute or two. Occasionally, these headaches are associated with cough or exercise. Many of these patients do not have focal neurologic signs, but frequently a disturbance of orientation or consciousness occurs. The physical examination may show nuchal rigidity resulting from meningeal irritation, but if the insult is relatively recent, it may not yet be pronounced. Occasionally, the examiner can see perivenous or subhyaloid hemorrhages in the eye, resulting from high ICP and the extravasation of subarachnoid blood. Intense headaches of acute onset without physical findings again often do not have intracranial pathology, but if this attack is the first one, obtaining a scan is mandatory, and performing a lumbar puncture often is desirable.

A lumbar puncture should be considered if a fever without a cause accompanies the headache or if meningismus and new neurologic signs or abnormal behaviors are present, despite normal neuroimaging results. If a child is febrile with meningismus and without evidence of focal signs or elevated ICP, proceeding with a lumbar puncture before obtaining a CT or MRI scan may be appropriate. If a scan shows acute sinusitis, that infection must be treated vigorously.

The presence of abnormal findings on lumbar puncture or an acute or subacute abnormality on neuroimaging dictates that the child be hospitalized. If these tests are normal, the child still may need to be hospitalized if clinical evidence of elevated ICP or new neurologic signs are present. In the face of pernicious vomiting, a child may have to be hospitalized for rehydration. Children also may require hospitalization for the treatment of intractable pain or, rarely, for acute psychiatric care.

If the child has no evidence of having an intracranial lesion and has a prior history of headache that indicates migraine or tension headache, pain sometimes can be relieved by the intramuscular administration of 1 to 2 mg/kg of meperidine and 1 mg/kg of hydroxyzine. The use of morphine or morphine derivatives to relieve pain rarely is necessary. If the child is agitated, sedation with pentobarbital or chloral hydrate may be necessary. This therapy usually requires hospital admission

for observation. However, the use of these analgesics is not the most satisfactory way of treating acute attacks of migraine that have not responded to analgesics at home. If this diagnosis is substantiated, other methods of treating the acute pain and vomiting are available and include the intravenous administration of 0.1 to 0.2 mg/kg of chlorpromazine or 0.2 mg/kg of prochlorperazine, with up to 1 mg of dihydroergotamine. Dyskinetic and dystonic movements may occur, and sedation frequently occurs. However, the vomiting and headache often stop. Five hundred milligrams of intravenous valproate may help. Adolescents may respond to a 10-mg intravenous dose of ketorolac tromethamine (Toradol) to relieve pain. Older children also may be given up to 6 mg of sumatriptan subcutaneously (approximately 0.1 mg/kg) or other triptans orally if they are not vomiting. If the headache cannot be broken by these means, the child may require hospitalization to be given dihydroergotamine, administered intravenously at 0.02 mg/kg up to 1.0 mg. every 8 hours for 48 to 72 hours, or until the headache has subsided for 8 hours. Patients usually are pretreated with metoclopramide administered intravenously at 0.2 mg/kg up to 10 mg. An initial test dose of 20% of the final calculated dose should be given to test the patient's tolerance to the drug. Sedation with other narcotics may be required.

Acute headaches also can occur after the patient undergoes lumbar puncture. These headaches usually vary markedly with position, virtually disappearing when the patient is flat. Treatment is 24 to 48 hours of bed rest. If this treatment fails, an epidural blood patch may be needed. The best treatment is prevention by using a small-bore needle.

Suggested Readings

Al-Twaijri WA, Shevell M. Pediatric migraine equivalents: Occurrence and clinical features in practice. *Pediatr Neurol* 2002;26:365.

Bigal ME, Sheftell FD, Rapoport AM, et al. Chronic daily headache: Identification of factors associated with induction and transformation. *Headache* 2002;42:575.

Bille B. Migraine in school children. *Acta Pediatr* 1962;51(Suppl 136):14.

Bolay H, Reuter U, Dunn AK, et al. Intrinsic brain activity triggers trigeminal meningeal afferents in a migraine model. *Nature Medicine* 2002;8:136.

Cutrer MF, Silberstein SD, Matthew NT, et al. Antiepileptic drugs in migraine, cluster headache, and mood disorders. *Headache* 2001;41(Suppl 1):S1.

DeVeber G, Andrew M, Adams C, et al. Cerebral sinovenous thrombosis in children. *N Engl J Med* 2001;354:417.

Diamond S, London L. Psychological management of headaches. *Headache Q* 2000;11:263.

Ferrari MD, Roon KI, Lipton RB, et al. Oral triptans (serotonin 5-HT (1D/1B) agonists) in acute migraine treatment: a meta-analysis of 53 trials. *Lancet* 2001;358:1668.

Headache Classification Committee of the International Headache Society. Classification and diagnostic criteria for headache disorders, cranial neuralgias and facial pain. *Cephalgia* 1988;8(Suppl 7):9.

Hershey AD. Chronic daily headaches in children. *Expert Opin Pharmacother* 2003;4:485.

Kesler A, Fattal-Valevski A. Idiopathic intracranial hypertension in the pediatric population. *J Child Neurol* 2002;17:745.

Lewis DW, Ashwal S, Dahl G, et al. Practice parameter: evaluation of children and adolescents with recurrent headaches. *Neurology* 2002;59:490.

Martelletti P. Inflammatory mechanisms in cervicogenic headache: an integrative view. *Curr Pain Headache Rep* 2002;6:315.

Matthew NT, Stubits E, Migram MR. Transformation of episodic migraine into daily headache. *Headache* 1982;22:66.

Olesen J. The ischemic hypotheses of migraine. *Arch Neurol* 1987;44:321.

Ott NL, O'Connell EJ, Hoffman AD, et al. Childhood sinusitis. *Mayo Clin Proc* 1991;66:1238.

Prensky AL. Migraine and migrainous variants in pediatric patients. *Pediatr Clin North Am* 1976;23:461.

Stillman MJ. Pharmacotherapy of tension-type headaches. *Curr Pain Headache Rep* 2002;6:408.

Thilander B, Rubio G, Pena L, et al. Prevalence of temporomandibular dysfunction and its association with malocclusion in children and adolescents: an epidemiologic study related to specified stages of dental development. *Angle Orthod* 2002;72:146.

Weiss HD, Stern BJ, Goldberg J. Post-traumatic migraine: chronic migraine precipitated by minor head or neck trauma. *Headache* 1991;31:451.

CHAPTER 418 ■ UNCLASSIFIED NERVOUS SYSTEM DISORDERS: ALPERS DISEASE

MARVIN A. FISHMAN

The term *Alpers disease* (progressive poliodystrophy) tradition-ally has been used to refer to a progressive degenerative disease that begins in early infancy and is characterized by a rapid deterioration associated with intractable seizures, loss of de-velopmental skills, stupor, and death within several years of onset. The diagnosis was based on the examination of brain tissue obtained at biopsy or necropsy. Therefore, whether sev-eral different diseases have similar pathology and should be grouped together as Alpers disease or whether the pathol-ogy is specific and unique to a single disease entity remains unclear.

PATHOGENESIS AND PATHOLOGY

In the past, Alpers disease had been considered to be of un-known etiology. Studies of patients, however, have provided information that points to a metabolic basis for the condi-tion. Familial cases have been reported, and the inheritance pattern has suggested an autosomal recessive disorder. The ex-amination of tissues (including muscle and brain) has revealed the presence of abnormal mitochondria in some patients. Also, fatty infiltration of the liver has been noted in some children and is thought not to result from the effects of antiepileptic drug therapy but to be related to the primary disease.

Intermittent elevations in lactate and pyruvate levels have been found in the serum and, more important, in the cere-brospinal fluid (CSF) of some affected individuals. An increased ratio of lactate to pyruvate has been noted. The finding of in-creased concentrations of these metabolites in the CSF sug-gests an abnormality in the metabolism of pyruvate within the brain. The study of various tissues from involved patients has suggested various abnormalities in the metabolism of pyruvate. These abnormalities have included disturbances in the pyruvate dehydrogenase complex; in the second part of the citric acid cycle; and in oxidation of the reduced form of nicotinamide adenine dinucleotide, cytochrome aa_3, and pyruvate carboxy-lase. Thus, what previously was thought to be a degenerative disease of unknown etiology may represent an autosomal dis-order associated with pyruvate dysmetabolism.

A hallmark of Alpers disease in the brain is status spongio-sus, with neuronal degeneration and loss. Glial proliferation resulting in astrocytosis often is present, and capillaries ap-pear prominent and dilated. The disease involves primarily the cerebral gray matter; little, if any, change is found in the white matter. In severe cases, the thalamus, hippocampus, and cere-bellum also may be involved. In patients in whom the liver is affected, the findings are those of subacute hepatitis with massive fatty degeneration, hepatocyte loss, bile duct prolifer-ation, and fibrous scarring with or without cirrhosis. Changes in the muscle have included lipid infiltration, type grouping of fibers, or evidence of mitochondrial or lipid myopathies. Elec-tron microscopy has revealed abnormal mitochondria in some cases.

CLINICAL MANIFESTATIONS AND COMPLICATIONS

Two forms of Alpers disease—infantile and juvenile—have been described. The infantile form usually has its onset in chil-dren who are between 1 and 3 years of age and are either normal or have had previous mild developmental delays. The course is rapid, and death usually occurs when the child is between 2 and 6 years of age. The initial symptoms may be vomiting and failure to thrive; these symptoms are followed by a severe seizure disorder that often presents with bouts of sta-tus epilepticus. The seizures may be focal or generalized, and myoclonus also is noted. Once the epilepsy becomes manifest, psychomotor development stops and previously mastered skills are lost. Affected children often have hypotonia and paresis, which eventually may change to spasticity. Ataxia, visual dis-turbances, and deafness commonly develop. The clinical man-ifestations usually are exacerbated by intercurrent infections and stress. Clinical signs of liver disease, if they occur, develop late in the illness and may be manifest by hepatomegaly and as-cites. Occasionally, the liver disease may progress rapidly and cause fatal hepatic failure.

The juvenile form of Alpers disease has its onset in children between 4 and 10 years of age and follows a protracted, slow course, with death occurring when these patients reach between 12 and 20 years of age. The findings are similar to those of the infantile form, but the juvenile form also involves muscle wast-ing and evidence of a polyneuropathy. Visual disturbances may include hemianopia and blindness. Optic atrophy and retinal pigmentary degeneration occur in some patients.

The two clinical presentations just described are the most common forms of the disease. However, a prenatal onset has been described in some families. The affected infants had mi-crocephaly, intrauterine growth retardation, and typical mani-festations of fetal akinesia. Neonatal seizures were present. The brain pathology was characteristic of Alpers syndrome. No de-fects in energy metabolism were found, and the livers were nor-mal. Another unusual presentation occurs in teenaged patients and has a clinical picture similar to that of MELAS syndrome (*m*itochondrial *e*ncephalopathy, *l*actic *a*cidosis, and *s*trokelike episodes). Liver involvement is present.

DIAGNOSIS AND THERAPY

The diagnosis of Alpers disease is suggested from the clinical findings. Certain laboratory tests help to confirm the clinical suspicion. Examination of the CSF often reveals a significantly increased protein content, frequently greater than 200 mg/dL. The protein electrophoresis and oligoclonal banding patterns are normal. Lactate and pyruvate levels should be ascertained; elevated levels or a lactate-to-pyruvate ratio greater than 15 in the CSF suggest an abnormality of energy metabolism within the brain. Liver function test results often are abnormal, even before antiepileptic drug therapy is initiated. The results of computed tomography may be normal or may consist of slight generalized atrophy. The atrophy has been noted to be more prominent in the occipital region, and hypodensity may be present in that area. Magnetic resonance imaging (MRI) may show T2 prolongation in the cerebral cortex, white matter, and deep nuclei such as the thalamus. The results of electroencephalography are abnormal, and high-amplitude slow wave activity often is seen with polyspikes. Evoked potentials often are abnormal. In some patients, muscle biopsies have demonstrated the subsarcolemmal aggregation of mitochondria. The mitochondria frequently are enlarged and contain paracrystalline inclusions. In other patients, muscle biopsies have shown evidence of lipid myopathy or fiber type grouping. Biochemical studies of muscle biopsy show abnormalities in respiratory chain function. Similar findings have been found in the liver.

Other diseases that involve brain and liver dysfunction include Wilson disease, fructosemia, galactosemia, glycogen storage disease, Niemann-Pick disease, and Gaucher disease. The clinical and laboratory features readily distinguish these entities from progressive poliodystrophy. Subacute necrotizing encephalomyelitis (Leigh disease) also may be associated with energy dysmetabolism. The clinical symptoms of patients with Leigh disease are more diverse and progress at a variable rate. Brainstem signs, including nystagmus, abnormal eye movements, and abnormal respiratory patterns, are prominent. These findings are not major features of Alpers disease. MRI in Leigh disease may reveal abnormalities in the putamen, globus pallidum, caudate nucleus, periaqueductal region, and cerebral peduncle.

No specific treatment is available for patients with Alpers disease. The associated seizures often are refractory. Treatment with antiepileptic drugs may reduce their frequency but rarely achieves complete control. Valproic acid may accelerate the liver failure in Alpers disease and probably should be avoided. No data are available regarding the efficacy of vitamin therapy (including thiamine supplementation) or other dietary measures in the treatment of possible energy dysmetabolism.

Suggested Readings

Bicknese AR, May W, Hickey WF, Dodson WE. Early childhood hepatocerebral degeneration misdiagnosed as valproate toxicity. *Ann Neurol* 1992;32:767.

Boyd SG, Harden A, Egger J, Pampiglione G. Progressive neuronal degeneration of childhood with liver disease ("Alpers' disease"): characteristic neurophysiological features. *Neuropediatrics* 1986;17:75.

Canafoglia L, Franceschetti S, Antozzi C, et al. Epileptic phenotypes associated with mitochondrial disorders. *Neurology* 2001;56:1340.

Chow CW. Morphological correlates of mitochondrial dysfunction in children. *Hum Repro* 2000;15(Suppl 2):68.

Frydman M, Jager-Roman E, de Vries L, et al. Alpers progressive infantile neuronal poliodystrophy: an acute neonatal form with findings of the fetal akinesia syndrome. *Am J Med Genet* 1993;47:31.

Gabreels FJM, Prick MJJ, Trijbels JMF, et al. Defects in citric acid cycle and the electron transport chain in progressive poliodystrophy. *Acta Neurol Scand* 1984;70:145.

Harding BN, Alsanjari N, Smith SJ, et al. Progressive neuronal degeneration of childhood with liver disease (Alpers' disease) presenting in young adults. *J Neurol Neurosurg Psychiatry* 1995;58:320.

Harding BN, Egger J, Portmann B, Erdohazi M. Progressive neuronal degeneration of childhood with liver disease. *Brain* 1986;109:181.

Huttenlocher PR, Solitare GB, Adams G. Infantile diffuse cerebral degeneration with hepatic cirrhosis. *Arch Neurol* 1976;33:186.

Montine TJ, Powers JM, Vogel FS, et al. Alpers' syndrome presenting with seizures and multiple stroke-like episodes in a 17-year-old male. *Clin Neuropathol* 1995;14:322.

Narkewicz MR, Sokol RJ, Beckwith B, et al. Liver involvement in Alpers disease. *J Pediatr* 1991;119:260.

Prick MJJ, Gabreels FJM, Trijbels JMF, et al. Progressive poliodystrophy (Alper's disease) with a defect in cytochrome in muscle: a report of two unrelated patients. *Clin Neurol Neurosurg* 1983;85:57.

Schwabe MJ. Valproate-induced liver failure in one of two siblings with Alpers disease. *Pediatr Neurol* 1997;16:4.

Sokol R. Expanding spectrum of mitochondrial disorders. *J Pediatr* 1996;125:5.

SECTION XI ■ ALLERGY AND IMMUNOLOGY

CHAPTER 419 ■ GENERAL CONSIDERATIONS OF ALLERGIES IN CHILDHOOD

HUGH A. SAMPSON AND PEYTON A. EGGLESTON

The prevalence of allergic disorders such as asthma, atopic dermatitis, and allergic rhinitis has doubled in the past 25 years. Ironically, during this same time, a virtual explosion has occurred in our knowledge of the immunologic and biochemical mechanisms responsible for allergic disorders. Data support the pathogenic role of allergy in many cases of asthma, allergic rhinitis, atopic dermatitis, urticaria and angioedema, adverse food reactions, drug and biologic agent reactions, and stinging-insect hypersensitivity. Information is available to approach the diagnosis and treatment of these disorders in a rational medical fashion.

Allergy may be defined as any untoward physiologic event caused by an immunologically mediated reaction. This definition has several components that restrict its scope. First, a demonstrable event or disease must occur that is both symptomatic and pathologic, and this event must be related to an antigen or environmental factor that could include airborne pollens, ingested foods, contactants such as latex, industrial chemicals, or parenterally administered drugs. In addition, the disease must have a demonstrable immunologic mechanism and must occur as a result of this immune mechanism. Atopy, a subtype of allergy comprising a constellation of chronic diseases provoked by IgE-mediated mechanisms, has a strong genetic predisposition. Coca and Cooke initially coined the term *atopy* in 1923, and later suggested that atopy was made up of asthma, allergic rhinitis, and atopic eczema (or atopic dermatitis). However, not all asthma, rhinitis, and eczema are IgE mediated, which results in considerable semantic confusion.

CLASSIFICATION OF ALLERGIC DISEASES

In 1963, Gell and Coombs classified allergic (hypersensitivity) reactions into four types. The first three are antibody mediated and are distinguished by the different type of antigen and antibody class involved. Type IV reactions can be subdivided into three types depending on the class of T cell involved, Th1, Th2, or cytotoxic lymphocyte (CTL). Although somewhat simplistic, this classification is helpful and is referred to frequently. This chapter focuses primarily on type I, IgE-mediated hypersensitivity reactions.

Type I (Anaphylactic Reactions)

Type I reactions are mediated by antigen-specific IgE antibodies. This class of antibody binds to the surface of mast cells, circulating basophilic granulocytes, and certain antigen-presenting cells (e.g., macrophages, dendritic cells, Langerhans cells). The exposure of IgE-coated mast cells and basophils to antigen results in rapid cell activation and the release of a variety of pharmacologically potent mediators and cytokines. The interaction of these mediators with blood vessels, bronchi, or mucus-secreting glands causes disease. Examples of this type of allergy include anaphylactic reactions to insect stings, food-induced urticaria, or allergic rhinitis. The generation of cytokines leads to the more chronic inflammation seen in allergen-induced asthma, allergic rhinitis, and atopic dermatitis.

Type II (Cytotoxic Reactions)

In type II reactions, antibodies of the IgG or IgM class are formed to cell-surface antigens that may be environmental antigens adsorbed to the surface of cells or to self-antigens (as in autoimmune disease). Antibodies bind to the cell and activate complement, which can damage or destroy the cell via the membrane attack complex. Common clinical examples of this type of allergic reaction include drug-induced leukopenia, hemolytic anemia, and thrombocytopenia.

Type III (Arthus or Immune Complex Reactions)

In type III reactions, as in type II responses, IgG and IgM antibodies to an environmental antigen are produced. In this type of reaction, however, the antigen does not bind to cells but circulates in a soluble form. The antigen–antibody complexes that are formed may be small, intermediate, or large. Small complexes may remain harmlessly in the circulation, whereas large complexes are cleared rapidly by the reticuloendothelial system. Intermediate-size complexes, however, may be deposited in vessel walls and tissues. Vascular damage is then initiated by activation of complement, granulocytes, platelets and, probably, basophils. The most common example of this reaction is classic serum sickness.

Type IV (Cell-Mediated Reactions)

Type IV reactions involve antigen-presenting cells (APCs, e.g., monocytes, macrophages, dendritic cells) and one of three types of T lymphocytes with specific receptors for an antigen. After primary exposure, T cells respond to subsequent exposure by proliferation and differentiation into cells capable of causing cytolysis (CTLs), or by recruiting other inflammatory cells; for example, Th1 cells attract and activate macrophages, and Th2 cells attract and activate eosinophils. Classic examples of these reactions are graft-versus-host reactions, contact dermatitis from poison ivy or other chemicals, and forms of chronic asthma and atopic dermatitis.

PATHOGENESIS OF IgE-MEDIATED DISORDERS

By definition, atopic disease is caused by type I, IgE-mediated reactions, although studies indicate that the classic mast cell–bound IgE allergen reaction is not the only means by which mast cells and basophils participate in inflammation. IgE is produced primarily by plasma cells in lymphoid tissues lining the respiratory and gastrointestinal tracts, and it constitutes 0.001% of circulating immunoglobulins in normal individuals. This immunoglobulin class does not activate complement, nor does it cross the placenta. It has the unique property of binding to high-affinity receptors (FcεRI) on the surface of mast cells, basophilic granulocytes and antigen-presenting cells, and to low-affinity receptors (FcεRII) on lymphocytes, monocytes and macrophages, eosinophils, and platelets. The IgE molecule is bound by the Fc-terminal end, so the antigen-specific N-terminal end Fab is exposed and confers antigen specificity to the mast cell or basophil (sensitizes); 40,000 to 90,000 IgE molecules may bind to the cell membrane of a mast cell or basophil. On antigen-presenting cells, the IgE molecule serves as a highly efficient receptor for focusing allergen-specific T-cell responses, especially of the Th2 type.

All mammalian species make IgE antibody, and much of the information regarding its production and regulation is derived from work with rodent models. IgE-producing plasma cells are found in all lymphoid organs, but they are in the highest concentration in the lymphoid tissue of the respiratory tract (tonsils and adenoids) and gut (Peyer's patches and lamina propria). IgE-bearing B cells are present in the human fetus by the eleventh week of gestation, but IgE production *in utero* is negligible.

As with other immunoglobulin classes, surface IgM-bearing, virgin B cells differentiate into surface IgE-bearing memory B cells under the influence of regulatory CD4$^+$ helper T lymphocytes (Th). Studies have shown the presence of three types of CD4$^+$ cells based on the profile of cytokines they generate: Th1 cells that promote cell-mediated reactions by secreting interleukin-2 (IL-2), interferon-gamma, and granulocyte-macrophage colony-stimulating factor (GM-CSF); Th2 cells that promote immunoglobulin synthesis, especially IgE synthesis, by secreting IL-4, IL-5, IL-6, IL-10, IL-13, and GM-CSF; and Th3 cells that appear to regulate the function of Th1 and Th2 cells by secreting IL-10 and transforming growth factor alpha (TGF-α). B cells differentiate and mature into IgE-secreting plasma cells in the presence of allergen, APCs, and the appropriate antigen-presenting cell- and T cell–derived cytokines. The nature of the antigen is an important component of the IgE antibody response. Certain antigens, such as penicillin, ovomucoid, ragweed antigen E, and parasitic proteins, stimulate the production of more IgE than IgG antibodies. In general, these proteins are glycoproteins in the 10,000- to 60,000-dalton molecular weight range. Immunization with low doses of these antigens favors IgE production. Antigens presented at mucosal surfaces initiate IgE production in most individuals, but the response normally is turned off rapidly by specific regulatory or suppressor T lymphocytes. Procedures that eliminate T-suppressor cells, such as irradiation or cyclophosphamide, promote the indefinite production of high-titer IgE antibodies in animal models.

The modulation of IgE antibody is genetically controlled, although the development of antigen-specific IgE immune responses occur only after appropriate environmental exposure. Analogous to individual humans, certain inbred strains of mice preferentially produce IgE antibodies when immunized, whereas others produce IgG. Control appears to reside primarily with a T-helper lymphocyte population that is regulated by IgE-enhancing or IgE-inhibitory factors (cytokines) produced by APCs and other Th2 or Th3 lymphocytes, respectively. The growing body of data available concerning human IgE regulation is compatible with information derived from rodent models. Data from family and twin studies suggest that elevated serum IgE concentrations (more than 100 IU/mL) are inherited as a simple recessive trait. Complex diseases, such as asthma and allergic rhinitis, are multifactorial in that they are the result of interactions between major and minor genes and involve nongenetic interactions for their expression. Atopic diseases have a strong familial tendency. In a study of college-aged persons, the prevalence of atopic disease was 15% when no first-degree relative had one of the diseases, 33% when one first-degree relative was affected, and 68% when two or more first-degree relatives were atopic. No clear pattern of inheritance has been found, suggesting that atopy is a complex genetic trait (diabetes is another example of a complex trait). Indeed, studies have identified associated areas on several chromosomes, including 11q13 (IgE receptor) and 5q31 (IL-4, beta-adrenergic receptor). A number of alleles for the beta-adrenergic receptor have been found, including one that rapidly becomes unresponsive during continued beta-adrenergic use. Exposure to several environmental factors such as cigarette smoke, air pollutants, and allergens (mites, foods, pollens, cockroaches, and molds) have been associated with an increased risk of atopic disease.

In addition, specific IgE antibody responses more frequently are associated with specific (human leukocyte antigens) HLA specificities. For example, the development of IgE antibody to the Ra5 antigen of ragweed frequently is associated with HLA-Dw2, whereas individuals with a response to rye grass pollen have a frequency of HLA-B8 three times higher than expected.

Elevated serum IgE concentrations are not restricted to allergic disorders. Many disease states are associated with elevated levels of IgE. With atopic disorders, the IgE concentration generally is elevated in only 60% to 70% of patients and correlates roughly with disease severity. Individuals with no detectable serum or cell-bound IgE are apparently healthy, which suggests that IgE is not essential in maintaining good health. Serum containing IgE antibody can transfer sensitivity, but not particular atopic disorders, to normal individuals. The first human example was reported in 1919, when a patient with pernicious anemia was transfused with blood from a donor who was allergic to horses. The patient subsequently developed wheezing for the first time while driving home behind horses. More recently, recipients of liver transplants from food-allergic donors have experienced food allergic reactions after ingesting the food to which the donor was sensitive. Before the advent of radioimmunoassays, circulating IgE antibody was detected by its ability to sensitize normal skin (Prausnitz-Küstner reaction); the technique is still useful in animal experiments (passive cutaneous anaphylaxis). Passive sensitization occurs when IgE molecules bind with high avidity on tissue mast cells and blood basophils. In allergic individuals, a similar process occurs when mast cells and basophils are sensitized by the IgE molecules produced endogenously by plasma cells and released into the circulation.

Sensitization confers on the mast cell or basophil the ability to respond to an allergen. Once sensitization occurs, allergen

TABLE 419.1

PHARMACOLOGICALLY ACTIVE MEDIATORS AND CYTOKINES FROM MAST CELLS AND BASOPHILS

Preformed
Histamine
Eosinophil chemotactic factor of anaphylaxis
Neutrophil chemotactic factor
Kallikrein
Prekallikrein activator
Hageman's factor cleaver
Heparin
Tryptase

Newly formed
Leukotriene B_4, C_4, D_4, E_4
Prostaglandin D_2
Thromboxane B_2
Hydroxyeicosatetraenoic acid
Platelet-activating factor

Secondary
Bradykinin (serum)
Serotonin (platelets)
Major basic protein (eosinophils)

Cytokines
IL-4, IL-13 (stimulate and amplify Th2 cell responses)
IL-3, IL-5, GM-CSF (attract and activate eosinophils)
TNF-α (promote inflammation, activate endothelial cells, enhance cytokine production by other cells)

Chemokines
MIP-1α (attract monocytes, macrophages, and neutrophils)

exposure causes rapid (in seconds) changes in mast cell phospholipid and calcium metabolism, which results in an energy-dependent secretion of numerous pharmacologically active mediators, listed in Table 419.1. The release of these mediators results in an immediate response (within 15 to 30 minutes), which may include vasodilation, increased vascular permeability, and smooth-muscle constriction and mucus secretion in the respiratory and gastrointestinal tracts. In addition, thromboxanes and at least two proteins with chemotactic activity (IL-5 and GM-CSF) are secreted during the immediate phase, which may contribute to the infiltration of inflammatory cells. In addition to the immediate response, mast-cell activation may result in what is termed a *late-phase reaction* (LPR). As shown in Figure 419.1, the injection of an allergen causes an immediate wheal-and-flare reaction within 10 to 20 minutes. During the next 2 to 4 hours, the site may remain somewhat erythematous and edematous, but generally is not symptomatic. After 6 to 8 hours, the test site becomes pruritic (sometimes tender), warm, and more edematous and erythematous. This LPR may last 12 to 48 hours, although discoloration caused by extravasation of erythrocytes in severe reactions may persist for days. Histologically, lesions of LPRs show edema and perivascular infiltration of eosinophils and neutrophils. After 48 hours, mononuclear cells predominate in the cellular infiltrate, and the histology appears similar to the classic type IV, cell-mediated response. Studies have demonstrated that infiltrating lymphocytes are allergen-specific CD4+ Th2 cells (as opposed to CD4+ Th1 cells in type IV responses), which would promote further IgE synthesis and upregulation of IgE receptors on many cell types and would attract inflammatory cells. In addition to cytokines secreted by lymphocytes, it has been shown that tissue macrophages, mast cells, and eosinophils secrete a variety of

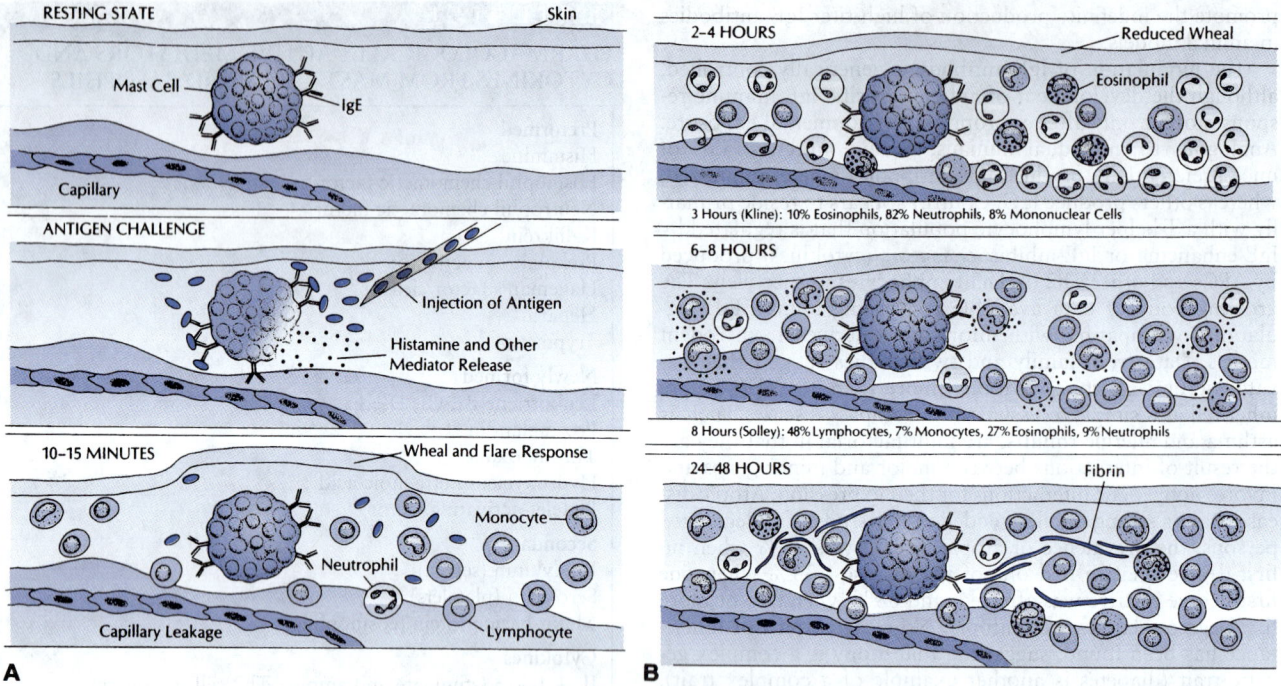

FIGURE 419.1. Bisphasic cutaneous response. **A:** Injected antigen activates mast cells by binding surface-bound IgE. Degranulation with release of histamine and activation of arachidonic acid metabolism with generation of inflammatory mediators occur in the immediate phase. **B:** In the late phase, neutrophils and eosinophils initially, and then lymphocytes and monocytes, infiltrate the area. (Reproduced with permission from Sampson HA. Late-phase response to food in atopic dermatitis. *Hosp Prac* 1987;22:112. Illustration by I. Arbel.)

cytokines (interleukins) that promote the IgE allergen-driven inflammatory response. In the nose, the LPR causes persistent nasal obstruction and hypersecretion. In the lung, LPR is associated with a persistent airflow obstruction that responds only partially to bronchodilator therapy. Airway bronchial hyperresponsiveness (propensity of the airways to obstruct secondary to nonimmunologic stimuli) may be measured by the concentration of histamine or methacholine required to cause significant airflow obstruction. This hyperresponsiveness may remain increased for weeks after initiation of the LPR (Fig. 419.2). Histologic examination of the lung in animal models and bronchial biopsies in man demonstrate an infiltrate similar to that seen in the LPR in human skin.

CLINICAL PRESENTATION OF THE ATOPIC SYNDROME

Atopy is a syndrome including specific chronic disorders of the skin and respiratory tree associated with type I mechanisms. These disorders often present sequentially—the "atopic march"—and include atopic dermatitis, allergic rhinitis, and

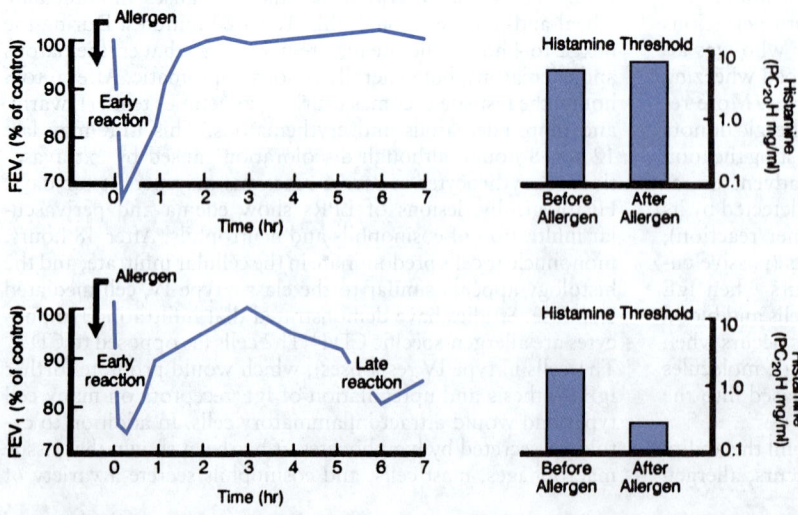

FIGURE 419.2. The effect of early and late reactions on bronchial hyperresponsiveness. Some asthmatic patients only had early asthmatic reactions to allergen challenges (*upper panels*); their bronchial reactivity to histamine did not change. Other asthmatic patients (*lower panels*) who developed both an early and a late reaction to allergen challenge had a rapid worsening of their bronchial reactivity 24 hours later. (Reprinted with permission from Cockcroft DW, Ruffin RE, Dolovich J, et al. Allergen-induced increase in nonallergic bronchial reactivity. *Clin Allergy* 1977;7:503.)

asthma. A number of allergic disorders are not included in the atopic syndrome, although some occur frequently in atopic individuals. These include food allergy, drug allergy, insect hypersensitivity, urticaria, angioedema, and contact dermatitis. Although food allergy is much more prevalent in atopic individuals, epidemiologic studies have not confirmed the suggestion that insect hypersensitivity or drug allergy, especially allergy to penicillin, occur more frequently in atopic individuals. The atopic disorders constitute a syndrome, because each has a similar, underlying IgE-dependent mechanism, and therefore each frequently is associated with one or more of the other disorders. For instance, asthma occurs in 40% to 60% children with atopic dermatitis, and 80% to 90% of children with asthma have concomitant allergic rhinitis. Moderate to severe atopic dermatitis, especially in the presence of egg sensitivity (i.e., positive skin test to egg or serum egg-specific IgE), is highly predictive of future asthma. Atopic dermatitis often represents the beginning of the "atopic march," a term coined to describe the natural history of atopic disease in childhood, including the progression of specific sensitization from food allergens to indoor environmental allergens to pollens. The progression of atopic diseases is discussed in more detail in the section on Natural History.

Prevalence and Natural History

A recent international survey using a standardized questionnaire found that the prevalence of atopic disorders varies dramatically worldwide, with prevalences as high as 35% in westernized countries and as low as 4% in far eastern and central European countries. These differences may be related to environmental factors. The incidence of atopic diseases is low (less than 1%) in West Indian populations, but quickly increases to levels comparable with western Europeans when West Indians emigrate and adopt European lifestyles. Allergic diseases affect more than 55 million people in the United States, or approximately 20% of the population. The cumulative prevalence of asthma among pre-teenaged children is considered to be 10% to 12%. Allergic rhinitis is more frequent in boys than girls at a young age; one study of 7-year-old children found a prevalence of 6% in boys and 1.5% in girls. Atopic dermatitis occurs in 10% to 12% of children, with more than 85% of cases presenting before age 5 years (Fig. 419.3).

The natural history of atopic diseases is complex. Each disorder generally appears for the first time at a characteristic age, frequently becomes more severe over a period of months to years, then undergoes a period of prolonged remission. For example, in children having an onset of asthma before age 3 years, about 50% outgrow it by late adolescence, but about

one-half have a recurrence in their mid-twenties. On the other hand, allergic rhinitis more commonly appears late in the first decade and remits less frequently. Atopic dermatitis and food allergy appear in the first several months of life and frequently resolve midway through the first decade of life.

PREDICTION AND PREVENTION

The development of atopic disease depends on sufficient contact between a genetically predisposed host and an allergen. Sensitization may take weeks or years and depends on host genetic factors, allergen dose and time of exposure, and adjuvant factors such as infection, cigarette smoke, and environmental pollutants (e.g., diesel exhaust particles). Because external factors are important in the sensitization of a predisposed individual, attempts to identify subjects at risk and modify their environment have been attempted.

Several historical and laboratory parameters may be used to determine a child's likelihood of developing atopic disease. The incidence of atopy in a child when neither parent has atopic disease is approximately 10%, approximately 40% when one parent is atopic, and 60% to 80% when both parents are atopic. Atopy tends to affect the same organ system within families (e.g., lung, skin, nasal passages), but this is not consistent. A history of recurrent bronchitis or multiple episodes of croup during infancy is associated with an increased risk of asthma, although these episodes actually may be early manifestations of asthma. Infantile colic with proven food intolerance is associated with atopy in approximately 50% of infants. Approximately 35% of infants with IgE-mediated cow's milk allergy develop other food allergies, and 15% retain cow's milk allergy beyond the first decade. Up to 80% of children with atopic dermatitis and egg sensitivity (2 kU/L or greater of egg-specific IgE) develop respiratory allergy and asthma. Peripheral blood eosinophilia (greater than 500 cells per microliter) at the time of "bronchitis" is associated with the development of atopic disease in 75% of infants. In children undergoing adenoidectomy, two-thirds of children with peripheral eosinophilia and elevated serum IgE concentrations developed atopic disease. Several studies have investigated the predictive value of cord-blood serum IgE. In one large series, 70% of infants with a cord-blood IgE level of more than 1.3 IU/mL developed atopic symptoms by 1.5 years of age, and 82% developed symptoms by 4.5 years of age. In another series, approximately 50% of healthy infants and children with serum IgE concentrations greater than one standard deviation above age-matched controls developed atopic disease within 18 months. The presence of antigen-specific IgE, as determined by radioallergosorbent test (RAST) or skin testing, also may predict future allergic disease. In one study of wheezing infants, a positive RAST result was found in 44% of infants who developed asthma or other allergic symptoms and in only 3% who remained healthy on follow-up.

Although genetic constitution appears to be of primary importance in developing atopic disease, several environmental factors are major contributors. Because allergen exposure induces specific IgE, avoidance of allergen exposure early in life may reduce the incidence of atopic disease, although recent studies looking at exposure to house pets raise some doubt about this strategy. A meta-analysis of well-controlled prospective studies found that breast-feeding exclusively for the first 4 to 6 months of life can affect the natural history of atopic disease and postpone allergic symptoms until after the first or second year of life. Recent studies have reported conflicting findings on the benefit of placing the lactating mother of a high-risk infant on a diet free of major allergens (eggs, milk, peanuts). However, once a food allergy is identified, the food should be removed from the mother's diet, because food

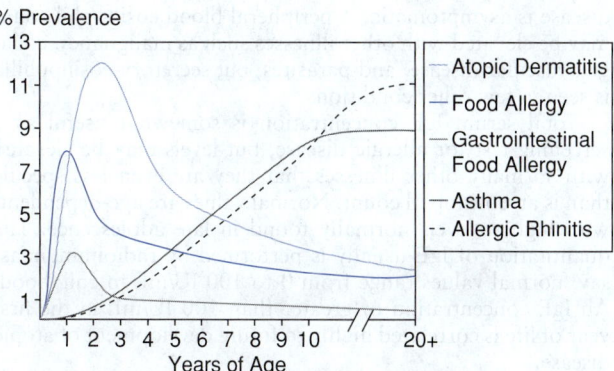

FIGURE 419.3. Prevalence of atopic disorders.

allergens are transmitted in maternal breast milk. The addition of solid foods to an infant's diet in the first 4 months of life has been directly correlated with increased risk of developing food allergy and atopic disease.

In earlier studies, exposure to inhalant allergens such as dust mites, molds, and pollens in the first 6 months of life was shown to be associated with an increased risk for developing atopic disorders. Consequently, measures to diminish exposure to animal products, dust mites, and molds seem justified in high-risk infants. Unlike earlier reports, recent studies investigating the effect of pet exposure suggest that early exposure to dogs and cats may actually have a protective effect against atopy. However, if a child becomes allergic to the pet, removal of the animal from the environment is recommended. Exposure to irritants or infection also may increase the risk of atopy. Several studies show that infants exposed to tobacco smoke develop higher serum IgE levels, have more positive skin test results to pollens, and develop respiratory disease at an earlier age than do infants in a nonsmoking environment. Furthermore, maternal smoking during pregnancy is associated with a twofold increased risk of atopy in offspring. Exposure to bacterial products, especially endotoxin, may actually reduce the risk of sensitization and of asthma. A few studies suggest that certain viral infections (e.g., respiratory syncytial virus, parainfluenza) may act as adjuvants for increased IgE responses to environmental allergens. Further study is needed before strong recommendations can be made about avoiding likely settings of infectious exposures.

Multiple atopic disorders (asthma, allergic rhinitis, atopic dermatitis), one of which is severe, and markedly elevated serum IgE levels (greater than 600 IU/mL) make it less likely that a child will outgrow the atopic condition. If patients remove themselves from pertinent allergens by controlling their environment or moving to an area of the country free of offending pollens or allergens, they often experience remission. However, many develop sensitivities to new local allergens, so moving is not frequently recommended.

DIAGNOSIS

No single historical, physical, or laboratory finding is diagnostic of atopic disease. In fact, practically every symptom or sign of atopic disease can be seen in nonatopic disorders. Although clinical history provides the majority of information, a firm diagnosis must be based on the accumulation of historical, physical, and laboratory data.

Developing a clear understanding of the age of onset and progression of symptoms is important in terms of increasing or decreasing severity. A patient with relatively severe disease that is worsening warrants a more aggressive diagnostic approach than does someone with mild or remitting disease. Symptoms sometimes are related to allergen exposure, but more frequently overt symptoms do not follow contact with an isolated allergen. Studies suggest that the immediate symptoms experienced by an allergic subject may go unrecognized as distinct from the chronic disease state, due to "down-regulation" of the immediate component of the allergic response. Instead, the LPR, which is largely unresponsive to beta agonists, sets up a state of hyper-irritability that causes the child to respond to a variety of nonspecific and often minor stimuli. For example, an egg-allergic child ingesting small amounts of egg protein may experience no immediate pruritus or rash, but develops chronic worsening of his atopic dermatitis. Similarly, a pollen-sensitive asthmatic may be hyperresponsive to a histamine bronchoprovocation challenge for up to 4 to 6 weeks after a single allergen exposure.

A variety of allergens may affect the atopic patient. Outdoor allergens, such as pollens, are most often associated with allergic rhinitis, whereas indoor allergens, such as dust mites and pets, are more frequently associated with asthma and chronic allergic rhinitis. Pollen-sensitive subjects generally experience seasonal difficulty, so knowledge of local flora helps in making the appropriate diagnosis. In general, most tree pollens are released during early spring (February to March) and, in most parts of the country, grass pollens are released from late spring through midsummer. In the eastern and midwestern United States, ragweed is a major source of pollen in late summer and early fall. Although pollens are wind-borne during dry weather and are cleared from the air during rainy periods, mold spores are found in high counts in clouds and mist. High humidity provides favorable conditions for mold growth. House dust (composed of dust mites, animal danders, molds, pollens) is nonseasonal and may be increased to high concentrations when cleaning or when a child plays in a closet or under a bed. Domestic animals are common sources of potent allergens, but families often deny that their pet causes symptoms, suggesting that the problem is actually pets in the neighborhood. Molds, especially in the high concentrations frequently found in basements or around vegetation (hay, cut grass, barns, forests), can be a major source of difficulty. Foods, especially cow's milk, eggs, and peanuts, are frequent causes of allergic symptoms. A complete accounting of a patient's environment (indoors and outdoors), daily activities, and eating habits is necessary to assess potential allergen exposure.

Several features in the physical examination suggest atopy. Characteristic features of specific atopic disorders are covered more thoroughly in Chapters 420 (Asthma), 423 (Atopic Dermatitis), and 424 (Allergic Rhinitis and Associated Disorders). Atopic children without overt atopic dermatitis may have dry skin with follicular prominence, mild scaling, and white dermographism. Children with nasal symptoms frequently have characteristic allergic facies, with allergic shiners and Dennie-Morgan folds below the eyes because of venous congestion; a transverse crease across the bridge of the nose secondary to the "allergic salute;" and persistent mouth breathing with adenoid facies characterized by deepened nasolabial folds, high-arched palate, and some degree of malocclusion and overbite. Tonsils and adenoids frequently are enlarged in children with atopic disease, presumably in response to allergic inflammation and more frequent infection. Otitis media with effusion also is a common finding in atopic children. Chest deformities are uncommon except in severe, long-standing asthma.

Laboratory tests help substantiate the clinical impressions formed from a careful history. Peripheral blood eosinophilia (greater than 500 cells per microliter) often occurs in atopic patients with asthma and atopic dermatitis, but is seen less commonly in patients with allergic rhinitis. Eosinophilia in respiratory or gastrointestinal secretions highly suggests allergic disease. Secretions may be collected, dried on a microscope slide, and stained with Hansel stain, which stains eosinophils in a few minutes. Both circulating and secretory eosinophils are related directly to the severity of disease and may be absent when the disease is asymptomatic. A peripheral blood eosinophil count may be elevated with other illnesses such as malignancy, collagen vascular disease, and parasites, but secretory eosinophilia is seen in few other conditions.

Total serum IgE concentration is somewhat useful as a screening test for allergic disease, but levels may be elevated with so many other illnesses that they are even less specific than is an eosinophil count. Normal values are age-dependent, with highest levels normally found in late adolescence. The quantitation of IgE usually is performed by radioimmunoassay; normal values range from 0 to 100 IU/mL in childhood. An IgE concentration of greater than 100 IU/mL in the first year of life is correlated highly to future development of atopic disease.

Specific sensitivity may be confirmed with immediate wheal-and-flare skin test results. These are performed using various epicutaneous methods, such as prick, puncture, or scratch techniques: The skin is lightly abraded by catching it with the tip of a needle, pressing a needle onto the skin, or scratching the skin through a drop of allergen solution. An intracutaneous (intradermal) technique, used predominantly in the evaluation of drug or insect-sting allergy, involves injecting a solution into the skin. The size of the resulting wheal is determined in approximately 15 minutes and is compared with sizes of a positive [histamine] and a negative [saline] control. A positive response simply denotes the presence of allergen-specific IgE, although the magnitude of the wheal-and-flare response roughly correlates with the likelihood that symptoms will be produced by natural exposure to the same allergens. Furthermore, a positive skin test result does not necessarily reflect current clinical reactivity. The intradermal skin test is more sensitive but much less specific than the epicutaneous methods. Skin tests provide a rapid readout and are relatively inexpensive. Disadvantages include moderate patient discomfort, minor risk of anaphylaxis, and suppression by antihistamines (for up to 1 week in some patients taking hydroxyzine and other long-lasting antihistamines).

As an alternative to the skin tests, several serologic assays used to measure allergen-specific IgE are available. The RAST was developed first and is used most widely. Other methods are variations of the RAST: enzyme allergosorbent test, fluorescent allergosorbent test, and a multiple-thread allergosorbent test. Although these assays measure circulating allergen-specific IgE antibodies that did not fix to mast cells, blood levels correlate with skin tests quite well. The tests are performed by incubating sera with allergens chemically coupled to a solid matrix. Nonspecific antibody is washed away, and adherent (allergen-specific) antibody is detected by incubation with a radiolabeled (enzyme-linked or fluorescein-linked) anti-human IgE antibody. The amount of radioactivity (enzyme activity or fluorescence) bound to the solid material directly correlates to the quantity of allergen-specific IgE present in the serum. A slightly more sensitive RAST, CAP System Fluorescent Enzyme Immunoassay (CAP-FEIA; Pharmacia & Upjohn, Kalamazoo, MI), has become available, and this test provides quantitative levels of allergen-specific IgE. Studies indicate that high levels of allergen-specific IgE antibodies are more predictive of symptomatic sensitivity. A multi-allergen RAST, Phadiatop Pediatric (Pharmacia & Upjohn, Kalamazoo, MI), has been shown to be 90% predictive of atopic disease. The advantages of *in vitro* studies include the fact that serum can be drawn anywhere and sent to a competent technical facility, allergens are better standardized, no risk of anaphylaxis exists, and patient medications do not interfere with the test. However, the tests are more expensive than skin tests, are slightly less sensitive, and results are not available immediately.

THERAPY

The treatment of allergic diseases falls into three categories: allergen avoidance, symptomatic drug intervention, and allergen immunotherapy. Allergen avoidance is the treatment of choice and is the most effective. Although highly effective for food allergens, compliance is difficult to obtain for indoor allergens and impossible to implement for outdoor allergens. Use of drug intervention and allergen immunotherapy are alternatives when avoidance is not effective. Effective drug therapy usually is available and practical, but treatment merely provides symptomatic relief. Immunotherapy is time-consuming, expensive, and has risks, but it may abrogate specific hypersensitivities. In some allergic disorders (e.g., life-threatening stinging-insect allergy), immunotherapy is the preferred treatment.

Allergen avoidance not only reduces symptoms, but sometimes reverses allergic disease activity. Specific IgE antibody production frequently diminishes over time without continued allergen exposure (stimulation). When total avoidance is possible for long periods (penicillin allergy, food allergy, insect-sting hypersensitivity), loss of reactivity ("outgrowing") the allergy frequently occurs. For example, in a large series of patients with atopic dermatitis and food hypersensitivity, approximately one-third of food allergies were lost after 1 to 2 years on a food allergen–elimination diet.

Animal dander from household pets such as cats and dogs are potent allergens that frequently lead to allergic symptoms. Removal of the pet from the household is the most effective form of therapy, although it may take months for the allergen content to drop to insignificant levels. Dust mites, the major allergen in house dust, also are a major cause of allergic symptoms. To date, no measures are known to eradicate dust mites completely, but exposure can be reduced. Mite-impermeable barriers (encasings) for pillows and mattresses, removal of carpeting from the bedroom, frequent washing of all bedcovers in hot water and drying in a hot dryer, and removal of non-washable stuffed animals and dolls ("dust mite farms") have been shown to be highly effective in minimizing atopic symptoms in dust mite–sensitive children. Because mites thrive in humid environments, room humidifiers can aggravate the problem. Dust mite avoidance practices should be directed primarily at the child's bedroom, because children spend so much time there. When household molds are a problem, they are best dealt with by installing a dehumidifier, because most available fungicides are only partially effective. Exposure to outdoor allergens is difficult to avoid. Using air conditioning instead of leaving windows open during pollen season decreases exposure significantly.

Drug intervention is the second arm of allergy therapy. Certain drugs prevent the IgE-mediated activation of mast cells and basophils. Corticosteroids inhibit mast-cell activation and interleukin production and also interfere with the LPR through direct effects on granulocyte chemotaxis. These drugs are especially important in treating chronic atopic diseases, because topically active agents with minimal toxicity are available for use in the airway. Cromolyn interferes with allergen-induced immediate-phase reactions and LPRs, but is much less effective in the chronic management of allergic disease. Antihistamines are competitive antagonists that interfere with immediate reactions by blocking the effects of histamine released from mast cells and basophils. Beta-adrenergic drugs, atropinic drugs, leukotriene antagonists, and decongestants largely attempt to reverse the effects of mast-cell and basophil mediators. These are discussed in more detail in sections on specific allergic disorders.

Immunotherapy is the only means to modify the immune mechanisms involved in allergic disease. Immunotherapy, or allergy-injection therapy, consists of repeated injections of allergenic material to increase the patient's tolerance of those allergens. Numerous studies have validated the effectiveness of immunotherapy for stinging-insect hypersensitivity and for allergic rhinitis and asthma (where allergen-related symptoms are implicated by history and laboratory testing). The treatment solutions may contain various extracts of wind-borne pollens, mold spores, or dust mites. No evidence exists to substantiate the effectiveness of food or bacterial proteins for use in immunotherapy. Although immunotherapy with animal dander extracts can be effective, it is not generally recommended because removal of the pet from the household is the preferred treatment. Immunotherapy with any allergen extract begins with the subcutaneous injection of very dilute solutions of allergen extracts. The concentration is gradually increased in weekly intervals until doses approximately 10,000 times higher are tolerated. At these levels, the therapy is extremely effective for allergy to venom of stinging insects and has been shown to be efficacious in treating seasonal allergic rhinitis (hay fever), perennial allergic rhinitis, and extrinsic asthma. The mechanism of this beneficial effect is not clearly delineated, but may relate to the IgG-blocking antibodies produced, generation of specific regulatory cells, and subsequent decreased IgE production or decreased mediator release by mast cells and basophils. Immunotherapy carries a small (1% to 5%) risk of systemic anaphylaxis. Its effectiveness should be analyzed critically, because some individuals do not respond; treatment showing no significant clinical benefit within 2 to 3 years should be discontinued. One of the most intriguing new findings is that immunotherapy in younger atopic children, those younger than 4 to 6 years of age, can prevent further sensitization to other unrelated allergens and the development of asthma.

UNPROVEN DISEASES AND THERAPY

A variety of disorders affecting every system of the body are attributed to allergy, although most allergists doubt their association. Examples include learning disorders, behavioral problems (especially hyperactivity), depression, schizophrenia, fatigue, insomnia, myalgia, inability to concentrate or think clearly, arthralgia and arthritis, assorted gastrointestinal complaints, obesity, pounding heart, and enuresis. A subspecialty has emerged, clinical ecology, whose proponents believe that the previously mentioned symptoms are caused by an accumulation of low-dose exposures to chemicals and substances in the environment and in our food supply. An evaluation includes a variety of unproven tests (e.g., sublingual or subcutaneous provocation, leukocyte cytotoxic tests, tests for IgG antibodies or antigen–antibody complexes, and trace-metal hair analysis). Although the concept that environmental exposure causing human disease is similar to the concept of allergy, no scientific basis exists for clinical ecology, and the methods have never been validated by objective clinical trials. The tension-fatigue syndrome has received considerable attention in pediatric literature. Proponents consider that a large number of emotional symptoms (anxiety, inattention, fatigue, headaches, hyperactivity) are caused by exposure to food or food additives. Many children with severe atopic disorders become irritable, moody, and fatigued secondary to the physical discomfort or sleep deprivation caused by their disease. The concept of tension-fatigue syndrome, however, is that symptoms are a direct consequence of allergy. Attempts to validate this syndrome in controlled, blinded clinical trials have failed.

Several therapeutic methods are practiced under the guise of allergy therapy, despite a lack of adequate experimental support or clear experimental evidence that the method is not effective. These include the administration of low doses of inhalant allergens to reduce allergic rhinitis (Rinkle therapy). Another example is the administration of small doses of food extracts (sublingual food drops or subcutaneous neutralization) to treat symptoms caused by food allergy. Certain chiropractic techniques also have been promoted as being able to eliminate allergies, but scientific validation is lacking.

Finally, several widely practiced therapeutic approaches are simply irrational. These include injection of the patient's urine to reduce symptoms, enzyme-potentiated transepidermal desensitization, extreme and arbitrary dietary manipulation such as rotational diets, the use of nystatin to eliminate intestinal *Candida albicans,* and confinement to aluminum foil–lined rooms.

Suggested Readings

Bieber T, Leung DYM, eds. *Atopic dermatitis.* New York: Marcel Dekker, Inc., 2002.
Holloway JW, Cakebread JA, Holgate ST. The genetics of allergic disease and asthma. In: Leung DYM, Sampson HA, Geha RS, Szefler SJ, eds. *Pediatric allergy: principles and practice.* St. Louis: Mosby, 2003:23.
Liu AH, Martinez FD, Taussig LM. Natural history of allergic diseases and asthma. In: Leung DYM, Sampson HA, Geha RS, Szefler SJ, eds. *Pediatric allergy: principles and practice.* St. Louis: Mosby, 2003:10.
Metcalfe DD, Sampson HA, Simon RA, eds. *Adverse reactions to foods and food additives,* 3rd ed. Oxford: Blackwell Scientific Publications, 2003.
Oettgen HC, Geha RS. Regulation and biology of Immunoglobulin IgE. In: Leung DYM, Sampson HA, Geha RS, Szefler SJ, eds. *Pediatric allergy: principles and practice.* St. Louis: Mosby, 2003:39.
Shearer W, eds. Primer on allergic and immunologic diseases. *J Allergy Clin Immunol* 2003;111(2 Suppl).
Szefler SJ. Asthma. In: Leung DYM, Sampson HA, Geha RS, Szefler SJ, eds. *Pediatric allergy: principles and practice.* St. Louis: Mosby, 2003:337.
Wood RA. Environmental control. In: Leung DYM, Sampson HA, Geha RS, Szefler SJ, eds. *Pediatric allergy: principles and practice.* St. Louis: Mosby, 2003:269.

CHAPTER 420 ■ ASTHMA

PEYTON A. EGGLESTON

Asthma is a chronic inflammatory airways disorder that causes recurrent episodes of wheezing, breathlessness, chest tightness, and coughing. Usually, these episodes are associated with widespread but variable airflow obstruction that is reversible either spontaneously or in response to treatment. The inflammation also causes an associated increase in the existing bronchial hyperresponsiveness to a variety of stimuli.

A leading cause of morbidity among children throughout the world, annually, asthma accounts for 3 million physician visits, 28 million restricted activity days, and one-third of all school days lost in the United States. In most urban hospitals, it is the most frequent cause for the hospitalization of children. In most Western countries, between 2% and 10% of children younger than age 16 are affected. In tropical and Third-World countries, the prevalence is significantly lower.

The prevalence of asthma in the United States has increased in children aged 5 to 14 years from 4.2% in 1980 to 8.7% in 2001. The reason for this increase is not clear, but it has been seen throughout the Western world and likely is related to increasing urbanization in these populations, increasing pollution, and more accurate diagnosis of asthma. Risk factors for increased prevalence and mortality in the United States primarily include urbanization and poverty. Definite pockets of increased mortality are seen in cities, especially among those in lower socioeconomic groups. Recently, it has been shown that children with frequent respiratory infections or with heavy exposure to bacterial products, such as endotoxin, have lower rates of asthma and atopy. This has led to a "hygiene hypothesis," which proposes that early childhood infection modifies the immune response and reduces the tendency to produce IgE antibodies to environmental allergens.

Deaths from asthma have been increasing steadily since the 1970s. The U.S. general population mortality rate due to asthma, 1.4 per 100,000, compares to 2.0 per 100,000 in Canada, 3.8 per 100,000 in Great Britain, 5.7 per 100,000 in Australia, and 6.0 per 100,000 in Sweden. At the same time, death from asthma is uncommon in children. In 2001, for example, the rate was 0.30 per 100,000 children for ages 5 to 14 in the United States, as compared to 11.6 per 100,000 for accidents in the same age group and 3.3 per 100,000 for cancer.

EPIDEMIOLOGY

The median age of onset of asthma is 4 years; more than 20% of children develop symptoms within the first year of life. Risk factors for incident asthma include a personal or family history of atopy, especially multiple positive skin tests or radioallergosorbent tests (RAST). The association with parental smoking is weaker, but is consistent, especially if the mother smokes during pregnancy.

Respiratory infections, especially due to respiratory syncytial virus (RSV), increase the risk for persistent wheezing, and between 40% and 50% of children with RSV bronchiolitis develop chronic asthma.

In 60% of cases, asthma beginning in childhood resolves by young adult life. Fifty percent of those who undergo remission in adolescence become symptomatic again as young adults, and tests of airway hyperactivity show that, even in asymptomatic young adults, the airways have not returned to normal. In general, those in whom the disorder resolves have less severe, intermittent asthma; usually do not have multiple positive skin tests to inhalant allergens; and do not have persistent wheezing or rhonchi. Studies demonstrate that heavy exposure to pollution, allergens, or cigarette smoke makes resolution less likely.

PATHOPHYSIOLOGY

As shown in the pathologic specimen in Figure 420.1, asthma is an inflammatory disease. Characteristically, the infiltrate in the airway wall and the surrounding parenchyma is rich in eosinophils, but neutrophils, basophils, and mononuclear cells also are common, without organized lymphoid nodules or granulomas. Large areas of respiratory epithelium are desquamated, and collagen is deposited in the area of the basement membrane. Bronchial smooth muscle is hypertrophied and hyperplastic. Frequently, respiratory epithelium and inflammatory cells fill large mucus plugs in the airway lumen.

The best defined pathway leading to this pattern of inflammation is through mast-cell activation. Mast cells are fixed tissue cells activated by either lymphokines or IgE-dependent mechanisms; they produce a variety of proinflammatory substances. IgE-dependent inflammation is described in more detail in Chapter 419 but here we should note that activation leads to the rapid release of chemical mediators and rapid airway obstruction—the "immediate response." This immediate response evolves into a late-phase reaction (LPR) within 2 to 4 hours after antigen exposure. In addition, an important physiologic element of asthma (i.e., airway hyperresponsiveness) has been found to increase for days to weeks after LPR.

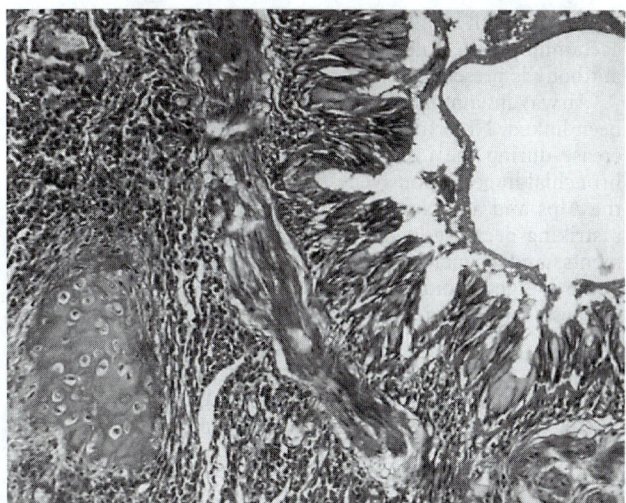

FIGURE 420.1. Pathology of asthma. Hematoxylin-eosin–stained specimen of cross-section of a small bronchus of an asthmatic patient.

It is important to recognize that all the classic airway pathology and bronchial hyperresponsiveness seen in asthma may occur without evidence of IgE-dependent sensitization. The mechanisms responsible for nonallergic or "intrinsic" asthma are not known.

Airway Hyperresponsiveness

Highly variable airway obstruction is characteristic of asthma. This *airway hyperresponsiveness* is illustrated best in Figure 420.2, which shows the record of daily peak expiratory flow rate (PEFR) measurements in two patients with asthma. With milder asthma, PEFR may be normal, but daily measures vary by more than 20%. With severe asthma, PEFR is frequently abnormal and daily variations are more than 60%. These variations in obstruction may be seen in response to many "precipitants" of bronchospasm, including exercise, irritants (cigarette smoke, odors, pollution, sulfite preservatives), weather changes, common colds, certain drugs (beta-adrenergic antagonists,

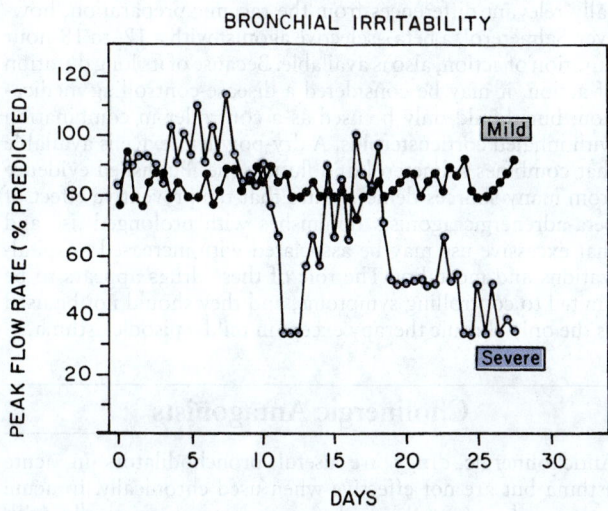

FIGURE 420.2. Daily peak expiratory flow rate measurement in two children with asthma.

aspirin, and all nonsteroidal antiinflammatory agents except acetaminophen). Allergens cause attacks when specific IgE antibody is present.

Airway inflammation and airway hyperresponsiveness have been linked. Not only does bronchial hyperresponsiveness increase during the LPR, but allergen avoidance can decrease bronchial hyperresponsiveness. Allergic children who move to the Alps and adults who are confined to hospital experience a striking decrease in airway symptoms, medication requirements, and bronchial hyperresponsiveness. Clinical trials of home allergen avoidance also decrease bronchial hyperresponsiveness, but to a smaller extent.

PHARMACOTHERAPY FOR ASTHMA

Beta-Adrenergic Agonists

Beta-adrenergic agonists are the symptomatic therapy of choice, acting through specific airway receptors to reverse obstruction quickly; using short-acting agents, bronchodilation is maximal within 5 to 10 minutes. In addition to being effective bronchodilators, beta-adrenergic agonists inhibit immediate asthmatic responses to allergens, exercise, and many inhaled irritants when given just before exposure. They have little effect on the LPR or on the resulting increase in reactivity. Toxicity includes tachycardia, palpitations, and central nervous system excitement and muscular tremor. All are dose-dependent and rarely are a problem with appropriate inhalation dosing. Whenever possible, beta-adrenergic agonists should be inhaled, because effective bronchodilation can be achieved using doses 10 to 20 times lower than those using oral dosing. Nebulized drugs may be given in solution from a nebulizer, from a hand-held metered-dose inhaler, or from a dry-powder inhaler. Infants may be treated using a metered-dose inhaler using an AeroChamber and a face mask. Adolescents must be cautioned against overuse of the inhalers and over-reliance on its brief bronchodilatory effects.

Epinephrine, the first available beta agonist, still is prescribed but is no longer the treatment of choice. The current drug of choice is albuterol, which is beta$_2$-selective and longer acting than epinephrine. Albuterol is a racemic mixture. Lev-albuterol, the R-isomer of albuterol, became available recently and has the theoretical advantage of greater bronchodilation with fewer side effects. Clinical trials have shown few clinically relevant differences from the racemic preparation, however. Salmeterol, a beta$_2$-selective agonist with a 12- to 18-hour duration of action, also is available. Because of its long duration of action, it may be considered a disease-controlling medication, but should only be used as a controller in combination with inhaled corticosteroids. A dry-powder device is available that combines salmeterol and fluticasone. Published evidence from many sources demonstrates that the preventive effect of beta-adrenergic agonists diminishes with prolonged use and that excessive use may be associated with increased hospitalizations and mortality. The role of these drugs appears to be limited to controlling symptoms, and they should not be used as the only chronic therapy except in mild, episodic asthma.

Cholinergic Antagonists

Anticholinergic drugs are useful bronchodilators in acute asthma but are not effective when used chronically. In acute asthma, they have been shown to act synergistically with beta adrenergic agonists. They are much less effective than beta-adrenergic agonists in the chronic management of asthma, and toxic effects (xerostomia, mydriasis, tachycardia, and abdominal pain) are annoying. Representative compounds in clinical use include atropine and ipratropium.

Cromolyn

Cromolyn was the first drug without bronchodilator properties shown to prevent allergen-induced asthma in humans. It is the only available drug that effectively inhibits both early- and late-phase asthma caused by allergen exposure. In chronic use, it reduces airway hyperreactivity slightly, and disease activity is decreased. Compared with other medications that control asthma, it is much less effective. Except for a rare allergic reaction, cromolyn is nontoxic.

Theophylline

Theophylline is a weak bronchodilator with antiinflammatory properties comparable to cromolyn; the mechanism for either of these effects is not known. Toxic effects include both mild symptoms (nausea, vomiting, abdominal pain, headache, irritability) and severe and life-threatening reactions (intractable convulsions, tachyarrhythmia). Both therapeutic and toxic effects are dose dependent, and it is difficult to maintain therapeutic effects without some toxicity. The drug was once the only orally effective agent; now it is used as a supplemental drug for chronic asthma in severe cases.

Leukotriene Modifiers

Leukotrienes, released from mast cells, eosinophils, and basophils, are potent bronchoconstrictors and pro-inflammatory mediators. The leukotriene modifiers act either to decrease the production of inflammatory agents or to inhibit tissue effects to those agents. The most useful clinical agents, montelukast and zafirlukast, are competitive inhibitors that have been shown to decrease airflow obstruction in mild asthma within an hour of dosing and to be effective as antiinflammatory agents. Chronically, they decrease bronchial hyperresponsiveness and inhibit bronchoconstriction from exercise and allergen exposure. Beta-adrenergic agents are more effective bronchodilators, and inhaled corticosteroids are more effective in chronic persistent asthma in clinical trials, but the low toxicity of the leukotriene modifiers and their effectiveness when taken orally has allowed them to become widely used alternatives for the daily therapy of mild persistent asthma. They also have been shown to increase the chronic benefits of inhaled corticosteroids.

Corticosteroids

Corticosteroids are the most effective therapy available for the acute and chronic treatment of asthma. They have broad antiinflammatory effects on most inflammatory cells and are capable both of reversing acute exacerbations of asthma and reducing bronchial hyperresponsiveness when used chronically, so that airway response to many triggers such as exercise, allergen (late phase), and irritants are reduced. For chronic use, inhaled corticosteroids are an important new advance in asthma therapy. By modifying the glucocorticoid molecule, these compounds have been rendered approximately 100 times more potent than prednisone. In addition, they are absorbed poorly from the respiratory tract and are cleared rapidly when absorbed from the gastrointestinal tract. These pharmacokinetic properties provide a wide therapeutic ratio, leading to the current recommendation that they be used as first-line therapy for persistent

TABLE 420.1

INHALED CORTICOSTEROIDS DAILY DOSES

	Low Dose*	Medium Dose	High Dose
Beclomethasone CFC[†]	84–336	336–672	>672
HFA	80–160	160–320	>320
Budesonide DPI	200–400	400–800	>800
Nebulized suspension	500	1,000	2,000
Fluticasone MDI	88–176	176–440	>660
DPI	100–200	200–400	>400
Flunisolide MDI	500–750	1,000–1,250	>1,250
Triamcinolone MDI	400–800	800–1,200	>1,200

*Total daily dose in μg per day.
[†]MDI, metered-dose inhaler; CFC, chlorinated fluorocarbon-powered metered-dose inhaler; HFA, halofreon-powered metered-dose inhaler; DPI, dry-powder inhaler.

asthma of any severity. Available agents and their dose ranges are listed in Table 420.1.

Corticosteroids have important toxicities, including inhibition of the hypothalamic-pituitary axis (HPA), suppressed immunity, bone demineralization, and impaired growth; all these effects are dose dependent and usually can be avoided or minimized. HPA suppression is seen routinely with systemic dosing, but the effects reverse quickly after 10 to 14 days of treatment. Cases of severe varicella infection have been reported in children treated with high systemic doses of corticosteroids for acute asthma, but not in those treated with the inhaled corticosteroids used in chronic therapy. Children may be exposed to systemic doses repeatedly to treat exacerbations related to upper respiratory tract infections; limited data suggests that systemic toxicity does not occur. Bone demineralization does not seem to occur with chronic inhaled steroid treatment in children. Growth is sensitive to chronic corticosteroid therapy, but reassuring studies have demonstrated that low-dose therapy using inhaled corticosteroids is not associated with growth delay, and that medium- to high-dose therapy only has effects for the first year or two of treatment.

CHRONIC ASTHMA MANAGEMENT

The goals of chronic management are to normalize pulmonary function, decrease peak flow variability, and allow normal or near-normal activity with infrequent night symptoms and no absences from school. Essential steps begin with establishing the diagnosis of asthma, then reducing airway inflammation by reducing exposure to precipitants and prescribing appropriate drug therapy, monitoring disease activity over time, and treating acute episodes promptly. The National Asthma Education Program of the National Institutes of Health has published *Guidelines for the Diagnosis and Management of Asthma*, a consensus of a number of experts in the field. This section relies heavily on their recommendations.

A diagnosis of asthma is based on a history of recurrent episodes of coughing or wheezing, especially if these episodes are related to typical precipitants and are relieved by beta-adrenergic agents. A family history of asthma or a personal history of eczema, food allergy, or allergic rhinitis is strongly supportive of the diagnosis. In most cases, little medical evaluation is needed to confirm the diagnosis of asthma, especially when a history of acute reaction to appropriate stimuli and quick relief by appropriate therapy is elicited. Additional history is primarily focused on excluding other causes of recurrent chronic respiratory symptoms such as cystic fibrosis, foreign-body aspiration, gastroesophageal reflux, and anatomic abnormalities. The physical examination may reveal wheezes even if the child is asymptomatic. Other findings, such as growth delay, digital clubbing, hypoxia, or localized crackles, should suggest other diagnoses. In most cases, laboratory tests in patients with asthma are normal. Eosinophilia (more than 400 eosinophils per cubic millimeter in blood; more than 10% in secretions), an elevated serum IgE or a positive Phadeotope test result (Pharmacia) are supportive of a diagnosis of asthma. If the child is cooperative, a measurement of PEFR or forced expired volume in one second (FEV_1) before and after inhaled bronchodilator administration may confirm the diagnosis.

Once a diagnosis is established, assessment of current severity is based on the NIH Guidelines. These are summarized in Table 420.2 and depend on the answers to two questions: "In the past 2 weeks, how many days has your child had symptoms of cough, wheeze, or tightness in the chest" and "In the past month, how many nights has your child had chest symptoms?" The child's measured PEFR or FEV_1 before bronchodilator administration is an essential objective measure. The child's asthma then is categorized according these factors as mild intermittent, mild moderate, or severe persistent. The category assigned depends on the most severe components. For example, a child with a history of exercise-induced wheezing each day but no night symptoms or lung-function abnormality would be categorized as having persistent asthma, as would a child with night symptoms several times a week or another with abnormal PEFR or FEV_1. These are functional categories that will determine the appropriate level of treatment, provide treatment goals, and be reassessed at each subsequent visit. It is also important to determine how much school loss, decreased activity, and family disruption is caused by the disease, because the control of these aspects will be a major goal of therapy.

TABLE 420.2

SEVERITY CLASSIFICATION FOR CHRONIC ASTHMA

	Days with Symptoms	Nights with Symptoms	PEFR/FEV_1 % Predicted	PEFR Variability
Mild intermittent	≤2/week	≤2/month	≥80%	≤20%
Mild persistent	3–6/week	3–4/month	≥80%	20–30%
Moderate persistent	Daily	≥5/month	60–80%	>30%
Severe persistent	Continuous	Frequent	≤60%	>30%

FEV_1, forced expiratory volume over 1 second; PEFR, peak expiratory flow.
Adapted from the National Heart, Lung and Blood Institute. National Asthma Education and Prevention Program. *Expert panel report 2: Guidelines for the diagnosis and management of asthma*, publication no. 97-4051. Bethesda, MD: National Institutes of Health, 1997.

TABLE 420.3

RECOMMENDED CHRONIC MEDICATIONS FOR DIFFERENT SEVERITY LEVELS OF ASTHMA

	Preferred Controller Medication	Alternative Controller Medications
Mild intermittent	No daily medications needed	None
Mild persistent	■ Inhaled corticosteroids-low dose	■ Leukotriene modifiers ■ Cromolyn ■ Sustained-release theophylline
Moderate persistent	■ Inhaled corticosteroids-low to medium dose plus long acting beta₂-agonists	■ Inhaled corticosteroids, medium dose ■ Inhaled corticosteroids, low to medium dose plus leukotriene modifiers or theophylline
Severe persistent	■ Inhaled corticosteroid-high dose plus long acting beta₂-agonists	■ Leukotriene modifiers, theophylline or oral steroids as needed

Treatment consists of reducing exposure to precipitants, controlling airway inflammation using medications, monitoring asthma disease activity, and treating asthma episodes promptly. A very important step is to establish a partnership with the family, to allow them to agree on treatment goals, and to monitor home treatment and asthma activity.

Avoiding Precipitants

Some precipitants, such as indoor allergens and irritants, can be avoided, whereas others, such as infection, are difficult to avoid, and still others, such as exercise, should be controlled using preventive medication.

Over 80% of asthmatic children are allergic to environmental allergens. However, the relationship of a given allergen to symptoms depends on a child's individual sensitivity. It is therefore important to establish sensitivity either from a history or appropriate testing before urging specific allergen avoidance. The most common allergen sources associated with chronic asthma are dust mites, furry animals, dogs, various molds, cockroaches, and various foods. Dust-mite allergy is caused by pteroglyph mites that infest bedding, rugs, and other fabrics. The allergen is carried on fecal particles that are relatively large and settle quickly after disturbance. To avoid mite allergen, airtight covers must be installed to cover mattresses and pillows completely and bedding must be washed frequently. Approximately one-third of patients with asthma are allergic to cats or dogs. Pets should be removed from households with sensitized children. Compromises short of this have not proven to be effective. Mold problems are worse in the moist environments encountered with bedroom vaporizers, in basements, and in homes without air conditioning in warm southern climates. The most effective way to remove mold and mildew is to remove contaminated material, wash with 2% chlorine bleach solutions or benzalkonium, and reduce home moisture content. Cockroaches have been found to contribute important allergens in urban environments, especially in the middle Atlantic and southeastern states. Elimination requires pest control treatment and careful clean-up of the remaining insect parts and feces.

Another approach to modifying the allergic response to environmental allergens is allergen immunotherapy, in which small amounts of aqueous extracts of source-allergen vectors (pollens, dust mites, mold spores) are injected regularly over a period of months to years. Allergen immunotherapy reduces the symptoms of allergic rhinitis, but it is less useful for asthma.

Environmental tobacco smoke is the irritant most strongly associated with increased asthma morbidity, especially in preschool children. Any person who lives with an asthmatic child should be urged to stop smoking. The physician's advice is the most important incentive, but community resources are available to help smokers stop.

Medication for Asthma

The first goal in selecting medications is to establish the severity of asthma using a schema shown in Table 420.2. The appropriate medications for each level of severity are summarized in Table 420.3. Mild intermittent asthma requires no daily antiinflammatory therapy. However, any child who meets the criteria for persistent asthma should receive daily therapy. Currently, inhaled corticosteroids are the treatment of choice for any child with persistent asthma. In treating mild persistent asthma, inhaled steroids may be started at low doses (Table 420.4). With moderate persistent asthma, the dose may be increased or a second daily medication may be added; alternatives include long-acting beta-adrenergic agents and leukotriene modifiers. Controlled clinical trials show that adding a second medication is more effective than increased doses of inhaled steroids.

Objective measurements of pulmonary function are essential in managing asthma on a day-to-day basis. Home peak expiratory flow meters should be used to help patients assess symptoms, establish a baseline for measuring exacerbations,

TABLE 420.4

PREDICTING CHILDHOOD ASTHMA IN WHEEZING INFANTS

Major Criteria	■ MD diagnosed eczema ■ MD diagnosed asthma in a parent
Minor Criteria	■ MD diagnosed allergic rhinitis ■ Wheezing apart from a cold ■ Eosinophilia ($\geq 4\%$)

Stringent predictive index: ≥ 3 wheezing episodes **plus** 1 major or 2 minor criteria.
This has positive predictive value of 77% for asthma sometime during childhood.

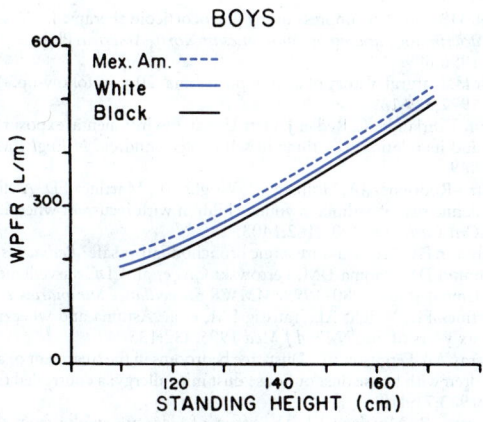
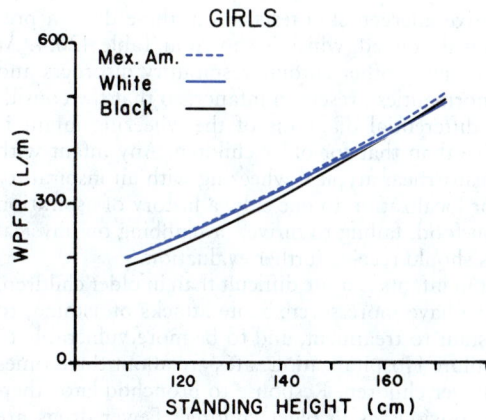

FIGURE 420.3. Prediction curves for peak expiratory flow rate measurements in children. Mex. Am., Mexican American; WPFR, Wright peak flow rate. (Reproduced with permission from Hsu KHK, Jenkins DE, Hsi BP, et al. Ventilatory functions of normal children and young adults—Mexican American, white and black: II. Wright peak flow meter. *J Pediatr* 1979;95:192.)

and adjust medications. Normal values are shown in Figure 420.3. Peak flows are within the normal range in mild asthma and never drop more than 20% during symptomatic episodes.

Regular follow-up visits are an essential component of good management. Guidelines recommend that therapy be reviewed every 1 to 6 months, especially in newly diagnosed patients, because they usually evolve from one stage of severity to another and require medication adjustment. At a typical visit, disease severity should be reassessed, and environmental avoidance and medication effects should be reviewed. Medications should be adjusted, the written acute action plan should be reviewed, and additional education should be provided regarding inhaler techniques, environmental avoidance, and control expectations.

Even mild asthmatics are susceptible to acute severe attacks of asthma that may be life threatening. It is essential that each patient receive a written acute action plan that explains appropriate medication for increasingly severe symptoms and PEFR changes. It should include emergency medical contact information and indications for calling or going to an emergency room. A copy of this plan should be available to the child's school or day-care provider.

TREATMENT OF ACUTE ASTHMA

The goal of acute asthma therapy is to normalize pulmonary functions rapidly and to prevent the progression of the attack. Essential to this process are early recognition of acute changes; prompt communication between patient and physician; removal of the allergen, irritant, or other trigger; and appropriate intensification of asthma medications.

Home management is based on a brief written action plan, so that treatment begins immediately and families gain some control of the disease. In mild to moderate attacks, with symptoms of coughing or wheezing and PEFR in the range of 50% to 80% of the child's personal best, albuterol should be given by nebulization or metered-dose inhaler. Albuterol may be repeated every 3 to 4 hours, and severity should be reassessed frequently. If the response is not complete, or if signs of a severe attack are present (marked symptoms, inability to talk, cyanosis, PEFR less than 50% of personal best), the family should contact the physician or go to the office or a hospital emergency room. In severe or persistent attacks, the physician may give oral prednisone (1 to 2 mg/kg per dose) and beta-agonist treatment should continue. If severity subsides to mild

over the next 4 hours, continued home treatment is appropriate. If moderate asthma continues, affected patients should be seen in the physician's office or in a hospital emergency department.

Certain patients are at risk for life-threatening severe attacks. These patients should be treated more aggressively than outlined above and sometimes cannot be treated at home at all. High-risk patients include those with prior intubation for asthma, two or more hospitalizations for asthma in the last year, three or more emergency department visits for asthma in the last year, hospitalization or emergency department use within the last month, a requirement for oral steroid therapy, a history of syncope or hypoxic seizures during an asthma attack, and a history of serious psychiatric or psychosocial problems.

The decision to treat in a physician's office or a hospital emergency department depends on many factors, including accessibility of the emergency department, ability and interest of the physician to manage severe asthma in the office, and the physician's previous relationship with such patients.

In the office, a reassessment should determine severity and rule out such complications as atelectasis, pneumomediastinum, and pneumothorax. Oxygen should be administered together with nebulized albuterol every 20 minutes for 1 hour. Prednisone should be given, unless the patient responds immediately to a nebulized dose. If treatment is required for more than 4 hours, hospitalization should be considered; if the response to treatment is poor, the patient should be admitted. Generally, patients who have responded will be discharged on continued medication, which usually includes prednisone, and with a follow-up plan.

Hospital management offers little pharmacologically that cannot be provided on an outpatient basis. The major indication for hospitalization is to observe for continued deterioration so that more intensive treatment can be given, in an intensive care unit if necessary.

WHEEZING INFANTS

Asthma is difficult to diagnose in infants because wheezy respiratory infections occur so commonly. In a prospective study, 49% of infants wheezed at least once with a respiratory infection, but this was usually transient, and only 27% of these infants went on to develop persistent wheezing at age 6 years. The most important risk factors predicting the development of asthma were a mother with asthma, elevated IgE levels, and multiple positive allergen skin tests. From these data, a predictive index was created, which is shown in Table 420.4. At the same time, many other chronic respiratory disorders and anatomic abnormalities present in infancy, so that the consideration of a differential diagnosis of the wheezing infant is more extensive than that for older children. Any infant with significant steatorrhea, atypical wheezing with an inspiratory component or localization to one side, a history of aspiration or choking on food, failing to thrive, or clubbing on physical examinations should receive further evaluation.

Treatment in infants is more difficult than in older children. Infants tend to have more severe acute attacks of asthma, to be more resistant to treatment, and to be more vulnerable to respiratory failure Hospitalization rates are about three times higher in younger children. Response to bronchodilator therapy is not as obvious as in older children. Fewer drugs are available that have undergone clinical trials and are approved by the U.S. Food and Drug Administration (FDA). For example, only one inhaled corticosteroid, budesonide, is approved in infants, and leukotriene modifiers have only recently been created in appropriate form for infants.

A spacer device, the AeroChamber, is available with a face mask, allowing some infants to be treated with metered-dose inhalers. Studies have demonstrated that these devices are as effective in acute asthma as administering aerosol therapy using a nebulizer, although none of these devices has received FDA approval.

Suggested Readings

Alden ER. The field of pediatrics. In: McMillan JA, DeAngelis CD, Feigen RD, et al., eds. *Oski's Pediatrics: Principles and practice*, 3rd ed. Philadelphia: Lippincott Williams and Wilkins, 1999:7.

Allen DB. Growth suppression by glucocorticoid therapy. In: Vassalo J, ed. *Endocrinology and metabolic clinics in North America*. Philadelphia: Saunders, 1996:699.

Blair H. Natural history of childhood asthma: 20-year follow-up. *Arch Dis Child* 1977;52:613.

Braun-Fahrlander C, Redler J, Herz U et al. Environmental exposure to endotoxin and its relation to asthma in school age children. *N Engl J Med* 2002;347:869.

Castro-Rodriguez JA, Holberg CJ, Wright AL, Martinez FD. A clinical index to define risk of asthma in young children with recurrent wheezing. *Am J Resp Crit Care Med* 2000;162:1403.

Eggleston PA. Are beta-adrenergic bronchodilators safe? *Pediatrics* 1997;99:729.

Mannino DM, Homa DM, Pertowski CA, et al. CDC surveillance for asthma-United States 1980–1999. *MMWR Surveillance Summaries* 2002;51:1.

Martinez FD, Wright AL, Taussig LM, et al. Asthma and wheezing in the first six years of life. *N Engl J Med* 1995;332:133.

Murray AB, Ferguson AC. Dust-free bedrooms in the treatment of asthmatic children with house dust or house dust mite allergy: a controlled trial. *Pediatrics* 1983;71:418.

Murray AB, Morrison BJ. The effect of cigarette smoke from the mother on bronchial responsiveness in severity of symptoms in children with asthma. *J Allergy Clin Immunol* 1986;77:575.

National Heart, Lung and Blood Institute. National Asthma Education and Prevention Program. *Expert panel report 2: guidelines for the diagnosis and management of asthma*, publication no. 97-4051. Bethesda, MD: National Institutes of Health, 1997.

Potsma DS, Bleecker ER, Amelung PJ, et al. Genetic susceptibility to asthma-bronchial hyperresponsiveness coinherited with a major gene for atopy. *N Engl J Med* 1995;333:894.

Rosenstreich DL, Eggleston PA, Kattan M, et al. The role of cockroach allergy and exposure to cockroach allergen in causing morbidity among inner-city children with asthma. *N Engl J Med* 1997;336:1356.

Sears MR. Worldwide trends in asthma mortality. *Bull Int Union Tuberc Lung Dis* 1991;66:79.

Strachan DP, Cook DG. Parental smoking and childhood asthma: longitudinal and case control studies. *Thorax* 1998;53:204.

Strunk RC. Asthma deaths in childhood: identification of patients at risk and intervention. *J Allergy Clin Immunol* 1987;80:472.

Tabachnik E, Levison H. Infantile bronchial asthma. *J Allergy Clin Immunol* 1981;67:339.

Weiss KB, Wagener DK. Changing patterns of asthma mortality: identifying target populations at high risk. *JAMA* 1990;264:1683.

CHAPTER 421 ■ URTICARIA AND ANGIOEDEMA

THOMAS B. CASALE AND JEFFREY R. STOKES

Urticaria (hives) is characterized by erythematous, edematous wheals of the superficial layers of the skin or mucous membranes. The lesions blanch with pressure, often are pruritic, and usually are distributed symmetrically. Usually, individual urticarial lesions are evanescent, commonly lasting less than 4 hours but occasionally persisting for 24 to 48 hours. If the lesions persist, underlying vasculitis may be the cause. Angioedema is a similar process, occurring in deeper layers of the skin and subcutaneous tissues. Angioedema is characterized by well-demarcated areas of swelling that are nonpitting, nondependent and, usually, not hot. Whereas urticaria may occur on any part of the body, angioedema often involves the extremities, face (especially the perioral and periorbital areas), or genitalia.

Pruritus or a chronic itch does not equal urticaria. Pruritus without visible lesions can be caused by a number of different diseases unrelated to urticaria, such as renal failure and lymphoproliferative diseases. Affected patients have severe pruritus and no evidence of urticaria. Although urticarial lesions often are pruritic, the presence of pruritus without urticaria is cause to formulate a distinct list of differential diagnoses.

Traditionally, the duration of urticaria has defined whether the disease is acute or chronic. Urticarial lesions that are either continuous or frequent for 6 weeks or longer are defined as chronic. Acute urticaria lesions are present for less than 6 weeks. Physical urticarias fall into a separate group and may last for several years but are manifested by recurrent episodes of acute lesions in relation to a physical stimulus, such as cold, exercise, or pressure. Chronic urticaria may be distinguished histologically. Biopsy samples show a nonnecrotizing perivascular infiltrate generally not noted during acute episodes of urticaria or physical urticarias. In most studies, an etiologic agent in chronic urticaria is found in only 5% to 10% of patients. Thus, most cases of chronic urticaria are labeled *idiopathic*. The success rates for identifying specific causes of acute urticaria are higher.

The incidence of urticaria and angioedema is extremely high. Between 15% and 20% of the population is estimated to experience an episode of urticaria or angioedema at some time in life. Acute urticaria may occur at any age and is the form seen most commonly in children. Chronic urticaria occurs more frequently in young adults (peak incidence occurring in the third and fourth decades) than in the pediatric population. Chronic urticaria may be persistent. In one long-term follow-up of pediatric and adult patients with chronic idiopathic urticaria or angioedema, the average duration of urticaria alone was 6 months, angioedema alone was 1 year, and urticaria with angioedema was 5 years. The effect of chronic urticaria on quality of life can be quite severe, causing disruption of sleep and simple daily living routines, and its impact has been comparable to adults with ischemic heart disease.

PATHOPHYSIOLOGY

Urticarial lesions are caused by dilation of blood vessels in the superficial dermis (erythema or flare) and by increased vascular permeability, with leakage of fluid into surrounding connective tissue (wheal). Histologically, urticaria is characterized by the dilation of small blood vessels and by edema, which leads to flattened rete pegs, widened dermal papillae, and swollen collagen fibers. Angioedema shows similar changes but is confined to the deeper dermis and subcutaneous tissue.

On the basis of varied evidence, many pathogenic factors and cells are seen to be involved in the development of urticaria (Box 421.1). These factors include mast cells and mast-cell mediators, autoantibodies, neuropeptides, and inflammatory (especially mononuclear) cells other than mast cells.

Mast Cells and Mast-Cell Mediators

Mast cells and mast-cell mediators long have been implicated as being important in the pathogenesis of urticaria. Evidence includes the morphologic and histologic definition of mast-cell degranulation after specific physical stimuli in patients with physical urticarias; wheal and flare formation after intracutaneous injection of mast-cell mediators; identification of mediators in biological fluids collected during urticarial reactions; and the ability to suppress the urticarial tissue response with specific mediator antagonists (e.g., antihistamines). Moreover, evidence of mast-cell degranulation is seen in chronic urticarial lesions, and the skin of patients with chronic urticaria often contains increased numbers of mast cells.

Overall, mast cells and mast cell–dependent mediators play a prominent role in the pathogenesis of urticaria and angioedema. A number of mediators other than histamine, however, are important in causing urticaria and angioedema (see Box 421.1). Therefore, selective H_1 antihistamines seldom are entirely effective in treating urticarial reactions. Studies of the role of mediators other than histamine in the pathogenesis of urticaria should aid in the development of new and better treatment modalities for this disorder. For example, because leukotrienes can induce wheal and flare responses and have chemotactic activity, leukotriene modifiers have been used in treating chronic urticaria.

Although mast cells and mast-cell mediators are central to the pathogenesis of urticaria and angioedema, the presence of IgE antibodies to specific allergens is not necessary. A number of mechanisms other than classic allergic reactions may lead to mast-cell degranulation. The activation of either the classic or alternative complement pathways may cause urticaria by producing anaphylatoxins (C3a, C4a, C5a), which can degranulate mast cells. A number of drugs, including opioids, some antibiotics, and nonsteroidal antiinflammatory agents, may lead to nonimmunologic mast-cell mediator release. Neuropeptides (discussed later) also can cause mast-cell degranulation. Inflammatory reactions resulting in the production of histamine-releasing factors from lymphocytes, macrophages, and neutrophils may cause mast-cell mediator release as well. Such physical stimuli as heat, cold, and pressure can cause mast-cell mediator release and urticaria in susceptible individuals. Thus, many potential mechanisms lead to mast-cell mediator release and urticaria.

Histamine-Releasing Factors

Studies have shown that the intradermal injection of autologous serum produces a wheal and flare reaction in approximately 60% of patients with chronic idiopathic urticaria, implying a role for circulating histamine-releasing factors. These patients can be subdivided into two groups of similar size. One group has heat-stable nonimmunoglobulin mediators that release histamine from mast cells but not from basophils. Another group has IgG autoantibodies to the high-affinity IgE receptors or IgE, or both, that are capable of inducing histamine release from both mast cells and basophils. Patients with this autoantibody have been shown to have an increased incidence of HLA-DR4, Hashimoto's thyroiditis, and antimicrosomal antibodies, thus implying that, in a subset of patients, chronic idiopathic urticaria is an autoimmune disorder. Patients often have a positive skin test to autologous serum injected intradermally and read at 30 minutes. Novel therapies for this subgroup of patients have included plasmapheresis, intravenous immune globulin, and cyclosporine.

Neuropeptides

The exact role of neuropeptides in chronic urticaria and physical urticarias is unclear. However, the proximity of mast cells to sensory nerves favors their involvement. The intradermal injection of many neuropeptides results in erythema and a wheal or induration that closely resembles an urticarial lesion. These neuropeptides are present in skin and have direct effects on cutaneous vasculature, including vasodilation and edema. The physical urticarias exhibit some evidence that neuropeptides might be important. The provocative stimuli in these conditions

---

> **BOX 421.1**   Pathogenic Factors in Urticaria and Angioedema
>
> **Mast Cells and Mast-Cell Mediators**
> Histamine
> Bradykinin
> Prostaglandins (e.g., PGD_2)
> Leukotrienes C_4, D_4, E_4
> Platelet-activating factor
> Cytokines
>
> **Histamine-Releasing Factors**
> Nonimmunoglobulin mediators
> IgG autoantibodies
>
> **Neuropeptides of Unmyelinated Sensory Fibers**
> Substance P
> Calcitonin gene–related peptide
> Vasoactive intestinal peptide
> Others
>
> **Inflammatory Cells**
> Monocytes
> T lymphocytes
> Neutrophils (rarely)

include such factors as cold, heat, and pressure, which are expected to activate neuropeptide-containing sensory nerve fibers in the skin. The release of these neuropeptides then can cause vasodilation and edema directly. Several neuropeptides, including substance P, also can degranulate cutaneous mast cells. Repeated topical application of capsaicin, a substance that depletes neuropeptides from afferent nerves, has prevented the urticarial response to thermal challenge in patients with cold- and heat-induced urticaria.

Cells

Numerous biopsy studies suggest that inflammatory cells other than mast cells play important roles in urticaria as well. Often, chronic urticarial lesions are characterized by a non-necrotizing perivascular infiltrate composed of CD4+ T lymphocytes and monocytes. Neutrophils are predominant in a minority of lesions. Because lymphocytes, monocytes, and other cells release histamine-releasing factors, and mast cells may produce substances that activate T cells and monocytes, one might envision a cyclic propagation of an event initiated by mast-cell degranulation. Corticosteroids work, in part, because T lymphocytes and monocytes likely play a role in the pathogenesis of chronic urticaria. Corticosteroids have not been shown convincingly to inhibit cutaneous mast-cell degranulation and, therefore, generally have not been shown to be effective in the immediate-onset physical urticarias in which cellular infiltrates usually are not noted by biopsy. In general, chronic urticarial lesions contain no evidence of complement or immunoglobulin deposition.

CAUSES OF URTICARIA AND ANGIOEDEMA

Because a number of mechanisms may lead to mast-cell mediator release, a variety of etiologic factors have been found to cause urticaria and angioedema. The major etiologic factors producing acute urticaria and angioedema are listed in Box 421.2. Most frequently, acute urticaria is caused by a food or drug and usually dissipates within days to several weeks. As stated, the cause of chronic urticaria usually is not determined. The incidence of atopy in patients with chronic idiopathic urticaria does not appear to be higher than that found in the general population.

Drugs and Therapeutics

Drug reactions are one of the most common causes of urticaria and angioedema. The reactions are mediated by type I or type III immune mechanisms or by direct nonimmunologic mast-cell mediator release. Depending on the mechanisms involved, the urticaria may occur immediately or at days to weeks after drug exposure (e.g., serum sickness syndrome with urticaria). Many drugs are associated with urticaria. Antibiotics, especially penicillin and related compounds, remain the leading causes of drug-induced urticaria. Aspirin and other nonsteroidal antiinflammatory agents are common causes of urticaria. Some data indicate that aspirin and nonsteroidal antiinflammatory drugs may exacerbate chronic urticaria in selected patients. Some drugs, such as the opioids, can cause mast-cell degranulation directly. Other classes of drugs frequently associated with urticaria include diuretics, radiocontrast dyes, muscle relaxants, and sedatives or barbiturates. All drugs taken by affected patients must be identified, because any drug can be a potential cause of urticaria. Vitamins, lotions, contracep-

---

> **BOX 421.2**   **Major Causes of Acute Urticaria and Angioedema (less than 6 weeks)**
>
> **Drugs**
> Antibiotics (especially beta-lactams)
> NSAIDs
> Opiates
> Sedatives
> Contrast Dyes
>
> **Food**
> Peanuts
> Milk
> Soybeans
> Tree nuts
> Wheat
> Eggs
> Fish and shellfish
> Food additives
>
> **Physical Triggers**
> Dermatographism
> Cholinergic urticaria
> Exercise-induced
> Delayed pressure urticaria
> Solar urticaria
> Vibratory urticaria
> Aquagenic urticaria
>
> **Infections**
> Viral hepatitis
> Mononucleosis
> Coxsackievirus
> Mycoplasma
> Helminthic parasites
> Beta-hemolytic streptococcus
> Fungal infections
>
> **Insect Stings**
> Hymenoptera
> Fleas
> Mosquitoes
> Chiggers
> Lice
>
> **Contactants**
> Animal saliva
> Plants
> Latex

---

tives, laxatives, and various over-the-counter drugs represent possible offenders. When a drug reaction is suspected, all unnecessary drugs should be eliminated, and an attempt should be made to switch to alternative, chemically distinct forms of necessary drugs. Blood products may cause urticaria through complement-mediated effects.

Foods

Foods are a common cause of acute urticaria, but also may cause chronic urticaria in a small percentage of patients. Daily hives suggest foods eaten regularly, whereas sporadic, recurrent hives suggest foods eaten intermittently. The most common offenders include tree nuts, peanuts, milk, eggs, soybeans, wheat, and fish. Food dyes (tartrazine) and additives (benzoate derivatives, sulfates) also may cause urticaria infrequently. Patients with respiratory allergies to pollen may develop urticaria or angioedema after the ingestion of certain foods with "cross-reactive" antigens. Reported examples include ragweed and bananas and melons; birch and celery, nuts, and certain fruits; and grass and tomatoes.

Infection

Many types of infections have been associated with urticaria. Viral infections are common causes of acute urticaria in children and adolescents. Although undetected infections have been considered a cause of chronic urticaria, the incidence is probably low. The infections known to be associated most commonly with urticaria include upper respiratory tract infections, infectious hepatitis, infectious mononucleosis, coxsackievirus infection, mycoplasma infection, helminthic parasites, and acute beta-hemolytic streptococcal infection. The association of urticaria with *Candida* or tinea infections still is not clear, but a careful examination of hands and feet should be performed. If an infection is found, it should be treated. However, extensive evaluation or empiric antimicrobial therapy for undetected infection is not warranted.

Inhalants

Infrequently, inhalant allergens (including pollen, animal dander, and spores) are associated with urticaria. Generally, respiratory allergic symptoms to the inhalant occur concomitantly.

Insects

Children may experience a hive-like reaction to such biting insects as fleas, mosquitoes, chiggers, lice, and mites, which is termed *papular urticaria*. These lesions are characterized by pruritic, papular lesions usually found on exposed skin surfaces, especially the extremities or where clothing fits snugly. Acute systemic urticaria and angioedema also may follow stings or bites from *Hymenoptera* in allergic individuals.

Contactants

Hive-like reactions can occur in response to skin contact with an allergen or irritant substance. For example, patients allergic to cats or dogs may develop urticaria where they have been licked by such animals. Another example of allergen-induced contact urticaria is latex. Children with spina bifida and urogenital abnormalities often are sensitized to latex early in life. Exposure to latex and other allergens in sensitized individuals can result in asthma and a generalized allergic reaction (anaphylaxis), in addition to urticaria and angioedema.

Systemic Diseases

A number of systemic diseases are associated with urticaria and angioedema. If the urticarial lesions are accompanied by fever, arthralgia, or elevated sedimentation rate, cutaneous vasculitis in association with an underlying connective tissue disorder should be considered. Systemic lupus erythematosus, rheumatic fever, and rheumatoid arthritis may be accompanied by urticaria-like lesions. The rash associated with juvenile rheumatoid arthritis may appear before other signs of the disease. In patients with connective tissue disorders, a biopsy of lesions usually reveals vasculitis.

Urticaria has been observed also in adults and children with lymphoreticular malignancies and in adults with carcinoma of the lung, rectum, or colon. However, several studies rule out a higher incidence of malignancies in patients with chronic urticaria. Unless evidence suggests malignancy, an exhaustive search for cancer is not indicated.

Thyroid disease (especially Hashimoto thyroiditis) and both hyperthyroidism and hypothyroidism are associated with chronic urticaria. A higher incidence of antimicrosomal antibodies is seen in patients with chronic idiopathic urticaria. Often, patients with thyroid autoantibodies have worse urticaria.

Exacerbations of chronic urticaria and cyclic urticaria have been noted during menses, suggesting a relationship between hormone levels and urticaria.

CLINICAL MANIFESTATIONS AND COMPLICATIONS

Urticaria Pigmentosa and Systemic Mastocytosis

Typically, urticaria pigmentosa occurs during childhood and is characterized by persistent, pigmented, maculopapular lesions that urticate when stroked (Darier sign). A biopsy of these lesions reveals mast-cell infiltrations of the skin. Systemic mastocytosis is a generalized form of mast-cell infiltration, with involvement of the skin, bone marrow, long bones, liver, spleen, or lymph nodes.

Hereditary Disorders

Several rare, inherited disorders are associated with urticaria and angioedema. (Familial cold urticaria and hereditary vibratory angioedema are discussed later.) Familial urticaria has been seen in combination with amyloidosis, nerve deafness, and limb pain. This syndrome appears to be inherited as an autosomal dominant condition.

Hereditary angioedema (HAE) is an autosomal dominant disorder caused by the absence of functional C1 esterase inhibitor (see also Chapter 429, Complement Deficiencies). Clinically, HAE is characterized by recurrent episodes of angioedema (without urticaria) precipitated spontaneously and variably after trauma. Multiple parts of the body may be involved, including and especially the face, extremities, and gastrointestinal tract. Edema of the bowel wall may result in crampy abdominal pain, obstipation, vomiting, and abdominal rigidity. The most severe complication is laryngeal edema, which may result in asphyxiation and death. Most cases of HAE manifest in childhood but often worsen during adolescence. The severity and frequency of attacks vary greatly among patients. Only minor trauma is necessary to induce an attack, with common triggers including contact sports and dental work. Sometimes, an erythematous rash (erythema marginatum) may accompany attacks. The diagnosis of HAE is made by examining patients' history and by evaluating complement levels (low C4 [best screening test], C2, and antigenic or functional C1 esterase–inhibitor levels). Usually, patients with HAE respond to androgen therapy.

Physical Urticarias

The physical urticarias are a unique subgroup of chronic urticarias in which wheals can be induced reproducibly by a physical stimulus. Variously, cold, heat, pressure, vibration, light,

TABLE 421.1

PHYSICAL URTICARIAS

Type of Urticaria	Key Features	Diagnostic Test
Dermatographism	2%–5% of general population Linear, pruritic wheals "scratch" hives	Light stroking with narrow object (fingernail, tongue-blade) causes wheal and flare within 15 minutes
Cholinergic urticaria	5%–7% of all urticarias due to elevated core body temperature causing small, papular, pruritic wheals with large erythema	Challenge by exercise for 10 to 15 minutes (especially in warm environment) with resultant small punctuate wheals surrounded by prominent erythema
Exercise-induced anaphylaxis	Associated with exercise and sometimes prior food ingestion	Exercise challenge, but still may have negative test
Cold urticaria	Essential (acquired), 1%–3% of all urticarias can have swelling of lips and tongue after cold drink	Ice cube on forearm for 10 minutes causes wheal within 5 minutes after removal
Pressure urticaria	<1% of urticaria 3–12 hours after pressure with diffuse tender swelling and erythema	Application of 5–15 lbs of weight over the forearm or shoulder for 15 minutes with resultant swelling 1 to 4 hours later
Solar urticaria	<1% of urticaria with pruritic wheals or morbilliform erythema over exposed areas	Irradiation with solar simulator (290–690 nm) for up to 2 minutes
Vibratory urticaria	Rare, angioedema proportional to intensity and duration of stimulus	Vibration with laboratory vortex for 4 minutes on forearm with rapid swelling of arm
Aquagenic urticaria	Rare, typically over upper torso	Challenge with a compress of tap water for 30 minutes

water, exercise, and increases in core body temperature are provoking stimuli. Physical urticarias make up as much as 17% of chronic urticarias and occur most frequently in young adults. Moreover, chronic idiopathic urticaria can coexist with physical urticaria. The physical urticarias are distinguished by episodic lesions often limited to the areas of physical stimuli. In some patients, more than one type of physical urticaria may be present. The urticarial lesions likely are caused, in part, by mast-cell activation and mediator release. Mast-cell mediators, especially histamine, have been demonstrated in draining venous blood and in tissue fluids obtained from urticated areas in patients with various forms of physical urticarias. The mechanism by which a physical stimulus to the skin releases mast-cell mediators is not understood fully, but may involve neuropeptides. In some forms of physical urticaria, a passive transfer factor (usually IgE) in the serum has been reported. (Only the more common physical urticarias are discussed here and listed in Table 421.1).

Symptomatic Dermatographism

Between 2% and 5% of the general population may have dermatographism, but only a subgroup have symptomatic dermatographism. *Dermatographism* means "writing on the skin" and is manifest by transient wheal and erythematous responses occurring within minutes after stroking the skin with pressure greater than 36 g/mm². Often, patients have increased pruritus

that leads to scratching and subsequent hiving of the skin. A transferable factor (probably IgE) has been identified in some patients. Usually, the disease can be treated effectively with antihistamines.

Cholinergic Urticaria

Cholinergic urticaria is fairly common, and it occurs most frequently in teenagers and young adults. The skin lesions are often distinctive and appear as 2- to 4-mm pruritic wheals surrounded by extensive areas of macular erythema, occurring most prominently on the upper trunk and arms. Systemic manifestations, including confluent urticaria, angioedema, hypotension, wheezing, and gastrointestinal complaints, have been reported in patients with cholinergic urticaria after exercise. An elevation in core temperature, induced by either exercise or passive heating (e.g., hot bath) but not by endogenous pyrogen, has elicited symptoms in susceptible subjects. The cholinergic nervous system effector mechanisms involved in the compensatory responses in thermoregulation are postulated to lead ultimately to mast-cell degranulation. Sometimes, attacks can be aborted by prompt cooling of affected patients (e.g., by cold bath). Some patients have a refractory period after a severe attack. This effect can be used to develop a program to induce tolerance by subjecting such patients to carefully graded increasing stimuli.

Exercise-Induced Anaphylactic Syndrome

Exercise-induced anaphylactic syndrome (EIA) is manifested clinically by urticaria and the signs and symptoms of a classic anaphylactic reaction, especially hypotension. The disease appears to be more common among young adults. Some reports have cited a family tendency in some subjects. Some subjects have symptoms only if exercise occurs postprandially. Celery, wheat, and shellfish are the foods implicated most commonly as precipitants, but any food may be associated with attacks. Subjects with postprandial EIA may avoid attacks by not eating for 4 to 6 hours before exercise. EIA and cholinergic urticaria can be clinically similar in their presentation, and both diseases may occur after exercise. However, passive heat challenges are positive only in those subjects with cholinergic urticaria. A single negative exercise challenge does not rule out the diagnosis of EIA, because exercise does not always reproduce symptom development in these subjects.

Cold Urticaria

Familial cold urticarias are autosomal dominant disorders characterized by burning erythematous papules with inflammatory cell infiltrates occurring after cold exposure. Two forms of familial cold urticaria are identified: an immediate form with onset of symptoms at 30 minutes to 3 hours and a rare, delayed form with onset of symptoms at 9 to 18 hours. The immediate familial form may be accompanied by a flu-like syndrome.

Essential (acquired) cold urticarias are more common than are the familial forms. Essential cold urticaria appears within minutes of cold contact and rewarming and is manifested by pruritic wheals. In the essential form, syncope and anaphylaxis may occur after intensive cold exposure. Indeed, swimming has resulted in massive mediator release and drowning. Provocative testing for the familial forms involves cold-air exposure. The essential forms (but not the familial forms) may be elicited by placing a plastic-wrapped ice cube on the skin. Occasionally, connective tissue disorders, malignancies, syphilis, and other diseases associated with abnormal immunoglobulins with cold-dependent properties are associated with acquired cold urticaria. Cold-dependent dermatographism leads to hive formation if the skin is scratched and then chilled.

Delayed Pressure Urticaria-Angioedema

Delayed pressure urticaria-angioedema is manifested by deep, tender swelling with or without urticaria. The lesions are localized and occur 3 to 12 hours after exposure to sustained pressure. Flu-like symptoms may accompany these lesions. Common precipitating events include walking (foot swelling), clapping (hand swelling), sitting (buttock swelling), and swelling under belts or tight articles of clothing. This disease may respond to nonsteroidal antiinflammatory drugs.

Solar Urticaria

Solar urticaria can occur at all ages, but is more common in the fourth and fifth decades. The disease is characterized by pruritic wheals or morbilliform erythema occurring within minutes on sun-exposed areas. Anaphylactic symptoms may occur when large body areas are exposed. If patients react only to the 400- to 500-nm wavelength, erythropoietic protoporphyria should be excluded. Therapy for solar urticaria includes antihistamines and avoidance of sunlight, wearing protective garments, and using topical agents to block or reflect light.

Vibratory Angioedema

Vibratory angioedema is characterized by the rapid onset of localized angioedema proportional to the intensity and duration of the vibratory stimulus and body surface area involved. Common precipitators include vigorous toweling, lawn mowing, and motorcycling. A familial autosomal dominant form of this disease exists. Delayed pressure urticaria-angioedema and dermatographism should be excluded with appropriate tests.

DIAGNOSIS

As with most diseases, the history and physical examination are key to the evaluation of patients with urticaria and angioedema. A detailed history of drug and new food exposure is essential. Drugs that have been taken for several months or drugs that have just been added can cause urticaria. A diary containing information about urticarial outbreaks in relation to time of day, food ingestion, activity, and exposure to possible precipitants can be helpful. A thorough physical examination should be performed. Signs and symptoms of systemic diseases and infections should be followed up with appropriate diagnostic tests. Provocative testing should be performed on patients thought to have a physical urticaria (Box 421.3).

Because chronic urticaria in children usually is a benign disorder, and most diagnostic tests are negative, extensive testing is indicated only when a systemic disease is suspected. Generally, skin testing is not indicated for chronic urticaria and should be reserved for patients with histories suggesting an allergen-induced disorder. If the cause is not obvious, recommended investigation includes urinalysis, complete blood cell count, differential white blood cell count, and erythrocyte sedimentation rate. Thyroid functions and thyroid autoantibodies should be checked in patients with chronic urticaria. Stool screens for ova and parasites, complement assays, antinuclear antibody levels, hepatitis B and C screen, and immunoglobulin levels are not obtained routinely unless a specific diagnosis is suspected (Box 421.4).

| BOX 421.3 | Work-Up for Urticaria and Angioedema |

Generally, for acute urticaria, no work-up is needed if cause identified

- Consider skin test or blood RAST for confirmatory testing of allergen-induced causes
- Can perform provocative testing for physical urticaria

Chronic urticaria

- CBC with manual differential
- Urinalysis
- Liver function tests
- Sedimentation rate
- Consider thyroid function tests including antithyroglobulin antibody and antimicrosomal antibody
- Consider antinuclear antibody
- Angioedema alone, C4 levels initially
- Skin biopsy if suspect urticarial vasculitis or refractory to treatment
- Skin testing to autologous serum

BOX 421.4   **Management of Chronic Urticaria or Angioedema**

Avoidance or treatment of underlying cause
Avoidance of potentiating factors (e.g., alcohol)
Epinephrine (for acute relief)
H_1 antihistamines
    Classic (e.g., hydroxyzine)
    Second-generation (preferred)
    Tricyclic antidepressants
Combinations of H_1 antihistamines
Combinations of H_1 and H_2 antihistamines
For recalcitrant symptoms consider:
    Addition of leukotriene antagonists
    Addition of sympathomimetics (e.g., terbutaline)
    Corticosteroids (rarely)
    Immunomodulators (experimentally)

Generally, skin biopsy tests are not helpful. However, skin biopsy tests should be performed when individual urticarial lesions persist for more than 24 to 48 hours or when the lesions suggest cutaneous vasculitis or urticaria pigmentosa. Biopsy tests may be helpful if the lesions are purpuric or present in postinflammatory hyperpigmented areas. Another indication is refractoriness to therapy.

THERAPY

The general principles of treatment of urticaria or angioedema are outlined in Box 421.4. When a causative agent is identified, the treatment of choice (if feasible) is avoidance. Generally, this rule applies when a specific allergen is identified or when the patient has a physical urticaria. If an associated systemic disease is found, treatment of the underlying condition is necessary. Patients should be advised also to avoid such potentiating factors as alcohol, opioids, angiotensin-converting enzyme inhibitors, aspirin and nonsteroidal antiinflammatory drugs, tight fitting clothes, and heat. Induction of tolerance may be attempted for some forms of physical urticaria (cholinergic, solar, cold, and localized heat urticaria and vibratory angioedema). Immunotherapy (allergy shots) is not indicated for urticaria without accompanying respiratory symptoms.

Drug therapy to relieve symptoms should be instituted while the cause is investigated. Therapy should be aimed at relieving most symptoms while keeping drug side effects to a minimum. The patient may have some lesions despite therapy. To minimize side effects, additional drug therapy is not indicated when remaining lesions are not physically or emotionally disturbing to the patient.

In acute severe urticaria or angioedema, intramuscular epinephrine is the drug of choice (0.01 mL of 1:1,000 epinephrine per kilogram of body weight, up to 0.3 mL). Oral antihistamines of the H_1 class are used in conjunction with epinephrine.

Antihistamines used on a daily basis remain the treatment of choice for recurrent or chronic urticaria. Specific dosage recommendations are somewhat arbitrary. Therapy should begin with low doses and should be titrated upward to relieve symptoms without causing significant adverse side effects. Performance in the classroom, learning, driving, and general awareness and work skills have been shown to be impaired by the sedating, first-generation antihistamines even at levels that do not lead to recognized drowsiness. In addition, second-generation antihistamines were superior to first-generation antihistamines in obtaining maximum skin and plasma levels, and in suppressing histamine-induced skin wheal and flare responses. Thus, although they may be more expensive, second-generation antihistamines with less or no sedation should be used, especially for patients requiring prolonged treatment. Currently, desloratadine (6 months and older), fexofenadine (6 years and older), loratadine (2 years and older), and cetirizine (6 months and older) are approved for pediatric use. If symptoms continue, the addition of a second, chemically distinct class of H_1 antihistamines or the concomitant use of an H_2 antihistamine may be beneficial. Tricyclic antidepressants, such as doxepin and amitriptyline, are potent antihistamines and are effective antiurticarial agents, but these agents have many side effects. Sympathomimetics also may be useful adjuncts to H_1 antihistamine therapy. Recently, leukotriene antagonists have demonstrated marginal effectiveness in treating urticaria.

For severe urticaria-angioedema unresponsive to these measures and disabling to the patient, corticosteroids may be tried. A short "burst" of corticosteroids (e.g., 0.5 mg/kg/day for 5 days) usually relieves symptoms. Rarely, patients require low daily or alternate-day corticosteroids for a longer time. Prolonged treatment using large doses of corticosteroids should be avoided because of the potential side effects. Antihistamines should not be discontinued during corticosteroid treatment. Newer drugs capable of antagonizing mediators other than histamine (e.g., leukotriene antagonists) or inhibiting mast-cell degranulation may prove effective as adjuncts to traditional antihistamines and corticosteroids. In patients who have a neutrophil-predominant urticaria by biopsy, therapy using dapsone or colchicine (in adults) can be considered. In the severely affected patient with autoimmune chronic urticaria, cyclosporine has been shown to be effective, but potential side effects must be monitored.

Suggested Readings

Casale TB, Keahey TM, Kaliner M. Exercise-induced anaphylactic syndromes. *JAMA* 1986;255:2049.

Casale TB, Sampson HA, Hanifin J, et al. Guide to physical urticarias. *J Allergy Clin Immunol* 1988;82:758.

Champion RH, Roberts SDB, Carpenter RG, et al. Urticaria and angioedema: a review of 554 patients. *Br J Dermatol* 1969;81:588.

Charlesworth EN. Urticaria and angioedema: a clinical spectrum. *Ann Allergy Asthma Immunol* 1996;76:484.

Kaplan AP. Chronic urticaria and angioedema. *N Engl J Med* 2002;346:175.

Kaplan AP. Urticaria and angioedema. In: Kaplan AP, ed. *Allergy*, 2nd ed. Philadelphia: Saunders, 1997:573.

Kobza-Black A. The physical urticarias. In: Champion RH, Greaves MW, Kobza-Black A, Pye RJ, eds. *The urticarias*. Edinburgh: Churchill Livingstone, 1985:168.

Paul E, Greilich KD, Dominante G. Epidemiology of urticaria. *Monogr Allergy* 1987;21:87.

Sabroe RA, Greaves MW. The pathogenesis of chronic idiopathic urticaria. *Arch Dermatol* 1997;133:1003.

Tharp MD. Chronic urticaria: pathophysiology and treatment approaches. *J Allergy Clin Immunol* 1996;98:S325.

Twarog FJ. Urticaria in childhood: pathogenesis and management. *Pediatr Clin North Am* 1983;30:887.

Wanderer AA, Berstein IL, Goodman DL, et al., eds. The diagnosis and management of urticaria: a practice parameter. *Ann Allergy Asthma Immunol* 2000;85:521.

CHAPTER 422 ■ FOOD ALLERGIES

HUGH A. SAMPSON

Adverse food reactions may be divided into *toxic* and *nontoxic reactions*. Toxic reactions may occur in anyone, provided a sufficient dose is ingested (e.g., histamine in scombroid fish poisoning, toxins secreted by *Salmonella*, *Shigella*, and *Campylobacter*). Nontoxic reactions depend on individual susceptibilities and may be the result of immune mechanisms (*allergy* or *hypersensitivity*) or nonimmune mechanisms (*intolerances*). Food intolerance makes up the majority of adverse food reactions and may be secondary to pharmacologic substances found in some foods, chemical or microbial contaminants, or metabolic disorders of the host (e.g., lactose intolerance). Although IgE-mediated mechanisms are the most well-characterized forms of hypersensitivity response, other less well-defined immunologic mechanisms are responsible for such disorders as food-induced enterocolitis syndrome, benign eosinophilic proctocolitis, allergic eosinophilic esophagitis and gastroenteritis, and celiac disease.

EPIDEMIOLOGY

Frequently, the term *food allergy* is used to denote any adverse food reaction, a misnomer that leads to considerable confusion in this field. In addition, the perceived prevalence of food allergy is far greater than actual prevalence. Household surveys indicate that one-third of American families alter their eating patterns in the belief that at least one family member suffers from a food allergy. In Bock's survey of a general pediatric practice involving 480 babies followed from birth until their third birthday, 28% of the infants were reported to have experienced adverse food reactions. However, symptoms were confirmed by oral food challenge in only 6% to 8% of infants. In four prospective studies from four different countries using appropriately performed milk challenges, 2.2% to 2.5% of infants were found to have cow's milk allergy in the first 1 to 2 years of life. Follow-up studies indicated that approximately 80% of these milk-allergic infants lost their reactivity to cow's milk by their fourth to fifth birthday. Similarly, about 1.3% of young children develop egg allergy and 0.8% develop peanut allergy. While approximately 80% of egg-allergic children lose their reactivity to egg by their fifth or sixth birthday, only about 15% to 20% of peanut allergic children "outgrow" their allergy. Adverse reactions to food additives also have been demonstrated in children, although these reactions are fairly rare. Children with atopic disorders tend to have a higher prevalence of food allergy. In a study of children who were referred to a dermatology clinic because of moderate to severe atopic dermatitis, approximately 40% were found to have skin symptoms provoked by food hypersensitivity; the more severe the atopic eczema, the more likely they were to have food allergy. Studies of asthmatic children attending general pulmonary clinics suggest that 8% to 10% of such patients have food-induced wheezing, and surveys of emergency department visits for anaphylaxis indicate that food allergy is the single leading cause of anaphylaxis outside of the hospital in the United States.

PATHOGENESIS

The pathogenesis of food allergy involves three main factors: the food (or allergen), the gastrointestinal barrier and its handling of food, and the affected individuals' genetic predisposition to developing an allergic response. Despite the existence of a widely varied diet, relatively few foods account for the majority of allergic responses. In children, egg, peanut, milk, soy, wheat, and fish account for 85% to 90% of reactions. The allergenic fractions of these foods have several features in common: They are glycoproteins of approximately 10,000 to 60,000 daltons, they are largely heat- and acid-stable, and they are water-soluble.

The gastrointestinal tract uses both nonimmunologic and immunologic mechanisms to prevent intact foreign antigens from gaining access to the body while processing ingested food into forms that can be absorbed and used for energy and cell growth. IgA secreted into the gastrointestinal tract lumen binds foreign antigens, such as food, and impedes their absorption. IgA food antigen complexes become "hung up" in the glycocalyx, where enzymes in the mucosal cell brush border can break down these complex proteins. Food antigen–specific IgA and IgG in the blood may be involved in clearing antigens that enter the circulation. Although more than 98% of ingested protein is blocked by the gastrointestinal barrier, minute amounts of intact food antigens are absorbed and gain access to immune reactive cells. Such factors as decreased stomach acidity (as with antacids) or the ingestion of alcohol or aspirin increases antigen absorption. However, antigenically intact food proteins entering the circulation normally do not cause allergic reactions, because most individuals develop "tolerance" to ingested food antigens.

Oral tolerance in humans has been studied to a very limited extent. Husby demonstrated that feeding keyhole limpet hemocyanin to normal human volunteers resulted in systemic T-cell tolerance but led to B-cell priming, with detection of keyhole limpet hemocyanin antibodies in serum and saliva. The extent of T-cell tolerance depended on the antigen, dosage, and immunization schedule used. The suppression of systemic immunity to foods after oral ingestion does not have a major suppressive effect on human B cells, because antibody production against food proteins is a universal phenomenon in both infants and adults and generally is not associated with hypersensitivity. Most low-level antibodies to foods in clinically tolerant individuals are of the IgG class, with high levels of IgE or IgA antibodies more likely to be an indicator of a pathologic process (e.g., cow's-milk allergy or celiac disease, respectively).

The increased susceptibility of young infants to food-allergic reactions appears to be the result of immunologic immaturity and, to some extent, immaturity of the gastrointestinal tract. Newborns lack IgA and IgM in exocrine secretions, and salivary secretory IgA (sIgA) is absent at birth and remains low during the early months of life. The relatively low concentration of sIgA in the intestine of young infants, together with the relatively immense quantities of ingested proteins, contributes to the large amount of food antigens confronting gut-associated lymphoid tissue. In genetically predisposed infants, these antigens may fail to appropriately activate regulatory T cells and may stimulate an excessive production of IgE antibodies or other abnormal immune responses.

Several prospective studies have indicated that exclusive breast-feeding may promote the development of oral tolerance and may prevent some food allergy, atopic dermatitis, and asthma. The protective effect of breast-feeding may be due to several factors: decreased exposure to foreign proteins, breast-milk sIgA that provides passive protection against foreign proteins and pathogens, and soluble factors, such as cytokines, in breast milk that may induce the earlier maturation of the gastrointestinal tract barrier and the infant's immune response. Resistance of sIgA to proteolytic digestion and decreased proteolytic activity in the infant gastrointestinal tract allows sIgA antibodies to reach sites in the infant's intestine where foreign antigens and microorganisms may be encountered. In addition to the passive protection provided by sIgA, soluble factors in human milk may stimulate lymphocytes to mature and to produce IgA. The antibacterial activity of human milk is well established, but the ability of breast-milk sIgA to prevent food antigen penetration is less clear.

CLINICAL MANIFESTATIONS AND COMPLICATIONS

A variety of food-allergic reactions have been confirmed by controlled trials. These are listed in Box 422.1.

BOX 422.1	**Symptoms Substantiated by Controlled Food Challenges**

Generalized Anaphylaxis with Cardiovascular Collapse (sometimes exercise-associated)

Respiratory Symptoms
Upper airway (rhinoconjunctivitis, laryngeal edema)
Lower airway (wheezing, asthma)

Cutaneous
Urticaria-angioedema
Atopic dermatitis
Exercise-associated urticaria
Dermatitis herpetiformis

Gastrointestinal Symptoms
IgE-mediated (lip swelling, palatal itching, tongue swelling, nausea, abdominal pain, cramps, emesis, diarrhea)
Celiac disease and dermatitis herpetiformis
Protein-induced enterocolitis (vomiting, diarrhea, rarely shock)
Protein gastroenteropathy, especially to soy and milk (diarrhea, gross or occult blood loss, malabsorption, failure to thrive)
Protein-induced colitis (diarrhea, gross blood loss)
Heiner syndrome (pulmonary infiltrates, iron-deficiency anemia, emesis, diarrhea, and failure to thrive)
Colic (cow's milk-induced, allergen in breast milk)
Allergic eosinophilic gastroenteritis

Neurologic Symptoms
Migraine

Gastrointestinal Food Hypersensitivity

A number of gastrointestinal syndromes are associated with both IgE-mediated and non–IgE-mediated food allergies.

Oral Allergy Syndrome

Pruritus and edema of the lips, tongue, palate, and throat may be the first symptoms of a generalized food-allergic reaction or may be the sole manifestations of ingesting a food allergen. The oral allergy syndrome occurs in patients with allergic pollenosis and is associated with the ingestion of various fresh fruits and raw vegetables. Symptoms are due to "conserved homologous proteins" in plant pollens and certain fruits and vegetables and are isolated to a contact reaction in the oropharynx. Oral symptoms developing during the ingestion of raw potatoes, carrots, celery, apples, and hazelnuts are associated with birch pollen allergy; and symptoms secondary to bananas and melons (e.g., watermelon, cantaloupe, honeydew) are associated with ragweed sensitivity. In addition, many children will experience symptoms when ingesting raw, pitted fruit (e.g., cherries, peaches, plums). No symptoms occur when such fruits and vegetables have been cooked, because these conserved proteins are not heat-stable.

Gastrointestinal Anaphylaxis

Nausea, abdominal pain, cramps, vomiting, and (less frequently) diarrhea develop within minutes to 2 hours of ingesting a food allergen in IgE-mediated gastrointestinal allergy. However, repeated ingestion of a food allergen in allergic infants may result in the partial desensitization of gastrointestinal mast cells and subclinical symptoms, such as poor appetite, periodic abdominal pain, and poor weight gain. Malabsorption has been demonstrated using various absorption markers (e.g., lactulose, rhamnose, mannitol, polyethylene glycol). Improved appetite and catch-up weight gain may follow the elimination of the responsible food allergen.

Eosinophilic Esophagitis and Gastroenteritis

Non–IgE-mediated food hypersensitivity appears to be responsible for symptoms in most patients with allergic eosinophilic esophagitis and gastroenteritis but, in a subset, IgE-mediated food allergy is responsible for symptoms. Typically, patients present with postprandial nausea and vomiting (or "spitting up"), gastroesophageal reflux, abdominal pain, diarrhea, and weight loss (in older children) or failure to thrive (in infants). Approximately one-half of patients will have peripheral blood eosinophilia and, less commonly, iron-deficiency anemia and hypoalbuminemia. Generally, patients with IgE-mediated food-induced symptoms have other atopic symptoms, elevated serum IgE levels, and positive skin-prick tests to a variety of foods and inhalants. In one study, approximately 40% of referred infants younger than 1 year of age experiencing gastroesophageal reflux were found to have milk-induced allergic eosinophilic esophagitis and reflux. The elimination of cow's-milk formula led to a resolution of symptoms, with normalization of biopsy findings. Blinded challenge with cow's milk provoked symptoms and abnormal biopsy findings. In rare infants, generalized edema develops secondary to marked protein-losing enteropathy and hypoalbuminemia, often in the presence of minimal gastrointestinal symptoms. Rarely, allergic eosinophilic gastroenteritis presents in infants as pyloric stenosis with outlet obstruction. Elimination of the responsible food allergen from the diet for 6 to 8 weeks may be necessary to bring about a resolution of symptoms and a normalization of intestinal histology.

Food-Induced Proctocolitis

Unlike the other eosinophilic gastroenteropathies, food-induced proctocolitis presents in the first few months of life and is generally secondary to cow's-milk or soy-protein hypersensitivity. The majority of affected infants presenting with this disorder are breast-fed and reacting to antigens passed in maternal breast milk. Typically, such infants appear healthy, and their disorder is discovered because of the presence of gross or occult blood in their stool. Mucosal lesions are confined to the distal large bowel. Sigmoidoscopic findings are variable but range from areas of patchy mucosal injection to severe friability, with small aphthoid ulcerations and bleeding. Biopsies reveal mucosal edema and a prominent eosinophilic infiltrate in the surface and crypt epithelium and lamina propria. Generally, gross hematochezia resolves within 72 hours of appropriate food-allergen elimination (or, in the case of a breast-fed infant, elimination of the food allergen from the mother's diet), but resolution of the mucosal lesions may take several weeks. Reintroduction of the responsible food leads to resumption of symptoms within several hours to days. Often, food-induced proctocolitis resolves after 6 months to 2 years of allergen avoidance.

Food-Induced Enterocolitis Syndrome

Young infants who are between ages 1 week and 3 months and have food hypersensitivity may present with protracted vomiting and diarrhea, resulting frequently in dehydration. Most often, cow's milk or soy proteins are responsible, but rice- and cereal grain–induced enterocolitis are being reported more frequently. Some infants appear to be sensitized by exposure to food proteins passed in maternal breast milk, but do not react until ingesting the actual food. Generally, the stools of affected infants contain occult blood, eosinophils, and polymorphonuclear neutrophils. IgE food-specific antibodies are absent. Jejunal biopsies reveal flattened villi, edema, and increased numbers of lymphocytes, eosinophils, and mast cells. Generally, the elimination of the responsible food leads to a resolution of symptoms within 72 hours. The diagnosis is established by oral food challenge, which consists of administering up to 0.3 to 0.6 g/kg body weight of the suspected protein allergen. A positive challenge results in vomiting and diarrhea within 1 to 6 hours, and occasionally it may be accompanied by shock. Monitoring the peripheral blood cell count reveals a rise in the absolute neutrophil count (greater than 3,500 cells per cubic millimeter) 4 to 6 hours after symptoms develop. Neutrophils, eosinophils, and occasionally red blood cells may be found in the stools. Once their disorder is diagnosed, children with cow's-milk sensitivity should be placed on a hypoallergenic formula (Alimentum, Nutramigen, or Pregestimil) until approximately 9 to 12 months of age, because as many as 50% may develop a similar sensitivity to soy if placed on a soy-based formula. Exposure to other foods probably should be limited until after 6 months of age. The majority of these children appear to outgrow their hypersensitivity in 1 to 3 years.

Food-Induced Enteropathy (Malabsorption) Syndromes

In the absence of celiac disease, diarrhea (frequently steatorrhea) and poor weight gain in the first few months of life may be secondary to a variety of food proteins, including those in cow's milk, soy, wheat and other cereal grains, and egg. Symptoms include protracted diarrhea, vomiting, and failure to thrive. Frequently, increased fecal fat and secondary carbohydrate malabsorption are present. Cow's-milk sensitivity appears to be the most frequent cause of this syndrome. Eliminating the responsible food from the diet brings about resolution of symptoms, but this process may require several days to weeks. A patchy villous atrophy similar to celiac disease, but generally less se-

vere, is seen on endoscopy, and biopsy reveals a prominent mononuclear round cell infiltrate of the epithelium and lamina propria, with a small number of eosinophils. Complete resolution of the intestinal lesions may require 6 to 18 months of food allergen avoidance. The natural history of this disorder has not been well studied.

Celiac disease is a more extensive enteropathy leading to malabsorption. Total villous atrophy and extensive cellular infiltrate are associated with sensitivity to gliadin, a component of gluten found in wheat, rye, and barley. Often, patients present with diarrhea or frank steatorrhea, abdominal distention and flatulence, weight loss, and (rarely) nausea and vomiting. Oral ulcers and other extraintestinal symptoms secondary to malabsorption are common. Quantitation of IgA antigliadin and IgA anti-tissue transglutaminase (anti-tTG) antibodies are useful screening tests for celiac disease. Surveys utilizing serologic screening for celiac disease have demonstrated a much higher prevalence than previously believed (1 in 300 to 400 patients) and revealed many minimal or "silent" cases. The gold standard of diagnosis remains the demonstration of biopsy evidence of villous atrophy and inflammatory infiltrate while the patient is ingesting gluten, resolution of biopsy findings after 6 to 12 weeks of gluten elimination, and recurrence of biopsy changes after reinstitution of gluten. Although some patients tolerate small amounts of gluten as they get older, a life-long elimination of gluten-containing foods is necessary to avoid an increased risk of gastrointestinal malignancy and lymphoma.

Infantile Colic

Double-blind crossover trials implicate food hypersensitivity as a pathogenic factor in approximately 15% of colicky infants. However, most infants "outgrow" their sensitivity within 1 to 2 years.

Respiratory Reactions

Both upper and lower respiratory reactions have been provoked during double-blind placebo-controlled oral food challenges (DBPCFC). Within minutes to 2 hours of ingestion, food allergens may induce the typical signs and symptoms of rhinoconjunctivitis, although isolated upper airway symptoms are uncommon. These symptoms include tearing and periocular pruritus and erythema, nasal congestion, pruritus, sneezing, and rhinorrhea. Nasal lavage fluid histamine levels rise significantly with the onset of nasal symptoms during DBPCFCs, indicating a pathogenic role for nasal mast-cell activation. Similarly, pulmonary function studies during DBPCFCs demonstrate significant drops in forced ventilatory capacity (FVC), forced expiratory volume over 1 second (FEV$_1$), and maximal midexpiratory flow (MMEF) in some patients experiencing a positive food challenge. More recent studies have demonstrated significant increases in airway hyperreactivity after positive food challenges, indicating a pathogenic role for food allergy in some patients with persistent asthma.

The consumption of food allergens rarely is the main aggravating factor in chronic rhinoconjunctivitis and asthma. Two large series of asthmatic patients followed in pulmonary clinics were evaluated for food allergy. In one survey of 140 children with asthma, eight patients (6%) had wheezing induced by oral food challenge. In most cases, asthmatic children with food-induced wheezing either had atopic dermatitis or a history of eczema.

Food-induced pulmonary hemosiderosis is a syndrome of chronic or recurrent pulmonary disease (with hemosiderosis), chronic rhinitis, gastrointestinal blood loss, and iron-deficiency anemia and failure to thrive secondary to milk ingestion. The pathogenic mechanism(s) responsible for this disorder, which was described initially by Heiner, remain unknown. Other foods rarely have been implicated.

Cutaneous Reactions

The skin is the most common target organ in IgE-mediated food hypersensitivity. The ingestion of food allergens may provoke a rapid onset of cutaneous symptoms or aggravate more chronic conditions.

Urticaria-Angioedema

Acute urticaria and angioedema are among the most common symptoms of food-allergic reactions. The exact prevalence of these reactions is unknown. In most cases, patients do not seek medical assistance (or even report the reaction) because the onset of hives or swelling occurs within minutes of ingesting the responsible food allergen, rendering the cause-and-effect nature of the reaction obvious to the patient. The foods incriminated most commonly include eggs, milk, peanuts, and nuts in children, and fish, shellfish, nuts, and peanuts in adults. Occasionally, food hypersensitivity is incriminated in chronic urticaria and angioedema (symptoms lasting longer than 6 weeks). In one series of 163 children with chronic or recurrent urticaria, food allergy was implicated in only 10% of patients.

Atopic Dermatitis

The pathogenic role of food allergy in atopic dermatitis has been debated since the turn of the twentieth century. In one study of children referred to a pediatric dermatology clinic for the evaluation of moderate to severe atopic dermatitis, IgE-mediated food allergy was found in approximately 40% of the children. In a more general population of patients seen by dermatologists and allergists, food hypersensitivity probably plays an etiologic role in approximately 25% of patients, with the incidence of food allergy being higher in younger patients with more severe atopic dermatitis. As in the gastrointestinal tract, the repeated ingestion of food allergens leads to a partial desensitization of skin mast cells, and a single ingestion of food allergen may not provoke obvious cutaneous symptoms. Repeated ingestion of food allergen leads to chronic inflammation and the typical eczematous lesions (see Chapter 423, Atopic Dermatitis).

Dermatitis herpetiformis is an erythematous, papulovesicular eruption sometimes mistaken for atopic dermatitis; it is associated with gluten-sensitive enteropathy in some patients. Unlike atopic dermatitis, the distribution of skin lesions is typically on extensor surfaces.

Generalized Anaphylactic Reaction

Systemic anaphylaxis is an acute, occasionally fatal, IgE-mediated reaction involving many organ systems. Systemic symptoms may include tongue swelling and itching, palatal itching, throat itching and tightness, nausea, abdominal pain, emesis, diarrhea, dyspnea, wheezing, cyanosis, chest pain, urticaria, angioedema, hypotension, and shock. Food-induced anaphylaxis is the leading single cause of anaphylaxis treated in U.S. emergency departments, twice as common as anaphylaxis due to bee stings. Peanuts, tree nuts, and seafood are responsible most often for severe, life-threatening reactions. In addition to the direct induction of anaphylaxis, food ingestion is implicated as a cofactor in some cases of exercise-induced anaphylaxis.

A variety of symptoms are attributed to "food allergy," but the connection has not been substantiated in controlled trials. Such symptoms include various behavioral disturbances,

learning disorders, fatigue, sleep disorders, enuresis, arthralgia-arthritis, and myalgia. The Feingold Diet has been promoted by its supporters for children with hyperactivity and learning disorders, but several well-done controlled trials have failed to verify any consistent therapeutic effect from the diet.

DIAGNOSIS

Symptoms that are secondary to food hypersensitivity and have been confirmed by appropriate controlled studies are listed in Box 422.1. Other symptoms often attributed to food allergy have not been substantiated in controlled trials. Some of these symptoms may be due to the pharmacologic properties of certain foods, such as sleep disturbances in children who drink caffeinated beverages. The differential diagnosis of food sensitivity is broad (Box 422.2), but a careful history often suggests the appropriate diagnostic category to pursue.

Although history can be verified in only 30% to 40% of cases, it remains the foundation of the evaluation. History should reveal types of symptoms, when symptoms occurred after ingestion, severity of symptoms, whether symptoms occurred more than once, and whether cofactors (e.g., exercise) are necessary to elicit symptoms. In general, symptoms occurring soon after ingestion are more likely to be due to food hypersensitivity than are those that take hours or days to develop. Physical examination may exclude some disorders in the differential diagnosis, but nothing in the physical examination is unique for individuals with food hypersensitivity.

Various diagnostic studies (e.g., radiographic studies, breath hydrogen, biopsy studies) exclude many anatomic and metabolic abnormalities. Such laboratory studies as skin-prick tests and tests for IgE-specific food antibodies (e.g., radioallergosorbent test [RAST], fluorescein allergosorbent test [FAST]) are of some value in discriminating among the foods responsible for immediate, IgE-mediated hypersensitivity reactions. Measuring the quantity of food-specific IgE antibody levels is more diagnostic than are skin tests or standard radioallergosorbent tests (Table 422.1). No evidence supports the use of

---

| BOX 422.2 | Differential Diagnosis of Adverse Food Reactions |

Gastrointestinal Disorders
Structural abnormalities (pyloric stenosis, hiatal hernia, tracheoesophageal fistula)
Enzyme deficiencies: primary versus secondary (lactase deficiency, sucrase deficiency, etc.)
Malignancy (lymphoma)
Other (cystic fibrosis, gallbladder disease)

Pharmacologic Agents
Caffeine (coffee, tea, soft drinks, cocoa)
Theobromine (chocolate, tea)
Tyramine (cheese, banana, tomato)
Tryptamine (tomato, blue plum)
Histamine (fish, beer, wine)
Phenylethylamine (chocolate)

Contaminants and Additives
Flavorings and preservatives
Dyes
Toxins (bacterial, seafood-associated)
Infectious organisms

Psychological Reactions

TABLE 422.1

FOOD-SPECIFIC IGE LEVELS MORE THAN 95% PREDICTIVE OF CLINICAL REACTIVITY

Allergen	Decision Point [kU$_A$/L]	PPV	NPV
Egg	7	98	38
Infants ≤2 years*	2	95	
Milk	15	95	53
Infants ≤2 years†	5	95	
Peanut	14	100	36
Fish	20	100	89
Soybean	30	73	82
Wheat	26	74	87
Tree nuts‡	15	95	

Decision Point, food-specific IgE level above which it is more than 95% likely that a child would experience an allergic reaction. PPV, positive predictive value; NPV, negative predictive value.
*Boyano MT, et al. *Clin Exp Allergy* 2001;31:1464.
†Garcia-Ara C, et al. *J Allergy Clin Immunol* 2001;107:185.
‡Clark AT, Ewan P. *Clin Exp Allergy* 2003;33:1019.
Adapted with permission from Sampson HA. Food allergy. *J Allergy Clin Immunol* 2003;111:540.

IgG-specific food antibodies or food antigen–antibody complexes in the diagnosis of food sensitivity.

Generally, to establish whether a patient has food hypersensitivity, a provocative oral food challenge is necessary. Food challenges may be performed openly, when both the patient and the physician know the contents of the challenge; may be single-blind, when only the physician is aware of the contents of the challenge; or may be double-blind, when neither the patient nor the physician knows the contents of the challenge. Placebo controls are necessary in the blinded challenges if they are to be truly blind. Only the double-blind procedure is free of psychological factors and inherent bias on the part of the patient and the physician. Several studies comparing the results of single-blind and double-blind challenges in the same patient population have demonstrated the necessity of removing observer bias.

For research purposes, the DBPCFC should be the gold standard for diagnosing food allergy. In some cases, such as celiac disease, open challenge followed by intestinal biopsy is the diagnostic approach of choice. Although the DBPCFC provides a scientifically acceptable means of diagnosing food hypersensitivity, often it is not practical in the office practice setting. Box 422.3 outlines an approach that should be more useful to the pediatrician in the office setting. The initial evaluation consists of a careful history and physical examination, and laboratory studies suggested by the history or physical. If immediate hypersensitivity is suspected, the results of skin-prick testing or testing of food-specific IgE antibody levels to a battery of six to eight foods (egg, milk, peanuts, fish, shellfish, nuts, soy, and wheat) or other foods suggested by history could be helpful. Negative skin-prick tests (i.e., a wheal diameter less than 3 mm larger than the negative control wheal) render immediate hypersensitivity extremely unlikely and preclude the need for further evaluation, unless the history highly suggests otherwise. Such skin testing is valuable only when an IgE-mediated mechanism is suspected.

Foods suspected by history should be eliminated from affected patients' diets for 2 weeks when IgE-mediated hypersensitivity is suspected (urticaria, atopic dermatitis, asthma) or for up to 8 weeks for some non–IgE-mediated disorders (allergic eosinophilic gastroenteritis, food-induced enteropathy syndrome). If symptoms have improved unequivocally, the diet

may be continued unless it requires the elimination of more than one major food (egg, milk, soy, wheat) or two or more minor foods (any food other than major food). If symptoms persist unabated, and food sensitivity is still contemplated, a brief trial (no longer than 2 weeks for suspected IgE-mediated disorders and 8 weeks for non–IgE-mediated disorders) of a severely restricted diet may be warranted. The following diets may be used:

- For patients younger than 4 months, milk substitute (extensive hydrolysates, such as Nutramigen, Pregestimil, and Alimentum; or amino-acid formulas such as Neocate or Elecare)
- For patients aged 4 to 8 months, milk substitute, rice cereal (many infant cereals contain more than one grain), and pears
- For patients aged 9 to 24 months, Neocate 1 Plus and rice, carrots, squash, and lamb
- For patients older than 2 years, the same diet as for 9- to 24-month-old patients plus fresh lettuce, potato, sunflower oil, tea, and sugar.

If symptoms fail to improve, an adverse food reaction can be ruled out.

When improvement is not clear, or several foods appear to be incriminated, a single-blind (or even open) challenge should be performed in the office setting under observation. Because food challenges are time-consuming and may result in severe anaphylaxis, many pediatricians prefer to refer affected patients to a qualified allergist to perform these studies. When immediate hypersensitivity reactions or food-induced enterocolitis is suspected, challenges never should be performed at home by parents. If challenges are performed in the office, appropriate equipment and personnel should be available in the office to deal with an emergency. If the office challenges reveal positive responses to only one major food or less than four foods in total, an appropriate elimination diet may be instituted. Such a diet would not be overly restrictive, and the results of such challenges would be acceptable.

Positive challenges to more than one major food or more than four foods in total should raise concern about the accuracy of the office challenges and should suggest the need to refer affected patients for DBPCFCs. Embarking on a diet restricted in a large number of foods without sound documentation subjects such patients to a diet that renders compliance extremely difficult and that may be nutritionally deficient.

If clinicians follow the protocol outlined in Box 422.3, the DBPCFC will be necessary in only a minority of patients. However, the need for the sound documentation of food sensitivity by challenge procedures cannot be overemphasized. Overly restricted diets in young children can lead to various eating disorders and can create family conflict, especially around mealtime. When various subjective complaints are ruled out (e.g., vague abdominal complaints, behavioral problems) or when symptoms are reported to take several hours or days to develop, DBPCFCs may be conducted at home. However, extreme caution should be exercised when recommending that parents administer a food at home. Only foods that are thought to be unlikely to elicit an immediate-type allergic reaction should be tested at home.

Other procedures advocated as useful in making the diagnosis of food hypersensitivity but *not* substantiated by controlled studies include leukocyte cytotoxicity tests, sublingual provocation with drops of antigen extracts, subcutaneous provocation with varying concentrations of food extracts, and measurement of IgG- or IgG4-specific antibody.

THERAPY

Strict avoidance of the offending food allergen is the only proven therapy for food sensitivity. Drugs may modify symptoms in some cases, but such measures should be considered only palliative. Corticosteroids alleviate symptoms in some food-induced hypersensitivities, such as allergic eosinophilic esophagitis and gastroenteritis, atopic dermatitis, and asthma, and may be life-saving in some fulminant secretory diarrheas but, generally, the side effects of long-term therapy are unacceptable. Antihistamines may modify some symptoms of immediate hypersensitivity, such as oral or cutaneous symptoms, but rarely, if ever, block them completely. Oral cromolyn sodium, rotational diets, immunotherapy, and sublingual or subcutaneous neutralization never have been shown to be efficacious in carefully controlled trials. Recently, monthly injections of anti-IgE antibodies have been shown to reduce the likelihood of anaphylaxis secondary to accidental peanut ingestion in peanut-allergic individuals.

Generally, infants sensitive to cow's milk can be managed adequately using such hypoallergenic formulas as Alimentum or Nutramigen. Most infants with IgE-mediated cow's-milk allergy can be given soy formulas, but infants with cow's milk–induced enterocolitis syndrome develop sensitivity to soy in as many as 50% of cases. Many infants develop diarrhea and localized skin rashes after ingesting various fruits and fruit juices (citrus, apple, grape, tomato). These reactions appear to represent a maturational "intolerance" to fructose or sorbitol and generally are short-lived. Most infants with food sensitivity can have their diets expanded appropriately (i.e., addition of fruits, vegetables, and meats) without difficulty. Adding only one new food every 3 to 5 days, however, probably is a useful practice.

Children older than 2 years rarely, if ever, require an elemental diet for the treatment of food sensitivity, except for some children with allergic eosinophilic esophagitis and gas-

troenteritis. Generally, appropriate oral challenge studies reveal only one or two specific food sensitivities in more than 90% of cases. The most practical method for implementing strict allergen avoidance diets is to teach parents (and older patients) to read food labels. Following long lists of foods that patients may or may not eat is difficult, and the list is readily outdated. Educating patients to recognize key words—ingredient listings that indicate the presence of a specific food—allows the least restrictive diet and results in good dietary compliance. For example, the presence of milk may be indicated by any of the following key words: milk, dried milk solids, whey, casein, lactalbumin, caseinate, cheese, butter, or curds. A dietitian's assistance in suggesting alternative food preparation techniques and assuring a nutritionally sufficient diet is invaluable.

The parents and caregivers of children with IgE-mediated food allergies should be instructed in the care of allergic reactions in case of accidental ingestions. Children who have experienced severe allergic reactions in the past, or who are at increased risk for severe reactions (for example, children with asthma, regardless of the severity, and older children with allergy to peanuts, tree nuts, or seafood), should have injectable epinephrine (EpiPen and Twinject) available at all times. In addition, a formal emergency plan should be developed in case of an accidental ingestion. The Food Allergy & Anaphylaxis Network (Fairfax, VA; tel. 800-929-4040; or www.foodallergy.org) has excellent educational material for patients, schools, and physicians dealing with food-allergy diets and emergency treatment plans.

Frequently, the implementation of strict allergen avoidance leads to the development of clinical tolerance to foods eliciting adverse responses. Most young infants experiencing diarrhea in response to cow's milk or soy protein hypersensitivity lose their sensitivity in 2 to 5 years. Several studies demonstrate the loss of immediate hypersensitivity reactions in approximately one-third of patients after 1 year of antigen avoidance. Although infants more consistently lose their food sensitivity, loss of hypersensitivity is not confined to younger children. In addition, the clinical severity of the initial adverse reaction does not necessarily influence the longevity of the hypersensitivity. Infants who are younger than 2 years and experience mild reactions may be rechallenged every 6 to 12 months to ascertain whether symptoms persist. Older patients may be rechallenged every 1 to 3 years, depending on the degree of difficulty in avoiding the food in question. Because loss of sensitivity varies with the antigen (e.g., peanuts, tree nuts, and seafood remaining persistent in about 80% of children), rechallenging with some foods should be undertaken no sooner than every 3 to 5 years. In certain disorders, such as celiac disease or dermatitis herpetiformis, restricted diets should be continued indefinitely.

Clinical reactivity to a food appears to be highly specific, and rarely are children sensitive to more than one or two foods, except in allergic eosinophilic esophagitis and gastroenteritis. Although the results of skin tests and *in vitro* tests of specific IgE commonly demonstrate cross-reactivity among members of a botanical family or animal species, clinically relevant intrabotanical cross-reactivity and intraspecies cross-reactivity is rare. Consequently, little evidence appears to warrant the avoidance of all foods within a botanical family when one member is suspected of provoking allergic symptoms. By avoiding this practice, patient compliance with elimination diets is improved, and a nutritionally deficient diet is less likely to be implemented.

Several contradictory reports discuss the role of breast-feeding in the prevention of food allergy. Several prospective studies suggest that exclusive breast-feeding for 6 months can reduce an infant's risk of developing food hypersensitivity and atopic dermatitis, only to postpone development of other atopic disorders. The avoidance of highly allergenic foods (peanuts and tree nuts) by lactating mothers may be beneficial, but dietary manipulation in the third trimester of pregnancy appears to offer no advantage and may compromise pregnant mothers' nutritional status.

CONCLUSION

Food intolerance reactions probably represent the majority of food sensitivities in children, are more common in the young infant, and are short-lived. Both food intolerance and food hypersensitivity should be treated by strict avoidance of the inciting food. Repeated challenges should be conducted at varying intervals, depending on the age of the child, the type of reaction provoked, and the food involved, to ascertain whether the sensitivity persists. Studies to document accurately the presence of food sensitivity will simplify the management of this disorder

by reducing the number of foods that need to be eliminated from the patient's diet and the length of time they must be avoided.

Suggested Readings

Leung DYM, Sampson HA, Yunginger JW, et al. Effect of anti-IgE therapy (TNX-901) in patients with severe peanut allergy. *N Engl J Med* 2003;348:986.

Metcalfe DD, Sampson HA, Simon RA, eds. *Adverse reactions to foods and food additives*, 3rd ed. Oxford: Blackwell Scientific Publications, 2003.

Sampson HA. Food allergy. *J Allergy Clin Immunol* 2003;111:540.

Sampson HA, ed. Food allergy. In: Leung DYM, Sampson HA, Geha RS, Szefler SJ, eds. *Pediatric allergy: principles and practice*. St. Louis: Mosby, 2003: 473.

Sicherer SH. Food allergy. *Lancet* 2002;360:701.

Sicherer SH, Munoz-Furlong A, Murphy R, et al. Pediatric food allergy. *Pediatrics* 2003;111:1591.

CHAPTER 423 ■ ATOPIC DERMATITIS

HUGH A. SAMPSON

The French physician, Besnier, presented the first comprehensive description of atopic dermatitis over a century ago. He emphasized its hereditary nature, chronically recurring course, and association with hay fever and asthma. Wise and Sulzberger later coined the term *atopic dermatitis* to further emphasize the relationship between atopic eczema, hay fever, and asthma (the allergic triad). Like asthmatics, patients with atopic dermatitis may be divided into those with extrinsic and intrinsic forms of the disorder. Approximately 80% of children younger than 10 years have the "allergic or extrinsic" form of atopic dermatitis, with flares of eczema exacerbated by specific food or airborne allergens, whereas older patients tend to have intrinsic atopic dermatitis and show no evidence of allergen-induced flares.

EPIDEMIOLOGY

A recent epidemiologic study in Portland, Oregon found that 17% of school-age children had had atopic dermatitis, indicating a three-fold increase in prevalence since the 1970s. Approximately 60% of affected patients develop symptoms within the first year of life, and approximately 90% develop symptoms within the first 5 years. More than 20% of pediatric dermatology visits and approximately 1% of pediatric visits are related to atopic dermatitis.

Etiology

The etiology of atopic dermatitis is not fully known. Food and airborne allergens, entering through mucosal surfaces or breaks in the skin, may exacerbate eczematous lesions after reaching cutaneous mast cells, monocytes, and Langerhans cells (antigen-presenting cells) by way of the circulation. The interaction of allergens with allergen-specific IgE on the surface of mast cells and Langerhans cells leads to the release

of a variety of inflammatory mediators. Mast cells release histamine, leukotriene C_4 (LTC_4), platelet-activating factor, tryptase, cytokines (IL-4 and IL-13 promote IgE synthesis, upregulation of $Fc\varepsilon I$ receptors on mast cells and antigen-presenting cells, and vascular cell adhesion molecule 1 [VCAM-1] expression on vascular endothelial cells; IL-5 attracts and activates eosinophils), and other factors that attract and activate inflammatory cells (e.g., lymphocytes and monocytes). IgE-bearing Langerhans cells have been shown to be highly efficient in activating Th2-type lymphocytes. Repeated allergen exposure provokes chronic inflammation, secondary to IgE-mediated mast cell and lymphocytic responses and contributes to the pathogenesis of atopic dermatitis. $CD4^+$ T_h2 lymphocytes specific for various allergens (e.g., milk, peanuts, dust mites, grass pollen) have been cloned from the eczematous lesions of patients with atopic dermatitis, implicating these allergens in the pathogenesis of lesional skin.

Skin biopsies from the chronic eczematous lesions of patients with atopic dermatitis also reveal large quantities of major basic protein, secreted by eosinophils, in the superficial dermis; this indicates that eosinophils were in the area, whereas actual eosinophils may be seen in more acute lesions. Major basic protein is not seen in uninvolved skin sites in these same patients or in the lesions of patients with contact dermatitis. In one study, food-allergic subjects developed a pruritic, erythematous, morbilliform rash and elevation of plasma histamine levels after double-blind, placebo-controlled food challenges. Skin biopsy specimens obtained 4 to 14 hours later revealed an infiltration of eosinophils and major basic protein deposition, which indicated that food allergen–induced mast-cell activation triggered both an immediate and a late-phase response in the skin. Another eosinophil product, eosinophil-derived neurotoxin, may be responsible for the demyelination of nerves in the dermal layer seen in eczematous skin.

Inhalant allergens (pollens, molds, and dust mites) also may play a role in IgE-induced pathology. Normal individuals passively sensitized to ragweed absorb sufficient pollen allergen via nasal challenge to produce a wheal-and-flare response at a distal skin site. In addition, eczematous skin changes have been provoked by bronchial challenges in some dust mite–sensitive patients. Using a modified patch technique with dust mite antigen, the infiltration of antigen-specific CD4+ Th2 lymphocytes, eczematous changes and, later, increased mast-cell numbers have been induced in patients with IgE antibodies to dust mites.

In addition to allergen IgE–initiated immediate and late-phase hypersensitivity responses, histamine-releasing factors (e.g., lymphokines, monokines) have been discovered that bind to surface-bound IgE molecules and activate mast cells and basophils, leading to the release of various cytokines and inflammatory mediators. IgE autoantibodies also have been found in approximately 80% of patients with atopic disorders. Because low-affinity IgE receptors (FcεII) have been found on B cells, T cells, monocytes, macrophages, eosinophils, and platelets, histamine-releasing factors and IgE autoantibody immune complexes may affect a number of immunologic responses and provoke inflammation.

Definition and Clinical Features

Atopic dermatitis is a chronic cutaneous inflammatory disorder that typically begins in early infancy. The skin symptoms generally present as an erythematous, papulovesicular eruption that progresses to a scaly, lichenified dermatitis over time. The distribution of the rash typically varies with age:

- In infancy (3 to 6 months to 2 years), the cheeks, wrists, and extensor surfaces of the arms and legs typically develop papulovesicular, often weeping lesions that occasionally develop fine scaling or lichenification. The scalp and postauricular area frequently are affected with dermatitis. The eczematous dermatitis may involve the entire body, but generally the diaper area is spared. Frequent scratching results in obvious traumatic lesions and secondary infection.
- In children (2 to 12 years), flexor surfaces, neck, wrists, and ankles generally are involved, with dry maculopapular lesions being a more prominent feature. Pruritus and scratching lead to excoriations, hyperpigmentation, and lichenification.
- In the teenaged patient and young adult, flexural surfaces, face (especially periorbital), hands, and feet frequently are involved. Extreme xerosis, marked papulation, and lichenification are characteristic of this stage. Older patients often have symptom-free periods that last for months but, even during remission, these patients retain a tendency toward dry, sensitive skin.

Unlike most dermatoses, atopic dermatitis has no primary skin lesion but is identified by a constellation of symptoms. The classification system proposed by Hanifin and Rajka (Box 423.1) remains an internationally accepted criterion for diagnosing atopic dermatitis. A modification of this criterion for the young infant is outlined in Box 423.2. Emphasis is placed on the extremely pruritic nature of the rash, its typical morphology and distribution, and its tendency toward a chronic or relapsing course. Some features, such as anterior subcapsular cataracts, nipple eczema, and upper lip cheilitis are uncommon but more specific for the diagnosis of atopic dermatitis. Other symptoms such as allergic shiners, Dennie-Morgan infraorbital folds, and hyperlinearity of the palms are common but less specific.

No single, routine laboratory test exists that indicates the diagnosis of atopic dermatitis. Peripheral blood eosinophilia (5% to 20%) and elevated total serum IgE concentrations are present in approximately 80% of patients. Test results for specific IgE antibodies to foods and inhalants (e.g., prick tests, *in vitro* tests of IgE) are positive in at least 80% of pediatric

---

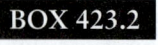

BOX 423.1 — **Diagnostic Features of Atopic Dermatitis**

Major Features*
Pruritus
Typical morphology and distribution
  Flexural lichenification or hyperlinearity in adults
  Facial and extensor involvement in infants and children
Chronic or chronically relapsing course
Personal or family history of atopy (asthma, allergic rhinitis, or atopic dermatitis)

Minor Features*
Xerosis
Ichthyosis, palmar hyperlinearity, keratosis pilaris
Immediate (type I) skin test reactivity
Elevated serum IgE
Early age of onset
Tendency toward cutaneous infections (especially *Staphylococcus aureus* and herpes simplex), impaired cell-mediated immunity
Tendency toward nonspecific hand or foot dermatitis
Nipple eczema
Cheilitis
Recurrent conjunctivitis
Dennie-Morgan infraorbital fold
Keratoconus
Anterior subcapsular cataracts
Orbital darkening
Facial pallor, facial erythema
Pityriasis alba
Itch when sweating
Intolerance to wool and lipid solvents
Perifollicular accentuation
Food hypersensitivity
Course influenced by environmental/emotional factors
White dermographism, delayed blanch

---
*Must have three or more major and three or more minor criteria.

BOX 423.2 — **Diagnostic Features of Atopic Dermatitis for Infants**

Major Features*
Family history of atopic disease
Typical facial or extensor eczematous or lichenified dermatitis
Evidence of pruritus

Minor Features*
Xerosis, ichthyosis, hyperlinear palms
Perifollicular accentuation
Postauricular fissures
Chronic scalp scaling

---
*Must have three or more of both major and minor criteria.

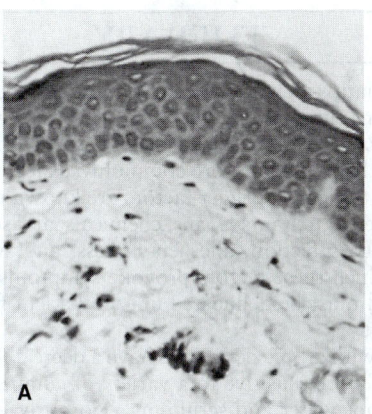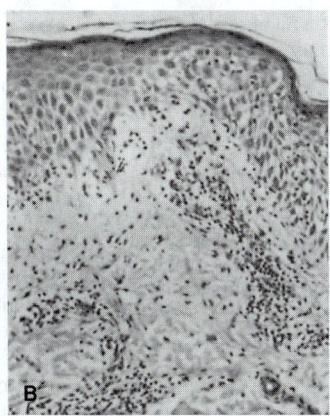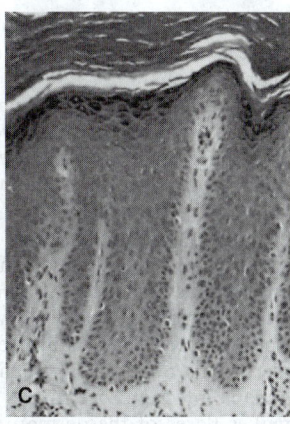

FIGURE 423.1. Skin biopsy section from **A:** normal skin compared with sections from **B:** acute and **C:** chronic atopic dermatitis lesions at the same magnification. Acute lesions are characterized by epidermal spongiosis and prominent mononuclear cell infiltrate. Chronic lesions have prominent hyperkeratosis, marked epidermal hyperplasia, and a mononuclear round cell infiltrate. (Courtesy of Dr. Antoinette B. Hood, Department of Dermatology, Johns Hopkins University, Baltimore.)

patients. The intracutaneous injection of acetylcholine (0.1 mL of 1:1,000) leads to increased sweating and delayed blanching at the injection site (normal response, erythema, sweating, and piloerection). It was shown that cutaneous mast cells bear FcεI receptors lacking the beta chain, a finding unique to this form of dermatitis. In addition, Langerhans cells in individuals with atopic dermatitis express high levels of FcεI receptors, and also high levels of CD86, as compared to CD80.

PATHOLOGY

Histologic changes in atopic dermatitis may appear similar to those of contact dermatitis, id reactions, acute photoallergic reactions, vesicular dermatophytosis, and others. Dermal pathology varies with the nature of the clinical lesion (Fig. 423.1). The acute lesion is characterized by spongiosis (intercellular edema) and ballooning of the keratinocytes (intracellular edema) and by slight psoriasiform hyperplasia of the epidermis with hyperkeratosis. Normal numbers of mast cells are present, and lymphocytes, rare monocytes, and macrophages infiltrate around venous plexes in the dermis. The chronic lesion is characterized by moderate to marked hyperplasia of the epidermis with elongation of the rete ridges and prominent hyperkeratosis. Varying degrees of intercellular edema are present. The acute inflammatory infiltrate consists of monocytes, macrophages, and lymphocytes (predominantly CD4 Th2-type) in both the perivenular and intervascular areas. Mast cells and Langerhans cells (skin dendritic cells) are significantly increased in chronic lesions. Langerhans cells bear high-affinity receptors (FcεI) for IgE molecules on their surface and may be activated through surface-bound IgE allergen interaction. Rarely, eosinophils are seen. Capillary number often is increased, and capillary walls may be thickened. The demyelination and fibrosis of cutaneous nerves are seen at all levels of the dermis.

CLINICAL MANIFESTATIONS AND COMPLICATIONS

Physiologic abnormalities described in patients with atopic dermatitis include decreased itch threshold, increased transepidermal water loss, abnormal cutaneous vascular responses, and abnormal pharmacologic responses including alpha-adrenergic

blockade. Itch is the dominant symptom in atopic dermatitis and the major cause of damaging excoriations, erosions, and lichenification, which are characteristic of atopic dermatitis. The etiology of increased pruritus is unknown. Vasodilatation precedes pruritus, suggesting that the local release of mediators is responsible for increased pruritus. The increased number of mast cells and elevated tissue histamine in chronically involved areas supports this hypothesis.

Increased transepidermal water loss is believed to be secondary to decreased sebum production. Sweating is abnormal in these patients, although studies evaluating the amount of sweating are contradictory. In general, sweating is believed to be increased. A variety of abnormal vascular responses include exaggerated constrictor response of cutaneous vessels and poor adaptability (vascular hyperactivity), white dermatographism, delayed blanch to cholinergic stimuli, and paradoxical response to the application of nicotinic acid. None of these responses is specific for atopic dermatitis.

Patients with atopic dermatitis have several features suggesting the presence of alpha-blockade. Their skin lacks the expected inhibition of DNA synthesis after treatment with beta-adrenergic agonists, and their leukocytes show functional responses that correlate with subnormal cellular cyclic adenosine monophosphate (cAMP) levels after beta-adrenergic stimulation. Some studies show a consistent increase in cAMP phosphodiesterase activity in untreated mononuclear leukocytes from patients with atopic dermatitis, but not in patients with contact dermatitis. This increased phosphodiesterase activity could account for the reduced cAMP levels seen in patients with atopic dermatitis.

Immunologic Abnormalities

Evidence suggests an underlying abnormality in some bone marrow–derived cells or factors. Latent atopy has been transferred by successful bone marrow transplantation of children from their atopic siblings. Abnormalities of both humoral and cellular immunity have been described in patients with atopic dermatitis. These include elevated serum IgE concentrations in approximately 80% of children; defective delayed-type skin responsiveness to various antigens; variably decreased lymphocyte responses to mitogens, recall antigens, and alloantigens *in vitro*; defective generation of cytotoxic T-lymphocyte response *in vitro*; and variably decreased phagocytic capacity and chemotaxis of neutrophils and monocytes. These defects generally fluctuate with disease activity and may revert to normal during long remissions.

Clinically, patients with atopic dermatitis experience increased numbers of skin infections. *Staphylococcus aureus* colonizes the skin of more than 90% of patients with atopic dermatitis, with high concentrations of the organism in areas of active dermatitis. The nearly constant presence of *S. aureus* suggests a microbicidal dysfunction, most likely due to the deficient expression of "defensins," important components of the primitive innate immune system, or to an abnormal fatty acid content of sebum. Superficial pustules, which are extremely pruritic and rapidly excoriated, usually are associated with active or flaring dermatitis. Septicemia generally is not a problem, and deep cutaneous infections are rare. The means by which *S. aureus* provokes flares of the dermatitis is not completely clear. However, many patients possess IgE antibodies to *Staphylococcus* exotoxins (staphylococcal exotoxins A and B and toxic shock syndrome toxin 1) that can activate mast cells, leading to further pruritus and inflammation. In addition, these exotoxins act as "superantigens," capable of activating large numbers of inflammatory cells. Application of *Staphylococcus* exotoxins to the skin has been shown to produce eczematous lesions.

Both clinical and laboratory findings indicate depressed cell-mediated Th1-type functions in patients with atopic dermatitis. Cutaneous anergy is most striking, with increased susceptibility to certain viral infections: herpes simplex (eczema herpeticum), verruca vulgaris (common warts), molluscum contagiosum and, rarely, vaccinia. Dermatophyte infections also are reportedly more common in patients with atopic dermatitis. Patients are less easily sensitized to *Rhus* (poison ivy) and dinitrochlorobenzene, and they show decreased delayed skin test reactivity to a variety of antigens.

Immunohistochemical studies of acute eczematous lesions in atopic dermatitis revealed an infiltration of primarily CD4+ Th2-type lymphocytes (lymphocytes expressing interleukin [IL]-4, -5 and -13) that was markedly different from that seen in classic delayed-type (type IV) hypersensitivity. These ThH2-type lymphocytes are seen in IgE-mediated hypersensitivity reactions and they antagonize Th1-type responses, probably accounting for the depressed cell-mediated function seen in the skin of patients with atopic dermatitis.

DIAGNOSIS

The diagnosis of atopic dermatitis is based on the presence of sufficient major and minor criteria (see Boxes 423.1 and 423.2). The absence of typical features, including pruritus, typical morphology or distribution, symptoms before 5 years of age, or a history of a chronic or relapsing course, should raise serious question as to the accuracy of the diagnosis. Seborrheic dermatitis and allergic contact dermatitis are confused most frequently with atopic dermatitis. Seborrheic dermatitis may be indistinguishable from atopic dermatitis in some cases, but often may be differentiated by seborrhea's more frequent distribution in the axillae and diaper area, less prominent pruritus, and general absence of elevated serum total IgE and positive skin test results to foods and inhalants. Other less common disorders may be mistaken for atopic dermatitis: hyper-IgE syndrome, Wiskott-Aldrich syndrome, and a variety of genetic disorders such as phenylketonuria, biotinidase deficiency, erythrokeratoderma variabilis, and histiocytosis X.

No consistent and distinctive laboratory abnormalities are associated with atopic dermatitis. Skin biopsies are not specific, except for the absence of FcεI beta chains and the expression of CD86 on cutaneous Langerhans cells. Consequently, no routine tests exist to evaluate atopic dermatitis.

THERAPY

Atopic dermatitis is characterized by intermittent inflammatory exacerbations superimposed on skin that is dry and easily irritated. The exacerbations may be infrequent, with prompt resolution and healing, but more commonly, exacerbations occur regularly. A variety of trigger factors are known to exacerbate flares of eczema: irritants (soaps, chemicals, and so forth), heat and humidity, infection, allergens, stress, and sweating. The extent to which these factors provoke symptoms vary among patients and must be delineated in each patient for successful management.

Patients with atopic dermatitis have a decreased itch threshold and are more sensitive to a variety of cutaneous irritants. Bathing in hot water and scrubbing vigorously with soap are the most frequent sources of irritation. Patients should be encouraged to bathe in tepid water (especially for hydration), avoid soap, and pat dry with soft absorbent towels. Clothing should be double-rinsed after washing to remove all residual detergent.

Most patients recognize that sweating causes pruritus. Whether thermal change, exercise, or anxiety induces sweating, it generally leads to cutaneous pruritus, scratching, and the subsequent skin changes characteristic of atopic dermatitis. Avoiding excessive room temperature; wearing light, nonocclusive clothing (e.g., cotton instead of polyester); keeping the bedroom cool; and avoiding excessive bed clothing help reduce sweating. Cutaneous infections are a frequent cause of acute flares in atopic dermatitis. *S. aureus* is implicated most frequently, although streptococcal infections may be seen. Infection typically is suspected in the presence of acute weeping or crusted lesions and small superficial pustules, but it also should be suspected in recalcitrant cases lacking these lesions. *Staphylococcus* organisms typically are resistant to first-generation penicillins, and many (approximately 50%) are resistant to erythromycin. Increasingly, community-acquired infections due to *Staphylococcus aureus* are methicillin resistant (MRSA) and have acquired resistance to other commonly used oral antibiotics, including the cephalosporins. Skin culture and antibiotic susceptibility tests are increasingly important in guiding therapy. Mupirocin, a topical antibiotic effective for superficial *Staphylococcus* infections, may be used when infection is localized. The nose may be a reservoir of *S. aureus*; therefore, in patients with recurrent *Staphylococcus* infection, mupirocin applied in the nose twice daily may be helpful.

When lesions fail to respond to oral antibiotics, herpes simplex infection should be considered. A Giemsa-stained Tzanck smear or culture indicates the presence of the viral infection. Patients at risk for ocular involvement or serious dissemination and systemic involvement of herpes simplex should be treated with intravenous acyclovir. Others may be treated with povidone iodine compresses and ointment, or topical acyclovir. Occasionally, patients experience a flare from superimposed dermatophyte infections. These infections respond readily to either locally applied dacarbazine (Imidazole) creams or oral griseofulvin daily for 1 month.

Despite a long-standing debate on the significance of food allergens in the pathogenesis of atopic dermatitis, a study of patients with moderate to severe atopic dermatitis referred to a university-based pediatric dermatology clinic demonstrated that food allergy was a causative factor in 37% of patients. Eggs, milk, peanuts, soy, and wheat are the most common offenders. The evaluation of possible food allergies has been discussed in Chapter 422, Food Allergies. A second study using dust-mite bronchoprovocation clearly demonstrated the role of inhalant allergens in the pathogenesis in some sensitized patients with atopic dermatitis. Nevertheless, no studies support the use of immunotherapy in the management of atopic dermatitis. In many cases, the dermatitis flares when allergy shots are initiated. Some attempt to reduce dust-mite exposure appears warranted. Stuffed animals, stuffed furniture, and throw rugs should be removed, mattresses and pillows should be encased in impermeable covers, and bedding should be laundered weekly in hot water and dried in a hot dryer.

Allergic contact dermatitis is not uncommon in patients with atopic dermatitis. Patients may become sensitized to topical medications or preservatives. Patch testing sometimes is useful in detecting the offending contact allergen.

Patients or their parents generally are aware that stress, anxiety, anger, and frustration provoke pruritus and flares of atopic dermatitis. Patients should be encouraged to verbalize their emotional conflicts and, occasionally, psychological counseling may be sought. In children, potentially stressful situations in the home or school should be assessed and discussed.

Several general measures may be taken to reduce pruritus and consequent skin damage secondary to scratching. Fingernails should be trimmed short and cotton gloves may be worn at night. Because dry skin is prone to itch, efforts to obtain maximal skin hydration are mandatory. Bathing for hydration (i.e., soaking in tepid water for 20 to 30 minutes) followed by the immediate application of an emollient ointment or cream is the most effective form of therapy. Lubricant creams and ointments (Aquaphor, Cetaphil, Eucerin, Lubriderm, petrolatum, Vanicream, etc.) should be applied within 3 minutes of the child getting out of the tub to seal in moisture so that water absorbed into the stratum corneum does not evaporate. For patients with marked excoriations or weeping lesions, initial wet wraps with Burrow's solution (1:40) avoids the stinging or burning sensation sometimes seen with bathing. Adding oil to bath water is generally ineffective but, if used, should not be applied until minutes before the child is to leave the bath.

Topical corticosteroids and, more recently, topical calcineurin inhibitors (tacrolimus [0.03%] and pimecrolimus) are the mainstay of therapy for atopic dermatitis. For general management, mid strength corticosteroids, such as 0.1% triamcinolone cream or ointment, are optimal. Occasionally, more potent fluorinated corticosteroids are required to suppress an acute flare. The use of these potent agents should be limited because of their accompanying major side effects. In general, the least potent corticosteroid that controls a patient's symptoms should be used. Topical nonsteroidal calcineurin inhibitors have been shown to be effective in controlling eczematous flares. Unlike topical steroids, calcineurin inhibitors do not cause cutaneous atrophy and are safe for use in facial and eyelid eczema. Systemic corticosteroids should be avoided, except in the most severe cases, because many patients experience a rebound flare after a short course, which only leads to further requests for systemic therapy. A course of anti-*Staphylococcus* antibiotics always should be considered before using systemic corticosteroids.

Most patients experience some symptomatic relief with antihistamines; whether this relief is because of an antipruritic or soporific effect is debated. Patient response to antihistamines varies, but hydroxyzine and doxepin appear most effective. Antihistamines are competitive antagonists and are best used on a regular basis. Daily large doses of hydroxyzine (2 mg/kg up to 75 to 100 mg before bedtime) or doxepin before bedtime generally circumvent daytime sedation and facilitate nighttime sleep.

Tar preparations provide a useful nonsteroidal approach to therapy. However, gel preparations frequently irritate dry skin, and the smell is unacceptable except to the most motivated patients. UV light (UVA and UVB) therapy is beneficial in some recalcitrant cases, but should be undertaken with extreme caution and careful professional supervision. Psoralen plus UVA (PUVA) therapy has been beneficial in some severe cases. The dangers of squamous cell carcinomas and skin damage make these UV therapies unacceptable in most cases. Several trials with immunomodulatory agents, high-dose intravenous gamma globulin, phosphodiesterase inhibitors, thymopentin, and interferon-gamma have shown marginal effects in moderate to severe cases of atopic dermatitis. A Chinese herbal tea was shown to be an effective form of treatment in moderate to severe cases, but unfortunately serious hepatic side effects have been seen with some herbal treatment regimens.

Hospitalization, or a simulated hospitalization at home, should be considered as a therapeutic modality. Whether removal from daily stresses or environmental factors is the goal, a brief period of bed rest often leads to considerable symptomatic improvement.

PROGNOSIS

The course of atopic dermatitis is somewhat capricious and marked by unexplained exacerbations and remissions. A lack of distinct diagnostic criteria has interfered with epidemiologic studies of atopic dermatitis. Figures for persistent dermatitis vary from 10% to 83% of affected children; although more recent studies indicate that the majority of patients "outgrow" their eczema, most retain some stigmata of the disorder throughout life. Less favorable prognostic signs include late onset and reverse pattern (involvement of extensor surfaces instead of flexors), severe widespread dermatitis in childhood, family history of atopic dermatitis, and associated allergic rhinitis or asthma. In general, the more severe the symptoms, the less likely is a permanent remission.

Suggested Readings

Bieber T, Leung DYM, eds. *Atopic dermatitis.* New York: Marcel Dekker, Inc., 2002.

Boguniewicz M, Eichenfield LF, Hultsch T. Current management of atopic dermatitis and interruption of the atopic march. *J Allergy Clin Immun* 2003; 112:S140.

Hanifin JM, Rajka G. Diagnostic features of atopic dermatitis. *Acta Dermatol Venereol* 1984;92(Suppl):44.

Leung DYM. *Atopic dermatitis.* In: Leung DYM, Sampson HA, Geha RS, Szefler SJ, eds. *Pediatric allergy: principles and practice.* St. Louis: Mosby, 2003:561.

Leung DYM, Boguniewicz M. Advances in allergic skin diseases. *J Allergy Clin Immun* 2003;111:S805.

Sampson HA. The evaluation and management of food allergy in atopic dermatitis. *Clin Dermatol* 2003;21:183.

CHAPTER 424 ■ ALLERGIC RHINITIS AND ASSOCIATED DISORDERS

F. ESTELLE R. SIMONS

Allergic rhinitis, or inflammation of the nasal mucosa, is the most common chronic disease of the respiratory tract and the most common of all allergic diseases, with physician-diagnosed allergic rhinitis occurring in up to 42% of 6-year-olds in the United States. It may be associated with allergic conjunctivitis, and also may be associated with chronic sinusitis or otitis media with effusion; moreover, 40% of young individuals with allergic rhinitis have concomitant asthma.

EPIDEMIOLOGY

Risk factors for allergic rhinitis include genetic susceptibility, early sensitization to allergens (total serum immunoglobulin E [IgE] of greater than 100 IU/mL before age 6 years), atopic dermatitis, high socioeconomic status, heavy exposure to indoor allergens, maternal tobacco smoking, and/or early introduction to cow's milk formula or solid foods in infancy.

Allergic rhinitis is often underdiagnosed, undertreated, and trivialized because it is not life-threatening; however, it may affect appearance and behavior, and may impair cognitive and psychomotor performance. It is a major cause of school absenteeism and diminished quality-of-life in the pediatric population.

Seasonal (intermittent) allergic rhinitis is commonly caused by nonflowering, wind-carried plant pollens. In temperate climates, symptoms are caused by tree pollens during the early spring, grass pollens during the late spring and early summer, ragweed and other weed pollens during the late summer and autumn, and outdoor molds during both the spring and the autumn. Due to a priming effect on the nasal mucosa during continued daily allergen exposure, less allergen is required to trigger severe nasal symptoms late in the pollen season than is required early in the season. Perennial (persistent) allergic rhinitis is triggered by indoor allergens such as animal danders, house dust mites, and indoor molds. In subtropical and tropical climates, pollens and outdoor molds cause perennial, rather than seasonal, rhinitis. Food allergens do not trigger allergic rhinitis as such, although they may trigger nasal symptoms during full-blown anaphylaxis, a severe acute allergic reaction involving many body systems.

PATHOPHYSIOLOGY

Allergic rhinitis involves the overexpression of IgE and the interaction of specific IgE with airborne allergens. Mucosal inflammation is characterized by an epithelial accumulation of eosinophils, mast cells, and basophils, along with endothelial and epithelial cell activation, up-regulation of dendritic (antigen-presenting cells) and, in persistent disease, CD4$^+$ T lymphocyte accumulation and activation. The release of chemical mediators of inflammation, including histamine and leukotrienes, from activated effector cells (primarily mast cells

and basophils); the synthesis and release of T helper (Th2) cytokines (interleukin [IL]-4, IL-5, IL-9, and IL-13); and the coordinate expression of chemokine and cell adhesion molecules characterize the immediate and late allergic response.

DIAGNOSIS

The cardinal symptoms of allergic rhinitis are paroxysmal sneezing, itching (sometimes manifest as grimacing or "picking" the nose), watery, profuse rhinorrhea (nasal discharge), and nasal congestion/stuffiness. The diagnosis is based on characteristic symptoms and signs in the absence of upper respiratory tract infections, and the exclusion of other, less common disorders in the differential diagnosis (Box 424.1). Allergic rhinitis symptoms may occur not only on exposure to airborne allergens, but also on exposure to irritants such as tobacco smoke, strong odors (paint fumes, perfumes), car exhaust fumes, and other pollutants, and may be triggered by physical factors such as cold air exposure or the ingestion of hot or spicy liquids

---

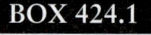 **BOX 424.1   Differential Diagnosis of Rhinitis**

Allergic: seasonal (intermittent) or perennial (persistent)
Infectious: usually viral (if bacterial, consider the possibility of immune deficiency disease)
Eosinophilic nonallergic rhinitis
Vasomotor rhinitis
Sinusitis (acute, subacute, recurrent, or chronic)
Adenoid hypertrophy
Foreign body
Anatomic variations: nasal septum deviation, unilateral choanal atresia
Trauma: septal hematoma, fracture of nasal bones, synechiae
Benign tumors: nasal polyps, dermoid cysts, meningomyelocele
Malignant tumors: nasal glioma
Granulomatous disease: Wegener's granulomatosis, sarcoid
Rhinitis medicamentosa: topical decongestants
Medications: nonsteroidal antiinflammatory agents, cocaine, some antihypertensives, beta-adrenergic blockers, oral contraceptives
Hormonal changes: hypothyroidism, pregnancy
Cerebrospinal fluid rhinorrhea
Ciliary dyskinesia

and foods. Associated symptoms include noisy or hypernasal breathing, oronasal breathing, snoring, loss of olfaction or taste, halitosis, itching of the palate or pharynx, and repeated throat clearing or cough secondary to postnasal drip or drainage of nasal secretions into the pharynx. Ocular symptoms such as redness, itching, or tearing also may be present (see the section, Allergic Conjunctivitis). Systemic symptoms include malaise and disturbed nocturnal sleep with or without sleep apnea, and subsequent daytime fatigue.

In children with allergic rhinitis, an examination of the nose sometimes reveals a transverse external wrinkle, secondary to rubbing and dorsal manipulation, also known as the "allergic salute." Inspection through an otoscope or a flexible fiberoptic rhinoscope usually reveals edema of the nasal mucosa, which may be pale, violaceous, or red in color. Watery, opaque, or mucoid secretions may be noted in the nasal cavity or on the posterior pharyngeal wall, and there may be evidence of recent epistaxis. Nasal polyps are uncommon in children; if they are observed, the diagnosis of cystic fibrosis must be considered.

Children with allergic rhinitis may have "allergic shiners," a term used to describe the dark discoloration of the infraorbital regions secondary to obstruction of venous drainage. If they are chronic oronasal breathers, they may have hypertrophied gingival mucosa, a gaping expression, a long, retrognathic facies with a high, narrow palate, and orthodontic anomalies such as posterior dental crossbite. Lymphoid tissue associated with the upper airways, including adenoids and tonsils, may be hypertrophied, and anterior cervical lymph nodes may be enlarged. If adenoid hypertrophy is severe, alveolar hypoventilation, hypoxemia, hypercarbia, hypoxic pulmonary vasoconstriction, and cor pulmonale may be present.

Diagnostic Tests

The diagnosis of allergic rhinitis is based on clinical history and physical examination, and it can be confirmed by the identification of eosinophils as the predominant cells in nasal secretions. Supportive evidence is provided by positive epicutaneous (prick) tests to airborne allergens such as tree, grass, and weed pollens; molds; house dust mites; and cat, dog, and other animal danders, performed along with histamine (positive) and diluent (negative) control tests. If severe atopic dermatitis precludes skin testing, or if withdrawal of an H_1-antihistamine for the requisite 7 days before skin testing is not feasible, allergen-specific IgE can be measured in serum using radioallergosorbent tests or enzyme-linked allergosorbent tests. Positive skin tests to allergen(s) and/or elevated allergen-specific IgE alone *cannot* be used to "diagnose" allergic rhinitis, because sensitization to allergens may occur in the absence of symptoms. Other tests, which are not necessary for the clinical diagnosis, but are useful in research, include the measurement of peak inspiratory flow, and intranasal allergen challenge under controlled conditions in the laboratory, followed by quantitation of mediators such as histamine and leukotrienes in nasal secretions and of immunochemically identified inflammatory cells in the nasal mucosa.

THERAPY

Treatment involves both pharmacologic and nonpharmacologic approaches (Table 424.1). Allergic rhinitis itself never

TABLE 424.1

MANAGEMENT OF ALLERGIC RHINITIS

Medication Class	Examples	Route of Administration	Symptoms Relieved	Safety
Corticosteroids	Fluticasone propionate, mometasone furoate	Intranasal	Congestion, itching, rhinorrhea, sneezing	Generally safe for long-term use
H_1-antihistamines*	Cetirizine, fexofenadine, loratadine	Oral	Itching, rhinorrhea, sneezing, and congestion	Second-generation drugs are nonsedating and safe for long-term use
H_1-antihistamines	Azelastine, ketotifen	Intranasal	Itching, rhinorrhea, sneezing, and congestion	Safe for short-term use
Leukotriene modifiers	Montelukast	Oral	Congestion, itching, rhinorrhea, sneezing	Safe for long-term use
Decongestants* (alpha-adrenergic agonists)	Pseudoephedrine	Oral	Congestion	Safe for short-term use
Decongestants* (alpha-adrenergic agonists)	Oxymetazoline, xylometazoline	Intranasal	Congestion	Use for 5 days maximum
Antiallergics*	Cromolyn sodium, lodoxamide tromethamine, nedocromil sodium, pemirolast	Intranasal	Modest efficacy in prevention of symptoms	Safe for long-term use
Anticholinergics	Ipratropium bromide	Intranasal	Rhinorrhea	Safe for short-term use

*One or more medications in this class is available over-the-counter in the United States.
Nonpharmacologic Interventions:
    Child and family education with regard to triggers for symptoms, recurrent or persistent inflammatory nature of allergic rhinitis; concomitant disorders; treatment options.
    Avoidance of airborne allergens and irritants such as cigarette smoke: easier said than done and easier done than maintained.
    Allergen-specific immunotherapy: selected children with moderate-severe disease.
The efficacy and safety of complementary and alternative treatments, which are widely used for children with allergic rhinitis and associated disorders, remains to be determined.
See *Physicians' Desk Reference* or other current resource for information about doses and formulations, and the youngest age for which a drug has received U.S. Food and Drug Administration (FDA) approval for use.

causes mortality, and it is therefore essential that the medications used to treat this disease are safe for long-term use in children; specifically, that they do not adversely affect linear growth, cognitive or psychomotor development, behavior, or sleep. Pharmacologic management must be individualized: requirements range from an antihistamine as-needed in a child with mild seasonal allergic rhinitis, to an intranasal glucocorticoid used daily in a child with severe perennial rhinitis and supplemented with additional medications from other classes when symptoms exacerbate. Polypharmacy should be avoided. This may be difficult to accomplish in children who express many different allergic phenotypes concurrently; for example, a child with allergic rhinitis, allergic conjunctivitis, asthma, and atopic dermatitis.

The most commonly used medications for allergic rhinitis are orally administered H_1-antihistamines, which decrease sneezing, itching, and rhinorrhea but are somewhat less effective for the relief of nasal congestion. The first-generation, potentially sedating H_1-antihistamines such as chlorpheniramine or diphenhydramine have not been adequately studied in young children, and these agents have never been documented to be safe for long-term use in the pediatric population. Compared with these older medications, the second-generation, nonsedating antiallergic antihistamines such as cetirizine, fexofenadine, and loratadine have a greatly improved benefit-to-risk ratio and can be administered once daily. They lack anticholinergic effects such as dry mouth. They do not cross the blood–brain barrier readily, and they do not interfere with the neurotransmitter effects of histamine, or cause central nervous system adverse effects such as sedation and impaired cognitive and psychomotor performance. They are free from cardiovascular adverse effects. Topical intranasal H_1-antihistamines such as azelastine or levocabastine are also available, and these have the advantage of a rapid onset of action; however, they require twice-daily administration.

The orally administered leukotriene D4 antagonist montelukast, well-studied in adolescents and adults with allergic rhinitis, relieves itching, sneezing, rhinorrhea, and congestion and has similar efficacy to the H_1-antihistamine loratadine. Extrapolating from asthma studies in children, it is safe for long-term use in the pediatric population. Cromolyn sodium, lodoxamide tromethamine, and nedocromil sodium applied to the nasal mucosa prophylactically have modest efficacy in preventing itching, sneezing and rhinorrhea, but are not very effective for congestion. They are minimally absorbed after topical administration and are relatively free from both systemic and local toxicity. Pseudoephedrine, an orally administered sympathomimetic, has a short elimination half-life and is best used for the intermittent relief of nasal congestion rather than for long-term therapy. When administered alone, or in combination with a nonsedating H_1-antihistamine, it may cause adverse effects including restlessness, insomnia, hallucinations, and hypertension. Topical intranasal alpha-1-adrenergic agents such as xylometazoline and oxymetazoline increase nasal patency and relieve congestion. If used for more than a few days, they may cause rebound congestion and, with long-term use, rhinitis medicamentosa occurs. In infants, they occasionally cause systemic symptoms, including central nervous system depression and coma.

Intranasal glucocorticoids, such as beclomethasone dipropionate, flunisolide, triamcinolone, budesonide, fluticasone propionate, and mometasone furoate, are the most effective medications available for the relief of sneezing, itching, nasal discharge, and congestion. They act locally to restore the normal histology of the nasal mucosa, down-regulate cytokine gene expression and modulate the dendritic (antigen-presenting) cell, Th2 lymphocyte, IgE, basophil, mast cell, and eosinophil axis of the allergic inflammatory response. They increase interferon-gamma and other antiinflammatory cytokines; they decrease IL-4 and other proinflammatory cytokines, cell adhesion pro-

teins; and they down-regulate activated endothelial and epithelial cells. Intranasal glucocorticoids have a faster onset of action than is generally realized (days, not weeks), although they may take weeks to achieve peak effects. Children with seasonal allergic rhinitis should begin using them before the pollen season starts. Once-daily dosing is possible with most medications in this class. Intranasal glucocorticoids have a high ratio of topical-to-systemic activity. When used in the lowest doses that control nasal mucosal inflammation, they do not generally affect hypothalamic-pituitary-adrenal axis function or linear growth. Careful instruction and regular monitoring of inhalation technique are essential; the spray should always be directed laterally, away from the nasal septum.

Although major advances have occurred recently in the pharmacologic treatment of allergic rhinitis, nonpharmacologic treatments remain important. These involve education of the child and family about the recurrent or persistent nature of the disease, avoidance of trigger allergens and irritants where possible and, in selected children, down-regulation of the immune response to airborne allergens using allergen-specific immunotherapy (allergy shots) (Table 424.1).

Well-maintained air-conditioning units are effective in reducing pollen and mold counts in homes and vehicles and in decreasing symptoms in children sensitized to these allergens. Similar beneficial effects are claimed for high-efficiency particulate air filter units. Avoiding nonspecific environmental stimuli such as tobacco smoke, paint fumes, perfumes, and other irritants, and physical factors such as breathing cold air or ingesting hot liquids or spicy foods also may be relevant.

Allergen-specific immunotherapy (allergy shots) consists of subcutaneous injections of increasing concentrations of allergen(s) to which a child is sensitized. It may reduce morbidity and medication requirements in selected children with allergic rhinitis whose symptoms are poorly controlled by a reduction of airborne allergens and irritants in the environment and by optimal pharmacologic management, including an intranasal glucocorticoid. The clinical response is dose-dependent. Successful immunotherapy is associated with down-regulation of the early and late response to specific allergen challenge in the nose and decreased allergen-specific IgE and increased IgG4 blocking antibody in the serum. There also occurs a loss of basophil responsiveness; decreased lymphocyte proliferation; the generation of allergen-specific suppressor T cells, including $CD8^+$ T lymphocytes; a decreased release of proinflammatory cytokines, including IL-4 and IL-5; and an increased release of antiinflammatory cytokines, such as interferon-gamma. During immunotherapy, the most common adverse effects are large local reactions at the injection sites. Rarely, generalized systemic reactions, such as anaphylaxis or serum sickness, occur. Standardized allergens should be used in preference to nonstandardized ones. New routes of allergen administration (sublingual) are being investigated, and new approaches to immunotherapy (allergen peptides, and allergen DNA vaccine conjugates) are being studied with regard to improving efficacy and safety.

DISORDERS ASSOCIATED WITH ALLERGIC RHINITIS

Allergic Conjunctivitis

Allergic conjunctivitis, the most common form of ocular allergy, often seasonal disorder, involves an IgE-mediated conjunctival reaction to airborne allergen(s). Symptoms and signs include intense itching, bilateral conjunctival erythema and swelling (chemosis), watery discharge, and eyelid edema. Conjunctival scrapings show eosinophils, and skin tests to airborne allergens are positive. The differential diagnosis includes palpebral or limbal *vernal conjunctivitis*, a potentially sight-threatening condition with male predominance, in which photophobia and intense eyelid and conjunctival itching occur. In palpebral vernal conjunctivitis, giant papillary reactions produce a cobblestone appearance in the everted tarsal conjunctivae, accompanied by a thick, white, ropy discharge. In limbal vernal conjunctivitis, yellow-gray gelatinous limbal masses are observed. Corneal complications, such as superficial keratitis and ulceration or secondary bacterial conjunctivitis, may occur. The differential diagnosis of allergic conjunctivitis also includes *giant papillary conjunctivitis*, which has been linked to chronic exposure to ocular foreign bodies such as contact lenses, and *contact allergy of the conjunctivae and eyelids*, which is associated with the use of contact lens solutions, topical medications, or preservatives such as benzalkonium chloride in these solutions. *Atopic kerato-conjunctivitis*, which typically occurs in adolescents with atopic dermatitis, is a chronic inflammation of the lower tarsal conjunctiva and the skin around the eye. Symptoms, which are usually perennial, include severe itching, burning, and tearing. If the cornea is involved, sight may be threatened.

The most important therapeutic goal in the management of all forms of ocular allergy is relief of itching. Oral, nonsedating H_1-antihistamines with antiallergic properties, such as cetirizine, fexofenadine, and loratadine, are the cornerstone of treatment. Topical ophthalmic medications for allergic conjunctivitis include the antiallergic antihistamines azelastine, emedastine, ketotifen, levocabastine, and olopatadine, antihistamine–vasoconstrictor combinations (pheniramine/naphthazoline), mast-cell stabilizers (cromolyn, lodoxamide, nedocromil, pemirolast), and nonsteroidal antiinflammatory drugs such as ketorolac. Topical glucocorticoid treatment should be prescribed only for severely affected children, who should be monitored regularly by an ophthalmologist during treatment, because of the possibility of increased intraocular pressure or cataract formation. The refrigeration of topical medications may decrease the stinging or burning that sometimes occurs when they are applied to the conjunctivae.

Nonpharmacologic treatment consists of avoidance of exposure of the conjunctivae to allergens and irritants, if possible. The application of cold compresses or the instillation of artificial tears may be helpful in reducing itching. In children with severe allergic conjunctivitis or vernal keratoconjunctivitis, allergen-specific immunotherapy may be considered.

Chronic Sinusitis

Chronic sinusitis, defined as inflammation of one or more of the paranasal sinuses lasting more than 90 days, may have an infectious or noninfectious basis. It is an easily overlooked cause of morbidity in children with allergic rhinitis. The ethmoid and the maxillary sinuses are present at birth. The sphenoid sinuses develop by age 5 years; the frontal sinuses, which appear at age 7 to 8 years, continue to develop until adolescence. In chronic sinusitis due to allergic inflammation, the appearance of the sinus mucosa on endoscopic and histologic examination is similar to that of the inflamed nasal mucosa with which it is contiguous. Partial or complete obstruction of the ostiomeatal complex is present, with subsequent hypo-oxygenation of the involved sinus, disturbance of ciliary function, and diminished local host-resistance factors.

Symptoms of chronic sinusitis include nasal discharge, persistent nasal congestion, halitosis, diminished sense of smell or taste, postnasal drip, and frequent cough. Facial pain, pressure, or fullness over the sinuses is infrequent. Sore throat, headache, sore neck, dental pain, malaise, nausea, decreased appetite, irritability, fatigue, and low-grade fever may be reported. The nasal mucosa may be red and swollen. Mucopurulent material may be present in the nose and on the posterior pharyngeal wall. Adenoids may be enlarged. The differential diagnosis of chronic sinusitis is similar to that of allergic rhinitis (Box 424.1); in addition, barotrauma, cystic fibrosis, gastroesophageal reflux, and immune deficiency diseases such as hypogammaglobulinemia deserve consideration.

Chronic sinusitis is diagnosed by history, endoscopic examination of the nose using flexible rhinoscopy, radiographs, and computed tomography (CT). Radiographs reveal sinus opacification, air fluid levels, or a greater than 6 mm thickening of the mucosa. Occipitomental (Waters) views facilitate optimal visualization of the maxillary sinuses, and occipitofrontal (Caldwell) views, of the ethmoid and frontal sinuses. Coronal CT scans (method of choice in school age children) provide a detailed image of sinus anatomy, including the ostiomeatal complex; however, imaging technology does not differentiate inflammation due to viral or bacterial infection from inflammation due to allergy. In children with chronic sinusitis, allergy skin tests or investigations for cystic fibrosis, or immune deficiency disease may be indicated. Paranasal sinus involvement with or without nasal polyposis is almost universal in cystic fibrosis, and it also may occur in children with mutations in the cystic fibrosis transmembrane conductance regulator gene who have a normal sweat chloride test.

Bacterial infection as a primary cause of chronic sinusitis is likely relevant in fewer than one-half of children with the disease. If antibiotic treatment is indicated, amoxicillin/clavulanate, cefuroxime or a third-generation cephalosporin, or for the penicillin/cephalosporin-allergic child, clarithromycin or trimethoprim/sulfamethoxazole should be administered for 3 to 6 weeks. In children with cystic fibrosis and sinusitis, in whom *Pseudomonas aeruginosa* is a frequent pathogen, topical tobramycin is useful. To reduce mucosal inflammation around the ostiomeatal complex and facilitate drainage, intranasal glucocorticoids, intranasal or oral decongestants, intranasal or oral antihistamines, mucolytics, and nasal washes often are recommended; however, there is little published evidence for the efficacy of any of these therapies. Functional endoscopic sinus surgery or other surgical intervention is sometimes deemed necessary. Surgical approaches are more likely to be beneficial in children older than age 6 years than in younger children. Those who undergo repeated endoscopic surgeries may derive diminishing benefit with each successive procedure. Potential complications include interference with facial skeletal growth.

Otitis Media with Residual or Persistent Effusion

Residual middle ear effusion lasting for up to 3 months occurs in the majority of children with acute otitis media, and this does not require any treatment. Persistent effusion is defined as an effusion lasting more than 3 months after an acute otitis media episode. When the eustachian tube is blocked, air cannot enter the middle ear. The residual air in the middle ear is absorbed, and serous fluid collects because of the resulting negative pressure. The role of allergy is controversial in otitis media with persistent effusion. Proposed mechanisms include allergic inflammation of the eustachian tube mucosa, resulting in direct obstruction; inflammation of the nasopharyngeal mucosa, causing indirect obstruction of the eustachian tube orifice; and inflammation of the middle ear mucosa itself. Otitis media is associated with a variety of genetic factors, including young age, male sex, Down syndrome, craniofacial abnormalities, immotile cilia syndrome, and hypogammaglobulinemia. It also is associated with a variety of environmental factors, including low socioeconomic status, bottle- rather than breast-feeding, pacifier use, chronic exposure to maternal tobacco smoke, daycare attendance, and recurrent upper respiratory tract infections.

Most children who have otitis media with effusion are asymptomatic. Rarely, a child may have plugging or popping of the ears, a sense of fullness in the head, balance problems, or loss of hearing which, if undetected, may lead to school or behavior problems. Physical findings include tympanic membrane opacification, bubbles, or an air-fluid interface, and diminished or absent mobility. Negative pressure is suggested by prominence of the lateral process and a horizontal orientation of the malleus. Signs of concomitant allergic rhinitis may be present. Complications of otitis media with effusion include atrophy of the tympanic membrane, retraction pockets, cholesteatoma, persistent membrane perforation, or tympanosclerosis.

A sensitive method for determining the presence or absence of middle ear effusion is acoustic immittance testing (tympanometry), in which the compliance of the tympanic membrane is measured at various positive and negative pressures. A low-admittance (flat) tympanogram is characteristic of both acute otitis media and otitis media with residual or persistent effusion. Pneumatic otoscopy may be used to check for middle ear effusion, which is likely present when insufflation creating negative pressure is observed to improve tympanic membrane mobility. Acoustic reflectometry also may be helpful in making the diagnosis. Middle ear effusions are associated with a conductive hearing loss in the range of 20 to 50 dB.

Persistent otitis media with effusion has a favorable spontaneous resolution rate, and treatment of this disorder is becoming increasingly conservative. Currently, a broad-spectrum antimicrobial for 2 to 4 weeks is recommended only for the occasional child with ear discomfort, tinnitus, balance or speech problems, developmental delay, or a bilateral conductive hearing loss of greater than 20 dB. A recent meta-analysis has confirmed that intranasal or oral glucocorticoid treatment, combined with an antibiotic, led to a more rapid resolution of otitis media with effusion in the short term, but offered no long-term benefit. Antihistamine–decongestant combinations, although often prescribed, have no documented efficacy; moreover, they have not been specifically tested in allergic children who have otitis media with persistent effusion. Myringotomy with tympanostomy tube insertion should be considered only after 6 months or more of continuous bilateral effusion, and this could be extended to even 9 or 12 months during the spring and summer, when otitis media with persistent effusion tends to resolve spontaneously. For children 2 years of age and older, adenoidectomy or adeno-tonsillectomy at the time of initial tympanostomy tube insertion reduces the likelihood of additional hospitalizations and surgery related to otitis media. The complications of tube insertion include tube blockage, early extravasation, otorrhea, and residual perforation of the tympanic membrane. The nonspecific treatment of otitis media with effusion includes breast-feeding, reduced pacifier use, avoidance of tobacco smoke, avoidance of upper respiratory tract infections whenever possible, and in allergic children, avoidance of relevant airborne allergens.

Asthma

At least 40% of young patients with allergic rhinitis have concurrent asthma, described in detail in Chapter 420, Asthma.

In some children, the rhinitis predominates and the asthma is undiagnosed or subclinical; in others, the asthma predominates and the rhinitis is undiagnosed or subclinical. A strong epidemiologic association exists between allergic rhinitis and asthma which, in the same patient, often have similar provoking factors and similar seasonal exacerbations. Anatomically, both the upper and lower airways are lined with ciliated columnar epithelium containing mucus-secreting goblet cells. Physiologically, the airways are connected not only by the nasobronchial reflex, but also by the adverse effects on the lower airways produced when nasal congestion results in loss of the nasal air-conditioning functions (warming, humidification, and filtration of the inspired air). The underlying immunopathologic process is similar in allergic rhinitis and asthma, involving not only an early response to allergen, but also a late response (persistent allergic inflammation) and a systemic immunologic response. Moreover, pharmacologic treatment of the disorders is similar with regard to relief of allergic inflammation using intranasal or inhaled glucocorticoids and other drug classes. The obvious exception to this is that vasoconstrictors (alpha-adrenergic agonists) are useful only in allergic rhinitis, and beta$_2$-adrenergic agonists are useful only in asthma. Nonpharmacologic treatments also are similar in both disorders and include education about the recurrent or persistent inflammatory nature of the disorders, allergen avoidance and, in selected children, allergen-specific immunotherapy. Phrases such as "combined allergic rhinitis–asthma syndrome," "allergic rhinobronchitis," "united airways," "one airway, one disease," and others in current use have led to an increased awareness that allergic inflammation occurs throughout the airways in many patients with allergic rhinitis.

PROGNOSIS

Allergic rhinitis and associated comorbidities, such as allergic conjunctivitis, chronic sinusitis, otitis media with persistent effusion, and asthma, are common in childhood. They decrease quality of life and are often underdiagnosed and undertreated. Physicians providing primary care for children should be vigilant in identifying these disorders and aware of the relief that optimal management can provide. They also should be mindful of the need to refer children who are unresponsive to conventional medical management, especially those concurrently expressing multiple allergic phenotypes, to a board-certified allergist or other appropriate specialist.

Suggested Readings

Bousquet J, Van Cauwenberge PB, Khaltaev N, in collaboration with the World Health Organization. Allergic rhinitis and its impact on asthma. *J Allergy Clin Immunol* 2001;108:1A,S147.

Dykewicz MS. Rhinitis and sinusitis. *J Allergy Clin Immunol* 2003;111: S520.

Lack G. Pediatric allergic rhinitis and comorbid disorders. *J Allergy Clin Immunol* 2001;108(Suppl 1):S9.

Plaut M, Valentine MD. Allergic rhinitis. *N Engl J Med* 2005;353:1934.

Simons FER. Advances in H$_1$-antihistamines. *N Engl J Med* 2004;351:2203.

CHAPTER 425 ■ INSECT STING ALLERGY

KENNETH C. SCHUBERTH

For most children and adults, insect stings are common, painful, but not particularly hazardous. However, in approximately 1% of the general population, stings trigger systemic anaphylactic reactions that account for approximately 50 fatalities in the United States each year. Although the risk of a fatal reaction is much lower in children than in adults, insect-allergic children are the source of much parental and pediatrician anxiety because children are more likely to be stung and may not be able to handle emergencies and provide self-treatment. Since the late 1970s, major advances in understanding insect venom biochemistry and immune response pathophysiology have led to the development of safe and effective venom immunotherapy for highly allergic individuals. At the same time, long-term studies of the epidemiology and natural history of insect allergy have provided reassuring evidence that, for most children, the allergic state is a transient, self-limited process that may not require treatment.

THE INSECTS

The true stinging insects that account for the majority of allergic reactions belong to the order Hymenoptera (Box 425.1). The females of each species have a modified ovipositor stinger through which an injection of venom is delivered. Biting insects such as mosquitoes, flies, and bugs only rarely produce systemic reactions and are not considered in this discussion.

Honeybees are the most common members of the apid family. They are small, fuzzy, relatively docile insects that usually live in domestic hives and often are seen gathering nectar and pollinating clover and flowering plants. They usually sting only when sat on or caught underfoot, and they leave their barbed stinger embedded in the victim. Bumblebees are large, slow-flying, yellow-and-black-striped bees that are usually solitary and only rarely sting. Honeybees and bumblebees survive the winter and are present throughout the summer.

The vespid family includes yellow jackets, hornets, and wasps. In most areas of the United States, these insects account for the majority of stings. Yellow jackets are common in the Northeast, whereas wasps are dominant in the South and Southwest. Yellow jackets are small, black-and-yellow-striped insects that usually nest in the ground or in decaying logs. They scavenge for food, are often seen around picnics and garbage, and become particularly aggressive late in the summer, when their nests are crowded. White-faced hornets are large black insects with white faces that build teardrop-shaped paper nests suspended in trees. The thin-bodied brown-and-yellow-striped Polistes wasp typically creates open-faced nests under the eaves of buildings.

Imported fire ants are less common members of the order. They inhabit the coastal areas of the Southeast and live in large dirt mounds. They attach themselves to the skin and deliver multiple stings that result in sterile pustules. Although their stings are a cause of systemic reaction, their venom has been less well studied. Current diagnosis and immunotherapy uses whole body extract, which appears quite successful.

REACTION TYPES

After a sting, 90% of children experience a normal reaction consisting of transient redness, swelling, and pain localized to the sting site, usually less than 2 in. in diameter and lasting for less than 24 hours (Box 425.2). Hymenoptera venoms contain a variety of enzymes (phospholipase A, hyaluronidase), cytotoxic proteins (apamine, mellitin), and vasoactive compounds (histamine and kinins) that, in the normal individual, induce local vasodilatation, edema, and tissue damage.

In 10% of children, the sting results in a large local reaction that is extensively swollen and tender, is larger than several

---

> **BOX 425.1** — **Classification of Common Stinging Insects (Order Hymenoptera)**
>
> **Apid Family**
> Honeybee
> Bumble bee
>
> **Vespid Family**
> Yellow jacket
> White-faced hornet
> Yellow hornet
> Polistes wasp
>
> **Imported Fire Ant**

> **BOX 425.2** — **Classification of Reactions to Insect Stings**
>
> **Normal**
> Swelling less than 2 inches in diameter
> Duration less than 24 hours
>
> **Large Local**
> Swelling greater than 2 inches in diameter
> Duration of 1 to 7 days
>
> **Systemic**
> Non–life-threatening: immediate-type generalized reaction confined to the skin (urticaria, angioedema, erythema, pruritus)
> Life-threatening: immediate-type generalized reaction that may include cutaneous symptoms but also has respiratory (laryngeal edema or asthma) or cardiovascular (hypotension/shock) symptoms

inches in diameter, and peaks in 3 to 7 days. Although the exact mechanism of this reaction is unknown, 75% of these individuals demonstrate venom-specific IgE, suggesting that immediate hypersensitivity may play some role in this exaggerated sting response.

True systemic anaphylactic reactions are less common. Estimates of their incidence in the general population range from 0.5% to 5.0%. Anaphylaxis is caused by the activation of mast cells sensitized by venom-specific IgE. This triggers the release of large quantities of vasoactive mediators, including histamine, leukotrienes, and other cytokines, and leads to vasodilatation and increased vascular permeability. Most of these reactions (70% to 80%) are not life-threatening. They begin several minutes to several hours after the sting and consist of simple generalized urticaria, erythema, pruritus, and angioedema. Life-threatening reactions begin within 5 to 10 minutes. Airway obstruction may occur secondary to laryngeal edema (tickle in the throat, gagging, difficulty in swallowing, or voice change) or bronchospasm (chest tightness or wheezing). Hypotension (dizziness or fainting) and frank cardiovascular collapse are accompanied by metabolic acidosis, clotting abnormalities, and evidence of complement activation. Although approximately 50 deaths per year are attributed to insect allergy, almost all of these occur in adults, particularly the elderly. Fatal outcome in children is extremely rare, averaging only one death per year in the United States.

Several types of non–IgE-mediated reactions include serum sickness, renal disease, neurologic manifestations, and delayed hypersensitivity phenomenon. Their pathophysiology remains unknown. When a child is stung many times simultaneously, a toxic, nonallergic reaction consisting of delayed fever, nausea, vomiting, and other systemic symptoms sometimes occurs. With an extremely large number of stings, such as may occur with Africanized honeybees or "killer bees," this type of nonallergic reaction occasionally is fatal.

ETIOLOGY AND NATURAL HISTORY

Systemic reactions are produced by venom-specific IgE directed against a variety of venom protein antigens. Phospholipase A is the major antigen in honeybee venom, whereas antigen 5, a protein of unknown function, is the most common in vespid sensitivity. Yellow jacket, hornet, and wasp venoms share a variety of common antigens, and a sting by one species often results in sensitivity to all vespids. Cross-reactivity is negligible between honeybee and vespid venoms. Nevertheless, almost 50% of children exhibit combined honeybee and vespid sensitivity, presumably as a result of previous stings from a variety of insects that did not result in unusual reactions. Although venom-specific IgE can be demonstrated in more than 90% of patients experiencing systemic reactions, it is present also in 75% of patients with large local reactions and approximately 15% to 20% of the general population, especially in the 12 to 24 months after an acute sting. Exposure to venom proteins in the general atopic population may produce a transient period of subclinical sensitivity that usually disappears. In a small percentage of those patients, another sting during that period of hypersensitivity results in systemic reactions.

More recent studies in the epidemiology and natural history of insect-sting allergy demonstrate several characteristics of the disease that were previously unrecognized. Children with a history of large local reactions only rarely go on to experience systemic reactions to subsequent stings (less than 3%). Children with a history of mild systemic reactions have only approximately a 10% chance of experiencing subsequent sys-

temic reactions, almost all of which are less severe than the prior ones. These two pieces of information suggest that, for most children, insect allergy is not a progressive problem and is outgrown. Much of the anxiety and sense of panic relating to insect allergy in the past were the result of anecdotal reports and poorly controlled studies.

DIAGNOSIS

The initial step in managing insect sting allergy is an attempt, by careful history taking, to identify the insect culprit and clearly define the reaction by category, extent, and time course. The critical distinction to make is between local and systemic reactions. If the reaction is systemic, particularly if life-threatening, referral for skin test evaluation is necessary.

Venom Skin Testing

For children with a history of a prior systemic reaction, venom skin testing is the quickest and most sensitive way to determine the presence of venom-specific IgE and identify which insect is responsible. Testing may be done as soon as 2 weeks after the reaction and has been useful in children as young as 9 months old. A panel of purified processed venoms, including those of honeybee, yellow jacket, white-faced hornet, yellow hornet, and Polistes wasp, is available for intradermal testing at concentrations from 0.001 to 1.0 μg/mL. Although testing identifies the sensitive state, no good correlation exists among the intensity of skin test reactivity, the severity of the previous reaction, and the likelihood of reaction to subsequent stings. Because children who have had normal or large local reactions only, without systemic symptoms, also may have positive skin tests, the results always must be interpreted in light of clinical history A negative skin test result in a patient with a history of systemic reactions suggests non–IgE-mediated anaphylactoid mechanisms, but this must be confirmed with follow-up skin tests and radioallergosorbent testing (RAST).

Radioallergosorbent Testing

Venom RAST detects the presence of venom-specific IgE in serum. Because it is slightly less sensitive and more expensive than skin testing, RAST is not used routinely as a screening test, but may be helpful in those situations in which skin testing is equivocal or negative.

THERAPY

Treatment of the Acute Episode

Systemic reactions in children most often consist of mild urticaria or angioedema occurring within minutes up to several hours after a sting. Pharmacologic treatment is guided by the severity of the reaction, but epinephrine is the cornerstone of therapy and should be administered promptly (Box 425.3). Some mild, slow-onset reactions may be observed carefully and treated with oral antihistamines. Rarely, more serious reactions may warrant the administration of nebulized beta-agonists, corticosteroids, intravenous fluids, oxygen, and full support in an intensive care unit. Some dramatic hypotensive episodes may be epinephrine resistant and respond only to rapid volume expansion and pressor agents. Large local reactions may

BOX 425.3	Treatment of Acute Anaphylactic Reaction

Epinephrine: 1:1,000 aqueous 0.01 mL/kg IM up to
   0.3 mL; may be repeated at 15-minute intervals
Diphenhydramine: 1 mg/kg up to 50 mg, IV, IM, or orally
Prednisone: 1 mg/kg/day for 3 to 5 days
In the event of a severe reaction:
   Nebulized beta-agonist
   Oxygen/respiratory support
   Intravenous volume expanders and vasopressor
      infusion

respond to the application of ice, elevation of the affected site, administration of antihistamine to control itching, and a short course of oral prednisone.

Emergency Self-Treatment

Children at risk for serious systemic reactions who have not yet reached maintenance immunotherapy should carry an epinephrine auto-injector for self-treatment. Epi-Pen (0.3 mg for children 40 pounds or more) or the Epi-Pen Jr. (0.15 mg for children less than 40 pounds) are preferred because of their ease of use. The use of these devices should be practiced in the doctor's office, and be available at home, school, or wherever insect contact is likely. Use of the auto-injector is advised only if signs of a serious systemic reaction occur, followed immediately by transport to a medical facility. Oral antihistamine may be used for mild reactions, but should never be substituted for epinephrine. In most cases, once the patient reaches maintenance immunotherapy, they are advised to carry epinephrine only if they are far from medical care. Those with mild cutaneous reactions also may choose carry the device, although their risk of systemic reaction is low.

Avoidance Measures

Careful sanitation and the extermination of vespid nests can significantly reduce the chance of a yellow jacket sting. For children especially, wearing shoes while walking in grass eliminates the most common cause of honeybee sting. The usual insect repellents are not effective against Hymenoptera. In severely allergic children, wearing a Medic-Alert bracelet or necklace provides quick and useful information in case of accidental sting reaction.

Venom Immunotherapy

In 1979, the U.S. Food and Drug Administration (FDA) licensed the use of purified extracts of insect venoms to prevent future systemic reactions in children and adults. The five venoms used in immunotherapy correspond to those used in skin testing. The selection of venoms for therapy is based on the demonstration of venom-specific IgE, either by skin testing or by RAST. The regimen usually consists of rapid advancement to maintenance doses at 4- to 8-week intervals for as long as 3 to 5 years. Children tolerate this regimen extremely well, although almost all of them sometimes experience local red-

ness or swelling at the injection site. Approximately one-fourth sometimes experience a large local reaction at the injection site, and an approximately 5% risk exists of a systemic reaction at some time during the immunotherapy regimen. These are similar to risks encountered with other high-dose immunotherapy regimens using pollens or other inhalants. No evidence exists of any long-term adverse effects. Studies using in-hospital challenge stings after 15 weeks of venom immunotherapy, and at yearly intervals thereafter, demonstrate a 97% to 98% nonreaction rate in various groups of adults and children.

The duration of therapy is governed by several factors. After 3 years, venom sensitivity, as measured by positive skin tests or RAST, disappears in approximately 20% of patients; for these patients, immunotherapy can be safely discontinued. For most of the remainder, 3 to 5 years of treatment confers a high degree of long-term protection after discontinuation. A few patients with very severe initial reactions, sting reactions while on therapy, or increasing venom skin test sensitivity should continue longer than 5 years.

Patient Selection for Venom Immunotherapy

Only those patients who have experienced a significant systemic reaction and who have positive skin test or RAST results are candidates for venom immunotherapy. The more severe the prior reaction, the more likely the subsequent reaction will be serious. Although positive skin test results identify sensitive individuals, they do not predict the risk of future reactions. As many as 40% to 60% of adults who have had a systemic reaction and have positive skin test results do not experience any systemic reaction if they are stung again. Children have an even lower risk, as evidenced by the high frequency of mild cutaneous systemic reactions and the extreme rarity of fatalities. For children who have had mild non–life-threatening systemic reactions and have positive skin test results, the risk of systemic reaction on being stung again is less than 10%, and the risk of progression to more serious reactions is much less. For these children, observation and emergency precautions, without venom immunotherapy, appear to be sufficient. For children with life-threatening systemic reactions and positive skin test or RAST results, referral to a specialist for venom immunotherapy is mandatory, as it is in all adults, regardless of the severity of prior systemic reactions. Although the guidelines for treatment (Table 425.1) are specific, the decision for or against venom immunotherapy must be made for each

TABLE 425.1

GUIDELINES FOR VENOM IMMUNOTHERAPY IN CHILDREN

Reaction	Skin Test/ RAST	Venom Therapy	Other
Systemic			
Life-threatening	Positive	Yes	
	Negative	No	Repeat ST/ RAST Carry Epi
Cutaneous only	Positive	No (usually)	May carry Epi
	Negative	No	
Large local	Not indicated		
Toxic	Not indicated		
Normal local	Not indicated		

patient after careful discussion of risks, benefits, and individual concerns between the physician and family.

Suggested Readings

Golden DBK, Kagey-Sobotka A, Norman PS, et al. Insect allergy with negative venom skin tests. *J Allergy Clin Immunol* 2001;107:897.

Golden DBK, Kwiterovich KA, Kagey-Sobotka A, Lichtenstein LM. Discontinuing venom immunotherapy: extended observations. *J Allergy Clin Immunol* 1998;101:298.

Graft DF, Schuberth KC, Kagey-Sobotka A, et al. A prospective study of the natural history of large local reactions after hymenoptera stings in children. *J Pediatr* 1984;104:664.

Portnoy DM, Moffitt JE, Golden DBK, et al. Stinging insect hypersensitivity: a practice parameter. *J Allergy Clin Immunol* 1999;103:963.

Reisman RE. Insect Sting Anaphylaxis. In: Leung DY, Sampson HA, Geha RS, Szefler SJ, eds. *Pediatric allergy*. St. Louis: Mosby, 2003:633.

Stafford CT. Hypersensitivity to fire ant venom. *Ann Allergy Asthma Immunol* 1996;77:87.

Valentine MD, Schuberth KC, Kagey-Sobotka A, et al. The value of immunotherapy with venom in children with allergy to insect stings. *N Engl J Med* 1990; 323:1601.

CHAPTER 426 ■ THE IMMUNE SYSTEM

HOWARD M. LEDERMAN

The immune system is composed of a variety of cells (B lymphocytes, T lymphocytes, monocytes, and neutrophils) and their secretory products (antibodies, complement, and cytokines), which recognize foreign antigens and react to them. This chapter reviews the normal physiology of the immune system.

NORMAL IMMUNE SYSTEM

Components of the immune system are found in all parts of the body, but are concentrated in the thymus, bone marrow, lymph nodes, spleen, liver, and blood (Fig. 426.1). Successfully integrated and functioning together, phagocytes, the complement system, and B and T lymphocytes form an important homeostatic mechanism necessary for the host's defense against infection and the generation of a normal inflammatory response. In conceptual terms, the components of the immune system can be divided into two compartments—innate and adaptive—each having fundamentally different modes of action (Table 426.1).

The Innate Immune System

The components of the innate immune system (neutrophils, macrophages, natural killer [NK] cells and complement) recognize foreign antigens through receptors encoded by intact germline genes (e.g., toll-like receptors and mannose binding lectin). These receptors bind to the pathogen-associated molecular patterns (PAMPs) that are shared by many microorganisms (e.g., bacterial lipopolysaccharide). The receptors for PAMPs are displayed nonclonally on cells of the innate immune system. For example, all neutrophils display one set of PAMP receptors, whereas all NK cells display a different set of PAMP receptors. Repeated exposure to an antigen does not alter the activity of the components of the innate immune system to that antigen.

Phagocytic Cells

Phagocytic cells ingest foreign antigens and microorganisms. Although many phagocytic cells are mobile and can move from the bloodstream through tissues to the site of microbial invasion or inflammation, other phagocytic cells are fixed in the sinusoids of the bloodstream and the lymphatic system where they clear microorganisms and other particulate matter from the circulation. A variety of cells possess phagocytic activity, but neutrophils, monocytes, and macrophages are the most critical to the functions of the immune system.

Neutrophils are large, polymorphonuclear leukocytes that arise in the bone marrow, circulate in the bloodstream, and migrate into tissues, where they are the first line of defense against local infections and the principal phagocytic cells of the acute inflammatory response. Monocytes also arise from stem cells in the bone marrow, circulate in the bloodstream, and migrate to the tissues, where they undergo morphologic and functional maturation to become macrophages. Monocytes and macrophages participate as effector cells in host defense and inflammation, but also can present antigen to lymphoid cells and secrete a variety of proinflammatory substances (including cytokines and complement components, among many others). Monocytes and macrophages thus play an important role in the generation of innate and adaptive immune responses.

Phagocytic Cell Movement and Binding. To function properly, phagocytic cells must attach to a substrate (adherence), move through tissues toward the site of microbial invasion (chemotaxis), attach and ingest microbes (phagocytosis), and finally kill them (intracellular killing).

Adherence to a substrate is a prerequisite before phagocytic cells can move. For example, phagocytes circulating in the bloodstream must adhere to vascular endothelium before they egress from the bloodstream. Similarly, once in the tissues, phagocytic cells adhere to connective tissue substrate as they crawl toward the site of microbial invasion or inflammation. The adherence of phagocytic cells is mediated by a family of cell-surface glycoproteins (integrins) including CR3, LFA-1, and p150,95. This adherence is enhanced by a number of soluble mediators, including C5a, thromboxane A2, leukotrienes, and platelet-activating factor.

Phagocytes also recognize microorganisms using the PAMP receptors that are expressed on bacteria and viruses but not by host cells (Table 426.2). For example, the macrophage mannose receptor binds specific sugar molecules found on the surface of many bacteria and viruses. A family of transmembrane receptors called Toll-like receptors (TLR) have specificity for

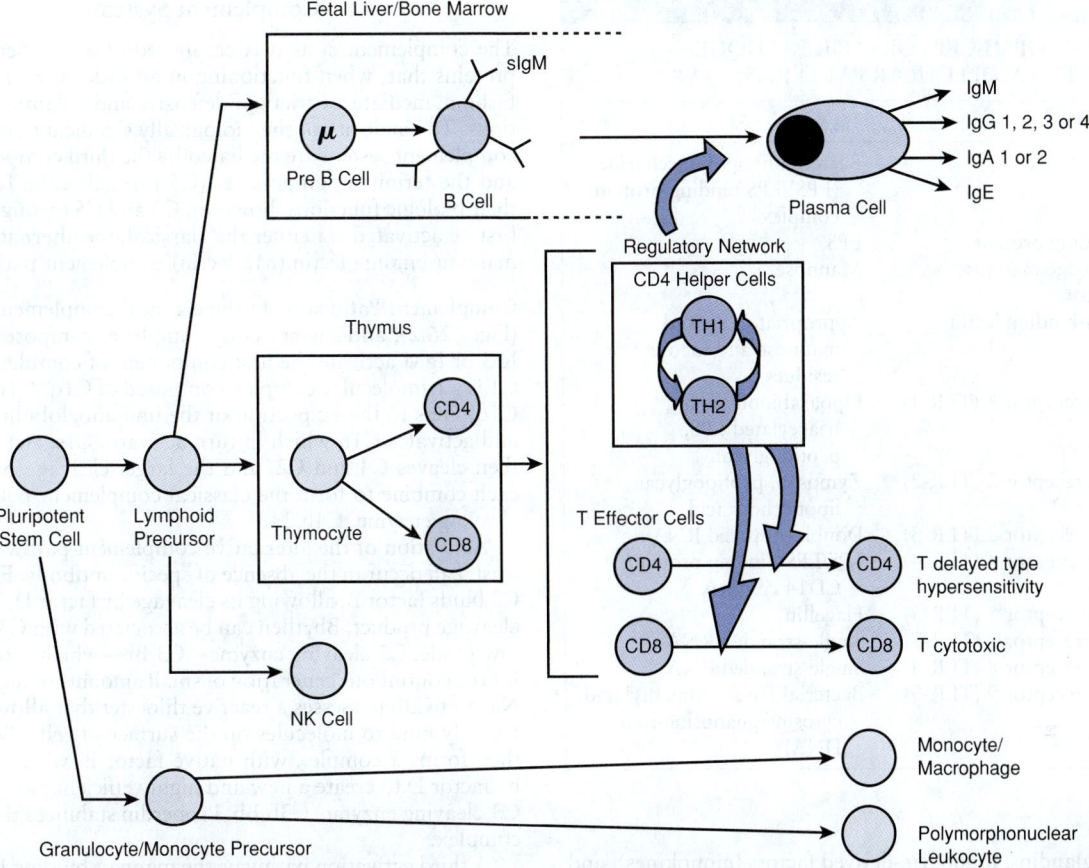

FIGURE 426.1. The cells of the immune system.

a variety of PAMPs. Binding to these receptors triggers a signalling cascade, with the induction of transcription factors and the activation of proinflammatory genes. One particularly important role for TLRs is to trigger macrophage responses to bacterial lipopolysaccharide (LPS). Bacterial LPS in body fluids is bound by the circulating LPS-binding protein, and this complex then binds to CD14 on the macrophage surface. When the LPS/LPS-binding protein/CD14 complex binds to TLR-4, the transcription factor NF-κB is translocated into the nucleus, where it activates genes involved in host defense such as tu-

mor necrosis factor-alpha (TNF-α) and inducible nitric oxide synthetase.

The directed movement of phagocytic cells toward a chemical stimulus is termed chemotaxis. The phagocytic cell senses chemical gradients across its length, and it moves in the direction of the higher concentration (i.e., the source of the chemotactic stimulus). A variety of substances act as chemoattractants. One of the more important stimuli is C5a, which is produced by activation of the complement system. Bacteria can release their own chemotactic peptides. In addition, a variety

---

TABLE 426.1

COMPONENTS OF THE IMMUNE SYSTEM

Feature	Innate Immunity	Adaptive Immunity
Cells	Neutrophils Monocytes/macrophages Natural killer cells	B lymphocytes T lymphocytes
Receptors	Expressed by all cells of a particular type (e.g., macrophages) Recognize broad classes of pathogens	Clonal distribution on individual cells Highly specific
Soluble factors	Complement Mannose-binding lectin Chemokines Cytokines (including IL-1, TNF-α)	Antibody Cytokines (including IL-2, IL-4, IL-5, IL-6, IL-10)
Change with repeated exposure to antigen	No	Yes (clonal expansion, memory lymphocytes)

TABLE 426.2

EXAMPLES OF RECEPTORS FOR PATHOGEN-ASSOCIATED MOLECULAR PATTERNS

Receptor	Ligands
CD14	Bacterial lipopolysaccharide (LPS)/LPS binding protein complex
LPS-binding protein	LPS
Macrophage mannose receptor	Mannose
Mannan-binding lectin	Appropriately spaced mannose and fucose residues
Toll-like receptor 1 (TLR-1)	Lipoarabinomannan, triaceylated LPS, peptidoglycan
Toll-like receptor 2 (TLR-2)	Zymosan, peptidoglycan, lipoteichoic acid
Toll-like receptor 3 (TLR-3)	Double-stranded RNA
Toll-like receptor 4 (TLR-4)	LPS/LPS-binding protein/CD14 complex
Toll-like receptor 5 (TLR-5)	Flagellin
Toll-like receptor 7 (TLR-7)	Single-stranded RNA
Toll-like receptor 8 (TLR-8)	Single-stranded RNA
Toll-like receptor 9 (TLR-9)	Bacterial DNA (unmethylated cytosine-guanosine-rich DNA)

of prostaglandins, monocyte-derived factors (monokines), and lymphocyte-derived factors (lymphokines) possess chemotactic activity. Together, these chemotactic stimuli cause phagocytic cells to migrate to and accumulate at sites of infection and inflammation.

Once phagocytic cells reach the site of infection, they ingest the microbes. The process is facilitated if the microbes have been coated with IgG antibody and/or the larger cleavage product of the third component of complement, C3b (opsonization). Receptors for these opsonins exist on phagocytic cells, thus allowing them to serve as ligands to bind the microbe to the phagocytic cell. C3b favors attachment of the opsonized particle to the phagocytic cell, whereas IgG favors its ingestion. Ingestion occurs by a process in which the phagocytic cell membrane circumferentially surrounds the opsonized particle, leading to its internalization in a phagocytic vacuole or phagosome.

Intracellular Killing. The process of intracellular killing begins soon after the phagosome is internalized. Both primary (azurophilic) and secondary (specific) granules can fuse with the phagosome, and a number of antimicrobial substances are thereby introduced into the phagosome. These substances include lysozyme, lactoferrin, acid hydrolases, and cationic proteins. Perhaps the most important, however, is the myeloperoxidase-H_2O_2-halide system. On ingestion of microorganisms, molecular oxygen is reduced to superoxide by a series of reactions involving nicotinamide-adenine dinucleotide phosphate (NADPH, reduced form) oxidase. The superoxide, in turn, undergoes further reactions, leading to the generation of reduced oxygen derivatives such as hydrogen peroxide and hydroxyl radicals. Myeloperoxidase catalyzes the reaction of hydrogen peroxide with chloride to create hypochlorite ions. The net effect of these toxic derivatives of reduced molecular oxygen is to kill microorganisms within the phagocytic vacuole.

Complement System

The complement system is composed of a number of serum proteins that, when functioning in an ordered and integrated fashion, mediate a variety of defensive and inflammatory reactions. The majority of the biologically significant effects of the complement system are mediated by the third component (C3) and the terminal components (C5 through C9). To subserve their biologic functions, however, C3 and C5 through C9 must first be activated via either the classical, the alternative, or the mannan-binding lectin (MB lectin) complement pathway.

Complement Pathways. In the classical complement pathway (Fig. 426.2), antigen–antibody complexes composed of either IgG or IgM activate the first component of complement (C1). C1 is a trimolecular complex composed of C1q, C1r, and C1s. C1q binds to the Fc portion of the immunoglobulin molecule and activates C1r, which in turn activates C1s. Activated C1s then cleaves C4 and C2, and the larger cleavage products of each combine to form the classical complement pathway C3-cleaving enzyme, C4b,2a.

Activation of the alternative complement pathway, in contrast, can occur in the absence of specific antibody. Fluid phase C3 binds factor B, allowing its cleavage by factor D. The larger cleavage product, Bb, then can be associated with C3 to form a low-grade, C3-cleaving enzyme—C3,Bb—which is responsible for the continuous generation of small amounts of nascent C3b. Nascent C3b possesses a reactive thioester that allows it to covalently bind to molecules on the surface of cells. Bound C3b then forms a complex with native factor B, which is cleaved by factor D to create a new and highly efficient particle-bound C3-cleaving enzyme, C3b,Bb. Properdin stabilizes this C3b,Bb complex.

A third activation pathway, the mannan-binding lectin (MB lectin) pathway, uses a molecule homologous to C1q to trigger the complement cascade. MBL binds to mannose residues on microbial surfaces, but does not bind mannose on host cells because it is blocked by sialic acid. When MBL binds to the surface of a pathogen, it forms a trimolecular complex with two serine proteases, MASP-1 and MASP-2. Together, this complex can cleave C4 and C2 in a manner analogous to that of the C1qrs complex.

Products of Complement Activation. Whether C3 is activated via the classical or alternative complement pathway, two fragments of unequal size are produced, C3a and C3b. In either case, the activation of C3 represents an amplification step because hundreds of C3 molecules can be cleaved by a single C3-convertase. C3a is released into the fluid phase, where it can act as an anaphylatoxin. Most of the C3b also is released into the fluid phase, where it is rapidly inactivated by hydrolysis. Some C3b, however, binds covalently to the surface of the activating cells or to the immunoglobulins of the activating immune complex, thereby acting as an opsonin or combining with either of the C3-convertases to create a C5-convertase. The classical pathway C5-convertase is C4b,2a,3b, whereas the alternative pathway C5-convertase is (C3b)2,Bb.

Activation of C5 creates a small cleavage product, C5a, and a large cleavage product, C5b. C5a is released into the fluid phase where, like C3a, it can act as an anaphylatoxin. In addition, C5a possesses potent chemotactic activity. C5b can combine with native C6. If it does so while still attached to the C5-convertase, it initiates the formation of a membrane attack complex, a multimolecular assembly of C5b, C6, C7, C8, and C9. This complex is inserted into cell membranes and is responsible for the cytolytic and bactericidal actions of complement.

The uncontrolled activation of C3 and C5 through C9 could result in the generation of excessive amounts of the phlogistic fragments of complement and immunopathologic damage to

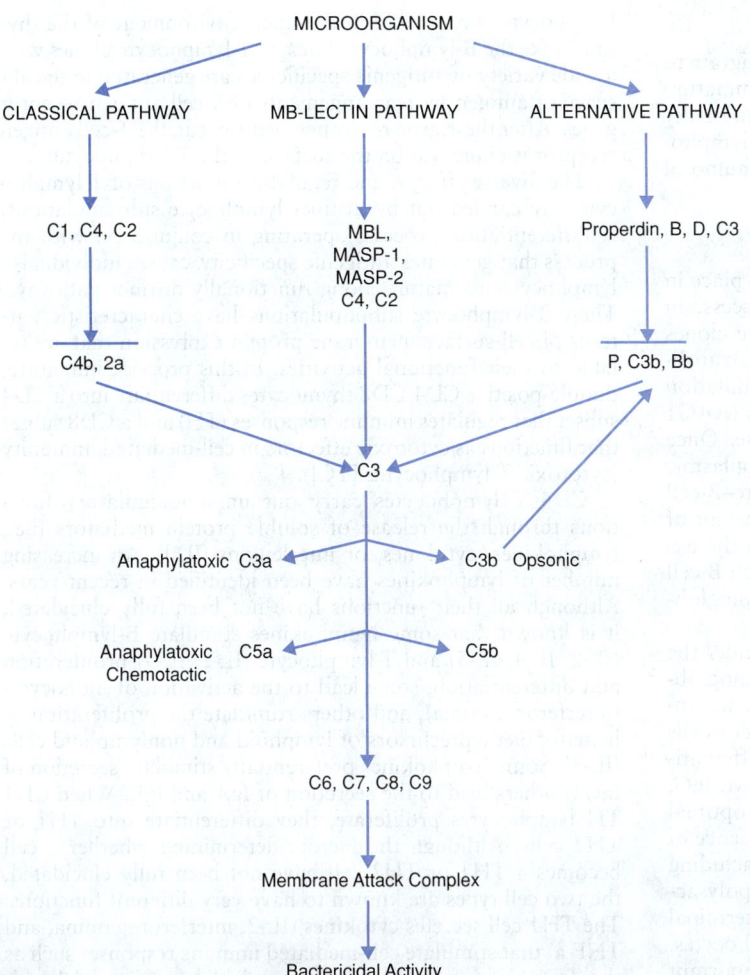

MICROORGANISM

CLASSICAL PATHWAY   MB-LECTIN PATHWAY   ALTERNATIVE PATHWAY

C1, C4, C2   MBL,
MASP-1,
MASP-2
C4, C2   Properdin, B, D, C3

C4b, 2a   P, C3b, Bb

C3

Anaphylatoxic C3a   C3b Opsonic

Anaphylatoxic
Chemotactic C5a   C5b

C6, C7, C8, C9

Membrane Attack Complex

Bactericidal Activity

FIGURE 426.2. The complement pathway.

the host. A number of mechanisms, however, control the assembly and expression of the C3 and C5 convertases. With respect to the classical complement pathway, the enzymatic actions of C1r and C1s are inhibited by a control protein, C1 esterase inhibitor. A second inhibitor, C4 binding protein, inhibits the C4b,2a enzyme by limiting the uptake of C2 by C4b, by accelerating the dissociation and decay of the C2a, and by enhancing the ability of yet another regulatory protein, factor I (C3b/C4b inactivator), to cleave and inactivate C4b. With respect to the alternative pathway, two control proteins, factor H and factor I, inhibit the generation, expression, or both generation and expression of the C3 and C5 convertases. Factor H competes with B for binding to C3b and can displace Bb from the (C3b)2,Bb complex. Factor I inhibits the alternative pathway C3 convertase by inactivating cell-bound C3b through proteolytic cleavage; its rate of C3b inactivation is accelerated by factor H. Thus, the assembly and expression of the C3-cleaving enzymes usually proceeds in a controlled fashion and is limited to the immediate vicinity of the initiating substance.

Natural Killer Cells

Natural killer (NK) cells are derived from the common lymphoid progenitor cell. However, unlike other lymphocytes, NK cells have invariant receptors that are not expressed clonally. One type are activating receptors that bind a variety of cell-surface carbohydrates. A second type are inhibitory receptors that bind major histocompatibility (MHC) class I alleles. NK cells can kill targets that express a net excess of activating versus inhibitory signals. This can occur, for example, if a viral-infected host cell has decreased expression of MHC class I molecules. NK cells also have receptors for the Fc portion of IgG (FcγR), so that they can bind to host cells expressing viral or tumor antigens to which IgG antibodies have attached. Once an NK cell has attached to a target, it can release cytotoxic granules that penetrate the target cell and induce programmed cell death (apoptosis). The cytotoxic activity of NK cells can be enhanced by prior exposure to interferons and the macrophage-derived cytokine IL-12.

The Adaptive Immune System

The cells of the adaptive immune system (B and T lymphocytes) recognize antigen via receptors assembled from rearranged gene segments, and each lymphocyte expresses a unique antigen receptor. Repeated exposure to an antigen selects those cells with the highest-affinity receptors for that antigen, induces proliferation of that clonal population, and induces differentiation into effector and long-lived memory cells. The net effect is to increase the kinetics and magnitude of the response to subsequent exposures of the same antigen.

Lymphoid System

Lymphoid stem cells arise in the fetal yolk sac, then migrate to the bone marrow, liver, and spleen. Their progeny of immature lymphoid precursors differentiate along one of two mutually exclusive pathways to become B or T lymphocytes. B lymphocytes are the effector cells of antibody-mediated or humoral immunity.

B Lymphocytes

Differentiation of B lymphocytes, which largely takes place in the bone marrow and fetal liver, is a two-stage process. In the first stage, an enormous number of B-lymphocyte clones are generated by a series of immunoglobulin gene rearrangements. This process occurs irrespective of antigenic stimulation and is mediated by two recombinase activation genes (RAG1 and RAG2) and terminal deoxynucleotide transferase. Once the immunoglobulin heavy-chain genes rearrange, cytoplasmic immunoglobulin is expressed, and the cells reach the pre–B-cell stage. Further differentiation, including the rearrangement of immunoglobulin light-chain genes, is associated with the expression of surface membrane IgM and IgD. Each such B cell has a unique antigenic specificity, marked by the immunoglobulin receptor on its cell membrane.

The second stage of B-cell differentiation occurs under the influence of antigen. When antigen binds to the immunoglobulin (antibody) expressed on the surface of one of the B lymphocytes, that cell proliferates to form a clone of progeny cells with identical antibody specificity. These cells then differentiate into plasma cells that secrete immunoglobulins IgM, IgG, IgA, IgE, or IgD. Most antigens are T dependent (i.e., optimal B-cell differentiation into plasma cells requires the presence of T-lymphocyte helper cells). A few antigens, however, including such clinically important ones as bacterial capsular polysaccharides, are T independent and are able to trigger terminal B-cell differentiation even in the absence of T lymphocytes. In all cases, CD4 helper T lymphocytes (TH) are important modulators of B-cell function, influencing the degree, duration, and quality (affinity and class distribution) of the antibody response.

Immunoglobulins

The five major classes of immunoglobulins are IgG, IgM, IgA, IgE, and IgD. Each class has unique structural and functional characteristics. Depending on the class, immunoglobulins function in host defense by opsonization of foreign microorganisms, activation of serum complement, neutralization of toxins and viruses, and inhibition of microbial attachment to mucosal surfaces. IgM is the first immunoglobulin produced in an immune response and is the most efficient activator of complement. IgG is the predominant serum immunoglobulin, is actively transported across the placenta, possesses opsonic activity, and activates complement. IgA, which is the major immunoglobulin secreted onto mucosal surfaces, is largely silent as an inflammatory mediator, but does prevent microbial adherence and penetration across the mucosa and clears and disposes of antigens. IgE is a mediator of allergic disease. By means of interactions with mast cells and eosinophils, IgE also can play a role in host defense against parasitic infections. Most IgD is expressed on the surface of naïve B lymphocytes, although limited amounts are secreted. It has no known role in host defense.

T Lymphocytes

T lymphocytes are the effectors for cell-mediated immunity. They also serve as important regulators of both the humoral and cell-mediated immune systems and modulate the activities of nonlymphoid cells such as monocytes. Differentiation of T lymphocytes occurs within the microenvironment of the thymus. Like the B-lymphocyte lineage, T-lymphocyte clones with a wide variety of antigenic specificities are generated in the absence of antigen by rearrangements of T-cell antigen receptor genes. After these gene rearrangements occur, the T-cell antigen receptor is expressed on the surface of the T lymphocyte.

The diverse effector and regulatory functions of T lymphocytes are carried out by distinct lymphocyte subpopulations. A differentiation process, operating in conjunction with the process that generates antigenic specificity, causes individual T lymphocytes to mature along functionally distinct pathways. These T-lymphocyte subpopulations have characteristic patterns of cell-surface membrane protein expression that are related to their functional activities. In this process, immature, double-positive CD4/CD8 thymocytes differentiate into a CD4 subset that regulates immune responses (TH) and a CD8 subset that functions as cytotoxic effectors in cell-mediated immunity (cytotoxic T lymphocytes [TC]).

CD4 T lymphocytes carry out immunoregulatory functions through the release of soluble protein mediators (i.e., lymphokines, cytokines, or interleukins [ILs]). An increasing number of lymphokines have been identified in recent years. Although all their functions have not been fully elucidated, it is known that some lymphokines stimulate B-lymphocyte (IL-2, IL-4, IL-5) and T-lymphocyte (IL-2, IL-4) proliferation and differentiation, some lead to the activation of monocytes (interferon-gamma), and others stimulate the proliferation of hematopoietic precursors of lymphoid and nonlymphoid cells (IL-3). Some lymphokines preferentially stimulate secretion of IgG1; others lead to the secretion of IgA and IgE. When CD4 TH lymphocytes proliferate, they differentiate into TH1 or TH2 cells. Although the factors determining whether a cell becomes a TH1 or TH2 cell have not been fully elucidated, the two cell types are known to have very different functions. The TH1 cell secretes cytokines (IL-2, interferon-gamma, and TNF-a) that stimulate cell-mediated immune responses such as the activation of macrophage bactericidal function, delayed-type hypersensitivity, and cytotoxicity. The TH2 cell secretes cytokines (IL-4, IL-5, IL-6, and IL-10) that drive B-cell proliferation and differentiation, resulting in antibody synthesis. These TH subsets are not mutually exclusive, but most infectious pathogens induce a response that is predominantly TH1 or TH2. In addition, cross-regulation of TH1 and TH2 cells occurs. The TH1 cytokine IFN-gamma down-regulates TH2 cells, whereas the TH2 cytokine IL-10 down-regulates TH1 cells.

TC cells can kill target cells such as virus-infected host cells, tumor cells, or the cells of a histoincompatible tissue graft. TC cells reversibly bind to their targets by means of the T-cell antigen receptor as well as several other cell-surface molecules. Once a TC-target conjugate is formed, the TC cell reorganizes its cytoplasm to concentrate cytoplasmic granules for attack at the point of contact. Two classes of cytotoxins are released: granzymes, which have proteolytic activity, and perforin, which can polymerize to generate pores in the target cell membrane.

Suggested Readings

Abreu MT, Arditi M. Innate immunity and toll-like receptors: clinical implications of basic science research. *J Pediatr* 2004;144:421.

Alam R, Gorska M. B Lymphocytes. *J Allergy Clin Immunol* 2003;111:S476.

Borish LC, Steinke JW. Cytokines and chemokines. *J Allergy Clin Immunol* 2003;111:S460.

Chaplin DD. Overview of the immune system. *J Allergy Clin Immunol* 2003;111:S442.

Parkin J, Cohen B. An overview of the immune system. *Lancet* 2001;357:1777.

Stiehm ER, Ochs HD, Winkelstein JA, eds. *Immunologic disorders in infants and children*, 5th ed. Philadelphia: WB Saunders, 2004.

CHAPTER 427 ■ CLINICAL PRESENTATION OF PRIMARY IMMUNODEFICIENCY DISEASES

HOWARD M. LEDERMAN

The primary immunodeficiency diseases were originally viewed as rare disorders, presenting early in life, with severe clinical symptoms. It has become increasingly clear, however, that these diseases are not as uncommon as originally suspected, that their clinical expression can sometimes be mild, and that they may present at any age. Furthermore, although the initial description of patients with primary immunodeficiency diseases focused on their increased susceptibility to infection, these patients may present with a variety of other clinical manifestations. These include autoimmune or chronic inflammatory disorders and syndrome complexes in which immunodeficiency may occur but is often not the presenting feature.

INCREASED SUSCEPTIBILITY TO INFECTION

Children with primary immunodeficiency diseases most commonly present with an increased susceptibility to infection. Respiratory tract infections and diarrhea are characteristic, but sepsis, meningitis, and osteomyelitis can occur as well. Individual infections may not be more severe than in a normal host, but the striking clinical feature of immunodeficiency is the chronic or recurrent nature of infections. It is difficult to provide specific guidelines about the number of infections that should prompt an evaluation for immunodeficiency, because a wide range of normal occurrence exists, and because the frequency of infections depends in part on the history of exposure. For example, first-born children whose care is provided by a parent who stays at home usually will have fewer infections than a child living with multiple other children in the household or one who is enrolled at a young age in a large day-care facility. Suggestions for when to consider an evaluation for immunodeficiency are provided in Box 427.1. Not all patients with immunodeficiency are diagnosed after a long series of recurrent infections. In some instances, the initial infection is so severe (e.g., pneumonia with empyema) or is caused by such an unusual organism (e.g., *Pneumocystis jerovicii*) that the diagnosis of immunodeficiency is made.

Because each functional compartment of the immune system plays a specialized role in host defense, infections with certain microorganisms characteristically are found in specific immunodeficiency diseases. For example, patients with abnormalities of cell-mediated immunity characteristically develop pneumocystic pneumonia, disseminated fungal infections, mucocutaneous candidiasis, overwhelming viral infections, and severe mycobacterial disease. Patients with defects of antibody or complement more often have infections with pyogenic encapsulated bacteria. Patients with phagocytic defects develop bacterial and fungal infections of the skin and reticuloendothelial system. These distinctions may be blurred, however, because the host's defense against any given microorganism depends on the successful integration of all components of the immune system. Thus, a rare patient with an antibody deficiency develops pneumocystic pneumonia or chronic enteroviral meningitis, whereas patients with deficiencies of cell-mediated immunity can develop pyogenic bacterial infections. Recurrent infections at a single anatomic site always should prompt consideration of other predisposing conditions, such as ciliary dyskinesia, cystic fibrosis, or bronchial obstruction. Patterns of illness and screening tests for primary immunodeficiency disorders are outlined in Table 427.1.

AUTOIMMUNE AND INFLAMMATORY DISORDERS

Children with primary immunodeficiency diseases sometime present with clinical manifestations that do not appear to relate directly to their increased susceptibility to infection. Just as immunodeficiency can lead to defects in the protective functions of the immune system and an increased susceptibility to infection, immunodeficiency also can lead to abnormal immunoregulatory mechanisms, with the result being autoimmune or chronic inflammatory diseases. Thus, patients with primary immunodeficiency diseases sometime present with autoimmune hemolytic anemia or immune thrombocytopenia, autoimmune endocrinopathy, juvenile rheumatoid arthritis, a lupus-like illness, or inflammatory bowel disease. This type of presentation is seen most often in patients with common variable immunodeficiency, selective IgA deficiency, chronic mucocutaneous candidiasis, and deficiencies of the classical complement pathway. Occasionally, a disorder that appears to be autoimmune may be caused by an infectious agent (e.g., the dermatomyositis syndrome that is sometimes seen in patients

---

BOX 427.1 — **History that Suggests Immunodeficiency**

- Frequent or chronic infections without other explanation
  - Otitis media increasing in frequency after age 2 years
  - Two or more pneumonias in a 3-year period
  - Infections associated with failure to thrive
- Severe or unusual infections
  - Bacterial meningitis in an immunized child
  - Meningococcemia
  - Pneumonia with empyema
- Infection with an opportunistic pathogen
  - *Pneumocystis jerovicii*
  - *Aspergillus* species
  - *Mycobacterium avium intracellulare*

TABLE 427.1

PATTERNS OF ILLNESS AND SCREENING TESTS FOR PRIMARY IMMUNODEFICIENCY

Disorder	Illnesses Infection	Other	Diagnostic Tests
Antibody	Sinopulmonary (pyogenic bacteria, viruses) Gastrointestinal (enterovirus, Giardia)	Autoimmune disease (autoantibodies, inflammatory bowel disease)	Quantitative immunoglobulin levels (IgG, IgA, IgM) Antibody responses to immunization
Cell-mediated immunity	Pneumonia, (pyogenic bacteria, *Pneumocystis jerovicii*, viruses) Gastrointestinal (viruses) Skin, mucous membranes (fungi)		Lymphocyte count Delayed type hypersensitivity tests T-lymphocyte subset numbers (CD4, CD8)
Complement	Sepsis and other blood-borne (streptococci, pneumococci, neisseria)	Autoimmune disease (systemic lupus erythematosus, glomerulonephritis)	Total hemolytic complement (CH50)
Phagocytes	Skin, reticuloendothelial system (staphylococcus, enteric bacteria, fungi, mycobacteria)		White blood count and differential; Nitroblue tetrazolium (NBT) dye test

with X-linked agammaglobulinemia is really a manifestation of a chronic enteroviral infection and is not an autoimmune disease).

IMMUNODEFICIENCY SYNDROMES

Immunodeficiency also can be seen as one part of a constellation of signs and symptoms in a syndrome complex (Table 427.2). Recognition that a patient has a syndrome in which immunodeficiency occurs allows a diagnosis of immunodeficiency to be made before any clinical manifestations of that immunodeficiency occur. For instance, children with the DiGeorge anomaly usually are identified initially because of the neonatal presentation of congenital heart disease or hypocalcemic tetany. This leads to the recognition that they have a T-lymphocyte defect before any infections occur that are attributable to that immunodeficiency. Similarly, a diagnosis of Wiskott-Aldrich syndrome can be made in young boys with eczema and thrombocytopenia, and they may be identified as immunodeficient before they develop infections attributable to their immunodeficiency. Recognition of any part of a syndrome complex should prompt a thorough investigation for other manifestations before they become symptomatic.

DIAGNOSIS

One of the most important aspects of the diagnostic work-up for immunodeficiency is deciding which patients should be screened, rather than how to proceed with the evaluation. As discussed previously, indications for screening include the history of severe, chronic, or recurrent infections; infection caused by an opportunistic organism; autoimmune disorders; or recognition of specific syndromes that have been associated with immunodeficiency. In addition, a diagnostic evaluation should be considered for any child in whom problems with infection exceed the norm for the clinician's own experience with children of the same age. The selection of screening tests for immunodeficiency should be based on the spectrum of problems in a given patient and the relative frequencies of primary immunodeficiencies in the population. Finally, whenever immunodeficiency

disease is suspected, consideration also must be given to secondary causes for immunodeficiency (e.g., human immunodeficiency virus infection [HIV] or complications of therapy using corticosteroids, cyclosporin A, and antineoplastic drugs).

Examination of the Peripheral Blood Smear

The complete blood count with examination of the blood smear is an inexpensive, readily available test that provides important diagnostic information relating to a number of immunodeficiency diseases.

Neutropenia may occur secondary to immunosuppressive drugs, infection, malnutrition, autoimmunity, or as a primary problem (congenital or cyclic neutropenia). A persistent neutrophilia with a predominance of immature forms is characteristic of leukocyte adhesion molecule deficiency, and abnormal cytoplasmic granules may be seen in the peripheral blood smear of patients with Chédiak-Higashi syndrome.

The blood is predominantly a "T-cell organ" (i.e., the majority [50% to 70%] of peripheral blood lymphocytes are T cells, whereas only 5% to 15% are B cells). Therefore, lymphopenia may be a presenting feature of T-cell or combined immunodeficiency disorders such as severe combined immunodeficiency disease or DiGeorge syndrome. Lymphocyte counts less than 2500/cu mm in the first year of life should be considered indicative of immunodeficiency untill proven otherwise.

Thrombocytopenia may occur as a secondary manifestation of immunodeficiency, but is often a presenting manifestation of the Wiskott-Aldrich syndrome. A unique finding in the latter group of patients is an abnormally small platelet volume, a measurement that is made easily by automated blood counters.

An examination of red blood cell morphology yields important clues about splenic function. Howell-Jolly bodies may be visible in peripheral blood in cases of splenic dysfunction or asplenia. The converse is not always true, and absence of Howell-Jolly bodies does not guarantee that splenic function is normal.

Evaluation of Humoral Immunity

The measurement of serum immunoglobulin levels is an important screening test to detect immunodeficiency for three reasons:

TABLE 427.2

EXAMPLES OF SYNDROMES IN WHICH IMMUNODEFICIENCY OCCURS

Syndrome	Clinical Presentation	Immunologic Abnormality
Acrodermatitis enteropathica	Dermatitis Alopecia Diarrhea	Variable B- and T-lymphocyte deficiency
Ataxia-telangiectasia	Ataxia Telangiectasia	Variable B- and T-lymphocyte deficiency
Cartilage hair hypoplasia	Short-limbed dwarfism Sparse hair	Neutropenia T-lymphocyte deficiency
Centromeric instability syndrome	Dysmorphic facies Mental retardation Developmental delay	Variable B- and T-lymphocyte deficiency
Chédiak-Higashi syndrome	Oculocutaneous albinism	Abnormal neutrophil function
DiGeorge anomaly	Congenital heart disease Dysmorphic facies Hypoparathyroidism	T-lymphocyte deficiency
Hyperimmunoglobulin E syndrome	Coarse facies Eczematoid rash Elevated IgE	Neutrophil chemotactic defect

Ivemark syndrome	Heterotaxia
	  Bilateral 3-lobed lungs
	  Midline liver
	  Discordance of cardiac
	    and abdominal situs
	Congenital heart disease
		Asplenia

Polyendocrinopathy syndrome	Endocrine organ dysfunction	Mucocutaneous candidiasis
Wiskott-Aldrich syndrome	Thrombocytopenia Eczema	Variable B- and T-lymphocyte deficiency

■ More than 80% of patients with primary disorders of immunity have abnormalities of serum immunoglobulins.

■ These measurements yield indirect information about several disparate aspects of the immune system, because immunoglobulin synthesis requires the coordinated function of B lymphocytes, T lymphocytes, and macrophages.

■ The measurement of serum immunoglobulin levels is readily available, highly reliable, and relatively inexpensive.

The initial screening test for humoral immune function is the quantitative measurement of serum immunoglobulins. Neither serum protein electrophoresis nor immunoelectrophoresis is sufficiently sensitive or quantitative to be useful for this purpose. Quantitative measurements of serum IgG, IgA, and IgM identify patients with panhypogammaglobulinemia as well as those with deficiencies of an individual class of immunoglobulins, such as selective IgA deficiency. Measurements of serum IgE and IgD may be useful in specific circumstances (e.g., IgE levels for suspected hyper-IgE syndrome, which can cause severe atopic disease and increased susceptibility to infection by *Staphylococcus aureus*; IgD levels for suspected hyper-IgD syndrome, which can cause recurrent fevers). The interpretation of results must be made in view of the marked variations with age in normal immunoglobulin levels. Therefore, age-related normal values always must be used for comparison.

Four subclasses of IgG exist, and selective deficiencies of these have been described. IgG1 and IgG3 are the principal subclasses used for responses to protein antigens; IgG2 is the principal subclass used for responses to polysaccharide antigens. In some instances, the total serum IgG may be normal or near-normal, but the patient still may have an IgG subclass deficiency. Thus, quantitative measurements of individual IgG subclasses should be performed when total serum IgG is normal in a child strongly suspected of humoral immunodeficiency.

In addition to measurement of immunoglobulin levels, an assessment of antibody function always should be included as part of the evaluation of humoral immunity. Antibody titers generated in response to childhood immunization with diphtheria and tetanus toxoids are usually the most convenient to measure. In children older than 18 to 24 months, the antibody response to polysaccharide antigens also should be assessed, because these responses may be deficient in some patients who can respond normally to protein antigens (e.g., Wiskott-Aldrich syndrome or IgG2 subclass deficiency). Antibody can be measured in response to immunization with pneumococcal or meningococcal capsular polysaccharide vaccines. Alternatively, because the ABO blood-group antigens are polysaccharides, antipolysaccharide antibody can be assessed by quantitating isoagglutinin titers. Their value in the young child is limited, however, because even normal children of this age may not have significant isoagglutinins.

If immunoglobulin levels and antibody titers are decreased, the evaluation should proceed with an enumeration of B lymphocytes in the peripheral blood. Further specialized tests may be necessary to delineate specifically the functional B-cell defect and may include *in vitro* studies of mitogen or antigen-driven B-cell proliferation and immunoglobulin secretion.

Evaluation of Cell-Mediated Immunity

Testing for defects of cell-mediated immunity is difficult because of the lack of good screening tests. Because T lymphocytes make up 50% to 80% of peripheral blood mononuclear cells, lymphopenia is suggestive of T-lymphocyte deficiency. However, lymphopenia is not always present in patients with T-lymphocyte functional defects. Similarly, the lack of a thymus silhouette on a chest radiograph is a helpful sign in some

T-lymphocyte disorders, but the thymus of normal children may involute after stress and give the appearance of thymic hypoplasia.

Delayed-type hypersensitivity skin testing using a panel of antigens is a screening method for older children. A standardized panel of antigens prepared for delayed-type hypersensitivity testing should be used. The presence of one or more positive delayed-type skin test results generally is indicative of intact cell-mediated immunity. However, significant limitations exist to this testing:

- Prior exposure to antigen is a prerequisite.
- A positive skin test result to some antigens does not ensure that the patient has normal cell-mediated immunity to all antigens (e.g., patients with chronic mucocutaneous candidiasis may have a lacunar defect in which cell-mediated immunity is generally intact except for their response to *Candida*).
- Normal patients may have transient depression of delayed-type hypersensitivity with acute viral infections.
- Normal children younger than 12 months frequently are unresponsive to all the antigens in the panel.

Therefore, the test is least helpful when it is most needed, namely in young infants in whom a congenital abnormality of T lymphocytes (e.g., severe combined immunodeficiency) is suspected. Overall, delayed-type hypersensitivity testing has poor positive or negative predictive value when applied to young children for the evaluation of immunodeficiency.

Indirect information about T-cell function may be obtained by enumerating peripheral blood T lymphocytes, using fluorescein-conjugated monoclonal antibodies to cell surface determinants. Total T ($CD2^+$ or $CD3^+$), TH ($CD4^+$), and TC ($CD8^+$) cells can be quantitated using the appropriate monoclonal antibodies. Patients with severe combined immunodeficiency and DiGeorge anomaly generally have decreased numbers of both $CD4^+$ and $CD8^+$ T lymphocytes. Patients infected with HIV have decreased numbers of $CD4^+$ lymphocytes, whereas patients infected with the Epstein-Barr virus have elevated numbers of $CD8^+$ cells.

Other specialized tests of cell-mediated immunity include the measurement of lymphocyte proliferation *in vitro* after stimulation with mitogens, antigens, or allogeneic cells; production of lymphokines; and cytotoxic effector function.

Evaluation of Phagocytic Cells

The evaluation of phagocytic cells usually entails an assessment of both their number and function. Disorders that are characterized by a deficiency in phagocytic cell number, such as congenital agranulocytosis or cyclic neutropenia, usually can be detected using a white blood cell count and differential.

An assessment of phagocytic cell function depends on a variety of assays. *In vitro* measurement of directed cell motility (chemotaxis), ingestion (phagocytosis), and intracellular killing (bactericidal activity) can be performed. In addition, assays exist that indirectly assess bactericidal activity by measuring the metabolic changes in those cells that are responsible for intracellular killing. The most readily available tests assess the oxidative metabolic responses of phagocytes by measuring the reduction of nitroblue tetrazolium to formazan (NBT test), the production of reduced forms of molecular oxygen (perox-

ide, superoxide, hydroxyl radicals), and chemiluminescence. Each of these functions is reduced markedly in disorders of intracellular killing, such as chronic granulomatous disease.

Evaluation of the Complement System

Most of the genetically determined deficiencies of the classical activating pathway of C3 (C1, C4, and C2), of C3 itself, and of the terminal components (C5, C6, C7, C8, and C9) can be detected using antibody-sensitized sheep erythrocytes in a total serum hemolytic complement (CH50) assay. Because this assay depends on the functional integrity of C1 through C9, a severe deficiency of any of these components leads to a marked reduction or absence of total hemolytic complement activity. Deficiencies of factor H, factor I, and properdin of the alternative pathway can be detected using a hemolytic assay that assesses the lysis of rabbit erythrocytes. The serum of patients with deficiencies of C3 or C5 through C9 is abnormal when tested in the rabbit erythrocyte assay (as well as in the CH50 assay), because the lysis of rabbit erythrocytes depends on these components as well as components of the alternative activating pathway.

The identification of the specific deficient component usually rests on both functional and immunochemical tests, and highly specific assays have been developed for each of the individual components. In most cases, both functional and immunochemical assessments of the specific component demonstrate the deficiency. Some exceptions exist. For example, one form of C1 inhibitor deficiency and one form of C1q deficiency are characterized by dysfunctional proteins that can be detected by using immunochemical assays but are markedly reduced in functional activity.

Suggested Readings

Bonilla FA, Geha RS. Primary immunodeficiency diseases. *J Allergy Clin Immunol* 2003;111:S571.

Buckley RH. Primary cellular immunodeficiencies. *J Allergy Clin Immunol* 2002;109:747.

Conley ME, Notarangelo LD, Etzioni A. Diagnostic criteria for primary immunodeficiencies. Representing PAGID (Pan-American Group for Immunodeficiency) and ESID (European Society for Immunodeficiencies). *Clin Immunol* 1999;93:190.

Fischer A. Human primary immunodeficiency diseases: a perspective. *Nat Immunol* 2004;5:23.

Fischer A. Primary immunodeficiency diseases: an experimental model for molecular medicine. *Lancet* 2001;357:1863.

Folds JD, Schmitz JL. Clinical and laboratory assessment of immunity. *J Allergy Clin Immunol* 2003;111:S702.

Immune Deficiency Foundation. *IDF Patient and Family Handbook for the Primary Immune Deficiency Diseases*, 3rd ed. Towson, MD: Immune Deficiency Foundation, 2001. (http://www.primaryimmune.org/pubs/book_pats/book_pats.htm).

Lindegren ML, Kobrynski L, Rasmussen SA, et al. Applying public health strategies to primary immunodeficiency diseases: a potential approach to genetic disorders. *MMWR Recomm Rep* 2004 Jan 16;53:1.

Rosenzweig SD, Holland SM. Phagocyte immunodeficiencies and their infections. *J Allergy Clin Immunol* 2004;113:620.

Shearer WT, Rosenblatt HM, Gelman RS, et al; Pediatric AIDS Clinical Trials Group. Lymphocyte subsets in healthy children from birth through 18 years of age: the Pediatric AIDS Clinical Trials Group P1009 study. *J Allergy Clin Immunol* 2003;112:973.

Stiehm ER, Ochs HD, Winkelstein JA, eds. *Immunologic disorders in infants and children*, 5th ed. Philadelphia: WB Saunders, 2004.

Wen L, Atkinson JP, Giclas PC. Clinical and laboratory evaluation of complement deficiency. *J Allergy Clin Immunol* 2004;113:585.

CHAPTER 428 ■ DISORDERS OF HUMORAL IMMUNITY

HOWARD M. LEDERMAN

Antibodies play a critical role in the host's defense against infection. Many of the protective functions of antibody, such as neutralization of viruses and toxins and inhibition of microbial adherence, can be performed without the participation of other components of the immune system. In addition, antibody-mediated functions exist, such as the activation of complement and the ability to opsonize foreign particles for phagocytosis, that depend on the recruitment of nonspecific host defense mechanisms. Together, these effector mechanisms form a defense network that is particularly effective against a variety of extracellular pathogens. Most notably, these include encapsulated bacteria such as *Haemophilus influenzae* and *Streptococcus pneumoniae*. Antibody also participates in the host defense against many viruses. Humoral immunity generally is not as important in the host's defense against intracellular bacteria (e.g., mycobacteria), fungi, or protozoa. The biologic significance of antibody in host defense against microorganisms is defined largely by the recognition of the specific infections that occur in patients with inborn errors of humoral immunity. This chapter discusses six such disorders.

X-LINKED AGAMMAGLOBULINEMIA

Pathophysiology

X-linked agammaglobulinemia (X-LA) is the prototypic disorder of humoral immunity. Male patients with this disease have severe panhypogammaglobulinemia, with little or no humoral immune function, but they have normal cell-mediated immunity. These patients have B-lymphocyte precursors (pre–B cells), but do not have mature B lymphocytes or plasma cells. T lymphocytes and all other components of the immune system are normal.

X-LA is caused by a mutation of the gene encoding a cytoplasmic tyrosine kinase (Bruton's tyrosine kinase). This protein is essential for the process by which B cells differentiate, and the absence of Bruton's tyrosine kinase results in a developmental arrest of B-lymphocyte maturation at the pre–B cell stage. The defective gene has been mapped to the X chromosome and, interestingly, an effect on B-lymphocyte differentiation is observed in female carriers of X-LA, all of whom are immunologically normal. Generally, the inactivation of one X chromosome occurs at random in female cells. However, among carriers for X-LA, all mature B lymphocytes have inactivated the abnormal X chromosome, because lack of expression of the normal gene blocks B-cell differentiation. In fact, an analysis of X chromosome activation patterns of peripheral blood can be used to determine carrier status.

Differential Diagnosis

The differential diagnosis of panhypogammaglobulinemia in infancy includes transient hypogammaglobulinemia of infancy, common variable immunodeficiency, immunoglobulin deficiency with increased IgM, combined immunodeficiency disorders, and rare cases of human immunodeficiency virus (HIV) infection. A quantitation of B and T lymphocytes in peripheral blood helps distinguish among these possibilities. Boys with X-LA have normal numbers of T lymphocytes but have no detectable B lymphocytes. In contrast, infants with transient hypogammaglobulinemia or common variable immunodeficiency generally have normal numbers of B and T lymphocytes; children with severe combined immunodeficiency have decreased numbers of T lymphocytes with normal, decreased, or increased numbers of B cells; and children with HIV infection have decreased numbers of CD4+ T lymphocytes.

Clinical Manifestations and Complications

Boys with X-LA usually are protected by transplacentally acquired maternal IgG for the first 3 to 4 months of life. Thereafter, chronic and recurrent infections are the predominant clinical manifestation of X-LA. Otitis media, pneumonia, diarrhea, and sinusitis occur most often, usually in combination. Clues to the diagnosis of immunodeficiency include the chronic or recurrent nature of infections and the occurrence of those infections at more than one anatomic site. *S. pneumoniae, H. influenzae,* and *Staphylococcus aureus* are the most frequently identified bacterial pathogens, but nontypeable, unencapsulated *H. influenzae, Salmonellae, Pseudomonas,* and *Mycoplasma* infections occur with increased frequency, as do certain specific viral infections. Infections are not limited to mucosal surfaces. Bacterial meningitis, sepsis, and osteomyelitis occur in as many as 10% to 15% of untreated patients. Other sentinel symptoms that should prompt consideration of X-LA include the presentation of oligoarticular arthritis or dermatomyositis in a young boy. A helpful sign on physical examination, related to the absence of B lymphocytes, is the finding of hypoplastic or absent tonsils, adenoids, and lymph nodes.

Enterovirus infections are a particularly difficult problem in patients with X-LA. This group of viruses (coxsackie, enteric cytopathogenic human orphan [ECHO], and polio) tends to cause chronic diarrhea, hepatitis, pneumonitis, and meningoencephalitis in patients with X-LA. In some instances, the infection takes the form of a dermatomyositis-like syndrome consisting of rash, edema of subcutaneous tissue, and muscle weakness. Enterovirus infections often are fatal in patients with X-LA, although therapy with extremely high doses of gamma globulin containing virus-specific antibodies has been helpful.

Therapy

The management of patients with X-LA includes the use of gamma globulin prophylaxis and an aggressive approach to the diagnosis and therapy of febrile or inflammatory illnesses. Early recognition of the disease and adequate gamma globulin replacement leads to a good prognosis in most patients. Although no controlled studies exist, gamma globulin prophylaxis appears to be most effective in patients who have not yet incurred structural damage to target organs of the respiratory or gastrointestinal tract, and when trough IgG levels are in the physiologic range. Nevertheless, chronic infections of paranasal sinuses and/or the lungs develop in approximately 50% of X-LA patients, particularly those who had severe, recurrent, or chronic infections before the recognition of immune deficiency and initiation of gamma globulin prophylaxis. Gamma globulin therapy should allow normal or near-normal growth velocity. Persistently impaired linear growth should prompt an evaluation of growth hormone levels because X-LA has occurred in association with growth hormone deficiency in a few kindreds. Most reported deaths of X-LA patients are attributed to recurrent lower respiratory tract infections with resulting chronic pulmonary disease or to chronic enterovirus infections. Early diagnosis is critical, so that gamma globulin therapy can be initiated before the onset of any of these problems and to provide families with appropriate genetic counseling. Bone marrow stem-cell transplants without a preparative regimen generally have not been successful.

COMMON VARIABLE IMMUNODEFICIENCY

Pathophysiology

The phrase *common variable immunodeficiency* (CVID) describes a heterogeneous group of disorders characterized by hypogammaglobulinemia. In distinction from X-LA, B lymphocytes frequently are found in the peripheral blood of patients with CVID, and the hypogammaglobulinemia may be less profound. Additional immunologic abnormalities, such as T-cell dysfunction and autoimmune diseases, are expressed variably. Many patients with CVID appear to have defects intrinsic to the B lymphocyte, but other patients have excessive T-lymphocyte suppressor function, inadequate T-lymphocyte helper function, or anti–B-lymphocyte antibodies. Most patients do not manifest symptoms until after the first decade of life, but some patients present in early childhood or infancy. It has long been assumed that patients with CVID have acquired hypogammaglobulinemia, although only a few reports exist in which the transition from normal gamma globulin levels to hypogammaglobulinemia is documented. No recognizable pattern of inheritance exists in most patients, but other disorders of humoral immunity (e.g., IgA deficiency and transient hypogammaglobulinemia of infancy) occur at higher frequency among family members of patients with CVID than among the general population.

It has become increasingly apparent that the clinical phenotype of CVID can be the result of a wide variety of immunologic abnormalities. For example, genetic analyses have identified mutations of *Btk* (the gene causing XLA), *SH2D1A* (the gene causing the X-linked lymphoproliferative syndrome) and *ICOS* (the "inducible stimulator" on activated T cells) among small numbers of individuals previously identified as having CVID. It is likely that such analyses will help to define subgroups of CVID patients who differ in presentation and outcome, and perhaps lead to novel therapies.

Clinical Manifestations and Complications

As in X-LA, the most frequent manifestations of CVID are chronic or recurrent infections of the upper and lower respiratory tracts. Recurrent pneumonia, chronic bronchitis, and sinusitis occur in the majority of patients and some eventually develop chronic pulmonary dysfunction. Most of the identified respiratory tract pathogens are encapsulated bacteria. An almost equal incidence of obstructive and restrictive lung disease occurs. Somewhat in contrast to patients with X-LA, in patients with CVID, disease of the gastrointestinal tract occurs with almost equal frequency as disease of the respiratory tract. As many as 30% to 60% of patients with CVID have chronic diarrhea. An infectious agent is identified in approximately one-half of patients; many of the others have idiopathic inflammatory bowel diseases. The most frequently documented gastrointestinal pathogen is *Giardia lamblia*. Bacterial overgrowth of the small bowel is an important cause of chronic diarrhea in patients with CVID; enteroviruses are a problem less frequently.

Patients with CVID have a variety of associated disorders for which no infectious etiology has been established. These disorders may be the result of infections caused by unidentified pathogens, but many are believed to be autoimmune in origin, perhaps the result of the same disordered immunoregulation that is presumed to be responsible for the development of hypogammaglobulinemia. Gastrointestinal and hematologic disorders predominate. Chronic idiopathic diarrhea is the single biggest problem. Intestinal biopsy samples typically demonstrate nodular lymphoid hyperplasia as well as villous blunting and epithelial atrophy in the small bowel. Inflammatory bowel diseases, achlorhydria, and pernicious anemia occur with significant frequency. Hematologic abnormalities include the development of persistent splenomegaly, immune thrombocytopenia, leukopenia, and autoimmune hemolytic anemia. Curiously, a few patients have developed a clinical picture typical of sarcoidosis, with granulomatous lesions and elevated angiotensin-converting enzyme levels, although without the hypergammaglobulinemia typically found in patients with sarcoidosis. Patients who present with CVID in infancy and early childhood often have particularly severe problems with autoimmune and chronic inflammatory disorders, resulting in a mortality rate that exceeds 50%. An increased susceptibility to malignancy (particularly thymoma and lymphoma) is present in adults with CVID, but the risk in children is not known.

Therapy

The treatment of the immunodeficiency is the same as for those individuals with X-LA: replacement with gamma globulin and aggressive management of infections. The management of autoimmune disease through the use of antiinflammatory and immunosuppressive drugs is necessary, but may complicate the problems that these individuals have with infections.

SELECTIVE IgA DEFICIENCY

By convention, the diagnosis of selective IgA deficiency is established when a patient has a serum IgA level of less than 5 mg/dL, with normal levels of other immunoglobulin classes, normal serum antibody responses, and normal cell-mediated immunity. Selective IgA deficiency is the most prevalent primary immunodeficiency disease, occurring in approximately 1 of 600 individuals. Usually, no recognized pattern of inheritance occurs, although the incidence of selective IgA deficiency is higher in families with other disorders of lymphocyte function. IgA deficiency also has been associated with certain HLA haplotypes and the 18q deletion syndrome.

Pathophysiology

IgA has several unique biologic features. Although IgA makes up only 15% of the immunoglobulin in serum, it is the predominant immunoglobulin class on the mucosal surfaces of the gastrointestinal and respiratory tracts. IgA is secreted onto mucosal surfaces as a macromolecular complex consisting of two IgA molecules joined to a J chain and a secretory component. The majority of patients with IgA deficiency lack both serum and secretory IgA, but rare cases occur in which a deficiency of secretory, but not serum, IgA occurs. Unlike the other major serum immunoglobulin classes, IgG and IgM, IgA is largely silent as a mediator of inflammatory responses. IgA provides an antimicrobial defense by inhibiting microbial adherence and neutralizing viruses and toxins. It also has an important role in antigen clearance, thus excluding soluble antigens from penetrating the mucosa and entering the systemic circulation. The unique biologic features of IgA may help to explain the clinical associations of IgA deficiency with infection, atopic disease, and rheumatic disorders.

Clinical Manifestations and Complications

Some patients with selective IgA deficiency are more susceptible to infection, although disagreement exists about the relative risk of infection that IgA deficiency imposes on the host. Among patients referred to tertiary-care centers for the evaluation of recurrent sinopulmonary infections, the incidence of IgA deficiency is significantly higher compared with that of the general population. However, many apparently asymptomatic individuals have been identified as IgA deficient using population-based screening. As might be expected by its role as the predominant secretory immunoglobulin, the most common infections in IgA-deficient patients occur on mucosal surfaces. Otitis media, sinusitis, bronchitis, pneumonia, and diarrhea are common; meningitis and bacterial sepsis are rare. In some series, as many as 50% of patients with selective IgA deficiency have chronic respiratory tract infections. A subgroup of IgA-deficient patients have additional deficiencies of the IgG subclasses IgG2 and IgG4. Studies suggest that these IgA-deficient patients tend to experience the most severe and chronic sinopulmonary infections. Because IgG subclass deficiencies are treatable (see following section), IgG subclass determinations and the measurement of IgG antibody responses should be included in the evaluation of all IgA-deficient patients. The second major target for infections in IgA-deficient patients is the gastrointestinal tract. Chronic diarrhea is often idiopathic; *Giardia* is the most frequently identified pathogen.

Atopic diseases such as allergic rhinitis, asthma, urticaria, eczema, and food allergy have been reported to occur in as many as 50% of patients with selective IgA deficiency. Lack of secretory IgA has been postulated to allow inhaled and ingested antigens to penetrate the mucosal epithelium and to elicit antibody responses in the bronchial and gastrointestinal lymphoid tissues. The development of anaphylactic reactions after the infusion of plasma or gamma globulin is a particularly hazardous allergic reaction in IgA-deficient patients.

A variety of autoimmune and rheumatic diseases have been associated with selective IgA deficiency. These include juvenile rheumatoid arthritis, systemic lupus erythematosus, thyroiditis, gluten-sensitive enteropathy, ulcerative colitis, Crohn disease, and pernicious anemia, among others. A unifying etiology to explain the association of these disorders with selective IgA deficiency has not been established. It has been hypothesized that penetration of environmental antigens may lead to the production of antibodies with specificity for self, or that disordered immunoregulation underlies both IgA deficiency and autoimmune disease.

Children with low but not absent IgA (5 to 10 mg/dL) share many of the same disease manifestations, but they tend to be less severely affected. Furthermore, in longitudinal studies, it has been observed that serum IgA levels increase to within the normal range in more than one-half of these less severe cases and, concomitantly, symptoms cease.

Therapy

Immunoglobulin therapy generally is contraindicated in selective IgA deficiency. Commercial gamma globulin preparations contain trace amounts of IgA, which are insufficient to provide replacement therapy but are sufficient to sensitize the patient to IgA, thereby inducing an IgG or IgE anti-IgA antibody response. This development is a relative and not an absolute contraindication to gamma globulin therapy. Patients with IgA deficiency and associated IgG subclass deficiencies who have recurrent infections may benefit from immunoglobulin prophylaxis. In such cases, an intravenous gamma globulin preparation that contains less than 0.01 g/L of IgA can be used, but with caution.

IgG SUBCLASS DEFICIENCIES

Pathophysiology

Four subclasses of IgG exist that differ somewhat in their biologic activities. IgG1, IgG2, and IgG3 fix complement, bind to Fc receptors on monocytes, and participate in antibody-dependent cellular cytotoxicity; IgG4 does not. The IgG response to protein antigens occurs predominantly within the IgG1 and IgG3 subclasses, whereas the IgG response to polysaccharide antigens generally is restricted to the IgG2 and IgG4 subclasses. Because antibodies to the polysaccharide capsules of bacteria such as *S. pneumoniae* and *H. influenzae* are important for host defense, deficiencies of IgG2 and IgG4 may predispose the host to infections caused by these and other encapsulated bacteria.

Clinical Manifestations and Diagnosis

Deficiencies of IgG subclasses have been described in association with other primary immunodeficiency diseases, such as selective IgA deficiency, ataxia-telangiectasia, and Wiskott-Aldrich syndrome. Isolated IgG subclass deficiencies have been identified only fairly recently. The clue to the diagnosis is often the presence of borderline or low-normal total serum IgG levels in a patient with recurrent sinopulmonary infections. In such individuals, further tests should include a quantitation of IgG subclasses and a measurement of antibody responses to T-dependent (e.g., diphtheria and tetanus toxoids) and T-independent (e.g., pneumococcal polysaccharide) vaccines.

Protein-polysaccharide conjugated vaccines (e.g., those currently used to immunize infants and young children to *H. influenzae* type b and *S. pneumoniae*) induce antibody responses in the same subclasses as protein antigen and cannot be used in place of pure polysaccharide vaccines for this purpose.

Therapy

Some patients with selective deficiency of IgG2, IgG3, or IgG4, or deficiencies of IgG2 and IgG4, have recurrent pyogenic infections of the respiratory tract. They may benefit from antibiotic prophylaxis or therapy with gamma globulin, but formal studies documenting efficacy are lacking. In general, gamma globulin therapy should be reserved for those patients who have a documented deficiency of antibody production and should not be used for patients with an IgG subclass deficiency and normal antibody responses to T-dependent and T-independent vaccine antigens.

HYPER-IgM SYNDROMES

Pathophysiology

Naïve B lymphocytes express IgM and IgD at the cell surface, and antibodies of the IgM class are the first to be produced during a humoral immune response. Under normal circumstances, prolonged or repeated exposure to antigen induces B lymphocytes to undergo class switch and somatic hypermutation. These processes lead to the secretion of high-affinity IgG, IgA, and/or IgE antibodies, and to the generation of memory B lymphocytes. Patients with the hyper-IgM syndrome (HIGM) have an inability to undergo class switch and somatic hypermutation. As a result, they have normal or elevated serum IgM and IgD levels but generally are deficient in other immunoglobulin classes, and they have few, if any, memory B cells. In infancy, it may be difficult to distinguish HIGM from X-LA or CVID because IgM is not consistently elevated in the first few months of life. Later, the marked elevation in IgM may mask the IgG deficiency if total gamma globulin is measured only by serum protein electrophoresis. Patients have peripheral blood B cells bearing immunoglobulin on their surface, and plasma cells are present in bone marrow and lymphoid tissues. However, most such cells express surface IgM; IgG- and IgA-bearing B lymphocytes are severely decreased. Antibody responses to immunization may be present, but are predominantly or exclusively of the IgM class.

Four genetically determined causes for HIGM are known, and each has slightly different clinical features that can be explained by the differences in underlying pathophysiology.

Hyper-IgM Types 1 and 3

One X-linked form of hyper-IgM deficiency (HIGM1) is caused by mutations of CD40 ligand (a membrane protein expressed on the surface of activated T lymphocytes) and one autosomal recessive form (HIGM3) is caused by mutations of CD40 (a membrane protein expressed on B lymphocytes, monocytes, dendritic cells, and myeloid precursor cells). Under normal circumstances, the mutual interaction of B and T lymphocytes via CD40–CD40 ligand binding causes a class switch of the B lymphocyte and facilitates the activation of the T lymphocyte. Neither process occurs efficiently in the absence of CD40 or CD40 ligand. Because antibody production is severely impaired, patients with HIGM1 and HIGM3 suffer from infections with the same pyogenic bacteria and viruses that cause problems in patients with X-LA. However, the added problem with T lymphocyte activation predisposes patients to a significant incidence of infections caused by opportunistic pathogens such as *Pneumocystis carinii, Cryptococcus neoformans, Cryptosporidium,* and *Mycobacteria.* Patients with HIGM1 and HIGM3 also have a significant risk for developing neutropenia, sclerosing cholangitis, lymphoid hyperplasia, and malignancy, but the mechanisms for these abnormalities are not fully understood.

Hyper-IgM Type 2

An autosomal recessive form of hyper-IgM deficiency (HIGM2) is caused by mutations of activation-induced cytidine deam-

inase, an enzyme expressed only in germinal-center B lymphocytes undergoing class switch and somatic hypermutation. These patients develop severe or recurrent pyogenic bacterial and viral infections, lymphoid hyperplasia, and problems with autoimmune disease. They do not exhibit T lymphocyte abnormalities in laboratory studies, and they do not develop opportunistic infections.

Hyper-IgM Type 4

HIGM4 is caused by hypomorphic mutations of NEMO-IKKγ, a protein involved in the regulation of the cytokine gene transcription factor NFκB. This immunodeficiency is associated with hypohidrotic ectodermal dysplasia and is inherited as an X-linked recessive trait. Antibody responses to bacterial polysaccharides and natural killer cell cytotoxicity are impaired, and the clinical features resemble those of HIGM1 and HIGM3.

TRANSIENT HYPOGAMMAGLOBULINEMIA OF INFANCY

Pathophysiology

Transient hypogammaglobulinemia is an ill-defined disorder of infants in whom the delayed acquisition of normal serum immunoglobulin levels occurs. Transient hypogammaglobulinemia is a diagnosis that can be established only in retrospect, after immunoglobulin levels become normal. Some patients who initially appear to have transient hypogammaglobulinemia in infancy continue to have persistent abnormalities of humoral immunity and eventually are classified as having CVID, immunodeficiency with increased IgM, or selective IgA deficiency.

Clinical Manifestation and Complications

Two broad groups of infants have been identified with transient hypogammaglobulinemia. The first includes children who have had serum immunoglobulins measured because they have recurrent infections, chronic diarrhea, or other symptoms attributable to immunodeficiency. The second group includes infants who may have had no symptoms attributable to hypogammaglobulinemia, but were evaluated prospectively because they had first-degree relatives with immunodeficiency. Other asymptomatic babies without a family history of immunodeficiency may not be recognized as having hypogammaglobulinemia but have a somewhat delayed acquisition of serum immunoglobulin levels. A controversy exists as to whether transient hypogammaglobulinemia of infancy should be considered an immunodeficiency disease or a developmental variant.

Most symptomatic patients with transient hypogammaglobulinemia have chronic or recurrent infections of the respiratory and gastrointestinal tracts. Bacterial sepsis, meningitis, and other systemic infections are rare. Atopic diseases, including eczema and asthma, also have been reported in some but not all series.

The immunologic evaluation of infants with transient hypogammaglobulinemia discloses a variable degree of panhypogammaglobulinemia and reduced antibody responses, but normal numbers of peripheral blood B lymphocytes. For a period of months or as long as 3 to 4 years, immunoglobulin levels remain low, then eventually increase to within the normal range. Antibody titers to previously administered vaccines (e.g., diphtheria and tetanus toxoids) often become detectable and indicate a resolution of the transient defect before serum immunoglobulin levels increase. Invasive infection or low tetanus antibody responses at presentation may be predictive of a persistent immunologic defect.

Therapy

Almost all children with transient hypogammaglobulinemia of infancy can be managed symptomatically, without the need for gamma globulin. Prophylactic antibiotics are sometimes useful for managing recurrent sinopulmonary infections. Chronic diarrhea often is caused by malabsorption, presumed to be the result of a previous acute infection, and is treated most quickly with dietary management. In the rare patient in whom symptoms do not respond to conservative measures, gamma globulin therapy may be considered. More important, the diagnosis should be reconsidered for that patient.

GENERAL PRINCIPLES OF THERAPY

As a general rule, the mainstay of therapy for disorders of humoral immunity is the replacement of the missing antibody by gamma globulin. Several limitations exist, however, on the extent to which pooled exogenous gamma globulin can replace antibody actively produced by the host. First, the antibodies provided are related to the previous antigenic exposure of the donor pool and do not necessarily reflect the exposure of a particular patient to a particular microorganism. For common organisms such as *H. influenzae*, this may have little therapeutic importance, but for organisms encountered infrequently in the general community, it may represent a major deficiency. The second limitation is inherent in the purification process used to prepare gamma globulin, which results in preparations containing virtually IgG only. These preparations contain insufficient amounts of IgA or IgM to provide replacement, and they contain almost no secretory IgA. Although insufficient IgA exists to provide replacement, enough IgA exists to serve as an antigen in IgA-deficient patients, thus making repeated gamma globulin infusions difficult or dangerous for some patients with selective IgA deficiency.

Administration of Gamma Globulins

Different gamma globulin preparations are available for intravenous, slow subcutaneous, and intramuscular administration. No one form is inherently more effective than another; efficacy appears to be a function of the serum level attained, regardless of the route or preparation used. Virtually all patients should be managed with intravenous or subcutaneous infusions, because the volume limitations of intramuscular injections prevents the delivery of adequate gamma globulin by this route. No universally accepted standard dose of gamma globulin exists. The minimum dosage is 300 to 400 mg/kg/month, but many patients require larger or more frequent doses. Both the dose and dosing interval should be adjusted for each patient to provide adequate prophylaxis of symptoms. For some patients, maintaining a trough serum IgG concentration of 400 mg/dL may be sufficient to control symptoms, but others may require substantially higher levels. In this regard, control of symptoms should be defined in the pediatric population as prophylaxis against infections and maintenance of normal growth velocity.

Most differences among gamma globulin preparations relate to the composition of the final product for infusion, such as sugar and sodium content, osmolality, pH level, and IgA content. These differences are sometimes clinically important. For example, the use of high osmolality intravenous Ig (IVIG) products has been associated with acute renal failure and thrombosis. This has been a particular problem among patients with pre-existing renal disease or coagulation disorders, and in those receiving rapid infusions of high-dose IVIG. In addition, individual patients have variable tolerability for one product versus another, for reasons that are generally not defined.

Risks of Gamma-Globulin Therapy

The major risk in the use of gamma globulin is the possibility of transmitting a blood-borne pathogen. The plasma fractionation process used to prepare gamma globulin has been tested and approved with regard to its ability to inactivate HIV at concentrations far exceeding those that have been found in any patient's serum. To date, no cases of HIV transmission have been linked to use of a gamma globulin product. However, outbreaks of hepatitis C have been caused by contaminated lots of intravenous gamma globulin preparations. New procedures, such as the addition of a solvent or detergent or the process of pasteurization, have been introduced to decrease this problem, but the possibility of disease transmission always must be considered when weighing the potential risks and benefits of gamma globulin use.

Complications

It is important to note that, despite what is currently considered optimal gamma globulin replacement therapy and aggressive treatment of acute infections, a significant percentage of antibody-deficient patients eventually develop chronic lung and/or sinus disease. The onset of these problems often is insidious. Therefore, pulmonary status should be monitored using spirometry and/or high-resolution computed tomography (CT) every 1 to 2 years, even in asymptomatic individuals.

Suggested Readings

Conley ME, Howard V. Clinical findings leading to the diagnosis of X-linked agammaglobulinemia. *J Pediatr* 2002;141:566.

Conley ME, Park CL, Douglas SD. Childhood common variable immunodeficiency with autoimmune disease. *J Pediatr* 1986;108:915.

Cunningham-Rundles C, Bodian C. Common variable immunodeficiency: clinical and immunological features of 248 patients. *Clin Immunol* 1999;92:34.

Cunningham-Rundles C. Physiology of IgA and IgA deficiency. *J Clin Immunol* 2001;21:303.

Dalal I, Reid B, Nisbet-Brown E, Roifman CM. The outcome of patients with hypogammaglobulinemia in infancy and early childhood. *J Pediatr* 1998;133:144.

Gulino AV, Notarangelo LD. Hyper IgM syndromes. *Curr Opin Rheumatol* 2003;15:422.

Hausser C, Virelizier JL, Buriot D, Griscelli C. Common variable hypogammaglobulinemia in children: clinical and immunologic observations in 30 patients. *Am J Dis Child* 1983;137:833.

Plebani A, Soresina A, Rondelli R, et al; Italian Pediatric Group for XLA-AIEOP. Clinical, immunological, and molecular analysis in a large cohort of patients with X-linked agammaglobulinemia: an Italian multicenter study. *Clin Immunol* 2002;104:221.

Quartier P, Debre M, De Blic J, et al. Early and prolonged intravenous immunoglobulin replacement therapy in childhood agammaglobulinemia: a retrospective survey of 31 patients. *J Pediatr* 1999;134:589.

Shackelford PG. IgG subclasses: Importance in pediatric practice. *Pediatr Rev* 1993;14:291.

Stiehm ER. Human intravenous immunoglobulin in primary and secondary antibody deficiencies. *Pediatr Infect Dis J* 1997;16:696.

Winkelstein JA, Marino MC, Ochs H, et al. The X-linked hyper-IgM syndrome: clinical and immunologic features of 79 patients. *Medicine* 2003;82:373.

CHAPTER 429 ■ COMPLEMENT DEFICIENCIES

JERRY A. WINKELSTEIN

The complement system is composed of a series of plasma proteins and cellular receptors that, when functioning in an ordered and integrated fashion, serve as important mediators of host defense and inflammation. Although the complement system was first described at the turn of the twentieth century, it was not until 1960 that the first patient with a genetically determined complement deficiency was identified. Since then, deficiencies have been described for nearly all components of the complement system (Table 429.1).

CLINICAL MANIFESTATIONS AND COMPLICATIONS

Individuals with genetically determined complement deficiencies have a variety of clinical presentations. Most patients present with an increased susceptibility to infection, some with a variety of rheumatic diseases, others with angioedema and, in some instances, some patients may be asymptomatic.

Increased Susceptibility to Infection

An increased susceptibility to infection is a prominent clinical finding in most patients with complement deficiencies. The kinds of infections relate to the biologic functions of those components that are missing. For example, the third component of complement (C3) is an important opsonic ligand. Therefore, patients with a deficiency of C3, or of a component of either of the two pathways that activate C3, are more susceptible to infections caused by encapsulated bacteria for which opsonization is the primary host defense (e.g., *Streptococcus pneumoniae, Streptococcus pyogenes,* and *Haemophilus influenzae*).

Similarly, C5 through C9 form the membrane attack complex and are responsible for the bactericidal functions of complement. Thus, patients with deficiencies of C5, C6, C7, C8, or C9 are susceptible to gram-negative bacteria, notably *Neisseria* species, because serum bactericidal activity is an important host defense against these organisms.

A number of studies have examined groups of patients with specific infectious diseases to determine the frequency of complement deficiencies in these infections and to evaluate the utility of screening for complement deficiencies. Between 5% and 15% of unselected patients with systemic meningococcal infections have a genetically determined complement deficiency. The differing estimates may reflect differences in populations examined. In general, the prevalence is higher if the patient has had recurrent meningococcal disease, has a positive family history for meningococcal disease, or is infected with an uncommon meningococcal serotype. Therefore, it seems reasonable to screen children with systemic meningococcal infections for the presence of a complement deficiency. In contrast, although many patients with complement deficiencies present with systemic pneumococcal or *H. influenzae* infections, the prevalence of complement deficiencies in patients with these specific infections appears to be quite low. Therefore, recommending routine screening for complement deficiencies in patients with bacteremia or meningitis caused by pneumococcus or *H. influenzae* is more difficult to justify.

Rheumatic Diseases

Patients with complement deficiencies also have a variety of clinical conditions that can be described best as rheumatic diseases. These include disorders that resemble systemic lupus

TABLE 429.1

GENETICALLY DETERMINED COMPLEMENT DEFICIENCIES

Deficiency	Inheritance	Major Clinical Manifestation
C1q	Autosomal recessive	Rheumatic disorders and pyogenic infections
C1r/s	Autosomal recessive	Rheumatic disorders
C4	Autosomal recessive	Rheumatic disorders and pyogenic infections
C2	Autosomal recessive	Rheumatic disorders and pyogenic intections
C3	Autosomal recessive	Pyogenic infections
C5	Autosomal recessive	Meningococcal sepsis and meningitis
C6	Autosomal recessive	Meningococcal sepsis and meningitis
C7	Autosomal recessive	Meningococcal sepsis and meningitis
C8	Autosomal recessive	Meningococcal sepsis and meningitis
C9	Autosomal recessive	Meningococcal sepsis and meningitis
Factor I	Autosomal recessive	Pyogenic infections
Factor H	Autosomal recessive	Hemolytic uremic syndrome
Properdin	X-linked recessive	Meningococcal sepsis and meningitis
C1 esterase inhibitor	Autosomal dominant	Angioedema

erythematosus (SLE) as well as glomerulonephritis, dermatomyositis, anaphylactoid purpura, and vasculitis. The prevalence of these inflammatory disorders is highest in those patients with deficiencies of the classical activating pathway (C1, C4, and C2) and of C3. The pathophysiologic basis for the occurrence of these diseases in complement-deficient patients may relate in part to the physiologic role of the complement system in processing immune complexes or its role in the clearance of apoptotic cells.

Some important differences exist between the rheumatic diseases seen in complement-deficient patients and their counterparts in non–complement-deficient individuals. For example, the SLE-like illness seen in complement-deficient individuals often is characterized by onset in childhood, skin lesions resembling discoid lupus, and relatively limited renal and pleuropericardial involvement. In addition, complement-deficient individuals with the lupus-like syndrome may have absent or low titers of antinuclear antibodies and negative lupus preparations. In contrast, their incidence of anti-Ro antibodies is significantly higher than in non–complement-deficient patients with lupus. Thus, complement-deficient patients with the lupus-like syndrome resemble a subgroup of lupus patients who have subacute, cutaneous lupus.

Angioedema

Patients with a deficiency of one of the control proteins of the classical pathway, C1 esterase inhibitor, usually present with angioedema of the skin or mucous membranes (see following discussion). No large studies have examined the prevalence of C1 esterase inhibitor deficiency in patients with angioedema.

Asymptomatic

Some patients with genetically determined complement deficiencies are relatively asymptomatic, never having developed a serious infection or a rheumatic disorder. These asymptomatic patients usually are ascertained as a consequence of screening family members of complement-deficient patients who themselves have been ascertained because of clinically significant problems.

SPECIFIC DISORDERS

Complement Deficiencies

C1q Deficiency

Two distinct forms of C1q deficiency exist. In one form, C1q cannot be detected through either functional or immunochemical analysis. In the other form, immunochemical C1q is present, but it lacks functional activity (i.e., it is dysfunctional). The dysfunctional C1q is antigenically deficient, and it does not interact with either IgG or C1r and C1s. The most common clinical presentation of either form of C1q deficiency has been a lupus-like syndrome. Some patients also have had an increased susceptibility to infection, manifested by bacterial sepsis or meningitis.

C1r/C1s Deficiency

Genetically determined deficiency of C1r is characterized by a marked reduction of C1r (less than 1% of normal) and a moderate reduction of C1s (20% to 50% of normal). The basis for the association of the moderately reduced levels of C1s with

the absence of C1r in these patients is unknown. C1r and C1s are structurally and functionally similar and have close genetic linkage. The clinical presentation of C1r/C1s deficiency has included both a lupus-like illness and glomerulonephritis.

C4 Deficiency

Two loci (C4A and C4B) within the major histocompatibility complex (MHC) encode for C4. Although the products of the two loci share some functional, structural, and antigenic characteristics that identify them as C4, they each possess unique epitopes and differences in electrophoretic mobility and specific functional activity. Patients with total C4 deficiency are homozygous deficient at both loci and have severely depressed serum levels of both antigenic and functional C4 (less than 1%). Those serum activities that depend on C3 and C5 through C9 and can be mediated via activation of the alternative pathway, such as opsonic, chemotactic, and bactericidal activities, are present but reduced, because of a lack of an intact classical pathway. The predominant clinical manifestation of complete C4 deficiency has been an SLE-like illness, characterized by photosensitive skin rashes, renal disease, and occasionally arthritis. Although some patients are more susceptible to infection, these are patients in whom the SLE-like illness also is present.

Although complete C4 deficiency is rare, individuals who are homozygous deficient for either C4A or C4B are relatively common. Approximately 1% of the population is homozygous deficient in C4A and 3% of the population is deficient in C4B. As mentioned, C4A and C4B differ somewhat; C4A interacts more efficiently with proteins, and C4B interacts more efficiently with carbohydrates. Because of these functional differences, it has been suggested that individuals who are deficient in one isotype might be predisposed to certain illnesses. For example, individuals who lack C4A might not be able to clear protein-containing immune complexes normally and may be more susceptible to immune-complex diseases, such as SLE. In fact, the prevalence of homozygous C4A deficiency in SLE is between 10% and 15%, a prevalence at least ten times higher than that in the general population. Individuals who are deficient in C4B lack the isotype that is most efficient in interacting with polysaccharides. They might not be able to assemble the classical pathway C3-cleaving enzyme on bacterial polysaccharide capsules and may be more susceptible to blood-borne bacterial infections. In fact, the prevalence of C4B deficiency is increased in children with bacteremia and meningitis.

C2 Deficiency

A deficiency of C2 is the most common of the inherited complement deficiencies. Homozygous deficiency of C2 occurs as frequently as 1 in 10,000 individuals. Complement-mediated serum activities such as opsonization and chemotaxis are present in patients with C2 deficiency, presumably because their alternative pathway is intact, although these activities are not generated as quickly or to the same degree as in individuals with an intact classical pathway. The clinical manifestations of C2 deficiency vary from individuals who are asymptomatic to individuals who are clinically affected with either an increased susceptibility to infection, rheumatic diseases, or both. The infections are mostly blood-borne and systemic (e.g., sepsis, meningitis, arthritis, and osteomyelitis) and caused by encapsulated bacteria. A variety of rheumatic diseases are associated with C2 deficiency. The most common are disorders that resemble SLE and discoid lupus. Glomerulonephritis, dermatomyositis, anaphylactoid purpura, and vasculitis also have been seen.

C3 Deficiency

Patients with C3 deficiency generally have less than 1% of the normal amount of C3 in their serum. Those serum activities either directly dependent on C3 (opsonization) or indirectly dependent on C3 because of its role in the activation of C5 through C9 (chemotaxis and bactericidal activity) also are markedly reduced. The clinical manifestations of C3 deficiency in humans include increased susceptibility to infection and rheumatic disorders. Patients with C3 deficiency have a variety of infections, including pneumonia, bacteremia, meningitis, and osteomyelitis, caused by encapsulated pyogenic bacteria. A number of patients have presented with arthralgias and vasculitic skin rashes and a clinical picture consistent with SLE. Renal disease also has been seen in C3-deficient patients. Histologically, the lesions most closely resemble membranoproliferative glomerulonephritis.

C5 Deficiency

Genetically determined C5 deficiency has been identified in a number of different families. The sera of patients with C5 deficiency have markedly reduced levels of C5 and are unable, therefore, to generate normal amounts of chemotactic or bactericidal activity. Serum opsonic activity is intact because activation of C3 can proceed without participation of C5. Although the initial patient identified as C5 deficient had SLE and membranoproliferative glomerulonephritis, subsequent patients have had either meningococcal meningitis or disseminated gonococcal infections.

C6 Deficiency

The only abnormality relating to the complement system in C6-deficient patients is a marked deficiency of serum bactericidal activity. The major clinical manifestation of C6 deficiency has been systemic neisserial infections. Although most patients have had meningococcal sepsis and meningitis, a few have had disseminated gonococcal infections.

C7 Deficiency

Only a few patients with C7 deficiency have been identified. Serum bactericidal activity has been markedly reduced in those patients in whom it has been tested. As with other deficiencies of terminal components, systemic meningococcal infections or disseminated gonococcal infections are predominant.

C8 Deficiency

Native C8 is composed of three chains (alpha, beta, and gamma). The alpha and gamma chains are covalently joined to form one subunit (C8 alpha-gamma), which is joined to the other subunit composed of the beta chain (C8 beta) by noncovalent bonds. In one form of C8 deficiency, patients lack the C8 alpha-gamma subunit, whereas in the other form, the C8 beta subunit is deficient. In either case, C8 activity is markedly reduced (less than 1% of normal). The only functional defect in C8-deficient sera is a marked reduction in bactericidal activity. The clinical presentation of C8 deficiency consists of meningococcemia, meningococcal meningitis, and disseminated gonococcal infections. SLE also has been seen rarely.

C9 Deficiency

Only a few patients with C9 deficiency have been identified. Serum hemolytic activity can be generated by a membrane attack complex composed only of C5b-8, albeit more slowly and to a lesser degree than the C5b-9 complex. Thus, patients with C9 deficiency possess some serum hemolytic and bactericidal activity. Patients with C9 deficiency have an increased susceptibility to systemic meningococcal infections, although probably not to the same degree as patients with deficiencies of the other terminal components.

Factor I Deficiency

Factor I controls the assembly and expression of the alternative pathway C3-cleaving enzyme. Factor I deficiency is characterized by uncontrolled activation of C3 via the alternative pathway because, in the absence of factor I, no control is imposed on the formation and expression of the alternative pathway C3 convertase. Patients with factor I deficiency, therefore, have a secondary consumption of C3 resulting in markedly reduced levels of native C3 in their serum. Most of the C3 is not in its native form, but rather in the form of its cleavage product, C3b. Those serum activities that directly or indirectly depend on C3 (opsonic activity, chemotactic activity, and bactericidal activity) are reduced in patients with factor I deficiency. The most common clinical expression of factor I deficiency is an increased susceptibility to infection. Organisms most commonly responsible for these infections are encapsulated, pyogenic bacteria, organisms for which C3 is an important opsonic ligand.

Factor H Deficiency

Factor H is a control protein of the alternative pathway. A deficiency of factor H has been described in only a few families. Factor H levels in the serum generally are reduced to less than 10% of normal. Both rheumatic disorders and an increased susceptibility to infection have been described in factor H deficiency.

Properdin Deficiency

Properdin stabilizes the alternative pathway enzymes that activate C3 and C5. Properdin deficiency is inherited as an X-linked recessive disorder. At least two forms of properdin deficiency occur. In one form, patients lack both antigenic and functional properdin in their serum; in the second form, antigenic properdin is present but has no functional activity. The only reported clinical manifestation of properdin deficiency is a marked increased susceptibility to systemic meningococcal infections.

C1 Esterase Inhibitor Deficiency

Pathophysiology. A genetically determined deficiency of C1 esterase inhibitor (C1-INH) is responsible for the clinical disorder hereditary angioedema (HAE). C1-INH deficiency is inherited in an autosomal dominant fashion. At least two forms of C1-INH deficiency occur. In the most common form (type I), which accounts for approximately 85% of patients, the serum of affected individuals is deficient in both C1-INH protein (5% to 30% of normal) and C1-INH activity. In the less common form (type II), a dysfunctional protein is present in normal or elevated concentrations, but its functional activity is markedly reduced. In either case, the level of C4 in serum is reduced both during and between attacks, making it a useful diagnostic clue.

The pathophysiologic mechanisms by which the absence of C1-INH activity leads to the angioedema characteristic of the disorder are still incompletely understood. Neither the mediators responsible for producing the edema nor the mechanisms initiating their production have been identified clearly, although evidence implicates both the complement system and the kinin system in the pathogenesis of the edema.

Clinical Manifestations and Complications. The clinical symptoms of HAE are the result of submucosal or subcutaneous edema. The lesions are characterized by noninflammatory edema associated with capillary and venule dilation. The three most prominent areas of involvement are the skin, respiratory tract, and gastrointestinal tract.

Attacks involving the skin may involve an extremity, the face, or genitalia. The edema may vary in size from a few centimeters to involvement of a whole extremity. The lesions are pale rather than red, usually are not warm, and are characteristically nonpruritic, although there may be a feeling of tightness in the skin caused by the accumulation of subcutaneous fluid. Attacks usually progress for 1 to 2 days and resolve over an additional 2 to 3 days.

Attacks involving the upper respiratory tract represent a serious threat to the patient with HAE. Pharyngeal edema occurs at least once in nearly two-thirds of the patients. The patients may initially experience a tightness in the throat, and swelling of the tongue, buccal mucosa, and oropharynx follow. In some instances, laryngeal edema, accompanied by hoarseness and stridor, progresses to respiratory obstruction and represents a life-threatening emergency.

The gastrointestinal tract can be affected by HAE. Symptoms are secondary to edema of the bowel wall and may include anorexia, dull aching of the abdomen, vomiting, and crampy abdominal pain. Abdominal symptoms can occur in the absence of concurrent cutaneous or pharyngeal involvement. The onset of symptoms referable to HAE occurs in more than one-half of the patients before adolescence but, in some patients, symptoms do not occur until adulthood. Although trauma, anxiety, and stress frequently are cited as events that initiate attacks, more than one-half of patients cannot clearly identify an event that initiated an attack. Dental extractions and tonsillectomy can initiate edema of the upper airway, and cutaneous edema may follow trauma to an extremity.

Therapy. The therapy of HAE is divided into two categories: prophylaxis of attacks and treatment of attacks. Long-term prevention of attacks may be indicated in those patients who have had laryngeal obstruction or have suffered frequent and debilitating attacks. Antifibrinolytic agents, such as epsilon aminocaproic acid or its cyclic analogue, tranexamic acid, have been used with some success in the long-term prevention of attacks. Impeded androgens, such as danazol and stanozolol, which have attenuated androgenic potential, have been found to be very useful in the long-term prophylaxis of HAE. These agents have not been used extensively in children, however, because of their androgenic effects. Apparently, they act by stimulating the synthesis of functionally intact C1-INH by the normal gene. In some instances, patients may need short-term prophylactic therapy (e.g., before oral surgery). In these circumstances, danazol therapy may be initiated 1 week before surgery, or epsilon aminocaproic acid may be used the day before surgery.

A number of drugs have been used in an attempt to interrupt an attack of HAE once it has begun. Epinephrine, antihistamines, and corticosteroids are of no proven benefit. Trials using partially purified C1-INH have been encouraging. The infusion of C1-INH has been accompanied by resolution of edema and symptoms within a few hours.

Suggested Readings

Figueroa JE, Densen P. Infectious diseases associated with complement deficiencies. *Clin Microbiol Rev* 1991;4:359.

Frank MM, Gelfand JA, Atkinson JP. Hereditary angioedema: the clinical syndrome and its management. *Ann Intern Med* 1976;84:580.

Kolble K, Reid KBM. Genetic deficiencies of the complement system associated with disease—early components. *Int Rev Immunol* 1993;10:17.

Ross SC, Densen P. Complement deficiency states and infections: epidemiology, pathogenesis, and consequences of neisserial and other infections in an immune deficiency. *Medicine* 1984;63:243.

Tedesco F, Nurnberge W, Perissulti S. Inherited deficiency of the terminal complement components. *Int Rev Immunol* 1993;10:51.

Walport MJ. Complement. Part I. *N Engl J Med* 2001;344:1058.

Walport MJ. Complement. Part II. *N Engl J Med* 2001;344:1140.

Waytes AT, Rosen FS, Frank MM. Treatment of hereditary angioedema with a vapor-heated C1 inhibitor concentrate. *N Engl J Med* 1996;334:1630.

Winkelstein JA, Sullivan K, Colten H. Genetically determined disorders of the complement system. In: Schriver CR, Beaudet AL, Sly WS, Valle D, eds. *The metabolic basis for inherited disease,* 8th ed. New York: McGraw-Hill, 1999.

CHAPTER 430 ■ FUNCTIONAL DISORDERS OF GRANULOCYTES

C. WAYNE SMITH AND M. MICHELE MARISCALCO

Mobile blood granulocytes and monocytes and fixed phagocytic cells function as a first-line defense against invasion by bacterial or fungal microorganisms. Impaired granulocyte production, as well as the functional abnormalities of granulocytes or other professional phagocytes, may significantly compromise host defense, thus increasing susceptibility to infection. Early animal studies demonstrated a critical 2- to 4-hour period after cutaneous invasion by pathogenic bacteria during which phagocytes must localize at a site of invasion to prevent or suppress the process of infection. Recurrent bacterial or fungal infections of the skin or mucous membranes are prominent in patients with quantitative deficiencies of blood granulocytes and in patients with functional deficits of granulocytic cells.

Two broad categories of functional disorders have been delineated: those typified by impaired motility, recruitment, or localization of granulocytes at or to sites of infection, and those resulting from the defective ingestion or intracellular killing of microorganisms by granulocytes and other phagocytic cells. In this latter group of patients, granulocytes accumulate normally in inflamed tissues but are unable to eradicate invading microorganisms. Laboratory studies of representative patients of both categories can be used to define abnormalities of one or more cellular functions (e.g., directed migration or chemotaxis, adhesion, ingestion, degranulation, oxidative intracellular killing, or all) *in vitro*. In selected disorders, molecular deficits have been defined, which allows important new approaches to the diagnosis or clinical management of disease.

DISORDERS OF ADHERENCE AND MOTILITY

Leukocyte Adhesion Deficiency Type I

Leukocyte adhesion deficiency type I (LAD I) is an autosomal recessive trait characterized by recurrent bacterial infections, impaired pus formation and wound healing, and a spectrum of functional abnormalities in granulocytes, monocytes, and lymphoid cells (Box 430.1).

Clinical Manifestations and Complications

The clinical hallmarks of this disease are recurrent, necrotic, and indolent infections of soft tissues, primarily involving skin, mucous membranes, and the intestinal tract. Superficial infections of body surfaces may invade locally or systemically. Typical small, erythematous, nonpustular skin lesions often progress to large, well-demarcated, ulcerative craters (or pyoderma gangrenosa), which heal slowly or with dysplastic eschars. Staphylococcal or gram-negative enteric bacterial organisms may be cultured from such lesions for several weeks, despite antimicrobial therapy. Septicemia progressing from omphalitis associated with delayed umbilical cord severance has been observed in several families. Perirectal abscess or cellulitis leading to peritonitis or septicemia has been reported in multiple patients, and facial or deep neck cellulitis has been observed to progress from ulcerative mucous membrane lesions of the oral cavity. Recurrent invasive candidal esophagitis, erosive gastritis, acute appendicitis, and necrotizing enterocolitis have been reported in multiple patients. Recurrent otitis media occurs commonly, and progression to mastoiditis and facial nerve paralysis has been reported. Other common respiratory infections include severe bacterial (pseudomonal) laryngotracheitis, recurrent pneumonitis, and sinusitis. Severe gingivitis or periodontitis is a major feature among all patients who survive infancy. Acute gingivitis has appeared in all cases upon the eruption of the primary dentition. Subsequently, these patients develop characteristic features of progressive generalized prepubescent periodontitis, including gingival proliferation, defective recession, mobility, pathologic migration, and advanced alveolar bone loss associated with periodontal pocket formation and the partial or total loss of both the deciduous and permanent dentition.

The recurrent infections observed in affected patients appear to reflect a profound impairment of leukocyte mobilization into extravascular inflammatory sites. Skin windows and biopsy samples of infected tissues demonstrate inflammatory infiltrates totally devoid of neutrophils. The histopathologic feature is particularly striking, because marked peripheral blood leukocytosis (9 to 20 times normal values) is a constant feature of this disorder. Transfusions of leukocytes result in the appearance of donor neutrophils and monocytes in skin windows and skin chambers. The dysregulated healing of traumatic or surgical wounds observed in several patients represents a clinical feature not generally observed in patients with neutropenia or dysfunctional neutrophils. Unusual, paper-thin or dysplastic cutaneous scars have been found in some patients and, in one patient with a unique CD18 mutation, hypertrophic scars occurred.

The severity of infectious complications among LAD patients appears to be related directly to the degree of glycoprotein deficiency. Severely affected patients have essentially undetectable expression of all three alpha–beta ($\alpha\beta$) complexes in their neutrophils. Moderately deficient patients express 2% to 25% of all three $\alpha\beta$ complexes. Patients with severe deficiency have either died in infancy or have demonstrated a susceptibility to severe, life-threatening systemic infections (peritonitis, septicemia, pneumonitis, aseptic meningitis). In contrast, among the patients expressing some functional CD11/CD18 integrins, life-threatening infections have been observed infrequently despite a relatively prolonged survival (greater than 50 years). In some moderately affected patients, skin lesions may disappear after the first few years of life, recurring only with occasional infections. Severe gingivitis always is observed in these patients and may be the presenting symptom. Delayed umbilical cord separation occurs more frequently in patients with the severe phenotype, but it is not universally found.

Therapy

Suggested therapeutic guidelines for LAD are based on limited clinical experience. Although infectious complications generally are observed on body surfaces, life-threatening systemic infections may occur at any time, especially in individuals who fail to express any CD18 integrins. Superficial inflammatory lesions must be managed aggressively, with local care and antibiotic therapy. This is of special importance, because inflammatory signs may be minimal before the development of septicemic episodes. Moreover, the impaired healing of superficial

---

BOX 430.1   Leukocyte Adhesion Defect

The molecular basis of LAD has been found to involve a family of structurally and functionally related glycoproteins on the surface of myeloid cells. These glycoproteins occur as noncovalently associated alpha and beta subunits with alpha$_1$-beta$_1$ stoichiometry. They share an identical beta subunit (Mr = 95,000) and are distinguished by distinct alpha subunits designated Mac-1-alpha (aM) (Mr = 165,000), LFA-1-alpha (αL) (Mr = 177,000), p150,95-alpha (αX) (Mr = 150,000), and alpha-D (Mr = 160,000). The World Health Organization designation for these glycoproteins is CD18 for the beta subunit, CD11a for the alpha-L subunit, CD11b for the alpha-M subunit, CD11c for the alpha-X subunit, and CD11d for the alpha-D subunit. The entire complex is designated CD11/CD18. Biosynthetic studies show that these patients possess heterogeneous abnormalities of the beta (CD18) but not alpha subunits of the CD11/CD18 glycoproteins. These findings suggested distinct mutations in the CD18 gene, which has been mapped to chromosome 21. Such mutations have been defined in several patients and include point mutations, deletions, or insertions, as identified by the nucleotide sequence analysis of patient or heterozygote CD18 cDNA or genomic DNA. Although most LAD phenotypes are not defined at the nucleotide level, it is probable that all include mutations of the CD18 gene and that CD18 mutants vary in their ability to complex with the different alpha subunits, thus determining the relative deficiency of the alpha-beta ($\alpha\beta$) protein complexes expressed on cell surfaces.

wounds appears to allow indolent colonization and subsequent reinfection. Early use of empiric combination therapy with a staphylocidal agent and an aminoglycoside is justified in acutely ill or febrile patients, in the absence of localizing findings. The use of prophylactic antibiotics may be advised. Limited clinical experience suggests that the number of systemic infections in patients with LAD is considerably diminished through the use of prophylactic regimens. Leukocyte transfusions have been used successfully in several patients with LAD; enhancement of inflammatory functions and clinical resolution of even life-threatening infections have been achieved in a clinical setting in which systemic antibiotic or surgical interventions were ineffective.

Bone marrow transplantation (BMT) with successful engraftment and apparent clinical recovery from disease has been achieved in several patients. Because of the inherent risks and expense, this approach should be considered only for patients with the severe phenotype of disease. Among patients undergoing transplantation, recipients of HLA-identical as well as HLA-mismatched (e.g., haplotype match) bone marrow have shown successful engraftment. In some cases, mixed but stable chimerism between donor and recipient cells is apparent 3 to 5 years after transplantation. In these cases, normal or slightly diminished blood granulocyte function is observed *in vitro*, and the patients demonstrate no clinical complications.

The identification in LAD patients having CD18 mutations raises the possibility that the introduction of a normal CD18 gene into hematopoietic cells could cure this disease, especially in light of the encouraging results of BMT. Some reports document the successful transfection or retroviral-mediated infection of LAD cells or cell lines with a normal CD18 cDNA, resulting in normal CD18 protein expression and normal cell adherence properties. Thus, the stage is set for future attempts at somatic cell gene therapy in LAD.

Leukocyte Adhesive Deficiency Type II

Leukocyte adhesive deficiency type II (Rambon-Hasharon syndrome, LAD II) is a rare condition characterized by the defective formation of ligands for the selectin adhesion molecule family. The syndrome is complex in that developmental abnormalities, mental retardation, and recurrent infections occur. It has been described in three kindreds, two of Middle Eastern descent and one of Brazilian origin. Each of the kindreds has distinct mutations in the GDP-fucose transporter and, functionally, a marked reduction in GDP-fucose transport into the Golgi apparatus. The distinctive clinical features of these patients include craniofacial dysmorphism, neurologic deficits (central hypotonia, seizures, developmental delay), recurrent respiratory infections, and constant peripheral blood leukocytosis and neutrophilia. An autosomal recessive genetic basis for this syndrome in these patients is supported by the finding that all lack the erythrocyte H antigen and manifest the Bombay (hh) phenotype that, in turn, is caused by a homozygosity for a rare recessive (h) allele. Individuals with the Bombay phenotype lack the H antigen, an intermediate in the production of erythrocytic A and B antigens, but do not share any other clinical features of LAD II.

The finding of markedly elevated neutrophil counts and recurrent respiratory infections in these patients prompted studies of leukocyte functions. These studies revealed diminished neutrophil emigration into skin windows and significant defects of random and directed migration and diminished homotypic aggregation of neutrophils *in vitro*. Studies of phagocytosis and intracellular bacterial killing, as well as lymphocyte proliferation and natural killer (NK) cell function, showed no abnormalities. In contrast to those of patients with LAD I, the

leukocytes of these patients demonstrated normal levels of surface CD11/CD18.

LAD II patients have a generalized fucosylation defect that affects the alpha-1,2-, alpha-1,3-, alpha-1,4- and alpha-α1,6-linkages of fucose in glycoconjugates. These apparently result from mutations in a GDP-fucose transporter in the Golgi membrane. Two specific mutations have been discovered: the replacement of arginine 147 by cysteine (R147C) functionally inactivates the transporter and represents the defect in one kindred, and replacement of threonine 308 by arginine (T308R) results in the defective transporter in another kindred.

Dietary supplementation of fucose has been shown to reverse effectively the deficit of selectin ligands in two of the kindreds, with resulting improvement is some of the manifestations of the syndrome (e.g., normalization of the blood neutrophil count). It remains unclear whether oral fucose will significantly alter the developmental aspects of the syndrome, and it appears that one of the defined mutations is unresponsive to fucose supplementation. In addition, in one of the patients, a complication of inducing fucosylation was the appearance of neoantigens on the surface of leukocytes and erythrocytes. This patient exhibited an autoimmune neutropenia.

Leukocyte Adhesion Deficiency Type III

Leukocyte adhesion deficiency type III is a category of rare syndromes exhibiting the normal expression of the leukocyte adhesion molecules but abnormal functioning (previously referred to as LAD I variants). Several patients have been described with reduced adhesive functions in leukocyte integrins of the beta$_1$, beta$_2$, and beta$_3$ families. One patient exhibited a disorder in the multistep process of leukocyte adhesion to endothelial cells; this disorder was associated with functional defects in multiple leukocyte integrins, recurrent infections, marked leukocytosis, and a bleeding tendency. This syndrome was associated with an impaired ability of neutrophil and lymphocyte beta$_1$ and beta$_2$ integrins to generate high-avidity adhesion to endothelial ligands and arrest cells on vascular endothelium in response to endothelial chemoattractant signals. In this patient, a defect occurred in the regulation of the small Ras-related GTPase, Rap1, activation that resulted in an inability of ligand-occupied integrins to generate high-avidity binding to ligands under shear flow. Another patient exhibited clinical features of both Glanzmann thrombasthenia and LAD I. The patient had normal expression of beta$_1$, beta$_2$, and beta$_3$ integrins, but all were dysfunctional. The key findings were that signaling pathways leading to integrin activation were defective, and this defect was associated with abnormal integrin clustering. Although this group of patients likely represents several distinct molecular deficits, they share the characteristic of a dysfunctional family or families of leukocyte integrins that variably affect all leukocytes, sometimes including platelets. The fact that they express normal levels of integrins distinguishes them from LAD I patients.

Specific Granule Deficiency

The first example of a primary deficiency of neutrophil-specific granules was recognized in 1972. Other cases have subsequently been reported by several laboratories. One patient appears to have had an acquired deficiency (associated with a myeloproliferative syndrome), whereas all others appear to have genetically determined disease. Each demonstrated susceptibility to recurrent and severe infections of the skin, mucous membranes, and lung, most commonly caused by *Staphylococcus aureus, Pseudomonas aeruginosa,* other enteric pathogens, and *Candida albicans*. Infections may progress from superficial sites; otitis media with associated mastoiditis was reported in one patient, and lung abscess formation caused by *S. aureus* followed the onset of pneumonia in another individual. The occurrence of necrotic oral lesions caused by *Escherichia coli* and species of *Pseudomonas* and *Klebsiella* were reported in another individual, but the severe neutropenia recognized in that patient may have accounted for the development of these mucous membrane lesions. Another patient with severe scalp infections caused by *Proteus mirabilis* and *S. aureus* required prolonged intravenous antibiotic therapy in addition to surgical débridement. Detailed descriptions of the histopathology of infected tissues in all patients are not reported, but skin window studies have demonstrated diminished pus formation in the tissues of some individuals who were not neutropenic.

Clinical Manifestations and Complications

Neutrophils from each patient studied have demonstrated morphologic abnormalities, including a severe or total deficiency of specific granules and a variety of nuclear abnormalities, such as bilobed or multilobed nuclei or nuclear blebs, clefts, or pockets. Diminished or absent neutrophil lactoferrin content has been confirmed in only three cases, and the membrane marker alkaline phosphatase has been shown to be diminished or absent in the neutrophils of all but one reported case. Total cellular content and release of the secondary granule markers (lactoferrin, B12 transport protein, cytochrome b, and lysozyme) have been shown to be diminished when assessed in selected patients, although the levels of primary granule constituents (myeloperoxidase, beta-glucuronidase) generally are normal. Among recognized cases, somewhat heterogeneous abnormalities in cellular functions have been observed. Chemotaxis and intracellular microbial activity represent the most consistently reported functional deficits.

The deficiency of specific granules is suggested by a history of recurrent cutaneous, subcutaneous, mucous membrane, or pulmonary infections caused by *S. aureus*, virulent gram-negative enteric bacteria, or species of *Candida*. Findings of abnormal morphology and abnormally weak cytochemical reactions for alkaline phosphatase are highly suggestive of this disorder. Cytochemical and ultrastructural studies to confirm the diminished numbers or abnormal morphology of specific granules and their specific constituents establishes a diagnosis.

Sequence analysis of DNA from a patient with secondary granule deficiency revealed a five base-pair deletion in the second exon of the transcription factor *CCAAT/enhancer binding protein–ε* (C/EBPε) locus. A second patient had a one base-pair insertion, and the predicted frame shifts resulted in truncations of the 32-kD major C/EBPε isoform, with loss of the dimerization domain, DNA binding region, and transcriptional activity. The phenotypic and functional defects of neutrophils from C/EBPε-deficient mice closely parallel those of the human syndrome of specific granule deficiency. The multiple functional defects observed in early neutrophil progenitor cells are apparently the consequence of C/EBPε deficiency. Specific granule deficiency is thus a defect in myelopoiesis, because C/EBPe is required for the promyelocyte–myelocyte transition in myeloid differentiation.

Functional Abnormalities in Neonatal Neutrophils

Because specific immunity is limited severely in the immediate postpartum period, the inflammatory functions of phagocytic cells are especially important for host defense against microbial invasion. Both quantitative and qualitative abnormalities of phagocytic cells contribute to enhanced susceptibility of neonates to infections. Neutropenia is commonly observed

in systemically infected neonates, and studies in neonatal animals indicate that the exhaustion of a limited reserve pool of bone marrow granulocytes contributes to a depletion of circulating or marginating pools when tissue demand is increased. Among the most consistently observed functional abnormalities thought to contribute to impaired inflammation in neonates are those related to the motility of leukocytes. As shown with skin windows, the inflammatory responses in newborns differ from those in older children and adults in two respects: The shift from the early granulocyte predominance to a predominance of mononuclear cells is slower and less pronounced, and a marked eosinophilia is observed in some infants aged 2 to 21 days. Strikingly diminished leukocyte mobilization in neonatal rats inoculated intraperitoneally with bacteria or chemotactic agents has been demonstrated.

Neonatal neutrophils exhibit impaired chemotactic responses to numerous chemotactic factors, including those released by replicating *S. aureus* and *E. coli* and those generated in plasma by antigen–antibody complexes (e.g., C5a). Visual assays demonstrate that neonatal cells not only have depressed migration but also are impaired significantly in their ability to orient toward a gradient of chemotactic factors. Depressed chemotaxis has been found in healthy neonates aged 1 to 5 days. In addition, diminished generation of chemotactic activity (chemotaxigenesis) by virulent type III group B streptococci occurs in neonatal sera, an abnormality directly related to diminished levels of both type-specific anticapsular antibody and serum complement activity. Thus, the impaired generation of chemotactic stimuli, as well as abnormal cellular responses, appear to account for the diminished inflammatory responses observed in even healthy term neonates.

The basis for abnormal neonatal granulocytic migratory functions is not defined fully but appears to involve defects of stimulated cell adhesion. The induction of CD11b/CD18 (Mac-1) surface expression by chemotactic agonists is diminished, and basal levels of the L-selectin adherence protein are markedly diminished on cord blood or neonatal granulocytes. The importance of these observations is suggested by findings of diminished transendothelial migration by neonatal neutrophils *in vitro*. This defect reflects impaired Mac-1–adhesive interactions with the endothelial ligand intracellular adhesion molecule 1 (ICAM-1) and deficits of L-selectin interactions with another endothelial adherence molecule, E-selectin. Studies of inflammation in neonatal animal models support a role for both neutrophil adhesion determinants in diminished inflammation.

Because multiple host defense mechanisms are defective or developmentally delayed in human neonates, no precise cause-and-effect relationship between impaired cellular migration and the occurrence of infectious complications is established. However, neonates are particularly susceptible to the development of cutaneous inflammatory lesions or abscesses at sites of local trauma (e.g., circumcision wounds, umbilicus, intertriginous areas, or sites of electrode-monitoring devices). Microorganisms such as *S. aureus*, gram-negative enteric organisms, and species of *Candida* are the most common agents infecting cutaneous or mucous membrane lesions in human neonates. The propensity for systemic invasion and the development of neonatal septicemia by endogenous respiratory or gastrointestinal flora may be related to insufficient infiltration of granulocytes or monocytes into submucosal tissues.

Chédiak-Higashi Syndrome

Chédiak-Higashi syndrome (CHS) is an autosomal recessive disorder of mink, cattle, beige mice, rats, and humans. This condition is characterized clinically by partial oculocutaneous albinism, the presence of giant lysosomal granules in all granular cell types, susceptibility to bacterial infection, variable occurrence of neutropenia and thrombocytopenia, and an accelerated lymphoma-like proliferative phase generally occurring in the first decade of life. Infectious complications are attributable to both neutropenia and functional deficits of neutrophils, monocytes, and NK cells. A comprehensive review in 1972 documented the significance of infectious morbidity and mortality in this syndrome. Among 56 cases reviewed, 33 individuals died before age 10 years; among 27 cases for which a cause of death was determined, infections were the sole cause in 17 and a contributing factor in nine more cases. Pulmonary, cutaneous, subcutaneous, and upper respiratory infections were observed most frequently. *S. aureus* accounted for approximately 70% of all infections for which an etiologic agent was determined; group A streptococcus, gram-negative enteric organisms (*Klebsiella, Pseudomonas, Proteus, Shigella* species), *Aspergillus,* and *Candida* species represented occasional etiologic agents.

Clinical Manifestations and Complications

Several functional abnormalities of the neutrophils, monocytes, and NK cells of these patients have been identified. Defective neutrophil and monocyte chemotaxis has been reported consistently, but the molecular determinants of these abnormalities are undefined. Neutrophils demonstrate delayed and diminished intracellular killing of both gram-positive and gram-negative bacterial organisms, despite a normal capacity to ingest these organisms and a normal or elevated oxidative burst. Microbicidal abnormalities are attributed to impaired post-phagocytic phagolysosomal fusion. A selective impairment of NK-cell functions (as opposed to other lymphocyte functions) has been reported. Dysfunction of the NK cell system may account for the ultimate development of an aggressive lymphoproliferative syndrome in most patients.

A diagnosis of CHS is made by identifying the characteristic clinical features of the disorder in addition to the characteristic large cytoplasmic inclusions in all granular cells, including peripheral blood granulocytes. Giant melanosomes can be demonstrated in the hair of patients. Neutropenia and thrombocytopenia are most characteristic during the accelerated phase of disease. When bone marrow aspirates are examined, common abnormalities include hypercellularity, with extensive vacuolization and inclusions in myeloid precursors. Elevated serum lysozyme levels probably reflect intramedullary granulocyte destruction. The accelerated phase of CHS is characterized by widespread tissue infiltrates of lymphoid and histiocytic cells, usually without malignant histologic characteristics. Splenomegaly and associated hypersplenism contribute to neutropenia. Although viral agents and immunologic mechanisms may contribute to the pathogenesis of the accelerated phase, the precise mechanisms are undefined. Most patients with CHS die from infectious or infiltrative complications within the first decade of life. Early BMT is the treatment of choice. Some patients with relatively mild forms of the disease survive into adulthood (Box 430.2).

Type 1b Glycogen Storage Disease

The association of neutropenia, impaired neutrophil migration, and recurrent infection in type 1b glycogen storage disease was first reported in 1980. Most clinical features of type 1b glycogen storage disease are similar to those of type 1a glycogen storage disease, including hepatomegaly, fasting hypoglycemia, lactic acidosis, short stature, hyperlipidemia, and the occurrence of hepatomas with a potential for malignant degeneration. Patients with type 1a glycogen storage disease demonstrate a deficiency of glucose-6-phosphatase activity in liver, kidney, and intestine. In contrast, patients with type 1b glyco-

---

| BOX 430.2 | Molecular Basis of Chédiak-Higashi Syndrome |

Homology between the disease in beige mice and Chédiak-Higashi syndrome (CHS) was recently supported by mapping of the CHS locus to chromosome 1q42–q43 in a segment corresponding to the beige locus region on mouse chromosome 13. It was confirmed by the sequence homology shared between the CHS and the beige coding sequence gene (LYST). Pathologic mutations in this gene have been reported in a substantial number of patients. In the severe form of childhood CHS, functionally null mutant *CHS1* alleles were present, whereas patients with the adolescent and adult forms of CHS were found to have missense mutant alleles that likely encoded CHS1 polypeptides with partial function. Thus, there appears to be allelic genotype–phenotype relationships within the clinical forms of CHS. Relatively little known is known about the functions of the CHS/beige protein, although it is clearly necessary for normal vesicle trafficking.

---

gen storage disease demonstrate normal glucose-6-phosphatase activity, but several mutations in the microsomal glucose-6-phosphate translocase (*G6PT1*) gene have been reported in different patients.

Clinical Manifestations and Complications

A review of the clinical and laboratory features of 21 patients with type 1b glycogen storage disease indicated that most had a variety of moderate to severe bacterial infections, including pneumonitis, recurrent otitis media, subcutaneous abscesses, generalized pyoderma, cellulitis, wound infections, and osteomyelitis, most commonly secondary to *S. aureus.* Most patients exhibited chronic neutropenia, which, in some patients, was associated with demonstrable serum inhibitors of myeloid stem-cell proliferation, abnormalities of myeloid maturation, and decreased peripheral marginating pools. Treatment with granulocyte colony-stimulating factor (G-CSF) has been reported to reduce the incidence of infections. Functional abnormalities, including diminished random or directed migration of neutrophils *in vitro,* were documented in eight of 11 patients tested, and deficient chemotactic modulation of adherence by chemotactic factors was observed in two patients. In contrast, the microbicidal activity of neutrophils and phagocytosis-associated oxidative metabolic activity are normal in most patients with type 1b glycogen storage disease (GSD1b) (Box 430.3).

Periodontitis Syndromes

Individuals who have developmental, genetic, or acquired disorders are characterized by quantitative deficiencies of peripheral blood phagocytes or functional abnormalities of neutrophils, and these patients commonly present with oral complications. Primary or secondary agranulocytosis and cyclic neutropenia syndromes are typified by severe ulceration, necrosis, or chronic inflammation of gingival or periodontal tissues. Patients with severe leukocytopathies, such as chronic granulomatous disease (CGD), CHS, and LAD, present with systemic as well as oral infections, whereas those demonstrating less profound functional deficits, such as in localized juvenile periodontitis, postlocalized juvenile periodontitis, or generalized juvenile periodontitis, present exclusively with periodontal manifestation.

Pathogenesis

The defective chemotactic responsiveness of neutrophils is thought to represent a major pathogenic mechanism in individuals with periodontitis syndromes. Of 183 patients with localized juvenile periodontitis studied by multiple investigators, 71% are reported to exhibit defective chemotaxis. Most exhibit intrinsic cellular defects, but cell-directed serum inhibitors, chemotactic factor inactivators, or abnormalities of chemotaxigenesis are reported in a small proportion of patients tested. The pathogenic mechanisms accounting for impaired chemotaxis have not been defined. The epidemiologic or clinical associations of certain periodontopathic bacterial organisms with some periodontitis syndromes suggest the possibility that cellular constituents or extracellular factors elaborated by these microorganisms may secondarily alter leukocyte functions. The pathogenic roles of gram-negative oral bacteria such as *Actinobacillus actinomycetemcomitans*, species of *Bacteroides*, and species of *Capnocytophaga* have been increasingly appreciated. Among the potentially pathogenic products of *A. actinomycetemcomitans*, a leukocytotoxin has been identified *in vitro* that may contribute to diminished chemotactic function. Sera from patients contain IgG antibodies that neutralize the leukotoxic activity of *A. actinomycetemcomitans*, and serum and gingival crevicular fluids from such patients contain high titers of antibodies to *A. actinomycetemcomitans* antigens. Other poorly defined inhibitors of chemotaxis are found in culture filtrates or sonicates of *Bacteroides gingivalis*, *Fusobacterium nucleatum*, and species of *Capnocytophaga*.

Shwachman-Diamond Syndrome

Shwachman-Diamond syndrome (SDS) is an autosomal recessive condition, with multisystemic abnormalities including exocrine pancreatic insufficiency, bone marrow hypoplasia with associated neutropenia, metaphyseal chondrodysplasia, growth retardation, and recurrent soft-tissue infections. The *SBDS* (Shwachman-Bodian-Diamond syndrome) gene in the region of the centromere, 7q11, is affected, most often with a loss-of function. While the function of the *SBDS* gene currently is unknown, it is a member of a highly conserved protein family found in diverse eukaryotic species. The diagnosis of SDS is based on the presence of exocrine pancreatic dysfunction and hematologic abnormalities. In the largest series of patients to date, steatorrhea was present in 86% of children, with 91% displaying a low serum trypsinogen. Patients older than 4 years more often had pancreatic insufficiency. Neutropenia occurred in 98% of patients, with anemia and thrombocytopenia in 42% and 34%, respectively. A heterogeneous occurrence was noted in skeletal abnormalities, including short stature in 56% of affected individuals. In addition, children were severely weight restricted; however when weight was expressed as percentage of ideal weight for height, a measure of nutritional status, patients were "normal." Recurrent sinusitis, otitis media, or both were noted in 20% of patients, with 24% having lower respiratory tract infections. Severe systemic or deep tissue infections were reported in 20% of patients. Urinary tract infections occurred in less than 2% of the series. Four children died in this series, two from infection, and two as a consequence of BMT.

Patients with SDS are at increased risk for severe bone marrow aplasia, myelodysplasia, and leukemic transformation. In fourteen patients who met the criteria of SDS, a neutrophil chemotaxis defect was identified in all fourteen, in that all were incapable of orienting and chemotaxing up a gradient of chemotactic factor in a spatial distribution. It is thought that a combination of both the neutropenia and the diminished chemotaxis results in the severe recurrent infection in this syndrome.

DISORDERS OF INTRACELLULAR MICROBIAL KILLING

Opsonophagocytosis mediated by specific membrane receptors initiates a sequence of metabolic, biophysical, and cytoskeletal events that promote the rapid, efficient killing of intracellular microorganisms by phagocytes. Phagocytosis is associated with a burst of oxidative metabolic activity, including the consumption of molecular oxygen and the evolution of superoxide, hydrogen peroxide, or other oxygen radicals. This respiratory burst requires a series of electron transfers using nicotinamide-adenine dinucleotide phosphate (NADPH) as the electron donor. It involves a flavin-adenine dinucleotide-containing flavoprotein and a unique cytochrome b. This oxidase system is associated with the plasma membrane of granulocytes or mononuclear phagocytes. Thus, lethal oxygen radicals are concentrated together with ingested microbes in phagosomes or the extracellular environment of neutrophils. Neutrophil myeloperoxidase in the presence of H_2O_2 and halide further catalyzes the formation of additional oxidants such as hypochlorous acid and free chlorine in phagolysosomes. Constituents of both primary and secondary lysosomal granules, including defensins, elastase, cathepsin G, lactoferrin, and other proteins, significantly contribute to nonoxidative microbial activity within phagosomes. An increased understanding of the molecular biology of phagocytes allows the delineation of several clinical disorders of intracellular microbicidal functions that are characterized by enhanced susceptibility to recurrent bacterial or fungal infections.

Chronic Granulomatosis Disease

The chronic granulomatosis diseases (CGDs) are a genetically heterogeneous group of disorders of the oxidative metabolism of phagocytes. CGD results in the impairment of intracellular killing of catalase-positive bacteria, fungi, or other microbes. CGD occurs at a frequency of 1 in 1 million and is identified most often in boys. Most patients with CGD develop recurrent soft-tissue infections during the first year of life; a high proportion of these become clinically ill before age 3 months. Rarely, individuals may be clinically well until early adolescence or adulthood, possibly reflecting less deleterious genetic phenotypes. Disease-free intervals may increase in some patients with increasing age, but older individuals are still at high risk for life-threatening infections. Improved prophylactic or therapeutic antibiotic, immunologic, or surgical regimens may have diminished mortality rates in CGD. Among 168 cases reviewed by Johnston in 1977, 95 deaths were reported, 45 before the age of 7 years and 50 before the age of 12 years. In some cases, however, considerable longevity has been documented (e.g., four brothers with CGD were reported to range in age from 28 to 40 years). The routine use of prophylactic antibiotics and the more recent introduction of interferon-gamma in the clinical management of CGD is likely to affect significantly the severity of this disease.

The basis for abnormal oxygen-dependent microbicidal activity in CGD cells is related directly to the impaired generation of superoxide anion, H_2O_2, and other oxygen intermediates. This abnormality is expressed in a number of cell types, including neutrophils, macrophages, eosinophils, and lymphocytes. Abnormal NADPH oxidase activity caused by one of several molecular defects recognized among CGD patients represents the fundamental basis for diminished microbicidal function.

Distinct forms of CGD are defined to involve quantitative or functional deficits of each of the components of the NADPH oxidase complex of neutrophils and other cell types. This multicomponent enzyme is inactive in resting neutrophils and is assembled and active on neutrophil ingestion or agonist exposure (Box 430.4).

Historically, three genetic forms of CGD were described, based on inheritance patterns and the spectrophotometric detection of the cytochrome b in phagocytes of affected patients: X-linked (approximately 70%), autosomal recessive (approximately 30%), and autosomal dominant (rare cases). Current evidence indicates that molecular defects underlying X-linked CGD include heterogeneous mutations in the gp91 *phox* gene that account for quantitative deficiency or functional abnormalities of this glycoprotein, in turn resulting in total or partial deficiency of neutrophil oxidase activity (65% of total). These include gross deletions (in chromosome Xp21.1) or subtle mutations in regulatory elements or in the reading frame of the gp91 gene that impair mRNA expression or stability or the functional assemblage of this protein together with other oxidase components. Autosomal recessive CGD includes patients with generally normal gp91 *phox* and cytochrome b levels. These comprise heterogeneous mutations of p22 *phox* (approximately 6% of total), p47 *phox* (approximately 23% of total), or p67 *phox* (approximately 6% of total). Genotypic heterogeneity appears to account for the considerable range of clinical severity among CGD kindreds. Precise definition of the molecular lesions in individual patients may even allow prognostic information or unique insights concerning novel therapeutic approaches (e.g., somatic-cell gene therapy).

Patients with CGD demonstrate a specific predilection for infection caused by catalase-positive microorganisms that generally do not elaborate H_2O_2 (Box 430.5).

Clinical Manifestations and Complications

Clinical infections in CGD largely reflect an inability of circulating phagocytes to kill invading bacteria or fungi at sites of heavy colonization on or beneath the skin or mucous membranes. Predictable clinical features in CGD are infections on body surfaces, including inflammatory lesions of skin or subcutaneous tissues, ulcerative stomatitis, pneumonitis, perianal abscesses, and conjunctivitis. More widespread and deep-seated infections in CGD further reflect the persistence of invading organisms within circulating phagocytes, which allows localized or generalized seeding of tissue macrophages throughout the reticuloendothelial system. As a result, typical granulomas,

---

| BOX 430.4 | The NADPH Oxidase Complex of Neutrophils |

The NADPH oxidase complex includes a unique membrane-associated cytochrome b, a heme-containing glycoprotein that exists as a heterodimer composed of a 22-kd alpha subunit (also termed *p22 phox*) and a 91-kd beta subunit (also termed *gp91 phox*). This cytochrome is associated with a low-molecular-weight guanosine triphosphate-binding protein (Raplo) and a flavin adenine dinucleotide-containing flavoprotein. Cystolic components of the oxidase complex include the p47 *phox* and p67 *phox* that exist in a preformed complex of 260-kd and a low-molecular-weight G protein (Rac1 or Rac2). The p47/p67 *phox* complex translocates to the plasma membrane of activated cells, where it associates with the cytochrome b complex to facilitate the catalysis of electron transfer from NADPH to molecular oxygen through its flavin adenine dinucleotide heme-redox centers. These events are regulated in part by the phosphorylation of p47 and p67 *phox*. Definition of the molecular phenotype of CGD patients is now possible because of the availability of cDNAs or monoclonal antibody reagents specifically reactive with patient DNA, mRNA, or protein components of the NADPH oxidase.

| BOX 430.5 | Infectious Agents that Cause Infections in Patients with Chronic Granulomatous Disease |

- *S. aureus* represents the most common infecting agent, accounting for 30% to 56% of clinical isolates in reported series of patient.
- Catalase-positive, gram-negative bacteria such as *E. coli, Klebsiella, Enterobacter* species, *Serratia marcescens, Salmonellae,* and *Pseudomonas* species account for approximately 30% of infections overall.
- In specific geographic locations, *Chromobacterium violaceum* infections have been recognized in several patients with CGD.
- Fungal pathogens also represent frequent and important etiologic agents. Fungal infections occurred in 20% of 245 cases reviewed in one report.
- *Aspergillus* species accounted for 78% of these; *C. albicans* and species of *Torulopsis* accounted for most of the remaining isolates.
- Other reports document the pathogenic importance of obligate intracellular pathogens such as *Pneumocystis jarovici* and *Mycobacterium* species.

Thus, patients with CGD are susceptible to infection by a variety of endogenous flora, as well as by ubiquitous organisms.

which constitute the histopathologic hallmark of this disorder, commonly develop in lymph nodes, lungs, liver, spleen, gastrointestinal tract, bone, and other tissues. Once established, these infections generally remain localized but may overwhelm the reticuloendothelial barriers, leading to the development of septicemia or meningitis. Prolonged intracellular microbial residence in tissue abscesses or granulomas accounts for the indolent nature of observed clinical infections, the considerable difficulties encountered in identifying specific infecting agents, and the delayed or refractory response to antimicrobial, surgical, or other therapeutic regimens commonly observed in patients with CGD.

Diagnosis

A diagnosis of CGD should be considered when a history of recurrent systemic infections or other clinical features beginning in infancy is elicited. Patients with CGD often are referred to tertiary-care centers with histories of recurrent or chronic illness or inflammatory disease for which no etiology has been determined despite extensive diagnostic evaluations. They frequently present with fever of unknown origin or carry a presumptive diagnosis of rheumatoid disease, and they may be misdiagnosed as examples of other granulomatous inflammatory disorders such as Crohn disease or tuberculosis. Particularly typical is a history of sterile tissue aspirates of superficial or deep-seated abscesses. The identification of unusual etiologic agents such as *S. marcescens* or *Pseudomonas maltophilia*, the occurrence of infections in unusual locations such as osteomyelitic involvement of small bones of hands or feet, and the occurrence of characteristic types of infections such as liver or other deep-seated abscesses should alert the clinician to the possibility of CGD.

Laboratory findings suggestive of CGD include leukocytosis, elevation of erythrocyte sedimentation rate, abnormal chest radiographs, and hypergammaglobulinemia. Serum levels of IgG, IgA, and IgM generally are elevated, whereas IgE levels are variably increased or normal. Specific antibody synthesis and delayed hypersensitivity skin test responses generally are normal. Microscopic evaluations of postmortem or biopsy tissues almost uniformly reveal granulomas at sites of infection. Commonly, histiocytes contain pigmented (yellow or tan) lipid material that may result from the persistent residence of microorganisms within macrophages.

A definitive diagnostic test for CGD is the demonstration of impaired intracellular bactericidal activity by neutrophils, eosinophils, or mononuclear phagocytes. Because bactericidal assays require special laboratory facilities and experience, other screening tests such as the nitroblue tetrazolium (NBT) dye test are applicable for use in the general diagnostic laboratory. Oxidized NBT is colorless. When reduced by superoxide, it precipitates in the cytosol as blue formazan, which can be identified histochemically. An absence of superoxide evolution by CGD neutrophils or monocytes precludes their reduction of formazan in response to soluble oxidative stimulants or during phagocytosis. A modified qualitative NBT slide test using the stimulant phorbol myristate acetate was originally developed by Newberger to allow a prenatal diagnosis of CGD using fetal blood. This rapid, inexpensive, and highly accurate assay is useful for both the identification of patients and family studies. Using this technique, essentially no CGD leukocytes demonstrate a normal reduction of NBT, whereas essentially all those of normal individuals have positive results for NBT. Heterozygous carriers of X-linked recessive CGD have nearly equal proportions of NBT-positive and NBT-negative cells.

Other laboratory techniques can be used to demonstrate impairment of the respiratory burst and thereby confirm a diagnosis of CGD. During phagocytosis, normal neutrophils or monocytes produce highly energized and unstable oxygen radicals, which return to more stable intermediates through the emission of light energy, or chemiluminescence. Chemiluminescence associated with phagocytosis or after stimulation by soluble stimulants can be measured conveniently in a scintillation counter. Leukocytes from patients with CGD generate no or markedly diminished chemiluminescence under most experimental conditions. The chemiluminescence assay may allow the recognition of heterozygous CGD carriers in family studies, and it may be used to detect other heritable disorders of leukocyte oxidative metabolism, including myeloperoxidase deficiency, glucose-6-phosphate dehydrogenase (G6PD) deficiency, and abnormalities of glutathione metabolism, each of which can be confirmed by more specific biochemical assays. Because molecular heterogeneity has been recognized increasingly among identified patients with CGD and their kindreds, more detailed investigations to delineate a precise molecular lesion in selected cases should be performed in specialized laboratories.

Therapy

The major clinical objectives in the management of CGD include prevention of infection, early identification of infection, and antimicrobial or surgical treatment. Superficial lesions such as furuncles, paronychia, and areas of cellulitis warrant concern, even with no fever or other systemic symptoms. Vigorous efforts should be made to isolate etiologic agents from involved tissues and to promptly initiate antimicrobial therapy. For recognized acute infections, appropriate antibiotics (based on susceptibility studies) should be administered for at least 10 to 14 days, even if the clinical response is prompt and favorable. Longer intervals of administration may be required when delayed defervescence is observed or when leukocytosis, an elevated sedimentation rate, or local inflammatory signs persist. Fever without an obvious site of infection is common. Noninvasive diagnostic procedures, such as ultrasonography or radionucleotide scans, should be considered early in the management of febrile episodes. The early administration of parenteral antibiotics is justified in febrile patients without localizing findings.

When possible, aggressive and early surgical intervention, including the incision and drainage of abscesses, should be considered. Antibiotic administration should be continued for approximately 1 to 2 weeks after complete wound healing, even if a specific and highly sensitive etiologic agent is recovered. The administration of oral antibiotics may be justified for several weeks to several months longer, even in the complete absence of clinical signs or laboratory abnormalities. The general rationale for this prolonged therapeutic interval is based on the knowledge that microorganisms are sequestered and not killed within phagocytes defective in microbicidal mechanisms and on the high incidence of relapsing infections in these patients.

The use of leukocyte transfusions in selected clinical settings of severe infection without adequate response to antibiotics should be considered. Even though several investigators have reported beneficial effects in managing infectious complications, comparative evaluations of the efficacy or possible complications associated with leukocyte transfusions in these patients are lacking. The possible benefits of transfused leukocytes must be weighed against possible complications associated with their use. Foremost is the possibility of sensitization to granulocyte or monocyte antigens in patients who have the McLeod phenotype. Three clinical indications for leukocyte transfusions in CGD include failure of conventional medical and surgical therapy to control infection or inflammation, rapidly progressive or life-threatening infection, and failure to appropriately localize an infectious process or focus, thereby obviating the possibility of conventional medical or surgical approaches.

In addition to the management of infections, patients with CGD must be evaluated carefully with respect to their erythrocyte phenotype. Some individuals with CGD lack known antigens from Kell series, a phenotype termed Ko, whereas others have the McLeod phenotype, characterized by erythrocytes that react weakly with those antibodies defining some Kell antigens. Because both phenotypes are rare, these patients are at risk of forming antibodies to the antigens on the erythrocytes of most blood donors. Thus, transfusion should be avoided in patients who have these rare Kell-associated phenotypes, or their erythrocytes should be stored for possible future use. Additional management involves the identification of a carrier state among family members and the provision of appropriate genetic counseling.

The ubiquitous nature of agents infecting patients with CGD precludes measures to diminish or eliminate exposure to most potential pathogens. One preventive measure, however, is for the patient to not smoke marijuana, which may be contaminated heavily with *Aspergillus* or *Salmonella* organisms. The management of patients with CGD traditionally has relied on antibiotic prophylaxis, although no randomized control trials support this approach. However, in two reviews of patients followed at the University of Minnesota Medical Center and the National Institutes of Health (NIH), disease-free periods were significantly greater for those who received prophylactic medications compared with those who did not. In general, prophylaxis has included trimethoprim-sulfamethoxazole (TMP-SMX) and/or antistaphylococcal agents (dicloxacillin or oxacillin), as were used in these two studies. In a subsequent study from the NIH, prophylaxis using TMP-SMX alone decreased the incidence of nonfungal infections by 50% to 75% without causing an increase in fungal disease. Prophylactic parenteral antibiotics generally are recommended for patients with CGD before elective surgical or dental procedures. A combination of an antistaphylococcal drug, based on community drug-resistance patterns, along with an aminoglycoside administered 30 to 60 minutes before and 8 to 16 hours after the procedure has been suggested.

Because invasive fungal disease, in particular *Aspergillus*, is particularly difficult to treat in CGD patients, a trial of itraconazole to prevent fungal infections was performed over a 10-year period at the NIH. Because of the rarity of this disorder, and the toxicity that may occur with the use of itraconazole, a novel trial design was employed. Patients received randomly, in a double-blind manner, alternate years of either itraconazole or placebo. The incidence of severe infection was significantly less when patients received itraconazole compared to placebo. Whereas no serious toxic effects occurred with itraconazole in this study, monitoring for long-term toxic effects is warranted.

In addition to the therapeutic and supportive measures described, the availability of recombinant interferon-gamma provides an important advantage in the clinical management of CGD. A number of *in vitro* and small *in vivo* studies suggested that interferon-gamma could enhance the killing of staphylococci and promote some superoxide production in phagocytic cells. These findings prompted the International CGD Cooperative Study of interferon-gamma prophylaxis in all forms of CGD. This study comprehensively evaluated the efficacy of subcutaneous interferon-gamma in decreasing the severity or frequency of serious infections in 128 patients, 67 of whom had X-linked CGD. Although no improvement in neutrophil staphylococcal killing or superoxide production by patient neutrophils was shown, a significant clinical benefit was noted in the treatment group. In subjects younger than 10 years, as much as a fourfold increase in the risk for significant infection was noted in the placebo-treated controls, when compared with the subjects treated with interferon-gamma. The long-term follow-up of these patients (3 to 5 years later) continued to demonstrate diminished infection rates and few complications, which were minor. The ameliorative effects of interferon-gamma in CGD likely involve immunologic mechanisms unrelated to (or in addition to) the NADPH oxidase complex.

BMT has become a valid therapeutic option in CGD patients who have an HLA-identical donor. The European experience from 1985 through 2000 has demonstrated that 22 of 27 patients who received a BMT from an HLA-identical donor after a myeloablative regimen achieved a "cure." Survival was especially good in patients without infection. In the United States, five adult and five pediatric patients received nonmyeloablative conditioning, followed by a T-cell–depleted allograft from an HLA-identical family donor. During the follow-up period, of those who engrafted, four patients had serious infections.

The successful *in vitro* replacement of gp91 *phox* or p47 *phox* proteins in CGD CD34$^+$ peripheral blood has been accomplished using retroviral vectors containing gp91 *phox* or *phox* DNA. Transient expression (up to 6 months) and some resulting functional restoration (enhanced superoxide generation) in these cells was observed. However, a very minor fraction of cells were oxidase positive (i.e., had normal oxidative burst). Although these early-phase studies show promise, they suggest that marrow conditioning prior to the infusion of transduced cells will be important to achieve higher levels of engraftment. In addition, for gene therapy to succeed, more efficient gene transfer techniques must be developed.

Glucose-6-Phosphate Dehydrogenase Deficiency

Most variants of heritable G6PD deficiency are characterized clinically by chronic nonspherocytic hemolytic anemia with no features related to leukocyte dysfunction. Rare examples have been described of severe or total deficiency of both erythrocyte and leukocyte G6PD activity associated with impaired leukocyte function and susceptibility to severe and life-threatening infectious complications. The leukocytes of individuals severely deficient (1% to 5% of normal) in G6PD share many characteristics of CGD. The cells of both groups demonstrate diminished intracellular killing of catalase-positive organisms and a failure to reduce NBT or generate chemiluminescence, superoxide anion, or H_2O_2; both also demonstrate an impaired activation of the hexose monophosphate shunt (HMPS) during phagocytosis. Methylene blue does not normalize HMPS shunt activation by G6PD-deficient leukocytes, as it does with CGD cells. This occurs because G6PD-deficient leukocytes contain limited pools of reduced pyridine nucleotides (NADPH), which serve as substrates for methylene blue, although they do contain normal NADPH oxidase activity.

Patients with severe variants of G6PD deficiency are susceptible to a variety of infectious agents and complications similar to those observed in individuals with CGD. A fatal episode of septicemia caused by *E. coli* and *Klebsiella* pneumonia was reported in a 52-year-old woman with total G6PD deficiency. In another report, the granulocytes of three G6PD-deficient male siblings of a single kindred demonstrated moderately diminished NBT reduction, HMPS activity, and microbicidal activity for *S. aureus*. One sibling experienced recurrent granulomatous lymphadenitis caused by *S. aureus* and required multiple drainage procedures and prolonged antibiotic therapy. A second sibling experienced a single episode of cervical lymphadenitis, and a third reportedly had no history of infections. One report described a Texas child with total G6PD deficiency who died of an overwhelming septicemia shock syndrome secondary to *Chromobacterium violaceum*. The granulocytes of an identical twin demonstrated severely impaired NBT reduction, HMPS activation, superoxide generation, and impaired microbicidal activity for *S. aureus* and *C. violaceum*. This unique infectious complication probably reflected both host defense deficits in this child as well as the selective endemic occurrence of *C. violaceum* in the southeastern United States. Individuals with mild to moderate G6PD deficiency (20% to 50% of normal G6PD) do not demonstrate susceptibility to infections.

Suggested Readings

Alon R, Etzioni A. LAD-III, a novel group of leukocyte integrin activation deficiencies. *Trends Immunol* 2003;24:561.

Anderson DC, Smith CW. Leukocyte adhesion deficiencies In: Scriver CR, Beaudet AL, Sly WS, et al., eds. *The metabolic and molecular bases of inherited disease*, 8th ed. New York: McGraw-Hill, 2001:4829.

Deas DE, Mackey SA, McDonnell HT. Systemic disease and periodontitis: manifestations of neutrophil dysfunction. *Periodontol 2000* 2003;32:82.

Dinauer MC, Lekstrom-Himes JA, Dale DC. Inherited neutrophil disorders: molecular basis and new therapies. *Hematology (Am Soc Hematol Educ Program)* 2000;303.

Gallin JI, Alling DW, Malech HL, et al. Itraconazole to prevent fungal infections in chronic granulomatous disease. *N Engl J Med* 2003;348:2416.

Ginzberg H, Shin J, Ellis L, et al. Shwachman syndrome: phenotypic manifestations of sibling sets and isolated cases in a large patient cohort are similar. *J Pediatr* 1999;135:81.

Gombart AF, Kwok SH, Anderson KL, et al. Regulation of neutrophil and eosinophil secondary granule gene expression by transcription factors C/EBP epsilon and PU.1. *Blood* 2003;101:3265.

Ho CM, Vowels MR, Lockwood L, Ziegler JB. Successful bone marrow transplantation in a child with a X-linked chronic granulomatous disease. *Bone Marrow Transplant* 1996;18:213.

Karim MA, Suzuki K, Fukai K, et al. Apparent genotype-phenotype correlation in childhood, adolescent, and adult Chédiak-Higashi syndrome. *Am J Med Genet* 2002;108:16.

Kim SK, Keeney SE, Alpard SK, Schmalstieg FC. Comparison of L-selectin and CD11b on neutrophils of adults and neonates during the first month of life. *Pediatr Res* 2003;53:132.

Kuijpers TW, Maianski NA, Tool AT, et al. Apoptotic neutrophils in the circulation of patients with glycogen storage disease type 1b (GSD1b). *Blood* 2003;101:5021.

Visser G, Rake JP, Labrune P, et al. Granulocyte colony-stimulating factor in glycogen storage disease type 1b. Results of the European Study on Glycogen Storage Disease Type 1. *Eur J Pediatr* 2002;161:S83.

Wild MK, Luhn K, Marquardt T, Vestweber D. Leukocyte adhesion deficiency II: therapy and genetic defect. *Cells Tissues Organs* 2002;172:161.

CHAPTER 431 ■ COMBINED IMMUNODEFICIENCY DISEASES

REBECCA H. BUCKLEY

Genetic defects in T-cell function lead to an increased susceptibility to infections or to other clinical problems that are more serious than in those disorders characterized by antibody deficiency alone. Those affected usually present during infancy with either common or opportunistic infections; they rarely survive beyond infancy or childhood. Except for the DiGeorge anomaly, no isolated defects of T-cell development occur. B cells require T-cell help for antibody production; therefore, a T-cell defect must of necessity also result in B-cell deficiency, even when the B cells themselves are completely competent. The spectrum of combined immunodeficiency ranges from the syndrome of severe combined immunodeficiency (SCID), in which T-cell function is absent, to those with combined immunodeficiency disorders (CID) in which some T-cell function is present, but not an adequate amount for a normal life span. Recent discoveries of the molecular causes of many of these defects have led to a new understanding of the flawed biology underlying this ever-growing number of defects (Table 431.1). This chapter reviews the current information on some, but by no means all, of these defects.

DIGEORGE SYNDROME

Pathophysiology and Comorbidity

Thymic hypoplasia results from dysmorphogenesis of the third and fourth pharyngeal pouches during early embryogenesis; this leads to hypoplasia or aplasia of the thymus and parathyroid glands. Other structures forming at the same age also are affected frequently, resulting in anomalies of the great vessels (right-sided aortic arch), esophageal atresia, bifid uvula, up-

per limb malformations, congenital heart disease (conotruncal, atrial, and ventricular septal defects), a short philtrum of the upper lip, hypertelorism, an anti-mongoloid slant to the eyes, mandibular hypoplasia, and low-set, often notched ears. A variable degree of hypoplasia of the thymus and parathyroid glands (partial DiGeorge syndrome) is more frequent than total aplasia. Those with complete DiGeorge syndrome are highly susceptible to infections by opportunistic pathogens and to graft-versus-host disease (GVHD) from nonirradiated blood transfusions.

DiGeorge syndrome has occurred in both males and females; rare cases of autosomal dominant inheritance have been reported. Microdeletions of specific DNA sequences from chromosome 22q11.2 (the DiGeorge chromosomal region) have been shown in a majority of, but certainly not all, patients with the clinical features of this syndrome. There appears to be an excess of 22q11.2 deletions of maternal origin. Another deletion associated with DiGeorge and velocardiofacial syndromes is on chromosome 10p13.

Clinical Manifestations and Complications

Patients with DiGeorge syndrome may be mildly to severely lymphopenic, due to the fact that the decrease in the number of circulating $CD3^+$ T cells depends on the degree of thymic deficiency. Immunoglobulin concentrations are usually normal, although sometimes IgE is elevated and IgA may be low. Responses of blood lymphocytes after mitogen stimulation have been absent, reduced, or normal. Thymic tissue, when found in the partial form, contains Hassall's corpuscles and a normal density of thymocytes; corticomedullary distinction is present.

TABLE 431.1

LOCATIONS OF FAULTY GENES IN CELLULAR IMMUNODEFICIENCY DISORDERS

Chromosome	Disease
1q21	MCH class II antigen deficiency caused by RFX5 mutation*
1q42–43	Chédiak-Higashi syndrome*
2q12	CD8 lymphocytopenia caused by ZAP70 deficiency*
5p13	SCID due to IL-7 receptor alpha chain deficiency*
6p21.3	MHC class I antigen defect caused by mutations in *TAP 1* or *TAP2**
6q22–q23	Interferon-R1 mutations*
8q21	Nijmegan breakage syndrome due to mutations in *Nibrin**
9p13	Cartilage hair hypoplasia due to mutations in endoribonuclease *RMRP**
10p13	SCID (Athabaskan, radiation sensitive) due to mutations in the *Artemis* gene*
10p13	DiGeorge syndrome/velocardiofacial syndrome
11p13	Il-2 receptor alpha chain deficiency*
11p13	SCID caused by RAG-1 or RAG-2 deficiencies*
11q22.3	Ataxia-telangiectasia (AT), attributable to AT mutation, causing deficiency of DNA-dependent kinase*
11q23	CD3 delta, gamma- or epsilon-chain deficiency*
13q	MHC class II antigen deficiency caused by RFXAP mutation*
14q13.1	Purine nucleoside phosphorylase (PNP) deficiency*
16p13	MHC class II antigen deficiency caused by CIITA mutation*
17	Human nude defect*
19p13.1	SCID caused by Janus kinase 3 (Jak3) deficiency*
20q13.11	SCID caused by adenosine deaminase (ADA) deficiency*
22q11.2	DiGeorge syndrome
Xp11.23	Wiskott-Aldrich syndrome (WAS) caused by WAS protein (WASP) deficiency*
Xq13.1	X-linked SCID caused by common gamma-chain γc deficiency*
Xq24-26	X-linked lymphoproliferative syndrome caused by mutations in the *SH2D1A* gene*

*Gene cloned and sequenced; gene product known. (Reproduced with permission, but updated from Buckley RH: Primary cellular immunodeficiencies. *JACI* 2004;109:747.)

Lymphoid follicles usually are present, but lymph-node paracortical areas and thymus-dependent regions of the spleen show variable degrees of depletion.

Therapy

Treatment of the complete form of DiGeorge syndrome should begin as soon as possible after diagnosis. Transplantation of cultured, mature thymic epithelial explants has successfully reconstituted the immune function of several infants with the complete DiGeorge syndrome. A few patients with complete DiGeorge syndrome have developed T-cell function after hu-

man leukocyte antigen (HLA)-identical bone marrow transplantation by adoptive transfer of donor T cells, but this treatment cannot correct the thymic defect. No immunologic treatment is needed for the partial form. If patients with the partial DiGeorge syndrome do not have a severe cardiac lesion, they have few clinical problems except that some experience seizures and developmental delay.

SEVERE COMBINED IMMUNODEFICIENCY

Pathophysiology

Severe combined immunodeficiency, or SCID, is a fatal syndrome of diverse genetic cause characterized by profound deficiencies of T- and B-cell (and sometimes natural killer [NK] cell) function. These infants also lack the ability to reject foreign tissue and are, therefore, at risk for GVHD from maternal T cells that cross into the fetal circulation while the SCID infant is *in utero*, or from T lymphocytes in nonirradiated blood products (Fig. 431.1) or allogeneic bone marrow.

In the five decades since the initial description of SCID, it has become evident that the genetic origins of this condition are extremely diverse (Fig. 431.2). X-linked SCID (SCID-X1) is the most common form, accounting for approximately 46% of cases in the United States (Fig. 431.2). In addition, mutated genes on autosomal chromosomes have been identified in nine genetic types of SCID: adenosine deaminase (ADA) deficiency, Janus kinase 3 (Jak3) deficiency, interleukin-7 receptor alpha-chain deficiency (IL-7R), recombinase-activating gene (*RAG-1* or *RAG-2*) deficiencies, *Artemis* deficiency, CD45 deficiency, and CD3 delta (CD3δ) chain and epsilon (CD3ε) deficiencies; and there are likely other causes yet to be discovered (Table 431.2).

Clinical Manifestations and Complications

Affected infants present within the first few months of life with frequent episodes of diarrhea, pneumonia, otitis, sepsis, and cutaneous infections. Persistent infections with opportunistic organisms such as *Candida albicans*, *Pneumocystis jiroveci*,

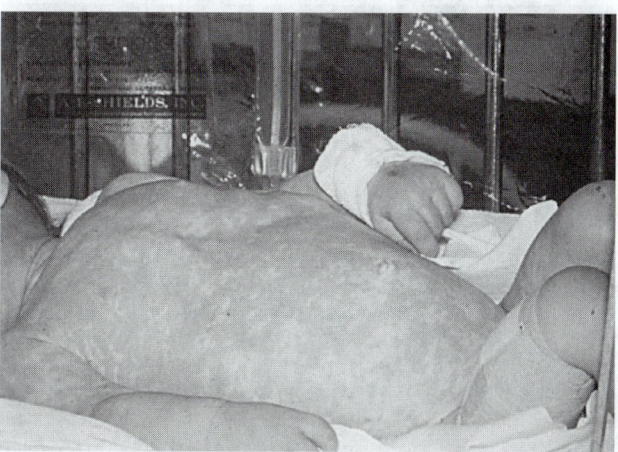

FIGURE 431.1. An infant with SCID who developed lethal graft-versus-host disease from a non-irradiated packed red blood cell transfusion. (Reproduced with permission from Buckley RH. A historical review of bone marrow transplantation for immunodeficiencies. *JACI* 2004;113:792.)

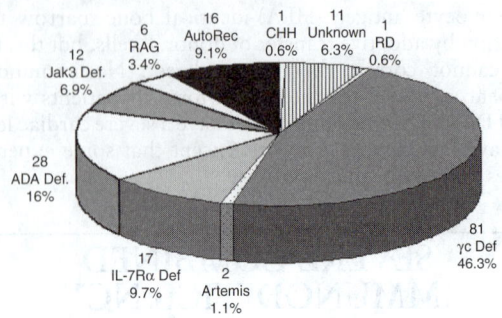

FIGURE 431.2. Relative frequencies of the different genetic types of SCID among 175 patients seen consecutively by the author.

TABLE 431.2
TEN ABNORMAL GENES IN SCID

Cytokine Receptor Genes
IL2RG
JAK3
IL7Rα
Antigen Receptor Genes
RAG1
RAG2
ARTEMIS
CD3δ and epsilon
Other Genes
ADA
CD45

varicella-zoster virus (Fig. 431.3), parainfluenza 3 virus, respiratory syncytial virus, adenovirus, cytomegalovirus, Epstein-Barr virus, and bacillus Calmette-Guérin lead to death. Infants with SCID are lymphopenic due to the fact that they lack T cells. They have an absence of lymphocyte proliferative responses to mitogens, antigens, and allogeneic cells *in vitro*, even on blood samples collected *in utero* or from the cord blood.

Diagnosis

Physicians caring for newborns must be aware of the normal range for the cord blood absolute lymphocyte count (2,000 to 11,000/mm³) and arrange for T-cell phenotypic and functional studies to be performed on blood from neonates with values below 2,500/mm³. Unfortunately, most SCIDs are not diagnosed until 6 to 7 months of age, when they present with serious infections. At that age, the normal absolute lymphocyte count is much higher, with the mean being 7,500/mm³ and the lower limit of normal 4,000/mm³. Serum immunoglobulin concentrations are diminished to absent, and no antibody formation occurs after immunization. Typically, all SCID patients have very small thymuses (usually less than 1 g), which fail to

descend from the neck, contain no thymocytes, and lack corticomedullary distinction and Hassall's corpuscles. However, the thymic epithelium is normal, and the results of bone marrow stem cell transplantation have shown that these tiny thymuses are capable of supporting the maturation of stem cells into normal T cells. Thymus-dependent areas of the spleen are depleted of lymphocytes in SCID patients, and lymph nodes, tonsils, adenoids, and Peyer's patches are absent or extremely underdeveloped.

AUTOSOMAL RECESSIVE SEVERE COMBINED IMMUNODEFICIENCY DISEASE CAUSED BY ADENOSINE DEAMINASE DEFICIENCY

Pathophysiology

An absence of the enzyme adenosine deaminase (ADA) was the first discovered molecular cause of SCID. It was first reported in 1972, and has since been observed in approximately 16% of patients with SCID, being the second most common cause of SCID (Table 431.2, Fig. 431.2). The gene encoding ADA is on chromosome 20q13-ter.

Clinical Manifestations and Complications

Certain distinguishing features of ADA deficiency can be noted, including the presence of multiple skeletal abnormalities of chondroosseous dysplasia on radiographic examination; these occur predominantly at the costochondral junctions, at the apophyses of the iliac bones, and in the vertebral bodies (causing a "bone-in-bone" effect). ADA deficiency results in pronounced accumulations of adenosine, 2′-deoxyadenosine, and 2′-O-methyladenosine. These toxic metabolites directly or indirectly lead to apoptosis of thymocytes and circulating lymphocytes, which causes the immunodeficiency. ADA-deficient infants usually have a much more profound lymphopenia than those with other types of SCID, with mean absolute lymphocyte counts of less than 500/mm³. They thus have a T-B-NK-lymphocyte phenotype (Table 431.3).

Therapy

As with other types of SCID, ADA deficiency can be cured by HLA-identical or haploidentical T cell–depleted bone marrow

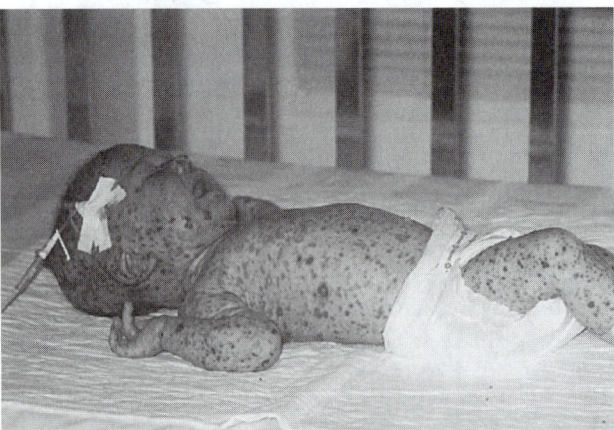

FIGURE 431.3. Infant with X-linked SCID who experienced varicella three times before the diagnosis of SCID was made. The child survived because of the availability of acyclovir and the ability to give a haploidentical bone marrow transplant from his mother. (Reproduced with permission from Buckley RH. A historical review of bone marrow transplantation for immunodeficiencies. *JACI* 2004;113:792.)

TABLE 431.3

LYMPHOCYTE PHENOTYPES IN THE DIFFERENT FORMS OF SCID

T⁻B⁺NK⁻	γc-deficient
	Jak 3-deficient
	CD45-deficient
T⁻B⁺NK⁺	IL-7Ra-deficient
	CD3δ-deficient
T⁻B⁻NK⁻	ADA or ε deficient
T⁻B⁻NK⁺	RAG1/RAG2-deficient
	Artemis-deficient

transplantation, which remains the treatment of choice. Enzyme replacement therapy using polyethylene glycol-modified bovine ADA (PEG-ADA) administered subcutaneously once or twice a week has resulted in both clinical and immunologic improvement. However, the immunocompetence achieved is not nearly so great as with bone marrow transplantation. In view of this, PEG-ADA therapy should not be initiated if bone marrow transplantation is contemplated, because it will confer graft-rejection capability upon the infant. After T-cell function is corrected by bone marrow transplantation (without pretransplantation chemotherapy), infants with ADA deficiency usually have adequate B-cell function.

X-LINKED RECESSIVE SEVERE COMBINED IMMUNODEFICIENCY DISEASE (SCID-X1)

Pathophysiology

After 1972, an X-linked pattern of inheritance was recognized in some families with SCID. These infants resembled those with non–X-linked SCID in their extreme susceptibility to infection and early demise from such. In 1989, the abnormal gene in SCID-X1 was mapped by restriction fragment length polymorphism (RFLP) analysis to the Xq13 region. In 1993, the faulty gene was identified as IL2RG, the gene encoding a common gamma γc chain shared by six cytokine receptors, including those for IL-2, IL-4, IL-7, IL-9, IL-15, and IL-21 (Table 431.2).

Clinical Manifestations and Complications

Despite the uniformly profound lack of T- or B-cell function, patients with SCID-X1 usually have few or no T or NK cells but a normal or elevated number of B cells. This results in a T-B⁺NK⁻ lymphocyte phenotype (Table 431.3). However, SCID-X1 B cells do not produce immunoglobulin normally, even after T-cell reconstitution through HLA-identical or T cell–depleted haploidentical bone marrow stem cell transplantation. In addition, they lack NK cells and function and do not maintain sustained production of NK cells after transplantation. The finding that the mutated gene results in faulty signaling through multiple cytokine receptors explains how many cell types can be affected by a mutation in a single gene. Of the first 136 patients studied, 95 distinct mutations spanning all eight IL2RG exons were identified, most of them consisting of small changes at the level of one to a few nucleotides. These mutations resulted in abnormal gamma chains in two-thirds of the cases and absent gamma protein in the remainder.

AUTOSOMAL RECESSIVE SEVERE COMBINED IMMUNODEFICIENCY DISEASE CAUSED BY JANUS KINASE 3 (JAK3) DEFICIENCY

Pathophysiology

Because Janus kinase 3 (Jak3) is the primary signal transducer from γc, the gene encoding it was considered a candidate for mutations leading to autosomal recessive SCID of unknown molecular type. Thus far, more than 40 patients with mutations in the Jak3 gene have been identified (Table 431.2, Fig. 431.2).

Clinical Manifestations and Complications

SCID patients with autosomal recessive SCID caused by Jak3 deficiency have clinical problems similar to those of all other types of SCID, but they have a lymphocyte phenotype identical to those of patients with X-linked SCID (that is, an elevated percentage of B cells and very low percentages of T and NK cells (T⁻B⁺NK⁻, Table 431.3). Because mutations in this gene abrogate signaling through the same six cytokine receptors affected by IL2RG mutations, Jak3-deficient SCID infants also often fail to develop normal B-cell function after T-cell function is corrected by HLA-identical or T cell–depleted haploidentical bone marrow transplantation. Moreover, in further similarity to SCID-X1 patients, they also fail to develop a sustained production of NK cells after transplantation.

AUTOSOMAL RECESSIVE SEVERE COMBINED IMMUNODEFICIENCY CAUSED BY INTERLEUKIN 7 RECEPTOR ALPHA CHAIN (IL-7Rα) DEFICIENCY

Because mice whose genes for either the alpha chain of the IL-7 receptor or of IL-7 itself have been mutated are profoundly deficient in T- and B-cell function but have normal NK-cell function, naturally occurring mutations in these genes were sought in some of the author's patients who had T⁻B⁺NK⁺ SCID (Table 431.3) and who had previously been shown not to have either γc or Jak3 deficiency. Mutations in the gene for IL-7Rα on chromosome 5p13 have thus far been found in seventeen (10%) of the author's patients, making it the third most common cause of human SCID (Fig. 431.2). These findings imply that the T-cell, but not the NK-cell defect, in SCID-X1 and Jak3-deficient SCID results from an inability to signal through the IL-7 receptor. The fact that these patients have developed normal B-cell function after nonablative T cell–depleted haploidentical bone marrow stem cell transplantation despite lacking donor B cells also suggests that the B-cell defect in SCID-X1 is not due to failure of IL-7 signaling.

AUTOSOMAL RECESSIVE SEVERE COMBINED IMMUNODEFICIENCY CAUSED BY RECOMBINASE-ACTIVATING GENE (RAG-1 OR RAG-2) DEFICIENCIES

Infants with autosomal recessive SCID caused by mutations in recombinase activating genes, RAG-1 and RAG-2, resemble all others in their infection susceptibility and complete absence of T- or B-cell function. However, their lymphocyte phenotype differs from those of patients with SCID caused by γc, Jak3, IL-7Rα, or ADA deficiencies in that they lack both B and T lymphocytes and have only NK cells in their circulation (i.e., a T⁻B⁻NK⁺ phenotype, Table 431.3). This particular phenotype suggested a possible problem with their antigen receptor genes, leading to the discovery of mutations in *RAG-1* and *RAG-2* in some (but not all) such SCID infants (Table 431.2). These genes, on chromosome 11p13, encode the proteins necessary for somatic rearrangement of antigen receptor genes on T and B cells. The proteins recognize recombination signal sequences (RSSs) and introduce a DNA double-stranded break, permitting V, D, and J gene rearrangements. *RAG-1* or *RAG-2* mutations result in a functional inability to form antigen receptors through genetic recombination, thus explaining the absence of both T and B cells in the circulation.

Patients with Omenn syndrome also have mutations in *RAG1* or *RAG2* genes, resulting in partial and impaired V(D)J recombinational activity. Omenn syndrome is characterized by the development soon after birth of a generalized erythroderma and desquamation, diarrhea, hepatosplenomegaly, hypereosinophilia, and markedly elevated serum IgE levels. The latter are caused by circulating, activated, oligoclonal T lymphocytes that do not respond normally to mitogens or antigens *in vitro*. Circulating B cells are not found, and lymph node architecture is abnormal due to a lack of germinal centers. The condition is fatal unless corrected by bone marrow transplantation.

AUTOSOMAL RECESSIVE SEVERE COMBINED IMMUNODEFICIENCY CAUSED BY DEFICIENCIES OF THE ARTEMIS GENE PRODUCT

Another cause of SCID characterized by absence of B and T cells but the presence of NK cells (a T⁻B⁻NK⁺ phenotype (Table 431.3) is a deficiency of a novel V(D)J recombination/DNA repair factor that belongs to the metallo-lactamase superfamily. It is encoded by a gene on chromosome 10p called *Artemis* (Table 431.2). A deficiency of this factor results in an inability to repair DNA after double-stranded cuts have been made by *RAG1* or *RAG2* gene products in rearranging antigen receptor genes from their germline configuration. In addition, increased radiation sensitivity is present in both the skin fibroblasts and bone marrow cells of those affected with this type of SCID. This defect also causes so-called Athabaskan SCID.

AUTOSOMAL RECESSIVE SEVERE COMBINED IMMUNODEFICIENCY CAUSED BY CD3 DELTA (CD3δ) AND EPSILON (CD3ε) CHAIN DEFICIENCIES

The most recently discovered causes of human SCID are deficiencies of the CD3 delta (CD3δ) chain a component of the T-cell antigen receptor (TCR) (Table 432.2). Infants with this type of SCID resemble those patients presenting with all the other types of SCID in their extreme infection susceptibility and complete absence of T-cell function. They had a normal or elevated number of B cells and a normal number of NK cells. Their lymphocyte phenotypes thus resembles that of IL-7Rα–deficient SCID (Table 431.3). Their blood lymphocytes failed

to proliferate in response to mitogens, and their thymi lacked corticomedullary distinction and Hassall's corpuscles. These infants contrast sharply with individuals who have mutations in genes encoding the CD3-gamma chain, who have only a partial arrest in T-cell development and much milder forms of immunodeficiency. The findings suggest that CD3δ and CD3ε are essential for T-cell development.

AUTOSOMAL RECESSIVE SEVERE COMBINED IMMUNODEFICIENCY CAUSED BY CD45 DEFICIENCY

Mutations in the gene encoding the common leukocyte surface protein CD45 have been identified in infants with human SCID who did not have any of the previously described mutations (Table 432.2). This hematopoietic-cell–specific transmembrane protein, a tyrosine phosphatase, functions to regulate the Src kinases required for T- and B-cell antigen receptor signal transduction. A 2-month-old male infant presented with a clinical picture of SCID and was found to have a very low number of T cells but a normal number of B cells. The T cells failed to respond to mitogens, and serum immunoglobulins diminished with time. He was found to have a large deletion at one *CD45* allele and a point mutation causing an alteration of the intervening sequence 13 donor splice site at the other. Two more cases of SCID due to CD45 deficiency have been reported.

THERAPY AND PROGNOSIS OF SEVERE COMBINED IMMUNODEFICIENCIES

Bone Marrow Transplantation

SCID is a pediatric emergency. Replacement therapy with intravenous immunoglobulin (IVIG) fails to halt the progressively downhill course. Unless bone marrow transplantation from HLA-identical or haploidentical donors can be performed, death usually occurs before the patient's first birthday and almost invariably before the second. On the other hand, transplantation in the first 3.5 months of life offers a greater than 97% chance of survival (Fig. 431.4). Therefore, early diagnosis is essential. Recent studies have shown that the immune reconstitution effected by stem cell transplants is due to thymic education of the transplanted allogeneic stem cells. The thymic output appears to occur sooner and to a greater degree in those infants transplanted in the neonatal period, as opposed to those transplanted after that time. Currently, more than 400 SCID patients are surviving worldwide as a result of successful bone marrow transplantation.

Gene Therapy

ADA deficiency was the first genetic defect in which gene therapy was attempted; these early efforts were unsuccessful. However, beginning in 1999, a normal γc cDNA was successfully transduced into the autologous marrow cells of nine infants with SCID-X1 using retroviral gene transfer, with subsequent full correction of their T- and NK-cell defects. This offered hope that gene therapy would eventually be the treatment of choice for all patients with SCID or other genetically determined immunodeficiency diseases for whom the molecular basis is known. Unfortunately, three of the recipients of the successful

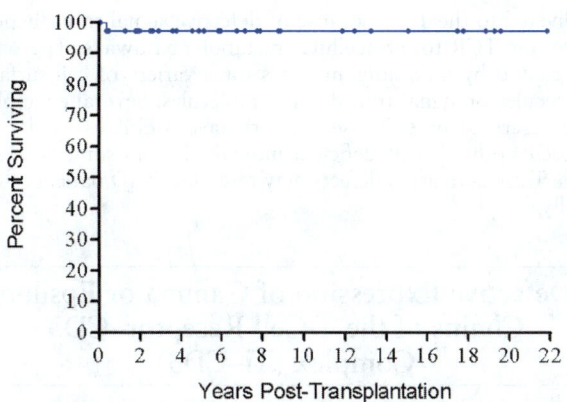

FIGURE 431.4. Kaplan-Meier survival curve for 38 consecutive infants with SCID who received bone marrow transplants at the author's institution from HLA-identical (n = 5) or haploidentical (n = 33) donors before they were 3.5 months of age without pretransplantation chemoablation or posttransplantation GVHD prophylaxis. Thirty-seven (97%) infants survive for periods of 2 months to 22 years after transplantation. The one death occurred from a cytomegalovirus infection.

gene therapy developed a leukemic-like process 3 years later due to a process called insertional oncogenesis. The γc cDNA was found to have integrated into the infants' DNA in or near the *LMO-2* oncogene. The *LMO-2* gene is aberrantly expressed in acute lymphoblastic leukemia of childhood. Because of these serious adverse events, gene therapy trials were halted until means to avoid this problem could be found.

COMBINED IMMUNODEFICIENCY

The term combined immunodeficiency (CID) is used to distinguish patients with low but not absent T-cell function from those with SCID. Three examples are given below.

Purine Nucleoside Phosphorylase Deficiency

Pathophysiology

More than 40 patients with CID have been found to have purine nucleoside phosphorylase (PNP) deficiency. The gene encoding PNP is on chromosome 14q13.1 (Table 431.1), and a variety of mutations in it have been found in patients with PNP deficiency. Unlike ADA deficiency, serum and urinary uric acid are deficient, because PNP is needed to form the urate precursors hypoxanthine and xanthine.

Clinical Manifestations and Complications

Deaths have occurred from generalized vaccinia, varicella, lymphosarcoma, and GVHD mediated by T cells from non-irradiated allogeneic blood or bone marrow. Two-thirds of patients have had neurologic abnormalities ranging from spasticity to mental retardation. One-third of patients developed autoimmune diseases, the most common of which is autoimmune hemolytic anemia. Most patients have normal or elevated concentrations of all serum immunoglobulins. PNP-deficient patients are as profoundly lymphopenic as those with ADA deficiency, with absolute lymphocyte counts of usually less than 500/mm³. T-cell function is low but not absent and is variable with time.

Therapy

Prenatal diagnosis is possible. PNP deficiency is invariably fatal in childhood unless immunologic reconstitution can be achieved. Bone marrow transplantation is the treatment of choice, but has thus far been successful in only a few such patients.

Ataxia-Telangiectasia

Pathophysiology

The inheritance of AT follows an autosomal recessive pattern. The mutated gene (*ATM*) responsible for this defect was mapped by restriction fragment-length polymorphism analysis to the long arm of chromosome 11 (11q22–23) and was cloned (Table 431.1). The gene product is a DNA-dependent protein kinase localized predominantly to the nucleus and believed to be involved in mitogenic signal transduction, meiotic recombination, and cell cycle control. No satisfactory definitive treatment has been found. The most common causes of death are lymphoreticular malignancy and progressive neurologic disease.

Clinical Manifestations and Complications

Ataxia-telangiectasia (AT) is a complex combined immunodeficiency syndrome with associated neurologic, endocrinologic, hepatic, and cutaneous abnormalities. The most prominent features are progressive cerebellar ataxia, oculocutaneous telangiectasias, chronic sinopulmonary disease, a high incidence of malignancy, and variable humoral and cellular immunodeficiency. The ataxia typically becomes evident shortly after the child begins to walk, and progresses until he is confined to a wheelchair, usually by 10 to 12 years of age. The telangiectasias develop at between 3 and 6 years of age. Recurrent, usually bacterial, sinopulmonary infections occur in roughly 80% of these patients. Fatal varicella has occurred, and transfusion-associated GVHD also has been reported. Selective IgA deficiency is found in from 50% to 80% of those affected. IgE concentrations are usually low, and IgG2 or total IgG may be decreased. Specific antibody titers may be decreased or normal. Impaired (but not absent) cell-mediated immunity is present *in vivo*, as evidenced by delayed skin test anergy and prolonged allograft survival. The percentages of CD3+ and CD4+ T cells are only modestly low, and *in vitro* tests of lymphocyte function have generally shown moderately depressed proliferative responses to T- and B-cell mitogens. The thymus is hypoplastic, exhibits poor organization, and is lacking in Hassall's corpuscles. Cells from patients, as well as those from heterozygous carriers, have an increased sensitivity to ionizing radiation, defective DNA repair, and frequent chromosomal abnormalities. The malignancies reported in this condition usually have been of the lymphoreticular type, but adenocarcinoma and other forms also have been seen; an increased incidence of malignancy also is noted in unaffected relatives.

Immunodeficiency with Thrombocytopenia and Eczema (Wiskott-Aldrich Syndrome)

Pathophysiology

The mutated gene responsible for this defect is on the short arm of the X chromosome at position 11.22–11.23 (Table 431.1); it was isolated in 1994, and it was found to be limited in expression to lymphocytic and megakaryocytic lineages. The gene product, a 501–amino-acid proline-rich protein that lacks a hydrophobic transmembrane domain, was designated WASP (WAS protein). It has been shown to bind CDC42H2 and rac, members of the Rho family of GTPases, which are important in actin polymerization. A large and varied number of mutations in the WASP gene have been identified in WAS patients. Isolated X-linked thrombocytopenia (XLT) also is caused by mutations in (usually) a different part of the WASP gene. Carriers of WAS or XLT can be detected and prenatal diagnosis made by chorionic villous sampling or amniocentesis, if the mutation is known in that family. Two families with apparent autosomal inheritance of a clinical phenotype similar to WAS have been reported and, in one case, a girl was shown to have this as an X-linked defect.

Clinical Manifestations and Complications

The Wiskott-Aldrich syndrome (WAS) is an X-linked recessive syndrome characterized by eczema, thrombocytopenic purpura with normal-appearing megakaryocytes but small defective platelets, and undue susceptibility to infection. Patients usually present during infancy with prolonged bleeding from the circumcision site, bloody diarrhea, or excessive bruising. Atopic dermatitis and recurrent infections usually also develop during the first year of life. Infections are usually those produced by pneumococci and other encapsulated bacteria, resulting in otitis media, pneumonia, meningitis, or sepsis. Later, infections with opportunistic agents such as *Pneumocystis carinii* and the herpesviruses become more problematic. Autoimmune cytopenias and vasculitis are common in those who live beyond infancy. Survival beyond the teens is rare. Infections, vasculitis, and bleeding are major causes of death, but the most common cause of death in WAS patients currently is Epstein-Barr virus (EBV)-induced lymphoreticular malignancy.

Patients with WAS have an impaired humoral immune response to polysaccharide antigens, as evidenced by absent or greatly diminished isohemagglutinins and poor or absent antibody responses to polysaccharide antigens. In addition, antibody titers to protein antigens fall with time. Most often, patients have a low serum IgM, elevated IgA and IgE, and a normal or slightly low IgG concentration. Flow cytometry of blood lymphocytes has shown a moderately reduced percentage of T cells, and lymphocyte responses to mitogens are depressed moderately.

Therapy

After being conditioned with irradiation or busulfan and cyclophosphamide, numerous patients with WAS have had complete corrections of both the platelet and the immunologic abnormalities using HLA-identical sibling bone marrow transplants. Success has been minimal with T cell–depleted haploidentical stem cell transplants in WAS, primarily because of resistance to engraftment. Recently, some success has been achieved in the treatment of WAS using matched unrelated donor (MUD) transplants when done in those under 5 years of age. It is likely that matched cord blood transplants will be similarly successful because, in both cases, T cells can be left in the donor-cell suspension. Several patients who required splenectomy for uncontrollable bleeding had impressive rises in their platelet counts and did well clinically while being administered prophylactic antibiotics and IVIG.

T-CELL ACTIVATION DEFECTS

These conditions are characterized by the presence of normal or elevated numbers of blood T cells that appear phenotypically normal but fail to proliferate or produce cytokines in response to stimulation with mitogens, antigens, or other signals delivered to the TCR because of defective signal transduction from the TCR to intracellular metabolic pathways. They can be caused by mutations in genes for a variety of cell surface molecules or signal transduction molecules. Several examples are described here. These patients have problems similar to those of other T cell–deficient individuals, and some with severe T-cell activation defects may resemble SCID patients clinically.

Defective Expression of Gamma or Epsilon Chains of the T-Cell Receptor–CD3 Complex (Ti–CD3)

Defective expression of CD3 on the surface of T cells was found in two male siblings in a Spanish family. The proband presented with severe infections and died at 31 months of age, with autoimmune hemolytic anemia and viral pneumonia. His lymphocytes had responded poorly to mitogens and to anti-CD3 *in vitro* and could not be stimulated to develop cytotoxic T cells. However, his antibody responses to protein antigens had been normal, indicating normal helper T-cell function. His 12-year-old brother was healthy, but he had almost no CD3-bearing T cells and had an IgG2 deficiency similar to his sibling. The defect in this family was shown to be attributable to mutations in the CD3 chain (Table 431.1).

The second form of this disorder was found in a 4-year-old French boy who had recurrent *Haemophilus influenzae* pneumonia and otitis media in early life but is now healthy. He had a partial defect in expression of Ti–CD3, resulting in an about half the normal percentage of CD3+ cells, all with very low CD3 staining on flow cytometry. His T cells did not proliferate in response to anti-CD3; however, they did respond normally to stimulation with anti-CD28. The defect was shown to be due to two independent CD3 gene mutations, leading to defective CD3 chain synthesis and preventing normal association and membrane expression of the Ti–CD3 complex (Table 431.1).

Zeta Chain-Associated Protein (ZAP-70) Deficiency

Pathophysiology

This condition is caused by mutations in the gene on chromosome 2 at position q12 that encodes ZAP-70, a non-src family protein tyrosine kinase important in T-cell signaling (Table 431.1). ZAP-70 has been shown to have an essential role in both positive and negative selection in the thymus. It is hypothesized that normal numbers of CD4+ T cells are present because thymocytes can use the other member of the same tyrosine kinase family, Syk, to facilitate positive selection of CD4+ cells. In addition, a stronger association of Lck with CD4+ is present than with CD8+ cells. Syk is present at fourfold higher levels in thymocytes than in peripheral T cells, possibly accounting for the lack of normal responses by the CD4+ blood T cells.

Clinical Manifestations

Patients with CD8 lymphocytopenia caused by ZAP-70 deficiency present during infancy with severe, recurrent, and sometimes fatal infections; however, they often live longer and present later than SCID patients. More than eight cases have been reported, and a majority were Mennonites. They have normal, low, or elevated serum immunoglobulin concentrations and normal or elevated numbers of circulating CD4+ T lymphocytes, but essentially no CD8+ cells. These CD4+ T cells fail to respond to mitogens or to allogeneic cells *in vitro* or to generate cytotoxic T lymphocytes. By contrast, NK activity is normal. The thymus may exhibit normal architecture, with normal numbers of CD4:CD8 double-positive thymocytes, but an absence of CD8 single-positive thymocytes.

Defective Expression of Major Histocompatibility Complex (MHC) Antigens
MHC Class I Antigen Deficiency

Pathophysiology

Mutations have been found in two genes within the MHC locus on chromosome 6 that encode the peptide transporter proteins, TAP1 and TAP2. TAP proteins function to transport peptide antigens from the cytoplasm across the Golgi apparatus membrane to join the chain of MHC class 1 molecules and B_2-microglobulin. The complex then can move to the cell surface; if the assembly of the complex cannot be completed because no peptide antigen is present, the MHC class I complex is destroyed in the cytoplasm. A newly discovered cause of MHC Class I antigen deficiency is a mutation in the gene encoding tapasin, another component of the peptide loading complex. Tapasin serves to link TAP1 and TAP2 to the MHC Class I heavy chain; its absence results in the impaired transport of MHC Class I antigens with peptides to the cell surface. The deficiency is somewhat less severe than in TAP1 and TAP2 mutations.

Clinical Manifestations and Complications

An isolated deficiency of MHC class I antigens is rare, and the resulting immunodeficiency is milder than that in SCID, resulting in a later age of presentation. A deficiency of CD8+ T cells is present, but not of CD4+ T cells. Sera from affected contain normal quantities of class I MHC antigens and B_2-microglobulin, but class I MHC antigens are not detected on any cells in the body.

MHC Class II Antigen Deficiency

Pathophysiology

Four different molecular defects resulting in impaired expression of MHC class II antigens have been identified (Table 431.1). In one, a mutation occurs in the gene on chromosome 1q that encodes a protein called RFX5, a subunit of RFX, a multiprotein complex that binds the X-box motif of MHC-II promoters. A second form is caused by mutations in a gene on chromosome 13q that encodes a second 36-kD subunit of the RFX complex, called *RFX-associated protein (RFXAP)*. The most common cause of MHC Class II defects are mutations in *RFXANK*, the gene encoding a third subunit of RFX. In a fourth type, a mutation occurs in the gene on chromosome 16p13 that encodes a novel MHC class II transactivator (CIITA), a non–DNA-binding coactivator that controls the cell-type specificity and inducibility of MHC-II expression. All these defects cause impairment in the coordinate expression of MHC class II molecules on the surface of B cells and macrophages.

Clinical Manifestations and Complications

Many patients affected with this autosomal recessive syndrome are of North African descent. More than 70 patients have been identified. They present in infancy with persistent diarrhea, often associated with cryptosporidiosis, *P. carinii* or bacterial pneumonia, septicemia, and viral or monilial infections. Nevertheless, their immunodeficiency is not as severe as in SCID, as

evidenced by their failure to develop bacille Calmette Guérin reactions (BCG-osis) or GVHD from nonirradiated blood transfusions. MHC class II–deficient patients have a very low number of CD4+ T cells, but normal or elevated numbers of CD8+ T cells. Lymphopenia is only moderate.

The MHC class II antigens, HLA-DP, DQ, and DR, are undetectable on blood B cells and monocytes. These patients have impaired antigen-specific responses caused by the absence of these antigen-presenting molecules. In addition, MHC antigen-deficient B cells fail to stimulate allogeneic cells in mixed leukocyte culture. Lymphocytes respond normally to mitogens but not to antigens. The thymus and other lymphoid organs are severely hypoplastic. The lack of Class II molecules results in abnormal thymic selection, because the recognition of HLA molecules by thymocytes is required for both positive and negative selection. The latter results in circulating CD4+ T cells that are not normally diverse. The associated defects of both B- and T-cell immunity and of HLA expression emphasize the important roles of HLA determinants in effective immune cell cooperation.

Suggested Readings

Arnaiz-Villena A, Timon M, Corell A, et al. Brief report: primary immunodeficiency caused by mutations in the gene encoding the CD3-γ subunit of the T lymphocyte receptor. *N Engl J Med* 1992;327:529.

Buckley RH. Molecular defects in human severe combined immunodeficiency and approaches to immune reconstitution. *Ann Rev Immunol* 2004;55:625.

Buckley RH. Primary cellular immunodeficiencies. *J Allerg Clin Immunol* 2002;109:747.

Buckley RH, Fischer A. Bone marrow transplantation for primary immunodeficiency diseases. In: Ochs HD, Smith CIE, Puck JM, eds. *Primary immunodeficiency diseases: a molecular and genetic approach*. New York and Oxford: Oxford University Press, 1999:459.

Buckley RH, Schiff SE, Schiff RI, et al. Hematopoietic stem-cell transplantation for the treatment of severe combined immunodeficiency. *N Engl J Med* 1999;340:508.

Cavazzana-Calvo M, Hacein-Bey S, deSaint Basile G, et al. Gene therapy of human severe combined immunodeficiency (SCID)-X1 disease. *Science* 2000;288:669.

Corneo B, Moshous D, Gungor T, et al. Identical mutations in RAG1 or RAG2 genes leading to defective V(D)J recombinase activity can cause either T-B-severe combined immune deficiency or Omenn syndrome. *Blood* 2001;97:2772.

Dadi HK, Simon AJ, Roifman CM. Effect of CD3-delta deficiency on maturation of alpha/beta and gamma/delta T-cell lineages in severe combined immunodeficiency. *N Engl J Med* 2003;349:1821.

de la Salle H, Hanau D, Fricker D. Homozygous human TAP peptide transporter mutation in HLA class I deficiency. *Science* 1994;265:237.

Driscoll DA, Sullivan KE. DiGeorge syndrome: a chromosome 22q11.2 deletion syndrome. In: Ochs HD, Smith CIE, Puck JM, eds. *Primary immunodeficiency diseases: a molecular and genetic approach*. New York and Oxford: Oxford University Press, 1999:198.

Elder ME, Lin D, Clever J, et al. Human severe combined immunodeficiency due to a defect in ZAP-70, a T cell tyrosine kinase. *Science* 1994;264:1596.

Gatti RA. Ataxia-telangiectasia. In: Stiehm ER, ed. *Immunological diseases in infants and children*, 4th ed. Philadelphia: Saunders, 1996:368.

Hacein-Bey-Abina S, Le Deist F, Carlier F, et al. Sustained correction of X-linked severe combined immunodeficiency by ex vivo gene therapy. *N Engl J Med* 2002;346:1185.

Hacein-Bey-Abina S, Von Kalle C, Schmidt M, et al. LMO2-associated clonal T cell proliferation in two patients after gene therapy for SCID-X1. *Science* 2003;302:415.

Hirschhorn R. Immunodeficiency diseases due to deficiency of adenosine deaminase. In: Ochs HD, Smith CIE, Puck JM, eds. *Primary immunodeficiency diseases: a molecular and genetic approach*. New York and Oxford: Oxford University Press, 1999:121.

Jawad AF, McDonald-McGinn DM, Zackai E, Sullivan KE. Immunologic features of chromosome 22q11.2 deletion syndrome (DiGeorge syndrome/velocardiofacial syndrome). *J Pediatr* 2001;139:715.

Klein C, Lisowska-Grospierre B, LeDeist F, et al. Major histocompatibility complex class II deficiency: clinical manifestations, immunologic features, and outcome. *J Pediatr* 1993;123:921.

Markert ML. Purine nucleoside phosphorylase deficiency. *Immunodefic Rev* 1991;3:1991.

Markert ML, Sarzotti M, Ozaki DA, et al. Thymus transplantation in complete DiGeorge syndrome: immunologic and safety evaluations in 12 patients. *Blood* 2003;102:1121.

Masternak K, Barras E, Zufferey M, et al. A gene encoding a novel RFX-associated transactivator is mutated in the majority of MHC class II deficiency patients. *Nat Genet* 1998;20:273.

Myers LA, Patel DD, Puck JM, Buckley RH. Hematopoietic stem cell transplantation for severe combined immunodeficiency (SCID) in the neonatal period leads to superior thymic output and improved survival. *Blood* 2002;99:872.

Ochs HD, Rosen FS. The Wiskott-Aldrich syndrome. In: Ochs HD, Smith CIE, Puck JM, eds. *Primary immunodeficiency diseases: a molecular and genetic approach*. New York and Oxford: Oxford University Press, 1999:292.

Patel DD, Gooding ME, Parrott RE, et al. Thymic function after hematopoietic stem-cell transplantation for the treatment of severe combined immunodeficiency. *N Engl J Med* 2000;342:1325.

Puel A, Ziegler SF, Buckley RH, Leonard WJ. Defective IL7R expression in T(−)B(+)NK(+) severe combined immunodeficiency. *Nat Genet* 1998;20:394.

Roberts JL, Lengi A, Brown SM, et al. Janus kinase 3 (JAK3) deficiency: clinical, immunologic and molecular analyses of 10 patients and outcomes of stem cell transplantation. *Blood* 2004;103:2009.

Schwarz K, Notarangelo L, Spanopoulou E, et al. Recombination defects. In: Ochs HD, Smith CIE, Puck JM, eds. *Primary immunodeficiency diseases: a molecular and genetic approach*. New York and Oxford: Oxford University Press, 1999:155.

Thoenes G, Soudais C, Le Deist F, et al. Structural analysis of low TCR-CD3 complex expression in T cells of an immunodeficient patient. *J Biol Chem* 1992;267:487.

SECTION XII ■ BONE AND JOINT DISEASES

CHAPTER 432 ■ BONE, JOINT, AND MUSCLE PROBLEMS

PAUL D. SPONSELLER

Most children's musculoskeletal problems present first to the pediatrician. She/he is entrusted to triage them and sort out those needing observation from those requiring active treatment. This chapter is designed to help in the initial understanding of this broad range of orthopedic conditions. Conditions limited to one body region are presented first, followed by generalized musculoskeletal conditions. Table 432.1 lists the differential diagnosis of certain signs and symptoms and is meant to aid in the formulation of a diagnostic plan.

Because some orthopedic terminology may be a "new language," a few definitions are in order. The term *congenital* refers to a condition that is present at birth, regardless of whether it is genetic. *Developmental* refers to problems that occur or increase with time and growth, irrespective of their causes. The regions of a long bone have specific names. *Physis* refers to the growth plate (Fig. 432.1); therefore, the *epiphysis* is that portion of a bone "on top of" the physis (i.e., nearer to the joint), the *metaphysis* is the widened portion of the shaft adjacent to and arising from the growth plate, and the *diaphysis* is the narrow portion of a tubular bone midway between two physes. Another set of terms refers to joints and their geometric relationships. The Greek root words *genu*, *coxa*, and *pes* refer to the knee, hip, and foot, respectively. They are used in such terms as genu recurvatum (hyperextensible knee), coxa plana (flat femoral head [i.e., Perthes disease]), and pes planus (flat feet). When two bones or two fracture fragments form an angle, they are in *varus* when the apex of the angle points away from the midline of the body, and they are in *valgus* when it points toward the midline (Fig. 432.2). Alternatively, angulation may be stated by the direction of the apex (i.e., genu valgus is a medial angulation of the lower extremity at the knee). *Dislocation* refers to complete loss of contact of two joint surfaces, and it is specified by the direction of displacement of the most distal part. For example, most shoulder dislocations are anterior because the humeral head comes out in front of the scapula. *Subluxation* is an incomplete dislocation. *Abduction* refers to movement away from the midline of the body; *adduction* denotes movement toward the midline.

One of the themes of this chapter is the changing nature of the skeleton with growth. Many clinical findings improve with time, due to the normal remodeling processes under the influence of growth and muscle forces: genu valgum, metatarsus adductus, tibial torsion, and fracture angulation. Others may get worse, such as Blount disease, neuromuscular hip dysplasia, and severe idiopathic scoliosis. Experience and judgment are needed to make these distinctions.

REGIONAL ABNORMALITIES

Hip and Femur

Developmental Dysplasia of the Hip

The normal hip develops from a single area of cartilage that then forms a joint cavity. Its characteristic spherical shape results from reciprocal contact and movement between the femoral head and acetabulum during *in utero* development. Loss of this contact may occur as a result of abnormal *in utero* positioning; such neuromuscular abnormalities as cerebral palsy, arthrogryposis, and Larsen syndrome; or intrinsic underdevelopment of the otherwise normal hip. The earlier an abnormal positioning occurs, the more marked are the femoral and acetabular abnormalities that result; the later it is corrected, the less is the remodeling potential.

The cause of congenital dislocation of the hip in an otherwise normal child is multifactorial. Mechanical factors play a role; thus, the frequency is increased greatly in fetuses with breech presentation, a factor in 30% of all cases of developmental dysplasia of the hip (DDH) in firstborn children and in infants with oligohydramnios. The left hip is involved more commonly than is the right. These factors cause positioning in adduction and hyperflexion, leading the femur to be directed out over the edge of the acetabulum. Hormonal factors may play a role, because generalized ligamentous laxity occurs around the time of birth, caused by an increase in circulating estrogens and relaxin. Probably for this reason, the incidence of DDH is sixfold greater in girls than in boys. More than 20% of patients have a positive family history.

TABLE 432.1

DIFFERENTIAL DIAGNOSIS OF COMMON PEDIATRIC SYMPTOMS

Limp
Pain
  Septic arthritis-osteomyelitis
  Transient synovitis
  Juvenile rheumatoid arthritis
  Migratory polyarthritis (immunologic)
  Legg-Calvé-Perthes disease
  Slipped capital femoral epiphysis
  Meniscus tear
  Idiopathic chondrolysis of the hip
  Osgood-Schlatter disease
  Impacted fracture
  Spinal disorder
Weakness
  Congenital dislocation of the hip
  Myopathy
  Polio
  Cerebral palsy–myelomeningocele
  Spinal cord compression
Limitation of motion
  Legg-Perthes disease–slipped capital femoral epiphysis (old)
  Posttraumatic muscle contracture
  Posttraumatic joint contracture
Leg-length inequality
  Idiopathic hemihypertrophy
  Posttraumatic malunion or growth-plate closure
  Neuromuscular
    Cerebral palsy
    Polio
  Neurofibromatosis
  Congenital limb deficiency
  Ollier disease
  Arteriovenous malformation

Knee Pain
Musculotendinous
  Patellofemoral stress syndrome
  Osgood-Schlatter disease
  Patellar-quadriceps tendinitis
  Iliotibial band syndrome
Bony-cartilaginous
  Meniscus tear
  Discoid meniscus

  Osteochondritis dissecans
  Tibial spine fracture–physeal injury
Miscellaneous
  Infection
  Tumor
  Connective tissue disorder
  Hip disorder

Childhood Back Pain
Developmental-acquired
  Scheuermann kyphosis
  Spondylolysis-spondylolisthesis
  Herniated nucleus pulposus
  Fracture of vertebral body
  Muscle strain
Infectious
  Vertebral body osteomyelitis
  Discitis
  Tuberculosis
Neoplastic
  Osteoid osteoma
  Osteoblastoma-osteosarcoma
  Leukemia-lymphoma
  Eosinophilic granuloma
  Ewing sarcoma–neuroblastoma
  Spinal cord tumor

Internal Rotation of the Lower Extremity: Toeing-In
Femoral
  Anteversion
  Muscular-capsular
Tibial torsion
Metatarsus adductus
Clubfoot, partially treated
Neuromuscular disorder

Flatfoot
Flexible-idiopathic
Tarsal coalition
Juvenile rheumatoid arthritis
Congenital vertical talus
Marfan syndrome
Neuromuscular disorders

In order of their increasing severity, the three degrees of hip dysplasia are subluxable, dislocatable, and dislocated. In the subluxatable hip, the femoral head rests in the acetabulum and can be dislocated partially during the examination. The dislocatable hip can be dislocated fully with manipulation but is located normally when a baby is at rest. In the dislocated hip, the femoral head rests in the dislocated position. The combined incidence of these three conditions is 1 in 60 births; the incidence of true dislocation is only 1 to 2 per 1,000 births. The term dysplasia describes the spectrum of severity of this disorder, which ranges from slight malformation to full dislocation of the hip. The term developmental acknowledges that some cases cannot be detected at birth and may occur later. The pathologic anatomy includes capsular laxity. Also, the acetabulum becomes shallow as a result of lack of contact with the femoral head. A false acetabulum may form where the femoral head contacts the pelvis above the normal location. The outer rim of the acetabulum becomes rounded during the period when the femoral head is able to slide in and out of the acetabulum. The movement over this ridge is felt as the "clunk"

of the Ortolani and Barlow tests. The femur remains rotated anteriorly (anteverted) as the head rests against the lateral iliac wall.

Physical examination remains the key to the diagnosis of DDH. The signs in the newborn period usually include instability without significant fixed deformity; in later months, untreated dislocation becomes more fixed, and less instability and more limitation of certain motions occur. Specifically, Barlow and Ortolani signs should be sought in newborns. These signs are defined as positive when the hip can be dislocated and relocated, respectively. Infants should be relaxed when the tests are performed, and only one hip should be examined at a time. The pelvis should be stabilized with one hand while the femur is controlled with the other hand, with fingers placed on the greater and lesser trochanters (Fig. 432.3). With adduction and pressure directed posteriorly, the femur can be felt to slide "out" in a posterosuperior direction in the abnormal hip (Barlow sign; see Fig. 432.3A) and then back in with abduction, causing a dull clunk to be heard (Ortolani sign; see Fig. 432.3B). Thus, the Barlow and Ortolani signs, which are the

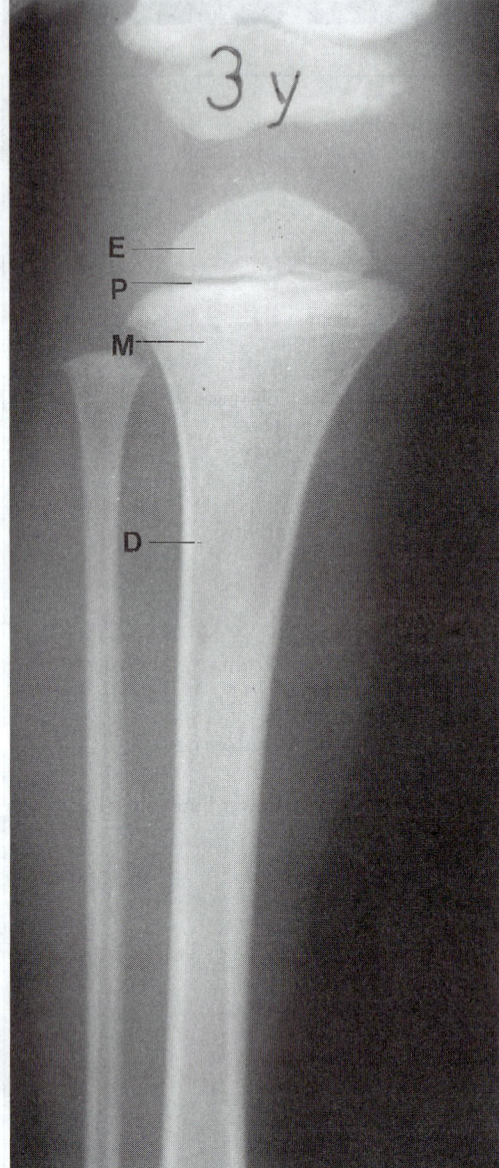

FIGURE 432.1. Regions of a long bone. D, diaphysis; E, epiphysis; M, metaphysis; P, physis.

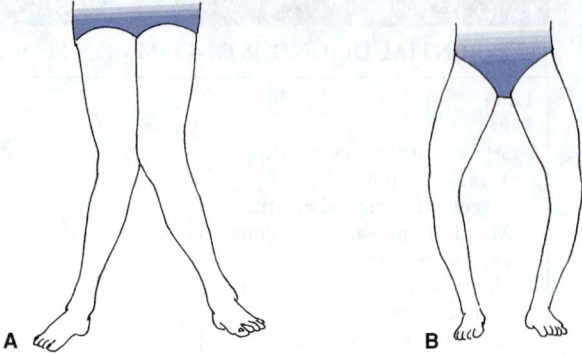

FIGURE 432.2. Examples of varus and valgus. **A:** Genu valgus, because apex of angulation is toward midline. **B:** Genu varus.

sensations of dislocation and relocation, are alternate phases of the same process of hip instability.

A common error made in DDH diagnosis is examining both hips at once, which impairs sensitivity. Another error is mistaking insignificant soft tissue "clicks" for the more important and palpable "clunk." These innocent clicks may result from movement of fascia over the greater trochanter or may originate from the meniscus of the knee or the patella. Routine screening of neonates in the last three decades has resulted in a dramatic increase in the early diagnosis of DDH and, thus, more successful treatment of the disorder.

Approximately 60% of all unstable hips seen in newborns normalize spontaneously within the first 2 to 4 weeks after birth as the baby is free of the constraints of the womb and perinatal laxity resolves. Not all hips can be reduced at birth, however, presumably because of fixed joint contracture. Some cases of dysplasia are believed to develop after birth. For this reason, most large series have shown that not all abnormal hips can be detected by screening, even when it is performed by skilled examiners. Neonatal ultrasonography is a useful tool in examining a newborn's hip, but it does not provide the precise image that we are accustomed to see in a radiograph or magnetic resonance imaging (MRI). It is much less clear than a prenatal ultrasound, because of the lack of a uniform fluid medium. It may result in overdiagnosis of dysplasia if performed on all newborns. Recommended indications for ultrasonography vary from region to region, but they usually involve some combination of abnormal physical examination or presence of risk factors.

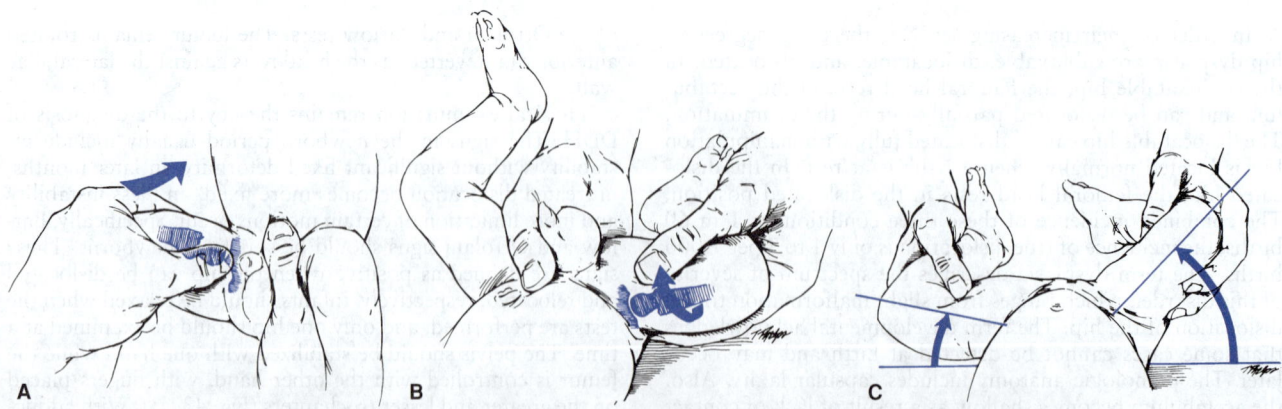

FIGURE 432.3. Barlow and Ortolani tests, performed with fingers on the lesser and greater trochanters, examining only one hip at a time. **A:** Barlow test: adduction and posterior pressure may produce a "clunk" of subluxation or dislocation. **B:** Ortolani test: abducting and "lifting" hip back into place. **C:** In children older than 3 to 6 months, Barlow and Ortolani tests often will be negative despite dislocation because of diminished laxity; the most important finding in this age group may be limitation of abduction.

The signs of a dysplastic hip change with time. If the hip remains dislocated, usually it cannot be relocated in the awake state by the time an affected baby is 6 months old. Findings of asymmetry, such as a limitation of abduction (see Fig. 432.3C) and apparent shortening of the thigh, are more sensitive at this time. This last sign, known as Allis sign or the Galeazzi sign, is best noted by comparing the lengths of the two flexed thighs when they are held together. Asymmetry of skin folds by itself is an unreliable finding. When children begin to walk, a positive Trendelenburg sign is noted: When weight is borne on the unstable side, the pelvis drops to the other side.

Radiographs are not the preferred imaging method before age 6 months because of a lack of easily detectable bony changes during this time, except in infants with teratologic conditions. Many centers use ultrasonography, but the accurate interpretation of these studies requires extensive experience and should be done by a pediatric radiologist or orthopedist. Ultrasonography is indicated if the neonatal examination is abnormal or questionable, and it may be used later to guide treatment. After age 6 months, the increasing ossification of the femur renders ultrasonography less reliable, and plain films are preferred. Anteroposterior (AP) radiography of the pelvis may show cephalad and lateral migration of the femur with a break in Shenton's line (Fig. 432.4), delayed appearance of the femoral ossific nucleus, a shallow and more vertical acetabulum, and later formation of a false acetabulum.

Treatment is more complex as age increases. The aim of all therapy is to restore contact between the femoral head and the acetabulum. Because a high percentage of patients experience spontaneous improvement of lax hip capsules in the early perinatal period, most orthopedists recommend observing a hip that is subject to subluxation and reexamining it at age 3 to 4 weeks. Dislocated hips should be treated at the time of diagnosis. Usually, the initial treatment is a brace that holds the hip in flexion and abduction, such as the Pavlik harness, which allows some motion while it holds the hip reduced. The alignment should be checked by ultrasound in 1 to 2 weeks. The brace is worn until the clinical and radiologic examinations are normal, an interval equal to approximately one to two times an affected child's age at diagnosis. If treatment is begun after affected children have reached age 6 months, usually they are too large and strong to tolerate the brace. At that point, reduction is performed under general anesthesia. Sometimes this procedure has been preceded by a period of traction to stretch out the soft tissues. Closed reduction is attempted first and checked with an arthrogram. If it is successful, the reduction is held in a spica cast for a number of months. If closed reduction is unsuccessful, open reduction should be performed.

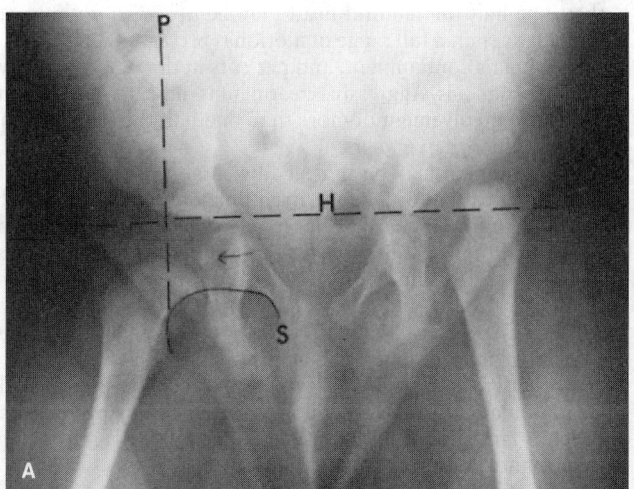

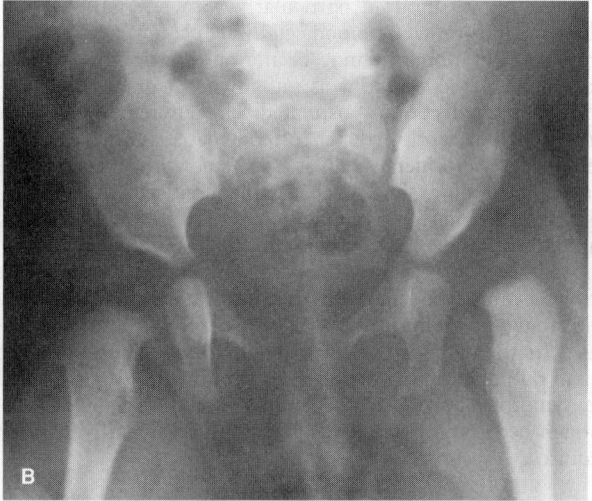

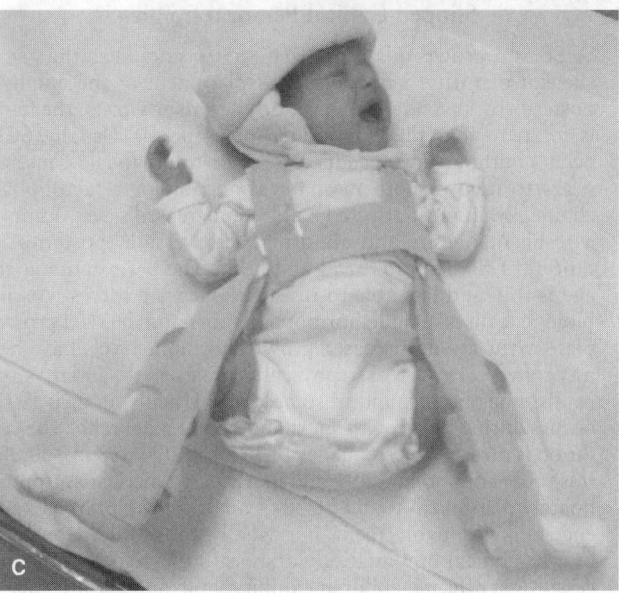

FIGURE 432.4. A: Illustrations of a congenitally dislocated hip. The femoral head ossific nucleus should be within the lower inner quadrant formed by Perkin's vertical line (*P*) at the outer edge of the acetabulum and Hilgenreiner's horizontal line (*H*). The nucleus appears at age 5 months, on the average. Shenton's line (*S*) is the arc of the femoral neck, which should continue smoothly into the superior pubic ramus. This is a teratologic hip dislocation; note extreme height and rounded false acetabulum. B: A subtler example of congenital dislocation of the left hip. C: Infant with congenital hip dislocation treated in a Pavlik Harness.

Open reduction involves releasing the tight psoas tendon and inferior capsule, thus allowing the femoral head to be brought down to its appropriate location.

If extensive distortion of the bones (i.e., a shallow acetabulum or a rotated femur) has occurred, a femoral or pelvic osteotomy and open reduction might be indicated. This condition is more common in patients who are older than 2 years.

Possible complications include persistent dysplasia from failure of normal development, recurrent dislocation, and avascular necrosis of the femoral head. The latter condition, which is the most serious complication of DDH, is caused by obstruction of the epiphyseal vessels by excess pressure or capsular stretch.

The earlier that treatment is carried out, the better is the resultant hip development and the safer is each of the steps in treatment. Thus, careful, methodical early screening can decrease the need for complex orthopedic procedures later.

Transient (Toxic) Synovitis of the Hip

Transient (toxic) synovitis of the hip is a diagnosis of exclusion; this self-limited condition is the most common cause of an irritable hip in children. The usual clinical presentation is a painful limp or hip pain of acute or insidious onset, usually occurring unilaterally. The most common age range for the condition is 2 to 6 years, but it has been described in patients ranging from ages 1 to 15. Spasm occurs on testing of hip range of motion, particularly with internal rotation. The temperature, white blood cell (WBC) count, and erythrocyte sedimentation rate may be normal or slightly elevated. The cause of the condition is unknown; an immune mechanism or viral infection is postulated. The differential diagnosis should include septic arthritis, osteomyelitis, and Legg-Calvé-Perthes disease, which usually is associated with changes in the femoral head on radiography. Juvenile monoarthritic rheumatoid arthritis and slipped capital femoral epiphysis (SCFE) also should be considered. Admission to the hospital, observation, and possible early aspiration should be undertaken if septic arthritis cannot be ruled out. Treatment consists of bed rest, with analgesic agents provided as needed for 2 to 7 days. Sometimes, if the diagnosis is clear, therapy can be accomplished on an outpatient basis with frequent follow-up. Persistence of the symptoms beyond 1 week should prompt reevaluation, although bed rest for as long as 1 month occasionally has been required.

Legg-Calvé-Perthes Disease (Coxa Plana)

The cause of Legg-Calvé-Perthes disease still is unknown. More recent evidence indicates that some cases may be caused by a subclinical hypercoagulable state, such as a deficiency of antithrombotic factors S or C or a decrease in fibrinolysis. The condition is characterized by ischemic necrosis of the proximal femoral epiphysis, with later resorption and eventual healing. The amount of the femur that is rendered ischemic varies and affects the outcome. Ischemia is followed by reossification, with or without collapse of the femoral head. Legg-Calvé-Perthes disease usually, but not exclusively, affects children between ages 4 and 8. Boys are affected four times as often as are girls. As a group, affected patients have slightly shorter stature and delayed bone age as compared to their peers. Fifteen percent of all cases are bilateral.

Usually, the clinical presentation of this disorder is a limp (i.e., an abductor lurch) with minimal pain of either short or long duration. The pain is not as acute or severe as that of transient synovitis or septic arthritis. In some patients the pain may be referred to the thigh or the knee. Motions that are especially limited include internal rotation and abduction. Internal rotation is tested with the patient supine and the hip flexed, and the angle to which the leg may be rotated laterally is measured.

These movements may be resisted by mild spasm or guarding. In the earliest stage, radiographic results may be normal or reveal that the affected femoral epiphysis is slightly smaller when compared with the contralateral side, as a result of its failure to grow after becoming avascular. Later, a narrow crescentic lucency, seen best on the lateral view, may be observed; it is the result of a tiny fracture of the subchondral bone. This view reveals the extent of bone involved (Fig. 432.5A). In some cases, revascularization may occur without collapse; in others, revascularization of the femoral head is accompanied by progressive resorption and deformation, often with lateral and superior migration (Fig. 432.5B). Reossification follows, and the femoral head continues to grow (Fig. 432.5C). Whether this further growth occurs spherically depends on the patient's age, the amount of collapse, and the method of treatment.

The differential diagnosis should include transient synovitis, septic arthritis, hematogenous osteomyelitis, various types of hemoglobinopathy, hypothyroidism, and the epiphyseal dysplasias. Often, the latter two conditions are temporally symmetric bilaterally, whereas Legg-Calvé-Perthes disease is not.

Treatment follows two principles: containment of the femoral head within the acetabulum and maintenance of range of motion. During the vulnerable phase, the avascular portion of the femoral head is less likely to become deformed severely and is more likely to reconstitute spherically if it is contained within the "mold" of the acetabulum by abduction. Children younger than 6 years or those who have involvement of less than one-half the femoral head may be observed without active treatment if a full range of motion is preserved, because this range signals containment, and patients in this age group have a good prognosis. Aggressive treatment is indicated for patients who have involvement of more than one-half the femoral head and are older than 6 years.

Containment may be achieved by surgery. Either a femoral osteotomy to redirect the involved portion within the acetabulum or an innominate osteotomy or shelf procedure may be performed (Fig. 432.6). The two procedures produce approximately equal results. Surgery does not speed the healing of the femoral head, but causes it to reossify in a more spherical fashion. Generally, children with Legg-Calve-Perthes disease have intermittent mild aching in the hip for 1.5 to 2 years, until reossification is complete, but then they are virtually asymptomatic throughout childhood. Arthritic symptoms may develop later in adulthood, depending on the degree of this deformation.

Slipped Capital Femoral Epiphysis

SCFE is a growth-plate disorder that occurs near the age of skeletal maturity; it involves a displacement of the epiphysis posteriorly, medially, and inferiorly. In other words, the femur is rotated externally from under the epiphysis. Usually, SCFE occurs without severe sudden force or trauma. The cause appears to involve both mechanical and biologic factors. Mechanically, in most affected children, increased stress occurs as a result of obesity and abnormal retroversion (posterior rotation) of the femoral head and neck. The periosteum at this age is thin and less able to resist the shearing forces. Possible biologic causes include hormonal factors and delayed growth-plate maturation. Increased growth hormone levels have been associated with decreased physeal shear strength, and hypothyroidism has been found in some cases. Usually, in girls, SCFE occurs during the growth spurt and before menarche. The condition is rare, with a frequency of 1 in 100,000 to 8 in 100,000. It is more common in boys and in African Americans. Approximately one-fourth to one-third of all affected children experience bilateral involvement, but usually not simultaneously.

The clinical presentation varies with the acuity of the process. Most affected children exhibit a limp and endure varying

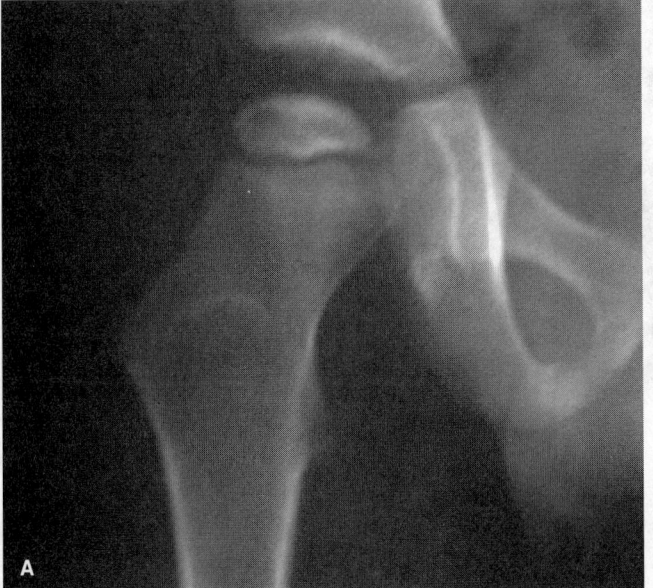

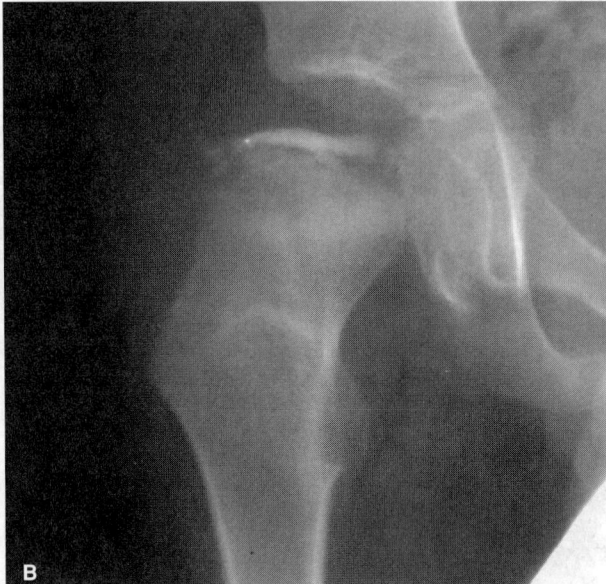

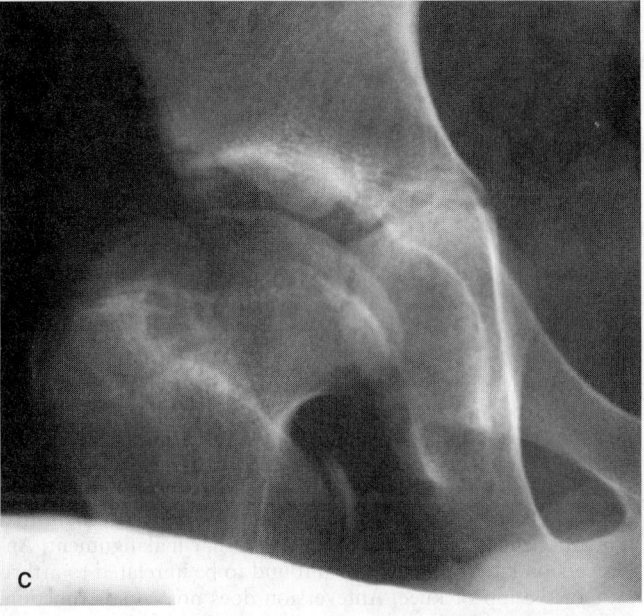

FIGURE 432.5. A: Early Legg-Calvé-Perthes disease, showing early flattening of the femoral head. B: Later, further resorption and apparent collapse of the femoral head are evident. C: Finally, restoration of a slightly ovoid but fully ossified femoral head is seen here at age 13, although the femoral neck is slightly short.

degrees of aching or pain. The discomfort may be in the groin, but often it is referred to the thigh or knee. This variation may cause confusion: Many patients are dismissed for an apparent knee complaint with no obvious cause, only to have the true hip pathology discovered later with worsening of the slip. This paradoxic distribution of pain is attributed to referral within the femoral nerve distribution, which involves both the hip and knee joints. Abduction, internal rotation, and flexion are the motions that are most limited. A characteristic finding is external rotation of the hip with flexion, which is caused by the preexisting retroversion and the slip itself (Fig. 432.7). Some patients have acute, severe pain and an inability to walk or move the hip. This is termed an "unstable" slip and indicates an increased risk of avascular necrosis.

The earliest radiographic findings are widening and irregularity of the growth plate and osteopenia of the femur. Later, displacement of the epiphysis occurs and is seen best on the frog-leg lateral view of the pelvis. On the AP view, a line drawn through the upper margin of the narrowest portion of the neck should intersect at least 20% of the epiphysis (Fig. 432.8). This

point is important because, with remodeling during chronic slipping, a step-off at the junction of the epiphysis and metaphysis may be absent. The severity of the slip is graded as mild (less than 33%), moderate (33% to 50%), or severe (greater than 50%). Later changes may include avascular necrosis of the epiphysis or chondrolysis (i.e., joint-space narrowing).

Treatment centers on preventing further slippage, usually by placing affected patients immediately at bed rest and obtaining a prompt orthopedic consultation. Surgery is intended to stabilize the upper femur and to cause the growth plate to close, thereby eliminating the weakened zone. Realignment of the slip is not safe in chronic cases, because the forces necessary to accomplish realignment may produce avascular necrosis by disrupting the blood supply to the epiphysis. The standard treatment is screw fixation *in situ*. The screw should not penetrate the joint. Osteotomy of the proximal or distal neck to correct the deformity has been performed occasionally, but it carries a high risk of avascular necrosis.

The contralateral side should be monitored by affected patients' parents for symptoms of SCFE and should be pinned

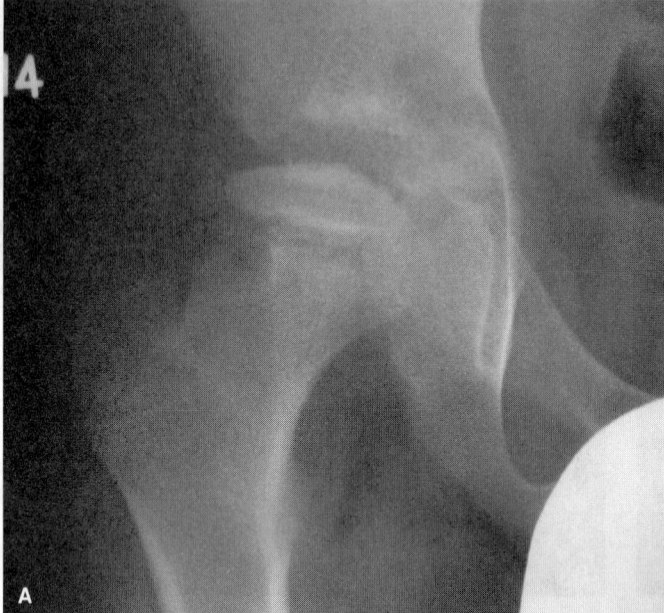
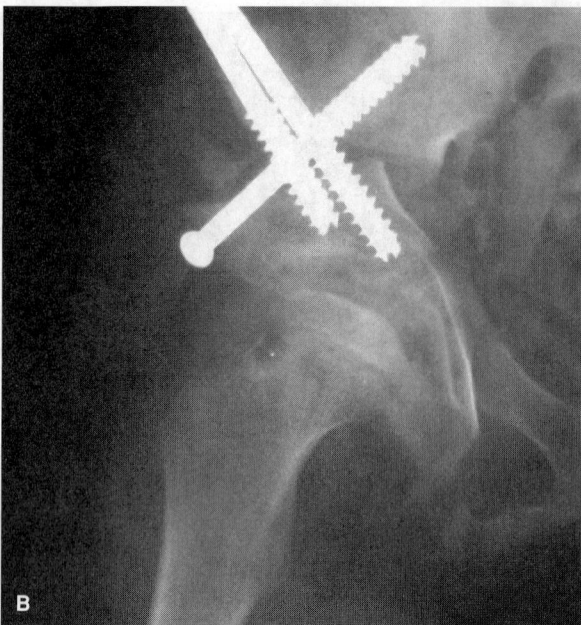

FIGURE 432.6. Operative containment for Perthes disease in an older child. **A:** Preoperative radiograph shows resorption of bone from femoral epiphysis and partial extrusion from acetabulum. **B:** postoperative radiograph shows acetabulum rotated to cover femoral head. This is an example of an iliac osteotomy.

early if such symptoms occur. Long-term follow-up reveals no early degenerative change unless chondrolysis or avascular necrosis occurs; each has an incidence of 1% to 5% and produces disability during adolescence. However, even in the absence of these complications, degenerative joint disease may occur in middle age.

Increased Femoral Anteversion

Increased femoral anteversion causes toeing-in and is one of a spectrum of torsional deformities that affect the alignment of the knee and foot. The differential diagnosis of toeing-in includes this disorder and internal tibial torsion and foot deformities, such as metatarsus adductus (see Table 432.1). Increased anteversion of the femur is defined as an increase in the angle between the plane of the femoral neck and the plane of the knee (posterior femoral condyles; Fig. 432.9). Normally, this angle is approximately 30 degrees at birth and declines to 15 degrees by age 10. Femoral anteversion persists in some neuromuscular conditions, presumably as a result of lack of re-

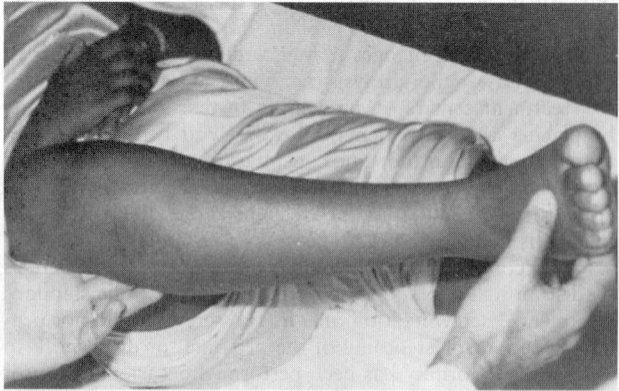

FIGURE 432.7. In slipped capital femoral epiphysis, the hip rotates externally as it is flexed by the examiner.

modeling forces. The type discussed here is isolated idiopathic femoral anteversion.

On physical examination, affected patients appear to toe in unless compensatory external tibial torsion is present. The patellae also face medially ("squint"). Internal rotation of the hip is much greater than is external rotation in both flexion (supine) and extension (prone). Usually, anteversion is not clinically significant unless external rotation at the hip is less than 15 degrees.

Radiographically, the femoral head and neck appear to be relatively straight on an AP film, with the patella forward. This is a one-plane projection of a two-plane deformity. Computed tomography (CT) is the best device for measuring femoral anteversion directly.

The natural history of femoral anteversion is benign. In a few patients, it may contribute to patellar malalignment. Anteversion later in life has been found to be unrelated to arthritis of the hip or knee. Anteversion does not impair function. Treatment of increased anteversion consists of observation, at least until affected patients are age 8, and restriction from prolonged W-sitting (with the knees touching and the legs folded under), which may impair remodeling. Instead, affected children should sit in the tailor position (with the feet tucked under and the knees out to the side). Braces and bars are not effective in derotating the femur, and no orthotic method of treatment affects anteversion. In fact, most cases need no treatment.

Femoral osteotomy, proximally or distally, is the only way to realign the femur. It should be performed rarely, however, and only in children who are older than 8 and have functional disability as a result of patellar malalignment or, rarely, a persistent concern regarding their appearance.

Knee

Extensor Mechanism Disorders (Patellofemoral Problems)

The patellofemoral joint is subject to repeated high loads of laterally and posteriorly directed forces. Numerous conditions

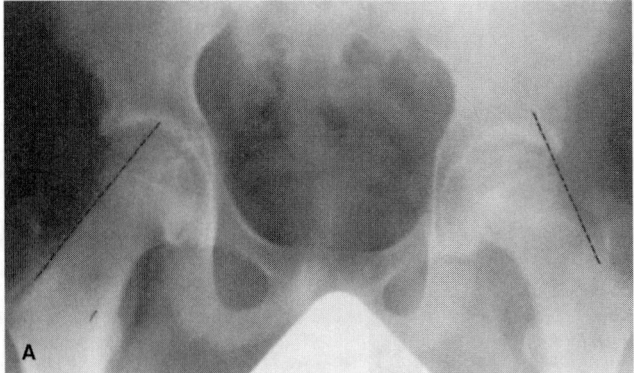

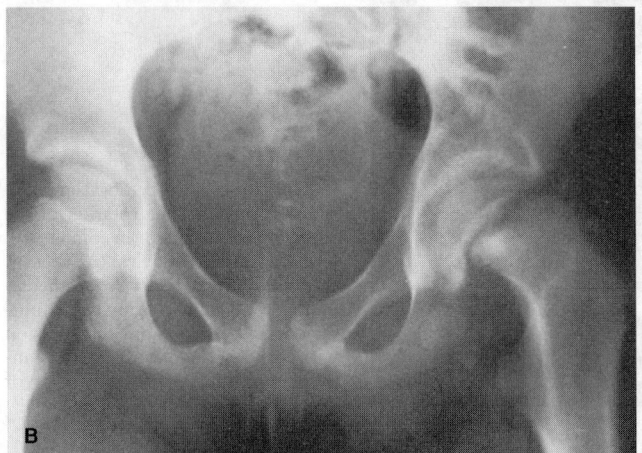

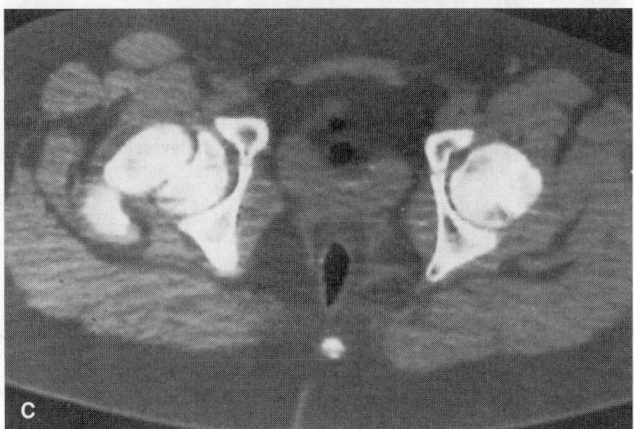

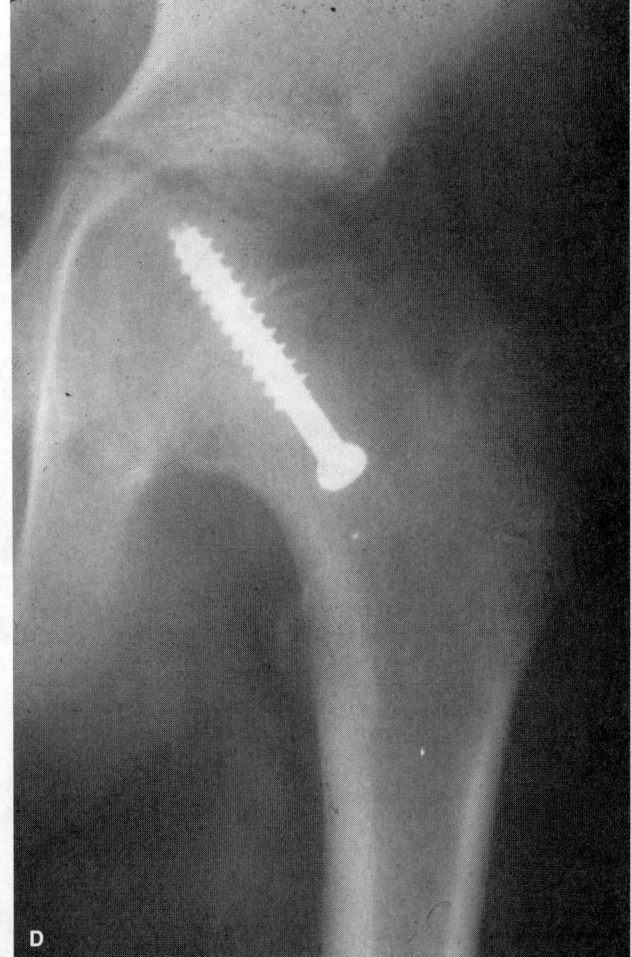

FIGURE 432.8. Radiographic findings in slipped capital femoral epiphysis. **A:** A line drawn along the superior-lateral femoral neck intersects less than the normal 20% of the epiphysis on the left (affected) side. **B:** A more severe slip, showing that the femoral neck subluxates laterally and superiorly with respect to the epiphysis. **C:** Computed tomographic scan most clearly shows the direction of the slip. **D:** This figure shows *in situ* fixation of slipped capital femoral epiphysis with a single screw, the preferred method for slips of mild to moderate degree and even many cases of severe degree.

involving this joint have been described in children and adolescents, and they are treated by attempting to improve the basic forces.

Chondromalacia refers specifically to the appearance of softening and degeneration of the patellar cartilage. Patellar subluxation refers to partial lateral displacement of the patella. The terms patellofemoral stress syndrome, patellar malalignment, and excessive lateral pressure syndrome refer to the abnormal mechanics causing stress concentration and pain.

The patellofemoral force may be as great as 2.5 times body weight and is greatest with the knee in flexion. The average tibiofemoral angle is approximately 6 degrees outward, which the patella must follow. The quadriceps-patella mechanism itself is angled away from the midline of the body, as measured by the Q (quadriceps) angle from the anterosuperior spine to the patella to the tibial tubercle (Fig. 432.10A). These high forces and asymmetric loads cause minor variations to become

significant, especially when repeated over the high numbers of cycles that occur as a part of daily living. Possible factors contributing to patellar pathology (Fig. 432.10B) include increased outward angulation of the knee, abnormal rotation in the form of increased anteversion of the femur or external torsion of the tibia, a high patella ("alta"), abnormal shape or development of the quadriceps, or flattening of the femoral groove. Laxity of the medial side of the patellar restraints contributes to subluxation or dislocation. Normally, women have slightly greater genu valgum than do men. Usually, the aforementioned factors cause greater stress on the lateral side of the patella and, sometimes, decreased medial patellofemoral contact. Cartilage degeneration occurs as a result of the decreased contact.

Clinically, problems with the patella cause aching that is greatest in the anteromedial knee region, on the medial side or center of the patella. Usually, this pain is worse with stair climbing or prolonged sitting, as flexion increases patellofemoral

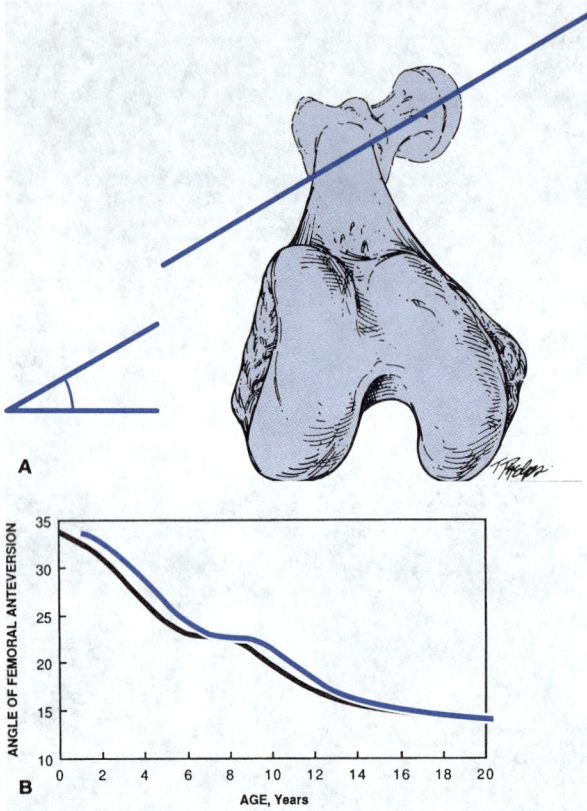

A

B

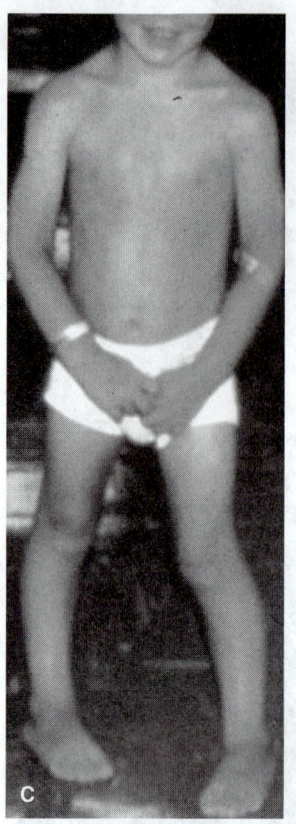

C

FIGURE 432.9. A: Femoral anteversion is defined as the rotation of the femoral neck forward (in comparison with the distal condyles), as seen in this view down the axis of the femur. B: The curve shows the normal decrease in femoral anteversion with age. C: Child with femoral anteversion, showing inward position of knees as well as feet.

force. Crepitus may be felt, but it may be painless in some patients and is not pathologic in itself. "Catching" or "locking" may be noted and might represent pain-induced inhibition or mechanical phenomena. A feeling of "giving way" may be described by the patient, especially with subluxation of the patella.

On physical examination, the most reliable way to test patellar tenderness is by direct compression of each facet against the femur. Palpation under the patella is not diagnostic. Contraction of the quadriceps and patella against resistance is nonspecific because it may be painful even in normal persons. Effusion is present only if patellar degenerative changes or extreme overuse has occurred. Reproducing patellar subluxation with laterally directed pressure may cause apprehension. The Q angle, femoral anteversion, and tibial torsion should be checked. Usually, radiographic results are nonspecific, but lateral displacement or tilt of the patella may be seen occasionally on the sunrise view.

The natural history of patellofemoral stress disorders is that they are common in patients between the ages of 10 and 20, but often they become less symptomatic later. Usually, they do not progress to osteoarthritis.

The differential diagnosis includes a synovial fold or "plica" that may snap over the medial femoral condyle, a medial meniscus tear, tendinitis of the quadriceps or patellar tendon, or osteochondritis dissecans of the patella or distal femur.

Treatment consists of altering the abnormal stresses that are occurring. Patients should refrain from activities performed with the knees flexed, especially those that cause pain (i.e., stair climbing, prolonged sitting, and bicycling). Temporary rest from sports and the use of nonsteroidal antiinflammatory agents may be necessary. Exercises to strengthen the medial (stabilizing) part of the quadriceps include resisted extension from 0 degrees to 30 degrees, most practically by lifting weights within this range or extending the knee on a pillow, flattening it. Hamstrings and rectus femoris muscles, if they are tight,

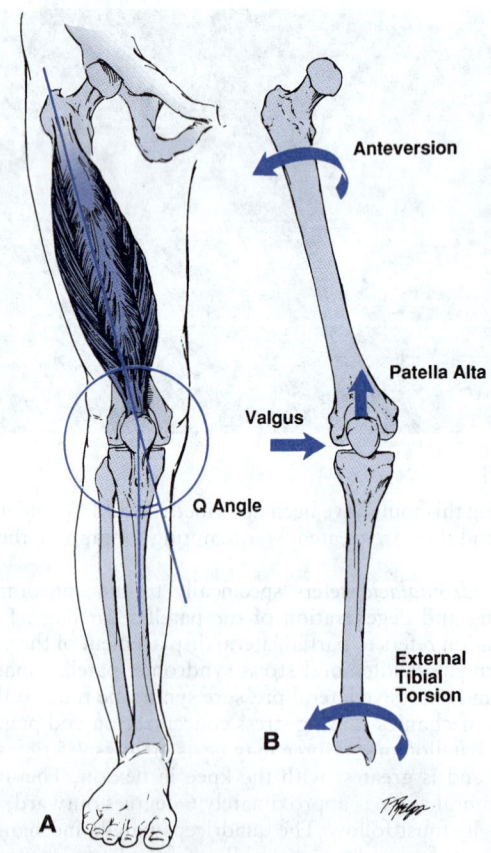

A   B

FIGURE 432.10. A: The Q angle, measured from anterior superior iliac spine to center of patella to tibial tubercle. B: Factors that may contribute to excess patellofemoral stress.

should be stretched to decrease preload on the extensors. Arch supports may help if severe flexible flatfoot is contributing to tibial torsion. Surgical measures include release of a tight lateral patellar retinaculum, medial soft tissue tightening, tibial tubercle transfer, or correction of genu valgum, knee anteversion, or patella alta if it is severe; all produce satisfactory pain relief in 75% to 90% of patients.

Patellar dislocations may be acute, recurrent or, rarely, habitual. Almost always, they occur in the lateral direction. Acute dislocations are associated with significant swelling and medial knee pain and with a history of significant outward or rotating force. They should be treated with a lateral knee immobilizer until symptom-free, except in skeletally mature patients with bony avulsion. Recurrent subluxation is common, causes less pain and swelling, and often occurs with minimal force. Usually, an associated extensor mechanism abnormality is present. A realignment operation (as described) is the only effective way to stop frequent and bothersome episodes.

Variously, Osgood-Schlatter disease, patellar tendinitis (jumper's knee), and quadriceps tendinitis are manifestations of excessive, repetitive stresses on the extensor mechanism. They are listed here in order of decreasing frequency in children.

Osgood-Schlatter Disorder. Osgood-Schlatter disorder is a traction-induced inflammation of the tibial tubercle. It is a reaction of the bone and cartilage of this region to high stress. The tibial tubercle is a downward extension of the proximal tibial epiphysis. It develops an ossification center in patients between ages 9 and 13 years, but it does not ossify completely until they are 15 to 17 years old. Within this age range, repetitive stresses gradually can deform the outer surface of the tubercle, causing it to enlarge and become locally inflamed (Fig. 432.11). Tenderness and swelling are localized to this region. Symptoms are worse with running, jumping, or kneeling. Treatment involves decreasing activity to a tolerable level and occasionally using a knee immobilizer, crutches, and ice after activity in severe cases. The patient may be vulnerable to recurrence of symptoms for up to 2 years until the tubercle matures. If affected children and their families are informed of this likelihood, individual regulation of activities can be effective. Usually, activities of daily living and even some sports are tolerated, using daily stretching of tight quadriceps and hamstrings and occasional antiinflammatory agents. Complete avulsion of the tubercle is extremely rare and seems to be related more to sudden stress than to apophysitis.

Patellar Tendinitis. Inflammation at the origin of the patellar tendon (which is at the inferior pole of the patella) is known as patellar tendinitis and is related to the same type of overuse as that seen in Osgood-Schlatter apophysitis. Most often, it is seen in basketball players and also is called jumper's knee. The duration of pain serves as a guide to the severity of involvement. Pain that is present during both rest and activity is more worrisome than is pain that occurs only after activity. Treatment is the same as that for Osgood-Schlatter disorder. Warm packs before and cold packs after activity also may be beneficial. Rarely, pain may occur at the proximal pole of the patella; in this case, the condition is termed quadriceps tendinitis. Treatment is the same as that described for Osgood-Schlatter apophysitis.

Tibiofemoral Disorders

Popliteal Cysts. Popliteal cysts in children are localized behind the knee on the medial side (Fig. 432.12). They are firm and nontender, vary in size with activity, and transilluminate in a darkened room. They occur most commonly in boys younger than age 9. The origin of these cysts is a slitlike communication between the knee joint and the gastrocnemio-semimembranous bursa. Unlike those in adults, in children, usually these cysts are not associated with any intraarticular pathology, and they tend

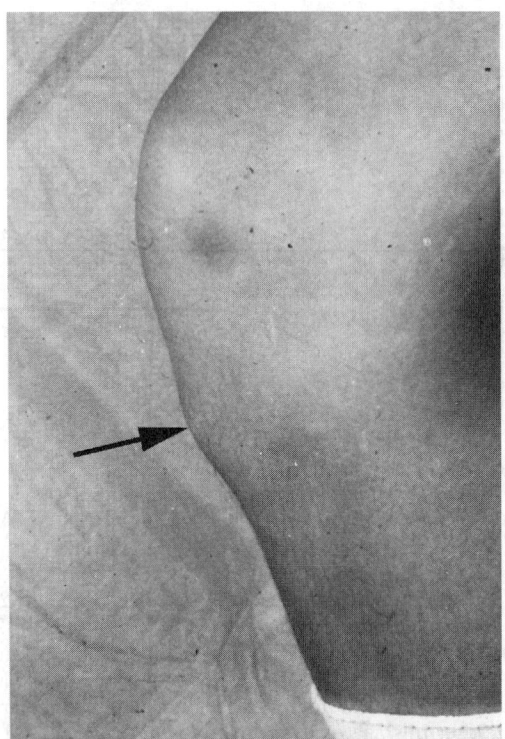

FIGURE 432.11. Osgood-Schlatter disease often produces an enlargement of the tibial tubercle (*arrow*).

to resolve spontaneously with time. Actually, the recurrence rate is higher after surgical excision.

Discoid Meniscus. An acquired flattening of the lateral meniscus is known as discoid meniscus. In some cases, this flattening occurs as a result of the absence of normal peripheral attachments. Often, such symptoms as pain, clicking, and locking develop in the absence of trauma in children from the age of 2 to adulthood. The meniscus should be trimmed or excised if symptoms become severe. If the attachments are intact, no removal is necessary unless a tear is seen.

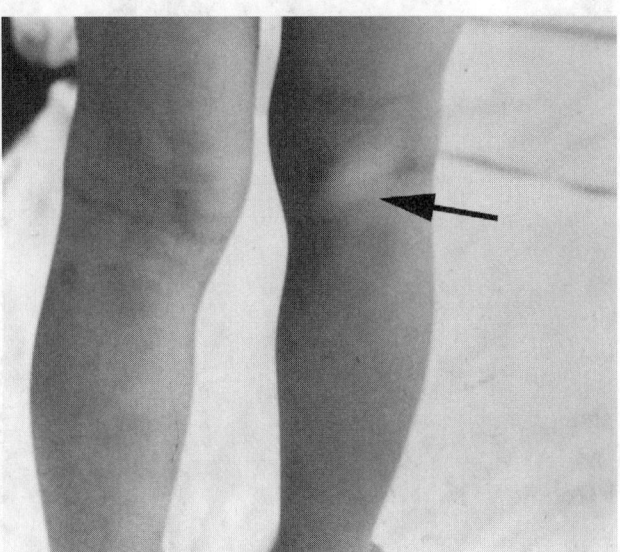

FIGURE 432.12. Popliteal cyst (*arrow*) in typical (medial) location behind right knee of this child.

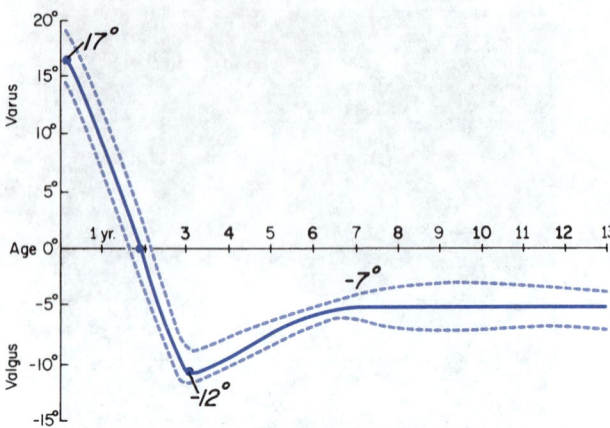

FIGURE 432.13. Normal change in the tibiofemoral angle during growth. (Reproduced with permission from Salenius P. Development of the tibiofemoral angle in children. *J Bone Joint Surg* 1975;57A:260.)

Genu Varum. Genu varum, or a "bowed leg" of up to 20 degrees, is normal in children until age 18 months (Fig. 432.13). Normally, it does not increase significantly after walking begins. After the child reaches the age of 24 months, genu valgum normally develops. Radiographs are indicated if genu varum is present after this age or is progressive after the age of 1 year, if it appears to be severe, or if it occurs in a high-risk group, such as obese children who walk early. Radiographic findings of benign genu varus include symmetric bowing of the tibia and femur, a normal-appearing growth plate without narrowing or step-off, and a generalized, rather than focal, outward bowing (Fig. 432.14).

Treatment involves observation to verify resolution. Objective assessment may be accomplished by measuring the distance between the femoral condyles. This method is not as accurate as are radiographs, but these measurements are a practical way of observing change in patients when the presumptive diagnosis is physiologic genu varum.

The differential diagnosis of physiologic genu varum includes Blount disease, rickets, posttraumatic growth-plate disturbance, enchondromatosis, achondroplasia, and other skeletal dysplasias. The ratio of physiologic bowing to Blount disease is more than 1,000:1.

Tibia Vara (Blount Disease). Tibia vara, also known as Blount disease, is an idiopathic, probably mechanical deficiency in the medial tibial growth plate that may be unilateral or bilateral. Initially, it may present in two different age groups: infants and adolescents.

Almost always, untreated infantile tibia vara is progressive and, in addition to exhibiting outward angulation, includes flexion, internal rotation and, often, abnormal lateral knee laxity. Radiography demonstrates progressive depression of the medial metaphysis, the growth plate, and the epiphysis and, eventually, fusion of the medial metaphysis to the epiphysis in severe cases. A helpful early distinction in tibia vara is the focal nature of the change, with sharp angulation of the proximal tibial metaphysis resulting in a metaphyseal-diaphyseal angle of 11 to 16 degrees or more, measured as shown in Figure 432.15. It is a specific sign, because such localized angulation occurs in fewer than 5% of children with physiologic varus but is seen in essentially all those with Blount disease.

Brace treatment usually is used for mild but definite cases of Blount disease. Valgus rotational osteotomy of the tibia is indicated if the angulation persists beyond 3 years. Recurrence is common if treatment begins after age 4, if the epiphysis is fragmented, or if an affected child is obese. Persistent tibia vara leads to early degenerative changes.

Adolescent tibia vara has its onset in children older than age 9. It is most common in obese boys. Probably, it is caused by decreased growth of the medial tibial physis resulting from excessive medial stresses. Radiography shows medial femoral and tibial bowing. Bracing is not practical in these obese adolescents. Treatment involves osteotomy to realign the limb or lateral growth-plate closure to allow growth to "catch up" medially.

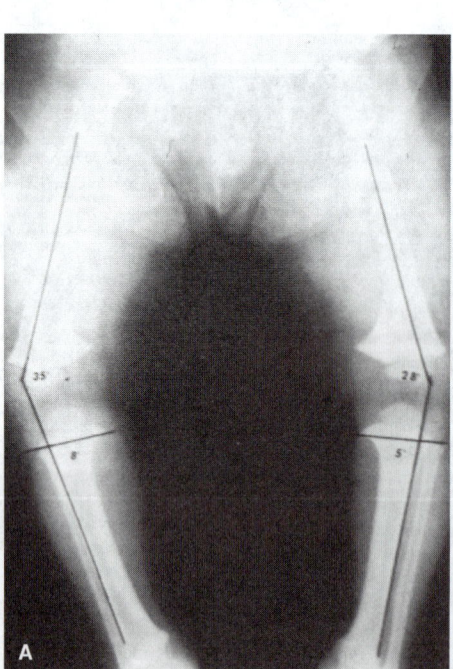

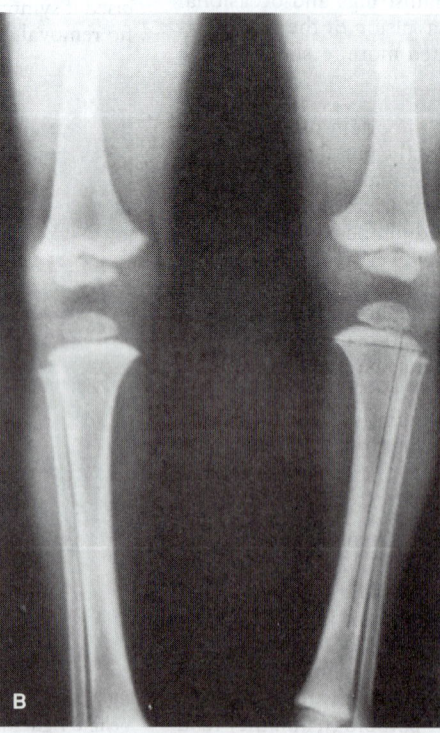

FIGURE 432.14. Note improvement in physiologic bowing between **A:** age 18 months and **B:** 24 months without treatment.

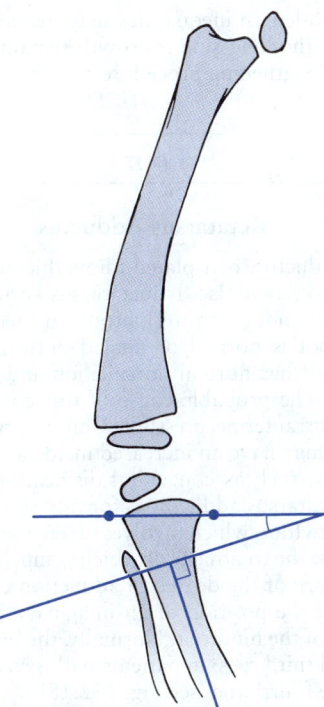

FIGURE 432.15. Metaphyseal-diaphyseal angle. The angle is formed by the line of the tibial shaft and the line between the medial and lateral beaks of the proximal tibial metaphysis. (Redrawn with permission from Levine AM. Physiologic bowing and tibia varum. *J Bone Joint Surg* 1982;64A:1159.)

Genu Valgum. Genu valgum is normal in children older than age 2, reaches a mean of 12 degrees at age 3, and remains approximately constant at a mean of approximately 7 degrees in boys and 9 degrees in girls after age 8. If the angle remains greater than 15 degrees when the child reaches age 10, early growth-plate stapling or later osteotomy of the affected region may be indicated. Valgus of the proximal tibia often follows medial metaphyseal fractures, but frequently it corrects spontaneously.

Tibia

Internal Tibial Torsion. Internal tibial torsion is the most common cause of toeing-in in children between ages 1 and 3. The child with tibial torsion typically has knees that point outward while the feet point inward. Tibial torsion is determined by measuring the angle between the foot and the thigh, with the ankle and knee positioned at 90 degrees. Normally, the foot rotates externally with age (Fig. 432.16). The differential diagnosis includes metatarsus adductus, femoral anteversion, and neuromuscular disorders. To make these distinctions, the foot as well as the hip should be examined (see Fig. 432.16A–C). Tibial torsion improves naturally with growth, but this improvement often takes years. Because of our improved knowledge of the benign natural history of this condition, bracing with such devices as the Denis-Browne bar is used only rarely. Studies have shown that braces cannot apply significant rotational force to the tibia, because the corrective force is taken up in the foot, knee, and hip joints. The improvement that previously was attributed to the brace is primarily the result of normal growth patterns. Correction is a slow process and often frustrates parents. Knowledge that braces were used heavily in the past, reinforced by grandparents and friends, often drives anxious parents to visit the doctor to ensure that they are not missing a golden opportunity to avoid problems. At-

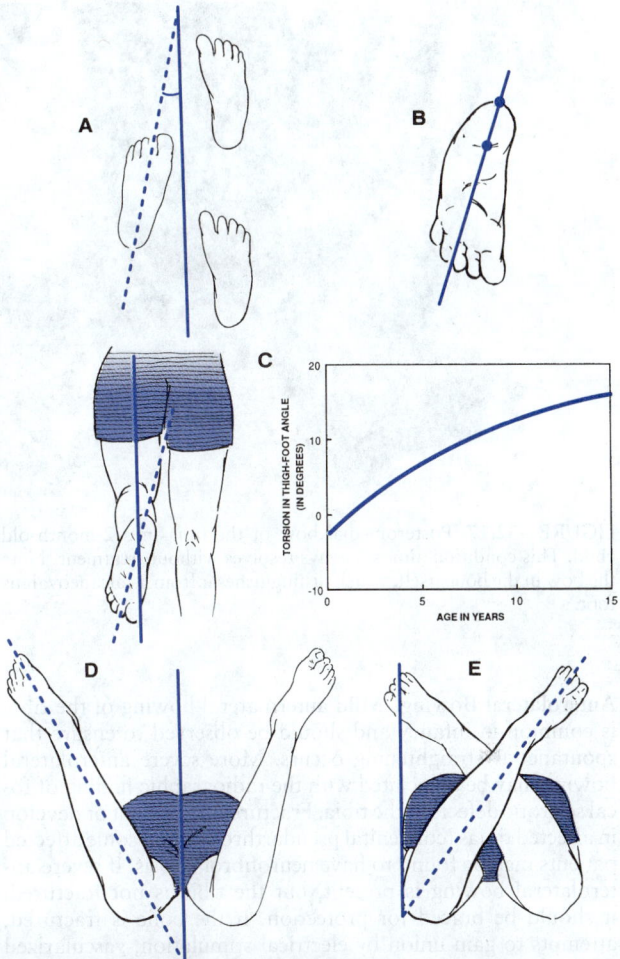

FIGURE 432.16. Assessment of torsional deformities. **A:** Angle of progression (the angle between the foot and the line of gait)—summation of femoral, knee, tibial, and foot relationships. **B:** Assessment of metatarsus adductus. Normally, the heel bisector falls between the second and third toe space. **C:** Thigh-foot angle and its variation with age. This is a reflection of tibial torsion. Measurement of **D:** internal and **E:** external rotation of the hip. If external rotation is less than 20 degrees, "in-toeing" may come from femoral anteversion or hip capsular contractures. (Redrawn with permission from Staheli LT, et al. Lower-extremity rotational problems in children. *J Bone Joint Surg* 1985;67A:41.)

tendant physicians should be confident in allaying such anxiety and should advise them in some such fashion as, "Your child is toeing-in because of inward twisting of the tibia, or leg bone. This is a normal stage in resolution of the position in the womb. Some children have more toeing-in than others. Although such children occasionally may catch a foot when they run, this will improve. As the bone grows longer, it will grow straighter. It may take a few years to correct. Doctors used to use braces for this, but we found that children were getting better by themselves. You can reassure friends and relatives that the child will outgrow it." Use of the graph shown in Figure 432.16C may prove convincing. Although very little evidence substantiates the efficacy of a brace or of any orthotic method, it has been a very widely used treatment that now is declining. Minor persistent internal torsion has not been shown to be detrimental.

External Tibial Torsion. External tibial torsion is less common. Few data address the course of the condition, no treatment is indicated, and some spontaneous improvement can be expected.

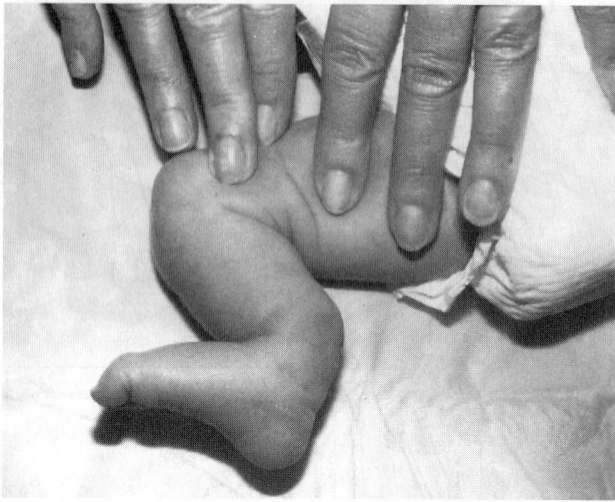

FIGURE 432.17. Posteromedial bow of the tibia in a 2-month-old child. This condition almost always resolves without treatment. Note the bow in the bone itself, which distinguishes it from a calcaneovalgus foot.

Anterolateral Bowing. Mild anterolateral bowing of the tibia is common in infancy and should be observed to ensure that spontaneous straightening occurs. More severe anterolateral bowing may be associated with the radiographic finding of focal sclerotic defects in the tibia. Fractures are present or develop in affected tibias (congenital pseudarthrosis), and some affected patients may be found to have neurofibromatosis. If severe anterolateral bowing is present, but the tibia is not fractured, it should be braced for protection. If the bone is fractured, attempts to gain union by electrical stimulation, vascularized fibula grafting, and bone grafting with rod stabilization have success rates that range from 50% to 75%. Anterolateral bowing may be seen also with congenital absence of the fibula.

Posteromedial Bowing. Posteromedial bowing (Fig. 432.17) of the tibia is more benign, usually straightens by the time the child reaches age 4 years, and is not associated with fracture. Commonly, between 2 and 6 cm of shortening is seen by maturity, however. Treatment involves stretching the tight dorsiflexor muscles and the use of length equalization as indicated.

Limb-Length Inequality

Limb-length differences are screened best by palpating the heights of the iliac crests with the hips and knees straight. Any discrepancy may be confirmed with a tape measure held between the anterior superior iliac spine and the inferior edge of the medial malleolus. Most commonly, apparent differences in the lengths of the lower limbs in children are due to measurement error, because patients have difficulty in lying still and in holding hips and knees straight. In the normal population, differences of 1 cm between the two sides are not uncommon findings.

Discrepancies of up to 2 cm in adults (or a proportionately smaller amount in children) have been shown to have no ill effects on gait or joints and do not need treatment. Larger discrepancies should be confirmed with a radiographic film (scanogram) or with a CT scan. Causes of true, significant discrepancy greater than 2 cm may include hemihypertrophy, hemiatrophy, coxa vara, hip dysplasia, or growth-plate damage, to name a few. Because hemihypertrophy has been associated with Wilms tumor in some cases, these patients should be examined with abdominal ultrasonography two to three times per year until the age of 8 to 10 years. The treatment of

significant limb-length inequalities may include a lift, an epiphysiodesis of the long side if growth remains, or a surgical shortening or lengthening procedure.

Foot

Metatarsus Adductus

Metatarsus adductus, or isolated idiopathic adduction of the metatarsals, is known also as metatarsus varus or C-foot. In contrast to the findings in a clubfoot, in metatarsus adductus the hindfoot is normal or angled outward slightly. The ankle joint itself has normal dorsiflexion and plantar flexion (Fig. 432.18). The probable cause of this condition is medially directed intrauterine pressure. Children with metatarsus adductus also may have an increased incidence of other molding deformities, such as congenital dislocation of the hip or torticollis. Metatarsus adductus deformity should be differentiated from skewfoot, which involves severe outward deviation of the hindfoot, the treatment of which is much more difficult. A rough measure of the degree of adduction can be obtained by determining the position of an imaginary line that would bisect the sole of the hindfoot. Normally, the line falls between the second and third toes; in patients with severe adduction, it is lateral to the fourth toe (see Fig. 432.18B).

The natural history of untreated metatarsus adductus is spontaneous correction in 85% of children, with the persistence of mild adduction in 10% and more pronounced adduction in 5%. In one longitudinal study of 2,000 feet in newborns followed until maturity, no patients had symptomatic adduction in adulthood. Those cases that will resolve spontaneously cannot be predicted, even on the basis of severity or rigidity.

The author's preferred treatment is observation, with stretching for the first 6 to 12 months, followed by corrective casts or special shoes for the very few patients in whom the condition persists beyond this time. The casts are changed every 1 to 2 weeks until the adduction is corrected clinically. Osteotomy for very late-presenting adduction in children older than age 3 rarely is necessary.

Clubfoot

Talipes equinovarus congenita, or clubfoot, is a more complex disorder involving not only metatarsal adduction but abnormalities of the hind part of the foot, including malrotation of the calcaneus under the talus and equinus (plantar flexion) of the ankle. The incidence is 1 in 1,000, and it is more common in boys than in girls. Clubfoot may be unilateral or bilateral. Its cause is unknown, but appears to be related to a primary defect of local connective tissue or a very early insult to the leg muscles or tarsal bones.

Physical examination reveals a small foot, and the combination of deformities often results in a 90-degree rotation of the forefoot in all planes, so that the leg and foot truly resemble the shape of a club. A deep crease is present on the medial border of the foot. The deformity is not completely correctible by manual manipulation in the neonatal period, and the range of motion in all planes is limited. Radiographs are not necessary in the typical case.

Neuromuscular disorders (especially lipomeningocele, myelomeningocele, Larsen syndrome, or arthrogryposis) may produce similar deformities. Also, the genetic conditions of Mobius syndrome, diastrophic dwarfism, and Freeman-Sheldon ("whistling face") syndrome include a deformity similar to clubfoot.

Clubfoot ranges from a mild, "postural," and easily correctable condition to one that is severe and resistant to treatment.

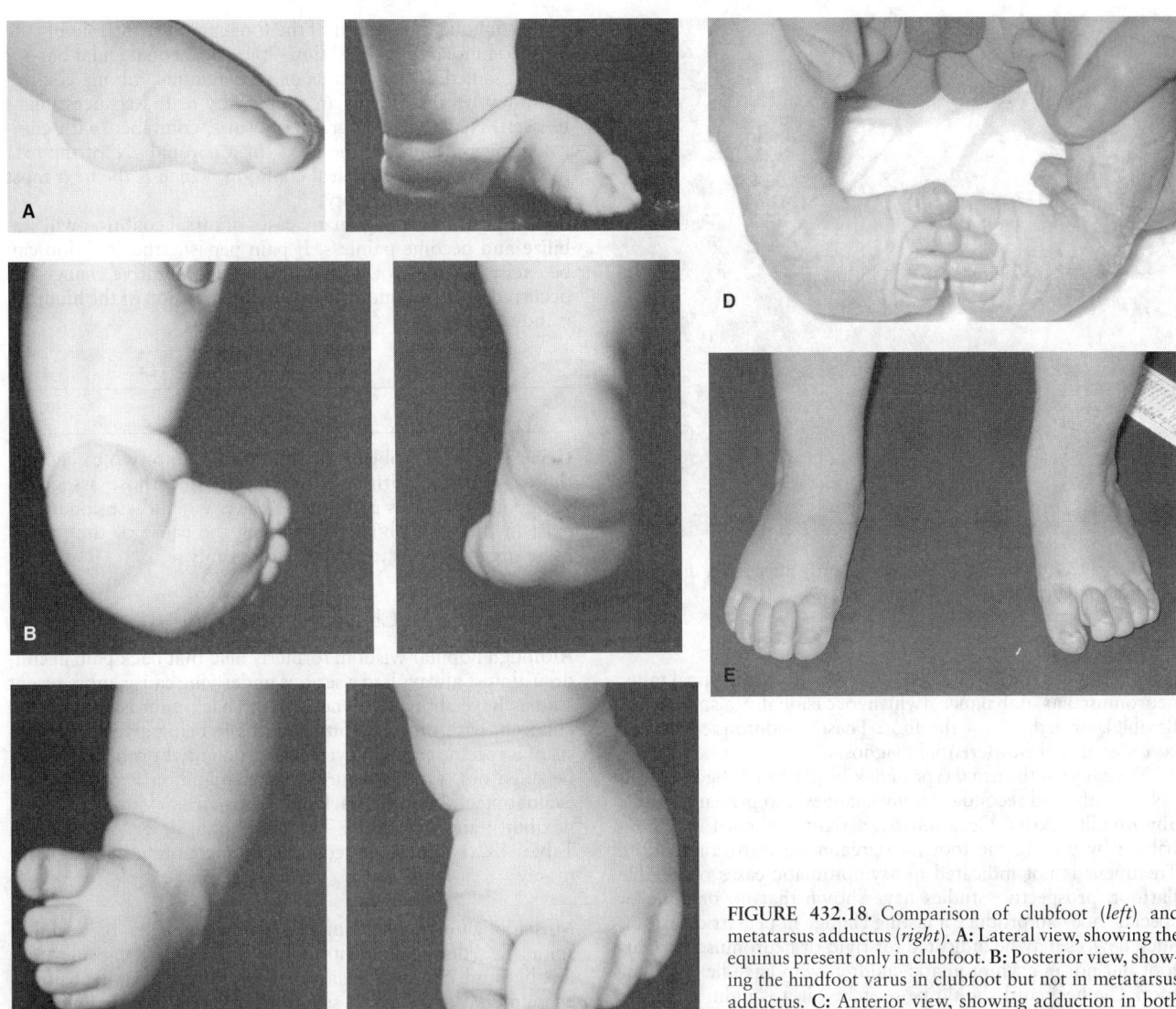

FIGURE 432.18. Comparison of clubfoot (*left*) and metatarsus adductus (*right*). **A:** Lateral view, showing the equinus present only in clubfoot. **B:** Posterior view, showing the hindfoot varus in clubfoot but not in metatarsus adductus. **C:** Anterior view, showing adduction in both feet, with the varus also present in clubfoot. **D:** Bilateral clubfeet before and **E:** after treatment.

A trial of cast correction is indicated in all cases, however. This treatment is most successful when started in the perinatal period, when ligamentous laxity is greatest, with the casts being changed once to twice per week. The residual tight heel cord may be corrected by an Achilles tenotomy in the office. After the feet are corrected by casts, corrective shoes with a bar between the shoes to turn them outward, are then worn for approximately 2 years. This treatment program is commonly known as "the Ponseti method." This method of nonoperative treatment produces better long-term results: more movement in the feet and less late pain than operative treatment. It represents a change in practice from the more operative approach taken by orthopaedic surgeons even 10 years ago. Overall, casting is effective in approximately two-thirds to three-quarters of all patients. Surgery is indicated in the others, and it involves a complete release of all bony malalignments and tendon contractures; it is performed most commonly between the ages of 6 and 12 months.

Calcaneovalgus Foot

A calcaneovalgus foot is seen commonly in newborns; it appears dramatic but is in fact benign and self-resolving. In this condition, the foot is dorsiflexed so extremely that the dorsum of the foot is pressed against the tibia (Fig. 432.19). The cause of the disorder is intrauterine molding. Actually, the alignment of the bones of the foot internally is fine and can be verified by observing the presence of an arch and by bringing the foot to a neutral position, a movement that should not require much pressure. The toes should have normal movement. This condition should be differentiated from posteromedial bowing of the tibia, which causes the foot to assume the same direction but with a more proximal apex to the deformity and a bowing in the distal tibia. The natural history is benign. The ankle and foot stretch out naturally with time, and no cast is needed. No known sequelae accompany this condition.

Flatfoot (Pes Planovalgus)

The condition called flatfoot must be divided into flexible and rigid types. The flexible type is very common in children and usually causes no symptoms. Development of the arch of the foot occurs spontaneously during the first 8 years of life in most children. The arch of the foot is restored when weight bearing is relieved. Inward-outward motion is normal. In contrast,

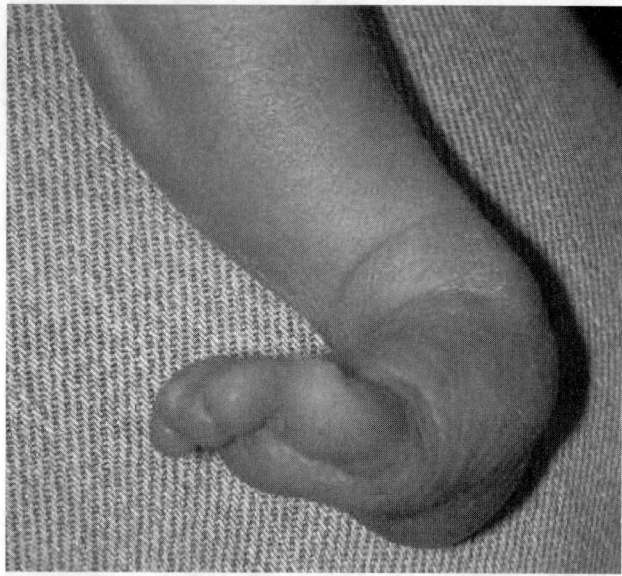

FIGURE 432.19. Calcaneovalgus foot shortly after birth, displaying significant valgus and dorsiflexion.

rigid flatfoot may be caused by tarsal coalition, a vertical talus, neuromuscular imbalance (which occasionally also may be flexible), or arthritis of the foot. These conditions should be considered in the differential diagnosis.

The cause of the usual type of flexible flatfoot is ligamentous laxity, with mild secondary bony changes. No primary muscle abnormality exists. Occasionally, a tight heel cord may contribute by pulling the foot into greater outward angulation. Treatment is not indicated in asymptomatic cases of flexible flatfoot; prospective studies have shown that no orthotic or special shoe can produce a lasting change in pediatric flatfoot. Such devices may be indicated for rigid or neuromuscular flatfoot but not in asymptomatic children who have flexible flatfoot. The heel cord should be stretched if it is tight. Rarely is surgery indicated.

The general principles that a physician should stress to parents when asked about shoes are summarized in an article by Staheli. In short, shoes are primarily for protection; "corrective shoes" have no effect on flatfoot; and shoes should be flat, flexible, porous, and high-topped to prevent them from slipping off the foot. These characteristics are available in most reasonably priced footwear found in regular shoe stores.

Tarsal Coalition

Tarsal coalition is the failure of complete separation of hindfoot bones, with persistence of a fibrous or bony bridge or coalition between two of them. This anomaly is transmitted in an autosomal dominant fashion and is present in approximately 5% of the population. Many individuals with tarsal coalition are asymptomatic. The presence of symptoms seems to be related to the degree of outward angulation that is present, which places more shear strain on the abnormal junction.

Usually, the diagnosis is made during the second decade after an ankle "sprain," with persistent pain or the spontaneous onset of pain in the ankle. The probable reason for this presentation is that the ossification that occurs at this time, near the point of skeletal maturity, renders the coalition stiffer. The hindfoot shows limitation of the inward-outward motion, but it is tender to palpation. Sometimes pain is manifested over the peroneal muscles, which contract excessively to stabilize the foot.

An oblique radiograph of the foot can illustrate reliably the most common type of coalition—the calcaneonavicular bar—if it has ossified. If it is fibrous or cartilaginous, a bony connection may be absent, but an irregularity of the cortices might be seen. Negative radiographic results, combined with clinical suspicion, indicate the need for a coronal CT of the foot to search for a talocalcaneal coalition, which is the next most common type of deformity.

With rest or casting, many cases of tarsal coalition will stabilize and become painless. If pain persists, the coalition can be excised, if it is not large and if no degenerative change has occurred. If these conditions are not met, fusion of the hindfoot is indicated.

Spine

Generally, back problems in children fall into two categories: those associated with spinal deformity and those associated with pain in various parts of the back. When these conditions exist in the same child, determining the cause of the pain is more urgent than is treating the deformity.

Childhood Back Pain

Although popular wisdom formerly held that back pain in children almost always had a serious underlying cause, more recent studies have shown that nonspecific back pain is common in children, with only one-fifth eventually being given a diagnosis of a specific cause. Nevertheless, potential problems should be ruled out. Careful neurologic examination is necessary in evaluating children for back pain, as is an assessment of spinal flexibility and deformity. The differential diagnoses listed in Table 432.1 are those conditions encountered most commonly.

Musculoligamentous Pain. All the components of a child's spine (i.e., discs, ligaments, muscles, and joint capsules) are flexible and conform easily to the extreme spinal positions encountered daily in the school yard or on the playing field. After the child reaches approximately 12 years, generally the spine loses some of its flexibility and, during the teenage years, further "stiffening" may take place. Muscular or ligamentous back pain almost never is observed in children who are younger than 10 years. This diagnosis should be reserved for an older child (often involved in a new physical activity) who has lumbar area pain for which no other specific cause can be elucidated. To warrant this diagnosis, affected children should have pain localized to the lumbar area, a normal neurologic examination, normal results on radiography of the lumbar spine and, in some instances, normal bone scan results.

Once the diagnosis has been made, the treatment of musculoligamentous pain involves rest from any activity that causes the pain. The use of ice in the first 24 hours after onset is helpful; thereafter, usually heat is more efficacious. Once the pain has resolved, exercises should be used to strengthen the abdominal musculature and the lumbar muscles before sports activity is resumed. Often, a lumbosacral corset is helpful in the acute stage and for a few months thereafter, while affected children are participating in sports, to protect the low back and its muscles from the extremes of spinal movement. The long-term use of a corset or other brace rarely is needed if the diagnosis of musculoligamentous back pain is correct. Once low-back pain has resolved, attendant physicians should stress to affected children that warming up before participating in sports activities is more important for them than for their teammates. The persistence of pain requires further investigation for unusual causes of back pain.

Spondylolysis and Spondylolisthesis. Spondylolysis is the most common cause of back pain to yield an anatomic diagnosis in children. Usually, it is a stress fracture of the pars interarticularis segment of the vertebra. This thin segment of bone between the facet joints is subjected to high forces, especially with marked lordosis of the lumbar spine or with heavy lifting. The overall incidence in the general population is approximately 6%. Most of these stress fractures likely occur in the early school years, though symptoms occur most frequently when children are in their early teenage years. A much higher frequency of spondylolysis occurs in children who participate in gymnastics, wrestling, and weight-lifting activities, at times approaching 20% for participants in these sports.

Most commonly, symptoms include pain in the lumbar area after or during a sports activity and a concomitant limitation of lumbar spine motion. If affected children have a chronic spondylolysis, often the pain is intermittent; if the spondylolysis is acute, the pain is more severe the first time it is noted. Occasionally, pain may radiate along the sciatic nerve distribution into the lateral calf or dorsum of the foot.

The physical examination may not be remarkable. Usually, limitation of lateral spine flexion toward the side of the spondylolysis occurs; often, it is associated with limited forward flexion from back pain, not only hamstring tightness, as in some other conditions. Back pain may be produced by straight-leg raising, but radiation of pain into the legs with this maneuver is rare. The results of the neurologic examination are normal.

Often, the diagnosis can be made by lumbar spine radiographs (Fig. 432.20). The most common location of spondylolysis is at L5, with L4 being the next most frequent site. Often, spondylolysis can be visualized by AP and lateral radiographic views, but usually oblique views are more definitive. In addition, oblique views reveal the unilateral or bilateral nature of the defect. If a lytic defect is observed, the age of the lesion should be determined. Generally, the spondylolysis is old if the defect has sclerotic edges. A technetium Tc^{99m} bone scan

with single-photon emission CT (SPECT) or pinhole collimator views is helpful to determine the age of the stress fracture. If the spondylolysis is old and sclerotic edges are present on radiography, obtaining bone union nonoperatively will not be possible. If the scan shows increased uptake at the lytic area and radiography reveals no sclerotic edges, however, the stress fractures might heal if the child is placed in a body jacket brace or cast.

If the scan shows no increased uptake, the treatment of spondylolysis is similar to that of a musculoligamentous problem. Initially, the patient should rest from activity. Often, a lumbosacral corset is helpful for a few weeks until pain resolves. Some teenagers with spondylolysis prefer to wear the corset during sports activities as added protection even after acute back pain resolves. Children should be followed with serial radiography during the growing years to rule out the development of a progressive slip. Generally, fusion for spondylolysis without spondylolisthesis is not needed. With the exception of occasional episodes of low-back pain, teenagers are able to participate in any sport that does not lead repetitively to back pain after playing.

Spondylolisthesis occurs in some children who have spondylolysis. This condition results from forward slipping of a superior vertebra on the inferior vertebra, most commonly slipping of L5 on the sacrum (Fig. 432.21). Worsening of this slip coincides with growth of the spine and generally subsides once growth is completed. As the vertebra slips forward, the posterior elements (i.e., the spinous process and inferior facets) remain behind, attached to the adjacent vertebrae by ligaments. The combination of excessive motion of the posterior elements and forward vertebral slipping may lead to irritation of L5 or S1 nerve roots. Because this slipping usually is slow, the nerve root irritation may present only as progressive tightening of the hamstrings. Affected children may note difficulty in touching their toes or reaching objects on the floor. If one side of the spine is affected more than the other, scoliosis also may be present.

On physical examination, the most striking finding is limitation in straight-leg raising because of the hamstring spasm. Radiation of pain into the calf or foot with straight-leg raising may indicate more advanced nerve root irritation. At times, the ankle jerk reflex is diminished.

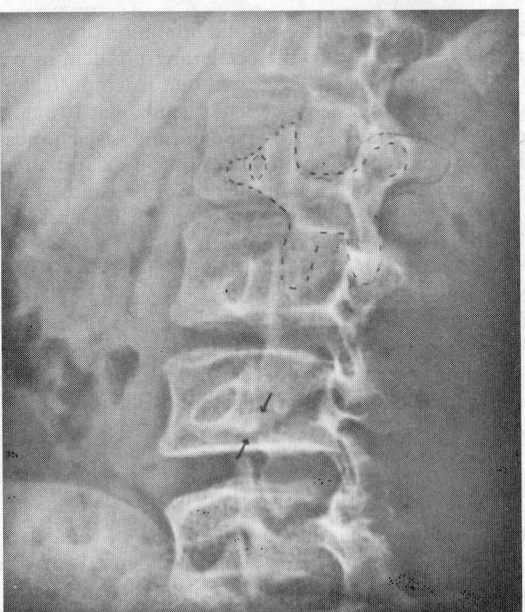

FIGURE 432.20. Spondylolysis. Oblique film of lumbar spine shows defect in pars interarticularis of L4 (*arrows*). Note that the posterior elements of a vertebra resemble a Scottie dog in this view, as outlined. The nose, eyes, ears, neck, and body are the transverse process, pedicle, pedicle superior articular process, pars interarticularis, and lamina, respectively. Spondylolysis appears as a break in the "neck" region.

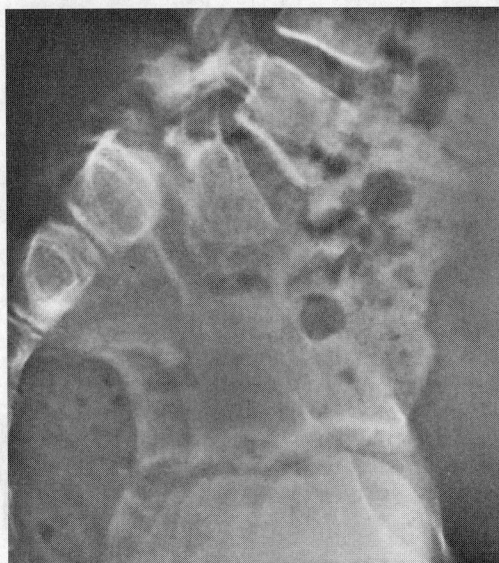

FIGURE 432.21. Severe vertebral slips, as shown here, lead to hamstring spasm and leg pain as well as to back pain. Surgery is needed.

A definite diagnosis can be made on the basis of plain radiography, most easily in the lateral view. The extent of slip is graded from 1 to 4 (i.e., grade 1, up to 25%; grade 2, up to 50%; etc.). If the slip is greater than 50%, posterior lumbosacral fusion is indicated. If the slip is less than 50%, initial management is directed toward relief of back pain and hamstring spasm, using rest and corset therapy, as with spondylolysis. If the pain does not respond to conservative treatment, fusion may be needed. If the pain improves with conservative treatment, a corset may be used for sports activities, and follow-up lateral lumbosacral radiography at 6- to 9-month intervals is recommended until growth is complete or a worsening slip can be identified. If progression of the slip occurs, fusion is indicated.

The use of a brace may prevent further slipping. If affected children do not have hamstring tightness and are pain-free, usually activities do not need to be restricted, provided such children and their parents are aware that periodic back pain is likely to occur. No evidence exists that increased physical activity causes an increase in vertebral slip.

Intervertebral Disc Herniation. Herniation of the intervertebral disc is a common cause of back and leg pain in middle-aged adults. In this age group, disc protrusion occurs posteriorly, with the protruded disc compressing the nerve roots or the cauda equina. If similar forces are applied to the spine of skeletally immature children, the disc will not always rupture posteriorly, but a fracture of the growth plate of the vertebral body may occur, causing the extrusion of disc material anteriorly (Fig. 432.22) or into the vertebral body itself (Schmorl nodes). Most affected children have back pain without radiation into the leg or calf. If nerve-root pain also occurs, a small avulsion fracture of the growth plate posterolaterally might be present in a position that causes nerve-root compression. The diagnosis of an old disc injury in children can be confirmed by radiographic findings of a narrowed lumbar disc adjacent to a vertebral end plate that has some irregular pattern of ossification.

If no neurologic defect is present, treatment consists of symptomatic care, usually rest until the pain resolves. If both leg pain and back pain are present, MRI should be performed to localize any neural compression, which could be relieved by surgical treatment.

Discitis. Discitis (inflammation of the disc space) may present in a wide variety of ways. Severe back pain with limitation of back movements is common in older children, whereas younger children simply may refuse to walk or may limp. Usually, the cause of this disc inflammation is bacterial infection. The vascular anatomy of the growing disc varies from that of the adult, and the common bacteremias of childhood can infect the disc more readily than the vertebral body itself. Approximately 50% of affected children have positive blood culture results at the time of their acute pain, with *Staphylococcus aureus* being the organism identified most commonly. Despite this finding, milder forms of discitis often appear to resolve without the need for antibiotics.

In discitis patients, the most striking finding on physical examination is marked stiffness of the spine that is notable with attempts at flexion. Often, fever is present. The results of the neurologic examination are normal. In the early stages, radiographs of the spine appear normal. Usually, a few weeks after the onset of pain, narrowing of a single disc may be seen on radiography. Often, the sedimentation rate and WBC count are elevated. Virtually always, an MRI or technetium Tc^{99m} bone scan reveals abnormality at the involved level and should be performed whenever discitis is suspected. If the scan results are positive, and the age and clinical presentation are typical, needle aspiration or open biopsy of the involved disc generally is not necessary.

The treatment of discitis involves antibiotics and immobilization. Antibiotics for *S. aureus* may be given orally for mild cases or intravenously for severe cases and should be used for 3 to 6 weeks. Bed rest should be instituted at the time of presentation if significant spasm is present. If the spasm persists for more than a few days, a body jacket brace or cast will allow for immobilization and ambulation on a limited basis. Rarely does discitis develop into vertebral osteomyelitis with local bone destruction. Usually, the involved vertebral bodies fuse together eventually after the infection resolves.

Spinal Cord Tumors. Back pain and limitation of spinal movement may be seen also as the presenting problem in patients with spinal cord tumors, even without a demonstrable neurologic deficit. In one large series of spinal cord tumors, the presenting complaint was back pain or scoliosis in almost one-third of the children. The hallmark of the physical examination is severe limitation of forward flexion of the spine. Pain may be worsened by neck flexion. Neurologic changes may be very subtle, and detection may be difficult.

In patients with back pain and marked limitation of spinal motion, especially if scoliosis also is present, MRI or CT-myelography is needed if the bone scan and plain radiography do not elucidate the cause. The most common tumor is an ependymoma. Treatment is neurosurgical. If the tumor is benign and can be removed, the pain, scoliosis, and back stiffness generally resolve.

Spinal Deformity

Approximately 5% of children will experience some degree of spinal deformity as they grow. Scoliosis, a lateral curvature of the spine, is the most common condition, and increased thoracic kyphosis or "round back" is the next. School screening programs for spinal deformity, which are mandated in many states, have served to increase the public's awareness of these conditions. Whereas formal school programs generally are targeted toward children in the fifth or sixth grades, routine evaluation of the back should be a feature of each child's annual examination.

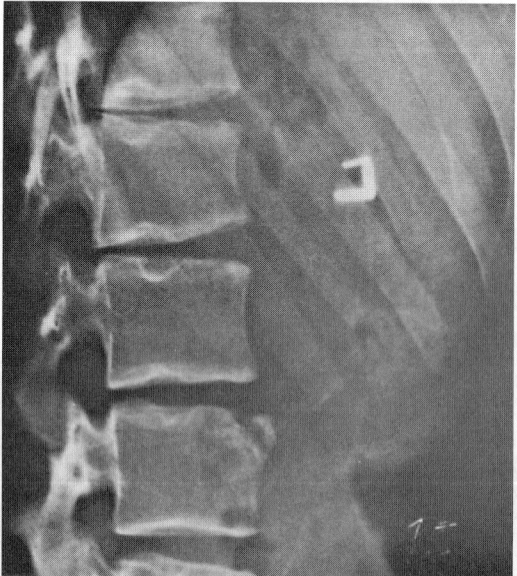

FIGURE 432.22. Excessive stress or pressure in susceptible skeletally immature children will lead to disruption of the apophysis or vertebral growth area, as shown here.

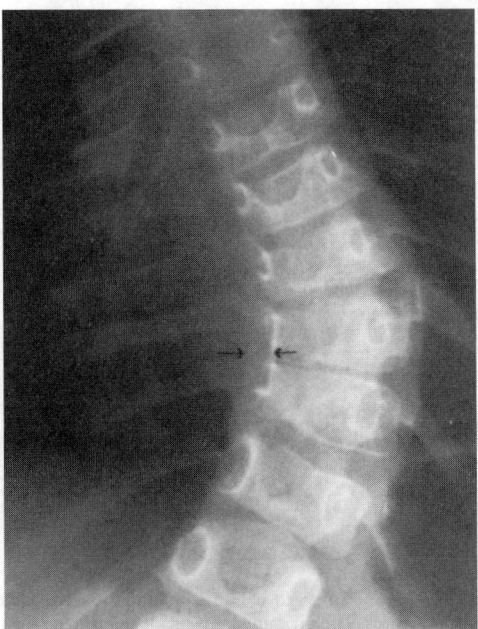

FIGURE 432.23. Congenital scoliosis results from incomplete vertebral segmentation *in utero* (*arrows*). Frequently, genitourinary abnormalities are associated with these bony deformities.

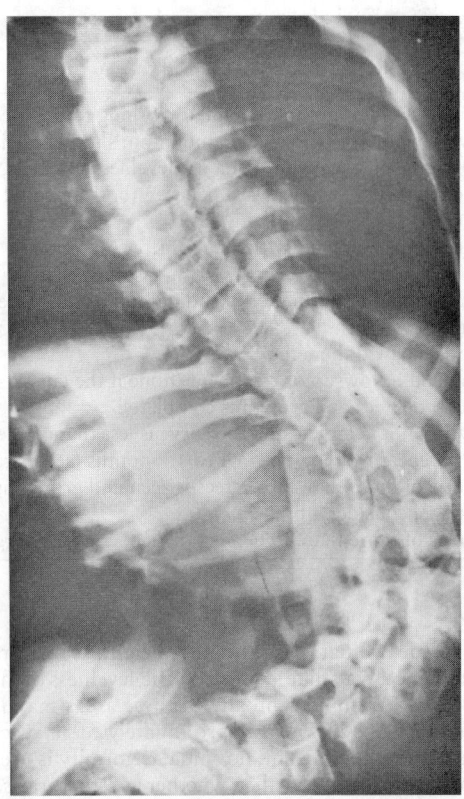

FIGURE 432.24. Sitting anteroposterior radiograph of a child with cerebral palsy and severe scoliosis. Note the C-shaped curve and the pelvic tilt characteristic of neuromuscular scoliosis.

Scoliosis. Scoliosis is a lateral curvature of the spine. The two forms of scoliosis are postural and structural. Postural scoliosis results from spinal factors outside the spine, such as leg-length discrepancy or hip disorders. In these cases, if the leg lengths are equalized or when the child sits, the spine becomes straight, indicating that no structural change has occurred. Structural scoliosis is of greater concern, because it may be progressive.

Although numerous conditions are associated with scoliosis, the most common groups include idiopathic (80%), congenital (5%), neuromuscular (10%), and miscellaneous (5%) disorders. The miscellaneous disorders encompass connective tissue disorders, genetic diseases, and other, less common, conditions.

Congenital scoliosis results from a misshapen vertebra and is present at birth, though often the diagnosis is not made at that time (Fig. 432.23). It may be associated with other birth defects or may present as an isolated condition. Because the genitourinary system arises embryologically from the same region as that of the spine, approximately 30% of children with a congenital spinal deformity have an associated genitourinary abnormality. The most common anomaly is unilateral renal agenesis. Ultrasonography or intravenous pyelography should be performed on all patients who have congenital scoliosis or kyphosis. Although active treatment of unilateral kidney absence may not be necessary, an important adjunct is appropriate cautioning against the child's participation in contact sports that may lead to kidney injury. The treatment of congenital scoliosis consists of serial radiographic follow-up to determine whether the deformity is worsening. If the curve does not increase, generally further treatment is not needed. If a worsening of 5 to 10 degrees or more is documented, surgical fusion is recommended, regardless of an affected child's age. Brace treatment is not indicated for congenital scoliosis.

Neuromuscular scoliosis is a spinal deformity associated with a wide variety of neurologic or muscular diseases, such as cerebral palsy, muscular dystrophy, myelomeningocele, and poliomyelitis. Spinal curvature secondary to muscular imbalance classically is C-shaped and extends to include the pelvis (Fig. 432.24), which usually is not the case in idiopathic scol-

iosis. Scoliosis is present more often and tends to worsen most quickly in patients who do not walk because of their neuromuscular disease. With continued progression, sitting balance becomes impaired further, and the child may need to use one arm or hand to assist in sitting. Treatment centers on preservation of sitting ability and pulmonary function. Although wearing a brace often is useful, frequently surgical fusion is indicated to improve sitting or standing.

Generally, idiopathic scoliosis is found in otherwise healthy children. Although idiopathic scoliosis requiring treatment is approximately eight times more frequent in girls than in boys, the incidence of mild curves is approximately equal between the genders.

A family history of curvature of the spine is found in as many as 70% of all children with scoliosis, though the exact mode of inheritance has not been determined definitely. Although the cause of idiopathic scoliosis remains elusive, a combination of growth asymmetry and postural imbalance is believed to be important. Minor abnormalities in the postural control center in the brainstem have been demonstrated in children with mild scoliosis. Once the curve begins to develop in response to this impaired postural feedback, growth asymmetry likely occurs. Growth is slower when increased pressure is exerted on the growth areas. Because more pressure is exerted on the concave growing areas than on the convex side, the convexity grows more quickly, leading to increasing curve size. This theory accounts for the observation that curves worsen most during the rapid adolescent growth spurt, which is the time when most of these curves are diagnosed. Muscles, discs, and bone appear to be normal in the young patient with idiopathic scoliosis.

The key to early detection of scoliosis is careful assessment of the entire trunk for asymmetry. Affected children should be examined with their back clearly exposed. The examination

TABLE 432.2

SPINAL DEFORMITY EVALUATION

Examine in swimming suit or similar clothing to expose back.
Observe asymmetry on trunk examination: shoulder height, scapular height, waistline equality, levelness of pelvis, leg-length difference, forward bending (both side and front-back).
Measure rib prominence with inclinometer (optional).
Assess skeletal maturity (e.g., age of menses onset).
Obtain standing posteroanterior radiograph of the spine if asymmetry is seen.
Measure using Cobb method.
Recommend follow-up or treatment (none if the curve is less than 25 degrees and growth is complete).
If growth is not complete and the curve is less than 25 degrees, obtain repeat radiographs in 4 to 15 months (see text).
If scoliosis of more than 25 degrees is seen and growth is not complete, consider a brace.
If scoliosis of more than 40 degrees is seen, consider surgery.

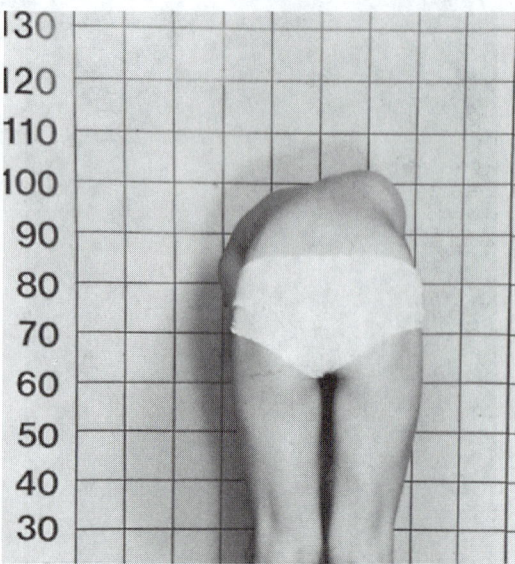

FIGURE 432.26. The forward-bending examination will detect even very small curvatures. The prominence is produced by chest-wall asymmetry, the result of vertebral-body rotation in the curved segment of the spine.

should include evaluation of shoulder height, scapula position and prominence, waistline symmetry, and levelness of the pelvis (Table 432.2). Asymmetry in any of these areas may indicate a scoliosis (Fig. 432.25). In approximately 50% of children with uneven shoulder height, no spinal deformity is present on radiography. To define further whether a structural scoliosis is present, affected children should be examined bending forward (Fig. 432.26). The view from the caudal aspect allows ready detection of prominence of the thoracic ribs, whereas

further bending or viewing from the head down is better for suspected lumbar curves. Both thoracic and lumbar regions should be checked. This "forward-bending" test is very sensitive in demonstrating the vertebral rotation that takes place in a structural scoliotic curve. However, it is not highly specific, and small degrees of rotation occur in patients without any significant scoliosis. A means of quantitating the trunk rotation is needed. The amount of rib hump can be measured by means of an inclinometer ("scoliometer") placed at the apex of the curve with an affected child bending forward. If the scoliometer measurement is 6 degrees or less, the scoliosis rarely is significant and radiographs usually are not needed. If the inclinometer reading exceeds 6 to 7 degrees, standing posteroanterior radiography is indicated for better assessment.

The magnitude of the scoliosis is measured radiographically using the Cobb method (Fig. 432.27). This measurement always should be performed on an erect posteroanterior spine radiograph. The error of measurement for this method is approximately 5 degrees. Because no treatment is needed until the curve reaches 25 degrees, the time estimate for a follow-up radiograph, once the diagnosis has been made, is 25 minus the present curve magnitude. This result provides an estimate of the number of months that may pass until another radiograph is indicated. For example, if an affected child has a scoliosis of 15 degrees, a repeat radiograph should be made in approximately 10 months to check for progression. This time estimate is based on the premise that, during the adolescent growth spurt, annual curve progression is 5 to 10 degrees, or approximately 1 degree per month. From the clinical standpoint, girls who have been menstruating for 2 years essentially have completed their spinal growth.

The treatment of scoliosis is based on three fundamental principles:

- Curves of more than 25 degrees are likely to increase if an affected child still is growing.
- Curves of 40 to 50 degrees are likely to increase even after growth is complete, and to cause more back pain than in patients without scoliosis.
- Some degree of clinical pulmonary restriction may begin to be noticeable in thoracic curves of more than approximately 75 degrees.

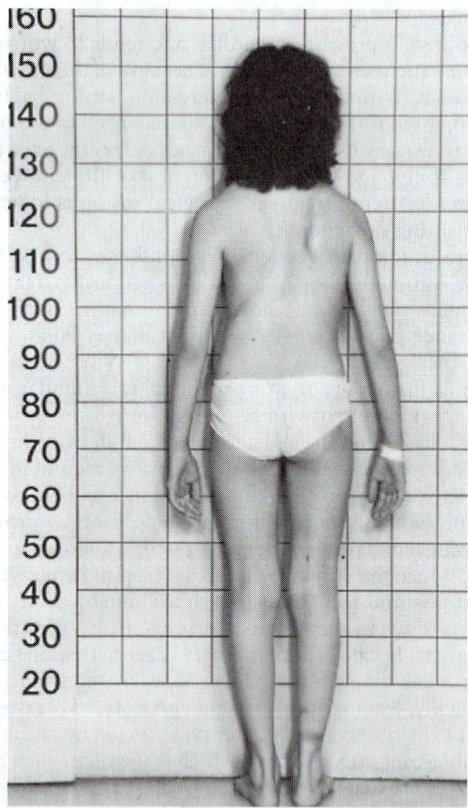

FIGURE 432.25. In examining for scoliosis, asymmetry of the trunk (shoulders, scapular height, waist area, pelvic height) should be noted carefully.

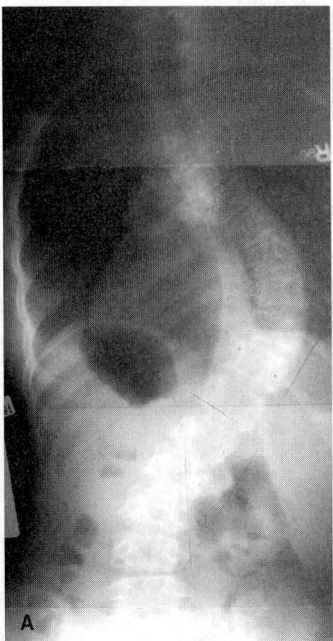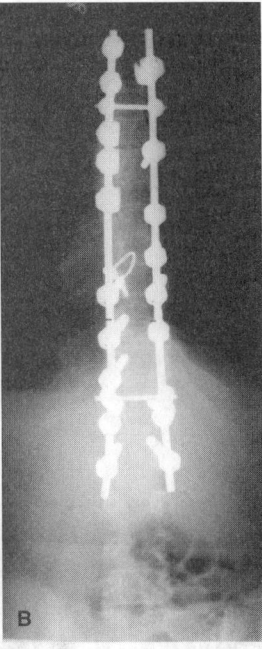

FIGURE 432.27. A standing posteroanterior radiograph of the spine is the correct film to use in quantitating the magnitude of scoliosis. **A:** The Cobb method of measurement is used routinely and is obtained as shown on this radiograph. **B:** The postoperative result after spinal correction and fusion in the same patient.

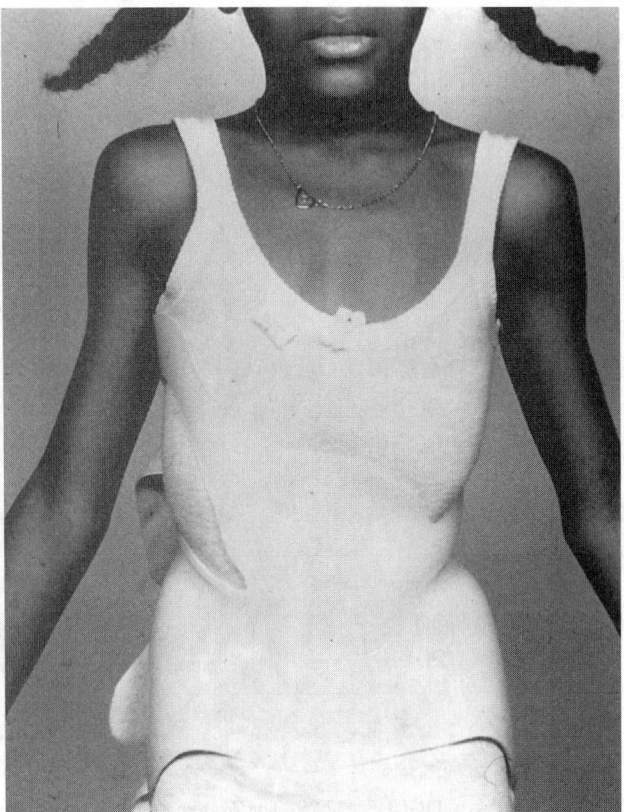

FIGURE 432.28. This child is wearing a low-profile brace currently recommended for most types of curves. It is worn under clothing and is not noticeable.

If affected children are skeletally mature and have a curvature of less than 25 degrees, no further evaluation or treatment of scoliosis is needed. If the scoliosis is 25 degrees or more, and such children still are growing, generally brace treatment is recommended and is successful in approximately 80% of the patients who actually wear the brace as prescribed (Fig. 432.28). Spinal exercises alone will not be successful in stopping curve progression. Once the brace treatment begins, it is continued until growth is complete. Usually, the brace is worn 18 to 23 hours daily. Physical activity is not limited by scoliosis, and affected children often can participate in sports activities while wearing their brace. Brace treatment is considered successful if it prevents further progression rather than providing correction of the curve, because long-term follow-up studies have shown that the final size of the curve is virtually the same as before brace treatment begins. Despite some earlier controversy about the efficacy of bracing, prospective randomized studies published within the last few years have shown bracing to be an effective treatment method.

Although children and parents often are dismayed by our inability to straighten the spine nonoperatively, if curves can be kept at less than 35 to 40 degrees by the time growth is completed, most cases of scoliosis will not worsen in adult life. If the thoracic curve is greater than 50 degrees, or the lumbar curve is greater than 40 degrees at the time growth is completed, usually progression will continue at a rate of approximately 1 degree annually, and often surgery will be recommended.

Surgical treatment is recommended for curves that are greater than 40 to 45 degrees, particularly in children who are not fully grown. Usually, the surgical treatment used consists of instrumentation of the curved area of the spine, combined with posterior spinal fusion of the instrumented area (see Fig. 432.27). Generally, correction of the scoliosis is at least 50%. Failure of fusion occurs in only approximately 1% of affected teenagers. Fusion is complete by 6 months after surgery, at which time such teenagers can return to almost all physical activities, except wrestling, and gymnastics. Teenagers should be encouraged to return to activity, including physical education class in school, to de-emphasize the psychological potential for disability after this surgery.

If the thoracic scoliosis exceeds 50 degrees, patients commonly have diminished vital capacity and residual lung volumes on pulmonary function testing. Arterial blood gas levels and forced expiratory volume in 1 second are normal except in children with severe curves. Vital capacity is decreased further if a thoracic lordosis is associated with the scoliosis. Even with surgical correction of the scoliosis, pulmonary function postoperatively will change little because of the persistence of chest wall or rib deformities that have occurred as a result of the scoliosis. Therefore, scoliosis should be prevented from progressing to this point if possible.

Pain is rare in adolescents who have idiopathic scoliosis. Although it may result from degenerative changes that are present by the time such patients are middle-aged, pain that occurs during adolescence is an indication for further evaluation. Such patients should be questioned in detail about the nature of the pain. If it is severe, limits activities, or requires frequent analgesics, a workup is indicated. If the neurologic examination is normal, a technetium Tc^{99m} bone scan should be performed to screen for discitis, stress fracture, osteoid osteoma, or other bone tumors. If spinal flexion is limited and a neurologic deficit is discovered, MRI or CT-myelography is necessary to rule out intraspinal pathology. Although all these conditions may cause scoliosis, the curvature will straighten as soon as its underlying cause is treated. Therefore, physicians should evaluate patients thoroughly for treatable causes of scoliosis before making a diagnosis of idiopathic scoliosis and instituting brace treatment or recommending spinal fusion.

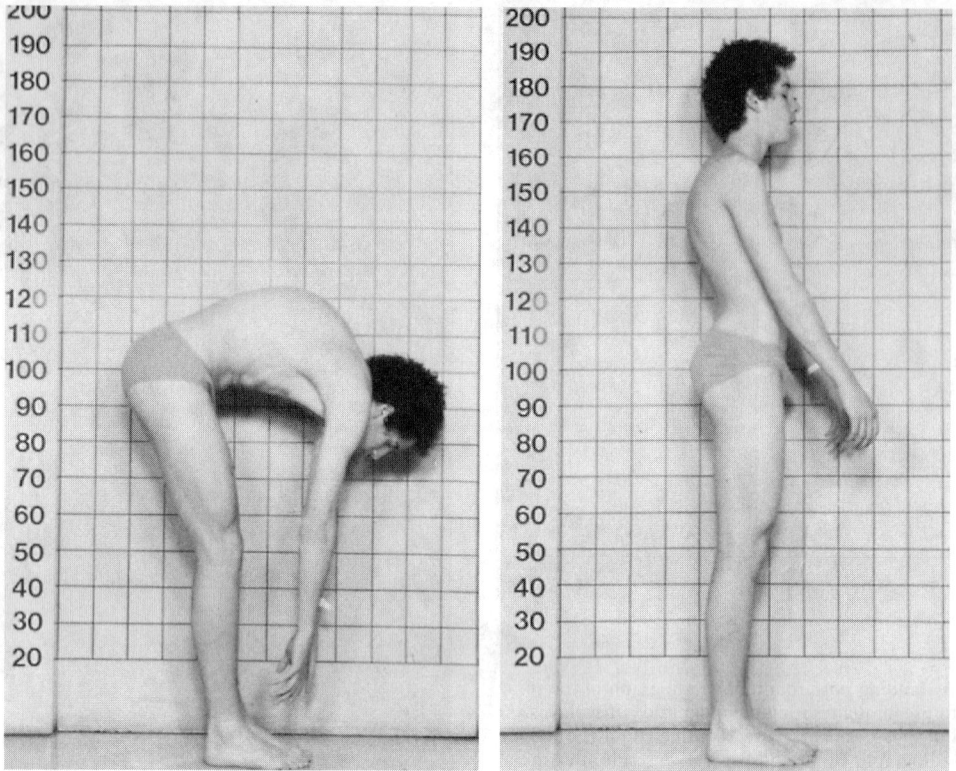

FIGURE 432.29. The examination for kyphosis also should include a forward-bending test to help to determine the rigidity and severity of the kyphosis, which may be hidden more easily in the upright position.

Kyphosis. Normal spinal sagittal contours consist of lordosis in the cervical and lumbar spinal segments to balance the kyphosis that is present in the thoracic area. Sometimes, the term kyphosis is used to describe those abnormal conditions in which increased rounding of the back is present in the thoracic or thoracolumbar area. Usually, parents complain about a child's posture. Assessment of apparent excessive kyphosis should include a forward-bending examination, viewed from the side, to determine whether the back is flexible or rigid in the rounded segment (Fig. 432.29). The kyphosis may be discovered to be a rib prominence associated with a scoliosis. Similarly, mild to moderate scoliosis is seen commonly with moderate and marked kyphosis, so careful examination for both conditions is necessary.

The least serious of these conditions is postural round back. This is seen most commonly in the preadolescent years. It occurs more often in children who are taller than their peers and in girls whose breasts have developed earlier than have their friends'. This condition is a flexible, increased kyphosis that can be straightened voluntarily by the child and can be corrected well with hyperextension positioning. This group of spinal deformities can be treated with exercises alone. Active hyperextension of the trunk and sit-ups to decrease lumbar lordosis are useful in improving trunk control. As long as no fixed deformity is established, as an affected teenager's body image improves, so will the rounding of the upper back.

Usually, a more fixed and less flexible thoracic or thoracolumbar kyphosis is called Scheuermann kyphosis. This condition occurs most commonly in teenage boys. Attempts to correct this kyphosis passively are unsuccessful, and often a large lumbar lordosis is associated with it. Lateral radiography of the spine will demonstrate irregularity of numerous disc spaces and anterior vertebral body wedging (Fig. 432.30). To establish the diagnosis of Scheuermann kyphosis radiographi-

cally, at least 5 degrees of wedging in three adjacent vertebrae should be demonstrated. The Cobb method also is used to measure the amount of kyphosis present. Normally, the amount of kyphosis from T3 to T12 is between 20 and 45 degrees. If the

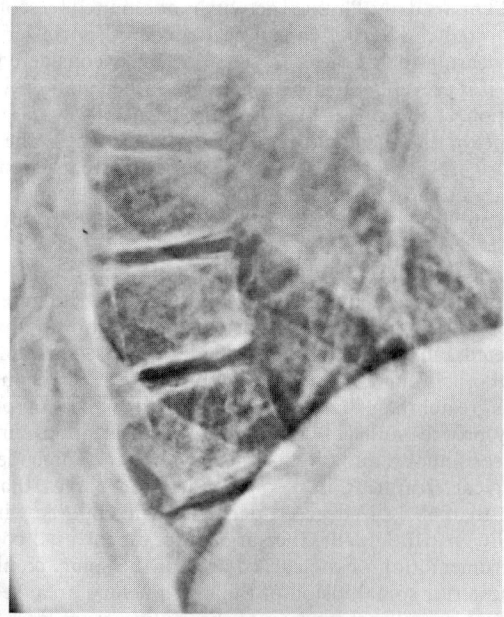

FIGURE 432.30. Lateral spine radiograph demonstrating the disc irregularities and anterior vertebral body wedging seen in Scheuermann disease.

kyphosis is present in the thoracolumbar area, which normally appears straight on lateral radiography, measurements greater than 10 degrees are abnormal.

If wedging is present, little correction can be achieved with thoracic spine hyperextension; if the lateral thoracic kyphosis is 55 to 60 degrees, bracing is indicated while the child is still growing. A Milwaukee brace, which uses a neck ring in addition to trunk pads, is the gold standard, but for kyphoses low in the thoracic spine, a more unobtrusive underarm brace may be used. Unlike scoliosis, in which little correction results from bracing, in kyphosis, approximately 50% improvement can be anticipated after 1 year of full-time brace wear. Once this degree of correction is obtained, nighttime brace wear generally is sufficient until growth is complete.

Increased thoracic kyphosis does not cause abnormalities in pulmonary function. The principal problem seen later in Scheuermann disease is pain in the low thoracic spine after an affected patient has been standing for some time. If the kyphosis exceeds 70 degrees by the time such a patient has stopped growing, spinal instrumentation and fusion, as with scoliosis, can provide excellent correction with a significant improvement in appearance.

Congenital kyphosis is less common than is congenital scoliosis but almost always requires early spinal fusion surgery. If the congenital kyphosis progresses unchecked, spinal cord compression at the apex of the kyphosis is common. As with congenital scoliosis, an evaluation for associated genitourinary abnormalities should be performed.

Cervical Spine

Evaluation of the cervical spine, because of its many normal variations on radiography, often is confusing. As seen on lateral cervical spine radiography, the anterior and superior corner of each vertebral body normally is the last part to ossify, sometimes giving the appearance of a small compression fracture. Full ossification and the development of the odontoid process are not complete in young children and may give the appearance of a spine being maldeveloped. The spine of children younger than age 10 is much more flexible than that of teenagers or older adults. As much as 3 mm of anterior movement of C2 on C3 with flexion is normal in this group, whereas no such movement should be present in adults. In fact, under experimental conditions, the newborn spine can stretch about 5 cm (2 in.) before it fails, whereas the adult spinal cord can stretch only 1.25 cm (0.5 in.) before it ruptures. Because of this difference in elasticity, infants who are involved in automobile accidents may sustain spinal cord injury without apparent spinal fracture. The proper use of car-seating supports for these very young children decreases the risk of these devastating injuries (see Chapter 16, Injury Prevention and Control).

Children with Down syndrome comprise a special group that commonly has instability of the atlantoaxial region. If this instability persists unrecognized, spinal cord compression with myelopathy may result, leading to leg weakness and lessened walking ability. Lateral cervical flexion–extension radiography should be performed at age 5 years in all children who have Down syndrome and are involved in activities involving forceful flexion of the neck or impact to the head. Although approximately 15% of such children will have some evidence of atlantoaxial instability, the majority do not need fusion surgery, but should have periodic follow-up by neurologic examination. If the first radiograph reveals increased laxity (greater than 5 mm distance between the odontoid and the atlas), films should be repeated every 2 years. If no laxity is seen, repeat radiography is not recommended as long as no signs of spasticity or symptoms of neck pain occur. Atlantoaxial posterior fusion is recommended if a neurologic deficit or excessive instability (greater than 8 mm) is present.

Instability of the upper cervical spine also may result from os odontoideum or from odontoid hypoplasia. Os odontoideum is a separation of the odontoid process from the body of the second cervical vertebra. It occurs most commonly as the result of an early childhood trauma that causes a fracture through the synchondrosis of the odontoid process. This unrecognized fracture develops into a fibrous nonunion that gradually becomes unstable over the ensuing months and years. Usually, the diagnosis is made when an affected patient is being evaluated for neck pain or other head or neck trauma. Neurologic symptoms rarely are present, but generally atlantoaxial fusion is indicated to stabilize this region and to protect the spinal cord from sudden, catastrophic injury that may result in death. After fusion is accomplished, such children will be able to participate in normal activities, although mild to moderate limitation of head rotation will be present. Odontoid dysplasia occurs periodically, but it is associated most often with genetic disorders, such as Morquio syndrome and spondyloepiphyseal dysplasia congenita. Generally, fusion is necessary.

Torticollis

Torticollis is present at or near the time of birth and results from a contracture of one of the sternocleidomastoid muscles. An affected child's head will be tilted toward the side of the contracture, with the chin rotated away from the contracted side because the origin of the contracted muscle is on the mastoid process. The cause of torticollis is not well defined, but the incidence is higher in children with breech presentation and forceps delivery. Commonly, a fusiform, firm mass is palpable in the body of the contracted muscle. Often, affected children have plagiocephaly, or asymmetry of face and skull development. If the neck range of motion can be returned to normal by age 1 year, this facial asymmetry will disappear. If the torticollis is untreated until later in childhood, the eyes and ears never will become level.

Cervical spine radiography should be evaluated to ensure that the position of the head is not the result of congenital spine abnormalities, such as hemivertebrae. If the bony cervical spine is normal, stretching exercises should be instituted shortly after birth. These exercises are designed to stretch the contracted sternocleidomastoid muscle and should be taught to parents of affected children by a knowledgeable physical therapist. Although one of the parents should be asked to do these stretching exercises at home, initial weekly checkups by the therapist or the physician can help to ensure compliance. If a significant contracture persists by the time such patients reach age 1, despite stretching exercises, surgical treatment to lengthen the sternocleidomastoid muscle is appropriate. Even after surgical release, some stretching and (at times) bracing will continue to be needed as the child grows.

Torticollis may present later in childhood after an upper respiratory infection or trauma. Torticollis that occurs after an upper respiratory infection is thought to result from retropharyngeal edema that leads to fixed malrotation of the vertebrae at the atlantoaxial level, causing a rotatory deformity. Similarly, after muscular neck trauma, affected children may have a persistent torticollis for several days or weeks, secondary to an unsuspected rotatory subluxation at the atlantoaxial level. A combination of plain radiographs with CT is the best means to demonstrate this problem. (Fig. 432.31). If torticollis from either of these causes persists, affected children should be treated with stretching or traction, followed by bracing. The likelihood that surgical fusion will be necessary increases with the duration of symptoms, so prompt treatment is required.

Klippel-Feil Syndrome

Failure of normal vertebral segmentation in the cervical spine is known as Klippel-Feil syndrome, defined as congenital

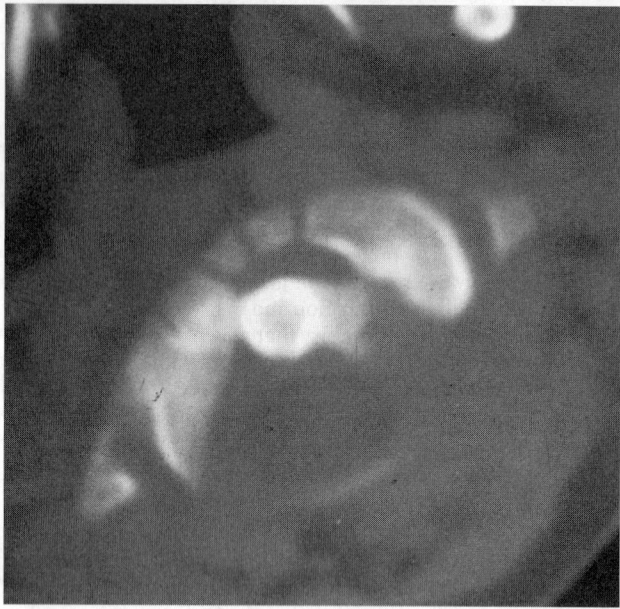

FIGURE 432.31. Torticollis due to atlantoaxial rotatory subluxation is best demonstrated by CT scan. Note the rotation of one side of C1 (outer ring vertebra) from C2 (inner vertebra).

fusion of at least two cervical vertebrae (Fig. 432.32). In the milder forms, when only one or two levels are involved, diagnosis may be delayed until the teenage years and, even then, may be made only when the neck is examined radiographically for other reasons. In more severely involved children, however, the neck is very short, and webbing appears to be present. Often, Klippel-Feil syndrome is associated with Sprengel deformity, which is failure of the normal descent of the scapulae. Associated genitourinary abnormalities may be present, and sonography or intravenous pyelography is indicated when the diagnosis of Klippel-Feil syndrome is made. Little specific treatment is available for this syndrome. Because of the congenital fusion of several segments of the cervical spine, instability may occur at the levels that do move. If this instability is excessive, or if neurologic deficits are present, fusing the unstable segment is necessary. Surgical fusion may be needed also in adult life, to treat degenerative changes at the moveable segments.

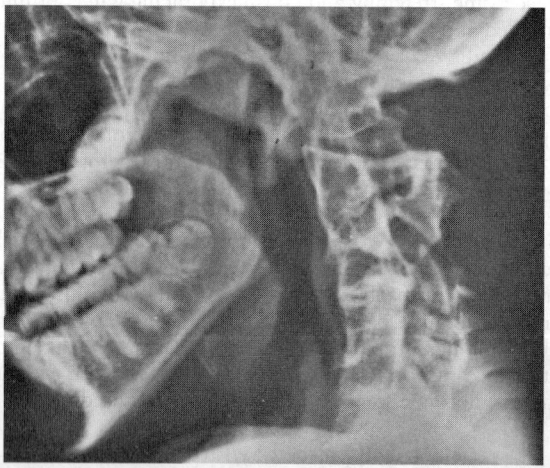

FIGURE 432.32. Klippel-Feil syndrome results from incomplete segmentation of the cervical vertebrae. Often, Sprengel deformity of the scapulae is associated with this syndrome.

Particularly in more involved cases, contact sports should be avoided, because any neck injury in a child with Klippel-Feil syndrome is more likely to be serious, as a result of the limited flexibility of the cervical area.

Upper Extremity

Congenital and developmental abnormalities of the upper extremities of children are less common than those of the lower extremities, perhaps partly because of the greater stresses that are imposed on the lower extremity *in utero* and later during standing.

Obstetric (Brachial Plexus) Palsy

The brachial plexus is composed of contributions from nerve roots C5 to T1. Most severe injuries to the area involve lateral flexion of the neck or downward pressure on the shoulder, such as may occur during a difficult delivery. Therefore, the upper portions of the plexus (C5 to C7) are stretched most commonly in a manner similar to that which causes the "burners" that occur during blocking maneuvers made in sports activities. This stretching causes denervation of the shoulder abductors and elbow flexors, which results in gradual joint contractures if not treated. These brachial plexus injuries are known as Erb-Duchenne palsies. The lower plexus (C7 to T1) can be affected by excessive abduction-traction and has a poorer prognosis; this is the rarest occurrence, and it is called Klumpke palsy. Such cases result in loss of function of the elbow extensors, wrist flexors, and finger muscles and possibly a Horner syndrome. Occasionally, the entire plexus may be involved.

Factors associated with brachial plexus palsy include shoulder dystocia, breech position, high birth weight, and prolonged labor. The incidence is 1 to 3 in 1,000 births. The incidence and severity of this condition have declined gradually as obstetric care has improved. The site of injury may be at any level from the origin of the nerve roots to the plexus itself, but even root lesions may resolve spontaneously. On physical examination, the early typical Erb palsy appears as an arm that is rotated internally at the shoulder, extended at the elbow, and flexed at the fingers. Initially, passive range of motion should be full.

Such skeletal injuries as clavicle fractures and proximal humerus separations should be ruled out radiographically, although often they can be differentiated by guarding on testing of passive motion and the presence of Moro response. Because of the trauma, palsy and skeletal injury may coexist.

Treatment involves the maintenance of motion and transfers of nerve or tendon in those rare, severe cases in which function does not return. With current obstetric practice, 92% of palsies resolve completely by the time affected infants reach 3 months of age, and 95% of such infants eventually recover fully. Physical therapy should be used initially to maintain range of motion. Splinting in most cases results in contractures, although later functional splinting of the hand may have a role. For patients with persistent weakness at age 3 months, electromyography and possibly myelography may help to identify those rare cases in which nerve grafting is required. Cases detected later may benefit from osteotomy or contracture release and tendon transfer, especially to restore shoulder external rotation.

Sprengel Deformity

Sprengel deformity, or congenital elevation of the scapula, actually represents embryonic failure of complete descent, rotation, and development of the scapula. Normally, this realignment occurs predominantly between the ninth and twelfth weeks of gestation. The cause is unknown.

On physical examination, the upper pole of the scapula may be visible in the base of the neck. Abduction is limited. The pectoralis major muscle may be underdeveloped. Such associated congenital anomalies as cervical or thoracic vertebral fusions, anal abnormalities, or cardiac abnormalities may coexist. Treatment is indicated in moderate and severe cases to improve abduction and appearance. The most effective means of treatment involves detaching and lowering the midline origins of the rhomboid and trapezius muscles (Woodward procedure), combined with a clavicular osteotomy.

Congenital Pseudarthrosis of the Clavicle

Congenital pseudarthrosis of the clavicle is a defect in bone continuity presumably caused by pressure from the more cephalad position of the right subclavian artery. The ends of the bone are sclerotic and tapered, like an old fracture. Almost always, the disorder involves the right clavicle, unless the patient has dextrocardia or a cervical rib. Bone grafting and pin fixation before the age of 6 years may be indicated.

Radial Clubhand

Longitudinal failure of the formation of many tissues on the radial side of the forearm and hand is known as radial clubhand. The severity of this condition varies. Approximately 50% of cases are bilateral. Associated abnormalities may include VATER (vertebral defects, imperforate anus, tracheoesophageal fistula, radial and renal dysplasia) syndrome, hydrocephalus, and clubfoot. The upper arm also may be short, and the shoulder girdle may be underdeveloped. The radial-sided muscles, radial carpal bones, thumb, and radial artery may be absent. The hand is deviated radially up to 90 degrees, because it lacks its normal radial support, and the ulna may be bowed. Treatment involves centralization of the wrist on the ulna, transfer of tendon, and possible straightening of the ulna and creation of a thumb, as long as reasonable elbow flexion is present. Untreated cases are problematic cosmetically, although surprisingly they pose less functional difficulty. Congenital absence of the ulna is only one-third as common. In most cases, some remnant of the proximal ulna provides elbow stability.

Radioulnar Synostosis

Often inherited, radioulnar synostosis (fusion) results in a fixed position of forearm rotation, usually in pronation. Usually, diagnosis is delayed because affected children use other joints to compensate for the lack of forearm motion. At times, the synostosis may be only fibrous. Usually, shoulder and wrist motion can compensate for the lack of rotation. Motion to the forearm cannot be restored surgically. Rotational osteotomy to alter the position of the fused forearm should be performed only if clear-cut functional deficit can be demonstrated.

Congenital Constriction Bands (Streeter's Bands)

Congenital constriction bands most likely are the result of intrauterine encirclement by amniotic bands or the umbilical cord. They may be located anywhere, and they also may cause nerve palsies or the amputation of parts (Fig. 432.33). The bands can be released with Z-plasties after the patient reaches age 2 or urgently if they are associated with neurocirculatory compromise.

Polydactyly

Polydactyly, or the presence of an extra digit, varies in spectrum from a hypoplastic addition of soft tissue to a fully developed digit with all phalanges and metacarpals. Fifth-finger polydactyly is ten times more common in black than in white individuals. Therefore, a white child with this finding should be examined for other abnormalities, especially of the cardiovascular system. The simple, small, nonskeletal duplications can be excised or tied off. If significant skeletal stability is present,

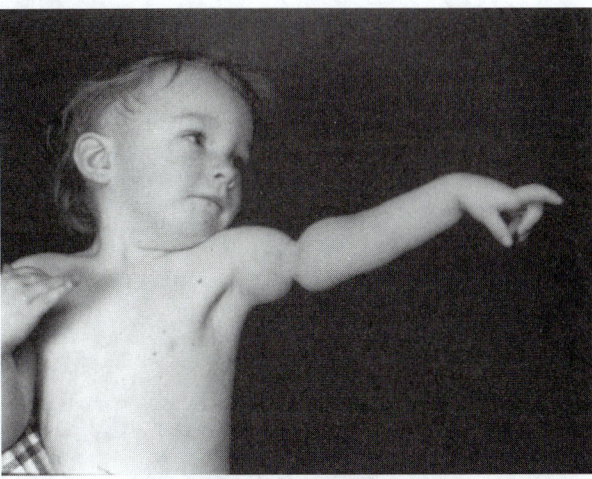

FIGURE 432.33. Child showing three sequelae of congenital constriction bands: deep ring around the left upper arm, paresis of the nerves to the tendons controlling the fingers, and amputation of the tips of the right fingers.

all the digits should be reexamined to determine which is the least functional, and this should be excised.

Congenital Trigger Thumb

Congenital trigger thumb presents as a flexed thumb and is not always recognized at birth. Usually, it is the result of excessive tightness of the annular ligament that encircles the flexor tendon at the metacarpal head. This tightness causes swelling of the tendon, which later becomes firm. Treatment consists of 6 to 8 weeks of stretching if the condition is diagnosed early and (usually) surgical release if it persists.

Nursemaid's Elbow

Annular ligament entrapment, known as nursemaid's elbow, consists of elbow pain after longitudinal traction on a pronated, extended elbow in children between the ages of 2 and 7. A snap may or may not be heard. Usually, radiography shows no bony abnormality or displacement. Only one case report describes actual exploration of this pathology (Salter, 1971). This report and laboratory studies suggest that the annular ligament of the radial head slips partially over the radial head, the narrowest portion being prominent when pronated (Fig. 432.34). An elbow fracture or septic arthritis should be ruled out, especially if the mechanism of injury is a fall rather than traction. Usually, treatment is reduction through stabilizing the elbow with one hand, with a finger placed over the radial head for palpation, followed by gentle firm flexion until a click is felt. Affected children should begin using the elbow within minutes. Usually, immobilization is not carried out and is not necessary in first-time cases. It can be accomplished with 2 to 3 weeks in a cast if the episode recurs. Parent education regarding the mechanism of this condition is most important.

GENERALIZED ABNORMALITIES

Bone Dysplasias

Osteocartilaginous Exostoses (Osteochondromas)

Osteochondromas, which can be single or multiple, are sessile or pedunculated bony masses that are located on the metaphysis, are directed away from the growth plate, and appear to move away from it over time (Fig. 432.35). These outgrowths

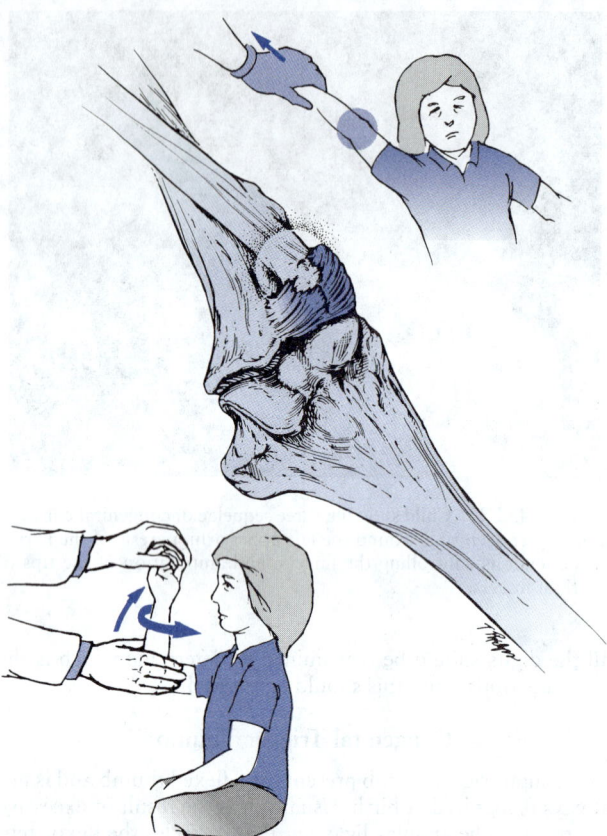

FIGURE 432.34. "Pulled elbow" represents subluxation of the radial head through a partially torn annular ligament. Method of injury (*above*) and method of reduction (*below*).

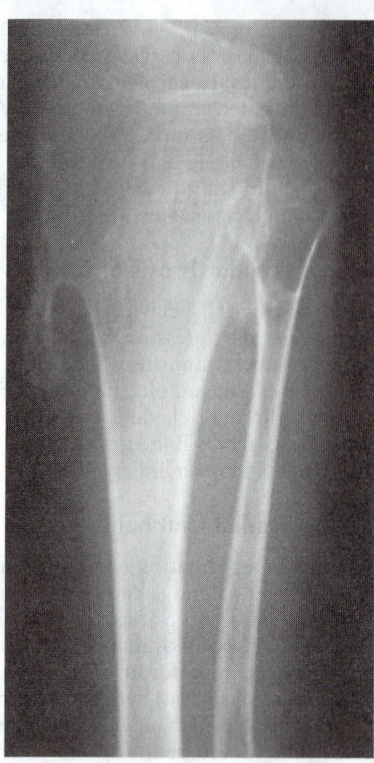

FIGURE 432.35. Osteocartilaginous exostoses are metaphyseal pedunculated or sessile lesions directed away from the growth plate.

have their own growth plates. Osteochondromas are thought to arise from defects in the perichondrial ring that encircles the growth plate, permitting lateral growth rather than the usual organized distal growth. Usually, the condition of multiple exostoses is distinct and is transmitted in an autosomal dominant manner; affected persons frequently are somewhat short. Three different genetic mutations (EXT) are know to cause this condition.

Any bone with endochondral growth may be affected, but the long bones of the extremities are involved most often. Because of asymmetric growth-plate activity, angular growth often ensues, resulting in outward angulation of the knees and ankles and in ulnar deviation of the forearm and wrist. These conditions should be corrected by partial epiphyseal stapling in young children or by osteotomy in older patients. Leg-length inequality is significant in 50% of patients.

The indication for excision of the lesions themselves is pain or compromise resulting from pressure on the tendons, nerves, or spinal cord. Malignant transformation should be suspected if continued growth occurs after skeletal maturity is reached or if new onset of pain occurs. A bone scan may be helpful in skeletally mature individuals because absence of uptake indicates a benign lesion; however, increased uptake does not always mean malignant change.

Fibrous Dysplasia

Fibrous dysplasia is a disorder exhibiting altered bone formation in the medulla and cortex and much fibrous tissue in the marrow. It has been linked to a mutation in G protein (GNAS1). Radiographically, the bone has a uniform "ground glass" consistency and the cortex is thin, soft, and tends to deform with growth and load. One bone (in the monostotic form) or several bones (in the polyostotic form) can be affected. Pathologic fractures occur often, but usually heal within a normal period. Management of proximal femoral ("shepherd's crook") bowing (Fig. 432.36) is the most difficult. Usually, deformities

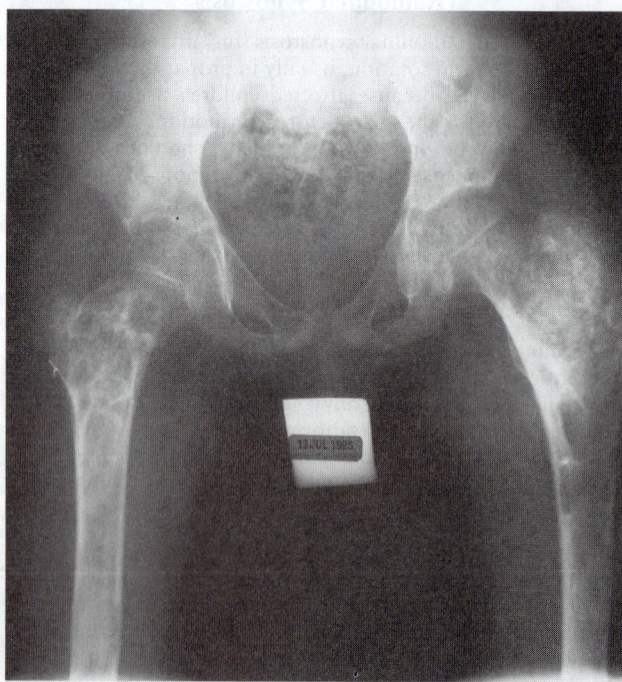

FIGURE 432.36. Polyostotic fibrous dysplasia produces loss of the normal trabecular pattern and thinning of the cortex, and often involves the proximal femur.

and fractures of the lower extremities require internal fixation, whereas those in the upper extremities require casting.

Irregular café au lait spots occur in 30% of patients with the polyostotic form of fibrous dysplasia. When polyostotic lesions and café au lait spots are associated with precocious puberty, the condition is called Albright syndrome. Other types of endocrinopathies (thyroid, parathyroid, or adrenal problems) may occur. Malignant transformation to fibrosarcoma or osteosarcoma is rare.

Osteogenesis Imperfecta

Osteogenesis imperfecta encompasses a spectrum of diseases that are the end result of defects in type I collagen synthesis (see Chapter 433, Skeletal Dysplasias). These diseases result in bones that have thin cortices and multiple fractures. Short stature, blue sclerae, middle-ear deafness, abnormal dentition, and thin skin may coexist. Usually, inheritance is dominant, occasionally is recessive, but frequently is the result of spontaneous mutation. Tiny fractures occur that cause a bowing of long bones and scoliosis. Child abuse should be considered in the differential diagnosis, and the absence of pelvic deformities or wormian cranial bones in children who are subjected to abuse may be helpful.

Using aids to mobility and preventive bracing can be very helpful in preventing fractures. Occasionally, intramedullary rods that elongate with growth are needed. Fortunately, the frequency of fractures diminishes with age.

TUMORS

A complete discussion of musculoskeletal tumors is beyond the scope of this section (see Chapter 311, Malignant Bone Tumors); instead, an attempt is made to describe an appropriate differential diagnosis and evaluation.

Benign or malignant musculoskeletal tumors can be classified according to their tissue of origin (Table 432.3). The history and physical examination rarely are definitive. Many tumors become evident after trauma, when a new prominence is noted, or when pathologic fracture occurs through weakened bone. For example, osteoid osteoma, a benign condition, frequently produces pain that is relieved by nonsteroidal antiinflammatory agents. Very early sarcoma may be painless. Unexpected presentations may occur, such as Ewing sarcoma, various types of histiocytoses, and leukemia, each of which may present with fever and malaise.

Some idea of the benign or malignant nature of a tumor can be gained from the following principles used in interpreting radiographic features. Lesions associated with rapid spread and lack of local containment should heighten the suspicion of malignancy. A vague zone of transition between the lesion and normal bone is worrisome, as is a soft tissue mass in the presence of a bone tumor. Periosteal lamellar change is a response to trauma or spread outside the cortex and may occur with benign or malignant tumors or with infection. Rapid growth is suggested when periosteal lamellation is extensive and no formation of definite new cortex occurs. Thinning of the cortex itself is not pathognomonic of malignancy; this condition occurs also with fibrous cortical defects and unicameral cysts. Internal stippling suggests calcification of a cartilage matrix; usually, fluffy opacification represents new bone formation, as in osteosarcoma. Usually, lesions crossing the epiphyseal plate are infections or malignant tumors. Leukemia presents with musculoskeletal complaints 20% of the time, and radiographic findings include osteopenia, sclerotic or lytic lesions, lucent metaphyseal bands, or periosteal new bone.

Certain general radiographic studies can be helpful. Radiographic studies must be tailored to the differential diagnosis. CT may show internal consistency, soft tissue spread, and extent of the lesion. Technetium^{Tc99m} bone scans reveal lesions in the remainder of the skeleton, bony involvement with soft tissue lesions, and bone turnover or activity of questionable lesions. MRI, magnetic resonance angiography (MRA), or angiograms may be helpful to determine whether the tumor involves a vascular bundle. MRI is also invaluable in assessing soft tissue involvement.

The location of a lesion is meaningful, and a diagram of the location of common bone lesions is presented in Figure 432.37. Generally, laboratory studies are not specific; the sedimentation rate and complete blood count are abnormal in several of the aforementioned tumors, and the alkaline phosphatase level often is elevated in patients with osteogenic sarcoma.

The treatment of musculoskeletal tumors defies simplification. The most important generalization is that any patient requiring surgery should be under the care of a surgeon who has had experience in this area. Errors related to biopsy placement or specimen adequacy are three to five times more frequent in centers where the surgeons do not specialize in tumor treatment.

TABLE 432.3

MUSCULOSKELETAL NEOPLASMS

Origin	Benign	Malignant
Cartilage	Chondroblastoma Enchondroma Chondromyxoid fibroma Osteochondroma	Chondrosarcoma*
Bone	Osteoid osteoma Osteoblastoma	Osteosarcoma
Marrow elements	Lipoma	Ewing sarcoma Reticulum cell sarcoma Liposarcoma* Plasma cell myeloma
Fibrous connective tissue	Desmoplastic fibroma	Fibrosarcoma
Skeletal muscle	Fibrous cortical defect	Rhabdomyosarcoma
Neurogenous tissue	Neurilemma Neurofibroma	Neuroblastoma
Unclear	Giant cell tumor*	Adamantinoma

*Rarely occurs in children.

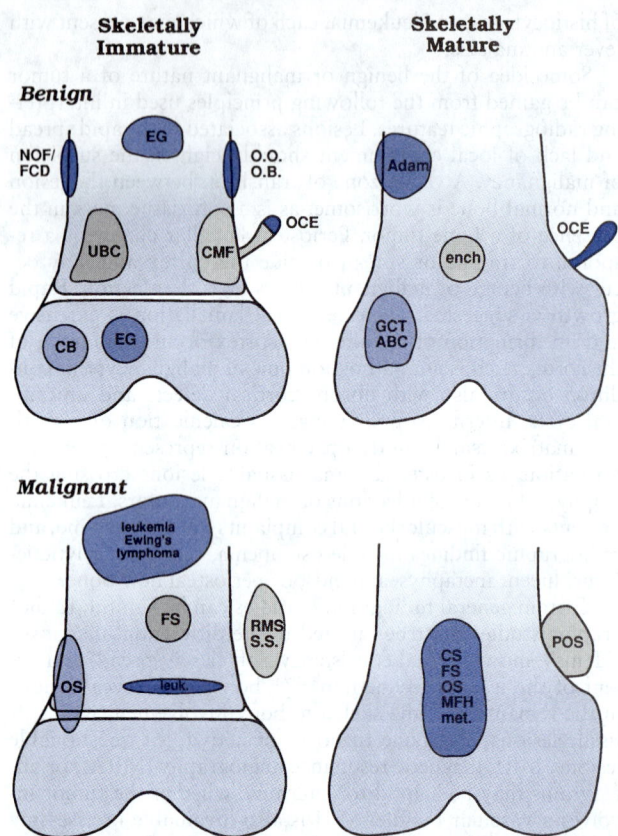

FIGURE 432.37. Location of tumors in immature and mature skeletons. Adam, adamantinoma; ABC, aneurysmal bone cyst; CB, chondroblastoma; CMF, chondromyxoid fibroma; CS, chondrosarcoma; EG, eosinophilic granuloma; ench, enchondroma; FCD, fibrous cortical defect; FS, fibrosarcoma; GCT, giant cell tumor; leuk., leukemia; met., metastasis; MFH, malignant fibrous histiocytoma; NOF, nonossifying fibroma; O.B., osteoblastoma; OCE, osteocartilaginous exostosis; OO, osteoid osteoma; OS, osteogenic sarcoma; P, parosteal; RMS, rhabdomyosarcoma; SS, synovial sarcoma; UBC, unicameral bone cyst.

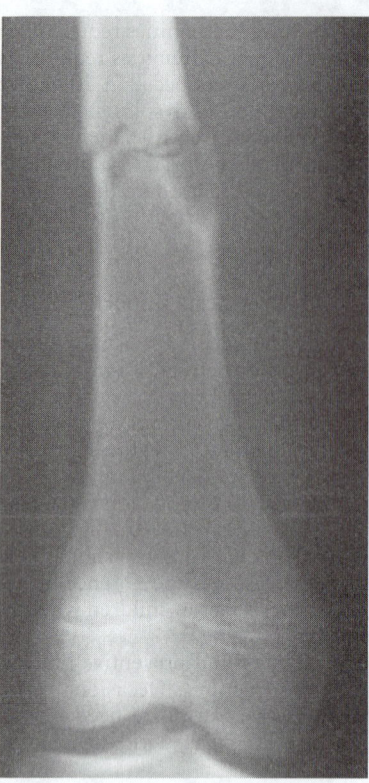

FIGURE 432.38. Fibrous cortical defects with pathologic fracture. Note two lesions on the medial side, within one wall of the cortex and expanding it.

Benign Bone Tumors

Two common, benign bone tumors deserve brief mention. A unicameral bone cyst is a smooth, well-marginated lucency that is located fairly centrally in the metaphysis of children between ages 2 and 15 (Fig. 432.38). The proximal humerus is the most common location, followed by the proximal femur. Usually, it is not recognized until a fracture occurs through the cyst. The fracture should be allowed to heal, and the lesion can be observed if it is small and is located in a bone that does not bear weight; otherwise, it can be injected with steroids or bone-inducing substance. The latter two treatments produce results equal to or better than open bone grafting. The natural history of this defect is spontaneous regression during late adolescence.

Fibrous cortical defects are well-marginated lucencies located in (and occasionally slightly expanding) the cortex. Usually, one radiographic view can show that these lesions are not central in bone (Fig. 432.39). They are present in as many as one-third of all young children at some time and disappear with age. In a weight-bearing bone, the risk of fracture is appreciable if the lesion is greater than approximately 3 cm in length and more than one-half the width of the bone. Lesions this large should be protected by limiting activities if possible or by performing bone grafting.

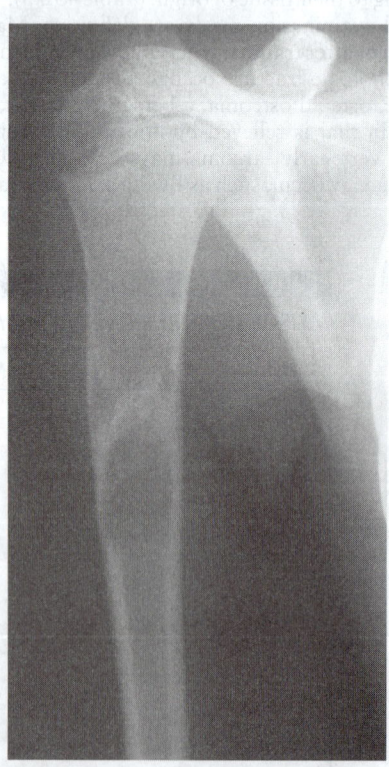

FIGURE 432.39. Unicameral bone cyst in the proximal humerus of a 9-year-old. Often, it is located closer to the growth plate.

NEUROMUSCULAR DISORDERS

Cerebral Palsy

Cerebral palsy is a collective term for a group of nonprogressive afflictions of the upper central nervous system. Two types of musculoskeletal problems result: disorders of control, for which little can be done, and bone and joint deformities resulting from continued muscle imbalance, which can be treated. Modifying the athetoid features that predominate in a few children is difficult, except with supportive bracing, but the more common spastic features are more amenable to modification. Discussion of such patients always should include identification of current functional problems and goals. Gait, if present, may be marked by a crouched position as a result of knee or hip flexion contractures. The ankle may tend toward plantar flexion or dorsiflexion.

Trial bracing or gait studies may help to determine the primary problem. Often, ankle plantar flexion can be controlled with bracing if the foot can be brought up to a right angle with the tibia when the knee is extended. If this is not possible, the tight heel cord should be lengthened; tight hamstring and hip flexors also may be lengthened when indicated. The "scissoring" of the legs seen with walking or lying down may be caused by tight adductor muscles.

Hip dislocation occurs with increasing frequency as the severity of disease involvement increases. It is the result of imbalance between the strong adductors and flexors and the weak abductors and extensors. The imbalance is acquired, rather than congenital, and usually occurs after affected patients reach several years of age. It should be checked every 6 to 12 months in diplegic or quadriplegic patients. Affected children are at risk for progressive hip subluxation if abduction is less than 30 degrees with the hip extended. Dislocation and subluxation cause difficulty with perineal care, balanced sitting, degenerative joint disease, pain, and increased spasm. Consequently, they should be prevented. Even in patients with severe involvement, dislocations and subluxations can be prevented through early muscle release or later osteotomy.

Scoliosis also is encountered more frequently with increasing severity of cerebral palsy. It is present in as many as 69% of severely affected children because of persistent primitive reflexes, an inclined pelvis, or asymmetric muscle tone. A brace may be prescribed if affected children have difficulty in sitting, but it is less effective in preventing worsening of the curve than it is in idiopathic scoliosis. Surgery may be necessary.

The upper extremity may be flexed at the elbow, wrist, and fingers. The decision to correct this condition is based on patients' intelligence, ability to control the hand voluntarily, and degree of sensation. The thumb may be clenched, and early bracing may be helpful, with surgery performed later if the digit has potential for use.

The benefits of physical therapy in general for children with cerebral palsy are debated. Positioning and hand and heel-cord stretching may produce increased range of motion. However, the severity of involvement probably is more important than is therapy in determining patients' ability to walk.

Myelodysplasia

Myelodysplasia or spinal dysraphism (spina bifida) involves a malformation of the neural tube, with paralysis below a certain thoracic or lumbar level of innervation. Usually, the functioning muscles allow more control than is possible in cerebral palsy patients. The goal of orthopedic treatment is optimizing mobility and socialization, which does not always mean enabling the patient to walk. The quadriceps are the most important muscles for mobility. Severely affected children with poor intelligence and weak quadriceps muscles are unable to walk and are more mobile in wheelchairs. In some cases, joint deformities are treated by surgical release and bracing. In contrast to cerebral palsy, usually hip dislocations are not painful and should not be reduced unless they are unilateral or affected children have good quadriceps muscles. Scoliosis also may occur, especially with higher-level spinal defects. One of the most important roles of the primary physician is to observe affected children for loss of lower extremity muscle power as they grow. As these children grow, this loss may be caused by tethering of the cord distally or by a disturbance of cerebrospinal fluid pressure.

INFECTIONS

Hematogenous Osteomyelitis

The incidence and presentation of hematogenous osteomyelitis is changing after the introduction of newer imaging and treatment methods, but certain principles remain constant. The summary presented here should be coupled with that provided in Chapter 73, Osteomyelitis and Septic Arthritis, to illustrate the spectrum of treatment philosophies.

By definition, acute hematogenous osteomyelitis includes processes that have been operating for a week or less at the time of diagnosis. After infancy, this condition occurs more frequently in boys than in girls, presumably because trauma plays a role in increasing susceptibility. The peak ages of occurrence are infancy (younger than 1 year) and preadolescence (9 to 11 years). The incidence declines in adulthood because of the change in the vascular supply of bone. The sites affected most commonly are the femur and tibia, each of which accounts for one-third of all cases, followed by the humerus, calcaneus, and pelvis. Any bone may be affected, however. The metaphysis is the region involved most often, and spread may occur from this point to involve any other portion. Rarely, the process may begin in the epiphysis.

The pathophysiology of acute hematogenous osteomyelitis explains some features of this disease. The metaphyseal vascular channels form loops near the growth plate. Blood flow is slowed, and the capillary basement membrane and reticuloendothelial system are deficient in these regions. Experimental bacteremias have been shown to produce foci of infection only in these areas. Trauma likely plays more than a circumstantial role, because experimentally traumatized areas are more susceptible to the development of osteomyelitis. Only approximately one-fourth of all cases have a demonstrable source, such as cutaneous, aural, or respiratory seeding. Direct traumatic inoculation is a different disease process.

After a focus of infection is initiated, local inflammation is followed by spread up and down the medullary canal. The growth plate in children has no bridging vessels after infancy and acts as a barrier to spread in most cases. The germinal cells are on the epiphyseal side and, therefore, are spared. In the first year of life, however, the transphyseal vessels that exist allow spread to proceed up to the epiphysis and into the joint. These facts have two implications. First, growth-plate damage is more likely during the first year of life. Second, in children of this age, septic arthritis may follow osteomyelitis in any metaphyseal location, whereas in older children without transphyseal vessels, it occurs only in locations where the joint capsule extends over the growth plate (i.e., the shoulder, elbow, and hip). At skeletal maturity, with growth-plate closure, this barrier again is eliminated, although hematogenous osteomyelitis is rare after this point. As intramedullary pressure

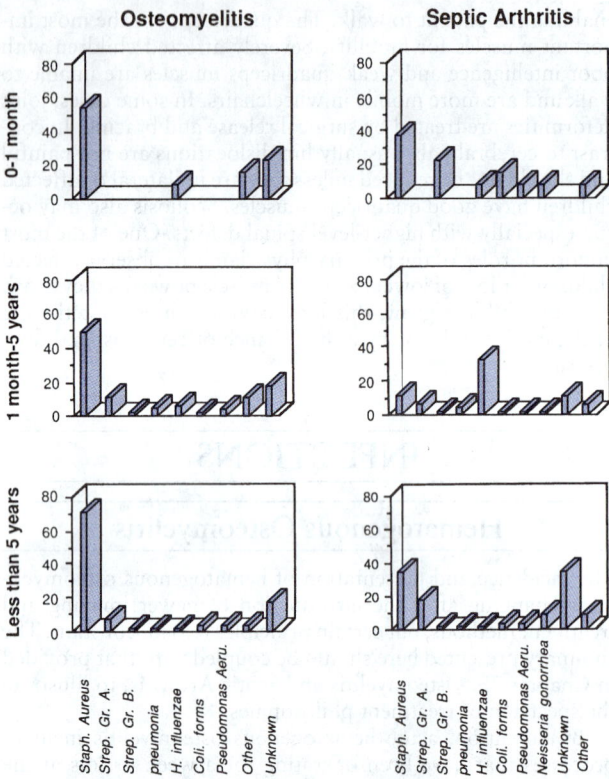

FIGURE 432.40. Frequency of occurrence of organisms involved in acute hematogenous osteomyelitis and septic arthritis in three age groups. (Drawn with permission from table from Jackson MA. Management of the bone and joint infections. *Pediatr Orthop* 1982;2:315.)

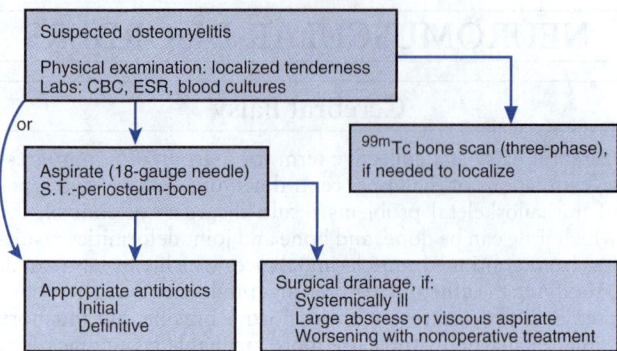

FIGURE 432.41. Diagnosis and treatment algorithm for hematogenous osteomyelitis. Complete blood count, CBC; ESR, erythrocyte sedimentation rate; ST, soft tissue.

increases, pus dissects through the haversian system, elevating the periosteum and producing a subperiosteal, then soft tissue, abscess. The elevated periosteum may be radiographically apparent within 1 to 2 weeks.

Unlike septic arthritis, the organisms involved in hematogenous osteomyelitis vary little with the age of affected patients (Fig. 432.40). In all age groups, the predominant organism is *S. aureus*, although *Streptococcus pneumoniae* and *Haemophilus* species must be considered. *S. aureus* infection is associated with a higher recurrence rate than other organisms. *Salmonella* should be considered in patients with sickle cell anemia, although in some studies, *S. aureus* infection still is more common in these patients. *Streptococcus pyogenes* should be considered in patients with or recovering from varicella. Blood culture results during the acute phase are positive approximately 40% to 50% of the time, and direct cultures of pus or bone are positive only 60% to 80% of the time, which may be the result of prior antibiotic use, errors in sampling or processing, or autoeradication of the organism.

Clinical diagnosis remains key, despite the availability of new imaging techniques. Affected children may appear well or may have systemic involvement ranging from malaise to shock. Often, refusal to bear weight is an early symptom. The very earliest sign is fever and local bone tenderness, followed later by a fluctuant mass if a subperiosteal or soft tissue abscess has developed. Spread to adjacent joints should be ruled out by palpation and range of motion evaluation. Usually, passive motion of the extremity is not resisted significantly unless a soft tissue abscess or joint involvement is present. Increased suspicion should be aroused with neonates, who more often are afebrile and first may be noted to have a swollen or motionless limb. Vertebral or pelvic osteomyelitis may present as abdominal pain and can resemble the more common septic arthritis of the hip.

The differential diagnosis primarily includes neoplasm, contusion, nondisplaced fracture, and sickle cell crisis. Elevated WBC counts and sedimentation rates are helpful but not diagnostic. Radiography at the earliest stage may show soft tissue swelling. Osteopenia or lysis may appear after 7 to 10 days, followed by new bone formation at the borders of the process. MRI is able to demonstrate early changes and anatomic detail, if the site of the process can be localized. For regions such as the axial skeleton, in which localization may be difficult, bone scanning has been used widely in the last two decades, but the subtleties of its use have been recognized only recently. The tracer used most widely is technetium Tc^{99m} methylene diphosphonate because of its speed, cost, and sensitivity (Fig. 432.41). Immediate scans for flow and blood pool should be obtained, as should later skeletal images. Results of the scan may be normal in the very early stages, but the procedure should be repeated after 48 hours if clinically indicated.

Cold or photopenic areas are important because they may indicate avascular sites, especially when they are accompanied by adjacent areas of increased uptake. Cellulitis may cause confusion, but usually does not show bony localization on delayed images. The overall accuracy of nuclear imaging is approximately 60% to 90%. It may be much lower in neonates, however, according to some reports. Gallium citrate may be sensitive, but results are not available for a minimum of 24 hours; indium-labeled WBC studies require similar amounts of time, including preparation of the tracer. Because of the aforementioned limitations, radionuclide scans are not reliable in some instances, especially when the clinical diagnosis is clear. These studies have their greatest value when localization in preparation for aspiration is difficult.

Aspiration is indicated when it is necessary to identify the pathogen and, in some cases, to decompress localized purulence. It should be performed with a large-diameter needle. The anesthetic may be local, intravenous, or general, as indicated. In sequence, the extraosseous soft tissues, periosteum, and (if necessary) intramedullary canal should be assessed for purulent localization. Fluoroscopy or ultrasound may be useful in deep lesions if radiographic changes are evident. Experiments in animals have shown that aspiration of bone alone does not cause a bone scan result to become positive.

Treatment involves the delivery of an appropriate antibiotic to all infected tissue. Therefore, avascular abscesses may require surgical decompression if aspiration cannot accomplish drainage. Antibiotic therapy can be divided into initial and definitive periods. In the initial phase, broad-spectrum antibiotics, including such antistaphylococcal agents as nafcillin or oxacillin (150 to 200 mg/kg/day), are indicated. Vancomycin should be used if resistance is suspected. In neonates, an aminoglycoside should be added because of the possibility of gram-negative infection. In children who are younger than 3 years and have not been vaccinated, ceftriaxone may be used to cover *Haemophilus influenzae*. During the definitive period, the most effective, least toxic antibiotic effective against the isolated organism should be given for 4 to 6 weeks. It may be administered by the oral route if affected patients are clinically improved and compliant and if adequate blood levels can be documented.

Surgery is reserved for cases in which affected children are systemically ill or worsening under medical treatment or in which an abscess has been demonstrated. An abscess or avascular tissue should be removed to allow antibiotic penetration, and usually the wound is closed over a drain. Complications include recurrence (5% overall), minor growth acceleration, growth-plate damage, and fracture through weakened bone.

Subacute Osteomyelitis

Subacute osteomyelitis is a more subtle condition. No systemic signs may be evident and, in Roberts' series, fewer than one-fifth of all patients had a fever, an elevated WBC count, or a positive blood count result. Abnormal radiographic and bone scan results, however, were more common than in the acute form. Treatment follows the principles discussed. Chronic osteomyelitis is seen almost exclusively in patients who did not have access to proper antibiotic treatment initially or who have an underlying disorder (such as sickle cell anemia), or in those areas of the body with impaired perfusion, such as traumatized extremities. In these cases, surgical debridement of devitalized and infected bone, as well as long-term antibiotics, is necessary.

Chronic Recurrent Multifocal Osteomyelitis

Chronic recurrent multifocal osteomyelitis is a rare syndrome involving low-grade systemic manifestations that are ongoing for several years, with reports of up to 12 areas of lytic-sclerotic juxtaepiphyseal involvement. No organism has been isolated, and treatment is supportive.

Fungal Osteomyelitis

Fungal osteomyelitis may be disseminated (sporotrichosis, candidiasis) or direct (eumycetoma). Aggressive débridement in these conditions is more important than that in bacterial infections.

Puncture Wounds

Puncture wounds to the foot are significant in that they may involve *Pseudomonas* infection, which occurs with colonization of a sock or a sneaker by this organism. The wound should be inspected, and foreign material should be removed. If the bone or joint is contaminated, débridement and antibiotic therapy for recovered organisms should be begun. Otherwise, affected patients should be instructed to return if symptoms of infection occur.

Septic Arthritis

Slightly more common than hematogenous osteomyelitis, septic arthritis may have more disastrous long-term consequences if effective treatment is delayed. Most cases occur in infants and younger children, with nearly one-half of all affected patients being younger than 3 years of age. A high index of suspicion for septic arthritis should be maintained in sick neonatal patients, because they show few signs. The hip joint is involved most commonly in infants, as compared to the knee in older children. The spread may be from the bloodstream or from an adjacent osteomyelitis, especially in the hip and shoulder, where the capsular insertion extends over the growth plate onto the metaphysis. Many theories, including alteration of joint fluid by toxins from both the neutrophils and the bacteria, have been advanced to explain the pathogenesis of joint destruction.

The spectrum of causative organisms in septic arthritis is somewhat broader than in that of hematogenous osteomyelitis (see Fig. 432.40), which may be related to the greater frequency of this condition. Overall, *S. aureus* remains the most common causative organism. In patients between ages 1 month and 5 years, however, *H. influenzae* also is common. The use of the vaccine against this organism appears to have reduced, although not eliminated, this organism as a cause of septic arthritis in the toddler. The streptococci, *Kingella kingii*; *Escherichia coli*, *Proteus*, and other organisms also should be considered. The yield of organisms from aspiration is approximately 60% to 80%.

Clinical findings vary with the age of affected patients. In infants, fever, failure to feed, and tachycardia may be present. Subtle changes in position, unilateral swelling of an extremity or a joint, asymmetry of soft-tissue folds, and pain with range of motion may serve as clues. In older children, the signs are more localized.

Aspiration with a large needle should be performed if any reasonable suspicion of septic arthritis exists, both for diagnosis and, in some cases, for treatment. In such deep joints as the hip, ultrasound or the injection of radio-opaque dye should be used to confirm the position of the needle, especially if the aspirated fluid is normal. This ensures that joint fluid actually was obtained, and it also helps to distinguish joint infection from septic involvement of the bursa underneath the nearby psoas muscle. Usually, the WBC count in fluid obtained from patients with septic arthritis ranges from 50,000 to 250,000, with 95% polymorphonuclear leukocytes. Elevated lactate levels may be helpful in cases in which WBC counts are borderline.

The differential diagnosis includes toxic synovitis of the hip, in which pain, fever, leukocytosis, and spasm are more moderate and do not escalate on serial observations. Clinical research has shown that the most useful parameters to distinguish septic arthritis from synovitis are refusal to bear weight, temperature greater than 38.5°C, white blood count over 12,000, and erythrocyte sedimentation rate greater than 40 mm/hour. If all four features are present, septic arthritis is 99% likely. However, at times, the two conditions are indistinguishable, and in such situations, aspiration should be performed. Lyme arthritis, rheumatoid arthritis, cellulitis, traumatic synovitis, and the migratory multiple arthralgias of rheumatic fever should be considered. A sympathetic effusion also may occur from adjacent osteomyelitis.

The role of arthrotomy versus aspiration in confirmed cases of septic arthritis is controversial. The key feature is the removal of deleterious enzymes and the restoration of effective synovial perfusion. Because the decision not to operate requires the ability to monitor and aspirate repeatedly as needed, the use of arthrotomy probably is preferable in deep joints that are difficult to assess, such as the hip and shoulder; in young patients in whom examination is difficult; and when the fluid obtained is viscous or has a very high WBC count. In septic arthritis of the hip, arthrotomy is mandatory to prevent vascular compromise and ensure prompt resolution.

The surgical procedure should include irrigation, drainage, and closure, which may be performed arthroscopically in the knee, shoulder, and ankle. The direct instillation of antibiotics has no benefit. Some investigators feel that the femoral metaphysis should be drilled whenever the hip is aspirated, to decompress any possible femoral osteomyelitis.

Early, effective treatment is very important. The chance of achieving good results declines dramatically if treatment is initiated after the symptoms have been present for 4 days. Antibiotics should be continued for 4 to 6 weeks. Whether the joint should be immobilized or treated with continuous passive motion is controversial; however, the latter modality is practiced less commonly. Contractures should be prevented, and abduction of the hip decreases the likelihood of dislocation. Complications include permanent destruction of cartilage and, in the hip, avascular necrosis with resorption or overgrowth of the femoral head. Complications are more frequent in young infants.

Gonococcal arthritis also occurs in children. Usually, it becomes evident after the systemic and febrile phase of the illness and should be distinguished from the more common gonococcal migratory multiple arthralgia or tenosynovitis. An average of two to three joints, most commonly the wrists and knees, are affected. Treatment is aspiration and closed irrigation followed by 3 days of intravenous antibiotic (usually ceftriaxone) and 4 days of oral therapy (a fluoroquinolone). Oral treatment alone with one of these drugs for 7 days is acceptable in compliant patients after a loading dose has been given.

INJURIES

A comprehensive discussion of musculoskeletal trauma is beyond the scope of this chapter. The reader is referred to the works by Rockwood and by Rang for further information. The basic principles of injury evaluation and common injuries and emergencies are discussed here.

Children's bones differ from those of adults both biomechanically and physiologically. Mechanically, immature bone is more porous, and the pores serve to limit crack propagation. Instead of complete fractures, children often have involvement of only part of the cortex, such as in a buckle fracture from compression or a greenstick fracture from tension. The most extreme example is plastic deformation of bone without fracture. This deformity should be corrected if it is 20 degrees or greater.

Another biomechanical feature of children's skeletons is that the ligaments are stronger than is either the bone or the growth plate. Injuries that would produce dislocations or sprains in adults (e.g., elbow dislocation or medial collateral ligament tear of the knee, respectively) produce different patterns in children (i.e., supracondylar humeral fractures or femoral physeal separations, respectively; Fig. 432.42). Thus, the presence of nondisplaced fractures and separations should be sought on physical examination and radiography in children. Coned and oblique films may be helpful. In the knee, gentle stress radiography may show a nondisplaced separation, which should be immobilized.

Physiologic differences include union rates, remodeling, overgrowth, and growth-plate injuries. Nonunion is nearly nonexistent in children, occurring only in open fractures with extensive soft tissue loss and periosteal stripping. Bone union times range from 3 weeks in infants to 3 months in adolescents. Remodeling of angulation and displacement is an impressive tendency until the early teenage years. It occurs through alterations in physeal growth and through local periosteal resorption on the convex side and deposition on the concave side. It is most effective in the metaphysis, where angulation does not create as much deformity as in the midshaft.

Compensation for any residual deformity is much better if it is in the plane of joint motion. For example, posterior angulation of a distal femur fracture can be compensated by knee flexion, whereas the knee has no ability to compensate outward

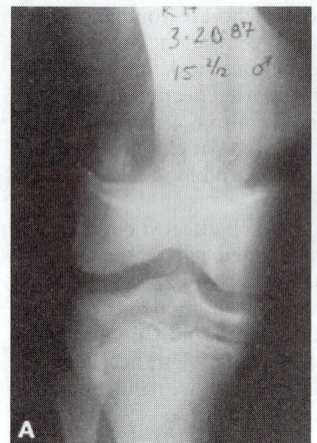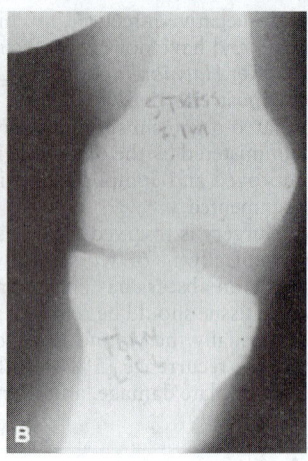

FIGURE 432.42. A valgus stress to the knee produces failure at the weakest spot. **A:** Growth plate in a child. **B:** The medial collateral ligament in an adult.

(varus) angulation at this site. In the upper extremity, overlap of fracture segments is acceptable as long as the angulation is not excessive.

Another physiologic feature of children's fractures is growth stimulation, which occurs because of hyperemia and continues for approximately 18 months after the fracture occurs. It is most significant in the femur, where it averages 1 cm, but occasionally it becomes significant in the tibia. In contrast, growth arrest may occur if the growth plate is crushed or crossed by the fracture. The Salter-Harris classification (Fig. 432.43) was developed to predict the risk for growth arrest. It is helpful also

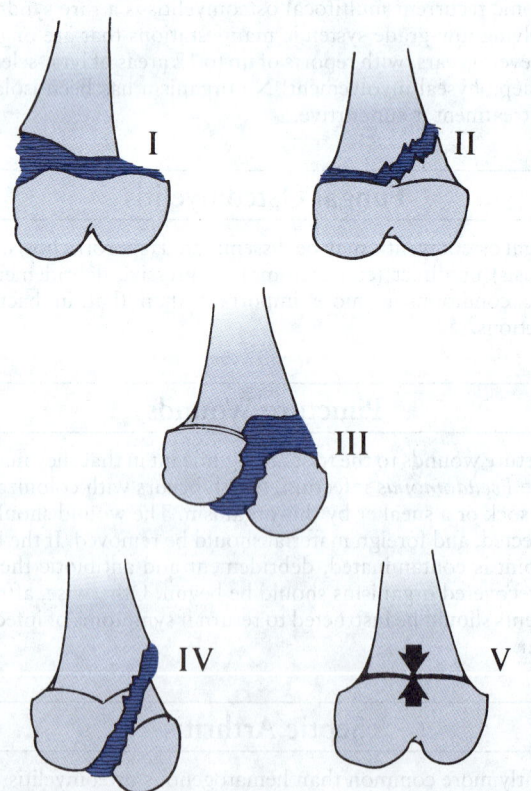

FIGURE 432.43. Salter-Harris classification of fractures involving the growth plate.

in communicating with consulting physicians. Because types I and II do not cross the germinal layers, the risk of growth-plate damage in these injuries is minimal. In types III and IV, the fracture crosses the plate, but anatomic reduction may diminish the risk of plate closure. In type V, the crushing cannot be reversed. Combinations of types may occur, especially with irregular growth plates. Such injuries should be observed carefully because, if a limited growth-plate bar forms, it can be resected to restore normal growth.

A basic evaluation of specific injuries should include three features: (a) assessment of the entire limb to rule out other fractures or dislocation above or below the joint; (b) assessment of neurovascular status, including sensation and motor function and pulses, capillary refill, and temperature (the possibility of compartment syndrome—tissue pressure greater than capillary perfusion pressure—should be considered in the forearm or leg); and (c) assessment of the site of injury. A surprising amount can be learned regarding skeletal structures (e.g., growth plates, ligaments) by palpating carefully in an attempt to identify the injured area. For example, lateral ankle swelling may be caused by fibular growth-plate injury, ligament sprain, or peroneal tendon subluxation, and all these conditions can be differentiated by palpation. Typically, ankle sprains have tenderness around the lateral ligaments of the ankle. A mild sprain has no bony tenderness, no laxity on forward pull of the foot, and no medial tenderness. Patients with mild ankle sprain may be treated with ice, elastic wrap, and range-of-motion exercises, as tolerated.

Hand Injuries

Injuries to the hand are common in children. Fractures of the phalangeal and metacarpal shafts can be splinted if they are minimally angled and stable, but rotational alignment should be checked by observing the fingernails with the fingers flexed and extended. They should be aligned similarly if no malrotation is present. "Buddy taping" helps to minimize malrotation. Growth-plate or epiphyseal fractures may be splinted if they are nondisplaced, but should be referred if they are displaced. Dorsally dislocated interphalangeal joints may be reduced and viewed radiographically to rule out fracture. If they are stable enough to allow active range of motion, they should be splinted for 3 weeks with an aluminum splint. Immobilization of the metacarpophalangeal joints should be in 50 to 90 degrees of flexion to minimize stiffness, and the interphalangeal joints should be in mild flexion of approximately 20 degrees.

One problematic injury is an avulsion of the base of the nail bed, often associated with open separation of the nearby phalangeal growth plate, which may become infected and stop growing. This condition should be distinguished from a Kirner deformity, which is a bilateral, idiopathic irregularity of the distal phalangeal growth plate.

Scaphoid Fractures

The scaphoid bone ossifies when a child is 6 years old. Scaphoid fractures may occur in children and develop nonunion if they are not recognized. They occur less often in children than in adults, however. Laceration of the palm and digits may sever a flexor tendon, and the active range of motion of each joint should be checked to ensure that this has not occurred.

Forearm Fractures

Forearm fractures are very common in children. Nondisplaced buckle fractures of one or both bones should be treated with a short arm cast for 3 or 4 weeks. Greenstick fractures represent tension or rotational failures with less intrinsic stability, and they should be held in a long arm cast for 6 weeks. Completion of the greenstick fracture is not necessary as long as angulation can be controlled. With any forearm fracture, the wrist and elbow joints should be checked, because dislocation may occur at one of these locations to compensate for fracture malalignment (Fig. 432.44A).

Clavicle Fractures

Usually, the clavicle fractures at the junction of the middle and distal thirds. Neurovascular damage to the underlying brachial plexus and subclavian vessels is rare, but should be considered. Usually, the periosteal sleeve is intact, and remodeling is excellent. Treatment consists of preventing movement with a sling for 4 weeks in children and 6 weeks in teenagers.

Knee Ligament Injuries

Knee ligament injuries are rare in children. Usually, femoral growth-plate separation occurs instead of collateral ligament damage. The tibial growth plate is protected, because the collateral ligaments insert distal to it. Any trauma resulting in a swollen knee in a growing child (i.e., ages 7 to 13 years) should be examined to rule out avulsion of the tibial intercondylar eminence, because this eminence represents the insertion of the anterior cruciate ligament and is a serious injury. It is seen best on the lateral view but may be pulled up and overlapped by the femoral condyles (Fig. 432.44B). Oblique views or positioning in extension may help.

Partial fractures of the medial proximal tibial metaphysis are notorious for later developing outward (valgus) angulation as a result of medial tibial growth-plate overactivity. Care should be taken to obtain good initial fracture alignment, and parents will accept this outward angulation better if they are forewarned that it may occur despite adequate care. Some of the angulation may decrease with time, but osteotomy may be performed near maturity if significant deformity persists (Fig. 432.44C, D). The ossification patterns of the elbow and wrist are complex. If a radiographic text is not available, comparison films of the contralateral side may clarify abnormalities (Fig. 432.44E).

Ankle Injuries

Several types of ankle injuries are common, with injuries of the distal fibula predominating. If a bone fragment is nondisplaced, diagnosis is made by palpating for tenderness at the growth plate, not by obtaining stress films. Three weeks in a short leg cast is the usual treatment; the intent is more to increase patient mobility than to decrease instability. On the tibial side, the anterolateral quadrant of the distal tibial physis is the last to close, and this area may be avulsed with rotation. It should be reduced if it is displaced.

Soft Tissue Injuries

Soft tissue trauma of the extremities may be encountered in the emergency department, and foreign penetration should be considered. Occasionally, palpation and radiography at soft tissue

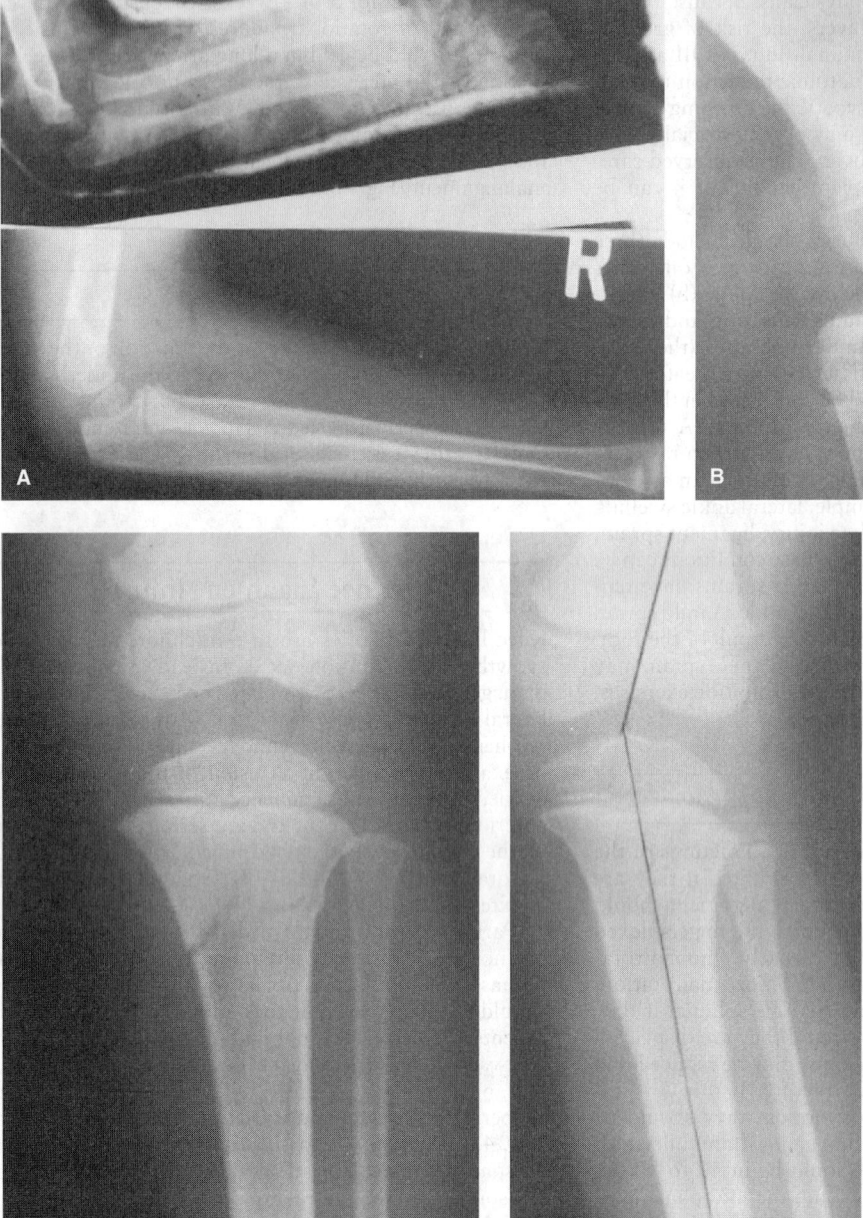

FIGURE 432.44. Avoiding five common pitfalls in evaluating musculoskeletal trauma. **A:** Always check the joint above and below a fracture. This Monteggia fracture of the ulna is reduced, but the radial head fracture was missed. The radial head should line up with the capitellum, as it does in the elbow on the right. **B:** In a child's swollen knee, check the lateral film for a tibial spine avulsion fracture. It may be obscured partially by the overlying femoral condyles. **C,D:** A proximal tibial fracture may result in valgus deformity even when initially reduced well. (Continued)

settings may help. Glass is seen only if it has a high lead content. Exploration for deeper foreign bodies may be very frustrating unless it is done surgically under adequate regional or general anesthesia. Contusions to areas with thick subcutaneous fat may produce permanent depression of the area secondary to fat necrosis; the families of affected children should be so counseled. Injuries involving large amounts of soft tissue loss might possibly be covered with a patient's skin, which can serve as a split-thickness graft, if it can be saved in cool storage.

Open Fractures, Dislocations, and Compartment Syndromes

Open fractures, dislocations, and compartment syndromes (the last in particular) should be treated as quickly as possible for best results. Open fractures allow bacteria to come in contact with damaged tissue, which is an ideal culture medium. They should be irrigated down to bone within 6 hours to decrease

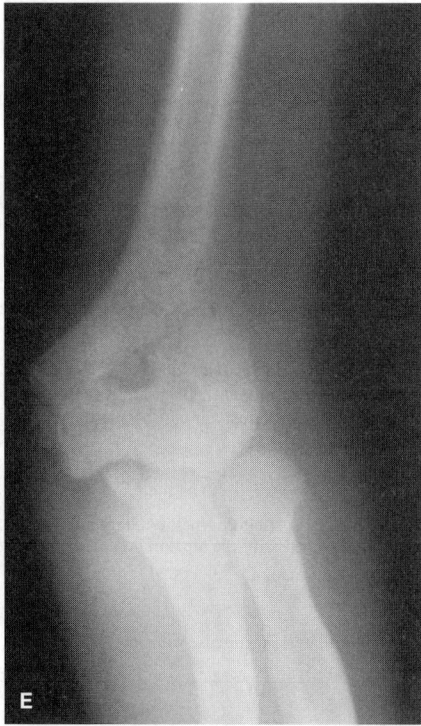
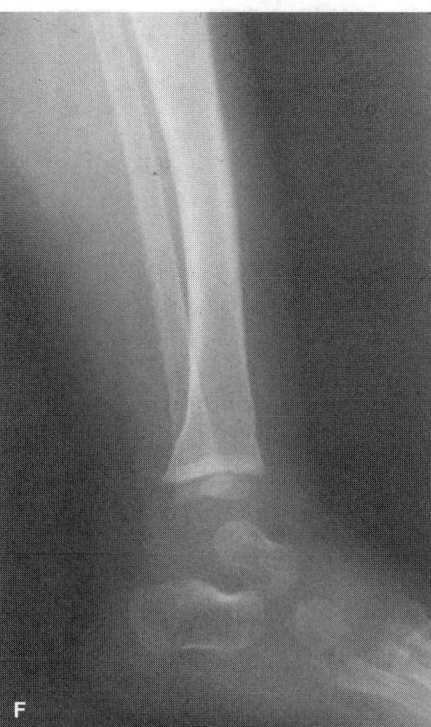

FIGURE 432.44. (Continued). **E:** Obtain comparison views when uncertain. This round ossicle in the medial joint space appears to belong there and was missed by an orthopedist, but actually, it represents the medial epicondyle trapped inside the joint. **F:** Note distal tibial irregularity just above joint. Careful examination of plain radiographs will sometimes reveal a toddler's fracture (buckle fracture) to be cause of a child's limp.

the rate of infection and, if extensive, should be left open for several days for drainage and further débridement unless they are small and clean.

Dislocations of almost all major joints constitute emergencies because nerves and vessels are stretched, and further swelling can add to the problem. The ulnar, median, and radial nerves and the brachial artery are involved at the elbow, the sciatic nerve is involved at the hip, and the popliteal artery is involved at the knee. Fractures that occur near these areas have similar implications.

Compartment syndromes have been recognized increasingly in the last two decades. Such syndromes occur when injury increases the tissue pressure within a closed fascial compartment, such as the forearm, or leg, above the capillary perfusion pressure (usually 30 to 45 mm Hg), resulting in ischemia and swelling. The earliest sign is excessive pain on passive stretch of the involved muscles within the compartment, followed by sensory loss and paresthesias of the involved nerves, and weakness of the muscle. Loss of pulses is a very late sign, and it indicates that pressure has risen above large arteriolar systolic pressure. Confirmation is obtained by measurement of the pressures using an electronic apparatus. Treatment involves emergent release of the tight fascia, with later skin closure when swelling resolves (if possible) or skin grafting (if not possible).

Fractures with Malposition

Fractures with malposition may have to be stabilized so that an affected child can be transported to a consultant. Materials used for this purpose may be improvised, or plaster splints over soft wadding may be used. In general, fractures should be splinted in the position in which they present, with the exception of femur fractures, which can be placed in longitudinal traction with a splint.

Muscle Contusions

Muscle contusions occur most frequently in the quadriceps, upper arm, or shoulder muscles. They may be intensely painful. Compartment syndromes are rare in these regions. Treatment consists of limitation of hemorrhage by rest, ice packing, and elastic bandage wrapping. Active range of motion should be instituted in 1 to 3 days, but passive range of motion (i.e., stretching) should be avoided because it may cause further damage. Strength rehabilitation is instituted after motion is regained. Myositis ossificans (i.e., intramuscular calcification and ossification) may follow this injury but usually does not limit function.

Child Abuse

Approximately 1% of all children in the United States are abused. Most victims are younger than 3 years of age. In children younger than 1 year, fracture often may be nonaccidental. One-third of victims are reinjured if the initial diagnosis is missed. Fractures occur in approximately one-third to one-half of all abused children. The most common sites include the long bones, skull, and ribs. Most fractures that are specific for abuse are those of the metaphysis near the growth plate, the posterior ribs, the scapula, or the sternum. No radiographic signs are completely diagnostic of abuse. The use of radiographs to look for inconsistency compared to the history of the mechanism of injury and to guide the investigation into the mechanism of fracture is helpful. Although long-bone fractures may occur from a spontaneous fall out of bed or from a counter, this is a rare mechanism for such injuries. Obtaining an idea of the "age" of a fracture by radiography also is useful. Periosteal new bone forms 6 to 10 days after a fracture in infants. At 10 to 14 days, blurring of the fracture lines and soft, mobile (poorly defined) callus is present. Hard callus occurs at 14 to

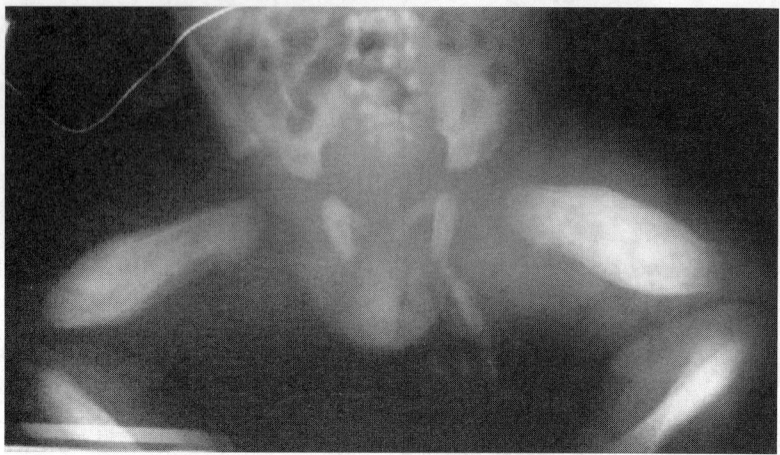

FIGURE 432.45. Caffey's disease (infantile cortical hyperostosis) may present with periosteal reaction in multiple bones simultaneously. It can be confused with nonaccidental injury.

21 days. The differential diagnosis includes osteogenesis imperfecta, Caffey disease (Fig. 432.45), syphilis, scurvy, rickets, leukemia, and congenital insensitivity to pain.

If abuse is suspected, reporting is mandatory, and the reporter is protected by law. The initial search for other fractures should be done by skeletal survey (AP and lateral views of the skull and spine, an AP view of the extremities), with bone scanning in selected cases. Usually, admission to the hospital is the best means of protecting affected children and further evaluating the family. Keeping careful records and being willing to advocate for such children may be the most important contributions physicians can make.

Suggested Readings

General

Flynn JM, Widmann RF: The limping child: evaluation and diagnosis. *J Am Acad Orthop Surg* 2001;9:89.

Lincoln TL, Suen PW. Common rotational variations in children. *J Am Acad Orthop Surg* 2003;312.

Morrissy RT, Weinstein SL. *Lovell and Winter's pediatric orthopaedics*, vol. 2, 5th ed. Philadelphia: Lippincott, 2001.

Rang M. *Children's fractures*. Philadelphia: Lippincott, 1983.

Rockwood CA, Wilkins KE, King RE, et al. *Fractures in children*. Philadelphia: Lippincott, 1997.

Sponseller PD, Multhopp-Stephens H. *Handbook of pediatric orthopaedics*. Boston: Little, Brown, and Company, 1996.

Staheli LT. *Fundamentals of pediatric orthopaedics*, 3rd ed. Philadelphia: Lippincott Williams and Wilkins, 2003.

Brachial Plexus Birth Injuries

Geutjens G, Gilbert A, Helsen K. Obstetrical brachial plexus palsy associated with breech delivery: a different pattern of injury. *J Bone Joint Surg Br* 1996;78:303.

Laurent JP, Lee RT. Birth-related upper brachial plexus injuries in infants: operative and nonoperative approaches. *J Child Neurol* 1994;9:109.

Waters PM. Comparison of natural history, outcome of microsurgical repair, and operative reconstruction in brachial plexus birth palsy. *J Bone Joint Surg* 1999;81:649.

Clubfoot

Roye DP, Roye BD. Idiopathic congenital talipes equinovarus. *J Am Acad Orthop Surg* 2002;10:239.

Congenital Dislocation or Developmental Dysplasia of the Hip

Aronsson DD, Goldberg MJ, Kling TR, Roy DR. Developmental dysplasia of the hip. *Pediatrics* 1994;94:201.

Darmonov AV, Zagoa S. Clinical screening for congenital dislocation of the hip. *J Bone Joint Surg* 1996;78A:383.

Harcke HT, Kumar SJ. Role of ultrasound in diagnosis and management of congenital dislocation and dysplasia of the hip. Current concepts. *J Bone Joint Surg* 1991;73A:622.

Mubarak S. Pitfalls in use of Pavlik harness for treatment of congenital dysplasia, subluxation and dislocation of the hip. *J Bone Joint Surg* 1981;63A:1239.

Rosendahl K, Markestad T, Lie RT, et al. Cost-effectiveness of alternative screening strategies for developmental dysplasia of the hip. *Arch Pediatr Adolesc Med* 1995;149:643.

Discoid Meniscus

Dickhaut SC, DeLee JC. The discoid lateral meniscus syndrome. *J Bone Joint Surg* 1982;64A:1068.

Fibrous Dysplasia

Harris WH, Dudley R, Barry RJ. The natural history of fibrous dysplasia. *J Bone Joint Surg* 1962;44A:207.

Flatfoot

Staheli LT. Shoes for children [review]. *Pediatrics* 1991;88:371.

Genu Varum, Tibia Vara, Genu Valgum

Feldman MD, Schoenecker PL. Use of the metaphyseal-diaphyseal angle in the evaluation of bowed legs. *J Bone Joint Surg* 1993;75A:1602.

Salenius P, Vankka E. The development of the tibiofemoral angle in children. *J Bone Joint Surg* 1975;57A:259.

Injuries

McMahon P, Grossman W, Gaffney M, et al. Soft-tissue injury as an indication of child abuse. *J Bone Joint Surg Am* 1995;77:1179.

Merrell GA, Driscoll JC, Degutis LC, Renshaw TS. Prevention of childhood pedestrian trauma: a study of interventions over six years. *J Bone Joint Surg* 2002;84:863.

Schwned RM, Werth C, Johnston A. Femur shaft fractures in children: rarely from child abuse. *J Pediatr Orthop* 2000;20:475.

Wissow LS. Child abuse and neglect. *N Engl J Med* 1995;332:1425.

Legg-Calvé-Perthes Disease

Glueck CJ, Crawford A, Roy D, et al. Association of antithrombotic factor deficiencies and hypofibrinolysis with Legg-Perthes disease. *J Bone Joint Surg* 1996;78A:3.

Herring JA. The treatment of Legg-Calvé-Perthes disease. A critical review of the literature. *J Bone Joint Surg* 1994;76A:448.

Metatarsus Varus

Churgay CA. Diagnosis and treatment of pediatric foot deformities. *Am Fam Physician* 1993;47:883.

Farsetti P, Weinstein SL, Ponseti IV. Long-term functional and radiographic outcomes of untreated and nonoperatively treated metatarsus adductus. *J Bone Joint Surg* 1994;76:257.

Widhe T. Foot deformities at birth: A natural history study over a 16 year period. *J Pediatr Orthop* 1997;17:20.

Musculoskeletal Tumors

Rogalsky RJ, Black GB, Reed MH. Orthopaedic manifestations of leukemia in children. *J Bone Joint Surg* 1986;68A:494.

Disorders

Dormans JP, Pellegrino L. *Caring for children with cerebral palsy: a team approach*. Baltimore: Brooks Publishing, 1998.

Sarwark JF, Lubicky JP. *Caring for the child with spina bifida*. Rosemont IL: American Academy of Orthopedic Surgery, 2001.

Osgood-Schlatter Disease

Peck DM. Apophyseal injuries in the young adult. *Am Fam Physician* 1995;
51:1891.
Rosenberg ZS, Kaweblum M, Cheung YY, et al. Osgood-Schlatter lesion: fracture or tendonitis? Scintigraphic, CT and MR imaging features. *Radiology*
1992;185:853.

Osteogenesis Imperfecta

Falk MF, Heeger S, Lynch KA et al. Intravenous bisphosphonate therapy in
children with osteogenesis imperfecta. *Pediatrics* 2003;111:573.

Osteomyelitis

Green NE. *Pseudomonas* infections of the foot following puncture wounds. In:
American Academy of Orthopaedic Surgeons Instructional Course Lectures,
1983:43.
Jansen BR, Hart W, Schreuder O. Discitis in childhood: 12–35 year follow-up of
35 patients. *Acta Orthop Scand* 1993;64:33.
Mazur JM, Ross G, Cummings J, et al. Use of magnetic resonance imaging for the
diagnosis of acute musculoskeletal infections in children. *J Pediatr Orthop*
1995;15:144.
Schreck P, Bradley J, Chambers H. Musculoskeletal complications of varicella.
J Bone Joint Surg 1996;78A:1713.
Song KM, Sloboda JF. Acute hematogenous osteomyelitis in children. *J Am Acad
Orthop Surg* 2001:166.

Popliteal Cysts

Dinham JM. Popliteal cysts in children. *J Bone Joint Surg* 1975;57B:69.

Pulled Elbow

Salter RB, Zaltz C. Anatomic investigations of the mechanism of injury and
pathologic anatomy of "pulled elbow" in young children. *Clin Orthop* 1971;
77:134.

Radial Clubhand

Bora FW. Radial clubhand deformity. *J Bone Joint Surg* 1981;63A:741.

Radioulnar Synostosis

Cleary JE, Omer GE. Congenital radioulnar synostosis. *J Bone Joint Surg* 1985;
67A:539.

Septic Arthritis

Kocher M, Mandinga R, Murphy JM, et al. A clinical practice guideline for
treatment of septic arthritis of the hip: efficacy in improving the process of
care and outcome of septic arthritis of the hip. *J Bone Joint Surg* 2003;85:
994.

Slipped Capital Femoral Epiphysis

Carney BT, Weinstein SL, Noble J. Long-term follow-up of slipped capital
femoral epiphysis. *J Bone Joint Surg* 1991;73A:667.

Loder RT, Richards BS, Shapiro PS, et al. Acute slipped capital femoral epiphysis: the importance of physeal stability. *J Bone Joint Surg Am* 1993;75:
1134.

Spinal Disorders

Nachemson AL, Peterson LE. Effectiveness of treatment with a brace in girls who
have adolescent idiopathic scoliosis. A prospective, controlled study based
on data from the brace study of the Scoliosis Research Society. *J Bone Joint
Surg Am* 1995;77:815.
Salminen JJ, Pentti J, Terho P. Low back pain and disability in 14-year-old
schoolchildren. *Acta Paediatr* 1992;81:1035.
Skaggs DL, Bassett GS. Adolescent idiopathic scoliosis: an update. *Am Fam Physi-
cian* 1996;53:2327.
Sponseller PD. Evaluating the child with back pain. *Am Fam Physician* 1996;
54:1933.
Sponseller PD. Sizing up scoliosis. *JAMA* 2003;289:608.
Tredwell SJ, et al. Instability of the upper cervical spine in Down syndrome.
J Pediatr Orthop 1990;10:602.
Weinstein SL, Dolan LA, Spratt KF. Health and function of patients with un-
treated idiopathic scoliosis. A 50-year natural history study. *JAMA* 2003;
289:559.

Sprengel Deformity

Carson WF, Lovell WW, Whitesides TE Jr. Congenital elevation of the scapula.
J Bone Joint Surg 1981;63A:1199.

Tarsal Coalition

Mosier KM, Asher M. Tarsal coalitions and peroneal spastic flat foot. *J Bone
Joint Surg* 1984;66A:976.

Tibial Deformities

Morrissy RT. Congenital pseudarthrosis of the tibia. *J Bone Joint Surg* 1981;
63B:367.
Pappas AM. Congenital posteromedial bowing of the tibia and fibula. *J Pediatr
Orthop* 1984;4:525.
Staheli LT, Corbett M, Wyss C, et al. Lower extremity rotational problems in
children. *J Bone Joint Surg* 1985;67A:39.

Transient Synovitis of the Hip

Fink AM, Berman L, Edwards K, et al. The irritable hip: immediate ultrasound
guided aspiration and prevention of hospital admission. *Arch Dis Child*
(England) 1995;72:110.
Haueisen DC, Weiner DS, Weiner SD. The characterization of transient synovitis
of the hip in children. *J Pediatr Orthop* 1986;6:11.

Upper Extremity

Bora WF. *Pediatric upper extremity*. Philadelphia: Saunders, 1986.
Dobyns JH, Wood V, Bayne LG. Congenital hand deformities. In: Green D, ed.
Textbook of hand surgery. New York: Churchill-Livingstone, 1982.

CHAPTER 433 ■ SKELETAL DYSPLASIAS

PATRICIA G. WHEELER AND DAVID D. WEAVER

Skeletal dysplasias are conditions presenting primary problems in growth resulting from defective formation of bone or carti-lage. This category of diseases includes a heterogenous group of disorders with a wide variety of clinical and radiographic manifestations. Much of the variation stems from the differ-ent combinations of involved bones and the ways in which these bones are affected in their shape, length, and density. Most skeletal dysplasias are genetically determined, can be in-herited, and result in disproportionately short stature. Because of the last problem, the term *dwarfism* frequently is applied to

these disorders. Other names include *chondrodysplasias*, *osteo-chondrodysplasias*, and *bone dysplasias*.

More than 200 recognized types of skeletal dysplasias ex-ist. The incidence of any single dysplasia is relatively low. Col-lectively, however, they are relatively frequent (1 in 3,000 to 5,000 births). Because of this frequency and the diversity of these conditions, it is essential that the practitioner be able to recognize a fetus, newborn, or child with a skeletal dysplasia so that the diagnosis can be established, the prognosis determined, and a treatment plan developed. Genetic counseling should be available to the individual, parents and family in regards to recurrence risks.

This chapter provides the primary-care physician with a basic understanding of skeletal dysplasias and presents the major clinical and radiographic features and complications of the more commonly encountered disorders. When encountering one of these disorders, the responsibilities of the primary-care physician are to treat any immediate medical problems, become familiar with the particular skeletal dysplasia present in the patient, and obtain appropriate and timely consultation. In all cases in which the patient survives the neonatal period, a long-term treatment program should be established.

EPIDEMIOLOGY

Most skeletal dysplasias are uncommon, and often their exact incidence is unknown. Osteogenesis imperfecta (OI or brittle bone disease), type I, which is one of the milder forms of the disorder, has an estimated frequency of 1 in 20,000 births. OI type II, the more severe and normally lethal form, is less common and affects approximately 1 in 50,000. Thanatophoric dysplasia, the most frequently encountered lethal skeletal dysplasia, is seen in approximately 1 in 30,000 births. Classic or heterozygous achondroplasia, the most common nonlethal skeletal dysplasia, occurs with a frequency of 1 in 25,000.

On the other hand, the incidence of some skeletal dysplasias in certain ethnic groups may be much higher. For instance, the McKusick type of metaphyseal chondrodysplasia (cartilage-hair hypoplasia) is rare in the general population, but is found in approximately 1 in 500 live births among the Amish population of North America. The higher incidence of certain bone dysplasias in some ethnic groups normally is the result of inbreeding or other factors that have increased the gene frequency in that group.

PATHOGENESIS

Development and Anatomy of Bone

Bone is formed from either mesodermal or neural crest cells. These cells form mesenchyme, which in turn forms embryonic connective tissue. For cartilaginous bone, cartilage is formed within the embryonic connective tissue, which then changes to bone. For membranous bone, the bone is formed directly within the connective tissue. The cartilage in cartilaginous bone is formed by chondroblasts, whereas the mineral portion of the bone is derived from osteoblasts in both bone types. The skull (except for its base), maxilla, mandible, squamous portion of the temporalis, nasal bones, and clavicles are membranous bone; all the rest of the skeleton is cartilaginous bone.

The anatomy of long bones is depicted in Figure 433.1. When long bones are growing, the growing end is known as the *epiphysis*. Below the epiphyseal center is the metaphysis. Longitudinal growth actually occurs at the junction between the epiphysis and the metaphysis, an area called the *physis* or *growth plate*. During puberty, the growth plate is obliterated, the epiphysis and metaphysis fuse, and lengthening of the bone ceases. The shaft of the bone is called the *diaphysis*. Molding of the diaphysis takes place as the bone becomes longer. The diaphysis also thickens with age and in response to increased stress exerted on the bone.

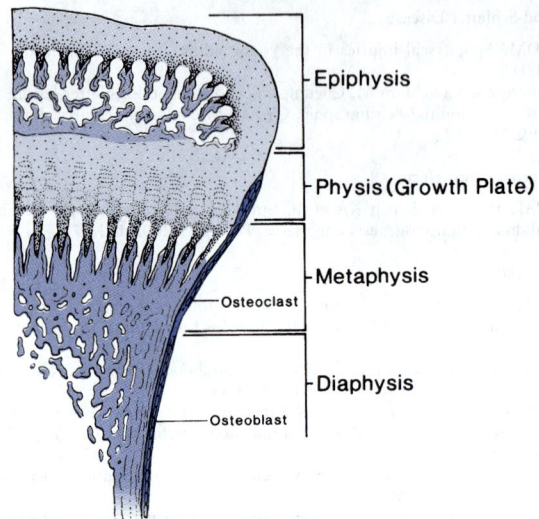

FIGURE 433.1. Anatomy of normal prepubertal tubular bone. Note that the bone is divided into four segments, each of which may be involved in skeletal dysplasias either separately or in combination.

Nomenclature and Classification of Skeletal Dysplasias

Skeletal dysplasias in general are named after the anatomic parts of the bones that are affected, after the appearance of the bone, or after the individual(s) who originally described the condition (Fig. 433.2). In some cases, a combination of these methods is used.

An example of the anatomic naming of bone dysplasias is *multiple epiphyseal dysplasia* (Fig. 433.3). In this condition,

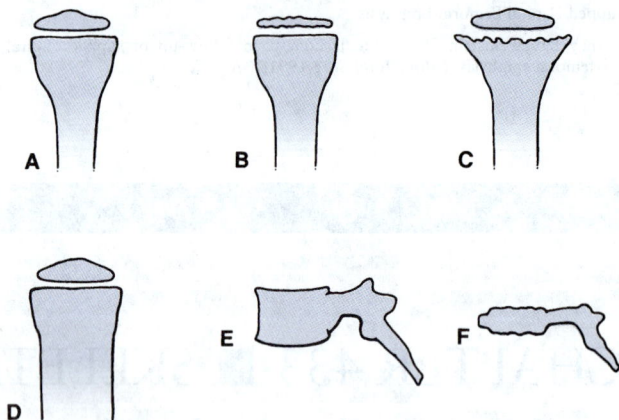

FIGURE 433.2. Diagrammatic representation of various types of bone dysplasias. **A:** Normal shape of growing long bones. **B:** Epiphyseal involvement such as in multiple epiphyseal dysplasia; note flattened and irregular epiphysis. **C:** Metaphyseal involvement that might be seen in achondroplasia; note widening and irregular surface of metaphysis. **D:** Diaphyseal involvement as seen in craniodiaphysial dysplasia. **E:** Normal lateral view of vertebra. **F:** Vertebral involvement that can be found in spondyloepiphyseal dysplasia congenita; note vertebral body flattening and surface irregularities. (Modified with permission from Rimoin DL, Lachman RS. The chondrodysplasias. In: Emery AEH, Rimoin DL, eds. *Principles and practice of medical genetics.* New York: Churchill Livingstone, 1990:895.)

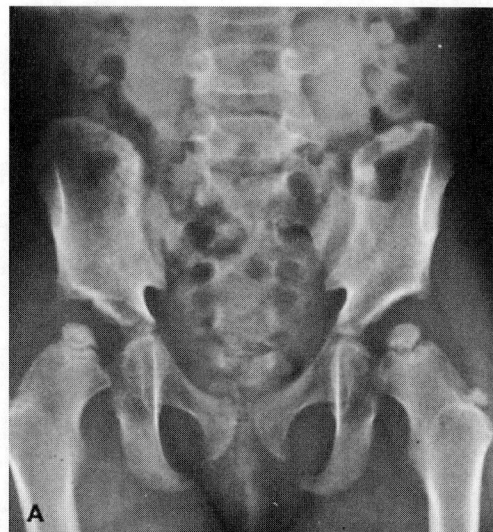
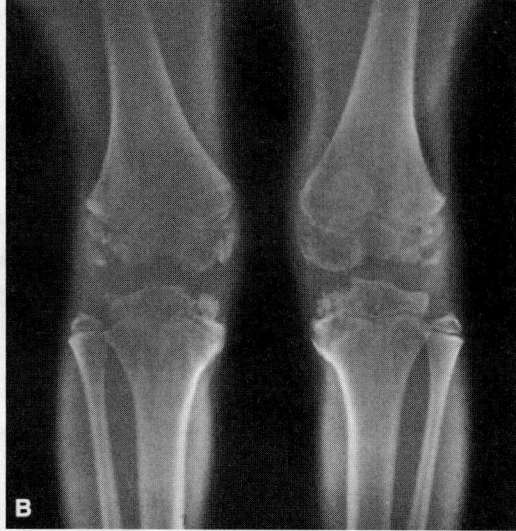

FIGURE 433.3. Radiographs of a patient with multiple epiphyseal dysplasia. **A:** Pelvis and hips at age 8 years; note small irregular proximal femoral epiphyses and poorly developed acetabular roof. **B:** Knees of patient at age 10 years; note irregular and mottled epiphyses of the long bones.

numerous epiphyses (see Fig. 433.2B) are involved, whereas the spine is affected only minimally. As a result of the involvement of multiple epiphyses, the individual usually has short stature and, with age, may develop significant arthritis in the involved joints. Another example of anatomic nomenclature is *spondyloepiphyseal dysplasia congenita*, in which many of the epiphyses, including those of the spine (spondylo-), are abnormal. The clinical picture is one of small, irregular epiphyses, flattened vertebral bodies (platyspondyly; see Fig. 433.2E, F) and, in some cases, kyphoscoliosis.

Other bone dysplasias are named after the appearance of the bone. An example is *campomelic* (or *camptomelic*) *dysplasia*. In this disorder, a characteristic bowing of the long bones of the lower extremities occurs. The term *camptomelic* is coined from the Greek *campo*, which means bent or curved. In OI, the term *imperfecta* refers to poorly mineralized bone. In a newly described disorder, schneckenbecken dysplasia, the pelvis is shaped like a snail shell; *schneckenbecken* is German for "snail-shaped."

The third mechanism for naming bone dysplasias involves the use of eponyms. For example, Kniest dysplasia is a rare, autosomal dominant disorder characterized by short stature and dumbbell-shaped femurs with extremely broad and shortened femoral necks. Kniest first reported the condition in 1952.

Frequently, eponyms are used in combination with one of the first two methods of naming skeletal dysplasias, most often to delineate the particular subtype of dysplasia. For instance, two types of achondrogenesis exist, one known as *Parenti-Fraccaro achondrogenesis* (type I) and the other as *Langer-Saldino achondrogenesis* (type II; Fig. 433.4). These two subtypes are not based on differences in the clinical appearance of the affected children (both types have nearly identical clinical phenotypes), but on radiographic variations. Type I has been subdivided further into type IA, with rib fractures and spike-shaped femurs; and type IB, without the rib fractures but with a pelvis that appears to be turned upside down. Type IA also has been denoted as the *Houston-Harris type* and type IB as the *Fraccaro type*.

Various systems for classifying the skeletal dysplasias have been devised. One of the earliest of these was based on the relative shortening of the limb or spine: For example, was the short stature of the child caused by primary shortening of the extrem-

ities, with relatively normal spinal length, or was the spine relatively short compared with the length of the arms and legs?

Achondroplasia is one example of a short-limbed skeletal dysplasia. In this condition, the sitting height—that is—the length of the trunk and head of an individual when she is sitting, is nearly normal, but the standing height is far less than normal. This reflects the very short legs in this condition. On the other hand, patients with Morquio syndrome (mucopolysaccharidosis, type IV) have the opposite characteristics. They have short trunk and, in relationship to the spinal length, long extremities. The shortening of the spine in Morquio syndrome is primarily a result of platyspondyly.

Another classification system is based on the age at which the first manifestation of the skeletal dysplasia appears. Some disorders can be detected prenatally or at birth (congenita), whereas others do not have clinical or radiographic manifestations until months or years after birth (tarda). Yet another system is based on the pattern of bone involvement and the types of skeletal changes seen in a particular disorder. The International Nosology and Classification of Constitutional Disorders of the Bone (Table 433.1) use this approach.

Yet another approach has been put forth by Kornak and Mundlos. Utilizing recent advances in molecular genetics, these authors have presented a classification based on a combination of molecular pathology and embryology. Bones develop first by the formation of a pattern: the determination of the location, size and shape of individual bones. Next, mesenchymal cells differentiate and condense into cartilage. Third, growth occurs in the cartilaginous growth plates at the ends of long bones. Finally, remodeling and homeostasis occurs. These authors have classified bone disorders according to how these disorders affect these four phases of bone development and maintenance. Bone disorders also may be classified as lethal and nonlethal.

Dysostoses

Dysostoses are conditions predominately affecting individual bones, either singly or a few in combination. A specific bone may be absent, hypoplastic, or malformed. Further dysostoses are distinguished from more generalized skeletal dysplasias

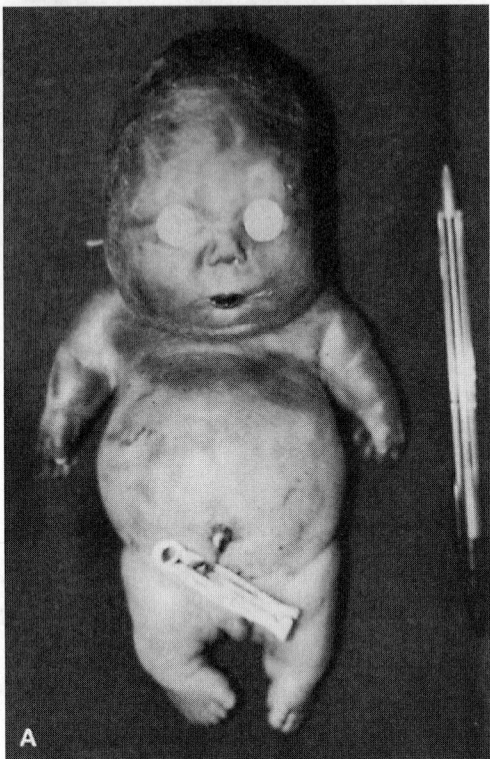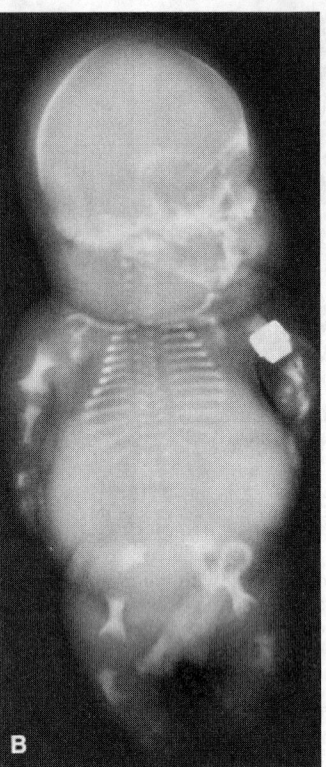

FIGURE 433.4. Achondrogenesis, type II in a term newborn. **A:** Note severe growth deficiency (standard ballpoint pen alongside for comparison), small chest and extremities, and protruding abdomen. This was a postmortem picture. **B:** Radiograph of the same patient; note the very short, irregularly shaped bones of the extremities, short and horizontal ribs, and poorly calcified vertebral bodies.

by being formed during embryogenesis (the third through the eighth week post conception), whereas skeletal dysplasias generally develop throughout intrauterine development and childhood.

Delineation of Skeletal Dysplasias

The discovery of new skeletal dysplasias has been an ongoing process since the 1940s. As noted already, a bewildering number of different disorders are recognized, making diagnosis problematic for the average clinician. The recognition of a specific disorder further is complicated by the similar appearances of many of these conditions. Furthermore, a spectrum of severity may exist within a single entity, or two conditions may have overlapping features, making arrival at a correct diagnosis exasperating even for the experts. A further characteristic of many skeletal dysplasias is that these conditions often become more severe with time. The condition may manifest prenatally, and may be severe, if not lethal, at birth. If the disorder is not lethal or not expressed at birth, it invariably worsens with age. If a child is seen early in the course of the condition, when the features often are not expressed fully, one may find it difficult or impossible to make the diagnosis.

During the 1940s, most individuals with disproportionately short stature were classified as having achondroplasia if the extremities were relatively short, or as having Morquio disease if the trunk was shortened disproportionately. Since then, numerous different skeletal dysplasias with similar appearances have been delineated from each of these disorders. This demarcation has been accomplished by the careful study of clinical, radiographic, and pathologic features, and noting the inheritance patterns of each. A newer trend in the grouping of skeletal dysplasias involves categorizing each skeletal dysplasia based on the specific protein, enzyme, or gene defect involved, if known.

The biochemical and/or genetic delineation of numerous skeletal dysplasias has made it clear that many previously de-

scribed and well-characterized conditions are, in actuality, the result of mutations at different locations within the same gene. The opposite also is true; individuals with the same apparent clinical condition may be biochemically and molecularly distinct. This heterogeneity in part accounts for the difference in severity of the "same" clinical condition.

Molecular Genetics and Biochemistry of Skeletal Dysplasias

During the last two decades, much has been learned about the molecular genetics and biochemistry of many skeletal dysplasias. Biochemical errors have been found in the structural proteins of cartilage (specifically different types of collagen), enzymes of cartilage metabolism (lysosomal enzymes), and regulators of cartilage growth (fibroblast growth factor receptors). As other genes and biochemical pathways in bone formation and function are found, one would expect to find additional errors in the bone matrix, osteoid (the mineral portion of the bone), and other components of cartilage. In addition, problems may be found in the function of the osteoblasts (those cells that form bone) or the osteoclasts (those cells that degrade and reshape bone).

One of the first skeletal dysplasias to be understood on the molecular and biochemical levels was OI. This disorder is characterized by bone fragility resulting in fractures. OI is divided into four main types based on clinical and radiographic findings. Type II is normally a perinatal or neonatal lethal, with multiple fractures occurring *in utero,* and the affected newborn typically having marked respiratory distress because of a small and excessively flexible chest and short and curved long bones. OI type III also presents at birth with multiple fractures, but respiratory complications are not as severe as in type II. Individuals with OI type III typically have multiple broken bones occurring throughout their life, progressive bone deformation, and marked short stature. OI types I and IV are less severe, with fewer fractures and most fractures occurring postnatally;

TABLE 433.1

SKELETAL DYSPLASIAS

A. Osteochondrodysplasias (Defects of tubular [and flat] bones and/or axial skeleton)
1. *Achondroplasia group*
   Achondroplasia
   Hypochondroplasia
   SADDAN (*severe achondroplasia, developmental delay, acanthosis nigricans*)
   Thanatophoric dysplasia, type I
   Thanatophoric dysplasia, type II (cloverleaf skull, straight femur)
2. *Severe spondylodysplastic dysplasias*
   Achondrogenesis, type IA
   Lethal platyspondylic skeletal dysplasias (Torrance and Luton types)
   Opsismodysplasia
   Spondylometaphyseal dysplasia, Sedaghatian type
3. *Metatropic dysplasia group*
   Fibrochondrogenesis
   Metatropic dysplasia (various forms)
   Schneckenbecken dysplasia
4. *Short-rib dysplasia with or without polydactyly*
   Asphyxiating thoracic dysplasia (Jeune syndrome)
   Chondroectodermal dysplasia (Ellis-van Creveld dysplasia)
   Short-rib dysplasia, type 1/III (Saldino-Noonan/Verma-Naumoff types)
   Short-rib dysplasia, type II (Majewski type)
   Short-rib dysplasia, type IV (Beemer type)
   Thoracolaryngopelvic dysplasia (Barnes syndrome)
5. *Atelosteogenesis-omodysplasia group*
   Atelosteogenesis type I (includes "boomerang dysplasia")
   Atelosteogenesis, type III
   de la Chapelle dysplasia
   Omodysplasia I, Maroteaux type
   Omodysplasia II, Borochowitz type
6. *Diastrophic dysplasia group*
   Achondrogenesis, type 1B
   Diastrophic dysplasia
   Multiple epiphyseal dysplasia, autosomal recessive type
7. *Dyssegmental dysplasia group*
   Dyssegmental dysplasia, Rolland-Desbuquois type
   Dyssegmental dysplasia, Silverman-Handmaker type
8. *Type II collagenopathies*
   Achondrogenesis, type II (Langer-Saldino type)
   Hypochondrogenesis
   Kniest dysplasia
   Mild spondyloepidysplasia with premature onset arthrosis
   Spondyloepimetaphyseal dysplasia
   Spondyloepiphyseal dysplasia congenita
   Spondyloepiphyseal dysplasia, Namaqualand type
   Spondyloperipheral dysplasia
   Stickler syndrome, type I
   Strudwick type
9. *Type XI collagenopathies Stickler syndrome, type II (with or without ocular involvement)*
   Marshall syndrome
   Otospondylomegaepiphyseal dysplasia
   Stickler syndrome, type III (without ocular involvement)
10. *Other spondyloepi (meta) physeal dysplasias*
    Anauxetic dysplasia
    Dyggve-Melchior-Clausen dysplasia
    Immunoosseous dysplasia (Schimke immunoosseous dysplasia)
    Progressive pseudorheumatoid dysplasia
    Schwartz-Jampel syndrome
    SPONASTRIME dysplasia

Spondyloepimetaphyseal dysplasia short limb-abnormal calcification type
Spondyloepimetaphyseal dysplasia with joint laxity
Spondyloepimetaphyseal dysplasia with multiple dislocations, Hall type
Spondyloepimetaphyseal dysplasia, Handigodu type
Spondyloepimetaphyseal dysplasia, Pakistani type
Wolcott-Rallison dysplasia
X-linked spondyloepiphyseal dysplasia tarda
11. *Multiple epiphyseal dysplasias and pseudoachondroplasia*
    Familial hip dysplasia, Beukes type
    Multiple epiphyseal dysplasia, Fairbanks and Ribbing types
    Pseudoachondrodysplasia
12. *Chondrodysplasia punctata (stippled epiphyses group)*
    CHILD (limb-reduction ichthyosis)
    Chondrodysplasia punctata, X-linked dominant, Conradi-Hünermann type
    Chondrodysplasia punctata, X-linked dominant, rhizomelic type 1
    Chondrodysplasia punctata, X-linked dominant, rhizomelic type 2
    Chondrodysplasia punctata, X-linked dominant, rhizomelic type 3
    Chondrodysplasia punctata, X-linked dominant, tibia-metacarpal type
    Chondrodysplasia punctata, X-linked recessive type (brachytelephalangic)
    Dappled diaphyseal dysplasia
    Hydrops-ectopic calcification-moth-eaten appearance (Greenberg dysplasia)
13. *Metaphyseal dysplasias*
    Acroscyphodysplasia (various types)
    Adenosine deaminase deficiency
    Cartilage hair hypoplasia (metaphyseal chondrodysplasia, McKusick type)
    Metaphyseal anadysplasia (various types)
    Metaphyseal chondrodysplasia, Jansen type
    Metaphyseal chondrodysplasia, Schmid type
    Metaphyseal chondrodysplasia, Spahr type
    Metaphyseal dysplasia with pancreatic insufficiency and cyclic neutropenia (Shwachmann-Diamond syndrome)
14. *Spondylometaphyseal dysplasias*
    Spondylometaphyseal dysplasia (Sutcliffe corner fracture type)
    Spondylometaphyseal dysplasia with severe genu valgum (including Schmidt and Algerian types)
    Spondylometaphyseal dysplasia, Kozlowski type
15. *Brachyolmia spondylodysplasias*
    Brachyolmia spondylodysplasias, autosomal dominant type
    Brachyolmia spondylodysplasias, Hobaek and Toledo types
    Brachyolmia spondylodysplasias, Maroteaux type
16. *Mesomelic dysplasias*
    Leri-Weill dyschondrosteosis
    Mesomelic dysplasia with synostoses
    Mesomelic dysplasia, Kantaputra type
    Mesomelic dysplasia, Kozlowski-Reardon type
    Mesomelic dysplasia, Langer type (homozygous Leri-Weill dyschondrosteosis)
    Mesomelic dysplasia, Nievergelt type
    Mesomelic dysplasia, Reinhardt-Pfeiffer type
    Mesomelic dysplasia, Robinow type, dominant
    Mesomelic dysplasia, Robinow type, recessive

(Continued)

TABLE 433.1

(CONTINUED)

Mesomelic dysplasia, Savarirayan type
Mesomelic dysplasia, Verloes type
Mesomelic dysplasia, Werner type

17. *Acromelic dysplasias*
Acrodysostosis
Acromicric dysplasia
Angel-shaped phalangoepiphysea dysplasia
Brachydactyly, type A1
Brachydactyly, type A2
Brachydactyly, type A3
Brachydactyly, type B
Brachydactyly, type C
Brachydactyly, type D
Brachydactyly, type E
Brachydactyly-hypertension dysplasia (Bilginturan syndrome)
Camptodactyly arthropathy coxa vara pericarditis
Christian brachydactyly
Craniofacial conodysplasia
Geleophysic dysplasia
Myhre dysplasia
Pseudohypoparathyroidism (Albright hereditary osteodystrophy)
Saldino-Mainzer dysplasia
Trichorhinophalangeal dysplasia type II (Langer-Giedion syndrome)
Trichorhinophalangeal dysplasia types I/III
Weill-Marchesani dysplasia

18. *Acromesomelic dysplasias*
Acromesomelic dysplasia, Campailla-Martinelli type
Acromesomelic dysplasia, Ferraz/Ohba type
Acromesomelic dysplasia, Maroteaux type
Acromesomelic dysplasia, type Osebold-Remondini
Cranioectodermal dysplasia
Grebe dysplasia

19. *Dysplasias with predominant membranous bone involvement*
Cleidocranial dysplasia
Parietal foramina (isolated)
Yunis-Varon dysplasia

20. *Bent-bone dysplasia group*
Camptomelic dysplasia
Cummins syndrome
Stuve-Wiedemann dysplasia (neonatal Schwartz-Jampel)

21. *Multiple dislocations with dysplasias*
Desbuquois syndrome
Larsen syndrome
Larsen-like syndromes (including La Reunion Island)
Pseudodiastrophic dysplasia

22. *Dysplasias with decreased bone density*
Bruck dysplasia, types I–II
Cole-Carpenter dysplasia
Geroderma osteodysplasticum
Idiopathic juvenile osteoporosis
Osteogenesis imperfecta, types I–IV
Osteopenia with radiolucent lesions of the mandible
Osteoporosis with pseudoglioma
Singleton-Merten syndrome

23. *Dysplasias with defective mineralization*
Hypophosphatasia, adult form
Hypophosphatasia, autosomal recessive perinatal lethal and infantile forms
Hypophosphatemic rickets
Neonatal hyperparathyroidism
Transient neonatal hyperparathyroidism with hypocalciuric hypercalcemia

24. *Increased bone density without modification of bone shape*
Cranial osteosclerosis with bamboo hair (Netherton syndrome)
Dysosteosclerosis
Melorheostosis
Mixed sclerosing bone dysplasia
Osteomesopyknosis
Osteopathia striata with cranial sclerosis
Osteopathia striata, isolated
Osteopetrosis
Delayed form, type I
Delayed form, type II
Infantile form
Intermediate form
With ectodermal dysplasia and immune defect
With infantile neuroaxonal dysplasia
Osteopoikilosis
Osteosclerosis, Stanescu type
Pyknodysostosis

25. *Increased bone density with diaphyseal involvement*
Craniodiaphysial dysplasia
Diaphyseal dysplasia (Camurati-Engelmann syndrome)
Diaphyseal dysplasia with anemia (Ghosal hematodiaphseal dysplasia)
Diaphyseal medullary stenosis with bone malignancy
Kenny-Caffey dysplasia, type I
Kenny-Caffey dysplasia, type II
Lenz-Majewski dysplasia
Endosteal hyperostosis
Scleroosteocerebellar dysplasia
Sclerosteosis
van Buchem type
Worth type
Oculodentoosseous dysplasia
Osteoectasia with hyperphosphatasia (juvenile Paget disease)
Trichodento-osseous dysplasia

26. *Increased bone density with metaphyseal involvement*
Pyle dysplasia
Craniometaphyseal dysplasia
Mild type
Severe type

B. **Disorganized development of cartilaginous and fibrous components of the skeleton**
Carpotarsal osteochondromatosis
Cherubism
Cherubism with gingival fibromatosis
Dysplasia epiphysealis hemimelica
Dysspondyloenchondromatosis
Enchondromatosis (Ollier disease)
Enchondromatosis with hemangiomata (Maffucci syndrome)
Fibrodysplasia ossificans progressiva
Fibrous dysplasia (McCune-Albright and other types)
Genochondromatosis
Jaffe-Campanacci type
Metachondromatosis
Multiple cartilaginous exostoses
Osteoglophonic dysplasia
Spondyloenchondromatosis
Spondyloenchondromatosis with basal ganglia calcification

Modified with permission from Hall CM. International nosology and classification of constitutional disorders of bone (2001). *Am J Med Genet* 2002;113:65.

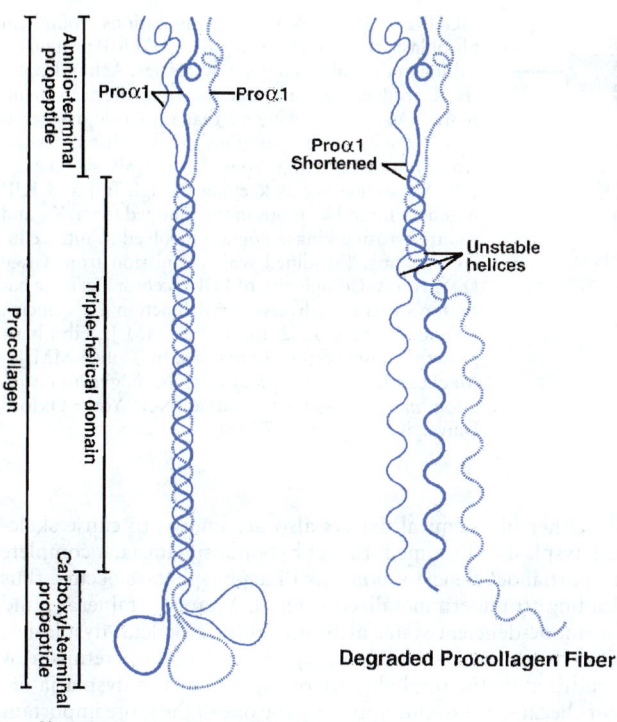

FIGURE 433.5. Normal type I procollagen molecule on the left showing normal helical formation. The figure on the right depicts the lack of coiling of the polypeptides when a change in or deletion of one or more amino acids occurs in both pro-alpha$_1$ chains, leading to degradation of the molecule. One pro-alpha$_1$ chain in each figure has been thickened for clarity.

short stature and teeth abnormalities also may be present. All four types of OI are produced by a defect in either the procollagen pro-alpha$_1$ gene (*COL1A1*) or the procollagen pro-alpha$_2$ gene (*COL1A2*). These genes normally produce the polypeptides pro-alpha$_1$ and pro-alpha$_2$, respectively. Under normal circumstances, two pro-alpha$_1$ chains combine with one pro-alpha$_2$ procollagen in a helical structure to form type I procollagen (Fig. 433.5). The end portions of the type I procollagen molecules then are cleaved to form mature procollagen molecules that are then secreted into the extracellular matrix and incorporated into the definitive type I collagen fibril. Deletions of one or more amino acids, or the substitutions of amino acids in the pro-alpha$_1$ or pro-alpha$_2$ chains, have been found in most patients with OI.

When these defects occur in the pro-alpha$_1$ or pro-alpha$_2$ chains, the formation of the normal helical structure of the type I procollagen molecule frequently is disrupted (see Fig. 433.5). If the disruption is significant enough, the abnormally formed procollagen is degraded within the cell, a process called *protein suicide*. The end result of protein suicide is a deficiency of type I collagen, but the type I collagen that is formed is normal. When the disruption of the helical formation is less severe, intracellular degradation of the procollagen fiber may not occur, and the abnormal procollagen is secreted from the cell and incorporated into the collagen fiber, thus making the collagen abnormal. Studies have shown that individuals who have more severe mutations (for example, premature stop codons or a substitution of a glycine) that prevent a pro-alpha$_1$ or a pro-alpha$_2$ chain from being formed typically have a milder form of OI (OI type I or IV), whereas those who have less disruptive mutations (single base-pair changes leading to substitution of a

nonglycine amino acid) that allow the abnormal protein to be incorporated into the procollagen strand tend to have a more severe form of OI (type II or III). The clinical phenotype appears to be milder if only 50% of the normal collagen protein is present, as opposed to having a normal amount of abnormally formed collagen. In reality, OI is a continuous spectrum of severity with type II being at one end and normally an early lethal condition, and types I and IV being at the other, with some individuals having few problems and a normal lifespan. This spectrum in part is due to the fact that over 200 mutations have been reported in *COL1A1* and *COL1A2* genes. However, the severity in any one family is frequently often similar, because affected individuals normally possess the identical mutations (the exception being type IV, in which striking intrafamilial variability may be present).

Until recently, isolated cases of possible OI were evaluated by looking for the abnormal or reduced production of procollagen in tissue samples, usually through skin biopsy from affected individuals. This evaluation detected approximately 85% of individuals with OI. However, direct gene testing of *COL1A1* or *COL1A2* now is available. Testing for these genes can be done on a blood sample and involves sequencing of both the *COL1A1* and *COL1A2* genes. This testing finds a mutation in 95% of individuals with clinical OI.

Another bone dysplasia that has been studied in detail is achondroplasia, the most common nonlethal skeletal dysplasia causing short stature. The genetic defect in achondroplasia has been isolated to a specific mutation in the fibroblast growth factor receptor 3 (*FGFR3*) gene (Figs. 433.6 and 433.7). In more than 99% of analyzed achondroplastic cases, a glycine-to-arginine substitution has been found at amino acid position 380 of the receptor. On the other hand, mutations in other areas of the *FGFR3* gene result in a lethal bone dysplasia, thanatophoric dysplasia, and a milder skeletal dysplasia,

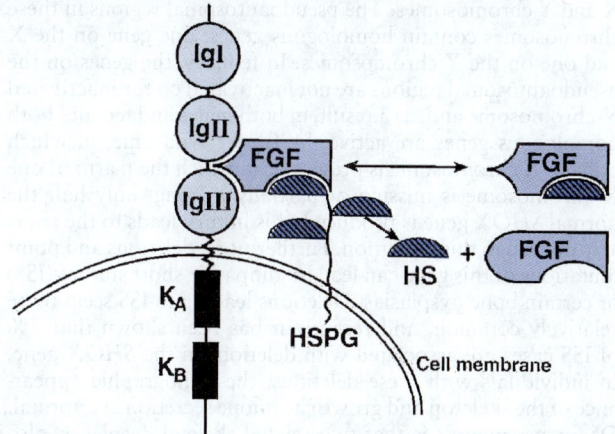

FIGURE 433.6. Model of fibroblast growth factor receptor 3 (FGFR3). The ligand, fibroblast growth factor (FGF), first binds to heparan sulfate proteoglycan (HSPG) (hashed half ovoids attached to the cell membrane), or heparan sulfate (HS). The complex then forms a trimolecular complex with FGFR3, resulting in structural changes in the tyrosine kinase parts of the molecules (K_A and K_B) and sequences genetic regulation of the cell. The IgI, IgII, and IgIII regions represent immunoglobin-like loops involved in the attachment of the FGF-HS/FGF-HSPG complex. The 23 recognized FGFs are structurally related polypeptides that play various roles in bone embryogenesis, growth, and homeostasis by inducing differentiation and mitogenesis, and stimulating chemotaxes, cell survival, and angiogenesis. Tyrosine kinase domains are involved in intracellular signalling. (Modified with permission from Givol D, Yayon A. Complexity of FGF receptors: genetic basis for structured diversity and functional specificity. *FASEB J* 1992;6:3362.)

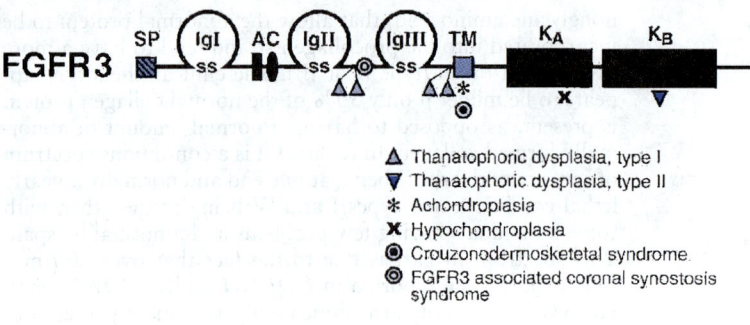

FIGURE 433.7. Location of mutations found in fibroblast growth factor receptor 3 (FGFR3) protein resulting in the indicated bone dysplasias. Achondroplasia is produced at only one location, the transmembrane TM domain, whereas thanatophoric dysplasia, type I results from mutations at five different sites. Abbreviations starting from the left: SP, signal peptide; SS, sulfide bonds keeping the IgI, IgII and IgIII immunoglobin-like loops in their looped form. K_A and K_B are tyrosine kinase domain involved in intracellular signaling. (Modified with permission from Givol D, Yayon A. Complexity of FGF receptors: genetic basis for structured diversity and functional specificity. *FASEB J* 1992;6:3362 and Cohen MM Jr. Fibroblast growth factor receptor mutations. In: Cohen MM Jr., MacLean RE, eds. *Craniosynostosis: diagnosis, evaluation, and management*, 2nd ed. New York: Oxford University Press, 2000:77.)

hypochondroplasia. The location of these and other mutations in the *FGFR3* gene are depicted in Fig. 433.7.

One current hypothesis to explain why different mutations in the *FGFR3* gene cause different bone dysplasias is based on the mutations causing a range of tyrosine kinase activity (referred to as a *gain of function mutation*). Tyrosine kinase acts as a negative regulator for endochondral bone growth. The more "turned on" the tyrosine kinase, the greater the reduction in bone length, and thus the greater the severity of the bone dysplasia. Different mutations in the *FGFR3* gene lead to a varying degree of up-regulation of the tyrosine kinase and result in the various dysplasias associated with this gene.

Another recent advance in the understanding of normal and abnormal bone growth and the cause of certain bone dysplasias has been the discovery of the *SHOX* gene. *SHOX* is the abbreviation for short stature homeobox-containing gene. This gene is located in the pseudoautosomal region of the p-arm of the X and Y chromosomes. The pseudoautosomal regions in these chromosomes contain homologous genes, one gene on the X and one on the Y chromosomes. In females, the genes on the pseudoautosomal regions are not inactivated on the inactivated X-chromosome and, as a result, in both males and females both homologous genes are active. In Turner syndrome, in which only an X chromosome is present or in which the p arm of one X chromosome is missing or partially missing, only half the normal *SHOX* gene is produced; this in turn leads to the short stature seen in this condition. Furthermore, deletions and point mutations of this gene can lead to idiopathic short stature (ISS) or certain bone dysplasias. Deletions leading to ISS seem to be relatively common, and recently it has been shown that 7% of ISS cases are associated with deletions in the *SHOX* gene. In individuals with these deletions, the radiographic appearance of the skeleton and growth hormone secretion are normal. Of further interest is that two related skeletal dysplasias also have been found to have mutations or deletions in this gene. The first condition is Leri-Weill dyschondrosteosis, an autosomal dominant disorder, characterized by Madelung deformity of the wrists (bowing of the radius and distal hypoplasia of the dorsally dislocated ulna) and short stature, with most of the shortening in the forearms (mesomelic shortening). In roughly 80% of Leri-Weill dyschondrosteosis cases, a deletion of the gene occurs; in about 20% of cases, a point mutation occurs. A second, rare disorder is mesomelic dysplasia, Langer type, which is the homozygous dominant state of the Leri-Weill dyschondrosteosis; it is caused by mutations in or deletion of both *SHOX* genes. Why this range in phenotypic expression is associated with the various mutations and deletions of this gene has not been unraveled.

Other biochemical defects also are known to cause skeletal dysplasias. In some forms of hypophosphatasia, a complete or partial deficiency of bone alkaline phosphatase occurs, thus leading to undermineralized osteoid. Vitamin-, mineral-, and hormone-deficient states also can produce skeletal dysplasias. One of the most severe bone dysplasias known (cretinism) is produced by the total absence of thyroxine. The dysplasia occurs because thyroxine appears to be one of the more important hormones involved in normal bone growth, and its deficiency produces a severe delay in osseous maturation.

With the continued application of DNA technologies, the identification of more of the defective genes producing bone dysplasias has been possible. Table 433.2 lists selected genes causing bone dysplasias, their chromosomal locations, and the gene products. In the future, the identification of additional genes will lead to further elucidation of the various biochemical defects, more reliable and specific methods of diagnosing bone dysplasias prenatally and postnatally and, ultimately, methods of treating or preventing these disorders.

DIAGNOSIS

The diagnosis of a skeletal dysplasia should be considered in any patient who has disproportionately short stature or abnormal development of one or more bones. When one encounters such an individual, that individual should be evaluated fully to determine whether a skeletal dysplasia is present and, if so, which one. The history should include a pregnancy history, with particular reference to any fetal evaluation; birth length, weight, and head circumference; postnatal growth and development; and medical problems. With regard to the family history, one should inquire about short stature and orthopedic problems in other family members and determine if consanguinity exists between the parents. While performing the physical examination, one should take care to search for nonosseous abnormalities such as cataracts, cleft palate, and congenital heart disease that would be useful in establishing the diagnosis and be helpful in formulating a treatment plan. Basic measurements should be obtained, including height, weight, head circumference, arm span, and upper segment–to–lower segment ratio. The lower segment length is determined by measuring the distance from the anterior-superior edge of the pubic symphysis to the floor while the patient is standing, or to the bottom of the feet in infants. The upper segment length is obtained by subtracting the lower segment length from the total body length. The upper segment–to–lower segment ratio is obtained by dividing the upper segment length by the

TABLE 433.2

GENES, CHROMOSOMAL LOCI, AND PEPTIDES, PROTEINS, AND ENZYMES INVOLVED IN SKELETAL DYSPLASIAS

	Gene	Chromosomal Locus	Peptide/Protein/Enzyme
Disorders of Collagen			
Type I collagenopathies			
Osteogenesis imperfecta			
Types I-IV	COL1A1	17q21.31q22.05	α (1) I procollagen
Types I-IV	COL1A2	7q22.1	α (2) I procollagen
Type II collagenopathies	COL2A1 *(multiple mutations)*	12q13.1q13.2	α (II) collagen
Achondrogenesis, type II			
Hypochondrogenesis			
Kniest dysplasia			
Osteoarthrosis, precocious			
Spondyloepiphyseal dysplasia congenita			
Spondyloepimetaphyseal dysplasia, Strudwick type			
Spondyloepiphyseal dysplasia with brachydactyly			
Mild spondyloepiphyseal dysplasia with premature onset arthrosis			
Stickler syndrome, type I			
Wagner syndrome, type II			
Type IX collagenopathies			
Multiple epiphyseal dysplasia	COL9A1	6q13	Type IX collagen
Multiple epiphyseal dysplasia, type 2	COL9A2	1p32.2p33	Type IX collagen
Multiple epiphyseal dysplasia, type 3	COL9A3	20ql3.3	Type IX collagen
Type X collagenopathies			
Metaphyseal dysplasia, Schmid type	COL10A1	6q21q22.3	COL10 α chain
Type XI collagenopathies			
Marshall syndrome	COL11A1	1p21	Collagen II α1, α2 chains
Otospondylomegaepiphyseal dysplasia	COL11A2	6p21.3	Collagen II α1, α2 chains
Stickler syndrome, type II	COL11A2	6p21.3	Collagen II α1, α2 chains
Stickler syndrome, type III	COL11A1	1p21	Collagen II α1, α2 chains
Dysplasias with Significant Membranous Bone Involvement			
Cleidocranial dysplasia	CBFA1	6p21	Core binding factor transcription factor α1 subunit
Disorders with Ectopic Bone Formation			
Fibrodysplasia ossificans progressiva	BMP4	14q22q23	Bone morphogenetic protein 4
Multiple cartilaginous exostoses	EXT1	8q23q24.1	Exostosin-1
	EXT2	11p12p11	Exostosin-2
Trichorhinophalangeal syndrome, type 2 (Langer-Giedion syndrome)	EXT1 & TRPS1	8q	
Disorders of Fibroblast Growth Factor Receptor 3			
Achondroplasia	FGFR3 *(G1138A & G1138C mutations)*	4p16.3	Fibroblast growth factor receptor protein
Hypochondroplasia	FGFR3 *(C1620A)*	4p16.3	Fibroblast growth factor receptor protein
Platyspondylic lethal skeletal dysplasia, San Diego type	FGFR3	4p16.3	Fibroblast growth factor receptor protein
SADDAN (*severe achondroplasia with developmental delay and acanthosis nigricans*)	FGFR3 *(A1949T)*	4p16.3	Fibroblast growth factor receptor protein
Thanatophoric dysplasia, type I	FGFR3 *(C742T, A1118G & others)*	4p16.3	Fibroblast growth factor receptor protein
Thanatophoric dysplasia, type II	FGFR3 *(A1948G)*	4p16.3	Fibroblast growth factor receptor protein
Chondrodysplasia Punctatas			
Chondrodysplasia punctata, rhizomelic type 1	PEX7	6q22–q24	PTS2 receptor
Chondrodysplasia punctata, rhizomelic type 2	DHAPAT	1q42	Dihydroxy-acetonphosphate acyltransesterase

(Continued)

TABLE 433.2

(CONTINUED)

	Gene	Chromosomal Locus	Peptide/Protein/Enzyme
Chondrodysplasia punctata, rhizomelic type 3	AGPS	2q31	alkyl-diahydroxy-diacetonphosphate synthase
Chondrodysplasia punctata, X-linked dominant Conradi-Hünermann type	EBP	Xp11.22p11.23	3β-hydroxy-steriod-Δ^8, Δ^7-isomerase
Chondrodysplasia punctata, X-linked recessive type (brachytelephalangic)	ARSE	Xp22.3	arylsulfatase E
Defects in Cartilage Oligomeric Matrix Protein			
Multiple epiphyseal dysplasia	MATN3		matrilin-3
Multiple epiphyseal dysplasia, Fairbanks and Ribbing types	COMP	19p	cartilage oligomeric matrix protein
	COL9A2	1p32.2p33	type IX collagen
	COL9A3	20q13.3	type IX collagen
	MATN3	2p23p24	matrilin 3
Pseudoachondroplasia	COMP	19p	cartilage oligomeric matrix protein
Defects in Diastrophic Dysplasia Sulfate Transporter			
Achondrogenesis, type 1B	DTDST	5q32q23	defect in diastrophic dysplasia sulfate transporter
Atelosteogenesis, type II	DTDST	5q32q23	defect in diastrophic dysplasia sulfate transporter
de la Chapelle dysplasia	DTDST	5q32q23	defect in diastrophic dysplasia sulfate transporter
Diastrophic dysplasia	DTDST	5q32q23	defect in diastrophic dysplasia sulfate transporter
Multiple epiphyseal dysplasia, autosomal recessive type	DTDST	5q32q23	defect in diastrophic dysplasia sulfate transporter
Dysplasias with Abnormal Mineralization			
Hypophosphatasia, adult form	ALPL	1p36.1p34	tissue nonspecific alkaline phosphatase
Hypophosphatasia, autosomal recessive perinatal lethal and infantile forms	ALPL	1p36.1p34	tissue nonspecific alkaline phosphatase
Hypophosphatemic rickets	PHEX	Xp22.2p22.1	phosphate regulating neutral endopeptidase
Hypophosphatemic rickets, autosomal dominant type	FGF23	12p13.3	fibroblast growth factor 23
Osteopetrosis, infantile form	TC1RG1	16q13	osteoblast proton pump subunit
	CLCN7	11q13.4q13.5	chloride channel 7 pump
		8q	carbonic anhydrase II
Osteopetrosis with renal tubular acidosis	CTSK	1q21	cathespin K
Pyknodysostosis	VDDR1	12q14	25-α-hydroxycholecalciferol-1-hydroxylase
Vitamin D-dependent rickets, type 1	VDDR2	12q12q14	
Vitamin D-resistant rickets with end-organ unresponsiveness to vitamin D3			1,25-α-dehydroxy-vitamin D3 receptor
Mesomelic Dysplasias			
Leri-Weill dyschondrosteosis	SHOX	Xpterp22.32	SHOX protein
Mesomelic dysplasia, Langer type (homozygous Leri-Weill dyschondrosteosis)	SHOX	Xpterp22.32	SHOX protein
Metaphyseal Chondrodysplasias			
Cartilage-hair hypoplasia (metaphyseal chondrodysplasia, McKusick type)	RMRP	9p13	RNA component mitochondrial RNA processing endoribonuclease
Metaphyseal chondrodysplasia, Jansen type	PTHR	3p22p21.1	parathyroid hormone receptor
Miscellaneous Disorders			
Camptomelic dysplasia	SOX9	17q24.3q25.1	SRY-box 9
Cherubism	SH3BP2	4p16.3	SH3 domain-binding protein 2

(Continued)

TABLE 433.2

(CONTINUED)

	Gene	Chromosomal Locus	Peptide/Protein/Enzyme
Chondroectodermal dysplasia (Ellis-van Creveld dysplasia)	EVC	4p16	
Craniometaphyseal dysplasia	ANKH	5p15.2p14.1	pyrophosphate transporter
Dyggve-Melchior-Clausen dysplasia	FLJ90130	18q12q21.1	SH3 domain-binding protein 2
Dyssegmental dysplasia, Silverman-Handmaker type	PLC (HSPG2)	1q36q34	perlecan
Grebe dysplasia	CDMP1	20q11.2	cartilage derived morphogenic protein 1
McCune-Albright fibrous dysplasia	GNAS1	20q13	guanine nucleotide protein α subunit
Nail-patella dysplasia	LMX1B	9q34.1	LIM homeodomain
Pseudohypoparathyroidism (Albright hereditary osteodystrophy)	GNAS1	20q13	guanine nucleotide binding protein of edenylate cyclase α–subunit
Robinow syndrome, autosomal recessive	ROR2	9q22	orphan receptor tyrosine kinase anhydrase II
Schwartz-Jampel syndrome	PLC (HSPG2)	1q36q34	perlecan
Spondylocostal dysplasia	DLL3	19q13	delta-like 3 signaling protein
Spondyloepiphyseal dysplasia tarda	SEDL	Xp22.2p22.1	SEDLIN

Modified with permission from Cohen MM Jr. Merging the old skeletal biology with the new. II Molecular aspects of bone formation and bone growth. *J Craniofac Gene Dev Biol* 2000;20:94. Hall CM. International nosology and classification of constitutional disorders of bone (2001). *Am J Med Genet* 2002;113:65. Superti-Furga A, et al. *Am J Med Genet (Semin Med Genet)* 2001;106:282.

lower segment length. The upper segment–to–lower segment ratio in normal children varies from 1.6 at birth to 0.93 in older teenagers and adults. Many children with bone dysplasias have ratios that are greater than normal for their age as a result of having short lower extremities, whereas children with values less than normal for their age usually have short trunks.

In addition to the clinical evaluation, a complete skeletal radiographic series also is essential, because the diagnosis of many skeletal dysplasias can be made only on the basis of the radiographic findings. A complete survey is crucial, because an inadequate study may not allow for the diagnosis to be established. Films should be obtained for the anteroposterior and lateral views of the skull and the entire spine; anteroposterior views of the chest, hands, and pelvis; and views of all the long bones, including the elbows, knees, and ankles. In patients at risk for atlantoaxial instability, lateral extension and flexion views of the cervical vertebrae must be obtained. If present, atlantoaxial instability may lead to spinal cord compression and loss of nerve function in some individuals, if not detected and treated. Osseous maturation (bone age) should be determined from radiographs of the hand or the left hemiskeleton. Finally, other radiographs must be taken as indicated by the history and findings in the individual patient.

Laboratory testing is important as an aid in the diagnosis of some skeletal dysplasias and to determine the health status of affected patients. Serum calcium, phosphorus, protein, and alkaline phosphatase levels should be obtained to rule out hypophosphatasia, vitamin D–resistant rickets, vitamin D–dependent rickets, and other disorders. Urine screening for storage disorders and other metabolic diseases should be considered. A serum thyroxine level must be determined on any youngster with short stature, large fontanelles, and retarded bone age to diagnose unrecognized hypothyroidism. Other laboratory testing also should be obtained as dictated by the clinical situation.

Classification of Skeletal Dysplasias

An extensive list of skeletal dysplasias is presented in Table 433.1. This table groups skeletal dysplasias into families based primarily on the radiographic appearance of the bones.

From the management standpoint, however, skeletal dysplasias first should be divided into lethal and nonlethal types. A lethal bone dysplasia means that most affected infants die as a result of the condition shortly after birth or during the first year or two of life. A nonlethal skeletal dysplasia implies that the dysplasia usually does not lead to the death of the affected child. The major significance of distinguishing between lethal and nonlethal skeletal dysplasias is that the lethal dysplasias frequently require a decision to be made whether to medically support the affected infant during the newborn period. If the decision is made to support the newborn having a lethal skeletal dysplasia, often extensive and long-term ventilator care may be required. For instance, it is not uncommon for patients with less severe "lethal" skeletal dysplasias to be placed on assisted ventilation after birth and for them to become ventilator-dependent, requiring support for months or years before their eventual death. Thus, it is important for physicians to recognize when newborns have lethal skeletal dysplasias that they probably will not survive despite extensive treatment efforts. In these situations, proper evaluation to establish the diagnosis and subsequent appropriate genetic counseling of the parents are essential. On the other hand, physicians also must be aware that some patients with typically lethal skeletal dysplasias, for example, asphyxiating thoracic dysplasia, may have milder forms of the condition and survive with appropriate respiratory and other medical support.

Lethal Skeletal Dysplasias

The more common lethal skeletal dysplasias are listed in Table 433.3. Usually, these conditions are lethal because the infant

TABLE 433.3

INHERITANCE AND FEATURES OF SELECTED LETHAL SKELETAL DYSPLASIAS

Name of Condition	Mode of Inheritance	Head and Neck	Trunk	Limbs	Other	Radiographic Features
				Clinical Features		
Conditions That Usually Are Lethal in the Neonatal Period						
Achondrogenesis, type I (Parenti-Fraccaro type; subtypes: Houston-Harris, type IA; Fraccaro, type IB)	AR (type IB due to mutation in *DTDST* gene)	Short, flat nose; low-set ears; cleft lip or palate	Short, rounded, protruding abdomen	Very short	Hydrops fetalis, growth failure, congenital heart defects	Poor ossification of cranium, vertebral bodies, pelvis, and sacrum; very short tubular bones; platyspondyly; short, thin, beaded, fractured ribs; short ilia; no pubic ossification
Achondrogenesis, type II (Langer-Saldino type)	AD (due to mutation in *COL2A1* gene)	Same as above	Same as above	Same as above	Same as above	Same as above except almost absent ossification of vertebrae and sacrum, less severe shortening of tubular bones, and well-developed calcification of cranium
Atelosteogenesis, type I (includes boomerang dysplasia)	AD, sporadic	Midface hypoplasia with depressed nasal bridge and micrognathia	Narrow chest, scoliosis	Short limbs, primarily rhizomelic; large joint dislocation; talipes	Polyhydramnios	Vertebral hypoplasia; platyspondyly; absent, short or clubbed humeri; shortened femora with round metaphyses; shortened bowed radius, ulna and tibia; absent fibula
Atelosteogenesis, type II	AR (due to a mutation in *DTDST* gene)	Same as above	Same as above	Same as above, with hitch-hiker thumb	Cleft palate and polyhydram-nios	Coronal and sagittal clefting platyspondyly; short dumbbell-shaped humeri (bifid distally); enlarged second and third metacarpals; hypoplastic, formed fibulae; rounded hypoplastic middle phalanges, short ribs

Fibrochondrogenesis	AR	Flat face, prominent eyes, short neck	Narrow chest	Short, enlarged joints	Cleft palate and occasional omphalocele	Short, dumbbell-shaped tubular bones; short ribs with cupping at anterior ends; platyspondyly, marked coronal cleft of vertebrae; small ilia with narrow sacrosciatic notches
Osteogenesis imperfecta, type II (osteogenesis imperfecta congenita)	AD, with 5–7% recurrence risk from germline mosaicism (mutation in COL1A1 or COL1A2 gene)	Soft calvaria, blue sclerae, pinched nose	Small chest	Short, bent limbs; multiple fractures	CNS hemorrhage, respiratory distress secondary to small chest	Generalized deficiency of bone; wormian bones of the skull; thin ribs with multiple fractures (beading); broad, ribbon-shaped tubular bones with multiple fractures
Schneckenbecken dysplasia (German for snail-shaped)	AR	Macrocephaly, short neck, flat midface	Narrow thorax	Short limbs, brachydactyly	Polyhydramnios	Dumbbell-shaped long bones; platyspondyly with wide vertebral bodies; characteristic snail-shaped pelvis; wide fibula
Short rib-polydactyly, type 1 (Saldino-Noonan type)	AR	Round, flattened face	Narrow chest, protuberant abdomen	Markedly short limbs, postaxial polydactyly	Hydrops fetalis; imperforate anus; defects of heart, lungs, kidneys, and GI tract	Very short long bones; metaphyseal spurs; very short horizontal ribs; platyspondyly, wide intervertebral spaces; small ilia, flat acetabulum
Short rib-polydactyly, type 2 (Majewski type)	AR	Short, flat nose; low-set ears; cleft lip or palate	Same as above	Moderately short limbs, preaxial or postaxial polydactyly	Dysplastic kidneys, respiratory tract anomalies, ambiguous genitalia, PDA	Stippled epiphyses; short, horizontal ribs; wide coronal clefts of vertebrae; trapezoid ilia; hypoplastic, oval shaped tibias

(Continued)

TABLE 433.3

(CONTINUED)

Name of Condition	Mode of Inheritance	Clinical Features					Radiographic Features
		Head and Neck	Trunk	Limbs	Other		
Spondyloepiphyseal dysplasia congenita (severe lethal form)	AD, sporadic (mutation in COL2A1 gene)	Flat face, cleft palate, short neck	Short trunk, barrel-shaped chest	Short limbs	Respiratory distress		Delayed osseous maturation, platyspondyly, coronal cleft of the vertebrae
Thanatophoric dysplasia, type 1 (curved femurs) and type 2 (straight femur with cloverleaf skull)	AD, sporadic (mutation in FGFR3 gene in both types)	Large head, depressed nasal bridge, prominent eyes, large fontanels, small foramen magnum	Narrow thorax, relatively long trunk	Short extremities, extra creases around arms and legs, short fingers with prominent finger creases	Congenital heart defects, respiratory distress		Flat vertebrae that are U-shaped in the thoracic region and inverted U-shaped in the lumbar region; short, bowed long bones; metaphyseal flaring; short ribs; hypoplastic pelvis with narrow sacrosciatic notch
Conditions That May Be Lethal in the Neonatal Period							
Achondroplasia, homozygous form	Homozygous dominant, both parents usually have heterozygous achondroplasia (FGFR3 gene mutation)	Large head with frontal bossing, depressed nasal bridge, large anterior fontanel	Small thorax, protuberant abdomen	Disproportionately short limbs, extra skin folds, trident hand	Respiratory distress		Large calvaria; short narrow base of skull; calvarial thickening; short mandibular rami; short ribs with wide, cupped ends; narrow, flat vertebral bodies; wide intervertebral distances; short, bowed long bones with more proximal shortening
Asphyxiating thoracic dysplasia (Jeune syndrome)	AR	Craniosynostosis occasionally reported (sagittal suture)	Long very narrow thorax, respiratory insufficiency	Extremity shortening variable, short hands and feet, ± postaxial polydactyly	Growth of the chest can occur, and long-term survival is possible		Short horizontal ribs; squared, short ilia; flat acetabulum with spur projecting from end; short middle and distal phalanges with markedly cone-shaped epiphyses

Disorder	Inheritance (gene)	Facies	Thorax	Limbs	Other	Radiographic features
Camptomelic dysplasia	AR (mutation in SOX9 gene)	Large skull; small, flat face; shallow orbits; micrognathia; short palpebral fissures	Small, narrow chest	Short and bowed femurs and tibias, dimples at point of maximum curvature, talipes equinovarus	Sex reversal in some males, cleft palate, generalized hypotonia	Narrow, wavy ribs; hypoplastic cervical vertebral bodies; long, slender, bowed femurs and tibias; short clavicles; hypoplastic scapulas
Chondrodysplasia punctata, rhizomelic forms (types 1, 2 and 3-all due to peroxisomal abnormalities)	AR (all types) (type 1 PEX7 defect, type 2 DHAPAT defect, type 3 AGPS defect)	Flat face, depressed nasal bridge and tip of nose		Rhizomelic shortening of extremities, joint contractures	Ichthyosiform erythroderma, cataracts, mental retardation	Stippled calcification in multiple epiphyses, wide clefts of vertebral bodies, trapezoid ilia, stippling of ischiopubis, calcification of larynx and trachea
Chondroectodermal dysplasia (Ellis-van Creveld dysplasia)	AR (mutation in EVC or EVC2 gene)	Notching or tenting of the upper lip, natal teeth, teeth abnormalities	Long, narrow chest and abdomen	Postaxial polydactyly of the hands and sometimes feet; shortening of arms and hands; hypoplastic nails; short, bowed limbs	Congenital heart defects (atrial septal defect and single atrium most common), long-term survival possible	Short ribs and narrow chest, squared ilia with hook-like spurs from the acetabulum, acromesomelic shortening, cone-shaped epiphyses, fused hamate and capitate bones
Dyssegmental dysplasia, Silverman-Handmaker type	AR [mutation in PCL (HSPG2) gene]	Flat face, orbital hypoplasia, micrognathia	Small thorax	Short, bowed limbs	Encephalocele or occipital defect	Coronal vertebral clefts, marked variation in the size of the vertebral bodies, bowed long bones, advanced carpal maturation

(Continued)

TABLE 433.3
(CONTINUED)

Name of Condition	Mode of Inheritance	Clinical Features					Radiographic Features
		Head and Neck	Trunk	Limbs	Other	
Hypochondrogenesis	AD, usually sporadic (defect in *COL2A1*)	Midface hypoplasia with depressed nasal bridge	Ribs not fractured, abdomen prominent	Very short extremities	Respiratory distress	Short, relatively well-proportioned long bones and vertebrae; small but well-sculptured ilia; partial ossification of ischia; femur straight with flat metaphyseal ends
Hypophosphatasia, congenital lethal form	AR, (mutation in *ALPL* gene)	Soft calvaria, globular-shaped head		Short, bowed flaccid extremities	Low levels of serum alkaline phosphatase and raised levels of phospho-ethanolamine, death hours or days after birth	Poor mineralization of the calvaria; short, thin ribs and tubular bones; irregular ossification of metaphyses; poor mineralization of other bones

AD, autosomal dominant; ALPL, alkaline phosphatase; AR, autosomal recessive; COL, collagen; DHAPAT, dihydroxy-acetonphosphate acyltransferase; DTSD, diastrophic dysplasia sulfate transporter; EVC, Ellis-van Creveld; FGFR, fibroblast growth factor receptor; FGFR3, fibroblast growth factor receptor 3; HSPG2, heparin sulfate proteoglycan of basement membrane 2; PCL, perlecam; PDA, patent ductus arteriosus PEX7, peroxisome biogenesis factor 7; SOX9, SRY-related HMB-box gene 9.

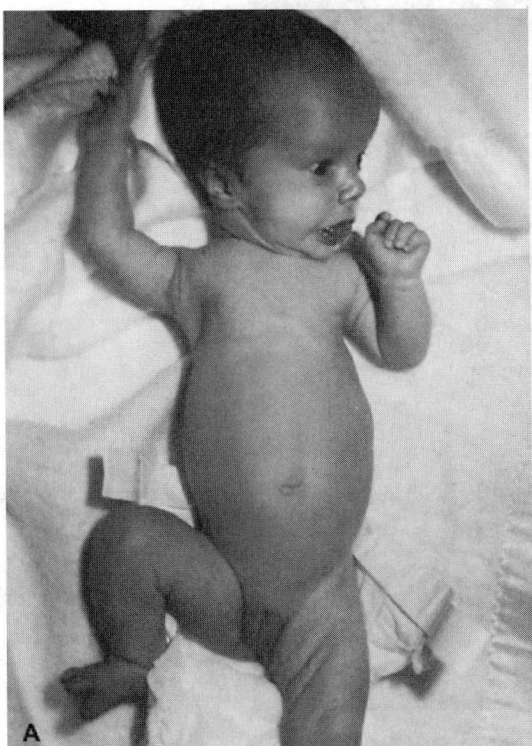

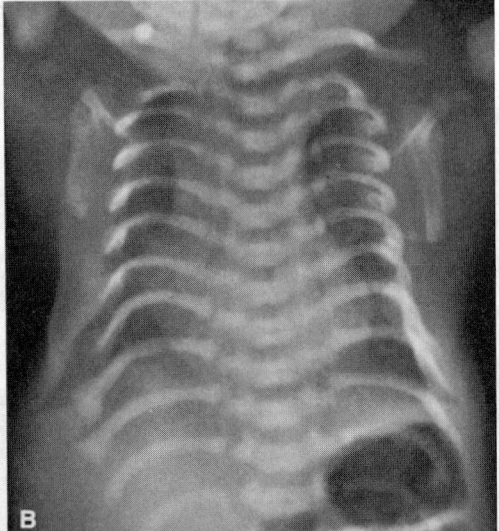

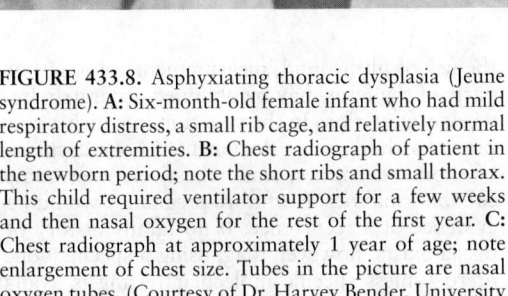

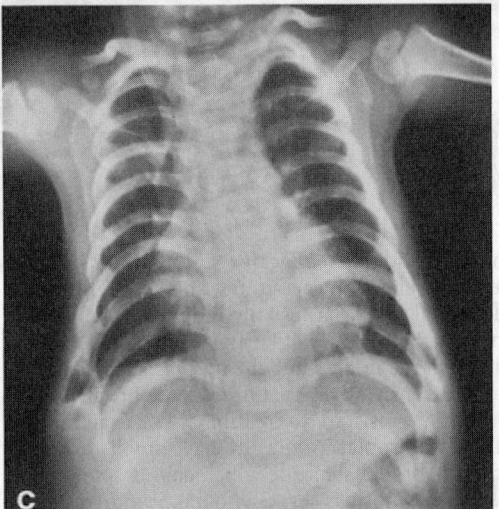

FIGURE 433.8. Asphyxiating thoracic dysplasia (Jeune syndrome). A: Six-month-old female infant who had mild respiratory distress, a small rib cage, and relatively normal length of extremities. B: Chest radiograph of patient in the newborn period; note the short ribs and small thorax. This child required ventilator support for a few weeks and then nasal oxygen for the rest of the first year. C: Chest radiograph at approximately 1 year of age; note enlargement of chest size. Tubes in the picture are nasal oxygen tubes. (Courtesy of Dr. Harvey Bender, University of Notre Dame, South Bend, IN.)

possesses a small thoracic cage as a direct result of having short ribs. The small chest cage leads to respiratory insufficiency and death in most cases. The chest circumference–to–abdominal circumference ratio in most of these cases usually is less than 0.85 and reflects the reduction of the chest size. However, the exact chest size that is consistently lethal has not been fully documented.

Clinically, lethal bone dysplasias are encountered in three time frames. The first is in the prenatal period, when fetuses are detected with short limbs and reduced chest circumferences. When a suspected lethal bone dysplasia is detected in the second trimester, the pregnancy termination option should be discussed with the parents. The second situation is when the child is stillborn or is live-born but dies within minutes or hours after birth, regardless of the effort put forth to support the neonate. The last situation, which generally causes the greatest distress for everyone involved, entails a child who is born with a skeletal dysplasia and who survives when placed on ventilator care. Some of these patients eventually can be weaned from the ventilator, but many cannot. Those children who are weaned successfully tend to survive long term without much, if any, respiratory difficulty. For example, no children with asphyxiating thoracic dysplasia (Fig. 433.8) who have managed to live beyond the age of 2 years have been reported to die of respiratory failure. The reason for their survival appears

to be the growth of the thoracic cage, resulting in adequate respiratory function. On the other hand, only a few children with thanatophoric dysplasia (Fig. 433.9) are known to have lived beyond 2 years, with the oldest reported individual living to age 10. Those who have survived beyond a few days have done so with full respiratory support, and long-term survivors have had growth and neurologic deficiencies, including seizure, hydrocephalus, strabismus, hearing loss, and mental retardation. Thus, when dealing with a newborn with a bone dysplasia, it is critical to establish the diagnosis quickly and then decide if a child should receive long-term ventilator care. If the decision is made to support the child, the parents must be aware of the prolonged nature of the therapy, what the therapy may involve, and the possibility that the child probably will not survive long-term even if he receives full respiratory support.

Nonlethal Skeletal Dysplasias

In contrast to lethal bone dysplasias, the nonlethal dysplasias (Table 433.4) usually do not require intensive neonatal respiratory care, although other problems may be present such as cleft palate, congenital heart defects, or fractures that require medical intervention. These latter individuals are more likely to require medical, orthopedic, and neurosurgical care

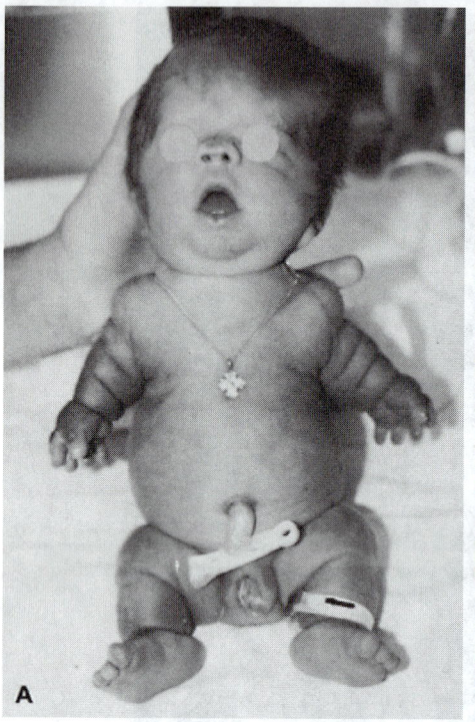
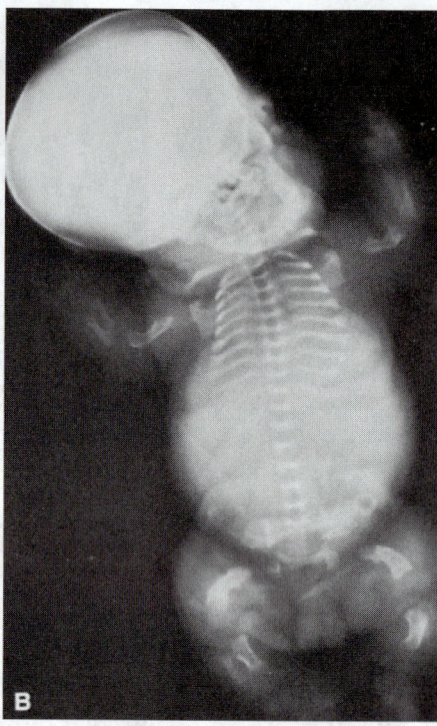

FIGURE 433.9. Thanatophoric dysplasia. **A:** Newborn delivered at 32 weeks' gestation. Note depressed nasal bridge, short extremities with extra skinfold creases, small chest, and prominent abdomen. The patient died a few hours after the picture was taken. **B:** Radiograph of another newborn with thanatophoric dysplasia; note the shortened, bowed long bones, the short horizontal ribs, the U-shaped vertebral bodies, and the tiny pelvis.

as infants, children, and adults. Because of long-term survival and associated problems, the spectrum of problems found in the nonlethal skeletal dysplasias usually is quite different from that found in the lethal disorders. Further, many of the problems encountered in the nonlethal bone dysplasias are chronic and may require extensive therapy. Often, these problems are difficult to treat or are resistant to treatment. For example, individuals with achondroplasia typically have small foramina magna and cervical spinal stenosis, which causes spinal cord compression. If the stenosis is severe enough, it may result in cord necrosis, apnea and sudden infant death (SIDS) during infancy, or hydrocephalus. In addition, many children and adults with nonlethal skeletal dysplasias have orthopedic problems, either in the form of malalignment of the legs or back, or in the form of arthritis that eventually requires total joint replacement.

When providing care for a patient with a nonlethal skeletal dysplasia, the primary-care physician must become familiar not only with the features of the condition, but also with the associated complications. The physician further should educate the parents with regard to these problems and advise them to watch for these complications. Furthermore, the primary-care physician also must assess the affected child periodically for medical problems. A qualified pediatrician or clinical geneticist and an orthopedic surgeon, who are knowledgeable about and experienced in the evaluation and management of skeletal dysplasias and their complications, also should see these children on a regular basis. It should be recognized that when individuals with nonlethal bone dysplasias are managed properly, they can live relatively normal and productive lives.

Prenatal Diagnosis of Skeletal Dysplasias

A prenatal diagnosis of bone dysplasias can be accomplished for many of the disorders by the use of high-resolution ultrasound scans, and molecular and other testing methods. With

the use of ultrasound, measurements of long bones and other parts of the fetus may be obtained accurately by the sixteenth week of gestation. In the situation in which a couple has had a previous child with a documented bone dysplasia, the finding of short extremities, small chest, or other compatible physical abnormalities in a future pregnancy would be presumptive evidence of a recurrence. If no family history of a bone dysplasia exists, however, diagnosing a specific bone dysplasia *in utero* (unless specific molecular testing is available) often is difficult.

Although prenatal ultrasound evaluation is reliable for detecting shorter than normal long bones and raising the suspicion of the bone dysplasia, currently this technique is not completely adequate for making specific diagnoses. In fact, in a recent study, the accuracy rate of prenatal ultrasound for diagnosing specific skeletal dysplasias was 65% and for predicting lethal outcomes was 100%. The latter figure probably is not realistic, and predicting a lethal result without molecular testing to confirm the diagnosis should be done cautiously.

The prenatal diagnosis of achondroplasia, OI, thanatophoric dysplasia, and certain other skeletal dysplasias is possible through DNA testing. In the future, the prenatal diagnosis of most skeletal dysplasias will be accomplished by a combination of more refined ultrasound and molecular techniques, and will be less equivocal than that obtained using current methods. For more specific information on the latest techniques used for the prenatal diagnosis of these disorders, including ultrasound techniques, one should consult a clinical geneticist or perinatologist.

CLINICAL MANIFESTATIONS AND COMPLICATIONS

Tables 433.3 and 433.4 list the relevant features of the common lethal and nonlethal skeletal dysplasias, respectively. (See the Electronic Database Information and Suggested Readings

TABLE 433.4

INHERITANCE AND FEATURES OF SELECTED NONLETHAL SKELETAL DYSPLASIAS

Name of Condition	Mode of Inheritance	Clinical Features				Other/Complications	Radiographic Features
		Head and Neck	Trunk	Limbs			
Conditions Identifiable at Birth							
Achondroplasia, heterozygous type (classic form)	AD, 80% represent new mutations (due to mutation in *FGFR3* gene)	Large head, depressed nasal bridge, prominent forehead and mandible, small foramen magnum	Stocky, prominent buttocks and abdomen	Short extremities with major shortening proximally, trident hands		Spinal stenosis, sudden infant death, hydrocephalus, bowed legs, kyphosis, otitis media, nerve root compression, normal intelligence	Short vertebral pedicles, decreasing lumbosacral distance between pedicles, square-shaped pelvis, ice cream cone-shaped proximal femur and humerus in infancy, relative overgrowth of fibula
Cleidocranial dysplasia	AD (mutation in *CBFA1* gene)	Large head with large fontanels and open sutures, delayed closure of fontanels, persistence of deciduous teeth	Droopy shoulders and narrow chest	Hyperextensible joints; short, squared fingers		Scoliosis; respiratory distress; dislocations of shoulders, head of radius, and hips; adult height normal or slightly reduced; wide variability in expression of disorder	Absence or hypoplasia of clavicles, decreased ossification of skull, multiple wormian bones, delayed ossification of many bones
Chondrodysplasia punctata, dominant type (Conradi-Hunermann disease; CDPX2)	XLD (mutation in *EBP* gene)	Flat face, depressed nasal bridge and tip of nose	Scoliosis	Asymmetrical shortening of limbs, joint contractures		Ichthyosiform erythroderma, alopecia, cataracts, lethal in hemizygous males	Flat facial bones; cleft of vertebral bodies; multiple but variable stippling of epiphyses, vertebrae, and ischiopubis; asymmetry of long bones
Chondrodysplasia punctata, X-linked recessive type; (CDPX1)	XLR (mutation in arylsulfatase E gene)	Nasal hypoplasia		Hypoplasia of distal phalanges, no limb asymmetry, mild short stature		Failure to thrive in infancy, hearing loss, mental retardation, ichthyosis, primarily affects males	Punctate calcifications (epiphyseal, paravertebral, laryngeal, tracheal), short distal phalanges in hands and feet, delayed ossification of calcanei

(Continued)

2523

TABLE 433.4 (CONTINUED)

Name of Condition	Mode of Inheritance	Clinical Features			Other Complications	Radiographic Features
		Head and Neck	Trunk	Limbs		
Diastrophic dysplasia	AR (mutation in *DTDST* gene)	Acute swelling of the pinnae leading to a cauliflower-like ear, cleft palate (50%)	Scoliosis, respiratory distress, kyphosis	Short limbs with club feet, progressive joint contractures, hitchhiker thumbs, symphalangism	Severe limitation of joint movement making feeding and walking difficult, congenital heart defects	Calcium deposits in external ears; precocious ossification of rib cartilage; scoliosis, kyphosis, and lumbar interpedicular narrowing; shortened long bones; broad metaphyses; delayed epiphyseal ossification
Kniest dysplasia	AD, sporadic (mutation in *COL2A1* gene)	Flat face, widely spaced and prominent eyes, depressed nasal bridge	Short trunk, kyphosis, scoliosis, accentuated lordosis, short broad thorax with sternal prominence	Short stature and extremities, prominent joints, joint contractures	Chronic otitis media, hearing loss, retinal detachment, cleft palate, occasionally lethal in the neonatal period	Frontal flattening, hypoplasia of maxilla, platyspondyly, small ilia, club-like metaphyses
Larsen syndrome (multiple congenital dislocations)	AD and AR	Prominent forehead with flat face, depressed nasal bridge, ocular hypertelorism	Laxity of chest wall during early infancy, kyphosis	Multiple dislocated joints (elbows, hip and knees), abnormal hands, pes equinovarus	Hypermobility of small vertebral joints; cervical spinal cord compression producing apnea and death; cleft palate	Multiple joint dislocations, abnormal curvature of the spine, supernumerary carpal bones
Mesomelic dysplasia, Langer type	AR (mutation in *SHOX* gene) homozygous form of Leri-Weill dyschondrosteosis	Micrognathia		Severe mesomelic (forearm and lower leg) shortening	Usually normal intelligence, short stature	Mandibular hypoplasia; shortening of long bones; more severe shortening of radius, ulna, and tibia; severe hypoplasia or absence of fibular epiphyses
Mesomelic dysplasia, Nievergelt type	AD	Nondysmorphic features		Severe mesomelic shortening of legs and sometimes arms	Clubfoot deformities, limited extension of elbows, walking delayed, normal intelligence	Short, triangular and rhomboid-shaped tibia; sometimes shortened fibula and ulna; radioulnar and tarsal synostosis

Condition	Inheritance/Genetics	Head/Face	Chest/Trunk	Limbs/Joints	Clinical Features	Radiographic Findings
Metatropic dysplasia	AD and AR	Normal skull and face	Relatively long trunk with narrow chest, frequently tail-like appendage over sacrum	Prominent joints with restricted range of motion, hyperextensibility of finger joints	Progressive kyphoscoliosis	Marked platyspondyly; hypoplastic, crescent-shaped ilia; short, broad, club-shaped long bones; marked metaphyseal flaring of long bones; epiphyseal dysplasia
Osteogenesis imperfecta, type III	AD, most cases sporadic (mutations in COL1A1 or COL1A2 gene)	Frontal bossing and triangular facies, blue sclerae often	Conical thorax, malaligned spine	Bowed and short limbs (more so in the lower extremities)	Multiple fractures present at birth and throughout life, often wheelchair bound	Severe generalized osteoporosis, wormian bones, mild shortening of long bones, overmodeling
Spondyloepiphyseal dysplasia congenita (Spranger-Wiedemann type)	AD, mostly sporadic (mutation in COL2A1 gene)	Flat face, occasionally ocular hypertelorism, short neck, myopia	Short, barrel-shaped chest, pectus carinatum	Short limbs, neck, and spine; genu valgum; clubfeet; normal sized hands	Subluxation of C1-C2 with cord compression, detached retina, hearing loss, cleft palate	Pear-shaped vertebrae, odontoid hypoplasia, retarded osseous maturation, shortened long bones, moderate kyphoscoliosis with lumbar lordosis
Conditions Identifiable Later in Life						
Arthro-ophthalmopathy (Stickler syndrome)	AD, (mutations in COL2A1, COL11A1 or COL11A2 genes)	Flat face with ocular hypertelorism, epicanthal folds, micrognathia; myopia; cleft of hard or soft palate		Hypotonia; hyperextensible knees; prominent joints; later in life, joint pain and morning stiffness	Pierre Robin sequence, blindness (risk for retinal detachment), cataracts, glaucoma, uveitis, normal to mild short stature, hearing loss. Individuals with a COL11A2 mutation do not have ocular findings.	Wedging of thoracic vertebrae; mild epiphyseal dysplasia; degenerative arthropathy, especially of weight-bearing joints
Cartilage hair hypoplasia (metaphyseal chondrodysplasia, McKusick type)	AR (mutation in MRMP gene)	Fine, sparse hair, eyebrows, and lashes; hair usually is lightly pigmented		Short limbs; short, pudgy hands and feet; laxity of ligaments	Malabsorption, immune deficiency (sometimes lethal reaction to varicella infection), Hirschsprung disease, increased risk of skin cancer	Metaphyseal flaring and irregularities, shortened long bones, disproportionately long fibula, moderate flattening of vertebral bodies during childhood

(Continued)

TABLE 433.4
(CONTINUED)

Name of Condition	Mode of Inheritance	Clinical Features				Other Complications	Radiographic Features
		Head and Neck	Trunk	Limbs			
Dyggve-Melchior-Clausen dysplasia (Smith-McCort dysplasia is allelic to DMC and has identical features except normal intelligence)	AR, (mutations in FLJ90130 gene)	Short neck	Short trunk, prominent sternum, excessive lumbar lordosis, scoliosis	Small hands and feet, claw-like hands, waddling gait, enlarged joints		Mental retardation in most patients	Platyspondyly, pear-shaped vertebrae; C1–C2 subluxation; short broad ilia; late ossification of femoral epiphyses; shortening of the tubular bones with irregular epiphyseal and metaphyseal ossification
Hypochondroplasia	AD (mutation in FGFR3 gene)	Macrocephaly with frontal prominence (in 56%)	Normal, with mild lumbar lordosis	Rhizomelic shortening of extremities, limited elbow extension, broad hands, bowed legs		Mild short stature, muscular appearance	Lumbosacral interpedicular narrowing; short pedicles of vertebrae; short, wide long bones; elongated fibula; short, broad femoral neck
Leri-Weill dyschondrosteosis	AD (mutation in SHOX gene) found in pseudoautosomal region of the X and Y chromosomes	Normal skull and face		Mild forearm shortening, subluxation of distal end of ulna (Madelung's deformity)		Mild short stature in some individuals, occasional pain in wrist, normal intelligence	Radius short in relation to ulna, dorsal subluxation of ulna, short tibia
Metaphyseal chondrodysplasia, Jansen type	AD (mutation in PTHR-parathyroid hormone receptor gene)	Large, broad head with prominent forehead		Short limbs, enlarged joints, clubfeet, osseous, restriction of mobility, ligamentous hyperlaxity		Hypercalcemia	Generalized demineralization; widened, splayed, frayed metaphyses; severe shortening and abnormal curvature of tubular bones; hyperostosis of skull; sclerosis of the base of the skull

Disorder	Inheritance (gene)	Facial/Cranial features	Spine/Trunk features	Limb/Clinical features	Stature/Onset	Radiographic features
Metaphyseal chondrodysplasia, Schmid type	AD (mutation in COL10A1 gene)			Short stature with short extremities; waddling gait; bowed legs		Metaphyseal splaying with cupping of all long bones, shortening of long bones, short femoral necks, coxa vara, genu varum
Multiple epiphyseal dysplasia, Fairbanks (severe) and Ribbing (mild) types	AD (severe type: COMP mutation, mild type: COL9A2, 3 or MATN3 mutation)		Kyphoscoliosis, may have back pain later in life	Pain or arthritis of hips, knees, and ankles; waddling gait; occasionally short hands	Mild short stature in some adults; some may need total hip replacement	Small irregularly ossified epiphyses of all joints (some may have more severe hip involvement); end plates of vertebrae irregular
Osteogenesis imperfecta, types I and IV	AD (mutation in COL1A1 or COL1A2)	Triangular face with a broad, tall forehead; dentinogenesis imperfecta; blue sclerae (type I)	Kyphoscoliosis; pectus carinatum or excavatum	Frequent fractures with often minimal trauma; anterior bowing of femur and tibia may occur in some	Short stature (more severe in type IV); hearing loss in adults	Wormian bones
Pseudoachondroplasia	AD (mutation in COMP gene)	Normal skull and face	Disproportionately long trunk; accentuated lumbar lordosis, mild scoliosis	Shortening of limbs similar to achondroplasia, hypermobility of joints except for elbows; genu valgum or varum; small broad hands	Onset 2 years or later; at risk for osteoarthroses especially of hips and knees; waddling gait	Epiphyseal and metaphyseal dysplasia with striking involvement of the hands and feet; shortened long bones; platyspondyly, tongue-like projection from vertebrae anteriorly; hypoplastic ischium and pubis; irregular acetabulum
Spondyloepiphyseal dysplasia tarda	XLR (mutation in SEDL gene)		Short trunk, prominent sternum, broad thorax, small hips	Osteoarthropathy of hips and knees	Short stature; pain in back, hips, and knees	Hypoplastic or enlarged epiphyses; premature osteoarthrosis of hips; platyspondyly with hump-shaped central portion of body; hypoplastic iliac wings

(Continued)

TABLE 433.4
(CONTINUED)

Name of Condition	Mode of Inheritance	Clinical Features			Other Complications	Radiographic Features
		Head and Neck	Trunk	Limbs		
Spondylometaphyseal dysplasia	AD	Occasional hyperopia	Short trunk, pectus carinatum, kyphoscoliosis	Limitation of movement of larger joints, knee and hip pain, waddling gait	Short stature, cesarean section for affected females because of narrow pelvis	Platyspondyly, kyphosis, scoliosis; narrow sacrosciatic notches; metaphyseal irregularities; delayed carpal ossification; short tubular bones
Spondylo-epimetaphyseal dysplasia, Strudwick type	AD (mutation in COL2A1)	Occasional cleft palate	Pectus carinatum, scoliosis	Short long bones, genu valgum	Short stature, risk for retinal detachment	Short tubular bones; small epiphyses of proximal femur, humerus, and radius; enlarged epiphyses of knees, mild metaphyseal irregularities; excessive down-slanting of ribs; platyspondyly; narrow ilia, hypoplastic acetabulum

AD, autosomal dominant inheritance; AR, autosomal recessive inheritance; CBFA1, core binding factor transcription factor ●1; CDPX1, chondrodysplasia punctate X-linked 1; CDPX2, chondrodysplasia punctate X-linked 2; COL, collagen; COMP, cartilage oligomeric matrix protein; DTDST, diastrophic dysplasia sulfate transporter; EBP, emopamil-binding protein; FGFR, fibroblast growth factor receptor; FLJ90130, unknown meaning; MATN3, matrilin 3; MRMP, RNA component mitochondrial RNA-processing endoribonuclease; PTHR, parathyroid hormone receptor; SEDL, spondyloepiphyseal dysplasia, late; SEDL, spondyloepiphyseal dysplasia, late; SHOX, short stature homeobox-containing gene; XLD, X-linked dominant inheritance; XLR, X-linked recessive inheritance.

TABLE 433.5

MEDICAL COMPLICATIONS OF BOTH LETHAL AND NONLETHAL SKELETAL DYSPLASIAS

Intrauterine	Polyhydramnios, edema, fractures, hydrocephalus, fetal demise
Respiratory	Respiratory distress secondary to small chest and hypoplastic lungs, asphyxiating thoracic dysplasia, small or collapsing trachea, narrowed upper airway and obstruction, snoring, hypoxic episodes, apnea
Central nervous	Hydrocephalus, spinal cord compression, nerve system damage secondary to instability of cervical vertebrae and stenotic vertebral foramina
Skeletal	Kyphosis, scoliosis, excessive lordosis, instability of vertebrae C1 and C2, various vertebral abnormalities, hip dysplasia and dislocated hips, tight and loose joints, joint contracture, osteoarthritis, bowed legs, fractures
Muscular	Truncal hypotonia, muscle disease, contractures of the muscles
Otolaryngologic	Frequent otitis media, hearing loss (conductive and neurosensory)
Dental	Malocclusions, dental crowding, structural abnormalities of teeth
Ophthalmologic	Cataracts, severe myopia, retinal detachment, blindness
Nutritional	Obesity
Obstetric	Constricted birth canal, cephalopelvic disproportions; cesarean section may be required for delivery

Modified with permission from Hall JG, Rimoin DL. Medical complications of dwarfing syndromes. *Growth Genet Horm* 1988;4:6.

sections of this chapter for additional information about these disorders. For in-depth discussions of the three most common bone dysplasias, see the articles and chapters by Francomano and Pauli on achondroplasia, Cohen on thanatophoric dysplasia, and Byers on osteogenesis imperfecta.)

THERAPY

Because of the many complications that can arise with the various skeletal dysplasias, a number of specialists should be available for consultation, including a pediatrician, clinical geneticist, and orthopedic surgeon, as well as an ophthalmologist, otolaryngologist, psychologist, neurologist, neurosurgeon, dentist, orthodontist, dietitian, and physical and occupational therapists. The primary pediatrician or family practitioner caring for the child should coordinate the management and treatment of the child in most cases.

Complications

Essentially, each bone dysplasia has its own set of recognized complications. However, the same complications may be encountered in a number of different skeletal dysplasias. Table 433.5 lists many of these common medical complications, whereas Table 433.6 delineates the specific respiratory problems in these disorders.

Genetic Counseling

Parents of children and adults with skeletal dysplasias must be informed of the mode of inheritance of their particular disorder and the risk of having a recurrence in subsequent pregnancies. Depending on the inheritance pattern of the condition and whether one or both of the parents is affected, the risk varies from the general background risk (which is usually less than 1%) to close to 100%. Normal parents of a child with an autosomal dominant bone dysplasia most likely do not have an increased risk of having another affected child, because their affected child probably is the result of a new mutation. In this situation, however, it is possible that one parent has germline mosaicism. This mosaicism occurs when a percentage of germ cells (usually 5% to 10% of all of the

TABLE 433.6

RESPIRATORY COMPLICATIONS THAT MAY BE ENCOUNTERED IN SKELETAL DYSPLASIAS

Pathology	Conditions
Small, mechanically abnormal chest	Achondrogenesis, types I and II Achondroplasia Achondroplasia, homozygous form Asphyxiating thoracic dystrophy Hypochondrogenesis Short rib-polydactyly syndromes Spondyloepiphyseal dysplasia congenita Thanatophoric dysplasia
Upper airway obstruction, secondary to micrognathia (Robin sequence)	Camptomelic dysplasia Diastrophic dysplasia Stickler syndrome
Upper airway obstruction secondary to basicranial malformations and pharyngeal obstruction	Achondroplasia
Laryngeal stenosis	Atelosteogenesis
Laryngomalacia	Camptomelic dysplasia Diastrophic dysplasia Larsen syndrome
Tracheobron-chomalacia	Camptomelic dysplasia Larsen syndrome Spondyloepiphyseal dysplasia congenita
Central apnea caused by medullary compression from foramen magnum stenosis	Achondroplasia Achondroplasia, homozygous form
Central apnea caused by cervical or medullary compression caused by cervical spine instability or kyphosis	Diastrophic dysplasia Kniest syndrome Larsen syndrome Morquio disease Pseudoachondroplasia Spondyloepiphyseal dysplasia congenita

Modified with permission from Harding CO, Gree CG, Perloff WH, Pauli RM. Respiratory complications in children with spondyloepiphyseal dysplasiacongenita. *Pediatr Pulmonol* 1990;9:49.

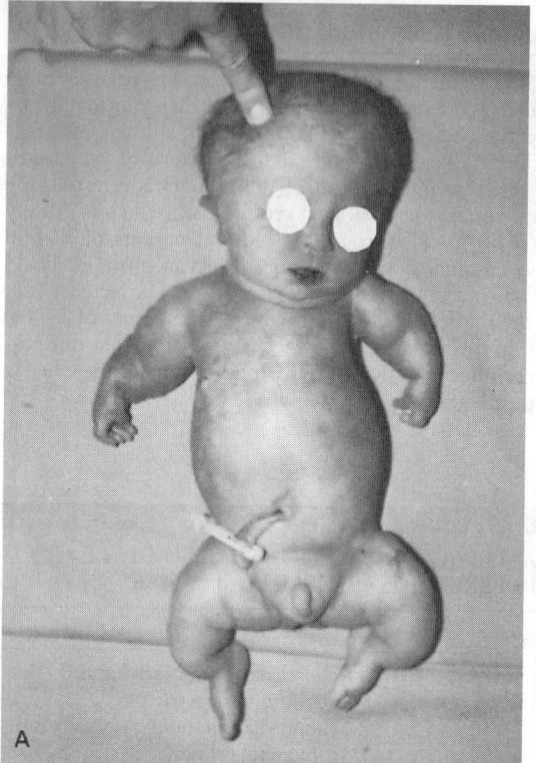 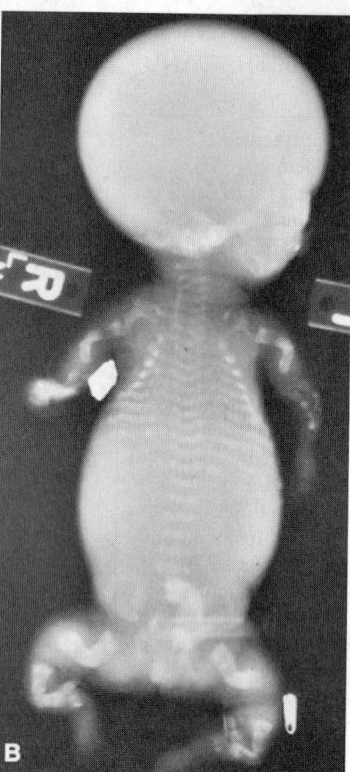

FIGURE 433.10. Osteogenesis imperfecta, type II. **A:** Newborn who died immediately after birth from respiratory insufficiency; note lack of calcified calvaria (finger easily indenting skull) and bowed arms and legs. **B:** Radiograph of another patient with this condition; note the demineralization of all bones (particularly the skull), the ribbon shape of the long bones, the marked bowing of the femora and tibiae, and the multiple fractures (particularly those of the ribs).

germ cells) contains a specific mutation, even though the somatic cells of the parent do not; therefore, that parent is at increased risk for having another child with the same genetic condition as the previous child. For example, OI type II, a lethal neonatal disorder (Fig. 433.10), previously was thought to be an autosomal recessive disorder. We now know that individuals with this disease normally represent new autosomal dominant mutations in the heterozygous state. However, the observed recurrence risk for parents of affected children is 5% to 7%, instead of the much less than 1% expected risk for a new autosomal dominant mutation. The recurrence of OI type II in some of these families has been shown to be the result of germline mosaicism for this autosomal dominant trait.

If the skeletal dysplasia in a particular family is inherited in an X-linked recessive mode, and the mother is a carrier, the recurrence risk in subsequent children of that mother is 25%. If the child's condition is inherited in an autosomal recessive manner, the parent's risk of having future affected children is 25%. In the latter case, the affected child's risk of having an affected offspring is less than 1%, assuming that his or her mate is not a relative. On the other hand, if one parent has an autosomal dominant skeletal dysplasia, the couple has a 50% risk of having an affected offspring.

Psychosocial Counseling

As one would predict, parents who have given birth to a child with a lethal bone dysplasia often need a great deal of emotional support. After the birth of the affected child, they may go through the various stages of grief that are usually observed with the birth of any child with significant abnormalities. Caregivers in these situations must be concerned, sympathetic, and

available to spend time with the parents to discuss the child's condition and parent's feelings.

Parents who deliver a child with a nonlethal dysplasia also may have similar emotional reactions. In addition, they may have numerous questions, such as how tall their child will be, what problems he will have, and whether he will be intellectually normal. If the answers are known, they should be empathically provided. Furthermore, at some time, the parents may wish to become involved in a support group, such as a local chapter of the Little People of America (Little People of America, Inc., 9289 NE Elam Young Parkway, Suite F-700, Hillsboro, OR 97124; e-mail, "mailto:info@lpaonline.org"). This organization was founded to provide answers, support, and fellowship for parents of children with bone dysplasias, their affected children, and adults with these disorders. From the physician's standpoint, the goals of parent counseling are to have them make the best possible adjustment to their child's condition and to encourage their children to foster age-related—not size-related—behavior, social interaction, and independence.

General Medical Management

Appropriate respiratory support, if it is needed, should be undertaken when the decision is made to support a neonate with a severe skeletal dysplasia. Long-term respiratory therapy most likely will be managed better with a tracheostomy. If the child is weaned from the ventilator and survives, she probably will require long-term respiratory management, even if it is only in the form of supplemental nasal oxygen. During infancy, children with skeletal dysplasias, particularly those with achondroplasia, should be evaluated for the development of hydrocephalus. This evaluation should be done by periodic measurement of the head circumference (see Horton for head circumference graphs for achondroplasia) and, if excessive head growth occurs, assessment of the brain by computed tomographic (CT) scanning or magnetic resonance imaging (MRI) should be undertaken. If apnea or other unexplained neurologic problems occur in any child with a bone dysplasia, the size of the foramen magnum should be assessed. Doing so is important, because the foramen magnum may be excessively small and thus the basis of the problems. If this problem is found, neurosurgical decompression by enlarging the foramen should be discussed. Routinely, all newborns or neonates with achondroplasia should be assessed for pathologic spinal cord compression by doing a careful neurologic exam, polysomnography, and CT scan or MRI of the foramen magnum and cervical spine. Abnormal findings in any of these tests may mean abnormal cord compression and a neonate at increased risk of SIDS from spinal cord necrosis; such an infant should be referred to a neurosurgeon for consideration of decompression. Other skeletal dysplasias, such as camptomelic dysplasia, diastrophic dysplasia, Larsen syndrome, and spondyloepiphyseal dysplasia congenita, have an increased risk of cervical spinal cord compression from C1-C2 subluxation. To detect these latter problems, asymptomatic individuals with these conditions should have lateral flexion and extension radiographs of the neck, looking for abnormal slippage of C1 or C2 vertebrae; if the child is neurologically abnormal, then a MRI evaluation of the cervical spine should be performed. In fact, because of the increased incidence of cervical spine abnormalities in many skeletal dysplasias, if a child with any type of skeletal dysplasia has apnea or neurologic abnormalities, the possibility of foramen magnum stenosis and cervical cord compression should be considered. For further information, Lachman has summarized many of the neurologic abnormalities found in bone dysplasias.

In infancy and childhood, recurrent upper airway infections and otitis media are common. These infections should be treated as one would in children without bone dysplasias, and the child's hearing should be checked periodically. Skeletal deformities and malalignment problems also are frequent in skeletal dysplasias. These skeletal problems normally are not amenable to bracing, and at some point, surgical correction often is required. Because of their smaller stature, those with bone dysplasias need fewer calories, and because they are often served portions designed for normal-sized persons, obesity also is common. Good dietary and nutritional habits should be encouraged starting in early childhood.

Previously, it was thought that it was impossible to increase the ultimate height of an individual with short stature resulting from a skeletal dysplasia. However, surgical techniques and equipment are available that can increase bone length. The procedure (Ilizarov procedure) involves breaking one or more of the long bones of the legs (or arms), and then daily separating the ends of the bone over a period of months. The continuous separating of the ends of the bones allows new bone growth between the broken ends. The procedure has resulted in increases of up to 25 to 30 cm of height in some individuals. However, the complication rate of the procedure is high, most commonly infections, and nerve damage can occur. Supplemental growth hormone therapy also has been tried to gain additional height in individuals with a variety of different skeletal dysplasia, most commonly achondroplasia and hypochondroplasia. Studies reporting on growth hormone use in individuals with achondroplasia have found increased growth velocities (0.3 to 0.7 SD), with the greatest gains in the first 1 to 2 years of treatment. Whether these results will translate to long-term gains in height still is uncertain. In addition, at least one study has shown a disproportionate increase in torso length in comparison to leg length in individuals with achondroplasia on long-term growth hormone therapy, which is concerning because this exacerbates the disproportionality in this condition.

Exercise should be promoted in children with bone dysplasias to assist in weight control and to develop strength and good muscle tone. These children, however, should avoid physical activities and contact sports that can damage their joints, opting instead for low-impact activities such as swimming and bicycling. Arthritis and neurologic problems are common in teenagers and adults with bone dysplasias. Frequently, these problems are more severe in overweight individuals or in those who have been unusually active.

Because medical problems are relatively common and often have major consequences in individuals with bone dysplasias, both during childhood and later in life, medical personnel should take complaints by these people seriously and investigate these complaints thoroughly. When significant problems are detected, appropriate management must be undertaken to prevent life-long disabilities and death.

Specific Management for Skeletal Dysplasias with Osteoporosis

The bisphosphonates are a group of medications that selectively decrease osteoclastic function. Decreasing osteoclastic function reduces bone breakdown, thus resulting in increased bone density. Bisphosphonate treatment of children (and adults) with osteoporosis and OI results in increased bone density and decreased bone pain and fractures. The improvement is significant enough that we recommend treatment with bisphosphonates for all individuals with moderate to severe OI. Currently, most children who are treated with bisphosphonates receive it intravenously. Oral forms of the bisphosphonates also are available, and their efficacy in children is being evaluated. Growth hormone therapy also has been studied in children with OI, and its use has resulted in increased growth velocity. The affect on fractures when using growth hormone therapy is not clear, with at least one study reporting increased fractures. Bone marrow transplant also has been attempted to treat severe OI and has resulted in increased bone density in those with successful engraftment. However, bone marrow transplant is not considered first-line therapy for OI at this time, because similar results can be achieved using bisphosphonates, without the risk of bone marrow rejection. One can find a more extensive discussion of the management of OI in the publication by Marini and Chernoff.

Surgical Management

Nonosseous birth defects, such as cleft lip and congenital heart disease, can occur in infants with skeletal dysplasias, and these problems in themselves may require treatment. Those medical problems directly related to the skeletal dysplasia frequently develop with age and should be treated at appropriate times and by appropriate means. For example, bowing of the legs in children with achondroplasia is common and results from the fibulas growing more rapidly than the tibias. The recommended treatment for this problem is osteotomy of the tibias and fibulas, with appropriate alignment of these bones. Bracing for this bowing is ineffective.

Other skeletal problems commonly found in individuals with skeletal dysplasias that may require surgical intervention include scoliosis, kyphosis, hip dysplasia, coxa vara, coxa valga, genu valgum, atlantoaxial instability, arthritis, and spinal or nerve root compression. If arthritis is present, and severe enough to cause significant pain or immobility, joint replacement may be appropriate treatment. Many neurologic problems encountered in skeletal dysplasias result from the abnormal size or shape of the vertebrae or small vertebral

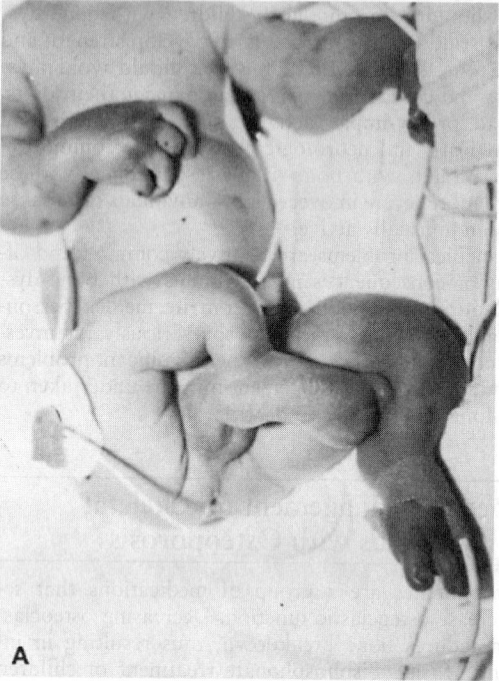 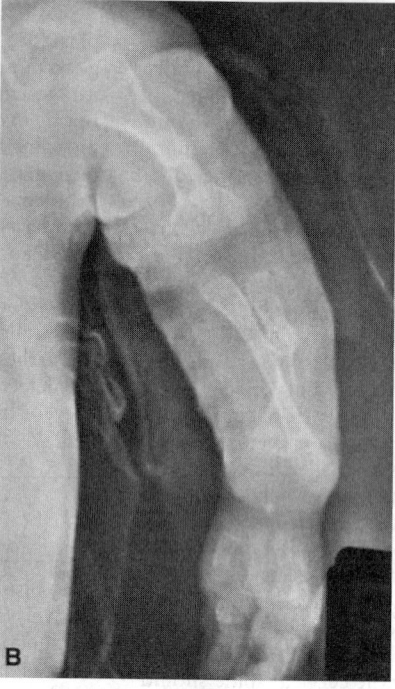

FIGURE 433.11. Osteogenesis imperfecta, type III. **A:** Extremities and trunk of a newborn who survived; note marked bowing of the extremities. **B:** Radiograph of another patient (aged 1 month) with this condition; observe the marked osteoporosis, relative thinness, and fractures of the bones.

foramina. Surgical intervention may preserve function or be life-saving in these situations.

Surgeons who treat children with bone dysplasias should be experienced in the treatment of these disorders. Often, the surgical management of bone dysplasias differs from the management of similar orthopedic problems in other patient populations. For example, in diastrophic dysplasia, an exaggerated inflammatory response to joint trauma occurs, which in turns leads to marked joint stiffness and fusion. As a result, severe limitation of movement in children with diastrophic dysplasia is common. However, treatment is not directed at making the foot mobile, but rather at keeping the foot in a functional position, to allow weight bearing and ambulation.

Death and Autopsy

Because many skeletal dysplasias are lethal during the neonatal or early childhood period, and because of pregnancy terminations from skeletal dysplasias, the practitioner is likely to become involved with a dead fetus or a child with a bone dysplasia. In one study, 30% of recognized skeletal dysplasias were lethal or terminated. The two most common neonatal lethal conditions are thanatophoric dysplasia and OI type II. These two conditions usually are not difficult to diagnose to the knowledgeable or experienced physician and, in questionable cases, the diagnosis can be confirmed by biochemical or molecular testing. The problem with lethal bone dysplasias arises when the diagnosis has not been established prior to the time of death. If adequate radiographs have not been obtained, these should be taken. If the case involves a newborn, a "babygram" may suffice; that is, an anterior-posterior radiograph of the dead child placed on a large cassette without clothing or wrappings. In others, particularly older infants and children, a complete skeletal survey should be obtained. To document the physical findings, and to share with a clinical geneticist later, color photographs or digital pictures also should be taken. Finally, an autopsy, if possible, should be performed. During the autopsy, bone and cartilage must be obtained and later histologically

analyzed, because the histologic appearance of these tissues may be diagnostic. In addition, skin, lung, or Achilles tendon for culturing fibroblasts also should be acquired. This tissue should be placed immediately in transport medium and sent to the tissue culture lab for culturing. From these fibroblasts, biochemical and molecular testing can be performed. Consideration also should be given to collecting blood before death, or tissue after death, to extract and store DNA for later genetic testing.

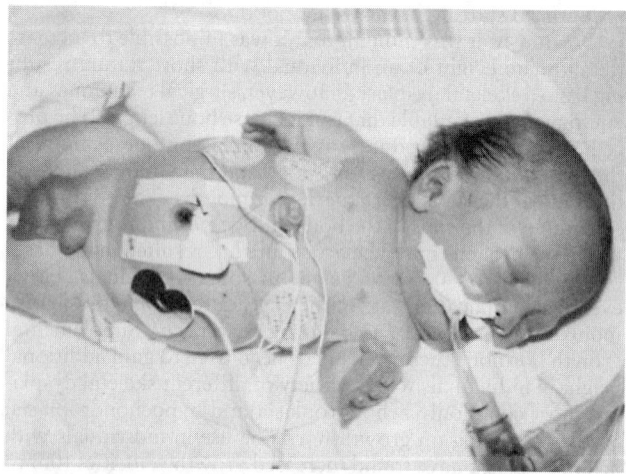

FIGURE 433.12. Diastrophic dysplasia in a term newborn. Note the remarkably short extremities, the position of the thumbs (hitch-hiker thumbs), relatively normal chest size, and normal ears. The ears became inflamed at about 2 weeks of age and developed the typical cauliflower appearance seen in this disorder. The patient had tracheomalacia and respiratory distress during infancy, but now has no significant respiratory problems.

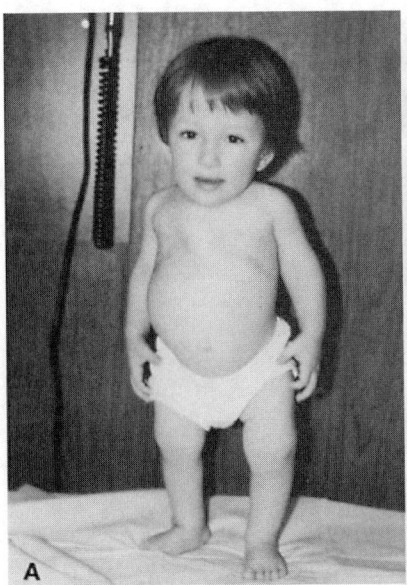
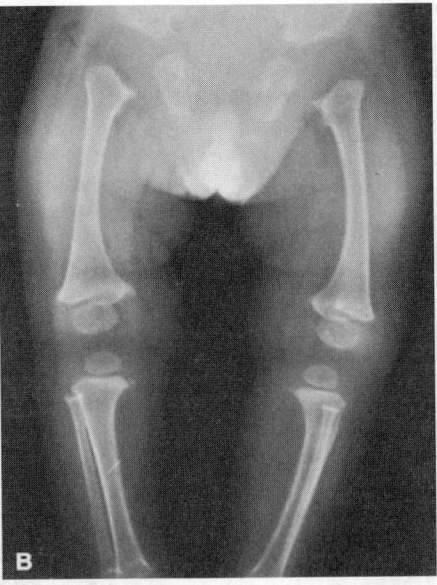
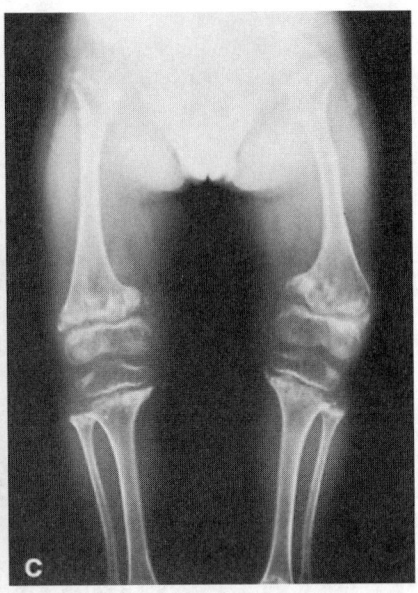

FIGURE 433.13. Spondyloepiphyseal dysplasia congenita. **A:** Boy (2.5 years old) with the disorder; note short stature, chest deformity, lordosis, and prominent abdomen. **B:** Radiograph of hips and lower extremities of patient at 9 months of age; observe mild epiphyseal and metaphyseal involvement. **C:** Radiograph of patient's hips and legs at 9.5 years of age; note the marked involvement of both the epiphyses and metaphyses at this age.

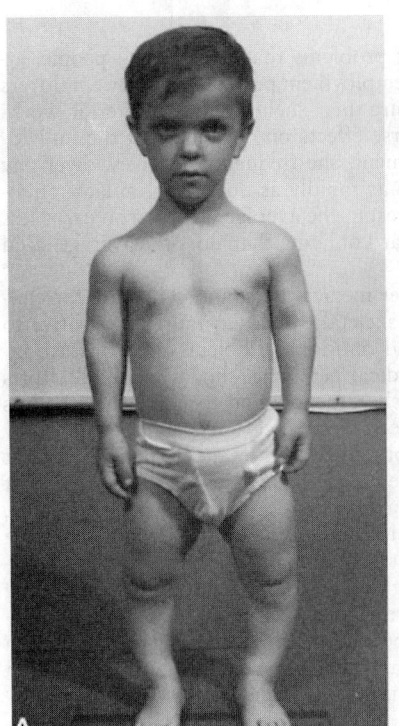
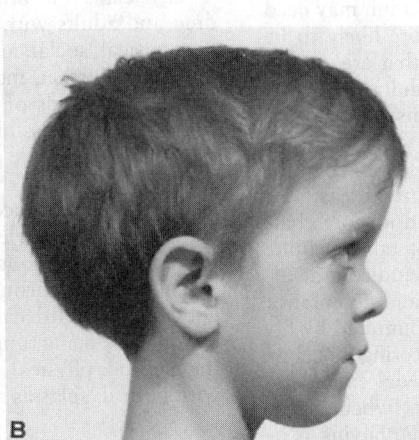
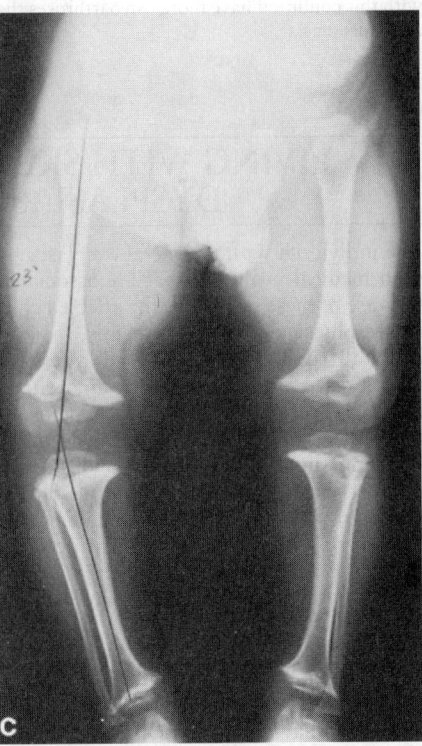

FIGURE 433.14. Achondroplasia in a 7-year-old boy. **A:** Note short arms and legs, particularly in the proximal portions (rhizomelia), and bowing of lower extremities. **B:** Note larger than normal dolichocephalic head, frontal bossing, and mildly depressed nasal bridge. **C:** Radiograph of lower extremities; note angulation of right leg and widening of the metaphyses.

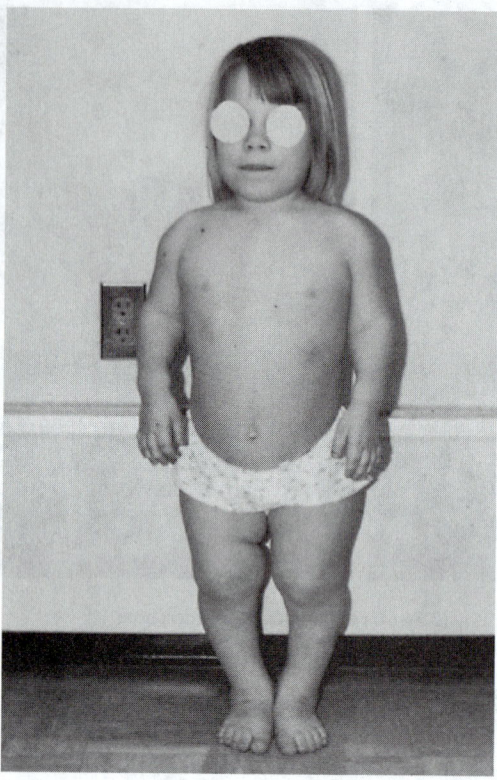

FIGURE 433.15. Pseudoachondroplasia in an 11-year-old child; note short stature, short extremities, and normal face. Children and adults with this condition have more osteoarthroses than do individuals with achondroplasia.

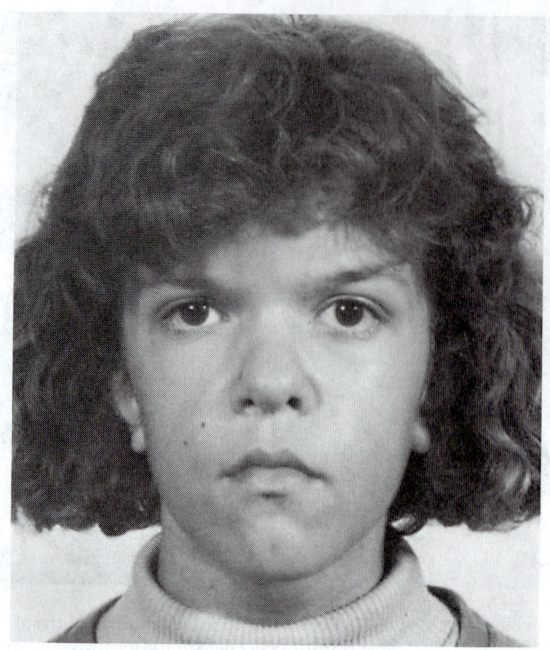

FIGURE 433.16. Facial view of a 13-year-old child with achondroplasia; note mild depression of the nasal bridge, shortening of the nose, and mild malar hypoplasia.

LIVING WITH SKELETAL DYSPLASIAS

The individual with a skeletal dysplasia frequently must cope with medical problems that are associated with his disorder. Because of these problems, the affected child or adult may need to see physicians more frequently, may be more likely to be hospitalized, and may have medical expenses that are greater than most. Furthermore, older children and adults with bone dysplasias often have more aches, pains, and discomfort than do those without these conditions.

Being short also poses other disadvantages. Living space in most societies is designed for persons who are at least 152 cm (5 ft) tall. As a result, short individuals find it more challenging to live in an environment designed for taller people. In addition, many short people experience prejudice that directly affects their self-image, earning power, and acceptance in society. Examples of specific difficulties encountered by little people include being unable to reach the steering wheel or pedals of an automobile without pillows or pedal extenders; being unable to touch the floor with their feet when sitting in a chair; having to hem or alter most clothing; having people bump into them in crowded public places because they are not seen; and being unable to reach light switches, window latches, or curtain pulls. Negative emotional reactions may result from being teased about their height, being stared at by both children and adults, being placed in embarrassing situations such as being the "class dwarf," feeling smothered (unable to get enough air) when in crowds where everyone is taller, and being leaned on or patted on top of the head like a pet.

The most devastating problems that many small people encounter, however, are employment prejudices. Many employers hesitate or refuse to hire them, believing them inferior workers or as having adverse effects on customers. If the individual does find employment, she frequently receives lower pay and does not advance as rapidly as do other, similarly qualified individuals. As a result, the average little person earns less and has a lower standard of living than does the average-sized individual.

Physicians and other medical personnel who care for children and adults with skeletal dysplasias must be sensitive to the physical, social, and emotional problems faced by these individuals. Further, medical personnel should make all efforts to meet the needs of short people and to make them feel as comfortable as possible in the medical environment where they receive care, be it the physician's office, the outpatient clinic at a medical center, or the hospital. Despite all the difficulty that most little people encounter, they learn to accept being short, adjust their living style to compensate for their height, and have a sense of humor about their size. Most are well-adjusted individuals who get through life just fine. In addition to providing good quality health care, the pediatrician also can help these individuals by being supportive and by attempting to break down the medical, physical, and psychological barriers that children with bone dysplasias and their families face.

ELECTRONIC DATABASE INFORMATION

Numerous web-based databases are available for additional and specific information on skeletal dysplasias. Listed here are several of these web sites and their web addresses:

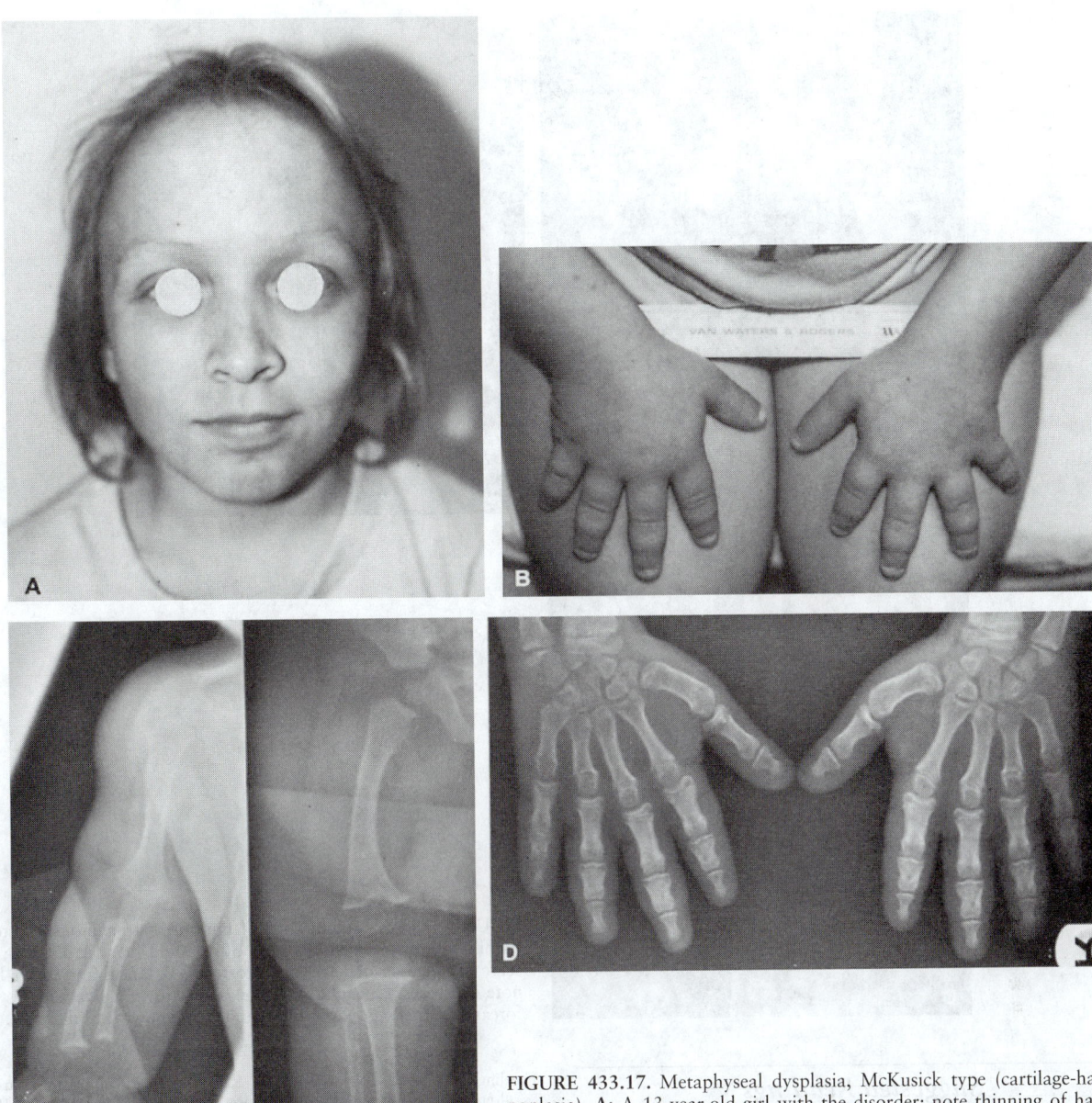

FIGURE 433.17. Metaphyseal dysplasia, McKusick type (cartilage-hair hypoplasia). **A:** A 13-year-old girl with the disorder; note thinning of hair and normal facial appearance. **B:** Hands of the same patient; note short fingers. **C:** Radiographs of the patient at age 9 months; observe bowing of femur and widening of the metaphyses. **D:** Radiographs of the hands of the patient at age 13 years; observe shortening of all tubular bones.

American Academy of Pediatrics, http://aappolicy. aappublications.org (health supervision for children with achondroplasia)

- GeneTests, http://www.genetests.org/(review articles on a number of skeletal dysplasias)
- Online Mendelian Inheritance in Man (OMIM), http://www.ncbi.nlm.nih.gov/Omim/(information on most inherited skeletal dysplasias)
- Osteogenesis Imperfecta Foundation, http://www.oif.org (information on osteogenesis imperfecta)

In addition to the above web-site databases, GeneTests (http://www.genetests.org/) also lists laboratories that do gene testing for many bone dysplasias. However, GeneTests only lists disorders for which gene testing is available, and it separates those laboratories doing commercial testing that charge for their service from those doing research. Although research laboratories normally do not charge for testing, they often will not state when results will be available.

Finally, three databases are only available by purchasing them. The first two, *Pictures of Standard Syndromes and Undiagnosed Malformations (POSSUM)* and *London Dysmorphology Database (LDD)* contain information on and pictures of numerous dysmorphic disorders, including most bone dysplasias, whereas the third, *Radiological Electronic Atlas of Malformation Syndromes and Skeletal Dysplasias (REALM)*, contains information primarily on skeletal dysplasias. The last database provides numerous radiographs to illustrate the over 200 skeletal dysplasias listed.

Figures 433.11 through 433.18 provide examples of other skeletal dysplasias.

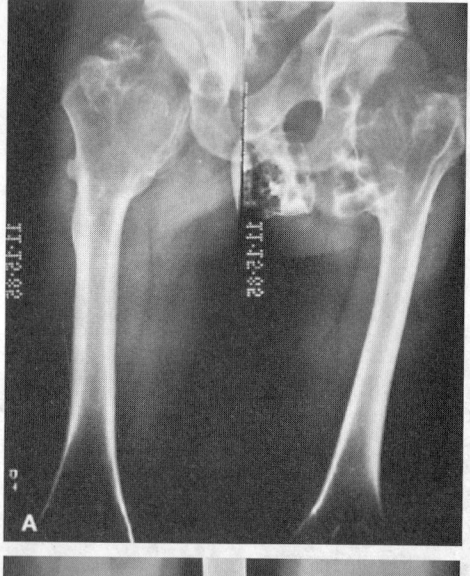

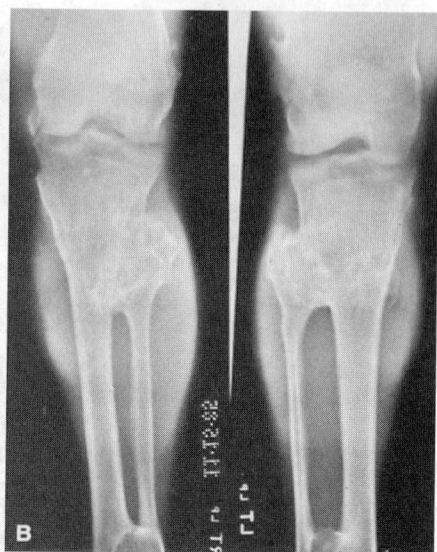

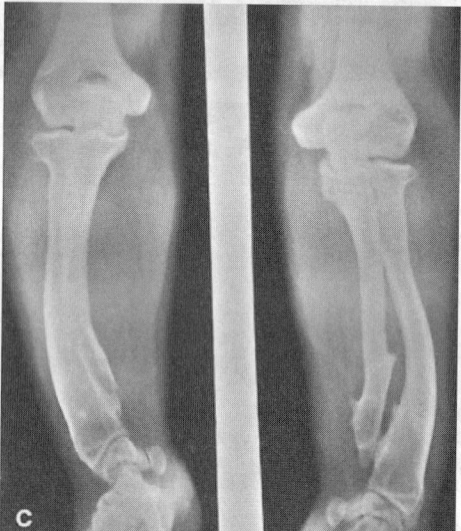

FIGURE 433.18. Radiographs of multiple cartilaginous exostoses (familial multiple exostoses) in a 30-year-old man. **A:** Femurs; observe broadening of neck and exostoses. **B:** Knees and lower legs; note exostoses. **C:** Right (*left side*) and left (*right side*) elbows and forearms; note hypoplasia of the ulnae and bowing of the radii.

Suggested Readings

Baker ER, Goldberg MJ. Diagnosis and management of skeletal dysplasias. *Semin Perinatol* 1994;18:283.

Beighton P. *McKusick's heritable disorders of connective tissue.* St. Louis: Mosby, 1993.

Byers PH. Disorders of collagen biosynthesis and structure. In: Scriver CR, Beaudet AL, Sly WS, Valle D, eds. *The metabolic and molecular bases of inherited diseases,* 8th ed. New York: McGraw-Hill Medical Publishing Division, 2001:5241.

Cohen MM Jr. Fibroblast growth factor receptor mutations. In: Cohen MM Jr., MacLean RE, eds. *Craniosynostosis: diagnosis, evaluation, and management,* 2nd ed. New York: Oxford University Press, 2000:77.

Cohen MM Jr. Merging the old skeletal biology with the new. II Molecular aspects of bone formation and bone growth. *J Craniofac Gene Dev Biol* 2000;20:94.

Cohen MM Jr. Some chondrodysplasias with short limbs: molecular perspectives. *Am J Med Genet* 2002;112:304.

Cohen MM Jr. Thanatophoric dysplasia. In: Cohen MM Jr., MacLean RE, eds. *Craniosynostosis: diagnosis, evaluation, and management,* 2nd ed. New York: Oxford University Press, 2000:366.

De Moerlooze L, Dickson C. Skeletal disorders associated with fibroblast growth factor receptor mutations. *Curr Opin Genet Dev* 1997;7:378.

Francomano CA. Achondroplasia. At GeneTests (http://www.genetests.org/), 2003.

Givol D, Yayon A. Complexity of FGF receptors: genetic basis for structured diversity and functional specificity. *FASEB J* 1992;6:3362.

Hall CM. International nosology and classification of constitutional disorders of bone (2001). *Am J Med Genet* 2002;113:65.

Hall JG, Rimoin DL. Medical complications of dwarfing syndromes. *Growth Genet Horm* 1988;4:6.

Harding CO, Gree CG, Perloff WH, Pauli RM. Respiratory complications in children with spondyloepiphyseal dysplasia congenita. *Pediatr Pulmonol* 1990;9:49.

Horton WA, Rotter JI, Rimoin DL, et al. Standard growth curves for achondroplasia. *J Pediatr* 1978;93:435.

Kornak U, Mundlos S. Genetic disorders of the skeleton: a developmental approach. *Am J Hum Genet* 2003;73:447.

Lachman RS. Neurologic abnormalities in skeletal dysplasias. *Am J Hum Genet* 1997;69:33.

Marini JC, Chernoff EJ. Osteogenesis imperfecta. In: Cassidy SB, Allanson JE, eds. *Management of genetic syndromes.* New York: Wiley-Liss, 2001:281.

Pauli RM. Achondroplasia. In: Cassidy SB, Allanson JE, eds. *Management of genetic syndromes.* New York: Wiley-Liss, 2001:9.

Pauli RM, Horton VK, Glinski LP, Reiser CA. Prospective assessment of risks for cervicomedullary-junction compression in infants with achondroplasia. *Am J Hum Genet* 1995;56:732.

Rimoin DL. Molecular defects in the chondrodysplasias. *Am J Med Genet* 1996;63:106.

Rimoin DL, Lachman RS. The chondrodysplasias. In: Emery AEH, Rimoin DL, eds. *Principles and practice of medical genetics.* New York: Churchill Livingstone, 1990:895.

Scott CI Jr. Dwarfism. *Clin Symp* 1988;40:2.

Spranger JW, Brill PW, Poznanski A. *Bone dysplasias: an atlas of genetic disorders of skeletal development,* 2nd ed. New York: Oxford University Press, 2002.

Spranger JW, Maroteaux P. The lethal osteochondrodysplasias. *Adv Hum Genet* 1990;19:1.

Superti-Furga A, Bonafe' L, Rimoin DL. *Am J Med Genet (Semin Med Genet)* 2001;106:282.

Weaver DD. Molecular-pathogenetic classification of genetic disorders of the skeleton. *Catalog of prenatally diagnosed disorders,* 3rd ed. Baltimore: Johns Hopkins University Press, 1998.

SECTION XIII ■ CONNECTIVE TISSUE DISEASES

CHAPTER 434 ■ RHEUMATIC DISEASES OF CHILDHOOD

JAMES T. CASSIDY

The rheumatic diseases of childhood comprise a group of heterogeneous disorders that result in inflammation of the connective tissues of the body. A frequent manifestation of these diseases is arthritis: the objective inflammation of a joint. Although the etiologies of these disorders are unknown, many have an immunogenetic predisposition and are characterized by prominent autoimmune phenomena: circulating autoantibodies such as antinuclear antibodies (ANAs) and rheumatoid factors (RFs) and, in some cases, the deposition of immunoglobulins in affected tissues. Often, tissue accumulation of lymphocytes and plasma cells occurs. Usually, these rheumatic diseases are chronic and seemingly self-perpetuating, although many respond to nonsteroidal antiinflammatory drugs (NSAIDs), glucocorticoids, antiinflammatory drugs, or immunosuppressive agents.

Data on the prevalence of the rheumatic diseases in children are incomplete. Juvenile rheumatoid arthritis (JRA) is the most common disorder for which reasonable estimates of frequency have been published. A study from Minnesota cited an incidence of 13.9 per 100,000 children per year (95% confidence limits: 9.9 to 18.8) and a prevalence of 113.4 per 100,000 children (95% confidence limits: 69.1 to 196.3). A Finnish investigation estimated its incidence to be 18.2 per 100,000 children per year, and the incidence of all forms of arthritis in childhood to be 108.5 per 100,000.

The prevalence of the other rheumatic diseases can be estimated by noting their relative frequency of referral to pediatric rheumatology clinics. Table 434.1 includes data from children referred to these clinics in North America from 1992 to 2002.

Table 434.2 is a condensed diagnostic classification of juvenile arthritis. Each of the major types of rheumatic diseases

TABLE 434.1

FREQUENCY OF THE PEDIATRIC RHEUMATIC DISEASES

Disease	Number of Cases (%)
Juvenile rheumatoid arthritis	7,368 (12.8)
Connective tissue diseases	3,861 (6.7)
Spondyloarthropathy and reactive arthritis	2,973 (5.1)
Psoriatic arthropathy	173 (0.3)
Infectious arthritis and osteomyelitis	1,620 (2.8)
Malignancy/hematologic	290 (0.5)
Chronic pain syndromes	4,483 (7.8)
Hypermobility and overuse syndromes	2,745 (4.7)
Other diseases	34,216 (59.3)

57,729 diagnoses from 48,934 consecutive patients with definite diagnoses entered into the Pediatric Rheumatic Disease Registry of the Pediatric Rheumatology Database Research Group 1992–2002. Courtesy of Suzanne Bowyer, M.D., Pediatric Rheumatology Database Research Group.

TABLE 434.2

DIAGNOSTIC CLASSIFICATION OF JUVENILE ARTHRITIS

Connective tissue diseases
Juvenile rheumatoid arthritis
Systemic lupus erythematosus
Dermatomyositis
Scleroderma
Vasculitis

Psoriatic arthritis

Seronegative spondyloarthropathies
Juvenile ankylosing spondylitis
Inflammatory bowel disease

Infectious arthritis
Bacterial arthritis (including staphylococcal, gonorrhea, tuberculosis)
Viral arthritis
Fungal arthritis
Lyme disease

Reactive arthritis
Rheumatic fever
Post-*Yersinia* arthritis

Rheumatic diseases associated with immunodeficiency

Congenital anomalies and genetically determined abnormalities of the musculoskeletal system
Constitutional diseases of bone
Lysosomal storage diseases
Heritable disorders of collagen and fibrous connective tissue
Amyloidosis

Nonrheumatic conditions of bones and joints
Traumatic arthritis
Reflex neurovascular dystrophy
Legg-Calvé-Perthes disease
Slipped capital femoral epiphysis
Toxic synovitis of the hip
Osteochondritis dissecans
Patellofemoral pain syndromes
Plant-thorn synovitis

Hematologic diseases
Sickle cell disease
Hemophilia
Thalassemia
Leukemia and lymphoma

Neoplastic diseases
Neuroblastoma
Malignant and benign tumors of cartilage, bone, and synovium
Histiocytosis

Arthromyalgia
Growing pains
Idiopathic pain syndromes

is included, but only selected subtypes pertinent to pediatric practice are provided for each category. As in all other areas of medicine, the correct diagnosis of a disease without a pathognomonic finding or known etiology requires the careful exclusion of similar disorders. Most of the rheumatic diseases occur more commonly in girls than in boys. However, exceptions occur, such as for polyarteritis and ankylosing spondylitis.

In JRA, the primary focus of the clinical disease is on arthritis: synovitis of the joints of the appendicular skeleton. Arthritis must be distinguished from arthralgia, which is pain in a joint without objective findings of inflammation on physical examination. Many more children have transient episodes of arthralgia, or even of arthritis, than can be categorized as JRA. One study estimated that only approximately 15% of children with unexplained arthralgia go on to develop chronic arthritis that meets the classification criteria for JRA.

Although arthritis is a frequent characteristic of the other rheumatic diseases, often they have more prominent manifestations of inflammation in other organ systems (Table 434.3). In systemic lupus erythematosus (SLE), the primary focus is immune-complex vasculitis of the arterioles that underlie the cutaneous, mucosal, and serosal surfaces of the body and involvement of internal organs, such as the kidneys and central nervous system (CNS). In dermatomyositis, the affected organs primarily are the skeletal muscles, skin, and gastrointestinal tract. In scleroderma, the skin, gastrointestinal tract, and cardiopulmonary system primarily are involved. In idiopathic or primary vasculitis, blood vessels are the predominant target organs, with multisystem disease involving the CNS; cardiopulmonary, gastrointestinal, and renal systems; and the skin, depending on the specific type of vasculitis in the child.

JUVENILE RHEUMATOID ARTHRITIS

JRA is the most common pediatric rheumatic disease having arthritis as the principal manifestation. It is one of the more frequent chronic childhood illnesses and a leading cause of disability and blindness.

Pathogenesis

The etiology of JRA is unknown. It likely does not represent a single disorder but rather a spectrum of diseases of diverse pathogenesis. An immunogenetic predisposition is present in certain children: the HLA antigens DR5 (DRB1*1104), DRw6, DRw8, DQw1 (DQA1*0501), and DPw2.1 (DPB1* 0201) are associated with the development of persistent oligoarthritis at an early age in young girls with ANA seropositivity, and DR4 (DRB1*0401 and 0404) is increased in frequency in older children with polyarthritis who are seropositive for RFs. The risk associated with these immunogenetic profiles appears to be age-related. A JRA-like arthritis is a manifestation of

---

TABLE 434.3
CLINICAL MANIFESTATIONS OF CONNECTIVE TISSUE DISEASES

Features	Juvenile Rheumatoid Arthritis	Systemic Lupus Erythematosus	Dermatomyositis	Systemic Scleroderma	Polyarteritis
Female-to-male ratio	2:1	5:1	2:1	2:1	1:3
Constitutional symptoms	+++	+++	+++	++	+++
Arthritis	+++	++	+	+	+
Dermatitis	+	+++	+++	++	+
Photosensitivity	−	++	+	−	−
Mucocutaneous ulcerations	−	++	+	−	−
Subcutaneous nodules	+	+	−	+	+
Calcinosis	−	−	++	++	−
Alopecia	−	++	+	+	−
Raynaud phenomenon	−	++	+	+++	+
Vasculitis	+	+++	++	+	+++
Myositis	−	+	+++	++	+
Cardiac involvement	+	+++	±	++	++
Pleuritis	++	+++	+	−	+
Pulmonary involvement	+	++	+	+++	++
Gastrointestinal disease	+	++	+++	+++	+++
Hepatomegaly	+	+	−	−	−
Splenomegaly	+	++	−	−	−
Lymphadenopathy	+	++	+	−	−
Renal disease	+	+++	±	++	+++
Hypertension	−	++	−	+++	+++
Ocular involvement	++	++	+	−	++
Nervous system disease	−	+++	+	−	+++
Anemia	++	+++	+	+	+
Leukocytosis	+	−	+	+	++
Leukopenia	−	++	−	−	−
Eosinophilia	−	−	+	−	++
Thrombocytopenia	−	++	−	−	−
Hypergammaglobulinemia	++	+++	+	+	+
Rheumatoid factors	+	++	−	+	+
Antinuclear antibodies	++	+++	+	++	+

−, absent; ±, rare; +, minimal; ++, moderate; +++, severe.

immunodeficiency in children with selective IgA deficiency, agammaglobulinemia or hypogammaglobulinemia, and C2 complement component deficiency. In children with oligoarthritis, T-lymphocyte proliferative responses to heat-shock protein 60 are associated with a remission of the inflammatory disease. A study of 144 families has established the association of several tumor necrosis factor-alpha (TNFα) single nucleotide polymorphisms (SNPs) with juvenile oligoarthritis. Interleukin-6 (IL-6) is increased in the circulation of children with systemic-onset disease. In systemic-onset disease, IL-6-174G is over-represented in the transcriptional regulation of the IL-6 gene and is associated with resistance to glucocorticoid therapy. Also in systemic-onset disease, high levels of macrophage inhibitory factor (MIF) in serum and synovial fluid are associated with a G to C SNP at position-173 of the MIF gene that leads to glycocorticoid resistance, persistence of arthritis, and a relatively poor outcome.

Pathology

The synovial membrane in JRA is characterized by villous hypertrophy and hyperplasia of the synovial lining layer. Edema and hyperemia are present, along with vascular endothelial hyperplasia and the infiltration of lymphocytes and plasma cells. Pannus formation eventually occurs in severely affected joints and leads to the destruction of articular cartilage and contiguous bone.

Infiltrates of inflammatory cells occur also in parenchymal organs, such as the liver, and along serosal surfaces of the pericardium, pleura, and peritoneum. Rheumatoid nodules result from a small-blood-vessel vasculitis but are rare findings in affected children. The rash of JRA is characterized histologically by a neutrophilic perivasculitis and infiltration of round cells surrounding capillaries and subdermal venules.

Clinical Manifestations and Complications

Although the onset of JRA occurring before a child reaches 6 months of age is unusual, the mean age at onset characteristically is young (1 to 3 years), with a substantial number of cases beginning throughout childhood and young adolescence. Girls are affected at least twice as frequently as are boys.

Fatigue, low-grade fever, anorexia, weight loss, and failure to grow are common findings at onset of the disease in moderate to severely affected children. Morning stiffness, musculoskeletal gelling after inactivity, and night pain often are associated with incompletely controlled disease. Affected children may not, however, always communicate these symptoms to their parents. Instead, the child may present with increased irritability, a posture of guarding the joints, a limp, or refusal to walk.

Tenosynovitis also is a component of active disease. A stenosing synovitis of the flexor tendon sheaths may lead to loss of extension of the fingers or to a trigger finger. Rheumatoid nodules may occur on the tendons or subcutaneously over pressure points. They are found particularly in children who have widespread polyarthritis, are older at onset, and have prominent small-joint disease, an unrelenting course with early development of bony erosions, and RF seropositivity.

Types of Onset

The classification of JRA is based on recognition of at least three distinct types of onsets of disease (Table 434.4): polyarthritis, oligoarthritis (pauciarticular disease), and systemic disease. These types of onsets are characterized by specific signs and symptoms at presentation and during the first 6 months of illness.

Polyarthritis is disease that begins in five or more joints. This onset occurs in one-third of affected children and may be acute or insidious. Systemic manifestations are not severe or persistent. The arthritis generally involves large joints, such as the knees, wrists, elbows, and ankles, and usually is symmetric. However, the smaller joints of the hands or feet may be affected early or late. Younger children may not complain of pain, although the joints are tender and appear painful on motion. The cervical spine often is involved in this type of onset, although onset of JRA solely in the cervical spine is a rare occurrence. The neck may be painful or stiff, with an alarmingly rapid loss of extension and rotation. Atlantoaxial subluxation may occur early and places a child at risk for incurring an injury of the cervical cord in an accident or with attempted intubation before general anesthesia. Temporomandibular joint disease is a relatively common occurrence in children with polyarthritis and leads to limitation or asymmetry of bite and micrognathia.

The onset of JRA in one-half of affected children involves four or fewer joints. Oligoarthritis or pauciarticular disease often is confined to the knees or ankles, or it may involve a single joint, such as a knee, at onset and throughout the course. The hips usually are spared at onset. Extra-articular systemic disease, except for chronic uveitis, is a distinctly unusual finding unless the child goes on to develop polyarticular involvement (approximately 10%).

TABLE 434.4

CLASSIFICATION OF TYPES OF ONSETS OF JUVENILE RHEUMATOID ARTHRITIS

Sign/Symptom of Onset	Polyarthritis	Oligoarthritis (Pauciarticular Disease)	Systemic Disease
Frequency of cases	30%	60%	10%
Number of joints involved	≥5	≤4	Variable
Female:male ratio	3:1	5:1	1:1
Systemic involvement	Moderate	Not present	Prominent
Occurrence of chronic uveitis	5%	5%–15%	Rare
Frequency of seropositivity			
Rheumatoid factors	10% (increases with age)	Rare	Rare
Antinuclear antibodies	40%–50%	75%–85%*	10%
Course	Systemic disease generally mild; possible unremitting articular involvement	Systemic disease absent; major cause of morbidity is uveitis	Systemic disease often self-limited; arthritis is chronic and destructive in 50%
Prognosis	Guarded to moderately good	Excellent, except for eyesight	Moderate to poor

*In girls with uveitis.

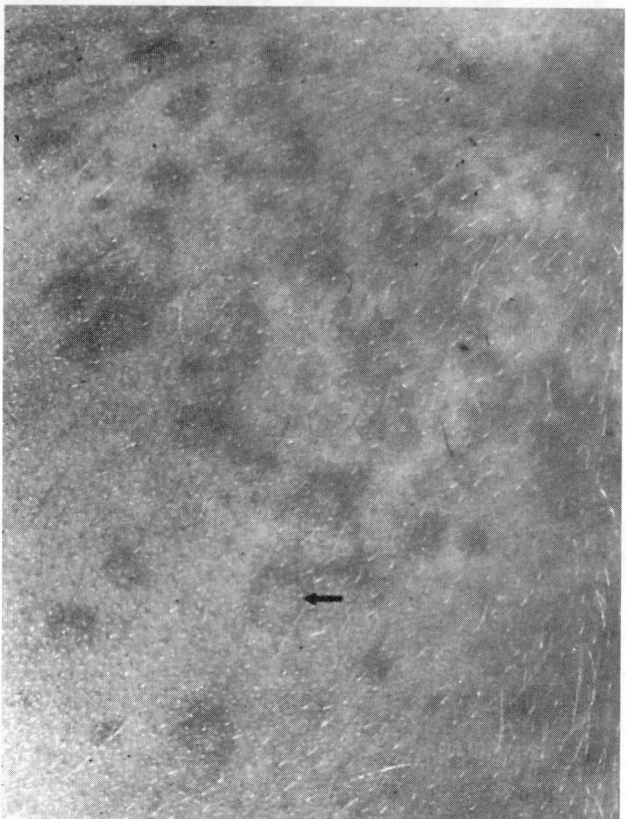

FIGURE 434.1. Rash of systemic-onset JRA. This 4-year-old girl presented with high-spiking fever that occurred once a day, accompanied by a transient nonpruritic rash. The arrow points to central clearing in a lesion. (Reprinted with permission from Cassidy JT. Juvenile rheumatoid arthritis. In Ruddy S, Harris ED Jr., Sledge CB, eds. *Kelley's textbook of rheumatology.* Philadelphia: WB Saunders, 2001.)

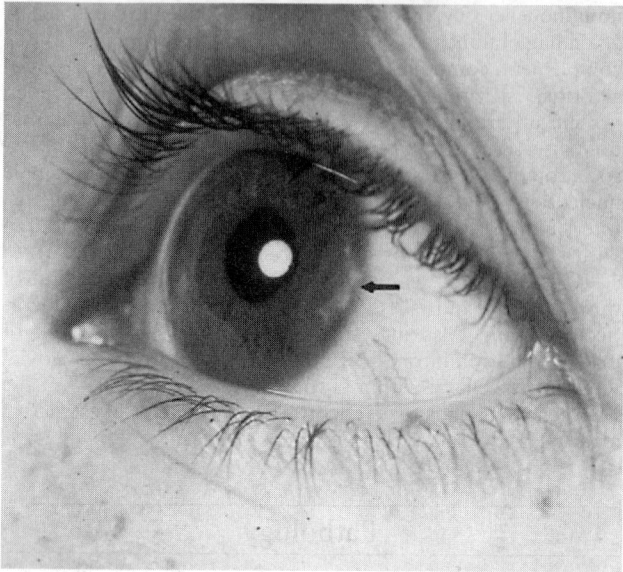

FIGURE 434.2. The arrow points to an area of band keratopathy just inside the corneal limbus in a girl who had ANA-positive oligoarticular JRA. Her chronic uveitis was bilateral and had resulted in a decrease in vision to 20/400 in the right eye.

A small number of children have onset of JRA with severe constitutional and systemic disease. These systemic signs and symptoms may precede the appearance of overt arthritis by weeks, months, or even years. A hallmark of this type of disease is a high-spiking fever, often combined with a rheumatoid rash. Elevations in temperature occur once or twice a day, often in late afternoon or evening, to a level of 39°C or higher, with a quick return to baseline temperature or lower. This quotidian pattern is highly suggestive of a diagnosis of JRA.

The rash of JRA develops often with this fever and consists of 2- to 5-mm erythematous morbilliform macules (Fig. 434.1). It is seen most commonly on the trunk and proximal extremities, and over pressure areas, but it may occur on the face, palms, or soles. Generally, it is not pruritic. The most characteristic feature is its transient nature. Usually, any single lesion does not persist for longer than an hour. Sometimes, the rash can be elicited in a child by rubbing or scratching the skin: the isomorphic response or Koebner phenomenon. This rash never occurs in children with oligoarthritis.

Children with systemic onset usually have concurrent hepatosplenomegaly and lymphadenopathy. Pericarditis, hepatitis, and other visceral disease may develop. Pulmonary involvement consists of a wide spectrum of abnormalities, such as pleuritis and effusion, interstitial fibrosis, and hemosiderosis. The CNS may be affected, but distinguishing encephalopathy from drug toxicity, viral infection, or other complications of the systemic illness and fever may be difficult.

Complications

Chronic Uveitis. One of the most serious complications of JRA is the development of a chronic nongranulomatous uveitis involving the iris, ciliary body, and occasionally the posterior choroid (Fig. 434.2). Involvement usually is bilateral and can lead to blindness. Chronic uveitis characteristically has an insidious, asymptomatic onset and is diagnosed only by ophthalmologic and slit-lamp examinations at the time of diagnosis; these examinations must be repeated at frequent intervals during the first years after onset. Chronic uveitis is confined to children with polyarthritis or oligoarthritis. It tends to occur particularly in young girls with an early age of onset, limited joint disease, and ANA seropositivity.

Growth Retardation. Disturbances of growth and normal development are complications of any chronic disease and often are prominent in children with JRA. Linear growth is retarded during periods of active disease or with the use of glucocorticoid drugs. Localized growth retardation also may occur in specific areas such as the jaw (micrognathia). Unequal leg or arm lengths develop with monarticular disease. Often, the development of secondary sexual characteristics is delayed. Psychosocial retardation may be a frequent, persistent, and potentially severe complication. Psychological regression to a more infantile pattern is present in most children with moderate to severe disease. Osteopenia is an almost universal occurrence and, if persistent, is a risk factor later in life for fractures and premature osteoporosis. Children with chronic arthritis have elevated levels of osteoprotegerin, a decoy receptor, that inhibits the differentiation and activation of osteoclasts. This abnormality is related to a TC that correlates with low bone mass and bone erosions.

Laboratory Examination

Children with active disease develop a normocytic, hypochromic anemia characteristic of the chronic anemia of inflammation. Often, it is moderately severe, with the hemoglobin concentration in the range of 7 to 10 g/dL. Leukocytosis and thrombocytosis are common findings with active disease, but they are much less pronounced in children with oligoarthritis.

The acute-phase reactants often are elevated at the onset of disease and are moderately useful in following the course of the inflammation. The Westergren erythrocyte sedimentation rate (ESR), C-reactive protein level, and immunoglobulin concentrations reflect inflammatory activity if increased. Serum complement components usually are elevated at onset and with exacerbations. The serum amyloid-like protein (SAA) is increased in concentration in children with active disease. Soluble immune complexes can be detected in the sera of some children, particularly in those with systemic onset.

Tests for RFs are positive in children with JRA less frequently than in adults with rheumatoid arthritis, although approximately 10% of children eventually become seropositive. RFs are IgM macroglobulins with antigenic specificity directed against the unfolded H-chains of IgG. Seropositivity seldom is observed in a child younger than 7 years of age; RFs tend to be present in children who are older at onset and in those who have symmetric polyarthritis with involvement of the small joints, subcutaneous rheumatoid nodules, articular erosions, and a poor functional outcome.

ANA seropositivity is present in at least 45% of children with JRA. The pattern of fluorescent staining usually is homogeneous or speckled; the titer generally is low to moderate. The presence of these antibodies is a significant risk factor for the development of chronic uveitis. They are found less commonly in older boys and in children with systemic disease. A positive ANA determination is a valuable diagnostic measure in a child suspected of having JRA because this antibody activity is not found frequently in other childhood illnesses, except for the rheumatic diseases and transient acute viral infection.

The synovial fluid white cell count in JRA is elevated moderately, in the range of 10,000 to 20,000/mm^3. Synovial glucose concentration is low. Complement levels may be depressed, as evidence for intrasynovial complement activation.

Urinalysis generally is normal in children with JRA except for those few who have a mild glomerulitis at onset. Proteinuria also may occur with fever. Persistent proteinuria may be the first evidence of drug toxicity or amyloidosis. Renal papillary necrosis may develop related to NSAID therapy and dehydration during the course of the disease.

Radiologic Examination

Children with JRA exhibit a wide range of distinctive radiologic findings. Early changes consist of soft-tissue swelling, juxta-articular osteoporosis, and periosteal new-bone apposition. Development of the ossification centers may be accelerated, or premature epiphyseal closure may be present, leading to stunting of bone growth. In children with polyarthritis or systemic disease, especially later in the course, marginal erosions may develop, along with narrowing of the cartilaginous spaces.

Cervical spine disease is characteristic of JRA. The upper cervical segments principally are affected with apophyseal joint fusion and atlantoaxial subluxation (Fig. 434.3). The lower vertebrae also may be involved, with failure to grow normally. Sacroiliac arthritis in children with JRA is not characterized by the degree of involvement and reactive sclerosis that would be seen in ankylosing spondylitis. Fractures, particularly of the long bones and vertebrae, occur in children who develop generalized osteopenia.

Routine radiographic studies generally are sufficient to document this progression of abnormalities in evaluating a child's response to a management program. Newer methods of objectively evaluating joint disease (e.g., bone scans, computed tomography [CT], and magnetic resonance imaging [MRI]) can be useful diagnostically. MRI is more precise than is routine

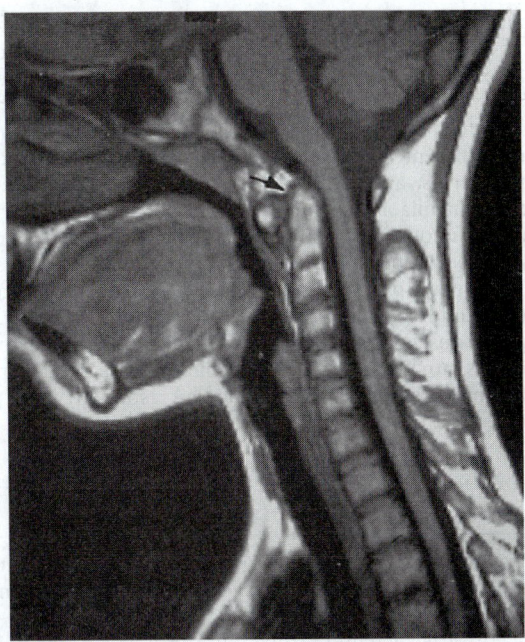

FIGURE 434.3. Magnetic resonance image of the cervical spine of a child with 7 mm of atlantoaxial subluxation. The arrow points to the odontoid, which is beginning to impinge on the upper cervical cord.

radiographic examination in delineating soft-tissue abnormalities in response to abnormal bone growth or fusion and in detecting early cartilage or bone destruction.

Diagnosis

The classification criteria for JRA of the American College of Rheumatology (ACR) and for juvenile idiopathic arthritis of the International League for Arthritis and Rheumatism (ILAR) are compared in Table 434.5. JRA was defined by the ACR as onset of arthritis in a child younger than 16 years. Arthritis is defined clinically by swelling or effusion or the presence of two or more of the following signs: limitation of range of motion, tenderness or pain on motion, and increased heat in one or more joints. JRA often is a diagnosis of exclusion and, therefore, similar diseases must be considered (see Table 434.2). The differential diagnosis generally includes other rheumatic

TABLE 434.5

COMPARISON OF ACR AND ILAR CRITERIA FOR ARTHRITIS IN CHILDREN

Entity	ACR (JRA)	ILAR (JIA)
Age at onset	<16 years	<16 years
Definition of arthritis	Yes	No
Duration of disease	≥6 weeks	≥6 weeks
Onset types	3	6
Course subtypes	9	1
Inclusion of JAS, psoriatic arthritis, and IBD	No	Yes
Exclusion of other forms of juvenile arthritis	Yes	Yes

ACR, American College of Rheumatology; ILAR, International League of Associations for Rheumatology; IBD, inflammatory bowel disease; JAS, juvenile ankylosing spondylitis; JCA, juvenile chronic arthritis; JRA, juvenile rheumatoid arthritis.

and connective tissue diseases, especially acute rheumatic fever, SLE, and ankylosing spondylitis. In our experience, other forms of arthropathy, such as reactive and psoriatic arthritis, are uncommon findings. Particular attention must be accorded, however, to infectious arthritis, serum sickness, Henoch-Schönlein purpura, the enteropathies such as ulcerative colitis and regional enteritis, and hematologic diseases such as leukemia, sickle-cell anemia, and hemophilia. The concurrence of arthritis and immunodeficiency already has been mentioned. Certain viral illnesses, especially rubella, mumps, and Lyme disease, have an associated arthritis. Tumors, especially neuroblastoma in young children, may present as bone pain or arthritis. Although the onset of JRA in the hip is an uncommon occurrence, transient synovitis, Legg-Calvé-Perthes disease, and slipped capital femoral epiphysis may mimic JRA, especially if the pain is referred to the knee, as it often is.

Therapy

Conservative management attempts to control the clinical manifestations of the disease and prevent or minimize deformity. Ideally, this approach involves a multidisciplinary team that follows the affected child throughout the course of the illness. Management should be family-centered, community-based, and coordinated. The long-term therapeutic program must be accepted by the child and family and judged to have a favorable risk-benefit ratio by the pediatric rheumatologist.

Prognosis is reasonably satisfactory for most children with JRA, so the philosophy of management initially should stress the simplest, safest, and most conservative measures. If this program of treatment proves inadequate, other therapeutic modalities should be chosen (Table 434.6).

NSAIDs are moderately effective in suppressing inflammation and fever. Aspirin seldom is used in North America at this time, and drugs such as naproxen, ibuprofen, and tolmetin are preferred. The first two drugs can be prescribed also as a suspension, which is particularly useful for younger children. All children with JRA should receive yearly influenza vaccines and should be immune to varicella.

Hydroxychloroquine is a useful adjunctive agent for treating the child with more progressive disease. Because of concern over retinopathy as a toxic reaction, a relatively low dose

is chosen, (e.g., 5 mg/kg/day), and every 6-month ophthalmologic examinations, especially for color vision, are monitored during its administration. Intramuscular gold compounds and D-penicillamine were used previously for children whose polyarthritis was unresponsive to conservative management. Toxicities from these drugs primarily are hematologic, renal, or hepatic.

Methotrexate has become the most accepted approach to the advanced drug treatment of severe or resistant polyarthritis. In a large, multinational, double-blind, randomized trial, a dose of 10 mg/m^2 once a week markedly reduced the articular severity index, compared with placebo. This drug is attractive for pediatric use because it is given only once a week orally as a pill or liquid, and it has no proven oncogenic potential or untoward risk of causing sterility. Toxicity is monitored clinically and by periodic complete blood cell counts and liver enzyme determinations.

Additional therapy can include etanercept, a TNFα blocker. It consists of two TNFα receptor monomer chains fused to the Fc domain of human IgG$_1$. The drug binds TNFα in the vascular and extracellular compartments and inhibits its activity. A controlled trial of etanercept in children with polyarticular JRA who had failed therapy with methotrexate indicated that 74% demonstrated improvement at 3 months on a subcutaneous dose of 0.4 mg/kg twice a week. A 2-year follow-up indicated that the overall rate of improvement was 79% and remissions occurred in 37%.

Infliximab is a monoclonal antibody that has the capacity to bind TNFα in both the extracellular and vascular compartments, and also on the cell surface. A pediatric trial is currently in progress to evaluate the safety and efficacy of this drug in JRA. Another biologic response modifier is anakinra (r-metHuIL-1ra), which interferes with the actions of IL-1 in the inflammatory response.

The long-term safety of cytokine blockade is unknown. Potentially, it is associated with an increased frequency of systemic infection and should not be used in children with recurrent or chronic infections. Tuberculosis always should be excluded before beginning therapy.

Glucocorticoid drugs should be reserved for treatment of the severely involved child who is recalcitrant to more conservative therapeutic regimens or for those with life-threatening disease and its complications, such as pericarditis. Many toxicities (e.g., Cushing syndrome) and growth retardation are associated with their use. Ophthalmic administration is indicated for treatment of chronic uveitis. Intra-articular steroid often is used to achieve the specific goals of a physical therapy program or for persistent monarticular or oligoarticular involvement.

Other immunosuppressive agents seldom are required in the long-term treatment of JRA. However, some children have failed to improve on all other therapies and are candidates for experimental protocols involving agents such as azathioprine or cyclophosphamide. Critical considerations are the oncogenic potential of these agents, potential sterility, and bone marrow suppression. Intravenous immunoglobulin, cyclosporin A, and other biologic response modifiers are additional approaches to experimental therapy.

Physical and Occupational Therapy

The maintenance of function and prevention of deformity cannot be overemphasized in the total management of the child with JRA. Appropriate prescriptions for physical and occupational therapy, a balanced program of rest and activity, and selective splinting are indicated. Normal play should be encouraged. Only unacceptable levels of stress on inflamed weight-bearing joints should be limited. Children with cervical spine disease should wear a padded collar when traveling in an automobile or studying.

TABLE 434.6

MANAGEMENT OF CHILDREN WITH JUVENILE RHEUMATOID ARTHRITIS

Medication program: suppression of inflammation
Nonsteroidal antiinflammatory drugs
Hydroxychloroquine
Methotrexate
Glucocorticoid drugs
Immunosuppressive drugs

Preservation of function and prevention of deformities
Local and general rest
Physical therapy
Occupational therapy
Orthopedic surgery: preventive and reconstructive

Psychosocial development
Peer group relationships and schooling
Counseling of patients and families
Involvement of community agencies

Maintenance of adequate nutrition
Coordinated care

Reconstructive Surgery

Synovectomy or tenosynovectomy sometimes is indicated in the course of management. Total joint replacement generally is delayed until after growth has ceased and the epiphyses have closed. Cosmetic surgery and orthodontic reconstruction for micrognathia or destruction of the temporomandibular joint are useful late approaches when indicated.

Prognosis

In general, more than half of the children who develop JRA have a satisfactory recovery from their disease and enter adult life without serious functional disability, although as many as 45% may have continuing low-grade activity for some years. A small percentage of patients whose disease has gone into remission will have a recurrence of arthritis during the adult years. As many as 15% of children with JRA, however, enter adulthood with significant functional disability. The child most at risk has had polyarthritis of later age of onset, early symmetric involvement of the small joints of the hands or feet, unremitting activity of the joint disease, early appearance of erosions, prominent systemic manifestations, and development of RF seropositivity and subcutaneous nodules. Progressive hip disease also is a major cause of long-term disability.

Serious functional disability is an uncommon development in children who have oligoarthritis and pursue a course of limited joint disease. The prognosis for sight in children with chronic uveitis has improved dramatically, a development probably related to earlier detection and better management of this complication. Blindness, however, still occurs in as many as 15% of affected eyes.

Approximately one-half of children with systemic onset eventually will recover completely; however, most JRA-related deaths in the United States have been associated with this type of disease. Death occurs in fewer than 1% of children with JRA, and it often is a result of overwhelming infection. In Europe, renal failure secondary to amyloidosis is a leading cause of death. Amyloidosis seldom occurs as a complication of JRA in North America.

Estimates of prognosis should remain optimistic, and, in many children, prognosis is excellent. Of importance is that both the child and parents understand the disease and share in its long-term management. The nature of JRA, the goals of therapy, and the expected course of the disease should be discussed in detail. A carefully selected program of coordinated care, initiated by the pediatric rheumatologist, must be reinforced constantly by the team nurse and social worker. Some families of children with JRA display psychiatrically important disruptions (e.g., divorce, separation, and depression). Thus, a priority in the management of a child with this chronic illness is to foster normal psychological and social development and peer group activities. A child's unceasing potential for physical and psychological growth is a critical factor working in favor of the therapeutic program and team management. This natural endowment for future physical and psychological development is what enables so much to be accomplished in most children with JRA.

SYSTEMIC LUPUS ERYTHEMATOSUS

SLE is a multisystemic disease in which widespread inflammatory involvement of the connective tissues and immune-complex vasculitis occur. It is a prototypic example of autoimmunity in humans that results from abnormal immunologic hyperreactivity and an immunogenetic predisposition to the disease.

Pathogenesis

Numerous environmental, hereditary, and immunogenetic factors are implicated in the pathogenesis of this autoimmune disorder. The F1 hybrid of New Zealand white and black mice develops an SLE-like disease with early onset of renal failure that is more marked in females than in males. Household dogs also develop an SLE-like illness and, identical to their mouse counterparts, have circulating antibodies to native DNA and immune-complex deposition in tissues.

Environmental triggers, such as excessive exposure to the sun, a drug reaction, or an infection, may precipitate the onset of SLE. The basic pathogenesis of SLE appears to be immunologic abnormalities of homeostatic control affecting nuclear and cytoplastic antigens. Antibodies found in children with SLE include those that are tissue-specific as well as those related to nuclear antigens. These antibodies participate in specific manifestations of the disease, such as acute hemolytic anemia, thrombocytopenia, leukopenia, and thrombosis, and in the antigen–antibody complex deposition that results in systemic vasculitis and lupus nephritis, as well as impaired cell-mediated immunity and T-suppressor cell dysfunction.

Another connective tissue disease or an abnormal marker of immunologic function (e.g., ANA) is present in approximately 10% of family members. SLE has occurred in identical twins (concordance 24%). It is associated with sporadic or familial immunodeficiency, such as selective IgA deficiency, and inherited disorders of complement components, such as homozygous C2, C1q, C1r, or C1 esterase inhibitor deficiency. In many affected children, a marked immunogenetic predisposition is evident in the extended haplotype for genes located on chromosome 6: HLA-B8, DR2 or DR3, DQw1 or DQw2, and C4A null.

Pathology

An immune-complex vasculitis with fibrinoid necrosis is the basic inflammatory lesion. Vascular lesions are widespread throughout the parenchymal organs, in subdermal tissues, and on the mucosal and serosal surfaces. Soluble immune complexes can be demonstrated beneath the vascular endothelium and along the dermal-epidermal junction in the lupus-band test.

In the kidney, immune complexes are deposited initially in the mesangium and then in subendothelial areas beneath the basement membrane. This type of immunologic involvement is characteristic of focal proliferative glomerulitis and, when more extensive and severe, of diffuse proliferative glomerulonephritis. In membranous disease, immune complexes are deposited or form along the epithelial side of the glomerular basement membranes.

Clinical Manifestations and Complications

Although SLE can develop at any age, onset in children usually occurs after they reach the age of 5 years and is increasingly more commonly during the adolescent years. The female-to-male ratio is approximately 8:1 except in the youngest children, when relatively more boys are affected.

The manifestations of SLE are variable (Table 434.7) and present with any degree of severity from an acute, rapidly fatal illness to insidious, chronic disability with multisystemic exacerbations. In more than three-fourths of affected children, SLE

TABLE 434.7

CLINICAL PRESENTATION AND COURSE OF SYSTEMIC LUPUS ERYTHEMATOSUS IN CHILDREN

Presentation	At Onset (%)	During Course (%)
Nephritis	84	86
Hypertension	10	28
Arthritis	72	76
Dermatitis	69	76
Malar erythema	51	56
Photosensitivity	16	16
Alopecia	16	20
Oral or nasopharyngeal ulcerations	12	16
Pericarditis	40	47
Pleuritis	31	36
Central nervous system disease	9	31
Raynaud phenomenon	16	24
Hepatomegaly	43	47
Splenomegaly	20	20
Anemia	43	47
Leukopenia	60	71
Thrombocytopenia	22	24

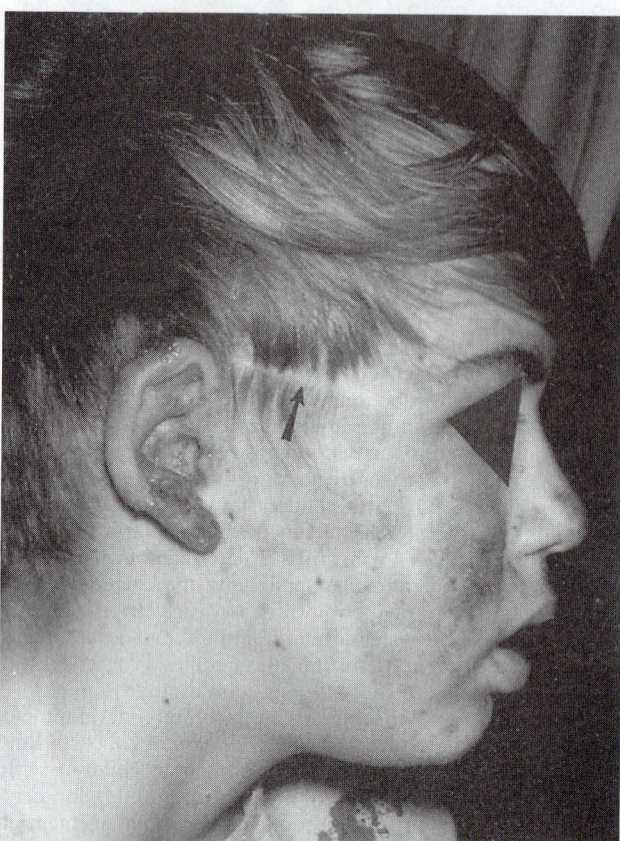

FIGURE 434.4. Excoriating erythematous facial rash of acute SLE in a 14-year-old boy. The crusting lesions are present over the nose, malar areas, cheeks, and earlobes. The arrow points to a clear area corresponding to the eyeglass frame, confirming the role of photosensitivity in the genesis of this lesion.

is diagnosed within the first 6 months after onset because of the acute nature of the illness, but diagnosis sometimes is delayed by 4 to 5 years in a few patients.

Fever, malaise, and weight loss are common findings. Each exacerbation of the disease tends to mimic previous episodes. If serious renal disease develops, it usually does so within 2 years after onset. The major exception to the predictability of the course of SLE is in the occurrence of CNS illness, which may intervene at any time in approximately one-third of the children.

A malar erythematous rash in a butterfly distribution across the bridge of the nose and over each cheek is characteristic of an acute onset or exacerbation (Fig. 434.4). Other forms of cutaneous and mucocutaneous involvement are common findings and vary in character and distribution. Raynaud phenomenon is a frequent occurrence. It may progress to serious digital ulceration and gangrene. The risk of developing osteonecrosis, particularly of the femoral heads, is common and is worsened by glucocorticoid therapy.

Arthritis affects most children and commonly involves the small joints of the hands, wrists, elbows, shoulders, knees, and ankles. This arthritis characteristically is transient and may be migratory. Pain often is more severe than is supported by objective changes. The arthritis of SLE almost never is erosive, nor does it often result in permanent deformity.

Pericarditis is the most common manifestation of cardiac involvement. The child with SLE also may develop congestive heart failure, arrhythmias, or myocardial infarction. Valvular insufficiency develops in a few cases, and a sterile verrucous endocarditis (Libman-Sacks) is particularly characteristic. Echocardiography is a sensitive method of confirming valvular abnormalities. Pleuritis also is a common finding and may involve the diaphragmatic pleurae along with a basilar pneumonitis. Pulmonary hemorrhage rarely occurs, but can be fatal.

Abdominal pain often presents a diagnostic dilemma in a child with SLE, especially in those who are being treated with glucocorticoids and in whom peptic ulcer disease is a consideration. Mesenteric thrombosis and acute pancreatitis are life-threatening events. Hepatomegaly and splenomegaly are common occurrences, and splenic infarction may occur.

Disease of the CNS and peripheral nervous system is a common cause of morbidity. Pseudotumor cerebri may be a complication of SLE or of glucocorticoid therapy. Recurrent headaches, seizures, chorea, or frank psychosis all are encountered. Intracranial hemorrhage may result from hypertension, thrombocytopenia, or thrombosis associated with antiphospholipid antibodies. The so-called cytoid body of retinal vasculitis often is seen in disease involving the CNS or in lupus crisis. Systemic polyneuropathy, the Guillain-Barré syndrome, transverse myelopathy, or involvement of the specific cranial nerves has been reported.

Some degree of renal involvement is present in virtually all children with SLE. Even moderately severe nephritis may not be detected early by the presence of an abnormal urinary sediment, proteinuria, or changes in the creatinine clearance. Evidence of active immune-complex disease, such as increased levels of antinative DNA antibodies or hypocomplementemia, correlates with active nephritis in most patients.

In the diagnosis of lupus nephritis, the microscopic interpretation of a renal biopsy is categorized by the World Health Organization (WHO) as type I, normal; type II, mesangial; type III, focal proliferative; type IV, diffuse proliferative; type V, membranous; and type VI, sclerosing disease. The relation of these specific types of involvement to prognosis and eventual renal failure, although not universally accepted, is depicted in Table 434.8. Thus, renal biopsy to delineate the type of nephritis is warranted in most children with SLE, unless no clinical evidence of significant involvement of the kidneys is found because the safest approach to long-term therapy usually is based

TABLE 434.8

CLASSIFICATION OF LUPUS NEPHRITIS

Type of Renal Disease	Remission	Nephrotic Syndrome	Renal Failure	Uremic Deaths
Glomerular lesions				
Mesangial	+	−	−	−
Focal proliferative	++	+	+	+
Diffuse proliferative	+	++	++	+++
Membranous	+	+++	++	+
Extraglomerular lesions	+	+	++	++

−, absent; +, minimal; ++, moderate; +++, severe.

TABLE 434.9

CRITERIA FOR CLASSIFICATION OF SYSTEMIC LUPUS ERYTHEMATOSUS*

Malar (butterfly) rash
Discoid-lupus rash
Photosensitivity
Oral or nasal mucocutaneous ulcerations
Nonerosive arthritis
Nephritis
  Proteinuria >0.5 g/day
  Cellular casts
Encephalopathy
  Seizures
  Psychosis
Pleuritis or pericarditis
Cytopenia
Positive immunoserology
  Antibodies to nDNA
  Antibodies to Sm nuclear antigen
  Biological false-positive test for syphilis
Positive antinuclear antibody test

*Four of 11 criteria provide a sensitivity of 96% and a specificity of 96% for systemic lupus erythematosus.

on careful evaluation of the renal status. Serious renal lesions are thought to occur more commonly in children with SLE than in adults, and prognosis for renal disease is more guarded.

Laboratory Examination

The acute-phase reactants generally are increased in active systemic disease. Otherwise unexplained leukopenia is particularly characteristic. Most affected children are leukopenic at onset, with neutrophils predominating in the peripheral count. During the course of the illness, the white blood cell (WBC) count often does not become elevated to an appropriate degree even with serious infection or bacteremia. Thrombocytopenia and acute hemolytic anemia also may be present. Coombs tests often are positive in these children. Besides systemic disease, other causes of anemia include menorrhagia, septicemia, and gastrointestinal bleeding. SLE may present as thrombocytopenic purpura.

ANAs are present in virtually all children with SLE. They generally occur in high titer, with a homogeneous pattern. A peripheral nuclear pattern virtually is synonymous with the presence of antinative DNA antibodies. Well-standardized assays for DNA antibodies are critical to evaluating the degree of activity of this systemic immune-complex disease. Anti-Ro antibodies are characteristic of the neonatal lupus syndromes and subacute cutaneous lupus, and they are associated with the development of pulmonary disease and nephritis. Anti-Sm antibodies also are diagnostic of SLE or of an associated syndrome, and these correlate with isolated CNS disease.

RFs and other antitissue antibodies, such as antithyroglobulin, often are positive. Cold agglutinins or cryoglobulins may result in peripheral anoxia and Raynaud phenomenon. Antiphospholipid antibodies or circulating lupus anticoagulants that cross-react with phospholipid antigens predispose the affected child to repeated episodes of chorea or thrombosis. The presence of a biologic false-positive serologic test for syphilis is a risk factor for future development of SLE.

Components of both the classic and alternative complement pathways are consumed in the presence of active immune-complex vasculitis. The hemolytic complement determination or CH_{50} reflects the status of the total complement cascade; C3 concentration appears to be depressed less frequently, but usually a falling concentration of C4 is a reliable indicator of active disease. Rarely, the determination of circulating immune complexes, such as C1q binding or Raji cell assays, are useful in selected patients.

Diagnosis

Diagnostic suspicion of SLE in children depends on recognizing an episodic, multisystemic constellation of characteristic clinical disease that is associated strongly with persistent ANA seropositivity. Eleven criteria have been evaluated by the American College of Rheumatology for the classification of SLE. These are listed in Table 434.9.

A differential diagnosis should include JRA, other forms of acute glomerulonephritis, hemolytic anemia, leukemia, allergic or contact dermatitis, an idiopathic seizure disorder, mononucleosis, acute rheumatic fever with carditis, and septicemia. SLE remains the great masquerader.

Therapy

Long-term supportive care of a child with SLE includes providing adequate nutrition, maintaining fluid and electrolyte balance, recognizing and treating infections early, and controlling hypertension. A fever that might be an early sign of potential infection should be evaluated promptly and thoroughly. Pneumonitis, septicemia, and pyelonephritis are of particular concern.

Because SLE is a serious illness, an affected child benefits from contact with the same medical team over the course of the illness. This team should emphasize the rationale supporting the treatment program and encourage the prophylactic measures of avoiding excessive sunlight, unnecessary drug exposure, or transfusion. Appropriate photoprotective clothing and sunscreens are indicated. The child's general activities and interactions with peer groups should not be restrained unnecessarily.

NSAIDs (e.g., naproxen) are useful in treating minor manifestations of SLE, such as arthralgia and myalgia. Hydroxychloroquine is an important adjunctive medication that helps to control photosensitive dermatitis and moderates glucocorticoid dosage. Glucocorticoid drugs are the mainstay of the basic regimen, however, and prednisone is the preferred analogue. A negative purified protein derivative (PPD) test for tuberculosis should be verified before a child is started on prednisone if at all possible. The minimum prednisone dose to achieve the goals of the treatment program is initiated at onset and maintained during the course of the disease. Low-dose therapy, defined as 0.5 mg/kg/day in divided doses, is used to treat noninfectious fever, dermatitis, arthritis, or serositis. Usually, these manifestations are suppressed promptly. Weeks often are required to see an improvement in anemia or the serologic tests reflecting active immune-complex disease. Low-dose glucocorticoid programs often control clinical disease in children with mesangial or focal glomerulonephritis.

High-dose prednisone therapy, defined as 1 to 2 mg/kg/day in divided doses, is used for lupus crisis, CNS disease, acute hemolytic anemia, or the more severe forms of nephritis. Hypertension, azotemia, and preexisting psychosis are relative contraindications to prolonged high-dosage regimens. The results of treatment are monitored by the clinical course of the disease in the child and by a periodic assessment of antinative DNA antibodies and serum complement levels. Exacerbation of the disease during a steroid taper is signaled by a deterioration of the serologic indices. Although still a controversial matter, the precise glucocorticoid program and consideration of specific immunosuppressive drugs often are predicated on the WHO classification of the renal disease.

Intravenous methylprednisolone pulse therapy may be indicated in an acute exacerbation of the disease to avoid increasing the daily steroid prescription. Immunosuppressive agents, in addition to prednisone, are necessary for some children. Although azathioprine has been used extensively, current data suggest that intravenous pulse cyclophosphamide is preferable, especially in children with severe nephritis. Dialysis and kidney transplantation have been used successfully in end-stage renal disease.

Prognosis

Prognosis in children with SLE has improved substantially since the 1960s; therefore, a guardedly optimistic attitude toward this disease is warranted. An estimated 85% to 90% of children will survive over a 10-year period, but survivorship in children with diffuse proliferative glomerulonephritis is less favorable (70%). Infection has replaced severe nephritis and CNS disease as the leading cause of death. Malignant hypertension, gastrointestinal bleeding or perforation, acute pancreatitis, and pulmonary hemorrhage also are serious complications of the disease or its treatment.

SLE is characterized by repeated exacerbations and remissions; often, active disease is prolonged over the course of many years. Generalizations concerning prognosis for a specific child are especially unwise during the first 1 to 2 years after diagnosis. Later, a more reliable estimate can be offered the family based on the degree of systemic activity and its response to therapy and on the severity of accompanying nephritis, systemic vasculitis, and parenchymal organ involvement. Prognosis for life or function is poorest in diffuse proliferative nephritis or the organic brain syndrome; it is best in minimal systemic disease and mesangial nephritis and with a prompt sustained response to glucocorticoid therapy.

DRUG-INDUCED SYSTEMIC LUPUS ERYTHEMATOSUS

In some children, acute SLE is precipitated or preceded by a drug reaction. Agents that have been implicated most frequently are hydralazine, isoniazid, penicillin, minocycline, sulfonamides, and anticonvulsants. The most frequent clinical manifestations in drug-induced SLE are cutaneous and pleuropericardial. CNS disease and nephritis are uncommon findings. In most instances, drug-induced SLE is a self-limited illness that abates on withdrawal of the offending agent. Antibodies to native DNA are not present, but antihistone reactivity characteristically is present in 95% of affected children. The serum complement concentration remains normal. Although the precise immunologic mechanisms have not been elucidated, some of these medications (e.g., hydralazine) may sensitize cutaneous DNA to degradation by ultraviolet (UV) light. A drug reaction also may precipitate clinical manifestations of SLE that are indistinguishable from idiopathic disease.

LUPUS PHENOMENA IN THE NEWBORN PERIOD

A child born of a mother with active SLE may develop a transient neonatal lupus-like syndrome within the first few days of life. This condition results from the transplacental passage of maternal IgG ANAs with anti-Ro (SS-A) activity. In most of these infants, no associated clinical disease is present, and the serologic abnormalities (ANA seropositivity and depressed complement levels) abate within the first few months of life. Thrombocytopenia may be present, along with mild hemolytic anemia or leukopenia. In some infants, malar erythema or discoid lupus-like lesions develop. SLE may recur in young adults who have had transient manifestations of neonatal lupus.

Another permanent neonatal lupus syndrome is the development in utero of complete congenital heart block; other cardiac abnormalities, including endomyocardial fibroelastosis, may be present. Approximately one-third of infants with congenital heart block are born of mothers who have SLE or who eventually will develop an SLE-like disorder. The primary immunologic abnormality is, again, the presence of anti-Ro antibody that is directed against a small cytoplasmic RNA-protein complex that binds to fetal cardiac epitopes and, in some cases, antibody to La (SS-B) has been present in every child and mother studied with this syndrome.

MIXED CONNECTIVE TISSUE DISEASE

Mixed connective tissue disease (MCTD) is an overlap syndrome that combines clinical elements of JRA, dermatomyositis, scleroderma, and SLE with the presence of very high titers of ANAs to an extractable nuclear antigen (ENA). This autoimmune reactivity is related to a ribonucleoprotein specificity (RNP) that is RNAse-sensitive and specifically to antibodies to small nuclear U_1RNP and U_1RNA.

This disorder originally was described in adults as an autoimmune disease of unknown etiology with a consistently good prognosis. Rarely did life-threatening systemic disease involving the lungs, heart, gastrointestinal tract, or kidneys develop. An excellent response to low-dose glucocorticoid therapy was expected. A long-term follow-up of children, however, suggests that the outcome was not so favorable. Severe thrombocytopenia occurred in many of them, and the disorder progressed into a more scleroderma-like disease (with sclerodactyly, gastrointestinal involvement, and pulmonary disease) in some or, in others, it evolved into a course more typical of SLE. Even in the late stages of the disease, nephritis may occur, albeit infrequently, but more severely in children than in adults.

SJÖGREN SYNDROME

The diagnosis of Sjögren syndrome (SS) is based on a triad of findings: (a) the sicca syndrome (dry eyes and dry mouth), (b) a connective tissue disease (usually SLE or scleroderma), and (c) high titers of autoantibodies (usually RFs or ANAs). SS can be divided into two forms: primary disease, in which a defined connective tissue disease is not present, and secondary disease, in which a connective tissue disease is clinically present. The secondary form of the disorder occurs far less commonly in children than in adults. The primary disorder is very rare but has been reported in children as young as 5 years of age. SS occurs much more commonly in girls than in boys.

Pathogenesis

Pathophysiologically, SS is an extreme example of uncontrolled B-cell hyperactivity to a variety of antigens, in conjunction with decreased T-cell suppression and responsiveness. Skin tests for delayed hypersensitivity are impaired, and *in vitro* measures of lymphocyte transformation are decreased. HLA-B8 and -DR3 are associated with development of this syndrome.

Pathology

Histopathologically, a widespread infiltration by lymphocytic and mononuclear cells and, to a lesser extent by plasma and reticulum cells, is present in parenchymal organs and the salivary and lacrimal glands. In some cases, germinal follicle formation is present within the glands, and atrophy and obliteration of secretory acini develop. An important diagnostic feature in salivary glands is the proliferation of ductal lining cells to form epimyoepithelial islands. Often, the presence of this feature aids in distinguishing benign involvement from malignant infiltration. SS *per se*, however, is not always a clinically benign disorder. At least in adults, pseudolymphoma and lymphoma may develop during its course, and these are particularly prone to occur in patients who do not have an overt connective tissue disease.

Clinical Manifestations and Complications

SS is a multisystem disorder that often involves many organ systems (Table 434.10). It often is insidious in onset, slowly progressive, and may present as recurrent bilateral parotid swelling. The sicca component is the dominant symptomatic feature of SS and is related directly to lymphocytic infiltration of the lacrimal and salivary glands, although more widespread involvement of the entire upper respiratory tract, larynx, stomach, and genitourinary systems may be present. Patients with SS also may have achlorhydria or develop pancreatitis, hepatobiliary disease, chronic active hepatitis, or evidence of active vasculitis. Renal tubular abnormalities related to hypergammaglobulinemia or lymphocytic infiltration may be present and can result in renal tubular acidosis. Hyposthenuria unresponsive to vasopressin occurs with decreased permeability of the distal convoluted tubules and collecting ducts to water. Some patients develop a chronic interstitial nephritis.

Laboratory Examination

Anemia, thrombocytopenia, and persistent leukopenia may be present in approximately one-third of the children. A striking polyclonal hypergammaglobulinemia almost always is found. All patients have high titers of RFs or other autoantibodies, such as ANAs, in which a speckled or nucleolar pattern frequently is found.

Most individuals with SS also have circulating antibodies directed against small nuclear or cytoplasmic ribonucleoprotein antigens that are termed *SS-A (Ro)* and *SS-B (La)*. Rheumatoid arthritis precipitin (RAP) often is present. Approximately 15% of patients have positive LE cell preparations, even in the absence of overt SLE. Other antitissue antibodies, including

TABLE 434.10

ASSOCIATED FEATURES OF SJÖGREN SYNDROME

Sicca complex
Bilateral parotid enlargement
Hashimoto thyroiditis
Lymphoid myositis
Achlorhydria
Hyposthenuria and renal tubular acidosis
Hepatomegaly
Pancreatitis
Celiac syndrome

Connective tissue disease
Systemic lupus erythematosus
Vasculitis
Raynaud phenomenon
Nonthrombocytopenic purpura
Chronic active hepatitis

Autoantibodies
Rheumatoid factors
Antinuclear antibodies
Antibodies to SS-A, SS-B, and rheumatoid arthritis
    precipitin
Antisalivary duct antibodies
Antitissue antibodies

Malignancy
Pseudolymphoma
Lymphoma
Macroglobulinemia

antiparietal cell and antithyroid antibodies, are found in 40% of children.

Diagnosis

Diagnosis is secured by demonstrating the cardinal features of the sicca complex. The mucous membranes are dry to inspection. Inadequate tearing is documented by a positive Schirmer test, which demonstrates decreased wetting of a filter paper strip placed in the conjunctival sac. Sialography using contrast media or scintigraphy of the salivary glands using ^{99m}Tec is positive. Diagnosis may be confirmed in difficult cases by biopsy of the labial mucosa to demonstrate the characteristic round-cell infiltration in the minor salivary glands.

Therapy

Treatment of the sicca complex primarily is symptomatic. Affected children may benefit from the use of artificial tears, saline nasal douches, or sour-lemon drops to provide some relief from the xerostomia. Glucocorticoid and immunosuppressive agents can be considered if life-threatening complications occur. When SS is secondary to an established connective tissue disease, treatment is directed toward that disorder.

DERMATOMYOSITIS

A classification of idiopathic inflammatory myositis is presented in Table 434.11. Dermatomyositis in children is characterized by the nonsuppurative inflammation of striated muscle and skin. These multisystemic findings are accompanied early in the course by an immune-complex vasculitis and later by the development of calcinosis.

TABLE 434.11

CLASSIFICATION OF INFLAMMATORY MYOSITIS

Polymyositis
Dermatomyositis
Dermatomyositis or polymyositis with malignancy
Dermatomyositis with onset in childhood
Acute rhabdomyolysis
Polymyositis with Sjögren or overlap syndrome

Dermatomyositis occurs in approximately 5% of children newly referred to a pediatric rheumatology clinic. The disease is seen slightly more commonly in girls than in boys in a ratio of 1.6 to 1.0. The disease can present at any age, but onset is especially common between the ages of 4 and 10 years.

Pathogenesis

Current investigations demonstrate that dermatomyositis is autoimmune in pathogenesis, with both humoral and cell-mediated abnormalities. Immune-complex vasculitis may be an initiating or perpetuating event as immunoglobulins and complement are deposited in the walls of small blood vessels and in skeletal muscles. An immunogenetic predisposition for the development of dermatomyositis may be present. HLA-DQA1*0501 is increased in frequency in white children with dermatomyositis, a specificity also associated with an increase in the TNFα-308A allele. Dermatomyositis also has occurred in children with selective IgA deficiency and C2 complement component deficiency. It has developed after vaccination and as a hypersensitivity reaction to drugs, sunburn, or infections (e.g., coxsackie B-virus or toxoplasmosis). An acute transient inflammatory myositis occurs after certain viral infections, especially influenza A and B, in otherwise normal children. Myositis has been described in a few children with agammaglobulinemia in association with echovirus infection.

Pathology

The initial lesion is an acute, patchy, inflammatory, round-cell infiltration in striated muscle, skin, or the gastrointestinal tract. Degeneration of striated muscle of all fiber types and accompanying regeneration follow, with a moderate variation in fiber size. During healing, interstitial connective tissue and fat replace areas of focal necrosis. Smooth muscle is not affected primarily in dermatomyositis. The heart seldom is involved, although a few children have been described with focal myocardial fibrosis and contraction-band necrosis.

The nature and extent of the immune-complex necrotizing vasculitis are important prognostic factors in the survival of children with dermatomyositis. Arterioles, capillaries, and venules are affected and lead to infarction, ulceration, and diffuse bleeding, especially in the gastrointestinal tract. The presence on electron microscopy of a noninflammatory obliterative vasculopathy in muscle is related to a poorer prognosis associated with cutaneous ulcerations. Diffuse linear and occasionally granular deposits of IgM, C3d, and fibrin are found in these lesions.

Distinctive nail-fold capillary loop abnormalities are present in one-half of children with dermatomyositis and show the simultaneous dilation of isolated loops, dropout of surrounding vessels, and an arborized cluster of peripheral capillary loops. These changes, like the noninflammatory vasculopathy, correlate with more severe, chronic, steroid-unresponsive disease.

TABLE 434.12

CLINICAL FEATURES ASSOCIATED WITH DERMATOMYOSITIS IN CHILDHOOD

Muscle weakness
   Proximal pelvic girdle (95%)
   Proximal shoulder girdle (75%)
   Neck flexors (60%)
   Pharyngeal muscles (30%)
   Distal muscles of the extremities (30%)
   Facial and extraocular muscles (5%)
Muscle contractures and atrophy (60%)
Muscle pain and tenderness (50%)
Skin lesions (85%)
   Heliotrope rash of eyelids
   Malar rash
   Subcutaneous and periorbital edema
   Periungual and articular rash (Gottron papules)
Raynaud phenomenon (20%)
Arthritis and arthralgia (25%)
Dysphagia, other gastrointestinal symptoms (10%)
Calcinosis (40%)
Pulmonary fibrosis (5%)

Clinical Manifestations and Complications

Table 434.12 lists the characteristic clinical features of this disease in childhood. Most children have prominent constitutional symptoms of fatigue, malaise, weight loss, anorexia, and low-grade fever. The proximal limb-girdle muscles of the lower extremities are affected initially, the next most frequently involved being the shoulder girdle and proximal arm muscles. The affected muscles occasionally are edematous and indurated. The child may be unable to hold the head upright or to maintain a sitting posture, because of weakness of the anterior neck flexors and back muscles. The distal muscles of the extremities may be involved later in the disease or in children in whom the disease has an acute onset. The affected child may stop walking, may be unable to dress or climb stairs, or may complain of muscle pain. The child usually has a pronounced inability to get up from the floor unaided (Gower sign) or to rise from bed unaided.

Involvement of the pharyngeal, hypopharyngeal, and palatal muscles develops in 10% of children. Dysphonia and difficulty swallowing may be related to this involvement or to esophageal hypomotility. Palatal speech or regurgitation of liquids through the nose are early signs of impending respiratory difficulty and aspiration. Profound involvement of the thoracic and respiratory muscles occurs in a few children and leads to increasing dyspnea at rest, aspiration, or even death.

The classic rash of dermatomyositis is seen in most of these children, and it may be the first sign of the disease; in the remainder, it is less characteristic but usually suggestive of the diagnosis (Fig. 434.5). The rash is most distinctive over the upper eyelids, malar areas, and the dorsal surfaces of the knuckles, elbows, and knees. The severity of cutaneous involvement is variable. Often, at onset of the disease, indurative edema of the skin and subcutaneous tissues is present. Later, manifestations include thinning and atrophy of the accessory epidermal structures, with loss of hair and development of telangiectases. Vasculitic ulcers at the corners of the eyes, around the axillae, and over stretch marks are serious complications, especially if they become infected.

Laboratory Examination

The acute-phase reactants, such as the ESR and the C-reactive protein, tend to correlate with the degree of clinical

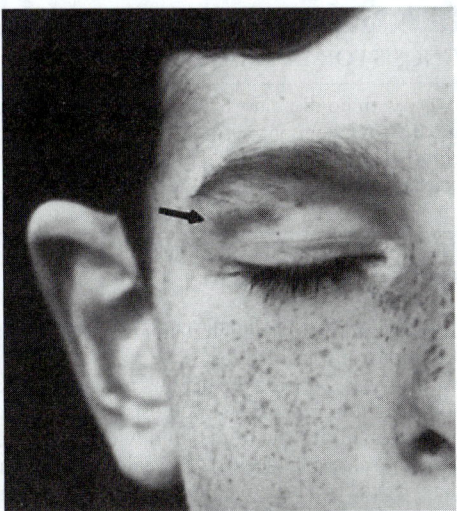

FIGURE 434.5. The arrow points to the violaceous suffusion of the upper eyelid in a boy with active dermatomyositis.

TABLE 434.13

DIAGNOSTIC CRITERIA FOR DERMATOMYOSITIS

Progressive symmetric weakness of proximal limb-girdle and anterior neck flexor muscles

Classic dermatitis of eyelids, metacarpophalangeal and proximal interphalangeal joints, elbows, knees, and medial malleoli

Elevation of serum muscle enzymes

Electromyographic demonstration of myopathy and denervation

Muscle biopsy confirming inflammatory myositis

inflammation. Anemia is an uncommon finding at onset, except in children with gastrointestinal bleeding. Urinalysis generally is normal, except in the few children with microscopic hematuria at onset. ANAs are variably present, and specific antibodies, such as those to the PM antigen, have been described (although rarely). At onset, one-half of the children have positive tests for circulating immune complexes.

The three most important diagnostic laboratory abnormalities are elevated serum muscle enzyme levels, which are present in 98% of the children; abnormal electromyographic changes in 96%; and specific histopathologic abnormalities on muscle biopsy in 79%. The levels of the serum muscle enzymes are important for establishing the diagnosis and in monitoring effective therapy. Generally, a panel checking the levels of creatine kinase (CK), aspartate transaminase (AST), alanine transaminase (ALT), and aldolase is followed initially. The degree of increase in serum concentrations ranges from 20 to 40 times normal for the CK or AST. The appearance of MB bands on the isozyme pattern of the CK usually is interpreted as evidence of regenerative striated muscle and not of cardiac damage. The serum concentration of von Willebrand factor VIII antigen is elevated in active disease, as evidence of vasculitis, as is the serum neopterin level.

Electromyography (EMG) aids in confirming the diagnosis in a few selected children and helps to determine the best site for a muscle biopsy, but it often is fraught with difficulty in obtaining cooperation in children. Abnormalities on EMG are those of myopathy and denervation. Magnetic resonance imaging (MRI) also is abnormal and distinguishes between unaffected and affected muscles; it often is a better guide to the site for muscle biopsy than is the EMG.

Although seldom necessary for diagnosis, generally a muscle biopsy is indicated in the initial assessment of a child to support long-term glucocorticoid therapy (or, eventually, immunosuppressive drugs) and to provide an assessment of prognosis. The muscle to be examined should be involved clinically but not atrophied. The best sites generally are a deltoid or quadriceps. An open surgical biopsy should be generous (2 cm); however, experience is increasing with closed-needle biopsy.

Diagnosis

Dermatomyositis is diagnosed on the basis of an acute onset of proximal limb-girdle muscle weakness accompanied by a characteristic dermatitis (Table 434.13). Polymyositis, or in-

flammatory myositis without dermatitis, rarely is encountered in children. The differential diagnosis entails little confusion with the acute systemic onset of JRA or with SLE. However, mild forms of dermatomyositis with a prominent degree of arthritis may be confused with either of these two diseases. Scleroderma presents unique diagnostic problems because approximately one-fifth of affected children present with a primary myositis not unlike that of dermatomyositis. An occasional child develops an overlap syndrome with varying features of the other connective tissue diseases. Eosinophilic fasciitis and mixed connective tissue disease are distinctive syndromes within this category.

The muscular dystrophies are diagnostic considerations at onset. In these disorders, an insidious onset, progressive or remitting disease, a positive family history, and a selective and predictable pattern of muscle involvement are present. Dermatitis and nail-fold capillary abnormalities are absent. The serum CK is increased in the first-degree relatives of children with muscular dystrophy and especially in mothers of children with X-linked disorders. Other congenital myopathies, myotonias and hypotonic syndromes, the metabolic and endocrine myopathies, paroxysmal myoglobulinuria, thyrotoxic myopathy, and myasthenia gravis also must be considered.

Poliomyelitis and the Guillain-Barré syndrome, in addition to influenza, coxsackievirus, and echovirus, are other diagnostic possibilities in children with an acute onset of severe pain and muscle weakness. Trichinosis and toxoplasmosis cause myositis of varying severity, and severe pustular acne may be associated with inflammation of muscle and an arthropathy. Rhabdomyolysis may develop after an acute infection, trauma, or extreme muscular excretion, with an acute onset characterized by profound weakness, myoglobinuria and, occasionally, oliguria and renal failure.

Therapy

General supportive care and a coordinated team approach are necessary to manage this serious disease. Treatment should include a program of graduated rest and positioning, along with physical therapy to minimize contractures. Generally, the use of prednisone in a dosage of approximately 2 mg/kg/day in divided doses is necessary for at least the first month after diagnosis. If clinical response is acceptable, and the serum muscle enzyme concentrations decrease, then a lower dosage in the range of approximately 1 mg/kg/day is instituted. Thereafter, the daily dose is tapered slowly by frequent monitoring the child's improvement in the clinical status, the degree of muscle weakness documented by objective testing, and the serum muscle enzyme concentrations. Myositis is not controlled satisfactorily until the serum muscle enzymes return to normal (or nearly normal) levels and remain there while the steroid is tapered, concomitant with an increase in the child's level of physical activity. Because the long-term administration of glucocorticoid is accompanied by significant toxicity in growing children, the steroid dose should be lowered as quickly as possible, consistent with continued improvement in indices of the disease. The initial or early use of intravenous methylprednisolone pulse therapy may minimize steroid toxicity and eventual calcinosis.

Acute gastrointestinal complications occur in a minority of children and may not be controlled adequately by glucocorticoid therapy. These complications have been an important cause of death. Respiratory insufficiency, with or without aspiration, also often is a preterminal event. Cutaneous ulcerations develop in many children and likewise are poor prognostic signs. These acute complications, along with disease that is steroid-unresponsive, are indications for the use of immunosuppressive agents. Methotrexate has been effective adjuvant therapy in some resistant children. Intravenous cyclophosphamide, cyclosporin A, and repeated steroid-pulse therapy also have been used.

Prognosis

The course of dermatomyositis can be divided into four characteristic clinical phases (Table 434.14). Approximately three-fourths of affected children follow a uniphasic course that lasts from 8 months to 2 years. The remainder continue to have acute exacerbations and remissions; some of these patients eventually develop a clinical disease more typical of systemic vasculitis. Late in the course of the disease, a small number of children assume more of the characteristics of scleroderma, with profound sclerodactyly and cutaneous atrophy. Lipoatrophy, acanthosis nigricans, insulin resistance, or a recurrence of arthritis may develop. During the course of the disease, progressive healing of the myositis and the extent of the rash may not correlate. Even years after onset, other affected children have persistent (if only moderate) elevations of serum muscle enzymes and demonstrate characteristic histopathologic features of the disease on muscle biopsies.

Long-term survival in dermatomyositis approaches 90%. If death occurs, it often is within the first years after onset. This observation suggests that the major factors to be assessed in estimating prognosis are the basic nature of the inflammatory disease, its early effective treatment and response, and whether obstructive vasculopathy is present or the involvement of other organ systems, such as the gastrointestinal or pulmonary tracts, is present.

The average child with dermatomyositis is expected to improve progressively to an acceptable level of functional recovery (Table 434.15). During this period of clinical improvement, physical therapy is intensified to normalize function and minimize the development of contractures secondary to muscle weakness or atrophy. Muscle strengthening exercises should be added to the program only when acute inflammation subsides. Functional outcome appears best in children who have been seen early and treated vigorously. Most survivors function

TABLE 434.14

CLINICAL PHASES OF CHILDHOOD DERMATOMYOSITIS

Prodromal period with nonspecific symptoms (weeks to months)
Progressive muscle weakness and rash (days to weeks)
Persistent weakness, rash, and active myositis (up to 2 years)
Recovery with residual muscle atrophy and contractures with or without calcinosis

Adapted with permission from Hanson V. Dermatomyositis, scleroderma, and polyarteritis nodosa. *Clin Rheum Dis* 1976;2:445.

TABLE 434.15

PROGNOSIS FOR DERMATOMYOSITIS

Recovery with no disability	65%
Minimal atrophy or contractures	25%
Calcinosis*	20%
Wheelchair dependence	5%
Death	7%

*Children with calcinosis also are included in the other categories.

independently as adults, although many of them have residual atrophy of skin or muscle groups.

Late in the disease, during the healing phase, approximately one-half of the children develop calcinosis of the skin and subcutaneous tissues, about the joints, and within the interfascial planes of the muscles (Fig. 434.6). The calcium salts have been identified as hydroxyapatite or fluorapatite. Many approaches to the therapy of calcinosis have been reported; none has been uniformly successful. Surgical excision of calcific tumors in areas of ulceration or pressure can be performed if necessary.

SCLERODERMA

The sclerodermas are systemic or localized connective tissue diseases of unknown etiology. The development of scleroderma in a child often is unrecognized initially because the disorder is so rare. The localized forms of the disease, such as morphea or linear scleroderma, often are regarded as more dermatologic than rheumatologic. A classification of the sclerodermas is presented in Table 434.16. In all these disorders, girls are affected more often than are boys, and no peak age of onset during childhood exists.

Diffuse Scleroderma

An idiopathic angiitis is the basic lesion of scleroderma and involves the lungs, heart, and kidneys in addition to the skin and gastrointestinal tract. Arterioles undergo eventual hyalinization and fibrosis. Perivascular infiltrates of mononuclear cells are predominantly T lymphocytes. In systemic scleroderma, thinning of the epidermis and atrophy of the dermal

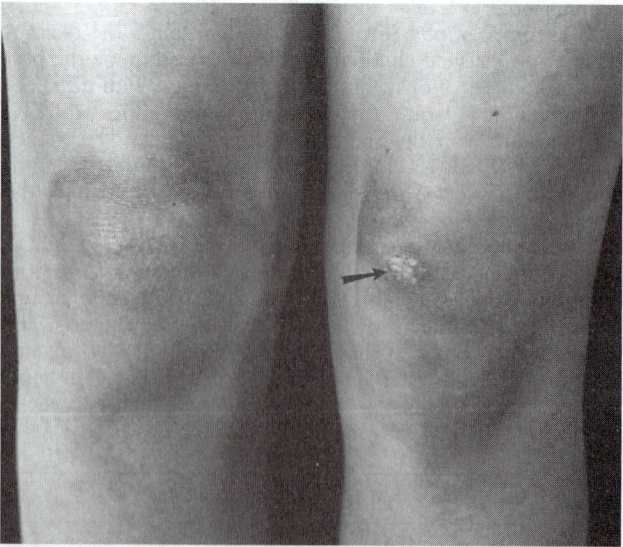

FIGURE 434.6. Knees of a girl with the erythematous prepatellar lesions of dermatomyositis. The arrow points to an area of calcinosis cutis.

TABLE 434.16

CLASSIFICATION OF SCLERODERMA

Systemic disease
Scleroderma
  Diffuse
  Limited
Localized disease
Morphea
Linear scleroderma

appendages, an increased density and thickness of collagen deposition, and a predominance of embryonal fibers are present.

Clinical Manifestations and Complications. Often, a diagnosis of scleroderma is delayed for years because of the subtle and insidious nature of the onset. Presentation is characterized by the appearance of Raynaud phenomenon; thinning and atrophy of the skin of the hands or face; or the development of cutaneous telangiectases about the face, upper trunk, and over the hands (Table 434.17). Dysphagia or symptoms of reflux esophagitis and other disturbances of gastrointestinal motility may be present even early in the course. Malabsorption may be minimal or become severe.

Tightening and thickening of the skin is virtually universal at onset and becomes gradually more generalized. Acrosclerosis of the hands and feet and distal extremities is characteristic. Hypopigmentation and hyperpigmentation are present, along with later development of subcutaneous calcifications. Ulcerations may occur over the fingers, elbows, and malleoli. Raynaud phenomenon with a two- or three-color change occurs in most children and may antedate the onset of cutaneous abnormalities. It is characterized by obstructive digital arterial disease and sympathetic hyperactivity that often are progressive. Digital gangrene may supervene, with small atrophic pits on the fingertips. Acro-osteolysis of the digital tufts often accompanies this abnormality and can be documented on radio-

graphs of the hands or feet. This resorption of bone may be accompanied by small areas of soft-tissue calcification.

Many children have arthralgia, and a few present with objective arthritis or contractures. Muscle pain and tenderness are present in approximately 20%. Elevation of the serum muscle enzyme levels, however, tends to be only mild to moderate. Cardiac involvement with arrhythmias may develop during the course of the disease, and congestive heart failure often is a terminal event. Dyspnea on exertion may be related to skin tightness, intercostal muscle weakness, or intrinsic pulmonary disease.

Laboratory Examination. Routine laboratory studies often are normal. ANAs occur in most affected children and are characterized by high-titered speckled patterns. Distinct antigenic specificity may be present: anticentromere in localized systemic scleroderma, anti-Scl 70 (tropoisomerase 1) in diffuse systemic scleroderma, or nucleolar antibodies.

Plethysmography is abnormal in affected digits in Raynaud phenomenon and documents both the obstructive vascular disease and involvement of the sympathetic nervous system. Arteriography should not be performed as a diagnostic procedure because it may exacerbate digital anoxia.

Pulmonary diffusion and spirometry are sensitive measures of involvement of the respiratory tract. These studies are abnormal in many children at onset and are progressive. Usually, upper gastrointestinal films document disordered motility of the distal esophagus (Fig. 434.7). Balloon esophageal motility and pH probe studies are more sensitive indicators of the degree of abnormality in these children.

Diagnosis

Diagnosis is based on demonstration of the classic cutaneous findings: skin tightening of the face, hands, and feet, telangiectases, Raynaud phenomenon, and the presence of visceral

TABLE 434.17

CLINICAL MANIFESTATIONS IN CHILDREN WITH SYSTEMIC SCLERODERMA

Organ System	Frequency of Involvement (%)
Skin	
Digital arteries (Raynaud phenomenon)	75
Subcutaneous calcification	60
Telangiectases	30
Ulceration	30
Pigmentation	20
Musculoskeletal	
Contractures	75
Resorption of digital tufts	60
Muscle weakness	40
Muscle atrophy	40
Gastrointestinal tract	
Abnormal esophageal motility	75
Colonic sacculations	20
Duodenal dilatation	5
Pulmonary tract	
Abnormal diffusion	75
Abnormal vital capacity	70
Heart	
Electrocardiographic abnormalities	30
Cardiomegaly	15
Congestive failure	15

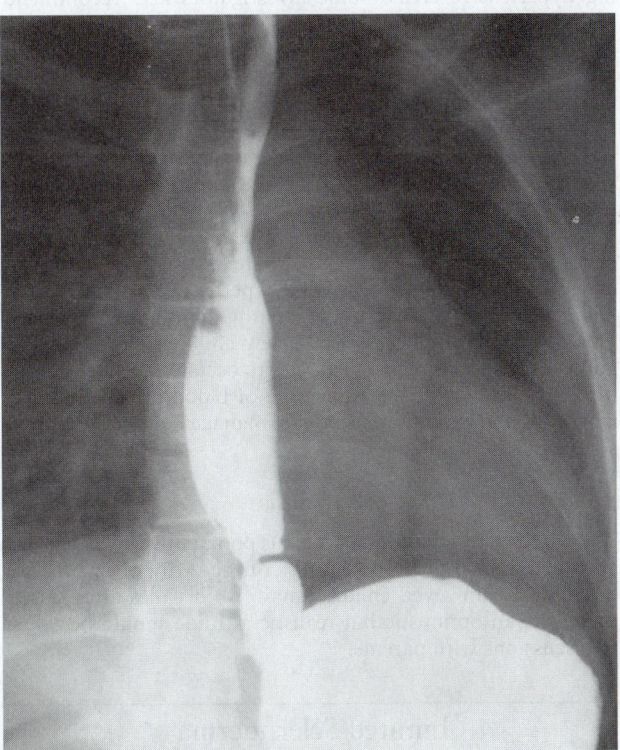

FIGURE 434.7. A barium swallow examination in the supine position of a 14-year-old girl who presented with severe dysphagia and scleroderma. The barium column collected in the patulous esophagus, which was virtually without peristaltic movement.

disease, usually gastrointestinal or pulmonary. Diagnostic abnormalities of the nail-fold capillaries are virtually universal at onset of the disease. Viewed through the +40 lens of an ophthalmoscope, a reduction in the number of vessels, thickening of vascular walls, and a marked tortuosity of the remaining vessels are seen. Scattered fibrotic clear areas without capillaries are prominent.

The differential diagnosis includes dermatomyositis, SLE, overlap syndromes, and, less frequently, JRA. Children with localized systemic scleroderma have prominent *c*alcinosis, *R*aynaud phenomenon, *e*sophageal abnormalities, *s*clerodactyly, and *t*elangiectases (CREST syndrome). This variant once was thought to have a more favorable prognosis; however, evidence for this judgment has not been confirmed in more recent studies.

Numerous other entities mimic or duplicate abnormalities found in scleroderma. Scleroderma-like disease has developed as a toxic reaction to vinyl chloride, bleomycin, and pentazocine. It also occurred in epidemic proportions, with many deaths occurring in Spain secondary to contaminated cooking oil (rapeseed oil). It is encountered as a component of graft-versus-host disease in bone marrow transplantation recipients. Scleroderma-like changes also may occur in children with phenylketonuria or progeria.

Therapy

Of the connective tissue diseases, scleroderma is one of the most difficult to treat. NSAIDs are useful to relieve the musculoskeletal stiffness and aching. Colchicine also may be beneficial. Children who present with gastrointestinal problems demand special therapeutic considerations for esophageal stricture or obstruction, reflux esophagitis, or malabsorption.

Raynaud phenomenon is managed with alpha-blocking agents such as phenoxybenzamine or with calcium-channel blockers such as nifedipine or verapamil. Angiotensin-converting enzyme (ACE) inhibitors, such as captopril, are crucial in treating hypertensive crisis. Some investigators also recommend early treatment of the angiitis of scleroderma with these drugs. Children with prominent Raynaud phenomenon need to dress seasonally and avoid cold liquids and exposure that exacerbate not only the peripheral arteriolar constriction but also vascular spasm within viscera. If prescribed early, D-penicillamine may be useful in managing cutaneous manifestations of the disease. Vigorous physical therapy to prevent contractures is important.

Glucocorticoid drugs probably are contraindicated in most children. These agents may exacerbate small blood vessel disease and renal involvement with hypertension. Renal failure and acute hypertensive encephalopathy may supervene as potentially fatal complications in a few children. As studied in adults, these events seem most likely to occur early in the course of the disease. Emergency lowering of blood pressure to normal levels and expert intensive care management are critical to survival.

Prognosis

The outcome of scleroderma often is poor, but survival has not been determined precisely because of the rarity of the disease in children. However, children may live decades after onset; therefore, an optimistic but realistic attitude should be taken in discussions with parents.

Limited Scleroderma

Localized scleroderma occurs much more commonly than does systemic disease. Fibrosis of connective tissues in morphea is limited to the dermis, subdermis, and superficial striated muscles. This variant is subcategorized into single or multiple plaques, guttate morphea consisting of small lesions in a generalized distribution, bullous morphea, or extensive coalescent involvement in deep morphea. Morphea is characterized by one or more circumscribed cutaneous lesions of varying size marked by hypopigmentation and induration surrounded by hyperpigmented skin. Erythema and acute inflammatory edema are present, especially at the margins of the lesions. These distinct and localized lesions are located anywhere on the trunk or extremities. The affected child also may complain of paresthesia or pain over the involved areas. Each area of involvement may enlarge centrifugally or coalesce and involve larger areas of skin.

Hide-binding from fibrosis of the involved skin and subcutaneous tissues may become extensive and result in marked contractures of an extremity. Active disease may undergo exacerbations and remissions for many months to years, although lesions tend to regress slowly with time. The application of local emollients and glucocorticoid ointments may result in some improvement. D-Penicillamine may be effective if used early in the more generalized form of morphea. Systemic antibiotics have been reported to be effective in a few studies.

Linear scleroderma (or linear morphea) develops primarily in the patient's first two decades of life. This disorder is characterized by the presence of one or more areas of linear involvement of the skin of the head, trunk, or extremities. Because lesions of the face or scalp may look like scars from dueling, the term *en coup-de-sabre* has been used to describe them. Often, underlying muscle and bone are involved in the pattern of fibrosis and inflammation in this form of the disease, with localized growth abnormalities, deformities, or contractures of joints occurring. Linear scleroderma often affects only one side of the body, producing hemiatrophy of the involved parts (Fig. 434.8). It is this lack of normal growth and development that produces the most severe disabilities (e.g., hemifacial atrophy, failure of an extremity to grow in proportion to its opposite member, severe joint contractures).

Localized scleroderma has few laboratory abnormalities. ANAs are positive in approximately 50% of patients. Antibodies to centromere or Scl-70 generally are not present in the localized forms of the disease.

Linear scleroderma also may regress without treatment or with time. Although individual lesions may improve, significant abnormalities of local growth persist, particularly if deep tissues and bone have been involved. Occasionally, visceral disease or a seizure in a child with involvement of the skull develops late in the course of the disease. In a few children, the disease evolves into an overlap syndrome with another connective tissue disease, such as SLE.

EOSINOPHILIC FASCIITIS

Eosinophilic fasciitis originally was described in young adults who presented with acute painful inflammation and induration of cutaneous and subcutaneous tissues. This involvement occurred in upper and lower extremities, was often bilateral, and occasionally spread to the trunk or face. Raynaud phenomenon, nail-fold capillary abnormalities, and visceral disease were absent. An acute onset of the disease often was preceded by unusual degrees of physical exertion.

Although the condition rarely occurs in childhood, affected children present acutely with marked induration of the cutaneous and subcutaneous tissues resembling that seen in scleroderma or dermatomyositis. Controversy continues whether eosinophilic fasciitis is a distinct clinicopathologic entity or an unusual variant of localized scleroderma (deep morphea). Morphea *per se* also may accompany or precede the disorder. A remarkable eosinophilia and hypergammaglobulinemia occur in

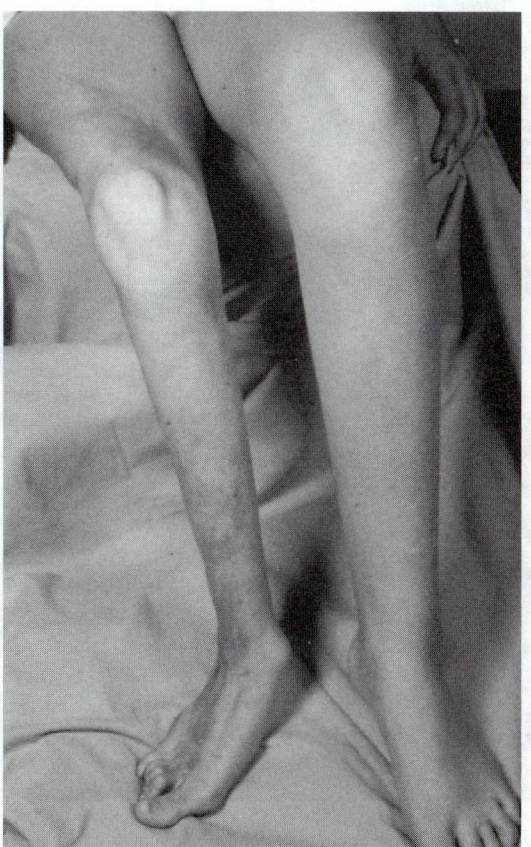

FIGURE 434.8. Linear scleroderma affecting the right leg of an adolescent girl. This lesion involves not only the skin but the deeper subcutaneous tissues, fascia, muscle, and bone. It had resulted in a severe deformity and a 7.5 cm shortening of that limb. (Reprinted with permission from Cassidy JT. SLE, juvenile dermatomyositis, scleroderma, and vasculitis. In Ruddy S, Harris ED Jr., Sledge CB, eds. *Kelley's textbook of rheumatology.* Philadelphia: WB Saunders, 2001.)

approximately one-half of the children. The eosinophilia may reach 40% to 60% of the peripheral WBC count. The ESR and other acute-phase reactants also are increased.

Diagnosis of eosinophilic fasciitis is established by microscopic examination of a deep biopsy of skin, fascia, and muscle

---

TABLE 434.18

CLASSIFICATION OF IDIOPATHIC VASCULITIS

Necrotizing vasculitis of medium and small arteries
Polyarteritis nodosa
Kawasaki disease

Necrotizing arteritis of small vessels
Leukocytoclastic vasculitis
Hypersensitivity angiitis
Henoch-Schönlein purpura

Granulomatous vasculitis
Allergic necrotizing granulomatosis
Wegener granulomatosis

Giant cell arteritis
Systemic giant cell arteritis
Takayasu arteritis
Cranial arteritis
Behçet syndrome

---

in an area of involvement. Inflammation is present in all layers, but the most characteristic feature is thickened fascia with round-cell infiltration of histiocytes and often eosinophils and a prominent perivascular infiltrate of lymphocytes and plasma cells. IgG, IgM, and C3 may be deposited in these lesions.

Originally, eosinophilic fasciitis was noted to be a self-limited disorder with spontaneous resolution after months to years, or a marked, satisfactory response to low doses of glucocorticoids. Occasionally, a more prolonged and steroid-resistant course developed, or a more severe form of the disease evolved with serious hematologic abnormalities.

IDIOPATHIC VASCULITIS

Although vasculitis is a prominent and almost universal component of the various connective tissue diseases, distinct types of idiopathic vasculitis are encountered in children (Table 434.18). All forms of vasculitis, except for Henoch-Schönlein purpura and Kawasaki disease rarely occur in children. Several attempts have been made to classify the various forms of vasculitis: Table 434.19 presents a classification that accounts for the most significant features of histopathology and clinical findings. This schema is derived from the classification proposed by Zeek, in 1953, and the reexamination of these

---

TABLE 434.19

PATHOLOGIC CLASSIFICATION OF IDIOPATHIC VASCULITIS

Classification	Size of Vessels	Location of Lesions and Organ Involvement	Histopathologic Features
Polyarteritis	Small to medium muscular arteries, adjacent veins	Widespread near bifurcations; kidneys, gastrointestinal tract, mesentery, pancreas	Fibrinoid necrosis, aneurysms, lesions of various ages
Hypersensitivity angiitis	Arterioles, venules, and capillaries	Widespread; kidneys, heart, lungs, spleen, skin, serosa	Necrosis, lesions at same state of development, eosinophilic infiltration
Allergic granulomatosis	Small arteries and veins	Widespread; lungs, heart, spleen	Necrotizing granulomas, lesions of various ages, eosinophilic infiltration
Giant cell arteritis	Large arteries	Aorta and major branches; temporal arteries	Granulomatous inflammation, no necrosis, multinucleated giant cells
Wegener granulomatosis	Medium to small arteries and veins	Respiratory tract and kidneys	Necrotizing granulomas, giant cells

diseases by a committee of the American College of Rheumatology in 1990. Classification is based on the size of the vessel involved, the distribution of visceral involvement, and whether the predominant histopathology is necrosis of a vessel wall or a granulomatous response. In necrotizing arteritis, destruction of the vascular wall often is a direct consequence of immune-complex deposition. In most cases, the responsible antigen is unknown; however, in a few instances of classic polyarteritis nodosa (PAN), a causal relationship between hepatitis B infection and immune-complex disease has been established. The predominant pathologic features of giant cell arteritis involve larger blood vessels and giant cells in the lesions. In Wegener granulomatosis, the principal finding is a necrotizing granuloma.

Necrotizing Vasculitis of Medium-sized Arteries

In this type of necrotizing vasculitis, the medium and small muscular arteries are involved predominantly and the characteristic histologic abnormality is fibrinoid necrosis of the entire thickness of the vessel wall in all stages of development from acute to chronic. The inflammatory lesions are segmental, with a predilection for areas of bifurcations. Angiography often demonstrates small aneurysms in the celiac and renal vessels. Although each form of this disorder has characteristic features, distinguishing among polyarteritis, hypersensitivity angiitis, and allergic granulomatosis is not always possible clinically.

Polyarteritis Nodosa

Establishing diagnosis early and correctly classifying PAN often are difficult. The course and progression of this disease is highly variable, and multisystemic involvement leads to diagnostic confusion with other entities.

Clinical Manifestations and Complications

No single pattern of clinical presentation is characteristic. Frequently, the onset is insidious. Constitutional symptoms of fever and weight loss may be the presenting complaints (Table 434.20). Renal, gastrointestinal, nervous system, and cardiac disease often occur initially separately or together (Fig. 434.9). Dermatitis, although characteristic, includes a spectrum of lesions of purpura, gangrene of the distal parts of the extremities, and erythematous, painful nodules. The initial clinical diagnosis of PAN may be renovascular hypertension or an acute ab-

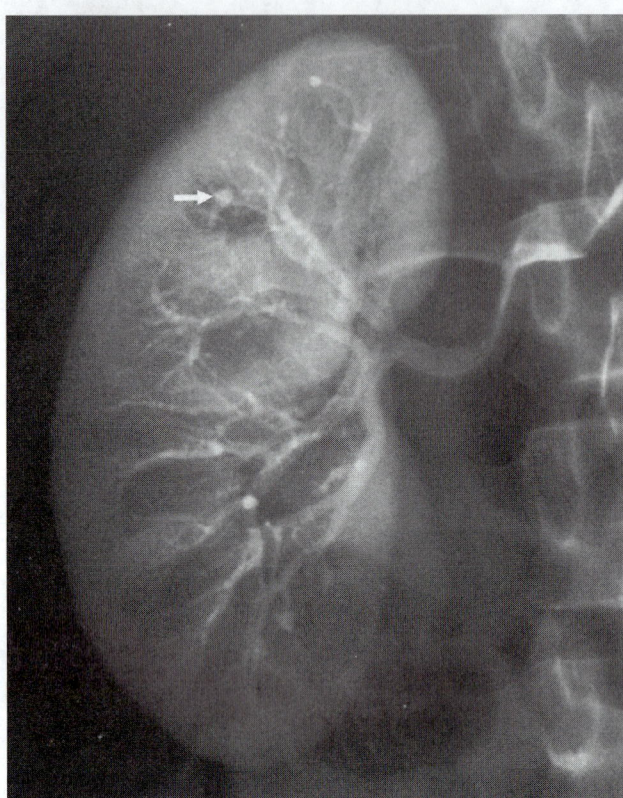

FIGURE 434.9. Renal angiogram of an adolescent boy with polyarteritis nodosa (PAN) who presented with musculoskeletal aching, hypertension, and hematuria. The arrow points to an aneurysm that is characteristic of this disease.

domen. Severe, symmetric sensorimotor peripheral neuropathy (mononeuritis multiplex) frequently is present.

Laboratory Examination

The level of anemia, leukocytosis, elevation of the ESR, concentration of the serum immunoglobulins, and urinary sediment changes often reflect the extent of multisystem involvement. A firm diagnosis is based, however, on characteristic histologic changes in a biopsy specimen or an angiogram demonstrating multiple aneurysms.

Therapy

The administration of glucocorticoid is the primary approach to management. Prednisone is prescribed initially in suppressive amounts in the range of 1 to 2 mg/kg/day in divided doses. The degree of cardiac or renal involvement, or the presence of hypertension, modulates therapeutic aggressiveness. Extensive systemic involvement, particularly of the intra-abdominal vessels with aneurysms or thrombosis, generally is an indication for the addition of cyclophosphamide.

Prognosis

Although the course of PAN is highly variable, most commonly death is secondary to renal failure, myocardial infarction, or hypertensive encephalopathy. Children with more restricted organ involvement have a better prognosis. Cogan syndrome is a very rare occurrence in childhood and is characterized by ocular and inner-ear vasculitis. Affected patients present with interstitial keratitis, vertigo, tinnitus, and deafness. Serous otitis media also may be seen in children in association with PAN.

TABLE 434.20

CLINICAL MANIFESTATIONS OF POLYARTERITIS

Manifestation	Percentage of Children
Constitutional signs and symptoms	75
Musculoskeletal involvement	75
Leukocytosis, eosinophilia	75
Dermatitis	60
Peripheral neuropathy	40
Mesenteric involvement	40
Central nervous system disease	30
Pulmonary disease	25
Nephritis and hypertension	25
Myocardial infarction	20

Necrotizing Vasculitis of Small Vessels

Leukocytoclastic Vasculitis

Leukocytoclastic vasculitis is a form of necrotizing vasculitis that involves the smaller blood vessels and post-capillary venules. Polymorphonuclear leukocytes infiltrate the entire vessel wall, and nuclear debris is present around the lesions. This form of vasculitis may be idiopathic or occur secondary to drug hypersensitivity, infectious endocarditis, or malignancy.

Hypersensitivity Angiitis

Smaller blood vessels, including arterioles, capillaries, and venules, are the principal sites of involvement in hypersensitivity angiitis. The inflammatory lesions of angiitis are at a similar stage of histologic development, and eosinophiles often are prominent. This disorder may develop as a hypersensitivity reaction to the administration of a therapeutic drug or in conjunction with another systemic illness. Serum sickness is a form of this type of vasculitis in which immune complexes can be demonstrated in the circulation of many affected children and by fluorescent histopathology at the site of vascular inflammation. Experimental serum sickness in animals and soluble immune-complex disease are laboratory counterparts of hypersensitivity angiitis.

Pulmonary and cutaneous disease are common findings in hypersensitivity vasculitis. Dermatologic lesions consist of palpable purpura or superficial hemorrhagic infarcts. The disease is characterized by a variable course, and often outcome is determined in large part by the extent and severity of cardiac or renal abnormalities. Glucocorticoids usually are effective in suppressing the clinical vasculitis and in preventing severe complications or death. Classically, this disease runs its course in approximately 6 weeks.

Other Types of Small Blood Vessel Vasculitis

Isolated cutaneous vasculitis presents with palpable purpura, painful nodules, or ridges that develop along the course of involved vessels. Otherwise, the affected child is well, without systemic or constitutional symptoms. The clinical course is variable and characterized by remissions and exacerbations, often over the course of many years. Although each crop of lesions may respond to glucocorticoids or occasionally to NSAIDs, this disease frequently is of such long duration that treating the growing child with prednisone during the entire course is difficult. Alternate-day dosage may be preferable therapy for such children.

Hypocomplementemic urticarial vasculitis also has been described in a rare child. Girls are more at risk. The pathogenesis is unknown, but an immune-complex process is suggested. The eruption affects principally the face, upper extremities, and trunk. The urticarial lesions last for only a few days with each exacerbation, then fade without scarring. Systemic features may accompany the cutaneous disease. The degree of hypocomplementemia parallels the severity of the illness. Some of these children warrant treatment with glucocorticoids.

Cryoglobulinemia, either essential or secondary to another disease, results in an immune-complex vasculitis that can mimic any of the entities discussed earlier. Cryoglobulins can be demonstrated in plasma chilled to 4°C to 22°C. Depending on the disease (e.g., hepatitis C) and the nature of the involvement, therapy consists of the specific treatment of the underlying problem, the use of prednisone or immunosuppressive agents, or plasmapheresis.

GRANULOMATOUS VASCULITIS

Allergic Necrotizing Granulomatosis

Allergic necrotizing granulomatosis is a rare systemic vasculitis that occurs predominantly in young males with a history of chronic asthma. The histopathology is that of a necrotizing vasculitis with an eosinophilic infiltrate and extravascular necrotizing granulomata. Peripheral eosinophilia often is prominent. Other manifestations are identical to those seen in polyarteritis, especially in the gastrointestinal tract, CNS, and musculoskeletal system. Pulmonary disease often is the most important manifestation, with prominent radiologic abnormalities. Renal disease may be seen less frequently. Administration of glucocorticoids is the main approach to treatment. Prognosis is variable; often death involves cardiopulmonary failure.

Wegener Granulomatosis

Wegener granulomatosis is a very rare syndrome in children, although it has been described in infants as young as 3 months of age. It is characterized by a necrotizing granulomatous angiitis involving both the respiratory tract (sinuses, nasal passages, and lungs) and the kidneys. Characteristic granulomata also may be found in skin, heart, CNS, gastrointestinal tract, and synovia. Constitutional symptoms almost always are prominent.

Unexplained sinopulmonary pain, rhinorrhea, mucosal ulceration, or bleeding from the upper respiratory tract may be a presenting sign. Hemoptysis and pleuritic pain are frequent manifestations. The pulmonary disease may progress to hemorrhage, obstruction, atelectasis, or repeated episodes of infection. Chest films demonstrate multiform pulmonary infiltrates and nodules. CT scans may document erosion of nasal cartilage and bone. Most of the affected children have moderate to severe renal disease that may progress if untreated. Hypertension may occur less commonly than in other types of nephritis.

The differential diagnosis includes the other forms of vasculitis, sarcoidosis, berylliosis, Loeffler syndrome, tuberculosis, disseminated fungal disease, syphilis, or lymphoma. Clinically, Goodpasture syndrome and other rare forms of granulomatous arteritis are confused easily with this disorder. Diagnosis is established by microscopic examination of a biopsy of an affected organ, usually the nasal mucosa, or an open-lung biopsy. Granulomata and necrotizing vasculitis with leukocytic, lymphocytic, and giant-cell infiltration are present.

Historically, death from renal or pulmonary disease occurred with only rare long-term survival. Treatment with glucocorticoids had some effect early in the disease, but more recent trials support therapy with cyclophosphamide. A dramatic response to its use has altered the outcome of this otherwise fatal disease to one of remission, if not cure, in the adult series reported from the National Institutes of Health (NIH). More recent investigations have considered other agents with less toxicity, such as methotrexate or trimethoprim-sulfamethoxazole.

Giant Cell Arteritis

Giant cell arteritis characteristically involves the aorta or its major branches. Histologically, disruption of the internal elastic lamina, intimal proliferation, and infiltration of the wall with mononuclear cells and giant cells occur.

Systemic Giant Cell Arteritis

Systemic giant cell arteritis involves major branches or segments of the thoracic or abdominal aorta at single or multiple locations. The affected child may present with constitutional symptoms such as weight loss, malaise, fatigue, fever of unknown origin, or hypertension. Vascular occlusion leads to the development of peripheral anoxia, cyanosis, and gangrene. The recanalization of involved vessels may occur spontaneously or during treatment with glucocorticoid drugs. Diagnosis is established by arteriography, occasionally combined with the histologic examination of a biopsy of an accessible vessel.

Takayasu Arteritis

Takayasu arteritis is a giant cell arteritis that occurs predominantly in teenage girls. Stenosis, occlusion, dilation, and formation of an aneurysm are confined to the aorta, its major branches, and the pulmonary arteries. This disease has been called *pulseless disease* because of the obliteration of the radial pulses or reverse coarctation. Hypertension frequently occurs. The acute-phase reactants and the WBC count usually are elevated. Takayasu arteritis appears to be more common in Asians, Latinos, blacks, and Sephardic Jews. The female-to-male ratio is 8:1. Unidentified environmental or genetic factors may play a role in its pathogenesis. Occasionally, it develops in the families of children with other connective tissue diseases; it also has been reported in monozygotic twin sisters.

The course of Takayasu arteritis may be limited, lasting 3 to 6 months, or be prolonged over many years. Establishing the diagnosis early often is difficult because of its insidious onset, and an erroneous diagnosis (e.g., systemic onset JRA, acute rheumatic fever) may be made. Eventually, signs of vascular insufficiency suggest the correct diagnosis, which then can be confirmed by angiography or MRI. Calcification in the affected vessels may be present on plain-film radiography.

NSAIDs are useful in managing the symptoms of these patients during the acute early phases of the illness. Generally, glucocorticoid drugs are indicated for the suppression of early disease, along with consideration of weekly methotrexate pulse therapy. Aggressive control of hypertension is essential. Anticoagulants or antiplatelet agents may be required if widespread chronic occlusion of vessels is present. Vessel grafts have been successful late in the course of the disease.

Cranial Arteritis

Cranial or temporal arteritis generally is found only in the older adult. However, it may present rarely in childhood. It is characterized by a severe, persistent headache and localized pain or tenderness directly over a cranial or temporal vessel. The ESR is very high. The threat of blindness (amaurosis fugax) occurring from involvement of the ophthalmic and central retinal arteries is an important consideration and an indication for prompt initiation of glucocorticoid therapy. Diagnosis is established by the microscopic examination of a generous biopsy from an involved superficial vessel.

Behçet Syndrome

Behçet syndrome consists of a triad of recurrent uveitis, mucocutaneous ulcerations, and genital ulcerations. However, establishing with certainty the diagnosis in a child is difficult unless involvement of the CNS is present. Additional features include arthritis, gastrointestinal disease, and cardiovascular involvement.

This disorder is an uncommon occurrence in North America. It originally was described in the Middle East and has occurred especially frequently in geographic areas characterized by immigration from those areas of the world. That this disorder arose along the silk road from the Orient to the Adriatic Sea is well-documented.

No etiology has been identified. An infectious cause has been advanced because of the geographic foci of the disease. Inclusion bodies have been noted in exudative cells in some studies. The mucocutaneous lesions may represent lesions of delayed hypersensitivity. Superficial trauma reproduces typical cutaneous lesions when active disease is present (pathergy).

Pathology

The basic pathologic lesion is a vasculitis of small- and medium-sized arteries and veins with a mononuclear cell infiltrate, fibrinoid necrosis, and narrowing and obliteration of the vessel lumen. Venous thromboses of the terminal vascular beds or vena cava are especially common findings. Immunofluorescent microscopy demonstrates C3, C4, and the terminal components of the complement cascade in vessel walls along with IgG and fibrinogen. Circulating immune complexes often are present.

Clinical Manifestations

Males are affected more frequently than are females. The most common age at onset is 18 to 40 years. Occurrence of the disease in children as young as 2 years of age has been reported. A nondestructive polyarthritis occurs in approximately 75% of those children. The peripheral joint disease may be either symmetric or asymmetric. Large joints, such as the knees, are affected most frequently, but small joints may be involved. Multiple recurrences of synovitis, particularly in the knees and ankles, develop during a period of several years, although bony erosions and functional disability are uncommon occurrences. Fever and erythema nodosum frequently accompany the arthritis.

Aphthous stomatitis is a common finding, as are ulcerative lesions of the mucous membranes of the upper and lower gastrointestinal tracts. The oral ulcerations are quite painful and interfere with swallowing and speech. Similar ulcerations occur in the genitourinary tract and are accompanied by a sterile pyuria. These lesions may resemble herpes simplex or the Stevens-Johnson syndrome. An incorrect diagnosis of regional enteritis or ulcerative colitis may have been made in these children. Behçet syndrome can be confused clinically with reactive arthritis with conjunctivitis and urethritis or cervicitis.

Involvement of the eye includes photophobia, pain, conjunctivitis, and blurred vision. Uveitis is a common finding. Scleritis, retinal vasculitis, and optic neuritis also may develop and lead to blindness.

CNS involvement ranges from trivial neurologic signs to overt confusion to papilledema and pseudotumor cerebri. These complications occur in approximately one-fourth of the patients and are divided into five syndromes: pseudotumor cerebri, meningoencephalitis, brain-stem involvement, dementia, and changes in personality and behavior.

Laboratory Examination

This condition has no specific laboratory findings. Cerebral spinal fluid abnormalities include pleocytosis and increased concentrations of protein. Hypergammaglobulinemia is characteristic. Autoantibodies reacting with mucosal cells have been demonstrated in some patients. HLA associations include B5 in North American studies and an increased prevalence of

B27 elsewhere, although the frequency of spondylitis does not appear to be increased.

Therapy

Treatment is difficult and puzzling because the prolonged course is punctuated by spontaneous remissions. Reports suggest that immunosuppressive or alkylating agents (chlorambucil) may be indicated along with glucocorticoid drugs.

Prognosis

The course of Behçet syndrome is highly variable from patient to patient. Active disease may span a period of a few weeks or extend to several years, and the typical pattern of involvement is characterized by frequent remissions and exacerbations. Prognosis often is related directly to the extent of CNS disease.

Suggested Readings

Ansell BA, Rudge S, Schaller JG. *Color atlas of pediatric rheumatology*. St. Louis: Mosby-Year Book, 1992.
Athreya B, ed. Pediatric rheumatology. *Rheum Dis Clin North Am* 1997;23:491.
Cassidy JT, Levinson JE, Bass JC, et al. A study of classification criteria for a diagnosis of juvenile rheumatoid arthritis. *Arthritis Rheum* 1986;29:274.
Cassidy JT, Petty RE, eds. *Textbook of pediatric rheumatology*, 4th ed. Philadelphia: WB Saunders, 2001.
Lovell D, White P, eds. Pediatric rheumatology into the '90s. *J Rheumatol* 1992; 19(Suppl 33):1.
Miller ML. Pediatric rheumatology. *Pediatr Clin North Am* 1995;42:999.

CHAPTER 435 ■ AMYLOIDOSIS

PATRICIA WOO

Amyloidosis is characterized by the deposition of a homogenous eosinophilic material in the parenchyma and around blood vessels. Amyloidosis was originally divided into two types: primary amyloidosis in association with plasma cell disorders, which occurs as an idiopathic or familial disease, and secondary amyloidosis, found in conjunction with another inflammatory disease (e.g., juvenile rheumatoid arthritis, familial Mediterranean fever [FMF], chronic pulmonary disease, or osteomyelitis). A classification of different types of amyloidoses is summarized in Table 435.1.

In primary or amyloid-containing immunoglobulin light-chain amyloidosis (see Table 435.1), the principal sites of involvement are the skin and gastrointestinal tract. The patient may present with macroglossia, carpal tunnel syndrome or arthritis, congestive heart failure, malabsorption, or gastrointestinal bleeding. In secondary or amyloid A (AA) amyloidosis (see Table 435.1), the patient develops hepatomegaly, splenomegaly, and nephrotic syndrome. Secondary amyloidosis is a rare occurrence in children, but it is seen in association with Hodgkin disease or renal carcinoma, in addition to the inflammatory diseases mentioned previously. In young adults, it increases in frequency in chronic suppurative conditions, with the infectious complications of intravenous drug use, and in diseases such as leprosy or malaria. Amyloidosis has also been described in endocrine organs, in association with diabetes and thyroid disease and as localized cutaneous deposits (see Table 435.1).

PATHOLOGY

All amyloid deposits display a green birefringence when stained with Congo red dye and viewed under a polarizing microscope. These deposits appear microscopically homogenous. The major component of amyloid deposits by electron microscopy is a 100-Å fibril that is thin, nonbranching, and rigid. Although the ultrastructural appearances of the fibrils in the various types of amyloidoses are nearly identical, their biochemical compositions are distinct. These fibrils assume a predominantly antiparallel beta-pleated sheet conformation by x-ray crystallography. In primary or AL amyloidosis, the amino acid sequence is homologous with the variable region of immunoglobulin light chains.

In secondary or AA amyloidosis, the major fibrillar protein is not immunoglobulin light chains. A serum component that circulates normally in very low concentrations, serum amyloid A (SAA), is the precursor protein for these amyloid fibrils. SAA is an acute-phase protein, and a chronic elevation of SAA is part of the prerequisite for the pathogenesis of AA amyloidosis. A serum P component exists that is an $alpha_1$-glycoprotein that is adsorbed onto the fibrillar structure. This pentagonal component is common to all types of amyloids, but it constitutes only approximately 5% of the deposits. The serum amyloid P (SAP) component is a doughnut-shaped structure composed of five identical subunits closely related in structure and function to C-reactive protein. The remainder of the fibrils are composed of glycosaminoglycans and small amounts of matrix proteins.

Hereditary Amyloidosis

The most common type of hereditary amyloidosis is that associated with FMF, a periodic disease inherited as an autosomal recessive trait. FMF is particularly common in Jews, Turks, Armenians, and Levantine Arabs. The onset of disease occurs generally in individuals between the ages of 5 and 15 years. Each stereotypic exacerbation is characterized by fever, abdominal and pleuropericardial pain, and arthritis. An attack begins acutely and may last for 1 week before slowly subsiding. The gene (*pyrin*) for FMF has been described and is located on chromosome 16; patients with FMF have mutations of this gene. FMF-associated amyloidosis occurs in certain ethnic groups only (e.g., North African Jews), affecting children and resulting

TABLE 435.1

CLASSIFICATION OF AMYLOIDOSIS

Amyloid Protein	Protein Precursor	Clinical
AA	Serum amyloid A	Reactive (secondary); familial Mediterranean fever; familial amyloid nephropathy with urticaria and deafness (Muckle-Wells syndrome)
AL	Immunoglobulin light chains	Idiopathic (primary), myeloma, or macroglobulinemia-associated
ATTR	Transthyretin (prealbumin)	Familial amyloid polyneuropathy, Portuguese type; familial amyloid cardiomyopathy, Danish type
ApoAI	Apolipoprotein A-I	Familial amyloid polyneuropathy, Iowa type; hereditary nonneuropathic systemic amyloidosis (Ostertag type)
AGel	Gelsolin	Familial amyloidosis, Finnish type
ACys	Cystatin C	Hereditary cerebral hemorrhage with amyloidosis, Icelandic type
ALys	Lysozyme	Hereditary nonneuropathic systemic amyloidosis (Ostertag type)
AFib	Fibrinogen	Hereditary renal amyloidosis
Aβ	Beta protein precursor	Alzheimer disease; Down syndrome; hereditary cerebral hemorrhage with amyloidosis, Dutch type 2
Aβ2M	Beta$_2$-microglobulin	Associated with chronic dialysis
AScr	Scrapie protein precursor	Creuzfeldt-Jakob disease, etc.; Gerstmann-Straüssler-Scheinker syndrome
ACal	(Pro)calcitonin	In medullary carcinomas of the thyroid
AANF	Atrial natriuretic factor	Isolated atrial amyloid
AAPP	Islet amyloid polypeptide	In islets of Langerhans, diabetes type II, insulinoma

Adapted from EG Husby. *Reactive amyloidosis and the acute phase response.* London: Bailliere Tindall, 1994.

TABLE 435.2

HEREDITARY AMYLOIDOSES

Name	Mutant Protein
Familial amyloid polyneuropathy	
Portuguese	Transthyretin
Iowa	Apolipoprotein A-I
Hereditary systemic amyloidosis (Ostertag)	Lysozyme
Alzheimer disease	Beta protein
Familial Finnish amyloidosis	Gelsolin
Icelandic hereditary cerebral hemorrhage	Cystatin C

addition to visceral involvement. Familial amyloid polyneuropathy has been well described in Portuguese and Japanese kindreds and is caused by mutations in transthyretin. Onset of the clinical disease is often not observed until the patient is in the third decade of life. The various types are shown in Table 435.2.

DIAGNOSIS

The diagnosis of amyloidosis is histologic, using Congo red stain and polarizing microscopy. A noninvasive method has been shown to be a valuable aid in diagnosing the disease and monitoring its progression. Radiolabelled serum P component can be used to visualize amyloid deposits, using a gamma camera, which is particularly useful in AA amyloidosis. Regression of amyloid deposits has been shown to occur when the inflammatory disease is abolished.

THERAPY

Human trials of new drugs are in progress that will remove the glycosaminoglycans or SAP from the fibrils. Meanwhile, in AL and AA amyloidosis, the principle of treatment to date has been to lower the SAA levels by treating the underlying disease. SAP scintigraphy has shown that the amyloid load can be reduced if the underlying disease is in remission. In children with known malignant disease, treatment involves cytotoxic drugs. AA amyloidosis is a relatively common complication of juvenile rheumatoid arthritis in some northern European countries (7%), and chlorambucil has been used with good result, causing a remission of juvenile rheumatoid arthritis. A long-term increase in the risk of malignancy is a major problem with this treatment. More recent drugs, such as anti-TNF, may be a better option, although the long-term effects of its use are unknown at this point.

Recent analysis of the gene mutations in the periodic fever syndrome showed that mutations of the cryopyrin gene in Muckle-Well syndrome and chronic infantile neurologic cutaneous arthropathy (CINCA) syndromes predispose to an inflammatory state through an elevation of serum interleukin-1 (IL-1) and a concomitant chronic elevation of SAA, thus leading to systemic AA amyloidosis. In these patients, preliminary trials of a recombinant IL-1 antagonist (IL-1 receptor antagonist, anakinra) had very good results. For patients with FMF, no form of treatment is universally successful. Nonsteroidal antiinflammatory drugs are useful for relieving symptoms, and colchicine reduces the frequency and severity of attacks. Colchicine has been shown to prevent the development of renal failure due to amyloidosis, if given before proteinuria occurs, and to retard the onset of renal failure, if given early in the nephritic syndrome caused by FMF-associated amyloidosis.

in the nephrotic syndrome and eventual death from renal failure. FMF and amyloidosis may be inherited separately.

Most other familial forms of amyloidosis are inherited as autosomal dominant diseases. Each family presents characteristic clinical features and geographic distribution. These hereditary forms are rare and often have neuropathic elements in

Suggested Readings

Cassidy JT, Levinson JE, Bass JC, et al. A study of classification criteria for a diagnosis of juvenile rheumatoid arthritis. *Arthritis Rheum* 1986;29:274.

Cassidy JT, Petty RE. *Textbook of paediatric rheumatology*, 4rd ed. WB Saunders, Philadelphia: 2001.

Hawkins PN. Serum amyloid P component scintigraphy for diagnosis and monitoring amyloidosis. *Curr Opin Nephrol Hypertens* 2002;11:649.

Hawkins PN, Lachmann HJ, McDermott MF. Interleukin-1-receptor antagonist in the Muckle-Wells syndrome. *N Engl J Med* 2003;348:2583.

Lachmann HJ, Hawkins PN. Novel pharmacological strategies in amyloidosis. *Nephron Clin Pract* 2003;94:c85.

Woo P. Amyloidosis in children. *Baillieres Clin Rheumatol* 1994;8:691.

CHAPTER 436 ■ HENOCH-SCHÖNLEIN SYNDROME

LESLIE M. HIGUCHI AND ROBERT P. SUNDEL

Henoch-Schönlein syndrome (HSP) is the most common vasculitis in children, occurring in 20 children per 100,000 per year. It is a multisystem disorder that principally involves the skin, gastrointestinal tract, joints, and kidneys. Heberden is credited with describing the first case in 1801. Other names for the syndrome include *anaphylactoid, rheumatoid* or *allergic purpura, leukocytoclastic vasculitis,* and *Henoch-Schönlein purpura*. Most cases of HSP occur in children younger than 7 years, with a peak age range between 4 and 7 years. In adults, an inflammatory vasculopathy sharing features with HSP is typically diagnosed as hypersensitivity vasculitis, although this is increasingly thought to be the same condition. The male-to-female ratio is 1.5–2:1. Peak seasonal incidence has been reported in the fall, winter, and spring.

ETIOLOGY

Although the etiology of HSP remains unknown, several predisposing factors have been suggested. Upper respiratory infections precede the onset of illness in at least 50% of children with the syndrome. Streptococcal infections are most common, although numerous others have been reported including parvovirus, adenovirus, *Mycoplasma pneumoniae, Yersinia, Legionella,* Epstein-Barr virus, and varicella. Insect bites, exposure to cold, and vaccination against measles, cholera, yellow fever, typhoid, and paratyphoid A and B preceded HSP in other cases.

All the conditions known to incite HSP are far more common than the vasculitis itself, so additional factors related to host susceptibility also must play a role in the condition. Reports of the familial occurrence of HSP suggest a genetic connection, but because families also may have similar environmental exposures, such evidence is only circumstantial. Additional support for an inherited predisposition comes from children transplanted for end-stage renal failure associated with HSP. In one report, nine histologic renal recurrences of HSP occurred among 12 living related donor grafts, but no recurrences developed in the five cadaveric kidneys. The specific genetic loci involved are not known, although HSP has been associated with genes of the major histocompatibility complex (MHC) located on chromosome 6, including a weak relationship to HLA-B35 and HLA-DR4, as well as aberrant expression of the fourth component (C4) of the complement system.

PATHOPHYSIOLOGY

HSP is thought to be an immune-mediated vasculitic disorder. Abnormalities in patients include the deposition of immunoglobulin A (IgA) in affected organs and elevated serum IgA concentrations. *In vitro* studies of lymphocytes from patients with HSP demonstrate an increased number of IgA-bearing and -secreting B cells, with altered T-cell regulation of antibody synthesis. Both IgA and IgG immune complexes and IgA rheumatoid factor have been described, and unconfirmed reports also have pointed to a possible contribution of autoantibodies of the IgA isotype. IgA is able to activate the alternative pathway of complement; and C3, properdin, and membrane attack complexes (C5 through C9) may be demonstrated within the glomerular mesangium of children with HSP. In addition, total serum hemolytic complement (CH_{50}) and properdin levels may be depressed, and levels of C3d, a C3 breakdown product, may be elevated. Thus, plasma proteins may form aggregates that activate the alternative pathway of the complement system, thus leading to deposition within target organs, release of a cascade of inflammatory mediators and, eventually, tissue injury.

The centrality of any of these findings is, however, controversial. The IgA "complexes" actually may represent IgA aggregates or IgA complexed to complement-fixing proteins such as IgG or fibronectin, and many patients have no evidence of autoantibodies. Recently, therefore, some authors have suggested that abnormal O-glycosylation of IgA leads to deposition in the renal mesangium and development of HSP. Alternatively, some evidence points to a role for factor XIII in the pathogenesis of HSP. The disease is characterized by bleeding into affected organs, despite a normal platelet count and normal prothrombin and partial thromboplastin times. Factor XIII, also known as *fibrin-stabilizing factor,* is decreased in these patients. According to this alternate hypothesis, proteases released during the local tissue inflammatory response may degrade factor XIII, resulting in tissue fibrin deposition and contributing to the development of vasculitis. Interestingly, the gene encoding the factor XIII A chain, containing the catalytic function, is found on chromosome 6, near MHC genes potentially associated with HSP.

Whatever the trigger, histopathologic features of HSP are typical of other leukocytoclastic vasculitides. Small vessels have a perivascular infiltrate consisting of neutrophils and mononuclear cells. Deposits of IgA, C3, and fibrin may be detected using immunofluorescence and electron microscopy. Renal biopsies typically show an endocapillary proliferative glomerulonephritis involving endothelial and mesangial cells, with deposition of IgA, C3, fibrin or fibrinogen, properdin, IgG and, less commonly, IgM. Proliferation of extracapillary cells also may occur, resulting in variable degrees of crescent formation.

CLINICAL MANIFESTATIONS AND COMPLICATIONS

The typical clinical presentation is that of a previously well child who develops malaise and low-grade fever followed by palpable purpura, colicky abdominal pain, and arthritis. The manifestations may occur simultaneously or sequentially over a period of several days or weeks. About half of the children with HSP present with a skin rash (Fig. 436.1). The classic eruption of HSP begins as localized or generalized urticarial wheals that are replaced by erythematous macules or maculopapules. Subsequently, petechiae and larger purpuric areas form. Often, the purpuric lesions are palpable and described as raised papules or plaques that, similar to the stages of ecchymoses, evolve over several days from red-purple to yellow and then to purple-brown before fading. The lesions usually arise in crops, and new crops may arise at different times, resulting in a polymorphic appearance with varying stages of eruption simultaneously present.

Typically, the rash is nonpruritic and favors pressure-dependent areas, with a characteristic distribution on the lower extremities and the buttocks in toddlers and older children. Younger patients who are not ambulatory may show involvement of the upper extremities, face, and trunk. The rash may be transient or persist for weeks, and it may recur. In addition to the classic rash, various forms of erythema multiforme, with central hemorrhage or ulceration, vesicular eruptions, and bullae, have been described. Additionally, nonpitting edema

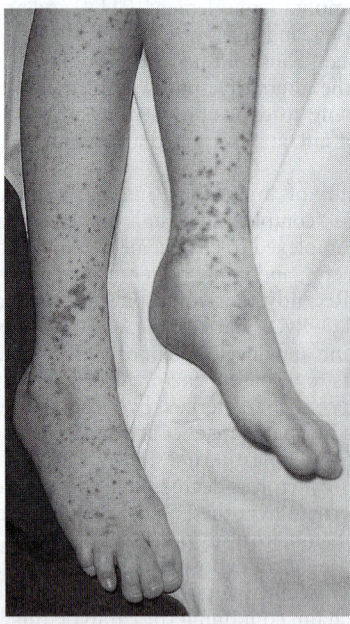

FIGURE 436.1. This patient demonstrates the classic appearance of the rash over the lower distal extremity. (Reproduced with permission from Fleisher GR, Ludwig S, Baskin MN. *Atlas of pediatric emergency medicine.* Philadelphia: Lippincott Williams & Wilkins, 2004:311.)

occurs in 35% to 70% of patients, more commonly in children younger than 3 years. Affected areas are tender and distorted, with localized swelling having a predilection for the scalp, ears, periorbital region, and the dorsum of the hands and feet. More diffuse swelling of dependent areas and the periorbital regions also may occur as a secondary complication of nephrosis.

The second clinical feature that makes up the diagnostic triad of HSP is joint involvement. Arthralgia or arthritis develops in 65% to 85% of patients and is the presenting symptom or sign of the illness, preceding the rash, in 17% to 25% of patients. The joint involvement is nonmigratory, and both articular and periarticular tissues are affected. Whereas joints may be extremely painful, erythema and warmth are uncommon. Joint involvement more commonly affects the knees and ankles than the smaller joints of the fingers and wrists and usually is self-limited, never resulting in residual sequelae.

The final cardinal manifestation of HSP, gastrointestinal involvement, occurs in as many as three-fourths of patients. The colicky abdominal pain frequently causes tenderness, but rebound is uncommon. Gastrointestinal complaints may precede the rash in 15% of cases, creating particular difficulty in differentiating the condition from appendicitis or other abdominal pathology. Often, gastrointestinal bleeding occurs, manifesting as melena or guaiac-positive stools (56%) or hematemesis (10%). Massive gastrointestinal hemorrhage (5%) is rare. Vomiting and ileus are reported in 25% and 40% of cases, respectively.

The typical abdominal pain of HSP is intermittent or waxing and waning. An acute change in the nature, intensity, or pattern of abdominal pain is often a sign of secondary intestinal complications such as intussusception, bowel infarction, perforation, pancreatitis, or hydrops of the gallbladder. Of these, intussusception is the most common, occurring in 3% of patients. It is more common in older children, and is ileoileal in 65% of cases, in contrast, to sporadic cases of intussusception which tend to be ileocolic and frequently occur in children younger than 3 years. Other rare gastrointestinal complications include protein-losing enteropathy and late-onset ileal stricture formation. Hepatomegaly, of uncertain significance, is noted in 10% of patients.

Renal involvement develops in 20% to 60% of patients, depending on the particular criteria used and the method of examination. Typically, renal manifestations occur after other signs of the disease, usually within 3 months of the onset of rash. In 3% of patients, however, renal manifestations may appear before the onset of other symptoms. Renal involvement may be manifest as a wide range of findings, from microscopic hematuria (60%), gross hematuria (40%), nephrotic syndrome (30%), mild proteinuria (25%), and acute nephritis with hypertension (15%), to rapidly progressive glomerulonephritis (fewer than 1%). Children older than 9 years and adults tend to develop more significant nephropathy than their younger peers.

As with all vasculitides, the manifestations of HSP may be protean, involving virtually any organ system. Among the more characteristic findings are acute scrotal inflammation, which occurs in 2% to 38% of male subjects with HSP. Clinical features include pain, tenderness, and swelling of the involved testicle or scrotum. The presentation may mimic the symptoms and signs of testicular torsion, and surgical evaluation may be unavoidable, although testicular ultrasound and technetium^{99m} imaging is often sufficient to distinguish between the two entities. In HSP, normal or increased Doppler and radionuclide flow are expected, whereas in testicular torsion, both Doppler flow and radionuclide scan are decreased on the affected side. When it is necessary, surgical exploration typically demonstrates localized vasculitis and bleeding into the affected testes.

Central nervous system involvement in HSP is uncommon, although headaches and behavioral changes develop in as many as 31% of patients. Other neurologic findings, such as seizures, focal neurologic deficits, and peripheral neuropathies, are reported in only 2% to 8% of patients. Seizures may be associated with hypertension, metabolic disturbances, or intracranial hemorrhage, including subarachnoid, subdural, cortical, or intraparenchymal hemorrhages. Electroencephalographic changes have been described. Most neurologic symptoms are transient, although permanent deficits may remain after hemorrhage or infarction.

Despite the fact that respiratory symptoms are uncommon, occult pulmonary involvement is actually the rule in HSP. Impairment of pulmonary lung diffusion capacity has been reported in 97% of children during the acute phase of HSP, although none of these children exhibited pulmonary symptoms. Pulmonary hemorrhage has been reported in severe cases of HSP, as have other rare complications, such as intramuscular hemorrhage, ureteral vasculitis with stenosis, and carditis.

DIAGNOSIS

The diagnosis of HSP rests on clinical characteristics, not laboratory, imaging, or histopathologic results. Thus, whereas no pathognomonic laboratory tests are available to confirm the clinical impression, laboratory evaluation can assist with the exclusion of other diagnoses and the assessment of specific organ involvement.

A leukocytosis of 10,000 to 20,000 cells per microliter is noted in two-thirds of patients, with an accompanying left shift seen in one-half of patients. Anemia may occur, possibly resulting from intestinal blood loss. The erythrocyte sedimentation rate and platelet count may be normal or elevated, often depending on the condition that triggered the HSP. The prothrombin time and partial thromboplastin time are normal, but factor XIII (fibrin-stabilizing factor) usually is decreased and normalizes with resolution of the disease. Reportedly, concentrations of factor XIII that are less than 50% of normal may herald gastrointestinal or renal complications. Serum IgA is elevated during the acute illness in approximately 50% of patients, and serum IgG and IgM may be normal or elevated. Assay results for antinuclear antibodies and rheumatoid factor are negative. Approximately one-third of patients develop a low total hemolytic complement level (CH_{50}) associated with normal C3 and C4 levels and low properdin levels.

Urinalysis should be performed on all patients with HSP because of the centrality of renal involvement in determining prognosis and therapy. The urine may demonstrate red or white blood cells, cellular casts, or protein. Onset of renal involvement may be delayed for weeks, months, or years, so that any child who has had HSP probably warrants urinanalyses at routine office visits. Serum creatinine and blood urea nitrogen levels may be elevated, suggesting renal insufficiency associated with glomerulonephritis. Indications for a renal biopsy include the presence of nephrotic syndrome, renal insufficiency or a rapid deterioration in renal function, or persistent nephritis with macroscopic hematuria or hypertension. Electrolyte abnormalities and hypoalbuminemia may be present secondary to renal disease or protein-losing enteropathy. Stool examination will reveal evidence of gross or microscopic blood loss in at least half of affected children.

When gastrointestinal symptoms are present, contrast radiologic studies of the gastrointestinal tract usually demonstrate small-bowel involvement, with thickened folds, pseudotumors, hypomotility, and "thumbprinting," representing submucosal hemorrhages. Abnormalities of the terminal ileum resembling those of Crohn disease may be seen, but colonic findings are unusual. Ultrasound evaluation for intussusception may be helpful, given its noninvasive nature and its ability to identify intussusceptions proximal to the terminal ileum, which are often missed by air or liquid contrast enemas. The ultrasound appearance of intussusception is that of a rounded mass with echocentric structures resembling a target. Ultrasound also may demonstrate intestinal wall thickening and abnormal peristalsis, which are suggestive of gastrointestinal vasculitis. A small number of reports describe endoscopy findings in children who developed hematemesis, melena, or severe abdominal pain. Abnormalities include gastritis and duodenitis with erythema, edema, petechiae or hemorrhage, and erosions or ulcerations of the mucosa. Colonic aphthous lesions and rectal ulcers also have been reported in a few cases.

Differential Diagnosis

In the presence of the characteristic constellation of clinical findings of HSP, the diagnosis is generally apparent. However, when the presentation is incomplete, other causes of palpable purpura, abdominal pain, nephritis, and arthritis must be considered.

Petechiae or purpuric rashes may be associated with septicemia and disseminated infections, idiopathic thrombocytopenic purpura, hemolytic uremic syndrome, bacterial endocarditis, acute poststreptococcal glomerulonephritis, leukemia, and coagulopathies. Laboratory evaluation with positive blood culture results, abnormal platelet and coagulation study results, or low C3 levels may differentiate these disorders from HSP. Other systemic vasculitides, including systemic lupus erythematosus, polyarteritis nodosa, Wegener granulomatosis, and cryoglobulinemia, may similarly cause a purpuric rash. In addition to the clinical course, assays for serum complement, antinuclear antibodies, and antineutrophil cytoplasmic antibodies may be helpful. Rheumatoid arthritis and rheumatic fever may present with joint pain accompanied by skin rashes, but these generally may be differentiated from HSP on the basis of characteristic clinical features.

Patients with IgA nephropathy or Berger disease present with a glomerulonephritis having immunologic and histopathologic findings similar to those seen in HSP. In fact, whether these two illnesses actually represent differing manifestations of the same underlying condition is controversial. Similarities between HSP and IgA nephropathy include elevated serum IgA levels, increased circulating immune complexes and polymeric IgA, decreased Fc receptor–mediated immune clearance, and IgA deposition in dermal vessels. Observations of both disorders occurring in the same patient or in close relatives, or in identical twins in whom one developed HSP and the other IgA nephropathy, support the hypothesis that these two entities are variants of the same disease. Nonetheless, differing age distributions and clinical presentations between IgA nephropathy and HSP lead some authorities to consider these two conditions to be distinct entities, perhaps sharing a common pathogenic basis.

THERAPY

For the most part, the treatment of HSP is supportive; convincing evidence that therapy improves symptoms or prognosis is sparse. The majority of HSP cases are mild, and affected children may be followed as outpatients. Nonetheless, admission to the hospital may be indicated if children develop concerning signs such as severe abdominal pain suggestive of intussusception or surgical conditions, frank gastrointestinal hemorrhage, significant renal disease, or changes in mental status.

In the acute care of the ill patient with HSP, management includes adequate hydration and monitoring for potential complications. Optimal nutrition should be maintained, especially if the course is prolonged. Frequent assessment of vital signs, including blood pressure, physical examination findings, hematocrit, urinalysis, and stool guaiac, often will provide an early indication of clinical deterioration. Determining when a child with abdominal complaints warrants further evaluation is difficult. In general, any sudden worsening of gastrointestinal symptoms may signify intussusception, perforation of the bowel, or pancreatitis. Acute changes in behavior or level of consciousness may be secondary to intracranial complications. Some authors suggest nonsteroidal antiinflammatory drugs for relief of joint and soft-tissue discomfort, but caution should be exercised in the setting of prominent abdominal symptoms or renal insufficiency.

The use of corticosteroid therapy to manage the manifestations and complications of HSP is controversial. Steroids are the treatment of choice for other types of vasculitis, and many clinicians believe that they help mitigate the severity of HSP as well. However, the paucity of randomized, placebo-controlled studies has precluded establishing any formal consensus on the indications or effectiveness of corticosteroids. Favorable anecdotal evidence suggests a role for a short course of prednisone, 1 to 2 mg/kg/day, to hasten improvement of abdominal pain, and steroids seem to have a role in the treatment of severe nephritis as well (as discussed in later paragraphs). However, other retrospective studies have shown that the abdominal pain in children with HSP tends to resolve within 3 to 7 days with or without treatment, and the duration of illness is not altered by corticosteroids. If steroids are used, it is important to taper them gradually, because symptoms often flare as therapy is withdrawn.

Apart from corticosteroids, case reports claim that gastrointestinal manifestations improve after intravenous immunoglobulin or factor XIII administration but, again, no formal studies have confirmed their efficacy. Further investigation is sorely needed.

Renal damage is the most important cause of long-term morbidity in HSP. Complicating a determination of the efficacy of therapy is the fact that severe nephritis and renal insufficiency may develop decades after an episode of HSP. Accordingly, although it is difficult to identify a suitable target population for prospectively assessing the effectiveness of medications to prevent severe renal involvement, those children who are clearly at high risk of having a poor outcome do warrant aggressive treatment. Different groups advocate various regimens, generally including corticosteroids plus potent immunosuppressive agents, such as cyclophosphamide or azathioprine. Children who may require such therapies should generally receive a renal biopsy, and should be managed by specialists familiar with these medications.

PROGNOSIS

In the absence of significant renal, gastrointestinal, or neurologic complications, the clinical course usually is self-limited and has an excellent prognosis. Symptoms may persist for an average of 4 weeks, with a duration ranging from 3 days to 2 years. Up to 33% of children have a recrudescence (typically milder than the initial episode), and half of these will have at least one additional recurrence. Recurrences usually occur within 6 weeks of onset, but they have been reported up to years later. Children younger than 2 years generally follow a milder, shorter clinical course, with fewer recurrences and renal and gastrointestinal manifestations than their older peers.

The reported long-term morbidity is almost exclusively secondary to renal complications. Microscopic hematuria alone

or in combination with mild proteinuria usually is associated with a good renal outcome. On the other hand, in patients with nephritis, nephrosis, or both, 44% develop long-term impairment of renal function. Children with both hematuria and nephrotic-range proteinuria have a 15% risk of developing renal failure, and those with diffuse crescentic glomerulonephritis, uremia, and nephrotic syndrome have a 50% chance of developing renal failure within 10 years. Overall, in some series, end-stage renal failure is reported to develop in as many as 2% to 5% of patients. Given that the progression of renal disease may not develop for years, long-term follow-up is necessary in patients with renal involvement. Mortality in HSP is less than 1%, and is caused by severe gastrointestinal, renal, pulmonary, or neurologic involvement.

Suggested Readings

Agraharkar M, Gokhale S, Le L, et al. Cardiopulmonary manifestations of Henoch-Schönlein purpura. *Am J Kidney Dis* 2000;35:319.

Allen DM, Diamond LK, Howell DA. Anaphylactoid purpura in children (Schönlein-Henoch syndrome). *Am J Dis Child* 1960;99:833.

Besgas N, Duzova A, Topaloglu R, et al. Pulmonary hemorrhage in a 6-year old boy with Henoch-Schonlein purpura. *Clin Rheumatol* 2001;20:293.

Choong CK, Beasley SW. Intra-abdominal manifestations of Henoch-Schonlein purpura. *J Paediatr Child Health* 1998;34:405.

Couture A, Veyrac C, Baud C, et al. Evaluation of abdominal pain in Henoch-Schönlein syndrome by high frequency ultrasound. *Pediatr Radiol* 1992;22:12.

Dalens B, Travade P, Labbé A, et al. Diagnostic and prognostic value of fibrin stabilising factor in Schönlein-Henoch syndrome. *Arch Dis Child* 1983;58:12.

Davin JC, Ten Berge IL, Weening JJ. What is the difference between IgA nephropathy and Henoch-Schonlein purpura nephritis? *Kidney Int* 2001;59:823.

Davin JC, Weening JJ. Henoch-Schonlein purpura nephritis: an update. *Eur J Pediatr* 2001;160:689.

Garcia-Fuentes M, Martin A, Chantler C, et al. Serum complement components in Henoch-Schönlein purpura. *Arch Dis Child* 1978;53:417.

Gardner-Medwin JM, Dolezalova P, Cummins C, et al. Incidence of Henoch-Schonlein purpura, Kawasaki disease, and rare vasculitides in children of different ethnic origins. *Lancet* 2002;360:1197.

Gunasekaran TS. Henoch-Schonlein purpura: what does the "rash" look like in the gastrointestinal mucosa? *Pediatr Dermatol* 1997;14:437.

Hasegawa A, Kawamura T, Ito H, et al. Fate of renal grafts with recurrent Henoch-Schönlein purpura nephritis in children. *Transplant Proc* 1989;21:2130.

Kassutto S, Wolf MA. Clinical problem-solving. A wrinkle in time. *N Engl J Med* 2003;349:597.

Knight JF. The rheumatic poison: a survey of some published investigations of the immunopathogenesis of Henoch-Schönlein purpura. *Pediatr Nephrol* 1990;4:533.

Oner A, Tinaztepe K, Erdogan O. The effect of triple therapy on rapidly progressive type of Henoch-Schonlein nephritis in children. *Pediatr Nephrol* 1995;9:6.

Østergaard JR, Storm K. Neurologic manifestations of Schönlein-Henoch purpura. *Acta Paediatr Scand* 1991;80:339.

Paolini S, Ciapetta P, Piattella MC, et al. Henoch-Schonlein syndrome and cerebellar hemorrhage: report of an adolescent case and literature review. *Surg Neurol* 2003;60:339.

Reif S, Jain A, Santiago J, et al. Protein losing enteropathy as a manifestation of Henoch-Schönlein purpura. *Acta Paediatr Scand* 1991;80:482.

Rosenblum ND, Winter HS. Steroid effects on the course of abdominal pain in children with Henoch-Schönlein purpura. *Pediatrics* 1987;79:1018.

Saulsbury FT. Henoch-Schonlein purpura in children. Report of 100 patients and review of the literature. *Medicine* (Baltimore) 1999;78:395.

Singh S, Devidayal, Kumar L, et al. Severe Henoch-Schonlein nephritis: resolution with azathioprine and steroids. *Rheumatol Int* 2002;22:133.

Szer IS. Gastrointestinal and renal involvement in vasculitis: management strategies in Henoch-Schönlein purpura. *Cleve Clin J Med* 1999;66:312.

Tönshoff B, Momper R, Schweer H, et al. Increased biosynthesis of vasoactive prostanoids in Schönlein-Henoch purpura. *Pediatr Res* 1992;32:137.

Trygstad CW, Stiehm ER. Elevated serum IgA globulin in anaphylactoid purpura. *Pediatrics* 1971;47:1023.

White RHR, Yoshikawa N. Henoch-Schönlein nephritis. In: Holliday MA, Barratt TM, Avner ED, eds. *Pediatric nephrology*. Baltimore: Williams & Wilkins, 1994:729.

Wyatt RJ, Hogg RJ. Evidence-based assessment of treatment options for children with IgA nephropathies. *Pediatr Nephrol* 2001;16:156.

Zickerman AM, Allen AC, Talwar V, et al. IgA myeloma presenting as Henoch-Schonlein purpura with nephritis. *Am J Kidney Dis* 2000;36:E19.

SECTION XIV ■ THE SERIOUSLY ILL CHILD

CHAPTER 437 ■ INTENSIVE CARE: PHYSICAL ENVIRONMENT

NATHAN RODGERS AND FERNANDO STEIN

The pediatric intensive care unit (ICU) is only as good as the people who work in it. Although having excellent equipment is important, the major emphasis always should be placed on the quality of the staff. An area of 150 to 200 square feet per child or adolescent patient is a minimum; 250 square feet per patient is ideal. This area is necessary because of recent innovations and additions in equipment, such as ventilators, dialysis machines, suction and infusion pumps, continuous electroencephalographic monitoring, and other computerized equipment that can be brought to the bedside. Adequate space in the patient's area also will allow staff to access the patient for routine ICU procedures such as central line insertion or intubation.

According to the Center for Health Design, designers of ICUs should consider the importance of privacy, security, patient demographics, noise control, natural and artificial light, artwork, color schemes, and efficient layouts. Designers should create a facility that is flexible and sensitive to the needs of the population. For example, hospitals should adapt their facilities and services to better serve the prominent culture within their populations. The positive effect of natural light on establishing circadian rhythms has been documented, and code regulations now require a window for every bed in an ICU. The proximity of patients to natural light can aid in promoting regular sleep patterns. Additionally, evidence shows that softer colors, such as pastels, have a calming, restful effect on patients and staff. An ICU that promotes an environment of healing and support, while minimizing stress, will increase patient satisfaction and significantly influence patient outcomes.

Each bedside should be equipped with continuous display monitors with at least four channels: one each for heart rate and respiratory rate and two for other aspects of monitoring, such as pressure, carbon dioxide level, temperature, and respiratory patterns. The headboard should have sufficient outlets for oxygen, compressed air, and suction, and three different sets of electrical outlets, as well as 12 or more electrical outlets of standard amperage. At least two 220-amp outlets and sufficient grounding sockets also should be available. In areas where patients are being ventilated with an endotracheal tube, a person who is capable of intubating should be immediately available. Thus, a call room located inside or in immediate proximity to the ICU is strongly suggested.

CHAPTER 438 ■ ELECTROCARDIOGRAPHIC AND RESPIRATORY MONITORS

CARMEN C. COSIO AND THOMAS A. VARGO

The monitoring of cardiorespiratory parameters is an integral part of the care of critically ill children. Life-threatening cardiopulmonary derangements occur frequently as a result of respiratory and cardiac failure from acute respiratory distress syndrome, congenital heart diseases, cardiac surgery, electrolyte disturbances, systemic infections, toxic ingestions, cardiomyopathies, trauma, and shock states. The routine use of continuous oscillographic electrocardiographic (ECG) monitoring and the concurrent measurement of respiratory bioimpedance, pulse oximetry, and capnography greatly facilitate the detection of deleterious changes in heart rate and rhythm and in respiratory function. Once such abnormalities have been identified, interventions directed toward their correction and prevention can be undertaken.

ELECTROCARDIOGRAPHIC MONITORING

Continuous ECG monitoring of the hospitalized patient usually is accomplished by using a simplified system of three electrodes placed on the right and left upper chest and the left hip. The electrodes function as bipolar leads that measure the potential between two points, one positive and one negative. In so doing, they record ECG leads I, II, and III, which by standard convention are calibrated to a 1-mV deflection equaling 10 mm on the strip-chart recorder with paper speed set at 25 mm/second. The electrode pads themselves should be moist and not outdated. They should be placed on skin that has been cleaned to remove all sources of electrical resistance. Electrodes may need to be moved if an adequate ECG tracing is not obtained. The lead that gives the best visualization of the P, QRS, and T waves should be chosen for display, especially when monitoring for arrhythmias. Most bedside ECG systems feed to a standard oscillographic display at the bedside and to a remote display screen at a central location for additional surveillance. Monitors in the intensive care unit (ICU) should allow permanent graphic recording of the ECG.

A common error in the interpretation of monitoring ECGs is to diagnose atrial enlargement from an oscilloscopic tracing displaying data from a single lead, without realizing that the tracing has a high sensitivity that gives the P waves an exaggerated height. Similarly, ST-segment abnormalities sometimes are diagnosed erroneously from these electrographic strip recordings. Artifact waveform recordings caused by loose or broken leads, leads placed on bony prominences, or patient movement (particularly during rhythmic chest physiotherapy) also can produce misleading ECG tracings. Whenever the morphologic characteristics of a monitor recording are in question, a standard 12- or 15-lead ECG should be obtained for precise diagnosing. Continuous ECG monitoring is extremely helpful in detecting arrhythmias such as sinus tachycardia, sinus bradycardia, supraventricular tachycardia, and ventricular tachycardia.

RESPIRATORY MONITORING

The routine monitoring of the respiratory rate and depth of respiration is performed using transthoracic bioimpedance. This technique involves placing one electrode on either side of the thorax and a reference electrode over the hip or the apex of the heart. In pediatric ICUs, the same electrodes and oscilloscope used for ECG surveillance are used to monitor respiratory parameters. Changes in both intrathoracic lung and blood volumes cause proportional changes in electrical resistance. This change in resistance causes the bioimpedance changes that are used to measure the respiratory rate and depth of respiration. Alarm systems are incorporated to identify respirations that are abnormally high, low, or absent. This technology has gained acceptance for monitoring apnea in both the hospital and home settings. Like oscilloscopic ECG monitors, respiratory monitors are subject to mechanical interference by ventilator breaths, patient movements, and loose or inappropriate lead placement.

PULSE OXIMETRY

Pulse oximetry has become the standard of care that provides an easy, noninvasive, and reliable method to monitor oxygenation. A disposable probe containing a light source and a photodetector is placed, in order of the most frequently used sites, on a finger, toe, ear lobe, or nasal bridge. Most of the light is absorbed by connective tissue, skin, bone, and venous blood. This absorption of light is constant with time and does not vary during the cardiac cycle. With each heartbeat, a small increase in the arterial blood occurs, which results in an increase in light absorption. The light source consists of two light emitting diodes (LEDs) that emit light in the 660 nm (red) and 940 nm (infrared) wavelengths. These wavelengths are used because oxyhemoglobin and reduced hemoglobin have different absorptions at these two wavelengths. Pulse oximetry calculates the oxygen saturation by comparing the percentage of oxyhemoglobin to the sum of oxyhemoglobin and reduced hemoglobin.

Pulse oximetry may yield misleading or inaccurate information in certain situations, such as carbon dioxide poisoning, methemoglobinemia, severe anemia with a hemoglobin level of less than 5 g/dL, elevation of fetal hemoglobin, or low perfusion-pressure states. Treatment with methylene blue, and the use of blue or green nail polishes, in addition to excessive light from a number of sources, including surgical, infrared, or bilirubin lamps, can interfere with oximetric accuracy. Pulse oximetry is relatively accurate in the 70% to 100% saturation range, and it is less accurate in lower ranges. In addition to its use in the ICU, monitoring by pulse oximetry provides immediate feedback on oxygen changes and early warning of ventilator malfunction in the operating room and recovery rooms. Continuous pulse oximetric measurements in these settings allows for the earlier detection of desaturation, which leads to the earlier initiation of corrective measures and the prevention of adverse consequences. Pulse oximetry should be used to monitor the cardiorespiratory status of patients at risk of developing hypoxemia under a variety of conditions, such as in children receiving general anesthesia or deep sedation, children with acute lung diseases or on mechanical ventilation, newborns, and children with cyanotic heart disease.

CAPNOGRAPHY

Capnography is both the measurement of expired carbon dioxide tension (CO_2) and the display of CO_2 waveform from breath to breath. Capnography operates on the principle that CO_2 molecules absorb infrared light; this absorption is measured by a sensor attached to the endotracheal tube. The sensor consists of an infrared source and a detector. Infrared light is passed through gas in a reference chamber and through the expired gas, and the absorption of light by each gas is measured. The comparison of absorption of light by the expired gas to absorption by the reference gas determines the amount of CO_2 in the expired gas and defines end-tidal CO_2 ($ETCO_2$). $ETCO_2$ is a continuous indirect measure of alveolar carbon dioxide (P_aCO_2), with the assumption made that $ETCO_2$ is equal to P_aCO_2. However, due to dilution by dead space ventilation, the normal values for $ETCO_2$ (33 to 43 mm Hg) are slightly lower than P_aCO_2. The primary uses for capnography in the critically ill patient are to verify the correct position of an endotracheal tube and to monitor the effectiveness of cardiopulmonary resuscitation. It also can be used to decrease arterial blood gas sampling and to provide an indirect measure to monitor severity of lung disease.

The set-up of a capnogram requires time to warm up for calibration and, therefore, it cannot be used emergently. For emergent situations, colorimetric CO_2 detectors containing a pH-sensitive dye are used. They are inexpensive, disposable devices for estimating $ETCO_2$ semiquantitatively, and they are easily attached to an endotracheal tube. The colorimeter's purple color changes to yellow with the detection of CO_2, thus verifying the correct position of the endotracheal tube. Colorimetric CO_2 detectors have become a standard of care to confirm the correct placement of an endotracheal tube. Colorimetric CO_2 detectors are used mostly on transports and in cardiopulmonary resuscitation in a nonintensive care setting, and they should be available on transport packs and emergency ("crash") carts.

Suggested Readings

Kouffman RE, Banner W Jr., et al. Guidelines for monitoring and management of pediatric patients during and after sedation for diagnostic and therapeutic procedures. *Pediatrics* 1992;89:1110.

Nichols DG, Cameron DE, et al. Perioperative monitoring. In: Nichols DG, ed. *Critical heart disease in infants and children.* St. Louis: Mosby, 1995.

Rodriguez RM, Light RW. Capnography in the ICU: when and how to monitor carbon dioxide levels noninvasively. *J Crit Ill* 1998;13:372.

Schnapp LM, Cohen NH. Pulse oximetry. uses and abuses. *Chest* 1990;98;5:1244.

CHAPTER 439 ■ INFUSION DEVICES

FERNANDO STEIN AND JOSE C. CORTES

A standard practice of pediatric intensive care is to give intravenous fluids and medication through an infusion device. These devices guarantee the constant and accurate delivery of the pre-established volume within a given period. They also help to maintain the viability and patency of catheters such as central lines, pulmonary artery catheters, or arterial pressure lines.

In addition to the infusion device, a fluid reservoir should ensure the accurate recording of infused fluids. This type of receptacle is available in different sizes for patients of different ages. The five types of infusion devices are controller, multiple-rate programmable pump, dual- or multiple-channel pump, syringe pump, and computer-controlled infusion pump (Table 439.1).

Because many of the pumps are insensitive to obstruction of flow, the insertion site of a catheter or needle should be monitored to avoid the complications of extravasation and infiltration. Research in this area has found that the dynamic hydraulic properties of an intravenous line can be used to detect infiltration and extravasation, as well as other fluid-flow faults such as a kinked line or an occluded catheter, and the line is more than 90% reliable.

Modern infusion devices can deliver increments of 0.01 mL in volumes up to 999 mL/hour. This type of electronic device offers the advantage of allowing maximum concentration of fluids and drugs to be administered under special patient circumstances.

TABLE 439.1

TYPES OF INFUSION DEVICES

Infusion Device	Pushing Mechanism	Control
Controller	Gravity	Electronic drop-counter
Multiple-rate, programmable pump	Syringe or pulsatile flow	Electronic measuring device
Dual- or multiple-channel pump	Syringe or pulsatile flow	Electronic measuring device
Syringe pump	Turning infinitive screw	Speed-to-syringe ratio
Computer-controlled infusion pump	Syringe or pulsatile flow	Electronic hydraulic sensing device

CHAPTER 440 ■ TEMPERATURE-CONTROLLING AND TEMPERATURE-SENSING DEVICES

FERNANDO STEIN AND JOSE C. CORTES

Four types of temperature-controlling devices are used commonly in the intensive care unit (ICU): the cooling/heating blanket, the heated water-filled mattress, the radiant warmer, and the incubator. The cooling/heating blanket can be placed between the patient and the bed, thereby controlling the temperature while maintaining easy access to the patient. The blanket is particularly useful for children who weigh more than 6 kg because radiant warming devices are not made to fit children this size. New, safe, and effective blankets that circulate heated or cooled air are available; these blankets are placed over the child. The radiant warming device is an electronic heating apparatus. A heated coil placed above the patient radiates heat toward the child; the temperature can be preset or regulated through a servomechanism connected to the child.

Research has shown that a heated water–filled mattress is superior to a radiant warmer in preventing heat loss. The standard incubator provides warming by circulating humidified warm air.

All four devices must be checked regularly by the hospital's biomedical instrumentation department for accuracy in the delivered temperature. Patients must be monitored when connected to a warming or cooling device, and temperature checks should be performed every hour. Overheating is the most serious complication of any type of warming device. Specific recommendations from the manufacturer always should be observed, and personnel should be thoroughly familiar with the operating details of all warming and cooling devices used in their units.

Because changes in temperature are characteristic of many pathophysiologic processes, temperature monitoring is crucial in the ICU. Four basic temperature-sensing devices exist. The most common is the thermal-expansive thermometer, a standard glass thermometer filled with mercury, which is applied to the mouth, axilla, or rectum. It continues to be the most consistently reliable device for monitoring body temperature. When temperature is being monitored hourly, irritation may occur in the area where the thermometer is being applied, particularly the rectum.

Another commonly used device is the thermal-resistive electronic thermometer. It produces a reading in approximately one-third to one-tenth the time required by the standard mercury thermometer (depending on the patient's temperature), and it has a digital display. This device must be calibrated and checked regularly, and it must be approved by the biomedical instrumentation department.

The infrared tympanic thermometer measures temperature better than digital axillary models do, and it is reliable in estimating core temperature.

The temperature probe is a thermally sensitive device used to monitor changes in temperature on a minute-by-minute basis. This thermal-resistive thermometer is connected to the rectum or the esophagus; it also can be applied to the axilla.

The main pitfall of temperature monitoring in the ICU is inaccuracy in performing the technique. False elevations may occur when the probe is placed in the axilla or too close to a warming blanket, or when the probe is located near a large blood vessel. An esophageal probe may read the temperature of the cool or warm gases that are being circulated in the trachea through the respirator. Meticulous attention must be given to detail to maintain an appropriate standard in measuring temperature in the ICU setting.

CHAPTER 441 ■ VASCULAR CATHETERS

CARMEN C. COSIO AND THOMAS A. VARGO

PERIPHERAL VENOUS CATHETERS

Venous cannulation is the most common procedure performed in a pediatric hospital. It is indicated for administering therapeutic drugs and intravenous fluids to the infant or child for whom oral therapy is inadequate or contraindicated. In infants, favored sites for placing peripheral intravenous lines include scalp, external jugular, hand, antecubital, foot, and saphenous veins. In older children and adolescents, catheter placement in the lower extremities generally is avoided so that ambulation is not hindered. In infants, 22- and 24-gauge catheters are large enough for most purposes. Larger-bore catheters are used in children and adolescents. Care should be taken not to compromise the patient's airway when restricting patient movements during the placement of scalp or external jugular catheters. Preparation of the site is dictated by the patient's immune status and the purpose for the placement of the peripheral catheter. If the patient is immunocompromised or the catheter is needed for the administration of total parenteral nutrition fluids, site preparation should include swabbing with a povidone-iodine solution or other antiseptic that is allowed to air dry. For the routine short-term administration of fluids and medications, or when emergency venous access is required, preparation of the skin with denatured alcohol is considered adequate. The dressing should not impede inspection of the cannula and the surrounding area. In children with right-to-left intracardiac shunts, intravenous lines ordinarily are equipped with microfilters inserted distally to all administered fluids, to reduce the risk of systemic air and particulate matter embolization.

Hypertonic medications and solutions should not be given through peripheral catheters. However, if the emergency administration of hypertonic medications is absolutely necessary, and a central venous line access is unavailable, the peripheral catheter can be used. In such situations, the peripheral catheter should flush easily, and the skin must be observed for any evidence of extravasation over the catheter site. Peripheral catheters used to deliver hypertonic drugs or solutions should be replaced by central venous access, when feasible, to avoid the risk of a subsequent occurrence of extravasation. In situations in which an adrenergic agonist extravasates, subcutaneous dilute phentolamine mesylate is injected into the site through the extravasated catheter and to the leading edges of the extravasation. Risks associated with peripheral venous catheter placement are related to the patient's underlying illness, to difficulty in making the insertion, and to the duration of cannulation. A patient with an underlying coagulopathy is at risk for the formation of a hematoma, which can be life-threatening. Such a case could occur after jugular venous punctures, with the development of a hematoma in the neck, which could impinge on the airway. Sepsis can occur from peripheral venous catheters; this complication is seen more commonly in children who are immunocompromised or have an untreated systemic infection before the catheter is placed. Catheter-related infections can be reduced if the catheter is removed when it no longer is needed medically or when the site is erythematous or tender. In many infants and children, the need for a peripheral catheter can be longer than 2 or 3 days and, therefore, the catheter should be inserted in a sterile fashion, and meticulous attention should be paid to the site.

ARTERIAL CATHETERS

Arterial catheter placement is used in the neonatal and pediatric intensive care units (ICUs) for continuous systemic blood pressure monitoring and arterial blood gas sampling. The most frequent indications are labile blood pressure and hemodynamic instability and for frequent monitoring of gas exchange in children with respiratory insufficiency or failure.

One should avoid cannulating an artery in a limb that has a compromised arterial supply. Examples include limbs affected by arteritis, coarctation of the aorta, or previous arterial cut-downs and any arm that has had a classic Blalock-Taussig shunt on the same side. The preferred sites of arterial cannulation in newborns are the umbilical and radial arteries. In children, the radial, posterior tibial, and dorsalis pedis arteries are used because of the collateral circulation supplied by the ulnar, dorsalis pedis, and posterior tibial arteries, respectively. The femoral artery is an alternative site used in children and adolescents. The brachial artery has limited collateral circulation and is used only in those situations in which other sites are not available. Any limb that has an arterial catheter in place should be observed for evidence of compromised arterial supply, with extra attention given to an arm with a brachial arterial line. Catheters are inserted using a sterile percutaneous or direct cutdown technique; the percutaneous technique is used most frequently. To decrease the obstruction of arterial blood flow by the catheter itself, the smallest-bore catheter that allows easy sampling and gives a good pressure waveform is used. A 24-gauge cannula is adequate in the extremities of premature infants, a 22-gauge cannula in full-term infants, and a 20-gauge catheter in children weighing more than 10 kg.

CENTRAL VENOUS CATHETERS

The placement of central venous lines (CVLs) is indicated for the management of hypovolemic shock, septic shock, and myocardial failure or cardiogenic shock. Other indications are for the administration of hypertonic solutions or drugs such as 3% normal saline solution, mannitol, calcium chloride infusions, total parenteral nutrition fluids, and inotropic agents. Also, a CVL usually is used for placing a transvenous pacing wire within the heart. The placement of CVLs also may be needed in those children in whom peripheral access is impossible to obtain.

In the newborn, the umbilical vein is the central vein used most frequently. The tip of an umbilical vein catheter often is in the left atrium, even though the catheter may appear to be in the right atrium on an anteroposterior chest radiograph. This situation occurs because the left atrium is essentially behind the right atrium, rather than to the left of it. To help prevent the occurrence of systemic embolization, the umbilical vein catheter tip should be at the junction of the right atrium and inferior vena cava, which is approximately 0.5 to 1 cm cephalad of the right diaphragm.

After the newborn period, in infants and young children, the internal jugular and femoral veins are the sites most frequently used. In older children and adolescents, the subclavian veins can be used, in addition to the internal jugular, brachial, median, basilic, and femoral veins. Complications occasionally occur from the accidental puncture of various adjacent structures. In a child with severe coagulation abnormalities, the femoral or peripheral veins usually are the preferred sites for the insertion of a CVL. In older children and adolescents, large-bore central catheters often can be inserted through an antecubital vein.

Before the CVL is placed, the patient should be placed in a position that favors cannulation. The Trendelenburg position is used during the insertion of catheters into the jugular or subclavian veins. The insertion techniques used most frequently are the percutaneous and cutdown methods. The percutaneous method usually is preferred, but direct cutdown occasionally is used for catheterization of the superficial saphenous, median basilic, or femoral veins. Arteries and nerves in the cutdown site should be identified to avoid accidental puncture. After the catheter is inserted, blood return by aspiration with a syringe usually is necessary to confirm the location of the catheter inside the vessel. After all CVLs have been inserted, a chest radio-graph should be obtained to confirm an appropriate intrathoracic location. In our pediatric ICU, the catheter tip usually is positioned at the level of the right atrium–superior vena cava junction if the line is inserted in the neck or the chest, or 1 cm cephalad to the diaphragm if placed from the femoral vein.

Central catheters placed in the umbilical, internal jugular, brachial, and other peripheral veins have been associated with the development of pericardial effusions and tamponade. Several cases of intravenous solution extravasation into the pericardial space have been seen, and some of these extravasations have led to the development of pericardial tamponade within a few hours to days after the insertion of a CVL. This complication has been seen in children of all ages; we have seen it most often in infants receiving total parenteral nutrition fluids through central catheters, when the tip of the catheter is located inside the cardiac silhouette and is likely abutting or wedged into the wall of the heart or vena cava. Therefore, checking on the position of the tip by a chest radiograph and withdrawing the line to a proper position is important. To assess for tamponade, an echocardiogram should be performed in all patients who have unexpected hemodynamic deterioration after the placement of a CVL.

Other complications that can occur with CVLs include local site cellulitis, systemic infection, hemorrhage, thrombus formation, arrhythmias, and accidental arterial or nerve puncture. The insertion of internal jugular and subclavian vein catheters can cause a pneumothorax, hemothorax, or cardiac tamponade. Catheter-related infection can be reduced by decreasing manipulation and by applying dressing changes using a rigorous protocol. Studies have shown that if CVLs are to remain in place for weeks, the incidence of infection is lower with weekly dressing changes, using an antibiotic-laden patch placed at the insertion site at the time of the dressing.

The incidence of endocarditis and thrombi in infants and children with CVLs seems to be increasing. The increase of these complications may be attributed to the increased use of CVLs or to the higher index of suspicion and to the improvements that have been made in detecting thrombi by echocardiography.

The life of a CVL depends on the indications for placement. At times, a catheter must remain in place for weeks or months for total parenteral nutrition or antibiotic administration. Changing catheter sites often is impractical in the chronically ill infant and child in whom venous access is limited, and it is not necessary if strict adherence to sterile technique with dressing changes is maintained.

PERIPHERALLY INSERTED CENTRAL CATHETERS

In premature and older infants, children, and adolescents who are hemodynamically stable and have a need for the long-term administration of total parenteral nutrition, antibiotics, or other drugs, the use of a peripherally inserted central catheter (PICC) is helpful. A PICC usually is placed in the basilic or cephalic veins of the arm, with the basilic vein above the elbow considered by many physicians to be the ideal position. The insertion site does not impede use of the arm, which is advantageous for the usually active child. However, movement of the arm can cause displacement of the catheter tip, which could result in pericardial effusion or arrhythmias; these patients should be monitored for the development of these complications and also for migration of the catheter tip to an inappropriate position. PICC insertions may be done in the interventional radiology unit or in the operating room under fluoroscopy, but they also can be done using sedation in a properly equipped procedure room or at the bedside without sedation in older children and adolescents. PICC insertion may be blind or guided by ultrasound, with confirmation obtained by plain radiograph or fluoroscopy. The incidence of infection is low, and, like other central venous catheters, changes of dressing can be done once a week if an antibiotic-laden patch is used at the insertion site. Blood samples can be drawn through a PICC, and the child foregoes painful venipunctures. A PICC is unsuitable for rapid fluid bolus or rapid contrast injection because the catheter can rupture under high-pressure flow. In the smaller child, PICCs also are limited to single-lumen catheters, although smaller catheters with more lumens are being developed.

If the site develops clinical evidence of infection with erythema, swelling, or induration, the PICC may need to be removed. However, these symptoms also may be caused by an acute inflammatory reaction. If the latter is thought to be the case, warm towels placed on the extremity and administration of an antiinflammatory drug for 24 hours will alleviate the discomfort. If the symptoms persist, or evidence of bloodstream infection is present, the PICC usually is removed and blood cultures are obtained. Intravenous antibiotic therapy can be given empirically until the culture results are available. An advantage of a PICC is that a visiting nurse often can complete the child's therapy at home, allowing the child to return more quickly to a normal environment.

INTRAOSSEOUS INFUSIONS

In life-threatening situations in which fluid replacement or drugs must be given and an intravascular line cannot be obtained, fluids and resuscitative drugs can be given through an intraosseous infusion (IO). In most children, this access is obtained by inserting a spinal or bone-marrow needle into the tibia. However, as soon as intravenous access is obtained, the fluids and drugs should be given intravascularly rather than intraosseously.

PULMONARY ARTERY CATHETERS

Pulmonary artery (PA) catheters provide data defining hemodynamic, respiratory, and metabolic functions. Most commonly, they are used to monitor hemodynamic indices in children who have undergone corrective cardiac procedures or in children with septic shock, congestive heart failure, or acute respiratory distress syndrome. Information that can be gained with a diagnostic PA catheter includes a direct measurement of PA pressure, pulmonary capillary wedge pressure, right atrial pressure, and central venous pressure. With a thermodilution catheter, cardiac output, vascular resistances, and ventricular function can be estimated. The simultaneous determination of cardiac output and paired mixed venous and arterial blood oxygen contents can be used to calculate intrapulmonary shunt fraction, oxygen consumption, oxygen extraction ratio, and the arterial mixed venous oxygen difference. These data assist in making bedside interpretations of cardiopulmonary and metabolic interrelationships in patients with serious illnesses and in gauging the success of cardiotonic agents, afterload reduction, mechanical ventilation, and positive end-expiratory pressure.

The PA catheter most commonly used is a balloon-tipped, four-lumen catheter with a thermistor at the tip for measuring cardiac output. This catheter is available in a 5- or 7-French size. The four lumens consist of a distal port for the measurement of PA pressure and pulmonary capillary wedge pressure, a proximal port for measuring right atrial or central venous pressure, a thermistor for determining cardiac output, and a port for inflating the balloon. Two- and three-lumen catheters also are available and usually are easier to manipulate into the PA; however, they are limited in the amount of physiologic information that can be obtained because they do not have a thermistor at the tip for measuring cardiac output. The size of the catheter is determined by the patient's weight. The 5-French catheter typically is used in children with a body weight of 25 kg or less, whereas the 7-French catheter is used in larger children and adolescents. In the pediatric ICU, PA catheters usually are placed through the subclavian or femoral vein. When the femoral vein is used, the catheter may cross the foramen ovale to enter the left side of the heart, but this is not common. The internal jugular and brachial veins are other routinely used insertion sites.

Catheters typically are inserted at the bedside. Portable fluoroscopy rarely is needed to guide the placement of a catheter. The PA catheter insertion is placed by using the flow-directed approach, with monitoring of the characteristic pressures and waveforms recorded from the bedside oscilloscope as the catheter passes through the systemic veins, right atrium, right ventricle, and finally into the main PA. The final position for the catheter tip is in the PA, where near-maximal balloon inflation produces damping of the PA pressure, and the wedge pressure is obtained. The wedge pressure reflects left atrial pressure. Complications of PA catheter placement include the puncture of major systemic vessels or cardiac chambers, ventricular arrhythmias, PA rupture, pneumothorax, catheter knotting, and bacteremia. A chest radiograph should be obtained to verify the location of the catheter, and this procedure should be repeated frequently enough to ensure that the catheter has not migrated. The duration of a catheter placement is dictated by the need for hemodynamic monitoring and the difficulty of performing subsequent reinsertions of a PA catheter. If practical, PA catheters should be changed every 3 to 5 days.

Suggested Readings

Nowlen TT, Rosenthal GL, Johnson GL, Tom DJ, Vargo TA. Pericardial effusion and tamponade in infants with central catheters. *Pediatrics* 2002;110:137.
Ponamem ML, White L. Intraosseous infusions. In: Levin DL, Morriss FC, eds. *Essentials of pediatric intensive care.* St. Louis: Quality Medical Publishing, 1990.
Pope J. Pulmonary artery catheters. In: Blumer JL, ed. *A practical guide to pediatric intensive care.* St. Louis: Mosby-Year Book, 1990.

CHAPTER 442 ■ MEASUREMENT OF CARDIAC OUTPUT

CARMEN C. COSIO AND THOMAS A. VARGO

Cardiac output is an important hemodynamic variable in the assessment of cardiovascular function. Cardiac output (liters per minute) equals the product of the heart rate (beats per minute) and average effective stroke volume (liters per beat). In pediatrics, it usually is indexed to body surface area in square meters (liters per minute per square meter). If cardiovascular anatomy is normal, and the systemic and pulmonary circulations are in series, the systemic and pulmonary blood flows are equal to each other, and each equals the cardiac output. However, for some patients in the intensive care unit (ICU), the two circulations are not in series because of left-to-right or right-to-left shunting. In these cases, separate determinations of the systemic blood flow ($\dot{Q}s$) and pulmonary blood flow ($\dot{Q}p$) may be necessary to evaluate hemodynamic intricacies. The thorough evaluation of $\dot{Q}s$ and $\dot{Q}p$ is best performed in the cardiac catheterization laboratory.

Serial determinations of cardiac output made in the ICU can be useful in guiding fluid management, vasoactive drug therapy, and ventilator management in patients with compromised myocardial function, abnormal pulmonary or systemic vascular resistance, or elevated mean airway pressures. Several methods are available to estimate cardiac output, but only a few are applicable to the critically ill child. In an ICU patient, the methods used most frequently to estimate cardiac output are indicator-dilution methods, the Fick method, and echocardiographic volumetric flow analysis.

Indicator Dilution Methods

Thermodilution and dye-dilution techniques for determining cardiac output are indicator-dilution methods. The dye-dilution method to determine cardiac output rarely is used, even in the cardiac catheterization laboratory. The thermodilution method is the method used most commonly in an ICU to determine cardiac output. This method requires the placement of a pulmonary artery catheter with a proximal injection port and a distal thermistor for continuous temperature measurement. Thermodilution measurements are fairly accurate, reproducible, and easy to perform. The technique requires minimal subjective interpretation of collected data, and serial estimates can be obtained rapidly. The variance of cardiac output estimates by the thermodilution method range from 10% to 15%, so that the average of three to five successive measurements usually is taken to provide the best estimate of cardiac output.

A 3- to 10-mL volume of iced normal saline or a 5% dextrose solution is injected into the proximal port. The thermistor in the pulmonary artery measures body temperature at baseline, and this temperature drops as the cool, injected solution passes the distal tip of the pulmonary artery catheter. Less cooling of the thermistor occurs as the cardiac output increases. A cardiac-output computer can construct the thermal dilution (time–temperature) curve and calculate the cardiac output quickly.

Fick Method

The Fick method is considered the gold standard for determining cardiac output, with the most common application being in the cardiac catheterization laboratory and not in an ICU. The Fick method requires an indwelling pulmonary catheter and systemic arterial catheter for the simultaneous sampling of mixed venous and arterial blood. Oxygen consumption ($\dot{V}O_2$) can be measured directly by the analysis of expired air over a defined period of time, or it can be estimated using published standards that are specific for the patient's size, gender, and heart rate. Arterial oxygen content (C_aO_2) and venous oxygen content (C_vO_2) are determined using the oxygen saturation data of blood gas samples and the hemoglobin concentration (which is the primary determinant of oxygen content). Cardiac index is determined by using the Fick method, which is $\dot{V}O_2$ divided by the difference between C_aO_2 and C_vO_2.

The Fick principle can be used at the bedside to estimate changes in cardiac output, given certain assumptions. If $\dot{V}O_2$ is constant, cardiac output is inversely proportional to the difference between C_aO_2 and C_vO_2. When C_aO_2 also is essentially constant, cardiac output is proportional to C_vO_2. If these assumptions hold, decreases in mixed venous saturation correspond to decreases in cardiac output.

Echocardiographic Volumetric Flow Analysis

Echocardiography often can be used in the ICU to estimate cardiac output, $\dot{Q}p$, or $\dot{Q}s$. One method requires accurate two-dimensional and Doppler echocardiograms of the ascending aorta or main pulmonary artery. Using the diameter of a vessel, obtained by two-dimensional echocardiogram measurements, one can estimate its cross-sectional area (in square centimeters). The mean velocity (in centimeters per second) of blood passing through the vessel during systole is assessed using Doppler echocardiography. The stroke volume (in milliliters per beat) can be calculated from the product of the mean systolic velocity and the cross-sectional area of the vessel. Multiplying stroke volume by the heart rate (in beats per minute) yields the volume of blood that flows through the vessel per minute. Another echocardiographic method of estimating cardiac output relies on estimates of left ventricular end-systolic and end-diastolic volume. The difference of these volumes equals the stroke volume. Several methods exist for estimating the left ventricular chamber volume using echocardiographic measurements. Inaccuracies in estimating left ventricular volume can distort greatly those estimates of cardiac output determined by this method.

Suggested Reading

Vargo TA. Cardiac catheterization—hemodynamic measurements. In: Garson A Jr., Bricker JT, Fisher DJ, Neish SR, eds. *The science and practice of pediatric cardiology.* Baltimore: Williams & Wilkins, 1998.

CHAPTER 443 ■ ECHOCARDIOGRAPHY

JASON T. SU AND THOMAS A. VARGO

Echocardiography is the diagnostic gold standard for the evaluation of cardiac anatomy and myocardial function in most pediatric patients in the intensive care setting. Echocardiography is the imaging modality of choice because of its safety, portability, and ease of use. Furthermore, recent advances in technology have enabled the miniaturization of ultrasound machines, thus allowing for improved portability, battery operation, and digital storage capability.

In the intensive care unit (ICU), echocardiography can quickly and accurately identify valvular abnormalities (including valvular stenosis and regurgitation), evaluate intracardiac shunting, identify pericardial effusions, and evaluate cardiac function. The use of echocardiography has given cardiologists a noninvasive means to diagnose most congenital heart diseases; many infants and children are able to proceed directly to surgical cardiac repair without cardiac catheterization being performed.

In some patients, making an echocardiographic diagnosis may be more difficult because of poor acoustic windows (e.g., obesity, marked chest-wall abnormalities, surgical scar formation, pneumopericardium, pneumothoraces, or hyperaeration of the lungs). For the critically ill child in the ICU, routine echocardiographic examination may be difficult to perform because of the need for mechanical ventilation, the acuity and nature of the underlying diseases (renal failure requiring hemodialysis), and certain postoperative conditions (open chest after cardiac surgery).

In children who are difficult to image using standard echocardiographic techniques, transesophageal echocardiography (TEE) can be performed. TEE almost always allows excellent imaging of intracardiac structures. Transesophageal probes are relatively large (requiring that the child weigh at least 4 kg), and special considerations also must be made regarding the patient's gastrointestinal status (esophageal stricture, active gastrointestinal bleeding, a perforated viscus, presence of a tracheoesophageal fistula) and respiratory status. At our institution, general anesthesia almost always is used for children requiring TEE.

Cardiac function can be defined easily by echocardiography because ventricular wall motion is seen relatively well in children, as compared with adults. Almost all ventricular muscle abnormalities, such as depressed contractility, ventricular dilatation, or regions of infarction, usually can be well visualized. Because precise and accurate measurements of ventricular volume and ejection fraction are difficult to obtain in children, the typical method of measuring contractility is to determine the shortening fraction (the difference between left ventricular systolic and diastolic diameters). Normally, the left ventricular systolic diameter is at least two-thirds that of the diastolic diameter (i.e., a shortening fraction of 33%). Shortening fractions of less than 25% suggest a marked reduction in left ventricular function.

Pericardial effusions usually are well visualized by echocardiography. Pericardial effusions are associated with a range of systemic diseases (e.g., autoimmune disorders, neoplasms, and infections), may occur after cardiac surgery (postpericar-

diotomy syndrome), and occasionally are seen after the insertion of a central venous catheter. An echocardiogram should be done in any sick child who has unexplained cardiomegaly demonstrated on the chest radiograph. Echocardiography also can be used during the pericardiocentesis to monitor the drainage of the pericardial space.

Echocardiography also frequently is performed to evaluate for abnormal intracardiac masses such as (a) intracardiac thrombi in the patient with prolonged central venous line placement, a history of a cerebrovascular accident, cardiomyopathy, or an atrial arrhythmia and (b) intracardiac vegetations in the patient with persistent fever or positive blood cultures. The yield on studies performed for any of the above reasons often is low. In many of these patients, a TEE may be indicated. Children with an arrhythmia (especially a chronic atrial arrhythmia) almost always should be evaluated by TEE for the presence of a thrombus because of the increased incidence of intracardiac thrombus formation in arrhythmias. A definite risk of embolization of the thrombus occurring during the arrhythmia exists, and an even higher risk exists during cardioversion.

Doppler echocardiography can be used to estimate the pressures in cardiac chambers and the pressure gradients across various cardiac defects. The following modified Bernoulli equation formula is used:

$$PG = 4 \times V^2$$

where PG is the pressure gradient in mm Hg and V is the velocity of the flow in the heart in meters per second. The Doppler technique usually estimates intracardiac pressures accurately. For example, the left ventricular pressure can be estimated in a patient with aortic stenosis (AS). Suppose that the mean velocity of the flow across the AS is 4 m/second and the systemic blood pressure using a sphygmomanometer is 104/60 mm Hg. Using the modified Bernoulli equation, a 64 mm Hg [$4 \times (4$ m/second)^2] gradient exists between the left ventricle and aorta. Assuming the aortic systolic pressure is the same as the arterial systolic pressure obtained by sphygmomanometry, an estimate of left ventricular pressure is calculated by adding 64 to 104. In this case, the left ventricular systolic pressure is $104 + 64 = 168$ mm Hg.

In most cases, echocardiography can establish diagnoses immediately and can identify cardiac diseases that may require emergent therapy. We contend that echocardiography should be considered in the intensive care setting for the critically ill child with clinical instability that potentially may be exacerbated or caused by cardiac disease. In fact, we recommend that an echocardiogram should be considered in any critically ill infant or child in whom the cause of the illness is not known.

Suggested Reading

Geva T. Echocardiography and Doppler ultrasound. In: Garson A, Bricker JT, McNamara DG, Neish SR, eds. *The science and practice of pediatric cardiology*, 2nd ed. Baltimore: Williams & Wilkins, 1998.

CHAPTER 444 ■ INTRACRANIAL PRESSURE MEASUREMENTS

FERNANDO STEIN

An elevation of intracranial pressure (ICP) is a common complication in patients with head injury, neoplasia, cerebral vascular accidents, infections, or metabolic disorders. ICP is monitored in the pediatric intensive care unit (ICU) when one or more of the indications listed in Table 444.1 is present.

Normal ICP in children is 15 mm Hg or less. However, the goal in controlling ICP is not necessarily to preserve this ideal number but to preserve cerebral perfusion pressure (CPP). CPP

TABLE 444.1

INDICATIONS FOR INTRACRANIAL PRESSURE (ICP) MONITORING

Acute shifting of the midline brain structures, indicated by computed tomography of the brain
Traumatic injury with evidence of brain edema
Traumatic injury with Glasgow coma score of less than 8 points
Evidence of increased ICP by physical examination in a condition that consistently leads to brain edema
Presence of space-occupying lesions with increased ICP
Hydrocephalus under certain circumstances
Other individual cases in which monitoring of the ICP is necessary for accurate and successful treatment

is the difference between the mean arterial pressure (MAP) and the ICP: CPP = MAP − ICP. In a normal child, a CPP of 40 mm Hg or more is sufficient to maintain normal blood flow and the appropriate delivery of nutrients.

Three basic types of ICP monitors are hydrodynamic monitors, electronic fiberoptic monitors, and cuff-pressure monitors. Hydrodynamic monitors contain a fluid-filled column connected to a transducer that in turn connects to an oscilloscope or digital display. The fluid-filled column usually is a catheter implanted in the ventricle or it is a bolt that sits in the subarachnoid or epidural space. The intraventricular cannula allows cerebrospinal fluid to be withdrawn in case of an extreme increase in ICP. Emphasis should be placed on the early insertion of the ventricular cannula, because once edema of the brain has progressed, the ventricles of the brain become small and, therefore, difficult to locate percutaneously. In an electronic fiberoptic monitor, a sensor sits directly in the brain and measures the pressure by fiberoptic oscillation. Cuff-pressure monitors use an air- or fluid-filled bag that transmits the pressure by compression of the bag or cuff. These monitors must be implanted through a burr hole and usually are large and cumbersome to insert and remove.

Regardless of the type of ICP monitor used, equipment failure may occur. Close neurologic observation with frequent pupillary checks is mandatory whenever ICP is monitored.

CHAPTER 445 ■ INTUBATION

FERNANDO STEIN AND JORGE M. KARAM

Because most instances of cardiac arrest in children are caused by respiratory failure, the ability to intubate the trachea is a skill every pediatrician should have. Except in cases of acute upper airway obstruction with arrest, intubation of the trachea should be a carefully planned and preconceived procedure. All the necessary equipment should be kept available and should be checked regularly. Box 445.1 lists the minimal equipment necessary for intubation.

Ventilatory assistance can be provided for most children with a bag and mask, and while such assistance is being instituted, the physician should give clear, concise commands regarding the orderly performance of procedures and the administration of medications. Semiconscious or alert patients who require endotracheal intubation should receive appropri-

ate sedation and cardiovascular protection, and they should be paralyzed for the procedure (Table 445.1). Use of an intravenous line is recommended with rare exceptions. Typically, the sequence of medications used is as described in the following sections.

CARDIOVASCULAR PROTECTION

Cardiovascular protection is provided by administering atropine sulfate at 0.01 mg/kg/dose; the drug should be given intravenously and is recommended in patients beyond the neonatal age. The use of atropine is contraindicated specifically in patients with glaucoma.

BOX 445.1	Minimal Intubation Equipment

1. Suction device (wall or portable unit) with suction tube and suction catheter, all appropriate sizes to fit endotracheal tubes
2. Ambu bags, several sizes (infant, child, adult) and appropriately sized masks (infant, child, adult)
3. Oxygen source (tank or central)
4. Endotracheal tubes, several sizes (2.5–8.0)
5. Laryngoscopes, at least two, preferably one straight blade, one curved blade; *check lights*
6. Malleable metal stylet, with lubrication
7. Oropharyngeal airways, six sizes
8. Adhesive tape
9. Carbon dioxide monitoring device
10. Ventilation system
11. McGill forceps
12. Bite lock

RESPIRATORY PROTECTION

This involves oxygenation with an inspired fraction of oxygen of 100% without manual ventilatory assistance and allowing for 3 minutes of spontaneous breathing of 100% oxygen.

SEDATION, ANALGESIA, AND CONTROL OF MOVEMENT

Various sedatives are available, and the administration of anesthetic or sedative-analgesic agents is an individualized decision that depends on the patient's condition.

TABLE 445.1

DRUGS USED IN INTUBATION*

Drug	Dose
Cardiovascular Protection	
Atropine sulfate (use if bradycardia is probable)	0.01 mg/kg
Sedation	
Ketamine (asthmatic patients)	0.5–2 mg/kg
Morphine	0.1–0.3 mg/kg
Diazepam	0.1–0.3 mg/kg
Barbiturates	
Thiopental (short acting) (cardiovascular stability)	5–10 mg/kg
Pentobarbital (intermediate acting)	3–5 mg/kg
Etomidate (cardiovascular instability)	0.2–0.3 mg/kg
Paralyzation	
Succinylcholine (depolarizing; short acting)	1 mg/kg
Dimethyltubocurarine (nondepolarizing)	0.2–0.4 mg/kg
Pancuronium (nondepolarizing)	0.1 mg/kg
Rocuronium	1.2 mg/kg
Atracurium	0.4–0.5 mg/kg
Vecuronium	0.1 mg/kg
Pancuronium	0.1–0.3 mg/kg

*The physician should be thoroughly familiar with the action, half-life, pharmacologic interactions, and pharmacokinetics of all drugs administered.

Opiates are a satisfactory alternative because they provide both analgesia and narcosis; an antagonist drug (naloxone) is available, if required. Barbiturates are used commonly, and either the short-acting or the intermediate-acting type is suitable for intubation of the trachea. Some of the benzodiazepines are also acceptable, but in sporadic reports they have been associated with elevation of pulmonary artery pressure.

Administration of a rapidly acting neuromuscular relaxant requires that every case be individualized in reference to the use of neuromuscular blocking agents. *A word of caution: When a paralyzing agent is used, physicians may not know prospectively whether or not they will be able to ventilate the patient with upper airway obstruction by mask and bag.*

Therefore, physicians who infrequently perform endotracheal intubations are advised to call for expert help immediately while the child is observed continuously. Physicians should ensure that all the necessary equipment is available and that the patient is monitored appropriately.

LAYNGOSCOPE INTUBATION

Laryngoscope intubation is performed under direct visualization with an oral tube and stylet inside the endotracheal tube. The patient's head is placed over a 1- to 2-inch pillow or folded piece of cloth; initially, the airway should be cleared of debris, blood, and secretions; and an artificial oral airway is inserted to remove the tongue from the normal anatomic air passages. An oral (Guedel) or nasopharyngeal airway may be necessary to maintain patency until a definitive airway is secured; it should be opened using the jaw-thrust or chin-lift maneuver. The position for standard tracheal intubation flexes the lower cervical spine and extends the occiput on the atlas. Then the bag and mask are applied. A tight seal should be created between the mask and the patient's face, and the bag should be compressed at a rate no slower than 15 times/minute. Expansion of the chest should be noted, and a stethoscope should be used to determine that breath sounds are satisfactory. After 2 to 3 minutes of bag and mask ventilation with 100% oxygen (except in neonates), the laryngoscope is inserted into the patient's mouth and is lifted to a 45-degree angle in reference to the horizontal axis. The technique used should be the one with which the operator is most familiar. If intubation is performed with a straight blade, the blade should be moistened, inserted through the right side of the mouth, and advanced toward the epiglottis on the right side of the tongue. The epiglottis then is visualized, and the laryngoscope blade tip lifts the epiglottis, thus providing visualization of the larynx with a lift forward at a 45-degree angle, as described earlier. Visualization should not be forced by angling the laryngoscope blade against the teeth; doing so is a leading cause of dental trauma. The endotracheal tube then is inserted with the concavity lateral to the angle of the mouth. The tube is advanced toward the larynx until it disappears beyond the vocal cords. Sometimes the tube must be rotated 90 to 150 degrees. After intubation is accomplished, the tube is advanced 3 to 5 cm beyond the vocal cords, depending on the patient's size and age.

The technique used when intubation is performed with a curved blade is slightly different in that the epiglottis is not elevated. With the curved blade, the tip is positioned in the fold between the base of the tongue and the epiglottis (volecula). An upward motion stretches the ligaments and folds the epiglottis upward, so the vocal cords can be visualized. After intubation has been accomplished, bilateral and equal breath sounds should be noted. The endotracheal tube is secured, a mouth block or oral airway is applied, and a chest radiograph is obtained to check for satisfactory position of the tip of the tube.

If the procedure cannot be performed, time should not be wasted with repeated attempts at intubation while the patient is desaturating. As soon as the problem is recognized, other methods of securing the airway should be considered.

LARYNGEAL MASK AIRWAY

The laryngeal mask airway (LMA) is gaining wider support in maintaining the airway; a tracheal tube (size 6 or less) may be placed, either blindly or via flexible fibreoptic laryngoscopy. The LMA does not, however, protect the airway from aspiration, and by acting as a bolus in the pharynx, it actually may relax the lower esophageal sphincter and increase reflux. Use of the LMA probably should be limited to maintenance of the airway after a failed attempt at intubation.

COMBITUBE

The Combitube is a double-lumen tube inserted blindly into the esophagus or trachea. The position of the tube is confirmed by the presence of breath sounds or capnography. By inflating one of the two cuffs present, the lungs then may be ventilated. Problems arise after positioning with definitive securing of a tracheal tube has been achieved and again with protection of the airway from aspiration, although stomach suctioning is possible through the gastric port.

CRICOTHYROIDOTOMY

A surgical airway should be recognized and performed quickly by an experienced person. It may be used as a primary airway, in patients with injuries to the pharynx, for example, or after failure of orotracheal intubation. It may be approached via a percutaneous needle cricothyroidotomy with high-flow oxygen or in a full surgical manner. The patient may present with carbon dioxide retention with this technique, so we monitor the levels in arterial samples.

Suggested Readings

Benumof JL. Laryngeal mask airway and the ASA difficult airway algorithm. *Anesthesiology* 1996;84:686.

Brimacombe JR, Brain AIJ. *The laryngeal mask airway: a review and practical guide.* Philadelphia: WB Saunders, 1997.

Gregory GA. *Pediatric anesthesia,* 4th ed. New York: Churchill Livingstone, 2002.

Hunter JM. Rocuronium: the newest aminosteroid neuromuscular blocking drug. *Br J Anaesth* 1996;2:184.

Miller RD. *Anesthesia,* 5th ed. Philadelphia: Churchill Livingstone, 2000:412.

Natalini G, Rosano A. Resistive load of laryngeal mask airway and proseal laryngeal mask airway in mechanically ventilated patients. *Acta Anaesthesiol Scand* 2003;47:761.

Pennant JH, White PF. The laryngeal mask airway: its uses in anesthesiology. *Anesthesiology* 1993;79:144.

CHAPTER 446 ■ EXTUBATION

FERNANDO STEIN AND JORGE M. KARAM

When the indications that prompted endotracheal intubation no longer exist, extubation should be executed carefully. Three major concerns in the removal of a tube are avoiding laryngospasm, maintaining airway patency, and ensuring adequate ventilatory function.

The tube should be removed when the patient has adequate reflex control. Therefore, paralyzing agents, sedatives, and narcotics must be discontinued or weaned before extubation is performed.

Laryngospasm occurs when the patient is in a state of semialert-semiasleep consciousness and droplets of secretions fall on the vocal cords, which in turn approximate and occlude the airway. Although this situation may be short-lived, it is potentially fatal, so extubation should be conducted as if the patient were to require intubation at the same time, which implies having the equipment and medications immediately available.

Laryngospasm is better prevented than treated. The treatment includes administering oxygen under pressure using a reservoir bag and mask and perhaps paralyzing the patient completely. Laryngospasm is prevented best by keeping the patient as alert as possible and by providing attention to the aspiration of secretions. Before the tube is removed, the lungs should be inflated with 100 percent oxygen for 1 to 3 minutes; after removal of the tube, the patient should be given oxygen.

In infants and small children, the administration of racemic epinephrine has been shown to be helpful in the control of postintubation subglottic edema. After the endotracheal tube has been removed, a chest radiograph should be obtained to check for postintubation atelectasis.

A randomized controlled trial comparing the administration of corticosteroids with placebo on the prevalence of reintubation or postextubation stridor in infants or children showed that the prophylactic administration of dexamethasone before elective extubation is performed reduces the prevalence of postextubation stridor in neonates and children and may reduce the rate of reintubation.

SEQUENCE OF ACTIONS FOR EXTUBATION

1. Suction oropharynx, suction trachea via ETT.
2. Confirm that an air leak exists around the ETT. The air leak should occur at less than 20 cm H_2O. If no leak is present, an increased risk of stridor and airway obstruction due to tracheal edema may be present. Consider administering dexamethasone (Decadron), 0.5 to 1.0 mg/kg/dose, 24 hours before extubation, generally continued for three to four doses q6, after extubation.
3. Confirm that the patient is sufficiently awake, breathing spontaneously, and able to sustain adequate oxygenation.
4. The patient should have been NPD for at least 4 hours prior to extubation. Every extubation is a planned reintubation.
5. Obtain all supplies at bedside for intubation.

6. Untape ETT and remove.
7. Have epinephrine aerosol available if a concern exists that the patient will have stridor.
8. Observe for ventilation and oxygenation, air movement, stridor, or weakness.

Suggested Readings

Anene O, Meert KL, Uy H, et al. Dexamethasone for the prevention of pos-textubation airway obstruction: a prospective, randomized, double-blind, placebo-controlled trial. *Crit Care Med* 1996;24:1666.

Bach JR, Saporito LR. Criteria for extubation and tracheostomy tube removal for patients with ventilatory failure. A different approach to weaning. *Chest* 1996;110:1566.

Khan N, Brown A, Venkataraman ST. Predictors of extubation success and failure in mechanically ventilated infants and children. *Crit Care Med* 1996; 24:1568.

Markovitz BP, Randolph AG. Corticosteroids for the prevention and treatment of post-extubation stridor in neonates, children and adults. *Cochrane Database Syst Rev* 2000;2:CD001000.

Markovitz BP, Randolph AG. Corticosteroids for the prevention of reintubation and postextubation stridor in pediatric patients: a meta-analysis. *Pediatr Crit Care Med* 2002;3:223.

Scott K Epstein. Extubation. *Respir Care* 2002;47:483.

CHAPTER 447 ■ TRACHEOSTOMY

FERNANDO STEIN, JORGE M. KARAM, AND NADEEM I. SHAFI

A tracheostomy is an opening created surgically through the neck and into the trachea (windpipe). A tracheostomy tube usually is placed through this opening to provide a permanent airway and to remove secretions from the lungs. The indications for tracheostomy in children are divided into three categories: airway obstruction, pulmonary toilet, and mechanical ventilation (Table 447.1).

A tracheostomy can help in managing patients with chronic lung disease, pulmonary fibrosis, interstitial lung disease, bronchiolitis obliterans, bronchopulmonary dysplasia, and certain neonatal conditions by decreasing airway dead space and facilitating pulmonary toilet.

In a 12-year review of indications for tracheostomy at Children's Hospital of Pittsburgh, Pennsylvania, the indications for 80% of the procedures were assisted ventilation and pulmonary toilet; the remaining procedures were performed for upper airway obstruction. With small variations, the same is true for most children's hospitals in the United States.

The assessment of urgency is the most important factor in choosing and planning the most appropriate and safest technique of securing the airway. Whenever time and conditions allow, a tracheostomy should be performed by the most expert personnel available, and the procedure should be undertaken in the operating room.

An endotracheal tube should be in place before the tracheostomy procedure begins, except in case of extreme obstructive emergencies. This procedure should be performed with the patient under general controlled anesthesia; use of local anesthesia usually is inappropriate. The neck is cleaned and draped. Surgical cuts are made to expose the tough cartilaginous rings that make up the anterior wall of the trachea. The surgeon cuts two of these rings and inserts a tracheostomy tube. After the tracheostomy has been performed, provision of warmed, filtered, and humidified air is important because the tube bypasses the nasopharynx. Most patients require 24 to 72 hours to adapt to breathing through a tracheostomy tube.

Some of the most serious complications that develop after tracheostomy can be divided in two groups: early complications and late complications. Table 447.2 summarizes the possible complications after tracheostomy. Any of these problems can be fatal; most can be prevented.

When the patient returns to the intensive care unit after undergoing tracheostomy, the equipment required to perform a new tracheostomy should be placed at the bedside and should remain there in a sterile package for 3 to 5 days. An appropriate light source for the performance of emergency surgery should be available at the bedside. Physical and pharmacologic restraint of the patient is necessary to avoid accidental extubation or dissection of air between superficial and deep tissue planes. Suctioning and ventilation with a mask should be performed by personnel who are trained appropriately regarding the complications of recent tracheostomy.

TABLE 447.1

INDICATIONS FOR TRACHEOSTOMY

Types of Airway Obstruction	
Static	**Dynamic**
Choanal atresia	Vocal cord paralysis
Macroglossia	Physical trauma of the face
Micrognathia	Epiglottitis
Subglottic and laryngeal stenosis	Laryngotracheobronchitis
Laryngomalacia	Paralysis of the muscles that affect swallowing
Tracheomalacia	Foreign body
	Neck or mouth injuries
	Intubation
	Inhalation of toxic gases or steam
	Burns by corrosive chemicals

Conditions Requiring Mechanical Ventilation	
Neuromuscular	**Pulmonary**
Brain damage	Preterm neonate
Long-term unconsciousness or coma	Cardiac surgery
	Critical illness
Poliomyelitis	Short-term intubation (<3 weeks)
Tetanus	Long-term intubation (>3 weeks)
Guillain-Barré syndrome	
Paraneoplastic neurologic syndromes	
Duchenne muscular dystrophy	

TABLE 447.2

COMPLICATIONS OF TRACHEOSTOMY

Early Complications (First Week)	Late Complications
Apnea: more common in smaller children with chronic airway obstruction	All complications seen in the first postoperative week also possible later
Air leak: surgical emphysema possible after the operation	Accidental decannulation: less dangerous in the later period because the tract is well formed; risk of stenosis of the tract within 10 minutes of decannulation
Accidental decannulation: serious complication in the first 2 to 3 days because the fistulous tract will not have formed	Obstruction: may be caused by a granuloma or by a mucous plug; granulations may cause bleeding during recannulation
Creation of a false passage: changing of the tube or its reinsertion may lead to creation of a false passage that may lead to obstruction or pneumothorax	Hemorrhage: serious hemorrhage a possible result of erosion of a large vessel; rarely occurs in the first week
Obstruction: most common cause of obstruction is accumulation of mucus and crusts in the tube or in the lumen of the trachea	Chest infections: more common in tracheostomized children than in other children
Hemorrhage: bleeding from the dissection field is usually trivial	Tracheitis: bacterial tracheitis common after a recent viral upper respiratory infection
Chest infections: more common in infants with previous pulmonary disease	

Dislodgment of the tracheostomy tube is a constant risk in a patient who has a tracheostomy tube. Nursing personnel, respiratory therapists, and eventually all home caretakers should be trained to replace a tracheostomy tube. The procedure is described here briefly. Two persons are strongly recommended to perform this procedure. An infant or small child may require physical restraint. All equipment is prepared and made readily accessible beforehand. An Ambu bag with supplemental oxygen is readied if available, and suction apparatus is preassembled and turned on. The new tracheostomy tube is unpackaged, and its patency is ensured. Integrity of the cuff is confirmed if present, the obturator is placed, and the tip is lubricated with a water-soluble lubricant or saline. Ties can be inserted into the tracheostomy tube or passed behind the neck of the child with the ends placed to either side of the head for easy access. A roll is placed beneath the shoulders to assist in exposing the tracheostomy site adequately. The airway is suctioned before tube removal to optimize airway patency while the tracheostomy tube is not in use. Old ties are carefully undone or cut while the tube is held in place. The tube is then removed with an up-and-out motion, following the angle of the tube. The new tube is inserted, taking care to follow the epithelialized ostomy tract. The tracheostomy tube is stabilized, and the obturator is removed promptly so the child can breathe. The tube then is secured using the ties. The child should be observed closely after a tracheostomy tube has been changed so problems may be addressed swiftly and professional assistance can be sought if necessary.

Suggested Readings

Amin RS, Fitton CM. Tracheostomy and home ventilation in children. *Semin Neonatol* 2003;8:127.

Bleile KM, ed. *The care of children with long-term tracheostomies.* San Diego: Singular Publishing, 1993.

Brook I. Treatment of aspiration or tracheostomy-associated pneumonia in neurologically impaired children: effect of antimicrobials effective against anaerobic bacteria. *Int J Pediatr Otorhinolaryngol* 1996;35:171.

Kremer B, Botos-Kremer AI, Eckel HE, Schlondorff G. Indications, complications, and surgical techniques for pediatric tracheostomies: an update. *J Pediatr Surg* 2002;37:1556.

MacEntee MV, Khan TZ, Stenmark KS, et al. Airway inflammation and bacterial colonization in stable pediatric patients with tracheostomies. *Am J Respir Crit Care Med* 1995;151:A95.

Meyer CM, Cotton RT, Shott SR, eds. *The pediatric airway: an interdisciplinary approach.* Philadelphia: JB Lippincott, 1995.

Stool SE, Eavey R. Tracheostomy. In: Bluestone CD, Stool SE, eds. *Pediatric otolaryngology.* Philadelphia: WB Saunders, 1983.

CHAPTER 448 ■ ABDOMINAL PARACENTESIS

EILEEN D. BREWER

Abdominal paracentesis is a useful procedure to obtain diagnostic information for evaluation of ascites, peritonitis, and intraperitoneal hemorrhage or to initiate therapeutic interventions, such as decompression of ascites for relief of respiratory compromise or the instillation of fluid to promote internal cooling during heat stroke. Diagnostic peritoneal lavage once was the procedure of choice for the early detection of intraabdominal trauma in children, but it has been supplanted by careful serial clinical and laboratory observation and computed tomography (CT) in centers where abdominal CT is readily available. Diagnostic peritoneal lavage still is indicated for the unconscious or intoxicated patient in whom physical observation may be unreliable, in the child who has multiple organ trauma and needs emergent surgery for intracranial or skeletal injuries, or in the presence of a penetrating abdominal wound and uncertainty about bowel integrity or perforation. No absolute contraindications to abdominal paracentesis exist, but relative contraindications necessitate prudent judgment before undertaking the procedure. Relative contraindications include previous abdominal surgery, pregnancy, bleeding disorders, disruption of the abdominal wall, and marked distention of the bowel, which predisposes to puncture and leakage of bowel contents into the peritoneum.

TECHNIQUE

The technique for abdominal paracentesis is as follows:

1. To avoid puncture of organs, be sure the stomach is decompressed and the bladder is empty before starting. Use a nasogastric or orogastric tube, if needed, to decompress the stomach. Have the patient empty the bladder spontaneously or use in-and-out straight catheterization. In the young child, a full bladder is positioned more in the lower abdomen than pelvis and is at greater risk for puncture.

2. Place the patient in the supine position with the head elevated at least 30 degrees to assure the ascites is dependent in the lower abdomen. Verify the presence of ascites by physical examination.

3. Choose a puncture site on the abdominal wall. The most commonly used entry site is infraumbilical, in the midline below the umbilicus, approximately one-third of the distance from the umbilicus to the symphysis pubis (Fig. 448.1, site P). A midline supraumbilical approach rarely is used in pediatrics, but is recommended for the patient who is pregnant or has a pelvic fracture (Fig.

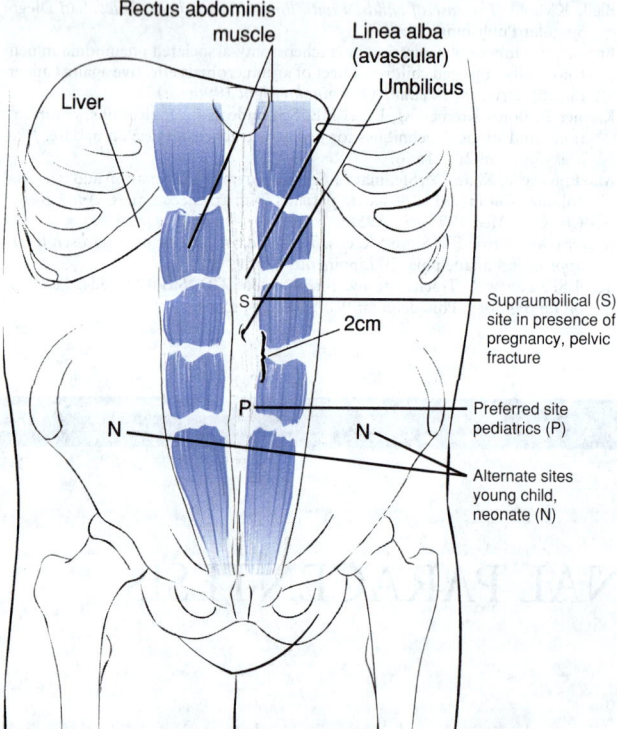

Rectus abdominis muscle
Linea alba (avascular)
Umbilicus
Liver
S
2cm
Supraumbilical (S) site in presence of pregnancy, pelvic fracture
P
N
N
Preferred site pediatrics (P)
Alternate sites young child, neonate (N)

FIGURE 448.1. Insertion sites for paracentesis. Midline infraumbilical (P) is the most common site for pediatric insertion. Lateral lower quadrants (N) are best for young children and neonates, to avoid accidental bladder puncture because the bladder is located more in the abdomen in these patients. Midline supraumbilical (S) insertion is used rarely, but recommended for the pregnant teenager or patient with a pelvic fracture.

448.1, site S). The midline location allows the needle to pass through the relatively avascular linea alba and avoids bleeding complications. If an abdominal scar, local skin infection, or abdominal wall hematoma is present in the midline, an alternative puncture site is the right or left lower quadrant of the abdomen, halfway between the umbilicus and iliac crest, in line with the nipples; the lateral edge of the rectus sheath must be avoided to minimize bleeding complications (Fig. 448.1, sites N). The lower quadrant approach also may be used for young children and neonates, to reduce the possibility of accidental bladder puncture in the midline. Avoid choosing a puncture site near a scar from a previous abdominal surgery, where the bowel may be adherent to the abdominal wall and easily punctured. If concerns arise about the location of viscera, presence of adhesions, or the location of a specific loculated fluid collection to be sampled, use ultrasound guidance for needle insertion.

4. Prepare a large area of skin around the planned puncture site with a standard antiseptic solution and sterile drapes.

5. Using sterile technique, infiltrate the site of abdominal wall entry with 1% lidocaine for local anesthesia.

6. Choose either a 16- to 20-gauge needle with internal or over-the-needle catheter set, or a peritoneal lavage catheter with needle and wire for placement using the Seldinger technique. Introduce the needle at the chosen puncture site with steady pressure and advance until the peritoneum is entered, which usually will be indicated by a "popping sensation" or loss of resistance. If using a needle with catheter set, advance the catheter a short way into the peritoneum, then withdraw the needle and advance the catheter further, as needed for adequate sampling of fluid (at least 10 to 20 mL) through a syringe attached to the catheter. If using the Seldinger technique to place a peritoneal lavage catheter, insert the needle into the peritoneum, then pass the wire through the needle into the abdomen, directed to either pelvic gutter, remove the needle with the wire remaining in place, pass the lavage catheter over the wire, and finally remove the wire. The lavage catheter has multiple side holes that improve flow through the catheter to ensure adequate sampling of ascitic fluid and make it easy to instill and drain fluid for peritoneal lavage or to remove ascites for therapeutic purposes.

7. Sample the contents of the peritoneal cavity for the appropriate diagnostic tests indicated by the condition being evaluated. Diagnostic tests include cell count with differential, Gram stain, culture and sensitivity (aerobic, anaerobic, acid-fast, fungal, viral), chemical analysis (glucose, total protein, albumin, creatinine, amylase, lactate dehydrogenase, cholesterol, triglycerides), or cytology for cancer evaluation.

8. If performing diagnostic peritoneal lavage, infuse 20 mL/kg of fluid (normal saline, lactated Ringer's, or other balanced salt solution). Then drain the abdomen and send the entire contents for cell count with differential and amylase.

9. When paracentesis or lavage is completed, pull the catheter out, firmly apply a sterile gauze to the site, then apply a pressure dressing to stop any further leakage.

FLUID ANALYSIS

Appearance

Peritoneal fluid normally is clear and straw colored. A cloudy fluid suggests infectious or chemical peritonitis. A milky appearance is characteristic of chylous ascites. Green-stained fluid may indicate pancreatitis or gallbladder or common duct perforation. Red-brown or brown fluid suggests hemorrhagic pancreatitis. Feculent material or cloudy greenish yellow fluid is characteristic of bowel perforation with peritonitis. Blood-tinged or bright red fluid is associated with abdominal organ injury and intraperitoneal hemorrhage or a traumatic tap.

Cell Count and Differential, Cytology

Infectious peritonitis is defined as the presence of more than 500 white blood cells per milliliter, with 50% or greater neutrophils by differential count. A predominance of lymphocytes and monocytes may be seen with chylous ascites or tuberculous peritonitis. Diagnostic peritoneal lavage for abdominal trauma and intraperitoneal hemorrhage is positive if more than 100,000 red blood cells per milliliter are present. Special cytology is needed for the detection of malignant cells.

Chemical Analysis

The classification of ascitic fluid as transudate or exudate may be helpful in determining the etiology of the ascites. A total protein concentration less than 2.5 g/dL and a fluid-to-serum total protein ratio of 0.5 or less are consistent with a transudate. A serum-to-ascites albumin gradient greater than 1.1 g/dL is diagnostic of portal hypertension. Decreased fluid glucose concentration to less than 60 mg/dL or less than two-thirds the serum glucose value is associated with tuberculous peritonitis, but also with bacterial peritonitis and malignancy. A fluid creatinine concentration greater than serum concentration is diagnostic of urine leak into the peritoneum. Elevated fluid amylase levels greater than in the serum occur in patients with pancreatitis, pancreatic pseudocyst, intestinal perforation, or bowel

strangulation. An elevated fluid triglyceride level is characteristic of chylous ascites. Increased fluid lactate dehydrogenase and cholesterol levels are associated with malignant ascites.

COMPLICATIONS

The complications of abdominal paracentesis are few and rarely serious. Intestinal perforation usually seals rapidly after withdrawal of the needle. Perforation of a blood vessel into the peritoneal cavity leads to a bloody tap, but rarely leads to intraperitoneal hematoma. Extraperitoneal hematoma in the abdominal wall may occur secondary to perforation of the deep epigastric vessels in the lateral aspect of the rectus muscle. Bacterial contaminants may be introduced and lead to infection, if sterile technique is not maintained. During therapeutic paracentesis, the rapid removal of a large volume of ascites may result in hypotension from intravascular volume depletion after re-equilibration.

Suggested Readings

Dzakovic A, Notrica DM, Smith EO, Wesson DE, Jaksic T. Primary peritoneal drainage for increasing ventilatory requirements in critically ill neonates with necrotizing enterocolitis. *J Pediatr Surg* 2001;36:730.

Foltin GL, Cooper A. Abdominal trauma. In: Barkin RG, ed. *Pediatric emergency medicine*, 2nd ed. St. Louis: Mosby, 1997:345.

Kramer RE, Sokol RJ, Yerushalmi B, et al. Large volume paracentesis in the management of ascites in children. *J Pediatr Gastroenterol Nutr* 2001;33:245.

Meyer DM, Thal ER, Coln D, Weigelt JA. Computed tomography in evaluation of children with blunt abdominal trauma. *Ann Surg* 1993;217:272.

Rice TB, Pontus SP. Diagnostic and therapeutic centeses. In: Fuhrman BP, Zimmerman JJ, ed. *Pediatric Critical Care*, 2nd ed. St. Louis: Mosby, 1998:147.

Towers HM. Neonatal ascites. In: Burg FD, Ingelfinger JR, Polin RA, Gershon AA, ed. *Current pediatric therapy*, 17th ed. Philadelphia: WB Saunders, 2002:280.

CHAPTER 449 ■ ACUTE PERITONEAL DIALYSIS

EILEEN D. BREWER AND ARUNDHATI S. KALE

Peritoneal dialysis (PD) therapy has been used for decades to treat acute and chronic renal failure in children because it is technically easier to perform than hemodialysis, requires no vascular access or anticoagulation, and avoids rapid hemodynamic changes in the critically ill child. Technical advances have led to the development of the automated cycler, but PD is still done by manual exchanges in most parts of the world.

PD is possible because of the characteristics of the peritoneal membrane that lines the intra-abdominal wall and viscera. This membrane is a very thin mesothelial monolayer overlying a layer of loose connective tissue separated by an intervening basement membrane. The space between the parietal and visceral surfaces of the peritoneum normally contains only a small amount of fluid, but can hold a large volume of solution if needed. During PD, the peritoneal membrane functions as a semipermeable dialysis membrane, allowing water and permeable solutes to pass freely, through osmosis, diffusion, and convection, between the capillaries and venules comprising the

vasculature of the peritoneal membrane and the dialysis solution instilled into the peritoneal cavity. In general, permeable solutes travel from areas of high concentration to lower concentration, but transfer also is affected by the permeability characteristics of the membrane itself. The surface area of the peritoneal membrane is roughly equal to the body surface area in older children and adults. Infants and small children have a greater peritoneal surface area–to–body weight ratio than adults, so PD is more efficient in these patients. On average, the peritoneal membrane is a little more permeable in infants and young children relative to adults, so equilibration occurs more rapidly and exchange times should be shorter (1 hour or less) in these patients.

During the PD procedure itself, a specific volume (dwell volume) of specialized dialysis solution is instilled into the peritoneal cavity via a peritoneal dialysis catheter (PD access) for a specified period of time (dwell time) during which equilibration occurs. After the desired period of equilibration, the dialysis effluent containing waste products and excess fluid (ultrafiltrate) is drained out, and fresh dialysis solution is instilled again to continue the process. Small molecules like urea, creatinine, potassium, and phosphorus pass freely from their higher concentration in the blood into the peritoneal fluid, while larger particles like blood cells and large proteins remain in the vascular space. Albumin and smaller proteins are filtered and removed in the PD fluid and may exacerbate hypoalbuminemia in critically ill patients. Normal concentrations of the essential electrolytes and minerals are maintained by using dialysis solution with a desired concentration of these solutes.

Commercially available dialysis solutions contain physiologic concentrations of sodium, chloride, and magnesium; slightly higher than physiologic concentrations of calcium; and no potassium or phosphorus. Potassium can be added to the solution in low or physiologic concentration if clinically indicated at the time of dialysis. Phosphorus should not be added, because of the risk of precipitation with calcium and magnesium already present in the solution. Lactate, which can be converted rapidly by the liver to bicarbonate and is stable in stored solution with the other salts and minerals, is used to provide alkali to treat the acidosis of renal failure. Bicarbonate-based solutions, which are not commercially available currently in the United States, can be made up specially if needed, but should not contain calcium because of the risk of precipitation. When liver function is poor, or in critically ill children with persistent lactic acidosis, a bicarbonate-containing solution may be required. If so, serum ionized calcium levels should be monitored closely and supplemental doses of calcium administered as needed or provided as a continuous intravenous drip or part of total parenteral nutrition.

The removal of excess fluid by ultrafiltration during PD requires an osmotic gradient that favors the movement of water from vascular space into the peritoneal fluid. High concentrations of dextrose are used for this purpose in commercial dialysis solutions approved for use in the United States. Commercially available PD solutions contain 1.5, 2.5, or 4.25 g/dL of dextrose, which is 10 to 50 times higher than the usual range of blood glucose concentration (75 to 150 mg/dL). In infants and small children, because they have a larger surface area to body weight, the rapid absorption of dextrose from the dialysate solution may result in rapid equilibration and poor ultrafiltration with extended dwell times. For this reason, dwell times of 1 hour or less are usually preferred for acute peritoneal dialysis.

PD can be performed technically either manually or with an automated cycler. Each technique requires specialized supplies and equipment and should be performed by trained personnel to avoid complications. Manual PD is simple to perform utilizing a heating bag to warm the dialysis fluid and a two-bag, Y-tubing set for older children or the Gesco Dialy-Nate system (Utah Medical Products, Midvale, UT) with a buretrol contained in the tubing to allow for the accurate measurement of small-volume exchanges (less than 100 mL) for infants. Pediatric cyclers usually have the capability to deliver exchange volumes of 50 mL or more per exchange, using programmed increments as small as 10 mL. The newer cyclers are small, portable devices that are easy to accommodate in small bedside spaces.

In critically ill children, when continuous fluid removal is necessary, frequent small-volume exchange cycles performed hourly or more often, throughout the 24-hour period, are prescribed. In more stable acute conditions, the duration may be limited to 8 to 12 hours/day. The recommended starting exchange volume is 10 mL/kg or 250 mL/m². If the patient has no respiratory or myocardial instability, the volume may be increased gradually to a maximum of 40 mL/kg or 1,100 mL/m². The time components of each exchange include a fill time, dwell time, and drain time. Fill time through a properly functioning PD catheter should take no more than 5 to 10 minutes, and drain time should take only 10 to 20 minutes. Drain time

may be extended if outflow is sluggish. Dwell time for continuous manual or cycler exchanges is usually 30 to 120 minutes, with shorter dwell times used to attain higher ultrafiltration rates. Dwell times of less than 30 minutes are less efficient, both for the clearance of solutes and ultrafiltration, and these short dwell times are not recommended. The fill time, dwell time, and drain time together constitute one exchange cycle.

The efficacy of acute PD can be determined by monitoring the improvement in blood chemistries and the adequate removal of fluid overload. Blood chemistry values should be checked at least once or twice daily during acute PD, to avoid electrolyte or mineral imbalances or poor correction of acidosis. Body weight should be measured at least twice daily, if possible, at the beginning and end of the PD procedure. Ultrafiltration volume is automatically recorded for each exchange and as a total by the automated cycler. For manual exchanges, ultrafiltration must be calculated by hand from the total drain fluid minus the instilled fluid volume; this value should be recorded on a flow sheet that includes the amount for each exchange as well as a daily running total. Blood pressure should be monitored frequently during acute PD.

INDICATIONS

PD used to be the modality of choice for acute renal failure in children, but advances in hemodialysis and continuous renal replacement therapy (CRRT) technology have changed clinical practice (Box 449.1). In a 1999 survey, pediatric nephrology centers in the United States ranked PD and CRRT equally as their primary initial modality for acute renal failure. Even neonates can be treated effectively, with few technical complications, using newer hemodialysis and continuous venovenous hemofiltration (CVVH) machinery. Outcome may be improved by more intense CRRT in the setting of sepsis and multiorgan failure than with slower PD. When a rapid correction of fluid overload, hyperkalemia, severe acidosis, tumor lysis syndrome, hyperammonemia, or intoxication with a dialyzable drug or poison is desired, hemodialysis is a better initial choice. If patients are hemodynamically unstable, but still need rapid correction, CRRT is preferred. In children who are too small for reliable vascular access or who can tolerate a slower removal of fluid and waste products and a slower correction of electrolyte abnormalities, acute PD still is desirable. In neonates and infants with oliguria after surgery to correct congenital heart disease, the early initiation of low-volume continuous PD has

---

BOX 449.1	Acute Renal Failure: Indication for Peritoneal Dialysis

Uremic syndrome
Blood urea nitrogen of greater than 100 mg/dL
Persistent hyperkalemia (serum potassium level of greater than 6.5 mEq/L)
Persistent metabolic acidosis (serum bicarbonate of less than 10 mEq/L)
Persistent congestive heart failure
Oliguric acute renal failure secondary to hemolytic uremic syndrome or rhabdomyolysis with myoglobinuria

been used effectively to promote fluid removal with few dialysis complications and improved patient outcome, compared with treatment using high-volume PD or other dialysis modalities later in the postoperative course.

Absolute contraindications for PD include abdominal wall defects such as omphalocele or gastroschisis, diaphragmatic hernia, and multiple abdominal adhesions from previous infection or abdominal surgery. Relative contraindications include ventriculo-peritoneal shunt, colostomy or ileostomy, bowel perforation or infarction, necrotizing enterocolitis, and recent abdominal surgery. The presence of a urinary diversion, including nephrostomy, ureterostomy, or vesicostomy, is not a contraindication to PD, but does demand that careful attention be paid to positioning the PD catheter exit site where it will not be chronically wet or bathed with infected urine.

PD CATHETER ACCESS

PD catheter access usually can be placed simply and quickly. If the duration of acute PD is anticipated to be a few days, an uncuffed temporary catheter may be placed emergently at the bedside. Temporary catheters made of Teflon are more likely to leak or become infected with prolonged use and are too rigid to remain in place for longer than about 5 days. A single, cuffed silicon catheter can be used as a temporary catheter by positioning the cuff just outside the skin at the exit site. When the duration of PD is anticipated to be longer than a few days, a cuffed silicon catheter with a protective skin tunnel placed in the operating room by an experienced surgeon is preferred. Because PD catheters come in a limited number of sizes for the many different sizes and shapes of children, finding the best fit may be a challenge and usually will be more successful in the hands of a surgeon who does these procedures often. Complications of catheter placement include poor flow, outflow occlusion by omentum or fibrin plugs, peritonitis or tunnel/exit site infection, and leakage. Complications can be minimized by partial omentectomy, heparin added to the dialysis fluid for the first 48 hours to prevent fibrin plugs, perioperative antibiotics to prevent contamination with normal skin flora, and the use of low-volume (10 mL/kg body weight) exchanges for the first week.

COMPLICATIONS

Infection is the most common complication of PD and may involve the peritoneum (peritonitis) or the PD access catheter (exit site or tunnel infections). Infection is more likely with a temporary catheter left in place for longer than 72 hours or if there is leakage around the catheter. Signs and symptoms of peritonitis include cloudy effluent, abdominal pain, and sometimes fever, vomiting, or diarrhea. Dialysate effluent containing greater than 100 white blood cells per mL and greater than 50% neutrophils is diagnostic of peritonitis during PD. A culture of the effluent always should be sent before starting antibiotic therapy. The most common organisms encountered are *Staphylococcus aureus* or *epidermidis*, but other skin flora, such as streptococci as well as gram-negative organisms, including *Escherichia coli*, *Klebsiella*, *Serratia*, and *Pseudomonas*, and fungi, notably *Candida* species, may be the causative agent. Peritonitis associated with PD is treated with intraperitoneal antibiotics. Exit site and tunnel infections are infections of the skin around the catheter exit site and in the subcutaneous tunnel. The usual manifestations are erythema, pain, and purulent drainage.

Because of the chronically high intra-abdominal pressures associated with PD exchanges, hernias may occur or worsen during PD. Types of hernias include inguinal hernias, umbilical hernias, ventral hernias, and hernias at the catheter insertion site. Rarely, fluid from the peritoneum may migrate through the diaphragm and cause hydrothorax, especially on the right side, and respiratory distress. Chylous ascites, a rare condition reported mostly in neonates undergoing PD, should be considered when cloudy dialysis effluent appears milky in character. Hyperglycemia may be a consequence of glucose absorption from PD fluid, especially when the dextrose concentration is high (4.25 g/dL) to promote fluid removal.

Cardiorespiratory instability may worsen with acute PD. A large volume of dialysis fluid instilled into the abdomen can compromise cardiac output by decreasing venous return. An increase in intra-abdominal volume and pressure also may cause an elevation of the diaphragm, with a decline in the functional residual capacity and expiratory reserve volume. This situation may lead to atelectasis and a decline in P_aO_2, with an increased alveolar–arterial oxygen gradient. Low-volume, continuous PD exchanges (10 to 20 mL/kg) may be used to treat or prevent cardiorespiratory instability and still provide acceptable dialysis and fluid removal.

Suggested Readings

Brandt ML, Brewer ED. Peritoneal catheter placement in children. In: Nissenson AR, Fine RN, ed. *Dialysis therapy*, 3rd ed. Philadelphia: Hanley & Belfus, 2002:468.

Chadha V, Warady BA, Blowey DL, et al. Tenckhoff catheters prove superior to Cook catheters in pediatric acute peritoneal dialysis. *Am J Kidney Dis* 2000;35:1111.

Daugirdas JT. Peritoneal dialysis in acute renal failure—why the bad outcome? *N Engl J Med* 2002;347:933.

Flynn JT. Choice of dialysis modality for management of pediatric acute renal failure. *Pediatr Nephrol* 2002;17:61.

Kale AS, Brewer ED. Peritoneal dialysis. In: Burg FD, Ingelfinger JR, Polin RA, Gershon AA, ed. *Current pediatric therapy*, 17th ed. Philadelphia: WB Saunders, 2002:818.

Goldstein SL. Overview of pediatric renal replacement therapy in acute renal failure. *Artif Organs* 2003;27:781.

Golej J, Kitzmueller, Hermon M, et al. Low-volume peritoneal dialysis in 116 neonatal and paediatric critical care patients. *Eur J Pediatr* 2002;161:385.

Neu AM. Infant and neonatal peritoneal dialysis. In: Nissenson AR, Fine RN, ed. *Dialysis therapy*, 3rd ed. Philadelphia: Hanley & Belfus, 2002:480.

Quan AH. Peritoneal dialysis. In: Levin DL, Morris FC, ed. *Essentials of pediatric intensive care*, 2nd ed. New York: Churchill Livingstone, 1997:1576.

Sorof JM, Stromberg D, Brewer ED, et al. Early initiation of peritoneal dialysis after surgical repair of congenital heart disease. *Pediatr Nephrol* 1999;13:641.

Strazdins V, Watson AR, Harvey B. Renal replacement therapy for acute renal failure in children: European guidelines. *Pediatr Nephrol* 2004;19:199.

CHAPTER 450 ■ ACUTE HEMODIALYSIS

STUART L. GOLDSTEIN

Hemodialysis is a treatment used to augment or replace renal excretory function. Most water-soluble substances that are not protein- or tissue-bound in the extracellular fluid can be effectively removed through hemodialysis. In general, the management of acute renal failure consists of supportive care until the kidney recovers from the acute renal insult. Acute renal replacement therapy in the form of intermittent dialysis or continuous renal replacement therapy is indicated when pharmacologic management is insufficient to treat or prevent the following situations: volume overload with pulmonary edema or hypertension, hyperkalemia, metabolic acidosis, uremia, calcium–phosphorus imbalance, or neurologic symptoms secondary to uremia or electrolyte imbalance. Acute hemodialysis also is indicated in certain clinical situations that are not accompanied by renal failure, such as tumor lysis syndrome in patients with newly diagnosed leukemia or lymphoma, hyperammonemia in patients with inborn errors of metabolism and drug intoxications (Table 450.1). In such clinical cases, close attention to and supplementation of the patient's serum phosphorus and potassium is required, because hemodialysis can lead rapidly to hypophosphatemia and hypokalemia in a patient with normal renal function. Hemodialysis is indicated for the elimination of a toxin if there is a potential clinical benefit to the patient of removing the toxin more quickly than the endogenous clearance rate, a significant amount of the toxin can be removed, and a clear relationship exists between the blood levels of an agent and its toxic effects. Toxins that can be removed successfully through dialysis are distributed in body water, have low molecular weights, and are not bound to plasma or tissue proteins.

TABLE 450.1

MOST COMMON INDICATIONS FOR ACUTE HEMODIALYSIS

Condition	Underlying Illnesses
Hyperkalemia	Acute renal failure
	New onset end-stage renal disease
	Tumor lysis syndrome
	Rhabdomyolysis
Hypertension	Fluid Overload associated with Acute Renal Failure
Hyperphosphatemia/ hypocalcemia	Acute renal failure
	New onset end-stage renal disease
	Tumor lysis syndrome
Hyperammonemia	Inborn Errors of Metabolism (e.g., Urea cycle defects)
Drug overdose	Lithium toxicity
	Ethylene glycol poisoning
	Valproic acid overdose
	Phenobarbital overdose

Solute clearance during hemodialysis occurs through two physiologic mechanisms: diffusion and convection. Diffusion refers to solute migration across a semipermeable membrane. The factors governing the rate of transfer are membrane permeability (i.e., the number and size of the pores in the membrane), solute size and charge, membrane surface area, and magnitude of concentration gradient across the membrane. Solute transfer rates are inversely proportional to particle size—smaller particles diffuse more rapidly than do larger particles. On the other hand, solute transfer rates are directly proportional to membrane surface area and concentration gradient, both of which can be manipulated by prescription to improve clearance.

Convection refers to the phenomenon of solute movement (or solute drag) across the membrane, independent of concentration gradient. The main determinant of solute drag is the osmotic gradient achieved by the amount of plasma water pushed across the membrane (ultrafiltrate). The amount of convective transfer of a particular solute is proportional to both the amount of ultrafiltrate achieved during the treatment and the sieving properties of particular dialyzers. A sieving coefficient for each solute–dialyzer pair reflects the interaction between the size and charge of the solute, combined with the pore number and size of the dialyzer.

Most acute dialysis access occurs via a temporary, uncuffed dual-lumen catheter placed in the femoral, internal jugular, or subclavian vein. Infants often require dialysis via two separate single-lumen venous catheters, for example through the via umbilical vessels, because dual-lumen catheters may not be of appropriate size for the smaller vessel diameters of these patients. Many patients with acute renal failure (ARF) are too ill to be transported to a chronic hemodialysis unit, so water treatment is accomplished using commercially available portable reverse-osmosis machines. Many medications, including antimicrobials, anticonvulsants, sedatives, and chemotherapeutic agents are removed by hemodialysis. Therefore, additional doses of these medications may be required during or after the hemodialysis treatment to maintain therapeutic serum concentrations. Patients who require two or more pressors to maintain normotension may be too unstable for intermittent hemodialysis and attendant intermittent ultrafiltration, and these patients might be treated more appropriately using continuous renal replacement therapy.

The availability of pediatric dialysis tubing and dialyzers of small volume has made hemodialysis feasible even in neonates. The volume of the dialyzer and connecting tubes must approximate no more than 10% of the child's blood volume, to prevent the removal of too much volume, which can result in cardiovascular instability. The appropriate rate at which to pump the patient's blood through the artificial kidney is determined by the rate at which the blood can be returned, by the membrane characteristics of each artificial kidney, and by the patient's hemodynamic status. In general, a minimum blood flow of 2 to 3 mL/kg/minute provides an adequate clearance rate of urea or creatinine.

Although all pediatric hemodialysis requires specialized nursing and medical expertise, hemodialysis for neonates is an especially complicated procedure. Neonatal-sized blood tubing is available to minimize the blood volume of the extracorporeal circuit. The neonatal tubing is one-fourth the diameter of standard tubing, so the blood pump flow rate must be quadrupled to deliver the same blood volume per minute (e.g., a Qb of 160 mL/minute on the dialysis machine yields an actual blood flow of 40 mL/minute through the dialyzer when neonatal tubing is used). Even with smaller neonatal tubing, the extracorporeal volume is usually greater than 10% of patient blood volume, so the circuit should be primed with packed red blood cells mixed to a concentration of 35%. Current volumetric hemodialysis machines produce an ultrafiltration accuracy of 50 to 100 mL, which is acceptable for most pediatric patients but is not tolerable for neonates. Digital scales, which are accurate to within 10 g, can be placed under an infant warmer and help guide ultrafiltration during a neonatal hemodialysis treatment.

Complications that may occur in association with hemodialysis include hemorrhagic hypotension secondary to blood loss during machine malfunction, circulatory shock secondary to rapid changes in intravascular volume, tissue ischemia, air embolism, hemolysis, and wide variation in body temperature.

Suggested Readings

Brittinger WD, Walker G, Twittenhoff WD, Konrad N. Vascular access for hemodialysis in children. *Pediatr Nephrol* 1997;11:87.

Bunchman TE, McBryde KD, Mottes TE, et al. Pediatric acute renal failure: outcome by modality and disease. *Pediatr Nephrol* 2001;16:1067.

Donckerwolcke RA, Bunchman TE. Hemodialysis in infants and small children. *Pediatr Nephrol* 1994;8:103.

Evans ED, Greenbaum LA, Etlenger RB. Principles of renal replacement therapy in children. *Pediatr Clin North Am* 1995;42:1579.

Gaudio KM, Siegel NJ. Pathogenesis and treatment of acute renal failure. *Pediatr Clin North Am* 1987;34:771.

Goldstein SL, Jabs K: Hemodialysis. InAvner ED, Harmon WE, Niaudet P, eds. *Pediatric nephrology* 5th ed. Philadelphia: Lippinicott Williams & Wilkins, 2004:1395.

Goldstein SL, Macierowski CT, Jabs K. Hemodialysis catheter survival and complications in children and adolescents. *Pediatr Nephrol* 1997;11:74.

CHAPTER 451 ■ CONTINUOUS RENAL REPLACEMENT THERAPY

STUART L. GOLDSTEIN

When acute renal failure occurs in critically ill patients, severe cardiovascular, respiratory, and metabolic instability may contraindicate standard intermittent dialysis techniques. In such situations, patients generally are monitored in intensive care units, and continuous renal replacement therapy (CRRT) may be required to minimize cardiovascular instability. Under these conditions, effective renal replacement must (a) provide adequate blood purification from uremic toxins; (b) correct fluid, electrolyte, and acid–base derangements; (c) maintain homeostasis; and (d) protect the kidneys from further injury.

Transition from the use of adaptive continuous renal replacement therapy (CRRT) equipment to hemofiltration machines with volumetric control that allows for accurate ultrafiltration flows has likewise led to a change in pediatric renal replacement therapy modalities. Accurate ultrafiltration (UF) and blood flow rates are crucial for pediatric CRRT, because the extracorporeal circuit volume can comprise more than 15% of a small pediatric patient's total blood volume, and small UF inaccuracies may represent a large percentage of a small pediatric patient's total body water. Polls of U.S. pediatric nephrologists demonstrate increased CRRT use over peritoneal dialysis as the preferred modality for treating pediatric acute renal failure (ARF). In 1995, 45% of pediatric centers ranked PD and 18% ranked CRRT as the most common modality used for initial ARF treatment. In 1999, 31% of centers chose PD versus 36% of centers reporting CRRT as their primary initial modality for ARF treatment.

Continuous venovenous hemofiltration (CVVH) is performed using blood pumps and double-lumen venous catheters to avoid the complications found in previous arteriovenous treatments. The use of countercurrent dialysate flow can be used alone (CVVH-D) or in combination with hemofiltration (CVVH-DF) and is subject to local standards of care, because no data to date demonstrate improved patient outcome using one form of therapy versus another. High clearances can be obtained during continuous therapy, and adequate blood purification can be achieved in severely catabolic patients. The difficulties and complications encountered with these techniques are related to anticoagulation practices, the establishment of adequate vascular access, and the selection of an appropriate hemofilter for the system. The ideal machine should have a small volume, an interface that is easy to use, and high flexibility. The machine must be freestanding and easily transportable to the bedside.

The overall reported survival for critically ill children requiring CRRT ranges from 34% to 42%. A recent pediatric study suggests that initiating early CRRT to prevent worsening fluid overload in critically ill patients may improve survival, because early initiation may allow for more optimal nutrition and blood-product provision, without further accumulation of fluid or catabolic waste products. Other pediatric studies suggest that the early initiation of CRRT for critically ill children with bone marrow transplantation improves survival. Because CRRT mitigates the solute rebound that can occur with acute intoxications or syndromes that generate super-physiologic solute levels, CRRT use may be the optimal renal replacement therapy option for certain drug intoxications, tumor lysis syndrome, and hyperammonemia. A multicenter collaborative group of 11 U.S. pediatric centers, The Prospective Pediatric CRRT Registry Group, is examining potential factors that may affect CRRT patient survival and machine functioning.

Suggested Readings

Bunchman TE, Donckerwolcke RA. Continuous arterial-venous diahemofiltration and continuous veno-venous diahemofiltration in infants and children. *Pediatr Nephrol* 1994;8:96.

DiCarlo JV, Alexander SR, Agarwal R, et al. Continuous veno-venous hemofiltration may improve survival from acute respiratory distress syndrome after bone marrow transplantation or chemotherapy. *J Pediatr Hematol Oncol* 2003;25:801.

Goldstein SL. Overview of pediatric renal replacement therapy in acute renal failure. *Artif Organs* 2003;27:781.

Goldstein SL, Currier H, Graf C, et al. Outcome in children receiving continuous venovenous hemofiltration. *Pediatrics* 2001;107.

Goldstein SL, Somers MJ, Brophy PD, et al. The Prospective Pediatric Continuous Renal Replacement Therapy (ppCRRT) Registry: design, development and data assessed. *Int J Artif Organs* 2004;27:9.

Michael M, Kuehnle I, Goldstein SL. Fluid overload and acute renal failure in pediatric stem cell transplant patients. *Pediatr Nephrol* 2004;19:91.

Pascual JF, Lopez JD, Molina M. Hemofiltration in children with renal failure. *Pediatr Clin North Am* 1987;34:803.

Ronco C, Barbacini S, Digito A, Zoccali G. Achievements and new directions in continuous renal replacement therapies. *New Horiz* 1995;3:708.

Symons JM, Brophy PD, Gregory MJ, et al. Continuous renal replacement therapy in children up to 10 kg. *Am J Kidney Dis* 2003;41:984.

Warady BA, Bunchman T. Dialysis therapy for children with acute renal failure: survey results. *Pediatr Nephrol* 2000;15:11.

CHAPTER 452 ■ CONTINUOUS DRIP FEEDING

FERNANDO STEIN

Continuous drip feeding is used in those patients who cannot tolerate boluses of food or in those patients in whom the presence of a large volume of material in the stomach is deemed inadvisable. The continuous infusion of liquid nutrients or formula can be achieved through a nasogastric, gastrostomy, or duodenal tube.

Because of circadian rhythms, bowel function is not optimal during the late hours of the evening and early hours of the morning (11 PM to 5 AM). For this reason, some practitioners administer the 24-hour continuous drip requirement over a 16-hour period.

Because formula and liquefied foods that remain at room temperature longer than 4 hours may become contaminated with pathogenic organisms, they should not hang in the bag longer than 4 hours. The bag and the connecting tubes should be changed at least every 8 hours, and residuals should be checked by aspirating the stomach contents every 2 to 4 hours. No universal agreement exists as to what constitutes an acceptable residual. The author recommends that residuals greater in volume than the amount of nutrients given in the previous 3 to 4 hours of continuous feeding should be noted carefully, and reasons for these findings should be sought. Aspirates that are the same in quantity as those of the previous 1 or 2 hours probably are insignificant in children beyond the neonatal period.

The head of the bed or crib sometimes is elevated between 15 to 30 degrees to prevent gastroesophageal reflux in patients receiving continuous feedings.

CHAPTER 453 ■ SHOCK

M. MICHELE MARISCALCO

PATHOPHYSIOLOGY

Shock is a clinical syndrome that has been characterized in cardiovascular terms. Shock states reflect a disruption in and eventual loss of normal metabolic function at the cellular level. Cellular derangement occurs because of the inadequate delivery or impaired use of oxygen, termed *cellular hypoxia*, and of other essential substrates. Cellular hypoxia causes the cell to shift to anaerobic metabolism; this shift causes the accumulation of lactic acid and other metabolic by-products, which can lead to further cell dysfunction. Shock can be recognized clinically by evidence of acute disruption of circulatory or other organ function, particularly of the brain, lungs, and kidneys.

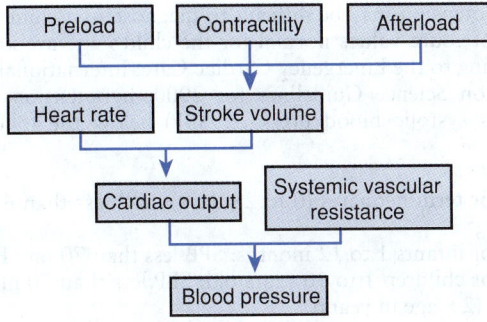

FIGURE 453.1. Regulation of blood pressure.

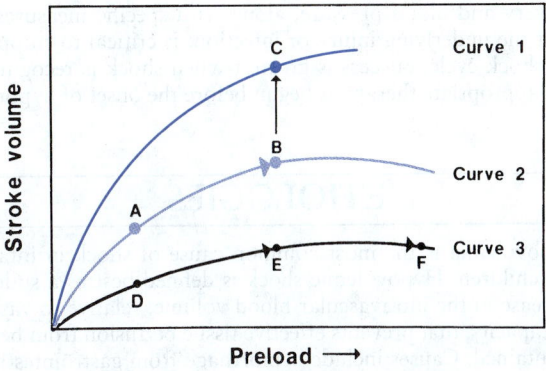

FIGURE 453.2. Frank-Starling curve. *Curve 1:* Increased contractility or decreased afterload. Stroke volume can increase from B to C with same preload by increasing contractility or decreasing afterload. *Curve 2:* Normal heart. Moving from A to B, stroke volume increases with an increase in preload. *Curve 3:* Depressed contractility or increased afterload. Stroke volume can increase if preload is increased from D to E. Further preload increase to F does not increase stroke volume and may lead to increased hydrostatic pressure and pulmonary edema.

Hypotension is a late manifestation of shock. The body has a host of mechanisms to maintain adequate perfusion to the central vascular bed. If a logical treatment plan is to be developed, the dynamics of the shock state must be understood.

The cardiovascular system can be likened to a pump that generates pulsatile flow through a series of tubes. The pressure (blood pressure) generated by the pump (the heart) depends on the amount of fluid flowing through the tubes (cardiac output) and the resistance to that flow (systemic vascular resistance). Thus, as in Figure 453.1,

Blood pressure = cardiac output × systemic vascular resistance

If a decrease in cardiac output occurs (as in cardiogenic shock or hypovolemic shock), a compensatory increase in systemic vascular resistance occurs to maintain blood pressure. This increase is mediated by the sympathetic nervous system and endogenous catecholamines. Clinically, the patient's periphery appears cool and mottled. In patients with septic shock, one of the primary defects is loss of systemic vascular resistance; the periphery is warm and appears vasodilated. To maintain blood pressure, cardiac output must increase to compensate for the decrease in systemic vascular resistance.

According to the model, the pulsatile flow generated by the pump depends on the rate and volume of each stroke:

Cardiac output = stroke volume × heart rate

Therefore, tachycardia should be present in most forms of shock as a compensatory mechanism to increase cardiac output. Severe bradyarrhythmias or tachyarrhythmias may themselves result in shock if the stroke volume is insufficient to compensate for the reduced cardiac output.

Stroke volume, the amount of blood ejected with each heartbeat, is determined by three factors (see Fig. 453.1): (a) ventricular preload, the volume of blood in the ventricle at the end of diastolic filling, which reflects venous return to the right side of the heart; (b) ventricular afterload, the impedance to the ejection of blood; and (c) intrinsic myocardial contractility. According to Frank-Starling mechanisms, the stroke volume is directly proportional to the preload (Fig. 453.2). For the myocardium to contract, the contractile proteins of the myocardial fibril, actin and myosin, must overlap. The greater the degree of stretch of the myocardial fibrils at the end of diastolic filling (i.e., increased preload), the greater the overlap of the contractile proteins and the greater the increase in stroke volume. Stroke volume decreases with increased preload if the myofibrils are stretched to the point where the contractile proteins no longer overlap.

At a given preload and afterload, the force that a myocardial fibril can generate depends on its intrinsic contractility. Contractility can be increased by the release of endogenous catecholamines, increased sympathetic stimulation of the nervous system, and the infusion of exogenous inotropic agents such

as epinephrine, dopamine, and dobutamine (see Fig. 453.2). Afterload is the composite of factors that oppose ventricular ejection. These factors include resistance to flow by the arterial tree, as reflected by aortic blood pressure, and left ventricular cavity size. Afterload is inversely proportional to stroke volume. An increase in afterload decreases stroke volume, unless either preload or contractility increases concomitantly. Because blood pressure is a clinical estimate of afterload, increases in blood pressure may decrease cardiac output in certain hemodynamic states. Thus, support of blood pressure does not guarantee adequate delivery of blood and oxygen to the tissues.

Oxygen delivery to the tissues is defined as:

Oxygen delivery = hemoglobin level × saturation
× cardiac output

In addition to cardiac output, the hemoglobin content of the blood and the oxygen saturation of the hemoglobin are important in oxygen delivery. If delivery is inadequate for cellular needs, cellular hypoxia results. Examples of inadequate oxygen delivery from decreased cardiac output include cardiogenic and hypovolemic shock. In contrast, in septic shock, cellular dysfunction occurs secondary to an intrinsic inability to use oxygen and/or increased needs above baseline, as well as a decrease in oxygen availability from peripheral vasodilation and decreased preload.

With these basic principles in mind, the practitioner can understand and treat the initial hemodynamic derangements seen in various shock states. In cardiogenic shock, the underlying hemodynamic dysfunction is in cardiac contractility; in hypovolemic shock, a decrease in preload volume occurs; and in septic shock, the initiating event is a decrease in systemic vascular resistance and hypovolemia. Hypoxia (absolute oxygen deficit) and ischemia (oxygen and substrate deficit) occur at some time in all types of shock. Either of these insults leads to lactic acidosis and the release of vasoactive metabolites and other mediators that are responsible for a host of cellular injuries. Some metabolites and mediators can cause an increase in capillary permeability that leads to a decrease in intravascular volume; others are direct depressants of myocardial contractility, which leads to further hemodynamic compromise and multiorgan dysfunction. Thus, the shock cycle perpetuates itself.

Unfortunately, the clinician can do little to interrupt the action of the mediators of cellular injury. Support of oxygen delivery and blood pressure, along with specific measures to treat the underlying injury or infection, is critical to stopping the shock cycle. Success is greatest when shock is recognized and appropriate therapy is begun before the onset of hypotension.

ETIOLOGIES

Hypovolemia is the most common cause of shock in infants and children. Hypovolemic shock is defined best as a sudden decrease in the intravascular blood volume, relative to vascular capacity, that prevents effective tissue perfusion from being maintained. Causes include hemorrhage from gastrointestinal loss or trauma, plasma loss from burns, and fluid and electrolyte loss, such as occurs from vomiting and diarrhea or endocrinologic disease (e.g., adrenal insufficiency, diabetes insipidus, diabetic ketoacidosis).

Cardiogenic shock is the state in which an abnormality of cardiac function is responsible for the failure of the cardiovascular system to meet the metabolic needs of tissues. Common to all causes of cardiogenic shock is depressed cardiac output. In most cases, the depressed output is caused by decreased myocardial contractility. Decreased myocardial contractility may be caused by an idiopathic cardiomyopathy, by metabolic processes or inflammation of the myocardial muscle itself, or by hypoxic-ischemic events. In other cases, acute heart rate changes may result in inadequate preload (such as occurs with supraventricular tachycardia or ventricular dysrhythmias). Severe bradycardia may lead to shock if stroke volume cannot increase to maintain cardiac output.

Distributive shock is caused by a maldistribution of blood flow to the tissues. Such maldistribution of flow results from widespread abnormalities of vasomotor tone. Profound inadequacies in tissue oxygenation can occur, even in the face of a normal or high cardiac output. Distributive shock can occur with anaphylaxis, spinal or epidural anesthesia, or disruption of the spinal cord.

Septic shock is the most complex and controversial type of shock. It comprises a cascade of metabolic, hemodynamic, and clinical changes resulting from invasive infection and the release of microbial toxins into the bloodstream and the host's response to them. Septic shock often is the combination of multiple problems, including hypovolemia with maldistribution of blood flow, myocardial depression, and multiple metabolic and endocrine derangements. Initially, in the early stage of sepsis, adult patients present in a hyperdynamic state characterized by elevated cardiac output, decreased systemic vascular resistance, widened pulse pressure, and warm extremities. If sepsis progresses, steady deterioration in cardiovascular performance occurs, marked by a decline in cardiac output, hypotension, and metabolic acidosis. In children with sepsis after fluid resuscitation, only about 20% demonstrated low systemic vascular resistance and increased cardiac output. Almost 60% had increased systemic vascular resistance and low cardiac output, and another 20% had low systemic vascular resistance and low cardiac output. Thus, children need specific therapies to address each of these states.

DIAGNOSIS

The key to making an early diagnosis of shock is to have a high index of suspicion and a knowledge of which conditions predispose children to shock. A correct diagnosis can be made only after a patient history has been obtained. Given the exigencies of the case, the history may be brief initially, but it is crucial in providing optimal stabilization.

Hypotension may be difficult to diagnose in a child unless blood pressure values normal for the child's age are known. According to the Emergency Cardiac Care: International Consensus on Science Guidelines for 2000, hypotension is defined as systolic blood pressure (SBP) below the following limits:

- For term neonates (0 to 28 days): SBP less than 60 mm Hg
- For infants 1 to 12 months: SPB less than 70 mm Hg
- For children 1 to 10 years old: SBP less than 70 mm Hg + (2 × age in years)

An observed drop of 10 mm Hg in SBP should prompt a careful serial evaluation for additional signs of shock. In the adult, a SBP lower than 90 mm Hg or a fall of 30 to 40 mm Hg from baseline is considered hypotension. In addition, the adequacy of perfusion to the core circulation must be assessed because inadequate perfusion precedes hypotension. Oliguria (0.5 to 1.0 mL/kg/hour) accompanies diminished renal perfusion from insufficient cardiac output. Altered mental states, such as confusion and agitation, occur in patients in early shock. With advanced hypoperfusion, patients classically exhibit obtundation and stupor. Vasoconstriction and diminished flow to the skin manifest as pallor, mottling, and poor capillary refill. In septic shock, if systemic vascular resistance decreases, the skin is warm, often flushed, and one must rely on other signs, symptoms, and laboratory tests to make the diagnosis.

Tachycardia and tachypnea almost invariably are present in patients with shock. As discussed, tachycardia is a compensatory mechanism to increase cardiac output. If cardiac output is diminished, the pulses are rapid, weak, and thready. In patients in early septic shock with low systemic vascular resistance, cardiac output initially is increased; the pulses are bounding. In patients in advanced shock, bradycardia results from severe hypoxia and acidosis. It usually heralds circulatory arrest unless appropriate and timely interventions are made. Because of limited reserves in stroke volume, the younger child is more dependent on heart rate to increase cardiac output. Extremely rapid heart rates can be seen in neonates, infants, and small children before hypotension occurs.

Lactic acidosis, the consequence of tissue hypoxia and ischemia, elicits a compensatory increase in alveolar ventilation, which results in a fall in P_aCO_2. The patient exhibits tachypnea (rapid breathing) or hyperpnea (deep breathing). The ensuing respiratory alkalosis compensates for the metabolic acidosis. However, the rise in minute ventilation increases the proportion of the cardiac output that must be supplied to the respiratory muscles. This increase occurs at a time when cardiac output is limited. Relative hypoventilation occurs as the respiratory muscles tire. The acidosis worsens, and the patient decompensates with increasingly shallow and ineffective respirations, and respiratory arrest occurs.

Several laboratory investigations can assist in the further assessment of the severity and cause of shock states. Probably the most common and most useful investigation is the blood gas analysis. The adequacy of ventilatory function can be evaluated by monitoring the arterial oxygen and carbon dioxide content. The degree of metabolic acidosis can be a useful indicator of tissue hypoxia or ischemia and of the efficacy of therapeutic support. Other laboratory investigations, such as serum electrolyte levels, blood cell counts, platelet counts, and hematocrit levels, are important in detecting the extent of metabolic disturbances. Calcium levels should be determined in all shock states because hypocalcemia occurs frequently and can compromise further myocardial, respiratory muscle, and metabolic function. Ionized calcium determinations are preferable to measurement of serum calcium levels.

MONITORING

The most effective and sensitive physiologic monitoring available is the frequent, repeated examination of the child by a competent, careful observer. Minimal monitoring of the child in shock or at risk for developing shock should include performing continuous electrocardiographic monitoring, obtaining frequent blood pressure and temperature measurements, and measuring blood glucose levels in younger infants. The monitoring of such patients should occur in the intensive care unit (ICU). Noninvasive blood pressure monitoring performed with the correct size cuff placed at the brachial pulse usually suffices, but critically ill children often require continuous intraarterial pressure monitoring. Urine production is a sensitive indicator of core perfusion; hourly monitoring of urine output is essential. Central venous catheters also can be useful in patients who require close monitoring and a manipulation of ventricular filling pressures and cardiac contractility, but they must be used as an adjunct to the physical examination, never as a replacement for it.

THERAPY

For all forms of shock, the cornerstones of therapy are the treatment of the underlying cause and optimization of oxygen and substrate delivery to critical vascular beds (i.e., cerebral, renal, and coronary vascular beds). The ultimate goal is to prevent or reverse the defects in cellular metabolism until homeostasis is restored and adequate nutritional support can be instituted to allow healing to begin.

As discussed in previous paragraphs, the provision of an adequate airway, oxygenation, and ventilation are crucial to maximizing oxygen delivery. The hemoglobin saturation (percent saturation) at a given P_aO_2 level is shown by the oxyhemoglobin dissociation curve (Fig. 453.3). Acidosis, hyperthermia, and hypercarbia shift the curve to the right and decrease hemoglobin oxygen affinity or hemoglobin saturation, thereby releasing more oxygen to the tissues. Because of the shape of the curve, increases in P_aO_2 above 65 mm Hg have little effect in increasing oxygen saturation of the hemoglobin, but P_aO_2 of less than 60 mm Hg can cause large decreases in hemoglobin saturation. Therefore, providing supplemental oxygen is part of the initial management of the child in shock.

The respiratory effects of shock can tax an already compromised cardiovascular system. Assisted ventilation decreases pulmonary oxygen transport needs, thereby allowing available oxygen to be delivered to other organs. In addition, positive pressure ventilation helps decrease left ventricular afterload and thus may be useful in the patient with myocardial compromise. However, positive pressure ventilation also may increase intrathoracic pressure enough to decrease venous return to the right side of the heart, thus decreasing preload and ultimately compromising cardiac output and oxygen delivery. Thus, the effects of mechanical ventilation must be monitored closely.

The most important maneuver in reestablishing circulation is to place an intravenous catheter of an adequate bore for the child's size or an intraosseous catheter. Cardiac output and blood pressure are optimized based on the principles outlined in the Pathophysiology section. Preload augmentation often is adequate to restore perfusion and blood pressure in children. Rapid intravascular expansion is guided by clinical examination and urine output. Volume expansion of 20 mL/kg over 10 minutes generally is safe. Controversy continues as to the type of volume to use (i.e., isotonic crystalloid such as normal saline or lactated Ringer's solution versus albumin-containing solutions). Although the controversy is far from solved, a recent trial in adult patients in the ICU did not demonstrate that either saline or 4% albumin was superior for multiple end-points, including mortality. When a volume resuscitation of greater than 50 to 70 mL/kg in the first 4 to 6 hours is required, more invasive monitoring should be considered. Modifications must be made to fluid resuscitation to replace ongoing losses caused by excessive urine output, excessive stool output, or hemorrhage. In pediatric trauma patients or those with acute blood loss, red blood cell transfusion (typically 10 to 15 mL/kg) is recommended when signs of shock or hemodynamic instability persist despite the provision of 2 to 3 boluses of isotonic crystalloid. In patients with sepsis, large volumes often are required to maintain adequate preload; volumes of more than 70 to 100 mL/kg are not uncommon.

Preload augmentation is limited in children when evidence is seen of an elevated ventricular filling pressure without an increase in cardiac output. Clinically, this condition can be monitored by observing for signs of cardiac congestion: jugular venous distention, liver enlargement associated with a previously undetected cardiac gallop rhythm, and continued evidence of hypoperfusion. The placement of central venous pressure lines may be helpful to prevent further volume overload in these patients. A central venous pressure that is rising or exceeds 7 to 10 mm Hg indicates myocardial dysfunction, volume overload, or increased right ventricular afterload. In these cases, further management may require more invasive monitoring and the use of inotropic or afterload-reducing agents. Aggressive fluid administration in patients who are on the downward slope of the Frank-Starling curve (see Fig. 453.2) results in increased venous pressure and the decreased perfusion of several critical beds. Increased venous pressure may worsen vascular leak, leading to increased tissue edema (most notably pulmonary edema) and contributing to the likelihood that adult respiratory distress syndrome will develop. In such patients, the use of agents to increase contractility, such as dopamine or milrinone, or decrease afterload, such as nitroprusside, are indicated and are discussed further in the section on myocarditis. Cardiac dysfunction can occur with any shock state, and the physician must be prepared to intervene at its occurrence. The inotropic agents commonly used have variable effects on heart rate and vascular tone, depending on the dose used, the child's age, and the physiologic disturbance. Given this fact, to label these agents vasopressors is misleading; indeed, one rarely wishes to use a pure vasopressor in most forms of shock (Table 453.1).

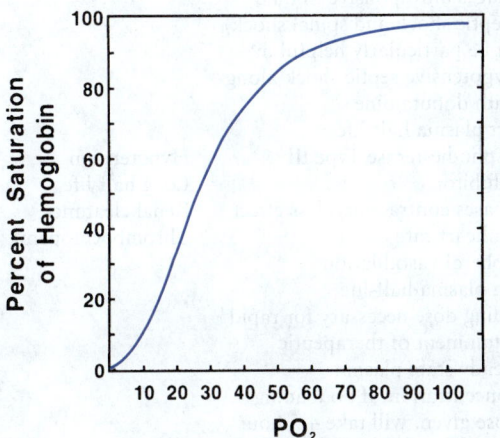

FIGURE 453.3. Oxyhemoglobin dissociation curve.

TABLE 453.1

DRUGS TO SUPPORT CARDIAC OUTPUT

Name	Dose	Indications	Pharmacology	Precautions
Dopamine	2–20 μg/k/minute	Inadequate cardiac output Hypotension Low doses (0.2–5 μg/kg/minute) may enhance renal and splanchnic blood flow, not consistent and controversial	Dopaminergic effects at lowest doses (vasodilation) Intermediate doses, with direct cardiac stimulation, stimulate release of norepinephrine in cardiac sympathetic nerves; beta effects predominate including vasodilation High dose: alpha effects predominate with vasoconstriction Widespread variability in plasma clearance and pharmacodynamics; therefore titrate to desired effect Short plasma half life	Tachycardia Arrhythmia Hypertension Depresses release of thyroid stimulating hormone and prolactin during prolonged administration
Dobutamine	2–20 μg/kg/minute	Myocardial dysfunction Inadequate cardiac output, particularly in patients with elevated systemic or pulmonary vascular pressure	Relatively selective beta$_1$; increase heart rate and contractility with dilation of peripheral vascular bed Widespread variability in plasma clearance and pharmacodynamics; therefore titrate to desired effect Short plasma half-life	Tachycardia Tachyarrhythmias Ectopic beats
Epinephrine	0.1–1 μg/kg/minute	Inadequate cardiac output Hypotension Symptomatic bradycardia Pulseless cardiac arrest Septic shock	Beta effects at lower doses Alpha effects at higher doses with increase in systolic and diastolic blood pressure and narrowing of pulse pressure Short plasma half life	Tachyarrhythmias Supraventricular and ventricular tachycardia Profound vasoconstriction (high dose)
Norepinephrine	0.1–2 μg/kg/minute	Hypotension (especially due to vasodilation) Inadequate cardiac output Spinal shock α-Adrenergic blockade	Potent inotrope Potent peripheral alpha and beta adrenergic effects, alpha effects predominate at doses used clinically with vasoconstriction Preferable to dopamine for those with depleted myocardial norepinephrine stores (chronic congestive heart failure) Most useful in those with slow systemic vascular resistance that is unresponsive to fluid (septic shock and spinal shock) May be particularly helpful in hypotensive septic shock along with dobutamine Short plasma half-life	Hypertension Organ ischemia, including digital and renal Arrhythmias
Milrinone	Loading dose: 50–75 μg/kg Continuous infusion 0.5–0.75 μg/kg/minute	Inadequate cardiac output with high systemic vascular resistance Cardiogenic shock Septic shock	Phosphodiesterase Type III inhibitor Increases contractility; less effect on heart rate Peripheral vasodilation Long plasma half-life Loading dose necessary for rapid attainment of therapeutic steady state plasma concentration. If no loading dose given, will take 4.5 hours to reach steady state concentration	Hypotension Long half-life Renal clearance Thrombocytopenia

Note: All agents should be infused through a large bore cannula. Extravasation has high potential of leading to tissue ischemia and necrosis (less likely with dobutamine). Catecholamines are inactivated in alkaline solutions.

Recently, guidelines have been developed for the management of severe sepsis and shock in adults and children. Whereas some of the guidelines are developed from randomized controlled trials, others are determined on the basis of consensus. The basis of resuscitation for sepsis in both adults and children is fluid challenges up to 60 mL/kg to achieve an acceptable blood pressure. In adults, a mean arterial pressure greater than or equal to 65, urine output greater than or equal to 0.5 mL/kg/hour, and a central venous pressure of 8 to 12 mm Hg with a central venous oxygen saturation of 70% or more is recommended within the first 6 hours. If central venous oxygen saturation of 70% is not achieved with fluid resuscitation, then packed red blood cells should be transfused to achieve a hematocrit of greater than or equal to 30% and/or dobutamine should be administered up to a maximum of 20 μg/kg/minute to achieve this goal. The use of "vasopressors" includes norepinephrine or dopamine as first-line therapy, when fluid alone is insufficient to achieve adequate blood pressure and organ perfusion. Early, goal-directed therapy in adults has demonstrated improved survival.

Guidelines for children differ from those of adults. Ventilation should be considered earlier in children, due to respiratory muscle fatigue. Vasopressors should be used only after adequate volume resuscitation has occurred. Therapeutic endpoints in children are based more on physical examination, including capillary refill in less than 2 seconds, normal pulses with no differential between peripheral and central pulses, warm extremities, urine output greater than 1 mL/kg/hour, normal mental status, decreased lactate and base deficit, and superior vena cava or mixed venous saturation of 70% or more. In a retrospective study, the practice of resuscitation was consistent with the consensus guidelines in only 30% of the patients. However, when practice was in agreement with guideline recommendations, a lower mortality rate was noted.

Managing the multisystem deterioration that accompanies shock states is as important as treating the underlying condition. Renal, gastrointestinal, hematologic, and central nervous system derangements should be anticipated, searched for, and treated. Coagulation abnormalities are common occurrences to some extent in all forms of septic shock, but they also are likely to occur in hypoperfusion states due to any cause. It is crucial to monitor prothrombin time, partial thromboplastin time, fibrinogen level, level of fibrin split products, and platelet count and to monitor for evidence of excessive bleeding. The use of vitamin K, fresh-frozen plasma, and platelet transfusions corrects most abnormalities.

Gastrointestinal disturbances include paralytic ileus and bleeding from gastritis or ulcer. The ileus may lead to a severe fluid and electrolyte disorder, complicating the management of the shock. Gastrointestinal blood loss may be prevented by the use of antacids or H_2 receptor blockers, such as cimetidine and ranitidine hydrochloride. Liver dysfunction often accompanies shock. Monitoring liver enzymes indicates the severity of injury, but elevations in the levels of these enzymes usually occur after the first 24 hours of presentation. A modification of drug therapy should be considered when evidence of liver involvement is present. Renal support is essential to avoid prolonged periods of anuria or oliguria during hypoperfusion states. The management of acute renal insufficiency is discussed in Chapter 456, Acute Renal Failure.

Acid-base disturbances can be severe. The primary treatment for metabolic acidosis is increased minute ventilation and a compensatory respiratory alkalosis. Respiratory failure ensues if the patient cannot compensate for the acidosis from shock. A base deficit of greater than 10 mEq/L with a pH of less than 7.15 probably should be corrected in acute shock states. Acidosis itself can be an acute, life-threatening event because the hepatic conversion of lactate or acetate to correct acidosis is inadequate. Primary correction is accomplished by increasing minute ventilation. However, if severe acidosis (pH less than 7.15 and P_aCO_2 less than 30 mm Hg) continues after minute ventilation is increased, bicarbonate supplementation can be given. This supplementation is accomplished by the repeated slow infusion of boluses of sodium bicarbonate, 1 to 2 mEq/kg. In infants, 0.5 mEq/mL of solution is used to decrease the risk of developing an intraventricular hemorrhage. Large amounts of bicarbonate may be required. The major limitations to bicarbonate replacement are sodium overload and hyperosmolarity. The overzealous administration of bicarbonate can lead to alkalosis, which shifts the oxyhemoglobin curve to the left, increases oxygen-hemoglobin affinity, and thereby worsens oxygen delivery at the tissue level. A close monitoring of serum sodium level, pH, and P_aCO_2 is indicated.

A fall in the serum ionized calcium level occurs commonly as the pH returns to normal. Decreased serum ionized calcium levels can lead to alterations in the level of consciousness, tremors, seizures, hypotension, myocardial depression, and acidosis. Serum ionized calcium bears little relationship to total serum calcium. The administration of either calcium gluconate, 100 mg/kg, given intravenously as a slow-infusion bolus, or calcium chloride, 20 mg/kg, rapidly restores serum levels of ionized calcium.

Hyperglycemia or hypoglycemia can accompany severe stress states in children. Hypoglycemia is a common occurrence in the small or malnourished child. It can be corrected by bolus injection of 25% dextrose, 0.5 to 1.0 mL/kg, or a continuous infusion of glucose, 4 to 8 mg/kg/minute. Hyperglycemia can cause difficulties with osmotic diuresis. Correcting the underlying stress usually resolves the hyperglycemia without the use of insulin.

Suggested Readings

Balk RA. Optimum treatment of severe sepsis and septic shock: evidence in support of the recommendations. *Dis Mon* 2004;50:163.

Carcillo JA. Pediatric septic shock and multiple organ failure. *Crit Care Clin North Am* 2003;19:413.

Ceneviva G, Pachall JA, Maffei F, Carcillo JA. Hemodynamic support in fluid-refractory pediatric septic shock. *Pediatrics* 1998;102:e19.

Dillinger RP, Carlet JM, Masur H. Surviving sepsis campaign guidelines for management of severe sepsis and septic shock. *Crit Care Med* 2004;32:858.

Han YY, Carcillo JA, Dragotta MA. Early reversal of pediatric-neonatal septic shock by community physicians is associated with improved outcome. *Pediatrics* 2003;112:793.

Hazinksi MF, ed. PALS Provider Manual. Dallas: American Academy of Pediatrics and American Heart Association, 2002.

McConnell MK, Perkin RM. Shock states. In: Furhman BP, Zimmerman JJ, eds. *Pediatric critical care*. St. Louis: Mosby–Year Book, 1998:293.

Notterman DA. Pharmacology of the cardiovascular system. In: Furhman BP, Zimmerman JJ, eds. *Pediatric critical care*. St. Louis: Mosby–Year Book, 1998:329.

Spivey WH. Interosseous infusion. *J Pediatr* 1987;111:639.

The SAFE Study Investigators. A comparison of albumin and saline for fluid resuscitation in the intensive care unit. *N Engl J Med* 2004;350:2247.

CHAPTER 454 ■ ACUTE RESPIRATORY DISTRESS SYNDROME

M. MICHELE MARISCALCO

Acute lung injury (ALI) is a syndrome of lung inflammation and increased vascular permeability. It is associated with clinical, radiologic, and physiologic abnormalities that cannot be explained by left atrial hypertension. The term *acute respiratory distress syndrome* (ARDS), formerly known as adult respiratory distress syndrome, is reserved for the most severe end of the spectrum of acute lung injury. It can occur in adults, children, and infants. The syndrome first was described in 1967, by Ashbaugh and Petty, who reported a series of 12 patients (one 11-year-old) suffering from a syndrome similar to hyaline membrane disease in newborns. In 1994, the American-European Consensus Conference (AECC) recommended the following definition for ARDS: (a) acute onset of respiratory distress; (b) hypoxemia (P_aO_2/F_IO_2 of 200 mm Hg or less, regardless of the level of positive end-expiratory pressure [PEEP]); (c) detection of bilateral pulmonary infiltrates on the frontal chest radiograph; and (d) no clinical evidence of left atrial hypertension or a pulmonary capillary wedge pressure of no more than 18 mm Hg. Patients who have a P_aO_2/F_IO_2 level of 300 mm Hg or less are considered to have ALI.

EPIDEMIOLOGY

A determination of the incidence of ALI, ARDS, and acute respiratory failure (ARF) has been problematic even in adult patients because of the difficulty in defining ALI, ARDS, and ARF in population-based studies. At present, the incidence of ALI is estimated at 22 to 87 cases per 100,000 each year, of which 75% of such cases fit the AECC definition of ARDS. The data are more limited in children and, therefore, even more problematic. In a study using the 1999 hospital discharges from six large states (22% of the U.S. population), the overall average incidence of mechanical ventilation in children (a surrogate marker for ARF) is 47 cases per 100,000 population each year, with 73 cases per 100,000 each year in the 1- to 4-year-old group and 30 cases per 100,000 in the 5- to 9-year-old group. In this study, 64% of these cases were nonsurgical. Note that defining ALI or ARDS in this patient population was not possible. Of the nonsurgical cases, 35% were caused by severe sepsis, 57% by pneumonia, and 10% by asthma. In a 24-month surveillance study conducted in the pediatric intensive care unit (ICU) at the Children's Hospital of Pennsylvania in the early 1990s, 2.7% of children admitted had ARDS diagnosed during their stay in the ICU. ARDS occurred in approximately 12% of children admitted to the pediatric ICU for sepsis, viral pneumonia, smoke inhalation, or drowning. A low incidence (less than 3%) was observed in children admitted for pulmonary contusion or multiple trauma.

In adult studies, shock from any cause has been associated with ARDS, as have surface burns, smoke inhalation, infectious and aspiration pneumonia, and disseminated intravascular coagulopathy. Current evidence supports that 115,000 people with sepsis each year will develop ARDS. Sepsis is the primary etiology in adults for ARDS. Other causes include drug overdose, cardiopulmonary bypass, fat embolism, high-altitude exposure, toxic gas inhalation, pancreatitis, and massive transfusion. At present, death rates from ARDS are less than 40%, although one recent study of 17,000 adult ventilated patients demonstrated a 52% mortality rate. Important to highlight is that those with ARDS who die, do so from their underlying illness, sepsis, or multiorgan dysfunction and not from their lung injury. The ARDS mortality rate in adults in the late 1970s was 90%. Death from ALI is calculated to amount to 17,000 to 43,000 deaths per year (deaths from acute myocardial infarction and breast cancer are approximately 200,000 and 40,000, respectively, in comparison). Mortality rates in children who are ventilated have been reported to be between 1.6% and 14%, depending on whether rates were based on patients who were followed prospectively for respiratory failure or were based on epidemiologic data. This rate is quite low compared with 30% in adult patients in a 2002 prospective study. Mortality rates in children with ARDS range from 40% to 75%, although more recent reports suggest that it may be as low as 30%.

PATHOGENESIS

No unifying hypothesis for the pathogenesis of ARDS exists. Experimental data from various studies indicate that the activation of complement causes granulocytes to adhere to and damage pulmonary microvascular endothelial cells via the release of lysozymes and toxic oxygen radicals. Increased permeability of pulmonary capillaries results. Studies of humans with ARDS using bronchoalveolar lavage have demonstrated large concentrations of neutrophils, along with the presence of such inflammatory cytokines as tumor necrosis factor and interleukin-1. Other mediators, such as the metabolites of arachidonic acid, prostaglandins, thromboxanes, and leukotrienes, also have been implicated in the increase in vascular permeability and pulmonary artery changes. Evidence does suggest that pulmonary endothelial injury can occur via neutrophil-independent mechanisms, as is the case in oxygen toxicity or endotoxin-induced ARDS models. Clearly, many complex permutations underlie the phenomenon of ARDS, and therapy must be directed at more than one mechanism if morbidity and mortality are to improve further. Despite a number of clinical trials using "antiinflammatory" therapies, none has proved to ameliorate the course of the disease. Only the use of ventilation strategies has demonstrated improved benefit.

CLINICAL MANIFESTATIONS AND COMPLICATIONS

The clinical course of the patient with ARDS varies, depending on the inciting event. Once direct or indirect injury has occurred, the affected patient usually experiences a latent period during which the respiratory status appears stable. Tachypnea and tachycardia develop primarily during the first 12 to 24 hours. As the syndrome progresses, the work of breathing increases dramatically, with nasal flaring and intercostal and accessory respiratory muscle activity developing. Lung compliance worsens. Auscultation of the chest reveals either no abnormality or high-pitched end-expiratory crackles throughout the lung fields. In some patients, ARDS resolves completely in the acute phase. In others, it progresses to fibrosing alveolitis with persistent hypoxemia, increased alveolar dead space, and a further decease in lung compliance. Pulmonary hypertension secondary to obliteration of the pulmonary capillary bed may be severe and lead to right ventricular failure. Once ARDS and respiratory failure occur, affected patients require a prolonged course of mechanical ventilation (mean of 8.8 days) and have a prolonged length of stay in the ICU (14.3 days) and in the hospital. (24.5 days). Patients may develop severe fibrotic lung disease requiring prolonged mechanical ventilation.

DIAGNOSIS

An early study of extracorporeal membrane oxygenation (ECMO) in ARDS, completed in the 1970s, was critical to furthering our understanding of the histopathology of the disease. ARDS often is progressive and is characterized by distinct stages having different histopathologic, clinical, and radiographic findings. In the acute phase, interstitial and then alveolar edema develops within the first 24 to 96 hours after injury. Erythrocytes, neutrophils, and macrophages begin to move into the interstitium and alveolus (Fig. 454.1). The thin, type I alveolar cells that form the normal epithelial lining of the lung are destroyed, leaving denuded basement membranes. The epithelial damage appears to be more severe at this stage than is the damage to the capillary endothelium. Within 72 hours of the injury, type II alveolar cells proliferate dramatically

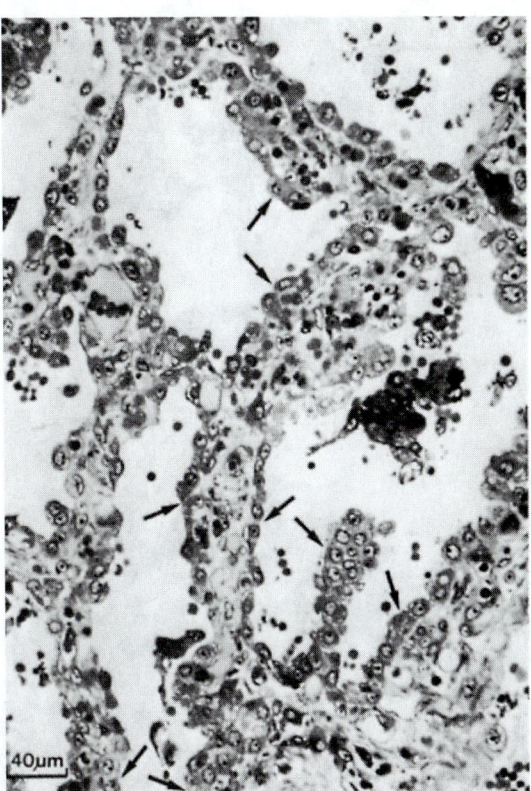

FIGURE 454.2. Light-microscopic view showing proliferation of type II alveolar cells and a markedly thickened septum with cellular proliferation. Pronounced epithelial transformation (*arrows*). (Reproduced with permission from Bachofen M, Weibel ER. Structural alterations of lung parenchyma in the adult respiratory distress syndrome. *Clin Chest Med* 1982;3:35.)

(Fig. 454.2). These cells are thick, enzymatically active, and responsible for the production of surfactant. Hyaline membranes form over the denuded alveolar surface (Fig. 454.3). In the proliferative phase, during the next 3 to 10 days, the alveolar septum becomes markedly thickened and is infiltrated by proliferating fibroblasts, plasma cells, leukocytes, and histiocytes. The first endothelial changes can be seen as irregularities of the luminal surface. However, significant capillary injury can occur with little morphologic change in the endothelial cells. By the end of the first week, fibrotic changes may develop in both the alveolar septa and the hyaline membranes. The alveolar structure no longer is recognizable (Fig. 454.4). This diffuse alveolar damage is the pathologic hallmark of ARDS.

Noncardiogenic pulmonary edema is a central feature of ARDS. On gross inspection, the lungs of patients with ARDS appear red, heavy, and airless. Both ultrastructural studies and the elevated protein content of the edema fluid in patients with ARDS support the hypothesis that the restrictive properties of the capillary membrane are disrupted. Noncardiogenic pulmonary edema floods the lungs more rapidly than occurs with hydrostatic pulmonary edema because an increase in capillary permeability occurs and the protective osmotic gradient between the capillary and interstitium subsequently is compromised.

Patients with ARDS demonstrate reduced lung volumes, large intrapulmonary shunt fractions, and hypoxemia (decreased P_aO_2). Alveolar flooding with fluid, proteinaceous debris, and inflammatory cell infiltrate, in concert with surfactant abnormalities, decreases alveolar volume and leads to widespread atelectasis in the exudative phase of ARDS. Areas

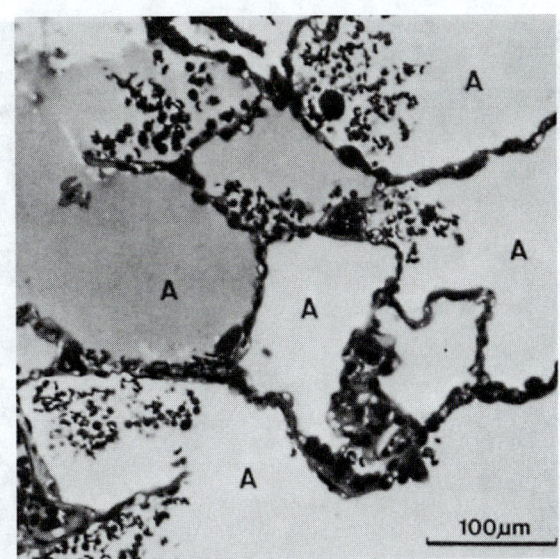

FIGURE 454.1. Light-microscopic view showing pulmonary edema and alveolar spaces. (A) inhomogeneously filled with proteinaceous fluid. The alveolar walls are edematous, and the capillaries are congested. Red blood cells and leukocytes have spilled into the alveolar spaces. (Reproduced with permission from Bachofen M, Weibel ER. Structural alterations of lung parenchyma in the adult respiratory distress syndrome. *Clin Chest Med* 1982;3:35.)

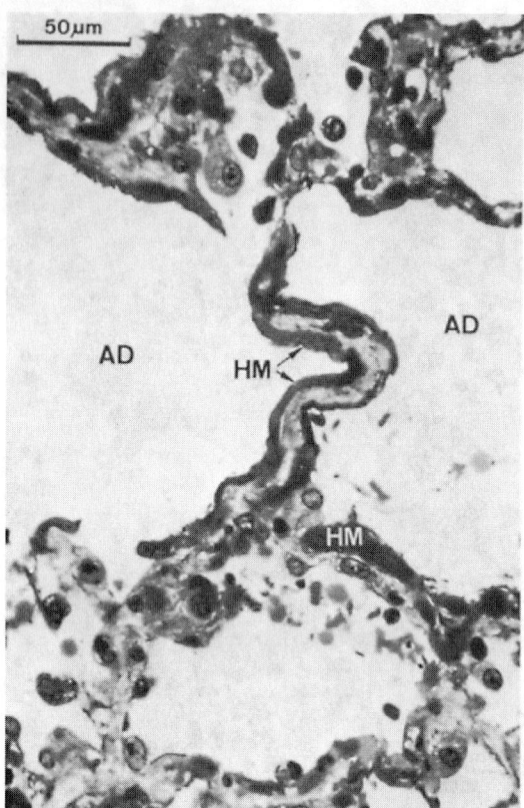

FIGURE 454.3. Light-microscopic view of hyaline membranes (*HM*) lining alveolar ducts (*AD*). (Reproduced with permission from Bachofen M, Weibel ER. Structural alterations of lung parenchyma in the adult respiratory distress syndrome. *Clin Chest Med* 1982;3:35.)

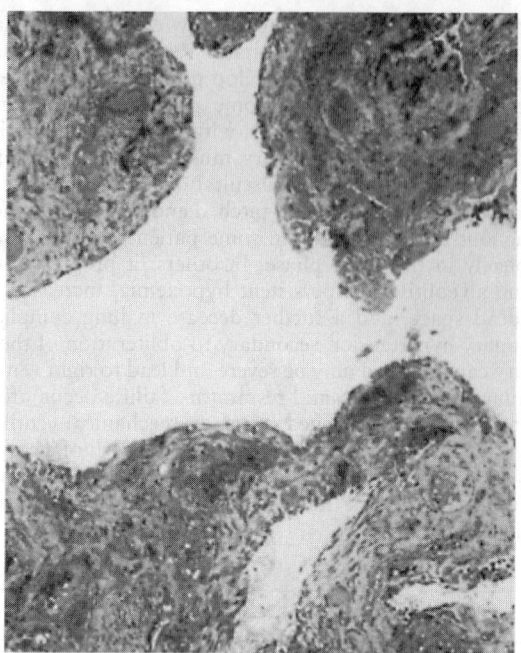

FIGURE 454.4. Light-microscopic view demonstrating markedly distorted pulmonary architecture. The alveolar septa are markedly thickened, and the alveolar spaces are almost obliterated. (Hematoxylin and eosin, low-power view.) (Reproduced with permission from Bachofen M, Weibel ER. Structural alterations of lung parenchyma in the adult respiratory distress syndrome. *Clin Chest Med* 1982;3:35.)

of the lung that are perfused either are not ventilated (intrapulmonary shunt) or are ventilated inadequately (i.e., have ventilation-perfusion inequalities), both of which lead to hypoxemia. Decreases in lung volume are reflected by decreases in functional residual capacity and lung compliance. Radiographically, the findings in the exudative phase may be indistinguishable from those of cardiogenic pulmonary edema, and infiltrates can be patchy or asymmetric and may include pleural effusions (Fig. 454.5). Computed tomography (CT) demonstrates that alveolar filling, consolidation, and atelectasis occur predominantly in dependent lung zones, whereas other areas may be spared.

In the proliferate phase of ARDS, only as much as one-half to one-third of the lung may be functioning. Chest radiographs show linear opacities, consistent with the presence of evolving fibrosis. CT of the chest shows diffuse interstitial opacities and bullae. On the basis of CT scan, Gattinoni described a three-zone lung model consisting of healthy, diseased, and recruitable lung in what appear to be areas of diffuse disease on plain lung radiography. The decreased lung compliance in severe ARDS may, in fact, be more a function of small lung volume than a "stiff lung." The work of breathing is elevated markedly because of the change in lung compliance. In patients in whom the disease course is protracted, marked pulmonary artery hypertension and lung fibrosis develop. Often, patients with ARDS also have multiple organ failure, which has led to the hypothesis that ARDS is part of a spectrum of diseases of diffuse organ injury.

Data support the hypothesis that ARDS occurring as a result of direct pulmonary injury, ARDSp (pneumonia, aspiration of gastric contents, pulmonary contusion, inhalation

injury, fat emboli), is different from that caused by extrapulmonary etiologies, ARDSexp (sepsis, trauma, drug overdose, acute pancreatitis, cardiopulmonary bypass). In ARDSp, during the acute exudative phase, in which alveolar collapse, fibrinous exudate, and alveolar wall edema occur, a fibroproliferative response also occurs that leads to alveoli obliteration.

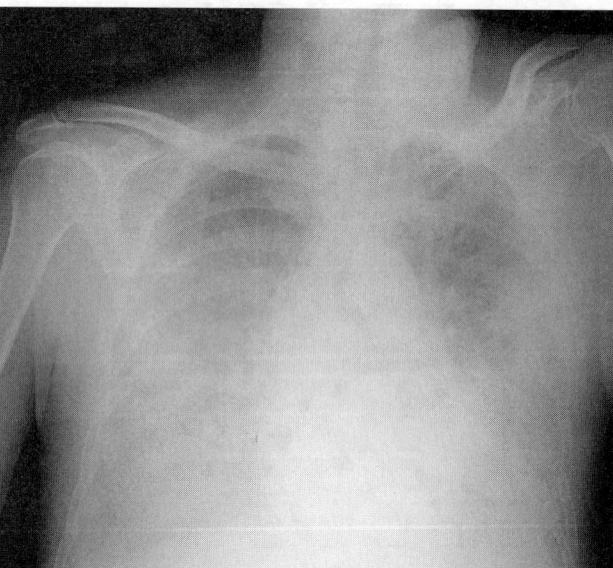

FIGURE 454.5. Bilateral pulmonary infiltrates consistent with, although not diagnostic of, acute respiratory distress syndrome (ARDS). (Courtesy of Mark Silverberg, MD.) (Reused with permission from Bailey H. Acute respiratory distress syndrome. In: Greenberg MI, ed. *Greenberg's text-atlas of emergency medicine.* Philadelphia: Lippincott Williams & Wilkins, 2005:670.)

In addition, in the acute exudative phase, increased collagen, but not elastic fiber content, appears to occur in those patients with ARDSp compared with ARDSexp. Thus, in the ARDSp, early extracellular matrix remodelling appears to occur. On chest radiographics, patients with ARDSp have an increased amount of "patchy" densities likely representing pulmonary consolidations. This finding is in contrast to the rather "hazy" and "diffuse" lung densities representing interstitial edema and compression atelectasis, which is seen more often in patients with ARDSexp.

THERAPY

Treatment of the underlying etiology is the first step in the management of ARDS. Currently, no therapeutic modality can halt or reverse either the capillary leak or the pulmonary fibrosis. The basis of therapy is supportive at present, with a view to minimize the occurrence of harm from therapies. The goal of supportive care in patients with ARDS is to deliver sufficient oxygen to satisfy the metabolic demands of the tissue while minimizing complications to the lungs from the therapy. Oxygen delivery depends on the percent saturation of hemoglobin by oxygen, the hemoglobin content of the blood, and the cardiac output. Therapy is directed at increasing the saturation of oxyhemoglobin without compromising cardiac output or causing pulmonary toxicity. All patients with respiratory insufficiency require supplemental oxygen, which may be supplied by face mask or nasal prongs. However, when oxygen concentrations of up to 50% to 60% no longer is sufficient to prevent hypoxemia, or affected patients have evidence of respiratory muscle fatigue, endotracheal intubation and positive-pressure ventilation are indicated.

The primary mode of respiratory support is mechanical ventilation with a tidal volume and respiratory rate adequate to provide an "acceptable" amount of minute ventilation and titrated FIO_2 and PEEP to support oxygenation. With the understanding that (a) patients with ARDS have small lung volumes, (b) the lungs of patients with ARDS have "patchy" involvement, and (c) alveolar overdistention and cyclic reopening of collapsed alveoli have been implicated in the lung damage termed *volutrauma*, several ventilatory strategies have been suggested. In general, certain generally consensus-derived principles determine ventilatory strategy. As a general rule, the desired goal is to use the least PEEP and tidal volume necessary to achieve acceptable gas exchange while avoiding tidal collapse and the reopening of an unstable lung unit. This is called the *open lung approach*. Several small studies and a large randomized control trial have demonstrated improved outcome in patients with ARDS when a low tidal volume strategy is utilized. In the ARDS Network Trial, patients who were ventilated with a tidal volume of 6 mL/kg and maintained at a plateau pressure of less than 30 had a 25% decrease in death rate and a 25% increase in their organ failure-free days compared with those who had a higher tidal volume (11 cc/kg). Oxygenation was maintained with increasing levels of PEEP in attempts to decrease FIO_2. At present, no consensus exists on the optimum level of PEEP in patients with ARDS. The ARDS Network ALVEOLI study, comparing 60-day mortality, using higher PEEP/lower FIO_2 versus lower PEEP/higher FIO_2, was discontinued prematurely because of lack of efficacy.

Although no studies in children have been performed, in general, most centers adjust the FIO_2 to maintain an SaO_2 between 88% and 95%, with a partial pressure of oxygen less than or equal to 70% and a partial pressure of carbon dioxide between 45 and 55 mm Hg. However, many experts advocate adjusting ventilation to keep the pH level at 7.2 or greater, thus allowing carbon dioxide to accumulate. This procedure is known as *permissive hypercapnia*. Often, the strategy entails optimizing oxygen delivery by maintaining normal hemoglobin values and cardiac output. Permissive hypercapnia may minimize volutrauma. Small tidal volumes and higher ventilator rates may be needed, and P_aCO_2 is allowed to increase slowly (at least to 55 mm Hg, though some advocate levels of 100 mm Hg or less). Marked acidosis can be corrected by chemical means (provision of bicarbonate, lactate, or tromethamine). If an increase in oxygenation is desired, mean airway pressure may be increased. Mean airway pressure can be altered by changes in waveform, PEEP, peak inspiratory pressure, or the ratio of the inspiratory-expiratory time. However, an important consideration is that continued increases in mean airway pressure may result in decreases in cardiac output. In addition, the application of PEEP does not retard or reverse the development of pulmonary edema. Thus, increased mean airway pressure may improve the hemoglobin saturation but might decrease cardiac output, with the resultant decrease in oxygen delivery and tissue hypoxia.

Several unconventional ventilatory strategies have been advocated for use in patients with ARDS. High-frequency positive-pressure ventilation (e.g., jet ventilation) has been shown to have no advantage over conventional ventilation. However, one trial in children with ARDS demonstrated that high-frequency oscillatory ventilation improved outcomes (i.e., decreased mortality and decreased barotrauma), when compared to conventional ventilatory strategies. Such strategies also may benefit neonates who are treated with surfactant and develop hyaline membrane disease. Other therapies, such as inverse-ratio ventilation and airway pressure release, variously have been advocated as salvage techniques or as routine alternatives to conventional ventilation, although no controlled trials support their use. A 1979 study using ECMO in adult patients demonstrated no improvement in survival rates compared to the non-ECMO group; both groups had a survival rate of 10%. More recently, an adult ARDS study using extracorporeal CO_2 removal ($ECCO_2R$) demonstrated that conventional therapy and $ECCO_2R$ had equal survival rates (50%). Although ECMO is used in some centers in children with ARDS, and some physicians have claimed that it improves survival rates, again, no controlled trial supports its routine use.

Changes in position improve gas exchange in patients with ARDS because lung infiltrates are not distributed evenly. Putting patients in the prone position has been advocated but was shown to be of no benefit in a large randomized trial. Prone positioning, however, is complicated and cumbersome. This approach should be used only in centers experienced with its application. Neither the use of liquid ventilation with agents that can carry oxygen nor the use of inhaled nitric oxide has been proved to improve outcome in either adult or pediatric patients with ARDS.

Meticulous fluid and blood-product management remains key to the stabilization of patients with ARDS. Whether crystalloid or colloid replacement should be used remains controversial. At present, volume expansion using blood products seems to be preferable to crystalloid because the delivery of oxygen is improved by increases in both hematocrit and cardiac output. Because of the permeability of the alveolar–capillary membrane, some fluid will leak into the pulmonary interstitium or alveoli, ultimately worsening the intrapulmonary shunt. Although colloid also ultimately will leak into the injured lung unit, it will occur more distant to the time of infusion than will crystalloid. In addition, the use of colloidal products may reduce the amount of volume required to stabilize affected patients by one-half, as compared to crystalloid. Cardiac filling pressures should be monitored so that overhydration can be avoided scrupulously. Patients with ARDS have increased pulmonary edema at normal filling pressures. In the management of fluids and support of cardiac output, right atrial pressure catheters or pulmonary artery catheters are helpful to measure pulmonary capillary wedge pressure. Inotropic agents also are used to maximize cardiac output. An ongoing trial is examining which strategies (fluid restrictive or loose) and which monitors of central pressure are beneficial in ARDS. Until then, it seems prudent to maintain cardiac output through initial judicious fluid administration and then the addition of inotropic agents or vasoactive agents as indicated.

Nutritional support is vital in patients with ARDS and should be instituted as early as possible in the clinical course. Often, gastrointestinal motility is impaired in ARDS, usually from a variety of factors, including positive pressure ventilation, inactivity, and sedatives. It may result in the patient's requiring parenteral nutrition. Calories are maximized, whereas the administration of fluids is minimized. Excessive intake of carbohydrates is avoided because carbohydrates are metabolized into fat in the liver, leading to large amounts of CO_2 production. Patients with respiratory failure may not be able to increase minute ventilation sufficiently to excrete this excess CO_2 load. Other supportive measures include diligent surveillance for secondary infections and the use of sedatives and, occasionally, muscle relaxants to ventilate such patients effectively.

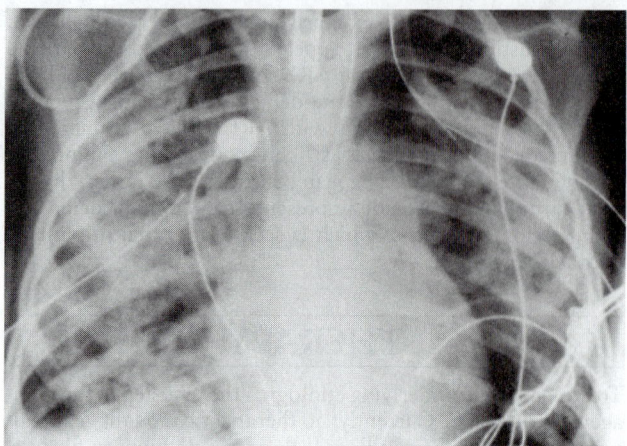

FIGURE 454.6. Severe adult respiratory distress syndrome and pneumothoraces in a 4-year-old boy who required multiple chest-tube drainage.

Complications of Therapy

The main complications of therapy for ARDS include volutrauma and oxygen toxicity to the lungs. For those patients treated with prolonged mechanical ventilation, alveolar rupture from overdistention can lead to pneumothorax, pneumoperitoneum, pneumomediastinum, pneumopericardium, and subcutaneous air. Pneumothorax should be suspected whenever patients with ARDS who are on positive pressure ventilation exhibit an unexplained sudden deterioration in clinical appearance, arterial oxygen tension, or hemodynamic stability (Fig. 454.6). The successful management of the pneumothorax almost always requires closed-chest thoracostomy tube evacuation of air to an underwater seal. Other complications include the acquisition of nosocomial pneumonia and the development of other organ injury. In particular, the risk of developing acute renal failure is greater in patients with ARDS than in those with ALI, worsening the prognosis of survival.

PROGNOSIS

Adult long-term survivors of ARDS are likely to have normal chest radiography and minimal respiratory symptoms. Data suggest that the gas-exchanging surface area of the lung is adequate to meet oxygen requirements of affected patients at rest; during exercise, however, efficient oxygenation is impaired and P_aCO_2 may fall. Although existing follow-up data on children who have had severe ARDS are limited, they tend to support the premise that such children are more likely than are adults to be left with significant respiratory abnormalities, including resting hypoxemia, cough, and exertional dyspnea. Twenty-five percent of adult patients ventilated for more than 7 days are at

risk of developing acquired paresis, which can result in long-term disability. The incidence in children is 5% of all children ventilated for more than 5 days.

Suggested Readings

Arnold JH, Hanson JH, Toro-Figuero LO, et al. Prospective randomized comparison of high-frequency oscillatory ventilation and conventional mechanical ventilation in pediatric respiratory failure. *Crit Care Med* 1994;22:1530.

Banwell BL, Mildner RJ, Hassall AC, et al. Muscle weakness in critically ill children. *Neurology* 2003;61:1779.

Davis SL, Furman DP, Costarino AT. Adult respiratory distress syndrome in children: associated disease, clinical course, and predictors of death. *J Pediatr* 1993;123:35.

Esteban A, Anzueto A, Frutos F, et al. Characteristics and outcomes in adult patients receiving mechanical ventilation. *JAMA* 2002;287:345.

Green TP, Moler FW, Goodman DM, for the Extracorporeal Life Support Organization. Probability of survival after prolonged extracorporeal membrane oxygenation in pediatric patients with acute respiratory failure. *Crit Care Med* 1995;23:1132.

Morris AH, Wallace CJ, Menlove RL, et al. Randomized clinical trial of pressure-controlled inverse ratio ventilation and extracorporeal CO_2 removal for adult respiratory distress syndrome. *Am J Respir Crit Care Med* 1994;149:295.

Pelosi P, D'Onofrio D, Chiumello D, et al. Pulmonary and extrapulmonary acute respiratory distress syndrome are different. *Eur Respir J* 2003;22:48s.

Randolph AG, Meert KL, O'Neil ME, et al. The feasibility of conducting clinical trials in infants and children with acute respiratory failure. *Am J Respir Crit Care Med* 2003;167:1334.

Rubenfeld GD. Epidemiology of acute lung injury. *Crit Care Med* 2003;31:s276.

The Acute Respiratory Distress Syndrome Network. Ventilation with lower tidal volume as compared with traditional tidal volumes for acute lung injury and the acute respiratory distress syndrome. *N Engl J Med* 2000;342:1301.

Timmons OD, Havens PL, Fackler JC, and the Pediatric Critical Care Study Group and the Extracorporeal Life Support Organization. Predicting death in pediatric patients with acute respiratory failure. *Chest* 1995;108:789.

Ware LB, Matthay MA. The acute respiratory distress syndrome. *N Engl J Med* 2000;342:1334.

CHAPTER 455 ■ ACUTE HEPATIC FAILURE

PENELOPE TERHUNE LOUIS

Acute hepatic failure is a clinical syndrome that occurs within weeks to a few months of the onset of liver disease in patients in whom liver function is presumed to have been normal before the illness. Acute hepatic failure is a rare but devastating event, with a mortality rate of 80% or higher. However, full recovery to normal hepatic structure and function is possible, even after massive injury. In view of this potential for full recovery, all patients with acute hepatic failure should receive intensive support.

Acute hepatic failure implies the occurrence of either acute massive destruction of liver tissue or other processes that cause rapid deterioration in function. Hepatic encephalopathy with hyperammonemia is necessary for establishing the diagnosis of acute hepatic failure, as is coagulopathy with prolongation of the prothrombin time (PT) and partial thromboplastin time (PTT).

EPIDEMIOLOGY

The cause of acute hepatic failure is age-dependent. Usually, acute liver failure in patients in the pediatric intensive care unit is associated with viral hepatitis, drugs, or toxins. Viral hepatitis accounts for more than 80% of cases of acute hepatic failure in children of all age groups. Acute hepatic failure in the neonate may result from infection with viruses that characteristically do not cause severe hepatitis in older patients. Herpes simplex virus (HSV) infections usually are associated with systemic symptoms. Cytomegalovirus (CMV) hepatitis does not cause acute hepatic failure in this age group but rather a chronic or chronic progressive hepatitis; it is usually associated with other systemic features. Epstein-Barr virus (EBV) rarely causes acute hepatic failure in neonates.

Excepting neonates and immunocompromised patients, most cases of viral hepatitis resulting in acute hepatic failure are the result of infection with hepatitis virus type A or B or sporadic non-A-G hepatitis. Acute hepatitis type A is a relatively frequently diagnosed cause of acute hepatic failure, but the risk of hepatic failure developing in patients symptomatic with hepatitis A virus is very low. The prevalence of acute hepatitis B infection in a large series of acute hepatic failure ranges from 25% to 75%, rendering it the leading cause, overall. Hepatitis B is an uncommon finding in pediatric series in places where hepatitis B virus is not endemic. The overall rate of hepatic failure in hepatitis B infection is estimated to be approximately 1%. Hepatitis C is a very unusual cause of acute hepatic failure. Hepatitis D virus infection can be acquired as a coinfection with hepatitis B virus or as superinfection in patients previously infected with hepatitis B. Hepatitis D virus infection probably plays little role in the etiology of acute hepatic failure in children. No cases of hepatitis E virus involving children have been reported from western Europe or the United States. Sporadic non-A-G hepatitis is diagnosed if the patient has evidence of acute hepatitis in the absence of markers for hepatitis virus infection and in the absence of clinical or serologic evidence of systemic infection with other viral agents. Non-A-G hepatitis causes very severe hepatitis. It is the most important cause of acute hepatic failure in children in developed countries, comprising the majority of pediatric acute hepatic failure cases. Non-A-G hepatitis rarely is seen outside the setting of acute hepatic failure. A high case fatality rate is characteristic of acute hepatic failure secondary to non-A-G hepatitis.

HSV, varicella-zoster virus, CMV, and EBV have been reported to cause acute hepatic failure, almost always in immunocompromised hosts.

Drug-induced fulminant hepatic failure may be related to toxic effects or may be immune-related. Hepatic necrosis is associated with the ingestion of acetaminophen, phenytoin, valproic acid, isoniazid, halothane, or carbon tetrachloride. In children, the three most common drugs that cause acute hepatic failure are acetaminophen, isoniazid, and propylthiouracil. Halothane toxicity is seen more frequently in adults, but it has been observed in children. A systemic hypersensitivity reaction characterized by fever, rash, arthralgias, and hepatocellular damage may result from treatment with sulfamethoxazole, sulfasalazine, carbamazepine, and phenytoin. The ingestion of toxic amounts of iron and vitamin A also may cause acute hepatic failure.

Children who present with hepatic failure may have end-stage chronic liver disease or previously undiagnosed liver disease. Patients with biliary atresia may have hepatic failure before or after undergoing portoenterostomy. Metabolic diseases, such as tyrosinemia, alpha$_1$-antitrypsin deficiency, Wolman disease, errors in fatty oxidation defects, Wilson disease, Niemann-Pick disease, hereditary fructose intolerance, and cystic fibrosis, may result in hepatic failure.

CLINICAL MANIFESTATIONS AND COMPLICATIONS

Mild to moderate nausea, anorexia, and fatigue occur commonly with acute hepatitis. The presence of protracted vomiting, altered behavior, bruisability, or ascites alerts clinicians that the case may be associated with acute hepatic failure. Other associated symptoms include jaundice, abdominal pain, fever, and rash. Throughout the course of the illness, the degree of neurologic deterioration is one of the most reliable means of assessing and following the severity of the hepatic failure.

Monitored liver function tests include measurements of liver enzymes, alkaline phosphatase, bilirubin, albumin, and PT. The liver enzymes become elevated with altered hepatocellular integrity. The absolute height of their elevation does not correlate with the severity of the disease. The pattern of change in liver enzyme levels with time can be useful in following the activity of the disease, as long as the liver still can produce the enzymes. The destruction of hepatocytes may be so rapid that the enzymes can fall precipitously as a premorbid event.

Alkaline phosphatase is produced in the bile canaliculus in response to increased pressure within the canaliculus. Thus, alkaline phosphatase of liver origin rises with any extrahepatic or intrahepatic obstruction to bile flow. An assay of 5'-nucleotidase may be useful to differentiate between bone and liver alkaline phosphatase.

Gamma-glutamyl transpeptidase, an enzyme distributed throughout the biliary tree, may be increased in biliary tract disease. It also is present in other organs, including the pancreas, seminal vesicles, lungs, kidneys, and heart.

Neither the liver enzymes nor alkaline phosphatase defines liver function as well as serum bilirubin, albumin, or PT. In the face of acute hepatic failure, the prolonged PT observed is more than 3 seconds beyond control and is not responsive to parenteral vitamin K. Often, the albumin level is less than 4 g/dL, despite the long half-life of this protein. Mixed hyperbilirubinemia is variable, with levels ranging from 15 to 40 mg/dL.

Hepatic Encephalopathy and Cerebral Edema

Hepatic encephalopathy is a multifactorial syndrome with symptoms ranging from drowsiness to coma. Elevated ammonia levels often (but not always) are found in patients with hepatic encephalopathy. The degree of ammonia elevation does not correlate with the severity of the encephalopathy. Therapeutic interventions that decrease ammonia levels, such as trapping ammonia in the gastrointestinal tract (with lactulose) or decreasing urea-producing gastrointestinal tract organisms (with lactulose and antibiotics), may be associated with some improvement in the encephalopathy. The mechanism by which ammonia may cause the encephalopathy is not understood. One theory is that ammonia converts to glutamine, a compound that blocks excitatory transmission. Ammonia also depresses cerebral blood flow and oxygen consumption. Cerebral edema is the apparent cause of death in 25% to 80% of patients with hepatic failure. As with the encephalopathy, the cause of cerebral edema is poorly understood.

Coagulopathy

By definition, an elevated PT is present in acute hepatic failure. This coagulopathy is the result of the inadequate synthesis of factors V, VII, and X. Patients with acute hepatic failure given a trial of vitamin K may show little or no change in the PT. Low-grade, disseminated intravascular coagulation; prolonged PT, PTT, and thrombin time; lowered fibrinogen and platelet counts; and the presence of fibrin split products variously are common in acute hepatic failure.

Gastrointestinal Bleeding

As many as 70% of patients with acute hepatic failure may experience gastrointestinal bleeding, and as many as 30% of those die from this complication. Bleeding is the result of stress gastritis and portal hypertension exacerbated by the coagulopathy of liver disease. The incidence of stress gastritis can be reduced by maintaining gastric pH levels at 4.5 or higher. Complications of portal hypertension include esophageal or gastric varices.

Renal Failure

Renal insufficiency complicates the course of children with acute hepatic failure. Oliguria poses a particular problem because of the fluid volume frequently needed to support these patients. These patients may require hemodialysis or hemofil-

tration. Few patients recover spontaneously, although renal function returns quickly to normal after successful liver transplantation has been performed. Therefore, renal failure has prognostic significance.

One complication of acute hepatic failure is an oliguric form of renal failure described as the *hepatorenal syndrome*. This condition is characterized by a urine sodium concentration of less than 20 mEq/L, normal urinary sediment, and reduced urinary output. The cause of the hepatorenal syndrome is unknown. Functionally, patients with acute hepatic failure behave as if they have depletion in the intravascular volume, rendering them particularly sensitive to any further decrease, such as that associated with septic shock, diuresis, or gastrointestinal hemorrhage. Any of these events can result in progressive renal failure in these patients. The kidney in such patients is histologically normal and can function normally when transplanted into another patient.

Electrolyte Imbalance

Profound alterations in serum sodium and potassium levels are common occurrences. Patients with acute hepatic failure may require large doses of intravenous potassium to maintain a normal serum level because of the kaliuresis associated with secondary hyperaldosteronism. Decreased serum sodium is noted because of an antidiuretic-like activity combined with increased total body sodium and fluid retention caused by a hyperaldosterone-like activity. Additionally, in some patients, a shift of sodium into intracellular compartments occurs. Profound hypoglycemia is found in as many as 40% of the children with acute hepatic failure. Severe hypoglycemia occurs because of the liver's impaired ability to store glycogen. Respiratory alkalosis also is a common phenomenon, occurring in the presence of central hyperventilation.

Infection

Fifty percent of children with acute hepatic failure have courses complicated by infection. The frequency of infection in patients with acute hepatic failure exceeds that observed in similarly ill patients in intensive care settings. Both the cellular and humoral immune systems are impaired in the patient with acute hepatic failure. Neutropenia is observed commonly, and neutrophil function may be affected. Opsonization is defective because of low plasma levels of complement and fibronectin. Gram-positive organisms, presumably of skin origin, are implicated most frequently in infections in these patients. Occasionally, infection in patients with liver disease consists of bacteremia from gastrointestinal tract organisms caused by poor hepatic clearing of these organisms seeded from the edematous bowel of portal hypertension, urinary tract infections, and aspiration pneumonia. Worsening encephalopathy, sudden development of hepatorenal syndrome, and new onset of fever and leukocytosis should raise suspicion of infection.

Respiratory Failure

Many reasons for respiratory failure and the need for respiratory support in fulminant hepatic failure exist. Neurologic dysfunction in hepatic coma may warrant intubation and mechanical ventilation, independent of respiratory failure. Encephalopathic changes produce an inappropriate secretion of antidiuretic hormone and potentiate the development of pulmonary edema. Hepatic failure has been implicated also in the production of respiratory failure through intrapulmonary shunting secondary to the effect of vasoactive substances normally metabolized by the liver.

cision to transplant in a child with acute hepatic failure is complex, with many factors to consider.

THERAPY

Initial, specific therapy for treatable conditions that cause hepatic failure must be instituted as rapidly as possible. Otherwise, the aim of therapy in patients with acute hepatic failure is to maintain cerebral, renal, cardiac, and pulmonary function until hepatic regeneration can occur. Basic maintenance includes monitoring, intravenous alimentation, respiratory support, control of cerebral edema, prevention of and intervention for hepatorenal syndrome, prevention of bleeding disorders (including gastrointestinal bleeding), and aggressive therapy during infectious complications.

Generally, attempting to correct the coagulopathy associated with fulminant hepatic failure is nonproductive. The exception is in the presence of active bleeding or in preparation for an invasive procedure.

The high rate of mortality for all cases of fulminant hepatic failure, despite the administration of intensive medical therapy, has led to the investigation of several methods and devices to support affected patients until hepatic function returns. Double-volume exchange transfusion, charcoal hemoperfusion, plasmapheresis, liver-assist devices containing cultured hepatocytes, and hemodialysis have been used to provide support until the liver recovers. These therapies have not been found to improve survival. At present, liver transplantation seems to provide the greatest life-saving potential, but the de-

Suggested Readings

Bhadieri BR, Mieli-Vergani G. Fulminant hepatic failure: pediatric aspects. *Semin Liver Dis* 1996;16:349.
Bismuth H, Samuel D, Gugenheim J, et al. Emergency liver transplantation for fulminant hepatitis. *Ann Intern Med* 1987;107:337.
Chapman RW, Forman D, Peto R, et al. Liver transplantation for acute hepatic failure? *Lancet* 1990;335:32.
Chowdhury JR, Chowdhury NR, Strom SC, et al. Human hepatocyte transplantation: gene therapy and more? *Pediatrics* 1998;102:647.
Clemmenson JO, Lasen FS, Kondup J, et al. Cerebral herniation in patients with acute liver failure is correlated with arterial ammonia concentration. *Hepatology* 1999;29:648.
Dedray D, Cullufi P, Devictor D, et al. Liver failure in children with hepatitis A. *Hepatology* 1997;26:1018.
Lee WM. Acute liver failure. *N Engl J Med* 1993;329:1862.
O'Brady JG, Alexander GJM, Hayllar KM, et al. Early indicators of prognosis in fulminant hepatic failure. *Gastroenterology* 1989;97:439.
Mackenjee MKR, Keipiela P, Cooper R, et al. Clinically important immunological processes in acute and fulminant hepatitis, mainly due to hepatitis B virus. *Arch Dis Child* 1982;57:277.
Nicolette L, Bilmire D, Faulkenstein K, et al. Transplantation for acute hepatic failure in children. *J Pediatr Surg* 1998;33:998.
Partin JC. Acute hepatic failure in children. *Pediatr Ann* 1985;14:446.
Pereira SP, Langley PG, Williams R. The management of abnormalities of hemostasis in acute liver failure. *Semin Liver Dis* 1996;16:403.
Psachanopolous HT, Mowat AP, Davies M, et al. Fulminant hepatic failure in childhood. *Arch Dis Child* 1980;55:252.
Riely CA. Acute hepatic failure in children. *Yale J Biol Med* 1984;57:161.
Whitington PF, Soriano HE, Alonso EM. Fulminant hepatic failure in children. In: Suchy FJ, Sokol RJ, Balistreri WF, eds. *Liver disease in children*. Philadelphia: Lippincott Williams & Wilkins, 2001:63.

CHAPTER 456 ■ ACUTE RENAL FAILURE

M. MICHELE MARISCALCO

Acute renal failure (ARF) is defined as an abrupt decline in the renal regulation of water, electrolytes, and acid-base balance of a magnitude sufficient to result in the retention of nitrogenous waste. Often, acute oliguria is the earliest sign of impaired renal function. Oliguria in adults is defined as an output of less than 400 mL of urine per day. In infants and children, oliguria is based on body size. Most sources use a urine volume of less than 0.5 mL per kilogram of body weight per hour in infants and urine volumes of less than 500 mL/m^2/day in children. The occurrence of nonoliguric renal failure in adults is recognized increasingly. It is thought to be secondary to the increased use of nephrotoxic drugs (in particular, aminoglycosides and nonsteroidal antiinflammatory agents), improved resuscitation, and the improved survival of trauma victims. The pediatric series reflect a very low incidence of nonoliguric renal failure, with most cases occurring in postoperative patients.

In the clinical setting, the terms acute renal failure (ARF) and acute tubular necrosis (ATN) are used interchangeably. ATN was described first during World War II as acute loss of kidney function that occurred in severely injured crush victims. Histologically, patchy necrosis of renal tubules was noted at autopsy. However, subsequent studies have demonstrated that tubular necrosis often is seen only in occasional tubule cells

and, in some cases, tubular necrosis is not demonstrated at all. What is clear is that the glomeruli are morphologically normal. In this chapter, ARF is differentiated from reversible vasoconstriction, such as occurs with prerenal azotemia or urinary obstruction (post renal azotemia). Here, ARF will include the entity of ATN, as it often is called in the clinics.

The process of ARF can be divided into three phases:

- Initiation phase. Ischemia or a toxin sets in motion a sequence of events that produces an injury to tubular epithelial cells, and glomerular filtration rate (GFR) declines.
- Maintenance phase. The GFR remains relatively low for several days or weeks, depending on the severity of the initiating insult.
- Recovery phase. Recovery is characterized by gradual and progressive restoration of GFR and tubule function.

During an acute renal injury, both renal vascular and tubular abnormalities occur. Increasing evidence indicates that inflammation also is involved in the pathogenesis of the decreased GFR. With ischemic injury and that due to sepsis, nephron autoregulation occurs. With ischemia, rather than the normal autoregulatory vasodilation that occurs as a result of decreased renal perfusion, autoregulation appears to be lost, and renal vasoconstriction occurs. Increased vasoconstrictor response to endogenous norepinephrine occurs. In adult patients with sepsis, renal arteriolar vasodilation occurs at a time when perfusion is compromised because of systemic vasodilation. The afferent arteriole may not be responsive to endogenous norepinephrine, leading to decreased transglomerular pressure and ischemia.

With ARF, tubular epithelial injury results in altered reabsorption of solute and water in the proximal nephron. In ARF, proximal tubule brush border membranes and epithelial tubule cells are shed and excreted into the urine, and this debris ultimately can obstruct the lumen. Concomitantly, a loss of tubular integrity occurs. Solute and fluid that should be retained within the tubule lumen leak back across the damaged membrane into the peritubular fluid and eventually into the plasma. The progressive necrosis of epithelial cells can result in the obstruction of some nephrons and the loss of tubular integrity in others. However, the "backleak" hypothesis can account for only about a 10% decrease in GFR in ARF. The other mechanisms for decreased GFR that result from tubular injury remain to be elucidated. Vasoactive compounds, such as the renin-angiotensin-aldosterone system, nitric oxide, vasodilatory prostaglandins, and adenosine, have been implicated as the mediators in this cycle.

EPIDEMIOLOGY

A relative paucity of published reports exists covering ARF in pediatrics. In work by Williams, encompassing the years 1989 to 1998, the age distribution of 125 children with ARF was 37%, younger than 1 year old; 20%, 2 to 4 years old; and 43%, 5 to 15 years old. The overall survival rate was 73%. Survival rates for the three age groups were 60%, 96%, and 80%, respectively. Forty-one percent of the patients received renal replacement therapies. In developing countries, the most common causes of ARF include hemolytic uremic syndrome (HUS, 31%), glomerulonephritis (23%), and postoperative sepsis and ischemic/prerenal events (18% each). In work by Williams from the United States, hemolytic-uremic syndrome (HUS) accounts for only 16% of cases of ARF. The other etiologies include heart surgery (18%), hematologic-oncologic complications (17%), sepsis (15%), ischemic/prerenal causes (5%), pulmonary (3%), and "others" (24%).

The most frequent cause of ARF in newborns is perinatal asphyxia, which results in underperfusion of the kidneys. Other causes in the newborn include hemorrhage, necrotizing enterocolitis, and increased insensible fluid loss through the skin, especially while under radiant warmers and during bilirubin phototherapy. Oliguria does not result from occlusion of the artery, the vein, or the ureter of a single kidney unless the contralateral kidney is absent or not functioning. Renal artery stenosis and renal vein thrombosis are rare findings in children, but they do occur in the newborn period. Usually, renal artery stenosis occurs as a complication of umbilical artery catheterization and presents with hypertension. Renal vein thrombosis should be suspected in neonates with hematuria, proteinuria, or an enlarging abdominal mass. An early ultrasonographic diagnosis is imperative in establishing this diagnosis and other causes of obstruction, such as bilateral ureteral obstruction or bladder outlet obstruction. One should rule out obstruction of these anatomic sites before considering other medical reasons for ARF.

ARF can be caused by renal or other intrinsic events, including small-vessel vasculitis or acute glomerulonephritis caused by connective-tissue disease, poststreptococcal glomerulonephritis, and rapidly progressive glomerulonephritis. Other causes include interstitial nephritis caused by drugs, infection,

or cancer. ARF may result from exposure to nephrotoxic antibiotics, heavy metals, solvents, radiographic contrast dyes, intratubular crystals (uric acid or oxalate), or intratubular pigments (hemoglobinuria or myoglobinuria).

HUS is defined by the presence of anemia (hemolysis), thrombocytopenia, and impaired renal function. The most common form has been associated with diarrheal prodromes, especially hemorrhagic colitis, caused by *Escherichia coli* (O157:H7). In the classic form of the disease, toxins are released by those infectious agents that cause glomerular endothelial damage. A thrombotic microangiopathy develops, with platelet aggregation and fibrin deposition in small vessels of the kidney but also in other sites such as the gastrointestinal tract and central nervous system. Other infectious agents (i.e., *Streptococcus pneumoniae*, *Shigella*, and *Salmonella*, human immunodeficiency virus [HIV]) also have been associated with the development of HUS.

Acute poststreptococcal glomerulonephritis and HUS also occur in adults. Thrombotic thrombocytopenic purpura is a syndrome with features similar to those of HUS. Thrombotic thrombocytopenic purpura occurs in adults to a greater extent than in children. Other clinical syndromes that occur in all ages, but more commonly in adults, include crescentic rapidly progressive glomerular nephritis, renal vasculitic diseases (polyarteritis nodosa, Wegener granulomatosis), and immune-mediated diseases (Goodpasture disease and systemic lupus erythematosus).

Drugs can induce kidney injury in all age groups. Several mechanisms of drug-induced injury have been described. The most common pattern is tubular toxicity, which occurs with many medications, including antibiotics, cisplatinum, certain anesthetics, and radiocontrast agents. Tubular injury may occur either via direct toxicity or via changes in intrarenal blood flow patterns. Acute tubulointerstitial nephritis is characterized by inflammation of the renal interstitium accompanied by interstitial edema and renal tubular injury. Although drugs often are associated with this type of nephritis, it also may be caused by infectious agents. The usual toxicity profile of a drug may be enhanced in critically ill patients because of the use of multiple, potentially nephrotoxic, medications in addition to hemodynamic insults.

Finally, oligoanuria may be the result of an anatomic obstruction of the kidneys. Unilateral obstruction rarely causes ARF unless only one kidney is present or the other kidney is diseased. Unrelieved obstruction results in changes in renal blood flow characteristics that ultimately redistribute blood flow from the outer to the inner cortex, with resultant relative ischemia of the renal medulla. Causes of urinary tract obstruction include tumors, cystic disease, calculi, prune belly syndrome, and neurogenic bladder.

DIAGNOSIS

The renal failure indices listed in Table 456.1 can be helpful in distinguishing between oliguric patients with decreased perfusion to the kidneys and those with intrinsic renal failure. Clinical conditions associated with a decreased effective intravascular volume in children include dehydration secondary to vomiting, diarrhea, or nasogastric drainage in addition to that caused by peripheral pooling of fluid from sepsis or third-spacing from acute abdominal processes. In such a clinical setting, repletion of the intravascular volume through appropriate fluid therapy results in an increased urine output. Occasionally, children with the nephrotic syndrome become oliguric because of a decreased circulating volume secondary to a reduced plasma oncotic pressure. Conversely, children with myocardial failure may have an adequate blood volume but diminished cardiac output, with a consequent decrease in their renal blood

TABLE 456.1

CLINICAL EVALUATION OF ACUTE RENAL FAILURE IN ADOLESCENTS, CHILDREN, AND NEONATES

	Prerenal (Hypovolemia or Decreased Perfusion)	Acute Renal Failure
U_{Na} (mEq/L)	<10 (<30 in neonate)	>50
$FE_{Na}\%^*$	<1 (<2.5 in preterm infants)	>2 (>2.5 in preterm infants)
U_{osm} (mOsm/L)	>500 (>400 in neonate)	<350 (<400 in neonate)
U/P_{osm}	>2 (>1.5 in neonate)	<1
BUN/Cr	>20	Progressive increases in both BUN and Cr

BUN, blood urea nitrogen; U, urea; p, plasma; Cr, creatinine; FE_{Na}, percent fractional excretion of sodium.
$^*FE_{Na}\% = (U/P)_{Na} \div (U/P)_{(Cr)} \times 100$.

flow. Therapy in such children is aimed at improving cardiac function.

Patients with intrinsic renal failure manifest an acute decrease in glomerular filtration rate, as reflected in a decrease in creatinine clearance and in paralysis of tubular function. Creatine clearance can be calculated using a timed urine collection, the time recommended being 24 hours. Creatine clearance also can be estimated using the Schwartz formula (Box 456.1). One should recognize that GFR that is either estimated or calculated from timed creatine clearance may lead to an overestimation of the GFR. In addition, this method is particularly problematic in neonates and young infants. The GFR changes with age, with a range of 40 to 65 mL/1.73m^2/minute in full term, newborn infants to 89 to 165 mL/1.73m^2/minute in children 2 to 12 years old.

In patients with ARF, the rate of blood urea nitrogen (BUN) change is not a specific index of the level of the GFR because it can be affected by a variety of factors, including catabolic rate, protein load, and medications. With diminished tubular function, the small volume of urine that is produced has a high level of urine sodium (usually greater than 50 mEq/L), and an elevated fractional excretion of sodium (greater than 2%) occurs. The urine is isotonic, as compared to plasma, with a urine osmolality of 280 to 300 mOsm/L and a urine–plasma osmolality of 0.8 to 1.2.

Nonoliguric ARF has been described in association with the use of nephrotoxic aminoglycoside antibiotics. The presentation is that of a gradual onset of nonoliguric renal failure that frequently is preceded by polyuria and decreased urine osmolality. In patients with nonoliguric renal failure, clinical studies show more normal urinary indices, a lower BUN, a higher measured GFR, fewer complications, and lower mortality rates.

THERAPY

Once the diagnosis of ARF is made, all aspects of patient care must be monitored closely. Survival and return of renal function in 1 to 3 weeks are likely to occur if affected patients do not die from the underlying disease process or develop infectious, metabolic, or hemorrhagic complications of ARF or its treatment. The basis of therapy is careful monitoring of fluid and electrolyte balances, nutritional management directed at preventing a catabolic state, and meticulous care to avoid the development of infections. The physiologic consequences of ARF include edema; pericarditis; electrolyte abnormalities, including acidosis, anemia, thrombocytopenia, coagulopathy, gastrointestinal bleeding, and poor nutrition; and sepsis.

The first step in caring for an oliguric patient is a careful assessment of volume status. Physical examination may reveal hypovolemia (dry mucous membranes, tachycardia, "tenting" of the skin) or volume overload (peripheral edema, rales, gallop rhythm, hypertension, liver enlargement). Chest radiography should be performed to evaluate for cardiomegaly, and an electrocardiogram (ECG) should be obtained if hyperkalemia is a concern. If no evidence of hypervolemia is present, a fluid challenge of 10 to 20 mL/kg of normal saline should be given. Central venous pressure catheters are invaluable in monitoring the adequacy of blood volume when it is in question. Neither diuretics nor vasopressors should be given until the adequacy of circulating volume has been ascertained.

No therapies have been identified specifically in reversing or preventing ARF. Although initial studies using a synthetic form of human atrial natriuretic peptide (h-ANP) were beneficial in both animal and human studies in reversing ARF, subsequent large trials in humans were negative. However, recently, in a trial using 50 ng/kg/minute of h-ANP, one quarter of the dose used in the previous studies, the rates of need for dialysis decreased by 75% and that of mortality by 50% in critically ill, postoperative cardiac patients. Until further studies are performed, however, the use of h-ANP remains experimental. The use of diuretics, such as furosemide, has been advocated to convert "oliguric" ARF to "polyuric" ARF. Although loop diuretics, such as furosemide, can and do function in this regard, no data establish that their use will alter the outcome of patients with renal failure; its use can though simplify fluid and nutritional management. The use of diuretics, however, may worsen the renal function, presumably by decreasing renal perfusion. Likewise, the use of low-dose dopamine (less than 5 μg/kg/minute) has been postulated as being "renal protective" in the intensive care unit (ICU) population. Subsequent

BOX 456.1

Creatinine Clearance Estimation Using Schwartz Formula

Creatinine clearance = k × height/serum creatinine.
  k = 0.45 (age younger than 2)
  k = 0.55 (2 to 13 years of age)
  k = 0.55 female; k = 0.7 for male (13 to 20 years of age)
Units:
  Creatinine clearance (mL/1.73m^2/minute)
  Height (cm)
  Serum creatinine (mg/dL)
Ranges:
  Age: 6 months to 20 years
  Height: 40 to 200 cm
  Serum creatinine: 0.22 to 9 mg/dL

studies have not supported these initial observations, and recent work suggests that low-dose dopamine in fact may be harmful in select patient groups. Thus, the mounting body of evidence is that the routine use of low-dose dopamine has little place in the treatment of patients in the ICU.

Despite these controversies, however, recommendations may be made. Of primary importance is the identification of patients at risk for developing iatrogenic renal failure, with rapid evaluation to rule out prerenal or postrenal causes of oliguria. Nephrotoxic drugs should be discontinued when possible. As reviewed earlier, a fluid challenge is appropriate if no evidence of volume overload is present. The use of diuretics, although controversial, clearly is indicated if a sign of volume overload is present. Data support the conversion from oliguric to nonoliguric renal failure with diuretic use. Diuretics *can* increase urine flow in human ischemic and nephrotoxic renal failure; however, increased urine flow is not the equivalent of *improved* renal function. The rapid intravenous administration of 0.5 g/kg of mannitol should result in a urine output of more than 0.5 mL/kg within 1 hour. Mannitol may cause hypervolemia and pulmonary edema in patients who cannot excrete it, so avoiding its use is best if any question of incipient volume overload or congestive heart failure occurs. Mannitol may be particularly useful in patients who have a risk or presence of ARF due to myoglobinuria and/or hemoglobinuria. Furosemide should be given in a dose of 1 mg/kg intravenously to adequately or overly hydrated patients. If no response occurs within 30 minutes, incrementally higher doses up to 10 mg/kg have been used, although the risk of developing ototoxicity increases dramatically. The use of these agents may have deleterious effects on renal blood flow and GFR if intravascular volume is inadequate. In critically ill patients, or those refractory to bolus doses, the use of continuous furosemide infusion results in increased diuresis, often requiring less drug than would be used if dosed intermittently. For continuous infusions, the initial dose is 3 to 4 mg/hour in adults and 0.05 to 0.1 mg/kg/hour in children.

In critically ill children with ARF or evidence of worsening renal function, it is imperative to ensure adequate perfusion to the kidney. In the past, after normovolemia was assured, the drug of first choice was dopamine. Dopamine has been used extensively in patients with "distributive" shock with hypotension (i.e., septic shock) and was thought to work as a pressor. However, recent work suggests that in patients with septic shock, dopamine's effect well may be primarily as an inotrope. In addition, norepinephrine at moderate doses with adequate volume resuscitation will increase vascular resistance and provide increased perfusion to the kidney, and it may in fact shorten the time to resuscitation, when compared with dopamine. If an inotrope is required to improve myocardial function, it is theoretically advantageous to add dobutamine, which has more selective beta-agonists effects, while avoiding the side effects of dopamine. Again, it is critical that any drug that has a pressor effect, such as norepinephrine, high-dose dopamine (greater than 10 μg/kg/minute), or vasopressin, be monitored closely because any additional vasoconstriction to the kidney in the face of inadequate perfusion will compromise renal function further.

Once renal failure occurs, conservative management should be followed. This includes normalizing intravascular volume, systemic blood pressure and renal blood flow, sodium and potassium levels, and acid–base balance; and minimizing the accumulation of nitrogenous wastes by restricting protein intake moderately while maximizing caloric intake. Prophylaxis for gastrointestinal bleeding should be initiated. Special care must be taken to preclude the development of infectious complications.

Strict attention given to physical examination, an accurate record of input and output, and daily weight and serum sodium determinations will maintain correct fluid balance. Fluid administration, both oral and parenteral, should be restricted to the sum of insensible losses (400 mL/m^2/day) plus measured urine output and any other losses (e.g., gastrointestinal, respiratory, evaporative loss secondary to burns). Hyponatremia can occur in patients with volume overload. If it does occur, management entails further fluid restriction. Hyponatremia also can be seen in patients who experience increased urinary sodium excretion and are in the diuretic phase of recovering ARF. In this case, sodium replacement is indicated.

Often, hyperkalemia is encountered in patients with ARF. Serum potassium does not reflect total body potassium content adequately because potassium may move into or out of cells in exchange for hydrogen ions. Therefore, serum potassium must be interpreted in the context of the affected patient's acid–base status. Hyperkalemia is a life-threatening complication of ARF, and it must be treated promptly to avoid cardiac toxicity. Electrocardiographic changes range from the mild (peaked T waves) to the ominous, including widened QRS complex and arrhythmias. Measures to decrease serum potassium levels rapidly include sodium bicarbonate, 1 to 2 mEq/kg given over the course of 15 to 30 minutes; glucose, 0.5 to 1.0 g/kg; insulin, 0.1 to 0.2 U/kg; and 10% calcium gluconate solution (0.5 mL/kg) given over the course of 5 to 10 minutes. These measures will drive potassium into the cells and will antagonize the effects of hyperkalemia, but they will not remove potassium from the body. Care must be taken not to induce hypoglycemia; thus, frequent checks of blood sugar levels are warranted. Sodium polystyrene sulfonate (Kayexalate) is an ion-exchange resin that reduces the total body burden of potassium by exchanging equal, milliequivalent amounts of sodium and potassium. The dose is 1 g/kg in 70% sorbitol by mouth or in 30% sorbitol by rectum. Dialysis may be necessary to control hyperkalemia. Continuous ECG monitoring and repeated glucose and potassium determinations should be performed as therapy proceeds.

A consequence of impaired renal function is the retention of hydrogen ions, sulfate, and phosphate, with the development of an increased anion gap metabolic acidosis. Usually, respiratory compensation is adequate, and no intervention is required. If acidosis is severe, contributing to the development of hyperkalemia, or if the affected patient's respiratory compensation is impaired, sodium bicarbonate can be given. Sodium bicarbonate is effective as a buffer only if the carbon dioxide produced can be removed by adequate ventilation. Also, the rapid correction of acidosis in affected patients, who often have hypocalcemia, limits the availability of ionized calcium and may induce tetany or seizures.

Frequently, hypertension is a complication in children with ARF. Hypertensive encephalopathy may present as headache, irritability, or seizures. Papilledema is not necessarily present in affected patients. Often, volume overload is an inciting event and must be addressed early in the management. Acutely, a rapid-onset, short-acting agent, such as labetalol, nitroprusside, or hydralazine, may be used. Diazoxide also may be used, but its availability may be limited, especially in the United States. Labetalol is an excellent first-line drug because it has a rapid onset of action. It can be given as a bolus in adolescents as 1 mg/kg (maximum 20 mg) over the course of 10 minutes initially, then repeated up to a dose of 40 to 80 mg every 10 minutes until 300 mg total is administered. Alternatively, in children or adolescents, administration can begin with a bolus of 0.2 to 1 mg/kg. Infusion is begun at 1 mg/kg/hour. The infusion rate is increased at 10 to 15 minute intervals until an effect is achieved. If no effect occurs at a dose of 2.5 mg/kg/hour, another agent should be chosen. Other agents that are useful include hydralazine, 0.1 to 0.2 mg/kg IV every 4 to 6 hours, and nifedipine by mouth or sublingual, 0.25 mg to 0.50 mg/kg.

Usually, children with ARF are catabolic. High rates of catabolism lead to an increased accumulation of potassium, phosphate, and urea and may necessitate the earlier initiation of dialysis. If calories are supplied, and the breakdown of endogenous proteins is spared, the need for dialysis may be delayed. One concern was that the administration of parenteral amino acids to patients with ARF worsens the degree of azotemia, but current data do not support this concern. No study performed to date has shown that hyperalimentation leads to an increase in rates of morbidity or mortality. Because of fluid restriction in affected patients, providing adequate calories without the use of parenteral hypertonic glucose, amino acids, and intralipids often is difficult. The protein requirements of such patients may range from 0.5 g/kg to 1.5 g/kg in the severely catabolic patient. Hypertonic glucose can be given relatively safely through central venous catheters. Such complications as sepsis, acidosis, and hyperglycemia may occur. Once affected patients no longer are oligoanuria or are on an artificial kidney, fluid administration may be liberalized, and nutritional management becomes easier and safer to maintain. Enteral alimentation should be initiated as soon as clinically feasible.

The six indications for dialysis are (a) volume overload with evidence of pulmonary edema or hypertension refractory to pharmacologic therapy; (b) hyperkalemia despite conservative measures; (c) severe persistent metabolic acidosis; (d) BUN exceeding 150, or lower if rising rapidly; (e) neurologic symptoms secondary to uremia or electrolyte imbalance; and (f) calcium–phosphorus imbalance (hypocalcemia with tetany or seizures in the presence of a high serum phosphate). During the last few years, in critically ill adult patients, it has become increasingly clear that: (a) ARF is an important independent risk factor for mortality; critically ill adults die *of*, not *with*, ARF as previously thought; and (b) the amount of dialysis used will determine outcome (i.e., those patients who have more dialysis do better than those with less). Whether this difference is due to improved fluid removal and/or the removal of metabolites or mediators of injury is unclear. Both peritoneal dialysis and intermittent hemodialysis have been used for many years in adults and children with ARF. However, these modes of therapy may be inadequate or may be impossible to initiate due to cardiovascular instability. Intermittent modes of administration render difficult the removal of extravascular fluid without causing further fluctuations in blood pressure. Effective peritoneal dialysis also requires an adequate cardiac output, which may not be present in these children. Peritoneal dialysis also can lead to respiratory embarrassment.

During the past years, a shift has occurred toward the increasing use of continuous renal replacement therapy (CRRT) in both adults and children. These modes include continuous arteriovenous hemofiltration (CAVH) and continuous venovenous hemofiltration (CVVH). Both CAVH and CVVH can be combined with dialysis for the removal of toxic metabolites. With increasingly sophisticated technology, children as small as 3 kg may successfully receive CRRT with CVVH dialysis. Use of CRRT in patients who are oligoanuria will permit the administration of drugs and nutrients without fear of causing fluid excess. In addition, these modes are characterized by ease of application and hemodynamic stability, so therapy may be instituted earlier in the clinical course. CAVH requires the insertion of arterial and venous catheters. The driving pressure supplied by the arterial bed provides the flow through the dialysis membrane. In CVVH, a two-lumen catheter is inserted into the venous system and, because of the absence of an artery-to-vein pressure gradient to drive the blood flow, these circuits require additional tubing to accommodate a blood pump that drives the blood across the dialysis membrane. With both CAVH and CVVH, fluid and electrolyte balances can be maintained because hemofiltration of plasma water can be replaced with sterile fluid and parenteral or enteral nutrition. Countercurrent dialysis can be added to either circuit to increase the clearance to control uremia, improve electrolyte and mineral imbalances, and treat inborn errors of metabolism. In some clinical situations, ultrafiltration without the replacement of fluid or dialysis may be desired and is known as *slow continuous ultrafiltration*. However, unrestrained ultrafiltration can result in rapid fluid removal and hypotension; therefore, ultrafiltration rate control is crucial. For this reason, slow continuous ultrafiltration seldom is used.

In most series of childhood ARF, the mortality rate is approximately 30%. The irreversible nature of the underlying disease, rather than the renal failure itself, has been suggested to be the cause. However, given the observations in critically ill adult patients, critically ill children also possibly may be dying because of ARF. Whether this is, indeed, the case and whether the early institution of extracorporeal kidney support will be beneficial remain to be determined.

Suggested Readings

Badr KF, Ichikawa I. Prerenal failure: a deleterious shift from renal compensation to decompensation. *N Engl J Med* 1988;319:623.

Chan JSM, Williams DM, Roth KS. Kidney failure in infants and children. *Ped Rev* 2002;23:47.

Debaveye YA, Van den Berghe GH. Is there still a place for dopamine in the modern intensive care unit? *Anesth Analg* 2004;98:461.

du Cheyron D. Atrial natriuretic peptide to prevent acute renal failure: old concept with new promise. *Crit Care Med* 2004;32:1421.

Goldstein SL. Overview of pediatric renal replacement therapy in acute renal failure. *Artif Organs* 2003;27:781.

Jones DP, Chesny RW, Friedman AL. Glomerular dysfunction and acute renal failure. In: Fuhrman BP, Zimmerman JJ, eds. *Pediatric critical care*. St. Louis: Mosby–Year Book, 1998;741.

Flynn JT. Causes, management approaches, and outcome of acute renal failure in children. *Curr Opin Pediatr* 1998;10:184.

Klahr S, Miller SB. Acute oliguria. *N Engl J Med* 1998;338:671.

Schrier RW, Wang W. Acute renal failure and sepsis. *N Engl J Med* 2004;351:159.

Schrier RW, Wang W, Poole B, Mitra A. Acute renal failure: definitions, diagnosis, pathogenesis and therapy. *J Clin Invest* 2004;114:5.

Schwartz GJ, Haycock GB, Edelmann CM Jr., Spitzer A. A simple estimate of glomerular filtration rate in children derived from body length and plasma creatinine. *Pediatrics* 1976;58:259.

Stewart CL, Barnett R. Acute renal failure in infants, children and adults. *Crit Care Clin* 1997;13:575.

Williams DM, Sreedhar SS, Mickell JJ, Chan JCM. Acute kidney failure: a pediatric experience over 20 years. *Arch Pediatr Adolesc Med* 2002;156:893.

CHAPTER 457 ■ HEMOLYTIC-UREMIC SYNDROME

RITA D. SHETH

The hemolytic-uremic syndrome (HUS), first described in 1955, is characterized by the triad of nephropathy, thrombocytopenia, and microangiopathic hemolytic anemia. HUS is a heterogeneous group of disorders that have a common end result. To differentiate the pathogenesis and clinical outcome, the following classification has been proposed (Fig. 457.1):

- *Typical or diarrhea-associated (D+ HUS):* This is the classic HUS syndrome that presents in infants or small children after a prodrome of bloody diarrhea. The most common infectious agent associated with D+ HUS is the verotoxin-producing strain of *Escherichia coli*. Other enterotoxin producing bacteria such as enteropathic *E. coli*, *Shigella*, or *Salmonella* also have been associated with D+ HUS. Neuraminidase-producing streptococcal infections also can be associated with a typical HUS picture in the absence of a diarrheal illness. In these cases, the prodrome is often a respiratory illness with *Streptococcus pneumoniae*.
- *Atypical or D− HUS:* This category includes those patients with HUS who usually are not associated with an infectious illness or prodrome, hence the absence of diarrhea (D−). The etiology of HUS in this category includes familial cases with genetic mutations.
- *Secondary:* Secondary HUS occurs secondary to drugs (calcineurin inhibitors, cytotoxic agents, antiplatelet agents, and oral contraceptives) or is associated with certain conditions (bone marrow transplantation, pregnancy, lupus, or the antiphospholipid syndrome).

D+ HUS

Epidemiology

D+ HUS is largely a disease of infants and children. The syndrome is endemic in Argentina, southern Africa, and the western United States. It has no predilection for either gender or ethnic background. Post diarrheal HUS occurs more frequently during warmer months. Epidemics of HUS have been associated with the contamination of a variety of food products. The summer disease incidence peak correlates with the higher incidence of positive enterohemorrhagic *E. coli* fecal cultures in cattle during the warmer months.

HUS associated with streptococcal infections is less common and occurs in younger children, typically after a respiratory illness, such as lobar pneumonia.

Pathogenesis

The inciting event is thought to be direct endothelial damage by toxins produced by the infectious organism (Fig. 457.2). These toxins are released in the gut, absorbed in the blood stream, and bind to neutrophil surfaces in the systemic circulation. These toxins then bind to those specific receptors (Gb3) found in high concentration in renal microvasculature endothelial cells, and the result is cellular damage and death. Verotoxins also induce the release of proinflammatory cytokines and procoagulant factors. Endothelial cell damage secondary to enterotoxins and proinflammatory cytokines causes a cascade of events that results in cell wall damage and the formation of platelet and fibrin clots in the small capillaries and arterioles of the kidney. Circulating red cells are deformed and fragmented, resulting in the microangiopathic hemolytic anemia seen in HUS. The ongoing formation of microthrombi in the damaged vessels results in platelet consumption and thrombocytopenia. The occlusion of the renal microvasculature with platelet and fibrin thrombi results in glomerular damage and renal failure.

In patients with *Streptococcus pneumoniae*–associated HUS, normally occurring Thomsen-Friedenreich antigens are exposed by streptococcal neuraminidase. These antigens bind with preformed IgM antibodies and cause subsequent erythrocyte, platelet, and endothelial injury, and thus begins the cascade of events leading to microangiopathic vascular injury.

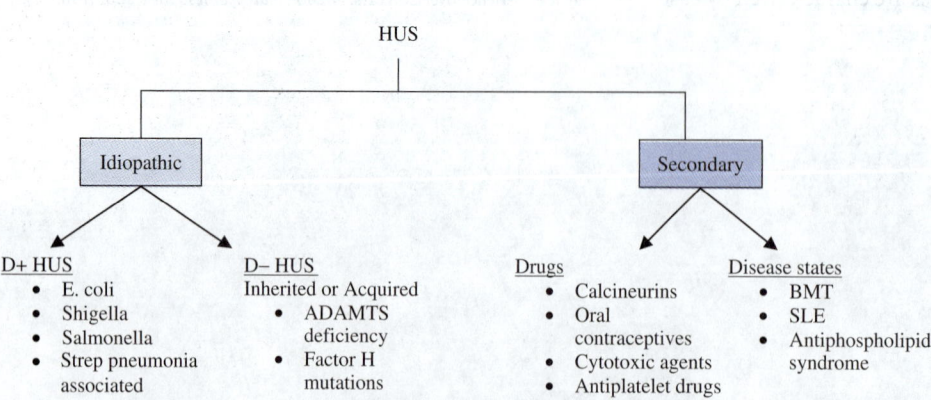

FIGURE 457.1. Classification of childhood HUS.

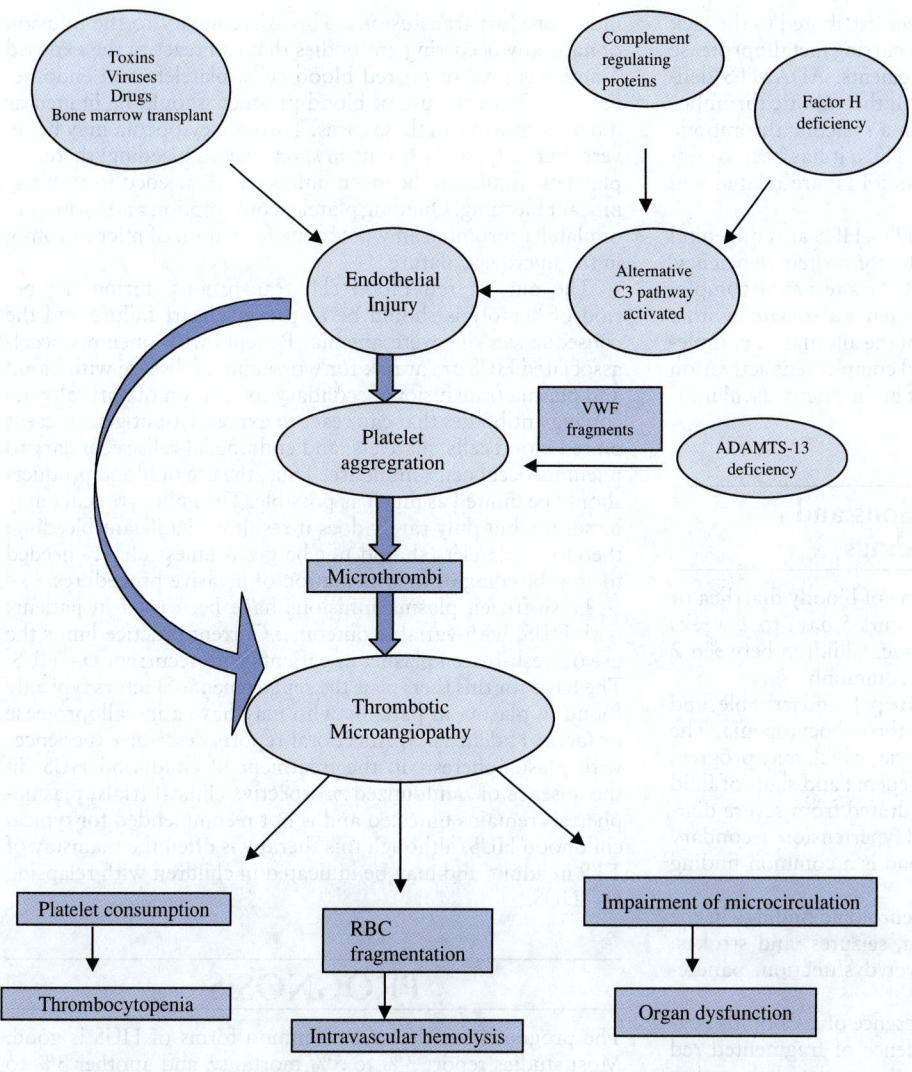

FIGURE 457.2. Schematic of HUS pathogenesis.

Pathology

The hallmark of HUS is the presence of small-vessel endothelial damage in the form of endothelial cell swelling, with an accumulation of fibrin-rich material in the vessel wall (thrombotic microangiopathy; Fig. 457.3). The lumen are occluded and filled with cellular debris, red blood cell fragments, and platelet thrombi. Glomerular changes are nonspecific and may show mild cellular proliferation, mesangial degeneration with mesangiolysis, fibrin deposition, and subsequent sclerosis if severe damage is present. Immunofluorescence usually is negative except for fibrin.

D—HUS

This more unusual presentation may present acutely with no prodromal illness or symptoms. It also may occur after an inciting event or in association with medication use. No gender or racial predisposition is noted. Rarely, a family history of similar conditions may be present. These patients often have a relapsing course, featuring multiple episodes of clinical HUS.

Pathogenesis

Although the hallmark of HUS is endothelial injury and platelet and fibrin formation, the inciting event in the cascade leading to HUS is different in this category of patients. In some patients,

a congenital or acquired condition that causes an inability to break down von Willebrand factor (vWF) multimers has been described. This pathologic abnormality results in large numbers of circulating vWF fragments with resultant platelet

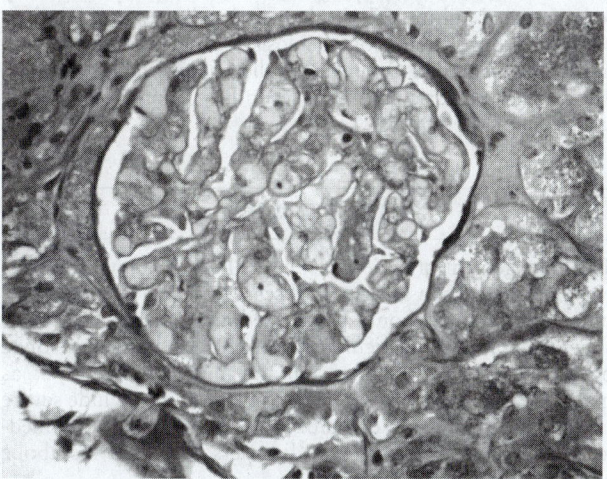

FIGURE 457.3. Fibrin deposition within the glomerular capillaries (pink homogenous material) and mesangiolysis due to ischemic injury characterize the histopathologic features of hemolytic uremic syndrome (PAS stain, original magnification 400×). (Courtesy of Dr. John Hicks, Department of Pathology, Baylor College of Medicine and Texas Children's Hospital.)

aggregation and clumping. This has been attributed to the lack of ADAMTS 13, which is a naturally occurring metalloprotease that normally breaks down vWF fragments. ADAMTS deficiency has been described in adults with thrombotic thrombocytopenic purpura (TTP), and result in a systemic thrombotic microangiopathy similar to D− HUS. Thus, it has been recognized that certain types of D− HUS and TTP are related and may represent a single disease entity.

Other abnormalities described with D− HUS are congenital or acquired factor H or membrane cofactor protein deficiency, both of which are proteins that regulate the alternative complement pathway. This type of D− HUS often is associated with a low C3 value. This altered regulation of the alternative complement cascade can result in uncontrolled complement activation and endothelial damage that can result in the microvascular injury seen in HUS.

Clinical Manifestations and Laboratory Findings

Typically, the syndrome has a prodrome of bloody diarrhea or a respiratory illness. The prodrome occurs 5 days to 2 weeks before the onset of the classic syndrome. Children between 2 months and 8 years are affected most commonly.

On presentation, affected children are pale and irritable, and they may have petechiae secondary to thrombocytopenia. The onset of renal failure manifests as oliguria, which may progress to anuria. Affected children may have edema and signs of fluid overload or may be significantly dehydrated from severe diarrhea, vomiting, or poor oral intake. Hypertension secondary to acute renal failure and fluid overload is a common finding in these children.

Extrarenal involvement includes neurologic findings in the form of irritability, altered sensorium, seizures, and strokes. Other organ involvement includes liver dysfunction, pancreatitis, or cardiac failure.

Laboratory findings include the presence of a Coombs negative hemolytic anemia with the evidence of fragmented red blood cells (schistocytes) on peripheral smear and thrombocytopenia. PT/PTT values usually are normal but may be prolonged with evidence of abnormal fibrin degradation products. Biochemical evaluation reveals findings consistent with uremia in the form of elevated blood urea nitrogen (BUN) and serum creatinine levels. Electrolyte abnormalities usually secondary to acute renal failure include abnormal sodium and potassium concentrations, a metabolic acidosis, and hypocalcemia with hyperphosphatemia. Other metabolic findings include an elevated LDH and uric acid level secondary to ongoing cell destruction and hemolysis.

THERAPY

The management of patients with D+ HUS is mainly supportive. Patients vary in severity of disease and clinical manifestations, and therapy should be directed accordingly. The mainstay of therapy is a meticulous control of fluid and electrolyte balance, control of hypertension and initiation of dialysis as needed. The indications for initiation of dialysis include severe uremia, volume overload and/or hyperkalemia and other medically unresponsive electrolyte disorders such as a metabolic acidosis or hypocalcemia.

Judicious use of red blood cell transfusions is advocated. The aim of red blood cell transfusions during *ongoing* hemolysis should be to prevent hypoxemia, cardiac dysfunction and the consequences of severe anemia. Patients with pneumococcal associated HUS are at risk for worsening of disease with blood product transfusions. This is secondary to the infusion of naturally occurring antibodies that can react to the exposed T-antigens present on red blood cells, platelets and endothelial cells. Thus the use of blood products should be limited as much as possible in these cases. Thrombocytopenia may be severe, but only rarely results in *spontaneous* bleeding; therefore platelets should not be given unless clearly needed to stop significant bleeding. Ongoing platelet consumption and formation of platelet thrombi can worsen the formation of microthrombi in the microvasculature.

The aim of red blood cell transfusions during the period of hemolysis should be to prevent heart failure and the consequences of severe anemia. Patients with pneumococcal-associated HUS are at risk for worsening of disease with blood and plasma transfusions secondary to infusion of naturally occurring antibodies that can react to exposed T-antigens present on red blood cells, platelets, and endothelial cells secondary to pneumococcal neuraminidase. Thus, the use of blood products should be limited as much as possible. Thrombocytopenia may be severe, but only rarely does it result in significant bleeding; therefore, platelets should not be given unless clearly needed to stop bleeding or in anticipation of invasive procedures.

Fresh-frozen plasma infusions have been used in patients with HUS, with variable outcome. Current practice limits the use of fresh-frozen plasma in patients with recurrent D− HUS. The basis for this therapy is the replacement of factors typically found in plasma in patients who may have a metalloprotease or factor H deficiency. Anecdotal reports describe experiences with plasmapheresis in the treatment of childhood HUS. In the absence of randomized prospective clinical trials, plasmapheresis remains untested and is not recommended for typical childhood HUS, although this therapy is often the mainstay of TTP in adults and may be indicated in children with relapsing D− HUS.

PROGNOSIS

The prognosis for the most common forms of HUS is good. Most studies report 3% to 5% mortality, and another 3% to 5% of patients experience chronic renal disease. The long-term follow-up of patients has reported a high incidence of long-term sequelae (proteinuria, hypertension, and renal insufficiency), especially in patients with severe HUS. Thus, the long-term monitoring of these patients is advisable. D− HUS may have a recurrent or relapsing form, often with a poor renal prognosis and progression to end-stage renal disease, as well as a risk for recurrence in a transplanted kidney.

Suggested Readings

Corrigan JJ, Boineau FG: Hemolytic-uremic syndrome. *Pediatr Rev* 2001;22:365.

Kaplan BS. Another step forward in our understanding of the hemolytic uremic syndromes: tying up some loose ends. *Pediatr Nephrol* 1995;9:30.

Kaplan BS, Ceary TG, Obrig TG. Recent advances in understanding the pathogenesis of HUS. *Pediatr Nephrol* 1990;4:276.

Liu J, Hutzler M, Li C, Pechet L. Thrombotic thrombocytopenic purpura (TTP) and hemolytic syndrome (HUS): the new thinking. *J Thromb Thrombol* 2001; 11:261.

Loirat C, Taylor MC. Hemolytic uremic syndromes. In: Avner ED, Harmon WE, Niaudet P, ed. *Pediatric nephrology*, 5th ed. Philadelphia: Lippincott Williams and Wilkins, 2004:887.

Moake JL. Mechanism of disease: thrombotic microangiopathies. *N Engl J Med* 2002;347:589.

Renaud C, Niaudet P, Gagnadoux MF, et al. Haemolytic uraemic syndrome: prognostic factors in children over 3 years of age. *Pediatr Nephrol* 1995;9:24.

Ruggenti P, Noris M, Remuzzi G. Thrombotic microangiopathy, hemolytic uremic syndrome, and thrombotic thrombocytopenia purpura. *Kidney Int* 2001;60:831.

Siegler RL. The hemolytic uremic syndrome. *Pediatr Clin North Am* 1995;42: 1505.

CHAPTER 458 ■ SYNDROME OF INAPPROPRIATE SECRETION OF ANTIDIURETIC HORMONE

ARUNDHATI S. KALE

Hyponatremia occurring as a result of the release of antidiuretic hormone (ADH) that is not attributable to osmolar- or baroreceptor-mediated stimuli is called the syndrome of inappropriate secretion of ADH (SIADH).

NORMAL PHYSIOLOGY

Normally, ADH is released from the posterior pituitary in response to changes in plasma osmolality and effective circulating blood volume. Serum osmolality is maintained in a very narrow range, with only a 1% to 2% change altering the secretion of ADH via the osmoreceptors, whereas a larger change in volume (approximately 10%) is needed to affect the carotid and left atrial stretch receptors to stimulate or inhibit ADH release.

PATHOGENESIS

The initial event leading to SIADH is ADH-induced water retention, leading to volume expansion and natriuresis. The mediator of natriuresis may be atrial natriuretic peptide (ANP), together with suppression of the renin-angiotensin-aldosterone system. The continued ingestion or infusion of fluids in the presence of persistent antidiuretic activity leads to dilutional hyponatremia. Excess water reabsorption decreases serum osmolality, causing water shifts into the intracellular fluid (ICF) and cell swelling (Fig. 458.1). No visible edema is apparent because of the expansion of both the intracellular and extracellular spaces. Patients with SIADH continue to drink fluids despite

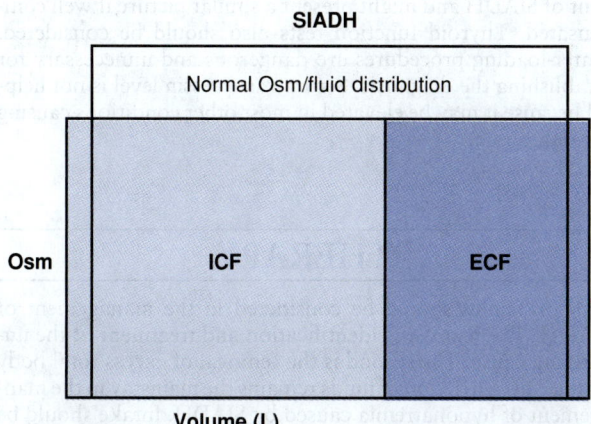

SIADH

Normal Osm/fluid distribution

Osm

ICF

ECF

Volume (L)

FIGURE 458.1. Excess water reabsorption causes ECF expansion and decreases serum osmolality, thus causing water shifts into the ICF and cell swelling.

the presence of hypotonic hyponatremia because the inhibitory effect of osmoregulated thirst is not sufficiently strong to halt drinking.

CLINICAL MANIFESTATIONS AND COMPLICATIONS

The physical findings in SIADH are related to the associated disease process. Despite mildly increased total body water, the formation of edema typically is not seen. Symptoms are related to the presence and duration of hyponatremia. Anorexia, nausea, changes in mental status, and convulsions are more likely to occur with the acute onset of a serum osmolality of less than 240 mOsm/kg H_2O and a serum sodium concentration of less than 120 mEq/L; the faster the rate of fall, and the lower the serum sodium concentration, the more severe the symptoms. Most patients will remain asymptomatic if serum sodium concentration is greater than 120 to 125 mEq/L over a long period of time (greater than 3 days).

Associated Disorders

In children, SIADH occurs most often in association with central nervous system (CNS) disorders. Laboratory evidence of SIADH was noted in almost 60% of children presenting with bacterial meningitis. ADH levels in patients with meningitis also were elevated significantly in comparison with normal and febrile controls. The duration and degree of hyponatremia was shown to correlate significantly with the subsequent development of seizures and subdural effusions. A leak of endogenous ADH across inflamed meninges has been suggested to explain these findings, but laboratory markers of inflammation did not show a correlation with arginine vasopressin (AVP) levels. SIADH occurs with other CNS infections, including brain abscesses and encephalitis, and with Rocky Mountain spotted fever, most likely secondary to the hypothalamic involvement from rickettsial vasculitis. Such CNS disturbances as head trauma, perinatal hypoxia, brain tumors, subarachnoid hemorrhage, anatomic defects, and Guillain-Barré syndrome may produce SIADH.

Intrathoracic disturbances are less common causes of SIADH in children. Pulmonary tuberculosis is well recognized, but viral, fungal, bacterial, and mycoplasma pneumonias also have been cited. Disorders that lead to decreased left atrial pressure, such as positive-pressure ventilation or pneumothoraces, can induce an excessive release of ADH by diminishing venous return. This condition is perceived inappropriately by stretch receptors as evidence of decreased circulating blood volume. Levels of ADH probably are elevated by a similar mechanism in status asthmaticus, leading one to reconsider the vigorous use of intravenous fluids often recommended in initial management.

TABLE 458.1

DISORDERS AND AGENTS ASSOCIATED WITH THE SYNDROME OF INAPPROPRIATE ANTIDIURETIC HORMONE SECRETION

Central Nervous System
Meningitis, encephalitis
Head trauma
Brain tumor
Hypoxia-ischemia
Guillain-Barré syndrome
Subarachnoid hemorrhage
Acute intermittent porphyria
Cavernous sinus thrombosis
Anatomic abnormalities
Vasculitis
Brain abscess
Hydrocephalus
Acute psychosis
Rocky Mountain spotted fever
Spinal fusion
Craniopharyngioma (triphasic postoperative response)

Drugs
Enhancement of antidiuretic hormone release
Morphine
Vincristine
Beta-adrenergic agonists
3,4-methylenedioxymethamphetamine (MDMA, Ecstasy)
Cyclophosphamide
Carbamazepine
Barbiturates
Halothane
Clofibrate
Nicotine
Phenothiazines

Adenine arabinoside
Potentiation of antidiuretic hormone action
Chlorpropamide
Indomethacin

Lung Disease
Tuberculosis
Viral, bacterial, fungal pneumonia
Mycoplasmal pneumonia
Empyema
Asthma
Pneumothorax
Cystic fibrosis
Positive-pressure ventilation
Positive end-expiratory pressure
Tumor

Neoplasia
Leukemia
Lymphoma
Sarcoma
Mesothelioma
Carcinoma of lung, pancreas, bladder

Miscellaneous
Pain
Stress (postoperative)
Nausea, vomiting
Bacterial endocarditis
Glucocorticoid deficiency
Severe hypothyroidism
Idiopathic

Many drugs have been implicated in the production of SIADH, acting either by increasing endogenous central release of ADH or by enhancing its renal tubular effects (Table 458.1). Frequently used agents include chemotherapeutic agents, morphine, beta-adrenergic agonists, and indomethacin. Reportedly, carbamazepine-induced SIADH was reversed by the concomitant use of phenytoin, which inhibits ADH secretion. Phenytoin may minimize SIADH, while treating seizures associated with CNS insult. Illicit drugs such as 3,4-methylenedioxymethamphetamine (MDMA, Ecstasy) also may have a similar effect.

Many other disorders can induce SIADH. The ectopic production of ADH may occur in adults with bronchogenic carcinoma, leukemia, and thymoma. Transient increases in the secretion of ADH also occur as part of the triphasic ADH response after the resection of craniopharyngiomas. The secretion of ADH caused by the effects of increased epinephrine release from pain or stress, nausea and vomiting, the use of morphine, or the surgical procedure itself may be excessive in the general postoperative setting; posterior spinal fusion for scoliosis is a common association. A syndrome of hyponatremia with water intoxication has been described in otherwise normal infants receiving dilute formula at home; levels of AVP that were increased inappropriately were found in some of these infants.

DIAGNOSIS

The diagnosis of SIADH is made by the following criteria: (a) low plasma sodium and osmolality, (b) urine osmolality in excess of plasma osmolality, (c) normal renal and adrenal function, (d) increased renal sodium excretion, and (e) absence of edema or volume depletion.

SIADH must be differentiated from the many clinical conditions that cause hyponatremia in children. A physical examination and the evaluation of simultaneous urine and serum sodium concentrations and osmolalities, urine specific gravity, and serum electrolytes will help to exclude such disorders as hyponatremic dehydration, congestive heart failure, and renal insufficiency. Serum cortisol levels may be considered if adrenal insufficiency is suspected; patients may demonstrate a component of SIADH and might present a similar picture if well compensated. Thyroid function tests also should be considered. Water-loading procedures are dangerous and unnecessary for establishing the diagnosis. Serum vasopressin level is not helpful because it may be elevated in most other conditions causing hyponatremia.

THERAPY

Two principles should be considered in the management of SIADH. The first is the identification and treatment of the underlying cause. The second is the removal of excess total body water. The restriction of fluids remains the mainstay in the management of hyponatremia caused by SIADH. Intake should be limited to insensible losses (400 to 800 mL/m²/day), with appropriate sodium content to allow the slow excretion of excess fluid to diminish extracellular volume and thus decrease the urinary excretion of sodium.

The management of fluids in patients with meningitis has undergone increasing scrutiny. Although SIADH may occur in this setting, many affected patients may be volume-depleted and may have associated hyponatremic dehydration. In a study by Powell et al., children with meningitis were assigned randomly to receive either fluids restriction (two-thirds maintenance) or maintenance fluid therapy, plus estimated deficit replacement during the initial 24 hours of therapy. Initially, plasma concentrations of AVP were elevated in both groups, but these concentrations returned to normal after 24 hours of therapy in those patients who received maintenance and deficit therapy; levels were unchanged in fluid-restricted patients. The reduction of ADH was presumed to be secondary to the correction of hypovolemia and sodium deficits. The restriction of fluids in an animal model of bacterial meningitis also produced decreased cerebral flow and increased cerebrospinal fluid lactic acidosis. Therefore, probably an appropriate approach is to give maintenance plus replacement fluids to patients with meningitis who initially do not demonstrate laboratory evidence of SIADH. Close monitoring of electrolytes should continue during the first 24 to 48 hours of therapy, and the presence of hyponatremia should prompt the evaluation of urine osmolality and sodium concentration to rule out SIADH.

Drugs have no established place in the management of SIADH. Scattered reports in the literature describe the use of antidiuretic antagonists known as *aquaretics*, which are still in different research study phases. Recently, a synthetic non-peptide antidiuretic antagonist has been shown to increase the excretion of solute free water in patients with SIADH. Lithium and demeclocycline may have an effect, but they are associated with significant toxicity, thus limiting their use in children.

Hypertonic (3%) saline infusion should be used only in patients whose hyponatremia has induced seizures or coma. Care should be taken not to increase the serum sodium concentration by more than 10 to 12 mEq/L/day, to avoid central pontine myelinolysis. The concomitant use of furosemide can act to increase the excretion of free water relative to the excretion of sodium and can diminish the volume expansion induced by hypertonic saline. The use of furosemide alone, with replacement of measured urine electrolyte losses, also has been suggested. Corticosteroids have been used in combination to increase sodium retention, but their use remains controversial.

Suggested Readings

Bartter FC, Schwartz WB. SIADH. *Am J Med* 1967;42:790.
Baylis PH. The syndrome of inappropriate antidiuretic hormone secretion. *Int J Biochem Cell Biol* 2003;35:1495.
Burrows FA, Shutack JG, Crone RK. Inappropriate secretion of ADH in a post-surgical pediatric population. *Crit Care Med* 1983;11:527.
David R, Ellis D, Gartner JC. Water intoxication in normal infants: role of ADH in pathogenesis. *Pediatrics* 1981;68:349.
Janicic N, Verbalis JG. Evaluation and Management of hypo-osmolality in hospitalized patients. *Endocrinol Metab Clin North Am* 2003;32:459.
Powell KR, Sugarman LI, Eskenazi AE, et al. Normalization of plasma AVP concentrations when children with meningitis are given maintenance plus replacement fluid therapy. *J Pediatr* 1990;117:515.
Rascher W, Tulassay T, Lang RE. Atrial natriuretic peptide in plasma of volume-overloaded children with chronic renal failure. *Lancet* 1985;2:303.
Saito T, Ishikawa SE, Abe K, et al. Acute aquaresis by the non-peptide vasopressin antagonist OPC-31260 improves hyponatremia in patients with SIADH. *J Clin Endocrinol Metabol* 1997;82:1054.
Trachtman H. Sodium and water homeostasis. *Pediatr Clin North Am* 1995;42:1343.
Tureen JH, Tauber MG, Sande MA. Effect of hydration status on cerebral blood flow and CSF lactic acidosis in rabbits with experimental meningitis. *J Clin Invest* 1992;89:947.

CHAPTER 459 ■ CARE OF CHILDREN WITH SOLID-ORGAN TRANSPLANTS

WILLIAM F. BALISTRERI, THOMAS R. WELCH, AND STEPHEN R. DANIELS

Isolated attempts at transplanting kidneys were undertaken more than 100 years ago, but the modern era of solid-organ transplantation began with the recognition, in the middle of the twentieth century, that the immune system could be modified pharmacologically. Parallel advances in surgical techniques and drug development have rendered possible the routine offering of renal, cardiac, hepatic, and small-bowel replacement in children. In most cases, significant rehabilitation and a high quality of life are realistic goals. With thousands of children and adolescents now living with transplanted organs, most primary-care physicians are likely to have contact with such patients. As the interval from transplant lengthens, more and more routine care is directed by generalists.

GENERAL CARE

Despite the nuances particular to specific organs, all children with solid-organ transplants present common issues. These issues should be kept in mind when providing well-child or acute-illness care.

Infections and Immunizations

Ideally, immunizations should be completed *before* transplantation. Although the response may be attenuated in the immune-suppressed transplant recipient, most transplantation centers recommend the usual schedule of age-appropriate immunizations after stabilization, with some important modifications. In general, live-virus vaccines (e.g., measles-mumps-rubella) are withheld, although some transplant physicians are using the varicella vaccine in susceptible children. Annual influenza immunization should be provided.

The two-edged sword of immunosuppressive therapy renders organ transplantation possible but subjects recipients to an increased risk of acquiring serious infection. In the first months after operation, the management of febrile illness in transplant recipients is complex and, therefore, always within the province of the transplantation center. Gradually, however, the intensity of immunosuppression is decreased, and the likelihood of overwhelming opportunistic infection is diminished.

In the assessment of an acute febrile illness in children who received a solid-organ transplant more than 3 years previously, the differential diagnosis is weighted heavily toward the common diseases of childhood. The primary-care physician must be aware, however, of concerns specific to individual patients. Urosepsis, for example, is a consideration in a kidney transplant recipient who had undergone lower urinary tract reconstruction. Children with a surgical or functional splenectomy are at risk for infection with encapsulated organisms. Some heart recipients may be susceptible to bacterial endocarditis, and liver recipients are at risk for biliary tract infection. These infections are often a reflection of underlying problems, such as graft rejection or anatomic issues. In the absence of such established risk factors or evidence of bacterial infection, empiric antibiotic therapy rarely is recommended.

Growth

As with any children with chronic disease, transplant recipients may be at risk for significant growth delay. Early on, this deficiency may be a consequence of the disorder that necessitated the transplant. After transplantation, growth failure may represent the residue of original disease, graft dysfunction, malnutrition, the complications of drug therapy (e.g., corticosteroids), or behavioral issues.

Primary physicians should monitor statural and ponderal growth very carefully. An alteration in growth velocity, if confirmed, should prompt careful dietary analysis and contact with the transplantation center.

Some children may display excessive weight gain after transplantation. Although this response probably is multifactorial, corticosteroid therapy, increased caloric intake, and low physical activity variously are likely to be operative. Although dietary counseling is provided in the transplantation center, involved primary physicians may wish to identify local resources for dealing with this troublesome issue.

Development and School Problems

Especially when end-stage kidney, heart, or liver disease has its onset in the first year of life, developmental delay and subsequent school difficulties are very common. Local resources, such as early intervention programs, should be identified, and early referral should be effected. Local physicians can be very helpful in facilitating the school entry (or reentry) of children with organ transplants.

Complications of Drug Therapy

Today, most children with organ transplants will receive two or three different immunosuppressive drugs as maintenance therapy. Many of these agents have the potential for serious interactions with commonly prescribed agents. A review of prescribing decisions with the affected child's transplantation center always is prudent.

Immunosuppressive agents also have the potential of inducing a variety of side effects. Some (hirsutism, acne, gum hypertrophy, weight gain) are largely cosmetic but may be troubling enough to compromise medication compliance. Other complications are potentially life-threatening and include hyperten-

sion, renal or hepatic dysfunction, glucose intolerance, cytopenias, and neurologic complaints. The possibility of drug effect must be entertained whenever a new complaint or finding occurs in children with an organ transplant.

Finally, noncompliance with immunosuppressive agents can result in accelerated graft loss, even years after transplantation. The primary-care physician should assess and reinforce medication compliance at every visit. For this to be effective, of course, communication between the transplant center and primary physician must be current with respect to medication regimens.

Pregnancy and Contraception

With well-functioning allografts, pituitary–ovarian function usually is normal, and pregnancy is possible. Sizable numbers of solid-organ transplant recipients have completed uneventful pregnancies. Thus, counseling with regard to issues of sexuality and contraception is as appropriate for the transplant recipient as for any similarly aged adolescent. Specific transplantation centers vary in their contraception recommendations, so contact with the transplant physician is critical.

Pregnancies do present very complex management issues. They are high-risk and should be supervised from the outset by a perinatal center with a close relationship to the transplant program.

Neoplasia

Although the introduction of more potent immunosuppressive drugs definitely has improved the success of solid-organ transplantation, another problem has emerged. Transplanted patients have a life-long increased risk of a variety of malignancies. In some situations, these cancers are biologically indistinguishable from those occurring in patients without transplants. In others, the tumors are unique to those with immunosuppression. Of the latter, a lymphoproliferative syndrome associated with Epstein-Barr virus infection is the most important; the features of the syndrome are summarized in Box 459.1. The possibility of occult malignancy must be kept in mind when investigating any enigmatic new complaint in a child with a solid-organ transplant.

Skin cancer, ranging from squamous or basal cell carcinomas to melanomas, are actually the most common tumors occurring in transplant recipients. As for any child, careful prevention of sun exposure through the use of clothing and sunscreen is a vital component of care.

BOX 459.1

Presenting Symptoms of Epstein-Barr Virus–Related Posttransplantation Lymphoproliferative Disorder

Fever, diarrhea
Headache, visual disturbance, seizures
Lymphadenopathy; tonsillar and adenoidal hypertrophy
Hepatosplenomegaly
Infiltrate on chest radiograph
Abdominal pain, gastrointestinal ulceration/bowel perforation, gastrointestinal bleeding

KIDNEY TRANSPLANTATION

Nearly 1,000 pediatric kidney transplantations are performed annually in the United States. In adults, the majority of grafts are undertaken because of acquired nephropathies, such as that seen with diabetes mellitus. On the other hand, congenital disorders account for approximately one-half of pediatric end-stage renal disease. This difference raises some very specific management issues for the generalist.

Renal failure with onset in early infancy, for example, may have irreversible long-term effects on cognitive and motor developmental attainments. Whether this outcome is a function of prolonged hospitalization at a critical period, central nervous system development in the uremic milieu, or other unrecognized factors currently is not clear. Regardless of specific etiology, affected children are at an extraordinarily high risk for developmental delay.

Associated features of the disorder resulting in the need for kidney transplantation may develop and may evolve despite excellent graft function. For example, successful kidney transplantation corrects the otherwise terminal uremia of cystinosis. The operation does nothing to correct the sequelae of cystine deposits in the rest of the body: hypothyroidism, myopathy, corneal injury, and the like. Similarly, transplantation for autosomal recessive polycystic kidney disease does not alter the course of the associated congenital hepatic fibrosis.

Transplanted kidneys do not have unlimited survival, and a recipient may receive several in the course of a lifetime. In the intervals between transplantations, occasional returns to dialysis are not uncommon. Importantly, physicians should try to minimize procedures that could compromise later dialysis access. Catheterization of the great vessels, for example, may complicate later use of the upper extremity for hemodialysis.

The glomerular filtration rate in many children with kidney transplants, even those with apparently normal serum creatinine concentration, frequently is impaired. This must be considered in prescribing any drug the excretion of which is predominantly renal. Even with a graft exhibiting seemingly excellent function, the renal reserve probably never is normal. Therefore, the important precaution is to avoid any interventions that could compromise renal function further. The routine use of nonsteroidal antiinflammatory drugs for fever and pain control, for example, may not be wise in children with kidney transplants.

LIVER TRANSPLANTATION

The most important factor determining survival is the severity of illness at the time of transplantation. Posttransplantation survival rates for infants are lower than those reported for older children or adults. Infants younger than 1 year or weighing less than 10 kg have reported survival rates of 65% to 88% overall; however, these rates improve yearly as the field advances. The use of reduced-size liver allograft and living donors are the most significant factors contributing to this improved survival. A major challenge is the high frequency of viral disease in children, especially cytomegalovirus and Epstein-Barr virus disease.

Variously, hepatic synthetic function, gastrointestinal tract absorption, and appetite improve after successful pediatric liver transplantation. Despite these improvements, growth disturbances do not resolve immediately. Most children have significant pretransplantation growth abnormalities, placing them below the median for height and weight. In the first year after transplantation, very little catch-up growth occurs. The etiol-

---

BOX 459.2   **Presenting Symptoms and Signs of Rejection**

Kidney
Fever, irritability, and graft pain and tenderness
Elevation in serum creatinine
Sudden change in urine output
Development of new abnormalities on urinalysis
    (e.g., proteinuria)

Liver
Fever, elevated white blood cell count
Anorexia
Jaundice (late)
Elevated serum levels of aminotransferases

Heart
Irritability, fever, malaise, and poor feeding
Symptoms and signs of congestive heart failure, including
    dyspnea, tachypnea, diaphoresis, rales, hepatomegaly
Increased heart rate or new arrhythmias (usually atrial
    arrhythmia)

---

ogy of the growth disturbance is multifactorial. A reduction in steroid dosage is the key element in management.

Rejection is an ongoing concern (Box 459.2), thus periodic monitoring via the measurement of serum levels of aspartate aminotransferase (AST), alanine aminotransferase (ALT), and gamma-glutamyltransferase (GGT) is required. Similarly, the monitoring of immunosuppressive drug levels is the only way to ensure adequate protection against both rejection and drug toxicity. As the survival rates after liver transplantation in children have increased, health care providers have begun to measure the overall health status of liver transplant recipients as a complement to traditional measures of medical outcomes. The overriding objective of hepatic transplantation in children is complete rehabilitation with improved quality of life. Factors contributing to the attainment of this goal include improved nutritional status, with appropriate growth and development, and enhanced motor and cognitive skills, allowing social reintegration.

Many infants with chronic liver disease have significant developmental delay (especially motor skills) before transplantation, owing in part to malnutrition and prolonged hospitalization; usually, this condition is reversed after transplantation. However, the long-term impact of liver transplantation on the psychosocial and financial health of the entire family unit is the subject of much concern. Compliance, especially in adolescent patients, is a major problem. In long-term pediatric liver transplantation survivors, in-depth, multicenter, longitudinal studies will be necessary to clarify the issues.

HEART TRANSPLANTATION

Since the early 1980s, survival after heart transplantation has improved markedly. A number of reasons are posited for this finding, including better donor organ preservation and improved immunosuppressive management. At present, approximately 400 pediatric heart transplantation procedures are performed each year in the United States. Pediatric patients with severe, uncontrollable heart failure from a variety of causes may be candidates for heart transplantation. Overall survival rates are better that 75% at 1 year and over 50% at 10 years.

Like the care of other pediatric posttransplantation patients, the care of children after cardiac transplantation is a team effort including primary-care pediatricians, pediatric cardiologists, cardiac surgeons, and others with expertise in immunosuppression, infectious disease, nephrology, and oncology.

Many issues after heart transplantation are common to patients with other types of solid-organ transplants. However, the recognition of certain differences is important for the primary-care physician.

All children and adolescents undergo frequent clinical evaluations after cardiac transplantation. This assessment usually includes physical examination and noninvasive testing using electrocardiography and echocardiography. Much research has been accomplished in an attempt to identify noninvasive approaches for recognizing rejection. However, the endomyocardial biopsy remains the most accurate method for determining whether rejection is present. For this reason, routine surveillance endomyocardial biopsies are performed frequently in the first year after transplantation and less often during subsequent follow-up. Transplantation centers differ in their frequency and timing of surveillance endomyocardial biopsy and echocardiography. Biopsy is usually performed to confirm clinically suspected rejection.

The clinical diagnosis of rejection can be difficult, because the signs may be subtle and nonspecific (see Box 459.2). Laboratory tests that may be helpful include chest radiography, which may show increased heart size and pulmonary edema; electrocardiography, which may show a reduction in voltage, a change in the QRS axis, or arrhythmias; echocardiography, which may show diminished function, increased chamber size, effusion or increased wall thickness; and cardiac muscle enzyme level determinations, which may be elevated.

The major morbidities following heart transplantation include rejection, infection, renal dysfunction, diabetes, hypertension, hyperlipidemia, and coronary vasculopathy. A unique form of coronary artery disease may develop in the transplanted heart, and this is a leading cause of death after the first year following transplantation. The mechanism of this disease is not well understood. One component appears to be immunologic and may represent a form of chronic rejection. Other nonimmunologic factors also influence the development of posttransplantation coronary artery disease, including dyslipidemia, infection, and the use of corticosteroid medication.

The most difficult problem in posttransplantation coronary artery disease is the difficulty in detecting its presence and severity. For some patients, the first and only sign may be sudden death. The diagnosis of coronary artery disease can be made using coronary angiography, intracoronary ultrasonography, and dobutamine stress echocardiography.

Augmented immunosuppression, vigorous lipid-lowering therapy, and antiinflammatory therapy may provide some improvement in patients with coronary artery disease in the transplanted heart. Patients with coronary artery disease in the transplanted heart may require retransplantation.

SUMMARY

The involvement of primary-care physicians is instrumental in the care of children after solid-organ transplantation. Such involvement is predicated on comprehensive, bidirectional communication between the involved physicians and transplantation centers. Frequently, transplantation centers provide guidelines to primary physicians to aid this communication (Box 459.3). Finally, physicians caring for children who have

| BOX 459.3 | Issues Prompting Consultation with the Transplantation Center |

Fever: Temperature higher than 38.5°C for more than 24 hours without obvious explanation; fever associated with abdominal pain, headache, or other neurologic complaints

Medication: Addition of any new prescription or over-the-counter medication not previously discussed with the transplantation center

Hypertension: Systolic or diastolic blood pressure consistently above the 95th percentile for age, unless already known by the transplantation center

Neurologic: Atypical headaches, visual disturbances, seizures

Respiratory: Persistent cough, abnormal chest roentgenogram, respiratory distress

Gastrointestinal: Diarrhea for more than 24 hours, vomiting for more than 12 hours, gastrointestinal bleeding, severe persistent abnormal pain

Liver function: Any acute change in liver function tests

Renal function: Any acute change in serum creatinine or electrolytes

Hematologic: Persistent leukopenia or unexplained leukocytosis

Surgery: Before *any* elective surgery, including dental procedures; as soon as possible or before or after emergency surgery

Other: Any time questions arise

Adapted with permission from Shaw B, Stratto R, Donovan E, et al. Care after liver transplantation. *Semin Liver Dis* 1989;9: 225.

undergone successful organ transplantation are in a strong position to promote organ donation.

Suggested Readings

Alonso EM, Neighbors K, Mattson C, et al. Functional outcomes of pediatric liver transplantation. *J Pediatr Gastroenterol Nutr* 2003;37:155.

Bereket G, Fine RN. Pediatric renal transplantation. *Pediatr Clin North Am* 1995;42:1603.

Boucek MM, Edwards LB, Keck BM, et al. The Registry of the International Society for Heart and Lung Transplantation: Fifth Official Pediatric Report 2001–2002. *J Heart Lung Transplant* 2002;21:827.

Bucuvalas JC, Britto M, Krug S, et al. Health-related quality of life in pediatric liver transplant recipients: a single-center study. *Liver Transpl* 2003;9:62.

Chinnock RE, Pearce FB. Pediatric Heart Transplantation. In: Kirklin JK, Young JB, McGriffin DC, eds. *Heart transplantations*. New York: Churchill Livingston, 2002:717.

Fishman JA, Rubin RH. Medical progress: infection in organ-transplant recipients. *N Engl J Med* 1998;338:1741.

Guthery SL, Heubi JE, Bucuvalas JC, et al. Determination of risk factors for Epstein-Barr virus-associated posttransplant lymphoproliferative disorder in pediatric liver transplant recipients using objective case ascertainment. *Transplantation* 2003;75:987.

Guthery SL, Pohl JF, Bucuvalas JC, et al. Bone mineral density in long-term survivors following pediatric liver transplantation. *Liver Transpl* 2003;9:365.

Whitington PF, Balistreri WF. Liver transplantation in pediatrics: indications, contraindications, and pre-transplant management. *J Pediatr* 1991;118:169.

CHAPTER 460 ■ MULTIPLE TRAUMA

M. MICHELE MARISCALCO

As therapeutic measures for patients with congenital anomalies and serious infections have become increasingly successful, trauma has become the leading cause of death and disability during childhood and adolescence. In 2001, 22,000 children and adolescents (age 1 to 21 years) died from traumatic injury. Traumatic injury accounts for 57% of all deaths in children aged 1 to 4 years and 81% of all deaths in children aged 5 to 21. In infants, deaths from injury are due to child abuse, suffocation, choking, motor vehicle accidents, and fires. For the preschool-age group, fires, drowning, and motor vehicle accidents are the leading causes, whereas cycling and pedestrian injuries become more common among school-aged children. Motor vehicle injuries, suicide, and homicide become the leading causes of death during the adolescent years. Each year, an estimated 300,000 children are hospitalized for the treatment of injuries in the United States, and 16 million are treated in emergency departments.

Because the causes of injury in children differ from those in adults, reflecting the differences in activities, size, and intellectual maturity, the patterns of injury in children also differ from those in adults. Head trauma occurs in 80% or more of severely injured children. Abdominal injuries occur more frequently because poorly developed abdominal muscles offer little protection to the viscera. Both the spleen and the duodenum are more likely to be injured. Elasticity of the chest wall renders rib and sternal fractures rare events but also permits severe crush injuries of the heart and lungs without apparent deformation of the chest wall.

PHYSIOLOGY OF TRAUMA

Restoring and preserving adequate tissue perfusion and oxygenation is the highest priority in the care of the injured patient. Although, as in all cases of hypoperfusion, the restoration of blood pressure, urine output, and heart rate are adequate endpoints, as many as 85% of patients may have continued evidence of poor tissue perfusion. However, in the era of nonoperative management of solid organ injuries, concerns regarding the "overexpansion" of circulating volume, which could lead to excessive bleeding and "blowing the clot," render resuscitation end-points even more critical. No perfect end-point exists; however, many clinicians use base deficits and serum lactate levels as indicators of ongoing tissue perfusion deficits. Clinicians familiar with the injured, multiple-trauma victim recognize that the combination of a cool patient, bleeding from multiple sites, and metabolic acidosis represents the "triad of death."

Blunt trauma accounts for 80% to 90% of pediatric trauma. It differs from other forms of injury in that multiple organ injuries are common findings, as is occult head injury. Progressive organ damage occurs frequently in blunt trauma because of continuing hemorrhage or the formation of edema. Often, acidosis and hypoxia are more prominent than is the dysfunction from the primary injury.

Children's physiologic responses also differ from those of adults. The vascular system can compensate for a greater loss of blood volume (20% to 25%) before hypotension occurs, but tachycardia presents earlier than in adults. The maintenance of normal blood pressure masks impaired tissue perfusion and may lead to a delay in providing treatment. Young children become hypothermic easily, which greatly increases the difficulty of resuscitation. Because children are growing organisms, uncorrected injury may lead to progressive deformity and disability.

PREHOSPITAL CARE

The treatment of multiple trauma begins at the scene, rendered by prehospital attendants. A fundamental difference between the medical delivery and surgical delivery of prehospital emergency care exists. In medical prehospital care, in which the vast majority of patients are adults with cardiac dysfunction, the working premise is to take time to stabilize affected patients and to achieve a stable rhythm, then slowly transport the patient to the hospital. For trauma patients, the definitive management is available only in the hospital. Once the airway is stabilized, such patients are ventilated adequately; patients should be transported to the hospital as soon as possible after bony injuries are stabilized.

In children, the concept of stabilization should be confined to airway control and immobilization of the cervical spine and long bones. Control of hemorrhage can be obtained by primary pressure. Peripheral intravenous access is the preferred route but may be technically difficult in children. Intraosseous infusion is technically easy and safe to perform and is recommended in children younger than 8 years old, although it may be used in older children and adults. Once vascular access is established, care must be taken to avoid the overtransfusion of crystalloid. Transport must not be delayed while vascular access is established in pediatric trauma patients. Notable is the paradigm shift from treatment with intravenous fluids *before* control of hemorrhage to treatment only *after* hemorrhage has been managed. A large clinical trial of hypotensive patients with penetrating trauma demonstrated that delayed resuscitation (i.e., only on arrival to the operating room) improved outcome, when compared to immediate resuscitation preoperatively. Importantly, these studies involved adult patients with penetrating injuries. The role for this scheme in blunt trauma patients is not as clear. Because children predominantly have blunt traumatic injuries, the relevance of these paradigms to children with trauma remains unproven.

PRIMARY SURVEY

The successful initial management of critically injured, multiple-trauma pediatric patients depends on the expertise of a well-coordinated team consisting of physicians—often headed by surgeons familiar with pediatric trauma—and emergency medical personnel. The primary survey systematically evaluates the essential components of ABCDE (*a*irway, breathing, circulation, neurologic disability, and exposure) for life-threatening injuries. Within the first 20 to 30 minutes at the hospital, affected patients should receive a primary survey with initial resuscitation, a secondary survey consisting of a complete examination from head to toe, and a plan for definitive care.

The initial focus of the primary survey is the airway. The goals are to relieve anatomic obstruction, to prevent the aspiration of gastric contents, and to promote adequate gas exchange with protection of the cervical spine. Any child with significant trauma is assumed to have cervical spine injury. These goals may be met by maneuvers as simple as a chin lift or a jaw thrust, with careful attention given to avoiding hyperextension of the cervical spine. Use of a rigid collar, sandbags, and tape or use of manual immobilization with the head in a neutral position prevents those manipulations of the cervical spine that may result in spinal cord injury with quadriplegia. The mouth may be suctioned for retained secretions, but care must be taken to avoid precipitating vomiting and regurgitation. Artificial nasopharyngeal and oropharyngeal airways are tolerated poorly and often induce gagging. Usually, children who tolerate them have compromised protective reflexes and require definitive airway management using an endotracheal tube.

The second goal of the primary survey is to maintain breathing. Affected patients should receive 100% inspired oxygen. If ventilation is inadequate or absent, if arterial hypoxemia unresponsive to increased inspired oxygen is present, if the face and neck are burned, or if such patients are hemodynamically unstable, the airway should be secured. Oral tracheal intubation is the preferred route. Such patients are at high risk for vomiting and aspirating. Also, their airways may be rendered more inaccessible by traumatic injury to the bones and soft tissue. Intubation is performed by the most experienced personnel and under controlled conditions using rapid sequence and cricoid pressure to prevent passive regurgitation. Manual, cervical in-line immobilization is performed to counter the flexion and extension caused during intubation if cervical injury is suspected.

Once the patient is intubated, ventilation is begun using 100% inspired oxygen at rates of 10 to 20 breaths per minute. If head injury is suspected, the minute ventilation rate should be increased to lower the arterial carbon dioxide pressure. If ventilation is impaired, malposition of the endotracheal tube or tube plugging with secretions is suspected. If inadequate ventilation continues, a pneumothorax, hemothorax, or other thoracic injury is suspected, evaluation is completed, and treatment is given. Usually, treatment entails the use of needle thoracentesis or tube thoracostomies.

The third goal of the primary survey is to ensure effective circulation. Initially, it may be accomplished by artificial support with chest compressions. At the same time, basic steps for hemorrhagic shock, including control of active hemorrhage, placement of intravenous lines, and aggressive crystalloid and blood replacement, are undertaken. The control of obvious hemorrhage is most important. In most situations, direct pressure is adequate. Fractures of the pelvis or long bones produce hidden blood loss that can be massive in both adults and children.

In patients with hemorrhage and shock, no substitute for volume and blood replacement exists. The debate about the use of crystalloid versus colloid for volume replacement continues. In the few studies of young-adult, previously healthy trauma patients, no differences in the development of pulmonary edema and pulmonary dysfunction were noted when either crystalloid or colloid was used. Some physicians prefer the use of lactated Ringer's solution over the use of normal saline because the chloride concentration more closely approximates that found in normal plasma and the lactate serves as

a source of buffering base. The volume infused should be 20 to 30 mL/kg initially, with an observation for improvement in circulatory status; if no improvement is noted, another 20 to 30 mL/kg is given. Balanced salt solution is not intended as a substitute for blood. A loss in excess of 30% of total circulating blood volume must be replaced with red blood cells in addition to fluid. Blood volume is 60 to 80 mL/kg of optimal body weight. In the emergent phase of resuscitation, time may not allow for a full type and crossmatch to be obtained. When uncrossmatched blood is used, obtaining at least an ABO-Rh type and a partial crossmatch is best. This combination is preferable to the use of type O, Rh-negative uncrossmatched blood, although it may be used if type-specific uncrossmatched blood is unavailable. If large amounts of crystalloid and red blood cells are required, hemostatic defects occur. Fresh-frozen plasma should be given to replete circulating coagulation factors and platelets when 100% to 200% of the circulating blood volume has been replaced.

If children with blunt trauma are in cardiorespiratory arrest despite having an adequate airway and ventilation, immediate insertion of bilateral thoracostomy tubes and a large fluid bolus are indicated. This step is followed by pericardiocentesis if improvement does not result. Failure to respond indicates irreversible shock, traumatic myocardial injury with pump failure, or severe central nervous system failure.

An assessment of the patient's disability necessitates performing a rapid neurologic examination to evaluate the level of consciousness and presence of abnormal pupillary findings. The neurologic examination may be carried out using the AVPU system (alert, responds to verbal stimuli, responds to painful stimuli, unresponsive). Alternatively, the Glasgow Coma Scale and its modification for infants can be used (Table 460.1). The final component of the primary survey involves fully undressing an affected patient and examining under cervical collars and bandages. Because of the increased surface area–to–mass ratios in children, increased minute ventilation with accompanying heat of vaporization loss, and (usually) resuscitation in a cold environment, affected children may become fairly hypothermic, thus further complicating resuscitation. Temperature can be supported by warming administered fluid and blood, by using external heating elements, and by wrapping all exposed areas in plastic once the full evaluation is accomplished.

SECONDARY SURVEY

The secondary survey begins with a systematic and careful assessment of organ systems in an organized manner. Additional history, including AMPLE (allergies, medications, past medical history, last meal, and events), should be obtained at this point. Specifics of the head examination include pupillary size and reactivity, funduscopic evaluation, palpation of the skull, and careful assessment of the cervical spine (with an affected patient in full restraint). Assessment of the chest and internal structures involves inspection for wounds and flail segments, palpation for tenderness and crepitation, and auscultation for asymmetry or poorly transmitted breath sounds. Examination of the abdomen is most reliable when performed on cooperative patients. A focused assessment sonography for trauma (FAST) is standard of care in the multiply injured patient. It permits the examination of the pericardium and pleural cavities, as well as the intraabdominal area for contents and blood. This examination, along with computed tomography (CT), which can be done quickly (usually in 10 minutes for the complete torso with the latest generation of spiral CT), clearly is emerging as a valued tool to evaluate the presence of blunt and penetrating injuries of the chest and abdomen. A rectal examination provides information regarding sphincter tone, prostatic position, and the presence of blood in the stool. Examination of

TABLE 460.1

GLASGOW COMA SCALE MODIFIED FOR PEDIATRIC PATIENTS

Score	>1 year	<1 year	
Eye response			
4	Spontaneous	Spontaneous	
3	To verbal command	To shout	
2	To pain	To pain	
1	None	None	

Score	>1 year	<1 year	
Motor response			
6	Obeys commands	Spontaneous	
5	Localizes pain	Localizes pain	
4	Withdraws to pain	Withdraws to pain	
3	Abnormal flexion to pain (decorticate)	Abnormal flexion to pain (decorticate)	
2	Abnormal extension to pain (decerebrate)	Abnormal extension to pain (decerebrate)	
1	None	None	

Score	>5 years	2–5 years	0–2 years
Verbal response			
5	Oriented and converses	Appropriate words and phrases	Babbles, coos
4	Confused conversation	Inappropriate words	Cries but is consolable
3	Inappropriate words	Persistent crying or screaming to pain	Persistent crying or screaming to pain
2	Incomprehensible sounds	Grunts or moans to pain	Grunts or moans to pain
1	None	None	None

Scoring: severe, <9; moderate, 9–12; mild, 13–15.

the extremities is directed toward evaluating any deformities, penetrations, or decreased perfusion.

By now, affected children should be either hemodynamically stable, with a controlled airway, or rapidly on the way to the operating room because of continued instability. With the recognition of the lethal triad of hypothermia, acidosis, and coagulopathy, the concept of damage-control surgery has become the approach now advocated. The first stage is a direct surgical approach and is targeted at true damage control. It consists of focused surgery to control hemorrhage and alleviate contamination. Definitive reconstruction is delayed, and rapid, simple closure is encouraged. Fractures are immobilized, not definitively set or reduced. During the second stage, the child is taken to the intensive care unit for further resuscitation and stabilization. This phase may be protracted and very complicated. Patients may return to the operating room multiple times during the third phase, during which definitive repair occurs. Often phase II and III overlap. With the use of damage-control surgery, a new challenge has arisen for the critical care practitioners: the increasing occurrence of the abdominal compartment syndrome. Edema, ascites, tissue swelling, and ongoing bleeding may lead to increased intraabdominal pressure. This elevated pressure leads to further respiratory compromise and difficulty in ventilating the patient, requiring very elevated pressures on the respirator. In addition, increased intraabdominal pressures will compromise renal and gut flow, thus putting these organs at risk for further damage.

THORACIC INJURIES

Thoracic injuries are less common occurrences than are intraabdominal injuries in children. In children with multiple trauma, only 4.5% have isolated thoracic injuries; however, the associated mortality rate is 25%. Children's chest injuries differ from those of adults in two ways. The more compliant chests of children contribute to a low incidence of rib fracture, although serious intrathoracic injury may be present in the absence of obvious chest wall injury. In addition, the mediastina of children are more mobile, which contributes to a low overall incidence of major vessel and airway injury; however, cardiovascular and ventilatory compromise can occur rapidly with excessive mediastinal shifting.

The following five immediately life-threatening injuries can involve the chest wall and parenchyma. Each should be diagnosed in the initial primary assessment.

- Either penetrating or blunt trauma can produce an *open pneumothorax*. The inability to generate negative intrathoracic pressure causes lung collapse and ventilatory insufficiency. In addition, a to-and-fro movement occurs in the mediastinum, with interference of venous return to the right side of the heart. Treatment consists of immediately covering any hole in the chest with an airtight dressing and inserting a chest tube through a separate incision.
- *Flail chest* results from the paradoxical movement of a portion of the chest wall because of multiple rib fractures. As in open pneumothorax, the generation of negative intrathoracic pressure is prevented. The chest wall is unstable, moving inward with inspiration and outward with expiration. Definitive treatment is positive-pressure ventilation for internal stabilization of the chest wall. Often, flail chest is complicated by underlying pulmonary contusion.
- *Massive hemothorax* occurs from injuries to the aortic arch, pulmonary hilum, or systemic vessels, such as the internal mammary or intercostal arteries (Fig. 460.1). Most of the bleeding that occurs with thoracic injuries is not from the lung but from the systemic arteries in the chest. Chest tubes must be placed early in any patient with

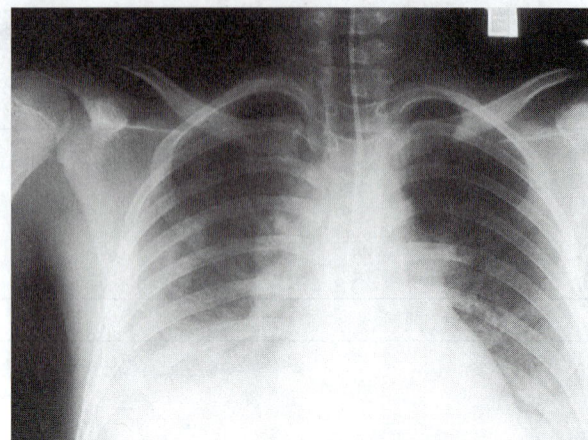
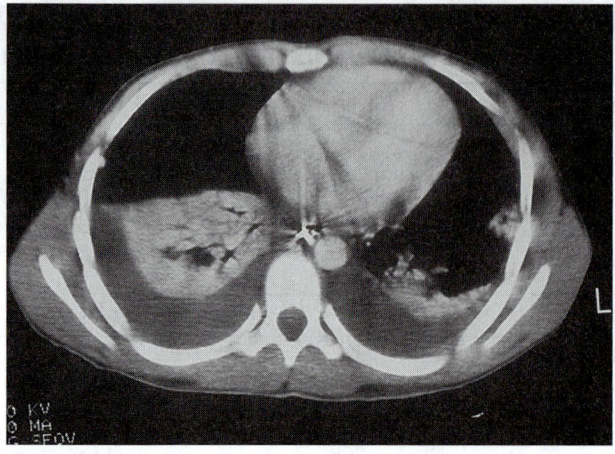

FIGURE 460.1. A 15-year-old child involved in an auto–pedestrian accident. Vital signs were stable at the scene, but the child had decreased breath sounds bilaterally. **A:** The chest radiograph shows bilateral hemothorax and pulmonary contusions. **B:** Computed tomography confirmed and better delineated hemothorax and pulmonary contusions. (Reproduced with permission from Fleisher GR, Ludwig S, Baskin MN. *Atlas of pediatric emergency medicine*. Philadelphia: Lippincott Williams & Wilkins, 2004:357.)

intrathoracic blood loss. Usually, total blood loss of more than 20% or 30% of total blood volume or more than 2 to 3 mL/kg/hour indicates the need for surgery.

■ A laceration in the pulmonary parenchyma may act to allow the ingress of air into the chest cavity with no egress, creating a *tension pneumothorax*. Pleural pressure rises, the lung collapses, the mediastinum shifts into the opposite hemithorax, the opposite lung becomes compressed, and venous return to the heart is compromised. Treatment is immediate tube thoracostomy.

■ Children with *pericardial tamponade* present with paradoxical pulse, distended neck veins, and muffled heart sounds. Lethal hypotension may result from inadequate filling of the ventricles. Pericardiocentesis is used as temporizing treatment and to establish a definitive diagnosis. Ultimately, treatment requires surgical exploration.

Usually, several common occult and potentially serious injuries to the chest and its contents are diagnosed on the secondary survey. *Pulmonary contusion* with or without laceration or hemorrhage is the most common serious chest injury. Pulmonary contusion from blunt injury is a common finding and often is associated with both pulmonary edema and atelectasis. Pulmonary contusion presents almost immediately with respiratory distress, hypoxemia, atelectasis, and roentgenogram changes. Small areas of lung involvement require no specific therapy other than pulmonary toilet, but extensive injuries usually mandate mechanical ventilation. If a laceration is associated with the contusion, chest tube insertion is required for evacuation of the pneumothorax.

Tracheobronchial rupture is characterized by respiratory distress, subcutaneous emphysema, and hemoptysis. Depending on the nature of the injury, some patients have airway obstruction, some have a tension pneumothorax, many have a simple pneumothorax, and all have mediastinal air on chest roentgenography. A chest tube is inserted to evacuate the pneumothorax. Usually, thoracotomy is required to control the tear.

Myocardial contusion is a bruise or intramural hematoma of the myocardium occurring after blunt trauma of the anterior chest. The diagnosis is made on the basis of arrhythmias or on routine electrocardiography. Because affected children may be at risk of developing life-threatening arrhythmias, they require cardiac monitoring.

Diagnosing *rupture of the diaphragm* may be difficult unless the physician has a high index of suspicion. The disorder occurs more often on the left side. Treatment is urgent diaphragmatic repair.

Occasionally, *esophageal injury* may result from penetrating trauma. Esophageal perforation produces mediastinitis, a potentially lethal, rapidly progressive infection in the mediastinal space. Treatment consists of primary repair and drainage.

Most patients who have rupture or *injury of the great vessels* die at the scene of the accident. If such patients have a wide mediastinum or obliteration of the aortic knob on roentgenography, prompt angiographic diagnostic studies are required. Unlike this injury in adults, associated fractures of the first and second ribs do not correlate with injury to the great vessels in children.

Traumatic asphyxia is a dramatic but rare complication of blunt chest trauma. It results from a sudden, intense compression of the chest wall with the glottis closed. The intrathoracic pressure is increased suddenly, and this increase is reflected in the veins of the upper torso. Affected children present with petechial hemorrhages in the sclerae, conjunctiva, and skin of the upper extremities and head. The hemorrhages resolve over the course of several days. Traumatic asphyxia implies severe, blunt forces to the chest wall.

ABDOMINAL TRAUMA

Intraabdominal injuries account for a significant percentage of the traumatic deaths in children. The liver and spleen are the two organs injured most commonly. The main purpose of the primary and secondary survey is not to obtain a specific diagnosis of organ injury but to determine the next course of action. Immediate laparotomy is indicated in patients with frank peritonitis or signs of massive hemorrhage. Again, damage-control surgery becomes most important.

Approximately 85% to 90% of all patients with blunt hepatic and splenic injuries have relatively low grade (grade I to III) injuries and can be managed nonoperatively. With a recognition of the problems of postsplenectomy infection, nonoperative management of splenic injuries and splenic preservation is preferred. Nonoperative management of splenic injury includes close observation of affected patients in the intensive care unit, with frequent measurement of hematocrit. Observation without operative treatment is not contraindicated by the need to administer a blood transfusion. Evidence that angiographic embolization can be used to control hemorrhage is increasing. In adults, the use of angiographic techniques to control liver injuries has reduced mortality rates from 40% to 80% down to 8% to 22%. Patients too unstable to undergo angiography or CT should undergo early but abbreviated laparotomy, which then is closed expeditiously. They then should be transported to the angiography suite with the resuscitation team for further treatment.

Small-intestine and pancreatic injuries in children occur secondary to high-speed deceleration—when affected children crash against the handlebars of a bicycle—or after blunt injury from nonaccidental trauma. The injuries include duodenal hematoma, traumatic rupture of the jejunum near the ligament of Treitz, and pancreatic contusion or transection. Pancreatic trauma is the most common cause of pancreatitis and pseudocyst formation in children. Serum amylases or lipases (or both) should be monitored for several hours after presentation and for several days after the event. The symptoms of duodenal hematoma may develop gradually, with abdominal pain, bilious vomiting, epigastric tenderness, and leukocytosis occurring hours to even days after the initial event. Expectant therapy with bowel rest, nasogastric tube placement, and parenteral nutrition is required for 7 to 10 days. Occasionally, expectant therapy fails, and evacuation of the hematoma is indicated. Usually, diagnosis of traumatic jejunal rupture is based on clinical signs of peritonitis; abdominal roentgenography shows free air in fewer than one-half of cases.

Injury to the urinary tract occurs in approximately 5% of pediatric trauma patients. A catheter should not be passed in patients with pelvic fracture until gentle retrograde urethrography has excluded the presence of a urethral tear. Other contraindications for catheter insertion are blood at the urethral meatus; a high-riding prostate; gross hematuria; and labial, scrotal, or perianal ecchymosis or hematoma. CT scanning has replaced intravenous pyelography for the evaluation of renal trauma. Most renal injuries do not require operation. Ureteral injuries are rare events in children but should be suspected if extravasation of contrast material occurs in the presence of good renal function and an intact pelvicaliceal system.

INJURIES TO THE SPINE AND CRANIUM

Vertebral column and spinal cord trauma must be presumed to have occurred in any child rendered unconscious with a head injury. As many as 10% of patients with spinal cord injuries develop cord compression during the initial period of emergency care. Great care must be taken during transport and during in-hospital resuscitation to minimize head movement until fractures and dislocations have been excluded by appropriate films. The initial workup incorporates lateral cervical spine films that include the C7–T1 junction. Often, in pediatric trauma, spinal cord injury can exist without radiographic abnormality. Whereas fractures below the C3 level account for only 30% of spinal lesions among children younger than 8 years old, spinal cord injury can exist without radiographic abnormality and has been estimated to be found in 10% to 20% of children. The prognosis for spinal cord injury is poor if the lesion remains complete 24 hours after the initial injury. Recent work supports the use of high-dose methylprednisolone in adults with spinal cord injury. There is no data in children.

The management of children with closed-head injury begins, as for any child with trauma, with attention to essential (ABCDE) evaluative components. The evaluation of such children during the primary survey focuses on the Glasgow Coma Scale (see Table 460.1). The scale briefly evaluates best eye, motor, and verbal responses, giving a score that is reproducible and of prognostic significance. Severe head injury is found in patients with a Glasgow Coma score of 8 or less. These patients should have control of their airway and ventilatory support provided. A more thorough examination is performed in the secondary survey, with documentation of the level of consciousness, spontaneous reactions, and response to stimuli. Cranial nerve examination should concentrate on movements of the eyes and face, particularly pupillary size and reactivity. Doll's-eye maneuvers or caloric responses should not be attempted because of the possibility that the patient has an unstable cervical spine or ruptured eardrums.

If the affected child has a significant head injury (GCS $\leq$ 8), initial treatment should be directed at maintaining normal blood pressure and intracranial pressure (ICP). An intraventricular pressure monitor should be placed in these children. Intravenous fluid should be isoosmolar and nonhypotonic and should be given at baseline infusion rates, unless such children have associated injuries requiring fluid resuscitation. Frequently, mannitol is given to seriously head-injured children to reduce ICP. It should be reserved for patients with acute neurologic dysfunction or transtentorial herniation and should be used as a life-saving measure while definitive diagnostic or surgical options are being carried out. The dose of mannitol is 0.25 to 1.00 g/kg, given via rapid intravenous infusion.

CT scanning is the most important diagnostic modality in the management of pediatric head injury. CT scanning can render possible the establishment of a diagnosis of a surgically treatable mass lesion (epidural or subdural hematoma), diffuse cerebral swelling, or increased cerebrospinal fluid volume. While definitive diagnostic studies are undertaken, hyperventilation to a P_{CO_2} in the 25- to 30-mm Hg range will decrease ICP by decreasing cerebral blood volume. The control of seizures is essential for the management of acute head injury. Other treatments will be predicated best on the results of diagnostic studies.

Suggested Readings

Bayir H, Kochanek PM, Clark RSB. Traumatic brain injury in infants and children. *Crit Care Clin* 2003;19:529.

Bliss D, Silen M. Pediatric thoracic trauma. *Crit Care Med* 2002;30:S409.

Gains BA, Ford HR. Abdominal and pelvic trauma in children. *Crit Care Med* 2002;30:S416.

Garcia VF, Brown RL. Pediatric trauma: beyond the brain. *Crit Care Clin* 2003; 19:551.

PALS Provider Manual. *Trauma resuscitation and spinal immobilization.* Hazinski MF, ed. Dallas: American Heart Association, 2002.

Pepe PE, Eckstein M. Reappraising the prehospital care of the patient with major trauma. *Emerg Clin North Am* 1998;16:1.

Proctor MR. Spinal cord injury. *Crit Care Med* 2002;30:S489.

Wetzell RC, Burns RD. Multiple trauma in children: critical care overview. *Crit Care Med* 2002:S468.

APPENDICES: PEDIATRICIAN'S COMPANION:
THINGS YOU FORGET TO REMEMBER

APPENDIX A ■ LABORATORY VALUES

MICHAEL A. BARONE

The following reference values for laboratory tests have been drawn from the sources listed at the end of the chapter. They represent guidelines as the reference range varies from one institution to the next, depending on the laboratory method used. Where applicable, conventional units and International System (SI) units are provided. Conversion factors are also listed.

SI PREFIXES

Factor	Prefix	Symbol
10^3	kilo	k
10^{-1}	deci	d
10^{-2}	centi	c
10^{-3}	milli	m
10^{-6}	micro	μ
10^{-9}	nano	n
10^{-12}	pico	p
10^{-15}	femto	f

ABBREVIATIONS

CI	confidence interval
F	female
Hb	hemoglobin
M	male
MCHC	mean corpuscular hemoglobin concentration
MCV	mean corpuscular volume
RBC	red blood cell
SD	standard deviation
WBC	white blood cell

BLOOD

Test	Conventional Units Reference Range	Conversion Factor	SI Units Reference Range
Adrenocorticotropic hormone (ACTH)	Cord: 130–160 pg/mL 1st wk: 100–140 Adult 0800 hr: 25–100 1800 hr: <50		Cord: 130–160 ng/L 1st wk: 100–140 Adult 0800 hr: 25–100 1800 hr: <50
Alanine aminotransferase (ALT)	0–5 yr: 7–46 U/L >5 yr: 6–39		0–5 yr: 7–46 U/L >5 yr: 6–39
Albumin	Premature, 24 hr: 1.5–3.0 g/dL Term, 6 d: 2.5–3.4 1–3 yr: 3.4–4.2 4–6 yr: 3.5–5.2 7–19 yr: 3.7–5.6	g/dL × 10 = g/L	Premature, 24 hr: 15–30 g/L Term, 6 d: 2.5–3.4 1–3 yr: 34–42 4–6 yr: 35–52 7–19 yr: 37–56
Aldolase	10–24 mo: 3.4–11.8 U/L 2–16 yr: 1.2–8.8 U/L Adult: 1.7–4.9 U/L		10–24 mo: 3.4–11.8 U/L 2–16 yr: 1.2–8.8 U/L Adult: 1.7–4.9 U/L
Aldosterone	Full Term Infants: 3 d: 7–184 ng/dL 1 wk: 5–175 1–12 mo: 5–90 Children: 1–2 yr: 7–54 2–10 yr (supine): 3–35 2–10 yr (upright): 5–80 10–15 yr (supine): 2–22 10–15 yr (upright): 4–48 Adults: Supine: 3–16 Upright: 7–30	ng/dL × 0.0277 = nmol/L	Full Term Infants: 3 d: 0.19–5.10 nmol/L 1 wk: 0.14–4.85 1–12 mo: 0.14–2.49 Children: 1–2 yr: 0.19–1.50 2–10 yr (supine): 0.08–0.97 2–10 yr (upright): 0.14–2.22 10–15 yr (supine): 0.06–0.61 10–15 yr (upright): 0.11–1.33 Adults: Supine: 0.08–0.44 Upright: 5.54–22.16
Alkaline phosphatase	Infant 150–420 U/L 2–10 yr: 100–320 11–18 yr (M): 100–390 11–18 yr (F): 100–320 Adult: 30–120		Infant 150–420 U/L 2–10 yr: 100–320 11–18 yr (M): 100–390 11–18 yr (F): 100–320 Adult: 30–120

(continued)

	BLOOD (Cont.)		
Test	Conventional Units Reference Range	Conversion Factor	SI Units Reference Range
Alpha₁-antitrypsin	0–5 d: 143–440 mg/dL 1–13 yr: 147–259 >13 yr: 152–317	mg/dL × 0.01 = g/L	0–5 d: 1.43–4.40 g/L 1–13 yr: 1.47–2.59 >13 yr: 1.52–3.17
Alpha-fetoprotein	Fetal peak: 200–400 mg/dL Cord: <5 mg/dL >1 yr: <30 ng/mL	mg/dL × 0.01 = g/L	Fetal peak: 2–4 g/L Cord: <0.05 g/L >1 yr: <30 μg/L
Ammonia nitrogen	Newborn: 90–150 μg/dL 0–2 wk: 79–129 >1 mo: 29–70 Thereafter 0–50	μg/dL × 0.714 = μmol/L	Newborn: 64–107 μmol/L 0–2 wk: 56–92 >1 mo: 21–50 Thereafter: 0–35.7
Amylase	Newborn: 5–65 U/L Thereafter: 0–130		Newborn: 5–65 U/L Thereafter: 0–130

Androstendione	Male and Female (Preterm):
	26–28 weeks to day of life 4:
	  92–892 ng/dL
	31–35 weeks to day of life 4:
	  80–446 ng/dL
	Male and Female (Full-term):
	1–7 days: 20–290 ng/dL
	1–12 mo: 6–68 ng/dL
	Male and Female (prepubertal):
	  8–50 ng/dL
	Male:
	Tanner II: 31–65 ng/dL
	Tanner III: 50–100
	Tanner IV: 48–140
	Tanner V: 65–210
	Adult: 78–205
	Female:
	Tanner II: 42–100 ng/dL
	Tanner III: 80–190
	Tanner IV: 77–225
	Tanner V: 80–240
	Adult: 85–275
		ng/dL × 0.03492
		= nmol/L
			Male and Female (Preterm):
			26–28 weeks to day of life 4:
			  3.21–31.15 nmol/L
			31–35 weeks to day of life 4:
			  2.79–15.57 nmol/L
			Male and Female (Full-term):
			1–7 days: 0.70–10.13 nmol/L
			1–12 mo: 0.21–2.37 nmol/L
			Male and Female (prepubertal):
			  0.28–1.75 nmol/L
			Male:
			Tanner II: 1.08–2.27 nmol/L
			Tanner III: 1.75–3.49
			Tanner IV: 1.68–4.89
			Tanner V: 2.27–7.33
			Adult: 2.72–7.16
			Female:
			Tanner II: 1.47–3.49 nmol/L
			Tanner III: 2.79–6.63
			Tanner IV: 2.69–7.86
			Tanner V: 2.79–8.38
			Adult: 2.97–9.6

Angiotensin converting enzyme (ACE)	<1 yr: 10.9–42.1 U/L 1–2 yr: 9.4–36 3–4 yr: 7.9–29.8 4–9 yr: 9.6–35.4 10–12 yr: 10.3–37 13–16 yr: 9–33.4 17–19 yr: 7.2–26.6 >19 yr: 6.1–21.1		<1 yr: 10.9–42.1 U/L 1–2 yr: 9.4–36 3–4 yr: 7.9–29.8 4–9 yr: 9.6–35.4 10–12 yr: 10.3–37 13–16 yr: 9–33.4 17–19 yr: 7.2–26.6 >19 yr: 6.1–21.1
Anion gap	7–14 mEq/L		7–14 nmol/L
Aspartate amino-transferase (AST)	Newborn: 25–75 U/L Infant: 15–60 1–3 yr: 20–60 4–6 yr: 15–50 7–9 yr: 15–40 10–11 yr: 10–60 12–19 yr: 15–45		Newborn: 25–75 U/L Infant: 15–60 1–3 yr: 20–60 4–6 yr: 15–50 7–9 yr: 15–40 10–11 yr: 10–60 12–19 yr: 15–45
Bicarbonate	Premature: 18–26 mEq/L <2 yr: 20–25 >2 yr: 22–26		Premature: 18–26 mmol/L <2 yr: 20–25 >2 yr: 22–26

Bilirubin (total)	*Preterm*	*Term*	mg/dL × 17.1 = μmol/L	*Preterm*	*Term*
	Cord: <2 mg/dL	<2		Cord: <34 μmol/L	<34
	0–1 day: <8	<8		0–1 day: <137	<137
	1–2 days: <12	<11.5		1–2 days: <205	<197
	3–5 days: <16	<12		3–5 days: <274	<205
	>1 month: <2	<1.2		>1 month: <34	<21

(continued)

	BLOOD (Cont.)		
Test	Conventional Units Reference Range	Conversion Factor	SI Units Reference Range
Bilirubin (conjugated)	0–0.2 mg/dL	mg/dL × 17.1 = μmol/L	0–3.4 μmol/L
C-peptide	8 AM fasting 0.4–2.2 ng/dL 2 hr post prandial 1.2–3.4 2 hr postglucose 2–4.5		8 AM fasting 0.4–2.2 μg/L 2 hr post prandial 1.2–3.4 2 hr postglucose 2–4.5
C-reactive protein	0–0.5 mg/dL (varies based on individual lab standards)		
Calcitonin	Newborn: 70–348 pg/mL Children Males: 3–19 Females: 2–14	pg/mL × 0.28 = pmol/L	Newborn: 70–348 pmol/L Children Males: 0.84–5.32 Females: 0.56–3.92
Calcium (ionized)	<7 d: 4.52–6.32 mg/dL Adult: 4.68–5.28	mg/dL × 0.25 = nmol/L	<7 d: 1.13–1.58 nmol/L Adult: 1.17–1.32
Calcium (total)	Preterm <1 wk: 6–10 mg/dL Term <1 wk: 7–12 Child: 8.0–10.5 Adult: 8.5–10.5	mg/dL × 0.25 = mmol/L	Preterm <1 wk: 1.5–2.5 mmol/L Term <1 wk: 1.75–3.0 Child: 2.0–2.6 Adult: 2.1–2.6
Carbon dioxide (CO_2 content)	Cord blood: 14–22 mEq/L Infant/child: 20–24 Adult: 24–30		Cord blood: 14–22 mmol/L Infant/child: 20–24 Adult: 24–30
Carbon monoxide (carboxyhe-moglobin)	*Percent of Hb saturation* Nonsmoker: <2% Smoker: <10% Toxic: >20% Lethal: >50%		*Fraction of HbCO* Nonsmoker: <0.02 Smoker: <0.1 Toxic: >0.2 Lethal: >0.5
Carotene	Infant: 20–70 μg/dL Child: 40–130 Adult: 50–250	μg/dL × 0.01862 = μmol/L	Infant: 0.37–1.3 μmol/L Child: 0.74–2.42 Adult: 0.95–4.69
Ceruloplasmin	1–12 yr: 30–65 mg/dL 7–12 yr: 15–60	mg/dL × 10 = mg/L	1–12 yr: 300–650 mg/L >12 yr: 150–600
Chloride	Pediatric: 99–111 mEq/L Adult: 96–109		Pediatric: 99–111 mmol/L Adult: 96–109
Cholesterol (total)	mg/dL 5th–95th percentile Cord Blood: Male: 44–103 Female: 50–108 0–4 yr Male: 114–203 Female: 112–200 5–9 yr Male: 121–203 Female: 126–205 10–14 yr Male: 119–202 Female: 124–201 15–19 yr Male: 113–197 Female: 119–200	mg/dL × 0.0259 = mmol/L	mmol/L 5th–95th percentile Cord Blood: Male: 1.14–2.66 Female: 1.29–2.79 0–4 yr Male: 2.95–5.25 Female: 2.90–5.18 5–9 yr Male: 3.13–5.25 Female: 3.26–5.30 10–14 yr Male: 3.08–5.23 Female: 3.21–5.20 15–19 yr Male: 2.93–5.10 Female: 3.08–5.18
Complement, C_3	Cord blood: 57–116 mg/dL 1–3 mo: 53–131 3 mo to 1 yr: 62–180 1–10 yr: 77–195 Adult: 83–177	mg/dL × 10 = mg/L	Cord blood: 570–1,160 mg/L 1–3 mo: 530–1,310 3 mo to 1 yr: 620–1,800 1–10 yr: 770–1,950 Adult: 830–1,770
Complement, C_4	Cord blood: 6.6–23.0 mg/dL 1–3 mo: 7–28 3 mo to 1 yr: 7–42 1–10 yr: 9.2–40.0 Adult: 15–45	mg/dL × 10 = mg/L	Cord blood: 66–230 mg/L 1–3 mo: 70–280 3 mo to 1 yr: 70–420 1–10 yr: 92–400 Adult: 150–450

(continued)

BLOOD (Cont.)			
Test	**Conventional Units Reference Range**	**Conversion Factor**	**SI Units Reference Range**
Complement, total hemolytic (CH$_{50}$)	75–160 U/mL		75–160 U/mL
Copper	0–6 mo: 20–70 μg/dL 6 yr: 90–190 12 yr: 80–160 Adult (M): 70–140 Adult (F): 80–155	μg/dL $\times$ 0.157 = μmol/L	0–6 mo: 3.1–11.0 μmol/L 6 yr: 14–30 12 yr: 12.6–25.0 Adult (M): 11–22 Adult (F): 12.6–24.0

Cortisol	0800 hr or pre-ACTH:
	  5.7–16.6 μg/dL
	1 hr post-ACTH: 16–36 μg/dL
		μg/dL $\times$ 27.59 = nmol/L	0800 hr or pre-ACTH:
			  157–458 nmol/L
			1 hr post-ACTH: 441–993 nmol/L

Creatine kinase	Newborn: 76–600 U/L Adult (M): 38–174 Adult (F): 96–140		Newborn: 76–600 U/L Adult (M): 38–174 Adult (F): 96–140
Creatine kinase isoenzymes	*Percent activity* CK–BB: trace CK–MB: 4–6 CK–MM: 94–96		*Fraction of total activity* CK–BB: trace CK–MB: 0.04–0.06 CK–MM: 0.94–0.96
Creatinine	Cord blood: 0.6–1.2 mg/dL Newborn: 0.3–1.0 Infant: 0.2–0.4 Child: 0.3–0.7 Adolescent: 0.5–1.0 Adult (M): 0.6–1.3 Adult (F): 0.5–1.2	mg/dL $\times$ 88.4 = μmol/L	Cord blood: 53–106 μmol/L Newborn: 27–88 Infant: 18–35 Child: 27–62 Adolescent: 44–88 Adult (M): 53–115 Adult (F): 44–106

Dehydroepiandrosterone (DHEA)

Age	M (ng/dL)	F (ng/dL)
<6 yr	26–72	19–42
6–8 yr	29–66	73–165
8–10 yr	53–135	74–180
10–12 yr	183–383	234–529
12–14 yr	240–520	224–611
>14 yr	307–835	282–771

ng/dL $\times$ 0.0347 = nmol/L

Age	M (nmol/L)	F (nmol/L)
<6 yr	0.9–2.5	0.66–1.66
6–8 yr	1.01–2.29	2.53–5.73
8–10 yr	1.84–4.69	2.57–6.25
10–12 yr	6.35–13.29	8.12–18.36
12–14 yr	8.33–18.04	7.77–21.20
>14 yr	10.65–28.98	9.79–26.75

Test	Conventional Units Reference Range	Conversion Factor	SI Units Reference Range
Dehydropiandrosterone sulfate (DHEA-S)	1–5 yr: <30 μg/dL 6–11 yr: 10–150 12–17 yr: 30–550	μg/dL $\times$ 0.026 = μmol/L	1–5 yr: <0.78 μmol/L 6–11 yr: 0.26–3.90 12–17 yr: 0.78–14.30
Erythrocyte sedimentation rate	Newborn (0–48 hr): 0–4 mm/hr Child: 4–20 mm/hr Adult (M): 0–10 mm/hr Adult (F): 0–20 mm/hr		

Estradiol

Tanner stage, M (ng/dL)

I: 0.5–1.1
II: 0.5–1.6
III: 0.5–2.5
IV: 1.0–3.6
V: 1.0–3.6
Adult: 0.8–3.5

ng/dL $\times$ 36.71 = pmol/L

Tanner stage, M (pmol/L)

I: 18–40
II: 18–59
III: 18–92
IV: 37–132
V: 37–132
Adult: 29–128

Tanner stage, F (ng/dL)

I: 0.5–2.0
II: 1.0–2.4
III: 0.7–6.0
IV: 2.1–8.5
V: 3.4–17.0
Adult: follicular, 3–10; luteal, 7–30

Tanner stage, F (pmol/L)

I: 18–73
II: 37–88
III: 26–220
IV: 77–312
V: 125–624
Adult: follicular, 110–367;
  luteal, 257–1,100

Free fatty acids	Child: <31 mg/dL Adult: 8–25	mg/dL $\times$ 0.035 = mmol/L	Child: <1.10 mmol/L Adult: 0.3–0.9

(continued)

BLOOD (Cont.)			
Test	Conventional Units Reference Range	Conversion Factor	SI Units Reference Range
Ferritin	Newborn: 25–200 ng/mL 1 mo: 200–600 2–6 mo: 50–200 6 mo to 15 yr: 7–140 Adult (M): 15–200 Adult (F): 12–150		Newborn: 25–200 μg/L 1 mo: 200–600 2–6 mo: 50–200 6 mo to 15 yr: 7–140 Adult (M): 15–200 Adult (F): 12–150
Fibrinogen	Newborn: 125–300 mg/dL Adult: 200–400	×0.01	Newborn: 1.25–3 g/L Adult: 2–4 g/L
Folate	Newborn: 7–32 ng/mL Thereafter: 1.8–9.0	ng/mL × 2.265 = nmol/L	Newborn: 15.9–72.4 nmol/L Thereafter: 4–20
Folate (RBC)	150–450 ng/mL RBC	ng/mL × 2.265 = nmol/L	340–1,020 nmol/L RBC
Follicle-stimulating hormone	*Tanner stage, M (mlU/mL)* I: 0.26–3.0 II: 1.8–3.2 III: 1.2–5.8 IV: 2.0–9.2 V: 2.6–11.0 Adult: 2.0–9.2 *Tanner stage, F (mlU/mL)* I: 1.0–4.2 II: 1.0–10.8 III: 1.5–12.8 IV: 1.5–11.7 V: 1.0–9.2 Adult: follicular, 1.8–11.2; midcycle, 6–35; luteal, 1.8–11.2		*Tanner stage, M (U/L)* I: 0.26–3.0 II: 1.8–3.2 III: 1.2–5.8 IV: 2.0–9.2 V: 2.6–11.0 Adult: 2.0–9.2 *Tanner stage, F (U/L)* I: 1.0–4.2 II: 1.0–10.8 III: 1.5–12.8 IV: 1.5–11.7 V: 1.0–9.2 Adult: follicular, 1.8–11.2; midcycle, 6–35; luteal, 1.8–11.2
Fructose	1–6 mg/dL	mg/dL × 55 = μmol/L	55–330 μmol/L
Galactose	Newborn: 0–20 mg/dL Thereafter: <5	mg/dL × 0.055 = mmol/L	Newborn: 0–1.11 mmol/L Thereafter: <0.28
Gamma glutamyl transferase	Cord blood: 19–270 U/L 0–3 wk: 0–130 3 wk to 3 mo: 4–120 3 mo to 1 yr (M): 5–65 3 mo to 1 yr (F): 5–35 1–15 yr: 0–23 Adult (M): 11–50 Adult (F): 7–32		Cord blood: 19–270 U/L 0–3 wk: 0–130 3 wk to 3 mo: 4–120 3 mo to 1 yr (M): 5–65 3 mo to 1 yr (F): 5–35 1–15 yr: 0–23 Adult (M): 11–50 Adult (F): 7–32
Gastrin	Cord: 20–290 pg/mL 0–4 d: 120–183 Child: <10–125 Adult (16–60 yr): 25–90	×1	Cord: 20–290 ng/L 0–4 d: 120–183 Child: <10–125 Adult (16–60 yr): 25–90
Glucagon	Cord: 0–215 pg/mL 1–3 d: 0–1,750 4–14 yr: 0–148 Adult: 20–100	×1	Cord: 0–215 ng/L 1–3 d: 0–1,750 4–14 yr: 0–148 Adult: 20–100
Glucose	Preterm: 20–60 mg/dL Newborn (<1 d): 40–60 Newborn (>1 d): 50–80 Child: 60–100 >16 yr 75–105	mg/dL × 0.0555 = mmol/L	Preterm: 1.1–3.3 mmol/L Newborn (<1 d): 2.2–3.3 Newborn (>1 d): 2.8–4.5 Child: 3.3–5.6 >16 yr 4.1–5.9
Growth hormone (somatotropin)	1 d: 5–53 ng/mL 1 wk: 5–27 1–12 mo: 2–10 Fasting Child/adult: <0.7–6.0		1 d: 5–53 μg/L 1 wk: 5–27 1–12 mo: 2–10 Fasting Child/adult: <0.7–6.0
Haptoglobin	40–180 mg/dL	mg/dL × 0.01 = g/L	0.4–1.8 g/L

(continued)

BLOOD (Cont.)			
Test	Conventional Units Reference Range	Conversion Factor	SI Units Reference Range
Hemoglobin A1C	3.0–7.7% of total Hb		0.030–0.077 fraction of total Hb
beta-Hydroxybutyrate	<1 mg/dL	mg/dL × 96 = μmol/L	<96 μmol/L
17-Hydroxyprogesterone	Premature Infant: 26–568 ng/dL	ng/dL × 0.03 = nmol/L	Premature Infant: 0.8–1.7 nmol/L
	Term Infant (<3 d): 7–77		Term Infant (<3 d): 0.2–2.3
	Prepubertal Child: 3–90		Prepubertal Child: 0.1–2.7
	Tanner I:		Tanner I:
	M: 3–90		M: 0.1–2.7
	F: 3–82		F: 0.1–2.5
	Tanner II:		Tanner II:
	M: 5–115		M: 0.2–3.5
	F: 11–98		F: 0.3–3
	Tanner III:		Tanner III:
	M: 10–138		M: 0.3–4.2
	F: 11–155		F: 0.3–4.7
	Tanner IV:		Tanner IV:
	M: 29–180		M: 0.9–5.4
	F: 18–230		F: 0.5–7
	Tanner V:		Tanner V:
	M: 24–175		M: 0.7–5.3
	F: 20–265		F: 0.6–8
	Adult Male: 27–199		Adult Male: 0.8–6
	Adult Female (premenopausal):		Adult Female (premenopausal):
	Follicular: 15–70		Follicular: 0.4–2.1
	Luteal: 35–290		Luteal: 1–8.7

Immunoglobulin G, M, A (95% CI)	IgG	IgM	IgA
Cord blood	636–1,606 mg/dL	6.3–25 mg/dL	1.4–3.6 mg/dL
1 mo	251–906	20–87	1.3–53
2 mo	206–601	17–105	2.8–47
3 mo	176–581	24–89	4.6–46.0
4 mo	196–558	27–101	4.4–73.0
5 mo	172–814	33–108	8.1–84.0
6 mo	215–704	35–102	8.1–68.0
7–9 mo	217–904	34–126	11–90
10–12 mo	294–1,069	41–149	16–84
1 yr	345–1,213	43–173	14–106
2 yr	424–1,051	48–168	14–123
3 yr	441–1,135	47–200	22–159
4–5 yr	463–1,236	43–196	25–154
6–8 yr	633–1,280	48–207	33–202
9–10 yr	608–1,572	52–242	45–236
Adult	639–1,349	56–352	70–312

Immunoglobulin G subclasses (mg/dL) 95% Cl

Age	IgG1	IgG2	IgG3	IgG4
0–1 yr	190–620	30–140	9–62	6–63
1–2 yr	230–710	30–170	11–98	4–43
2–3 yr	280–830	40–240	6–130	3–120
3–4 yr	350–790	50–260	9–98	5–180
4–6 yr	360–810	60–310	9–160	9–160
6–8 yr	280–1,120	30–630	40–250	11–620
8–10 yr	280–1,740	80–550	22–320	10–170
10–13 yr	270–1,290	110–550	13–250	7–530
13 yr to adult	280–1,020	60–790	14–240	11–330

(continued)

BLOOD (Cont.)			
Test	Conventional Units Reference Range	Conversion Factor	SI Units Reference Range
Immunoglobulin E (IU/mL) (95% CI)			
0 d	0.04–1.28		
6 wk	0.08–6.12		
3 mo	0.18–3.76		
6 mo	0.44–16.3		
9 mo	0.76–7.31		
1 yr	0.80–15.2		
2 yr	0.31–29.5		
3 yr	0.19–16.9		
4 yr	1.07–68.9		
7 yr	1.03–161.3		
10 yr	0.98–570.6		
14 yr	2.06–195.2		
17–85 yr	1.53–114.0		
Insulin (fasting)	1.8–24.6 μU/mL		1.8–24.6 mU/L

Insulin-like growth factor–1 (IGF-1/somatomedin-C)	*Age*	*Male ng/mL (μg/L)*	*Female ng/mL (μg/L)*
	2 mo–6 yr	17–248 ng/mL (17–248 μg/L)	17–248 ng/mL (17–248 μg/L)
	6–9 yr	88–474 (88–474)	88–474 (88–474)
	9–12 yr	110–565 (110–565)	117–771 (117–771)
	12–16 yr	202–957 (202–957)	261–1096 (261–1096)
	16–26 yr	182–780 (182–780)	182–780 (182–780)
	>26 yr	123–463 (123–463)	123–463 (123–463)

Test	Conventional Units Reference Range	Conversion Factor	SI Units Reference Range
Iron	Newborn: 100–250 μg/dL Infant: 40–100 Child: 50–120 Adult (M): 65–170 Adult (F): 50–170	μg/dL × 0.179 = μmol/L	Newborn: 18–45 μmol/L Infant: 7–18 Child: 9–22 Adult (M): 12–30 Adult (F): 9–30
Iron-binding capacity	Newborn: 150–240 μg/dL Infant: 200–400 Thereafter: 250–400	μg/dL × 0.179 = μmol/L	Newborn: 26.9–43.0 μmol/L Infant: 35.8–71.6 Thereafter: 44.8–71.6
Lactate	Venous: 5–20 mg/dL Arterial: 5–14	mg/dL × 0.111 = mmol/L	Venous: 0.55–2.2 mmol/L Arterial: 0.55–1.6
Lactate dehydrogenase	0–4 d: 290–775 U/L 4–10 d: 545–2,000 10 d–24 mo: 180–430 24 mo–12 yr 110–295 >12 yr: 100–190		0–4 d: 290–775 U/L 4–10 d: 545–2,000 10 d–24 mo: 180–430 24 mo–12 yr 110–295 >12 yr: 100–190
Lactate dehydrogenase-isoenzymes		*Percent of Total:* LD-1: 18–33 LD-2: 28–40 LD-3: 18–30 LD-4: 6–16 LD-5: 2–13	
Lead	<10 μg/dL	μg/dL × 0.0483 = μmol/L	<0.48 μmol/L
Lipase	1–5 yr: 18–98 U/L 6–12 yr: 21–120 13–18 yr: 26–144 Adult: 30–160		1–5 yr: 18–98 U/L 6–12 yr: 21–120 13–18 yr: 26–144 Adult: 30–160

LIPIDS high density lipoprotein (HDL) cholesterol	*Age*	*Males mg/dL (mmol/L) 95% CI*	*Females mg/dL (mmol/L) 95% CI*
	6–11 yr:	30–70 (0.77–1.80)	34–65 (0.88–1.68)
	12–14 yr:	30–65 (0.77–1.80)	30–65 (0.77–1.68)
	15–19 yr:	30–60 (0.77–1.80)	33–65 (0.85–1.68)

(continued)

	BLOOD (Cont.)		
Test	**Conventional Units Reference Range**	**Conversion Factor**	**SI Units Reference Range**
LIPIDS low density lipoprotein (LDL) cholesterol	*Age*	*Males mg/dL (mmol/L) 95% CI*	*Females mg/dL (mmol/L) 95% CI*
	6–11 yr:	60–140 (1.6–3.7)	60–150 (1.6–4)
	12–14 yr:	60–140 (1.6–3.7)	60–150 (1.6–4)
	15–19 yr:	60–140 (1.6–3.7)	60–150 (1.6–4)
LIPIDS very low density lipoprotein (VLDL) cholesterol	*Age*	*Males mg/dL (mmol/L) 95% CI*	*Females mg/dL (mmol/L) 95% CI*
	5–9 yr:	18 (0.47)	24 (0.62)
	10–13 yr:	22 (0.57)	23 (0.59)
	14–17 yr:	26 (0.67)	24 (0.62)
Luteinizing hormone	*Male:* Tanner I: 0.02–0.3 mIU/mL Tanner II: 0.2–4.9 Tanner III: 0.2–5 Tanner IV–V: 0.4–7.0 Adult: 1.5–9 *Female:* Tanner I: 0.02–0.18 mIU/mL Tanner II: 0.02–4.7 Tanner III: 0.10–12 Tanner IV–V: 0.4–11.7 Adult: Follicular: 29 Midcycle: 18–49 Luteal: 2–11	×1	*Male:* Tanner I: 0.02–0.3 U/L Tanner II: 0.2–4.9 Tanner III: 0.2–5 Tanner IV–V: 0.4–7.0 Adult: 1.5–9 *Female:* Tanner I: 0.02–0.18 U/L Tanner II: 0.02–4.7 Tanner III: 0.10–12 Tanner IV–V: 0.4–11.7 Adult: Follicular: 29 Midcycle: 18–49 Luteal: 2–11
Magnesium	1.3–2.0 mEq/L	mEq/L × 0.411 = mmol/L	0.53–0.82 mmol/L
Methemoglobin	<0.3 g/dL	g/dL × 154 = µmol/L	<46 µmol/L
Osmolality	285–295 mOsm/kg		285–295 mmol/kg
Partial thromboplastin time (activated) (APTT)	Preterm: 80–168 sec Term: 31.3–54.3 Child/adult: 26.6–40.3		
Phosphorus (inorganic)	0–5 d: 4.8–8.2 mg/dL 1–3 yr: 3.8–6.5 4–11 yr: 3.7–5.6 12–15 yr: 2.9–5.4 16–19 yr: 2.7–4.7	mg/dL × 0.323 = mmol/L	0–5 d: 1.55–2.65 mmol/L 1–3 yr: 1.25–2.1 4–11 yr: 1.2–1.8 12–15 yr: 0.95–1.75 16–19 yr: 0.90–1.50
Phytanic acid	<0.3% of total serum fatty acids		<0.003 fraction of total serum fatty acids
Potassium	<10 d: 4–6 mEq/L ≥10 d: 3.5–5.0		<10 d: 4–6 mmol/L ≥10 d: 3.5–5.0
Prealbumin	<5 days: 6–21 mg/dL 1–5 yrs: 14–30 6–9 yrs: 15–33 10–13 yrs: 20–36 14–19 yrs: 22–45		
Progesterone	*Tanner stage, M (ng/dL)* I: <10–33 II: <10–33 III: <10–48 IV: 10–108 V: 21–82 Adult: 13–97 *Tanner stage, F (ng/dL)* I: <10–33 II: <10–55 III: 10–450 IV: 10–1,300 V: 10–950 Adult: follicular, 15–70; luteal, 200–2,500	ng/dL × 0.032 = nmol/L	*Tanner stage, M (nmol/L)* I: <0.32–1.05 II: <0.32–1.05 III: <0.32–3.43 IV: 0.32–3.43 V: 0.67–2.61 Adult: 0.410–3.08 *Tanner state, F (nmol/L)* I: <0.32–1.05 II: <0.32–1.75 III: 0.32–14.31 IV: <0.32–41.34 V: <0.32–30.21 Adult: follicular, 0.48–2.23; luteal, 6.36–79.50

(continued)

BLOOD (Cont.)			
Test	**Conventional Units Reference Range**	**Conversion Factor**	**SI Units Reference Range**
Prolactin	Newborn: <200 ng/mL Adult (M): 3–18 Adult (F): 3–24	ng/mL × 0.0426 = nmol/L	Newborn: <8.52 nmol/L Adult (M): 0.13–0.77 Adult (F): 0.13–1.02
Protein, total	Preterm: 4.3–7.6 g/dL Term: 4.6–7.4 1–3 mo: 4.7–7.4 3–12 mo: 5.0–7.5 1–15 yr: 6.5–8.6	g/dL × 10 = g/L	Preterm: 43–76 g/L Term: 46–74 g/L 1–3 mo: 47–74 3–12 mo: 50–75 1–15 yr: 65–86
Prothrombin time (PT)	Preterm: 11–17 sec Term: 10–16 sec Adult: 10 sec		
Pyruvate	0.3–0.9 mg/dL	mg/dL × 0.11 mmol/L	0.03–0.10 mmol/L
Renin, plasma activity (PRA)	ng/mL/hr: Cord: 4–32 1–7 d: 2–35 Child, normal Na diet, supine: 1–12 mo: 2.4–37 1–3 yr: 1.7–11.2 3–5 yr: 1–6.5 5–10 yr: 0.5–5.9 10–15 yr: 0.5–3.3 Adult, normal Na diet: Supine: 0.2–1.6 Standing (4 hr): 0.7–3.3		μg/L/hr: Cord: 4–32 1–7 d: 2–35 Child, normal Na diet, supine: 1–12 mo: 2.4–37 1–3 yr: 1.7–11.2 3–5 yr: 1–6.5 5–10 yr: 0.5–5.9 10–15 yr: 0.5–3.3 Adult, normal Na diet: Supine: 0.2–1.6 Standing (4 hr): 0.7–3.3
Sodium	Premature: 130–140 mEq/L Older: 135–146		Premature: 130–140 mmol/L Older: 135–146
Testosterone, free	Prepubertal Children: 0.15–0.6 pg/mL Men: 52–280 Women: 1.1–6.3		
Testosterone, total	Prepubertal Children: 0.15–0.6 pg/mL Men: 275–875 Women: 23–75 Pregnant Women: 35–195		
Thyroid-stimulating hormone (TSH)	Cord blood: <2.5–17.4 mlU/mL 1–3 d: <2.5–13.3 1–4 wk: 0.6–10.0 1–12 mo: 0.6–6.3 1–15 yr: 0.6–6.3 16–50 yr: 0.2–7.6		Cord blood: <2.5–17.4 μU/mL 1–3 d: <2.5–13.3 1–4 wk: 0.6–10.0 1–12 mo: 0.6–6.3 1–15 yr: 0.6–6.3 16–50 yr: 0.2–7.6
Thyroxine (T_4), total	Cord: 7.4–13.0 μg/dL <1 mo: 7.0–22.6 1 mo to 1 yr: 7.2–16.5 1–5 yr: 7.3–15.0 5–10 yr: 6.4–13.3 10–15 yr: 5.6–11.7 Adult: 4.3–12.5	μg/dL × 12.9 = nmol/L	Cord: 95–168 nmol/L <1 mo: 90–292 1 mo to 1 yr: 93–213 1–5 yr: 94–194 5–10 yr: 83–172 10–15 yr: 72–151 Adult: 55–161
Thyroxine (T_4), free	1–10 d: 0.6–2.0 ng/dL >10 d: 0.7–1.7	ng/dL × 12.9 = pmol/L	1–10 d: 7.74–25.8 pmol/L >10 d: 9.03–21.9
Transferrin	Newborn: 130–275 mg/dL 3 mo–10 yr: 203–360 Adult: 215–380	mg/dL × 0.1 = g/L	Newborn: 1.30–2.75 g/L 3 mo–10 yr: 2.03–3.60 Adult: 2.15–3.80

(continued)

BLOOD (Cont.)			
Test	**Conventional Units Reference Range**	**Conversion Factor**	**SI Units Reference Range**
Triglycerides (fasting)	Cord Blood: (M): 10–98 mg/dL (F): 10–98 0–5 yr: (M): 30–86 (F): 32–99 6–11 yr: (M): 31–108 (F): 35–114 12–15 yr: (M): 36–138 (F): 41–138 16–19 yr: (M): 40–163 (F): 40–128 20–29 yr: (M): 44–185 (F): 40–128	mg/dL × 0.1 = g/L	Cord Blood: (M): 0.10–0.98 g/L (F): 0.10–0.98 0–5 yr: (M): 0.30–0.86 (F): 0.32–0.99 6–11 yr: (M): 0.31–1.08 (F): 0.35–1.14 12–15 yr: (M): 0.36–1.38 (F): 0.41–1.38 16–19 yr: (M): 0.40–1.63 (F): 0.40–1.28 20–29 yr: (M): 0.44–1.85 (F): 0.40–1.28
Triiodothyronine (T_3)	Cord: 15–75 ng/dL <1 mo: 32–240 1 mo to 1 yr: 110–280 1–5 yr: 105–269 5–10 yr: 94–241 10–15 yr: 83–215 Adult: 70–204	ng/dL × 0.0153 = nmol/L	Cord: 0.23–1.16 nmol/L <1 mo: 0.49–3.70 1 mo to 1 yr: 1.70–4.31 1–5 yr: 1.62–4.14 5–10 yr: 1.45–3.71 10–15 yr: 1.28–3.31 Adult: 1.08–3.14
Triiodothyronine resin uptake (T_3RU)	25%–35%		0.25–0.35 fractional uptake
Urea nitrogen	Premature (<1 wk): 3–25 mg/dL Newborn: 4–12 Infant/Child: 5–18 Adult: 6–20	mg/dL × 0.357 = mmol/L	Premature (<1 wk): 1.1–8.9 mmol/L Newborn: 1.4–4.3 Infant/Child: 1.8–6.4 Adult: 2.1–7.1
Uric acid	0–2 yr: 2.4–6.4 mg/dL 2–12 yr: 2.4–5.9 12–14 yr: 2.4–6.4 Adult (M): 3.5–7.2 Adult (F): 2.4–6.4	mg/dL × 0.058 = mmol/L	0–2 yr: 0.14–0.38 mmol/L 2–12 yr: 0.14–0.35 12–14 yr: 0.14–0.38 Adult (M): 0.20–0.43 Adult (F): 0.14–0.38
Vitamin A (retinol)	Preterm: 13–46 μg/dL Full-term: 18–50 1–6 yr: 20–43 7–12 yr: 20–49 13–19 yr: 26–72	μg/dL × 0.0349 = μmol/L	Preterm: 0.46–1.61 μmol/L Full-term: 0.63–1.75 1–6 yr: 0.7–1.5 7–12 yr: 0.9–1.7 13–19 yr: 0.9–2.5
Vitamin B_1 (thiamine)	5.3–7.9 μg/dL	μg/dL × 0.03 = μmol/L	0.16–0.23 μmol/L
Vitamin B_2 (riboflavin)	3.7–13.7 μg/dL	μg/dL × 26.5 = μmol/L	98–363 μmol/L
Vitamin B_6	3.6–18.0 ng/mL	ng/mL × 4.06 = nmol/L	14.6–72.8 nmol/L
Vitamin B_{12} (cobalamin)	Newborn: 160–1,300 pg/mL Child/Adult: 200–835	pg/mL × 0.74 = pmol/L	Newborn: 118–959 pmol/L Child/Adult: 148–616
Vitamin C	0.2–2.0 mg/dL	mg/dL × 56.8 = μmol/L	11.4–113.6 μmol/L
Vitamin D (1,25 dihydroxy)	25–45 pg/mL	pg/mL × 2.4 = pmol/L	60–108 pmol/L
Vitamin E	<11 yr: 3–15 mg/L >11 yr: 5–20	mg/L × 2.32 = μmol/L	<11 yr: 7–35 μmol/L >11 yr: 11.6–46.4
Zinc	1–5 yr: 67–118 μg/dL 6–9 yr: 77–107 10–14 yr: 76–118 14–19 yr: 60–117	μg/dL × 0.153 = μmol/L	1–5 yr: 10.3–18.1 μmol/L 6–9 yr: 11.8–16.4 10–14 yr: 11.6–18.0 14–19 yr: 9.2–17.9

URINE			
Test	Conventional Units Reference Range	Conversion Factor	SI Units Reference Range
Albumin	4–16 yr (M): 3.35–13.15 mg/24 hr/1.73 m² 4–16 yr (F): 3.75–18.34 mg/24 hr/1.73 m²		
Aminolevulinic acid	1–7 mg/24 hr	mg/24 hr × 7.63 = μmol/24 hr	8.53 μmol/24 hr
Calcium	<6 mg/kg/24 hr	mg/kg/24 hr × 0.025 = mmol/kg/24 hr	<0.15 mmol/kg/24 hr
Catecholamines	*Epinephrine:* 0–1 yr: 0–2.5 μg/24 hr 1–2 yr: 0–3.5 2–4 yr: 0–6 4–10 yr: 0.2–10 10–15 yr: 0.5–20 Adult: 0–20	μg/24 hr × 5.46 = nmol/24 hr	*Epinephrine:* 0–1 yr: 0–14 nmol/24 hr 1–2 yr: 0–19 2–4 yr: 0–33 4–10 yr: 1–55 10–15 yr: 3–109 Adult: 0–109
	Norepinephrine: 0–1 yr: 0–10 μg/24 hr 1–2 yr: 1–17 2–4 yr: 4–29 4–7 yr: 8–45 7–10 yr: 13–65 10–15 yr: 15–80 Adult: 15–80	μg/24 hr × 5.91 = nmol/24 hr	*Norepinephrine:* 0–1 yr: 0–59 nmol/24 hr 1–2 yr: 6–100 2–4 yr: 24–171 4–7 yr: 47–266 7–10 yr: 77–384 10–15 yr: 89–473 Adult: 89–473
	Dopamine: 0–1 yr: 0–85 μg/24 hr 1–2 yr: 10–140 2–4 yr: 40–260 4–15 yr: 65–400 Adult: 65–400	μg/24 hr × 6.53 = nmol/24 hr	*Dopamine:* 0–1 yr: 0–555 nmol/24 hr 1–2 yr: 65–914 2–4 yr: 261–1,697 4–15 yr: 424–2,612 Adult: 424–2,612
Copper	5–18 yr: 0.36–7.56 mg Cu/mol Cr	mg Cu/mol Cr × 15.7 = μmol Cu/mol Cr	5–18 yr: 6–119 μmol Cu/mol Cr
Coproporphyrin	<200 μg/24 hr	μg/24 hr × 1.527 = nmol/24 hr	<300 nmol/24 hr
Cortisol (free)	Child: 2–27 μg/24 hr Adolescent: 5–55 Adult: 10–100	μg/24 hr × 2.759 = nmol/24 hr	Child: 5.5–7.4 nmol/24 hr Adolescent: 14–152 Adult: 27–276
Creatinine	Premature: 8.1–15.0 mg/kg/24 hr Full term: 10.4–19.7 1–6 yr: 10–15 7–15 yr (M): 5.2–41 7–15 yr (F): 11.5–29.1	mg/kg/24 hr × 8.84 = μmol/kg/24 hr	Premature: 72–132 μmol/kg/24 hr Full term: 92–174 1–6 yr: 88–132 7–15 yr (M): 46–362 7–15 yr (F): 101–257
Cystine	5–31 mg/24 hr	mg/24 hr × 8.33 = μmol/24 hr	40–260 μmol/24 hr
Dehydroepiandosterone	<5 yr: <0.1 mg/24 hr 6–9 yr: <0.2 10–15 yr: <0.4 Adult (M): <2.3 Adult (F): <1.2	mg/24 hr × 3.5 = μmol/24 hr	<5 yr: <0.3 μmol/24 hr 6–9 yr: <0.7 10–15 yr: <1.4 Adult (M): <8.0 Adult (F): <4.2
Fluoride	<1 mg/24 hr	mg/24 hr × 52.63 = μmol/24 hr	<53 μmol/24 hr

Homovanillic acid (values are per 24 hr)	Age	*95th percentile* mg/g Cr (mmol/mol Cr)	*100th percentile* mg/g Cr (mmol/mol Cr)
	0–1 yr	32.6 (20)	76.9 (48)
	2–4 yr	22 (14)	58.8 (37)
	5–9 yr	15.1 (9)	33.2 (21)
	10–19 yr	12.8 (8)	44.2 (27)
	>19 yr	7.6 (5)	9.4 (6)

(continued)

URINE (Cont.)			
Test	Conventional Units Reference Range	Conversion Factor	SI Units Reference Range
Metanephrines (free plus conjugated)	0–3 mo: 202–708 μg/g creatinine 4–6 mo: 156–572 7–9 mo: 150–526 10–12 mo: 148–651 1–2 yr: 40–526 2–6 yr: 74–504 6–10 yr: 121–319 10–16 yr: 46–307	μg/g creatinine × 0.574 = mmol/mol creatinine	0–3 mo: 116–407 mmol/mol creatinine 4–6 mo: 89–328 7–9 mo: 86–302 10–12 mo: 85–374 1–2 yr: 23–302 2–6 yr: 42–289 6–10 yr: 69–183 10–16 yr: 26–176

Osmolality	50–1,200 mOsm/kg H_2O
	On average fluid intake:
	  300–900
	After 12 hr fluid restriction:
	  >850		

Oxalate	20–60 mg/24 hr	mg/24 hr × 11 = μmol/24 hr	220–660 μmol/24 hr
Porphobilinogen	0–2 mg/24 hr	mg/24 hr × 4.42 = μmol/24 hr	0–8.8 μmol/24 hr
Potassium	6–10 yr: Male: 17–54 mEq/24 hr Female: 8–37 10–14 yr: Male: 22–57 Female: 18–58 Adult: 25–125	mEq/24 hr × 1 = mmol/24 hr	6–10 yr: Male: 17–54 mmol/24 hr Female: 8–37 10–14 yr: Male: 22–57 Female: 18–58 Adult: 25–125
Pregnanetriol	2 wk–2 yr: 0.02–0.2 mg/24 hr 2–5 yr: <0.5 5–15 yr: <1.5 >15 yr: <2	mg/24 hr × 2.97 = μmol/24 hr	2 wk–2 hr: 0.06–0.6 μmol/24 hr 2–5 yr: <1.5 5–15 yr: <4.5 >15 yr: <5.9
Protein, total	1–14 mg/dL 50–80 mg/24 hr (at rest) <250 mg/24 hr after intense exercise	×10	10–140 mg/dL 50–80 mg/24 hr (at rest) <250 mg/24 hr after intense exercise
Steroids 17-OH-corticosteroid	0-1 yr: 0.5–1 mg/24 hr Child: 1–5.6 Adult Male: 3–10 Adult Female: 2–8 OR 2–6.6 mg/g creatinine	mg/24 hr × 2.76 = μmol/24 hr mg/g creatinine × 0.312 = mmol/mol creatinine	0–1 yr: 1.4–2.8 μmol/24 hr Child: 2.8–15.5 Adult Male: 8.3–27.6 Adult Female: 5.5–22.1 OR 0.62–2.03 mmol/mol creatinine
17-ketosteroids	1–4 yr: <2 mg/24 hr 5–9 yr: <3 10–12 yr: 1–5 12–14 yr: 1–6 14–16 yr (M): 3–13 14–16 yr (F): 2–8 Adult (M): 10–25 Adult (F): 6–14	mg/24 hr × 3.47 = μmol/24 hr	1–4 yr: <7 μmol/24 hr 5–9 yr: <10 10–12 yr: 3–17 12–14 yr: 3–21 14–16 yr (M): 10–45 14–16 yr (F): 8–28 Adult (M): 35–87 Adult (F): 21–49
Uric acid	250–750 mg/24 hr	mg/24 hr × 0.0059 = mmol/24 hr	1.48–4.43 mmol/24 hr

Vanillylmandelic acid	Age	95th percentile mg/g Cr (mmol/mol Cr)	100th percentile mg/g Cr (mmol/mol Cr)
	0–1 yr	18.8 (11)	59. (34)
	2–4 yr	11 (6)	20.8 (12)
	5–9 yr	8.3 (5)	9.4 (5)
	10–19 yr	8.2 (5)	13.9 (8)
	>19 yr	6 (3)	8.3 (5)

AGE-SPECIFIC INDICES FOR HEMATOLOGY

Age	Hgb (g/dL) Mean	Hgb (g/dL) −2SD[a]	Hematocrit (%) Mean	Hematocrit (%) −2SD[a]	MCV (fl) Mean	MCV (fl) −2SD[a]	MCHC (g/dL, RBC) Mean	MCHC (g/dL, RBC) −2SD[a]	Reticulo-cyte (%)	Platelets (1,000 per mm³) Mean (±SD) [Range]
18–21 wk gestation[b]	11.69	9.2	37.3	28.7	131.1	109.2				234 (±57)
22–25 wk gestation[b]	12.2	9	38.59	30.7	125.1	109.4				247 (±59)
26–29 wk gestation[b]	12.91	10.2	40.88	32	118.5	102.6				242 (±69)
>30 wk gestation[b]	13.64	9.2	43.55	29.2	114.4	95.7				232 (±87)
Term (cord blood)	16.5	13.5	51	42	108	98	33	30	3–7	290
1–3 days	18.5	14.5	56	45	108	95	33	29	1.8–4.6	192
1 wk	17.5	13.5	54	42	107	88	33	28	0–1	248
2 wk	16.5	12.5	51	39	105	86	33	28	0–1	252
1 mo	14	10	43	31	104	85	33	29	0–1	
2 mo	11.5	9	35	28	96	77	33	29	0–2	280
3–6 mo	11.5	9.5	35	29	91	74	33	30	0.7–2.3	
6–24 mo	12	10.5	36	33	78	70	33	30		[150–300]
2–6 yr	12.5	11.5	37	34	81	75	34	31	0.5–1.0	[150–300]
6–12 yr	13.5	11.5	40	35	86	77	34	31	0.5–1.0	[150–300]
12–18 yr (male)	14.5	13	43	37	88	78	34	31	0.5–1.0	[150–300]
12–18 yr (female)	14	12	41	36	90	78	34	31	0.5–1.0	[150–300]

[a]At −2 SD from mean, approximately 95% of the population is encompassed.
[b]Forestier F, Daffos F, Catherine N, Renard M, Andreaux JP. Developmental hematopoiesis in normal human fetal blood. *Blood* 1991;77:2360. Data compiled from normal reference values in Nathan DG, Orkin SH, Ginsburg D, Look AT. *Nathan and Oski's hematology of infancy and childhood*, 6th ed. Philadelphia: Saunders, 2003.

AGE-SPECIFIC WHITE BLOOD CELL DIFFERENTIAL

Age	Total Leukocytes[a] Mean	Total Leukocytes[a] Range[c] (±SD)	Neutrophils[b] Mean	Neutrophils[b] Range[c]	Neutrophils[b] Percent	Lymphocytes Mean	Lymphocytes Range[c]	Lymphocytes Percent	Monocytes Mean	Monocytes Percent	Eosinophils Mean	Eosinophils Percent
18–21 wk gestation[d]	2.57[e]	(0.42)			6			88		3.5		2
22–25 wk gestation[d]	3.73[e]	(2.17)			6.5			87		3.5		3
26–29 wk gestation[d]	4.08[e]	(0.84)			8.5			85		3.5		4
>30 wk gestation[d]	6.4[e]	(2.99)			23			68.5		3.5		5
Birth	18.1	9–30	11	6–26	61	5.5	2–11	31	1.1	6	0.4	2
12 hr	22.8	13–38	15.5	6–28	68	5.5	2–11	24	1.2	5	0.5	2
24 hr	18.9	9.4–34.0	11.5	5–21	61	5.8	2.0–11.5	31	1.1	6	0.5	2
1 wk	12.2	5–21	5.5	1.5–10.0	45	5	2–17	41	1.1	9	0.5	4
2 wk	11.4	5–20	4.5	1.0–9.5	40	5.5	2–17	48	1	9	0.4	3
1 mo	10.8	5.0–19.5	3.8	1–9	35	6	2.5–16.5	56	0.7	7	0.3	3
6 mo	11.9	6.0–17.5	3.8	1.0–8.5	32	7.3	4.0–10.5	61	0.6	5	0.3	3
1 yr	11.4	6.0–17.5	3.5	1.5–8.5	31	7	4.0–10.5	61	0.6	5	0.3	3
2 yr	10.6	6–17	3.5	1.5–8.5	33	6.3	3.0–9.5	59	0.5	5	0.3	3
4 yr	9.1	5.5–15.5	3.8	1.5–8.5	42	4.5	2–8	50	0.5	5	0.3	3
6 yr	8.5	5.0–14.5	4.3	1.5–8.0	51	3.5	1.5–7.0	42	0.4	5	0.2	3
8 yr	8.3	4.5–13.5	4.4	1.5–8.0	53	3.3	1.5–6.8	39	0.4	4	0.2	2
10 yr	8.1	4.5–13.5	4.4	1.8–8.0	54	3.1	1.5–6.5	38	0.4	4	0.2	2
16 yr	7.8	4.5–13.0	4.4	1.8–8.0	57	2.8	1.2–5.2	35	0.4	5	0.2	3
21 yr	7.4	4.5–11.0	4.4	1.8–7.7	59	2.5	1.0–4.8	34	0.3	4	0.2	3

[a]Leukocytes in thousands per cubic millimeter.
[b]Neutrophils include band cells at all ages and a small amount of metamyelocytes and myelocytes in the first few days of life.
[c]Ranges are 95% Cl.
[d]Forestier F, Daffos, F, Catherine N, Renard M, Andreaux JP. Developmental hematopoiesis in normal human fetal blood. *Blood* 1991;77:2360.
[e]Corrected for nucleated red blood cells.
Data compiled from normal reference values in Nathan DG, Orkin SH, Ginsburg D, Look AT. *Nathan and Oski's hematology of infancy and childhood*, 6th ed. Philadelphia: Saunders, 2003.

CEREBROSPINAL FLUID								
Cell Count Range								

Preterm: 0–25 WBC × 10^6 cells per liter (57% polymorphonuclears)
Term: 0–22 WBC × 10^6 cells per liter (61% polymorphonuclears)
Child: 0–7 WBC × 10^6 cells per liter (5% polymorphonuclears)

	Cell Count Percentiles							
	Total WBC			Polymorphonuclears			Monocytes		
Age	25%	50%	75%	25%	50%	75%	25%	50%	75%
<6 wk	0.50	2.57	5.16	0	0	2.42	0	0.83	2.71
6 wk to 3 mo	0.34	1.86	3.75	0	0	0.66	0	0.96	2.78
3–6 mo	0	1.11	2.31	0	0	0.40	0	0.43	1.64
6–12 mo	0.41	1.47	3.25	0	0	0.52	0.03	0.93	2.32
>12 mo	0	0.68	1.82	0	0	0	0	0.25	1.45

Test	Conventional Units References Range	SI Reference Range
Glucose	Preterm: 24–63 mg/dL Term: 34–119 Child: 40–80	Preterm: 1.3–3.5 mmol/L Term: 1.9–6.6 Child: 2.2–4.4
Protein	Preterm: 65–150 mg/dL Term: 20–170 Child: 5–40	Preterm: 0.65–1.50 g/L Term: 0.20–1.70 Child: 0.05–0.40
Pressure	<200 mm H_2O	<200 mm H_2O

Suggested Readings

Berman RE, Kliegman RM, Jenson HB, *Nelson Textbook of Pediatrics,* 17th ed. Philadelphia: Saunders, 2004.

Burtis A, Ashwood ER. *Tietz textbook of clinical chemistry,* 3rd ed. Philadelphia: Saunders, 1999.

Gunn VL, Nechyba C, eds. *The Harriet Lane handbook,* 16th ed. Philadelphia: Mosby, 2002.

Joliff CR, Cost KM, Stivrins PC, et al. Reference intervals for serum IgG, IgA, IgM, C3, and C4 as determined by rate nephelometry. *Clin Chem* 1982;28: 126.

Kjellman NM, Johansson SG, Roth A. Serum IgE levels in healthy children quantified by a sandwich technique (PRIST). *Clin Allergy* 1976;6:51.

Meites S, ed. *Pediatric clinical chemistry,* 3rd ed. Washington, DC: American Association for Clinical Chemistry, 1989.

Metric Commission Canada Sector 9.10 Health and Welfare. *SI manual in health care,* 2nd ed. Ottawa: Metric Commission Canada, 1982.

Nathan DG, Orkin SH, Ginsburg D, Look AT. *Nathan and Oski's hematology of infancy and childhood,* 6th ed. Philadelphia: Saunders, 2003.

Schur PH. IgG subclasses—a review. *Ann Allergy* 1987;58:89.

Tietz NW. *Clinical Guide to Laboratory Tests,* 3rd ed. WB Saunders. Philadelphia, PA, 1995.

Johns Hopkins Medical Laboratories, Department of Pathology, March 2002.

Wallach J. *Interpretation of Diagnostic Tests,* 7th ed. Lippincott, Williams and Wilkins. Philadelphia, 2000.

Zetterstrom O, Johansson SG. IgE concentrations measured by PRIST in serum of healthy adults and in patients with respiratory allergy. *Allergy* 1981;36:537.

APPENDIX B ■ DYSMORPHOLOGY: GENETIC SYNDROMES AND ASSOCIATIONS

AMY FELDMAN LEWANDA, SIMEON A. BOYADJIEV, AND ETHYLIN WANG JABS

A pediatrician is often called on to evaluate a child with congenital abnormalities. Knowledge of patterns of anomalies or malformations is essential in making a syndromic diagnosis. A *syndrome* is a constellation of features that occur together and have a common cause. An *association* describes the sporadic occurrence of two or more features more often than their individual frequencies would suggest. The underlying cause of such associations is unknown. A *sequence* defines a condition that results from a single initiating defect leading to a series of subsequent abnormalities. Most of the conditions reviewed in this appendix have a genetic basis and are caused by chromosomal abnormalities or single-gene defects. Several other conditions are caused by environmental effects *in utero.* As more becomes known about their molecular etiology, the distinctions between traditional groupings will change.

An accurate diagnosis allows the practitioner to identify organ systems that may be involved, monitor for potential complications, and predict the prognosis for a patient, as well as identify other family members at risk. For example, recognition of trisomy 18 in a newborn alerts the pediatrician to the poor outcome associated with this condition. The diagnosis of Marfan syndrome allows for timely screening for heart disease.

This appendix provides information and illustrations for 66 representative conditions; these are followed by a listing of conditions with similar system involvement as an aid for differential diagnosis. Many additional conditions not detailed in this chapter are included in these lists. More extensive compendiums and descriptions are available in Jones's *Smith's Recognizable Patterns of Human Malformation* (Saunders), Gorlin et al.'s *Syndromes of the Head and Neck* (Oxford University Press), and Online Mendelian Inheritance in Man (http://www.ncbi.nlm.nih.gov/Omim/).

Amniotic Band Sequence, or Disruption Complex

Key Features

Facial clefting
Annular constriction of limbs or digits
Limb or digital amputations
Pseudosyndactyly
Strands of amnion on infant or placenta

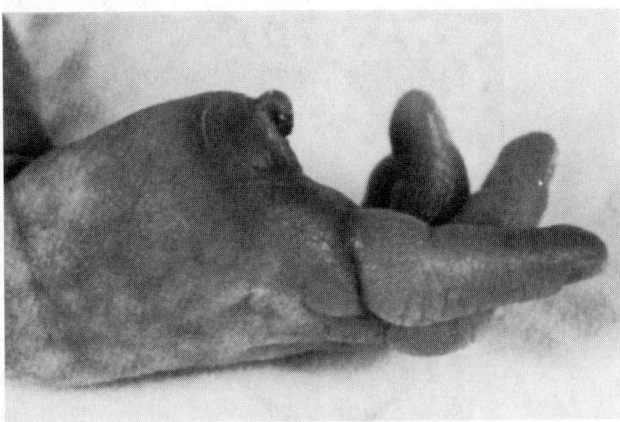

Other Finding

Features of fetal akinesia caused by constriction

Comments. Amniotic band sequence occurs in 1 in 1,200 to 15,000 newborns. Elevated amniotic alpha-fetoprotein levels often are found. Due to the variable nature of this disruption sequence, findings may be quite disparate between patients. Findings depend on the degree of entanglement, the body part(s) involved, and the timing of insult.

Performance. Affected individuals usually have normal intelligence. However, cases with cranial constriction and central nervous system defects would be expected to have some intellectual impairment.

Etiology. Occurrence of amniotic band sequence or disruption complex is usually sporadic, with a low risk of recurrence. Rare cases have been associated with maternal trauma during pregnancy. Amniotic bands have been released fetoscopically to relieve limb constriction *in utero*, and spontaneous resolution also has been reported.

Suggested Readings

Bodamer OA, Popek EJ, Bacino C. Atypical presentation of amniotic band sequence. *Am J Med Genet* 2001;100:100.
Keswani SG, et al. In utero limb salvage: fetoscopic release of amniotic bands for threatened limb amputation. *J Pediatr Surg* 2003;38:848.
Pagon RA. Congenital anomalies and aberrant tissue bands. *Am J Med Genet* 1987;27:491.
Pedersen TK, Thompsen SG. Spontaneous resolution of amniotic bands. *Ultrasound Obstet Gynecol* 2001;18:673.

Diabetic Embryopathy (Infant of a Diabetic Mother)

Key Features

Macrosomia
Cardiac septal hypertrophy
Other congenital heart disease (ventricular septal defect [VSD])
Caudal regression (hypoplasia of sacrum and lower extremities)
Hypoglycemia, hypocalcemia in the newborn period

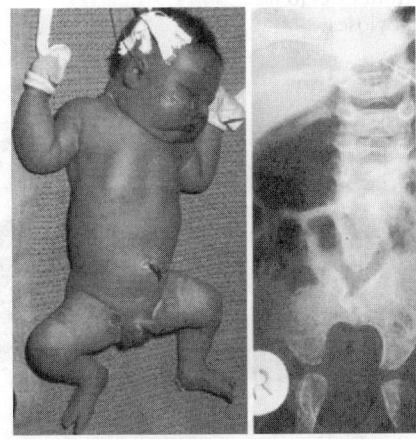

Other Findings

Malformation of external ear
Cleft lip, palate, or both
Rib and vertebral defects
Single umbilical artery
Central nervous system abnormalities

Comments. The rate of fetal complications appears to be higher in constitutional diabetics than in women who become diabetic only during pregnancy (gestational diabetics). Because of the macrosomia, these infants are at higher risk for birth trauma and birth asphyxia, which occurs in 25%.

Performance. Mental retardation is not significantly increased; however, an increased risk exists for cerebral palsy and epilepsy. Such impairments are believed to be on the basis of birth trauma, asphyxia, pregnancy complications, or central nervous system defects.

Etiology. Maternal hyperglycemia during pregnancy is the cause.

Suggested Readings

Grix A. Malformations in infants of diabetic mothers. *Am J Med Genet* 1982; 13:131.
Kousseff BG. Diabetic embryopathy. *Curr Opin Pediatr* 1999;11:348.
Martinez-Frias ML. Epidemiological analysis of outcomes of pregnancy in diabetic mothers: identification of the most characteristic and most frequent congenital anomalies. *Am J Med Genet* 1994;51:108.
Neave C. Congenital malformation in offspring of diabetics. *Perspect Pediatr Pathol* 1984;8:213.
Schwartz R, Teramo KA. Effects of diabetic pregnancy on the fetus and newborn. *Semin Perinatol* 2000;24:120.

Fetal Akinesia Deformation Sequence (Pena-Shokeir Syndrome)

Key Features

Polyhydramnios
Growth retardation
Hypertelorism
Low-set, malformed ears
Micrognathia
Pulmonary hypoplasia
Camptodactyly
Rocker-bottom or club feet
Multiple ankyloses

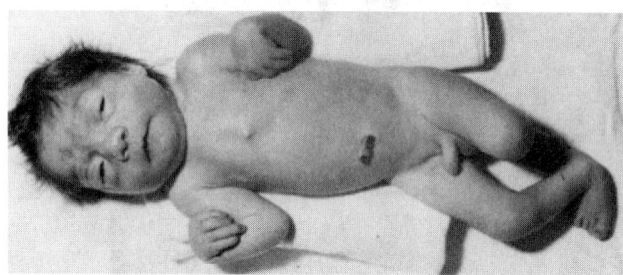

Other Findings

Decreased flexion creases on fingers and palms
Short umbilical cord
Cryptorchidism

Comments. Almost one-third of fetuses with fetal akinesia deformation sequence are stillborn, and the pulmonary hypoplasia is a cause of significant mortality in live-born infants. Physical features may be confused with those seen in trisomy 18.

Performance. High morbidity and mortality occur. Performance prognosis depends in part on the etiology of this phenotype in the particular patient, because multiple causes exist for decreased *in utero* movement (see following discussion).

Etiology. Heterogeneous causes of decreased fetal movement include neuromuscular disorders, severe prenatal anoxic insult, cortical or cerebellar abnormalities, and fetal constraint. Asymptomatic maternal myasthenia also has been reported as a cause. The recurrence risk varies, but should be considered to be as high as 25% in the case of autosomal recessive etiologies. An autosomal dominant variant has been reported in an unaffected man who had four affected children by two wives, presumably caused by germinal mosaicism.

Suggested Readings

Brueton LA, et al. Asymptomatic maternal myasthenia as a cause of the Pena-Shokeir phenotype. *Am J Med Genet* 2000;92:1.
Hageman G, Willemse J, Van Ketel BA, et al. The heterogeneity of the Pena-Shokeir syndrome. *Neuropediatrics* 1987;18:45.
Ho NC. Monozygotic twins with fetal akinesia: the importance of clinicopathological work-up in predicting risks of recurrence. *Neuropediatrics* 2000; 31:252.
Vlaanderen W, Manschot TAJM, Vermuelen-Meiners C. A dominant-heredity variation of the Pena-Shokeir syndrome: a case report. *Eur J Obstet Gynecol Rep* 1991;40:163.
Witters I, Moerman P, Fryns JP. Fetal akinesia deformation sequence: a study of 30 consecutive in utero diagnoses. *Am J Med Genet* 2002;113:23.

Fetal Alcohol Syndrome

Key Features

Growth retardation
Microcephaly
Small palpebral fissures
Short nose
Smooth philtrum
Thin upper lip
Cardiac defects (VSD, atrial septal defect [ASD])
Hypoplastic fifth fingernails

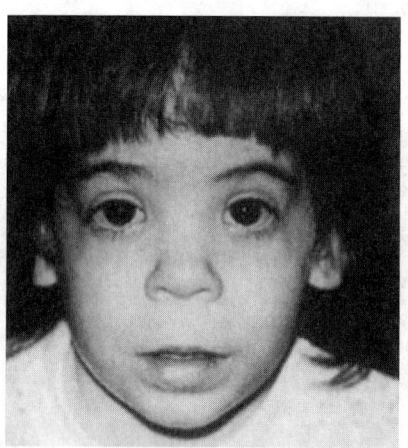

Other Findings

Ptosis
Microphthalmia
Optic nerve hypoplasia
Cleft lip or cleft palate
Cervical spine defects
Joint abnormalities
Short fourth and fifth metacarpals
Central nervous system abnormalities

Comments. Fetal alcohol syndrome is estimated to occur in 1 in 500 to 1,000 live births. Features of this condition range from mild (referred to as fetal alcohol effects) to severe (fetal alcohol syndrome). The degree of involvement depends in part on the amount of alcohol consumed during pregnancy, as well as the timing of exposure. Thirty percent to 50% of children of chronic alcoholic women (consumers of 6 to 8 drinks or more per day) are estimated to have mental retardation. Infants may present with tremulousness and irritability, and children may have fine motor dysfunction and hyperactivity.

Performance. Mental retardation, behavioral abnormalities, and language delays are common, and range in severity depending on the degree of prenatal exposure. The average IQ of an individual with fetal alcohol syndrome is 67.

Etiology. The maternal ingestion of alcohol during the pregnancy is the cause.

Suggested Readings

Johnson VP, Swayze W II, Sato Y, Andreasen NC. Fetal alcohol syndrome: craniofacial and central nervous system manifestations. *Am J Med Genet* 1996; 61:329.
Lewis DD, Woods SE. Fetal alcohol syndrome. *Am Fam Physician* 1994;50:1025.
Mattson SN, Schoenfeld AM, Riley EP. Teratogenic effects of alcohol on brain and behavior. *Alcohol Res Health* 2001;25:185.
Moore ES, et al. New perspectives on the face in fetal alcohol syndrome: what anthropometry tells us. *Am J Med Genet* 2002;109:249.

Fetal Rubella Syndrome/TORCH Infections

Key Features

Growth retardation
Microcephaly
Cataracts
Glaucoma
Deafness
Hepatomegaly
Thrombocytopenia

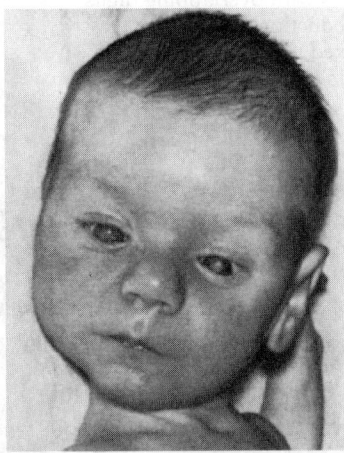

Other Findings

Corneal opacities and chorioretinitis
Interstitial pneumonia
Cardiac defects (patent ductus arteriosus [PDA], peripheral
  pulmonic stenosis, septal defects)
Obstructive jaundice
Hypospadias, cryptorchidism
Osteolytic metaphyseal lesions
Anemia
Diabetes mellitus

Comments. Fetal rubella syndrome is due to intrauterine rubella infection passed to the fetus during maternal infection. Other TORCH infections, including toxoplasmosis, cytomegalovirus (CMV), herpes simplex, and lymphocytic choriomeningitis virus can cause similar fetal damage, particularly involving the central nervous system. The most serious consequences of fetal rubella syndrome seem to occur with a first-trimester infection, and fetal death may occur. The risk of fetal infection in the first trimester is approximately 50%. Infection later in pregnancy is still a significant concern and is associated with growth deficiency, deafness, cardiac effects, and mental retardation. The incidence has been greatly reduced by widespread immunization for rubella. The clinical manifestations of severe fetal cytomegalovirus or toxoplasmosis infection may overlap those of fetal rubella syndrome.

Performance. Affected individuals have mild to moderate mental deficiency, with 60% having an IQ of less than 90, and 20% having an IQ of less than 70.

Etiology. Maternal infection with the rubella virus during pregnancy is the cause. A rare, autosomal recessive form of intracranial calcification and microcephaly mimicking the TORCH syndrome, called pseudo-TORCH syndrome or Baraitser-Reardon syndrome, also been described.

Suggested Readings

Hardy JB. Clinical and developmental aspects of congenital rubella. *Arch Otolaryngol* 1973;98:230.
Stegmann BJ, Carey JC. TORCH infections. Toxoplasmosis, other (syphilis, varicella-zoster, parvovirus B-19), rubella, cytomegalovirus (CMV), and *Herpes* infections. *Curr Womens Health Rep* 2002;2:253.
Vivarelli R, et al. Psuedo-TORCH syndrome or Baraitser-Reardon syndrome: diagnostic criteria. *Brain Dev* 2001;23:18.

Retinoic Acid Embryopathy (Accutane Embryopathy)

Key Features

Anotia, microtia
Ipsilateral facial nerve paralysis
Conotruncal heart defects (transposition of the great vessels, tetralogy of Fallot [TOF], double-outlet right ventricle, truncus arteriosus)
Central nervous system abnormalities (neuronal migration abnormalities, hypoplasia of posterior fossa structures)

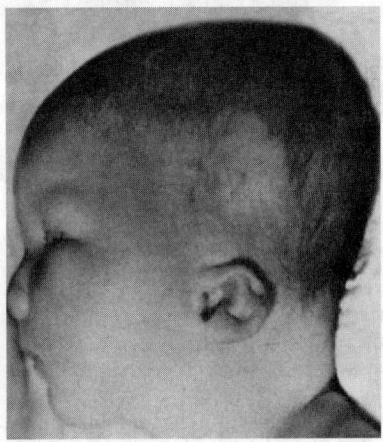

Other Findings

Microcephaly
Facial asymmetry
Hypertelorism
Depressed nasal bridge
Internal ear and temporal bone anomalies

Comments. Retinoic acid is highly teratogenic, with a 35% risk of embryopathy if the medication is continued past 15 days postconception. Teratogenic effects of the related topical compound, tretinoin (Retin-A) also have been reported.

Performance. Approximately 50% have an IQ of less than 85.

Etiology. A daily dose of Accutane from 0.5 to 1.5 mg/kg of maternal body weight is thought to be teratogenic.

Suggested Readings

Adams J, Lammer EJ. Neurobehavioral teratology of isotretinoins. *Reprod Toxicol* 1993;7:175.
Lammer EJ, Hayes EM, Schunior A, Holmes LB. Risk for major malformation among human fetuses exposed to isotretinoin (13-*cis*-retinoic acid). *Teratology* 1987;35:68A.
Moerike S, Pantzar JT, De Sa D. Temporal bone pathology in fetuses exposed to isotretinoin. *Pediatr Dev Pathol* 2002;5:405.
Selcen D, Seidman S, Nigro MA. Otocerebral anomalies associated with topical tretinoin use. *Brain Dev* 2000;22:218.

Trisomy 13 Syndrome (Patau Syndrome)

Key Features

Microcephaly with sloping forehead
Cutis aplasia of scalp (localized scalp defects)
Microphthalmia
Cleft lip, palate, or both
Postaxial polydactyly
Fingers flexed and overlapping
Nails hyperconvex
Cardiac malformations (VSD, PDA, ASD, dextrocardia)

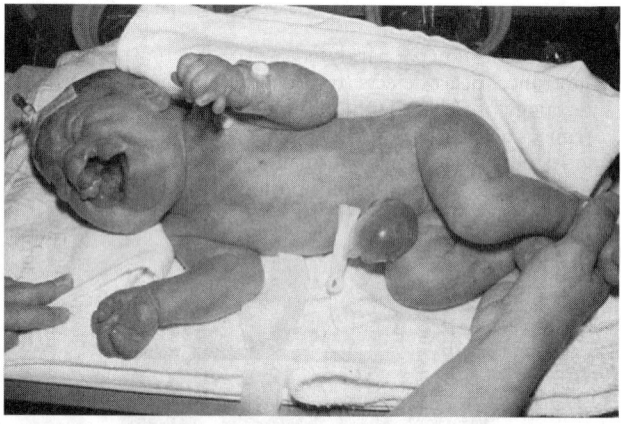

Other Findings

Low birth weight
Holoprosencephaly
Iris coloboma
Dysplastic ears
Omphalocele
Genital abnormalities (cryptorchidism, bicornuate uterus)
Polycystic kidney or other renal defects
Seizures, agenesis of corpus callosum

Comments. Trisomy 13 syndrome occurs in approximately 1 in 5,000 to 12,000 live births.

Performance. Prognosis is extremely poor, with 82% mortality within the first month and 5% survival at 6 months. Survivors have severe mental retardation, failure to thrive, and often have seizures.

Etiology. Trisomy for all or most of chromosome 13 is present. More than three-fourths of cases result from chromosomal nondisjunction and are associated with advanced maternal age. Trisomy 13 due to a translocation is another cause and imparts a higher recurrence risk for the parents (approximately 10% for a carrier). Five percent of all cases are mosaic (in which another normal cell line is present in addition to the trisomic cell line). Trisomy 13 constitutes approximately 1% of all recognized spontaneous abortions.

Suggested Reading

Baty BJ, Blackburn BL, Carey JC. Natural history of trisomy 18 and trisomy 13: I. Growth, physical assessment, medical histories, survival, and recurrence risk. *Am J Med Genet* 1994;49:175.

Trisomy 18 Syndrome (Edwards Syndrome)

Key Features

Low birth weight
Lack of subcutaneous fat
Prominent occiput
Narrow bifrontal diameter of forehead
Small palpebral fissures
Low-set, malformed ears
Micrognathia
Short sternum
Clenched hands with overlapping digits
Limited hip abduction
Short dorsiflexed halluces
Cardiac defects (VSD, ASD, PDA)

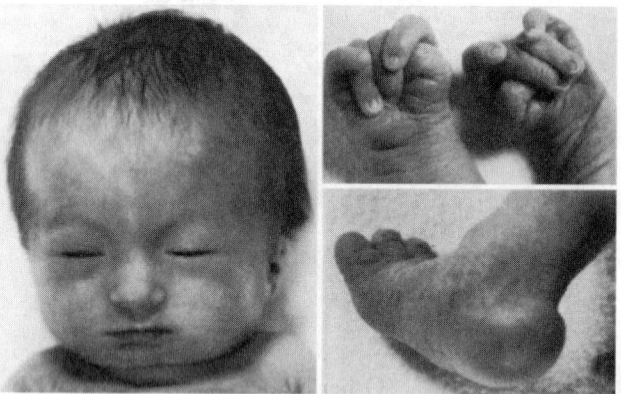

Other Findings

Microcephaly
Clefting of lip, palate, or both
Rocker-bottom feet
Cardiac valvular abnormalities, coarctation of the aorta
Abdominal, inguinal, or diaphragmatic hernia
Renal abnormalities
Genital abnormalities

Comments. Trisomy 18 syndrome occurs in approximately 1 in 3,000 to 7,000 live births. In the newborn period, babies have a poor suck and hypotonia, which is followed by failure to thrive and hypertonia.

Performance. Mortality is 50% in the first weeks of life, with less than 10% surviving the first year. Survivors have severe mental retardation.

Etiology. Trisomy for all or most of chromosome 18 is present. Eighty percent of cases are caused by chromosomal nondisjunction and are associated with advanced maternal age. If the trisomy is found to be caused by a translocation, parental karyotypes should be obtained to rule out an inherited defect. Trisomy may be partial (involving only a portion of the chromosome) or mosaic. Both would be expected to show a variable and generally less severe phenotype.

Suggested Reading

Carey JC. Health supervision and anticipatory guidance for children with genetic disorders (including specific recommendations for trisomy 21, trisomy 18 and neurofibromatosis I). *Pediatr Clin North Am* 1992;39:25.

Trisomy 21 Syndrome (Down Syndrome)

Key Features

Brachycephaly
Upslanting palpebral fissures*
Epicanthal folds
Flattened facial profile*
Small, rounded ears*
Excess nuchal skin*
Congenital cardiac anomalies in 40% to 50% (endocardial
    cushion defect, VSD, PDA)
Dysplasia of pelvis*
Hyperflexibility of joints*
Brachydactyly
Clinodactyly of fifth fingers (dysplasia of mid phalanx)*
Single transverse palmar crease (simian crease)*
Hypotonia,* poor Moro reflex*

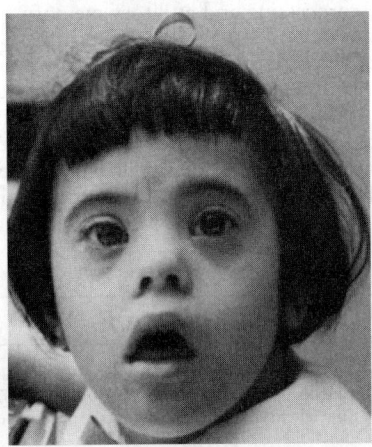

Other Findings

Short stature
Brushfield spots (speckling of the iris)
Wide gap between first and second toes

Comments. Trisomy 21 is the most common autosomal
chromosome abnormality in live-born infants and occurs in
approximately 1 in 700 to 800 newborns, with frequencies
increasing with advanced maternal age. In 90% of neonates
with Down syndrome, ten key features (indicated by asterisks)
are found. These features designate the Hall criteria for diagnosis. Also, an increased risk exists for duodenal atresia,
Hirschsprung disease, leukemia, hypothyroidism, atlantoaxial
instability, and premature aging.

Performance. All individuals are mentally retarded, although a considerable range of severity occurs (average IQ of
30 to 50). Early intervention programs have been beneficial
in helping these children to achieve to their maximum potential.

Etiology. Trisomy for all or part of chromosome 21 is
present. The majority of cases (almost 95%) are caused by
full trisomy, usually caused by maternal meiosis I nondisjunction, with the remainder made up of translocation cases (2%)
and mosaic Down syndrome (3%). Each parent of a child with
translocation Down syndrome should have karyotype analysis

to rule out the small possibility of being a translocation carrier,
which could carry as high as a 100% risk of recurrence for a
translocation involving both chromosomes 21.

Suggested Readings

American Academy of Pediatrics Committee on Genetics. Health supervision for
    children with Down syndrome. *Pediatrics* 1994;93:855.
Cooley WC, Graham JM. Down syndrome—an update and review for the pri-
    mary pediatrician. *Clin Pediatr* 1991;30:233.
Leonard S, Bower C, Petterson B, Leonard H. Medical aspects of school-aged
    children with Down syndrome. *Dev Med Child Neurol* 1999;41:683.

Turner Syndrome (XO)

Key Features

Short stature
Prominent or low-set ears
Excess nuchal skin (broad-based neck), low posterior hairline
Broad chest with widely spaced nipples
Cubitus valgus (increased carrying angle of arms)
Dorsal lymphedema of hands and feet (most evident in the
    newborn period)
Congenital heart disease (bicuspid aortic valve, coarctation
    of aorta)
Ovarian dysgenesis (primary or secondary amenorrhea)
Renal abnormalities (horseshoe kidney)
Hypertension

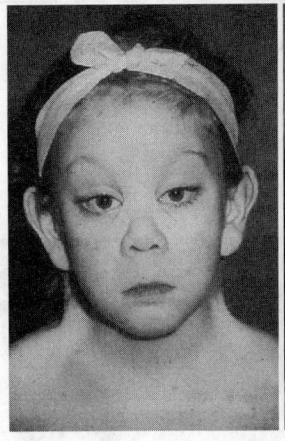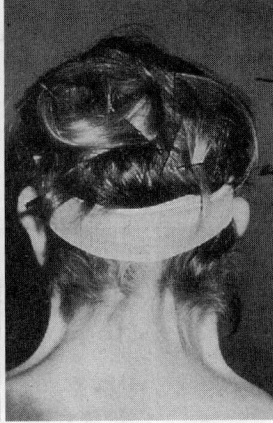

Other Findings

Ptosis, epicanthal folds
Narrow palate
Poor breast development
Hypoplastic, hyperconvex nails
Short fourth metacarpal/metatarsal
Pigmented nevi
Hearing impairment
Hypothyroidism

Comments. The attrition rate of Turner syndrome fetuses is
extremely high, with only approximately 5% to 10% surviving
to birth. The occurrence of Turner syndrome is 1 in 2,000 to

6,000 live births. The adult height when untreated is usually less than 144 cm. Ultimate height achievement has been improved greatly by combination therapy using growth hormone and oxandrolone. Additional hormonal treatment with estrogen may allow for menstrual cycling, although fertility remains greatly reduced.

Performance. Turner syndrome individuals are usually of normal intelligence, with a mean IQ of 90. They may have specific deficits in the areas of visual-spatial organization, psychomotor coordination, and social interaction.

Etiology. The loss of one X chromosome, leading to a 45,X chromosome complement, with the paternal sex chromosome most commonly lost, occurs in 50% of cases. Mosaicism may lead to more complex karyotypes, including 46,XX/45,X or 46,XY/45,X. A ring chromosome X, with loss of some associated genes, as well as isochromosome Xp, with loss of genetic material from the long arm, can lead to similar phenotypes depending on the amount of the deleted material. The finding of any Y chromosome material is significant because of the increased risk of gonadoblastoma.

Suggested Readings

Halac I, Zimmerman D. Coordinating care for children with Turner syndrome. *Pediatr Ann* 2004;33:189.
Saenger P, et al. Recommendations for the diagnosis and management of Turner syndrome. *J Clin Endocrinol Metab* 2001;86:3061.

Klinefelter Syndrome (XXY)

Key Features

Eunuchoid habitus
Gynecomastia
Hypogonadism
Long limbs

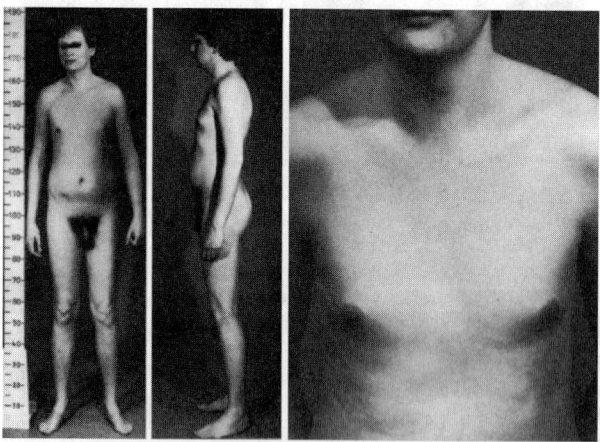

Other Findings

Scoliosis
Infertility

Comments. Klinefelter syndrome affects approximately 1 in 600 to 800 male infants. Individuals with the syndrome have a mean height of 177.4 cm and a reduced upper to lower segment ratio. Prepubertal males have no significant dysmorphism, but minor anomalies, such as clinodactyly or other skeletal defects and small penis may provide a clue to the diagnosis. Most boys have inadequate or partial puberty, and they should be considered for testosterone replacement therapy beginning in the early teen years. A delay in treatment with testosterone may lead to decreased muscle and bone mass, with subsequent risk of osteoporosis. This replacement therapy has traditionally been given intramuscularly, although transdermal delivery systems are now available. A relationship seems to exist with germ cell tumors and breast cancers. The frequency of breast carcinoma in men with Klinefelter syndrome is 66 times that of normal men and approaches the risk in women. The incidence of mediastinal teratomas is 34 to 40 times that of the general population.

Performance. IQ usually ranges from 85 to 95; with 12.8 mean years of education. Delayed speech and language development persists during childhood. Behavior problems, particularly immaturity and insecurity, are common, as are difficulties with auditory processing and auditory memory.

Etiology. The presence of an extra X chromosome is noted in boys and men. Most human trisomies originate from errors at maternal meiosis I. Klinefelter syndrome is an exception, because nearly one-half of all cases are due to paternal nondisjunction. Chromosomal mosaicism also may be seen, in which the XXY cell line is found in conjunction with a normal XY cell line, leading to an improved prognosis for testicular function.

Suggested Readings

Bojesen AS, et al. Prenatal and postnatal prevalence of Klinefelter syndrome: a national registry study. *J Clin Endocrinol Metab* 2003;88:622.
Simpson, JL et al. Klinefelter syndrome: expanding the phenotype and identifying new research directions. *Genet Med* 2003;5:460.

Fragile X Syndrome

Key Features

Macrocephaly
Long face
Large ears
High arched palate
Macroorchidism (after puberty)

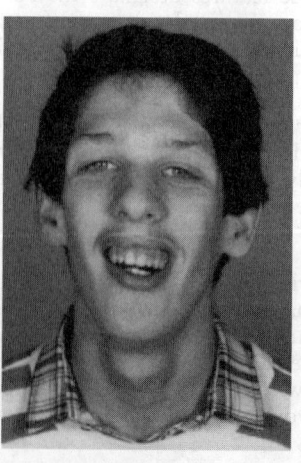

Other Findings

Prominent nasal bridge extending to the nasal tip
Prominent jaw
Joint laxity

Comments. Fragile X syndrome is believed to be the most common form of heritable mental retardation. Cytogenetic estimates of the prevalence of fragile X syndrome were as high as 1 in 1,039 males. However, population-based studies have established that the prevalence is probably between one in 6,000 to one in 4,000 in Caucasians males. Female heterozygotes have an increased risk for developmental delay and behavioral abnormalities, but are usually less affected than males. Fragile X syndrome should be considered in the differential diagnosis of developmental delay and early overgrowth in both sexes. The clinical diagnosis of fragile X mental retardation is unreliable, because dysmorphic features before puberty are subtle. Molecular diagnosis by polymerase chain reaction (PCR) and Southern blot is the confirmatory test and makes carrier detection and prenatal diagnosis possible.

Performance. All males affected with the fragile X syndrome have developmental delays, speech delays, or both. The IQs of affected boys usually range from 30 to 55. Hyperactivity and autistic behaviors are frequent, as are poor motor coordination and temper tantrums.

Etiology. Fragile X was first detected as a gap or constriction in the X chromosome when cells from patients were grown in folate-deficient media and karyotyped. This chromosomal abnormality is caused by an expansion of the familial mental retardation 1 (*FMR1*) gene at chromosome Xp27.3. The gene normally contains fewer than 59 trinucleotide CGG repeats. Individuals who carry 59 to 200 repeats are said to have the premutation and are at an increased risk for having affected children. It has been estimated that 1 in 259 females and 1 in 813 males in the general population are carriers of the fragile X premutation. Clinical symptoms of the fragile X syndrome become apparent when the repeat length has expanded to 200 or more repeats or when these repeats are methylated. The increased methylation of a gene can cause the gene to be inactivated.

Suggested Readings

Chiurazzi P, et al. Understanding the biological underpinnings of fragile X syndrome. *Curr Opin Pediatr* 2003;15:559.
Committee on Genetics, American Academy of Pediatrics. Health supervision for children with fragile X syndrome. *Pediatrics* 1996;98:297.
Crawford DC, et al. Prevalence of the fragile X syndrome in African Americans. *Am J Med Genet* 2002;110:226.
Dombrowski C, et al. Premutation and intermediate-size FMR1 alleles in 10572 males from the general population: loss of an AGG interruption is a late event in the generation of fragile X syndrome alleles. *Hum Mol Genet* 2002;11:371.

Cri du Chat Syndrome (5p-, deletion 5p)

Key Features

Low birth weight and growth retardation
Microcephaly
Rounded face
Epicanthal folds
Hypertelorism
High-pitched, catlike cry
Single transverse palmar crease
Hypotonia

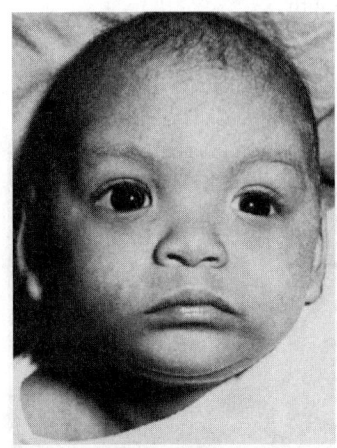

Other Findings

Dysplastic ears
Malocclusion
Congenital heart disease
Scoliosis

Comments. Cri du chat syndrome occurs in 1 in 20,000 to 50,000 live births. The cat-like cry characteristic of this disorder is believed to be caused by abnormal laryngeal development and tends to disappear with age.

Performance. Patients with cri du chat syndrome are profoundly mentally retarded. They have significant behavioral abnormalities including self-injurious and aggressive tendencies, hypersensitivity to sound, and repetitive movements. In general, they can, with appropriate intervention, learn to communicate their needs, interact with others, and become independently mobile.

Etiology. Deletion of the short arm of chromosome 5 is present. The critical region for the high-pitched cry appears to be at 5p15.3, with the remaining features caused by deletion of 5p15.2. In *de novo* deletions (which account for 85% of cases), the vast majority are paternal in origin. The remaining 15% of cases are caused by inherited unbalanced translocation from a carrier parent.

Suggested Readings

Cornish K, Bramble D. Cri du chat syndrome: genotype-phenotype correlations and recommendations for clinical management. *Dev Med Child Neurol* 2002;44:494.
Cornish KM, Pigram J. Developmental and behavioral characteristics of cri du chat syndrome. *Arch Dis Child* 1996;75:448.
Van Buggenhout GJ, et al. Cri du chat syndrome: changing phenotype in older patients. *Am J Med Genet* 2000;90:203.

Wolf-Hirschhorn Syndrome (4p-, deletion 4p)

Key Features

Growth retardation
Microcephaly

"Greek helmet" facies
High-arched eyebrows
Hypertelorism
Low-set, simple ears
Downturned mouth
Cleft lip, palate, or both
Short philtrum
Hypospadias/cryptorchidism

Progressive narrowing of lumbar interpedicular distance
Lumbar lordosis
Rhizomelic limb shortening
Trident hand (fingers cannot appose one another)

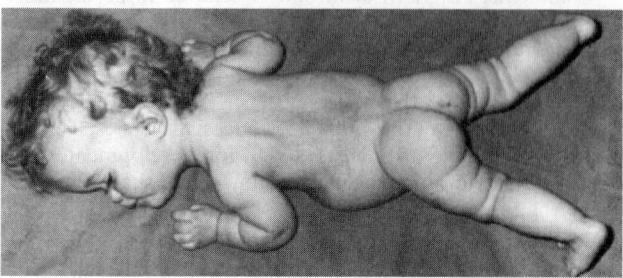

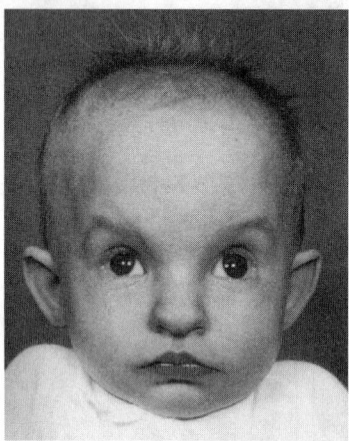

Other Findings

Midline posterior scalp defects
Craniofacial asymmetry
Ptosis
Cardiac anomalies (ASD, VSD)
Scoliosis
Hypotonia

Comments. Wolf-Hirschhorn syndrome occurs in 1 in 50,000 live births. Patients have slow growth, frequent respiratory infections, and increased mortality.

Performance. These patients have profound mental retardation, usually with a severe seizure disorder.

Etiology. Partial deletion of the short arm of chromosome 4 (including band 4p16.3) is present. Almost 90% are caused by *de novo* deletions, with the remainder caused by an unbalanced form of a parental translocation.

Suggested Readings

Battaglia A, et al. Wolf-Hirschhorn (4p-) syndrome. *Adv Pediatr* 2001;48:75.
Katz DS, Smith TH. Wolf syndrome. *Pediatr Radiol* 1991;21:369.
Zankl A, et al. A characteristic EEG pattern in 4p-syndrome: case report and review of the literature. *Eur J Pediatr* 2001;160:123.

Achondroplasia

Key Features

Short stature (mean adult height for men is 131 cm and for women is 124 cm)
Macrocephaly, frontal bossing
Narrowed foramen magnum
Depressed nasal bridge

Other Findings

Hydrocephalus
Cuboid-shaped vertebral bodies
Small iliac wings and narrow sciatic notches
Bowed legs

Comments. Achondroplasia is the most common skeletal dysplasia in humans, occurring in 1 in 15,000 live births. Early motor progress may be delayed. Because of the small foramen magnum and narrowed lower spinal canal, patients are predisposed to neurosurgical complications.

Performance. Intelligence usually is normal.

Etiology. Achondroplasia is an autosomal dominant condition. Mutations of the fibroblast growth factor receptor 3 (*FGFR3*) gene at chromosome 4p16.3 are responsible for achondroplasia, as well as related conditions hypochondroplasia (mild) and thanatophoric dysplasia (severe and lethal). A single mutation accounts for almost all cases of achondroplasia. Eighty percent to 90% of cases represent new mutations, all occurring in the father's sperm, and are associated with advanced paternal age.

Suggested Readings

Committee on Genetics. Health supervision for children with achondroplasia. *Pediatrics* 1995;95:443.
Gordon N. The neurological complications of achondroplasia. *Brain Dev* 2000;22:3.
Hunter AG, et al. Medical complications of achondroplasia: a multicentre patient review. *J Med Genet* 1998;35:705.
Shiang R, et al. Mutations in the transmembrane domain of *FGFR3* cause the most common genetic form of dwarfism, achondroplasia. *Cell* 1994;78:335.

Alagille Syndrome (Arteriohepatic Dysplasia)

Key Features

Broad forehead
Deep-set eyes
Ocular abnormality (posterior embryotoxon)
Long straight nose with flattened tip
Prominent chin
Peripheral pulmonic stenosis

Intrahepatic biliary atresia
Butterfly vertebrae

Seizures
Absence of speech

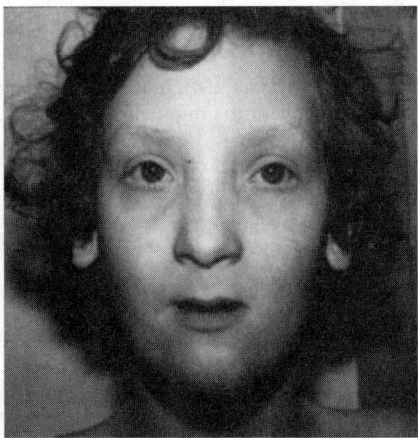

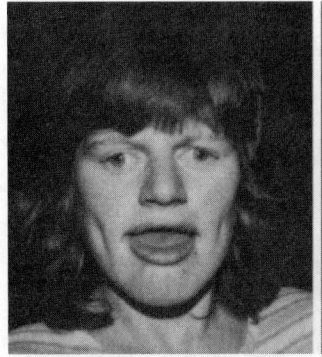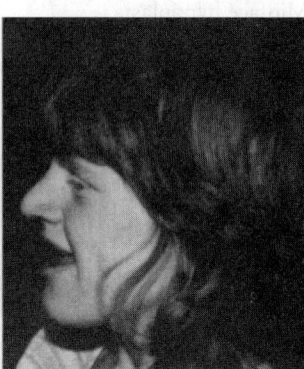

Other Findings

Strabismus
Scoliosis
Unprovoked bursts of laughter
Electroencephalographic abnormalities

Comments. Angelman syndrome also has been called the *happy puppet syndrome* because of the unusual gait and unprovoked laughter. Affected individuals usually are unable to communicate verbally, but some may communicate by sign language.

Performance. Patients have severe mental retardation.

Etiology. An interstitial deletion of chromosome 15q11–q13 accounts for 60% to 80% of cases. This region is known to show genomic imprinting, meaning that the parental origin of the deleted material affects the phenotypic expression. In Angelman syndrome, the deleted material is always maternal in origin, as opposed to the Prader-Willi syndrome, in which the same deleted segment is paternal. Deletions may be large enough to detect cytogenetically, or may require molecular methods (fluorescent *in situ* hybridization [FISH]) to detect.

A much less frequent cause of Angelman syndrome is lack of the maternal genetic material via paternal uniparental disomy. In this case, the individual inherits both chromosomes 15 from the father, with no genetic contribution from the mother. Although two copies of the genetic information is present, a lack of maternal genetic input still exists.

Mutations of the E6-AP ubiquitin-protein ligase gene is another cause of Angelman syndrome.

Other Findings

Growth retardation
Retinal degeneration
Cardiac defects
Renal abnormalities

Comments. Patients usually present with direct hyperbilirubinemia in the neonatal period, and a number have undergone liver transplantation.

Performance. A few individuals have mild mental retardation.

Etiology. Alagille syndrome is an autosomal dominant condition. Mutations have been found in the *JAGGED1* gene, which is located at chromosome 20p12.

Suggested Readings

Alagille D, et al. Syndromic paucity of interlobular bile ducts (Alagille syndrome or arteriohepatic dysplasia): review of 80 cases. *J Pediatr* 1987;110:195.
Krantz ID, Piccoli DA, Spinner NB. Clinical and molecular genetics of Alagille syndrome. *Curr Opin Pediatr* 1999;11:558.
Li L, et al. Alagille syndrome is caused by mutations in human *JAGGED1*, which encodes a ligand for *NOTCH1*. *Nature Genet* 1997;16:243.
Piccoli DA, Spinner NB. Alagille syndrome and the *Jagged1* gene. *Semin Liver Dis* 2001;21:525.

Angelman Syndrome

Key Features

Microbrachycephaly
Hypopigmentation, blond hair, pale blue eyes
Large mouth with tongue protrusion
Prognathism
Awkward gait with arms upheld and flexed at the wrists and elbows

Suggested Readings

Clayton-Smith J, Laan L. Angelman syndrome: a review of the clinical and genetic aspects. *J Med Genet* 2003;40:87.
Matsuura T, et al. De novo truncating mutations in E6-AP ubiquitin-protein ligase gene (*UBE3A*) in Angelman syndrome. *Nature Genet* 1997;15:74.
Molfetta GA, Silva-Jr WA, Pina-Neto JM. Clinical, cytogenetical and molecular analyses of Angelman syndrome. *Genet Couns* 2003;14:45.
Nicholls RD. Genomic imprinting and uniparental disomy in Angelman and Prader-Willi syndrome: a review. *Am J Med Genet* 1993;46:16.

Apert Syndrome

Key Features

Craniosynostosis
Brachycephaly with flat occiput
Wide, late-closing anterior fontanelle

Frontal bossing
Downslanting palpebral fissures
Shallow orbits with proptosis
Midface hypoplasia
High-arched, narrow palate
"Mitten-type" syndactyly of hands and feet

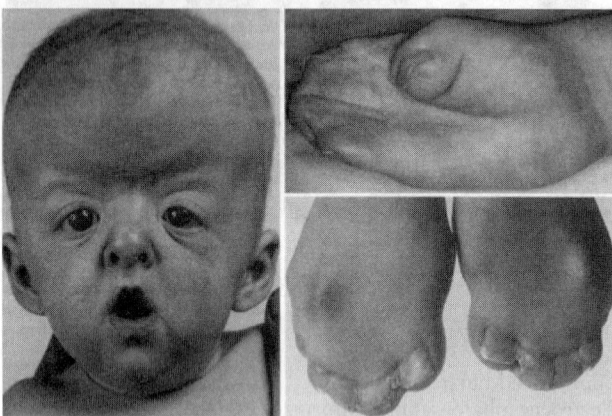

Other Findings

Cervical fusions
Progressive ankyloses of elbows, shoulders, hips
Cardiac defects
Genitourinary defects
Gastrointestinal or respiratory abnormalities
Hearing loss secondary to chronic otitis media
Central nervous system abnormalities
Moderate to severe acne (trunk and arms at adolescence)

Comments. Birth prevalence is estimated to be 1 in 160,000. Affected individuals are typically born with fused coronal sutures and a large patent midline skull defect where the sagittal and metopic sutures would normally form. Because this gap takes 2 to 3 years to fill in with bone, the incidence of increased intracranial pressure is low in the first years of life. Some patients have complete osseous and cutaneous fusion of digits. Most patients undergo multiple cranial and hand and feet reconstruction procedures.

Performance. A significant percentage of patients have mental retardation, which is not believed to be solely caused by increased intracranial pressure and may reflect in part the increased incidence of central nervous system malformations.

Etiology. Apert syndrome is an autosomal dominant condition caused by mutations in the fibroblast growth factor receptor 2 (*FGFR2*) gene on chromosome 10q25–q26. The majority of cases result from new mutations, although at least one three-generation family has been reported. Sporadic cases are associated with *de novo* mutations in the father's sperm and with increased paternal age.

Suggested Readings

Cohen MM Jr, Kreiborg S. An updated pediatric perspective on the Apert syndrome. *Am J Dis Child* 1993;147:989.
Lajeunie E, et al. Clinical variability in patients with Apert's syndrome. *J Neurosurg* 1999;90:443.
Park WJ, et al. Analysis of phenotypic features and *FGFR2* mutations in Apert syndrome. *Am J Hum Genet* 1995;57:321.

Bardet-Biedl Syndrome

Key Features

Obesity
Short stature
Retinal dystrophy
Other ocular defects (myopia, astigmatism, nystagmus, cataracts, glaucoma, retinitis pigmentosa)
Postaxial polydactyly
Renal abnormalities (abnormal calyces, communicating cysts, fetal lobulations)
Hypogonadism

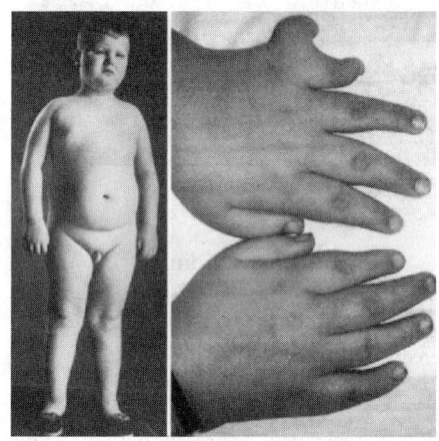

Other Findings

Brachydactyly
Short, broad feet
Hearing deficit
Asthma
Psychological and neurologic disorders

Comments. The highest incidence of Bardet-Biedl syndrome has been reported in the Middle East (1 in 13,500), with much less frequent occurrence in Switzerland (1 in 160,000). Retinal dystrophy is present in 100% of patients, with visual disturbances beginning in childhood. More than 70% are blind by age 20. Early visual changes can be detected by electroretinography. Renal failure develops in a small but significant number. The Lawrence Moon syndrome is another autosomal recessive condition with pigmentary retinopathy, hypogonadism, spastic paraplegia, mental retardation, but no polydactyly.

Performance. Mental deficiency occurs in more than three-fourths of patients. Delay of gross and fine motor skills is common, as are both dyspraxia and clumsiness. Speech delay also is seen in the majority of patients and appears amenable to speech therapy. Inappropriate mannerisms and affect are common.

Etiology. Bardet-Biedl syndrome can be inherited as an autosomal recessive condition with heterogeneity. Eight loci have been identified to date. *BBS1* is located on chromosome 11q13, *BBS2* at 16q21, *BBS3* at 3p13–p12, *BBS4* at 15q22–q23, *BBS5* at 2q31, *BBS6* (also responsible for the McKusick-Kaufman syndrome [hydrometrocolpos, post-axial polydactyly and congenital heart defects]) at 20q12, *BBS7* at 4q27, and *BBS8* at 14q32. The clinical manifestation of some forms of Bardet-Biedl syndrome requires recessive mutations in one of the loci plus an additional mutation in a second locus. A number of families do not show linkage to any of these sites, indicating that still other causative loci exist. Significant interfamilial and intrafamilial variation in phenotype exists, attributable to various genes defects and probably related to a dysfunction of the basal body of ciliated cells.

Suggested Readings

Beales PL, Elcioglu N, Woolf AS, et al. New criteria for improved diagnosis of Bardet-Biedl syndrome: results of a population survey. *J Med Genet* 1999; 36:437.

Beales PL, Warner AM, Hitman GA, et al. Bardet-Biedl syndrome: a molecular and phenotypic study of 18 families. *J Med Genet* 1997;34:92.

Eichers ER, Lewis RA, Katsanis N, Lupski JR. Triallelic inheritance: a bridge between Mendelian and multifactorial traits. *Ann Med* 2004;36:262.

Sheffield VC, Nishimura D, Stone EM. The molecular genetics of Bardet-Biedl syndrome. *Curr Opin Genet Dev* 2001;11:317.

Beckwith-Wiedemann Syndrome

Key Features

Macrosomia
Nevus flammeus of forehead and eyelids
Linear ear creases
Indentations on posterior pinnae
Macroglossia
Abdominal wall defects (diastasis recti, umbilical hernia, or omphalocele)
Organomegaly
Hypoglycemia in the newborn period

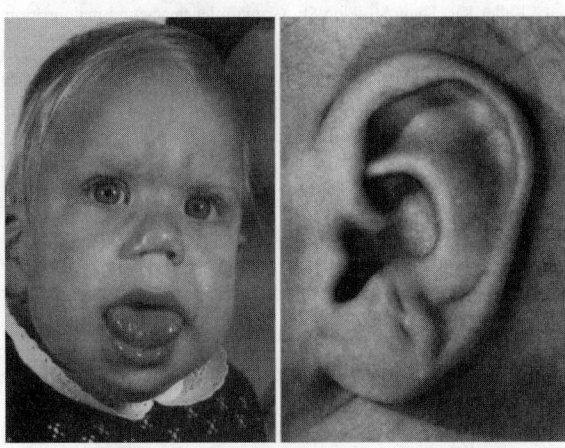

Other Findings

Hemihypertrophy
Large fontanelles
Diaphragmatic hernia
Advanced bone age
Polycythemia in the newborn period

Comments. Beckwith-Wiedemann syndrome (BWS) occurs in approximately 1 in 15,000 live births. An increased rate of both polyhydramnios and prematurity exists. Babies are usually large at birth (average weight, 4 kg; average length, 52.6 cm), but tend to level off closer to upper normal ranges as they get older. Advanced bone age similarly is more pronounced in the first few years of life. These children are at increased risk of malignancy, specifically Wilms tumor, hepatoblastoma, and gonadoblastoma, and should be followed with serum alpha-fetoprotein levels and abdominal ultrasounds. The serum alpha-fetoprotein level normally decreases by the first year of life, and level checks are recommended every 6 weeks until the age of 3 to 4 years. Abdominal ultrasounds have been recommended every 3 months until the age of 8 years, then every 6 months until skeletal growth is complete. The risk of malignancy is more significantly increased in those patients who also have hemihypertrophy.

Performance. Intellect is normal in most cases, but a minority of patients have intellectual impairment ranging from mild to severe. It is thought that some of these cases are explainable by the prematurity, hypoglycemic insult, or chromosome abnormalities documented in a few patients.

Etiology. Most cases are sporadic, but a significant percentage are inherited in an autosomal dominant manner. The gene has been localized to chromosome 11p15. The maternal copy of the gene is normally imprinted, or inactive, so the single paternal gene provides normal function. Beckwith-Wiedemann syndrome results if the paternal copy is duplicated or a translocation causes activation of the normally quiescent maternal gene. Evidence exists for the insulin-like growth factor–2 gene and a tumor-suppressor gene in this chromosomal region. Some evidence recently has emerged of an increased rate of BWS in pregnancies achieved through assisted reproductive technology.

Suggested Readings

Elliott M, Bayly R, Cole T, et al. Clinical features and natural history of Beckwith-Wiedemann syndrome: presentation of 74 new cases. *Clin Genet* 1994; 46:168.

Elliott M, Maher ER. Beckwith-Wiedemann syndrome. *J Med Genet* 1994; 31:560.

Gosden R, Trasler J, Lucifero D, Faddy M. Rare congenital disorders, imprinted genes, and assisted reproductive technology. *Lancet* 2003;361:1975.

Hatada I, Mukai T. Genomic imprinting and Beckwith-Wiedemann syndrome. *Histol Histopathol* 2000;15:309.

Weng EY, Mortier GR, Graham JM Jr. Beckwith-Wiedemann syndrome. An update and review for the primary pediatrician. *Clin Pediatr (Phila)* 1995; 34:317.

Blepharophimosis-Ptosis-Epicanthus Inversus Syndrome (BPES)

Key Features

Small palpebral fissures
Eyelid ptosis
Epicanthus inversus

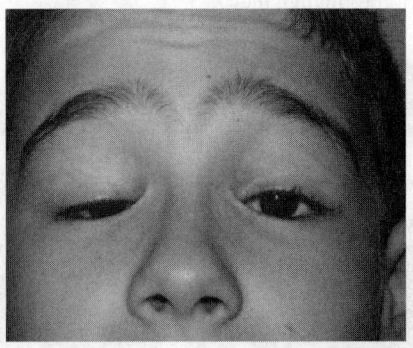

Other Findings

Eyelid dysplasia
Depressed nasal bridge

Hypoplastic nares
Low, posteriorly rotated ears
Oral anomalies (clefts, hypodontia)
Premature ovarian failure with secondary amenorrhea and infertility defines BPES type I

Comments. BPES patients have complex eyelid anomalies and flattened expressionless face due to taut facial skin. The epicanthal folds run characteristically upward and inward rather than downward, hence the term epicanthus inversus. The supraorbital ridges are flattened and eyebrows are highly arched. The head is tilted backward to compensate for the ptosis. BPES is an autosomal dominant syndrome with over 180 reported families, but many cases are sporadic. Nonpenetrance may cause counseling problems. Associated anomalies and/or developmental delay may indicate associated chromosomal abnormality and require karyotype analysis.

Performance. Affected individuals generally have normal intelligence. Microdeletions are associated with mental retardation.

Etiology. FOXL2 mutations cause both BPES types I and II. It is believed that BPES type I is generally caused by loss of function mutations, while BPES type II is due to mutations generating FOXL2 protein products with an elongated polyalanine tract. However, phenotype–genotype correlations are not precise as recent reports show that both BPES types may be caused by the same mutation.

Suggested Readings

De Baere E, et al. FOXL2 and BPES: mutational hotspots, phenotypic variability, and revision of the genotype-phenotype correlation. *Am J Hum Genet* 2003; 72:478.
Temple IK, Baraitser M. Pitfalls in counselling of the blepharophimosis, ptosis, epicanthus inversus syndrome (BPES). *J Med Genet* 1989;26:517.

Bloom Syndrome

Key Features

Prenatal-onset growth deficiency
Small, narrow facies
Facial erythema and telangiectasia (exacerbated by sunlight)
Protruding ears
High-pitched voice
Predisposition to malignancy

Other Findings

Absence of upper lateral incisors
Café au lait spots
Immunoglobulin deficiency

Comments. Bloom syndrome is most common in Ashkenazi Jewish individuals, with a carrier frequency believed to be at least 1 in 100 in that population. Skin lesions present on the nose, lips, malar areas, forearms, dorsa of hands, and back of neck and ears. Malignancy occurs in approximately 25% of those with Bloom syndrome and is the major cause of death. Leukemias are frequent, and a variety of solid tumor types have been described. Men are usually infertile because of insufficient spermatogenesis.

Performance. Patients may show mild mental retardation or learning disabilities, although the majority are of normal intelligence.

Etiology. Bloom syndrome is an autosomal recessive condition, and its gene, *BLM*, which encodes the DNA helicase RecQ protein-like-3, is located at chromosome 15q26.1. Chromosome analysis shows increased sister chromatid exchange, considered diagnostic of this condition.

Suggested Readings

Cohen MM, Levy HP. Chromosome instability syndromes. Bloom syndrome. *Adv Hum Genet* 1989;18:103.
Ellis NA, et al. The Bloom's syndrome gene product is homologous to RecQ helicases. *Cell* 1995;83:655.
Keller C, Keller KR, Shew SB, Plon SE. Growth deficiency and malnutrition in Bloom syndrome. *J Pediatr* 1999;134:472.
Van Kerckhove CW, Ceuppens JL, Vanderschueren-Lodeweyckx M, et al. Bloom's syndrome. Clinical features and immunologic abnormalities of four patients. *Am J Dis Child* 1988;142:1089.

Branchio-Oto-Renal Syndrome (BOR, Melnick-Fraser Syndrome)

Key Features

Hearing loss (sensorineural, conductive or mixed)
Preauricular pits
Anomalous pinnae
Inner ear malformations
Branchial pits or sinuses
Renal dysplasia

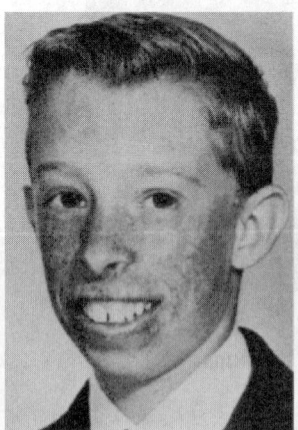
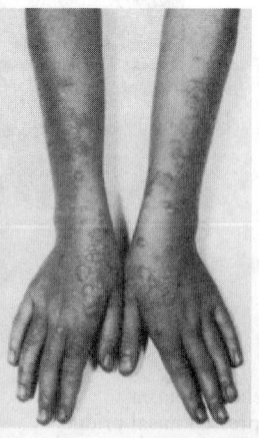
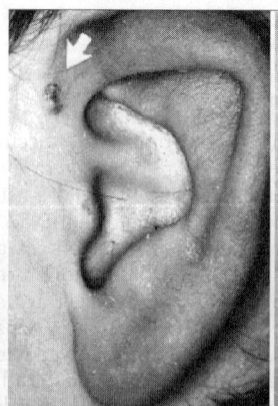
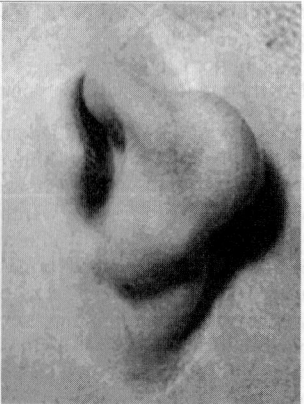

Other Findings

Lacrimal duct stenosis or aplasia
Cleft palate
Ossicular malformations
Functional renal abnormalities (vesicoureteral reflux)

Comments. The findings in BOR are highly variable even within a family. The three major areas of involvement (branchial anomalies, ear/hearing loss, and renal dysplasia) may range from mild enough to go unnoticed to very severe. Due to this variability, all family members of an affected individual should be carefully evaluated. If an individual is found to have even mild manifestations, it implies that they, too are affected and have a 50% risk of passing the condition on to offspring. It has been reported that the diagnosis of BOR is associated with 2% of all cases of profound hearing loss.

Performance. Patients are generally of normal intelligence but may have speech and language delays due to hearing impairment.

Etiology. BOR syndrome is an autosomal dominant condition caused by mutations of the *EYA1* gene at chromosome 8q13.3.

Suggested Readings

Abdelhak S, et al. Clustering of mutations responsible for branchio-oto-renal (BOR) syndrome in the eyes absent homologous region (eyaHR) of EYA1. *Hum Mol Genet* 1997;6:2247.
Bellini C, et al. Branchio-oto-renal syndrome: a report on nine family groups. *Am J Kidney Dis* 2001;37:505.
Chen A, et al. Phenotypic manifestations of branchio-oto-renal syndrome. *Am J Med Genet* 1995;58:365.
Millman B, Gibson WS, Foster WP. Branchio-oto-renal syndrome. *Arch Otolaryngol Head Neck Surg* 1995;121:922.

Cockayne Syndrome

Key Features

Profound postnatal growth deficiency
Loss of adipose tissue
Microcephaly
Sunken eyes
Retinal degeneration
Large ears
Sensorineural hearing loss
Beaklike nose
Dental abnormalities
Photosensitive dermatitis
Hypertension

Other Findings

Thickened calvarium
Corneal opacity, cataracts
Slender nose
Kyphosis
Cryptorchidism in boys, menstrual irregularities and underdevelopment of breasts in girls
Cool hands and feet, may be cyanotic
Ataxia, dysarthria, incoordination

Comments. Affected individuals usually appear normal at birth, but the growth retardation and striking loss of adipose tissue become evident by 2 to 4 years of age. Life expectancy is approximately 12 years. A more severe, early-onset form has been described (Cockayne syndrome II) with average life expectancy of 6 to 7 years.

Performance. Patients have mild to moderate mental retardation.

Etiology. This *premature aging syndrome* is an autosomal recessive condition, and two causative genes have been identified. The excision-repair cross-complementing group 8 gene (*ERCC8*) at chromosome 5 has been designated *CKN1* and is responsible for "classic Cockayne" syndrome. *CKN2* (*ERCC6*) is located at chromosome 10q11, and is responsible for the congenital/earlier onset form.

Suggested Readings

Friedberg EC. Cockayne syndrome—a primary defect in DNA repair, transcription, both or neither? *Bioessays* 1996;18:731.
Henning KA, et al. The Cockayne syndrome group A gene encodes a WD repeat protein that interacts with CSB protein and a subunit of RNA polymerase II TFIIH. *Cell* 1995;82:555.
Nance MA, Berry SA. Cockayne syndrome: review of 140 cases. *Am J Med Genet* 1992;42:68.
Ozdirim E, Topcu M, Ozon A, Cila A. Cockayne syndrome: review of 25 cases. *Pediatr Neurol* 1996;15:312.

Coffin-Lowry Syndrome

Key Features

Short stature
Coarse facies
Bulbous nose
Tapering fingers

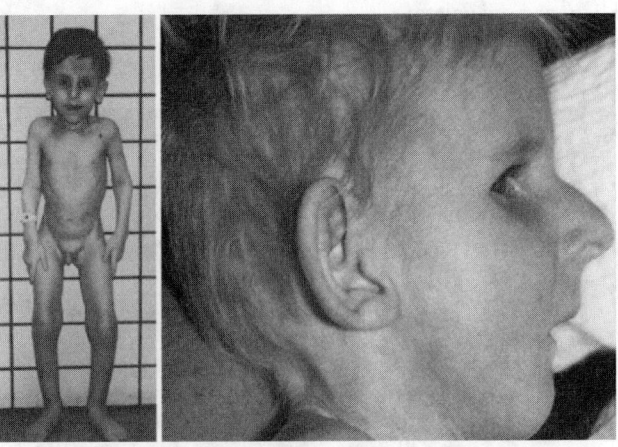

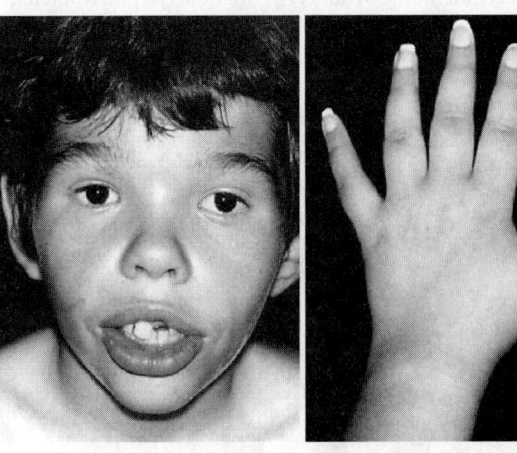

Other Findings

Prominent brow
Heavy, arched eyebrows
Downslanting palpebral fissures
Prominent pinnae
Anteverted nares
Maxillary hypoplasia
Large open mouth with everted lower lip
Dental abnormalities
Abnormal sternum
Vertebral abnormalities
Small fingernails
Loose skin

Comments. In addition to postnatal growth deficiency, the face coarsens with age and the vertebral dysplasia and kyphoscoliosis usually develops after 6 years. Occasional cases have rectal and uterine prolapse, mitral insufficiency, sensorineural hearing loss, and seizures. Some phenotypic overlap occurs with Williams syndrome.

Performance. Mental retardation is usually severe, with absent or significant speech delay in males. IQ is 60 to normal in female carriers.

Etiology. Most cases are new mutations. Inheritance is X-linked with severely affected males and carrier females with mild facial changes, tapered fingers, and short stature. Some obligate females are completely normal. Mutations have been found in ribosomal protein S6 kinase, 90kD, polypeptide 3 gene, which is a growth factor that regulates serine-threonine protein kinase, that is located at chromosome Xp22.2.

Suggested Readings

Gilgenkrantz S, et al. Coffin-Lowry syndrome: a multicenter study. *Clin Genet* 1988;34:230.
Hunter AGW. Coffin-Lowry syndrome: a 20-year follow-up and review of long-term outcomes. *Am J Med Genet* 2002;111:345.

Cornelia de Lange Syndrome (Brachmann–de Lange Syndrome)

Key Features

Microbrachycephaly
Bushy eyebrows with synophrys
Long, curly eyelashes
Depressed nasal bridge, anteverted nares
Thin upper lip, long philtrum
Downturned corners of mouth
Hirsutism, low posterior hairline
Limb defects including syndactyly, oligodactyly, micromelia, phocomelia
Cryptorchidism

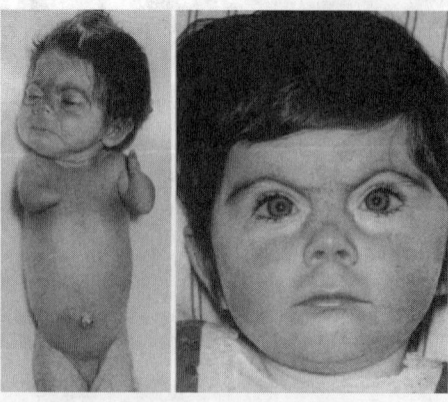

Other Findings

Ocular abnormalities (myopia, nystagmus)
High-arched palate
Hearing loss
Mandibular spur, 13 ribs
Cardiac defect (VSD)
Gastrointestinal abnormalities (reflux, malrotation, pyloric stenosis)
Delayed osseus maturation
Low-pitched, growling cry
Hypertonicity
Seizures

Comments. Cornelia de Lange syndrome occurs in approximately 1 in 10,000 to 20,000 live births. In addition to prenatal onset growth deficiency, feeding difficulties are frequent, and affected individuals often fail to thrive because of persistent vomiting and other gastrointestinal disturbances. Those followed beyond 13 years of age had normal onset of puberty.

Performance. Average IQ is 53, with the range being 30 to 86. Some individuals have autistic or self-destructive behaviors.

Etiology. Usually, Cornelia de Lange syndrome occurs sporadically. Cases of autosomal dominant inheritance through either parent have been reported. Mutations have been found in the *Nipped-B*-like gene that is located at chromosome 5p13. Patients with abnormalities of the chromosome 3q26.3 region show features similar to the syndrome.

Suggested Readings

Berney TP, Ireland M, Burn J. Behavioral phenotype of Cornelia de Lange syndrome. *Arch Dis Child* 1999;81:333.
Jackson L, et al. De Lange syndrome: a clinical review of 310 individuals. *Am J Med Genet* 1993;47:940.

Crouzon Syndrome

Key Features

Craniosynostosis, usually coronal synostosis
Brachycephaly
Proptosis due to shallow orbits
Hypertelorism
Strabismus
Beaked nose
Midface hypoplasia
High, narrow palate
Prognathism

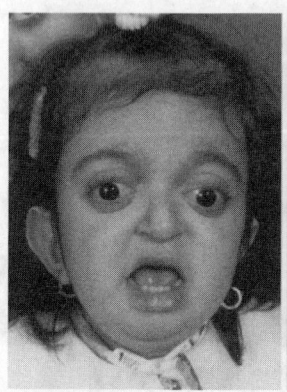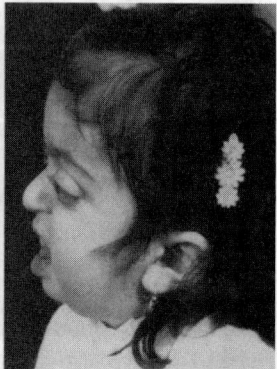

Other Findings

Conductive hearing loss
Dental malocclusion
Acanthosis nigricans

Comments. Birth prevalence has been estimated at 1 in 25,000 live births. The phenotype is highly variable, and some patients are only diagnosed after the birth of a more severely affected child.

Performance. Mental retardation has been reported in a small percentage of patients. Surgical correction of increased intracranial pressure caused by craniosynostosis is indicated to avoid intellectual compromise.

Etiology. Crouzon syndrome is inherited as an autosomal dominant condition. Crouzon syndrome is caused by mutations of the fibroblast growth factor receptor gene family. In sporadic cases, these mutations have been proven so far to be paternal, and they are associated with advanced paternal age. Most mutations have been reported in the *FGFR2* gene; however, some patients with Crouzon syndrome with the additional finding of acanthosis nigricans have a mutation in *FGFR3*. Pfeiffer syndrome (craniosynostosis and broad thumbs and toes) is a similar autosomal dominant condition that can be caused by mutations in the *FGFR1*, *FGFR2*, or *FGFR3* gene. Some patients with Pfeiffer syndrome carry an identical *FGFR2* mutation to that seen in Crouzon patients. Different *FGFR2* mutations cause Apert syndrome.

Suggested Readings

Jabs EW, et al. Jackson-Weiss and Crouzon syndromes are allelic with mutations in fibroblast growth factor receptor 2. *Nature Genet* 1994;8:275.
Koler JC, Munro IR, Farkas LG. Patterns of dysmorphology in Crouzon syndrome: an anthropometric study. *Cleft Palate J* 1988;25:235.
Vajo Z, Francomano CA, Wilkin DJ. The molecular and genetic basis of fibroblast growth factor receptor 3 disorders: the achondroplasia family of skeletal dysplasias, Muenke craniosynostosis, and Crouzon syndrome with acanthosis nigricans. *Endocr Rev* 2000;21:23.

Ectodermal Dysplasia Syndromes

Key Features

Sparse, fine hair
Hypodontia/anodontia
Conically shaped teeth
Decreased number of sweat and mucous glands
Thin and hypoplastic skin
Hyperthermia with increase in ambient temperature

Other Findings

Decreased tear production
Dysplastic nails
Hoarse voice

Comments. At least 170 ectodermal dysplasia syndromes are known. The most notable is the hypohidrotic form. These patients are at considerable risk of heat-related illness (i.e., heat stroke) because of the inability to cool themselves adequately by sweating. Avoiding overexertion and exposure to hot weather are important preventive measures, and cooling with water is imperative in an overheated patient. Climate-controlled suits similar to those used by astronauts for maintenance of body temperature in hot environments have been used. Ectrodactyly–ectodermal dysplasia–clefting (EEC) is a condition of autosomal dominant inheritance and heterogeneity with varying manifestations of lobster-claw deformity (ectrodactyly) of the hands and feet, nasolacrimal duct obstruction, and cleft lip and palate, as well as the skin and hair manifestations.

Performance. Mental deficiency has been reported, but may be the result of central nervous system exposure to high temperatures.

Etiology. The hypohidrotic form is X-linked, due to mutations in the *ED1* gene (Xq12.2–q13.1), encoding ectodysplasin-A. The majority of female carriers can be identified by dental examination and sweat testing. The EEC condition has been mapped to more than one locus at chromosome 7q11.2–q21.3, 3q27 (a p63 encoding gene), and chromosome 19. Autosomal recessive forms of ectodermal dysplasia also have been noted. Recent animal studies have suggested that the phenotype of an affected fetal mouse can be corrected by treating the mother with recombinant EDA1 protein.

Suggested Readings

Gaide O, Schneider P. Permanent correction of an inherited ectodermal dysplasia with recombinant EDA. *Nat Med* 2003;9:614.
Kere J, et al. X-linked anhidrotic (hypohidrotic) ectodermal dysplasia is caused by mutation in a novel transmembrane protein. *Nature Genet* 1996;13:409.
Priolo M, Lagana C. Ectodermal dysplasias: a new clinical-genetic classification. *J Med Genet* 2001;38:579.

Ehlers-Danlos Syndrome

Key Features

Skin hyperextensibility and easy bruising
Joint hypermobility, leading to sprains and joint dislocations
Increased tissue fragility (leading to formation of widened, atrophic scars)
Velvety feel to skin
Thin, translucent skin and hollow organ (aorta, intestine, uterus) fragility and rupture (type 4 Ehlers-Danlos syndrome)

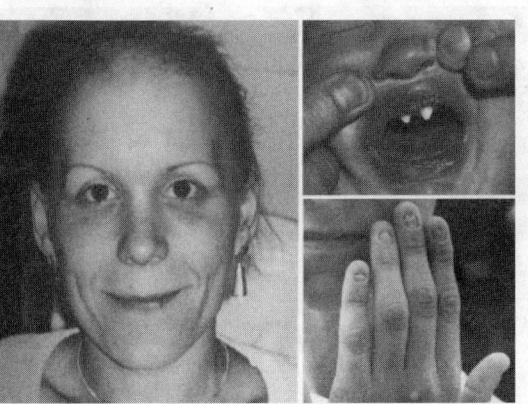

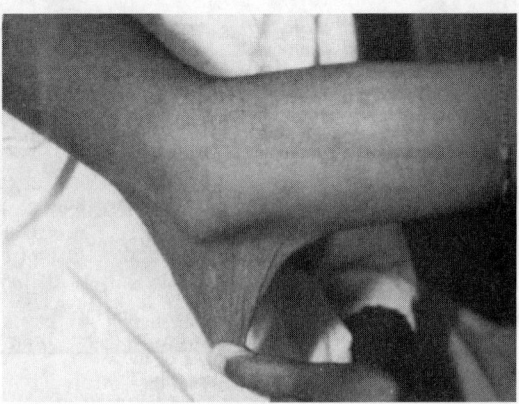

Other Findings

Small, mobile subcutaneous nodules (may represent adipose or mucinous material)
Mitral valve prolapse
Chronic joint and limb pain
Postsurgical complications (incisional hernias)
Preterm birth caused by premature rupture of membranes

Comments. The Ehlers-Danlos syndromes are a group of inherited connective tissue disorders. Previously, ten forms were named, but revised nosology now recognizes six separate conditions: type 1 (classic), type 2 (hypermobility), type 3 (vascular), type 4 (kyphoscoliosis), type 5 (arthrochalasia), and type 6 (dermatosparaxis). The latter three types are considerably less common. The vascular form carries the highest risk of early death from rupture of the aorta and may have significant morbidity from rupture of intestines or midsized arteries.

Performance. Intelligence usually is normal, although some mental deficiency has been reported. Psychosocial functioning is affected, with increased incidence of anxiety and depression.

Etiology. Ehlers-Danlos syndrome types are thought to be distinct from one another, and some forms have shown further genetic heterogeneity. The classic form is autosomal dominant, and is caused by a defect in type V (or in some cases, type I) collagen. The vascular form is also dominant and is caused by defects of type III collagen.

Suggested Readings

Beighton P, et al. Ehlers-Danlos syndromes: revised nosology, Villefranche, 1997. *Am J Med Genet* 1998;77:31.
Rowe PC, et al. Orthostatic intolerance and chronic fatigue syndrome associated with Ehlers-Danlos syndrome. *J Pediatr* 1999;135:494.
Stanitski DF, et al. Orthopaedic manifestations of Ehlers-Danlos syndrome. *Clin Orthop* 2000;1:213.
Yeowell NH, Pinnell SR. The Ehlers-Danlos syndrome. *Semin Dermatol* 1993; 12:229.

Fanconi Pancytopenia Syndrome

Key Features

Short stature
Microcephaly
Radial ray defects (hypoplastic/aplastic thumbs and radii; supernumerary thumbs)
Irregular brown skin pigmentation most notable on groin, axillae, trunk, and anogenital area
Pancytopenia developing in childhood (5 to 10 years of age)

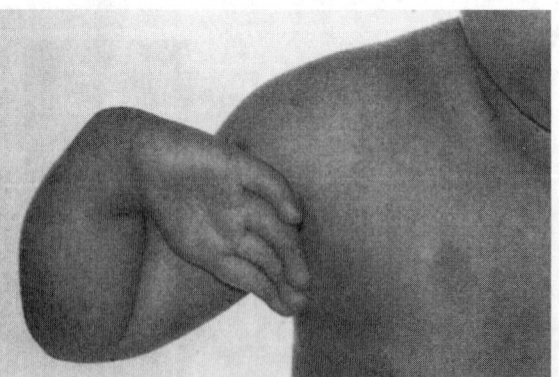

Other Findings

Ptosis, strabismus, nystagmus
Renal malformations, double ureters
Hypogenitalism
Skeletal defects, including rib abnormalities, congenital hip dislocation, scoliosis, talipes equinovarus, clinodactyly, syndactyly
Leukemia, myelodysplastic syndrome

Comments. Less common features of Fanconi pancytopenia syndrome include abnormalities of the central nervous system and gastrointestinal tract. The pancytopenia usually improves with high-dose androgen therapy, although the only curative treatment is a bone marrow transplant. This condition can be distinguished from thrombocytopenia-absent radius (TAR) syndrome because radial hypoplasia or aplasia occurs only with aplasia of the thumb in Fanconi pancytopenia syndrome, while thumbs are always present in TAR.

Performance. Mental retardation occurs in approximately 25% of patients.

Etiology. Fanconi pancytopenia syndrome is an autosomal recessive condition. Genetic heterogeneity has been shown by the presence of nine complementation groups: A, B, C, D1, D2, E, F, G, and L. Chromosome studies show a high rate of diepoxy-butane–induced breakage (DEB), which is used for both prenatal and postnatal diagnosis. Due to the spectrum of anomalies, some clinical overlap occurs with the VACTERL association; DEB testing in these individuals would likely lead to identification of additional cases.

Suggested Readings

Dokal I. The genetics of Fanconi's anemia. *Baillieres Best Pract Res Clin Haematol* 2000;13:407.
Esmer C, et al. DEB test for Fanconi anemia detection in patients with atypical phenotypes. *Am J Med Genet* 2004;124A:35.
Glanz A, Fraser FC. Spectrum of anomalies in Fanconi anemia. *J Med Genet* 1982;19:412.
Gordon-Smith EC, Rutherford TR. Fanconi anemia—constitutional aplastic anemia (review). *Semin Hematol* 1991;28:104.

Holt-Oram Syndrome

Key Features

Defects of upper limbs and shoulder girdle
Narrow, sloping shoulders
Thumb anomalies (bifid, hypoplastic, absent)
Frequent asymmetric involvement
Hypoplastic radius
Cardiac septal defects (ASD and VSD most common)
Cardiac arrhythmias
Hypoplastic distal blood vessels

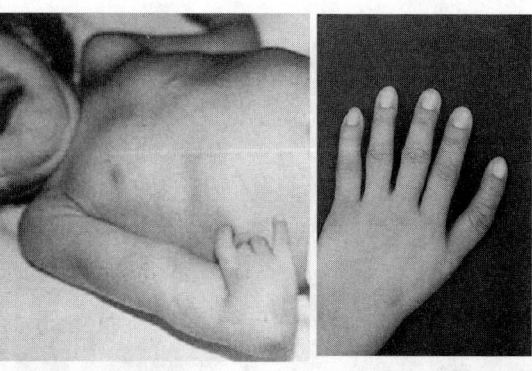

Other Features

Other cardiovascular defects (patent ductus arteriosus, pulmonic stenosis)
Absent pectoralis major muscle
Scoliosis and vertebral defects

Comments. Although affected individuals show upper limb and cardiac anomalies, a wide range of severity occurs with these findings. Limb effects may be as mild as clinodactyly and sloping shoulders or as severe as phocomelia; and cardiac defects may range from EKG changes only to AV canal defect. Because absent pectoralis major muscle has been reported in Holt-Oram syndrome, it should be considered in the differential diagnosis of Poland syndrome (absent pectoralis major muscle and ipsilateral hand defects). The latter condition is considered to be sporadic, and possibly due to hypoplasia of the subclavian artery or its branches.

Performance. Mentation generally is considered to be normal.

Etiology. Holt-Oram syndrome is a dominant condition caused by mutations in the *TBX5* gene on chromosome 12q24.1. This gene is critical for limb and heart development and is a member of the T-box transcription factor family. A related gene, *TBX3*, is responsible for the ulnar-mammary syndrome.

Suggested Readings

Basson CT et al. Mutations in human TBX5 [corrected] cause limb and cardiac malformation in Holt-Oram syndrome. *Nat Genet* 1997;15:30.
Huang T. Current advances in Holt-Oram syndrome. *Curr Opin Pediatr* 2002; 14:691.
Li QY et al. Holt-Oram syndrome is caused by mutations in TBX5, a member of the Brachyury (T) gene family. *Nat Genet* 1997;15:21.
Newbury-Ecob RA, Leanage R, Raeburn JA, Young ID. Holt-Oram syndrome: a clinical genetic study. *J Med Genet* 1996;33:300.

Hurler Syndrome (Mucopolysaccharidosis Type I)/Hunter Syndrome (MPS Type II)

Key Features

Short stature
Macrocephaly
Coarse facies
Cloudy corneas
Anteverted nares
Clawhand deformity
Decreased joint mobility
Hepatosplenomegaly

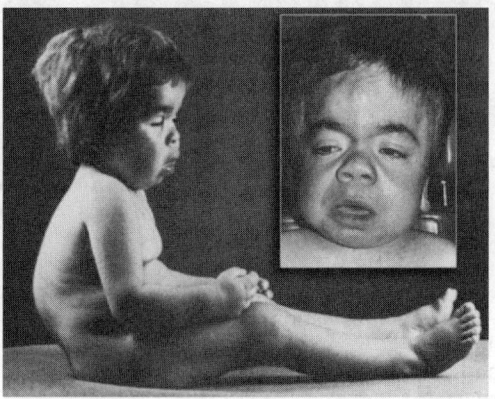

Other Findings

Hirsutism
Umbilical hernia
Kyphoscoliosis and thoracolumbar gibbus deformity of spine
Radiographic features (dysostosis multiplex)
Deafness
Dermal melanocytosis

Comments. Affected infants may appear normal at birth, but the coarse clinical features develop over time. Patients usually die in childhood as the result of respiratory or cardiac compromise. A related condition, Hunter syndrome (mucopolysaccharidosis type II) has similar physical features but is more gradual in onset, presents with clear corneas, and has X-linked inheritance.

Performance. Increasing developmental delay occurs with age. Children have severe mental retardation.

Etiology. Hurler syndrome is an autosomal recessive condition caused by deficiency of alpha-L-iduronidase (IDUA) and leads to the deposition of mucopolysaccharides in body tissues. Dermatan sulfate and heparan sulfate are excreted in the urine. The IDUA gene is found at chromosome 4p16.3. Available treatments include bone marrow transplant or enzyme replacement therapy with recombinant human alpha-L-iduronidase.

Suggested Readings

Hanson M, Lupski JR, Hicks J, Metry D. Association of dermal melanocytosis with lysosomal storage disease: clinical features and hypotheses regarding pathogenesis. *Arch Dermatol* 2003;139:916.
Kakkis ED, et al. Enzyme replacement therapy in mucopolysaccharidosis I. *N Engl J Med* 2001;344:182.
Roubicek M, Gehler J, Spranger J. The clinical spectrum of alpha-L-iduronidase deficiency. *Am J Med Genet* 1985;20:471.
Weisstein JS, et al. Musculoskeletal manifestations of Hurler syndrome: long-term follow-up after bone marrow transplantation. *J Pediatr Orthop* 2004; 24:97.

Jeune Syndrome (Asphyxiating Thoracic Dystrophy)

Key Features

Short stature
Long, narrow, bell-shaped thorax
Lung hypoplasia
Hepatic fibrosis and proliferation of bile ducts
Progressive nephropathy
Hypoplastic iliac wings
Short limbs

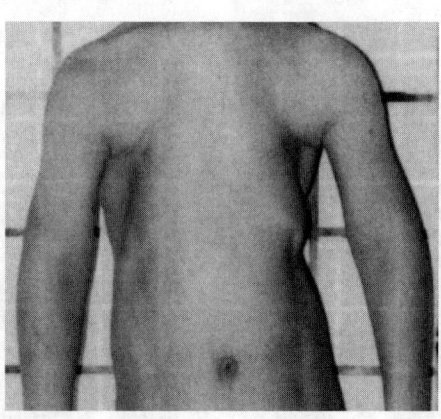

Other Findings

Retinal degeneration
Dental abnormalities
Pancreatic defects
Polydactyly

Comments. Jeune syndrome occurs in approximately 1 in 100,000 to 130,000 live births. These patients usually die early as a result of pneumonia or asphyxia, although milder cases with longer survival (into the fourth decade) are known. Surgical expansion of the thoracic cage has been done in some patients. It has been diagnosed prenatally by ultrasound examination in the second trimester. This disorder shares many physical features with Ellis–van Creveld syndrome. In the latter condition, however, polydactyly of the hand is a common feature, and upper lip and cardiac anomalies are seen.

Performance. Intelligence is usually normal, although mental retardation has been reported.

Etiology. Jeune syndrome is an autosomal recessive condition that has been mapped to chromosome 15q13. This condition and short-rib polydactyly type III (Verma-Naumoff) have occurred in the same family, and are felt to be variants of the same disorder.

Suggested Readings

Ho NC, Francomano CA, van Allen M. Jeune asphyxiating thoracic dystrophy and short-rib polydactyly type III (Verma-Naumoff) are variants of the same disorder. *Am J Med Genet* 2000;90:310.

Lachman RS. Skeletal dysplasias. In: Taybi H, Lachman RS, eds. *Radiology of syndromes, metabolic disorders and skeletal dysplasias,* 4th ed. St. Louis: Mosby, 1996:765.

Morgan NV, et al. A locus for asphyxiating thoracic dystrophy, ATD, maps to chromosome 15q13. *J Med Genet* 2003;40:431.

Ozcay F, et al. A family with Jeune syndrome. *Pediatr Nephrol* 2001;16:623.

Todd DW, et al. A thoracic expansion technique for Jeune's asphyxiating thoracic dystrophy. *J Pediatr Surg* 1986;21:161.

Marfan Syndrome

Key Features

Skeletal*: Pectus excavatum or carinatum requiring surgery, reduced extension at elbow, scoliosis, protrusio acetabulae, pes planus, reduced upper to lower segment ratio or arm span to height ratio, Walker-Murdoch wrist sign (the ability of the fifth finger and thumb to overlap when encircling the opposite wrist), and Steinberg thumb sign (the ability of the nail of the thumb to project beyond the ulnar aspect of the palm when the hand is clenched without assistance)
Ocular*: Lens subluxation (typically upward)
Cardiac*: Ascending aorta dilatation, dissection, or both
Dural ectasia*

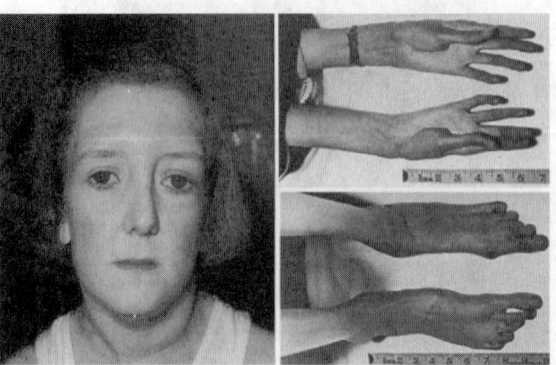

Other Findings

Dolichocephaly, narrow high-arched palate, joint hypermobility, tall stature, arachnodactyly
Mitral valve prolapse
Spontaneous pneumothorax
Skin striae, hernias

Comments. Marfan syndrome occurs in approximately 1 in 10,000 individuals in the United States. Expression is highly variable. The most severely affected individuals present with cardiac abnormalities in early infancy (neonatal Marfan syndrome). Individuals with Marfan syndrome are at risk for early death caused by aortic dissection and may be treated with beta-blockers to prevent further aortic dilatation or with surgical replacement of the aortic root if dilatation is severe. Diagnosis requires positive findings in two major categories marked by asterisks and one minor (some are listed under Other Findings); or findings in one major category and one minor with positive family history or fibrillin mutation.

Performance. Intelligence is normal, although some neuropsychological deficits (including learning disabilities and attention deficit disorder) occur with increased frequency.

Etiology. Marfan syndrome is inherited as an autosomal dominant condition with wide variation of expression. The disorder is caused by mutations in the *fibrillin* gene located at chromosome 15q21.1. Approximately 25% to 30% of new cases are sporadic. A paternal age effect has been demonstrated.

Suggested Readings

De Paepe A, et al. Revised diagnostic criteria for the Marfan syndrome. *Am J Med Genet* 1996;62:417.

Giampietro PF, Raggio C, Davis JG. Marfan syndrome: orthopedic and genetic review. *Curr Opin Pediatr* 2002;14:35.

Van Karnebeek CD, Naeff MS, Mulder BJ, et al. Natural history of cardiovascular manifestations in Marfan. *Arch Dis Child* 2001;84:129.

Meckel-Gruber Syndrome

Key Features

Occipital encephalocele
Polycystic kidneys
Postaxial polydactyly

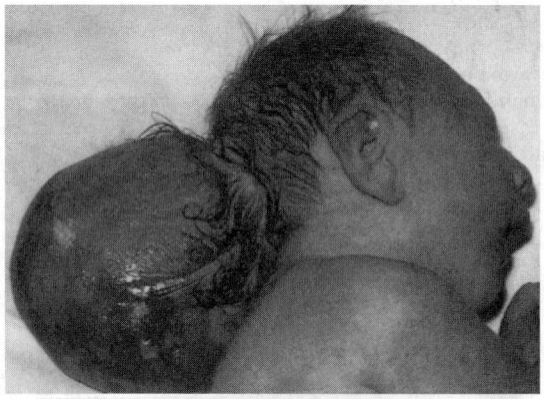

Other Findings

Microcephaly, cerebral and cerebellar hypoplasia
Dandy-Walker malformation
Sloping forehead
Microphthalmia
Cleft palate
Pulmonary hypoplasia

Cardiac anomalies (VSD, ASD, aortic coarctation)
Genital abnormalities
Short, bowed limbs

Comments. Considerable phenotypic variability is described. Oligohydramnios and breech presentation occur in approximately 50% to 60% of cases. Prenatal diagnosis can be accomplished by high-resolution ultrasound or alpha-fetoprotein screening if an encephalocele is present.

Performance. Patients with the full syndrome usually survive only days to weeks.

Etiology. Meckel-Gruber syndrome is inherited as an autosomal recessive condition with genetic heterogeneity. Several loci have been mapped to chromosome 17q22–q23, 11q13, and 8q24.

Suggested Reading

Salonen R. The Meckel syndrome: clinicopathological findings in 67 patients. *Am J Med Genet* 1984;18:671.

Miller-Dieker Lissencephaly Syndrome

Key Features

Lissencephaly ("smooth brain")
Heterotopias
Absent/hypoplastic corpus callosum
Microcephaly with bitemporal narrowing
Vertical furrowing of forehead with crying
Small, anteverted nose
Long philtrum
Thin prominent upper lip

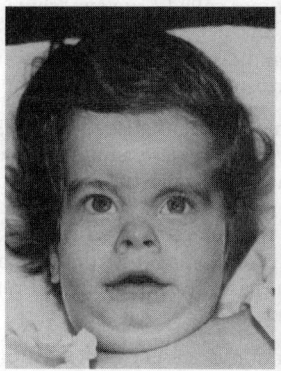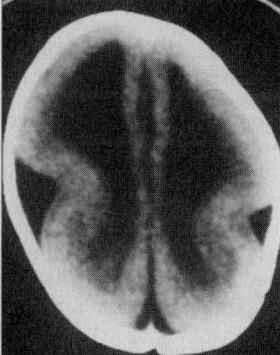

Other Findings

Cardiac defects
Cryptorchidism

Comments. Lissencephaly is pachygyria/agyria resulting from deficiency of neuronal migration. Patients have significant seizures, failure to thrive, and feeding problems. Survival is reduced greatly and death usually occurs before 2 years of age.

Performance. Patients have severe mental retardation.

Etiology. Miller-Dieker lissencephaly syndrome is caused by deletion of several genes at chromosome 17p13.3, which can be detected in 90% of patients by FISH. Isolated lissencephaly sequence is caused by point mutations in the *LIS1* gene.

Suggested Readings

Cardoso C, et al. Refinement of a 400-kb critical region allows genotypic differentiation between isolated lissencephaly, Miller-Dieker syndrome, and other phenotypes secondary to deletions of 17p13.3. *Am J Hum Genet* 2003;72:918.

Dobyns WB, et al. Clinical and molecular diagnosis of Miller-Dieker syndrome. *Am J Hum Genet* 1991;48:484.

Möbius Syndrome (Congenital Facial Diplegia)

Key Features

Sixth (abducens) and seventh (facial) nerve palsy
Mask-like facies
Limb malformation (syndactyly, brachydactyly, oligodactyly, talipes equinovarus)
Sequelae of palsy/paralysis of other facial nerves

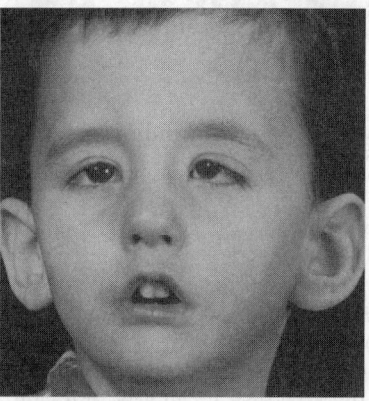

Other Findings

Micrognathia
Klippel-Feil anomaly (primary defect of cervical vertebrae)
Poland sequence (absence or hypoplasia of pectoral musculature and ipsilateral upper limb defects)
Rib defects

Comments. Other facial nerves in addition to VI and VII may be involved in Möbius syndrome. Ocular nerve palsies may result when nerves VI, III (oculomotor), or IV (trochlear) are affected. The tongue may be hypoplastic because of hypoglossal nerve (XII) paralysis. Speech and swallowing difficulties may result, with involvement of the trigeminal (V), glossopharyngeal (IX), or vagus (X) nerves.

Performance. Mental retardation is present in 10% to 15% of patients. Autistic spectrum disorder and learning disability may occur in one-third of patients.

Etiology. Möbius syndrome is heterogeneous because a similar phenotype may result from aplasia, hypoplasia, neuropathy, or myopathy. Several studies have indicated that transient hypoxic or ischemic events during pregnancy may be causative. One locus has been mapped to chromosome 13q12.2-13.

Suggested Reading

Stromland K, et al. Mobius sequence—a Swedish multidiscipline study. *Eur J Paediatr Neurol* 2002;6:35.

Neurofibromatosis Syndrome

Key Features

Café au lait spots (six measuring at least 5 mm before puberty or 15 mm after puberty*)
Lisch nodules (hamartomas of the iris)*
Neurofibromas (two cutaneous or one plexiform type*)
Optic glioma*
Inguinal or axillary freckling*
Bony lesions (pseudoarthrosis, sphenoid wing dysplasia)*

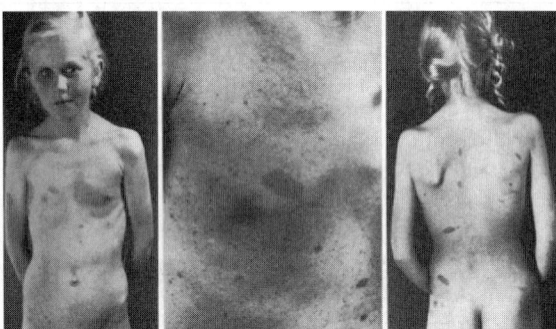

Other Findings

Macrocephaly
Scoliosis
Pheochromocytoma
Tumors of the central nervous system

Comments. Neurofibromatosis type 1 (NF1), also called *von Recklinghausen disease*, occurs in approximately 1 in 3,000 live births. The diagnosis of NF1 is considered to be established in anyone having two key features (positive family history and those marked by an asterisk). Skin findings may or may not be present at birth and tend to progress during childhood. Neurofibromas may become more numerous and prominent during puberty and pregnancy. Each neurofibroma has a 5% lifetime risk for malignant degeneration, so vigilance is advised for any pain, bleeding, or changes in color or size of an existing growth. Neurofibromatosis type 2 (NF2) is a distinct disorder marked by bilateral acoustic neuromas, multiple intracranial tumors, and less prominent skin findings.

Performance. A small percentage (5% to 8%) of patients are mentally retarded; a greater number (25% to 50%) have more subtle difficulties such as learning disabilities, hyperactivity, or speech problems.

Etiology. Neurofibromatosis syndrome is inherited as an autosomal dominant condition caused by mutations of the neurofibromin gene, *NF1*, at chromosome 17q11.2. Approximately one-half of individuals with NF1 represent a new mutation, and a paternal age effect has been noted in these cases. The risk for an affected individual to have an affected child is 50%; however, expression is quite variable, and offspring may be affected to a greater or lesser extent than the parent. Several young children with some features of NF1, and hematologic malignancies have been identified with homozygous mutations in the mismatch repair genes MLH1 and MSH2. NF2 is caused by mutations of the merlin gene on chromosome 22.

Suggested Readings

Castle B, Baser ME, Huson SM, et al. Evaluation of genotype-phenotype correlations in neurofibromatosis type 1. *J Med Genet* 2003;40:e109.
DeBella K, Szudek J, Friedman JM. Use of the National Institutes of Health Criteria for diagnosis of neurofibromatosis 1 in children. *Pediatrics* 2000;105:608.
Friedman JM. Neurofibromatosis 1: clinical manifestations and diagnostic criteria. *J Child Neurol* 2002;17:548.

Noonan Syndrome

Key Features

Short stature
Downslanting palpebral fissures
Ptosis
Low-set, malformed ears
Short or broad-based (webbed) neck
Shield chest
Cardiac abnormalities (pulmonic stenosis)
Cryptorchidism

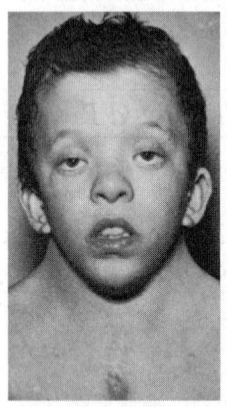

Other Findings

Pectus excavatum or carinatum
Cubitus valgus
Edema of dorsal aspects of hands and feet
Hearing loss
Malignant hyperthermia (sometimes called *King syndrome* when present)
Bleeding diathesis (von Willebrand disease, platelet dysfunction, or defects of intrinsic pathway)

Comments. Noonan syndrome has been referred to as *male Turner syndrome* because many features are similar in these two conditions. However, Noonan syndrome can occur in both sexes and is a separate entity from Turner syndrome. It is thought to be fairly common, with a frequency of approximately 1 in 1,000 to 2,500. Most cases are sporadic with advanced paternal age. In familial cases, a significant sex-ratio bias favors transmission to males.

Performance. Mental retardation is present in at least one-fourth of patients. However, learning disabilities, language delay, and articulation problems are frequent.

Etiology. Noonan syndrome is usually sporadic; however, autosomal dominant transmission has been described. Mutations in the *PTPN11* gene are present in about half of the patients. Mutations in the *NF1* gene, which is the site of mutations causing classic neurofibromatosis type I, have been found in neurofibromatosis-Noonan syndrome.

Suggested Readings

Chakraborty A. Noonan syndrome: a brief overview. *Hosp Med* 2002;63:743.
Ranke MB, et al. Noonan syndrome: growth and clinical manifestations in 144 cases. *Eur J Pediatr* 1988;148:220.
Zenker M, et al. Genotype-phenotype correlations in Noonan syndrome. *J Pediatr* 2004;144:368.

Oculo-Auriculo-Vertebral Dysplasia (Facioauriculovertebral Spectrum, Goldenhar Syndrome, Hemifacial Microsomia)

Key Features

Hypoplasia of malar, maxillary, mandibular region, or all three
Hypoplasia of associated musculature
Ear abnormalities (aplasia, hypoplasia, pits or tags that may lie anywhere from tragus to the corner of the mouth)
Hearing loss
Vertebral abnormalities (hypoplastic or hemivertebrae most common in, but not limited to, cervical spine)

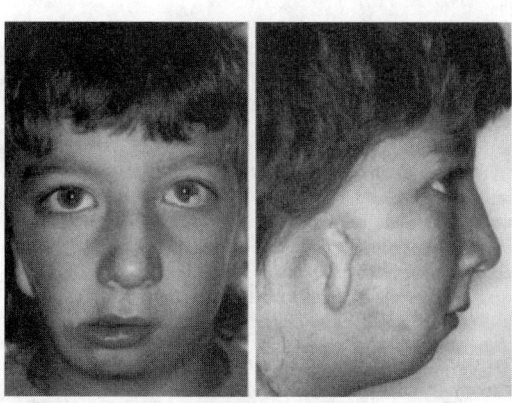

Other Findings

Epibulbar or lipodermoid of eye
Microphthalmia
Cleft of lip or palate
Cardiac defects (VSD, PDA, TOF, or coarctation of aorta)
Renal defects (ectopic or fused kidneys, renal agenesis, ureteral duplication, multicystic dysplastic kidney)
Imperforate anus

Comments. Frequency is estimated at 1 in 3,000 to 5,000 births and has a slight male predominance. The phenotypic spectrum ranges from unilateral hypoplasia of facial bones and musculature (hemifacial microsomia) to a more specific combination of these features with epibulbar dermoid and lateral facial clefts (Goldenhar syndrome). Features that tend to be asymmetric are most often (70%) unilateral and are more commonly right sided.

Performance. Intelligence is usually normal, but some individuals have mental deficiency (13% have an IQ of less than 85).

Etiology. Oculo-auriculo-vertebral dysplasia is usually sporadic, most likely because of vascular interruption during development of the first and second branchial arches. Autosomal dominant inheritance and genetic heterogeneity have been reported. Estimated recurrence risk for first-degree relatives is approximately 2%; family members should be examined for facial asymmetry or minor features of the spectrum.

Suggested Reading

Rollnick BR, et al. Oculoauriculovertebral dysplasia and variants: phenotypic characteristics of 294 patients. *Am J Med Genet* 1987;26:361.

Oculodentodigital Dysplasia (ODDD)

Key Features

Microophthalmia
Thin nose
Hypoplastic alae nasi
Abnormalities of enamel hypoplasia and tooth loss
Syndactyly
Spastic bladder or gait disturbances
Progressive leukodystrophy

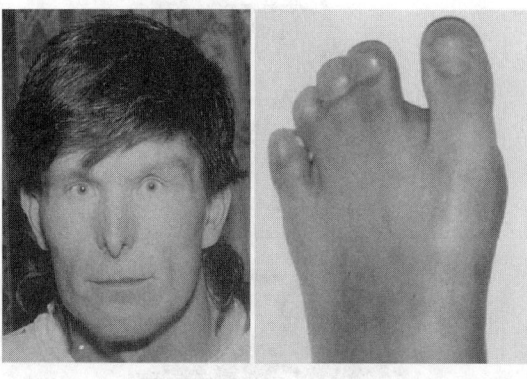

Other Findings

Hypotrichosis
Microcephaly
Dysplastic ears
Conductive hearing loss
Cleft palate
Fifth-finger camptodactyly
Brittle nails
Skeletal abnormalities

Comments. All but a few cases have been reported in the Caucasian population. Syndactyly type III with involvement of the fourth and fifth fingers occurs. The neurologic manifestations are evident by the second decade of life.

Performance. Intelligence usually is normal.

Etiology. Oculodentodigital dysplasia usually is sporadic and can be inherited as an autosomal dominant condition. Mutations in the gap junction alpha 1 or connexin 43 gene at chromosome 6q22–q23 are the cause of the condition.

Suggested Readings

Gorlin RJ, Miskin LH, Gene JW. Oculodentodigital dysplasia. *J Pediatr* 1963; 63:69.
Loddenkemper T, et al. Neurological manifestations of the oculodentodigital dysplasia syndrome. *J Neurol* 2002;249:584.
Paznekas WA, et al. Connexin 43 (GJA1) mutations cause the pleiotropic phenotype of oculodentodigital dysplasia. *Am J Hum Genet* 2003;72: 408.

Opitz Syndrome (BBB Syndrome, G Syndrome)

Key Features

Hypertelorism
Upslanting or downslanting palpebral fissures
Epicanthal folds
Posteriorly rotated ears
Micrognathia
Cleft lip with or without cleft palate
Hypospadias, cryptorchidism

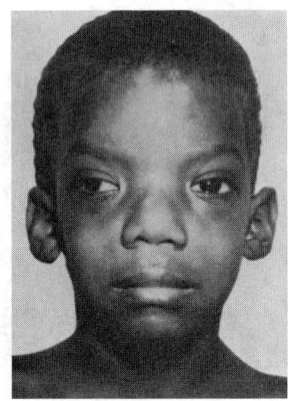

Other Findings

Laryngotracheoesophageal defects
Cardiac defects
Renal abnormalities
Structural central nervous system abnormalities

Comments. Considerable overlap exists between what Opitz and colleagues described as the BBB and G syndromes; both entities are considered the same and bear Opitz's name. Male infants are usually more severely affected, and female infants have normal genitalia. Hypertelorism may be the only distinguishing feature in affected females. Feeding and swallowing problems (stridor, aspiration, wheezing) may indicate a laryngotracheoesophageal defect, such as clefting of the upper gastrointestinal or respiratory tract, and esophageal dysmotility may prove lethal if not corrected.

Performance. Mild to moderate mental deficiency is present in the majority of patients.

Etiology. Two genetic loci, one at Xp22 and another at 22q11.2, have been identified, indicating genetic heterogeneity. Both show dominant inheritance and are clinically indistinguishable. The gene on chromosome X is *MID1*.

Suggested Readings

Quaderi NA, et al. Opitz G/BBB syndrome, a defect of midline development, is due to mutations in a new RING finger gene on Xp22. *Nature Genet* 1997; 17:285.
Robin NH, et al. Opitz syndrome is genetically heterogeneous with one locus on Xp22 and a second locus on 22q11.2. *Nat Genet* 1995;11:459.
Verloes A, et al. BBBG syndrome or Opitz syndrome. *Am J Med Genet* 1989; 34:313.

Oral-Facial-Digital Syndrome

Key Features

Dystopia canthorum (lateral displacement of inner canthi)
Broad nasal root
Midface hypoplasia
Midline cleft of upper lip that can extend through frenula and palate
Multiple frenula
Malposition, supernumerary teeth, and dental caries
Hypoplasia of the mandible ramus
Clinodactyly of fingers
Syndactyly of fingers
Brachydactyly of fingers and toes
Preaxial polysyndactyly of hallux

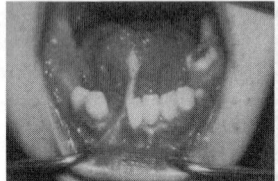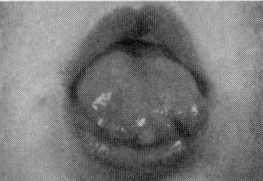

Other Findings

Dryness, alopecia of scalp hair
Milia of the face and ears, seborrheic skin
Respiratory infections
Adult polycystic kidneys
Central nervous system structural anomalies

Comments. Oral-facial-digital syndrome has an incidence of 1 in 50,000 and has been subdivided into types I through IX. Type I is characterized by oral frenula and clefts, hypoplasia of alae nasi, and digital asymmetry. Type II has the key features of cleft tongue with hamartomas and ankyloglossia, deafness, and partial reduplication of hallux. Type II is distinguished from type I in that in the former skin and hair are normal; broad bifid tip of nose, absent lower central incisors, conductive hearing loss caused by a defect of the incus, bilateral polysyndactyly, and mild short stature are present; and hyperplastic frenula are absent. Additional features observed in the other types include alternating eyelid winking, retinal abnormalities, postaxial polydactyly, growth hormone deficiency, hypogonadotrophic hypogonadism, hypothalamic hamartoma, cardiac anomalies, and hydronephrosis.

Performance. Approximately one-third of type I patients die in early infancy, and mild mental retardation has been noted in approximately one-half of the surviving patients, with their IQs ranging from 70 to 90. Treatment is directed to surgical correction of oral clefts, dental care and speech therapy.

Etiology. Oral-facial-digital syndrome type I is inherited as an X-linked disorder in female infants and is lethal in male infants. Mutations in the OFD1 gene (*CXORF5*) at Xp22 were found to underlie OFD1. Type II has autosomal recessive inheritance.

Suggested Readings

Toriello HV. Heterogeneity and variability in the oral-facial-digital syndromes. *Am J Med Genet* 1988;4(Suppl):149.
Toriello HV. Oral-facial-digital syndromes, 1992. *Clin Dysmorphol* 1993;2:95.

Osteogenesis Imperfecta Syndrome

Key Features

Increased bone fragility with multiple fractures
Short stature
Blue sclerae
Hearing loss
Dentinogenesis imperfecta (translucent/opalescent teeth with increased susceptibility to caries)
Bowing of limbs
Joint hyperextensibility

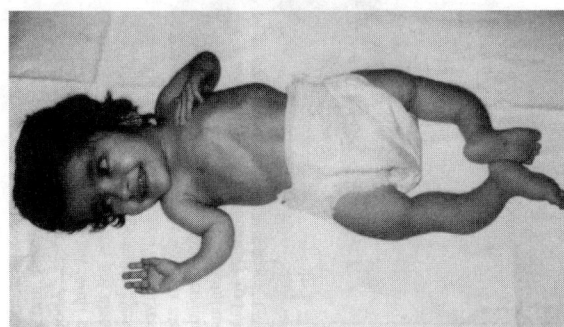

Other Findings

Wormian bones of skull
Scoliosis
Easy bruisability

Comments. Osteogenesis imperfecta syndrome represents a group of disorders with increased bone fragility. These disorders are divided into four types, and each type is divided into subtypes that indicate the presence or absence of features such as blue sclerae and dental abnormalities. Type I is generally mild to moderate in severity, type II is the severe perinatal lethal form, type III is described as progressively deforming, and type IV involves bone fragility without characteristic features of type I.

Performance. Infants with type II disease usually are stillborn or die in the early perinatal period. In types I, III, and IV, intelligence is generally normal.

Etiology. Mutations in the genes contributing to the formation of type I collagen have been found in all forms. Mutations in both *COL1A1* and *COL1A2* have been identified in all types. These conditions usually are dominant, and many represent new mutations with a paternal age effect. However, recessive inheritance has been described for some of the rarer type II and III subtypes.

Suggested Readings

McLean KR. Osteogenesis imperfecta. *Neonatal Netw* 2004;23:7.
Rauch F, Glorieux FH. Osteogenesis imperfecta. *Lancet* 2004;363:1377.

Prader-Willi Syndrome

Key Features

Obesity
Almond-shaped palpebral fissures
Hypogonadism
Small hands and feet
Hypotonia in infancy

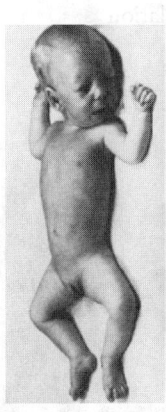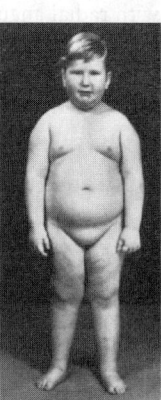

Other Findings

Narrow bifrontal diameter
Strabismus
Frequent skin picking, leading to scabs and scars

Comments. The incidence of Prader-Willi syndrome is approximately 1 in 16,000 live births. These patients are hypotonic at birth. They often have failure to thrive in infancy and may require tube feedings. However, by 6 months to 6 years of age, appetite increases, and they rapidly begin to put on weight, leading to obesity.

Performance. Mild to moderate mental retardation is present. Behavior problems are frequent and include excessive eating, rage behaviors (especially when denied food), and eating unusual foodstuffs. Psychiatric problems may develop in adolescents.

Etiology. Deletion of chromosome 15q11–q13 is detectable by high-resolution chromosome analysis or FISH in 70%. The deleted segment is always paternal, in contrast to the Angelman syndrome, in which the maternal copy of the same chromosome segment is deleted. In a small percentage of cases, the patient has inherited both copies of chromosome 15 from the mother (uniparental disomy), leading to a functional deletion of paternal information. This contiguous gene syndrome results from inactivity of the paternal copies of the imprinted small ribonucleoprotein N gene (*SNRPN*), the necdin gene, and possibly other genes on 15q11.

Suggested Readings

Gunay-Aygun M, Schwartz S, Heeger S, et al. The changing purpose of Prader-Willi syndrome clinical diagnostic criteria and proposed revised criteria. *Pediatrics* 2001;108:E92.
Whittington J, Holland A, Webb T, et al. Relationship between clinical and genetic diagnosis of Prader-Willi syndrome. *J Med Genet* 2002;39:926.

Rubinstein-Taybi Syndrome

Key Features

Short stature (postnatal onset)
Downslanting palpebral fissures
Low-set, dysplastic ears
Beaked nose
Narrow palate with maxillary hypoplasia
Broad great toes
Broad thumbs with radial angulation

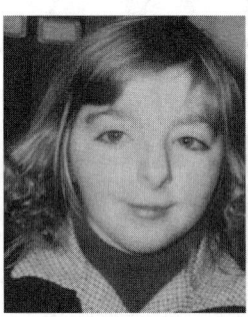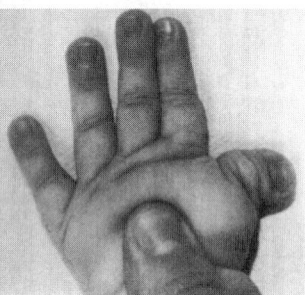

Other Findings

Long eyelashes
Ptosis, strabismus
Cardiac defects (PDA, VSD, ASD)
Cryptorchidism
Broad fingers (in addition to thumb)
Excessive keloid formation

Comments. Feeding difficulties, obstipation, and respiratory infections are common in infants affected with Rubinstein-Taybi syndrome. The majority have speech difficulties and a stiff gait. Affected children require speech and physical therapy. Significant variability occurs in this condition.

Performance. Mental retardation is present, with an average IQ of approximately 50.

Etiology. Rubinstein-Taybi syndrome usually occurs sporadically. The *CREBBP* (cAMP-regulated enhancer binding protein) gene at chromosome 16p13.3 has been found to be deleted or mutated in a number of cases. Approximately one-fourth of cases are caused by submicroscopic deletions detectable by FISH.

Suggested Readings

Petri F, et al. Rubenstein-Taybi syndrome caused by mutations in the transcriptional co-activator CBP. *Nature* 1995;346:348.
Stevens CA, et al. Rubenstein-Taybi syndrome. A natural history study. *Am J Med Genet* 1990;6(Suppl):30.

Russell-Silver Syndrome

Key Features

Short stature of prenatal onset
Normal head circumference
Small triangular facies
Asymmetry of limbs or trunk
Incurving of fifth fingers (clinodactyly)
Café au lait spots

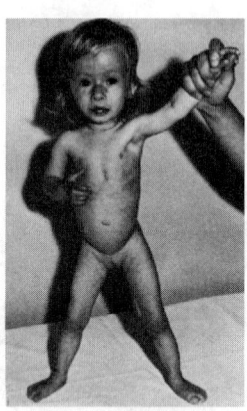

Other Findings

Frontal bossing
Delayed closure of anterior fontanelle
Downturned corners of mouth
Gastroesophageal reflux
Renal or genital abnormalities
Metacarpal and phalangeal abnormalities
Immature osseous maturation
Tendency toward fasting hypoglycemia in early childhood

Comments. Newborns with Russell-Silver syndrome are usually quite small at full term and have proportional short stature in the early years. There tends to be some improvement in growth during childhood and adolescence, and some adults have achieved height within the normal range. Growth hormone deficiency has been noted in some patients.

Performance. Developmental delay or mental retardation is present in approximately one-third of patients.

Etiology. The genetic basis of this condition is unknown. Genetic heterogeneity with several different chromosomal abnormalities exists, including reported cases of chromosome 17q25 aberrations. Several affected individuals have been reported with maternal uniparental disomy of chromosome 7, although it has been excluded in others.

Suggested Readings

Kotzot D, et al. Maternal uniparental disomy 7—review and further delineation of the phenotype. *Eur J Pediatr* 2000;159:247.
Prince SM, Stanhope R, Garrett C, et al. The spectrum of Silver-Russell syndrome: a clinical and molecular genetic study and new diagnostic criteria. *J Med Genet* 1999;36:837.

Smith-Lemli-Opitz Syndrome

Key Features

Microcephaly
Ptosis
Anteverted nares and broad nasal tip
Syndactyly of second and third toes
Genital abnormalities (hypospadias, cryptorchidism, bifid or
   hypoplastic scrotum)
Renal abnormalities

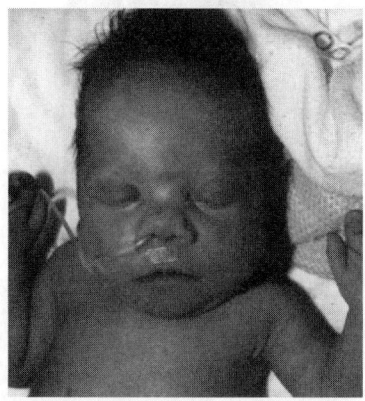

Other Findings

Cardiac defects (ASD and VSD)
Seizures
Short thumbs
Polydactyly
Aggressive behavior

Comments. Babies with Smith-Lemli-Opitz syndrome have severe failure to thrive, irritability, and abnormalities of muscle tone (initially hypotonic, with hypertonicity developing with time). Approximately 20% die within the first year of life, and 50% die by age 18 months.

Performance. Moderate to severe mental retardation is present.

Etiology. Smith-Lemli-Opitz syndrome is inherited in an autosomal recessive manner. The disorder is caused by a defect in cholesterol biosynthesis, leading to low blood cholesterol levels and dramatic elevations of the cholesterol precursor 7-dehydrocholesterol (which is the basis for diagnostic blood testing). Cholesterol supplementation is used to ameliorate some of the symptoms (such as irritability), but not cognitive development. Prenatal cholesterol supplementation of women carrying affected fetuses has been attempted, although no formal studies have been conducted to assess its effectiveness.

Suggested Readings

Merkens LS, Connor WE, Linck LM, et al. Effects of dietary cholesterol on plasma lipoproteins in Smith-Lemli-Opitz syndrome. *Pediatr Res* 2004;56: 726.

Ryan AK, et al. Smith-Lemil-Opitz syndrome: a variable clinical and biochemical phenotype. *J Med Genet* 1998;35:558.

Sikora DM, Ruggiero M, Petit-Kekel K, et al. Cholesterol supplementation does not improve developmental progress in Smith-Lemli-Opitz syndrome. *J Pediatr* 2004;144:783.

Sotos Syndrome (Cerebral Gigantism Syndrome)

Key Features

Large size
Macrocephaly
Dolichocephaly
Hypertelorism
Prominent jaw
Large hands and feet
Advanced osseous maturation
Poor coordination

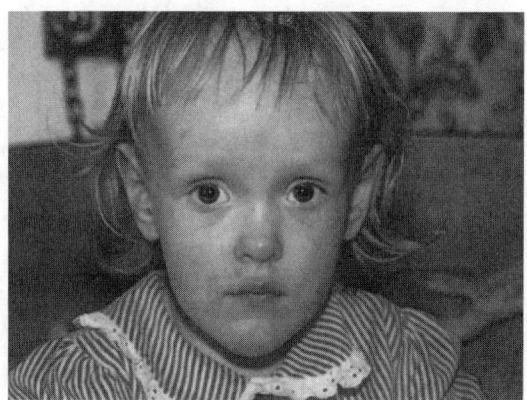

Other Findings

Sparse hair in the frontoparietal region
Premature eruption of teeth
High-arched palate
Genu valgum
Pes planus
Thin, brittle nails
Cardiac defects
Kyphoscoliosis
Seizures
Abnormal glucose tolerance test result
Malignancy
Central nervous system structural abnormalities (prominence
   of the trigone and occipital horns, ventriculomegaly)

Comments. Large size is of prenatal onset and remains at 97% or higher during childhood and early adolescence. Final height is often within the normal range. Neonatal respiratory and feeding difficulties occur. Increased otitis media has been noted. Sotos syndrome can be confused with other overgrowth conditions: Weaver syndrome, which has a distinctive facial appearance including a prominent and long philtrum and micrognathia, widened distal long bones, and more accelerated osseous maturation; and Bannayan-Riley-Ruvalcaba syndrome, which has distinctive pigmentary spotting of the penis and intestinal polyposis. As with other overgrowth syndromes Sotos is associated with a risk of malignancies.

Performance. Patients present with variable mental deficiency, with mean IQ of 72. Behavioral problems are significant. Excessive size with poor coordination leads to problems of social adjustment, often with undue aggression and temper tantrums.

Etiology. The majority of cases are sporadic. Several families have been reported with autosomal dominant inheritance. More than 60% of cases are caused by mutations in the *NSD1* gene and submicroscopic deletions of chromosome 5q35, including *NSD1*.

Suggested Reading

Visser R, Matsumoto N. Genetics of Sotos syndrome. *Curr Opin Pediatr* 2003; 15:598.

Stickler Syndrome (Hereditary Arthroophthalmopathy)

Key Features

Flat facies, maxillary hypoplasia
Severe, progressive myopia (may lead to retinal detachment)
Deafness (conductive or sensorineural)
Robin sequence (micrognathia and rounded palatal cleft)
Rhizomelic limb shortening
Enlargement of wrist, knee, and ankle joints at birth

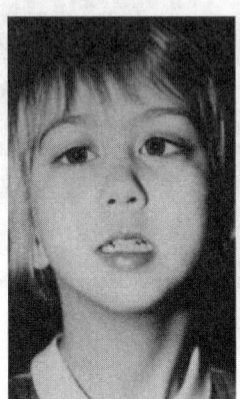 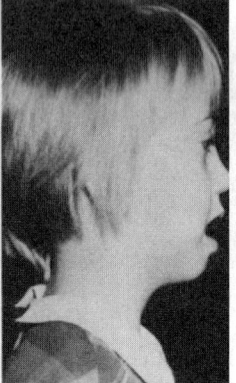

Other Findings

Mitral valve prolapse
Scoliosis
Arthritis
Hyperextensible joints
Mild spondyloepiphyseal dysplasia

Comments. Any newborn with the Robin sequence should be evaluated to rule out the Stickler syndrome. Ocular involvement is progressive and severe. Arthritis becomes a problem in young adulthood.

Performance. Mental retardation has been reported in some patients, but is not considered a frequent finding.

Etiology. Stickler syndrome is an autosomal dominant condition. Most patients with Stickler syndrome have mutations in the gene for type II collagen (*COL2A1*) located at chromosome 12q13.11–q13.2. A minority of Stickler syndrome families have mutations in *COL11A1* (chromosome 1p21) and *COL11A2* (chromosome 6p21.3) genes. Several other syndromes with similar features are associated with mutations in these genes and may represent clinical variants of Stickler syndrome: Wagner syndrome (*COL2A1*), Marshall syndrome (*COL11A1*), and Weissenbacher-Zweymuller syndrome (*COL11A2*).

Suggested Readings

Donoso LA, et al. Clinical variability of Stickler syndrome: role of exon 2 of the collagen COL2A1 gene. *Surv Ophthalmol* 2003;48:191.
Zlotogora J, et al. Variability of Stickler syndrome. *Am J Med Genet* 1992; 42:337.

Thrombocytopenia–Absent Radius Syndrome (TAR Syndrome)

Key Features

Thrombocytopenia with absence or hypoplasia of megakaryocytes
Bilateral absence of radius
Thumbs are present

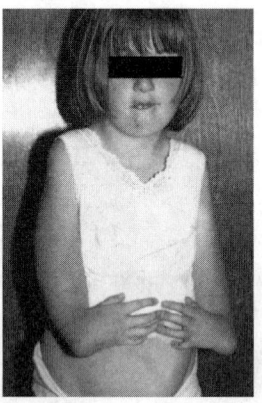

Other Findings

Congenital heart disease (TOF, ASD)
Meckel's diverticulum, pancreatic cysts
Ulnar, humeral, shoulder, or all three joint abnormalities
Lower limb abnormalities
Renal anomalies
Leukemoid granulocytosis
Eosinophilia
Anemia
Central nervous system structural abnormalities

Comments. Hematologic abnormalities are most severe in early infancy, and vigorous early management is indicated. Severity of the hematologic disorder lessens with age. Bracing and stabilization of the wrist are central to care. Arthritis of wrist and knee is a late complication. Cow's milk allergy is common. Initial evaluation should include echocardiogram and abdominal/renal ultrasound. Thrombocytopenia–absent radius syndrome can be distinguished from Fanconi anemia by the absence of thumbs, late onset of hematologic manifestations, and chromosomal changes in the latter condition. Patients with Holt-Oram syndrome have normal platelets and other distinguishing characteristics.

Performance. Forty percent of patients die during early infancy as a result of hemorrhage. Seven percent have mental retardation that usually is related to intracranial bleed. Delayed motor development is caused by skeletal abnormalities.

Etiology. Thrombocytopenia–absent radius syndrome is an autosomal recessive condition. Prenatal diagnosis can be made by demonstrating the defect of the upper limb on ultrasonography.

Suggested Readings

Greenhalgh KL, et al. Thrombocytopenia-absent radius syndrome: a clinical genetic study. *J Med Genet* 2002;39:876.
Hall JG, et al. Thrombocytopenia and absent radius (TAR) syndrome. *J Med Genet* 1987;24:79.

Treacher Collins Syndrome (Mandibulofacial Dysostosis)

Key Features

Downslanting palpebral fissures
Lower eyelid coloboma
Dysplastic ears
Malar hypoplasia
Micrognathia
Conductive hearing loss

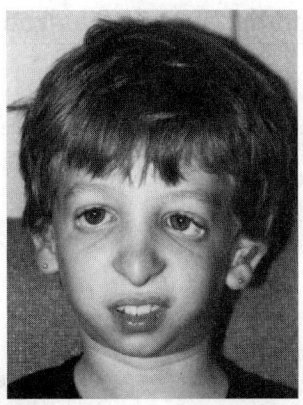

Other Findings

Partial to absent lower eyelashes
Blind fistulas and skin tags between auricle and angle of the mouth
External ear canal defect
Macrostomia
Cleft palate
Projection of scalp hair onto lateral cheek

Comments. Treacher Collins syndrome occurs in 1 in 50,000 live births. Patients have early respiratory and feeding difficulties because of their narrow airway, micrognathia, cleft palate, or all three features. Early recognition of deafness is important for treatment with hearing aids and surgery. Hemifacial microsomia (Oculo-auriculo-vertebral dysplasia or Goldenhar syndrome) presents with similar, but asymmetric or unilateral facial involvement and epibulbar dermoids. Nager and Miller syndromes, with acrofacial dysostosis, share some facial features with Treacher Collins syndrome, but have limb abnormalities and are recognized as separate disorder.

Performance. Mental retardation has been reported in only 5% of cases.

Etiology. Treacher Collins syndrome is an autosomal dominant condition. Treacher Collins syndrome is caused by mutations in *TCOF1* located at chromosome 5q32–q33.

Suggested Readings

The Treacher Collins Syndrome Collaborative Group. Positional cloning of a gene involved in the pathogenesis of Treacher Collins syndrome. *Nature Genet* 1996;12:130.
Wise C, et al. *TCOF1* gene encodes a putative nucleolar phosphoprotein that exhibits mutations in Treacher Collins syndrome throughout its coding region. *Proc Natl Acad Sci USA* 1997;94:3110.

Tricho-Rhino-Phalangeal Syndrome (TRP Syndrome)

Key Features

Sparse hair
Bulbous nose
Epiphyseal coning

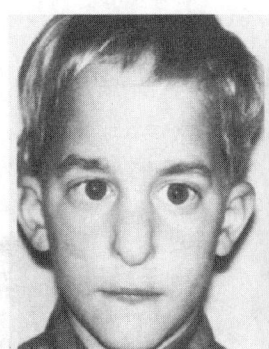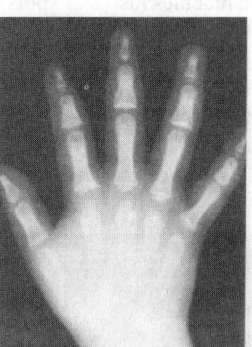

Other Findings

Large prominent ears
Long, prominent philtrum
Thin upper lip
Small carious teeth
Short metacarpals and metatarsals

Comments. In Type I, hair is usually sparse at birth. Phalangeal changes, split distal radial epiphyses, and winged scapula may develop in childhood and worsen until adolescence. Degenerative hip disease can present in adulthood. Some cases have increased respiratory infections. Type II (Langer-Giedion syndrome) patients resemble that of Type I, but they also have multiple exostoses (especially of the long bones), loose redundant skin in infancy, nevi, laxity of joints, microcephaly, growth deficiency, hearing deficit, and other dental and bony abnormalities. Type III is the severe end of the spectrum of Type I, presenting with severe brachydactyly (due to short metacarpals) and severe short stature, but without exostoses.

Performance. Intelligence is normal for Type I, and mild to severe retardation occurs in 70% for Type II.

Etiology. Tricho-rhino-phalangeal syndrome is an autosomal dominant condition due to a genetic alteration at chromosome 8q24.11–q24.13. Types I and III can be caused by different subclasses of mutations in the zinc finger transcription factor gene *TRPS1*. In Type II, the exostoses can occur with mutations in the exostosin 1 gene *EXT1*. Type I and II can result from different sized deletions in 8q and may be considered a contiguous gene syndrome. Deletion of 8q24.12 accounts for features in common to Type I and II, and deletion 8q24.13 results in exostoses.

Suggested Readings

Ludecke H-J, et al. Genotypic and phenotypic spectrum in tricho-rhino-phalangeal syndrome types I and III. *Am J Hum Genet* 2001;68:81.
Ludecke H-J, et al. Molecular dissection of a contiguous gene syndrome: localization of the genes involved in the Langer-Giedion syndrome. *Hum Molec Genet* 1995;4:31.

Tuberous Sclerosis Syndrome

Key Features

Hamartomas in multiple organ systems
Glioma-angioma lesions in the cortex and white matter*
Fibrous plaque on forehead*
Hamartomas of the retina*
Fibrous-angiomatous lesions of the cheeks*
White macules (ash leaf spots)
Shagreen patch
Café au lait spots
Pit-shaped enamel defects of labial premolar surface
Ungual fibromas*
Cyst-like areas of phalanges
Seizures

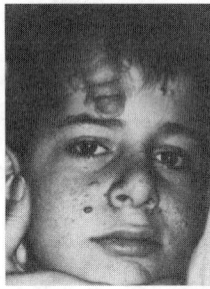 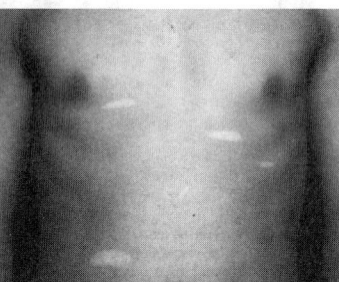

Other Findings

Infantile spasms
Intracranial mineralization in basal ganglia and
  periventricular region
Cardiac rhabdomyoma
Renal angiomyolipomas or cysts

Comments. The occurrence of tuberous sclerosis syndrome is 1 in 10,000 live births. Only one of the features with an asterisk or two or more other features are required for diagnosis. Facial nodular lesions are present in 50% of children by 5 years of age, whereas white macules are present at birth or in early infancy. Proper skin inspection requires examination with Wood's lamp. An estimated 51% to 86% of patients diagnosed with cardiac rhabdomyoma may have tuberous sclerosis. Malignant transformation may occur, and approximately 6% of patients develop a brain tumor. Patients have behavioral problems and autism.

Performance. The most significant morbidity associated with tuberous sclerosis is related to CNS involvement, which can be profoundly debilitating. Seizures occur in more than 80% of patients (including infantile spasms in approximately one-third) and developmental delay (including autistic spectrum disorders) in more than 60%. The severity of these symptoms is related to the extent of hamartomatous involvement of the brain.

Etiology. Tuberous sclerosis syndrome is an autosomal dominant condition, with 60% to 80% of cases representing *de novo* mutations. Two genes causing tuberous sclerosis syndrome have been identified: *TCS1* on chromosome 9q34 and *TCS2* on chromosome 16p13.3. Contiguous to the *TCS2* gene on chromosome 16q13 is the autosomal dominant polycystic kidney disease gene. In angiomyolipomas and lymphangiomyomatosis, loss of heterozygosity (a germline mutation in one gene is already present, followed by the loss of the second gene of the pair) of *TCS1* or *TCS2* occurs.

Suggested Readings

Jones AC, et al. Comprehensive mutation analysis of TSC1 and TSC2- and phenotypic correlations in 150 families with tuberous sclerosis. *Am J Hum Genet* 1999;64:1305.

Roach ES, et al. Diagnostic criteria: tuberous sclerosis complex. Report of the diagnostic criteria committee of the National Tuberous Sclerosis Association. *J Clin Neurol* 1992;7:221.

van Slegentenhorst M, et al. Identification of the tuberous sclerosis gene *TSC1* on chromosome 9q34. *Science* 1997;277:805.

Van der Woude Syndrome

Key Features

Lower lip pits and sinuses that may drain accessory or
  heterotopic salivary glands
Cleft lip
Cleft palate
Bifid uvula

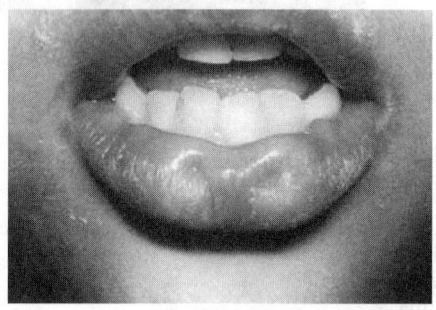

Other Finding

Hypodontia

Comments. Van der Woude syndrome is the most common syndromic form of cleft lip and/or palate, accounting for about 2% of all patients with oral clefts. It is almost completely penetrant, but severity of the individual features is highly variable within and between families. Lip pits occur in 86% of the affected and are the only manifestation in 44% of the cases. Cleft lip and/or palate with or without lip pits occur in more than 50% of the cases. Careful examination for minor manifestations in relatives who are thought to be "unaffected" is necessary. Bifid uvula may be a minimal clinical manifestation of this syndrome. Popliteal pterygium syndrome has a similar orofacial phenotype and also includes skin and genital anomalies. Van der Woude and popliteal pterygium syndromes are thought to represent a clinical spectrum of the same genetic disorder.

Performance. The individuals with either van der Woude or popliteal pterygium syndrome have normal intelligence. Exceptions occur with large deletions of the *IRF6* gene region.

Etiology. Both van der Woude syndrome and popliteal pterygium syndrome can be caused by mutations in the gene encoding interferon regulatory factor-6, *IRF6*. Diagnostic genetic testing is available and should be considered also for families with more than one individual with cleft lip and/or palate, even in the absence of lip pits.

Suggested Readings

Burdick AB, Bixler D, Puckett CL. Genetic analysis in families with van der Woude syndrome. *J Craniofac Genet Dev Biol* 1985;5:181.

Kondo S, et al. Mutations in IRF6 cause Van der Woude and popliteal pterygium syndromes. *Nat Gene* 2002;32:285.

Suggested Readings

Emanuel BS, McDonald-McGinn D, Saitta SC, Zackai EH. The 22q11. 2 deletion syndrome. *Adv Pediatr* 2001;48:39.

Goldberg R, et al. Velo-cardio-facial syndrome: a review of 120 patients. *Am J Med Genet* 1993;45:313.

McDermid HE, Morrow BE. Genomic disorders on 22q11. *Am J Hum Genet* 2002;70:1077.

Morrow B, et al. Molecular definition of the 22q11 deletions in velo-cardio-facial syndrome. *Am J Hum Genet* 1995;56:1391.

Perez E, Sullivan KE. Chromosome 22q11. 2 deletion syndrome (DiGeorge and velocardiofacial syndromes). *Curr Opin Pediatr* 2002;14:678.

Velo-Cardio-Facial Syndrome (Shprintzen Syndrome, chromosome 22q11 deletion)

Key Features

Cleft of the secondary palate
Velopharyngeal incompetence
Prominent nose
Narrow palpebral fissures
Retruded mandible
Microcephaly
Slender and hyperextensible hands and fingers
Cardiac defects (VSD, TOF, right aortic arch)

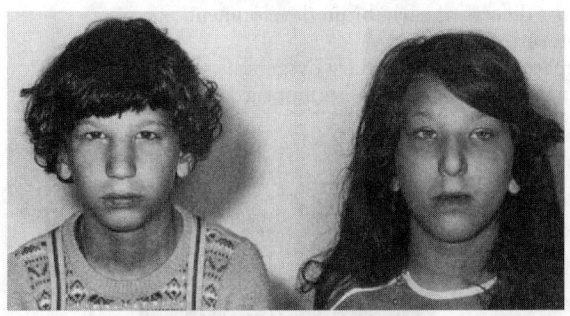

Other Findings

Minor auricular anomalies
Hypoplastic and elongated malar area
Medial displacement of the internal carotid arteries
Scoliosis
Hypernasal speech
Psychiatric disorders

Comments. Hypotonia in infancy is frequent, with transient hypocalcemia.

Performance. Learning disabilities and mild intellectual impairment (IQ of 70 to 90) is present. Speech development often is delayed, and language is impaired. Socialization skills may surpass intellectual skills.

Etiology. Velo-cardio-facial syndrome is inherited as an autosomal dominant condition with an estimated frequency of 1 out of 4,000 to 5,000 live births. Affected individuals have an interstitial deletion of chromosome 22q11.21–q11.23 and are monosomic for this region. The deletion is detected by FISH in approximately 85% of the patients and is inherited in approximately 28% of the cases. The same region is deleted in some cases of DiGeorge syndrome, a condition that variably includes lateral displacement of inner canthi with short palpebral fissures, short philtrum, micrognathia, ear anomalies, and defects of development of the thymus, parathyroids, and great vessels.

Waardenburg Syndrome

Key Features

Partial albinism
White forelock
Heterochromia of irises
Telecanthus (lateral displacement of medial canthi)
Deafness

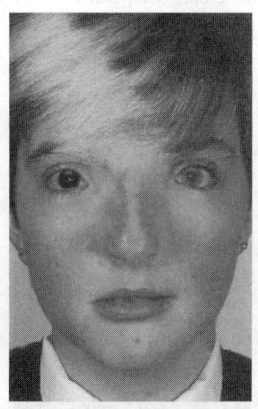

Other Findings

Broad nasal bridge
Hypoplastic alae
Medial flare of bushy eyebrows
Aplasia of posterior semicircular canal
Cardiac anomaly (VSD)
Intestinal aganglionosis

Comments. Four clinical types of Waardenburg syndrome have been described (WS1-4). Pigmentary defects and deafness are the cardinal symptoms for all forms. The white forelock may be present at birth and become pigmented early in life; the hair may become prematurely gray. Telecanthus is known to occur in WS1, but not in WS2. Limb defects are considered characteristic for WS3. WS4 is also known as Hirschsprung disease type II and is characterized by intestinal aganglionosis.

Performance. Intelligence is normal. Deafness is the most significant burden of the disorder. Waardenburg syndrome accounts for 2% to 5% of cases of congenital deafness.

Etiology. Waardenburg syndrome is inherited as an autosomal dominant condition. WS1 and WS3 are caused by loss of function mutations in the *PAX3* gene at chromosome 2q35. WS2 is genetically heterogeneous, and mutations in *MITF* and *SLUG* genes have been found in some but not all patients. Mutations in the *EDN3, EDNRB*, and *SOX10* genes result in WS4.

Suggested Readings

McCallion AS, Chakravarti A. EDNRB/EDN3 and Hirschsprung disease type II. *Pigment Cell Res* 2001;14:161.

Pardono E, et al. Waardenburg syndrome: clinical differentiation between types I and II. *Am J Med Genet* 2003;117A:223.

Sanchez-Martin M, Rodriguez-Garcia A, Perez-Losada J, et al. SLUG (*SNAI2*) deletions in patients with Waardenburg disease. *Hum Mol Genet* 2002; 11:3231.

Williams Syndrome
(William-Beuren Syndrome)

Key Features

Periorbital soft tissue fullness
Blue irides with stellate pattern
Medial eyebrow flare
Anteverted nares
Long philtrum
Prominent, thick lips with mouth held open
Cardiac abnormalities (supravalvular aortic stenosis, peripheral pulmonic stenosis, pulmonary valve stenosis, ASD, VSD)

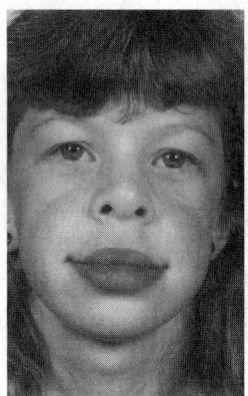

Other Findings

Mild short stature
Hoarse, husky voice
Renal anomalies, artery stenosis
Hypoplastic nails
Friendly, "cocktail party" personality
Hypercalcemia in infancy
Dental abnormalities, agenesis of permanent teeth

Comments. Feeding difficulties are frequent in infants with the Williams syndrome. Adults are at risk for additional medical problems, including hypertension, gastrointestinal difficulties (gastrointestinal bleeding, constipation, diverticulosis), urinary tract infections, and joint contractures. A detailed cardiac evaluation must be performed in all patients due to the high incidence of cardiovascular abnormalities.

Performance. Mental retardation occurs, with an IQ usually in the 50s. Language skills are less affected than cognitive skills and may hide the extent of the patient's mental impairment.

Etiology. Cases of Williams syndrome are usually sporadic, although dominant inheritance has been reported. This condition is a contiguous gene syndrome that is due to a deletion at chromosome 7q11.23. At least twenty-four genes have been assigned to the deleted region. Deletions and mutations in the *elastin* gene are associated with the cardiovascular phenotype. Loss of *LIM-kinase-1*, is possibly responsible for the impaired visuospatial cognition, whereas loss of *CYLN2* has been associated with the neurologic phenotype.

Suggested Readings

Lashkari A, et al. Williams-Beuren syndrome: an update and review for the primary physician. *Clin Pediatr (Phila)* 1999;38:189.

Tassabehji M. Williams-Beuren syndrome: a challenge for genotype-phenotype correlations. *Hum Mol Genet* 2003;12:R229.

Zellweger Syndrome
(Cerebrohepatorenal Syndrome)

Key Features

Macrocephaly with large fontanelles
High forehead
Flat occiput
Flat facies
Gross defects of early brain development
Anteverted nares
Hepatomegaly with biliary dysgenesis
Renal microcysts with albuminuria

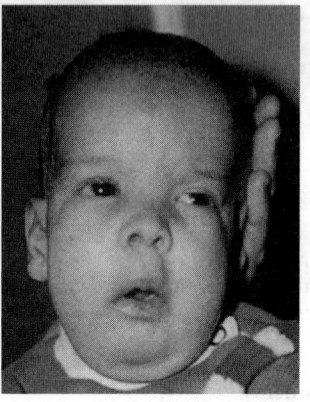

Other Findings

Congenital cataracts
Retinal pigmentary changes
Failure to thrive
Hypotonia
Cardiac defects (PDA, septal changes)
Variable contractures
Stippling of patellae

Comments. Most infants with Zellweger syndrome are born with breech presentation and present with failure to thrive. They are found to have variable elevated serum iron levels and evidence of iron storage, pipecolic acidemia, abnormal bile acids, and absent liver peroxisomes. Diagnosis is based on biochemical studies, including decreased dihydroxyacetone phosphate acyltransferase activity in fibroblasts and blood cells, a lowered plasmalogen biosynthesis, accumulation of unmetabolized very long-chain fatty acids, and an absence of catalase-containing subcellular particles in fibroblasts.

Performance. The vast majority of infants die within the first year of life. Survivors have severe mental retardation and seizures.

Etiology. Zellweger syndrome is inherited as an autosomal recessive condition. The condition is heterogeneous and is caused by mutations in any of several different genes involved in peroxisome biogenesis. Peroxin (*PEX*) genes can be mutated and have been mapped to chromosomes 12, 8, and 6. Mutations have been found in the peroxisomal membrane protein PMP70 at chromosome 1p22–p21. Another locus is suspected at chromosome 7q11.23, where chromosomal aberrations have been detected.

Suggested Readings

FitzPatrick DR. Zellweger syndrome and associated phenotypes. *J Med Genet* 1996;33:863.

Weller S, Gould SJ, Valle D. Peroxisome biogenesis disorders. *Annu Rev Genomics Hum Genet* 2003;4:165.

Arthrogryposis

Key Features

Joint contractures
Club foot
Skin dimpling over joints
Decreased spontaneous movement

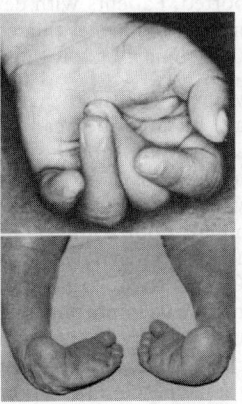

Other Findings

Congenital hip dislocation
Radial or ulnar deviation of fingers
Altered creasing patterns

Comments. Arthrogryposis describes the finding of congenital joint contractures. They range from mild involvement of limited joints (as in distal arthrogryposis) to more severe involvement of a greater number of joints (as in amyoplasia congenita) with lifelong implications. Spinal muscular atrophy and nemaline myopathy should be considered in the differential diagnosis. Physical therapy is of great importance to maximize joint function, and in more severe cases, orthopedic intervention is required.

Performance. Usually, intelligence is normal unless the arthrogryposis is part of a larger genetic syndrome with known intellectual compromise (such as trisomy 18 or Freeman-Sheldon syndrome).

Etiology. Arthrogryposis results from prolonged decrease of fetal movement *in utero*. Many forms of arthrogryposis exist and can be subdivided in four main pathogenetic categories: myopathies, neuropathies, connective tissue disorders, and exogenous effects, such as limitation of space due to uterine constraint or extrauterine pressure. Discerning the etiology of the individual's impairment is essential for recurrence risk counseling. Arthrogryposis occurs as part of syndromes that are chromosomal, dominant, and recessive. Distal arthrogryposis has been associated with mutations in genes encoding proteins of the contractile apparatus specific to fast-twitch myofibers, such as *TNNI2*, *TNNT3*, and *TPM2*. It is not possible on the basis of only clinical characteristics to distinguish which gene may be responsible. Sporadic forms that occur because of external factors carry a lower recurrence risk.

Suggested Readings

Gordon N. Arthrogryposis multiplex congenita. *Brain Dev* 1998;20:507.

Hall JG, et al. The distal arthrogryposis. Delineation of new entities—review and nosologic discussion. *Am J Med Genet* 1982;11:185.

Hall JG, et al. Part I: amyoplasia: a common sporadic condition with congenital contractures. *Am J Med Genet* 1983;15:571.

Sung SS, et al. Mutations in genes encoding fast-twitch contractile proteins cause distal arthrogryposis syndromes. *Am J Hum Genet* 2003;72:681.

Cleft Lip with or without Cleft Palate/Robin Sequence

Key Features

Cleft lip
Cleft palate

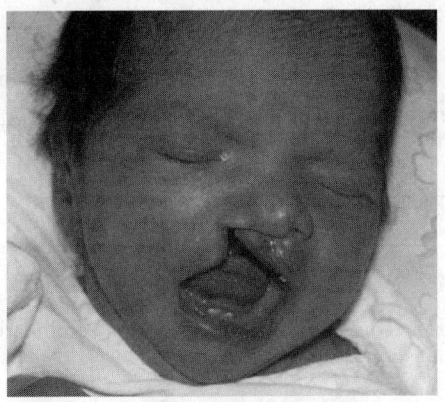

Other Findings

Dental anomalies (missing or malpositioned teeth)
Hearing loss (caused by frequent otitis media)
Articulation problems
Feeding difficulties

Comments. Overall frequency of cleft lip with or without cleft palate in the white population is approximately 1 in 1,000. A significant racial predilection exists; clefting occurs most frequently in the Native American and Asian populations, and least often in blacks. Male infants are generally affected more often than female infants. The differential diagnosis for cleft lip and palate includes Van der Woude syndrome, and for cleft palate includes Robin sequence and velo-cardio-facial syndrome. Robin sequence (also referred to as Pierre Robin sequence) involves a small, underdeveloped jaw during gestation. The small jaw affects the position of the tongue and interferes with the normal closure of the palate. It may be seen alone or as part of one of several genetic syndromes.

Performance. Individuals with isolated cleft lip with or without cleft palate (not associated with a genetic syndrome) are usually of normal intelligence. Speech or articulation problems may give a false impression of intellectual compromise.

Etiology. Cleft lip with or without cleft palate (CLP) is etiologically distinct from isolated cleft palate. The defect in lip closure occurs at approximately 5 to 7 weeks of gestation, with failure of the maxillary and medial nasal prominences to fuse. The medial nasal prominences form the primary (anterior) palate; therefore, defective lip closure may in turn lead to an anterior palatal cleft. Isolated cleft palate results from failure of fusion of maxillary shelves, which form the secondary palate.

Nonsyndromic cleft lip or palate follows multifactorial inheritance. More than twenty candidate genes have been suggested, and linkage to multiple chromosomal regions has been established. Variations in the *IRF6* gene are responsible for 12% of the genetic contribution to nonsyndromic cleft lip or palate, and these variations triple the risk of recurrence in families that already have one affected child. Mutations of *PVRL1* are associated with both sporadic, nonsyndromic CLP in northern Venezuela and with syndromic form of cleft lip and palate known as Zlotogora-Ogur syndrome. This suggests that genes for rare developmental syndromes also might play roles in common birth defects.

The recurrence risk for CLP (approximately 3% to 5%) increases when the defect is severe or bilateral and when multiple family members are affected.

Suggested Readings

Jones MC. Facial clefting: etiology and developmental pathogenesis. *Clin Plast Surg* 1993;20;599.

Murray JC. Gene/environment causes of cleft lip and/or palate. *Clin Genet* 2002; 61:248.

Shprintzen RJ, et al. Anomalies associated with cleft lip, cleft palate, or both. *Am J Med Genet* 1985;20:585.

Zucchero TM, et al. Interferon regulatory factor 6 (*IRF6*) gene variants and the risk of isolated cleft lip or palate. *N Engl J Med* 2004;351:769.

Craniosynostosis

Key Feature

Premature fusion of an isolated suture or a combination of calvarial sutures

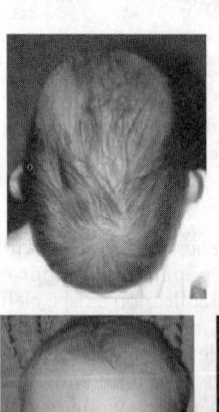
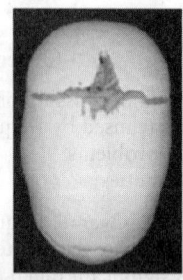
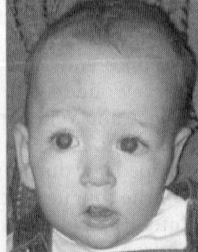
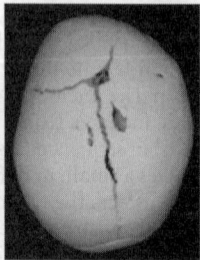

Other Findings

Eye or vision abnormalities (strabismus, hypo- or hypertelorism, amblyopia)
Oral anomalies (high arched palate, malocclusion)
Facial asymmetry
Symptoms of increased intracranial pressure (headaches, vomiting)

Comments. Craniosynostosis can present as an isolated malformation in about 1 out of 2,000 live-born babies. The type of skull shape deformity is based on the sutural involvement. An elongated skull (dolichocephaly) is the most common and is caused by sagittal synostosis (top row of photos). A boxed shaped skull (brachycephaly) is caused by bilateral coronal synostosis and an asymmetric skull shape of plagiocephaly can be caused by unilateral lambdoid or coronal fusion (bottom row of photos). Trigonocephaly is due to metopic synostosis. A complex deformity may be due to multiple suture fusion.

Craniosynostosis should be differentiated from positional plagiocephaly. Often, premature infants have dolichocephaly, and infants have occipital flattening because of positioning, but no synostosis on CT scan. When craniosynostosis is associated with other congenital anomalies, the differential diagnosis should include Crouzon, Pfeiffer, and Saethre-Chotzen syndromes. Molecular analysis of the *FGFR1, FGFR2, FGFR3,* and *TWIST* genes in which mutations causing syndromic craniosynostosis have been found are recommended for patients with coronal and multiple suture craniosynostosis.

Performance. Children with nonsyndromic craniosynostosis are usually of normal intelligence, although learning problems have been reported. Patients with developmental and/or neurologic problems should be evaluated for increased intracranial pressure and Chiari I malformation.

Etiology. Nonsyndromic craniosynostosis is believed to be a multifactorial trait. Intrauterine head constraint is believed to be a risk factor. Fetal exposure to sodium valproate is associated with metopic craniosynostosis. Most commonly, nonsyndromic craniosynostosis occurs sporadically, but about 8% of the cases are familial. Approximately fifteen to 50% of the patients with presumable nonsyndromic coronal craniosynostosis may have a FGFR3 Pro250Arg mutation. Testing for this mutation and others may be important because the presence of the Pro250Arg mutation can predict a poorer surgical outcome than cases without the mutation. In addition to craniosynostosis, patients may have subtle limb anomalies, hearing loss, and/or developmental delay.

Suggested Readings

Cohen MM Jr, MacLean RE. *Craniosynostosis: diagnosis, evaluation, and management.* New York: Oxford University Press, 2000.

Renier D, Lajeunie E, Arnaud E, Marchac D. Management of craniosynostoses. *Childs Nerv Syst* 2000;16:645.

Shipster C, Hearst D, Somerville A, et al. Speech, language, and cognitive development in children with isolated sagittal synostosis. *Dev Med Child Neurol* 2003;45:34.

Holoprosencephaly

Key Features

Inadequate midfacial and incomplete forebrain development resulting in varying degrees of hypotelorism and lack of the philtrum or nasal septum
Anomalies of brain development

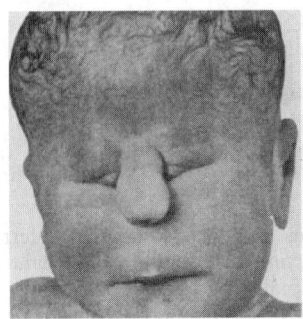
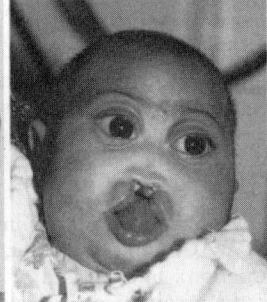

Other Findings

Cyclopia (synophthalmia, fusion of the eyes) with failure of cleavage of prosencephalon
Proboscis, olfactory placodes consolidate into a single tube-like structure located superior to the eyes
Absence of the ethmoid and other midline facial bones
Cleft lip and palate, median or bilateral
Endocrine abnormalities

Comments. Holoprosencephaly occurs in 1 in 15,000 live births and is present in as many as 1 in 250 spontaneous abortions. During the third to fourth week of development, incomplete migration of the prechordal mesoderm to an area anterior to the notochord occurs, resulting in dysmorphogenesis of the midface and failure of division of the forebrain into cerebral hemispheres. Wide intrafamilial variability appears, with clinical manifestations ranging from simple hypotelorism and/or single central maxillary incisor to alobar brain with cyclopia.

Performance. The prognosis for central nervous system function in individuals with alobar defect is extremely poor, whereas children with semilobar forms exhibit moderate to severe mental retardation, and minimally affected individuals may have normal cognition.

Etiology. Holoprosencephaly is heterogeneous and can be caused by genetic or environmental insults. It is usually sporadic, although dominant inheritance has been reported. It can be associated with several chromosomal abnormalities. At least 12 different chromosomal loci have been associated with holoprosencephaly, and mutations in several distinct genes have been identified—sonic hedgehog (*SHH*) and its receptor (*PTCH*), *GLI2, ZIC2, SIX3,* and *TGIF.*

Suggested Readings

Hahn JS, Pinter JD. Holoprosencephaly: genetic, neuroradiological, and clinical advances. *Semin Pediatr Neurol* 2002;9:309.
Wallis D, Muenke M. Mutations in holoprosencephaly. *Hum Mutat* 2000;16:99.

CHARGE

Key Features

Coloboma of retina, lens, choroid, or optic nerve
Heart defect (TOF, PDA, VSD, ASD)
Atresia choanae
Retardation of growth, development, or both

Genital abnormalities in male infants (cryptorchidism, microphallus)
Ear abnormalities or deafness

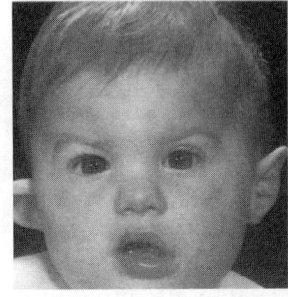
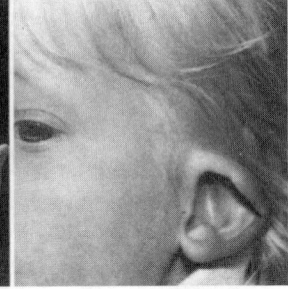

Other Findings

Cleft lip or cleft palate
Micrognathia
Multiple cranial nerve abnormalities
Facial palsy
Tracheoesophageal fistula
Hypocalcemia

Comments. In infants with CHARGE, feeding problems are frequent, and some patients die in infancy. Coloboma (79%) and choanal atresia (57%) are among the most specific diagnostic clues, and at least three other cardinal malformations (heart, ear, and genital) should be present. Growth retardation is not a necessary diagnostic criterion.

Performance. Almost all patients have some degree of mental retardation, ranging from mild to profound. Concomitant central nervous system malformations may be found, including holoprosencephaly.

Etiology. CHARGE is usually sporadic. About 8% of cases are familial. This association was redefined as a syndrome because mutations involving the chromodomain helicase DNA-binding protein-7 (*CHD7*) or semaphorin-3E (*SEMA3E*) gene were found in patients. The pathogenesis of this condition is thought to involve a defect in neural crest cell migration and deficiency of mesoderm formation during the second month of gestation.

Suggested Readings

Davenport SLH, et al. The spectrum of clinical features in CHARGE syndrome. *Clin Genet* 1986;29:298.
Oley CA, et al. A reappraisal of the CHARGE association. *J Med Genet* 1988; 25:147.
Tellier AL, et al. CHARGE syndrome: report of 47 cases and review. *Am J Med Genet* 1998;76:402.

VATER/VACTERL

Key Features

Vertebral defects
Anal atresia (imperforate anus)
Cardiac defects
Tracheoesophageal fistula
Renal, radial, or both kinds of dysplasia
Limb abnormality

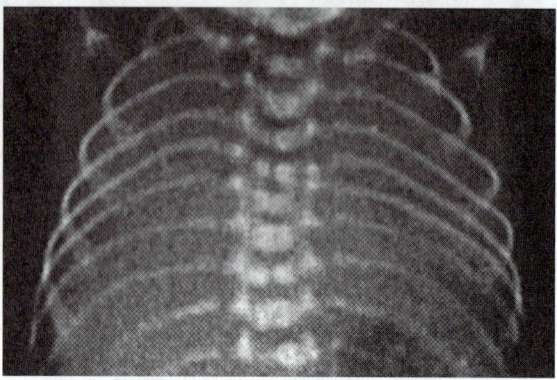

Other Findings

Single umbilical artery
Genital abnormalities
Growth retardation
Ear abnormalities

Comments. The nonrandom association of vertebral defects, anal defects, tracheoesophageal fistula, and renal and radial abnormalities was initially designated as *VATER association*, but has been expanded to *VACTERL* to recognize the increased incidence of cardiac and limb defects. These patients usually do not show facial dysmorphism. The presence of at least three of the features is considered necessary for diagnosis.

Performance. Intelligence usually is normal.

Etiology. The association usually is sporadic, with increased occurrence in infants of diabetic mothers. Possible associations with deletion of chromosome 13q22 or defective *Shh* signaling during human embryogenesis have been suggested.

Suggested Readings

Walsh LE, Vance GH, Weaver DD. Distal 13q Deletion Syndrome and the VACTERL association: case report, literature review, and possible implications. *Am J Med Genet* 2001;98:137.
Weaver DD, Mapstone CL, Pao-lo Y. The VATER association: analysis of 46 patients. *Am J Dis Child* 1986;140:225.

Aniridia-Wilms Tumor (WAGR)

Key Features

Aniridia with associated foveal hypoplasia
Wilms tumor
Genital abnormalities (cryptorchidism, hypospadias)
Growth retardation

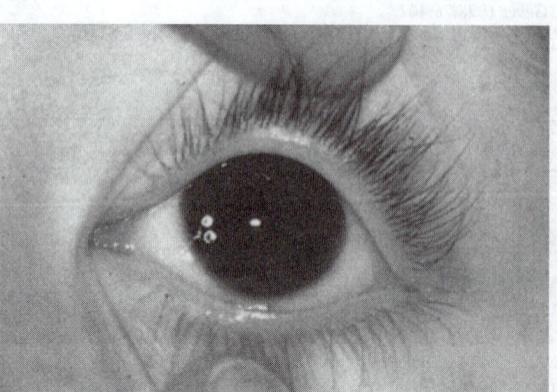

Other Findings

Microcephaly
Additional ocular abnormalities (congenital cataracts, nystagmus, ptosis, blindness)
Low-set, dysplastic ears
Gonadoblastoma (rare)

Comments. Aniridia-Wilms tumor is sometimes referred to as *WAGR* (*W*ilms tumor, *a*niridia, *g*enital abnormalities, *r*etardation). In contrast to isolated occurrences of Wilms tumor, the involvement is likely to be bilateral and to occur at an earlier age. High-resolution cytogenetic testing is used for diagnostic purposes. If the chromosome 11q13 band is found to be deleted in a patient with aniridia, the risk of developing Wilms tumor is up to 50%. Children with obvious or cryptic (detectable by FISH) deletion of 11p13 band require regular renal ultrasound examinations every 3 months until they reach 8 years of age. Those with aniridia, but without 11p13 deletion are at very low risk of Wilms tumor and do not require such examinations.

Performance. Moderate to severe mental retardation is present in most patients.

Etiology. Most cases of aniridia-Wilms tumor are sporadic; however, a familial form can be found that is caused by a balanced chromosome translocation in the parent. This condition is a contiguous gene syndrome. Most cases are associated with a chromosome 11p13 deletion, which may vary in size from patient to patient. Within this critical region are the deleted genes *PAX6*, which causes aniridia, and *WT1*, which causes Wilms tumor.

Suggested Readings

Breslow NE, et al. Characteristics and outcomes of children with the Wilms tumor-Aniridia syndrome: a report from the National Wilms Tumor Study Group. *J Clin Oncol* 2003;21:4579.
Gronskov K, et al. Population-based risk estimates of Wilms tumor in aniridia. A comprehensive procedure of PAX6 identifies 80% of mutations in aniridia. *Hum Genet* 2001,109:11.

DISORDERS LISTED BY KEY FEATURES

Cranium

Craniosynostosis

Apert syndrome
Baller-Gerold syndrome (craniosynostosis, radial aplasia)
Carpenter syndrome (acrocephaly, lateral displacement of inner canthi, polydactyly and syndactyly of feet, autosomal recessive)
Crouzon syndrome
Greig cephalopolysyndactyly syndrome (frontal bossing, preaxial and postaxial polydactyly, syndactyly)
Jackson-Weiss syndrome (craniosynostosis, foot anomalies)
Pfeiffer syndrome (brachycephaly, broad thumbs and toes)
Saethre-Chotzen syndrome (brachycephaly, prominent ear crus, maxillary hypoplasia, and syndactyly)

Thanatophoric dysplasia type II (cloverleaf skull deformity, short bowed limbs, short lifespan)

Eyes

Hypertelorism

Aarskog syndrome (hypertelorism, brachydactyly, shawl scrotum)
Apert syndrome
Cat-eye syndrome (iris coloboma, anal atresia)
Crouzon syndrome
Frontonasal dysplasia (primary defect in midface development, lateral displacement of eyes, broad nasal tip)
Greig cephalopolysyndactyly syndrome
Noonan syndrome
Opitz syndrome
Fetal akinesia deformation sequence
Pfeiffer syndrome
Retinoic acid embryopathy
Saethre-Chotzen syndrome
Sotos syndrome

Hypotelorism

Holoprosencephaly
Fetal effects of maternal phenylketonuria
Trisomy 13 syndrome

Coloboma

Aniridia-Wilms tumor association
Cat-eye syndrome
CHARGE association
Trisomy 13

Ears

Ear Tags or Pits

Beckwith-Wiedemann syndrome
Branchio-oto-renal syndrome (BOR syndrome)
Cat-eye syndrome
Cri du chat syndrome
Frontonasal dysplasia
Oculo-auriculo-vertebral dysplasia
Retinoic acid embryopathy
Townes-Brocks syndrome (auricular, thumb, and anal anomalies)
Treacher Collins syndrome

Hearing Loss

Apert syndrome
Baller-Gerold syndrome
Branchio-oto-renal syndrome
Carpenter syndrome
CHARGE association
Cleft palate (secondary hearing loss)
Cleidocranial dysplasia
Cockayne syndrome
Cornelia de Lange syndrome
Crouzon syndrome
Fetal rubella syndrome
Mucopolysaccharidoses (Hurler and Hunter syndromes)
Noonan syndrome
Oculo-auriculo-vertebral dysplasia
Osteogenesis imperfecta syndrome
Pfeiffer syndrome
Saethre-Chotzen syndrome

Stickler syndrome
Treacher Collins syndrome
Waardenburg syndrome

Mouth

Cleft Lip with or without Cleft Palate

Amniotic band sequence
Ectrodactyly–ectodermal dysplasia–clefting syndrome
Oral-facial-digital syndrome
Roberts-SC phocomelia syndrome (cleft lip with or without cleft palate, hypomelia, severe growth retardation)
Trisomy 13 syndrome
Van der Woude syndrome (cleft lip, lip pit)
Wolf-Hirschhorn syndrome

Cleft Palate

Oral-facial-digital syndrome
Retinoic acid embryopathy
Robin sequence (Pierre-Robin sequence)
Stickler syndrome
Treacher Collins syndrome
Velo-cardio-facial syndrome

Neck

Broad Neck or Excess Nuchal Skin

Aarskog syndrome
Klippel-Feil sequence (primary defect of cervical vertebrae)
Noonan syndrome
Trisomy 13 syndrome
Trisomy 21 syndrome
Turner syndrome
Zellweger syndrome

Heart

Cardiac and Great Vessel Malformations

Alagille syndrome
Carpenter syndrome
Cat-eye syndrome
CHARGE association
Diabetic embryopathy
DiGeorge syndrome (defects of the thymus, parathyroids, great vessels)
Ellis–van Creveld syndrome (atrial septal defect, short distal extremities, polydactyly, nail hypoplasia)
Fetal alcohol syndrome
Fetal effects of maternal phenylketonuria
Fetal rubella syndrome
Holt-Oram syndrome (atrial septal defect, narrow shoulders, upper limb defect)
Kartagener syndrome (dextrocardia, situs inversus, sinusitis, bronchiectasis)
Marfan syndrome
Pallister-Hall syndrome (endocardial cushion defect, hypothalamic hamartoblastoma, hypopituitarism, imperforate anus, postaxial polydactyly)
Noonan syndrome
Retinoic acid embryopathy
Rubinstein-Taybi syndrome
Stickler syndrome
Thrombocytopenia–absent radius syndrome

Trisomy 13 syndrome
Trisomy 18 syndrome
Trisomy 21 syndrome
Turner syndrome
VATER/VATERL association
Velo-cardio-facial syndrome
Williams syndrome
Wolf-Hirschhorn syndrome

Abdomen

Abdominal Wall Defects/Umbilical Abnormalities

Beckwith-Wiedemann syndrome
Meckel-Gruber syndrome
Mucopolysaccharidoses (Hurler and Hunter syndromes)
Trisomy 13 syndrome
Trisomy 18 syndrome
Trisomy 21 syndrome

Kidney

Renal Malformations

Aniridia-Wilms tumor association
Bardet-Biedl syndrome
Beckwith-Wiedemann syndrome
Branchio-oto-renal syndrome
Cat-eye syndrome
CHARGE association
Ectrodactyly–ectodermal dysplasia–clefting syndrome
Fanconi pancytopenia syndrome
Jeune syndrome
Meckel-Gruber syndrome
MURCS association (*m*üllerian duct, *r*enal aplasia, and *c*ervicothoracic *s*omite dysplasia)
Noonan syndrome
Oral-facial-digital syndrome
Pallister-Hall syndrome
Townes-Brocks syndrome
Trisomy 13 syndrome
Trisomy 18 syndrome
Tuberous sclerosis syndrome
Turner syndrome
VATER/VACTERL association
Williams syndrome
Zellweger syndrome

Genitalia

Genital Anomalies

Aarskog syndrome
Aniridia-Wilms tumor association
Carpenter syndrome
CHARGE association
Fetal akinesia deformation sequence
Hand-foot-uterus syndrome
Klinefelter syndrome
Meckel-Gruber syndrome
Miller-Dieker lissencephaly syndrome
MURCS association
Noonan syndrome
Opitz syndrome
Prader-Willi syndrome
Robinow syndrome (flat facies, short forearms, hypoplastic genitalia)

Rubinstein-Taybi syndrome
Smith-Lemli-Opitz syndrome
Trisomy 13 syndrome
Trisomy 18 syndrome
Wolf-Hirschhorn syndrome

Anus

Imperforate Anus

Cat-eye syndrome
Pallister-Hall syndrome
Townes-Brocks syndrome
VATER/VACTERL association

Limbs

Syndactyly

Amniotic band sequence
Apert syndrome
Carpenter syndrome
Cornelia de Lange syndrome
Greig cephalopolysyndactyly syndrome
Holt-Oram syndrome
Jackson-Weiss syndrome
Oral-facial-digital syndrome
Oculodentodigital syndrome
Pfeiffer syndrome
Poland sequence (syndactyly and brachydactyly of the hand, unilateral defect of pectoralis muscle)
Roberts-SC phocomelia syndrome
Saethre-Chotzen syndrome
Smith-Lemli-Opitz syndrome

Polydactyly

Bardet-Biedl syndrome
Carpenter syndrome
Ellis–van Creveld syndrome
Grebe syndrome (polydactyly, severe distal limb reduction)
Greig cephalopolysyndactyly syndrome
Meckel-Gruber syndrome
Pallister-Hall syndrome
Townes-Brocks syndrome
Trisomy 13 syndrome

Limb Reduction

Amniotic band disruption sequence
Baller-Gerold syndrome
Cornelia de Lange syndrome
Fanconi pancytopenia syndrome
Holt-Oram syndrome
Poland sequence
Roberts-SC phocomelia syndrome
Thrombocytopenia–absent radius syndrome

Limb Overgrowth

Klippel-Trenaunay-Weber syndrome (asymmetric limb hypertrophy, hemangiomata)
Maffucci syndrome (enchondromatosis, hemangiomata)
Proteus syndrome (hemihypertrophy, subcutaneous tumors, macrodactyly)

Joint Restriction

Achondroplasia
Amyoplasia congenita disruptive sequence

Arthrogryposis
Cockayne syndrome
Congenital contractural arachnodactyly syndrome (Beals syndrome)
Fetal akinesia deformation sequence
Fetal alcohol syndrome
Mucopolysaccharidoses (Hunter and Hurler syndromes)
Pallister-Hall syndrome
Pseudoachondroplasia
Saethre-Chotzen syndrome
Trisomy 18 syndrome
Zellweger syndrome

Skin

Pigmentary Abnormalities

Angelman syndrome
Bloom syndrome
Ectrodactyly–ectodermal dysplasia–clefting syndrome
Fanconi pancytopenia syndrome
Hypohidrotic ectodermal dysplasia
Hypomelanosis of Ito (streaked, whorled, mottled hypopigmentation)
Incontinentia pigmenti syndrome (blisters followed by hyperpigmentation, dental anomalies, patchy alopecia)
McCune-Albright syndrome (hyperpigmentation, polyostotic fibrous dysplasia, sexual precocity)
Neurofibromatosis syndrome
Peutz-Jeghers syndrome (mucocutaneous hyperpigmentation, intestinal polyposis)
Prader-Willi syndrome
Russell-Silver syndrome
Sturge-Weber syndrome (facial and meningeal hemangiomata with seizures)
Tuberous sclerosis syndrome
Turner syndrome
Waardenburg syndrome
Xeroderma pigmentosa syndrome (sunlight sensitivity, atrophic skin changes, actinic skin tumors)

Growth Patterns

Overgrowth/Obesity

Bardet-Biedl syndrome
Beckwith-Wiedemann syndrome
Carpenter syndrome
Cohen syndrome (obesity, hypotonia, prominent incisors)
Prader-Willi syndrome
Sotos syndrome
Weaver syndrome (accelerated growth and maturation, macrosomia, craniofacial anomalies, camptodactyly)

Tall Stature

Homocystinuria syndrome
Klinefelter syndrome
Marfan syndrome
XYY syndrome

Small Stature

Aarskog syndrome
Achondroplasia
Bloom syndrome
Hypochondroplasia
Jeune syndrome

Mucopolysaccharidoses (Hurler and Hunter syndromes)
Noonan syndrome
Opitz syndrome
Osteogenesis imperfecta syndrome
Robinow syndrome
Russell-Silver syndrome
Rubinstein-Taybi syndrome
Seckel syndrome (severe short stature, microcephaly, prominent nose)
Turner syndrome

Craniofacial and Limb Abnormalities

Apert syndrome
Baller-Gerold syndrome
Carpenter syndrome
Coffin-Lowry syndrome
Cornelia de Lange syndrome
Ectrodactyly–ectodermal dysplasia–clefting syndrome
Fanconi pancytopenia syndrome
Greig cephalopolysyndactyly syndrome
Jackson-Weiss syndrome
Meckel-Gruber syndrome
Oculodentodigital syndrome
Oral-facial-digital syndrome
Otopalatodigital syndrome
Pfeiffer syndrome
Popliteal pterygium syndrome
Rubinstein-Taybi syndrome
Saethre-Chotzen syndrome
Tricho-rhino-phalangeal syndrome
Trisomy 13 syndrome
Trisomy 18 syndrome
Trisomy 21 syndrome

Cardiac and Limb Abnormalities

Carpenter syndrome
Ellis–van Creveld syndrome
Holt-Oram syndrome
Marfan syndrome
Thrombocytopenia–absent radius syndrome
Trisomy 13 syndrome
VATER/VACTERL association

Cardiac and Renal Abnormalities

Cat-eye syndrome
Noonan syndrome
Trisomy 13 syndrome
Trisomy 18 syndrome
Turner syndrome
VATER/VACTERL association
Williams syndrome

Ear and Renal Abnormalities

Beckwith-Wiedemann syndrome
Branchio-oto-renal syndrome
Cat-eye syndrome
CHARGE association
Oculo-auriculo-vertebral dysplasia
Turner syndrome
Trisomy 13 syndrome
Trisomy 18 syndrome

PHOTOGRAPH CREDITS

Teratogens and Uterine Factors

Amniotic Band Sequence

Reprinted with permission from Wiedemann HR, Kunze J, with contributions from FR Grosse, eds. *Clinical syndromes*, 3rd ed. London: Mosby-Wolfe, 1997.

Diabetic Embryopathy

Reprinted with permission from Mann TP, ed. *Colour atlas of paediatric facial diagnosis*. New York: Macmillan, 1990; reprinted with permission from Wiedemann HR, Kunze J, with contributions from FR Grosse, eds. *Clinical syndromes*, 3rd ed. London: Mosby-Wolfe, 1997.

Fetal Akinesia Deformation Sequence

Reprinted with permission from Punnett HH, Kistenmacher ML, Valdes-Dapena M, Ellison RT Jr. Syndrome of ankylosis, facial anomalies, and pulmonary hypoplasia. *J Pediatr* 1974;85:375.

Fetal Alcohol Syndrome

Reprinted with permission from Clarren SK, Smith DW. The fetal alcohol syndrome. *N Engl J Med* 298:1063, 1978.

Fetal Rubella Syndrome

Reprinted with permission from Wiedemann HR, Kunze J, with contributions from FR Grosse, eds. *Clinical syndromes*, 3rd ed. London: Mosby-Wolfe, 1997.

Retinoic Acid Embryopathy

Reprinted with permission from Gorlin RJ, Cohen M Jr, Levin SL, eds. *Syndromes of the head and neck*, 3rd ed. New York: Oxford University Press, 1990.

Chromosomal Syndromes

Trisomy 13 Syndrome

Reprinted with permission from Moore KL, Persaud TVN, Shiota K, eds. *Color atlas of clinical embryology*. Philadelphia: Saunders, 1994.

Trisomy 18 Syndrome

Reprinted with permission from Wiedemann HR, Kunze J, with contributions from FR Grosse, eds. *Clinical syndromes*, 3rd ed. London: Mosby-Wolfe, 1997.

Trisomy 21 Syndrome

Reprinted with permission from Bergsma D, ed. *Birth defects compendium*, 2nd ed. New York: Alan R. Liss, 1979.

Turner Syndrome (XO)

Reprinted with permission from Mann T, ed. *Colour atlas of paediatric facial diagnosis*. New York: Macmillan, 1990.

Klinefelter Syndrome (XXY)

Reprinted with permission from Wiedemann HR, Kunze J, with contributions from FR Grosse, eds. *Clinical syndromes*, 3rd ed. London: Mosby-Wolfe, 1997.

Fragile X Syndrome

Reprinted with permission from Tewfik TL, Der Kaloustian VM, eds. *Congenital anomalies of the ear, nose, and throat*. New York: Oxford University Press, 1997.

Cri du Chat Syndrome (5p-, deletion 5p)

Reprinted with permission from Gorlin RJ, Cohen MM Jr, Levin SL, eds. *Syndromes of the head and neck*, 3rd ed. New York: Oxford University Press, 1990.

Wolf-Hirschhorn Syndrome (4p-, deletion 4p)

Reprinted with permission from Schinzel A, Schmid W. Partial deletion of the short arm of chromosome 4 (Wolf's syndrome). Two further cases. *Arch Genet* 1972;45:88.

Genetic Syndromes

Achondroplasia

Reprinted with permission from Buyse ML, ed. *Birth defects encyclopedia*. Cambridge, MA: Blackwell Science, 1990.

Alagille Syndrome

Reprinted with permission from Baraitser M, Winter RM, eds. *Color atlas of congenital malformation syndromes*. London: Mosby-Wolfe, 1996.

Angelman Syndrome

Reprinted with permission from Buyse ML, ed. *Birth defects encyclopedia*. Cambridge, MA: Blackwell Science, 1990.

Apert Syndrome

Reprinted with permission from Tewfik TL, Der Kaloustian VM, eds. *Congenital anomalies of the ear, nose, and throat*. New York: Oxford University Press, 1997; reprinted with permission from Mann T, ed. *Colour atlas of paediatric facial diagnosis*. New York: Macmillan, 1990.

Bardet-Biedl Syndrome

Reprinted with permission from Wiedemann HR, Kunze J, with contributions from FR Grosse, eds. *Clinical syndromes*, 3rd ed. London: Mosby-Wolfe, 1997; reprinted with permission from Baraitser M, Winter RM, eds. *Color atlas of congenital malformation syndromes*. London: Mosby-Wolfe, 1996.

Beckwith-Wiedemann Syndrome

Reprinted with permission from Mann T, ed. *Colour atlas of paediatric facial diagnosis*. New York: Macmillan, 1990; reprinted with permission from Wiedemann HR, Kunze J, with contributions from FR Grosse, eds. *Clinical syndromes*, 3rd ed. London: Mosby-Wolfe, 1997.

Blepharophimosis-Ptosis-Epicanthus Inversus Syndrome (BPES)

Reprinted with permission from Crisponi L, et al. The putative forkhead transcription factor *FOXL2* is mutated in blepharophimosis/ptosis/epicanthus inversus syndrome. *Nat Genet* 2001;27:165.

Bloom Syndrome

Reprinted with permission from German J. Bloom's syndrome. I. Genetical and clinical observations in the first twenty-seven patients. *Am J Hum Genet* 1969;21:196; reprinted with permission from Wiedemann HR, Kunze J, with contributions from FR Grosse, eds. *Clinical syndromes*, 3rd ed. London: Mosby-Wolfe, 1997.

Branchio-oto-renal Syndrome (BOR)

Reprinted with permission from Pennie BH, Marres HAM. Shoulder abnormalities in association with branchio-oto-renal dysplasia in a patient who also has familial joint laxity. *Int J Pediatr Otorhinolaryngol* 1992;23:269–273; reprinted with permission from Stratakis CA, Lin JP, Rennert OM. Description of a large kindred with autosomal dominant inheritance of branchial arch anomalies, hearing loss, and ear pits, and exclusion of the branchio-oto-renal (BOR) syndrome gene locus (Chromosome 8q13.3). *Am J Med Genet* 1998;79:212.

Cockayne Syndrome

Reprinted with permission from Gorlin RJ, Cohen MM Jr, Levin SL, eds. *Syndromes of the head and neck*, 3rd ed.

New York: Oxford University Press, 1990; reprinted with permission from Baraitser M, Winter RM, eds. *Color atlas of congenital malformation syndromes*. London: Mosby-Wolfe, 1996.

Coffin Lowry Syndrome

Reprinted with permission from Hanauer A, Young ID. Coffin-Lowry syndrome: clinical and molecular features. *J Med Genet* 2002;39:707 & 709.

Cornelia de Lange Syndrome

Reprinted with permission from Gorlin RJ, Cohen MM Jr, Levin SL, eds. *Syndromes of the head and neck*, 3rd ed. New York: Oxford University Press, 1990; reprinted with permission from Baraitser M, Winter RM, eds. *Color atlas of congenital malformation syndromes*. London: Mosby-Wolfe, 1996.

Crouzon Syndrome

Reprinted with permission from Tewfik TL, Der Kaloustian VM, eds. *Congenital anomalies of the ear, nose, and throat*. New York: Oxford University Press, 1997.

Ectodermal Dysplasia Syndromes

Reprinted with permission from Buyse ML, ed. *Birth defects encyclopedia*. Cambridge, MA: Blackwell Science, 1990; reprinted with permission from Baraitser M, Winter RM, eds. *Color atlas of congenital malformation syndromes*. London: Mosby-Wolfe, 1996; reprinted with permission from Bergsma D, ed. *Birth defects compendium*, 2nd ed. New York: Alan R. Liss, 1979.

Ehlers-Danlos Syndrome

Reprinted with permission from Buyse ML, ed. *Birth defects encyclopedia*. Cambridge, MA: Blackwell Science, 1990.

Fanconi Pancytopenia Syndrome

Reprinted with permission from Baraitser M, Winter RM, eds. *Color atlas of congenital malformation syndromes*. London: Mosby-Wolfe, 1996.

Holt-Oram Syndrome

Reprinted with permission from Hurst JA, Hall CM, Baraitser M. The Holt-Oram syndrome. *J Med Genet* 1991;28:406-410; reprinted with permission from Bohm M. Holt-Oram syndrome. *Circulation* 1998;98:2636.

Hurler Syndrome

Reprinted with permission from Gorlin RJ, Cohen MM Jr, Levin SL, eds. *Syndromes of the head and neck*, 3rd ed. New York: Oxford University Press, 1990.

Jeune Syndrome

Reprinted with permission from Bergsma D, ed. *Birth defects compendium*, 2nd ed. New York: Alan R. Liss, 1979.

Marfan Syndrome

Reprinted with permission from Mann T, ed. *Colour atlas of paediatric facial diagnosis*. New York: Macmillan, 1990.

Meckel-Gruber Syndrome

Reprinted with permission from Baraitser M, Winter RM, eds. *Color atlas of congenital malformation syndromes*. London: Mosby-Wolfe, 1996.

Miller-Dieker Lissencephaly Syndrome

Reprinted with permission from Dobyns WB, Stratton RF, Parke JT, Greenberg F, Nussbaum RL, Ledbetter DH. Miller-Dieker syndrome: lissencephaly and monosomy 17p. *J Pediatr* 1983;102:552; reprinted with permission from Baraitser M, Winter RM, eds. *Color atlas of congenital malformation syndromes*. London: Mosby-Wolfe, 1996.

Möbius Syndrome

Reprinted with permission from Sogg R. Congenital facial diplegia syndrome of Möbius: a case report. *Arch Ophthalmol* 1961;65:16.

Neurofibromatosis Syndrome

Reprinted with permission from Wiedemann HR, Kunze J, with contributions from FR Grosse, eds. *Clinical syndromes*, 3rd ed. London: Mosby-Wolfe, 1997.

Noonan Syndrome

Reprinted with permission from Gorlin RJ, Cohen MM Jr, Levin SL, eds. *Syndromes of the head and neck*, 3rd ed. New York: Oxford University Press, 1990.

Oculo-Auriculo-Vertebral Dysplasia

Reprinted with permission from Tewfik TL, Der Kaloustian VM, eds. *Congenital anomalies of the ear, nose, and throat*. New York: Oxford University Press, 1997.

Oculodentodigital Syndrome

Reprinted with permission from Paznekas WA, et al. Connexin 43 (GJA1) mutations cause the pleiotropic phenotype of oculodentodigital dysplasia. *Am J Hum Genet* 2003;72:409.

Opitz Syndrome

Reprinted with permission from Opitz JM, Summitt RL, Smith DW. The BBB syndrome: familial telecanthus with associated congenital anomalies. In: Bergsma D, ed. *Birth defects: original article series*. Baltimore: The National Foundation–March of Dimes, 1969;5:86.

Oral-Facial-Digital Syndrome

Reprinted with permission from Mann T, ed. *Colour atlas of paediatric facial diagnosis*. New York: Macmillan, 1990.

Osteogenesis Imperfecta Syndrome

Reprinted with permission from Tewfik TL, Der Kaloustian VM, eds. *Congenital anomalies of the ear, nose, and throat*. New York: Oxford University Press, 1997.

Prader-Willi Syndrome

Reprinted with permission from Wiedemann HR, Kunze J, with contributions from FR Grosse, eds. *Clinical syndromes*, 3rd ed. London: Mosby-Wolfe, 1997.

Rubinstein-Taybi Syndrome

Reprinted with permission from Baraitser M, Winter RM, eds. *Color atlas of congenital malformation syndromes*. London: Mosby-Wolfe, 1996; reprinted with permission from Wiedemann HR, Kunze J, with contributions from FR Grosse, eds. *Clinical syndromes*, 3rd ed. London: Mosby-Wolfe, 1997.

Russell-Silver Syndrome

Reprinted with permission from Schumacher G, Niederhoff H. The Russell and Silver syndromes. Description of 2 more children. *Helv Paediatr Acta* 1967;22:404.

Smith-Lemli-Opitz Syndrome

Reprinted with permission from Baraitser M, Winter RM, eds. *Color atlas of congenital malformation syndromes*. London: Mosby-Wolfe, 1996.

Sotos Syndrome

Reprinted with permission from Baraitser M, Winter RM, eds. *Color atlas of congenital malformation syndromes*. London: Mosby-Wolfe, 1996.

Stickler Syndrome

Reprinted with permission from Jones KL, ed. *Smith's recognizable patterns of human malformation,* 5th ed. Philadelphia: Saunders, 1997.

Thrombocytopenia–Absent Radius Syndrome

Reprinted with permission from Baraitser M, Winter RM, eds. *Color atlas of congenital malformation syndromes.* London: Mosby-Wolfe, 1996.

Treacher Collins Syndrome

Reprinted with permission from Cohen MM Jr, Baum BJ, eds. *Studies in stomatology and craniofacial biology.* Amsterdam: IOS Press, 1997.

Tricho-Rhino-Phalangeal Syndrome

Reprinted with permission from KL Jones, ed. *Smith's recognizable patterns of human malformation,* 5th ed. Philadelphia: WB Saunders Company, 1997 (Courtesy of D. Weaver, University of Indiana, Indianapolis, IN).

Tuberous Sclerosis Syndrome

Reprinted with permission from Cohen MM Jr. In: Stewart RE, Prescott GH, eds. *Orofacial genetics.* St. Louis: Mosby, 1988; reprinted with permission from Mann T, ed. *Colour atlas of paediatric facial diagnosis.* New York: Macmillan, 1990.

Van Der Woude Syndrome

Reprinted with permission from Kantaputra PN, Sumitsawan Y, Schutte BC, Tochareontanaphol C. Van der Woude syndrome with sensorineural hearing loss, large craniofacial sinuses, dental pulp stones, and minor limb anomalies: report of a four-generation Thai family. *Am J Med Genet* 2002;108:277.

Velocardiofacial Syndrome

Reprinted with permission from Meinecke P, Beemer FA, Schinzel A, Kushnick T. The velo-cardio-facial (Shprintzen) syndrome. Clinical variability in eight patients. *Eur J Pediatr* 1986;145:539.

Waardenburg Syndrome

Composite photos reprinted with permission from Mann T, ed. *Colour atlas of paediatric facial diagnosis.* Hingham, MA: Kluwer, 1989; Gorlin RJ, Cohen MM Jr, Levin SL, eds. *Syndromes of the head and neck,* 3rd ed. New York: Oxford University Press, 1990.

Williams Syndrome

Reprinted with permission from Mann T, ed. *Colour atlas of paediatric facial diagnosis.* New York: Macmillan, 1990.

Zellweger Syndrome

Reprinted with permission from Baraitser M, Winter RM, eds. *Color atlas of congenital malformation syndromes.* London: Mosby-Wolfe, 1996.

Multifactorial Conditions

Arthrogryposis

Reprinted with permission from Wiedemann HR, Kunze J, with contributions from FR Grosse, eds. *Clinical syndromes,* 3rd ed. London: Mosby-Wolfe, 1997; reprinted with permission from Moore KL, Persaud TVN, Shiota K, eds. *Color atlas of clinical embryology.* Philadelphia: Saunders, 1994.

Cleft Lip with or without Cleft Palate

Reprinted with permission from Moore KL, Persaud TVN, Shiota K, eds. *Color atlas of clinical embryology.* Philadelphia: Saunders, 1994.

Craniosynostosis

Courtesy of J. Panchal, Oklahoma.

Holoprosencephaly

Reprinted with permission from Davis WB. Congenital deformities of the face. Types found in a series of one thousand cases. *Surg Gynecol Obstet* 1935;61:209; reprinted with permission from Baraitser M, Winter RM, eds. *Color atlas of congenital malformation syndromes.* London: Mosby-Wolfe, 1996.

Associations

CHARGE

Reprinted with permission from Baraitser M, Winter RM, eds. *Color atlas of congenital malformation syndromes.* London: Mosby-Wolfe, 1996.

VATER/VACTERL

Reprinted with permission from Wiedemann HR, Kunze J, with contributions from FR Grosse, eds. *Clinical syndromes,* 3rd ed. London: Mosby-Wolfe, 1997.

Aniridia-Wilms Tumor (WAGR)

Reprinted with permission from Baraitser M, Winter RM, eds. *Color atlas of congenital malformation syndromes.* London: Mosby-Wolfe, 1996.

APPENDIX C ■ PEDIATRIC PROCEDURES

MICHAEL A. BARONE

The general pediatrician must have proficiency in both diagnostic and emergency procedures. This chapter addresses preparatory steps for all procedures and describes some common procedures in detail.

Preparation of the Child and Family

Except in life-threatening emergencies, any procedure should optimally begin with an explanation to the parents (and, when appropriate, the child) of why the procedure is necessary. This discussion should include a clear description of the steps involved, a realistic outline of the potential therapeutic or diagnostic benefits, a consideration of alternatives to performing the procedure, and a discussion of any possible risks. Documentation of this discussion should then be included in the medical record. This important process is known as *obtaining informed medical consent* and while it generally is not performed in detail for such procedures as simple phlebotomy and IV catheter insertion, its importance is relevant to all procedures. When obtaining consent for a procedure, take time to ensure that the parent or guardian truly understands the procedure and possible risks. Studies have shown that, even when doctors feel they have provided adequate information, 20% to 40% of subjects did not fully understand the necessary details. A full discussion of informed medical consent can be found in guidelines issued by the American Academy of Pediatrics.

Whenever possible, the *assent* of the patient should be obtained. After explaining the procedure to the child in a manner appropriate to his developmental level, one should attempt to solicit some indication of the child's willingness to undergo the procedure. Avoid, however, presenting the child with the suggestion that he has a choice as to whether an essential procedure is performed. Virtually any healthy child will respond with a resounding "No" to the question, "Would you like to have your bone marrow aspirated now?" In many instances, it is possible to offer the child appropriate choices: "Do you want the IV started in your left hand or in your right hand?"

If possible, procedures performed in inpatient settings should be carried out in a neutral environment, separate from the child's room. This reinforces a sense that she is secure during at least some part of the hospitalization. Some studies have demonstrated that parental presence during procedures does not increase physician anxiety and does not negatively impact procedure success rates. Physicians should feel comfortable in encouraging (but never forcing) parents to comfort their child during the procedure. Hospital policies prohibiting parental involvement are outdated.

Begin the procedure with a description of the process for the child. Demonstrating the procedure on a procedure doll sometimes is helpful. Set limits for the child, with the understanding that you will tell him when to expect discomfort. Because many procedures may be too painful to expect the necessary cooperation, careful consideration must be given to analgesia and sedation. Many behavioral strategies can decrease the child's anxiety. These techniques should be specific to the developmental age of the child. For example, toddlers respond well to distraction, whereas preschool children, who may engage in "magical thinking," often are helped by using vivid imagery in which, for example, they might be asked to imagine themselves in the midst of an exciting adventure. School-aged children and adolescents often can be taught effective relaxation techniques.

It is important to inform assistants of what is expected of them and to gather all necessary equipment beforehand. Position the child to provide adequate restraint. Be aware of your own comfort as well. Success is much more likely if the clinician is concentrating on the task at hand rather than, for example, the cramp in her lower back. Finally, because pediatric procedures may be a source of frustration or anger when success is not immediate, it is worth recalling a time-honored clinical rule: If an individual has been unsuccessful in two or three attempts, it is time for another person to try. Persistent efforts by a frustrated operator rarely are successful.

Analgesia and Sedation

The need for sedation varies with the procedure, and the age, developmental level, and temperament of the patient. The most crucial aspect of administering sedatives and analgesics to children is understanding the drugs' ability to cause cardiorespiratory depression. To this end, sedation for procedures should be carried out by experienced, credentialed individuals who are prepared to resuscitate a compromised patient. Most hospitals and emergency department settings have strict policies regarding prior time with no oral intake (generally 4 to 6 hours), number of care providers for the sedation (at least two), and recovery guidelines. Cardiorespiratory monitoring is essential throughout the procedure until the patient recovers to baseline consciousness.

The continuum from conscious sedation to deep sedation to general anesthesia must be understood. The achievement of conscious sedation yields a child who tolerates a noxious procedure but maintains airway protective reflexes and responds to commands. Should the patient progress toward deep sedation, the risk of airway compromise becomes much greater. Table C.1 lists some common agents used for sedation, only some of which also provide analgesia. The physician must avoid the common misconception that some medications such as chloral hydrate and midazolam provide analgesia merely because they provide sedation.

Local Anesthetics

Depending on the nature of the procedure, consideration should be given to the use of a local anesthetic. Lidocaine 1% is a suitable choice for injectable local anesthesia. If injected slowly with a 25- to 30-gauge needle, its burning sensation is usually tolerable. Combining lidocaine with 8.4% sodium bicarbonate in a 1:10 solution (1 mL $NaHCO_3$:9 mL lidocaine)

TABLE C.1

SEDATION FOR PROCEDURES

Drug	Dose	Comments
Chloral hydrate	PO/PR: 25–100 mg/kg per dose (max: 2 g per dose)	Requires same monitoring as other sedatives; not analgesic; contraindicated in hepatic or renal disease.
Diazepam	IM/IV: 0.04–0.20 mg/kg per dose q2–4 hour (max: 0.6 mg/kg in 8 hour) PO: 0.12–0.80 mg/kg/24 hours divided q6–8 hour	Infuse no faster than 2 mg/minute. Hypotension and respiratory depression may occur, especially in combination with narcotics or other sedatives.
Fentanyl	IM/IV: 1–2 μg/kg per dose q30–60 minutes	Respiratory depression may persist beyond period of analgesia.
Ketamine	IV: 0.5–1 mg/kg per dose IM: 2–5 mg/kg per dose PO: 3–4 mg/kg/dose	May cause hypotension, hypertension, emergence reactions, laryngospasm. Increases intracranial pressure. Use in combination with antisialagogue (atropine) and midazolam to reduce impact of emergence reactions.
Lorazepam	IM/IV: 0.05 mg/kg per dose	Similar side effects to diazepam. Shorter-acting agents may be more appropriate for procedures.
Midazolam	IV: 0.05–0.10 mg/kg over 2 minutes (may repeat 0.05 mg/kg q2–3 minutes to max dose of 0.2 mg/kg) PO: 0.50–0.75 mg/kg per dose (onset 20–30 minutes) Intranasal 0.2–0.5 mg/kg (onset 20–30 minutes)	Not analgesic. Has amnestic effect. May cause respiratory depression, hypotension, bradycardia, especially when used in combination with other sedatives and narcotics.
Pentobarbital	IV: 1–3 mg/kg per dose (max: 150 mg) PO/PR/IM: 2–6 mg/kg per dose (max: 150 mg)	May cause cardiovascular and respiratory depression. Not analgesic.
Reversal agents		
Flumazenil (for reversal of benzodiazepine sedation)	IV: 0.01 mg/kg (max dose 0.2 mg) given over 15 sec. May repeat q1 min to max cumulative dose of 0.05 mg/kg or 1 mg.	Onset of action in 1–3 minutes. Reversal effects may be shorter-lived than benzodiazepine effect. Does not reverse narcotics
Naloxone (for reversal of narcotic sedation)	IM/IV/SC/IT: <20 kg: 0.1 mg/kg per dose; may repeat q2–3 minutes ≥20 kg: 2 mg per dose; may repeat q2–3 minutes	Short duration of action. Multiple doses may be necessary. Does not cause respiratory depression.

reduces the burning. Lidocaine has a rapid onset of action (2 to 3 minutes), and anesthesia may last up to 2 hours. The maximum dose recommended for lidocaine infiltration is 5 to 7 mg/kg. Bupivacaine has a slower onset of action (3 to 5 minutes), but the duration of analgesia can last as long as 5 to 6 hours, making it useful for some procedures in which prolonged discomfort is expected. The recommended maximum dose is 2.5 mg/kg of bupivacaine.

Transdermal anesthesia with EMLA cream (eutectic mixture of local anesthetics; lidocaine 2.5% with prilocaine 2.5%) is very effective for many procedures. It is applied under Tegaderm dressings (supplied in the packaging) and should remain on the skin for at least 60 minutes. Broad guidelines for maximum application area are designed to prevent systemic toxicity: 100 cm^2 for less than 10 kg, 600 cm^2 for 10 to 20 kg, 2,000 cm^2 for more than 20 kg. Care should be taken to prevent the infant or young child from ingesting the cream. Another topical anesthetic is L.M.X.4, 4% lidocaine (formerly ELA-Max, Ferndale Laboratories). Available without a prescription, L.M.X.4 may be used with or without an occlusive dressing. Time to onset for analgesia is 30 minutes. Side effects of lidocaine toxicity are uncommon.

Two topical anesthetics that may also be used for procedures such as wound closure are TAC (tetracaine 0.5%, adrenaline 1:2,000, cocaine 11.8%) and LET (lidocaine 4%, epinephrine 1:2,000, tetracaine 0.5%). TAC is used infrequently due to concerns for cost and toxicity due to cocaine. LET is less expensive, safer, and provides equal analgesia. These mixtures are typically made up by hospital pharmacies in either aqueous or viscous preparations to be applied directly to the area of concern. LET can be applied to intact or damaged skin (lacerations). For each preparation, a 3- to 5-mL aliquot may be used per 3-cm segment of wound edge. Neither should be used on mucosa or on end-artery areas such as digits, the nose, or earlobes because both contain epinephrine.

Restraint

Manual restraint is the standard method of immobilization for most procedures, especially in infants. When assistants are unavailable, restraint ("papoose") boards are a convenient means of safely stabilizing young children. If these are not available, or if the patient is too large for the board, suitable restraints can be fashioned using hospital sheets (Fig. C.1).

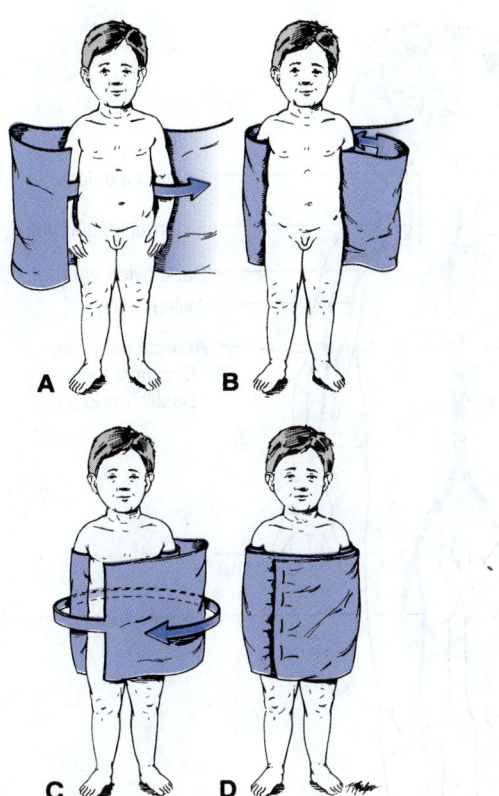

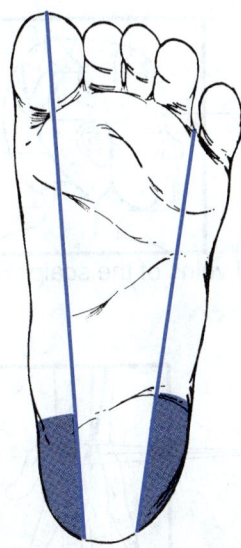

FIGURE C.2. Preferred sites for heel blood sampling in infants (*shaded areas*). The limits of the calcaneus are defined by two lines, one drawn parallel to the lateral margin of the heel from the space between the fourth and fifth toes and the other drawn parallel to the medial margin of the heel from the center of the great toe.

FIGURE C.1. Method for restraining the upper body using a hospital sheet.

Blood Sampling and Intravascular Access

Skin-Puncture Phlebotomy

In infants and children, skin-puncture blood sampling helps conserve sites of venous access and may be less distressing for the patient than venipuncture. Warming the sampling site first increases local blood flow and improves the ease of collection and the validity of the sample. A cloth towel or disposable diaper soaked in warm water suffices for this purpose (water temperatures of more than 44°C [111°F] may cause burns). Also available are infant heel warmers, which heat to approximately 104°F. The preferred sites for skin-puncture sampling are the palmar surface of the distal phalanx of the second, third, and fourth fingers or, in infants, the heel. Avoid penetrating the calcaneus by using a lancet puncture smaller than 2.5 mm and by performing the puncture on the medial or lateral plantar surface (Fig. C.2). Cleanse the puncture site with 70% alcohol, and wipe the surface dry with a sterile gauze pad (alcohol can cause hemolysis). Use either a short lancet (less than 2.5 mm) or an automated lancet to penetrate skin. Wipe away the first drop of blood, which may contain excessive interstitial and intracellular fluid. Hold the child's finger or heel below the level of the heart when possible and massage to express blood, allowing enough time for capillaries to refill. Avoid excessive squeezing of the area, which can increase interstitial and intracellular fluid content of the specimen as well as cause red-cell hemolysis. Samples may be inaccurate when the child is polycythemic, edematous, or poorly perfused.

Venipuncture

Venipuncture for blood sampling is most successful when the patient is adequately immobilized, the vein is maximally dis-

tended, and all supplies for blood collection or intravenous (IV) infusion are arranged beforehand. Immobilization for simple venipuncture is preferably performed by an assistant, although with rambunctious children, the limb may need to be taped to an arm board. Maximal venous distention is best achieved by applying a tourniquet snugly enough to restrict venous return but not arterial flow. Many children prefer a cloth or gauze pad under the tourniquet to prevent pinching of the skin. Other simple measures to increase distention and visibility of the vein include warming the site to increase blood flow, keeping the site dependent, tapping or flicking the vein, swabbing the vein with alcohol or iodine or, if the site is in the arm, asking the patient to alternately make a fist and relax the hand.

The usual sites for venipuncture are in the hands and the antecubital fossa. Infants younger than 1 year may have accessible scalp veins. Figure C.3 shows the most accessible peripheral veins. Attempting distal veins first will conserve sites if the previous tries are unsuccessful. Most venipunctures in children and adolescents can be performed using a 23-gauge butterfly needle, which allows maneuverability for the operator and causes minimal discomfort for the child.

The tourniquet should be applied as briefly as possible. The syringe (or Vacutainer attachment) can be attached to the butterfly tubing before or after entering the vein. Once the vein is distended, cleanse the overlying skin with 70% alcohol. Apply traction to the skin to help immobilize the vessel. Warn the patient, then insert the needle into the skin at about a 30-degree angle with the bevel up. Enter the vein with a quick motion to prevent it from rolling. Slowly aspirate the required amount of blood; excessive suction can cause the vein to collapse. When blood flow is slow, some samples can be collected by removing the syringe and allowing blood to drip directly into the collection tube. This is obviously not appropriate when a sterile sample is needed. When the collection is complete, release the tourniquet and remove the needle. Manual pressure with a gauze pad controls further bleeding.

External Jugular Venipuncture

The external jugular vein occasionally is the most accessible site for venipuncture in infants and young children. Special

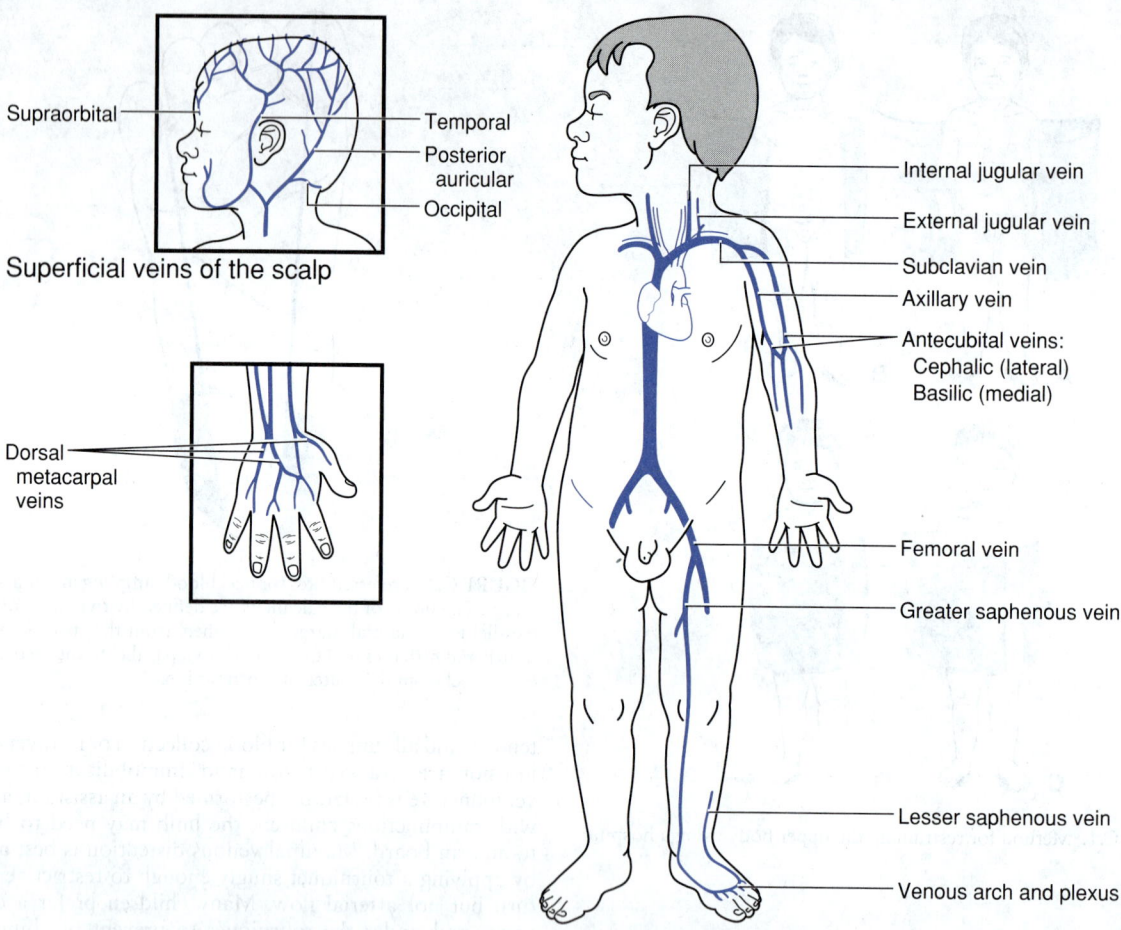

FIGURE C.3. Accessible peripheral veins for venipuncture and cannulation.

positioning ensures good visibility of the vein (Fig. C.4). The vein can be accessed for simple venipuncture or IV placement, or the Seldinger technique may be used for central venous line placement (for a description of the Seldinger technique, see the section Central Venous Catheter Placement). With the patient supine, an assistant holds the child's head and neck over the edge of a table (approximately 15 to 20 degrees) and rotates the head to the contralateral side to be punctured. An alternative to positioning the head over the edge of the table is to elevate the shoulders by placing pillows or a rolled blanket underneath them. To distend the external jugular vein, occlude the proximal segment of the vein or provoke the infant to cry. Cleanse the skin with povidone-iodine. Enter the skin at a 30-degree angle, about one-half the distance between the angle of the jaw and the clavicle. Keep constant suction on the syringe. When the procedure is completed, sit the child upright and apply pressure for 5 minutes. Complications of the procedure are bleeding, infection and, rarely, the creation of a pneumothorax. In the trauma patient, consider the possibility of a cervical spine injury before attempting this procedure.

Intravenous Infusions

When selecting a site for IV infusions, consider the age and hand preference of the patient, whether underlying injuries are present, the degree of restraint required to keep the catheter in place, whether the infusate burns or is damaging to surrounding tissues if extravasation occurs, and whether prolonged IV access is required. In general, select the most distal vein that is large enough to accommodate the catheter, and spare the larger

proximal veins for use if initial attempts fail or if prolonged IV access is anticipated. Veins are most easily cannulated if they are well anchored, such as at the site where two vessels meet (Fig. C.5).

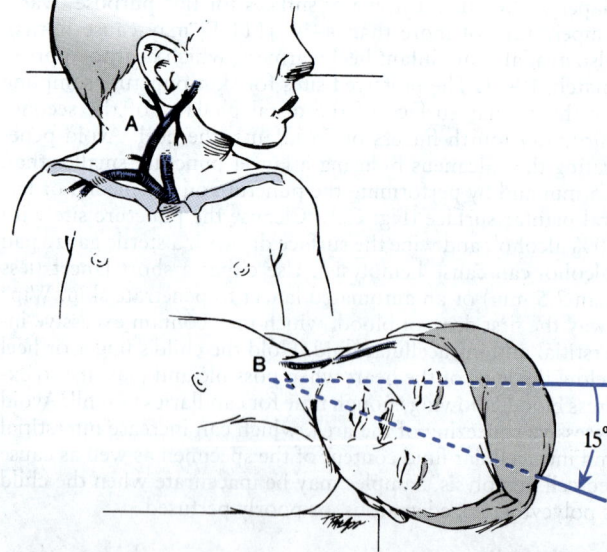

FIGURE C.4. External jugular venipuncture. **A:** Anatomy. **B:** Visibility of the vein is improved if the head is turned to the opposite side and lowered 15 degrees from the level of the table.

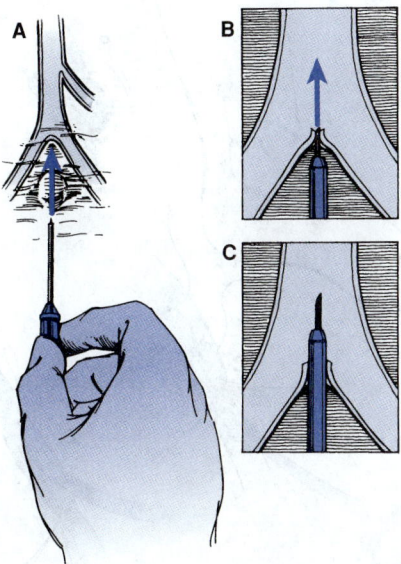

FIGURE C.5. Insertion of an intravenous catheter.

When using over-the-needle catheters, several different needleless safety systems exist. Be sure to be familiar with the operation of the system you select. Some children prefer that the site be anesthetized with an intradermal bleb of 1% lidocaine or a topical anesthetic (see the section, Local Anesthetics). At times, puncturing the skin with a needle larger than the gauge of the catheter prevents damage to the plastic sheaths, which can occur when the smaller, 22- and 24-gauge catheters are inserted directly through the skin. Insert the catheter directly or through the skin-puncture site, and enter the vein with a quick

stab (see Fig. C.5). Blood should appear in the needle hub. Advance the catheter a few millimeters to ensure that the plastic catheter tip sits inside the lumen. Then, holding the stylet needle in place, advance the catheter into the vein; it should advance completely without resistance. Remove the stylet, release the tourniquet, and flush with normal saline to assess patency. If the catheter flushes normally, apply antibacterial ointment and secure the IV catheter with gauze and tape as needed. Alternatively, transparent adhesives (Tegaderm, 3M Company, Minnesota), which are often used in dressing central IV catheters, permit visualization of the skin entry site. Protect the catheter from being dislodged by covering it with a protective dressing or a medicine cup.

Intraosseous Infusions

Intraosseous infusions are used as a means of emergency vascular access in situations of circulatory collapse or cardiopulmonary arrest in the infant or child. Although they are occasionally appropriate as a primary means of vascular access in these situations, as a general rule, the intraosseous route should be used after three failed peripheral IV attempts or after 90 seconds of attempting IV access. Any crystalloid, blood product, or medication (as a single dose or continuous infusion) may be given via the intraosseous route. Access to the general circulation is via the intramedullary veins.

Three sites are commonly used in children: the anteromedial surface of the proximal tibia (2 cm below the tibial tuberosity), the medial surface of the distal tibia (2 to 3 cm above the medial malleolus), and the distal femur along the midline (3 cm above the lateral condyle) (Fig. C.6A). After determining the site to be used, cleanse the skin with povidone-iodine, then with 70% alcohol. If time permits, infiltrate the skin and down to the periosteum with 1% lidocaine. Use a commercially available intraosseous needle. Other types of needles, such as

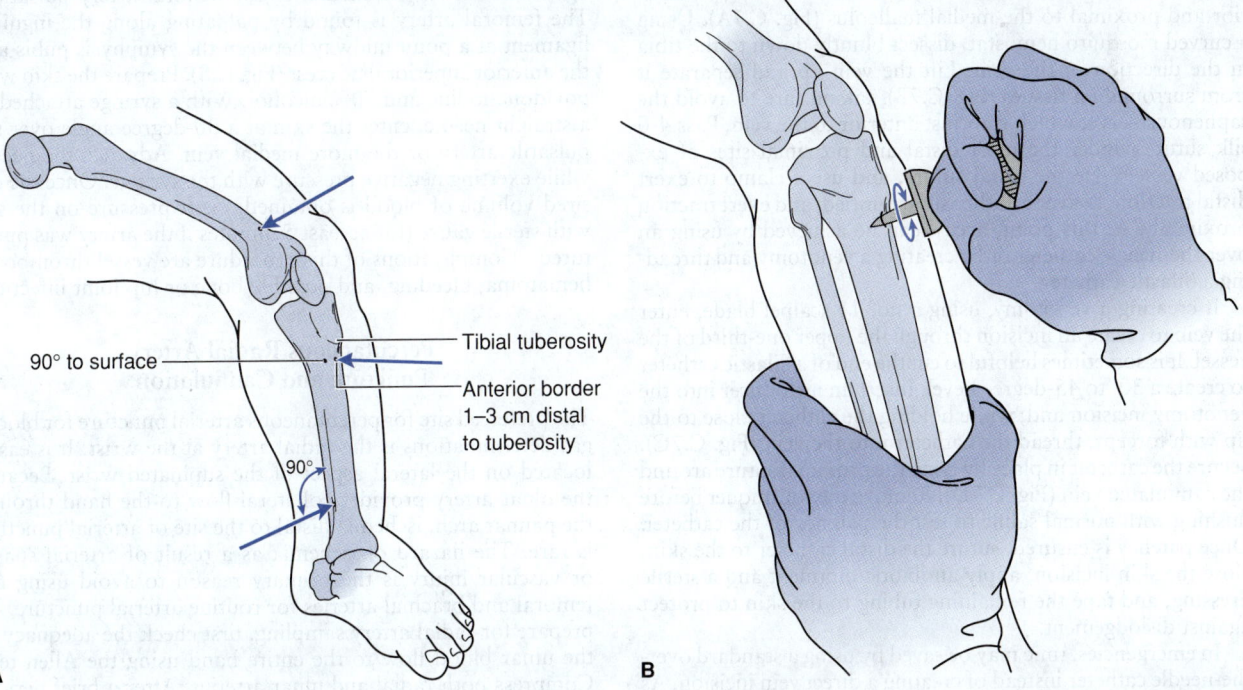

90° to surface

Tibial tuberosity

Anterior border
1–3 cm distal
to tuberosity

90°

A

B

FIGURE C.6. Intraosseous needle insertion. **A:** Three commonly used sites in children are (a) the anteromedial surface of the proximal tibia (2 cm below the tibial tuberosity), (b) the medial surface of the distal tibia (2 to 3 cm above the medial malleolus), and (c) the distal femur, along the midline (3 cm above the lateral condyle). **B:** Once the needle reaches the periosteum, the marrow space is entered by exerting downward force in a boring motion through the cortex.

butterflies, may become plugged with bone. Insert the needle through the skin, aiming slightly away from the growth plate. When the needle reaches the periosteum, exert firm downward pressure in a boring rotary manner (Fig. C.6B). As the needle enters the marrow space with a "pop," it becomes anchored by bone, and resistance suddenly drops. At this point, remove the inner stylet and flush with saline. It is not necessary to aspirate marrow. Connect IV tubing to the needle and allow fluid to drip in. The rapid administration of large volumes of fluid will need to be given under pressure to overcome the resistance of emissary veins. The infusion site must be monitored for extravasation of fluids. If this occurs, a different site in the opposite leg should be used. Complications of this procedure include fat or bone embolism, growth plate injury, soft-tissue necrosis due to fluid extravasation (similar to IV infiltrate), and soft tissue abscess or osteomyelitis. To reduce the small risk of osteomyelitis, remove the intraosseous needle after obtaining more permanent IV access, preferably within 3 hours.

Greater Saphenous Vein Cutdown

When percutaneous venous cannulation or intraosseous infusions are unsuccessful, cutdowns can provide a means of emergency venous access. The greater saphenous vein at the ankle is the preferred peripheral site for cutdown in infants and children. It is easily identified, and placement of the cutdown at that site does not interfere with resuscitative measures around the neck and chest.

The vein is located midway between the distal anterior tibia and the medial malleolus. Most hospitals and emergency departments have cutdown trays available with a supply of minor surgical instruments. Immobilize the lower leg by taping the foot onto a padded restraint board with the ankle externally rotated. Gently apply a tourniquet to the calf to help distend the vein. After cleansing the area around the medial malleolus using sterile technique, apply drapes and, if time allows, infiltrate the incision site and subcutaneous tissues with 1% lidocaine. Make a 1- to 2-cm transverse incision just anterior and proximal to the medial malleolus (Fig. C.7A). Using a curved mosquito hemostat, dissect bluntly down to the tibia in the direction of the vein. Lift the vein up and separate it from surrounding tissues (Fig. C.7B), taking care to avoid the saphenous nerve, which runs just anterior to the vein. Pass 4-0 silk sutures under the most distal and proximal sites of exposed vessels. Tie the distal suture, and use a clamp to exert distal traction. Leave the other suture untied, and exert traction proximally. At this point, access can be achieved by using an over-the-needle catheter or by creating a venotomy and threading a Silastic catheter.

If creating a venotomy, using a no. 11 scalpel blade, enter the vein to create an incision through the upper one-third of the vessel. It is sometimes helpful to cut the end of a Silastic catheter to create a 30- to 45-degree bevel. Insert an introducer into the venotomy incision and, while holding the catheter close to the tip with forceps, thread the catheter into the vein (Fig. C.7C). Secure the catheter in place by tying the proximal suture around the cannulated vein (Fig. C.7D). Remove the tourniquet before flushing with normal saline to test the patency of the catheter. Once patency is ensured, suture the distal catheter to the skin, close the skin incision, apply antibiotic ointment and a sterile dressing, and tape the remaining tubing to the skin to protect against dislodgement.

In emergencies, time may be saved by using a standard over-the-needle catheter instead of creating a direct vein incision. As soon as the vein is exposed, insert the over-the-needle catheter directly into the vein as if performing a percutaneous IV line placement. It is not necessary to tie the distal end of the vein in this case. Secure the catheter as described above. Complications of this procedure include bleeding, infection, catheter loss in the vessel, and sensory nerve laceration.

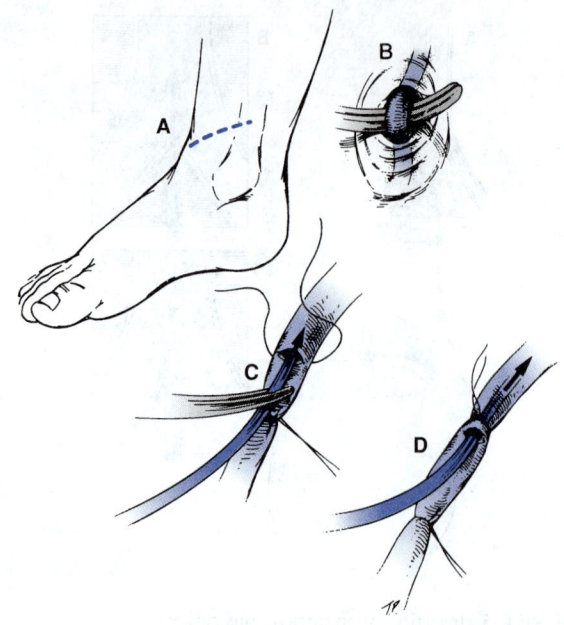

FIGURE C.7. Technique for venous cutdown at the greater saphenous vein. **A:** A 1- to 2-cm incision is made anterior and proximal to the medial malleolus. **B:** After the vein is isolated and a venotomy incision is made, **C:** the catheter is threaded into the vein. **D:** The proximal suture secures the catheter.

Femoral Artery and Vein Puncture

Puncture of the femoral vessels may be particularly useful in an emergency situation when peripheral vessels are not adequate. With the patient positioned supine, an assistant holds the child's hips flexed and abducted (in a frog-leg position). The site for femoral vein puncture is 2 cm distal to the inguinal ligament and 0.5 cm medial to the femoral artery pulsation. The femoral artery is found by palpating along the inguinal ligament at a point midway between the symphysis pubis and the anterior superior iliac crest (Fig. C.8). Prepare the skin with povidone-iodine and 70% alcohol. With a syringe attached to a straight needle, enter the skin at a 30-degree angle over the pulsatile artery or the more medial vein. Advance the needle while exerting negative pressure with the syringe. Once the desired volume of blood is obtained, exert pressure on the site with sterile gauze (for at least 5 minutes if the artery was punctured). Complications of this procedure are vessel thrombosis, hematoma, bleeding, and possible bone or hip joint infection.

Percutaneous Radial Artery Puncture and Cannulation

The preferred site for percutaneous arterial puncture for blood-gas determinations is the radial artery at the wrist. It is easily located on the lateral aspect of the supinated wrist. Because the ulnar artery provides collateral flow to the hand through the palmar arch, ischemia distal to the site of arterial puncture is rare. The hazard of ischemia as a result of arterial spasm or vascular injury is the primary reason to avoid using the femoral and brachial arteries for routine arterial puncture. To prepare for radial artery sampling, first check the adequacy of the ulnar blood flow to the entire hand using the Allen test. Compress both radial and ulnar arteries. After a brief period, release the ulnar artery compression. If the entire hand flushes while the radial artery is still compressed, the procedure can be performed safely. Next, secure the hand to a restraint board, with the wrist extended 20 to 30 degrees by placing it over a gauze padding. Leave the fingers exposed, so that any color change is seen quickly. If time permits, consider the options for

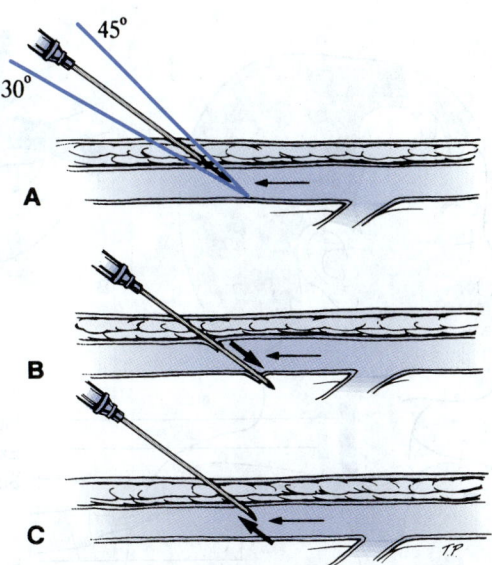

FIGURE C.9. Percutaneous arterial puncture. **A:** Insert the needle or catheter at a 30- to 45-degree angle, just far enough to enter the lumen of the vessel. **B:** Alternatively, the needle can be advanced through the opposite wall of the artery. **C:** The needle then is withdrawn slowly as one watches for blood return.

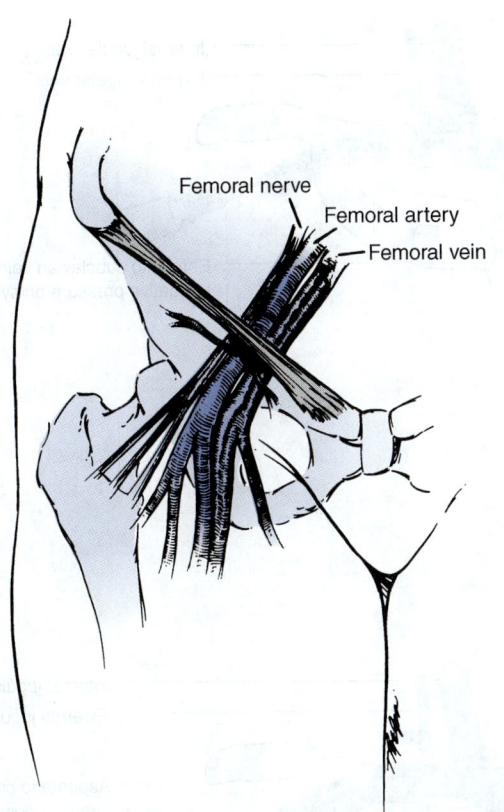

FIGURE C.8. The femoral vessels.

topical or injectable local anesthesia. After cleansing the wrist area with povidone-iodine, the artery may be palpated using sterile technique. At times, palpating the pulse is difficult with a gloved finger. Therefore, it is helpful to make a small skin impression with an object (e.g., end of a cotton swab, pen cap) before sterilizing the skin. In small infants, transillumination may help locate the artery. Using a 22- to 25-gauge needle, puncture the skin at a 30- to 45-degree angle (Fig. C.9), then insert the needle just far enough to enter the lumen but not transfix the vessel. An alternative maneuver is to pierce through the artery to transfix it, then withdraw the needle slowly, observing for blood flow into the syringe or tubing (see Fig. C.9). When the desired amount of blood has been withdrawn, apply pressure to the area for 5 minutes.

For radial artery cannulation, only a few modifications are necessary. After infiltrating the area with 1% lidocaine, use a 18- to 20-gauge needle to puncture the skin over the point of maximal impulse (about 0.5 to 1.0 cm proximal to the distal wrist crease). This will protect the plastic over-the-needle catheter from being damaged as it passes through the skin. Arterial puncture is then performed with a 20- to 24-gauge catheter. It can be done via transfixation or direct technique (see Fig. C.9). The direct technique is similar to peripheral venous catheter placement. To perform the transfixation technique, insert the catheter through the skin-puncture site at a 30-degree angle until it pierces through the artery, transfixing it. Remove the stylet, and slowly withdraw the catheter. At the first sign of blood return, redirect the catheter toward the horizontal plane, and advance the catheter to the hub. This maneuver is more difficult to perform with 24-gauge catheters, which tend to buckle. When it is advanced fully, the catheter then should be sutured in place. Apply antibiotic ointment and a dressing over the catheter site to prevent contamination. Complications of these procedures are vessel laceration, vessel occlusion by hematoma or thrombosis, hemorrhage, infection, or distal ischemia if collateral circulation is inadequate.

Central Venous Catheter Placement

Central venous access in children is useful in emergency settings when peripheral attempts fail or for stable vascular access for prolonged therapies such as antibiotic administration and parenteral nutrition. The most commonly used sites are the femoral, subclavian, and external and internal jugular veins. A technique using an introducer and a guidewire, the Seldinger technique, is effective for accessing these vessels. (The anatomic approach to the femoral vessels and the external jugular vein has been previously discussed. The approach to subclavian and internal jugular vessels, as well as the Seldinger technique, is described below.)

The placement of a central venous catheter in any site requires adequate analgesia and possibly sedation. For this reason, as well as because of the potential for cardiac dysrhythmia as a catheter enters the heart from the central circulation, cardiac and respiratory monitoring is essential during the procedure. For placement of a central venous catheter in the subclavian vein, position the child supine in a 20- to 30-degree Trendelenburg position with a towel roll underneath the shoulder to hyperextend the thoracic spine (Fig. C.10). The child's head should be turned opposite of the side to be cannulated. A povidone-iodine solution is used to prepare the neck and upper chest. The site of insertion is just below the clavicle, at the junction between the distal third and the medial third, aiming toward the midline (see Fig. C.10A). First, anesthetize this intended path with 1% lidocaine. Using an introducer needle with syringe, puncture in the desired location with gentle negative pressure on the syringe. Aim under the clavicle and toward the sternal notch (see Fig. C.10B). When blood is obtained, remove the syringe, taking care not to introduce air by covering the distal end of the needle with a gloved finger. Advance the guidewire as described below.

For placement of an internal jugular catheter, place the patient in a 15- to 20-degree Trendelenburg position with a towel roll under the shoulders to hyperextend the neck and, thus, tense the sternocleidomastoid muscle. Turn the neck slightly away from the side to be punctured. Prepare and drape the site in sterile fashion (Fig. C.11). Locate the sternal and clavicular heads of the sternocleidomastoid muscle and enter the skin

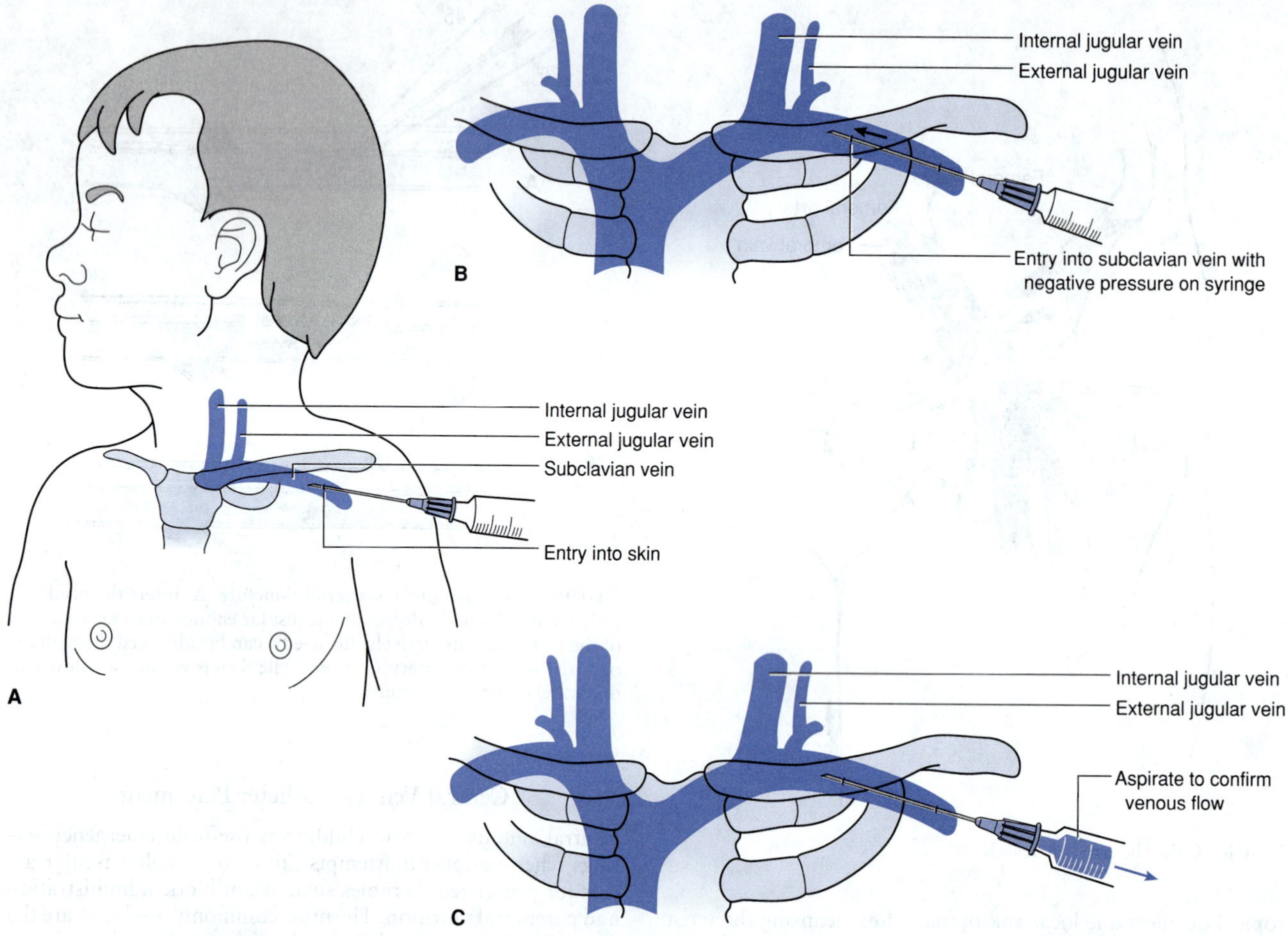

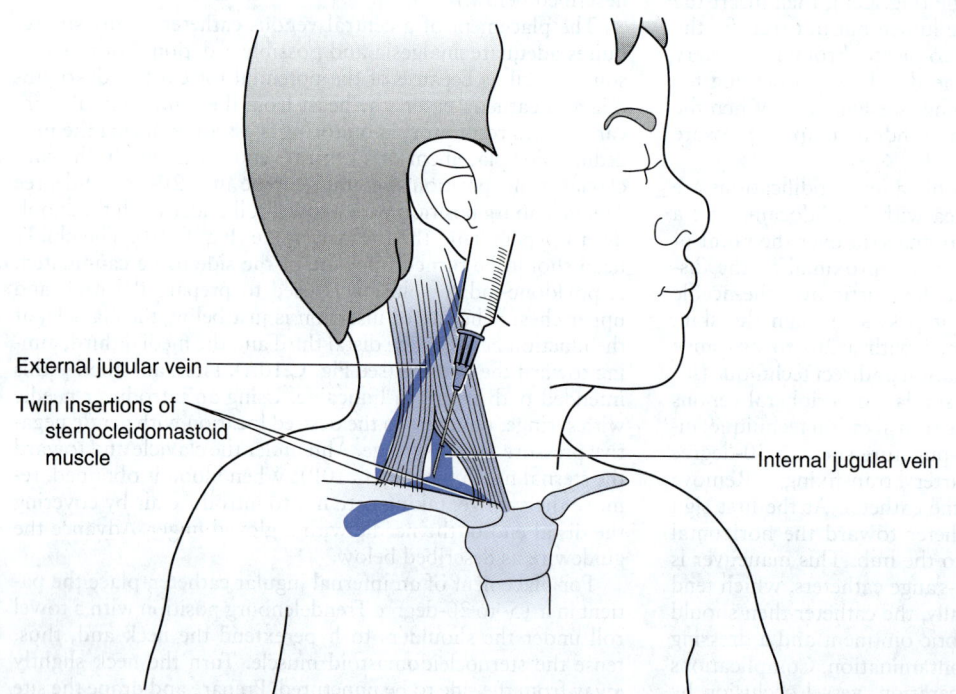

B

- Internal jugular vein
- External jugular vein
- Entry into subclavian vein with negative pressure on syringe

A

- Internal jugular vein
- External jugular vein
- Subclavian vein
- Entry into skin

C

- Internal jugular vein
- External jugular vein
- Aspirate to confirm venous flow

FIGURE C.10. Placement of a subclavian catheter. **A:** The patient is supine in a 20- to 30-degree Trendelenburg position. The needle insertion site is at the junction of the medial and distal one-third of the clavicle. **B:** Negative pressure is maintained on the syringe during insertion. **C:** Once blood is aspirated, the Seldinger over-the-wire technique can be performed.

- External jugular vein
- Twin insertions of sternocleidomastoid muscle
- Internal jugular vein

FIGURE C.11. Placement of an internal jugular catheter. The patient is supine in a 15- to 20-degree Trendelenburg position. The insertion site for this central approach is at the apex of the triangle formed by the sternal and clavicular heads of the sternocleidomastoid and the clavicle. Aim toward the ipsilateral nipple.

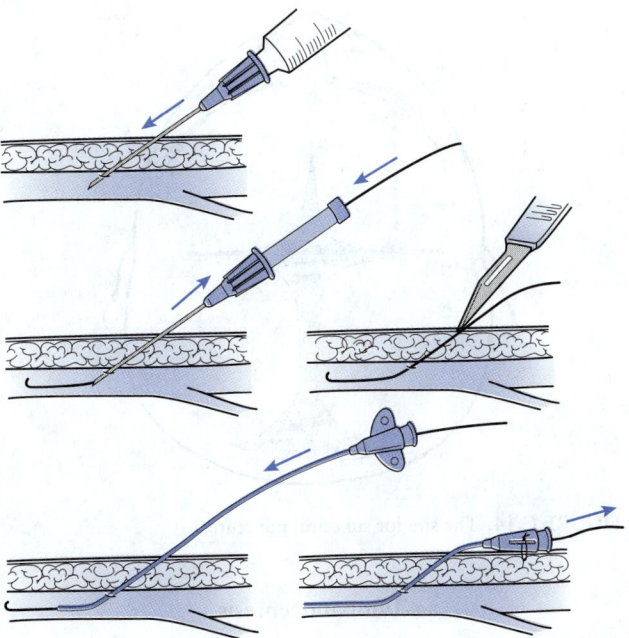

FIGURE C.12. Seldinger technique for percutaneous venous access (see text).

with an introducer needle at the apex of the triangle formed, aiming caudally for the ipsilateral nipple. Gentle suction should be applied to the syringe as the needle is advanced. When blood is obtained, remove the syringe, taking care not to introduce air by covering the distal end of the needle.

To proceed with the Seldinger technique for the subclavian or internal jugular approach, insert the soft tip of the guidewire through the metal needle, advancing it into the vein (Fig. C.12). Do not force against resistance. Observe the cardiac monitor for ectopy. Carefully remove the introducer needle, holding the guidewire in place. To enlarge the skin opening, a small skin incision can be made or dilators may be passed over the wire. Carefully thread a preflushed catheter of appropriate size over the guidewire, twisting it gently while advancing it into the vein. Withdraw the guidewire and secure the catheter. Confirm placement of the catheter by obtaining a radiograph. Complications of central venous catheter placement are vessel laceration or thrombosis (arterial or venous), bleeding, infection, air or catheter embolus, and cardiac arrhythmias. Subclavian and jugular punctures add the risk of pneumothorax, hemothorax, and pneumomediastinum.

Selected Diagnostic and Therapeutic Procedures

Lumbar Puncture

Although lumbar puncture generally is a safe procedure, its performance under certain conditions is associated with serious complications. Children with thrombocytopenia or bleeding diathesis are at risk for epidural hematoma after lumbar puncture. Infants with compromised cardiorespiratory function may experience further deterioration when restrained for the procedure. Most important, cerebral herniation can occur after lumbar puncture in the setting of elevated intracranial pressure, even when the fontanelle is open. Although it is important to examine the patient for evidence of papilledema, this physical finding may not be present despite significant intracranial hypertension. Only needles with stylets should be used; the use of open or butterfly needles is contraindicated because of the late development of intraspinal epidermoid tumors.

A key component of a successful lumbar puncture is adequate restraint of the patient. Children most often are restrained in the lateral recumbent position, with their backs at the edge of and perpendicular to the examining table (Fig. C.13). The lumbar spine must be flexed as much as possible to maximize the interlaminar distance. The position of the child's head relative to the performer's dominant side is a matter of personal preference. The sitting position is an alternative to the lateral recumbent position when the patient is either capable of remaining still or incapable of offering resistance. This method may be preferable in preterm infants, in whom neck flexion and the knee-chest position may cause airway compromise.

The spinal cord generally ends about the level of L1, with the filum terminate flowing caudally. A line connecting the superior portions of the posterior iliac crests passes through the spinous process of L4, conveniently identifying the L3–4 and L4–5 interspaces, which are the preferred sites for lumbar puncture (see Fig. C.13). Before sterile preparation, gently imprint a thumbnail into the child's skin at the anticipated site of needle insertion. Topical or injectable local anesthetic options may be considered. Don sterile gloves, and cleanse the site three times with a povidone-iodine solution, starting at the site of skin puncture (imprint) and working outward in a circular manner. Drape the area with a sterile towel.

Recheck the child's position, ensuring that the needle will enter directly in the midline and in the sagittal plane. Using a 22-gauge needle and stylet with the bevel pointed up to the ceiling (the length of the needle depends on the size of the patient), puncture the skin midway between the spinous processes of the L3–4 or L4–5 interspace and aim slightly cephalad

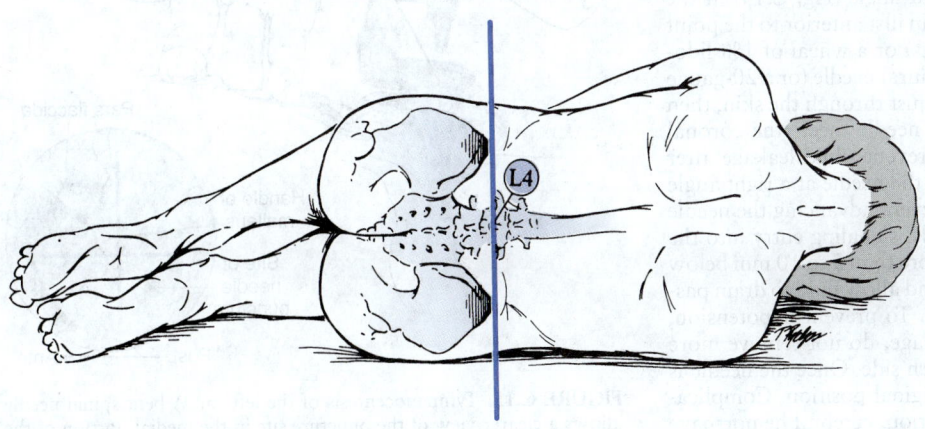

FIGURE C.13. Positioning of a child for lumbar puncture.

(toward the umbilicus). Advance the needle slowly, removing the stylet frequently to check for cerebrospinal fluid (CSF). This process is more important in smaller infants, because a "pop" may not always be felt as the needle penetrates the dura. If the needle does not advance, withdraw it and redirect its angle. Once the needle enters the subarachnoid space and CSF is flowing freely, turning the bevel toward the patient's head may improve CSF flow. If desired, connect the manometer to measure CSF pressure (an inaccurate procedure when the patient is struggling or when the neck and thighs are highly flexed). Collect the smallest volume of CSF necessary, controlling the rate of CSF flow using the stylet. Allow the CSF to drip into collection tubes for diagnostic studies. Never aspirate CSF with a syringe, because even a small amount of negative pressure can cause subdural hemorrhage or herniation. Replace the stylet before withdrawing the needle, then cover the site with an adhesive bandage. Many patients may complain of occipital and/or frontal headache after a lumbar puncture. This well-described post–lumbar puncture phenomenon is attributable to the lowering of intracranial pressure. The pain is usually more severe in the upright position and can be relieved by recumbent positioning for 4 to 6 hours after the procedure, IV hydration, and analgesics.

Ventriculoperitoneal Shunt Tap

A pediatrician may be required to tap a ventriculoperitoneal shunt for diagnostic or potentially life-saving therapeutic purposes. The area over the shunt bulb is shaved using a razor. After donning surgical gloves, cleanse the skin with povidone-iodine and 70% alcohol. Insert a 23- or 25-gauge butterfly needle through the bulb of the shunt, attaching a pressure manometer if desired. Fluid under pressure should flow out readily. Gentle suction on the syringe may be necessary if the ventricular end of the shunt is partially obstructed, whereas excessive suction may lead to aspiration of brain tissue. If no fluid is obtained in the setting of intracranial hypertension, emergent neurosurgical consultation is necessary.

Subdural Puncture

Occasionally, drainage of subdural fluid (blood or effusion) is necessary as a diagnostic or therapeutic procedure in infants. Position the child supine with the head at the edge of the table; monitor cardiorespiratory status. Proper restraint is essential, even in the unconscious child. The site of puncture is near the junction of the lateral aspect of the anterior fontanelle and the coronal suture. Shave the scalp and, after donning surgical gloves, cleanse the skin with povidone-iodine and 70% alcohol. A helpful landmark for the site of puncture is the point at which a line drawn from the ipsilateral pupil would intersect the coronal suture at a perpendicular angle (Fig. C.14). If the child is conscious, anesthetize the skin just anterior to the point of entry with EMLA (if time permits) or a wheal of 1% lidocaine. Insert an 18- to 20-gauge subdural needle (or a 20-gauge lumbar puncture needle with stylet) just through the skin, then pull the scalp posteriorly until the needle meets the coronal suture. This "Z-track" technique prevents fluid leakage after the needle is removed. Slowly insert the needle at a right angle to the surface. Brace the hand to prevent advancing the needle too far. Advance until resistance falls, signaling entry into the subdural space. This is usually no more than 5 to 10 mm below the skin surface. Remove the stylet and allow fluid to drain passively; never aspirate subdural fluid. To prevent hypotension, shift of the brain, or fresh hemorrhage, do not remove more than 15 to 20 mL at a time from each side. Once the needle is removed, the scalp returns to its original position. Complications of this procedure include infection, cerebral hemorrhage or contusion, and fluid or blood collection under the galea.

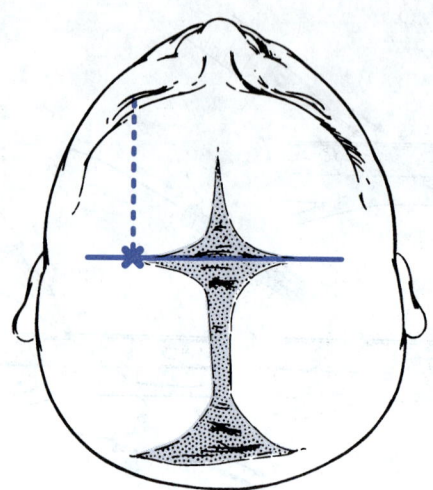

FIGURE C.14. The site for subdural puncture.

Tympanocentesis

Pediatricians should be familiar with this technique, but rarely is this procedure taught in pediatric residency training programs. Indications for tympanocentesis include otitis media thought to be due to resistant organisms, neonatal otitis media, otitis media in the immunocompromised patient, and those suppurative complications of otitis media such as mastoiditis or brain abscess. For this procedure, an otoscope with an operating head or an operating microscope is required. Remove cerumen from the external canal with a curette or by irrigation (see the next section). Restrain and, if necessary, sedate the patient. Sterilize the external canal by instilling a povidone-iodine solution or 70% alcohol; wait 45 to 60 seconds, then remove any of this fluid before tympanocentesis. A prepackaged tympanocentesis needle may be used or, alternatively, a 22-gauge spinal needle bent 30 degrees at a point 4 to 5 cm from the distal tip is effective for puncture with visualization. Attach a 1-mL tuberculin syringe to the end of the spinal needle (Fig. C.15). Applying negative pressure to the syringe, pass the needle briefly through the medial portion of the posterior inferior quadrant. The aspirate can be retrieved for culture and Gram

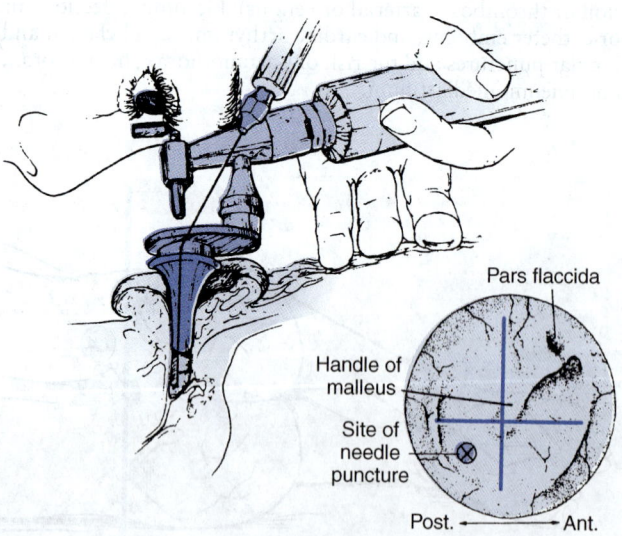

FIGURE C.15. Tympanocentesis of the left ear. A bent spinal needle allows a clearer view of the puncture site in the medial portion of the posterior inferior quadrant.

staining by flushing the needle with a small volume of non-bacteriostatic saline after removing it. A contaminated culture may be obtained if, while removing the needle, the external ear canal is contacted. Complications of this procedure are bleeding (from tympanic membrane or laceration of the external canal) and damage to the ossicles.

Removing Impacted Cerumen or Otic Foreign Body

The methods for removal of an otic foreign body include curettage, forceps removal, and irrigation. Irrigation and curettage are also very useful for impacted cerumen removal. Irrigation is performed by drawing lukewarm water into a 30- to 60-mL syringe. Next, attach the syringe to the tubing of a 23-gauge butterfly device after the needle has been removed. Insert the tubing 1 to 2 cm into the external auditory canal, and inject the water with moderate force, enabling the water to drain out the foreign body or impacted cerumen. If the patient experiences pain, discontinue irrigation and examine the tympanic membrane for perforation. Irrigation also may be successful using a Water-Pik device, using a low-pressure setting. Cerumen or foreign bodies may be removed with one of many curette devices (wire or plastic loop). This procedure is best done by experienced hands or under direct visualization, because one must advance beyond the object and slowly withdraw it. Foreign body removal with alligator forceps should be done only under direct visualization in the cooperative or sedated patient.

Nasogastric Tube Insertion

The length required for a nasogastric (NG) tube can be estimated by extending the tubing from the tip of the patient's nose to the earlobe to the xiphoid process. Small (5 to 8 Fr.) tubes are used for continuous enteral alimentation in neonates; larger tubes (12 to 16 Fr. in young children) are necessary for abdominal decompression.

Before inserting the NG tube, lubricate the tip to make passage through the nose less traumatic. If the tube is excessively pliable, it can first be immersed in ice water. Have suction available in the event the patient has emesis. With the patient sitting upright, tilt the head back slightly and slide the tube into the nostril along the base of the nose, advancing the tube slowly in a horizontal plane. Infants and unconscious children should be lying supine with head turned toward the side. If performing this procedure on a patient with a depressed level of consciousness, serious consideration should be given to protecting the airway prior to NG placement. Once the NG tube has reached the nasopharynx, several maneuvers can be used to ensure that the tube is directed away from the trachea and into the esophagus. One maneuver is to tilt the head forward, thereby opening the esophagus. Another is to rotate the NG tube 180 degrees, so that the curve in the tube faces the posterior pharynx. A third is to ask the patient to swallow or drink from a straw, because this maneuver closes the epiglottis. Once past the pharynx, advance the tube to the premeasured distance and check its position, either by attempting to aspirate gastric contents or by listening with a stethoscope over the stomach as a small volume of air is instilled into the tube. If these maneuvers seem equivocal, examine the tube placement via radiograph. Tape the tube in place when the position is judged to be adequate. Withdraw the tube if excessive coughing or choking occurs during placement, suggesting tracheal intubation. To reduce the unpleasantness of NG tube removal, kink or clamp the tube and withdraw it slowly.

Endotracheal Intubation

The indications for orotracheal intubation include the need for mechanical ventilation (such as respiratory failure), critical airway obstruction, and altered level of consciousness with

TABLE C.2

ENDOTRACHEAL TUBE SIZE

Age	Internal Diameter (mm)
Preterm infant	2.5–3.0
Term infant	3.0–3.5
2 months to 1 year	3.5–4.0
2 years	4.0–4.5
2–15 years	[16 + age (years)]/4

improper control of airway protective reflexes. The preparation for orotracheal intubation is involved, so excellent skills for opening the airway and supporting ventilation via bag-valve and mask should be the first priority. When intubation is determined to be necessary, some rules are useful for obtaining equipment of proper size. All laryngoscope handles are useful for all blades; straight blades are preferred in neonates and infants, whereas curved blades are preferred in older children. Have at least two blades available, and ensure the light is functional on attaching the blade to the laryngoscope handle. Table C.2 estimates endotracheal tube sizes based on age. In addition to the intended tube, have one size larger and one size smaller available. Cuffed tubes should be used in children aged 8 years or older, because the airway narrowing at the cricoid cartilage serves as a "cuff" in the younger child. Prepare oxygen, Yankauer suction, and cardiorespiratory monitoring devices. Maintain secure venous access. Have precut tape ready for securing the tube once it has been placed.

The procedure and medications for rapid sequence-intubation are outlined in Table C.3. The patient should be positioned supine on a firm surface. Extend the patient's neck slightly, and pull the jaw forward; a rolled towel or pillow under the shoulder may assist in this maneuver. Always, however, consider the possibility of a neck injury; in these settings, the neck must remain in in-line traction. Next, preoxygenate the patient using bag-valve and mask ventilation and 100% oxygen. Pretreatment with atropine often eliminates the reflex bradycardia caused by laryngoscopy. To occlude the esophagus, compression of the cricoid ring with the thumb and index finger (the Sellick maneuver) may be performed by an assistant. Drugs for sedation and paralysis vary in differing clinical situations; Table C.3 provides some broad guidelines. Regardless of the physician's dominant hand, the laryngoscope should always be held in the left hand. Introduce the laryngoscope blade on the right side of the mouth, and push the tongue to the left, out of the line of vision. This should leave an unobstructed passageway in the right side of the mouth for easy placement of the endotracheal tube. Proper laryngoscope blade position is important. The distal tip of the straight blade should be used to lift the epiglottis anteriorly, thus visualizing the vocal cords. The distal tip of the curved blade should fit in the vallecula, between the base of the tongue and the epiglottis. Traction is then exerted up and away, along the axis of the laryngoscope handle. This motion, instead of an improper levering motion, moves soft tissues anteriorly without damaging the patient's teeth and gums. Insert the endotracheal tube down the right corner of the mouth, maintaining visualization as the tube penetrates the vocal cords. Insert uncuffed tubes 2 to 3 cm or to the level of the tube's glottic marker. Cuffs on endotracheal tubes should lie entirely beneath the cords. The overall depth of insertion may be estimated by multiplying the inner diameter of the endotracheal tube by three; this gives an approximate distance from midtrachea to the teeth and gums. As an example, a 3.5-mm endotracheal tube should be placed so that the distance marker measures 10.5 cm at the gumline.

After the tube has been placed, an examination of the chest for equal bilateral breath sounds should take place. Other methods of assessing tube placement are noting equal bilateral

TABLE C.3

RAPID-SEQUENCE INTUBATION

Step	Drug	Dose (IV)	Comments
1	Preoxygenate	Bag-valve-mask 100%	
2	Vagolytic		
	Atropine	0.01–0.02 mg/kg (min.): 0.1 mg; max: 1 mg)	Prevents bradycardia and reduces oral secretions.
3	Anesthetic (optional)		
	Lidocaine	1–2 mg/kg	Blunts rise in intracranial pressure (ICP) and cough reflex. Useful in situations of elevated ICP.
4	Cricoid pressure		
5	Sedative/hypnotic		
	Thiopental	2–6 mg/kg	May cause hypotension, myocardial depression. Reduces ICP. Use low doses in hypotension.
	OR		
	Ketamine	1–4 mg/kg	May cause elevated ICP, hypertension, tachycardia, and excess oral secretions. Causes bronchodilator effect. May cause emergence phenomena.
	OR		
	Midazolam	0.05–0.1 mg/kg	May cause cardiorespiratory depression.
	Fentanyl	1–5 μg/kg	May cause cardiorespiratory depression. Chest wall rigidity with high dose or rapid administration. May be reversed by naloxone.
6	Paralytic		
	Succinylcholine	1–2 mg/kg	Onset in 30–60 seconds; duration of 3–10 minutes. Contraindicated in burns, severe crush injury, and neuromuscular disease. Elevates ICP. Not reversible.
	OR		
	Pancuronium	0.04–0.1 mg/kg	Onset in 70–120 seconds; duration of 45–90 minutes. Contraindicated in renal failure and tricyclic antidepressant use. May reverse in 45 minutes with neostigmine.
	OR		
	Vecuronium	0.1–0.2 mg/kg	Onset in 70–120 seconds; duration of 30–90 minutes. Minimal effect on blood pressure and heart rate. May reverse in 30–45 minutes.
	OR		
	Rocuronium	0.6–1.2 mg/kg	Rapid onset of 30–45 seconds; duration of 30–90 minutes. May crystallize in IV tubing, particularly with thiopental. Little to no effect on heart rate or blood pressure. May reverse in 30–45 minutes.

Modified with permission from Neuhaus EM. Emergency management. In: Barone MA, ed. *The Harriet Lane handbook*, 14th ed. St. Louis: Mosby–Year Book, 1996:4.

chest rise, observing mist in the endotracheal tube, or detecting the presence of end-tidal carbon dioxide with a colorimetric or other type of device attached to the endotracheal tube. Confirmation of placement can be done using chest radiography. If doubt exists as to tube placement, remove the endotracheal tube and begin to oxygenate the child with bag-valve and mask ventilation in preparation for another intubation attempt. Each attempt to intubate the patient should take no longer than 30 to 45 seconds, shorter if significant hypoxemia results. Secure the tube with tape to prevent unintentional extubation.

Thoracentesis

Aspiration of the pleural space, or thoracentesis, can be useful diagnostically and therapeutically. Symptomatic pleural effusions may be drained and the fluid analyzed. In addition, aspiration of air in the stable patient with a pneumothorax may relieve symptoms. For either pneumothorax or pleural effusion, if the fluid or air is expected to reaccumulate, a chest tube should be inserted (see next section). If a patient is hemodynamically compromised by a tension pneumothorax, the most effective way to evacuate air is by inserting a needle or plastic catheter into the second intercostal space in the midclavicular line anteriorly. A stopcock attached to the catheter then allows a release of further tension, if necessary. It is not advisable to evacuate all air in the pleural space before inserting a chest tube because this removes the "cushion" of air between the chest wall and the lung and increases the risk of injury to the lung during the procedure.

Because thoracentesis requires a cooperative patient, the need for sedation should be assessed. Position the patient sitting backward on a chair or leaning over a medical stand, with arms and head supported on a pillow. In this position, the lower tip of the scapula lies in the posterior axillary line just above the usual site for puncture—the seventh intercostal space (Fig. C.16A). In infants and supine patients, the site of puncture is generally between the fourth and seventh intercostal spaces, between the midaxillary and posterior axillary lines.

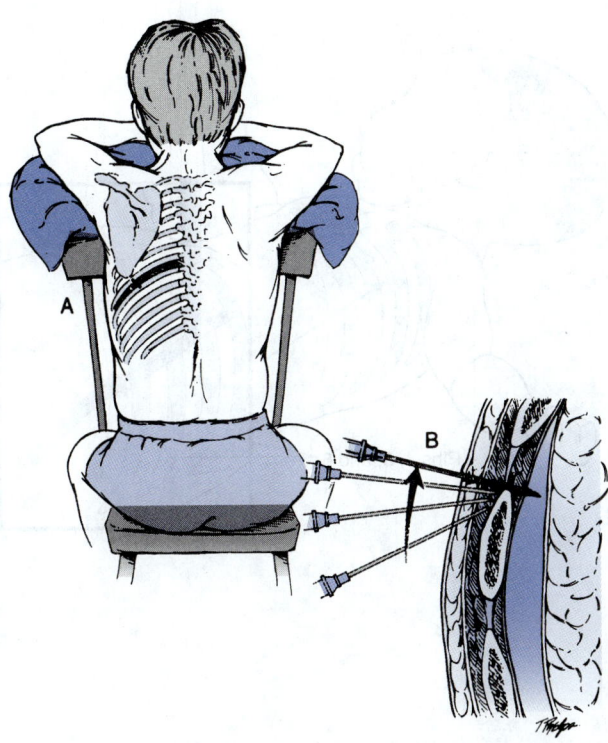

FIGURE C.16. Positioning a child for thoracentesis. **A:** The customary site for needle insertion is in the seventh intercostal space, just inferior to the lower tip of the scapula. **B:** After the catheter is inserted through the skin overlying the body of the eighth rib, it is gradually advanced over the superior margin of the rib into the interspace.

After preparing the skin using standard sterile technique, raise a wheal with 1% lidocaine over the rib below the interspace selected for the thoracentesis. Anesthetize the underlying periosteum as well as the pleura in the interspace above that rib. Using a plastic over-the-needle catheter (16- to 20-gauge), penetrate the skin at the site of the wheal, then "walk" the needle over the superior edge of the rib (Fig. C.16B). This process is meant to avoid the neurovascular bundle traveling on the underside of the rib above. Maintain continuous suction and gradually advance the needle until a "pop" is noted on entry of the pleural space. Advance the catheter an additional 2 to 3 mm to ensure that the plastic sheath is in the pleural space. Remove the needle, attach a syringe with a stopcock to the hub of the catheter, and slowly withdraw the desired volume of fluid or air. If nothing is aspirated, the catheter may be advanced a few millimeters or redirected. At the end of the procedure, quickly withdraw the needle, and apply an occlusive dressing to the site. Obtain a chest radiograph to assess the results of the procedure or the presence of an iatrogenic or residual pneumothorax.

Chest Tube Insertion

The most common indications for chest tube insertion in pediatrics are reaccumulating pneumothorax or pleural effusion, hemothorax, or empyema. When inserting a chest tube in a conscious child, consider the need for systemic analgesia or sedation, because it is a painful procedure. The patient is positioned supine with the arm restrained above the head. Positioning neonates with the affected side up may improve maneuverability. The site of chest tube entry into the pleural space is in the fourth or fifth intercostal space, at the level of the nipple, between the anterior and midaxillary lines. Avoid the nipple area, a landmark that may be less obvious in preterm infants. After preparing the site using aseptic technique, raise a skin

wheal with 1% lidocaine at the site of the intended skin incision. It is desirable to make this incision over a rib two levels below the intended entry site into the pleural cavity, at the sixth or seventh rib. Next, the entire track from skin to pleura should be anesthetized with lidocaine. Then, using a curved hemostat, bluntly dissect, creating a subcutaneous tunnel directed over the rib to the thoracic entry in the fourth or fifth intercostal space (Fig. C.17). This tunnel helps to provide an airtight seal while the tube is in place and after its removal. A moderate amount of pressure is required to force the clamp through the chest wall as intercostal muscles are being penetrated. A rush of air may be audible as the clamp enters the pleural space (see Fig. C.17). Spread the hemostat to enlarge the pleural opening, then remove it and place the chest tube in the curved portion of the clamp. Appropriately sized chest tubes are 8 and 10 Fr. for preterm infants, 12 Fr. for term infants and children up to age 3 years, 16 Fr. for children 3 to 10 years of age, and 20 to 28 Fr. for older children and adolescents. Insert the clamp and chest tube through the subcutaneous tunnel created earlier, and advance the tube into the pleural space (see Fig. C.17). Condensation in the lumen of the tube indicates that it has entered the pleural space. Its entry site should be palpated to ensure that it is not in the subcutaneous tissues. In most instances, the tube should be directed anteriorly and superiorly and advanced so that all side holes are in the pleural space. Secure the chest tube with nonabsorbable suture material in a purse-string fashion. Wrap petrolatum-soaked gauze around the tube at the skin entry site, and cover with a sterile dressing and tape. Confirm the position of the chest tube with a chest radiograph.

Pericardiocentesis

At times, circulation can be compromised by an accumulation of air, blood, or other fluid in the pericardium. Drainage by pericardiocentesis can be life-saving as well as diagnostic. Continuous electrocardiographic monitoring is essential. The conscious patient should be sedated unless contraindicated. Position the patient in a 30-degree sitting-up position, then prep and drape a large area centered at the subxiphoid. The preferred site for pericardiocentesis is just to the left of the xiphoid process, 1 cm inferior to the bottom rib. Infiltrate this area with 1% lidocaine. Select an 18- to 20-gauge angiocatheter or pericardial needle, the length of which depends on the age of the child. Kits are available with needle sizes of 7 cm and 15 cm. Attach a syringe and a three-way stopcock. Maintaining negative pressure on the syringe, insert the needle at a 45-degree angle to the skin, advancing in the direction of the patient's left shoulder (Fig. C.18). Observe closely for ventricular ectopy (a sign of myocardial contact) while advancing the needle. If this is noted, the needle should be withdrawn 1 to 2 cm. Once air or fluid begins to fill the syringe, clamp the needle at the skin edge with a hemostat to prevent further advancement. If using an angiocatheter, advance an additional 1 to 2 mm, ensuring that the plastic over-the-needle catheter is in the pericardial space. Withdraw the needle and quickly occlude the hub of the angiocatheter; then reattach the stopcock and syringe. Aspirate the pericardial fluid slowly. Pericardiocentesis has many potential complications, the most serious being hemopericardium (from laceration of the heart wall or coronary artery), cardiac arrhythmias, pneumothorax, and pneumopericardium.

Abdominal Paracentesis

Abdominal paracentesis is the removal of peritoneal fluid for therapeutic or diagnostic purposes. To minimize the risk of bladder puncture, it is important that the patient's bladder be empty before the procedure begins. Sedation may be necessary, but respiratory depressants should be used with extreme caution, because most children with ascites have a degree of respiratory compromise due to elevation of the diaphragm.

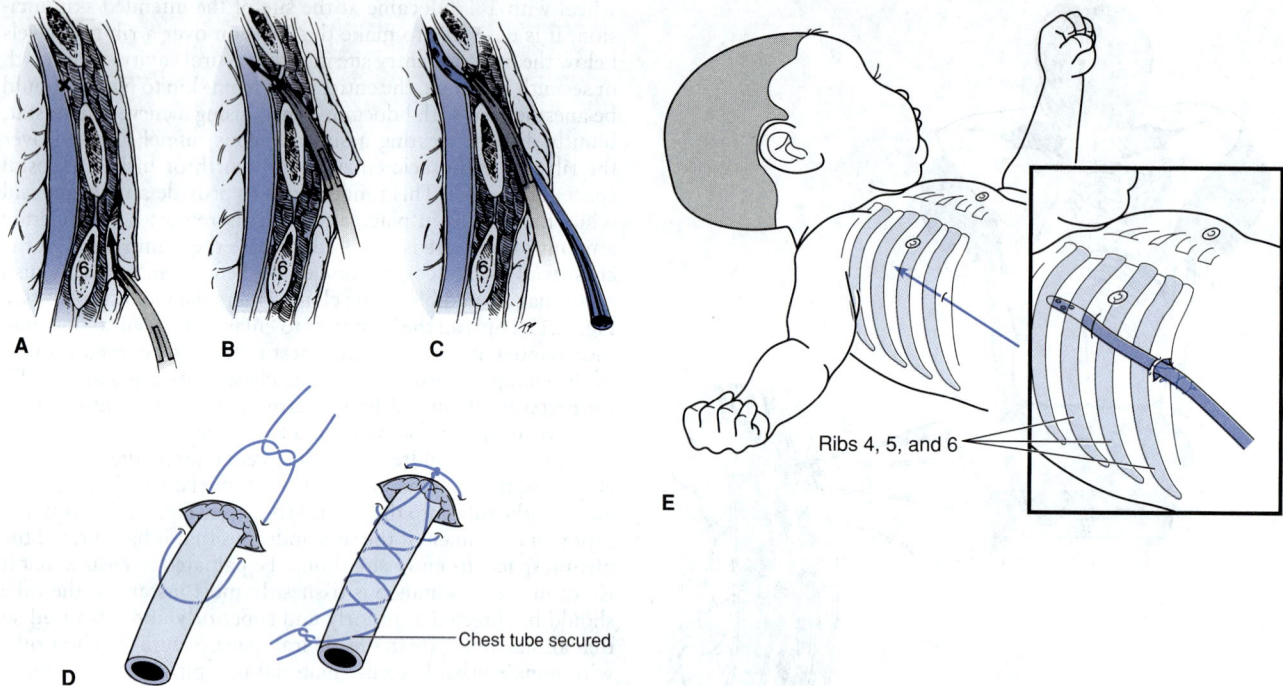

Chest tube secured

FIGURE C.17. Chest tube insertion. **A:** A curved hemostat inserted through a skin incision (at the sixth or seventh rib) is advanced through the subcutaneous tissues to the thoracic entry site at the fourth or fifth intercostal space. **B:** The clamp is forced through the chest wall. **C:** The chest tube is guided into the pleural space by placing it in the curved portion of the clamp. **D:** Securing the chest tube with suture. **E:** Chest tube placement with skin entry site at sixth intercostal space and entry into the pleural cavity at fourth intercostal space.

Position the patient in the sitting or lateral decubitus position. Sites for paracentesis are in the midline, halfway between the umbilicus and the symphysis pubis, or in either lower quadrant several centimeters above the inguinal ligament, lateral to the rectus muscle and in a line with the nipples. Avoid scars from previous surgery, because bowel tissue may adhere to the abdominal wall at these sites.

Cleanse the abdomen with povidone-iodine, then drape with sterile towels. Infiltrate the site of skin puncture with 1% lidocaine, and puncture the skin with a 14- to 16-gauge needle. Use a 14- to 20-gauge intravascular plastic catheter for the paracentesis. Choose the gauge by considering the size of the patient and by estimating the viscosity of the peritoneal fluid (e.g., pick a larger catheter when malignancy is suspected). Pull the skin to create a Z-track and, with a syringe attached to create negative pressure, insert the catheter through the puncture site, advancing just into the peritoneum. Remove the stylet, and slowly withdraw the desired volume of fluid. Rapid removal of large volumes of ascitic fluids can lead to hypotension. When the collection is complete, remove the catheter and apply a sterile dressing. Air aspirated from the peritoneal cavity is a sign of the penetration of a hollow viscus and is an indication to remove the needle immediately.

Bone Marrow Aspiration

The degree of discomfort children experience during the first bone marrow aspiration influences the anxiety they feel before subsequent examinations. With appropriate explanation, excellent local anesthesia, and sedation if necessary, bone marrow aspiration need not be painful or frightening. Behavioral techniques discussed earlier in this appendix may be especially helpful during this procedure.

The standard site for bone marrow aspiration in children of all ages is from the posterior superior iliac crest (Fig. C.19); the

tibia is an alternative site in children younger than 3 months. For aspiration at the posterior superior iliac crest, position the patient prone, with pillows under the pelvis to elevate it. Cleanse the skin with povidone-iodine and 70% alcohol, then raise a skin wheal with 1% lidocaine. After the skin is anesthetized, infiltrate the subcutaneous tissues and gradually anesthetize a wide area of periosteum at the site of aspiration. Test the adequacy of the local anesthesia before proceeding.

A 16- or 18-gauge bone-marrow needle usually is used for the procedure. Steady downward pressure in a boring rotary motion is exerted on the needle in a direction perpendicular to the surface of the bone. One hand should hold the needle in place over the bone. When the needle enters the marrow space, resistance decreases as the needle becomes anchored in place. Remove the obturator, and attach a 20-mL syringe. Aspirate rapidly for 1 to 2 seconds, taking care not to dilute the marrow specimen with sinusoidal blood (0.2 mL of marrow is sufficient). The patient may complain of pain at the time of negative pressure on the syringe. If no marrow is obtained, advance the needle further; change sites if this is not productive. Once the marrow specimen is obtained, remove the syringe from the needle hub, and prepare smears on glass slides. At the conclusion of the procedure, remove the needle, apply pressure to the site for 5 minutes, then apply a pressure dressing.

Suprapubic Bladder Puncture

Because the distended bladder is located intra-abdominally in infants, suprapubic aspiration is a common method of obtaining sterile urine specimens in patients younger than 2 years. The bladder must be distended for aspiration to be both safe and productive. The procedure should not be attempted until 60 minutes after the child's last void. It is often helpful but not necessary to obstruct urine outflow during the procedure by compressing the penile urethra in the male or by exerting

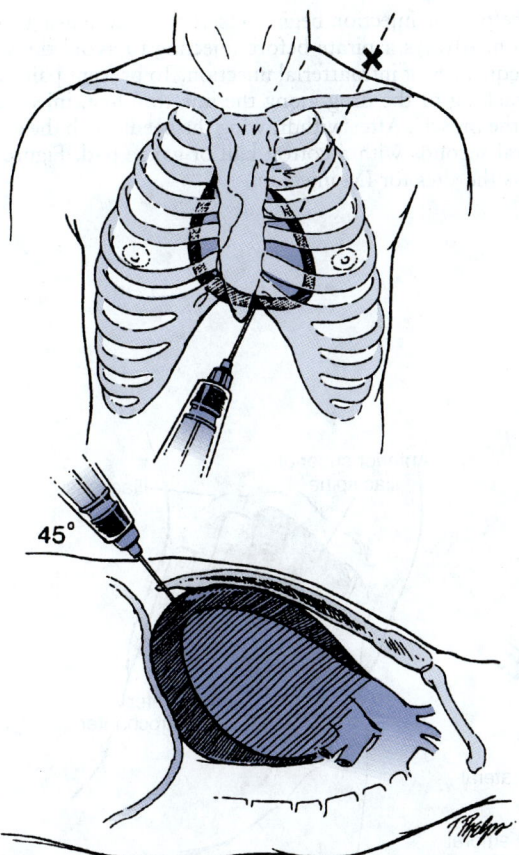

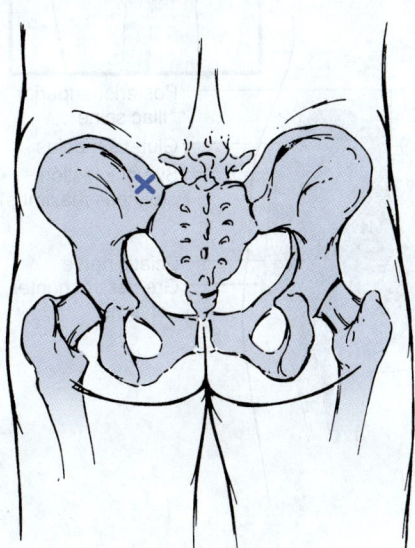

FIGURE C.18. Pericardiocentesis. (Reprinted with permission from Nichols DG, Yaster M, Lappe DG, Haller JA, eds. *Golden hour: the handbook of pediatric advanced life support*, 2nd ed. St. Louis: Mosby–Year Book, 1996.)

anterior rectal pressure on the female urethra via digital examination. Because manual pressure is not always successful in preventing urination, be prepared to obtain urine by bag or midstream catch. This may be useful for urinalysis, but culture results may be dubious. Position the child supine in a frog-leg position, and palpate to determine the position of the bladder.

FIGURE C.19. The site for bone marrow aspiration at the posterior superior iliac crest.

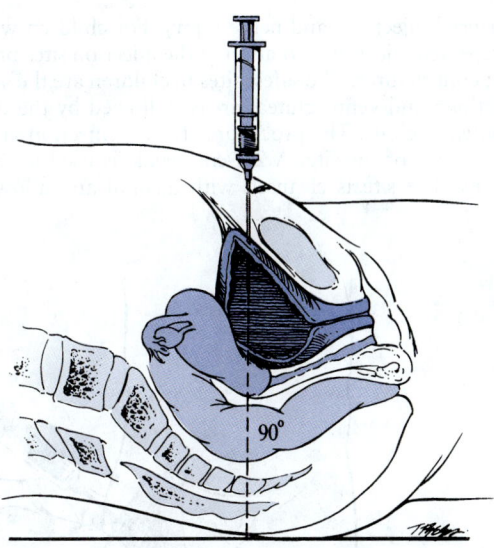

FIGURE C.20. Suprapubic bladder puncture.

After cleansing the suprapubic area with povidone-iodine and 70% alcohol, attach a syringe to a 22-gauge 1-inch needle. Insert the needle in the midline, 1 to 2 cm above the symphysis pubis, directed along the perpendicular to the abdominal wall (Fig. C.20). Excessive inferior angulation can result in injury to the bladder neck. Exert gentle negative pressure on the syringe while advancing slowly to a depth of no more than 2.5 cm. Urine appears in the syringe when the bladder is punctured. Once the specimen is collected, withdraw the needle and cover the site with an adhesive bandage. Complications of this procedure include hematuria (generally microscopic), bowel perforation, and abdominal wall infection.

Bladder Catheterization

Urinary bladder catheterization is a safe, quick method for obtaining a sterile urine specimen. Position the patient supine, in the frog-leg position. As with suprapubic bladder puncture, the child often may begin to urinate spontaneously before the catheter is inserted, so it is wise to have a sterile container on hand to collect a midstream specimen. In boys who have not been circumcised, the foreskin may be gently retracted to visualize the urethra. In girls, it is helpful to have an assistant use cotton swabs to spread the labia apart or to move redundant tissue at the introitus slightly posteriorly. Cleanse the urethral opening thoroughly with povidone iodine. Insert a well-lubricated catheter or feeding tube into the urethra until urine flow begins. In boys, extending and straightening the penis may simplify catheter insertion. Mild pressure on the catheter overcomes external sphincter spasm. Withdraw the catheter slowly at the end of the procedure.

Before inserting an indwelling urinary catheter, inflate the balloon to assess for leakage. Follow the procedure outlined above for catheter insertion. Once urine flow begins, advance the catheter further before inflating the balloon to ensure that the balloon is in the bladder and not in the proximal urethra. After the balloon is inflated, exert traction on the catheter to position the balloon at the trigone. Tape the catheter to the medial thigh, leaving sufficient slack so that movement of the leg does not create tension on the catheter.

Intramuscular Injections

Intramuscular (IM) injections are generally safe, but improper technique can lead to muscle contractures, abscess formation, intraarterial injection, and nerve injury. For children who receive repeated injections, rotation of the injection sites protects against contractures. The safest sites in children are the anterolateral thigh and ventrogluteal areas, followed by the deltoid and gluteal regions. The procedures for IM injection are similar regardless of the site. A 2.5-cm needle is used for all IM injections. The site is cleansed with alcohol and allowed to dry before the injection begins. Insert the needle using a quick motion. Always aspirate before injecting to avoid the serious consequences of intraarterial injection. To prevent pain caused by tracking of the drug along the injection line, inject slowly into the muscle. After withdrawing the needle, rub the area for several seconds with a cotton ball or gauze pad. Figure C.21 shows the sites for IM injection.

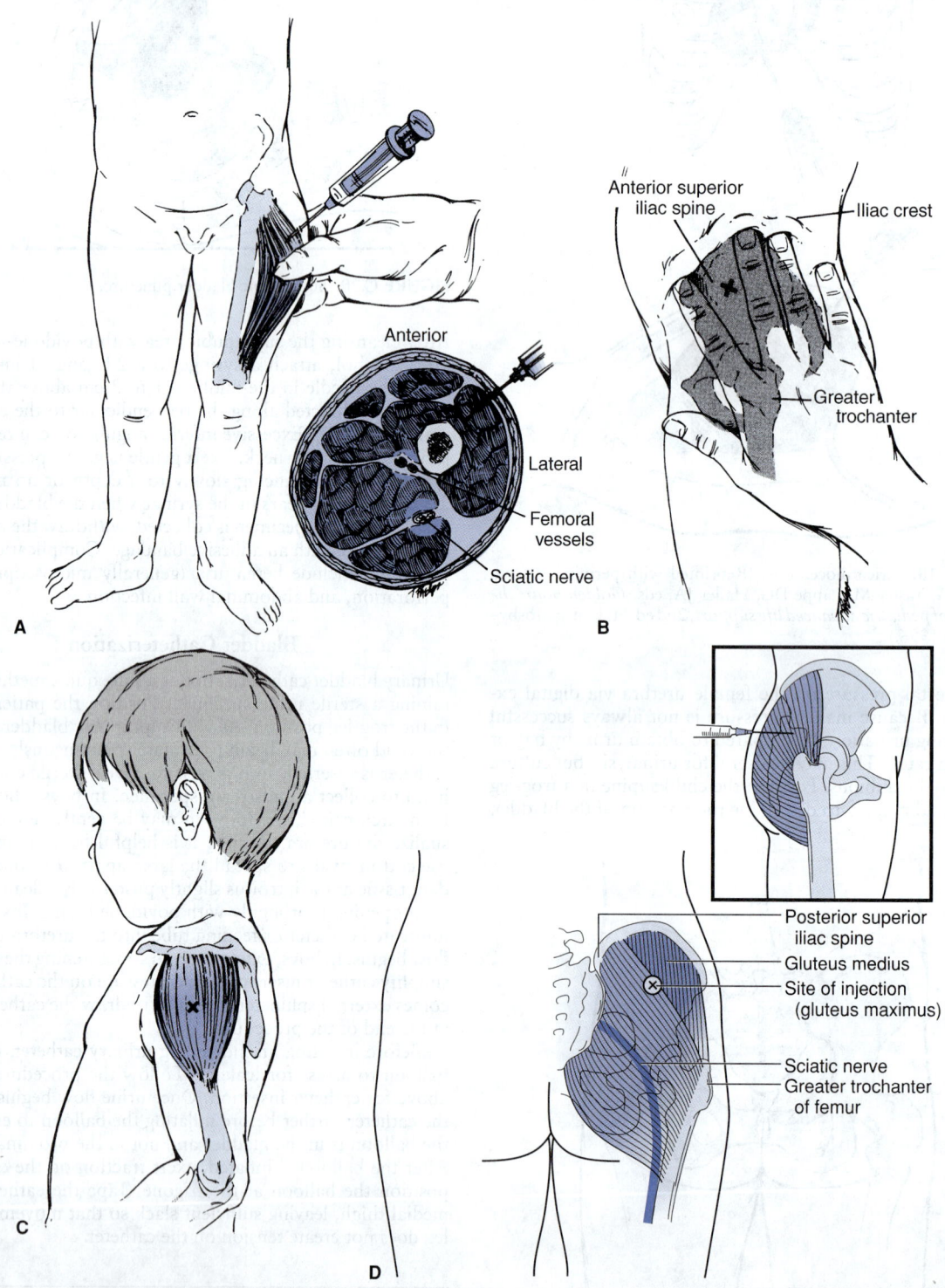

FIGURE C.21. Intramuscular injections. **A:** Anterolateral thigh injections are made in the midthigh. The needle should be directed inferiorly and at a 45-degree angle to the tabletop, which avoids injury to the femoral vessels and sciatic nerve (*highlighted areas*). **B:** Site for ventrogluteal injections. **C:** Site for deltoid injections. **D:** Site for dorsogluteal injections.

Anterolateral Thigh

The anterolateral thigh (see Fig. C.21A) is popular for IM injections because the sciatic nerve and femoral vessels are distant from the injection site. The operator compresses a wide area of thigh muscle together to increase muscle mass at the site. A 2.5-cm needle is inserted in the upper lateral quadrant of the midthigh. The needle is directed posteriorly at a 45-degree angle to the tabletop and inferiorly at a 45-degree angle to the long axis of the leg.

Ventrogluteal Area

Although many health professionals are unfamiliar with the ventrogluteal area (see Fig. C.21B), it is useful because it is free of major nerves and vessels. With the patient supine, the injection site is located by placing the operator's palm over the greater trochanter and the index finger over the anterior superior iliac spine, with the middle finger as close as possible to the tubercle of the iliac crest. The needle is inserted perpendicular to the skin, below the iliac crest in the center of this triangle, to a depth of 2.5 cm.

Deltoid Area

The injection site in the deltoid muscle (see Fig. C.21C) should be halfway between the acromion and the insertion of the deltoid muscle at the deltoid tuberosity of the humerus.

Gluteal Area

Injection into the gluteal area (see Fig. C.21D) involves a greater risk of sciatic nerve injury. This site should be avoided in children younger than 2 years, because muscle mass in this area is small. Inject in the upper outer quadrant, but lateral and superior to a line between the greater trochanter and posterior superior iliac spine, making sure to direct the needle perpendicular to the examining table with the patient prone. Injection in the medial direction (at a 90-degree angle to the skin) can result in sciatic nerve injury.

Taking the Temperature

Rectal measurements are the usual method of assessing body temperature in the child younger than 3 to 4 years. The child is placed prone on the parent's lap or the examining table. A lubricated rectal thermometer is inserted in a slightly anterior direction, no greater than 2.5 cm in children and 1.5 cm in infants. Placement of the thermometer more than 2.5 cm into the rectum increases the risk of rectal perforation. The time required for accurate measurements with electronic thermometers varies. Mercury thermometers should remain in place for approximately 3 minutes. Rectal temperatures should not be taken in neutropenic children or in those who have had recent anorectal surgery.

Oral temperature readings may be used in the older child who is able to keep her mouth closed. Make sure the patient has not recently had a hot or cold drink. Place the thermometer as far under the tongue as possible. For accurate measurements using mercury thermometers, leave in place at least 3 minutes.

For axillary temperatures, the axillae must be patted dry (rubbing the skin may falsely elevate the temperature). With the thermometer facing anteriorly, place the tip high in the axilla and bring the arm down to the patient's side. Again, 3 minutes is an acceptable time frame for measurement using a mercury thermometer.

Infrared auditory-canal thermometers have become the standard method in many office settings, hospital wards, and emergency departments. The readings represent an average of the temperature of the ear canal and the tympanic membrane. Although initially controversial, auditory canal thermometers, if calibrated appropriately, have been shown to closely track body core temperature. The measurement takes only a few seconds and is usually very well tolerated regardless of patient age. Position the ear canal to direct the probe toward the tympanic membrane. Middle-ear effusions, cerumen, or foreign bodies (even myringotomy tubes) do not affect measurements, because they are in thermal equilibrium with the auditory canal or tympanic membrane.

Temporal artery thermometers also are becoming widely available. These devices take multiple measurements (as many as 1,000 per second) of both ambient air temperature and skin temperature while they are swept over the area of the temporal artery. The method is desirable because it is completely noninvasive. Some studies have shown that temporal artery thermometers more closely reflect rectal temperatures than do tympanic temperatures. Other investigators have determined that these temple measurements are not reliably predictive of rectal temperatures in young infants. Because the technology is emerging, one must keep in mind that, when considering the use of an infrared auditory-canal thermometer or temporal artery thermometer, most studies to date examining disease outcome based on body temperature have used other methods (e.g., rectal temperatures and rates of serious bacterial illness in children younger than 28 days). Therefore, until further studies are performed, it does not seem appropriate to use these less invasive measures in all clinical situations.

Suggested Readings

American Academy of Pediatrics Committee on Bioethics. Informed consent, parental permission and assent in pediatric practice. *Pediatrics* 1995;95:314.

American Academy of Pediatrics Committee on Pediatric Emergency Medicine. Consent for medical services for children and adolescents. *Pediatrics* 1993;92:290.

Baucher H, Vinci R, Bak S, et al. Parents and procedures: a randomized clinical trial. *Pediatrics* 1996;98:861.

Bergeson PS, Singer SA, Kaplan AM. Intramuscular injections in children. *Pediatrics* 1982;70:944.

Chameides L, Hazinski MF, eds. *Textbook of pediatric advanced life support.* Dallas: American Heart Association, 1994.

Flood RG, Krauss B. Procedural sedation and analgesia for children in the emergency department. *Emerg Med Clin North Am* 2003;21:121.

Greenes DS, Fleisher GR. Accuracy of a noninvasive temporal artery thermometer for use in infants. *Arch Pediatr Adolesc Med* 2001;155:376.

Hughes WT, Buescher ES. *Pediatric procedures,* 2nd ed. Philadelphia: Saunders, 1980.

L.M.X.4. Product information. Accessed via the World Wide Web on 12/10/03 at http://www.ferndalelabs.com.

Meites S, Levitt MJ. Skin-puncture and blood-collecting techniques for infants. *Clin Chem* 1979;25:183.

Mohamed Tahir MA, Mason C, Find V. Informed consent: optimism versus reality. *Br Dent J* 2002;193:221.

Nichols DG, Yaster M, Lappe DG, Haller JA, eds. *Golden hour: the handbook of pediatric advanced life support,* 2nd ed. St. Louis: Mosby–Year Book, 1996.

O'Grady DM. Procedures. In: Barone MA, ed. *The Harriet Lane handbook,* 14th ed. St. Louis: Mosby–Year Book, 1996.

Rodriguez E, Jordan R. Contemporary trends in pediatric sedation and analgesia. *Emerg Med Clin North Am* 2002;20:199.

Ruddy RM. Illustrated techniques of pediatric emergency procedures. In: Fleisher GR, Ludwig S, eds. *Textbook of pediatric emergency medicine,* 3rd ed. Baltimore: Williams & Wilkins, 1993.

Schuman AJ. Infrared ear thermometry: an update for the clinician. *Contemp Pediatr* 1997;14(Suppl):1.

Siberry GK, Diener-West M, Schappell E, Karron RA. Comparison of temple temperatures with rectal temperatures in children under two years of age. *Clin Pediatr* 2002;41:405.

Walsh-Sukys MC, Krug SE, eds. *Procedures in infants and children.* Philadelphia: Saunders, 1997.

APPENDIX D ■ PRESENTING SIGNS AND SYMPTOMS

JANE A. OSKI

This chapter contains a group of common signs and symptoms. Each sign or symptom is followed by a list of possible causes, which are classified as common, uncommon, and rare. Common causes are those diseases that, collectively, are responsible for the given sign or symptom in approximately 90% of patients who have it; the term is not meant to imply that the disease itself is necessarily common. The uncommon causes category suggests that 1% to 10% of patients with the sign or symptom are found in that category. Rare causes are those diseases that represent less than 1% of the causes of the symptom or sign under discussion. When confronted with a given symptom or sign, common causes should always be considered first, but the rare causes should not be neglected.

Every attempt has been made to update and expand these differentials for the Fourth Edition of *Oski's Pediatrics: Principles and Practice*. A thorough discussion of each diagnostic category is beyond the scope of this chapter, but can be found in the recommended Suggested Readings. This appendix is an ongoing tribute to the life and work of Walter W. Tunnessen, Jr. M.D., whose encyclopedic text *Signs and Symptoms in Pediatrics, Third Edition* will provide the interested reader with great detail.

Suggested Reading

Tunnessen WW Jr. *Signs and Symptoms in Pediatrics,* 3rd ed. Philadelphia: Lippincott Williams & Wilkins, 1999.

Abdominal Masses

Common Causes
Appendiceal abscess
Bladder distention
Ectopic or horseshoe kidney
Fecal collection
Hepatomegaly (any etiology)
Hydronephrosis
Multicystic dysplastic kidney
Neuroblastoma
Polycystic kidney disease (with or without liver involvement)
Pregnancy (with or without ectopic location)
Pyloric stenosis
Splenomegaly (any etiology)
Wilms tumor

Uncommon Causes
Adrenal hemorrhage
Congenital mesoblastic nephroma (usually present at birth)
Hernia (with or without incarceration)
Intestinal duplication
Intussusception
Leukemia
Lymphadenopathy

Ovarian cyst
Renal vein thrombosis
Ureterocele

Rare Causes
Abscess
Anterior meningocele
Aortic aneurysm
Benign cystic causes
   Urachal cyst
   Mesenteric cyst
   Omental cyst
   Pancreatic cyst/pseudocyst
Bezoar
Bladder diverticulum
Hepatobiliary causes
   Cholecystitis/ascending cholangitis
   Choledochal cyst
   Hemangioendothelioma
   Hydrops of the gallbladder
Hydrometrocolpos
Intestinal causes
   Intestinal atresia (proximal dilatation)
   Intestinal stenosis (proximal dilatation)
   Malrotation with volvulus
   Meconium plug/ileus
   Regional enteritis
Solid tumors
   Granulosa-theca cell tumor
   Hepatoblastoma
   Hepatocellular carcinoma
   Lymphoma
   Mesoblastic nephroma
   Nephroblastomatosis
   Rhabdomyosarcoma
   Retroperitoneal lymphangioma
   Teratoma (abdominal/ovarian/retroperitoneal)

Suggested Readings

Merten DF, Kirks DR. Diagnostic imaging of pediatric abdominal masses. *Pediatr Clin North Am* 1985;32:1397.
Vane DW. Left upper quadrant masses in children. *Pediatr Rev* 1992;13:25.
Wilson DA. Ultrasound screening for abdominal masses in the neonatal period. *Am J Dis Child* 1982;136:147.

Abdominal Pain

Acute

Common Causes
Appendicitis
Bacterial enterocolitis

Campylobacter
Escherichia coli
Salmonella
Shigella
Yersinia
Dietary indiscretion
Food poisoning
Mesenteric lymphadenitis
Pharyngitis (streptococcal)
Pregnancy (with or without ectopic location)
Urinary tract infection
Viral gastroenteritis

Uncommon Causes
Cholecystitis/cholangitis
Diabetes mellitus/diabetic ketoacidosis
Dietl syndrome/crisis
Hepatitis
Herpes zoster
Incarcerated hernia
Infectious mononucleosis
Intussusception
Meckel diverticulum
Obstruction (adhesions)
Pelvic inflammatory disease
Peptic ulcer disease caused by *Helicobacter pylori*
Peritonitis
    Posttrauma/instrumentation
    Spontaneous
Pneumonia
Pyelonephritis
Sepsis
Trauma
    Bowel perforation
    Intramural hematoma
    Intraperitoneal blood
    Liver/spleen laceration or hematoma
    Musculocutaneous injury
    Pancreatic pseudocyst
Volvulus

Rare Causes
Abdominal abscess
Acute arrhythmia
Acute rheumatic fever
Adynamic ileus
    Drugs
    Metabolic
    Postsurgery/trauma
Ascites
Black Widow spider bite
Cat scratch disease
Eosinophilic gastroenteritis
Epididymitis
Erythromycin-induced cholestasis
Glomerulonephritis
Hemolysis
Hernia, incarcerated
Hypoglycemia
Malignancy
    Leukemia/lymphoma
    Solid tumor (with or without rupture/hemorrhage)
Menetrier syndrome
Mesenteric arterial insufficiency/obstruction
Nephrolithiasis
Nephrotic syndrome
Obstructive nephropathy
Pancreatitis
Paroxysmal cold hemoglobinuria
Pericarditis

Renal colic
Testicular torsion or neoplasm
Vasculitis
    Henoch-Schönlein purpura
    Kawasaki disease
    Polyarteritis nodosa
    Systemic lupus erythematosus

Recurrent

Common Causes
Carbohydrate malabsorption (hereditary or postinfectious)
Chronic nonspecific abdominal pain of childhood
Esophagitis (secondary to nonsteroidal antiinflammatory drugs
    or reflux)
Gastroesophageal reflux
Peptic ulcer disease
Psychophysiologic
    Conversion hysteria
    Anxiety reaction
    Depression
    Idiopathic recurrent pain
    Secondary gain
    Task-induced phobia (e.g., school, sports)

Uncommon Causes
Aerophagia
Collagen vascular disease
Constipation
Drugs
    Antibiotics
    Anticonvulsants
    Aspirin/nonsteroidal antiinflammatory drugs
    Bronchodilators
Dysmenorrhea
Enzymatic deficiency (e.g., lactose intolerance)
Food allergy: allergic-tension fatigue syndrome
Hepatosplenomegaly (any etiology)
Hiatal hernia
Inflammatory bowel disease
Irritable bowel syndrome
Mittelschmerz
Parasitic infection
    Ascariasis
    Giardiasis
    Strongyloidiasis
    Trichinosis
Sickle cell disease
Urinary tract infection

Rare Causes
Abdominal angina
Abdominal epilepsy
Abdominal masses/malignancies
    Lymphoma
    Neuroblastoma
    Ovarian lesions
    Wilms tumor
Abdominal migraine equivalent
Acute intermittent porphyria
Addison disease
Angioneurotic edema
Bowel anomaly with obstruction
    Duplication
    Malrotation with or without volvulus
    Stenosis
    Web
Choledochal cyst
Cystic fibrosis (meconium plug/ileus equivalent)
Diskitis
Endometriosis

Familial Mediterranean fever
Heavy metal intoxication
Hematocolpos
Hirschsprung disease
Hyperlipoproteinemia
Hyperthyroidism
Hypoperfusion states
   Coarctation of the aorta
   Familial dysautonomia
   Superior mesenteric artery syndrome
Linea alba hernia
Mesenteric cyst
Neurologic
   Central nervous system (CNS) mass lesion
   Radiculopathy
   Spinal cord injury/tumor
Recurrent/chronic arrhythmia
Recurrent pancreatitis
Slipping rib syndrome
Tuberculosis of spine
Wegener granulomatosis

Suggested Readings

Alford BA, McIlhenny J. The child with acute abdominal pain and vomiting. *Radiol Clin North Am* 1992;30:441.

Apley J. *The child with abdominal pains,* 2nd ed. Oxford: Blackwell Scientific Publications, 1975.

Barr RG. Abdominal pain in the female adolescent. *Pediatr Rev* 1983;4:281.

Barr RG, Levine MD, Watkins JB. Recurrent abdominal pain of childhood due to lactose intolerance. *N Engl J Med* 1979;300:1449.

Boyle JT. Recurrent abdominal pain: an update. *Pediatr Rev* 1997;18:310.

David EA, Werman HA, Rund DA. Use of leukocyte count and differential in the evaluation of abdominal pain. *Am J Emerg Med* 1986;4:482.

Dimson SB. Transit time related to clinical findings in children with recurrent abdominal pain. *Pediatrics* 1971;47:666.

Edwards NH. The accuracy of a Bayesian computer program for diagnosis and teaching in acute abdominal pain of childhood. *Computer Methods Programs Biomed* 1986;23:155.

Faro S, Maccato M. Pelvic pain and infections. *Obstet Gynecol Clin North Am* 1990;17:441.

Farrell MK. Abdominal pain. *Pediatrics* 1984;75(Pt 2):955.

Feuerstein M, Barr RG, Francoeur TE, et al. Potential biobehavioral mechanisms of recurrent abdominal pain in children. *Pain* 1982;13:287.

Hatch EI. The acute abdomen in children. *Pediatr Clin North Am* 1985;32:1151.

Lake AM. Acute abdominal pain in childhood. *Postgrad Med J* 1979;65:119.

Lebenthal E. Recurrent abdominal pain in childhood. *Am J Dis Child* 1980;134:347.

Michener WM. An approach to recurrent abdominal pain in children. *Primary Care* 1981;8:277.

Muse KN. Cyclic pelvic pain. *Obstet Gynecol Clin North Am* 1990;17:427.

Poole SR. Recurrent abdominal pain in childhood and adolescence. *Am Fam Physician* 1984;30:131.

Ryan NM. Recurrent abdominal pain among school-aged children. *MCN Am J Matern Child Nurs* 1986;11:102.

Silverberg M. Chronic abdominal pain in adolescents. *Pediatr Ann* 1991;20:179.

Alopecia

Common Causes
Alopecia areata
Distal trichorrhexis nodosa
Physiologic (newborns)
Temporal recession at puberty
Tinea capitis
Traction alopecia/traumatic alopecia
Trichotillomania

Uncommon Causes
Acute bacterial infections
   Cellulitis
   Folliculitis decalvans
   Pyoderma

Burns
Cancer therapy
   Antimetabolites
   Radiation
Chemical injury
Kerion
Proximal trichorrhexis nodosa
Psoriasis
Seborrhea
Viral infections
   Herpes simplex
   Varicella

Rare Causes
Circumscribed alopecia
   Androgenic alopecia
   Aplasia cutis
   Conradi-Hunermann disease
   Epidermal nevi, organoid
   Follicular aplasia
   Goltz syndrome
   Hair follicle hamartoma
   Incontinentia pigmenti
   Infections
      Leprosy
      Tuberculosis
   Inflammatory etiologies
      Keratosis follicularis
      Lichen planus
      Morphea
      Porokeratosis of Mibelli
      Sarcoid
      Systemic lupus erythematosus
   Myotonic dystrophy
   Triangular alopecia of the frontal scalp
Diffuse alopecia
   Anagen effluvium
      Cytostatic agents in plants
         Mimosine
         Selenocystothionine
      Radium
      Thallium
   Anhidrotic ectodermal dysplasia
   Atrichia congenita
   Cartilage-hair hypoplasia
   Chondroectodermal hypoplasia (Ellis-van Creveld syndrome)
   Congenital hypothyroidism
   Clouston syndrome
   Hair shaft deformities
      Monilethrix
      Pili torti
         Classic form
         Trichopoliodystrophy (Menkes syndrome)
      Trichorrhexis invaginata
      Trichorrhexis nodosa
         Argininosuccinic aciduria
   Hallermann-Streiff syndrome
   Hidrotic ectodermal dysplasia
   Langer-Giedion dysplasia
   Loose Anagen syndrome
   Marinesco-Sjögren syndrome
   Oculodentodigital dysplasia
   Oral-facial-digital syndrome type 1
   Progeria
   Rothmund-Thomson syndrome
   Seckel syndrome
   Telogen effluvium
      Childbirth

Chronic infection/illness
Drugs
    Anticoagulants
    Anticonvulsants
    Antikeratinizing drugs
    Antithyroid drugs
    Beta blockers (Propranolol)
    Heavy metals
    Hormones
Endocrine disorders
    Androgenetic alopecia
    Diabetes mellitus
    Hyperthyroidism
    Hypoparathyroidism
    Hypopituitarism
    Hypothyroidism
Excessive dieting
High fevers
Nutritional disorders
    Acrodermatitis enteropathica
    Celiac disease
    Hypervitaminosis A
    Iron deficiency
    Kwashiorkor and marasmus (severe)
    Rickets
Stress
Surgery
Werner syndrome

Suggested Readings

Atton AV, Tunnessen WW Jr. Alopecia in children: the most common causes. *Pediatr Rev* 1990;12:25.

Bergfeld WF. Hair disorders. *Major Prob Clin Pediatr* 1978;19:347.

Clore ER, Corey A. Hair loss in children and adolescents. *J Pediatric Health Care* 1991;5:245.

Hurwitz S. *Clinical pediatric dermatology*, 2nd ed. Philadelphia: Saunders, 1993: 491.

Levy ML. Disorders of the hair and scalp in children. *Pediatr Clin North Am* 1991;38:905.

Olsen EA. Alopecia: evaluation and management. *Primary Care* 1989;16:765.

Price VH. Disorders of the hair in children. *Pediatr Clin North Am* 1978;25: 305.

Price VH. Office diagnosis of structural hair anomalies. *Cutis* 1975;15:231.

Stroud JD. Hair loss in children. *Pediatr Clin North Am* 1983;30:641.

Weston WL. *Practical pediatric dermatology*. Boston: Little, Brown, 1979:269.

Anorexia

Common Causes
Acute infection
Apparent anorexia
    Dieting/fear of obesity
    Manipulative behavior
    Unrealistic expectations of caregivers
Constipation

Uncommon Causes
Appendicitis
Chronic infection
Drugs
    Aminophylline
    Amphetamines
    Anticonvulsants
    Antihistamines
    Antimetabolites
    Digitalis
    Narcotics
Esophagitis/gastroesophageal reflux

Food aversion in athletes
Iron deficiency
Irritable bowel syndrome
Pregnancy
Psychosocial deprivation (neglect/abuse)
Psychosocial factors
    Chronic mental/environmental stress
        Anxiety
        Fear
        Loneliness/boredom
    Depression
    Grief
    Mania

Rare Causes
Acquired immunodeficiency syndrome (AIDS)
Acute rheumatic fever
Alcohol/drug abuse
Anorexia nervosa
Chronic disease
Collagen vascular disease: JRA, SLE, sarcoidosis
Congestive heart failure
Cyanotic heart disease
Electrolyte disturbances
    Hypercalcemia
    Hypochloremia
    Hypokalemia
Endocrine disease
    Addison disease
    Adrenogenital syndrome
    Diabetes insipidus
    Hyperparathyroidism
    Hypothyroidism
    Panhypopituitarism
    Pseudohypoaldosteronism
Hypervitaminosis A
Hepatitis
Inborn errors of metabolism
Inflammatory bowel disease
Kwashiorkor
Lead poisoning
Liver failure
Malignancies (occult)
Neurologic
    Congenital degenerative disease
    Diencephalic syndrome
    Hypothalamic lesions
    Increased intracranial pressure
    Mental retardation/cerebral palsy
Pain avoidance
    Gastrointestinal obstruction
    Inflammatory bowel disease
    Pancreatitis
    Superior mesenteric artery syndrome
Polycystic ovary syndrome
Polycythemia
Postsurgery
Pulmonary insufficiency
Renal failure
Renal tubular acidosis
Schizophrenia
Zinc deficiency

Suggested Readings

Bernstein IL, Sigmundi RA. Tumor anorexia: a learned food aversion? *Science* 1980;209:416.

Brobeck JR. Nature of satiety signals. *Am J Clin Nutr* 1975;28:806.

Bryant-Waugh RJ, Lask BD, Shafran RL, Fosson AR. Do doctors recognize eating disorders in children? *Arch Dis Child* 1992;67:103.

Nussbaum MP, Shenker IR, Shaw H, Frank S. Differential diagnosis of anorexia nervosa. *Pediatrician* 1983;12:110.

Pugliese MT, Lifshitz F, Grad G, et al. Fear of obesity: a cause of short stature and delayed puberty. *N Engl J Med* 1983;309:513.

Smith NJ. Excessive weight loss and food aversion in athletes simulating anorexia nervosa. *Pediatrics* 1980;66:139.

Yates A, Leehey K, Shisslak CM. Running—an analogue of anorexia? *N Engl J Med* 1983;308:251.

Boltshauser E, Lange B, Dumermuth G. Differential diagnosis of syndromes with abnormal respiration (tachypnea-apnea). *Brain Dev* 1987;9:462.

Guilleminault C, Ariagno R, Korobkin R, et al. Mixed and obstructive sleep apnea and near-miss for sudden infant death syndrome: 2. Comparison of near-miss and normal control infants by age. *Pediatrics* 1979;64:882.

McBride JT. Infantile apnea. *Pediatr Rev* 1984;5:275.

Spitzer AR, Fox WW. Infant apnea. *Pediatr Clin North Am* 1986;33:561.

Torrey SB. Apnea. *Pediatr Emerg Care* 1985;1:219.

Valdes-Dapena MA. Sudden infant death syndrome: a review of the medical literature 1974–1979. *Pediatrics* 1980;66:597.

Apnea

Common Causes
Breath-holding spells
Bronchiolitis
Extrinsic suffocation
Gastroesophageal reflux/aspiration
Idiopathic (CNS immaturity?)
Prematurity
Seizure

Uncommon Causes
Arrhythmia
Asthma
Bronchopulmonary dysplasia spells
CNS hypoperfusion
CNS trauma/bleed
Congenital airway anomaly
Hypoglycemia
Hypoxemia/hypercarbia (severe)
Infection
    Croup
    Encephalitis/meningitis
    Epiglottitis
    Pertussis
    Pneumonia
    Sepsis
Laryngospasm
Laryngotracheobronchomalacia
Obstructive sleep apnea
Toxins/drugs

Rare Causes
Anemia
Glossoptosis
Guillain-Barré syndrome
Hypocalcemia
Increased intracranial pressure
Infantile botulism
Macroglossia
Metabolic disease
    Hyperammonemia
    Inborn errors
    Metabolic alkalosis
Micrognathia
Ondine's curse
Spinal cord injury
    Cervical spine instability
    Down syndrome
    Dwarfism
Trauma
Tumor (CNS, airway)

Back Pain

Common Causes
Back pain with no organic cause
    Anxiety/adjustment disorders
    Depression
    Drug abuse
    Physical abuse
    Pregnancy
    Sexual abuse
Lordotic mechanical back pain
Mechanical derangement (muscle strain or poor posture)
Myalgias
Scheuermann disease
Scoliosis
Spondylolysis/spondylolisthesis
Urinary tract infection

Uncommon Causes
Ankylosing spondylitis
Disc space infection (discitis)
Rheumatic disorders
Sacroiliac joint infections
Spina bifida occulta
Spinal cord tumors (lipomas, teratomas)
Vertebral osteomyelitis

Rare Causes
Aneurysmal bone cyst
Arteriovenous malformation of cord
Aseptic necrosis of vertebrae
Benign osteoblastoma
Diastematomyelia
Eosinophilic granuloma of vertebrae
Hemangioma of bone
Hematocolpos
Hemolytic anemia, chronic
Herniated nucleus pulposus
Herpes zoster
Limb-girdle muscular dystrophy
Malignancy involving bone (neuroblastoma, metastatic leukemia)
Multiple epiphyseal dysplasia
Neurenteric cyst
Osteomalacia of the spine
Osteoporosis
Paraspinal tumor or infection
Secondary hyperparathyroidism
Sickle cell disease
Spinal/epidural abscess
Tuberculosis of the spine
Vertebral osteoid osteoma

Suggested Readings

Anders TF, Weinstein P. Sleep and its disorders in infants and children. A review. *Pediatrics* 1972;50:312.

Suggested Readings

Abram SR, Tedeschi AA, Partain CL, Blumenkopf B. Differential diagnosis of severe back pain using MRI. *South Med J* 1988;81:1487.

Aiken BM, Cohen BS. The role of congenital anomalies in low back pain. *Md Med J* 1983;32:38.

Bunnell WP. Back pain in children. *Orthop Clin North Am* 1982;13:587.

Combs JA, Caskey PM. Back pain in children and adolescents: a retrospective review of 648 patients. *South Med J* 1997;90:789.

Gonzales R, Marino RV. A diagnostic approach to childhood back pain. *J Am Osteopath Assoc* 1986;86:454.

Williams HJ, Pugh DG. Vertebral epiphysitis: a comparison of the clinical and roentgenologic findings. *AJR Am J Roentgenol* 1963;90:1236.

Chest Pain

Common Causes

Costochondritic
  Arthritis
  Infectious costochondritis
  Tietze syndrome
Cough
Herpes zoster
Idiopathic
Indigestion (heartburn, esophagitis)
Mitral valve prolapse
Musculoskeletal (strain, occult trauma)
Pneumonitis/pneumonia
Psychogenic
  Conversion reaction
  Globus hystericus
  Hyperventilation
Reactive airway disease
Sickle cell disease
Trauma

Uncommon Causes

Arrhythmias
Congenital heart disease
    Aortic stenosis
    Mitral valve prolapse
    Pulmonic stenosis
Congestive heart failure
Esophageal (trauma associated with vomiting, foreign body)
Pleuritis/pleurisy
Pneumothorax
Precordial catch syndrome

Rare Causes

Cholecystitis
Cocaine abuse
Costoclavicular compression syndrome
Diaphragmatic irritation
  Abscess
  Fitz-Hugh–Curtis syndrome
  Peritonitis
  Ruptured viscus
  Tumor
Endocarditis
Epidemic pleurodynia (devil's grip)
Hiatal hernia
Juvenile ankylosing spondylitis
Juvenile rheumatoid arthritis
Mediastinitis
Myocardial ischemia (e.g., anomalous coronary artery)
Myocarditis
Osteomyelitis (vertebrae, ribs)
Peptic ulcerative disease
Pericarditis
Pneumomediastinum
Pubertal breast development
Pulmonary embolism
Rheumatic fever
Slipping rib syndrome
Spinal cord compression
Tracheitis
Xiphoid process syndrome

Suggested Readings

Asnes RS, Santulli R, Bemporad JR. Psychogenic chest pain in children. *Clin Pediatr* 1981;20:788.

Brenner JI, Berman MA. Chest pain in childhood and adolescence. *J Adolesc Health Care* 1983;3:271.

Calabro JJ, Jeghers H, Miller KA, Gordon RD. Classification of anterior chest wall syndromes. Letter. *JAMA* 1980;243:1420.

Calabro JJ, Marchesano JM. Tietze's syndrome: report of a case with juvenile onset. *J Pediatr* 1966;68:985.

Driscoll DJ, Glicklich LB, Gallen WJ. Chest pain in children: a prospective study. *Pediatrics* 1976;57:648.

Milov DE, Kantor RJ. Chest pain in teenagers. When is it significant? *Postgrad Med* 1990;88:145.

Porter GE. Slipping rib syndrome: an infrequently recognized entity in children: a report of three cases and a review of the literature. *Pediatrics* 1985;76:810.

Reynolds JL. Precordial catch syndrome in children. *South Med J* 1989;82:1228.

Selbst SM, Ruddy RM, Clark BJ, et al. Pediatric chest pain: a prospective study. *Pediatrics* 1988;82:319.

Sparrow MJ, Bird EL. "Precordial catch:" a benign syndrome of chest pain in young persons. *N Z Med J* 1978;88:325.

Coma

Common Causes

CNS trauma
  Cerebral edema
  Concussion
  Hemorrhage
    Epidural
    Subarachnoid
    Subdural
  Increased intracranial pressure
Drug intoxication
  Acetaminophen
  Anticonvulsants
  Antihistamines
  Benzodiazepines
  Digoxin
  Ethanol
  Heavy metals
  Hydrocarbons
  Hypnotics
    Barbiturates
  Insulin
  Lithium
  Narcotic analgesics
  Organophosphates
  Phencyclidine
  Phenothiazines
  Salicylate
  Tricyclic antidepressants

Uncommon Causes

Cardiorespiratory
  Cardiopulmonary arrest
  Hypercapnca
  Hypotension/shock
  Hypoxemia
Infection
  Abscess
  Encephalitis
  Meningitis

Metabolic
  Hypercalcemia/hypocalcemia
  Hypermagnesemia/hypomagnesemia
  Hypernatremia
  Hypoglycemia
  Hyponatremia
    Water intoxication
  Metabolic acidosis
  Metabolic alkalosis
Postictal state
Postoperative
  General anesthesia
  Hypotension/hypoxemia
Sepsis

Rare Causes
Cardiac
  Arrhythmia
  Hypertension
  Hypoperfusion
    Aortic stenosis
    Coarctation of the aorta
Cerebral tumors/metastases
  Ewing sarcoma
  Wilms tumor
Cerebrovascular
  Hemorrhage
  Thrombophlebitis
  Vasculitis
  Venous thrombosis
Dehydration
Diabetic ketoacidosis
Electric shock
Endocrine disorders
  Addison disease
  Congenital adrenal hyperplasia
  Cushing disease
  Pheochromocytoma
Esophageal foreign body
Inborn errors of metabolism
  Hyperammonemia
  Hypoglycemia
Intussusception
Heat stroke
Hepatic failure
  Alpha$_1$-antitrypsin deficiency
  Biliary atresia
  Cystic fibrosis
  Fulminant hepatitis
  Wilson disease
Hypothermia
Malignant hyperthermia
Porphyria
Postinfectious encephalomyelitis
  Measles
  Other viral infections
Psychiatric disturbances
  Fugue state
  Hysteria
Reye syndrome
Sudden infant death syndrome
Uremia
  Hemolytic-uremic syndrome

Suggested Readings

Dean JM, Kaufman ND. Prognostic indicators in pediatric near-drowning: the Glasgow Coma Scale. *Crit Care Med* 1981;9:536.

Helliwell M, Hampel G, Sinclair E, et al. Value of emergency toxicological investigations in differential diagnosis of coma. *BMJ* 1979;2:819.

Levy DE, Bates D, Caronna JJ, et al. Prognosis in nontraumatic coma. *Ann Intern Med* 1981;94:293.

Mickell JJ, Reigel DH, Cook DR, et al. Intracranial pressure: monitoring and normalization therapy in children. *Pediatrics* 1977;59:606.

Seshia SS, Seshia MMK, Sachdeva RK. Coma in childhood. *Dev Med Child Neurol* 1977;19:614.

Constipation

Constipation is defined here as stools less frequent than expected by the caretaker.

Common Causes
Appendicitis
Breast-feeding (begins at approximately 6 weeks of age)
Chronic idiopathic constipation
Cow's milk ingestion/allergy
Deficient fluid intake
Drugs
  Anticholinergics
  Antihistamines
  Narcotics
  Phenothiazines
Dysfunctional toilet training
Emotional disturbances
Functional ileus
Immobility
Inappropriate expectations of the caretaker
Intentional withholding
Intestinal abnormalities
  Atresia
  Hirschsprung disease
  Microcolon
  Volvulus
  Web
Low dietary fiber
Meconium plug/ileus
Meningomyelocele
Mental retardation/cerebral palsy
Painful defecation (hemorrhoids, fissure, sexual abuse, skin irritation)

Uncommon Causes
Diabetes mellitus
Electrolyte disturbances
  Hypercalcemia/hypocalcemia
  Hypokalemia
Hypothyroidism
Imperforate anus/anal stenosis
Intestinal pseudo-obstruction
Lead poisoning
Meconium ileus equivalent, cystic fibrosis
Salmonellosis
Spinal cord injury/tumor
Starvation

Rare Causes
Anal stenosis/rectal stenosis
Acute intermittent porphyria
Amyloidosis
Anteriorly located anus
Botulism
Chagas disease
Dolichocolon
Graft versus host disease
Multiple endocrine neoplasia
Myopathies/myotonias
Pheochromocytoma

Sacral malformations
Scleroderma
Small left colon syndrome
Tetanus
Tethered cord

Suggested Readings

Barr RG, Levine MD, Wilkinson RH, Mulvihill D. Chronic and occult stool retention: a clinical tool for its evaluation in school-aged children. *Clin Pediatr* 1979;18:674.
Bentley JFR. Constipation in infants and children. *Gut* 1971;12:85.
Davidson M, Kugler MM, Bauer CH. Diagnosis and management in children with severe and protracted constipation and obstipation. *J Pediatr* 1963;62:261.
Fleisher DR. Diagnosis and treatment of disorders of defecation in children. *Pediatr Ann* 1976;5:700.

Cough

Common Causes
Allergic disease
Aspiration (direct or indirect)
Atelectasis
Bacterial infection
   Bronchiectasis
   Bronchitis
   Pneumonia
   Sinusitis
   Tracheitis
Congestive heart failure
Cough variant asthma
Environmental irritants/pollution
   Dry Air
   Fumes
   Passive/active smoke
Foreign body
Gastroesophageal reflux
Infections, other
   Chlamydia
   Mycoplasma
   Pertussis
Postnasal drip
Reactive airway disease
Smoking/passive smoking
Viral infection
   Bronchiolitis
   Croup
   Pneumonitis
   Upper respiratory infection

Uncommon Causes
Bronchopulmonary dysplasia
Cystic fibrosis
Exercise-induced bronchospasm
Fungal infection
Malformation of the airway
Malignancy (primary or metastatic)
Mediastinal adenopathy
Psychogenic
Tracheobronchomalacia
Tracheoesophageal fistula
Tuberculosis
Vascular ring

Rare Causes
Allergic bronchopulmonary aspergillosis
Anomalous blood vessels

Auricular nerve stimulation
Bronchogenic cyst
Congenital lobar emphysema
Drug-induced
   Angiotensin-converting enzyme inhibitors
   Metoclopramide
Elongated uvula
Gilles de Tourette syndrome
Immotile cilia syndrome (Kartagener syndrome)
Lymphocytic interstitial pneumonitis
Neuromuscular disorders
Opportunistic infections (*Pneumocystis carinii*, cytomegalovirus, *Mycobacterium avium-intracellulare*)
Papilloma of trachea and/or bronchi
Parasitic infection
Pulmonary embolism
Pulmonary hemosiderosis
Pulmonary sequestration
Sarcoidosis

Suggested Readings

Cloutier MM. Finding the cause of chronic cough in children. *J Respir Dis* 1980;1:20.
Cloutier MM, Loughlin GM. Chronic cough in children: a manifestation of airway hyperactivity. *Pediatrics* 1981;67:6.
Eigen H. The clinical evaluation of chronic cough. *Pediatr Clin North Am* 1982;29:67.
Godfrey RC. Diseases causing cough. *Eur J Respir Dis* 1980;110(Suppl):57.
Irwin RS, Corrao WM, Pratter MR. Chronic persistent cough in the adult: the spectrum and frequency of causes and successful outcome of specific therapy. *Am Rev Respir Dis* 1981;123:413.
Irwin RS, Rosen MJ, Braman SS. Cough: a comprehensive review. *Arch Intern Med* 1977;137:1186.
Mellis CM. Evaluation and treatment of chronic cough in children. *Pediatr Clin North Am* 1979;26:553.
Stein MT. Chronic cough in infants younger than 3 months. *West J Med* 1982;136:505.
Wilmott RW. Pursuing the cause of persistent cough. *Contemp Pediatr* 1987;4:26.

Cyanosis

Common Causes
Acrocyanosis (especially cold stress)
Apnea of prematurity
Aspiration
   Direct (swallowing disorders, neuromuscular disease)
   Indirect (gastroesophageal reflux, emesis)
Atelectasis
Breath holding
Bronchiolitis
Congenital heart disease
   Decreased pulmonary blood flow (no pulmonary hypertension)
      Anomalous systemic venous return
      Ebstein's anomaly
      Hypoplastic right ventricle
      Pulmonary stenosis/atresia
      Tetralogy of Fallot
      Tricuspid stenosis/atresia/insufficiency
   Eisenmenger's physiology
   Increased pulmonary blood flow
      Atrioventricular canal
      Coarctation (preductal)
      Hypoplastic left heart
      Total anomalous pulmonary venous return
      Transposition
      Truncus arteriosus
      Ventricular septal defect (large)

Pump failure
  Aortic stenosis
  Coarctation (postductal)
  Patent ductus arteriosus
  Ventricular septal defect
Croup
Crying
Drugs, respiratory depressants (e.g., narcotics,
  benzodiazepines)
Hyaline membrane disease
Mucus plug
Nasal obstruction
Pneumonia
Pulmonary edema
Reactive airway disease
Seizures
Sepsis
Shock, various causes
Sleep apnea (tonsillar/adenoidal hypertrophy)

Uncommon Causes
Abdominal distention
Arterial thrombosis
Bronchopulmonary dysplasia
Chest wall abnormalities
  Congenital bone/cartilage abnormalities
  Pectus
  Flail chest
Cystic fibrosis
Dysrhythmias
Foreign body
Hypoglycemia
Hypovolemia
Mediastinal mass
Persistent fetal circulation
Pickwickian syndrome/obesity
Pleural effusion
Pneumothorax
Polycythemia
Pulmonary hemorrhage
Retropharyngeal/peritonsillar abscess
Scoliosis
Tracheal compression
  Abscess
  Adenopathy
  Congenital goiter
  Hemorrhage
  Tumor
  Vascular ring
Tracheobronchomalacia
Venous stasis

Rare Causes
Alveolar proteinosis
Angioedema
Atrial myxomas
Bronchogenic cyst
CNS disease
  Edema
  Hemorrhage
  Infection
  Trauma
Constrictive pericarditis
Chylothorax
Cystic adenomatoid formation
Diaphragmatic hernia
Endocardial fibroelastosis
Epiglottitis
Factitious (blue paint/dyes/makeup)

Familial dysautonomia
Glossoptosis
Hemoglobinopathy (M, low oxygen affinity)
Hypoplastic lungs
Laryngeal web
Lobar emphysema
Methemoglobinemia
  Methemoglobin reductase deficiency
  Oxidant stress
    Acetophenetidin
    Antimalarials
    Benzocaine
    Crayons
    Disinfectants
    Ethylenediaminetetraacetic acid (EDTA)
    Hydralazine
    Marking dyes
    Naphthalene
    Nitrites
      Amyl/butyl nitrate
      Nitrate-contaminated well water
      Nitrate food additives
      Nitroglycerin
      Plant nitrates (e.g., carrots grown in contaminated
        soil)
    Nitroprusside
    Prilocaine
    Pyridium
    Sulfonamides
    Vitamin K analogues
Ondine's curse
Primary pulmonary hypertension
Pulmonary arteriovenous malformation/fistula
Pulmonary embolism/thrombosis
Pulmonary hemosiderosis
Pulmonary fibrosis
Pulmonary sequestration
Pulmonary tumor (primary or metastatic)
Reflex sympathetic dystrophy
Respiratory muscle dysfunction
  Botulism
  Muscular dystrophy
  Myasthenia gravis
  Neuromuscular blockade
  Phrenic nerve damage
  Werdnig-Hoffmann disease
Subglottic cyst
Superior vena cava syndrome
Tracheoesophageal fistula
Tumor
Vocal cord paralysis

Suggested Readings

Engle MA. Cyanotic congenital heart disease. *Am J Cardiol* 1976;37:283.
Jaffe ER. Methemoglobinemia in the differential diagnosis of cyanosis. *Hosp Pract (Off Ed)* 1985;20:92,101,108.
Lees MH. Cyanosis of the newborn infant. *J Pediatr* 1970;77:484.
Levin AR. Management of the cyanotic newborn. *Pediatr Ann* 1981;10:16.
Vichinsky EP, Lubin BH. Unstable hemoglobins, hemoglobins with altered oxygen affinity, and M-hemoglobins. *Pediatr Clin North Am* 1980;27:421.

Diarrhea, Chronic

Common Causes
Antibiotic-induced
Carbohydrate malabsorption, lactose

Acquired, postinfectious
Developmental
Hereditary
Chemotherapy-induced
Cystic fibrosis
Dietary
   Allergy (milk, soy, other)
   Inadequate dietary fat
   Overfeeding
Infection
   Bacterial
   Human immunodeficiency virus (HIV)
   Parasitic
   Viral, especially rotavirus

Uncommon Causes
Anatomic lesions
   Hirschsprung disease
   Malrotation
Celiac disease
Constipation with encopresis
Gastrointestinal bleeding
Irritable bowel syndrome
Malnutrition, starvation
Necrotizing enterocolitis
Parenteral infections
   Otitis media
   Urinary tract infections
Regional enteritis
Toddlers' diarrhea (chronic nonspecific diarrhea of
   childhood)
Ulcerative colitis

Rare Causes
Abetalipoproteinemia and hypobetalipoproteinemia
Acrodermatitis enteropathica
Adrenal insufficiency
Biliary atresia
Blind loop syndrome
Carbohydrate malabsorption
   Sucrose, isomaltose, glucose, galactose
Chronic hepatitis
Chronic pancreatitis
Clostridium Difficile toxin
Enterokinase deficiency
Familial chloride diarrhea
Familial protein intolerance
Ganglioneuroma
Hyperthyroidism
Immune deficiency
   Ataxia-telangiectasia
   Combined immune deficiency
   Hypogammaglobulinemia
   IgA deficiency
   Wiskott-Aldrich syndrome
Intestinal ischemia
Intestinal lymphangiectasia
Intestinal pseudoobstruction
Liver abscess
Maternal deprivation
Mesenteric artery insufficiency
Microvillus inclusion disease
Neuroblastoma
Pancreatic insufficiency and neutropenia (Shwachman-
   Diamond-Oski syndrome)
Pancreatic tumors
Radiation-induced
Scleroderma
Short bowel syndrome

Small bowel tumors; lymphosarcoma
Well water
   Contamination
   Mineral content
Whipple disease
Wolman disease

Suggested Readings

Cohen SA, Hendricks KM, Mathis RK, et al. Chronic nonspecific diarrhea: dietary relationships. *Pediatrics* 1979;64:402.
Dewitt TG, Humphrey KF, McCarthy P. Clinical predictors of acute bacterial diarrhea in young children. *Pediatrics* 1985;76:551.
Drossman DA, Powell DW, Sessions JT Jr. The irritable bowel syndrome. *Gastroenterology* 1977;73:811.
Gall DG, Hamilton JR. Chronic diarrhea in childhood. *Pediatr Clin North Am* 1974;21:1001.
Gryboski JD. Chronic diarrhea. *Curr Probl Pediatr* 1979;9:5.
Hirschhorn N. The treatment of acute diarrhea in children: an historical and physiological perspective. *Am J Clin Nutr* 1980;33:637.
Larcher VF, Shepherd R, Francis DEM, Harries JT. Protracted diarrhoea in infancy. *Arch Dis Child* 1977;52:597.
Phillips SF. Diarrhea: a current view of the pathophysiology. *Gastroenterology* 1972;63:495.

Dysphagia/Odynophagia

Common Causes
Chemical mucositis
   Caustic ingestion
   Gastroesophageal reflux with esophagitis
   Radiation/chemotherapy
Immature sucking/swallowing mechanism
Oropharyngeal infections
   Cervical adenitis
   Gingivitis
   Herpetic stomatitis
   Peritonsillar abscess
   Pharyngitis
   Retropharyngeal abscess
   Sinusitis
   Tooth abscess
Physiologic expulsion reflux

Uncommon Causes
Cerebral palsy
Cleft palate
Esophageal spasm
Esophageal stricture
External compression of the esophagus
   Esophageal diverticula
   Esophageal duplication
   Mediastinal masses/tumors
   Vascular anomalies
Foreign body
Infectious esophagitis
   Candida
   Herpes
Macroglossia (any cause)
Micrognathia
Pharyngeal diverticula
Physiologic (globus hystericus)
Submucosal cleft
Tracheoesophageal fistula

Rare Causes
Angioneurotic edema
Brain tumors
Choanal atresia

Collagen vascular disease
  Dermatomyositis
  Scleroderma
Diphtheria
Encephalitis/meningitis
Epiglottitis
Esophageal atresia, web, cyst
Laryngeal cyst, cleft
Muscular hypertrophy of the esophagus
Neuromuscular causes
  Arnold-Chiari malformation
  Botulism
  Bulbar and suprabulbar palsy
    Möbius syndrome
  Chalasia/achalasia of the esophagus
  Congenital laryngeal stridor
  Cranial nerve palsy
  Demyelinating disease
  Dystonia musculorum deformans
  Familial dysautonomia
  Guillain-Barré syndrome
  Hypotonias
  Muscular dystrophy
  Myasthenia gravis
  Myotonic dystrophy
  Pharyngeal or cricopharyngeal incoordination
  Spinal muscular atrophy(Werdnig Hoffman syndrome)
  Tetanus
Opitz Frias syndrome
Pharyngeal cyst, cleft
Regional enteritis
Rumination
Stevens-Johnson syndrome
Temporomandibular ankylosis/hypoplasia
Tumors (oropharynx, esophagus)
Wilson disease

Suggested Readings

Eklof O, Ekstrom G, Eriksson BO, et al. Arterial anomalies causing compression of the trachea and/or oesophagus. *Acta Paediatr Scand* 1971;60:81.
Illingworth RS. Sucking and swallowing difficulties in infancy: diagnostic problem of dysphagia. *Arch Dis Child* 1969;44:655.
Kato S, Komatsu K, Haroda Y. Medication induced esophagitis in children. *Gastroenterol Jpn* 1990;25:485.

Dysrhythmia

Common Causes
Acidemia
Congenital heart disease
Drugs
  Antiarrhythmics
  Antihistamines, nonsedating
  Beta blockers
  Caffeine
  Cocaine
  Psychotropics
  Sympathomimetics
  Tricyclic antidepressants
Hypoxemia
Idiopathic
Postoperative (cardiac procedures)

Uncommon Causes
Cardiomyopathy (dilated, hypertrophic, infiltrative)
Electrical injury
Electrolyte disturbances (especially K, Ca, Mg)

Myocarditis
Sickle cell disease
Sick sinus syndrome
Wolff-Parkinson-White syndrome (or other accessory
  bypass tracts)

Rare Causes
Anomalous coronary artery
CNS
  Hemorrhage
  Infection
  Trauma
Collagen vascular disease
Complete congenital heart block
Endocrine (thyrotoxicosis, secondary electrolyte
  disturbances)
Kawasaki disease
Myocardial ischemia
Myocardial trauma
Myocardial tumors
Neonatal lupus
Prolonged QT syndrome
Rheumatic fever

Suggested Readings

Bailey B, Gaudreault P, Thigvierge RL, Turgeon JP. Cardiac monitoring of children with household electrical injuries. *Ann Emerg Med* 1995;25:612.
Giardina ACV, Ehlers KH, Engle MA. Wolf-Parkinson-White syndrome in infants and children. *Br Heart J* 1972;34:839.
Morady F, Scheinman MM. Paroxysmal supraventricular tachycardia. Part I. Diagnosis. *Mod Concepts Cardiovasc Dis* 1982;51:107.
Morady F, Scheinman MM. Paroxysmal supraventricular tachycardia. Part II. Treatment. *Mod Concepts Cardiovasc Dis* 1982;51:113.
Pfammatter JP. Cardiac arrhythmias mimicking primary neurologic disorders. *Acta Paediatr* 1995;84:569.

Dysuria

Common Causes
Candidal dermatitis/vaginitis
Chemical urethritis (bubble bath/shampoo)
Contact dermatitis/vulvitis
Diarrhea: perineal irritation
Urethritis
Urinary tract infection
Viral cystitis

Uncommon Causes
Balanitis
Foreign body
Herpes simplex
Meatitis
Phimosis
Pinworms
Urethral trauma

Rare Causes
Appendicitis
Bladder diverticulum
Bladder outlet obstruction
  Posterior urethral valves
Bladder stones
Constipation
Drugs
  Amitriptyline
  Antihistamines
  Cyclophosphamide (Cytoxan)

Heparin
Imipramine
Isoniazid
Sulfonamides
Hemorrhagic cystitis
Hematospermia
Interstitial cystitis
Meatal stenosis
Posthitis
Prostatitis
Reiter syndrome
Schistosomiasis
Stevens-Johnson syndrome
Tuberculosis
Urethral diverticulum
Urethral prolapse
Urethral stricture
Varicella
Wilms tumor

Suggested Readings

Brock WA, Kaplan GW. Voiding dysfunction in children. *Curr Probl Pediatr* 1980;10:4.

Fleisher GR. Pain-dysuria. In: Fleisher GR, Ludwig S, eds. *Textbook of pediatric emergency medicine*. Baltimore: Williams & Wilkins, 1993:366.

Heldrich FJ. Dysuria. In: Hoekelman RA, Friedman SB, Nelson NM, Seidel HM, Weitzman ML, eds. *Primary Pediatric Care*. St. Louis: Mosby, 1997:929.

Spencer JR, Schaeffer AJ. Pediatric urinary tract infections. *Urol Clin North Am* 1986;13:661.

Encopresis

Common Causes
Chronic constipation
Diarrheal disorders
Emotional disturbance
Failure to achieve control
Regressive behavior

Uncommon Cause
Hirschsprung disease

Rare Causes
Diastematomyelia
Epidural abscess
Muscular dystrophies
Myelomeningoceles
Poliomyelitis
Postanorectal surgery
Osteomyelitis of the vertebral body
Regional enteritis
Sacral agenesis
Seizures
Sexual abuse: pain avoidance
Spinal cord tumor
Syringomyelia
Transverse myelitis

Suggested Readings

Bellman M. Studies on encopresis. *Acta Paediatr Scand* 1966;(Suppl 170):7.

Davidson M, Kugler MM, Bauer CH. Diagnosis and management in children with severe and protracted constipation and obstipation. *J Pediatr* 1963;62:261.

Johns C. Encopresis. *Am J Nurs* 1985;85:153.

Levine MD. Children with encopresis: a descriptive analysis. *Pediatrics* 1975;56:412.

Levine MD. Encopresis: its potentiation, evaluation, and alleviation. *Pediatr Clin North Am* 1982;29:315.

Levine MD. The schoolchild with encopresis. *Pediatr Rev* 1981;2:285.

Loening-Baucke VA, Cruikshank BM. Abnormal defecation dynamics in chronically constipated children with encopresis. *J Pediatr* 1986;108:562.

Rappaport LA, Levine MD. The prevention of constipation and encopresis: a developmental model and approach. *Pediatr Clin North Am* 1986;33:859.

Silber DL. Encopresis. *Clin Pediatr* 1969;8:225.

Enuresis

Common Causes
"Busy little girl" syndrome: micturition deferral
Developmental delay of bladder function and capacity
Psychological

Uncommon Causes
Chronic constipation
Diabetes mellitus
Emotional stress
Food allergy
Giggle incontinence
Obstructive abnormalities of the urinary tract
Polydipsia/polyuria associated
Stress incontinence
Urge syndrome (unstable bladder)
Urinary tract infection

Rare Causes
Compulsive water drinking
Diabetes insipidus, central or nephrogenic
Diverticulum of anterior urethra
Ectopic ureter
Hydrocolpos/hematocolpos
Labial fusion
Lumbosacral anomalies
    Spinal dysraphisms
    Diastematomyelia
    Sacral agenesis
Obesity (trapping of urine)
Obstructive sleep apnea
Occult neuropathic bladder
Seizure disorder
Sickle cell disease
Sickle cell trait
Spinal cord tumors

Suggested Readings

Cohen MW. Enuresis. *Pediatr Clin North Am* 1975;22:545.

Friman PC. A preventive context for enuresis. *Pediatr Clin North Am* 1986;33:871.

Hinman F. Urinary tract damage in children who wet. *Pediatrics* 1974;54:142.

Maizels M, Firlit C. Guide to the history in enuretic children. *Am Fam Physician* 1986;33:205.

McLain LG. Childhood enuresis. *Curr Probl Pediatr* 1979;9:1.

Palmisano PA. Enuresis: causes, cures, and cautions. *West J Med* 1976;125:347.

Robson WLM. Diurnal enuresis. *Pediatr Rev* 1997;18:407.

Starfield B. Enuresis: its pathogenesis and management. *Clin Pediatr* 1972;11:343.

Starfield B. Functional bladder capacity in enuretic and nonenuretic children. *J Pediatr* 1969;70:777.

Werry JS. Enuresis—an etiologic and therapeutic study. *J Pediatr* 1965;67:423.

Epistaxis

Common Causes
Allergic rhinitis
Exercise/exertion
Low humidity/dryness
Repeated sneezing

Trauma
  External
    Self-inflicted (nose picking)
Upper respiratory infection

Uncommon Causes
Factor XI deficiency
Hypertension
Platelet dysfunction syndromes
Sickle cell disease
Thrombocytopenia (any cause)
Von Willebrand disease

Rare Causes
Angiofibroma
Ataxia-telangiectasia
Barometric changes
Beta thalassemia
Congenital syphilis
Ehlers-Danlos syndrome
Foreign body (unilateral)
Hemangiomas
Lethal midline granulomas
Malaria
Measles
Nasal angiomas
Nasal diphtheria
Nasal polyp
Oral contraceptives
Osler-Weber-Rendu disease
Pertussis
Rhabdomyosarcoma
Rheumatic fever
Scarlet fever
Scurvy
Streptococcosis
Superior vena cava syndrome
Syphilis
Typhoid fever
Varicella
Wegener granulomatosis

Suggested Readings

Beran M, Petruson B. Occurrence of epistaxis in habitual nose-bleeders and analysis of some etiological factors. *ORL J Otorhinolaryngol Relat Spec* 1986;48:297.

Juselius H. Epistaxis: a clinical study of 1,727 patients. *J Laryngol Otol* 1974;88:317.

McDonald TJ. Nosebleed in children: background and techniques to stop the flow. *Postgrad Med* 1987;81:217.

Okafor BC. Epistaxis: a clinical study of 540 cases. *Ear Nose Throat J* 1984;63:153.

Stevens M. Management of epistaxis. *Aust Fam Physician* 1986;15:707.

Failure to Thrive

Common Causes
Neglect
  Inadequate ingestion/metabolism of calories
    Depression with anorexia
    Manipulative behavior
    Rumination as self-stimulation
    Secondary malabsorption
      Self-induced (vomiting, laxative abuse)
      Specific deficiency (e.g., zinc, biotin)
      Starvation
    Secondary neuroendocrine abnormalities
      Abnormal cycling of growth hormone
      Cortisol deficiency

Physical neglect/abuse
Psychosocial deprivation
Withholding of food as neglect/abuse
  Intentional withholding of food
  Unintentional withholding of food
    Overwhelmed caretaker
      Lack of support systems (financial/social)
      Primary personal needs (e.g., drug/alcohol abuse)
      Psychotic or depressed caretaker
      Time constraints (e.g., unsupervised eating, bottle propping)
Nonorganic failure to thrive
  Inadequate volume of feeds
    Too few feeds per day
    Too little per feed
      Colic
      "Difficult" feeder
      Financial factors
      Ignorance
      Inexperienced/impatient caretaker with or without compounding child factors
  Inappropriate foods for age
    Cultural factors
    Fad diets
    Financial factors
    Ignorance
  Incorrect preparation of formula
    Chronic dilution
    Financial factors
    Ignorance
    Prolonged use after gastroenteritis
  Inappropriate additives
Normal variants
  Delayed adolescent growth spurt
  Early-onset growth retardation
  Familial short stature
  Shifting linear growth
Organic failure to thrive
  CNS etiologies
    Mental retardation/cerebral palsy
    Neurodevelopmental retardation
  Gastrointestinal etiologies
    Chronic gastroenteritis
    Gastroesophageal reflux
    Pyloric stenosis
Prematurity
Small for gestational age

Uncommon Causes
Defective utilization of calories
  Chronic hypoxemia: upper airway obstruction
  Diabetes mellitus
  Hyperthyroidism
Defects in absorption
  Cystic fibrosis
  Enzymatic deficiencies
  Food sensitivity/intolerance
  Hepatitis
  HIV infection
  Inflammatory bowel disease
  Milk allergy
  Starvation
Inadequacy of food intake
  Cleft lip/palate
  Dyspnea of any cause
    Congenital heart disease
    Respiratory disease/insufficiency

Fetal alcohol syndrome
Immature suck/swallow
Pharyngeal incoordination
Increased metabolism
  Chronic anemia
  Chronic/recurrent infections
    Otitis, sinusitis, pneumonia
    Parasites
    Tuberculosis
    Urinary tract infections
  Chronic respiratory insufficiency
  Congenital heart disease
  HIV infection
  Malignancies

Rare Causes
Defective utilization of calories
  Adrenal insufficiency
  Chromosomal syndromes
  Diabetes insipidus
  Diencephalic syndrome
  Drugs/toxins
  Dysmorphogenic syndromes
  Fetal exposure syndromes
  Growth hormone deficiency
  Hypopituitarism
  Hypothyroidism
  Metabolic disorders
    Aminoacidopathies
    Galactosemia
    Organic acidurias
    Storage diseases
  Parathyroid disorders
  Renal tubular acidosis
Defects in absorption
  Acrodermatitis enteropathica
  Biliary atresia/cirrhosis
  Celiac disease
  Hirschsprung disease
  Immunologic deficiency
  Necrotizing enterocolitis
  Pancreatic insufficiency
  Short bowel syndrome
Inadequacy of food intake
  Choanal atresia
  CNS disorders
    Cerebral insults
    Degenerative diseases
    Drugs/toxins
    Subdural hematoma
  Diaphragmatic hernia/hiatal hernia
  Esophageal atresia
  Fetal hydantoin syndrome
  Generalized muscle weakness
    Congenital hypotonia
    Myasthenia gravis
    Werdnig-Hoffmann disease
  Micrognathia/glossoptosis
  Smith-Lemli-Opitz syndrome
  Tracheoesophageal fistula
Increased metabolism
  Acquired heart disease
  Adrenocortical excess
  Chronic inflammation (e.g., JRA, SLE)
  Chronic seizure disorder
  Drugs/toxins
  Hyperaldosteronism
  Hyperthyroidism

Intoxications
  Hypervitaminosis A
  Lead
  Mercury
Nonorganic
  Deprivation dwarfism

Suggested Readings

Baertl JM, Adrianzen B, Graham GG. Growth of previously well-nourished infants in poor homes. *Am J Dis Child* 1976;130:33.

Barbero GJ, Shaheen E. Environmental failure to thrive: a clinical view. *J Pediatr* 1967;77:639.

Berwick DM. Nonorganic failure-to-thrive. *Pediatr Rev* 1980;1:265.

Bithoney WG. Elevated lead levels in children with nonorganic failure to thrive. *Pediatrics* 1986;78:891.

Casey PH, Bradley R, Wortham B. Social and nonsocial home environments of infants with nonorganic failure-to-thrive. *Pediatrics* 1984;83:348.

Cupoli JM, Hallock JA, Barness LA. Failure to thrive. *Curr Probl Pediatr* 1980;10:5.

Ellerstein NS, Ostrov BE. Growth patterns in children hospitalized because of caloric-deprivation failure to thrive. *Am J Dis Child* 1985;139:164.

Hannaway PJ. Failure to thrive: a study of 100 infants and children. *Clin Pediatr* 1970;9:96.

Homer C, Ludwig S. Categorization of etiology of failure to thrive. *Am J Dis Child* 1981;135:848.

Mitchell WG, Gorrell RW, Greenberg RA. Failure-to-thrive: a study in a primary care setting. Epidemiology and follow-up. *Pediatrics* 1980;65:971.

Rosenn DW, Loeb LS, Jura MB. Differentiation of organic from nonorganic failure to thrive syndrome in infancy. *Pediatrics* 1980;66:698.

Sills RH. Failure to thrive. *Am J Dis Child* 1978;132:967.

Sills RH, Sills IN. Don't overlook environmental causes of failure to thrive. *Contemp Pediatr* 1986;3:25.

Zenel JA. Failure to thrive: a general pediatrician's perspective. *Pediatr Rev* 1997;18:371.

Fatigue

Common Causes
Acute recovery from surgery, trauma, most illnesses
Anemia
Caloric deficiency (young children)
Chronic atopy
Eating disorders
  Excessive dieting (with or without anorexia nervosa, bulimia)
Excessive exercise
Mononucleosis (and most viral infections)
Obesity
Pregnancy
Psychosocial
  Chronic boredom
  Chronic depression/anxiety
  Grief
  Stress (prolonged and severe)
Sedentary lifestyles
Sleep disorders
  Insomnia
  Sleep pattern disruption (lack of REM sleep)

Uncommon Causes
Acute bacterial infections
  Bacteremia
  Meningitis
Allergy
Chronic hypoxemia
  Asthma
  Cardiomyopathy
  Chronic pulmonary disease
  Congenital heart disease
  Congestive heart failure
  Cystic fibrosis

Heart disease
Pericarditis
Pulmonary hypertension
Chronic infections
  Brucellosis
  Cytomegalic inclusion disease
  Histoplasmosis
  Osteomyelitis
  Parasitic infestations
  Pyelonephritis
  Sinusitis
  Subacute bacterial endocarditis
  Toxoplasmosis
  Tuberculosis
  Urinary tract infection
Dehydration
Hepatitis
Upper airway obstruction (sleep apnea)
  Pickwickian syndrome
  Tonsillar-adenoidal hypertrophy

Rare Causes
AIDS
Allergic tension fatigue syndrome
Chronic Epstein-Barr virus infection
Chronic fatigue syndrome
  Neurally mediated hypotension
Connective tissue diseases
  Dermatomyositis
  Juvenile rheumatoid arthritis
  Mixed connective tissue disease
  Scleroderma
  Systemic lupus erythematosus
Endocrine disorders
  Diabetes insipidus
  Diabetes mellitus
  Hyperadrenalism/hypoadrenalism
  Hyperparathyroidism
  Hyperpituitarism/hypopituitarism
  Hyperthyroidism/hypothyroidism
  Primary aldosteronism
Hepatic insufficiency
Hypoglycemia
Inborn errors of metabolism
Inflammatory bowel disease
Intussusception
Malignancy
  Leukemia
  Lymphoma
  Solid tumors
Metabolic disturbances
  Hypermagnesemia/hypomagnesemia
  Hypokalemia
  Hyponatremia
Neurologic
  Intracranial hematomas
  Myasthenia gravis
  Narcolepsy
Polycythemia
Renal tubular acidosis
Toxins and drugs
  Alcohol
  Analgesics and salicylates
  Anticonvulsants
  Antihistamines
  Barbiturates
  Carbon monoxide
  Corticosteroids
  Digitalis
  Heavy metals

Insulin
Nicotine
Pesticides
Progesterones
Sedatives
Tetracycline
Vitamin A
Vitamin D
Uremia

Suggested Readings

Cavanaugh RM Jr. Evaluating adolescents with fatigue. *Am Fam Physician* 1987;
  35:163.
Rockwell DA, Burr BD. The tired patient. *J Fam Pract* 1977;5:853.
Solberg LI. Lassitude: a primary care evaluation. *JAMA* 1984;251:3272.

Fever of Unknown Origin

Fever is defined here as a temperature higher than 38.5°C lasting more than 2 weeks.

Common Causes
Collagen vascular disease
  Juvenile rheumatoid arthritis
  Lupus erythematosus
  Polyarteritis nodosa
Factitious
Infections
  Atypical mycobacterial infections
  Epstein-Barr virus infections
  Indwelling catheter infection
  Osteomyelitis
  Sinusitis, mastoiditis
  Urinary tract infections
  "Viral syndromes"
Inflammatory bowel disease
  Regional enteritis
  Ulcerative colitis
Malignancy
  Acute lymphoblastic leukemia
  Neuroblastoma
  Hodgkin disease
  Non-Hodgkin lymphoma

Uncommon Causes
Collagen vascular diseases
  Henoch-Schönlein purpura
  Rheumatic fever
Drug-induced
Infections
  Appendiceal abscess
  Cat-scratch disease
  Cytomegalic inclusion disease
  Hepatitis (anicteric, chronic)
  Histoplasmosis
  Lung abscess
  Lyme disease
  Pelvic inflammatory disease
  Pharyngitis, chronic
  Salmonellosis
Kawasaki disease
Lyme disease

Rare Causes
Atrial myxoma
Behçet syndrome
Cyclic neutropenia
Dermatomyositis

Diabetes insipidus
 Central
 Nephrogenic
Diencephalic syndrome
Ectodermal dysplasia
Familial dysautonomia
Familial Mediterranean fever
Hepatoma
Hyperthyroidism
Ichthyosis
Infection
 Blastomycosis
 Brucellosis
 Campylobacter
 Ehrlichiosis
 Endocarditis
 HIV infection
 Leptospirosis
 Liver abscess
 Lymphogranuloma venereum
 Malaria
 Perinephric abscess
 Psittacosis
 Q fever
 Rocky Mountain spotted fever
 Streptococcosis
 Subdiaphragmatic abscess
 Toxoplasmosis
 Tuberculosis
 Tularemia
 Viral encephalitis
 Visceral larva migrans
 Visceral leishmaniasis
 Yersiniosis
Myelogenous leukemia
Pancreatitis
Periodic disease (familial fever)
Reticulum cell sarcoma
Sarcoidosis
Serum sickness
Subdural hematoma, chronic
Syndrome of periodic fever, pharyngitis and aphthous
 stomatitis
Thyrotoxicosis

Suggested Readings

Arnow PA, Flaherty JP. Fever of unknown origin. *Lancet* 1997;350:575.

Feigin RD, Shearer WT. Fever of unknown origin in children. *Curr Probl Pediatr* 1976;6:3.

Kleiman MB. The complaint of persistent fever: recognition and management of pseudo-fever of unknown origin. *Pediatr Clin North Am* 1982;29:201.

Lohr JA, Hendley JO. Prolonged fever of unknown origin: a record of experiences with 54 childhood patients. *Clin Pediatr* 1977;16:768.

McCarthy PL, Lembo RM, Baron MA, et al. Predictive value of abnormal physical examination findings in ill-appearing and well-appearing febrile children. *Pediatrics* 1985;76:167.

McClung HJ. Prolonged fever of unknown origin in children. *Am J Dis Child* 1972;124:544.

Musher DM, Fainstein V, Young EJ, Pruett TL. Fever patterns. *Arch Intern Med* 1979;139:1225.

Petersdorf RG, Beeson PB. Fever of unexplained origin: report on 100 cases. *Medicine* 1961;40:1.

Pizzo PA, Lovejoy FH, Smith DH. Prolonged fever in children: review of 100 cases. *Pediatrics* 1975;55:468.

Gastrointestinal Bleeding

In the Neonate

Common Causes
Esophagitis
Gastritis

Ingested maternal blood
Ingested blood, epistaxis
Necrotizing enterocolitis
Stress ulcer (gastric)

Uncommon Causes
Acquired coagulopathy
Gastroenteritis (*Campylobacter* infections)
Hemophilia
Renal trauma or gastrointestinal trauma
Thrombocytopenia
Vitamin K deficiency
Volvulus

Rare Causes
Acute ulcerative colitis
Gastric polyp
Gastrointestinal duplication cyst
Intussusception
Leiomyoma
Milk allergy
Nasal or pharyngeal bleeding
Severe cyanotic congenital heart disease
Spontaneous rupture of esophagus
Vascular malformation of the gut (hemangioma,
 telangiectasia, arteriovenous malformation)

In Infancy

Common Causes
Anal fissure
Cow's milk protein sensitivity
Esophagitis
Gastritis
Gastroenteritis
Gastroesophageal reflux

Uncommon Causes
Acute intestinal ischemia
Drug ingestion, such as aspirin or caustic
Esophageal varices
Hemophilia
Intussusception
Meckel diverticulum
Peptic ulcer
Thrombocytopenia

Rare Causes
Disseminated intravascular coagulation
Duplication of the bowel or esophagus
Gangrenous bowel
Hemangioma of the bowel
Henoch-Schönlein purpura
Mallory-Weiss syndrome
Polyps
Swallowed blood in breast-fed infants; maternal nipple
 fissure

In Childhood

Common Causes
Anal fissures
Esophagitis
Gastritis (possibly caused by corrosive agents or drug
 ingestion)
Gastroenteritis
Polyps

Uncommon Causes
Acquired coagulation disturbance
H. Pylori gastritis

Hemophilia
Henoch-Schönlein purpura
Inflammatory bowel disease
Mallory-Weiss syndrome
Meckel diverticulum
Parasitism
Peptic ulcer
Thrombocytopenia

Rare Causes
Aplastic anemia
Chronic granulomatous disease
Diverticulitis
Ehlers-Danlos syndrome
Esophageal varices
Hemangiomas and telangiectasias
Hemolytic-uremic syndrome
Hemorrhoids
Intestinal foreign body
Leiomyoma, leiomyosarcoma
Lymphosarcoma
Münchhausen syndrome by proxy
Peutz-Jeghers syndrome
Pseudoxanthoma elasticum
Rendu-Osler-Weber
Scurvy
Trauma

Suggested Readings

Berman WF, Holtzapple PG. Gastrointestinal hemorrhage. *Pediatr Clin North Am* 1975;22:885.

Cox K, Ament ME. Upper gastrointestinal bleeding in children and adolescents. *Pediatrics* 1979;63:408.

Hillemeier C, Gryboski JD. Gastrointestinal bleeding in the pediatric patient. *Yale J Biol Med* 1984;57:135.

Hyams JS, Leichtner AM, Schwartz AN. Recent advances in diagnosis and treatment of gastrointestinal hemorrhage in infants and children. *J Pediatr* 1985;106:1.

Oldham KT, Lobe TE. Gastrointestinal hemorrhage in children: a pragmatic update. *Pediatr Clin North Am* 1985;32:1247.

Silber G. Lower gastrointestinal bleeding. *Pediatr Rev* 1990;12:85.

Stanley-Brown EG, Stevenson SS. Massive gastrointestinal hemorrhage in the newborn infant. *Pediatrics* 1965;35:482.

Stevenson RJ. Gastrointestinal bleeding in children. *Surg Clin North Am* 1985; 65:1455.

Wagner ML. Acute gastrointestinal bleeding in infants and children. *Pediatr Ann* 1975;4:663.

Headache

Common Causes
Extracranial infection
  Otitis/mastoiditis
  Pharyngitis
  Sinusitis
  Tooth abscess
Febrile illness
Migraine
Tension
  Anxiety
  Environmental stress

Uncommon Causes
Depression
Exertion
Eye strain
Meningitis/encephalitis

Temporomandibular joint disease
Trauma
  Concussion
  Occipital neuralgia

Rare Causes
Allergy
Allergic tension-fatigue syndrome
Arnold-Chiari malformation
Basilar impression
Cervical osteoarthritis
Chronic paroxysmal hemicrania
Chronic renal disease
Congenital erythropoietic porphyria
Cranial bone disease
Decreased intracranial pressure
  Postlumbar puncture
Drugs/toxins
  Amphetamines
  Carbon monoxide
  Corticosteroids
  Heavy metals
  Indomethacin
  Nalidixic acid
  Nitrates/nitrites
  Oral contraceptives
  Sulfa
  Tetracycline
  Vitamin A
Epilepsy
Hyperventilation
Increased intracranial pressure
  Hydrocephalus
  Mass/tumor/abscess
  Pseudotumor cerebri
Leukemic infiltration
Mastocytosis
MELAS syndrome (*mitochondrial encephalopathy, lactic acidosis, stroke-like episodes*)
Metabolic
  Hyperammonemia
  Hypercarbia
  Hypoglycemia
  Hyponatremia
  Hypoxia
  Metabolic acidosis
Myositis
Obstructive sleep apnea
Orbit
  Glaucoma
  Orbital tumor
Psychogenic
  Conversion reaction
  Mimicry
  Secondary gain
Pheochromocytoma
Vascular
  Anemia
  Aneurysm
  Arteritis
    Giant cell
    Periarteritis nodosa
    Subacute bacterial endocarditis
    Systemic lupus erythematosus
  Arteriovenous malformation
  Cerebral infarct
    Embolus
    Thrombosis
  Cluster headache

Hemorrhage
  Epidural
  Parenchymal
  Subdural
Hypertension
Phlebitis
Venous sinus thrombosis

Suggested Readings

Diamond S. Severe headaches—understanding types and treatments. *Drug Ther* 1975;3:81.

Ferry PC. Diagnosis and office management of headaches in children. *Clin Pediatr* 1972;11:195.

Ferry PC. Office management of headaches in children. *Drug Ther* 1973;1:78.

Hanson RR. Headaches in childhood. *Semin Neurol* 1988;8:51.

Honig PJ, Charney EB. Children with brain tumor headaches. *Am J Dis Child* 1982;136:121.

Ling W, Oftedal G, Weinberg W. Depressive illness in childhood presenting as severe headache. *Am J Dis Child* 1970;120:122.

MacDonald JT. Childhood migraine: differential diagnosis and treatment. *Postgrad Med* 1986;80:301.

McIntre SC. Recurrent and Chronic headaches. In: Gartner JC Jr., Zitelli BJ. *Common and chronic symptoms in pediatrics.* St. Louis: Mosby, 1997:51.

Meloff KL. Headache in pediatric practice. *Headache* 1973;13:125.

Prensky AL. Differentiating and treating pediatric headaches. *Contemp Pediatr* 1984;1:12.

Prensky AL. Migraine and migrainous variants in pediatric patients. *Pediatr Clin North Am* 1976;23:461.

Rossi LN, Vassella F. Headache in children with brain tumors. *Child Nerv Syst* 1989;5:307.

Singer HS, Rowe S. Chronic recurrent headaches in children. *Pediatr Ann* 1992; 21:369.

Swaiman KF, Frank Y. Seizure headaches in children. *Dev Med Child Neurol* 1978;20:580.

Hematuria

Common Causes
Benign causes
  Benign recurrent hematuria
  Familial hematuria
  Idiopathic recurrent gross hematuria
  Postural hematuria
Contamination
  Menstrual
  Münchhausen syndrome
  Münchhausen syndrome by proxy
  Pregnancy-related bleeding
Hemoglobinopathies
  Hgb C
  Hgb SC
  Sickle cell disease/trait (Hgb SS/SA)
  Sickle thalassemia trait
Hypercalciuria
  Distal renal tubular acidosis
  Diuretic therapy
  Endocrine disorders
    Diabetes mellitus
    Hyperadrenocorticism
    Hyperparathyroidism
    Hypothyroidism
  Hypercalcemia
  Hyperphosphatemia
  Hypertension
  Immobilization
  Juvenile rheumatoid arthritis
  Medullary sponge kidney
  Metabolic acidosis
  Neoplasm
  Renal tubular dysfunction

Sarcoidosis
  Vitamin D excess
Hypoxia, asphyxia, and circulatory compromise
  Acute tubular necrosis
  Cortical and medullary necrosis
Infections
  Cystitis (viral, bacterial)
  Pyelonephritis
  Urethritis
Meatal stenosis
Meatal ulceration
Noninfectious cystitis
  Cyclophosphamide (Cytoxan)
  Radiation
Perineal irritation
Phimosis
Postinfectious glomerulonephritis
Trauma
  Fractured pelvis
  Postcatheterization
  Post circumcision
  Postsurgery
  Renal contusion
  Renal fracture
  Urethral trauma
Urethral ulceration

Uncommon Causes
Bladder diverticula/polyps
Coagulopathies
Drug-induced
  Analgesic nephropathy
  Cephalosporins
  Cyclophosphamide (Cytoxan)
  Penicillin
  Sulfonamides
Exercise
Glomerular disorders
  IgA nephropathy
  Mesangioproliferative
  Minimal change disease
Hydronephrosis
Infections
  Epididymitis
  Prostatitis
Masturbation (with or without instrumentation)
Periureteritis (appendicitis, ileitis)
Polycystic disease
Reflux nephropathy
Renal calculi
Renal vein thrombosis
Thrombocytopenia
Ureteropelvic junction obstruction
Urethral foreign body
Wilms tumor

Rare Causes
Allergy
Apparent
  "Beeturia"
  Betadine
  Biliuria
  Deferoxamine
  Dyes
    Aniline
    Congo red
  Hemoglobinurias
  Myoglobinuria
  Phenothiazines

Porphyria
Urate crystals
Appendicitis
Autoerythrocyte sensitization
Diabetic nephropathy
Epidemic nephropathy
Glomerular disorders
   Amyloidosis
   Crescentic glomerulonephritis
   Familial nephritis (Alport)
   Focal segmental proliferative glomerulonephritis
   Focal segmental sclerosis
   Goodpasture syndrome
   Membranous glomerulonephritis
   Mesangiocapillary glomerulonephritis
   Subacute bacterial endocarditis
   Systemic lupus erythematosus
   Wegener granulomatosis
Hemangioma
Klippel-Trenaunay-Weber syndrome
Hematospermia
Immunologic
   Hemolytic-uremic syndrome
   Henoch-Schönlein purpura
   Polyarteritis nodosa
   Systemic lupus erythematosus
Infections
   Leptospirosis
   Malaria
   Schistosomiasis
   Toxoplasmosis
   Tuberculosis
   Varicella
Malignant hypertension
Medullary sponge kidney
Neoplasms
   Bladder cancer
   Prostate cancer
Renal infarction
Retroperitoneal fibrosis
Vitamin deficiency
   Scurvy
   Vitamin K deficiency

Suggested Readings

Birch DF, Fairley KF. Haematuria: glomerular or nonglomerular? [letter]. *Lancet* 1979;2:845.

Daeschner CW. Screening for renal diseases. *J Pediatr* 1976;88:369.

Dodge WF, West EF, Smith EH, Bunce H. Proteinuria and hematuria in schoolchildren: epidemiology and early natural history. *J Pediatr* 1976;88:327.

Fassett RG, Horgan BA, Mathew TH. Detection of glomerular bleeding by phase-contrast microscopy. *Lancet* 1982;1:1432.

Fitzwater DS, Wyatt RJ. Hematuria. *Pediatr Rev* 1994;15:102.

Given GZ. Hematuria in children. A guide in differential diagnosis. *Urol Clin North Am* 1974;1:561.

Ingelfinger JR, Davis AE, Grupe WE. Frequency and etiology of gross hematuria in a general pediatric setting. *Pediatrics* 1977;59:557.

James JA. Proteinuria and hematuria in children. Diagnosis and assessment. *Pediatr Clin North Am* 1976;23:807.

Jones DP, Stapleton FB. Hypercalciuria: an important cause of childhood hematuria. *Contemp Pediatr* 1987;4:69.

Northway JD. Hematuria in children. *J Pediatr* 1971;78:381.

Ruley EJ. Hematuria. In: Hoekleman RA, Friedman SB, Nelson NM, Seidel HM, Weitzman ML, eds. *Primary pediatric care.* St. Louis: Mosby, 1997:996.

Vehaskari VM, Rapola J, Koskimies O, et al. Microscopic hematuria in schoolchildren: epidemiology and clinicopathologic evaluation. *J Pediatr* 1979;95:676.

West CD. Asymptomatic hematuria and proteinuria in children. Causes and appropriate diagnostic studies. *J Pediatr* 1976;89:173.

Wyatt RJ, McRoberts JW, Holland NH. Hematuria in childhood: significance and management. *J Urol* 1977;117:366.

Hemoptysis

Common Causes
Aspiration
   Blood
      Epistaxis
      Gingivitis
      Tonsillitis
      Upper airway trauma (e.g., intubation)
   Corrosives
   Foreign body
   Gastric contents
   Oral lesions
Cystic fibrosis
Pulmonary infection (bacterial)
   Bronchiectasis
   Bronchitis
   Pneumonia
   Tracheitis
Pulmonary infection (viral)
   Laryngitis
   Laryngotracheobronchitis
   Pneumonitis
Pulmonary trauma
   Contusion
   Penetrating injury

Uncommon Causes
Lung abscess
Pertussis
Pulmonary hemorrhage (barotrauma)
Pulmonary tuberculosis
Sickle cell disease

Rare Causes
Arteriovenous malformation/fistula
   Rendu-Osler-Weber syndrome
Bronchogenic cysts
Cardiac disease
   Endomyocardial fibrosis
   Mitral stenosis
   Pulmonary hypertension
Coagulopathy
Heiner syndrome
Idiopathic pulmonary hemosiderosis
Laryngotracheal papilloma
Münchhausen syndrome
Münchhausen syndrome by proxy
Pulmonary embolus
Pulmonary infection
   Aspergillosis
   Blastomycosis
   Coccidiomycosis
   Echinococcosis
   Hemorrhagic fevers
   Paragonimiasis
   Stachybotrys atra
Pulmonary vasculitis
   Antiphospholipid syndrome
   Goodpasture syndrome
   Henoch-Schönlein purpura
   Polyarteritis nodosa

Systemic lupus erythematosus
   Wegener granulomatosis
Pulmonary venous thrombosis
Tumors

Suggested Readings

Beckerman RC, Taussig LM, Pinnas JL. Familial idiopathic pulmonary hemosiderosis. *Am J Dis Child* 1979;133:609.

Coss-Bu JA, Sachdeva RC, Bricker JT, Harrison GM, Jefferson LS. Hemoptysis: a 10-year retrospective study. *Pediatrics* 1997;100:E7.

Etzel RA, Montana E, Sorenson WG, et al. Acute pulmonary hemorrhage in infants associated with exposure to *Stachybotrys atra* and other fungi. *Arch Pediatr Adolesc Med* 1998;152:757.

Pianosi P, Al-Sadoon H. Hemoptysis in children. *Pediatr Rev* 1996;17:344.

Sherman JM. When you see red. *Contemp Pediatr* 1997;14:79.

Smiddy JF, Elliott RC. The evaluation of hemoptysis with fiberoptic bronchoscopy. *Chest* 1973;64:158.

Tom LWC, Weisman RA, Handler SD. Hemoptysis in children. *Ann Otol Rhinol Laryngol* 1980;89:419.

Hepatomegaly

Common Causes

Benign cystic disease
Benign transient hepatomegaly (usually with viral
   gastrointestinal illness)
Biliary tract obstruction
   Alagille disease
   Ascending cholangitis
   Biliary atresia
   Choledochal cyst
Congestive heart failure
Cystic fibrosis
Diabetes mellitus
Hyperalimentation
Iron deficiency anemia
Leukemia, lymphoma
Malnutrition
Maternal diabetes (infant of diabetic mother)
Neonatal hepatitis
Pulmonary hyperinflation ("apparent" hepatomegaly)
Septicemia
Sickle cell disease
Toxin/drug reactions (hepatitis, cholestasis, fatty
   infiltration)
   Acetaminophen
   Oral contraceptives
   Corticosteroids
   Hydantoins
   Phenobarbital
   Sulfonamides
   Tetracycline
Viral hepatitis
   Cytomegalovirus, Epstein-Barr virus, coxsackievirus
   Hepatitis A, hepatitis B, hepatitis C, hepatitis E

Uncommon Causes

Chronic active hepatitis
Chronic anemias
Erythroblastosis fetalis
Hamartoma
Hemangioma
Hemolytic anemias
Hepatic abscess (pyogenic)
Hepatoblastoma
Inflammatory bowel disease
Liver hemorrhage
Metastatic tumors

Pericarditis
Rocky Mountain spotted fever
Systemic inflammatory disease (e.g., juvenile rheumatoid
   arthritis, systemic lupus erythematosus)
Visceral larva migrans

Rare Causes

Alpha$_1$-antitrypsin deficiency
Amyloidosis
Ascariasis
Babesiosis
Beckwith-Wiedemann syndrome
Brucellosis
Budd-Chiari syndrome
Candidiasis
Carnitine deficiency
Chédiak-Higashi syndrome
Congenital lipodystrophy
Crigler-Najjar syndrome
Echinococcosis
Familial intrahepatic cholestasis
Farber disease
Fucosidosis
Galactosemia
Gangliosidosis M$_1$
Gaucher disease
Glycogen storage disease
Granulomatous hepatitis
   Chronic granulomatous disease
   Sarcoidosis
   Tuberculosis
Hemangioendotheliomas
Hemochromatosis
Hemophagocytic syndromes
Hepatic porphyrias
Hepatocellular carcinoma
Hereditary fructose intolerance
Histiocytic syndromes
Histoplasmosis
Homocystinuria
Hyperlipoproteinemia 1
Hypervitaminosis A
Infantile pyknocytosis
Infantile sialidosis
Klippel-Trenaunay-Weber syndrome
Leptospirosis
Malaria
Mannosidosis
Methylmalonic acidemia
Moore-Federmann syndrome
Mucolipidosis
Mucopolysaccharidoses
Mulibrey nanism
Niemann-Pick disease
Parasitic infections
   Amebiasis
   Flukes
   Schistosomiasis
Rendu-Osler-Weber syndrome
Reye syndrome
Rickets
Tangier disease
Tyrosinemia
Urea cycle defects
Venoocclusive disease
Wilson disease
Wolman disease
Zellweger syndrome

Suggested Readings

Goldenring JM, Flores M. Primary liver abscesses in children and adolescents. Review of 12 years' clinical experience. *Clin Pediatr* 1986;25:153.

Lawson EE, Grand RJ, Neff RK, Cohen LF. Clinical estimation of liver span in infants and children. *Am J Dis Child* 1978;132:474.

Reiff MI, Osborn LM. Clinical estimation of liver size in newborn infants. *Pediatrics* 1983;71:46.

Walker WA, Mathis RK. Hepatomegaly: an approach to differential diagnosis. *Pediatr Clin North Am* 1975;22:929.

Weisman LE, Cagle N, Mathis R, Merenstein GB. Clinical estimation of liver size in the normal neonate. *Clin Pediatr* 1982;21:596.

Younoszai MK, Mueller S. Clinical assessment of liver size in normal children. *Clin Pediatr* 1975;14:378.

Hirsutism

Common Causes
Familial or racial factors
Idiopathic hirsutism
Obesity
Physiologic hirsutism
    Pregnancy
    Puberty

Uncommon Causes
CNS injury
Drugs
    Anabolic steroids
    Cyclosporine
    Diazoxide
    Dilantin
    Minoxidil
    Oral contraceptives
    Progesterones
    Testosterone
Polycystic ovarian disease
Precocious puberty (physiologic hirsutism)
Severe malnutrition

Rare Causes
Achard-Thiers syndrome
Acromegaly
Adrenal disorders
    Adrenal carcinoma
    Congenital adrenal hyperplasia
    Cushing syndrome
    Virilizing adrenal adenoma
Congenital erythropoietic porphyria
Dysmorphogenic syndromes (many)
Hypothyroidism
Male pseudohermaphroditism
Ovarian disorders
Pure gonadal dysgenesis
Stein-Leventhal syndrome
Virilizing ovarian tumors
    Arrhenoblastoma
    Granulosa-theca cell tumors

Suggested Readings

Bates GW. Hirsutism and androgen excess in childhood and adolescence. *Pediatr Clin North Am* 1981;28:513.

Bransome ED Jr. Hirsutism and virilization. *Resident Staff Physician* 1979;25:118.

Braunstein GD. Hirsutism in adolescents. *West J Med* 1979;131:522.

Givens JR. Hirsutism and hyperandrogenism. *Adv Intern Med* 1976;21:221.

Hatch R, Rosenfield RL, Kim MH, Tredway D. Hirsutism: implications, etiology, and management. *Am J Obstet Gynecol* 1981;140:815.

Hurwitz S. *Clinical pediatric dermatology.* Philadelphia: Saunders 1993:503.

Jones JR, Brandeis VT. Hirsutism in puberty—how serious is it? *Contemp Pediatr* 1985;2:47.

Kustin J, Rebar RW. Hirsutism in young adolescent girls. *Pediatr Ann* 1986;15:522.

Rittmaster RS, Loriaux DL. Hirsutism. *Ann Intern Med* 1987;106:95.

Hoarseness

Common Causes
Allergy
Caustic ingestion
Excessive use of the voice
Foreign body
Infectious mononucleosis
Instrumentation (nasogastric/orogastric tube)
Laryngitis
Laryngotracheitis
Laryngotracheobronchitis
Postintubation hoarseness
Postnasal drip
Vocal cord nodules
Vocal cord paralysis (postsurgical trauma)

Uncommon Causes
Congenital vocal cord paralysis
Epiglottitis
Hypocalcemia (e.g., hyperparathyroidism)
Hypothyroidism
Laryngeal trauma
Laryngomalacia
Sicca syndrome
Toxins (chemotherapy, lead, mercury, irradiation, smoke)
Tracheitis (bacterial)
Vocal cord polyps

Rare Causes
Amyloidosis
Angioneurotic edema
Chromosomal abnormalities
    Achondroplasia
    Bloom syndrome
    Cockayne syndrome
    Cri du chat syndrome
    Cornelia de Lange syndrome
    Diastrophic dwarfism
    Dysautonomia
    Williams syndrome
Congenital abnormalities
    Arytenoid cartilage displacement
    Clefts
    Cysts
    Webs
Cricoarytenoid arthritis (juvenile rheumatoid arthritis)
Diphtheria
Gastroesophageal reflux
Recurrent laryngeal nerve impingement
    Aberrant great vessels
    Cardiomegaly
    Hemorrhage
    Hilar adenopathy
    Neoplasm
Recurrent laryngeal nerve dysfunction
    CNS disease
    Arnold-Chiari malformations

Chédiak-Higashi disease
Encephalitis
Hallervorden-Spatz disease
Huntington chorea
Infection
Ischemia
   Idiopathic
   Sickle cell disease
   Moyamoya disease
Kernicterus
Meningitis
Metabolic disease
Multiple sclerosis
Polyneuritis
Pseudobulbar palsy
Ramsay Hunt syndrome
Storage disease
Syphilis
Syringobulbia
Toxin
Trauma
Tumor
Wilson disease
Motor unit dysfunction
   Botulism
   Bulbar poliomyelitis
   Muscular dystrophy
   Myasthenia gravis
   Toxins
   Werdnig-Hoffmann disease
Sarcoidosis
Storage diseases (e.g., lysosomal)
Tetany
Tuberculosis
Tumors of the larynx
   Adenoma
   Carcinoma
   Chondroma
   Ectopic thyroid
   Fibroangioma
   Fibroma
   Fibrosarcoma
   Hamartoma
   Hemangioma
   Hygroma
   Leukemia
   Lymphoma
   Myoma
   Myxoma
   Neuroblastoma
   Neurofibroma
   Papilloma
   Rhabdomyosarcoma
   Xanthoma
Vocal cord hemorrhage (nontraumatic)
Wegener granulomatosis

Suggested Readings

Baker BM, Baker CD, Le HT. Vocal quality, articulation, and audiological characteristics of children and young adults with diagnosed allergies. *Ann Otol Rhinol Laryngol* 1982;91:277.

Cohen SR, Geller KA, Birns JW, Thompson JW. Laryngeal paralysis in children: a long-term retrospective study. *Ann Otol Rhinol Laryngol* 1982;91:417.

Cohen SR, Thompson JW, Geller KA, Birns JW. Voice change in the pediatric patient: a differential diagnosis. *Ann Otol Rhinol Laryngol* 1983;92:437.

Cotton RT, Richardson MA. Congenital laryngeal anomalies. *Otolaryngol Clin North Am* 1981;14:203.

Kenna MA. Hoarseness. *Pediatr Rev* 1995;16:69.

Newman B, Flom L, Rivero HJ, Oh KS. Vocal cord paralysis and cardiovascular disease in children. *Ann Radiol* 1986;29:697.

Hyperhidrosis

Common Causes
Emotional stimuli
Exercise
Fever, recovery from fever
Increased environmental temperature
Ingestion of spicy foods

Uncommon Causes
Atopic predisposition
Chronic illness
   Brucellosis
   Malaria
   Pulmonary tuberculosis
Cluster headaches
Congestive heart failure
Drug withdrawal
Hypoglycemia
Respiratory failure
Salicylate intoxication

Rare Causes
Acrodynia
Acromegaly
Auriculotemporal syndrome
Benign positional vertigo
Carbon monoxide poisoning
Carcinoid syndrome
Chédiak-Higashi syndrome
Citrullinemia
Diencephalic syndrome
Familial dysautonomia
Familial periodic paralysis
Hyperthyroidism
Insulin overdose
Ipecac ingestion
Juvenile rheumatoid arthritis
Myocardial infarction
Organophosphate poisoning
Phenylketonuria
Pheochromocytoma
Pyridoxine deficiency
Raynaud phenomenon
Spinal cord injury
Syncope
Thrombocytopenia–absent radius syndrome
Vasoactive intestinal peptide–secreting tumor

Suggested Readings

Cloward RB. Hyperhidrosis. *J Neurosurg* 1969;30:545.

O'Donoghue G, Finn D, Brady MP. Palmar primary hyperhidrosis in children. *J Pediatr Surg* 1980;15:172.

Hyperkalemia

Hyperkalemia is defined here as a serum potassium level higher than 5.5 mEq/L.

Common Causes
Artifactual, "pseudohyperkalemia"
  Fist clenching during venipuncture
  Hemolysis during venipuncture
Acidosis
Renal failure
Severe dehydration

Uncommon Causes
Artifactual, "pseudohyperkalemia"
  Severe thrombocytosis (platelets greater than
    1,000 K/mL)
  Severe leukocytosis (white blood cell count greater than
    100 K/mL)
Drugs
  Amiloride
  Spironolactone
  Triamterene
Excessive intake
  Excessive potassium infusion
  High-potassium diet: bananas, orange juice, carrots,
    celery, broccoli
  Potassium replacement therapy
  Potassium salts of antibiotics
  Salt substitutes
Insulin deficiency
Shock

Rare Causes
Addison disease (adrenal insufficiency)
Cell lysis syndromes (tissue necrosis, rhabdomyolysis,
  burns)
Crush injury
Familial hyperkalemic periodic paralysis
Malignant hyperthermia
Renal tubular acidosis
Theophylline intoxication
Tubular unresponsiveness to aldosterone (e.g., sickle cell
  disease, systemic lupus erythematosus)

Suggested Reading

Don BR, Sebastian A, Cheitlin M, et al. Pseudohyperkalemia caused by fist clenching during phlebotomy. *N Engl J Med* 1990;322:1290.

Hypernatremia

Hypernatremia is defined here as a serum sodium level higher
than 145 mEq/L.

Common Causes
Excessive loss of free water
  Diarrhea
  Diuretics
  High environmental temperature
  Hyperpnea
  Sweating
  Vomiting

Uncommon Causes
Nephrogenic diabetes insipidus
Postobstructive diuresis
Salt poisoning
Sickle cell nephropathy

Rare Causes
Cushing disease

Diuretic phase of acute tubular necrosis
Hypercalcemic nephropathy

Hypertension

Common Causes
Agitation
Anxiety
Coarctation of the aorta
Essential hypertension
Immobilization
Inappropriate cuff size
Obesity
Orthopedic manipulation
Pain
Renal causes
  Acute tubular necrosis
  Congenital anomalies
    Hydronephrosis
    Nephrophthisis
    Polycystic kidneys
    Renal aplasia/hypoplasia/dysplasia
    Segmental hypoplasia
  Glomerulonephritis (acute and chronic)
    Membranoproliferative, and so forth
    Postinfectious
  Miscellaneous nephropathy
    Diabetes mellitus
  Nephrolithiasis
  Nephrotic syndrome
    Idiopathic
    Minimal change disease
  Obstructive uropathy
  Other nephritides
    Familial nephritis
    Hemolytic-uremic syndrome
    Henoch-Schönlein purpura
    Hypersensitivity/transfusion reaction
    Radiation
    Systemic lupus erythematosus
  Pyelonephritis
  Renal failure (acute and chronic)
  Renal transplantation
  Renal vascular disease
    Renal artery
      Aneurysm
      Arteritis
      Embolic disease
      External compression
      Fibromuscular dysplasia
      Fistula
      Stenosis
      Thrombosis
      Trauma
    Renal vein thrombosis
Retroperitoneal fibrosis
Trauma
Tumors
  Extrinsic tumors
    Adrenal carcinoma
    Neuroblastoma
    Renin-secreting tumors (J-G cell)
    Wilms tumor

Uncommon Causes
Cardiovascular etiologies
  Anemia
  Aortic insufficiency

Aortic aneurysm/thrombosis
Arteriovenous fistula
  Aorticopulmonary window
Bacterial endocarditis
Iatrogenic hypervolemia
Leukemia
Patent ductus arteriosus
Polycythemia
Pseudoxanthoma elasticum
Radiation aortitis
Takayasu arteritis
Williams syndrome
Drugs and chemicals
  Anabolic steroids
  Cocaine
  Glucocorticoids
  Glycyrrhizic acid (licorice)
  Heavy metals (lead, cadmium, mercury)
  Methysergide
  Mineralocorticoids
  Monoamine-oxidase inhibitors
  Oral contraceptives
  Phencyclidine
  Sodium salts
  Sympathomimetics (decongestants)
  Tricyclic antidepressants
Periarteritis nodosa

Rare Causes
Acute intermittent porphyria
Amyloidosis
Burns
CNS
  Dysautonomia (Riley-Day syndrome)
  Encephalitis
  Guillain-Barré syndrome
  Increased intracranial pressure
    Pseudotumor cerebri
    Trauma
    Vascular accidents
  Meningitis
  Neurofibromatosis
  Poliomyelitis
Chronic hypoxia
Collagen vascular disease
  Dermatomyositis
  Scleroderma
Cystinosis
Endocrine
  Congenital adrenal hyperplasia
    11-Alpha-hydroxylase deficiency
    17-Hydroxylase deficiency
  Cushing syndrome
  Hyperaldosteronism
    Primary
    Conn syndrome
    Dexamethasone-suppressible
    Idiopathic nodular hyperplasia
    Secondary
  Hyperthyroidism
  Pheochromocytoma
Fabry disease
Gout
Liddle syndrome
Malignant hyperthermia
Metabolic
  Hypercalcemia
  Hypernatremia
  Renal tubular acidosis with nephrocalcinosis

Neurofibromatosis
Sickle cell disease
Stevens-Johnson syndrome
Tuberous sclerosis

Suggested Readings

Bailie MD, Mattioli LF. Hypertension: relationships between pathophysiology and therapy. *J Pediatr* 1980;96:789.

Balfe JW, Rance CP. Recognition and management of hypertensive crises in childhood. *Pediatr Clin North Am* 1978;25:159.

Daniels SR. The diagnosis of hypertension in children: an update. *Pediatr Rev* 1997;18:131.

de Swiet M, Fayers P, Shinebourne EA. Systolic blood pressure in a population of infants in the first year of life: the Brompton study. *Pediatrics* 1980;65:1028.

Hohn AR, Riopel DA, Loadholt B. Which blood pressure? *J Pediatr* 1984;104:89.

Hypertension: more than ever, a pediatric concern. *Contemp Pediatr* 1985;2:30.

Kaplan MR, Hernandez LG. The pathogenesis and diagnosis of hypertension in children. *Pediatr Ann* 1982;11:592.

Klein AA, McCrory WW, Engle MA. Hypertension in children. *Cardiovasc Clin* 1981;11:11.

Lauer RM, Burns TL, Clarke WR. Assessing children's blood pressure—considerations of age and body size: the Muscatine study. *Pediatrics* 1985;75:1081.

Lieberman E. Essential hypertension in children and youth: a pediatric perspective. *J Pediatr* 1974;85:1.

Loggie JMH, Horan MJ, Hohn AR, et al. Juvenile hypertension: highlights of a workshop. *J Pediatr* 1984;104:657.

Loggie JMH, New MI, Robson AM. Hypertension in the pediatric patient: a reappraisal. *J Pediatr* 1979;94:685.

Londe S. Causes of hypertension in the young. *Pediatr Clin North Am* 1978;25:55.

Londe S, Bourgoignie JJ, Robson AM, Goldring D. Hypertension in apparently normal children. *J Pediatr* 1971;78:569.

National High Blood Pressure Working Group on Hypertension Control in Children and Adolescents. Update on the 1987 Task Force report on high blood pressure in children and adolescents: a working group report from the National High Blood Pressure Education Program. *Pediatrics* 1996;98:649.

Piazza SF, Chandra M, Harper RG, et al. Upper- vs lower-limb systolic blood pressure in full-term normal newborns. *Am J Dis Child* 1985;139:797.

Rosen PR, Treves S, Ingelfinger J. Hypertension in children. *Am J Dis Child* 1985;139:173.

Sinaiko AR. Hypertension in children. *N Engl J Med* 1996;335:1968.

Hypokalemia

Hypokalemia is defined here as a serum potassium level lower than 3.5 mEq/L.

Common Causes
Chronic diarrhea
Diuretics
Malnutrition
Metabolic alkalosis
Vomiting/gastric suction

Uncommon Causes
Excessive corticosteroids
Renal tubular disorders

Rare Causes
Amphotericin B therapy
Bartter syndrome
Colon cancer
Cushing syndrome
Familial hypokalemic periodic paralysis
Laxative abuse
Primary aldosteronism
Pseudoaldosteronism
Ureterosigmoidostomy
Villous adenoma
Zollinger-Ellison syndrome

Hyponatremia

Hyponatremia is defined here as a serum sodium level lower than 130 mEq/L.

Common Causes
Diarrhea
Excessive salt-free infusions
Syndrome of inappropriate antidiuretic hormone secretion
Water intoxication

Uncommon Causes
Acute renal failure
Chronic renal failure
Congestive heart failure
High environmental temperatures
Spurious
   Hyperglycemia

Rare Causes
Adrenal insufficiency
Cirrhosis
Cystic fibrosis and excessive sweating
Spurious
   Hyperlipidemia

Hypotonia, Neonatal

Common Causes
Asphyxia/anoxia
Benign, congenital
Congenital infections
   Cytomegalovirus
   Herpes
   Rubella
   Syphilis
   Toxoplasmosis
Sepsis
Trauma

Uncommon Causes
Congenital joint laxity
Down syndrome
Hypermobility syndrome
Hypothyroidism
Neonatal myasthenia
Spinal cord injury
Werdnig-Hoffmann disease

Rare Causes
Achondroplasia
Cerebrohepatorenal syndrome
Congenital hypomyelination neuropathy
Congenital lactic acidosis
Congenital myopathies
   Central core disease
   Myotubular myopathy
   Nemaline myopathy
Cri du chat syndrome
Ehlers-Danlos syndrome
Familial dysautonomia
Generalized gangliosidosis
Glycogen storage disease (type II)
Hyperammonemia
Hyperlysinemia
Mannosidosis
Maple syrup urine disease
Marfan syndrome

Myotonic dystrophy
Nonketotic hyperglycinemia
Oculocerebrorenal syndrome (Lowe syndrome)
Osteogenesis imperfecta
Prader-Willi syndrome
Pseudodeficiency rickets
Thanatophoric dwarfism
Toxins and drugs
   Botulism
   Fetal aminopterin syndrome
   Fetal warfarin syndrome
   Hypermagnesemia (secondary maternal magnesium-sulfate
     therapy)
   Kernicterus
   Lidocaine toxicity
Trisomy 13
Williams syndrome (idiopathic hypercalcemia)

Suggested Readings

Fishman MA, Finegold M. Progressive neurologic deterioration in a hypotonic infant. *J Pediatr* 1985;107:634.
Hanson PA. "Floppy baby" (Oppenheim's disease, amyotonia congenital). *Pediatr Ann* 1977;6:98.
Low NL. Spinal muscular atrophy syndromes. *Pediatr Ann* 1977;6:35.
Sarnat HB. Diagnostic value of the muscle biopsy in the neonatal period. *Am J Dis Child* 1978;132:782.
Slater GE, Swaiman KF. Muscular dystrophies of childhood. *Pediatr Ann* 1977; 6:50.
Spiro AJ. Approach to diagnosis in the child with muscle weakness. *Pediatr Ann* 1977;6:11.
Thompson CE. Pitfalls in muscle biopsies of hypotonic children. *Dev Med Child Neurol* 1985;27:675.

Jaundice, Beyond the Neonatal Period

Common Causes
Acute or chronic hemolytic anemias
Gilbert disease
Hepatitis A, hepatitis B, hepatitis C, Epstein-Barr virus

Uncommon Causes
Bacterial infections: pyelonephritis, sepsis, liver abscess, cholangitis
Cholelithiasis
Chronic active hepatitis
Cirrhosis
Cystic fibrosis
Drug-induced hepatitis
Sepsis
Total parenteral nutrition

Rare Causes
Alagille syndrome
Alpha$_1$-antitrypsin deficiency
Apparent jaundice
   Carotenoderma
   Drugs, especially antimalarials
   Lycopenoderma
Benign recurrent cholestasis
Biliary atresia
Byler disease
Caroli disease
Chemical injury
Cholecystitis: posttraumatic or autoimmune
Choledochal cyst
Crigler-Najjar syndrome
Dubin-Johnson syndrome

Fibrosing pancreatitis
Galactokinase deficiency
Galactosemia
Glycogen storage disease (types III and IV)
Hemophagocytic syndromes
Hereditary fructose intolerance
Intestinal obstruction
  Annular pancreas
  Hirschsprung disease
  Pyloric stenosis
Niemann-Pick disease
Parasitic infection
Pheochromocytoma
Primary sclerosing cholangitis
Reye syndrome
Rotor syndrome
Trisomy 18
Tyrosinemia
Wilson disease

Suggested Readings

Balistreri WF. Neonatal cholestasis. *J Pediatr* 1985;106:171.

Fung KP, Lau SP. Gamma-Glutamyl (γ-Glutamyl) transpeptidase activity and its serial measurement in differentiation between extrahepatic biliary atresia and neonatal hepatitis. *J Pediatr Gastroenterol Nutr* 1985;4:208.

Johnston GS, Rosenbaum RC, Hill JL, Diaconis JN. Differentiation of jaundice in infancy: an application of radionuclide biliary studies. *J Surg Oncol* 1985;30:206.

Kaye R. Abdominal pain, constipation, and melena. In: Kaye R, Oski FA, Barness LA, eds. *Core textbook of pediatrics.* Philadelphia: Lippincott–Raven, 1982: 109.

Lubin BH, Baehner RL, Schwartz E, et al. The red cell peroxide hemolysis test in the differential diagnosis of obstructive jaundice in the newborn period. *Pediatrics* 1971;48:562.

Maisels MJ. Bilirubin: on understanding and influencing its metabolism in the newborn infant. *Pediatr Clin North Am* 1972;19:447.

Mathis RK, Andres JM, Walker WA. Liver disease in infants. *J Pediatr* 1977;90: 864.

Melhorn DK, Izant RJ Jr. The red cell hydrogen peroxide hemolysis test and vitamin E absorption in the differential diagnosis of jaundice in infancy. *J Pediatr* 1972;81:1082.

Seligman JW. Recent and changing concepts of hyperbilirubinemia and its management in the newborn. *Pediatr Clin North Am* 1977;24:509.

Thaler MM. Jaundice in early infancy. *Pediatr Ann* 1977;6:286.

Tunnessen WW Jr. *Sign & Symptoms in Pediatrics*, 3rd edition. Lippincott, Williams & Wilkins, 1999.

Joint Pain

Common Causes
Growing pains
Osteomyelitis
Overuse
Retropatellar pain syndrome (chondromalacia patellae)
Septic arthritis
Sickle cell disease
Sympathetic effusion
Tietze syndrome
Transient synovitis
Trauma
  Contusion
  Fracture
  Hemarthrosis
  Sprain/strain
Viral arthritis
  Adenovirus
  Epstein-Barr virus
  Hepatitis
  Varicella

Uncommon Causes
Attention-seeking behavior
Child abuse
Foreign body
Legg-Calvé-Perthes disease
Mycoplasma
Osgood-Schlatter disease
Osteochondritis dissecans
Popliteal cyst (Baker cyst)
Psoriatic arthritis
Reactive arthritis
  Brucella
  Campylobacter
  Neisseria gonorrhoeae
  Salmonella
  Shigella
  Yersinia
Referred pain (retroperitoneal/intraperitoneal inflammation)
Slipped capital femoral epiphysis
Subluxation of the patella

Rare Causes
Bone tumors
Carpal-tarsal osteolysis
Congenital joint laxity
  Ehlers-Danlos syndrome
  Marfan syndrome
  Stickler syndrome
Cystic fibrosis
Fabry disease
Familial Mediterranean fever
Gaucher disease
Giardia
Gout
Homocystinuria
Hyperlipoproteinemia
Hyperparathyroidism
Idiopathic chondrolysis
Immunodeficiency
  Complement deficiency
  Hypogammaglobulinemia
Immunologic
  Acute rheumatic fever
  Ankylosing spondylitis
  Behçet syndrome
  Dermatomyositis
  Giant cell arteritis
  Henoch-Schönlein purpura
  Hepatitis
  Inflammatory bowel disease
  Juvenile rheumatoid arthritis
  Kawasaki disease
  Mixed connective tissue disease
  Polyarteritis nodosa
  Reiter syndrome
  Scleroderma
    Serum sickness
    Sjögren syndrome
    Systemic lupus erythematosus
Leukemia
Lipogranulomatosis
Lyme disease
Mucopolysaccharidoses
Mycobacterial disease
Neuropathic arthropathy
Psychogenic rheumatism
Reflex sympathetic dystrophy
Rickets
Sarcoidosis

Stevens-Johnson syndrome
Subacute bacterial endocarditis
Syphilis
   Charcot joint
   Infection
Thorn-induced arthritis
Thyroid disease
Villonodular disease
Viral arthritis
   Mumps
   Rubella
Whipple disease

Suggested Readings

Fulkerson JP. The etiology of patellofemoral pain in young active patients: a prospective study. *Clin Orthop* 1983;179:129.

Kunnamo I, Kallio P, Pelkonen P, Hovi T. Clinical signs and laboratory tests in the differential diagnosis of arthritis in children. *Am J Dis Child* 1987;141:34.

Kunnamo I, Pelkonen P. Routine analysis of synovial fluid cells is of value in the differential diagnosis of arthritis in children. *J Rheumatol* 1986;13:1076.

Morrissy RT, Shore SL. Bone and joint sepsis. *Pediatr Clin North Am* 1986;33:1551.

Phillips PE. Viral arthritis in children. *Arthritis Rheum* 1977;20(Suppl 2):584.

Schaller JG. Arthritis in children. *Pediatr Clin North Am* 1986;33:1565.

Limb Pain

Common Causes

Growing pains
Hypermobility syndrome
Infection
   Cellulitis
   Osteitis
   Osteomyelitis
   Postrubella vaccination
   Septic arthritis
   Soft tissue abscess
   Toxic synovitis
   Viral myositis
Sickle cell disease, vasoocclusive crisis
Trauma
   Compartment syndrome
   Dislocation and subluxation
   Fracture
   Joint strain, sprain, internal damage
   Myositis ossificans
   Patellofemoral pain syndrome (chondromalacia patellae)
   Pathologic fractures
      Bone cysts
      Fibrous dysplasia
   Postimmunization, postinjection
   Shin splints
   Soft tissue contusion or hemorrhage
   Stress fracture
   Tendonitis, bursitis, fasciitis
   Traumatic periostitis

Uncommon Causes

Accessory tarsal ossicle
Collagen vascular disease (dermatomyositis, lupus)
Conversion reactions
Henoch-Schönlein purpura
Juvenile rheumatoid arthritis
Legg-Calvé-Perthes disease
Osgood-Schlatter disease
Osteochondritis dissecans
Rheumatic fever
Tarsal coalition

Rare Causes

Acute poststreptococcal polymyalgia
Bone tumors
   Benign
      Benign osteoblastoma
      Osteoid osteoma
   Malignant
      Ewing sarcoma
      Osteogenic sarcoma
      Chondrosarcoma
Cushing syndrome
Ehlers-Danlos syndrome
Familial Mediterranean fever
Fibromyalgia
Gaucher disease
Goldbloom syndrome
Hemophilia
Histiocytosis X
Hyperparathyroidism
Hypervitaminosis A
Inflammatory bowel disease
Leukemia
Lymphoma
Mucopolysaccharidosis
Multiple epiphyseal dysplasia
Myopathies
Neuroblastoma
Osteoporosis
Popliteal cyst (Baker cyst)
Reflex sympathetic dystrophy
Renal tubular acidosis
Rickets
Scurvy
Slipped capital femoral epiphysis
Soft tissue tumors (rhabdomyosarcoma, fibrosarcoma)
Stickler syndrome
Syphilis
Trichinosis

Suggested Readings

Bowyer SL, Hollister JR. Limb pain in childhood. *Pediatr Clin North Am* 1984;31:1053.

Groshar D, Lam M, Even-Sapir E, et al. Stress fractures and bone pain: are they closely associated? *Injury* 1985;16:526.

Naish JM, Apley J. "Growing pains:" a clinical study of non-arthritic limb pains in children. *Arch Dis Child* 1951;26:134.

Oster J, Nielsen A. Growing pains. *Acta Paediatr Scand* 1972;61:329.

Park HM, Rothschild PA, Kernek CB. Scintigraphic evaluation of extremity pain in children: its efficacy and pitfalls. *AJR Am J Roentgenol* 1985;145:1079.

Passo MH. Aches and limb pain. *Pediatr Clin North Am* 1982;29:209.

Peterson H. Growing pains. *Pediatr Clin North Am* 1986;33:1365.

Shapiro MJ. Differential diagnosis of nonrheumatic "growing pains" and subacute rheumatic fever. *J Pediatr* 1939;14:315.

Sherry DD. Limb pain in childhood. *Pediatr Rev* 1990;12:39.

Szer IS. Musculoskeletal pain syndromes that affect adolescents. *Arch Pediatr Adolesc Med* 1996;150:740.

Limp

Common Causes

Attention-seeking behavior (usually after minor trauma)
Calluses/corns/ingrown toenails
Contusion
Foreign body (especially plantar surface)
Fracture (may be occult)
Growing pains
Hemophilia (hemarthroses, soft tissue bleeds)

Hypermobility syndrome
Immunization (local pain)
Leg length discrepancy
Mimicry
Myositis (acute viral)
Patellofemoral pain syndrome (chondromalacia patellae)
Poorly fitting shoes (tight or loose)
Shin splints
Sickle cell disease (painful crisis, infarction)
Soft tissue/cutaneous infection
Sprain/strain
Tendonitis
Torsion deformities
Toxic synovitis

Uncommon Causes
Arthritis (septic)
Blount disease
Bone tumor (benign or malignant; see Limb Pain)
Calcaneal spurs
Child abuse
Congenital contractures
Coxa vera
Developmental dysplasia of the hip
Erythema nodosum
Legg-Calvé-Perthes disease
Leukemia
Neuromuscular disease
    Ataxia
    CNS bleed
    CNS infection
    Flaccid paralysis
    Migraine
    Muscular dystrophy
    Peripheral neuropathy
        Causalgia
        Diabetes mellitus
        Guillain-Barré syndrome
        Heavy metal intoxication
        Periodic paralysis
        Poliomyelitis
        Tick paralysis
    Radiculopathy
    Spastic paralysis
Osgood-Schlatter disease
Osteochondritis dissecans
Osteomyelitis
Phlebitis
Plantar wart
Popliteal cyst (Baker cyst)
Referred pain
    Discitis
    Epidural/paraspinal abscess
    Iliac adenitis
    Intraperitoneal infection/inflammation
    Pelvic inflammatory disease
    Retroperitoneal fibrosis
    Retroperitoneal mass
Slipped capital femoral epiphysis
Subluxation of the patella

Rare Causes
Arthritis/arthralgia
    Acute rheumatic fever
    Dermatomyositis
    Henoch-Schönlein purpura
    Inflammatory bowel disease
    Juvenile rheumatoid arthritis
    Kawasaki disease

Lyme disease
Polyarteritis nodosa
Serum sickness
Systemic lupus erythematosus
Brucellosis
Caffey disease
Congenital joint laxity (Ehlers-Danlos syndrome)
Erythromelalgia
Freiberg disease
Hepatitis
Herniated nucleus pulposus
Hypervitaminosis A
Hysteria
Intervertebral disc herniation
Köhler disease
Larsen-Johansson disease
Neuroblastoma
Postmeningococcal skeletal dystrophy
Pott disease
POH's disease
Psoas abscess
Pyomyositis
Rickets
Scurvy
Sever disease
Sinding-Larsen disease
Spinal tumor
Trichinosis

Suggested Readings

Chung SMK. Identifying the cause of acute limp in childhood: some informal comments and observations. *Clin Pediatr* 1974;13:769.
Hensinger RN. Limp. *Pediatr Clin North Am* 1986;33:1355.
Illingworth CM. 128 limping children with no fracture, sprain, or obvious cause. *Clin Pediatr* 1978;17:139.
McIntre SC, Farrell JD. The limping child. In: Gartner JC Jr., Zitelli BJ, eds. *Common and chronic symptoms in pediatrics.* St. Louis: Mosby, 1997:63.
Phillips WA. The child with a limp. *Orthop Clin North Am* 1987;18:489.
Renshaw TS. The child who has a limp. *Pediatr Rev* 1995;16:458.
Singer J, Towbin R. Occult fractures in the production of gait disturbances in childhood. *Pediatrics* 1979;64:192.
Steere AC. Lyme disease. *N Engl J Med* 1989;321:586.

Lymphadenopathy (Generalized)

Common Causes
Benign lymphoid hypertrophy
Infection
    Bacterial
        Sepsis
        Syphilis
    Fungal
        Candida
    Viral
        Enteroviruses
        Hepatitides
        Infectious mononucleosis
Juvenile rheumatoid arthritis
Serum sickness

Uncommon Causes
Atopic dermatitis
Drug reactions
    Antibacterials (penicillins, tetracyclines, sulfonamides)
    Anticonvulsants
    Antithyroid
    Aspirin
    Isoniazid

HIV infection
Hodgkin disease
Infection
  Bacterial
    Leptospirosis
    Salmonellosis
    Scarlet fever
    Streptococcosis
  Viral
    Cytomegalovirus
  Other
    Malaria
    Mycoplasma
    Tuberculosis
Leukemia
Lyme disease
Non-Hodgkin disease
Systemic lupus erythematosus

Rare Causes
Angiofollicular lymph node hyperplasia
Angioimmunoblastic lymphadenopathy
Chédiak-Higashi syndrome
Chronic granulomatous disease
Gaucher disease
Gianotti-Crosti syndrome
Hemophagocytic syndromes
Histiocytosis
Hyperthyroidism
Infections
  Bacterial
    Brucellosis
    Plague
    Typhoid fever
  Viral
    Rubella
    Rubeola
  Other
    Histoplasmosis
    Toxoplasmosis
    Trypanosomiasis
Metastatic neuroblastoma
Niemann-Pick disease
Sarcoidosis
Tangier disease

Suggested Readings

Barton LL, Feigin RD. Childhood cervical lymphadenitis: a reappraisal. *J Pediatr* 1974;84:846.
Bedros A, Mann JP. Lymphadenopathy in children. *Adv Pediatr* 1981;28:341.
Canale VC, Smith CH. Chronic lymphadenopathy simulating malignant lymphoma. *J Pediatr* 1967;70:891.
Carithers HA. Lymphadenopathy. *Am J Dis Child* 1978;132:353.
Frizzera G, Moran EM, Rappaport H. Angio-immunoblastic lymphadenopathy. *Am J Med* 1975;59:803.
Herzog LW. Prevalence of lymphadenopathy of the head and neck in infants and children. *Clin Pediatr* 1983;22:485.
Kissane JM, Gephardt GN. Lymphadenopathy in childhood. *Hum Pathol* 1974;5:431.
Knight PJ, Mulne AF, Vassy LE. When is lymph node biopsy indicated in children with enlarged peripheral nodes? *Pediatrics* 1982;69:391.
Lake AM, Oski FA. Peripheral lymphadenopathy in childhood. *Am J Dis Child* 1978;132:357.
Musiej-Nowakowska E, Rostropowicz-Denisiewicz K. Differential diagnosis of neoplastic and rheumatic diseases in children. *Scand J Rheumatol* 1986;15:124.
Rieger CHL, Lustig JV, Justman RA, Rothberg RM. Immunologic function of patients with chronic benign lymphadenopathy. *Eur J Pediatr* 1976;124:51.
Slap GB, Connor JL, Wigton RS, Schwartz S. Validation of a model to identify young patients for lymph node biopsy. *JAMA* 1986;255:2768.
Steere AC. Lyme disease. *N Engl J Med* 1989;321:586.
Zuelzer WW, Kaplan J. The child with lymphadenopathy. *Semin Hematol* 1975;12:323.

Odors of Disease

Common Causes
Diabetes mellitus: fruity, acetone-like
Tonsillitis/pharyngitis: Group A beta hemolytic strep odor
Uremia: fishy (trimethylamine ammonia)
Urinary tract infection: ammoniacal

Uncommon Causes
Intestinal obstruction: feculent, foul
Intranasal foreign body: fetid
Lung abscess: foul, putrid
Vaginal foreign body: foul

Rare Causes
Beta-methylcrotonyl CoA carboxylase deficiency: cat urine
Diphtheria: mousey odor
Fish odor syndrome: fishy (impaired *N*-oxidation of trimethylamine)
Glutaric acidemia (type III): sweaty feet
Hepatic failure: musty fish or raw liver
Hypermethioninemia and hypertyrosinemia (rancid butter syndrome): fish, rancid butter, boiled cabbage
Isovaleric acidemia (sweaty sock syndrome): sweaty feet
Maple syrup urine disease: maple syrup, caramel-like
Oasthouse syndrome: dried malt or hops (methionine malabsorption)
Phenylketonuria: musty, wolflike, stale
Scurvy: putrid
Trimethylaminuria: rotting fish
Tyrosinemia: yeastlike

Suggested Readings

Hayden GF. Olfactory diagnosis in medicine. *Postgrad Med* 1980;67:110.
Hnekin RI. Body Odor. *JAMA* 1995;273:1171.
Liddell K. Smell as a diagnostic marker. *Postgrad Med J* 1976;52:136.
Mace JW, Goodman SI, Centerwall WR, Chinnock RF. The child with an unusual odor. *Clin Pediatr* 1976;15:57.
Moriarty RA. Nasal foreign body presenting as an unusual odor. *Am J Dis Child* 1978;132:96.
Rizzo WB, Roth KS. On 'being led by the nose': rapid detection of inborn errors of metabolism. *Arch Pediatr Adolesc Med* 1994;148:869.

Polyuria

Common Causes
Diabetes mellitus
Diuretic abuse
  Alcohol
  Caffeine
  Medications
Iatrogenic
  Aggressive parenteral hydration
  Diuretic use
Pregnancy
Psychogenic polydipsia
Renal failure
Sickle cell disease
Urinary tract infection

Uncommon Causes

Diabetes insipidus (central)

Interstitial nephritis
  Analgesic abuse
  Diphenylhydantoin
  Mercury poisoning
  Methicillin reaction
  Sulfonamides

Renal calculi/hypercalcemia

Renal tubular acidosis

Rare Causes

Bartter syndrome

Cystinosis

Medullary cystic disease of the kidney

Nephrogenic diabetes insipidus

Neuroblastoma/ganglioneuroblastoma

Pheochromocytoma

Suggested Readings

Czernichow P, Pomarede R, Basmaciogullari A, et al. Diabetes insipidus in children. III. Anterior pituitary dysfunction in idiopathic types. *J Pediatr* 1985; 106:41.

Kohn B, Norman ME, Feldman H, et al. Hysterical polydipsia (compulsive water drinking) in children. *Am J Dis Child* 1976;130:210.

Scherbaum WA, Czernichow P, Bottazzo GF, Doniach D. Diabetes insipidus in children. IV. A possible autoimmune type with vasopressin cell antibodies. *J Pediatr* 1985;107:922.

Proteinuria

Common Causes

Chronic pyelonephritis

Isolated transient/intermittent proteinuria
  Cold exposure
  Congestive heart failure
  Exercise
  Febrile illness
  Idiopathic proteinuria
  Orthostatic proteinuria
  Pregnancy
  Trauma
  Urinary tract infection

Uncommon Causes

Nephritic sediment
  Membranoproliferative glomerulonephritis
  Postinfectious glomerulonephritis

Nephrotic sediment
  Minimal change disease
  Preeclampsia

Tubular proteinuria
  Acute tubular necrosis
  Obstructive uropathy
  Polycystic kidney disease

Rare Causes

Drugs
  Captopril
  Fenoprofen
  Gold
  Penicillamine
  Probenecid

Nephritic sediment
  Hereditary nephritis

IgA nephropathy

Mixed cryoglobulinemia

Rapidly progressive glomerulonephritis

Subacute bacterial endocarditis

Systemic lupus erythematosus

Nephrotic sediment
  Amyloidosis
  Diabetes mellitus
  Focal glomerulonephritis
  Membranous nephropathy
  Miscellaneous infections
    Hepatitis B
    Malaria
    Syphilis

Overflow proteinuria
  Bence Jones proteinuria
  Lysozymuria (in leukemia)

Tubular proteinuria
  Analgesic abuse
  Chronic hypertension
  Hypercalciuria
  Hyperuricemia
  Radiation nephritis

Suggested Readings

Burke EC, Stickler GB. Proteinuria in children. *Clin Pediatr* 1982;21:741.

Daeschner CW. Screening for renal diseases. *J Pediatr* 1976;88:369.

Dodge WF, West EF, Smith EH, Bunce H III. Proteinuria and hematuria in schoolchildren: epidemiology and early natural history. *J Pediatr* 1976;88:327.

Houser M. Assessment of proteinuria using random urine samples. *J Pediatr* 1984;104:845.

James JA. Proteinuria and hematuria in children: diagnosis and assessment. *Pediatr Clin North Am* 1976;23:807.

Pollak VE, Ooi BS. Just what is the significance of proteinuria? *Resident Staff Physician* 1971;11:89.

Robinson RR. Isolated proteinuria in asymptomatic patients. *Kidney Int* 1980; 18:395.

Sinniah R, Law CH, Pwee HS. Glomerular lesions in patients with asymptomatic persistent and orthostatic proteinuria discovered on routine medical examination. *Clin Nephrol* 1977;7:1.

Stewart DW, Gordon JA, Schoolwerth AC. Evaluation of proteinuria. *Am Fam Physician* 1984;29:218.

Vehaskari VM, Rapola J. Isolated proteinuria: analysis of a school-age population. *J Pediatr* 1982;101:661.

West CD. Asymptomatic hematuria and proteinuria in children. Causes and appropriate diagnostic studies. *J Pediatr* 1976;89:173.

Pruitus

Common Causes

Atopic dermatitis

Cholestasis of pregnancy

Contact allergens (plants, cosmetics, dyes, medications, jewelry [nickel])

Contact irritants (bubble bath, soaps, chemicals, citrus juices, excrement, wool, urine)

Drugs
  Aminophylline
  Aspirin
  Barbiturates
  Erythromycin
  Gold
  Griseofulvin
  Isoniazid
  Opiates
  Phenothiazines
  Vitamin A

Dry skin
  Excess bathing/strong detergents
  Low humidity
Foreign body: fiberglass, cactus spine, hair
Hepatitis
High humidity
Insect bites/infestations
  Fleas, mosquitoes, scabies, lice, mites, chiggers
Iron deficiency anemia
Parasitic infections
  Pinworms
  Toxocara canis
Pityriasis rosea
Psoriasis
Seborrheic dermatitis
Skin infections (bacterial/viral/fungal)
Urticaria

Uncommon Causes
Acquired immunodeficiency syndrome
Biliary obstruction
  Drug-induced
  Extrahepatic biliary obstruction
  Primary biliary cirrhosis
Chronic renal failure
Hematopoietic malignancies
  Hodgkin disease
  Leukemia
  Lymphoma
Neurodermatitis
Parasitic infections
  Cercaria: Swimmer's itch
  Hookworm
  Trichinosis
Pleomorphic light eruption (Hispanic and Native American
  populations)

Rare Causes
Autoimmune
  Juvenile rheumatoid arthritis
  Systemic lupus erythematosus
Congenital ectodermal disorders
Endocrine diseases
  Carcinoid syndrome
  Diabetes mellitus
  Hypercalcemia
  Hyperthyroidism/hypothyroidism
  Hypoparathyroidism
Erythropoietic protoporphyria
Hematopoietic malignancies
  Mastocytosis
  Polycythemia vera
Malignant solid tumors
Neurofibromatosis
Neurologic syndromes
Psychosis
Seabather's eruption: jellyfish larvae
Urticaria pigmentosa

Suggested Readings

Denman St. A review of pruritus. *J Am Acad Dermatol* 1986;14:375.
Edwards AE, Shellow WVR, Wright ET, Dignam TF. Pruritic skin disease, psychological stress, and the itch sensation. *Arch Dermatol* 1976;112:339.
Gilchrest BA. Pruritus: pathogenesis, therapy, and significance in systemic disease states. *Arch Intern Med* 1982;142:101.
Shelley WB, Arthur RP. The neurohistology and neurophysiology of the itch sensation in man. *Arch Dermatol* 1957;76:296.

Purpura (Petechiae and Ecchymoses)

Common Causes
Thrombocytopenia
  Idiopathic thrombocytopenic purpura
  Infection: bacterial infections, bacterial sepsis
  Drugs
  Autoimmune disease
    Systemic lupus erythematosus
    Acquired hemolytic anemia
    Neoplastic disease, acute leukemia
Trauma
Viral infections: Coxsackieviruses, echoviruses

Uncommon Causes
Abnormal platelet function
  Uremia
Drug-induced (aspirin, antihistamines, nonsteroidal
  antiinflammatory drugs, penicillins, phenothiazines,
  sulfonamides)
Maternal drug ingestion (warfarin, barbiturates, phenytoin)
Child abuse
Cupping and coin rubbing
Factitious
Hemolytic-uremic syndrome
Henoch-Schönlein purpura
Hereditary coagulation disturbance
Infection
TORCHS (*toxoplasmosis, rubella, cytomegalovirus, herpes
  simplex, and syphilis*)
  Meningococcemia
  Bacterial septicemia
  Parvovirus B19: papular-purpuric "gloves and socks"
    syndrome
Septic emboli
Thrombocytopenia in the newborn
  Isoimmune thrombocytopenia
  Maternal autoimmune thrombocytopenia
Vasculitis
  Autoimmune
  Rickettsial
Violent coughing

Rare Causes
Adenosine diphosphate storage pool disease
Aplastic anemia
Autoerythrocyte sensitization
Bernard-Soulier disease
Cushing syndrome
Cyanotic congenital heart disease
Dysproteinemias
Ehlers-Danlos syndrome
Exercise
Fanconi syndrome
Glanzmann thrombasthenia
Hermansky-Pudlak syndrome
Hereditary hemorrhagic telangiectasia
Hypersplenism
Kasabach-Merritt syndrome
Lyme disease
Maculae caeruleae
May-Hegglin anomaly
Osteogenesis imperfecta
Osteopetrosis
Phototherapy-induced purpura
Polyurethane exposure
Protein C deficiency

Protein S deficiency
Purpura fulminans
Schamberg disease (progressive pigmentary dermatosis)
Scurvy
Thrombocytopenia–absent radius syndrome
Trisomy 13 and 18 syndromes
Wiskott-Aldrich syndrome
Vitamin K deficiency

Suggested Readings

Mandl KD, Stack AM, Fleisher GR. Incidence of bacteremia in infants and children with fever and petechiae. *J Pediatr* 1997;131:398.

Oski FA, Naiman JL. *Hematologic problems of the newborn*, 3rd ed. Philadelphia: Saunders, 1982.

Paller AS, Eramo LR, Farrell EE, et al. Purpuric phototherapy-induced eruption in transfused neonates: relation to transient porphyrinemia. *Pediatrics* 1997;100:360.

Pramanik AK. Bleeding disorders in neonates. *Pediatr Rev* 1992;13:163.

Rasmussen JE. Puzzling purpuras in children and young adults. *J Am Acad Dermatol* 1982;6:67.

Ratnoff OD. The psychogenic purpuras: a review of autoerythrocyte sensitization, autosensitization to DNA, "hysterical" and factitial bleeding, and the religious stigmata. *Semin Hematol* 1980;17:192.

Saulsbury FT, Hayden GF. Skin conditions simulating child abuse. *Pediatr Emerg Care* 1985;1:147.

Sorensen RU, Newman AJ, Gordon EM. Psychogenic purpura in adolescent patients. *Clin Pediatr* 1985;24:700.

Scrotal Swelling

Common Causes
Painless
  Hernia
  Hydrocele
  Varicocele
Painful
  Epididymitis
  Testicular torsion
  Torsion of appendix testis

Uncommon Causes
Contact dermatitis
Edema
Epididymitis
Henoch-Schönlein purpura
Idiopathic scrotal edema
Insect bites
Orchitis
Secondary to ascites
Trauma

Rare Causes
Adrenal hemorrhage in the newborn
Angiomas
Arteriovenous malformation
Cysts
Elephantiasis
Familial Mediterranean fever
Healed meconium peritonitis
Hypertriglyceridemia
Leukemia
Regional enteritis
Sarcoidosis
Scrotal cellulitis
Spermatocele
Testicular tumors

Suggested Readings

Bartsch G, Marberger FH, Mikuz G. Testicular torsion: late results with special regard to fertility and endocrine function. *J Urol* 1980;124:375.

Brosman SA. Testicular tumors in prepubertal children. *Urology* 1979;13:581.

Dresner ML. Torsed appendage. *Urology* 1973;1:63.

Hermann D. The pediatric acute scrotum. *Pediatr Ann* 1989;18:198.

Kaplan GW. Acute idiopathic scrotal edema. *J Pediatr Surg* 1977;12:647.

Kaplan GW, King L. Acute scrotal swelling in children. *J Urol* 1970;104:219.

Kappahn C. Male reproductive health: part 1. Painful scrotal masses. *Adolesc Health Update* 1992;4:1.

Kappahn C. Male reproductive health: part 2. Painless scrotal masses. *Adolesc Health Update* 1992;5:1.

Pedersen JF, Holm HH, Hald T. Torsion of the testis diagnosed by ultrasound. *J Urol* 1975;113:66.

Rabinavitz R. The importance of the cremasteric reflex in acute swelling in children. *J Urol* 1984;132:89.

Skoglund RW, McRoberts JW, Ragde H. Torsion of testicular appendages: presentation of 43 new cases and a collective review. *J Urol* 1970;104:598.

Skoog SJ, Toberts KP, Goldstein M, Pryor JL. The adolescent varicocele: what's new with an old problem in young patients? *Pediatrics* 1997;100:112.

Seizures

Common Causes
Febrile seizures
Idiopathic seizures
Unknown cause

Uncommon Causes
CNS infections
  Aseptic meningitis
  Bacterial meningitis
  Mosquito/tick-borne encephalitides
  Viral encephalitis
CNS injury
  Anoxic encephalopathy
  Child abuse
  Concussion
  Hemorrhage: subdural, subarachnoid, intracerebral, intraventricular
  Hypoxic-ischemic encephalopathy
Hypoglycemia
Juvenile myoclonic epilepsy (Janz syndrome)

Rare Causes
CNS infection
  Cat scratch disease
  Congenital infection
  Parasitic infection
    Cysticercosis
    Toxoplasmosis
  Postinfectious
  Syphilis
  Tetanus
  Tuberculosis
Congenital CNS malformation
  Aicardi syndrome
  Agenesis/dysgenesis
    Holoprosencephaly
    Porencephaly
    Hydrocephalus
Drugs/toxins
  Aminophylline
  Amphetamines
  Antihistamines
  Atropine
  Camphor
  Carbon monoxide

Drug withdrawal: heroin, methadone, barbiturates, propoxyphene
Heavy metals
Hexachlorophene
Hydrocarbons
Local anesthetics
Narcotics
Organophosphates
Penicillin
Pertussis toxoid
Phencyclidine
Scabicides
Steroids
Tricyclic antidepressants
Inborn errors of metabolism
Aminoacidopathy
Galactosemia
Organic aciduria
Urea cycle defects
Storage disease
Metabolic
Hypernatremia
Hypocalcemia
Hypomagnesemia
Hyponatremia
Miscellaneous
Arrhythmia
Dysmorphogenic syndromes (many)
Eclampsia
Gelastic seizures
Infantile spasms
Kernicterus
Lowe syndrome
Metachromatic leukodystrophy
Myoclonic epilepsy and ragged red fibers (MERRF)
Neonatal adrenoleukodystrophy
Postmaturity: various reasons
Pyridoxine deficiency
Rett syndrome
Reye syndrome
Subacute sclerosing panencephalitis (SSPE)
Tay-Sachs disease
Video-game related seizures
Neurocutaneous syndromes
Incontinentia pigmenti
Linear sebaceous nevi
Neurofibromatosis
Sturge-Weber disease
Tuberous sclerosis
Seizure mimics
Breath-holding spells
Episodic dyscontrol syndrome
Hyperekplexia: "stiff baby" or "startle disease"
Hyperventilation
Malingering
Masturbation
Migraine
Myoclonus
Narcolepsy
Orthostatic hypotension
Paroxysmal torticollis of infancy
Pavor nocturnus: night terrors
Pseudoseizures
Sandifer syndrome
Shivering on urination
Shuddering attacks
Spasmus nutans
Syncope
Tetany

Tics
Vertigo
Systemic infection
Roseola
Shigella
Tumors
Vascular
Arteriovenous malformation
Embolic phenomenon
Hemorrhage
Hypertension
Hyperviscosity
Sickle cell disease
Thrombosis
Vasculitis

Suggested Readings

Golden GS. Nonepileptic paroxysmal events in childhood. *Pediatr Clin North Am* 1992;39:715.
Haslam RHA. Nonfebrile Seizures. *Pedaitr Rev* 1997;18:39.
Rothner AD. "Not everything that shakes is epilepsy." The differential diagnosis of paroxysmal nonepileptiform disorders. *Cleve Clin J Med* 1989;56: PS206.
Snyder CH. Conditions that simulate epilepsy in children. *Clin Pediatr* 1972;11: 487.

Splenomegaly

Common Causes
Acute infections (bacterial, viral, rickettsial, protozoal, spirochetal, mycobacterial)
Congenital hemolytic anemias
Hemoglobinopathies
Hereditary spherocytosis
Thalassemia major, thalassemia intermedia

Uncommon Causes
Acquired immunodeficiency syndrome
Chronic infections (bacterial, viral, protozoal, fungal, mycobacterial, spirochetal)
Congestive splenomegaly
Cirrhosis
Extrahepatic lesions
Constrictive pericarditis
Cyanotic congenital heart disease
Hodgkin disease
Iron deficiency anemia, severe
Juvenile rheumatoid arthritis
Leukemia
Lymphoma
Non-Hodgkin disease
Pseudosplenomegaly: low diaphragm
Rickettsial infection
Systemic lupus erythematosus

Rare Causes
Acquired autoimmune hemolytic anemia
Amyloidosis
Beckwith-Wiedemann syndrome
Brucellosis
Chediak-Hegashi syndrome
Chronic granulomatous disease
Congenital erythropoietic porphyria
Dysgammaglobulinemia
Familial lipochrome histiocytosis

Hemophagocytic syndromes
Hemosiderosis
Histiocytosis
Hurler syndrome and other mucopolysaccharidoses
Malaria (rare in United States, most common worldwide)
Metastatic neuroblastoma
Myelofibrosis
Osteopetrosis
Sarcoidosis
Serum sickness
Splenic cyst or hemangioma
Storage disease (e.g., Gaucher, Niemann-Pick, sea blue
    histiocyte disease, amyloidosis)
Wolman disease

Suggested Readings

Gartner JC Jr. Hepatosplenomegaly. In: Gartner JC Jr., Zitelli BJ, eds. *Common and chronic symptoms in pediatrics.* St. Louis: Mosby, 1997:355.
Mimouni F, Merlob P, Ashkenazi S, et al. Palpable spleens in newborn term infants. *Clin Pediatr* 1985;24:197.
Silverstein MN, Maldonado JE. Asymptomatic splenomegaly. *Postgrad Med* 1970;8:80.

Stridor (See Also Hoarseness)

Common Causes
Allergic reactions
Croup
Foreign-body aspiration
Hypertrophied tonsils/adenoids
Laryngomalacia
Peritonsillar abscess
Postinstrumentation edema
Retropharyngeal abscess
Secretions
Spasmodic croup
Subglottic stenosis (congenital, postintubation)
Vocal cord nodules

Uncommon Causes
Corrosive ingestion
Granuloma (postintubation/tracheostomy)
Laryngeal trauma
Psychogenic stridor
Tracheitis (bacterial)
Tracheomalacia
Vocal cord paralysis (congenital, postsurgical)
Vocal cord polyps

Rare Causes
Angioneurotic edema
Aryepiglottic cyst
Asthma (severe)
Bronchogenic cyst
Cartilage ring abnormalities ("segmental malacia")
Congenital goiter
Cricoarytenoid arthritis (juvenile rheumatoid arthritis)
Dermoid cyst
Diphtheria
Ectopic thyroid
Epiglottitis
Esophageal foreign body
External tracheal compression
    Hemorrhage
    Infection
    Tumors

Farber disease
Floppy epiglottis
Gastroesophageal reflux
Glossoptosis
Hemangioma
Hypoplastic larynx
Internal laryngocele
Laryngeal papilloma
Laryngeal tumors
Laryngeal web
Laryngismus stridulus (rickets)
Macroglossia
Marshall-Smith syndrome
Opitz-Frias syndrome
Pierre Robin syndrome
Posttracheostomy stricture
Psychogenic stridor
Sarcoidosis
Subglottic cyst
Tetany
Thyroglossal duct cyst
Tracheoesophageal fistula
Tracheolaryngoesophageal cleft
Vascular ring/aberrant vessels

Suggested Readings

Frey EE, Smith WL, Grandgeorge S, et al. Chronic airway obstruction in children—evaluation with Cine-CT. *AJR Am J Roentgenol* 1987;148:347.
Gonzales C, Reilly JS, Bluestone CD. Synchronous airway lesions in infancy. *Ann Otol Rhinol Laryngol* 1987;96:77.
Mancuso RF. Stridor in neonates. *Pediatr Clin North Am* 1996;43:1339.
McBride JT. Stridor in childhood. *J Fam Pract* 1984;19:782.
Milner AD. Acute stridor in the preschool child. *Br Med J* 1984;1:811.
Nielson DW, Heldt GP, Tooley WH. Stridor and gastroesophageal reflux in infants. *Pediatrics* 1990;85:1034.
Quinn-Bogard AL, Potsic WP. Stridor in the first year of life. *Clin Pediatr* 1977;16:913.
Ryckman F, Rodgers BM. Obstructive airway disease in infants and children. *Surg Clin North Am* 1985; 65:1663.
Smith RJH, Catlin FI. Congenital anomalies of the larynx. *Am J Dis Child* 1984;138:35.

Torticollis

Common Causes
Congenital muscular
    Sternocleidomastoid hematoma
Vertebral anomalies
    Arnold Chiari
    Down syndrome
    Failure of segmentation of vertebrae
    Hemivertebrae
    Klippel-Feil syndrome

Uncommon Causes
Cervical adenopathy
Congenital nystagmus
Drug-induced (e.g., phenothiazines, haloperidol,
    metoclopramide, trimethobenzamide)
Mastoiditis
Otitis Media
Paroxysmal
Pharyngitis
Retropharyngeal abscess
Sandifer syndrome (secondary to reflux esophagitis)
Superior oblique muscle weakness

Torticollis following upper respiratory infection
Trauma (congenital or acquired)
  Subluxation
  Dislocation
  Fractures
  Ligamentous injuries
  Muscle injuries

Rare Causes
Brachial plexus palsy
Calcification of intervertebral discs
Cervical diskitis
Dystonia musculorum deformans
Eosinophilic granuloma of cervical vertebrae
Fibromyositis
Fibrodysplasia ossificans progressiva
Focal myositis
Functional torticollis
Hepatolenticular degeneration (Wilson disease)
Juvenile rheumatoid arthritis
Kernicterus
Lemierre syndrome
Ligamentous laxity
Myasthenia gravis
Neuritis of spinal accessory nerve
Osteoid osteoma
Osteomyelitis of the cervical vertebrae
Pneumonia of an upper lobe
Poliomyelitis
Polymyositis
Posterior fossa tumor
Spasmus nutans
Spinal tumor
Trauma
  Subluxation
  Dislocation
  Fracture
Tuberculosis

Suggested Readings

Ballock RT, Song KM. The prevalence of nonmuscular causes of torticollis in children. *J Pediatr Orthop* 1996;16:500.

Bray PF, Herbst JJ, Johnson DG, et al. Childhood gastroesophageal reflux: neurologic and psychiatric syndromes mimicked. *JAMA* 1977;237:1342.

Hanukoglu A, Somekh E, Fried D. Benign paroxysmal torticollis in infancy. *Clin Pediatr* 1984;23:272.

Hensinger RN. Orthopedic problems of the shoulder and neck. *Pediatr Clin North Am* 1986;33:1495.

Kiwak KJ. Establishing an etiology for torticollis. *Postgrad Med* 1984;75:126.

Klassen AC. Torticollis. *Postgrad Med* 1984;75:124.

Lipson EH, Robertson WC Jr. Paroxysmal torticollis of infancy: familial occurrence. *Am J Dis Child* 1978;132:422.

Murphy WJ, Gellis SS. Torticollis with hiatus hernia in infancy. *Am J Dis Child* 1977;131:564.

Plagiocephaly and torticollis in young infants [editorial]. *Lancet* 1986;2:789.

Sanner G, Bergstrom B. Benign paroxysmal torticollis in infancy. *Acta Paediatr Scand* 1979;68:219.

Vertigo and Syncope

Vertigo (dizziness) and syncope (light-headedness, fainting) may be difficult symptoms for a child to distinguish with certainty. Many entities that are traditionally thought to cause syncope also may cause vertigo. Syncope, therefore, is discussed as a subheading of causes of vertigo.

Common Causes
Benign paroxysmal vertigo
Drugs
  Alcohol
  Anticonvulsants
  Antihypertensives
  Aspirin
  Dilantin
  Gentamicin
  Narcotics
  Sedatives
  Streptomycin
Ear disease
  External canal impaction
    Cerumen
    Foreign body
  Inner ear disease
    Cholesteatoma (with extension)
    Fistula
    Mastoiditis (with extension)
    Suppurative labyrinthitis
    Vestibular neuronitis
    Viral (acute) labyrinthitis
  Middle ear disease
    Chronic suppurative otitis (with extension)
    Hemotympanum (basilar skull fracture)
    Otitis media (rare as isolated finding)
    Serous otitis media
    Tympanic membrane perforation
Headache
  Basilar artery migraine complex
  Migraine
Hyperventilation syndrome
Paroxysmal torticollis of infancy
Seizure
  Aura/recovery phase
  Reflex seizure
Trauma
  Postconcussion syndrome
Visual impairment

Uncommon Causes
Basilar skull fracture
Cerebellar lesion/hemorrhage
CNS infection
  Abscess
  Encephalitis
  Meningitis
Hypotension
Trauma
  Labyrinthine trauma
  Temporal bone fracture

Rare Causes
Anemia
Arnold-Chiari malformation
Benign positional vertigo
Brainstem ischemia
Breath-holding spells
Central causes
  Vertebrobasilar artery ischemia
  Vestibulocerebellar ataxia
CNS tumors
  Acoustic neuroma
  Brainstem glioma
  Cerebellar glioma
  Ependymoma
  Medulloblastoma

Demyelinating disease
  Multiple sclerosis
Endocrine disorders
  Adrenal insufficiency
  Diabetes mellitus
  Thyrotoxicosis
Hypertension
Hypoglycemia
Increased intracranial pressure
Ménière disease
Pellagra
Perilymphatic fistula
Psychosomatic illness
Ramsay Hunt syndrome
Syncope (many causes previously discussed)
  Anterior mediastinal tumors
  Cardiovascular etiologies
    Arrhythmia
    Atrioventricular block
    Cardioauditory syndrome
    Emery-Dreifuss muscular dystrophy
    Mitral valve prolapse
    Paroxysmal atrial tachycardia
    Paroxysmal ventricular tachycardia
    Prolonged QT syndrome
    Sick sinus syndrome
  Cardiac anomalies
    Aortic stenosis
    Pulmonary stenosis
    Tetralogy of Fallot
    Transposition
    Truncus arteriosus
  Carotid sinus syncope
  Coronary artery spasm
  Dysautonomia (Riley-Day syndrome)
  Idiopathic hypertrophic subaortic stenosis
  Left atrial myxoma
  Myocardial infarction
  Orthostatic hypotension
  Pulmonary hypertension
  Vasovagal stimulation
Cough
Micturition
Swallowing
Vestibulocerebellar ataxia

Wheezing

Common Causes
Aspiration
  Direct (e.g., defective swallow, neuromuscular disease)
  Indirect (gastroesophageal reflux, emesis)
Asthma (reactive airway disease)
Atopic disease
Bronchiectasis
Bronchiolitis
Bronchitis
Foreign-body aspiration
Pneumonitis

Uncommon Causes
Anaphylaxis
Bronchopulmonary dysplasia
Congestive heart failure
Cystic fibrosis
Hypersensitivity pneumonitis
  Allergic bronchopulmonary aspergillosis
Mediastinal mass/adenopathy
Pulmonary edema
Tracheobronchomalacia
Vocal cord dysfunction/psychogenic airway obstruction

Rare Causes
Aberrant vessels
Alpha$_1$-antitrypsin deficiency
Angioneurotic edema
Carcinoid syndrome
Factitious wheezing
Immotile cilia syndrome (Kartagener syndrome)
Lobar emphysema
Neoplasm/tumor
Psychogenic airway obstruction
Pulmonary hemosiderosis (idiopathic, cow's milk allergy,
  myocarditis associated, Goodpasture disease)
Pulmonary sequestration
Pulmonary vasculitis
Sarcoidosis
Tracheobronchomegaly
Tracheobronchostenosis
Tracheoesophageal fistula
Vascular ring/sling
Visceral larva migrans

Suggested Readings

Benditt DG, Remole S, Milsteins, Bailin S. Syncope: causes, clinical evaluation, and current therapy. *Annu Rev Med* 1992;43:283.
Busis SN. Vertigo. In: Bluestone CD, Stool SE, Kenna MA, eds. *Pediatric otolaryngology*, 3rd ed. Philadelphia: WB Saunders, 1996:285.
Chang-Sing P, Peter CT. Syncope: evaluation and management. A review of current approaches to this multifaceted and complex clinical problem. *Cardiol Clin* 1991;9:641.
Drachman DA, Hart CW. An approach to the dizzy patient. *Neurology* 1972;22:323.
Dunn D. Dizziness: when is it vertigo? *Contemp Pediatr* 1987;4:67.
Eviatar L, Eviatar A. Vertigo in children: differential diagnosis and treatment. *Pediatrics* 1977;59:833.

Suggested Readings

Barnes SD, Grob CS, Lachman BS, et al. Psychogenic upper airway obstruction presenting as refractory wheezing. *J Pediatr* 1986;109:1067.
Clayton D. Catching up with the ABCs of sneezing, wheezing, and itching. *Can Med Assoc J* 1984;130:1609.
Kemper KJ. Chronic asthma: an update. *Pediatr Rev* 1996;17:111.
Leffert F. Asthma: a modern perspective. *Pediatrics* 1978;62:1061.
Morgan WJ, Martinez FD. Risk factors for developing wheezing and asthma in childhood. *Pediatr Clin North Am* 1992;39:1185.
Rachelefsky GS. The wheezing child. *Pediatrics* 1984;74(Suppl 5):941.
Richard W. Differential diagnosis of childhood asthma. *Curr Probl Pediatr* 1974;4:3.

Page numbers followed by f indicate figures; page numbers followed by t indicate tables; page numbers followed by b indicate boxes.